HARRISON'S
PRINCIPLES OF INTERNAL MEDICINE

THIRTEENTH EDITION

THIRTEENTH EDITION

HARRISON'S
PRINCIPLES
OF
INTERNAL
MEDICINE

Editors

KURT J. ISSELBACHER, A.B., M.D.

Mallinckrodt Professor of Medicine, Harvard Medical School; Physician and Director, Cancer Center, Massachusetts General Hospital, Boston

EUGENE BRAUNWALD, A.B., M.D., M.A. (Hon.), M.D. (Hon.), Sc.D. (Hon.)

Hersey Professor of the Theory and Practice of Medicine, Harvard Medical School; Chairman, Department of Medicine, Brigham and Women's Hospital, Boston

JEAN D. WILSON, M.D.

Charles Cameron Sprague Distinguished Chair and Professor of Internal Medicine; Chief, Division of Endocrinology and Metabolism, The University of Texas Southwestern Medical Center, Dallas

JOSEPH B. MARTIN, M.D., Ph.D., F.R.C.P. (C), M.A. (Hon.)

Professor of Neurology and Chancellor, University of California, San Francisco

ANTHONY S. FAUCI, M.D.

Director, National Institute of Allergy and Infectious Diseases; Chief, Laboratory of Immunoregulation; Director, Office of AIDS Research, National Institutes of Health, Bethesda

DENNIS L. KASPER, M.D.

William Ellery Channing Professor of Medicine, Harvard Medical School; Chief, Division of Infectious Diseases, Beth Israel Hospital; Co-Director, Channing Laboratory, Brigham and Women's Hospital, Boston

McGRAW-HILL
Health Professions Division

New York   St. Louis   San Francisco   Auckland   Bogotá   Caracas   Lisbon   London   Madrid
Mexico City   Milan   Montreal   New Delhi   San Juan   Singapore   Sydney   Tokyo   Toronto

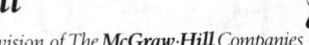

McGraw-Hill

A Division of The **McGraw·Hill** *Companies*

Note: Dr. Fauci's work as editor and author was performed outside the scope of his employment by the U.S. government. This work represents his personal and professional views and not necessarily those of the U.S. government.

HARRISON'S
PRINCIPLES OF INTERNAL MEDICINE
Thirteenth Edition

4 5 6 7 8 9 0 DOW DOW 9 8 7 6

Foreign Language Editions

ARABIC (Thirteenth Edition)—McGraw-Hill Libri Italia srl (Est. 1996)
CHINESE (Twelfth Edition)—McGraw-Hill Book Company-Singapore © 1994
CROATIAN (Thirteenth Edition)—McGraw-Hill Libri Italia srl (Est. 1996)
FRENCH (Thirteenth Edition)—McGraw-Hill Libri Italia srl © 1995
GERMAN (Thirteenth Edition)—McGraw-Hill Libri Italia srl © 1995
GREEK (Twelfth Edition)—Parissianos © 1994
ITALIAN (Thirteenth Edition)—McGraw-Hill Libri Italia srl © 1995
JAPANESE (Eleventh Edition)—Hirokawa © 1991
PORTUGUESE (Thirteenth Edition)—McGraw-Hill/Nueva Editorial Interamericana © 1995
SPANISH (Thirteenth Edition)—McGraw-Hill Interamericana de España © 1994
TURKISH (Thirteenth Edition)—McGraw-Hill Libri Italia srl (Est. 1996)

This book was set in Times Roman by Monotype Composition Company.
The editors were J. Dereck Jeffers and Stuart D. Boynton. The indexer was Irving Tullar; the production supervisor was Roger Kasunic; the designer was Marsha Cohen; R. R. Donnelley & Sons Company was printer and binder.

Library of Congress Cataloging-in-Publication Data

Harrison's principles of internal medicine—13th ed./editors,
    Kurt J. Isselbacher . . . [et al.]
        p.   cm.
    Includes bibliographical references and index.
    ISBN 0-07-032370-4 (1-vol. ed.) : 98.00 — ISBN 0-07-911169-6 (2
vol. ed. set) : 127.00 — ISBN 0-07-032371-2 (bk. 1). — ISBN
0-07-032372-0 (bk. 2)
    1. Internal medicine.   I. Harrison, Tinsley Randolph, 1900–
II. Isselbacher, Kurt J.   III. Title: Principles of internal
medicine.
    [DNLM: 1. Internal Medicine.   WB 115 P957 1994]
RC46.H333   1994
616—dc20
DNLM/DLC
for Library of Congress   93-47393

A SALUTE TO ROBERT G. PETERSDORF

By The Editors Of Harrison's.

We dedicate this thirteenth edition of *Harrison's Principles of Internal Medicine* to Robert G. Petersdorf, who became an editor of *Harrison's* in 1968 for the preparation of the sixth edition and served as Editor-in-Chief of the tenth edition. He was a powerful force for six editions and more than 20 years in establishing the pivotal role of this book in the education of students, residents and practitioners of medicine.

Dr. Petersdorf is a graduate of Brown University and of Yale University Medical School. His postgraduate training included residencies in medicine at Yale and at the Peter Bent Brigham Hospital and a research fellowship at Johns Hopkins. As Chair of the Department of Medicine at the University of Washington he fashioned one of the truly great departments of internal medicine in the nation, with well-balanced and great strengths in education, clinical care, and research. His interests and contributions broadened steadily and he served successively as the first President of the newly merged Brigham and Women's Hospital in Boston, as Vice Chancellor for Health Sciences and Dean of the School of Medicine, University of California, San Diego, and most recently as President of the Association of American Medical Colleges.

Dr. Petersdorf has, from the beginning of his career, made notable and outstanding contributions in a number of areas in the field of Infectious Disease. He carried out a series of classic studies on the pathogenesis of fever, of pneumococcal meningitis and of infective endocarditis, and on the chemoprophylaxis and epidemiology of gram-negative infections, especially of the urinary tract.

Dr. Petersdorf is a remarkably inspiring and effective teacher. Many students, interns, and residents at the medical schools and teaching hospitals where he has served considered him to be the most outstanding teacher they had *ever* encountered. At the bedside he is an exemplary clinician and demonstrates by personal example how to care for the sick. His lectures are models of clarity and precision. His effectiveness as a teacher is reflected in the fact that he has been one of the most sought-after Visiting Professors of Medicine in the country.

Robert Petersdorf is a unique figure in contemporary American medicine, having played a leadership role in virtually every important organization shaping the role of academic medicine in the United States. He has been an active proponent of the need to expand the scope of undergraduate medical education and to restructure graduate medical education in innovative ways that can better benefit the public. He was among the very first to point out the crisis in the availability of primary care internists and took active measures to help solve this problem. Dr. Petersdorf has been recognized for his creative thinking on undergraduate and graduate medical education, as well as on the organization and management of departments of internal medicine and of academic health centers. He has been dedicated to the ideals of the humanist-physician and has forcefully emphasized to a wide audience that medicine must be both a caring and a learned profession.

Robert Petersdorf brought a unique perspective to *Harrison's*. His personal involvement in clinically relevant laboratory research, his extensive experience as a broadly based clinician and teacher, as well as his unparalleled understanding of medical education and health care policy shaped not only the Infectious Diseases section, for which he had primary responsibility, but indeed the entire book. His influence will continue to permeate the book for many editions. At meetings of the editors, Dr. Petersdorf was usually the first to insist that the reader must never be allowed to lose sight of the clinical implications of the fundamental biological science presented, that descriptions of disease states must be of practical value to physicians, and that writing must be precise and show economy of expression.

Robert Petersdorf has been an inspiration to students of medicine—undergraduate, graduate, and postgraduate—as well as to others interested in health care, both in and outside the profession. Among those who have benefitted the most from his remarkable talents are his co-editors of *Harrisons,* who affectionately dedicate this edition to him.

NOTICE

Medicine is an ever-changing science. As new research and clinical experience broaden our knowledge, changes in treatment and drug therapy are required. The editors and the publisher of this work have checked with sources believed to be reliable in their efforts to provide information that is complete and generally in accord with the standards accepted at the time of publication. However, in view of the possibility of human error or changes in medical sciences, neither the editors, nor the publisher, nor any other party who has been involved in the preparation or publication of this work warrants that the information contained herein is in every respect accurate or complete. Readers are encouraged to confirm the information contained herein with other sources. For example and in particular, readers are advised to check the product information sheet included in the package of each drug they plan to administer to be certain that the information contained in this book is accurate and that changes have not been made in the recommended dose or in the contraindications for administration. This recommendation is of particular importance in connection with new or infrequently used drugs. Readers should also consult their own laboratories for normal values.

ABBREVIATED CONTENTS

CONTENTS

PART SIX
INFECTIOUS DISEASE

Section 1: Basic Considerations in Infectious Disease

Section 2: Clinical Syndromes—Community Acquired

Section 3: Clinical Syndromes—Nosocomial Infections

Section 4: Bacterial Disease: General Considerations

Section 5: Diseases Caused by Gram-Positive Bacteria

Section 6: Diseases Caused by Gram-Negative Bacteria

**PART ELEVEN
DISORDERS OF THE IMMUNE SYSTEM,
CONNECTIVE TISSUE, AND JOINTS**

Section 1: Disorders of the Immune System

Section 2: Disorders of Immune-Mediated Injury

Section 3: Disorders of the Joints

**PART TWELVE
HEMATOLOGY AND ONCOLOGY**

**Section 1: Disorders of the Hematopoietic
System**

PART THIRTEEN
ENDOCRINOLOGY AND METABOLISM

Section 1: Endocrinology

Section 2: Disorders of Intermediary Metabolism

COLOR PLATES

ATLAS OF DERMATOLOGY *Stephen F. Templeton / Thomas J. Lawley*

1 Common skin diseases and lesions

2 Cutaneous neoplasms

3 Pigmented lesions—benign and malignant

4 Infectious disease and the skin

5 Immunologically mediated skin disease

6 Skin manifestations of internal disease

ATLAS OF ENDOSCOPIC FINDINGS

ATLAS OF FUNDOSCOPIC EXAMINATION

ATLAS OF HEMATOLOGY

LIST OF CONTRIBUTORS

ELIAS ABRUTYN, M.D.

Professor and Associate Chairman, Medicine, and Vice-Dean for Veterans Affairs, Medical College of Pennsylvania; Chief, Infectious Diseases, Veterans Administration Medical Center, Philadelphia

RAYMOND D. ADAMS, B.A., M.A., M.D., M.A. (Hon.), D.Sc. (Hon.), M.D. (Hon.)

Bullard Professor of Neuropathology, Emeritus, Harvard Medical School; Consultant Neurologist, Massachusetts General Hospital; Emeritus Director, Eunice K. Shriver Research Center, Boston; Médicin Adjoint L'Hôpital, Cantonale de Lausanne, Lausanne

MICHAEL J. AMINOFF, M.D.

Professor of Neurology; Director, Clinical Neurophysiology Laboratories, University of California, San Francisco

MICHAEL A. APICELLA, M.D.

Professor and Head, Department of Microbiology, University of Iowa College of Medicine, Iowa City

GORDON LEE ARCHER, M.D.

Professor of Medicine and Microbiology/Immunology and Chairman, Division of Infectious Diseases, Medical College of Virginia, Virginia Commonwealth University, Richmond

ARTHUR K. ASBURY, M.D.

Ruth Wagner Van Meter and J. Ray Van Meter Professor of Neurology; Vice Dean for Research, University of Pennsylvania School of Medicine and Hospital of the University of Pennsylvania, Philadelphia

K. FRANK AUSTEN, M.D.

Theodore Bevier Bayles Professor of Medicine, Harvard Medical School; Chairman, Department of Rheumatology and Immunology, Brigham and Women's Hospital, Boston

ROBERT AUSTRIAN, M.D., D.Sci. (Hon.)

John Herr Musser Professor and Chairman Emeritus, Department of Molecular and Cellular Engineering, University of Pennsylvania School of Medicine, Philadelphia

BERNARD BABIOR, M.D., Ph.D.

Head, Division of Biochemistry, Department of Molecular and Experimental Medicine and Member, Division of Hematology and Oncology, Department of Medicine, Scripps Clinic and Research Foundation, La Jolla

KAMAL F. BADR, M.D.

Professor of Medicine, Emory University; Chief, Division of Nephrology, Atlanta Veteran's Medical Center; Attending Physician, Emory University Hospital, Atlanta

DONALD S. BAIM, M.D.

Associate Professor of Medicine, Harvard Medical School; Chief, Interventional Cardiology Section, Beth Israel Hospital, Boston

ANN SULLIVAN BAKER, M.D.

Associate Professor of Medicine, Harvard Medical School; Director, Infectious Diseases Service, Massachusetts Eye and Ear Infirmary; Physician, Infectious Disease Service, Massachusetts General Hospital, Boston

ANDREA BALLABIO, M.D.

Associate Professor, Institute for Molecular Genetics and Human Genome Center, Baylor College of Medicine, Houston

KENNETH J. BART, M.D., M.P.H.

Director, National Vaccine Program, Office of the Assistant Secretary of Health, Department of Health and Human Services, Rockville

ROBERT C. BAST, Jr., M.D.

R. Wayne Rundle Professor of Medicine and Director, Duke Comprehensive Cancer Center, Duke University Medical Center, Durham

M. FLINT BEAL, M.D.

Associate Professor of Neurology, Harvard Medical School; Assistant Neurologist, Massachusetts General Hospital, Boston

ARTHUR L. BEAUDET, M.D.

Professor, Institute for Molecule Genetics and Departments of Pediatrics and Cell Biology, Baylor College of Medicine; Investigator, Howard Hughes Medical Institute, Houston

JOHN E. BENNETT, M.D.

Head, Clinical Mycology Section, Laboratory of Clinical Investigation, National Institute of Allergy and Infectious Diseases, National Institutes of Health, Bethesda

ANDREW BERCHUCK, M.D.

Associate Professor, Division of Gynecologic Oncology, Duke University Medical Center, Durham

MICHAEL S. BERNSTEIN, M.D.

Assistant Professor of Medicine and Anesthesia, Division of Pulmonary and Critical Care Medicine, University of California at San Francisco Medical Center, San Francisco

DANIEL G. BICHET, M.D.

Associate Professor of Medicine, University of Montreal; Director, Clinical Research Unit, Hôpital du Sacre-Coeur de Montréal, Montreal

DAVID R. BICKERS, M.D.

Professor and Chairman, Department of Dermatology, Case Western Reserve University School of Medicine; Director, Department of Dermatology, University Hospitals of Cleveland, Cleveland

EDWIN L. BIERMAN, M.D.

Professor of Medicine and Head, Division of Metabolism, Endocrinology and Nutrition, University of Washington School of Medicine, Seattle

NEIL R. BLACKLOW, M.D.

Richard M. Haidack Professor of Medicine and Chairman, Department of Medicine, University of Massachusetts Medical School, Worcester

MARTIN J. BLASER, M.D.

The Addison B. Scoville Professor of Medicine; Director, Division of Infectious Diseases and Professor of Microbiology and Immunology, Vanderbilt University School of Medicine; Staff Physician, Veterans Affairs Medical Center, Nashville

JEAN L. BOLOGNIA, M.D.

Associate Professor of Dermatology, Department of Dermatology, Yale University School of Medicine, New Haven

LAWRENCE F. BORGES, M.D.

Associate Professor of Surgery (Neurosurgery), Harvard Medical School; Associate Visiting Neurosurgeon, Massachusetts General Hospital, Boston

RICHARD C. BOUCHER, Jr., M.D.

Professor of Medicine and Director, Division of Pulmonary Diseases, Critical Care and Occupational Medicine, University of North Carolina at Chapel Hill; University of North Carolina Hospitals, Chapel Hill

AUBREY E. BOYD III, M.D.

Professor of Medicine and Neuroscience; Chief, Division of Endocrinology, Diabetes, Metabolism and Molecular Medicine, New England Medical Center, Boston

WALTER G. BRADLEY, D.M., F.R.C.P.

Professor and Chairman, Department of Neurology, University of Miami School of Medicine, Miami

HUGH R. BRADY, M.D., Ph.D., F.R.C.P.I.

Assistant Professor of Medicine, Harvard Medical School; Chief, Renal Section, Brockton/West Roxbury Veteran's Affairs Medical Center; Associate Physician, Brigham and Women's Hospital, Boston

DAVID L. BRAFF, M.D.

Professor of Psychiatry, University of California at San Diego; Director of Psychiatry, UCSD Medical Center, San Diego

KENNETH D. BRANDT, M.D.

Professor of Medicine and Head, Rheumatology Division, Indiana University School of Medicine, Indianapolis; Director, Multipurpose Arthritis and Musculoskeletal Diseases Center, Indiana University School of Medicine, Indianapolis

EUGENE BRAUNWALD, A.B., M.D., M.A. (Hon.), M.D. (Hon.), Sc.D. (Hon.)

Hersey Professor of the Theory and Practice of Medicine, Harvard Medical School; Chairman, Department of Medicine, Brigham and Women's Hospital, Boston

IRWIN M. BRAVERMAN, M.D.

Professor, Department of Dermatology, Yale University School of Medicine, New Haven

JAMES L. BREELING, M.D.

Associate Chief, Medical Service, West Roxbury VA Medical Center, Boston

JOEL G. BREMAN, M.D., D.T.P.H.

Deputy Chief, Malaria Branch, Division of Parasitic Diseases, National Center for Infectious Diseases, Centers for Disease Control and Prevention, Atlanta; Visiting Lecturer, Harvard School of Public Health, Boston

BARRY M. BRENNER, M.D., A.M. (Hon.), D.Sc. (Hon.), D.M.Sc. (Hon.)

Samuel A. Levine Professor of Medicine, Harvard Medical School; Senior Physician and Director, Renal Division, Brigham and Women's Hospital, Boston

KENNETH R. BRIDGES, M.D.

Assistant Professor of Medicine, Harvard Medical School; Brigham and Women's Hospital, Boston

KAREN THATCHER BRITTON, M.D., Ph.D.

Professor of Psychiatry, University of California at San Diego, La Jolla

CLAIRE V. BROOME, M.D.

Associate Director for Science, Centers for Disease Control and Prevention, Atlanta

MARTIN M. BROWN, M.A., M.D., M.R.C.P.

Senior Lecturer in Neurology, St. George's Hospital Medical School, London

MICHAEL S. BROWN, M.D.

Paul J. Thomas Professor, Department of Molecular Genetics, The University of Texas Southwestern Medical Center, Dallas

ROBERT H. BROWN, Jr., M.D., D.Phil.

Associate Professor, Harvard Medical School; Associate Neruologist and Director, Cecil B. Day Laboratory for Neuromuscular Research, Massachusetts General Hospital, Boston

H. FRANKLIN BUNN, M.D.

Professor of Medicine, Harvard Medical School; Senior Physician and Director, Hematology Research, Brigham and Women's Hospital, Boston

RONALD M. BURDE, M.D.

Isidor Tachna Professor and Chairman, Department of Ophthalmology; Ophthalmologist and Neuro-ophthalmologist, Albert Einstein College of Medicine/Montefiore Medical Center, New York

JOAN R. BUTTERTON, M.D.

Clinical and Research Fellow, Infectious Diseases Unit, Massachusetts General Hospital, Boston

ALFRED E. BUXTON, M.D.

Professor of Medicine and Cardiology, Temple University School of Medicine; Associate Chief, Cardiology Section, Temple University Hospital, Philadelphia

STEPHEN B. CALDERWOOD, M.D.

Associate Professor of Medicine, Harvard Medical School; Chief, Infectious Diseases Unit, Massachusetts General Hospital, Boston

CHARLES B. CARPENTER, M.D.

Professor of Medicine, Harvard Medical School; Director, Laboratory of Immunogenetics and Transplantation, Brigham and Woman's Hospital, Boston

BRUCE R. CARR, M.D.

Paul C. MacDonald Professor and Director, Division of Reproductive Endocrinology, Department of Obstetrics and Gynecology, The University of Texas Southwestern Medical Center, Dallas

AGUSTIN CASTELLANOS, M.D.

Professor of Medicine, University of Miami School of Medicine; Director, Clinical Electrophysiology, Jackson Memorial Hospital, Miami

VERNE S. CAVINESS, Jr., M.D., Ph.D.

Joseph P. and Rose F. Kennedy Professor of Child Neurology and Mental Retardation, Harvard Medical School; Chief, Pediatric Neurology Service, Massachusetts General Hospital, Boston

JOHN S. CHILD, M.D.

Professor of Medicine, School of Medicine, University of California at Los Angeles; Associate Chief, Division of Cardiology and Director, Adult Cardiac Imaging and Hemodynamics Laboratories, UCLA Medical Center, Los Angeles

WALLACE A. CLYDE, Jr., M.D.

Professor of Pediatrics and Microbiology, University of North Carolina, Chapel Hill

FREDRIC L. COE, M.D.

Professor of Medicine and Physiology and Chief, Nephrology Program, University of Chicago Pritzker School of Medicine, Chicago

ALAN S. COHEN, M.D.

Distinguished Professor of Medicine and Rheumatology; Director, Arthritis Center at Boston University School of Medicine, Boston University School of Medicine, Boston

WILSON COLUCCI, M.D.

Associate Professor of Medicine, Harvard Medical School; Physician, Brigham and Women's Hospital

PATRICIA C. COME, M.D.

Associate Professor of Medicine, Harvard Medical School; Harvard Community Health Plan, Boston

JOEL D. COOPER, M.D.

Professor of Surgery and Head, Section of General Thoracic Surgery, Washington University School of Medicine; Barnes Hospital, St. Louis

MAX D. COOPER, M.D.

Professor of Medicine, Pediatrics and Microbiology and Howard Hughes Medical Institute Investigator, University of Alabama at Birmingham, Birmingham

LAWRENCE COREY, M.D.

Professor of Laboratory Medicine, Microbiology and Medicine, University of Washington, Seattle

MARK A. CREAGER, M.D.

Associate Professor of Medicine, Harvard Medical School; Director, Vascular Diagnostic Laboratory, Brigham and Women's Hospital, Boston

RONALD G. CRYSTAL, M.D.

Webster Professor of Medicine, Cornell University Medical College; Attending Physician, New York Hospital; Chief, Division of Pulmonary and Critical Care Medicine, New York Hospital-Cornell Medical Center, New York

JOHN J. CUSH, M.D.

Associate Professor of Internal Medicine, Rheumatic Diseases Division University of Texas Southwestern Medical Center at Dallas, Dallas

CHARLES A. CZEISLER, Ph.D., M.D.

Associate Professor of Medicine, Harvard Medical School; Physician and Director, Laboratory for Circadian and Sleep Disorders Medicine, Brigham and Women's Hospital, Boston

THOMAS M. DANIEL, M.D.

Professor of Medicine and International Health, Center for International Health, CWRU School of Medicine, Cleveland

GILBERT H. DANIELS, M.D.

Associate Professor of Medicine, Harvard Medical School; Physician and Co-Director, Thyroid Clinic, Massachusetts General Hospital, Boston

ROBERT B. DAROFF, M.D.

Gilbert W. Humphrey Professor and Chairman, Department of Neurology, Case Western Reserve University School of Medicine; Director, Department of Neurology, University Hospitals of Cleveland; Neurology Service, Cleveland Veteran's Administration Medical Center, Cleveland

JOHN R. DAVID, M.D.

Richard Pearson Strong Professor and Chairman, Department of Tropical Public Health, Harvard School of Public Health, Boston

CHARLES EDWARD DAVIS, M.D.

Professor of Pathology and Medicine, School of Medicine, University of California, San Diego; Director, Microbiology Laboratory, UCSD Medical Center, San Diego

KENNETH DAVIS, M.D., F.A.C.R.

Professor of Radiology, Harvard Medical School; Department of Neuroradiology, Massachusetts General Hospital, Boston

ROBERT L. DERESIEWICZ, M.D.

Instructor in Medicine, Harvard Medical School; Associate Physician, Brigham and Women's Hospital, Boston

ROBERT J. DESNICK, Ph.D., M.D.

Professor and Chairman, Department of Human Genetics, Mount Sinai School of Medicine; Attending Physician, Mount Sinai Hospital, New York

MARC A. DICHTER, M.D., Ph.D.

Professor of Neurology and Pharmacology, University of Pennsylvania School of Medicine and Graduate Hospital, Philadelphia

JULES L. DIENSTAG, M.D.

Associate Professor of Medicine, Harvard Medical School; Associate Physician, Massachusetts General Hospital, Boston

ALAN R. DIMICK, M.D.

Professor of Surgery, University of Alabama at Birmingham; Director, Burn Center, University of Alabama Hospital, Birmingham

CHARLES A. DINARELLO, M.D.

Professor of Medicine, Tufts University School of Medicine; Division of Geographic Medicine and Infectious Diseases, New England Medical Center, Boston

ROBERT G. DLUHY, M.D.

Associate Professor of Medicine, Harvard Medical School; Associate Program Director of the Clinical Research Center, Brigham and Women's Hospital, Boston

RAPHAEL DOLIN, M.D.

Charles A. Dewey Professor of Medicine; Chair, Department of Medicine, University of Rochester School of Medicine and Dentistry, Rochester

DANIEL B. DRACHMAN, M.D.

Professor of Neurology and Neurosciences and Director, Neuromuscular Unit, The Johns Hopkins University School of Medicine, Baltimore

JEFFREY M. DRAZEN, M.D.

Parker B. Francis Professor of Medicine, Harvard Medical School; Chief, Pulmonary Division, Brigham and Women's and Beth Israel Hospitals, Boston

JOHANNA T. DWYER, D.Sc., R.D.

Professor of Medicine and Community Health, Tufts University School of Medicine; Professor of Nutrition, Tufts University School of Nutrition; Senior Scientist, USDA Human Nutrition Research Center on Aging, Tufts University; Director, Frances Stern Nutrition Center, New England Medical Center Hospital, Boston

VICTOR J. DZAU, M.D.

William G. Irwin Professor of Medicine and Chief, Division of Cardiovascular Medicine, Stanford University School of Medicine; Stanford University Hospital, Stanford

BARRY I. EISENSTEIN, M.D.

Professor of Medicine, Indiana University School of Medicine; Vice President, Lilly Research Laboratories, Indianapolis

VIRGINIA L. ERNSTER, Ph.D.

Professor and Chair, Department of Epidemiology and Biostatistics, University of California, San Francisco

KENNETH H. FALCHUK, M.D.

Associate Professor of Medicine, Harvard Medical School; Physician, Brigham and Women's Hospital, Boston

FERRIC C. FANG, M.D.

Assistant Professor of Medicine and Pathology, University of Colorado Health Sciences Center; Director, Clinical Microbiology Laboratory, University Hospital, Denver

ANTHONY S. FAUCI, M.D.

Director, National Institute of Allergy and Infectious Diseases; Chief, Laboratory of Immunoregulation; Director, Office of AIDS Research, National Institutes of Health, Bethesda

MURRAY J. FAVUS, M.D.

Professor of Medicine, Sections of Endocrinology and Nephrology, Department of Medicine, University of Chicago Pritzker School of Medicine, Chicago

THOMAS F. FERRIS, M.D.

Nesbitt Professor and Chairman, Department of Medicine, University of Minnesota; University of Minnesota Hospital and Clinics, Minneapolis

BERNARD N. FIELDS, M.D.

Adele Lehman Professor of Microbiology and Molecular Genetics, Professor of Medicine and Chairman, Department of Microbiology and Molecular Genetics, Harvard Medical School, Boston

HOWARD L. FIELDS, M.D., Ph.D.

Professor of Neurology and Physiology and Vice Chairman, Department of Neurology, University of California, San Francisco

GREGORY A. FILICE, M.D.

Associate Professor of Medicine and Chief, Infectious Disease Section, University of Minnesota VA Medical Center, Minneapolis

ROBERT W. FINBERG, M.D.

Associate Professor of Medicine, Harvard Medical School; Chief, Laboratory of Infectious Diseases, Dana-Farber Cancer Institute, Boston

STUART C. FINCH, M.D.

Professor of Medicine, University of Medicine and Dentistry of New Jersey-Robert Wood Johnson Medical School and the Cooper Hospital/University Medical Center, Camden

J. STEPHEN FINK, M.D.

Associate Professor, Harvard Medical School; Assistant Neurologist, Massachusetts General Hospital, Boston

DANIEL W. FOSTER, M.D.

Donald W. Seldin Distinguished Chair in Internal Medicine and Chairman, Department of Internal Medicine, The University of Texas Southwestern Medical Center, Dallas

MICHAEL M. FRANK, M.D.

Professor and Chairman, Department of Pediatrics, Duke University Medical Center; Professor of Medicine, Department of Medicine, Duke University Medical Center, Durham

ARNOLD S. FREEDMAN, M.D.

Assistant Professor of Medicine, Harvard Medical School; Division of Tumor Immunology, Dana-Farber Cancer Institute, Boston

STANLEY D. FREEDMAN, M.D.

Clinical Professor of Medicine, University of California at San Diego; Head, Division of Infectious Diseases, Scripps Clinic and Research Foundation, La Jolla

MICHAEL FREISSMUTH, M.D.

Lecturer, Department of Pharmacology, University of Vienna, Vienna

GERALD H. FRIEDLAND, M.D.

Director, AIDS Program, Yale University School of Medicine, New Haven

HARVEY MICHAEL FRIEDMAN, M.D.

Chief, Infectious Disease Division, Department of Medicine, University of Pennsylvania School of Medicine, Philadelphia

LAWRENCE S. FRIEDMAN, M.D.

Associate Professor of Medicine, Harvard Medical School; Associate Physician, Massachusetts General Hospital, Boston

PAUL J. FRIEDMAN, M.D.

Professor of Radiology, University of California, San Diego

WILLIAM F. FRIEDMAN, M.D.

J.H. Nicholson Professor of Pediatrics (Cardiology) and Executive Chairman, Department of Pediatrics, University of California, Los Angeles School of Medicine; University of California, Los Angeles Medical Center, Los Angeles

LAWRENCE A. FROHMAN, M.D.

Edmund F. Foley Professor and Head, Department of Medicine, University of Illinois at Chicago, Chicago

ROBERT F. GAGEL, M.D.

Professor of Medicine and Chief of Endocrinology Section, The University of Texas, M.D. Anderson Cancer Center, Houston

JOHN I. GALLIN, M.D.

Director, Division of Intramural Research, National Institute of Allergy and Infectious Diseases, National Institutes of Health, Bethesda

ROBERT C. GALLO, M.D.

Chief, Laboratory of Tumor Cell Biology, National Cancer Institute, National Institutes of Health, Bethesda

MARC B. GARNICK, M.D.

Associate Clinical Professor of Medicine, Dana-Farber Cancer Institute and Harvard Medical School; Vice President for Clinical Development, Genetics Institute, Cambridge

JEFFREY A. GELFAND, M.D.

Sara Murray Jordan Professor and Vice Chairman, Department of Medicine, Tufts University School of Medicine; Associate Physician-in-Chief, New England Medical Center, Boston

JAMES L. GERMAN III, M.D.

Professor of Pediatrics, Cornell University Medical College; Director, Laboratory of Human Genetics, New York Blood Center, New York

BRUCE C. GILLILAND, M.D.

Professor of Medicine, Professor of Laboratory Medicine and Adjunct Professor of Microbiology, and Associate Dean, Clinical Affairs, University of Washington School of Medicine, Seattle

ALFRED G. GILMAN, M.D., Ph.D.

Raymond Willie Distinguished Chair in Molecular Neuropharmacology; Department of Pharmacology, The University of Texas Southwestern Medical Center, Dallas

SID GILMAN, M.D.

Professor and Chairman, Department of Neurology, University of Michigan, Ann Arbor

RICHARD J. GLASSOCK, M.D.

Professor and Chairman, Department of Internal Medicine, University of Kentucky College of Medicine, Lexington

ROBERT M. GLICKMAN, M.D.

Herrman Ludwig Blumgart Professor of Medicine, Harvard Medical School; Physician-in-Chief, Beth Israel Hospital, Boston

MARK A. GOLDBERG, M.D.

Assistant Professor of Medicine, Harvard Medical School; Associate Physician, Brigham and Women's Hospital, Boston

ARY GOLDBERGER, M.D.

Associate Professor of Medicine, Harvard Medical School; Physician, Beth Israel Hospital, Boston

DAVID W. GOLDE, M.D.

Professor of Medicine, Cornell University Medical College; Professor of Molecular Pharmacology and Therapeutics, Sloan-Kettering Division of the Cornell Graduate School of Medical Sciences; Member, Attending Physician, and Head, Division of Hematologic Oncology, Memorial Sloan-Kettering Cancer Center, New York

LEE GOLDMAN, M.D.

Professor of Medicine, Harvard Medical School; Vice-Chairman, Department of Medicine and Chief, Division of Clinical Epidemiology, Brigham and Women's Hospital, Boston

JOSEPH L. GOLDSTEIN, M.D.

Paul J. Thomas Professor and Chairman, Department of Molecular Genetics, The University of Texas Southwestern Medical Center, Dallas

RAJ K. GOYAL, M.D.

Rabb Professor of Medicine, Harvard Medical School; Chief, Division of Gastroenterology, Beth Israel Hospital, Boston

JOHN W. GRAEF, M.D.

Associate Clinical Professor of Pediatrics, Harvard Medical School; Director, The Lead/Toxicology Clinic, The Children's Hospital, Boston

HARRY B. GREENBERG, M.D.

Professor of Medicine and Microbiology and Immunology, Stanford University Medical Center, Stanford

NORTON J. GREENBERGER, M.D., M.A.C.P.

Peter T. Bohan Professor and Chairman, Department of Medicine, University of Kansas Medical Center, Kansas City

JOHN S. GREENSPAN, B.D.S., Ph.D., F.R.C.Path.

Professor and Chairman, Department of Stomatology, University of California School of Dentistry, San Francisco

JAMES E. GRIFFIN, M.D.

Professor of Internal Medicine, The University of Texas Southwestern Medical Center, Dallas

J. McLEOD GRIFFISS, M.D.

Professor of Lab Medicine and Medicine, University of California at San Francisco VA Medical Center, San Francisco

ROBERT C. GRIGGS, M.D.

Edward A. and Alma Vollertsen Rykenboer Professor of Neurophysiology, Professor of Neurology and Medicine, and Chairman, Department of Neurology, University of Rochester School of Medicine and Dentistry, University of Rochester Medical Center, Rochester

WILLIAM GROSSMAN, M.D.

Dana Professor of Medicine, Harvard Medical School; Chief, Cardiovascular Division, Beth Israel Hospital, Boston

JOHN H. GROWDON, M.D.

Professor of Neurology, Harvard Medical School; Neurologist and Director, Memory Disorders Unit, Massachusetts General Hospital, Boston

SUBHASH C. GULATI, M.D., Ph.D.

Associate Professor of Medicine, Cornell University Medical College; Associate Member and Associate Attending Physician, Memorial Sloan-Kettering Cancer Center, New York

VLADIMIR HACHINSKI, M.D.

Richard and Beryl Ivey Professor and Chairman, Department of Clinical Neurological Sciences, University of Western Ontario, University Hospital, London, Ontario

BEVRA HANNAHS HAHN, M.D.

Professor of Medicine, Department of Medicine; Chief of Rheumatology, University of California, Los Angeles, Los Angeles

ROBERT I. HANDIN, M.D.

Associate Professor of Medicine, Harvard Medical School; Director, Hematology Oncology Division, Brigham and Women's Hospital, Boston

H. HUNTER HANDSFIELD, M.D.

Professor of Medicine, University of Washington School of Medicine; Director, STD Control Program, Seattle-King County Department of Public Health, Seattle

STEPHEN L. HAUSER, M.D.

Betty Anker Fife Professor and Chairman, Department of Neurology, University of California, San Francisco

BARTON F. HAYNES, M.D.

Director, Arthritis Center; Chief, Division of Rheumatology and Immunology; Frederic M. Hanes Professor of Medicine; Director, Basic Research, Center for AIDS Research, Duke University School of Medicine, Durham

STEVEN C. HERBERT, M.D.

Associate Professor of Medicine, Harvard Medical School; Physician, Brigham and Women's Hospital, Boston

I. CRAIG HENDERSON, M.D.

Professor of Medicine; Chief of Medical Oncology; Director, Clinical Oncology Program, Moffitt-Long Hospitals, San Francisco

CHARLES B. HIGGINS, M.D.

Professor of Radiology and Chief, Magnetic Resonance Imaging, University of California School of Medicine, San Francisco

RAYMOND L. HINTZ, M.D.

Professor of Pediatrics and Head, Division of Pediatric Endocrinology, Stanford University School of Medicine, Stanford

MARTIN S. HIRSCH, M.D.

Professor of Medicine, Harvard Medical School; Massachusetts General Hospital, Boston

FRED HOCHBERG, M.D.

Associate Professor of Neurology, Harvard Medical School; Neurologist, Massachusetts General Hospital, Boston

GARY S. HOFFMAN, M.D.

Chairman, Department of Rheumatic and Immunologic Diseases, Cleveland Clinic Foundation, Cleveland

JOHN H. HOLBROOK, M.D.

Professor of Internal Medicine, University of Utah School of Medicine, Salt Lake City

MICHAEL F. HOLICK, Ph.D., M.D.

Professor of Medicine, Physiology and Dermatology; Chief of Endocrinology, Diabetes and Metabolism; Director of the General Clinical Research Center, Boston University School of Medicine, Boston

KING K. HOLMES, M.D., Ph.D.

Professor of Medicine and Director, Center for AIDS and Sexually Transmitted Diseases, University of Washington School of Medicine, Seattle

RANDALL K. HOLMES, M.D., Ph.D.

Chairman, Department of Microbiology and Immunology, Uniformed Services University of the Health Sciences, Bethesda

THOMAS H. HOSTETTER, M.D.

Professor of Medicine, University of Minnesota School of Medicine; Director, Division of Renal Disease, University Hospital, Minneapolis

LYN J. HOWARD, B.M., D.Ch., F.R.C.P.

Professor of Medicine and Associate Professor of Pediatrics; Head, Division of Clinical Nutrition, Albany Medical College, Albany

HOWARD HU, M.D., M.P.H., Sc.D.

Assistant Professor of Medicine, Harvard Medical School; Associate Physician, Channing Laboratory, Brigham and Women's Hospital, Boston

GARY W. HUNNINGHAKE, M.D.

Professor of Internal Medicine and Director, Pulmonary and Critical Care Medicine, University of Iowa College of Medicine, Iowa City

EDWARD P. INGENITO, M.D., Ph.D.

Assistant Professor of Medicine, Harvard Medical School; Director, Medical Intensive Care Unit, Brigham and Women's Hospital, Boston

ROLAND H. INGRAM, Jr., M.D.

Professor of Medicine, Emory University School of Medicine; Chief of Medicine, Emory-Crawford Long Hospital, Atlanta

CHARLES E. IRWIN, Jr., M.D.

Professor of Pediatrics; Director, Division of Adolescent Medicine, Department of Pediatrics School of Medicine, University of California, San Francisco, San Francisco

KURT J. ISSELBACHER, M.D.

Mallinckrodt Professor of Medicine, Harvard Medical School; Physician and Director, MGH Cancer Center, Massachusetts General Hospital, Boston

MARK E. JOSEPHSON, M.D.

Professor of Medicine, Harvard Medical School; Director, Harvard-Thorndike Electrophysiology Institute and Arrhythmia Service, Beth Israel Hospital, Boston

LEWIS L. JUDD, M.D.

Mary Gilman Marston Professor and Chairman, Department of Psychiatry, University of California at San Diego, La Jolla

LEE M. KAPLAN, M.D., Ph.D.

Assistant Professor of Medicine, Harvard Medical School; Assistant in Medicine, Gastrointestinal Unit, Massachusetts General Hospital, Boston

DENNIS L. KASPER, M.D.

William Ellery Channing Professor of Medicine, Harvard Medical School; Chief, Division of Infectious Diseases, Beth Israel Hospital; Co-Director, Channing Laboratory, Brigham and Women's Hospital, Boston

LLOYD H. KASPER, M.D.

Professor of Medicine, Neurology and Microbiology, Dartmouth Medical School, Hanover

SATISH KATHPALIA, M.D., F.A.C.P.

Associate Professor of Medicine, University of Illinois School of Medicine; Attending Physician, Renal Division, Department of Medicine, Michael Reese Hospital and Medical Center, Chicago

DONALD KAYE, M.D.

Klinghoffer Professor and Chairman, Department of Medicine, The Medical College of Pennsylvania, Philadelphia

GERALD T. KEUSCH, M.D.

Professor of Medicine and Chief, Division of Geographic Medicine and Infectious Diseases, New England Medical Center Hospitals, Boston

MICHAEL B. KIMMEY, M.D.

Associate Professor of Medicine and Director of GI Endoscopy, University of Washington School of Medicine, Seattle

LOUIS V. KIRCHHOFF, M.D.

Associate Professor of Internal Medicine and Staff Physician, Department of Veterans Affairs Medical Center, Iowa City

J. PHILLIP KISTLER, M.D.

Associate Professor of Neurology, Harvard Medical School; Associate Neurologist and Director of Stroke Service, Massachusetts General Hospital, Boston

HARVEY G. KLEIN, M.D.

Chief, Department of Transfusion Medicine, Clinical Center, National Institutes of Health, Bethesda

JAMES P. KNOCHEL, M.D.

Professor of Internal Medicine, The University of Texas Southwestern Medical Center; Chairman, Department of Medicine, Presbyterian Hospital, Dallas

HOWARD K. KOH, M.D.

Associate Professor of Dermatology, Medicine, and Public Health; Co-Director, Skin Oncology Program; Director, Cancer Prevention and Control Center, Boston University Schools of Medicine and Public Health, Boston

ANTHONY KOMAROFF, M.D.

Professor of Medicine, Harvard Medical School; Director, Division of General Medicine, Brigham and Women's Hospital, Boston

STANLEY J. KORSMEYER, M.D.

Professor, Howard Hughes Medical Institute, Washington University School of Medicine, Saint Louis

WILLIAM J. KOVACS, M.D.

Associate Professor of Medicine, Division of Endocrinology, Vanderbilt University School of Medicine, Nashville

STEPHEN M. KRANE, M.D.

Persis, Cyrus, and Marlow B. Harrison Professor of Medicine, Harvard Medical School; Physician and Chief, Arthritis Unit, Massachusetts General Hospital, Boston

DONALD KUFE, M.D.

Professor of Medicine, Harvard Medical School and Dana-Farber Cancer Institute, Boston

HELENA KUIVANIEMI, M.D., Ph.D.

Research Assistant Professor, Department of Biochemistry and Molecular Biology, Jefferson Medical College of Thomas Jefferson University, Philadelphia

J. THOMAS La MONT, M.D.

Chief, Section of Gastroenterology, The University Hospital, Boston

LEWIS LANDSBERG, M.D

Irving S. Cutter Professor and Chairman, Department of Medicine, Northwestern University Medical School; Physician-in-Chief, Northwestern Memorial Hospital, Chicago

H. CLIFFORD LANE, M.D.

Clinical Director, National Institute of Allergy and Infectious Diseases, National Institutes of Health; Chief, Clinical Molecular Retrovirology Section, Laboratory of Immunoregulation, National Institute of Allergy and Infectious Diseases, NIH, Bethesda

THOMAS J. LAWLEY, M.D.

Professor and Chairman, Department of Dermatology, Emory University School of Medicine, Atlanta

ALEXANDER R. LAWTON III, M.D.

Edward C. Stahlman Professor in Pediatric Physiology and Cell Metabolism; Professor of Pediatrics and Microbiology; Head, Division of Pediatric Immunology and Rheumatology, Vanderbilt University School of Medicine, Nashville

J. MICHAEL LAZARUS, M.D.

Associate Professor of Medicine, Harvard Medical School; Senior Physician and Director of Clinical Services, Nephrology Division, Brigham & Women's Hospital, Boston

ROBERT SAMUEL LEBOVICS, M.D., F.A.C.S.

Chief, Otolaryngology, National Institute on Deafness and Other Communication Disorders, National Institutes of Health, Bethesda

RICHARD T. LEE, M.D.

Assistant Professor of Medicine, Harvard Medical School; Director, Noninvasive Cardiac Laboratory, Brigham and Women's Hospital, Boston

PHILLIP I. LERNER, M.D.

Professor of Medicine, Case Western Reserve University School of Medicine; Chief, Division of Infectious Diseases, The Mount Sinai Medical Center, Cleveland

NORMAN G. LEVINSKY, M.D.

Wade Professor and Chairman, Department of Medicine, Boston University School of Medicine; Physician-in-Chief, Boston City Hospital and Boston University Medical Center Hospital, Boston

MATTHEW E. LEVISON, M.D.

Professor of Medicine and Chief, Division of Infectious Diseases, Medical College of Pennsylvania, Philadelphia

RICHARD W. LIGHT, M.D.

Professor of Medicine, University of California, Irvine; Physician, Veterans Administration Hospital, Long Beach

CHRISTOPHER H. LINDEN, M.D., F.A.C.E.P.

Associate Professor of Medicine; Associate Director, Toxicology Service and Associate Clinical Director, Department of Emergency Medicine, University of Massachusetts Medical Center, Worcester

PETER E. LIPSKY, M.D.

Professor of Internal Medicine and Microbiology; Director, Rheumatic Diseases Division; Director, Harold C. Simmons Arthritis Research Center, The University of Texas Southwestern Medical Center at Dallas, Dallas

LEO X. LIU, M.D., D.T.M.H.

Assistant Professor of Medicine, Harvard Medical School; Division of Infectious Diseases, Department of Medicine, Beth Israel Hospital, Boston

BERNARD LO, M.D.

Professor of Medicine; Director, Program in Medical Ethics; Co-Director, Robert Wood Johnson Clinical Scholars Program; Physician, Moffitt-Long Hospitals, University of California, San Francisco

RICHARD M. LOCKSLEY, M.D.

Associate Professor of Medicine and Microbiology and Immunology and Chief, Division of Infectious Diseases, Department of Medicine, University of California, San Francisco

DAN L. LONGO, M.D.

Director, Biological Response Modifiers Program, Division of Cancer Treatment, National Cancer Institute, Frederick Cancer Research and Development Center, Frederick

FREDERICK H. LOVEJOY, Jr., M.D.

William Berenberg Professor of Pediatrics, Harvard Medical School; Associate Physician-in-Chief, The Children's Hospital, Boston

SHEILA A. LUKEHART, Ph.D.

Research Associate Professor, Department of Medicine, Division of Infectious Diseases, University of Washington School of Medicine, Seattle

LAWRENCE C. MADOFF, M.D.

Assistant Professor of Medicine, Harvard Medical School; Channing Laboratory, Brigham and Women's Hospital; Division of Infectious Diseases, Beth Israel Hospital, Boston

JAMES HARVEY MAGUIRE, M.D.

Associate Professor of Medicine, Harvard Medical School; Physician, Brigham and Women's Hospital, Boston

HENRY J. MANKIN, M.D.

Edith M. Ashley Professor of Orthopaedic Surgery, Harvard Medical School; Chief, Orthopaedic Services, Massachusetts General Hospital, Boston

FRANCIS E. MARCHLINSKI

Clinical Professor of Medicine, University of Pennsylvania School of Medicine; Co-Director, Philadelphia Heart Institute, Philadelphia

JOSEPH B. MARTIN, M.D., Ph.D., F.R.C.P. (C), M.A. (Hon.)

Professor of Neurology and Chancellor, University of California, San Francisco

JOEL B. MASON, M.D.

Assistant Professor, Divisions of Clinical Nutrition and Gastroenterology; Scientist, USDA Human Nutrition Research Center on Aging, Tufts University, Boston

HENRY MASUR, M.D.

Chief, Critical Care Medicine Department, National Institutes of Health, Bethesda

ROBERT J. MAYER, M.D.

Professor of Medicine and Clinical Director, Department of Medicine, Dana-Farber Cancer Institute, Boston

JOHN D. McCONNELL, M.D.

Associate Professor of Surgery, Division of Urology, The University of Texas Southwestern Medical Center, Dallas

E. R. McFADDEN, Jr., M.D.

Argyl J. Beams Professor of Medicine and Director, Division of Pulmonary and Critical Care Medicine, Case Western Reserve University School of Medicine, Cleveland

JAMES E. McGUIGAN, M.D.

Chairman, Department of Medicine, University of Florida College of Medicine, Gainesville

NANCY K. MELLO, Ph.D.

Professor of Psychology, Department of Psychiatry (Neuroscience), Harvard Medical School, Boston; Co-Director, Alcohol and Drug Abuse Research Center, McLean Hospital, Belmont

JERRY R. MENDELL, M.D.

Professor and Chairman, Department of Neurology, The Ohio State University College of Medicine, Columbus

JOHN MENDELSOHN, M.D.

Winthrop Rockefeller Chair in Medical Oncology and Chairman, Department of Medicine, Memorial Sloan-Kettering Cancer Center

JACK H. MENDELSON, M.D.

Professor of Psychiatry (Neuroscience), Harvard Medical School, Boston; Co-Director, Alcohol and Drug Abuse Research Center, McLean Hospital, Belmont

RICHARD A. MILLER, M.D.

Associate Professor of Medicine, University of Washington School of Medicine; Chief, Infectious Disease Section, Seattle VA Medical Center, Seattle

JOHN D. MINNA, M.D.

Professor of Medicine and Pharmacology and Director, Simmons Cancer Center, The University of Texas Southwestern Medical Center, Dallas

JEROME H. MODELL, M.D.

Professor of Anesthesiology, College of Medicine, University of Florida; Senior Associate Dean for Clinical Affairs; Associate Vice President for University of Florida Health Science Center Affiliations, Gainesville

J. P. MOHR, M.D.

Sciarra Professor of Clinical Neurology, College of Physicians and Surgeons of Columbia University Neurological Institute, New York

STEPHEN MORSE, Ph.D.

Director, Division of Sexually Transmitted Diseases Laboratory Research, National Center for Infectious Diseases, Centers for Disease Control and Prevention, Atlanta

KENNETH M. MOSER, M.D.

Professor of Medicine, School of Medicine, University of California at San Diego; Director, Pulmonary/Critical Care Division, UCSD Medical Center, San Diego

ARNOLD M. MOSES, M.D.

Professor of Medicine and Director, Clinical Research, Unit, State University of New York Health Science Center, Syracuse

HARALAMPOS M. MOUTSOPOULOS, M.D.

Professor and Head of Medicine, Department of Internal Medicine, University of Ioannina Medical School, Ioannina, Greece

ROBERT F. MUNFORD, M.D.

Professor of Internal Medicine and Microbiology, University of Texas Southwestern Medical Center, Dallas

DANIEL M. MUSHER, M.D.

Chief, Infectious Disease Section, Veterans Affairs Medical Center; Professor of Medicine and Professor of Microbiology and Immunology, Baylor College of Medicine, Houston

ROBERT J. MYERBURG, M.D.

Professor of Medicine and Physiology and Director, Division of Cardiology, University of Miami School of Medicine, Miami

LEE M. NADLER, M.D.

Professor of Medicine, Harvard Medical School; Division of Tumor Immunology, Dana-Farber Cancer Institute, Boston

THEODORE ELLIOT NASH, M.D.

Senior Scientist, Laboratory of Parasitic Diseases, National Institutes of Health, Bethesda

LAURENCE NEEDLEMAN, M.D.

Associate Professor of Radiology and Associate Director, Division of Diagnostic Ultrasound, Thomas Jefferson University Hospital, Philadelphia

THOMAS B. NUTMAN, M.D.

Senior Investigator, Laboratory of Parasitic Diseases, National Institute of Allergy and Infectious Diseases, National Institutes of Health, Bethesda

JOHN OATES, M.D.

Professor and Chairman, Department of Medicine, Vanderbilt University School of Medicine; Physician-in-Chief, Vanderbilt University Hospital, Nashville

JERROLD M. OLEFSKY, M.D.

Professor of Medicine and Head, Division of Endocrinology and Metabolism, School of Medicine, University of California at San Diego, La Jolla

ANDREW B. ONDERDONK, Ph.D.

Associate Professor of Pathology, Harvard Medical School; Director, Clinical Microbiology Laboratory, Brigham and Women's Hospital, Boston

STUART H. ORKIN, M.D.

Leland Fikes Professor of Pediatric Medicine, Harvard Medical School; Children's Hospital, Boston

ROBERT A. O'ROURKE, M.D.

Charles Conrad Brown Distinguished Professor of Medicine, The University of Texas Health Science Center at San Antonio; Director of Cardiology, The University of Texas Health Science Center Teaching Hospitals, San Antonio

DARWIN L. PALMER, M.D.

Professor of Medicine and Chief, Division of Infectious Diseases, University of New Mexico School of Medicine, Albuquerque

JOSEPH E. PARRILLO, M.D.

James B. Herrick Professor of Medicine, Rush Medical College; Chief, Section of Cardiology; Chief, Section of Critical Care Medicine and Medical Director, Rush Heart Institute, Rush-Presbyterian-St. Luke's Medical Center, Chicago

RICHARD C. PASTERNAK, M.D.

Assistant Professor of Medicine, Harvard Medical School; Director of Preventive Cardiology and Cardiac Rehabilitation, Massachusetts General Hospital, Boston

PETER L. PERINE, M.D.

Professor of Epidemiology, Center for AIDS and STD, University of Washington, Seattle; Professor of Tropical Public Health and Medicine Emeritus, Uniformed Services University of the Health Sciences, Bethesda

ROBERT G. PETERSDORF, M.D.

President, Association of American Medical Colleges, Washington, D.C.

ELIOT A. PHILLIPSON, M.D.

Sir John and Lady Eaton Professor of Medicine and Chair, Department of Medicine, University of Toronto; Physician-in-Chief, Mount Sinai Hospital, Toronto

GERALD B. PIER, Ph.D.

Associate Professor of Medicine, Harvard Medical School; Channing Labatory, Brigham and Women's Hospital, Boston

DANIEL K. PODOLSKY, M.D.

Associate Professor of Medicine, Harvard Medical School; Chief, Gastrointestinal Unit, Massachusetts General Hospital, Boston

RONALD J. POLINSKY, M.D.

Senior Associate Director, Human Pharmacology, Drug Safety Department, Sandoz Research Institute, Sandoz Pharmaceuticals Corporation, East Hanover, New Jersey

RONALD E. POLK, Pharm.D.

Professor of Pharmacy and Medicine, School of Pharmacy, Medical College of Virginia, Virginia Commonwealth University, Richmond

MATTHEW POLLACK, M.D.

Professor of Medicine, Uniformed Services University of the Health Sciences, F. Edward Hebert School of Medicine, Bethesda

JOHN T. POTTS, Jr., M.D.

Jackson Professor of Clinical Medicine, Harvard Medical School; Physician-in-Chief, Massachusetts General Hospital, Boston

LAWRIE W. POWELL, M.D.

Professor of Medicine, The University of Queensland; Director, Queensland Institute of Medical Research, Brisbane

DARWIN J. PROCKOP, M.D.

Professor and Chairman, Department of Biochemistry and Molecular Biology, Jefferson Medical College of Thomas Jefferson University; Director, Jefferson Institute of Molecular Medicine, Philadelphia

AMY PRUITT, M.D.

Assistant Professor of Neurology, University of Pennsylvania School of Medicine and Graduate Hospital, Philadelphia

LOUIS J. PTÁČEK, M.D.

Department of Neurology, The University of Utah School of Medicine, Salt Lake City

JOEL M. RAPPEPORT, M.D.

Professor of Medicine, Yale University School of Medicine; Director, Bone Marrow Transplantation Program, Yale New Haven Hospital, New Haven

NEIL H. RASKIN, M.D.

Professor of Neurology, University of California, San Francisco

C. GEORGE RAY, M.D.

Professor and Chairman, Department of Pediatrics, St. Louis University School of Medicine, St. Louis

SHARON LEE REED, M.D.

Associate Professor of Pathology and Medicine and Associate Director, Microbiology Laboratory, Division of Infectious Diseases, UCSD Medical Center, San Diego

ANTONIO J. REGINATO, M.D.

Head, Division of Rheumatology; Professor of Medicine, Cooper Hospital/University Medical Center, University of Medicine and Dentistry of New Jersey/Robert Wood Johnson Medical School at Camden, Camden

RICHARD C. REICHMAN, M.D.

Professor of Medicine and Head, Infectious Disease Unit, University of Rochester School of Medicine and Dentistry, Rochester

NEIL M. RESNICK, M.D.

Assistant Professor of Medicine, Harvard Medical School; Chief, Division of Gerontology, Brigham and Women's Hospital; Geriatric Research Education and Clinical Center, Brockton-West Roxbury Veterans Administration Medical Center, Boston

HERBERT Y. REYNOLDS, M.D.

Chairman, Department of Medicine and J. Lloyd Huck Professor of Medicine, The Pennsylvania State University; University Hospital, The Milton S. Hershey Medical Center, Hershey

STUART RICH, M.D.

Professor of Medicine and Chief, Section of Cardiology, University of Illinois at Chicago College of Medicine, Chicago

GARY S. RICHARDSON, M.D.

Instructor in Medicine, Harvard Medical School; Associate Physician, Brigham and Women's Hospital, Boston

HAL B. RICHERSON, M.D.

Professor of Internal Medicine, University of Iowa College of Medicine; University of Iowa Hospitals and Clinics, Iowa City

JAMES M. RICHTER, M.D.

Assistant Professor of Medicine, Harvard Medical School; Chief, Gastrointestinal Clinic, Massachusetts General Hospital, Boston

R. PAUL ROBERTSON, M.D.

Professor of Medicine and Cell Biology; Director, Division of Diabetes, Endocrinology and Metabolism, University of Minnesota, Minneapolis

ALLAN H. ROPPER, M.D.

Professor of Neurology, Tufts University School of Medicine; Chief, Division of Neurology, St. Elizabeth's Medical Center, Boston

IRWIN H. ROSENBERG, M.D.

Professor of Medicine, Nutrition and Physiology; Director, USDA Human Nutrition Research Center on Aging, Tufts University, Boston

LEON E. ROSENBERG, M.D.

President, Bristol-Myers Squibb Pharmaceutical Research Institute, Princeton

WENDELL F. ROSSE, M.D.

Florence Reynaud McAlister Professor of Medicine and Medical Research, Duke University School of Medicine; Duke University Medical Center, Durham

DANIEL ROTROSEN, M.D.

Medical Office, Laboratory of Host Defenses, National Institute of Allergy and Infectious Diseases, National Institutes of Health, Bethesda

JODI ROY, M.S., R.D.

Frances Stern Nutrition Center, New England Medical Center Hospital, Boston

ARTHUR H. RUBENSTEIN, M.D.

Lowell T. Coggeshall Professor; Chairman, Department of Medicine, University of Chicago Pritzker School of Medicine, Chicago

JEREMY N. RUSKIN, M.D.

Associate Professor of Medicine, Harvard Medical School; Director, Cardiac Arrhythmia Service, Massachusetts General Hospital, Boston

ARTHUR I. SAGALOWSKY, M.D.

Professor of Urology and Surgical Director of Renal Transplantation, The University of Texas Southwestern Medical Center, Dallas

MATTHEW SAMORE, M.D.

Instructor in Medicine, Harvard Medical School; New England Deaconess Hospital, Boston

JAY P. SANFORD, M.D.

Professor of Internal Medicine, University of Texas Southwestern Medical School; Dean Emeritus, Uniformed Services University of the Health Sciences, Dallas

DAVID A. SCHEINBERG, M.D., Ph.D.

Chief, Leukemia Service, Memorial Sloan-Kettering Cancer Center, New York

I. HERBERT SCHEINBERG, M.D.

Senior Lecturer in Medicine, College of Physicians and Surgeons, Columbia University; Senior Research Associate, St. Luke's/Roosevelt Hospital, New York

W. MICHAEL SCHELD, M.D.

Professor of Internal Medicine and Neurosurgery and Associate Chair for Residency Programs, University of Virginia School of Medicine, Charlottesville

ALAN L. SCHILLER, M.D.

Irene Heinz Given and John LaPorte Given Professor and Chairman of Pathology, Mount Sinai School of Medicine; Chairman of Pathology, The Mount Sinai Hospital, New York

ROBERT T. SCHOOLEY, M.D.

Professor of Medicine and Head, Infectious Disease Division, University of Colorado Health Sciences Center, Denver

JOHN SPEER SCHROEDER, M.D.

Professor of Medicine (Cardiology), Stanford University School of Medicine; Stanford Hospital, Stanford

ANNE SCHUCHAT, M.D.

Medical Epidemiologist, Meningitis and Special Pathogens Branch, Division of Bacterial and Mycotic Diseases, National Center for Infectious Diseases, Centers for Disease Control and Prevention, Atlanta

MARC A. SCHUCKIT, M.D.

Professor of Psychiatry, School of Medicine, University of California at San Diego; Director, Alcohol Research Center, San Diego Veteran's Administration Medical Center, La Jolla

PETER H. SCHUR, M.D.

Professor of Medicine, Harvard Medical School; Department of Rheumatology, Brigham and Women's Hospital, Boston

DAVID S. SEGAL, Ph.D.

Professor of Psychiatry, University of California at San Diego, La Jolla

JULIAN I. SEIFTER, M.D.

Associate Professor of Medicine, Harvard Medical School; Physician, Brigham and Women's Hospital, Boston

ANDREW P. SELWYN, M.D.

Associate Professor of Medicine, Harvard Medical School; Director of Cardiac Catheterization, Brigham and Women's Hospital, Boston

PETER A. SELWYN, M.D., M.P.H.

Associate Professor of Internal Medicine, Epidemiology and Public Health, and Associate Director, AIDS Program, Yale University School of Medicine, New Haven

MARY-ANN SHAFER, M.D.

Professor of Pediatrics; Associate Director, Division of Adolescent Medicine, Department of Pediatrics, School of Medicine, University of California, San Francisco

GORDON C. SHARP, M.D.

Curators' Professor and Michael Einbender Distinguished Professor of Medicine; Director, Division of Immunology and Rheumatology; Director, Arthritis Center; Director, Missouri Arthritis Rehabilitation Research and Training Center; Associate Chairman for Research, Department of Internal Medicine, University of Missouri-Columbia School of Medicine; Director, Antinuclear Antibody Laboratory, University of Missouri Hospital & Clinics, Columbia

ELIZABETH M. SHORT, M.D.

Associate Chief Medical Director for Academic Affairs, Department of Veteran's Affairs, Washington, DC

GEORGE R. SIBER, M.D.

Associate Professor of Medicine, Harvard Medical School; Director, Massachusetts Public Health Biologic Laboratories, Jamaica Plain

WILLIAM SILEN, M.D.

Johnson and Johnson Professor of Surgery, Harvard Medical School; Surgeon-in-Chief; Beth Israel Hospital, Boston

FRED E. SILVERSTEIN, M.D.

Professor of Medicine and Director, Gastrointestinal Endoscopy Fellowship Training, University of Washington School of Medicine, Seattle

KARL L. SKORECKI, M.D., F.R.C.P.(C)

Director, Division of Nephrology, Department of Medicine and Pediatrics, University of Toronto, Toronto

THOMAS L. SLAMOVITS, M.D.

Professor and Vice Chairman, Department of Ophthalmology and Professor of Neurology and Neurosurgery, Albert Einstein College of Medicine/Montefiore Medical Center, New York

CHRISTOPHER A. SLAPAK, M.D.

Assistant Professor of Medicine, Harvard Medical School and Dana-Farber Cancer Institute, Boston

JAMES B. SNOW, JR., M.D.

Director, National Institute on Deafness and Other Communication Disorders, National Institutes of Health, Bethesda

ARTHUR J. SOBER, M.D.

Associate Professor of Dermatology, Harvard Medical School; Associate Chief of Dermatology, Massachusetts General Hospital, Boston

FRANK E. SPEIZER, M.D.

Edward H. Kass Professor of Medicine, Harvard Medical School; Co-Director, Channing Laboratory, Brigham and Women's Hospital, Boston

ANDREW SPIELMAN, SD

Professor of Tropical Public Health, Harvard School of Public Health, Boston

WALTER E. STAMM, M.D.

Professor of Medicine, University of Washington School of Medicine; Head, Infectious Diseases, Harborview Medical Center, Seattle

ALLEN C. STEERE, M.D.

Professor of Medicine and Chief, Rheumatology/Immunology, New England Medical Center and Tufts University School of Medicine, Boston

ROBERT S. STERN, M.D.

Professor, Department of Dermatology, Beth Israel Hospital, Boston

DENNIS L. STEVENS, M.D., Ph.D.

Professor of Medicine, University of Washington School of Medicine, Seattle; Chief, Infectious Diseases, VA Medical Center, Boise

GENE H. STOLLERMAN, M.D.

Professor of Medicine and Public Health, Boston University; University Hospital, Boston

RICHARD M. STONE, M.D.

Assistant Professor of Medicine, Harvard Medical School and Dana-Farber Cancer Institute, Boston

STEPHEN E. STRAUS, M.D.

Chief, Laboratory of Clinical Investigation, National Institute of Allergy and Infectious Diseases, National Institutes of Health, Bethesda

DAVID H.P. STREETEN, M.D.

Professor of Medicine and Head, Section of Endocrinology, State University of New York Health Science Center, Syracuse

ROBERT A. SWERLICK, M.D.

Associate Professor, Department of Dermatology, Emory University School of Medicine, Atlanta

RUP TANDAN, M.D., M.R.C.P.

Associate Professor of Neurology, University of Vermont College of Medicine; Attending Neurologist, Medical Center Hospital of Vermont, Burlington

JOEL D. TAUROG, M.D.

Associate Professor, Department of Internal Medicine and Investigator, Harold C. Simmons Arthritis Research Center, The University of Texas Southwestern Medical Center; Attending Physician, Parkland Memorial Hospital, Sale Lipshy University Hospital, Veterans Administration Medical Center, Dallas

BAYU TEKLU, M.D.

Professor and Chairman, Department of Internal Medicine, College of Medicine, King Saud University, Abha Branch; Consultant Physician, Asir Central Hospital, Saudi Arabia

STEPHEN F. TEMPLETON, M.D.

Assistant Professor of Dermatology and Pathology, Emory University School of Medicine, Atlanta

E. DONNALL THOMAS, M.D.

Professor of Medicine Emeritus, University of Washington; Member, Fred Hutchinson Cancer Research Center, Seattle

LUCY STUART TOMPKINS, M.D.

Associate Professor of Medicine (Infectious Diseases and Geographic Medicine) and Microbiology and Immunology, Stanford University School of Medicine; Director, Clinical Microbiology Laboratory, Stanford University Medical Center, Stanford

PHILLIP P. TOSKES, M.D.

Professor of Medicine and Chief, Division of Gastroenterology, University of Florida, Gainesville

GERARD TROMP, M.D.

Research Assistant Professor, Department of Biochemistry and Molecular Biology, Jefferson Medical College of Thomas Jefferson University, Philadelphia

E. P. TRULOCK, M.D.

Associate Professor of Medicine, Washington University School of Medicine; Barnes Hospital, St. Louis

KENNETH L. TYLER, M.D.

Associate Professor of Neurology, Medicine and Microbiology, University of Colorado Health Sciences Center; Chief, Neurology Service, VA Medical Center, Denver

DAVID VALLE, M.D.

Professor of Pediatrics and Molecular Biology and Genetics, Johns Hopkins University School of Medicine; Investigator, Howard Hughes Medical Institute, Baltimore

MAURICE VICTOR, M.D.

Professor of Medicine (Neurology), Dartmouth Medical School, Hanover; Distinguished Physician of the Veterans Administration, White River Junction

JAMES F. WALLACE, M.D.

Professor of Medicine, University of Washington School of Medicine; Associate Physican-in-Chief, University of Washington Medical Center, Seattle

RICHARD J. WALLACE, Jr., M.D.

Chairman, Department of Microbiology, University of Texas Health Center, Tyler

PETER D. WALZER, M.D.

Professor of Medicine, University of Cincinnati College of Medicine; Chief, Infectious Disease Section, VA Medical Center, Cincinnati

LEONARD WARTOFSKY, M.D.

Professor of Medicine and Physiology, Uniformed Services University of the Health Sciences; Chairman, Department of Medicine, Washington Hospital Center, Washington, DC

CARL V. WASHINGTON, Jr. M.D.

Assistant Professor of Dermatology, Emory University School of Medicine, Atlanta

STEVEN E. WEINBERGER, M.D.

Associate Professor of Medicine, Harvard Medical School; Associate Chairman for Education, Department of Medicine, and Clinical Director, Pulmonary and Critical Care Division, Beth Israel Hospital, Boston

LOUIS WEINSTEIN, M.D., Ph.D.

Senior Physician (Emeritus), Department of Medicine, Brigham and Women's Hospital

ROBERT A. WEINSTEIN, M.D., F.A.C.P.

Professor of Medicine and Program Director, Joint University of Illinois/University of Chicago Infectious Disease Fellowship Training Program, Department of Medicine, Michael Reese Hospital and Medical Center, Chicago

PETER F. WELLER, M.D.

Associate Professor of Medicine, Harvard Medical School; Division of Infectious Diseases, Department of Medicine, Beth Israel Hospital, Boston

MICHAEL R. WESSELS, M.D.

Associate Professor of Medicine, Harvard Medical School; Associate Physician, Beth Israel Hospital; Division of Infectious Diseases, Channing Laboratory, Brigham and Women's Hospital, Boston

NICHOLAS J. WHITE, M.B., B.S., B.Sc., M.R.C.P.

Wellcome Mahidol University, Oxford Tropical Medicine Research Programme, Faculty of Tropical Medicine, Mahidol University, Bangkok

RICHARD J. WHITLEY, M.D.

Loeb Eminent Scholar in Pediatrics and Professor of Pediatrics, Medicine and Microbiology, University of Alabama at Birmingham, Birmingham

GRANT R. WILKINSON, Ph.D.

Professor of Pharmacology, Vanderbilt University School of Medicine, Nashville

GORDON H. WILLIAMS, M.D.

Professor of Medicine, Harvard Medical School; Chief, Endocrine-Hypertension Division, Brigham and Women's Hospital, Boston

JEAN D. WILSON, M.D.

Charles Cameron Sprague Distinguished Chair and Professor of Internal Medicine; Chief, Division of Endocrinology and Metabolism, The University of Texas Southwestern Medical Center, Dallas

BRUCE U. WINTROUB, M.D.

Professor and Chairman, Department of Dermatology, University of California at San Francisco; Associate Dean, UCSF/Mt. Zion Medical Center, San Francisco

SHELDON M. WOLFF, M.D.

Endicott Professor and Chairman, Department of Medicine, Tufts University School of Medicine; Physician-in-Chief, New England Medical Center, Boston

BEVERLY WOO, M.D.

Assistant Professor of Medicine, Harvard Medical School; Physician, Brigham and Women's Hospital, Boston

ALASTAIR J. J. WOOD, M.B.Ch.B., FRCP (Edin)

Professor of Medicine and Professor of Pharmacology, Vanderbilt University School of Medicine; Attending Physician, Vanderbilt University Hospital, Nashville

THEODORE E. WOODWARD, M.D., M.A.C.P.

Professor of Medicine Emeritus, University of Maryland School of Medicine and Hospital, Baltimore

ROBERT L. WORTMANN, M.D.

Professor and Chairman, Department of Medicine, East Carolina University School of Medicine; Chief Medical Service, Pitt County Memorial Hospital, University Medical Center of Eastern Carolina-Pitt County, Greenville

SHIRLEY H. WRAY, M.D., Ph.D., F.R.C.P.

Associate Professor of Neurology, Harvard Medical School; Director, Unit for Neurovisual Disorders, Department of Neurology, Massachusetts General Hospital, Boston

PAUL W. WRIGHT, M.D.

Professor of Family Practice, University of Texas Health Center, Tyler

JOSHUA WYNNE, M.D.

Professor of Internal Medicine and Chief, Division of Cardiology, Wayne State University School of Medicine; Chief, Section of Cardiology, Harper Hospital, Detroit

KIM B. YANCEY, M.D.

Senior Investigator, Dermatology Branch, National Cancer Institute, National Institutes of Health, Bethesda

JAMES B. YOUNG, M.D.

Professor of Medicine, Northwestern University Medical School; Attending Physician, Northwestern Memorial Hospital, Chicago

DORI F. ZALEZNIK, M.D.

Assistant Professor of Medicine, Harvard Medical School; Hospital Epidemiologist, Beth Israel Hospital, Boston

PREFACE

Since the first edition of *Harrison's Principles of Internal Medicine* was published nearly 50 years ago, each subsequent edition has built upon the solid clinical foundation and scientific advances occurring in the interim. In the present 13th edition of *Harrison's*, the Editors have extensively revised the text to reflect important advances in our understanding of the biology and pathophysiology of disease and at the same time to build appropriate links between the extraordinary advances in basic science and clinical medicine, and to emphasize these advances while retaining those facts which, while not new, remain clinically useful and important. Every chapter in the 13th edition has been revised or substantially rewritten, and major new ones have been added. In this preface, we cannot describe all of these revised sections. However, we would like to call to the reader's attention some of the most important ones:

Part One, "Introduction to Clinical Medicine," contains new chapters dealing with medical ethics and the impact of social factors on disease, including the effects of age, gender, genetic background, geography, and ethnic origin. These factors importantly influence the incidence and clinical expression of human disease. Examples of women's health issues discussed in Chap. 5 include screening for ischemic heart disease and discussions of osteoporosis and immunologically mediated diseases in women. Important medical disorders during pregnancy are dealt with in a new Chap. 6. A new Chap. 8, "Geriatric Medicine," describes age-related changes in each organ system and their clinical consequences. There is also a detailed discussion of the management of common geriatric conditions, including intellectual impairment, mobility, incontinence, and iatrogenic drug reactions. Two timely chapters (9 and 10) focus on cost awareness and the quantitative aspects of medicine.

Part Two, "Cardinal Manifestations of Disease," remains the mainstay of this edition, and serves as a comprehensive introduction to clinical medicine. Major patient symptoms are reviewed by organ systems and correlated with specific disease states—the basis of differential diagnosis. The 13th edition also contains chapters on headache, back and neck pain, fever, including fever of unknown origin, and disturbances of smell, taste, and hearing. There is an entirely new and extensively rewritten chapter on diarrhea and constipation, as well as a completely new chapter on jaundice.

Part Three, "Genetics and Disease," has been extensively updated, including a new chapter on genes and neoplasia.

Part Four, "Clinical Pharmacology" and Part Five, "Clinical Nutrition," have been reorganized and updated. The chapters on clinical pharmacology include principles of drug therapy and a new chapter on adverse reactions to drugs. Up-to-date coverage of the physiology and pharmacology of the autonomic nervous system explores its key role in many disease states and the various ways in which drugs interact with this system. Included here also is an updated chapter on G proteins and the regulation of second messengers.

Coverage of nutrition in clinical medicine encompasses nutritional requirements, the assessment of nutritional status, important eating disorders such as anorexia nervosa and bulimia, and obesity. New discussions are presented on diet therapy, including enteral and parenteral nutrition.

A primarily etiologically oriented review in Part Six, "Infectious Disease," has been extensively revised and updated under the aegis of our new editor, Dennis L. Kasper. Here the reader will find the latest approaches to the diagnosis, prevention, and treatment of bacterial, viral, and fungal infections and parasitic infestations. New chapters include "Infections (Excluding AIDS) in Injection Drug Users," "Infections in the Immunocompromised Host," and "Infec-

tions of Skin, Muscle, and Soft Tissues." There have also been major revisions of chapters covering host-organism interaction, the laboratory diagnosis of infectious diseases, septicemia and septic shock, nosocomial infections, and molecular mechanisms of bacterial pathogenesis. There is an important and up-to-date chapter on the human retroviruses.

We believe that the chapter on HIV disease and AIDS by Anthony S. Fauci and H. Clifford Lane is one of the most comprehensive and up-to-date treatises on AIDS. It covers the areas from the natural history and epidemiology to a scholarly treatise on the immunopathogenic mechanisms of HIV disease. In addition, the chapter contains both an organ system by organ system approach as well as an infection breakdown of the major complications of HIV disease.

The core of *Harrison's*, disorders of the organ systems, encompasses Parts Seven through Fourteen, and includes succinct accounts of the pathophysiology of the major human diseases, with emphasis on disease manifestations, diagnostic procedures, differential diagnosis, and treatment strategies. This comprehensive review of organ system disorders includes new chapters on electrocardiography, with excellent new illustrations on the electrocardiographic recognition of acute myocardial infarction. There are updated chapters on cystic fibrosis, lung transplantation, glomerulopathies associated with multisystem diseases, acid-peptic disease (with special focus on *H. pylori*), acute and chronic hepatitis, and liver transplantation.

The section on hematology and oncology includes chapters on oncogenes and tumor suppressor genes, with thorough discussions of p53, the tumor suppressor gene most commonly lost or mutated in human cancers. There is an important new chapter on cancer therapy, with emphasis on immunotherapy and the potential role of gene therapy. There are also new chapters on disorders affecting multiple endocrine systems, porphyrias, and gout. The chapter on diabetes includes a discussion of the impact of tight control on the development of diabetic complications.

In the Part Fourteen, "Neurological Diseases," there are new chapters on the impact of neurobiology on both neurology and psychiatry. There is also a detailed tabulation of the recent molecular genetic discoveries in neurology. There are new chapters on clinical electrophysiology, demyelinating diseases like multiple sclerosis, bacterial meningitis and brain abscess, viral diseases of the central nervous system, and disorders of the autonomic nervous system. For the first time there is a chapter on chronic fatigue syndrome, an entity which has created great interest because of its relationship to psychosomatic medicine.

Finally, Part Fifteen, "Environmental and Occupational Hazards," has been expanded and reorganized.

In the 12th edition of *Harrison's*, the editors decided to identify laboratory data using the International System (SI) of units for clinical laboratory values, plus the conventional system of laboratory nomenclature used in most hospitals in the United States. We felt this was important, since SI units are in frequent use in many countries other than the United States. In the 12th edition and in the present 13th edition, we have listed the SI units first and the conventional units in parentheses for all measurements except blood pressure, which is given only in millimeters of mercury, and for those measurements in which the numbers are the same for both systems. As the readers of the medical literature may be aware, in 1992 the *New England Journal of Medicine*, having previously endorsed SI units, decided to "retreat" to the use of only conventional units. However, the *Harrison's* editors have concluded that, at least for the 13th edition, we should continue to use the SI units, with technologic advances and computerization for many aspects of diagnosis and treatment, (3) the increased geographic mobility of both patients and physicians, (4) the growing number of health-maintenance organizations, in which the patient may have little choice in selecting a physician, (5) the need for more than a single physician to be involved in the care of most patients who are seriously ill, and (6) an increasing reliance by patients to express their disappointments with the health care system by legal means (i.e., by malpractice litigation). Given these changes in the medical care system, maintaining the humane aspects of medical care and the empathetic qualities of the physician is a major challenge. It is now more important than ever that the physician consider each patient to be a unique individual deserving of humane treatment, regardless of personal or financial circumstances.

The American Board of Internal Medicine has defined humanistic qualities as encompassing integrity, respect, and compassion. Availability, the expression of sincere concern, the willingness to take the time to explain all aspects of the patient's illness, and an attitude of being nonjudgmental with patients who have lifestyles, attitudes, and values different from those of the physician and which he or she may in some instances even find repugnant are just a few of the characteristics of the humane physician. Every physician will, at times, be challenged by patients who evoke strongly negative (and occasionally strongly positive) emotional responses. Physicians should be alert to their own reactions to such patients and situations and consciously monitor and control their behavior so that the patients' best interests remain the principal motivation for their actions at all times.

The famous statement of Dr. Francis Peabody is even more relevant today than when delivered more than a half century ago:

The significance of the intimate personal relationship between physician and patient cannot be too strongly emphasized, for in an extraordinarily large number of cases both the diagnosis and treatment are directly dependent on it. One of the essential qualities of the clinician is interest in humanity, for the secret of the care of the patient is in caring for the patient.

CLINICAL SKILLS   History taking   The written history of an illness should embody all the facts of medical significance in the life of the patient. If the history is recorded in chronologic order, recent events should be given the most attention. Likewise, if a problem-oriented approach is used, the problems that are clinically dominant should be listed first. Ideally, the narration of symptoms or problems should be in the patient's own words. However, few patients have sufficient powers of observation or recall to give a history without some guidance from the physician, who must be careful not to suggest the answers to the questions being posed. Often a symptom which has concerned a patient has little significance, while a seemingly minor complaint may be of considerable importance. Therefore, the physician must be constantly alert to the possibility that any event related by the patient, however trivial or apparently remote, may be the key to the solution of the medical problem.

An informative history is more than an orderly listing of symptoms. Something is always gained by listening to patients and noting the way in which they talk about their symptoms. Inflections of voice, facial expression, and attitude may betray important clues to the meaning of the symptoms to the patient. In listening to the history, the physician discovers not only something about the disease but also something about the patient.

With experience, the pitfalls of history taking become apparent. What patients relate for the most part consists of subjective phenomena colored by past experience. Patients obviously differ widely in their responses to the same stimuli and in their coping mechanisms. Their attitudes are variably influenced by fear of disability and death and by concern over the consequences of their illness to their families. Sometimes the accuracy of the history is affected by language or sociologic barriers, by failing intellectual powers that interfere with recall, or by disorders of consciousness that make them unaware of their illness. It is not surprising, then, that even the most careful

physician may at times despair of collecting factual data and be forced to proceed with evidence that represents little more than an approximation of the truth. It is in obtaining the history that the physician's skill, knowledge, and experience are most clearly in evidence.

The family history serves several functions. First, in rare single-gene defects a positive family history of a similarly affected individual or a history of consanguinity may have important diagnostic implications. Second, in diseases of multifactorial etiology that have a familial aggregation, it may be possible to identify patients at risk for disease and to intervene prior to development of overt manifestations. For example, recent weight gain may be a more ominous development in a woman who has a family history of diabetes than in one who does not. In certain situations the family history has major implications for preventive medicine. When a diagnosis of a hereditary condition known to predispose to cancer is made, it is the physician's obligation to follow up this possibility carefully in the patient, to survey the family, and to educate them about the need for long-term follow-up.

However accurate and complete, the medical history does much more than provide facts of critical importance. The very act of taking the history provides the physician with the opportunity to establish or enhance the unique bond that is the basis for the critically important patient-physician relationship. An effort should be made to place the patient at ease, regardless of the circumstances of the encounter. The patient should, at some point, have the opportunity to tell his or her own story of the illness without frequent interruption and, when appropriate, should receive expression of interest, encouragement, and empathy from the physician. It is often enlightening to develop an appreciation of the patient's own perception of the illness, the patient's expectations of the physician and the medical care system, and the financial and social implications of the illness to the patient. The confidentiality of the patient-physician relationship should be emphasized, and the patient should be given the opportunity to identify those aspects of the history which he or she wishes not to be disclosed to anyone else.

Physical examination   Physical signs are the objective and verifiable marks of disease and represent solid, indisputable facts. Their significance is enhanced when they confirm a functional or structural change already suggested by the patient's history. At times, the physical signs may be the only evidence of disease, especially when the history has been inconsistent, confused, or lacking altogether.

The physical examination should be performed methodically and thoroughly, with due regard for the patient's comfort and modesty. Although attention has often been directed by the history to the diseased organ or part of the body, the examination of a new patient must extend from head to toe in an objective search for abnormalities. Unless the examination procedure is systematic, important parts of it may be omitted, a common error even among the most skilled clinicians. The results of the examination, like the details of the history, should be recorded at the time they are elicited, not hours later when they are subject to the distortions of memory. Many inaccuracies stem from the careless practice of writing or dictating notes long after the examination has been concluded. Skill in physical diagnosis is acquired with experience, but it is not merely technique that determines success in eliciting signs. The detection of a few scattered petechiae, a faint diastolic murmur, or a small mass in the abdomen is not a question of keener eyes and ears or more sensitive fingers but of a mind alert to these findings. Skill in physical diagnosis reflects a way of thinking more than a way of doing. Physical findings are subject to change. Just because the examination is normal on one occasion does not guarantee that this will be the case on subsequent examinations. Likewise, abnormal findings may disappear in the course of illness. It is important, therefore, to repeat the physical examination as frequently as the clinical situation warrants.

Laboratory tests   The increase in the number and availability of laboratory tests has resulted in increasing reliance on these studies in the solution of clinical problems. It is essential, however, to bear in mind the limitations of such procedures, which by virtue of their impersonal quality and complexity often gain an aura of authority regardless of the fallibility of the tests themselves, of the individuals doing or interpreting them, or of their instruments. More important, the accumulation of laboratory data cannot relieve the physician from the responsibility of careful observation and study of the patient. Physicians also must weigh carefully the hazards and expense involved in the laboratory procedures they order. Moreover, laboratory tests are rarely ordered and reported singly. Rather, they are produced as "batteries." Some laboratories now perform batteries of 24 and even 40 tests. The various combinations of laboratory tests are often useful. For example, they may provide the clue to such nonspecific symptoms as generalized weakness and increased fatigability by revealing abnormalities of hepatic function together with elevated levels of serum IgG, which, in turn, would suggest the diagnosis of chronic liver disease. Sometimes a single abnormality, such as an elevated serum calcium level, points to a specific disease, such as hyperparathyroidism.

The thoughtful use of screening tests should not be confused with indiscriminate laboratory testing. The use of screening tests is based on the fact that a group of laboratory determinations can be carried out conveniently on a single specimen of blood at relatively low cost. Biochemical measurements, together with simple laboratory examinations such as blood count, urinalysis, and sedimentation rate, often provide the major clue to the presence of a pathologic process. At the same time, the physician must learn to evaluate occasional abnormalities among the screening tests that may not necessarily connote significant disease. There is nothing more wasteful and unproductive than an in-depth workup following a report of an isolated laboratory abnormality in a patient who is otherwise well. Among the more than 40 tests that are performed on many patients, one or two are often slightly abnormal. If there is no suspicion of an underlying illness, these tests are ordinarily repeated to ensure that the abnormality does not represent a laboratory error. If an abnormality is confirmed, it is important to distinguish a minor one (less than two standard deviations) from a major one (more than two standard deviations). Even in the case of the latter, the decision of whether to proceed with further workup is a test of the physician's clinical judgment.

Imaging techniques The past two decades have seen the arrival of ultrasonography, a variety of scans that employ isotopes to visualize organs heretofore inaccessible, computed tomography with its varying permutations, magnetic resonance imaging, and positron emission tomography. Aside from opening up new diagnostic vistas, this new technology benefits patients because it has frequently supplanted invasive techniques that require surgical biopsy or the insertion of tubes, wires, or catheters into the body—procedures that are often painful and sometimes risky. While the enthusiasm for noninvasive technology is understandably justified, all too often the results of these tests have not been validated properly before they are disseminated as clinical dogma. Moreover, the expense entailed in performing these imaging tests is often substantial and is not always considered when ordering them. Nevertheless, these examinations should be used judiciously, preferably in lieu of, not in addition to, the invasive maneuvers they are meant to replace.

THE DIAGNOSIS OF DISEASE Clinical diagnosis requires both aspects of logic—analysis and synthesis—and the more difficult the clinical problem, the more important is a logical approach to it. Such an approach requires that the physician list carefully each problem suggested by the symptoms and physical and laboratory findings and seek answers to each. Most physicians attempt consciously or unconsciously to fit a given problem into one of a series of syndromes. *The syndrome is a group of symptoms and signs of disordered function related to one another by means of some anatomic, physiologic, or biochemical peculiarity.* It embodies a hypothesis concerning the deranged function of an organ, organ system, or tissue. Congestive heart failure, Cushing's syndrome, and dementia are examples. In congestive heart failure, dyspnea, orthopnea, cyanosis, dependent edema, engorged neck veins, pleural effusion, rales, and hepatomegaly are known to be connected by a single pathophysiologic mechanism—insufficiency of the cardiac pump mechanism. In Cushing's syndrome, moon facies, hypertension, diabetes mellitus, and osteoporosis are recognized effects of excess glucocorticoids acting on many target organs. In dementia, deterioration of memory, incoherent thinking, impaired language functions, visual-spatial disorientation, and faulty judgment are related to destruction of the association areas of the cerebrum.

A syndrome usually does not identify the precise cause of an illness, but it narrows the number of possibilities and often suggests certain special clinical and laboratory studies. The derangements of each organ system in humans are reducible to a relatively small number of syndromes. The diagnosis is simplified greatly if a clinical problem conforms neatly to a well-defined syndrome, because only a few diseases need to be considered in the differential diagnosis. In contrast, the search for the cause of an illness that does not conform to a syndrome is more difficult because a much greater number of diseases have to be considered. Even here an orderly approach which proceeds from symptom to sign to laboratory findings will usually result in the diagnosis.

CARING FOR THE PATIENT Patient care begins with the development of a personal relationship between the patient and the physician. In the absence of a sense of trust and confidence on the part of the patient, the effectiveness of most therapeutic measures is diminished. In many instances, when there is confidence in the physician, reassurance is the best treatment and is all that is needed. Likewise, in those cases which do not lend themselves to easy solutions and for which no effective treatment is available, a feeling on the part of the patient that the physician is doing all that is possible is one of the most important therapeutic measures that can be provided. An important aspect of clinical decision making and patient care involves the "quality of life," a subjective assessment of what each patient values most. Such an assessment requires detailed, sometimes intimate knowledge of the patient, which can usually be obtained only through deliberate, unhurried, and often repeated conversation. In situations where complete freedom from signs and symptoms of disease is impossible, enhancement of the quality of life is the major goal of therapy.

Assessing the outcome of treatments Clinicians generally use *objective* and readily measurable parameters to judge the outcomes of a therapeutic intervention. For example, findings on physical or laboratory examination—such as the level of blood pressure, the patency of a coronary artery on an angiogram, the size of a mass on a radiologic examination, or the titer of an antibody—can provide information of critical importance. However, patients usually seek medical attention for *subjective* reasons; they wish relief from pain, to preserve or regain function, and to enjoy life. Although these goals are often nebulous and differ among individuals, the field of "medical outcomes research" has suggested that a patient's health status or quality of life can be separated into a number of categories, including bodily comfort, physical activity, social activity, personal and professional role function, sexual function, cognitive function, sleep, vitality, and overall perception of health. Function in each of these important areas can be assessed by means of structured interviews or specially designed questionnaires. However, in a less formal way these categories also provide useful parameters by which the physician can judge the patient's view of his or her disability and the response to treatment, particularly of chronic illness. The intelligent practice of medicine requires consideration and integration of both objective and subjective outcomes.

Drug therapy With each succeeding year, more drugs are released, every one with the hope and the promise that it is an improvement over its predecessor. Although the pharmaceutical industry must be given most of the credit for advances in drug therapy, it is also true that many new drugs have only a marginal advantage over the agents they are aimed to replace. The barrage of new information with which practitioners are deluged does little to provide a clear picture of clinical pharmacology; on the contrary, to most physicians new drugs are confusing. With some exceptions, however, the approach to a new drug should be one of caution. Unless the new agent is established beyond doubt to be a real advance, it is wiser to use agents the efficacy and safety of which have been well established.

Care of the elderly   Over the next several decades, the practice of medicine will be greatly influenced by the health care needs of the elderly, whose numbers are increasing rapidly. It is estimated that in the United States the population over age 65 will almost triple over the next 30 years. It is therefore essential that we understand and appreciate the physiologic processes associated with aging; the different responses of the elderly compared with younger patients to common diseases or disease mechanisms such as acute infections, hyperthyroidism, and uncontrolled diabetes mellitus; and disorders that occur commonly with aging such as depression, dementia, urinary incontinence, and falls. The elderly have more trouble with medications in large part due to altered pharmacokinetics and pharmacodynamics. Adverse reactions increase steadily above age 50. In the elderly, commonly used drugs such as digoxin have prolonged half-lives in part because of the decreased renal function that accompanies aging and in part because tissues such as the central nervous system become more sensitive to certain drugs, such as the benzodiazepines and narcotics.

Diseases in men versus women   There are significant gender differences in diseases that afflict both men and women. These have not been clearly evident because in the past most epidemiologic studies and clinical research have been carried out in adult men rather than women. There is now increasing evidence that in ischemic heart disease, mortality rates are higher in women. Hypertension is more prevalent in African-American women than in their male counterparts; diseases involving the immune system such as lupus erythematosus, multiple sclerosis, and primary biliary cirrhosis occur more frequently in women; and women have a greater longevity than men. The reason for these differences is not yet clear, and it is all too evident that more research in women's health issues is badly needed.

Iatrogenic disorders   An *iatrogenic disorder* occurs when the deleterious effects of a therapeutic or diagnostic regimen produce pathology independent of the condition for which the regimen is given. No matter what the clinical situation, it is the responsibility of the physician to use powerful therapeutic measures wisely, with due regard to their action, potential dangers, and cost. Every medical procedure, whether diagnostic or therapeutic, has the potential for harm, but it would be impossible to afford the patient the benefits of modern scientific medicine if reasonable steps in diagnosis and therapy were withheld because of possible risks. *Reasonable* implies that the physician has weighed the pros and cons of a procedure and has concluded that it is advisable or essential for the relief of discomfort or the cure or amelioration of disease. For example, the use of glucocorticoids to arrest progressive systemic lupus erythematosus may produce Cushing's syndrome. In this instance, the benefits usually exceed the untoward side effects. However, much harm can result when the deleterious effects of a procedure or a drug exceed any possible advantages that might have been anticipated. Examples include the dangerous or fatal drug reactions that occasionally follow the use of antibiotics given for minor respiratory infections, the gastric hemorrhage or perforation caused by glucocorticoid administration for mild arthritis, and the occurrence of fatal liver disease that may follow needless transfusions of blood or plasma.

However, the harm that a physician can do to a patient is not limited to the imprudent use of medication or procedures. Equally important are ill-considered or unjustified remarks. Many a patient has developed a cardiac neurosis because the physician ventured a grave prognosis on the basis of a misinterpreted finding of a heart murmur on auscultation. Not only the treatment itself but the physician's words and behavior are capable of causing injury.

The physician must never become so absorbed in the disease as to forget the patient who is its victim. As the science of medicine advances, it is all too easy to become so fascinated by the manifesta-tions of disease that one disregards the ailing person's fears and concerns about suffering and death, job and family, the cost of medical care, and the specter of economic insecurity. Treatment of a patient consists of more than the dispassionate confrontation of a disease. It embodies also the expression of warmth, compassion, and understanding.

Informed consent   In an era of rapidly advancing technology, patients will require diagnostic and therapeutic procedures that are painful and that pose some risk. These include all surgical procedures, e.g., biopsies of tissues, endoscopy, radiographic maneuvers involving the insertion of catheters, and many others. In most hospitals and clinics, patients undergoing such procedures are required to sign a form consenting to them. More important, however, is the notion that the patient must understand clearly the risk entailed in these procedures; this is the definition of *informed consent*. It is incumbent on the physician to explain to the patient, in a clearly understandable manner, the procedures which he or she faces. By doing this conscientiously, much of the dread of the unknown that is inherent in hospitalization will be mitigated.

Accountability   Throughout the world, physicians, once licensed to practice medicine, have not had to account for their actions except to their peers. In the United States, however, during the past two decades there have been increasing demands for physicians to account for the way in which they practice medicine by meeting certain standards prescribed by federal and state governments. The hospital-ization of patients whose health care is reimbursed by the government (Medicare and Medicaid) and other third parties is subjected to utilization review. This means that the physician must defend the cause for and duration of a patient's hospitalization if it falls outside certain "average" standards. In some instances, a second opinion is necessary before a patient can have elective surgery. The purpose of these regulations is to contain spiraling health care costs. It is likely that this type of review will be extended to all phases of medical practice and will alter the practice of medicine even more profoundly.

Physicians also may be expected to give account of their continuing competence by mandatory continuing education, patient-record audit, recertification by examination (time-limited certification), or relicens-ing. While these measures probably enhance the physician's factual knowledge, there is no evidence that they have a similar effect on the quality of practice.

Practice guidelines   Physicians are faced with a large, often bewildering array of potentially useful diagnostic techniques and therapeutic measures from which to choose as they deal with individual patients. The intelligent and cost-effective practice of medicine consists of selecting those most appropriate to a particular patient and clinical situation. To aid physicians and other care-givers in making these selections, professional organizations and government agencies are developing formal clinical practice guidelines. These guidelines may be viewed as double-edged swords. On the one hand, when they are current and properly applied, they can provide a useful framework for managing patients with particular diagnoses or symptoms. They also offer practice standards that protect patients—particularly those with inadequate health care benefits—from receiving substandard care. They can also protect conscientious caregivers from inappropriate charges of malpractice, and they can protect society from the excessive costs associated with the overuse of medical resources. On the other hand, clinical guidelines tend to oversimplify the practice of medicine. Different groups with differing perspectives may develop divergent recommendations regarding issues as basic as the need for a periodic sigmoidoscopy in middle-aged persons. Furthermore, guidelines do not—and cannot be expected to—take into account the complex interplay between genetic and environmental influences that are responsible for the uniqueness of each individual and of his or her illness. The practice of medicine strictly according to guidelines carries with it the danger of transforming medicine from a learned profession rooted in the biologic and behavioral sciences to a tech-nical vocation. The challenge for the physician is to accept and incor-porate into clinical practice the valuable recommendations offered by the knowledgeable individuals who prepare clinical practice guidelines without accepting them blindly or being inappropriately constrained.

Cost-effectiveness in medical care As the cost of medical care continues to rise, it is becoming necessary to establish stringent priorities in the expenditure of money for health care. In some instances, preventive measures offer the greatest return for the expenditure; outstanding examples include vaccination, immunization, reduction in accidents and occupational hazards, improved environmental control, and biochemical and molecular biologic screening of newborns. For example, the detection of phenylketonuria by newborn screening may result in a net saving of many thousands of dollars.

As resources become increasingly constrained, it will be necessary to weigh the justification of performing costly procedures that provide only a limited life expectancy against the pressing need for more primary care for those persons who do not have adequate access to medical services. At the level of the individual patient, it is important to reduce costly hospital admissions as much as possible if total health care is to be provided at a cost that most can afford. This, of course, implies and depends on a close cooperative effort between patients, their physicians, their employers, third-party carriers, and government, along with constant surveillance of those types of procedures which can be conducted safely and effectively on an ambulatory basis. Equally important in reducing total health care expenditures is the need for individual physicians to know the cost of medicines that they prescribe and to monitor both the cost and effectiveness of those drugs. In the last analysis, the medical profession should provide leadership and guidance to the public in matters of cost control, and physicians must take this responsibility seriously without being or seeming to be self-serving. It is important, however, that the socioeconomic aspects of health care delivery not be permitted to interfere with the concern of physicians for the welfare of their patients. The patient must be able to rely on the individual physician as his or her principal advocate in matters of health care.

Research and teaching The title *doctor* is derived from the Latin *docere*, "to teach," and the physician should share information and medical knowledge with others and be willing to teach what he or she has learned to colleagues as well as to students of medicine and related professions. The practice of medicine is dependent on the sum total of medical knowledge, which in turn is based on an unending chain of scientific discovery, clinical observation, analysis, and interpretation. Advances in medicine depend on the acquisition of new information, i.e., on research, which must often involve patients; improved medical care requires the transmission of this information. As part of broader societal responsibilities, the physician should encourage patients to participate in ethical and properly approved clinical investigations if they do not impose undue hazard, discomfort, or inconvenience.

Incurability and death No problem is more distressing than that presented by the patient with an incurable disease, particularly when premature death is inevitable. What should the patient and family be told, what measures should be taken to maintain life, and how is death to be defined?

Although some would argue otherwise, there is no ironclad rule that the patient must immediately be told "everything," even if the patient is an adult and the head of a family. How much the patient is told should depend on the patient's ability and capacity to deal with the possibility of imminent death; often this capacity grows with time, and whenever possible, gradual rather than abrupt disclosure is the best strategy. This decision also may take into consideration the patient's religious beliefs, financial and business status, and to some extent the wishes of the family. The patient must be given an opportunity to talk with the physician and ask questions. Patients may find it easier to share their feelings about death with their physician, who is likely to be more objective and less emotional than family members.

One thing is certain; it is not for you to don the black cap and, assuming the judicial function, take hope away from any patient . . . hope that comes to us all.

William Osler

Even when the patient directly inquires, "Doctor, am I dying?" the physician must attempt to determine whether this is a request for information, a demand for reassurance, or even an expression of hostility. Most would agree that only open communication between the patient and the physician can resolve these questions and guide the physician in what to say and how to say it.

The physician should provide or arrange for emotional, physical, and spiritual support and must be compassionate, unhurried, and open. There is much to be gained by the laying on of hands. Pain should be adequately controlled, human dignity maintained, and isolation from family avoided. The last two in particular tend to be overlooked in hospitals, where the intrusion of life-sustaining apparatuses can so easily detract from attention to the whole person and encourage concentration instead on the life-threatening disease. The physician also must prepare to deal with guilt feelings on the part of the family when a member becomes gravely or hopelessly ill. It is important for the doctor to reassure the family that everything possible has been done.

The President's Committee for the Study of Ethical Problems in Medicine defined death as (1) irreversible cessation of circulatory and respiratory function or (2) irreversible cessation of all functions of the entire brain, including the brainstem. Clinical and electroencephalographic criteria permit the reliable diagnosis of cerebral death. According to the criteria adopted by the staff of the Massachusetts General Hospital and the Harvard Committee on Brain Death, death occurs when all signs of receptivity and responsivity are absent, including all brainstem reflexes (pupillary reactions, ocular movement, blinking, swallowing, breathing), and the electroencephalogram is isoelectric. Occasionally, intoxications and metabolic disorders may simulate this state; hence the diagnosis requires expert evaluation. Under the aforementioned circumstances, to continue with heroic, highly costly supportive measures merely for the purpose of preserving cardiac function is against the best interests of patient, family, and society. In such instances, the dilemma of continuing care could be avoided if the medical profession, in accord with social sanction, can be brought to redefine life and death by these criteria.

The following guidelines are deserving of consideration:

1 The diagnosis of brain death, based on the preceding criteria, should be corroborated by another physician and confirmed by clinical examination and EEG, repeated one or more times.

2 The family should be informed of the irreversibility of loss of brain function but should not be requested to ratify the decision whether the medical treatment should be discontinued. An exception to this limited decision-making power of the family might apply where the patient has directed the family that he or she wishes them to make the decision.

3 The physician, after consultation with a professional colleague, may withdraw supportive measures, assuming that nothing more can be offered.

4 The possibility that such patients may become sources of organs for grafting should not enter into the aforementioned decisions, although prior to the cessation of heart action the family may be asked whether this would be their wish, or the family may suggest that organs be used for this purpose. In many states, laws now require physicians to request organ donations. A question arises when the patient has indicated in advance a wish to be an organ or tissue donor whether the family must be approached, since many believe the patient's prior wishes carry overriding weight. This issue is controversial.

"Do not resuscitate" orders and cessation of therapy When carried out in a timely and expert manner, cardiopulmonary resuscitation is often useful in the prevention of sudden, unexpected death.

However, unless there are reasons to the contrary, it should not be carried out when it merely prolongs life in a patient with terminal, incurable disease. The decision not to resuscitate a patient and decisions about the intensity of therapy and, indeed, whether or not treatment is to be delivered or continued to patients who are incurably and terminally ill must be reviewed frequently and must take into consideration any unexpected changes in the patient's condition. In this context the administration of fluids and food are considered therapies that may be withdrawn or withheld. These decisions also must take into account both the underlying medical condition and the wishes of the patient or, if these cannot be or have not been ascertained directly, those of a close relative or other surrogate who can be relied on to transmit the patient's feelings and to be guided by the patient's best interests and wishes. The patient's autonomy—whether the choice is to continue or discontinue treatment or to be resuscitated in the event of a cardiopulmonary arrest—is paramount. The courts have ruled that competent patients may be able to refuse therapy and that an incompetent patient's previously stated wishes regarding life support should be respected. The issues involving death and dying are among the most difficult in medicine. In approaching them rationally and consistently, the physician must combine both the art and the science of medicine.

2 ETHICAL ISSUES IN CLINICAL MEDICINE

BERNARD LO

Physicians frequently confront ethical issues in clinical practice that are perplexing, time-consuming and emotionally draining. Experience, common sense, and simply being a good person do not guarantee that physicians can identify or resolve ethical dilemmas. Knowledge about common ethical dilemmas is also essential.

FUNDAMENTAL ETHICAL GUIDELINES

In patient care, physicians should follow two fundamental but frequently conflicting ethical guidelines: respecting patient autonomy and acting in the patient's best interests.

RESPECTING PATIENT AUTONOMY Competent, informed patients have the right to be free of unwanted medical interventions. They may exercise their self-determination by refusing recommended interventions and choosing among the available alternatives.

Informed consent Physicians are required to obtain patients' agreement to care and to provide them with pertinent, comprehensible information about the nature of the proposed care, the alternatives, the risks and benefits of each, and the likely consequences. At the same time, physicians must avoid overwhelming patients with medical jargon, complicated explanations, or too much information at once. Informed consent involves more than obtaining patients' signatures on consent forms; physicians also need to discuss options with patients, educate them about their condition, answer questions, and help them deliberate. Patients and physicians need to share decision-making. Physicians have expertise about the benefits and risks of each option, which must be weighed according to patients' values and goals.

Nondisclosure of information Physicians may consider withholding a serious diagnosis, misrepresenting it, or limiting discussions of prognosis or risks because they fear that a patient will develop severe anxiety or depression or reject needed care. Patients should not be forced to receive information against their will. Surveys show,

however, that most people want to know their diagnosis and prognosis, even if they are terminally ill. Without such information, patients cannot make informed decisions. Generally physicians should provide relevant information, while offering empathy and hope and helping patients cope with bad news.

Emergency care Informed consent is not required when patients cannot give consent and delaying treatment would place their life or health in peril. People are presumed to want such emergency care, unless they have indicated otherwise.

Futile interventions Respect for patient autonomy does not entitle patients to insist on whatever care they want. Physicians are not obligated to provide futile interventions that offer no physiologic benefit or have no prospect of achieving the goals of care. For example, cardiopulmonary resuscitation would be futile in a patient with multisystem failure that is worsening despite maximal therapy. But physicians should be wary of using the term ''futile'' in looser senses to justify unilateral decisions to withhold interventions because they believe the probability of success is too low, the patient's goals inappropriate, or the costs too high. If patients insist on ''futile'' care, physicians should check for misunderstandings and unaddressed psychosocial issues. Discussions with an ethics committee may also be helpful.

ACTING IN THE BEST INTERESTS OF PATIENTS The guideline of *beneficence* requires physicians to take actions for patients' benefit, not just to avoid harming them. Laypeople do not possess medical expertise and may be vulnerable because of their illness. Thus patients rely on physicians to provide sound advice and to promote their well-being. Physicians encourage such trust. For these reasons, physicians have a fiduciary duty to act in the best interests of their patients. The guideline of ''do no harm'' forbids physicians from providing ineffective therapies or from acting selfishly or maliciously. This precept, while often cited, provides only limited guidance, because many beneficial interventions also have serious risks.

CONFLICTS BETWEEN BENEFICENCE AND AUTONOMY Patients' refusals of care may thwart their own goals or cause them serious harm. For example, a young man with asthma may refuse mechanical ventilation for reversible respiratory failure. Physicians can approach such conflicts using a series of questions.

1 *What is the patient's diagnosis and prognosis?* Resolving ethical issues requires sound medical information.
2 *Is the patient competent and informed?* Simply to accept such refusals, in the name of respecting autonomy, would fail to show caring. Physicians can elicit patients' expectations and concerns, correct misunderstandings, and try to persuade them to accept beneficial therapies. If disagreements persist after discussions, the patient's informed choices and view of best interests should prevail.
3 If the patient lacks decision-making capacity, two further questions need to be asked. *Has the patient provided advance directives?* Trustworthy advance directives should be respected. *Who is the appropriate surrogate for the patient?* The following section addresses these latter two questions.

PATIENTS WHO LACK DECISION-MAKING CAPACITY

Patients may not be able to make informed decisions because of illness or the effects of medications. Such patients may not express any choices, or their uninformed decisions may jeopardize their health. Generally surrogates need to make decisions for such patients.

ASSESSING CAPACITY TO MAKE MEDICAL DECISIONS All adults are considered legally competent unless declared incompetent by a court. In practice, however, physicians usually determine that patients lack the capacity to make health care decisions and arrange for surrogates to make them, without involving the courts. By definition, competent patients can express a choice and appreciate the medical situation, the nature of the proposed care, the alternatives, and the risks, benefits, and consequences of each. Their choices should be consistent with their values and should not result from delusions or hallucinations. Assessing decision-making capacity is difficult when patients can understand some important aspects of their situation but not others. Psychiatrists may help in hard cases because they are skilled at interviewing mentally impaired patients and can identify treatable depression or psychosis. When impairments are fluctuating or reversible, decisions should be postponed if possible until the patient recovers decision-making capacity.

CHOICE OF SURROGATE   Physicians routinely ask family members to serve as surrogates, presuming that they know the patient's preferences and have the patient's best interests at heart. While most patients want their family members to be surrogates, some may prefer a close friend. Patients' designation of surrogates for health care decisions should be respected. In a few cases, the courts have already named a surrogate for the patient.

STANDARDS FOR SURROGATE DECISION MAKING Advance directives   These are statements by competent patients that indicate (1) what interventions they would refuse or accept or (2) who should serve as surrogate if they lose decision-making capacity. Following advance directives respects patients' autonomy.

Oral conversations are the most frequent form of advance directives. While such conversations are generally followed in clinical practice, casual or vague comments may not be trustworthy.

Living wills direct physicians to withhold or withdraw life-sustaining interventions if the patient becomes terminally ill and incapable of making decisions. Generally patients may refuse only interventions that "merely prolong the process of dying." In some states, living wills also apply in persistent vegetative states or allow patients to appoint surrogates.

The durable power of attorney for health care allows patients to appoint surrogates to make health care decisions if they lose decision-making capacity. It is more flexible and comprehensive than the living will, applying whenever the patient is unable to make decisions.

Physicians should encourage patients to provide advance directives and to discuss their preferences with family members or surrogates. In discussions with patients, physicians can ensure that advance directives are informed, up-to-date, and address likely clinical scenarios. The federal Patient Self-Determination Act requires hospitals to inform patients of their right to make health care decisions and to provide advance directives.

Substituted judgment   In the absence of clear advance directives, surrogates and physicians should try to decide as the patient would under the circumstances, using all information that they know about the patient. While such substituted judgments try to respect the patient's values, they may be problematic. Surrogates may be mistaken about the patient's preferences, particularly when they have not been discussed explicitly. In some cases, so little is known about the patient's values that substituted judgments would be mere speculation.

Best interests   When the patient's preferences are unclear or unknown, decisions should be based on the patient's best interests. Best interests are controversial, especially when quality as well as duration of life are considered. Judgments about quality of life are appropriate if they reflect the patient's own values. Bias or discrimination may occur, however, if others project their values onto the patient. For instance, most patients with chronic illness rate their quality of life higher than their family members and physicians do.

Legal issues   Physicians need to know pertinent state laws regarding patients who lack decision-making capacity. A few state courts allow life-sustaining treatments to be withheld only if patients have provided written advance directives or very specific oral ones.

Problems   Disagreements may occur among potential surrogates or between the physician and surrogate. Physicians can remind everyone to base decisions on what the patient would want, not what they would want for themselves. Consultation with the hospital ethics committee or with another physician often helps resolve disputes. Such consultation is also helpful when patients have no surrogate and no advance directives. The courts should be used as a last resort when disagreements cannot be resolved in the clinical setting.

DECISIONS ABOUT LIFE-SUSTAINING INTERVENTIONS

While medical technology can save lives, it can also prolong the process of dying or be imposed against patients' wishes. Competent, informed patients may refuse life-sustaining interventions. Such interventions may be withheld from patients who lack decision-making capacity on the basis of advance directives or decisions by appropriate surrogates. Patients need not be terminally ill or comatose. Courts have ruled that foregoing life-sustaining interventions is neither suicide nor murder.

MISLEADING DISTINCTIONS   People commonly draw distinctions that are intuitively plausible but prove untenable on closer analysis.

Extraordinary and ordinary care   Some physicians are willing to forego "extraordinary" or "heroic" interventions, such as surgery, mechanical ventilation, or renal dialysis, but insist on providing "ordinary" ones, such as antibiotics, intravenous fluids, or feeding tubes. However, this is not a logical distinction. All medical interventions, however, have both risks and benefits. Any intervention may be withheld, if the burdens for the individual patient outweigh the benefits.

Withdrawing and withholding interventions   Many people feel more responsible for a patient's death if they withdraw an intervention than if they had withheld it. Such reluctance to withdraw treatments needs to be acknowledged. There is no logical distinction, however, between the two acts. Reasons that justify withholding interventions also justify withdrawing them, and additional reasons may emerge after starting treatment: it may prove unsuccessful or new information about the patient's preferences or condition may become available. Patients and surrogates might not start potentially beneficial treatments if they could not be discontinued later.

DO NOT RESUSCITATE (DNR) ORDERS   Because cardiopulmonary resuscitation (CPR) must be initiated emergently, decisions to withhold it need to be discussed in advance. While CPR can restore people to vigorous health, it can also disrupt a peaceful death, particularly one that is anticipated. After CPR is attempted on a general hospital service, only 14 percent of patients survive to discharge, and even fewer in certain subgroups. Standard practice is to initiate CPR unless a DNR order has been made. To prevent misunderstandings, DNR orders should be written, not given orally. DNR orders are appropriate if the patient or surrogate requests them or if CPR would be futile. "Slow" or "show" codes that merely appear to provide CPR are deceptive and therefore unacceptable. Strictly speaking, a DNR order signifies only that CPR will be withheld. Concerns that DNR orders may cause other care to be withheld inappropriately need to be worked out among the health care team.

ASSISTED SUICIDE AND ACTIVE EUTHANASIA   Proponents of these controversial acts believe that competent, terminally ill patients should have control over the end of life and that physicians should help them end their suffering. Opponents assert that life is sacred, that suffering can generally be relieved in other ways, that abuses are inevitable, that such actions are outside the physician's proper role, and that current prohibitions should continue. Whatever their personal views, physicians need to respond to patients' inquiries with compassion and concern. Physicians need to elicit and address any underlying problems, such as unrelieved suffering, loss of control, or depression. Distress usually can be relieved more effectively and patients in turn may withdraw their requests for these acts. Patients need to be reassured that life-prolonging interventions will not be imposed against their wishes.

CARE OF DYING PATIENTS   Relieving pain in terminal illness and alleviating dyspnea when patients forego mechanical ventilation enhances patient comfort and dignity. Spending time with dying patients, listening to them, and paying attention to their psychological distress can ease their suffering. In some cases, relief of symptoms may require doses of narcotics or sedatives that may suppress respiratory drive and hasten death. Administering such doses should be distinguished from active euthanasia and is ethically appropriate if lower doses have failed to relieve suffering.

AVOIDING CONFLICTS OF INTEREST

Acting in the patient's best interests may conflict with the physician's self-interest or the interests of third parties such as insurers. The ethical ideal is to keep the patient's interests paramount. Otherwise physicians violate their fiduciary duty to patients and undermine trust in the profession.

FINANCIAL INCENTIVES In managed care systems, primary care physicians may serve as gatekeepers who authorize hospitalizations and referrals and who may be financially liable for expenditures. Such arrangements need to be disclosed to patients. The ethical concern is that physicians may withhold beneficial care in order to control costs. In contrast, physicians have incentives to provide more care than indicated when they receive fee-for-service reimbursement or when they refer patients to medical facilities in which they have invested. Regardless of financial incentives, physicians should recommend available care that is in the patient's best interests—no more and no less.

GIFTS FROM PHARMACEUTICAL COMPANIES Physicians often receive gifts ranging from pens and notepads to lavish entertainment. Some people worry that any gift from drug companies may render physicians less objective. Physicians may underestimate the influence of commercial information on their patient care decisions. Even the appearance of bias and conflict of interest may be deleterious. In accepting gifts from drug companies, physicians may contribute to higher drug prices that patients ultimately must pay.

OCCUPATIONAL RISKS Some health care workers, fearing fatal occupational infections, refuse to care for persons with human immunodeficiency virus (HIV) infection or multidrug-resistant tuberculosis. Such fears about personal safety need to be acknowledged and addressed. Institutions need to reduce occupational risk by providing proper training, equipment, and supervision. Professional organizations enjoin physicians to provide appropriate care within their clinical expertise, despite personal risk. Employment contracts of antidiscrimination laws also may require the provision of such care.

MISTAKES Mistakes are inevitable in clinical medicine. They may seriously harm patients or require substantial changes in management. Physicians and students may fear that disclosing such mistakes could damage their careers or heighten legal liability. Without disclosure, however, patients or surrogates cannot understand their clinical situation or make informed choices about subsequent care. Similarly, attending physicians need to know about trainees' mistakes to provide optimal care and to help them learn.

AVOIDING MISREPRESENTATION Patients may ask physicians to misrepresent their condition to help them obtain such benefits as insurance coverage and disability. While physicians understandably want to help patients, they also have countervailing duties to third parties who rely on the information provided and to other people who would pay higher premiums or taxes. Misrepresentation also violates physicians' integrity.

Misrepresentation may be an issue for trainees. Educational activities, such as learning invasive procedures, may present inconvenience or even risk to patients. Some patients refuse permission for trainees to work on their case. To increase patient cooperation, students may be introduced as physicians, or the experience of trainees performing invasive procedures may be misrepresented. But it is ethically preferable to persuade patients to participate in teaching programs by providing more information, not less, particularly about how closely trainees are supervised.

UNETHICAL BEHAVIOR BY OTHERS Students and house officers may observe flagrantly unethical behavior by others that seriously harms patients. Fulfilling their ethical duty to protect their patients may provoke retaliation from those accused of wrongdoing. Discussing such dilemmas with a sympathetic senior physician or with the ethics committee can help trainees check their interpretation of the situation and obtain advice and assistance.

ADDITIONAL ETHICAL ISSUES

MAINTAINING CONFIDENTIALITY Maintaining the confidentiality of medical information respects patients' autonomy and privacy, encourages them to seek treatment and to discuss their problems candidly, and prevents discrimination. Physicians need to guard against inadvertent breaches of confidentiality, e.g., by discussing patients in elevators. Maintaining confidentiality is not an absolute rule. The law may require physicians to override confidentiality in order to protect third parties. Physicians must warn persons whom psychiatric patients threaten with serious physical violence and report persons with specified conditions, such as tuberculosis and syphilis, to public health officials.

ALLOCATING RESOURCES JUSTLY Allocation of health care resources is unavoidable. Some physicians attempt to control costs by rationing medical care at the bedside. Such ad hoc rationing by an individual physician, however, may be inconsistent, discriminatory, and ineffective. Ideally, allocation decisions should be made as public policy, with physician input. At the bedside, physicians generally should act as patient advocates within constraints set by society and sound practice. In some cases, however, two patients may compete for the same limited resources, such as physician time or a bed in intensive care. When this occurs, physicians should ration their time and resources according to patients' medical needs and the probability of benefit.

ASSISTANCE WITH ETHICAL ISSUES Discussing perplexing ethical issues with other members of the health care team, colleagues, or the hospital ethics committee often clarifies ethical issues and suggests ways to improve communication and to deal with strong emotions. When struggling with difficult ethical issues, physicians may need to reevaluate their basic convictions, tolerate uncertainty, and maintain their integrity while respecting the opinions of others.

REFERENCES

AMERICAN COLLEGE OF PHYSICIANS: *American College of Physicians Ethics Manual.* Ann Intern Med, 117:947,1992

APPELBAUM PS et al: *Informed Consent: Legal Theory and Clinical Practice.* New York, Oxford University, 1987

BUCHANAN AE, BROCK DW: *Deciding for Others.* Cambridge, Cambridge University, 1989

EMERGENCY CARDIAC CARE COMMITTEE AND SUBCOMMITTEES, AMERICAN HEART ASSOCIATION: Guidelines for cardiopulmonary resuscitation and emergency cardiac care, VIII: Ethical considerations in resuscitation. JAMA 268:2282, 1992

LO B: *Resolving Ethical Dilemmas in Adult Medicine.* Baltimore, Williams & Wilkins, 1993, in press

JONSEN AR et al: *Clinical Ethics,* 3d ed. New York, Macmillan, 1991

PELLOGRINO ED: The metamorphosis of medical ethics—A 30-year retrospective. JAMA 269:1158, 1993

PRESIDENT'S COMMISSION FOR THE STUDY OF ETHICAL PROBLEMS IN MEDICINE AND BIOMEDICAL AND BEHAVIORAL RESEARCH: *Deciding to Forego Life-sustaining Treatment.* Washington, U.S. Government Printing Office, 1983

---

3   HOST AND DISEASE: INFLUENCE OF DEMOGRAPHIC FACTORS

EUGENE BRAUNWALD / JEAN D. WILSON

The enormous diversity of the human race profoundly influences the susceptibility to as well as the incidence and clinical expression of disease. Major components of this diversity are age, gender, sexual orientation, genetic background, geography, and ethnic and cultural factors. As we begin to understand more about how these demographic factors affect illness, they must be considered increasingly in the assessment and care of the individual patient.

AGE Since the biologic characteristics and clinical expressions of disease differ dramatically between children and adults, the separate specialty of Pediatrics was developed in the nineteenth century to focus on caring for the young. Similarly, the subspecialties of Adolescent Medicine and Geriatrics evolved to deal with the unique problems that affect patients at the two extremes of the adult age spectrum. Aspects of the biologic, medical, and sociologic characteristics of persons in these two age groups are discussed in Chaps. 7 and 8, respectively. However, it is important to recognize that age can influence disease prevalence even within the adult range. For example, a testicular tumor in a man in his twenties is most likely to be a nonseminomatous germinoma, whereas in the forties, seminoma is by far the most frequent tumor of the testicle. Likewise, symptoms of urethral obstruction (hesitancy, urgency, frequency) in a young man are likely due to infectious agents or urethral causes, whereas in a 60-year-old man prostatic disease is the most common cause of such symptoms. The onset of recurrent unilateral headaches in a young woman likely denotes migraine, whereas onset of new headaches after age 50 necessitates ruling out a serious cause such as brain tumor.

GENDER Although most illnesses affect both men and women, there are notable exceptions. By definition, disorders affecting the reproductive tract occur exclusively in one gender. Others, such as carcinoma of the breast, rarely occur in men, whereas recessive disorders linked to the X chromosome, such as hemophilia and Duchenne's muscular dystrophy, are far more common in males. A much larger number of conditions are seen regularly in both sexes but predominate or tend to be more severe in one or the other. Examples include diabetes mellitus, connective tissue diseases, iron deficiency anemia, and osteoporosis in women; coronary atherosclerosis in young and middle-aged men; and gout in men of all ages.

Major illnesses that affect women and other aspects of women's health are discussed in Chap. 5.

SEXUAL ORIENTATION Certain diseases are much more common in groups of individuals depending on their sexual orientation and practices. This is particularly true in the case of infectious diseases. For example, homosexual men have a much higher incidence of AIDS, gonorrhea, and syphilis than do heterosexual men. Hepatitis B infection, which can be transmitted sexually, also is more common in non-intravenous drug-using homosexual men than in non-intravenous drug-using heterosexual men. Colitis due to a variety of parasites ("gay bowel syndrome") and carcinomas of the anus and the oropharynx occur with greater frequency in homosexual men. The large numbers of sexual partners and the nature of the sexual practices among some homosexual men and not homosexuality itself are responsible for these high incidences and prevalences.

GENETIC BACKGROUND While only a small proportion of serious illnesses are the result of chromosomal disorders (Table 62-1) or simple Mendelian inheritance (Table 60-3), many of the major chronic disorders of adults—coronary artery disease, hypertension, diabetes mellitus, many forms of thyroid disease, epilepsy, schizophrenia, and manic-depressive psychosis—result from an interaction between mutations at different loci and environmental factors (Table 60-5). Therefore, it is often essential to elicit a detailed family history, frequently supplemented by physical and laboratory examinations and occasionally by specialized genetic testing. The family history is particularly important in two settings. The first is in the situation when one is faced with rare or baffling symptoms and signs in which knowledge of affected family members with similar problems or a history of parental consanguinity may provide clues that may lead the physician to establish a specific diagnosis. A specific example is the early onset of dementia due to familial Alzheimer's disease. The other is when common disorders occur in unusual combinations or inappropriate situations and in which a positive family history may suggest the possibility of an inborn error of metabolism, for example, the patient with premature atherosclerosis or unusual peripheral

neuropathy (familial amyloid polyneuropathy). Sometimes it is necessary to extend the examination to members of the patient's family. The genetic basis for disease is discussed in Chaps. 60 to 65.

GEOGRAPHY This impacts on disease in at least two different ways. Certain disorders occur only in persons who have resided for long periods in specific areas. For example, iodine insufficiency (and hence iodine-deficient goiter) occurs predominantly in people who live in areas previously covered by glaciers; toxic waste syndromes usually require prolonged residence in an area exposed to chemical toxins; pulmonary hypertension is more likely to develop in people residing at high altitudes; sarcoidosis is more common in residents of the coniferous belt in the southern United States; multiple sclerosis is more common in individuals who reside in temperate climates.

Some infectious diseases also occur primarily in people who have been dwelling in specific geographic regions for more than brief periods of time. Melioidosis, leprosy, leishmaniasis, Chagas' disease, and filariasis tend to occur in such populations. Other infectious diseases can occur in persons with only transient but well-defined exposures in endemic areas, although these diseases still affect indigenous populations primarily. Malaria, cholera, coccidioidomycosis, histoplasmosis, amebiasis, various types of equine encephalitis, and other insect vector–borne viral infections generally develop in people with distinctive geographic exposures. In an era of widespread international travel, refugee resettlement, and immigration, differential diagnosis must encompass a wide array of diseases previously unknown in most developed countries. In dealing with patients who are immigrants, it is always appropriate to inquire about exposure to endemic diseases, although these patients may well have the same diseases affecting the poor in the United States, including tuberculosis, AIDS, other sexually transmitted diseases, and chronic pulmonary diseases.

ETHNIC ORIGIN Ethnicity also has an important effect on the expression of disease. Despite considerable heterogeneity among people of the same ethnic origin, such individuals share many genes in common. Table 60-1 lists examples of simple (Mendelian) inherited diseases that are found with increased frequency in various ethnic groups. In addition to genetic influences, persons with similar ethnic backgrounds also share cultural, nutritional, environmental, economic, and social characteristics that influence disease. (The impact of social factors on disease is discussed in Chap. 3.) With the exception of the diseases inherited as simple Mendelian traits, such as the hemoglobinopathies or glucose-6-phosphate dehydrogenase (G6PD) deficiency, it is often difficult to determine the relative importance of inheritance and environment in the disease profile of persons of the same ethnic origin.

The following focuses on a few examples of how ethnic background can affect the risk, incidence, and expression of disease.

Hematologic disorders Sickle cell anemia and other hemoglobinopathies are found almost exclusively in persons of African, Arabic, Indian, Greek, and Italian ancestry. Beta thalassemia occurs primarily in descendants of persons from the Mediterranean basin, central Africa, Asia, and parts of India. There are three principal forms of G6PD deficiency (Chap. 307): one affects primarily blacks originating from central Asia, the second affects Sephardic Jews and other peoples of the eastern Mediterranean, while the third is seen among the Chinese.

Hypertension The age-adjusted prevalence of hypertension in African-Americans is two to four times that in whites, with the highest rates occurring among black women. This high frequency is associated with a parallel increase in end-stage renal disease secondary to hypertension. African-Americans tend to have low-renin hypertension associated with a volume excess and a greater responsiveness to diuretics. The mechanism for this type of hypertension is not clear. However, it may be related to the selective survival of individuals who were able to conserve sodium under conditions in which sodium intake was restricted and whose descendants, who now have a much higher intake of sodium, continue to retain salt. In contrast, hypertension (like coronary artery disease, discussed below) appears to be uncommon among blacks residing in rural Africa. Environmental factors may also play a role in the pathogenesis of hypertension in blacks, in that a high level of social stress, instability, and occupational insecurity may worsen hypertension. Other ethnic differences in the control of blood pressure include the correlation between insulin resistance or hyperinsulinemia and hypertension in whites but not in blacks or Pima Indians, a group with a very high incidence of hyperinsulinemia (see below). Cerebrovascular complications of hypertension (particularly intracerebral hemorrhage) are more frequent in African-Americans than in other ethnic groups.

Diabetes mellitus   The prevalence of non-insulin–dependent diabetes mellitus is approximately twice as high in African-Americans and Native Americans as in whites. It is especially high in the Pima Indians, approximately half of whom now develop this disease by age 35. This prevalence has increased dramatically during the past 30 years and appears to parallel the increase in obesity in this population during this period. On the other hand, insulin-dependent diabetes mellitus occurs less frequently in African-Americans than in whites and is apparently even less common among blacks born and residing in Africa.

Coronary and cerebral arterial disease   In the United States, the age-adjusted mortality rates for stroke and sudden death are higher in blacks than in whites; the rates for symptomatic coronary artery disease are also higher in black women than white women. Such racial differences are probably related to the aforementioned higher prevalence among African-Americans of hypertension and diabetes mellitus, both of which are major risk factors for coronary and cerebral atherosclerosis. These differences may also be related to cultural factors, such as the high prevalence of obesity in African-American women. Indeed, coronary artery disease is quite uncommon in South African blacks, who tend to be lean and who may be protected by a low-fat, low-sodium diet. Coronary vascular disease is also less common in Asians than in white Americans, especially in Asians living in their native lands, probably because they have lower circulating levels of total cholesterol and low-density lipoproteins.

Neoplastic disease   Overall, cancer is somewhat more frequent in blacks than whites in the United States. In particular, deaths caused by cancer of the esophagus and stomach, pancreas, lung, cervix, and prostate are more common in African-Americans. Some of these variations may be related to differences in smoking, diet, and alcohol consumption. However, when adjustments are made for the stage of the disease at the time of diagnosis, these interracial differences diminish. Hepatocellular carcinoma occurs more frequently in Chinese and Southeast Asians and those residing in sub-Saharan Africa, while colorectal, breast, and prostate cancers are less common in Asian than in white Americans.

Tuberculosis   Both the prevalence and incidence of tuberculosis are approximately twice as high in blacks as in whites. At first, these differences were ascribed to overcrowding, poor nutrition, and other consequences of economic deprivation. However, the fact that blacks are infected about twice as frequently as whites when exposed under comparable conditions to *M. tuberculosis* in prisons and nursing homes suggests that genetic factors also play a role—perhaps a dominant role. Consonant with this concept, tubercle bacilli grow faster in macrophages harvested from black than from white subjects.

Osteoporosis   Both osteoporosis and one of its principal complications, vertebral fractures, occur more frequently in women than in men and in white than in black women. The latter observation correlates with bone density, which is greater in black (and Polynesian) than in white women. These differences may be explained, in part, by the hormonal and metabolic changes that occur during puberty, a time when black women undergo substantially greater increases in vertebral bone density than do white women. On the other hand, Asians have lower bone densities than whites.

Gastrointestinal disorders   Both cancer of the stomach and cirrhosis occur more frequently in Hispanics than in whites; which may be related to a high incidence of alcoholism in Hispanics. Lactose intolerance is more common in Africans, African-Americans, Asians,

and Mexicans than in whites. Episodic bouts of peritonitis, a cardinal manifestation of familial Mediterranean fever, occur predominantly in persons of Sephardic Jewish, Armenian, and Arabic ancestry. Inflammatory bowel disease is more common in the Jewish population.

Arthritis and connective tissue disorders   Since the histocompatibility antigen HLA-B27 is found more often in white populations, disorders linked to this antigen, such as ankylosing spondylitis and Reiter's syndrome, are more prevalent among whites. In contrast, systemic lupus erythematosus and polymyositis are more common and usually more severe in blacks.

CONCLUSIONS   Appropriate understanding and consideration of demographic and ethnic factors in dealing with the individual patient is of diagnostic as well as therapeutic importance. As the practice of medicine and the postgraduate training of physicians grow highly specialized, consideration of these factors is frequently underemphasized. A broad view of the context of the illness is important.

REFERENCES

BOWMAN JE, MURRAY RF JR: *Genetic Variation and Disorders in Peoples of African Origin*. Baltimore, Johns Hopkins University, 1990
CRUICKSHANK JK, BEEVERS DG: *Ethnic Factors in Health and Disease*. Boston, Wright, 1989
FRASER PA: Epidemiology of rheumatic diseases in selected non-European populations, in *Oxford Textbook of Rheumatology*, PJ Maddison et al (eds). Oxford, Oxford University, 1993, in press
KEIL JE et al: Mortality rates and risk factors for coronary disease in black as compared with white men and women. N Engl J Med 329:73, 1993
LEIGH H, REISER MF: *The Patient: Biological, Psychological and Social Dimensions of Medical Practice*, 3d ed. New York, Plenum, 1992.
Report of the Secretary's Task Force on Black and Minority Health. U.S. Department of Health and Human Services, vol. I, Executive Summary. Washington DC, 1985

4   THE IMPACT OF SOCIAL FACTORS ON DISEASE

VIRGINIA L. ERNSTER

Marked variations in health exist among different subgroups of the population, and social factors are major determinants of disease occurrence and survival. Broadly interpreted, social factors include *socioeconomic status, culture and acculturation, religion, and psychosocial factors* (e.g., life events, social mobility, and social networks), as well as aspects of the environment that are the result of human activity. The focus here is on the influence of socioeconomic status (SES) and racial/ethnic factors on health indicators in the United States. Though individual physicians have limited impact on the social world of patients, it is critical to recognize the role of SES and racial/ethnic factors in determining environmental exposures, behavioral risk factors, access to health care, and compliance with recommended regimens, all of which influence disease etiology and prognosis.

The key points of this chapter are that (1) marked improvements have occurred in mortality and life expectancy during this century; (2) individuals of lower SES experience greater morbidity and mortality than individuals of higher SES; (3) the differences in disease occurrence and survival across racial/ethnic groups diminish considerably or disappear entirely once SES is controlled; and (4) behavioral risk factors play a major role in disease etiology but do not entirely explain differences in disease prevalence across SES and racial groups.

IMPROVEMENTS IN MORTALITY AND LIFE EXPECTANCY   In 1900, approximate life expectancies at birth in the United States were

TABLE 4-1 Life expectancy in years at birth by race and sex, United States 1900–1989

	White		Black	
	Male	Female	Male	Female
1900	46.6	48.7	32.5	33.5
1940	62.1	66.6	—	—
1950	66.5	72.2	58.9	62.7
1960	67.4	74.1	60.7	65.9
1970	68.0	75.6	60.0	68.3
1980	70.7	78.1	63.8	72.5
1987	72.2	78.9	65.2	73.6
1988	72.3	78.9	64.9	73.4
1989	72.7	79.2	64.8	73.5

SOURCE: U.S. Department of Health and Human Services: Advance report of final mortality statistics, 1989. CDC Monthly Vital Statistics Report 40:1, 1992. U.S. Department of Health and Human Services: *Health United States and Prevention Profile 1989.* DHHS Pub No(PHS)90-1232, Hyattsville, MD, 1990.

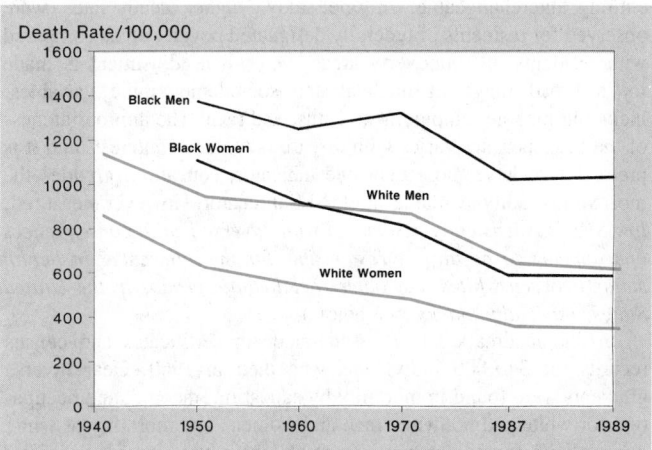

FIGURE 4-1 Death rates per 100,000, 1940–1989, for white and black men and women, age-adjusted to the 1940 U.S. population. *(From U.S. Department of Health and Human Services: Advance report of final mortality statistics, 1989. CDC Monthly Vital Statistics Report 40:1, 1992.)*

47 years for white men, 49 for white women, 32 for black men, and 34 for black women. In less than a century, those figures have increased by nearly 60 percent for whites and doubled in blacks. By 1989, average life expectancy at birth approximated 73 and 79 years, respectively, for white men and women and 65 and 74 years for black men and women (Table 4-1). These gains in life expectancy are the result of declines in age-adjusted mortality rates (Fig. 4-1). Improved environmental conditions in the first half of the century led to declines in infectious diseases and resulted in improvements in infant and early childhood survival. Infant mortality rates have continued to decline largely because of improvements in medical care; between 1950 and 1989, rates decreased from 27 to 8 per 1000 births among whites and from 44 to 18 per 1000 births among blacks. Simply put, at the turn of the century 30 percent of children died before the age of 5 years compared with only 2 percent today. Since the mid-1960s, most of the decline in mortality rates has been due to reductions in death from cardiovascular disease and stroke, affecting primarily the older age groups. Age-adjusted death rates from cardiovascular disease have declined by more than 40 percent since 1970; between 1980 and 1988 alone, age-adjusted ischemic heart disease mortality rates in the population aged 35 and older declined 24 percent—from 588 to 449 per 100,000. Whereas life expectancy at birth increased 8 percent between 1950 and 1980, life expectancy at age 45 increased by 12 percent. By 1988, 12 percent of the U.S. population was over the age of 65, compared with only 4 percent in 1900.

Although overall trends are positive, there was a slowing of life expectancy gains in blacks compared with whites in the mid-1980s

and there remains a continuing gap in life expectancy between blacks and whites and a twofold excess in infant mortality among blacks. The male-female gap in life expectancy has widened and then narrowed during this century, a trend that correlates with the adoption of cigarette smoking first by men and later by women (see Chap. 5). Among whites, life expectancy was on average 2 years longer for women than men in 1900, 8 years longer in 1970, and 6 years longer in 1989. Nonetheless, for all of the leading causes of death in the United States, there is a male excess in the ratio of male-to-female age-adjusted death rates; the excess is more than twofold for deaths due to accidents, suicide, chronic liver disease and cirrhosis, homicide, and HIV-infection (Table 4-2).

HIGHER MORTALITY AND MORIBIDITY IN LOWER SOCIOECONOMIC GROUPS Numerous population-based studies demonstrate that, despite dramatic improvements over time in life expectancy and death rates for all major subgroups of the population, SES is still a major determinant of health status. The existence of overall mortality differentials by occupational status is especially well documented in the United Kingdom, and social class differences in mortality there may be widening.

Socioeconomic status is measured in various ways, including education, income, occupation, population density, nature of residence, and combined indices. Different measures of SES are not

TABLE 4-2 Ratio of age-adjusted death rates* for the leading causes of death by sex and race: United States 1989†

All causes	Male to female	White men to white women	Black men to black women	Black to white	Black men to white men	Black women to white women
Heart disease	1.9	1.9	1.6	1.4	1.3	1.6
Malignant neoplasms	1.5	1.4	1.8	1.3	1.5	1.2
Cerebrovascular diseases	1.2	1.2	1.2	1.9	1.9	1.9
Accidents and adverse effects	2.6	2.6	3.1	1.3	1.4	1.2
Motor vehicle accidents	2.4	2.3	3.2	1.0	1.1	0.8
All other	3.0	3.0	3.0	1.7	1.8	1.8
Chronic obstructive pulmonary diseases	1.8	1.8	2.3	0.8	0.9	0.7
Pneumonia and influenza	1.7	1.6	2.0	1.5	1.6	1.3
Diabetes mellitus	1.1	1.1	0.9	2.3	2.0	2.3
Suicide	4.1	4.1	5.2	0.6	0.6	0.5
Chronic liver disease and cirrhosis	2.3	2.4	2.4	1.7	1.7	1.7
Homicide and legal intervention	3.6	2.9	5.0	6.6	7.6	4.5
Human immunodeficiency virus infection	8.7	14.6	5.0	3.3	3.1	9.0
All causes	1.7	1.7	1.8	1.6	1.6	1.6

* Per 100,000 population, age-adjusted to the 1940 U.S. population.
† SOURCE: U.S. Department of Health and Human Services: Advance report of final mortality statistics, 1989. CDC Monthly Vital Statistics Report 40:1, 1992

entirely interchangeable; in one study, higher death rates were observed for residents of federally designated poverty areas compared with residents of nonpoverty areas even when adjustment is made for a broad range of medical and sociodemographic variables, including income, employment status, and race. The appropriateness of the SES measure varies with disease outcome of interest, and it is preferable to have more than one indicator; education provides the most valid readily available single SES indicator. However measured, *low SES is consistently associated with adverse health consequences and appears to be largely responsible for the differences in health status between whites and other racial/ethnic groups in the United States, especially blacks* (see below).

In one landmark study based on death certificates and census records for 340,000 individuals who died in 1960, clear inverse gradients were found in mortality by education, income, and occupation for white and nonwhite men and women. The mortality of white women with four or more years of college education, for example, was only 71 percent of the overall rate for white women, whereas those with less than five years of education had a mortality ratio of 127 percent. Similarly, remaining life expectancy for white women aged 25 with at least one year of college education was almost 10 years greater (56.4 years) than for those with less than five years of schooling. Likewise, in Alameda County, California, death rates in individuals with inadequate family income were twice as high as in those with adequate income. Findings in other areas of the United States and in other developed countries have been similar. Even the onset of the decline in coronary heart disease rates among white women occurs earliest in those areas with the highest average income, education, and occupational levels. Similarly, the 1960 Matched Records Study and the National Health and Nutrition Examination Survey (NHANES I) showed that the decline in heart disease mortality among men between 1960 and 1971-84 was sharpest for those with more years of education.

Morbidity is also inversely related to income. In the United States in 1988, 23 percent of individuals whose family income was less than $10,000 reported limitation of activity due to chronic conditions compared with only 8 percent of those whose income was $35,000 or greater (Table 4-3). Other analyses using a combination of education and income to measure social class show that most preventable morbidity and functional limitation in the U.S. population before age 75 occurs in the lower SES strata. The adverse effect of income on disability is apparent even among children. In 1980, the average number of disability days was 9 for children whose families had annual incomes of $5000, compared with 4 for those whose families had incomes of $25,000 or more, and the incidence of lower respiratory illness among infants is inversely related to educational level of the head of household. Patients of lower SES (whether measured by income, occupation, or education) also have longer and more costly hospitalizations.

A notable exception to the inverse gradient between SES and disease is the fact that the incidence of breast cancer is higher in upper SES groups. However, the inverse gradient of social class correlates with many seemingly unrelated causes of disease, e.g., heart disease death rates, survival of patients with coronary artery disease following cardiac catheterization, incidence and survival for many cancers, visual impairment, childhood accidents, overall childhood mortality, and prevalence of migraine headache. Known risk factors account for some of these patterns but not for the broad effects across disparate conditions. To cite just one study, even after control for baseline medical characteristics related to survival of patients with coronary artery disease, those with annual household incomes of $40,000 or greater were about half as likely to die within 5 years of entering the study as patients with lower incomes.

Considering that about one in eight Americans lives in a family whose income is below the poverty level as defined by the federal government, and realizing that nearly one in four children under age 6 falls into this category, social inequity represents a compelling challenge for the nation's health.

TABLE 4-3   Limitation of activity due to chronic conditions by family income, United States, 1988

Family income, $	Percent of population
<10,000	23.2
10,000–14,999	15.4
15,000–19,999	13.1
20,000–34,999	10.7
≥35,000	8.1

SOURCE: U.S. Department of Health and Human Services: *Health United States and Prevention Profile 1989.* DHHS Pub No(PHS)90-1232, Hyattsville, MD, 1990.

Attention is being given to understanding the reason for the impressive relationship of SES to disease. Differences in disease severity are explained only in part by differences in the prevalence of known risk factors across SES groups, even in the United Kingdom, where a national health system diminishes inequities in health services. Gradients in health status correlate with relative privilege, even among individuals whose absolute levels of income or occupation indicated they are not deprived. In Britain, for example, among individuals in nonmanual occupations who are homeowners, mortality is lower in those with two cars when compared with those with only one car. Nearly two-thirds of the variation in mortality rates among member nations of the Organization for Economic Cooperation and Development may be attributable to *within*-country differences in income distribution, i.e., the relative gap between rich and poor. Similarly, across the 12 countries of the European Community, income distribution correlates with life expectancy.

DIFFERENCES IN DISEASE OCCURRENCE AND SURVIVAL ACROSS RACIAL/ETHNIC GROUPS   Mortality rates have traditionally been presented in the United States for all races combined or for whites and blacks (or nonwhites) separately (Table 4-2). Overall age-adjusted mortality rates are 60 percent higher for blacks, with notable excesses for cerebrovascular diseases, diabetes mellitus, and homicide. Lung cancer incidence rates are 50 percent higher, and rates for AIDS are three times higher in blacks, although there is considerable variation by sex, age, and risk group. An examination of U.S. deaths for 1980-86 from 12 causes considered preventable by medical intervention (tuberculosis, cervical cancer, Hodgkin's disease, rheumatic heart disease, hypertensive heart disease, acute respiratory disease, pneumonia and bronchitis, influenza, asthma, appendicitis, hernias, and cholecystitis) found that mortality rates for the 12 causes combined were 4.5 times higher in blacks than whites, with highest relative differences for tuberculosis, hypertensive heart disease, and asthma. In New York's Harlem, where the population is 96 percent black, the age-adjusted overall mortality rate for the period 1979-81 was more than twice that of U.S. whites; in the population under age 65, the ratio of deaths in Harlem to the number expected was 2.9 for men and 2.7 for women, and black men in Harlem were less likely to survive to age 65 than men in Bangladesh. National morbidity data are consistent with the mortality data. In 1988, 16 percent of blacks compared with 13 percent of whites reported limitation of their activity due to chronic conditions.

Attempts are now being made to collect national mortality and morbidity data for racial/ethnic groups other than whites and blacks. However, the actual disease experience of a group is accurate only if the coding of race/ethnicity is accurate. Moreover, broad categories such as "Hispanic," "Asian," or "Native American" include diverse populations with diverse disease risks. For example, Mexican-Americans appear to have a low risk of cerebrovascular disease, whereas Puerto Ricans have a high risk of stroke, so that statistics for "Hispanics" should not be based on the combined experience. Some precise ethnic categories, particularly for Asians and Pacific Islanders, may have too few individuals for reliable calculation of cause-specific death rates. Finally, increasing interracial admixture makes traditional racial categories less meaningful.

Recognizing these limitations, attempts have been made to characterize the disease experience of minorities in the United States. The results indicate that (1) overall death rates are lowest among Asians; (2) blacks have the highest overall death rates for all age groups except ages 15 to 24, when rates are slightly higher for American Indian/Alaskan Natives; (3) in all age groups under 65, death rates among whites and Hispanics are intermediate between those of Asians and blacks; (4) in young people aged 15 to 24, blacks are seven times more likely and Hispanics and American Indians are three to four times more likely to die of homicide than Asians and whites; (5) in the age groups under 45, injury rates are particularly excessive among American Indian/Alaskan Natives; (6) in the age groups 25 to 64, heart disease rates in blacks are much higher, and rates in Hispanics and especially in Asians are considerably lower than those of whites; and (7) among the population 65 years and older, cancer death rates among Asians, American Indians, and Hispanics are only half or less those of whites, and death rates in blacks are about 20 percent higher than in whites.

Racial/ethnic differences in rates for many diseases are due to differences in socioeconomic status. When SES is controlled, black/white differences in the incidence of some but not all cancers, such as invasive cervical cancer and lung cancer in men, are reduced or disappear. In fact, overall cancer rates are higher in blacks in the United States, but when adjusted for SES rates are higher in whites than in blacks. Though black women have lower survival from breast cancer than white women, race is not significant if SES is controlled. Similarly, although infant mortality rates are twice as high among normal birthweight black babies, no differences are found in comparisons of normal birthweight infants born to black and white college-educated parents. Furthermore, no significant differences have been found in overall mortality or in coronary heart disease mortality by race *within* the low (less than eight years of education and lower occupational group) or high (some college education and occupation of proprietor or professional) SES groups. Differences in heart disease rates across occupational groups in the United States are much greater than differences between blacks and whites. It is of particular concern that social class disparities, as measured by income, are widening.

In addition to social class, other sociocultural factors undoubtedly affect health-related behaviors and outcomes. Even when income, health status, age, sex, and history of chronic disease are taken into account, blacks in the United States have fewer ambulatory visits and are less likely to see a physician, suggesting disadvantages in access to care. In one study, black patients with ischemic heart disease underwent coronary angiography and coronary artery bypass grafting less often than whites, even when age, sex, income, source of payment, primary diagnosis, and the number of secondary diagnoses were controlled. Among Medicare patients, sex- and age-adjusted incidence of coronary artery bypass grafting were about three times higher among whites in 1986 and were not related to admission rates for acute myocardial infarction. Even among college-educated parents, blacks are more likely than whites to have low birthweight babies, which accounts for the higher overall black infant mortality in this group, despite the similarity in mortality rates for normal birthweight infants. Yet in the face of SES adversity, cultural factors may play a protective role. U.S.-born Hispanic infants, with the exception of those of Puerto Rican descent, have infant mortality rates similar to those of whites, i.e., about half those of blacks.

Of course, many racial differences in morbidity and mortality cannot be explained by SES, culture, or racism. Hypertensive end-stage renal disease rates in blacks are higher than in whites, adjusting for age, prevalence of hypertension, diabetes mellitus, and education level. On the other hand, malignant melanoma is more common in whites. It is obviously important to distinguish between genetic and social differences in disease risk across racial/ethnic groups.

KNOWN RISK FACTORS EXPLAIN ONLY PART OF THE DIFFER-ENCES Differences in health status across SES and racial groups are partially explained by differences in the distribution of known disease risk factors. Cigarette smoking, the leading cause of preventable death in the United States, shows a strong inverse relationship

TABLE 4-4 Prevalence of cigarette smoking in persons aged 25 and over, by sex, race, and education, United States, 1987

Education, years	Men White	Men Black	Women White	Women Black
<12	45.3	49.4	37.0	35.0
12	34.6	43.6	29.4	28.1
13–15	28.0	32.4	26.2	27.2
≥16	17.4	20.9	16.4	19.5
Total	30.6	41.9	27.0	28.6

SOURCE: U.S. Department of Health and Human Services: *Health United States and Prevention Profile 1989.* DHHS Pub No(PHS)90-1232, Hyattsville, MD, 1990.

to SES. In the population 18 years of age and older, 37 percent of men and 27 percent of women with less than a high school education were smokers in 1990, compared with only 14.5 percent and 12 percent, respectively, of college graduates (Table 4-4). By the year 2000 smoking prevalence among those with a high school education or less is projected to be about 30 percent, whereas it will be less than 10 percent among college graduates. In California, between 1984 and 1989, smoking, infrequent use of seat belts, not exercising outside of work, being overweight, and hypertension were more common among women with a high school education or less compared to those with more education (Table 4-5). Self-reports of mammogram screening and having had a Pap smear within the previous year are also positively associated with income. Finally, the proportion of children vaccinated for measles, rubella, diphtheria-tetanus-pertussis, poliomyelitis, and mumps is 15 to 20 percent higher among white children (Table 4-6).

For many diseases, however, controlling for differences in known risk factors does not eliminate differences across SES and racial groups. Controlling for serum cholesterol, systolic blood pressure, smoking, physical activity, body mass, and other factors accounted for only about 60 percent of the differential in coronary heart disease mortality across different employment grades in the British Civil Services. Similarly, adjustment for age, smoking, body weight, blood pressure, and serum cholesterol levels accounted for only a modest proportion of the elevated risks of heart disease death among the least educated men and women aged 45 to 74 in the National Health and Nutrition Examination Survey (NHANES). Approximately a third of excess mortality in blacks is due to identified risk factors and a third to family income, leaving a third unexplained. On the other hand, lower cardiovascular disease mortality has been observed among Mexican-American compared with non-Hispanic white men, despite higher cardiovascular risk factors.

Still, behavioral and other avoidable risk factors account for a large part of differences in disease status in all SES groups, even

TABLE 4-5 Prevalence of behavioral risk factors* by education level in California ages 35–44, 1984-89

Risk factor	Men ≤ High-school, %	Men > High-school, %	Women ≤ High-school, %	Women > High-school, %
Current smoking	40.7	25.6	30.1	19.1
Irregular/nonuse of seatbelts	29.6	17.8	20.9	10.9
No exercise outside of work	39.4	14.4	31.9	20.2
Overweight	33.1	19.6	21.6	14.1
Hypertension	13.1	20.0	15.9	10.9
Chronic drinking	13.9	12.8	4.0	2.5
Drinking and driving	6.7	5.2	1.1	1.3

* Based on responses to telephone interviews conducted as part of the CDC's ongoing Behavioral Risk Factor Survey. N = 10,650 California participants during 1984-89.
SOURCE: Ackermann SP et al: Cancer screening behaviors among U.S. women: breast cancer 1987–1989, and cervical cancer, 1988–1989. MMWR 41:17, 1992.

TABLE 4-6 Vaccination of children aged 1 to 4 for selected diseases, by race, United States, 1985

	% of population	
	White	All other
Measles	63.6	48.8
Rubella	61.6	47.7
DTP*	68.7	48.7
Polio	58.9	40.1
Mumps	61.8	47.0

* Diphtheria-tetanus-pertussis.
SOURCE: U.S. Department of Health and Human Services: *Health United States and Prevention Profile 1989.* DHHS Pub No(PHS)90-1232, Hyattsville, MD, 1990.

among the elderly. Priority areas for health promotion (individual behaviors), health protection (environmental and regulatory measures), and prevention (counseling, screening, immunization, or chemoprophylactic intervention in clinical settings) are documented in *Healthy People 2000: National Health Promotion and Disease Prevention Objectives.* In this landmark reference, the health consequences and current status of the U.S. population are reviewed, and goals are proposed for the year 2000. Attempts to promote healthy lifestyles among the socially disadvantaged deserve high priority. Unfortunately, such efforts may not be a high priority for the individuals in greatest need. Intensive education about risk factors (tobacco, diet, alcohol, drugs) is needed but will have little impact unless accompanied by adequate income, employment, and housing.

Disadvantaged segments of our population have yet to approximate the purported maximum lifespan, and attempts to change established behavioral risk factors, while critically important, will not be sufficient to improve morbidity for the population as a whole. Improvements in socioeconomic status and recognition of the continuing impact of race and/or racism on health outcomes are fundamental to achieving that goal.

REFERENCES

Mortality, morbidity, and socioeconomic status

EPSTEIN AM et al: Do the poor cost more? A multihospital study of patients' socioeconomic status and use of hospital resources. N Engl J Med 322:1122, 1990

FELDMAN JJ et al: National trends in educational differentials in mortality. Am J Epidemiol 129:919, 1989

KAPLAN GA et al: Socioeconomic status and health, in *Closing the Gap: The Burden of Unnecessary Illness,* RW Amler, HB Dull (eds). New York, Oxford University, 1987, pp 125–129

KITAGAWA EM, HAUSER PM (eds): *Differential Mortality in the United States: A Study in Socioeconomic Epidemiology.* Cambridge, MA, Harvard University, 1973

MARMOT MG et al: Social/economic status and disease. Ann Rev Public Health 9:111, 1987

PAPPAS G et al: The increasing disparity in mortality between socioeconomic groups in the United States, 1960 and 1986. JAMA 329:103, 1993

SMITH GD et al: The Black report on socioeconomic inequalities in health 10 years on. Br Med J 301:373, 1990

WILKINSON RG: National mortality rates: The impact of inequality? Am J Public Health 82:1082, 1992

WILLIAMS RB et al: Prognostic importance of social and economic resources among medically treated patients with angiographically documented coronary artery disease. JAMA 267:520, 1992

Disease occurrence and survival by race/ethnicity

BARKER JC: Cultural diversity—Changing the context of medical practice, In Cross-cultural Medicine—A Decade Later. West J Med 157:248, 1992

BLENDON RJ et al: Access to medical care for black and white Americans. JAMA 261:276, 1989

GOLDBERG KC et al: Racial and community factors influencing coronary artery bypass graft surgery rates for all 1986 Medicare patients. JAMA 267:1473, 1992

GURALNIK JM: Educational status and active life expectancy among older blacks and whites. JAMA 329:110, 1993

KEIL JE et al: Does equal socioeconomic status in black and white men mean equal risk of mortality? Am J Public Health 82:1133, 1992

MCCORD C, FREEMAN HP: Excess mortality in Harlem. N Engl J Med 322:173, 1990

NAVARRO V: Race *or* class or race *and* class: Growing mortality differentials in the United States. Int J Health Serv 21:229, 1992

SCHOENDORF KC et al: Mortality among infants of black as compared with white college-educated parents. N Engl J Med 326:1522, 1992

SCHWARTZ E et al: Black/white comparisons of deaths preventable by medical intervention: United States and the District of Columbia 1980–1986. Int J Epidemiol 19:591, 1990

US DEPARTMENT OF HEALTH AND HUMAN SERVICES: *Health, United States, 1990.* Hyattsville, MD, National Center for Health Statistics, 1991

WENNEKER MB, EPSTEIN AM: Racial inequalities in the use of procedures for patients with ischemic heart disease in Massachusetts. JAMA 261:253, 1989

WHITTLE JC et al: Does racial variation in risk factors explain black-white differences in the incidence of hypertensive end-stage renal disease? Arch Intern Med 151:1359, 1991

Socioeconomic status and race

DAVEY SMITH G et al: The magnitude and causes of socio-economic differentials in mortality: Further evidence from the Whitehall study. J Epidemiol Community Health 44:265, 1990

OTTEN MW JR et al: The effect of known risk factors on the excess mortality of black adults in the United States. JAMA 263:845, 1990

PIERCE JP et al: Trends in cigarette smoking in the United States. Projections to the Year 2000. JAMA 261:61, 1989

5 WOMEN'S HEALTH

ANTHONY L. KOMAROFF / BEVERLY WOO

In recent years, there has been a growing appreciation that the health problems of women require increased attention. Although certain diseases that occur primarily in women (e.g., breast cancer) have been the subject of considerable research, most illnesses that can affect men and women have not been as well studied in women. Many research studies of disease prevention and pathophysiology have included only male subjects; the findings may not be generalizable to female subjects. There are poorly understood differences in the expression of diseases in the two sexes. For example, several immunologically mediated diseases occur predominantly in women, for reasons that are uncertain. Furthermore, women receive different care than men for health problems that are common to both sexes. Finally, there are differences in morbidity and mortality between men and women. The causes for these differences are only partly understood.

This chapter summarizes some of the issues regarding the health of women that require special attention. Detailed discussions of specific diseases (those that occur predominantly or exclusively in women, as well as those that are not gender-specific) are found in other chapters.

PREVENTION Primary and secondary prevention are crucial elements in improving health. One general risk factor, cigarette smoking, has been well studied in women. In the United States during the 1930s, over 50 percent of men vs. only 20 percent of women smoked. By 1960, the rate had stayed about level in men but had risen to over 30 percent in women. In 1990, 28 percent of men vs. 23 percent of women were regular smokers. Thus, over the past 60 years there has been a sharp decline in smoking among men but not among women. "Low-yield" cigarettes are marketed heavily to women; however, the risk of myocardial infarction is equal for users of "low-yield" and higher-yield brands. Although it is of obvious importance to diminish smoking rates in both men and women (see Chap. 393), different interventions and educational strategies aimed at women may well be required.

Particularly in the past decade, a large number of important case-control and prospective cohort observational studies have been published that concentrate on the prevention of disease in women. A prime example is the Nurses' Health Study, in which more than 100,000 women have been followed prospectively. In this study, women aged 34–45 who used one to six aspirins per week had a 25 percent lower rate of developing a first myocardial infarction than women who reported no aspirin use, a statistically significant difference after adjusting for known cardiovascular risk factors. The study also found that postmenopausal estrogen therapy is associated with a

40 to 50 percent reduction in deaths due to ischemic heart disease (IHD), a finding supported by several case-control studies, as well.

At the same time, the major prospective, randomized controlled trials of primary prevention of cardiovascular disease—the Multiple Risk Factor Intervention Trial (MRFIT), the Physician's Health Study of aspirin and beta-carotene, the Cholesterol-Lowering Atherosclerosis Study (CLAS), the Helsinki Heart Study, and the Lipid Research Clinics Coronary Primary Prevention Trial—have included only male subjects. This is because cardiac endpoints are more common in men, allowing smaller and less costly studies. Now that these studies have contributed valuable information about several interventions in men, it becomes more important to perform studies in women, since IHD is the most common cause of death in women. Indeed, large randomized trials in women now are being organized by the United States National Institutes of Health to study the benefits and risks of postmenopausal hormone replacement therapy, and the value of low-dose aspirin and antioxidants in preventing cardiovascular disease and cancer in healthy women.

GENDER DIFFERENCES IN DISEASE   Obviously, some conditions and diseases occur exclusively (or nearly exclusively) in women—e.g., the menopause and various breast and gynecologic disorders (see Chaps. 340, 341). In this chapter, we seek primarily to highlight some interesting gender differences in diseases that occur in both women and men.

Ischemic heart disease   Many persons think of IHD as primarily a problem of men, perhaps because men have about twice the total incidence of cardiovascular morbidity and mortality of women from ages 35–84. However, in the United States, IHD is the leading cause of death among women as well as men; nearly 400,000 women die annually from IHD (Table 5-1). This mortality rate is five- to sixfold higher than the mortality rate for either lung or breast cancer, the two most common causes of death from cancer in women. On average, women develop IHD 10 years later than men and have myocardial infarction and sudden death 20 years after men.

LDL cholesterol levels and the ratios of total/HDL cholesterol are lower for women than men until age 60 to 70 years. In all age groups, HDL cholesterol levels are, on average, about 10 mg/dL higher in women than men. Some studies suggest that in women HDL cholesterol is more closely related to IHD risk than LDL cholesterol level.

There is a growing body of knowledge about IHD risk factors in women. However, more information is needed about the relative power of these risk factors and whether interventions can change an individual's risk. Large observational studies suggest that, in women,

obesity is an independent risk factor for nonfatal myocardial infarction and IHD mortality. As mentioned earlier, smoking is an important risk factor for IHD in women. Current use of oral contraceptives is associated with a two- to fourfold increase in the risk of myocardial infarction, independent of other known risk factors, in older premenopausal women. Past use of oral contraceptives does not appear to affect the risk of myocardial infarction. In women who use oral contraceptives, smoke, and have hypertension, the risk of myocardial infarction is especially high.

IHD presents differently in men and women. In the Framingham cohort, myocardial infarction was the first manifestation of IHD in 43 percent of men vs. 29 percent of women. In contrast, angina pectoris was the presenting symptom of IHD in 55 percent of women vs. 39 percent of men. The exercise ECG appears to have a lower specificity for IHD in women than men.

Finally, it has been suggested that women, particularly African-American women, have higher risks of morbidity and mortality than men following a myocardial infarction, coronary artery bypass graft surgery, and percutaneous transluminal coronary angioplasty. Whether this is true after adjusting for age and severity of disease remains uncertain. While women and men apparently experience a similar *relative* benefit with thrombolytic therapy following an acute myocardial infarction, the mortality rates remain higher in women.

Hypertension   Although population-based epidemiologic studies in the United States show a higher prevalence of uncontrolled hypertension in men compared to women, the overall prevalence of hypertension (uncontrolled plus successfully treated) is about equal or slightly higher in women. The prevalence of hypertension appears to be the same for white women and men; however, African-American women have a higher prevalence of hypertension than African-American men. The risk of cardiovascular diseases that is attributable to hypertension appears to be the same or greater in women as compared to men, among the largely white subjects in the Framingham Study.

Immunologically mediated diseases   Several diseases thought to be immunologically mediated—e.g., rheumatoid arthritis, systemic lupus erythematosus, multiple sclerosis, Graves' disease, and thyroiditis—occur much more frequently in women than in men. Although it is not entirely clear why this is so, estrogens appear to play an important role in pathogenesis. In animal models of rheumatoid arthritis, lupus, and multiple sclerosis, for example, the females of the species are predominantly affected.

Osteoporosis   Endogenous levels of estrogen appear to play an important role in osteoporosis. The risk of osteoporosis in postmenopausal women is much greater than in men of the same age, and postmenopausal estrogen supplementation is associated with a decreased incidence of osteoporosis. The mechanisms by which estrogen exerts its protective effects remain to be fully elucidated.

Psychological disorders   Depression, anxiety disorders, bulimia, and anorexia nervosa are diagnosed more often in women. However, there is a disagreement as to whether the actual prevalence of these disorders is different in the two sexes. Men may be more reluctant to bring emotional problems to the attention of a physician and may develop substance abuse disorders in response to underlying depression and anxiety more often, causing the former but not the latter to be diagnosed. Similarly, physicians may be more prone to diagnose mood or anxiety disorders when the patient who seeks medical care for vague symptoms with no obvious organic basis is a woman.

Social factors may account for the greater prevalence of some disorders in women. It has been suggested that the traditionally subordinate role of women in society may have generated a greater sense of vulnerability in women than in men. Bulimia and anorexia nervosa are believed, at least in part, to be an exaggerated distortion of the 20th century Western ideal of female beauty: the lean woman. In addition, it is possible that biological factors, including hormonally influenced neurochemical changes, may also play a role in what may be the greater prevalence of psychological disorders and eating

---

TABLE 5-1   Death rates (per 100,000) for the leading causes of death in U.S. women, 1988

Age 25–34 Total: 74.0	Age 45–54 Total: 350.9	Age 65–74 Total: 2056.1	All ages Total: 826.9
1. Motor vehicle accidents (11.6)	1. Breast cancer (45.3)	1. Ischemic heart disease (453.1)	1. Ischemic heart disease (194.4)
2. Homicide (7.3)	2. Ischemic heart disease (36.8)	2. Lung cancer* (164.1)	2. Cerebrovascular disease (72.0)
3. Suicide (5.7)	3. Lung cancer* (35.0)	3. Cerebrovascular disease (137.3)	3. Lung cancer* (36.8)
4. Nonmotor vehicle accidents (5.0)	4. Cerebrovascular disease (17.4)	4. Breast cancer (109.4)	4. Breast cancer (33.5)

* Cancer of respiratory and intrathoracic organs, predominantly lung cancer.

SOURCE: Adapted from National Center for Health Statistics. *Vital Statistics of the United States, 1988.* Volume II, Mortality, Part A. Washington: Public Health Service, 1991. DHHS Publication No. (PHS)91-1101, pp. 40–52.

disorders in women. For example, the limbic system and hypothalamus, areas of the brain thought to subserve appetite, satiety, and emotion, have recently been shown to contain estradiol and testosterone receptors.

Alcohol abuse Blood alcohol levels are higher in women than in men after drinking equivalent amounts of alcohol (adjusted for body weight). This greater bioavailability of alcohol in women is probably due to decreased gastric "first pass metabolism" of alcohol, associated with lower activity of gastric alcohol dehydrogenase. On average, alcoholic women drink less than alcoholic men but exhibit the same degree of impairment. In addition, alcoholic women are more likely than alcoholic men to abuse tranquilizers, sedatives, and amphetamines. These findings have important implications in women for suggested "safe" levels of drinking with regard to driving and other activities.

Women alcoholics have a higher mortality rate than both nonalcoholic women and alcoholic men. Compared to men, women also appear to develop alcoholic liver disease and other alcohol-related diseases with shorter drinking histories and lower levels of alcohol consumption.

HIV infection This is a major health issue for women (as it is for men). There is a rapidly growing number (and percentage) of women who are HIV-infected but who do not yet have AIDS. An anonymous survey of the prevalence of HIV infection, the Sentinel Hospital study, found that as many as 8 percent of women in some urban areas who were felt not to be at high risk for HIV infection were, in fact, HIV-positive.

In the United States, AIDS is now the leading cause of death in young African-American women. Eleven percent of the reported cases of AIDS in the United States are in women, and the rate of increase in the incidence of AIDS is greater for women than men. About half of AIDS cases in women are associated with intravenous drug use and the other half appear to result from infection acquired by heterosexual transmission. A recent study indicates that death occurs sooner after the diagnosis of AIDS in women than in men. Worldwide, during the 1990s, an estimated 3 million women will die of AIDS.

The presentation of HIV infection in women has some special features. Vaginal candidiasis and pelvic inflammatory disease are prominent. Other sexually transmitted diseases as well as preneoplastic and neoplastic disease occur more frequently, and with greater severity, in HIV-infected women than in uninfected women.

Violence against women During the past 20 years, there has been a growing awareness of the enormous problem of violence against women, particularly involving family members and social acquaintances.

Rape has recently been redefined in many statutes as "nonconsensual sexual penetration of an adolescent or adult obtained by physical force, by threat of bodily harm, or when the victim is incapable of giving consent by virtue of mental illness, mental retardation, or intoxication." Epidemiologic studies in the United States suggest that at least 20 percent of adult women have experienced sexual assault during their lifetimes. Nearly 100,000 cases of rape are reported annually in the United States, and this undoubtedly represents only a fraction of the actual number of cases. Adult women are much more likely to be raped by a spouse, ex-spouse, or acquaintance than by a stranger.

In addition, every year in the United States more than 2 million women receive severe physical injury and more than 1000 women are killed by their current or former male partner. Domestic violence is the most common cause of physical injury in women, exceeding all injuries due to rape, mugging, and auto accidents combined. Surveys of women seeking medical care for any reason in internal medicine and emergency room practices have reported that the prevalence of domestic violence is an astonishing 15–20 percent. Domestic violence is a major health problem in women from all age, ethnic, and socioeconomic groups.

Women who have been raped or injured, as well as women who have been molested during childhood, frequently seek medical care for headaches, sleep and eating disorders, abdominal or pelvic pain, vaginal discharge, or musculoskeletal symptoms. They may also present to physicians with depression, suicidal ideation, and substance abuse. Given this indirect presentation of the consequences of violence, and the high prevalence of violence, clinicians should readily consider the possibility of violence in patients with vague symptoms and psychological disorders.

The immediate treatment of rape and domestic violence is focused on assessing and treating physical injury, providing emotional support, evaluating and dealing with the risks of sexually transmitted infection and pregnancy, assessing the safety of the patient and other family members, and documenting the patient's history and findings on physical examination. In addition to dealing with the medical and psychological issues, appropriate care includes providing information about legal services, shelters and safe houses, hotlines, support groups, and counseling services.

GENDER DIFFERENCES IN RESEARCH As noted earlier, relatively few women have been involved in studies of the prevention and pathophysiology of major diseases that involve both women and men. The same is also true for research related to treatment. Over $30 billion of pharmaceuticals are sold each year in the United States, and the great majority are used by women. Yet most clinical pharmacologic studies involving diseases that occur frequently in both sexes have been conducted in men. Even clinical pharmacologic studies in animals often concentrate on the males of the species. Two reasons are commonly given for conducting most clinical pharmacologic studies in men. First, cyclic hormonal changes in females could make experiments more difficult to control and interpret. Second, particularly with new drugs, concern about unsuspected pregnancy and subsequent teratogenic effects have discouraged the recruitment of female subjects.

Those studies that have included women indicate that there are clinically significant differences in the way women respond to a number of frequently prescribed pharmaceuticals, including sedative-hypnotics, antidepressants, antipsychotics, anticonvulsants, and beta-adrenoceptor blockers. Some studies have found that women have a higher frequency of adverse drug reactions than men, even after adjusting for several factors, including age, number of drugs being administered simultaneously, and duration of hospitalization. Women have more drug-induced gastrointestinal disturbances and cutaneous allergic reactions than men. Other studies suggest that the efficacy of many drugs may be lower in women. For example, women may be less responsive than men to antidepressant drugs. As another example, it has been shown that women require lower doses of neuroleptics than men to control schizophrenia. The reasons for these differences are not clear. Estrogens may reduce drug clearance via the cytochrome P450 oxidase system, an observation that could be of great practical importance given that millions of women regularly use estrogens. In some instances, drug pharmacokinetics may change during the menstrual cycle. For example, there is reasonable evidence that some anticonvulsants and lithium may be metabolized more rapidly in the premenstrual period, resulting in an increased frequency of premenstrual ("catamenial") seizures and increased symptoms of bipolar disorder, respectively, in women treated with these drugs.

DIFFERENCES IN THE MEDICAL EVALUATION OF MEN AND WOMEN In recent years, there has been growing evidence that gender, as well as race, may be an important factor in determining the care a patient receives. This has been most extensively studied with regard to IHD and end-stage renal disease. With regard to gender, several studies indicate that women with known IHD or with symptoms that might be secondary to IHD are less likely to undergo coronary angiography and revascularization. Further research is needed to determine why these gender differences exist. For example, do clinicians think that such procedures are of lesser benefit or greater risk in women (and, if so, on what basis do they take this position)? Are women less likely than men to ask about or consent to these diagnostic and therapeutic procedures? Finally, is the current use of coronary angiography and revascularization at the optimal level, in women and men?

Inequalities based on gender and race also have been observed with regard to the treatment of end-stage renal disease in the United States as well as other countries. Women with this condition are only 70 percent as likely to receive dialysis compared to men. In addition, women receiving long-term dialysis have only 75 percent the chance that men have of receiving a kidney transplant. The result of these two gender-related differences in care is that women aged 45 to 60 years receive a transplant less than half as often as men of the same age and race. Biological factors do not appear to explain these differences. Further research is needed to determine what role the beliefs of patients or doctors may play in creating this difference in the utilization of technology related to end-stage renal disease, and whether these beliefs are valid.

MORBIDITY AND MORTALITY IN WOMEN   There are substantial differences in the rates of morbidity and mortality between men and women. A number of psychosocial and biological factors have been identified that clearly influence these differences, but much remains to be learned.

Morbidity   Women may well experience greater morbidity than men. In 1980, females experienced a 26 percent higher rate of restricted activity and a 40 percent higher rate of bed disability adjusted across all ages. Women also make more visits to physicians, particularly for acute self-limited illnesses. The age-adjusted male/female ratio of the frequency of acute conditions of different types is summarized in Table 5-2. Except for injuries, acute conditions are diagnosed more frequently in women than men. It is unclear whether these differences in the incidence of acute conditions, and the associated increased disability and utilization of medical care, reflect real differences in the prevalence of morbidity, differences in concern about and reporting of symptoms, or differences in care-seeking behavior following the development of symptoms. Interestingly, in children less than age 15, it is the males that have higher rates of acute conditions, acute disability, and physician visits.

Mortality differences   As shown in Table 5-1, among young women in the United States almost half of all deaths are violent and are due to accidents, homicide, and suicide. During the middle years, breast cancer is a slightly more common cause of death than IHD and lung cancer. In women between ages 65 and 74, IHD and lung cancer overtake breast cancer as the leading causes of death. Across the entire age spectrum IHD is the leading cause of death in women by a substantial margin.

In the developed nations, women live longer than men. In the United States, the current average life expectancy from birth is 78.8 years for females, and 72.0 years for males. Although there are more male fetuses conceived than female fetuses, females have a survival advantage when compared to males, in all age groups both before and after birth. As shown in Table 5-3, age-adjusted death rates for the 15 leading causes of death in the United States are all greater in men than in women. From age 15 to 44 years, males are more than twice as likely to die than females.

TABLE 5-3   Ratio of age-adjusted death rates for the 15 leading causes of death, United States, 1988: Male/Female

Rank	Cause of death	Male/female ratio
1	Diseases of the heart	1.9
2	Malignant neoplasms	1.5
3	Cerebrovascular diseases	1.2
4	Accidents	2.7
5	Chronic obstructive pulmonary diseases	2.0
6	Pneumonia and influenza	1.7
7	Diabetes mellitus	1.1
8	Suicide	4.0
9	Chronic liver disease and cirrhosis	2.3
10	Nephritis, nephrotic syndrome, and nephrosis	1.5
11	Atherosclerosis	1.3
12	Homicide	3.3
13	Septicemia	1.3
14	Infant perinatal conditions	1.3
15	Human immunodeficiency virus infection	8.6

SOURCE: Adapted from: *MMWR* (40)494, 1991.

Social factors and women's health   Gender differences in morbidity and mortality may be explained in part by psychosocial factors such as socially defined gender roles, poverty, participation in the workforce, health insurance, and lifestyle factors.

In the past 30 years in the United States there has been a ''feminization of poverty''—a rapid growth in the relative percentage of people in female-headed households who are living in poverty. One-third of families headed by women currently live in poverty, and the fraction is greater than one-half for African-American and Latino women. Almost a fifth of women over age 65 live below the poverty level. Lack of adequate health insurance is a major problem for many women, especially minority women, poor and low-income women, and women of reproductive age. Women in general are more likely than men to have low-paying, part-time, nonunion jobs that do not provide health insurance. Women are more likely than men to lose health insurance, as a consequence of being divorced or widowed.

Women's increasing participation in the workforce could affect their health, although data on this question are limited and controversial. The 20th century has witnessed a striking social change in this regard. Whereas at the beginning of the century only about 20 percent of U.S. women were in the workforce, that figure has risen to about 75 percent, and is expected to continue to rise. Fewer than 10 percent of U.S. families currently consist of a father working outside the home and a mother working at home caring for children.

As discussed earlier, gender differences in lifestyle can explain some differences in morbidity and mortality. Substance abuse (including not only illicit drugs but also cigarettes and alcohol), reckless driving, and armed physical conflict (military and civilian) are more common in men. Men die from homicide approximately four times as often as women. These factors account for a part of the higher mortality rate in men, compared to women, particularly in the adolescent and young adult age groups.

Biological factors influencing morbidity and mortality   There also may be biological differences that contribute to the greater longevity of women. The most obvious is the exposure to estrogen that most women experience for about 40 years of their lives. As discussed earlier, premenopausal women are ''protected'' from IHD, perhaps related to high estrogen levels or other factors. It is hoped that further research on biological differences between the sexes will produce much-needed knowledge in this area.

CONCLUSION   Research has demonstrated important differences in the natural history, prevention, evaluation, and treatment of diseases in men and women. Studies are urgently needed of the important health problems of women mentioned above, as well as others not mentioned, including lung, breast, and other major cancers of women;

TABLE 5-2   Incidence of acute conditions for males and females, United States, 1980

Type of condition	Male/female ratio*
Infective and parasitic diseases	0.88
Respiratory conditions	0.81
Digestive conditions	0.92
Injuries	1.39
All other acute conditions, excluding pregnancy-related ones	0.66

* Calculated as incidence per 100 persons per year, adjusted for age.
SOURCE: Adapted from Verbrugge & Wingard, 1987; and Jack SS: Current estimates from the National Health Interview Survey: United States, 1980. In *Vital and Health Statistics*, Ser. 10, No. 139, National Center for Health Statistics, DHHS Publ. (PHS) 82-1567, 1982.

common disorders such as dysmenorrhea and premenstrual syndrome; contraception; and infertility.

REFERENCES

Anastos K et al: Hypertension in women: What is really known? Ann Intern Med 115:287, 1991

Ayanian JZ, Epstein AM: Differences in the use of procedures between women and men hospitalized for coronary heart disease. N Engl J Med 325:221, 1991

Blume SB: Women and alcohol. A review. JAMA 256:1467, 1986

Blumenthal SJ et al: *Towards a Women's Health Research Agenda. Findings of the Scientific Advisory Meeting.* Washington, Bass and Howes, Inc. 1991

Council on Scientific Affairs, American Medical Association: Violence against women. Relevance for medical practitioners. JAMA 267:3184, 1992

Fiebach NH et al: Differences between women and men in survival after myocardial infarction. Biology or methodology? JAMA 263:1092, 1990

Gijsbers van Wijk CMT et al: Symptom sensitivity and sex differences in physical morbidity: A review of health surveys in the United States and the Netherlands. Women and Health 17:91, 1991

Manson JE et al: A prospective study of aspirin use and primary prevention of cardiovascular disease in women. JAMA 266:521, 1991

Minkoff HL, DeHovitz JA: Care of women infected with the human immunodeficiency virus. JAMA 266:2253, 1991

Rodin J et al: Women's health. Review and research agenda as we approach the 21st century. Amer Psychol 45:1018, 1990

Verbrugge LM, Wingard DL: Sex differentials in health and mortality. Women & Health 12:103, 1987

6   MEDICAL DISORDERS DURING PREGNANCY

THOMAS F. FERRIS

Pregnancy may be complicated by chronic disease or a new illness. In the past, many disorders were considered contraindications to pregnancy, but now, with appropriate care, excellent outcomes for both mother and child are the rule.

HYPERTENSION

Systemic vascular resistance is reduced in pregnancy. In spite of a 40 percent increase in cardiac output during the second trimester, blood pressure falls (usually to 100/70 mmHg or lower). Although a modest rise may occur during the last month of normal pregnancy, an increase in systolic pressure of 30 mmHg or diastolic pressure of 15 mmHg at any time during gestation is abnormal. Perinatal mortality increases with blood pressure levels that would be normal in nonpregnant women. For example, when mean arterial blood pressure (diastolic plus one-third of the pulse pressure) is 90 mmHg or higher during the second trimester, there is greater risk for stillbirth, fetal growth retardation, and preeclampsia.

Hypertension during pregnancy usually has one of four causes: (1) preeclampsia (toxemia), (2) chronic essential hypertension, (3) gestational hypertension, or (4) renal disease.

PREECLAMPSIA (TOXEMIA)   Preeclampsia is a disease of late pregnancy in which hypertension is associated with hepatic, neurologic, hematologic, or renal involvement. Rapid development of edema, particularly of the face and hands, along with a rise in blood pressure, usually signals the onset of this condition. Jaundice and abnormal liver function may be present. Hyperreflexia, visual disturbances, and headache indicate neurologic involvement and convulsions indicate the presence of eclampsia. Hematologic manifestations of preeclampsia include thrombocytopenia with elevated lactate dehydrogenase (LDH), microangiopathic hemolytic anemia, and

thrombocytopenia. In fulminant preeclampsia, disseminated intravascular coagulation may cause a reduction in plasma fibrinogen and elevated circulating fibrin degradation products (Chap. 316).

Proteinuria indicates renal involvement, and since the glomerular filtration rate (GFR) increases by about 50 percent in normal gestation, a reduction in GFR heralds the onset of preeclampsia even with normal levels of blood urea nitrogen (BUN) and serum creatinine. Indeed, a BUN of 6.4 mmol/L (18 mg/dL) or a creatinine of 90 μmol/L (1 mg/dL) during pregnancy may reflect a 50 percent decline in GFR. In preeclampsia, urate clearance decreases, because of increased proximal tubular reabsorption of urate, which in turn is probably due to the reduction of vascular volume. Hyperuricemia usually precedes the rise in serum creatinine and BUN; in fact, a plasma uric acid above 270 μmol/L (4.5 mg/dL) in a hypertensive pregnant woman suggests preeclampsia. Volume contraction is similar to that in some other hypertensive states in which venoconstriction causes capillary pressure to rise, with expansion of interstitial volume at the expense of intravascular volume.

Fibrin deposits in the glomeruli, with characteristic swelling of the glomerular endothelial cells, are evident in renal biopsies; peripheral necrosis with fibrin deposits in the sinusoids may be present in the liver. Tomographic scanning techniques (CT or MRI) reveal hypodense areas consistent with small cerebral infarctions in approximately half of the women with eclampsia.

An abnormality in endothelial integrity may be the cause of the widespread fibrin deposits. Increased synthesis of two vasodilator prostaglandins—prostaglandin E_2 (PGE_2) and prostacyclin (PGI_2)—may explain the vasodilation and resistance to angiotensin II in normal pregnancy. In preeclampsia, synthesis of PGI_2 decreases, and sensitivity to angiotensin II increases, and the balance that normally exists between the platelet aggregatory and vasoconstrictor effects of thromboxane A_2 (produced by platelets) and the counteracting antiaggregatory and vasodilating effects of PGI_2 (produced by endothelial cells) may be lost, contributing to hypertension and platelet aggregation. The likelihood of preeclampsia may be reduced in women at risk when low-dose aspirin (an inhibitor of thromboxane A_2 synthesis) is administered throughout pregnancy.

Management   Once preeclampsia is diagnosed, hospitalization is indicated, since the disease can rapidly progress to eclampsia, characterized by convulsions. The definitive treatment of preeclampsia and eclampsia is delivery of the conceptus, which should be carried out promptly if fetal size and maturity are adequate. If the fetus is immature, bed rest, restriction of sodium intake to 2 g/d or less, and antihypertensive therapy are indicated. Beta blockers, calcium antagonists, hydralazine, and central sympathetic antagonists are all useful agents. Angiotensin converting enzyme (ACE) inhibitors are *contraindicated in pregnancy* since they increase the risk for fetal loss.

If an immediate reduction in blood pressure is needed, as in other forms of severe, uncontrolled hypertension (Chap. 209), several agents are useful. These include intravenous hydralazine (10-mg doses every 15 minutes until the desired effect is maintained); 500 mg alpha-methyldopa over 30 minutes; and labetalol, 1 mg/kg IV, followed by a continuous infusion of 20 mg/h. Obstetricians have long relied upon intravenous magnesium sulfate, which has mild antihypertensive properties and which increases synthesis of PGI_2 by endothelial cells.

CHRONIC ESSENTIAL HYPERTENSION   Like normal women, women with chronic essential hypertension experience a reduction in peripheral resistance during pregnancy. Indeed, a "normal" blood pressure may be obtained for the first time during pregnancy. Women with chronic hypertension are at higher risk for preeclampsia. Careful monitoring for proteinuria and of serum creatinine and uric acid are important in detecting the onset of this complication. There is no evidence that pregnancy has an adverse effect on the course of chronic essential hypertension. Thus antihypertensive medication (other than ACE inhibitors) should be continued throughout pregnancy in women with essential hypertension. Alpha-methyldopa has been used extensively in pregnancy, and children born to mothers who have taken this drug throughout pregnancy develop normally.

GESTATIONAL HYPERTENSION Hypertension that develops late in pregnancy (with no evidence of preeclampsia) and disappears after delivery is termed gestational hypertension. Usually women with this condition are overweight; others have a family history of hypertension, eventually develop chronic essential hypertension later in life, and have a high incidence of recurrence during subsequent pregnancies. Attention must be directed toward detecting increases in urinary protein and serum uric acid, creatinine, or BUN, since these remain normal in gestational hypertension and become elevated in preeclampsia. A beta blocker or alpha-methyldopa are usually effective in lowering blood pressure.

RENAL DISEASE

The increase in GFR during normal pregnancy is due to a rise in renal plasma flow without a concomitant rise in glomerular pressure. However, in renal disease, any rise in GFR depends on an elevation in glomerular pressure, which can increase proteinuria and worsen the underlying disease. Hypertension becomes more severe during pregnancy in most women with chronic renal disease, and proteinuria increases in approximately 20 percent. Since autoregulation of renal blood flow may be impaired in renal disease, any increase in blood pressure is more apt to raise glomerular pressure. The development or worsening of hypertension during pregnancy in patients with renal disease may be due to preeclampsia superimposed on renal disease.

It is desirable to maintain blood pressure below 120/80 mmHg in pregnant women with chronic renal disease. Twenty-four-hour urine protein excretion should be assessed throughout pregnancy, and an increase in proteinuria with no clinical evidence of toxemia usually reflects elevated glomerular pressure. Antihypertensive drugs other than ACE inhibitors should be utilized.

Many women have had successful pregnancies after renal transplantation. Although these patients receive chronic immunosuppressive therapy throughout gestation, the incidence of congenital malformations does not appear to be increased.

If systemic lupus erythematosus (SLE) (Chap. 284) is quiescent for 12 to 18 months prior to conception, pregnancy does not appear to activate the disease. In nonpregnant women, flare-ups of lupus nephropathy are usually associated with extrarenal manifestations of the disease, i.e., arthritis, rash, and fever, accompanied by a reduction in serum complement and a rise in anti-DNA antibodies. In contrast, pregnant women with SLE may manifest an increase in blood pressure and proteinuria along with a reduction in renal function in the absence of extrarenal manifestations. The renal exacerbations may be due to superimposed preeclampsia or the effect of hypertension on the nephropathy, since there is no clinical evidence of lupus activity and no increase in anti-DNA antibodies. This is an important distinction because these women may be treated inappropriately with higher doses of glucocorticoids or immunosuppressive agents (which may exacerbate hypertension) when antihypertensive therapy or delivery (depending on gestational age and maternal condition) is indicated instead. Conversely, women with active SLE who could be treated with glucocorticoids are often delivered inappropriately early for the mistaken diagnosis of preeclampsia.

CARDIAC DISEASE

As noted above, pregnancy is associated with a reduction in systemic vascular resistance. Normally, increases occur in stroke volume, heart rate, and cardiac output; these changes often produce systolic (flow) murmurs and third heart sounds. The rise in cardiac output exceeds the increase in oxygen consumption, so the arteriovenous oxygen difference falls. Four cardiac disorders are adversely affected by pregnancy: (1) valvular heart disease, (2) primary pulmonary hypertension, (3) the Eisenmenger syndrome, and (4) the Marfan syndrome.

VALVULAR HEART DISEASE (See also Chap. 201) The increased cardiac output associated with pregnancy may cause deterioration in women with *mitral stenosis*. If severe mitral stenosis is identified *prior* to pregnancy, valvulotomy should be carried out before conception, if possible. Asymptomatic pregnant women with mitral stenosis require close observation but not definitive therapy. However, if symptoms of pulmonary congestion develop, diuretics and restriction of activity are indicated. Atrial fibrillation should be treated with oral digoxin to slow the ventricular rate. Thromboembolism associated with mitral stenosis requires anticoagulation with intravenous heparin; warfarin is *contraindicated* in pregnancy because of its teratogenic effects. A closed mitral valvulotomy (surgical or, preferably, by balloon mitral valvuloplasty) can be carried out during pregnancy, when symptoms of mitral stenosis are severe; open-heart surgery is associated with an increase in fetal loss.

Mitral regurgitation is usually well tolerated during pregnancy, presumably because peripheral resistance is lower. Aortic stenosis is a contraindication for pregnancy until the lesion has been corrected. A maternal mortality of 15 percent has been reported in women with critical aortic stenosis.

Artificial heart valves in pregnant women are associated with many problems. It is mandatory to continue full anticoagulation in patients with mechanical valvular prostheses. Warfarin is contraindicated because of its teratogenic effects; heparin is preferable but may cause bleeding and fetal loss. Tissue valves are less thrombogenic, but their limited durability in young adults is a serious disadvantage. Therefore in women with serious valvular heart disease every effort should be made to allow pregnancy to go to completion prior to valve replacement, and subsequent pregnancies avoided once a mechanical valve has been implanted.

In women with prosthetic valves, antibiotic prophylaxis with agents effective against genitourinary organisms is mandatory during the peripartum period.

PULMONARY HYPERTENSION AND EISENMENGER SYNDROME (See Chaps. 225 and 199) Pulmonary hypertension of all causes is a strong contraindication for pregnancy. If moderate or severe pulmonary hypertension (systolic pulmonary artery pressure >45 mmHg) is detected during the first trimester, termination of the pregnancy is advisable. In women with congenital heart disease, pulmonary hypertension, and a right-to-left shunt, i.e., the Eisenmenger syndrome, both maternal and fetal mortality are high, the latter increasing with the severity of maternal cyanosis.

MARFAN SYNDROME (See Chap. 351) Cardiovascular manifestations of the Marfan syndrome include mitral valve prolapse, mitral and aortic valve abnormalities, and aortic regurgitation due to enlargement of the aortic root. When the aortic root diameter measured by echocardiography exceeds 40 mm, the risk of aortic dissection and rupture during pregnancy is increased. Women with the Marfan syndrome, especially those with a dilated aortic root, should avoid pregnancy; however, if such women become pregnant and refuse abortion, beta-adrenoceptor blocker therapy should be instituted to reduce the force of myocardial contraction and the resultant shear stress on the aorta.

OTHER FORMS OF CARDIAC DISEASE In the absence of pulmonary hypertension, atrial septal defect (p. 1040) is well tolerated by pregnant women, although the risk of fetal loss is increased. Patients with ventricular septal defect (p. 1041) without pulmonary hypertension also tolerate pregnancy well, but this lesion may be complicated by infective endocarditis, so antibiotic prophylaxis at the time of delivery is mandatory. Mitral valve prolapse (p. 1058), which is common among pregnant women, does not appear to complicate the pregnancy, nor does pregnancy complicate prolapse, although antibiotic prophylaxis is warranted. Women with hypertrophic cardiomyopathy (p. 1092) generally tolerate pregnancy well; indeed, the gestational hypervolemia may be associated with a reduction of the intraventricular pressure gradient and thus ameliorate symptoms. Because of its poor prognosis, chronic dilated cardiomyopathy (p. 1090) accompanied by heart failure is a contraindication to pregnancy.

Peripartum cardiomyopathy, a form of acute dilated cardiomyopathy that may be associated with a myocarditis, appears around the time of delivery, most frequently during the first 6 weeks postpartum, is sometimes associated with preeclampsia, and may actually be caused by pregnancy (p. 1090). Infant mortality is high if congestive heart failure ensues, and maternal mortality may be as high as 30 percent within the first few months. About one-third of patients show functional recovery and the remaining third have persistent severely impaired left ventricular function. Subsequent pregnancies should be avoided.

Premature atrial or ventricular systoles during pregnancy can be treated by the elimination of stimulants, avoidance of excessive fatigue, and reassurance. Drug therapy should be avoided, if possible, but cardioversion has been used safely for tachyarrhythmias during pregnancy.

PULMONARY EMBOLISM (See also Chap. 226)

In pregnancy all of the coagulation factors are increased, except factors XI and XIII, and antithrombin III, a major inhibitor of coagulation, is reduced. Pulmonary embolism occurs about once in 750 pregnancies. Because of the immediate need to prevent embolism and the other long-term complications of deep vein thrombosis (DVT), it is important to recognize the latter. DVT may occur during pregnancy owing to compression of the iliac veins by the enlarged uterus as well as changes in the coagulation and fibrinolytic systems that favor thrombosis. This complication also occurs in the postpartum period. Impedance plethysmography and Doppler ultrasonography are noninvasive nonradiologic techniques useful in documenting DVT. When pulmonary embolism is suspected, perfusion lung scanning can be accomplished with smaller quantities of isotope, and pulmonary angiography can be carried out if the abdomen is shielded. Despite the potential small hazard of fetal irradiation posed by these latter procedures, it is extremely important to diagnose pulmonary embolism.

Anticoagulant therapy is indicated in pregnant women with DVT to prevent pulmonary embolism. Heparin, which does not cross the placenta and therefore does not cause fetal complications, can be administered at a dose of 1000 units per hour by continuous infusion until early during labor. Protamine can then be used to reverse the drug's effects, and heparin can be restarted within 2 h of delivery and continued for 3 to 4 days after which subcutaneous heparin or oral warfarin therapy may be instituted for 6 months. When venous thrombosis or pulmonary embolism occur in the early postpartum period, heparin treatment should be instituted for 7 to 10 days, followed by warfarin for about 3 months.

DIABETES MELLITUS (See also Chap. 337)

From a metabolic standpoint, pregnancy resembles starvation—that is, blood sugar and amino acids are low while plasma free fatty acids, ketones, and triglycerides are increased. Plasma glucose is 0.8–1.1 mmol/L (15 to 20 mg/dL) lower after an overnight fast than in nonpregnant women; when fasting lasts longer than 12 h, plasma glucose may fall to 2.2–2.5 mmol/L (40 to 45 mg/dL) while plasma hydroxybutyrate and acetoacetate levels rise to levels two to four times higher than in nonpregnant women. As a consequence, ketoacidosis develops in the absence of striking hyperglycemia in pregnant diabetics. Maternal insulin and glucagon do not cross the placenta, but acetoacetate and beta-hydroxybutyrate are readily transferred and oxidized by the fetal brain and liver.

In spite of the fetal demand for glucose, pregnancy is also a diabetogenic state by virtue of the development of insulin resistance. Elevation of several hormones in pregnancy may be responsible for insulin resistance, including progesterone, estrogen, prolactin, and human placental lactogen.

Pregnancy in diabetics is associated with a higher perinatal mortality (3 to 5 percent vs. 1 to 2 percent in nondiabetic women) and a higher incidence of congenital anomalies (6 to 12 percent vs. 2 to 3 percent in nondiabetics). Glucose control, particularly during organogenesis, reduces the incidence of congenital anomalies. Counseling should emphasize the importance of home monitoring of glucose levels and the need to adjust the insulin dose to maintain fasting blood sugar at a normal level and postprandial glucose no higher than 7.8 mmol/L (140 mg/dL). Glycosylated hemoglobin should also be monitored during pregnancy. Ultrasound evaluation of the fetus should be carried out during the second trimester, and alpha-fetoprotein levels should be assessed in the 20th week to detect neural tube defects.

Women with diabetic nephropathy have an excellent chance of a normal pregnancy, with perinatal survival of approximately 90 percent. As with other renal diseases, hypertension can worsen late in pregnancy, with increased proteinuria and decreased creatinine clearance that represents either superimposed preeclampsia or a rise in glomerular pressure. There is no evidence that pregnancy worsens diabetic nephropathy, but care of pregnant women with diabetic nephropathy requires management by obstetricians skilled in high-risk pregnancies, neonatologists, diabetologists, and nephrologists. Hypertension should be treated as described earlier in this chapter.

GESTATIONAL DIABETES   The insulin resistance of normal pregnancy may also contribute to gestational diabetes in women in whom the capacity for insulin secretion is not sufficient to meet the increased insulin demands of pregnancy. The overall prevalence of gestational diabetes is between 1 and 3 percent. An important reason for recognizing the disorder early is that it induces excessive fetal insulin secretion, which in turn can cause fetal macrosomia and increase the risk for birth trauma and the need for cesarean section.

There are no universally accepted criteria for the diagnosis or screening for gestational diabetes if the fasting glucose is normal. The 1990 Workshop-Conference on Gestational Diabetes recommended the screening of pregnant women with normal fasting blood sugar levels between the 24th and 28th weeks of gestation using a 50-g oral glucose load. If the 1-h glucose level exceeds 7.8 mmol/L (140 m/dL) a 100-g oral glucose test is performed after an overnight fast. Gestational diabetes is defined as any two of the following values: 1 h >10.5 mmol/L (>190 ng/dL), 2 h >9.2 mmol/L (>165 ng/dL), and 3 h >8.0 mmol/L (>145 ng/dL). In contrast, the American College of Obstetricians and Gynecologists recommends screening only for women at high risk, namely women over age 30; women with previous macrosomic, malformed, or stillborn infants; and those with obesity, hypertension, or glycosuria.

Gestational diabetes is treated with diet; if fasting glucose remains elevated insulin therapy should be started. Following delivery, carbohydrate tolerance may return to normal, but 30 percent or more of women with gestational diabetes develop diabetes mellitus within 5 years of pregnancy.

THYROID DISEASE (See also Chap. 334)

The diagnosis of thyroid disease in pregnancy is complicated by the increases in thyroid size, radioactive iodine uptake, basal metabolic rate, and thyroxine-binding globulin during normal pregnancy. Plasma T_3 and T_4 are elevated, but free T_3, T_4, and thyroid-stimulating hormone (TSH) remain normal, while the T_3 resin uptake is in the hypothyroid range. Maternal thyrotoxicosis occurs about once in 500 pregnancies, and the diagnosis may be difficult because the increase in cardiac output, tachycardia, skin warmth, and heat intolerance typical of pregnancy can mimic hyperthyroidism. Values of T_4 above 154 mmol/L (12 μg/dL) with a resin T_3 uptake in the euthyroid range (25 to 35 percent) suggests hyperthyroidism in a pregnant woman. Pregnant women can tolerate mild degrees of hyperthyroidism without difficulty, and thyrotoxicosis does not increase fetal loss. Gestation does not worsen thyrotoxicosis; indeed, hyperthyroidism is often more easily controlled during pregnancy. The treatment of gestational thyrotoxicosis involves a choice between antithyroid drugs and ablative surgery. Propylthiouracil is the drug of choice, since methimazole may cause aplasia cutis in the fetus. Maternal T_4 concentration should be maintained in the upper range of normal, using as low a dose of propylthiouracil as possible. Since this drug crosses the placenta and blocks fetal synthesis of thyroxine, fetal goiter occasionally develops due to stimulation of fetal TSH. When surgery is planned for the treatment of thyrotoxicosis, propylthiouracil should be administered preoperatively to control the hyperthyroid state.

Hypothyroidism during pregnancy should be treated with hormone replacement as in the nongravid state.

DISORDERS OF CALCIUM METABOLISM (See also Chap. 357)

Although serum calcium normally falls in pregnancy because of the decrease in serum albumin, the concentration of ionized calcium remains unchanged. Parathyroid hormone (PTH) levels increase in pregnancy with no change in phosphate clearance. This increase in PTH may be the cause of the higher plasma 1,25-dihydroxyvitamin D in pregnancy, resulting in an increase in intestinal calcium absorption and hypercalciuria. Urinary calcium excretion is approximately 7.5 mmol/d (300 mg/d), compared with 2.5 mmol/d (100 mg/d) in nonpregnant women, and urinary calculi develop in about one of 2000 pregnancies. When hyperparathyroidism with hypercalcemia occurs during pregnancy, the neonate may exhibit tetany because of the suppression of fetal PTH secretion.

HEMATOLOGIC DISORDERS

During pregnancy, plasma volume increases more than does red cell mass, so that a fall in hemoglobin concentration of 10 to 20 g/L (1 to 2 g/dL) is usual. Two potential causes of anemia during pregnancy are deficiencies of iron or folate. Since the developing fetus utilizes these substances in large amounts, these deficiencies may be prevented by providing iron and folate supplements. Pregnancy also results in a leukocytosis that can sometimes reach 18,000 per cubic millimeter.

Sickle cell anemia (Chap. 306) may be complicated by pregnancy, and vasoocclusive crises become more frequent, particularly during labor and the postpartum period. The risks for spontaneous abortion, prematurity, and neonatal death are high.

Thrombocytopenia in pregnancy is most often due to preeclampsia, although sepsis and idiopathic thrombocytopenic purpura may also be responsible. In the last-named condition, antiplatelet antibodies cross the placenta and can cause thrombocytopenia in the fetus as well. Cesarean section is indicated if the fetal platelet count obtained by percutaneous umbilical cord sampling performed at 36 to 37 weeks is less than 50,000 per milliliter.

Stillbirth, often associated with placental venous thrombosis, occurs in women with the so-called lupus anticoagulant (Chap. 284), an immunoglobulin that binds to negatively charged phospholipids and interferes with vitamin K–dependent coagulation factors. The lupus anticoagulant is actually more apt to cause thrombosis than bleeding, and treatment with low dose aspirin and prednisone throughout pregnancy may reduce the rate of fetal loss.

Disseminated intravascular coagulation may occur due to abruptio placentae, a retained dead fetus, amniotic fluid embolism, saline induced abortion, or fulminant preeclampsia and can be cured by treating the underlying cause.

GASTROINTESTINAL AND LIVER DISEASES

Nausea and vomiting occur in approximately 90 percent of women between the 6th and 16th weeks of pregnancy. When severe, the problem can be treated with oral dimenhydrinate, 50 to 100 mg every 4 h, or D-oxylamine, 12.5 mg every 4 h. In its severe form *hyperemesis gravidarum* can cause dehydration that requires parenteral feeding. Heartburn, which may be due to relaxation of the lower esophageal sphincter, is usually responsive to treatment with antacids and H-2 receptor blocking agents.

Pregnancy in women with inflammatory bowel disease may be uncomplicated, but it is difficult to anticipate the course in advance. Most patients do well but in some the pregnancy may exacerbate the disease; rarely the pregnancy may need to be terminated. If the disease is active at the time of conception, the incidence of spontaneous abortion is higher than in normal pregnancy.

Although pregnancy is associated with supersaturation of the bile with cholesterol, the incidence of cholelithiasis in a first pregnancy does not appear to be increased. However, the risk for this complication increases with multiparity. Serum triglycerides and cholesterol are elevated during pregnancy; although serum bilirubin remains normal, there is a striking rise in alkaline phosphatase (which originates from the placenta) that may reach a peak 2 to 4 times normal at term.

Although total serum protein concentration declines by approximately 20 percent in midpregnancy because of a decrease in albumin, hepatic synthesis of other plasma proteins increases. In a normal pregnancy, serum gamma-glutamyl transpeptidase and serum lactate dehydrogenase (LDH) are increased, whereas serum aminotransferases and aspartate aminotransferase are normal.

Intrahepatic cholestasis of pregnancy usually appears in the third trimester and is manifested by pruritus, with bilirubin levels usually less than 100 μmol/L (6 mg/dL). Although bilirubin levels usually remain in the range of 34 to 86 μmol/L (2 to 5 mg/dL), there is a striking increase in alkaline phosphatase. The cholestasis and pruritus disappear promptly after delivery, but the syndrome may recur with subsequent pregnancies. Aside from pruritus, the mother does not suffer any adverse effect. However, there appears to be an increase in stillbirths thought to be secondary to the toxicity of bile acids to the fetus. Therefore, fetal surveillance should be carried out once the diagnosis of intrahepatic cholestasis of pregnancy is established. Treatment of pruritus consists of antihistamine and cholestyramine, 4 g four times a day.

Acute fatty liver of pregnancy, with histologic changes showing hepatocytes with increased microvesicular fat and fibrin deposits in the hepatic sinusoids, may occur late in pregnancy and may be associated with preeclampsia. Serum bilirubin may exceed 170 μmol/L (10 mg/dL), and AST and ALT are in the range of 5 to 8 μkat/L (300 to 500 U/L). Prothrombin time may be prolonged, and disseminated intravascular coagulation may cause depressed fibrinogen levels, an increase in fibrin degradation products, and thrombocytopenia. Maternal deaths may occur, but this condition is usually ameliorated following delivery.

Hepatitis B (Chap. 266) during pregnancy increases prematurity and fetal death with a high risk of transmission to the infant, particularly in mothers who are HBe antigen-positive at the time of the delivery. Women who are HBs antigen-positive and HBe antigen-negative transmit the disease less frequently. Approximately 5 to 10 percent of infants infected with hepatitis B acquire the disease by the transplacental route. Infants born to mothers with hepatitis B should be treated with both hepatitis B immune globulin and hepatitis B vaccine.

The severity of viral hepatitis A is not altered by pregnancy and the risk of transmission to the neonate is small.

INFECTIONS

Infectious diseases constitute serious risk to both the pregnant woman and the fetus.

BACTERIAL INFECTIONS Urinary tract infections (see Chap. 90) are the most common type of bacterial infection in pregnancy. Asymptomatic bacteriuria occurs in up to 7 percent of pregnancies.

Physiologic changes in pregnancy such as hormone-induced dilatation of the urinary tract, hydroureter, and vesicoureteral reflux predispose to asymptomatic bacteriuria, and one-third of patients with these conditions develop pyelonephritis, usually during the last trimester. Since over 75 percent of pregnancy-associated acute pyelonephritis can be avoided by treating asymptomatic bacteriuria, screening for bacteriuria at the first prenatal visit is recommended. *Escherichia coli* is the most commonly isolated organism, and treatment for asymptomatic bacteriuria for 3 days with ampicillin, cephalexin, nitrofurantoin, or sulfisoxazole is appropriate, although the last drug should not be used during the final month of gestation because it may cause jaundice in the infant.

Intrauterine infection occurs in up to 4 percent of pregnancies and is associated with increased morbidity and mortality in the prenatal period. Intraamniotic infection is most common when ascending infection follows rupture of the membranes, but it is also seen with intact membranes, especially in preterm labor. Infection is usually polymicrobial, involving both aerobes and anaerobes, genital mycoplasmas, *Gardnerella vaginalis*, and group B streptococci. Since early clinical signs may be subtle, diagnosis requires a high degree of suspicion. Clinical clues include fever, maternal or fetal tachycardia, uterine tenderness, foul-smelling amniotic fluid, and leukocytosis. Delivery of the fetus is indicated. Antibiotic therapy should begin during labor, rather than afterward. Antibiotics with broad coverage are indicated, such as ampicillin and gentamicin.

Postpartum infections remain the most common cause of maternal mortality in the United States. The majority of deaths are related to postpartum endometrial infections complicated by pelvic abscess, peritonitis, or pelvic thrombophlebitis. Rates of endometritis vary from 1 to 3 percent after vaginal delivery and from 6 to 18 percent after cesarean section. Endometritis should be suspected when a patient has a fever after delivery. Few patients exhibit all of the classical manifestations such as fever, abdominal pain, malaise, and purulent or foul-smelling lochia. Work-up should include complete blood count, blood cultures, and a genital tract culture. The most common bacterial pathogens responsible for postpartum endometritis are group B streptococci, mixed anaerobic and aerobic organisms, *E. coli*, and *Staphylococcus aureus*. Treatment depends upon the organism cultured, but broad-spectrum antibiotics or combinations such as ampicillin, an aminoglycoside, and clindamycin are usually used.

Group B *Streptococcus* (Chap. 103) has become a major cause of postpartum bacteremia, accounting for 10 to 20 percent of blood culture isolates from women admitted to obstetrical services. Although most of these patients have an uncomplicated course following appropriate antibiotic therapy, complications such as endocarditis and meningitis are occasionally seen. In contrast to bacteremia with no identifiable source, most severe Group B *Streptococcus* infections in pregnancy are associated with an identifiable source such as endometritis or a urinary tract infection.

Listeria monocytogenes (see Chap. 105) is another bacterial infection which has specific pregnancy-related morbidity. Infection can occur at any time during pregnancy, but is most common during the third trimester. Symptoms are frequently suggestive of a urinary tract infection, but urine cultures are sterile. Diagnosis is made by a positive blood culture. Clinical severity of infection can range from a mild febrile to severe illness. This infection can precipitate labor and result in premature birth of a dead or infected infant.

Neisseria gonorrhoeae (see Chap. 110) can be transmitted from mother to infant in utero, during delivery, or in the postpartum period. The most common clinical problem caused by this transmission is gonococcal conjunctivitis of the newborn. Conjunctival installation of a 1% aqueous solution of silver nitrate is effective in preventing blindness caused by this infection. Congenital syphilis (see Chap. 133) occurs by infection of the fetus in utero. Transmission of *Treponema pallidum* to the fetus, most common in the early stages of syphilis, can occur at any time during pregnancy. Infection of the fetus before the fourth month is rare. Syphilis can have severe effects on the offspring, including stillbirth, neonatal disease, or latent infection.

VIRAL INFECTIONS   These are of major concern during pregnancy because of the consequences to the fetus. Since transplacental transmission may occur, maternal infections with cytomegalovirus (CMV), rubella, varicella zoster, and herpes simplex virus have the greatest teratogenic potential, particularly during the first trimester. Perinatal infection can result from transmission of the virus to the infant during passage through an infected uterine cervix.

CMV infection (see Chap. 146) is the most common cause of congenital viral infection. The virus is ubiquitous; 35 to 100 percent of the adult population have evidence of prior infection, with the highest prevalence among lower socioeconomic groups. CMV is usually acquired by the oral-respiratory route, through sexual contact, or by blood transfusion. CMV infection establishes a lifelong latent infection in the host which can be reactivated later by immunosuppression. Rates of cervical infection with CMV increase in later stages of pregnancy. Although during pregnancy CMV can be shed with no evidence of clinical disease in the mother, high numbers of CMV in the cervix suggest the neonate is at risk during birth. Approximately 1 to 2 percent of all newborn infants in the United States are infected with CMV in utero, but the vast majority of these are normal. Clinically apparent congenital infections are most common in the first infant of mothers with primary infection during pregnancy. CMV disease occurs in infants whose mothers are not immune. Cytomegalic inclusion disease is characterized by jaundice, hepatosplenomegaly, a petechial rash, and multiple system and organ involvement. Other manifestations range from subtle neurologic sequelae to severe microcephaly.

Rubella (see Chap. 156) can have severe outcomes in the fetus, including fetal death and premature delivery, if the mother is infected during early pregnancy. A variety of congenital defects are caused by rubella, including cataracts, cardiac abnormalities, deafness, and mental retardation. Fetal abnormalities are greatest when maternal rubella occurs during the first trimester, with 80 percent of children affected; the percentage falls to about 25 percent when infection occurs at the end of the second trimester. Congenital infection can be diagnosed prenatally by detecting rubella IgM antibody in fetal blood under ultrasound guidance. In places where immunization programs have been widely used, the problem has been eliminated. The vaccine can be administered during pregnancy without harm to the fetus. Infection during pregnancy with varicella zoster virus (VZV) represents a health risk to the mother (see Chap. 144). There is nearly a 10 percent risk for severe pneumonia. Early antiviral therapy should be instituted if there is any suspicion of chickenpox-related pneumonia. Although most infants born to VZV-infected mothers are normal, there is a risk to the unborn child of developing congenital teratogenic infection.

Infection of the newborn with herpes simplex virus (HSV) can range from mild localized infection to fatal dissemination (see Chap. 143). Retrograde infection or birth through a maternal genital tract infected with HSV-2 can result in serious disseminated neonatal infection.

OTHER INFECTIONS OF PREGNANCY   *Vulvovaginal candidiasis* (see Chap. 166) is more common in pregnant than nonpregnant women. High estrogen levels apparently encourage growth of this organism. Infection rates increase as the gestational period progresses, with up to 55 percent of third-trimester women being colonized and with symptomatic disease developing in the majority of those colonized.

Toxoplasmosis (see Chap. 177) causes symptoms in only 10 to 20 percent of women infected during pregnancy. Unfortunately, the fetus is at risk whether or not the mother is symptomatic. Transmission to the fetus can occur transplacentally or at birth. One-third of infants born to mothers infected during pregnancy become infected. The risk for congenital infection is greater when maternal infection occurs during the third trimester than the first, although the risk of spontaneous abortion is highest when infection is acquired in the first trimester.

Most infected newborns have no symptoms at birth but develop symptoms, particularly chorioretinitis, by adolescence. Less-common manifestations include strabismus, epilepsy, and psychomotor retardation. Toxoplasmosis does not cause fetal malformation.

HUMAN IMMUNODEFICIENCY VIRUS INFECTION

Approximately 80 percent of women with AIDS are of childbearing age. The incidence of infection with HIV will increase in women in the United States during the 1990s (see also Chap. 279). Worldwide, particularly in developing countries, HIV infection is predominantly spread heterosexually with the male-to-female ratio in certain countries approaching 1. The majority of the current cases of AIDS among women in the United States are those who are intravenous drug users (IVDUs) or who are the heterosexual partners of IVDUs. The geographic distribution of HIV infection among women closely parallels the geographic distribution of HIV infection among IVDUs, with the highest incidence in the Northeast and Southeast seaboard states and Puerto Rico. In New York City, approximately 10,000 women of childbearing age developed AIDS by 1993.

EFFECT OF HIV INFECTION ON PREGNANCY   Although earlier studies suggested that HIV-positive women were at a higher risk of delivering infants with an unfavorable outcome, at the present time accumulating evidence indicates that HIV infection alone does not impose a significant negative effect on pregnancy outcome, particularly when the infection is in the asymptomatic stage. Further, an acceleration of HIV disease during pregnancy is uncommon and may be due to other factors associated with confounding issues present in the women most likely to be infected such as IV drug use and inadequate access to prenatal care.

Primary infection is generally associated with a burst of viremia with or without an acute HIV syndrome, the latter occurring in approximately 50 to 70 percent of individuals following initial infection. It is unclear what effect this burst of viremia has on the pregnancy itself or the chances of the fetus becoming infected during the pregnancy, if a previously uninfected mother develops a primary infection during the pregnancy.

TRANSMISSION OF HIV TO THE FETUS/INFANT   The rate of transmission of HIV from mother to fetus/infant averages approximately 30 percent, with a range of 13 percent in a European collaborative study to 45 percent in Central Africa (see Chap. 279). Higher rates of transmission have been associated with the symptomatic stage in the mother and with low maternal CD4+ T lymphocyte counts. Although infection of the fetus can occur throughout pregnancy, it is felt that maternal transmission occurs most commonly during the perinatal period. Nonetheless, caesarean sections are not currently recommended unless there are other obstetrical reasons for doing so. Postnatal transmission from mother to infant has been documented, and colostrum and breast milk have been implicated. Where possible, breast feeding by an infected mother should be avoided.

TREATMENT OF HIV INFECTION DURING PREGNANCY   Despite the fact that the effects of the commonly employed antiretroviral drugs on the pregnant woman and the fetus have not been fully delineated, most physicians treat HIV-infected pregnant women according to the same guidelines as for nonpregnant HIV-infected individuals. Treatment and/or prophylaxis of opportunistic infections should also be approached according to existing guidelines for HIV-infected patients except for those situations in which a drug is clearly contraindicated in pregnancy.

NEOPLASTIC DISEASES

Transmission of leukemia or lymphoma to the fetus has not been reported, and there is no clear evidence that pregnancy adversely affects the course of any type of malignancy; however, it is possible that the high estrogen levels of pregnancy accelerate the course of breast cancer.

Deciding whether the pregnancy should be terminated in women with neoplastic disease requires judgment about whether the pregnant state presents a significant obstacle to effective therapy and whether the fetus will be harmed as a result of such therapy. Although most antineoplastic agents are potentially teratogenic or cause fetal wastage, many healthy full-term infants have been born despite active maternal chemotherapy at the time of conception or during the first trimester. Thus while it would be safer to avoid fetal exposure, the decision to terminate a pregnancy must take into account the parents' desire to have a child. Pregnant women with leukemia who are given the usual chemotherapy for this condition have done surprisingly well; in some studies maternal survival rates have been 100 percent, and the incidence of congenital abnormalities in the newborn is less than 10 percent.

REFERENCES

BARRON WM, LINDHEIMER MD: *Medical Complications in Pregnancy*. St. Louis, Mosby-Year Book Publishers, 1991

BRIGGS GG, FREEMAN RK, YAFFE SJ: *Drugs in Pregnancy and Lactation*, 3d ed. Baltimore, Williams & Wilkins, 1990

BURROW GN, FERRIS TF: *Medical Complications During Pregnancy*, 4th ed. Philadelphia, Saunders, 1994, in press

NANDA D, MINKOFF HL: HIV in pregnancy—transmission and immune effects. Clin Obst Gyn 32:456, 1989

SELWYN PA et al: Prospective study of human immunodeficiency virus infection and pregnancy outcomes in intravenous drug users. JAMA 261:1289, 1989

7   ADOLESCENT HEALTH PROBLEMS

CHARLES E. IRWIN, JR / MARY-ANN SHAFER

APPROACH TO THE ADOLESCENT PATIENT

Adolescence is the period between childhood and adulthood. This period is usually defined by rapid onset of biological and psychological growth and development prior to or at the second decade of life and terminating before age 20. Major social and environmental factors influence the onset, duration, and termination of adolescence. Over the next decade, the numbers of adolescents will increase, adolescents will include more ethnic and racial minorities than the general population, and the adolescent population will become more impoverished, thereby decreasing their access to health care. Currently, the adolescent population in the United States is the group least likely to have health insurance. Physicians need a careful understanding of the biological and psychosocial changes of adolescence, the associated environmental changes, and the legal and ethical issues that affect the provision of health care services to adolescents.

BIOLOGICAL MATURATION   Puberty (See also Chaps. 339 and 340)   Puberty is defined as the biological processes that ultimately lead to reproductive capacity. The onset and tempo of puberty vary by sex, population group, and individual. During puberty, major alterations in the hormonal regulatory systems in the central nervous system, gonads, and adrenals cause changes in skeletal growth and in body composition and the acquisition of secondary sexual characteristics. The mechanisms responsible for the initiation of puberty through activation of the hypothalamic-pituitary-gonadal axis remain undefined.

The sexual maturity ratings (SMRs) of Marshall and Tanner are helpful in monitoring the development of secondary sexual

TABLE 7-1   Sexual maturity rating for females*

A Pubertal development in size of female breasts
   Stage 1: Prepubertal. Elevation of the papilla only.
   Stage 2: Breast bud stage. A small mound of breast tissue is formed by
   the elevation of the breast and papilla. Areolar diameter enlarges.
   Stage 3: Further enlargement of breast and areola with no separation of
   their contours.
   Stage 4: Projection of the areola and papilla to form a secondary mound
   above the level of the breast.
   Stage 5: Adult. The breasts resemble those of a mature female. The
   areola has recessed to the general contour of the breast.

B Pubertal development of female pubic hair
   Stage 1: Prepubertal. There is no pubic hair.
   Stage 2: Sparse growth of long, slightly pigmented, downy hair, straight
   or only slightly curled, primarily along the labia.
   Stage 3: The hair is considerably darker, coarser, and more curled, and
   spreads sparsely over the junction of the pubes.
   Stage 4: The hair, now adult in type, covers a smaller area than in the
   adult and does not extend onto the medial surface of the thighs.
   Stage 5: Adult. The hair is adult in quantity and type, with extension
   onto the thighs.

*Modified from van Wieringen JC et al: *Growth Diagrams*. Gronigen, Neth., Woplter-Noorhoff Publishing, 1971.

characteristics of pubertal maturation, which are the somatic manifestations of adrenal and gonadal activity. These ratings correlate more closely with bone age than chronologic age. The SMRs for girls are based upon breast and pubic hair development, each in five stages (Table 7-1). The ratings for boys are based upon genital and pubic hair development each also in five stages (Table 7-2).

The mean age of onset of puberty for girls as defined by breast budding is 11.2 ± 1.6 years, whereas the mean age of onset for boys as defined by enlargement of testes is 11.6 ± 1.1 years. The mean age of menarch in the United States is 13.3 ± 1.3 years, and the mean age for spermarche is between 13.5 and 14.5 years. The average duration of puberty for girls is 4 years with a range of 1.5 to 8 years, and the average duration of puberty for boys is 3 years with a range of 2 to 5 years. Even though the timing and duration of the events vary, each adolescent follows an orderly sequence in somatic growth and development (Figs. 7-1 and 7-2). Monitoring these events through a careful history and physical examination is helpful in identifying medical conditions that become manifest during adolescence (Table 7-3).

Skeletal growth (See also Chap. 332)   The pubertal height spurt accounts for approximately 25 percent of final adult height and occurs at an average age of 12 years for girls (SMR 2–3) and 14 years for

TABLE 7-2   Sexual maturity ratings for males*

A Pubertal development in size of male genitalia
   Stage 1: Prepubertal. Penis, testes, and scrotum are of childhood size.
   Stage 2: The scrotum and testes enlarge with testicular measurement
   greater than 2.5 cm in length (testicular volume, 4–7 mL). Penis
   usually show no growth. Scrotal skin reddens or darkens.
   Stage 3: Further growth of testes (testicular volume, 8–10 mL) and
   scrotum with enlargement of penis, mainly in length.
   Stage 4: Continued growth of the testes (testicular volume, 10–15 mL)
   and scrotum with increased size of the penis, especially in breadth.
   Stage 5: Adult. The genitalia are adult in size (testicular volume, 20–25
   mL) and shape.

B Pubertal development of male pubic hair
   Stage 1: Prepubertal. Pubic hair is absent.
   Stage 2: Sparse growth of long, slightly pigmented, downy hair, straight
   or only slightly curled, primarily at the base of the penis.
   Stage 3: The hair is considerably darker, coarser, and more curled. The
   hair spreads sparsely over the junction of the pubes.
   Stage 4: The hair, now adult in type, covers a smaller area than in the
   adult and does not extend onto the medial surface of the thighs.
   Stage 5: Adult. The hair is adult in quantity and type, with extension
   onto the thighs.

*Modified from van Wieringen JC et al: *Growth Diagrams*. Gronigen, Neth. Woplter-Noorhoff Publishing, 1971.

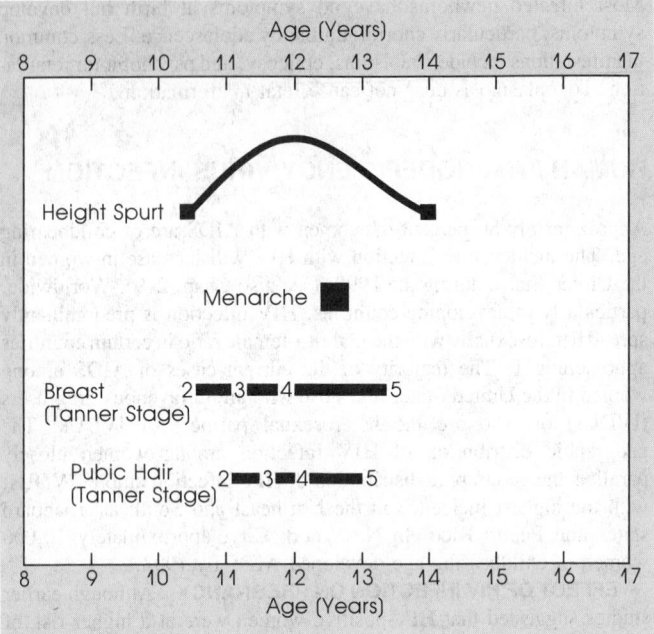

FIGURE 7-1   Pubertal events in females.

boys (SMR 3–4). During this spurt, females gain 9.0 cm ± 1.03 cm/year and reach a final mean adult height of 163 cm at 16 years; males gain 10.3 ± 1.54 cm/year and reach a final mean adult height of 177 cm at 18 years. Assessment of skeletal growth during adolescence should be done through a height velocity curve with consideration of the sexual maturity rating. Bone age can be determined through the utilization of hand roentgenograms.

Changes in body composition   Weight gain during the growth spurt accounts for 40 percent of ideal body weight. Lean body mass increases in males from 80 to 90 percent and decreases in girls from 80 to 75 percent. In males mean body fat increases from 4.3 to 11.2 percent by late puberty and is distributed primarily in the truncal area. In females, mean body fat increases from 15.7 to 26.7 percent and is deposited in the pelvic, breast, upper back, and arm areas. Shortly after the growth spurt is completed, muscle mass peaks and is greater in boys than in girls.

FIGURE 7-2   Pubertal events in males.

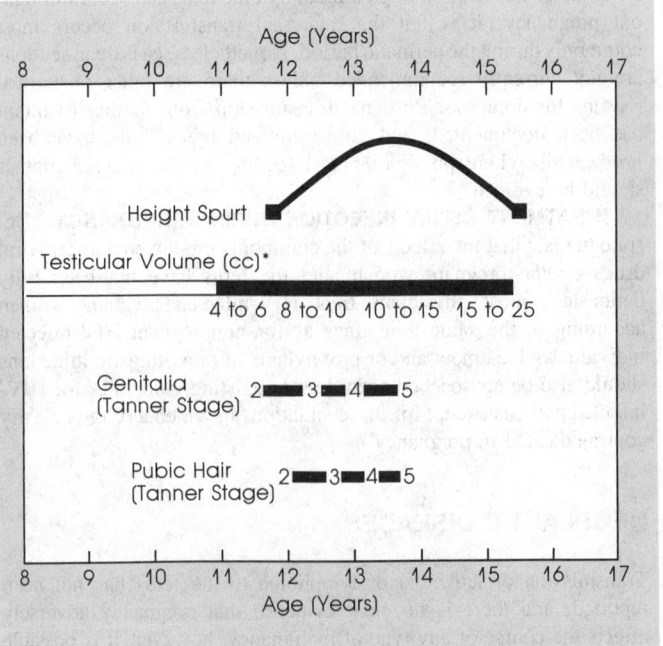

TABLE 7-3   Relation between development of features of maturation and sexual maturity ratings (SMR)*

Clinical feature	SMR
Hematocrit rise (male)	2–5
Alkaline phosphatase peak (male)	3
Alkaline phosphatase peak (female)	2
Adolescent hormonal levels (rise in estrogen for females, testosterone for males)	2–5
Peak height velocity (male)	3–4
Peak height velocity (female)	2–3
Usual timing of menarche	3–4
Slipped capital femoral epiphysis	2–3
Acute worsening of idiopathic adolescent scoliosis	2–4
Osgood-Schlatter disease	3
Appearance of "normal" gynecomastia	2–3
Usual appearance of acne vulgaris	2–3
Increased levels of serum uric acid in males	2–5

*After Daniel WA.

Cardiorespiratory changes   At puberty heart rate decreases and stroke volume, cardiac output, and blood pressure increase. The lungs increase in size. The male larynx, under the influence of androgens, develops an acute 90-degree angle in the anterior thyroid cartilage, and the male vocal cords are three times the length of those in females. These changes account for the deepening of vocal quality.

PSYCHOLOGICAL DEVELOPMENT   Adolescence is often viewed as a tumultuous period (Table 7-4). However, most adolescents pass through puberty without disruption in their lives. The clinician must assess whether psychosocial development of the adolescent is normal. The adolescent is confronted with a series of changes, which,

if mastered, allow function as an adult. These changes include separation from the family, maturation of sexual identity, planning for education and career, and development of the capacity for intimacy. Adolescents also undergo cognitive changes with behavioral and social sequelae. The functional and cognitive changes do not necessarily correlate with physical maturation. The early adolescent (ages 10 to 13) tends to focus on the physical changes in his/her body and may have concerns about the maturational process.

Middle adolescence (ages 14 to 16 years) is the period of rapid cognitive growth when formal operational thinking emerges. Adolescents begin to understand abstract concepts and may question the judgment of adults. The individual then shifts from the egocentric world of the early adolescent to the sociocentric world of the middle and late adolescent and begins to modulate impulsive behavior.

Late adolescence (ages 17 to 21 years) is the period of establishment of personal identity with intimate relationships and a function in society. The late adolescent views life in a more sociocentric view, characteristic of adulthood. The late adolescent may be altruistic, and conflicts with the family and society may center on moral issues rather than egocentric considerations.

Families can facilitate adolescence by providing a graduated increase in independence and in responsibilities. Adolescents need both individuality and involvement with family and society to facilitate development of identity and of rational competence. Clinicians should support this process by encouraging adolescents to make their own appointments, assisting the chronically ill adolescent in assuming more responsibility for his/her health care, and encouraging parents to decrease their role in clinical management issues.

PSYCHOLOGICAL CHANGES ASSOCIATED WITH PUBESCENCE   Hormones and behavior   Specific behavioral changes are

TABLE 7-4   Biopsychosocial development during adolescence

Characteristics	Impact
EARLY ADOLESCENCE (Age 10 to 13 Years)	
Onset of puberty, becomes concerned with developing body	Major questions concerning normality of physical maturation; often concerned about the stages of sexual development and how the process relates to peers of same gender. Masturbation begins.
Begins to expand social radius beyond family and concentrate on relationships with peers	Encourage some external responsibilities alone in consultation with parents, i.e., visit with health care provider, contacts with school counselors.
Cognition is usually concrete	Concrete thinking requires dealing with most health situations in a simple, explicit manner using visual and verbal cues.
MIDDLE ADOLESCENCE (Age 14 to 16 Years)	
Pubertal development usually complete and sexual drives emerge	Explores ability to attract opposites. Sexual behavior and experimentation (same and opposite sex) begin. Masturbation increases.
Peer group sets behavioral standards, although some family values persist	Peer group affects compliance, and peers rather than parents offer key support.
Conflicts over independence	Increased assumption of independent action, together with continued need for parental support and guidance; able to discuss and negotiate changes in rules; ambivalence on part of adolescent in discussion and negotiation.
Cognition begins to be abstract	Begins to consider full range of possibilities with poor ability to integrate into real life because of immaturity and incomplete cognitive development.
LATE ADOLESCENCE (Age 17 to 21 Years)	
Physical maturation complete. Body image and gender role definition are secured	Begins to feel comfortable with relationships and decisions regarding sexuality and preference. Individual relationships become more important than peer group.
Narcissism declines; there is a process of giving and sharing	More open to specific questioning regarding behavior.
Idealism	Idealism may lead to conflicts with family and other authority figures.
Emancipation is nearly secured	With emancipation, more awareness about consequences of person actions.
Cognitive development is complete	Most are capable of understanding a full range of options for health issues.
Functional role begins to be defined	Often interested in significant discussion of life goals because this is the primary function of this stage.

*After Shafer MAB, Irwin CE, Jr.

associated with puberty and its timing. Androgens have been implicated in this process. During peak height velocity (stages 3 to 4), boys tend to have more conflict with their mothers, and as boys complete puberty mothers tend to defer more to their sons. Girls also tend to have more conflict with their mothers and to decrease interactions with their fathers. Other activities associated with changes in androgens include heterosexual behavior. Boys with rising levels of testosterone tend to initiate sexual intercourse and are reported to be more impatient, irritable, and aggressive. Rising levels of adrenal androgens correlate with increased masturbatory activity and heterosocial behavior in girls.

Timing of maturation Timing of puberty is associated with psychological and behavioral sequelae. Earlier physical maturation in girls is associated with more dissatisfaction with their bodies, lower self esteem, and general unhappiness. Early-developing girls also receive less support from peer groups and may associate with older adolescents. The earlier developing girl initiates sexual behavior earlier than her age peers, experiences an early identity crisis, has greater interest in independence and decision making and tends to have more behavioral problems and less interest in academic activities. For boys, early physical maturation is also associated with earlier initiation of sexual behavior, but late maturation in boys seems to be more often associated with negative psychological sequelae. The late-maturing boy tends to have a negative self-concept and body image and an increased frequency of identity crises.

ENVIRONMENTAL CHANGES Social environment Changes in the social environment during the second decade may affect health status. The family tends to provide less supervision and allow for more freedom in choices regarding free time, often providing the adolescent an opportunity to engage in risky behaviors. Schools are transformed from supportive elementary schools to the large, impersonal, and unstructured environments of middle/junior high schools, high schools and colleges. Work environments provide even less supervision and on-the-job guidance for the adolescent. With the economic crisis of the 1990s fewer nurturing programs are available for youth after school, and the increase in poverty has had a negative effect on the health status of children.

Legal environment The law in most states requires consent of a parent for medical care for children younger than 18. In general, the involvement of parents is not a barrier to the provision of health services, but some sensitive health issues (e.g., sexual behavior and substance use) may interfere with access to health care for adolescents. The Mature Minor Doctrine generally allows adolescents to seek health care independently if they are capable of understanding the risks and benefits of the proposed treatment and therefore capable of informed consent. There is generally little risk of liability in providing health care to the older mature minor (14 years or older) if the care is for the adolescent's benefit or is an emergency. In many states adolescents can seek care without parental permission for sensitive issues such as sexually transmitted diseases, contraception, pregnancy, substance use, and some mental health problems. Adolescents may also be treated without parental permission if the condition is an emergency and a delay in treatment would be detrimental to well being. Emancipated minors (adolescents who live away from home, are no longer subject to parental control, are economically self-supporting, are married, or are members of the military service) may also consent to their own health care.

MORBIDITY AND MORTALITY

The concept that adolescence is the healthiest period of life is based on measures of mortality and morbidity that do not include functional assessment of health status or the effects of behaviors initiated during adolescence on adult mortality and morbidity.

Mortality Mortality rates are low, but since 1985, there has been an increase in mortality for adolescents and young adults. Mortality (per 100,000) increases from 28 10 to 14 year olds to 88 15 to 19

year olds to 115 20 to 24 year olds. Most adolescent mortality is due to violence, particularly motor vehicle accidents, homicide, and suicide. In 1988, injuries accounted for most deaths between ages 10 and 24, and mortality rates for males are double those of females. Ethnic groups differ in respect to the cause of death: black males of 15 to 19 years old have a fivefold greater rate of homicide and the lowest life expectancy of all adolescents. In contrast, white male adolescents have higher suicide and motor vehicle accident death rates. Unintentional injuries account for more than half of deaths in the second decade. Risky driving habits account for half of fatal crashes, and adolescent drivers have the highest rates of motor vehicle fatalities. Alcohol is also implicated in other fatal injuries including bicycle, boating, skateboard, and swimming accidents. Suicide is responsible for 13 percent of deaths between ages 15 and 24. Native American males have higher rates, and black adolescents have lower rates of suicide. Between ages 15 and 24 homicide accounts for 14 percent of deaths. Homicide is the leading cause of death in late black male adolescents and young adults, accounting for 40 percent and 37 percent of the deaths, respectively. Adolescents in impoverished metropolitan areas are more likely victims of homicide. Cardiovascular diseases account for 1.4 to 4.8 deaths and malignancies for 3.1 to 5.7 deaths per 100,000 persons aged 10 to 24.

Morbidity Most morbidity during adolescence originates from substance abuse, sexual activity, and accidents. Additional causes include mental health problems and those associated with changes in the skeletal and reproductive systems.

Skeletal system (See also Chap. 332) Rapid growth of the long bones and closure of the epiphyses by age 21 are associated with several orthopedic problems. Slipped capital femoral epiphyses occurs primarily at the time of rapid growth spurt and is more common in the obese. Osgood-Schlatter disease (osteochondrosis of the tibial tuberosity) and idiopathic scoliosis are disorders of adolescence, and neoplasms of osseous origins peak during adolescence. Fractures due to injuries are also common throughout adolescence.

Female reproductive health problems Reproduction health problems are a common cause of morbidity in young women.

ANOVULATORY CYCLES (See also Chap. 340) Dysfunctional uterine bleeding (DUB) is common. Primary DUB results from anovulatory cycles, i.e., oscillations of estrogen levels that lack the characteristic LH surge and subsequent corpus luteum development, progesterone production, and endometrial maturation of a mature cycle. Without progesterone, the endometrial lining becomes thickened and fragile, resulting in intermittent sloughing and irregular, frequently excessive menstrual bleeding. The differential diagnosis includes pregnancy, disorders of coagulation, and disorders of the vagina, cervix, uterus and ovary. Anovulatory cycles may persist for 5 years following menarche.

DYSMENORRHEA Dysmenorrhea, both primary and secondary, is a major complaint of menstruating adolescents and a major cause of school absenteeism. Primary dysmenorrhea is due to prostaglandin-stimulated myometrial contractions during ovulatory cycles. Secondary dysmenorrhea is associated with pelvic infections, intrauterine and extrauterine pregnancy, intrauterine devices and congenital anomalies. Primary dysmenorrhea is treated by suppressing production of the prostaglandins and/or inhibiting ovulation. If the girl fails to respond to oral contraceptives and prostaglandin inhibitors, further evaluation must be undertaken.

SEXUALLY TRANSMITTED DISEASES (STD) (See also Chap. 80) Sexually active adolescents have the highest rates of STD of any age group in the United States. Complications include cervical intraepithelial neoplasia, pelvic inflammatory disease, ectopic pregnancy, infertility, genital cancers, and AIDS. As of September 1992, 912 cases of AIDS have been diagnosed in 13 to 19 year olds and 9270 cases in the 20- to 24-year-old cohort. The extent of HIV seroprevalence in adolescents is unknown. When one STD is diagnosed, the clinician must screen for other STDs.

Male reproductive health problems (See also Chap. 339) Testicular masses and varicoceles may become evident during puberty. Most varicoceles are discovered during a routine physical examination. Surgical repair may be indicated to enhance fertility and in the following situations: genital discomfort, testicular volume loss, abnormal semen analysis, or abnormal luteinizing hormone-releasing hormone stimulation test. Testicular cancer is rare in adolescents, but teaching young adults and adolescents to perform self testicular examinations may increase early identification of tumors.

RISK-TAKING BEHAVIORS

SUBSTANCE USE AND ABUSE Adolescent use of substances has declined in the United States since the 1970s. In 1991, only 29 percent of high school seniors reported illicit substance abuse at any time. The declining rates of marijuana and cocaine use have been accompanied by an increasing perception of harm associated with these substances. Rates of lifetime use of LSD and heroin among high school seniors have remained essentially stable at 9 percent and 1 percent respectively, and only 1.5 percent of high school seniors report use of crack cocaine. Nevertheless, lifetime alcohol and tobacco use approximated 88 percent and 63 percent, respectively, among high school seniors in 1991. Binge drinking (the consumption of at least five drinks or more in a row at least once in the past 2 weeks) was reported by 30 percent of high school seniors and by 43 percent of college students. Substance abuse during adolescence has major negative health consequences in adulthood. Girls consistently report greater use of cigarettes, whereas males have a higher use of alcohol. Approximately 18 percent of adolescents leave high school as smokers, and 14 percent of college students are regular smokers. The lower rates of cigarette smoking in boys may be due to the increase in use of smokeless tobacco (snuff and chewing tobacco).

Surveys may underestimate the true prevalence of substance use, but it is clear that patterns of substance use vary by region, age, gender, and ethnicity. Substance use generally increases with age. Native American adolescents have the highest prevalence rates for cigarettes, alcohol, and most illicit drugs, followed by rates for whites, Hispanics, African-Americans, and Asian-Americans.

UNINTENTIONAL INJURIES Injuries, particularly motor vehicle accidents, account for more than half of deaths in adolescents, and hospitalization for injury accounts for the largest number of hospital days. Alcohol, high speed, and reckless behavior play important roles in these injuries, and are also implicated in injuries with bicycles, skateboards, swimming, and boating. Males outnumber females by greater than 2 to 1 in all injury situations.

SEXUAL BEHAVIOR Adolescents now initiate heterosexual behavior earlier than cohorts of previous generations. By age 15, 26 percent of white females and males, 24 percent of black females, and 69 percent of black males experience coitus. These figures increase by age 19 to 76 percent of white females, 85 percent of white males, 83 percent of black females and 96 percent of black males. White adolescent females report more frequent sexual intercourse and more partners than their age-related black cohorts. Adolescent females with earlier menarche begin to have intercourse earlier than those with a later menarche. Adolescents who initiate sexual behavior early tend to have more sexual partners and are more likely to acquire a sexually transmitted disease or become pregnant. Use of contraceptives among adolescents is increasing, but fewer than half of sexually active adolescents use condoms. Reported rates of unprotected heterosexual anal intercourse are from 12 percent to 26 percent. Reliable data on same-sex behavior during adolescence are not available, but rates may approximate 5 to 10 percent. Retrospective data from adult homosexual and bisexual men indicate that half of these men initiated same-sex sexual behavior by age 16.

Overall birth rates have declined over the past decade; however, the number of births to unmarried adolescent females has increased, and there were an estimated 416,170 abortions in adolescents in 1988. Sexually transmitted diseases are more frequent among sexually active adolescents than any other age group in the United States.

COVARIATION OF RISK BEHAVIORS The onset of one risk behavior is associated with a greater likelihood for initiation of another in the near future. The association between alcohol abuse and injury is well established. Other activities that predispose to injury include reckless driving and failure to use seat belts and helmets.

The strongest evidence for covariation is in substance abuse, sexual activity, and delinquent behavior. The major risk for initiation of cigarette, alcohol, and marijuana use is by age 20 and for illicit substance use is by age 21. Young adults who have not used these substances are unlikely to do so thereafter. During early and middle adolescence, less serious substance use predicts subsequent use of more serious substances. Alcohol use precedes marijuana use, and marijuana use precedes other illicit drugs (including psychedelics, cocaine, heroin, and nonprescribed stimulants, sedatives, and tranquilizers). In girls, cigarette use is predictive of subsequent substance use. The influence of alcohol and tobacco use on subsequent marijuana use is independent of age. The earlier adolescents begin using marijuana the more likely the use of other illicit substances. Substance use is also correlated with delinquent behavior, early sexual debut, and less effective contraceptive use.

MENTAL HEALTH PROBLEMS

Approximately 10 percent of adolescents have symptoms of psychological distress. Psychiatric conditions that may begin in childhood include anxiety and panic disorders, personality disorders, schizophrenia, suicide, and eating disorders. Three common problems encountered by the primary care physician during adolescence are suicide, depression, and eating disorders.

SUICIDE Suicide is the fourth leading cause of death in early adolescence (10 to 14 years old) and the second leading cause in late adolescence and young adulthood. The greatest increase in rates of suicide during the past 20 years is among 15- to 24-year-old males. Suicide is relatively uncommon before puberty and increases after age 16 with most occurring among 18 to 24 year olds. White and Native American late adolescents boys and young men have the highest rates of suicide. The relation between male sex and substance abuse and conduct disorders may be responsible for this predominance. For every completed suicide, there may be 50 to 120 attempted suicides with a female preponderance. Differences in methods may be responsible for the sex differences between fatal and attempted suicides. Methods for fatal suicide include firearms, hanging, and jumping from heights. Drug ingestion, which rarely causes fatality, is the most common method for suicide attempts in adolescents.

Etiology of suicide Common factors in suicidal adolescents include a history of suicide in family members, alcohol and substance abuse, conduct disorders, depressive disorders, anxiety states, and knowing someone who has committed or attempted suicide. Precipitating factors include acute stress, trouble with the law, trouble at school such as cheating or being truant, substance abuse, pregnancy or fear of pregnancy, hypochondriasis, social isolation, and anxiety. In occasional girls perfectionism and anxiety about academic performance (in the presence of average intelligence) or environmental change appear to be causal. Many suicide victims are intoxicated at the time of death.

Recognition of the at-risk suicidal adolescent Recognition of the suicidal or depressed adolescent may be difficult. The most common underlying psychiatric factor in suicidal adolescents is depression, manifested by feelings of hopelessness, low self-esteem, despair, and somatic complaints. In the younger adolescent, depressive equivalents of school problems and acting out behavior may include legal problems. The younger adolescent may also have difficulty in characterizing his/her feelings. In the older adolescent, substance abuse is more common. Injured adolescents should be queried about the cause of the injury to rule out suicidal behavior. Adolescents with a family history of suicide, a history of psychiatric disorders, or a past history of suicidal behavior need to be screen for suicide risk.

A depressed adolescent contemplating suicide generally welcomes the opportunity to communicate his/her feelings.

Once a suicidal adolescent is identified, an extensive evaluation is required to assess the problem. Comprehensive workup should include evaluation of the adolescent, the family, and the family together with the adolescent. Parents and/or guardians should be informed immediately about the suicidal behavior. Confidentiality is immaterial in the face of potential suicide. Suicidal intent is as important as the lethality of the method. Many adolescents have little knowledge of lethality. Evaluation should focus on mental health disorders in the family, past history of mental health problems in the adolescent, sexual abuse, and sexual behavior including same-sex behavior, since homosexual adolescents appear to be at greater risk for suicide. All suicidal adolescents need evaluation by a psychiatrist as soon as possible.

In emergencies, the physician must decide if outpatient or inpatient care is appropriate. If immediate treatment is needed, psychiatric consultation is sought when the patient is stable medically. If the patient is medically stable, the clinician must decide whether he/she is at ongoing risk for suicide. Some programs recommend hospitalization for all suicidal adolescents, and hospitalization is always advisable for the following groups: (1) those still intent on suicide; (2) those with previous suicide attempts; (3) all males; (4) all severely depressed patients; (5) those impaired by substance abuse; (6) those whose attempt was with a lethal method (e.g., firearm, hanging, or jumping from high place); and (7) those without a supportive environment at home or through residential care.

When the patient is discharged, the clinician needs to monitor the compliance with the mental health treatment program and to query the family about the availability of firearms at home. Adolescents who are depressed or suicidal are difficult to engage in treatment programs and a follow-up appointment with the primary care physician is the best way to monitor compliance. If the adolescent fails to keep the appointment, the physician should telephone and reschedule it.

Depression (See also Chap. 389)   Depression is the most common feature in patients who attempt suicide. The prevalence of major depressive disorders in adolescence is between 4 to 6 percent with a slight preponderance of females to males. The diagnostic criteria for depression during adolescence are the same as in adulthood (Table 7-5) and include changes in mood and relationships, cognitive functioning and bodily functioning. Depressive equivalents in the adolescent include hypochondriasis, substance abuse, decrements in school functioning, problems with the law, and major family conflicts.

EATING DISORDERS (See also Chap. 74)   Eating disorders generally have their onset in postpubertal adolescents, and adolescents may fulfill the DSM-IIIR criteria for anorexia nervosa or bulimia nervosa prior to the completion of puberty (Table 74-1). Adolescents with subclinical eating disorders may need the same treatment as adolescents with full-fledged disorders. The warning signs of emerging eating disorders are listed in Table 7-6 and include major body image problems, difficulty establishing autonomy from the family, perfectionism, and family history of eating disorders including obesity.

TABLE 7-5   DSM-III-R criteria for diagnosis of major depression*

Diagnosis requires symptom 1 or 2 and at least four other symptoms for a 2-week period

1 Depressed or irritable mood
2 Diminished interest or pleasure
3 Weight loss or weight gain
4 Insomnia or hypersomnia
5 Psychomotor agitation or retardation
6 Fatigue or loss of energy
7 Feelings of worthlessness or excessive guilt
8 Decreased concentration or indecisiveness
9 Thoughts of death, suicidal ideation, or suicide attempt

*After American Psychiatric Association, p 217.

TABLE 7-6   Possible warning signs for anorexia nervosa or bulimia nervosa*

Anorexia nervosa	Bulimia nervosa
EATING AND RELATED BEHAVIORS	
Caloric intake < 100 kcal/d	Binge eating > twice/week
Calorie counting	Eating used as coping strategy
Denial of hunger cues	Fasting or restrictive dieting
Extreme physical activity	Feels lack of control over eating
Fasting or restrictive dieting	Frequent meal skipping
Feels controlled by food	Frequent sweets, starches, cravings
Food avoidances or hoarding	Frequent thoughts about food
Food seen as good or bad	Guilt after eating/secret eating
Frequent meal skipping	Purging behavior
Frequent thoughts about food	Regular alcohol use
	Wide variation in caloric intake
BODY IMAGE AND BODY SATISFACTION	
Body image disturbance	Current or previous obesity
Fear of weight gain	Fear of weight gain
Previously overweight	Overconcern with weight/shape
Thinness as valued goal	Thinness as valued goal
Weight goal < 85% expected weight	Unrealistic weight goal
HEALTH STATUS	
Amenorrhea (< 3 months w/no menses)	Bloating/nausea/abdominal pain
Bloating/nausea	Constipation
Cold intolerance	Frequent weight fluctuations
Constipation	Irregular menses (< 21 days or > 45 days)
Weight < 85% expected weight	
PERSONAL FUNCTIONING	
Delayed psychosexual development	Depressed affect
Depressed affect	Negative self-identity
Individuation difficulties	Perfectionistic
Negative self identity	Poor coping with life event
Perfectionistic	Recent withdrawal from friends
Poor coping with life events	Substance use/early sexual activity
Recent withdrawal from friends	
ENVIRONMENTAL INFLUENCES	
Enmeshed or overinvolved family	Chaotic or uninvolved family
Family history of obesity, eating disorder, or weight focus	Family history or obesity, eating disorder, weight or fitness focus
Few close friends	High achievement expectations
High achievement expectations	Participation in body-focused activity
Participation in body-focused activity	

*Adapted from Adams LB, Shafer MA.

While the eating patterns in many adolescents appear abnormal, and adolescent girls commonly have dissatisfaction with weight and shape and some fear of gaining weight, these feelings and fears are extreme in the adolescent with an eating disorder.

Anorexia nervosa (See also Chap. 74)   Anorexia now involves approximately 1 percent of white girls between ages 14 and 24 (Table 7-6), generally from middle to upper socioeconomic families. The disorder also occurs in Asian-Americans, African-Americans, Hispanics, and Native Americans. Approximately 5 to 10 percent of cases are boys, but the disorder in boys may be more severe and associated with gender disturbances.

The disorder generally begins shortly after the completion of puberty, but some girls develop the disease after graduation from high school when they begin college or employment. The cause is unclear. Some adolescents appear to have the onset with the increased deposition of adipose tissue with puberty and concern generated by parents and peers. Hypothalamic abnormalities may occur prior to weight loss; up to 40 percent of girls with anorexia nervosa have secondary amenorrhea prior to weight loss. The psychological profile is one of low self-esteem, high anxiety, and normal cognitive functioning. Generally, the girls are overachievers and perfectionists.

Associated psychiatric illnesses include depression and other affective disorders. The families tend to be enmeshed: overprotective, rigid, and with little ability to resolve conflicts. Subpopulations at risk include ballet dancers and gymnasts.

The findings depend on the degree and method of starvation. The weight should be measured with the adolescent undressed and in a gown after voiding. Laboratory data are generally not helpful except when vomiting has led to hypokalemia and metabolic alkalosis. With amenorrhea, LH and FSH levels are prepubertal, and serum estradiol levels are low. In boys, serum testosterone level is low. Triiodothyronine levels are low, and cortisol, endorphins, and cholesterol are elevated with an increase in high-density lipoproteins. ST-segment depression on exercise stress testing and prolonged QT intervals have been reported. These findings have been associated with ventricular tachycardia in adults with anorexia nervosa.

Successful treatment begins with early diagnosis and development of a comprehensive medical and psychiatric regimen. Mortality rates range from 2 to 10 percent in the 10 years following diagnosis. Early intensive therapy appears to improve the prognosis.

Bulimia nervosa (See also Chap. 74) Bulimia nervosa is diagnosed by the criteria listed in Table 7-7. The prevalence is approximately 2 to 5 percent of females and less than 1 percent for males. Individual patients may have both anorexia nervosa and bulimia nervosa at the same time or alternate between the two syndromes. The cause is not clear. Individuals with mild disease may function fairly well, whereas others are disabled by repeated binging, purging, suicide attempts, and substance abuse.

The typical patient is a middle to late adolescent who begins bulimic behavior to lose weight. Complaints include fatigue, bloating, or irregular menses, and sore throat or hoarseness secondary to vomiting. Most do not mention purging or binging behavior unless specifically queried. Physical findings include bilateral swelling of the parotid glands and calluses or scars on the dorsum of fingers used to induce vomiting. Teeth enamel may be lost to the acidic nature of vomitus. Reflex esophagitis, aspiration pneumonia, and cardiac abnormalities secondary to hypokalemia can occur. Use of syrup of ipecac to induce vomiting can also cause cardiotoxicity. Metabolic alkalosis and an elevated serum amylase may be present. Once the diagnosis is made, the effect of binging and purging must be dealt with prior to dealing with the underlying psychopathology. Pharmacotherapy may be helpful.

THE CLINICAL VISIT OF THE ADOLESCENT

TRANSITION INTERVIEW Establishing an effective doctor-patient relationship with the adolescent is a formidable task for the physician whose practice is primarily with adults. A transition interview for the adolescent and family helps to define the relationship between the physician and the emerging adult. Areas to be emphasized include the necessity for the physician to interview and examine the adolescent privately and the need for the patient to generate his/her own questions including initiating appointments. Normal adolescence and the continuing need for some decisions to be made with familial

guidance and support should be discussed. The payment mechanisms and responsibility for fees should be clarified. During this interview, the physician should inquire about the adolescent's previous source of health care and request authorization to contact the former physician.

CONFIDENTIALITY Fundamental to any doctor-patient relationship is confidentiality. All adolescents need to be able to discuss all matters with the physician openly, honestly, and confidentially, and the physician must provide assurance of the confidential nature of all information. Prior to queries about sexual behavior or substance use, it may be useful to restate the confidential nature of the questioning. With life-threatening behaviors or diseases (e.g., suicidal behavior or management of chronic disease), the physician generally has the right to intervene including identification of a parent, guardian, or supportive adult to assist in the management.

GATHERING THE HISTORY History taking should be guided by the developmental stage of the patient (Table 7-4). The adolescent may not disclose his/her primary concern until a secure and confidential relationship has been established. General screening should be undertaken for the major health-damaging behaviors of adolescence, including sexual activity, substance use, vehicle use, depression and its equivalents, and dietary changes suggestive of an eating disorder. Distinguishing between risk-taking behaviors that are temporary, even though dangerous, and those that are pathologic is a challenge. This judgment requires assessing the effects of risky behavior on the health status and the motivation for engaging in them and determining whether normal psychosocial development is impaired. Figure 7-3 summarizes the biopsychosocial and environmental factors that increase vulnerability for initiating risky behaviors. Male sex, positive

FIGURE 7-3 Principal factors in risk-taking behaviors. (Adapted from Irwin and Millstein.)

Predisposing Biopsychosocial (Endogenous) Factors	**Predisposing Environmental (Exogenous) Factors**
Sensation Seeking Aggressiveness Asynchrony of Biological/ Psychological & Social Development Cognition Developmental Drives During Adolescence Male Gender Hormonal Effects (in Boys) Internalization of Peer Engagement Low Self-Esteem	Family Factors: Authorization and Permissive Parenting Styles Maladaptive Family Situations Low Parental Support and Controls Parental Denial Parentals Involvement in Risk Behaviors Lack of knowledge of Consequences of Behavior Peer Behavior School Transitions Societal Denial and Unresponsiveness

Increased Vulnerability and/or Risk Situation

Precipitating Factors	**Precipitating Factors**
Lack of Experience/ Knowledge Substance Use/Multiple Substance Use Lack of Skills to Resist Peer Pressure	Peer Initiation School Transitions Social Pressure Substance Use/ Availability

Risk-Taking Behavior

TABLE 7-7 DSM-III-R criteria for diagnosis of bulimia nervosa*

A Recurrent episodes of binge eating (rapid consumption of a large amount of food in a discrete period).

B A feeling of lack of control over eating behavior during binges.

C The person regularly engages in self-induced vomiting, use of laxatives or diuretics, strict dieting or fasting, or vigorous exercise to prevent weight gain.

D A minimum average of two binge-eating episodes a week for at least 3 months.

E Persistent overconcern with body shape and weight.

* After American Psychiatric Association, pp 68–69.

attitudes toward risky behaviors, lack of parental supervision, contact with peers engaging in the behavior, and multiple school transitions are associated with an increased propensity for risky behaviors. The physician should be specific in questioning about individual behaviors, their frequency and their intensity. One behavior may serve as a warning sign for another risky behavior. For example, early substance abuse correlates with early sexual activity.

Frequently, adolescents do not want to disclose current behavior, and the physician may query instead about general risk-taking and the behavior of peer groups. The physical signs associated with risky behaviors are similar to the signs and symptoms in adult patients, but the behavioral consequences of risky behaviors may have a greater effect on the adolescent, including more family conflicts, impaired academic performance, unwise peer relationships and activities, and changes in extracurricular activities.

Immunization history needs to be reviewed. Previously immunized adolescents who received a complete series of immunizations prior to 5 years of age need to receive a second measles vaccination. This immunization may be for measles alone or MMR (measles, mumps, and rubella). Adolescents who have never been immunized and those for whom the immunization history is not available should receive a three-dose primary series of Td (tetanus, diptheria) and OPV (oral poliovirus) and a two-dose primary series of MMR. Hepatitis B vaccine should be given to sexually active adolescents.

The physical examination and laboratory assessment are guided by the general complaints and the associated physical stigmata of risky behaviors.

REFERENCES

ADAMS LB, SHAFER MA: Early manifestations of eating disorders in adolescents: Defining those at risk. J Nutr Ed 20:307, 1988

AMERICAN PSYCHIATRIC ASSOCIATION: *Diagnostic and Statistical Manual of Mental Disorders*, 3d ed, revised. Washington DC, The American Psychiatric Association, 1987

BACHMAN JAG et al: Racial/ethnic differences in smoking, drinking and illicit drug use among American high school seniors, 1976–89. Am J Public Health 81:372, 1991

BLUMENTHAL SJ, KUPFER DJ: *Suicide over the Life Cycle*. Washington DC, American Psychiatric Press, Inc., 1990

CENTERS FOR DISEASE CONTROL: HIV/AIDS Surveillance Report, October 1992, 11

————: Premarital sexual experience among adolescent women—United States, 1970–1988. MMWR 39:929, 1991

————: Weapon-carrying among high school students—United States, 1990. MMWR 40:681, 1991

COPELAND KC et al: Assessment of pubertal development. Ross Laboratories PREP series. Columbus, Ross Laboratories, 1986

DANIEL WA: Growth at adolescence: Clinical correlates. Semin Adolesc Med 1:15, 1985

ENGLISH A: Treating adolescents: Legal and ethical considerations. Med Clin North Am 74:1097, 1990

FELDMAN SS, ELLIOTT GR: *At the Threshold: The Developing Adolescent*. Cambridge, Harvard University, 1990

FRIEDMAN SB et al (eds): *Comprehensive Adolescent Health Care*. St. Louis, Quality Medical Publishing, Inc., 1992

GOLD PW et al: Abnormal hypothalamic-pituitary-adrenal function in anorexia nervosa. N Engl J Med 314:1335, 1986

GREULICH WW, PYLE SI: *Radiographic Atlas of Skeletal Development of the Hand and Wrist, 2d ed.* Stanford, Stanford University, 1959

IRWIN CE JR: The theoretical concept of at-risk adolescents. Adolesc Med: State Art Rev 1:1, 1990

————, MILLSTEIN SG: Biopsychosocial correlates of risk taking behavior during adolescence: Can the physician intervene? J Adolesc Health Care 7:82S, 1986

————, SHAFER MA: Adolescent sexuality: Negative outcomes of a normative behavior, in *Adolescents at Risk: Medical and Social Perspectives*, DE Rogers, E Ginzberg (eds). Boulder, Westview Press, 1992, pp 35–79

JOHNSTON LD et al: *Monitoring the Future Substance Use Data for 1991*. Ann Arbor, University of Michigan Institute for Social Research: Press release, 27 January 1992

KASS EJ: Adolescent varicocele: Current concepts. Semin Urol 6:140, 1988

MARSHALL WA, TANNER JM: Variation in the pattern of pubertal changes in boys. Arch Dis Child 45:13, 1970

————: Variation in the pattern of pubertal changes in girls. Arch Dis Child 44:291, 1969

MCANARNEY ER et al: *Textbook of Adolescent Medicine*. Philadelphia, Saunders, 1992

MILLSTEIN SG et al: Health risk behaviors among young adolescents. Pediatrics 89:422, 1992

NATIONAL CENTER FOR HEALTH STATISTICS: *Vital Statistics of the United States, 1988*, Vol 2, Mortality, part A. DHHS publication no (PHS) 91-1101, 1991, pp 14–38

NEWACHECK PW et al: Health insurance coverage of adolescents: A current profile and assessment of trends. Pediatrics 90:589, 1992

NOTTELMANN ED et al: Developmental processes in early adolescence: Relations between adolescent adjustment problems and chronologic age, pubertal stage and puberty-related hormones. J Pediatr 110:473, 1987

PALLA B, LITT IF: Medical complications of eating disorders in adolescents. Pediatrics 81:613, 1988

SHAFER MAB, IRWIN CE JR: The adolescent patient, in *Rudolph's Pediatrics*, 19th ed, A Rudolph (ed). Norwalk, Appleton and Lange, 1991, pp 39–81

SHAFFER D et al: Preventing teenage suicide: A critical review. J Am Acad Child Adolesc Psychiatry 27:675, 1988

STYNE D, GRUMBACH MM: Disorders of puberty in males and females, in *Reproductive Endocrinology*, SS Yen, RB Jaffee (eds). Philadelphia, W. Saunders, 1991, pp 511–54

TANNER JM, DAVIES PSW: Clinical longitudinal standards for height and weight velocity for North American Children. J Pediatr 107:317, 1985

UDRY JR: Biological predispositions and social control in adolescent sexual behavior. Am Soc Rev 53:709, 1988

US OFFICE OF TECHNOLOGY ASSESSMENT: *Adolescent Health, Volume III, Crosscutting Issues in the Delivery of Health and Related Services*, OTA-H-467, Washington DC, 1991

US PREVENTIVE SERVICES TASK FORCE: *Guide to Clinical Preventive Services: An Assessment of the Effectiveness of 169 Interventions*. Baltimore, Williams & Wilkins, 1989

8 GERIATRIC MEDICINE

NEIL M. RESNICK

Of all the people who have ever lived to age 65, more than half are now alive. This statistic has important demographic and economic implications, and its impact on medical care is also substantial.

BIOLOGY OF AGING

Numerous theories have been proposed to explain the biologic mechanisms of aging, but all have inherent difficulties. Moreover, most are not mutually exclusive, and at present there is no evidence for a *single* mechanism of aging. Instead, aging is likely to have multiple and interacting causes that are probably different in cells and organs that are postmitotic (such as neurons, cardiac, and skeletal muscle cells) as compared to those with renewable tissues (such as bone marrow, skin, and gastrointestinal cells). For example, damage due to free radicals might be more ominous in a nonreplicating organ, such as the nervous system, than in a continuously replicating organ such as bone marrow, and the mechanisms required to cope with such damage may also be differentially affected by age.

As interest in population-based, organism-based, and organ-based theories of aging has waned, interest in cellular models has increased for several reasons: (1) cells grown in culture universally senesce; that is, after a finite series of doublings they cease to replicate although they perform most metabolic functions and remain alive up to a year or longer; (2) the number of replications prior to senescence is directly proportional to the maximum lifespan of the species; (3) the number of cell doublings is inversely related to the age of the donor; (4) cells taken from patients with premature aging syndromes (e.g., Werner's and progeria) exhibit decreased lifespans in vitro.

Although the mechanism(s) responsible remain elusive, potentially important insights into aging have emerged from studies of cellular aging. For example, the failure of senescent cells to replicate in the presence of growth factors is associated with failure to induce the c-*fos* gene and with a block in the late G_1 phase of the cell cycle. This block can be overcome by fusing senescent cells with those from immortal cell lines. In addition, the block is associated with secretion of statin (a 57-kDa protein) and expression of a still uncharacterized protein located in the outer surface of the plasma membrane. When added to younger cells, this protein blocks DNA synthesis and replication at the same, late G_1 phase of the cell cycle.

Another factor implicated in cellular senescence is retinoblastoma gene product, an inhibitor of cell proliferation, that can be inactivated only by phosphorylation. Failure to induce kinases may be a general feature of aging cells, leading to alterations in phosphorylation such that they become unable to deactivate gene products that inhibit cell proliferation. There is no evidence that important genes coding for specific peptides are routinely deleted or inactivated during aging. However, noncoding DNA sequences, which may be important for cell division or transcription regulation, might be affected. There is also little consistent data that aging affects RNA transcription.

Many mechanisms previously postulated to be involved in aging have not been substantiated, such as somatic mutation (in which aging is due to cumulative spontaneous mutations), error catastrophe (in which aging results from errors in the synthesis of proteins) and intrinsic mutagenesis (in which aging is the result of ongoing DNA rearrangements). Other mechanisms, such as free radical damage, alterations in DNA methylation, and telomere attrition, remain the subjects of active investigation.

PRINCIPLES OF GERIATRIC MEDICINE

From a physiologic standpoint, aging can be described as the progressive constriction of the homeostatic reserve of every organ system. This decline, often referred to as *homeostenosis*, is evident by the third decade and is gradual and progressive although the rate and extent of decline vary. The decline of each organ system (Table 8-1) appears to occur independently of changes in other organ systems and is influenced by diet, environment, and personal habits, as well as by genetic factors.

TABLE 8-1 Selected age-related changes and their consequences

Organ/system	Age-related physiologic change*	Caused by age-related physiologic change	Caused by disease, not age
General	↑ Body fat	↑ Volume of distribution for fat soluble drugs	Obesity
	↓ Total body water	↓ Volume of distribution for water soluble drugs	Anorexia
Eyes/ears	Presbyopia	↓ Accomodation	
	Lens opacification	↑ Susceptibility to glare	Blindness
	↓ High-frequency acuity	Difficulty discriminating words if background noise is present	Deafness
Endocrine	Impaired glucose	↑ Glucose level in response to acute illness	Diabetes mellitus
	↓ Thyroxine clearance (and production)	↓ T_4 dose required in hypothyroidism	Thyroid dysfunction
	↑ ADH, ↓ renin, and ↑ aldosterone		↓ Na$^+$, ↑ K$^+$
	↓ Testosterone		Impotence
	↓ Vitamin D absorption and activation	Osteopenia	Osteoporosis, osteomalacia
Respiratory	↓ Lung elasticity and ↑ chest wall stiffness	Ventilation/perfusion mismatch and ↓ P_{O_2}	Dyspnea, hypoxia
Cardiovascular	↓ Arterial compliance and ↑ systolic BP →LVH	Hypotensive response to ↑ HR, volume depletion, or loss of atrial contraction	Syncope
	↓ β-adrenergic responsiveness	↓ Cardiac output and HR response to stress	Heart failure
	↓ Baroreceptor sensitivity and ↓ SA node automaticity	Impaired blood pressure response to standing, volume depletion	Heart block
Gastrointestinal	↓ Hepatic function	Delayed metabolism of some drugs	Cirrhosis
	↓ Gastric acidity	↓ Ca$^+$ absorption on empty stomach	Osteoporosis, B$_{12}$ deficiency
	↓ Colonic motility	Constipation	Fecal impaction
	↓ Anorectal function		Fecal incontinence
Hematologic/immune system	↓ Bone marrow reserve(?)		
	↓ T cell function	False-negative PPD response	Anemia
	↑ Autoantibodies	False-positive rheumatoid factor, antinuclear antibody	Autoimmune disease
Renal	↓ GFR	Impaired excretion of some drugs	↑ Serum creatinine
	↓ Urine concentration/dilution (see also "Endocrine")	Delayed response to salt or fluid restriction/overload; nocturia	↓ ↑ Na$^+$
Genitourinary	Vaginal/urethral mucosal atrophy	Dyspareunia, bacteriuria	Symptomatic UTI
	Prostate enlargement	↑ Residual urine volume	Urinary incontinence; urinary retention
Musculoskeletal	↓ Lean body mass, muscle		Functional impairment
	↓ Bone density	Osteopenia	Hip fracture
Nervous system	Brain atrophy	Benign senescent forgetfulness	Dementia, delirium
	↓ Brain catechol synthesis		Depression
	↓ Brain dopaminergic synthesis	Stiffer gait	Parkinson's disease
	↓ Righting reflexes	↑ Body sway	Falls
	↓ Stage 4 sleep	Early wakening, insomnia	Sleep apnea

* Changes generally observed in healthy elderly subjects free of symptoms and detectable disease in the organ system studied. The changes are usually important only when the system is stressed or other factors are added (e.g., drugs, disease, or environmental challenge); they rarely result in symptoms otherwise. Abbreviations: T_4 = thyroxine, BP = blood pressure, HR = heart rate, ADH = antidiuretic hormone, GFR = glomerular filtration rate.

Several important principles follow from these facts: (1) Individuals become more dissimilar as they age, belying any stereotype of aging; (2) an *abrupt* decline in any system or function is always due to disease and not to "normal aging"; (3) "normal aging" can be attenuated by modification of risk factors (e.g., increased blood pressure, smoking, sedentary lifestyle); and (4) "healthy old age" is not an oxymoron. *In fact, in the absence of disease, the decline in homeostatic reserve causes no symptoms and imposes few restrictions on activities of daily living regardless of age.*

Appreciation of these facts may make it easier to understand the striking increases that have occurred in life expectancy. Average life expectancy is now 17 years at age 65, 11 years at age 75, 6 years at age 85, 4 years at age 90, and 2 years at age 100. Moreover, the bulk of these years is characterized by a lack of significant impairment (Table 8-2)—only 35 percent of people over age 85 are impaired in any activity required for daily living, and only 20 percent reside in a nursing home. Yet, as individuals age they are more likely to suffer from disease, disability, and the side effects of drugs all of which, when combined with the decrease in physiologic reserve, make the older person more vulnerable to environmental, pathologic, and pharmacologic challenges.

The following concepts underlie the remainder of the chapter:

1. The onset of a new disease in the elderly (usually defined as over age 75 to 80) generally affects an organ system made vulnerable by prior physiologic and pathologic changes. Because this organ system often differs from the diseased organ system in the young, disease presentation in the elderly may be atypical. For example, less than one-fourth of older patients with hyperthyroidism present with goiter, tremor, and exophthalmos; more likely are atrial fibrillation, confusion, depression, syncope, and weakness. Significantly, because the "weakest link" is so often the brain, the lower urinary tract, or the cardiovascular or musculoskeletal system, a limited number of presenting symptoms predominate—acute confusion, depression, incontinence, falling, and syncope—no matter what the underlying disease. Thus for the most common geriatric syndromes, regardless of the presenting symptom, the differential diagnosis is often largely similar. The corollary is equally important: The organ system usually associated with a particular symptom is less likely to be the source of that symptom in older individuals than in younger ones. Compared with middle-aged individuals, for example, acute confusion in older patients is less often due to a new brain lesion, depression to a psychiatric disorder, incontinence to bladder dysfunction, falling to a neuropathy, or syncope to heart disease.

2. Because of impaired physiologic reserve, older patients often present at an earlier stage of their disease. For example, heart failure may be precipitated by mild hyperthyroidism, cognitive dysfunction by mild Alzheimer's disease, urinary retention by mild prostatic enlargement, and nonketotic hyperosmolar coma by mild glucose intolerance. Paradoxically, therefore, treatment of the underlying disease may be easier because it is often less advanced at the time of presentation. A corollary is that drug side effects can occur with drugs and drug doses unlikely to produce side effects in younger people (Chap. 67). For instance, an antihistamine may cause confusion, diuretics may precipitate urinary incontinence, digoxin may induce depression even with normal serum levels, and over-the-counter sympathomimetics may precipitate urinary retention in men with mild prostatic obstruction.

3. Since many homeostatic mechanisms may be compromised concurrently, there are usually multiple abnormalities amenable to treatment, and small improvements in each may yield dramatic benefits overall. For instance, cognitive impairment in patients with Alzheimer's disease may be exacerbated by hearing or visual impairment, depression, heart failure, and electrolyte imbalance. Similarly, urinary incontinence can be worsened by fecal impaction, medications, and excess urinary output. In each case, substantial functional improvement can result from treating the contributing factors even if—as in Alzheimer's disease—specific treatment is not possible.

4. Many findings that are abnormal in younger patients are relatively common in older people—e.g., bacteriuria, premature ventricular contractions, low bone mineral density, impaired glucose tolerance, and uninhibited bladder contractions. However, they may not be responsible for a particular symptom but only be incidental findings that result in missed diagnoses and misdirected therapy. For instance, the finding of bacteriuria should not end the search for a source of fever in an acutely ill older patient, nor should an elevated random blood sugar—especially in an acutely ill patient—be incriminated as the cause of neuropathy. On the other hand, certain other abnormalities must not be dismissed as due to old age—e.g., there is no anemia, impotence, depression, or confusion of old age.

5. Because symptoms in older people are often due to multiple causes, the diagnostic "law of parsimony" often does not apply. For instance, fever, anemia, retinal embolus, and a heart murmur prompt almost a reflex diagnosis of infective endocarditis in a younger patient but may reflect aspirin-induced blood loss, a cholesterol embolus, insignificant aortic sclerosis, or a viral illness in an older patient.

6. Because the older patient is more likely to suffer the adverse consequences of disease, treatment—and even prevention—may be equally or even more effective. For instance, the benefits of thrombolysis and beta-blocker therapy after a myocardial infarction are as impressive in older patients as in younger ones; and treatment of hypertension, and immunization against influenza and pneumococcal pneumonia, are more effective in older patients. In addition, prevention in older patients often must be seen in a broader context. For instance, although efforts to increase bone density may be futile in older patients, fracture still may be prevented by interventions that improve balance, strengthen legs, treat contributing medical conditions, repair nutritional deficits, remove adverse medications, and reduce environmental hazards.

HISTORY TAKING IN ELDERLY PATIENTS   Most older patients are able to provide a reliable medical history; however, a multitude of complaints may make obtaining a history more difficult. If the patient is unable to comprehend or communicate, data should be sought from family, friends, and caregivers. The history should include drug ingestion, a dietary history, history of falling, of incontinence, and of depression and anxiety.

Advance directives   All older patients should be asked whether they have drafted advance health care directives, and, if they have, a copy should be placed in the record. Such directives may consist of a health care proxy or durable power of attorney for health care, in which patients designate a surrogate decision-maker who makes health care decisions if the patient cannot; and/or a living will or medical directive, in which patients specify their desires for treatment in specific situations if they cannot communicate at the critical time.

Whether or not the patient has formally drafted these directives, it is useful to indicate in the record who should make health care decisions if the patient is no longer able to do so. Patients should then be encouraged to discuss with the physician as well as the designated proxy their feelings about resuscitation, intubation, feeding

TABLE 8-2   Life expectancy and number of remaining years free of dependency in ADL*

Age	Life expectancy*, av		Disability-free years remaining	
	Men	Women	Men	Women
65–69	13	20	9	11
70–74	12	16	8	8
75–79	10	13	7	7
80–84	7	10	5	5
≥85	7	8	3	3

* For independent noninstitutionalized elderly men and women in Massachusetts. Longevity and disability-free longevity are surprisingly long and must be incorporated into treatment decisions. ADL = activities of daily living. av = average. All figures rounded to nearest year. See text for more recent data on longevity alone.
SOURCE: Katz S et al: Active life expectancy. N Engl J Med 309:1218, 1983.

tubes, hospitalization, etc. in their current state of health and possible future declining states of health. The early elicitation of a patient's preferences and values can often help both physicians and families in subsequent difficult decisions by giving surrogate decision-makers the sense that they are doing as the patient would have wanted.

PHYSICAL EXAMINATION Certain features of the examination should receive special attention, depending in part on clues from the history. Weight and postural blood pressure should be measured at each visit. Vision and hearing should be checked; if hearing is impaired, excess cerumen should be removed from the external auditory canals. Denture fit should be assessed, and the oral cavity should be inspected with the dentures removed. Although thyroid disease becomes more common with age, the sensitivity and specificity of related findings are substantially lower than in younger individuals; consequently, the physical examination can rarely corroborate or exclude thyroid dysfunction in older patients. The breasts should not be overlooked, since older women are more likely to have breast cancer and less likely to do breast self-examination. In auscultating the chest, the physician must recall that the presence of a fourth heart sound in an elderly person does not imply significant cardiac disease. The systolic murmur of aortic sclerosis is common and may be difficult to differentiate from aortic stenosis.

In inactive patients and those with fecal or urinary incontinence, one should check for fecal impaction. In patients with urinary incontinence—especially men—a distended bladder must be looked for, since it may be the only finding in urinary retention; perineal sensation and the bulbocavernosus reflex also should be tested. Patients who fall should be observed standing up from a chair, walking 10 feet, turning, returning, and sitting again; abnormalities of gait and steadiness on standing should be evaluated with the patient's eyes open and closed and in response to a sternal push. It should be appreciated that "frontal release signs" (e.g., "snout," "glabellar," or palmomental reflexes) and absent ankle jerks and vibratory sense in the feet may be normal in the elderly.

MENTAL STATUS EXAMINATION In addition to evaluating mood and affect, some form of cognitive testing is desirable in all elderly patients, even if it involves only checking different components of the history for consistency. People with mild degrees of dementia usually retain their social graces and may mask intellectual impairment by a cheerful and cooperative manner (Chap. 25). Thus, the examiner should always probe for content. For patients who follow the news, one can ask what stories they are particularly interested in and why; the same applies to reading, social events—even the "soap operas" on television.

If there is any suspicion of a cognitive deficit after this kind of conversational probing, further questioning is indicated. An examination that tests only orientation as to person, place, and time is insufficient to detect mild or moderate intellectual impairment. As a quick screen, simply assessing orientation and asking the patient to draw a clock with the hands at a set time (e.g., 10 min before 2:00) can be very informative regarding cognitive status, visuospatial deficits, ability to comprehend and execute instructions in logical sequence, and presence or absence of perseveration. For slightly more detailed examinations, many practical mental status tests are available. The most widely used is the Mini-Mental Status Examination of Folstein (Chap. 25), which provides a numerical score that can be obtained in 5 to 10 min. Regardless of the test employed, the total score is less useful diagnostically than is knowledge of the specific domain of the deficit. As a general rule, disproportionate difficulty with immediate recall (e.g., of a list of three items) suggests depression, while predominant difficulty with recalling the items 5 min later suggests dementia. For patients with deficits of attention—recognized by inability to spell simple words backwards, repeat five digits, or recite the months of the year backwards—delirium is probably present, and the accuracy of the remainder of the test is dubious. However, the test can be interpreted accurately only in the context of a comprehensive evaluation.

EVALUATION OF FUNCTIONAL CAPACITY A clear description of the patient's degree of fitness or functional incapacity based on both medical and psychosocial problems is essential. The functional assessment includes determination of the patient's ability to perform basic activities of daily life (ADL), which are those needed for personal self-care, as well as the ability to perform more complex tasks required for independent living, the instrumental activities of daily living (IADL). ADLs include bathing, dressing, toileting, feeding, getting in and out of chairs and bed, and walking. IADLs include shopping, cooking, money management, housework, using a telephone, and traveling outside the home. For frail patients, an assessment in the home by a trained observer may be required, but for most patients a questionnaire dealing with these activities can be completed by the family or patient. In either case, the physician must determine the cause of any impairment and whether it can be treated. The assessment should conclude with determination of the socioeconomic circumstances and social support systems.

Since disease can present atypically in the elderly, acute functional decline may represent the first sign of serious acute illness. _Thus, acute functional decline presenting as the onset or worsening of falls, confusion, depression, or incontinence should prompt immediate medical evaluation._

MANAGEMENT OF COMMON GERIATRIC CONDITIONS

Diseases more common in the elderly are covered elsewhere in the text. The medical problems discussed below do not usually present as clear-cut organ-specific diagnoses and are most common in the frail elderly, especially those over 80 years of age.

INTELLECTUAL IMPAIRMENT The predominant causes of impaired mentation in older patients are delirium, dementia, and depression. Each condition is covered elsewhere in the text in detail (Chaps. 25 and 389), but their management in the elderly is discussed here.

The most important first step is to search for and correct all factors that may contribute to cognitive impairment. Evidence of dangerous behavior also should be sought (e.g., leaving the stove on, wandering, and getting lost) and plans should be devised to deal with it. Although there is no specific pharmacologic treatment for Alzheimer's disease, this does not mean that the physician has no further role in treating the patient and family. In addition to discontinuing all nonessential medications and treating new intercurrent illness, the physician should help the family and patient predict and deal with the disease; indeed, the family often needs the physician's support more than the patient does.

Community services should be suggested as needed. Support groups such as the Alzheimer's Association often are of value to the family and help them to anticipate problems. Signs of patient abuse by an overstressed caregiver should be watched for. Legal counsel should be recommended to help the patient and family devise plans for ongoing management and ultimate disposition of assets.

Finally, the onset of disruptive behavior should always prompt a search for new illness or medication. Exacerbation of cognitive dysfunction may occur with mild infections (e.g., subungual toe abscess or pressure ulcer); with "therapeutic" levels of many drugs; with use of nonprescribed drugs or alcohol; with modest abnormalities of serum sodium, calcium, or thyroxine; with borderline nutritional deficiencies; and even with the development of fecal impaction, urinary retention, pain, or change in environment, particularly in frail older patients. However, if a cause is not found and behavior does not respond to environmental manipulation, low doses of an antipsychotic medication may be helpful (e.g., haloperidol 0.25 to 2 mg per day orally; see below).

DEPRESSION Depression of significant degree occurs in 5 to 10 percent of community-dwelling elderly but is often overlooked. At highest risk are individuals with recent medical illness (e.g., stroke), bereavement, lack of social supports, recent nursing home admission, or psychiatric history (including alcohol abuse). The diagnosis requires the presence of a depressed mood for at least two consecutive weeks plus at least four of the following eight signs: sleep disturbance, lack of interest, feelings of guilt, decreased energy, decreased concentration, decreased appetite, psychomotor agitation/retardation, and suicidal ideation. Also helpful diagnostically are a personal or family history of depression and past response to an antidepressant. It is essential to bear in mind that depression in older patients is often caused or contributed to by drugs or a systemic illness.

Treatment   For the hospitalized patient in whom acute depression delays recovery or rehabilitation—when correction of medical and pharmacologic contributing factors is ineffective and there is no prior history of mania or major depression—methylphenidate, 5 to 10 mg at 8 A.M. and noon (to avoid insomnia) is often very effective, with benefits discernible within a few days. For many patients with major depression, there is no ideal antidepressant drug. All are about equally effective, but the side effects differ (see below and Chap. 389). Consequently, one should become familiar with one or two agents for patients with psychomotor retardation (e.g., desipramine, fluoxetine) and for those with agitation (e.g., nortriptyline or trazodone). Because of its potent anticholinergic and orthostatic side effects, amitriptyline should be avoided whenever possible in older patients. Initial low dosages should be increased slowly to avoid serious side effects; low doses of each medication (e.g., doxepin, 10 to 50 mg daily; desipramine, 25 to 75 mg daily) are often effective in the elderly. Careful follow-up is required to anticipate and minimize anticholinergic side effects, orthostatic hypotension, sedating effects, confusion, bizarre mental symptoms, cardiovascular complications, and drug overdose with suicidal intent. Adverse drug reactions should not be assumed to be due to the aging process.

Cautious use of the monoamine oxidase inhibitors is sometimes of benefit when other antidepressants are ineffective. Monoamine oxidase inhibitors should not be used in combination with the cyclic compounds. Electroconvulsive therapy has been successful and is usually well tolerated by elderly patients who remain severely depressed despite drug treatment.

URINARY INCONTINENCE   Transient incontinence (Table 8-3) Because urinary continence requires adequate mobility, mentation, motivation, and manual dexterity—in addition to integrated control of the lower urinary tract—problems outside the bladder can result in incontinence.

1 *Delirium.* A clouded sensorium impedes recognition of both the need to void and the location of the nearest toilet; once delirium clears, incontinence resolves.
2 *Infection.* Symptomatic urinary tract infection commonly causes or contributes to incontinence; asymptomatic infection does not.

TABLE 8-3   Classification of incontinence

TRANSIENT

Delirium/confusional state
Infection—urinary (symptomatic)
Atrophic urethritis/vaginitis
Pharmaceuticals
Psychological, especially depression
Excessive urine output (e.g., CHF, hyperglycemia)
Restricted mobility
Stool impaction

ESTABLISHED

Detrusor overactivity
Detrusor underactivity
Urethral obstruction
Urethral incompetence

SOURCE: Adapted from Resnick NM: Urinary incontinence in the elderly. Medical Grand Rounds 3:281, 1984.

TABLE 8-4   Medications that can potentially affect continence

Type of medication	Examples	Potential effects on continence
Potent diuretics	Furosemide	Polyuria, frequency, urgency
Anticholinergics	Antihistamines, trihexyphenidyl, benztropine, dicyclomine, disopyramide	Urinary retention, overflow incontinence, delirium, impaction
Psychotropics Antidepressants	Amitriptyline, desipramine	Anticholinergic actions, sedation
Antipsychotics	Thioridazine, haloperidol	Anticholinergic actions, sedation, rigidity, immobility
Sedatives/hypnotics	Diazepam, flurazepam	Sedation, delirium, immobility
Narcotic analgesics		Urinary retention, fecal impaction, sedation, delirium
Alpha-adrenergic blockers	Prazosin, terazosin	Urethral relaxation (stress incontinence in women)
Alpha-adrenergic agonists	Decongestants	Urinary retention in men
Calcium channel blockers	All	Urinary retention
Alcohol		Polyuria, frequency, urgency, sedation, delirium, immobility
Vincristine		Urinary retention

SOURCE: Resnick NM: Geriatric medicine and the elderly patient, in *Current Medical Diagnosis and Treatment*, LT Tierney et al (eds). Norwalk, Appleton & Lange, 1993 (in press).

3 *Atrophic urethritis/vaginitis.* Atrophic urethritis/vaginitis, characterized by the presence of vaginal telangiectasia, petechiae, erosions, erythema, or friability, commonly contributes to incontinence in women and responds to a short course of low-dose estrogen or vaginal estrogen creams.
4 *Pharmaceutical.* The drugs most commonly causing transient incontinence are listed in Table 8-4.
5 *Psychologic.* Depression and psychosis are uncommon but treatable causes.
6 *Excess urine output.* Excess urine output may overwhelm the ability to reach a toilet in time. Causes include diuretics, excess fluid intake, and metabolic abnormalities (e.g., hyperglycemia, hypercalcemia, diabetes insipidus); nocturnal incontinence may result from mobilization of peripheral edema.
7 *Restricted mobility.* If mobility cannot be improved, access to a urinal or commode may restore continence. (See Immobility below.)
8 *Stool impaction.* This is a common cause of urinary incontinence, especially in hospitalized or immobile patients. Although the mechanism is unknown, a clue to its presence is the coexistence of both urinary and fecal incontinence. Disimpaction restores continence.

Established incontinence   (Table 8-3)   The causes of established incontinence include irreversible functional deficits, such as end-stage Alzheimer's disease, and intrinsic lower urinary tract dysfunction. Lower urinary tract dysfunction should be sought after transient causes have been excluded.

DETRUSOR OVERACTIVITY   This disorder (uninhibited bladder contraction) accounts for two-thirds of geriatric incontinence in both sexes, regardless of whether patients are demented. Detrusor overactivity can be diagnosed presumptively in a woman when leakage occurs in the absence of stress maneuvers or urinary retention and is preceded by the abrupt onset of an intense urge to urinate that cannot be forestalled. In men, the symptoms are similar, but since detrusor overactivity coexists with urethral obstruction, urodynamic testing should be done if prescription of a bladder relaxant is planned. Because detrusor overactivity also may be due to bladder stones or tumor, the abrupt onset of otherwise unexplained urge incontinence—especially if accompanied by perineal/suprapubic discomfort or sterile hematuria—should prompt cystoscopy and cytologic examination.

The cornerstone of treatment is behavioral therapy. Patients should be instructed (or "prompted" if they are demented) to void every 1 to 2 h while awake and to suppress urgency in between; once daytime continence is restored, the interval between voiding can be progressively increased. When drugs are necessary, they should be added to these regimens and monitored to avoid inducing urinary retention. Effective drugs include anticholinergics (e.g., propantheline, 7.5 to 30 mg four to six times daily), oxybutynin (2.5 to 5 mg three or four times daily), imipramine or doxepin (25 to 100 mg at bedtime), and calcium channel blockers (in doses used for cardiac disease).

Indwelling catheterization is rarely indicated for detrusor overactivity. If all measures fail, an external collection device or protective pad or undergarment may be required.

STRESS INCONTINENCE This disorder, the second most common cause of established incontinence in older women (it is rare in men), is characterized by symptoms and evidence of *instantaneous* leakage of urine in response to stress. Leakage is worse or occurs only during the day unless another abnormality (e.g., detrusor overactivity) is also present. On examination, with the bladder full and the perineum relaxed, instantaneous leakage upon coughing strongly suggests stress incontinence, especially if it reproduces symptoms and if urinary retention has been excluded by a postvoiding residual determination; a several-second delay suggests that leakage is instead caused by an uninhibited bladder contraction induced by coughing.

Surgery is the most effective treatment with a cure rate of approximately 85 percent. For women who can comply, pelvic muscle exercises are an option for mild to moderate stress incontinence; if not contraindicated, an alpha-adrenergic agonist (e.g., phenylpropanolamine) is also helpful in such cases, especially if combined with estrogen. Occasionally, a pessary or even a tampon (for women with vaginal stenosis) provides some relief.

URETHRAL OBSTRUCTION Rarely present in women, urethral obstruction (due to prostatic enlargement, urethral stricture, bladder neck contracture, or prostate cancer) is the second most common cause of established incontinence in older men. It can present as dribbling incontinence after voiding, urge incontinence due to detrusor overactivity (which coexists in two-thirds of cases), or overflow incontinence due to urinary retention. Renal ultrasound is recommended to exclude hydronephrosis in men whose postvoiding residual volume exceeds 100 to 200 mL; in older men for whom surgery is planned, urodynamic confirmation of obstruction is usually required.

Surgical decompression is the most effective treatment for obstruction, especially if there is urinary retention. For a nonoperative candidate, intermittent or indwelling catheterization is used; a condom catheter is contraindicated when urinary retention is present. For a man with prostatic obstruction who is not in retention, treatment with an alpha-adrenergic antagonist (e.g., prazosin, 1 to 2 mg two to four times daily) may relieve symptoms, and the 5α-reductase inhibitor finasteride may partially relieve obstruction in a third or more of patients.

DETRUSOR UNDERACTIVITY Whether idiopathic or due to sacral lower motor nerve dysfunction, this is the least common cause of incontinence (<10 percent of cases). When it causes incontinence, detrusor underactivity is associated with urinary frequency, nocturia, and frequent leakage of small amounts. The elevated postvoiding residual volume (generally over 450 mL) distinguishes it from detrusor overactivity and stress incontinence, but only urodynamic testing (rather than cystoscopy or intravenous urography) differentiates it from urethral obstruction in men; such testing usually is not required in women, in whom obstruction is rare.

For the patient with a poorly contractile bladder, augmented voiding techniques (e.g., double voiding or applying suprapubic pressure) are often effective; pharmacologic agents (e.g., bethanechol) are rarely effective. If further emptying is needed or for the patient with an acontractile bladder, intermittent or indwelling catheterization is the only option. Antibiotics should be used for symptomatic upper tract infection or as prophylaxis for recurrent symptomatic infections only in a patient using intermittent catheterization; they should not be used as prophylaxis with an indwelling catheter.

FALLS Falls are a major problem for elderly people, especially women. Thirty percent of community-dwelling elderly fall each year; and one out of four of those who fall has serious injuries, including fractures in 5 percent. Falls are the sixth leading cause of death for older people and a contributing factor in 40 percent of admissions to nursing homes. Resultant hip problems and fear of falls are major causes of loss of independence. Nonetheless, falling must *not* be viewed as accidental, inevitable, or untreatable.

Causes of falls Balance and ambulation require a complex interplay of cognitive, neuromuscular, and cardiovascular function, and the ability to adapt rapidly to an environmental challenge. Balance becomes impaired and sway increases with age. The resulting vulnerability makes the older person predisposed to fall when challenged by an additional insult to *any* of these systems. Thus, a seemingly minor fall may be due to a serious problem, such as pneumonia or a myocardial infarction.

Much more commonly, however, falls are due to the complex interaction between a variably impaired patient and an environmental challenge. While a warped floorboard may pose little problem for a vigorous, unmedicated, alert person, it may be sufficient to precipitate a fall and hip fracture in the patient with altered balance, muscle tone, and cognition. Thus, falls in older people are rarely due to a single cause, and effective prevention entails a comprehensive assessment of the patient's intrinsic deficits (usually diseases and medications), the routine activities, and the environmental obstacles.

Intrinsic deficits are those that impair sensory input, judgment, blood pressure regulation, reaction time, and balance and gait (Table 8-5). Medications and alcohol use are among the most common, significant, and reversible causes of falling. Other treatable contributors include postprandial hypotension (which peaks 30 to 60 min after a meal), insomnia, urinary urgency, and peripheral edema (which can burden impaired leg strength and gait with an additional 5 to 10 pounds).

Environmental obstacles are listed in Table 8-6. Since most falls occur in or around the home, a visit by a visiting nurse, physical therapist, or physician often reaps substantial dividends.

Complications of falls and treatment The risk of falling and consequent injury, disability, and potential institutionalization can be reduced by modifying where possible those factors outlined above and in Tables 8-5 and 8-6.

Subdural hematoma is a treatable but easily overlooked complication of falls that must be considered in any elderly patient presenting with new neurologic signs, including confusion alone, even in the absence of a headache. Dehydration, electrolyte imbalance, pressure sores, and hypothermia also may occur and endanger the patient's life following a fall.

IMMOBILITY The main causes of immobility are weakness, stiffness, pain, imbalance, and psychological problems. Weakness may result from disuse of muscles, malnutrition, electrolyte disturbances, anemia, neurologic disorders, or myopathies. The most common cause of stiffness in the elderly is osteoarthritis; however, Parkinson's disease, rheumatoid arthritis, gout, pseudogout, and antipsychotic drugs such as haloperidol may also contribute. Pain, whether from bone (e.g., osteoporosis, osteomalacia, Paget's disease, metastatic bone cancer, trauma), joints (e.g., osteoarthritis, rheumatoid arthritis, gout), bursa, or muscle (e.g., polymyalgia rheumatica, intermittent claudication, or "pseudoclaudication"), may immobilize the patient.

Imbalance and fear of falling are major causes of immobilization.

TABLE 8-5 Intrinsic risk factors for falling and possible interventions

Risk factor	Interventions	
	Medical	Rehabilitative or environmental
Reduced visual acuity, dark adaptation, and perception	Refraction; cataract extraction	Home safety assessment
Reduced hearing	Removal of cerumen; audiologic evaluation	Hearing aid if appropriate (with training); reduction in background noise
Vestibular dysfunction	Avoidance of drugs affecting the vestibular system; neurologic or ear, nose, and throat evaluation, if indicated	Habituation exercises
Proprioceptive dysfunction, cervical degenerative disorders, and peripheral neuropathy	Screening for vitamin B$_{12}$ deficiency and cervical spondylosis	Balance exercises; appropriate walking aid; correctly sized footwear with firm soles; home safety assessment
Dementia	Detection of reversible causes; avoidance of sedative or centrally acting drugs	Supervised exercise and ambulation; home safety assessment
Musculoskeletal disorders	Appropriate diagnostic evaluation	Balance-and-gait training; muscle-strengthening exercises; appropriate walking aid; home safety assessment
Foot disorders (calluses, bunions, deformities, edema)	Shaving of calluses; bunionectomy; treatment of edema	Trimming of nails; appropriate footwear
Postural hypotension	Assessment of medications; rehydration; possible alteration in situational factors (e.g., meals, change of position)	Dorsiflexion exercises; pressure-graded stockings; elevation of head of bed; use of tilt table if condition is severe
Use of medications (sedatives: benzodiazepines, phenothiazines, antidepressants; antihypertensives; others: antiarrhythmics, anticonvulsants, diuretics, alcohol)	Steps to be taken: 1. Attempted reduction in the total number of medications taken 2. Assessment of risks and benefits of each medication 3. Selection of medication, if needed, that is least centrally acting, least associated with postural hypotension, and has shortest action 4. Prescription of lowest effective dose 5. Frequent reassessment of risks and benefits	

SOURCE: After Tinetti and Speechley.

TABLE 8-6 Environmental factors affecting the risk of falling in the home

Environmental area or factor	Objective and recommendations
All areas	
Lighting	Absence of glare and shadows; accessible switches at room entrances; night light in bedroom, hall, bathroom
Floors	Nonskid backing for throw rugs; carpet edges tacked down; carpets with shallow pile; nonskid wax on floors; cords out of walking path; small objects (e.g., clothes, shoes) off floor
Stairs	Lighting sufficient, with switches at top and bottom of stairs; securely fastened bilateral handrails that stand out from wall; top and bottom steps marked with bright, contrasting tape; stair rises of no more than 6 in; steps in good repair; no objects stored on steps
Kitchen	Items stored so that reaching up and bending over are not necessary; secure step stool available if climbing is necessary; firm, nonmovable table
Bathroom	Grab bars for tub, shower, and toilet; nonskid decals or rubber mat in tub or shower; shower chair with handheld shower; nonskid rugs; raised toilet seat; door locks removed to ensure access in an emergency
Yard and entrances	Repair of cracks in pavement, holes in lawn; removal of rocks, tools, and other tripping hazards; well-lit walkways, free of ice and wet leaves; stairs and steps as above
Institutions	All the above; bed at proper height (not too high or low); spills on floor cleaned up promptly; appropriate use of walking aids and wheelchairs
Footwear	Shoes with firm, nonskid, nonfriction soles; low heels (unless person is accustomed to high heels); avoidance of walking in stocking feet or loose slippers

SOURCE: After Tinetti and Speechley.

changes occur in skeletal muscle. At the cellular level, intracellular ATP and glycogen concentrations decrease, rates of protein degradation increase, and contractile velocity and strength decline, while at the whole-muscle level, atrophy, weakness, and shortening are seen. Pressure sores are a third serious complication; mechanical pressure, moisture, friction, and shearing forces all predispose to their development. As a result, within days of being confined to bed, the risk of postural hypotension, falls, and skin breakdown rises. Moreover, these changes usually take weeks to months to reverse.

Management The most important step is preventive—to avoid bedrest whenever possible. When it cannot be avoided, several measures can be employed to minimize its consequences. Patients should be positioned as close to the upright position as possible several times daily. Range of motion exercises should begin immediately, and the skin over pressure points should be inspected frequently. Isometric and isotonic exercises should be performed while the patient is in bed, and whenever possible patients should assist their own positioning, transferring, and self-care. As mobility becomes feasible, graduated ambulation should begin.

If a pressure ulcer develops, the multiplicity of topical therapies underscores the fact that no single one is clearly more effective than others. Surgical debridement may be required for severely undermined lesions. A special mattress (e.g., foam or static air mattress) or air-fluidized bed or water bed may be required for the very debilitated patient.

In addition to treating all identified factors that contribute to immobility, consultation with a physical therapist should be sought. Installing handrails, lowering the bed, and providing chairs of proper height with arms and rubber skid guards may allow the patient to be safely mobile in the home. A properly fitted cane or walker may be helpful.

IATROGENIC DRUG REACTIONS For several reasons, older patients are two or three times more likely to have adverse drug reactions (Chap. 67). Drug clearance is often markedly reduced. This

Imbalance may result from general debility, neurologic causes (e.g., stroke; loss of postural reflexes; peripheral neuropathy due to diabetes mellitus, alcohol, or malnutrition; and vestibulocerebellar abnormalities), orthostatic or postprandial hypotension, drugs (e.g., diuretics, antihypertensives, neuroleptics, and antidepressants), or may occur following prolonged bed rest. Psychologic conditions such as severe anxiety or depression also may contribute to immobilization.

Consequences The hazards of bed rest in the elderly are multiple, serious, quick to develop, and slow to reverse. Deconditioning of the cardiovascular system occurs within days and involves fluid shifts, fluid loss, decreased cardiac output, decreased peak oxygen uptake, and increased resting heart rate. Perhaps even more striking is due to a decrease in renal plasma flow and glomerular filtration rate and a reduced hepatic clearance. The last is due to a decrease in activity of the drug-metabolizing microsomal enzymes and an overall decline in blood flow to the liver with aging. The volume of distribution of drugs also is affected, since the elderly have a decrease in total body water and a relative increase in body fat. Thus, water-soluble drugs become more concentrated, and fat-soluble drugs have longer half-lives. In addition, serum albumin levels decline, especially in sick patients, so that there is a decrease in protein binding of some drugs (e.g., warfarin, phenytoin), leaving more free (active) drug available.

In addition to impaired drug clearance, which alters pharmacokinetics, older patients have altered responses to similar serum drug levels, a phenomenon known as altered pharmacodynamics. They are more sensitive to some drugs (e.g., opiates, anticoagulants) and less sensitive to others (e.g., beta-adrenergic agents). Finally, the older patient with multiple chronic conditions is likely to be taking several drugs, including nonprescribed agents. Thus, adverse drug reactions and dosage errors are more likely to occur, especially if the patient has visual, hearing, or memory deficits.

Precautions to avoid drug toxicity DRUG SELECTION AND ADMINISTRATION   Before initiating treatment, the physician should first ensure that the symptom requiring treatment is not itself due to another drug. For example, antipsychotic agents can cause symptoms that mimic depression (flat affect, restlessness, and pacing); such symptoms should prompt lowering of the dose rather than initiation of an antidepressant. In addition, drug therapy should be employed only after nonpharmacologic means have been considered or tried and only when the benefit clearly outweighs the risk.

Once pharmacotherapy has been decided upon, it should begin at less than the usual adult dosage (although many elderly patients require full doses), and the dose should be increased slowly. The dosage schedule should be kept as simple as possible and the number of pills should be kept as low as possible. Serum drug levels are often useful in older patients, especially for monitoring drugs with narrow therapeutic indices such as phenytoin, theophylline, quinidine, aminoglycosides, lithium, and psychotropic agents such as nortriptyline. However, toxicity can occur even with ''normal'' therapeutic levels of some drugs (e.g., digoxin, phenytoin).

SEDATIVE-HYPNOTICS   The effects of sedative-hypnotics persist much longer in the elderly and have been associated with confusional states, falls, fractures, driving accidents, and incontinence. The long acting agents in particular (e.g., flurazepam and diazepam) should be avoided whenever possible; however, even the shortest-acting benzodiazepines (e.g., triazolam) may have adverse effects. If nonpharmacologic treatment of insomnia is unsuccessful, short-term use of an intermediate-acting agent whose metabolism is not affected by age (e.g., oxazepam, 10 to 30 mg/d) may be useful.

ANTIBIOTICS   Serum creatinine is not a good index of renal function in old people; however, when it is elevated special care must be taken with the administration of drugs normally excreted by the kidneys. Concentrations of relevant antibiotics should be measured directly.

CARDIAC DRUGS   In older patients, digitalis, procainamide, and quinidine have prolonged half-lives and narrow therapeutic windows; toxicity is common at the usual dosages. For example, digoxin toxicity—especially anorexia, confusion, or depression—can occur even with therapeutic digoxin levels.

ANTIDEPRESSANTS AND ANTIPSYCHOTICS   These agents can produce anticholinergic side effects in old people (e.g., confusion, urinary retention, constipation, dry mouth). This can be minimized by switching to a nonanticholinergic agent (e.g., fluoxetine or trazodone) or one with less anticholinergic effect (e.g., desipramine). In general, the least potent agents for psychosis (e.g., chlorpromazine) have the most sedating and anticholinergic effects and are the most likely to induce postural hypotension. By contrast, the most potent antipsychotic agents (e.g., haloperidol) have the least sedating, anticholinergic, and hypotensive side effects but cause extrapyramidal

side effects, including dystonia, akathisia, rigidity, and tardive dyskinesia. Thus all of these agents are potentially toxic. Moreover, since both depression and agitation often remit spontaneously, cautious discontinuation of these drugs should be considered periodically.

GLAUCOMA MEDICATIONS   Both topical beta-blockers and carbonic anhydrase inhibitors can cause systemic side effects. The latter can cause malaise and anorexia independent of the induced metabolic acidosis.

ANTICOAGULANTS   Elderly patients benefit from anticoagulation as much as do younger individuals but are more vulnerable to serious bleeding. Hence, more careful monitoring and less aggressive anticoagulation are advisable.

AVOID OVERTREATMENT   Drugs are not necessarily indicated in some common clinical situations. For instance, antibiotics need not be given for asymptomatic bacteriuria unless obstructive uropathy, other anatomic abnormalities, or stones are also present. Ankle edema is often due to venous insufficiency, drugs such as NSAIDs or some calcium antagonists, or even inactivity or malnutrition in chairbound patients. Diuretics are usually not indicated unless edema is associated with heart failure. Fitted, pressure gradient stockings are often helpful. Finally, since older patients generally tolerate aspirin and other NSAIDs less well than do younger patients, localized pain should be treated when possible with local measures such as injection, physical therapy, heat, ultrasound, or transcutaneous electrical stimulation (see Chap. 11).

PREVENTION

Much can be done to prevent the progression and even the onset of disease in older people. Dietary inadequacies in the elderly should be corrected; for the patient with inadequate sun exposure and intake of vitamin D, a daily multivitamin capsule is recommended. Tobacco and alcohol use should be minimized, since the benefits of discontinuing these accrue even to individuals over age 65. The importance of reviewing all of a patient's medications and discontinuing them whenever feasible cannot be overemphasized.

The benefits of treating both isolated systolic hypertension and combined systolic and diastolic hypertension in ambulatory elderly have now been documented. Treatment reduces the risk of stroke and the risk of death due to cardiovascular causes in this age group. Conclusive results have been achieved using *low doses* of a thiazide-like diuretic (e.g., chlorthalidone, 12.5 to 25 mg/d) as the first step (alone effective in almost half of patients) and adding low-dose reserpine (0.05 to 0.1 mg/d) or atenolol (25 to 50 mg/d) only as needed. Benefits were dramatic, side effects were minimal, cost was trivial, and concerns about potential toxicity were not borne out.

Because of the prevalence, functional impact, and ease of treatment, glaucoma should be screened for, and visual and auditory impairment should be corrected. Dentures should be assessed for their fit, and oral lesions beneath them should be detected.

A Papanicolaou test should be done in women who have not had one before, since the incidence of both preventable cervical carcinoma and associated death increases with age, especially in this group. Immunizations (for influenza, pneumococcal pneumonia, tetanus) should be current because of the established benefit of prophylaxis in the elderly. PPD testing should be done on residents of chronic care facilities and on those at high risk of tuberculosis; those who have recently converted probably should be treated. Since responsiveness wanes with age, the test, if negative, should be repeated in a week to increase the chances of detecting all exposed patients. Screening mammography is indicated every 1 to 2 years at least until age 75 and thereafter if a positive finding would result in therapeutic intervention. The relative risks and benefits of low-dose aspirin and (for women) estrogen replacement therapy have not yet been elucidated sufficiently to warrant routine use, but they should be considered on an individual basis.

Exercise should be encouraged not only because of its beneficial effects on blood pressure, cardiovascular conditioning, glucose home-ostasis, bone density, and functional status, but also because it may improve mood and social interaction, reduce insomnia and constipation, and prevent falls. Spinal flexion exercises should be avoided in patients with osteopenia; consultation with a physical therapist may be helpful.

Measures should be taken to prevent falling, as outlined in Tables 8-5 and 8-6. Counseling about driving is important, especially for patients with cognitive impairment. But perhaps the most valuable procedure for prevention of disease in old people is to take a careful history, focusing not only on the "chief complaint" but also on common and often hidden conditions such as falls, confusion, depression, sexual dysfunction, and incontinence. In addition, one should always identify the complications for which the specific patient is at risk and take steps to avert them. For instance, a patient with cognitive impairment who smokes is at risk not only for lung cancer but also for starting a fire, and a patient who requires narcotics is at risk for fecal impaction, delirium, urinary retention, and confusion. Community-dwelling patients who are at highest risk of rapid deterioration and institutionalization and who should be monitored more closely include those over age 80, those who live alone, those who are bereaved or depressed, and those who are intellectually impaired.

REFERENCES

Biology of aging

ARKING R: *Biology of Aging: Observations and Principles.* Englewood Cliffs, NJ: Prentice-Hall, 1991
JOHNSON TE, LITHGOW GJ: The search for the genetic basis of aging: The identification of gerontogenes in the nematode *Caenorhabditis elegans.* J Amer Geriatr Soc 40:936, 1992
GOLDSTEIN S: Replicative senescence: The human fibroblast comes of age. Science 249:1129, 1990

Functional assessment

LACHS MS et al: A simple procedure for general screening for functional disability in elderly patients. Ann Intern Med 112:699, 1990

Dementia, delirium, depression

NIH CONSENSUS DEVELOPMENT PANEL: Diagnosis and treatment of depression in late life. JAMA 268:1018, 1992
FRANCIS J: Delirium in older patients. J Amer Geriat Soc 40:829, 1992
HOWELL T, WATTS DT: Behavioral complications of dementia: A clinical approach for the general internist. J Gen Intern Med 5:431, 1990
KATZMAN R, ROWE JW (eds): *Principles of Geriatric Neurology.* Philadelphia, Davis, 1992
SIU A: Screening for dementia and assessing its causes. Ann Intern Med 115:122, 1991

Urinary incontinence

RESNICK NM, OUSLANDER JG (eds): National Institutes of Health Consensus Development Conference on Urinary Incontinence. J Am Geriatr Soc 38:263, 1990
URINARY INCONTINENCE GUIDELINE PANEL: Urinary incontinence in adults: Clinical practice guideline. AHCPR Publication No. 92-0038. Rockville, MD, 1992

Falls/Immobility

TINETTI ME, SPEECHLEY M: Prevention of falls among the elderly. N Engl J Med 320:1055, 1989
WASSON JH et al: The prescription of assistive devices for the elderly. J Gen Intern Med 5:46, 1990

Geriatric pharmacology

MONTAMAT SC et al: Management of drug therapy in the elderly. N Engl J Med 321:303, 1989
SALZMAN C: *Clinical Geriatric Psychopharmacology,* 2d ed. Baltimore, Williams & Wilkins, 1992

Prevention

AMERY A, SCHAEPDRYVER AD: Introduction: The European Working Party on High Blood Pressure in the Elderly. Am J Med 90(Suppl 3A):3, 1991
HAYWARD RSA et al: Preventive care guidelines: 1991. Ann Intern Med 114:758, 1991
SHEP COOPERATIVE RESEARCH GROUP: Prevention of stroke by antihypertensive drug treatment in older persons with isolated systolic hypertension. Final results of the Systolic Hypertension in the Elderly Program (SHEP). JAMA 265:3255, 1991

Miscellaneous

HARRIS J: The treatment of cancer in an aging population. JAMA 268:96, 1992
LIBOW LS, STARER P: Care of the nursing home patient. N Engl J Med 321:93, 1989
MORLEY JE et al: Nutrition in the elderly: ULCA conference. Ann Intern Med 109:890, 1988
PRINZ PN et al: Sleep disorders and aging. N Engl J Med 323:520, 1990
RESNICK NM, GREENSPAN SL: "Senile" osteoporosis reconsidered. JAMA 261:1025, 1989

9   COST AWARENESS IN MEDICINE

LEE GOLDMAN

COSTS OF HEALTH CARE IN THE UNITED STATES

Health care expenditures in the United States are now about $900 billion per year. Through the 1980s and early 1990s, these expenditures rose at a rate of more than 10 percent per year, which exceeded the rates of inflation and of growth in the gross national product (GNP). As a consequence, the percentage of the GNP that is spent on health care increased from about 7 percent in 1970 to 9 percent in 1980 and is expected to be nearly 15 percent in 1995. As a percentage of the GNP, medical care expenditures in the United Kingdom are about four percentage points lower than in the United States. In Canada, expenditures as a percentage of GNP were similar to the United States until about 1970 but now are about two percentage points lower. Much of the difference between the United States and Canada is explained by higher physician fees rather than by a higher per capita use of services. The United States also spends substantially more on the administrative costs of health care than Canada or Great Britain.

The reasons for the increase in health care costs are multifactorial. The aging of the population and the availability of new diagnostic and therapeutic advances have increased the demand for health care. Furthermore, between 1970 and 1990, the supply of physicians in the United States increased from about 150 to 240 per 100,000 population. This increase in physicians provided Americans with easier access to medical services but raised concerns that a possible oversupply of physicians in portions of the country could contribute to an excessive escalation in costs. The costs of care are especially influenced by decisions regarding hospital admission and surgery and by decisions affecting the use of intensive care units, life-sustaining treatments, and long-term care facilities. Efforts at cost-containment have attempted to identify unnecessary services, such as routine preoperative electrocardiograms in healthy young patients, or situations in which extraordinary expenses occur, such as in the last 6 months of life. Although some services may represent "fat" in the health care system, it is likely that any future reduction in unnecessary care may be more than counterbalanced in costs by growth in the number and age of the population and by continued advances in technology.

Despite these rising costs, an estimated 31 million Americans, or about 13 percent of the population, do not have health care insurance of any kind, even though nearly half are in households in which someone is employed. This lack of insurance coverage and access to health care is often blamed for the fact that the United States, despite its high expenditures on health care, ranks about twentieth in the world in infant mortality and is not in the top ten in life expectancy.

HEALTH INSURANCE   Traditional fee-for-service insurance reimburses the hospital and the physician for services rendered but frequently does not cover preventive care. Even when insurance provides coverage for a service, the patient may be responsible for an initial "deductible" and a copayment, which is usually a fixed percentage of the entire amount charged.

Patients who must pay such out-of-pocket charges for some of their medical care seek less care than those whose care is fully covered by insurance. In the working poor this may result in reduced utilization of services and in an increase in the prevalence of serious disease. When adults of all socioeconomic classes lose health insurance coverage, they may use fewer medical services; as a result, their health status tends to decline.

Most alternatives to traditional fee-for-service medical care require enrolled persons to prepay a fixed premium, which, except when a relatively small copayment is required, usually covers acute, chronic, and preventive medical services and sometimes covers medications and other health care needs. Prepaid plans have varying organizational and financial structures. Early on in their development, staff-model HMOs were among the most popular formats. In this model, groups of salaried physicians practiced physically together in one or a few central facilities to provide prepaid care. In recent years, independent practice associations (IPAs) have shown the most rapid growth. IPAs provide prepaid care to the patient by contracting with office-based practitioners who agree to see patients on a prenegotiated fee schedule. To balance the normal fee-for-service incentives and control utilization, IPAs employ various forms of administrative controls and review. The rate of hospitalization can be reduced among enrollees in HMOs, and HMOs have been among the leaders in attempts to reduce hospital costs and lengths of stay.

REIMBURSEMENT OF HOSPITALS AND PHYSICIANS In 1983, Medicare introduced a system of prospective reimbursement using diagnosis-related groups (DRGs), whereby hospitals were paid a predetermined sum based on the patient's principal diagnosis, procedures, complications, and comorbidities regardless of the costs or charges that were actually generated by the hospital stay (Table 9-1). This reimbursement system was designed to reward hospitals for being more efficient, and hospitals could actually be paid more than their costs. In the first few years after the introduction of the DRG system, many hospitals, especially the large teaching hospitals, reported substantial operating surpluses. In response, Medicare kept the rate of annual increase in reimbursement below the rate of increase in hospital costs, and the extra payments for teaching hospitals were reduced. While the prospective reimbursement system has undoubtedly stimulated efficiency, it also has raised concerns about the practice of discharging patients prematurely or transferring them to other institutions if the projected cost of caring for them exceeds the expected reimbursement.

Since the introduction of federal prospective reimbursement, the number of inpatient hospital days has decreased. This reduction has been accompanied by a marked increase in ambulatory services, including a shift to the outpatient arena of services that previously were delivered only on an inpatient basis. This shift should lower the cost of delivering an individual unit of service, such as the cost of a

TABLE 9-2 Physician reimbursement: The relative value scale versus traditional fee for service

Average Medicare reimbursement	Method of calculating reimbursement	
	Traditional fee for service, $*	Relative value scale, $†
Office visit, limited service, established patient	23	22
Initial hospital consultation, comprehensive service	75	83
Repair of sliding inguinal hernia	524	335
Coronary artery bypass, three grafts	3700	2225

* Defined as an individual physician's customary fee for service, limited to a prevailing fee by third-party insurers.
† A service-specific reimbursement based on the resource inputs required to perform a service, including the physician's work involved and specialty differences in practice expenses and costs related to training. Reimbursements are also adjusted to account for local differences in the cost of practice.

breast biopsy, but the overall cost of medical care will rise if, for example, the breast biopsy is performed on an ambulatory basis *and* the inpatient resources that the breast biopsy patient would have used are now consumed by new services such as the treatment of a cancer patient with bone marrow transplantation.

Physician payment Methods of physician payment also have been revised. Physician reimbursement in the United States, whether by Medicare or by private insurers, traditionally was a direct payment based on the doctor's "usual and customary" fee. In recent years, the rate of annual increase in fees has been fixed by the payor so that relative payments really reflect fee patterns from a decade or more ago. Because of concerns that this traditional approach had led to inequities in reimbursement and especially to underreimbursement for nonprocedural tasks such as office visits, recent analyses have considered the resource inputs of physicians' services, including time, intensity, practice costs, and the investment in training, to propose a new and fairer approach to physician reimbursement. These analyses have been incorporated into a new Medicare reimbursement system for physicians using the *relative value scale* (Table 9-2), which is based on the concept that payment rates for medical services should, as with other economic "goods," reflect the costs of producing those services. This change suggests that procedural tasks were being reimbursed at rates exceeding those of nonprocedural tasks that require comparable time, skill, and experience. Medicare's new relative rates are similar to preexisting fee schedules in Canada.

Proponents of changes in the reimbursement system hope that more equitable pay for cognitive tasks will reduce the incentive to perform procedures and increase the incentive for physicians to spend more time with patients, including time for discussion of such issues as health screening, health promotion, and disease prevention. Opponents of a change in the physician reimbursement system argue, among other issues, that changes in the reimbursement system may limit access and fail to take into account the extent to which patients may value some services more than others. Although the consequences of this change in the reimbursement system will not be known for some time, the physician's diagnostic and therapeutic recommendations should be guided by the goal of promoting maximal well-being for the patient, tempered by an awareness of the relative cost that must be incurred to reap this benefit.

Control of health care costs Two different approaches have been suggested to control health care costs: regulation and competition. Regulations, such as per diem rate setting, attempt to control costs by setting and enforcing practice or reimbursement standards. Other regulatory means of attempting to reduce costs include mandatory second opinions prior to elective hospitalization or surgery, but such programs usually do not save more than the costs of administration of the programs themselves. It is vital that physicians work closely with third-party payors, government agencies and commissions, and

TABLE 9-1 Example of diagnosis-related groups (DRGs) for prospective payment by Medicare

DRG no.	Name	Approximate Medicare reimbursement for a large urban teaching hospital in 1992, $
89	Simple pneumonia and pleurisy with complications or comorbid conditions	5,000
121	Acute myocardial infarction with complications, discharged alive	6,800
148	Major small or large bowel procedure with complications or comorbid conditions	13,000
106	Coronary artery bypass surgery with catheterization on same admission	23,000

SOURCE: Prospective Payment Assessment Commission.

regulatory bodies such as the Joint Commission on Accreditation of Health Care Organizations that have assumed increasing responsibilities for setting reimbursement rates and for determining performance standards and conditions for payment.

The competitive approach encourages hospitals and providers to bid in a free-market atmosphere, in which consumers will presumably make rational choices based on the perceived cost and quality of the available alternatives. Insurance plans that utilize deductibles and copayments reflect this approach. It also has been proposed that physicians who practice inexpensively should be rewarded financially, but if physicians are paid to perform fewer services, the quality of care may suffer.

The reimbursement system differs in different countries. In the United Kingdom, for example, the National Health Service insurance program covers hospital and physician reimbursement on a non-fee-for-service basis, although patients can pay privately for services outside the system. Patients often must endure long delays for nonemergency procedures. In Canada, hospitals are paid an annual lump sum, and most physicians are paid on a fee-for-service basis via a fee schedule that is negotiated between the medical societies and the provincial governments. Private insurance, by law, can cover only services such as long-term care and dental care that are not covered by public insurance. New technology has diffused less rapidly in Canada, and the rates at which many procedures are performed are lower, but may not be less optimal, than in the United States. In Canada, delays for elective services have not been a major problem, life expectancy is higher than in the United States, and the prestige and relative income of physicians is analogous to those in the United States.

COSTS AND COST-EFFECTIVENESS

The costs of medical care include direct costs, such as the salaries of health personnel, and indirect costs, such as utilities, maintenance, and mortgage payments. Some costs are fixed (i.e., they do not vary with the volume of services provided), and other costs are variable (i.e., they depend on volume). For example, consider a situation in which a new instrument to perform a blood chemistry test costs $1000 and will last for 1 year. Also assume that each individual chemical analysis has an incremental cost of $10 in reagents, personnel time, and other resource inputs. If the laboratory utilizes the instrument to analyze 100 specimens in a year, the average cost per specimen is $20 ($10 each in fixed and variable costs), but if it analyzes 10,000 specimens, the average cost per specimen is $10.10 ($0.10 in fixed costs and $10.00 in variable costs) because the fixed costs are spread over more specimens.

The charges for medical services do not necessarily correspond to the true costs of providing the services. This occurs in part because the costs are difficult to measure and in part because charges are usually fixed regardless of volume, while costs vary with volume. Most analyses of cost and cost-effectiveness in medicine are based on charges rather than on true costs.

The net costs for a health care program include the costs of providing the program, costs that are generated by adverse side effects of treatment, and costs for treating disease that would not have occurred if the patient had not lived longer as a result of the original treatment. From these costs, the savings in health care, rehabilitation, or custodial costs due to prevention or alleviation of disease are subtracted to determine the net cost. For example, consider a program to perform mammography in women over age 40. The program would have its own direct costs related to advertising, screening, mammography, physician visits, breast biopsy, etc. Some women would have false-positive mammograms and would receive unnecessary breast biopsies. Other women would live longer as a result of early diagnosis and treatment of breast cancer, but they might develop other illnesses, such as coronary disease, in the interim. If they developed conditions such as Alzheimer's disease, the custodial costs

might be substantial. However, these costs would be countered by savings from hospitalizations for advanced cancer and by a potential increase in productive wage-earning years.

In all analyses of costs, it is important to consider *when* the costs will be incurred and *when* the effects in health benefits may be realized. Present dollars or health benefits are considered to have greater worth than a promise of future dollars or health benefits for several reasons. Other events may intercede so that a projected future cost or benefit may never occur, and there is always the possibility that money spent now will not achieve the desired effect at some time in the future. Furthermore, another illness may intervene, or there might be better ways to spend the money in the future. The principle by which future dollars and benefits are less highly valued than known immediate costs and benefits is termed *discounting*. It is independent of monetary inflation. By this concept, it is preferable to spend $1000 today to prevent someone from dying today than it is to spend $1000 today in the expectation that someone will not die 10 years from now.

It is unusual for any program simultaneously to achieve the greatest possible benefit and have the lowest possible cost. Instead, one usually either determines the desired benefit and then finds the lowest cost needed to achieve it or determines the resources available and then finds the greatest possible benefit that can be achieved.

Analyses of cost-effectiveness commonly examine the ratio of cost to effectiveness, i.e., the number of dollars required to save a life or a year of life. Such analyses are relevant to medicine because interventions only rarely both save lives and reduce costs. Hence it is important to estimate the tradeoff of costs for gains in health. Two strategies with the same ratio may have quite different absolute costs and absolute benefits. For example, a program that saves 100 lives for $100,000 has the same cost-effectiveness ratio as one that saves 1000 lives for $1 million, but the absolute costs and absolute benefits vary tenfold. The choice between these two programs may depend on how much money is available to spend. In assessing any program, it is important to measure incremental costs and effects rather than average costs and effects. For example, consider two programs to reduce death from lung cancer. If, on average, program A costs $100 million to save 100,000 years of life (average of $1000 per year of life) and program B costs $200 million to save 100,100 years of life (about $2000 per year of life), the *incremental* cost of program B versus program A is $1 million per year of life saved.

SOCIETAL ISSUES IN COSTS   It is rare to find a medical intervention, such as measles vaccination programs, that both saves lives and reduces overall costs because the savings from disease prevention more than outweigh the expenses of the treatment itself. More commonly, medical practices that are truly of benefit also cause an associated increase in medical care costs. Among the more cost-effective examples is coronary artery bypass surgery in patients with left main coronary artery disease, which costs under $10,000 per year of life saved.

The shift of services from the inpatient to the outpatient setting or from the hospital to the home generally reduces the expense of delivery of that aspect of medical care. For example, home dialysis is less expensive than dialysis in an outpatient center, which in turn is less expensive than dialysis in a hospital. Similarly, the administration of parenteral nutrition and intravenous antibiotics at home and the home care for patients with AIDS have greatly reduced the need for hospitalization for conditions in which skilled nursing care is otherwise not required. However, a by-product of this strategy is an increased percentage of severely ill hospital inpatients who require more intensive and expensive care than the less sick patients who otherwise might have occupied hospital beds.

To date, society has been reluctant to make ethical decisions regarding the amount of cost appropriate for any particular net benefit. Neither medicine nor society is accustomed to placing a dollar value on a life or a year of life. In many analyses, however, the projected annual costs of approximately $35,000 to $45,000 (in 1995 dollars) for renal dialysis for 1 year of useful life have been used as a benchmark of how much the United States is willing to spend to save a year of life, because such a program is supported with tax dollars and presumably is a reasonable reflection of national priorities.

The physician has a unique responsibility. On the one hand, the physician must serve as an advocate for the individual patient and recommend the course of action most likely to be beneficial to the patient. The overriding nature of the patient-physician relationship is the cornerstone of humane medical care. On the other hand, physicians must understand the costs as well as the benefits of medical interventions so that they can choose from among the wide range of options. The physician must serve as the advocate for providing the best options to the individual patient and should know which options are of little or no value or are more likely to do harm than good. The physician must, with the assistance and consent of the patient and the family, set priorities for the patient's management within any limits or restrictions imposed by society; such limits may be expressed, for example, in a finite number of dollars available for the treatment of a specific illness. In addition, physicians have a broad role in determining health costs. Individually and through various professional organizations, physicians have a responsibility to help set national priorities, based on their appreciation of the finite resources available for health care and their knowledge of the relative benefits and costs of various diagnostic and therapeutic options in particular types of patients. Inappropriate attempts to reduce costs, such as limiting Medicaid payments for effective medications, are counterproductive in that they worsen health and ultimately lead to increased overall costs.

HEALTH SCREENING *Screening* refers to the performance of a medical evaluation and/or diagnostic tests in asymptomatic persons in the hope that early diagnosis may lead to improved outcome. For such persons, it was initially assumed that a periodic health examination, often accompanied by multiphasic diagnostic testing, is beneficial. However, there is no definitive information regarding the value of such an approach and even less information regarding which aspects yield results that are worth the costs incurred. In fact, there is no universally accepted approach to screening in the asymptomatic adult, given the uncertainties about the benefits and cost-effectiveness of each intervention. Nevertheless, the recommendations in Table 9-3 represent a reasonable set of guidelines for the periodic health assessment of asymptomatic adults.

Another issue in screening concerns the choice of which routine tests to perform in a patient who is about to undergo an operation or who is admitted to the hospital. For example, routine preoperative chest radiography is not indicated in persons without signs, symptoms, or risk factors for pulmonary or cardiac disease. Routine preoperative electrocardiography is generally recommended in any person with cardiac signs or symptoms and in men over age 40 and women over age 50 because of the age-related increase in asymptomatic cardiac disease and the likelihood that the preoperative tracing may be helpful for comparison should any cardiac problems arise during the perioperative period. In these situations, appropriate tests must be performed to investigate specific symptoms and signs. In terms of screening tests for asymptomatic conditions, those tests and procedures which have not been performed under the guidelines in Table 9-3 normally should be performed while the patient is under medical care.

HEALTH PROMOTION AND DISEASE PREVENTION Health promotion and disease prevention require investment of time, energy, and resources in the hope that the yield in terms of improved health warrants this investment. Unfortunately, there is limited information on the effectiveness of health promotion and disease prevention efforts. Interventions that result in a specified *relative* reduction in adverse outcomes have a greater *absolute* effect in higher-risk populations. For example, the same relative reduction in serum cholesterol will be of greater absolute benefit in persons with higher serum cholesterol levels or other unfavorable risk factors. In general, interventions to alter risk factors have a diminishing effect as risk factors decrease in severity.

Both patients and society commonly expect physicians to play a leadership role in health promotion and disease prevention. Patients

TABLE 9-3 Guidelines for preventive medical services*

	Age of person		
	19–39 years	40–64 years	65+ years
HISTORY			
	Every 1 to 3 years†: diet; physical activity; tobacco, alcohol, drugs; sexual practices	Same as 19–39 years	Every year: same as 19–39 years; and also functional status and symptoms of transient ischemia attacks
PHYSICAL EXAMINATION			
	Every 1 to 3 years: height, weight, blood pressure	Every 1 to 3 years: height, weight, blood pressure, breast	Every year: as for 40–64 years and also hearing and visual acuity
	High risk: oral cavity, thyroid, breast, testes, skin	High risk: oral cavity, thyroid, skin, carotids	High risk: as for 40–64 years (but every year)
LABORATORY			
	Pap smear (every 1–3 years), total cholesterol	Pap smear (every 1–3 years), mammogram (every 1–2 years after age 50), total cholesterol	Mammogram (every 1–2 years until age 75), thyroid indices (women), dipstick urinalysis, total cholesterol
	High risk: fasting glucose, rubella antibodies, VDRL, urinalysis, *Chlamydia* testing, gonorrhea culture, HIV testing, hearing, PPD, ECG, mammogram, colonoscopy	High risk: fasting glucose, VDRL, urinalysis, *Chlamydia* testing, gonorrhea culture, HIV testing, hearing, PPD, ECG, fecal occult blood/sigmoidoscopy/colonoscopy, bone mineral content	High risk: fasting glucose, PPD, ECG, Pap smear (every 1–3 years), fecal occult blood/sigmoidoscopy/colonoscopy
SPECIAL COUNSELING			
	Injury prevention, dental health	Injury prevention, dental health, skin protection from ultraviolet light, discussion of aspirin therapy in men and estrogen replacement in women	As for 40–64 years and also glaucoma testing
	High risk: hemoglobin testing, skin protection from ultraviolet light		
IMMUNIZATIONS			
	Tetanus-diphtheria booster every 10 years	As for 19–39 years except not measles-mumps-rubella	Tetanus-diphtheria booster (every 10 years) influenza (every year), pneumococcal
	High risk: hepatitis B, pneumococcal, influenza (every year), measles-mumps-rubella		High risk: hepatitis B

* Except for the visit itself, the frequency is at clinical discretion unless otherwise specified.
† With counseling for any high-risk behaviors.
SOURCE: Adapted from U.S. Preventive Services Task Force (*Guide to Clinical Preventive Services.* Baltimore, Williams & Wilkins, 1989), whose official report lists full details, including the definition of high-risk situations.

expect and desire their physicians to make recommendations regarding physical activity, diet, and other lifestyle issues, and physicians often fail in this regard. If physicians do not become involved, patients seek advice elsewhere, risking the possibility that fads or other erroneous sources may influence their choices.

When physicians become actively involved in health promotion, patients respond frequently and make appropriate behavior changes. For example, a physician's encouragement to increase physical activity, especially if combined with explicit suggestions, is likely to lead to changes in behavior so that the time spent by the physician appears to be cost-effective. Advice by a physician that a patient should lose weight or discontinue smoking is successful in only a small minority of cases, but it is an excellent first step toward health promotion and disease prevention (Chap. 393).

Physician-directed dietary interventions commonly lower the serum cholesterol level by as much as 10 percent. Drug treatment may be more effective but is more expensive. For example, treatment with lovastatin in men for the primary prevention of coronary heart disease costs more than $50,000 per year of life saved except in very high risk persons. Treatment strategies for hypertension are more cost-effective; the approximate cost of screening and treating hypertension, given the average medication compliance rates and treatment with a generic beta-adrenergic antagonist, ranges from a projection of about $15,000 per year of life saved for a patient with a diastolic blood pressure of 105 mmHg or higher to about $25,000 to $30,000 for a person with a diastolic blood pressure of 95 to 104 mmHg. Costs would be higher with more expensive medications, although the cost could be warranted if a reduction in side effects led to an improvement in an individual's quality of life.

Immunizations, including pneumococcal and influenza vaccination in elderly and high-risk patients, are effective ways to reduce disease and its associated costs. Guidelines for immunizations in adults are indicated in Table 9-3 (see also Chap. 82).

DIAGNOSTIC TESTING   As detailed in Chap. 10, diagnostic tests are valuable only to the extent that they provide new, *incremental* information that cannot be obtained less expensively from the history, physical examination, or other less expensive tests. Although these tests may often be of psychological benefit in reassuring the patient or the physician, they commonly generate redundant information, often result in a needless expense, and may entail risk. For example, in the evaluation of left ventricular function, the physician must decide whether a two-dimensional echocardiogram is sufficient or the more precise but more expensive measurement by radionuclide ventriculography is worthwhile. The physician faces analogous choices when deciding whether to obtain both an abdominal ultrasound examination and an abdominal CT or, in a different case, whether CT and MRI of the head are both required.

Ideally, each test should be ordered in sequence only to the extent that it is expected to add to the data available. However, this iterative approach can be expensive in hospitalized patients, where the sequencing of tests may lead to delays in scheduling and performing them. In these situations, the expense of the additional days of waiting may more than offset the savings from possibly avoiding a particular test. Usually, careful consideration of the problem by a physician is one of the most cost-effective ways to evaluate the patient. Expert consultation may be more cost-effective and helpful than ordering more diagnostic tests. Although interventions designed to reduce test utilization have met with variable success, those which have been successful have generally included educational components, full endorsement by locally respected leaders, and frequent reinforcement.

TREATMENT CHOICES   In choosing among various treatments, physicians try to enhance the likelihood of an optimal outcome. It is important to consider whether an equivalent outcome could be achieved at a lower cost. For example, generic medications may be substituted for more expensive brand-name counterparts. Similarly, outcome is not usually compromised by interventions designed to encourage the use of less expensive antibiotic regimens. Endorsement by the medical profession of restricted indications for procedures such as pacemaker implantation and tonsillectomy have led to decreased utilization without any detectable reduction in life expectancy or quality of life. Whenever possible, diagnostic and therapeutic options should be subjected to strict evaluation of both benefit and cost-effectiveness, and physicians have responsibility to assist in such evaluations and to learn from their results.

INDIVIDUALIZATION

As already stated, the physician has a moral and legal responsibility to serve as an advocate for the patient, within the limits set by society. This requires an individual approach to the patient and an understanding of how the available resources of the health care system can best be applied to the person and the problem at hand. Nevertheless, the physician and the patient must recognize that expensive medicine is not necessarily better medicine, and physicians should not be induced by financial incentives to order tests that are not necessary.

Special consideration revolves around the use of expensive procedures in medical care, such as liver, heart, and bone marrow transplantation. In these situations, the limited availability of donors makes it necessary to choose the best possible recipients from among a wide range of potential candidates and to "ration." Although rationing is not pleasant, physicians have often responded well in situations with limited resources. For example, when faced with a reduction in intensive care unit availability, physicians are usually successful at maintaining normal admission rates for patients who most require intensive care so that little, if any, adverse effects occur in those excluded from intensive care.

There is marked variability in the rates at which various procedures are performed in different geographic areas, even though there are no obvious differences in the types or ages of patients. To date, little difference in health care outcomes can be detected despite wide differences in the rates of various procedures. These variations may in part be related to patients' preferences and in part to differing beliefs among physicians regarding optimal medical care choices. When the records of patients who have undergone such procedures are reviewed to determine how the indications for their procedure compared with the standards recommended by experts, a substantial proportion of procedures are deemed inappropriate. However, so far there is no close correlation between the percentage of cases deemed inappropriate and the rate at which the procedure is performed in a given location. There is no definitive evidence that high rates of performance can be equated with a high rate of unnecessary use.

The variations in rates of utilization, the proportion of cases in which some procedures seem not to be necessary, and the ability of physicians to respond to situations in which rationing is necessary suggest that in many situations the quality of medical care and the likelihood of a favorable outcome can be maintained while lowering costs. Society, with the input of physicians, must exercise this role without compromising the physician's responsibility to the individual patient and without restricting access on the basis of sex, socioeconomic status, or ethnic background.

REFERENCES

DETSKY AS, NAGLIE IG: A clinician's guide to cost-effectiveness analysis. Ann Intern Med 113:147, 1990

ENTHOVEN A, KRONICK R: A consumer-choice health plan for the 1990s: Universal health insurance in a system designed to promote quality and economy. N Engl J Med 320:29, 1989

FUCHS VR, HAHN JS: How does Canada do it? A comparison of expenditures for physicians' services in the United States and Canada. N Engl J Med 323:884, 1990

GOLDBERGER AL, O'KONSKI MS: Utility of the routine electrocardiogram before surgery and on general hospital admission: Critical review and new guidelines, in *Common Diagnostic Tests: Use and Interpretation*, 2d ed, HC Sox Jr (ed). Chicago, American College of Physicians, 1990, pp. 67–78

GOLDMAN L: Cost-effective strategies in cardiology, in *Heart Disease*, 4th ed, E Braunwald (ed). Philadelphia, Saunders, 1992, pp 1694–1707

HAYWARD RSA et al: Preventive care guidelines: 1991. Ann Intern Med 114:758, 1991

HEMENWAY D et al: Physicians' responses to financial incentives: Evidence from a for-profit ambulatory care center. N Engl J Med 322:1059, 1990

HSIAO WC et al: Assessing the implementation of physician-payment reform. N Engl J Med 328:928, 1993

——— et al: Special report: Results and policy implications of the resource-based relative-value study. N Engl J Med 319:881, 1988

IGLEHART JK: The American health care system. N Engl J Med 326:962, 1992

LEVY JM et al: Impact of the Medicare fee schedule on payments to physicians. JAMA 264:717, 1990

REDELMEIER DA, FUCHS VR: Health expenditures in the United States and Canada. N Engl J Med 328:772, 1993

SCHWARTZ WB, MENDELSON DN: Hospital cost containment in the 1980s: Hard lessons learned and prospects for the 1990s. N Engl J Med 324:1037, 1991

WOOLHANDLER S, HIMMELSTEIN DU: The deteriorating administrative efficiency of the U.S health care system. N Engl J Med 324:1253, 1991

10 QUANTITATIVE ASPECTS OF CLINICAL REASONING

LEE GOLDMAN

The process of clinical reasoning is poorly understood but is based on factors such as experience and learning, inductive and deductive reasoning, interpretation of evidence that itself varies in reproducibility and validity, and intuition that often is difficult to define. In an effort to improve clinical reasoning, a number of attempts have been made to analyze quantitatively the many factors involved, including defining the cognitive approaches that clinicians apply to difficult problems, devising computerized decision support systems that are designed to emulate certain features of decision making, and applying decision theory to understand how judgments should be reached. While each of these approaches has advanced the understanding of the diagnostic process, all have practical and/or theoretical problems that limit their direct applicability to the care of the individual patient.

Nevertheless, these preliminary attempts to apply the rigor and logic inherent in the quantitative method have provided significant insights into the process by which clinical reasoning is accomplished, have identified ways in which the process may be improved, and have made it possible to minimize certain features of the workup that are not cost-effective. Thus, while clinical reasoning cannot be reduced to probabilities or numbers, attempts at quantitative analysis of the process may improve the ways in which the problems of individual patients are approached and solved.

In a simplified model, quantitative clinical reasoning includes five phases. The *first* consists of an investigation of the chief complaint through key questions that are included in the history of the present illness (Table 10-1). These questions are supplemented by the past medical history and by a physical examination that emphasizes detailed investigation of potential key organ systems. In the *second* phase, the physician may select from an array of diagnostic tests, each with its own accuracy and usefulness for investigating the possibilities raised in the differential diagnosis. Since each test has its costs, and some entail risk and discomfort as well, the physician must ask whether the history and physical examination are sufficiently diagnostic before ordering tests. *Third*, the clinical data must be integrated with test results to estimate the likelihood of conditions in the differential diagnosis. *Fourth*, the comparative risks and benefits of further diagnostic and therapeutic options must be weighed to reach a recommendation for the patient. In the *fifth* and final phase, this recommendation is presented to the patient, and after appropriate discussion of the options, a therapeutic plan is initiated. Each of the five steps in this simplified model of the clinical reasoning process can be analyzed individually.

HISTORY AND PHYSICAL EXAMINATION It originally had been assumed that physicians begin investigating a patient's chief complaint by obtaining a comprehensive history, which includes many, if not most, of the questions included in a full review of systems, and by performing an all-inclusive physical examination. However, experienced clinicians begin to form hypotheses based on the chief complaint and on the responses to initial questioning, and they ask further questions in a sequence that allows them to evaluate the initial hypotheses and, if necessary, shorten or amend the list of possibilities. Only a limited number of diagnostic hypotheses can be entertained at any one time, and information is used to build a case for or against the most likely. In such a way, high-priority questions are selected from the almost limitless number that might be asked, and these specific questions are incorporated into the history of the present illness. Often, a key response, such as a history of melena, will be selected, a list of potential explanations for it will be formulated, and this list will then be trimmed, based on the response to more probing questions, so that a principal diagnosis can be selected and then tested. This process, termed *iterative hypothesis testing*, is an efficient approach to diagnosis and is preferable to attempts to gather every conceivable piece of information prior to formulating a differential diagnosis.

Advocacy of iterative hypothesis testing does not argue against the need for a systematic, thorough, and complete history of the present illness, past medical history, review of systems, family history, social history, and physical examination. For example, if a patient presents with abdominal pain, the physician should gather information regarding its location and quality as well as the factors that precipitate and/or relieve it. The physician then asks questions relating to the diagnoses that may be suspected based on the response to the initial questions. If the pain is suggestive of pancreatitis, the clinician would ask about alcohol intake, the use of thiazide diuretics or glucocorticosteroids, symptoms suggestive of concomitant gallbladder disease, a family history of pancreatitis, and questions aimed at uncovering the possibility of a posterior penetrating ulcer. Alternatively, if the discomfort seems more typical of reflux esophagitis, a different sequence of questions would be triggered. The use of iterative hypothesis testing encourages the physician to elicit detailed information in high-yield areas, without forgoing a systematic and thorough approach to the patient. Findings on the history and physical examination should influence each other. The history focuses the physical examination on certain organs, and findings on physical examination should encourage more detailed review of certain systems.

As physicians proceed through this reasoning process with both the history and physical examination, a variety of issues may influence the accuracy of the decision-making process. First is the potential for some historical information or physical findings to be poorly reproducible, either because the patient's responses vary or because different physicians elicit information differently or vary in the way they interpret the answers. The careful use of clear and, when possible, precise questions can increase the reproducibility and validity of the medical history but still cannot eliminate all variability.

When assessing the reproducibility of findings on the physical examination, two observers frequently agree that an uncommon abnormality such as an enlarged spleen is not present but agree less often when one of them thinks that it is present in a patient in whom it would not usually be expected. This principle can best be demonstrated by understanding that some agreement always occurs by chance, and the likelihood of chance agreement is higher if the finding is either very common or very uncommon. For example, if two physicians each consider 90 percent of patients to be abnormal in some manner, such as having a systolic heart murmur, they will agree 81 percent of the time by chance alone. In some studies of the reproducibility of common signs and symptoms, such as an enlarged liver, actual agreement rates have not been substantially better than chance. Disagreement rates may be reduced by emphasizing physical examination skills during medical training, by looking for other correlative physical findings, and by learning how physical findings correlate with the results of diagnostic tests. Therefore, when a clinician notes an unexpected and somewhat subjective abnormality for which there may be a high rate of interobserver disagreement, such as an unexpectedly enlarged spleen, other abnormalities that may often be associated with it, such as hepatomegaly or lymphadenopathy,

---

TABLE 10-1 Phases of clinical reasoning and decision making

1. Investigation of the complaint by means of clinical examination (history and physical examination)
2. Ordering of diagnostic tests, each with its own intrinsic accuracy and usefulness
3. Integration of clinical findings with test results to assess diagnostic probabilities
4. Weighing of comparative risks and benefits of alternative courses of action
5. Determination of patient's preferences and development of a therapeutic plan

should be sought to increase the likelihood that the spleen would be expected to be abnormal. In some situations, ordering a diagnostic test, such as an abdominal ultrasound, to assess the finding more objectively should be considered if the test is sufficiently reliable.

These comments about the factors that limit the reproducibility and validity of the medical history and physical examination do not denigrate their critical importance in clinical reasoning. Rather, they emphasize that care and diligence in the application of these skills are necessary. For example, careful auscultation of the heart during various bedside maneuvers (see Chap. 188) has been shown to be remarkably accurate in determining the cause of systolic murmurs.

When physicians use the history and the physical examination to arrive at a diagnosis, they are rarely certain of it. Therefore, it would be better to assess the likelihood of the diagnosis in terms of probabilities. All too frequently this probability is not expressed as an actual percentage but rather in such terms as "nearly always," "commonly," "sometimes," or "rarely." Since different physicians may assign different probabilities to the same terms, these imprecise words frequently lead to major misunderstandings among physicians or between the physician and the patient. Physicians should be as rigorous and quantitative as possible in their assessments, and when feasible, a quantitative expression of probability should be used. For example, rather than saying that it is unlikely that a radiographic pattern is indicative of a carcinoma of the colon, it would be preferable, if possible, to provide a more precise indication of the probability of carcinoma with this radiographic pattern. A 10 to 15 percent probability of carcinoma may be interpreted as "unlikely" but from a clinical perspective usually warrants further evaluation because of the serious consequences of missing a potentially resectable tumor.

Although such quantitative estimates would be desirable, they usually are not available in practice. Even experienced physicians often are unable to estimate accurately the likelihood of particular conditions. There is a tendency to overestimate the likelihood of relatively uncommon conditions, and physicians are especially poor at quantifying probabilities that are very high or very low. For example, a physician may not know whether the probability of bacterial meningitis or of another disease that could be diagnosed by a lumbar puncture in a patient with a severe headache is 1 in 20 or 1 in 2000. In both situations, the probability is low, but the decision as to whether a lumbar puncture should be performed may depend on this estimate.

As was emphasized in Chap. 1, the history and physical examination have other important purposes. They allow the physician to evaluate the emotional status of the patient and to understand how the present problems fit into the context of the patient's social and family life, and they encourage the development in the patient of confidence in the physician, which is so necessary for reaching an agreement on the coming plan of action.

DIAGNOSTIC TESTS: INDICATIONS, ACCURACY, AND USEFULNESS A diagnostic test should be ordered for specified clinical indications, be sufficiently accurate to be efficacious for such indications, and be the least expensive and/or risky of the available efficacious tests. No diagnostic test is totally accurate, and physicians often have difficulty interpreting test results. It is therefore critical to understand several commonly used terms in test analysis and epidemiology, including prevalence, sensitivity, specificity, positive predictive value, and negative predictive value (Table 10-2).

Although reports of the accuracies of diagnostic tests are commonly expressed in terms of positive and negative predictive values, these calculated values are dependent on the prevalence of the disease in the population being studied (Table 10-3). A test with a particular sensitivity and specificity has different positive and negative predictive values when used in groups of patients that have different prevalences of disease. For example, a mildly abnormal alkaline phosphatase level in a young adult with a known lymphoma suggests hepatic involvement by the tumor (i.e., it is likely to be a *true positive*), while the same alkaline phosphatase level as part of a routine screening

TABLE 10-2 Definitions of commonly used terms in epidemiology and decision making

Test result	Disease state		
	Present		Absent
Positive	a (true positive)		b (false positive)
Negative	c (false negative)		d (true negative)
Prevalence (prior probability)	=	$(a + c)/(a + b + c + d)$	= all patients with the disease/all patients tested
Sensitivity	=	$a/(a + c)$	= true-positive test results/all patients with the disease
Specificity	=	$d/(b + d)$	= true-negative test results/all patients without the disease
False-negative rate	=	$c/(a + c)$	= false-negative test results/all patients with the disease
False-positive rate	=	$b/(b + d)$	= false-positive test results/all patients without the disease
Positive predictive value	=	$a/(a + b)$	= true-positive test results/all positive test results
Negative predictive value	=	$d/(c + d)$	= true-negative test results/all patients with negative results
Overall accuracy	=	$(a + d)/(a + b + c + d)$	= true-positive + true-negative test results/all tests

battery of blood tests in an asymptomatic person of the same age is unlikely to be due to tumor (i.e., in this setting it is more likely to be a *false positive*).

Although the sensitivity and specificity of a test do not depend on the prevalence (or percentage of patients being tested who have the disease), they do depend on the spectrum of patients in whom the test is being evaluated. For example, measurement of a prostate-specific antigen for diagnosing carcinoma of the prostate (see Chap. 323) will appear to have a nearly perfect sensitivity and specificity if the diseased population has a palpable prostate nodule and an elevated serum acid phosphatase level while the nondiseased population is composed of normal medical students. If, however, without changing the prevalence of disease in the population being tested, the spectrum of the diseased and nondiseased patients is altered by including patients with other characteristics (i.e., if the population of patients with carcinoma of the prostate were composed principally of those without palpable nodules and with stage 1 disease, while the population without carcinoma of the prostate included elderly men with marked benign prostate hypertrophy), the sensitivity and specificity of the test would change dramatically. In the latter situation, the sensitivity and specificity of the prostate-specific antigen are not only lower than in the first example, because the spectrum of diseased and nondiseased patients has been changed, but more important, they may be so low that the test is of limited clinical value. This example also demonstrates the methodologic problems encountered when applying data from one study to a different type of patient or when pooling data from studies of different subsets of patients.

In some situations, uncertainty about the sensitivity and specificity of the test in the type of patient being assessed may limit its clinical value. Since the physician rarely knows (or can know) the population on which every test that is ordered has been standardized, the results provide information that is far less decisive than usually thought. Furthermore, it may be quite difficult to distinguish random laboratory errors from test results that might be falsely positive or negative because of coexistence of a process that can affect the test, such as the finding of an elevated level of CK in a patient who has undergone strenuous exercise and is being evaluated for chest pain.

Because no single value or cutoff point of an individual test can be expected to have both a perfect sensitivity and a perfect specificity,

TABLE 10-3 How the positive and negative predictive values of the same test vary depending on the prior probability of disease

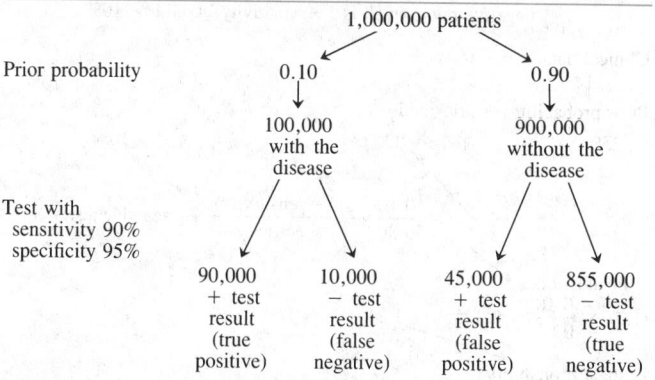

INTERPRETATION OF TEST RESULT WHEN 10% OF PATIENTS TESTED HAVE THE DISEASE (PRIOR PROBABILITY = 10%)

The probability of disease in a patient with a positive test result (positive predictive value) = 90,000/135,000 = 67%

The probability of no disease in a patient with a negative test result (negative predictive value) = 855,000/865,000 = 99%

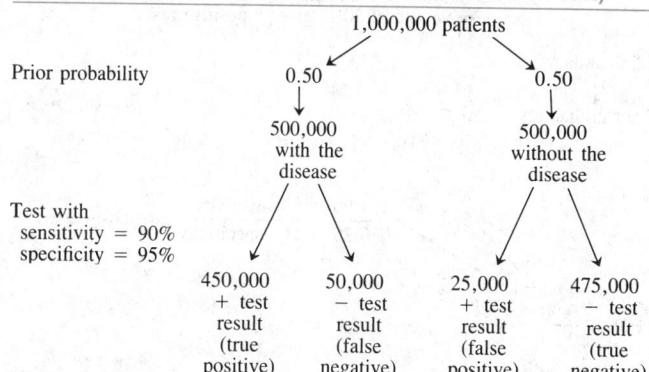

INTERPRETATION OF TEST RESULT WHEN 50% OF PATIENTS TESTED HAVE THE DISEASE (PRIOR PROBABILITY = 50%)

The probability of disease in a patient with a positive test result (positive predictive value) = 450,000/475,000 = 95%

The probability of no disease in a patient with a negative test result (negative predictive value) = 475,000/525,000 = 90%

it is often necessary to determine which value or cutoff point is the most appropriate to guide decision making. A graph (Fig. 10-1) of the test's *receiver operating characteristic curve*, which displays the inevitable trade-off between emphasizing a high sensitivity, such as defining an exercise electrocardiogram as abnormal if it shows ≥0.5 mm of ST-segment depression, versus emphasizing a high specificity, such as defining an exercise electrocardiogram as abnormal only if it shows ≥2.0 mm of ST-segment depression, can help the clinician understand the implications of various definitions of a "positive" test result. Such a graph demonstrates that different definitions of normal versus abnormal may be appropriate depending on whether one wishes to rule in the disease via a positive result on a test that has a high specificity or to exclude the disease via a negative result on a test that has a high sensitivity. Different tests may have different sensitivities and specificities, and better tests may have both a higher sensitivity and a higher specificity than poorer tests.

FIGURE 10-1 The inherent trade-off between sensitivity and specificity. For any diagnostic test, an increase in sensitivity will be associated with a decline in specificity. The closer this curve comes to the upper-left-hand corner, the more useful the test; the closer to the broken line, the less useful it is. When deciding on the cutoff between normal versus abnormal, one must determine what sensitivity and specificity are most useful clinically.

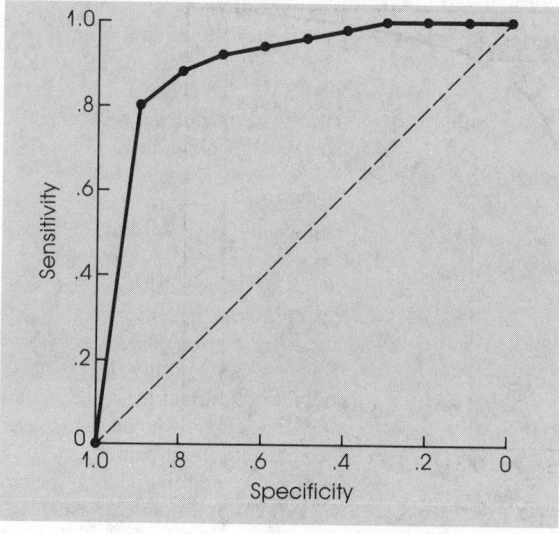

One example of a sensitive test is an enzyme-linked immunosorbent assay (ELISA) to test for the presence of antibodies to human immunodeficiency virus type 1 (HIV-1). This relatively inexpensive test has a high sensitivity for detecting HIV-1 antibodies but is not sufficiently specific to be used as the basis for making a firm diagnosis. Thus, if the ELISA assay is positive, it is commonly repeated. Confirmation of the diagnosis of HIV-1 antibody positivity requires a western blot, or an equivalently specific test, to exclude the possibility of a false-positive ELISA assay (see Chap. 279). A common example of a reasonably specific test would be an electrocardiogram to diagnose acute myocardial infarction. While the precise specificity depends on the spectrum of patients being tested, the presence of new ST-segment elevations exceeding 1.0 mm in two or more electrically contiguous leads in patients who present to an emergency department with prolonged acute chest pain consistent with myocardial ischemia is sufficiently specific, i.e., sufficiently unlikely to be a false-positive result, that admission to an intensive care unit is virtually always recommended. However, this test is not sensitive, and if admission to the unit were restricted to patients with this electrocardiographic finding, almost half of patients with myocardial infarctions presenting to hospital emergency departments would be missed.

To optimize the clinical value of a diagnostic test, it is helpful to obtain local experience with it; often its value will differ from that reported in the literature. Reports of the efficacy of a test should emphasize its accuracy when compared with an independent standard, and the test must be evaluated in a spectrum of patients with varying severities of the disease in question and in patients who have conditions that are part of the same differential diagnosis. The reproducibility of the test should be known, and the "normal limits" of the test should be clear and appropriate. In some instances, the test or procedure required to establish the validity of a diagnostic test is so risky that only a skewed sample of patients is included in a study, as, for example, in the analysis of the usefulness of the abdominal CT scan in patients with suspected pancreatic carcinoma. If patients with "negative" CT scan results never come to laparotomy or postmortem examination, neither the sensitivity nor specificity of the CT scan for pancreatic carcinoma can be assessed. In such situations, an estimated value of the diagnostic test may be inaccurate because it has not been validated.

INTEGRATION OF CLINICAL DATA AND TEST RESULTS Although, as we have seen, neither clinical data nor test results may be entirely accurate, the integration of the two can lead to better diagnostic predictions than either alone. By knowing the probability

TABLE 10-4   Example of the use of Bayesian analysis to integrate the pretest probability with the test result to calculate a posttest probability

Example 1: Prior probability of disease = 25%; a test with a sensitivity (true-positive rate) of 90% and a specificity of 80% (which implies a false-positive rate of 20%) gives a positive result

Example 2: Same pretest probability and test, but now the test gives a negative result. Here the true-negative rate would be 80% and the false-negative rate (which is 1 − sensitivity) would be 10%.

* Sensitivity = probability of a positive test result in a patient with the disease
† (1 − specificity) = probability of a positive test result in a patient without the disease

‡ (1 − sensitivity) = probability of a negative test result in a patient with the disease.
§ Specificity = probability of a negative test result in a patient without the disease.

that the patient has a particular condition before a test is performed (the prior, or pretest, probability), and by knowing the sensitivity and the specificity of the test, the posttest probability can be calculated. A common mathematical technique for integrating clinical data and a test result is the odds-likelihood form of Bayesian analysis (Table 10-4). A pretest probability can be expressed as odds (as in a horse race, for example) and multiplied by the likelihood ratio (which is the sensitivity of the test divided by 1 minus the specificity of the test) to yield the posttest odds, which may be transformed back into a posttest probability. This approach can be employed in any situation in which the physician can use clinical findings to estimate a pretest diagnostic probability and integrate this with the result as well as the sensitivity and specificity of the diagnostic test. Many clinical situations may be so complex that it is not practical to estimate the prior probabilities of all likely diagnoses or to know the sensitivities and specificities of each of the tests that might be performed individually or in sequence. Nevertheless, attempts in this direction will stimulate critical thinking, expose uncertainties, and generate ideas for original investigations or a review of past experiences to facilitate the application of Bayesian analysis to the integration of clinical data and laboratory tests.

The results of Bayesian analyses often can be expressed in graphic form, such as the value of exercise electrocardiograms for predicting the presence of coronary artery disease (Fig. 10-2; also see Chap. 203). This series of curves also demonstrates how to consider a test whose result may be in the "gray zone" rather than clearly positive or clearly negative.

One of the key assumptions inherent in most such analyses is that

FIGURE 10-2 How the exercise tolerance test affects the probability of coronary artery disease. The before-test probability of coronary artery disease (CAD) will be modified by the result of the exercise electrocardiogram to yield an after-test probability of CAD. Note that the finding of <1 mm of ST-segment depression will reduce the probability of CAD, whereas ≥1 mm of ST-segment depression will increase the probability. For example, if a patient with a before-test probability of CAD of 90 percent (about that of a middle-aged man with typical anginal symptoms) had 2 to 2.49 mm on ST-segment depression on exercise testing, the after-test probability of CAD would be 99.5 percent. In contrast, the same exercise test result in a patient with 30 percent before-test probability of CAD (about that of a patient with atypical anginal symptoms) would yield an after-test probability of about 90 percent. In an asymptomatic patient, with a before-test probability of about 5 percent, the same exercise test result would yield an after-test probability of 53 percent. Thus the same test yields different after-test probabilities in patients with different before-test probabilities. (*Adapted, with permission of the New England Journal of Medicine, from RD Rifkin, WB Hood, Bayesian analysis of electrocardiographic exercise stress testing. N Engl J Med 297:684, 1977.*)

the correlation between the pretest probability and the test result is no greater than expected by chance. If the diagnostic test simply duplicates information that has already been obtained by the clinical examination, it will not have any additional benefit for predicting whether or not the disease is present. For example, in trying to determine whether or not a patient with carcinoma of the colon has hepatic metastases, the finding of jaundice on physical examination should be a strong predictor. The degree of hyperbilirubinemia also can be measured, but the bilirubin level in a patient with clinical jaundice does not add substantial *independent* information to that obtained by a careful physical examination. When integrating a diagnostic test with clinical information, the test is helpful only when it adds incremental information to what can be inferred based on the history and physical examination and on prior, less costly or less risky diagnostic tests. If a diagnostic test (such as a retrograde cholangiogram in a patient with hyperbilirubinemia) provides information that cannot be inferred directly, it is less likely that its results are associated with pretest probabilities to an extent greater than would be expected by chance.

A diagnostic test has an impact on the evaluation of a specific patient only if it changes the diagnostic probability to the extent that the new probability dictates a change in the diagnostic strategy or therapeutic plans or if the test serves as part of a sequence of tests that moves the probability across such a threshold. An example is a patient suspected of having a pulmonary embolism, with an estimated probability of 50 percent based on clinical data alone. Performing a "low probability" pulmonary ventilation-perfusion scan may reduce the probability of pulmonary embolism, but if the goal is to exclude pulmonary embolism with the highest possible degree of certainty, a pulmonary angiogram would be required (Chap. 226).

Because diagnostic tests often do not provide important new information even when their results are accurate, several questions should be considered in deciding when to order diagnostic tests. First, how likely is the disease in question? Second, what would be the clinical consequences if the diagnosis were missed or if the patient were mistakenly treated for a disease that is not present? Third, what is the likelihood that the diagnostic test will change the probability sufficiently to have an effect on either diagnosis or therapy? The physician should consider the probabilities, the risks, the likelihood and costs of obtaining new information, and the adverse consequences of delay, because observation and follow-up are always among the available diagnostic options.

Since the establishment of valid diagnostic probabilities is a cornerstone to clinical reasoning, accumulated clinical experience, often in the form of computerized data banks, has been used to generate statistical approaches for improving diagnostic predictions. In such research, it is common to begin by identifying individual factors that have a univariate correlation with the diagnosis in question. Then these univariate correlates may be included in a multivariate analysis to determine which of them are significant independent predictors of the diagnosis. Some analyses may identify the important predictive factors and then assign them "weights," which can be transformed to calculate a probability. Alternatively, the analysis may result in a limited number of categories of patients, each with a discrete probability of the diagnosis.

These quantitative approaches to the estimation of various diagnostic probabilities, which are often termed "prediction rules," are especially helpful if they are in a format that is readily usable by the clinician and if they have been validated prospectively on a sufficient number and spectrum of patients. For example, by carefully defining the key historical questions, findings on physical examination, and electrocardiographic abnormalities that might predict the probability of acute myocardial infarction among emergency department patients with chest pain, a protocol was devised and shown in prospective validation testing to have the same sensitivity as physicians for identifying infarction and at the same time to have a significantly higher specificity.

For such prediction rules to be useful to the clinician, they must be derived from relevant patient populations and use tests that are reproducible and readily available so that the results can be extrapolated to local medical practice. Since only a minority of published prediction rules have adhered to rigid criteria as to the number and spectrum of patients examined and their prospective validation, most are not yet suitable for routine clinical application. Furthermore, many prediction rules cannot evaluate the probability of each of the diagnoses or outcomes that the clinician must consider.

COMPARING RISKS AND BENEFITS: DECISION ANALYSIS

Inherent in the concept that probabilities can guide decision making is the assumption that one can arrive at a reasonable threshold by knowing the relative risks (or costs) and benefits of various options and deciding at what probability this ratio changes to favor an alternative strategy. Decision analysis is an organized process for evaluating such situations and identifies the key issues and problems.

One problem with applying decision-analysis techniques to difficult clinical problems is that the decision analysis is no better than the data on which it is based. In some instances, an attempted decision analysis of a complex clinical problem may yield no more information than that the critical data required for the analysis are missing and that more research in the field needs to be performed. In addition, when clinicians are uncertain about diagnostic or therapeutic strategies, formal analyses may indicate that the differences in outcome among various strategies are very small. In such cases, the formal analysis may have such inherent error that it is not definitive. Even when decision analysis is potentially helpful, it may not be feasible to complete the detailed estimations and calculations within the time constraints of bedside decision making. Nevertheless, the value of the analytic approach to decision making is that it integrates available data, mandates rigorous thinking, and exposes areas of uncertainty or ignorance.

Decision analysis depicts graphically two types of issues in the decision-making process: first, the decisions (or choices) available to the physician and, second, the probabilities of all the events that may result from each decision. To illustrate how this process works, consider a very simplified decision analysis of whether to use an intravenous thrombolytic agent in a patient with a suspected acute myocardial infarction (see Chap. 202). Figure 10-3 depicts the simplified decision tree for this problem. The square box or "node" labeled *A* indicates a decision that the physician must make. The circular nodes, labeled *B* through *O*, indicate where different outcomes, each of which has an estimatable probability, could occur. In this analysis, the initial choices were to treat the patient with an intravenous thrombolytic agent or not to treat. The use of such an agent may or may not result in serious complications of therapy, especially bleeding and intracranial hemorrhage.

Each of the possible outcomes for a patient is typically assigned a "utility," which is the relative preference for the outcome, where 1.0 is a perfect outcome and 0 is the worst possible outcome. Each terminal branch of the decision tree is assigned the utility corresponding to its outcome, and the "expected value" of each terminal branch is calculated by multiplying its probability by its utility. To calculate the "expected value" of each of the two possible courses of action (see Fig. 10-3, node *A*), the expected values of each of the terminal branches that originate from it would be summed. The preferred course of action is the one which, when all possible outcomes are considered, including the risks and benefits of therapy, yields the highest expected value, which is the sum of the product of the probability multiplied by the utility for each of its possible outcomes.

In performing any decision analysis, the relevant probabilities must be known or estimated, a process that sometimes requires guesswork. Next, utilities could be assigned to each of these outcomes. A major practical limitation of decision analysis is the subjective judgment often required to estimate utilities. It is also difficult to adjust future years of life for their quality in any numerical fashion, e.g., in considering how treatment complications, such as an intracranial hemorrhage, or the advantages of treatment, such as congestive

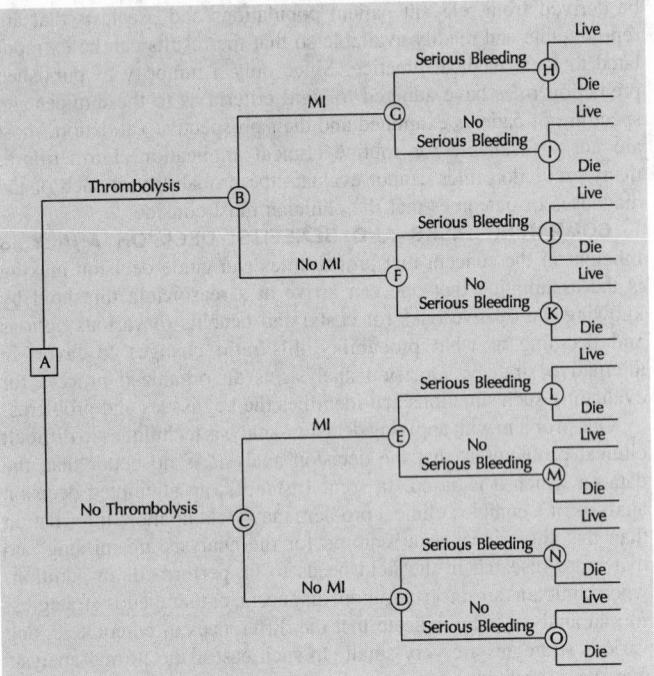

FIGURE 10-3 Simplified decision tree for the decision of whether or not to use an intravenous thrombolytic agent in a patient with a suspected acute myocardial infarction. The square node represents the decision point, and the round nodes denote chance events (see text for details).

heart failure averted because an infarction was smaller, affect the quality of future years of life.

The results and usefulness of a decision analysis depend on the probabilities and utilities that are used in the calculation, and it is imperative for decision analyses to include a *sensitivity analysis*, in which various estimates for each probability are included in the analysis to determine if the conclusions would be changed. For example, in the analysis in Fig. 10-3, some range of probabilities must be assumed for the risk of serious bleeding complications and for the likelihood that any particular patient is having an acute myocardial infarction. Because of the impressive benefit of thrombolysis for improving survival in patients with acute myocardial infarctions, decision analyses have shown treatment to be the preferred option even when an acute myocardial infarction is not certain and even in most elderly patients. If the conclusions of an analysis were altered by relatively minor changes in the assumptions on which it was based, the analysis would not be sufficiently reliable to become the basis for decision making.

Decision analysis sometimes demonstrates a clear and dramatic advantage with one particular option. In other circumstances, there may be little difference between two options; either option may be reasonable, or secondary issues that cannot be taken into account in the formal analysis, such as the patient's feelings about taking risks or the recent local experience with particular interventions, should be the final determinants in the decision. Physicians who perform a decision analysis therefore must determine the probabilities of each of the possible events by reviewing the pertinent patient experience at their own institution or practice or by reviewing the pertinent literature. Even when the outcome of the analysis seems clear, the physician or the patient may believe that the situation in question is

an exception to the rule. Furthermore, even the best analyses, like all clinical intuition, are based on assumptions that may be open to debate.

In the preceding example, dealing with whether or not to use a thrombolytic agent in a patient with a suspected acute myocardial infarction, decision analysis indicated the preferred strategy in terms of outcome but did not consider the costs at which such benefits might be achieved. In determining health policy, a formal cost-effectiveness analysis can be performed to determine how many dollars must be spent to achieve a unit of benefit, often defined as a life saved, a year of life saved, or a quality-adjusted year of life saved, in which the years are adjusted to take into account the quality of life during that time. For example, in 1994 dollars, 1 year of in-center hemodialysis can be estimated to cost about $35,000 to $45,000 per quality-adjusted year of life saved; this figure includes only the direct medical costs and not indirect costs related to issues such as time lost or travel or any benefits in terms of a patient's ability to work. In some situations, the ability of the patient to maintain gainful employment may offset some or all of the direct medical expenses. In other situations, such as with pneumococcal vaccine, the savings from episodes of pneumonia that are averted may more than offset the cost of the vaccine in high-risk persons.

ETHICS AND PATIENT INPUT   In both quantitative and nonquantitative clinical reasoning, the physician must consider ethical issues as well as the patient's values and preferences. While a detailed discussion of these issues is beyond the scope of this chapter, it is important to emphasize that patients' preferences for alternative therapies may not agree with the preferences that the physicians propose on the basis of their own clinical judgment or the results of a decision-analysis approach. For example, many patients with carcinoma of the larynx may prefer radiation therapy, with a lower cure rate but a higher likelihood of maintaining speech, to extirpative surgery. It is imperative that physicians assess those characteristics of life which the patient prizes most (the elusive ''quality of life'') prior to basing controversial decisions solely on quantitative approaches, the physicians' own subjective impressions of the likely medical benefits, their own personal preferences, or their assumptions about the patient's preferences. While quantitative analyses may apply to groups of patients, judgment must be exercised when adapting them to the individual patient. Therefore, the final plan should reflect an agreement between a well-informed patient and a sympathetic physician who has detailed knowledge of the relevant medical issues and of the impact of the various possible outcomes on the specific patient.

REFERENCES

AMERICAN COLLEGE OF PHYSICIANS: Guidelines for counseling postmenopausal women about preventive hormone therapy. Ann Intern Med 117:1038, 1993

GABLE CB et al: Pneumococcal vaccine: Efficacy and associated cost savings. JAMA 264:2910, 1990

GARNICK MB: Prostate cancer: Screening, diagnosis, and management, Ann Intern Med 118:804, 1993

GOLDMAN L et al: A computer protocol to predict myocardial infarction in emergency department patients with chest pain. N Engl J Med 318:797, 1988

KASSIRER JP: Diagnostic reasoning. Ann Intern Med 110:893, 1989

LEMBO NJ et al: Bedside diagnosis of systolic murmurs. N Engl J Med 318:1572, 1988

MANDEL JS et al: Reducing mortality from colorectal cancer by screening for fecal occult blood. N Engl J Med 328:1365, 1993

SACKETT DL et al: *Clinical Epidemiology: A Basic Science for Clinical Medicine*, 2d ed. Boston, Little, Brown, 1991

SLOAND EM et al: HIV testing: State of the art. JAMA 266:2861, 1991

SOX HC JR (ed): *Common Diagnostic Tests: Use and Interpretation*, 2d ed. Philadelphia, American College of Physicians, 1990

section 1 Pain

11 PAIN: PATHOPHYSIOLOGY AND MANAGEMENT

HOWARD L. FIELDS / JOSEPH B. MARTIN

The task of medicine is to preserve and restore health and to relieve suffering. Understanding pain is essential to both these goals. Because pain is universally understood as a signal of disease, it is the most common symptom that brings a patient to a physician's attention. The function of the pain sensory system is to detect, localize, and identify tissue-damaging processes. Since different diseases produce characteristic patterns of tissue damage, the quality, time course and location of a patient's pain complaint, and the location of tenderness provide important diagnostic clues and are used to evaluate the response to treatment.

THE PAIN SENSORY SYSTEM

Pain is an unpleasant sensation localized to a part of the body. It is often described in terms of a penetrating or tissue-destructive process (e.g., stabbing, burning, twisting, tearing, squeezing) and/or of a bodily or emotional reaction (e.g., terrifying, nauseating, sickening). Furthermore, any pain of moderate or higher intensity is accompanied by anxiety and the urge to escape or terminate the feeling. These properties illustrate the duality of pain: It is both sensation and emotion. When it is acute, pain is characteristically associated with behavioral arousal and a stress response consisting of increased blood pressure, heart rate, pupil diameter, and plasma cortisol levels. In addition, local muscle contraction (e.g., limb flexion, abdominal wall rigidity) is often seen and may produce secondary tenderness.

THE PRIMARY AFFERENT NOCICEPTOR A peripheral nerve consists of the axons of three different types of neurons: primary sensory afferents, motor neurons, and sympathetic postganglionic neurons (Fig. 11-1). The cell bodies of primary afferents are located in the dorsal root ganglia in the vertebral foramina. After emerging from its cell body, the primary afferent axon bifurcates to send one process into the spinal cord and the other to innervate bodily tissues. Primary afferents are classified by their diameter, degree of myelination, and conduction velocity. The largest-diameter fibers, A-beta, respond maximally to light touch and/or moving stimuli; they are present primarily in nerves that innervate the skin. In normal individuals, the activity of these fibers does not produce pain. There are two other classes of primary afferents: the small-diameter myelinated (A-delta) and the unmyelinated (C fiber) axons (see Fig. 11-1). These fibers are present in the nerves to the skin and to deep somatic and visceral structures. Some tissues, such as the cornea, are innervated only by A-delta and C afferents. Most A-delta and C afferents respond maximally only to intense (painful) stimuli and produce pain when they are electrically stimulated; this defines them as *primary afferent nociceptors (pain receptors)*. The ability to detect painful stimuli is completely abolished when A-delta and C axons are blocked.

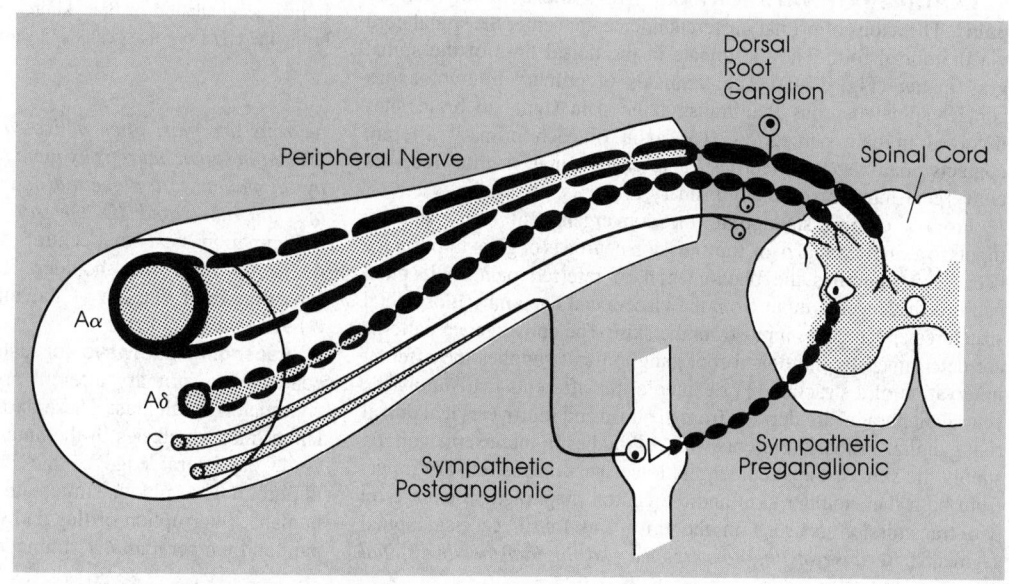

FIGURE 11-1 Components of a typical cutaneous nerve. There are two distinct functional categories of axons: primary afferents with cell bodies in the dorsal root ganglion and sympathetic postganglionic fibers with cell bodies in the sympathetic ganglion. Primary afferents include those with large-diameter myelinated (A-β), small-diameter myelinated (A-δ), and unmyelinated (C) axons. All sympathetic postganglionic fibers are unmyelinated.

Individual primary afferent nociceptors can respond to several different types of noxious stimuli. For example, most nociceptors respond to heating, intense mechanical stimuli such as a pinch, and application of irritating chemicals.

Sensitization   When intense, repeated, or prolonged stimuli are applied, if tissue is damaged or if inflammation is present, the threshold for activating primary afferent nociceptors is lowered and the frequency of firing is higher for all stimulus intensities. This process, called *sensitization*, produces a situation in which stimuli that are normally innocuous can produce pain. Sensitization is a clinically important process that contributes to tenderness, soreness, and hyperalgesia. A striking example of sensitization is sunburned skin in which severe pain can be produced by a gentle slap on the back or a warm shower.

Compared with superficial structures (e.g., skin, cornea), most deep tissues are relatively insensitive to noxious mechanical or thermal stimuli under normal conditions. In contrast, when affected by a disease process with an inflammatory component, deep structures such as joints or hollow viscera characteristically become exquisitely sensitive to mechanical stimulation. Inflammatory mediators such as bradykinin, some prostaglandins, and leukotrienes can activate and/or sensitize primary afferents. (For example, in experimental arthritis produced by Freund's adjuvant, A-delta and C joint afferents are sensitized, and many become active even without mechanical or thermal stimuli.)

Most A-delta and C afferents innervating viscera are completely insensitive in normal noninjured, noninflamed tissue. That is, they cannot be activated by known mechanical or thermal stimuli and are not spontaneously active. However, in the presence of inflammatory mediators, these afferents become sensitive to mechanical stimuli. Such afferents have been termed *silent nociceptors*, and their characteristic properties may explain how under pathologic conditions the relatively insensitive deep structures can become the source of severe and debilitating pain and tenderness.

Nociceptor-Induced Inflammation   One important concept to emerge in recent years is that afferent nociceptors also have a neuroeffector function. Most nociceptors contain polypeptide mediators that are released from their peripheral terminals when they are activated (Fig. 11-2). An example is substance P, an 11 amino acid peptide. Substance P is released from primary afferent nociceptors and has multiple biologic activities. It is a potent vasodilator, degranulates mast cells, is a chemoattractant for leukocytes, and increases the production and release of inflammatory mediators. Interestingly, depletion of substance P from joints reduces the severity of experimental arthritis. Primary afferent nociceptors are not simply passive messengers of threats to tissue injury but also play an active role in tissue protection through these neuroeffector functions.

CENTRAL PATHWAYS FOR PAIN   The spinal cord and referred pain   The axons of primary afferent nociceptors enter the spinal cord via the dorsal root. They terminate in the dorsal horn of the spinal gray matter (Fig. 11-3). The terminals of primary afferent axons contact spinal neurons that transmit the pain signal to brain sites involved in pain perception. The axon of each primary afferent contacts many spinal neurons, and each spinal neuron receives convergent inputs from many primary afferents.

From a clinical standpoint, the convergence of many sensory inputs to a single spinal pain-transmission neuron is of great importance because it underlies the phenomenon of referred pain. All spinal neurons that receive input from the viscera and deep musculoskeletal structures also receive input from the skin. The convergence patterns are determined by the dorsal root ganglion that supplies the afferent innervation of a structure. For example, the afferents that supply the central diaphragm are derived from the third and fourth cervical dorsal root ganglia. Primary afferents with cell bodies in these same ganglia supply the skin of the shoulder and lower neck. Thus sensory inputs from both the shoulder skin and the central diaphragm converge on pain-transmission neurons in the third and fourth cervical spinal segments. *Because of this convergence and the fact that the spinal*

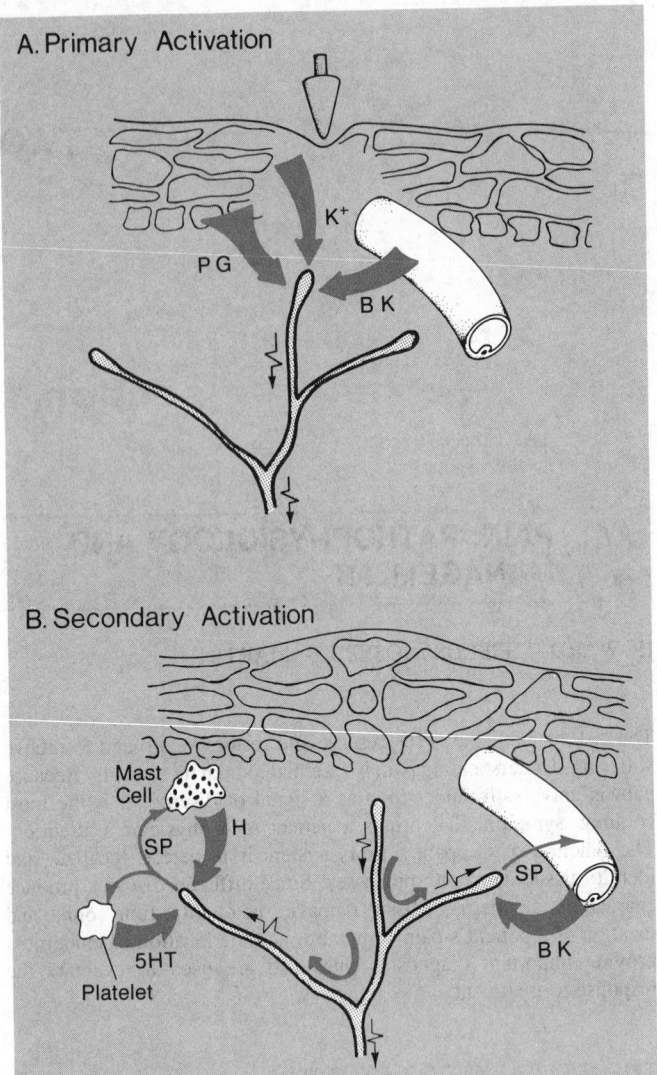

FIGURE 11-2 Events leading to activation, sensitization, and spread of sensitization of primary afferent nociceptor terminals. *A.* Direct activation by intense pressure and consequent cell damage. Cell damage leads to release of potassium (K^+) and to synthesis of prostaglandins (PG) and bradykinin (BK). Prostaglandins increase the sensitivity of the terminal to bradykinin and other pain-producing substances. *B.* Secondary activation. Impulses generated in the stimulated terminal propagate not only to the spinal cord but also into other terminal branches, where they induce the release of peptides, including substance P (SP). Substance P causes vasodilation and neurogenic edema with further accumulation of bradykinin. Substance P also causes the release of histamine (H) from mast cells and serotonin (5HT) from platelets.

neurons are most often activated by inputs from the skin, activity evoked in spinal neurons by input from deep structures is mislocalized by the patient to a place that is roughly coextensive with the region of skin innervated by the same spinal segment. For example, inflammation near the central diaphragm is usually reported as discomfort near the shoulder. This spatial displacement of pain sensation from the site of the injury that produces it is known as *referred pain.*

Ascending pathways for pain   A majority of spinal neurons contacted by primary afferent nociceptors send their axons to the contralateral thalamus. These axons form the contralateral spinothalamic tract which lies in the anterolateral white matter of the spinal cord, the lateral edge of the medulla, and the lateral pons and midbrain. The spinothalamic pathway is crucial for pain sensation in humans. Interruption of this pathway produces permanent deficits in pain and temperature discrimination.

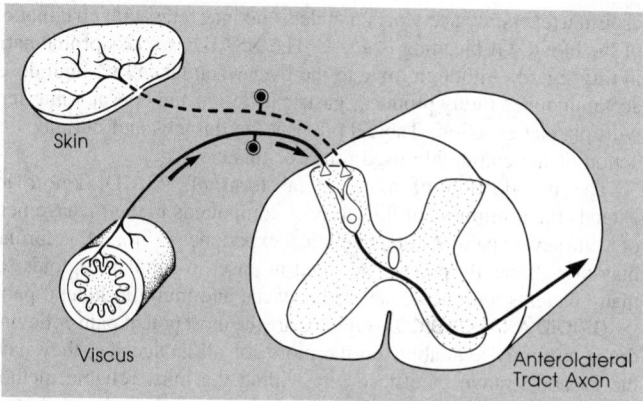

FIGURE 11-3 The convergence-projection hypothesis of referred pain. According to this hypothesis, visceral afferent nociceptors (S) converge on the same pain-projection neurons as the afferents from the somatic structures in which the pain is perceived. The brain has no way of knowing the actual source of input and mistakenly "projects" the sensation to the somatic structure.

One major target area for spinothalamic tract axons is the ventrobasal region of the thalamus (Fig. 11-4). Spinothalamic tract axons connect to thalamic neurons that project to somatosensory cortex. This pathway from spinal cord to thalamus to somatosensory cortex appears to be particularly important for the sensory aspects of pain, i.e., its location, intensity, and quality. Spinothalamic tract axons also connect to medial thalamic regions linked with the frontal cortex and the limbic system. This pathway is thought to subserve the affective or unpleasant emotional dimension of pain.

PAIN MODULATION The pain produced by similar injuries is remarkably variable in different situations and in different people. For example, athletes have been known to sustain serious fractures with only minor pain, and Beecher's classic World War II survey revealed that many men were unbothered by battle injuries that would

have produced agonizing pain in civilian patients. Furthermore, even the suggestion of relief (placebo) has a significant analgesic effect. On the other hand, many patients find even minor injuries (such as venipuncture) unbearable, and the expectation of pain has been demonstrated to induce pain *without a noxious stimulus*.

The powerful effect of expectation and other psychologic variables on the perceived intensity of pain implies the existence of brain circuits that can modulate the activity of the pain-transmission pathways. Although there are probably several circuits that can modulate pain, only one has been studied extensively. This circuit has links in the hypothalamus, midbrain, and medulla, and it selectively controls spinal pain-transmission neurons through a descending pathway (see Fig. 11-4).

There is good evidence that this pain-modulating circuit contributes to the pain-relieving effect of narcotic analgesic medications. Each of the component structures of the pathway contains opioid receptors and is sensitive to the direct application of opioid drugs. Furthermore, lesions of the system reduce the analgesic effect of systemically administered opioids such as morphine. Along with the opioid receptor, the component nuclei of this pain-modulating circuit contain endogenous opioid peptides such as the enkephalins and beta-endorphin.

The most reliable way to activate this endogenous opioid-mediated modulating system is by prolonged pain and/or fear. There is evidence that pain-relieving endogenous opioids are released following operative procedures and in patients given a placebo for pain relief.

Pain modulation is bidirectional. Pain-modulating circuits not only produce analgesia but are also capable of increasing pain. Both pain-inhibiting and pain-facilitating neurons in the medulla project to and control spinal pain-transmission neurons. Since pain-transmission neurons can be activated by modulatory neurons, it is theoretically possible to generate a pain signal with no peripheral noxious stimulus. Some such mechanism could account for the finding that pain can be induced by suggestion alone and may provide a framework for understanding how psychological factors can contribute to chronic pain.

FIGURE 11-4 *A*. Transmission system for nociceptive messages. Noxious stimuli activate the sensitive peripheral ending of the primary afferent nociceptor by the process of transduction (1). The message is then transmitted over the peripheral nerve to the spinal cord, where it synapses with cells of origin of the two major ascending pain pathways, the spinothalamic and spinoreticulothalamic. The message is relayed in the thalamus to both the frontal (F Cx) and the somatosensory cortex (SS Cx). *B*. Pain-modulation network. Inputs from frontal cortex and hypothalamus (Hyp.) activate cells in the midbrain, which control spinal pain-transmission cells via cells in the medulla.

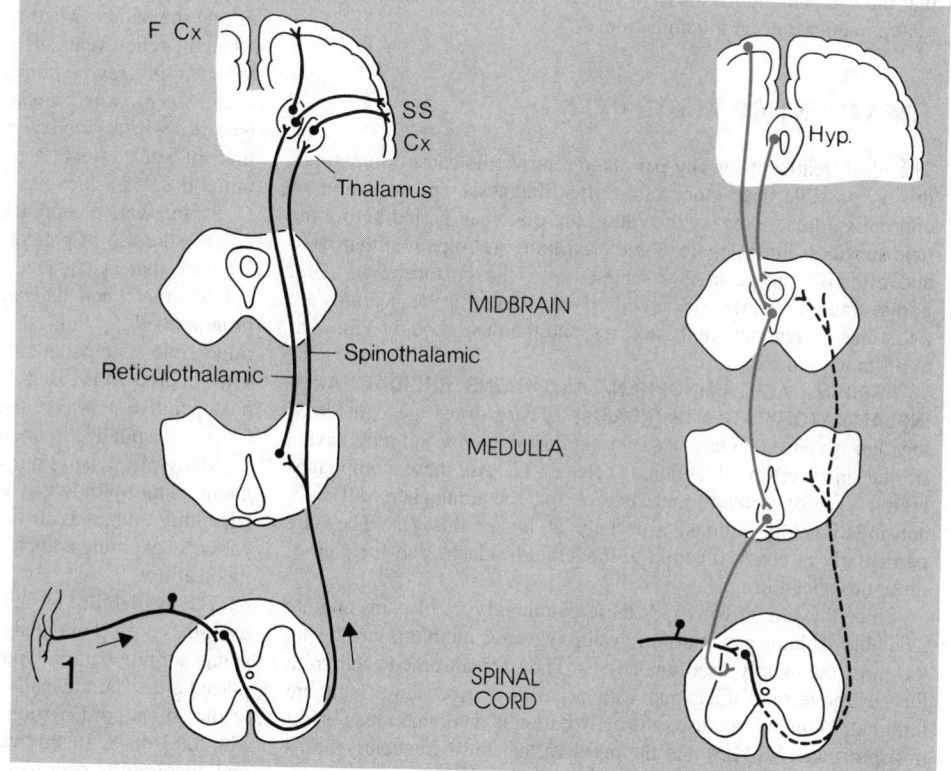

NEUROPATHIC PAIN   The normal nervous system transmits coded signals that result in pain. Thus lesions of the peripheral or central nervous system may result in a loss or impairment of pain sensation. Paradoxically, damage or dysfunction of the nervous system can produce pain. For example, damage to peripheral nerves, as occurs in diabetic neuropathy, or to primary afferents, as in herpes zoster, can result in pain that is referred to the body region innervated by the damaged nerves. Though rare, pain also may be produced by damage to the central nervous system, particularly the spinothalamic pathway or thalamus. Such neuropathic pains are often severe and are notoriously intractable to standard treatments for pain.

Neuropathic pains typically have an unusual burning, tingling, or electric shock–like quality and may be triggered by very light touch. These features are rare in other types of pain. On examination, a sensory deficit is characteristically present in the area of the patient's pain.

A variety of mechanisms contribute to neuropathic pain. Damaged primary afferents, including nociceptors, become highly sensitive to mechanical stimulation and begin to generate impulses in the absence of stimulation. Damaged primary afferents also may develop sensitivity to norepinephrine released by sympathetic postganglionic neurons. Interestingly, spinal pain-transmission neurons cut off from their normal input may become spontaneously active. Thus both central and peripheral nervous system changes may contribute to neuropathic pain.

Sympathetically maintained pain   A certain percentage of patients with peripheral nerve injury develop a severe burning pain (causalgia) in the region innervated by the nerve. The pain typically begins after a delay of hours to days or even weeks. The pain is accompanied by swelling of the extremity, periarticular osteoporosis, and arthritic changes in the distal joints. A similar syndrome called *reflex sympathetic dystrophy* can be produced without obvious nerve damage by a variety of injuries, including fractures of bone, soft tissue trauma, myocardial infarction, and stroke. Although the pathophysiology of this condition is poorly understood, the pain can be relieved within minutes by blocking the sympathetic nervous system. This implies that sympathetic activity activates nociceptors even if they are not obviously damaged. These results also suggest that the sympathetic nervous system can, under some circumstances, play an active role in inflammation.

TREATMENT OF ACUTE PAIN

The ideal treatment for any pain is to remove the cause. Sometimes this is possible, but more often after diagnosis and initiation of appropriate treatments for the cause, there is a lag period before the pain subsides. Furthermore, some conditions are so painful that rapid and effective analgesia is essential (e.g., the postoperative state, burns, trauma, cancer, sickle cell crisis). Analgesic medications are a first line of treatment in these cases, and their use should be familiar to all practitioners.

ASPIRIN, ACETAMINOPHEN, AND NONSTEROIDAL ANTI-INFLAMMATORY AGENTS (NSAIDs)   These drugs are considered together because they are used for similar problems and may have a similar mechanism of action (Table 11-1). All these compounds inhibit cyclooxygenase, and, except for acetaminophen, all have anti-inflammatory actions, especially at higher dosages. They are particularly effective for mild to moderate headache and for pain of musculoskeletal origin.

Since they are effective for these common types of pains and are available without prescription, cyclooxygenase inhibitors are by far the most commonly used analgesics. They are absorbed well from the gastrointestinal tract, and with occasional use, side effects are minimal. With chronic use, gastric irritation is a common side effect of aspirin and NSAIDs and the problem that most frequently limits the dose that can be given. Gastric irritation is most severe with aspirin, which may cause erosion of the gastric mucosa, and because

aspirin irreversibly acetylates platelets and interferes with coagulation of the blood, GI bleeding is a risk. The NSAIDs are less problematic in this regard. Although toxic to the liver when taken in a high dose, acetaminophen rarely produces gastric irritation and does not interfere with platelet function. Table 11-1 lists the dosages and durations of action of the commonly used drugs of this class.

The introduction of a parenteral form of NSAID, ketorolac, extends the usefulness of this class of compounds in the management of acute severe pain. Although clinical experience is limited, ketorolac may be sufficiently potent and rapid in onset to supplant opioids for many patients with acute severe headache and musculoskeletal pain.

OPIOID ANALGESICS   Opioids are the most potent pain-relieving drugs currently available. Furthermore, of all analgesics, they have the broadest range of efficacy, providing the most reliable method for rapidly relieving pain. Although side effects are common, except for respiratory depression, they are usually not serious and can be reversed rapidly with the narcotic antagonist naloxone. The physician should not hesitate in patients with acute severe pain to use opioid analgesics. Table 11-1 lists the most commonly used opioid analgesics.

Opioids produce analgesia by actions in the central nervous system. They activate pain-inhibitory neurons and directly inhibit pain-transmission neurons. Most of the commercially available opioid analgesics act at the same opiate receptor (mu receptor), differing mainly in potency, speed of onset, duration of action, and optimal route of administration. Although the dose-related side effects (sedation, respiratory depression, pruritus, constipation) are similar among the different opioids, some side effects are due to accumulation of nonopioid metabolites that are unique to individual drugs. One striking example of this is normeperidine, a metabolite of meperidine. Normeperidine produces hyperexcitability and seizures that are not reversible with naloxone. Normeperidine accumulation is much greater in patients with renal failure.

The most rapid relief with opioids is obtained by IV administration; relief with oral administration is significantly slower. Common acute side effects include nausea, vomiting, and sedation. These effects are dose-related, and there is great variability among patients in the doses that relieve pain and produce side effects. Because of this, initiation of therapy requires titration to optimal dose and interval. The most important principle is to provide adequate pain relief. This requires asking the patient whether the drug has relieved their pain and, if so, when the relief wears off. *The most common error made by physicians in managing severe pain with opioids is to prescribe an inadequate dose. Since many patients are reluctant to complain, this practice leads to needless suffering.* In the absence of sedation at the expected time of peak effect, a physician should not hesitate to repeat the initial dose to achieve satisfactory pain relief.

An innovative approach to the problem of achieving adequate pain relief is the use of patient-controlled analgesia (PCA). PCA requires a device that instantaneously delivers a programmed IV dose of an opioid drug when the patient pushes a button. The device can be programmed to limit the total hourly dose so that overdosing is impossible. The patient can then titrate the dose to the optimal level. This approach is used most extensively for the management of postoperative pain, but there is no reason why it should not be used for any hospitalized patient with persistent severe pain.

Many physicians, nurses, and patients have a certain trepidation about using opioids that is based on an exaggerated fear of patients becoming addicted. In fact, there is a vanishingly small chance of patients becoming addicted to narcotics as a result of their appropriate medical use.

The availability of new routes of administration has extended the usefulness of opioid analgesics. Most important is the availability of spinal administration. Opioids can be infused through a spinal catheter placed either intrathecally or epidurally. By applying opioids directly to the spinal cord, regional analgesia can be obtained at a relatively low total dose. In this way, such side effects as sedation, nausea, and respiratory depression can be minimized. This approach has been used extensively in obstetrical procedures and for lower-

TABLE 11-1 Drugs for relief of pain

NONNARCOTIC ANALGESICS: USUAL DOSES AND INTERVALS

Generic name	Dose, mg	Interval	Comments
Acetylsalicylic acid	650 PO	q 4 h	Enteric-coated preparations available
Acetaminophen	650 PO	q 4 h	Side effects uncommon
Ibuprofen	400 PO	q 4–6 h	Available without prescription
Naproxen	250–500 PO	q 12 h	Delayed effects may be due to long half-life
Fenoprofen	200 PO	q 4–6 h	
Indomethacin	25–50 PO	q 8 h	Gastrointestinal side effects common
Ketorolac	15–60 IM	q 4–6 h	Available for parenteral use (IM)

NARCOTIC ANALGESICS: USUAL DOSES AND INTERVALS

Generic name	Parenteral dose, mg	PO dose, mg	Comments
Codeine	30–60 q 4 h	30–60 q 4 h	Nausea common
Oxycodone	—	5–10 q 4–6 h	Usually available with acetaminophen or aspirin
Morphine	10 q 4 h	60 q 4 h	
Morphine sustained release		60–180 bid to tid	Oral slow-release preparation
Hydromorphone	1–2 q 4 h	2–4 q 4 h	Shorter acting than morphine sulfate
Levorphanol	2 q 6–8 h	4 q 6–8 h	Longer acting than morphine sulfate; absorbed well PO
Methadone	10 q 6–8 h	20 q 6–8 h	Delayed sedation due to long half-life
Meperidine	75–100 q 3–4 h	300 q 4 h	Poorly absorbed PO; normeperidine a toxic metabolite
Butorphanol	—	1–2 q 4 h	Intranasal spray
Fentanyl	—		Transdermal patch

ANTICONVULSANTS AND ANTIARRHYTHMICS

Generic name	PO dose, mg	Interval
Phenytoin	300	daily/qhs
Carbamazepine	200–300	q 6 h
Clonazepam	1	q 6 h
Mexiletine	150–300	q 6–12 h

TRICYCLIC ANTIDEPRESSANTS

Generic name	Uptake blockade		Sedative potency	Anticholinergic potency	Orthostatic hypotension	Cardiac arrhythmia	Average dose, mg/day	Range, mg/day
	5HT	NE						
Doxepin	+ +	+	High	Moderate	Moderate	Less	200	75–400
Amitriptyline	+ + + +	+ +	High	Highest	Moderate	Yes	150	25–300
Imipramine	+ + + +	+ +	Moderate	Moderate	High	Yes	200	75–400
Nortriptyline	+ + +	+ +	Moderate	Moderate	Low	Yes	100	40–150
Desipramine	+ + +	+ + + +	Low	Low	Low	Yes	150	50–300

body postoperative pain. Opioids also can be given intranasally (butorphanol), rectally, and transdermally (Fentanyl), thus avoiding the discomfort of frequent injections in patients who cannot be given oral medication.

OPIOID AND CYCLOOXYGENASE INHIBITOR COMBINATIONS When used in combination, opioids and cyclooxygenase inhibitors have additive effects. Because a lower dose of each can be used to achieve the same degree of pain relief and their side effects are nonadditive, such combinations can be used to lower the severity of dose-related side effects. It is important to recognize that fixed-ratio combinations of an opioid with acetaminophen carry a special risk. Dose escalation as a result of increased severity of pain or decreased opioid effect as a result of tolerance may lead to levels of acetaminophen that are toxic to the liver.

CHRONIC PAIN

PATIENT EVALUATION Managing patients with chronic pain is intellectually and emotionally challenging. The patient's problem is often difficult to diagnose; such patients are demanding of the physician's time and often appear emotionally distraught. Although it is always possible that a rare or obscure bodily disease is the cause of the pain, the traditional medical approach of seeking an obscure organic pathology is usually unhelpful. On the other hand, psychologi-

cal evaluation and behaviorally based treatment paradigms are frequently helpful, particularly in the setting of a multidisciplinary pain-management center.

There are several factors that can cause, perpetuate, or exacerbate chronic pain. First, of course, the patient may simply have a disease that is characteristically painful for which there is presently no cure. Arthritis, cancer, migraine headaches, fibromyalgia, and diabetic neuropathy are examples of this. Such diseases may be sufficient to explain chronic pain without invoking other factors. Second, there may be neural and somatic perpetuating factors that are initiated by a bodily disease and may persist after that disease has resolved. Examples include damaged sensory nerves, sympathetic efferent activity, and painful reflex muscle contraction. Finally, a variety of psychological conditions can exacerbate or even cause pain.

There are certain areas to which special attention should be paid in the medical history. Because depression is the most common emotional disturbance in patients with chronic pain, they should be questioned about their mood, appetite, sleep patterns, and daily activity. A simple standardized questionnaire, such as the Beck Depression Inventory, can be a useful screening device. It is important to remember that major depression is a common, treatable, and potentially fatal illness.

Other clues that a significant emotional disturbance is contributing to a patient's chronic pain complaint are the pain occurs in multiple unrelated sites; a pattern of recurrent, but separate, pain problems beginning in childhood or adolescence; pain beginning at a time of emotional trauma, such as the loss of a parent or spouse; a history of physical or sexual abuse; and past or present substance abuse.

On examination, special attention should be paid to whether the patient guards the painful area and whether certain movements or postures are avoided because of pain. Discovering a mechanical component to the pain can be useful both diagnostically and therapeutically. Painful areas should be examined for deep tenderness, noting whether this is localized to muscle, ligamentous structures, or joints. Chronic myofascial pain is very common, and in these patients, deep palpation may reveal highly localized trigger points that are firm bands or knots in muscle. If injection of local anesthetic into these trigger points relieves the pain, it supports the diagnosis. A neuropathic component to the pain is indicated by evidence of nerve damage, such as sensory impairment, exquisitely sensitive skin, weakness and muscle atrophy, or loss of deep tendon reflexes. Evidence suggesting sympathetic nervous system involvement is the presence of diffuse swelling, changes in skin color and temperature, and hypersensitive skin and joint tenderness compared with the normal side. Relief of the pain with a sympathetic block is diagnostic.

A guiding principle in evaluating patients with chronic pain is to assess both emotional and organic factors before initiating therapy. Addressing these issues together, rather than waiting to "rule out" organic causes of the pain, improves compliance in part because it assures patients that a psychological evaluation does not mean that the physician is questioning the validity of their complaint. Even when an organic cause for a patient's pain can be found, it is still wise to look for other factors. For example, cancer patients with painful bony metastases also may have pain due to nerve damage and significant depression. Optimal therapy requires that each of these factors be looked for and treated.

TREATMENT OF CHRONIC PAIN Once the evaluation process has been completed and the likely causative and exacerbating factors identified, an explicit treatment plan should be developed. An important part of this process is to identify specific and realistic functional goals for therapy, such as getting a good night's sleep, being able to go shopping, or returning to work. A multidisciplinary approach which utilizes medications, counseling, physical therapy, nerve blocks, and even surgery may be required to improve the patient's quality of life. This may require referral to a pain clinic; however, this is not necessary for all chronic pain patients. For some, pharmacologic management alone can provide significant help.

Antidepressant medications The tricyclic antidepressants (see Table 11-1) are extremely useful for the management of patients with chronic pain. Although developed for the treatment of depression, the tricyclics have a spectrum of dose-related biologic activities that include the production of analgesia in a variety of clinical conditions. Although the mechanism is unknown, the analgesic effect of tricyclics has a more rapid onset of action and occurs at a lower dose than is typically required for the treatment of depression. Furthermore, patients with chronic pain who are not depressed obtain pain relief with antidepressants. There is evidence that tricyclic drugs potentiate opioid analgesia, so they are useful adjuncts for the treatment of severe persistent pain such as occurs with malignant tumors. Table 11-2 lists some of the painful conditions that respond to tricyclics. Tricyclics are of particular value in the management of neuropathic pains such as painful diabetic neuropathy and postherpetic neuralgia, for which there are few other therapeutic options.

The tricyclics that have been shown to relieve pain have significant side effects. Unfortunately, some of the newer antidepressants such as fluoxetine (Prozac) that have fewer and less serious side effects have not been shown to provide pain relief.

Anticonvulsants and antiarrhythmics (See Table 11-1) These drugs are useful primarily for patients with neuropathic pain. Phenytoin (Dilantin) and carbamazepine (Tegretol) were first shown to relieve the pain of trigeminal neuralgia. This pain has a characteristic brief, shooting, electric shock–like quality. In fact, anticonvulsants seem to be helpful largely for pains that have such a lancinating quality.

TABLE 11-2 Painful conditions that respond to tricyclic antidepressants
Postherpetic neuralgia*
Diabetic neuropathy*
Tension headache*
Migraine headache*
Rheumatoid arthritis[†]*
Chronic low back pain[†]
Cancer

* Controlled trials demonstrate analgesia.
[†] Controlled studies indicate benefit but not analgesia.
SOURCE: Fields, 1987, p 291.

Antiarrhythmic drugs such as low-dose lidocaine and mexiletine (Mexitil) seem to be effective for pains that respond to anticonvulsants, as well as other conditions, including postoperative and burn pain. These drugs block the spontaneous activity of primary afferent nociceptors that appears when they are damaged. They should be considered for use in patients with pain associated with damage to peripheral nerves.

Chronic opioid medication The long-term use of opioids is accepted for patients with pain due to malignant disease. Although its use for chronic pain of nonmalignant origin is highly controversial, it is clear that for many such patients opioid analgesics are the only option available for obtaining effective relief. This is understandable since opioids are the most potent and have the broadest range of efficacy of any analgesic medications. Although addiction is rare in patients who first use opioids for pain relief, some degree of tolerance and physical dependence are likely to occur with long-term use. Therefore, before embarking on opioid therapy, other options should be explored, and the limitations and risks of opioids should be explained to the patient. It is also important to point out that some opioid analgesic medications have mixed agonist-antagonist properties (e.g., pentazocine and butorphanol). From a practical standpoint, this means that they may worsen pain by inducing an abstinence syndrome in patients who are physically dependent on other opioid analgesics.

With long-term outpatient use of orally administered opioids it is desirable to use long-acting compounds such as levorphanol, methadone, or sustained-release morphine (see Table 11-1). The pharmacokinetic profile of these drugs enables prolonged pain relief, minimizes side effects such as sedation that are associated with high peak plasma levels, and, perhaps, reduces the likelihood of rebound pain associated with a rapid fall in plasma opioid concentration. Constipation is a virtually universal side effect of opioid use and should be treated expectantly.

It is worth emphasizing, in conclusion, that many patients, especially those with chronic pain, seek medical attention primarily because they are suffering and because only physicians have access to the medications required for their relief. Clearly, it is a primary responsibility of all physicians to attempt to minimize the physical and emotional discomfort of their patients. Familiarity with pain mechanisms and analgesic medications is an important step toward accomplishing this aim.

REFERENCES

ARNER S: Intravenous phentolamine test: Diagnostic and prognostic use in reflex sympathetic dystrophy. Pain 46:17, 1991

BASBAUM AI, FIELDS HL: Endogenous pain control systems: Brainstem spinal pathways and endorphin circuitry. Ann Rev Neurosci 7:309, 1984

FIELDS HL (ed): *Pain Syndromes in Neurology*. London, Butterworth, 1990

————: *Pain*. New York, McGraw-Hill, 1987

GLAZER SAB, PORTENOY RK: Systemic local anesthetics in pain control. J Pain Symptom Manage 6:30, 1991

MAX MB et al: Effects of desipramine, amitriptyline, and fluoxetine on pain in diabetic neuropathy. N Engl J Med 326:1250, 1992

MELZACK R, CASEY KL: Sensory, motivational, and central control determinants of pain, in *International Symposium on the Skin Senses*, DR Kenshalo (ed). Springfield, Ill, Charles C Thomas, 1968, p 423

ROWBOTHAM MC et al: Both intravenous lidocaine and morphine reduce the pain of postherpetic neuralgia. Neurology 41:1024, 1991

WALL PD, MELZACK R (eds): *Textbook of Pain*. New York, Churchill Livingstone, 1989

WILLIS WD (ed): *Hyperalgesia and Allodynia*. New York, Raven Press, 1992

WILLIS WD, COGGESHALL RE: *Sensory Mechanism of the Spinal Cord*. New York, Plenum Press, 1991

12 CHEST DISCOMFORT AND PALPITATION

LEE GOLDMAN / EUGENE BRAUNWALD

CHEST DISCOMFORT

Chest discomfort is one of the most frequent complaints for which patients seek medical attention; the potential benefit (or harm) resulting from the proper (or improper) assessment and management of the patient with this complaint is enormous. Failure to recognize a serious disorder, such as ischemic heart disease, may result in the dangerous delay of much-needed treatment, while an incorrect diagnosis of a potentially hazardous condition such as angina pectoris is likely to have harmful psychological and economic consequences and may lead to unnecessary cardiac catheterization. There is little relation between the severity of chest discomfort and the gravity of its cause. Therefore, a frequent problem in patients who complain of chest discomfort or pain is distinguishing trivial complaints from coronary artery disease and other serious disorders (Table 12-1).

PATHOPHYSIOLOGY   Discomfort due to myocardial ischemia Discomfort due to myocardial ischemia occurs when the oxygen supply to the heart is deficient in relation to the oxygen need. Oxygen consumption is closely related to the physiologic effort made during

---

TABLE 12-1   Some causes of chest discomfort

I **Cardiac**
  A Coronary artery disease
  B Aortic stenosis
  C Hypertropic cardiomyopathy
  D Pericarditis

II **Vascular**
  A Aortic dissection
  B Pulmonary embolism
  C Pulmonary hypertension
  D Right ventricular strain

III **Pulmonary**
  A Pleuritis or pneumonia
  B Tracheobronchitis
  C Pneumothorax
  D Tumor
  E Mediastinitis or mediastinal emphysema

IV **Gastrointestinal**
  A Esophogeal reflux
  B Esophogeal spasm
  C Mallory-Weiss tear
  D Peptic ulcer disease
  E Biliary disease
  F Pancreatitis

V **Musculoskeletal**
  A Cervical disk disease
  B Arthritis of the shoulder or spine
  C Costochondritis
  D Intercostal muscle cramps
  E Interscalene or hyperabduction syndromes
  F Subacromial bursitis

VI **Other**
  A Disorders of the breast
  B Chest wall tumors
  C Herpes zoster

---

contraction, and coronary venous blood is normally much more desaturated than that draining other areas of the body. As a consequence, the removal of more oxygen from each unit of blood, which is one of the adjustments commonly utilized by exercising skeletal muscle, is already employed in the heart in the basal state. Therefore, the heart must rely primarily on an increase in the coronary blood flow for obtaining additional oxygen.

The blood flow through the coronary arteries is directly proportional to the pressure gradient between the aorta and the ventricular myocardium during systole and the ventricular cavity during diastole but is also proportional to the fourth power of the radius of the coronary arteries. A relatively slight alteration in coronary luminal diameter below a critical level can produce a large decrement in coronary flow, provided that other factors remain constant. Coronary blood flow occurs primarily during diastole, when it is unopposed by systolic myocardial compression of the coronary vessels.

When the epicardial coronary arteries are narrowed critically (>70 percent stenosis of the luminal diameter), the intramyocardial coronary arterioles dilate in an effort to maintain total flow at a level that will avert myocardial ischemia at rest. Further dilatation, which normally occurs during exercise, is therefore not possible. Hence any condition in which increased heart rate, arterial pressure, or myocardial contractility occurs in the presence of coronary obstruction tends to precipitate anginal attacks by increasing myocardial oxygen needs in the face of a fixed oxygen supply.

By far the most frequent underlying cause of myocardial ischemia is organic narrowing of the coronary arteries secondary to coronary atherosclerosis (see also Chap. 203). A *dynamic* component of increased coronary vascular resistance, secondary to spasm of the major epicardial vessels (often near an atherosclerotic plaque) or more frequently to constriction of smaller coronary arterioles, is present in many, perhaps the majority, of patients with chronic angina pectoris. There is no evidence that systemic arterial constriction or increased cardiac contractile activity (rise in heart rate or blood pressure or increase in contractility from liberation of catecholamines or adrenergic activity) due to emotion can precipitate angina unless there is also organic or dynamic narrowing of the coronary vessels. Acute thrombosis superimposed on an atherosclerotic plaque is frequently the cause of unstable angina and acute myocardial infarction.

Aside from conditions that narrow the lumen of the coronary arteries, the only other frequent causes of myocardial ischemia are disorders such as valvular aortic stenosis (Chap. 201) or hypertrophic cardiomyopathy (Chap. 205), which cause a marked disproportion between the coronary perfusion pressure and the heart's oxygen requirements. Under such conditions, the rise in left ventricular systolic pressure is not, as in hypertensive states, balanced by a corresponding elevation of aortic perfusion pressure. Epidemiologic studies indicate that chest pain is no more common in patients with mitral valve prolapse than in those without it.

An increase in heart rate is especially harmful in patients with coronary atherosclerosis or with aortic stenosis, because it both increases myocardial oxygen needs and shortens diastole relatively more than systole, thereby decreasing the total available perfusion time per minute. Tachycardia, a decline in arterial pressure, thyrotoxicosis, and diminution in arterial oxygen content (such as occurs in anemia or arterial hypoxia) are precipitating and aggravating factors rather than underlying causes of angina.

Discomfort due to pericarditis The visceral surface of the pericardium ordinarily is insensitive to pain, as is the parietal surface, except in its lower portion, which has a relatively small number of pain fibers carried in the phrenic nerves. The pain associated with pericarditis is believed to be due to inflammation of the adjacent parietal pleura. These observations explain why noninfectious pericarditis (e.g., that associated with uremia and with myocardial infarction) and cardiac tamponade with relatively mild inflammation are usually painless or accompanied by only mild pain, whereas infectious pericarditis, being nearly always more intense and spreading to the neighboring pleura, is usually associated with pain (Chap. 206).

Vascular causes of chest pain *Aortic dissection* develops as a result of a subintimal hematoma, which may start either because a tear has developed in the intima of the aorta or because of bleeding into the vasa vasorum. Antegrade movement of this hematoma can compromise major branches off the aorta, while retrograde spread can occlude a coronary artery, disrupt the aortic valve annulus, or rupture into the pericardial space.

Pulmonary emboli These commonly originate from thrombi in the venous circulation, especially in the lower extremities. Venous thrombosis is usually related to stasis or slowing of blood flow because of inactivity or impedance to venous return, to damage in the vessel wall, or to alterations in the coagulation system. When thrombi from any source embolize to the pulmonary arterial circulation, they can cause not only mechanical obstruction but also vasoconstriction and elevated pulmonary vascular resistance related to the release of humoral factors, such as histamine, serotonin, and prostaglandins. As a result, hypoxemia and, occasionally, right-sided heart failure can ensue, and an acute fall in cardiac output can lead to sudden death. The acute pain from massive pulmonary emboli is thought to be related to pulmonary hypertension and to distention of the pulmonary artery. Infarction of a segment of the lung that is adjacent to the pleura commonly irritates the pleural surface and causes chest discomfort hours or even days later (see Chap. 226).

Other pulmonary causes of chest discomfort A variety of diseases of the lung can cause chest discomfort. Pleural pain, which is usually brief, sharp pain that is precipitated by inspiration, is very common and generally results from stretching of an inflamed parietal pleura.

Gastrointestinal causes of chest discomfort Esophageal pain includes *esophageal reflux* and *esophageal spasm*. Esophageal discomfort usually results from chemical (acid) irritation of the esophageal mucosa because of acid reflux or spasm of the esophageal muscle. Injury of the esophagus, such as in a Mallory-Weiss tear that is caused by severe vomiting, can cause severe acute chest pain (Chap. 251).

Occasionally, other gastrointestinal diseases, including *peptic ulcer disease, biliary disease*, and *pancreatitis*, may present with chest discomfort as well as abdominal discomfort.

Neuromusculoskeletal causes of chest discomfort Neuromusculoskeletal chest discomfort can be caused by *cervical disk disease* because of compression of nerve roots, by *arthritis of the shoulder or spine*, or by *costochondritis*, which is an inflammation of the costochondral junctions. Inflammation of the subacromial bursa or, less commonly, the supraspinatus or deltoid tendon may cause pain that radiates to the chest. *Intercostal muscle cramps* may occur throughout the chest. Anterior scalene and hyperabduction syndromes also can cause chest discomfort.

Other causes of chest discomfort A variety of *disorders of the breast*, including inflammatory breast disease, benign and malignant tumors, and mastodynia, can cause chest discomfort, usually in association with local abnormalities of the breast. *Chest wall tumors*, including metastases from other organs or malignant disease in the ribs, also can present as chest discomfort. The pain of *herpes zoster* may antedate the typical rash by a day or more, making early diagnosis difficult (see Chap. 144).

DIFFERENTIAL DIAGNOSIS The key issue in the evaluation of the patient with chest discomfort is to distinguish potentially life-threatening conditions such as coronary artery disease, aortic dissection, and pulmonary embolism from other causes of chest discomfort. Even patients who have brief episodes of pain and are otherwise in apparently excellent health may have intermittent myocardial ischemia or even recurrent pulmonary emboli.

The radiation of pain arising in the thoracic viscera can usually be explained by known neuroanatomic relationships (see Chap. 11). Pain impulses which enter one cord segment may spill over and excite nearby cord segments.

The chest discomfort of myocardial ischemia, most commonly from coronary artery disease but also occasionally from the other causes of ischemia noted above, is angina pectoris. Myocardial ischemia from coronary atherosclerosis is more common in patients who have hypercholesterolemia, diabetes mellitus, hypertension, obesity, or who smoke cigarettes (Chap. 208). Toxins, including cocaine ingestion or withdrawal of chronic exposure to nitroglycerin, can cause sufficient coronary vasoconstriction to result in myocardial ischemia, and cocaine also can cause myocardial infarction.

Angina pectoris is usually described as a heaviness, pressure, or squeezing, or as a sensation of strangling or constriction in the chest, but also may be described as aching, burning, or even as indigestion. Some patients steadfastly deny pain but will admit to a discomfort or unusual feeling or may complain of difficulty in breathing.

Typically, angina pectoris develops gradually during exertion, after heavy meals, and with anger, excitement, frustration, and other emotional states; it is not precipitated by coughing, respiratory movements, or other motion. When angina is induced by walking, it often forces the patient to stop or to reduce speed. Angina occurs most typically in the substernal region, anteriorly across the midthorax; it may radiate to or rarely occur alone in the interscapular region, in the arms, shoulders, teeth, and abdomen. It rarely radiates to below the umbilicus, to the back of the neck, or to the occiput. The more severe the attack, the greater is the radiation from the substernal areas to the left arm, especially its ulnar aspect. Although the radiation of chest discomfort to the left arm increases the likelihood that myocardial ischemia or infarction is present, impulses from the skin and from visceral structures, such as the esophagus and heart, converge on a common pool of neurons in the posterior horn of the spinal cord. Their origin may be confused by the cerebral cortex; hence almost any condition capable of causing chest discomfort may induce radiation to the left arm. Also, stimulation of one of the thoracic nerves that also innervates the heart by, for example, protrusion of an intervertebral disk may be misinterpreted as pain originating from the heart.

When the history is atypical, as is often the case, the correct diagnosis of angina pectoris may be aided by noting that the pain disappears more rapidly (usually within 5 min) and more completely when sublingual nitroglycerin is used. The demonstration that the time required for a given exercise to produce pain is consistently and considerably longer when it is undertaken within a few minutes after a sublingual nitroglycerin pill than after a placebo may, in some instances, represent powerful clinical evidence for the diagnosis of angina pectoris. Angina is rarely relieved within a few seconds of lying down, nor is it precipitated by stooping forward.

Myocardial infarction is usually associated with a discomfort similar in quality and distribution to that of angina but of longer duration (usually 30 min) and usually of greater intensity. In contrast to angina, the pain of myocardial infarction is not rapidly relieved by rest or by coronary dilator drugs and may require large doses of narcotics. It may be accompanied by diaphoresis, nausea, and hypotension (see Chap. 202).

The physical examination in patients with myocardial ischemia frequently is totally normal. However, myocardial ischemia can cause a third or fourth heart sound because of an impairment of myocardial contraction or relaxation. Ischemic papillary muscle dysfunction can cause transient mitral regurgitation and its associated murmur. Myocardial infarction and, less commonly, severe and generalized ischemia can cause congestive heart failure.

The chest discomfort from myocardial ischemia that is caused by aortic stenosis, hypertrophic cardiomyopathy, and nonatherosclerotic causes of coronary artery disease is generally similar to that of angina pectoris from coronary atherosclerosis. However, the physical examination will usually reveal classic findings of an aortic systolic murmur in patients with aortic stenosis (see Chap. 201) and will reveal dynamic outflow obstruction in many patients with hypertrophic cardiomyopathy (see Chap. 205).

Pericarditis can cause pain in several locations (see Chap. 206). Since the central part of the diaphragm receives its sensory supply from the phrenic nerve (which arises from the third to fifth cervical segments of the spinal cord), pain arising from the lower parietal pericardium and central tendon of the diaphragm is felt characteristically at the tip of the shoulder, the adjoining trapezius ridge, and the neck. Involvement of the more lateral part of the diaphragmatic pleura, supplied by branches from the sixth to ninth intercostal nerves, causes pain not only in the anterior part of the chest but also in the upper part of the abdomen or corresponding region of the back, sometimes simulating the pain of acute cholecystitis or pancreatitis.

Pericardial pain commonly has a pleuritic component; i.e., it is related to respiratory movements and aggravated by cough and/or deep inspiration, because of pleural irritation. It is sometimes brought on by swallowing, because the esophagus lies just behind the posterior portion of the heart, and is often altered by a change of body position, becoming sharper and more left-sided in the supine position and reduced when the patient sits upright, leaning forward. It is frequently referred to the neck and lasts longer than the pain of angina pectoris.

In some patients, however, pericardial pain may be described as a steady substernal discomfort that can mimic the pain of acute myocardial infarction. The mechanism of this steady substernal pain is not certain, but it may arise from marked inflammation of the relatively insensitive inner parietal surface of the pericardium or from irritated afferent cardiac nerve fibers lying in the periadventitial layers of the superficial coronary arteries. Occasionally, both pleuritic and steady pain may be present simultaneously.

Patients with marked *right ventricular hypertension* may have exertional pain which is quite similar to that of angina. This discomfort probably results from relative ischemia of the right ventricle brought about by the increased oxygen needs and by the elevated intramural resistance, with reduction of the normally large systolic pressure gradient which perfuses this chamber.

The pain due to *acute dissection of the aorta* (Chap. 210) or to an expanding aortic aneurysm results from stimulation of nerve endings in the adventitia. The pain usually begins abruptly, reaches an extremely severe peak rapidly, is felt in the center of the chest and/or in the back depending on the site of the dissection, lasts for hours, and requires unusually large amounts of analgesics for relief. Patients commonly describe a true pain rather that the vague discomfort that is sometimes described with myocardial ischemia. The pain is not aggravated by changes in position or respiration.

The pain resulting from *pulmonary embolism* (Chap. 226) may resemble that of acute myocardial infarction, and in massive embolism it is located substernally. In patients with smaller emboli, the pain is located more laterally, is pleuritic in nature, and may be associated with hemoptysis.

Pleural pain from fibrinous pleurisy or any pneumonic process is very common. It generally results from stretching of inflamed parietal pleura and is similar in character to the pleural pain of pericarditis (see above). Pneumothorax and tumors involving the pleural space also may irritate the parietal pleura and cause pleural pain; the latter is sharp, knifelike, superficial in quality, and its aggravation by each breath and by coughing distinguishes it from the deep, dull, relatively steady pain of myocardial ischemia. Substernal discomfort also frequently occurs in the presence of *tracheobronchitis;* it is commonly described as a burning sensation accentuated by coughing.

The pain of *mediastinal emphysema* (Chap. 228) may be intense and sharp and may radiate from the substernal region to the shoulders; often a distinct crepitus is heard. The pain associated with *mediastinitis* and *mediastinal tumors* usually resembles that of pleuritis but is more likely to be maximal in the substernal region, and the associated feeling of constriction or oppression may cause confusion with myocardial infarction.

The several *abdominal disorders* which may at times mimic anginal pain may usually be suspected from the history. Esophageal pain commonly presents as a deep thoracic burning discomfort, which is the hallmark of acid-induced pain. Intake of aspirin, alcohol, or certain foods typically exacerbates this burning discomfort, and the discomfort may be relieved promptly by antacids or even by one or two swallows of food or water. Patients may have accompanying dysphagia, regurgitation of undigested food, or weight loss. The symptoms of a hiatus hernia tend to be exacerbated by lying down, and all forms of acid-peptic disease may be worse in the early morning when acidic secretions are not neutralized by food. Esophageal spasm, which may be induced by reflux of gastric acid into an esophagus in which the mucosa has been previously irritated, can cause a squeezing pain that may be indistinguishable from myocardial ischemia and that may even have a similar pattern of radiation. Pain resulting from gastric or duodenal ulcer (Chap. 252) is epigastric or substernal, usually commences about 1 to 1½ h after meals, and is usually relieved in several minutes by antacids or milk.

The discomfort caused by acute cholecystitis is more commonly described as an ache, which may be epigastric or substernal. It most commonly tends to occur an hour or so after meals and not in relation to exertion.

The presence of an abdominal disorder, such as a hiatus hernia or a duodenal ulcer, does not constitute proof that the patient's chest pain is related to it. Such disorders are frequently asymptomatic and are not at all uncommon in patients who also have angina pectoris.

Musculoskeletal pain   The *costochondral and chondrosternal articulations* are the most common sites of anterior chest pain. Objective signs in the form of swelling (Tietze's syndrome), redness, and heat are rare, but sharply localized tenderness is common. The pain may be darting and last for only a few seconds or may be a dull ache enduring for hours or days. An associated feeling of tightness due to muscle spasm (see below) is frequent. *Pressure on the chondrosternal and costochondral junctions and on the pectoralis muscles is an essential part of the examination of every patient with chest pain* and will reproduce the pain arising from these tissues. A large percentage of patients with costochondral pain, especially those who also have minor and innocent T-wave alterations, are erroneously labeled as having coronary disease.

Pain secondary to *subacromial bursitis, biceps tendonitis,* and *arthritis of the shoulder and spine* may be precipitated by motion but not by general exertion. Pain arising in the chest wall or upper extremity may develop as a result of muscle or ligament strains brought on by unaccustomed exercise and felt in the costochondral or chondrosternal junctions or in the chest wall muscles. Other causes are *osteoarthritis* of the dorsal or thoracic spine and *ruptured cervical disk disease.* Pain in the left upper extremity and precordium may be due to compression of portions of the brachial plexus by a cervical rib or by spasm and shortening of the scalenus anticus muscle because of high fixation of the ribs and sternum. Deep breathing, turning or twisting of the chest, and movements of the shoulder girdle and arm may elicit and duplicate the pain of which the patient complains. The pain may be very brief, lasting only a few seconds, or aching and persist for hours. The duration is therefore likely to be either longer or shorter than untreated angina pectoris, which usually lasts for only a few minutes.

Emotional disorders are also commonly associated with chest pain. Usually, the discomfort is experienced as a sense of "tightness," sometimes called "aching," and occasionally it may be sufficiently severe as to be designated a pain of considerable magnitude. Since the discomfort may be described as a tightness or constriction and is often localized at least in part beneath the sternum, it is not surprising that this type of discomfort is frequently confused with that of myocardial ischemia. Ordinarily, it lasts for a half hour or more, is unrelated to exertion, and with slow fluctuation of intensity. The association with fatigue or emotional strain is usually clear, although this may not be volunteered by the patient. Associated hyperventilation can cause innocent changes in the T waves and ST segments, which can be confused with coronary artery disease.

APPROACH TO THE PATIENT WITH CHEST DISCOMFORT   A detailed and *meticulous history* of the behavior of the pain is the cornerstone of the evaluation. The location, radiation, quality, intensity, and duration of the episodes are important. Even more so is the story of the aggravating and alleviating factors. A history of intense aggravation by breathing, coughing, or other respiratory movements will usually point toward the pleura and pericardium or mediastinum as the site, although chest wall pain is likewise affected by respiratory motion. Similarly, a pain that regularly appears on rapid walking, or with other exertion such as sexual activity, and vanishes a few minutes after stopping suggests the diagnosis of angina pectoris, although a similar story will occasionally be obtained from patients with skeletal disorders.

While data from the history are of cardinal importance in the assessment of chest discomfort, physicians should not be misled into overreliance on any single feature. For example, acute myocardial infarction sometimes presents with pain that may be described as burning or even as sharp and may not be principally located in the substernal area.

A thorough *physical examination* can provide important clues to the cause of chest discomfort. Blood pressure should be checked in both arms if aortic dissection is being considered. Examination of the skin may reveal cyanosis, which suggests hypoxemia from either diminished cardiac output or impaired respiratory function, or xanthelasthma, which would suggest hyperlipidemia and associated coronary disease. The finding of lymphadenopathy suggests a tumor. The examination of the chest wall should include both inspection and palpation to search for costochondritis and other musculoskeletal abnormalities. Lung examination may reveal a pleural rub, signs of pneumonic consolidation, or evidence of congestive heart failure. The physical examination may be totally normal in persons with severe myocardial ischemia, but it also may demonstrate abnormalities of vital signs, a third or fourth heart sound, or mitral regurgitation from papillary muscle dysfunction. Aortic stenosis will be accompanied by its typical murmur (Chap. 201). The cardiac examination also should search for an increased pulmonic second sound that may indicate elevated pulmonary artery pressure, such as is found in pulmonary embolism, and the pericardial friction rub that strongly suggests pericarditis. A careful upper abdominal examination may be the first clue to peptic ulcer disease or cholecystitis.

Critical information can often be obtained by attempts to produce or alleviate the pain, such as with nitroglycerin. Careful palpation of the chest wall, subacromial bursa, deltoid tendon, abdomen, and other structures may be very helpful if it reproduces the chest discomfort. Shoulder and arm motion commonly reproduces pain related to these structures. However, the finding that such maneuvers can cause chest discomfort does not mean that such musculoskeletal diseases are the cause of the presenting complaint unless one can be sure that the patient's syndrome is reproduced precisely. Alternatively, the demonstration that a localized pain can be completely relieved by infiltration of a local anesthetic will be conclusive in convincing both the patient and the physician. Evaluation of the patient at the time of a spontaneous episode, such as with an electrocardiogram during pain, is also extremely helpful.

APPLICATION OF THE PRINCIPLES OF CLINICAL REASONING
The assessment of the probability of the various causes of chest pain requires the integration of multiple pieces of data, because no single clinical feature can be considered decisive. Each of the conditions that can cause chest discomfort can have varied presentations, and the diagnostic tests upon which physicians often rely can also have false-positive or false-negative results. Thus the principles of clinical reasoning (Chap. 10) should be applied to the evaluation of the patient with chest discomfort.

History and physical examination   The information obtained from a careful medical history and physical examination can be used to develop a differential diagnosis of the causes of chest discomfort in an individual patient, to rank these diagnostic possibilities, and often to assign approximate percent probabilities to them. Although the various causes of chest discomfort have typical characteristics, these characteristics must be interpreted in light of the prior probability that a person with a given age and sex and with a particular past medical history would have such a cause of chest discomfort. For example, the possibility of angina pectoris as a cause of precordial or substernal discomfort must be seriously considered in a middle-aged man with coronary risk factors such as hypercholesterolemia

and smoking, even if the description of the discomfort is not perfectly typical for angina pectoris. Conversely, when a 20-year-old woman describes the onset of new discomfort in a way that is seemingly classic for angina pectoris, such a diagnosis is relatively unlikely because the prior probability of ischemic heart disease, given her age and sex, is so low.

Although it is not always possible to assign numerical probabilities to the various causes of chest discomfort in an individual patient, experienced clinicians either implicitly or explicitly assess the relative likelihoods of various potential explanations for any chest discomfort syndrome to help guide their future diagnostic evaluations and therapy. For example, a middle-aged or elderly man with typical characteristics for angina pectoris has about an 80 to 85 percent probability of having hemodynamically significant coronary artery disease. By comparison, the same man with a history of chest discomfort that has some characteristics that are typical for angina pectoris but other characteristics that are atypical will have a probability of important coronary disease ranging from about 30 to 60 percent. Even persons with chest pain that is decidedly unlikely to represent coronary disease still have some finite possibility of coronary disease, which may range from exceedingly unlikely in a young woman to the 10 percent range in a middle-aged man with many coronary risk factors.

Diagnostic tests   Although myocardial ischemia commonly is associated with electrocardiographic changes (Chap. 203), many patients have normal tracings between attacks, and some may even be normal during an episode of pain. However, depression of the ST segments, caused by myocardial ischemia, typically occurs during exertion and is accompanied by anginal discomfort; moreover, electrocardiographic evidence of myocardial ischemia may occur at rest and with or without accompanying chest discomfort. The finding of flat or down-sloping ST-segment depressions of 0.1 mV or greater during an attack of pain substantially increases the likelihood that the pain is anginal in origin. Exercise electrocardiography will show ischemic changes in about 50 to 80 percent of persons with symptomatic coronary disease but also in about 10 to 15 percent of patients who do not have coronary disease. The accuracy of ambulatory ischemia monitoring in the general population is less clear. Exercise thallium scintigraphy (Chap. 190) will demonstrate a perfusion defect in about 75 to 85 percent of patients with angina pectoris and will be falsely positive in about 10 percent of patients who have chest discomfort from noncoronary causes.

The evaluation of patients with suspected pulmonary embolism should usually focus on the documentation of deep venous thrombosis (Chap. 226) and the evaluation of pulmonary perfusion with a lung scintigram and/or pulmonary arteriography (Chap. 216). Aortic dissection is often suggested by the routine chest radiograph, and the diagnosis may be established by echocardiography (especially transesophageal echocardiography), computed tomography, or magnetic resonance imaging. Aortography is the definitive test, but because of its invasiveness, it is usually reserved for situations in which the suspicion of dissection is moderate or high and definitive anatomic documentation or localization is needed, often because of the need to consider a surgical repair.

Esophageal or peptic ulcer diseases can often be diagnosed by an upper gastrointestinal roentgenogram. Esophageal manometry and measurement of lower esophageal sphincter pressure are useful in identifying esophageal spasm. The Bernstein acid perfusion test, in which an attempt is made to reproduce the pain by infusing hydrochloric acid into the esophagus, can help establish acid reflux as the cause of pain (Chap. 251).

Integration of clinical data and test results   It is often useful to subdivide patients into those with an *acute* onset of a new or worsened chest pain syndrome versus those with more *chronic* pain. Acute chest pain, with a duration of minutes to hours prior to the patient's presentation to a physician, could be caused by many of the entities described in this chapter and would be especially suspicious for acute myocardial infarction, aortic dissection, pulmonary embolism, biliary colic, or acute musculoskeletal trauma. In many situations, the patient may have had prior pain that was similar to but less severe than the current discomfort; this prior pain may be an important clue to recurrent problems such as biliary colic or esophageal spasm. Some, but certainly not all, patients with acute myocardial infarctions will have had a prior history of angina pectoris.

Accumulated data from large numbers of patients who have presented to emergency departments with acute chest pain can aid the assessment of the probability that an individual is having an acute myocardial infarction. By integrating information from the history, physical examination, and electrocardiogram, such empirically derived algorithms have been able to predict which patients are having acute myocardial infarctions more accurately than are the physicians who actually saw the patients in the emergency department. For example, a person without a history of known coronary disease is unlikely to be having an acute myocardial infarction if the electrocardiogram is normal and the chest pain does not radiate to the neck or left shoulder or arm. Although no algorithm can be considered a perfect predictor that can be used in a vacuum, physicians have the opportunity to improve patient management by incorporating such information into their decision-making.

In patients with chronic or recurrent chest pain, the prior pain pattern is usually very helpful in establishing the current diagnosis. For patients with recurrent myocardial ischemia, a worsening of a stable pain pattern may herald unstable angina pectoris (Chap. 203). Unlike acute chest pain, where decision-making revolves around the need for immediate hospitalization and electrocardiographic monitoring to avoid sudden death, chronic chest pain, unless indicative of unstable angina pectoris, may be clarified by outpatient diagnostic testing, such as exercise electrocardiography and exercise thallium scintigraphy.

Although exercise electrocardiography and exercise thallium scintigraphy are of value in distinguishing between cardiac and noncardiac causes of chest discomfort, the results must be interpreted in light of the prior probability of coronary artery disease, which is the probability

FIGURE 12-2 Approximate probability of coronary artery disease before and after noninvasive testing of a patient with typical (*A*) and atypical (*B*) angina pectoris. The percentages demonstrate how the sequential use of an exercise electrocardiogram and an exercise thallium test may affect the probability of coronary artery disease. (*From L Goldman, in W Branch, Jr (ed): The Office Practice of Medicine, 2d ed, Philadelphia, Saunders, 1987.*)

FIGURE 12-1 The curves show the posterior (after-test) probability as a function of the prior (before-test) probability for positive versus negative exercise thallium scintiscans, defined as a perfusion defect that is produced by exercise and resolves with rest. The before-test probability could be estimated from the clinical presentation or could be a postexercise electrocardiogram probability derived from Fig. 10-2 (p. 46). (*From L Goldman, in W Branch, Jr (ed): The Office Practice of Medicine, 3rd ed, Philadelphia, Saunders, 1994.*)

that the patient has coronary disease based on the presenting clinical characteristics, age, and sex (see Fig. 10-2, p. 46). Since exercise thallium scintigraphy appears to provide information that is correlated with the standard exercise electrocardiogram no more than would be expected by chance, it can provide additional independent information (Chap. 10) and further change the probability of coronary artery disease (Fig. 12-1). If absolute diagnostic knowledge is required, cardiac catheterization with coronary angiography serves as the gold standard, i.e., the test that is considered definitive regarding the presence or absence of coronary disease, even though the presence of anatomic disease does not guarantee that the coronary stenoses are causing the chest discomfort.

A sequence of consistently negative cardiologic test results reduces the probability of coronary artery disease to below 10 percent in patients with atypical chest discomfort. However, even after a normal exercise electrocardiogram and exercise thallium scintigram, the probability of coronary disease will still be about 30 percent in a middle-aged or elderly patient with a typical history of angina pectoris (Fig. 12-2). By recognizing the potential change in probabilities that can be obtained with positive and negative results of the diagnostic tests that are planned, the physician can decide whether these potential changes in probability are sufficient to warrant the test. For example, the physician should commonly decide that a patient with typical angina pectoris and a positive exercise electrocardiogram does not require an exercise thallium scintigram to *diagnose* coronary disease, although under some circumstances it might aid in the estimation of the patient's subsequent prognosis.

A useful test result is commonly one that moves the likelihood of a diagnostic possibility across a threshold, so the test result would lead to a change in management, either by influencing the decision to order additional tests or by causing a change in treatment. In the case of chest discomfort, the decisions cannot be based on a 50 percent threshold: Probabilities of coronary artery disease, pulmonary embolism, or aortic dissection that are well below 50 percent may still demand further evaluation because of the dire consequences of missing one of these important diagnoses. The physician must be prepared to embark on an appropriate evaluation when the history and physical examination do not exclude these diagnoses with a reasonable degree of certainty. The degree of certainty must be determined for the individual condition and patient at hand, typically after an appropriately full and frank discussion between the patient and the physician.

PALPITATION

Palpitation is a common, disagreeable symptom that may be defined as an awareness of the beating of the heart, an awareness most commonly brought about by a change in the heart's rhythm or rate or by an augmentation of its contractility. Palpitation is not pathognomonic of any particular group of disorders; indeed, often it signifies not a primary physical disorder but rather a psychological disturbance. Even when it occurs as a more or less prominent complaint, the diagnosis of the underlying disease is made largely on the basis of other associated symptoms and data. Nevertheless, palpitation is frequently of considerable importance in the minds of patients, who fear that it may indicate heart disease. Concern is all the more pronounced in patients who have been told that they *may* have heart disease; to them palpitation may seem to be an omen of impending disaster. Since the resulting anxiety may be associated with increased activity of the autonomic nervous system, with consequent increases of the cardiac rate and rhythm and the vigor of contraction, the patient's awareness of these changes may then lead to a vicious cycle, which may ultimately be responsible for incapacitation.

Palpitation may be described by the patient in various terms, such as "pounding," "fluttering," "flopping," and "skipping," and in most cases it will be obvious that the complaint is of a sensation of disturbed heartbeat. The sensitivity to alterations in cardiac activity among different individuals varies widely. Some patients seem to be unaware of the most serious and chaotic dysrhythmias; others are seriously troubled by an occasional extrasystole. Patients with anxiety states often exhibit a lowered threshold at which disorders of rate and rhythm result in palpitation. The awareness of the heartbeat also tends to be more common at night and during introspective moments but is less marked during activity. Patients with organic heart disease and chronic disorders of cardiac rate, rhythm, or stroke volume tend to accommodate to these abnormalities and are often less sensitive than normal persons to such events. Persistent tachycardia and/or atrial fibrillation may not be accompanied by continuous palpitation, in contrast to a sudden, brief alteration in cardiac rate or rhythm, which often causes considerable subjective discomfort. Palpitation is particularly prominent when the precipitating cause for increased heart rate or contractility or arrhythmia is recent, transient, and episodic. Conversely, in emotionally well-adjusted individuals, palpitation commonly becomes progressively less disconcerting as it becomes more chronic.

PATHOGENESIS OF PALPITATION   Under ordinary circumstances, the rhythmic heartbeat is imperceptible to the healthy individual of placid or even average temperament. Palpitation may be experienced by normal persons who have engaged in strenuous physical effort or have been aroused emotionally or sexually. This type of palpitation is physiologic and represents the normal awareness of an overactive heart—i.e., a heart that is beating at a rapid rate and with an increased contractility. Palpitation due to overactivity of the heart also may occur in certain pathologic states, e.g., fever, acute or severe anemia, or thyrotoxicosis.

When palpitation is heavy and regular, it is usually caused by an augmented stroke volume. Pathologic states, such as aortic regurgitation or a variety of hyperkinetic circulatory states (e.g., anemia, arteriovenous fistula, and thyrotoxicosis) should be considered, as well as the benign so-called idiopathic hyperkinetic heart syndrome. Palpitation also may occur immediately after the onset of cardiac slowing, as with the sudden development of complete atrioventricular block, or upon the conversion from atrial fibrillation to sinus rhythm. Unusual movements of the heart within the thorax are also frequently the mechanism of palpitation. Thus the ectopic beat and/or the compensatory pause may be appreciated, since both are associated with alterations in cardiac motion.

IMPORTANT CAUSES OF PALPITATION (See also Chap. 198)
Extrasystoles   In most cases the diagnosis will be suggested by the patient's story. The premature contraction and postpremature beat are often described as a "flopping," or the patient may say that it feels as if "the heart were turning over." The pause following the premature contraction may be felt as an actual cessation of the heartbeat. The first ventricular contraction succeeding the pause may be felt as an unusually vigorous beat and will be described as "pounding" or "thudding."

When extrasystoles are numerous, clinical differentiation from atrial fibrillation can be made by any procedure that will bring about a definite increase in the ventricular rate. In persons without serious underlying heart disease, the extrasystoles usually diminish in frequency and then disappear at increasingly rapid heart rates, whereas the ventricular irregularity of atrial fibrillation increases.

Tachycardias   These conditions, which are considered in detail in Chap. 198, are common and medically important causes of palpitation. Ventricular tachycardia, one of the most serious arrhythmias, rarely is manifested as palpitation; this may be related to the abnormal sequence, and hence impaired coordination and vigor, of ventricular contraction. If the patient is seen between attacks, the diagnosis of ectopic tachycardia and its type will have to depend on the history, but the precise diagnosis can be made only when an electrocardiogram and observations on the effect of carotid sinus pressure are made during the episode. The mode of onset and offset gives the most important lead in distinguishing sinus from one of the various forms of ectopic tachycardias. Ectopic rhythms characteristically begin instantaneously, while sinus tachycardia has a more gradual onset and ending over seconds or minutes. Continuous ambulatory (Holter) electrocardiography and asking the patient to record the time of onset and cessation of the palpitations in a diary are extremely helpful in determining the cause of this symptom.

Other causes   These include thyrotoxicosis (Chap. 334), hypoglycemia (Chap. 338), pheochromocytoma (Chap. 336), fever (Chap. 16), and drugs. The relationship between the development of palpitation and the use of tobacco, coffee, tea, alcohol, epinephrine, ephedrine, aminophylline, atropine, or thyroid medication can usually be established from a careful medical history.

Palpitation as a manifestation of the anxiety state   Persons who are healthy physically and well adjusted emotionally may have palpitation under certain circumstances. During or immediately after vigorous physical exertion or during sudden emotional tension, palpitation is common and is usually associated with sinus tachycardia. In poorly conditioned persons without organic heart disease, the sinus tachycardia of exercise may be excessive and associated with palpitation.

In some persons, palpitation may be one of the outstanding manifestations of an episode of acute anxiety. In others, the palpitation may, with other symptoms, represent prolonged anxiety neurosis or a lifelong disorder characterized by volatile autonomic function. Whether these illnesses are simply an expression of a chronic, deep-seated anxiety state superimposed on a normal autonomic nervous system or whether they depend on instability of the autonomic nervous system is not clear. At any rate, the clinical significance of the differentiation between the transitory and the enduring forms is that the former is often dissipated by firm reassurance from the physician, whereas the latter is usually resistant even to the most thorough and expert psychiatric care. In the latter case, the patient must be treated

TABLE 12-2 Items to be covered in history of patient with palpitation	
Does the palpitation occur:	If so, suspect:
As isolated "jumps" or "skips"?	Extrasystoles
In attacks, known to be of abrupt beginning, with a heart rate of 120 beats per minute or over, with regular or irregular rhythm?	Paroxysmal rapid heart action
Independent of exercise or excitement adequate to account for the symptom?	
In attacks developing rapidly though not absolutely abruptly, unrelated to exertion or excitement?	Atrial fibrillation, atrial flutter, thyrotoxicosis, anemia, febrile states, hypoglycemia, anxiety state
In conjunction with the taking of drugs?	Hemorrhage, hypoglycemia, tumor of the adrenal medulla
	Tobacco, coffee, tea, alcohol, epinephrine, ephedrine, aminophylline, atropine, thyroid extract, monoamine oxidase inhibitors
On standing?	Postural hypotension
In middle-aged women, in conjunction with flushes and sweats?	Menopausal syndrome
When the rate is known to be normal and the rhythm regular?	Anxiety state

with most carefully planned psychological support and tranquilizing medications. This chronic form of palpitation is known by various names such as *Da Costa's syndrome, soldier's heart, effort syndrome, irritable heart, neurocirculatory asthenia,* and *functional cardiovascular disease.* Aside from palpitation, the chief symptoms are those of an anxiety state.

Physical examination usually reveals the typical findings of the hyperkinetic syndrome. These include a left parasternal lift, a precordial or apical systolic murmur, a wide pulse pressure, rapidly rising pulse, and excessive perspiration. The electrocardiogram may display minor depressions of the ST segment and inversion of T waves and so occasionally lead to a mistaken diagnosis of coronary disease; this is particularly likely to occur when these findings are associated with complaints by the patients of an aching feeling of substernal tightness, commonly present in emotional stress. The presence of any kind of organic disease is one of the most common causes of the underlying anxiety which frequently precipitates this functional syndrome. Thus, even when a patient presents undoubted objective evidence of organic cardiac disease, the possibility that a superimposed anxiety state may be responsible for the symptoms described above should be considered. Palpitation associated with organic cardiac disease is nearly always accompanied by arrhythmia or tachycardia, whereas the symptom may exist with regular rhythm and with a heart rate of 80 beats per minute or less in patients with the anxiety state. An anxiety state, in contrast to heart disease, causes a sighing type of dyspnea. Also, pain localized to the apex, either brief and lancinating in character or lasting for hours or days and accompanied by hyperesthesia, is due usually to an anxiety state, not to structural cardiac disease. Giddiness due to this syndrome usually can be reproduced by hyperventilation or by change from the recumbent to the erect posture.

The *treatment* of the anxiety state with palpitation is difficult and depends on removal of the cause. In many instances a thorough examination of the heart and a statement that it is normal will suffice. Instructions to take more rather than less physical exercise will reinforce these statements. When the anxiety state is a manifestation of chronic anxiety neurosis or related emotional disorder, the symptoms are more likely to persist.

Table 12-2 summarizes the main points of information to be ascertained in the history in elucidating the significance of palpitation. The recording of an ambulatory electrocardiogram and the precise temporal correlation of the cardiac rate and rhythm with the presence of palpitation are extremely useful in the identification or exclusion of an arrhythmia if the symptom does not occur when the patient is under direct observation. The effectiveness of antiarrhythmia treatment also can be assessed objectively in this manner, without the necessity of relying only on the patient's subjective symptoms. Beta-adrenergic blockade with propranolol, beginning with 40 mg/d in divided doses, and ranging as high as 400 mg/d, or with equivalent doses of longer-acting beta-adrenergic antagonists can be extremely effective in patients with palpitation and sinus rhythm or sinus tachycardia.

One point merits special emphasis. *As a rule, palpitation produces anxiety and fear out of all proportion to its seriousness.* When the cause has been accurately determined and its significance explained to patients, their concern is often ameliorated and may disappear entirely.

REFERENCES

GOLDMAN L et al: A computer protocol to predict myocardial infarction in emergency department patients with chest pain. N Engl J Med 318:797, 1988

KOTLER TS, DIAMOND GA: Exercise thallium-201 scintigraphy in the diagnosis and prognosis of coronary artery disease. Ann Intern Med 113:684, 1990

LAM HGT et al: Acute noncardiac chest pain in a coronary care unit: Evaluation by a 24-hour pressure and pH recording of the esophagus. Gastroenterology 102:453, 1992

POZEN MW et al: A predictive instrument to improve coronary care unit admission practices in acute ischemic heart disease: A prospective multicenter clinical trial. N Engl J Med 310:1273, 1984

RUSTGI AK, CHOPRA S: Chest pain of esophageal origin. J Gen Intern Med 4:151, 1989

RUTHERFORD JD, BRAUNWALD E: Chronic ischemic heart disease, in *Heart Disease,* 4th ed, E. Braunwald (ed). Philadelphia, Saunders, 1992, p 1292

SOX HC JR. et al: The role of exercise testing in screening for coronary artery disease. Ann Intern Med 110:456, 1989

WOLF MA: Palpitations and disturbances of cardiac rhythm, in *Office Practice of Medicine* 3rd ed, WT Branch Jr (ed). Philadelphia, Saunders, 1994

13 ABDOMINAL PAIN

WILLIAM SILEN

The correct interpretation of acute abdominal pain is one of the most challenging demands made of any physician. Since proper therapy may require urgent action, the luxury of the leisurely approach suitable for the study of other conditions is sometimes denied. Few other clinical situations demand greater experience and judgment, because the most catastrophic of events may be forecast by the subtlest of symptoms and signs. Nowhere in medicine is a meticulously executed, detailed history and physical examination of greater importance. The etiologic classification in Table 13-1, although not complete, forms a useful frame of reference for the evaluation of patients with abdominal pain.

The diagnosis of "acute or surgical abdomen" so often heard in emergency wards is not an acceptable one because of its often misleading and erroneous connotation. The most obvious of "acute abdomens" may not require operative intervention, and the mildest of abdominal pains may herald the onset of an urgently correctable lesion. Any patient with abdominal pain of recent onset requires early and thorough evaluation with specific attempts at accurate diagnosis.

SOME MECHANISMS OF PAIN ORIGINATING IN THE ABDOMEN

Inflammation of the parietal peritoneum The pain of parietal peritoneal inflammation is steady and aching in character and is

---

TABLE 13-1   Some important causes of abdominal pain

PAIN ORIGINATING IN THE ABDOMEN

A   Parietal peritoneal inflammation
    1   Bacterial contamination, e.g., perforated appendix, pelvic inflammatory disease
    2   Chemical irritation, e.g., perforated ulcer, pancreatitis, mittelschmerz
B   Mechanical obstruction of hollow viscera
    1   Obstruction of the small or large intestine
    2   Obstruction of the biliary tree
    3   Obstruction of the ureter
C   Vascular disturbances
    1   Embolism or thrombosis
    2   Vascular rupture
    3   Pressure or torsional occlusion
    4   Sickle cell anemia
D   Abdominal wall
    1   Distortion or traction of mesentery
    2   Trauma or infection of muscles
E   Distention of visceral surfaces, e.g., hepatic or renal capsules

PAIN REFERRED FROM EXTRAABDOMINAL SOURCE

A   Thorax, e.g., pneumonia, referred pain from coronary occlusion
B   Spine, e.g., radiculitis from arthritis
C   Genitalia, e.g., torsion of the testicle

METABOLIC CAUSES

A   Exogenous
    1   Black widow spider bite
    2   Lead poisoning and others
B   Endogenous
    1   Uremia
    2   Diabetic ketoacidosis
    3   Porphyria
    4   Allergic factors (C'1 esterase inhibitor deficiency)

NEUROGENIC CAUSES

A   Organic
    1   Tabes dorsalis
    2   Herpes zoster
    3   Causalgia and others
B   Functional

---

located directly over the inflamed area, its exact reference being possible because it is transmitted by somatic nerves supplying the parietal peritoneum. The intensity of the pain is dependent on the type and amount of foreign substance to which the peritoneal surfaces are exposed in a given period of time. For example, the sudden release into the peritoneal cavity of a small quantity of *sterile* acid gastric juice causes much more pain than the same amount of grossly contaminated neutral fecal material. Enzymatically active pancreatic juice incites more pain and inflammation than does the same amount of sterile bile containing no potent enzymes. Blood and urine are often so bland as to go undetected if exposure of the peritoneum has not been sudden and massive. In the case of bacterial contamination, such as in pelvic inflammatory disease, the pain is frequently of low intensity early in the illness until bacterial multiplication has caused the elaboration of irritating substances.

So important is the rate at which the irritating material is applied to the peritoneum that cases of perforated peptic ulcer may be associated with entirely different clinical pictures dependent only on the rapidity with which the gastric juice enters the peritoneal cavity.

The pain of peritoneal inflammation is invariably accentuated by pressure or changes in tension of the peritoneum, whether produced by palpation or by movement, as in coughing or sneezing. Consequently, the patient with peritonitis lies quietly in bed, preferring to avoid motion, in contrast to the patient with colic, who may writhe incessantly.

Another of the characteristic features of peritoneal irritation is tonic reflex spasm of the abdominal musculature, localized to the involved body segment. The intensity of the tonic muscle spasm

accompanying peritoneal inflammation is dependent on the location of the inflammatory process, the rate at which it develops, and the integrity of the nervous system. Spasm over a perforated retrocecal appendix or perforated ulcer into the lesser peritoneal sac may be minimal or absent because of the protective effect of overlying viscera. As in pain of peritoneal inflammation, a slowly developing process often greatly attenuates the degree of muscle spasm. Catastrophic abdominal emergencies such as a perforated ulcer have been repeatedly associated with minimal or occasionally no detectable pain or muscle spasm in obtunded, seriously ill, debilitated elderly patients or in psychotic patients.

Obstruction of hollow viscera   The pain of obstruction of hollow abdominal viscera is classically described as intermittent, or colicky. Yet the lack of a truly cramping character should not be misleading, because distention of a hollow viscus may produce steady pain with only very occasional exacerbations. Although not nearly as well localized as the pain of parietal peritoneal inflammation, some useful generalities can be made concerning its distribution.

The colicky pain of obstruction of the small intestine is usually periumbilical or supraumbilical and is poorly localized. As the intestine becomes progressively dilated with loss of muscular tone, the colicky nature of the pain may become less apparent. With superimposed strangulating obstruction, pain may spread to the lower lumbar region if there is traction on the root of the mesentery. The colicky pain of colonic obstruction is of lesser intensity than that of the small intestine and is often located in the infraumbilical area. Lumbar radiation of pain is common in colonic obstruction.

Sudden distention of the biliary tree produces a steady rather than colicky type of pain; hence the term *biliary colic* is misleading. Acute distention of the gallbladder usually causes pain in the right upper quadrant with radiation to the right posterior region of the thorax or to the tip of the right scapula, and distention of the common bile duct is often associated with pain in the epigastrium radiating to the upper part of the lumbar region. Considerable variation is common, however, so that differentiation between these may be impossible. The typical subscapular pain or lumbar radiation is frequently absent. Gradual dilatation of the biliary tree, as in carcinoma of the head of the pancreas, may cause no pain or only a mild aching sensation in the epigastrium or right upper quadrant. The pain of distention of the pancreatic ducts is similar to that described for distention of the common bile duct but, in addition, is very frequently accentuated by recumbency and relieved by the upright position.

Obstruction of the urinary bladder results in dull suprapubic pain, usually low in intensity. Restlessness without specific complaint of pain may be the only sign of a distended bladder in an obtunded patient. In contrast, acute obstruction of the intravesicular portion of the ureter is characterized by severe suprapubic and flank pain which radiates to the penis, scrotum, or inner aspect of the upper region of the thigh. Obstruction of the ureteropelvic junction is felt as pain in the costovertebral angle, whereas obstruction of the remainder of the ureter is associated with flank pain which often extends into the corresponding side of the abdomen.

Vascular disturbances   A frequent misconception, despite abundant experience to the contrary, is that pain associated with intraabdominal vascular disturbances is sudden and catastrophic in nature. The pain of embolism or thrombosis of the superior mesenteric artery or that of impending rupture of an abdominal aortic aneurysm certainly may be severe and diffuse. Yet, just as frequently, the patient with occlusion of the superior mesenteric artery has only mild continuous diffuse pain for 2 or 3 days before vascular collapse or findings of peritoneal inflammation appear. The early, seemingly insignificant discomfort is caused by hyperperistalsis rather than peritoneal inflammation. Indeed, absence of tenderness and rigidity in the presence of continuous, diffuse pain in a patient likely to have vascular disease is quite characteristic of occlusion of the superior mesenteric artery. Abdominal pain with radiation to the sacral region, flank, or genitalia should always signal the possible presence of a rupturing abdominal aortic aneurysm. This pain may persist over a period of several days before rupture and collapse occur.

Abdominal wall Pain arising from the abdominal wall is usually constant and aching. Movement, prolonged standing, and pressure accentuate the discomfort and muscle spasm. In the case of hematoma of the rectus sheath, now most frequently encountered in association with anticoagulant therapy, a mass may be present in the lower quadrants of the abdomen. Simultaneous involvement of muscles in other parts of the body usually serves to differentiate myositis of the abdominal wall from an intraabdominal process which might cause pain in the same region.

REFERRED PAIN IN ABDOMINAL DISEASES Pain referred to the abdomen from the thorax, spine, or genitalia may prove a vexing diagnostic problem, because diseases of the upper part of the abdominal cavity such as acute cholecystitis or perforated ulcer are frequently associated with intrathoracic complications. A most important, yet often forgotten dictum is that the possibility of intrathoracic disease must be considered in every patient with abdominal pain, especially if the pain is in the upper part of the abdomen. Systematic questioning and examination directed toward detecting the presence or absence of myocardial or pulmonary infarction, pneumonia, pericarditis, or esophageal disease (the intrathoracic diseases which most often masquerade as abdominal emergencies) will often provide sufficient clues to establish the proper diagnosis. Diaphragmatic pleuritis resulting from pneumonia or pulmonary infarction may cause pain in the right upper quadrant and pain in the supraclavicular area, the latter radiation to be sharply distinguished from the referred subscapular pain caused by acute distention of the extrahepatic biliary tree. The ultimate decision as to the origin of abdominal pain may require deliberate and planned observation over a period of several hours, during which time repeated questioning and examination will provide the proper explanation.

Referred pain of thoracic origin is often accompanied by splinting of the involved hemithorax with respiratory lag and decrease in excursion more marked than that seen in the presence of intraabdominal disease. In addition, apparent abdominal muscle spasm caused by referred pain will diminish during the inspiratory phase of respiration, whereas it is persistent throughout both respiratory phases if it is of abdominal origin. Palpation over the area of referred pain in the abdomen also does not usually accentuate the pain and in many instances actually seems to relieve it. The frequent coexistence of thoracic and abdominal disease may be misleading and confusing, so differentiation may be difficult or impossible. For example, the patient with known biliary tract disease often has epigastric pain during myocardial infarction, or biliary colic may be referred to the precordium or left shoulder in a patient who has suffered previously from angina pectoris. For an explanation of the radiation of pain to a previously diseased area, see Chap. 11.

Referred pain from the spine, which usually involves compression or irritation of nerve roots, is characteristically intensified by certain motions such as cough, sneeze, or strain and is associated with hyperesthesia over the involved dermatomes. Pain referred to the abdomen from the testicles or seminal vesicles is generally accentuated by the slightest pressure on either of these organs. The abdominal discomfort is of dull aching character and is poorly localized.

METABOLIC ABDOMINAL CRISES Pain of metabolic origin may simulate almost any other type of intraabdominal disease. Here several mechanisms may be at work. In certain instances, such as hyperlipemia, the metabolic disease itself may be accompanied by an intraabdominal process such as pancreatitis, which can lead to unnecessary laparotomy unless recognized. C'1 esterase deficiency associated with angioneurotic edema is also often associated with episodes of severe abdominal pain. Whenever the cause of abdominal pain is obscure, a metabolic origin always must be considered. Abdominal pain is also the hallmark of familial Mediterranean fever (Chap. 293).

The problem of differential diagnosis is often not readily resolved.

The pain of porphyria and of lead colic usually is difficult to distinguish from that of intestinal obstruction, because severe hyperperistalsis is a prominent feature of both. The pain of uremia or diabetes is nonspecific, and the pain and tenderness frequently shift in location and intensity. Diabetic acidosis may be precipitated by acute appendicitis or intestinal obstruction, so if prompt resolution of the abdominal pain does not result from correction of the metabolic abnormalities, an underlying organic problem should be strongly suspected. Black widow spider bites produce intense pain and rigidity of the abdominal muscles and of the back, an area infrequently involved in disease of intraabdominal origin.

NEUROGENIC CAUSES Causalgic pain may occur in diseases that injure nerves of sensory type. It has a burning character and is usually limited to the distribution of a given peripheral nerve. Normal stimuli such as touch or change in temperature may be transformed into this type of pain, which is also frequently present in a patient at rest. A helpful finding is the demonstration that cutaneous pain spots are now irregularly spaced, and this may be the only indication of an old nerve lesion underlying causalgic pain. Even though the pain may be precipitated by gentle palpation, rigidity of the abdominal muscles is absent, and the respirations are not disturbed. Distention of the abdomen is uncommon, and the pain has no relationship to the intake of food.

Pain arising from spinal nerves or roots comes and goes suddenly and is of a lancinating type (see Chap. 15). It may be caused by herpes zoster, impingement by arthritis, tumors, herniated nucleus pulposus, diabetes, or syphilis. Again, it is not associated with food intake, abdominal distention, or changes in respiration. Severe muscle spasm, as in the gastric crises of tabes dorsalis, is common but is either relieved or is not accentuated by abdominal palpation. The pain is made worse by movement of the spine and is usually confined to a few dermatome segments. Hyperesthesia is very common.

Psychogenic pain conforms to none of the aforementioned patterns of disease. Here the mechanism is hard to define. The most common problem is the hysterical adolescent or young person who develops abdominal pain and who frequently loses an appendix or other organs because of it. Ovulation or some other natural event that causes brief mild abdominal discomfort may sometimes be experienced as an abdominal catastrophe.

Psychogenic pain varies enormously in type and location but usually has no relation to meals. It is often at its onset markedly accentuated during the night. Nausea and vomiting are rarely observed, although occasionally the patient reports these symptoms. Spasm is seldom induced in the abdominal musculature and, if present, does not persist, especially if the attention of the patient can be distracted. Persistent localized tenderness is rare, and if found, the muscle spasm in the area is inconsistent and often absent. Restriction of the depth of respiration is the most common respiratory abnormality, but this is in the nature of a smothering or choking sensation and is part of an anxiety state. It occurs in the absence of thoracic splinting or change in the respiratory rate.

APPROACH TO THE PATIENT WITH ABDOMINAL PAIN There are few abdominal conditions that require such urgent operative intervention that an orderly approach need be abandoned, no matter how ill the patient. Only those patients with exsanguinating hemorrhage must be rushed to the operating room immediately, but in such instances, only a few minutes are required to assess the critical nature of the problem. Under these circumstances, all obstacles must be swept aside, adequate access for intravenous fluid replacement obtained, and the operation begun. Many patients of this type have died in the radiology department or the emergency room while awaiting such unnecessary examinations as electrocardiograms or films of the abdomen. *There are no contraindications to operation when massive hemorrhage is present.* Although exceedingly important, this situation fortunately is relatively rare.

Nothing will supplant an orderly, painstakingly *detailed history*, which is far more valuable than any laboratory or roentgenologic examination. This kind of history is laborious and time-consuming, making it not especially popular, even though a reasonably accurate diagnosis can be made on the basis of the history alone in the majority of cases. Recent studies of computer-aided diagnosis of abdominal pain indicate that this technique provides no advantage over clinical assessment alone. In cases of *acute* abdominal pain, a diagnosis is readily established in most instances, whereas success is not so frequently achieved in patients with *chronic* pain. Since the irritable bowel syndrome is one of the most common causes of abdominal pain, the possibility of this diagnosis must always be kept in mind (see Chap. 256). The *chronological sequence of events* in the patient's history is often more important than emphasis on the location of pain. If the examiner is sufficiently open-minded and unhurried, asks the proper questions, and listens, the patient will usually provide the diagnosis. Careful attention should be paid to the extraabdominal regions which may be responsible for abdominal pain. An accurate menstrual history in a female patient is essential. Narcotics or analgesics should be withheld until a definitive diagnosis or a definitive plan has been formulated, because these agents often make it more difficult to secure and to interpret the history and physical findings.

In the examination, simple critical inspection of the patient, e.g., of facies, position in bed, and respiratory activity, may provide valuable clues. The amount of information to be gleaned is directly proportional to the *gentleness* and thoroughness of the examiner. Once a patient with peritoneal inflammation has been examined brusquely, accurate assessment by the next examiner becomes almost impossible. For example, eliciting rebound tenderness by sudden release of a deeply palpating hand in a patient with suspected peritonitis is cruel and unnecessary. The same information can be obtained by gentle percussion of the abdomen (rebound tenderness on a miniature scale), a maneuver which can be far more precise and localizing. Asking the patient to cough will elicit true rebound tenderness without the need for placing a hand on the abdomen. Furthermore, the forceful demonstration of rebound tenderness will startle and induce protective spasm in a nervous or worried patient in whom true rebound tenderness is not present. A palpable gallbladder will be missed if palpation is so brusque that voluntary muscle spasm becomes superimposed on involuntary muscular rigidity.

As in history taking, there is no substitute for sufficient time spent in the examination. It is important to remember that abdominal signs may be minimal but nevertheless, if accompanied by consistent symptoms, may be exceptionally meaningful. Signs may be virtually or actually totally absent in cases of pelvic peritonitis, so careful *pelvic and rectal examinations are mandatory in every patient with abdominal pain.* The presence of tenderness on pelvic or rectal examination in the absence of other abdominal signs must lead the examiner to consider such important operative indications as perforated appendicitis, diverticulitis, twisted ovarian cyst, and many others.

Much attention has been paid to the presence or absence of peristaltic sounds, their quality, and their frequency. Auscultation of the abdomen is probably one of the least rewarding aspects of the physical examination of a patient with abdominal pain. Severe catastrophes, such as strangulating small intestinal obstruction or perforated appendicitis, may occur in the presence of normal peristalsis. Conversely, when the proximal part of the intestine above an obstruction becomes markedly distended and edematous, peristaltic sounds may lose the characteristics of borborygmi and become weak or absent even when peritonitis is not present. It is usually the severe chemical peritonitis of sudden onset which is associated with the truly silent abdomen. Assessment of the patient's state of hydration is important. The hematocrit and urinalysis permit an accurate estimate of the severity of dehydration so that adequate replacement can be carried out.

Laboratory examinations may be of enormous value in assessment of the patient with abdominal pain, yet with but a few exceptions they rarely establish a diagnosis. Leukocytosis should never be the single deciding factor as to whether or not operation is indicated. A white blood cell count greater than 20,000/mm^3 may be observed

with perforation of a viscus, but pancreatitis, acute cholecystitis, pelvic inflammatory disease, and intestinal infarction may be associated with marked leukocytosis. A normal white blood cell count is by no means rare in cases of perforation of abdominal viscera. The diagnosis of anemia may be more helpful than the white blood cell count, especially when combined with the history.

The urinalysis is also of great value in indicating to some degree the state of hydration or to rule out severe renal disease, diabetes, or urinary infection. Determination of the blood urea nitrogen, blood sugar, and serum bilirubin levels also may be helpful. The serum amylase determination is overrated. Since many diseases other than pancreatitis, e.g., perforated ulcer, strangulating intestinal obstruction, and acute cholecystitis, may be associated with very marked increase in the serum amylase, great care must be exercised in denying an operation to a patient solely on the basis of an elevated serum amylase level. The determination of the serum lipase may have a somewhat greater accuracy than the serum amylase.

Plain and upright or lateral decubitus roentgenograms of the abdomen may be of the greatest value. They are usually unnecessary in patients with acute appendicitis or strangulated external hernias. However, in cases of intestinal obstruction, perforated ulcer, and a variety of other conditions, films may be diagnostic. In rare instances, barium or water-soluble medium examination of the upper part of the gastrointestinal tract may demonstrate partial intestinal obstruction which may elude diagnosis by other means. If there is any question of obstruction of the colon, oral administration of barium sulfate should be avoided. On the other hand, barium enema is of inestimable value in cases of colonic obstruction and should be used with greater frequency where the possibility of perforation does not exist.

Peritoneal lavage is a safe and effective diagnostic maneuver in patients with acute abdominal pain. It is of special value in patients with blunt trauma to the abdomen, in whom evaluation of the abdomen may be difficult because of other multiple injuries to the spine, pelvis, or ribs and in whom blood in the peritoneal cavity produces only a very mild peritoneal reaction. In the absence of trauma, peritoneal lavage has been replaced by ultrasound and laparoscopy. Ultrasonography has proved to be useful in detecting an enlarged gallbladder or pancreas, the presence of gallstones, an enlarged ovary, or a tubal pregnancy. Laparoscopy is especially helpful in diagnosing pelvic conditions such as ovarian cysts, tubal pregnancies or salpingitis, and acute appendicitis. Radioisotopic scans (HIDA) may help differentiate acute cholecystitis from acute pancreatitis. A computed tomography (CT) scan may demonstrate an enlarged pancreas or a ruptured spleen, but it should be used only for *specific* questions such as these.

Sometimes, even under the best of circumstances with all available auxiliary aids and with the greatest of clinical skill, a definitive diagnosis cannot be established at the time of the initial examination. Nevertheless, despite lack of a clear anatomic diagnosis, it may be abundantly clear to an experienced and thoughtful physician and surgeon that on clinical grounds alone operation is indicated. Should that decision be questionable, watchful waiting with repeated questioning and examination will often elucidate the true nature of the illness and indicate the proper course of action.

REFERENCES

DAVIES AH et al: Ultrasonography in the acute abdomen. Br J Surg 78:1178, 1991
LEE PWR: The plain x-ray in the acute abdomen: A surgeon's evaluation. Br J Surg 63:763, 1976
LEEK BF: Abdominal and pelvic visceral receptors. Br Med Bull 33:163, 1977
SILEN W: *Cope's Early Diagnosis of the Acute Abdomen*, 18th ed. London, Oxford Press, 1991
SUTTON GC: How accurate is computer-aided diagnosis? Lancet 2:905, 1989
VALMAN HB: Acute abdominal pain. Br Med J 282:1858, 1981

14   HEADACHE

NEIL H. RASKIN

Few of us are spared the experience of head pain during our lifetimes; indeed, severe, disabling headache is reported to occur at least annually by 40 percent of individuals worldwide. This incidence occurs whether subjects live in large urban environments or in rural villages. The mechanism generating such "benign" headaches may be activated by stress and anxiety, but emotional factors are not necessary for the symptom to occur. The more severe the headache, the more likely it is to be associated with nausea and to be experienced as a pulsing or pounding discomfort; photo- and phonophobia are also more likely to be reported. Moreover, there does not appear to be any utility in having headache; most sufferers report the contrary.

Since headache is a ubiquitous symptom, it may properly be regarded as a *normal* aspect of living; it then follows that the mechanism for such a common phenomenon is more likely to be ordinary than extraordinary. This "ordinary" headache-generating mechanism appears to be influenced by hereditary factors that may "turn up the gain," resulting in susceptibility to more frequent or more severe head pain. The term *migraine* is used nowadays to refer to such a mechanism, in contrast to its prior usage referring to an aggregation of certain symptoms.

Headache is usually a benign symptom and only occasionally is the manifestation of a serious illness, such as brain tumor or giant cell arteritis. The first issue to resolve in confronting the patient who complains of headache is to make the distinction between benign and more ominous causes.

GENERAL CONSIDERATIONS   The quality, location, duration, and time course of the headache and the conditions that produce, exacerbate, or relieve it should be carefully reviewed with the patient.

Ascertaining the *quality* of cephalic pain is occasionally helpful. Most headaches are dull, deeply located, and of aching character. Superimposed on such nondescript pain may be other pain elements that have greater diagnostic value. It is useful to clarify to the patient that it is of interest to learn about *all* the pain elements that have been experienced regardless of their frequency or intensity. A throbbing quality and tight muscles about the head, neck, and shoulder girdle are common nonspecific accompaniments of headache, suggesting that intra- and extracranial arteries and skeletal muscle surrounding the head and neck are activated by a generic head pain–generating mechanism. It was formerly believed that tight "hat-band" headaches indicated anxiety or depression, but investigations have not supported this view. Jabbing, brief, sharp cephalic pain, often occurring multifocally (ice picklike pain), is the signature of a benign disorder.

Pain *intensity* seldom has diagnostic value—in the head or in any other somatic location. From the therapeutic perspective, it is, of course, the single aspect of pain that is most important. Physicians should be cautious about assessing pain intensity by visually inspecting a patient. People respond to pain in a variety of ways that range from overt histrionic behavior to stoicism. Inquiries as to how pain disturbs day-to-day function may extract more useful information. *Response to placebo medication or procedures produces no useful information*— either diagnostic or therapeutic. It simply identifies a "placebo responder," about 30 percent of the population. There is no evidence that placebo responders have lower pain levels than nonresponders or do not really have pain. Patients entering emergency departments with the most severe headache of their lives usually have migraine. Meningitis, subarachnoid hemorrhage, and cluster headache also produce intense cranial pain. Contrary to common belief, the headache produced by a brain tumor is not usually particularly or distinctively severe.

Data regarding *location* of headache may be informative. If the source is an extracranial structure, as in giant cell arteritis, the correspondence with the site of pain is fairly precise. Inflammation of an extracranial artery causes pain and extensive tenderness localized to the site of the vessel. Lesions of paranasal sinuses, teeth, eyes, and upper cervical vertebrae induce less sharply localized pain, but one that is still referred in a regional distribution that is quite constant. Intracranial lesions in the posterior fossa cause pain that is usually occipitonuchal, and supratentorial lesions most often induce fronto-temporal pain.

Duration and *time-intensity* curves of headaches are particularly useful. A ruptured aneurysm results in head pain that peaks in an instant, thunderclaplike; much less often, unruptured aneurysms may signal their presence in the same way. Cluster headache attacks reach their peak over 3 to 5 min, remain at maximal levels for about 45 min, and then taper off. Migraine attacks build up over hours, are maintained for several hours to days, and are characteristically relieved by sleep. Sleep disruption is characteristic of headaches produced by brain tumors.

Headaches that bear a relationship to certain biologic events or to physical environmental changes are essential data for triage of patients. The following exacerbating phenomena make the benign nature of the syndrome highly probable: provocation by red wine, sustained exertion, organic odors, hunger, lack of sleep, weather change, and menses. The association of diarrhea with attacks (Table 14-1) is pathognomonic of a benign disorder (migraine). The cessation or amelioration of headache during pregnancy, especially the second and third trimesters, is also pathognomonic of migraine. Patients with continuous benign headaches often observe a pain-free interlude of several minutes upon awakening before head pain commences. This phenomenon occurs with other centrally mediated pain syndromes, such as thalamic pain, but does not occur among patients with somatic disease as the cause of pain. In attempting to elicit this information, patients commonly respond negatively to initial inquiries in the mistaken belief that because the relationships are not consistent, the validity of the observation is in question. Activation of the mechanism by red wine and hunger, for example, is *always* inconsistent, for reasons that are unclear. It is important to make this context clear to the patient or else valuable information may be lost, resulting in unnecessary neuroimaging.

A history of amenorrhea or galactorrhea should lead one to question whether the polycystic ovary syndrome or a prolactin-secreting pituitary adenoma is the source of headache. Headache arising *de novo* in a patient with known malignancy suggests either cerebral metastases or carcinomatous meningitis. When there is striking accentuation of pain with eye movement, a systemic infection and particularly meningitis should be seriously considered. Head pain appearing abruptly after bending, lifting, or coughing can be the clue to a posterior fossa mass or the Arnold Chiari malformation. Orthostatic headache arises after lumbar puncture and also occurs with subdural hematoma and benign intracranial hypertension. The

TABLE 14-1   Symptoms accompanying severe migraine attacks in 500 patients

Symptom	Percentage affected
Nausea	87
Vomiting	56
Diarrhea	16
Photophobia	82
Visual disturbances	36
Fortification spectra	10
Photopsia	26
Paresthesias	33
Scalp tenderness	65
Lightheadedness	72
Vertigo	33
Alteration of consciousness	18
Seizure	4
Syncope	10
Confusional state	4

SOURCE: NH Raskin, *Headache*, 2d ed, New York, Churchill Livingstone, 1988.

eye itself is seldom the cause of acute orbital pain if the sclerae are white and not injected; a "red eye" is the sign of ophthalmic disease. Similarly, acute sinusitis nearly always declares itself through a dark green, purulent nasal exudate.

The analysis of facial pain requires a disparate approach. Trigeminal and glossopharyngeal neuralgia are common causes of facial pain, especially the former. "Neuralgias" are painful disorders characterized by paroxysmal, fleeting, often electric shocklike episodes that are caused by demyelinative lesions of nerves (the trigeminal or glossopharyngeal nerves in cranial neuralgias) that result in the activation of a CNS pain-generating mechanism. Certain maneuvers characteristically trigger paroxysms of pain. However, the most common cause of facial pain by far is dental; provocation by hot, cold, or sweet foods is typical. The application of a cold stimulus will repeatedly induce dental pain whereas in neuralgic disorders a refractory period usually occurs after the initial response so that pain cannot be repeatedly induced. The presence of refractory periods can nearly always be elicited in the history so that patients need not be put through a painful experience.

Mealtimes offer the physician an opportunity to gain needed insight into the mechanism of a patient's facial pain. Is it the chewing, the swallowing, or the taste of the food that elicits pain? Chewing points toward trigeminal neuralgia, temporomandibular joint dysfunction, or giant cell arteritis ("jaw claudication"), whereas swallowing *and* taste provocation points toward glossopharyngeal neuralgia. Pain upon swallowing is common among patients with carotidynia (facial migraine, see below) because the inflamed, tender carotid artery abuts the esophagus during deglutition.

Many patients with the complaint of facial pain do not describe stereotypic syndromes, in parallel with most painful conditions; such patients have sometimes had their syndromes categorized as "atypical facial pain" as if this were a well-defined clinical entity. There is only scant evidence that nondescript facial pain is caused by emotional distress, as has sometimes been alleged. Vague, poorly localized, continuous facial pain is *characteristic* of the condition that may result from nasopharyngeal carcinoma and other somatic diseases; a burning painful element often supervenes as deafferentation occurs and evidence of cranial neuropathy appears. Occasionally, the cause of a pain problem cannot be resolved promptly, necessitating periodic follow-up until further clues appear (and they usually do). "Facial pain of unknown cause" appears to be a more reasonable tentative diagnosis than "atypical facial pain."

PAIN-SENSITIVE STRUCTURES OF THE HEAD   The most common type of pain is that resulting from activation of peripheral nociceptors in the presence of a normally functioning nervous system, as in the pain resulting from scalded skin or appendicitis. Another type of pain is the result of injury or activation of the peripheral or central nervous system. Headache, formerly believed to originate peripherally, may originate from either mechanism. Headache may arise from dysfunction, displacement, or encroachment upon pain-sensitive cranial structures. The following are sensitive to mechanical stimulation: the scalp and aponeurotica, middle meningeal artery, dural sinuses, falx cerebri, and the proximal segments of the large pial arteries. The ventricular ependyma, choroid plexus, pial veins, and much of the brain parenchyma are pain-insensitive. On the other hand, electrical stimulation near midbrain dorsal raphe cells has resulted in migrainelike headaches. Thus most of the brain is insensitive to electrode probing, but a particular midbrain site is nevertheless a putative locus for headache generation.

Sensory stimuli from the head are conveyed to the central nervous system via the trigeminal nerves for structures above the tentorium in the anterior and middle fossae of the skull and via the first three cervical nerves for those in the posterior fossa and infradural structures. The ninth and tenth cranial nerves supply part of the posterior fossa and refer pain to the ear and throat.

Headache can occur as the result of (1) distention, traction, or dilation of intracranial or extracranial arteries; (2) traction or displacement of large intracranial veins or their dural envelope; (3) compression, traction, or inflammation of cranial and spinal nerves; (4) spasm, inflammation, and trauma to cranial and cervical muscles; (5) meningeal irritation and raised intracranial pressure; and (6) perturbation of intracerebral serotonergic projections. By and large, intracranial masses cause headache when they deform, displace, or exert traction on vessels, dural structures, or cranial nerves at the base of the brain; this often happens long before intracranial pressure rises. Such mechanical displacement mechanisms do not explain the headaches resulting from cerebral ischemia, or from benign intracranial hypertension after the pressure is reduced, or the headaches that are so common in febrile illnesses and systemic lupus erythematosus. Perturbation of intracerebral serotonergic projections has been posited as a possible mechanism for these phenomena.

PRINCIPAL CLINICAL VARIETIES OF HEADACHE

Normally there is little difficulty in diagnosing the headache of glaucoma, purulent sinusitis, bacterial meningitis, and brain tumor because of the clues provided by the associated symptoms and signs. Headache alone is nondescript. It is when headache is chronic, recurrent, and unattended by other important signs of disease that the physician faces a challenging but ultimately gratifying medical problem. The headache syndromes described below should be considered (see Table 14-2).

MIGRAINE   The term *migraine* stems from Galen's usage of *hemicrania* to describe a periodic disorder comprising paroxysmal blinding hemicranial pain, vomiting, photophobia, recurrence at regular intervals, and relief by dark surroundings and sleep. Hemicrania was later corrupted into low Latin as *hemigranea* and *migranea*; eventually the French translation, *migraine*, gained acceptance in the eighteenth century and has prevailed ever since. The passage of time has proved this to be a misleading designation for a condition manifested by lateralized head pain in less than 60 percent of those affected. Furthermore, undue emphasis on the dramatic features of migraine has often led to the illogical conclusion that periodic headache lacking such features is not migrainous in mechanism. It has become clear that severe headache attacks, regardless of cause, are more likely to be described as throbbing and associated with vomiting and scalp tenderness. Milder headaches tend to be nondescript—tight, bandlike discomfort often involving the entire head—the profile of "tension headache." These differing clinical profiles of headaches that are not caused by an intracranial structural anomaly or systemic disease probably represent different points on a continuum rather than disparate clinical entities. Whether a single common mechanism underlies these varying headache profiles is not entirely clear and remains to be investigated further. A working definition of migraine offered here is benign recurring headache and/or neurologic dysfunction usually attended by pain-free interludes and almost always provoked by stereotyped stimuli. It is by far more common in women; there is a hereditary predisposition toward attacks; and the cranial circulatory phenomena that attend attacks appear to be secondary to a primary CNS disorder.

Clinical subtypes   The designation *classic migraine* (migraine with aura) denotes the syndrome of headache associated with characteristic premonitory sensory, motor, or visual symptoms; *common migraine* (migraine without aura) denotes one in which there is no focal neurologic disturbance preceding the occurrence of headache. However, the latter is by far the most frequent clinical problem, and focal neurologic disturbances are more common during headache attacks than as prodromal symptoms. Focal neurologic disturbances without headache or vomiting have come to be known as *migraine equivalents* or *accompaniments* and appear to occur more commonly in patients between the ages of 40 and 70 years. The term *complicated migraine* has generally been used to describe migraine with dramatic focal neurologic features, thus overlapping with classic migraine; it has also been used to connote a persisting neurologic deficit that is a residuum of a migraine attack.

TABLE 14-2 Common types of headaches

Type	Usual site	Age and sex	Clinical features	Life profile
Migraine, with or without aura	Frontotemporal, uni- or bilateral.	All ages; highest incidence in children and young adults. Female > male in adults. Female = male in children.	Onset after awakening; quelled by sleep. Provoked by menses, odors, foods. Stops after 2d trimester of pregnancy. Duration: 6 h to 2 days.	Cycles of several months to years. Less frequent and less severe with aging.
Cluster headache	Lateralized, orbital or temporal.	All ages above 10; peaks at 30–50. Mainly men (90%). Provoked by alcohol.	Periodic attacks. 1–2 attacks per day, commonly awakens from sleep. Duration: 45 min. Associated with red eye and stuffy nose homolaterally.	Daily attacks for 6 weeks with annual recurrence of bout.
Tension headache	Generalized.	All ages; principally young adults. Female preponderance.	Nondescript, tight bandlike discomfort continuously. Exacerbations provoked by factors similar to migraine.	Cycles of several years.
Brain tumor	Variable.	All ages, both sexes.	Interrupts sleep, unrelieved by sleep. Exacerbated by orthostatic changes. Steadily worsening pain; may be preceded by days to weeks of nausea and vomiting.	Monophasic illness lasting weeks to months.
Giant cell arteritis	Lateralized, temporal or occipital.	Over 55 years, either sex.	Marked scalp tenderness with superimposed jabbing and jolting pain. Deep, intermittent throbbing. Associated with malaise and morning stiffness and pain in shoulders and hips.	Monophasic illness lasting weeks to months.
Lumbar puncture headache	Bifrontal and/or bioccipital.	Over 10 years, either sex.	Orthostatic; head pain present with patient sitting or standing and disappears in prone or supine positions.	Arises 1–2 days after lumbar puncture and persists for 3–4 days.

COMMON MIGRAINE Benign periodic headache of several hours duration, often attributed to "tension" by its sufferers, is the most liberal way of circumscribing common migraine. The fallacy intrinsic to most of the traditional definitions is that they are acceptable definitions of severe attacks but do not include those patients with more modest degrees of head pain; thus, pain unilaterality, attendant nausea or vomiting, positive family history, responsiveness to ergotamine, and scalp tenderness in varying combinations have been alleged to establish a diagnosis of migraine. However, each of these occur in roughly 60 to 80 percent of patients as *dependent* variables, and the validity of using such clinical features to diagnose migraine has never been established. Common migraine is the most frequent headache type reported by patients and includes the now anachronistic concept of periodic tension headache.

CLASSIC MIGRAINE The most common premonitory symptoms reported by migraineurs are visual, arising from dysfunction of occipital lobe neurons. Scotomas and/or hallucinations occur in about one-third of migraineurs and usually appear in the central portions of the visual fields. A highly characteristic syndrome occurs in about 10 percent of patients; it usually begins as a small paracentral scotoma, which slowly expands into a "C" shape. Luminous angles appear at the enlarging outer edge, becoming colored as the scintillating scotoma expands and moves toward the periphery of the involved half of the visual field. It eventually disappears over the horizon of peripheral vision, the entire process consuming 20 to 25 min. This phenomenon never occurs *during* the headache phase of an attack and is pathognomonic for migraine, never having been described in association with a cerebral structural anomaly. It is commonly referred to as a *fortification spectrum* because the serrated edges of the hallucinated "C" seemed to Dr. Hubert Airy to resemble a "fortified town with bastions all round it"; "spectrum" is used in the sense of an apparition or specter.

BASILAR MIGRAINE Symptoms referable to a disturbance in brainstem function such as vertigo, dysarthria, and diplopia occur as the only neurologic symptoms of the attack in about 25 percent of patients (Table 14-1). Bickerstaff called attention to a stereotyped sequence of dramatic neurologic events often comprising total blind-ness and sensorial clouding that is common among but not restricted to adolescent women. These episodes begin with total blindness accompanied or followed by admixtures of vertigo, ataxia, dysarthria, tinnitus, and distal and perioral paresthesia. In about one-quarter of patients, a confusional state supervenes. The neurologic symptoms usually persist for 20 to 30 min and are generally followed by a throbbing occipital headache. The basilar migraine syndrome is now known to occur in children as well as in adults over age 50. Sensorial alterations may last for as long as 5 days and may take the form of confusional states that may be mistaken for psychotic reactions.

CAROTIDYNIA The carotidynia syndrome, sometimes called lower half headache or facial migraine, is more prominent among an older population of patients, with peak incidence in the fourth through sixth decades. Pain is usually reported to be located at the jaw or neck, although sometimes periorbital or maxillary pain occurs; it may be continuous, deep, dull, and aching, and becomes pounding or throbbing episodically. There are often superimposed sharp, ice picklike jabs. Attacks occur one to several times per week, each lasting several minutes to hours. Tenderness and prominent pulsations of the cervical carotid artery, and soft tissue swelling overlying the carotid, are usually present homolateral to the pain; many patients also report throbbing ipsilateral headache concurrent with carotidynia attacks as well as interictally. Dental trauma is a common precipitant of this syndrome. Carotid artery involvement in the more traditional forms of migraine appears to be common as well; over 50 percent of patients with frequent migraine attacks are found to have carotid tenderness at several points homolateral to the cranial side preponderantly involved during their attacks.

Pathogenesis Modern orientations toward migraine began with the publication by Liveing in 1873 of the first major treatise devoted to the subject of migraine, *A Contribution to the Pathology of Nerve Storms*. Liveing believed that the analogy of migraine to epilepsy was obvious, and that the clinically apparent circulatory phenomena that occurred during migrainous attacks were secondary to cerebral discharges, or "nerve storms." Attention was focused on the vascular features of migraine by Graham and Wolff in the 1930s who showed that the administration of ergotamine reduced the amplitude of the pulsations of the temporal artery in patients with headache and that this effect was often, but *not consistently*, associated with a decrease in head pain. Because of these observations and other less substantial lines of evidence, it was widely held for many years that the headache phase of migrainous attacks was caused by extracranial vasodilatation and that neurologic symptoms were produced by intracranial vasoconstriction, the ''vascular'' hypothesis of migraine. A barrage of publications by Wolff and his coworkers followed in support of this hypothesis so that observations made during the 1940s nonresonant with it were ignored.

K. S. Lashley, neuropsychologist at Harvard, in 1941 was among the first to chart in detail his own migrainous fortification spectrum at brief intervals. He was able to estimate that the evolution of his own scotoma proceeded across the occipital cortex at a rate of 3 mm/min. He speculated that a wavefront of intense excitation followed by a wave of complete inhibition of activity were propagated across the visual cortex. Uncannily, in 1944, the phenomenon that has come to be known as *spreading depression* was described by a Brazilian physiologist, Leão, in the cerebral cortex of laboratory animals. It is a slowly moving (2- to 3-mm/min) potassium-liberating depression of cortical activity, preceded by a wavefront of increased metabolic activity that can be produced by a variety of experimental stimuli, including hypoxia, mechanical trauma, and the topical application of potassium.

These observations, striking in retrospect, could not possibly be incorporated into the aforementioned vascular model of migraine, which had been tenaciously grasped by the medical community. However, observations made over the past decade in Copenhagen have rendered untenable an hypothesis invoking a primary vascular mechanism, and lend support to the possibility that spreading depression, or more likely a neuronal phenomenon with similar characteristics, is important to the mechanism of classic migraine.

The pathogenesis of migraine as it is currently understood can be partitioned into three phases. The first is brain (stem) generation; the second may be expressed as ''vasomotor activation'' wherein arteries both within and outside brain may contract or dilate; the third is activation of cells of the medullary trigeminal nucleus caudalis (the brain's head and face pain-processing mechanism) and the subsequent release of vasoactive neuropeptides at vascular terminations of the trigeminal nerve. This last phase provides a reasonable mechanism for the soft-tissue swelling and tenderness of blood vessels that attend migraine attacks. It seems clear that activation of any of the phases is *sufficient* for headache production, and that one phase may appear to dominate in a particular migrainous syndrome. For example, the evolution of the fortification spectrum is probably entirely neurogenic, requiring only first phase activation (see below).

Regional cerebral blood flow studies have shown that in patients with classic migraine there is, during attacks, a modest cortical hypoperfusion that begins in the visual cortex and spreads forward at a rate of 2 to 3 mm/min. The decrease in blood flow averages 25 to 30 percent (too little to explain symptoms) and progresses anteriorly in a wavelike fashion independent of the topography of cerebral arteries. The wave of hypoperfusion persists for 4 to 6 h, appears to follow the convolutions of the cortex, and does not cross the central or lateral sulcus, progressing to the frontal lobe via the insula. Subcortical perfusion is normal. Contralateral neurologic symptoms appear during temporoparietal hypoperfusion; at times hypoperfusion persists in these regions after symptoms cease. More often frontal spread continues as the headache phase begins. A few patients with classic migraine show no flow abnormalities; an occasional patient has developed focal ischemia sufficient to cause symptoms. However, focal ischemia does not appear *necessary* for focal symptoms to occur. During common migraine, no flow abnormalities are seen. The cerebral blood flow changes are probably the manifestation of a derangement in cerebral neuronal function; moreover, these cortical events require a ''generator,'' presumably within the brainstem.

Neuromagnetic activity has been detected in the temporooccipital cortex of migraineurs during headache episodes. Spontaneous, long-duration (1- to 8-s) biphasic signals have been observed, consistent with a primary neuronal origin of migraine.

Pharmacologic data converge on serotonin receptors. About 35 years ago, methysergide was found to antagonize certain peripheral actions of serotonin (5-hydroxytryptamine) and was introduced as the first drug capable of preventing migraine attacks through stabilization of the mechanism. Subsequently, it was found that platelet levels of serotonin fall consistently at the onset of headache and that migrainous episodes may be triggered by drugs that release it. Such changes in circulating levels proved to be pharmacologically trivial, however, and interest in the humoral role of serotonin in migraine declined. Currently, there is renewed interest due almost entirely to the introduction of a new drug, sumatriptan, that is remarkably effective for migraine attacks. Of still greater interest is that sumatriptan is a designer drug, synthesized to activate selectively a particular subpopulation of serotonin receptors.

There are four main families of 5-hydroxytryptamine receptors—types 1, 2, 3, and 4—within each family of which receptor subtypes have been found. Sumatriptan interacts with serotonin 1A receptors and especially with 1D receptors. By contrast, dihydroergotamine, another drug that is highly effective in aborting migraine attacks, is most potent as an agonist of serotonin 1A receptors and is an order of magnitude less potent at 1D receptors. After systemic administration, dihydroergotamine in brain is found in highest concentrations in the midbrain dorsal raphe. The dorsal raphe is a good candidate for the generator of migraine and the main site of drug action; the highest concentration of serotonin receptors in brain tissue is found there. They are mainly of the 1A variety, but 1D receptors also are present.

As mentioned earlier, electrical stimulation near dorsal raphe neurons can result in migrainelike headaches. There are projections from the dorsal raphe that terminate on cerebral arteries and alter cerebral blood flow. There are also major projections from the dorsal raphe to important visual processing way stations, including the lateral geniculate body, superior colliculus, retina, and visual cortex. These various projections are the anatomic and physiologic matrices for the circulatory and visual characteristics of migraine. The dorsal raphe cells stop firing during deep sleep, and sleep is known to ameliorate migraine; the antimigraine drugs also stop the firing of the dorsal raphe cells through a direct or indirect agonist effect (Figure 14-1). The shutdown of an inhibitory system might be expected to enhance or stabilize neurotransmission, and there is evidence that this indeed occurs.

Migraine may represent, therefore, a hereditary perturbation of serotonergic neurotransmission. Such perturbation may underlie many types of head pain; ordinary periodic headaches may be the ''noise'' of the normally functioning system.

Treatment Several nonpharmacologic treatments have been advocated in recent years, but the most rigorously controlled trials have shown no benefit without concomitant drug treatment. Thus, the mainstay of therapy is the judicious use of one or more of the many drugs that are relatively specific for migraine.

ACUTE TREATMENT In general, an adequate dose of whichever agent is chosen should be used at the onset of an attack. If additional medication is requested in 30 to 60 min because symptoms return or have not abated, the initial dose should be increased for subsequent attacks. Drug absorption is impaired during migrainous attacks because of reduced gastrointestinal motility. Delayed absorption occurs in the absence of nausea and is related to the severity of the attack and not its duration. Therefore, when oral agents fail, the major considerations revolve about rectal ergotamine, subcutaneous sumatriptan, parenteral dihydroergotamine, and intravenous chlorpromazine and prochlorperazine.

For patients with a prolonged buildup of headache, oral agents may indeed suffice. When aspirin and acetaminophen fail, the addition of butalbital and caffeine to these analgesics is highly effective; ibuprofen (600 to 800 mg) and naproxen (375 to 750 mg) are often useful. Isometheptene compound, 1 to 2 capsules, is effective for

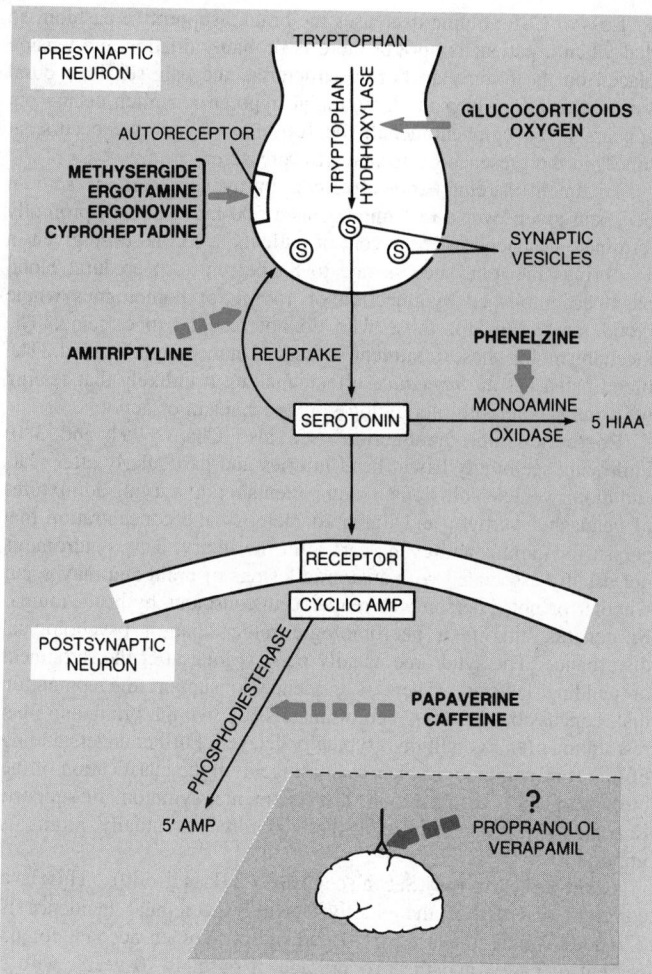

FIGURE 14-1 The actions of the antimigraine drugs at brainstem and forebrain synapses. The solid arrows indicate stimulative or agonist properties and the segmented arrows indicate inhibitory properties. (*From NH Raskin, Headache, 2d ed, New York, Churchill Livingstone, 1988.*)

mild-to-moderate "stress headaches." When these measures fail, more aggressive therapy should be considered.

A subnauseating dose of ergotamine, if possible, should be determined; a dose that provokes nausea—probably a centrally mediated side effect—is too high and may intensify head pain. The average oral dose is 3 mg (three 1-mg ergotamine-caffeine tablets); the average dose of the 2-mg suppository is one-half (1 mg). Many patients use one-quarter of a suppository (0.5 mg) with an optimal result. Sumatriptan may be given as an oral 100-mg dose or a 6-mg subcutaneous dose; there is a high recurrence rate because of the short half-life of this drug (2 h), so that a second dose may be necessary.

Dihydroergotamine is available presently only as a parenteral preparation. Peak plasma levels of dihydroergotamine are achieved 45 min after subcutaneous dosing, 30 min after intramuscular administration, and 3 min following intravenous dosing. If an attack has not already peaked, subcutaneous or intramuscular administration of 1 mg suffices for about 90 percent of patients. A common intravenous protocol is the mixture of prochlorperazine, 5 mg and 0.5 mg dihydroergotamine (they are miscible), administered over 2 min.

When patients' headache profiles transform into a chronic daily headache syndrome, opiate-type analgesics should be restricted to 2 days out of 7. The mainstay of therapy for these patients is daily amitriptyline (30 to 100 mg) or nortriptyline (40 to 120 mg). For recalcitrant individuals, valproate (500 to 2000 mg) or phenelzine (45 to 90 mg) may be necessary.

PROPHYLAXIS A substantial number of drugs are now available that have the capacity to stabilize migraine; they must be taken daily. When to implement this approach is contingent on the frequency of attacks and how well acute treatment is working. At least two or three attacks monthly could signal this approach. There is usually a lag of 2 weeks or so before an effect is seen, which may be the time necessary to down-regulate serotonin receptors. The major drugs and their daily dosage used in this setting are propranolol (60 to 240 mg), amitriptyline (30 to 100 mg), valproate (500 to 2000 mg), verapamil (120 to 480 mg), phenelzine (45 to 90 mg), and methysergide (4 to 12 mg). Phenelzine and methysergide are usually reserved for more recalcitrant patients because of serious potential side effects. Phenelzine is a monoamine oxidase inhibitor; therefore, tyramine-containing foods, decongestants, and meperidine are contraindicated. Methysergide may cause retroperitoneal or cardiac valvular fibrosis when it is used for more than 8 months, so monitoring is required for patients using this drug; the risk of the fibrotic complication is about 1:1500 and is likely to reverse after the drug is stopped.

The probability of success with any one of the antimigraine drugs is of the order of 60 to 75 percent; if one drug is assessed each month, there is the high likelihood that effective stabilization will be achieved within a few months. The large majority of patients are successfully managed with propranolol or amitriptyline; for more urgent resolution, valproate, methysergide, or phenelzine can be implemented. Once effective stabilization is achieved, the drug is continued for 5 to 6 months and then slowly tapered to assess its continued need. Many patients are able to discontinue medication and experience fewer and less severe attacks for long periods of time, suggesting that these drugs may alter the natural history of migraine.

CLUSTER HEADACHE Recognition of this clinical entity has been retarded by a variety of confusing names lent to this condition, including *Raeder's syndrome*, *histamine cephalalgia*, and *sphenopalatine neuralgia*. Cluster headache is now firmly established as a distinctive syndrome whose recognition is important since it is likely to be responsive to treatment. The episodic type, the most common, is characterized by one to three short-lived attacks of periorbital pain per day over a 4- to 8-week period, followed by a pain-free interval that averages 1 year. The chronic form, which may begin *de novo* or several years after an episodic pattern has become established, is characterized by the absence of sustained periods of remission. Each type may transform into the other. Men are affected more commonly than women in a proportion of 7–8:1; hereditary factors are usually absent. Although most patients begin experiencing headache between the ages of 20 and 50 years, the syndrome may begin as early as the first decade and as late as the eighth decade. The cluster syndrome is genetically, biochemically, and clinically different from migraine; propranolol and amitriptyline are largely ineffective. Lithium is beneficial for the cluster syndrome and ineffective in migraine. Nevertheless, the two disorders occasionally blend into one in occasional patients, suggesting that their mechanisms bear some degree of commonality.

Clinical features Periorbital, or less commonly, temporal pain begins without warning and reaches a crescendo within 5 min. It is often excruciating in intensity and is deep, nonfluctuating, and explosive in quality; only rarely is it pulsatile. Pain is strictly unilateral and usually affects the same side in subsequent months. Attacks last from 30 min to 2 h; there are often the associated symptoms of homolateral lacrimation, reddening of the eye, nasal stuffiness, lid ptosis, and nausea. Alcohol provocation of attacks occurs in about 70 percent of patients and ceases when the bout remits; this on-off vulnerability to alcohol is pathognomonic of the cluster headache syndrome. Only rarely do foods or emotional factors activate the mechanism, in contradistinction to migraine.

There is an uncanny periodicity of attacks in at least 85 percent of patients. At least one of the daily attacks of pain recurs at about the same hour each day for the duration of a cluster bout. This clock mechanism is set for the nocturnal hours in about 50 percent of the cases, and in such circumstances pain usually awakens patients within 2 h of falling asleep.

Pathogenesis   There are no consistent cerebral blood flow changes attending attacks of pain. Perhaps the strongest evidence pointing to a central mechanism is the ''periodicity''; reinforcing this conclusion is the observation that the autonomic symptoms that accompany the pain are bilateral, more severe on the painful side. The hypothalamus may be the site of activation in this disorder. The posterior hypothalamus contains cells that regulate autonomic functions and the anterior hypothalamus contains cells (the suprachiasmatic nuclei) that serve as the principal circadian pacemaker in mammals. Activation of both is necessary to explain the symptoms of cluster headache. The pacemaker is modulated serotonergically via dorsal raphe projections. The tentative conclusion may be reached that both migraine and cluster headache may result from abnormal serotonergic neurotransmission, albeit at different loci.

Treatment   The most satisfactory treatment is the administration of drugs to prevent cluster attacks until the bout is over. The major prophylactic drugs are prednisone, lithium, methysergide, ergotamine, and verapamil. Lithium (600 to 900 mg daily) appears to be particularly effective for the chronic form of the disorder. A 10-day course of prednisone, beginning at 60 mg daily for 7 days and rapidly tapering, appears to actually curtail the mechanism of a bout for many patients. When ergotamine is implemented, it is most effective when given 1 to 2 h before an expected attack; for patients with a single nocturnal episode, 1 mg ergotamine in suppository formulation taken at bedtime may be all that is necessary. Patients must be educated regarding the early symptoms of ergotism when ergotamine is used daily; a weekly limit of 14 mg should be adhered to.

For the attacks themselves, oxygen inhalation (9 L/min via a tight mask) is the most effective modality; 15 min inhalation of 100 percent oxygen is often necessary. The self-administration of intranasal lidocaine, either 4% topical or 2% viscous, to the most caudal aspect of the inferior nasal turbinate can deliver a sphenopalatine ganglionic block that is usually remarkably effective for the termination of an attack. Sumatriptan, 6 mg subcutaneously, will usually shorten an attack to 10 to 15 min.

TENSION HEADACHE   ''Tension'' headache is usually bilateral and occipitonuchal or bifrontal in localization. The sensation described by patients includes fullness, tightness, or pressure (as if the head is surrounded by a band or in a vise), on which waves of aching pain are superimposed. The onset of pain is more gradual than in classic migraine, but commonly a throbbing ''vascular'' type of headache is described. Tension headaches may occur acutely under conditions of emotional duress or intense worry and may last for hours or a day or two.

There is no evidence that the origin of the pain is sustained muscle activity. On the other hand, elicitation in some patients of headache after the administration of amyl nitrite, a vasodilator, or after histamine, indicates that there is a close link between tension headaches and migraine.

Treatment   For the common everyday headache due to fatigue, acute stress, or excessive use of alcohol or tobacco, the physician may recommend therapy with aspirin, 0.6 g, or acetaminophen, 0.6 g given every 4 to 6 h. Chronic headaches falling into the common migraine or tension category are much more difficult to manage.

OTHER HEADACHE SYNDROMES   Lumbar puncture headache   Headache following lumbar puncture usually begins within 48 h but may be delayed for up to 12 days. Its mean incidence is about 30 percent. Head pain is dramatically positional; it begins when the patient sits or stands upright; there is relief upon reclining or with abdominal compression. The longer the patient is upright, the longer the latency before head pain subsides. It is worsened by head shaking and jugular vein compression. The pain is usually a dull ache, but may be throbbing; its location is occipitofrontal. Nausea and stiff neck often accompany headache, and occasional patients report blurred vision, photophobia, tinnitus, and vertigo. The symptoms resolve over a few days but may on occasion persist for weeks to months.

Loss of CSF volume decreases the brain's supportive cushion, so that when a patient is upright there is probably dilation and tension placed on the brain's anchoring structures, the pain-sensitive dural sinuses, resulting in pain. Intracranial hypotension often occurs but appears to be epiphenomenal; the full-blown syndrome occurs, at times, in the presence of normal CSF pressure.

Treatment is remarkably effective. Intravenous caffeine sodium benzoate given over a few minutes as a 500-mg dose will promptly terminate headache in 75 percent of patients; a second dose given in 1 h brings the total success rate to 85 percent. An epidural blood patch accomplished by injection of 15 mL of homologous whole blood rarely fails for those who do not respond to caffeine. The mechanism for these treatment effects is not straightforward. The blood patch has an *immediate* effect, making it unlikely that sealing off a dural hole with blood clot is its mechanism of action.

Postconcussion headaches   (See also Chaps. 291 and 380) Following seemingly trivial head injuries and particularly after rear-end motor vehicle collisions, many patients report varying admixtures of headache, vertigo, and impaired memory and concentration that persist for months and even years after the injury. This syndrome is not usually associated with anatomic lesions of brain and may occur whether or not a person was rendered unconscious by head trauma. In general, this is a neurobiologic rather than a psychological disturbance. The syndrome usually persists long after the settlement of pending lawsuits. There is evidence to support the contention that concussion perturbs neurotransmission within brain and that restoration of this condition is typically delayed. Further understanding of this very common problem is contingent on the clarification of the biology of cerebral concussion. The treatment is symptomatic support. Repeated encouragement that the syndrome eventually remits is important.

Giant cell arteritis   (See also Chaps. 291 and 380) This is a common disorder of the elderly; its average annual incidence is 77:100,000 individuals aged 50 and older. Women account for 65 percent of cases, and the average age of onset is 70 years, with a range of 50 to 85 years. The involvement of cranial arteries by an inflammatory process may result in blindness in 50 percent of patients if glucocorticoid treatment is not instituted; indeed, the ischemic optic neuropathy induced by giant cell arteritis is the major cause of rapidly developing bilateral blindness in the patient over 60 years of age.

The most common initial symptoms are headache, polymyalgia rheumatica, jaw claudication, fever, and weight loss (see Chap. 291). Headache is the dominant symptom and often appears in a setting of malaise and muscle aches. Head pain may be unilateral or bilateral and is located temporally in 50 percent of patients but may involve any and all aspects of the cranium. Pain usually appears gradually over a few hours before peak intensity is reached; occasionally, it is explosive in onset. The quality of pain is only seldom throbbing; it is almost invariably described as dull and boring with superimposed episodic ice picklike lancinating pains similar to the sharp pains that appear in migraine. Most patients can recognize that the origin of their head pain is superficial, external to the skull, rather than originating deep within the cranium (the pain site for migraineurs). Scalp tenderness is present, often to a marked degree; brushing the hair or resting the head on a pillow may be impossible because of pain. Headache is usually worse at night and is often aggravated by exposure to cold. Reddened, tender nodules or red streaking of the skin overlying the temporal arteries is found in highest frequency in patients with headache, as is tenderness of the temporal, or less commonly, the occipital arteries. Curiously, temporal artery biopsy not infrequently coincides with the cessation of headache.

The erythrocyte sedimentation rate (ESR) is often but not always elevated; a normal ESR does not exclude giant cell arteritis. A temporal artery biopsy and the initiation of prednisone at 80 mg daily for the first 4 to 6 weeks should be instituted when clinical suspicion is high. Patients with migraine often report amelioration of their headaches with prednisone so that one must be cautious about interpreting the therapeutic response. Contrary to widespread notions, the prevalence of migraine among the elderly is substantial, considerably higher than giant cell arteritis.

Cough headache One of the male-dominated (4:1) syndromes, it is characterized by transient, severe head pain upon coughing, bending, lifting, sneezing, or stooping. Head pain persists for seconds to a few minutes. Many patients date the origins of the syndrome to a lower respiratory infection accompanied by severe coughing or to strenuous weight-lifting programs. Headache is usually diffuse but is lateralized in about one-third of patients. The incidence of serious intracranial structural anomalies causing this condition is about 25 percent; the Arnold-Chiari malformation is a common cause. Magnetic resonance imaging is indicated for most of these patients. The benign disorder may persist for a few years; it is inexplicably and remarkably ameliorated by indomethacin at doses ranging from 50 to 200 mg daily.

Many patients with migraine note that attacks of headache may be provoked by *sustained* physical exertion, such as during the third mile of a 5-mile run. Such headaches build up over hours, distinctly different from the cough headache syndrome. The term *effort migraine* has been used for this syndrome to avoid the ambiguous term *exertional headache*.

Coital headache Another male-dominated (4:1) syndrome, attacks occur periorgasmically, are very abrupt in onset, and subside in a few minutes if coitus is interrupted. These are nearly always benign events and usually occur sporadically; if they persist for hours or are accompanied by vomiting, subarachnoid hemorrhage must be excluded through a CSF examination and CT scanning.

Brain tumor headache About 30 percent of patients with brain tumors consider headache to be their chief complaint. The head pain syndrome is nondescript; a deep, dull aching quality, of moderate intensity, occurs intermittently, is worsened by exertion or change in position, and is associated with nausea and vomiting. This pattern of symptoms results from migraine far more often than from brain tumor. Headache disturbs sleep in about 10 percent of patients. Vomiting that precedes the appearance of headache by weeks is highly characteristic of posterior fossa brain tumors.

Headache caused by systemic illness There is hardly any illness that is never manifested by headache; however, some illnesses are *characteristically* associated with headache. These include infectious mononucleosis, systemic lupus erythematosus, chronic pulmonary failure with hypercapnia (early morning headaches), Hashimoto's thyroiditis, glucocorticoid withdrawal, oral contraceptives, ovulation-promoting medications, inflammatory bowel disease, many of the HIV-associated illnesses, and the acute blood pressure elevations that occur in pheochromocytoma and in malignant hypertension. The last two examples are the exceptions to the generalization that hypertension per se is a very uncommon cause of headache; diastolic pressures of at least 120 mmHg are requisite for hypertension to cause headache.

APPROACH TO THE PATIENT WITH HEADACHE Entirely different diagnostic possibilities are raised by a patient who presents with the first severe headache ever and a patient who has had recurrent headache over many years. In the first instance, the probability of finding a potentially serious cause is considerably greater than in the second; some of the causes that should be considered include meningitis, subarachnoid hemorrhage, epidural or subdural hematoma, glaucoma, and purulent sinusitis. In general, acute, severe headache with stiff neck and fever means meningitis and without fever means subarachnoid hemorrhage; when confronted with such a patient, lumbar puncture is mandatory. Acute persistent headache and fever is often the manifestation of an acute systemic viral infection; if the neck is supple in such a patient, lumbar puncture may be deferred. There is always the possibility of a first attack of migraine, but fever would be a rare associated feature.

When the signature of migraine has not clarified the cause of recurring headache, one should consider the investigation of cardiovascular and renal status by blood pressure and urine examination; eyes by fundoscopy, intraocular pressure measurement and refraction; the cranial arteries by palpation; the cervical spine by the

effect of passive movement of the head and imaging; and the nervous system by neurologic and psychological evaluation.

The adolescent with chronic daily frontal or holocephalic headache represents a special type of problem. Extensive diagnostic batteries are most often unrevealing, including the psychiatric assessment. Fortunately, the headaches tend to stop after a few years so that structured analgesic support can enable these teenagers to move through secondary school and enter college. By the time they reach the late teens, the cycle has usually ended.

The relationship of head pain to depression is not straightforward. Many patients in chronic daily pain cycles become depressed, a not unreasonable sequence of events; moreover, there is a greater-than-chance coincidence of migraine with both bipolar (manic depressive) and unipolar depressive disorders. Studies of large populations of depressed patients do not reveal headache prevalence rates that are different from the general population. The physician should be cautious about assigning depression as the cause of recurring headache; drugs with antidepressant actions are effective in migraine also.

Finally, a note on recurring headache that may be pain-driven. Temporomandibular joint dysfunction is an example; in general, it produces preauricular pain that is associated with chewing food. The pain may radiate to the head but is not easily confused with headache per se. On the other hand, headache-prone patients may observe that headaches are more frequent and severe in the presence of a painful temporomandibular joint problem. Similarly, headache disorders may be activated by the pain attending otological or endodontic surgical procedures. Treatment of the headache problem is largely ineffectual until the cause of the primary pain problem is dealt with. Thus pain about the head as the result of somatic disease or trauma may reawaken an otherwise quiescent migrainous mechanism.

REFERENCES

BICKERSTAFF ER: Basilar artery migraine. Lancet 1:15, 1961

BLAU JN: Migraine: Theories of pathogenosis. Lancet: 339:1202, 1992.

BOLES DB: Visual field effects of classical migraine. Brain Cogn 21:181, 1993

COUCH JR: Headache to worry about. Med Clin North Am 77:141, 1993

DECHANT KL, CLISSOLD SP: Sumatriptan. Drugs 43:776, 1992

GOADSBY PJ, EDVINSSON L: The trigeminovascular system and migraine—Studies characterizing cerebrovascular and neuropeptide changes seen in humans and cats. Ann Neurol 33:48, 1993

GOADSBY PJ, GUNDLACH AL: Localization of ³H-dihydroergotamine-binding sites in the cat central nervous system: Relevance to migraine. Ann Neurol 29:91, 1991

HARDEBO JE: Subcutaneous sumatriptan in cluster headache—A time study of the effect on pain and autonomic symptoms. Headache 33:18, 1993

HUGHES RL: Identification and treatment of cerebral aneurysms after sentinel headache. Neurology 42:1118, 1992

JENSEN R et al: Muscle tenderness and pressure pain thresholds in headache—A population study. Pain 52:193 1993

JOHNS D: Benign sexual headache within a family. Arch Neurol 43:1158, 1986

LANCE JW: *Mechanism and Management of Headache*, 5th ed. London, Butterworth Scientific, 1993

————: Headaches related to sexual activity. J Neurol Neurosurg Psychiatry 39:1226, 1976

MOSKOWITZ MA et al: Pain mechanisms underlying vascular headaches. Rev Neurol (Paris) 145:181, 1989

OLESEN J: Cerebral and extracranial circulatory disturbances in migraine: Pathophysiological implications. Cerebrovasc Brain Metab Rev 3:1, 1991

RANDO TA, FISHMAN RA: Spontaneous intracranial hypotension. Neurology 42:481, 1992

RASKIN NH: Pharmacology of migraine. Prog Drug Res 34:209, 1990

————: Lumbar puncture headache:. A review. Headache 30:197, 1990

————: *Headache*, 2d ed. New York, Churchill Livingstone, 1988

RASMUSSEN BK, OLESEN J: Symptomatic and nonsymptomatic headaches in a general population. Neurology 42:1225, 1992

SJAASTAD O: *Cluster Headache Syndrome*. London, Saunders, 1992

STANG PE et al: Incidence of migraine headache: A population-based study in Olmsted County, Minnesota. Neurology 42:1657, 1992.

VINKEN PJ, BRUYN GW, KLAWANS HL (eds): *Handbook of Clinical Neurology*, vol 48: Headache. Amsterdam, Elsevier Science, 1986

15　BACK AND NECK PAIN

HENRY J. MANKIN / LAWRENCE F. BORGES

ANATOMY AND PHYSIOLOGY OF THE LOWER PART OF THE BACK

The bony spine is anatomically divisible into two parts. The *anterior* part consists of a series of cylindrical vertebral bodies connected to one another by the intervertebral disks and held tightly together by the anterior and posterior longitudinal ligaments. The *posterior* part consists of more delicate elements that extend from the vertebral body as pedicles and broaden posteriorly to form laminae, which together with ligamentous structures form the vertebral canal. The posterior elements are joined to adjacent vertebrae by two small facetal synovial joints which allow a modest degree of motion between any two segments but in aggregate produce a rather extensive range (Fig. 15-1). Stout transverse and spinous bony processes project laterally and posteriorly and serve as the attachments of muscles which move, support, and protect the vertebral column. The stability of the spine depends on two types of support: that provided by the bony articulations (principally by the diskal joints and the synovial articulations of the posterior elements) and a second type provided by the ligamentous (passive) and muscular (active) supporting structures. The ligamentous structures are quite strong, but because neither they nor the vertebral body–disk complexes have sufficient integral strength to resist the enormous forces acting on the column during even simple movements, voluntary and reflex contractions of the sacrospinalis, abdominal, gluteal, psoas, and hamstring muscles afford much of the stability.

The vertebral and paravertebral structures are innervated by branches of the segmental spinal nerves that exit the neural foramina at each spinal level. The sinuvertebral nerve, which is considered the major sensory nerve supply to the structures of the lumbar spine, arises from the spinal nerve prior to its division into an anterior and posterior ramus. The sinuvertebral nerve reenters the spinal canal through the intervertebral foramen to provide sensory innervation to the posterior longitudinal ligament, external portions of the posterior annulus fibrosus, anterior dura, dura of the nerve root sleeve, and epidural veins, all within the spinal canal. The other major nerve supply to the spinal and paraspinal structures arises from the posterior primary ramus. The posterior primary ramus of the spinal nerve further divides into medial and lateral branches. Together these nerves supply the posterior parts of the spine, including the facet joints, as well as the paraspinal muscles and fascia. In addition, the upper three lumbar spinal nerves provide cutaneous sensation to the skin of the low back.

FIGURE 15-1 *Left:* Superior view of a stripped lumbar vertebra. *Right:* Lateral view of two articulated lumbar vertebrae. B = body; SC = spinal canal; IVF = intervertebral foramen; IF = inferior articular facet; SF = superior articular facet; P = pedicle; TP = transverse process; SP = spinous process; L = lamina. *(Adapted from DB Levine, in Arthritis and Allied Conditions: A Textbook of Rheumatology, 10th ed, DJ McCarty (ed). Philadelphia, Lea & Febiger, 1985.)*

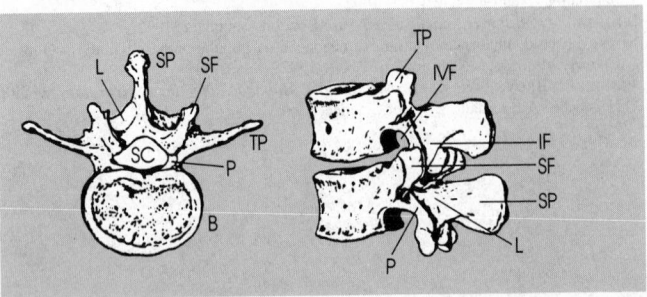

The parts of the back that possess the greatest freedom of movement, and hence are most frequently subject to injury, are the lumbar and cervical regions. In addition to the voluntary motions required for bending, twisting, and other movements, many actions of the spine are reflex in nature and are the basis of posture.

GENERAL CLINICAL CONSIDERATIONS

TYPES OF LOW BACK PAIN　Four types of pain may be differentiated: local, referred, radicular, and that arising from secondary (protective) muscular spasm.

Local pain is caused by any pathologic process that impinges on or irritates sensory endings. Involvement of structures that contain no sensory endings is painless. The central, medullary portion of the vertebral body, for example, may be destroyed by tumor, without evocation of pain, whereas cortical fractures or tears and distortions of the periosteum, synovial membranes, muscles, annulus fibrosus, and ligaments are often exquisitely painful. The latter structures are innervated by afferent fibers of the posterior primary rami and the sinuvertebral nerve. Although painful states are often accompanied by swelling of the affected tissues, this may not be apparent if a deep structure of the back is the site of disease. Local pain is often described as steady but may be intermittent, varying considerably with position or activity. The pain may be sharp or dull and although often diffuse is always felt in or near the affected part of the spine. Reflex splinting of the spine segments by paravertebral muscles is frequently noted and may produce deformity or postural abnormality. Certain movements or postures that alter the position of the injured tissues aggravate the pain. Firm pressure or percussion on superficial structures in the region involved usually evokes tenderness, which is of aid in identifying the site of the abnormality.

Referred pain is of two types: that projected from the spine into regions lying within the area of the lumbar and upper sacral dermatomes and that projected from the pelvic and abdominal viscera to the spine. Pain due to diseases of the upper part of the lumbar spine is usually referred to the anterior aspects of the thighs and legs; that from the lower lumbar and sacral segments is referred to the gluteal regions, posterior thighs, calves, and sometimes feet. Pain of this type, although of deep, aching quality and rather diffuse, tends at times to be superficially projected. In general, the referred pain parallels in intensity the local pain in the back. In other words, maneuvers that alter local pain have a similar effect on referred pain, though not with such precision and immediacy as in radicular, or "root," pain. Referred pain may be confused with pain from visceral disease, but the latter is usually described as "deep" and tends to radiate from the abdomen through to the back. Also, visceral pain is usually unaffected by movement of the spine, does not improve with recumbency, and may be modified by the activity of the involved viscus. An important exception to this is pain caused by an aortic aneurysm. A slowly enlarging aortic aneurysm may erode the anterolateral spine and produce discomfort that changes with movement or recumbency.

Radicular, or "root," *pain* has some of the characteristics of referred pain but differs in its greater intensity, distal radiation, circumscription to the territory of a root, and the factors which excite it (Table 15-1). The mechanisms are principally distortion, stretching, irritation, and compression of a spinal root, most often central to the intervertebral foramen. In addition, it has been suggested that in patients with spinal stenosis the "lumbar claudication" pattern may be due to a relative ischemia associated with compression. Although the pain itself is often dull or aching, various maneuvers which increase the irritation of the root or stretch it may greatly intensify the pain, eliciting a lancinating quality. Nearly always the radiation of pain is from a central position near the spine to some part of the lower extremity. Cough, sneeze, and strain are characteristic evocative maneuvers, but since they may also jar or move the spine, they may aggravate local pain as well. Forward bending with the knees extended

TABLE 15-1 Anatomic localization of pain referred by lumbar and sacral roots

Root	Region
L1, L5	Inguinal
L2	Lateral thigh
L2, L3	Anterior thigh
L3	Knee
L4	Anterior shin
L5, S1	Lateral calf
L5, S1	Posterior calf
L5	Dorsum of foot
S1	Heel
S1	Lateral foot
L5 ganglion	Anterior leg/foot

or "straight-leg raising" in disease of the lower part of the lumbar spine excites radicular pain on the basis of stretch; jugular vein compression, which raises intraspinal pressure and may cause a shift in the position of or pressure on the root, may have a similar effect. Irritation of the fourth and fifth lumbar and first sacral roots, which form the sciatic nerve, causes pain that extends mainly down the posterior aspects of the thigh and the posterior and lateral aspects of the leg. Typically, this pain radiation—which is termed *sciatica*—stops at the ankle and is associated with sensations of tingling or numbness—*paresthesias*—that radiate more distally into the foot. Tingling, paresthesias, and numbness or sensory impairment of the skin, soreness of the skin, and tenderness along the nerve also may accompany classic sciatic pain, and on physical examination, reflex loss, weakness, atrophy, fascicular twitching, and occasionally stasis edema may occur if the motor fibers of the anterior root are involved.

Pain resulting from muscular spasm is usually mentioned in relation to local pain, but the anatomic or physiologic basis is more obscure. Muscle spasm associated with many disorders of the spine can produce significant distortions of the normal posture; as a result, chronic tension in muscles may give rise to a dull and sometimes cramping ache. In this instance, one can feel the tautness of the sacrospinalis and gluteal muscles and demonstrate by palpation that the pain is localized to these structures.

Other pains often of undetermined origin are sometimes described by patients with chronic disease of the lower part of the back. Unilateral symptoms of drawing, pulling, cramping sensations (without involuntary muscle spasm), tearing, throbbing, or jabbing pains, or feelings of burning or coldness are difficult to interpret but, like paresthesias and numbness, should always suggest the possibility of nerve or root disease.

In addition to assessing the character and location of the pain, one should determine the factors that aggravate and relieve it, its constancy, and its relationship to recumbency and such stereotypical movements and maneuvers as forward bending, cough, sneeze, and strain. Frequently, the most important lead comes from the knowledge of the mode of onset and circumstances that initiated the pain. It cannot be overemphasized that a careful history provides the cornerstone of an accurate diagnosis. Inasmuch as many painful afflictions of the back are the result of injury incurred during work or in an accident, the possibility of exaggeration or prolongation of pain for purposes of compensation or other personal reasons, or because of hysteria or malingering, must always be kept in mind.

EXAMINATION OF THE LOWER PART OF THE BACK

Inspection of the normal spine shows a dorsal kyphosis and lumbar lordosis in the sagittal plane, which in some individuals may be exaggerated (swayback). Patients with spinal disorders may demonstrate excessive curvature, flattening of the normal lumbar arch, presence of a gibbus (a short, sharp, kyphotic angulation usually indicative of a fracture or congenital abnormality), lateral curvature

and/or rotation (scoliosis), pelvic tilt or obliquity, or asymmetry of the paravertebral or gluteal musculature. In severe sciatica, one may observe that the affected limb is held with the hip and knee flexed, presumably to reduce tension on the irritated part.

The spine, hips, and legs should be observed during certain motions, but no advantage accrues from trying to find out how much pain the patient can endure. It is more important to assess when and under what conditions the pain commences. Normally, the motion of forward bending produces flattening and reversal of the lumbar lordotic curve and exaggeration of the dorsal curve. With ruptured lumbar disks or lesions that involve the posterior ligaments, articular facets, or sacrospinalis muscle, protective reflexes prevent stretching of these structures; as a consequence, the sacrospinalis muscles remain taut and limit motion in the lumbar part of the spine, causing forward bending to occur at the hips and at the lumbar-thoracic junction. With disease principally affecting the spinal roots or the lumbosacral joints, forward bending occurs in such a way as to avoid tensing the hamstring muscles, which puts undue leverage on the pelvis. In unilateral "sciatica," with its increased curvature toward the side of the lesion, the lumbar and lumbosacral motions are splinted, and bending is mainly at the hips; at a certain point the knee on the affected side is flexed to relieve hamstring spasm, and tilting of the pelvis occurs to slacken the lumbosacral roots and sciatic nerve.

With lumbosacral lesions and sciatica, passive lumbar flexion in the supine position causes little pain and is not limited as long as the hamstrings are relaxed and the sciatic nerve is not stretched. With lumbosacral and lumbar spine disease (e.g., arthritis), passive flexion of the hips is free, whereas flexion of the lumbar spine may be impeded and painful. Passive straight-leg raising (possible in most normal individuals up to 80 to 90° except in those who have unusually tight hamstrings), like forward bending with the knees extended in the standing posture, places the sciatic nerve and its roots under tension, thereby producing pain. It also may cause an anterior rotation of the pelvis around a transverse axis, increasing stress on the lumbosacral joint, and thus causing pain if this segment is arthritic or otherwise impaired. Consequently, in diseases of the lumbosacral joints and lumbosacral roots, this movement is limited on the affected side and to a lesser extent on the opposite side. Evocation of such a response (pain and limitation of movement during flexion of the hip when the knee is extended) is known as *Lasègue's sign* and is considered to be a useful test of this condition. Straight-leg raising also may be tested by having the patient extend the knee while seated. This maneuver produces the same extent of sciatic nerve stretch as the Lasègue sign but does not stress the lumbosacral joint and thus may identify true nerve root irritation more accurately. A positive contralateral straight-leg raising sign is believed by some to be a sign of a more extensive lesion, such as an extruded disk fragment in the axilla of the nerve, rather than a simple prolapse or protrusion. It is important to remember, however, that the evoked pain is always referred to the diseased side, no matter which leg is flexed.

Hyperextension is best evaluated with the patient standing or lying prone. If the condition causing back pain is acute, it may be difficult to extend the spine in the standing position. A patient with lumbosacral strain or disk disease can usually extend or hyperextend the spine without aggravation of pain. If the lesion is in the upper lumbar segments or if an active inflammatory process, fracture of the vertebral body, or a very tight canal (vertebral stenosis) is present, hyperextension may be markedly limited.

Palpation and percussion of the spine are the last steps in the examination. It is preferable to palpate first those regions which are the least likely to evoke pain. At all times the examiner should know what structures are being palpated (see Fig. 15-2). Localized tenderness is seldom pronounced in disease of the spine because the involved structures are so deep that they rarely give rise to surface tenderness. However, spinal disease may give rise to intense spasm in the paraspinal muscles which could result in local tenderness. Mild superficial and poorly localized tenderness signifies only a disease process within the affected segment of the body, i.e., dermatome.

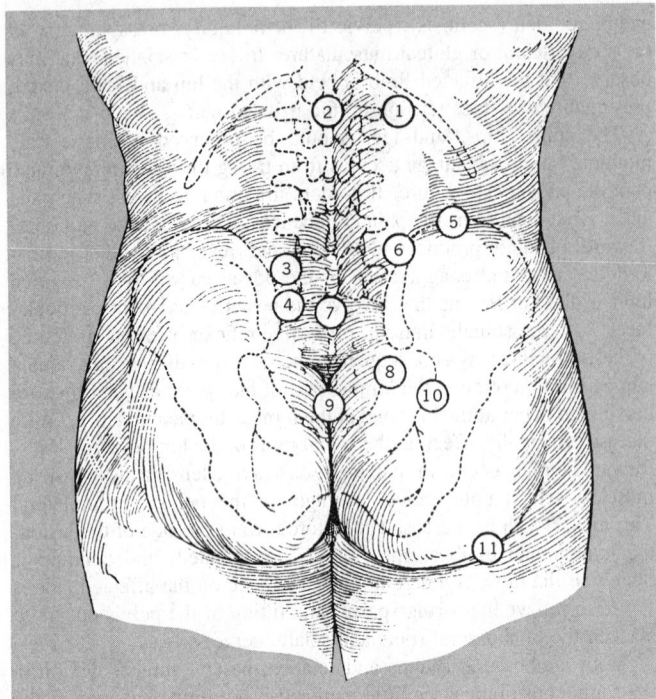

FIGURE 15-2 (1) Costovertebral angle. (2) Spinous process and interspinous ligament. (3) Region of the articular fifth lumbar to the first sacral facet. (4) Dorsum of sacrum. (5) Region of iliac crest. (6) Iliolumbar angle. (7) Spinous processes of fifth lumbar to first sacral vertebrae (tenderness = faulty posture or occasionally spina bifida occulta). (8) Region between posterior superior and posterior inferior spines. Sacroiliac ligaments (tenderness = sacroiliac sprain, often tender with fifth lumbar to first sacral disk). (9) Sacrococcygeal junction (tenderness = sacrococcygeal injury, i.e., sprain or fracture). (10) Region of sacrosciatic notch (tenderness = fourth to fifth lumbar disk rupture and sacroiliac sprain). (11) Sciatic nerve trunk (tenderness = ruptured lumbar disk or sciatic nerve lesion).

Tenderness over the costovertebral angle often indicates renal disease, adrenal disease, or an injury to the transverse processes of the first or second lumbar vertebra. Hypersensitivity on palpation of the transverse processes of the other lumbar vertebrae as well as the overlying sacrospinalis muscles may signify fracture of the transverse process or a strain of muscle attachments. Tenderness of a spinous process or aggravation of pain by the jarring of gentle percussion may be nonspecific but frequently indicates the presence of a disk lesion at the site deep to it, inflammation (as in disk space infection), or fracture. Tenderness in the region of the articular facets between the fifth lumbar and first sacral vertebrae is consistent with disease of a lumbosacral disk (Fig. 15-2). It is also frequent in rheumatoid arthritis.

In palpation of the spinous processes, it is important to note any deviation in the lateral plane (this may be indicative of fracture or arthritis) or in the anteroposterior plane. A "step-off" forward displacement of the spinous process may be an important clue to the presence of a spondylolisthesis one segment below the displaced level.

Abdominal, rectal, and pelvic examination and assessment of the status of the peripheral vascular system are important parts of the examination of the patient with complaints in the lower back and should not be omitted. They may provide evidence for vascular, visceral, neoplastic, or inflammatory disorders which may extend to the spine or cause pain to be referred to this region. Finally, a careful neurologic examination should be performed, with special attention given to motor, reflex, and sensory changes, particularly in the lower extremities. It is especially important when performing the neurologic examination to attempt to identify a pattern of nerve root involvement.

Table 15-2 correlates the motor and reflex components of each of the lumbar roots. It is important to note that isolated lesions of the L2 root do not usually cause identifiable weakness on examination. The L2 root provides innervation to the thigh adductors. However, dysfunction of more than just the L2 root is usually necessary to produce actual weakness in these muscles (see "Protrusion of Lumbar Intervertebral Disks," below).

SPECIAL LABORATORY PROCEDURES Useful laboratory tests, depending on the nature of the problem and the circumstances, include a complete blood count, erythrocyte sedimentation rate (especially helpful in screening for infection or myeloma), measurement of serum calcium, phosphorus, alkaline phosphatase, acid phosphatase, prostate-specific antigen (see Chap. 323) (the last two mentioned are of importance if one suspects metastatic carcinoma from the prostate), serum immunoelectrophoresis, and tests for rheumatoid factor. Roentgenograms of the lumbar part of the spine in the anteroposterior, lateral, and oblique planes should be obtained in every patient with low back pain and sciatica. Special spot views or stereoscopic or laminographic films may provide further information in certain cases. Bone scans are of particular aid in revealing some fractures and neoplastic and inflammatory lesions.

The most sensitive noninvasive imaging modality for examining the spine and paraspinal tissues is magnetic resonance imaging (MRI). Standard MRI scans are performed in the sagittal and axial planes. They provide remarkable anatomic detail of the vertebral bodies, disks, spinal canal, nerve roots, spinal cord, and paraspinal soft tissues. The high-field-strength instruments (1.5 T) often provide more detailed images of the spine than do the lower-field-strength instruments. In select instances, intravenous contrast (gadolinium) may allow additional anatomic details to be visualized (see Chap. 365). Initial MRI scans of the spine should be done without contrast infusion. This is particularly important when the scan is being performed to assess for metastatic disease in the spine. In this situation, contrast medium may actually obscure the difference between tumor tissue and normal vertebral body. Several important caveats surround the use of MRI scans. MRI does not provide an accurate assessment of bone detail in the spine. Computed tomography (CT) is a superior method of evaluating details of spinal bone structure and would be the preferred method of identifying a subtle fracture. Furthermore, MRI scans are so sensitive that they often reveal anatomic abnormalities that are clinically meaningless. Therefore, the data derived from an MRI scan *must* be interpreted by an experienced clinician who also has evaluated the patient's clinical problem.

Despite the sensitivity of the MRI scan, examination of the spinal canal with a contrast medium—myelography—continues to be important, particularly in the assessment of benign degenerative disease of the spine. When a myelogram is performed, a sample of cerebrospinal fluid should always be removed for cytologic and chemical examination prior to the instillation of the contrast medium. Except for special circumstances, a water-soluble contrast medium should be used for myelography. Water-soluble contrast medium is less irritating to the neural structures, is associated with a lower incidence of arachnoiditis, and does not have to be removed from the subarachnoid space because it is systemically absorbed and excreted by the kidneys. In addition, myelography should always include CT

TABLE 15-2 Motor examination of lumbar and sacral roots		
Root	Muscle	Reflex
L1	—	—
L2	—	—
L3	Quadriceps, iliopsoas	Knee absent
L4	Anterior tibialis	Knee reduced
L5	EHL,* EDB†	
S1	Foot evertors, gastrocnemius	Ankle reduced

* EHL = extensor hallucis longus.
† EDB = extensor digitorum brevis.

scanning of the affected area of the spine. CT/myelography can often provide the best definition of subtle compression of nerve roots by herniated disks or osteophytes.

Injection of contrast medium directly into the intervertebral disk (diskograms) has waxed and waned in popularity over the years and remains controversial. The technique of this procedure is more complicated than that of CT/myelography and carries a risk of infection of the disk.

Confirmation of proximal motor and sensory nerve and root disease can be obtained by nerve conduction studies, H and F responses, and electromyography (see Chap. 382).

PRINCIPAL CONDITIONS THAT GIVE RISE TO DISABLING PAIN IN THE LOWER PART OF THE BACK

CONGENITAL ANOMALIES OF THE LUMBAR SPINE One of the most common disorders is a failure of fusion of the laminae of the neural arch (spina bifida) of one or several of the lumbar vertebrae or of the sacrum. Hypertrichosis or hyperpigmentation in the sacral area may betray the condition, but in most patients the spine defect remains entirely occult until disclosed by x-ray. The anomaly has greater potential for causing pain if accompanied by malformation of vertebral joints, and usually the pain is induced by injury. Other congenital anomalies that affect the lower lumbar vertebrae, such as asymmetric facetal joints, abnormalities of the transverse processes, sacralization of the fifth lumbar vertebra (in which L5 is firmly fixed to the sacrum), or lumbarization of the first sacral vertebra (in which the first sacral segment resembles a sixth lumbar), are rarely the cause of specific symptomatology.

Spondylolysis consists of a bony defect probably caused by trauma to a congenitally abnormal segment in the pars interarticularis (a segment near the junction of the pedicle with the lamina) of the lower lumbar area. The defect is best visualized on oblique projections or with CT. In some individuals the defect is bilateral. In the circumstance of either a single injury or repeated minor injuries, the vertebral body, pedicles, and superior articular facets slip anteriorly, leaving the posterior elements behind. This latter abnormality, known as *spondylolisthesis*, more often results in symptoms, often proportional to the degree of forward slip. The patient may complain of pain in the low back radiating into the thighs, and a limitation of motion may be noted. Often tenderness is elicited near the segment which has "slipped" forward (most often L5 on S1 or occasionally L4 on L5), and one can feel a "step" on deep palpation of the posterior elements of the segment above the spondylolisthetic joint. In moderately severe displacements the pelvis is sometimes rotated and hip flexion limited by hamstring spasm. A variety of usually minor neurologic deficits indicative of radiculopathy may be present. In exceptionally severe degrees of spondylolisthesis the trunk may be shortened and the abdomen protuberant, both the result of the extreme forward displacement of L5 on S1.

TRAUMATIC AFFLICTIONS OF THE LOWER PART OF THE BACK Trauma constitutes the most frequent cause of acute low back pain, and such injured patients should be evaluated very carefully. In severe acute injuries that involve fracture or dislocation of the vertebral segments, the examining physician must be careful to avoid further damage, particularly to the neural structures. Tests of mobility and forceful manipulations should be avoided until a diagnosis has been made and adequate measures have been instituted for the proper care of the patient. A patient complaining of back pain and inability to move the legs may have a fractured spine. The neck should not be flexed, nor should the patient be allowed to sit up. (See Chap. 381 for further discussion of spinal cord injury.)

Sprains, strains, and derangements The terms lumbosacral *sprain* and *strain* are often used loosely by patients and their physicians and do not clearly relate to a known anatomic lesion. The authors prefer the term *low back derangement* or *strain* for minor, self-limited

injuries usually associated with lifting a heavy object, a fall, or a sudden deceleration, as may occur in an automobile accident. Occasionally, these syndromes are more chronic in nature, suggesting that diskal or arthritic factors may play a role. The patients with low back derangement are often acutely discomfited and may assume unusual postures related to spasm of the sacrospinalis muscles. The pain is usually confined to the lower back and is usually relieved by rest and analgesic medication within a few days. More extensive or longer-lasting problems, formerly classified as sacroiliac strain or sprain, are now known to be due in most instances to disk disease (see below).

Vertebral fractures Most fractures of the lumbar vertebral body result from flexion injuries and consist of anterior wedging or compression. With more severe trauma the patient may sustain a fracture dislocation, "bursting" fracture, or asymmetric fracture involving not only the body but the posterior elements as well. The initiating trauma which causes fractures of the vertebrae is usually a fall from a height (in which case the calcanei also may be fractured), sudden deceleration in an automobile accident, or other major violence. When fractures occur with minimal trauma (or even spontaneously), the bone is presumed to have been previously weakened by some pathologic process. Most of the time, particularly in older individuals, the cause of such an event is senile or postmenopausal osteoporosis (see Chap. 358), but there may be other underlying systemic disorders such as osteomalacia, hyperparathyroidism, hyperthyroidism, multiple myeloma, metastatic carcinoma, and a large number of local conditions that may play a role in weakening the vertebral body. Spasm of the lumbar muscles, limitation of motion of the lumbar segments, and the roentgenographic appearance of the damaged vertebra (with or without neurologic abnormalities) are the basis for the clinical diagnosis. The pain is usually immediate, though occasionally it may be delayed in onset for a few days, and the patient may develop a mild paralytic ileus or urinary retention during the acute period.

Fractures of the transverse processes are almost always associated with severe injury to the paravertebral muscles, principally the psoas. A significant retroperitoneal hemorrhage may be present (identified on CT or MRI) which can result in a marked depression in the hematocrit and, in extensive fractures, hypovolemic shock. Such injuries may be diagnosed by the finding of deep tenderness at the site of the injury, local muscle spasm on one side, and limitation of all movements which stretch the lumbar muscles. Radiologic evidence (especially CT or MRI) provides the final confirmation. Fractures of multiple transverse processes, although seemingly trivial, should be the object of considerable concern, and the patient should be carefully watched for internal hemorrhage.

Protrusion of lumbar intervertebral disks This condition is the major cause of severe chronic or recurrent low back and leg pain. It is most likely to occur between the fifth lumbar and first sacral vertebrae and, with lessening frequency, between the fourth and fifth lumbar, the third and fourth lumbar, the second and third lumbar, and, rarely, between the first and second lumbar vertebrae. Rare in the thoracic portion of the spine, it is next most frequent between the sixth and seventh and fifth and sixth cervical vertebrae. The cause is usually a flexion injury, but in many cases no trauma is recalled. Degeneration of the posterior longitudinal ligaments and the annulus fibrosus, which occurs in most adults of middle and advanced years, may have taken place silently or have been manifested by mild, recurrent lumbar ache. A sneeze, lurch, or other trivial movement may then cause the nucleus pulposus to prolapse, pushing the frayed and weakened annulus posteriorly. In more severe cases of disk disease, the nucleus may protrude through the annulus or become extruded to lie as a free fragment in the vertebral canal.

The fully developed syndrome of ruptured lumbar intervertebral disk consists of backache, abnormal posture, and limitation of motion of the spine (particularly flexion). Nerve root involvement is indicated by radicular pain, sensory disturbances (paresthesias, hyper- and hyposensitivity in dermatome pattern), coarse twitching and fasciculation, muscle spasms, and impairment of a tendon reflex. Motor abnormalities (weakness and muscle atrophy) also may occur but are usually less prominent than the pain and sensory disorder. Since herniation of the intervertebral lumbar disks most often occurs between the fourth and fifth lumbar vertebrae and the fifth lumbar and first sacral vertebrae with irritation and compression of the fifth lumbar and first sacral roots, respectively, it is important to recognize the clinical characteristics of lesions of these two roots. *Lesions of the fifth lumbar root* produce pain in the region of the hip, groin, posterolateral thigh, lateral calf to the external malleolus, dorsal surface of the foot, and the first or second and third toes. Paresthesias may be in the entire territory or in only the distal parts of these territories. The tenderness is in the lateral gluteal region and near the head of the fibula. Weakness, if present, involves the extensor of the great toe and less often of the foot. The knee and ankle reflexes are seldom altered, although occasionally the ankle jerk is moderately depressed. Walking on the heels may be more difficult, because of weakness of dorsiflexion of the foot, and more uncomfortable than walking on the toes. In *lesions of the first sacral root* the pain is felt in the midgluteal region, posterior part of the thigh, posterior region of the calf to the heel, and the plantar surface of the foot and fourth and fifth toes. Tenderness is most pronounced over the midgluteal region (sacroiliac joint), posterior thigh area, and calf. Paresthesias and sensory loss are mainly in the lower leg and outer toes, and weakness, if present, involves the flexor muscles of the foot and toes, evertors of the foot, abductors of the toes, and hamstring muscles. The ankle reflex is diminished or absent in the majority of cases. Walking on the toes is more difficult, because of weakness of plantar flexors, and more uncomfortable than walking on the heel. With lesions of either root there may be limitation of straight-leg raising during the acute, painful stages.

Degeneration of the intervertebral disk without frank extrusion of a fragment of disk tissue may give rise to low back pain, or the disk may herniate into the adjacent vertebral body, giving rise to a Schmorl's node, usually visualized by x-ray. Such cases often show no signs of nerve root involvement, though the back pain may be referred to the thigh and leg.

The rarer *lesions of the fourth and third lumbar roots* give rise to pain in the anterior part of the thigh and knee, with corresponding sensory loss. The knee jerk is diminished or abolished. An inverted Lasègue sign (pain with hypertension of the limb in relation to the trunk, best elicited with the patient in the prone position) is often positive when the third lumbar root is affected.

The lumbar disk syndromes are usually unilateral. Occasionally, with massive derangements of the disk or with the extrusion of a large, free fragment into the canal, the symptoms and signs are bilateral. Often one side is affected more than the other, and the pain and motor and sensory changes may be associated with paralysis of the sphincters. The pain of lumbar disk disease is variable and may be mild or severe. There may be back pain with little or no leg pain, and occasionally the patient experiences leg pain with little or no discomfort in the back. Some patients present with evidence of multiple disk ruptures affecting both cervical and lumbar segments, suggesting a diffuse disorder of the connective tissue of the disks, possibly including both the annulus fibrosus and the nucleus pulposus.

When all components of the syndrome are present, the diagnosis is easy; when only one part is present (particularly backache), it may be difficult, especially if there has not been a clearly remembered initiating traumatic event. Since similar symptoms may occur without demonstrable disk rupture, other diagnostic procedures are required. Plain roentgenograms usually show no abnormality or at most a narrowing of the intervertebral space, sometimes more on the side of the rupture. Traction spurs, which are indicative of disk degeneration, may be present; in extreme cases, there may be a "vacuum" disk sign, in which a gas-density shadow is present in the intervertebral space, usually on lateral roentgenogram. CT transverse images with or without contrast media sometimes show the herniated disk very clearly, and at times the MRI will demonstrate a remarkably sharp

image of cauda equina or nerve root compression by a bulging or extruded disk fragment. Less frequently than in the past do clinicians resort to myelography to demonstrate the disk herniation. The CT/myelogram remains the most reliable of the studies for demonstrating nerve root compression from disk herniation, and many surgeons are loathe to consider laminectomy without such a study. Occasionally, the electromyogram is helpful in showing denervation of paravertebral and leg muscles (see Chap. 382).

It should be noted in evaluating patients with herniated disks that epidural or intradural tumors of the spinal canal may produce a syndrome similar to that of ruptured disk. These lesions may present with unremitting pain even with bed rest and predominant sphincter disturbances even early in the course (see Chap. 381).

OTHER CAUSES OF LOW BACK PAIN AND SCIATICA   In a sizable number of patients, disk-rupture types of symptoms occur, but the problem has a different cause. Often these patients have had multiple operations for diskogenic disease with or without arthrodesis of the lumbar vertebrae, but the pain and disability have not remitted. The indications for the original surgery may have been questionable, with only a disk bulge noted on CT, MRI, or myelogram and no definite neurologic signs. To explain these chronic pain states, a number of pathologic entities have been introduced, some of uncertain status. Entrapment of one or more nerve roots may be the consequence not only of a disk rupture but also of spondylotic spurs with variable stenosis of the lateral recess and intervertebral canal, hypertrophy of apophyseal facets, or a more nebulous cause.

The syndrome that is caused by spondylotic spurs and stenosis of the lateral recess and intervertebral foramen has not been clearly distinguished from that of ruptured disk. Known variously as vertebral stenosis, lumbar claudication, degenerative spinal stenosis, and narrow canal, the cause appears to be related principally to an encroachment on roots of the cauda equina by bony excrescences usually attributed to osteoarthritis but possibly related to spondylolisthesis, old trauma, Paget's disease, or a congenital abnormality of the shape or size of the canal. Many of these patients are elderly, and the pattern must be clearly distinguished from the claudicatory pain associated with peripheral vascular disease. The pain, often bilateral along the sciatic distribution, becomes increasingly severe with standing and walking and is relieved by a short period of rest. Although some of the patients have no physical findings, motor, reflex, and sensory changes may be present. Some patients find sleeping in recumbency difficult and must sleep in a chair.

The *facet syndrome* is closely related to the above but tends to be unilateral. Reynolds et al. have reported 22 cases in which a lumbar monoradiculopathy had simulated a ruptured disk: 16 had an L5 radiculopathy, 3 an S1 radiculopathy, and 3 an L4 radiculopathy. Coexisting back pain was present in 15 of the cases. No disk rupture was found by myelography. At operation, the spinal root was compressed against the floor or roof of the intervertebral canal by an enlarged superior or inferior facet. Foraminotomy and facetectomy relieved the symptoms in 12 of the 15 operated cases.

Lumbar adhesive arachnoiditis with radiculopathy has waxed and waned over the years as an entity employed to explain low back pain persisting after treatment. Most often it is considered in patients who have had multiple lumbar operations and myelograms and are left with backache and leg pain in combination with mild to moderate motor, sensory, and reflex changes. On surgical exploration, the arachnoidal membrane is thickened and opaque, adherent to dura, and tightly bound to pia and roots. The contrast medium during myelography does not fill the root sheaths and tends to be irregularly loculated. Disk rupture, multiple Pantopaque myelograms, operative procedures, infection, and subarachnoid hemorrhage, in various combinations, are factors that favor its development. Treatment is unsatisfactory; lysis of adhesions and epidural steroid injections have been of only limited value.

In patients with persistent chronic low back pain and sciatica after failed disk surgery or due to spondylitic spurs, spondylolysis, facetal joint degeneration, or arachnoiditis, some surgeons have attributed the disability in part, at least, to "instability" of the lumbar segments and the perpetuation of the pain to excessive or abnormal movements of the lumbar vertebral segments. For such patients, spinal fusion is occasionally advocated and can in certain circumstances provide a measure of relief. A posterior arthrodesis of the fourth and fifth lumbar segments to the sacrum may reduce motion at these parts and decrease pressure on the nerve roots associated with abnormal movements. More often than not, however, the patient continues to have pain (although often reduced in degree), and the procedure should not be regarded as a panacea. The authors rarely advocate such an operative intervention, unless clear anatomic evidence exists for a mechanical problem that could be alleviated by stabilization of the spine.

ARTHRITIS Arthritis of the spine is a major cause of backache, cervical pain, and occipital headache.

Osteoarthritis (See also Chap. 296) This more frequent type of osteoarthritic spinal disease occurs usually in later life and may involve any part of the spine. It is most prevalent in the cervical and lumbar regions, however, and the exact location determines the localization of the symptoms. Patients often complain of pain centered in the spine that is increased by motion and is almost invariably associated with complaints of stiffness and limitation of motion. There is a notable absence of systemic symptoms such as fatigue, malaise, and fever, and the pain usually can be relieved by rest. The severity of the symptoms often bears little relation to the radiologic findings; pain may be present when there are minimal findings on an x-ray, and conversely, marked osteophytic overgrowth with spur formation, ridging, and bridging of vertebrae can be seen in asymptomatic patients in middle and later life. Osteoarthropathic changes in the cervical spine and to a lesser extent in the lumbar spine may by their location compress roots or even the cauda equina or spinal cord, giving rise to the spondylitic form of radiculopathy or myelopathy (see Chap. 381).

Rheumatoid arthritis and ankylosing spondylitis (See also Chaps. 285 and 289) Arthritic disease of the spine takes two distinct forms, ankylosing spondylitis (the more common) and rheumatoid arthritis.

Patients with *ankylosing spondylitis* (also called Marie-Strümpell arthritis) are usually young men who complain of mild to moderate pain which early in the course of the disease is centered in the middle or lower back and on occasion radiates to the back of the thighs. The symptoms may be vague at first, and the diagnosis may be overlooked for a considerable period. Although the pain is often intermittent, the finding of limitation of movement is constant and progressive and over a period of time tends to dominate the picture. Early in the course this finding is described as "morning stiffness" or increasing stiffness after periods of inactivity, and it may be present long before radiologic changes are manifest. Limitation of chest expansion, tenderness over the sternum, and decreased motion and flexion contractures of the hips also may be present early in the course. The radiologic hallmarks of the disease are periarticular destructive changes and subsequent obliteration of the sacroiliac joints, development of syndesmophytes on the margins of the vertebral bodies, followed by bridging by bone to produce the characteristic "bamboo spine." The entire spine becomes immobilized, often in a flexed position, and usually the pain then subsides. Patterns of restricted movement, indistinguishable from those of ankylosing spondylitis, may accompany Reiter's syndrome, psoriatic arthritis, and chronic inflammatory bowel diseases. Patients with these disorders rarely show the joint manifestations of peripheral rheumatoid arthritis, and seldom do they display involvement of the hips or knees. The rheumatoid factor is usually absent, but the sedimentation rate is often rapid, and many of the patients are found to have an HLA-B27 antigen.

Occasionally, ankylosing spondylitis is complicated by progressively destructive vertebral lesions. This complication should be suspected whenever the pain returns, after a period of quiescence, or becomes localized. The etiology of these lesions is not known, but they may represent an exaggerated healing response to fracture or

excessive production of fibrous inflammatory tissues. Rarely they may result in collapse of a segment of the spine and compression of the spinal cord. Another complication of severe ankylosing spondylitis is bilateral ankylosis of the ribs to the spine, which, coupled with a decrease in the height of axial thoracic structures, causes marked impairment of respiratory function.

Spinal rheumatoid arthritis tends to be localized to the cervical apophyseal joints and atlantoaxial articulation; the pain, stiffness, and limitation of motion are then in the neck and back of the head. Unlike ankylosing spondylitis, rheumatoid arthritis is rarely confined to the spine, and it does not lead to significant degrees of intervertebral bridging. Because of major affection of other joints, the diagnosis is relatively easy to make, but significant involvement of the neck may be overlooked. In the advanced stages of the disease, one or several of the vertebrae may be displaced anteriorly, or a synovitis of the atlantoaxial joint may damage the transverse ligament of the atlas, resulting in forward displacement of the atlas on the axis, i.e., atlantoaxial subluxation. In either instance, serious and even life-threatening compression of the spinal cord may occur gradually or suddenly (see Chaps. 285 and 381). Lateral roentgenograms in flexion and extension, performed cautiously, are sometimes necessary to visualize dislocation or subluxation.

OTHER DESTRUCTIVE DISEASES **Neoplastic, infectious, and metabolic diseases** Metastatic carcinoma (breast, lung, prostate, thyroid, kidney, gastrointestinal tract), multiple myeloma, and non-Hodgkin's and Hodgkin's lymphomas are the malignant tumors which most frequently involve the spine. Since the primary site may be overlooked or asymptomatic, the presenting complaint in such patients may be pain in the back. The pain tends to be constant and dull and is often unrelieved by rest. Indeed, it may be worse at night. Radiographic changes may be absent early in the disease, but when they appear, usually they are manifest as destructive lesions in one or several vertebral bodies with little or limited involvement of the disk space, even in the face of a compression fracture. A ^{99m}Tc diphosphonate bone scan is helpful in demonstrating "hot spots," indicating areas of increased blood flow and reactive bone formation associated with destructive, inflammatory, or arthritic lesions. It should be noted, however, that myeloma and sometimes metastatic thyroid carcinoma may fail to show increased activity on a bone scan.

Infection of the vertebral column is usually the result of pyogenic organisms (staphylococci or coliform bacilli) or, somewhat less commonly today, the tubercle bacilli. Patients complain of pain in the back of subacute or chronic nature that is exacerbated by motion but not materially relieved by rest. There is limitation of motion, tenderness over the spine of the involved segments, and pain with jarring of the spine, such as occurs with walking on the heels. Usually, these patients are afebrile and often do not have a leukocytosis, although the erythrocyte sedimentation rate is almost invariably elevated. Radiographs may demonstrate narrowing of a disk space with erosion and destruction of the two adjacent vertebrae. A paravertebral soft tissue mass evident on contrast CT or MRI may be present, indicating an abscess, which may in the case of tuberculosis drain spontaneously at sites quite remote from the vertebral column. In addition to a bone scan, a gallium scan is sometimes helpful in identifying a soft tissue inflammatory or infectious lesion even when overt bone destruction is not visible in x-rays.

Special mention should be made of the spinal *epidural abscess* (usually staphylococcal), which necessitates urgent surgical treatment. The symptoms are a localized pain, occurring spontaneously, aggravated by percussion and palpation. The patient is febrile and usually has severe radicular complaints, often bilateral, progressing rapidly to a flaccid paraplegia (see Chap. 381). Chronic drug abusers are particularly prone to this problem. Patients with AIDS also have been noted to have increased incidence of epidural abscess and of pyogenic and granulomatous osteomyelitis.

In metabolic bone diseases (hyperparathyroidism, osteoporosis, or osteomalacia), a considerable degree of loss of bone substance may occur without any symptoms whatsoever. Many patients with such conditions do, however, complain of aching in the lumbar or thoracic area. This is most likely to occur following an injury, sometimes trivial in nature, which leads to collapse or wedging of a vertebra. Certain movements greatly enhance the pain, while certain positions relieve it. One or more spinal roots may be involved. Paget's disease of the spine is readily identifiable on x-ray and is often painless. The disease may, however, lead to compression of the spinal cord or roots because of encroachment on the canal or foramina by the pagetoid bone. The recognition of these bone disorders is discussed in some detail elsewhere (Chaps. 358 and 361).

In general, patients thought to have neoplastic, infectious, or metabolic disease of the spine should be thoroughly evaluated by means of radiographs, bone scans, CT or MRI scans, and appropriate laboratory studies (see above). One of the most useful studies is measurement of bone density by dual-beam photon absorbitometry or quantitative digital radiography.

REFERRED PAIN FROM VISCERAL DISEASE The pain of disease of the pelvic, abdominal, or thoracic viscera is often felt in the region of the spine; i.e., it is referred to the posterior parts of the spinal segment that innervates the diseased organ. Occasionally, back pain may be the first and only sign. The general rule is that pelvic diseases are referred to the sacral region, lower abdominal diseases to the lumbar region (centering around the second to fourth lumbar vertebrae), and upper abdominal diseases to the lower thoracic spine (eighth thoracic to the first and second lumbar vertebrae). Characteristically, local signs or stiffness of the back are not elicited, and motion may be of full range without augmentation of the pain. However, some positions, e.g., flexion of the lumbar area of the spine in the lateral recumbent position, may be more comfortable than others.

Low thoracic and upper lumbar pain in abdominal disease Peptic ulceration or tumor of the wall of the stomach and of the duodenum most typically induces pain in the epigastrium (see Chaps. 252 and 275); but if the posterior wall is involved, and particularly if there is retroperitoneal extension, the pain may be felt in the region of the spine. The pain may be central in location or more intense on one side, or it may be felt in both locations. If very intense, it may seem to encircle the body. It tends to retain the characteristics of pain from the affected organ; e.g., if due to peptic ulceration, it appears about 2 h after a meal and is relieved by food and antacids.

Diseases of the pancreas (peptic ulceration with extension to the pancreas, cholecystitis with pancreatitis, cyst, or tumor) are apt to cause pain in the back, being more to the right of the spine if the head of the pancreas is involved and to the left if the body and tail are implicated.

Diseases of retroperitoneal structures, e.g., lymphomas, sarcomas, and carcinomas, may evoke pain in the adjacent part of the spine with some tendency toward radiation to the lower part of the abdomen, groin, and anterior thighs. A secondary tumor of the iliopsoas region on one side often produces a unilateral lumbar ache with radiation toward the groin, labia, or testicle; there also may be signs of involvement of the upper lumbar spinal roots. An aneurysm of the abdominal aorta may induce pain which is localized to this region of the spine but may be felt higher or lower, depending on the location of the lesion.

Sudden appearance of obscure lumbar pain in a patient receiving anticoagulants should arouse suspicion of retroperitoneal bleeding.

Lumbar pain with lower abdominal diseases Inflammatory diseases of segments of the colon (colitis, diverticulitis) or tumor of the colon cause pain which may be felt in the lower part of the abdomen between the umbilicus and pubis, in the midlumbar region, or in both places. If very intense, the pain may have a beltlike distribution around the body. A lesion in the transverse colon or first part of the descending colon may be central or left-sided, and its level of reference to the back is to the second to third lumbar vertebrae. If the sigmoid colon is implicated, the pain is lower, in the upper sacral region and anteriorly in the midline suprapubic region or left lower quadrant of the abdomen.

Sacral pain in pelvic (urologic and gynecologic) diseases The pelvis is seldom the site of a disease which causes obscure low back pain, although gynecologic disorders may manifest themselves in this manner. Of painful pelvic lesions, less than a third are due to inflammatory disease; other more hypothetical entities, such as relaxation of uterine supporting structures, retroversion of uterus, pelvic varicosities, and adnexal edema, have been largely discredited. Recently, CT, MRI, or diagnostic laparoscopy has been recommended as a valuable supplement to rectal and pelvic examinations, sigmoidoscopy, and intravenous pyelography for patients with obscure pelvic pain. The importance of psychiatric illness in the majority of undiagnosed cases has been stressed.

Menstrual pain itself may be felt in the sacral region. It is rather poorly localized, tends to radiate down the legs, and is often described as cramplike. The most important source of chronic back pain from the pelvic organs, however, is thought to be the uterosacral ligaments. Endometriosis or carcinoma of the uterus (body or cervix) may invade these structures, while malposition of the uterus may cause traction on them. The pain is localized centrally in the sacrum below the lumbosacral joint but may be more on one side than the other. In endometriosis, the pain begins during the premenstrual phase and often continues until it merges with menstrual pain. Malposition of the uterus (retroversion, descensus, and prolapse) is thought by some to lead to sacral pain, especially after the patient has been standing for several hours. One may observe the effect of postural influences here as when a fibroma of the uterus pulls on the uterosacral ligaments. Carcinomatous pain due to involvement of nerve plexuses is continuous and becomes progressively more severe; it tends to be more intense at night. The primary lesion may be overlooked on pelvic examination. Papanicolaou smears, pyelogram, CT scan, and laparoscopy are the most useful diagnostic procedures. X-ray therapy of these tumors may produce sacral pain from necrosis of tissue and injury to nerve roots. Low back pain with radiation into one or both thighs is common in the last weeks of pregnancy.

Chronic prostatitis, evidenced by prostatic discharge, burning and frequency of urination, and sometimes a reduction in sexual potency, may be attended by a nagging sacral ache; it may be mainly on one side, with radiation into one leg if the seminal vesicle is involved on that side. Carcinoma of the prostate with metastases to the lower part of the spine is another more common cause of sacral or lumbar pain. It may be present without urinary frequency or burning. Spinal nerves may be infiltrated by tumor cells, or the spinal cord itself may be compressed if the epidural space is invaded. The diagnosis is established by rectal examination, imaging studies and bone scans of the spine, and measurement of acid phosphatase (particularly the prostatic phosphatase fraction) and prostate-specific antigen. Lesions of the bladder and testes are usually not accompanied by back pain. When the kidney is the site of disease, the pain is ipsilateral, being felt in the flank or lumbar region.

Visceral derangements of whatever type may intensify the pain of arthritis, and the presence of arthritis may alter the distribution of visceral pain. With disease of the spine in the lumbosacral region, for example, distention of the ampulla of the sigmoid by feces or a bout of colitis may aggravate the arthritic pain. In patients with arthritis of the cervical or thoracic spine, the pain of myocardial ischemia may radiate to the back.

OBSCURE TYPES OF LOW BACK PAIN AND THE QUESTION OF PSYCHIATRIC DISEASE The practitioner is frequently consulted by persons who complain of low back pain of obscure origin. Usually the disorder is benign in nature and results from some minor derangement, muscular strain, or diskal prolapse. This is particularly true for those lesions which are of acute onset, aggravated by motion, and relieved by rest. Considerably more difficult are patients with chronic pain, especially those who have had prior back surgery or chronic visceral disease or those who have severe and progressive pain in which neoplasia or infection is considered.

Even when exhaustive studies have been performed, there remains a group of patients in whom no anatomic or pathologic lesion can be found. These patients generally fall into two categories: those with "postural" back pain and those with psychiatric illness.

"Postural" back pain   Some slender asthenic young individuals complain of a vague pain in the back, diffuse in nature, and most frequently noted with prolonged sitting or standing. Similarly, some obese middle-aged patients describe a discomfort in the back, either thoracic or lumbar in location. The physical examination in these patients is negative except for slack musculature and what may be best termed "poor posture." Imaging studies and laboratory evaluation usually show no abnormalities, and characteristically, the pain is relieved by bed rest. Exercises to strengthen the paraspinal and abdominal muscles are sometimes therapeutic.

Psychiatric illness   Low back pain may be encountered in compensation hysteria and malingering, in chronic anxiety states or depression, and in many individuals whose symptoms and complaints do not fall within any category of psychiatric illness. It is important to be certain that pain in the back in such patients does not signify disease of the spine and adjacent structures, and all such patients should be studied carefully. However, even when organic factors are found, the pain may be exaggerated, prolonged, or woven into a pattern of invalidism or disability because of coexistent psychological factors, especially when there is the possibility of secondary gain (notably compensation for a work-related injury) (see Chap. 11).

PAIN IN THE NECK AND SHOULDER

It is useful to distinguish three major categories of painful disease—of the spine, brachial plexus (thoracic outlet), and shoulder. Although pain in these three regions of the body may overlap, the patient can usually indicate the site of origin.

Cervical spine   Pain arising from the cervical spine is felt in the neck and back of the head (though it may often be projected to the shoulder, arm, and even forearm and hand), is evoked or enhanced by certain movements or positions of the neck, and is accompanied by tenderness and limitation of motions of the neck.

Osteoarthritis of the cervical spine may cause pains which radiate into the back of the head, shoulders, and arms on one or both sides of the thorax. Coincident involvement of nerve roots is manifested by paresthesias, sensory loss, weakness, or deep tendon reflex change. Should bony ridges form in the spinal canal (spondylosis), the spinal cord may be compressed (see Chap. 381). A myelogram, CT, or MRI may reveal the degree of encroachment on the spinal canal (narrowing of the canal to less than 11 mm in the anteroposterior diameter) at the level at which the spinal cord is affected. Difficulty may be experienced in distinguishing the syndrome associated with spondylosis with or without disk rupture and spinal cord dysfunction from primary neurologic diseases (syringomyelia, amyotrophic lateral sclerosis, or tumor) with an unrelated osteoarthritis of the cervical portion of the spine, particularly at the fifth to sixth and sixth to seventh cervical vertebrae, where the disk spaces are often narrowed in the adult. The newer imaging studies such as CT or MRI are helpful in this regard. A painful injury to ligaments and muscles after an accident in which the neck is forcibly extended and flexed (e.g., "whiplash" injury to spine) may be a difficult diagnostic problem, particularly if the patient has some ostensible spurring and especially if in the course of the injury a cerebral concussion has occurred. If the pain is persistent and limited to the neck, imaging studies will sometimes prove that the problem is due to disruption of a disk, but it is often complicated by psychological factors.

Thoracic outlet   Pain resulting from abnormalities of the thoracic outlet is experienced in and around the shoulder in the supraclavicular region or between the shoulders, is induced by the performance of certain tasks and by certain positions, and is associated with tenderness of structures above the clavicle. There may be a palpable abnormality above the clavicle (aneurysms of the subclavian artery, tumor, cervical rib). The combination of circulatory symptoms and signs referable to the lower part of the brachial plexus, manifested in the hand by obliteration of pulse when the patient holds a full breath with the head tilted back or turned (Adson's test), unilateral Raynaud's phenomenon, trophic changes in the fingers, and sensory loss over the ulnar side of the hand with or without interosseous atrophy complete the clinical picture. Roentgenograms and other imaging studies showing a cervical rib, deformed thoracic outlet, or superior sulcus tumor of the lung (Pancoast's syndrome) corroborate disease in this location. Electromyography and conduction studies along the plexus from points stimulated above and below the clavicle and studies of arterial and venous circulation (venograms, noninvasive Doppler techniques) are especially helpful in evaluating this problem.

Shoulder   Pain localized to the shoulder region is often worse at night and may be associated with local tenderness over the shoulder. The pain is characteristically aggravated by abduction, internal rotation, and extension. Most often shoulder lesions are in the form of a tendonitis or bursitis (sometimes calcific) usually affecting the supraspinatus tendon, the adjacent subdeltoid bursa, or the biceps tendon; occasionally, the lesion is more extensive and consists of a rupture of the rotator cuff, in which case the patient may have weakness on abduction and forward flexion. In some such patients there is an adhesive capsulitis, leading to profound limitation of motion, designated as a "frozen shoulder." Partial cuff tears, impingement of the cuff under the acromion, and slight subluxations produce a variety of symptoms about the shoulder particularly with exercise or maintaining the arm in abduction for long periods of time. The pain of shoulder disease may at times radiate into the arm or hand, but the sensory, motor, and reflex changes which indicate disease of nerve roots, plexus, or peripheral nerves are absent.

RUPTURED CERVICAL DISKS   One of the most common causes of neck, shoulder, and arm pain is disk herniation in the lower cervical region. As with rupture of the lumbar disks, the complete syndrome includes the disorder of spinal function and evidence of neural involvement. It may develop after trauma, either major or minor (sudden hyperextension of the neck, diving injuries, forceful manipulations, etc.). Virtually every patient exhibits a diminution in range of motion of the neck (often accompanied by intensification of pain). Hyperextension is the movement that most consistently aggravates the pain, although one occasionally sees patients whose principal limitation is in flexion. Rotation and lateral movements are often moderately restricted by pain. With laterally situated disk lesions between the fifth and sixth cervical vertebrae, the symptoms and signs are referred to the sixth cervical roots. The full syndrome is characterized by pain felt at the trapezius ridge, tip of the shoulder, anterior upper part of the arm, radial forearm, and often in the thumb; paresthesias and sensory impairment or hypersensitivity in the same regions; tenderness in the area above the spine of the scapula and in the supraclavicular and biceps regions; weakness in flexion of the forearm; and diminished to absent biceps and supinator reflexes (triceps retained or exaggerated). When the protruded disk lies between the sixth and seventh cervical vertebrae, the seventh cervical root is involved. Under these circumstances, in the patient with the complete syndrome, the pain is in the region of the shoulder blade, pectoral region and medial axilla, posterolateral upper arm, elbow and dorsal forearm, index and middle fingers, or all the fingers; tenderness is most pronounced over the medial aspect of the shoulder blade opposite the third to fourth thoracic spinous processes, in the supraclavicular area and triceps region; paresthesias and sensory loss are most pronounced in the second and third fingers or tips of all the fingers; weakness is seen in extension of the forearm, in the extension of the wrist, and in the hand grip; the triceps reflex is diminished to absent, and the biceps and supinator reflexes are preserved. Either of these syndromes may be incomplete in that only one of several of the typical findings (e.g., pain) is present. Usually the patient states that cough, sneeze, and downward pressure on the head in the hyperextension position exacerbate pain and that traction (even manual) tends to relieve it.

Unlike lumbar disks, the cervical ones, if large and centrally situated, may result in compression of the spinal cord (central disk, all the cord; paracentral disk, part of the cord). The central disk is often nearly painless, and the cord syndrome may simulate a degenerative disease (amyotrophic lateral sclerosis, combined system disease). A common error is to fail to think of a ruptured disk in the cervical region in patients with obscure symptoms in the legs. The diagnosis of ruptured cervical disk should be confirmed by the same laboratory procedures that were mentioned under "Spondylosis," above.

OTHER CONDITIONS   Metastases to the cervical spine are fortunately less common than to other parts of the vertebral column. They are frequently painful and the cause of disordered root function. Compression fractures or extension of the tumor posteriorly may lead to rapid development of quadriplegia.

Shoulder injuries (rotator cuff), subacromial or subdeltoid bursitis, the frozen shoulder (periarthritis or capsulitis), tendonitis, and arthritis may develop in patients who are otherwise well, but these conditions are also frequent in hemiplegics or in individuals suffering from coronary heart disease. The pain is often severe and extends toward the neck and down the arm into the hand. The dorsum of the latter may tingle without other signs of nerve involvement. Vasomotor and arthropathic changes may also occur in the hand (shoulder-hand syndrome, reflex dystrophy), and after a time, osteoporosis and atrophy of cutaneous and subcutaneous structures occur (Sudeck's atrophy or Sudeck-Leriche syndrome). These conditions fall more within the province of orthopedics than of medicine and are not discussed here in detail. The physician, however, must know that they can often be prevented by proper exercises.

The *carpal tunnel syndrome*, with paresthesias and numbness in palmar distribution of the median nerve and aching pain which extends up into the forearm, may be mistaken for disease of the shoulder or neck. Similarly, other less common forms of nerve entrapment may involve the ulnar, radial, or median nerves and lead to a mistaken diagnosis of brachial plexus lesion or cervical syndrome. Electromyography and conduction studies are especially helpful in such conditions (Chap. 382).

MANAGEMENT OF BACK AND NECK PAIN

Without doubt, the preventive aspects of back pain are important. There would be far fewer back problems if adults kept their trunk muscles in optimal condition by regular exercise such as swimming, bicycle riding, walking briskly, running, or calisthenic programs. A weight-reduction diet and a regular exercise program to strengthen abdominal and paraspinal muscles are frequently very beneficial for patients with chronic low back discomfort. Morning is the ideal time, since the back of the older adult tends to stiffen during the night because of inactivity. This happens regardless of whether a bed board or a stiff mattress is used. Sleeping with the back hyperextended and sitting for long times in an overstuffed chair or a badly designed auto seat commonly cause difficulties for the patient with low back problems. It is estimated that pressures between disks are increased 200 percent by changing from a recumbent to a standing position and 400 percent by sitting slumped in an easy chair. Correct sitting posture lessens this. Long trips in a car or plane without change in position put maximal strain on disk and ligamentous structures in the spine. Lifting from a position of flexed trunk, as in removing a suitcase from the trunk of a car, is dangerous (always lift with the object close to the body). Sudden strenuous activity without conditioning and warm-up also is likely to cause trouble to disks and their ligamentous envelopes (the most common sources of back pain).

Muscular and ligamentous strains and minor disk prolapses are usually self-limited, responding to simple measures in a relatively short period of time. The basic principle of therapy is rest in a recumbent position for several days to weeks. When weight bearing is resumed, a light lumbosacral support is occasionally helpful in continuing the immobilization until the patient is restored to full health. Physical measures such as heat, cold, diathermy, or massage are of limited value; of considerably greater importance are active exercises to both reduce the spasm and improve muscle tone. Analgesic medication should be given liberally during the first few days: codeine, 30 mg, and aspirin, 0.6 g, or pentazocine, 50 mg, propoxyphene, 65 mg, or meperidine, 50 mg. Muscle relaxants are often a valuable adjunct, particularly in that such drugs as diazepam, 8 to 40 mg in divided doses, may make bed rest more tolerable. If an inflammatory component is suspected, indomethacin, 75 mg/d (in divided doses), ibuprofen, 600 mg three or four times daily, or naproxen, 375 to 500 mg once or twice daily, may be helpful.

In the treatment of a clearly diagnosed acute or chronic rupture of a lumbar or cervical disk, complete bed rest is essential, at least initially, and analgesic medication may be required. Traction is of little value in lumbar disk disease, and it is best to permit the patient to find the most comfortable position. Cervical traction with a halter may be of considerable benefit to patients with cervical disk syndrome. It can be administered with the patient in recumbency or, after sufficient improvement to allow ambulation, can be performed intermittently in the erect, slightly forward flexed position using special equipment. During the recumbent phase of treatment of lumbar disk disease, exercises to reduce spasm, muscle relaxants, and anti-inflammatory agents as described above may be of considerable value. After 2 to 3 weeks in bed, the patient can be allowed to slowly resume activities, usually with the protection of a brace or light spinal support. Exercise programs designed to increase the strength of the abdominal and paraspinal muscles are helpful at this point. The patient may suffer some minor recurrence of the pain but be able to carry on his or her usual activities, and eventually most individuals will recover. If the pain and neurologic findings do not disappear on prolonged, conservative management, or if the patient suffers frequently recurring acute episodes, administration of epidural glucocorticoid may be indicated. For only those patients who fail to improve with a long trial of conservative care or those whose symptoms are worsening at a rapid rate, surgical management may be considered. This should always be preceded by a CT, MRI, and/or myelogram to localize the lesion (and rule out the presence of intra- or extradural tumors). The surgical procedure most often indicated is a partial hemilaminectomy with excision of the disk involved. Arthrodesis of the involved segments is indicated only in cases in which there is extraordinary instability usually related to an anatomic abnormality (such as spondylolysis) or in the cervical region when an extensive laminectomy has rendered the spine unstable. The result of conservative management of patients with diskal disease and sciatica is that approximately 80 percent improve at the end of 4 weeks regardless of whether traction, exercises, manipulation, or corset, or some combination thereof, is used. Therefore, only a small number of patients should be considered to require surgery.

Spondylosis of the cervical spine, if painful, is helped by bed rest and traction; if signs of spinal cord involvement are present, a collar to limit movement may lead to improvement. Decompressive laminectomy or anterior fusion is reserved for severe instances of the disease with advancing neurologic symptoms. The shoulder-hand syndrome may benefit from stellate ganglion blocks or ganglionectomy, but the basic treatment is physiotherapy, with or without medication, and surgical procedures are measures of last resort.

The management of patients with thoracic outlet syndrome is complex and requires first a careful study to be certain that the cause of the lesion is really a mechanical encroachment of the brachial plexus in the interspace between the clavicle and first rib. Exercises to reduce the tension in this region are mainly designed to strengthen the clavicular musculature and improve posture, thus opening the outlet. Many patients benefit from change of work circumstances, and for women with pendulous breasts, a better-designed brassiere is sometimes helpful. Nonsteroidal anti-inflammatory agents are sometimes beneficial, as are muscle relaxants such as diazepam. If the patient's difficulties are intractable or the root compression causes neurologic deficits, exploration of the anterior scalene triangle with resection of the first rib usually gives excellent results.

REFERENCES

BATES D, RUGGIERI P: Imaging modalities for evaluation of the spine. Radiol Clin North Am 29:675, 1991

BELL GR, PARKMAN RH: The conservative treatment of sciatica. Spine 9:54, 1984

BOGDUK N: The innervation of the lumbar spine. Spine 8:286, 1983

BUCHANAN JR ET AL: A comparison of the risk of vertebral fracture in menopausal osteopenia and other metabolic disturbances. J Bone Joint Surg 70:704, 1988

BUNDSCHUH CV et al: Epidural fibrosis and recurrent disk herniation in the lumbar spine: MR imaging assessment. AJR 150:923, 1988

CAPUTY AJ, LEUSSENHOP AJ: Long-term evaluation of decompressive surgery for degenerative lumbar stenosis. J Neurosurg 77:669, 1992

DEYO RA, DIEHL AK: Measuring physical and psychosocial function in patients with low back pain. Spine 8:635, 1983

ELGHAZAWI AK: Clinical syndromes and differential diagnosis of spinal disorders. Radiol Clin North Am 29:651, 1991

EL-KHOURY GY, RENFREW DL: Percutaneous procedures for the diagnosis and treatment of lower back pain: Diskography, facet-joint injection, and epidural injection. AJR 157:685, 1991

FRYMOYER JW: Back pain and sciatica. N Engl J Med 318:291, 1988

GRABIAS SL: The treatment of spinal stenosis. J Bone Joint Surg 62A:308, 1988

GRANT R ET AL: Metastatic epidural spinal cord compression. Neurol Clin 9:825, 1991

LEE C, DEAN BL: Contrast-enhanced magnetic resonance imaging of the spine. Top Magn Reson Imaging 3:41, 1991.

MASARYK TJ et al: High-resolution MR imaging of sequestered lumbar intervertebral disks. AJR 150:1155, 1988

MANELFE C: T1 imaging of degenerative processes of the spine. Curr Opin Radiol 4:63, 1992

MODIC MT, ROSS JS: Magnetic resonance imaging in the evaluation of low back pain. Orthop Clin North Am 22:283, 1991

——— et al: Imaging of degenerative disk disease. Radiology 168:177, 1988

MURPHY RW: Nerve roots and spinal nerves in degenerative disk disease. Clin Orthop 129:46, 1977

PLEATMAN CW, LUKIN RR: Lumbar spinal stenosis. Semin Roentgenol 23:106, 1988

REYNOLDS AV et al: Lumbar monoradiculopathy due to unilateral facet hypertrophy. Neurosurgery 10:480, 1982

RISCH SV et al: Lumbar strengthening in chronic low back pain patients—Physiologic and psychological benefits. Spine 18:332, 1993

WILSON ES, BRILL RF: Spinal stenosis: The narrow lumbar canal syndrome. Clin Orthop 122:244, 1977

section 2 Alterations in body temperature

16 FEVER, INCLUDING FEVER OF UNKNOWN ORIGIN

JEFFREY A. GELFAND / CHARLES A. DINARELLO / SHELDON M. WOLFF

Fever is an elevation of body temperature above the normal circadian variation as the result of a change in the thermoregulatory center, located in the anterior hypothalamus. A normal body temperature is maintained, despite environmental variations, due to the ability of the thermoregulatory center to balance heat production by the tissues, notably muscles and the liver, with heat dissipation. With fever, the balance is shifted to increase the core temperature. *Hyperthermia* is an elevation of body temperature above the hypothalamic set point due to insufficient heat dissipation (e.g., as is seen in exercise, perspiration-inhibiting drugs, hot environment, etc.).

While the "normal" temperature in humans has been said to be 37°C (98.6°F) based on Wunderlich's original observations over 120 years ago, the overall mean temperature for normal individuals aged 18 to 40 years is actually 36.8 ± 0.4°C (98.2 ± 0.7°F), with a nadir at 6 A.M. and a zenith at 4 to 6 P.M. The maximum normal oral temperature at 6 A.M. is 37.2°C (98.9°F), and the maximum normal oral temperature at 4 P.M. is 37.7°C (99.9°F), both defining the 99th percentile for normal individuals. Using these criteria, *an A.M. temperature greater than 37.2°C (98.9°F) or a P.M. temperature greater than 37.7°C (99.9°F) would define a fever*. Rectal temperatures are generally 0.6°C (1°F) higher. Lower esophageal temperatures closely reflect core temperature. The temperature of a freshly passed urine specimen is close to rectal values. The normal 24-h circadian temperature rhythm is associated with temperatures varying typically by 0.5°C (0.9°F) but occasionally as much as 1°C between the A.M. nadir and the P.M. peak. This morning low and evening high pattern is usually preserved in febrile diseases but is abolished in hyperthermia. In menstruating women, the A.M. temperature is generally lower in the 2 weeks prior to ovulation, rising to about 0.6°C (1°F) with ovulation, until menses occur. There may even be a seasonal variation in body temperature. Finally, such physiologic alterations as postprandial state, pregnancy, endocrine factors, and age may alter baseline temperatures.

PYROGENS Substances that cause fever are called *pyrogens* and may be either exogenous or endogenous. *Exogenous pyrogens* are from outside the host, whereas endogenous pyrogens are produced by the host, generally in response to initiating stimuli usually triggered by infection or inflammation. The majority of exogenous pyrogens are microorganisms, their products, or toxins. The best characterized exogenous pyrogen is the heterogeneous group of molecules common to all gram-negative bacteria referred to as *endotoxin* (lipopolysaccharide, LPS). LPS is found in the outer membrane of all gram-negative bacteria and comprises a lipid A and polysaccharide core, linked to an "O-polysaccharide" side-chain composed of repeating units of sugars which vary for each specific gram-negative organism. Gram-positive organisms also produce potent exogenous pyrogens. These include lipoteichoic acid, peptidoglycan, and various exotoxins and enterotoxins. In vivo, LPS is capable of producing fever in humans with as little as 1 ng/kg; while there are no in vivo data in humans, gram-positive cell wall constituents generally require a 2 to 3 log higher amount of material by weight when compared with LPS to induce the production of endogenous pyrogens in vitro. In general, exogenous pyrogens act primarily by inducing the formation of endogenous pyrogens by stimulation of the host's cells, generally monocytes and macrophages. However, the distinction between exogenous and endogenous pyrogens is sometimes blurred. For example, LPS may act directly on endothelial cells in the brain to generate fever, whereas many endogenous products result in the release of endogenous pyrogens, thereby causing fever. Such endogenous substances include antigen-antibody complexes with complement, complement cleavage products, steroid hormone metabolites, bile acids, and some cytokines.

Endogenous pyrogens are polypeptides produced by a variety of host cells, particularly monocytes/macrophages. Endogenous pyrogens, produced either systemically or locally, gain entrance to the circulation and produce fever at the level of the thermoregulatory center of the hypothalamus.

It was originally thought that there was a single endogenous pyrogen, or EP. The standard experimental model utilized injection of leukocyte supernatants or sera of febrile rabbits into normal rabbits. It was then realized that there are two leukocyte EPs, *interleukin 1α* (IL-1α) and *interleukin 1β* (IL-1β). They share a common molecular weight of approximately 17.5 kDa, have only 26 percent amino acid sequence homology, and bind to the same receptors. Originally thought to be produced only by phagocytic cells, IL-1α or IL-1β is produced also by endothelial cells, B lymphocytes, natural killer cells, fibroblasts, smooth-muscle cells, keratinocytes, and glial cells. Because of the ubiquitous production of these and other interleukins, cell-derived inflammatory polypeptides, and growth-promoting peptides, the more general term *cytokine* has been adopted to refer to these substances. Cytokines are regulatory polypeptides produced by a large variety of nucleated cells. Cytokines are produced by monocytes/macrophages, lymphocytes, endothelial cells, hepatocytes, epithelial cells, keratinocytes, and fibroblasts, as well as other cells. Cytokines typically act locally, initiating autocrine (self-stimulating) or paracrine (stimulating nearby) effects. Cytokines, when found in the circulation, are usually present in picogram per milliliter concentrations.

The major pyrogenic cytokines appear to be IL-1β, IL-1α, tumor necrosis factor α (TNFα), tumor necrosis factor β (TNFβ, lymphotoxin), interferon α (IFNα), and interleukin 6 (IL-6). When endogenous pyrogens IL-1α, IL-1β, TNFα, and IL-6 have been administered intravenously to humans, chills and fever occur within 1 h. IL-1α and IL-1β are the most pyrogenic, with febrile responses of 39°C taking place with doses of 10 to 30 ng/kg body weight. At doses of 100 ng/kg, higher fevers and rigors have been observed. TNFα produces chills and fever at 39°C at somewhat higher doses (50 to 100 ng/kg). IL-6 is the least pyrogenic of the three cytokines, producing fever of 39°C at 1 μg/kg. IFNα and IFNγ have been administered primarily by the subcutaneous route, and therefore chills and fever occur after 3 to 4 h. On a weight basis, the interferons are less potent than IL-1 or TNF and similar to IL-6.

HYPOTHALAMIC CONTROL OF TEMPERATURE The metabolic rate of humans consistently produces more heat than is necessary to maintain core body temperature at 37°C, assuming a neutral environment. Body temperature is controlled by the hypothalamus. Neurons in both the preoptic anterior hypothalamus and posterior hypothalamus receive two kinds of signals—one from peripheral nerves that reflect receptors for warmth and cold and the other from the temperature of the blood bathing the region. These two signals are integrated by the thermoregulatory center of the hypothalamus to maintain normal temperature. In addition, there are clusters of neurons in the preoptic/anterior hypothalamus supplied by a rich and highly permeable vascular network with reduced blood-brain barrier function. The specialized vascular network is called the *organum vasculosum laminae terminalis* (OVLT). It is likely that the endothelial cells of the OVLT release arachidonic acid metabolites when exposed to endogenous pyrogens from the circulation. Arachidonic acid metabolites, largely prostaglandin E_2 (PGE$_2$), then presumably diffuse into the preoptic/anterior hypothalamic region and initiate fever. It is possible that PGE$_2$ or other arachidonic acid products induce a second messenger such as cyclic AMP, which in turn raises the thermoregulatory set point. PGE$_2$ is the most potent of the fever-producing arachidonic acid derivatives when injected directly into the hypothalamus and is believed to mediate the rise in the thermoregulatory set point. With the new, higher "thermostatic setting," signals go to various efferent nerves, particularly those sympathetic fibers innervating the peripheral blood vessels, which in turn initiate vasoconstriction and promote heat conservation. The thermoregulatory center also sends signals to the cerebral cortex, initiating behavioral changes such as seeking a warm environment, clothes, special posturing. With the shunting of blood from the periphery, as well as behavioral changes, body temperature usually rises 2 to 3°C; if the hypothalamus calls for more heat, shivering (involuntary muscle contraction) is also triggered to increase heat production. The combination of heat conservation and increased heat production continue until the temperature of the blood bathing the

anterior hypothalamic neurons matches the new "setting." At that point, the hypothalamus maintains the new febrile temperature (Fig. 16-1).

If the hypothalamic set point is reset downward by the disappearance of stimulating endogenous pyrogens or by the inhibition of local prostaglandin synthesis by cyclooxygenase inhibitors such as aspirin, ibuprofen, or acetominophen, then vasodilation and sweating dissipate heat through radiation and conduction from the skin. Behavioral changes also may be triggered, such as the removal of insulating clothing or bedding. There are also endogenous antipyretic substances. These include arginine vasopressin, adrenocorticotropin, α-melanocyte stimulating hormone, and corticotropin-releasing hormone, each of which appears to alter the ability of endogenous pyrogens to stimulate prostaglandin production.

Several peptides only modulate responses in febrile diseases. These are the cytokine antagonists and inhibitory cytokines. The IL-1 receptor antagonist (IL-1Ra) is a 23- to 25-kDa protein that blocks the binding of IL-1 to its receptors. Whereas IL-1Ra blocks the hypotensive effects of IL-1 and gram-negative and gram-positive bacteremia in experimental animals, in human volunteers it failed to prevent fever in response to minute doses of LPS. Peak molar concentrations of IL-1Ra may exceed those of IL-1β by 100-fold, but these levels tend to occur 1 h after the IL-1β peak and may be part of the recovery process.

Endogenously produced binding proteins for TNF are produced by cleavage of the extracellular domains of the two TNF receptors. Circulating levels of these two soluble TNF receptor fragments (TNFR type I and TNFR type II) are higher than circulating levels of TNF. In addition, cytokines that inhibit the production of the major pyrogens IL-1 and TNF include transforming growth factor β (TGFβ), IL-4, and IL-10. There is very little information regarding the role of these cytokines in modulating the febrile response.

BIOLOGIC ACTIVITIES OF IL-1, TNF, AND IL-6 It is important to distinguish between the critical physiological roles of local IL-1 and TNF and the high systemic blood levels often seen with severe and life-threatening diseases. IL-1 and TNF mediate local phagocytic cell emigration and activation and the release of lipid-derived mediators such as PGE$_2$, thromboxane, and platelet-activating factor (PAF). IL-1 induces IL-8 synthesis, which in turn is a potent neutrophil and monocyte chemotactic factor. IL-8 stimulates the release of enzymes from neutrophils, further enhancing the host's attack on invading microbes. Vasodilation, the induction of adhesive glycoproteins, T and B lymphocyte activation, and enhanced phagocytic cell killing are directly or indirectly mediated by these pyrogenic cytokines. The acute phase response is stimulated, resulting in changes in protein synthesis in the liver. Serum albumin levels decrease, and the production of acute phase proteins, including antiproteases, complement components, fibrinogen, ceruloplasmin, ferritin, and haptoglobin, is increased. C-reactive protein, which in turn binds to damaged and necrotic cells and some microorganisms, may increase 1000-fold. Serum amyloid A (SAA) protein also may increase markedly and be deposited in various organs to cause secondary amyloidosis. Serum iron and zinc levels are decreased, depriving invading microbes of these critical growth factors. Although IL-1 and TNF can induce these hepatic changes, IL-6 is thought to be the prime mediator of the acute phase response.

Both IL-1 and TNF act synergistically to mediate local and systemic inflammatory effects. Amounts that cause little inflammation individually produce refractory hypotension and multiorgan system failure in combination. Suppression of either of these two cytokines may have a significant therapeutic effect by blocking this synergistic toxicity. Furthermore, IL-1–induced activation of T and B cells is greater at 39°C than at 37°C. Both IL-1 and TNF increase loss of mean body mass and cause anorexia, contributing to the cachexia of chronic febrile states. IL-1 and TNF are found in the circulation only briefly but nevertheless induce IL-6. IL-6 levels correlate better with the amount of fever and other pathologic findings in a variety of infectious diseases than IL-1 or TNF because of the persistence of

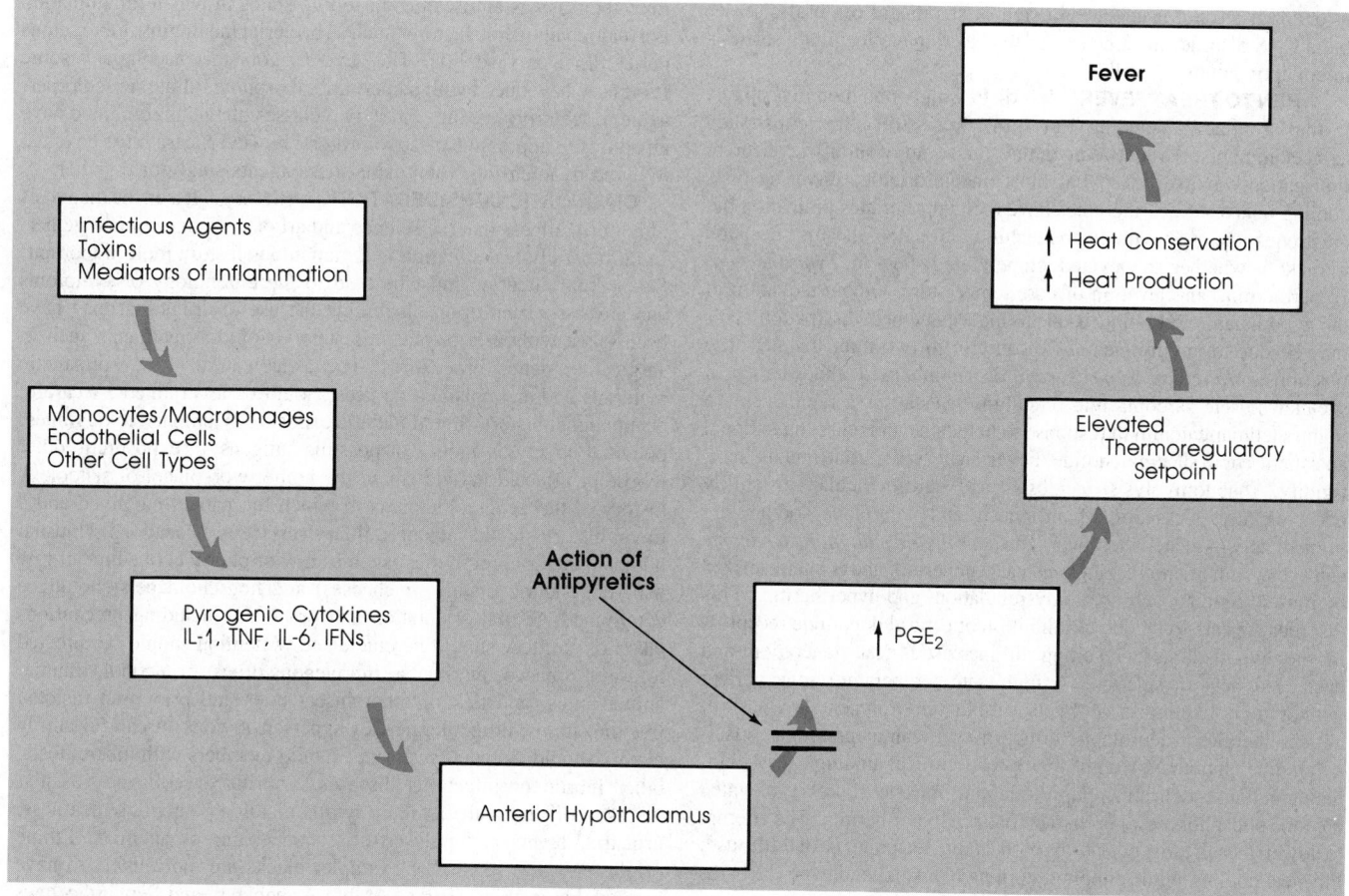

FIGURE 16-1   Chronology of events required for the induction of fever.

IL-6 in the circulation. Unlike IL-1 and TNF, however, there is little or no evidence that IL-6 is a lethal cytokine.

WHY FEVER?   Fever has been present for hundreds of millions of years in evolutionary terms. Fish, amphibians, and reptiles develop fever. When fish are injected with bacterial endotoxin or gram-negative bacteria, they raise their body temperature by swimming to warmer water. When lizards are injected with bacteria or pyrogens, they generate fever by basking in the sun to raise their core temperature to "febrile" levels. In many situations, the elevation of body temperature increases survival. The growth and virulence of several bacterial species are impaired at high temperatures, and fever therapy was used to treat neurosyphilis before antibiotics were available. Type III pneumococci are particularly sensitive to high temperature and at 41°C grow poorly and may autolyze. Inhibiting fever in rabbits infected with type III pneumococci increases the mortality rate. Temperatures in the febrile range appear to increase the phagocytic and bactericidal activity of neutrophils and the cytotoxic effects of lymphocytes. Thus fever probably enhances the ability to survive infection. The fact that there are redundancies among the pyrogens (IL-1β, IL-1α, TNF, IL-6, interferons) suggests that it is beneficial to preserve a number of pathways for eliciting this response.

However, there are considerable "costs" to the host in addition to discomfort. For each elevation of body temperature of 1°C, there is an increase in O_2 consumption of 13 percent and increased caloric and fluid requirements. The increased metabolic demand may stress the fetus during pregnancy and patients with marginal cardiac or cerebral vascular supply. IL-1 and TNF accelerate muscle catabolism, leading to a loss of body weight and negative nitrogen balance. Essentially, skeletal muscle is utilized as an energy source, with liberation of amino acids for gluconeogenesis and for the synthesis of acute phase proteins and formation of clones of immune cells. Fever reduces mental acuity and can produce delirium and stupor.

Children are prone to develop seizures with fevers, particularly if there is a prior history of seizures. A single episode of fever ≥37.8°C (100°F) in the first trimester of pregnancy doubles the risk of neural tube defects in the fetus.

ACCOMPANIMENTS OF FEVER   Not surprisingly, many of the associated features of fever can be reproduced by infusions of purified cytokines, including back pain, generalized myalgias, arthralgias, anorexia, and somnolence. These symptoms may be reduced by cyclooxygenase inhibitors. *Chills*, a sensation of cold occurring in most fevers, are part of the central nervous system (CNS) response to the thermoregulatory "set point" calling for more heat. A *rigor*, a profound chill, with piloerection ("goose flesh") associated with teeth chattering and severe shivering, is common in bacterial, rickettsial, and protozoal diseases and in influenza (but not in other viral diseases). Sepsis, systemic infections such as leptospirosis, brucellosis, rat bite fever, and endocarditis, malaria, and the intermittent sepsis seen with abscesses may all produce rigors, as can lymphomas, leukemias, renal cell carcinoma, and hepatoma. Rigors are also common with drug-induced fevers. *Sweats* occur with the activation of heat loss mechanisms, either due to antipyretics, reaching the new "thermal ceiling," or to the elimination of the febrile stimulus. The intermittent administration of antipyretics may exaggerate swings of temperature, leading to chilliness, discomfort, and exhaustion. Hypothalamic reflexes trigger sweating, allowing rapid dissipation of heat by evaporative loss.

Alterations of mental status and convulsions are common in the very young and very old and patients with dementia, hepatic failure, and chronic renal failure. There may be a progression from irritability to delirium to frank obtundation. This usually clears with the fever.

Febrile convulsions in infants and children less than 5 years old typically occur particularly at the onset of febrile disease and are more common at higher temperatures (>40°C). Febrile convulsions in children are not necessarily a sign of significant cerebral disease, but a CNS disorder must be excluded. Fever may precipitate seizures in epileptic adults as well.

WHEN TO TREAT FEVER   It is distressingly common in hospitals to find "routine," "standing," or "prn" orders for antipyretics (such as acetaminophen) for a temperature above an arbitrary level or to find patients awake, alert, but most uncomfortable, shivering on a cooling blanket. Such therapies have their appropriate application but are frequently used without therapeutic rationale. The first decision to make is whether an elevated temperature is *fever* or *hyperthermia*. Hyperthermia, an elevation of core temperature without elevation of the hypothalamic set point, is due to inadequate heat dissipation. This may be due to environmental exposure or to two rare, distinct drug reactions. *Malignant hyperthermia* is an inherited abnormality of skeletal muscle sarcoplasmic reticulum that causes a rapid increase in intracellular calcium in response to halothane and other inhalational anesthetics or to succinylcholine. Fever, increased muscle metabolism, rigidity, rhabdomyolysis, acidosis, and cardiovascular instability occur rapidly. Cessation of anesthesia and dantrolene sodium are immediately indicated therapies. The *neuroleptic malignant syndrome* can occur with phenothiazines such as haloperidol and is characterized by muscle rigidity, autonomic dysregulation, and hyperthermia. This disorder appears to be due to inhibition of central dopamine receptors in the hypothalamus, resulting in increased heat generation and decreased heat dissipation. A high core temperature in a patient with a high likelihood of hyperthermia (environmental exposure, anticholinergic or neuroleptic drugs, tricyclic antidepressants, succinylcholine, halothane) with appropriate clinical findings (dry skin, hallucinations, delirium, pupil dilation, muscle rigidity, elevated creatine phosphokinase) is characteristic of hyperthermia. The attempt to lower the already normal hypothalamic set point is of little use. Physical cooling with sponging, cooling blankets, and even ice baths should be initiated immediately, in conjunction with appropriate pharmacologic agents (such as dantrolene for malignant hyperthermia and the neuroleptic malignant syndrome or physostigmine for tricyclic antidepressant overdose). With hyperpyrexia (fever ≥41°C), antipyretics are clearly indicated, and physical cooling while "resetting" the hypothalamic set point with antipyretics will speed the process. Antipyretics also suppress the constitutional symptoms that accompany fever (myalgias, chills, headache, etc.). However, with "low-grade" or moderate temperatures, there is little evidence that fever is harmful or that antipyretic therapy is beneficial. Exceptions include the aforementioned situations of children with febrile seizures, pregnant women, and patients with impaired cardiac, pulmonary, or cerebral function. Temperature is often suppressed needlessly, and "routine" antipyretic orders may obscure the important clinical information to be gained from following the upward, or downward, course of a temperature. In addition, NSAIDs and glucocorticoids may mask the inflammatory features of a localized infection, preventing its detection and even encouraging its spread. In addition, the drugs themselves may cause side effects. Aspirin is to be avoided in children with viral diseases because of the possibility of Reye's syndrome, which occurs in association with influenza and varicella and occasionally with enteroviruses. In addition, the antiplatelet and even antiphagocytic effects of aspirin have led to the general use of acetaminophen. Acetaminophen is a poor cyclooxygenase inhibitor in peripheral tissue and thus lacks anti-inflammatory activity; in the CNS, acetaminophen is oxidized, converting it to an active cyclooxygenase inhibitor, thus explaining its antipyretic effect. Ibuprofen may be safe for children, with possibly greater temperature reduction and duration of effect at similar doses as acetaminophen. Ibuprofen does not appear to pose a risk of Reye's syndrome, but the caveat about bacterial infections remains. Other NSAIDs, particularly indomethacin and naproxen, are also useful as antipyretics.

Glucocorticoids are potent antipyretics. They inhibit PGE_2 synthesis by inhibiting phospholipase A_2 and block both mRNA transcription for IL-1 and TNF and translation of these cytokines. The potent immunosuppressive and antiphagocytic effects of glucocorticoids limit their use as antipyretics to febrile states in which inflammation is a major pathogenic factor—such as bacterial meningitis, tuberculous pericarditis, or vasculitis. The severe rigors that accompany some fevers can be reduced with meperidine, morphine sulfate, prochlorperazine, or chlorpromazine. These two classes of agents combined have an additive suppressive effect on rigors; however, care must be taken to avoid hypotension when using these agents singly or together.

DIAGNOSTIC CONSIDERATIONS   **History**   It is in the diagnosis of a febrile illness that the science and art of medicine come together. In no other clinical situation is a meticulous history more important. Painstaking attention must be paid to the chronology of symptoms and any associated drugs, including the use of drugs that may have been taken without a physician's supervision, or treatments such as surgical or dental procedures. The exact nature of any prosthetic materials and/or implanted devices should be ascertained. A careful occupational history should include exposure to animals, toxic fumes, potential infectious agents, or possible antigens, or exposure to other febrile or infected individuals in the home, workplace, or school. A history of the geographic areas in which the patient has lived and a travel history should include military service and locations. Unusual hobbies, dietary proclivities (such as raw or poorly cooked meat, raw fish, unpasteurized milk or cheeses) and household pets should be determined. Sexual orientation and practices, including precautions taken or omitted, should be elucidated. Attention should be directed to use of tobacco, marijuana, intravenous drugs, or alcohol, trauma, animal bites, and tick or other insect bites and prior transfusions, immunizations, drug allergies, or hypersensitivities. A careful family history should include a history of family members with tuberculosis, other febrile or infectious diseases, arthritis or collagen vascular disease, or unusual familiar symptomatology such as deafness, urticaria, fevers and polyserositis, bone pains or anemias. Ethnic origin may be critical. For example, blacks are more likely to have hemoglobinopathies. Turks, Arabs, Armenians, and Sephardic Jews are more likely to have familial Mediterranean fever.

Patterns of fever   The widespread use of antipyretics, glucocorticoids, and antibiotics can alter fever patterns so that "classic" fever patterns are not seen. Some patterns are clinically useful, however. Whereas the circadian temperature pattern is preserved and in fact exaggerated with most fevers, a reversal of this pattern may be seen with typhoid fever and disseminated tuberculosis. Temperature-pulse dissociation (relative bradycardia) is seen with typhoid fever, as well as brucellosis, leptospirosis, some drug fevers, and many factitious fevers. Bradycardia in the presence of fever also may signify cardiac conduction abnormalities, as with acute rheumatic fever, Lyme disease, viral myocarditis, or valve ring abscess complicating bacterial endocarditis.

Fever may be sustained, intermittent, remittent, or relapsing. A *sustained* fever is one in which temperature elevation is persistent, with minimal variation. With *intermittent* fever, there is an exaggeration of the normal circadian rhythm; when this variation is extremely large, the fever is termed *hectic* or *septic*. When hectic fevers occur daily, the term *quotidian* is sometimes used. With *relapsing* fevers, febrile episodes are separated by intervals of normal temperature; when paroxysms occur on the first and third days, the fever is called *tertian*. *Plasmodium vivax* causes tertian fevers. *Quartan* fevers are associated with paroxysms on the first and fourth day and are seen with *P. malariae*. Other relapsing fevers are seen with *Borrelia* infections and rat bite fever. Both are associated with days of fever followed by a several-day afebrile period and then relapses of days of fevers. Pel-Ebstein fever, with fevers lasting 3 to 10 days followed by afebrile periods of 3 to 10 days, is classic for Hodgkin's disease and other lymphomas. Another characteristic fever is that of cyclic neutropenia, in which fevers occur every 21 days and accompany the neutropenia. *Intermittent, hectic,* and *septic* fevers are common with deep-seated or systemic infections, malignancy, and drug fevers. *Remittent* fever, in which the temperature falls each day but not to normal is typical for tuberculosis, viral diseases, many bacterial infections, and noninfectious causes of fever. It should be emphasized that newborns, the elderly, patients with chronic renal or hepatic failure, and patients on glucocorticoids or with bacteremic shock may fail to generate fever altogether, and in these individuals, *hypothermia* may be a sign of severe infection.

Physical examination A meticulous physical examination should be repeated on a regular basis. All the vital signs are relevant. Temperature may be taken orally or rectally, but the specific site used should be kept consistent. Axillary temperatures are notoriously unreliable, as are oral temperatures obtained after recent hot or cold drinks, smoking, or hyperventilation.

In some cases, patients are thoroughly examined at the time of initial evaluation, but the diagnostic emphasis then shifts to laboratory data and other diagnostic procedures. Particular attention should be paid to daily physical examination, sometimes more often, until the diagnosis is certain and the anticipated response has been achieved. Special attention should be paid to the skin, lymph nodes, eyes, nailbeds, cardiovascular system, chest, abdomen, musculoskeletal system, and nervous system. Rectal examination is imperative. The penis, prostate, scrotum, and testes should be examined carefully, and the foreskin, if present, retracted. Pelvic examination is part of every complete physical examination of a female.

Laboratory tests There are few signs and symptoms in medicine with as many diagnostic possibilities as fever. If the history, epidemiologic circumstances, or physical examination suggests more than a simple viral illness or streptococcal pharyngitis, then laboratory testing is indicated. The tempo and complexity of the workup will depend on the pace of the illness, diagnostic considerations, and the immune status of the host. If findings are focal or if the history, epidemiologic considerations, or physical examination suggests certain diagnoses, the laboratory examination can be focused. If fever is undifferentiated, the "diagnostic nets" must be cast farther, and certain guidelines are then indicated, which follow.

CLINICAL PATHOLOGY Workup should include a complete blood count, a differential count performed manually or with an instrument sensitive to the identification of eosinophils, juvenile or band forms, toxic granulations, and Döhle bodies, the last three suggestive of bacterial infection. Neutropenia may be seen with some viral infections, particularly parvovirus B19, drug reactions, systemic lupus erythematosus (SLE), typhoid, brucellosis, and infiltrative diseases of the bone marrow, including lymphoma, leukemia, tuberculosis, and histoplasmosis. Lymphocytosis may be seen with typhoid, brucellosis, tuberculosis, and viral disease. Atypical lymphocytes are seen with many viral diseases, including Epstein-Bar virus (EBV), cytomegalovirus (CMV), human immune deficiency virus (HIV), dengue, rubella, varicella, measles, viral hepatitis, serum sickness, and toxoplasmosis. Monocytosis is seen in typhoid, tuberculosis, brucellosis, and lymphoma. Eosinophilia may be found in hypersensitivity drug reactions, Hodgkin's disease, adrenal insufficiency, and certain metazoan infections. If the febrile illness appears severe or prolonged, the smear should be examined carefully, and an erythrocyte sedimentation rate (ESR) should be performed. Urinalysis, with examination of urinary sediment, is indicated. It is axiomatic that any abnormal fluid accumulation (pleural, peritoneal, joint, etc.), even if previously sampled, merits reexamination in the presence of undiagnosed fever. Joint fluids should be examined for crystals. Bone marrow biopsy (not simple aspiration) for histopathology (as well as culture) is indicated when marrow infiltration by pathogens or tumor cells is possible. Stool should be inspected for occult blood; an inspection for fecal leukocytes, ova, or parasites also may be indicated.

CHEMISTRY Electrolytes, glucose, blood urea nitrogen, and creatinine determinations should be done. Liver function tests are usually indicated if the cause of fever does not point to another organ. Additional chemistries (creatine phosphokinase, etc) can be added as the workup progresses.

MICROBIOLOGY Smears and cultures of the throat, urethra, anus, cervix, and vagina should be obtained in appropriate situations. Sputum evaluation (Gram stain, AFB stain, cultures) is indicated for any patient with fever and cough. Blood cultures and cultures of abnormal fluid collections and urine are indicated when fever is thought to be more than uncomplicated viral illness. Cerebrospinal fluid should be examined and cultured if meningismus, severe headache, or mental status changes are present.

RADIOLOGY A chest x-ray is usually part of the evaluation for any significant febrile illness.

In most patients with fever, the history, physical examination, and initial screening laboratory studies lead to a diagnosis, or the patient recovers spontaneously. In the latter case, a viral illness is usually considered the source of the fever. When fever continues for 2 to 3 weeks, during which time repeat physical examinations and laboratory tests are unrevealing, patients are provisionally diagnosed as having fever of unknown origin (FUO).

FEVER OF UNKNOWN ORIGIN *Fever of unknown origin* (FUO) was defined by Petersdorf and Beeson in 1961: (1) fevers higher than 38.3°C (101°F) on several occasions, (2) a duration of more than 3 weeks, and (3) failure to reach a diagnosis after 1 week of inpatient investigation. While this classification has stood for more than 30 years, Durack and Street have proposed a new classification of FUO: (1) "classical FUO," (2) nosocomial FUO, (3) neutropenic FUO, and (4) HIV-associated FUO (Table 16-1).

Classic FUO This category corresponds closely to the prior definition of FUO and is modified only with regard to the prior requirement for 1 week's study in hospital to encompass three outpatient visits or 3 days in the hospital without a cause having been determined. In our opinion, 2 weeks of fever is sufficient to entertain the diagnosis when other criteria have been met.

Nosocomial FUO Nosocomial FUO is used when fever of ≥38.3°C (101°F) occurs on several occasions in a hospitalized patient receiving acute care and in whom infection was not present or incubating on admission. Three days of investigation, including at least 2 days' incubation of cultures is the minimum duration for this diagnosis. In hospitalized patients, occult nosocomial infections, infected intravascular lines, recurrent pulmonary embolism, transfusion-related viral infection, and drug fever are possible diagnoses. In this setting, the approach is to focus on sites where occult infections

TABLE 16-1 Categories of FUO*

	Nosocomial	Neutropenic	HIV-associated	Classic
Patient circumstance	Hospitalized, acute care, no infection when admitted	Has ≤500 neutrophils/mm³ or anticipated 1 to 2 days	Confirmed HIV-positive	All others with fevers ≥3 weeks
Duration of illness while under investigation	3 days†	3 days†	3 days† or 4 weeks as outpatient	3 days† or 3 outpatient visits
Examples of cause	Septic thrombophlebitis, sinusitis, *C. difficile* colitis, drug fever	Perianal infection, aspergillosis, candidemia	MAI, tuberculosis, non-Hodgkin's lymphoma, drug fever	Infections, malignancy, inflammatory diseases, drug fever

* All require fevers ≥ 38.3°C (101°F) on several occasions.
† Includes at least 2 days' incubation of microbiology cultures
SOURCE: After Durack and Street.

TABLE 16-2   Classic FUO in adults

Authors	Years of study	No. of cases	Infections (%)	Neoplasms (%)	Collagen vascular diseases (%)	Miscellaneous (%)	Undiagnosed (%)
Petersdorf and Beeson	1952–57	100	36	19	13	25	7
Jacoby and Swartz	1957–71	128	40	20	15	17	8
Howard et al.	1969–76	100	37	31	19	8	5
Larson et al.	1970–80	105	30	31	16	10	12
Knockaert et al.	1980–89	199	22.5	7	21.5*	26.5*	22.5*

* Authors' raw data retabulated to conform to prior diagnostic categories.

might be sequestered (such as the sinuses of intubated patients, infections of prosthetic devices) or on nosocomial complications such as acalculous cholecystitis, *Clostridium difficile* toxin in the stool (if diarrhea is present), and drug reactions. Blood cultures are mandatory. Appropriate diagnostic maneuvers include ultrasonography and computed tomography (CT) of the abdomen, indium 111–labeled white blood cell or immunoglobulin scans, sinus x-rays, and the cessation of suspect drugs.

Neutropenic FUO   This is defined as fever of ≥38.3°C (101°F) on several occasions in a patient with less than 500 neutrophils per cubic millimeter (or expected to fall below that level within 1 to 2 days). The diagnosis of neutropenic FUO is invoked if a specific cause is not identified after 3 days of investigation, including at least 2 days' incubation of cultures. Neutropenic patients are susceptible to focal bacterial and fungal and bacteremic infections and to infections involving catheters, including septic thrombophlebitis, as well as to perianal infections. *Candida* and *Aspergillus* infections are common. Viral infections due to herpes simplex or CMV are sometimes causes of FUO in this group. While the duration of illness is far shorter in these patients, the consequences of untreated infection may be catastrophic.

HIV-associated FUO   This disorder is defined by fever of ≥38.3°C (101°F) on several occasions over a period of more than 4 weeks for outpatients or more than 3 days' duration in the hospital in a patient with HIV infection. This diagnosis is invoked if 3 days of appropriate investigation, including 2 days' incubation of cultures, reveals no source. In this group of patients, HIV infection alone may be a cause. *Mycobacterium avium intracellulare* (MAI), toxoplasmosis, CMV, tuberculosis, *Pneumocystis carinii*, salmonellosis, cryptococcosis, histoplasmosis, non-Hodgkin's lymphoma, and importantly, drug fever are all possible causes.

Adaptation of these categories of FUO on a wide scale in the literature would allow a more rational compilation of data regarding these disparate groups. In the remainder of this chapter, the discussion will be focused on classic FUO, unless otherwise designated.

CAUSES OF CLASSIC FUO   Table 16-2 summarizes the findings of a number of large studies of FUO since the advent of the antibiotic era. Coincident with the widespread use of antibiotics, increasingly useful diagnostic technologies, both noninvasive and invasive, have been developed. Newer studies reflect not only changing patterns of disease but also the impact of diagnostic techniques that make it possible to eliminate many patients with specific illness from the FUO category. The ubiquitous use of microbiologic cultures and widespread use of potent broad-spectrum antibiotics may have decreased the number of infections causing FUO. The wide availability of ultrasonography, CT, and magnetic resonance imaging (MRI) has enhanced detection of occult neoplasms and lymphomas that previously were thought to be FUO. Likewise, the widespread availability of highly specific and sensitive immunologic testing has reduced the numbers of undetected cases of SLE and other autoimmune diseases. Several generalizations can be however. Infections remain the leading cause of FUO. Tuberculosis, especially extrapulmonary tuberculosis, remains an important cause. Prolonged mononucleosis syndromes with EBV, CMV, or HIV are considerations, sometimes confounded by

delayed antibody responses. Intraabdominal abscesses, sometimes poorly localized, and renal, retroperitoneal, and paraspinous abscesses continue to be difficult to diagnose. Osteomyelitis, especially where prosthetic devices have been implanted, and infective endocarditis must be considered. Although true culture-negative infective endocarditis is rare, one may be misled by slow-growing organisms of the HACEK group (*Haemophilus aphrophilus, Actinobacillus actinomycetemcomitans, Eikenella corrodens, Kingella kingii*) or by fungal, chlamydial, or rickettsial infections. Prostatitis, dental abscesses, sinusitis, and cholangitis continue to be sources of occult fever.

Fungal disease, most notably histoplasmosis involving the reticuloendothelial system, may cause FUO. FUO with headache should prompt examination of spinal fluid for *Cryptococcus neoformans*. Malaria continues to be a cause of FUO, particularly when nonsynchronized. Malaria may result from transfusion, the failure to take prescribed prophylaxis, or drug resistance.

In most early series, neoplasms were the next most common cause of FUO, after infections (Table 16-3). In a series by Knockaert and associates, of 199 patients studied between 1980 and 1989, the percentage of FUO due to malignancy was reduced, a decrease attributed to the improvement in diagnostic technologies. This does not diminish the importance of suspecting neoplasia in the initial diagnostic evaluation of a patient with fever. This series noted a large number of patients with diseases such as temporal arteritis, adult Still's disease, drug-related fever, and factitious fever. In most series, undiagnosed FUOs account for approximately 10 percent of cases. The general category of "collagen vascular diseases" is used somewhat loosely to apply not only to SLE and temporal arteritis but also to systemic rheumatologic or vasculitic diseases such as polymyalgia rheumatica and adult Still's disease.

Many diseases have been grouped in the various studies as "miscellaneous." At the top of this list are the granulomatous diseases, including sarcoidosis, Crohn's disease, and granulomatous hepatitis. Additional diagnoses include drug fever, erythema multiforme, pulmonary embolism, factitious fever, familial Mediterranean fever (FMF), Behçet's syndrome, Fabry's disease, and Whipple's disease (now attributed to a bacillus named *Tropheryma whippelii*).

Drug fever must be considered in anyone with prolonged fever. Any febrile pattern may be seen, and both relative bradycardia and hypotension are uncommon. Eosinophilia and/or rash are seen in only one-fifth of such patients. Fever usually begins 1 to 3 weeks from the start of the drug and remits 2 to 3 days after the drug is stopped. Virtually all classes of drugs cause fever, but antimicrobials (especialy β-lactam antibiotics), cardiovascular drugs (e.g., quinidine), antineo-

TABLE 16-3   Malignancies that commonly cause FUO

Hodgkin's disease
Non-Hodgkin's lymphoma
Leukemia (includes preleukemic and aleukemic phases)
Renal cell carcinoma
Hepatoma

TABLE 16-4 Causes of FUO lasting more than 6 months

	Percent of cases
No cause determined	19
Miscellaneous	13
Factitious	9
Granulomatous hepatitis	8
Neoplasm	7
Still's disease	6
Infection	6
Collagen-vascular disease	4
Familial Mediterranean fever	3
No fever*	27

* No acutal fever observed during 2 to 3 weeks inpatient observation; includes patients with exaggerated circadian rhythm.
SOURCE: From a study of 347 patients referred to the National Institutes of Health from 1961 to 1977 with a presumptive diagnosis of FUO >6 months (Aduan et al).

plastic drugs, and CNS drugs (e.g., phenytoin) are especially common as causes.

It is axiomatic that as the duration of fever increases, the likelihood of an infectious cause decreases (Table 16-4). In a series of 347 patients referred to one of us (S.M.W.) at the National Institutes of Health from 1961 to 1977, only 6 percent had infection. A significant number (9 percent) had *factitious fevers*, due either to false elevations of temperature or self-induced disease. A substantial number of these factitious cases were young women in the health professions. It is worth noting that 8 percent of the patients with prolonged fevers had granulomatous hepatitis, some of whom had completely normal liver function studies, and 6 percent had adult Still's disease. After prolonged investigation, 19 percent had no specific diagnosis. A total of 27 percent either had no actual fever observed during the weeks of inpatient observation or had an exaggerated circadian temperature rhythm without chills, elevated pulse, or other abnormalities. A differential diagnosis for classic FUO in adults is offered in Table 16-5. While this list is restricted to the United States, the frequency of global travel underscores the need for a detailed travel history.

Specialized diagnostic studies in classic FUO Certain specific diagnostic maneuvers become critical in dealing with prolonged fevers. If factitious fever is suspected, numbered thermometers should be used, temperature-taking should be supervised, and simultaneous urine and body temperatures should be measured. Any tissue removed in prior relevant surgery should be reexamined; slides should be requested and, if need be, the "paraffin blocks" of fixed pathologic material should be reexamined and additional special studies performed. Any relevant x-rays should be requested and reexamined; reviewing prior reports may be insufficient. Serum should be set aside in the laboratory as soon as possible and retained for future examination of rising antibody titers. *Febrile agglutinins* is a vague term that normally means, in most laboratories, serologic studies for salmonellosis, brucellosis, and rickettsial diseases. They are seldom useful, of low sensitivity, and variable specificity. Rising titers for *Brucella* are usually diagnostic, but false-positive titers may occur in typhoid fever, tularemia, and yersinial infections. Infection with *B. canis* may be missed with standard antibody tests for *Brucella*. *Salmonella* infection elevates antibody titers to the H and O antigens. High titers of antibody to the O antigen persist for years and may reflect previous infection or immunization. Specific antirickettsial titers should be requested for diagnosing Rocky Mountain spotted fever and Q fever. Multiple blood cultures, no less than three, rarely more than six, should be obtained. These should be cultured in the laboratory for at least 2 weeks to ensure growth of HACEK-group organisms. Lysis-centrifugation blood culture techniques should be employed in cases where prior antimicrobial therapy or fungal or atypical mycobacterial infection is suspected. Blood culture media should be supplemented with L-cysteine or pyridoxal to assist in the isolation of nutritional variant streptococci. It should be noted that sequential cultures positive for multiple organisms may be found when fever is caused by self-injection of contaminated substances. Urine cultures, including

cultures for mycobacteria, fungi, and CMV, are indicated. Liver biopsy, even in the absence of abnormal liver function studies, should be considered and pursued if the diagnosis remains elusive. Specimens should be cultured for mycobacteria and fungus. Likewise, bone marrow biopsy (not simple aspiration) should be performed for histology and culture. The blood smear should be examined for malaria, babesia, trypanosomes, leishmania, and *Borrelia*.

In an FUO workup, an ESR should be obtained. Striking elevation of the ESR and anemia of chronic disease are frequently seen in association with giant cell arteritis or polymyalgia rheumatica, common causes of FUO in patients over 50 years of age. Still's disease is also suggested by elevations of ESR, leukocytosis, and anemia and is often accompanied by arthralgias, polyserositis (pleuritis, pericarditis), lymphadenopathy, splenomegaly, and rash. Antinuclear antibody should be measured to rule out other collagen vascular diseases. Another cause of extremely high ESR may be a "false-positive" ESR, from a "cold agglutinin" with a broad thermal amplitude. The ESR is a nonspecific test that depends on certain serum proteins, most notably fibrinogen, that interfere with the zeta-potential that keeps erythrocytes from clumping. When fibrinogen levels go up, the zeta-potential is inhibited, erythrocytes clump, and the ESR is high. A cold agglutinin, by binding to the erythrocyte, can produce a "false-positive" agglutinin that mimics an acute phase response; cold agglutinins may be seen with *Mycoplasma* and EBV infection and lymphomas.

With rare exceptions, the intermediate-strength purified protein derivative (PPD) skin test should be done for tuberculosis in patients with classic FUO. Concurrent controls should be performed. The CMI test (Connaught Labs, Swiftwater, Pa.) is an especially effective control. It should be kept in mind that a negative PPD skin test in the face of negative controls may be seen with miliary tuberculosis, sarcoidosis, Hodgkin's disease, malnutrition, or AIDS. Noninvasive procedures should include an upper gastrointestinal contrast study with small-bowel follow-through and barium enema to include the terminal ileum and cecum. Chest x-rays should be repeated if new symptoms arise. In some cases it may be necessary to do pulmonary function studies. A diminished carbon monoxide diffusing capacity (DL_{CO}) may be present in restrictive lung diseases such as sarcoidosis, even in the face of a normal chest x-ray. In such cases, transbronchial biopsy may prove diagnostic. It may be advisable to perform flexible colonoscopy, since colon carcinoma is a cause of FUO, and these tumors easily escape detection by ultrasound and CT.

CT scan of the chest and abdomen should be performed. If a spinal or paraspinal lesion is suspected, MRI is preferred. MRI may be superior to CT in demonstrating intraabdominal abscesses and aortic dissection, but the comparative utility of MRI and CT in FUO is unknown. At present, it would appear that the use of abdominal CT should be the routine, unless there is a more specific indication for MRI. Ultrasonography of the abdomen is useful for the investigation of the hepatobiliary tract, kidneys, spleen, and pelvis. An echocardiogram also may be useful for bacterial endocarditis, pericarditis, nonbacterial thrombotic endocarditis, and atrial myxomas. Transesophageal echocardiography is especially sensitive for these lesions.

Radionuclide scanning procedures using technetium (Tc) 99m sulfur colloid, gallium (Ga) citrate, or indium (In) 111–labeled leukocytes or immunoglobulin may be useful in identifying and/or localizing inflammatory processes. Technetium bone scans should be undertaken to look for osteomyelitis or bony metastases; gallium scans may be used to identify sarcoidosis or *P. carinii* in the lungs, or Crohn's disease in the abdomen. ^{111}In-labeled white blood cell scans may be used to locate abscesses. ^{111}In-labeled immunoglobulin scanning also shows promise in this regard. With both gallium and indium WBC scans, false-positive and false-negative findings are common.

Biopsy of the liver and bone marrow should be considered routine in the workup of FUO if the studies mentioned above are unrevealing or if fever is prolonged. It goes without saying that areas of suspected abnormality should be pursued for pathologic examination, where

TABLE 16-5   Diseases causing FUO in adults in the United States

Infections
A Localized pyogenic infections
  Appendicitis
  Cat-scratch disease
  Cholangitis
  Cholecystitis
  Dental abscess
  Diverticulitis/abscess
  Lesser sac abscess
  Liver abscess
  Mesenteric lymphadenitis
  Osteomyelitis
  Pancreatic abscess
  Pelvic inflammatory disease
  Perinephric/intrarenal abscess
  Prostatic abscess
  Sinusitis
  Subphrenic abscess
  Suppurative thrombophlebitis
  Tuboovarian abscess
B Intravascular infections
  Bacterial aortitis
  Bacterial endocarditis
  Vascular catheter infections
C Systemic bacterial infections
  Brucellosis
  Campylobacter
  Gonococcemia
  Legionella
  Leptospirosis
  Listeriosis
  Lyme disease
  Melioidosis
  Meningococcemia
  Rat bite fever
  Relapsing fever
  Salmonellosis
  Syphilis
  Tularemia
  Typhoid
  Vibriosis
  Yersinia
D Mycobacterial infections
  MAI
  Other atypical mycobacteria
  Tuberculosis
E Fungal infections
  Aspergillosis
  Blastomycosis
  Candidiasis
  Coccidioidomycosis
  Cryptococcosis
  Histoplasmosis
  Mucormycosis
  Paracoccidioidomycosis
  Sporotrichosis
F Other bacteria
  Actinomycosis
  Cat-scratch disease
  Nocardiosis
  Whipple's bacillus
G Rickettsial infections
  Cat-scratch disease/bacillary angiomatosis (*Rochalimaea henselae*)
  Ehrlichiosis
  Murine typhus
  Q-fever
  Rickettsialpox
  Rocky Mountain Spotted Fever
H Mycoplasma
I Chlamydial infections
  LGV
  Psittacosis
  TWAR
J Viral infections
  Colorado tick fever
  Coxsackie group B
  CMV
  Dengue
  EBV
  Hepatitis A, B, C, D, and E
  HIV
  LCM
  Parvovirus B-19

K Parasitic
  Amebiasis
  Babesia
  Chagas' disease
  Leishmaniasis
  Malaria
  Pneumocystis carinii
  Strongyloides
  Toxoplasmosis
  Toxocariasis
  Trichinosis
L Presumed infections, agent undetermined
  Kawasaki's disease (mucocutaneous lymph node syndrome)
  Kikuchi's disease (necrotizing lymphadenitis)
Neoplasms
A Malignant
  Colon
  Hodgkin's lymphoma
  Immunoblastic lymphadenopathy
  Kidney
  Leukemia
  Liver
  Lymphomatoid granulomatosis
  Malignant histiocytosis
  Non-Hodgkin's lymphoma
  Pancreas
  Sarcoma
B Benign
  Atrial myxoma
  Renal angiomyolipoma
Collagen vascular diseases/hypersensitivity diseases
Adult Still's disease
Behçet's disease
Erythema multiforme
Erythema nodosum
Giant cell arteritis/polymyalgia rheumatica
Hypersensitivity pneumonitis (e.g., "metal fume fever," "farmer's lung," "air-conditioner lung")
Hypersensitivity vasculitis
Mixed connective tissue disease
Polyarteritis nodosa
Relapsing polychondritis
Rheumatic fever
Rheumatoid arthritis
Systemic lupus erythematosus
Takayasu's aortitis
Weber-Christian disease
Wegener's granulomatosis
Granulomatous diseases
Crohn's disease
Idiopathic granulomatous hepatitis
Midline granuloma
Sarcoidosis
Miscellaneous diseases
Aortic dissection
Drug fever
Gout
Hematomas
Hemolytic diseases/hemoglobinopathies
Laennec's cirrhosis
Postmyocardial infarction syndrome
Recurrent pulmonary emboli
Subacute thyroiditis (deQuervain's)
Tissue infarction/necrosis
Inherited and metabolic diseases
Adrenal insufficiency
Cyclic neutropenia
Deafness, urticaria and amyloid
Fabry's disease
Familial Mediterranean fever
Hyperimmunoglobulinemia D and periodic fever
Type V hypertriglyceridemia
Thermoregulatory disorders
A Central
  Brain tumor
  Cerebrovascular accident
  Encephalitis
  Hypothalamic dysfunction
B Peripheral
  Hyperthyroidism
  Pheochromocytoma
Factitious fevers
"Afebrile" FUO (<38.3°C)
Habitual hyperthermia (exaggerated circadian rhythm)

SOURCE: After RK Root, RG Petersdorf, in JD Wilson et al (eds): *Harrison's Principles of Internal Medicine*, 12th ed. New York, McGraw-Hill, 1991.

practical. Where possible, a section of the tissue block should always be retained for further sections or stains. The polymerase chain reaction (PCR) technology makes it possible to identify and speciate mycobacterial DNA in paraffin-embedded, fixed tissues. Thus, in some cases, it is possible to diagnose long-fixed pathologic tissues retrospectively. In a patient over age 50 (occasionally younger) with the appropriate symptoms and laboratory findings, "blind biopsy" of one or both temporal arteries may yield a diagnosis of arteritis. If present, tenderness or decreased pulsation should guide the location of the biopsy. Lymph node biopsy may be helpful if nodes are enlarged, but inguinal nodes are often palpable and seldom diagnostically useful.

Exploratory laparotomy has been performed when all other diagnostic procedures failed, but modern imaging and guided-biopsy techniques have largely replaced laparotomy.

THERAPEUTIC APPROACH TO THE FEBRILE PATIENT The advantages and disadvantages of antipyretic therapy have been discussed earlier in this chapter. More specific therapy is directed on the basis of the differential diagnosis for a given patient, the relative probabilities of these diagnoses, the risks of not treating, and the risks of treatment itself.

Sepsis is defined as evidence of infection with a systemic response. *Sepsis syndrome* refers to a systemic response sufficient to produce organ dysfunction, and *septic shock* is the sepsis syndrome with documented hypotension. In a nonimmunocompromised adult with sepsis, gram-positive infection, gram-negative rod infection, and meningococcal infection can be "covered" by a variety of antibiotic combinations, including imipenem, ticarcillin/clavulanate, or a third-generation cephalosporin. Suspicion of a methicillin-resistant *Staphylococcus aureus* would dictate the addition of vancomycin. If the patient has had a splenectomy, then ampicillin/sulbactam, ceftriaxone, cefotaxime, or cefuroxime would be indicated. Suspicion of *Legionella* would dictate the addition of erythromycin (possibly with rifampin) or, alternatively, clarithromycin or azithromycin. In appropriate settings, rickettsia should be suspected, and either doxycycline or chloramphenicol would be indicated. If septic shock is present without an evident source, the differential diagnosis should include meningococcemia, staphylococcal and streptococcal toxic shock syndromes and, rarely, gram-negative bacteremia. A combination of high-dose penicillin and penicillinase-resistant synthetic penicillins (nafcillin, oxacillin) would "cover" these cocci; a third-generation cephalosporin would treat the gram-negative bacteremia. If a typhoidal syndrome is suspected, then a fluoroquinolone such as ciprofloxacin or ofloxacin would be indicated. Intravenous penicillin should be used if leptospirosis is suspected. Suspected endocarditis should be treated with either penicillin, oxacillin/nafcillin, or vancomycin, plus gentamicin, depending on the type of patient and the suspected origin of infection. In IV drug users, methicillin-sensitive or -resistant *S. aureus* and gram-negative bacilli also would be considerations.

Patients with neutropenic FUO may be treated by a variety of empirical protocols, which usually combine an aminoglycoside plus antipseudomonal β-lactam antibiotic or, alternatively, imipenem or ceftazidime alone. Vancomycin should be added if intravenous catheter-associated infection is suspected. If vancomycin is included and fever continues, the addition of amphotericin B should be considered.

Empirical therapy for nosocomial FUO must be guided by the clinical situation. While empirical antibiotic therapy might be indicated, it should be remembered that complications of drug therapy, including *C. difficile* colitis and drug fever, may be causes.

The treatment of HIV-associated FUO depends on many factors and is discussed in Chap. 279. MAI, CMV, drug fever, and HIV itself are probably the most common causes of FUO, after *P. carinii*, cryptococcosis, toxoplasmosis, tuberculosis, and bacterial sinusitis have been ruled out. Discontinuing or changing drugs is often necessary, and empirical therapy for these infections may be indicated.

The emphasis in patients with classic FUO is on continued observation and examination, with the avoidance of "shotgun" empirical therapy. Empirical therapy for endocarditis, for example, should be avoided unless there are specific reasons to invoke this diagnosis beyond fever. Every patient with FUO should have an exhaustive examination to prove, or disprove, tuberculosis. If the PPD skin test is positive, or if granulomatous hepatitis or other granulomatous disease is present with anergy (and sarcoid seems unlikely), then a therapeutic trial with isoniazid and rifampin (or possibly three drugs) should be undertaken, usually for up to 6 weeks. A failure of the fever to respond over this period should suggest an alternative diagnosis.

A dramatic response to aspirin and NSAIDs may be seen with rheumatic fever and Still's disease. The effect of glucocorticoids on temporal arteritis, polymyalgia rheumatica, and granulomatous hepatitis are equally dramatic. Colchicine is highly effective in preventing attacks of FMF but is of little use once an attack is well under way. The ability of glucocorticoids and NSAIDs to mask fever while permitting the spread of infection dictates that their use be avoided unless infection has been largely ruled out and unless inflammatory disease is both probable and debilitating or threatening.

When no underlying source is identified after prolonged observation (>6 months), the prognosis is generally good, however vexing to the patient. Under such circumstances, debilitating symptoms are treated with NSAIDs, and glucocorticoids are the last resort. It is axiomatic that the initiation of empirical therapy does not dictate the end of the diagnostic workup; rather, it commits the physician to continued thoughtful reexamination and evaluation. Patience, compassion, equanimity, and intellectual flexibility are indispensable attributes for the successful clinician dealing with FUO.

REFERENCES

Fever: pathophysiology

ATKINS E: Fever: Historical aspects, in *Interleukin-1, Inflammation, and Disease*, Bomford R, Henderson B (eds). New York, Elsevier Science Publishers, 1989, pp 3–15

CANNON JG et al: Circulating interleukin-1 and tumor necrosis factor in septic shock and experimental endotoxin fever. J Infect Dis 161:79, 1990

DINARELLO CA: Interleukin-1 and interleukin-1 antagonism. Blood 77: 1627, 1991

——, WOLFF SM: Pathogenesis of fever, in *Principles and Practice of Infectious Diseases,* 3d ed, GL Mandell et al (eds). New York, Wiley, 1990, pp 462–467

—— et al: New concepts on the pathogenesis of fever. Rev Infect Dis 10:168, 1988

MACKOWIAK PA et al: A critical appraisal of 98.6°F, the upper limit of the normal body temperature, and other legacies of Carl Reinhold August Wunderlich. JAMA 268:1578, 1992

MILUNSKY A et al: Maternal heat exposure and neural tube defects. JAMA 268:882, 1992

Fever of unknown origin

ADUAN R et al: Prolonged fever of unknown origin. Clin Res 26:558A, 1978

—— et al: Factitious fever and self-induced infection. Ann Intern Med 90:230, 1979

DATA FL, THORNE DA: Gastrointestinal tract radionuclide activity on In-111 labeled leukocyte imaging: Clinical significance in patients with fever of unknown origin. Radiology 160:635, 1986

DINARELLO CA, WOLFF SM: Fever of unknown origin, in *Principles and Practice of Infectious Diseases,* 3d ed, GL Mandell et al (eds). New York, Wiley, 1990, pp. 468–479

DURACK DT, STREET AC: Fever of unknown origin—reexamined and redefined, in *Current Clinical Topics in Infectious Diseases,* JS Remington, MN Swartz (eds). Cambridge, MA, Blackwell, 1991

GRANOWITZ EV et al: Interleukin-1 receptor antagonist production during experimental endotoxaemia. Lancet 338:1423, 1991

HOWARD P JR et al: Fever of unknown origin: A prospective study of 100 patients. Tex Med 73:56, 1977

HUGHES WT et al: Guidelines for the use of antimicrobial agents in neutropenic patients with unexplained fever. J Infect Dis 161:381, 1990

ISAAC B et al (eds): *Unexplained Fever.* Boca Raton, CRC Press, 1991

JACOBY GA, SWARTZ MN: Fever of undetermined origin. N Engl J Med 289:1407, 1973

KNOCKAERT DC, VANNESTE LJ: Fever of unknown origin in the 1980s. Arch Intern Med 152:51, 1992

LARSON EB, FEATHERSTONE HJ: Fever of undetermined origin: Diagnosis and follow-up of 105 cases, 1970–80. Medicine 61:269, 1982

MEYERS SP, WIENER SN: Diagnosis of hematogenous pyogenic vertebral osteomyelitis by magnetic resonance imaging. Arch Intern Med 151:683, 1991

PETERSDORF RG, BEESON PB: Fever of unexplained origin. Medicine 40:1, 1961

ROSENBERG MR, GREEN M: Neuroleptic malignant syndrome. Arch Intern Med 149:1927, 1989

ROWLAND MD, DEL BENE VE: Use of body computed tomography to evaluate fever of unknown origin. J Infect Dis 156:408, 1987

RUBIN RH et al: ¹¹¹In-labeled nonspecific immunoglobulin scanning in the detection of focal infection. N Engl J Med 321:935, 1989

SABBOOR SA et al: Detection of mycobacterial DNA in sarcoidosis and tuberculosis with polymerase chain reaction. Lancet 339:1012, 1992

SCHMIDT KG et al: Indium-111 granulocyte scintigraphy in the evaluation of patients with fever of undetermined origin. Scand J Infect Dis 19:339, 1987

SIMON HB, WOLFF SM: Granulomatous hepatitis and prolonged fever of unknown origin: A study of 13 patients. Medicine 52:1, 1973

SMITH JW: Southwestern internal medicine conference: Fever of undetermined origin: Not what it used to be. Am J Med Sci 292:56, 1986

WEINSTEIN L: Clinically benign fever of unknown origin: A personal retrospective. Rev Infect Dis 7:692, 1985

WILSON ME: A World Guide to Infections: Diseases, Distribution, Diagnosis. New York, Oxford University Press, 1991

WOLFF SM et al: A syndrome of periodic hypothalamic discharge. Am J Med 36:956, 1964

——— et al: Unusual etiologies of fever and their evaluation. Annu Rev Med 26:277, 1975

section 3　Nervous system dysfunction

17　FAINTNESS, SYNCOPE, AND SEIZURES

JOSEPH B. MARTIN / JEREMY RUSKIN[1]

Episodic faintness, light-headedness, and reduced alertness are frequently difficult to distinguish, tending to shade into one another. The difference between faintness and frank syncope is often only quantitative. Types of episodic weakness, such as myasthenia gravis, cataplexy, and familial periodic paralysis, which cause striking reduction of muscular strength but no impairment of consciousness, should be set apart (see Chaps. 386 and 387). Seizures, an important cause of altered consciousness, usually differ from syncope, but in some instances distinguishing the two may be difficult. The features that distinguish seizures from syncope are discussed at the end of this chapter and in Chap. 367.

SYNCOPE AND FAINTNESS

Syncope comprises a generalized weakness of muscles, with loss of postural tone, inability to stand upright, and a loss of consciousness. The term *faintness*, in contrast, refers to lack of strength, with sensation of impending loss of consciousness (*presyncope*). At the beginning of a syncopal attack the patient is nearly always in the upright position, either sitting or standing [the Stokes-Adams attack (see Chap. 197) is exceptional in this respect]. Usually the patient is warned of the impending faint by a sense of "feeling bad." A sense of giddiness and movement or swaying of the floor or surrounding objects ensues. The senses become confused; the patient yawns or gapes, there are spots before the eyes, vision may dim, and the ears may ring. Nausea and sometimes vomiting accompany these symptoms. There is a striking pallor or ashen gray color of the face, and very often the face and body are bathed in cold perspiration. In some patients, a deliberate onset may allow time for protection against injury; in others, the occurrence of syncope is sudden and without warning.

The depth and duration of unconsciousness vary. Sometimes the patient is not completely oblivious of the surroundings, or there may be profound coma with complete lack of awareness and of capacity to respond. The patient may remain in this state for seconds to minutes or even as long as half an hour. Usually the patient lies motionless with skeletal muscles relaxed, but a few clonic jerks of the limbs and face may occur shortly after the beginning of the unconsciousness. In some situations there may be a brief tonic-clonic seizure. Sphincter control is usually maintained. The pulse is feeble or cannot be felt, the blood pressure may be low to undetectable, and breathing may be almost imperceptible. Once the patient is in a horizontal position, gravitation no longer hinders the flow of blood to the brain. The strength of the pulse may then improve, color begins to return to the face, breathing becomes quicker and deeper, and consciousness is regained. There is usually an immediate recovery of consciousness. Some patients may, however, be keenly aware of physical weakness, and rising too soon may precipitate another faint. In other patients, particularly those with transient tachyarrhythmias, there may be no residual symptoms following the initial syncope. Headache and drowsiness, which, with mental confusion, are the usual sequelae of a convulsion, do not follow a syncopal attack.

ETIOLOGY　The list of causes in Table 17-1 is based on established or assumed physiologic mechanisms. The more common types of faint are reducible to a few simple mechanisms. Syncope results from a sudden impairment of brain metabolism usually brought about by hypotension with reduction of cerebral blood flow.

Several mechanisms subserve circulatory adjustments to the upright posture. Approximately three-fourths of the systemic blood volume is contained in the venous bed, and any interference with venous return may lead to a reduction in cardiac output. Cerebral blood flow may still be maintained, as long as systemic arterial vasoconstriction occurs, but when this adjustment fails, serious hypotension with resultant cerebral underperfusion to less than half normal results in syncope. Normally, the pooling of blood in the lower parts of the body is prevented by (1) pressor reflexes which induce constriction of peripheral arterioles and venules, (2) reflex acceleration of the heart by means of aortic and carotid reflexes, and (3) improvement of venous return to the heart by activity of the muscles of the limbs. Placing a normal person on a tilt table to relax the muscles and tilting upright slightly diminish cardiac output and allow the blood to accumulate in the legs to a slight degree. This may then be followed by a slight transitory fall in systolic arterial pressure and, in patients with defective vasomotor reflexes, may be a means of producing faints.

TYPES OF SYNCOPE　**Vasodepressor (vasovagal) or neurocardiogenic syncope**　This form of syncope is the common faint that may be experienced by normal persons. It is frequently recurrent and commonly precipitated by emotional stress (especially in a warm, crowded room), fear, extreme fatigue, injury, or pain. Many episodes, however, occur without obvious antecedent cause. In its classic form, vasodepressor neurocardiogenic syncope comprises a constellation of symptoms including hypotension, bradycardia, nausea, pallor, and diaphoresis. Syncope typically occurs in the setting of diminished venous return which leads to reduced stroke volume and a reflex increase in sympathetic activity. In susceptible individuals, this increase in sympathetic activity causes cardiac hypercontractility and excessive stimulation of ventricular mechanoreceptors (afferent vagal C fibers), which, in turn, leads to sympathetic withdrawal and activation of the parasympathetic nervous system via a centrally mediated vasomotor reflex. The net result is a vicious cycle of inappropriate peripheral vasodilatation and relative bradycardia leading to progressive hypotension and syncope which can be reversed by assumption of supine posture and elevation of the legs. Orthostatic

---

[1] Raymond D. Adams was senior author of this chapter in an earlier edition.

TABLE 17-1 Causes of recurrent weakness, faintness, and disturbances of consciousness

I **Circulatory (reduced cerebral blood flow)**
  A Inadequate vasoconstrictor mechanisms
    1 Vasovagal (vasodepressor)
    2 Postural hypotension
    3 Primary autonomic insufficiency
    4 Sympathectomy (pharmacologic, due to antihypertensive medications such as methyldopa and hydralazine, or surgical)
    5 Diseases of central and peripheral nervous systems, including autonomic nerves (Chaps. 379 and 383)
    6 Carotid sinus syncope (see also ''Bradyarrhythmias,'' below)
    7 Hyperbradykininemia
  B Hypovolemia
    1 Blood loss—gastrointestinal hemorrhage
    2 Addison's disease
  C Mechanical reduction of venous return
    1 Valsalva maneuver
    2 Cough
    3 Micturition
    4 Atrial myxoma, ball valve thrombus
  D Reduced cardiac output
    1 Obstruction to left ventricular outflow: aortic stenosis, hypertrophic subaortic stenosis
    2 Obstruction to pulmonary flow: pulmonic stenosis, primary pulmonary hypertension, pulmonary embolism
    3 Myocardial: massive myocardial infarction with pump failure
    4 Pericardial: cardiac tamponade
  E Arrhythmias (Chaps. 197 and 198)
    1 Bradyarrhythmias
      a Atrioventricular (AV) block (second- and third-degree), with Stokes-Adams attacks
      b Ventricular asystole
      c Sinus bradycardia, sinoatrial block, sinus arrest, sick-sinus syndrome
      d Carotid sinus syncope (see also inadequate vasoconstrictor mechanisms, above)
      e Glossopharyngeal neuralgia (and other painful states)
    2 Tachyarrhythmias
      a Episodic ventricular tachycardia with or without associated bradyarrhythmias
      b Supraventricular tachycardia without AV block
II **Other causes of weakness and episodic disturbances of consciousness**
  A Altered state of blood to the brain
    1 Hypoxia
    2 Anemia
    3 Diminished carbon dioxide due to hyperventilation (faintness common, syncope seldom occurs)
    4 Hypoglycemia (episodic weakness common, faintness occasional, syncope rare)
  B Cerebral
    1 Cerebrovascular disturbances (cerebral ischemic attacks, see Chap. 368)
      a Extracranial vascular insufficiency (vertebral-basilar, carotid)
      b Diffuse spasm of cerebral arterioles (hypertensive encephalopathy)
    2 Emotional disturbances, anxiety attacks, and hysterical seizures

stress induced by prolonged upright tilt testing at 60 to 80° is a sensitive technique for reproducing syncope in many patients with this syndrome. The use of low-dose isoproterenol infusion enhances the sensitivity of upright tilt testing but may lead to false-positive tests when used in high doses. Because of the critical role of beta-adrenergic stimulation and hypercontractility in this syndrome, effective prophylaxis can usually be achieved with the use of beta-adrenergic receptor blocking agents or disopyramide. Since neurocardiogenic syncope usually occurs in patients with normal left ventricular systolic function, the use of these agents is usually well tolerated. Other pharmacologic agents which have been used to treat neurocardiogenic syncope include theophylline, scopolamine, and ephedrine. Cardiac pacing alone is rarely indicated or effective in the prevention of neurocardiogenic syncope. However, this modality may be necessary in a small minority of patients in whom profound bradycardia or asystole predominates over peripheral vasodilatation as the primary mechanism of syncope.

Postural hypotension with syncope This type of syncope affects persons who have a chronic defect in, or variable instability of, vasomotor reflexes. The fall in blood pressure on assumption of upright posture is due to a loss of vasoconstriction reflexes in resistance and capacitance vessels of the lower extremities. Though the character of the syncopal attack differs little from that of the vasovagal or vasodepressor type, the effect of posture is its cardinal feature; sudden arising from a recumbent position or standing still are precipitating circumstances.

Postural syncope tends to occur under the following conditions:

1 In otherwise normal persons who for some unknown reason have defective postural reflexes (this may be familial). In such individuals, fainting may occur when they are tilted on a table. Under such circumstances it has been found that the blood pressure at first diminishes slightly and then stabilizes at a lower level. Shortly thereafter, the compensatory reflexes suddenly fail and the arterial pressure falls precipitously.

2 In *primary autonomic insufficiency* and in the *dysautonomias*. At least three syndromes have been delineated:

ACUTE OR SUBACUTE DYSAUTONOMIA In this disease an otherwise healthy adult or child develops over a period of a few days or weeks a partial or complete paralysis of the parasympathetic and sympathetic nervous systems. Pupillary reflexes are lost, as are lacrimation, salivation, and sweating, and there is impotence, paresis of bladder and bowel musculature, and orthostatic hypotension. The CSF protein is increased. Sensory and motor nerve fibers are demonstrably intact, but nonmedullated autonomic ones have degenerated. Recovery occurs within a few months, possibly hastened by prednisone therapy. The disease is believed to represent a variant of acute idiopathic polyneuritis, akin to Guillain-Barré syndrome.

CHRONIC POSTGANGLIONIC AUTONOMIC INSUFFICIENCY This is a disease of middle-aged and elderly individuals who gradually develop chronic orthostatic hypotension, sometimes in conjunction with impotence and sphincter disturbances. Upon standing for 5 to 10 min, the blood pressure decreases at least 35 mmHg and the pulse pressure narrows, both without increase in pulse rate, pallor, or nausea. Men are more often affected than women. The condition is relatively benign and seemingly irreversible.

CHRONIC PREGANGLIONIC AUTONOMIC INSUFFICIENCY In this condition, orthostatic hypotension with variable anhidrosis, impotence, and sphincter disturbances is combined with a disorder of the central nervous system. The disorders include (1) tremor, extrapyramidal rigidity, and akinesia (Shy-Drager syndrome), (2) progressive cerebellar degeneration, some instances of which are familial, and (3) a more variable extrapyramidal and cerebellar disorder (striatonigral degeneration). These syndromes lead to disability and often death within a few years (see Chaps. 371 and 379.)

The differentiation of the chronic peripheral postganglionic and central preganglionic insufficiency is based on pathologic and pharmacologic evidence. In the postganglionic type, neurons of the sympathetic ganglia degenerate, whereas in the central type, the lateral horn cells of the thoracic spinal cord degenerate. In the postganglionic peripheral type, the resting levels of norepinephrine are subnormal because of failure to release norepinephrine from postganglionic endings, and there is hypersensitivity to injected norepinephrine. In the central type, resting levels of norepinephrine are normal. On standing, unlike the reaction in the normal individual, there is little, if any, rise in norepinephrine levels in either type. And in both types, the levels of plasma dopamine β-hydroxylase (the enzyme that converts dopamine to norepinephrine) are subnormal.

The distinction between the various types of orthostatic hypotension has therapeutic significance. In the peripheral postganglionic type, the most effective treatment is 9α-fluorohydrocortisone (oral dose 0.1 to 0.2 mg/d) and salt loading to increase blood volume, supplemented by mechanical devices to prevent pooling of blood in the legs and lower trunk (g suit). However, salt together with mineralocorticoids may induce serious supine hypertension, and the dose of the drug must be adjusted for this. For the central preganglionic type, there has been greater success with use of a sympathomimetic amine such as tyramine (which releases norepinephrine from intact postganglionic endings) supplemented by a monoamine oxidase inhibitor (to prevent destruction of the amine) and possibly propranolol. Levodopa has been effective in some cases. In the postganglionic type, judicious use of phenylephrine or ephedrine may be beneficial. Initial reports of the effectiveness of indomethacin in chronic orthostatic hypotension have not been substantiated.

OTHER CAUSES OF POSTURAL SYNCOPE   (1) After physical deconditioning, e.g., after prolonged illness with recumbency, especially in elderly individuals with reduced muscle tone. (2) After a sympathectomy that has abolished vasopressor reflexes. (3) In diabetic, alcoholic, and other neuropathies; syringomyelia; and diseases of the nervous system which cause muscular atrophy and paralysis of vasopressor reflexes. The most common form of neurogenic orthostatic hypotension is that which accompanies diseases of the peripheral nervous system. Diabetic polyneuropathy, beriberi, amyloid polyneuropathy, and the Adie syndrome are examples. Usually the orthostatic hypotension is associated with disturbances in sweating, impotence, and sphincter difficulties. Presumably the lesion involves postganglionic, nonmedullated fibers in peripheral nerves. (4) In patients receiving antihypertensive and vasodilator drugs as well as those who may be hypovolemic because of diuretics, excessive sweating, or adrenal insufficiency.

Micturition syncope, a condition usually seen in the elderly during or after urination, particularly after arising from the recumbent position, is probably a special type of vasodepressor syncope. It has been suggested that release of intravesicular pressure causes sudden vasodilatation, augmented by standing, and that vagally mediated bradycardia is a contributory factor.

Hyperbradykininemia   Deficient kinin-inactivating enzymes with apparently normal sympathetic function may result in symptoms of faintness or syncope on assumption of upright posture. Hyperbradykininemia causes arteriolar and venular dilatation, giving rise to postural hypotension and syncope with tachycardia. The pathophysiology of this condition remains uncertain. Treatment with beta-receptor antagonists has been beneficial.

Syncope of cardiac origin (cardiac syncope)   Cardiac syncope results from a sudden reduction in cardiac output, caused most commonly by a cardiac arrhythmia. In normal individuals, slow ventricular rates, but above 35 to 40 beats per minute, and fast ones not exceeding 180 beats per minute do not reduce cerebral blood flow, especially if the person is in the supine position. However, changes in pulse rate outside these limits may impair cerebral circulation and function. Upright posture, cerebrovascular disease, anemia, and coronary, myocardial, or valvular disease all reduce the tolerance to alterations in rate.

High-degree atrioventricular block is one of the most common arrhythmias that leads to fainting, and syncopal episodes associated with this arrhythmia are known as the *Stokes-Adams-Morgagni syndrome*. The etiology of disturbances in atrioventricular conduction is considered elsewhere (Chap. 197), but in patients with these attacks the block may be persistent or intermittent and is often preceded or followed by disturbed conduction in one or more of the three fascicles through which the ventricles are normally activated. When the block is high-grade or complete and the pacemaker below the block fails to function, syncope occurs. Stokes-Adams attacks occur usually without more than a momentary sense of weakness, the patient suddenly losing consciousness. After cardiac standstill of more than several seconds, the patient turns pale, falls unconscious, and, as in other types of fainting, may exhibit a few clonic jerks. With longer periods of asystole, the ashen gray pallor gives way to cyanosis, stertorous breathing, fixed pupils, incontinence, and bilateral Babinski signs. While recovery following a Stokes-Adams attack is usually prompt and complete, prolonged confusion and neurologic signs due to cerebral ischemia may occur in some patients, and permanent impairment of mental function may occasionally result, although focal neurologic signs are rare. Cardiac faints of this type may recur several times a day. Commonly the heart block is transitory, and the ECG taken later may not show any arrhythmia. In some patients, ventricular tachycardia or fibrillation may follow a period of asystole, resulting in syncope or sudden death.

Disorders of sinus node automaticity or sinoatrial conduction also may result in asystole or bradycardia of sufficient severity to cause presyncope or syncope. This disorder is most frequently detected with ambulatory ECG monitoring. Findings consistent with a diagnosis of sinus node dysfunction include symptomatic sinus pauses (>3 s) resulting from sinus arrest or sinoatrial block and severe unexplained sinus bradycardia (<40 beats per minute). The *bradycardia-tachycardia syndrome* is a common form of sinus node dysfunction in which syncope generally occurs as a result of marked sinus pauses following termination of paroxysmal supraventricular tachycardia. In occasional patients with syncope and suspected sinus node dysfunction in whom the diagnosis is not established by ambulatory ECG recording, electrophysiologic testing may be helpful in unmasking diagnostic abnormalities.

Recurrent paroxysmal tachyarrhythmias also may cause presyncope and syncope as a result of a sudden reduction in cardiac output. The magnitude of tachycardia-induced hypotension is dependent on the interaction of several variables, including the rate and mechanism of the tachycardia, the type and severity of underlying cardiac disease, the patient's posture and activity level at the onset of the tachycardia, the sensitivity of the tachycardia to catecholamines, and the integrity of compensatory autonomic reflexes. Supraventricular tachyarrhythmias are not commonly associated with syncope. However, even in the absence of structural heart disease, the combination of extremely high heart rates and loss of atrial transport may impair cardiac filling and output sufficiently to cause loss of consciousness. These tachycardias result most commonly from the occurrence of paroxysmal atrial flutter, atrial fibrillation, or reentry involving the atrioventricular node or accessory pathways which bypass part or all of the atrioventricular conduction system. Patients with the Wolff-Parkinson-White syndrome are susceptible to several forms of supraventricular tachycardia, the most dangerous of which is atrial fibrillation with rapid antegrade conduction to the ventricles over an accessory atrioventricular connection which may result in syncope and, in rare instances, sudden death. When supraventricular tachycardia is suspected as a cause of syncope, electrophysiologic testing is indicated to define the mechanism and pathway of the tachycardia and to facilitate the selection of an effective antiarrhythmic intervention (see also Chap. 197).

Paroxysmal ventricular tachycardia is a relatively common cause of syncope, particularly in patients with structural heart disease. Typically, the tachycardias are rapid and associated with abrupt loss of consciousness without premonitory symptoms. More often than not the patient is unaware of palpitations, and recovery following an episode is usually prompt and complete without residual neurologic or cardiac sequelae. The occurrence of unexplained syncope in a patient with structural heart disease is a potentially ominous finding and merits careful evaluation. The presence of pathologic Q waves on the ECG indicative of a prior transmural myocardial infarction is strongly associated with ventricular tachycardia as a cause of syncope in patients with ischemic heart disease. Other forms of heart disease such as hypertrophic and dilated cardiomyopathy, right ventricular dysplasia, and the long-QT-interval syndromes are also frequently associated with paroxysmal ventricular tachycardia and syncope.

In another form of cardiac syncope, the heart block is reflexive and is due to irritation of the vagus nerves. Examples of this phenomenon have been observed in patients with esophageal diverticula, mediastinal tumors, gallbladder disease, carotid sinus disease, glossopharyngeal neuralgia, and pleural and pulmonary irritation. However, in these conditions, reflex bradycardia is more commonly of the sinoatrial than the atrioventricular type.

Cardiac syncope also may result from *acute massive myocardial infarction*, particularly when associated with cardiogenic shock. *Aortic stenosis* often sets the stage for exertional syncope, most commonly by limiting cardiac output in the face of peripheral vasodilatation, with resultant myocardial and cerebral ischemia and occasionally arrhythmias. *Idiopathic hypertrophic subaortic stenosis* also may lead to exertional syncope because of intensified obstruction and/or ventricular arrhythmias (Chap. 205). In *primary pulmonary hypertension*, a relatively fixed cardiac output and bouts of acute right ventricular failure may be associated with syncope (Chap. 204). However, vagal reflexes may be involved in this condition as well as in the syncope that occurs with *pulmonary embolism*. Ball-valve thrombus in the left atrium, left atrial myxoma, or thrombosis or malfunction of a prosthetic valve may produce sudden mechanical obstruction of the circulation and syncope. *Tetralogy of Fallot* is the congenital cardiac malformation most commonly responsible for syncope. In this condition, systemic vasodilatation, perhaps associated with infundibular spasm, greatly increases the right-to-left shunt and produces arterial hypoxia, which leads to syncope (Chap. 199).

Carotid sinus syncope The carotid sinus is normally sensitive to stretch and gives rise to sensory impulses carried via the nerve of Hering, a branch of the glossopharyngeal nerve, to the medulla oblongata. Massage of one or both of the carotid sinuses, particularly in elderly persons, causes (1) a reflex cardiac slowing (sinus bradycardia, sinus arrest, or even atrioventricular block), the so-called vagal type of response, and (2) a fall of arterial pressure without cardiac slowing, the so-called depressor type of response. Both types of carotid sinus response may coexist.

Syncope due to carotid sinus sensitivity may be initiated by turning of the head to one side, by a tight collar, or, as in a few reported cases, by shaving over the region of the sinus. Spontaneous attacks also may occur. The attack nearly always begins when the patient is in an upright position, usually when standing. The period of unconsciousness seldom lasts longer than a few minutes. Full consciousness is regained immediately. Most reported cases have been in men. In a patient displaying faintness on compression of one carotid sinus, it is important to distinguish between the benign disorder (hypersensitivity of one carotid sinus) and a much more serious condition—atheromatous narrowing of the opposite carotid or of the basilar artery (see Chap. 368).

Other forms of vasovagal syncope have been described. Exceptionally intense pain of visceral origin may inhibit cardiac action through vagal stimulation, e.g., cardiac standstill during an attack of gallbladder colic, a lesion of the esophagus or mediastinum, bronchoscopy, pleural or peritoneal taps, intense vertigo from labyrinthine or vestibular disease, and needling of body cavities. Occasionally, a patient with a severe migraine attack will sustain a syncopal episode.

Vagal and glossopharyngeal neuralgia Occasionally this induces a reflex type of fainting. Again, the sequence is always pain, then syncope; in this instance the pain is localized to the base of the tongue, pharynx or larynx, tonsillar area, and ear. It may be triggered by pressure at these sites. Section of the appropriate branches of the ninth or tenth cranial nerve relieves the condition. The cardiovascular effects are attributable to excitation of the dorsal motor nucleus of the vagus via collateral fibers from the nucleus of the tractus solitarius.

Tussive syncope (laryngeal vertigo) This is a rare condition that results from a paroxysm of coughing, usually in men with chronic bronchitis. After hard coughing the patient suddenly becomes weak and loses consciousness momentarily. The intrathoracic pressure becomes elevated and interferes with the venous return to the heart, as does the Valsalva maneuver (exhaling against a closed glottis).

Syncope associated with cerebrovascular disease This is usually caused by partial or complete occlusion of the large arteries in the neck. Physical activity may then critically reduce blood flow to the upper part of the brainstem, causing abrupt loss of consciousness (see Chap. 368).

PATHOPHYSIOLOGY OF SYNCOPE The loss of consciousness in each type of syncope is caused by reduction of oxygenation to those parts of the brain which subserve consciousness. There are demonstrable reductions in cerebral blood flow, cerebral oxygen utilization, and cerebrovascular resistance. If the ischemia lasts only a few minutes, there are no lasting effects on the brain. Prolonged ischemia may result in necrosis of brain tissue in the border zones of perfusion between the vascular territories of the major cerebral arteries.

In a patient with faintness or syncope attended by bradycardia, one has to distinguish that due to failure of neurogenic reflexes from that due to a cardiogenic (Stokes-Adams) attack. The ECG is decisive, but even without it, the Stokes-Adams attacks can be recognized clinically by their longer duration, by the greater constancy of the slow heart rate, by the presence of audible sounds synchronous with atrial contractions, by atrial contraction (A) waves in the jugular venous pulse, and by marked variation in intensity of the first sound despite the regular rhythm (Chap. 197).

DIFFERENTIAL DIAGNOSIS OF CONDITIONS INVOLVING EPISODIC WEAKNESS AND FAINTNESS BUT NOT SYNCOPE **Anxiety attacks and the hyperventilation syndrome** These symptoms are discussed in Chap. 389. The giddiness of anxiety is frequently interpreted as a feeling of faintness without actual loss of consciousness. Such symptoms are not accompanied by facial pallor and are not relieved by recumbency. The diagnosis is made on the basis of the associated symptoms, and part of the attack can be reproduced by hyperventilation. Two of the mechanisms known to be involved in the attacks are reduction in carbon dioxide as a result of hyperventilation and the release of epinephrine. Hyperventilation results in hypocapnia, alkalosis, increased cerebrovascular resistance, and decreased cerebral blood flow.

Hypoglycemia When severe, hypoglycemia is usually traceable to a serious disease, such as a tumor of the islets of Langerhans or advanced adrenal, pituitary, or hepatic disease, or to excessive administration of insulin. The clinical picture is one of confusion or even a loss of consciousness. When mild, as is usually the case, hypoglycemia is often of the reactive type (Chap. 338), occurring 2 to 5 h after eating, and is not usually associated with a disturbance of consciousness. The diagnosis depends on the history and the documentation of reduced blood sugar during an attack.

Acute hemorrhage Acute hemorrhage, usually within the gastrointestinal tract, is an occasional cause of syncope. In the absence of pain and hematemesis, the cause of the weakness, faintness, or even unconsciousness may remain obscure until the passage of a black stool.

Cerebral transient ischemic attacks Such attacks occur in some patients with arteriosclerotic narrowings or occlusion of the major arteries of the brain. The main symptoms vary from patient to patient and include dim vision, hemiparesis or sudden drop attacks, numbness of one side of the body, dizziness, and thick speech. In any one patient all attacks are of identical type and indicate a temporary deficit of function in a certain region of the brain due to inadequate circulation (see Chap. 368).

Hysterical fainting Fainting usually occurs under dramatic circumstances. The attack is unattended by any outward display of anxiety. The evident lack of change in pulse and blood pressure or color of the skin and mucous membranes distinguishes it from the vasodepressor faint. The diagnosis is based on the bizarre nature of the attack in a person who exhibits the general personality and behavioral characteristics of the hysteric.

Type of onset When the attack begins over the period of a few seconds, carotid sinus syncope, postural hypotension, sudden atrioventricular block, asystole, or ventricular tachycardia is likely. When the symptoms develop gradually during a period of several minutes, hyperventilation or hypoglycemia should be considered. Onset of syncope during or immediately after exertion suggests aortic stenosis, idiopathic hypertrophic subaortic stenosis or excessive bradycardia, and, in elderly subjects, postural hypotension. Exertional syncope is seen occasionally in persons with aortic insufficiency and with severe occlusive disease of cerebral arteries. In patients with ventricular standstill or ventricular fibrillation, loss of consciousness occurs several seconds later, followed rapidly by cessation of electroencephalographic activity and then often by brief clonic muscle contractions.

Position at onset of attack Epilepsy and syncopal attacks due to hypoglycemia, hyperventilation, or heart block are likely to be independent of posture. Faintness associated with a decline in blood pressure (including carotid sinus attacks) and with ectopic tachycardia usually occurs only in the sitting or standing position, whereas faintness resulting from orthostatic hypotension is apt to set in shortly after change from the recumbent to the standing position.

Associated symptoms Symptoms such as palpitation may be present when the attack is due to anxiety or hyperventilation, to ectopic tachycardia, or to hypoglycemia. Numbness and tingling in the hands and face are frequent accompaniments of hyperventilation. Genuine convulsions during the attack may occasionally occur with heart block, asystole, or ventricular tachycardia. When *duration of attack* is very brief, i.e., a few seconds to a few minutes, carotid sinus syncope or one of the several forms of postural hypotension is most likely. A duration of more than a few minutes but less than an hour suggests hypoglycemia or hyperventilation.

SPECIAL METHODS OF EXAMINATION In many patients who complain of recurrent weakness or syncope but who do not have a spontaneous attack while under observation, an attempt to reproduce attacks is of great assistance in diagnosis.

When hyperventilation is accompanied by faintness, the pattern of symptoms can be reproduced readily by having the subject breathe rapidly and deeply for 2 to 3 min. This test is often of therapeutic value also, because the underlying anxiety tends to be lessened when the patient learns that the symptoms can be produced and alleviated at will simply by controlling breathing.

Among other conditions in which the diagnosis is commonly clarified by reproducing the attacks are carotid sinus hypersensitivity (massage of one or the other carotid sinus), orthostatic hypotension and orthostatic tachycardia (observations of pulse rate, blood pressure, and symptoms in the recumbent and standing positions), and tussive syncope (by inducing the Valsalva maneuver). In all these instances, the crucial point is not whether symptoms are produced (the procedures mentioned frequently induce symptoms in healthy persons) but whether the exact pattern of symptoms that occurs in the spontaneous attacks is reproduced in the artificial ones. Continuous ambulatory ECG monitoring may be extremely useful in identifying an arrhythmia responsible for the syncopal episode, particularly in patients with frequently recurring symptoms. Monitoring is most helpful if it shows that the syncopal episode is characterized by a bout of asystole, extreme bradycardia, or tachyarrhythmia.

In cases of recurrent syncope of unknown cause in which ambulatory ECG monitoring is unrevealing, the use of intracardiac electrophysiologic techniques with programmed stimulation can be helpful in detecting cardiac rhythm abnormalities and in establishing effective treatment. During stimulation, up to two-thirds of such patients can be shown to have rapid ventricular tachycardia, His bundle conduction delays, atrial flutter, sick-sinus syndrome, or hypervagotonia. The technique is particularly useful in patients with ischemic heart disease and prior myocardial infarction, a common clinical setting for recurrent ventricular tachycardia. The diagnostic yield of electrophysiologic testing is lower with patients with nonischemic heart disease and patients with structurally normal hearts than with patients with ischemic heart disease. Recently, the signal-averaged surface ECG has proved to be useful in identifying patients with unexplained syncope who are likely to have ventricular tachycardia induced by electrophysiologic study.

Head-up tilt testing is a useful provocative technique for the diagnosis of vasodepressor syncope. Upright tilt to a maximum of 60 to 70° usually precipitates symptomatic hypotension or syncope within 10 to 30 min in patients with this syndrome. In normal subjects, passive tilting to 60° causes a small decrease in systolic blood pressure and an increase in diastolic blood pressure and heart rate. Recently, tilt testing has been used in conjunction with electrophysiologic testing to assess the efficacy of prophylactic pacing in selected patients with vasodepressor syncope and to evaluate the impact of posture on the hemodynamic consequences of some tachyarrhythmias.

The electroencephalogram may be helpful in differentiating syncope from seizures. In the interval between epileptic seizures it may show some degree of abnormality in 40 to 80 percent of cases. In the interval between syncopal attacks it should be normal.

TREATMENT In most instances fainting is relatively benign. In dealing with patients who have fainted, the physician should think first of those causes of fainting which constitute a therapeutic emergency. Among them are massive internal hemorrhage and myocardial infarction, which may be painless, and cardiac arrhythmias. In elderly persons, a sudden faint, without obvious cause, should arouse the suspicion of complete heart block or a tachyarrhythmia, even though all findings are negative when the patient is seen.

Patients seen during the preliminary stages of fainting or after they have lost consciousness should be placed in a position which permits maximal cerebral blood flow, i.e., with head lowered between the knees, if sitting, or in the supine position. All tight clothing and other constrictions should be loosened and the head turned so that the tongue does not fall back into the throat, blocking the airway. Peripheral irritation, such as sprinkling or dashing cold water on the face and neck or the application of cold moist towels, is helpful. If the temperature is subnormal, the body should be covered with a warm blanket. Since emesis is frequent, aspiration should be prevented. The head should be turned to the side and nothing given by mouth until the patient has regained consciousness. Patients should not be permitted to rise until the sense of physical weakness has passed and should be watched carefully for a few minutes after rising.

The *prevention* of fainting depends on the mechanisms involved. In the usual vasovagal faint of adolescents, which tends to occur in periods of emotional excitement, fatigue, hunger, etc., it is enough to advise the patient to avoid such circumstances. In postural hypotension, patients should be cautioned against arising suddenly from bed. Instead, they should first exercise their legs for a few seconds and then sit on the edge of the bed and make sure they are not light-headed or dizzy before starting to walk. Sleeping with the headposts of the bed elevated on wooden blocks 8 to 12 in high and wearing a snug elastic abdominal binder and elastic stockings are often helpful. Drugs of the ephedrine group may be useful if they do not cause insomnia. If there are no contraindications, a high intake of sodium chloride, which expands the extracellular fluid volume, may be beneficial.

In the syndrome of chronic orthostatic hypotension, special mineralocorticoid preparations (fludrocortisone acetate tablets, 0.1 to 0.2 mg/d in divided doses) have given relief in some cases. Binding of the legs (g suit) and sleeping with head and shoulders elevated are helpful.

The treatment of carotid sinus syncope involves first of all instructing the patient in measures that minimize the hazards of a fall (see below). Loose collars should be worn, and the patient should learn to turn the whole body, rather than the head alone, when looking to one side. Atropine or the ephedrine group of drugs should be used, respectively, in patients with pronounced bradycardia or hypotension during attacks. If atropine is not successful, a demand pacemaker should be inserted into the right ventricle. Radiation or surgical denervation of the carotid sinus has apparently yielded favorable results in some patients, but it is rarely necessary. Once it has been concluded that the attacks are due to a narrowing of major cerebral arteries, some of the surgical measures discussed in Chap. 368 must be considered.

The treatment of the various cardiac arrhythmias which may induce syncope is discussed in Chap. 197. The treatment of hypoglycemia is found in Chap. 338.

The chief hazard of a faint in most elderly persons is not the underlying disease but fracture or other trauma due to the fall. Therefore, patients subject to recurrent syncope should cover the bathroom floor and bathtub with rubber mats and should have as much of their home carpeted as is feasible. Especially important is the floor space between the bed and the bathroom, because faints are common in elderly persons when walking from bed to toilet. Outdoor walking should be on soft ground rather than hard surfaces, and the patient should avoid standing still, which is more likely than walking to induce an attack.

SEIZURES

A *brain seizure* or *convulsion* is defined as an abrupt alteration in cortical electrical activity manifested clinically by a change in consciousness or by a motor, sensory, or behavioral symptom. Seizures, which may be due to a variety of causes, become important in the differential diagnosis of syncope when the episode occurs with minimal or no warning and results in only a brief loss of consciousness. *Epilepsy* (discussed in Chap. 367) is the term used to describe recurrent seizures present over months or years, often with a stereotyped clinical pattern.

CLINICAL CHARACTERISTICS OF SEIZURES   A detailed account of the types of seizures, of their pathophysiology, and of their treatment is found in Chap. 367. The purpose here is to recount briefly the varieties of seizures that occur and to outline their clinical presentation, particularly with respect to their distinction from syncope. A single seizure may occur during the course of many medical illnesses; its importance derives from the fact that it signifies involvement of the central nervous system by the disease process.

Partial seizures (focal seizures)   The appearance of focal motor or sensory manifestations provides clinical documentation of the localization of the cerebral lesion. Deviation of the eyes and head to one side (aversive seizure) usually points to an irritative focus in the opposite prefrontal region. A Jacksonian seizure begins as a clonic movement in one portion of the body, often the thumb, the corner of the mouth, or the great toe, and spreads to adjacent muscular groups over a few seconds or minutes. The seizure may progress to involve the entire side or become generalized with attendant loss of consciousness. Jacksonian seizures almost always are accompanied by an abnormal interictal EEG.

Complex partial seizures (temporal lobe or psychomotor seizures)   These differ from simple partial seizures. They may begin with an aura that arises from discharges in the autonomic, visceral, and olfactory portions of the temporal lobe and limbic system and are often associated with behavioral or complex motor movements for which the patient is amnesic after the attack. Subjective experiences of the aura include hallucinations (olfactory, gustatory, visual, or auditory), illusions (spatial distortions, shrinkage, or angulation), aberrations in cognition (déjà vu, a sense of familiarity; jamais vu, a sense of unfamiliarity; or recurrent memory), and affective changes (anxiety, fear, and, very rarely, rage). The seizure may terminate with only the subjective component or may progress to the motor phase, which is often evident by repetitive motor acts such as smacking the lips, swallowing, undressing, and incoherent or dysphasic speech.

Tonic-clonic (grand mal) seizure   The abrupt presentation, without warning, of a generalized motor seizure is one of the most common indications of involvement of the cerebral cortex by a disease process. Grand mal seizures usually begin with opening of the eyes and mouth, flexion and abduction of the arms, and extension of the legs. The *tonic* phase of the seizure is often heralded by contraction of the respiratory muscles resulting in a vocalization. These motor signs are followed by closure of the jaw, often with laceration of the tongue, respiratory arrest with plethora and cyanosis, and urinary or, less commonly, fecal incontinence. The tonic phase of the seizure, which usually persists for only 15 to 30 s, is followed immediately by the *clonic* phase, characterized by violent rhythmic muscular contractions affecting the whole body, including the muscles of respiration. Eye movements, facial grimacing, and persistence of respiratory apnea are evident. The clonic movements subside in amplitude and frequency, and the seizure terminates, usually within 1 to 2 min. Normal respiration resumes, and the patient falls asleep; arousal may occur in a few minutes, but lethargy, fatigue, and postseizure (postictal) confusion are common and may persist for several hours. Postictal headache is also common.

The generalized seizure occurring in the course of a major medical illness signifies involvement of the central nervous system by the disorder and requires careful assessment and investigation. Such a seizure may accompany high fever, hyponatremia, metabolic acidosis, alcohol or drug withdrawal, and renal or liver failure, indicating the presence of a *metabolic encephalopathy* without requiring the postulation of another separate neurologic illness. The determination that a metabolic encephalopathy may be responsible is dependent on documentation of the systemic illness and careful attention to the

exclusion of an additional infectious, vascular, or neoplastic lesion in the nervous system. Central nervous system evaluation should include a careful history, a detailed neurologic examination searching for focal neurologic deficit, and, in many cases, electroencephalography computed tomography (CT) or MRI. If infection is suspected, an examination of the cerebrospinal fluid is mandatory. Recurrent seizures (status epilepticus) indicate a serious compromise of cerebral cortical function and require vigorous treatment to prevent hypoxic damage to the brain and, following termination of the seizures, a thorough investigation of the cause.

An isolated generalized seizure occurring in an otherwise healthy, asymptomatic patient when observed by family or other bystanders is not difficult to distinguish from syncope. More difficult to assess is the circumstance of sudden loss of consciousness occurring without warning and unwitnessed by an observer or an akinetic "drop-seizure." The latter may be indistinguishable from syncope. Postictal confusion or drowsiness, injury such as laceration of the tongue, urinary or fecal incontinence, or muscle soreness suggests that a convulsion has occurred. One common clinical presentation is the sudden occurrence of a brief clonic seizure during a minor surgical or dental procedure. The patient is usually in a seated position, and the episode is considered to be due to cerebral ischemia associated with systemic hypotension and bradycardia accompanying vasovagal syncope. There are usually only two or three clonic movements, without a prior tonic phase, and recovery is rapid without postictal symptoms. Such patients should have a neurologic examination and an EEG and, if these are normal, be treated with reassurance and not given anticonvulsants. There is no evidence to indicate an underlying cerebral lesion in such patients.

Generalized seizures may be preceded by a specific warning or *aura*, and attention to these symptoms may be important in aiding in the localization of the seizure focus and can assist in distinguishing the episode from syncope. Tingling or numbness in one extremity points to involvement of the parietal lobe, and visual or auditory sensations suggest occipitotemporal localization. However, as mentioned, tingling in both hands or a variety of visual "greying out" phenomena may precede syncopal episodes. More complex psychological and cognitive sensations may accompany temporal lobe seizures and also transient cerebral ischemic attacks (see Chap. 368), but in the latter symptoms usually persist for many minutes or hours.

Absence (petit mal) seizures   Absence seizures, in contrast to grand mal, are noted for their brevity and for the degree of loss of awareness accompanied by minimal motor manifestations. They are abrupt in onset and are often evident only by a stare or cessation of ongoing behavior; they may be accompanied by fluttering of the eyelids or by a few facial twitches. Full recovery occurs in 5 to 10 s, and the episode may go unnoticed by the patient, the family, or the teacher. Loss of postural tone (atonic or akinetic seizure) with falling is uncommon but, when present, requires distinction from syncope. The EEG is diagnostic in such cases, consisting of three-per-second spike and wave discharges. This condition, which indicates a specific generalized disorder of cerebral electrical activity, is responsive to specific drug treatments (see Chap. 367).

DIFFERENTIAL DIAGNOSIS OF SEIZURES AND SYNCOPE
Syncope must be distinguished from disturbances of cerebral function caused by a seizure. A seizure may occur day or night, regardless of the position of the patient; syncope rarely appears when the patient is recumbent, the only common exception being the Stokes-Adams attack. The patient's color may not change in seizures, though there may be cyanosis; pallor is an early and invariable finding in all types of syncope, except chronic orthostatic hypotension and hysteria, and it precedes unconsciousness. Seizures are often heralded by an aura, which is caused by a focal seizure discharge and hence has brain-localizing significance. It is usually followed by rapid return to normal or by loss of consciousness. The onset of syncope is usually more deliberate and without aura. Injury from falling is frequent in a seizure and rare in syncope for the reason that only in seizures are protective reflexes abolished instantaneously. Tonic-convulsive movements with upturning eyes are a feature of seizures and usually do not occur with

syncope, although, as stated above, brief tonic clonic seizure-like activity can accompany fainting episodes. The period of unconsciousness tends to be longer in seizures than in syncope. Urinary incontinence is frequent in seizures and rare in syncope. The return of consciousness is prompt in syncope, slow after a seizure. Mental confusion, headache, and drowsiness are common sequelae of seizures; physical weakness with a clear sensorium characterizes the postsyncopal state. Repeated spells of unconsciousness in a young person at a rate of several per day or month are more suggestive of epilepsy than of syncope. No one of these points will absolutely differentiate a seizure from syncope, but taken as a group and supplemented by electroencephalograms, they provide a means of distinguishing the two conditions.

REFERENCES

ABI-SAMRA F et al: The usefulness of head-up tilt testing and hemodynamic investigations in the workup of syncope of unknown origin. PACE 11:1202, 1988

ALMQUIST A et al: Provocation of bradycardia and hypotension by isoproterenol and upright posture in patients with unexplained syncope. N Engl J Med 320:346, 1989

BROOKS R et al: Evaluation of the patient with unexplained syncope, in *Cardiac Electrophysiology*, DP Zipes and J Jalife (eds). Philadelphia, Saunders, 1990

CHEN MY et al: Cardiac electrophysiologic and hemodynamic correlates of neurally mediated syncope. Am J Cardiol 63:66, 1989

DAY SC et al: Evaluation and outcome of emergency room patients with transient loss of consciousness. Am J Med 73:15, 1982

DELGADO-ESCUETA AV et al: The treatable epilepsies (2 parts). N Engl J Med 308:1508 and 1576, 1983

DIMARCO JP et al: Approach to the patient with syncope of unknown cause. Mod Concepts Cardiovasc Dis 52:11, 1983

EAGLE KA et al: Evaluation of prognostic classifications for patients with syncope. Am J Med 79:455, 1985

ECTOR H et al: Bradycardia, ventricular pauses, syncope, and sports. Lancet 1:591, 1984

EWING DJ et al: The natural history of diabetic autonomic neuropathy. Q J Med 49:95, 1980

GRUBB BP et al: Differentiation of convulsive syncope and epilepsy with head-up tilt testing. Ann Int Med 115:871, 1991

HICKLER R: Fainting, in *Signs and Symptoms*, 6th ed, RS Blacklow (ed). Philadelphia, Lippincott, 1977, chap 33

JOHNSON RH, SPAULDING JMK: *Disorders of the Autonomic Nervous System*. Philadelphia, Davis, 1974

KAPOOR WN et al: Diagnostic and prognostic implications of recurrences in patients with syncope. Am J Med 83:700, 1987

———— et al: A prospective evaluation and follow-up of patients with syncope. N Engl J Med 309:197, 1983

KENNY RA et al: Head-up tilt: A useful test for investigating unexplained syncope. Lancet 1:1352, 1986

LEE JE et al: Episodic unconsciousness, in *Diagnostic Approaches to Presenting Syndromes*, JA Barondess (ed). Baltimore, Williams & Wilkins, 1971, pp 133–167

MCLEOD JG, TUCK RR: Disorders of the autonomic nervous system. 1. Pathophysiology and clinical features. Ann Neurol 21:419, 1987

————, ————: Disorders of the autonomic nervous system: 2. Investigation and treatment. Ann Neurol 21:519, 1987

POLINSKY RJ et al: Pharmacologic distinction of different orthostatic hypotension syndromes. Neurology 31:1, 1981

RICHARDS AM et al: Syncope in aortic valvular stenosis. Lancet 1:1113, 1984

SILVERSTEIN MD et al: Patients with syncope admitted to medical intensive care units. JAMA 248:1185, 1982

STREETER DHP et al: Hyperbradykininism: A new orthostatic syndrome. Lancet 2:1048, 1972

SUTHERLAND JM, EADIE MJ: *The Epilepsies*, 3d ed. Edinburgh, Churchill Livingstone, 1980

WEISSLER AM, WARREN JV: Syncope and shock, in *The Heart*, 4th ed, JW Hurst et al (eds). New York, McGraw-Hill, 1978, p 705

WINTERS SL et al: Signal averaging of the surface QRS complex predicts inducibility of ventricular tachycardia in patients with syncope of unknown origin: A prospective study. J Am Coll Cardiol 10:775, 1987

YOUNG RR et al: Pure pandysautonomia with recovery: Description and discussion of diagnostic criteria. Brain 98:613, 1975

18   DIZZINESS AND VERTIGO

ROBERT B. DAROFF

Dizziness is a common and often vexing symptom. Patients use the term to encompass a variety of sensations, including those which seem semantically appropriate (e.g., lightheadedness, faintness, spinning, giddiness, etc.) and those which are misleadingly inappropriate, such as mental confusion, blurred vision, headache, tingling, "walking on cotton." Moreover, some patients with gait disturbances and no abnormal cephalic sensations will describe their problem as "dizziness." A careful history is necessary to determine exactly what a patient who states, "Doctor, I'm dizzy," is experiencing.

After eliminating the misleading symptoms such as confusion, "dizziness" usually means either *faintness* (analogous to the feelings that precede syncope) or *vertigo* (an illusory or hallucinatory sense of environmental or self-movement). In other instances, neither of these terms accurately describes a patient's symptoms, and the explanation may only become apparent when the neurologic examination reveals spasticity, parkinsonism, or other ambulation disturbances as the cause of the complaint. Operationally, dizziness is classified into four categories: (1) faintness, (2) vertigo, (3) miscellaneous head sensations, and (4) gait disturbances.

FAINTNESS   Fainting (syncope) is a loss of consciousness secondary to cerebral ischemia, more specifically ischemia to the brainstem (see Chap. 17). Prior to the actual faint, there are often prodromal symptoms (*faintness*) reflecting ischemia to a degree insufficient to impair consciousness. The sequence of symptoms is reasonably stereotyped and includes increasing lightheadedness, visual blurring proceeding to blindness, diaphoresis, and heaviness in the lower limbs progressing to postural sway. The symptoms increase in severity until consciousness is lost or the ischemia is corrected, often by assuming the recumbent position. True vertigo almost never occurs during the presyncopal state.

The causes of faintness are described in Chap. 17 and include the multiple etiologies of decreased cardiac output, postural (orthostatic) hypotension, and mimics such as vertebrobasilar insufficiency and seizures.

VERTIGO   Vertigo is a hallucination of self- or environmental movement, most commonly a feeling of spinning, usually due to a disturbance in the vestibular system. The end organs of this system, situated in the bony labyrinths of the inner ears, consist of the three semicircular canals and the otolithic apparatus (utricle and saccule) on each side. The canals transduce angular acceleration, while the otoliths transduce linear acceleration and static gravitational forces, the latter providing a sense of head position in space. The neural output of the end organs is conveyed to the vestibular nuclei in the brainstem via the eighth cranial nerve. The principal projections from the vestibular nuclei are to the nuclei of cranial nerves III, IV, and VI, the spinal cord, the cerebral cortex, and the cerebellum. The vestibuloocular reflex (VOR) serves to maintain visual stability during head movement and depends on direct projections from the vestibular nuclei to the sixth cranial nerve (abducens) nuclei in the pons and, via the medial longitudinal fasciculus, to the third (oculomotor) and fourth (trochlear) cranial nerve nuclei in the midbrain (see Fig. 26-1). These connections account for the nystagmus (to-and-fro oscillation of the eyes) which is an almost invariable accompaniment of vestibular dysfunction. The vestibulospinal pathways assist in the maintenance of postural stability. Projections to the cerebral cortex, via the thalamus, provide conscious awareness of head position and movement. The vestibular nerves and nuclei project to areas of the cerebellum (primarily the flocculus and nodulus) which modulate the VOR.

The vestibular system is one of three sensory systems subserving spatial orientation and posture; the other two are the visual system (retina to occipital cortex) and the somatosensory system that conveys peripheral information from skin, joint, and muscle receptors. The three stabilizing systems overlap sufficiently to compensate (partially or completely) for each other's deficiencies. Vertigo may represent either physiologic stimulation or pathologic dysfunction in any of the three systems.

Physiologic vertigo This occurs when (1) the brain is confronted with a mismatch among the three stabilizing sensory systems, (2) the vestibular system is subjected to unfamiliar head movements to which it has never adapted, such as in seasickness, or (3) unusual head/neck positions, such as the extreme extension when painting a ceiling. Intersensory mismatch explains carsickness, height vertigo, and the visual vertigo most commonly experienced during motion picture chase scenes; in the latter, the visual sensation of environmental movement is unaccompanied by concomitant vestibular and somatosensory movement cues. *Space sickness*, a frequent transient effect of active head movement in the weightless zero-gravity environment, is another example of physiologic vertigo.

Pathologic vertigo This results from lesions of the visual, somatosensory, or vestibular systems. Visual vertigo is caused by new or incorrect spectacles or by the sudden onset of an extraocular muscle paresis with diplopia; in either instance, central nervous system compensation rapidly counteracts the vertigo. Somatosensory vertigo, rare in isolation, is usually due to a peripheral neuropathy which reduces the sensory input necessary for central compensation when there is dysfunction of the vestibular or visual systems.

The most common cause of pathologic vertigo is vestibular dysfunction. The vertigo is frequently accompanied by nausea, jerk nystagmus, postural unsteadiness, and gait ataxia.

LABYRINTHINE DYSFUNCTION This causes severe rotational or linear vertigo. When rotational, the hallucination of movement, whether of environment or self, is directed away from the side of the lesion. The fast phases of nystagmus beat away from the lesion side, and the tendency to fall is toward the side of the lesion.

When the head is straight and immobile, the vestibular end organs generate a tonic resting firing frequency which is equal from the two sides. With any rotational acceleration, the anatomic positions of the semicircular canals on each side necessitate an increased firing rate from one and a commensurate decrease from the other. This change in neural activity is ultimately projected to the cerebral cortex, where it is summed with inputs from the visual and somatosensory systems to produce the appropriate conscious sense of rotational movement. After cessation of movement, the firing frequencies of the two end organs reverse; the side with the initially increased rate decreases, and the other side increases. A sense of rotation in the opposite direction is experienced; since there is no actual head movement, this hallucinatory sensation is *vertigo*. Any disease state that changes the firing frequency of an end organ, producing unequal neural input to the brainstem and ultimately the cerebral cortex, causes vertigo. The symptom can be conceptualized as the cortex inappropriately interpreting the abnormal neural input from the brainstem as indicating actual head rotation. Transient abnormalities produce short-lived symptoms. With a fixed unilateral deficit, central compensatory mechanisms ultimately diminish the vertigo. Since compensation depends on the plasticity of connections between the vestibular nuclei and the cerebellum, patients with brainstem or cerebellar disease have diminished adaptive capacity, and symptoms may persist indefinitely. Compensation is always inadequate for severe fixed bilateral lesions despite normal cerebellar connections; these patients are permanently symptomatic.

Acute unilateral labyrinthine dysfunction is caused by infection, trauma, and ischemia. Often, no specific etiology is uncovered, and the nonspecific term *acute labyrinthitis* or, preferably, *acute peripheral vestibulopathy* is used to describe the event. It is impossible to determine whether a patient recovering from the first bout of vertigo will have recurrent episodes.

Acute bilateral labyrinthine dysfunction is usually the result of toxins such as drugs or alcohol. The most common offending drugs are the aminoglycoside antibiotics.

TABLE 18-1 Differentiation of peripheral and central vertigo

Sign or symptom	Peripheral (labyrinth)	Central (brainstem or cerebellum)
Direction of associated nystagmus	Unidirectional; fast phase opposite lesion*	Bidirectional or unidirectional
Purely horizontal nystagmus without torsional component	Uncommon	Common
Vertical or purely torsional nystagmus	Never present	May be present
Visual fixation	Inhibits nystagmus and vertigo	No inhibition
Severity of vertigo	Marked	Often mild
Direction of spin	Toward fast phase	Variable
Direction of fall	Toward slow phase	Variable
Duration of symptoms	Finite (minutes, days, weeks) but recurrent	May be chronic
Tinnitus and/or deafness	Often present	Usually absent
Associated central abnormalities	None	Extremely common
Common causes	Infection (labyrinthitis), Ménière's, neuronitis, ischemia, trauma, toxin	Vascular, demyelinating, neoplasm

* In Ménière's disease, the direction of the fast phase is variable.

Schwannomas involving the eighth cranial nerve (*acoustic neuroma*) grow slowly and produce such a gradual reduction of labyrinthine output that central compensatory mechanisms prevent or minimize the vertigo; auditory symptoms of hearing loss and tinnitus are the most common manifestations. While lesions of the brainstem or cerebellum can cause acute vertigo, associated signs and symptoms usually permit distinction from a labyrinthine etiology (Table 18-1). Rarely, an acute lesion of the vestibulocerebellum may present with monosymptomatic vertigo indistinguishable from a labyrinthopathy.

Recurrent unilateral labyrinthine dysfunction, in association with signs and symptoms of cochlear disease (progressive hearing loss and tinnitus), is usually due to Ménière's disease. When auditory manifestations are absent, the term *vestibular neuronitis* denotes recurrent monosymptomatic vertigo. Transient ischemic attacks of the posterior cerebral circulation (vertebrobasilar insufficiency) almost never cause recurrent vertigo without concomitant motor, sensory, visual, cranial nerve, or cerebellar signs.

Positional vertigo is precipitated by a recumbent head position, either to the right or to the left. Benign paroxysmal positional vertigo (BPPV) is particularly common. Although the condition may be due to head trauma, usually no precipitating factors are identified. It generally abates spontaneously after weeks or months. The vertigo and accompanying nystagmus have a distinct pattern of latency, fatigability, and habituation that differs from the less common central positional vertigo (Table 18-2) due to lesions in and around the fourth ventricle. Moreover, the pattern of nystagmus in BPPV is often distinctive. The lower eye displays a large-amplitude torsional nystagmus, and the upper eye has a lesser degree of torsion combined with upbeating nystagmus. If the eyes are directed to the upper ear, the vertical nystagmus in the upper eye increases in amplitude.

Position*al* must be distinguished from position*ing* vertigo. The latter is provoked by head movement rather than head position and is a feature of *all* vestibulopathies, central or peripheral. Since vertigo increases with rapid head movements, patients tend to hold their heads still.

Vestibular epilepsy, vertigo secondary to temporal lobe epileptic activity, is rare and almost always intermixed with other epileptic manifestations.

TABLE 18-2   Benign paroxysmal positional vertigo (BPPV) and central positional vertigo

Features	BPPV	Central
Latency*	3–40 s	None: immediate vertigo and nystagmus
Fatigability[†]	Yes	No
Habituation[‡]	Yes	No
Intensity of vertigo	Severe	Mild
Reproducibility[§]	Variable	Good

* Time between attaining head position and onset of symptoms.
[†] Disappearance of symptoms with maintenance of offending position.
[‡] Lessening of symptoms with repeated trials.
[§] Likelihood of symptom production during any examination session.

Psychogenic vertigo, usually a concomitant of agoraphobia (fear of large open spaces, crowds, or leaving the safety of home), should be suspected in patients so "incapacitated" by their symptoms that they adopt a prolonged housebound status. Despite their discomfort, most patients with organic vertigo attempt to function. Organic vertigo is accompanied by nystagmus; a psychogenic etiology is almost certain when nystagmus is absent during a vertiginous episode.

EVALUATION OF PATIENTS WITH PATHOLOGIC VESTIBULAR VERTIGO
The evaluation depends on whether a central etiology is suspected (see Table 18-1). If so, magnetic resonance imaging (MRI) of the head or, if unavailable, computed tomography (CT), with emphasis on the posterior fossa, is mandatory. Such an examination is rarely helpful in cases of recurrent monosymptomatic vertigo with a normal neurologic examination. Typical BPPV requires no investigation after the diagnosis is made (see Table 18-2).

Vestibular function tests serve to (1) demonstrate an abnormality when the distinction between organic and psychogenic is uncertain, (2) establish the side of the abnormality, and (3) distinguish between peripheral and central etiologies. The standard test is electronystagmography (ENG), where warm and cold water (or air) is applied, in a prescribed fashion, to the tympanic membranes, and the slow-phase velocities of the resultant nystagmus from the right and left ears are compared. A velocity decrease from one side indicates hypofunction ("canal paresis"). An inability to induce nystagmus with ice water denotes a "dead labyrinth." Some institutions have the capability of quantitatively determining various aspects of the vestibuloocular reflex using computer-driven rotational chairs and precise oculographic recording of eye movements.

Treatment of acute vertigo consists of bed rest and vestibular suppressant drugs such as antihistaminics (meclizine, dimenhydrinate, promethazine), centrally acting anticholinergics (scopolamine), or a tranquilizer with GABA-ergic effects (diazepam). If the vertigo persists beyond a few days, most authorities advise ambulation in an attempt to induce central compensatory mechanisms, despite the short-term discomfiture to the patient. Chronic vertigo of labyrinthine origin may be treated with a systematized exercise program to facilitate compensation.

Prophylactic measures to prevent recurrent vertigo are variably effective. Antihistamines are commonly utilized. Ménière's disease may respond to a very low salt diet (1 g/day). The unusual examples of persisting (beyond 4 to 6 weeks) BPPV respond dramatically to specific exercise programs.

There are a variety of surgical procedures for all forms of refractory chronic or recurrent vertigo, but these are only rarely necessary.

Miscellaneous head sensations This designation is used, primarily for purposes of initial classification, to describe dizziness which is neither faintness nor vertigo. However, cephalic ischemia or vestibular dysfunction may be of such low intensity that the usual symptomatology is not clearly identified. For example, a small decrease in blood pressure or a slight vestibular imbalance may cause sensations different from distinct faintness or vertigo but which may be identified properly during provocative testing techniques. Other causes of dizziness in this category are hyperventilation syndrome, hypoglycemia, and the somatic symptoms of a clinical depression. All these patients should have normal neurologic examinations and vestibular function tests.

Gait disturbances Some individuals with gait disorders complain of dizziness despite the absence of vertigo or other abnormal cephalic sensations. The causes include peripheral neuropathy, myelopathy, spasticity, parkinsonian rigidity, and cerebellar ataxia. In this context, the term *dizziness* is being used to describe disturbed mobility. There may be mild associated lightheadedness, particularly with impaired sensation from the feet or poor vision; this is known as *multiple-sensory-defect dizziness* and occurs in elderly individuals who complain of dizziness only during ambulation. Decreased position sense (secondary to neuropathy or myelopathy) and poor vision (from cataracts or retinal degeneration) create an overreliance on the aging vestibular apparatus. A less precise, but sometimes comforting, designation is *benign dysequilibrium of aging*.

EVALUATION OF THE DIZZY PATIENT The most important diagnostic tool is a careful history focused on the meaning of "dizziness" to the patient. Is it faintness? Is there a sensation of spinning? If either of these is affirmed and the neurologic examination is normal, appropriate investigations for the multiple etiologies of cephalic ischemia or vestibular dysfunction are undertaken.

When the source of the dizziness is uncertain, provocative tests may be helpful. These office procedures simulate either cephalic ischemia or vestibular dysfunction. Cephalic ischemia is obvious if the dizziness is duplicated during orthostatic hypotension. Further provocation involves the Valsalva maneuver, which decreases cerebral blood flow and should reproduce ischemic symptoms.

The simplest provocative test for vestibular dysfunction is rapid rotation and abrupt cessation of movement in a swivel chair. This always induces vertigo which the patients can compare with their symptomatic dizziness. The intense induced vertigo may be unlike the spontaneous symptoms, but shortly thereafter, when the vertigo has all but subsided, a lightheadedness supervenes which may be identified as "my dizziness." When this occurs, the dizzy patient, originally classified as suffering from "miscellaneous head sensations," is now properly diagnosed as having mild vertigo secondary to a vestibulopathy.

Patients with symptoms of positional vertigo should be appropriately tested (see Table 18-2); positional testing is more sensitive with special spectacles that preclude visual fixation (Frenzel lenses).

A final provocative test, requiring the use of Frenzel lenses, is vigorous head shaking in the horizontal plane for about 10 s. If nystagmus develops after the shaking stops, even in the absence of vertigo, vestibular dysfunction is demonstrated. The maneuver can then be repeated in the vertical plane. If the provocative tests establish the dizziness as a vestibular symptom, the previously described evaluation of vestibular vertigo is undertaken.

Hyperventilation is the cause of dizziness in many anxious individuals; tingling of the hands and face may be absent. Forced hyperventilation for 1 min is indicated for patients with enigmatic dizziness and normal neurologic examinations. Similarly, depressive symptoms (which patients usually insist are "secondary" to the dizziness) must alert the examiner to a clinical depression as the *cause*, rather than the effect, of the dizziness.

Central nervous system disease can produce dizzy sensations of all types. Consequently, a neurologic examination is always required even if the history or provocative tests suggest a cardiac, peripheral vestibular, or psychogenic etiology. Any abnormality on the neurologic examination should prompt appropriate neurodiagnostic studies.

REFERENCES

BRANDT T: Man in motion: Historical and clinical aspects of vestibular function. *Brain* 114:2159, 1991

DELL'OSSO LF et al: Nystagmus and saccadic intrusions and oscillations, in *Neuro-Ophthalmology*, 2d ed, JS Glaser (ed). Philadelphia, Lippincott, 1990, chap 11

LEIGH RJ, ZEE DS: *The Neurology of Eye Movements*, 2d ed. Philadelphia, Davis, 1991, chaps 2 and 10

SMITH GDP et al: Post-exertion dizziness as the sole presenting symptom of autonomic failure. Brit Heart J 69:359, 1993

TROOST BT: Dizziness and vertigo, in *Neurology in Clinical Practice*, WG Bradley et al (eds). Boston, Butterworth-Heinemann, 1991, chap 17

——, Patton JM: Exercise therapy for positional vertigo. Neurology 42:1441, 1992

19   DISTURBANCES OF VISION AND OCULAR MOVEMENTS

SHIRLEY H. WRAY / THOMAS L. SLAMOVITS / RONALD M. BURDE

THE HUMAN VISUAL SYSTEM

The visual system functions to form color images instantly over a wide range of background illumination. In addition, the image is placed simultaneously on the foveas of both eyes, producing a three-dimensional construct of the image (stereopsis).

Light entering the eye is focused first by the cornea, which has a fixed refractile power throughout adult life, and then by the lens, which can change focal length to form a sharp image on the retina. The variation in lens shape allows objects to be seen clearly at both near and far distances. Focusing an image on the retina is called *refraction*, and optical aberrations can be corrected by spectacles or contact lenses.

The lens is fully pliable at birth. It becomes more spherical when the zonules arising from the ciliary body relax, allowing an increase in its refractive power and a clear near image. With age the lens becomes less malleable, its protein changes, and by the fifth decade it can no longer focus near objects. This accommodative loss (presbyopia) leads to the need for reading glasses. Progressive change in lenticular protein with age also can cause opacification and impaired vision (cataract).

The retina is a multilayered structure lining the posterior wall of the globe. Light reaches the retina after passing through the cornea, aqueous humor, lens, and vitreous humor. Light also must pass through all layers of the retina to reach the photoreceptor cells. Photoreceptors are specialized neurons whose most distal segment consists of a stack of membranes containing wavelength-specific photopigments (vitamin A congeners) connected to a neuron-specific protein. The particular photopigment and the structural anatomy of the cell (whether rod or cone) determine its function. Since each photoreceptor connects with multiple ganglion cells, the photoreceptor cell participates in more than one function.

The retina is divided into a system of rods, dealing with light detection and motion, and a system of cones, dealing with higher visual function (acuity and color perception). Rods contain one photopigment (rhodopsin) and are achromatic; cones contain one of three photopigments (red, blue, yellow) which respond to chromatic stimuli producing color vision. Incoming light is perceived by the photoreceptors as present or absent. The signals are then integrated by a network of neurons, including horizontal, bipolar, and amacrine cells, before reaching the ganglion cells. In the periphery of the retina (containing mostly rods) there is considerable convergence of information; hundreds of thousands of rods influence the response of one ganglion cell. In the foveamacular area, which subserves central vision, there is much less convergence, and for some bipolar cells there is a one-to-one relationship: one photoreceptor is connected to one bipolar cell to one ganglion cell.

Ganglion cells are of several types, each with specialized functions. Large ganglion cells, A cells (M cells, phasic), project to the magnocellular layers of the lateral geniculate body. They respond to contrast and motion. Small ganglion cells, C cells (P cells, tonic), project to the parvocellular layers of the lateral geniculate nucleus and deal with chromatic stimuli (chromaticity). Ganglion cell axons project to the brain through the optic nerve, optic chiasm, and optic tracts. The majority of axons project to the lateral geniculate body. Axon collaterals, which form proximal to the lateral geniculate body, project to suprachiasmatic nucleus of the hypothalamus, pupillomotor centers in the pretectum, and to ocular, sensory, and motor centers in the superior colliculus. Second-order neurons in the lateral geniculate nucleus project to the occipital cortex via the optic radiations.

The image formed by the retina is inverted and reversed. The temporal retina images the nasal visual field, while the nasal retina images the temporal field. Similarly, the superior retina perceives the inferior visual field and the inferior retina the superior field.

The fovea-macula projection (papillomacular bundle) is the major ocular-cortical outflow. The central 5° of retina is subserved by 25 to 27 percent of the axons, and the central 20° by 90 percent of the axons. The temporal field axons (nasal retina), which account for 52 percent of axons in the optic nerve, cross in the chiasm to project to the contralateral lateral geniculate nucleus, where they synapse and project to the striate cortex in the occipital lobe.

CLINICAL ASSESSMENT OF DISTURBANCES OF VISION

ACUITY   Acuity is a perceptual response of a subject to a stimulus of minimal magnitude. There are many different types of visual acuity in addition to that determined by the standard Snellen chart, such as resolution, orientation, motion, color, contrast sensitivity, and stereopsis. Visual disturbances are characterized by subnormal visual acuity (less than 20/20 Snellen acuity; see below) and by abnormalities of visual field, color vision, contrast sensitivity, and depth perception. A corrected visual acuity of less than 6/60 metric (20/200 conventional) bilaterally constitutes legal blindness. Refractive errors (myopia, hyperopia, astigmatism) commonly cause subnormal visual acuity and must be assessed for by measuring *best corrected* (i.e., best refracted) visual acuity. A pinhole can be used for a reasonable approximation of best corrected visual acuity. Visual acuity at distance is measured with a Snellen chart [normal 6/6 m (20/20 ft)]. In the fractional denotation—e.g., 6/60 metric (20/200 conventional)—the numerator 6 (or 20) stands for the testing distance (in meters or feet), and the denominator 60 (or 200) stands for the test letter's size normally seen at that denominator distance. Near acuity is measured with a near card (Jaeger chart). Bifocals or near spectacles must be worn by presbyopes (who have difficulties with accommodation) when testing near vision.

COLOR VISION   Acquired color vision abnormalities in red/green perception usually imply optic neuropathy. Bedside testing may consist of gross recognition or comparison of prime colors or the use of a series of color charts (Ishihara pseudoisochromatic or American Optical Hardy-Rand-Rittler plates). Color desaturation tests rely on a comparison of the subjective perception of a colored target (e.g., red bottle top) in the right and left eyes or in the nasal and temporal half-fields of a single eye. The test detects unilateral or hemianopic abnormalities.

CONTRAST SENSITIVITY   Testing of this acuity requires manipulation of both contrast and spatial frequency by measuring the minimum contrast necessary to see patterns of various sizes. Contrast sensitivity plates (Arden or American Optical) can be used at the bedside.

STEREOPSIS   There is a linear relationship between stereoacuity and Snellen visual acuity. Individuals with normal 6/6 (20/20) vision in each eye and binocular fixation (no manifest strabismus) have an average stereopsis of 40 seconds of arc. Stereoacuity is reduced with decreasing acuity down to 6/60 (20/200), at which level monocular and binocular responses become identical. The Titmus stereoacuity test is used in children and adults who have been corrected for presbyopia and is suitable for bedside use. This linearity may not exist in the presence of optic nerve damage even if visual acuity returns to normal.

VISUAL FIELDS   It is possible to perform a visual field test using any perceptual stimulus. The bedside exam is performed by confrontation. Two types of "formal" field testing are in common use:

1. On *kinetic perimetry* (Goldmann, tangent screen), the patient is instructed to look at a central fixation target while test objects of varying brightness and size (white or chromatic) are moved from the periphery toward the fixation point until the patient signals that the test object is visualized. The normal field using white objects is approximately 90° temporally, 50° nasally, 50° superiorly, and 65° inferiorly. Concentric contraction of the visual field binocularly to less than 10° constitutes legal blindness.

2. On *automated static perimetry* (Humphrey, Octopus), the patient fixes on a central target in a hemisphere with a homogeneous white background while a nonmoving light of fixed size and brightness is presented at various points in the hemisphere. Brightness is increased until the patient recognizes the presence of the stimulus above background. Thus static perimetry measures brightness sensitivity of various retinal points.

Visual field defects are localizable on the basis of the anatomy of the visual pathway. Retinal and optic nerve lesions affect one of three types of nerve fiber bundles, leading to blind spots (scotomas) termed (1) central/cecocentral, (2) arcuate, or (3) radial. Loss of nerve fibers between the optic nerve and macula (maculopapillary bundle) leads to central or cecocentral scotomas, i.e., involving the center of the visual field or extending between the center and the physiologic blind spot (cecum) (Fig. 19-1D and E). Temporal retinal lesions above and below the maculopapillary bundle or those involving the superotemporal or inferotemporal optic nerve affect the *arcuate* bundles and cause inferonasal or superonasal visual field defects, respectively. Because such field defects abut the horizontal midline, they are at times referred to as *altitudinal* (Fig. 19-1B). Lesions involving the nasal retinal or optic nerve fibers (radial nerve fiber bundle defects) lead to inferotemporal and superotemporal visual field defects that extend toward the physiologic blind spot (Fig. 19-1A).

Retinal field defects frequently correspond to lesions seen with the ophthalmoscope, i.e., areas of infarction, inflammation, or degenerative change. Macular lesions produce central scotomas. Retinitis pigmentosa usually produces constricted fields and equatorial ring scotomas.

Discrete lesions, frequently ischemic, primarily in the anterior optic nerve may produce *arcuate field defects*. Such lesions include anterior ischemic optic neuropathy, glaucoma, and optic atrophy secondary to papilledema. The central/cecocentral scotoma is a specific and common sign of optic nerve disease. It occurs in a variety of conditions both intrinsic (demyelinating, infiltrative, metabolic-toxic) and compressive in nature.

At the chiasm, the visual afferents become divided into a right and left half so that the right brain sees left visual space and the left brain sees right visual space. A discrete vertical midline is the hallmark of all visual pathway disorders at or posterior to the chiasm. A chiasmal lesion most often causes bitemporal hemianopsia (Fig. 19-2B), but several different patterns can occur: junctional scotoma, superior or inferior bitemporal quadrantanopsia, or monocular temporal hemianopsia. Each type can occur with chiasmal compression due to a pituitary tumor, craniopharyngioma, or aneurysm. Pseudochiasmal or ocular syndromes that can mimic chiasmal lesions include tilted optic discs, drug toxicity (chloroquine), sector retinitis pigmentosa, and bilateral retinal detachments. A mass in the retrochiasmatic region impinging on or displacing the optic tract results in homonymous hemianopsia of two types: an incongruous homonymous hemianopsia or a complete homonymous hemianopsia.

Homonymous field defects due to lesions of the anterior optic radiation tend to be incongruous. Those due to damage to the

FIGURE 19-1   Types of monocular visual field loss in left eye. *A.* Superior arcuate scotoma (inferior nerve fiber bundle defect). *B.* Inferior altitudinal field defect respecting the horizontal meridian (superior nerve fiber bundle defect). *C.* Enlargement of the blind spot in the left eye. *D.* Central scotoma, normal blind spot. *E.* Centrocecal scotoma. *F.* Temporal hemianopsia respecting the vertical meridian but with involvement of central vision. *G.* Generalized constriction of the visual field to 2 isopters. *H.* Nonorganic "corkscrew" field defect to 1 isopter. *(From Wray, 1985; by permission.)*

radiations close to the visual cortex are congruous. (Congruity is said to be present when the edge of the field defect in each eye is identical in shape.) Depending on its site, the lesion may involve only the upper or lower fibers of the radiation and thus cause a lower or upper quadrant defect in the opposite half-field; e.g., temporal lobe radiation lesion causes "pie in the sky" (Fig. 19-2E), whereas a parietal lobe radiation lesion causes "pie on the floor" (Fig. 19-2G). A complete hemianopic defect to bilateral simultaneous visual stimulation (attention defect) may, however, be the only detectable sign of visual dysfunction in lesions of the parietal area. Left temporoparietal lesions are associated with defective recognition of visual symbols, alexia, and agraphia; lesions of the right temporoparietal area are manifested by impaired judgment of spatial relationships, as in topographic agnosia and constructional apraxia (see Chap. 27).

Destruction of the visual cortex of one occipital lobe produces a contralateral congruous homonymous hemianopsia. This is the most common type of cortical field defect and is frequently the result of embolic occlusion of the posterior cerebral artery. Other patterns of visual loss permit precise localization of the deficit. These defects

PUPILLARY EXAMINATION Normal pupillary responses consist of prompt, symmetric constriction (miosis) on exposure to light or on attempted near convergence. Diminished response to a direct light stimulus, combined with a normal consensual pupillary response following stimulation of the contralateral eye, is termed a *relative afferent pupillary defect* (RAPD). The RAPD is an important objective sign of ipsilateral optic neuropathy. The best way to elicit the RAPD is to perform a swinging flashlight test (Fig. 19-3). Anisocoria (unequal pupil size) and abnormal pupillary reflexes are two clinically important pupillary abnormalities. Comparing pupil size in the dark and in room light and observing direct light responses help to determine whether the smaller or larger pupil is the abnormal one. With parasympathetic anisocoria, the difference in pupil size will be accentuated in room light, since the affected (large) pupil constricts subnormally. With oculosympathetic paresis, the anisocoria is more marked in dim light because the affected (small) pupil dilates subnormally.

FIGURE 19-2 Nerve fiber anatomy of the visual pathways from retina to occipital cortex. The effect of the fields of vision produced by lesions at various points along the optic pathway is shown on the right. *A*. Complete blindness in left eye. *B*. Bitemporal hemianopsia. *C*. Nasal hemianopsia of left eye. *D* and *E*. Right incongruous homonymous hemianopsia. *F* and *G*. Right upper and lower homonymous quadrantanopsia. *H*. Complete right homonymous hemianopsia. *Courtesy of DD Donaldson. (From Wray, 1985; by permission.)*

FIGURE 19-3 Swinging flashlight test demonstrates a right relative afferent pupillary defect (RAPD) in a patient with a traumatic right optic neuropathy. The patient is fixating on a distant target to avoid near effort and related accommodative miosis. *A*. Pupils in a dimly lit room. *B*. Flashlight illuminates right eye, leading to minimal direct constriction of right pupil and minimal consensual constriction of left pupil. *C*. Flashlight is swung to the left eye, causing obvious pupillary constriction directly on left and consensually on right. *D*. Flashlight is again swung to right eye, leading to bilateral pupillary dilation—a result of the right optic nerve conduction deficit.

are congruous homonymous hemianopic scotoma, congruous homonymous hemianopsia sparing the temporal crescent, or, rarely, a monocular field defect due to loss of the temporal crescent, bilateral homonymous hemianopsia, bilateral altitudinal scotoma, cortical blindness, and tunnel or keyhole vision.

Isolated chronic pupillary dilation (mydriasis) is almost never caused by a lesion in the oculomotor nerve; it may be constitutional (physiologic, "benign"), pharmacologic (induced by local instillation of mydriatics), traumatic, or a result of a parasympathetic lesion at or distal to the ciliary ganglion (tonic pupil, Adie's pupil). The diagnostic workup utilizes changes in pupil size in response to topical agents (Table 19-1).

Unilateral mydriasis with impaired direct-light and near response, ipsilateral ptosis, and extraocular muscle paresis of the superior, medial, and inferior rectus and inferior oblique muscles constitutes an oculomotor nerve palsy. Unilateral miosis with normal direct-light response and mild ipsilateral ptosis constitutes an oculosympathetic lesion or Horner syndrome. The diagnosis of the Horner pupil can be confirmed by pharmacologic testing (Table 19-1).

Light-near dissociation (LND) of the pupillary response is bilateral and characterized by an impaired response to light with an intact response to near vision. When LND is bilateral and symmetric, it occurs with dorsal midbrain lesions (hydrocephalus, pineal region tumors). Argyll-Robertson pupil is a special form of LND caused by syphilis; the pupils are miotic and usually irregular in shape. LND also can occur in diabetes mellitus. LND accompanied by bilaterally poor vision is generally due to anterior visual pathway disease. Unilateral LND is most commonly seen in patients with ipsilateral retinal or optic nerve disease. Bilateral pupillary enlargement with subnormal direct and near responses occurs with pharmacologic blockade, botulism, or diphtheria. Bilaterally miotic pupils are produced by the use of parasympathomimetics for glaucoma; a pontine lesion (pinpoint pontine pupils) or narcotic (heroin) overdose should be considered in a comatose patient with bilateral miosis.

OCULAR DISEASES

THE CONJUNCTIVA AND CORNEA   Diseases of the conjunctiva and cornea can produce loss of visual acuity, pain, and discharge.

Examination should first be directed to the lids and lid margins as well as to the lashes. Chronic infectious processes are often characterized by scaling around the lashes or pointing of the ducts of the meibomian glands. It is to be noted that basal cell and squamous cell carcinomas often involve the lids. Evidence of discharge from the conjunctiva can frequently be observed as crusting, either nasally or temporally, on the lids.

The eyes are ordinarily white and quiet. When a patient complains of discomfort or discharge, the upper and lower fornix as well as the palpebral conjunctiva should be inspected, by pulling the lower lid out and down or everting the upper lid on the tarsus. Discharge, foreign bodies, and Kaposi's sarcoma may go undetected without such an examination.

The presence of perilimbal injection is indicative of anterior uveal inflammation, and such patients should be referred for ophthalmologic evaluation.

Diseases of the conjunctiva and cornea may occur as a result of direct trauma, drying associated with disorders of tearing, exposure to radiant energy (ultraviolet light, sun, and welding guns), allergens (pollen, mold), infectious agents (bacteria, viruses, fungi, and ameba), and inflammatory, metabolic, and neoplastic processes.

Neonatal infection of the cornea or conjunctiva is usually due to staphylococci or gonococci or, in some geographic areas, to chlamydiae. Prophylactic silver nitrate treatment in the newborn is effective against gonococci but may itself cause a chemical conjunctivitis. Tetracycline or erythromycin ointment is equally effective for gonococcal prophylaxis. Congenital syphilis can produce interstitial keratitis late in the last decade of life, resulting in bilateral corneal vascularization, photophobia, and visual loss. Herpes simplex infections cause dendritic keratitis. Failure to recognize herpetic keratopathy and its inappropriate treatment with topical glucocorticoids can lead to corneal "melting" and perforation. Treatment with acyclovir topically or systemically can suppress herpetic keratopathy (see Chap. 143). Herpesvirus can become latent in the trigeminal ganglia, allowing recurrent keratitis to occur in some patients.

TABLE 19-1   Characteristics of pupils encountered in neuroophthalmology

	General characteristics	Responses to light and near stimuli	Room condition in which anisocoria is greater	Response to mydriatics	Response to miotics	Response to pharmacologic agents
Essential anisocoria	Round, regular	Both brisk	No change	Dilates	Constricts	Normal and rarely needed
Horner's syndrome	Small, round, unilateral	Both brisk	Darkness	Dilates	Constricts	Cocaine 4%, poor dilation; Paredrine 1%, no dilation if third-order neuron damage
Tonic pupil syndrome (Holmes-Adie syndrome)	Usually larger* in bright light; sector pupil palsy, vermiform movement Unilateral or, less often, bilateral	Absent to light, tonic to near; tonic redilation	Light	Dilates	Constricts	Pilocarpine 0.1% or 0.125% constricts; Mecholyl 2.5% constricts
Argyll Robertson pupils	Small, irregular, bilateral	Poor to light, better to near	No change	Poor	Constricts	
Midbrain pupils	Middilated; may be oval; bilateral	Poor to light, better to near (or fixed to both)	No change	Dilates	Constricts	
Pharmacologically dilated pupils	Very large†, round, unilateral	Fixed‡	Light		No‡	Pilocarpine 1% will not constrict
Oculomotor palsy (nonvascular)	Middilated (6–7 mm), unilateral (rarely bilateral)	Fixed	Light	Dilates	Constricts	

* Tonic pupil may appear smaller following prolonged near-effort or in dim illumination; affected pupil is initially large, but with passing time gradually becomes smaller.
† Atropinized pupils have diameters of 8 to 9 mm. No tonic, midbrain, or oculomotor palsy pupil ever is this large.
‡ Pupils may be weakly reactive, depending on interim after instillation.
SOURCE: TL Slamovits and JS Glaser in *Clinical Ophthalmology*, vol 2, T Duane (ed). Philadelphia, Lippincott, 1988

Adenovirus infection is the leading cause of keratoconjunctivitis in adults; it is usually self-limiting and benign. In sexually active young adults, inclusion conjunctivitis is common. In developing countries, trachoma and onchocerciasis are leading causes of corneal scarring and blindness.

Chronic indolent amebic ulcers of the cornea can occur in soft contact lens wearers who have a break in the corneal epithelium; such ulcers are difficult to treat. However, this complication is rare in those who remove and clean contact lenses daily. Debilitated patients can develop keratitis due to gram-negative bacteria (*Klebsiella, Pseudomonas*) or fungi. Malnutrition and avitaminosis A can lead to conjunctival and corneal scarring with keratinization (xerosis) and severe visual loss.

Keratoconjunctivitis also can occur in patients with Stevens-Johnson syndrome (Chap. 52), Wegener's granulomatosis (Chap. 291), rheumatoid arthritis (Chap. 285), atopic dermatitis (Chap. 51), and cicatricial pemphigoid (Chap. 53). These processes are often associated with corneal ulceration. Band keratopathy is caused by corneal deposition of calcium salts, especially within the palpebral fissure (Fig. A8-10). It occurs as a result of chronic inflammation (keratouveitis) or of systemic hypercalcemia (see Chap. 357).

Corneal clouding is prominent in G_{M1} gangliosidosis (Chap. 349), in certain of the mucopolysaccharidoses (Chap. 349), and in aminoaciduria [cystinosis (Chap. 352)]. In Wilson's disease (Chap. 348) and in chronic biliary cirrhosis, copper deposits form a golden-brown ring (Kayser-Fleischer ring) (Fig. A8-16) in the cornea at the level of Descemet's membrane. Corneal drug deposition may occur following systemic use of chloroquine, phenothiazine, gold, silver, or amiodarone.

THE LENS AND CATARACTS Opacification of the normally clear and transparent crystalline lens is termed a *cataract*. Visual symptoms are blurred vision, glare, altered color perception, and monocular diplopia. *Congenital* cataracts occur as a complication of intrauterine rubella, herpes simplex, herpes zoster, syphilis, and cytomegalic inclusion disease. The majority are idiopathic or inherited. Acquired cataracts result from trauma, radiation, drugs, metabolic disorders, ocular inflammatory disorders, or aging (senile cataract). Cataracts develop earlier in patients with diabetes mellitus (type I and type II) and in some patients with a strong family history of cataract formation. Metabolic disorders complicated by cataract include galactosemia (Chap. 354), chronic hypercalcemic states (Chap. 357), Fabry's disease, Wilson's disease (Chap. 348), and Lowe's syndrome (Chap. 244). More than a third of patients with myotonic dystrophy have multicolored crystalline opacities scattered throughout the lens. Cataracts also may be associated with chromosomal disorders; with the Alport, cri-du-chat, Conradi, Crouzon, and Down syndromes; and with gonadal dysgenesis. Inflammatory ocular diseases, and drugs and toxic substances such as haloperidol, glucocorticoids, and iron also can cause cataracts. Cataract extraction is performed by removing the lens nucleus and cortex from within the lens capsule. In most adults, a plastic lens is then implanted within the capsule.

The zonules holding the lens may be broken in one region, allowing the lens to move eccentrically, often leaving its edge in the pupillary axis (subluxation), or totally broken, allowing the lens to move into the anterior chamber or into the vitreous cavity (luxation). The most common cause of subluxation or luxation is trauma. Others include homocystinuria (Chap. 352), Marfan's syndrome, spherophakia, and sulfite oxidase insufficiency.

UVEAL DISEASES The uvea consists of the iris and ciliary body anteriorly and the choroid posteriorly. Anatomically, the choroid has three layers of vessels and a cellular matrix including pigmented cells. Common diseases of the uvea are inflammatory or neoplastic. Inflammation can involve the iris (iritis), ciliary body (cyclitis), or choroid (choroiditis) or any combination of the three (uveitis). Uveitis causes photophobia, ocular discomfort, and visual blurring. Chronic uveitis can cause cystoid macular edema with decreased central acuity, cataract formation, and secondary glaucoma. The most common form of uveitis is idiopathic. Systemic diseases causing uveitis include pauciarticular juvenile rheumatoid arthritis (rheumatoid factor nega-

tive), juvenile nevoxanthogranuloma, rheumatoid arthritis, sarcoidosis, Lyme disease, and relapsing polychondritis. Treatment of uveitis (dependent on severity) includes cycloplegic drops and glucocorticoids (topically or systemically) and sometimes immunosuppressive drugs (chlorambucil, azathioprine, cyclophosphamide, and cyclosporin A).

Ocular malignant melanoma is a primary neoplastic disease of the choroid. Choroidal involvement also occurs as a result of metastases (lung, breast, prostate) and in association with lymphoma of the central nervous system (reticulum cell sarcoma)—conditions that are sometimes responsive to low-dose radiation.

RETINAL DISEASES Retinal abnormalities are best seen by performing a dilated fundus examination. Retinal diseases involving the macula cause distortion of straight lines (metamorphopsia), loss of central acuity, and visual field abnormalities. Nonmacular retinal disorders cause scotomata involving the peripheral or paracentral visual field, correlating with the site of retinal pathology. Retinopathies can be due to diseases of the retinal vessels, neurosensory retina, or the retinal pigment epithelium.

Retinal vasculopathies These changes occur in many systemic conditions. In hypertensive retinopathy, the severity of retinal changes correlates closely with the level of systemic hypertension (see Chap. 209). Grade I consists of arteriolar narrowing; grade II includes arteriovenous nicking, minimal exudation, and splinter hemorrhages; grade III includes retinal edema, hemorrhages, and cotton-wool spots (focal ischemia in the nerve fiber layer); grade IV includes grade III changes plus papilledema, often with a macular star produced by deposition of cellular debris (hard exudates). Hypertensive retinopathy can be seen with all forms of hypertension—essential and secondary. Cotton-wool spots, a common feature of malignant hypertension, also may occur in anemia, leukemia, collagen vascular disease, dysproteinemia, infective endocarditis, and diabetes mellitus. They are the most common ophthalmic lesions in acquired immunodeficiency syndrome (AIDS) (see Chap. 279). Other ocular manifestations of AIDS include cytomegalovirus (CMV) retinitis (Fig. A8-14) and toxoplasmic and fungal retinal infections. Nonretinal ocular manifestations of AIDS include optic neuropathy, Kaposi's sarcoma of the conjunctiva, and orbital lymphoma.

Diabetic retinopathy is classified into two groups: (1) background retinopathy (Fig. A8-12), characterized by microaneurysms, dot-blot hemorrhages, cotton-wool spots, hard exudates, intraretinal microvascular shunt vessels, and venous beading, sometimes with related macular edema, and (2) proliferative retinopathy (Fig. A8-13), characterized by neovascularization, proliferation of fibrous tissue into the vitreous cavity, and eventually traction retinal detachments with visual loss (see Chap. 337). Panretinal photocoagulation is beneficial in maintaining vision in early proliferative retinopathy. The progression of diabetic retinopathy correlates best with the concentration of hemoglobin A_{lc}, reflecting the long-term metabolic control. The lower the hemoglobin A_{lc} concentration, the slower is the progression. The acute induction of so-called tight control is often associated with a short-term aggravation of the retinopathic process (e.g., insulin infusion pump or multiple injection regime).

Other proliferative retinopathies Somewhat similar retinal vascular changes (''sea fan'' proliferation) occur in sickle cell diseases (S-S, S-C, S-Thal) and in the retinopathy of prematurity. In sickle cell disease focal photocoagulation is helpful. Focal retinal cryotherapy is of benefit in a subset of infants with acute retinopathy of prematurity.

Retinopathy of prematurity (ROP) Retinopathy of prematurity (formerly retrolental fibroplasia) is now classified according to the following criterion: *location* (zones I to III), *extent* (hours of the clock), *stage* (1 to 5), and *plus disease* (marked vascular shunting). Risk factors for the development of ROP are birth weight and gestational age. Neonates less than 28 weeks and weighing less than 1250 g are especially at risk. Initial fundus examination of these infants should be at 4 to 6 weeks, with subsequent examinations determined by the fundus findings or every 2 to 3 weeks until maturity. Care must be taken in dilating the eyes of these patients owing to the potential side effects of mydriatics and cycloplegic drops. A large multicenter trial has demonstrated the efficacy of transscleral cryotherapy in decreasing the incidence of retinal detachment and retinal folding from 43 to 22 percent in patients with stage 3+ ROP with plus disease. Currently, the effectiveness of laser ablation is being studied.

Occlusive retinal vasculopathies Permanent blindness occurs with *infarction* of the inner retina due to occlusion of the central retinal artery (CRA). Funduscopic examination shows rectangular "box car" segmentation of venous blood flow and an opaque white retina due to axoplasmic stasis in ganglion cell axons. A central cherry-red spot is due to visualization of the choroid in the macular area devoid of axons (Fig. A8-2). CRA occlusion may be embolic (ipsilateral internal carotid artery, aorta, or heart) or thrombotic due to giant cell arteritis, arteriosclerosis, collagen vascular disease, or hyperviscosity states. CRA occlusion is an ophthalmic emergency. Treatment may include ballotement of the globe, retrobulbar anesthetic block, and paracentesis of aqueous humor in an attempt to move embolic material into peripheral arterioles.

Monocular transient blurring of vision (amaurosis fugax) lasting seconds to minutes may herald CRA occlusion but, more important, may be a precursor of a stroke. Most cases of amaurosis fugax are caused by presumed embolic phenomena. In younger patients a cardiac source is more likely, but with increasing age carotid atheromatous disease becomes a more frequent source. Depending on the physical examination, these patients require an evaluation of the aortic arch and carotid circulation as well as the heart (see Chap. 368). Based on recent studies, patients in both North America and Europe with high-grade stenosis (>70 percent) benefit from carotid endarterectomy by reducing the risk of subsequent stroke by 33 to 66 percent as compared with patients on medical therapy.

Central (Fig. A8-3) and branch retinal vein occlusion may occur spontaneously or in association with hypertension or elevated intraocular pressure. Venous stasis retinopathy mimics early vein occlusion with venous dilatation, hemorrhages, and cotton-wool spots; it is due to impaired retinal perfusion produced by severe carotid occlusive disease and Takayasu's disease. Systemic coagulopathies such as thrombocytopenia, disseminated intravascular coagulopathy, and systemic lupus erythematosus with circulating anticoagulants (cardiolipin) may cause retinal hemorrhages, clotting in the submacular choriocapillaris, choroidal hemorrhages, and detachment of the retina. Perivenous sheathing occurs in primary retinal vasculitis (Eales disease), leukemia, and optic nerve demyelination. Fundus changes may be the mark of an abused child presenting with multiple retinal hemorrhages (subhyaloid lakes, blot and flame hemorrhages) and cotton-wool spots. This retinopathy is caused by severe shaking or choking of the child.

Retinal vascular anomalies are rare and among them are to be found retinal telangiectasia (Coat's disease), retinal angiomatosis [von Hippel-Lindau syndrome (Chap. 378)], direct arteriovenous connections (Wyburn-Mason syndrome), miliary aneurysms, cavernous retinal hemangiomas.

Nonvascular diseases of the retina These include infections such as congenital and acquired toxoplasmosis, herpes retinitis, and *Monilia* and nematode infestations. Inflammatory diseases of the outer retina and choroid include the presumed ocular histoplasmosis syndrome, acute multifocal placoid pigment epitheliopathy, serpiginous retinopathy, "bird-shot" chorioretinopathy, multiple evanescent white dot syndrome, and neoplastic diseases such as retinoblastoma.

Retinal degenerative disease These may involve the retinovitreal interface with focal capillary sclerosis and hole formation (lattice degeneration) or may appear as isolated areas of retinovitreal adhesion and vitreous liquefaction (syneresis) leading to retinal traction, retinal horseshoe-shaped tears, and detachment. Lightning-like flashes and/or an acute vitreous hemorrhage producing a spiderweb-like shadow and blurred vision may herald detachment. These patients must be examined by an ophthalmologist utilizing an indirect ophthalmoscope. Emergency surgery (laser, cryotherapy) is required to seal the tears. Degeneration of the outer retina and pigment epithelium is characteristic of retinitis pigmentosa (Fig. A8-9) which occurs in

sporadic, X-linked, autosomal recessive, and autosomal dominant forms. Several mutations have been shown to be associated with the genetic forms of retinitis pigmentosa. Some involve point mutations in rhodopsin, which may present as either an autosomal dominant or autosomal recessive phenotype. Symptoms are loss of night vision, progressive concentric contraction of the visual field, and eventually, loss of central vision.

Multisystem disorders Several disorders may cause retinal degeneration, including abetalipoproteinemia (Bassen-Kornzweig syndrome, Chap. 344), neuronal ceroid lipofuscinosis (Batten-Mayou disease), Refsum's disease (Chap. 383), certain mucopolysaccharidoses, and the Kearns-Sayre syndrome (Chap. 385).

Certain lysosomal storage diseases, including G_{M1} and G_{M2} gangliosidosis and the sphingolipidoses, affect ganglion cell function, leading to blindness; cherry-red spots are invariably present (Chap. 349). Toxic retinopathy may follow the use of phenothiazine derivatives, especially thioridazine (Mellaril), chloroquine, and hydroxychloroquine. Long-term therapy with these agents should be monitored at regular intervals with static perimetry or kinetic perimetry with red and white targets.

DISEASES OF THE RETINAL PIGMENT EPITHELIUM Bruch's membrane is a multilayered structure formed by the choriocapillaris and the pigment epithelium of the retina. With aging, the pigment epithelium may accumulate intracellular material, leading to age-related macular degeneration. Visual loss is slowly progressive, associated with metamorphopsia, and rarely causes less than 6/120 (20/400) Snellen acuity. A second type of age-related macular degeneration can occur in the paramacular foveal area and cause visual loss. It results from degeneration of Bruch's membrane with the formation of large or small breaks in its integrity and subretinal neovascularization. Subsequent exudation and hemorrhage cause a further elevation of the sensory or pigment epithelium of the retina. Visual loss is often acute and catastrophic in nature, decreasing acuity to less than 6/120 (20/400) with a large central scotoma that is defined by the anatomic detachment. Laser ablation of the neovascular net may delay blindness. Angioid streaks are large breaks in Bruch's membrane (Fig. A8-8). They are associated with Paget's disease, acromegaly, pseudoxanthoma elasticum, sickle cell disease, and severe myopia.

DISEASES OF THE OPTIC NERVE

The optic disc is the exit site of all retinal ganglion cell axons. The axons leave the globe in the optic nerve by passing through the lamina cribrosa. Just posterior to the lamina, the nerve fibers become myelinated. The blood supply of the nerve head is primarily derived from choroidal and posterior ciliary branches of the ophthalmic artery.

GLAUCOMA Glaucoma is characterized by progressive field loss due to nerve damage from elevated intraocular pressure. It is an important cause of blindness worldwide and in the United States occurs in 1 to 2 percent of patients above age 60. The disease may be asymptomatic with painless, slow loss of peripheral and paracentral visual fields. Early detection depends on a routine eye examination with intraocular pressure measurement (tonometry), funduscopy with attention to optic disc appearance, and visual field testing. In the normal eye, the optic cups are symmetric and the neural rim is pink (Fig. A8-1). In glaucoma, either localized notching or generalized enlargement of the optic cup can be seen (Fig. A8-11). The rim, although thinned, remains pink until late. The central optic cup diameter can be compared with the diameter of the disc, and a ratio of the horizontal and vertical dimensions can be recorded. The normal cup-disc ratio is less than 0.2 to 0.3. Vertical disparity in one or both eyes is an early sign of glaucoma. Glaucoma is often asymmetric, and the finding of asymmetry of the cup-disc ratio implies glaucoma. Early visual field loss includes nonspecific constriction and small paracentral scotomas. Eventually, arcuate nerve fiber bundle defects develop with a characteristic *nasal step* (e.g., arcuate bundle defect extending to the nasal horizontal raphe forms a steplike configuration on kinetic visual field testing). The papillomacular bundle and acuity are spared until late in the disease. Intraocular pressure reflects the balance between the production and outflow of aqueous humor, and the normal range is 2.09 ± 0.33 kPa (15.8 ± 2.5 mmHg) measured by applanation tonometry. (Schiotz tonometers measure intraocular pressure by indentation of the cornea, whereas most tonometers measure by planating the corneal surface, hence applanation.)

Glaucoma is an appellation for many disease states. It results from decreased outflow of aqueous humor through the pupil, trabecular meshwork, and Schlemm's canal, leading to elevated intraocular pressure. Chronic or *primary open-angle glaucoma*, the most common of adult glaucomas, is asymptomatic and detected only by routine eye examination. It is associated with a relative obstruction to aqueous outflow through the trabecular meshwork and is of unknown cause. Treatment includes the use of topical agents including cholinergic (pilocarpine, carbachol, echothiophate) or adrenergic agonists (epinephrine dipivefrin) or antagonists, i.e., beta-adrenergic blockers (timolol, levobunalol, betaxolol). If topical agents do not reduce the intraocular pressure satisfactorily, systemic carbonic anhydrase inhibitors (acetazolamide or methazolamide) are added. Laser trabeculoplasty or filtration surgery, to improve aqueous outflow, is indicated when medical therapy fails.

Secondary open-angle glaucoma may develop in patients with ocular inflammatory or neoplastic disease, with mature cataracts or elevated episcleral venous pressure, or during a course of long-term glucocorticoid therapy, either topical or systemic.

Angle-closure glaucoma occurs when the iris blocks egress of aqueous humor through the trabecular meshwork. In the primary form, an anatomic abnormality of the eye leads to pupillary block and obstruction of the trabecular meshwork. An acute rise in intraocular pressure occurs, with dilation of the pupil causing severe eye and face pain, nausea, vomiting, colored halos around lights, and loss of visual acuity. Conjunctival hyperemia, corneal edema, and a fixed middilated pupil are common signs. Urgent reduction of the intraocular pressure is best accomplished by the use of hyperosmotic agents, including oral glycerine and sorbitol or intravenous mannitol. Laser or surgical iridotomy is curative in most cases.

Secondary angle-closure glaucoma can occur when the lens or ciliary body becomes swollen, pushing the iris against the trabecular meshwork or sealing the iris to the trabecular meshwork as a result of the formation of a neovascular network. This process occurs in patients with diabetic retinopathy, advanced ocular ischemic syndrome due to severe occlusive carotid disease, or inflammatory adhesions (synechiae).

OPTIC NEUROPATHIES Diseases of the optic nerve cause acuity loss, subjective color and brightness desaturation, changes in contrast sensitivity, and visual field loss. There is almost always a relative afferent pupillary defect (RAPD) with a unilateral or asymmetric optic nerve process. (Fig. 19-3). Papilledema (optic disc edema secondary to elevated intracranial pressure) and infiltration of the optic nerve sheath cause visual dysfunction late in the course of the disease. In acute optic neuropathy the optic disc may be normal or swollen. In chronic optic neuropathy the disc is swollen or pale (atrophy).

Optic neuritis most commonly afflicts patients in their twenties or thirties, women more than men, and can either be a primary demyelinating disease of unknown etiology or associated with past, present, or future manifestations of multiple sclerosis (see Chap. 373). Acute optic neuritis is usually unilateral. There is acute visual acuity or visual field loss, an RAPD, and more than 90 percent of the time ocular pain, typically exacerbated by eye movement. In the acute phase, the nerve appearance is normal (retrobulbar optic neuritis) in two-thirds or swollen (anterior optic neuritis or papillitis) in one-third of cases. Of patients with acute optic neuritis, about half have brain abnormalities on MRI consistent with demyelination. Prognosis for visual acuity recovery is excellent, even without treatment, but some residual visual dysfunction generally persists, such as abnormal

color vision or visual field or contrast sensitivity. Within a decade and a half of the onset of acute optic neuritis, about three-quarters of women and one-third of men will develop multiple sclerosis.

Treatment of acute idiopathic or demyelinating optic neuritis with oral prednisone in standard doses alone is not indicated because it appears to increase the risk of subsequent episodes of optic neuritis. Treatment with intravenous methylprednisolone (1 g/d for 3 days) followed by a short course of oral prednisone does not appear to increase recurrence risk and, compared with no treatment, hastens reversal of visual loss. However, methylprednisolone therapy only leads to slightly better vision after 6 months in adults, and therefore, the appropriateness of treatment has to be weighed for the individual patient. Treatment benefit may be greater when visual loss is relatively more profound (worse than 20/40) within the first week of onset of visual symptoms.

Anterior ischemic optic neuropathy (AION) occurs most often in patients over 40 years of age. Typically, sudden visual loss and altitudinal field loss occur, i.e., a superior or inferior visual field defect with one border along the horizontal midline, associated with disc swelling due to infarction of the nerve head (Fig. A8-6). It occurs in two forms: (1) nonarteritic (median age 56 years), in which the risk factors are diabetes mellitus in younger patients and hypertension in older patients, and (2) an arteritic (giant cell arteritis) variety (median age 74 years). Symptoms of giant cell arteritis (anorexia, malaise, proximal arthralgia, myalgia, headache, and jaw claudication) and an elevated erythrocyte sedimentation rate are indications for prompt systemic glucocorticoid therapy and a temporal artery biopsy. Untreated, arteritic ischemic optic neuropathy may affect the contralateral eye and cause blindness in 40 percent of cases.

Compression (intrinsic or extrinsic) of the optic nerve causes insidious progressive acuity and field loss. The disc may be normal, swollen, or atrophic (Fig. A8-7). Intrinsic tumors include optic nerve sheath meningioma and glioma. In Graves' ophthalmopathy, the optic neuropathy is due to compression of the nerve in the orbital apex by the enlarged extraocular muscles. Benign or malignant orbital tumors, metastatic lesions, tumors arising from the adjacent paranasal sinuses and middle cranial fossa, and giant pituitary adenomas can each lead to compressive optic neuropathy.

Infiltrative and toxic optic neuropathies are rare. Progressive disc swelling and visual loss characterize infiltration by inflammatory disease (sarcoidosis), infection (cryptococcosis), or neoplasia (leukemia, lymphoma, metastatic carcinoma). Toxic agents (methanol, ethambutol) cause a more acute visual loss with normal or swollen discs, whereas nutritional amblyopias are associated with a more insidious course.

Leber hereditary optic neuropathy This condition, which affects males primarily (Western populations), is transmitted mitochondrially, i.e., through the female line. Leber's hereditary optic neuropathy probably represents the pure neurologic end of the spectrum of the encephalomyelopathies in contrast to Kearns-Sayre's syndrome (progressive external ophthalmoplegia, pigmentary retinopathy, and cardiac conduction block), which is midspectrum. At least six mutations in the DNA of mitochondria have been identified. Between 50 and 60 percent have a mitochondrial point mutation at the nucleotide position 11,778, where there is a guanine-adenine substitution. This converts a highly conserved arginine to a histidine in complex I of the mitochondrial redox system. This is believed to cause a relative metabolic deficiency, but how or why this produces the clinical complex is uncertain.

This mutation can be demonstrated using *Mae* III or *Sfa* NI restriction probes. The 11,778 mutation has not been found in healthy human beings. As mentioned previously, at least five other mutations have been found. Pedigree studies have demonstrated that 50 percent of men and 20 percent of women who have inherited the 11,778 defect develop an optic neuropathy. This penetrance cannot be explained on the basis of heteroplasmy, and it has been suggested that the mitochondrial DNA mutation can only be expressed when matched with a specific X chromosome allele.

Leber hereditary optic neuropathy is characterized by rapid loss of central vision during early adult life. Both eyes are affected either simultaneously or sequentially. The visual fields contain scotomas that are initially central and rapidly become cecocentral in location. In acute Leber hereditary optic neuropathy, the ophthalmoscopic findings are (1) circumpapillary telangiectatic microangiopathy, (2) swelling of the nerve fiber layer around the disc, and (3) absence of leakage from the disc or peripapillary region on fluorescein angiography with arteriovenous shunting present in the area of telangiectatic vessels. Late in the course of the disease, optic atrophy develops. About 15 percent of patients recover useful vision in one or both eyes many years after the ictus; however, those with the 11,778 mutation have been reported to have a uniformly poor visual prognosis.

Papilledema   Optic disc swelling resulting from elevated intracranial pressure (Fig. A8-4) is typically bilateral, often asymmetric, and associated with transient visual loss lasting seconds (visual obscurations) and horizontal diplopia. Optic atrophy, impaired vision, and field loss may ensue if papilledema becomes chronic. Increased intracranial pressure may be caused by mass lesions, inflammatory disease, or idiopathic pseudotumor cerebri (benign intracranial hypertension), but the immediate obligation is to exclude an intracranial mass lesion with appropriate neuroimaging tests (see Chap. 369).

Pseudopapilledema   Pseudopapilledema is usually due to congenital disc anomalies, giving rise to apparent rather than true disc swelling. Small or absent optic cups, abnormal branching of the major retinal vessels, and calcific excrescences [optic disc drusen (Fig. A8-5)] may be seen.

DISORDERS OF EYE MOVEMENT

Disorders of eye movement in the adult usually present with diplopia. The diagnostic approach to determine the cause is based on a series of specific questions and a step-by-step analysis of the eye movements to establish first whether the double vision is monocular or binocular. If diplopia is present with one eye covered, the patient has monocular diplopia. Monocular diplopia almost never signals a neurologic disorder but is most often due to an optical problem (refractive error, keratoconus, or cataract). It may be psychogenic or functional. Binocular diplopia resolves with occlusion of vision to either eye and is due to ocular misalignment, whether caused by disorders of the ocular motor nerves, of the myoneural junction (myasthenia gravis; see Chap. 386), or of the extraocular muscles themselves. Myasthenia gravis can usually be diagnosed with the edrophonium or prostigmine test. Restriction of extraocular muscle function can result from inflammation (orbital myositis), infiltration (thyroid ophthalmopathy or metastatic disease), or entrapment (blowout fracture of the orbital floor). Restriction of movement of the globe can be confirmed with a positive forced duction test. Topical proparacaine is used to anesthetize the eye, especially over the insertion of the rectus muscles to be manipulated. While the patient looks in the direction of gaze limitation, the physician, using a cotton-tipped applicator or toothed forceps, attempts to move the globe in the direction of gaze deficit. The inability to overcome the eye movement limitation signifies the presence of a restrictive process.

Once restrictive disease and myasthenia gravis are excluded, the major cause of binocular diplopia is a cranial nerve lesion. The type of binocular diplopia—horizontal, vertical, or oblique—provides clues in determining which muscle is affected. A red glass test allows a more exact documentation of the type of diplopia.

ISOLATED OCULAR MOTOR NERVE PALSIES   Oculomotor nerve (third cranial nerve)   The oculomotor (third nerve) nuclear complex is a compact midline structure in the rostral midbrain containing somatic motor and visceral nuclei. Motor neurons project ipsilaterally to the medial rectus, inferior rectus, and inferior oblique muscles and contralaterally to the superior rectus muscle. One central caudal nucleus innervates the levator palpebrae superioris bilaterally. Axons from the visceral nuclei project ipsilaterally as the pregangli-

onic, parasympathetic outflow to the sphincter of the pupil and the ciliary ganglion, controlling pupillary sphincter function and accommodation. A complete lesion of the nucleus of the oculomotor nerve (e.g., midbrain infarction) would be expected to produce a unilateral third nerve palsy, paralysis of the contralateral superior rectus muscle, and bilateral ptosis. Subnuclear (i.e., partial nuclear) or fascicular (i.e., intramesencephalic) oculomotor lesions lead to partial third nerve palsies with single or multiple extraocular muscle weakness with or without pupillary involvement. High-resolution magnetic resonance imaging (MRI) of the midbrain, especially with gadolinium enhancement, may demonstrate such focal lesions, which usually are vascular or metastatic in origin.

The fascicular portion of the third nerve courses through the red nucleus and ventral mesencephalon to emerge in the interpeduncular fossa. It then runs forward beneath the posterior cerebral artery and lateral to the posterior communicating artery, pierces the dura, and enters the cavernous sinus. The pupillary fibers travel superficially in the dorsomedial portion of the nerve. At the superior orbital fissure, where the nerve enters the orbit, it divides into a superior branch (supplying the levator and superior rectus) and an inferior branch (supplying medial and inferior rectus, inferior oblique, and pupillomotor fibers).

A complete third nerve lesion causes ptosis and inability to turn the eye upward, downward, or inward. At rest, the eye is deviated down and temporally. The iris sphincter may be involved or spared, as determined by pupillary size and reactivity.

Lesions at various sites along the course of the nerve from the nucleus to the muscle give characteristic patterns of loss of function. As the fascicles of the third nerve traverse the midbrain, they pass through important structures that enable precise localization of fascicular third nerve palsies. Aside from isolated partial third nerve palsies with or without pupillary involvement, four syndromes can be recognized. When the third nerve palsy is accompanied by involvement of the red nucleus, a contralateral cerebellar ataxia and slow "rubral" tremor occur—Claude syndrome. If the oculomotor nerve is damaged as it traverses the cerebral peduncle, a contralateral hemiparesis results—Weber syndrome. More extensive lesions (tumor or infarct) may affect the third nerve, red nucleus, and cerebral peduncle—Benedikt syndrome—and additionally cause vertical gaze palsy—Nothnagel syndrome.

After the third nerve leaves the brainstem, it is susceptible to meningeal processes (infection, tumor, blood) or compression. When the nerve is compressed against the tentorial edge, petroclinoid ligament, or clivus by the uncus of the temporal lobe during cerebral herniation, the pupil fibers are affected first, and the pupils dilate and become unresponsive to light. Compression of the third nerve by aneurysm (posterior communicating artery or posterior cerebral artery) produces an acute, total, isolated painful third nerve palsy and a dilated nonreactive pupil. Initial pupil sparing can be found in 8 to 15 percent of aneurysms, but pupillary involvement usually occurs within 5 to 7 days. Prompt consideration of cerebral angiography and surgery is indicated in all third nerve palsies with pupil involvement at all ages.

Within the cavernous sinus, the oculomotor nerve may be compressed by aneurysm or tumor (pituitary tumor, meningioma, nasopharyngeal carcinoma), or the nerve may be affected by thrombosis, local infection, or inflammation. Pain in the face and paresis of the abducens and/or trochlear nerves also may be present.

Pupillary sparing (normal size and reflex response) is the hallmark of an isolated painful third nerve palsy due to microinfarction in association with diabetes mellitus, hypertension, or collagen vascular disease. Patients over age 50 with an isolated third nerve palsy and pupil sparing without signs of subarachnoid hemorrhage can be followed expectantly. Recovery following microinfarction of the nerve is usually complete within a 3-month follow-up period. In the absence of recovery, the patient should be reinvestigated.

Head trauma, with or without skull fracture, is also a major cause of oculomotor nerve palsy. Mild head trauma causing a third nerve palsy, however, should suggest the presence of a tumor at the base of the skull.

Aberrant regeneration of the third nerve may occur after trauma, aneurysm, congenital third nerve palsy, and migraine. The clinical signs of aberrant regeneration often include abnormal lid movements, most commonly lid elevation with attempted ipsilateral adduction or depression of the eye. If aberrant regeneration is encountered without a history of preceding oculomotor palsy (primary aberrant regeneration), then slowly growing intracavernous mass lesions (meningioma, carotid aneurysm, etc.) are likely, although sometimes no cause can be found.

Isolated lesions (trauma, neurofibroma) of the branches of the third nerve produce partial third nerve palsies involving the structures innervated by the superior or inferior branch.

Trochlear nerve (fourth cranial nerve) The neurons of the fourth nerve nucleus lie dorsally in the rostral brainstem at the level of the inferior colliculi, contiguous to the caudal end of the oculomotor complex. The axons run dorsally and decussate in the anterior medullary velum (the roof of the fourth ventricle), where they are vulnerable to head trauma. The nerve exits the brainstem dorsally, crosses the superior cerebellar artery, runs forward in the cavernous sinus, and enters the orbit through the superior orbital fissure to innervate the superior oblique muscle.

A superior oblique palsy causes vertical diplopia with hypertropia and excyclotorsion of the eye. Many patients compensate for this by adapting a head tilt toward the uninvolved side (i.e., a patient with a right superior oblique palsy will often have a left head tilt). Some patients who have a congenital fourth nerve palsy may be asymptomatic until later in life, when the ability to fuse is lost. Such patients generally have a head tilt documented on childhood and adult photographs.

Damage to the trochlear nerve nucleus by intrinsic brainstem disease (medulloblastoma, ependymoma, metastatic tumor, multiple sclerosis, arteriovenous malformation) cannot be readily distinguished from fascicular nerve palsies. Paresis of the superior oblique muscle with pontine lesions can be obscured by associated conjugate or internuclear gaze defects. In such patients, recognition of a trochlear nerve palsy becomes possible only after the horizontal gaze difficulties have resolved.

Bilateral trochlear nerve pareses may occur with fascicular involvement of both trochlear nerves in the anterior medullary velum by compression, ischemia, hemorrhage, and, most commonly, trauma. Computed tomography (CT) and MRI aid in the topographic diagnosis of such lesions. Neuroimaging has demonstrated an intrinsic lesion in the mesencephalon producing a trochlear paresis and contralateral Horner's syndrome. This is consistent with the known anatomy, in which the sympathetic pathways run through the dorsolateral tegmentum of the mesencephalon adjacent to the trochlear fascicles.

Head trauma, especially blunt frontal injury (motorcycle accidents, vertex blows), is the most common cause of unilateral and bilateral trochlear nerve palsy. Contracoup forces transmitted to the brainstem by the free tentorial edge may injure the nerves in the anterior medullary velum. The second most common cause of a trochlear nerve palsy is ischemic neuropathy, often associated with small-vessel disease such as diabetes (mononeuritis multiplex). Recovery usually occurs within 3 months. Trochlear nerve palsies are also observed with tentorial meningioma, pinealoma, sphenoid sinusitis, encephalitis, and migraine. Management is usually conservative, using vertical prism glasses or unilateral patching to alleviate symptoms. A variety of surgical procedures on the superior oblique or inferior oblique muscle can be performed if conservative treatment is unsatisfactory.

Abducens nerve (sixth nerve) The abducens nucleus is located beneath the floor of the fourth ventricle and lateral to the midline of the pons at the junction of the pons and medulla. The genu of the facial nerve curves over the dorsal and lateral surfaces. The medial longitudinal fasciculus lies adjacent and medial to it. The abducens nucleus contains motor neurons that innervate the ipsilateral lateral rectus muscle and a pool of interneurons whose axons cross the

midline and ascend in the medial longitudinal fasciculus to reach the contralateral oculomotor subnucleus innervating the medial rectus muscle of the opposite eye. The abducens nucleus thus participates in control of horizontal gaze.

The abducens nucleus is susceptible to abnormalities of development or injury in early life. Mobius syndrome consists of a disturbance of horizontal eye movements and facial diplegia. Many cases of Mobius syndrome display a horizontal gaze palsy rather than a simple lateral rectus paralysis, suggesting a failure of development of the abducens nuclei. In cases where only a lateral rectus weakness is apparent, the lesion may be in the abducens nerve or lateral rectus muscle. Failure of normal development of the abducens nucleus is also associated with Duane retraction syndrome; there is an absence of motor neurons innervating the lateral rectus muscle, but preservation in the abducens nucleus of interneurons projecting via the contralateral medial longitudinal fasciculus to the contralateral third nerve subnucleus of the medial rectus muscle. It is postulated that during the developmental stage in these patients, oculomotor neurons intended for various muscle groups innervated by the third cranial nerve are misdirected and innervate the lateral rectus muscle. As a result, patients with Duane syndrome often have a complete abduction deficit but preserved adduction on the affected side. The accompanying retraction of the globe and palpebral fissure narrowing on adduction are due to cofiring of muscles innervated by the oculomotor nerve due to the aberrant developmental oculomotor innervation.

The fascicular portion of the sixth nerve traverses the pons ventrally, laterally, and caudally and passes medial to the olivary nucleus, to exit the brainstem in a groove between the pons and the medulla. The proximity of the sixth nerve nucleus and its fascicular portion to the motor nucleus of the facial nerve, facial nerve fascicle, vestibular nucleus, and descending sympathetic fibers within the brainstem explains the association of sixth nerve deficits with a multitude of disease states.

Causes of nuclear and fascicular sixth nerve lesions include pontine and cerebellar tumors, Wernicke's encephalopathy, and demyelinating disease. Infarction of the pons is an important cause of fascicular sixth nerve palsies, and infarction of the medial inferior pons may produce an ipsilateral abducens palsy, ipsilateral facial weakness, and contralateral hemiplegia—Millard-Gubler syndrome.

After emerging from the brainstem, the nerve runs along the face of the bony clivus to penetrate the dura below the crest of the petrous bone to enter the cavernous sinus. The sixth nerve is not situated within the sinus wall, like the third and fourth cranial nerves, but instead lies within the body of the sinus itself. It enters the orbit through the superior orbital fissure within the annulus of Zinn to innervate the lateral rectus muscle. A sixth nerve palsy causes an inward deviation of the eye and paresis of abduction. Causes of sixth nerve palsy include infarction, aneurysm, tumor, trauma, leptomeningitis, and multiple sclerosis. Papilledema is usually present with a sixth nerve palsy due to raised intracranial pressure. However, despite improved diagnostic techniques, many cases of monocranial nerve palsy remain unexplained (idiopathic).

MULTIPLE OCULAR MOTOR NERVE PALSIES The localization of lesions that cause combinations of third, fourth, or sixth nerve palsies depends on accurate assessment of the various combinations of associated neurologic deficits.

Lesions producing ophthalmoplegia involving the functions of more than one ocular motor nerve and associated with pain or hypesthesia in the distribution of the trigeminal nerve (fifth nerve) can be localized depending on the extent of fifth nerve involvement. The lesion is at the superior orbital fissure or anterior cavernous sinus region if only the first division of nerve V is involved, at the middle to posterior cavernous sinus region if the first (V1) and second (V2) divisions are involved, and in the parasellar region if all three divisions are involved. If the ipsilateral optic nerve is affected, the lesion must be in the orbital apex. Causes of these syndromes include nasopharyngeal carcinomas, granulomatous inflammatory processes (pseudotumor of the orbit or "Tolosa Hunt" syndrome), and lymphoma. Pituitary tumors, meningiomas, chordomas, and other, rarer tumors can produce cavernous sinus–orbital apex syndromes. The diagnosis is aided by neuroimaging of the suspected area, including the nasopharynx.

SUPRANUCLEAR DISORDERS   The bedside diagnosis of brainstem disorders is aided by an understanding of the neuroanatomy of ocular motor control. There are two classes of eye movements, rapid or saccadic movements and slow or pursuit movements. Both systems alter the direction of gaze (eye position in space). Rapid eye movements are used to bring new images onto the fovea. Pursuit eye movements are used to hold the object's image stationary on the moving retina.

Saccadic eye movements are tested by observation of eye movements on command, refixation saccades between two targets, and quick phases of optokinetic nystagmus and/or vestibular stimulation. Saccades and quick phases share the same immediate premotor neural circuitry within the brainstem. The descending pathways transmitting saccadic signals for gaze control are part of a corticobulbar pathway with connections between visual, frontal, and brainstem structures. All decussate in the midbrain to terminate in the contralateral pontine paramedian reticular formation (PPRF) in the brainstem, just rostral to the sixth nerve nucleus. Pursuit eye movements are tested by observation of the eyes tracking a target horizontally and vertically. Three visual cortical areas in the temporal-occipital junction are concerned with control of pursuit eye movements. They are the middle temporal and medial superior temporal cortex and the fundus of the superior temporal cortex. Pursuit pathways descend ipsilaterally to the dorsal lateral pontine nuclei, the Purkinje P cells in the cerebellar flocculus, to the vestibular nuclei and onward to the final common brainstem pathway, the PPRF.

Direct vertical gaze requires bilateral cortical activation. The rostral PPRF acts as the first brainstem center from which fibers project to the pretectal rostral interstitial nucleus of the median longitudinal fasciculus, which is the final vertical gaze center. Paralysis of horizontal and vertical gaze can be produced by lesions affecting cortical, mesencephalic, and pontine centers and their projections. Destruction of the ocular motor nuclei, fascicles, or nerves as well as myasthenia gravis can mimic a gaze palsy. Isolated upward gaze paralysis (Parinaud syndrome) and isolated downward gaze or complete vertical gaze paralysis are produced by lesions involving the mesencephalon and pretectum. Tumors in the region of the pineal gland produce Parinaud syndrome or the sylvian aqueduct syndrome; ocular signs include a supranuclear paralysis of upward gaze, light-near dissociation of the pupils, convergence paresis, skew deviation, and convergence retraction nystagmus. Brainstem infarction is possibly the only cause of selective paralysis of downward gaze, and is caused by occlusion of a single perforating vessel, the posterior thalamosubthalamic paramedian artery.

Degenerative diseases, e.g., progressive supranuclear palsy (see Chap. 371), may selectively or primarily involve the supranuclear structures of the brainstem. Vertical saccades are affected first, being slow and then small. Eventually there is complete loss of voluntary vertical refixations. With chronicity, the horizontal eye movements become similarly affected. Convergence may be impaired. The disease may progress to total ophthalmoplegia. Other degenerative diseases—Huntington chorea, abetalipoproteinema, amyotrophic lateral sclerosis, and olivopontocerebellar degeneration—may be associated with a supranuclear disorder of vertical as well as horizontal gaze. Supranuclear vertical gaze disorders also occur in multiple sclerosis, Whipple's disease, syphilis, brucellosis, tetanus, encephalitis, neurofibromatosis, and tuberculoma, as well as brainstem trauma, including neurosurgical procedures.

Opsoclonus is a striking disorder of saccadic eye movements reflecting the presence of unwanted saccades. It consists of involuntary, arrhythmic, multidirectional, high-amplitude, conjugate back-to-back saccades. The eye movements are usually continuous and persist during sleep. Opsoclonus can occur with encephalitis, trauma, intracranial tumors, hydrocephalus, thalamic hemorrhage, and toxic and metabolic encephalopathies. It occurs as a paraneoplastic or remote effect of neuroblastoma in children and, less commonly, of other carcinomas (ovary, lung, breast) in adults (Chap. 328). Paraneoplastic opsoclonus is accompanied by the presence of antibodies (anti-Purkinje cell or anti-Rhi) in the blood and spinal fluid.

INTERNUCLEAR OPHTHALMOPLEGIA   Clinically, internuclear ophthalmoplegia (INO) is characterized by (1) paresis or paralysis of adduction of the ipsilateral eye on attempted horizontal gaze to the contralateral side and (2) horizontal jerk nystagmus in the contralateral abducting eye. Typically, convergence is intact if the lesion does not extend to the mesencephalon; gaze-evoked vertical nystagmus on upward gaze is frequent. Unilateral INO is due to interruption of the ipsilateral medial longitudinal fasciculus (MLF) after fibers have crossed from the interneurons of the contralateral abducens nucleus projecting to the ipsilateral medial rectus subnucleus. Unilateral internuclear ophthalmoplegia is most commonly due to multiple sclerosis in young adults and to vascular infarction in the elderly. Prognosis for full recovery is good.

Bilateral INO is usually due to brainstem glioma in children and to multiple sclerosis in adults. Myasthenia gravis can mimic both unilateral and bilateral INO.

NYSTAGMUS AND OTHER ENTITIES THAT MIMIC NYSTAGMUS
Nystagmus is a repetitive, to-and-fro movement of the eyes. Pendular nystagmus consists of smooth sinusoidal oscillations, and jerk nystagmus consists of slow drift alternating with corrective quick phases. Normal subjects develop nystagmus in response to vestibular and optokinetic stimuli.

Normally, the vestibular, optokinetic, and pursuit systems each act to hold images steady on the retina, and a neural integrator allows maintenance of eccentric positions of gaze. Disorders of these systems create nystagmus. Identification of the cause of nystagmus requires historical information—especially about drug use (anticonvulsants, haloperidol, lithium) or alcohol abuse—and a complete ocular motor evaluation. The most important clinical types of nystagmus are discussed below.

Congenital nystagmus   Congenital nystagmus is a pendular or jerk nystagmus that remains horizontal in all positions of gaze, is dampened by convergence, and is associated with better vision at near rather than far distances. Patients with congenital nystagmus often have afferent visual system dysfunction.

Labyrinthine-vestibular nystagmus   Disease of the vestibular system causes constant-velocity slow-phase drifts with corrective quick phases that create a "saw-tooth" jerk nystagmus. By convention, the side of the nystagmus is designated by the direction of the quick corrective saccade (fast phase). Vestibular nystagmus may be due to a peripheral or central lesion. In peripheral vestibular disease, the nystagmus is usually of mixed type. For example, in benign positional nystagmus, a mixed vertical-torsional nystagmus is common. In unilateral labyrinthine destruction, a mixed horizontal-torsional nystagmus occurs. Peripheral vestibular nystagmus is suppressed by fixation and exacerbated by changes in head position. Peripheral nystagmus is often associated with severe vertigo, nausea, vomiting, and oscillopsia. Disturbances of central vestibular connections are associated with a central imbalance between semicircular canal inputs and disruption of ascending vestibular or cerebellovestibular connections. Mixed nystagmus can be caused by peripheral labyrinthine or central vestibular disease. Purely bilateral vertical (upbeat, downbeat), torsional, or horizontal nystagmus can only occur with central vestibular disease. Central vestibular nystagmus is poorly suppressed by fixation but exacerbated or induced by changes in head position (Chap. 18).

Four forms of primary position vestibular nystagmus have anatomic localizing value: downbeat, upbeat, horizontal, and torsional nystagmus. Downbeat nystagmus in the primary position and accentuated on lateral gaze occurs with cervicomedullary junction disorders, such as Arnold-Chiari malformation and basilar invagination; in multiple sclerosis, brainstem infarction, cerebellar atrophy, hydrocephalus, metabolic disorders, and familiar periodic ataxia; or as a toxic side effect of anticonvulsant drugs. Lesions associated with primary position upbeat nystagmus are in the tegmentum of the rostral medulla and caudal pons; causes include infarction, demyelination, myelinolysis, and diffuse infiltration with glioma. Horizontal primary position nystagmus is rare and is usually due to peripheral vestibular disease.

Primary position torsional nystagmus is common in the lateral medullary syndrome. With this lesion, the nystagmus may be horizontal or mixed with both torsional and vertical components. Typically, the horizontal nystagmus beats away from the side of the medullary infarction with the eyes in a primary position but beats ipsilaterally when gaze is directed toward •he lesion. Vertical nystagmus, if present, is usually upbeating.

Gaze-evoked nystagmus   Gaze-evoked nystagmus implies a weakness in holding the eyes in an eccentric position due to a defect in the integrator in the brainstem. It is commonly caused by drugs such as sedatives c: anticonvulsants. Asymmetric but conjugate horizontal gaze-evoked nystagmus occurs with unilateral cerebellar disease and cerebellopontine-angle tumors such as acoustic neuroma or meningioma.

REFERENCES

BECK RW et al: A randomized controlled trial of corticosteroids in the treatment of acute optic neuritis. N Engl J Med 326:581, 1992

BURDE RM et al: *Clinical Decisions in Neuro-ophthalmology*, 2nd ed. St. Louis, Mosby, 1992

CRYOTHERAPY FOR RETINOPATHY OF PREMATURITY COOPERATIVE GROUP: Multicenter trial of cryotherapy for retinopathy of prematurity. Arch Ophthalmol 106:471, 1988

DUANE T (ed): *Clinical Ophthalmology*. Philadelphia, Lippincott, 1988

GLASER JS: *Neuroophthalmology*, 2nd ed. Philadelphia, Lippincott 1989

HUMPHRIES P et al: On the molecular genetics of retinitis pigmentosa. Science 256:804, 1992

LEIGH RJ, ZEE DS: *The Neurology of Eye Movements*, 2nd ed. Philadelphia, Davis, 1991

MILLER NR: *Walsh and Hoyt's Clinical Neuroophthalmology*, 4th ed. Baltimore, Williams & Wilkins, 1982

NATHANS J: Rhodopsin: Structure, function, and genetics. Biochemistry 31:4923, 1992

NIKOSKELAINEN EK: Leber hereditary optic neuropathy. Curr Opin Ophthalmol 2:531, 1991

NORTH AMERICAN SYMPTOMATIC CAROTID ENDARTERECTOMY TRIAL COLLABORATORS: Beneficial effect of carotid endarterectomy in symptomatic patients with high-grade carotid stenosis. N Engl J Med 325:445, 1991

OPTIC NEURITIS STUDY GROUP: The clinical profile of optic neuritis: Experience of the optic neuritis treatment trial. Arch Ophthalmol 109:1673, 1991

QUIGLEY HA: Open-angle glaucoma. N Engl J Med 328:1097, 1993

20   DISTURBANCES OF SMELL, TASTE, AND HEARING

JAMES B. SNOW, JR. / JOSEPH B. MARTIN

SMELL   The sense of smell determines the flavor and palatability of food and drink. It serves along with the trigeminal system as a monitor of inhaled chemicals, including dangerous substances such as natural gas, smoke, and air pollutants. Although qualitative sensations of smell are subserved by the olfactory neuroepithelium, many substances are capable of producing somatic sensations of coolness, warmth, and irritation through the trigeminal, glossopharyngeal, and vagal afferents in the nose, oral cavity, tongue, pharynx, and larynx. The sense of smell should be considered as one of several chemosensory systems, since most chemical substances initiate olfactory, trigeminal, and taste perceptions.

The *olfactory neuroepithelium* is located in the superior part of the nasal cavities. It contains an orderly arrangement of bipolar olfactory receptor cells, microvillar cells, sustentacular cells, and basal cells. The dendritic process of the bipolar cell has a bulb-shaped knob or vesicle that projects into the mucous layer and bears six to eight cilia. The receptor sites for odorant molecules are located on the cilia. The microvillar cells are located adjacent to the receptor cells on the surface of the neuroepithelium. The sustentacular cells, unlike their counterparts in the respiratory epithelium, are not specialized to secrete mucus. Their function is unknown. The basal cells are progenitors of other cell types in the olfactory neuroepithelium, including the bipolar receptor cells. There is a regular turnover of the bipolar receptor cells, which function as the primary sensory neurons. In addition, with injury to the cell body or its axon, the receptor cell is replaced by a differentiated basal cell which reestablishes a central neural connection. *Hence these primary sensory neurons are unique among sensory systems in that they are regularly replaced and regenerate after injury.*

The unmyelinated axons of the receptor cells form the fila of the olfactory nerve, pass through the cribriform plate, and terminate within spherical masses of neuropil, termed *glomeruli*, in the olfactory bulb. The glomeruli are a focus of a high degree of convergence of information, since many more fibers enter than leave them. The main second-order neurons are the mitral cells. The primary dendrite of each mitral cell extends into a single glomerulus. Axons of the mitral cells project along with the axons of adjacent tufted cells to the limbic system, including the anterior olfactory nucleus, the prepiriform cortex, the periamygdaloid cortex, the olfactory tubercle, the nucleus of the lateral olfactory tract, and the corticomedial nucleus of the amygdala. Cognitive awareness of smell requires stimulation of the prepiriform cortex or the amygdaloid nuclei.

Odorants are absorbed into the mucus overlying the olfactory neuroepithelium, diffuse to the cilia, and reversibly bind to membrane receptor sites. The process causes conformational changes in the receptor proteins which induce a chain of biochemical events that results in generation of action potentials in the primary neurons. Intensity appears to be coded by the amount of firing in the afferent neurons. Indeed, a clear relationship exists in humans between psychophysical measures of intensity and the magnitude of the evoked potential from the olfactory neuroepithelium. The discovery of a large family of receptor genes suggests that there may be specific receptors for each odorant.

Disturbances of the sense of smell   Disturbances of the sense of smell are caused by conditions that interfere with the access of the odorant to the olfactory neuroepithelium (transport loss), injure the receptor region (sensory loss), or damage central olfactory pathways (neural loss).

Transport olfactory loss can result from swollen nasal mucous membrane in acute viral upper respiratory infections, bacterial rhinitis and sinusitis, and allergic rhinitis, with structural changes in the nasal cavity such as deviations of the nasal septum, polyps, and neoplasms. It is also likely that abnormalities of mucus secretion in which the olfactory cilia are immersed could result in a loss of olfactory sensitivity.

Sensory olfactory losses are caused by destruction of the olfactory neuroepithelium by viral infections, neoplasms, the inhalation of toxic chemicals, drugs that affect cell turnover, and radiation therapy to the head. *Neural olfactory losses* occur in head trauma, with or without fracture of the base of the anterior cranial fossa or cribriform plate area; Parkinson's disease, Alzheimer's disease, Korsakoff's psychosis, and vitamin B_{12} deficiency; neoplasms of the anterior cranial fossa; neurosurgical procedures; administration of neurotoxic agents (e.g., ethanol, amphetamines, topical cocaine, aminoglycosides, tetracycline, cigarette smoke); and in some congenital disorders such as Kallmann's syndrome. Other endocrine disorders, including Cushing's syndrome, hypothyroidism, and diabetes mellitus, can affect smell perception.

From the psychophysical point of view, disturbances of the sense of smell may be categorized by either the patient's complaint or the objective sensory measurements as *total anosmia* (general anosmia)—

inability to detect any qualitative olfactory sensations; *partial anosmia*—ability to detect some, but not all, qualitative olfactory sensations; *specific anosmia*—loss of ability to appreciate only one or a very limited number of odorants; *total hyposmia* (general hyposmia)—decreased sensitivity to all odorants; *partial hyposmia*—decreased sensitivity to some odorants; *dysosmia* (cacosmia or paraosmia)—distortion in the perception of an odor, i.e., the perception of an unpleasant odor when a pleasant odorant is being presented or the perception of an odor when there is no odorant in the environment; *total hyperosmia* (general hyperosmia)—increased sensitivity to all odorants; *partial hyperosmia*—increased sensitivity to some odorants; and *agnosia*—inability to classify, contrast, or identify odor sensations verbally, even though the ability to distinguish between odorants or to recognize them may be normal.

CLINICAL EVALUATION The history of the onset and development of the disturbance of the sense of smell may be of paramount importance in making an etiologic diagnosis. Unilateral anosmia is rarely a complaint. Only by separate testing of smell in each nasal cavity can it be recognized. Bilateral anosmia, on the other hand, does bring patients to medical attention. Anosmic patients usually complain of a loss of the sense of taste even though their taste thresholds may be within normal limits. In actuality, they are complaining of a loss of flavor detection, which is mainly an olfactory function. Flavor appreciation depends on the olfactory detection of volatile substances in food and beverages as well as the sense of taste. The physical examination should include a complete examination of the ears, upper respiratory tract, and head and neck. A neurologic examination emphasizing the cranial nerves is essential. CT scans of the head with enhancement are required to rule out neoplasms of the anterior cranial fossa, unsuspected fractures of the anterior cranial fossa, paranasal sinusitis, and neoplasms of the nasal cavity and paranasal sinuses.

The sensory evaluation of olfactory function is necessary for corroboration of the patient's complaint, evaluation of the efficacy of treatment, and determination of the degree of permanent impairment. The first step in the sensory evaluation is to determine the degree to which qualitative sensations are present. For this assessment, a smell identification test is used that consists of a 40-item, forced choice, microencapsulated odor, scratch-and-sniff paradigm. For example, one of the items reads, ''This odor smells most like (a) chocolate, (b) banana, (c) onion, or (d) fruit punch,'' and the patient is instructed to answer one of the alternatives. The test is highly reliable (short-term test-retest reliability $r = 0.95$) and is sensitive to age and sex differences (Fig. 20-1). It is an accurate quantitative determination of the relative degree of olfactory deficit. Persons with a total loss of smell function score in the range of 7 to 19 out of 40. The average score for total anosmics is slightly higher than that expected on the basis of chance because of the inclusion of some odorants which act by trigeminal stimulation.

The second step is to establish a detection threshold for the odorant phenyl ethyl alcohol, using a graduated stimulus. Sensitivity for each side of the nose is determined with a detection threshold for phenyl ethyl methyl ethyl carbinol. Nasal resistance is measured with anterior rhinomanometry for each side of the nose.

Techniques have been developed to biopsy the olfactory neuroepithelium, but in view of the widespread degeneration of the olfactory neuroepithelium and intercalation of respiratory epithelium in the olfactory area of adults with no apparent olfactory dysfunction, biopsy material must be interpreted cautiously.

DIFFERENTIAL DIAGNOSIS At the present time, there are no psychophysical methods to differentiate sensory from neural olfactory losses. Fortunately, the history of the disease provides important clues to the cause. The leading causes of olfactory disorders are head trauma and viral infections. Head trauma is a more frequent cause of anosmia in children and young adults, and viral infections are more important causes of anosmia in older adults.

Cranial trauma is followed by uni- or bilateral impairment of smell in 5 to 10 percent of cases. Frontal injuries and fractures disrupt the

FIGURE 20-1 Smell identification test. Scores for a group of male and female subjects 5 to 99 years in age are shown. *(Reprinted with permission from RL Doty et al. Copyright 1984 by the AAAS.)*

cribriform plate and olfactory axons which perforate it. Sometimes there is an associated cerebrospinal fluid (CSF) rhinorrhea resulting from a tearing of the dura overlying the cribriform plate and paranasal sinuses. Anosmia also may follow blows to the occiput. Once traumatic anosmia develops, it is usually permanent; only about 10 percent of patients ever improve or recover. Perversion of the sense of smell may occur as a phase in the recovery process.

Viral infections destroy the olfactory neuroepithelium, and it is replaced by respiratory epithelium. Congenital anosmias are rare but important. Kallmann's syndrome is a neuronal migration defect for which the X-linked gene (KAL) has been cloned. It is characterized by congenital anosmia and hypogonadotropic hypogonadism (see Chap. 331). The hypothalamic and olfactory bulb defects result from failure of migration from the olfactory placode of olfactory receptor neurons and neurons synthesizing gonadotropin-releasing hormone. Anosmia also can occur in albinos. The receptor cells are present but are hypoplastic, lack cilia, and do not project above the surrounding supporting cells.

Meningioma of the inferior frontal region is the most frequent neoplastic cause of anosmia; rarely, anosmia can occur with glioma of the frontal lobe. Occasionally, pituitary adenomas, craniopharyngiomas, suprasellar meningiomas, and aneurysms of the anterior part of the circle of Willis extend forward and damage olfactory structures. These tumors and hamartomas also may induce seizures with olfactory hallucinations, indicating involvement of the uncus of the temporal lobe.

Dysosmia, subjective distortions of olfactory perception, may occur with intranasal disease that partially impairs smell or may represent a phase in the recovery from a neurogenic anosmia. Most dysomic disturbances consist of disagreeable or foul odors, and they may be accompanied by distortions of taste. Dysosmia is associated with depression.

TREATMENT Therapy for patients with transport olfactory losses due to allergic rhinitis, bacterial rhinitis and sinusitis, polyps, neoplasms, and structural abnormalities of the nasal cavities can be undertaken rationally and with a high chance of improvement. Allergy management, antibiotic therapy, topical and systemic glucocorticoid therapy, and operations for nasal polyps, deviation of the nasal septum, and chronic hyperplastic sinusitis are frequently effective in restoring the sense of smell.

There is no treatment with demonstrated efficacy for sensorineural olfactory losses. Fortunately, spontaneous recovery often occurs. Zinc and vitamin therapy are advocated by some. Profound zinc deficiency can undoubtedly result in losses and distortion of the sense of smell, but it is not a clinical problem except in very limited geographic areas. Vitamin therapy has mainly been in the form of vitamin A. The epithelial degeneration associated with vitamin A deficiency can cause anosmia, but vitamin A deficiency is not a common clinical problem in the United States.

TASTE Many patients with a loss of olfactory sensitivity also complain of a loss of the sense of taste. On psychophysical testing, most of these patients have normal detection thresholds for taste. Disturbances of the sense of taste are far less frequent than disturbances of the sense of smell.

The taste receptor cells are located in the taste buds, spherical groups of cells arranged like the segments of a citrus fruit. At the surface, the taste bud has a pore into which microvilli of the receptor cells project. Taste buds have a similar appearance wherever they are located. Unlike the olfactory system, the receptor cell is not the primary neuron. Instead, gustatory afferent nerve fibers contact individual taste receptor cells.

The sense of taste is mediated through the facial, glossopharyngeal, and vagal nerves. The gustatory system consists of at least five receptor populations. Taste buds are located in the foliate papillae along the lateral margin of the tongue, in the fungiform papillae throughout the dorsum of the tongue, in the circumvallate papillae at the junction of the dorsum and the base of the tongue, and in the palate, epiglottis, larynx, and esophagus. The chorda tympani branch of the facial nerve subserves taste from the anterior two-thirds of the tongue. The posterior third of the tongue is supplied by the lingual branch of the glossopharyngeal nerve. Afferents from the palate travel with the greater superficial petrosal nerve to the geniculate ganglion and thence via the facial nerve to the brainstem. The internal branch of the superior laryngeal nerve of the vagus nerve contains the taste afferents from the larynx including the epiglottis and esophagus.

The central connections of the nerves terminate in the brainstem in the nucleus of the tractus solitarius. The fibers of the chorda tympani and greater superficial petrosal nerves go to the cephalic portion of the nucleus. The glossopharyngeal gustatory fibers go to the middle, and the superior laryngeal nerve fibers go to the caudal portion of the nucleus. The central pathway from the nucleus of the tractus solitarius projects to the ipsilateral parabrachial nuclei of the pons. Two divergent pathways project from the parabrachial nuclei. One ascends to the gustatory relay in the dorsal thalamus, synapses, and continues to the cortex of the insula. There is also evidence for a direct pathway from the parabrachial nuclei to the cortex. (Olfaction and taste appear to be unique among sensory systems in that at least some fibers bypass the thalamus.) The other pathway from the parabrachial nuclei goes to the ventral forebrain, including the lateral hypothalamus, substantia innominata, central nucleus of the amygdala, and the stria terminalis.

Tastants gain access to the receptor cells through the taste pore. Four classes of taste are recognized: sweet, salt, sour, and bitter. Individual gustatory afferent fibers almost always respond to a number of different chemicals. Response patterns of gustatory afferent axons can be grouped into classes based on the stimulus chemical that produces the largest response. For example, for sucrose-best response neurons, the second-best stimulus is almost always sodium chloride. The fact that individual gustatory afferent fibers respond to a large number of different chemicals led to the *across-fiber-pattern* theory of gustatory coding, while the best-stimulus analysis led to the concept of *labeled* afferents. It appears that labeled fibers are important for establishing gross quality, but the across-fiber pattern within a best-stimulus category, and perhaps among categories, is needed for discriminating chemicals within qualities. For example, sweetness may be carried by sucrose-best neurons, but the differentiation of sucrose and fructose may require a comparison of the relative activity among sucrose-best, salt-best, and quinine-best neurons. As with olfaction and other sensory systems, intensity appears to be encoded by the quantity of neural activity.

Disturbances of the sense of taste Disturbances of the sense of taste are caused by conditions that interfere with the access of the tastant to the receptor cells in the taste bud (transport loss), injure

receptor cells (sensory loss), or damage gustatory afferent nerves and central gustatory pathways (neural loss).

Transport gustatory losses result from xerostomia due to many causes, including Sjögren's syndrome, heavy-metal intoxication, and bacterial colonization of the taste pore. The salivary milieu of the receptors may prove to be important to diverse causes of gustatory loss.

Sensory gustatory losses are caused by inflammatory and degenerative diseases in the oral cavity; a vast number of drugs, particularly those which interfere with cell turnover such as antithyroid and antineoplastic agents; radiation therapy to the oral cavity and pharynx; viral infections; endocrine disorders; neoplasms; and aging.

Neural gustatory losses occur with neoplasms, trauma, and operations in which the gustatory afferents are injured. Taste buds degenerate when their gustatory afferents are transected but remain when their somatosensory afferents are severed.

CLINICAL MANIFESTATIONS From the psychophysical point of view, disturbances of the sense of taste may be categorized by either the patient's complaint or the objective sensory measurements as *total ageusia*—inability to detect the qualities of sweet, salt, bitter, or sour; *partial ageusia*—ability to detect some of but not all the qualitative gustatory sensations; *specific ageusia*—inability to detect the taste quality of certain substances; *total hypoguesia*—decreased sensitivity to all tastants; *partial hypoguesia*—decreased sensitivity to some tastants; and *dysgeusia*—distortion in the perception of a tastant, i.e., the perception of the wrong quality when a tastant is presented or the perception of a taste when there has been no tastant ingested. Confusions of sour and bitter are common and, at times, may be semantic misunderstandings. Frequently, however, they have physiologic or pathophysiologic bases.

It may be possible to differentiate between the loss of flavor recognition in patients with olfactory losses who complain of a loss of taste as well as smell by asking if they are able to taste sweetness in sodas, saltiness in potato chips, etc.

Patients who complain of loss of taste should be evaluated psychophysically for gustatory function in addition to being evaluated for olfactory function. The first step is to perform suprathreshold whole-mouth taste testing for quality, intensity, and pleasantness perception with sucrose, citric acid, caffeine, and sodium chloride. In the quantification of the sense of taste, detection thresholds are obtained by applying graduated dilutions to the tongue quadrants or by whole-mouth sips. Finally, suprathreshold magnitude estimation may be used to shed further light on the patient's complaint. Electric taste testing (*electrogustometry*) is used clinically to identify taste deficits in specific quadrants of the tongue.

Biopsy of the foliate or fungiform papillae for histopathologic study of taste buds remains experimental but holds promise of shedding light on the categorization of taste disorders.

DIFFERENTIAL DIAGNOSIS As with olfaction, psychophysical methods for differentiating transport, sensory, and neural gustatory losses are not available. Once there is objective evidence of a disorder of taste, it is important to establish, as is done in other neurologic deficits, an anatomic diagnosis before proceeding to an etiologic diagnosis. The history of the disease often provides important clues to the cause. For example, absence of taste on the anterior two-thirds of the tongue associated with a facial paralysis indicates that the lesion is proximal to the point of junction of the chorda tympani branch with the facial nerve in the mastoid.

TREATMENT Therapy for gustatory losses remains limited. Artificial saliva benefits some patients with a disturbed salivary milieu. Treatment for bacterial and fungal infections of the oral cavity is appropriate and may be helpful. Withdrawal of drugs affecting cell turnover is usually helpful if the patient's general condition permits. Zinc and vitamin therapy for gustatory losses is advocated by some but lacks demonstrated efficacy. No therapeutic strategies exist for the sensorineural disorders of taste.

HEARING Hearing occurs by air conduction and bone conduction. In air conduction, sound waves reach the ear by propagation in air, enter the external auditory canal, and set the tympanic membrane in motion, which in turn moves the malleus, incus, and stapes. Movement of the footplate of the stapes causes pressure changes in the fluid-filled inner ear eliciting a traveling wave in the basilar membrane of the cochlea. Hearing by bone conduction occurs when the sounding source, in contact with the head, results in vibration of the bones of the skull, including the temporal bone, producing a traveling wave in the basilar membrane. In either case, the traveling wave moves from the base to the apex of the cochlea. Hairs (stereocilia) of the hair cells of the organ of Corti, which rests on the basilar membrane, are imbedded in the tectorial membrane and are deformed by the traveling wave. A point of maximal displacement of the basilar membrane determined by the frequency of the stimulating tone occurs with each traveling wave. High-frequency tones cause maximal displacement of the basilar membrane near the base of the cochlea. As the frequency of the stimulating tone decreases, the point of maximal displacement moves toward the apex of the cochlea.

The inner and outer hair cells of the organ of Corti have different innervation patterns, but both are mechanoreceptors. The outer hair cells have an internal organization that is in certain respects similar to muscle cells. Not only does the organ of Corti respond to acoustic stimulation, it also produces acoustic energy that can be detected in the external auditory canal with sensitive microphones. These otoacoustic emissions occur spontaneously and can be evoked by acoustic stimulation. The sources of this acoustic energy are the outer hair cells.

Motility of outer hair cells occurs with mechanical (acoustical) and electrical stimulation, iontophoretically applied acetylcholine, and changes in their internal and external ionic milieu and is modulated by stimulation of the efferent olivocochlear bundle.

The outer hair cells are capable of slow and fast motility. Slow elongation and contraction occurs with increased intracellular calcium in the presence of ATP, the application of acetylcholine, and changes in the ionic environment (increased potassium, which depolarizes the cell), while rapid motility occurs with mechanical (acoustic) and direct-current electrical stimulation. The electrokinetic membrane is located in the outer or lateral wall of the outer hair cell. Fast contractile activity occurs with changes in the membrane potential. The electromotility is driven by a novel and perhaps unique membrane-based force generator which can achieve audible frequencies.

The motility of the outer hair cells alters the micromechanics of the inner hair cells and thereby satisfies the long-sought cochlear amplifier required to explain the exquisite sensitivity and frequency selectivity of the cochlea.

A resting direct-current potential, the *endocochlear potential*, exists in the scala media and at the stereocilia end of the hair cells. It is generated by the stria vascularis. It is present whether there is acoustic stimulation or not. It has a magnitude of 80 mV, not unlike the intracellular potential, but its polarity is positive within the endolymph relative to the perilymph. It increases the potential differential at the stereocilia end of the hair cell, which undoubtedly is of importance in transduction.

As the traveling wave moves along the basilar membrane, the stereocilia are deformed and several receptor potentials are produced: the cochlear microphonic and the positive and negative summating potentials. It is thought that these receptor potentials arise at the apical end of the stereocilia. It may be that the summating potentials are generated largely by the inner hair cells and the cochlear microphonic is generated by the outer hair cells. The summating potential represents a direct-current shift that approximates the "envelope" of the acoustical stimulus. The cochlear microphonic potential is an alternating-current response that faithfully represents the frequency and intensity of the stimulating tone.

The current concept of cochlear transduction is that displacement of the tips of the stereocilia allows potassium to flow into the cell, resulting in its depolarization. The potassium causes calcium channels near the base to open and allow calcium to enter the cell. The calcium ions stimulate transmitter release. The action potential in the eighth

nerve occurs 0.5 ms after the onset of the cochlear microphonic. This latency is taken as evidence for release of an as yet unidentified neurotransmitter at the hair cell and cochlear nerve dendrite interface. Each of the cochlear nerve neurons can be activated at a frequency and intensity specific for that cell. This phenomenon of the characteristic or best frequency occurs at each point of the central auditory pathway: dorsal and ventral cochlear nuclei, trapezoid body, superior olivary complex, lateral lemniscus, inferior colliculus, medial geniculate body, and auditory cortex. At low frequencies, individual auditory nerve fibers can respond more or less synchronously with the stimulating tone. At higher frequencies, phase-locking occurs so that neurons take turns in responding to particular phases of the cycle of the sound wave. Intensity is encoded by the amount of neural activity in individual neurons, the number of neurons that are active, and the specific neurons that are activated.

Disturbances of the sense of hearing   A loss of hearing can result from lesions in the external auditory canal, middle ear, inner ear, or central auditory pathways. Lesions in the external auditory canal or middle ear cause conductive hearing losses, while lesions in the inner ear or eighth nerve cause sensorineural hearing losses.

Conductive hearing losses result from obstruction of the external auditory canal by cerumen, debris and foreign bodies, swelling of the lining of the canal, and stenosis and neoplasms of the canal. Perforations of the tympanic membrane, as in chronic otitis media, disruption of the ossicular chain, as occurs with necrosis of the long process of the incus in trauma or infection, fixation of the ossicles as in otosclerosis, and fluid, scarring, or neoplasms in the middle ear also result in conductive hearing losses. *Sensory hearing losses* are due principally to damage to the hair cells of the organ of Corti caused by intense noise, viral infections, ototoxic drugs, fractures of the temporal bone, meningitis, cochlear otosclerosis, Ménière's disease, and aging. Neural hearing losses are due mainly to cerebellar angle tumors such as acoustic neuromas but also may result from any neoplastic, vascular, demyelinating, infectious, or degenerative disease or trauma affecting the central auditory pathways.

CLINICAL EVALUATION OF HEARING   The physical examination should evaluate the external ear canal and tympanic membrane. Careful inspection of the nose, nasopharynx, and upper respiratory tract is indicated. The other cranial nerves should be carefully evaluated. Conductive and sensorineural hearing losses can be differentiated by comparing the threshold of hearing by air conduction with that elicited by bone conduction. Testing the hearing by air conduction is accomplished by presenting the stimulus in air. Hearing by air conduction is affected by the patency of the external auditory canal, the efficiency of the middle ear, and the integrity of the inner ear, eighth nerve, and central auditory pathways. Testing the hearing by bone conduction is accomplished by placing the stem of a vibrating tuning fork or an oscillator of an audiometer in contact with the head. Hearing by bone conduction bypasses the external auditory canal and middle ear and tests the integrity of the inner ear, eighth nerve, and central auditory pathways. If air-conduction thresholds are elevated and bone-conduction thresholds are in the normal range, the lesion causing hearing loss is in the external auditory canal or middle ear. If both air-conduction and bone-conduction thresholds are elevated, the lesion is in the inner ear, eighth nerve, or central auditory pathways. Of course, conductive and sensorineural hearing losses can coexist, in which case both the air-conduction and bone-conduction thresholds are elevated, but in this case, air-conduction thresholds are elevated more than bone-conduction thresholds.

The Weber and Rinne tuning fork tests are used to differentiate conductive from sensorineural hearing losses. The Weber tuning fork test may be performed with a 256- or 512-Hz fork. The Rinne tuning fork test is most sensitive in detecting mild conductive hearing losses if a 256-Hz fork is used. Weber's test is performed by placing the stem of a vibrating tuning fork on the head in the midline and asking the patient whether the tone is heard in both ears or better in one ear than in the other. With a unilateral conductive hearing loss, the tone is perceived in the affected ear. With a unilateral sensorineural hearing loss, the tone is perceived in the unaffected ear. Rinne's test compares the ability to hear by air conduction with the ability to hear by bone conduction. The tines of a vibrating tuning fork are held near the opening of the external auditory canal, and then the stem is placed on the mastoid process. The patient is asked to indicate whether the tone is louder by air conduction or bone conduction. Normally, a tone is heard louder by air conduction than by bone conduction. With a conductive hearing loss, the bone-conduction stimulus is perceived as louder than the air-conduction stimulus. With sensorineural hearing losses, both air-conduction and bone-conduction perceptions are reduced, but the air-conduction stimulus is perceived as louder, as it is in normal hearing. The combined information from the Weber and Rinne tests permits a tentative conclusion as to whether a conductive or sensorineural hearing loss is present.

Measurement of hearing Quantification of hearing loss is obtained with an audiometer, an electronic device that allows the presentation of specific frequencies at specific intensities to each ear by either air or bone conduction. The testing is done in a sound-attenuated chamber, and masking, usually with broad-spectrum noise, is presented to the nontest ear so that responses are based on perception from the ear under test. Frequencies from 250 to 8000 Hz are used in clinical testing. The responses are measured in decibels. A decibel (dB) is equal to 10 times the logarithm of the ratio of the acoustic power required to achieve threshold in the patient to the acoustic power required to achieve threshold in a normal hearing person. An *audiogram* is a plot of intensity in decibels versus frequency.

The audiometric pattern of hearing loss is often of diagnostic value. Conductive hearing losses usually have a fairly equal threshold elevation for each frequency. Conductive hearing losses with a large mass component, as is often seen in middle ear effusions, have a greater elevation of thresholds in the higher frequencies. Conductive hearing losses with a large stiffness component, as in fixation of the footplate of the stapes in early otosclerosis, have a greater elevation of thresholds in the lower frequencies. In general, sensorineural hearing losses tend to have a greater threshold elevation at each higher frequency. Interesting exceptions to this generalization are noise-induced hearing loss, in which the loss at 4000 Hz is greater than it is at higher frequencies, and in Ménière's disease, particularly in the early stages of the disease, where thresholds are elevated more in lower than in higher frequencies.

Speech audiometry provides essential additional information. The *spondee threshold* is defined as the intensity at which speech is recognized as a meaningful symbol and is obtained by presenting through an audiometer two-syllable words with an equal accent on each syllable. The intensity at which the patient can repeat 50 percent of the words correctly is the spondee threshold and usually approximates the average threshold at the speech frequencies (500, 1000, and 2000 Hz). Once the spondee threshold is determined, the discrimination or word-recognition ability is tested by presenting one-syllable words at 25 to 40 dB above the spondee threshold. The words are phonetically balanced (PB) in that the phonemes (speech sounds) occur in the list of words at the same frequency that they occur in ordinary conversational English. An individual with normal hearing can repeat 90 to 100 percent of the PB words correctly. Likewise, individuals with a conductive hearing loss do well in discrimination testing. On the other hand, patients with a sensorineural hearing loss have a loss of discrimination attributable to the loss of peripheral analysis of sound in the inner ear or eighth nerve. With a lesion in the inner ear, the discrimination is moderately affected, usually in the 50 to 80 percent range, while with neural lesions, the discrimination is severely affected, often in the 0 to 50 percent range.

The discrimination testing may then be done at higher intensities than 25 to 40 dB above the spondee threshold to determine the performance-intensity function. A deterioration in discrimination ability at higher intensities suggests a lesion in the eighth nerve or central auditory pathways.

Tympanometry measures the impedance of the middle ear to sound. A sounding source and microphone are introduced into the ear canal with an airtight seal. The amount of sound that is absorbed through the middle ear or reflected from the middle ear is measured at the microphone. In conductive hearing losses, more sound is reflected than in the normal middle ear. The pressure in the ear canal can be increased or decreased from atmospheric pressure. Normally, the middle ear is most compliant at atmospheric pressure. With a negative pressure in the middle ear, as with eustachian tube obstruction, the point of maximal compliance occurs with negative pressure in the ear canal. With discontinuity of the ossicular chain, no point of maximal compliance can be obtained. Tympanometry is particularly useful in the identification and diagnosis of middle ear effusions in children.

During tympanometry, an intense tone (80 dB above the hearing threshold) elicits contraction of the stapedius muscle. The change in compliance of the middle ear with contraction of the stapedius muscle can be detected. The presence or absence of this *acoustic reflex* is important in the anatomic localization of facial nerve paralysis. The presence or absence of *acoustic reflex decay* helps differentiate sensory from neural hearing losses. In neural hearing loss, the reflex adapts or decays with time.

In order to evaluate a patient with a loss of hearing, the minimum audiologic assessment should include the measurement of pure tone air-conduction and bone-conduction thresholds, spondee threshold, discrimination score, performance-intensity function, tympanometry, acoustic reflexes, and acoustic-reflex decay. This information provides a comprehensive screening evaluation of the whole auditory system and allows one to determine whether further differentiation of a sensory (cochlear) from a neural (retrocochlear) hearing loss is indicated.

In addition to these tests, testing for recruitment, the short increment sensitivity index, tone decay, Békésy audiometry, and auditory brainstem evoked responses (ABR) help differentiate sensory from neural hearing losses. Of these, ABR is the most powerful means of differentiating the site of sensorineural hearing loss (see Chap. 366). In response to sound, five distinct waves can be recorded with computer averaging from scalp surface electrodes. Poor or absent waveforms, abnormal latency of waves, and abnormal interwave latency are evidence of lesions in the eighth nerve and brainstem. In addition, ABR is valuable in situations in which patients cannot or will not give reliable voluntary thresholds. It is also used to measure auditory function in neonates and young children and to monitor the integrity of the auditory nerve and brainstem in various clinical situations, including intraoperatively and in determination of brain death.

Otoacoustic emissions can be measured with sensitive microphones inserted into the external auditory canal in infants, children, and adults. The emissions may be spontaneous or evoked with sound stimulation. The presence of otoacoustic emissions indicates that the outer hair cells are intact and can be used as important evidence in distinguishing sensory from neural hearing losses. Otoacoustic emissions are particularly robust in infants.

The measurement of otoacoustic emissions can be done rapidly and with limited technical expertise in newborns. This technique promises to become the preferred method of screening neonates for hearing impairment. Currently, early identification of hearing impairment depends on the use of high-risk registries and testing of high-risk infants with ABR. High risk is indicated by a family history of hearing impairment, prenatal infection, prematurity, low birth weight, neonatal anoxia, a low Apgar score, neonatal jaundice, and neonatal infection. Unfortunately, 50 percent of infants with profound hearing impairment are not identified by use of ABR in high-risk infants. In the United States, the average age of identification of profound hearing impairment is 2½ years.

The natural acquisition and development of language depend on hearing language. The critical period for language acquisition is the first 2 years of life. Therefore, the early identification of hearing impairment in infants is of the greatest importance so that amplification with a hearing aid and special education can commence within the first several months of life.

In addition to the universal screening of infants for hearing impairment, the hearing should be assessed in all children before the first formal educational experience (preschool or kindergarten). Hearing also should be measured in the late teenage period when otosclerosis and noise-induced hearing loss begin to appear and in the sixth decade of life when presbycusis makes its appearance. Known causes of hearing impairment in addition to the risk factors already mentioned are meningitis, head trauma, middle ear infections and effusions, administration of ototoxic drugs (e.g., salicylates, quinine and its synthetic analogues, aminoglycoside antibiotics, loop diuretics such as furosemide and ethacrynic acid, and cancer chemotherapeutic agents such as *cis*-platinum), and noise exposure. At any time in life when one of these hearing risks is encountered, an audiologic assessment should be carried out.

Ten million Americans have noise-induced hearing loss, and 20 million are exposed to hazardous noise in their employment. Noise-induced hearing loss results from recreational as well as occupational activities and begins in adolescence, particularly among boys as they begin to engage in high-risk activities, such as wood and metal working with electrical equipment and target practice and hunting with small firearms. All internal-combustion and electric engines, including snow and leaf blowers, snowmobiles, outboard motors, and chain saws, require protection of the user with hearing protectors such as ear plugs or fluid-filled ear muffs. Virtually all noise-induced hearing loss is preventable through education, which should begin before the teenage years.

Programs of industrial conservation of hearing are required when the exposure over an 8-h period averages 85 dB on the A scale. Workers in such noisy environments can be protected with preemployment audiologic assessment, the mandatory use of hearing protectors, and annual audiologic assessments.

CLINICAL ASSESSMENT OF A COMPLAINT OF HEARING LOSS   In evaluating patients who complain of loss of hearing, associated symptoms of tinnitus, vertigo, difficulty with balance, earache, otorrhea, and aural fullness should be sought along with a careful reconstruction of the history of evolution of the hearing deficit. A sudden onset of unilateral hearing loss, with or without tinnitus, may represent a viral infection in the inner ear. Gradual progression in a hearing deficit is common with otosclerosis, noise-induced hearing loss, acoustic neurinoma, or Ménière's disease. In the latter case, intermittent tinnitus and vertigo are usual. Hearing loss can occur with demyelinative lesions in the brainstem.

One in 1000 infants is born with profound hearing impairment. At least 50 percent of congenital deafness has a genetic basis. A larger number of such individuals develop hereditary hearing impairment in childhood and later in life. Between 70 and 80 percent of hereditary hearing impairment is autosomal recessive, and between 15 and 20 percent is autosomal dominant. Less than 5 percent is X-linked. Approximately 25 percent of hereditary hearing impairment occurs in syndromes in which other organ systems are affected. Greater progress has been made in finding the genes for syndromes of hereditary deafness because of the ease of making the determination of the hereditary basis of the hearing impairment. The gene for Waardenburg's syndrome (failure of melanocytes to migrate from the neural crest, resulting in deafness and pigmentary and integumentary changes) type 1 has been mapped to chromosome 2, and the gene for Usher's syndrome (deafness, vestibular loss, and blindness due to retinitis pigmentosa) type 2 has been mapped to chromosome 1. The genes for one form of Alport's syndrome (deafness and glomerulonephritis leading to renal failure), albinism, and neurofibromatosis type 2 (bilateral acoustic neurinomas) have been found. The first nonsyndromic deafness gene has been found in a Costa Rican kindred with an autosomal dominant hearing impairment on the long arm of chromosome 5. It is likely that most forms of hearing impairment will be found to have a genetic basis, including the predisposition to noise-induced hearing loss and presbycusis.

Between 30 and 35 percent of individuals over 65 years of age have a hearing loss that is sufficiently great to require a hearing aid.

Presbycusis is characterized by a loss of discrimination for phonemes, recruitment (abnormal growth of loudness), and particular difficulty in understanding speech in noisy environments.

Tinnitus is defined as the perception of a sound when there is no sound in the environment. It may have a buzzing, roaring, or ringing quality and may be pulsatile (synchronous with the heartbeat). Tinnitus is usually associated with a conductive or sensorineural loss of hearing. The pathophysiology of tinnitus is not well understood. The cause of the tinnitus can usually be determined by finding the cause of the associated hearing loss. Tinnitus may be the first symptom of a serious condition such as a vestibular schwannoma. Pulsatile tinnitus requires evaluation of the vascular system of the head to exclude vascular tumors such as glomus jugulare tumors, aneurysms, and stenotic lesions.

DIFFERENTIAL DIAGNOSIS   Many patients with sensorineural hearing losses should have the vestibular system evaluated with electronystagmography and caloric testing (see Chap. 18). Most patients with conductive hearing losses should have CT of the temporal tones. Patients with unilateral or asymmetric sensorineural hearing losses should have magnetic resonance imaging of the head with gadolinium enhancement.

PREVENTION   Conductive hearing losses may be prevented by prompt and appropriate antibiotic therapy of adequate duration for acute otitis media and by reventilation of the middle ear with tympanostomy tubes in middle ear effusions lasting 6 weeks or longer. Loss of vestibular function and deafness due to aminoglycoside antibiotics can largely be prevented by careful monitoring of serum peak and trough levels. Noise-induced hearing loss can be prevented by avoidance of exposure to loud noise or by regular use of ear plugs or fluid-filled muffs to attenuate intense sound. Vaccination of infants against type B *Haemophilus influenzae* meningitis will prevent a major cause of acquired deafness, as has immunization for measles, mumps, and rubella.

TREATMENT   Most patients with conductive hearing losses can have the middle ear reconstructed using procedures such as tympanoplasty after chronic otitis media and trauma and stapedectomy for otosclerosis. Tympanostomy tubes allow the prompt return of hearing to normal in children and adults with middle ear effusions. Hearing aids are effective and well-tolerated for patients with conductive hearing losses. Patients with mild, moderate, and severe sensorineural hearing losses are regularly rehabilitated with hearing aids of varying configuration and strength. However, the problem of understanding conversation with a hearing aid in noise remains. Hearing aids have been improved to provide greater fidelity and have been miniaturized. High-frequency emphasis, needed for many sensorineural hearing losses, has been achieved principally by venting the ear mold and with filters. The augmentation of soft sounds and the nonamplification of intense sounds has been achieved. Digital hearing aids lend themselves to programming for the individual, and multiple and directional microphones at the ear level help some with difficulty of hearing with a hearing aid in noisy surroundings. Since all hearing aids amplify noise as well as speech, the only absolute solution to the problem found so far is to place the microphone closer to the speaker than the noise source. This arrangement is not possible with a self-contained, cosmetically acceptable device. It is cumbersome and requires a user-friendly environment.

In many situations, including lectures and the theater, hearing-impaired persons benefit from assistive devices that are based on the principle of having the speaker closer to the microphone than any source of noise. Assistive devices include infrared and FM transmission as well as an electromagnetic loop around the room for transmission to the individual's hearing aid. Hearing aids with telecoils also can be used with properly equipped telephones in the same way.

Cochlear implants are neural prostheses which convert sound energy to electrical energy and which can be used to stimulate the auditory division of the eighth nerve directly. Cochlear implants consist of electrodes that are inserted into the cochlea, speech processors that extract acoustical elements of speech for conversion to electric currents, and a means of transmitting the electrical energy through the skin. Most commonly for this purpose an induction coil is held over an implanted induction coil with magnets in each coil. In most causes of profound hearing impairment, the auditory hair cells are lost, but the ganglionic cells of the auditory division of the eighth nerve are preserved. Cochlear implants are appropriate for children and adults with hearing impairment that is so profound that they are not able to obtain any help with a hearing aid in understanding speech. Worldwide, more than 7000 deaf individuals, 1300 of whom are children, have had cochlear implants. They experience sound which helps with speech reading and allows some open-set word recognition. It is anticipated that improvements in the electrode design and speech processors will permit further improvement in understanding speech. The implant also allows the recipient to hear and identify environmental sounds and distinguish between men's and women's voices. It is also a help in modulating the person's own voice.

For individuals who have had both eighth nerves destroyed by trauma or bilateral acoustic neurinomas, a brainstem auditory implant has been placed into the cochlear nucleus on a limited, experimental basis. Recipients of the brainstem implant derive benefit similar to those with the cochlear implant.

The treatment of tinnitus is particularly problematic. The frequency range and intensity of tinnitus can often be matched with the use of an audiometer. Relief of the tinnitus may be obtained by masking it with background music. Hearing aids also are helpful in tinnitus suppression, as are tinnitus maskers, devices that present a sound to the affected ear which is more pleasant to listen to than the tinnitus. The use of a tinnitus masker is often followed by several hours of inhibition of the tinnitus.

COMMUNICATING WITH HARD-OF-HEARING INDIVIDUALS   First of all, unnecessary noise should be eliminated or reduced. The radio and television should be turned off. Persons with hearing impairment depend on speech reading. They should be allowed to see the face of the speaker at all times. Speaking directly into the ear is occasionally helpful, but usually more is lost in communication than gained when the speaker's face cannot be seen. The lighting of the face of the speaker should be considered. The hard-of-hearing person should sit with his or her back to the window so that the light will be on the speaker's face. Speech should be slow enough to make each word distinct, but overly slow speech is distracting and loses contextual benefits. Although speech should be in a loud, clear voice, one should be aware that in sensorineural hearing losses in general and in elderly hard-of-hearing persons in particular, recruitment (the ability to hear loud sounds normally loud) may be troublesome. Above all, optimal communication cannot take place without both parties giving it their full and undivided attention.

REFERENCES

ALBERTI PW, RUBEN RJ (eds): *Otologic Medicine and Surgery*. New York, Churchill Livingstone, 1988

BALDWIN CT et al: An exonic mutation in the HuP2 paired domain gene causes Waardenburg's syndrome. Nature 355:637, 1992

BALLENGER JJ: *Diseases of the Nose, Throat, Ear, Head and Neck*, 14th ed. Philadelphia, Lea & Febiger, 1991

BROWNELL WE et al: Evoked mechanical responses of isolated cochlear outer hair cells. Science 227:194, 1985

COLE P: Upper respiratory airflow, in *The Nose: Upper Airway Physiology and the Atmospheric Environment*, DF Proctor, IB Anderson (eds). Amsterdam, Elsevier, 1982, pp 163–189

DOTY RL: A review of olfactory dysfunctions in man. Am J Otolaryngol 1:57, 1979
—— et al: Smell identification ability: Changes with age. Science 226:1441, 1984
——: Presence of both odor identification and detection deficits in Alzheimer's disease. Brain Res Bull 18:597, 1987
——: Olfactory dysfunction in Parkinsonism: A general deficit unrelated to neurological signs, disease stage or disease duration. Neurology 38:1237, 1988

FRANCO B et al: A gene deleted in Kallmann's syndrome shares homology with neural cell adhesion and axonal path-finding molecules. Nature 353:529, 1991

GETCHELL TV et al: *Smell and Taste in Health and Disease*. New York, Raven Press, 1991

JERGER JR: *Modern Developments in Audiology*, 2d ed. New York, Academic Press, 1973

KACHAR B et al: Electrokinetic shape changes of cochlear outer hair cells. Nature 322:365, 1986

KEMP DT: Stimulated acoustic emissions from within the human auditory system. J Acoust Soc Am 64:1386, 1978

KONIGSMARK BW: Hereditary diseases of the nervous system with hearing loss, in *Handbook of Clinical Neurology*, PJ Vinken, GW Bruyn (eds). Elsevier, Amsterdam, 1975, vol 22, chap 23, pp 499–526

LEVINE SB, SNOW JB: Pulsatile tinnitus. Laryngoscope 97:401, 1987

LIM DJ: Functional structure of the organ of Corti: A review. Hearing Res 22:117, 1986

LOWELL MA et al: Biopsy of human olfactory mucosa: An instrument and a technique. Arch Otolaryngol 108:247, 1982

NAKASHIMA T et al: Structure of human fetal and adult olfactory neuroepithelium. Arch Otolaryngol 110:641, 1984

NORGREN R: The gustatory system in mammals. Am J Otolaryngol 4:234, 1983

RINTELMAN WF: *Hearing Assessment*. Baltimore, Baltimore University, 1979

RUBEN RJ et al: *Genetics of Hearing Impairment*. New York, New York Acad Science, 1991

SNOW JB, TELIAN SA: Sudden deafness, in *Otolaryngology*, 3rd ed, MM Paprella et al (eds). Philadelphia, Saunders, 1991, pp 1619–1628
—— et al: Central auditory imperception. Laryngoscope 87:1450, 1977
——: Clinical problems in chemosensory disturbances. Am J Otolaryngol 4:224, 1983

TALAMO BR et al: Pathological changes in olfactory neurons in patients with Alzheimer's disease. Nature 337:736, 1989

21 PARALYSIS AND MOVEMENT DISORDERS

JOHN H. GROWDON / J. STEPHEN FINK*

Impairments of motor function may be subdivided into (1) paralysis due to lesions of corticospinal, corticobulbar, or brainstem descending (subcorticospinal) neurons, (2) abnormalities of movement and posture due to disease of the extrapyramidal motor system, (3) apraxic or nonparalytic disturbances of purposive movement due to involvement of the cerebral hemispheres, (4) abnormalities of coordination (ataxia) due to lesions in the cerebellar system, including its inputs and outputs, and (5) paralysis due to disorders of the motor unit, including bulbar or spinal motor neurons, neuromuscular junction, and muscle. This chapter reviews signs and symptoms that result from lesions of lower motor neurons, descending corticospinal and other tracts, and the extrapyramidal system. It also includes consideration of apraxic disorders. The cerebellar system is discussed in Chap. 22. Signs and symptoms that result from lesions of the neuromuscular junction and muscle are discussed in Chaps. 385 and 386.

FUNCTIONAL ANATOMY OF PRINCIPAL MOTOR TRACTS AND THE MOTOR UNIT

PYRAMIDAL SYSTEM   The motor area of the cerebral cortex includes that part of the precentral convolution which contains Betz cells (area 4 of Brodmann, the *primary motor cortex*) (see Fig. 27A), but it also includes the premotor areas which extend rostrally into area 6 and the adjacent cortex along the banks of the cingulate cortex. In the primary motor cortex, the muscle groups of contralateral face, arm, trunk, and leg are somatotopically organized, with those of the face being at the lower end of the precentral convolution and those of the leg being in the paracentral lobule on the medial surface of the cerebral hemisphere. The parts of the body capable of the most delicate movements have, in general, the largest cortical representation. In humans, the premotor areas include the *premotor cortex*, located over the lateral surface of the hemispheres immediately rostral to the primary motor cortex, and the *supplementary motor area*, located on the medial surface of the hemisphere, rostral to the premotor cortex. The premotor areas are also organized somatotopically and appear to be important in the planning of volitional movements.

Neurons in cortical layer V of the primary motor cortex, the supplementary motor area, the premotor cortex, and the postcentral

*The authors acknowledge the contributions of Robert R. Young, coauthor in the 11th edition.

somatosensory cortex (areas 1, 2, 3, 5, and 7) contribute axons to the pyramidal system. The chief element of the pyramidal system, the corticospinal tract, is the only direct connection between the cortex and spinal cord. Corticospinal fibers descend in the internal capsule, where they intermingle with those destined to end in the striatum, globus pallidus, substantia nigra, red nucleus, and reticular substance, as well as others ascending from the thalamus. Fibers destined for cranial nerves separate in the midbrain and cross the midline to the contralateral cranial nerve nuclei. These fibers form the corticomesencephalic, corticopontine, and corticobulbar tracts and are included in the pyramidal system of motor neurons because they have functions similar to those of the corticospinal tract. The decussation of the corticospinal tract at the lower end of the medulla is variable. Most of the crossing fibers come to occupy a position in the posterolateral part of the lateral funiculus to form the lateral corticospinal tract; a few fibers cross to form an anterior funiculus. A small number of fibers, 10 to 30 percent, do not cross but descend ipsilaterally as the uncrossed corticospinal tract in the anterior funiculus of the spinal cord. Axons that travel in the lateral corticospinal tract terminate on (1) neurons of the dorsal horn, (2) interneurons in the intermediate zone of spinal gray matter, particularly those innervating distal muscles, and (3) motor neurons located dorsolaterally in the anterior horn. The corticospinal tract in the anterior funiculus terminates bilaterally on motor neurons located in the ventromedial anterior horn; these neurons innervate axial muscles. Most corticospinal tract neurons have direct connections with a small number of functionally related muscles, in some cases to muscles that are antagonistic (flexors and extensors of the same joint). The corticospinal tract is particularly important for the performance of highly fractionated movements (e.g., those involving the digits).

BULBOSPINAL SYSTEMS   In addition to the pyramidal (corticospinal and corticobulbar) tract, the spinal gray matter receives axons from two groups of descending pathways from the brainstem. Major contributions to the *ventromedial system* come from the lateral and medial vestibulospinal tracts originating in the lateral and medial vestibular nuclei, the reticulospinal tract originating in the reticular formation of the medulla and pons, and the teetospinal tract originating in the superior colliculus of the midbrain. Neurons originating in the raphe nuclei of the medulla (containing serotonin), in the region of the locus coeruleus in the dorsal brainstem (containing norepinephrine), and in the interstitial nucleus of Cajal also contribute axons to the ventromedial brainstem descending system. These descending ventromedial axons terminate largely on motor neurons located in the ventromedial anterior horn that innervate axial and proximal muscles; this pool of motor neurons is important in the maintenance of posture and balance. Neurons in the red nucleus of the midbrain contribute axons to the rubrospinal tract, which is the major component of the *dorsolateral system* of brainstem descending pathways. Other fibers in this system originate in the ventrolateral pontine tegmentum and the caudal raphe nuclei. Like the corticospinal tract in the lateral funiculus, the dorsolateral system terminates in the lateral portion of the intermediate zone and on motor neurons located dorsolaterally in the anterior horn; these motor neurons innervate distal muscles of the limbs.

ANATOMY AND PHYSIOLOGY OF THE MOTOR UNIT   Each motor nerve cell, through extensive arborization of the terminal part of its fiber, comes into contact with hundreds of muscle fibers; together they constitute the motor unit. Motor neuron excitability is modulated by segmental afferent and suprasegmental descending pathways. Descending corticospinal axons are believed to release excitatory amino acids (aspartate and glutamate) as neurotransmitters. Afferent modulation of motor unit activity is provided, in part, by axons of dorsal root ganglia cells which innervate most lamina of the dorsal horn, the intermediate zone, and some motor neurons directly. Substance P and glutamate are released by the primary afferent neurons and can modulate the gain of the reflex arc. Release of gamma-aminobutyric acid (GABA) and the neuropeptide enkephalin from interneurons in the dorsal spinal cord gray matter increases presynaptic inhibition of primary afferent neurons. The amino acid glycine is the major postsynaptic inhibitory neurotransmitter and is released by interneurons in the intermediate and ventral gray matter and Renshaw cells. Blockage of glycine receptors by strychnine or glycine release by tetanus toxin produces hyperreflexia. Descending serotonin and catecholamine pathways modulate spinal cord reflex mechanisms and flexor reflex afferents.

Motor nerve fibers of each anterior spinal root intermingle with those from adjacent roots and join to form plexuses and, ultimately, peripheral nerves. Innervation of muscles proceeds from corresponding segments of the spinal cord, and each large muscle is supplied by two or more roots. A single peripheral nerve contains several roots and usually provides the complete motor innervation of a muscle or group of muscles. For this reason, the distribution of paralysis due to disease of the anterior horn cells or anterior roots differs from that which follows a lesion of a peripheral nerve. Acetylcholine is the excitatory neurotransmitter released by axon terminals of anterior horn cells at the neuromuscular junction.

Muscle tone and tendon reflexes depend on muscle spindles and their afferent fibers. A tap on a tendon, by stimulating muscle spindles, activates stretch receptors which transmit impulses to alpha motor neurons in the spinal cord. The result is the familiar brief muscle contraction or tendon reflex. All variations in force and type of movement are determined by differences in the number and size of motor units called into activity, the frequency of their firing rates, and the patterns of activity in different muscles. Feeble movements recruit few units; the number and size of motor units increase in a stereotyped fashion with stronger movements. Motor units involved in tonic contractions have muscle fibers known as type I that are rich in oxidative enzymes and mitochondria; those controlling phasic contractions innervate muscle fibers that have anaerobic metabolism (type II fibers) (see also Chap. 382). When a motor neuron becomes diseased, as in progressive muscular atrophy, its axon may manifest increased irritability, and all the muscle fibers that it controls may discharge sporadically, in isolation from other units. The result of the contraction of one or several such units is a muscular twitch, or *fasciculation*, which can be observed visibly and recorded in the electromyogram (EMG). If the motor neuron or its axon is destroyed, all the muscle fibers to which it is attached undergo profound denervation atrophy. As a result, individual muscle fibers become hypersensitive to acetylcholine and contract spontaneously, although they are unresponsive to nerve impulses. Isolated activity of individual muscle fibers is called *fibrillation;* it is so fine that it cannot be seen through the intact skin and can be recorded only as a short-duration spike potential in the EMG (see Chap. 382).

All motor activity, even of the most elementary reflex type, requires the cooperation of several muscles. Analysis of a relatively simple movement, such as clenching the fist, affords some idea of the complexity of the underlying neural arrangements. In this act, the primary movement is a contraction of the flexor muscles of the fingers, the flexor digitorum sublimis and profundus, the flexor pollicis longus and brevis, and the adductor pollicis brevis. These muscles act as *agonists*, or *prime movers*, in this act. In order for flexion to be smooth and forceful, finger extensor muscles act as *antagonists* and must relax at the same rate at which the flexors contract. The muscles which flex the fingers also tend to flex the wrist, and since that weakens the grip, muscles which extend the wrist must be brought into play to prevent its flexion. The action of the wrist extensors is *synergic*, and these muscles are called synergists in this particular act. The elbow and shoulder must be stabilized by appropriate flexor and extensor muscles, which serve as *fixators*. The coordination of agonists, antagonists, synergists, and fixators involves reciprocal innervation and is managed entirely by segmental spinal mechanisms with guidance from proprioceptive input. Only the agonist movement in a voluntary act is believed to be initiated at a cortical level. There are many other basic motor activities, such as the maintenance of certain postures and stepping movements, where agonists and antagonists contract simultaneously (see Chap. 22). In general, the more delicate the movement, the more precise is the coordination between agonist and antagonist muscles.

CLINICAL MANIFESTATIONS OF MOTOR SYSTEM DISEASES

When applied to voluntary muscles, *paralysis* means loss of contraction due to interruption of one or more motor pathways from the cortex to the muscle fiber. It is preferable to use *paresis* for slight and *paralysis* or *plegia* for severe loss of motor strength. Motor paralysis may result from lesions of upper motor neurons (corticospinal, corticobulbar, or subcorticospinal neurons) or of the motor unit. In addition to weakness, impaired facility of movement is an important functional deficit.

PARALYSIS DUE TO DISEASES OF PYRAMIDAL AND SUBCOR-TICOSPINAL NEURONS Corticospinal paralysis may be due to lesions in the cerebral cortex, subcortical white matter, internal capsule, brainstem, or spinal cord. Lesions confined to one of these anatomic locations without damaging adjacent parts of the brain are rare but afford an opportunity to assess pure pyramidal tract function. In cases of unilateral pyramidal tract damage in the medulla, for example, initial paralysis may be striking, but there is a remarkable degree of recovery of motor function in the affected contralateral arm and leg, leaving only an extensor plantar reflex (Babinski's sign) and impaired fine finger movement. The extent of recovery is surprising and may be due to preservation of a few fibers in the pyramid or to preservation of lateral brainstem pathways. This picture of pure pyramidal tract damage is much different from the extensive deficits that generally accompany most spastic hemiplegic syndromes. In clinical practice, most lesions of the upper motor neurons interrupt descending fibers from the cerebral cortex (corticospinal, corticorubral, corticostriatal, corticopallidal, corticopontine, and corticoreticular) and from the brainstem (reticulospinal, vestibulospinal, and rubrospinal). These lesions produce the classic upper motor neuron syndrome consisting of weakness, hyperactivity of tendon reflexes, and spasticity (Table 21-1).

With corticospinal lesions in humans, the distribution of the paralysis varies with the lesion site, but there are certain common features. Paralysis due to a lesion of upper motor neurons always involves a group of muscles, never individual muscles. In general, hand, arm, and leg muscles are most affected after a corticospinal lesion; of the cranial musculature, only the lower face and tongue are involved to any significant degree. Whatever volitional movement remains, the maximum effort is attained more slowly than in the normal limb, fewer motor units are recruited, and the frequency of their discharge is reduced. Corticospinal paralysis never involves all the muscles on one side of the body, even with a complete hemiplegia. Movements that are invariably bilateral, such as those of the eyes, jaw, pharynx, larynx, neck, thorax, and abdomen, are usually unaffected.

Acute lesions of the corticospinal and subcorticospinal motor system below the medulla, such as the cervical cord, produce a distinctive picture of total paralysis and areflexia known as *spinal shock*. After a few days to weeks, flaccidity subsides, muscular tone reappears, and the affected limbs become spastic; paralysis persists unchanged. *Spasticity* is a feature of all lesions of the motor system at cerebral, capsular, midbrain, and pontine levels. Spasticity is defined as a motor disorder characterized by a velocity-dependent increase in tonic stretch reflexes (''muscle tone'') with exaggerated tendon jerks; it is one component of the upper motor neuron syndrome. Spasticity is related to excessive activity of motor neurons that are released from inhibition consequent to lesions of the corticospinal or descending brainstem pathways. With supraspinal lesions, certain spinal neurons are more active than others; the arm is maintained in a pronated, flexed position and the leg in an adducted, extended position. Attempts to extend the arm or flex the leg passively will elicit increasing resistance which abruptly subsides (*clasp-knife phenomenon*). When the limb is left in the new position, the resistance reappears (*lengthening and shortening reactions*). With combined lesions of corticospinal and other suprasegmental tracts, sustained resistance to movement (*hypertonus*) is more common than the clasp-knife type of spasticity. Upper motor neuron lesions also release the nocifensive spinal flexion reflexes, including Babinski's sign, and diminish or abolish the cutaneomuscular abdominal and cremasteric reflexes. Other signs of corticospinal or upper motor neuron lesions include exaggerated stretch and cutaneous reflexes in cranial as well as in limb and trunk muscles. If the corticospinal lesions are bilateral, there is *pseudobulbar paralysis* (dysarthria, dysphonia, and dysphagia with bifacial paralysis) accompanied by forced crying and laughing. Prolonged flexor and extensor spasms occur with lesions of the spinal cord; they are due to a release of cutaneous reflexes from suprasegmental modulation.

Spasticity is present with paresis as well as paralysis and can add to disturbances of voluntary movements. In general, all attempts by the patient to move the hemiparetic extremities appear to be hampered. Discrete movements of individual fingers and finely coordinated movements of the hand are lost, but voluntary control over proximal muscles is generally maintained. Synergies of movements eventually appear. For example, in the upper extremity a flexion synergy consisting of finger flexion, wrist flexion and pronation, elbow flexion, and shoulder elevation and abduction is produced in a slow, stereotyped fashion upon attempted grasp of an object. Attempts to push with the hand result in a weak pronation of the hand, extension or flexion of the fingers, extension of the wrist and elbow, adduction of the upper arm, and lowering of the shoulder. In the lower extremity the extensor synergy (thigh adduction, thigh and knee extension, and plantar flexion of the toes and foot) is more powerful than the flexor synergy of hip abduction, hip and knee flexion, and dorsiflexion and inversion of toes and foot. A bias toward extensor synergy facilitates weight bearing and walking, which are eventually achieved by nearly all hemiplegic patients. These synergies indicate that there is a diminution in voluntary anterior horn cell activation (the negative effect of a motor lesion) and excessive reflex and synergistic discharges in the same motor neuron pools (the positive effects of the lesion). Strong-willed effort to move the paretic limb also may evoke symmetric associated (mirror) movements in the normal limb.

In spasticity, where the neurons responsible for excitation of the extensor muscles of the leg and flexors of the arm are overactive, it is not known whether there is a functional excess of excitatory neurotransmitters or a deficiency of inhibitory transmitters or both. Current evidence indicates that drugs that decrease spasticity act at the spinal cord level to alter neurotransmitter function. Baclofen slows conduction in the spinal cord reflex arc, perhaps by interfering with the release of excitatory neurotransmitters, including glutamate and substance P, from primary afferent neurons. GABA and glycine interneurons are thought to be underactive in spasticity. Diazepam facilitates GABA-mediated presynaptic inhibition of primary afferent excitatory transmitter release, and enhanced glycinergic neurotransmission suppresses spasticity.

TABLE 21-1 Differences between paralysis due to lesions of upper versus lower motor neurons

Upper motor neuron paralysis	Lower motor neuron paralysis
Muscle groups affected diffusely, never individual muscles	Individual muscles may be affected
Atrophy slight	Atrophy pronounced, 70 to 80% of total bulk
Spasticity with hyperactivity of the tendon reflexes	Flaccidity and hypotonia of affected muscles with loss of tendon reflexes
Extensor plantar reflex, Babinski's sign	Plantar reflex, if present, is of normal flexor type
Fascicular twitches not produced	Fasciculations may be present
	EMG reveals reduced numbers of motor units and fibrillations

PARALYSIS DUE TO DISEASES OF THE MOTOR UNIT Damage to the lower motor neurons can produce paresis or paralysis as a direct result of physiologic block or destruction of anterior horn cells or their axons in anterior roots and nerves. The signs and symptoms of the lower motor neuron syndrome vary according to the location of the lesion: The most important question for clinical purposes is whether sensory changes coexist with muscular weakness. The combination of flaccid areflexic paralysis and sensory loss usually indicates involvement of mixed motor and sensory nerves or damage to both anterior and posterior roots. If sensory changes are absent, the lesion must be situated in the gray matter of the spinal cord, in the anterior roots, in a purely motor branch of a peripheral nerve, or in motor axons alone. The distinction between nuclear (spinal) and anterior root (radicular) lesions may at times be impossible to make.

If all or practically all peripheral motor nerves supplying a muscle are destroyed, voluntary, postural, and reflex movements are abolished. The muscle becomes soft and yields excessively to passive stretching, a condition known as *flaccidity*. Muscle tone—the slight resistance that normal relaxed muscle offers to passive movement— is reduced (*hypotonia* or *atonia*). The denervated muscles undergo extreme atrophy and lose 70 to 80 percent of their original bulk within 4 months. The reflex reaction of the muscle to sudden stretch, as by tapping its tendon, is lost. If only a few motor units in the muscles are affected, partial paralysis will ensue. With partial denervation, EMG evidence of fibrillations also may be obtained. Clinical features that distinguish lower motor and upper motor neuron lesions are summarized in Table 21-1.

APRAXIC OR NONPARALYTIC DISORDERS OF MOTOR FUNCTION Loss of learned movements can simulate paresis of a limb, even though the pyramidal tract and spinal cord motor units are intact. This condition is called *apraxia* and is defined as a disorder of learned movement that is not due to weakness, incoordination, sensory loss, or failure to comprehend commands. A failure to execute a designated action while retaining the ability to carry out the individual movements upon which such an act depends is the main feature of apraxia. A clinical test of motor deficits of this type is to observe a series of self-initiated actions such as using a comb, a razor, a toothbrush, or a common tool or gesturing, e.g., waving goodbye, saluting, shaking the fist as though angry, or blowing a kiss. These actions are usually elicited by a verbal command or a request to imitate the examiner. Of course, failure to follow a spoken or written request may be due to an aphasia that prevents understanding of what is asked or to an agnosia that prevents recognition of the tool or object to be used. But when these difficulties are excluded, there remains a peculiar motor deficit in which the patient appears to understand but has lost the memory of how to perform a given act, especially if it is called for in an unnatural setting. The patient may have the idea of what to do but cannot translate the idea of the sequence of movements into a precise, well-executed act. An apraxic deficit may be evident both after a spoken command and in requests to imitate the gestures of the examiner. Sometimes these two conditions may be dissociated; the patient, while not aphasic, cannot execute a gesture to a spoken command but can still imitate the act if it is called forth by gesture. Also, if merely given the tool, the patient may use it properly in an automatic fashion.

To understand the anatomic basis of apraxia, it is necessary to appreciate that the production of complex motor behavior results from association among several cortical brain areas. The motor response of right-handed (and most left-handed) persons to a command requires the integrity of the left parietal and temporal lobes, especially the region around the left supramarginal gyrus, and their connection with the left premotor regions for control of the right hand. Information flows through the corpus callosum from the left to the right motor cortex for control of the left side of the body. Disconnection of the supramarginal area from motor areas of the right hemisphere (most commonly by lesions of the midcallosum, dominant frontal association cortex, or posterior parietal lobe) results in apraxia of left limbs when tested by response to verbal commands.

EXAMINATION SCHEME FOR MOTOR PARALYSIS AND APRAXIA The first step in examination is to inspect the paralyzed limb, taking note of its posture and whether there are signs of muscular hypertrophy, atrophy, or fascicular twitchings. Slight atrophy may be due to disuse from any cause, i.e., pain, fixation as the result of a cast, or any type of paralysis. Pronounced atrophy usually occurs only with denervation of several weeks' or months' duration. The patient is then called on to move each muscle group, and the power and facility of movement are graded and recorded. The Medical Research Council scale provides a useful clinical measure of weakness:

0 = no contraction
1 = trace contraction
2 = active movement with gravity eliminated
3 = active movement against gravity
4 = active movement against gravity and resistance
5 = normal power

The examiner then determines the range of passive movement and the degree of resistance encountered moving all the joints. This provides information concerning alterations of muscle tone, i.e., hypotonia, spasticity, and rigidity. Dislocations, diseased joints, and ankyloses also may be revealed by these same maneuvers. The tendon reflexes are then tested. The usual routine is to try to elicit the jaw jerk (increased in pseudobulbar palsy) and the biceps, triceps, quadriceps, and Achilles tendon reflexes. Two cutaneous reflexes are then tested, the abdominal and plantar reflexes.

If there is no evidence of upper or lower motor neuron disease, but motor acts are nonetheless imperfectly performed, one should look for a disorder of postural control associated with cerebellar incoordination or consider that rigidity with abnormalities of posture and movement may be due to disease of the basal ganglia. In the absence of these disorders, the possibility of an apraxic disorder may be investigated by watching the patient's own movements and those called forth by specific command and gesture.

DIFFERENTIAL DIAGNOSIS OF PARALYSIS The diagnostic consideration of paralysis may be simplified by the following subdivisions, which relate to the location and distribution of weakness. Paralysis may result from dysfunction of upper motor neurons (corticospinal, corticobulbar, and subcorticospinal neurons) or of the motor unit (bulbar and spinal motor neurons, neuromuscular junction, and muscle). In general, the presence or absence of atrophy of muscles in a monoplegic limb can assist the clinician to arrive at an anatomic and clinical diagnosis.

Monoplegia It is necessary to determine carefully the distribution of muscle weakness. For example, patients who complain of weakness of one extremity often have unnoticed weakness in another limb, and the condition is actually hemiplegia or paraplegia. A comprehensive physical examination should be conducted in order to determine whether there is weakness of all the muscles in a limb or only isolated muscle groups. The examination also should exclude nonparalytic conditions such as ataxia, sensory disturbances, mechanical limitation resulting from arthritis, the rigidity of parkinsonism, or pain in an extremity; such conditions are often interpreted by the patient as weakness.

PARALYSIS WITH LITTLE OR NO ATROPHY The most frequent cause of monoplegia without muscular wasting is a lesion of the cerebral cortex; diseases that interrupt the corticospinal tract at the level of the internal capsule, brainstem, or spinal cord rarely cause monoplegia because corticospinal fibers to arm and leg are intermingled at subcortical levels. A cortical vascular lesion (thrombosis or embolus) is the most common cause of monoplegia, but a discrete traumatic lesion, tumor, or abscess may have the same effect. Multiple sclerosis and spinal cord tumor, early in their course, may cause isolated weakness of one extremity, usually the leg. Weakness due to damage of upper motor neurons is usually accompanied by spasticity, increased reflexes, and an extensor plantar reflex (Babinski's sign). In acute diseases affecting the lower motor neurons, such as poliomyelitis, the tendon reflexes are always reduced or abolished, but atrophy may not appear for several weeks. Hence one must take into account the mode of onset and the duration of the disease in evaluating the tendon reflexes, muscle tone, and degree of atrophy before reaching an anatomic diagnosis.

PARALYSIS WITH MUSCULAR ATROPHY Atrophy of muscles in a paralyzed limb usually indicates a lesion of some portion of the motor unit (spinal cord, spinal roots, peripheral nerve, or muscle). Disease of the neuromuscular junction (e.g., myasthenia gravis) is not associated with muscular atrophy. In addition to the paralysis, reduced or abolished tendon reflexes, and decreased tone, there may be visible fasciculations. The EMG shows decreased numbers of motor units (often of large size), fasciculations at rest, and fibrillations. The location of the lesion can usually be decided by the distribution of the palsied muscles (whether the pattern is one of muscles, nerve, spinal root, or spinal cord involvement), by the associated neurologic symptoms and signs, and by special tests (CSF examination, CT or magnetic resonance imaging scans of the spine, myelogram, serum muscle enzymes, EMG, sensory evoked responses, and biopsy). A clinical approach to the signs and symptoms that assist the clinician in arriving at an anatomic diagnosis of diseases of the motor unit (spinal cord, spinal motor nerves, neuromuscular junction, or muscle) are described in more detail in Chaps. 382 and 383.

The anatomic pattern of paralysis with atrophy may suggest the clinical diagnosis. Atrophic monoplegia affecting the arm should suggest brachial plexus trauma in an infant; poliomyelitis in a child; and poliomyelitis, syringomyelia, amyotrophic lateral sclerosis, or neuritis of the brachial plexus in an adult. Crural monoplegia (affecting the leg) is more frequent than brachial monoplegia and may be caused by any lesion of thoracic or lumber cord, including trauma, tumor, myelitis, or multiple sclerosis. Multiple sclerosis almost never causes atrophy, and ruptured intervertebral disk and the many varieties of neuritis rarely paralyze all or most of the muscles of a limb. Muscular dystrophy may begin in one limb, but by the time the patient is seen, the typical pattern of symmetric proximal limb and trunk involvement is usually evident. A unilateral retroperitoneal tumor may paralyze the leg by implicating the lumbosacral plexus. Prolonged disuse of a limb may lead to atrophy, but this is usually not so marked as in diseases that denervate muscles. In disuse atrophy, the tendon reflexes are normal, and the responses of the muscles to electric stimulation and on EMG are unaltered.

Hemiplegia Loss of strength in the arm, leg, and sometimes face on one side of the body is the most frequent distribution of paralysis. With rare exceptions (a few unusual cases of poliomyelitis or motor system disease), this pattern of paralysis is due to involvement of the descending motor tracts. The site or level of the lesion that produced hemiplegia can usually be deduced from the associated neurologic findings. Diseases localized in the cerebral cortex, cerebral white matter (corona radiata), and internal capsule usually produce weakness or paralysis of the face, arm, and leg on the side of the body contralateral to the brain lesion. The occurrence of convulsive seizures or the presence of a defect in speech (aphasia), a cortical type of sensory loss (astereognosis and loss of two-point discrimination), anosognosia, or defects in the visual fields suggest a cortical or subcortical rather than a capsular location. A pure, isolated motor hemiplegia affecting simultaneously the face, arm, and leg indicates a small, discrete lesion in the posterior limb of the internal capsule, cerebral peduncle, pons, or medullary pyramids. Damage to the corticospinal and corticobulbar tracts in the upper portion of the brainstem will cause paralysis of the face, arm, and leg in the side opposite the lesion, plus deficits in cranial nerve function on the same side as the lesion. These "crossed paralyses" that are so characteristic of brainstem diseases are described in Chap. 368.

Hemiplegia that spares cranial musculature may be caused by a lesion in the lateral column of the cervical spinal cord. At this level, however, the pathologic process often induces bilateral signs, with resulting quadriparesis or quadriplegia. Homolateral paralysis, if combined with a loss of vibratory and position sense on the same side and contralateral loss of pain and temperature (Brown-Séquard syndrome), signifies disease of the spinal cord (Chap. 381).

Muscle atrophy of minor degree is often associated with hemiplegia but never reaches the proportions seen in diseases of the lower motor neurons. Atrophy secondary to upper motor neuron damage is largely due to disuse. There is an important exception to this rule: When the motor cortex and adjacent parts of the parietal lobe are damaged in infancy or childhood, the normal development of the muscles and the skeletal system in the affected limbs is retarded, and the palsied limbs and even the trunk on one side are small. Developmental atrophy does not occur, however, if the paralysis begins after puberty, when the greater part of skeletal growth has been attained. In hemiplegia due to spinal cord injury, muscles at the level of the lesion may undergo atrophy if there is associated damage to anterior horn cells or ventral roots.

Vascular diseases of the cerebral hemispheres and brainstem are the most common causes of hemiplegia. Trauma (brain contusion, epidural and subdural hemorrhage) ranks second, followed by other diseases such as brain tumor, demyelinative disease, brain abscess, and encephalitis. Complications of meningitis, tuberculosis, and syphilis were common causes of hemiplegia in the past but are much less evident in current practice.

Paraplegia Paraplegia denotes a condition of weakness or paralysis of both lower extremities with sparing of the upper extremities. Paraplegia most commonly occurs in diseases of the spinal cord, spinal roots, or peripheral nerves. Among cerebral causes, parasagittal tumors and hydrocephalus cause leg weakness. If the onset is acute, it may be difficult to distinguish spinal from peripheral nerve or root causes of paralysis because sudden damage to either may result in flaccidity and abolition of reflexes. As a rule, in acute spinal cord diseases the paralysis affects all muscles below a given level; often, if the white matter is extensively damaged, sensory loss below a particular level (loss of pain and temperature sense from lateral spinothalamic tracts involvement and loss of vibratory and position sense from posterior columns damage) is conjoined. Also, in bilateral disease of the spinal cord the bladder and bowel sphincters are paralyzed. Alterations of CSF (dynamic block and increases in protein or cells) are frequent. In peripheral nerve diseases both sensory loss and motor loss tend to involve the distal muscles of the legs more than the proximal ones (an exception is acute idiopathic polyneuritis), and the sphincters are spared or only briefly deranged in function. Sensory loss, if present, is more likely to consist of distal impairment of touch, vibration, and position sense, with pain and temperature sense spared in many instances. The CSF protein level may be normal or elevated. Studies of nerve conduction through spinal roots (F waves) are always abnormal.

Acute paraplegia most commonly occurs after trauma or in association with metastatic neoplasia. Uncommon causes of acute paraplegia include a medial pontine lesion affecting the leg fibers which are near the midline (as in pontine infarction or central pontine myelinolysis), spontaneous hematomyelia with bleeding from a vascular malformation (angioma, telangiectasis), thrombosis of a spinal artery with infarction (myelomalacia), and dissecting aortic aneurysm or atherosclerotic occlusion of nutrient spinal arteries arising from the aorta with resulting infarction (myelomalacia). Postinfectious or postvaccinal myelitis, acute demyelinative myelitis (Devic's disease if the optic nerves are affected), necrotizing myelitis, and epidural abscess or hemorrhage with spinal cord compression tend to develop somewhat more slowly over a period of hours or days, but they may have an acute onset. Poliomyelitis, in those countries where immunization is incomplete, presents as a purely motor disorder with meningitis and must be distinguished from the other acute myelopathies.

Subacute or chronic paraplegia in adults results from such common diseases as cervical spondylosis and multiple sclerosis. Other causes are subacute combined degeneration, spinal cord tumor, ruptured cervical disk, syphilitic meningomyelitis, chronic epidural infections (fungus and other granulomatous diseases), motor system disease, and syringomyelia. Familial spastic paraparesis is a rare cause of paraplegia in which there is symmetric demyelination of the dorsolateral corticospinal tract. (See Chap. 381 for discussion of these spinal cord diseases.) The several varieties of polyneuritis, including Guillain-Barré syndrome and polymyositis, must be considered in the differential diagnosis of paraparesis. Friedreich's ataxia and familial spastic paraplegia, progressive muscular dystrophy, and the chronic varieties of polyneuritis tend to appear during late childhood and adolescence and are slowly progressive.

Paraplegia (or paraparesis) may be due to a lesion of the leg areas of the motor cortex. Arterial (anterior cerebral arteries) or venous (superior sagittal sinus and tributary cerebral veins) distribution cerebral infarctions are causes of acute paraplegia; parasagittal meningioma is a cause of asymmetric chronic paraplegia. Usually other signs such as confusion, stupor, or seizures indicate the cerebral localization, and differential diagnosis is not a problem.

Quadriplegia   All that has been written about the common causes of paraplegia applies to quadriplegia except that the lesion is in the cervical rather than the thoracic or lumbar segments of the spinal cord. If it is situated in the low cervical segments and involves the anterior half of the spinal cord, as in occlusion of the anterior spinal artery, the arm paralysis may be flaccid and areflexic and the leg paralysis spastic (anterior spinal syndrome). There are only a few points of difference between the common paraplegic and quadriplegic syndromes. One of the most common causes of subacute quadriplegia is the Guillain-Barré syndrome due to inflammatory demyelination of motor neuron axons in the anterior roots. Repeated cerebral vascular accidents may lead to bilateral hemiplegia, usually accompanied by pseudobulbar palsy. An unusual cause of quadriplegia is bilateral infarctions of the medullary pyramids.

Isolated paralysis   Paralysis of isolated muscle groups usually indicates a lesion of one or more peripheral nerves. The basis for diagnosing a lesion of an individual peripheral nerve is the presence of weakness or paralysis of the muscle or group of muscles and impairment or loss of sensation in the distribution of the nerve in question (Chap. 383). Complete transection or severe injury to a peripheral nerve is usually followed by atrophy of the muscles it innervates and by loss of their tendon reflexes. Trophic changes in the skin, nails, and subcutaneous tissue also may occur. It is of considerable importance to decide whether the lesion is only a temporary one (conduction block) or there has been a dissolution of axonal continuity, requiring nerve regeneration for recovery.

THE BASAL GANGLIA

The basal ganglia subserve motor functions that are distinct from those attributed to the pyramidal (corticospinal) tract. The term *extrapyramidal* underscores this distinction and calls attention to a set of neurologic illnesses caused by lesions that affect the basal ganglia.

ANATOMIC CONNECTIONS AND NEURONAL TRANSMITTERS IN THE BASAL GANGLIA   The basal ganglia are paired subcortical masses of gray matter that form anatomically distinct nuclear groups. The major nuclei are the caudate and the putamen (which together are called the *striatum*), the internal and external segments of the globus pallidus, the subthalamic nucleus, and the substantia nigra (Fig. 21-1). In contrast to the pyramidal system, the basal ganglia do not project directly to the spinal cord. The basal ganglia receive cortical input and project back to the frontal cortex through the thalamus. Together with parallel circuits originating in the cerebellum, the basal ganglia–thalamocortical circuit modulates activity in the corticospinal (pyramidal) motor system.

The striatum receives somatotopic cortical input from the frontal, sensory, motor, and parietotemporal-occipital association areas (see Fig. 21-1). Corticostriatal afferents release the excitatory amino acid glutamate. Another major afferent input to the striatum is from neurons in the substantia nigra pars compacta (SNc) which synthesize

FIGURE 21-1   Diagram of the major functional connections of the basal ganglia. The striatum receives afferents (glutamatergic) from the sensorimotor cortex; the other major afferent arises from the substantia nigra pars compacta and contains dopamine. The major output of the striatum flows through the internal globus pallidus and substantia nigra pars reticulata to ventral anterior and ventral lateral nuclei of the thalamus. Abbreviations: GABA = gamma-aminobutyric acid; ENK = enkephalin; SP = substance P; (+) = excitatory pathway; (-) = inhibitory pathway. *(Diagram courtesy of Dr. Douglas G. Cole.)*

and release dopamine (DA). Additional afferents to the striatum arise from the intralaminar thalamic nuclei and the brainstem raphe (containing serotonin). The striatum contains two distinct classes of cells: local circuit neurons, whose axons do not project beyond the confines of the nucleus, and other neurons, whose axons project to the globus pallidus and substantia nigra. Many neurotransmitters are present in striatal local circuit neurons, but their role in basal ganglia function are not well understood. The one exception is acetylcholine, which is present in large local circuit striatal neurons and appears to act in a manner which is functionally antagonistic to DA. The major output nuclei of the basal ganglia, the internal segment of the globus pallidus (GPi) and the substantia nigra reticulata (SNr), send GABA-containing inhibitory projections to the ventral anterior, ventral lateral, and intralaminar thalamic nuclei, including the centromedian nucleus (see Fig. 21-1). The influence of the basal ganglia circuits on the cortical motor areas is completed by means of the excitatory pathway from the thalamus to precentral cortex (see Fig. 21-1).

Basal ganglia output nuclei (GPi and SNr) are inhibitory to thalamic nuclei and are differentially modulated by two GABA-containing efferent projections from the striatum. A *direct pathway* consists of inhibitory striatal (putaminal) efferents containing substance P which projects to the SNr (see Fig. 21-1). A parallel *indirect pathway*, containing enkephalin, projects to the GPi by way of the external globus pallidus (GPe) and subthalamic nucleus (STN). The two striatal efferent systems appear to exert opposing effects on the basal ganglia output nuclei and, in turn, on the thalamic target nuclei. Activation of the direct pathway results in net excitation of the thalamocortical circuits and facilitation of cortically initiated movements. Activation of the indirect pathway increases excitatory drive to the STN and the basal ganglia output nuclei, resulting in inhibition of the thalamocortical circuit. The influence of DA-containing nigrostriatal afferents is to enhance transmission through the direct pathway and suppress transmission through the indirect pathway. The net effect of DA, then, is to enhance positive feedback to the cortical motor areas and facilitate volitional movements.

Alterations in the balance between the indirect and direct pathways' influence on thalamocortical activity may result in hypokinetic and hyperkinetic movements seen in disorders of the extrapyramidal system. Increases in transmission through the direct pathway decrease thalamic inhibition and produce hyperkinetic disorders, and enhanced transmission through the indirect pathway increases thalamic inhibition and results in hypokinetic disorders. Deficiency of DA, as occurs in Parkinson's disease, increases transmission through the indirect pathway and decreases transmission through the direct pathway; the net effect is to increase the output through the STN and GPi/SNr, thereby inhibiting the facilitatory thalamocortical influences on motor function and producing hypokinesia. Consistent with this model, lesions of the STN have been reported to ameliorate motor impairments in experimental parkinsonism. This model also provides an explanation for hyperkinetic movement disorders. Damage to the STN, for example, is the usual cause of hemiballismus. In early Huntington's disease, when chorea is prominent, there is a selective loss of striatal GABA/enkephalin neurons that give rise to the indirect pathway.

Like the basal ganglia, the cerebellum receives cortical inputs and modulates pyramidal tract function through the thalamus. The major cerebellar output, which exits the cerebellum through the superior cerebellar peduncle, terminates with the pallidothalamic fibers in the ventral anterior and ventral lateral thalamic nuclei. This region of the thalamus, therefore, forms an essential link in the ascending fiber systems from both the basal ganglia and the cerebellum to the motor cortex. Although parallel, the basal ganglia and cerebellar circuits influence cortically initiated motor activity through segregated thalamic and cortical regions. Despite the apparently crucial nature of these structures, lesions placed stereotaxically in the ventral thalamus can abolish essential-familial tremor or the rigidity and tremor in Parkinson's disease without producing functional deficits.

PHYSIOLOGY OF THE BASAL GANGLIA Recordings from neurons in the globus pallidus and substantia nigra in awake, performing primates confirm the main motor function of the basal ganglia. Cells within these regions clearly participate in the initiation of movement, because they increase their firing rates before movement is observed clinically or detected by EMG. Discharges in the basal ganglia are related principally to contralateral rather than ipsilateral limb movements. Many neurons increase their firing rates during slow (ramp) movements, but some others discharge during more rapid (ballistic) movements. There is somatotopic localization of leg, arm, and face within the internal segment of the globus pallidus and pars reticulata of the substantia nigra. This observation provides a possible explanation for the occurrence of restricted dyskinesias: Focal dystonia and buccal-lingual-masticatory tardive dyskinesia may result from localized pallidal or nigral lesions that affect only regions with hand or face representation.

Although the basal ganglia are motor nuclei, it is not possible to identify a specific type of basal ganglia movement. Hypotheses about the function of the basal ganglia in human beings derive from correlations between clinical signs and sites of pathologic lesions in patients with extrapyramidal diseases. The basal ganglia are a constellation of nuclei centered around the globus pallidus, through which impulses are channeled to the thalamus and onward to the cerebral cortex (see Fig. 21-1). Neurons in each satellite nucleus contribute excitatory and inhibitory impulses, and the sum of these influences on the main pathway from basal ganglia to thalamus and cerebral cortex, modified by the cerebellum, determines smooth motor

function as expressed through the corticospinal and other descending cortical tracts. If one or more of the supporting nuclei are damaged, the sum of the impulses to the globus pallidus changes, and disordered mobility can occur. Hemiballismus is the most dramatic of these; damage to the subthalamic nucleus results in violent, involuntary, rotatory flinging movements of the contralateral arm and leg. Similarly, dysfunction of the caudate nucleus often results in chorea, whereas the opposite phenomenon, akinesia, typically occurs when dopamine-producing cells in the substantia nigra degenerate. Lesions restricted to the globus pallidus often cause flexion dystonia and impaired postural reflexes.

CLINICAL MANIFESTATIONS OF LESIONS OF THE BASAL GANGLIA **Akinesia** When extrapyramidal diseases are analyzed into primary functional deficits (negative symptoms due to loss of connectivity) and secondary release effects (positive symptoms of excessive activity), akinesia stands as a principal negative or deficit symptom. *Akinesia* refers to the inability to initiate changes in activity and to perform ordinary volitional movements rapidly and easily. The terms *bradykinesia* and *hypokinesia* are employed to describe lesser degrees of impairment. In contrast to paralysis, which is the negative symptom of corticospinal tract lesions, strength is preserved, although there is a delay in achieving peak power. Akinesia is the most disabling feature of Parkinson's disease. Akinetic patients display severe immobility and underactivity. They sit motionless for long periods of time without shifting postures and take more than the time normally required to eat, dress, and bathe. There is general poverty of movement, including loss of automatic associated motions, such as eye blinks and freely swinging arms when walking. Akinesia probably accounts for such common symptoms in Parkinson's disease as facial immobility, vocal hypophonia, micrographia, and difficulty in arising from a chair and beginning to walk. Akinesia can affect the mind as well; slowed speed of thought is called *bradyphrenia*. Although pathophysiologic details remain uncertain, clinical analysis of akinesia supports the hypothesis that the basal ganglia are mainly responsible for initiation and automatic execution of learned motor plans. Neuropharmacologic evidence suggests that akinesia itself results from DA deficiency.

Rigidity Muscle tone is defined as the amount of resistance encountered when a relaxed limb is moved passively. In rigidity, the muscles are in continuous contraction, and resistance to passive movement is constant. Rigidity secondary to extrapyramidal disorders may superficially resemble spasticity due to corticospinal tract lesions in that both produce increases in muscular tone. A few clinical guidelines provide help in distinguishing these conditions at the bedside (Table 21-2). The distribution of increased tone often differs in rigidity and spasticity. Although rigidity is present in both flexor and extensor muscle groups, it tends to be more prominent in those which maintain a flexed posture. Rigidity is easy to detect in large muscle groups, but smaller muscles of the face, tongue, and larynx are also often affected. In contrast to rigidity, spasticity usually produces increased tone in the extensor muscles of the legs and the flexor musculature of the arms. The quality of hypertonus also can be used to distinguish the two conditions. Resistance to passive

TABLE 21-2 Clinical characteristics of altered muscle tone

	Hypertonia		Hypotonia
	Spasticity	Rigidity	
Resistance to stretch	Increased "clasp knife"	Increased; "lead pipe"	Decreased
Associated findings	Increased DTRs, Babinski's sign	Bradykinesia, resting tremor	Decreased DTRs, muscle atrophy, ataxia, intention tremor
Clinical conditions	Upper motor neuron lesions	Extrapyramidal syndromes	Lower motor neuron lesions, cerebellar syndromes

movements is constant and independent of movement speed in rigidity, accounting for terms such as "lead pipe" and "plastic" resistance. In spasticity, increased tone is velocity-dependent; there may be a free interval followed classically by the clasp-knife phenomenon; muscles do not contract until they are stretched a bit, and later, during stretch, the augmentation in muscle tone quickly subsides. Deep tendon reflexes are normal in rigidity but increased in spastic states. Spasticity results from hyperactivity of the stretch reflex arc due to central changes but without increased sensitivity of the muscle spindle; spasticity can be abolished by sectioning posterior spinal roots. Rigidity has less relationship with hyperactivity of segmental reflex arcs and depends more on heightened discharge of alpha motor neurons. A special type of rigidity is the cogwheel phenomenon, which is commonly associated with tremor in Parkinson's disease. When the hypertonic muscle is passively stretched, the resistance may be rhythmically jerky, as though the resistance of the limb were controlled by a ratchet.

Chorea   Derived from the Greek word meaning "dance," chorea refers to widespread arrhythmic movements of a forcible, rapid, jerky, restless type. Choreic movements are noted for their irregularity and variability; they are generally continuous, may be simple or quite elaborate, and affect any part of the body. They may resemble voluntary movement in complexity, but they are never combined into a coordinated act unless the patient incorporates them into a deliberate movement in order to make them less noticeable. Normal volitional movements are possible because there is no paralysis, but they may be excessively quick, poorly sustained, and deformed by choreic movements. Chorea may be generalized or limited to one side of the body. Generalized chorea is the predominant involuntary movement in Huntington's disease and in rheumatic (Sydenham's) chorea and usually involves the face, trunk, and limbs; it is often seen with levodopa toxicity in patients with Parkinson's disease. Another common choreiform disorder, tardive dyskinesia, occurs in association with chronic neuroleptic administration. Choreic movements in this disorder are generally restricted to the buccal, lingual, and mandibular musculature, although trunk and limbs may be involved in severe cases. Chorea may also occur in medical illnesses (e.g., systemic lupus erythematosus), cerebrovascular diseases, drug intoxications, and after infections (e.g., Sydenham's chorea). When alleviating the underlying disorder is not possible, benzodiazepines, reserpine, and neuroleptics may be moderately effective in suppressing chorea.

Athetosis   This term is from a Greek word meaning "unfixed" or "changeable." Athetosis is characterized by an inability to sustain the muscles of the fingers, toes, tongue, or any other muscle group in one position. The maintained posture is interrupted by continuous, slow, sinuous writhing movements. These are most pronounced in the digits and hands and consist of extension, pronation, flexion, and supination of the arm with alternating flexion and extension of the fingers. Athetotic movements are slower than those associated with chorea, but gradations are commonly seen and termed *choreoathetosis* when it is impossible to distinguish between the two. Generalized athetosis may be seen in children with static encephalopathy (cerebral palsy); it also can occur in Wilson's disease, in torsion dystonia, and following cerebral anoxia. Posthemiplegic athetosis is unilateral and occurs especially in children who have suffered a stroke. Patients whose athetosis is due to cerebral palsy or cerebral anoxia have variable degrees of additional motor deficit due to associated corticospinal tract disease. Discrete individual movements of the tongue, lips, and hands are often impossible, and attempts to perform such voluntary movements result in contraction of all the muscles in the limb and other parts of the body. Variable degrees of rigidity are generally associated with all forms of athetosis and may account for the slower quality of movement in this disorder in contrast to chorea. Treatment of athetosis is generally unsatisfactory, although some patients improve with the drugs used to suppress chorea and dystonia.

The dystonias   Dystonia refers to increased muscular tone that causes fixed abnormal postures. Some patients with dystonia also have shifting postures resulting from irregular, forceful twisting movements that affect trunk and extremities and produce bizarre, grotesque movements and positions of the body. The mobile spasms of dystonia are similar to those of athetosis but are generally slower. Dystonic movements increase during volitional motor activity, nervousness, and emotional stress; they diminish during relaxation and, like most extrapyramidal movement disorders, disappear completely during sleep.

Dystonias may be classified in two ways: by etiology or by the pattern of affected body parts. *Primary idiopathic torsion dystonia*, formerly known as dystonia musculorum deformans, is frequently inherited as an autosomal dominant characteristic due to an abnormal gene on chromosome 9. Spontaneous cases without family histories of dystonia are also common. Manifestations of dystonia usually begin in the first two decades of life, but adult forms are recognized. Torsion dystonia is classified as an extrapyramidal disease even though no pathologic lesions have been observed in the basal ganglia or elsewhere in the brain. *Secondary dystonias* are those which result from a known illness. Examples include Wilson's disease, posthemiplegic dystonia, perinatal brain injury, kernicterus, and sequelae of neuroleptic drugs (e.g., acute dystonic reactions and tardive dystonia).

Focal dystonias are more common than generalized dystonias and include such disorders as spasmodic torticollis, writer's cramp, blepharospasm, and spastic dysphonia. In the focal dystonias, a single area of the body is affected. Focal dystonias occur more frequently in adults than in children, remain stable, and rarely spread to involve other body parts. Spasmodic torticollis is the most common focal dystonia. There are intermittent or continuous spasms of the sternocleidomastoid, trapezius, and other neck muscles, usually more prominent on one side than on the other, that cause turning or tipping of the head. Torticollis is involuntary and cannot be inhibited and thereby differs from habit spasm or tic. Torticollis is worse when the patient sits, stands, or walks; placing a finger to the chin or side of the jaw often alleviates the muscle imbalance. Women are affected twice as often as men; the average age of onset is 40 years old. *Segmental dystonia* indicates involvement of two or more continuous body parts. Meige syndrome (oromandibular dystonia and blepharospasm) is a segmental cranial dystonia. In *generalized dystonia*, most body parts, including the legs, are involved. *Hemidystonia* involves an arm and leg on the same side of the body.

Development of rational pharmacologic therapy for dystonia is limited by the lack of information regarding neuroanatomic and neurochemical abnormalities. For generalized and segmental dystonias, symptomatic relief is sometimes achieved with high doses of anticholinergic drugs, benzodiazepines, baclofen, carbamazepine, and reserpine; levodopa has been helpful in some types of dystonia. Focal dystonias, such as blepharospasm, have been treated successfully by injecting a dilute solution of botulinum toxin into the affected musculature. When spasmodic torticollis is severe, surgical denervation of the affected muscles (C1–C3 bilaterally and C4 on one side) has given favorable results in most patients.

Myoclonus   This is a descriptive term for very brief, involuntary, random muscular contractions. Myoclonus can occur spontaneously at rest, in response to sensory stimuli, or with voluntary movements. Myoclonus may involve a single motor unit and simulate a fasciculation, or it may simultaneously involve groups of muscles that displace the limb or distort its voluntary movement. Myoclonus is a symptom that occurs in a wide variety of generalized metabolic and neurologic disorders collectively called the myoclonias. Posthypoxic intention myoclonus is a special myoclonic syndrome that occurs as a sequel to transient cerebral anoxia such as might occur, for example, during a brief cardiorespiratory arrest. Cognitive abilities are usually preserved; however, there are signs of cerebellar dysfunction, and voluntary movements are marred by action myoclonus involving the extremities, facial muscles, and even the voice. Action myoclonus deforms all movements and severely limits the patient's ability to eat, talk, write, or even walk. Myoclonus also may result from lipid storage disease, encephalitis, Creutzfeldt-Jakob disease, or metabolic

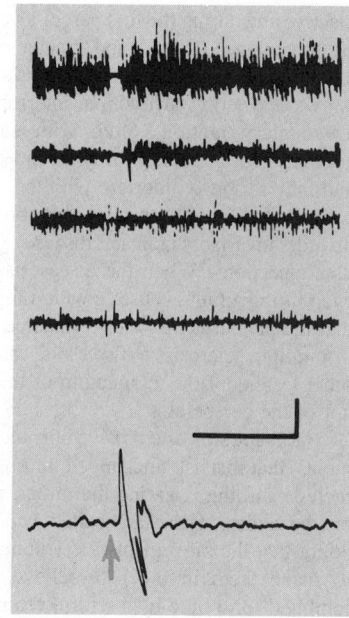

FIGURE 21-2 Asterixis recorded from the outstretched left arm of a patient with metrizamide-induced encephalopathy. The bottom trace is from an accelerometer on the dorsum of the hand. Calibration is 1 s. Note the continuous voluntary EMG interrupted at the arrow by a brief involuntary silent period in all four muscles. This silent period is followed by a lapse of posture and its jerky restitution, which is recorded by the accelerometer.

encephalopathies due to respiratory failure, chronic renal failure, hepatic failure, or electrolyte imbalance. Therapies for myoclonus include baclofen, clonazepam, and valproic acid.

Asterixis   Quick arrhythmic movements that occur due to brief interruptions in background tonic muscular contractions are called *asterixis*; in a sense, asterixis may be considered as negative myoclonus. Asterixis may be observed in any voluntary muscle during contraction but is usually demonstrated clinically as a brief lapse of posture with prompt restoration during voluntary extension of the limb with dorsiflexion of the wrist or ankle. Asterixis is characterized by 50- to 200-ms silent periods in ongoing EMG activity in all muscle groups in one limb (Fig. 21-2). This results in a downward movement of the wrist or ankle due to gravity before muscular activity resumes and restores the limb to its original position. Asterixis is commonly observed bilaterally in metabolic encephalopathies, and its description in hepatic failure accounted for the original term "liver flap." Asterixis may be caused by drugs, including all anticonvulsants and the radiographic contrast agent metrizamide. Unilateral asterixis can occur after brain lesions in the distributions of the anterior or posterior cerebral arteries. The smallest brain lesion that can cause unilateral asterixis involves structures that are destroyed during stereotactic ventrolateral thalamotomy.

Hemiballismus   Hemiballismus is a hyperkinetic movement disorder characterized by violent flinging motions in the arm contralateral to a lesion (usually vascular) in or near the subthalamic nucleus. The movements in ballism also have a rotary component at the shoulder and hip; there may be concomitant flexion and extension movements in the hand and foot as well. The involuntary motions persist throughout the day but generally attenuate during sleep. Strength and muscle tone may be slightly decreased in the affected extremities, and accurate movements are impaired, but patients with hemiballismus are not paralyzed. Both experimental and clinical observations indicate that the subthalamic nucleus probably exerts a controlling influence on the internal segment of the globus pallidus (see Fig. 21-1). Damage to the subthalamic nucleus destroys the excitatory input to the globus pallidus and thereby disinhibits thalamic facilitatory influences on motor cortex.

Tremor   This common symptom consists of a rhythmic oscillation of a part of the body around a fixed point. Tremors usually involve the distal parts of limbs; the head, tongue, or jaw; and rarely the trunk. There are several different types of tremor, and each has its own clinical setting, pathophysiology, and therapeutic requirements. Often several different tremors exist in the same patient and must be treated individually. In a general hospital, most patients who appear

tremulous actually have asterixis as a manifestation of a metabolic encephalopathy. Tremors may be subdivided clinically according to their distribution, amplitude, and relationship to volitional movement.

Tremor at rest is a coarse tremor with an average rate of four to five beats per second. It is most often localized in one or both hands and, occasionally, in the jaw or tongue. It is frequently a feature of Parkinson's disease. It characteristically occurs with postural (tonic) contraction of axial and limb girdle musculature when the limb is in an attitude of repose; willed movement temporarily suppresses it (Fig. 21-3). If the proximal muscles are completely relaxed, the tremor usually disappears, but the average patient rarely achieves this state. In some cases the tremor is constant; in others it varies from time to time and may extend from one group of muscles to another as the disease progresses. In some patients with Parkinson's disease there is no tremor; in others the tremor tends to be rather gentle and more or less limited to the distal muscles, whereas in a minority of parkinsonian patients and in patients with Wilson's disease, tremor has a large amplitude and involves proximal muscles. In many cases there is a variable degree of plastic rigidity in the tremulous limb or elsewhere. Although it is a source of great embarrassment and often is deemed responsible for all of a patient's motor difficulties, rest tremor interferes with voluntary movements surprisingly little: It is not uncommon to see a patient who has been trembling violently raise a full glass of water to the lips and drain the contents without spilling a drop. It is the combination of tremor at rest, slowness of movement, rigidity, flexed postures without true paralysis, and postural instability that constitutes Parkinson's syndrome. Often patients with Parkinson's disease also suffer from the tremor of stage fright (one of the enhanced physiologic tremors—see below) or from essential-familial tremor. Both may be exaggerated by increased levels of catecholamines in the bloodstream and may be suppressed by drugs, such as propranolol, that block beta-adrenergic receptors.

Tremor at rest almost always reflects idiopathic Parkinson's disease. Other conditions in which rest tremor may occur include Wilson's disease and severe essential tremor. Patients with titubation and a proximal tremor at rest (rubral tremor) as a symptom of cerebellar system dysfunction can be differentiated by the presence of ataxia and dysmetria from those with Parkinson's disease.

Action tremor refers to tremors present when the limbs are active, either when maintained in a certain position, as when outstretched, or throughout voluntary movement. Tremor amplitude may increase slightly as the action of the limbs becomes more precise, but it never approaches the degree of augmentation seen with cerebellar ataxia/dysmetria. In contrast to tremor at rest, action tremors disappear when the limbs are relaxed. Some of the action tremors are an exaggeration of normal *physiologic tremor;* such enhanced physiologic tremors are extremely common. They are experienced occasionally by all normal persons as well as by patients with essential-familial tremor or Parkinson's disease. They involve the outstretched hand as well as

FIGURE 21-3 Tremor at rest in a patient with Parkinson's disease. The upper two traces are surface EMG recordings from extensors and flexors of the left wrist; the lower trace is from an accelerometer attached to the left hand. The horizontal calibration denotes 1 s. Note the tremor at rest results from alternating contractions of antagonistic muscles at approximately 5 Hz. At the arrow, the patient is asked to dorsiflex the left wrist, and the tremor at rest disappears.

L. EXT.

L. FLEX.

L. ACC.

TABLE 21-3 Conditions that enhance physiologic tremors

HYPERADRENERGIC STATES

Anxiety
Bronchodilators and other beta agonists
Excitement
Hypoglycemia
Hyperthyroidism
Pheochromocytoma
Peripheral metabolites of levodopa
Stage fright

POSSIBLE HYPERADRENERGIC STATES

Amphetamines
Antidepressants
Withdrawal from alcohol or opiates
Xanthines in tea and coffee

STATES OF UNCERTAIN ETIOLOGY

Glucocorticoid therapy
Exercise
Fatigue
Lithium therapy

head, lips, and tongue. In general, they are due to a hyperadrenergic state and sometimes are iatrogenic (Table 21-3). Activation of beta₂ receptors in muscle alters the mechanical properties of muscle, eliciting action tremor. These alterations are reflected in discharges of muscle spindle afferents which modify the timing of activity around the stretch reflex arc and serve to augment the amplitude of preexisting physiologic tremor. Only patients without functional stretch reflex arcs are immune to these tremors. Peripherally active drugs that block beta₂-adrenergic receptors diminish enhanced physiologic tremors. This type of tremor is seen in numerous medical, neurologic, and psychiatric diseases and is therefore more difficult to interpret than tremor at rest.

Essential-familial tremor (Fig. 21-4) is a somewhat slower action tremor which may occur as the only neurologic abnormality either sporadically or in several members of a family. It may begin in childhood but usually comes on later and persists throughout adult life. It becomes a source of embarrassment because it suggests to the onlooker that the patient is nervous. A curious fact about this tremor is that one or two drinks of an alcoholic beverage may abolish it, but it will become worse after the effects of the alcohol have worn off. Essential-familial tremors are suppressed by primidone or CNS-active beta-adrenergic blocking agents such as propranolol.

Intention tremor is an ambiguous term: The abnormal movements are certainly not intentional, and the abnormality is best described as an oscillatory ataxia generated proximally rather than as tremor. True tremors tend to affect distal musculature, and the movements are more rhythmic and tend to be in one plane. Cerebellar ataxia, in which the direction of abnormal movement varies from second to second, requires for its full expression the performance of an exacting, precise, willed movement. Ataxia is absent when the limbs are

FIGURE 21-4 Action tremor in a patient with essential-familial tremor. Recordings from the right upper extremity are with the hand actively dorsiflexed. The horizontal calibration denotes 500 ms. Note that during this action tremor, bursts of EMG activity at approximately 8 Hz occur synchronously in antagonistic muscles.

inactive and during the first part of a voluntary movement but develops as the action continues and greater precision is demanded (e.g., in touching a target such as the patient's nose or the examiner's finger). Ataxia is a jerky, arrhythmic interruption of forward progression in a voluntary motion, often with side-to-side oscillations. Ataxia continues for a fraction of a second or so after the act is completed and may seriously interfere with the patient's performance of skilled acts. Sometimes the head is involved (titubation). This movement disorder invariably indicates disease of the cerebellar system, including its connections. When the disease is very severe, every movement, even lifting a limb, causes a wide-ranging oscillation of such violence that the patient is thrown off balance. This state is occasionally seen in multiple sclerosis, Wilson's disease, and vascular, traumatic, and other lesions of the tegmentum of the midbrain and subthalamus but not of the cerebellum.

Habit spasms and tics Many individuals develop habitual movements that persist unchanged throughout life. Common examples include sniffing, clearing the throat, protruding the chin, and pulling on the collar. These are called *habit spasms*. Affected individuals admit that the movements are voluntary but that they feel compelled to make them in order to relieve tension. Habit spasms can be inhibited for a time by a willful effort but reappear when attention is diverted. In certain cases they become so ingrained that the person is unaware of them and unable to control them. Children between 5 and 10 years of age are especially likely to have habit spasms.

Tics are characterized by stereotyped, purposeless, and irregularly repetitive movements. Gilles de la Tourette syndrome is the most common and severe form of multiple tic disorder. This syndrome is a neuropsychiatric disorder with motor and behavior abnormalities; it usually begins in the first two decades of life and affects boys four times more frequently than girls. Motor symptoms include multiple brief muscular spasms, known as *convulsive tics*, in the face, neck, and shoulders. Vocal tics, including grunts and barking sounds, are also common. Behavioral abnormalities include coprolalia (swearing and repeating other vile utterances) and repeating the words of others (echolalia). The cause of Tourette's syndrome is unknown, and its pathophysiology remains obscure. Treatment with neuroleptic drugs will decrease the severity and frequency of tics in 75 to 90 percent of patients with Tourette's syndrome, regardless of disease severity. The noradrenergic agonist clonidine also has been reported to suppress symptoms.

EXAMINATION OF EXTRAPYRAMIDAL SYNDROMES In broad terms, all the extrapyramidal disorders should be viewed in terms of primary deficit (negative symptoms) and of the new phenomena (abnormal postures and involuntary movements) that have appeared. The positive symptoms are ascribed to release from inhibition or disequilibrium of undamaged motor parts of the nervous system. The physician must cultivate the habit of accurately observing and describing abnormalities of movement and must not be content merely to give the condition a name or to force it into some superficial category. The fully developed extrapyramidal motor syndromes can be recognized without difficulty once the physician has become familiar with the typical pictures. A mental picture of Parkinson's disease, with its slowness of movement, poverty of facial expression, tremor at rest, and muscular rigidity, should be fixed in mind. Similarly, the gross distortions of posture found in dystonia, whether widespread in trunk muscles or involving only neck muscles as in spasmodic torticollis, should be easily recognized. Athetosis, with its instability of postures, ceaseless movements of finger and hands, and intention spasm; chorea, with its rapid and complicated movements; and myoclonus, with its abrupt movements that flit over the body, are other standard syndromes. There tends to be a mild defect in the voluntary use of the affected parts in all extrapyramidal syndromes.

Early or mild forms of these conditions, like all medical diseases, may offer special difficulties in diagnosis. Cases of Parkinson's disease seen before the appearance of tremor are often overlooked. Uncertainty of balance and short gait (*marche à petit pas*) in the elderly is often incorrectly attributed to loss of confidence and fear of falling. Patients may complain of being nervous and restless and describe a stiffness and aching in parts of the body. Because there is no weakness or change in reflexes, the disorder may then be considered rheumatic or even psychogenic. Parkinson's disease often begins in a hemiplegic distribution, and for this reason, the illness may be misdiagnosed as cerebral thrombosis or tumor. Facial immobility, a suggestion of a limp, mild rigidity, failure of an arm to swing naturally in walking, or loss of certain movements of cooperation will help in diagnosis at this time. Every patient presenting with atypical extrapyramidal symptoms should be surveyed for Wilson's disease in order to avoid missing a treatable illness. Mild or early chorea is often mistaken for simple nervousness. Observing the patient at rest as well as in action is critical to the diagnosis. There are instances, nonetheless, in which it is impossible to distinguish simple fidgets from early chorea, especially in children, and there are no laboratory tests to aid in the diagnosis. The first postural manifestations of dystonia may suggest hysteria, and it is only with repeated examinations that an accurate diagnosis is reached.

Motor disorders seldom appear in pure form, and extrapyramidal syndromes often coexist with lesions in the corticospinal tract or cerebellar systems. For example, syndromes such as progressive supranuclear palsy, olivopontocerebellar atrophy, and the Shy-Drager syndrome have many elements of Parkinson's disease but also have paralysis of voluntary eye movements, ataxia, apraxia, postural hypotension, or spasticity with bilateral Babinski's signs. Wilson's disease usually displays tremor at rest, rigidity, slowness of movement, and flexion dystonia of the trunk, but exceptionally there are athetosis, dystonia, and intention tremor. Emotional or cognitive abnormalities may be the presenting signs in Wilson's disease. Hallervorden-Spatz disease may take the form of universal rigidity and flexion dystonia, but choreoathetosis is sometimes observed. In some forms of Huntington's disease, particularly with juvenile onset, rigidity replaces choreoathetosis. Corticospinal and various extrapyramidal disorders may be associated in patients with cerebral diplegia. Some of the neurodegenerative diseases in which corticospinal tract and basal ganglia lesions coexist are described in Chap. 371.

REFERENCES

ALBIN RL et al: The functional anatomy of basal ganglia disorders. Trends Neurosci 12:366, 1989

ALEXANDER GE, CRUTCHER MD: Functional architecture of basal ganglia circuits: Neural substrates of parallel processing. Trends Neurosci 13:266, 1990

BERGMAN H et al: Renewal of experimental parkinsonism by lesions of the subthalamic nucleus. Science 249:1436, 1990

DUM RP, STRICK PL: Premotor areas: Nodal points for parallel efferent systems involved in the central control of movement, in *Motor Control: Concepts and Issues: Dahlem Konferenzen*, DR Humphrey, HJ Freund (eds). Chichester, Wiley, 1991, pp 383–411

FAHN S et al: Classification and investigation of dystonia, in *Movement Disorders 2*, CD Marsden, S Fahn (eds). London, Butterworths, 1987, pp 332–358

FREUND HJ, HEFTER H: The role of basal ganglia in rhythmic movement. Adv Neurol 60:88, 1993

GROWDON JH et al: L-Threonine in the treatment of spasticity. Clin Neuropharmacol 14:403, 1991

HALLET M: Classification and treatment of tremor. JAMA 266:1115, 1991

JAGIELLA WM, SUNG JH: Bilateral infarction of the medullary pyramids in humans. Neurology 39:21, 1989

JANKOVIC J, BRIN MF: Therapeutic uses of botulinum toxin. N Engl J Med 325:1186, 1991

JANKOVIC J, SCHWARTZ KS: Longitudinal experience with botulinum toxin injections for treatment of blepharospasm and cervical dystonia. Neurology 43:834, 1993

KUYPERS HGJM: Anatomy of the descending pathways, in *Handbook of Physiology*, sec 1: *The Nervous System*, vol 2: *Motor Control*, part 1, VB Brooks (ed). Bethesda, American Physiological Society, 1981, pp 597–666

OHYE C: Dynamic aspects of striatothalamic connection studies in cases with movement disorder. Adv Neurol 60:78, 1993

OZELIUS L et al: Human gene for torsion dystonia located on chromosome 9q32–q34. Neuron 2:1427, 1989

PAPAGNO C et al: Ideomotor apraxia without aphasia and aphasia without apraxia: The anatomical support for a double dissociation. J Neurol Neurosurg Psychiatry 56:286, 1993

PARENT A, HAZRATI LN: Anatomical aspects of information processing in primate basal ganglia. Trends Neurosci 16:111, 1993

POLO JM et al: Hereditary ''pure'' spastic paraplegia: A study of nine families. J Neurol Neurosurg Psychiatry 56:175, 1993

22   ATAXIA AND DISORDERS OF BALANCE AND GAIT

SID GILMAN

In the assessment of patients with neurologic disorders, it is important when taking the history to inquire about posture and gait and to examine these functions routinely as part of the neurologic examination. Abnormalities of posture and gait can result from disorders affecting several levels of the nervous system, and the type of abnormality observed clinically often indicates the site affected.

NEURAL STRUCTURES REQUIRED FOR STANDING AND WALKING   The structures in the central nervous system that control standing and walking are the basal ganglia, a "locomotor region" in the mesencephalon, the cerebellum, and the spinal cord. The cerebral cortex doubtless is important in many aspects of standing and walking, but in experimental animals, complete removal of the cerebral cortex during the neonatal period, preserving the basal ganglia, thalamus, and lower structures, leaves stance and locomotion essentially normal. In the adult animal, if the cerebral cortex, basal ganglia, and thalamus are removed, leaving the mesencephalon and lower brainstem intact, standing and walking are still possible. Electrical stimulation in a region of the mesencephalon termed the *locomotor region* evokes walking motions, and the speed and form of locomotion can be modified from a slow walk to a trot or gallop with changes in stimulation strength. This region receives projections from the basal ganglia, including the subthalamic and endopeduncular nuclei and the substantia nigra.

The spinal cord contains neural circuitry that coordinates the muscles for locomotion. After transection of the spinal cord in the midthoracic region in experimental animals, the hindlimbs maintain the capacity to perform coordinated walking movements when placed on a moving treadmill. With increased treadmill speed, walking movements can switch to simultaneous movements of the hindlimbs, as in a gallop. After a high spinal transection, both the forelimbs and the hindlimbs can generate alternating movements, and the sets of limbs remain coordinated. Thus neural circuitry in the spinal cord can coordinate movements among all four limbs. The cerebellum controls many of the movements required for walking. Ablation of the cerebellum in animals results in severe disorders of standing and walking.

In summary, walking is the result of integrated activity of the basal ganglia, mesencephalon, cerebellum, and spinal cord. Sensory inputs from movements of joints and muscle afferents provide important components for the control of walking. Without appropriate sensory feedback information, the pattern of walking is severely disrupted.

THE CEREBELLUM   The cerebellum functions in concert with the motor cortex, basal ganglia, and many brainstem structures in executing a variety of movements. The cerebellum is needed to maintain proper posture and balance for walking and running; to perform fine voluntary movements such as those needed for writing, dressing, and eating; to carry out rapidly alternating and repetitive movements such as in playing a musical instrument or working with a computer; and to coordinate smooth tracking movements of the eyes. The cerebellum controls certain properties of movements, including trajectory, velocity, and acceleration. Voluntary movements can be performed in the absence of cerebellar function, but the movements are clumsy and disorganized. The disturbances of movement from cerebellar dysfunction are termed *dyssynergia* (also *asynergia* or *ataxia*).

The cerebellum consists of a midline vermal region and two hemispheres, which are attached to the medulla, pons, and midbrain by three peduncles on each side. A layer of gray matter, the cerebellar cortex, covers the cerebellar surface and encloses an internal core of white matter. Three pairs of deep cerebellar nuclei are buried within the cerebellum. From medial to lateral these consist of the fastigial, interposed (globose and emboliform), and dentate nuclei.

The cerebellum consists of three lobes. The *flocculonodular lobe*, which is the oldest part of the cerebellum phylogenetically (archicerebellum), consists of the paired flocculi and the nodulus. This lobe receives input principally from the vestibular nuclei. The *anterior lobe*, the second oldest part (paleocerebellum), consists of vermal and paravermal structures in the anterosuperior portion of the cerebellum. The anterior lobe receives input chiefly from the spinal cord. The *posterior lobe* is the largest and phylogenetically newest part of the cerebellum (neocerebellum) and is located between the other two lobes. The posterior lobe receives projections from the cerebral hemispheres via the pontine nuclei.

The cerebellar cortex contains three layers: an outermost *molecular layer*, a middle *Purkinje cell layer*, and an inner *granular layer*. The afferent fibers reaching the cerebellar cortex send collateral projections to the deep cerebellar nuclei and terminate either in the granule cell layer as *mossy fibers* or on the dendrites of Purkinje cells as *climbing fibers*. Mossy fiber afferents are derived from the spinal cord, pontine nuclei, vestibular receptors and nuclei, trigeminal nuclei, reticular nuclei, and deep cerebellar nuclei. Climbing fiber afferents are derived exclusively from the inferior olive. Both mossy fiber and climbing fiber inputs are excitatory to the deep cerebellar nuclei and the cerebellar cortex. Purkinje cells provide the only route for all information exiting from the cerebellar cortex and are inhibitory to the deep cerebellar and vestibular nuclei.

Projections to the cerebellum also originate in the locus coeruleus and the raphe nuclei of the brainstem. The afferents to the cerebellum from the locus coeruleus are noradrenergic; those from the raphe nuclei are serotonergic; and both sets of afferents are inhibitory. Several amino acids have been identified as putative neurotransmitters in the cerebellum. These include glutamate, which is used by mossy fibers and the axons of granule cells (parallel fibers); aspartate, which is used by climbing fibers; and γ-aminobutyric acid, which is used by the axons of Purkinje cells, Golgi cells, and basket cells.

The *inferior cerebellar peduncle* (*restiform body*) consists chiefly of afferent fibers. The peduncle contains a single efferent tract, the fastigiobulbar tract, which projects from the fastigial nuclei to the vestibular nuclei and completes a vestibular circuit through the cerebellum. Afferent fibers enter the inferior cerebellar peduncle from at least six sources (Fig. 22-1): (1) fibers from the vestibular nerve and nuclei, (2) olivocerebellar fibers from the inferior olivary nuclei, (3) the dorsal spinocerebellar tract, (4) some of the fibers from the ventral spinocerebellar tract, (5) the cuneocerebellar tract from the accessory cuneate nuclei in the medulla, and (6) reticulocerebellar fibers. The *middle cerebellar peduncle* (*brachium pontis*) consists almost entirely of crossed afferent fibers from the pontine nuclei in the gray substance of the basal part of the pons (pontocerebellar or transverse pontine fibers) (Fig. 22-2). The major projections to the pontine nuclei originate within the cerebral cortex. The *superior cerebellar peduncle* (*brachium conjunctivum*) consists principally of efferent projections from the cerebellum. Fibers arising in the dentate and interposed nuclei project to the reticular formation, red nucleus, and thalamus. Some fibers of the fastigiobulbar tract also run with the superior peduncle for a short distance before entering the inferior cerebellar peduncle. The superior cerebellar peduncle contains afferent projections from the ventral spinocerebellar tract, a portion of the dorsal spinocerebellar tract, and trigeminocerebellar projections.

Except for direct projections of Purkinje cells onto vestibular nuclei, the efferent pathways of the cerebellum begin with the deep nuclei. The fastigial nucleus sends fibers to the reticular and vestibular nuclei of the brainstem. These nuclei project into the spinal cord and are concerned with posture and balance. The interposed nuclei of each side of the cerebellum project axons through the superior cerebellar peduncle to the red nucleus of the contralateral side. The red nucleus sends fibers into the rubrospinal tract (see Fig. 22-2), and this tract crosses the midline before descending into the spinal cord. The origin of this pathway in the interposed nuclei and the terminal

FIGURE 22-1   The central nervous system connections of the dorsal and ventral spinocerebellar tracts, the fastigial nuclei, and the vestibular nuclei. *(Adapted from S Gilman and S Winans Newman, Manter & Gatz's Essentials of Clinical Neuroanatomy and Neurophysiology, 8th ed, Philadelphia, Davis, 1992.)*

portion in the spinal cord are on the same side of the body. Both the dentate and the interposed nuclei send fibers through the superior cerebellar peduncle to the contralateral ventrolateral nucleus of the thalamus. The ventrolateral nucleus relays fibers to the motor regions of the ipsilateral frontal lobe. The thalamic endings in the cerebral cortex make connection with corticospinal neurons whose efferent fibers pass through the pyramidal tract and cross to the contralateral side of the spinal cord. Thus the origin of the cerebellothalamocortical

FIGURE 22-2   The central nervous system connections of the dentate nucleus and interposed (emboliform and globose) nuclei. *(Adapted from S Gilman and S Winans Newman, Manter & Gatz's Essentials of Clinical Neuroanatomy and Neurophysiology, 8th ed, Philadelphia, Davis, 1992.)*

pathway in the dentate and interposed nuclei and its termination in the spinal cord are on the same side of the body (see Fig. 22-2).

For clinical purposes, a useful method of describing the cerebellum is based on the existence of longitudinal sagittal zones. Each half of the cerebellum is subdivided into three longitudinal strips arranged from medial to lateral, including the cerebellar cortex, underlying white matter, and deep cerebellar nuclei: (1) a midline zone consisting of the vermal region with the fastigial nucleus, (2) an intermediate zone, the paravermal region, with the interposed nuclei, and (3) a lateral zone consisting of the cerebellar hemisphere with the dentate nucleus. Lesions of the midline zone cause disorders of stance and gait, truncal ataxia and titubation, and rotated or tilted postures of the head. Lesions of the lateral zone lead to disturbances in coordinated limb movement (ataxia), dysarthria, hypotonia, nystagmus, and kinetic tremor. Lesions of the intermediate zone cause symptoms characteristic of involvement of both the midline and lateral zones.

Ataxia is the result of dysmetria and decomposition of movement. *Dysmetria* is a disturbance of the trajectory or placement of a limb during active movement in which the limb falls short of its target (*hypometria*) or extends beyond its target (*hypermetria*). *Decomposition of movement* refers to errors in the sequence and speed of the component parts of a movement. The result is a lack of speed and skill in acts requiring the smoothly coordinated activity of several muscles. Movements previously fluid and accurate become halting and imprecise. *Ataxia* appears clinically as a disturbance in the rate and extent of an individual movement and commonly occurs from lesions of the cerebellum or of the sensory systems. Ataxia of gait consists of irregularities in the rate, length, and consistency of walking movements, with veering to one side or the other.

PHYSIOLOGIC RESPONSES IMPORTANT IN STANDING AND WALKING   Maintenance of the upright posture results from the actions of a number of postural reflex responses: (1) local static reactions acting on individual limbs, (2) segmental static reactions linking the extremities together, and (3) general static reactions resulting from the position of the head in space. *Local static reactions* include the stretch reflex and the positive supporting reaction. The simplest *stretch reflex* is illustrated by the muscle stretch response (deep tendon reflex), a brief muscle twitch evoked by rapid stretch of the muscle's tendon. Maintenance of muscle extension results in sustained contraction of that muscle through the stretch reflex. The *positive supporting reaction*, as elucidated in animal studies, results from a light cutaneous contact of the skin of the foot and also by proprioceptive stimulation owing to stretch of the interosseous muscles. The result of these stimuli is an extensor thrust by the limb.

The *segmental static reactions* include the crossed extension reflex and interlimb coordination. In the crossed extension reflex, application of noxious stimulation to an extremity results in flexion of that limb and simultaneous extension of the contralateral limb. With stronger stimulation, the crossed extension reflex triggered from a hindlimb can induce flexion in the contralateral forelimb and extension in the ipsilateral forelimb. Thus the whole body moves along a diagonal path through the extended contralateral hindlimb and ipsilateral forelimb, thereby removing the stimulated limb from the source of noxious stimulation. This diagonal pattern of interlimb coordination also provides postural adjustments in various situations.

The *general static reactions* consist of two general types. The first, the *tonic neck* and *labyrinthine reflexes*, function together to adjust body posture when the head moves relative to the trunk in space. The second, the *righting reflex*, is triggered by vestibular, neck proprioceptive, and visual stimuli and helps the animal to regain an upright position after a fall. The *grasp reflex* is a component of the righting reflex. Other forms of general static reactions include the placing and hopping reactions, as well as adjustment of body postures during limb movements.

CLINICAL APPROACH TO DISORDERS OF EQUILIBRIUM AND GAIT   When evaluating a disorder of gait, the physician should inquire whether the disturbance occurs more in the dark than in the light; whether vertigo, giddiness, or lightheadedness accompanies the

disorder; and whether there is pain, numbness, or tingling of the limbs. Inquiry should search for weakness, bowel and bladder dysfunction, and limb stiffness or rigidity. The physician should ask whether there is difficulty in the initiation or termination of walking and whether walking up or down stairs or on uneven surfaces worsens the disturbance in walking.

Examination of stance and gait is performed best in a setting in which the physician can observe the patient walk from the front, back, and sides. The patient should rise quickly from a chair, walk normally at a slow pace, then more rapidly, and then turn around. The patient should walk on the heels, on the toes, and in tandem, placing the heel of one foot directly in front of the toes of the opposite foot, attempting to progress in a straight line. The patient should stand erect with the feet together and the head straight, first with the eyes open and then with the eyes closed to determine whether balance can be maintained (Romberg's sign). It is often helpful to observe the gait initially as the patient comes into the examining room when the patient is unaware that gait and stance are being examined.

With normal walking the body should be held erect, the head should be straight, and the arms should hang loosely at the sides, each moving in rhythm with movement of the opposite leg. The shoulders and hips should be level, and the arms should swing equally. The steps should be straight and equal in length. The head should not be tilted, and there should be no appreciable scoliosis or lordosis. With each step the hip and knee should flex smoothly, the ankle should dorsiflex, and the foot should clear the ground easily. The heel should strike the ground first, and the weight of the body should be transferred successively onto the sole of the foot and then onto the toes. The head and body should rotate slightly with each step without lurching or falling movements. Each person walks in a characteristic fashion that is often familial. Some people walk with the toes turned inward, others with the toes turned outward. Some people stride with large steps, and others shuffle, making small steps. A person's gait is often a reflection of personality traits and can reflect shyness and timidity or aggressiveness and self-confidence.

Hemiparesis   The patient with weakness of the limbs on one side of the body from a lesion of the corticospinal tract usually develops a characteristic gait disorder. The severity of the disorder depends on the degree of weakness and stiffness of the affected limbs. The severely hemiparetic subject will stand and walk with the affected arm adducted at the shoulder and flexed at the elbow, wrist, and fingers and the affected leg stiffly extended at the hip, knee, and ankle. There is difficulty in flexing the hip and knee and dorsiflexing the ankle. Thus the paretic leg swings outward at the hip so that the foot does not scrape the floor. The leg is held stiffly and rotates in a semicircle, first away from and then toward the trunk in a circumduction movement. Often the upper body tilts slightly to the opposite side during the leg movement. The arm on the hemiparetic side usually swings little during walking. The loss of arm swing can be an early sign of a progressive hemiparesis. A person with a mild hemiparesis may show a gait disorder similar to that of the severely hemiparetic individual, but with a lesser degree of abnormality. In this case, a decrease in arm swing may be associated with subtle circumduction of the leg, without clear stiffness or weakness of the affected limbs.

Paraparesis   Diseases of the spinal cord that affect the function of both legs produce a characteristic gait resulting from a combination of spasticity and weakness of the lower extremities. Walking requires considerable effort and consists of slow, stiff movements at the hips and knees. The legs are usually maintained extended or slightly flexed at the hips and knees and adducted at the hips. In some people with paraparesis the legs may cross with each step, producing a scissoring motion. The steps usually are regular and short, and the patient may move the trunk from side to side, attempting to compensate for the stiff movements of the legs. The legs circumduct at the hips, and the feet scrape along the floor so that the soles of the shoes become worn at the toes.

Parkinsonism   Parkinson's disease produces a characteristic posture and gait. The severely affected individual stands in a posture of flexion, with the thoracic spine bent forward, the head bent downward, the arms moderately flexed at the elbows, and the legs slightly flexed at the hips and knees. The patient sits or stands with striking immobility, showing a fixed facial expression with infrequent blinking and making few automatic movements of the limbs. The patient seldom crosses the legs or adjusts body posture when seated in a chair. Although the arms are held immobile, often a tremor involves the fingers and wrists at four to five cycles per second. In some people the tremor also occurs at the elbows and even at the shoulders. In advanced cases there may be drooling and a rhythmic tremor of the jaw. The patient usually gets up slowly to walk, and with walking, the trunk bends even farther forward and the arms remain immobile at the sides of the body or become further flexed and are carried a bit ahead of the body. The arms fail to swing. As forward progression begins, the legs remain bent at the hips, knees, and ankles. Characteristically, the steps are short so that the feet barely clear the ground and the soles of the feet shuffle and scrape the floor. With forward locomotion the steps become successively more rapid, and the patient may fall unless assisted (*festination*). If the patient is pushed forward or backward, compensatory flexion or extension movements of the trunk fail to occur, and the patient is forced to make a series of propulsive or retropulsive steps.

Patients with Parkinson's disease often have great difficulty in rising from a chair or walking after standing still. The individual may initiate walking with several small steps before taking longer strides. Walking may stop involuntarily with attempts to pass through a doorway or into an elevator. Parkinsonian patients at times can walk with surprising speed and dexterity for brief intervals. In times of acute emergency, as in a fire, a person previously immobile can walk rapidly or even run briefly.

Cerebellar disease   Disease of the cerebellum causes difficulty in standing without support and in walking. The disorder may result from lesions intrinsic to the cerebellum or from lesions in the connecting pathways to and from the cerebellum. The difficulty is worsened by attempts to walk with a narrow base. The affected person usually stands with the legs apart, and standing may provoke *titubation*, a coarse forward and backward tremor of the trunk. Attempting to stand with the feet together provokes swaying or falling. The instability is the same whether the eyes are open or closed. The patient walks cautiously, taking steps of varying lengths, and lurches from side to side. The patient complains of difficulty with balance, is fearful of walking without support, and may insist on holding onto objects such as a bed or chair, moving cautiously between these objects. Frequently the individual does not need to be supported; simply touching a wall or an object in the room makes it possible to walk with a greater sense of security. When a mild gait disorder is present, walking may deteriorate with attempts to walk in tandem in a straight line. This causes the patient to lose balance and, in response, to place one foot to the side to avoid falling. With unilateral lesions of the cerebellum, balance is lost toward the side of the lesion.

When disease is restricted to the midline (vermal) portions of the cerebellum, as occurs in alcoholic cerebellar degeneration, disorders of stance and gait may develop without other signs of cerebellar dysfunction such as limb ataxia or nystagmus. In contrast, disease of the cerebellar hemispheres, either unilaterally or bilaterally, often causes marked limb ataxia and nystagmus in association with a gait disorder. With a lesion confined to one cerebellar hemisphere, ipsilateral disturbances of posture and movement commonly accompany the gait disorder. The patient usually stands with the shoulder on the side of the lesion lower than the other, and there may be an accompanying scoliosis. The limbs on the side of the cerebellar lesion show diminished resistance to passive manipulation (hypotonia). On walking the patient staggers and deviates toward the affected side. This can be demonstrated by asking the patient to walk around a chair. Rotation toward the affected side results in a fall into the chair,

and rotation toward the normal side causes movement away from the chair in a spiral. The affected arm and leg show marked ataxia in tests of coordinated movement such as successively touching the patient's nose and then the examiner's finger (the "finger-nose-finger test") or running the heel of the affected leg down the shin of the opposite leg (the "heel-knee-shin test").

Sensory ataxia   A characteristic gait disorder results from loss of sensation in the lower extremities due to disease processes in the peripheral nerves, dorsal roots, dorsal columns of the spinal cord, or medial lemnisci. The most disabling component of the sensory disorder is the loss of joint position sense, but loss of input from muscle spindle receptors, vibration detectors, and cutaneous receptors also contributes to the disability. People with sensory ataxia are unaware of the position of the lower extremities and consequently have difficulty in both standing and walking. The patient usually stands with the legs spread widely apart. The patient remains stable if asked to stand with the feet together and the eyes open but sways and often falls (positive Romberg's sign) when the eyes are closed. The test for Romberg's sign cannot be performed if the subject is unsteady when standing with the feet together and the eyes open, as may occur with cerebellar disease.

The patient with sensory ataxia walks with the legs spread widely apart, watching the ground carefully. The legs are lifted higher than necessary at the hips and are flung forward and outward in abrupt motions. The steps vary in length, and the feet make characteristic slapping sounds as they contact the floor. The patient usually holds the body somewhat flexed at the hips, often using a cane for support. If vision is impaired or the patient attempts to walk in the dark, the gait disturbance worsens. The patient becomes unsteady and often falls when attempting to wash the face because of the temporary loss of visual compensation occurring with closure of the eyes.

Cerebral palsy   This term encompasses a number of different motor abnormalities, most of them resulting from hypoxic-ischemic injury to the central nervous system in the perinatal period. The severity of the gait disturbance varies with the nature and extent of the lesion. Mild limited lesions can lead to increased deep tendon reflexes and extensor plantar responses with a slight degree of talipes equinovarus, without a clear gait disorder. More severe and extensive lesions commonly lead to bilateral hemiparesis. The patient stands and walks with a paraparetic posture and gait. The arms are adducted at the shoulders and flexed at the elbows and wrists.

Movement disorders commonly alter the gait in people with cerebral palsy. Athetosis occurs frequently and consists of slow or moderately rapid serpentine movements of the arms and legs, with postures alternating between the extremes of flexion with supination and extension with pronation. On walking, people with athetotic cerebral palsy show involuntary limb movements that are accompanied by rotary movements of the neck and frequent facial grimacing. The arms are usually flexed and the legs are extended, but asymmetric limb postures can occur with ambulation. For example, one arm may flex and supinate, and the other may extend and pronate. Asymmetric limb postures commonly occur as the head rotates from side to side. Usually when the chin turns to one side, the arm on that side extends and the opposite arm flexes.

Chorea   Individuals with choreic movements often develop a characteristic gait disorder. Chorea occurs most frequently in children with Sydenham's chorea, in adults with Huntington's disease, and occasionally in adults with Parkinson's disease treated with excessive amounts of dopamine agonist medications. Choreic movements consist of intermittent rapid movements of the face, trunk, neck, and limbs. Flexion, extension, and rotary movements of the neck occur along with grimacing movements of the face, twisting movements of the trunk and limbs, and rapid piano-playing movements of the digits. Frequently, in early chorea, flexion and extension movements of the hips occur so that the individual constantly seems to be crossing and uncrossing the legs. The patient may scowl, frown, and smile involuntarily. Walking usually accentuates the choreic movements. Sudden forward or sideward thrusting movements of the pelvis and rapid twisting movements of the trunk and limbs result in a gait that resembles a series of dance steps. The steps are usually irregular in size, and the patient has difficulty walking in a straight line. The rate of progression varies from slow to rapid owing to variability in the rate and amplitude of each step.

Dystonia This is an involuntary postural and movement disorder affecting children (dystonia musculorum deformans or torsion dystonia) and adults (dystonia of adult onset). The condition may occur sporadically without known cause, as a genetic disorder, or as part of another process such as Wilson's disease. In dystonia musculorum deformans, which commonly begins in childhood, the first symptom often consists of an abnormal gait. Characteristically, the patient will walk with one foot inverted at the ankle, placing weight on the lateral side of the foot; as the disease progresses, this problem worsens, and other postural abnormalities develop. These include elevation of one shoulder, elevation of a hip, twisted postures of the trunk, and excessive flexion of the wrist and fingers of one upper limb. Intermittent spasms of the trunk and limbs may interfere with walking. Eventually, torticollis, tortipelvis, lordosis, and scoliosis may supervene. In extreme cases, the patient becomes unable to walk. Adult-onset dystonia often results in a similar progression of movement disorders.

Muscular dystrophy Marked weakness of the muscles of the trunk and proximal portions of the legs causes a characteristic stance and gait. In attempting to rise from a seated position, the affected person bends forward, flexing the trunk at the hips, places the hands on the knees, and pushes the trunk upward by working the hands up the thighs. Standing occurs with exaggerated lumbar lordosis and a protuberant abdomen owing to weakness of the abdominal and paravertebral muscles. The patient walks with the legs spread widely apart and develops a waddling motion of the pelvis because of weakness of the gluteal muscles. The shoulders often slope forward, and winging of the scapulae may be seen with walking.

Frontal lobe disease Bilateral frontal lobe disease causes a characteristic gait disorder that is usually associated with dementia and frontal lobe release signs, including grasp, suck, and snout reflexes. The patient characteristically stands with the feet spread widely apart and takes a first step only after a long delay. This hesitancy is followed by very small shuffling steps and then by a few steps of moderate amplitude, after which time the patient freezes, unable to continue walking. The cycle then is repeated. Affected individuals usually do not show muscular weakness, abnormalities of the deep tendon reflexes, sensory changes, or extensor plantar reflex responses. Usually the patient can perform the individual limb movements required for walking if asked to mimic walking movements while lying supine. The gait disorder with frontal lobe disease is a form of apraxia, i.e., a disturbance in the performance of a motor function in the absence of weakness of the muscles required for the function.

Normal-pressure hydrocephalus Normal-pressure hydrocephalus (NPH) is a disorder characterized by dementia, gait apraxia, and urinary incontinence. Computed tomography reveals large cerebral ventricles, widening of the callosal angle, and lack of filling with cerebrospinal fluid of the subarachnoid space over the cerebral hemispheres. Injection of radioactive isotope into the lumbar subarachnoid space demonstrates pathologic reflux of the isotope into the ventricular system and inadequate penetration into the cortical subarachnoid spaces.

The gait in NPH resembles that seen in apraxia from frontal lobe disease, consisting of a series of small, shuffling steps, making it appear that the feet are glued to the floor. Initiation of walking is impaired, and slow and small angular displacements of the hip, knee, and ankle joints occur along with low clearance of the foot from the floor so that the patient appears to be sliding the feet along the floor. There is continuous contraction of the antigravity muscles of the legs but low muscle activity in the calf muscles. The gait disorder in NPH is thought to result from impaired function of the frontal lobes. In about half the patients with NPH the gait is improved by surgical shunting of cerebrospinal fluid from the cerebral ventricles into the venous system.

Aging Changes in gait and difficulties with balance occur with aging. Elderly men develop forward flexion of the upper portion of the trunk with flexion of the arms and knees, decreased arm swing, and shortening of step length. Elderly women develop a waddling gait with shortening of step length. Abnormalities of gait and balance predispose the elderly to falls. About half the falls in the aged result from environmental factors, including poor illumination, stairs, and uneven or slippery surfaces. Other causes of falls include drop attacks, orthostatic hypotension, turning movements of the head, and vertigo.

Lower motor neuron disorders Diseases of the lower motor neurons or peripheral nerves characteristically cause distal limb weakness. Foot drop is a common manifestation. In the case of lower motor neuron disease, the limb weakness occurs in association with fasciculations and muscle atrophy. The patient usually cannot dorsiflex the foot and compensates by raising the knees higher than usual, thereby walking with a "steppage gait." If proximal muscles are affected, the gait also can take on a waddling quality.

Hysterical gait disorders Hysterical disorders of gait commonly appear in association with hysterical paralysis of one or more limbs. Usually the gait is bizarre, easily recognized as hysterical, and unlike any disorder of gait evoked by organic disease. In other instances, however, hysterical gait disorders may resemble organic gait disorders and can be difficult to identify. Hysterical gait disorders can occur in men or women and can appear in youth, young adulthood, and middle age.

In hysterical hemiplegia, the patient drags the affected leg along the ground behind the body and does not circumduct the leg or use it effectively to support the body weight. At times the hemiplegic leg may be pushed ahead of the patient and used mainly for support. The arm on the affected side often remains limp, hanging uselessly beside the body, and does not develop the flexed posture commonly seen in hemiplegia from organic causes. The patient with hysterical hemiplegia usually shows "give way" weakness. This is tested by asking the patient to make a maximum contraction of a set of muscles in an affected limb. Initially, a strong contraction may occur, but as the examiner attempts to oppose the contracting muscles, the contraction suddenly gives way. Hysterical patients also commonly contract their muscles very slowly upon request, displaying great concentration and effort to evoke the contraction. Objective signs of neurologic disease are absent; the affected limbs show normal resistance to passive manipulation, the deep tendon reflexes are equal on the two sides of the body, and the plantar responses are downgoing.

In hysterical paraplegia, the patient usually walks with one or two crutches or lies in bed with the legs maintained either completely limp or stiffly extended. The term *astasia-abasia* refers to patients who cannot stand or walk but who can carry out natural movements of the limbs when lying in bed. Some patients with hysterical paraparesis walk with seeming difficulty but show normal power and coordination when lying in bed. On walking, the hysterical person clings to the bed or the furnishings of the room. If asked to walk without support, the patient may lurch forward dramatically, veering from side to side at regular intervals. The patient can manage feats of extraordinary balance to avoid falling and may assume a variety of postures, walking with the legs in stiff extension, as if the legs are granite pillars, or walking with the legs in flexion and teetering from side to side. The hysterical patient may fall with walking, but only when a nearby physician or family member can catch the patient or when soft objects are available to cushion the fall. The gait disturbance is usually dramatic when an audience is present, and the patient can display remarkable agility in the rapid postural adjustments that occur.

REFERENCES

Coles SK et al: The mesencephalic centre controlling locomotion in the rat. Neuroscience 28:149, 1989

GILMAN S: Cerebellar deficit, in *Diseases of the Nervous System*, vol. 1: *Clinical Neurobiology*, 2d ed, AK Asbury et al (eds). Philadelphia, Saunders, 1992

——— et al: *Disorders of the Cerebellum*. Philadelphia, Davis, 1981

HORE J et al: Cerebellar dysmetria at the elbow, wrist, and fingers. J Neurophysiol 65:563, 1991

ITO M: Structural-functional relationships in cerebellar and vestibular systems. Arch Ital Biol 129:53, 1991

LEMPERT T et al: How to identify psychogenic disorders of stance and gait. J Neurol 238:140, 1991

MAZZIOTTA J, GILMAN S (eds): *Clinical Brain Imaging: Principles and Applications*. Philadelphia, Davis, 1992

ROSS CA et al: Messenger molecules in the cerebellum. Trends Neurosci 13:216, 1990

SANES JN et al: Motor learning in patients with cerebellar dysfunction. Brain 113:103, 1990

23 MUSCLE SPASMS, CRAMPS, AND EPISODIC WEAKNESS

ROBERT C. GRIGGS

Spontaneous or exercise-related discomfort from muscles or joints is usually benign and does not signal neuromuscular disease. Such symptoms may, however, provide clues to disabling disorders that too often evade diagnosis. The terms *pain*, *spasm*, and *cramp* are often used interchangeably by patients to describe symptoms referable to muscles. Other terms, including *aching*, *heaviness*, *stiffness*, and *rheumatism*, are also used and usually connote less certainty about the source or localization of the discomfort. In clinical terminology, *spasm* refers to a brief, unsustained contraction of a single or multiple muscles. *Cramp* is a paroxysmal, spontaneous, prolonged, and painful contraction of one or more muscles. Muscle pain may be associated with fatigue (asthenia) or weakness. This chapter discusses both fatigue and episodic weakness. The usual causes of weakness are considered in Chaps. 21 and 22.

SPASMS   Abnormal movements of muscle may arise from abnormal electrical activity of the central nervous system (CNS) mediated via the motor neuron or occur within the motor neuron or muscle fiber itself. It may be difficult on clinical grounds alone to determine the precise site of origin of the abnormal motor activity. In general, movements originating in the CNS affect the entire side of the body, an entire limb, or a group of muscles. Central disorders may be rhythmic or intermittent; those arising in the periphery are usually random. The electroencephalogram (EEG) may provide evidence for altered cortical activity in some conditions with a CNS etiology. The electromyogram (EMG) is less helpful because it reflects motor activity from any cause. EMG evidence of an underlying nerve or muscle disease may, however, be helpful in diagnosis (see Chaps. 366 and 382).

Intermittent, nonrhythmic movements of an entire limb, of the trunk, or of a portion of the face may result from cerebral seizure activity (Chap. 366) or from myoclonus (Chap. 21). Flexor and extensor spasms of an entire side or of the lower limbs result from a loss of motor inhibition within the CNS (Chap. 21). *Segmental myoclonus* results from focal disease within the brainstem or spinal cord that causes an abnormal discharge of groups of motor neurons. Localized vascular disease, tumor, or another lesion may be implicated.

Abnormal facial movements   *Hemifacial spasm* results from paroxysmal facial nerve activity, sometimes triggered by pressure from a tortuous blood vessel adjacent to the facial nerve as it leaves the brainstem. Hemifacial spasm commonly occurs in muscles about the eye but also may involve or spread to the entire side of the face. Symptoms are often intermittent and intensified when patients are using facial muscles in activities such as speaking. Hemifacial spasm is painless but embarrassing, especially to individuals dealing with the public. Since it is often intensified and more severe when the patient is in stressful situations, an erroneous diagnosis of tic (habit spasm) is often made. Cerebellopontine angle lesions can occasionally produce a similar disorder. Neuroradiologic investigation is indicated in patients with hemifacial spasm. Injection of botulinum toxin into involved muscles alleviated spasm for up to 3 months; surgical exploration and shielding of the facial nerve from the adjacent vessel is often curative (Chap. 380).

Facial *tics* (habit spasms) are stereotyped movements of the face such as eye blinking, head turning, or grimacing that are under voluntary control but may be suppressed only by effort and anxiety on the part of the subject (see Chap. 21). Some tics are so frequently encountered as to be considered mannerisms, analogous to excessive clearing of the throat. The repetitive elevation of the eyebrows by frontalis muscle contraction is an example. Certain hereditary movement disorders such as Gilles de la Tourette syndrome are characterized by multiple tics. Tics usually can be controlled by neuroleptic agents (Chap. 21).

Synkinesias of the face result from aberrant regeneration of the facial nerve following facial paralysis from Bell's palsy or other facial nerve lesions. Nearly 50 percent of patients who recover from Bell's palsy display such movements; an example is *jaw winking*, where voluntary movements of the lower face elicit contraction of the orbicularis oculi muscle with eye closure (see Chap. 380).

Trigeminal neuralgia (tic douloureux) is characterized by brief, paroxysmal, lancinating pain in one side of the face (see Chap. 380). Although the portion of the nerve involved is almost exclusively sensory, the severity of the pain causes involuntary contraction of facial muscles; hence the name *tic*. Abnormal movements do not occur in the absence of pain.

Facial myokymia refers to a nearly continuous, fine or coarse rippling and fascicular twitching of facial muscles. Although often benign, it may result from lesions of the pons such as a neoplasm or multiple sclerosis. Similar movements occur in motor neuron diseases such as amyotrophic lateral sclerosis or occasionally as an isolated, hereditary condition.

Abnormal limb movements   No movement should be visible in totally relaxed muscles. Diseases of motor neurons or their proximal axons are often associated with *fasciculations*, the spontaneous firing of an entire motor unit. Fasciculations are visible on inspection of muscle or perceived by the patient as a pulsation or quivering within muscle. Fasciculations occur at times in most normal individuals, and unless weakness is present, they are seldom of any significance. Fasciculations are normal if observed in incompletely relaxed muscles. *Myokymia*, consisting of numerous, repetitive fasciculations, also may occur in limb muscles, giving a writhing appearance. Myokymia disappears with neuromuscular blockade, proving that the activity originates in anterior horn cells or in peripheral nerve. In patients with long-standing muscle denervation and reinnervation, motor unit size enlarges and fasciculations may be so large as to produce movement of the limbs, particularly of the fingers, a condition termed *minipolymyoclonus*.

Certain conditions are characterized by a compulsion to move the extremities. *Akathisia*, or motor restlessness, occurs in Parkinson's disease and other disorders of the basal ganglia, including drug-induced movement disorders. The *restless legs syndrome* describes an uncomfortable sensation in muscles, usually in the legs and thighs, which occurs most commonly in middle-aged women. Patients feel they need to move their legs to relieve the abnormal sensation. The restless leg syndrome is frequent in uremia and may occur in other neuropathies, suggesting that the sensation is caused by an underlying neuropathy. It also may be familial, and detailed study of such patients has failed to demonstrate any evidence of neuropathy. The restless sensation may be accompanied by myoclonic jerks of muscle. These myoclonic jerks are similar to the myoclonus observed in normal individuals entering REM sleep (see Chap. 29).

These forms of muscle spasm and myoclonus are somewhat similar to a group of unusual *startle* syndromes or *hyperexplexias* characterized by sudden jerking of limbs or occasionally of trunk muscles. Sudden noise or touch may cause a patient to jump or to fling an extremity. Hyperexplexias may result from an abnormality of gamma-aminobutyric acid (GABA) receptors.

SUSTAINED MUSCLE CONTRACTIONS Distinguishing central from peripheral causes of sustained muscle contraction is often difficult. Abnormal muscle contractions with increased muscle tone usually result from CNS disease. Thus loss or disturbance of CNS inhibition may lead to abnormal muscle contraction characteristic of spasticity, rigidity, or ''paratonic'' rigidity. In most instances there is other evidence of CNS disorder (Chap. 21). Diseases of the basal ganglia, presumably resulting from altered neurotransmitter release, may lead to dystonia (see Chaps. 21 and 22).

Abnormal muscle contractions also may arise from repetitive depolarization of the component portions of the motor unit: the motor neuron, the peripheral axon of the neuron, the neuromuscular junction, or muscle fibers. Electrically inactive contractions may arise from disorders of the muscle contractile system.

Motor neuron disorders *Cramp* is a term often used by patients to refer to a painful, involuntary contraction of a single muscle or a muscle group. Muscle cramps can arise from spontaneous firing of groups of anterior horn cells followed by contraction of many motor units. EMG recordings indicate that motor units fire at a rate of up to 300 per second, much higher than occurs with voluntary contraction. Cramps occur frequently in the legs in elderly patients and, when severe, are followed by residual tenderness and evidence of muscle fiber necrosis, including elevation of serum creatine kinase. Cramps in the calf muscles are so common as to be considered normal, but more generalized cramps may be a sign of chronic disease of the motor neuron, such as amyotrophic lateral sclerosis. They may be particularly troublesome during pregnancy, in patients with electrolyte disturbances (hyponatremia), and in patients on hemodialysis. When recurrent and localized to one muscle group, they suggest nerve root disease. In many instances, however, it is impossible to determine the cause of cramps. Benign cramps, occurring commonly at night, may be relieved by quinine sulfate. Other causes of contractions arising from the motor neuron include *tetanus* (Chap. 106) and the *stiff-man syndrome*. In both disorders, a loss of inhibitory neuronal input to anterior horn cells may result in repeated firing of motor neurons, producing severe, painful muscle contraction. Antibodies to glutamic acid decarboxylase are present in the stiff-man syndrome, and the disorder may respond to plasma exchange. A similar clinical picture may occur acutely with *strychnine poisoning*. Diazepam improves these spasms but may cause respiratory depression in doses sufficient to alleviate muscle contraction.

Peripheral nerve *Tetany* is characterized by contractions of predominantly distal muscles, particularly in the hand (carpal spasm) and feet (pedal spasm). Laryngospasm also may occur. Tetany results from increased excitability of peripheral nerves. The muscle contractions are initially painless, but if sustained, they may cause muscle damage with pain. Severe tetany may involve spine musculature to produce opisthotonus. Tetany is usually caused by hypocalcemia, but it may occur with hypomagnesemia or severe respiratory alkalosis (see Chap. 357). Idiopathic normocalcemic tetany, *spasmophilia*, occurs in both hereditary and acquired forms. The acquired disorder is similar to Isaac's syndrome (neuromyotonia), in which hyperexcitability of peripheral nerve leads to muscle cramps and twitching. Such patients have responded to plasma exchange and it may be mediated by IgG autoantibodies to nerve membrane ion channels.

Muscle MYOTONIA Repetitive depolarization of muscle cells can cause muscle contraction resulting in muscle stiffness and impaired relaxation. Myotonia is usually painless, but it may disable patients by interfering with fine hand movements or by slowing ambulation. Myotonic dystrophy is the most common disorder associated with myotonia, although other manifestations of the disease such as cataracts and muscle weakness are usually more symptomatic (see Chap. 385). Myotonia congenita and paramyotonia congenita are less

common but more troublesome in terms of severity of myotonia. Myotonia is often worsened by cold and characteristically is attenuated by repeated muscle activity. *Myotonia congenita* has both autosomal dominant and recessive variants; myotonia results from defects in chloride channel function. *Paradoxical myotonia* worsens with repeated activity and is characteristic of paramyotonia congenita; these patients also suffer from episodic and cold-induced weakness (see Chap. 387). Myotonia can often be alleviated by quinine, phenytoin, or mexilitine. Impaired muscle relaxation that is electrically inactive is characteristic of the delayed relaxation of myxedema. This delay produces the characteristic ''hung-up'' ankle reflexes but is essentially asymptomatic.

CONTRACTURE Muscle contracture is a painful shortening of a muscle unassociated with muscle membrane depolarization. It occurs in disorders where a metabolic defect such as myophosphorylase deficiency limits the production of high-energy phosphates. Contractures are precipitated by exercise, are usually intensely painful, and result in muscle damage; widespread muscle contractures may cause sufficient myoglobinuria to precipitate renal failure. This use of the term *contracture* is confusing because the same word is used to describe the unrelated limitation of joint movement by shortening of muscle tendons seen in rheumatologic disorders, cerebral palsy, or chronic myopathies. Muscle rigidity from metabolic contracture can occur in the malignant hyperthermia syndrome, usually associated with general anesthesia (see Chap. 398). In the neuroleptic malignant syndrome, muscle rigidity arises from CNS overactivity, and intense electrical activity is present in muscle (see Chap. 398).

MUSCLE PAIN, ACHING, AND TENDERNESS Painful muscles do not always imply muscle disease. Joint and bone disease frequently produces complaints of muscle pain and may further confuse the anatomic localization of symptoms by resulting in disuse atrophy and moderate muscle weakness. Pain from disease of overlying subcutaneous tissue or fascia and of tendons also may be referred to muscle. Additionally, disease of major peripheral nerves or of their small intramuscular branches may produce both muscle pain and weakness. Muscle pain may be a major symptom in inflammatory, metabolic, endocrine, and toxic myopathies (see Chaps. 384 and 385).

Muscle trauma Vigorous activity, even in conditioned athletes, may be associated with muscle and tendon tears which lead to temporary acute muscle pain, swelling, and tenderness. Rupture of muscle tendons such as the biceps or gastrocnemius muscle may produce visible muscle shortening.

The almost-pleasurable ache and fatigue of muscles after strenuous activity is separable only by degree from more severe, but still normal pain following severe, unaccustomed activity. Such symptoms are often associated with laboratory evidence of profound muscle damage, including a rise in serum enzymes (creatine kinase), focal edema on MRI, and widespread muscle necrosis on biopsy. Myoglobinemia and myoglobinuria may occur. Particularly likely to produce muscle pain and necrosis are certain types of exercise: brief periods of contracting a muscle while it is lengthening (eccentric contractions) and prolonged exercise such as marathon running. The point at which such symptoms become abnormal is not clear. Many patients have pain with moderate activity. Such exertional muscle pain is also characteristic of metabolic disorders of muscle such as carnitine palmitoyl transferase deficiency and myoadenylate deaminase deficiency; patients with partial defects in *dystrophin* may have recurrent exercise-induced myalgias. Complete deficiency of this protein causes Duchenne muscular dystrophy (see Chap. 385). Deficiencies of enzymes of glycolysis are more commonly associated with contractures (see Chap. 385). The majority of patients with exertional and postexertional muscle pain do not have a definable abnormality.

Diffuse myalgias Muscle pain in the absence of muscle weakness can occur in acute infections caused by influenza virus and coxsackievirus. Fibrositis, fibromyalgia, and fibromyositis are synonyms for a disorder associated with pain and tenderness of muscle and adjacent connective tissue. Focal ''trigger points'' of tenderness can be identified, and systemic symptoms such as fatigue, insomnia, and depression are frequently present (see Chap. 384). Although patients often identify painful swellings, histologic evaluation discloses no abnormality of muscle or connective tissue. Symptoms may respond partially to amitriptyline or nonsteroidal anti-inflammatory agents, but the disorder tends to be chronic and unrelenting. A supportive program of physical reconditioning is sometimes helpful. Patients whose symptoms persist for months or years are often considered to have a psychiatric disorder, but its nature has not been defined.

Polymyalgia rheumatica occurs in patients over age 50 and is characterized by stiffness and pain in shoulder and hip musculature. Despite symptoms of pain localized to muscles, there is convincing evidence that the disease includes a proximal, inflammatory arthritis; joint effusions are often present in knees and other peripheral joints as well. Patients often develop profound disuse atrophy of muscles and complain of weakness, giving rise to a suspicion of polymyositis. However, creatine kinase levels are usually normal, and muscle biopsy shows atrophy without evidence of muscle necrosis or inflammation. The erythrocyte sedimentation rate is elevated in most patients, and temporal arteritis may be present (see Chap. 291). Treatment with nonsteroidal anti-inflammatory agents is advocated except in patients with temporal arteritis, for whom prednisone (40 to 60 mg daily) is recommended. Patients with polymyalgia rheumatica who fail to respond to nonsteroidal anti-inflammatory agents may require low-dose prednisone (10 to 20 mg daily). Myalgias are also frequent in other rheumatologic disorders, including rheumatoid arthritis, systemic lupus erythematosus, polyarteritis nodosa, scleroderma, and the mixed connective tissue syndrome. Patients with polymyositis and dermatomyositis may have myalgias, although in the majority muscle pain is lacking or minimal (see Chap. 384).

EPISODIC WEAKNESS   The term *weakness* is often used by a patient to describe a loss of stamina or decreased "energy." Even careful efforts at eliciting a history of true as opposed to subjective weakness may fail to distinguish the two conditions. The most helpful strategy is to ask the patient to identify whether a discrete loss of function has occurred and to elicit the circumstances in which symptoms are noted.

Weakness, whether true or perceived, may be due to disorders of the central or peripheral nervous system. Weakness from CNS disorders such as transient cerebral ischemia is usually associated with a change in level of consciousness or cognition, with increased muscle tone and muscle stretch reflexes, and often with alterations of sensation. Most neuromuscular causes of intermittent weakness are associated with normal mental function but diminished muscle tone and muscle stretch reflexes. The major causes of intermittent weakness are listed in Table 23-1. Central causes are considered in Chaps. 21 and 368.

EPISODIC ASTHENIA   Patients who describe intermittent "weakness" as *fatigue* and loss of *stamina* suffer from asthenia, which can be separated from true weakness by the fact that patients do not lack the ability to do a task but rather the ability to perform it repetitively. Asthenia is a major problem in many patients with serious renal, hepatic, cardiac, or pulmonary disease. Examination of such patients usually confirms their ability to do all functional activities at least once, such as rising from a knee bend, climbing stairs, or rising from a chair. Fatigue is also characteristic of relatively selective damage to CNS descending motor tracts, in which signs of neurologic abnormality may be minimal. Fatigue that is worsened by activity is characteristic of the *chronic fatigue syndrome* (see Chap. 388).

Intermittent weakness due to peripheral neuromuscular disease may result from abrupt changes in peripheral nerve function, intermittent destruction of muscle, alterations of electrophysiologic properties of muscle from abnormalities of blood electrolytes, and intermittent failure of neuromuscular transmission.

FAILURE OF PERIPHERAL NERVE CONDUCTION   A number of uncommon peripheral neuropathies are associated with recurrent weakness. *Hereditary liability to pressure palsies*, often termed *tomaculous* neuropathy because of the sausage-like appearance of

TABLE 23-1   Causes of episodic generalized weakness

Electrolyte disturbances
  Hypokalemia: Primary aldosteronism (Conn's syndrome); barium poisoning; renal tubular acidosis; juxtaglomerular apparatus hyperplasia (Bartter's syndrome); villous adenoma of colon; alcoholism; diuretics; licorice; para-aminosalicylic acid; glucocorticoids
  Hyperkalemia: Addison's disease; chronic renal failure; hyporeninemic hypoaldosteronism
  Hypercalcemia
  Hypocalcemic tetany
  Hyponatremia
  Hypophosphatemia
  Hypermagnesemia
Neuromuscular junction disorders
  Myasthenia gravis
  Lambert-Eaton syndrome
Muscle disorders
  Periodic paralyses
  Metabolic defects of muscle (impaired carbohydrate or fatty acid utilization)
Central nervous system causes
  Cataplexy and sleep paralysis associated with narcolepsy
  Multiple sclerosis
  Transient ischemic attacks
Disorders with only subjective weakness: Hyperventilation, hypoglycemia

myelin on nerve biopsy, is an autosomal dominant disorder characterized by abrupt paralysis following compression of a peripheral nerve. The paralysis is usually self-limited, lasting days to weeks. Other types of peripheral neuropathy also may predispose to the development of reversible, compressive neuropathies (see Chap. 383).

DISORDERED NEUROMUSCULAR JUNCTION TRANSMISSION   *Myasthenia gravis*, particularly in its initial manifestations, is characterized by transient weakness. Cranial muscles are usually affected first, causing double vision, ptosis, dysphagia, and dysarthria. Rarely, limb weakness may herald the onset of myasthenia gravis and in the absence of cranial muscle dysfunction may escape diagnosis for months. Diurnal variation in strength is typical, and reflexes are preserved. Other, less-common defects of the neuromuscular junction such as the Lambert-Eaton syndrome also may present with intermittent weakness (see Chap. 386).

INTERMITTENT ALTERATIONS IN ELECTROLYTES   Transient shifts in serum potassium are associated with profound alterations in muscle strength. Although the primary periodic paralyses (hypo- and hyperkalemic periodic paralysis) spring to mind in a patient with weakness and an abnormality in serum potassium, other causes of abnormal serum potassium are more frequently behind episodic weakness (see Chap. 387). Familial periodic paralysis seldom presents after age 30; other causes are usually present in older patients. Hypokalemic periodic paralysis may occur in patients with hyperthyroidism. Episodic weakness due to hypokalemia may occur with renal or gastrointestinal potassium loss (see Table 23-1).

Hyperkalemic weakness usually occurs in the setting of chronic renal or adrenal disease. Other electrolyte disturbances may produce intermittent weakness as the initial clinical manifestation of a severe metabolic abnormality (see Table 23-1). Correction of the metabolic derangement improves the weakness.

METABOLIC MUSCLE DISEASE   A number of uncommon defects in glycogen and lipid utilization are associated with impaired energy production by muscle and cause intermittent weakness, usually accompanied by muscle pain and evidence of muscle damage. Carnitine palmitoyl transferase deficiency is one such condition. Mitochondrial disorders such as cytochrome oxidase deficiency may produce severe exercise intolerance with fatigue and weakness associated with lactic acidosis. Muscle pain and destruction seldom occur. (See also Chap. 385.)

Recurrent attacks of a feeling of "weakness" often occur in patients with the *hyperventilation syndrome;* such patients are, however, of normal strength when tested. Similarly, *recurrent hypoglycemic episodes* are associated with subjective weakness, although hypoglycemia is uncommon as the cause of this symptom.

Central nervous system disorders may cause generalized weakness without an associated alteration of consciousness. *Drop attacks* resulting from impaired blood supply to the motor pathways of the brainstem cause sudden paraparesis or quadriparesis, usually lasting only a few seconds. Patients with narcolepsy may have sudden loss of muscle strength and tone during episodes of *cataplexy*. A disorder of the reticular activating system is responsible for these episodes as well as for *sleep paralysis* that occurs as narcoleptic patients are falling asleep or awakening (see Chap. 29).

REFERENCES

ARGOV Z: Phosphorus magnetic resonance spectroscopy (³¹P MRS) in neuromuscular disorders. Ann Neurol 30:90, 1991

BARCHI RL, FURMAN RE: Pathophysiology of myotonia and periodic paralysis, in Diseases of the Nervous System, vol. 1: Clinical Neurobiology, AK Asbury et al (eds). Philadelphia, Saunders, 1992

BERTOLASI L et al: The influence of muscular lengthening on cramps. Ann Neurol 33:176, 1993

BROOKE MH: A Clinician's View of Neuromuscular Diseases. Baltimore, Williams & Wilkins, 1986

EDWARDS RHT et al: Muscle biochemistry and pathophysiology in postviral fatigue syndrome. Br Med Bull 47:826, 1991

FLECKENSTEIN JL et al: Magnetic resonance imaging of muscle injury and atrophy in glycolytic myopathies. Muscle Nerve 12:849, 1989

GEORGE AL et al: Molecular basis of Thomsen disease (autosomal dominant myotonia-congenita). Nature Genet 3:305, 1993

LAYZER RB: Muscle pain, cramps and fatigue, in Myology, AG Engel, BQ Banker (eds). New York, McGraw-Hill, 1986

24 NUMBNESS, TINGLING, AND SENSORY LOSS

ARTHUR K. ASBURY

Normal somatic sensation is a continuous process that commands considerable moment-to-moment nervous system activity. Little of the activity intrudes on consciousness or exacts notice. In contrast, disordered sensation, particularly pains and paresthesias, may be highly intrusive, alarming, and tenacious, and may dominate attention. Abnormalities of sensation tend to make patients seek medical attention quickly. When abnormal sensations are perceived as painful, medical advice is sought even more quickly. For a consideration of pain, see Chap. 11. The physician must have a framework of knowledge in order to assess abnormal sensations, estimate their likely site of origin, and recognize their implications.

POSITIVE AND NEGATIVE PHENOMENA It is useful to divide all abnormal sensory phenomena into two great categories, positive and negative. Positive phenomena include tingling, pins-and-needles, pricking, bandlike sensations, lightning-like shooting feelings (lancinations), aching, and knifelike, twisting, drawing, pulling, tightening, burning, searing, electrical, and raw sensations. These descriptors are frequently the actual words used by patients. Such sensations may or may not be experienced as painful. It is thought that the pathophysiologic basis of positive phenomena resides in the ectopic generation of volleys of impulses at some site of lowered neural threshold along the sensory pathways, either in peripheral or central sensory fibers. Such trains of ectopically generated afferent impulses arising from sites other than normal peripheral nerve receptors determine the quality of the abnormal sensation experienced, depending on the number, rate, and distribution of impulses and the type and function of nerve fibers in which they arise.

Positive phenomena represent heightened activity in sensory pathways; therefore, they are not necessarily associated with any demonstrable sensory deficit upon examination, an important point for the examiner to bear in mind.

Negative phenomena result from loss of sensory function and are characterized by numbness or diminution or absence of feeling in a particular distribution. Negative phenomena, in contrast to positive phenomena, are accompanied by abnormal findings on sensory examination. In disorders affecting peripheral sensation, it is estimated that at least half the afferent fibers innervating a given site must be lost or functionless in order for sensory deficit to be demonstrated. This estimate probably varies according to how rapidly sensory fibers have lost function. If the rate of loss is slow and chronic, lack of cutaneous feeling may be unnoticed by the patient and difficult to demonstrate on examination, even though few sensory fibers are functioning. Rapidly evolving sensory abnormality usually evokes positive phenomena of some type and is more readily recognized by patients than insidious deafferentation. Subclinical degrees of sensory dysfunction not demonstrable on clinical sensory examination may be revealed by sensory nerve conduction studies or somatosensory cerebral evoked potentials (see Chaps. 366 and 382).

Terminology Two general types of medical terms are used to characterize abnormal sensation, those referring to symptoms of which patients complain (both positive and negative phenomena) and those describing abnormalities found on examination (only negative phenomena). *Paresthesia* and *dysesthesia* are terms used to denote positive phenomena. Paresthesia carries the implication that the abnormal sensation is perceived without an apparent stimulus, whereas dysesthesia is a more general term used to describe all types of positive sensations whether a stimulus is evident or not. Abnormalities on examination are denoted by *hypesthesia* or *hypoesthesia* (reduction of cutaneous sensation to a specific type of testing such as pressure, light touch, and warm or cold stimuli), *anesthesia* (complete absence of skin sensation to the same stimuli plus pinprick), and *hypalgesia* (referring to loss of pain perception, i.e., nociception, such as the pricking quality elicited by a pin). *Hyperesthesia* connotes exaggerated perception of sensations in response to mild stimuli (light touch or stroking of the skin). Similarly, *allodynia* describes the situation in which an ordinarily nonpainful stimulus, once perceived, is experienced as painful, even excruciating. An example is elicitation of a painful sensation by application of a vibrating tuning fork. *Hyperalgesia* denotes an exaggerated response to a noxious stimulus, and *hyperpathia*, a broad term, encompasses all the phenomena described by hyperesthesia, allodynia, and hyperalgesia.

Disorders of deep sensation, arising from muscle spindles, tendons, and joints, deserve special comment. Normally these afferents subserve proprioception (position sense) and the moment-to-moment sense of the state of muscle contraction. If a significant number of these special nerve endings become denervated, the resulting manifestations include imbalance, particularly with eyes closed or in the dark, clumsiness of precision movements, and unsteadiness of gait, all of which is referred to as *sensory ataxia* (see Chap. 22). Other findings on examination include reduced or absent joint position and vibratory sensibility and absent deep tendon reflexes in the affected limbs. Romberg's sign is positive, which means that the patient sways or topples when asked to stand with feet close together and eyes closed.

In severe states of deafferentation involving deep sensation, the patient cannot walk or stand unaided or even sit unsupported. Continuous, sometimes wormlike involuntary movements, called *pseudoathetosis*, of the hands and arms occur, particularly with eyes closed. Such patients are severely disabled.

Normal sensation Cutaneous afferent innervation is subserved by a rich variety of receptors, both naked endings (nociceptors and thermoreceptors) and encapsulated terminals (mechanoreceptors). Each has its own set of sensitivities to specific stimuli, size and distinctness of receptive fields, and adaptational qualities. Much of the knowledge about these receptors has come from the development of techniques to study single intact nerve fibers intraneurally in alert unanesthetized human subjects. It is possible not only to record from single nerve fibers, large or small, but also to stimulate single fibers in isolation. A single impulse, whether elicited by a natural stimulus or evoked by electrical microstimulation, in a large myelinated afferent fiber may be both perceived and localized.

Afferent fibers in peripheral nerve trunks sort themselves into topographically coherent patterns as they approach the dorsal roots and enter the dorsal horn of the spinal cord. From there the polysynaptic projections of the smaller fibers (unmyelinated and small myelinated), which in general subserve nociception and temperature sensibility, cross and ascend in the contralateral spinothalamic tract through spinal cord, through brainstem, to the ventral posterolateral nucleus (VPL) of the thalamus, and ultimately project to the postcentral gyrus of the parietal cortex (see Chap. 11). This is the spinothalamic pathway. The larger fibers that subserve tactile and position sense and kinesthesia project rostrally in the ipsilateral posterior column of the spinal cord and finally make their first synapse in the gracile or cuneate nuclei of the lower medulla (see Fig. 24-1). The second-order neuron decussates and ascends in the medial lemniscus located medially in the medulla and in the tegmentum of the pons and midbrain and synapses in VPL. The third-order neuron projects to parietal cortex; this entire system is referred to as *lemniscal*.

Although the fiber types and functions that make up the spinothalamic and lemniscal systems are relatively well known, it has been found that many other fibers, particularly those associated with touch, pressure, and position sense, ascend in a diffusely distributed pattern both ipsilaterally and contralaterally in the anterolateral quadrants of the spinal cord. These anatomic facts explain why an individual with a known complete lesion of the posterior columns of the spinal cord may have little sensory deficit on examination.

EXAMINATION OF SENSATION   The initial step in examination of the somatosensory system is to do the tests of primary sensation, which by convention include the sense of pain, touch, vibration, joint position, and thermal sensation, both hot and cold. These tests have gradually become codified through tradition, but they do appear to assess, if crudely, the major afferent functions and pathways (see Table 24-1). Testing of both primary sensation and cortical sensory function can be carried out in the office or at the bedside with a minimum of special equipment.

Some general principles pertain to the sensory examination. First, it should be remembered that the examiner is depending on subjective patient response; therefore, discriminating responses depend on the level of alertness, motivation, and intelligence of the patient and also on the skill with which the examiner has made the task clear. In a stupefied or obtunded patient, the examiner is reduced to observing the briskness of withdrawal and the complexity of defensive movements of the patient in response to a pinch or other noxious stimulus. In the alert but uncooperative patient, it is often possible to get some idea of proprioceptive function by noting the patient's best performance in casually observed movements requiring balance and precision, but cutaneous sensation may be unexaminable.

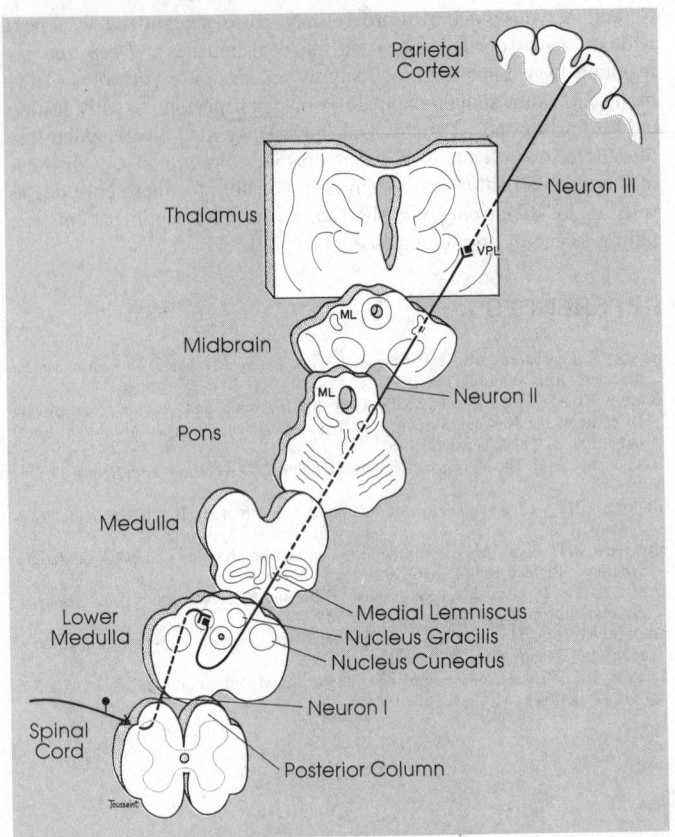

FIGURE 24-1   Schematic diagram of lemniscal system, which subserves proprioception and discriminative touch.

Second, sensory examination should not be pressed if the patient is fatigued. An abbreviated survey will suffice until a more extensive examination can be carried out when the patient has rested. Third, sensory examination in a patient who has no neurologic complaints should be quite abbreviated and may consist of pin, touch, and vibration testing in the hands and feet plus evaluation of station and gait, including Romberg's maneuver, which also tests the integrity of motor and cerebellar systems. Fourth, patients should be tested with their eyes closed or covered during both primary sensation and cortical sensory function examination.

Primary sensation (see Table 24-1)   The sense of pain is usually tested with a pin, asking the patient to focus on the pricking or unpleasant quality of the stimulus and not just the pressure or touch sensation elicited. Areas of hypalgesia should be mapped by

TABLE 24-1   Testing primary sensation

Sense	Test device	Endings activated	Fiber size mediating	Central pathway*
Pain	Pinprick	Cutaneous nociceptors	Small	SpTh, also D
Temperature, heat	Flask with warm water	Cutaneous thermoreceptors for hot	Small	SpTh
Temperature, cold	Flask with cold water	Cutaneous thermoreceptors for cold	Small	SpTh
Touch	Cotton wisp, fine brush	Cutaneous mechanoreceptors, also naked endings	Large and small	Lem, also D and SpTh
Vibration	Tuning fork, 128 Hz	Mechanoreceptors, especially pacinian corpuscles	Large	Lem, also D
Joint position	Passive movement of specific joints	Joint capsule and tendon endings, muscle spindles	Large	Lem, also D

*D = diffuse ascending projections in ipsilateral and contralateral anterolateral columns; SpTh = spinothalamic projection, contralateral; Lem = posterior column and lemniscal projection, ipsilateral.

proceeding from the most hypalgesic zones to less affected ones (see Figs. 24-2 and 24-3).

Temperature sensation, both to hot and to cold, is probably best tested by touching the skin for a couple of seconds with a water flask filled with water of the desired temperature, using a thermometer to verify the temperature. For most purposes, it is satisfactory if a patient can identify as warm the flask that is 35 or 36°C and as cool the one that is 28 to 32°C. Between 28 and 32°C, most individuals can distinguish temperature differences in 1°C steps. Both cold and warm should be tested because different receptors respond to each.

Touch is usually tested with a wisp of cotton or a fine camel's hair brush. In general, it is better to avoid testing touch on hairy skin because of the profusion of sensory endings that surround each hair follicle. The patients, whose eyes are covered, should be asked to say "now" each time they feel the stimulus. They also may be asked to point to the site where the stimulus was felt, although this tests not only the sense of touch but also touch localization (see cortical sensory testing below).

Joint position testing is a measure of proprioception, one of the most important functions of the sensory system. Joint position is usually tested first in the great toe and then in the fingers. Patients are asked to keep their eyes closed and to relax completely the part to be examined. In the case of the great toe, one starts with the toe in a neutral position and grasps it lightly between the thumb and the forefinger on either side of the toe (not top and bottom), and then the toe is moved a few degrees either in a dorsal or a plantar direction, and the patient is asked to say whether the movement was up or down. One must make sure that the patient understands that it is the

FIGURE 24-3 Posterior view of dermatomes (*left*) and cutaneous areas supplied by individual peripheral nerves (*right*). (*Modified from MB Carpenter and J Sutin, in Human Neuroanatomy, 8th ed, Baltimore, Williams & Wilkins, 1983.*)

FIGURE 24-2 Anterior view of dermatomes (*left*) and cutaneous areas supplied by individual peripheral nerves (*right*). (*Modified from MB Carpenter and J Sutin, in Human Neuroanatomy, 8th ed, Baltimore, Williams & Wilkins, 1983.*)

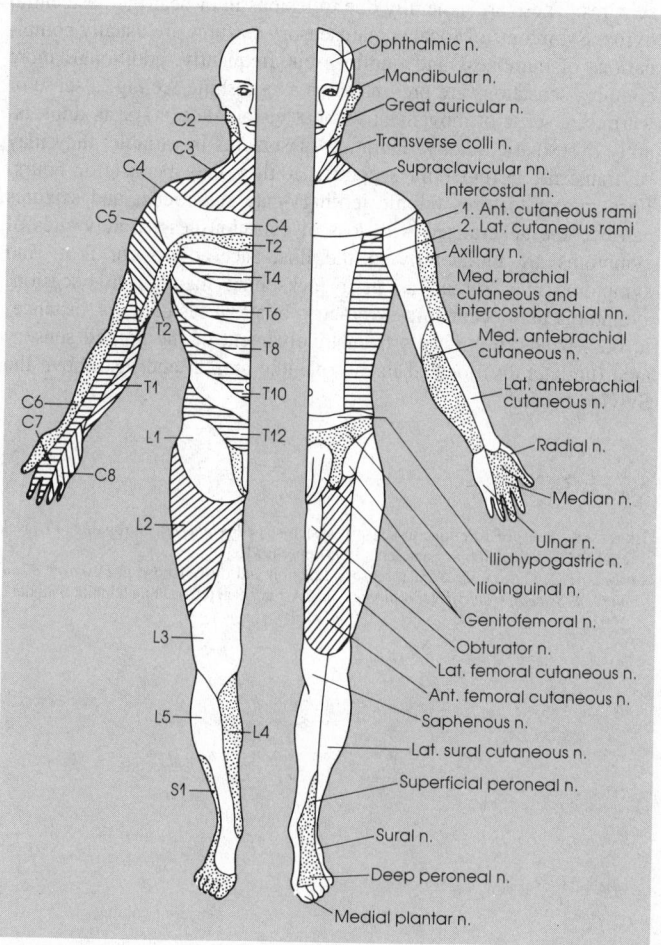

direction of movement which is being tested and not the direction the toe is pointing when it stops. A patient with absence of position sense in the part being tested will have a 50 percent error rate because only two choices are available. Answers that are consistently greater than 50 percent in error should be viewed with skepticism. If errors are made in recognizing the direction of passive movements of the toe, then passive movements of the ankle or even of the knee should be undertaken in the same way. Similarly, position sense at the proximal interphalangeal joint of the index finger may be tested, and if abnormal, other finger joints and the wrist and elbow joints also should be tested. A test of proximal joint position sense, primarily at the shoulder, can be carried out by asking the patient to bring the two index fingers together with the arms extended and the eyes closed. Normal individuals should be able to do this quite accurately with errors of a centimeter or less.

The sense of vibration is tested with a tuning fork, preferably a large one that vibrates at 128 Hz. The decay of vibration using this fork is slow enough to be of quantitative use because it requires between 15 and 20 s to decay below the threshold of perceptibility. Vibration is usually tested at bony prominences, specifically the malleoli at the ankles, the patella, the anterior iliac spine, the spinous processes of the vertebral bodies, the metacarpal-phalangeal joints (knuckles), the styloid process of the ulna, the elbow, and the acromion of the shoulder. Control sites at which to test vibration are the sternum and the forehead. The examiner can compare the threshold at a given site in both patient and self. A crude approximation of degree of vibratory sense loss can be made by counting the seconds that the examiner can feel the sense of vibration longer than the patient. It must be clear to the patient that it is the sense of vibration and not just the pressure of the end of the tuning fork to which attention is directed.

Cortical sensation   Cortical sensory testing includes two-point discrimination, touch localization, stereognosis, graphesthesia, and bilateral simultaneous stimulation, to name the most commonly used methods. Abnormalities of these sensory tests, in the presence of normal primary sensation and an alert cooperative patient, signify a lesion of the parietal cortex or thalamocortical projections to the parietal lobe. If primary sensation is altered, it is not possible to test for these cortical discriminative functions.

Two-point discrimination is tested by special calipers whose points may be set from 2 mm to several centimeters apart and then applied simultaneously to the site to be tested. The pulp of the fingertips is a common site to test; a normal individual can distinguish about 3-mm separation of points there. One can distinguish more closely set points on the tongue and lips, but the threshold for discriminating two points may be centimeters at other sites on the body. Comparisons should always be made between analogous sites on the two sides of the body, since the deficit, with a specific parietal lesion, is likely to be hemilateral. This point holds true for all cortical sensory testing.

Touch localization is usually carried out by light pressure with the examiner's fingertip, asking the patient, whose eyes are closed, to identify the site of touch. It is usual to ask the patient to touch the same site with a fingertip. Bilateral simultaneous stimulation at analogous sites (e.g., the dorsa of both hands) can be carried out to determine whether the perception of touch is extinguished consistently on one side or the other. The phenomenon is referred to as *extinction* on bilateral simultaneous stimulation.

Graphesthesia means the capacity to recognize letters or numbers drawn by the examiner's fingertip on various parts of the body while the patient maintains closed eyes. The usual comparison is the palm of one hand versus the palm of the other. Numbers should be drawn large enough to occupy most of the palm. Once again, the comparison of one side with the other is of prime importance. Failure to recognize numbers or letters is termed *agraphesthesia*.

Stereognosis refers to the ability to identify common objects by palpation, recognizing their shape, texture, and size. Common standard objects are the best test objects, such as a marble, a paper clip, a small rubber ball, or coins. Patients with normal stereognosis should be able to distinguish a dime from a penny and certainly a nickel from a quarter. Patients should only be allowed to feel the object with one hand at time. If they are unable to identify it in one hand, it should be placed in the other for comparison. Individuals unable to identify common objects and coins in one hand who can do so in the other are said to have *astereognosis* of the abnormal hand. Note that the major comparison is one side of the body with the other.

Localization of sensory abnormalities   Peripheral neuropathies are generally graded, distal, and symmetric in their distribution of deficit. Although most peripheral neuropathies are pansensory and affect all modalities of sensation, selective sensory dysfunction according to nerve fiber size may occur. In small fiber neuropathies, the hallmark is burning, painful dysesthesias with reduced pinprick and thermal sensation but with sparing of proprioception, motor function, and even deep tendon jerks. Touch is variably involved, but when spared, the sensory pattern is referred to as *sensory dissociation* (see below). In contrast to small fiber neuropathies, large-fiber neuropathies are characterized by position sense deficit, imbalance, absent tendon jerks, variable motor dysfunction, but preservation of most cutaneous sensation and few or no dysesthesias.

Paresthesias and dysesthesias may be of either peripheral nerve or spinal cord origin and probably can arise in the brainstem, but in every instance they are thought to represent abnormal showers of impulses generated from an ectopic focus or foci. By themselves, paresthesias may not be localizable, but when accompanied by other signs of neuropathy or of myelopathy, the correct site of origin may be deduced.

Dissociated sensory deficit patterns, in which pinprick and thermal sensation are lost but touch is spared, are usually a sign of spinothalamic tract involvement in the spinal cord, especially if the deficit is unilateral and has an upper level on the torso. Bilateral spinothalamic tract involvement occurs with lesions affecting the center of the spinal cord, such as happens with expansion of the central canal in hydromyelia or syringomyelia. Sensory dissociation also may occur in peripheral neuropathies in which afferent cutaneous nerve fibers of small diameter are preferentially affected. Neuropathies in which sensory dissociation may occur include leprous neuritis, hereditary sensory neuropathy, and certain cases of amyloid and diabetic polyneuropathy (see Chap. 383).

Hemisensory disturbance with tingling numbness from head to foot is usually thalamic in origin. If abrupt in onset, the thalamic lesion is likely to be due to a small stroke (lacunar infarction). Occasionally, with lesions affecting the posterolateral thalamus (VPL) or adjacent white matter, a syndrome of thalamic pain, also called *Déjerine-Roussy syndrome*, may ensue. This is a persistent unrelenting hemipainful state often described in dramatic terms such as ''like the flesh is being torn from my limbs'' or ''as though that side is bathed in acid'' (see Chap. 11). Harlequin patterns of sensory disturbance, in which one side of the face and the opposite side of the body are affected, localize to the lateral medulla, where a small lesion may damage both the ipsilateral descending trigeminal tract and ascending spinothalamic fibers (lateral lemniscus) subserving the opposite arm, leg, and hemitorso (see ''Lateral Medulla Syndrome'' in Chap. 368).

With lesions of the parietal lobe, either of the cortex or of subjacent white matter, the most prominent symptoms are contralateral hemineglect, hemi-inattention, and a tendency not to use the contralateral hand and arm. Tests of primary sensation are usually normal or minimally altered, but tests of cortical sensation are often severely abnormal (see Chap. 27). Dysesthesias, or even a sense of numbness, are unusual except in the special circumstance of focal sensory seizures. These are generally due to lesions in or near the postcentral gyrus. Symptoms of focal somatosensory seizures are usually combinations of numbness and tingling, but frequently, additional, more complex sensations are present, such as a rushing feeling, a sense of warmth, a sense of movement without visible motion, or an unpleasantly dysesthetic quality. Duration of seizures is variable; they may be transient, lasting only seconds, or they may persist for hours. Focal motor features (clonic jerking) may supervene, and seizures can become generalized with loss of consciousness. Likely sites of symptoms are unilaterally in the lips, face, digits, or foot, and symptoms may spread as in a Jacksonian march. On occasion, symptoms may occur in a symmetric bilateral fashion, for instance, in both hands; this results from involvement of the second sensory area (unilaterally) located in the rolandic area at and just above the Sylvian fissure.

REFERENCES

Light AR, Perl ER: Peripheral sensory systems, in *Peripheral Neuropathy*, PJ Dyck et al (eds). Philadelphia, Saunders, 1993, pp 149–165

Lindblom U, Ochoa JL: Somatosensory function and dysfunction, in *Diseases of the Nervous System: Clinical Neurobiology*, AK Asbury et al (eds). Philadelphia, Saunders, 1992

25   ACUTE CONFUSIONAL STATES, AMNESIA, AND DEMENTIA

MARTIN M. BROWN / VLADIMIR C. HACHINSKI

The complexity and vulnerability of neuronal function allow cognitive function to be easily disturbed. Many systemic and neurologic illnesses come to notice because of disruption of cognitive function, often without other symptoms or signs. Recognizing the patterns of the resulting syndromes avoids mistaken psychiatric diagnoses and allows early and appropriate management. Testing of individual cognitive functions allows identification of specific areas of abnormality and helps in establishing the cause of the disorder.

SYNDROME DEFINITION

CONFUSION   Any disorder of cognitive function may cause confusion, i.e., a lack of clarity and coherence of thought, perception, understanding, or action. Confusion is often the first feature of cognitive impairment noticed by relatives or the examiner. Confusion also may appear to be the presenting complaint in isolated focal disorders of cognitive function such as aphasia or visuospatial agnosia (see Chap. 27), but careful examination will show that the confusion is related to a single deficit.

The acute confusional state is a common syndrome, consisting of global impairment of cognitive function accompanied by deficits in attention and consciousness. The impairment of cognition usually includes disorientation, abnormal perception, disordered reasoning, and poor memory. A wide variety of causes may be responsible.

DELIRIUM   The term *delirium* is synonymous with the acute confusional state, although, strictly speaking, it describes a clinically distinct variety of acute confusional state characterized by periods of agitation, heightened mental activity, increased wakefulness, marked readiness to respond to certain stimuli (such as sudden noises), intrusive visual hallucinations, motor hyperactivity, and autonomic stimulation. Impairment of attention, essential to the acute confusional state, is present despite the apparent arousal (see "Consciousness," below). The agitation of delirium characteristically fluctuates and may alternate with or progress to a subdued confusional state. The clinical picture is exemplified by the excited hallucinatory state of *delirium tremens* which follows alcohol withdrawal. However, delirium may be seen in acute confusional states from any cause.

DEMENTIA   This is a syndrome of acquired global or multifocal impairment of cognitive function involving decline in intellect, memory, and personality in the presence of normal consciousness. Relatively normal alertness and attention distinguish dementia from the acute confusional state (see Table 25-1). The decline usually involves all intellectual functions, but the diagnosis may be established by impairment of any three of the following spheres: language, memory, visuospatial skills, emotion, personality, or cognition. Loss of a single intellectual function such as speech or memory, however devastating, is not sufficient. Dementia is not necessarily progressive, and in some instances it can be reversed or halted by appropriate treatment. It is therefore important to recognize dementia as a syndrome with many causes.

AMNESIA   This term describes an isolated disorder of memory characterized by inability to remember past events and to learn new information despite normal consciousness and attention. Amnesia has a variety of possible causes.

OBSERVABLE COMPONENTS OF COGNITION

Despite the complexity of mental activity, certain aspects can be assessed reliably at the bedside as part of the neurologic examination.

TABLE 25-1   Clinical features of the acute confusional state and dementia compared

	Acute confusional state	Dementia
Onset	Acute	Usually insidious
Duration	Transient (hours to weeks)	Persistent (months to years)
Course	Fluctuating over hours; diurnal variation common	Stable over days
Sleep-wake cycle	Disrupted	Normal
Consciousness level	Depressed	Normal
Attention	Impaired	Normal
Orientation	Impaired	Impaired
Language	Incoherent	Aphasia common
Memory		
Digit span	Shortened	Normal
Long-term memory	Impaired	Impaired
Perception	Impaired (illusions, delusions, hallucinations)	Normal early, agnosia later
Mood	Agitation or fear common	Apathy or disinhibition common
Autonomic changes	Common	Unusual
Psychomotor changes (depressed motor activity or restlessness)	Common	Uncommon
Involuntary movements	Common	Uncommon
EEG	Diffuse slow-wave activity	Mild slowing

CONSCIOUSNESS   Consciousness is the state of awareness of self and the environment and has various facets (see also Chap. 26). The *content* of consciousness represents the sum of cognitive and affective mental functions and can be assessed only by inference. *Arousal* is closely allied to the appearance of *alertness*, i.e., the readiness to respond to stimulation. *Attention* includes the capacity to attend selectively to relevant stimuli and to manipulate abstract ideas. Consciousness also includes the concepts of *insight* and recognition of self. *Clouding of consciousness* is an essential feature of acute confusional states and describes the mildest impairment of consciousness on the continuum from full consciousness to deep coma. In most instances, clouding of consciousness involves all facets of consciousness. In delirium the patient may appear aroused and excited, but the content of consciousness, awareness of the surroundings and self, and the capacity to attend selectively to relevant stimuli are all impaired.

PERCEPTION   Perception involves conscious awareness, selection, and identification of a stimulus from the environment. Even under normal conditions the perception of a stimulus depends on numerous factors, both physiologic (such as lighting) and psychological (such as mood and expectation). With clouding of consciousness, attention falters, and perception becomes more subject to these influences. For example, poor vision or deafness may make the elderly more prone to misperception, and the advent of darkness often contributes to delirium. Coherent perception requires intact visuospatial and language function. Disturbances of perception are frequent in acute confusional states and include *illusions* (misperceptions of actual sensory stimuli) and *hallucinations* (perceptions experienced without apparent sensory stimulation). In dementia, misperception commonly results from focal impairments of visuospatial or language function such as agnosia or aphasia.

MEMORY   Three classes of memory can be distinguished at the bedside depending on the length of recall. The *immediate memory* system holds information close to consciousness for a few seconds while it is used for mental activity. It can be tested by the reproduction of a string of numerals and has a finite capacity for information at around seven digits, which are retained for only seconds or minutes unless the information is rehearsed by internal repetition. Normal attention is required for immediate memory function, and impairment of immediate memory and a shortened digit span are diagnostic features of the acute confusional syndrome. Immediate memory is relatively normal in dementia and amnesic syndromes. Immediate memory appears to be mediated by a separate system that does not necessarily lead to longer-term storage. *Recent memory*, the recall of information presented within minutes, hours, or days, is distinguished from *remote memory*, the recall of events months or years earlier. Recall of information after a delay of a few minutes requires a process of consolidation or learning and is mediated by the *long-term*, or *secondary memory* system, with almost limitless capacity and durability. In contrast to immediate memory, recall of information from long-term memory is often selected by its relevance to the individual and usually incorporates the meaning of the information rather than exact words or pictures. Recent and remote memory probably both involve the same long-term memory system, but access to remote memories is less sensitive to interference (e.g., from the effect of head injury) than recent memory. Impaired recent memory is usual in dementia and acute confusional states and is the defining feature of amnesic syndromes.

MOOD AND PERSONALITY　*Mood* refers to the prevailing emotional state, while *affect* is the emotional experience evoked by a particular stimulus. Individual reactions to any situation are closely related to underlying personality, previous experience, expectations, and degree of insight. The prevailing mood may have a profound influence on all aspects of cognition, especially at the extremes of the continuum of mood. Hypomania may be accompanied by illusions, flight of ideas, and extreme motor and verbal output sometimes mimicking delirium. In contrast, depression may exhibit slowing of thought, speech, and activity (psychomotor retardation) which, if severe, may be mistaken for dementia. Extreme anxiety also may interfere with the organization and coherence of thought and speech. Many diseases of the brain alter mood and affect. Frontal lobe lesions, in particular, may cause either lack of drive and initiative (abulia) with indifference to outcome or sometimes fatuous euphoria with social and sexual disinhibition.

PROBLEM SOLVING　Thought is intangible and elusive. However, the processes of reasoning, logic, and the ability to solve problems using language or mathematics can be assessed more easily using tests of words or numbers. Disorder of these processes is an essential feature of the acute confusional states and dementia, but in contrast, reasoning is intact in the amnesic syndrome, except when recent memory is required. One manifestation of defective reasoning seen in acute confusional states and sometimes in dementia is the occurrence of delusions (false beliefs maintained in spite of convincing contradictory evidence). Delusions in psychiatric illnesses such as schizophrenia tend to be more organized and persistent than in acute confusional states.

APPROACH TO THE PATIENT WITH DISORDERS OF COGNITION

HISTORY　A careful history taken from close relatives or friends is essential and may provide important clues about the underlying pathology. Questioning should establish the first appearance of intellectual impairment and the subsequent tempo of the disease. Was the onset over hours or days, suggesting an acute confusional state, or over months or years, making dementia a more likely diagnosis? Was there an organic precipitating event such as a head injury, or did the confusion follow an emotional crisis, suggesting a psychiatric cause or a drug overdose? Questioning should include inquiries about impairment of memory, personality and mood change, and how the patient copes with work, driving, and the activities of daily life. The history should include questioning about symptoms which suggest raised intracranial pressure (headaches, nausea, vomiting, and ataxia), strokelike events, or seizures. Attention to past medical and family history, drugs, alcohol, and toxic exposure is important (see also Chap. 363). The handedness of the patient should be determined to assess the likelihood that the left hemisphere is dominant for speech.

EXAMINATION OF COGNITIVE FUNCTION　Careful examination of cognitive function is an important component of the neurologic examination. Cognitive impairment is frequently missed, especially in the elderly, because this part of the examination has been neglected. The main focus is to establish the level of consciousness and to determine whether the patient's deficit involves one aspect of intellectual function, suggesting a focal lesion at a single site, or more than one aspect, suggesting more global pathology. An initial step is to determine the patient's premorbid level of intellect. A rough indicator can be obtained from the patient's profession or occupation and the amount of schooling completed.

Examination of cognitive function needs to be adjusted according to the previous and current intellectual state, but it is useful to have a sequence of questions that the examiner has applied regularly to intellectually intact patients so as to have a good understanding of the normal range of replies. The Mini-Mental State Questionnaire provides an example of such a sequence that can be used to screen for cognitive impairment. However, the Mini-Mental State does not cover all aspects of intellectual function and does not always reveal mild or focal deficits, especially in younger or highly intelligent patients. It should therefore be supplemented by a fuller examination of cognitive function, as described below, if cognitive impairment is suspected. The patient's answers to questioning should be carefully recorded so that deterioration or improvement can be easily confirmed at a later evaluation. A number of pitfalls may cause the patient's intellectual function to be underestimated. Perseveration, usually a sign of frontal lobe disease, may cause the patient to repeat replies and have difficulty switching attention to a new task. Aphasia, with difficulty understanding commands or expressing the correct answer in response to questions, may cloud interpretation of the examination. The incoherence or mutism resulting from isolated expressive aphasia is commonly misinterpreted as a confusional state or dementia.

Orientation　Orientation to person, place, and time (including date, time of day, month, and year) should be tested first. Usually, the more severe the impairment of memory, the more inaccurate is the date. If the patient cannot name the place accurately, ask the patient to identify the type of place (e.g., hospital or home).

Consciousness　The normally alert individual engages in conversation or some other diversional activity, while the patient with impairment of consciousness remains quiet or engages in purposeless repetitive activities. Obtunded patients may drift into sleep when undisturbed but awaken promptly when questioned or examined. The demented patient may lack spontaneous activity or conversation but shows normal alertness and responsiveness to questioning.

Attention　Attention is assessed during history taking. Does the patient pay attention to questions, or is the patient easily distracted? The capacity for sustained attention and concentration can be tested by asking for sequential subtraction of 7 from 100 down to zero, but the response should be interpreted with caution, since immediate memory and mathematical ability are also required. Forward and reverse digit spans are also specific tests of attention as well as of immediate memory (see below).

Abnormalities of perception　Abnormalities of perception should be sought by specific questioning about perception of the environment. The presence of hallucinations may be betrayed by the patient brushing or picking nonexistent objects off the bed covers or turning to answer an imaginary question.

Language　Aphasia results in nonfluency of speech, hesitation, circumlocution, neologisms, or jargon and is usually appreciated during routine conversation and history taking (see Chap. 28). It is also useful to ask the patient to name common and uncommon objects to assess for nominal aphasia and to give a complex command to test for minor degrees of receptive dysphasia. (For example, "If I take my pen out of my pocket, please touch your left ear with your right index finger.") Agraphia should be sought by asking the patient to write his or her name and a short spontaneous sentence. Reading should be assessed using a standard text or newspaper article, asking for an explanation of its meaning by the patient. Simple sums are given to assess mathematical skills.

Visuospatial function The most useful test of visuospatial function is to ask the patient to copy a drawing, starting with a simple object such as a five-pointed star and progressing to a more difficult object such as a three-dimensional box. Constructional apraxia, or visuospatial agnosia, results in difficulty in drawing the lines required in the correct spatial orientation or position. Perseveration or visual neglect also may be revealed by this test. The visual recognition of common objects will have been tested when examining for nominal aphasia, but bedside testing for difficulty in recognition of faces (prosopagnosia) requires a newspaper or magazine containing photographs of famous people, unless individuals who should be well known to the patient can be presented without other clues such as voice to aid recognition.

Memory *Immediate memory* and attention are tested by determining *digit span*. The patient is asked to repeat a string of numerals after the examiner starting with a short string and working up to the normal digit span of six or seven consecutive numbers presented at about half-second intervals. A shorter string of numerals or a short word can be given to repeat or spell backwards. This test requires sustained attention as well as immediate memory. *Recent memory* should be assessed by asking the patient to learn the names of three common objects or a simple address. After confirming that the patient has registered the information, recall is tested after 2 and 5 min, depending on the degree of anticipated amnesia. If the patient fails to recall the information, then the severity of the amnesia can be gauged by giving the patient a clue, and if this fails, recognition can be tested by asking the patient to identify the correct answer from a choice. Recent memory for events over the last few days or weeks is assessed by asking for a description of events of personal or world importance. A relative or friend may need to corroborate the appropriateness of the description. *Remote long-term memory* can be tested by asking for items of common general knowledge such as the dates of important past events, names of important political figures, or the locations of major cities.

Mood and personality Judgments about personality, mood, affect, and insight should be made during history taking and examination. The appearance of the patient, content of conversation, and speed of movement provide the most useful clues to mood. Affect is signaled by language, facial expression, gestures, and posture, all of which should be studied closely. The presence of euphoria, disinhibition, or abulia should be noted.

Thought and problem solving Incoherence of reasoning and logical thought will usually have been detected during history taking or testing of language skills and mathematics. More subtle disorder of thought is sometimes revealed by asking the patient to explain the meaning of well-known proverbs or sayings.

Cognitive scales A number of scales (e.g., Blessed Dementia Scale; Mini-Mental State Examination) have been developed to make an approximate assessment of cognitive function. These are not true psychometric tests but questionnaires that can be completed fairly quickly by untrained staff to provide a score that roughly reflects the degree of intellectual and behavioral impairment. Another scale, the Ischemic Score, helps to distinguish multi-infarct from degenerative dementia. On the whole, these scales are less useful in diagnosis than a careful cognitive examination conducted in the manner described above.

ACUTE CONFUSIONAL STATES AND DELIRIUM

Acute confusional states occur in about 10 percent of all hospitalized patients and in 30 to 50 percent of hospitalized geriatric patients; patients with dementia are particularly vulnerable.

PATHOPHYSIOLOGY *Neurologic diseases* cause confusional states in a variety of ways, including depression of consciousness. Consciousness is normally maintained by the ascending reticular activating system in the brainstem and thalamic regions (see Chap. 26). Focal diseases (such as a brain tumor or subdural hematoma) may depress consciousness by compression of the brainstem or thalamus or by producing hydrocephalus. Diffuse impairment of neuronal function (e.g., concussion or encephalitis) and multifocal disease (e.g., multiple metastases or multiple infarcts) also may present with confusion if the loci of disease cause several separate deficits of cognitive function with impaired attention. Usually lesions in both hemispheres are necessary, but occasionally a single right nondominant hemispheric lesion (usually a parietal infarct) presents with an acute confusional state because of impairment of attention, a predominant right hemisphere function.

Systemic diseases result in confusion from diffuse impairment of neuronal function. This may be due to inadequate supply of oxygen (hypoxia), glucose (hypoglycemia), or other factors required for metabolism, including vitamins and hormones. In metabolic encephalopathy, the mechanisms include acid-base disturbance, electrolyte imbalance, and circulating toxins (e.g., ammonia in liver failure). In systemic infections, there are several possible factors, including high fever, hypoxia, dehydration, and circulating bacterial toxins. Most drug-induced confusional states result from direct interference with synaptic transmission. In delirium following drug withdrawal, the excited state may result from the sudden exposure of neurotransmitter receptor sites.

In many cases of acute confusion, multiple mechanisms can be identified, particularly in the elderly. At any age, the brain may be made more vulnerable by preexisting brain damage, sleep or sensory deprivation, the effects of drugs, mild organ failure, or an unfamiliar environment.

CLINICAL FEATURES Because most causes of the acute confusional state affect neuronal function diffusely, all aspects of intellectual function are impaired to a lesser or greater degree (see Table 25-1). The cardinal feature is *clouding of consciousness*, manifested by impaired alertness, awareness, and attention. This impairment is usually mild but can advance to coma if untreated. Depression of consciousness is distinguished from natural drowsiness by observing that the patient cannot be aroused easily. Reduced attentiveness can range from mild apathy and a failure to grasp complex details to reduced interaction with the examiner, lack of normal spontaneous comment or questions, and neglect of bodily needs. In delirium, arousal is evidenced by a readiness to respond to certain stimuli, insomnia, and excessive reactions to noise or bright lights. This is accompanied by a reduced ability to focus attention, distractibility, and inability to concentrate.

Variability in the level of arousal is a common feature of the acute confusional state. Reduced responsiveness may be interspersed with excited outbursts. Sleep-wake cycles are frequently disrupted or reversed, and confusion is often more marked during the night. The early symptoms of delirium often include insomnia and vivid, unpleasant dreams before a frank confusional state supervenes.

Impairment of memory with reduced digit span, poor recent memory, and defective recall for distant events is an important feature. One of the earliest signs of this impairment is disorientation for time and, later, disorientation for place. Knowledge of personal identity is usually retained if the patient can understand the question. The memory deficit is characteristically patchy so that distortions of memory (para-amnesia) and partially correct information may be incorporated into confabulatory answers or delusions. When the patient recovers, partial or total amnesia for the period of confusion is usual, although isolated events, especially vivid hallucinations, may be remembered in detail.

Impairment of cognitive function leads to difficulty performing tasks requiring logic, mathematics, or spatial organization. Thought processes are slowed, although the agitated delirious patient may have flight of ideas. Thinking is disorganized and disjointed. Speech is incoherent, rambling, and often inappropriate. Comprehension of complex material is impaired, and errors in the naming of objects or in writing may be elicited.

Impaired perception may compound confusion. The patient often misperceives surroundings and attendants as those more familiar to the patient. More concrete illusions and hallucinations are common, especially following drug withdrawal and in alcoholic delirium tremens. Hallucinations are most frequently visual but may involve any sensory modality.

Disturbances of emotion may include blunting of affect or emotional lability. Mood disturbances include dysphoria, depression, agitation, and fear, and these may be accompanied by appropriate autonomic responses. *Autonomic hyperactivity*, including tachycardia, diaphoresis, and anxiety, is marked in drug and alcohol withdrawal.

Psychomotor changes are common. In most patients, spontaneous motor activity is depressed, but hyperactivity and restlessness characterize delirium. Repetitive stereotyped motor behavior, such as plucking at the bed clothes or tossing from side to side, is frequent. *Involuntary movements*, including irregular tremor, asterixis, and myoclonus, are usually seen in drug withdrawal or metabolic encephalopathy. Rarely, patients show catatonic behavior.

DIFFERENTIAL DIAGNOSIS　The first essential distinction to be made is whether the confusional state results from primary neurologic disease or as a complication of systemic illness (see Table 25-2). This distinction can often be made on examination but may require laboratory investigation.

Neurologic causes　These can usually be recognized by the presence of focal neurologic signs in addition to disordered intellectual function. Examples include hemiparesis in *cerebral infarction*, neck stiffness in *meningitis* or *subarachnoid hemorrhage*, and gait disturbance in *hydrocephalus*. However, diffuse neurologic diseases such as *encephalitis*, *epileptic confusion*, or *small-vessel vasculitis* may cause no neurologic signs apart from the disorder of cognition. *Neoplasias* of the nervous system usually cause headache and focal signs, but midline tumors may present with a gradually evolving confusional state. Acute onset may be caused by brainstem compression or acute hydrocephalus.

Postictal confusion after a minor seizure lasts a few seconds and after a major seizure usually about an hour unless complicated by head injury, hypoxia, or status epilepticus. However, a persistent confusional state may occur with continuous or serial minor seizures (*minor epileptic status*) (see Chap. 367). Acute confusional states may accompany *encephalitis* or *brain abscess* without systemic signs of infection always being present.

Systemic causes　Systemic causes are usually characterized by absence of focal neurologic signs apart from cognitive disorders, although minor signs such as reflex asymmetry or extensor plantar responses may be seen. An exception to this rule is occasionally seen in hypoglycemia, which may be accompanied in the elderly by hemiparesis. In *metabolic encephalopathy*, acidotic hyperventilation, tremor, asterixis, or myoclonus may suggest the diagnosis. *Wernicke's encephalopathy* (see Chaps. 377 and 390) should be considered in patients with a history of alcoholism or malnutrition. *Drugs* often cause confusion, especially in the elderly and those on multiple medications. *Endocrine dysfunction* (see Chaps. 331 and 334) rarely causes acute confusional state but should always be considered, particularly if there is hyponatremia. *Systemic infections*, especially *septicemia* and *subacute bacterial endocarditis*, can cause acute confusional states, particularly in the elderly, in whom fever may not always be evident, as can meningitis or brain abscess complicating the systemic infection.

Psychiatric causes　In *anxiety*, extreme *grief*, or *depression*, orientation for person and place is usually preserved, and with encouragement, the patient can concentrate and improve cognitive performance. Hyperactivity, diminished need for sleep, pressure of speech, delusions, short attention span, and distractibility in *acute mania* may be confused with the hyperexcitability of delirium. Mania is characterized by a sustained elevation of mood and preservation of orientation. Hyperactivity persists throughout the manic episode in contrast to delirium, in which hyperactivity may be interspersed with somnolence. *Disassociative or hysterical disorders*, e.g., psychogenic

---

TABLE 25-2　Differential diagnosis of the acute confusional state

NEUROLOGIC (FOCAL SIGNS ARE COMMON)

Trauma
　Concussion
　Intracranial hematoma
　Subdural hematoma
Vascular disorders
　Multiple infarcts
　Right hemisphere or posterior circulation infarcts
　Hypertensive encephalopathy
　Vasculitis (e.g., systemic lupus erythematosus, polyarteritis nodosa, giant-cell arteritis)
　Air and fat embolism
　Subarachnoid hemorrhage
Neoplasia
　Multiple parenchymal metastases
　Meningeal carcinomatosis
　Midline brain tumors
　Brain tumors causing brainstem compression, edema, or hydrocephalus
　Paraneoplastic syndromes (limbic encephalitis)
Infections
　Meningitis and encephalitis (viral, bacterial, fungal, protozoal)
　Multiple abscesses
　Progressive multifocal leukoencephalopathy
Inflammations
　Acute disseminated encephalomyelitis
　Postinfectious encephalitis
Epilepsy
　Postictal state
　Temporal lobe status (complex partial status)

SYSTEMIC (FOCAL NEUROLOGIC SIGNS ARE UNCOMMON)

Substrate depletion
　Hypoglycemia
　Diffuse hypoxia
　　Pulmonary
　　Cardiac
　　Carbon monoxide poisoning
Metabolic encephalopathy
　Diabetic ketoacidosis
　Renal failure
　Liver failure
　Electrolyte, fluid, and acid-base imbalance (especially Na^+, Ca^{2+}, Mg^{2+})
　Hereditary metabolic disease, e.g., porphyria, metachromatic leukodystrophy, mitochondrial cytopathy
Vitamin deficiency
　Thiamine (Wernicke's encephalopathy)
　Nicotinic acid (pellagra)
　B_{12} deficiency
Endocrine; over- or underactivity
　Thyroid
　Parathyroid
　Adrenal
Infection
　Septicemia
　Malaria
　Subacute bacterial endocarditis
　Focal infection, e.g., pneumonia
Thermal injuries
　Hypothermia
　Heat stroke
Hematologic disorders
　Hyperviscosity syndrome
　Severe anemia
Toxic causes
　Drug and alcohol intoxication (therapeutic, social, or illegal)
　Drug withdrawal, e.g., alcohol, barbiturates, narcotics
　Chemical toxins, e.g., heavy metals, organic toxins

PSYCHIATRIC

Acute mania
Depression or extreme anxiety
Schizophrenia
Hysterical fugue states

---

amnesia and fugue states, are usually distinguished from organic confusional states by the focal nature of the amnesia. *Acute schizophrenia* may simulate the acute confusional state, but consciousness, normal sleep-wake cycles, orientation, and attention are usually preserved (see Chap. 389).

INVESTIGATION Investigation is an urgent procedure. A *biochemical profile*, including blood sugar level, readily diagnoses the common metabolic disorders. A *blood count* detects hematologic disorders, and a neutrophilia suggests infection. If in doubt, a raised *erythrocyte sedimentation rate* supports the diagnosis of an organic disorder. *Arterial blood gas analysis* is a useful screen for hypoxia, respiratory failure, and acidosis. *Chest x-ray* and *blood and urine cultures* should be performed even if there is no fever. A complete infectious disease screen is indicated if there is a stronger suspicion of infection. *Endocrine tests* and *vitamin B$_{12}$* measurement may be indicated in individual patients. *Drug and toxicologic screens* are indicated for suspicion of drug overdose or toxic exposure. *Cerebrospinal fluid (CSF) examination* is mandatory in all patients with fever or neck stiffness so long as raised intracranial pressure or intracranial mass is not suspected and is also helpful in distinguishing metabolic from neurologic disease. The CSF white cell count is usually normal in metabolic disease, whereas leukocytosis implies neurologic disease, usually meningitis or encephalitis. The *electroencephalogram* (EEG) is useful if the presence of encephalopathy is uncertain; it is almost always abnormal in organic causes but does not necessarily distinguish between neurologic and systemic causes. Certain patterns may suggest metabolic disorders (particularly liver failure), encephalitis (especially herpes simplex), or epileptic status; and focal abnormalities may point to a stroke, abscess, or tumor. *Magnetic resonance imaging (MRI)* or *computed tomography (CT)* is not an emergency procedure unless examination or the EEG suggests a focal lesion but should be considered if no systemic cause is found after initial investigation.

MANAGEMENT The patient with acute confusional state is often agitated, and before the appropriate examination and investigations can be completed, the cooperation of the patient is required. Patients can frequently be calmed by a sympathetic and friendly physician. A relative or friend can often help and should be encouraged to stay with the patient. Nursing care should be given in a well-lit, relatively quiet environment with facilities for frequent observation. Sedation is seldom required. However, some agitated, violent, or paranoid patients may require a long-acting oral or intramuscular major tranquilizer such as chlorpromazine or haloperidol. For short-term sedation, such as during a CT or MRI scan, an intravenous benzodiazapine may be required. However, psychopharmaceutical agents may exacerbate an abnormal mental state or disguise the neurologic signs of deterioration.

Management begins with identification and correction of hypoxia, hypoglycemia, hyperthermia, or dehydration. Parenteral thiamine should be given to all patients suspected of Wernicke's encephalopathy. Later treatment depends on the underlying cause. If the confusional state does not resolve quickly, attention to hydration and nutrition is required to prevent perpetuation of the confusional state.

AMNESIA

PATHOPHYSIOLOGY The anatomic basis of memory is only partly understood, but it clearly involves the temporal lobes. Most lesions cause impairment of learning and recent memory loss without affecting immediate memory or attention. As a rule, significant amnesia occurs only after bilateral lesions of the medial temporal lobes. Unilateral lesions of the speech-dominant temporal lobe cause deficits of verbal memory, and unilateral lesions of the nondominant temporal lobe result in deficits in visual or nonverbal recall, but these deficits are rarely significant in the absence of preexisting contralateral temporal lobe pathology. The minimum lesion required to produce amnesia has not been established, but involvement of limbic structures appears crucial. Cholinergic neurons may play an important role. For example, anticholinergic drugs disrupt memory storage, and cholinergic drugs may on occasion improve memory.

CLINICAL FEATURES The classic example of amnesia is *Korsakoff's syndrome*, secondary to chronic alcoholism (see Chap. 377 and Chap. 390). The cardinal feature is an inability to recall new information despite a normal level of consciousness. Immediate memory, digit span, and attention are normal. Memory of knowledge acquired before the onset of illness is relatively intact, but memory for new events is severely impaired. Patients are disoriented in place and time and incapable of recalling information for more than the duration of immediate memory. They are thus condemned to be brief visitors to the present; their inner world consists only of memories of their remote past. On first encounter, they may seem relatively normal, taking part in ward routine and engaging in conversation. Because of intact immediate memory, they retain information briefly but forget as soon as they are distracted. In the pure syndrome, tests of intelligence not requiring long-term memory may be normal. Compensation is by confabulation, giving more or less plausible answers incorporating some relevant information and sometimes fantastic elaboration. Although characteristic, confabulation is not universal in Korsakoff's syndrome and may be seen in amnesia due to other causes as well as in acute confusional states. Amnesic subjects can slowly and laboriously learn some tasks, such as tactile or visual mazes, tunes on the piano, and the use of a computer. Despite evidence that the subjects acquire and retain new skills, they do not recall learning and deny the new skills, demonstrating dramatically a disassociation between recollection and retention of information.

DIFFERENTIAL DIAGNOSIS The diagnosis of *Korsakoff's syndrome* is usually clear from its association with chronic alcoholism. It often follows an episode of Wernicke's encephalopathy, and the amnesic deficit becomes evident with recovery from the acute confusional state. Nonalcoholic causes of *thiamine deficiency* (see Chap. 377) may cause Korsakoff's syndrome. Similar clinical syndromes may occur after bilateral temporal lobe lesions resulting from *medial temporal lobectomy*, *head injury*, *herpes simplex encephalitis*, *strokes*, or *brain tumors*. *Alzheimer's disease* (see below) also may cause isolated amnesia before generalized dementia becomes evident.

Temporary amnesia is a common feature of *head injury* (see Chap. 376). The memory disturbance occurs both for events before *(retrograde amnesia)* and after *(posttraumatic amnesia)* the time of injury. *Anterograde amnesia* refers to impairment in learning new material, which accompanies posttraumatic amnesia. Almost invariably, retrograde amnesia causes permanent inability to recall the few minutes prior to the head injury, implying disruption of the immediate memory system and failure to register long-term memory. In severe head injuries, retrograde amnesia may extend back for hours or weeks. With recovery, the duration of retrograde amnesia shrinks and may resolve. During retrograde amnesia, remote memory is usually accessible. The length of posttraumatic amnesia generally corresponds to the length of postconcussive confusion and may continue despite normal immediate memory and digit span. The duration of posttraumatic amnesia indicates the severity of head injury, the ability to learn new material often being the last cognitive deficit to recover.

Transient global amnesia is a syndrome in which a previously well person suddenly becomes confused and amnesic. The attacks are usually spontaneous but occasionally follow immersion in cold or hot water, emotional stimuli, physical exertion, sexual intercourse, or travel in a motor vehicle. The patient appears bewildered and repeatedly asks questions about present and recent events. Orientation for person and sometimes place is preserved, but recent memory is impaired, and the patient cannot recall new information after a few minutes' delay. Behavior is otherwise normal and appropriate. Examination during an attack shows intact immediate memory but severe impairment of recall of recent and sometimes more distant events. General intellectual function is normal. By definition, no other neurologic signs are present. The attacks usually last 2 to 12 h. Headache, nausea, and vomiting may occur. Recovery is complete, and recurrence is unusual. The cause of transient global amnesia is a mystery. Similar symptoms may sometimes accompany migraine, temporal lobe ischemia or epilepsy. The disorder is usually benign; rarely, the attack is due to an underlying temporal lobe tumor.

Brief "blanks" in memory may cause difficulties in diagnosis. Occasionally, *complex partial seizures* may occur without the patient being conscious of any associated signs or loss of awareness, apart from the disruption of memory during the seizure. Amnesia also may rarely accompany *classical migraine*. A number of *drugs*, including alcohol and short-acting benzodiazepines, may impair memory and cause amnesia for events during the period of their use. *Electroconvulsive therapy* (ECT) causes temporary retrograde and anterograde amnesia.

Psychogenic amnesia for personally important memories is common, although whether this results from deliberate avoidance of unpleasant memories or from unconscious repression may be impossible to establish. This *event-specific amnesia* is particularly common after violent crimes such as homicide of a close relative or sexual abuse. It also may occur with severe drug or alcohol intoxication and sometimes with schizophrenia. More prolonged psychogenic amnesia occurs in *fugue states* that also commonly follow severe emotional stress. The patient with a fugue state suffers from a sudden loss of personal identity and may be found wandering far from home. In contrast to organic amnesia, fugue states are associated with amnesia for personal identity and events closely associated with the personal past. At the same time, memory for other recent events and the ability to learn and use new information are preserved. The episodes usually last hours or days and occasionally weeks or months while the patient takes on a new identity. On recovery, there is a residual amnesic gap for the period of the fugue.

MANAGEMENT   The cause of temporary amnesia is usually evident from the history. In patients with transient global amnesia, investigations to exclude an underlying structural cause (MRI or CT), epilepsy (EEG), and vascular risk factors are appropriate. Unless the investigations are positive, reassurance is the only further measure required. The management of persistent amnesia is more demanding. Although Wernicke's encephalopathy responds to thiamine, established Korsakoff's syndrome does not, and the amnesia is usually permanent. Nevertheless, a course of thiamine should be given in newly diagnosed cases to prevent further deterioration.

DEMENTIA

Dementia is common, affecting about 4 million people in the United States alone. It is the major cause of long-term disability in old age. The prevalence of dementia increases rapidly with age, afflicting about 2 percent of the population between ages 65 and 70 and 20 percent of people above 80. With increasing longevity of the population and decreasing birth rates, the prevalence will continue to rise.

PATHOPHYSIOLOGY   Some authorities separate dementia occurring before the age of 65 (presenile dementia) from that occurring after (senile dementia). This distinction was based on the assumption that the causes were different: rare neuronal degenerations in the young and vascular disease or senescence in the elderly. Although the expression of diseases may differ at different ages, the major findings in demented patients of all ages are similar, and the distinction is arbitrary.

Most diseases causing dementia are either widespread neuronal degenerations or multifocal disorders. The initial symptoms depend on where the dementing process starts, but the location and numbers of neurons lost that are required to cause dementia are difficult to establish. Aging results in a gradual loss of neurons and of brain mass, but this is not accompanied by significant intellectual decline in the absence of disease. Indeed, brain mass is a poor guide to intellectual function. Patients with a degenerative dementia in the sixth decade may have a greater brain mass than intellectually normal patients in their eighth decade. Consequently, documentation of generalized atrophy by CT scan is not a clear indication of dementia.

Dementia may result from cortical disease (e.g., Alzheimer's disease) or from disease of subcortical structures such as the basal ganglia, thalamus, and deep white matter (e.g., Huntington's disease or multiple sclerosis). Cortical dementia is characterized by loss of cognitive functions such as language, perception, calculation; in contrast, subcortical dementia exhibits slowing of cognition and information processing (''bradyphrenia''), flattening of the affect, and disturbances of motivation, mood, and arousal. Memory is impaired in both types. The features of subcortical dementia also occur in cortical processes affecting the frontal lobes and probably reflect damaged projections to and from the frontal lobes.

In Alzheimer's disease, which is the most common cause of dementia, the dementia results from loss of cortical tissue especially in the temporal, parietal, and frontal lobes. This is accompanied in most cases by increased space between the gyri and enlargement of the ventricles. The histologic hallmark is the presence of numerous neurofibrillary tangles and senile plaques (see Chap. 370). Plaques and tangles are found in normal elderly brains but are increased in number in Alzheimer's disease, especially in the hippocampus and temporal lobes. The hippocampal involvement probably accounts for the memory disorder, which may be partially mediated by a reduction in cholinergic activity. The activities of other neurotransmitters, including norepinephrine, serotonin, dopamine, glutamate, and somatostatin, are also reduced. These changes are accompanied by reductions in cerebral blood flow and decreased metabolism of oxygen and glucose.

DIFFERENTIAL DIAGNOSIS   The causes of dementia are numerous (Table 25-3). However, a small number of diseases account for most cases. In most of the western world, Alzheimer's disease is responsible for 50 to 90 percent and vascular disease for 5 to 10 percent of cases of dementia referred to hospital. In Japan and parts of Scandinavia, vascular disease appears to be more prevalent than Alzheimer's disease, at least in hospitalized patients. Cerebral infarction contributes to intellectual loss in a further 15 percent of patients with Alzheimer's disease documented at autopsy (*mixed dementia*). Dementia attributed to ethanol abuse may account for 5 to 10 percent of cases. Metabolic disturbances, cerebral neoplasms, subdural hematoma, and normal-pressure hydrocephalus account for around 10 percent of cases, and Huntington's chorea accounts for about 2 percent. The remainder of causes, including Creutzfeldt-Jakob disease, are rare, accounting for less than 1 percent of cases. In human immunodeficiency virus (HIV) infection, dementia occurs in 30 to 40 percent of patients and is an important cause in younger patients. Diffuse Lewy body disease increasingly is recognized as a cause of a degenerative dementia, although it remains unclear whether it is an entity or a variant of Alzheimer's disease (see Chap. 370).

The main aim of diagnosis is to identify treatable causes of dementia. The differential diagnosis depends primarily on a careful history and examination, supported by investigation. Illnesses that cause dementia can be divided into those in which dementia is the primary manifestation of the disease (other neurologic signs are absent), those in which dementia is secondary to other neurologic disorders (additional neurologic findings are usually present), and systemic diseases in which dementia is usually associated with signs outside the central nervous system.

In the elderly, dementia must be distinguished from the minor degree of forgetfulness that accompanies aging (*age-associated memory impairment* or *benign senescent forgetfulness*); the latter is often accompanied by slowing of physical and mental agility and rigidity of thinking. This is by no means universal with aging and may reflect an unidentified disease process. Benign senescent forgetfulness is not disabling in the activities of daily life and does not progress to more severe disability. Early on, dementias are often indistinguishable from benign senescence, and it is only the young age of the patient or progression of the symptoms that confirms the diagnosis of dementia.

Primary dementia   The diagnosis of *Alzheimer's disease* is only certain at autopsy but is suggested by the characteristic history and signs, supported by negative investigations excluding other causes of dementia. Series of well-investigated patients with dementia attributed to Alzheimer's disease always include cases with an alternative diagnosis established at autopsy. The term *dementia of Alzheimer type* is sometimes used for patients with the characteristic clinical

TABLE 25-3 Differential diagnosis of dementia

Primary dementia with no other signs
  Alzheimer's disease
  Pick's disease
  Frontal lobe degeneration
Dementia with signs of vascular disease
  Multi-infarct dementia*
  Thalamic infarction
  "Binswanger's disease"* and lacunar state*
  Vasculitis,* e.g., systemic lupus erythematosus, polyarteritis nodosa, granulomatous angiitis of the central nervous system, Behçet's disease
Dementia with evidence of chronic infection†
  Human immunodeficiency virus
  Syphilis*
  Papovavirus (progressive multifocal leukoencephalopathy)
  Subacute sclerosing panencephalitis
  Creutzfeldt-Jakob disease (subacute spongiform encephalopathy)
  Tuberculosis,* fungal and protozoal infections*
  Sarcoidosis*
  Whipple's disease*
Secondary dementia with signs of the underlying neurologic condition
  Neoplasia and mass lesions
    Primary and secondary tumors*
    Carcinomatous meningitis
    Paraneoplastic encephalitis
    Chronic subdural hematoma*
    Hydrocephalus*
  Movement disorders
    Parkinson's disease
    Lewy body dementia
    Huntington's chorea
    Progressive supranuclear palsy (Steele-Richardson syndrome)
    Multisystem degeneration (Shy-Drager syndrome)
    Hereditary ataxias
  Motor neuron disease (amyotrophic lateral sclerosis)
  Multiple sclerosis
Dementia following diffuse brain damage‡
  Acute head injury
  Pugilistic dementia
  Anoxia
  Encephalitis
Endocrine disorders and vitamin deficiency
  Hypothyroidism*
  B_{12} deficiency*
  Thiamine deficiency*
  Nicotinic acid deficiency* (pellagra)
  Adrenal insufficiency* and Cushing's syndrome*
  Hypo-* and hyperparathyroidism*
  Chronic hypoglycemia*
Toxic disorders
  Drug and narcotic poisoning*
  Alcoholic dementia*
  Heavy metal intoxication*
  Organic toxins*
  Dialysis dementia*
Psychiatric
  Chronic schizophrenia
  Pseudodementia*
Additional conditions to consider in adolescents or young adults
  Movement disorders
    Wilson's disease*
    Hallervorden-Spatz disease
  Tuberous sclerosis
  Progressive myoclonic epilepsy*
  Metabolic diseases, e.g., leukodystrophies, mitochondrial cytopathy, storage diseases, Leigh's disease, homocystinuria

---

* Condition in which treatment may reverse or prevent progression of dementia.
† Systemic, hematologic or CSF findings suggest infection except in Creutzfeldt-Jakob disease.
‡ History of acute injury with depression of consciousness usual, except in pugilistic dementia.

---

picture and negative investigations in whom pathologic confirmation has not been obtained.

The mean duration from the onset of symptoms to death is 8 years, with a range of 2 to 15 years. The course may be more rapid in younger patients. The early features vary according to the initial brain site involved. The onset is insidious and subtle and can rarely be pinpointed. In most cases, insight is lost early, and intellectual failures are attributed to old age or oversight. Some patients have no spontaneous complaints but become disturbed when unable to answer simple questions. The history is almost invariably given by a relative. Early loss of spontaneity and initiative is frequent. The patient may give up hobbies and lose interest in social contacts or conversation. Lapses of memory, difficulty learning new information, and failure to remember names and appointments are noticed. At this stage, the memory deficit is more likely to involve recent events. In the early stages, social graces are usually preserved, and routine behavior and simple conversation are normal so that friends and relatives may be unaware that anything is wrong, unless the patient is tested by an unfamiliar situation or by a formal examination of cognitive function. As the disease progresses, inexplicable mistakes are made in the activities of everyday life, and dress, appearance, and personal hygiene are neglected. Spatial disorientation may become evident, especially in unfamiliar surroundings. The patient may oscillate between apathy and unprovoked irritability or aggression.

Examination in the early stage usually shows impairment of memory for recent events with varying degrees of other deficits. The patient often appears puzzled in response to questioning. Primitive reflexes such as palmomental response or suck reflex may be present.

As the disease advances, the impairments of memory, speech, and behavior become so marked that patients are unable to care for themselves, repeat questions over and over again, and fail to recognize friends and relatives. Restlessness is common, especially at night, and patients become lost if allowed to wander. Delusions, paranoia, and hallucinations may occur. On examination at this stage, the patient remains alert but is disoriented to time and place and has poor memory for recent and distant events. Digit span is usually preserved. Speech lacks spontaneity and fluency and exhibits minor aphasic errors, and there is difficulty understanding complex commands. Nonfluent aphasia, especially in younger patients, may be striking. Motor and constructional apraxia and agnosia may be present. Extrapyramidal signs, including stooped posture, slow shuffling gait, generalized bradykinesia, and rigidity, are common. The tendon reflexes may be brisk, but extensor plantar responses are rare. Grasp reflexes may be elicited. In the last stage, the patient is immobile, mute, and incontinent. The patient no longer recognizes relatives, and testing of cognitive function is not possible. Seizures and myoclonus may become prominent. Weight loss and a shrunken appearance may precede death, often from intercurrent infection.

Pick's disease is characterized by circumscribed cortical atrophy, usually confined to the frontal and temporal lobes, associated with a characteristic histologic appearance of degenerative neurons in the cortex, basal ganglia, and brainstem, which contain Pick's bodies (see Chap. 370). The age at onset and course are similar to Alzheimer's disease. Patients with Pick's disease suffer slowly progressive dementia and in the early stages may show frontal-temporal lobe features uncommon in Alzheimer's disease, including personality and emotional changes, disinhibition, lack of restraint, poor social and inappropriate sexual conduct, and lack of foresight. Later, patients may appear euphoric or retreat into increasing apathy and abulia in association with nonfluent aphasia, which progresses to mutism. Some cases of Pick's disease are indistinguishable clinically from Alzheimer's disease, and some cases of Alzheimer's disease show a frontal predominance so that the distinction may only be made at autopsy. A similar picture of *frontal lobe dementia* may occur in association with primary neuronal degeneration in the frontal and anterior temporal lobes without the neuropathologic findings of either Alzheimer's or Pick's disease.

Vascular dementia Usually vascular dementia results from multiple areas of discrete infarction and not from chronic diffuse ischemia. The term *multi-infarct dementia* emphasizes this distinction. The diagnosis of vascular dementia is strongly suggested by an abrupt onset, especially if there is a history of previous stroke. The course characteristically fluctuates with periods of improvement and stepwise deterioration, in contrast to the steady progression of Alzheimer's disease. Hypertension is usual in vascular dementia but rare in Alzheimer's disease. Nocturnal confusion, relative preservation of personality, emotional lability, somatic complaints, and depression are more common in vascular dementia but not diagnostic. Focal neurologic signs (other than those of the cognitive deficits), including pseudobulbar palsy, visual-field deficits, hemiparesis, or extensor plantar responses, may suggest vascular dementia but also may be symptomatic of other neurologic causes such as a tumor.

Multi-infarct dementia can result from all types of cerebral vascular disease but is most likely to result from recurrent bilateral cerebral embolism from the heart or carotid arteries. It also can occur as a result of bilateral brain damage after a single episode of severe hypotension or cardiac arrest. Multi-infarct dementia may occur with widespread involvement of small vessels by vasculitis, from a few strategically placed large cortical infarcts, or from multiple small infarcts in subcortical structures, such as occurs in the *lacunar state* secondary to hypertensive small-vessel disease (see Chap. 368). Hypertensive or atherosclerotic disease with thickening of the perforating deep vessels and capillaries supplying the subcortical white matter also may cause *Binswanger's disease (subcortical arteriosclerotic encephalopathy)*, in which dementia is associated with diffuse loss of subcortical white matter and enlargement of the underlying ventricle. In contrast to multi-infarct dementia, major stroke is unusual in Binswanger's disease, and examination shows features of subcortical dementia (see above), a characteristic small-stepped, wide-based gait (*marche à petit pas*), pseudobulbar palsy, and corticospinal signs.

Chronic infections   Chronic infections are important to consider, since the dementia may be treatable. Infections of the CNS are usually associated with systemic manifestations, meningeal involvement, abnormal CSF, and abnormalities on MRI or CT scan. Cerebral *syphilis* was a major cause and should still be excluded in all patients (see Chap. 133). *HIV* infection is an important cause of dementia in young people (see Chaps. 279 and 375) but should be considered in all patients at risk. The dementia may be the first manifestation of the infection. Dementia also may arise from "slow" virus infections. *Subacute sclerosing panencephalitis* causes dementia in children and occasionally in adolescents due to persistent replication of the measles virus in the brain many years after initial infection (see Chap. 375). *Creutzfeldt-Jakob disease (subacute spongiform encephalopathy)*, a rare dementia, has been transmitted by a novel agent, known as a *prion protein*, to animals and to humans by corneal transplantation, neurosurgical instrumentation, or injections of growth hormone extracted from human pituitaries. In most cases, the route of infection is unknown. After incubating for several years, the illness occurs in middle or late life and progresses to death within months. The dementia is often combined with ataxia, corticospinal signs, abnormal movements, cortical blindness, and myoclonus (see Chap. 375). Bizarre behavior and hallucinations are sometimes striking. In contrast to most other infections of the nervous system, signs of intracranial inflammation are absent and the CSF is normal, but characteristic EEG abnormalities (repetitive complexes) may be helpful in diagnosis. A rare genetic disorder, Gerstmann-Schenker-Straussler disease, is caused by a mutation in the prion protein.

Neoplasia and mass lesions   *Primary or secondary brain tumors* may present with dementia, particularly slowly growing, deep, midline tumors of the corpus callosum or frontal lobe. Frontal meningiomas are the most important to consider in all patients because they are benign and the dementia is potentially curable. Other curable mass lesions include *chronic subdural hematoma*. The head trauma in such cases may have been remote, trivial, or forgotten, particularly in the elderly. Diffuse primary tumors and multiple secondary tumors also may cause dementia. Features of raised intracranial pressures (such as headaches or papilledema) and focal signs apart from the cognitive disorders may be absent, although minor signs such as a grasp reflex or extensor plantar response are often present. Most causes of dementia due to mass lesions or raised intracranial pressure are easily diagnosed from the MRI or CT scan.

Malignancy arising outside the nervous system also may cause dementia through *metastatic carcinomatous meningitis* or from a *nonmetastatic paraneoplastic encephalitis* (see Chaps. 328 and 369).

The latter condition usually begins insidiously and progresses slowly. Depression of consciousness is absent in the early stages, and psychiatric disturbances may be striking. The CSF is usually abnormal in these conditions.

Obstructive or communicating hydrocephalus in adults characteristically presents with subacute progressive dementia and is an important treatable cause. A history of headache may be obtained, and ataxia and gait disturbance are usual. Signs of raised intracranial pressure may be absent. The diagnosis is hampered in the elderly by the difficulty of distinguishing the scan appearances of hydrocephalus due to abnormal CSF dynamics from hydrocephalus ex vacuo secondary to atrophy. However, the combination of dementia, urinary incontinence, and gait disorder suggests the syndrome of *normal- or low-pressure hydrocephalus*. In this condition, routine measurements of CSF pressure at lumbar puncture or ventriculography are normal, but intermittent waves of increased CSF pressure may be detected if patients are monitored for several days. Such cases may respond to ventricular drainage.

Movement disorders   A number of degenerative neurologic diseases other than the primary dementias also may cause dementia, usually as a late manifestation. Movement disorders provide the largest group, of which the most common is *idiopathic Parkinson's disease*, where dementia develops in the late stages of the disease in 15 to 30 percent (see Chap. 371). Another important cause is Huntington's chorea, partly because the diagnosis has genetic implications (see Chap. 370). In these conditions, the cause of the dementia is usually evident from the history or clinical signs of the underlying neurologic disease, but very occasionally the dementia may be the only feature.

Diffuse brain damage   In dementia secondary to *head injury, anoxia, hypoglycemia,* or *encephalitis*, the cause is usually obvious from the history. The initial insult almost invariably causes loss of consciousness, and the dementia becomes evident when consciousness is regained after prolonged coma. If the patient recovers but then declines intellectually, the possibility of a secondary cause of dementia such as hydrocephalus should be considered. Repeated, less severe head trauma, such as occurs in boxers, may lead later in life to dementia associated with extrapyramidal signs, dysarthria, and ataxia (*dementia pugilistica*, or the "punch drunk" syndrome).

Endocrine disorders and vitamin deficiency   Imbalances sufficient to affect neuronal function usually cause an acute confusional state with disturbance of attention and consciousness, but on occasion the presentation may be more chronic and mimic dementia. These conditions are treatable and cause reversible dementia, and they must be excluded in all patients. *Hypothyroidism* is the most common endocrine condition to present with dementia.

Toxic disorders   Intoxications usually present with acute confusional state, often fluctuating according to the exposure. However, chronic intoxication may result in a reversible dementia. *Drugs* are an important cause, especially in the elderly, and the medication history should be carefully reviewed. The list of potential agents is large and includes drugs of abuse, psychotherapeutic agents (including barbiturates, sleeping tablets, tranquilizers, and antidepressants), drugs used in Parkinson's disease (levodopa and anticholinergics), and anticonvulsants. *Alcohol* is the most prevalent intoxicant implicated in dementia. Chronic inebriation results in reversible intellectual impairment but also may lead to a persistent deficit. In some cases, this is pure amnesia due to Korsakoff's psychosis, but in others it is a global dementia associated with cerebral atrophy. Factors accounting for dementia in alcoholics include vitamin deficiency, repeated head injury, anoxia or hypoglycemia during alcoholic stupor, chronic liver failure, or the rare complication of *Marchiafava-Bignami disease*, which causes widespread demyelination in the cerebral hemispheres.

Dementia in adolescents and young adults   This requires consideration of a further group of conditions in addition to those already mentioned (Table 25-3). Late presentation of *Wilson's disease* is another important example of a treatable dementia and should be excluded in all patients under the age of 40. Metabolic diseases are the largest group. There is usually evidence of a systemic disorder such as a peripheral neuropathy, myopathy, retinopathy, or hepatosplenomegaly. Specific diagnosis relies on special investigation.

Pseudodementias Nonorganic causes of apparent intellectual decline are not rare, although it is probably more frequent for organic dementia to be misdiagnosed initially as a psychiatric illness. A mistaken diagnosis is particularly common in the elderly, in whom the behavioral changes of dementia may be attributed to depression. Conversely, the severely depressed patient may appear disoriented and perform poorly in all aspects of intellectual function. These deficits are caused by the psychomotor retardation, apathy, and loss of interest that accompanies depression. Such intellectual impairments may be due to reversible neurochemical changes that mimic the irreversible changes of degenerative dementias. The distinction may be difficult, but the correct diagnosis of depression is often suggested by a history of sudden onset, marked sleep disturbance, a previous history of psychiatric illness, or precipitation by an emotional event. In addition, depressed patients often complain to a greater extent about difficulties with mentation that seem justified from their performance on tests of intellectual function. In contrast, the patient with true dementia rarely complains appropriately about deficits that are obvious on examination. Dementia due to depression also may be suggested by inconsistency during the history; for example, patients may give a clear account of some topic of interest to them or recount the history and details of their personal lives reasonably well but then show inconsistent difficulties with specific questions, often failing even to attempt an answer. Variability in performance during testing, particularly improvement with encouragement, is characteristic. Negative neurologic investigation supports the diagnosis of pseudodementia but also may be found in organic dementia. The only way to confirm the diagnosis is to demonstrate improvement in intellectual functioning with appropriate psychiatric treatment (see Chap. 389).

Pseudodementias also may occur as a *hysterical phenomenon*, when amnesia is often striking. In one variety, Ganser syndrome, the answers to simple questions are often inaccurate, but the patient may retain a sense of the purpose of the question (''approximate'' answers), indicating that, despite the absurdity of the answer, the question is understood and the correct answer is known to the patient. In hysterical pseudodementia and Ganser syndrome, the apparent severe disturbance of intellect is not reflected in the patient's behavior. Frank simulation of dementia is rare, although the distinction between hysteria and malingering is not always clear. Intellectual impairment is a feature of *mania* and *schizophrenia;* the diagnosis is made from the accompanying thought disorder (see Chap. 389).

INVESTIGATION   The age, history, and clinical findings will dictate the selection of screening tests. Investigations essential in all patients are aimed at excluding reversible causes of dementia. These include a full blood count, biochemical profile, thyroid function tests, serum vitamin B_{12}, and red cell folate. Syphilis and HIV serology also may be indicated. Ideally, every patient with dementia should have an *MRI* or *CT scan* to exclude treatable intracranial pathology, especially in the presence of focal clinical signs, a history of subacute illness, or a younger age of patient. Scanning is less likely to influence management if the patient is elderly and has a long history of degenerative dementia. In Alzheimer's disease, the scan may show progressive cortical atrophy and ventricular dilatation, but this is not invariable and also can be found in normal aging. The CT or MRI may show areas of low attenuation or abnormal signal in the deep white matter, particularly in the periventricular regions and centrum semiovale, referred to by the descriptive term *leukoaraiosis*. These findings are characteristic of Binswanger's disease but also can be seen in Alzheimer's disease, cerebrovascular disease, and in apparently normal subjects. The *EEG* may show features that support the diagnosis of Alzheimer's disease, subacute sclerosing panencephalitis, or Creutzfeldt-Jakob disease. *CSF examination* is normal in the primary degenerative dementias but may be useful if there is doubt about the diagnosis and is essential if there is a suspicion of intracranial infection. *Regional cerebral blood flow studies* (e.g., single-photon

or positron emission CT) may sometimes be useful in distinguishing between frontal lobe dementias and Alzheimer's disease or in demonstrating multifocal deficits in vascular dementia. *Cerebral angiography* is rarely helpful except for the investigation of suspected vascular dementia, vasculitis, or intracranial masses. *Neuropsychologic testing* (such as the Wechsler Adult Intelligence Scale) may help document intellectual decline or identify pseudodementia. *Meningeal and brain biopsy* may occasionally be justified when infection, vasculitis, or treatable tumor is suspected and occasionally in younger patients when etiology remains in doubt.

MANAGEMENT   The initial management includes treatment of any reversible cause of dementia or superimposed confusional state. About 10 percent of patients with dementia have a treatable neurologic or systemic illness, 10 percent have pseudodementia due to treatable psychiatric illnesses, and 10 percent have a modifiable contributory cause such as alcoholism or hypertension. Unfortunately, the remainder have irreversible dementia so that management aims to support the patient and the family.

The mildly demented patient may continue relatively normal activities at home but rarely at work. As the dementia progresses, more supervision is required. As the disorder deepens, the patient requires increasing help with the activities of daily life. Some fairly severely impaired patients can live alone if they have support from the community, including daily visits from family or friends, regular visits by a community nurse, the provision of meals, and help from neighbors. Many mildly demented individuals become disoriented and confused when removed to unfamiliar surroundings such as a hospital.

In the early stages the patient may be helped by treatment of associated depression, anxiety, agitation, psychotic symptoms, or insomnia with appropriate psychotropic medication. However, psychotropic drugs may make demented patients more confused, requiring reduction or withdrawal of the medication. The demands on relatives caring for a severely demented patient are high, especially if the patient is restless at night and requires constant supervision to prevent wandering or personal harm. The fact that individuals may live for many years in such a state increases the burden. The situation often becomes intolerable when incontinence develops. Sleep deprivation and physical exhaustion aggravate the stress of caring for a demented relative, who may appear ungrateful, cantankerous, aggressive, or disinhibited. Sympathetic attention to the relatives of the demented is therefore important. It may help to obtain a ''baby sitter'' to allow the caregiver regular time off. If the caregiver can do so without undue feelings of guilt, an annual holiday while the patient is placed temporarily in a nursing home is invaluable.

Eventually, many demented patients require full-time nursing care in a residential home or hospital. Relatives should be encouraged to plan for this and should be counseled not to regard this outcome as a personal failure. In the later stages, management aims at preserving the patient's dignity and comfort.

REFERENCES

BROWN MM, HACHINSKI VC: Vascular dementia. Curr Opinion Neurol Neurosurg 2:78, 1989

CUMMINGS JL: Subcortical dementia: Neuropsychology, neuropsychiatry, and pathophysiology. Br J Psychiatry 149:682, 1989

CONSENSUS CONFERENCE: Differential diagnosis of dementing diseases. JAMA 258:3411, 1987

DAVIES DC: Alzheimer's disease: Towards an understanding of the aetiology and pathogenesis, in *Current Problems in Neurology II*. London, Libbey, 1989

DOBKIN BH, HANLON R: Dopamine agonist treatment of antegrade amnesia from a mediobasal forebrain injury. Ann Neurol 33:313, 1993

ERICKSON KR: Amnestic disorders: Pathophysiology and patterns of memory dysfunction. West J Med 152:159, 1990

FIBIGER HC: Cholinergic mechanisms in learning, memory and dementia: A review of recent evidence. Trends Neurosci 14:220, 1991

GUSTAFSON L: Frontal lobe degeneration of non-Alzheimer type. Clinical picture and differential diagnosis. Arch Geront Geriat 6:209, 1987

HO DD et al: The acquired immunodeficiency syndrome (AIDS) dementia complex (clinical conference). Ann Intern Med 111:400, 1989

HODGES JR, WARLOW CP: The aetiology of transient global amnesia: A case-control study of 114 cases with prospective follow-up. Brain 113:639, 1990

KOPELMAN MD: Amnesia: Organic and psychogenic. Br J Psychiatry 150:428, 1987

KRITCHEVSKY M, SQUIRE LR: Permanent global amnesia with unknown etiology. Neurology 43:326, 1993

LIPOWSKI ZJ: Delirium in the elderly patient. N Engl J Med 320:578, 1989

LISHMAN WA: Organic Psychiatry: The Psychological Consequences of Cerebral Disorder, 2d ed. Oxford, Blackwell, 1987

MALETTA GJ: Treatment considerations for Alzheimer's disease and related dementing illnesses. Clin Geriatr Med 4:699, 1988

ROMAN GC: Senile dementia of the Binswanger type: A vascular form of dementia in the elderly. JAMA 258:1782, 1987

ROTH M, IVERSEN LL (eds): Alzheimer's disease and related disorders. Br Med Bull 42:1, 1986

SCHOLTZ CL: Dementia in middle and late life. Curr Top Pathol 76:105, 1988

TATEMICHI TK et al: Clnical determinants of dementia related to stroke. Ann Neurol 33:568, 1993

WADE JPH, HACHINSKI VC: Multi-infarct dementia, in Dementia (Medicine in Old Age), BM Pitt (ed). London, Churchill Livingstone, 1987, pp 209–228

26   COMA AND OTHER DISORDERS OF CONSCIOUSNESS

ALLAN H. ROPPER / JOSEPH B. MARTIN

Coma is a common problem in general medicine; it is estimated that up to 3 percent of admissions to the emergency ward of large municipal hospitals are due to diseases that cause a disorder of consciousness. The importance of this class of neurologic disorders requires acquiring a systematic approach to their diagnosis and management.

The increased availability of computed tomography (CT) and magnetic resonance imaging (MRI) has focused attention on lesions that are radiologically detectable (e.g., hemorrhages, tumors, or hydrocephalus) in the diagnosis of coma. This approach, although at times expedient, is often imprudent because most coma is metabolic or toxic in origin. The physician confronted with an unresponsive patient should formulate a differential diagnosis based on the history and the clinical signs. The findings on general and neurologic examination allow the physician to narrow the possibilities responsible for the comatose state. A rational approach to defining the precise diagnosis and planning subsequent management can then be initiated and clinical changes anticipated. This chapter describes a practical approach to coma based on the anatomy and physiology of consciousness, the general and neurologic examination, and neuroimaging.

Coma is characterized by unresponsiveness and as such is easily recognized. A narrative description of the clinical state of the patient and of responses evoked by various stimuli, precisely as they are observed at the bedside, remains the optimal way to characterize coma and related disturbances of consciousness. Such a description is preferable to summary terms such as *semicoma* or *obtundation*, which are often ambiguous and commonly differ between observers. *Stupor*, as currently used, implies a state from which the patient can be aroused by vigorous stimuli, but verbal responses are slow or absent and the patient makes some effort to avoid uncomfortable stimuli; *coma* suggests a state from which the patient cannot be aroused by stimulation, and no purposeful attempt is made to avoid painful stimuli.

Although the definition of consciousness is a psychological and philosophical matter, the distinction between *level* of consciousness, or wakefulness, and *content* of consciousness, or awareness, has physiologic significance. Wakefulness or alertness is maintained by a diffuse system of upper brainstem and thalamic neurons, the reticular activating system (RAS), and its connections to the cerebral hemispheres. Therefore, depression of either hemispheral or RAS activity may cause reduced wakefulness. *Awareness* is dependent on integrated and organized material thoughts, subjective experience, emotions, and mental processes, each of which resides to some extent in anatomically defined regions of the brain. The inability to maintain a coherent sequence of thoughts, accompanied usually by inattention, is called *confusion* and is a disorder of content of consciousness (see Chap. 25). In special cases confusion is accompanied by illusions (misperceptions of environmental sight, sound, or touch) or hallucinations (spontaneous endogenous perceptions). The confused patient is usually subdued, not inclined to speak, and less active physically than usual. Psychiatrists use the term *delirium* for any confusion, but neurologists prefer to use delirium as a description for an agitated, hypersympathotonic, frequently hallucinatory state most often due to alcohol or drug withdrawal. Many processes that ultimately lead to coma begin with confusion or delirium, and diagnostic considerations should address the primary problem as an alteration in the level of consciousness. Focal cerebral lesions that cause deficits in language, orientation, or memory may make the patient appear to be confused (see Chap. 27).

ANATOMIC CORRELATES OF CONSCIOUSNESS   A normal level of consciousness (wakefulness) depends on activation of the cerebral hemispheres by groups of neurons located in the brainstem RAS. All these components and the connections between them must be preserved for normal consciousness. The principal causes of coma are, therefore, (1) bilateral hemispheral damage or suppression by hypoxia, hypoglycemia, drugs, or toxins or (2) a brainstem lesion or metabolic derangement that damages or suppresses the RAS.

Reticular activating system   The RAS is defined as a physiologic system, not an anatomic one. It is contained within the rostral reticular formation, which consists of loosely grouped neurons located bilaterally in the medial tegmental gray matter of the brainstem and extending from the medulla to the diencephalon. These neurons have been shown in neuroanatomic studies to span long rostrocaudal distances within the reticular formation. Animal experiments and human cliniconeuropathologic observations have established that the *neurons located in the region extending from the rostral pons to the caudal diencephalon are of primary importance for maintaining wakefulness.* Lesions here that produce coma also commonly affect adjacent brainstem structures concerned with control of pupillary constriction and eye movements (Fig. 26-1). *Abnormalities in these systems on physical examination provide signposts of brainstem damage.* Lesions confined to the cerebral hemispheres do not directly affect the brainstem RAS, although secondary dysfunction of the upper brainstem often results from compression by a mass in a cerebral hemisphere (see transtentorial herniation below).

Brainstem RAS neurons project rostrally to the cortex, primarily via "nonspecific" thalamic relay nuclei that exert a tonic influence on the activity of the cerebral cortex. Experimental work in primates suggests that the brainstem RAS indirectly affects the level of consciousness by suppressing the activity of the nonspecific nuclei. The basis of behavioral arousal by environmental stimuli (somesthetic, auditory, and visual) depends on the rich innervation of the RAS by each of these sensory systems.

The relay between the RAS and thalamic and cortical areas is accomplished by neurotransmitters. Of these, the influences of acetylcholine and biogenic amines on arousal have been studied most extensively. Cholinergic fibers connect the midbrain to other areas of the upper brainstem, thalamus, and cortex. These pathways are thought to mediate the clinical and EEG arousal observed after administration of cholinergic drugs such as physostigmine. Serotonin and norepinephrine also subserve important functions in the regulation of the sleep-wake cycle (see Chap. 29). Their roles in arousal and coma have not been clearly established, although the alerting effects of amphetamines are likely to be mediated by catecholamine release.

Cerebral hemispheres and consciousness   The specialized functions of the cerebral cortex in language, control of movement, and perception are regionalized (see Chaps. 25, 27, and 28). In contrast, wakefulness is related in a semiquantitative way to the total mass of functioning cortex and is not focally represented in any region of the hemispheres, with the exception that large, purely unilateral

FIGURE 26-1   Brainstem reflexes in the coma examination. Midbrain and third nerve function are tested by pupillary reaction to light, pontine function by spontaneous and reflex eye movements and corneal responses, and medullary function by respiratory and pharyngeal responses.

Reflex conjugate, horizontal eye movements are dependent on the medial longitudinal fasciculus (MLF) interconnecting the sixth and contralateral third nerve nuclei. Eye movements are elicited by head rotation (oculocephalic reflex) or caloric stimulation of the labyrinths (oculovestibular reflex). These reflex movements are suppressed in the awake patient by the cerebral hemispheres via their connections to the brainstem.

hemispheral lesions, particularly on the left, may cause transient drowsiness even in the absence of damage to the opposite hemisphere or RAS. Hemispheral lesions may cause coma in one of two ways: (1) most commonly, bilateral, generalized hemispheral lesions or metabolic derangements such as occur in encephalitis, hyperammonemia, hypoglycemia, generalized epilepsy, drug ingestion, global brain ischemia, and widespread traumatic damage interfere with awareness in a graded fashion and (2) large lesions in one or both hemispheres may compress the upper brainstem and diencephalic RAS causing coma indirectly. *The degree of decrease in alertness is related to the acuteness of onset of the cortical dysfunction or RAS compression.*

The concept of *transtentorial herniation* with progressive brainstem compression has been used to explain neurologic signs in coma caused by supratentorial mass lesions. *Herniation* refers to displacement of brain tissue away from a mass, past a less mobile structure such as dura, and into a space that it normally does not occupy. The common herniations seen at postmortem examinations are transfalcial (displacement of the cingulate gyrus under the falx in the anterior midline), transtentorial (medial temporal lobe displaced into the tentorial opening), and foraminal (the cerebellar tonsils forced into the foramen magnum). Uncal transtentorial herniation, or impaction of the uncal gyrus into the anterior portion of the tentorial opening, is thought to cause compression of the third nerve with pupillary

dilation. Subsequent coma is due to midbrain compression by the parahippocampal gyrus. Central transtentorial herniation denotes downward movement of the diencephalon (thalamic region) through the tentorial opening in the midline and is heralded by miotic pupils and drowsiness. These shifts in brain can cause an orderly progression of rostral to caudal compression of first the midbrain, then the pons, and finally the medulla leading to the sequential appearance of neurologic signs corresponding to the level damaged and to progressively diminished alertness. However, some patients with supratentorial masses do not follow these stereotypic patterns; for example, an orderly progression of signs from midbrain to medulla is rarely seen in catastrophic lesions, where all brainstem functions are lost almost simultaneously. Furthermore, drowsiness and stupor typically occur with moderate lateral shifts at the level of the diencephalon when there is only minimal vertical displacement of structures near the tentorial opening and before downward herniation is evident on CT or MRI scan.

PATHOPHYSIOLOGY OF COMA   The pathophysiologic basis of coma is either mechanical destruction of crucial areas of the brainstem or cerebral cortex (anatomic coma) or global disruption of brain metabolic processes (metabolic coma). Coma of metabolic origin may be produced by interruption of energy substrate delivery (hypoxia, ischemia, hypoglycemia) or by alteration of the neurophysiologic responses of neuronal membranes (drug or alcohol intoxication, toxic endogenous metabolites, or epilepsy).

The brain is dependent on continuous cerebral blood flow (CBF), oxygen, and glucose. CBF is approximately 75 mL per 100 g/min in gray matter and 30 mL per 100 g/min in white matter (mean = 55 mL per 100 g/min). Oxygen consumption is 3.5 mL per 100 g/min, and glucose consumption is 5 mg per 100 g/min. Brain stores of glucose provide energy for approximately 2 min after blood flow is interrupted, and consciousness is lost within 8 to 10 s. When hypoxia occurs simultaneously with ischemia, available glucose is exhausted more rapidly. When mean CBF is below 25 mL per 100 g/min, the EEG becomes diffusely slowed (typical of metabolic encephalopathies), and at 15 mL per 100 g/min brain electrical activity ceases. If all other conditions such as temperature and arterial oxygenation remain normal, CBF less than 10 mL per 100 g/min causes irreversible brain damage. The duration of ischemia is a major determinant of irreversible damage.

Coma due to hyponatremia, hyperosmolarity, hypercapnia, and the encephalopathies of hepatic and renal failure are associated with a variety of metabolic derangements of neurons and astrocytes. The toxic effects of these conditions on the brain are not well understood but may be multifactorial, producing impaired energy supplies, changes in resting membrane potentials, neurotransmitter abnormalities, and in some instances morphologic changes (see Chap. 377). For example, the high brain ammonia concentration associated with hepatic coma has been theorized to interfere with cerebral energy metabolism and the Na^+,K^+-ATPase pump, increase the number and size of astrocytes, result in increased concentrations of potentially toxic products of ammonia metabolism, and result in abnormalities of neurotransmitters, including possible "false" neurotransmitters, which may act competitively at receptor sites. Ammonia or other metabolites also may bind to benzodiazepine–γ-aminobutyric acid receptors to cause central nervous system (CNS) depression.

The exact cause of the encephalopathy of renal failure is also poorly understood. Unlike ammonia, urea itself does not produce CNS toxicity. A multifactorial cause is likely, including increased permeability of the blood-brain barrier to toxic substances such as organic acids and an increase in brain calcium or cerebrospinal fluid (CSF) phosphate content.

Abnormalities of osmolarity are involved in the coma and seizures caused by several systemic medical disorders, including diabetic ketoacidosis, the nonketotic hyperosmolar state, and hyponatremia. Brain water volume correlates best with level of consciousness in hyponatremic–hypoosmolar states, but other factors probably also play a role. Sodium levels below 115 mmol/L are associated with coma and convulsions, depending on the rapidity with which the hyponatremia develops. Serum osmolarity is generally above 350 mosmol/L in hyperosmolar coma.

Hypercapnia produces a diminished level of consciousness proportional to the P_{CO_2} tension in the blood and to acuteness of onset. A relationship between CSF acidosis and severity of symptoms has been established. The pathophysiologies of other metabolic encephalopathies such as hypercalcemia, hypothyroidism, vitamin B_{12} deficiency, and hypothermia are incompletely understood but probably reflect derangements of CNS biochemistry.

Central nervous system depressant drugs, anesthetics, and some endogenous toxins produce coma by suppression of both the RAS and cerebral cortex. For this reason, combinations of cortical and brainstem signs occur in drug overdose and other metabolic comas, which may lead to a specious diagnosis of structural brainstem damage.

Although all metabolic derangements alter neuronal electrophysiology, the disturbance of brain electrical activity most commonly encountered in clinical practice is epilepsy. Continuous, generalized electrical discharges of the cortex are associated with coma even in the absence of epileptic motor activity. Coma following seizures (postictal state) may be due to exhaustion of energy metabolites or be secondary to locally toxic molecules produced during the seizures. Recovery from postictal unresponsiveness occurs when neuronal metabolic balance is restored. The postictal state produces a pattern of continuous, generalized slowing of the background EEG activity similar to that of metabolic encephalopathy.

Endogenous "excitatoxins" such as glutamate released after injury have been found to cause secondary neuronal damage in experimental models of ischemia. These endogenous "neurotoxins" act to allow calcium influx into cells, a mechanism thought to lead to neuronal death. This mechanism may play a role in the genesis of coma, or at least in its neuropathologic changes, after global ischemia.

PRACTICAL APPROACH TO THE COMATOSE PATIENT   The diagnosis and acute management of coma depend on understanding the pitfalls of examining the comatose patient, an interpretation of brainstem reflexes, and the efficient use of diagnostic tests. Acute respiratory and cardiovascular problems should be attended to prior to neurologic diagnosis. The complete medical evaluation, except for the vital signs, funduscopy, and examination for nuchal rigidity, may be deferred until the neurologic evaluation has established the severity and nature of coma.

History   In many cases, the cause of coma is immediately evident (e.g., trauma, cardiac arrest, and known drug ingestion). In the remainder, historical information about the onset of coma is often sparse. The most useful historical points are (1) the circumstances and temporal profile of the onset of neurologic symptoms, (2) the precise details of preceding neurologic symptoms (weakness, headaches, seizures, dizziness, diplopia, or vomiting), (3) the use of drugs or alcohol, and (4) history of liver, kidney, lung, heart, or other medical disease. Telephone calls to family and observers on the scene are an important part of the initial evaluation.

Physical examination and general observations   The temperature, pulse, respiratory rate and pattern, and blood pressure should be measured. Fever suggests systemic infection, bacterial meningitis, or a brain lesion that has disturbed the temperature-regulating centers. High body temperature, 42 to 44°C, associated with dry skin should arouse the suspicion of heat stroke or anticholinergic drug intoxication. Hypothermia is observed with bodily exposure to lowered environmental temperature; alcoholic, barbiturate, or phenothiazine intoxication; hypoglycemia; peripheral circulatory failure; or hypothyroidism. Hypothermia causes coma only when the temperature is below 31°C. Aberrant respiratory patterns that may reflect brainstem disorders are discussed below. A change of pulse rate combined with hyperventilation and hypertension may signal an increase in intracranial pressure. Marked hypertension occurs in patients with hypertensive encephalopathy, cerebral hemorrhage, hydrocephalus, and acutely after head trauma. Hypotension occurs in the coma of alcohol or barbiturate

intoxication, internal hemorrhage, myocardial infarction, septicemia, and Addisonian crisis. The funduscopic examination is useful in detecting subarachnoid hemorrhage (subhyaloid hemorrhages), hypertensive encephalopathy (exudates, hemorrhages, vessel-crossing changes), and increased intracranial pressure (papilledema). Generalized cutaneous petechiae suggest thrombotic thrombocytopenic purpura or a bleeding diathesis associated with intracerebral hemorrhage.

General neurologic assessment   An exact description of spontaneous and elicited movements in coma is of great value in establishing the level of neurologic dysfunction. The patient's state should be observed first without examiner intervention. The nature of respirations and spontaneous movements are observed. Patients who toss about, reach up toward the face, cross their legs, yawn, swallow, cough, or moan are closest to being awake. The only sign of seizures may be small excursion twitching of a foot, finger, or facial muscle. An outturned leg at rest or lack of restless movements on one side suggests a hemiparesis.

The terms *decorticate* and *decerebrate rigidity*, or "posturing," are used to describe stereotyped arm and leg movements, occurring spontaneously or elicited by sensory stimulation of the patient. Flexion of the elbows and wrists and arm supination (decortication) suggest severe bilateral damage in the hemispheres above the midbrain, whereas extension of the elbows and wrists with pronation (decerebration) suggests damage in the midbrain or caudal diencephalon. Arm extension with minimal leg flexion or flaccid legs has been associated with lesions in the low pons. Acute lesions, however, frequently cause limb extension regardless of location, and almost all extensor posturing becomes flexor in nature as time passes, so posturing alone cannot be depended on to make an accurate anatomic localization. Metabolic coma, especially after acute hypoxia, also may produce vigorous spontaneous extensor (decerebrate) rigidity. Posturing may coexist with purposeful limb movements, usually reflecting subtotal damage to the motor system. Multifocal myoclonus is almost always an indication of metabolic disorder, particularly azotemia, anoxia, or drug ingestion. In an awake, confused patient, asterixis is a certain sign of metabolic encephalopathy or drug ingestion, particularly phenytoin.

Elicited movements and level of arousal   If the patient is not aroused by conversational voice, a sequence of increasingly intense stimuli is used to determine the patient's best level of arousal and the optimal motor response of each limb. Nasal tickle with a cotton wisp is a strong arousal stimulus. Pressure on the knuckles or bony prominences is the preferred and humane form of noxious stimulus. Pinching the skin over the face, chest, or limbs causes unsightly ecchymoses and is not necessary.

Responses to noxious stimuli should be appraised critically. Abduction avoidance movement of a limb is usually purposeful and denotes an intact corticospinal system to that limb. Stereotyped posturing following stimulation of a limb indicates severe dysfunction of the corticospinal system. Adduction and flexion of the stimulated limbs may be reflex movements and imply corticospinal system damage. Brief clonic or twitching limb movements frequently occur at the end of extensor posturing excursions and should not be mistaken for seizures.

Brainstem reflexes   Brainstem signs are a key to localization of the causative lesion in coma (see Fig. 26-1). As a rule, coma associated with normal brainstem function indicates widespread and bilateral hemispheral disease or dysfunction. The brainstem reflexes that are convenient to examine are pupillary light responses, eye movements, both spontaneous and elicited, and respiratory pattern. Pupillary reaction should be examined with a bright, diffuse light and, if the response is absent, confirmed with a magnifying lens. Light reaction in pupils smaller than 2 mm is often difficult to appreciate. Excessive room lighting mutes pupillary reactivity. Symmetrically reactive round pupils (2.5 to 5 mm in diameter) usually exclude midbrain damage as the cause of coma. An enlarged (greater than 5 mm) and unreactive or poorly reactive pupil results either from an intrinsic midbrain lesion (on the same side) or, far more commonly, is secondary to compression or stretching of the third nerve from transtentorial herniation or horizontal brainstem displacement. Unilateral pupillary enlargement usually denotes an ipsilateral mass but rarely occurs contralaterally, possibly by compression of the midbrain or third nerve against the opposite tentorial margin. Oval and slightly eccentric pupils often accompany early midbrain–third nerve compression. Bilaterally dilated and unreactive pupils indicate severe midbrain damage, usually from secondary compression by transtentorial herniation or from ingestion of drugs with anticholinergic activity. The use of mydriatic eye drops by a previous examiner, self-administration by the patient, or direct ocular trauma may cause misleading pupillary enlargement. Reactive and bilaterally small but not pinpoint pupils (1 to 2.5 mm) are most commonly seen in metabolic encephalopathy or after deep bilateral hemispheral lesions such as hydrocephalus or thalamic hemorrhage. This has been attributed to dysfunction of sympathetic nervous system efferents emerging from the posterior hypothalamus. Profound barbiturate-induced coma may produce similar-sized pupils. Very small but reactive pupils (less than 1 mm) denote narcotic overdose but also occur with acute, extensive bilateral pontine damage, usually from hemorrhage. The response to naloxone and the presence of reflex eye movements (see below) distinguish these. The unilaterally small pupil of a Horner's syndrome is detected by failure of the pupil to enlarge in the dark. It is rare in coma but may occur ipsilateral to a large cerebral hemorrhage that affects the thalamus. Lid tone, tested by lifting the eyelids, palpating resistance to opening, and speed of closure, is reduced progressively as coma deepens.

Eye movements are the second foundation of physical diagnosis in coma because their examination permits exploration of a large portion of the rostrocaudal extent of the brainstem. The eyes are first observed by elevating the lids and noting the resting position and spontaneous movements of the globes. Horizontal divergence of the eyes at rest is normally observed in drowsiness. As patients either awaken or coma deepens, the ocular axes become parallel again. An adducted eye at rest indicates lateral rectus paresis (weakness) due to a sixth nerve lesion, and when bilateral, it is often a sign of increased intracranial pressure. An abducted eye at rest, often accompanied by ipsilateral pupillary enlargement, indicates medial rectus paresis due to third nerve paresis. With few exceptions, vertical separation of the ocular axes, or *skew deviation*, results from pontine or cerebellar lesions.

Spontaneous eye movements in coma generally take the form of conjugate horizontal roving. This motion exonerates the midbrain and pons and has the same meaning as normal reflex eye movements (see below). Cyclic vertical downward movements are seen in specific circumstances. "Ocular bobbing" describes a brisk conjugate downward and slow upward movement of the globes associated with loss of horizontal eye movements and is diagnostic of bilateral pontine damage. "Ocular dipping" is a slow, arrhythmic downward movement followed by a faster upward movement in patients with normal reflex horizontal gaze and denotes diffuse anoxic damage to the cerebral cortex. The eyes may turn down and inward in thalamic and upper midbrain lesions.

"Doll's eye," or *oculocephalic*, responses are reflex movements tested by moving the head from side to side or vertically, first slowly then briskly; eye movements are evoked in the opposite direction to head movement (see Fig. 26-1). These responses are mediated by brainstem mechanisms originating in the labyrinths and cervical proprioceptors. They are normally suppressed by visual fixation mediated by the cerebral hemispheres in awake patients but appear as the hemispheres become suppressed or inactive. The neuronal pathways for reflex horizontal eye movements require integrity of the region surrounding the sixth nerve nucleus and are yoked to the contralateral third nerve via the medial longitudinal fasciculus (MLF) (see Fig. 26-1). Two pieces of information can be obtained from the reflex eye movements. *First*, in coma resulting from bihemispheral disease or metabolic or drug depression, the eyes move easily or "loosely" from side to side in a direction opposite to the direction of head turning. The ease with which the globes move toward the opposite side is a reflection of disinhibition of brainstem reflexes by damaged cerebral hemispheres. In drowsy patients, the first two or three head rotations cause opposite conjugate eye movements, following which the maneuver itself usually causes arousal and the reflex movements stop. *Second*, full conjugate oculocephalic movements demonstrate the integrity of brainstem pathways extending from the high cervical spinal cord and medulla, where vestibular and proprioceptive input from head turning originates, to the midbrain, at the level of the third nerve. Thus full and conjugate oculocephalic induced eye movements demonstrate the functional integrity of a large segment of brainstem and assist in excluding a lesion in the brainstem as the cause of coma. Incomplete adduction indicates an ipsilateral midbrain (third nerve) lesion or, alternatively, damage to the pathways mediating reflex eye movements in the MLF (i.e., internuclear ophthalmoplegia). Third nerve damage is usually associated with an enlarged pupil and horizontal ocular divergence at rest, whereas MLF destruction shows neither. Adduction of the globes is by nature more difficult to obtain with head turning than abduction, and subtle symmetric abnormalities in the "doll's eye" maneuver should be interpreted with caution.

Caloric stimulation of the vestibular apparatus (*oculovestibular* or *vestibuloocular response*) is a useful adjunct to the oculocephalic test and acts as a stronger stimulus to reflex eye movements. Irrigation of the external auditory canal with cold water causes convection currents in the endolymph of the labyrinths of the inner ear. With the head at approximately 30° elevation from the supine position, endolymph movement is induced primarily in the horizontal semicircular canals. An intact brainstem response is indicated, with variable latency, by tonic deviation of both eyes (lasting 30 to 120 s) to the side of cold-water irrigation. Bilateral conjugate eye movements have the same significance as full oculocephalic responses. If the cerebral hemispheres are intact, a rapid corrective conjugate movement is generated away from the side of tonic deviation. The absence of this saccadic, nystagmus-like quick phase signifies damage to the cerebral hemispheres.

Conjugate horizontal ocular deviation at rest or incomplete conjugate eye movements with head turning indicate damage in the pons on the side of the gaze paresis or frontal lobe damage on the opposite side. This phenomenon may be summarized by the aphorism "the eyes look toward a hemispheral lesion and away from a brainstem lesion." It is usually possible to overcome the ocular deviation associated with frontal lobe damage by oculocephalic testing. Seizures also may cause aversive (opposite) eye deviation with rhythmic, jerky movements to the side of gaze. On rare occasions, the eyes may turn paradoxically away from the side of a deep hemispheral lesion ("wrong-way eyes"). In hydrocephalus with dilatation of the third ventricle, the globes frequently rest below the horizontal meridian. Two types of rapid rhythmic eye movements may occur in stupor or coma. *Ocular myoclonus* is a rapid horizontal oscillatory nystagmus usually associated with a similar movement of the palate and due to damage to the central tegmental fasciculus, a longitudinal gray matter tract in the brainstem. *Opsoclonus* is an irregular, jerky, saccadic movement varying in direction that results from cerebellar lesions.

A major pitfall in coma diagnosis may occur when reflex eye movements are suppressed by drugs. The eyes then move with the head as it is turned as if locked in place, thus spuriously suggesting anatomic brainstem damage. Overdoses of phenytoin, tricyclic antidepressants, and barbiturates are commonly implicated as well as, on occasion, alcohol, phenothiazines, diazepam, and neuromuscular blockers such as pancuronium. The presence of normal pupillary size and light reaction will distinguish most drug-induced comas from brainstem damage (except for pontine infarction or hemorrhage, in which the pupils remain small). Small to midposition, 1- to 3-mm nonreactive pupils also may occur with very high serum levels of barbiturates or secondary to hydrocephalus (see below).

Although the *corneal reflexes* are rarely useful alone, they may corroborate eye movement abnormalities because they also depend on the integrity of pontine pathways. By touching the cornea with a wisp of cotton, a response consisting of brief bilateral lid closure may be observed. The corneal response may be lost if the reflex connections between the fifth and seventh cranial nerves within the pons are damaged. The normal efferent response is bilateral, with closure of both eyelids. CNS depressant drugs diminish or eliminate the corneal responses soon after the reflex eye movements become paralyzed but before the pupils become unreactive to light.

Respiration   Respiratory patterns have received much attention in coma diagnosis but are of inconsistent localizing value. Shallow, slow, but well-timed regular breathing suggests metabolic or drug depression. Rapid, deep (Kussmaul) breathing usually implies metabolic acidosis but also may occur with pontomesencephalic lesions. Cheyne-Stokes respiration in its classic cyclic form, ending with a brief apneic period, signifies mild bihemispheral damage or metabolic suppression and commonly accompanies light coma. Agonal gasps reflect bilateral lower brainstem damage and are well known as the terminal respiratory pattern of severe brain damage. In brain-dead patients, shallow respiratory-like movements with irregular, nonrepetitive back arching may be produced by hypoxia and are probably generated by the surviving cervical spinal cord and lower medulla. Other cyclic breathing variations are not usually diagnostic of specific local lesions.

COMA-LIKE SYNDROMES AND RELATED STATES   The simple observation of inability to arouse a patient characterizes most comatose states. Several syndromes, however, render patients unresponsive or insensate but are considered separately because of their unusual features. The *vegetative state*, an unfortunate term, describes patients who were earlier comatose but whose eyelids have subsequently opened giving the appearance of being awake. There may be yawning, grunting, and random limb and head movements but a complete inability to respond to commands or communicate. These are associated with signs of extensive damage to both cerebral hemispheres, i.e., Babinski signs, decerebrate or decorticate posturing, and absence of response to visual stimuli. Corrective nystagmus on oculovestibular testing fails to occur. Autonomic nervous system functions such as cardiovascular and thermoregulatory and neuroendocrine control are preserved and may be subject to periods of overactivity. The syndrome results from global damage to the cerebral cortex, most often in practice from global ischemia or head injury (see Chap. 376). *Akinetic mutism* refers to a partially or fully awake patient who is immobile and silent. The state may result from hydrocephalus, from masses in the region of the third ventricle, or from large bilateral lesions in the cingulate gyrus or other portions of both frontal lobes. *Abulia* is a mild form of akinetic mutism in which the patient is hypokinetic and slow to respond but generally gives correct answers. Lesions in the periaqueductal or low diencephalic regions may cause a similar state in which hypophonia is prominent. The *locked-in syndrome* (pseudocoma) describes patients who are awake but selectively deefferented, i.e., have no means of producing speech or limb, face, or pharyngeal movements. This results from infarction or hemorrhage of the ventral pons, which transects all descending corticospinal and corticobulbar pathways but spares the RAS arousal system, vertical eye movements, and lid elevation. Such eye movements can be used by the patient to signal to the examiner. A similar awake state simulating unresponsiveness may occur in severe cases of acute polyneuritis as a result of total paralysis of limb, ocular, or bulbar musculature. Unlike basilar artery stroke, vertical eye movements are not selectively spared.

Certain psychiatric states mimic coma by producing apparent unresponsiveness. *Catatonia* is a term for peculiar hypomobile syndrome associated with major psychosis. In the typical form, catatonic patients appear awake with eyes open but make no voluntary or responsive movements, although they blink spontaneously and may not appear distressed. There may be associated "waxy flexibility," in which limbs maintain their posture when lifted by the examiner. Upon recovery, such patients have some memory of events that occurred during their catatonic stupor. Patients with *pseudocoma conversion* states have signs that indicate voluntary attempts to appear comatose. They may resist eyelid elevation, blink to threat when the lids are held open, and move the eyes concomitantly with head rotation, all signs belying brain damage.

LABORATORY EXAMINATION IN COMA   Four laboratory tests are used most frequently in the diagnosis of coma: chemical-toxicologic analysis of blood and urine, CT or MRI, EEG, and CSF examination.

Chemical blood determinations are made routinely to investigate metabolic, toxic, or drug-induced encephalopathies. The major metabolic aberrations encountered in clinical practice are those of electrolytes, calcium, blood urea nitrogen (BUN), glucose, plasma osmolarity, and hepatic dysfunction. Toxicologic analysis is of great value in any case of coma where the diagnosis is not immediately clear. However, the presence of exogenous drugs or toxins, especially alcohol, does not ensure that other factors, particularly head trauma, may not also contribute to the clinical state.

The notion that a normal CT scan excludes anatomic lesions as the cause of coma is erroneous. Early bilateral hemisphere infarction, small brainstem lesions, encephalitis, mechanical shearing of axons as a result of closed head trauma, absent cerebral perfusion associated with brain death, sagittal sinus thrombosis, and subdural hematomas that are isodense to adjacent brain are some of the lesions that may be overlooked by CT. Nevertheless, in coma of unknown etiology, a CT scan should be obtained early in the evaluation. In those cases in which the etiology is clinically apparent, the CT provides verification and defines the extent of the lesion. With acute mass lesions, 3 to 5 mm of horizontal displacement of the pineal calcification from the midline generally corresponds to drowsiness, 5 to 8 mm corresponds to stupor, and greater than 8 mm corresponds to coma. As a supratentorial mass enlarges, the opposite perimesencephalic cistern is first compressed from lateral movement of the brainstem, the ipsilateral cistern is widened, and finally, both are compressed from the lateral mass effect. The lateral ventricle opposite the mass becomes enlarged as the third ventricle is compressed. These radiologic features of tissue shifts near the tentorial opening are helpful in correlating the clinical state with the progress of a mass lesion on scans (Fig. 26-2). They also suggest that transtentorial herniation is not necessary for upper midbrain compression and diminished consciousness. For technical reasons, MRI is difficult to perform in comatose patients, and it also does not demonstrate hemorrhages as well as CT (see Chap. 365). As MRI becomes more widely available and practical in comatose patients, some of the anatomic causes of coma that are not appreciated by CT scan, such as widespread white matter damage from trauma, will become better recognized.

The EEG is rarely diagnostic in coma, with the occasional exceptions of coma due to ongoing clinically unrecognized seizures, herpes virus encephalitis, and Creutzfeldt-Jakob disease. The EEG, however, may suggest metabolic encephalopathy and provide important information about the general state of the cortex. The amount of background slowing of the EEG is useful for gauging and following the severity of any diffuse encephalopathy. The EEG pattern of "alpha coma" is defined by widespread, invariant 8- to 12-Hz activity superficially resembling the normal alpha rhythm of waking but is unresponsive to environmental stimuli. Alpha coma results from either high pontine or diffuse cortical damage and is associated with a poor prognosis. Coma due to persistent epileptic discharges that are not clinically manifested may be revealed by EEG recordings. Normal alpha activity on the EEG also may alert the clinician to the locked-in syndrome. Computed on-line EEG analysis and evoked potential recordings (auditory and somatosensory) are currently under investigation as additional methods of coma diagnosis and monitoring.

Lumbar puncture is now used more judiciously than previously because the CT scan excludes intracerebral hemorrhages and most subarachnoid hemorrhages. The use of lumbar puncture in coma is limited to diagnosis of meningitis-encephalitis, occasional cases of subarachnoid hemorrhage, and cases with normal CT in which the

FIGURE 26-2 *A*. Axial CT scans from a comatose patient with a large cerebral hemorrhage showing the main radiologic signs of a unilateral intracranial mass. There is enlargement of the perimesencephalic cistern on the side of the mass (*small arrow*), compression contralaterally, and early enlargement of the lateral ventricle opposite the mass (*large arrow*). The pineal is shifted 8 mm from the midline. *B*. Coronal MRI scans from the same patient showing displacement of brain tissue across the midline, above the tentorium (*left, arrow*). The manner of horizontal displacement of the upper brainstem from a mass is appreciated, and the right scan shows a small uncal herniation (*arrow*).

origin of coma is obscure. If the CT is normal or unavailable and suspicion of meningeal infection or subarachnoid hemorrhage remains, then the CSF should be examined for white cells, microorganisms, and blood. In no case should lumbar puncture be deferred if meningitis is a strong clinical possibility. Xanthochromia is documented by spinning the CSF in a large tube and comparing the supernatant to water. Yellow coloration indicates preexisting blood in the CSF and permits exclusion of a traumatic puncture. In addition, initial and final tubes should be inspected for a decrement in the number of erythrocytes, indicating traumatic puncture.

DIFFERENTIAL DIAGNOSIS OF COMA In most instances, coma is part of an obvious medical problem such as known drug ingestion, hypoxia, stroke, trauma, or liver or kidney failure. Attention is then appropriately focused on the primary illness. A complete listing of all diseases that cause coma would serve little purpose, since it would not aid diagnosis. Some general rules, however, are helpful. Illnesses that cause sudden or acute coma are due to drug ingestion or to one of the catastrophic brain lesions—hemorrhage, trauma, hypoxia, or, rarely, acute basilar artery occlusion. Coma which appears subacutely is usually related to preceding medical or neurologic problems, including the secondary brain swelling that surrounds a preexisting lesion. Coma diagnosis, therefore, requires familiarity with the common intracerebral catastrophes. These are described in more detail in Chap. 368 but may be summarized as follows: (1) basal ganglia and thalamic hemorrhage (acute but not instantaneous onset, vomiting, headache, hemiplegia, and characteristic eye signs), (2) subarachnoid hemorrhage (instantaneous onset, severe headache, neck stiffness, vomiting, third or sixth nerve lesions, transient loss of consciousness, or sudden coma with vigorous extensor posturing), (3) pontine hemorrhage (sudden onset, pinpoint pupils, loss of reflex eye movements and corneal responses, ocular bobbing, posturing, hyperventilation, and sweating), (4) cerebellar hemorrhage (occipital headache,

vomiting, gaze paresis, and inability to stand), and (5) basilar artery thrombosis (neurologic prodrome or warning spells, diplopia, dysarthria, vomiting, eye movement and corneal response abnormalities, and asymmetric limb paresis). The most common stroke, namely, infarction in the territory of the middle cerebral artery, does not cause coma acutely. The syndrome of acute hydrocephalus causing coma may accompany many intracranial catastrophes, particularly subarachnoid hemorrhage. Acute symmetric enlargement of both lateral ventricles causes headache and vomiting followed by drowsiness that may progress quickly to coma, with extensor posturing of the limbs, bilateral Babinski signs, small nonreactive pupils, and impaired vertical oculocephalic movements.

If the history and examination are not typical for any neurologic diagnosis and metabolic or drug causes are excluded, then information obtained from CT may be used as outlined in Table 26-1. The neurologic examination remains preeminent because it allows localization of lesions to one or both hemispheres or to the brainstem (with the exceptions noted above). The CT scan is useful to focus the differential diagnosis, and because of its accuracy and general availability, the diagnoses which it facilitates are listed in the table. The majority of medical causes of coma are established without a CT or with the study being normal.

COMA AFTER HEAD TRAUMA Concussion is a common form of transient coma that probably results from torsion of the hemispheres about the midbrain-diencephalic junction with brief interruption of RAS function. Persistent coma after head trauma presents a more complex and serious problem (Chap. 376).

EMERGENCY TREATMENT OF THE COMATOSE PATIENT The immediate goal in acute coma is prevention of further CNS damage. Hypotension, hypoglycemia, hypoxia, hypercapnia, and hyperthermia should be corrected rapidly and assiduously. An oropharyngeal airway is adequate to keep the pharynx open in drowsy patients who are

TABLE 26-1   Approach to the differential diagnosis of coma

NORMAL BRAINSTEM REFLEXES, NO LATERALIZING SIGNS

A   Bilateral hemispheral dysfunction without mass lesion (CT or MRI normal; primary test used for diagnosis is indicated in parentheses)
    1   Drug-toxin ingestion (toxicologic analysis)
    2   Endogenous metabolic encephalopathy (glucose, ammonia, calcium, osmolarity, P_{O_2}, P_{CO_2}, urea, sodium)
    3   Shock, hypertensive encephalopathy
    4   Meningitis (CSF analysis)
    5   Nonherpetic viral encephalitis (CSF analysis)
    6   Epilepsy (EEG)
    7   Reye's syndrome (ammonia, increased intracranial pressure)
    8   Fat embolism
    9   Subarachnoid hemorrhage with normal CT (CSF analysis)
    10   Acute disseminated encephalomyelitis (CSF analysis)
    11   Acute hemorrhagic leukoencephalitis (repeat MRI)
    12   Creutzfeldt-Jakob disease (EEG)
B   Anatomic lesions of hemisphere found by CT or MRI
    1   Hydrocephalus
    2   Bilateral subdural hematomas
    3   Bilateral contusions, edema, or axonal shearing of hemispheres due to closed head trauma, subarachnoid hemorrhage
    4   Subarachoid hemorrhage

NORMAL BRAINSTEM REFLEXES (WITH/WITHOUT UNILATERAL 3D NERVE PALSY), LATERALIZING MOTOR SIGNS (CT OR MRI ABNORMAL)

A   Unilateral mass lesion found
    1   Cerebral hemorrhage (basal ganglia, thalamus)
    2   Large infarction with surrounding brain edema
    3   Herpes virus encephalitis (temporal lobe lesion)
    4   Subdural or epidural hematoma
    5   Tumor with edema
    6   Brain abscess with edema
    7   Vasculitis with multiple infarctions
    8   Metabolic encephalopathy superimposed on preexisting focal lesions (i.e., stroke with hyperglycemia, hyponatremia, etc.)
    9   Pituitary apoplexy
B   Asymmetric signs accompanied by diffuse hemispheral dysfunction
    1   Metabolic encephalopathies with asymmetric signs (blood chemical determinations)
    2   Isodense subdural hematoma (MRI, CT with contrast)
    3   Thrombotic thrombocytopenic purpura (blood smear, platelet count)
    4   Epilepsy with focal seizures or postictal state (EEG)

MULTIPLE BRAINSTEM REFLEX ABNORMALITIES

A   Anatomic lesions in brainstem
    1   Pontine, midbrain hemorrhage
    2   Cerebellar hemorrhage, tumor, abscess
    3   Cerebellar infarction with brainstem compression
    4   Mass in hemisphere causing advanced bilateral upper brainstem compression
    5   Primary brainstem tumor, demyelination, or abscess
    6   Traumatic brainstem contusion-hemorrhage
B   Brainstem dysfunction without mass lesion
    1   Basilar artery thrombosis causing brainstem infarction (clinical signs, angiogram)
    2   Severe drug overdose (toxicologic analysis)
    3   Brainstem encephalitis (CSF)
    4   Basilar artery migraine

breathing normally. Tracheal intubation is indicated if there is apnea, upper airway obstruction, hypoventilation, or emesis, or if the patient is liable to aspirate. Mechanical ventilation is required if the patient is hypoventilating or if there is an intracranial mass and hypocapnia is therapeutically necessary. An intravenous access is established, and naloxone and dextrose are administered if narcotic overdose or hypoglycemia are even remote possibilities. Thiamine is generally administered with glucose in order to prevent an exacerbation of Wernicke's encephalopathy. The veins of intravenous drug abusers may be difficult to cannulate; in such cases, naloxone can be injected sublingually through a small-gauge needle. In cases of suspected basilar thrombosis with brainstem ischemia, intravenous heparin is administered after obtaining a CT scan, keeping in mind that cerebellar and pontine hemorrhages resemble the syndrome of basilar artery occlusion. Physostigmine, when used by experienced physicians with

careful monitoring, may awaken patients with anticholinergic-type drug overdose, but many physicians believe that this is justified only to treat associated cardiac arrhythmias. The use of benzodiazepine antagonists is promising for treatment of overdoses. Intravenous fluid should be monitored carefully in any serious acute CNS illness because of the potential for exacerbating brain swelling by excess water administration. Neck injuries must not be overlooked, particularly prior to attempting intubation or the oculocephalic maneuver. Headache accompanied by fever and meningismus indicates a need for examination of the CSF to diagnose meningitis, and *lumbar puncture should not be delayed while awaiting a CT scan*.

Enlargement of one pupil usually indicates secondary midbrain compression by a hemispheral mass and demands immediate reduction of intracranial pressure (ICP). Normal saline is the safest intravenous fluid because it is slightly hyperosmolar in most patients. Therapeutic hyperventilation may be used to achieve an arterial P_{CO_2} of 3.7 to 4.2 kPa (28 to 32 mmHg). This acts rapidly to reduce ICP, but the beneficial effect rarely lasts more than 1 to 2 h. The weak base and buffer THAM (tromethamine) may be a useful adjunct to keep the CSF alkalotic. Hyperosmolar therapy with mannitol or an equivalent is the mainstay of ICP reduction. It may be used simultaneously with hyperventilation in critical cases. It is generally best to administer mannitol before attempting to intubate a patient with impending herniation. A ventricular puncture is necessary to decompress hydrocephalus if medical measures fail to improve alertness. The use of high-dose barbiturates soon after cardiac arrest has not been shown in clinical studies to be beneficial, although they may still be useful in lowering intracranial pressure in other circumstances.

BRAIN DEATH   Brain death results from total cessation of cerebral blood flow and global infarction of the brain at a time when respiration is preserved with artificial support and the heart continues to function. It is the only type of irrevocable loss of brain function currently recognized by law as death. Many sets of roughly equivalent criteria have been advanced for the diagnosis of brain death, and it is essential to adhere to those approved locally and recognized as standard practice. Ideal criteria are ones that are simple, conducted at the bedside, and which allow no chance of diagnostic error. Widespread cortical destruction is usually shown by unresponsiveness to the environment, midbrain damage by absent pupillary light reaction, pontine damage by absent oculovestibular and corneal reflexes, and medullary dysfunction by complete apnea. The pulse rate is invariant and unresponsive to atropine. Most patients have diabetes insipidus, but in some it develops after the clinical signs of brain death. The pupils need not be fully dilated but should not be constricted. The absence of spinal reflexes is not required because the spinal cord remains functional in many cases. Many centers use an isoelectric EEG as a confirmatory test for cortical death. The possibility of profound drug-induced or hypothermic CNS depression should always be excluded. Some period of observation, usually 6 to 24 h, is desirable during which this state is shown to be sustained. It is often advisable to delay clinical testing for up to 24 h if a cardiac arrest has caused brain death or if the inciting disease is not known.

The demonstration of apnea generally requires that the P_{CO_2} be high enough to stimulate respiration. This can be accomplished safely in most patients by removal of the respirator and use of diffusion oxygenation sustained by a tracheal cannula connected to an oxygen supply. In brain-dead patients, CO_2 tension increases approximately 0.3 to 0.4 kPa/min (2 to 3 mmHg/min) during apnea. At the end of an appropriate interval, arterial P_{CO_2} should be at least above 6.6 to 8.0 kPa (50 to 60 mmHg) for the test to be valid. Large posterior fossa lesions that compress the brainstem, CNS–depressant drugs, and profound hypothermia can simulate brain death, but adherence to recognized protocols for diagnosis will prevent these errors. Radionuclide brain scanning, cerebral angiography, or transcranial Doppler measurements also may be used to demonstrate the absence of cerebral blood flow in brain death. These techniques have the virtue of rapidity but, with the exception of Doppler, are cumbersome and have not been correlated extensively with pathologic material.

There is no implicit reason to make the diagnosis of brain death except when organ transplantation or difficult resource-allocation (intensive care) issues are involved. Although it is commonly accepted that the respirator can be disconnected from a brain-dead patient, most problems arise because of inadequate explanation and preparation of the family by the physician.

PROGNOSIS OF COMA Interest in predicting the outcome of coma is oriented toward allocating medical resources and limiting the support of hopeless cases. To date, no collection of clinical signs except those of brain death assuredly predicts outcome of coma. Children and young adults may have ominous early clinical findings such as abnormal brainstem reflexes and yet recover. All schemes for prognosis should therefore be taken as only approximate indicators, and medical judgments must be tempered by other factors such as age, underlying disease, and general medical condition. In an attempt to collect prognostic information from large numbers of patients with head injury, a "Glasgow Coma Scale" has been devised that empirically has predictive value in cases of brain trauma (see Chap. 376). Major points include a 95 percent death rate in patients whose pupillary reaction or reflex eye movements are absent 6 h after onset of coma, and a 91 percent death rate if the pupils are unreactive at 24 h (although 4 percent make a good recovery).

Prognostication of nontraumatic coma is difficult because of the heterogeneity of contributing diseases. Unfavorable signs in the first hours after admission are the absence of any two of pupillary reaction, corneal reflex, or the oculovestibular response. One day after the onset of coma, the preceding signs, in addition to absence of eye opening and muscle tone, predict death or severe disability and the same signs at 3 days strengthen the prediction of a poor outcome. In many patients, precise combinations of predictive signs do not occur, and coma scales lose their value. The use of evoked potentials aids prognostication in head-injured and post–cardiac arrest patients. Bilateral absence of cortical somatosensory evoked potentials is associated with death or a vegetative state in most cases. Medical practitioners are becoming less reluctant to withdraw support from non-brain-dead but severely neurologically injured patients as predictions become more reliable and resources more limited.

REFERENCES

CELESIA GG et al: Persistent vegetative state—Report of the American Neurological Association Committee on Ethical Affairs. Ann Neurol 33:386, 1993

IVAN L, BRUCE D: Coma. Springfield, Ill., Charles C Thomas, 1982

JENNET B et al: Prognosis of patients with severe head injury. Neurosurgery 4:283, 1979

LEVY D et al: Prognosis in non-traumatic coma. Ann Intern Med 94:229, 1981

PLUM F, POSNER J: The Diagnosis of Stupor and Coma, 3d ed. Philadelphia, Davis, 1980

REICH JB et al: Magnetic resonance imaging measurements and clinical changes accompanying transtentorial and foramen magnum brain herniation. Ann Neurol 33:159, 1993

ROPPER AH: Lateral displacement of the brain and level of consciousness in patients with an acute hemispheral mass. N Engl J Med 314:953, 1986

———: Coma and acutely raised intracranial pressure, in Diseases of the Nervous System, 2d ed, A Asbury et al (eds). Philadelphia, Saunders, 1992

———: Neurological and Neurosurgical Intensive Care, 3d ed. New York, Raven, 1992

27 SYNDROMES DUE TO FOCAL CEREBRAL LESIONS

RAYMOND D. ADAMS / MAURICE VICTOR

In addition to the general syndromes described in Chap. 25, there are many others that relate to lesions of particular parts of the cerebrum. Recognition of the latter syndromes constitutes irrefutable evidence that all parts of the cerebrum are not functionally equivalent. Some of the symptoms and signs that make up these syndromes have the same diagnostic value as a hemiplegia and, once identified, require the same type of clinical analysis as to cause and pathophysiologic mechanism.

These focal syndromes will be described in terms of the conventional anatomic divisions of the cerebrum, but it will be obvious that most diseases do not respect these boundaries. Furthermore, cerebral functions are not localized to discrete aggregates of cerebral cortical neurons but are organized in fairly widespread networks. A lesion in a particular part will cause a loss of function (negative symptoms), but the positive symptoms arising from the lesion are attributable to the now disinhibited functions of closely related intact parts of the cerebrum.

FRONTAL LOBES In Fig. 27-1 it is seen that the frontal lobes lie anterior to the central (rolandic) sulcus and superior to the Sylvian fissure. They consist of several functionally different parts, which are conventionally designated in the neurologic literature by numbers (according to the scheme of Brodmann) or by letters (according to the scheme of von Economo and Koskinas).

The posterior parts, areas 4 and 6 of Brodmann, are specifically related to motor function. There is also a supplementary motor area, located in the posterior part of the superior frontal convolution and in close relationship to the anterior part of the cingulate gyrus. Voluntary movement in humans depends on the integrity of these

FIGURE 27-1 Diagram to show the cytoarchitectural zones of the human cerebral cortex (lateral surface) according to the scheme of Brodmann. Although the auditory association areas of Wernicke (areas 41 and 42) are shown on the lateral surface, they actually lie on the superior surface of the temporal lobe, deep within the sylvian fissure. *(From Adams and Victor.)*

areas, and lesions in them produce a spastic paralysis of the contralateral face, arm, and leg. This is discussed in Chap. 21. A lesion limited more or less to the *premotor area* (area 6 and the supplementary motor area) is accompanied by less paralysis and more spasticity, as well as by a contralateral grasp reflex, and bilateral lesions of these parts are accompanied by a suck reflex. A lesion in area 8 of Brodmann interferes with the mechanism for turning the head and eyes contralaterally. In addition, a lesion of the left supplementary motor area can result in mutism at its onset; in time the condition resolves to a state of transcortical motor aphasia, with reduced language output but preserved capacity for repetition and naming. Ideomotor apraxia is another manifestation of area 6 lesions observed in some patients. A lesion in area 44 (Broca's area) of the dominant (usually the left) cerebral hemisphere and the parts of motor areas superior and posterior to it results in at least a temporary loss of verbal expression. As speech returns, it is characterized by loss of inflection (dysprosody), a phonetic-articulatory defect (cortical dysarthria), agrammatism, retention of "content words," and omission of articles, prepositions, and conjunctions. More extensive lesions, including adjacent insular and motor cortex, result in a more severe and persistent motor speech disorder, agraphia, and apraxia of the face, lips, and tongue (see Chap. 28). Lesions of the anterior cingulate gyrus, in the acute stages, may cause a speechless, aphonic state; with recovery, speech returns through whispering and hoarseness rather than dysarthria and aphasia, according to Brown. Lesions in the medial limbic or piriform cortex (areas 23 and 24), where the mechanisms controlling respiration, circulation, and micturition are organized bilaterally, have relatively unclear clinical effects.

The remaining parts of the frontal lobes (areas 9 to 12 of Brodmann), sometimes called the *prefrontal areas*, have less specific and measurable functions. Their connections with other parts of the cerebral hemisphere and thalamus and, through the corpus callosum, with the opposite hemisphere have been well established by anatomic and physiologic studies (Denny-Brown). In contrast to the motor areas of the frontal lobes and other areas of the brain, electrical stimulation of the prefrontal areas in humans has yielded a paucity of findings.

Many patients with gunshot wounds of the prefrontal areas have shown only mild and inconsistent abnormalities of behavior. Nevertheless, the following groups of symptoms have been observed in patients with large lesions of one or both of the frontal lobes and of the central white matter and the anterior part of the corpus callosum by which they are joined:

1 Lack of initiative and spontaneity in conjunction with diminished speech and motor activity—variously called *apathetic*, *akinetic*, or *abulic* state. It is difficult to distinguish between lack of motivation or impulse and lack of emotional reactions; probably both are affected. Necessary daily activities are neglected. Interpersonal social reactions are reduced and shallow.

2 Change of personality, usually expressed as lack of concern over the consequences of any action, and an evident social disinhibition. Sometimes it may take the form of childish excitement, inappropriate joking and punning, thoughtless impulsivity, instability and superficiality of emotion, or irritability. The capacity for worry, anxiety, and depression (tortured self-concern) is reduced. These changes are especially prominent with orbital frontal lesions.

3 Slight impairment of intelligence, usually described as a lack of concentration and attention, inability to analyze a problem in all aspects and carry out planned activity, difficulty in changing from one activity to another, or perseveration. These cognitive impairments are more prominent with dorsolateral frontal lesions. Goldstein reduced the difficulty to a loss of capacity for abstract thinking, but we regard this tendency to concrete thinking as another manifestation of abulia and perseveration and the inability to sustain a sequence of mental activity. According to Luria, who views the frontal lobe as a regulating mechanism of the organism's activities, planned action is deficient with respect to steady control

and goal orientation. Brown conceives of this difficulty as a manifest failure in one or more stages in an action sequence—a failure of activation, a faulty integration or final implementation. With left frontal lesions, intelligence is reduced more (10 points on the IQ scale) than with right frontal lesions, probably because of reduced verbal skills. There is also an impairment of memory, usually slight, probably because the mental strategies needed for memorization and recall are impaired. Only with extensive posterior orbital, preamygdaloid lesions has a severe memory defect been reported.

4 A decomposition of gait and upright stance, consisting of a wide-based gait, flexed posture, and small shuffling steps, culminating in an inability to stand (Bruns' frontal lobe ataxia or gait apraxia), reflex grasping or sucking, and incontinence of sphincters.

Some differences have been noted between the dominant (left) and right prefrontal lobes. In psychological tests, left-sided lesions impair verbal fluency and cause a greater degree of perseveration, and right-sided ones impair the learning of visual spatial patterns and cause impersistence (see Hecaen and Albert and Luria for details).

From all the foregoing comments it should be evident that the frontal lobes do not have a unitary function but comprise a number of interconnected functional components, each subserving a different aspect of motor function, speech, and behavior.

TEMPORAL LOBES The boundaries of the temporal lobes are illustrated in Fig. 27-1. The Sylvian fissure separates the superior surface of each temporal lobe from the frontal lobe and anterior part of the parietal lobe. Posteriorly, there is no definite anatomic boundary between the temporal and the occipital and parietal lobes. The temporal lobe includes the superior, middle, and inferior temporal, fusiform, and hippocampal convolutions and the transverse convolutions of Heschl, which are the auditory receptive area on the superior surface, within the Sylvian fissure. The hippocampal convolution was once thought to be related to olfactory function, but lesions here do not cause anosmia. Only the medial and anterior parts of the temporal lobes (uncal regions) are related to smell. The lower fibers of the geniculocalcarine pathway (from the inferior retina) swing in a wide arc over the temporal horn of the ventricle into the white matter of the temporal lobe en route to the occipital lobes, and lesions that interrupt them characteristically produce a contralateral upper homonymous quadrantanopia. Hearing, localized in the superior surfaces of the temporal lobes (Heschl's gyri), is bilaterally represented, which accounts for the fact that both temporal lobes must be affected to cause deafness. Electrical stimulation (or a seizure discharge) of the superior surface of the temporal lobe, posterior to the auditory cortex, evokes vertigo. Disease in the superior convolution of the left temporal lobe and adjacent inferior parietal lobule in right-handed individuals results in Wernicke's aphasia. This syndrome, discussed in Chap. 28, consists of paraphasic speech or jargon aphasia and inability to read, write, repeat, or understand the meaning of spoken words.

Between the auditory and olfactory projection areas there is a large expanse of temporal lobe subserving three specific functional systems. In the inferolateral parts (areas 20, 21, and 37) are located some of the visual-associated projections from the striate and peristriate cortex of the occipital lobes. In the superolateral parts (areas 22, 41, and 42) are the primary and secondary areas for acoustic perception. In the mediobasal parts are the limbic structures (amygdaloid nuclei and hippocampi) containing the neural organizations for emotional and memory processes.

Bilateral lesions of the geniculocalcarine pathways result in cortical blindness; lesions of the visual cortex of the dominant temporal lobe result in a variety of agnosias, apparently based on a loss of visual memories: recognition of written words (alexia), visual naming (anomia), pattern discrimination, color recognition (achromatopsia), and object agnosia. Bilateral hippocampal/parahippocampal lesions produce a deficit in which the patient is unable to record events and information, i.e., has a loss of retentive memory (see Chap. 25). Also, the temporal lobes include a large part of the limbic system, which subserves the emotional and motivational aspects of behavior and vegetative functions ("visceral brain"). Lesions involving both the visual and limbic areas contribute to the Klüver-Bucy syndrome. This syndrome, first produced in monkeys by removal of both temporal lobes, has been observed only rarely in human beings, usually after an attack of herpes simplex encephalitis. It consists of apathy, impaired recognition of objects and persons, uncontrollable oral exploration, hypersexuality, amnesia, and bulimia. Usually the syndrome is incomplete.

Apart from aphasia, psychological studies have shown a difference between the effects of dominant and nondominant temporal lobe lesions. With dominant lesions there is impairment in learning auditorily presented verbal material; with nondominant lesions there is a failure in learning visually presented nonverbal material. In addition, about 20 percent of patients with either a right or left temporal lobectomy have shown an alteration of personality similar to that described after lesions in the prefrontal parts of the brain (see above).

The study of patients with uncinate seizures, with the characteristic dreamy state, olfactory or gustatory hallucinations, and masticatory movements, suggests that all these functions are organized through the temporal lobes. Stimulation of the posterior parts of the temporal lobes of fully conscious epileptic patients during surgical procedures arouses complex memories and visual and auditory images, some with strong emotional content. Stimulation of the amygdaloid nucleus, which is in the anteromedial part of the temporal lobe, may evoke symptoms like those of schizophrenia and mania. Complex emotional experiences may be revived. There are also autonomic effects: the blood pressure rises, pulse increases, respirations increase in frequency and depth, and the patient looks frightened. In temporal lobe epilepsy there may be an intensification of the patient's emotional reactions, vague preoccupation with moral and religious issues, a tendency to write excessively, and sometimes aggressiveness. Ablation of the amygdaloid nuclei has eliminated uncontrollable rage reactions in psychotic patients. Hippocampal and adjacent convolutions have been excised bilaterally, with a disastrous loss of ability to learn or to establish new memories (Korsakoff amnesic state).

The abnormalities consequent on lesions of the temporal lobes may be summarized as follows:

1 Effects of unilateral disease of the dominant temporal lobe:
   a Upper homonymous quadrantanopia
   b Wernicke's aphasia
   c Impairment in tests of verbal material presented through the auditory sense
   d Dysnomia or amnesic aphasia
   e Amusia (inability to name musical scores and to read and write music)
2 Effects of unilateral disease of nondominant temporal lobe:
   a Upper homonymous quadrantanopia
   b Inability to judge spatial relationships in rare cases
   c Impairment in tests of nonverbal visually presented material
   d Inability to recognize melodies and other nonlexical qualities of music
3 Effects of disease of either temporal lobe:
   a Auditory illusions and hallucinations
   b Psychotic behavior (aggressivity)
   c Upper homonymous quadrantanopia
4 Effects of bilateral disease:
   a Korsakoff amnesic defect
   b Apathy and placidity ⎫
   c Increased sexual activity ⎬ Klüver-Bucy syndrome
   d Sham rage ⎭
   e Cortical deafness
   f Loss of other unilateral functions

PARIETAL LOBES   This part of the brain lies between the fissure of Rolando and the parietooccipital notch. It includes Brodmann areas 1, 3, 5, 7, 31, 39, and 40.

The postcentral convolution is the terminus of somatic sensory pathways from the opposite half of the body. However, destructive lesions here do not abolish cutaneous sensation but cause mainly a defect in sensory discrimination with variable impairment of primary sensation. In other words, the perception of painful, tactile, thermal, and vibratory stimuli is affected little or not at all, whereas stereognosis (ability to recognize the size, shape, and texture of objects by touch), sense of position, distinction between single and double contacts (two-point threshold), and the localization of sensory stimuli are impaired or lost (atopognosia). There is also the phenomenon of extinction; i.e., if a stimulus (tactile, painful, visual) is delivered simultaneously to corresponding parts of the body or visual fields, only the stimulus on the normal side is perceived. This type of sensory disturbance, sometimes called *cortical sensory defect*, is really a disturbance of somatic sensory perception and is discussed in Chap. 24. Extensive lesions deep in the white matter of the parietal lobes produce an impairment of all forms of sensation contralaterally, and if these lesions encroach on the uppermost part of the temporal lobe, there may be a contralateral homonymous hemianopia, often incongruous and tending to be greater in the inferior quadrants. Lesions of the angular gyrus of the dominant hemisphere cause an inability to read (alexia).

In addition, the parietal lobes function in the perception of one's position in space, the interrelationships of objects in space, and the relationship of the various parts of the body to one another. Patients with large lesions of the minor parietal lobe are often unaware of their hemiplegia and hemianesthesia; Babinski called this condition *anosognosia*. Related psychological disorders are lack of recognition of the left arm and leg, neglect of the left side of the body (as in dressing) and of external space on the left side, and constructional apraxia (an inability to perceive and construct simple figures). While all these disorders may occur with left-sided lesions as well, they are observed less frequently, in part because the aphasia that occurs with lesions of the left hemisphere precludes adequate testing of other parietal lobe functions.

Another frequent constellation of symptoms, usually referred to as *Gerstmann's syndrome*, occurs only with lesions of the dominant parietal lobe. This consists of inability to write (agraphia), calculate (acalculia), distinguish right from left, and identify fingers (finger agnosia) and other parts of the body. This syndrome is a true *agnosia*, since it represents a defect in the formulation and use of symbolic concepts (including the significance of numbers and letters and the names of parts of the body) in which a unilateral (dominant) lesion evokes the defect bilaterally. An ideomotor apraxia may or may not be associated. *Apraxia* and *agnosia* are discussed in Chaps. 21 and 24.

The effects of disease of the parietal lobes may be summarized as follows:

1 Effects of unilateral disease of the parietal lobe, right or left:
   a Cortical sensory syndrome and sensory extinction (or total hemianesthesia with large acute lesions of white matter)
   b In children, mild contralateral hemiparesis and hemiatrophy
   c Visual inattention and sometimes anosognosia, constructional and dressing apraxias, and neglect of the opposite half of the body and extrapersonal space (all these defects are observed far more frequently with right than with left parietal lesions)
   d Abolition of optokinetic nystagmus to one side
2 Effects of unilateral disease of the dominant parietal lobe (left hemisphere in right-handed patients), additional phenomena:
   a Disorders of language (especially alexia)
   b Gerstmann's syndrome
   c Bimanual astereognosis (tactile agnosia)
   d Bilateral ideational or ideomotor apraxia

In all parietal lesions, if sufficiently extensive, there may be a bland mood, indifference to illness or neurologic defects, reduction in the capacity to think clearly, inattentiveness, and impaired memory.

OCCIPITAL LOBES　The occipital lobes, comprising Brodmann areas 17, 18, and 19, are the termini of the geniculocalcarine pathways and are essential for visual sensation and perception.

Destructive lesions in one occipital lobe result in a contralateral homonymous hemianopia, i.e., a loss of vision in part or all of the homonymous fields. Occasionally, patients complain of changes in the form and contour of visually perceived objects (metamorphopsia), as well as illusory displacement of images from one side of the visual field to another (visual allesthesia), or of abnormal persistence of the visual image after the object has been removed (palinopsia). Visual illusions and elementary (unformed) hallucinations also may occur. Bilateral lesions cause "cortical" blindness, a state of blindness without change in the optic fundi or pupillary reflexes.

Patients with lesions in Brodmann's areas 18 and 19 of the dominant hemisphere (see Fig. 27-1) are unable to recognize objects visually, even though by tests of visual acuity and perimetry they appear to see sufficiently well to do so—a state termed *visual object agnosia*; they are able to recognize objects by tactile or other nonvisual senses. In these terms, *alexia*, or inability to read, represents a visual verbal agnosia or "word blindness." Patients can see letters and words but do not know their meaning, although they can still recognize them through tactile or auditory senses. Several other types of agnosia are observed with bilateral occipital lesions: disorders of *spatial or topographic localization*, in which the patient cannot describe or find his or her way in familiar surroundings (usually due to bilateral occipitoparietal lesions); failure to identify a familiar face (*prosopagnosia*), often with achromatopsia (inferomesial occipitotemporal lesions); an inability to scan the peripheral field and to grasp an object under visual guidance, coupled with visual inattention (*Balint's syndrome*, due usually to bilateral occipitoparietal lesions); and a failure to perceive simultaneously all the elements of a scene (*simultanagnosia*). In actuality, these agnosias do not represent the effects of purely occipital lesions but of either occipitotemporal or occipitoparietal disconnections.

The details of these syndromes of the different lobes of the cerebrum can be found in the textbook of Adams and Victor and the monographs by Walsh and Mesulam.

CORPUS CALLOSUM AND THE DISCONNECTION SYNDROMES
Considerable attention has been devoted to the study of each of the two cerebral hemispheres in isolation. This is possible only when the corpus callosum, which forms a bridge between the two hemispheres, is absent (*agenesis*) or is surgically sectioned (for epilepsy) or destroyed by infarction or tumors. From these studies emerges the well-known fact that the left hemisphere is dominant in all language functions and auditory perception and the right hemisphere is superior in spatial and visual perception. Partial lesions of the corpus callosum or of the long tracts in the cerebral white matter are found to be associated with a number of interesting syndromes (commissural and intrahemispheric) described below.

When the corpus callosum is sectioned by a surgical procedure or destroyed by an anterior cerebral artery occlusion (anterior four-fifths), the language and perceptual areas of the left hemisphere are isolated from the sensory and motor areas of the right hemisphere. These patients, if blindfolded, are then unable to match an object held in one hand with an identical object in the other hand. Further, they cannot match an object seen in the right half of the visual field with one in the left half. If given verbal commands, they perform correctly with the right hand but not with the left. Without vision, objects placed in the right hand are named correctly, but not those in the left. In lesions confined to the posterior fifth of the corpus callosum (splenium), only the visual part of the disconnection syndrome occurs. Occlusion of the left posterior cerebral artery provides the best examples of the latter. Infarction of the left occipital lobe causes a right homonymous hemianopia, as a consequence of which all visual information needed for activating the speech areas of the left hemisphere must come from the right occipital lobe, across the splenium of the corpus callosum. If there is a lesion in the corpus callosum (or in other portions of the crossing fibers), the patient cannot read or name colors because the visual information cannot reach the left angular gyrus. There is no difficulty in copying words, although the patient cannot read what he or she has written (alexia without agraphia); matching colors without naming them is done without error. Apparently the visual information for activating the left motor area crosses the corpus callosum more anteriorly. A lesion that is limited to the anterior third of the corpus callosum does not result in a left-sided apraxia (a failure of the left hand to obey commands, the right one performing perfectly). A section of the entire corpus callosum does result in such an apraxia, indicating that the fiber systems connecting the left to the right motor areas cross posterior to the genu (but anterior to the splenium).

There are also intrahemispheric disconnections, of which the most important are the following:

1 *Conduction aphasia* (also called *central aphasia*). The patient has fluent but paraphasic speech and writing with nearly perfect comprehension of spoken or written language. Repetition of what is heard or read is, however, severely impaired. The lesion is presumably in the arcuate fasciculus, which connects Wernicke's area with Broca's area.
2 *Pure word deafness.* Although the patient is able to hear and identify nonverbal sounds, there is a loss of ability to comprehend spoken language. The patient's speech remains normal. The defect has been attributed to a subcortical lesion undercutting Wernicke's area.

PATIENTS WITH FOCAL CEREBRAL LESIONS　Diagnosis and management involve the same principles described in Chap. 25. Special tests, mostly of the psychological type, are available for each of the focal cerebral syndromes. The investigation and care of individual patients also will be governed by the underlying disease, of course.

REFERENCES

ABSHER JR, BENSON DF: Disconnection syndromes—An overview of Geschwind's contributions. Neurology 43:862, 1993
ADAMS RD, VICTOR M: *Principles of Neurology*, 5th ed. New York, McGraw-Hill, 1993
BRODAL A: *Neurological Anatomy in Relation to Clinical Medicine*, 3d ed. New York, Oxford University Press, 1981
BROWN JW: Frontal lobe syndromes, in *Handbook of Clinical Neurology*, JAM Frederiks (ed). Amsterdam, Elsevier Science, 1985, vol 45, chap 3
DIMOND SJ: The disconnection syndromes, in *Modern Trends in Neurology*, D Williams (ed). London, Butterworth, 1975
GESCHWIND N: Disconnection syndromes in animals and man. Brain 88:237, 585, 1965
HECAEN H, ALBERT ML: Disorders of mental functioning related to the frontal lobes, in *Modern Trends in Neurology*, D Williams (ed). London, Butterworth, 1975
HEILMAN KM, VALENSTEIN E (eds): *Clinical Neuropsychology*, 2d ed. Oxford, Oxford University Press, 1985
LURIA AR: *The Working Brain: An Introduction to Neuropsychology*. New York, Basic Books (trans Penguin Books Ltd), 1973
MARLOWE WH et al: Complete Klüver-Bucy syndrome in man. Cortex 11:53, 1975
MESULAM M-M (ed): *Principles of Behavioral Neurology*. Philadelphia, Davis, 1985
WALSH KW: *Neuropsychology: A Clinical Approach*, 2d ed. London, Churchill Livingstone, 1987

28　DISORDERS OF SPEECH AND LANGUAGE

J. P. MOHR

Impairments of language and speech are among the most important consequences of brain disease because they affect the interaction between the victim and other people. The spectrum of impairment in communication ranges widely, from loss of all interpersonal communication at the most severe end of the spectrum to minor disturbances in intonation of normally selected words or minor flaws in selection at the other end. The more gross disturbances are easily recognized as signs of brain disease, whereas the minor disturbances may pass unnoticed by all but the most probing of examinations.

DEFINITIONS The site, size, and temporal proximity of a brain lesion influence speech and language in distinctively different ways. Disturbance in the comprehension or production of language in written or spoken forms is known broadly as *aphasia*. The disorder is usually incomplete and hence is often described as *dysphasia*. Because of its more common use, aphasia will be employed in this chapter. The term *language* has wide connotations and refers to the selection and serial ordering of words according to learned rules by which a person can use spoken or written modalities to communicate with others and to express cerebral activities involved with thinking and learning.

Brain lesions also may compromise the capacity to comprehend or produce the sights and sounds needed to convey language. Injuries to the main sensory and motor pathways can affect the skills involved in scanning visual displays and the selection of those shapes learned earlier to be letters, numbers, or marks of grammatical notation, such as apostrophes; listening to strings of sounds and selecting from among them the distinctive cluster that makes up the sounds of letters and syllables; and the execution of acquired motor skills for the pronunciation of these same items and marking down their graphic equivalents. A brain lesion also can disturb efforts of noting whether word strings seen or heard are given special emphasis or intonation, the intonation of strings of words to make questions or statements, the grouping of words into phrases, and the production of the speech "melody" that is distinctive for given languages and regional dialects. The needs of the patient can be exquisitely sensitive to such seemingly minor patterns of disturbance; e.g., a lesion that disturbs skills in vocal timing and emphasis could ruin the career of an actor but have no impact on that of a typist. While no general term has emerged to classify these disturbances in the sensory discrimination and motor production of the shapes and sounds of language, they are commonly referred to as *speech sensory* or *motor modalities*, as opposed to the language that they convey, and have a wide variety of terms that emphasize the focal nature of the disturbance. *Dysarthria*, a defect in articulation usually related to poor pronunciation of consonants, occurs with flaccid or spastic paralysis, rigidity, repetitive spasms (stuttering), or ataxia of the oropharynx and respiratory apparatus. *Dysphonia*, a defect in phonation (voice), is due to disease of the larynx or its innervation, causing inability to produce the basic vowel sounds. *Dysgraphia*, faulty writing skills, is due to disturbances of motor skills in writing. More complex disorders in understanding the meaning of words heard (word deafness) and seen (word blindness) are discussed below.

GENERAL PRINCIPLES As a general orientation, most lesions that lead to aphasia occur in the perisylvian regions (frontal, temporal, and parietal) of the dominant cerebral hemisphere, i.e., the left side in right-handed individuals. When the lesion is due to infarction as a result of arterial occlusion, hemorrhage, masses from various causes, or other focal conditions that cause gross changes in tissue characteristics, the anatomic site of the lesion can usually be demonstrated by computed tomography (CT scan) or magnetic resonance imaging (MRI). Focal dysfunction caused by cell death, atrophy, or impairment of cortical microvascular regulation may be evaluated by measurement of regional cerebral blood flow (rCBF) or by single-photon-emission tomography (SPECT) or positron-emission tomography (PET) (see Chap. 365).

Diseases of the cerebral surface gray matter produce a more significant deficit than those confined to the white matter; tumors, located largely in the white matter, usually reach a large size before causing a speech or language deficit. Small infarcts or traumatic lesions of a few centimeters in diameter are usually associated with an evanescent deficit that fades to functional insignificance within weeks or months. Improvements over weeks to months occur in all but the largest vascular lesions, whereas those due to tumors show progression. The site of the lesion determines the qualitative features of the deficit, whereas size determines the severity of the syndrome. Furthermore, deficits in speech function predominate in smaller lesions, whereas major disturbances in language are superimposed on the speech disturbance with larger lesions.

The history of aphasiology has mirrored the notions of brain function popular at the time. Over a century ago, when sensory functions were thought to reside in the posterior half of the brain and motor in the anterior, it was popular to speak in broad terms of a sensory aphasia and a motor aphasia. When studies of the fiber pathways predominated, complex schemes were developed to show that aphasias could be cortical (brain surface, gray matter, centers), subcortical (affecting the pathways connecting the peripheral speech organs with the "cortical centers"), and transcortical (connecting various "cortical centers" with each other). PET studies have challenged these concepts. Most recently, awareness of the direct interactions between brain regions has led to the currently popular notion of neural networks. To date, however, the precise neural substrate of language continues to elude investigators, and it remains unknown what the brain does neurochemically and neurophysiologically when it is said to be thinking, comprehending words seen and heard, and formulating a reply. Even less is known about how improvements occur after lesions that destroy areas once thought essential for language function. It is not idle to speculate that the neurobiologic basis for language may prove as surprising and as clarifying as has research into the neural basis of vision.

CEREBRAL DOMINANCE: RELATION TO SPEECH AND HAND-EDNESS The side of the brain dominant for language is inferred to be the side opposite from the eye, hand, or foot preferentially used for intricate, complex acts. Over 90 percent of people are right-handed. The dominance is more complete in some persons than in others. Hereditary, anatomic, and developmental factors play a role, but there is considerable evidence of hemisphere specialization for certain types of tasks. In normal individuals, PET has shown the left hemisphere to be activated more for verbal tasks, whereas the right is more activated for spatial motor tasks. Left hemisphere dominance for language occurs in 95 percent of right-handed people and in 50 percent of those who are left-handed. Anatomic differences in size between the dominant and the nondominant cerebral hemispheres may explain the dominance: the planum temporale, adjacent to the auditory center of Heschl's transverse gyrus, is larger in the left hemisphere in right-handed individuals. Left-handedness may be hereditary or may result from disease of the left cerebral hemisphere in early life.

LESION LOCATION AND LANGUAGE DISTURBANCE Although language deficits are not always closely correlated with anatomic pathology, two large syndromic categories, recognized for over a century by the eponyms *Broca's* and *Wernicke's aphasia*, remain recognized by their distinctive clinical features. Large anterior lesions involving the bulk of the frontal operculum (that region that lies above the insula) and the insula itself result in Broca's aphasia, in which the main language disturbance is *agrammatism*. In its fully developed form, sentences have a sharply constricted structure, with absence of most small words and a preservation of words mainly serving predicative, interjectional, or substantive functions. The most severely affected patient may only be able to say *hi*, *no*, and *hello* or to use simple nouns, such as *ball*, *top*, and *key*.

Large posterior sylvian lesions cause Wernicke's aphasia, in which simple syllabic or word elements are missing or are replaced by substitutions so that the desired response is only approximated (*paraphasias*). These latter may consist of faulty pronunciations (*literal paraphasias*) or faulty word selections (*verbal paraphasias*). Verbal paraphasias may approximate the desired word with a similarity of sound or of spelling (formal verbal paraphasias), such as *stock* for *stop*, or by similarity of meaning (semantic verbal paraphasias), such as *slow* for *stop*. Disturbances in understanding language, both auditory and visual speech, occur in both types of major paraphasias and tend to be of the same type of disorder as that seen in language production.

LESION LOCATION AND DISTURBANCE IN SPEECH MODALITIES Focal left-sided sylvian lesions often disturb speech modalities. When small, the disturbance may occur with little or no accompanying aphasia, but when large, the aphasia often makes it difficult to determine the severity of the disturbances in speech. Anterior sylvian lesions, which lie close to the sensorimotor cortex for oropharyngeal movements, mainly disturb the act of speaking. These range from mutism through impaired articulation to disordered transitions from syllable to syllable to abnormalities in phrasing, intonation, and melody. Lesions just posterior to the lower rolandic region produce malpositioning of the tongue, lips, and other structures in the oropharynx, with anticipatory errors from some syllables occurring out of sequence. Lesions grouped around the posterior sylvian fissure, including the superior temporal lobe and its auditory gyri, are manifested by disordered understanding of spoken words, resulting in poor repetition of speech sounds. Those located more posteriorly over the left lateral parietal or occipital lobes interfere with reading.

Lesions well away from the sylvian region either fail to disturb human communicative skills or alter them only secondarily. A large lesion of the anterior frontal lobes, especially the medial and orbital parts, impairs all motor activities and often results in lack of attention and responsiveness (abulia), verging on the akinetic mute state (see Chap. 27). The speech is laconic, with long pauses between utterances, and there is an inability to sustain monologue and narrative, leaving an incorrect impression of aphasia. Extensive occipital lesions impair reading and reduce the utilization of all visual, lexical stimuli. Posterior thalamic and deep lesions in the adjacent temporal lobe impair alertness and cause fluctuating states of inattention and disorientation, thereby inducing fragmentation of words (*neologisms*) and phrases and protracted, uncontrollable talking (*logorrhea*). Strong stimulation to increase momentarily the level of awareness and alertness usually will show that such patients have intact language mechanisms. Lesions in the anterior thalamus, located beneath the genu of the internal capsule and the head of the caudate, may interrupt projection systems controlling rCBF over the convexity and produce short-lived reductions in the complexity and length of verbal responses. The deficit includes some elements of abulia but also disturbances in naming and in the proper use of grammatical forms. These syndromes usually improve within weeks or months, paralleling the improvement in rCBF. Recognition of these specific syndromes from isolated lesions separate from the more traditional aphasias has been increasing with improvements in brain imaging and may continue to proliferate.

The nondominant hemisphere provides the substratum for several types of behavior: motor responses of mimicry, social anticipation (smiling, handshaking, modesty reactions), and self-care (washing and feeding); avoidance behavior to noxious stimuli; and the capability of matching visually simple words with pictures.

APHASIA

TYPES OF APHASIA Disturbances of speech and language can result from several abnormalities. Classifications have been based on the predominant form, the presumed physiologic or psychological bases, and the anatomy of the underlying diseases. The classification utilized here has been formulated on the basis of the anatomic localization and the clinical presentation (see Table 28-1). The prognoses are helpful in management, particularly in the choice of therapy.

Aphasias also have been classified according to the severity of impediment to speech production and flow, the most obvious disturbance on brief personal contact with the patient. *Nonfluent aphasias* are characterized by slow, incorrectly articulated words and sentences; the lesion usually lies in the dominant frontal lobe. *Fluent aphasias* show runs of well-articulated speech, with basically normal rhythm and flow, although lacking in language meaning; the defect is usually a lesion in the dominant parietal or temporal lobe.

Total (global) aphasia The causative lesion is located in the left sylvian region, destroying a large part of the speech and language areas and leaving a severe aphasia with a poor prognosis for improvement. Most patients with total aphasia are initially mute or say few stereotyped words, such as *hi* and *yes*; they do not read or write even the simplest words, and they understand only a few words of the speech of others. Related signs include right hemiplegia, hemianesthesia, and homonymous hemianopsia. The alert patient may participate in common gestures of greeting, may show modesty and avoidance reactions, and is able to engage in self-help activities. Some improve months later with a persistent Broca's aphasia.

Infarction from occlusion of the left internal carotid or middle cerebral artery, a large hemorrhage, major tumor, or penetrating trauma is most often responsible for the deficit. In the rare instances of rapid improvement, the main cause is postconvulsive paralysis, posttraumatic edema, or transitory ischemia from a fragmenting embolus. Occasionally, hyperthermia, infection, or hyponatremia may cause temporary return of aphasia due to an old lesion.

Broca's aphasia (major motor aphasia) This term designates a complex syndrome with severely disturbed speech and writing, accompanied by simplified grammar skills (agrammatism) in speaking and writing and a less obvious impairment in language comprehension. It results from a large lesion involving cortex and subcortical structures in the anterior sylvian region and insula, including but usually extending beyond Broca's area (the inferior frontal convolution). The CT scan may underestimate the lesion because the angle of the imaged lesion may seem to merge with the sylvian fissure, but both coronal and true-axial MRI shows the real size. The lesion is smaller than that of total aphasia and usually involves the sensorimotor rolandic region, producing an accompanying persisting hemiparesis and hemisensory syndrome. Intitially, a transient ipsilateral deviation of the eyes is observed due to the frontal infarction.

In the acute phase, the entire language mechanism appears to be inactivated, and the helplessly mute, noncommunicative, and uncomprehending patient presents the syndrome of complete or global aphasia. Within weeks to years, the disorder of comprehension abates somewhat, and this improvement exceeds that found in speaking and writing, leaving the motor speech deficits that gave the syndrome its original name. For a time an apraxia of the lingual and oropharyngeal apparatus retards efforts to make purposeful movements. Imitation may be better performed than execution of acts on command. Certain stereotyped and simple phrases, such as *hi*, *good morning*, or curses are uttered more easily, and words of popular songs may be sung surprisingly well. The patient's efforts to speak and the facial expressions suggest an awareness of his or her ineptitudes and mistakes, and an accompanying exasperation and despair are common. Most patients with Broca's aphasia have a correspondingly severe impairment in communication by writing with either hand. However, communication by writing is superior to that of speaking, suggesting a certain independence between these two acts as vehicles of language.

As improvement occurs, words are enunciated slowly and laboriously, with greatly impaired melody of speech (prosody). Speech is sparse and consists mainly of nouns, transitive verbs, and important adjectives; many of the small words (articles, prepositions, conjunctions) are omitted, giving the speech an agrammatic and telegraphic character. The preservation of substantive words allows the patients to communicate despite the gross mechanical and agrammatic language difficulties. This hesitant, laconic speech has been termed *nonfluent aphasia*.

The syndrome is most often due to embolic occlusions of the upper division of the left middle cerebral artery; major putaminal hypertensive hemorrhage, huge frontal lobe tumor or abscess, metastatic lesions, subdural hematoma, and encephalitis are less common causes.

Minor motor aphasia More circumscribed focal lesions along the anterior and superior sylvian operculum and insula produce remarkably discrete effects on speech modalities which may resemble

TABLE 28-1   Classification of aphasic disorders

	Clinical manifestations	Anatomic location	Etiology	Associated clinical symptoms
MAJOR SYNDROMES				
Global aphasia	Minimal speech; nonfluent aphasia; comprehension poor for spoken and written language	Large lesion of dominant frontal, parietal, and superior temporal lobe	Infarction in distribution of internal carotid or middle cerebral artery; trauma; tumor	Contralateral hemiplegia; hemisensory loss; hemianopsia
Broca's aphasia	Nonfluent aphasia; agrammatic sentences; poor articulation; dysprosody; may be mute	Cortical and subcortical lesion of prefrontal and frontal regions	Infarction in distribution of superior frontal branch middle cerebral artery; hemorrhage; tumor	Contralateral hemiparesis; minor or no sensory loss; no visual field disturbance; oral dyspraxia; cortical dysarthria; severe impairment in writing
Wernicke's aphasia (central or sensory aphasia)	Fluent speech; total incomprehension of spoken speech; inability to read or to repeat sounds or words; alexia, agraphia, paraphasia common	Posterior perisylvian structures of the parietal and temporal lobe	Infarction in distribution of lower division of middle cerebral artery; tumor; herpes simplex encephalitis	Parietal lobe sensory deficits; hemianopsia; no motor disturbance
MINOR CENTRAL APHASIA SYNDROMES				
Conduction aphasia	Paraphasia; difficulty in repetition of speech and in reading aloud; aware of deficit; adequate comprehension of written and spoken words	Upper bank of sylvian fissure; inferior parietal lobule	Embolic occlusion of posterior branches of middle cerebral artery	Contralateral hemihypesthesia or homonymous hemianopsia; abnormal optokinetic nystagmus
Mainly auditory (pure word deafness)	Impaired auditory comprehension; inability to repeat a sentence or write a dictation	Lesion in superior temporal gyrus	Infarction; tumor; abscess	Rarely deafness
Mainly visual (dyslexia with dysgraphia)	Visual language compromised more than auditory; cannot read or write	Parietooccipital lesion	Infarction; tumor, lobar hemorrhage	Hemianopsia
OTHER SYNDROMES				
Pure word blindness	Normal spoken language and writing, with inability to read	Left occipitostriate cortex, adjacent association cortex, and posterior corpus callosum (splenium)	Infarction in distribution of posterior cerebral artery; tumor, lobar hemorrhage	Hemianopsia
Isolation of speech areas	Parrot-like speech; echolalia	Ischemic infarction in border (watershed) zones between anterior, middle, and posterior cerebral artery distributions	Systemic hypotension or hypoxia; cardiac arrest	Decreased alertness and responsiveness; bilateral leg weakness
Amnesic-dysnomic aphasia	Inability to recall names of objects or parts of objects; difficulty with recent memory	Deep temporal lobe lesions, parahippocampal, hippocampal gyrus	Tumor; Alzheimer's disease; infarction in distribution posterior cerebral artery; herpes simplex encephalitis	Apraxia; dementia; no motor or sensory abnormalities; upper quadrantic visual field defect

major motor aphasia except for the satisfactory understanding of spoken and written words. The prognosis for nearly full recovery is excellent. Indeed, none of these focal lesions produces significant or lasting deficits in language usage.

Broca's area infarction affects the lower premotor cortex adjacent to the primary motor cortex controlling the oropharynx, larynx, and respiratory apparatus. The infarct interrupts skilled movements of these muscle groups, and the resultant dyspraxia in speech causes impaired transitions between syllables in words and disruption of the melodic intonation of phrases (dysprosody). Involvement of this region alone is insufficient to produce the major syndrome referred to as *Broca's aphasia. Rolandic infarction* involves the sensorimotor cortex itself; either the syndrome of dysprosody occurs or speech has poor articulation and lowered volume and pitch, while a nasal quality to the voice reveals the paresis of the nasopharyngeal musculature. *Postcentral, anterior parietal infarction* is associated with errors in the positioning of the oral cavity for individual sounds, syllables, and whole words; the acoustic features of the utterance are often distorted by these malpositions of the oral cavity and strike the ear as literal paraphasias.

Lesions in the more anterior parts of the dominant frontal lobe (sparing Broca's area) in the medial frontal lobe in the anterior cerebral artery territory, or in the head of the caudate and anterior

limb of the internal capsule also may cause an aphasic disorder. Usually, the speech output is reduced and nonfluent, and auditory comprehension is intact. Repetition of words spoken by the examiner is preserved. This condition has been called *transcortical motor aphasia* but is usually part of frontal lobe syndromes in which spontaneous speech is lacking (mutism) and all motor activity is reduced (akinesia).

Almost all these syndromes are due to stroke, usually infarction from embolism into a single branch. Other diseases rarely produce such circumscribed lesions. Exceptions supporting this view are the rare instances of highly focal penetrating head wounds from missile fragments. Deeper, larger lesions or larger emboli involving the stem of the upper division of the middle cerebral artery can cause several types of deficit in a single patient, making these individual distinctions less clear and blending with the major syndrome of Broca's aphasia. Facial, lingual, and sometimes brachial paresis and ideomotor dyspraxia of the face and left, nondominant limbs commonly accompany the speech disorder. Most of these syndromes recede within weeks or months (see Chap. 27).

Wernicke's aphasia (major central or sensory aphasia)   This term encompasses syndromes that arise from lesions of the posterior perisylvian structures or the posterior temporal, parietal, and occipital regions supplied by the lower division of the middle cerebral artery.

When restricted to the temporal lobe, the main disturbance is in language tasks involving words heard; when more parietal and occipital, in words seen. Spoken and written communication, as well as auditory and visual comprehension, are affected, a combination that justifies the term *central aphasia*. Speech contains many language errors but is fluent, hence the term *fluent aphasia*.

In a severe or acute injury, the patient usually speaks easily in a series of incomprehensible syllables, makes illegible marks in attempts at writing, cannot repeat aloud or copy correctly, and treats the examiner's attempts at written and verbal communication as if they were in a wholly unfamiliar foreign language. Patients may seem puzzled that they are not communicating and may become angry and abusive. In less severe cases, the patient can repeat aloud and copy but echoes the words heard with faulty pronunciation or copies the words in a slavish manner, imitating even the examiner's handwriting style, as though the test words were unfamiliar. In the mildest cases, the deficits are manifested in errors in word comprehension and usage. The disturbance in language does not simply reflect a disturbance in hearing or vision. The patient may choose words that show approximation to the desired response, the words often belonging to the same functional class [i.e., *cow* for *pig*, but not *cow* for *yellow* (semantic verbal paraphasias)], or the words may be similar in sound or shape (formal verbal paraphasis) such as *flee* for *tree*; there may be errors in word structure, with improper tenses, prefixes, or suffixes (e.g., "beautifulling"), or other errors that resemble those of normal people unfamiliar with the language in question. Some patients pass for normal in brief or casual conversation. In its mildest form or later in the course of the illness, the speech resembles that of a person who is tired or distracted, and the abnormality is detected only on tests of complex language function.

Minor central aphasia syndromes   In time, Wernicke's aphasia improves, and a number of lesser syndromes appear. However, these latter syndromes may be present in comparatively pure form from the beginning when only a small, restricted lesion involves some part of the territory of the lower division of the middle cerebral artery. The posterior sylvian region, comprising posterosuperior temporal, opercular, supramarginal, and posterior insular gyri, appears to encompass a variety of language functions. Seemingly minor changes in size and locale of the lesion are associated with important variations in the elements of Wernicke's aphasia.

Depending on the location of the lesion, language behavior dependent on auditory function (hearing spoken words, echoing sounds and speech, relating the spoken to the written word, and finally, repeating and writing it) may be deranged partially or completely. The same is true of language behavior dependent on visual function when the left posterior parietal lobe is involved. These partial syndromes are termed *conduction aphasia*, *pure word deafness*, *dyslexia with dysgraphia*, *isolation of speech areas*, and *pure word blindness*.

CONDUCTION APHASIA   A clinical syndrome, which acquired its name for historical reasons not reflected in its pathoanatomy, conduction aphasia is characterized by disturbance in repeating words or sentences. This disturbance resembles that of Wernicke's aphasia; there is the same degree of paraphasia in self-initiated speech, in repeating what is heard, and in reading aloud. However, little or no difficulty is encountered in comprehending words that are heard or seen. Because the motor regions are unaffected, no element of dysarthria or dysprosody occurs. The patient is alert and fully aware of the deficit. The errors take the form of literal paraphasia, i.e., mispronunciations, many of which seem explained as errors in oropharyngeal positioning that produce detectably different sounds from those intended.

The lesion at autopsy is located in the cortex and subcortical white matter in the upper bank of the sylvian fissure, involving the supramarginal gyrus of the inferior parietal lobule. The posterior part of the superior temporal region is occasionally affected. The usual cause is an embolus in the ascending parietal or posterior temporal branch of the middle cerebral artery. Deeper, larger lesions that interrupt the arcuate fasciculus, once thought the explanation for the "disconnection" of the posterior and anterior language zones (hence the term *conduction aphasia*), rarely produce the syndrome.

PURE WORD DEAFNESS   This is considered to be the auditory form of Wernicke's aphasia. The most obvious findings are an impaired auditory comprehension and an inability to repeat what is said or to write to dictation. Spoken language is less impaired but rarely normal. Occasionally, the paraphasic speech leads to an initial diagnosis of Wernicke's aphasia. Little defect in hearing is found by audiometric testing. The patient frequently learns to use visual cues well enough to overcome much of the difficulty. Comprehension of visually presented material such as printed matter, although not normal, is better than auditory comprehension. When there is full preservation of reading skill, the traditional term *pure word deafness* can be applied. The syndrome is rare but has an excellent prognosis for functional recovery.

In most autopsy studies, the lesion has been focal and the result of embolism. The infarcts have been bilateral in the superior temporal gyrus in a position to damage the primary auditory cortex in the transverse gyrus of Heschl and to impair its relation to the associated areas of the superoposterior part of the temporal lobe. A unilateral infarct has rarely been found in this part of the major (dominant) temporal lobe, thought to encroach on those regions whose involvement precipitates the larger syndrome of Wernicke's aphasia.

DYSLEXIA WITH DYSGRAPHIA   This syndrome, often a late sequela of the larger syndrome of Wernicke's aphasia, is its visual form and thus is most evident in reading and writing. Errors occur in response to lexical stimuli. Auditory comprehension, while abnormal, is less impaired than visual comprehension. Since conversational testing is frequently the only type of clinical evaluation in such patients, satisfactory auditory comprehension, ability to repeat aloud, and mild paraphasic errors in spontaneous speech frequently lead to a misdiagnosis of mild Wernicke's aphasia. Detailed testing of reading aloud and reading for comprehension and tests of spontaneous writing and writing in response to dictated and visually presented material reveal a greater disturbance in these tasks.

The parietal and occipital regions are usually affected in the syndrome of dyslexia with dysgraphia. Although a discrete embolism is unusual, a small clot may pass through the more proximal territory and lodge distally. Tumors, abscess, and lobar hemorrhages usually disrupt other structures as well, and this syndrome is often a less conspicuous part of a larger clinical picture. Systemic hypotension and hypoxia may leave dyslexia with dysgraphia as a residual impairment, but more often they produce a more severe defect, described below under "Isolation of Speech Areas."

ISOLATION OF SPEECH AREAS   This rare syndrome is of importance to show that the act of repeating aloud can be accomplished without major portions of the parietal, temporal, and occipital lobes. Following prolonged hypoxia from cardiac arrest or other causes of hypotension, widespread cerebral ischemia can affect the vascular border zones linking the major cerebral arteries and their distal branches on the cerebral surfaces and can spread centripetally into their adjacent territories. The central fields of supply of these arteries are often spared. In the middle cerebral artery territory, this sparing leaves largely intact the sylvian region and its speech areas. Despite much of the rest of the brain that is inactive in patients who survive such episodes, spoken responses can be activated by words heard. The response is a parrot-like repetition of the sounds (*echolalia*) that is done well enough to indicate that the auditory-vocal loop is functional. Scant signs of comprehension or self-initiated conversation occur, reflecting the widespread injury outside the speech regions. The prognosis for full recovery is poor.

PURE WORD BLINDNESS   In the fully developed syndrome, victims lose the ability to read and usually to name colors. The patient is unable to name or point to a letter or word on command. However, understanding spoken language, repetition of what is heard, writing dictation, conversation, and writing are all intact. The condition is also sometimes termed *dyslexia without dysgraphia*. Because the victim may be unaware the deficit exists, the examiner is often required to test for its presence rather than simply assuming that the complaint will be volunteered. The errors may be minimal and the defect obscured if other visual cues are available, such as the bottle on which the words *Coca-Cola* appear. The naming of common colors presented singly and of objects is also impaired. When the syndrome is less severe, reading is impaired mainly in the affected visual field, producing a dyslexia for the letters on the affected side of the longer words (so-called hemidyslexia). Right homonymous hemianopsia, an amnesic defect, and a right hemisensory defect reflect respectively the involvement of the left occipital lobe and its callosal decussation, the left fornix, and the left thalamus. This combination nearly always signifies thrombosis or embolism of the left posterior cerebral artery, placing the origin of this syndrome rather remote from the main language zone supplied by the middle cerebral artery.

Autopsy usually demonstrates a lesion that destroys the left visual striate cortex (area 17) and visual association areas (18 and 19), as well as the connections of the right visual cortex and association areas with the temporoparietal region. This latter "disconnection" usually is due to interruption of the fibers passing through the posterior part (splenium) of the corpus callosum, which connect the visual association areas of the two hemispheres. Rarely, a lesion deep in the left parieto-occipital region prevents visual information from either occipital lobe from reaching the left language region. Right homonymous hemianopsia may be absent. Aside from infarction, the syndrome may occur from a primary or secondary tumor, multifocal leukoencephalopathy, or even multiple sclerosis.

In rare instances, the dyslexia has been found limited to the left side of space and to the initial letter or letters of a word. This partial left hemidyslexia has been explained by highly specific infarction or surgery done on the posterior end of the corpus callosum or fiber bundles passing through the callosum. The existence of such cases indicates the highly organized visual pathways serving reading.

Amnesic-dysnomic aphasia   This may be a relatively early or isolated syndrome in patients with CNS disease. The patient has difficulty recalling names on demand, not only nouns, but also adjectives and other descriptive parts of speech. There are usually pauses in speech, groping for words, and substitution of another word or phrase that conveys the meaning (circumlocution). The function of an object may be described, but its name forgotten. The difficulty applies not only to common objects seen but also to the names of things heard or felt. By contrast, other verbal tasks, including recall of the names of the letters and digits, reading, writing, spelling, etc., are far better performed.

The causative lesion is usually deep in the temporal lobe, presumably interrupting connections of sensory speech areas with the hippocampal-parahippocampal regions concerned with learning and memory (see Chap. 27). Masses such as a tumor or abscess are the most frequent causes; as they enlarge, an upper contralateral quadrantic visual field defect or Wernicke's aphasia is added. Dysnomia may be part of the syndromes produced by occlusion of the temporal branches of the posterior cerebral artery. Alzheimer's or Pick's disease may begin with a dysnomic or amnesic type of aphasia; by the time the patient's difficulty is fully recognized, other disorders of speech and indifference, apathy, and abulia are conjoined. When Alzheimer's or Pick's disease is the cause, rCBF, SPECT, or PET studies may reveal reduced activity of the posterolateral parietal or occipital regions, even when the CT or MRI shows no major abnormalities. Dysnomia also may be present in confusional states caused by metabolic, infectious, intoxicative, or other acute medical illnesses, but then it has no particular localizing value.

The combination of dysnomia and major impairment of auditory comprehension, with a remarkable retention of the ability to repeat what is heard, is called *transcortical sensory aphasia*. The causative lesion spares the auditory cortex and Wernicke area and involves the inferior temporal cortices, particularly area 37.

DISORDERS OF ARTICULATION AND PHONATION

The highly coordinated act of speaking involves the larynx, pharynx, palate, tongue, lips, and respiratory musculature, which are innervated by the hypoglossal, vagal, facial, and phrenic nerves. Their nuclei are controlled through the corticobulbar tracts by both motor cortices and extrapyramidal influences from the cerebellum and basal ganglia.

In speaking, the current of air is produced by expiration and is finely regulated by the activity of the various muscles engaged in speech. Phonation, or the production of vocal sounds, is a function of the larynx. Changes in the size and shape of the glottis and in the length and tension of the vocal cords are controlled by the laryngeal muscles, which transmit their vibrations to the column of air passing over the vocal cords. Sounds thus formed are modified as they pass through the nasopharynx and mouth, which act as resonators. Articulation consists of contractions of the tongue, lips, pharynx, and palate that interrupt or alter the vocal sounds. Vowels are of laryngeal origin, as are some consonants, but the latter are formed for the most part during articulation. The consonants *m*, *b*, and *p* are labial; *l* and *t* are lingual; and *k* and *g* are nasoguttural.

Disorders of phonation (aphonia, dysphonia) prompt examination of the vocal cords, tongue, palate, and pharynx. Paresis of the respiratory movements, as in poliomyelitis and acute infectious polyneuritis, or incoordination as part of extrapyramidal disease may affect the voice because insufficient air is provided for phonation and speech. Reduced volume of speech due to limited excursion of the breathing muscles is common; the patient is unable to speak above a whisper or is unable to shout. Paresis of both vocal cords causes complete aphonia, with no voice, and the patient only able to speak in whispers. If one vocal cord is paralyzed, the voice becomes hoarse, low-pitched, and rasping. Involvement of one of the tenth cranial nerves by tumor, for example, also may cause a nasal voice because the posterior nares do not close during phonation. Consonants such as *b*, *p*, *n*, and *k* are followed by escape of air into the nasal passages. *Spastic dysphonia* is a poorly understood neurologic disorder similar to dystonia. Many patients who are middle-aged or elderly and otherwise healthy gradually lose the ability to speak quietly and fluently. Any effort to speak results in contraction of the speech musculature so that the voice is strained and phonation is labored. The condition differs from the stridor caused by spasm of the laryngeal muscles in tetany. It is nonprogressive but may be combined with restricted extrapyramidal disorders such as blepharospasm and spasmodic torticollis. Surgical section of the superior laryngeal nerve on one side has been found to at least partially diminish the rigidity.

Defects in articulation can be subdivided into paretic dysarthria, spastic and rigid dysarthria, and choreic, myoclonic, and ataxic dysarthria. *Paretic dysarthria* is due to a neural or bulbar (medullary) weakness or paralysis of the articulatory muscles (lower motor neuron paralysis). There is a special difficulty in the correct utterance of vibratives, such as *r*; the voice develops a nasal quality due to palatal weakness; and as the paralysis becomes more complete, lingual and labial consonants are not pronounced. In the advanced stages, the shriveled tongue lies inert on the floor of the mouth, and the lips are relaxed and tremulous. Bulbar palsy, peripheral neuropathies, and muscle diseases including myasthenia gravis are common causes. *Spastic and rigid dysarthria* is a supranuclear weakness of articulation from diseases that involve the corticobulbar or subcortical tracts, usually brainstem stroke. Unlike bulbar paralysis due to lower neuron involvement, this condition entails no atrophy or fasciculation of the paralyzed muscles, the jaw jerk and other facial reflexes are exaggerated, the palatal reflexes are retained, emotional control is poor (pathologic laughter and crying), and sometimes breathing is periodic (Cheyne-Stokes). When the frontal operculum alone is involved, the speech deficit may be a pure dysarthria but usually without the impairment in emotional control. In the beginning, the patient may be totally anarthric and aphonic, but when improvement occurs or when the patient has a milder version of the same condition, speech is notably slow, thick, and indistinct, much like that of a patient with partial bulbar paralysis. Choreic, myoclonic, and ataxic dysarthria may occur in Huntington's disease, cerebellar syndromes, and palatal myoclonus (see Chaps. 21 and 371). Speech is irregular, explosive, inarticulate, and unpredictable.

CLINICAL APPROACH TO LANGUAGE DISORDERS

DIAGNOSIS For aphasia, conversational testing permits quick assessment of the motor aspects of speech (praxis and prosody), apparent language formulation, and auditory comprehension. Disabilities in the purely motor aspects of speech suggest a motor aphasia. This possibility can be pursued by tests of repeating from dictation and tests of praxis of the oropharyngeal and respiratory apparatus. Disabilities in language formulation, such as literal paraphasias with impaired comprehension, are indicative of Wernicke's aphasia. Disorders confined to naming, generally without paraphasias, when other language functions (reading, writing, spelling, etc.) are adequate, are diagnostic of amnesic dysnomia.

Dyspraxia of limbs and speech musculature in response to spoken commands or to visual mimicry is generally associated with Broca's aphasia and sometimes with Wernicke's aphasia. Bilateral or unilateral homonymous hemianopsia without motor weakness is often linked with pure word blindness (alexia or dyslexia) or to amnesic-dysnomic aphasia. Bilateral hemiplegias due to extensive frontal lesions are accompanied occasionally by pure word muteness.

When conversation indicates virtually no disabilities, other tests may be revealing. Reading aloud single letters, words, and text may reveal pure word blindness, whereas tests of writing in this syndrome are normal. Literal and verbal paraphasic errors may appear in milder cases of Wernicke's aphasia as the patient reads aloud from text or from words in the examiner's handwriting. Similar errors occur more frequently when the patient is asked to explain the text, read aloud, or give explanations in writing. Adequacy of response channels is determined by presenting tasks that permit a response physically identical with the test stimulus, such as copying visual stimuli and repeating aloud from auditory stimuli. Inadequacy of speech modality functions such as vision, hearing, phonation/articulation, or body-part movements for writing precludes further analysis of language function via that channel. If reception and response channels are adequate in these initial tests, they may then be used in tests requiring all types of language function, such as writing from dictation, vocal naming of visual stimuli, and matching physically dissimilar stimuli having a name in common (e.g., the word *cow* and a picture of a cow). By using the same test material as in the earlier tests, direct comparison of performances in spoken naming, written naming, and matching can be made from visual, auditory, and palpated stimuli. A performance profile can be constructed separately for each type of stimulus material tested (objects, pictures, words, letters, numbers, colors, etc.). The resultant profile can then be used to determine whether the main deficits fall across one or more input or response channels. These data provide a baseline against which later changes may be compared.

Disturbances of articulation point to involvement of a different set of neural structures, such as the motor cortices, the corticobulbar pathways, the seventh, ninth, and tenth nuclei, the brainstem, and extrapyramidal nuclei and tracts. It may be necessary to use other neurologic findings to decide which of these areas is involved. There is no special treatment for the dysarthric disturbance of speech.

PROGNOSIS The outcome depends on the underlying disease and the magnitude of the lesion within the speech areas. Global aphasias lasting more than a week or two usually have had a bad long-term outcome. Seldom is there enough recovery of communicative speech to permit resumption of occupation or profession. Partial aphasias frequently improve, sometimes to a gratifying degree, if they are of vascular or encephalitic origin. Aphasias due to embolism, whether global or restricted, may disappear in hours to days or may persist. Most aphasias are due to vascular disease of the brain, and

some degree of spontaneous improvement usually occurs over days to months after the stroke. Sometimes recovery is complete within hours or days; at times, not more than a few words are regained after a year or two of assiduous speech training. Nevertheless, many experts in the field believe that speech training is worthwhile. Some of the methods used by specially trained therapists include melodic intonation therapy, which helps those with agrammatism; special programs to improve skills in syntax; and some programs to improve abilities to relate words heard to those seen and improve auditory comprehension at the level of sentences. Thus far, all such therapies have been based on insights into underlying brain mechanisms. When these insights become more firmly grounded, methods may improve, but the daunting problem facing all therapists is not simply to improve partially damaged functions, but to assist the brain in developing brand-new skills using tissues which may have had only marginal roles to play in speech and language before the brain injury.

REFERENCES

ALBERT ML et al: *Clinical Aspects of Dysphasia*. New York, Springer-Verlag, 1981
ALESANDER MP et al: Broca's area aphasias: Aphasia after lesions including the frontal operculum. Neurology 50:353, 1990
CHASE TN et al: Wechsler adult intelligence scale performance cortical localization by fluorodeoxyglucose F18-positron emission tomography. Arch Neurol 41:1244, 1984
COSTELLO AL, WARRINGTON EK: Dynamic aphasia: The selective impairment of verbal planning. Cortex 25:103, 1989
DAMASIO AR: Aphasia. N Engl J Med 325:531, 1992
——— (ed): Behavioral neurology. Sem Neurol 4:117, 1984
HART J, GORDON B: Delineation of single word semantic comprehension deficits in aphasia, with anatomical correlation. Ann Neurol 27:226, 1990
KARBE H et al: Profiles of language impairment in primary progressive aphasia. Arch Neurol 50:193, 1993
KEMPLER D et al: A metabolic investigation of a disconnection syndrome: Conduction aphasia. Ann Neurol 22:134, 1987
KERTESZ A: *Localization in Neuropsychology*. New York, Academic Press, 1983
LECOURS AR et al: *Aphasiology*. London, Bailliere Tindall, 1983
LUDLOW CL et al: Brain lesions associated with nonfluent aphasia fifteen years following penetrating head injury. Brain 109:55, 1986
METTER EJ et al: Brain behavior relationships in aphasia studied by positron emission tomography. Ann NY Acad Sci 620:153, 1991
MOHR JP et al: Broca aphasia: Pathologic and clinical aspects. Neurology 28:311, 1978
OJEMANN G et al: Cortical language localization in left, dominant hemisphere: An electrical stimulation mapping investigation in 117 patients. J Neurosurg 71:316, 1989
PETERSEN SE et al: Positron emission tomography studies of the cortical anatomy of single-word processing. Nature 331:585, 1988
POSNER MI et al: Localization of cognitive operations in the human brain. Science 240:1627, 1988
SHAYWITZ S et al: Evidence that dyslexia may represent the lower tail of a normal distribution of reading ability. N Engl J Med 326:145, 1992
VIGNOLO LA et al: Unexpected CT-scan findings in global aphasia. Cortex 22:55, 1986

29 DISORDERS OF SLEEP AND CIRCADIAN RHYTHMS

CHARLES A. CZEISLER / GARY S. RICHARDSON / JOSEPH B. MARTIN

Disturbed sleep is among the most frequent health complaints physicians encounter. One-third of adults in the United States experience occasional or persistent sleep disturbances. Sleep deprivation or disruption of the circadian timing system can lead to serious impairment of daytime functioning. Sleep disorders may either contribute to or result from related medical or psychiatric conditions. Twenty years ago, many such complaints were treated with hypnotic medications without further diagnostic evaluation. A distinct class of sleep and arousal disorders has now been identified, and the field of sleep disorders is now an established clinical discipline. Two principal neurobiologic systems govern the sleep-wake cycle: one that actively generates sleep and sleep-related processes and another that times sleep within the 24-h day. Either intrinsic abnormalities in these systems or extrinsic disturbances (environmental, drug- or illness-related) can lead to sleep or circadian rhythm disorders.

PHYSIOLOGY OF SLEEP AND WAKEFULNESS

Most adults sleep 7 to 8 h per night, although the timing, duration, and internal structure of sleep vary among apparently healthy individuals and as a function of age. At the extremes, infants and the elderly have frequent interruptions of sleep. In the United States, adults of intermediate age tend to have one consolidated sleep episode per day, although in some cultures sleep may be divided into a midafternoon nap and a shortened night sleep. While there is a wide range of normal sleep lengths, adults with habitual sleep durations of fewer than 4 h or greater than 9 have increased mortality rates as compared to those who sleep 7 to 8 h per night.

STATES AND STAGES OF SLEEP States and stages of human sleep are defined on the basis of characteristic patterns in the electroencephalogram (EEG), the electrooculogram (EOG—a measure of eye-movement activity), and the surface electromyogram (EMG). The continuous recording of this array of electrophysiologic parameters to define sleep and wakefulness is termed *polysomnography* (see Table 29-1).

Polysomnographic profiles define two states of sleep: (1) rapid-eye-movement (REM) sleep (also known as dreaming, paradoxical, desynchronized, or "D" sleep) and (2) non-rapid-eye-movement (NREM) sleep (also known as orthodox, synchronized, or "S" sleep). NREM sleep is in turn subdivided into four stages. NREM stage 1 is the transition from wakefulness and is characterized by disappearance of the regular alpha pattern and emergence of a low-amplitude, mixed-frequency pattern, predominantly in the theta range (2 to 7 Hz) (Fig. 29-1) and slow "rolling" eye movements. NREM stage 2 is defined by the occurrence of K complexes and sleep spindles superimposed upon a background activity similar to that of stage 1. K complexes are slow, high-amplitude, negative (upward) discharges followed immediately by a positive (downward) deflection. Sleep spindles are high-frequency (12 to 14 Hz) discharges lasting 0.5 to 2.0 s with a characteristic waxing-waning amplitude. Rapid-eye-movement activity is absent, and the EMG is similar to stage 1. NREM stage 3 is sleep with at least 20 percent but less than 50 percent high-amplitude (≥ 75 μV) delta (0.5 to 2 Hz) activity. Sleep spindles may persist, eye-movement activity is absent, and EMG activity persists at a reduced level. In NREM stage 4, the high-voltage, slow EEG pattern of stage 3 comprises at least 50 percent of the record. NREM stages 3 and 4 are referred to, collectively, as "slow-wave," "delta," or "deep" sleep.

REM sleep is characterized by a low-amplitude, mixed-frequency EEG similar to that of NREM stage 1 (Fig. 29-1). Bursts of 3- to 5-Hz activity with sharp negative deflections are often superimposed on this pattern. The EOG shows bursts of REM similar to that seen

FIGURE 29-1 Electroencephalogram of human sleep stages. The first trace illustrates alpha activity seen in quiet wakefulness (eyes closed) and the beta activity of an alert subject. Stage 1 theta activity is seen in the second trace; stage 2 sleep (with associated sleep spindle and K complex) in the third. The fourth and fifth traces show slow-wave (stages 3 and 4) sleep, with prominent delta activity. This synchronous activity is absent in REM sleep (sixth trace), which resembles stage 1 EEG. However, REM sleep is accompanied by rapid eye movements and muscle paralysis. (*Reproduced from Horne.*)

during eyes-open wakefulness. EMG activity is absent, reflecting the complete brainstem-mediated muscle atonia that is characteristic of that state.

ORGANIZATION OF HUMAN SLEEP Normal nocturnal sleep in adults displays a consistent organization from night to night (Fig. 29-2). After sleep onset, sleep usually progresses through NREM stages 1 to 4 within 45 to 60 min. Slow-wave sleep predominates in

---

TABLE 29-1 Electrophysiologic correlates of human sleep states and stages

	Electroencephalogram	Electrooculogram	Electromyogram
Wake (eyes open)	Low amplitude, mixed, (high) frequency	Rapid	High, variable
Wake (eyes closed)	Low amplitude, alpha (8–13 Hz) dominates, particularly over occipital region	Absent, but slow "rolling" eye movements	Reduced
NREM stage 1	Low amplitude, mixed frequency (alpha absent)	Slow "rolling" eye movements	Reduced
NREM stage 2	Low amplitude with addition of characteristic EEG patterns (K complexes and sleep spindles)	Absent	Reduced
NREM stage 3	Increased amplitude, decreased frequency 20–50% of record dominated by delta (0.5–2.0 Hz)	Absent	Reduced
NREM stage 4	>50% of record dominated by delta EEG activity	Absent	Reduced
REM	Low amplitude, mixed frequency	Rapid, conjugate	Absent

SOURCE: Modified from: Rechtschaffen A, Kales A (eds): *A Manual of Standardized Terminology, Technique and Scoring System for Sleep Stages of Human Subjects.* Los Angeles, UCLA Brain Information Service/Brain Research Institute, 1968.

FIGURE 29-2 Plots of the stages of REM sleep (solid bars) and the four stages of NREM sleep over the course of the entire night for representative young (upper panel, age 23) and elderly (lower panel, age 68) adult men. The recording in the elderly subject illustrates the reduction of slow-wave sleep, frequent spontaneous awakenings, early sleep onset, and early morning awakening that are characteristic features of sleep in the aged, even in the absence of specific medical or psychiatric pathology. *(From the Center for Circadian and Sleep Disorders Medicine, Brigham and Women' Hospital.)*

the first third of the night and comprises 15 to 25 percent of total nocturnal sleep time in young adults. The percentage of slow-wave sleep is influenced by several factors, most notably age (see below). Prior sleep deprivation increases both the rapidity of slow-wave onset and its percentage of total sleep.

After the first slow-wave sleep episode, the progression of NREM stages reverses; the first REM sleep occurs, usually not less than 80 min after sleep begins, although REM latency shortens with advancing age. More rapid onset of REM sleep in a young adult may (particularly if less than 30 min) suggest pathology such as endogenous depression, narcolepsy, circadian rhythm disorders, or drug withdrawal. NREM and REM alternate through the night with an average cycle of 90 to 110 min (the "ultradian" cycle). As the sleep period lengthens, the portion of each cycle composed of slow-wave sleep decreases and that of REM sleep increases. Overall, REM sleep is 20 to 25 percent of total sleep, NREM stages (1 and 2) are 50 to 60 percent (increasing in elderly subjects).

BEHAVIORAL CORRELATES OF SLEEP STATES AND STAGES
Age has a large impact on sleep state organization (Fig. 29-2). Slow-wave sleep is most prominent during childhood, decreasing sharply at puberty and across the second and third decades of life. After age 30, there is a progressive, almost linear decline in the amount of slow-wave sleep, and the amplitude of delta EEG activity comprising slow-wave sleep is reduced. In the otherwise healthy elderly, slow-wave sleep may be completely absent, particularly in males.

A different age profile exists for REM sleep. In infancy, REM sleep may comprise 50 percent of total sleep time, and the percentage is inversely proportional to developmental age. The amount of REM sleep falls off sharply over the first postnatal year as a mature REM-NREM cycle develops. During the rest of life into extreme old age, REM occupies a more constant percentage of total sleep time than does slow-wave sleep.

Polysomnographic staging of sleep correlates with behavioral changes during specific states and stages. Sleep onset is associated with marked decrements in perception of both auditory and visual stimuli and lapses of consciousness. At stage 1 subjects may respond to faint auditory or visual signals without "awakening." Furthermore, although memory incorporation appears to be inhibited at the onset of NREM stage 1, subjects aroused from that stage frequently deny having been asleep. In contrast, subjective and objective assessments of sleep agree more closely for subjects awakened from NREM stage 2. This has led some investigators to define sleep onset as the occurrence of the first K complex or sleep spindle suggestive of NREM stage 2 and to define NREM stage 1 as a "transitional stage." The progression of subsequent NREM stages corresponds with increasing depth of sleep as measured by threshold for arousal with a variety of auditory stimuli.

Awakenings from REM sleep are associated with recall of vivid dream imagery more than 80 percent of the time. The reliability of dream recall increases with REM periods occurring later in the night.

Imagery may also be reported after NREM sleep interruptions, though these typically lack the detail and vividness of REM dreams. The incidence of NREM dream recall can be increased by selective REM sleep deprivation, suggesting that REM sleep and dreaming per se are not inexorably linked.

PHYSIOLOGIC CORRELATES OF SLEEP STATES AND STAGES
All major physiologic systems are influenced by sleep. In some cases, concomitant behavior changes such as supine posture or inactivity are the proximal causes of altered physiologic function, but in most cases the sleep state itself appears to be responsible. Changes in cardiovascular function include a decrease in blood pressure and heart rate during NREM and particularly during slow-wave sleep. During REM sleep, phasic activity (bursts of eye movements) is associated with variability in both blood pressure and heart rate mediated principally by the vagus. Cardiac dysrhythmias may occur selectively during REM sleep. Respiratory function also changes (see Chap. 229). Respiratory rate and minute ventilation decrease during NREM sleep and become variable during phasic REM sleep. The ventilatory response to carbon dioxide attenuates during NREM sleep, resulting in a higher P_{CO_2}. During REM sleep the ventilatory response to both hypercapnia and hypoxia shows marked variability. Respiratory musculature, including that responsible for upper airway patency, is hypotonic throughout sleep and more so during REM sleep, resulting in an increase in airway resistance. In addition, the cough reflex is attenuated or absent during sleep. These changes in respiratory function may be relevant to the pathogenesis of obstructive sleep apnea (OSA) and sudden infant death syndrome (SIDS) (see Chap. 229).

Endocrine function also varies with sleep. The most prominent changes are apparent in neuroendocrine parameters. Slow-wave sleep is associated with secretion of growth hormone in young men, while sleep in general is associated with augmented secretion of prolactin. Sleep has a complex effect on the secretion of luteinizing hormone (LH); during puberty sleep is associated with increased LH secretion, whereas sleep in the mature woman inhibits LH secretion in the early follicular phase of the menstrual cycle. Sleep onset (and probably slow-wave sleep) is associated with inhibition of thyroid-stimulating hormone (TSH) and of the adrenocorticotropic hormone (ACTH)–cortisol axis, an effect that is independent of the circadian rhythms in the two systems.

Sleep is also associated with alterations of thermoregulatory function. NREM sleep is associated with an attenuation of thermoregulatory responses to either heat or cold stress, and animal studies of thermosensitive neurons in the hypothalamus document a NREM-dependent reduction of the thermoregulatory set-point. REM sleep is associated with complete absence of thermoregulatory responsiveness, effectively resulting in poikilothermy. However, the potential adverse impact of this failure of thermoregulation is blunted by inhibition of REM sleep by extreme ambient temperatures.

Neuroanatomy of sleep   Lesion studies in animals and neurologic diseases in humans have suggested distinct neuroanatomic sites in the generation of normal sleep and wakefulness. The studies of von Economo of patients with encephalitis lethargica suggested that the anterior hypothalamus contained a "sleep center" while the posterior hypothalamus contained a "wake center." Experimental studies in animals have variously implicated the medullary reticular formation, the thalamus, and the basal forebrain in the generation of sleep, while the brainstem reticular formation, the midbrain, the subthalamus, the thalamus, and the basal forebrain have all been suggested to play a role in the generation of wakefulness or EEG arousal (see also Chap. 26).

Despite many studies, there is little evidence for either a single, discrete "sleep center" or a single, discrete "wake center." Current hypotheses suggest that the capacity for sleep and wake generation is distributed along an axial "core" of neurons extending from the brainstem rostrally to the basal forebrain. Complex commingling of neuronal groups occurs at many points along this basal forebrain axis.

Nonetheless, the neuroanatomic correlates of REM sleep appear to be discretely localized. Specific regions in the pons are associated with each of the neurophysiologic correlates of REM sleep. Small lesions in the dorsal pons produce REM sleep without the descending muscle inhibition normally associated with that state; microinjections of carbachol into the same area produce atonia without other features of REM sleep. These experimental manipulations are mimicked by pathologic conditions in humans and animals. In narcolepsy, for example, abrupt, complete or partial paralysis (cataplexy) occurs in response to a variety of stimuli. In dogs with this condition, physostigmine, a central cholinesterase inhibitor, increases the frequency of cataplectic attacks while atropine decreases their frequency. Conversely, in REM sleep behavior disorder (see below), patients suffer from incomplete motor inhibition during REM sleep resulting in involuntary, occasionally violent movement during REM sleep.

Neurochemistry of sleep Early experimental studies that focused on the raphe nuclei of the brainstem appeared to implicate serotonin as the primary sleep-promoting neurotransmitter, while catecholamines were considered to be responsible for wakefulness. Subsequent work has demonstrated that the raphe-serotonin system may facilitate sleep but is not necessary to its expression. The extensive pharmacology of sleep and wakefulness suggests roles for other neurotransmitters as well. The alerting influence of caffeine implicates adenosine, whereas the hypnotic effect of benzodiazepines and barbiturates suggests a role for endogenous ligands of the GABA-receptor complex.

A variety of sleep-promoting substances have been identified. These are principally peptides, and the hypnotic effect is commonly limited to NREM or slow-wave sleep, although peptides that increase REM sleep have also been reported. Many of these "sleep factors," including interleukin 1 and prostaglandin E_2, are immunologically active as well, suggesting a link between immune function and sleep-wake states.

PHYSIOLOGY OF CIRCADIAN RHYTHMICITY The sleep-wake cycle is the most evident of the many 24-h rhythms in humans. Prominent daily variations also occur in endocrine, thermoregulatory, cardiac, pulmonary, renal, gastrointestinal, and cognitive functions. However, in evaluating a daily variation, it is important to distinguish between those rhythmic components passively evoked by periodic environmental or behavioral changes (e.g., the increase in blood pressure and heart rate upon assumption of the upright posture), and those actively driven by an endogenous oscillatory process (e.g., the circadian variation in plasma cortisol that persists under a variety of environmental and behavioral conditions).

The suprachiasmatic nuclei (SCN) of the hypothalamus act as the central neural pacemakers of the circadian timing system in mammals. Bilateral destruction of these nuclei results in a loss of endogenous circadian rhythmicity that can only be restored by transplantation of the same structure(s) from a donor animal. The period and phase of the endogenous neural oscillator are normally synchronized to the 24-h period of the environmental light-dark cycle. Entrainment of mammalian circadian rhythms by the light-dark cycle is mediated via the retinohypothalamic tract, a monosynaptic pathway that links the retina to the SCN.

The principal properties characterizing an endogenous circadian pacemaker are its *intrinsic period, phase, amplitude,* and *resetting capacity*. In human subjects living in controlled laboratory environments free of time cues (*free-running*), the duration of the behavioral rest-activity cycle averages 25 h. However, the timing of the light-dark cycle has generally been uncontrolled in such free-running studies, with the subjects choosing to be exposed to light during their "subjective days" and to darkness during their "subjective nights." Recent work suggests that when the light-dark cycle is controlled, the observed period of the human circadian pacemaker is much closer to 24 h. Nonetheless, synchronization of the endogenous circadian pacemaker to the 24-h day requires that the pacemaker be reset each day, which is normally achieved by exposure to the environmental light-dark cycle.

Exposure to light can shift the phase of the endogenous circadian pacemaker, but both the magnitude and direction of the phase shifts induced by light depend on the timing and intensity of the light. Properly timed exposure to light of sufficient intensity can, within 2 to 3 days, reset the human circadian pacemaker (presumably the SCN) to any desired hour.

The timing and internal architecture of sleep are directly coupled to the output of the endogenous pacemaker. Spontaneous sleep duration, sleepiness, REM sleep propensity, and both the ability and the tendency to sleep vary with the circadian phase as marked by the endogenous circadian temperature cycle in humans. Sleep tendency, sleepiness, and REM sleep propensity all peak just after the nadir of the endogenous circadian temperature cycle (approximately 2 to 3 h before awakening). In addition, 85 percent of all spontaneous awakenings of subjects living in constant environmental conditions occur on the rising slope of the temperature cycle. Furthermore, there are certain times (wake maintenance zones) when it is very difficult to fall asleep, even for subjects who are sleep-deprived. Misalignment of the output of the endogenous circadian pacemaker with the desired sleep-wake cycle is thought to be responsible for certain types of insomnia, as well as for the decrements of alertness and performance in night-shift workers and after jet lag.

DISORDERS OF SLEEP AND WAKEFULNESS

An international classification of sleep disorders (Table 29-2) divides these conditions into three major groups: dyssomnias, parasomnias, and medical psychiatric sleep disorders. A detailed description of each of these disorders may be found in the publication of the American Sleep Disorders Association.

APPROACH TO THE PATIENT WITH A SLEEP COMPLAINT Patients may seek help from a physician because of: (1) an acute or chronic inability to sleep adequately at night; (2) chronic fatigue, sleepiness, or tiredness during the day; or (3) a behavioral manifestation associated with sleep itself. Disruption or disturbance of nocturnal sleep is directly related to decreased alertness and impairment of daytime cognitive and psychomotor performance, which is often of serious concern to the patient.

Taking a careful history is critical in the evaluation of the patient with a sleep complaint. In particular, the duration, severity, and consistency of the complaint are important, along with the patient's estimate—in the case of an insomnia complaint—of the consequences of reported sleep loss on subsequent waking function. Information from a friend or family member can be an invaluable aid in assessing the severity of the complaint on daytime functioning, as some patients will underreport such potentially embarrassing symptoms as heavy snoring or falling asleep while driving.

Retrospective completion by the physician and patient of a day-by-day sleep-work-drug log in reverse chronologic order can help the physician better understand the nature of the complaint. Work times should be specified each day, as one in six working men and one in

TABLE 29-2   International classification of sleep disorders

DYSSOMNIAS

A Intrinsic sleep disorders
  1 Psychophysiologic insomnia
  2 Idiopathic insomnia
  3 Narcolepsy
  4 Recurrent or idiopathic hypersomnia
  5 Posttraumatic hypersomnia
  6 Sleep apnea syndromes
  7 Periodic limb movement disorder
  8 Restless legs syndrome
B Extrinsic sleep disorders
  1 Inadequate sleep hygiene
  2 Environmental sleep disorder
  3 Altitude insomnia
  4 Adjustment sleep disorder
  5 Sleep-onset association disorder
  6 Food allergy insomnia
  7 Nocturnal eating (drinking) syndrome
  8 Drug- or alcohol-dependent sleep disorders
C Circadian rhythm sleep disorders
  1 Time-zone change (jet-lag) syndrome
  2 Shift-work sleep disorder
  3 Delayed sleep phase syndrome
  4 Advanced sleep phase syndrome
  5 Non-24-h sleep-wake disorder

PARASOMNIAS

A Arousal disorders
  1 Confusional arousals
  2 Sleepwalking
  3 Sleep terrors
B Sleep-wake transition disorders
  1 Rhythmic movement disorder
  2 Sleep talking
  3 Nocturnal leg cramps
C Parasomnias usually associated with REM sleep
  1 Nightmares
  2 Sleep paralysis
  3 Impaired sleep-related penile erections
  4 Sleep-related painful erections
  5 REM sleep-related cardiac arrhythmias
  6 REM sleep behavior disorder
D Other parasomnias
  1 Sleep bruxism
  2 Sleep enuresis
  3 Nocturnal paroxysmal dystonia

SLEEP DISORDERS ASSOCIATED WITH MEDICAL/PSYCHIATRIC DISORDERS

A Associated with mental disorders
B Associated with neurologic disorders
  1 Cerebral degenerative disorders
  2 Parkinsonism
  3 Fatal familial insomnia
  4 Sleep-related epilepsy
  5 Sleep-related headaches
C Associated with other medical disorders
  1 Sleeping sickness
  2 Nocturnal cardiac ischemia
  3 Chronic obstructive pulmonary disease
  4 Sleep-related asthma
  5 Sleep-related gastroesophageal reflux
  6 Peptic ulcer disease
  7 Fibrositis syndrome

SOURCE: Modified from *International Classification of Sleep Disorders*, prepared by the Diagnostic Classification Steering Committee, Thorpy MJ, Chairman. Rochester, MN, American Sleep Disorders Association, 1990.

eight working women in the United States have an irregular work schedule that includes both day and night/evening work. Drug and alcohol use, including caffeine and hypnotics, should be noted each day. This log should be compared with a prospective sleep-work-drug log (including daytime naps and nocturnal awakenings) as recorded by the patient for at least 2 weeks. The resultant data should be plotted to facilitate recognition of circadian rhythm sleep disorders such as delayed sleep phase syndrome (see below). With the advent of objective measurements of sleep tendency (see below), quantifica-

tion of the impairment of daytime alertness is a valuable adjunct in the assessment of sleep problems. As a rule, the clinical approach to a patient with disrupted sleep but without impaired daytime alertness should be conservative. Chronic treatment of isolated insomnia with hypnotic medications is rarely justified.

Laboratory investigation   In addition to the three electrophysiologic variables used to define sleep states and stages (see above), the standard clinical polysomnogram includes measures of respiration (respiratory effort, air flow, and oxygen saturation), anterior tibialis EMG, and ECG. Evaluation of penile tumescence during nocturnal sleep also can be used to help determine whether the cause of erectile dysfunction in a patient is psychogenic or organic (see Chap. 47).

Assessment of daytime functioning as an index of the adequacy of sleep can be made with the multiple sleep latency test (MSLT), which involves repeated measurement of sleep latency (time to onset of sleep) under standardized conditions during a day following quantified nocturnal sleep. The average latency across four to six tests (administered every 2 h across the waking day) is taken as an objective measure of daytime sleep tendency. Disorders of sleep that result in pathologic, daytime somnolence can be reliably distinguished with the MSLT. In addition, the multiple measurements of sleep onset identify direct transitions from wakefulness to REM sleep that are indicative of specific pathologic conditions (e.g., narcolepsy).

INSOMNIA   Insomnia is the complaint of inadequate sleep; it is classified according to the nature of sleep disruption and the duration of the complaint. The nature of the sleep disruption provides important information about the possible etiology of the insomnia and is also central to the selection of specific and appropriate treatment. Insomnia is subdivided into difficulty falling asleep (*sleep onset insomnia*), frequent or sustained awakenings (*sleep maintenance insomnia*), or persistent sleepiness despite sleep of adequate duration (*nonrestorative sleep*). Similarly, the duration of the symptom is an important determinant of the nature of appropriate treatment. An insomnia complaint lasting one to several nights (within a single episode) is termed *transient insomnia*. Transient insomnia is typically the result of situational stress or a change in work schedule or environment (jet lag). *Short-term insomnia* lasts from a few days to 3 weeks. Disruption of this duration is usually associated with more protracted stress, such as recovery from surgery or short-term illness. *Long-term* or *chronic insomnia* lasts for months or years and commonly reflects the effects of psychiatric or other chronic medical conditions, medications, or a primary sleep disorder (see below). It is now clear that chronic insomnia may present as recurrent episodes of insomnia, not necessarily associated with parallel variation in the underlying cause. Although some clinicians refer to this as recurrent insomnia, others suggest that this may be the typical pattern of all chronic insomniacs.

While an occasional night of poor sleep, typically in the setting of stress or excitement about external events, is both common and without lasting consequences, persistent insomnia can have important adverse consequences in the form of impaired daytime function, mood disturbances, and increased risk of injury due to accidents. A complaint of persistent insomnia warrants specific investigation as to cause and intervention with appropriately designed treatment for either the underlying mechanism and/or the sleep disruption.

Psychophysiologic insomnia   Persistent psychophysiologic insomnia is a behavioral disorder in which patients are preoccupied with a perceived inability to sleep at night. The sleep disturbance is often triggered by an emotionally stressful event; however, the poor sleep habits acquired during the stressful period persist long after the initial incident. Such patients become hyperaroused by their own persistent efforts to sleep, and the insomnia is a conditioned or learned response. Patients with psychophysiologic insomnia fall asleep more easily at unscheduled times (when not trying) or outside the home environment. In these cases, polysomnographic recording reveals an objective sleep disturbance, often with an abnormally long sleep latency, frequent nocturnal awakenings, and an increased amount of stage 1 transitional sleep. Behavioral therapy is often beneficial; relaxation training can improve the sleep of patients in whom physical tension is prominent. Limited use of hypnotic medications, which can serve as a catalyst for successful behavioral therapy, may be appropriate. Extrinsic factors may contribute to this condition (see below). Rigorous attention should be paid to sleep hygiene (see below) and correction of counterproductive, arousing behaviors before bedtime.

Extrinsic insomnia   A number of sleep disorders are the result of extrinsic factors that interfere with sleep. *Adjustment sleep disorder*, also called *transient situational insomnia*, can occur after a change in the sleeping environment (e.g., in an unfamiliar hotel or hospital bed) or before or after a significant life event, such as a change of occupation, loss of a loved one, illness, or anxiety over a deadline or examination. Increased sleep latency, frequent awakenings from sleep, and early morning awakening can all occur. Recovery generally occurs rapidly, certainly within 2 to 3 weeks. *Inadequate sleep hygiene* is characterized by a behavior pattern prior to sleep and/or a bedroom environment that is not conducive to sleep. On taking a careful history, physicians may learn that some insomniac patients are attempting to sleep with the television on throughout the night or are attempting to sleep just after coming home from work at midnight. Noise and/or light in the bedroom can interfere with sleep, as can a bed partner with periodic limb movements during sleep or one who snores loudly. Luminous clocks can arouse the patient, heightening anxiety about the time it has taken to fall asleep. Drugs that act on the central nervous system, large meals, vigorous exercise, or hot showers just before sleep may interfere with sleep onset. In preference to hypnotic medications, patients should be counseled to develop a soporific bedtime ritual and to prepare and reserve the bedroom environment for sleeping. Consistent, regular rising times should be charted daily; irregular naps should be avoided; total time in bed should be restricted to actual sleep time.

Altitude insomnia   Sleep disturbance is a common consequence of exposure to high altitude. Periodic breathing of the Cheyne-Stokes type occurs during NREM sleep about half the time at altitude, with restoration of a regular breathing pattern during REM sleep. Central rather than obstructive sleep apnea appears to be responsible, characterized by regular respiratory pauses. Both hypoxia and hypocapnia are thought to be involved in the development of periodic breathing. Frequent awakenings and poor quality sleep characterize altitude insomnia, which is generally worst on the first few nights at high altitude but may persist. The duration of sleep is unchanged, but there are more arousals after sleep onset and less time in slow-wave (stages 3 and 4) sleep. Pretreatment with acetazolamide can decrease time spent in periodic breathing and substantially reduce hypoxia during sleep. Medroxyprogesterone acetate (MPA) also reduces periodic breathing but does not significantly reduce hypoxia during sleep at altitude.

Drug- or alcohol-dependent sleep disorders   Disturbed sleep can result from ingestion of a wide variety of agents. Caffeine is perhaps the most common pharmacologic cause of insomnia in sensitive patients. It produces increased latency to sleep onset, more frequent arousals during sleep, and a reduction in total sleep time for up to 8 to 14 h after ingestion. Occasional patients are surprised to learn that their insomnia may be related to coffee consumption; a careful history will reveal that such patients may drink 15 to 20 cups per day. As few as 3 to 5 cups of coffee can significantly disturb sleep in some patients; therefore, a 1- to 2-month caffeine withdrawal period should be attempted in patients with these symptoms. Similarly, alcohol and nicotine can interfere with sleep, although many patients use them to relax and promote sleep. Although alcohol can increase drowsiness and shorten sleep latency, even moderate amounts of alcohol increase awakenings after sleep onset by interfering with the ability of the brain to maintain sleep. In addition, alcohol ingestion prior to sleep is contraindicated in patients with sleep apnea because of the inhibitory effects of alcohol on respiration. Acutely, amphetamines and cocaine suppress both REM sleep and total sleep time, which return to normal with chronic use. Withdrawal leads to a REM sleep rebound. Finally, rebound insomnia associated with the acute

withdrawal of hypnotics can be severe, especially following the use of benzodiazepines with a short half-life. For this reason, hypnotics should rarely be prescribed for habitual use; doses should be low to moderate, the total duration of hypnotic therapy should be limited to 2 to 3 weeks, and drug dosage should be reduced prior to withdrawal.

NARCOLEPSY   Excessive daytime sleepiness with involuntary daytime sleep episodes, disturbed nocturnal sleep, and cataplexy (sudden weakness or loss of muscle tone, often elicited by emotion) are the most common symptoms of narcolepsy. Some patients also experience muscular paralysis and/or hallucinations at sleep onset or upon awakening. The severity varies. Patients may have two to three cataplectic attacks per day or per decade, and the extent and duration of an attack may vary from a transient sagging of the jaw to flaccid paralysis of the entire voluntary musculature for up to 20 to 30 min, in rare cases.

Narcolepsy affects over 200,000 people in the United States and appears to have a genetic basis. Experiments in some canine models of narcolepsy suggest an autosomal recessive pattern of inheritance. First-degree relatives of narcoleptic patients commonly exhibit excessive daytime somnolence and have a much higher incidence of narcolepsy than the general population. In addition, nearly all narcoleptics are positive for the human leukocyte antigen DR2 (ordinarily found in 20 to 30 percent of the general population) (see Chap. 64).

Symptoms typically begin in the second decade, although the onset ranges from ages 5 to 50. An identifiable stress (e.g., sleep-wake cycle disruption, divorce, loss of a loved one) may precede symptom onset.

Diagnosis   Classically, the diagnosis of narcolepsy required the presence of the "narcolepsy tetrad," consisting of (1) excessive daytime somnolence, (2) cataplexy, (3) hypnogogic hallucinations (the occurrence of vivid hallucinatory dream imagery at sleep onset), and (4) sleep paralysis (an awareness that voluntary musculature is paralyzed coincident with the onset of sleep). The last three symptoms of the tetrad are all manifestations of the abnormal REM sleep regulation inherent in the syndrome. All patients with narcolepsy have objectively verifiable daytime somnolence, but the other three symptoms are variably present. At least half have cataplexy of some degree and smaller percentages report hypnogogic hallucinations and/or sleep paralysis. Other associated symptoms are useful but not specific. A history of "automatic behavior" during wakefulness (a trancelike state during which simple motor behaviors persist) serves principally to corroborate the presence of daytime somnolence but is not specific for mechanism. Older patients with narcolepsy also commonly report severe disruption of nocturnal sleep.

A family history is important in the evaluation of the patient with excessive daytime somnolence. Careful observation of the children and siblings of known narcoleptics, particularly at the typical age of onset (second decade), can lead to early diagnosis. The diagnosis of narcolepsy in a patient with a suggestive history depends upon (1) objective verification of excessive daytime somnolence, typically using the MSLT after nocturnal sleep recording, and (2) documentation of abnormal REM sleep regulation as evidenced by REM sleep onset within 10 min of sleep onset, either during the nocturnal recording or on one or more of the MSLT determinations.

Treatment   The treatment of narcolepsy is symptomatic. Somnolence is treated with stimulants. Methylphenidate is considered the drug of choice by most. Pemoline, a common second choice, has a longer half-life and is associated with fewer side effects but may not be as effective. Dextroamphetamine and methamphetamine are also frequently used, particularly when methylphenidate and pemoline are inadequate.

Treatment of cataplexy, hypnogogic hallucinations, and sleep paralysis requires antidepressants, which are effective, in part, because of potent REM-suppressive effects. Protriptyline is the most commonly used anti-cataplectic in the United States. Efficacy is limited largely by anticholinergic side effects. Compounds including viloxzine hydrochloride and fluoxetine are under evaluation for this condition.

Gamma-hydroxy-butyrate (GHB), a drug available in Europe and Canada but still under evaluation in the United States, appears to be particularly useful to reverse nocturnal sleep disruption.

SLEEP APNEA SYNDROMES Respiratory dysfunction during sleep is a common, serious cause of excessive daytime somnolence as well as of disturbed nocturnal sleep. An estimated 2 to 5 million people in the United States stop breathing for 15 to 150 s, from a dozen to several hundred times every night during sleep. These cessations of breathing may be due to either an occlusion of the airway (*obstructive sleep apnea*), absence of respiratory effort (*central sleep apnea*), or a combination of these factors (*mixed sleep apnea*). Failure to recognize and appropriately treat these conditions may lead to serious cardiovascular complications and increased mortality. This problem is particularly prevalent in overweight men and in the elderly and is often associated with hypertension. Occult sleep-related breathing disorders may result in significant impairment of daytime alertness and functioning in otherwise healthy elderly persons. Readers are referred to Chap. 229 for a comprehensive review of the diagnosis and treatment of patients with these conditions.

DYSSOMNIA ASSOCIATED WITH LIMB MOVEMENTS Restless legs syndrome Patients with dyssomnia associated with the restless legs syndrome report an irresistible urge to move their legs when awake and inactive, especially when lying in bed just prior to sleep. This interferes with the ability to fall asleep. They report a creeping or crawling sensation deep within the calves or thighs, or sometimes even in the upper limbs, that is only relieved briefly by movement, particularly walking. In contrast, paresthesia secondary to peripheral neuropathy persists with activity. The severity of this chronic, idiopathic disorder may wax and wane with time and can be exacerbated by caffeine, iron deficiency, anemia, renal failure, and pregnancy. Nearly all patients with restless legs also experience periodic limb movement disorder during sleep, although the reverse is not the case. Together, these conditions can be documented in one-eighth of patients with insomnia seen at sleep disorders centers, although they are often thought to be an incidental finding rather than the cause of disturbed sleep.

Periodic limb movement disorder Periodic limb movement disorder, also known as *nocturnal myoclonus*, is the principal objective polysomnographic finding in 17 percent of patients with insomnia and 11 percent of those with excessive daytime somnolence. Stereotyped, rhythmic, 0.5- to 5.0-s extensions of the great toe and dorsiflexion of the foot recur every 20 to 40 s during NREM stages 1 and 2 sleep, in episodes lasting from minutes to hours. Most such episodes occur during the first half of the night. The disorder occurs in a wide variety of sleep disorders (including narcolepsy, sleep apnea, and various forms of insomnia) and is associated with frequent arousals and an increased number of sleep-stage transitions. However, it has not been demonstrated that these sleep disturbances lead to insomnia. In fact, periodic limb movement may be secondary to chronic sleep-wake disturbance rather than the cause of it. The incidence increases with age; 44 percent of healthy subjects over age 65 without a sleep complaint and almost all patients with the restless legs syndrome have periodic limb movements (see below). The pathophysiology is not well understood. Polysomnography with bilateral surface EMG recording of the anterior tibialis, extensor carpi radialis, triceps and/or biceps is used to establish the diagnosis. Treatment options are limited; some patients may respond to a combination of carbidopa and levodopa, clonazepam, or levodopa alone.

PARASOMNIAS The term *parasomnia* refers to behavioral disorders during sleep that are associated with brief or partial arousals but not with marked sleep disruption or impaired daytime alertness. The presenting complaint is usually related to the behavior itself. Most are more common in children but may persist into adulthood when their occurrence may have more pathologic significance.

Sleepwalking (somnambulism) Patients affected by this disorder carry out automatic motor activities that range from minor to complex. Individuals may leave the bed, walk, urinate inappropriately, or exit from the house while remaining unconscious or uncommunica-

tive. Arousal is difficult, and untoward or even fatal activities can occur. Sleepwalking occurs in stage 3 or 4 NREM sleep. It is most common in children and adolescents. Episodes are usually isolated but may be recurrent in 1 to 6 percent of patients. The cause is unknown.

Sleep terrors This disorder, also called *pavor nocturnus*, occurs primarily in young children during the first several hours after sleep onset, in stages 3 and 4 of NREM sleep. The child suddenly screams, exhibiting autonomic arousal with sweating, tachycardia, and hyperventilation. The individual may be difficult to arouse and rarely recalls the episode on awakening in the morning. Recurrent attacks are rare, and treatment is usually by way of reassurance of parents. Both sleep terrors and sleepwalking represent abnormalities of arousal. In contrast, *nightmares* (dream anxiety attacks) occur during REM sleep and cause full arousal, with memory for the dream-associated unpleasant episode.

REM sleep behavior disorder This is a rare parasomnia arising from REM sleep instead of slow-wave sleep, as is characteristic of the other, more common parasomnias. It primarily afflicts men of middle age or older, many of whom have a history of prior neurologic disease (e.g., degenerative diseases, Guillain-Barré syndrome, dementia, subarachnoid hemorrhage, stroke). Presenting symptoms are of violent behavior during sleep, reported by a bed partner. In contrast to typical somnambulism, injury to patient or bystander is common, and, upon awakening, the patient reports vivid, often unpleasant dream imagery. The principal differential diagnosis is that of nocturnal seizures, which can be excluded with polysomnography. In REM sleep behavior disorder, seizure activity is absent, and the EEG/EOG REM sleep pattern exhibits a high-amplitude EMG. Complex, purposeful motor behavior occurs during REM sleep episodes. The pathogenesis is unclear, but the preexisting neurologic disease may have involved brainstem areas responsible for descending motor inhibition during REM sleep. In support of this hypothesis are the remarkable similarities between the REM sleep behavior disorder and the sleep of animals with bilateral lesions of the pontine tegmentum in areas controlling REM sleep motor inhibition. Treatment with clonazepam provides sustained improvement in almost all reported cases.

Sleep bruxism Bruxism is an involuntary, forceful grinding of teeth during sleep that affects 10 to 20 percent of the population. The patient is usually unaware of the problem, and data on this parasomnia come from roommates and bed partners, alarmed by the loud grinding noise, and from dentists who see evidence of destruction of tooth enamel and dentum. The typical age of onset is 17 to 20 years, and spontaneous remission usually occurs by age 40. Sex distribution appears to be equal.

Hypotheses about the pathophysiology suggest contributory roles for dental abnormalities, e.g., malocclusion, and for central neural mechanisms. Psychological factors may also play a role in that stress exacerbates the disorder. Treatment is dictated by the risk of dental injury. In many cases, the diagnosis is made during dental examination, damage is minor, and no treatment is indicated. In more severe cases, treatment with a rubber tooth guard is necessary to prevent permanent and disfiguring tooth injury. Stress management or, in some cases, biofeedback can be useful when bruxism is a manifestation of severe stress. Useful pharmacologic therapy has not been described.

Sleep enuresis Bedwetting, like sleepwalking and night terrors, is another parasomnia occurring during slow-wave sleep in the young. Before age 5 or 6, nocturnal enuresis should probably be considered a normal feature of development. The condition usually spontaneously improves at puberty, has a prevalence in late adolescence of 1 to 3 percent, and is rare in adulthood. The age threshold for initiation of treatment depends on parental and patient concern about the problem. Persistence of enuresis into adolescence or adulthood may reflect a variety of underlying conditions. In older patients with enuresis a distinction must be made between primary and secondary enuresis, the latter being defined as bedwetting in patients who have been fully continent for 6 to 12 months. Treatment of primary enuresis is reserved for patients of appropriate age (older than 5 or 6 years) and consists of bladder training exercises and behavioral therapy. Urologic abnormalities are more common in primary enuresis and must be assessed by urologic examination. Important causes of secondary enuresis include emotional disturbances, urinary tract infections, cauda equina lesions, epilepsy, sleep apnea, and urinary tract malformations. In the patient for whom enuresis may be a source of significant stress, symptomatic pharmacotherapy may be appropriate while attention is also paid to underlying causes. This is usually accomplished with oxybutynin chloride or imipramine. Intranasal desmopressin has been used in some patients.

Miscellaneous parasomnias Other clinical entities fulfill the definition of a parasomnia in that they occur selectively during sleep and are associated with some degree of sleep disruption. Examples include *jactatio capitis nocturna* (nocturnal headbanging), sleep talking, and nocturnal leg cramps.

SLEEP DISORDERS ASSOCIATED WITH MEDICAL/PSYCHIATRIC DISORDERS **Sleep disorders associated with mental disorders** Although some differences are present in sleep architecture and physiology in *schizophrenia* (such as a decreased amount of stage 4 sleep and a lack of augmentation of REM sleep following REM sleep deprivation), chronic schizophrenics usually sleep well. In contrast, patients with other psychiatric disorders (anxiety disorders, affective illness, obsessive-compulsive disorders, and chronic alcoholism) often sleep poorly. There is considerable heterogeneity, however, in the nature of the sleep disturbance both between conditions and among patients with the same condition.

Depression can be associated with sleep onset insomnia, sleep maintenance insomnia, and/or early morning wakefulness. However, hypersomnia occurs in some depressed patients, especially adolescents and those with either bipolar or seasonal (fall/winter) depression (see also Chap. 389). Indeed, sleep disturbance is an important vegetative sign of depression and may commence before any mood changes are perceived by the patient and then return to normal at the beginning of remission. Consistent polysomnographic findings in depression include decreased REM sleep latency, lengthened first REM sleep episode, and shortened first NREM sleep episode; however, these findings are not specific for depression and the extent of these changes varies with age and symptomatology.

In *mania* and *hypomania*, sleep latency is increased, and total sleep time can be reduced. Patients with *obsessive-compulsive disorders* have sleep disturbances similar to those of endogenously depressed patients. Finally, *chronic alcoholics* lack slow-wave sleep, have decreased amounts of REM sleep, and have frequent arousals throughout the night. This is associated with impaired daytime alertness. The sleep of chronic alcoholics remains disturbed for years after discontinuance of alcohol usage.

Sleep disorders associated with neurologic disorders A variety of neurologic diseases result in sleep disruption through both indirect, nonspecific mechanisms (e.g., pain in cervical spondylosis or low back pain) or by impairment of central neural structures involved in the generation and control of sleep itself.

For example, the dementias have long been associated with disturbances in the timing of the sleep-wake cycle, often characterized by nocturnal wandering and an exacerbation of symptomatology at night (so-called sundowning). Such clinical observations are consistent with the recent neuropathologic finding that 80 percent of the cells in the hypothalamic circadian pacemaker (the SCN) are lost in patients with senile dementia (Alzheimer's disease), though a causal association remains unproven.

Epilepsy may rarely present as a sleep complaint (see also Chap. 367). Often the history is of abnormal, occasionally violent activity during sleep, and the differential diagnosis includes REM sleep behavior disorder, sleep apnea syndrome, and periodic movements of sleep (see above). Diagnosis requires nocturnal EEG recording. Other neurologic diseases associated with abnormal movements, such as *Parkinson's disease, hemiballismus, Huntington's chorea*, and *Gilles de la Tourette syndrome*, are also associated with disrupted

sleep, presumably through secondary mechanisms. Headache syndromes may show sleep-associated exacerbations (*migraine* or *cluster headache*) (see also Chap. 14). The mechanism of association between sleep and headache is unknown.

Fatal familial insomnia is a rare hereditary disorder caused by bilateral degeneration of anterior and dorsomedial nuclei of the thalamus. Insomnia is a prominent early symptom. Progressively, the syndrome produces autonomic dysfunction, dysarthria, myoclonus, coma, and death. The pathogenesis of the thalamic destruction is unknown.

Sleep disorders associated with other medical disorders A number of medical conditions are associated with disruptions of sleep. The association may be nonspecific, for example, that between sleep disruption and chronic pain from rheumatologic disorders. Attention to this association is important in that sleep-associated symptoms are the presenting complaint of many such patients. In addition, sleep disruption may stem from the appropriate use of drugs such as steroids or from the symptoms of another illness.

Among the most prominent associations is that between sleep disruption and *asthma*. In many asthmatics there is a prominent daily variation in airway resistance, probably related to daily rhythms in catecholamine and histamine levels, which results in marked increases in asthmatic symptoms at night. In addition, treatment of asthma with theophylline-based compounds, adrenergic agonists, or glucocorticoids can independently disrupt sleep. When sleep disruption is a prominent side effect of asthma treatment, inhaled steroids (e.g., beclomethasone) that do not disrupt sleep may provide a useful alternative.

Cardiac ischemia may also be associated with sleep disruption. Variability in autonomic nervous system function during REM sleep may account for the association of sleep and angina, although this remains unproven. Patients may present with complaints of nightmares or vivid, disturbing dreams, with or without awareness of the more classical symptoms of angina. *Paroxysmal nocturnal dyspnea* can also occur as a consequence of sleep-associated cardiac ischemia that causes pulmonary congestion exacerbated by recumbent posture.

Chronic obstructive pulmonary disease is also associated with sleep disruption, the pathogenesis of which is presumed to be sleep-related exacerbation of hypoxia and hypercapnia secondary to alveolar hypoventilation. In addition, recumbent posture results in suboptimal ventilation-perfusion ratios. Other conditions associated with sleep disruption include *cystic fibrosis, menopause, hyperthyroidism, gastroesophageal reflux, chronic renal failure*, and *liver failure*.

CIRCADIAN RHYTHM SLEEP DISORDERS

A subset of patients presenting with either insomnia or hypersomnia may have a disorder of sleep *timing* rather than sleep *generation*. Disorders of sleep timing can either be organic (i.e., due to an intrinsic defect in the circadian pacemaker or its responsiveness to entraining stimuli) or environmental (i.e., due to a disruption of exposure to entraining stimuli from the environment). Regardless of etiology, the symptoms reflect the influence of the underlying circadian pacemaker on sleep-wake function. Thus, effective therapeutic approaches should aim to entrain the oscillator at an appropriate phase.

ENDOGENOUS CIRCADIAN PHASE ASSESSMENT Abnormal synchronization of the circadian pacemaker to the 24-h day can be assessed clinically by studying patients under standardized behavioral and environmental conditions. Exogenous factors (such as variations in light exposure, room temperature, activity level, posture, nutritional intake), which can evoke physiologic responses, must be held constant to assess the phase and amplitude of endogenous circadian rhythms. Patients are studied for 30 to 50 h of enforced semirecumbent wakefulness in constant indoor room light, with their daily nutritional and fluid intake equally divided into hourly snacks. During such a constant routine, the body temperature cycle serves as a reliable marker of the output of the endogenous circadian pacemaker. In normal young men, the endogenous component of the body temperature cycle under such conditions reaches its nadir about 2 to 3 h before the habitual waketime. The technique can be used to determine whether there is an organic basis consistent with a diagnosis of delayed sleep phase syndrome, non-24-h sleep-wake schedule, or advanced sleep phase syndrome.

RAPID TIME-ZONE CHANGE (JET LAG) SYNDROME   More than 60 million people experience transmeridian air travel annually, which is often associated with excessive daytime sleepiness, sleep onset insomnia, and frequent arousals from sleep, particularly in the latter half of the night. Gastrointestinal discomfort is common. The syndrome is transient, typically lasting 2 to 14 days depending on the number of time zones crossed, the direction of travel, and the traveler's age and phase-shifting capacity. Travelers who spend more time outdoors reportedly adapt more quickly than those who remain in hotel rooms, presumably due to bright (outdoor) light exposure.

SHIFT-WORK SLEEP DISORDER   About 7 million workers in the United States regularly work at night, either on a permanent or rotating schedule. Studies of shift workers indicate that the circadian timing system of the average night-shift worker fails to adapt successfully to such work schedules. This leads to a misalignment between the desired work-rest schedule and the output of the pacemaker and in disturbed daytime sleep. Consequent sleep deprivation and misalignment of circadian phase produce decreased alertness and performance and cause increased safety hazards among night-shift workers. In addition, shift workers are believed to have higher rates of cardiac, gastrointestinal, and reproductive disorders.

Treatment must be aimed at minimizing both circadian disruption and sleep deprivation. The work schedule should: (1) favor a phase delay (clockwise) direction of shift rotation; (2) minimize the frequency of shift rotation so that shifts do not rotate more than once every 2 to 3 weeks; and (3) reduce the number of consecutive days worked at night from 7 (which is typical) to 4 or 5. These steps can lead to marked improvements in employee health and performance and to reduced accident rates among shift workers. Future approaches may include strategic use of bright-light exposure to facilitate rapid adaptation to night shift work.

DELAYED SLEEP PHASE SYNDROME   Delayed sleep phase syndrome is characterized by: (1) reported sleep onset and wake times intractably later than desired; (2) actual sleep times at nearly the same clock hours daily; and (3) essentially normal all-night polysomnography except for delayed sleep onset. Patients exhibit an abnormally delayed endogenous circadian phase, with the temperature minimum during the constant routine occurring later than normal. This delayed phase could be due to: (1) an abnormally long intrinsic period of the endogenous circadian pacemaker; (2) an abnormally reduced phase-advancing capacity of the pacemaker; or (3) an irregular prior sleep-wake schedule, characterized by frequent nights when the patient chooses to remain awake well past midnight (for social, school, or work reasons). In most cases, it is difficult to distinguish among these factors, since patients with an abnormally long intrinsic period are more likely to ''choose'' such late-night activities because they are unable to sleep at that time. Patients tend to be young adults. This self-perpetuating condition can persist for years and does not usually respond to attempts to reestablish normal bedtime hours.

Patients respond to a rescheduling regimen in which bedtimes are successively delayed by about 3 h per day until the desired (and earlier) bedtime is achieved. Treatment methods involving bright-light phototherapy during the morning hours also show promise in these patients.

ADVANCED SLEEP PHASE SYNDROME   Advanced sleep phase syndrome is the converse of the delayed sleep phase syndrome and tends to occur in the elderly. Patients with this condition report excessive daytime sleepiness during the evening hours, when they have great difficulty remaining awake, even in social settings. The patients awaken from 3 to 5 A.M. each day, often several hours before their desired wake times. Although such patients have not been studied extensively, some of these patients may benefit from bright-light phototherapy during the evening hours, designed to reset the circadian pacemaker to a later hour.

NON-24-H SLEEP-WAKE DISORDER   This condition occurs when the maximal phase-advancing capacity of the circadian pacemaker is not adequate to accommodate the difference between the 24-h geophysical day and the intrinsic period of the pacemaker in the patient. Patients affected are not able to maintain a stable phase relationship between the output of the pacemaker and the 24-h day. Such patients typically present with an incremental pattern of successive delays in sleep onsets and wake times, progressing in and out of phase with local time. When the patient's endogenous rhythms are out of phase with the local environment, insomnia coexists with excessive daytime sleepiness. Conversely, when the endogenous rhythms are in phase with the local environment, symptoms remit. The intervals of alternation between symptomatic vs. asymptomatic intervals may last several weeks to several months. Blind subjects unable to perceive light are particularly susceptible to this disorder.

MEDICAL IMPLICATIONS OF CIRCADIAN RHYTHMICITY   Understanding the role of circadian rhythmicity in the pathophysiology of illness may lead to improvements in diagnosis and treatment. For example, prominent circadian variations have been reported in the incidence of *acute myocardial infarction*, *sudden cardiac death*, and *stroke*, the leading causes of death in the United States. Platelet aggregability is increased after arising in the early morning hours, coincident with the peak incidence of these cardiovascular events. A better understanding of the possible role of circadian rhythmicity in the acute destabilization of a chronic condition such as atherosclerotic disease could improve the understanding of the pathophysiology.

Diagnostic and therapeutic procedures may also be affected by the time of day at which data are collected. Examples include blood pressure, body temperature, the dexamethasone suppression test, and plasma cortisol levels. The timing of chemotherapy administration has been reported to have an effect on the outcome of treatment. Few physicians realize the extent to which routine measures are affected by the time (or sleep/wake state) when the measurement is made.

In addition, both the toxicity and effectiveness of drugs can vary during the day. For example, more than a fivefold difference has been observed in mortality rates following administration of toxic agents to experimental animals at different times of day. Anesthetic agents are particularly sensitive to time-of-day effects.

Finally, it should be noted that the risk of errors and accidents due to inattention and/or sleepiness varies markedly with the time of day. Single-vehicle truck accidents, industrial errors and accidents, and lapses of attention all peak during a critical zone of vulnerability that typically occurs during the latter half of the night, coincident with maximal sleep drive within the brain. The physician must be increasingly aware of the public health risks associated with the ever-increasing demands made by the duty-rest-recreation schedules in our round-the-clock society.

REFERENCES

ALDRICH MS: Narcolepsy. Neurology 42 (Suppl 6):34, 1992

ANCH AM et al: *Sleep: A Scientific Perspective*. Englewood Cliffs, NJ, Prentice Hall, 1988

BLIWISE DL et al: Prevalence of self-reported poor sleep in a healthy population aged 50–65. Soc Sci Med 34:49, 1992

BRODEUR C et al: Treatment of restless legs syndrome and periodic movements during sleep with L-dopa: A double-blind controlled study. Neurology 38:1845, 1988

COLEMAN RM et al: Sleep-wake disorders based on a polysomnographic diagnosis: A national cooperative study. JAMA 247:997, 1982

CULEBRAS, A: Neuroanatomic and neurologic correlates of sleep disturbances. Neurology 42 (Suppl 6):19, 1992

CZEISLER, CA et al: Association of sleep-wake habits in older people with changes in output of circadian pacemaker. Lancet 340:933, 1992

—— et al: Exposure to bright light and darkness to treat physiologic maladaptation to night work. N Engl J Med 322:1253, 1990

DIAGNOSTIC CLASSIFICATION STEERING COMMITTEE, Thorpy MJ (chairman): *International Classification of Sleep Disorders: Diagnostic and Coding Manual*. Rochester, MN, American Sleep Disorders Association, 1990

DINGES DF, BROUGHTON RJ (eds): *Sleep and Alertness*. New York, Raven, 1989

FINDLEY LJ et al: Drivers with untreated sleep apnea. A cause of death and serious injury. Arch Intern Med 151:1451, 1991

HOFFSTEIN V et al: Treatment of obstructive sleep apnea with nasal continuous positive airway pressure, patient compliance, perception of benefits, and side effects. Am Rev Respir Dis 145:841, 1992

HORNE J: *Why We Sleep: The Functions of Sleep in Humans and Other Mammals.* Oxford, Oxford University Press, 1988

KLEIN DC et al (eds): *Suprachiasmatic Nucleus: The Mind's Clock.* New York, Oxford University Press, 1991

KRYGER MH et al (eds): *Principles and Practice of Sleep Medicine.* Philadelphia, Saunders, 1989

LEVINSON PD, MILLMAN RP: Causes and consequences of blood pressure alterations in obstructive sleep apnea. Arch Intern Med 151:455, 1991

LYDIC R, BIEBUYCK JF (eds): *Clinical Physiology of Sleep.* Bethesda, MD, American Physiological Society, 1988

MEDORI R et al: Fatal familial insomnia, a prion disease with a mutation at codon 178 of the prion protein gene. N Engl J Med 326:444, 1992

PRINZ PM et al: Geriatrics: Sleep disorders and aging. N Engl J Med 323:520, 1990

SCHENCK CH et al: Rapid eye movement sleep behavior disorder: A treatable parasomnia affecting older adults. JAMA 257:1786, 1987

SCHWARTZ WJ: A clinician's primer on the circadian clock: Its localization, function, and resetting. Adv Intern Med 38:81m, 1993

SOMERS VK et al: Sympathetic-nerve activity during sleep in normal subjects. N Engl J Med 328:303, 1993

VITIELLO MV et al: Sleep in Alzheimer's disease and the sundown syndrome. Neurology 42 (Suppl 6):83, 1992

WALSH JK et al: Insomnia, in *Sleep Disorders Medicine: A Comprehensive Textbook,* S Chokroverty (ed). Stoneham, MA, Butterworth, 1992

WARE JC, MOREWITZ J: Diagnosis and treatment of insomnia and depression. J Clin Psychiatry 52 (Suppl):55, 1991

WILLIAMS RL et al (eds): *Sleep Disorders: Diagnosis and Treatment,* 2d ed. New York, Wiley, 1988

section 4 Alterations in circulatory and respiratory function

30 COUGH AND HEMOPTYSIS

EUGENE BRAUNWALD*

COUGH

Cough is an explosive expiration which provides a means of clearing the tracheobronchial tree of secretions and foreign bodies. It is one of the most frequent cardiorespiratory symptoms and one of the most common symptoms for which medical attention is sought. Reasons for the latter include exhaustion, insomnia, and concern for the cause of the cough, especially fear of cancer and AIDS.

MECHANISM Coughing may be initiated either voluntarily or reflexively. As a defensive reflex it has both afferent and efferent pathways. The *afferent limb* includes receptors within the sensory distribution of the trigeminal, glossopharyngeal, superior laryngeal, and vagus nerves. The *efferent limb* includes the recurrent laryngeal nerve (which causes glottic closure) and the spinal nerves (which cause contraction of the thoracic and abdominal musculature). The *sequence of a cough* includes an appropriate stimulus which initiates a deep inspiration. This is followed by glottic closure, relaxation of the diaphragm, and muscle contraction against a closed glottis so as to produce maximally positive intrathoracic and intraairway pressures. These positive intrathoracic pressures result in a narrowing of the trachea, produced by an infolding of its more compliant posterior membrane. Once the glottis opens, the combination of a large pressure differential between the airways and the atmosphere coupled with this tracheal narrowing produces flow rates through the trachea close to the speed of sound. The shearing forces which are developed aid in the elimination of mucus and foreign materials. A tracheostomy short-circuits and an endotracheal tube prevents glottic closure. Therefore, both decrease the effectiveness of the cough mechanism.

ETIOLOGY Cough is produced by inflammatory, mechanical, chemical, and thermal stimulation of the cough receptors. *Inflammatory* stimuli are initiated by edema and hyperemia of the respiratory mucous membranes, as in bacterial or viral bronchitis, the common cold, and excessive cigarette smoking. It also may be caused by irritation from exudative processes, such as postnasal drip and gastric reflux with aspiration. Such stimuli may arise either in the airways (as in laryngitis, tracheitis, bronchitis, and bronchiolitis) or in the alveoli (as in pneumonitis and lung abscess). *Mechanical* stimuli are produced by inhalation of particulate matter, such as dust particles, and by compression of the air passages and pressure or tension on these structures. Lesions associated with airway compression may be either extramural or intramural. The former include aortic aneurysms, granulomas, pulmonary neoplasms, and mediastinal tumors; intramural lesions include bronchogenic carcinoma, bronchial adenoma, foreign bodies, granulomatous endobronchial involvement, and contraction of airway smooth muscle (bronchial asthma). Pressure or tension on the air passages is usually produced by lesions associated with a decrease in pulmonary compliance. Examples of specific causes include acute and chronic interstitial fibrosis (Chap. 224), pulmonary edema, and atelectasis. *Chemical* stimuli may result from inhalation of irritant gases, including cigarette smoke and chemical fumes. Many other drugs can exert adverse effects on the respiratory system and thereby cause cough. However, cough *per se* is the major side effect of angiotensin converting enzyme inhibitors. Finally, *thermal* stimuli may be produced by inhalation of either very hot or cold air.

Cough is commonly associated with episodic wheezing secondary to bronchoconstriction in symptomatic patients with bronchial asthma (Chap. 217). Chronic, persistent cough may be the *sole* presenting manifestation of bronchial asthma ("cough asthma"). Such patients are characterized by (1) absence of a history of episodic wheezing and (2) no evidence of expiratory airflow obstruction by spirometry, but (3) hyperreactive airways (characteristic of asthma) when challenged with a cholinergic agent, methacholine.

DIAGNOSTIC EVALUATION The history is the most important aspect of the evaluation. It should address the following issues:

1 Is the cough acute or chronic?
2 Is it associated with fever? with wheezing?
3 Is it associated with sputum? If so, what is its character?
4 Is it seasonal?
5 Does the patient have important risk factors for disease? (e.g., homosexuality, cigarette smoking, intravenous drugs, immobilization, environmental exposures?)
6 What is the past medical history?

The physical examination, chest roentgenogram, sputum examination, and screening pulmonary function studies (static lung volumes and dynamic flow rates) may then indicate a specific cause. The *history* may indicate specific diagnoses. Acute episodes of cough may be associated with such viral infections as acute tracheobronchitis or pneumonitis or with bacterial bronchopneumonia. Cough associated with an acute febrile episode and associated with hoarseness is usually

---

* The late Gennaro M. Tisi was the senior author of this chapter in the eleventh and previous editions of this book, and this chapter represents a continuing revision of that work.

produced by viral laryngotracheobronchitis. Postnasal drip is also a common cause of chronic cough.

The character of the cough may suggest the anatomic site of involvement: The patient with a "barking" type of cough may have epiglottal involvement (i.e., "whooping cough" due to *Bordetella pertussis* infection in young children), while the cough associated with tracheal or major airway involvement is often loud and "brassy." Cough associated with generalized wheezing may be produced by acute bronchospasm. The time of occurrence of a cough may indicate a specific cause: A cough which occurs selectively at night suggests congestive heart failure; one related to meals suggests gastrointestinal reflux into the tracheobronchial tree or a tracheoesophageal fistula, a hiatal hernia, or an esophageal diverticulum; a cough precipitated by a change in position suggests a lung abscess or a localized area of bronchiectasis. The description of sputum or secretions produced in conjunction with the cough should include color, consistency, odor, and volume. Purulent sputum and/or large amounts of sputum suggest lung abscess and bronchiectasis; bloody sputum, bleeding (see "Hemoptysis," below); frothy and pink-tinged sputum, pulmonary edema; mucoid and massive sputum, alveolar cell carcinoma.

The general *physical examination* may point to a nonpulmonary cause of cough, such as heart failure, primary nonpulmonary neoplasm, acquired immunodeficiency disease, etc. The character of the auscultatory findings may suggest the site of disease. Inspiratory stridor and wheezing may be present in laryngeal disease, inspiratory and expiratory rhonchi favor involvement of the trachea and major bronchi; coarse subcrepitant inspiratory rales may indicate interstitial fibrosis and/or edema; fine crepitant rales may indicate a process such as pneumonitis or pulmonary edema, which fills the alveoli with fluid. The *chest roentgenogram* may reveal the cause of the cough; it may show an intrapulmonary mass lesion (Chap. 227), an alveolar filling process which may be pneumonic or nonpneumonic, an area of honeycombing and cyst formation which may indicate an area of localized bronchiectasis, or bilateral hilar adenopathy which may indicate sarcoidosis or a lymphoma.

A careful *sputum examination* may be more enlightening than the patient's description of the character of the sputum. Examination shows whether the sputum is thin or viscid, purulent, foul-smelling, blood-tinged, or scant or copious. In pneumococcal pneumonia the sputum has a "rusty" color, while in *Klebsiella* pneumonia it may look like "currant jelly." Gram stain and culture of deep-cough specimens may reveal a specific bacterial, fungal, or mycoplasmal causation, while sputum cytology may result in a positive diagnosis of a pulmonary neoplasm.

Bronchoscopy may reveal the cause of otherwise unexplained chronic cough. *Pulmonary function* studies (Chap. 214) also may be helpful. Significant expiratory obstruction to airflow (as determined from a forced expiratory flow maneuver), coupled with a history of cough and significant sputum production, suggests that irrespective of other lesions the patient has significant bronchitis. Decreased lung volume (as determined from the static lung volumes) suggests that a restrictive type of lung disease (Chap. 224) is present. Perhaps more important than providing a specific diagnosis, pulmonary function studies are useful in quantifying the severity of disease, its progression over time, and the efficacy of an intervention.

Two features of cough should be highlighted: (1) A cough is often so common in the cigarette smoker as to be ignored or minimized. *Any change in the nature or character of a chronic cigarette cough should initiate immediate diagnostic evaluation, with particular attention directed to detection of bronchogenic carcinoma.* (2) Female patients are inclined to swallow sputum and not to expectorate as male patients do. This tendency may lead to the incorrect conclusion that a cough in a female patient is irritative and nonproductive.

COMPLICATIONS   Three complications may be produced by the coughing mechanism: Paroxysms of coughing may precipitate syncope (cough syncope, Chap. 17), and strenuous coughing may produce rupture of an emphysematous bleb, rib fractures, and costochondritis. A potential mechanism for cough syncope includes the development of markedly positive intrathoracic and alveolar pressures which decrease venous return, producing a decrease in cardiac output and resultant syncope. Although cough fractures of the ribs may occur in otherwise normal patients, their occurrence should at least raise the possibility of pathologic fractures, which are seen in multiple myeloma, osteoporosis, and osteolytic metastases.

THERAPY   Definitive treatment of cough depends on determining its precise cause and then initiating specific therapy for the underlying cause. When this is done, specific therapy is usually effective, as in smoking cessation, antibiotic therapy of a specific bacterial infection, or eliminating gastroesophageal reflux.

Symptomatic or nonspecific therapy of cough should be considered when (1) the cause of the cough is not known or specific treatment is not possible and (2) the cough performs no useful function or represents a potential hazard or causes marked discomfort. An irritative, nonproductive cough may be suppressed by an antitussive agent, which increases the latency or threshold of the cough center. Such agents include codeine (15 mg qid) or nonnarcotics such as dextromethorphan (15 mg qid). These drugs provide useful symptomatic therapy by interrupting prolonged, self-perpetuating paroxysms. However, a cough productive of significant quantities of sputum should usually not be suppressed, since retention of sputum in the tracheobronchial tree may interfere with the distribution of ventilation, alveolar aeration, and the ability of the lung to resist infection.

When secretions are tenacious and thick, adequate hydration, expectorants, and humidification of the air with an ultrasonic nebulizer with ipratroprium bromide, a class of bronchodilator with antimuscarinic actions given as two inhalations (36 μg qid), may be helpful. Iodinated glycerol (30 mg qid) may be especially useful in patients with cough asthma or chronic bronchitis and guaifenesin (100 mg tid) in acute or chronic bronchitis. Mucociliary clearance can be increased by beta-adrenergic agonists such as ephedrine (12.5 mg qid), especially in patients with cystic fibrosis, and theophylline (100 mg tid) in patients with chronic obstructive pulmonary disease.

Protussive (cough-enhancing) treatment is designed to increase the effectiveness of useful but inadequate cough. Hypertonic saline aerosol can increase the clearance of particles from the lower airways during coughing in patients with bronchitis, while amiloride aerosol has been shown to have a similar effect in patients with cystic fibrosis.

HEMOPTYSIS

Hemoptysis includes the expectoration from the respiratory tract of both blood-streaked sputum and gross blood. This symptom is often quite frightening to the patient. Any patient with gross hemoptysis should be given appropriate diagnostic tests so that a specific cause may be found. The patient with blood-streaked sputum also should be studied unless one can be certain that this type of hemoptysis is due to a benign condition. Recurrent episodes of hemoptysis should not be automatically ascribed to a previously established diagnosis, such as chronic bronchitis. Such an approach may result in missing a serious but potentially treatable lesion.

ETIOLOGY AND INCIDENCE   Prior to embarking on an extensive diagnostic workup of hemoptysis, it is essential to determine that the blood is in fact coming from the respiratory tract, not from the nasopharynx or gastrointestinal tract. Distinguishing hemoptysis from hematemesis is difficult at times. In hemoptysis, the prodrome is usually a tingling in the throat or a desire to cough, the blood is coughed up, is usually bright-red and *frothy*, and may be mixed with sputum; the pH is usually alkaline; and microscopic examination may show hemosiderin-laden macrophages. In hematemesis, the prodrome includes nausea and abdominal discomfort, the blood is vomited, and it is usually *dark red* in color. It may contain partially digested food, and the pH is usually acidic. Once this point is established, the diagnostic tests for hemoptysis may proceed. Although there are numerous single case reports of diseases which have been associated with hemoptysis, Table 30-1 presents the more common disorders.

The incidence of the diagnoses listed in Table 30-1 depends on the nature of the series reported and whether one includes both gross bleeding and blood streaking of the sputum. If both types of bleeding are included, then the major cause is chronic bronchitis. If the definition is restricted to gross bleeding (greater than several tablespoons), then the incidence depends on the type of series reported. Surgical series favor the incidence of mass lesions and operable lesions such as carcinoma. Those from centers with a large tuberculosis population obviously favor this condition. Combined medical-surgical series include a wider representation of those lesions which present with hemoptysis (carcinoma, bronchiectasis, bronchitis, other inflammatory lesions including tuberculosis, other lesions including the vascular, traumatic, and hemorrhagic etiologies listed in Table 30-1). Despite the most extensive of evaluations, 5 to 15 percent of cases entailing gross hemoptysis remain undiagnosed.

Two points should be highlighted with reference to diseases associated with hemoptysis: (1) hemoptysis is rare in metastatic carcinoma to the lung, and (2) although hemoptysis may occur at some time during the course of a viral or pneumococcal pneumonia, it is usually scanty and its occurrence should always raise the question of a more serious underlying process.

DIAGNOSIS As is the case for cough, the *history* is of enormous value. Recurrent, chronic hemoptysis in a young, otherwise asymptomatic female favors the diagnosis of a bronchial adenoma; hemoptysis with chronic, marked sputum production [associated with ring shadows, tram lines (abnormal air bronchograms), and cyst formation on the roentgenogram, see below] suggests a diagnosis of bronchiectasis; putrid sputum production suggests lung abscess; weight loss and anorexia in a male smoker over age 40 raise the possibility of carcinoma of the lung; a recent history of blunt trauma to the chest suggests a lung contusion; and acute pleuritic chest pain raises the possibility of pulmonary embolism with infarction or some other pleurally based lesion (lung abscess, coccidioidomycosis cavity, and vasculitis). A history of a bleeding disorder or of anticoagulant drug administration should be sought.

Several findings on the *physical examination* of the patient with hemoptysis also may suggest a specific diagnosis: A pleural friction rub suggests those diagnoses just mentioned in connection with pleuritic pain; the findings of pulmonary hypertension raise the diagnostic possibilities of primary pulmonary hypertension, mitral stenosis, recurrent or chronic thromboembolism, and Eisenmenger's

---

TABLE 30-1 Major causes of hemoptysis

I **Inflammatory**
  A Bronchitis
  B Tuberculosis
  C Bronchiectasis
  D Cystic fibrosis
  E Lung abscess
  F Pneumonia, particularly *Kliebsiella*
  G Septic pulmonary embolism
  H Localized parenchymal disease caused by fungi and parasites
II **Neoplastic**
  A Lung cancer; squamous cell, adenocarcinoma, oat cell
  B Bronchial adenoma
III **Other**
  A Pulmonary thromboembolism
  B Mitral stenosis
  C Left ventricular failure
  D Tracheobronchial trauma, including foreign body and lung contusion
  E Bronchiolithiasis
  F Bronchovascular fistula
  G Primary pulmonary hypertension, arteriovenous malformation, Eisenmenger's syndrome
  H Idiopathic pulmonary hemosiderosis
  I Pulmonary vasculitis including Wegener's granulomatosis, Goodpasture's syndrome, connective tissue disorders
  J Hemorrhagic diathesis including anticoagulant therapy

---

syndrome; a localized wheeze over a major lobar airway suggests an intramural lesion such as a bronchogenic carcinoma or a foreign body; systemic arteriovenous communications or the presence of a murmur over the lung fields suggests the diagnosis of Osler-Rendu-Weber disease with pulmonary arteriovenous malformation; evidence of significant expiratory obstruction to airflow coupled with sputum production suggests that whatever other lesion may be present, the patient has significant bronchitis.

The *chest roentgenogram* is critical to identifying the cause of hemoptysis. The presence of ring shadows favors a diagnosis of bronchiectasis; an air-fluid level, the diagnosis of a lung abscess; enlargement of the left atrium, the diagnosis of mitral stenosis; and a mass lesion, the diagnosis of a central or peripheral pulmonary neoplasm. A mass lesion which may cause hemoptysis should be distinguished from an area of blood pneumonitis caused by aspiration of blood into contiguous areas. When the chest roentgenogram is normal, the airways are the usual site of bleeding.

A common challenging problem is the identification of the site of bleeding in a patient with normal findings on physical examination and a normal roentgenogram of the chest. A patient with hemoptysis tends to keep the bleeding side dependent and may report a burning or deep pain which may localize the side of bleeding; bronchoscopy may then be useful. This procedure generally is most helpful when the bleeding is scant and of least help when the bleeding is massive, since blood may be aspirated into contiguous airways. Such aspiration may produce alveolar filling (i.e., a "blood pneumonitis") that may obscure the etiology of the hemoptysis on the initial chest roentgenogram. Blood pneumonitis usually clears within a week, and once clearing has occurred, a repeat chest roentgenogram may disclose the origin of the hemoptysis.

Following the history and physical examination, the approach to a patient with hemoptysis includes whatever specialized studies and procedures are required to make a specific diagnosis. In patients who are not bleeding actively, the roentgenogram is followed by computed tomography and then bronchoscopy. In patients who are bleeding actively, bronchoscopy is carried out on an emergent or urgent basis. Rigid bronchoscopy permits visualization of the more central airways. It is of particular value when the source of bleeding is in this portion of the airway system, the degree of hemoptysis is massive, and selective endobronchial intubation is being considered. Fiberoptic bronchoscopy (Chap. 216) includes within the range of visualization airways as small as several millimeters in diameter. This endoscopic technique may provide definitive visual, biopsy, or cytologic information. Bronchography may be employed to (1) establish the presence of localized bronchiectasis (including a sequestered lobe) and (2) rule out the presence of more generalized bronchiectasis in a patient with localized disease who is regarded as a surgical candidate because of either repetitive hemoptysis or recurrent infections. The majority of patients with bronchiectasis have a normal chest roentgenogram, but the diagnosis can usually be established by computed tomography (Chaps. 215 and 216). A PPD and, if sputum is present, examination for acid-fast bacilli should be obtained. The laboratory evaluation also should rule out a bleeding disorder.

MANAGEMENT Since hemoptysis is such an alarming symptom, there is a tendency to overtreat the patient. Usually hemoptysis is scant and will stop spontaneously without specific therapy. Following identification of the site and establishment of an etiologic diagnosis, the underlying disorder is treated. If the hemoptysis is substantial, the mainstays of therapy include keeping the patient calm, instituting complete bed rest, excluding unnecessary diagnostic procedures until the hemoptysis has begun to subside, and suppressing cough if it is present and an aggravating feature of the hemoptysis. Emergency care demands that intubation and suctioning equipment be at the bedside. Control of the airways must be obtained by endotracheal intubation in patients with massive hemoptysis (>500 mL/24h) to avoid asphyxiation. In patients in danger of asphyxiation by flooding of the lung contralateral to the side of hemorrhage, intubation by a technique which isolates the hemorrhaging lung and prevents contralateral aspiration of blood should be carried out. This can be accomplished by strategic location of a balloon catheter the introduction of which into the bronchus in question is facilitated by direct bronchoscopic visualization.

The management of massive, potentially lethal hemoptysis remains controversial. The choice between surgical and nonsurgical interventions hangs on the words *potentially lethal*. Massive hemoptysis is an alarming clinical situation in which asphyxiation due to aspiration of blood represents the principal threat to life. In many patients with massive hemoptysis, resectional surgery is ultimately carried out, but a strong effort is made to carry this out on an elective rather than emergent basis.

Since the source of massive hemoptysis is usually the bronchial arterial system, nonsurgical control includes bronchial arterial catheterization and embolization, a technique which is especially useful in patients with nonresectable lung cancer. Coagulation by means of a laser (neodymium:YAG—yttrium aluminum garnet) delivered through a bronchoscope and tamponading a proximal bleeding site with a balloon catheter or packing material applied through a rigid bronchoscope are also useful techniques.

The choice between surgical and nonsurgical management relates most often to the anatomic basis for the *massive* hemoptysis and its prognosis. In patients with cavitary tuberculosis, anaerobic lung abscess, and lung cancer, the risk of mortality is far greater than when the cause of the massive hemoptysis is bronchitis or bronchiectasis. Operation may occasionally be necessary in the former, but virtually never in the latter group. In either case the initial management should include the conservative measures suggested above. With such management, spontaneous cessation of bleeding usually occurs. Emergency surgical intervention should be considered in that small group of patients with a definable lesion on chest roentgenogram (i.e., cavitary disease, lung abscess, lung cancer) who have evidence of uncontrollable respiratory or hemodynamic compromise and who are considered to have pulmonary function that is sufficient to permit resection. If a patient is a surgical candidate, bronchoscopy should be performed to identify the specific site of bleeding. Otherwise, bronchoscopy should be deferred for several days because of the tendency of this procedure to aggravate cough and thereby perpetuate the hemoptysis.

REFERENCES

BENNETT WD et al: The acute effect of ipratropium bromide bronchodilator therapy on cough clearance in COPD. Chest 103:488, 1993

BUTCHER BL et al: High yield of chest radiography in walk-in clinic patients with chest symptoms. J Gen Intern Med 8:115, 1993

FITZGERALD JM et al: Chronic cough and gastroesophageal reflux. Can Med Assoc J 140:520, 1989

FREITAG L: Development of a new ballon catheter for management of hemoptysis with bronchofiberscopes. Chest 103:593, 1993

HENDELES L: Efficacy and safety of antihistamines and expectorants in nonprescription cough and cold preparations. Pharmacotherapy 13:154, 1993

IRWIN RS et al: Chronic cough: The spectrum and frequency of causes, key components of the diagnostic evaluation, and outcome of specific therapy. Am Rev Respir Dis 141:640, 1990

IRWIN RS, CURLEY FJ: The treatment of cough: A comprehensive review. Chest 99:1477, 1991

JONES DK, DAVIES R: Massive hemoptysis. Br Med J 300:299, 1990

KNOTT-CRAIG CJ et al: Management and prognosis of massive hemoptysis. Recent experience with 120 patients. J Thorac Cardiovasc Surg 105:394, 1993

PETTY TL: The National Mucolytic Study: Results of a randomized, double-blind, placebo-controlled study of iodinated glycerol in chronic obstructive bronchitis. Chest 97:75, 1990

POE RH et al: Chronic persistent cough: Experience in diagnosis and outcome using an anatomic diagnostic protocol. Chest 95:723, 1989

TAMURA S et al: Embolotherapy for persistent hemoptysis. Cardiovasc Intervent Radiol 16:85, 1993

THOMPSON AB et al: Pathogenesis, evaluation, and therapy for massive hemoptysis. Clin Chest Med 13:69, 1992

31   DYSPNEA AND PULMONARY EDEMA

ROLAND H. INGRAM, JR. / EUGENE BRAUNWALD

DYSPNEA

The breathing pattern is controlled by a series of higher central and peripheral mechanisms which can increase ventilation appropriate to increased metabolic demands during physical activity. It can also increase ventilation in excess of metabolic demands in conditions such as anxiety and fear. A normal resting person is unaware of the act of breathing, and while he or she may become conscious of breathing during mild to moderate exertion, no discomfort is experienced. However, during and following exhausting exertion, an individual may become unpleasantly aware of breathing yet feel reasonably assured that the sensation will be transitory and is appropriate to the level of exercise. Therefore, as a cardinal symptom of diseases affecting the cardiorespiratory system, *dyspnea* is defined as an *abnormally uncomfortable awareness of breathing*.

Although dyspnea is not painful in the usual sense of the word, it is, like pain, involved with both the perception of a sensation and the reaction to that perception. Patients experience a number of uncomfortable sensations related to breathing and use an even larger number of verbal expressions to describe these sensations, such as "cannot get enough air," "air does not go all the way down," "smothering feeling or tightness or tiredness in the chest," and a "choking sensation." It may be necessary, therefore, to review meticulously the patient's history in order to ascertain whether the more abstruse descriptions do, in fact, represent dyspnea. Once it is established that a patient does have dyspnea, it is of paramount importance to define the circumstances in which it occurs and to assess associated symptoms. There are situations in which breathing appears labored but in which dyspnea does not occur. For example, the hyperventilation associated with metabolic acidemia is rarely accompanied by dyspnea. On the other hand, patients with apparently normal breathing patterns may complain of shortness of breath.

QUANTITATION OF DYSPNEA   The gradation of dyspnea may usefully be based on the amount of physical exertion required to produce the sensation. In actual practice, the major functional classifications of patients with heart or lung disease are based largely on dyspnea in relation to degree of exertion. However, in assessing the severity of dyspnea, it is important to obtain a clear understanding of the patient's general physical condition, work history, and recreational habits. For example, the development of dyspnea in a trained runner upon running 2 mi may signify a much more serious disturbance than a similar degree of breathlessness in a sedentary person upon running a fraction of this distance. Another variable to consider in assessing the degree of dyspnea as an index of the severity of underlying heart or lung disease is the interindividual variation in perception. Some patients with extremely severe disease may complain of only mild dyspnea; others with mild disease may experience more severe shortness of breath. Thus, rather like variations in pain thresholds, patients have different degrees of subjective tolerance to cardiopulmonary dysfunction. There is some evidence that persons with relatively blunted ventilatory drives tolerate their disease with less dyspnea than those who have a heightened level of ventilatory responsiveness. Some patients with lung or heart disease may have such reduced capabilities due to other disease (e.g., peripheral vascular insufficiency or severe osteoarthritis of the hips or knees) that exertional dyspnea is precluded despite serious impairment of pulmonary or cardiac function.

Some patterns of dyspnea are not directly related to physical exertion. Sudden and unexpected dyspneic episodes at rest can be associated with pulmonary emboli, spontaneous pneumothorax, hypercapnea secondary to breath holding, or anxiety. Nocturnal episodes of severe paroxysmal dyspnea are characteristic of left ventricular failure. Dyspnea upon assuming the supine posture, *orthopnea* (see below), thought to be mainly characteristic of congestive heart failure, also may occur in some patients with asthma and chronic obstruction of the airways and is a regular finding in the rare occurrence of bilateral diaphragmatic paralysis. *Trepopnea* is used to describe the unusual circumstance in which dyspnea occurs only in the left or right lateral decubitus position, most often in patients with heart disease, while *platypnea* is dyspnea which occurs only in the upright position. Positional alterations in ventilation-perfusion relationships (see Chap. 214) have been invoked to explain these patterns. Platypnea can be seen with deficient abdominal musculature, a deficiency that results in loss of diaphragmatic support due to anterior protrusion of abdominal viscera in the upright posture. Upon lying down, the viscera resume support of the diaphragm, stretching it to its optimal operational length. This form of platypnea is alleviated by use of an abdominal binder.

MECHANISMS OF DYSPNEA Physicians usually relate the symptom of dyspnea to a process such as obstruction of the airways or congestive heart failure and generally proceed with further diagnostic and/or therapeutic attempts, having satisfied themselves that they understand the mechanism of the dyspnea. In fact, elucidation of the *actual* mechanism(s) of dyspnea has eluded clinical investigators.

Dyspnea occurs whenever the work of breathing is excessive. Increased force generation is required of the respiratory muscles to produce a given volume change if the chest wall or lungs are less compliant or if resistance to airflow is increased. Increased work of breathing also occurs when the ventilation is excessive for the level of activity. Although an individual is more apt to become dyspneic when the work of breathing is increased, the work theory does not account for the perceptual difference between a deep breath with a normal mechanical load and a normal-sized breath with an increased mechanical load. The work might be the same with both breaths, but the normal one with the increased load will be associated with discomfort. In fact, with respiratory loading, such as adding a resistance at the mouth, there is an increase in respiratory center output, as gauged by newer indexes, that is disproportionate to the increase in the work of breathing. It has been postulated that whenever the force that muscles actually generate during breathing approaches some fraction of their maximal force-generating ability, which may vary among individuals, dyspnea ensues due to transduction of mechanical to neural stimuli. Such a theory would still not explain why patients who are completely paralyzed, either by cord transections or neuromuscular blockade, experience dyspnea although aided by a mechanical ventilator. It is probable, in these circumstances, that signals from the lungs and/or airways travel via the vagus nerve to the central nervous system to account for the sensation.

In all likelihood, several different mechanisms operate to different degrees in the various clinical situations in which dyspnea occurs. There is a correlation between sensory descriptors of dyspnea and the method by which dyspnea is induced in normal subjects. In addition, there are correlations between certain clusters of sensory descriptions and the disease processes causing dyspnea. For example, patients with restrictive lung diseases may complain of rapid breathing, those with congestive heart failure may describe a need to sigh, and those with asthma may be most distressed by wheezing. Perhaps, in some circumstances, dyspnea is evoked by stimulation of receptors in the upper respiratory tract; in others it may originate from receptors in the lungs, airways, respiratory muscles, or some combination of these structures. In any event, dyspnea is characterized by an excessive or abnormal activation of the respiratory centers in the brainstem. This activation comes about from stimuli transmitted from or through a variety of structures and pathways, including (1) intrathoracic receptors via the vagi, (2) afferent somatic nerves, particularly from the respiratory muscles and chest wall, but also from other skeletal muscles and joints, (3) chemoreceptors in the brain, aortic and carotid bodies, and elsewhere in the circulation, (4) higher (cortical) centers, and perhaps (5) afferent fibers in the phrenic nerves. In general,

despite the interindividual variations described above, there is a reasonable correlation between the severity of dyspnea and the magnitude of disturbances of pulmonary or cardiac function which are responsible.

DIFFERENTIAL DIAGNOSIS **Obstructive disease of airways** (See also Chaps. 217 and 223) Obstruction to airflow can be present anywhere from the extrathoracic airways out to the small airways in the periphery of the lung. Large extrathoracic airway obstruction can occur acutely, as with aspiration of food or a foreign body or with angioedema of the glottis. Circumstantial evidence or testimony from witnesses should cause the physician to suspect aspiration, and an allergic history together with a few scattered hives should raise the possibility of glottic edema. The acute form of upper airway obstruction is a medical emergency. More chronic forms can occur with tumors or with fibrotic stenosis following tracheostomy or prolonged endotracheal intubation. Whether acute or chronic, the cardinal symptom is dyspnea, and the characteristic signs are stridor and retraction of the supraclavicular fossae with inspiration.

Obstruction of intrathoracic airways can occur acutely and intermittently or can be present chronically with worsening during respiratory infections. Acute intermittent obstruction with wheezing is typical of *asthma*. Chronic cough with expectoration is typical of *chronic bronchitis* and *bronchiectasis*. Most often there is a prolongation of expiration and coarse rhonchi which are generalized in chronic bronchitis and may be localized in the case of bronchiectasis. Intercurrent infection results in worsening of the cough, increased expectoration of purulent sputum, and more severe dyspnea. During such episodes, the patient may complain of nocturnal paroxysms of dyspnea with wheezing relieved by cough and expectoration of sputum. Despite the fact that severe limitation of expiratory flow and hyperinflation of the lung are characteristic of these diseases, the sensory experience is often that of an inability to take in a sufficiently deep breath rather than difficulty in exhaling.

The patient with predominant *emphysema* is characterized by many years of exertional dyspnea progressing to dyspnea at rest (Chap. 223). Although a parenchymal disease by definition, emphysema is invariably accompanied by obstruction of airways.

Diffuse parenchymal lung diseases (See also Chap. 224) This category includes a large number of diseases ranging from acute pneumonia to chronic disorders such as sarcoidosis and the various forms of *pneumoconiosis*. History, physical findings, and radiographic abnormalities often provide clues to the diagnosis. The patients are often tachypneic with arterial P_{CO_2} and P_{O_2} values below normal. Exertion often further reduces the arterial P_{O_2}. Lung volumes are decreased, and the lungs are stiffer, i.e., less compliant than normal.

Pulmonary vascular occlusive diseases (See also Chap. 226) Repeated episodes of dyspnea at rest often occur with recurrent pulmonary emboli. A source for emboli, such as phlebitis of a lower extremity or the pelvis, is quite helpful in leading the physician to suspect the diagnosis. Arterial blood gases are almost invariably abnormal, but lung volumes are frequently normal or only minimally abnormal.

Diseases of the chest wall or respiratory muscles (See also Chap. 229) The physical examination establishes the presence of a chest wall disease such as severe kyphoscoliosis, pectus excavatum, or spondylitis. Although all three of these deformities may be associated with dyspnea, only severe kyphoscoliosis regularly interferes with ventilation sufficiently to produce chronic cor pulmonale and respiratory failure. Even though vital capacity, lung volumes, and airflow rates are normal with pectus excavatum, in the most severe cases cardiac compression from the posteriorly displaced sternum may interfere with diastolic filling of the ventricle during exercise. Hence a cardiogenic component to the dyspnea may be present in this condition.

Both weakness and paralysis of respiratory muscles can lead to respiratory failure and dyspnea (Chap. 229), but most often the signs and symptoms of the neurologic or muscular disorder are more prominently manifested in other systems.

Heart disease   In patients with cardiac disease, exertional dyspnea occurs most commonly as a consequence of an elevated pulmonary capillary pressure; aside from uncommon causes such as congenital or acquired obstructive disease of the pulmonary veins (Chap. 199), pulmonary capillary hypertension is a consequence of left atrial hypertension, which in turn may be due to left ventricular dysfunction (Chaps. 194 and 195), reduced left ventricular compliance, and mitral stenosis. The elevation of hydrostatic pressure in the pulmonary vascular bed tends to upset the Starling equilibrium (see "Pulmonary Edema," below) with resulting transudation of liquid into the interstitial space, reducing the compliance of the lungs and stimulating J (juxtacapillary) receptors in the alveolar interstitial space. When prolonged, pulmonary venous hypertension results in thickening of the walls of small pulmonary vessels and an increase in perivascular cells and fibrous tissue, causing a further reduction in compliance. The competition for space between vessels, airways, and increased liquid within the interstitial space compromises the lumina of small airways, increasing the airways' resistance. Diminution in compliance and an increase in the airways' resistance increase the work of breathing, which, to some degree, is minimized by a reduction in tidal volume; the latter, in turn, is compensated for by an increase in frequency of respiration. In severe heart disease, usually involving elevation of both pulmonary and systemic venous pressures, hydrothorax may develop, interfering further with pulmonary function and intensifying dyspnea. In patients with heart failure and a severely diminished cardiac output, dyspnea also may be related to fatigue of the respiratory muscles as a consequence of their reduced perfusion. The metabolic acidosis characteristic of severe heart failure may play a contributory role. Dyspnea also may be associated with severe systemic and cerebral hypoxia, as occurs during exertion in patients with congenital heart disease and right-to-left shunts.

Cardiac dyspnea usually begins as breathlessness on strenuous exertion and, over the course of months or years, progresses until the patient is dyspneic at rest. Occasionally, a nonproductive cough developing in the recumbent position, particularly at night, may be the first complaint.

Orthopnea, i.e., dyspnea in the recumbent position, and *paroxysmal nocturnal dyspnea*, i.e., attacks of shortness of breath which usually occur at night and awaken the patient from sleep, are characteristic of more advanced forms of heart failure associated with elevations of pulmonary venous and capillary pressures and are discussed in Chap. 195. Orthopnea is the result of the alteration of gravitational forces when the recumbent position is assumed. This augmentation of intrathoracic blood volume elevates pulmonary venous and capillary pressures, which increases the pulmonary closing volume (Chap. 214) and reduces the vital capacity. An additional factor associated with recumbency is elevation of the diaphragm, which results in a lower end-expiratory lung volume. This combination of lower end-expiratory lung volume and increase in closing volume results in a significant alteration of alveolar-capillary gas exchange.

PAROXYSMAL (NOCTURNAL) DYSPNEA   Also known as *cardiac asthma*, this condition is characterized by attacks of severe shortness of breath which generally occur at night and usually awaken the patient from sleep. The attack is precipitated by stimuli which aggravate the previously existing pulmonary congestion; frequently, the total blood volume is augmented at night because of the reabsorption of edema from dependent portions of the body during recumbency; the redistribution of blood volume which takes place results in an increase in intrathoracic blood volume and therefore produces pulmonary congestion. A sleeping patient can tolerate relatively severe pulmonary engorgement and may awaken only when actual pulmonary edema and bronchospasm have developed, with the feeling of suffocation and with wheezing respirations.

CHEYNE-STOKES RESPIRATION   See Chap. 195.

DIAGNOSIS   The diagnosis of cardiac dyspnea depends on the recognition of heart disease on the basis of the clinical examination supplemented by noninvasive testing. There may be a history of antecedent myocardial infarction, third and fourth heart sounds

may be audible, and/or there may be evidence of left ventricular enlargement, jugular neck vein distention, and/or peripheral edema. Often there are radiographic signs of heart failure, with evidence of interstitial edema, pulmonary vascular redistribution, and accumulation of liquid in the septal planes and pleural cavity. Cardiomegaly is often present, but the overall heart size may be normal, particularly in patients with dyspnea due to acute myocardial infarction or mitral stenosis; an enlarged left atrium is usually evident in the latter condition. The electrocardiogram (Chap. 189) is rarely specific for heart disease and cannot specifically indicate whether a patient's dyspnea is caused by heart disease; however, it is rarely normal in patients with cardiac dyspnea. Echocardiography (Chap. 191) is particularly useful in establishing the diagnosis of structural heart disease, which can be responsible for dyspnea. Specifically, left atrial and/or left ventricular dilatation, left ventricular hypertrophy, a reduced left ventricular ejection fraction, and disorders of left ventricular wall motion may be clues to the presence of a cardiac etiology of otherwise unexplained dyspnea.

Differentiation between cardiac and pulmonary dyspnea   In most patients with dyspnea there is obvious clinical evidence of disease of either the heart or lungs. The dyspnea of chronic obstructive lung disease tends to develop more gradually than that of heart disease; exceptions, of course, occur in patients with obstructive lung disease who develop an episode of infectious bronchitis, pneumonia, or pneumothorax or an exacerbation of asthma. Like patients with cardiac dyspnea, patients with chronic obstructive lung disease also may waken at night with dyspnea, but this is usually associated with sputum production; the dyspnea is relieved after these patients rid themselves of secretions.

The difficulty in the distinction between cardiac and pulmonary dyspnea may be compounded by the coexistence of diseases involving both organ systems. Patients with a history of chronic bronchitis or asthma who develop left ventricular failure tend to develop recurrences of bronchoconstriction and wheezing in association with bouts of paroxysmal nocturnal dyspnea and pulmonary edema. This condition, i.e., cardiac asthma, usually occurs in patients with overt clinical evidence of heart disease. Acute cardiac asthma is further differentiated from acute attacks of bronchial asthma by the presence of diaphoresis, more bubbly airway sounds, and the more common occurrence of cyanosis.

It is desirable to carry out pulmonary function testing in patients in whom the etiology of dyspnea is not clear, for these tests may be helpful in determining whether dyspnea is produced by heart disease, lung disease, abnormalities of the chest wall, or anxiety. In addition to the usual means of assessing patients for heart disease (Chap. 187), determination of the ejection fraction at rest and during exercise by echocardiography or radionuclide ventriculography (Chap. 191) is helpful in the differential diagnosis of dyspnea. The left ventricular ejection fraction is depressed in left ventricular failure, while the right ventricular ejection fraction may be low at rest or may decline during exercise in patients with severe lung disease. Both ejection fractions are normal at rest and during exercise in dyspnea due to anxiety or malingering. Careful observation during the performance of an exercise treadmill test will often help in the identification of the patient who is malingering or whose dyspnea is secondary to anxiety. Under these circumstances, the patient usually complains of severe shortness of breath but appears to be breathing either effortlessly or totally irregularly. In less than obvious cases, measurements of P_{O_2}, pH, and P_{CO_2} in arterial blood and CO_2 and O_2 levels in mixed expired gas may be helpful in establishing either that gas exchange is normal or that a significant abnormality that is not detectable at rest exists during exercise.

Anxiety neurosis   Dyspnea experienced by someone with an anxiety neurosis is a difficult symptom to evaluate. The signs and symptoms of acute and chronic hyperventilation do not serve to distinguish between anxiety neurosis and other processes, such as recurrent pulmonary emboli. Another potentially confusing situation is seen when chest pain and electrocardiographic changes accompany the hyperventilation syndrome. When present and attributable to this condition, often referred to as *neurocirculatory asthenia* (Chap. 12), the chest pain is often sharp, fleeting, and in various loci, and the electrocardiographic changes are most often seen during repolarization; yet occasional ventricular ectopic activity can be seen as well. A rather extensive series of pulmonary and cardiac function tests, carried out both at rest and during exercise, may be needed to be certain that anxiety is, in fact, the cause of the dyspnea. Certain clues are helpful in leading one to suspect a psychogenic origin. Frequent sighing respirations and an irregular breathing pattern are helpful. Often the breathing pattern returns to normal during sleep.

PULMONARY EDEMA (See Table 31-1)

CARDIOGENIC PULMONARY EDEMA (see Table 31-1, IA)   An increase in pulmonary venous pressure, which results initially in engorgement of the pulmonary vasculature, is common in most instances of dyspnea in association with congestive heart failure. The lungs become less compliant, the resistance of small airways increases, and there is an increase in lymphatic flow which apparently serves to maintain a constant pulmonary extravascular liquid volume. At this early stage there is usually mild tachypnea, and if arterial blood gases are measured, the arterial P_{O_2} and P_{CO_2} are both lowered modestly

---

TABLE 31-1   Classification of pulmonary edema based on initiating mechanism

I IMBALANCE OF STARLING FORCES

A Increased pulmonary capillary pressure
  1 Increased pulmonary venous pressure without left ventricular failure (e.g., mitral stenosis)
  2 increased pulmonary venous pressure secondary to left ventricular failure
  3 Increased pulmonary capillary pressure secondary to increased pulmonary arterial pressure (so-called overperfusion pulmonary edema)
B Decreased plasma oncotic pressure
  1 Hypoalbuminemia
C Increased negativity of interstitial pressure
  1 Rapid removal of pneumothorax with large applied negative pressures (unilateral)
  2 Large negative pleural pressures due to acute airway obstruction alone with increased end-expiratory volumes (asthma)

II ALTERED ALVEOLAR-CAPILLARY MEMBRANE PERMEABILITY (ADULT RESPIRATORY DISTRESS SYNDROME)

A Infectious pneumonia—bacterial, viral, parasitic
B Inhaled toxins (e.g., phosgene, ozone, chlorine, Teflon fumes, nitrogen dioxide, smoke)
C Circulating foreign substances (e.g., snake venom, bacterial endotoxins)
D Aspiration of acidic gastric contents
E Acute radiation pneumonitis
F Endogenous vasoactive substances (e.g., histamine, kinins)
G Disseminated intravascular coagulation
H Immunologic—hypersensitivity pneumonitis, drugs (nitrofurantoin), leukoagglutinins
I Shock lung in association with nonthoracic trauma
J Acute hemorrhagic pancreatitis

III LYMPHATIC INSUFFICIENCY

A After lung tranplant
B Lymphangitic carcinomatosis
C Fibrosing lymphangitis (e.g., silicosis)

IV UNKNOWN OR INCOMPLETELY UNDERSTOOD

A High-altitude pulmonary edema
B Neurogenic pulmonary edema
C Narcotic overdose
D Pulmonary embolism
E Eclampsia
F After cardioversion
G After anesthesia
H After cardiopulmonary bypass

SOURCE: Reproduced with permission from Ingram and Braunwald.

---

with an increase in the alveolar-to-arterial oxygen difference. Tachypnea itself, which might result from stimulation of receptors in the pulmonary interstitium, apparently increases lymphatic flow by augmenting ventilatory pumping of lymphatic vessels. The changes described are seen well in advance of auscultatory findings or radiographic signs pointing to congestive heart failure. If sufficient both in magnitude and duration, the increase in intravascular pressure results in a net gain of liquid in the extravascular space despite further increases in lymphatic flow. It is at this point that symptoms worsen, tachypnea increases, gas exchange deteriorates further, and radiographic changes, such as Kerley B lines and loss of distinct vascular margins, are seen. It has been shown, even at this intermediate stage, that the capillary endothelial intercellular junctions have widened and allow passage of macromolecules into the interstices. Up to and including this stage, the edema is purely *interstitial*.

Further elevations in intravascular pressure result in disruption of the tighter junctions between alveolar lining cells, and alveolar edema ensues with outpouring of liquid which contains both red blood cells and macromolecules. At this point *alveolar edema* is present. Although at one time considered an early and subtle radiographic sign of interstitial edema, current evidence suggests that an antigravity redistribution of pulmonary blood flow (from the lung bases to the apices) occurs only after the onset of alveolar edema. With yet more severe disruption of the alveolar-capillary membrane, edematous liquid floods the alveoli and airways. At this point, full-blown clinical pulmonary edema with bilateral wet rales and rhonchi will occur, and the chest radiograph may show diffuse haziness of the lung fields with greater density in the more proximal hilar regions. Typically, the patient is anxious and perspires freely, and the sputum is frothy and blood-tinged. Gas exchange is more severely compromised with worsening hypoxia. Without effective treatment (Chap. 195), progressive acidemia, hypercapnia, and respiratory arrest ensue.

The earlier sequence of liquid accumulation described above follows the Starling law of capillary–interstitial fluid exchange:

$$\text{Liquid accumulation} = K[(P_c - P_{IF}) - \sigma(\pi_{pl} - \pi_{IF})] - Q_{lymph}$$

where K = hydraulic conductance (directly proportional to membrane surface area and inversely proportional to membrane thickness)
P_c = mean intracapillary pressure
π_{IF} = oncotic pressure of interstitial liquid
σ = reflection coefficient of macromolecules
P_{IF} = mean interstitial liquid pressure
π_{pl} = oncotic pressure of the plasma
Q_{lymph} = lymphatic flow

The pressures tending to move liquid out of the vessel are $\dot{P}_c$ and π_{IF}, which are normally more than offset by pressures tending to move liquid back into the vasculature, i.e., the algebraic sum of P_{IF} and π_{pl}. Implicit in the preceding equation is that lymphatic flow can increase in the case of imbalance of forces and result in no net accumulation of interstitial liquid. Further elevations in P_c not only increase the outward movement of liquid in each capillary region but also recruit more of the capillary bed, which increases K. These two effects lead to liquid filtration that exceeds clearance capability by the lymphatics, and liquid accumulates in the loose interstitial spaces of the lung. Even greater increases in P_c open first the loose endothelial intercellular junctions and later the tight alveolar intercellular junctions with an increase in permeability to macromolecules. This secondary disruption of both the function and structure of the alveolar-capillary membrane leads to alveolar flooding.

NONCARDIOGENIC PULMONARY EDEMA (See Table 31-1, IB, IC, II, III, and IV)   Several clinical conditions are associated with pulmonary edema based on an imbalance of Starling forces other than through primary elevations of pulmonary capillary pressure. Although diminished plasma oncotic pressure in hypoalbuminemic states (e.g., severe liver disease, nephrotic syndrome, protein-losing enteropathy) might be expected to lead to pulmonary edema, the balance of forces normally so strongly favors resorption that even in these conditions some elevation of capillary pressure is necessary before interstitial edema develops. Increased negativity of interstitial pressure has been implicated in the genesis of unilateral pulmonary edema following rapid evacuation of a large pneumothorax. In this situation, the findings may be apparent only by radiography, but occasionally the patient experiences dyspnea with physical findings localized to the edematous lung. It has been proposed that large negative intrapleural pressures during acute severe asthma may be associated with the development of interstitial edema. If this proposal can be supported by sufficient clinical data, then asthma would represent an additional example of edema due to increased negativity of interstitial pressure. Lymphatic blockade secondary to fibrotic and inflammatory diseases or lymphangitic carcinomatosis may lead to interstitial edema. In such instances, both clinical and radiographic manifestations are dominated by the underlying disease process.

There are other conditions characterized by increases in the interstitial liquid content of the lungs which begin neither with an imbalance between intravascular and interstitial forces nor with alterations in lymphatics, but rather appear to be associated primarily with disruption of the alveolar-capillary membranes. Any number of spontaneously occurring or environmental toxic insults, including diffuse pulmonary infections, aspiration, and shock (particularly due to gram-negative septicemia and hemorrhagic pancreatitis and following cardiopulmonary bypass), are associated with diffuse pulmonary edema which clearly does not have a hemodynamic origin. These conditions, which may lead to the adult respiratory distress syndrome, are discussed in Chap. 230.

Other forms of pulmonary edema   There are three forms of pulmonary edema which have not been clearly related to increased permeability, inadequate lymphatic flow, or an imbalance of Starling forces; hence their precise mechanism remains unexplained. *Narcotic overdose* is a well-recognized antecedent to pulmonary edema. Although illicit use of parenteral heroin is the most frequent cause, parenteral and oral overdoses of legitimate preparations of morphine, methadone, and dextropropoxyphene also have been associated with pulmonary edema. Thus the earlier idea that injected impurities lead to the disorder is untenable. Available evidence suggests that there are alterations in the permeability of alveolar and capillary membranes rather than an elevation of pulmonary capillary pressure.

Exposure to high altitude in association with severe physical exertion is a well-recognized setting for pulmonary edema in unacclimatized, yet otherwise healthy persons. Recent data show that acclimatized high-altitude natives also develop this syndrome upon return to high altitude after a relatively brief sojourn at low altitudes. The syndrome is far more common in persons under the age of 25 years. The mechanism for high-altitude pulmonary edema remains obscure, and studies have been conflicting, some suggesting pulmonary venous constriction and others indicating pulmonary arteriolar constriction as the prime mechanisms. A role for hypoxia at altitude is suggested by the fact that patients respond to the administration of oxygen and/or return to lower altitudes. Hypoxia per se does not alter permeability of the alveolar-capillary membrane. Hence increased cardiac output and pulmonary arterial pressures with exercise combined with hypoxic pulmonary arteriolar constriction, which is more prominent in young persons, may combine to make this an example of prearteriolar, high-pressure pulmonary edema.

Neurogenic pulmonary edema has been suspected in patients with central nervous system disorders and without apparent preexisting left ventricular dysfunction. Although most experimental equivalents have implicated sympathetic nervous system activity, the mechanism whereby sympathetic efferent activity leads to pulmonary edema is a matter of speculation. It is known that a massive adrenergic discharge leads to peripheral vasoconstriction with elevation of blood pressure and shifts of blood to the central circulation. In addition, it is probable that a reduction in left ventricular compliance also occurs, and both factors serve to increase left atrial pressures sufficiently to induce pulmonary edema on a hemodynamic basis. Some experimental

evidence suggests that stimulation of adrenergic receptors increases capillary permeability directly, but this effect is relatively minor as compared with the imbalance of Starling forces.

TREATMENT OF PULMONARY EDEMA   See Chap. 195.

REFERENCES

COLICE GL: Detecting the presence and cause of pulmonary edema. Postgrad Med 93:161, 169, 1993

CRAPO JD: New concepts in the formation of pulmonary edema. Am Rev Respir Dis 147:790, 1993

DePASO WJ et al: Chronic dyspnea unexplained by history, physical examination, chest roentgenogram and spirometry. Chest 100:1293, 1991

ELLIOTT MW et al: The language of breathlessness: Use of verbal descriptors by patients with cardiopulmonary diseases. Am Rev Respir Dis 144:826, 1991

INGRAM RH JR, BRAUNWALD E: Pulmonary edema: Cardiogenic and noncardiogenic, in *Heart Disease*, 4th ed, E Braunwald (ed). Philadelphia, Saunders, 1992, p 551

MAHLER DA et al: Measurement of breathlessness during exercise in asthmatics. Am Rev Respir Dis 144:39, 1991

SCHWARTZSTEIN RM et al: Dyspnea: A sensory experience. Lung 169:543, 1991

WASSERMAN K, CASABURI R: Dyspnea: Physiological and pathophysiological mechanisms. Annu Rev Med 39:503, 1988

32   HYPOXIA, POLYCYTHEMIA, AND CYANOSIS

EUGENE BRAUNWALD

HYPOXIA

The fundamental purpose of the cardiorespiratory system is to deliver oxygen (and substrates) to the cells and to remove carbon dioxide (and other metabolic products) from them. Proper maintenance of this function depends on intact cardiovascular and respiratory systems and a supply of inspired gas containing adequate oxygen. Changes in oxygen and in carbon dioxide tension as well as changes in the intraerythrocytic concentration of certain *organic phosphate compounds*, especially 2,3-biphosphoglyceric acid (2,3-BPG), cause shifts in the oxygen dissociation curve. These are discussed in detail in Chap. 302 and are illustrated in Fig. 302-4. When hypoxia results as a consequence of respiratory failure, Pa_{CO_2} usually rises (Chap. 214), and the oxygen dissociation curve is displaced to the right. Under these conditions, the percentage saturation of the hemoglobin in the arterial blood at a given level of alveolar oxygen tension (Pa_{O_2}) declines. Thus arterial hypoxia and cyanosis are likely to be more marked in proportion to the degree of depression of Pa_{O_2} when such depression results from pulmonary disease than when the depression occurs as the result of a decline in the partial pressure of oxygen in the inspired air, in which case Pa_{CO_2} falls and the oxygen dissociation curve is displaced to the left.

DIFFERENTIAL DIAGNOSIS   Anemic hypoxia   Any decrease in hemoglobin concentration is attended by a corresponding decline in the oxygen-carrying capacity of the blood. The Pa_{O_2} remains normal, but the absolute amount of oxygen transported per unit volume of blood is diminished. As the anemic blood passes through the capillaries and the usual amount of oxygen is removed from it, the P_{O_2} in the venous blood declines to a greater degree than would normally be the case.

Carbon monoxide intoxication (Chap. 395)   This condition is analogous to anemic hypoxia in that the hemoglobin which is combined with the carbon monoxide (carboxyhemoglobin) is unavailable for oxygen transport. In addition, the presence of carboxyhemoglobin shifts the dissociation curve of hemoglobin to the left so that the oxygen can be unloaded only at lower tensions. By such formation of carboxyhemoglobin, a given degree of reduction in oxygen-carrying power produces a far greater degree of tissue hypoxia than the equivalent reduction in hemoglobin due to simple anemia.

Respiratory hypoxia Arterial unsaturation is a common finding in advanced pulmonary disease. As discussed in Chap. 214, it may be caused by hypoventilation when it is associated with an elevation of Pa_{CO_2}. A second cause is shunting of blood from right to left by perfusion of nonventilated portions of the lung, as in pulmonary atelectasis or through vascular abnormalities of the lung with arteriovenous connections. The low Pa_{O_2} is not correctable by inspiring 100% O_2. The most common cause of respiratory hypoxia is ventilation-perfusion mismatch, which results from perfusion of poorly ventilated alveoli. The low Pa_{O_2} is usually readily correctable by inspiring 100% O_2.

Hypoxia secondary to right-to-left extrapulmonary shunting This cause of hypoxia resembles physiologically intrapulmonary right-to-left shunting but is caused by congenital cardiac malformations such as tetralogy of Fallot, transposition of the great arteries, and Eisenmenger's complex (Chap. 199). As in pulmonary right-to-left shunting, the Pa_{O_2} cannot be brought to normal with inspiration of 100% O_2.

Circulatory hypoxia As in anemic hypoxia, Pa_{O_2} is normal, but venous and tissue P_{O_2} values are reduced as a consequence of reduced tissue perfusion in the face of normal tissue oxygen consumption. Generalized circulatory hypoxia occurs in heart failure (Chap. 195) and in most forms of shock (Chap. 34).

Specific organ hypoxia Decreased circulation to a specific organ resulting in localized circulatory hypoxia may be due to organic arterial obstruction or may occur as a consequence of vasoconstriction. The latter is seen in the upper extremities in Raynaud's phenomenon. Reduced circulation may occur in all limbs in patients with heart failure or hypovolemic shock in an attempt to maintain adequate perfusion to more vital organs. Ischemic hypoxia with accompanying pallor occurs in organic arterial obliterative disease. Localized hypoxia also may result from venous obstruction and the resultant congestion and reduced arterial inflow. Edema, which increases the distance through which oxygen diffuses before it reaches the cells, also can cause localized hypoxia.

Increased oxygen requirements If the oxygen consumption of the tissues is elevated without a corresponding increase in volume flow per unit of time, the P_{O_2} in venous blood (and hence capillary and tissue P_{O_2}) may be reduced. This will occur even if oxygen diffusion into blood perfusing the pulmonary capillary bed is normal and the hemoglobin is qualitatively and quantitatively normal. Such a situation may be encountered when fever or thyrotoxicosis occurs in patients in whom the cardiac output is fixed and cannot rise normally. Under these conditions, the circulation may be considered deficient relative to the metabolic requirements.

Ordinarily, the clinical picture of patients with hypoxia due to an elevated metabolic rate is quite different from that in other types of hypoxia; the skin is warm and flushed, owing to increased cutaneous blood flow which dissipates the excessive heat produced, and cyanosis is usually absent.

Exercise is a classic example of increased tissue oxygen requirements. These increased demands are normally met by several mechanisms: (1) increasing the cardiac output and ventilation and thus oxygen delivery to the tissues, (2) preferentially directing the blood to the exercising muscles and away from resting muscles, skin, and viscera (by changing vascular resistances in various circulatory beds, directly and/or reflexly), (3) increasing oxygen extraction from the delivered blood and widening the arteriovenous oxygen differences, and (4) reducing the pH of the tissues and capillary blood, thereby unloading more oxygen from hemoglobin. If the capacity of these mechanisms is exceeded, then hypoxia, especially of the exercising muscles, will result.

Improper oxygen utilization Cyanide (Chap. 395) and several other similarly acting poisons cause a paradoxic state in which the tissues are unable to utilize oxygen, and as a consequence, the venous blood tends to have a high oxygen tension. This condition has been termed *histotoxic hypoxia*. Cyanide produces cellular hypoxia by paralyzing the electron-transfer function of cytochrome oxidase so

that it cannot pass electrons to oxygen, whereas diphtheria toxin is believed to inhibit the synthesis of one of the cytochromes and thus interfere with oxygen consumption and energy production by the cells involved.

EFFECTS OF HYPOXIA Changes in the central nervous system, particularly the higher centers, are especially important. Acute hypoxia produces impaired judgment, motor incoordination, and a clinical picture closely resembling that of acute alcoholism. When hypoxia is long-standing, fatigue, drowsiness, apathy, inattentiveness, delayed reaction time, and reduced work capacity occur. As hypoxia becomes more severe, the centers of the brainstem are affected, and death usually results from respiratory failure. With reduction of Pa_{O_2}, cerebrovascular resistance decreases and cerebral blood flow increases, which tends to reduce the cerebral hypoxia. On the other hand, when the reduction of Pa_{O_2} is accompanied by hyperventilation and diminution of Pa_{CO_2}, cerebrovascular resistance rises, blood flow falls, and hypoxia is enhanced. Compared with the brain, the phylogenetically older spinal cord and peripheral nerves are relatively insensitive to hypoxia. Hypoxia also causes pulmonary arterial constriction, which serves the useful function of shunting blood away from poorly ventilated areas toward better-ventilated portions of the lung. However, it has the disadvantage of causing increased pulmonary vascular resistance and increased right ventricular afterload.

A complex disturbance of cellular functions results from the metabolic effects of severe acute hypoxia. In liver and muscles, the metabolism of the primary foodstuff, carbohydrate, normally proceeds anaerobically (i.e., without oxidation) to the stage of formation of pyruvic acid. The breakdown of pyruvate requires oxygen, and when this is deficient, increasing proportions of pyruvate are reduced to lactic acid, which cannot be broken down further (Chap. 46). Hence there is an increase in the blood lactate, with decrease in bicarbonate and a corresponding metabolic acidosis. Under these circumstances, the total energy obtained from foodstuff breakdown is greatly reduced, and the amount of energy available for continuing resynthesis of energy-rich phosphate compounds becomes inadequate, leading to a complex disturbance of cellular function.

Most of the useful respiratory response to hypoxia originates in special chemosensitive cells in the carotid and aortic bodies, although the respiratory center in the brainstem is also stimulated directly by oxygen lack. The resultant increase in ventilation, with loss of carbon dioxide, leads to respiratory alkalosis. On the other hand, the diffusion of additional quantities of lactic acid from the tissues into the blood tends to produce metabolic acidosis. In either case, the total amount of bicarbonate, and hence the carbon dioxide–combining power, tends to be diminished (Chap. 46).

Diminished oxygen tension in any tissue results in local vasodilatation, and the diffuse vasodilatation which occurs in generalized hypoxia causes an elevation of total cardiac output (Fig. 302-5). In patients with preexisting heart disease, the development of hypoxia and the requirements of the peripheral tissues for an increase of cardiac output may precipitate congestive heart failure. In patients with ischemic heart disease, a reduced Pa_{O_2} may intensify ischemia and further impair left ventricular function. Prolonged or severe hypoxia also may impair hepatic and renal function.

One of the important mechanisms of compensation for prolonged hypoxia is an increase in the hemoglobin concentration. This is due not to direct stimulation of the bone marrow but to the effect of erythropoietin (Chap. 302). Assayable levels of erythropoietin are increased by hypoxia, and its production has been found to be regulated by the balance between tissue oxygen supply and demand.

POLYCYTHEMIA (See also Chap. 309)

The term *polycythemia* signifies an increase above normal in the number of red blood cells in the circulating blood. This elevation is usually, although not always, accompanied by a corresponding increase in the quantity of hemoglobin and in the hematocrit. The

TABLE 32-1   Differential diagnosis of erythrocytosis

ABSOLUTE (↑ RED CELL MASS)

I **Autonomous erythroid proliferation** (↓ EP*); polycythemia vera
II **Secondary erythroid proliferation**
   A Autonomous or inappropriate increase in EP
     1 Neoplasm
     2 Renal lesions
     3 Familial erythrocytosis (autosomal recessive inheritance)
   B Secondary increase in EP
     1 Hypoxia (↓ arterial P_{O_2})
       a High altitude
       b Alveolar hypoventilation
       c Pulmonary disease
       d Cardiac right-to-left shunt
     2 Abnormal hemoglobin function (normal arterial P_{O_2})
       a High-affinity variants (autosomal dominant inheritance)
       b Congenital methemoglobinemia
       c Carboxyhemoglobin (smokers' polycythemia)
   C Hormonal stimulus to erythropoiesis
     1 Cushing's syndrome
     2 Androgen or corticosteroid administration

RELATIVE (REDUCED PLASMA VOLUME, NORMAL RED CELL MASS)

I **Dehydration**
II **Stress erythrocytosis**

* Erythropoietin.
SOURCE: Adapted from HF Bunn et al, *Human Hemoglobins*, Philadelphia, Saunders, 1988.

---

increase may or may not be associated with an elevation in the total quantity of red blood cells in the body. It is important to distinguish between *absolute* polycythemia (an increase in the total red cell mass) and *relative* polycythemia, which occurs when, through loss of blood plasma, the *concentration* of the red cells in the circulating blood becomes greater than normal. This may be the consequence of abnormally lowered fluid intake, of the loss of plasma into the interstitial fluid, or of the marked loss of body fluids, such as occurs in persistent vomiting, severe diarrhea, copious sweating, or acidosis.

Because the term *polycythemia* is used loosely to refer to all varieties of increase in the number of red corpuscles, the terms *erythrocytosis* and *erythremia* are preferred in referring to two forms of *absolute* polycythemia. *Erythrocytosis* denotes absolute polycythemia which occurs in response to some known stimulus, most commonly hypoxemia (secondary polycythemia); *erythremia* (polycythemia vera) refers to the disease of unknown etiology. Erythrocytosis develops as a consequence of a variety of factors and represents a physiologic response to conditions of hypoxia. An approach to the differential diagnosis of erythrocytosis should begin with a consideration of its mechanisms (Table 32-1).

SECONDARY POLYCYTHEMIA   Sojourn at high altitudes leads to defective saturation of arterial blood with oxygen and stimulates the production of more red cells. The oxygen saturation, rather than oxygen tension, appears to be the more important determinant of the erythropoietic response to chronic hypoxia (Fig. 32-1). A condition known as *chronic mountain sickness* or *soroche* (Monge's disease) may set in insidiously after several years of continued residence at high altitude. This condition appears to be caused by the development of alveolar hypoventilation superimposed on a lowered inspired O_2 concentration. Prominent manifestations are a florid color which turns to cyanosis on mild exertion, impaired mental acuity, fatigue, and headache. Those affected are usually in the fourth to sixth decades. Return to sea level promptly relieves the symptoms. Living at high altitudes also evokes a number of compensatory reactions which act to increase oxygen delivery to the tissues. These include hyperventilation, which reduces the oxygen gradient between inspired and alveolar air, erythrocytosis, an augmentation of pulmonary capillary blood volume, an increase of diffusing capacity, and an increase in cardiac output.

Any pulmonary disease which produces chronic hypoxia may lead to erythrocytosis. The increased blood viscosity secondary to the polycythemia elevates pulmonary arterial pressure and, combined with the elevation of pulmonary vascular resistance resulting from hypoxia, further elevates right ventricular pressure, contributing to the development or intensification of cor pulmonale (Chap. 204). The *abnormal ventilatory conditions* present in very obese individuals may cause alveolar hypoventilation and result in arterial unsaturation, erythrocytosis, hypercapnia, and somnolence (the Pickwickian syndrome; Chap. 229). This syndrome is also observed in nonobese persons (sleep-apnea syndrome) in whom decreased sensitivity of the respiratory center to CO_2 may play a role (Chap. 229).

The partial shunting of blood from the pulmonary circuit (right-to-left shunts), such as occurs in *congenital heart disease*, causes the most striking erythrocytosis resulting from abnormalities in the heart or lungs (Chap. 199). Erythrocyte counts as high as 12×10^6 per microliter, which are possible only when the red corpuscles are smaller than normal, have been observed in such patients, with a hematocrit as high as 86 percent. As the polycythemia develops, there is a progressive elevation of blood viscosity, which begins to rise logarithmically when the volume of packed red blood cells exceeds 55 percent. The most common defects producing such polycythemia in the adult are tetralogy of Fallot and Eisenmenger syndrome. Other congenital cardiac malformations commonly responsible for polycythemia, but occurring more commonly in neonates, include transposition of the great arteries, tricuspid atresia, and persistent truncus arteriosus.

Rarely, patients with hepatic cirrhosis will be hypoxemic secondary to intrapulmonary shunts, or right-to-left shunts from the portal to the pulmonary veins. The polycythemia of cyanotic congenital heart disease may lead to spontaneous thrombosis at any site, including the central nervous system.

The increase in hematocrit and the sharp increase in viscosity which occur when these patients become dehydrated are particularly hazardous. Symptoms due to increased blood viscosity include reduced mentation, headache, fatigue, visual disturbance, and dizziness. This condition also may be accompanied by a variety of blood coagulation defects, including reduced fibrinogen and prothrombin concentrations, as well as thrombocytopenia. Reduction in red blood cell volume (phlebotomy with reinfusion of the plasma) is sometimes performed

FIGURE 32-1   Relationship between mean arterial oxygen saturation (percent) and the mean hemoglobin content (grams per deciliter) in healthy male residents at various altitudes. (*From Hurtado, by permission of Annals of Internal Medicine.*)

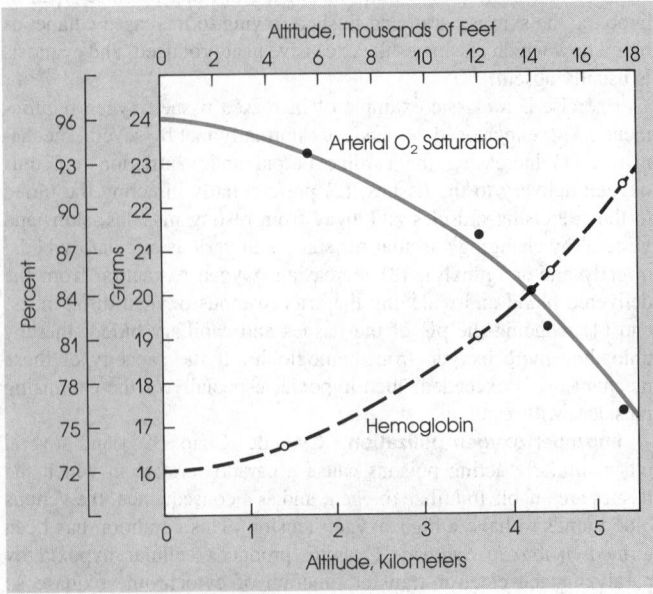

in severely symptomatic patients with extremely high hematocrit levels, usually exceeding 65 percent, but it must be carried out slowly, with caution, and with the realization that the polycythemia is, in fact, an important compensatory mechanism. However, reduction of red blood cell volume may result in a reduction of the elevated blood viscosity which improves blood flow.

The excessive use of coal-tar derivatives and other forms of chronic poisoning, by producing abnormal hemoglobin pigments such as *methemoglobin* and *sulfhemoglobin* (Chap. 306), also may cause erythrocytosis. Patients with abnormal hemoglobins which displace the oxygen dissociation curve to the left and interfere with oxygen unloading in the tissues stimulate the production of erythropoietin and a secondary erythrocytosis *unassociated* with leukocytosis or thrombocytosis (Chap. 306).

Mild erythrocytosis is sometimes found in *Cushing's syndrome* and can be produced by the administration of large amounts of adrenocortical steroids and androgens. Especially intriguing are the instances of erythrocytosis observed in association with various *tumors* which produce erythropoietin or an erythropoietin-like substance. These include vascular tumors (hemangioblastomas) in the posterior fossa, renal tumors (renal cell carcinoma, adenoma, and sarcoma), uterine myoma, hepatic carcinoma, and pheochromocytoma. Erythrocytosis also occurs occasionally in patients with solitary and polycystic disease of the kidneys, hydronephrosis, and renal artery stenosis. Plasma erythropoietin levels have been found to be elevated in a number of these patients with tumors and indeed all forms of secondary polycythemia. Erythropoietin-like activity has been demonstrated in tumor extracts and in renal cyst fluid, and erythrocytosis has disappeared after the associated tumor was removed.

Stress erythrocytosis This term has been applied to the polycythemia seen occasionally in active, hard-working, middle-aged white males who are typically hypertensive, overweight, and in a state of anxiety and who appear florid but have none of the other characteristic signs of polycythemia vera, i.e., no splenomegaly or leukocytosis with immature white blood cells. In such persons, the total red blood cell mass is normal, and the plasma volume is below normal. Thus they have a moderately elevated hematocrit, usually 50 to 60 percent, and *relative* polycythemia. *Smokers' polycythemia* is a closely related condition, but the high carboxyhemoglobin concentration may cause a small absolute increase in red cell mass which is often associated with a reduced plasma volume. Smoking should be discontinued.

CLINICAL FEATURES AND DIFFERENTIAL DIAGNOSIS Patients with polycythemia present with (in addition to the symptoms of the underlying condition) a characteristic ''ruddy'' cyanosis, dizziness, headache, epistaxes, and an increased incidence of thrombotic complications.

The *differential diagnosis* of absolute polycythemia is discussed in Chap. 309. In polycythemia vera, erythropoietin levels are usually absent or below normal, leukocyte alkaline phosphatase, vitamin B_{12} binding capacity, and vitamin B_{12} levels and platelet and total white blood cells are usually elevated, and splenomegaly is common. Serum uric acid and lactate dehydrogenase (LDH) levels may be increased. The bone marrow shows hyperplasia of all elements. In secondary polycythemia with hypoxia, Pa_{CO_2} is usually reduced, erythropoietin levels are elevated, while levels of leukocyte alkaline phosphatase, serum vitamin B_{12}, platelet, total white blood cell, and differential counts are all normal. The liver and spleen are not enlarged, and the bone marrow shows only erythroid hyperplasia. In the absence of features of either polycythemia vera or polycythemia secondary to hypoxia or to a tumor, a hemoglobin with a high affinity for oxygen should be sought.

Workup of patients with polycythemia should include a chest roentgenogram, electrocardiogram, and arterial oxygen saturation determination to search for disease of the heart and lungs. In addition, imaging of the spleen should be carried out to assess its size and of the kidney to look for an erythropoietin-producing lesion. In patients who do not appear to have polycythemia vera or hypoxemia, the oxygen affinity of the patient's hemoglobin, i.e., the P_{O_2} at which 50

percent of the hemoglobin is deoxygenated (P_{50}) should be measured to detect hemoglobins which fail to release oxygen normally.

CYANOSIS

Cyanosis refers to a bluish color of the skin and mucous membranes resulting from an increased amount of reduced hemoglobin, or of hemoglobin derivatives, in the small blood vessels of those areas. It is usually most marked in the lips, nail beds, ears, and malar eminences. The florid skin characteristic of polycythemia vera (Chap. 309) must be distinguished from the true cyanosis discussed here. A cherry-colored flush, rather than cyanosis, is caused by carboxyhemoglobin (Chap. 395). The degree of cyanosis is modified by the quality of cutaneous pigment and the thickness of the skin, as well as by the state of the cutaneous capillaries. The accurate clinical detection of the presence and degree of cyanosis is difficult, as proved by oximetric studies. In some instances, central cyanosis can be detected reliably when the arterial saturation has fallen to 85 percent; in others, particularly in dark-skinned persons, it may not be detected until the saturation has declined to 75 percent.

The increase in the quantity of reduced hemoglobin in the cutaneous vessels which produces cyanosis may be brought about either by an increase in the quantity of venous blood in the skin as the result of dilatation of the venules and venous ends of the capillaries or by a reduction in the oxygen saturation in the capillary blood. In general, cyanosis becomes apparent when the mean capillary concentration of reduced hemoglobin exceeds 5 g/dL. It is the *absolute* rather than the *relative* quantity of reduced hemoglobin which is important in producing cyanosis. Thus, in a patient with severe anemia, the relative amount of reduced hemoglobin in the venous blood may be very large when considered in relation to the total amount of hemoglobin. However, since the concentration of the latter is markedly reduced, the *absolute* quantity of reduced hemoglobin may still be small, and therefore patients with severe anemia and even *marked* arterial desaturation do not display cyanosis. Conversely, the higher the total hemoglobin content, the greater is the tendency toward cyanosis; thus patients with marked polycythemia tend to be cyanotic at higher levels of arterial oxygen saturation than patients with normal hematocrit values. Likewise, local passive congestion, which causes an increase in the total amount of reduced hemoglobin in the vessels in a given area, may cause cyanosis. Cyanosis also is observed when nonfunctional hemoglobin such as methemoglobin or sulfhemoglobin (Chap. 306) is present in blood.

Cyanosis may be subdivided into *central* and *peripheral* types. In the *central* type, there is arterial blood unsaturation or an abnormal hemoglobin derivative, and the mucous membranes and skin are both affected. *Peripheral* cyanosis is due to a slowing of blood flow to an area and abnormally great extraction of oxygen from normally saturated arterial blood. It results from vasoconstriction and diminished peripheral blood flow, such as occurs in cold exposure, shock, congestive failure, and peripheral vascular disease. Often in these conditions the mucous membranes of the oral cavity or those beneath the tongue may be spared. Clinical differentiation between central and peripheral cyanosis may not always be simple, and in conditions such as cardiogenic shock with pulmonary edema there may be a mixture of both types.

DIFFERENTIAL DIAGNOSIS (See Table 32-2) **Central cyanosis** Decreased arterial oxygen saturation results from a marked reduction in the oxygen tension in the arterial blood. This may be brought about by a decline in the tension of oxygen in the inspired air without sufficient compensatory alveolar hyperventilation to maintain alveolar oxygen tension. Cyanosis does not occur to a significant degree in an ascent to an altitude of 2500 m (8000 ft) but is marked in a further ascent to 5000 m (16,000 ft). The reason for this becomes clear on studying the *S* shape of the oxygen dissociation curve (Fig. 302-4). At 2500 m (8000 ft) the tension of oxygen in the inspired air is about 120 mmHg, the alveolar tension is approximately 80 mmHg, and the

---

TABLE 32-2   Causes of cyanosis

CENTRAL CYANOSIS

A Decreased arterial oxygen saturation
    1 Decreased atmospheric pressure—high altitude
    2 Impaired pulmonary function
      a Alveolar hypoventilation
      b Uneven relationships between pulmonary ventilation and perfusion
        (perfusion of hypoventilated alveoli)
      c Impaired oxygen diffusion
    3 Anatomic shunts
      a Certain types of congenital heart disease
      b Pulmonary arteriovenous fistulas
      c Multiple small intrapulmonary shunts
    4 Hemoglobin with low affinity for oxygen
B Hemoglobin abnormalities
    1 Methemoglobinemia—hereditary, acquired
    2 Sulfhemoglobinema—acquired
    3 Carboxyhemoglobinemia (not true cyanosis)

PERIPHERAL CYANOSIS

A Reduced cardiac output
B Cold exposure
C Redistribution of blood flow from extremities
D Arterial obstruction
E Venous obstruction

---

hemoglobin is nearly completely saturated. However, at 5000 m (16,000 ft) the oxygen tensions in atmospheric air and alveolar air are about 85 and 50 mmHg, respectively, and the oxygen dissociation curve shows that the arterial blood is only about 75 percent saturated. This leaves 25 percent of the hemoglobin in the reduced form, an amount likely to be associated with cyanosis in the absence of anemia. Similarly, a mutant hemoglobin with a low affinity for oxygen (e.g., Hb Kansas) causes lowered arterial oxygen saturation and resultant central cyanosis (Chap. 306).

Seriously *impaired pulmonary function*, through alveolar hypoventilation or perfusion of unventilated or poorly ventilated areas of the lung, is a common cause of central cyanosis (Chap. 214). This may occur acutely, as in extensive pneumonia or pulmonary edema, or with chronic pulmonary diseases (e.g., emphysema). In the last situation polycythemia is generally present, and clubbing of the fingers may occur. However, in many types of chronic pulmonary disease with fibrosis and obliteration of the capillary vascular bed, cyanosis does not occur because there is relatively little perfusion of underventilated areas.

Another cause of decreased arterial oxygen saturation is *shunting of systemic venous blood into the arterial circuit.* Certain forms of congenital heart disease are associated with cyanosis (Chap. 199). Since blood flows from a higher-pressure to a lower-pressure region, in order for a cardiac defect to result in a right-to-left shunt, it must ordinarily be combined with an obstructive lesion distal to the defect or with elevated pulmonary vascular resistance. The most common congenital cardiac lesion associated with cyanosis in the adult is the combination of ventricular septal defect and pulmonary outflow tract obstruction (tetralogy of Fallot). The more severe the obstruction, the greater the degree of right-to-left shunting and resultant cyanosis. The mechanisms for the elevated pulmonary vascular resistance which may produce cyanosis in the presence of intra- and extracardiac communications without pulmonic stenosis (Eisenmenger syndrome) are discussed elsewhere (Chap. 199). In patients with patent ductus arteriosus, pulmonary hypertension, and right-to-left shunt, *differential cyanosis* results; i.e., cyanosis occurs in the lower but not in the upper extremities.

Pulmonary arteriovenous fistulas may be congenital or acquired, solitary or multiple, microscopic or massive. The degree of cyanosis produced by these fistulas depends on their size and number. They occur with some frequency in hereditary hemorrhagic telangiectasia. Arterial oxygen unsaturation also occurs in some patients with

cirrhosis, presumably as a consequence of pulmonary arteriovenous fistulas or portal vein–pulmonary vein anastomoses.

In patients with cardiac or pulmonary right-to-left shunts, the presence and severity of cyanosis depend on the size of the shunt relative to the systemic flow as well as on the oxyhemoglobin saturation of the venous blood. In patients with central cyanosis due to arterial oxygen unsaturation, the severity of cyanosis increases with exercise. With increased extraction of oxygen from the blood by the exercising muscles, the venous blood returning to the right side of the heart is more unsaturated than at rest, and shunting of this blood or its passage through lungs incapable of normal oxygenation intensifies the cyanosis. Also, since the systemic vascular resistance normally decreases with exercise, the right-to-left shunt is augmented by exercise in patients with congenital heart disease and communications between the two sides of the heart. Secondary polycythemia occurs frequently in patients with arterial unsaturation and contributes to the cyanosis.

Cyanosis can be caused by small amounts of circulating methemoglobin and by even smaller amounts of sulfhemoglobin (Chap. 306). Although they are uncommon causes of cyanosis, these abnormal hemoglobin pigments should be sought by spectroscopy when cyanosis is not readily explained by malfunction of the circulatory or respiratory systems. Generally, clubbing does not occur with them. The diagnosis of methemoglobinemia can be suspected, if, on mixing the patient's blood in a test tube and exposing it to air, it remains brown.

Peripheral cyanosis   Probably the most common cause of peripheral cyanosis is generalized vasoconstriction resulting from exposure to cold air or water. This is a normal response. When cardiac output is low, as in severe congestive heart failure or shock, cutaneous vasoconstriction occurs as a compensatory mechanism, so blood is diverted from the skin to more vital areas such as the central nervous system and heart (Chap. 195), and intense cyanosis associated with cool extremities may result. Even though the arterial blood is normally saturated, the reduced volume flow through the skin and the reduced oxygen tension at the venous end of the capillary result in cyanosis.

Arterial obstruction to an extremity, as with an embolus, or arteriolar constriction, as in cold-induced vasospasm (Raynaud's phenomenon; Chap. 211), generally results in pallor and coldness, but there may be associated cyanosis. If there is venous obstruction and the extremity is congested, as with stagnation of blood flow, cyanosis is also present. Venous hypertension, which may be local (as in thrombophlebitis) or generalized (as in tricuspid valve disease or constrictive pericarditis), dilates the subpapillary venous plexuses and thereby intensifies cyanosis.

APPROACH TO THE PATIENT WITH CYANOSIS   Certain features are important in arriving at the proper cause of cyanosis:

1 The history, particularly the duration (cyanosis present since birth is usually due to congenital heart disease), and possible exposure to drugs or chemicals which may produce abnormal types of hemoglobin.
2 Clinical differentiation of central as opposed to peripheral cyanosis. Objective evidence by physical or radiographic examination of disorders of the respiratory or cardiovascular systems. Massage or gentle warming of a cyanotic extremity will increase peripheral blood flow and abolish peripheral but not central cyanosis.
3 The presence or absence of clubbing of the fingers (see below). Clubbing without cyanosis is frequent in patients with infective endocarditis and in association with ulcerative colitis; it may occasionally occur in healthy persons, and in some instances it may be occupational, e.g., in jackhammer operators. Slight cyanosis of the lips and cheeks, without clubbing of the fingers, is common in patients with mitral stenosis and is probably due to minimal arterial hypoxia resulting from fibrotic changes in the lungs secondary to long-standing congestion combined with reduction of cardiac output (Chap. 201). The combination of cyanosis and clubbing is frequent in patients with certain types of congenital cardiac disease and is seen occasionally in persons with pulmonary

disease such as lung abscess or pulmonary arteriovenous shunts. On the other hand, peripheral cyanosis or acutely developing central cyanosis is not associated with clubbed fingers.

4 Determination of arterial blood oxygen tension or oxygen saturation, spectroscopic and other examinations of the blood for abnormal types of hemoglobin.

CLUBBING The selective bullous enlargement of the distal segments of the fingers and toes due to proliferation of connective tissue, particularly on the dorsal surface, is termed *clubbing*; an increase occurs in the sponginess of the soft tissue at the base of the nail. Clubbing may be hereditary, idiopathic, or acquired and associated with a variety of disorders, including cyanotic congenital heart disease, infective endocarditis, and a variety of pulmonary conditions (among them primary and metastatic lung cancer, bronchiectasis, lung abscess, cystic fibrosis, and mesothelioma), as well as with some gastrointestinal diseases (including regional enteritis, chronic ulcerative colitis, and hepatic cirrhosis). Clubbing in patients with primary and metastatic lung cancer, mesothelioma, bronchiectasis, and hepatic cirrhosis may be associated with *hypertrophic osteoarthropathy*. In this condition, the subperiosteal formation of new bone in the distal diaphyses of the long bones of the extremities causes pain and symmetric arthritis-like changes in the shoulders, knees, ankles, wrists, and elbows. The diagnosis of hypertrophic osteoarthropathy may be confirmed by bone radiographs and scans. Although the mechanism of clubbing is unclear, it appears to be secondary to a (presumably humoral) substance which causes dilation of the vessels of the fingertip.

REFERENCES

DOLL DC, GREENBERG BR: Cerebral thrombosis in smokers' polycythemia. Ann Intern Med 102:786, 1985

ERSLEV AJ: Erythrocytosis (Chaps 73–75), in *Hematology*, 4th ed, WJ Williams et al (eds). New York, McGraw-Hill, 1990, p 705

HANSEN-FLASCHEN J, NORDBERG J: Clubbing and hypertrophic osteoarthropathy. Clin Chest Med 8:287, 1987

HURTADO A: Some clinical aspects of life at high altitudes. Ann Intern Med 53:247, 1960

MURPHY S: Polycythemia vera. Dis Mon 38:165, 1992

SCHWARCZ TH et al: Thromboembolic complications of polycythemia: Polycythemia vera vs. smokers' polycythemia. J Vasc Surg 17:518, 1993

SMITH JR, LANDAW SA: Smokers' polycythemia. N Engl J Med 298:6, 1978

SZIDON JP, FISHMAN AP: Cyanosis and clubbing, in *Pulmonary Diseases and Disorders*, 2d ed, A Fishman (ed). Philadelphia, Saunders, 1988, p 351

TERRITO MC, ROSOVE MH: Cyanotic congenital heart disease: Hematologic management. J Am Coll Cardiol 18:320, 1991

33 EDEMA

EUGENE BRAUNWALD

Edema is defined as an increase in the interstitial fluid volume, which may expand by several liters before the abnormality is apparent clinically. Therefore, a weight gain of several kilograms usually precedes overt manifestations of edema, and a similar weight loss from diuresis can be induced in a slightly edematous patient before ''dry weight'' is achieved. *Ascites* (Chap. 43) and *hydrothorax* refer to accumulation of excess fluid in the peritoneal and pleural cavities, respectively, and are considered to be special forms of edema. *Anasarca* refers to gross, generalized edema.

Depending on its cause and mechanism, edema may be localized or have a generalized distribution; it is recognized in its generalized form by puffiness of the face, which is most readily apparent in the periorbital areas, and by the persistence of an indentation of the skin following pressure; this is known as ''pitting'' edema. In its more subtle form, it may be detected by noting that after the stethoscope

is removed from the chest wall, the rim of the bell leaves an indentation on chest skin for a few minutes. When the ring on a finger fits more snugly than in the past or when a patient complains of difficulty in putting on shoes, particularly in the evening, edema may be present.

PATHOGENESIS (See also Chap. 45) About one-third of the total-body water is confined to the extracellular space. This compartment, in turn, is composed of the plasma volume and the interstitial space. Normally the plasma volume represents about 25 percent of the extracellular space, and the remainder is interstitial fluid. The forces that regulate the disposition of fluid between these two components of the extracellular compartment are frequently referred to as the Starling forces (see p. 177). The hydrostatic pressure within the vascular system and the colloid oncotic pressure in the interstitial fluid tend to promote movement of fluid from the vascular to the extravascular space. In contrast, the colloid oncotic pressure contributed by the plasma proteins and the hydrostatic pressure within the interstitial fluid, referred to as the *tissue tension*, promote the movement of fluid into the vascular compartment. Consequently there is a movement of water and diffusible solutes from the vascular space at the arteriolar end of the capillaries. Fluid is returned from the interstitial space into the vascular system at the venous end of the capillary and by way of the lymphatics, and unless these channels are obstructed, lymph flow tends to increase if there is net movement of fluid from the vascular compartment to the interstitium. These forces are usually balanced so that a steady state exists in the sizes of the intravascular and interstitial compartments, and yet a large exchange between them is permitted. However, should any one of the hydrostatic or oncotic forces be altered significantly, a net movement of fluid from one component of the extracellular space to the other will occur.

An increase in capillary pressure as a cause of edema may result from an elevation of venous pressure due to local obstruction in venous drainage. This increase may be generalized as occurs in congestive heart failure, or rarely it may result from the simple expansion of the vascular volume by the administration of large volumes of fluid at a rate in excess of the ability of the kidneys to excrete them. The colloid oncotic pressure of the plasma may be reduced, owing to any factor that may induce severe hypoalbuminemia, such as malnutrition, liver disease, loss of protein into the urine or into the gastrointestinal tract, or a severe catabolic state.

Edema may also result from damage to the capillary endothelium, which increases its permeability and permits the transfer of protein into the interstitial compartment. Injury to the capillary wall can result from chemical or bacterial agents as well as from thermal or mechanical trauma. Increased capillary permeability may also be a consequence of a hypersensitivity reaction and is characteristic of immune injury. Damage to the capillary endothelium is presumably responsible for inflammatory edema, which is usually nonpitting, localized, and accompanied by other signs of inflammation—redness, heat, and tenderness.

To formulate a hypothesis about the pathophysiology of an edematous state, it is important to discriminate between the *primary* events, such as venous or lymphatic obstruction, reduction of cardiac output, hypoalbuminemia, trapping of fluid in spaces such as the peritoneal cavity, or an increase in capillary permeability, and the predictable *secondary* consequences, which include the renal retention of salt and water in an attempt to restore the plasma volume. Both the primary event and the secondary consequences may contribute to the formation of edema.

The development of edema depends on one or more alterations in the Starling forces so that there is a net movement of fluid from the vascular system into the interstitium or into a ''third space'' or from the arterial compartment of the vascular space into the chambers of the heart or into the venous circulation itself. In many forms of edema the *effective arterial blood volume*, an as yet poorly defined parameter of the filling of the arterial tree, is reduced, and as a consequence a series of physiologic responses designed to restore it to normal are

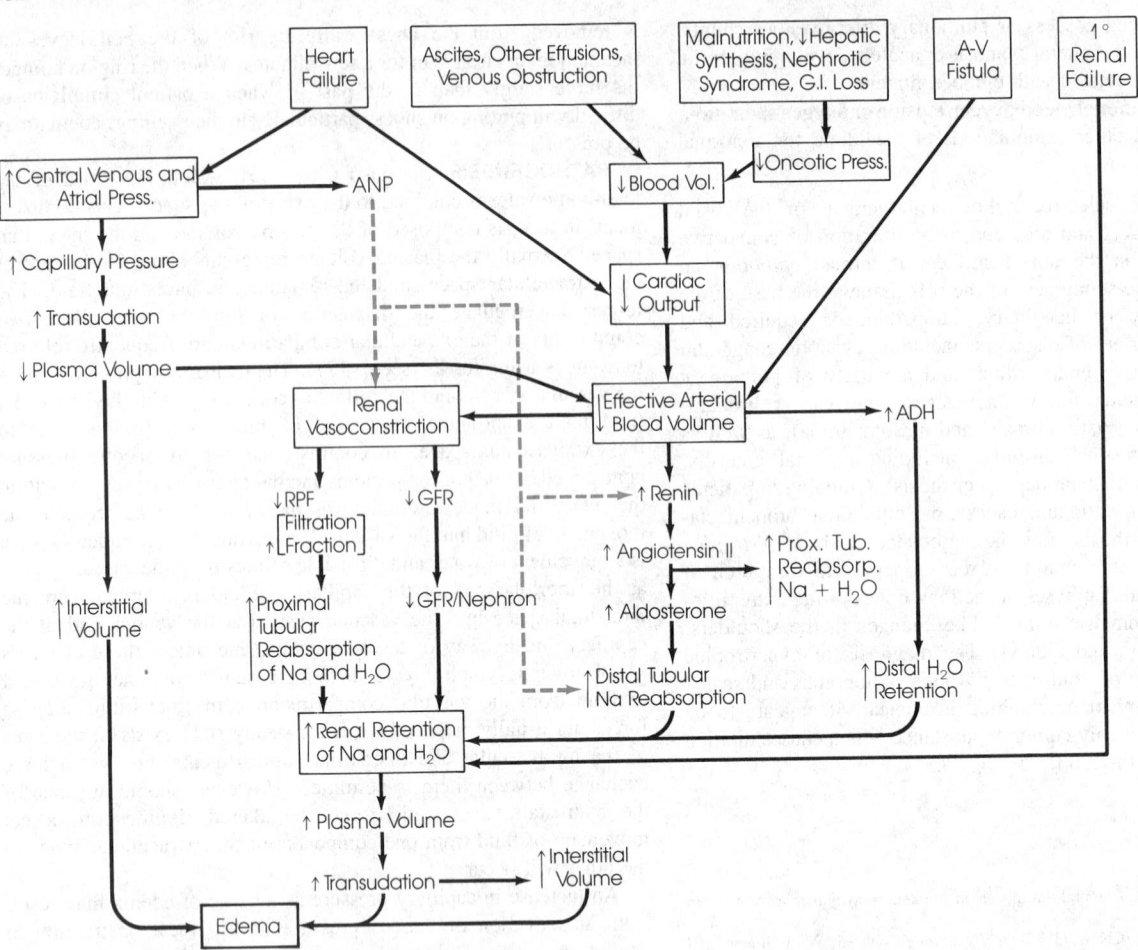

FIGURE 33-1   Sequence of events leading to the formation and retention of salt and water and the development of edema. ANP, atrial natriuretic peptide; RPF, renal plasma flow; GFR, glomerular filtration rate. Inhibitory influences are shown by colored dashed lines.

set into motion. A key element of these responses is the retention of an increment of salt and therefore of water, and in many instances this repairs the deficit of the effective arterial blood volume; often this occurs without the development of overt edema. If, however, the retention of salt and water is insufficient to restore and maintain the effective arterial blood volume, the stimuli are not dissipated, the retention of salt and water continues, and edema develops. This sequence of events is operative in dehydration and hemorrhage. Although in these conditions there is a reduction of effective arterial blood volume and activation of the entire sequence shown in the center of Fig. 33-1, including the diminished excretion of salt and water, edema does not occur because the net sodium and water balance is negative rather than positive. In most conditions that lead to edema the mechanisms responsible for maintaining a normal effective osmolality in the body fluids operate efficiently so that sodium retention promotes thirst and secretion of the antidiuretic hormone, which, in turn, lead to the ingestion and retention of approximately 1 L of water for each 140 mmol sodium retained. In edematous states, isotonic expansion of the extracellular fluid space may be massive, while the intracellular fluid volume is changed little or not at all.

Reduced cardiac output   A reduction of cardiac output, whatever the cause, is associated with a reduction of the effective arterial blood volume as well as of renal blood flow, constriction of the efferent renal arterioles, and an elevation of the filtration fraction, i.e., the ratio of glomerular filtration rate to renal plasma flow. In severe heart failure there is a reduction in the glomerular filtration rate. Activation of the sympathetic nervous system and of the renin-angiotensin systems are responsible for renal vasoconstriction. The finding that alpha-adrenergic blocking agents and/or angiotensin-converting enzyme inhibitors augment renal blood flow and induce diuresis supports the role of these two systems in elevating renal vascular resistance and salt and water retention.

Renal factors   Reduced cardiac output lowers effective arterial blood volume. This increases the tubular reabsorption of glomerular filtrate which, in turn, plays a principal role in the salt and water retention of heart failure. There is evidence for both proximal and distal increases in sodium reabsorption in heart failure. Alterations in intrarenal hemodynamics appear to play a significant role. Heart failure, by augmenting renal arteriolar constriction, reduces the hydrostatic pressure and raises the colloid osmotic pressure in the peritubular capillaries, thus enhancing salt and water reabsorption in the proximal tubule. The reduction of renal perfusion pressure may be responsible for augmentation of sodium reabsorption in the ascending limb of the loop of Henle.

In addition, the diminished renal blood flow characteristic of states in which the effective arterial blood volume is reduced is translated by the renal juxtaglomerular cells into a signal for increased renin release (Chap. 335). The mechanisms responsible for this release include a baroreceptor response: reduced renal perfusion results in incomplete filling of the renal arterioles and diminished stretch of the juxtaglomerular cells, a signal that provides for the elaboration or release, or both, of renin. A second mechanism for renin release involves the macula densa; as a result of reduced glomerular filtration the sodium chloride load reaching the distal renal tubules is reduced. This is sensed by the macula densa, which in an undefined manner signals the neighboring juxtaglomerular cells to secrete renin. A third mechanism involves the sympathetic nervous system and circulating catecholamines. Activation of the beta-adrenergic receptors in the juxtaglomerular cells stimulates renin release. These three mechanisms generally act in concert.

The renin-angiotensin-aldosterone (RAA) system (See Chap. 335) Renin, an enzyme with a molecular weight of about 40,000, acts on its substrate, angiotensinogen, an alpha$_2$ globulin synthesized by the liver, to release angiotensin I, a decapeptide, which is broken down to angiotensin II, an octapeptide. This has vasoconstrictor properties, especially on the efferent arterioles, and independently increases Na reabsorption in the proximal tubule. The intrarenal production of angiotensin II may also contribute to renal vasoconstriction and to the salt and water retention in heart failure. Angiotensin II also enters the circulation and stimulates the production of aldosterone by the zona glomerulosa of the adrenal cortex. In patients with heart failure, not only is aldosterone secretion elevated but the biologic half-life of aldosterone is prolonged, which further increases the plasma level of the hormone. A depression of hepatic blood flow, particularly during exercise, secondary to a reduction in cardiac output, is responsible for the reduced hepatic catabolism of aldosterone. The activation of the RAA system is most striking in the early phase of acute, severe heart failure and is less intense in patients with chronic, stable, compensated heart failure.

Although increased quantities of aldosterone are secreted in heart failure and in other edematous states and although blockade of the action of aldosterone by spironolactone often induces a moderate diuresis in edematous states, persistent augmented levels of aldosterone (or other mineralocorticoids) alone do not always promote accumulation of edema, as witnessed by the lack of striking fluid retention in most instances of primary aldosteronism (Chap. 335). Furthermore, although normal subjects retain some salt and water under the influence of a potent mineralocorticoid, such as deoxycorticosterone acetate or fludrocortisone, this accumulation is self-limiting, despite continued exposure to the steroid, a phenomenon known as mineralocorticoid escape. The failure of normal subjects receiving large doses of mineralocorticoids to accumulate large quantities of fluid and to develop edema is probably a consequence of an increase in glomerular filtration rate (pressure natriuresis) and through the action of natriuretic substance(s) (see below). The continued secretion of aldosterone may be more important in the accumulation of fluid in edematous states because patients with edema are generally unable to repair the deficit in effective arterial blood volume. As a consequence they do not develop pressure natriuresis nor do they elaborate normal quantities of atrial natriuretic peptide.

Blockade of the RAA system, by blocking angiotensin II receptors or inhibiting the angiotensin-converting enzyme (ACE) reduces efferent arterial resistance and increases renal blood flow. This action, combined with the rise in cardiac output secondary to afterload reduction as well as reduction in the secretion of aldosterone combine to cause diuresis. However, in patients with moderate or severe impairment of renal function interference with the RAA system can cause paradoxical sodium retention due to intensification of renal failure.

Atrial natriuretic peptide Atrial distention and/or a sodium load cause release into the circulation of atrial natriuretic peptide (ANP), a polypeptide; a high-molecular-weight precursor of ANP is stored in secretory granules within atrial myocytes. Release of ANP causes (1) excretion of sodium and water by augmenting glomerular filtration rate, inhibiting sodium reabsorption in the proximal tubule, and inhibiting release of renin and aldosterone; and (2) arteriolar and venous dilatation. Thus, ANP has the capacity to oppose sodium retention and arterial pressure elevation in hypervolemic states.

There is also some evidence for the existence of a distinctly different natriuretic factor, a low-molecular-weight substance that is activated or released as a result of the expansion of the extracellular fluid and causes natriuresis by inhibiting renal sodium reabsorption through inhibiting ouabain-sensitive Na^+,K^+-ATPase. The roles of the latter factor and of ANP in normal and pathophysiologic conditions requires clarification. For example, it is not yet clear why patients with heart failure and hepatic cirrhosis have low rates of sodium excretion and edema despite often having high circulating levels of ANP, but it is likely that abnormal resistance of the end-organ, i.e.,

the renal tubule to ANP, plays a key role. This resistance to ANP in edematous states makes it unlikely that pharmacologic elevation of ANP will be very helpful in the management of edema.

Obstruction of venous (and lymphatic) drainage of a limb In this condition the hydrostatic pressure in the capillary bed upstream to the obstruction increases so that more fluid than normal is transferred from the vascular to the interstitial space. Since the alternate route (i.e., the lymphatic channels) may also be obstructed, this event causes an increased volume of interstitial fluid in the limb, i.e., a trapping of fluid in the extremity, at the expense of the blood volume in the remainder of the body, thereby reducing effective arterial blood volume and leading to the consequences shown in Fig. 33-1.

As fluid accumulates in the interstitium of the limb in which venous and lymphatic drainage are obstructed, tissue tension rises until it counterbalances the primary alterations in the Starling forces, at which time no further fluid accumulates in that limb. When the additional accumulation of fluid has repaired the deficit in plasma volume the stimuli to retain more salt and water are dissipated. The net effect is a local increase in the volume of interstitial fluid, and the secondary responses repair the plasma volume deficit incurred by the primary event. This same sequence occurs in ascites and hydrothorax, in which fluid is trapped or accumulates in the cavitary space, depleting the intravascular volume and leading to secondary salt and fluid retention, as already described.

Congestive heart failure (See also Chap. 195) In this disorder the defective systolic emptying of the chambers of the heart and/or the impairment of ventricular relaxation promotes an accumulation of blood in the heart and venous circulation at the expense of the arterial volume, and the aforementioned sequence of events (Fig. 33-1) is initiated. In mild heart failure, a small increment of total blood volume may repair the deficit of arterial volume and establish a new steady state because, through the operation of Starling's law of the heart, an increase in the volume of blood within the chambers of the heart promotes a more forceful contraction and may thereby increase the cardiac output (Fig. 195-1). However, if the cardiac disorder is more severe, retention of fluid cannot repair the deficit in effective arterial blood volume. The increment accumulates in the venous circulation, and the increase in capillary and lymphatic hydrostatic pressure promotes the formation of edema.

Incomplete ventricular emptying (systolic heart failure), and/or inadequate ventricular relaxation (diastolic heart failure), both lead to an elevation of ventricular diastolic pressure. If the impairment of cardiac function involves the right ventricle, pressures in the systemic veins and capillaries may rise, thereby augmenting the transudation of fluid into the interstitial space and enhancing the likelihood of peripheral edema. The elevated systemic venous pressure is transmitted to the thoracic duct with consequent reduction of lymph drainage, further increasing the accumulation of edema.

If the impairment of cardiac function (incomplete ventricular emptying and/or inadequate relaxation) involves the left ventricle, then pulmonary venous and capillary pressures rise [leading in some instances to pulmonary edema (Chap. 31)], as does pulmonary artery pressure; this in turn interferes with the systolic emptying of the right ventricle, leading to an elevation of right ventricular diastolic and of central and systemic venous pressures, enhancing the likelihood of formation of peripheral edema. Pulmonary edema impairs gas exchange and may induce hypoxia, which embarrasses cardiac function still further, sometimes causing a vicious cycle.

Nephrotic syndrome and other hypoalbuminic states (See also Chap. 240) The primary alteration in this disorder is a diminished colloid oncotic pressure due to massive losses of protein into the urine. This promotes a net movement of fluid into the interstitium, causes hypovolemia, and initiates the edema-forming sequence of events described above, including activation of the RAA system. With severe hypoalbuminemia, the salt and water which are retained cannot be restrained within the vascular compartment, total and effective arterial blood volumes decline, and hence the stimuli to retain salt and water are not abated. A similar sequence of events occurs in other conditions which lead to *severe* hypoalbuminemia, including severe nutritional deficiency states, protein-losing enteropathy, congenital hypoalbuminemia, and severe, chronic liver disease. However, in the nephrotic syndrome, the impairment of renal function contributes to the retention of sodium.

Cirrhosis (See also Chaps. 43 and 268)   The *total* blood volume in hepatic cirrhosis is commonly increased when the disorder is accompanied by a system of dilated venous radicles and multiple small arteriovenous fistulas. On the other hand, tissue perfusion, the effective arterial blood volume, and the intrathoracic blood volume all are diminished, probably as a consequence of the passage of blood through these fistulas, as well as from the portal venous hypertension and the obstruction of the lymphatic drainage of the liver. Intrahepatic hypertension appears to be responsible for renal sodium retention. These alterations are frequently complicated by reduced serum albumin secondary to reduced hepatic synthesis, which reduces the effective arterial blood volume even further, leading to activation of the RAA system and other salt- and water-retaining mechanisms. The concentration of circulating aldosterone is elevated by the liver's failure to metabolize this hormone. Initially, the excess interstitial fluid is localized preferentially behind the congested portal venous system and obstructed hepatic lymphatics, i.e., in the peritoneal cavity. In later stages, particularly when there is severe hypoalbuminemia, peripheral edema may develop.

Idiopathic edema   This syndrome, which occurs almost exclusively in women, is characterized by periodic episodes of edema, frequently accompanied by abdominal distention. Fairly large, diurnal alterations in weight occur with orthostatic retention of sodium and water, so that the patient may weigh several pounds more after having been in the upright posture for several hours. Such large diurnal weight changes suggest an increase in capillary permeability which appears to fluctuate in severity and to be aggravated by hot weather. There is some evidence that a reduction in plasma volume occurs in this condition with secondary activation of the RAA system. Idiopathic edema should be distinguished from cyclical or premenstrual edema in which the sodium and water retention may be secondary to excessive estrogen stimulation. There are also some cases in which the edema appears to be "diuretic-induced." It has been postulated that in these patients, chronic diuretic administration leads to mild blood volume depletion which causes chronic hyperreninemia and juxtaglomerular hyperplasia. Salt-retaining mechanisms appear to overcompensate for the direct effects of the diuretics. *Acute* withdrawal of diuretics can then leave the sodium-retaining forces unopposed, leading to fluid retention and edema.

The treatment of idiopathic cyclic edema includes a reduction in salt intake, rest in the supine position for several hours each day, the wearing of elastic stockings which are put on before arising in the morning, and an attempt to understand any underlying emotional problems. A variety of pharmacologic agents including ACE inhibitors, progesterone, the dopamine receptor agonist bromocriptine, and the sympathomimetic amine dextroamphetamine have all been reported in observational studies to be useful when administered to patients who do not respond to simpler measures. Diuretics may be initially useful but may lose their effectiveness with continuous administration; accordingly, they should be employed sparingly, if at all. Persistent discontinuation of diuretics paradoxically leads to diuresis in "diuretic-induced" edema, described above.

DIFFERENTIAL DIAGNOSIS   As a rule, localized edema can be readily differentiated from generalized edema. The great majority of patients with generalized edema suffer from advanced cardiac, renal, hepatic, or nutritional disorders. Consequently, the differential diagnosis of generalized edema should be directed toward identifying or excluding these several conditions.

Localized edema (See also Chap. 211)   Edema originating from inflammation or hypersensitivity is usually readily identified. Localized edema due to venous or lymphatic obstruction may be caused by thrombophlebitis, chronic lymphangitis, resection of regional lymph nodes, filariasis, etc. Lymphedema is particularly intractable

because restriction of lymphatic flow results in increased protein concentration in the interstitial fluid, a circumstance which aggravates retention of fluid.

Edema of heart failure   Evidence of heart disease, as manifested by cardiac enlargement and gallop rhythm, together with evidence of cardiac failure, such as dyspnea, basilar rales, venous distention, and hepatomegaly, usually provides an indication on clinical examination that edema results from heart failure. Noninvasive tests such as echocardiography and radionuclide angiography may be helpful in establishing the diagnosis of heart failure (see also Chaps. 190 and 195).

Edema of the nephrotic syndrome   Marked proteinuria (>3.5 g/d), severe hypoalbuminemia (<2 g/dL), and in some instances hypercholesterolemia are present. This syndrome may occur during the course of a variety of kidney diseases, which include glomerulonephritis, diabetic glomerulosclerosis, and hypersensitivity reactions. A history of previous renal disease may or may not be elicited (see also Chap. 240).

Edema of acute glomerulonephritis and other forms of renal failure   The edema occurring during the acute phases of glomerulonephritis is characteristically associated with hematuria, proteinuria, and hypertension. Although some evidence supports the view that the fluid retention is due to increased capillary permeability, in most instances the edema in this disease results from primary retention of sodium and water by the kidneys owing to renal insufficiency. This state differs from congestive heart failure in that it is characterized by a normal or increased cardiac output and a normal arterial–mixed venous oxygen difference. Patients with edema due to renal failure commonly have evidence of pulmonary congestion on chest roentgenograms before cardiac enlargement is significant, but they usually do not develop orthopnea. Patients with chronic impairment of renal function (including some patients with the nephrotic syndrome *without* severe hypoalbuminemia) may also develop edema due to primary renal retention of sodium and water.

Edema of cirrhosis (Chap. 268)   Ascites and biochemical and clinical evidence of hepatic disease (collateral venous channels, jaundice, and spider angiomas) characterize edema of hepatic origin. The ascites is frequently refractory to treatment because it collects as a result of a combination of obstruction of hepatic lymphatic drainage, portal hypertension, and hypoalbuminemia. Edema may also occur in other parts of the body in these patients as a result of hypoalbuminemia. Furthermore, the sizable accumulation of ascitic fluid may increase intraabdominal pressure and impede venous return from the lower extremities; hence, it tends to promote accumulation of edema in this region as well.

Edema of nutritional origin   A grossly deficient diet over a prolonged period may produce hypoproteinemia and edema. The latter may be intensified by the development of beriberi heart disease, also of nutritional origin, in which multiple peripheral arteriovenous fistulas result in reduced effective systemic perfusion and effective arterial blood volume, thereby enhancing edema formation (Chap. 207). Edema may actually become intensified when these famished subjects are first provided with an adequate diet. The ingestion of more food may increase the quantity of salt ingested, which is then retained along with water. Refeeding edema may also be linked to increased release of insulin, which directly increases tubular sodium reabsorption. In addition to hypoalbuminemia, hypokalemia and caloric deficits may be involved in the edema of starvation.

Other causes of edema   These include hypothyroidism, in which the edema (myxedema) may be located typically in the pretibial region and which may also be associated with periorbital puffiness. Exogenous hyperadrenocortism, pregnancy, and administration of estrogens and vasodilators, particularly the calcium antagonist nifedipine, may also all cause edema.

Distribution   The distribution of edema is an important guide to the cause. Thus, edema of one leg or of one or both arms is usually the result of venous and/or lymphatic obstruction. Edema resulting from hypoproteinemia characteristically is generalized, but it is especially evident in the very soft tissues of the eyelids and face and tends to be most pronounced in the morning because of the recumbent posture assumed during the night. Less common causes of facial edema include trichinosis, allergic reactions, and myxedema. Edema associated with heart failure, on the other hand, tends to be more extensive in the legs and to be accentuated in the evening, a feature also determined largely by posture. When patients with heart failure have been confined to bed, edema may be most prominent in the presacral region. Unilateral edema occasionally results from lesions in the central nervous system affecting the vasomotor fibers on one side of the body; paralysis also reduces lymphatic and venous drainage on the affected side.

Additional factors in diagnosis The color, thickness, and sensitivity of the skin are significant. Local tenderness and increase in temperature suggest inflammation. Local cyanosis may signify a venous obstruction. In individuals who have had repeated episodes of prolonged edema, the skin over the involved areas may be thickened, indurated, and often red.

Measurement or estimation of the venous pressure is of importance in evaluating edema. Elevation in an isolated part of the body usually reflects localized venous obstruction. Generalized elevation of systemic venous pressure usually indicates the presence of congestive heart failure. Ordinarily, significant increase in venous pressure can be recognized by the level at which cervical veins collapse (Chap. 188); in doubtful cases and for accurate recording, the central venous pressure should be measured manometrically. In patients with obstruction of the superior vena cava, edema is confined to the face, neck, and upper extremities, where the venous pressure is elevated compared with that in the lower extremities. Measurement of venous pressure in the upper extremities is also useful in patients with massive edema of the lower extremities and ascites; it is elevated when the edema is on a cardiac basis (e.g., constrictive pericarditis or tricuspid stenosis) but is normal when it is secondary to cirrhosis. Severe heart failure may cause ascites that may be distinguished from the ascites caused by hepatic cirrhosis by the jugular venous pressure, which usually is elevated in heart failure and normal in cirrhosis.

Determination of the concentration of serum albumin aids importantly in identifying those patients in whom edema is due, at least in part, to diminished intravascular colloid oncotic pressure. The presence of proteinuria also affords useful clues. The total absence of protein in the urine is evidence against renal disease as a cause of edema. Slight to moderate proteinuria is the rule in patients with heart failure, whereas persistent massive proteinuria is characteristic of the nephrotic syndrome.

APPROACH TO THE PATIENT WITH EDEMA An important first question is whether the edema is localized or generalized. If it is localized, those phenomena that may be responsible should be concentrated upon. Localized edema includes hydrothorax, ascites, or both. Either may be a consequence of local venous or lymphatic obstruction, as in inflammatory disease or carcinoma.

If the edema is generalized, it should be determined, first, if there is hypoalbuminemia of significant degree, e.g., serum albumin concentration less than 2.5 g/dL. If there is, the history, physical examination, urinalysis, and other laboratory data will help evaluate the question of cirrhosis, severe malnutrition, protein-losing gastroenteropathy, or the nephrotic syndrome as the underlying disorder. If hypoalbuminemia is not present, it should be determined if there is evidence of congestive heart failure of a severity to promote generalized edema. Finally, it should be determined whether the patient has an adequate urine output, or if there is significant oliguria or even anuria. These abnormalities are discussed in Chaps. 44, 236, and 237.

REFERENCES

CODY RJ et al: Regulation of glomerular filtration rate in chronic congestive heart failure patients. Kidney Int 34:361, 1988

EDWARDS BS et al: Identification of atrial natriuretic factor within the tissue in hamsters and humans with congestive heart failure. J Clin Invest 81:82, 1988

GOLDEN MHN: Protein deficiency, energy deficiency, and the oedema of malnutrition. Lancet 1:1261, 1982

KELSCH RC, SEDMAN AB: Nephrotic syndrome. Pediatr Rev 14:30, 1993

MOE GW et al: Control of extracellular fluid volume and pathophysiology of edema formation, in The Kidney, 4th ed, BM Brenner, FC Rector Jr (eds). Philadelphia, Saunders, 1991, pp 623–676

MOORE J JR, CAROME MA: Proteinuria. Clin Lab Med 13:21, 1993

PACKER M: Neurohormonal interactions and adaptations in congestive heart failure. Circulation 77:721, 1988

ROSE BD: Edematous states, in Clinical Physiology of Acid-Base and Electrolyte Disorders. New York, McGraw-Hill, 1989, pp 416–463

SCHRIER RW: Pathogenesis of sodium and water retention in high-output and low-output cardiac failure, nephrotic syndrome, cirrhosis, and pregnancy. Part I. N Engl J Med 319:1065, 1988

STAUB NB, TAYLOR AE (eds): Edema. New York, Raven Press, 1984

STREETEN DHP: Idiopathic edema: Pathogenesis, clinical features, and treatment. Metabolism 27:353, 1978

34 SHOCK

JOSEPH E. PARRILLO

Shock may be defined as the state in which profound and widespread reduction in the effective delivery of oxygen and other nutrients to tissues leads first to reversible and then, if prolonged, to irreversible cellular injury.

CONTROL OF ARTERIAL BLOOD PRESSURE Maintenance of adequate perfusion of vital organs is critical for survival. Organ perfusion is dependent on an appropriate perfusion pressure, which, in turn, is determined by two variables, the cardiac output and the systemic vascular resistance. The latter is proportional to the vessel length and the viscosity of blood and inversely proportional to the fourth power of the vessel radius. Therefore, the cross-sectional area of a vessel is by far the most important determinant of the resistance to blood flow. Since vascular smooth-muscle tone regulates the cross-sectional area of the arteriolar bed (the major site of systemic resistance in the vascular tree), any variable that affects smooth-muscle tone has a profound effect on vascular resistance and, in turn, on perfusion pressure.

The second critical determinant of arterial pressure is the cardiac output, which itself is the product of stroke volume and heart rate. The stroke volume is a function of three major variables, as discussed in Chap. 194: (1) preload, generally reflected in the ventricular end-diastolic volume, (2) impedance to blood flow (afterload), which is related to the systemic vascular resistance, and (3) myocardial contractility.

Physiologic mechanisms can affect the arterial pressure by acting on one or more of the variables mentioned above. These mechanisms include the local release of vasodilator metabolites such as adenosine; the release from the endothelium of substances that relax (e.g., endothelium-derived relaxing factor, nitric oxide) or contract (e.g., endothelin) subjacent vascular smooth muscle; the activity of the autonomic (sympathetic and parasympathetic) nervous system and the modulation of this activity by baroreceptor reflexes and the vasomotor center in the brainstem, which, in turn, is acted on by higher centers in the nervous system; the release into the bloodstream of the catecholamines epinephrine or norepinephrine by the adrenal medulla and sympathetic nerve endings (Chap. 68); the activity of the renin-angiotensin system (Chap. 335); the release of vasopressin (Chap. 333); the release of vasodilators, including the kinins and prostaglandins; and alterations in intravascular volume via control of fluid and electrolyte balance (Chap. 33). All these mechanisms can affect the arterial pressure by altering the vascular resistance and/or cardiac output. Through the integrated operation of these several mechanisms, the mean arterial pressure (the average pressure throughout the cardiac

TABLE 34-1   Classification of forms of shock

CARDIOGENIC SHOCK

Myopathic (reduced systolic function)
    Acute myocardial infarction
    Dilated cardiomyopathy
    Myocardial depression in septic shock
Mechanical
    Mitral regurgitation
    Ventricular septal defect
    Ventricular aneurysm
    LV outflow obstruction (aortic stenosis, idiopathic hypertrophic subaortic
      stenosis)
Arrhythmic

EXTRACARDIAC OBSTRUCTIVE SHOCK

Pericardial tamponade
Constrictive pericarditis
Pulmonary embolism (massive)
Severe pulmonary hypertension (primary or Eisenmenger)
Coarctation of the aorta

OLIGEMIC SHOCK

Hemorrhage
Fluid depletion

DISTRIBUTIVE SHOCK

Septic shock
Toxic products, e.g., overdose
Anaphylaxis
Neurogenic shock
Endocrinologic shock

SOURCE: Adapted with permission from Parker and Parrillo.

cycle) in resting, young, healthy adults is maintained within a relatively narrow range of 90 to 100 mmHg.

CLASSIFICATION OF SHOCK   A classification of shock based on cause is shown in Table 34-1.

Oligemic or hypovolemic shock   Hemorrhage or a large loss of fluid secondary to vomiting, diarrhea, burns, or dehydration leads to inadequate ventricular filling, i.e., to severely decreased preload, reflected in decreased left and right ventricular end-diastolic volumes and pressures. These changes lead to shock by causing an inadequate stroke volume and inadequate cardiac output. This is probably the most frequent cause of shock and also the best studied, because all gradations of oligemic shock can be produced in animal models.

Cardiogenic shock (See Chap. 202)   This is due to a severe depression of systolic cardiac performance. Systolic arterial pressure is < 80 mmHg, the cardiac index is reduced below 1.8 L/min/m², and the left ventricular filling pressure is elevated, generally above 18 mmHg; pulmonary edema may or may not be evident. The patient is frequently obtunded, the urine output is less than 20 mL/h, and the extremities are cold and cyanotic. The most frequent cause is infarction involving 40 percent or more of the left ventricular myocardium, leading to a severe reduction in left ventricular contractility and failure of the left ventricular pump. Other causes include acute myocarditis and the depression of myocardial contractility following cardiac arrest and prolonged cardiac surgery.

Another form of cardiogenic shock is caused by mechanical abnormalities of the ventricle. Acute mitral or aortic regurgitation or acutely acquired ventricular septal defect or ventricular aneurysm, usually caused by acute myocardial infarction, can cause a severe reduction in *forward* cardiac output (blood flow throughout the aortic valve into the systemic arterial circulation) and thereby result in cardiogenic shock.

Extracardiac obstructive shock   This form of shock is best exemplified by pericardial tamponade (Chap. 206). Physiologically, the major abnormality is the inability of the ventricle to fill during diastole, markedly limiting the stroke volume and ultimately the cardiac output. Another cause of extracardiac obstructive shock is massive pulmonary embolism (Chap. 226). Although the mechanism responsible for the reduced cardiac output in extracardiac obstructive shock differs from that in cardiogenic shock, the actual cause of shock, i.e., the severe reduction in tissue perfusion, is similar.

Distributive shock   Examples of this form of shock are septic shock (Chap. 83), neurogenic shock, and anaphylactic shock (Chap. 282), all of which usually cause a profound decrease in peripheral vascular resistance; the first is now the most common cause of death in intensive care units in the United States. The pathogenesis of septic shock involves abnormalities of both the peripheral vascular system and the heart. It is considered in detail below.

Patients may suffer from more than one form of shock simultaneously. Thus septic and oligemic shock sometimes coexist. These two forms of shock may produce dissimilar, even opposing cardiovascular effects, and treatment of one form may unmask the presence of the other.

PATHOGENESIS   Some characteristics of the pathogenesis of shock are the same regardless of the underlying cause. The final pathway of shock is cell death. Once large numbers of cells from vital organs have reached this stage, shock becomes irreversible, and death occurs despite correction of the underlying cause. This concept of irreversibility is useful because it emphasizes the need to prevent the progression of shock.

The pathogenetic mechanism leading to cell death is incompletely understood. One of the common denominators of the first three forms of shock listed in Table 34-1 is a low cardiac output (see Fig. 34-1). Patients with oligemic shock, cardiogenic shock, and extracardiac obstructive shock and a minority of patients with distributive shock develop a severe decrease in cardiac output and hence in perfusion of vital organs. Initially, compensatory mechanisms such as vasoconstriction may maintain arterial pressure at near-normal level. However, if the process causing shock continues, these compensatory mechanisms ultimately fail, leading to the clinical manifestations of the shock syndrome. If shock persists, cell death will ensue and result in irreversible shock.

Of the forms of shock with low cardiac output, *oligemic shock* has been studied the most carefully, both in humans and in animal models, and it provides lessons applicable to other forms of low-output shock. A healthy adult can compensate for the sudden loss of 10 percent of total blood volume using the mechanisms described previously, principally sympathetically mediated vasoconstriction. However, if 20 to 25 percent of the blood volume is lost rapidly, the compensatory mechanisms usually begin to fail, and the clinical shock syndrome ensues. The cardiac output declines, and there is hypotension despite generalized vasoconstriction. Regulation of local blood flow maintains perfusion of the heart and brain until late in the course, when these mechanisms also fail. Vasoconstriction, which begins as a compensatory mechanism in shock, may become excessive in some tissues and cause destructive lesions such as ischemic necrosis of the intestines or digits. A myocardial depressant factor has been identified in the dog with hemorrhagic shock, but this factor has not been clearly related to clinical myocardial dysfunction. Ultimately, if shock continues, end-organ damage occurs, precipitating the adult respiratory distress syndrome (Chap. 230), acute renal failure (Chap. 236), disseminated intravascular coagulation (Chap. 316), and multiorgan failure leading to death.

Distributive shock has a different and more complicated pathogenesis. Septic shock (Chap. 83) is characterized, at least initially, by a low systemic vascular resistance and an elevated cardiac output. As shown in Fig. 34-2, septic shock usually begins with a nidus of infection that releases microbes and/or one or more mediators into the bloodstream. Many mediators [e.g., histamine, kinins, most prostaglandins, lipid A (the toxic component of endotoxin), endorphins, tumor necrosis factor, interleukin 1, and interleukin 2] produce vascular dilatation, while others (e.g., some prostaglandins and leukotrienes) produce vasoconstriction. The peripheral vasodilatation results in a reduced systemic vascular resistance and a high cardiac

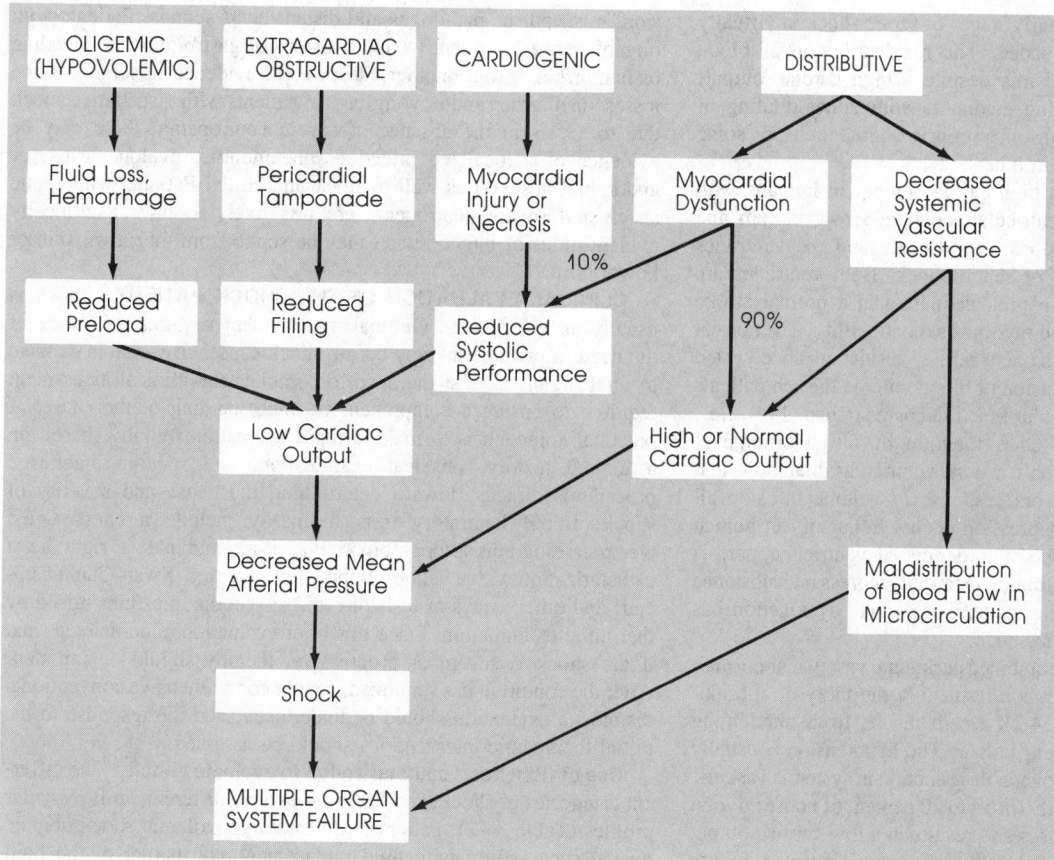

FIGURE 34-1 Pathogenesis of shock in humans. This schematic diagram depicts the present understanding of the pathogenetic relationships among the different types of shock and the cardiovascular abnormalities they usually produce.

FIGURE 34-2 Pathogenesis of human septic shock. This schematic diagram represents the present understanding of the interrelationships in the pathogenesis of septic shock in humans. (*From Parrillo et al, 1990.*)

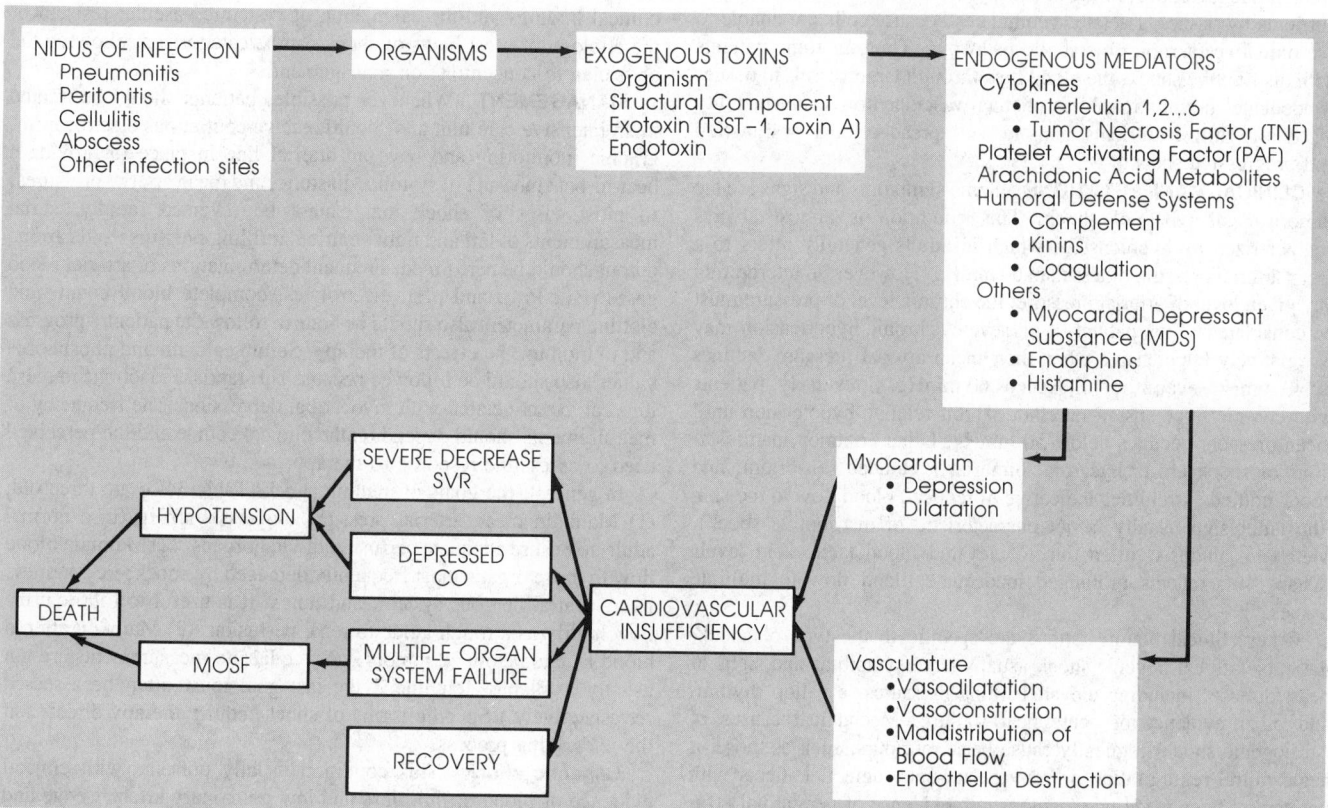

output; the latter occurs in the early stages of septic shock in virtually all patients who are volume-loaded. The maldistribution of blood flow, evidenced by lactic acidemia despite a high cardiac output, probably results from circulating mediators with either dilating or constricting properties, causing inappropriate dilatation in some vascular beds and constriction in others.

It has been argued that the high cardiac output in humans with septic shock indicates good ventricular function. However, left and right ventricular ejection fractions are reduced, and the ventricles dilate during the initial phase of septic shock. Both ventricles are usually dilated; the increase in preload maintains a normal stroke volume despite the depression of myocardial contractility. The normal stroke volume, combined with tachycardia, results in an elevated cardiac output. However, expansion of blood volume in such patients demonstrates depressed ventricular function curves (Chap. 194), i.e., the response of stroke work as a function of filling volume is subnormal. The reduced ejection fraction, ventricular dilatation, and decreased ventricular stroke work response to volume infusion all demonstrate that myocardial depression occurs frequently in human septic shock. The mechanism of this depressed ventricular performance is unknown; a circulating myocardial depressant substance probably plays a role. A similar pattern of cardiac dysfunction has been reported with anaphylactic shock.

If septic shock persists, the combined peripheral vascular abnormalities and the myocardial depression result in a mortality of approximately 50 percent (see Fig. 34-2). Death results from unrelenting hypotension and/or organ system failure. The hypotension is usually associated with a severe and irreversible reduction in systemic vascular resistance, although occasionally (in 10 to 20 percent of nonsurvivors) myocardial depression progresses and results in a low cardiac output that worsens the hypotension. Death from multiple-organ failure usually results from insufficiency of kidney, liver, brain, or lung function.

Other pathogenetic mechanisms in septic shock appear to relate to neutrophil aggregation, which produces microthrombi and endothelial cell injury; the latter, in turn, contribute to alterations in microvascular perfusion. In some forms of distributive shock, tissue blood flow appears adequate, but a mediator-induced "metabolic block" exists at the tissue level, preventing adequate utilization of oxygen and other nutrients by tissues. Lactate accumulates because cells are unable to use oxidative (aerobic) metabolic pathways. Thus, in some patients with distributive shock, the blood flow through large vessels to tissues is adequate, but abnormalities of microvascular flow or an inability of cells to utilize nutrients leads to widespread cellular dysfunction and progressive shock.

CLINICAL MANIFESTATIONS   Some symptoms and signs are the same for all types of shock. This condition is almost always characterized by hypotension, which in adults generally refers to a mean arterial pressure of less than 60 mmHg. However, in interpreting any given level of arterial pressure, the chronic level of pressure must be considered. Thus patients with severe, chronic hypertension may be relatively hypotensive when their mean arterial pressure declines by 40 mmHg, even if it still exceeds 60 mmHg. Conversely, patients with chronic hypotension may not exhibit relative hypotension until mean pressure declines below 50 mmHg. Other common manifestations of shock are tachycardia, oliguria, a clouded sensorium, and cool, mottled extremities indicative of reduced blood flow to the skin (the latter sign usually is not characteristic of distributive shock). Metabolic acidosis, often due to elevated blood lactic acid levels (Chap. 46), reflects prolonged inadequate blood flow to multiple tissues.

Other clinical manifestations are specific to the type of shock. Patients with cardiogenic shock usually have symptoms and signs of heart disease, including elevated filling pressures, a gallop rhythm, and other evidence of acute heart failure. Mechanical causes of cardiogenic shock frequently cause heart murmurs, such as those of acute mitral regurgitation or ventricular septal defect. Patients with pericardial tamponade may demonstrate evidence of pericardial effu-

sion, e.g., pulsus paradoxus and distant heart sounds. Patients with oligemic shock frequently have a history of gastrointestinal bleeding or hemorrhage from another site or clear evidence of large volume losses via diarrhea and/or vomiting. In patients with distributive shock due to sepsis in the absence of severe neutropenia, there may be evidence of a localized infection (pneumonitis, pyelonephritis, or abdominal abscess) as well as fever and chills. Patients with septic shock and severe neutropenia are less likely to have a clinically evident nidus of infection and may be septic from their own skin or bowel flora.

CLINICAL EVALUATION OF THE SHOCK PATIENT   Shock is usually an emergency. Optimal management requires a balance of the need to institute therapy before shock causes irreversible damage to vital organs against the need to complete the clinical assessment required to ensure a comprehensive understanding of the cause. A practical approach is to make a rapid evaluation initially, based on a limited history, physical examination, and specific diagnostic procedures directed toward determining the cause and severity of shock. Initial laboratory tests ordinarily include a chest x-ray; electrocardiogram; arterial blood P_{O_2}, P_{CO_2}, and pH; a right heart catheterization with a balloon-tipped flow-directed (Swan-Ganz) catheter; and other x-rays or tests directed at specific questions raised by the initial examination. Once this brief evaluation is completed, and if the shock is severe or progressive, therapy should be initiated. After the condition has stabilized, a more comprehensive conventional diagnostic evaluation should be undertaken, and the response to the initial therapeutic interventions should be assessed.

Use of right heart catheterization to evaluate shock   The different categories of shock (see Table 34-1) have different cardiovascular profiles (Table 34-2). Patients with mild hypovolemic shock may be treated successfully with fluid replacement, the nature of the fluid depending on the cause of the shock. However, in patients with moderate or severe shock, the flow-directed balloon-tipped pulmonary artery (Swan-Ganz) catheter is often useful for providing hemodynamic assessment and following the response to therapy, because clinical evaluation is frequently incorrect in estimating filling pressure and cardiac output.

Table 34-2 summarizes the usual hemodynamic profiles of patients with different forms of shock. When these profiles are combined with clinical findings and the calculation of systemic vascular resistance, the etiology of most bouts of shock can be categorized, allowing the physician to concentrate on management.

MANAGEMENT   Whenever possible, patients should be treated in an intensive care unit and should receive continuous electrocardiographic monitoring and have an arterial line in place to provide a beat-to-beat measure of systolic, diastolic, and mean arterial pressures. In most cases of shock that cannot be reversed rapidly, serial measurements of left and right ventricular filling pressures and cardiac output should be performed. Frequent determinations of arterial blood gases (P_{O_2}, P_{CO_2}, and pH), electrolytes, complete blood count, and clotting parameters also should be done to follow the patient's progress and to monitor the effects of therapy. Serum calcium and phosphorus values also should be followed because substantial reductions in these ions can be associated with myocardial depression. The frequency of measurements should depend on the clinical course and the perceived need to assess the response to therapy.

In general, the goals of treating shock (Table 34-3) are threefold: (1) Maintain mean arterial pressure above 60 mmHg (in a normal adult) to ensure adequate perfusion of vital organs. (2) Maintain blood flow to those organs most frequently damaged by shock, i.e., kidney, liver, central nervous system, and lungs. It is useful to follow urine flow hourly as a rough guide to renal perfusion. (3) Maintain arterial blood lactate below 22 mmol/L. (Since lactate measurements are not usually available "on line," the last goal must often be assessed retrospectively.) Specific forms of shock require therapy directed at the underlying process.

Oligemic shock   This condition usually presents with clinical evidence of blood or fluid loss and low pulmonary artery wedge and

TABLE 34-2 Use of right heart catheterization to diagnose the etiology of shock*

Diagnosis	Pulmonary capillary wedge pressure[†]	Cardiac output (CO)	Miscellaneous comments
Cardiogenic shock	↑ ↑	↓ ↓	
Cardiogenic shock due to myocardial dysfunction			Usually occurs with evidence of extensive myocardial infarction (>40% of left ventricular myocardium destroyed), severe cardiomyopathy, or myocarditis
Cardiogenic shock due to a mechanical defect			
Acute ventricular septal defect	↑ or nl	LVCO ↓ ↓ and RVCO > CO	If shunt is left to right, pulmonary blood flow is greater than systemic blood flow: oxygen saturation "step-up" occurs at right ventricular level
Acute mitral regurgitation	↑ ↑	Forward CO ↓ ↓	V waves in pulmonary capillary wedge pressure tracing
Right ventricular infarction	nl or ↓	↓ ↓	Elevated right atrial and right ventricular filling pressures with low or normal pulmonary capillary wedge pressures
Extracardiac obstructive forms of shock			
Pericardial tamponade	↑ ↑	↓ or ↓ ↓	Dip and plateau tracing in right and left ventricles. The right atrial mean, right ventricular end-diastolic, pulmonary artery end-diastolic, and pulmonary capillary wedge mean pressures are within 5 mmHg of one another
Massive pulmonary emboli	nl or ↓	↓ ↓	Usual finding is elevated heart pressure and with normal or low pulmonary capillary wedge
Oligemic shock (hypovolemia)	↓ ↓	↓ ↓	
Distributive forms of shock			
Septic shock	↓ or nl	↑ ↑ or nl, rarely ↓	
Anaphylactic shock	↓ or nl	↑ or nl	

* The hemodynamic profiles summarized in this table refer to patients with the diagnosis listed in the left column who are also in shock (MAP <60 mmHg).
[†] ↑ ↑ or ↓ ↓ designates a moderate-to-severe increase or decrease; ↑ or ↓ designates a mild-to-moderate increase or decrease; nl = normal; LV = left ventricular; RV = right ventricular.
NOTE: Systemic vascular resistance is increased, initially, in all forms of shock except distributive shock, in which it is usually reduced.
SOURCE: Modified from JE Parrillo, in *Major Issues in Critical Care Medicine*, JE Parrillo, SM Ayres (eds), Baltimore, William & Wilkins, 1984.

right atrial pressures. Rapid infusion of blood plasma or plasma expanders is the correct therapy while the source of blood or fluid loss is identified and corrected.

Cardiogenic shock When it is due to myocardial infarction, after mechanical causes have been excluded (see Tables 34-1 and 34-2 and Chap. 202), therapy should be directed toward reducing ischemia and salvaging severely ischemic but reversibly damaged

TABLE 34-3 Guidelines for managing shock

Parameter	Therapeutic goal
Hemodynamic	
Mean arterial pressure	At least 60 mmHg
Pulmonary capillary wedge pressure	Between 14 and 18 mmHg
Oxygen delivery	
Hemoglobin	Above 10 g/dL
Oxygen saturation	Above 92%
Cardiac index	Nonseptic shock: above 2.2 L/min/m² Septic shock: above 4.0 L/min/m²
Organ system function	Normalize values or otherwise reverse evidence of dysfunction
Renal—blood urea nitrogen and creatinine levels, urinary output	
Hepatic—bilirubin level	
Pulmonary—alveolar-arterial gradient	
Cardiovascular—mean arterial pressure, cardiac index	
Central nervous system—mental status	
Blood lactate level	Normalization

SOURCE: Adapted from Dixon AC, Parrillo JE, in *The Principles and Practice of Medical Intensive Care*, Carlson RW, Geheb MA (eds), Philadelphia, Saunders, 1992.

myocardium at the infarct border. This may be accomplished by administration of oxygen and nitrates, institution of intraaortic balloon pumping to unload the ventricle mechanically and augment coronary perfusion, and, perhaps most important, attempts to restore myocardial perfusion to salvage nonirreversibly damaged myocardium. Depending on the specific situation, the latter may include the administration of thrombolytic agents, cardiac catheterization and coronary arteriography to define coronary anatomy, and early coronary angioplasty or coronary bypass surgery in patients with appropriate anatomy. This aggressive approach may reduce the mortality of cardiogenic shock from approximately 90 percent to around 60 percent. Prospective, randomized studies are needed to document the true efficacy of this approach. Cardiogenic shock also occurs after a prolonged period of induced cardiac arrest, often during reparative cardiac surgery. The impaired (stunned) myocardium may require hours or days to recover sufficiently to support the circulation. Treatment consists of the combination of intraaortic balloon counterpulsation and sympathomimetic amines such as dopamine or dobutamine (Table 34-4; see also Chap. 68). In cardiogenic shock due to mechanical abnormalities, such as acute mitral regurgitation or ventricular septal defect, surgical correction is usually necessary.

Pericardial tamponade This is the prototype of extracardiac obstructive shock and may be recognized by clinical manifestations (hypotension, pulsus paradoxus, distended neck veins) and characteristic findings on electrocardiography (Chap. 206) or by echocardiography (Chap. 190). Although expansion of intravascular volume and the administration of inotropic agents, particularly sympathomimetic amines such as norepinephrine and/or dopamine, may temporarily improve hemodynamics and act as a "holding maneuver," pericardiocentesis or surgical pericardial drainage is the only effective treatment.

TABLE 34-4 Commonly used vasopressor agents (relative potency*)

Agent	Dose	Cardiac		Peripheral vasculature		
		Heart rate	Contractility	Vasoconstriction	Vasodilatation	Dopaminergic
Dopamine	1–4 (μg/kg)/min	2+	2+	0	2+	4+
	4–20 (μg/kg)/min	2+	2+	2–3+	0	0
Levarterenol (norepinephrine)	2–8 μg/min	2+	2+	4+	0	0
Dobutamine	1–10 (μg/kg)/min	1+	4+	1+	2+	0
Isoproterenol	1–4 μg/min	4+	4+	0	4+	0
Epinephrine	1–8 μg/min	4+	4+	4+	3+	0
Phenylephrine	20–200 μg/min	0	0	4+	0	0

* The 1 to 4+ scoring system represents an arbitrary quantitative scoring system to allow a judgment of comparative potency among these vasopressor agents.
SOURCE: Adapted from JE Parrillo, *Major Issues in Critical Care Medicine*, JE Parrillo, SM Ayres (eds), Baltimore, Williams & Wilkins, 1984.

Septic shock (See also Chap. 83) This condition can be considered in three broad categories. First, the nidus of infection must be identified and eliminated, using surgical drainage, antimicrobial therapy, or both. Rapid institution of appropriate antimicrobial therapy has been associated with improved survival; however, the specific organisms causing septic shock are frequently not identified when patients present with this illness. Thus broad-spectrum antimicrobial therapy must be instituted that will be effective against all the likely causative microorganisms given a patient's clinical presentation and a hospital's organism-sensitivity profile. An antimicrobial regimen should be chosen that has a very high likelihood of covering the organisms subsequently isolated.

Second, using cardiovascular monitoring and support, adequate organ system perfusion and function must be maintained while antibiotics (and surgery, if necessary) eradicate the source of sepsis. Since antibiotics usually require 48 h or more to reverse a septic focus, maintenance of cardiovascular support (blood pressure and tissue oxygen delivery) is critical to a favorable outcome. Since oxygen delivery is the product of blood hemoglobin concentration, oxygen saturation, and cardiac output, maintenance of a blood hemoglobin level at greater than 10 g/dL, an oxygen saturation of higher than 92 percent, and a cardiac index of greater than 4.0 L/min/m^2 are important therapeutic guidelines.

Electrocardiographic, arterial, and pulmonary artery monitoring should be instituted. Specific hemodynamic goals of therapy (see Table 34-3) are similar to those for shock in general: maintenance of a mean arterial pressure of 60 mmHg or greater (in adults); maintenance of oxygen delivery; frequent monitoring and normalization of kidney, liver, respiratory, and cardiac function; and normalization of blood lactate. Initial cardiovascular therapy should be to optimize preload by administering volume to attain a pulmonary artery wedge mean pressure of 14 to 18 mmHg. In patients with a low hemoglobin (<10 g/dL), blood should be used as a volume expander. If the serum albumin level is low (<2 g/dL), concentrated albumin infusions may be used to increase intravascular plasma oncotic pressure. In other instances, crystalloid is the most convenient and inexpensive method to achieve optimal preload.

If volume fails to achieve adequate blood pressure and organ perfusion, inotropic and vasopressor therapy should be initiated (see Table 34-4). For the persistently hypotensive patient, dopamine will frequently raise blood pressure and maintain or enhance blood flow to the renal and splanchnic circulations. Patients who remain hypotensive despite the aforementioned measures, including dopamine administration, may be treated with norepinephrine. As mentioned above, myocardial function is frequently abnormal in septic shock patients. To optimize oxygen delivery to tissues, raising a low cardiac index to 3.0 L/min/m^2 or higher with inotropic therapy is a logical therapeutic endpoint. Dobutamine is a useful inotropic agent in this setting (see Table 34-4).

Refractory hypotension and multiple-organ failure are the two major causes of mortality in septic shock. Support of dysfunctional organ systems represents an important therapeutic goal. Patients with respiratory failure due to adult respiratory distress syndrome may require oxygen therapy, mechanical ventilation, and institution of positive end-expiratory pressure to ensure adequate oxygenation while lung injury heals (Chap. 230). Disseminated intravascular coagulation (DIC) should be treated with replacement of clotting factors and platelets. Renal failure may require dialysis. Several retrospective trials have documented that intensive care monitoring and organ system support directed by specialized critical-care personnel has been associated with a reduced mortality in septic shock patients.

A third general therapeutic goal is to interrupt the pathogenic sequence leading to septic shock. Several multicenter trials have documented that early corticosteroid administration fails to improve morbidity or mortality in septic shock. Patients with documented or suspected adrenal insufficiency should receive corticosteroids.

Inhibition of endorphin receptors with naloxone has been shown to cause a mild transient rise in blood pressure but no sustained benefit in septic shock patients. Inhibition of arachidonic acid metabolites has shown some promise in reversing septic adult respiratory distress syndrome.

A human monoclonal antibody directed against the lipid A (toxic) portion of endotoxin is under investigation (see Chap. 83). Inhibitors of other sepsis mediators (e.g., tumor necrosis factor and the interleukins) are presently undergoing clinical trials. Such inhibitors may allow interruption of the pathogenetic pathways of sepsis at multiple key steps and thereby reduce the high mortality associated with this disease.

REFERENCES

ALPERT JS, BECKER RC: Cardiogenic shock: Elements of etiology, diagnosis, and therapy. Clin Cardiol 16:182, 1993

BECKOW EC, ASTIZ ME: Mechanisms and management of septic shock. Crit Care Clin 9:219, 1993

BONE RC et al and the Methylprednisolone Severe Sepsis Study Group: A controlled clinical trial of high-dose methylprednisolone in the treatment of severe sepsis and septic shock. N Engl J Med 317:653, 1987

CONNORS AF et al: Evaluation of right-heart catheterization in the critically ill patient without acute myocardial infarction. N Engl J Med 308:263, 1983

GIROIR BP: Mediators of septic shock: New approaches for interrupting the endogenous inflammatory cascade. Crit Care Med 21L780, 1993

GUYTON AC: Cardiac output and circulatory shock, in *Human Physiology and Mechanisms of Disease*, 5th ed. Philadelphia, Saunders, 1991, pp 187–200

LEOR J et al: Cardiogenic shock complicating acute myocardial infarction in patients without heart failure on admission: Incidence, risk factors, and outcome. Am J Med 94:265, 1993

MORITZ A, WOLNER E: Circulatory support with shock due to acute myocardial infarction. Ann Thorac Surg 55:238, 1993

MOULOPOULOS SD: Effect of protracted dobutamine infusion on survival of patients in cardiogenic shock treated with intraaortic balloon pumping. Chest 103:248, 1993

NATANSON C et al: Gram-negative bacteremia produces both severe systolic and diastolic cardiac dysfunction in a canine model that simulates human septic shock. J Clin Invest 77:259, 1986

OGNIBENE FP et al: Depressed left ventricular performance in response to volume infusion in patients with sepsis and septic shock. Chest 93:903, 1988

PARKER MM, PARRILLO JE: Septic shock and other forms of distributive shock, in *Current Therapy in Critical Care Medicine*. Toronto, B. C. Decker, 1987, pp 44–55

PARRILLO JE: Septic shock in humans: Clinical evaluation, pathogenesis, and therapeutic approach, in *Textbook of Critical Care*, 2d ed, WC Shoemaker et al (eds). Philadelphia, Saunders, 1989, pp 1006–1023

————: Management of septic shock: Present and future. Ann Intern Med 115:491, 1991

————: Pathogenetic mechanisms of septic shock. N Engl J Med 328:1471, 1993

———— et al: A circulating myocardial depressant substance in humans with septic shock: Septic shock patients with a reduced ejection fraction have a circulating factor that depresses in vitro myocardial cell performance. J Clin Invest 76:1539, 1985

PINSKY MR et al: Serum cytokine levels in human septic shock. Relation to multiple-system organ failure and mortality. Chest 103:565, 1993

ROCK P et al: Efficacy and safety of naloxone in septic shock. Crit Care Med 13:28, 1985

ROUMEN RM et al: Intestinal permeability after severe trauma and hemorrhagic shock is increased without relation to septic complications. Arch Surg 128:453, 1993

SANDIN R: Kidney function in shock. Acta Anesthesiol Scand Suppl 98:14, 1993

35 CARDIOVASCULAR COLLAPSE, CARDIAC ARREST, AND SUDDEN DEATH

ROBERT J. MYERBURG / AGUSTIN CASTELLANOS

OVERVIEW AND DEFINITIONS

Cardiac disorders account for the vast majority of natural sudden deaths. The magnitude of the problem of *cardiac* causes is highlighted by estimates that more than 300,000 sudden cardiac deaths (SCD) occur each year in the United States and that as many as 50 percent of all cardiac deaths are sudden and unexpected. Since techniques and systems are now available to save patients who have out-of-hospital cardiac arrest, which was uniformly fatal in the past, understanding the SCD problem has practical importance.

SCD must be defined carefully. In the context of time, "sudden" was previously defined as death within 24 h of the onset of the clinical event which led to a fatal cardiac arrest; this was subsequently shortened for most clinical and epidemiologic purposes to 1 h or less between the onset of the terminal illness and death. However, because of community-based interventions, victims may remain biologically alive for days or weeks after a cardiac arrest that has resulted in irreversible central nervous system damage. Confusion in terms can be avoided by adhering strictly to definitions of death, cardiac arrest, and cardiovascular collapse, as outlined in Table 35-1. Death is biologically, legally, and literally an absolute and irreversible event. Death may be delayed in a survivor of cardiac arrest, but "survival

after sudden death" is contradictory. Currently, the accepted definition of SCD is *natural death* due to *cardiac* causes, heralded by abrupt loss of consciousness within *1 h* of the onset of acute symptoms, in an individual who may have known *preexisting* heart disease but in whom the *time* and *mode* of death are *unexpected*. When biologic death of the cardiac arrest victim is delayed because of interventions, the relevant pathophysiologic event remains the sudden and unexpected cardiac arrest which leads ultimately to death, even though delayed by artificial methods. Thus the terminology used should reflect the fact that the index event was a cardiac arrest and that death was due to its delayed consequences.

ETIOLOGY, INITIATING EVENTS, AND CLINICAL EPIDEMIOLOGY

Extensive epidemiologic studies have identified populations at high risk for SCD. In addition, a large body of pathologic data provides information on the underlying *structural abnormalities* in victims of SCD, and clinical/physiologic studies have begun to identify a group of *transient functional factors* which may convert a long-standing underlying structural abnormality from a stable to an unstable state (Table 35-2). This information is developing into an understanding of the causes and mechanisms of SCD.

Cardiac disorders constitute the most common causes of sudden *natural* death. After an initial peak incidence of sudden death between birth and 6 months of age (the sudden infant death syndrome), the incidence of sudden death falls abruptly and then increases to a second

TABLE 35-2 Cardiac arrest and sudden cardiac death

I STRUCTURAL CAUSES

A Coronary heart disease
  1 Coronary artery abnormalities
    a Chronic atherosclerotic lesions
    b Acute (active) lesions
      (plaque fissuring, platelet aggregation, acute thrombosis)
    c Anomalous coronary artery anatomy
  2 Myocardial infarction
    a Healed
    b Acute
B Myocardial hypertrophy
  1 Secondary
  2 Hypertrophic cardiomyopathy
    a Obstructive
    b Nonobstructive
C Cardiomyopathy—dilated or infiltrative
D Myocarditis
E Valvular heart disease
F Electrophysiologic abnormalities, structural
  1 Anomalous pathways in Wolff-Parkinson-White syndrome
  2 Conducting system disease

II FUNCTIONAL CONTRIBUTING FACTORS

A Transient ischemia and reperfusion
  1 Loss of energy substrates
  2 Generation of injurious substances (e.g., superoxide radicals)
  3 Disturbed membrane electrical properties (e.g., channels, pumps, receptors)
B Low cardiac output states
  1 Heart failure
    a Chronic
    b Acute decompensation
  2 Shock
C Systemic metabolic abnormalities
  1 Electrolyte imbalance (e.g., hypokalemia)
  2 Hypoxemia, acidosis
D Neurophysiologic disturbances
  1 Autonomic fluctuations—central, neural, humoral
  2 Receptor function
  3 Long QT syndrome, congenital
E Toxic responses
  1 Proarrhythmic drug effects
  2 Cardiac toxins (e.g., cocaine, digitalis intoxication)

TABLE 35-1 Distinction between death, cardiac arrest, and cardiovascular collapse

Term	Definition	Qualifiers or exceptions
Death	Irreversible cessation of all biologic functions	None
Cardiac arrest	Abrupt cessation of cardiac pump function which may be reversible by a prompt intervention but will lead to death in its absence	Rare spontaneous reversions; likelihood of successful interventions relates to mechanism of arrest and clinical setting
Cardiovascular collapse	A sudden loss of effective blood flow due to cardiac and/or peripheral vascular factors which may reverse spontaneously (e.g., vasodepressor syncope) or only with interventions (e.g., cardiac arrest)	Nonspecific term which includes cardiac arrest and its consequences and also events which characteristically revert spontaneously

peak in the age range of 45 to 75 years. Moreover, increasing age is a powerful risk factor for sudden *cardiac* death. It follows that the *proportion* of *cardiac* causes among all sudden *natural* deaths increases dramatically with advancing years. From 1 to 13 years of age, only one of five sudden *natural* deaths is due to cardiac causes. Between 14 and 21 years of age, the proportion increases to 30 percent, and then to 88 percent in the middle-aged and elderly.

Men and women have very different susceptibilities to SCD, and the gender differences decrease with advancing age. The overall male/female ratio is approximately 4:1, but in the 45- to 64-year-old age group, the male SCD excess is nearly 7:1. It falls to approximately 2:1 in the 65- to 74-year-old age group. The difference in risk for SCD parallels the risks for other manifestations of coronary heart disease in men and women. As the gap for other manifestations of coronary heart disease closes in the seventh and eighth decades of life, the excess risk of SCD narrows. Despite the lower incidence in women, the classic coronary risk factors still operate in the proportionately smaller subgroup of women—cigarette smoking, diabetes, hyperlipidemia, hypertension.

Hereditary factors contribute to the risk of SCD, but largely in a nonspecific manner: They represent expressions of the hereditary predisposition to coronary heart disease. Except for a few specific syndromes, such as the genetic hyperlipoproteinemias (Chap. 344) and congenital long QT interval syndromes (Chap. 198), there are no *specific* hereditary risk factors for SCD. Higher levels of life stress, lower levels of education, social isolation, changes in life-style after myocardial infarction, cigarette use, alcohol consumption, obesity, and absence of regular exercise all have been *suggested* as contributors to risk of SCD. Among women, those who are unmarried and those who have fewer children or have greater educational disparity with their spouses appear to be at higher risk.

The major categories of structural causes of, and functional factors contributing to, the SCD syndrome are listed in Table 35-2. Worldwide, and especially in western cultures, coronary atherosclerotic heart disease is the most common structural abnormality associated with SCD. Up to 80 percent of all SCDs in the United States are due to the consequences of coronary atherosclerosis. The cardiomyopathies (dilated and hypertrophic, collectively, Chap. 205) account for another 10 to 15 percent of SCDs, and all the remaining diverse etiologies cause only 5 to 10 percent of these events. The relative role of various factors contributing to the initiation of cardiac arrest has not been quantitated as well as the structural basis. Transient ischemia in the previously scarred or hypertrophied heart, hemodynamic and fluid and electrolyte disturbances, fluctuations in autonomic nervous system activity, and transient electrophysiologic changes caused by drugs or other chemicals (e.g., proarrhythmia) have all been implicated as mechanisms responsible for transition from electrophysiologic stability to instability. In addition, spontaneous reperfusion of ischemic myocardium, caused by vasomotor changes in the coronary vasculature and/or spontaneous thrombolysis, may cause transient electrophysiologic instability and arrhythmias.

PATHOLOGY Data from necropsies of SCD victims parallel the clinical observations on the prevalence of coronary heart disease as the major structural etiologic factor. More than 80 percent of SCD victims have pathologic findings of coronary heart disease, and these commonly include ruptured atherosclerotic plaques and/or coronary thrombi. The most consistent *coronary artery* abnormality is extensive chronic coronary atherosclerosis. Seventy-five percent of the victims have two or more major vessels with ≥75 percent stenosis. In addition, in one study, atherosclerotic plaque fissuring, platelet aggregates, and/or acute thrombosis were observed in 95 of 100 individuals who had pathologic studies after SCD. Most of these acute changes were superimposed on preexisting chronic lesions. However, only 44 percent of the SCD victims had more than 50 percent luminal narrowing by recent coronary thrombi, raising issues about interactions between breakdown of preexisting noncritical lesions, local thrombus formation and spontaneous lysis, and acute coronary spasm with ischemia in the initiation of the terminal event.

The pathology of the *myocardium* in SCD reflects the extensive coronary heart disease which usually precedes the fatal event. As many as 70 to 75 percent of males who die suddenly have prior myocardial infarctions (MIs), and 20 to 30 percent have recent acute MIs. A high incidence of left ventricular (LV) hypertrophy coexists with prior MIs. Clinical, epidemiologic, and experimental data suggest that LV hypertrophy itself predisposes to SCD, and it is likely that coexistence with prior MI adds additional risk.

CLINICAL DEFINITION OF FORMS OF CARDIOVASCULAR COLLAPSE The definitions of the terms listed in Table 35-1 have important clinical applications. *Cardiovascular collapse* is a general term connoting loss of effective blood flow due to acute dysfunction of the heart and/or peripheral vasculature. Cardiovascular collapse may be caused by vasodepressor syncope (vasovagal syncope, postural hypotension with syncope, neurocardiogenic syncope—see Chap. 17), a transient severe bradycardia, or cardiac arrest. The latter is distinguished from the transient forms of cardiovascular collapse in that it usually requires an intervention to achieve resuscitation. In contrast, vasodepressor syncope and many primary bradyarrhythmic syncopal events are transient, and the patient will regain consciousness spontaneously.

The most common electrical mechanism for true cardiac arrest is ventricular fibrillation (VF), which is responsible for 65 to 80 percent of cardiac arrests. Severe persistent bradyarrhythmias, asystole, and electromechanical dissociation (organized electrical activity is present but there is no mechanical response) cause another 20 to 30 percent. Sustained ventricular tachycardia (VT) with hypotension is a less common cause. Acute low cardiac output states, having precipitous onset, also may present clinically as a cardiac arrest. The causes include massive acute pulmonary emboli, internal blood loss from ruptured aortic aneurysm, intense anaphylaxis, cardiac rupture after myocardial infarction, and unexpected fatal arrhythmia due to electrolyte disturbances.

CLINICAL CHARACTERISTICS OF CARDIAC ARREST

PRODROME, ONSET, ARREST, DEATH Long-term studies in both unselected and high-risk populations suggest that SCD may be presaged by days, weeks, or months of increasing angina, dyspnea, palpitations, easy fatigability, and other nonspecific complaints. However, these *prodromal complaints* are generally predictive of any major cardiac event; they are not specific for predicting SCD. In one study, nearly 50 percent of SCD victims saw a physician within the month prior to death, but the complaints generally appeared to be unrelated to the heart. Among survivors of out-of-hospital cardiac arrest, 28 percent retrospectively reported new onset of worsening angina pectoris or dyspnea prior to cardiac arrest. Prodromes are useful for identifying patients at risk for cardiovascular events but not for identifying the subgroup of SCD victims.

The *onset of the terminal event*, leading to cardiac arrest, is defined as an acute change in cardiovascular status preceding cardiac arrest by up to 1 h. When the onset is instantaneous or abrupt, the probability that the arrest is cardiac in origin and related to underlying coronary artery disease is >95 percent. Continuous ECG recordings, fortuitously obtained prior to a cardiac arrest, commonly demonstrate changes in cardiac electrical activity in the minutes or hours before the event. There is a tendency for the heart rate to increase and for advanced grades of premature ventricular contractions to evolve. Most cardiac arrests that occur by the mechanism of VF begin with a run of sustained or nonsustained VT which then degenerates into VF.

In the clinical classification proposed by Hinkle and Thaler, sudden unexpected loss of effective circulation was separated into "arrhythmic events" and "circulatory failure." Arrhythmic events are characterized by a high incidence of patients being awake and actively moving immediately prior to the event, are dominated by VF as the electrical mechanism, and have a short duration of terminal illness (<1 h). In contrast, circulatory failure deaths occur in patients who are inactive or comatose, have a higher incidence of asystole than VF, have a tendency to a longer duration of terminal illness, and are dominated by noncardiac events preceding the terminal illness.

The onset of cardiac arrest may be characterized by typical symptoms of an acute cardiac event, such as prolonged angina or the pain of onset of myocardial infarction, acute dyspnea or orthopnea, or the sudden onset of palpitations, sustained tachycardia, or lightheadedness. However, in many patients, the onset is precipitous, without forewarning.

Cardiac arrest is, by definition, abrupt. Mentation may be impaired in patients with sustained VT during the onset of the terminal event. However, complete loss of consciousness is a *sine qua non* in cardiac arrest. Although rare spontaneous reversions occur, it is usual that cardiac arrest progresses to death within minutes (i.e., SCD has occurred) if active interventions are not undertaken promptly.

The ability to resuscitate the victim of cardiac arrest is related to the time from onset to institution of resuscitative efforts, the setting in which the event occurs, the mechanism (VF, VT, electromechanical dissociation, asystole), and the clinical status of the patient prior to the cardiac arrest. Those settings in which it is possible to institute prompt cardiopulmonary resuscitation (CPR) provide a better chance of a successful outcome. However, the outcome in intensive care units and other in-hospital environments is more heavily influenced by the patient's preceding clinical status. The immediate outcome is good for cardiac arrest occurring in the intensive care unit in the presence of an acute cardiac event or transient metabolic disturbance, but the outcome for patients with far-advanced chronic cardiac disease or advanced noncardiac diseases (e.g., renal failure, pneumonia, sepsis, diabetes, cancer) is no more successful in hospital than in the out-of-hospital environment.

The success rate for initial resuscitation and ultimate survival from an out-of-hospital cardiac arrest depends in part on the mechanism of the event. When the mechanism is VT, the outcome is best (67 percent); VF is the next most successful (25 percent), and asystole and electromechanical dissociation have dismal outcome statistics (Fig. 35-1). Advanced age also adversely influences the chances of successful resuscitation.

Progression to biologic death is a function of the mechanism of

FIGURE 35-1 Initial electrophysiologic mechanisms recorded during out-of-hospital cardiac arrest. The figures highlighted by the boxes indicate the number of patients in each of three mechanism categories (ventricular fibrillation, ventricular tachycardia, and bradyarrhythmia/asystole). In each category, the data indicate the number of prehospital cardiac arrests (*top*), the number of patients successfully resuscitated in the field and transferred to the hospital alive (*middle*), and the number of patients who survived to be discharged from hospital (*bottom*). The percentages in parentheses indicate survivals between each level of care for each category. (*Modified from Myerburg RJ et al: Clinical, electrophysiologic, and hemodynamic profile of patients resuscitated from prehospital cardiac arrest. Am J Med 68:568, 1980, with permission*).

cardiac arrest and the length of the delay before interventions. VF or asystole, without CPR within the first 4 to 6 min, has a poor outcome, and there are few survivors among patients who had no life-support activities for the first 8 min after onset. Outcome statistics are dramatically improved by lay bystander intervention (basic life support—see below) prior to definitive interventions (advanced life support—defibrillation) and by early defibrillation. The most common causes of death during hospitalization after resuscitated cardiac arrests are related to the severity of injury to the central nervous system. Anoxic encephalopathy and infections subsequent to prolonged respirator dependence account for 60 percent of the deaths. Another 30 percent occur as a consequence of low cardiac output states which fail to respond to interventions. Paradoxically, recurrent arrhythmias are the least common cause of death, accounting for only 10 percent of in-hospital deaths.

Outcome during hospitalization, particularly in patients with acute MI, is very different for patients with primary and secondary cardiac arrests. *Primary* cardiac arrests refer to those which occur in the absence of hemodynamic instability, and *secondary* cardiac arrests are those which occur in patients in whom abnormal hemodynamics dominate the clinical picture before cardiac arrest. The success rate for immediate resuscitation in primary cardiac arrest during acute MI should approach 100 percent. In contrast, as many as 70 percent of patients with secondary cardiac arrest succumb immediately or during the same hospitalization.

IDENTIFICATION OF PATIENTS AT RISK FOR SUDDEN CARDIAC DEATH Primary prevention of cardiac arrest depends on the ability to identify individual patients at high risk. One must view the problem in the context of the total number of events and the population pools from which they are derived. In Fig. 35-2A, the inverted triangle demonstrates that the annual incidence of SCD among an unselected adult population is 1 to 2 per 1000 population, largely reflecting the prevalence of those coronary heart disease patients among whom SCD is the first clinically recognized manifestation (20 to 25 percent of first coronary events are SCD). The incidence (percent per year) increases progressively with addition of identified coronary risk factors to populations free of prior coronary events. The most powerful factors are age, elevated blood pressure, LV hypertrophy, cigarette smoking, elevated serum cholesterol level, obesity, and nonspecific electrocardiographic abnormalities. These coronary risk factors are not specific for SCD but rather represent increasing risk for all coronary deaths. The proportion of coronary deaths that are sudden remains at approximately 50 percent in all risk categories. Despite the marked *relative* increased risk of SCD with addition of multiple risk factors (from 1 to 2 per 1000 population per year in an unselected population to as much as 50 to 60 per 1000 in the highest risk subgroups), the *absolute* incidence remains relatively low when viewed in terms of the relationship between the number of individuals who have a preventive intervention versus the number of events which can be prevented. Specifically, a 50 percent reduction in annual SCD risk would be a huge *relative* decrease but would require an intervention in up to 200 unselected individuals to prevent one sudden death. These figures highlight the importance of primary prevention of coronary heart disease. Control of coronary risk factors may be the only practical method to prevent SCD in major segments of the population, since the majority of events occur in the large unselected subgroups rather than in the specific high-risk subgroups (compare "Events/Year" with "Percent/Year" in Fig. 35-2A). In addition to population and clinical determinants of risk, there also appears to be time-dependent modulation of risk (Fig. 35-2B). Under most conditions of higher level of risk, particularly those related to a recent major cardiovascular event (e.g., myocardial infarction, recent onset of heart failure, survival after out-of-hospital cardiac arrest), the highest risk of sudden death occurs within the initial 6 to 18 months and then decreases toward baseline risk of the underlying disease. Accordingly, preventive interventions are most likely to be effective when initiated early.

For patients with acute or prior clinical manifestations of coronary

	VENTRICULAR FIBRILLATION	VENTRICULAR TACHYCARDIA	ASYSTOLE / BRADY-ARRHYTHMIA	TOTAL
OUT-OF-HOSPITAL CARDIAC ARRESTS	220	24	108	352
	(40%) ↓	(88%) ↓	(9%) ↓	(33%) ↓
RESUSCITATED AND HOSPITALIZED	87	21	9	117
	(59%) ↓	(76%) ↓	(–) ↓	(57%) ↓
DISCHARGED	51	16	0	67

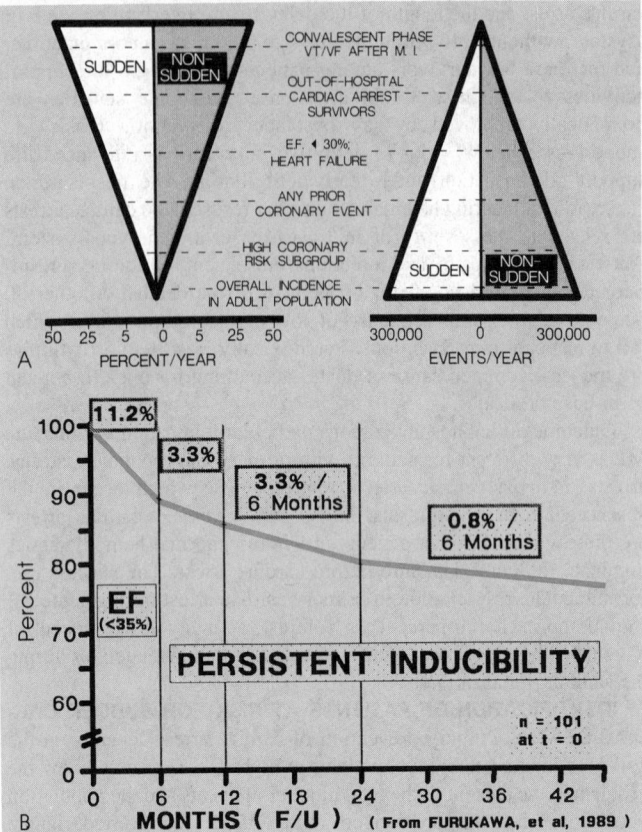

FIGURE 35-2 *A.* Incidence of sudden and nonsudden cardiac deaths in population subgroups, and the relation of total number of events per year to incidence figures. Approximations of subgroup incidence figures, and the related population pool from which they are derived, are presented. Approximately 50 percent of all cardiac deaths are sudden and unexpected. The incidence triangle on the left (''Percent/Year'') indicates the approximate percentage of sudden and nonsudden deaths in each of the population subgroups indicated, ranging from the lowest percentage in unselected adult populations (0.1 to 2 percent per year) to the highest percentage in patients with VT or VF during convalescence after an MI (approximately 50 percent per year). The triangle on the right indicates the total number of events per year in each of these groups, to reflect incidence in context with the size of the population subgroups. The highest risk categories identify the smallest number of total annual events, and the lowest incidence category accounts for the largest number of events per year. (EF = ejection fraction; VT = ventricular tachycardia; VF = ventricular fibrillation; MI = myocardial infarction.) *B.* Time dependence of risk among survivors of out-of-hospital cardiac arrest. Recurrence risk is highest in the first 6 months of the index event. Survival is expressed as a percentage. High risk is best predicted initially by an ejection fraction ≤ 35 percent during the first 6 months, and subsequently persistent inducibility of VT during electrophysiologic testing becomes an added major risk. (*Modified from Furukawa T et al, in Myerburg RJ et al. Reproduced with permission of the American Heart Association.*)

heart disease, high-risk subgroups having a much higher ratio of SCD risk to population base can be identified. The acute, convalescent, and chronic phases of MI provide large population subsets with more highly focused risk (Chap. 202). The potential risk of cardiac arrest from the onset through the first 72 h after acute MI (the acute phase) may be as high as 15 to 20 percent. The highest risk of SCD in relation to MI is found in the subgroup that has VT or VF during the convalescent phase (3 days to 8 weeks) after MI. A 50 to 80 percent mortality in 6 to 12 months has been observed among these patients, when managed with conventional therapy, and at least 50 percent of the deaths are sudden. Since the development of aggressive intervention techniques, the incidence has fallen dramatically to 15 to 20 percent in 18 months, or better.

Chronic premature ventricular complexes (PVCs) after the acute phase of MI identify a long-term risk for total cardiac mortality and SCD. Increasing *frequency* of PVCs, with a plateau above the range of 10 to 30 PVCs per hour on 24-h ambulatory monitor recordings, indicates increased risk, but advanced *forms* (salvos, nonsustained VT) are probably the more powerful predictor. PVCs interact strongly with the size of the MI, as reflected by decreased left ventricular ejection fraction (EF). The combination of frequent PVCs, salvos or nonsustained VT, and an EF ≤ 30 percent identifies patients who have an annual risk of 20 percent. The risk falls off sharply with decreasing PVC frequency and the absence of advanced forms, as well as with higher EF. Despite these risk implications of postinfarction PVCs, whether suppression of PVCs alters risk has not yet been determined. However, a large intervention trial, the Cardiac Arrhythmia Suppression Trial (CAST) demonstrated that, for the drugs studied, any potential benefit of suppression of PVCs was outweighed by a threefold increase in deaths among patients receiving the study drugs.

Beyond the specific problem of coronary heart disease, the general factors of extent of underlying disease due to any cause and a prior clinical expression of risk of SCD (i.e., survival after out-of-hospital cardiac arrest not associated with acute MI) identify very high risk patients. Survival after out-of-hospital cardiac arrest predicts a 30 percent 1-year recurrent cardiac arrest rate in the absence of specific interventions (see below) in this group of patients.

A general rule is that the risk of SCD is approximately one-half the total cardiovascular mortality rate. Thus the SCD risk is approximately 20 percent per year for patients with advanced coronary heart disease or dilated cardiomyopathy severe enough to result in a 40 percent 1-year total mortality rate. Figure 35-2*A* demonstrates a much more focused population fraction (''Percent/Year'') for identifying high-risk patients in the high-risk subgroups, but the impact on the overall population, indicated by the absolute number of preventable events (''Events/Year''), is considerably smaller.

MANAGEMENT OF CARDIAC ARREST

The individual who collapses suddenly is managed in five stages: (1) the initial response, (2) basic life support, (3) advanced life support, (4) postresuscitation care, and (5) long-term management. The initial response and basic life support can be carried out by physicians, nurses, paramedical personnel, and trained lay persons. There is a requirement for increasing skills as the patient moves through the stages of advanced life support, postresuscitation care, and long-term management.

INITIAL RESPONSE   The initial response will confirm whether a sudden collapse is indeed due to a cardiac arrest. Observations for respiratory movements, skin color, and the presence or absence of pulses in the carotid or femoral arteries will immediately determine whether a life-threatening cardiac arrest has occurred. Agonal respiratory movements may persist for a short time after cardiac arrest, but it is important to observe for severe stridor with a persistent pulse as a clue to aspiration of a foreign body or food. If this is suspected, a prompt Heimlich maneuver (see below) may dislodge the obstructing body. A precordial blow, or ''thump,'' delivered firmly by the clenched fist to the junction of the middle and lower third of the sternum may occasionally revert VT or VF, but there is concern about converting VT *to* VF. Therefore, it has been recommended to use precordial thumps only in monitored patients; this recommendation remains controversial. The third action during the initial response is to clear the airway. The head is tilted back and chin lifted so that the oropharynx can be explored to clear the airway. Dentures or foreign bodies are removed, and the Heimlich maneuver is performed if there is reason to suspect that a foreign body is lodged in the oropharynx. If respiratory arrest precipitating cardiac arrest is suspected, a second precordial thump is delivered after the airway is cleared.

BASIC LIFE SUPPORT   More popularly known as cardiopulmonary resuscitation (CPR), basic life support is intended to maintain organ perfusion until definitive interventions can be instituted. The elements of CPR are the establishment and maintenance of ventilation of the lungs and compression of the chest. Mouth-to-mouth respiration may be used if no specific rescue equipment is immediately available (e.g., plastic oropharyngeal airways, esophageal obturators, masked Ambu bag). Conventional ventilation techniques during CPR require the lungs to be inflated once every 5 s when two persons are performing the resuscitation and twice in succession every 15 s when one person is carrying out both ventilation and chest wall compression.

Chest compression is based on the assumption that cardiac compression allows the heart to maintain a pump function by sequential filling and emptying of its chambers, with competent valves maintaining forward direction of flow. The technique is illustrated in Fig. 35-3. The palm of one hand is placed over the lower sternum, with the heel of the other resting on the dorsum of the lower hand. The sternum is depressed, with the arms remaining straight, at a rate of approximately 80 per minute. Sufficient force is applied to depress the sternum 3 to 5 cm, and relaxation is abrupt. This conventional technique for CPR is currently being compared with a new technique based on simultaneous compression and ventilation. While measurable carotid artery flow can be achieved with conventional CPR, experimen-

tal data and theoretical considerations suggest that flow may be optimized by a pumping action produced by pressure changes in the entire thoracic cavity, as is achieved by simultaneous compression and ventilation. However, it is not yet clear whether this technique causes an unacceptable impedance of coronary blood flow and whether the increased *carotid flow* produces equivalent increases in *cerebral perfusion*. Until these issues are clarified, conventional CPR remains the generally accepted technique.

ADVANCED LIFE SUPPORT   Advanced life support is intended to achieve adequate ventilation, control cardiac arrhythmias, stabilize the hemodynamic status (blood pressure and cardiac output), and restore organ perfusion. The activities carried out to achieve these goals include (1) intubation with an endotracheal tube, (2) defibrillation/cardioversion and/or pacing, and (3) insertion of an intravenous line. Ventilation with O_2 (room air if O_2 is not immediately available) may promptly reverse hypoxemia and acidosis. The speed with which defibrillation/cardioversion is carried out is an important element for successful resuscitation. When possible, immediate defibrillation should precede intubation and insertion of an intravenous line; CPR should be carried out while the defibrillator is being charged. As soon as a diagnosis of VT or VF is obtained, a 200-J shock should be delivered. Additional shocks at higher energies, up to a maximum of 360 J, are tried if the initial shock does not successfully abolish VT or VF. If the patient is less than fully conscious upon reversion, or if two or three attempts fail, prompt intubation, ventilation, and arterial blood gas analysis should be carried out. Intravenous $NaHCO_3$, which was formerly used in large quantities, is no longer considered routinely necessary and may be dangerous in larger quantities. However, the patient who is persistently acidotic after successful defibrillation and intubation should be given 1 mmol/kg $NaHCO_3$ initially and an additional 50 percent of the dose repeated every 10 to 15 min.

After initial defibrillation attempts, whether successful or not, a bolus of 1 mg/kg lidocaine is given intravenously (Chap. 202), and the dose is repeated in 2 min in those patients who have persistent ventricular arrhythmias or remain in VF. This is followed by a continuous infusion at a rate of 1 to 4 mg/min. If lidocaine fails to provide control, intravenous procainamide (loading infusion of 100 mg/5 min to a total dose of 500 to 800 mg, followed by continuous infusion at 2 to 5 mg/min) or bretylium tosylate (loading dose 5 to 10 mg/kg in 5 min; maintenance dose 0.5 to 2 mg/min) may be tried. For persistent VF, epinephrine (0.5 to 1.0 mg) may be given intravenously every 5 min during resuscitation with attempts to defibrillate between each dose. The drug may be given by an intracardiac route if intravenous access is not available. Intravenous calcium gluconate is no longer considered safe or necessary for routine administration. It is used only in patients in whom acute hyperkalemia is known to be the triggering event for resistant VF, in the presence of known hypocalcemia, or in patients who have received toxic doses of calcium channel antagonists.

Cardiac arrest secondary to bradyarrhythmias or asystole are managed differently. Once it is known that this type of rhythm is present, there is no role for external shock. The patient is promptly intubated, CPR is continued, and an attempt is made to control hypoxemia and acidosis. Epinephrine and/or atropine are given intravenously or by an intracardiac route. External pacing devices are now available to attempt to establish a regular rhythm, but the prognosis is generally very poor in this form of cardiac arrest. The one exception is bradyarrhythmic/asystolic cardiac arrest secondary to airway obstruction. This form of cardiac arrest may respond promptly to removal of foreign bodies by the Heimlich maneuver or, in hospitalized patients, by intubation and suctioning of obstructing secretions in the airway.

POSTRESUSCITATION CARE   This phase of management is determined by the clinical setting of the cardiac arrest. *Primary VF in acute MI* (Chap. 202) is generally very responsive to life-support techniques and easily controlled after the initial event. Patients are maintained on a lidocaine infusion at the rate of 2 to 4 mg/min for

FIGURE 35-3 Major steps in cardiopulmonary resuscitation. *A.* Make certain the victim has an open airway. *B.* Start respiratory resuscitation immediately. *C.* Feel for the carotid pulse in the groove alongside the "Adam's apple" or thyroid cartilage. *D.* If pulse is absent, begin cardiac massage. Use 60 compressions a minute with one lung inflation after each group of 5 chest compressions. (*From J Henderson, Emergency Medical Guide, 4th ed, New York, McGraw-Hill, 1978.*)

"Adam's apple" (thyroid cartilage)

24 to 72 h after the event. In the in-hospital setting, respirator support is usually not necessary or is needed for only a short time, and hemodynamics stabilize promptly after defibrillation or cardioversion. In *secondary VF in acute MI* (those events in which hemodynamic abnormalities predispose to the potentially fatal arrhythmia), resuscitative efforts are less often successful, and in those patients who are successfully resuscitated, the recurrence rate is high. The clinical picture is dominated by hemodynamic instability. In fact, the outcome is determined more by the ability to control hemodynamic dysfunction than by electrophysiologic abnormalities. Bradyarrhythmias, asystole, and electromechanical dissociation are commonly secondary events in hemodynamically unstable patients and are less responsive to interventions.

The outcome after in-hospital cardiac arrest associated with *noncardiac* diseases is poor, and in the few successfully resuscitated patients, the postresuscitation course is dominated by the nature of the underlying disease. Patients with cancer, renal failure, acute central nervous system disease, and uncontrolled infections, as a group, have a survival rate of less than 10 percent after in-hospital cardiac arrest. Some major exceptions to the poor outcome of cardiac arrest due to noncardiac causes are patients with transient airway obstruction, electrolyte disturbances, proarrhythmic effects of drugs, and severe metabolic abnormalities, most of whom may have an excellent chance of survival if they can be resuscitated promptly and maintained while the transient abnormalities are being corrected.

LONG-TERM MANAGEMENT AFTER SURVIVAL OF OUT-OF-HOSPITAL CARDIAC ARREST   This form of care has evolved into a major area of specialized clinical activities since the development of community-based emergency rescue systems. Patients who do not suffer irreversible injury of the central nervous system and who achieve hemodynamic stability should have extensive diagnostic and therapeutic testing to guide long-term management. This aggressive approach is driven by the fact that statistics from the 1970s indicated survival after out-of-hospital cardiac arrest was followed by a 30 percent recurrent cardiac arrest rate at 1 year, 45 percent at 2 years, and a total mortality rate of almost 60 percent at 2 years. Historical comparisons suggest that these dismal statistics may be significantly improved by newer interventions, but the magnitude of the improvement is unknown because of the lack of concurrently controlled intervention studies.

Among those patients in whom a transmural, acute MI is the cause of out-of-hospital cardiac arrest, the management is the same as in any other patient who suffers cardiac arrest during the acute phase of a documented MI (see Chap. 202). For almost all other categories of patients, however, extensive diagnostic studies are carried out to determine etiology, functional impairment, and electrophysiologic instability as guides to future management. In general, patients who have out-of-hospital cardiac arrest due to chronic ischemic heart disease, without an acute MI, are evaluated to determine whether transient ischemia or chronic electrophysiologic instability was the more likely cause of the event. If there is reason to suspect an ischemic mechanism, anti-ischemic surgery or medical interventions (e.g., angioplasty, drugs) are used to reduce the ischemic burden. Electrophysiologic instability is best identified by the use of programmed electrical stimulation to determine whether sustained VT or VF can be induced in the patient (Chap. 198). If so, this information can be used as a baseline against which to evaluate drug efficacy for prevention of inducibility. It also can be used to determine suitability for map-guided antiarrhythmic surgery. Using this technique to establish drug therapy in patients with ejection fractions of 30 percent or more, the recurrent cardiac arrest rate is less than 10 percent during the first year of follow-up. The outcome is not as good for patients with ejection fractions under 30 percent but may be still better than the apparent natural history of survival after cardiac arrest. For patients for whom successful drug therapy cannot be identified by this technique, empiric treatment with amiodarone, insertion of an implantable cardioverter/defibrillator (ICD), or antiarrhythmic surgery (e.g., coronary bypass surgery, aneurysmectomy, cryoablation), can be considered options (Chap. 198). Primary surgical success, defined as surviving the procedure and reverting to a noninducible status without drug therapy, is better than 90 percent when patients are selected for ability to be mapped in the operating room. ICD therapy is also evolving into more sophisticated systems, including the ability to pace rather than shock out of some arrhythmias in selected patients. The array of interventions available for these patients, properly applied, is providing continuing improvement in long-term outcome.

PREVENTION OF SUDDEN CARDIAC DEATH

This remains a major unresolved challenge in modern medicine. Some progress appears to have been made in selected, very high risk subgroups. However, the majority of SCD cases, expressed in absolute numbers rather than relative risk, occur within those subgroups characterized by lesser degrees of risk (see Fig. 35-2). Major progress will therefore require effective measures for prevention of the underlying disease, plus the ability to identify and control transient initiating factors, and methods of identifying higher-risk clusters among the more general population groups.

REFERENCES

AKHTAR M et al: CAST and beyond: Implications of the Cardiac Arrhythmias Suppression Trial. Circulation 81:1123, 1990

AKHTAR M et al: Implantable cardioverter-defibrillator therapy for prevention of sudden cardiac death. Cardiol Clin 11:97, 1993

BEDELL SE et al: Survival after cardiopulmonary resuscitation in the hospital. N Engl J Med 309:569, 1983

BIGGER JT et al: The relationships among ventricular arrhythmias, left ventricular dysfunction, and mortality in the two years after myocardial infarction. Circulation 69:250, 1984

CRANDALL BG et al: Implantable cardioverter-defibrillator therapy in survivors of out-of-hospital sudden cardiac death without inducible arrhythmias. J Am Coll Cardiol 21:1186, 1993

ECHT DS et al: Mortality and morbidity in patients receiving encainide, flecainide, or placebo: The Cardiac Arrhythmia Suppression Trial. N Engl J Med 324:781, 1991

HEIMLICH HJ: A life-saving maneuver to prevent food choking. JAMA 234:398, 1975

HINKLE LA, THALER HT: Clinical classification of cardiac deaths. Circulation 65:457, 1982

JASTREMSKI MS: In-hospital cardiac arrest. Ann Emerg Med 22:113, 1993

JOSLYN ET AL: Survival from out-of-hospital cardiac arrest: Effects of patient age and presence of 911 Emergency Medical Services phone access. Am J Emerg Med 11:200, 1993

KANNEL WB, SCHATZKIN A: Sudden death: Lessons from subsets in population studies. J Am Coll Cardiol 5(suppl 6):141B, 1985

MYERBURG RJ, CASTELLANOS A: Cardiac arrest and sudden cardiac death, in *Heart Disease*, 4th ed, E Braunwald (ed). Philadelphia, Saunders, 1992, pp 756–789

—— et al: Sudden cardiac death: Structure, function and time dependence of risk. Circulation 85(suppl 1):2, 1992

ORNATO JP: Use of adrenergic agonists during CPR in adults. Ann Emerg Med 22:411, 1993

PACKER M: Sudden unexpected death in patients with congestive heart failure: A second frontier. Circulation 72:681, 1985

Standard and guidelines for cardiopulmonary resuscitation (CPR) and emergency cardiac care (ECC). JAMA 255:290, 1986

WILBER DJ et al: Out-of-hospital cardiac arrest: Use of electrophysiologic testing in the prediction of long-term outcome. N Engl J Med 318:19, 1988

WILLICH SN et al: Sudden cardiac death. Support for a role of triggering in causation. Circulation 87:1442, 1993

section 5   Alterations in gastrointestinal function

36   ORAL MANIFESTATIONS OF DISEASE

36   ORAL MANIFESTATIONS OF DISEASE

JOHN S. GREENSPAN*

A thorough oral examination, to include the oral and pharyngeal soft tissues as well as the teeth, is an important part of the physical examination. The common oral diseases are due to infection by bacteria, fungi, or viruses. The complex development of the orofacial structures leads to close interposition of a wide range of tissues, most of which are prone to developmental anomalies, growth disturbances, and neoplasia.

DISEASES OF THE TEETH

DENTAL CARIES, PULPAL AND PERIAPICAL DISEASE, AND COMPLICATIONS   Dental caries is a destructive disease of the hard tissues of the teeth due to infection with *Streptococcus mutans* and other bacteria. Formerly one of the most common human diseases, caries has shown marked changes in recent years. In the United States, fewer than half of those 17 years and younger now have carious lesions, although in many segments of the population and in developing countries this decrease has not occurred. Much of the decline is due to artificial fluoridation of drinking water to a level of 1 part per million, with additional effects due to fluoride-containing toothpastes and topical fluoride administration. Conversely, retention of teeth and the aging of the population have led to an increase in root caries. Increasing numbers of patients surviving with the consequences of cancer therapy and other special populations (diabetics and those with xerostomia due to Sjögren's syndrome or to medications) may experience severe caries unless appropriate topical fluoride prophylaxis is used. Treatment of caries involves removal of the softened and infected hard tissues, sealing of the exposed dentine, and restoration of the lost tooth structure with silver amalgam, composite plastic, gold, or porcelain.

If the carious lesion progresses, infection of the dental pulp may occur, causing *acute pulpitis*. The tooth may become sensitive to hot or cold, and then severe continuous throbbing pain ensues. At this stage, pulp damage is irreversible, and root canal therapy becomes necessary. The contents of the pulp chamber and root canals are removed, followed by thorough cleaning, antisepsis, and filling with an inert material. Alternatively, extraction of the tooth may be indicated.

If the pulpitis is not treated successfully, infection may spread beyond the tooth apex into the periodontal ligament. If the infection causes acute inflammation, pain on chewing or on percussion is present, and a *periapical abscess* may form, while chronic inflammation can produce a *periapical granuloma* within the alveolar bone. This may cause slight pain and tenderness or may be asymptomatic. Proliferation of epithelial cell rests may convert the granuloma into a *periapical cyst*. Both the granuloma and the cyst produce periapical radiolucencies, whereas the periapical abscess does not do so unless

it forms as a complication of one of the other two lesions. The pus in the periapical abscess may track through the alveolar bone into soft tissues, causing cellulitis and bacteremia, or may discharge into the oral cavity (*parulis* or *gumboil*), into the maxillary sinus, or through the skin of the face or submandibular area. A severe form of cellulitis, *Ludwig's angina*, originates from an infected mandibular molar, involves the submandibular space, and extends throughout the floor of the mouth, with elevation of the tongue, dysphagia, and difficulty in breathing. Glottal edema may occur, necessitating emergency tracheotomy.

EFFECT OF SYSTEMIC FACTORS ON TEETH   Systemic factors, occurring in utero or in infancy during the stages of crown formation, may influence the development and structure of the teeth. Enamel hypoplasia of the primary and/or permanent teeth, manifested by alterations ranging from white spots to gross defects in the surface structure of the crowns, may be caused by disturbances of calcium and phosphate metabolism such as are found in vitamin D–resistant rickets, hypoparathyroidism, gastroenteritis, and celiac disease. Premature birth or high fevers also may give rise to enamel hypoplasia. Tetracycline, when given during the second half of pregnancy, in infancy, and in childhood up to 8 years of age, causes both a permanent discoloration of the teeth and enamel hypoplasia. Daily ingestion of more than 1.5 mg fluoride can result in enamel discoloration (*mottling*). Prenatal factors appear to influence crown size. Larger teeth are associated with maternal diabetes, maternal hypothyroidism, and large birth size. Tooth size is reduced in Down syndrome. Premature loss of the deciduous dentition is frequently the first symptom in juvenile hypophosphatasia. Systemic disease may give rise to pain that simulates pulpal disease. Maxillary sinusitis is frequently manifested as pain in the maxillary teeth, including sensitivity to thermal changes and percussion. Cardiac disease with angina pectoris may result in pain referred to the lower jaw, probably through the vagus nerve.

PERIODONTAL DISEASES

In adults, chronic destructive periodontal disease becomes responsible for more loss of teeth than caries, particularly in the aged. However, the prevalence and incidence of periodontal disease also appears to be declining in the United States. The most common form of periodontal disease starts as inflammation of the marginal gingiva (*gingivitis*) which is painless, although the gingiva may bleed on brushing. The disease spreads to involve the periodontal ligament and alveolar bone. As the latter is slowly resorbed, there is loss of periodontal ligament attachment between tooth and bone. The soft tissue separates from the tooth surface, causing "pocket" formation with bleeding on probing and during chewing. Acute inflammation may become superimposed on this chronic process, with the production of pus and the formation of a *periodontal abscess*. Ultimately, extreme bone loss, tooth mobility, and recurrent abscess formation lead to tooth exfoliation or may mandate tooth extraction.

Gingivitis and periodontitis are infections associated with the accumulation of *bacterial plaque*, which may become mineralized (*calculus*) and which can be prevented by appropriate *oral hygiene* measures, including tooth brushing, flossing, antibacterial mouth rinses, and the removal of impacted food debris. Poorly fabricated or

* The author acknowledges the contribution of Dr. Paul Goldhaber in previous editions.

deteriorated restorations may contribute through overextended or inadequate margins, while the role of occlusal trauma is unclear. Therapy is directed at the causative microflora and consists of removal of plaque and calculus, debridement of the pocket lining and superficial infected cementum, and elimination of other contributing factors.

Periodontal disease appears to be a group of conditions, including *adult periodontitis*, associated with *Porphyromonas gingivalis, Prevotella intermedia*, and other gram-negative organisms. *Localized juvenile periodontitis* (LJP) causes rapid, severe pocketing and bone loss and is associated with *Actinobacillus actinomycetemcomitans* (*A.a*), *Capnocytophaga, Eikenella corrodens*, and other anaerobes. *Acute necrotizing ulcerative gingivitis* (ANUG) involves sudden inflammation of the gingivae with necrosis, tissue loss, pain, bleeding, and halitosis and is associated with *P. intermedia* and spirochetes. ANUG and an aggressive and rapid form of periodontitis (HIV-P) are seen in association with human immunodeficiency virus (HIV) infection. Some of these cases progress to a destructive gangrene-like lesion of oral soft tissues and bone (*necrotizing stomatitis*) resembling the *noma* formerly seen in severely malnourished populations. Therapy involves local antibacterial measures, debridement, and, in severe cases, systemic antibiotics effective against gram-negative anaerobes.

Host factors may be involved in the pathogenesis of periodontal disease in other populations as well. Thus familial defects in neutrophil chemotaxis are found in LJP, and these may predispose to tissue destruction caused by the toxins of *A.a.*, including leucotoxin, collagenase, endotoxin, and a factor further inhibiting neutrophil chemotaxis. Patients with IgA deficiency and agammaglobulinemia probably have less periodontal disease than matched healthy individuals, whereas in *Down syndrome* and *diabetes mellitus* severe periodon-

tal disease may occur. During pregnancy there may be severe gingivitis and the formation of localized *pyogenic granulomas*. Certain drugs, notably the anticonvulsant *phenytoin* and the antiangina calcium channel blocker *nifedipine*, cause *fibrous hyperplasia* of the gingiva which may cover the teeth, interfere with eating, and be unsightly. Similar clinical appearances can be due to *idiopathic familial gingival fibromatosis*. Surgical management is used for both conditions, although a change in medication may be appropriate for the drug-induced form.

Periapical and periodontal bacterial infections can cause transient bacteremia after tooth extraction and even routine dental prophylaxis. These can lead to bacterial endocarditis in patients with a history of rheumatic fever, other valvular disease, valvular graft, or heart or joint prostheses. Antibiotic coverage is appropriate in such cases.

DISEASES OF THE ORAL MUCOSA

INFECTIONS   Most oral mucosal diseases involve microorganisms (see Table 36-1).

PIGMENTED LESIONS (See Table 36-2)

DERMATOLOGIC DISEASES (See Tables 36-1, -2, and -3 and Chaps. 50 to 55)

DISEASES OF THE TONGUE (See Table 36-4)

HALITOSIS (See Table 36-5)

HIV DISEASE AND AIDS (See Table 36-6 and Chaps. 151 and 279)   Immunosuppression induced by HIV infection predisposes to numerous oral infections, neoplasms, and autoimmune and idiopathic lesions. Some of these, such as *oral candidiasis* (Fig. A1-41) and *hairy leukoplakia* (Fig. A1-40) (a benign epithelial hyperplasia

TABLE 36-1 Vesicular, bullous, or ulcerative lesions of the oral mucosa			
Condition	Usual location	Clinical features	Course
VIRAL DISEASES			
Primary acute herpetic gingivo-stomatitis (herpes simplex virus type 1, rarely type 2)	Lip and oral mucosa	Labial vesicles which rupture and crust, and intraoral vesicles which quickly ulcerate; extremely painful; acute gingivitis, fever, malaise, foul odor, and cervical lymphadenopathy; occurs primarily in infants, children, and young adults	Heals spontaneously in 10–14 days unless secondarily infected
Recurrent herpes labialis	Mucocutaneous junction of lip, perioral skin	Eruption of groups of vesicles which may coalesce, then rupture and crust; painful to pressure or spicy foods	Lasts about 1 week, but condition may be prolonged if secondary infection occurs
Recurrent intraoral herpes simplex	Palate and gingiva	Small vesicles which rupture and coalesce; painful	Heal spontaneously in about 1 week
Chickenpox (varicella-zoster virus)	Gingiva and oral mucosa	Skin lesions may be accompanied by small vesicles on oral mucosa that rupture to form shallow ulcers; may coalesce to form large bullous lesions that ulcerate; mucosa may have generalized erythema	Lesions heal spontaneously within 2 weeks
Herpes zoster (reactivation of varicella-zoster virus)	Cheek, tongue, gingiva, or palate	Unilateral vesicular eruption and ulceration in linear pattern following sensory distribution of trigeminal nerve or one of its branches	Gradual healing without scarring; postherpetic neuralgia is common
Infectious mononucleosis (Epstein-Barr virus)	Oral mucosa	Fatigue, sore throat, malaise, low-grade fever, and enlarged cervical lymph nodes; numerous small ulcers usually appear several days before lymphadenopathy; gingival bleeding and multiple petechiae at junction of hard and soft palates	Oral lesions disappear during convalescence
Warts (papillomavirus)	Anywhere on skin and oral mucosa	Single or multiple papillary lesions, with thick, white keratinized surfaces containing many pointed projections; cauliflower lesions covered with normal-colored mucosa or multiple pink or pale bumps (focal epithelial hyperplasia)	Lesions grow rapidly and spread

(Continued)

TABLE 36-1 Vesicular, bullous, or ulcerative lesions of the oral mucosa (*continued*)

Condition	Usual location	Clinical features	Course
VIRAL DISEASES			
Herpangina (coxsackievirus A; also possibly coxsackievirus B and echovirus)	Oral mucosa, pharynx, tongue	Sudden onset of fever, sore throat, and oropharyngeal vesicles, usually in children under 4 years, during summer months; diffuse pharyngeal congestion and vesicles (1–2 mm), grayish white surrounded by red areola; vesicles enlarge and ulcerate	Incubation period 2–9 days; fever for 1–4 days; recovery uneventful
Hand, foot, and mouth disease (type A coxsackieviruses)	Oral mucosa, pharynx, palms, and soles	Fever, malaise, headache with oropharyngeal vesicles which become painful, shallow ulcers	Incubation period 2–18 days; lesions heal spontaneously in 2–4 weeks
Primary HIV infection	Gingiva, palate, and pharynx	Acute gingivitis and oropharyngeal ulceration, associated with febrile illness resembling mononucleosis and including lymphadenopathy	Followed by HIV seroconversion, asymptomatic HIV infection and usually ultimately by HIV disease
BACTERIAL OR FUNGAL DISEASES			
Acute necrotizing ulcerative gingivitis ("trench mouth," Vincent's infection)	Gingiva	Painful, bleeding gingiva characterized by necrosis and ulceration of gingival papillae and margins plus lymphadenopathy and foul odor	Continued destruction of tissue followed by remission, but may recur
Prenatal (congenital) syphilis	Palate, jaws, tongue, and teeth	Gummatous involvement of palate, jaws, and facial bones; Hutchinson's incisors, mulberry molars, glossitis, mucous patches, and fissures of corners of mouth	Tooth deformities in permanent dentition irreversible
Primary syphilis (chancre)	Lesion appears where organism enters body; may occur on lips, tongue, or tonsillar area	Small papule developing rapidly into a large, painless ulcer with indurated border; unilateral lymphadenopathy; chancre and lymph nodes containing spirochetes; serologic tests positive by third to fourth weeks	Healing of chancre in 1–2 months, followed by secondary syphilis in 6–8 weeks
Secondary syphilis	Oral mucosa frequently involved with mucous patches, primarily on palate, also at commissures of mouth	Maculopapular lesions of oral mucosa, 5–10 mm in diameter with central ulceration covered by grayish membrane; eruptions occurring on various mucosal surfaces and skin accompanied by fever, malaise, and sore throat	Lesions may persist from several weeks to a year
Tertiary syphilis	Palate and tongue	Gummatous infiltration of palate or tongue followed by ulceration and fibrosis; atrophy of tongue papillae produces characteristic bald tongue and glossitis	Gumma may destroy palate, causing complete perforation
Gonorrhea	Lesions may occur in mouth at site of inoculation or secondarily by hematogenous spread from a primary focus elsewhere	Earliest symptoms are burning or itching sensation, dryness, or heat in mouth followed by acute pain on eating or speaking; tonsils and oropharynx most frequently involved; oral tissues may be diffusely inflamed or ulcerated; saliva develops increased viscosity and fetid odor; submaxillary lymphadenopathy with fever in severe cases	Lesions may resolve with appropriate antibiotic therapy
Tuberculosis	Tongue, tonsillar area, soft palate	A solitary, irregular ulcer covered by a persistent exudate; ulcer has an undermined, firm border	Lesions may persist
Cervicofacial actinomycosis	Swellings in region of face, neck, and floor of mouth	Infection may be associated with an extraction, jaw fracture, or eruption of molar tooth; in acute form resembles an acute pyogenic abscess, but contains yellow "sulfur granules" (gram-positive mycelia and their hyphae)	Acute form may last a few weeks; chronic form lasts months or years; prognosis excellent; actinomycetes respond to antibiotics (tetracyclines or penicillin) but not to antifungal drugs
Histoplasmosis	Any area in mouth, particularly tongue, gingiva, or palate	Numerous small nodules which may ulcerate; hoarseness and dysphagia may occur because of lesions in larynx, usually associated with fever and malaise	May be fatal
Candidiasis	Any area of oral mucosa	Pseudomembranous form has white patches which are easily wiped off leaving red, bleeding, sore surface; erythematous form is flat and red; rarely, candidal leukoplakia appears as white patch in tongue which does not rub off; angular cheilitis due to *Candida* involves sore cracks and redness at angle of mouth; *Candida* seen on KOH preparation in all forms	Responds to antifungals

(Continued)

TABLE 36-1   Vesicular, bullous, or ulcerative lesions of the oral mucosa *(continued)*

Condition	Usual location	Clinical features	Course
DERMATOLOGIC DISEASES			
Mucous membrane pemphigoid	Primarily mucous membranes of the oral cavity, but may also involve the eyes, urethra, vagina, and rectum	Painful, grayish white collapsed vesicles or bullae with peripheral erythematous zone; gingival lesions desquamate, leaving ulcerated area	Protracted course with remissions and exacerbations; involvement of different sites occurs slowly; glucocorticoids may temporarily reduce symptoms but do not control the disease
Erythema multiforme (Stevens-Johnson syndrome)	Primarily the oral mucosa and skin of hands and feet	Intraoral ruptured bullae surrounded by an inflammatory area; lips may show hemorrhagic crusts; the "iris," or "target" lesion, on the skin is pathognomonic; patient may have severe signs of toxicity	Onset very rapid; condition may last 1–2 weeks; may be fatal; acute episodes respond to steroids
Pemphigus vulgaris	Oral mucosa and skin	Ruptured bullae and ulcerated oral areas; mostly in older adults	With repeated recurrence of bullae, toxicity may lead to cachexia, infection, and death within 2 years; often controllable with steroids
Lichen planus	Oral mucosa and skin	White striae in mouth; purplish nodules on skin at sites of friction; occasionally causes oral mucosal ulcers and erosive gingivitis	Protracted course, may respond to topical steroids
NEOPLASTIC DISEASES			
Squamous cell carcinoma	Any areas in mouth, most commonly on lower lip, tongue, and floor of mouth	Ulcer with elevated, indurated border; failure to heal, pain not prominent; lesions tend to arise in areas of leukoplakia or in smooth or atrophic tongue	Invades and destroys underlying tissues and may metastasize to regional lymph nodes
Acute leukemia	Gingiva	Gingival swelling and superficial ulcerations followed by hyperplasia of gingiva with extensive necrosis and hemorrhage; deep ulcers may occur elsewhere on the mucosa complicated by secondary infection	Fatal if untreated
Lymphoma	Gingiva, palate, tongue, and tonsillar area	Elevated, ulcerated area which may proliferate rapidly, giving the appearance of a traumatic inflammatory lesion; swelling of regional lymph nodes	Fatal if untreated
Metastatic tumors	Deep in jaw bone, usually in premolar-molar area of mandible	May arise from carcinoma of distant organ such as breast, lung, or kidney; advanced lesion may expand and destroy bone, loosen and spread teeth, involve inferior alveolar nerve, cause pain and numbness of lower lip	Usually fatal
OTHER CONDITIONS			
Recurrent aphthous ulcers	Anywhere on nonkeratinized oral mucosa (lips, tongue, buccal mucosa, floor of mouth, soft palate, oropharynx)	Single or clusters of painful ulcers with surrounding erythematous border; lesions may be 1–2 mm in diameter in crops (herpetiform), 1–5 mm (minor), or 5–15 mm (major)	Lesions heal in 1–2 weeks but may recur monthly or several times a year; topical steroids give symptomatic relief; systemic glucocorticoids may be needed in severe cases; a tetracycline oral suspension may decrease severity of herpetiform ulcers
Behçet's syndrome	Oral mucosa, eyes, genitalia, gut, and CNS	Multiple aphthous ulcers in mouth; inflammatory ocular changes, ulcerative lesions on genitalia; inflammatory bowel disease and CNS disease	Ulcers may persist for several weeks and heal without scarring
Traumatic ulcers	Anywhere on oral mucosa; dentures frequently responsible for ulcers in vestibule	Localized, discrete ulcerated lesion with red border; produced by accidental biting of mucosa, penetration by a foreign object, or chronic irritation by a denture	Lesions usually heal in 7–10 days when irritant is removed, unless secondarily infected

associated with Epstein-Barr virus, or EBV), are common features of HIV disease and often precede or accompany full-blown AIDS. Some, such as oral Kaposi's sarcoma and lymphoma, are diagnostic of AIDS. Oral candidiasis is easily treated with topical or systemic antifungals. These include nystatin oral pastilles, clotrimazole oral troches, nystatin vaginal tablets used orally, fluconazole, and ketoconazole. While most oral lesions of HIV disease are also found in the general population, both hairy leukoplakia and HIV-P are strongly associated with HIV infection and are seen only very rarely in other

circumstances. Only small and variable amounts of HIV can be found in saliva, but blood, tissue fluid, and gingival crevicular exudate, found in the mouth as a result of lesions or of clinical manipulation, are certainly sources of other viruses, such as herpes simplex virus (HSV) and EBV, and the same may be true for HIV.

HEMATOLOGIC AND NUTRITIONAL DISEASE   Gingival bleeding, necrotic ulcers, and enlargement due to malignant infiltrates are seen in all forms of leukemia, particularly *monocytic leukemia*. In *agranulocytosis* severe oral mucosal ulcers are seen, while in

TABLE 36-2   Pigmented lesions of the oral mucosa

Condition	Usual location	Clinical features	Course
Oral melanotic macule	Any area of the mouth	Discrete or diffuse localized, brown to black macule	Remains indefinitely
Diffuse melanin pigmentation	Any area of the mouth	Diffuse pale to dark-brown pigmentation; may be physiologic ("racial") or due to smoking	Remains indefinitely
Nevi	Any area of the mouth	Discrete, localized, brown to black pigmentation	Remains indefinitely
Malignant melanoma	Any area of the mouth	Can be flat and diffuse, painless, brown to black, or can be raised and nodular	Expands and invades early; metastasis leads to death
Addison's disease	Any area in mouth but mostly on buccal mucosa	Blotches or spots of bluish-black to dark-brown pigmentation occurring early in the disease, accompanied by diffuse pigmentation of skin; other symptoms of adrenal insufficiency	Condition controlled by steroid therapy
Peutz-Jeghers syndrome	Any area in mouth	Dark-brown spots on lips, buccal mucosa, with characteristic distribution of pigment around lips, nose, eyes, and on hands; concomitant intestinal polyposis	Pigmented lesions remain indefinitely; polyps may become malignant
Drug ingestion (tranquilizers, oral contraceptives, antimalarials)	Any area in mouth	Brown, black, or gray areas of pigmentation	Disappears following cessation of drug
Amalgam tattoo	Gingiva and mucobuccal fold	Small blue-black pigmented areas associated with embedded amalgam particles in soft tissues; these may show up on radiographs as radiopaque particles in some cases	Remains indefinitely
Heavy metal pigmentation (bismuth, mercury, lead)	Gingival margin	Thin blue-black pigmented line along gingival margin; due to prior treatment for syphilis with bismuth or mercury or to accidental absorption of lead	Long-lasting
Black hairy tongue	Dorsum of tongue	Elongation of filiform papillae of tongue, which take on a brown to black coloration	Long-lasting but may disappear spontaneously
Fordyce's "disease"	Buccal and labial mucosa	Aggregation of numerous small yellowish spots just beneath mucosal surface; no symptoms; due to hyperplasia of sebaceous glands	Remains without apparent change indefinitely

thrombocytopenia oral petechiae, ecchymoses, and gingival bleeding occur. In *Plummer-Vinson syndrome* (see Chaps. 302 and 303), atrophy of oral mucosa, particularly the tongue papillae, causes redness and soreness as well as dysphagia. This is associated with increased susceptibility to oral cancer. A smooth tongue also can be seen in *pernicious anemia* (Chap. 304). Severe oral mucositis with ulcers, candidiasis, bacterial infections, and xerostomia complicate local radiotherapy for head and neck malignancies as well as chemotherapy for both local and other malignancies. Although now rarely seen in the United States, oral features of vitamin deficiency include oral mucositis and ulcers, glossitis, and burning sensations in the tongue (*B group vitamins*) and petechiae, gingival swelling, bleeding, and ulceration as well as loosening of teeth (*scurvy* of vitamin C deficiency).

ORAL CANCER

Oral *squamous cell carcinoma* accounts for 2 to 4 percent of malignancies in the United States (when skin carcinomas are excluded) and in most western countries but represents up to 50 percent of malignancies in India. Globally, oral cancer is fourth in incidence for men and sixth for women. The disease is age-related, occurring in those over 40 years of age and increasing in incidence with age. The male/female ratio is 3:1, but the incidence of lip and mouth cancer is decreasing in white males and increasing in black males and in females. However, both the overall incidence and death rate are fairly static. *Lip cancer* has shown significant decreases in incidence in recent years, probably because of changes in pipe-smoking habits, while *tongue cancer* has become more common. The lip is still the most common oral site for cancer, followed by tongue, floor of

mouth, and other intraoral locations. The etiology involves *tobacco* smoked in pipes, cigars, and cigarettes or chewed or "dipped." The role of pipe smoking in lip cancer also may include the effects of heat and other irritants. Other factors include *alcohol*, iron deficiency (Plummer-Vinson syndrome), and deficiencies of vitamins. Evidence linking oral *syphilitic* lesions and oral *candidiasis* with oral cancer is circumstantial, but a growing body of data indicates roles for *herpes simplex virus* and *human papillomavirus*. There are no data supporting the idea that irritation from sharp teeth or dental appliances causes oral cancer.

The most common precancerous lesion in the oral cavity presents as *leukoplakia*, a white patch on the mucosa that cannot be rubbed off. Histologically, such lesions show hyperkeratosis, acanthosis, and *atypia* (*dysplasia*). Leukoplakias include homogeneous and nonhomogeneous types. The nonhomogeneous nodular leukoplakias (white nodules on a red background) have a much higher potential for malignant transformation than homogeneous leukoplakia. Recent evidence suggests that the asymptomatic red velvety lesion (*erythroplasia*) of the floor of the mouth, ventrolateral aspect of the tongue, or soft palate–anterior pillar complex is more likely to be carcinoma in situ or invasive carcinoma than is the white lesion. All chronic ulcerative lesions that fail to heal within 1 to 2 weeks should be considered potentially malignant and must be biopsied in order to make a definitive diagnosis. It is noteworthy that in their early stages intraoral squamous cell carcinomas are rarely painful, in contrast to similar-appearing inflammatory lesions.

The prognosis for patients with carcinoma of the lip is usually good, since these malignant tumors are noted sooner and apparently metastasize later. Patients with carcinoma of the tongue have a poorer prognosis, particularly if the tumor occurs more posteriorly on the tongue. Intraoral carcinomas may spread by direct invasion to the

TABLE 36-3 White lesions of oral mucosa

Condition	Usual location	Clinical features	Course
Lichen planus	Buccal mucosa, tongue, gingiva, and lips; skin	Striae, white plaques, red areas, ulcers in mouth; purplish papules on skin; may be asymptomatic, sore, or painful; lichenoid drug reactions may look similar	Protracted; responds to topical steroids
White sponge nevus	Oral mucosa, vagina, anal mucosa	Painless white thickening of epithelium; adolescent/early adult onset; familial	Benign and permanent
Smoker's leukoplakia and smokeless tobacco lesions	Any area of oral mucosa, sometimes related to location of habit	White patch that may become firm, rough, or red-fissured and ulcerated; may become sore and painful but usually painless	Occasionally premalignant; may or may not resolve on cessation of habit
Nicotinic stomatitis	Palate in pipe smokers	White nodular elevations on hard palate with central red areas	Benign; usually resolves on cessation of pipe smoking
Frictional keratosis	Any area in mouth	Elevated white lesion due to hyperkeratosis and thickening of the oral epithelium secondary to chronic irritation	Removal of irritant leads to healing in 2–3 weeks
Candidiasis ("candidosis," "moniliasis")	Any area in mouth	*Pseudomembranous type* ("thrush"): creamy white curdlike patches that reveal a raw, bleeding surface when scraped; found in sick infants, debilitated elderly patients receiving high doses of glucocorticoids or broad spectrum antibiotics, or in patients with AIDS	Responds favorably to antifungal therapy and correction of predisposing causes where possible
		Erythematous type: flat, red, sometimes sore areas, same groups of patients	Course same as for pseudomembranous type
		Candidal leukoplakia: nonremovable white thickening of epithelium due to *Candida*	Responds to prolonged antifungals
		Angular cheilitis: sore fissures at corner of mouth	Responds to topical antifungals
Hairy leukoplakia	Usually lateral tongue, rarely elsewhere on oral mucosa	White areas ranging from small and flat to extensive and "hairy"; found in HIV carriers in all risk groups for AIDS; rarely causes discomfort	Due to EBV; many patients develop AIDS; responds to high dose acyclovir but recurs
Chemical burns	Any area in mouth	White slough due to necrosis of epithelium and underlying connective tissue caused by contact with agents (e.g., aspirin) applied locally or the use of undiluted sodium perborate or hydrogen peroxide as a mouthwash; removal of slough leaves a raw, painful surface	Lesion heals in several weeks if not secondarily infected

underlying bone. Depending on the site of origin of the intraoral carcinoma, metastases usually spread to the submaxillary or cervical lymph nodes. Death may result from recurrent or uncontrollable disease above the clavicles, metastatic disease beyond the neck, treatment complications, or a second primary cancer, usually in the oral cavity or the upper parts of the gastrointestinal or respiratory tract. Metastatic tumors to the jaw may occur from carcinomas of the lung, breast, kidney, or gastrointestinal tract.

DISEASES OF THE SALIVARY GLANDS

The major and minor salivary glands can be involved in mumps, sarcoidosis, tuberculosis, lymphoma, and Sjögren's syndrome (Chap. 288). The latter may cause dry eyes and dry mouth (*xerostomia*) and be associated with features of connective tissue diseases, including rheumatoid arthritis or systemic lupus erythematosus. Xerostomia also may be due to medications such as diuretics, antihistamines, or tricylic antidepressants as well as therapeutic irradiation for head and neck cancer. It may cause *cervical or incisal caries* and oral candidiasis. Management includes fluoride mouth rinses and topical applications, saliva substitutes, salivary stimulation with sugarless candies, and the avoidance of sugar-containing drinks or food. Candidiasis is treated with nystatin or other antifungals. Salivary stones (*sialolithiasis*), usually in the duct of a major salivary gland, cause *sialoadenitis* with pain and swelling, often on eating. Recurrent *parotitis* without apparent cause is seen in children.

The most common neoplasm of the salivary glands is the *pleomorphic adenoma*, which is benign but will recur unless fully enucleated; malignant tumors include *mucoepidermoid carcinoma*, *adenoid cystic carcinoma*, and *adenocarcinoma*. The pleomorphic adenoma causes a firm, slowly growing mass in the parotid, palate, or cheek, whereas malignant tumors grow faster and can cause ulceration and invade nerves, producing numbness or facial paralysis.

NEUROLOGIC DISTURBANCES AND OROFACIAL PAIN

The mouth and face may be the site of pain from a number of vascular, neurologic, muscle/connective tissue, or joint conditions. Interdisciplinary diagnosis and management programs involving neurologists, restorative dentists, oral surgeons, otorhinolaryngologists, and other specialists, together with new imaging techniques to diagnose or exclude organic lesions, have begun to clarify this complex field. *Temporal arteritis* causes pain in the face, jaws, and tongue and may mimic temporomandibular joint disease. Glucocorticoids may provide relief. *Myofascial pain* is a dull, constant ache with local tenderness in the muscles of the jaws and difficulty in opening the mouth. This may be related to clenching and grinding habits (*bruxism*). *Arthralgia* of the temporomandibular joint causes local pain which may extend to the face and head. Both myofascial pain and arthralgia can be relieved with heat, rest, and anti-inflammatory agents. Displacement of the meniscus or condyle may

TABLE 36-4 Alterations of the tongue

Type of change	Clinical features
SIZE OR MORPHOLOGY CHANGES	
Macroglossia	Enlarged tongue that may be part of a syndrome found in developmental conditions such as Down syndrome; may be due to tumor (hemangioma or lymphangioma), metabolic disease (such as primary amyloidosis), or endocrine disturbance (such as acromegaly or cretinism)
Fissured (''scrotal'') tongue	Dorsal surface and sides of tongue covered by painless shallow or deep fissures that may collect debris and become irritated
Median rhomboid glossitis	Congenital abnormality of tongue with ovoid, denuded area in median posterior portion of the tongue; may be associated with candidiasis and may respond to antifungals
COLOR CHANGES	
''Geographic'' tongue (benign migratory glossitis)	Asymptomatic inflammatory condition of the tongue, with rapid loss and regrowth of filiform papillae, leading to appearance of denuded red patches ''wandering'' across the surface of the tongue
Hairy tongue	Elongation of filiform papillae of the medial dorsal surface area due to failure of keratin layer of the papillae to desquamate normally; brownish-black coloration may be due to staining by tobacco, food, or chromogenic organisms
''Strawberry'' and ''raspberry'' tongue	Appearance of tongue during scarlet fever due to the hypertrophy of fungiform papillae plus changes in the filiform papillae
''Bald'' tongue	Atrophy may be associated with xerostomia, pernicious anemia, iron-deficiency anemia, pellagra, or syphilis; may be accompanied by painful burning sensation; may be an expression of erythmematous candidiasis and respond to antifungals

TABLE 36-5 Causes of halitosis

I **Upper respiratory infection**
 A Bronchiectasis
 B Lung abscess
II **Oral infection**
 A Acute primary herpetic gingivostomatitis
 B Acute necrotizing ulcerative gingivitis
 C Periodontal disease
 D Caries
III **Smoking**
IV **Hepatic failure (fishy odor)**
V **Azotemia (ammoniacal or urinary odor)**
VI **Diabetic ketoacidosis (sweet, fruity odor)**

TABLE 36-6 Oral lesions of HIV disease and AIDS

I **Fungal**
 A Candidiasis
  1 Pseudomembranous
  2 Erythematous
  3 Candidal leukoplakia
  4 Angular cheilitis
 B Histoplasmosis
 C Cryptococcosis
II **Bacterial**
 A Acute necrotizing ulcerative gingivitis
 B HIV-gingivitis
 C HIV-periodontitis
 D Necrotizing stomatitis
 E Mycobacterium avium intracellulare complex and tuberculosis
 F Stomatitis due to enteric organisms
III **Viral**
 A Herpes simplex
 B Herpes zoster
 C Hairy leukoplakia
 D Warts
IV **Neoplastic**
 A Kaposi's sarcoma
 B Lymphoma
V **Other**
 A Recurrent aphthous ulcers
 B Immune thrombocytopenic purpura
 C Xerostomia
 D Salivary gland enlargement

cause pain, clenching, or locking of the mandible in the open position. The joint may become involved in *osteoarthritis* with minimal symptoms, whereas *rheumatoid arthritis* causes pain and swelling in the joint, limitation of movement, and, in the *juvenile* form, severe malocclusion in children. *Ankylosis* may occur, necessitating condylectomy (see Chap. 285).

Trigeminal neuralgia (tic douloureux) causes sudden, severe, unilateral lancinating pain initiated by touching a ''trigger zone'' or occurring spontaneously. Confusion with pulpal or periapical pain is common, leading to inappropriate endodontic or surgical therapy. Many cases respond to carbamazepine and phenytoin, but for a few, surgical intervention to decompress the trigeminal nerve is indicated. Similar symptoms in the distribution of the ninth cranial nerve (tongue, pharynx, soft palate) are due to *glossopharyngeal neuralgia*, which may be triggered by swallowing and may produce referred pain in the temporomandibular joint. *Postherpetic neuralgia* may follow trigeminal herpes zoster (see Chap. 380) and cause burning, aching, and long-lasting pain. *Facial palsy* is usually unilateral and may be due to trauma, surgical intervention, tumor, or infection of the seventh cranial nerve. *Bell's palsy* is a form with acute onset and unknown cause, possibly viral infection such as herpes zoster. The corner of the mouth droops, and there may be difficulty in speech, eating, and in closing the eye. The symptoms usually disappear spontaneously, but residual facial immobility and lip drooping may persist. Abnormal or reduced *taste sensation* may be due to xerostomia, disturbances of the facial and glossopharyngeal nerves or their central connections, aging, or the wearing of dentures. Disease involving the hypoglossal nerve may cause atrophy of the tongue muscles with protrusion, if bilateral, or deviation toward the affected side, if unilateral.

REFERENCES

GENCO R et al: *Contemporary Periodontics.* St. Louis, Mosby, 1989
GREENSPAN D et al: *AIDS and the Mouth.* Chicago, Year Book, 1990
LYNCH MA et al: *Burket's Oral Medicine, Diagnosis and Treatment*, 8th ed. Philadelphia, Lippincott, 1983
NEWBRUN E: *Cariology*, 3d ed. Chicago, Quintessence, 1989
WRIGHT BA et al: *Oral Cancer: Clinical and Pathological Considerations.* Boca Raton, Fla, CRC Press, 1988

37   DYSPHAGIA

RAJ K. GOYAL

Dysphagia is defined as a sensation of "sticking" or obstruction of the passage of food through the mouth, pharynx, or the esophagus. It should be distinguished from other symptoms related to swallowing. *Aphagia* signifies complete esophageal obstruction, which is usually due to bolus impaction and represents a medical emergency. *Difficulty in initiating a swallow* occurs in disorders of the voluntary phase of swallowing. Once initiated, however, swallowing is completed normally. *Odynophagia* means painful swallowing. Frequently, odynophagia and dysphagia occur together. *Globus pharyngeous* is the sensation of a lump lodged in the throat. No difficulty, however, is encountered when actual swallowing is performed. *Misdirection of food*, resulting in nasal regurgitation and laryngeal and pulmonary aspiration of food during swallowing, is characteristic of oropharyngeal dysphagia. *Phagophobia*, meaning fear of swallowing, and *refusal to swallow* may occur in hysteria, rabies, tetanus, and pharyngeal paralysis due to fear of aspiration. Painful inflammatory lesions that cause odynophagia also may cause refusal to swallow. Some patients may feel the food as it goes down the esophagus. This esophageal sensitivity is not associated with sticking of the food or obstruction, however. Similarly, the *feeling of fullness in the epigastrium* that occurs after a meal or after swallowing air should not be confused with dysphagia.

PHYSIOLOGY OF SWALLOWING   The process of swallowing begins with a voluntary (oral) phase during which a bolus of food is pushed backward into the pharynx. The bolus activates oropharyngeal sensory receptors which initiate the involuntary (pharyngeal and esophageal) phase, or deglutition reflex. The deglutition reflex is a complex series of events which serves both to propel food through the pharynx and the esophagus and to prevent its entry into the airway. At the same time as the bolus is propelled backward by the tongue, the larynx moves forward and the upper esophageal sphincter opens. As the bolus moves into the pharynx, contraction of the superior pharyngeal constrictor against the contracted soft palate initiates a peristaltic contraction that proceeds rapidly downward to move the bolus through the pharynx and the esophagus. The lower esophageal sphincter opens as the food enters the esophagus and remains open until the peristaltic contraction has swept the bolus into the stomach. Peristaltic contraction in response to a swallow involves inhibition followed by sequential contraction of muscles along the entire swallowing passage and is called *primary peristalsis*. The inhibition that precedes the peristaltic contraction is called *deglutitive inhibition*. Local distention of the esophagus due to food activates intramural reflexes in the smooth muscle and results in *secondary peristalsis*, limited to the thoracic esophagus. *Tertiary contractions* are nonperistaltic as they occur simultaneously over a long segment of the esophagus. Tertiary contractions may occur in response to a swallow or esophageal distention, or they may occur spontaneously.

PATHOPHYSIOLOGY OF DYSPHAGIA   The normal transport of an ingested bolus through the swallowing passage depends on (1) the size of the ingested bolus, (2) the luminal diameter of the swallowing passage, (3) the peristaltic contraction, and (4) deglutitive inhibition, including normal relaxation of upper and lower esophageal sphincters during swallowing. Dysphagia caused by a large bolus or luminal narrowing is called *mechanical dysphagia*, whereas dysphagia due to incoordination or weakness of peristaltic contractions or to impaired deglutitive inhibition is called *motor dysphagia*.

Mechanical dysphagia   Mechanical dysphagia could be caused by a very large food bolus, intrinsic narrowing, or extrinsic compression of the lumen. In an adult, the esophageal lumen can distend up to a diameter of 4 cm because of the elasticity of the esophageal wall. When the esophagus cannot dilate beyond 2.5 cm in diameter, dysphagia can occur, but it is always present when it cannot distend

beyond 1.3 cm. Circumferential lesions produce dysphagia more consistently than do lesions that involve only a portion of circumferences of the esophageal wall, as uninvolved segments retain their distensibility. The causes of mechanical dysphagia are listed in Table 37-1. Common causes include (1) carcinoma, (2) peptic and other benign strictures, and (3) lower esophageal ring.

Motor dysphagia   Motor dysphagia may result from difficulty in initiating a swallow or abnormalities in peristalsis and deglutitive inhibition due to diseases of the esophageal striated or smooth muscle.

Diseases of the striated muscle involve the pharynx, upper esophageal sphincter, and upper part of the esophagus. The striated muscle is innervated by a somatic component of the vagus with cell bodies of the lower motor neurons located in the nucleus ambiguus. These neurons are cholinergic and excitatory and are the sole determinant of the muscle activity. Peristalsis in the striated muscle segment is due to sequential central activation of neurons innervating muscles at different levels along the esophagus. Motor dysphagia of the pharynx results from neuromuscular disorders causing muscle paralysis, simultaneous nonperistaltic contraction, or loss of opening of the upper esophageal sphincter. Loss of opening of the upper sphincter is caused by paralysis of geniohyoid and other suprahyoid muscles or loss of deglutitive inhibition of the cricopharyngeus muscle. Because each side of the pharynx is innervated by ipsilateral nerves, a lesion of motor neurons occurring only on one side leads to unilateral pharyngeal paralysis. Although lesions of striated muscle also involve the cervical part of the esophagus, the clinical manifestations of pharyngeal dysfunction usually overshadow the manifestations due to esophageal involvement.

Diseases of the smooth muscle segment involve the thoracic part of the esophagus and the lower esophageal sphincter. The smooth muscle is innervated by the parasympathetic component of the vagal preganglionic fibers and postganglionic neurons in the myenteric ganglia. These nerves exert a predominantly inhibitory influence on the lower esophageal sphincter and cause inhibition followed by contraction in the esophageal body. Peristalsis in this segment is due to neuromuscular mechanisms in the wall of the esophagus itself. Dysphagia results when the peristaltic contractions are weak or nonperistaltic or when the lower sphincter fails to open normally. Loss of contractile power occurs due to muscle weakness, as in scleroderma, or to loss of myenteric neurons, as in achalasia. The cause of nonperistaltic contractions, typically seen in diffuse esophageal spasm, is not understood. Impairment of deglutitive inhibition of the lower esophageal sphincter is associated with a defect in inhibitory nerves to the sphincter and is the major cause of dysphagia in achalasia.

The causes of motor dysphagia are also listed in Table 37-1. The important causes are pharyngeal paralysis, cricopharyngeal achalasia, scleroderma of the esophagus, achalasia, diffuse esophageal spasm and related motor disorders.

APPROACH TO THE PATIENT WITH DYSPHAGIA   History   The history can provide a correct presumptive diagnosis in over 80 percent of patients. The type of food causing dysphagia provides useful information. Difficulty only with solids implies mechanical dysphagia with a lumen that is not severely narrowed. The impacted bolus may be forced through the narrowed area by drinking liquids. In advanced obstruction, dysphagia occurs with liquids as well as solids. In contrast, motor dysphagia due to achalasia and diffuse esophageal spasm is equally affected by solids and liquids from the very onset. Patients with scleroderma have dysphagia to solids that is unrelated to posture and to liquids in the recumbent but not in the upright posture. When peptic stricture develops in these patients, dysphagia becomes more persistent.

The duration and course of dysphagia are helpful in diagnosis. Transient dysphagia of short duration may be due to an inflammatory process. Progressive dysphagia of a few weeks' to a few months' duration is suggestive of carcinoma of the esophagus. Episodic dysphagia to solids of several years' duration indicates a benign disease and is characteristic of a lower esophageal ring.

TABLE 37-1 Causes of dysphagia

Mechanical dysphagia	Motor (neuromuscular) dysphagia

I Luminal
  A Large bolus
  B Foreign body
II Intrinsic narrowing
  A Inflammatory condition causing edema and swelling
    1 Stomatitis
    2 Pharyngitis, epiglottitis
    3 Esophagitis
      a Viral (herpes simplex, varicella-zoster, cytomegalovirus)
      b Bacterial
      c Fungal (candidal)
      d Mucocutaneous bullous diseases
      e Caustic, chemical, thermal injury
  B Webs and rings
    1 Pharyngeal (Plummer-Vinson syndrome)
    2 Esophageal (congenital, inflammatory)
    3 Lower esophageal mucosal ring (Schatzki ring)
  C Benign strictures
    1 Peptic
    2 Caustic and pill-induced
    3 Inflammatory (Crohn's disease, candidal, mucocutaneous lesions)
    4 Ischemic
    5 Postoperative, postirradiation
    6 Congenital
  D Malignant tumors
    1 Primary carcinoma
      a Squamous cell carcinoma
      b Adenocarcinoma
      c Carcinosarcoma
      d Pseudosarcoma
      e Lymphoma
      f Melanoma
      g Kaposi's sarcoma
    2 Metastatic carcinoma
  E Benign tumors
    1 Leiomyoma
    2 Lipoma
    3 Angioma
    4 Inflammatory fibroid polyp
    5 Epithelial papilloma
III Extrinsic compression
  A Cervical spondylitis
  B Vertebral osteophytes
  C Retropharyngeal abscess and masses
  D Enlarged thyroid gland
  E Zenker's diverticulum
  F Vascular compression
    1 Aberrant right subclavian artery
    2 Right-sided aorta
    3 Left atrial enlargement
    4 Aortic aneurysm
  G Posterior mediastinal masses
  H Pancreatic tumor, pancreatitis
  I Postvagotomy hematoma and fibrosis
	I Difficulty in initiating swallowing reflex
	  A Oral lesions and paralysis of tongue
	  B Oropharyngeal anesthesia
	  C Lack of saliva (e.g., Sjögren's syndrome)
	  D Lesions of sensory components of vagus and glossopharyngeal nerves
	  E Lesions of swallowing center
	II Disorders of pharyngeal and esophageal striated muscle
	  A Muscle weakness
	    1 Lower motor neuron lesion (bulbar paralysis)
	      a Cerebrovascular accident
	      b Motor neuron disease
	      c Poliomyelitis, postpolio syndrome
	      d Polyneuritis
	      e Amyotrophic lateral sclerosis
	      f Familial dysautonomia
	    2 Neuromuscular
	      a Myasthenia gravis
	    3 Muscle disorders
	      a Polymyositis
	      b Dermatomyositis
	      c Myopathies (myotonic dystrophy, oculopharyngeal myopathy)
	  B Simultaneous onset contractions or impaired deglutitive inhibition
	    1 Pharynx and upper esophagus
	      a Rabies
	      b Tetanus
	      c Extrapyramidal tract disease
	      d Upper motor neuron lesions (pseudobulbar paralysis)
	    2 Upper esophageal sphincter (UES)
	      a Paralysis of suprahyoid muscles (causes same as paralysis of pharyngeal musculature)
	      b Cricopharyngeal achalasia
	III Disorders of esophageal smooth muscle
	  A Paralysis of esophageal body causing weak contractions
	    1 Scleroderma and related collagen vascular diseases
	    2 Hollow visceral myopathy
	    3 Myotonic dystrophy
	    4 Metabolic neuromyopathy (amyloid, alcohol?, diabetes?)
	    5 Achalasia (classical)
	  B Simultaneous-onset contractions or impaired deglutitive inhibition
	    1 Esophageal body
	      a Diffuse esophageal spasm
	      b Achalasia (vigorous)
	      c Variants of diffuse esophageal spasm
	    2 Lower esophageal sphincter
	      a Disorders of achalasia
	        (1) Primary
	        (2) Secondary
	          (a) Chagas' disease
	          (b) Carcinoma
	          (c) Lymphoma
	          (d) Neuropathic intestinal pseudoobstruction syndrome
	          (e) Toxins and drugs
	      b Lower esophageal muscular (contractile) ring

The localization of the site of dysphagia by the patient is helpful in determining the site of esophageal obstruction; the lesion is at or below the perceived location.

Associated symptoms provide important diagnostic clues. Nasal regurgitation and tracheobronchial aspiration with swallowing are hallmarks of pharyngeal paralysis or a tracheoesophageal fistula. Tracheobronchial aspiration unrelated to swallowing may be secondary to achalasia, a Zenker's diverticulum, or gastroesophageal reflux. Severe weight loss out of proportion to the degree of dysphagia is highly suggestive of carcinoma. When hoarseness precedes dysphagia, the primary lesion is usually in the larynx. Hoarseness following dysphagia may suggest involvement of the recurrent laryngeal nerve by extension of esophageal carcinoma beyond the walls of the esophagus. Sometimes hoarseness may be due to laryngitis secondary to gastroesophageal reflux. Association of laryngeal symptoms and dysphagia also occurs in various neuromuscular disorders. Hiccups suggest a lesion in the distal portion of the esophagus. Unilateral wheezing with dysphagia indicates a mediastinal mass involving the esophagus and a large bronchus. Chest pain with dysphagia occurs in diffuse esophageal spasm and in related motor disorders. Chest pain resembling diffuse esophageal spasms also may occur in acute aphagia due to a large bolus. A prolonged history of heartburn and reflux preceding dysphagia indicates peptic stricture. Similarly, a history of prolonged nasogastric intubation, ingestion of caustic agents, ingestion of pills without water, previous radiation therapy, or associated mucocutaneous diseases may provide the cause of esophageal stricture. If odynophagia is present, candidal or herpes esophagitis should be suspected. In patients with AIDS or other immunodeficiency states, esophagitis due to opportunistic infections such as *Candida*, herpes simplex virus, cytomegalovirus, and tumors such as Kaposi's sarcoma and lymphoma should be suspected.

Physical examination Physical examination is important in motor dysphagia due to skeletal muscle, neurologic, and oropharyngeal diseases. Signs of bulbar or pseudobulbar palsy, including dysarthria, dysphonia, ptosis, tongue atrophy, and hyperactive jaw jerk, in addition to evidence of generalized neuromuscular disease, should be carefully searched for. The neck should be examined for thyromegaly or a spinal abnormality. A careful inspection of the mouth and pharynx should disclose lesions that may cause interference with passage of food from the mouth or esophagus because of pain or obstruction. Changes in the skin and extremities may suggest a diagnosis of scleroderma and other collagen-vascular diseases, or mucocutaneous diseases such as pemphigoid or epidermolysis bullosa which may involve the esophagus. Metastatic diseases to lymph nodes and liver may be evident. Pulmonary complications of acute aspiration pneumonia or chronic aspiration may be present.

Diagnostic procedures   Dysphagia is one of the major symptoms of esophageal disease, and a cause for this symptom can invariably be determined. Therefore, all patients with dysphagia must be thoroughly investigated until a specific cause is determined. This is particularly important because the treatment depends on the underlying cause of dysphagia. Barium swallow with cineradiography, esophago-gastroscopy with biopsy and exfoliative cytology, and esophageal motility study are the main diagnostic procedures (see Chap. 251). The treatment is dependent on the cause of dysphagia.

REFERENCES

CASTELL DO (ed): *The Esophagus*. Boston, Little, Brown, 1992

ENTERLINE H, THOMPSON J: *Pathology of the Esophagus*. New York, Springer-Verlag, 1984

GOYAL RK, PATERSON WG: Esophageal motility, in *Handbook of Physiology: Gastrointestinal System I*. Bethesda, MD, American Physiological Society, 1989, pp 865–908

KRESPI YP, BLITZER A (guest eds): Aspiration and swallowing disorders. Otolaryngol Clin North Am 21:595, 1988

OTT DJ: Radiologic evaluation of esophageal dysphagia. Curr Probl Diagn Radiol 17:1, 1975

SONIES B, DALAKAS M: Dysphagia in patients with the postpolio syndrome. N Engl J Med 324:1162, 1991

TYTGAT GNJ: Dilation therapy of benign esophageal stenoses. World J Surg 13:142, 1989

WEBB WA: Management of foreign bodies of the upper gastrointestinal tract. Gastroenterology 94:204, 1988

YAMATO S et al: Role of nitric oxide in lower esophageal sphincter relaxation to swallowing. Life Sci 50:1263, 1992

38   ANOREXIA, NAUSEA, VOMITING, AND INDIGESTION

LAWRENCE S. FRIEDMAN / KURT J. ISSELBACHER

ANOREXIA

Anorexia is a loss of appetite or lack of desire to eat. It must be differentiated from specific food intolerances and early satiety, a sense of fullness after the ingestion of a small amount of food. Anorexia is a prominent symptom in a wide variety of intestinal and extraintestinal disorders but as an isolated symptom is of little specific diagnostic value.

The mechanisms whereby hunger and appetite are modified in various disease states are poorly understood. Food intake is regulated by two hypothalamic centers—a lateral "feeding center" and a ventromedial "satiety center." The latter inhibits the feeding center following a meal, leading to the sensation of satiety. The brain-gut peptide cholecystokinin (CCK) appears to have a satiety effect and may be involved in the regulation of feeding behavior.

Anorexia is commonly seen in *diseases of the gastrointestinal tract and liver*. For example, it may precede the appearance of jaundice in acute hepatitis, or it may be a prominent symptom in gastric carcinoma. In the setting of intestinal disease, anorexia should be clearly differentiated from *sitophobia* (fear of eating because of subsequent abdominal discomfort). In such circumstances, appetite may persist, but the ingestion of food is curtailed nonetheless.

Sitophobia may occur, for example, in regional enteritis (especially with partial obstruction) or in chronic mesenteric vascular insufficiency ("abdominal angina").

Anorexia also may be a prominent feature of *extraintestinal diseases*. Chronic pain from any source may lead to loss of appetite. Anorexia may be profound in severe congestive heart failure and may be a major symptom in patients with uremia, respiratory failure, and various endocrinopathies (e.g., hyperparathyroidism, Addison's disease, and panhypopituitarism). In patients with cancer, anorexia may result from anxiety, depression, pain, a decreased sense of taste and smell, the effect of the tumor on the gastrointestinal tract (e.g., partial intestinal obstruction) or liver (metastases), chemotherapeutic agents, and, possibly, the release of an anorectic substance by the tumor (possibly tumor necrosis factor). Medications such as antihypertensives, diuretics, digitalis, and narcotic analgesics may cause anorexia. Finally, anorexia often accompanies psychogenic disturbances such as depression and may result from emotional upset, boredom, or exposure to unpleasant sights, odors, or thoughts. For a discussion of anorexia nervosa, see Chap. 74.

NAUSEA AND VOMITING

Nausea and vomiting may occur independently of each other but generally are closely allied and are presumed to be mediated by the same neural pathways, so they may be considered together. *Nausea* denotes the feeling of an imminent desire to vomit, usually referred to the throat or epigastrium. *Vomiting* (or *emesis*) refers to the forceful oral expulsion of gastric contents. *Retching* denotes the labored rhythmic contraction of respiratory and abdominal musculature that frequently precedes or accompanies vomiting.

Nausea often precedes or accompanies vomiting. It is usually associated with diminished functional activity of the stomach (e.g., hypotonicity, hypoperistalsis, and hyposecretion) and altered small-intestinal motility (e.g., hypertonicity and reversed peristalsis of the duodenum). Often accompanying severe nausea is evidence of altered autonomic (especially parasympathetic) activity, such as skin pallor, increased perspiration, hypersalivation, defecation, and, occasionally, hypotension and bradycardia (vasovagal syndrome); anorexia is also usually present.

Nausea, retching, and hypersalivation frequently precede the act of vomiting, which is a highly integrated sequence of involuntary visceral and somatic motor events. The stomach plays a relatively passive role in the vomiting process, the major ejection force being provided by the abdominal musculature. With relaxation of the gastric fundus and gastroesophageal sphincter, a sharp increase in intraabdominal pressure is brought about by forceful contraction of the diaphragm and abdominal wall muscles. This, together with concomitant annular contraction of the gastric pylorus, results in the expulsion of gastric contents into the esophagus. Increased intrathoracic pressure results in the further movement of esophageal contents into the mouth. Reversal of the normal direction of esophageal peristalsis may play a role in this process. Reflex elevation of the soft palate during the vomiting act prevents the entry of the expelled material into the nasopharynx, whereas reflex closure of the glottis and inhibition of respiration help to prevent pulmonary aspiration.

Repeated emesis may have deleterious effects in a number of ways. The process of vomiting, if forceful, may lead to pressure rupture of the esophagus (Boerhaave's syndrome) or to linear mucosal (Mallory-Weiss) tears in the region of the cardioesophageal junction with resulting hematemesis. Prolonged vomiting may lead to dehydration, the loss of gastric secretions (especially hydrochloric acid) resulting in metabolic alkalosis with hypokalemia, malnutrition with various deficiency states, and dental caries. In states of central nervous system depression (e.g., coma), gastric contents may be aspirated into the lungs, with a resulting aspiration pneumonitis.

VOMITING MECHANISM   The act of vomiting is under the control of two functionally distinct medullary centers: the *vomiting center* in the dorsal portion of the lateral reticular formation and the *chemoreceptor trigger zone* in the area postrema of the floor of the fourth ventricle. The vomiting center controls and integrates the actual act of emesis. It receives afferent stimuli from the gastrointestinal tract and other parts of the body, from higher brainstem and cortical centers, especially the labyrinthine apparatus, and from the chemoreceptor trigger zone. Persons vary considerably in the threshold of their vomiting centers to different stimuli. The important efferent pathways in vomiting are the phrenic nerves (to the diaphragm), the spinal nerves (to the intercostal and abdominal musculature), and visceral efferent fibers in the vagus nerve (to the larynx, pharynx, esophagus, and stomach). The vomiting center is located near other medullary centers regulating respiratory, vasomotor, and autonomic functions that may be involved in the act of vomiting.

The chemoreceptor trigger zone by itself is incapable of mediating the act of vomiting; rather activation of this zone results in efferent impulses to the medullary vomiting center, which in turn initiates emesis. The chemoreceptor trigger zone is an emetic chemoreceptor that can be activated by a variety of stimuli or drugs, including apomorphine and other opiates, levodopa (after decarboxylation to dopamine), digitalis, bacterial toxins, radiation, and metabolic abnormalities as occur with uremia and hypoxia.

CLINICAL CLASSIFICATION Nausea and vomiting are common manifestations of many organic and functional disorders. The precise mechanisms triggering vomiting in various clinical conditions are not well understood, making classification of mechanisms difficult.

Many *acute abdominal emergencies* which lead to the ''surgical abdomen'' are associated with nausea and vomiting. Vomiting may be seen with inflammation of a viscus, as in acute appendicitis or acute cholecystitis, intestinal obstruction, or acute peritonitis (see Chap. 260).

Other *disorders of the alimentary tract*, including those associated with chronic indigestion (see below), are frequently accompanied by nausea and vomiting. In peptic ulcer, emesis may be either spontaneous or self-induced and may lead to relief of symptoms, particularly if antral or pyloric edema has resulted in gastric outlet obstruction. Nausea and vomiting are also prominent in patients with disordered gastrointestinal motility, including postvagotomy, diabetic, or idiopathic gastroparesis (gastric atony), other gastric ''dysrhythmias'' resulting from abnormal myoelectric activity, and intestinal pseudo-obstruction due to abnormal intestinal myogenic or neurogenic function. Gastroparesis may be demonstrated by gastric scanning after a radiolabeled meal or by radiography after ingestion of indigestible radiopaque solid markers. Experimentally, some patients with otherwise unexplained nausea and vomiting have been demonstrated to have accelerated (''tachygastria'') or irregular (''gastric tachyarrhythmia'') gastric electrical activity as measured by electrodes implanted surgically on the serosa of the stomach or placed on the abdominal surface (''electrogastrogram''). Typically, intestinal obstruction of any cause (e.g., adhesions, malignancy, hernia, volvulus) leads to vomiting, as do other disorders of the liver, pancreas, and biliary tract. Nausea and vomiting may accompany the distention and pain seen in the aerophagic syndromes (see below).

Viral, bacterial, and parasitic *infections of the intestinal tract* are typically associated with severe nausea and vomiting, often with diarrhea. *Acute systemic infections* with fever, especially in young children, are also frequently accompanied by vomiting and often by severe diarrhea. The mechanism whereby infections remote from the gastrointestinal tract produce these manifestations may relate to stimulation of the medullary chemoreceptor trigger zone by toxins or abnormal metabolites.

Central nervous system disorders which lead to increased intracranial pressure (e.g., neoplasms, encephalitis, hydrocephalus) may be accompanied by vomiting, which is often *projectile* (intensely forceful). Vertigo due to disorders of the labyrinthine apparatus, such as acute labyrinthitis and Ménière's disease, may be accompanied by vomiting with nausea and retching. Similarly, motion sickness is typically associated with anorexia, nausea, and vomiting as well as

apathy, increased salivation, cold sweating, and headache. Additionally, migraine headaches, tabetic crises, acute meningitis, and the reactive phase of hypotension with syncope may be associated with nausea and vomiting.

Nausea and vomiting may be present in *acute myocardial infarction*, especially when posterior in location or transmural in extent, and in *congestive heart failure*, perhaps in relation to congestion of the liver. The possibility that these symptoms also may be due to drugs (e.g., opiates or digitalis) should always be borne in mind in patients with cardiac disease. Nausea and vomiting are common in cancer patients, especially those who are terminally ill.

Nausea and vomiting commonly accompany several *metabolic and endocrinologic disorders*, including uremia, diabetic ketoacidosis, hypo- and hyperparathyroidism, hyperthyroid crisis, and adrenal insufficiency, especially adrenal crisis. The morning sickness of early pregnancy is another instance of nausea and vomiting possibly related to hormonal changes; the term *hyperemesis gravidarum* is applied when fluid and electrolyte disturbances or nutritional deficiency results.

The *side effects of many drugs and chemicals* include nausea and vomiting. In some cases, drugs have central emetic effects, as with digitalis, morphine, histamine, and some chemotherapeutic agents. In other cases, drug-induced gastric irritation leads to stimulation of the medullary vomiting center, as with salicylates, aminophylline, and ipecac. The ingestion of a toxin (e.g., food poisoning) also may cause acute vomiting.

Psychogenic vomiting refers to chronic or recurrent vomiting which may result from an emotional or psychological disturbance. Often patients with emotional disorders and chronic vomiting maintain a relatively normal state of nutrition because only a relatively small amount of the ingested food is vomited. In some cases regurgitation rather than vomiting may predominate, and the degree of weight loss may be out of proportion to the patient's description of the frequency and severity of vomiting. As discussed in Chap. 74, anorexia nervosa and bulimia are emotional disturbances which may be associated with vomiting and weight loss.

DIFFERENTIAL DIAGNOSIS Vomiting should be distinguished from *regurgitation*, which refers to the expulsion of food in the absence of nausea and without the abdominal diaphragmatic muscular contraction associated with vomiting. Regurgitation of esophageal contents may occur with esophageal strictures or diverticula. Regurgitation of gastric contents is generally seen in gastroesophageal reflux disease due to gastroesophageal sphincter incompetence, in pyloric spasm or obstruction due to peptic ulcer, or in gastroparesis. *Hiccups* are a distinctive sound caused by contractions of the inspiratory muscles terminated abruptly by closure of the glottis. Brief episodes of hiccups may be caused by gastric distention, a sudden change in temperature, ingestion of alcohol, excess smoking, or excitement, whereas persistent hiccups may signify a serious underlying disease, such as a structural lesion or infection of the central nervous lesion, diaphragmatic irritation by a tumor or inflammatory process, metabolic derangement, vascular lesion, intraabdominal process, or systemic infection. In addition, a variety of drugs, including barbiturates and sedatives, general anesthesia, and psychogenic factors may lead to hiccups.

The temporal relationship of vomiting to eating may be of help diagnostically. Vomiting that occurs predominantly in the morning is often seen early in pregnancy and in uremia. Alcoholic gastritis is also commonly accompanied by early-morning retching and emesis, the so-called dry heaves. Vomiting that occurs during or shortly after eating may suggest psychogenic vomiting or peptic ulcer with pylorospasm. Vomiting that occurs 4 to 6 h or longer after eating and involves the elimination of large quantities of undigested food often indicates gastric retention (e.g., pyloric obstruction, gastroparesis) or certain esophageal disorders (achalasia, Zenker's diverticulum). Vomiting that is projectile or without antecedent nausea suggests the possibility of a central nervous system lesion.

Associated symptoms also may provide diagnostic clues. For

example, vertigo and tinnitus indicate the possibility of Ménière's disease. A long history of vomiting with little or no weight loss suggests psychogenic vomiting. Relief of abdominal pain with vomiting is typical of peptic ulcer. Early satiety is typical of gastroparesis.

The character of the vomitus also offers clues to the diagnosis. If the vomitus contains large amounts of free hydrochloric acid, gastric outlet obstruction due to an ulcer or a hypersecretory state such as Zollinger-Ellison syndrome should be considered. Absence of free hydrochloric acid is more compatible with gastric malignancy. A feculent or putrid odor reflects the results of bacterial action on the intestinal contents and may occur with distal intestinal obstruction, peritonitis, or gastrocolic fistula. Bile is commonly present in gastric contents whenever vomiting is prolonged; it has no significance unless constantly present in large quantities, when it may signify an obstructing lesion below the ampulla of Vater. The presence of blood in the gastric contents usually denotes bleeding from the esophagus, stomach, or duodenum.

TREATMENT Effective therapy of nausea and vomiting usually depends on correction of the underlying cause. *Antiemetic agents* vary in their usefulness depending on the cause of the symptoms, responsiveness of the patient, and occurrence of side effects. *Antihistamines* such as dimenhydrinate and promethazine hydrochloride are effective for the control of nausea and vomiting due to motion sickness and other inner ear disturbances and may be effective in pregnancy, uremia, and postoperative vomiting; they do not act on the chemoreceptor trigger zone and are of little value in other causes of vomiting. *Anticholinergics* such as scopolamine block central muscarinic receptors in afferent pathways of the vomiting reflex and are also effective in motion sickness. *Phenothiazine* derivatives such as prochlorperazine and the structurally related butyrophenone haloperidol inhibit cerebral dopamine receptors and act principally at the chemoreceptor trigger zone. They are often ineffective for severe nausea and vomiting and have the potential for causing sedation, hypotension, and Parkinson-like effects. *Metoclopramide* is the prototype of selective dopamine antagonists called *substituted benzamides*. Metoclopramide is useful in all types of vomiting except motion sickness and inner ear dysfunction. In contrast to the phenothiazines, which have anticholinergic effects, metoclopramide has powerful peripheral cholinergic effects that enhance gastric emptying. Metoclopramide may be superior to phenothiazines in the treatment of severe nausea and vomiting and is particularly useful in the treatment of gastroparesis. The usual oral dosage is 5 to 20 mg four times daily, but intravenous doses up to 1 to 3 mg/kg, which also inhibit 5-hydroxytryptamine$_3$ receptors, may be effective as prophylaxis prior to potent chemotherapeutic agents (e.g., cisplatin). Unfortunately, neurologic side effects are frequent, including drowsiness, dystonic reactions, anxiety, insomnia, depression, parkinsonism, confusion, and a rise in prolactin level. Experimental agents (not yet licensed for use in the United States) such as *domperidone* and *cisapride* exert peripheral antiemetic effects without the central nervous system side effects of metoclopramide. *Corticosteroids* are often combined with metoclopramide to control nausea and vomiting due to cancer chemotherapy; the mechanism of action may involve inhibition of prostaglandin formation. The sedative *lorazepam* may be added to this regimen. *Tetrahydrocannabinol*, the active ingredient of marijuana, is marketed as dronabinol for the prevention of nausea and vomiting after cancer chemotherapy; the mechanism of action is unknown. *Ondansetron*, a serotonin antagonist which binds to 5-hydroxytryptamine$_3$ receptors in the chemoreceptor trigger zone and gut, is particularly effective in preventing chemotherapy-induced nausea and vomiting. The recommended dose is 0.15 mg/kg intravenously infused over 15 min and given three times 4 h apart, beginning 30 min before the start of chemotherapy. The antibiotic *erythromycin*, which binds to motilin receptors in the gut, has been shown to enhance gastric emptying in patients with gastroparesis; however, stimulation of antral contractility by erythromycin leads to abdominal cramps, nausea, and bloating and may limit its usefulness.

INDIGESTION

Indigestion, or *dyspepsia*, is a term frequently used by patients to describe a variety of symptoms generally appreciated as upper abdominal distress and often associated with the intake of food. The term is nonspecific and may not have the same meaning for the patient and physician. Thus, in approaching the patient with indigestion, it is important for the physician first to elicit a precise description of this complaint. To some patients, indigestion refers to actual abdominal pain, pressure, or heartburn. Others may use the term to describe either a vague feeling that digestion has not proceeded naturally or intolerances to specific foods exist. Still others may use it to describe belching, a feeling of excessive gas, or flatulence.

After having ascertained the patient's definition of indigestion, it is important to determine (1) the location and duration of the discomfort, (2) the temporal relation of the symptoms to the ingestion of food, and (3) the possible relation of the symptoms to the ingestion of specific types of food (e.g., milk, fatty foods) or drugs.

Indigestion may occur in association with diseases of the gastrointestinal tract or pathologic states in other organ systems. As a result of a systematic clinical and laboratory investigation, a definable pathophysiologic process sometimes can be shown to be responsible for the symptoms in a given case of indigestion. Frequently, however, a clear etiologic explanation for the patient's complaint of indigestion cannot be established, and descriptive designations are applied. For example, the term *nonulcer dyspepsia* is often used to describe ulcer-like symptoms when no ulcer is found. The term *flatulent dyspepsia* is used when belching, abdominal distention, and early satiety are prominent symptoms; the term *dysmotility-like dyspepsia* has been applied to the same constellation of symptoms. Unfortunately, these terms do not imply that the symptoms described are attributable to a particular pathogenic process. The term *functional dyspepsia* also has been used when clinical evaluation fails to reveal an explanation for indigestion. In some cases of functional dyspepsia, sophisticated testing of gastrointestinal electrical activity and manometric studies may reveal disturbances of gastrointestinal motility, although the cause-and-effect relationship between such findings and the patient's symptoms may be difficult to prove. Indeed, some patients with functional indigestion also have features of the irritable bowel syndrome, suggesting a diffuse intestinal motility disturbance (see Chap. 256).

SYNDROMES COMMONLY DESCRIBED AS INDIGESTION
Pain A careful elucidation of the pattern of pain may provide important diagnostic information. Visceral abdominal pain is mediated by visceral afferent nerves which accompany the abdominal sympathetic pathways (see Chap. 13). Visceral pain is described as dull and aching in nature, with a diffuse midline localization, or as fullness or pressure. The location of the discomfort generally corresponds to the segmental level of neural innervation of the affected organ. Abdominal visceral pain, which can be produced experimentally by artificially increasing pressure in a hollow viscus, results from distention or exaggerated muscular contraction of the viscus. Inflammation generally lowers the threshold for pain from such stimuli.

The visceral pain of indigestion should be distinguished from the sharp, localized pain patterns of many acute abdominal processes involving the peritoneum. In contrast to visceral pain, this somatic pain is mediated by cerebrospinal afferent nerves.

In view of the diffuse nature of visceral abdominal pain, the main clue to the cause comes from the *location* of the pain and the corresponding segmental level of neural innervation; however, in any given segmental region there is no way of determining which of several viscera is the source of the pain (Table 38-1). The following rules, already described in Chap. 13, are useful: *Substernal pain* of gastrointestinal origin usually arises from disorders of the esophagus or cardia of the stomach. Because pain in this area can emanate from the heart, cardiac disease must be carefully considered and excluded. *Epigastric pain* is generally of gastric, duodenal, biliary, or pancreatic origin. (The epigastrium is also a frequent location for "functional"

TABLE 38-1   Distribution of visceral pain and examples of disorders frequently involving the specific organ

Organ	Common location of pain	Examples of disorders
Esophagus	Substernum, epigastrium	Peptic esophagitis, stricture, esophageal spasm, carcinoma
Stomach	Epigastrium	Gastritis, gastric ulcer, carcinoma
Duodenum (first and second portions)	Epigastrium	Duodenal ulcer
Small intestine (excluding first and second portions of duodenum)	Periumbilical region	Infectious gastroenteritis, regional enteritis, lymphoma, intestinal obstruction
Gallbladder	Epigastrium, right upper quadrant, right upper back	Cholelithiasis, cholecystitis
Pancreas	Epigastrium, left upper quadrant, left side of back	Pancreatitis, pancreatic carcinoma
Liver	Right upper quadrant	Hepatitis, cirrhosis, passive congestion
Colon	Below umbilicus	Infectious colitis, ulcerative colitis, carcinoma, partial obstruction

pain.) As pathologic processes in the biliary tract or pancreas become more intense, pain may lateralize and localize, e.g., biliary pain to the right upper quadrant and tip of the scapula and pancreatic pain to the left upper quadrant and back. *Periumbilical pain* is generally associated with disease involving the small intestine. *Pain below the umbilicus* is often of appendiceal, colonic, or pelvic origin.

The unraveling of the *temporal relationships* of the patient's symptoms often provides additional diagnostic clues. It is important to ascertain whether the symptoms are *constant* (continually present over extended periods of time), as may occur with an infiltrating gastric carcinoma, or *intermittent*, as in acute gastritis or biliary colic. The symptoms may have a *diurnal* pattern, as in reflux esophagitis in which pain often occurs nocturnally and with recumbency. Pain that awakens the patient from a sound sleep may occur with duodenal ulcer. Occasionally symptoms are *seasonal*, as in peptic ulcer disease, in which some patients experience more discomfort in the spring and autumn than at other times.

Another helpful diagnostic feature is the relation of pain to *food ingestion*. Early postprandial symptoms may reflect esophageal disease, acute gastritis, or gastric carcinoma. Late postprandial indigestion, i.e., occurring several hours after eating, may reflect failure of the stomach to empty adequately, as in gastric outlet obstruction, gastroparesis and other disorders of gastric motility, or duodenal ulcer, in which case pain results from exposure of ulcerated mucosa to acid secreted by the stomach and unbuffered by food. Conversely, the relief of pain following ingestion of food or antacids is characteristic of duodenal ulcer and is presumably due to the neutralization of acid. Late postprandial indigestion also may result from impaired digestive and absorptive processes, as in pancreatic insufficiency.

It is important to recognize that the pain patterns and relationships to the intake of food described above are generalizations, and many cases do not conform to classic "textbook" descriptions. For example, although pain limited to the right upper quadrant is often caused by gallbladder disease, about half of patients with this condition experience only epigastric pain. Similarly, there are some patients with peptic ulcer whose pain is not relieved by food or antacids; there are other patients with functional indigestion and even gastric carcinoma whose pain improves with food or antacids.

Nonulcer dyspepsia   Nonulcer dyspepsia refers to symptoms that suggest a diagnosis of peptic ulcer despite the absence of an ulcer by endoscopy or barium x-ray studies and the absence of any other demonstrable organic disorder (e.g., biliary tract disease) or evidence of the irritable bowel syndrome to account for the symptoms. Nonulcer dyspepsia is twice as common as peptic ulcer and may affect up to 20 to 30 percent of the population. The pathogenesis is poorly understood; most patients with nonulcer dyspepsia have normal gastric acid secretion, and a relation between nonulcer dyspepsia and duodenitis or duodenal ulcer has not been demonstrated. Similarly, the role of *Helicobacter pylori* and associated chronic gastritis in causing dyspeptic symptoms in persons without peptic ulcer is uncertain (see Chap. 252). A role for disordered gastroduodenal and small-intestinal motility in nonulcer dyspepsia has been suggested but requires further investigation. In contrast to peptic ulcer, nonulcer dyspepsia improves inconsistently following antacids and other standard ulcer therapy.

Heartburn   Heartburn, or pyrosis, is a sensation of warmth or burning located substernally or high in the epigastrium with radiation into the neck and occasionally to the arms. Occasional heartburn is common in normal persons, but frequent and severe heartburn is generally a manifestation of esophageal dysfunction. Heartburn may result from abnormal motor activity or distention of the esophagus, reflux of acid or bile into the esophagus, or direct esophageal mucosal irritation (esophagitis).

Heartburn is most often associated with gastroesophageal reflux (see Chap. 251). In this setting, heartburn typically occurs after a large meal, with stooping or bending, or when the patient is supine. It may be accompanied by the spontaneous appearance in the mouth of fluid which may be salty ("water brash"), sour (gastric contents), or bitter and green or yellow (bile). Heartburn may arise following the ingestion of certain foods (e.g., citrus fruit juices) or drugs (e.g., alcohol and aspirin). Characteristically, heartburn is alleviated promptly, even if only temporarily, by antacids.

Heartburn also may occur in the absence of a demonstrable anatomic or physiologic condition. In this setting, it is frequently accompanied by aerophagia, which may represent an attempt by the patient to relieve discomfort, and is often attributed to psychological factors for lack of other explanations.

Food intolerance   In some persons, specific foods or types of foods appear to be related to indigestion. Careful documentation of this relationship is sometimes of great help in arriving at an etiologic diagnosis.

Some foods may be poorly tolerated because of their consistency. Patients with esophageal stricture or carcinoma may tolerate liquids well but may experience discomfort, especially substernal distress, after ingesting solids (see Chaps. 37 and 251). Citrus fruits, perhaps because of their relatively low pH, and spicy foods often provoke symptoms in patients with peptic ulcer disease or peptic esophagitis. Certain foods may be tolerated poorly because of impaired intestinal digestion or absorption, as with the ingestion of fatty foods in patients with pancreatic or biliary tract disease.

Patients may have a congenital or acquired *deficiency of a specific enzyme* required for intestinal absorption of a certain nutrient. One example is the deficiency of lactase, the intestinal mucosal enzyme which catalyzes the hydrolysis of lactose. In persons who are lactase-deficient, the ingestion of milk (which contains lactose) results in abdominal cramps, distention, diarrhea, and flatulence (Chap. 254). Sucrose may lead to similar symptoms in persons with hereditary sucrase-isomaltase deficiency. Certain nutrients may lead to profound systemic effects because of *biochemical defects* in the patient that render the substances particularly hazardous, as in galactose intolerance in persons with galactosemia (see Chap. 354).

Some foods or food additives may initiate *allergic reactions*, which should be suspected when symptoms occur after ingestion of a specific food, recur on challenge testing, and are associated with other features of an allergic reaction, such as lip swelling, urticaria, angioedema, asthma, or, rarely, anaphylactic shock. Acute IgE-mediated reactions are most commonly associated with cow's milk (in infants), shellfish, wheat, eggs, nuts, and chocolate and may be confirmed by the radioallergosorbent test (RAST) in some cases. Delayed hypersensitivity reactions also may occur; may be associated with less severe symptoms, including joint and muscle pain, fatigue, serous otitis, and altered spacial perception; and are more difficult to relate to specific foods. Some foods may exert *toxic effects* on the intestine in susceptible persons (e.g., gluten in patients with celiac sprue).

In many instances we do not understand the mechanism by which indigestion is associated with the ingestion of specific foods. Thus a history of fatty food intolerance or distress after eating spicy foods is commonly obtained from patients with indigestion; however, the mechanisms leading to these symptoms in these circumstances are often unclear.

Aerophagia   Patients with a complaint of *chronic, repetitive eructation* (belching) can usually be observed to precede each belch with a swallow of air, most of which passes only partway down the esophagus and is then regurgitated. Thus excessive eructation results from *aerophagia*, or air swallowing, not from excessive gas production in the stomach or the intestine. A degree of aerophagia occurs in normal persons, but some individuals gulp air excessively because of chronic anxiety, rapid eating, drinking carbonated beverages or through a straw, gum chewing, sucking on hard candy, smoking cigarettes, postnasal drip, poorly fitting dentures, or esophageal speech. Because eructation which follows aerophagia may provide temporary relief to the patient, a vicious cycle of aerophagia and eructation may ensue.

About 20 to 60 percent of intestinal gas represents swallowed air. Because nitrogen and oxygen are the only gases present in the atmosphere in appreciable concentrations, and because they are not produced in the gastrointestinal tract, their detection on chromatographic analysis of intestinal gas indicates that swallowed air is the source. Swallowed air that is not eructated passes into the stomach and intestine. Accumulation of swallowed air in the stomach may lead to postprandial fullness and pressure and the finding by x-ray of a large amount of air in the gastric fundus. This symptom complex, referred to as the *magenblase* (i.e., gastric bubble) *syndrome*, may occur when a patient lies supine after a large meal, thereby permitting gastric air to be "trapped" below the gastroesophageal junction by overlying fluid and unable to be eructated. Inability to eructate is also thought to underlie the "gas-bloat" syndrome observed after surgical repair of a hiatal hernia. Acute gastric distention by swallowed air can sometimes produce sharp pains which may mimic angina pectoris. Swallowed air which successfully passes the stomach may either produce diffuse abdominal distention or become trapped in the splenic flexure of the colon. The latter condition, or *splenic flexure syndrome*, is characterized by a sensation of left upper quadrant fullness and pressure with radiation to the left side of the chest. Relief of pain often follows defecation or the expulsion of flatus. The diagnosis is suggested by the finding of increased tympany in the extreme left lateral portion of the upper abdomen on physical examination or of large amounts of air in the splenic flexure of the colon on a plain abdominal radiograph.

Gaseousness, bloating, and flatulence   Despite the widely held belief that feelings of *diffuse abdominal pain and bloating* are often caused by excessive quantities of intestinal gas, studies employing an intestinal gas wash-out technique suggest that patients complaining of excessive gas have normal volumes of intestinal gas. The primary abnormality causing functional bloating and pain in such persons appears to be a motility disturbance that causes the patient to perceive pain with an intestinal gas volume that is well tolerated by normal subjects. Alternatively, intestinal motility may be normal in such persons, but they may be excessively responsive to normal impulses arising from the intestinal tract.

A major source of intestinal gas is the fermentative action of intestinal bacteria on carbohydrates and proteins within the lumen. Normally such bacteria are limited to the colon, and the principal

gases produced are carbon dioxide and hydrogen (in addition to minute quantities of odoriferous gases—indoles, skatols, and sulfur-containing compounds—which give flatus its characteristic odor). In the upper small bowel carbon dioxide is also produced when hydrochloric acid from the stomach or ingested fatty acids are neutralized by bicarbonate. (This may explain, in part, indigestion associated with fatty foods.) About one-third of adults produce appreciable quantities of methane in the colon; this appears to be a familial trait and unrelated to food ingestion.

An increase in intraluminal gas production resulting in *abdominal distention, bloating, and flatulence* occurs following the ingestion of certain foods, such as legumes and some grains, which contain significant quantities of nonabsorbable complex carbohydrates that pass into the colon where they supply gas-forming substrates for colonic bacteria. The best-studied example of this is beans, which contain oligosaccharides (stachyose and raffinose) that cannot be split by intestinal mucosal enzymes but are metabolized by colonic bacteria. Less well appreciated is that fructose, a natural or added sweetener in fruit, fruit juices, soft drinks, figs, dates, prunes, and grapes and present in oligosaccharides in onions, asparagus, and wheat, may be incompletely absorbed in the small intestine and thereby contribute to abdominal distention, bloating, and flatulence. [In contrast, intestinal absorption of fructose is more likely to be complete when fructose is mixed with glucose or ingested as sucrose (glucose-fructose).] Intestinal malabsorption of sorbitol may underlie symptoms of abdominal distention, gaseousness, and diarrhea associated with certain fruits or when sorbitol is used as a sweetener in "sugar-free" gums and candies or as an "inert" ingredient in some medications. Increased intraluminal gas production also may result from abnormal bacterial colonization of the small intestine (bacterial overgrowth syndrome) or infection with *Giardia lamblia*.

Indigestion due to extraintestinal disease   A number of extraintestinal diseases may lead to indigestion. Thus indigestion may be prominent in congestive heart failure, pulmonary tuberculosis, neoplastic disease, and uremia. Also, a variety of drugs such as aspirin, nonsteroidal anti-inflammatory agents, and glucocorticoids may cause indigestion because of their ulcerogenic properties.

DIAGNOSTIC APPROACH TO THE PATIENT WITH INDIGESTION
Indigestion represents a challenging and difficult diagnostic problem because of its nonspecific nature. It is essential to obtain a clear and detailed description of the specific symptoms, particularly the patient's definition of the term *indigestion*. The nature of the distress, its frequency and time of occurrence, its relationship to meals, and the special circumstances which lead to its exacerbation or relief should be elicited. Associated intestinal symptoms such as nausea and vomiting, abnormal bowel habits, diarrhea, steatorrhea, and melena should be sought, and an assessment of nutritional status, appetite, and changes in weight should be made. A careful history also should include an assessment of the patient's general health, including the possible presence of extraintestinal disorders which may produce indigestion. A careful dietary history is essential, and asking the patient to keep a diary of foods eaten may prove revealing. Similarly, the patient's medications should be reviewed, particularly for agents that may slow gut transit such as narcotics, anticholinergics, and calcium antagonists. Psychological factors may play an etiologic or contributory role, and the presence of anxiety, depressive symptoms, or hysteria should be noted.

Physical examination rarely establishes the specific diagnosis but may be useful in detecting diseases in other organ systems which can affect intestinal function (e.g., congestive heart failure). Stools should be examined for appearance and occult blood.

Whether further diagnostic studies are indicated depends on the specific nature of the patient's complaints and the patient's age (concern about the possibility of gastrointestinal malignancy being greater in older patients). Abdominal pain may be evaluated with radiologic and imaging studies of the esophagus, stomach, small intestine, colon, pancreas, and biliary tract. Esophagogastroscopy, endoscopic cholangiopancreatography, sigmoidoscopy, or colonoscopy may be considered depending on the specific symptoms. On the other hand, in patients under age 40 with epigastric pain typical of peptic ulcer, routine diagnostic studies are unlikely to disclose serious diseases (such as gastric carcinoma) and are often in fact negative; thus an empiric trial of antacids, H-2-receptor–blocking drugs, or sucralfate may be appropriate. Esophagogastroscopy may be reserved for patients with symptoms that persist despite therapy or that recur soon after therapy is discontinued. In patients with *H. pylori* on endoscopic antral biopsy and no other explanation for indigestion, eradication of *H. pylori*, which requires treatment with bismuth subsalicylate and two oral antibiotics, is cumbersome and of uncertain value but may be considered in selected cases. In individuals complaining of excessive eructation, the simple demonstration that aerophagia reproduces the symptoms may suffice to confirm the diagnosis and hopefully break the habit. Patients complaining of excessive gas, bloating, distention, and flatulence must be questioned carefully about dietary preferences and the relation of symptoms to ingestion of specific foods. In some cases, elimination of certain foods (e.g., milk, legumes) from the diet followed by rechallenge may be confirmatory. In other cases, a more detailed assessment, including stool examination for fat and muscle fibers and for parasites such as *G. lamblia*, breath tests to detect carbohydrate malabsorption or bacterial overgrowth, esophageal manometry and ambulatory pH monitoring, measurement of the rate of gastric emptying of a solid meal, and gastrointestinal motility studies, may be desirable. When no precise explanation for gaseousness can be identified, trials of activated charcoal to reduce gaseousness associated with carbohydrate malabsorption or simethicone to alter the elasticity of gas bubbles may be considered, although their value is uncertain.

In many cases of indigestion no clear explanation is obtained, even after careful diagnostic studies and therapeutic trials. Some cases represent nonulcer dyspepsia or intestinal motility disturbances, perhaps due to subtle physiologic derangements not detectable by currently available methods. In some such instances, an empiric trial of dopamine antagonists (e.g., metoclopramide) which augment gastrointestinal motility may be beneficial. Other cases represent early stages of actual disease processes which may only be diagnosed by conventional methods at a later date. Still others are psychogenic and may respond to appropriate psychiatric measures. The ultimate evaluation of indigestion requires, therefore, the utmost in sensitivity, diligence, and concern on the part of the examining physician.

REFERENCES

FELDMAN M: Nausea and vomiting, in *Gastrointestinal Disease*, 4th ed, MH Sleisenger, JS Fordtran (eds). Philadelphia, Saunders, 1989, pp 222–238

HANSON JS, MCCALLUM RW: The diagnosis and management of nausea and vomiting. Am J Gastroenterol 80:210, 1985

HEALTH AND PUBLIC POLICY COMMITTEE, AMERICAN COLLEGE OF PHYSICIANS: Endoscopy in the evaluation of dyspepsia. Ann Intern Med 102:266, 1985

LEVITT MD, BOND JH: Intestinal gas, in *Gastrointestinal Disease*, 4th ed, MH Sleisenger, JS Fordtran (eds). Philadelphia, Saunders, 1989, pp 257–263

MITCHELSON F: Pharmacologic agents affecting emesis: A review (part I). Drugs 43:295, 1992

OUYANG A: Approach to the patient with nausea and vomiting, in *Textbook of Gastroenterology*, T Yamada et al (eds). Philadelphia, Lippincott, 1991, pp 647–659

PERMAN JA, SALTZBERG DM: Approach to the patient with gas and bloating, in *Textbook of Gastroenterology*, T Yamada et al (eds). Philadelphia, Lippincott, 1991, pp 681–692

TALLEY NJ: Non-ulcer dyspepsia: Myths and realities. Aliment Pharmacol Ther 5(suppl 1):145, 1991

TYTGAT GNJ et al (eds): Towards understanding dyspepsia: An update and concensus from an International Working Party. Scand J Gastroenterol 26(suppl 182):1, 1991

39 DIARRHEA AND CONSTIPATION

LAWRENCE S. FRIEDMAN / KURT J. ISSELBACHER

NORMAL INTESTINAL FUNCTION

INTESTINAL FLUID ABSORPTION AND SECRETION On an average day, 9 L of fluid enters the gastrointestinal tract: 2 L by direct ingestion, 1 L as saliva, 2 L as gastric juice, and 4 L as biliary, pancreatic, and small intestine secretions. On passage through the small intestine, 4 to 5 L of fluid is reabsorbed in the jejunum and 3 to 4 L in the ileum. Therefore, approximately 1 L of residual enters the colon, where an additional 800 mL is reabsorbed before passage to the rectum and evacuation. Overall, the usual amount of fluid excreted in feces is approximately 200 mL/d.

In the intestine, water absorption follows active and passive sodium (Na^+) and nutrient absorption (Fig. 39-1). In the small intestine, Na^+ is cotransported with chloride (Cl^-) and nutrients such as glucose; in the terminal ileum, Na^+ is cotransported with bile salts; and in the colon, Na^+ is absorbed via Na^+ channels and by the electroneutral NaCl absorptive mechanism used in the small intestine. The cotransport mechanisms for Na^+ and nutrient absorption depend in part on Na^+ gradients across the apical membrane of intestinal epithelial cells created by the Na^+, K^+-ATPase pump of the basolateral membrane. The most important of these clinically is an Na^+-glucose cotransport carrier in the small intestine. Absorption of glucose by this mechanism results in accumulation of glucose in the epithelial cell, followed by its movement across the basolateral membrane by a facilitated transport mechanism, while Na^+ is actively pumped across the basolateral membrane by Na^+,K^+-ATPase. The absorption of Na^+ also promotes absorption of Cl^- through a paracellular pathway. Water absorption follows passively to maintain isoosmolality in the intercellular space. Because the Na^+-glucose cotransport mechanism remains unaffected by most diarrheal diseases, administration of a glucose-salt solution is useful clinically for the management of diarrhea and dehydration of most causes.

Other cotransport mechanisms exist. An Na^+-Cl^- cotransport mechanism is thought actually to be composed of an Na^+-H^+ exchange carrier and a Cl^--HCO_3^- exchange carrier. This mechanism permits entry of both Na^+ and Cl^- into a cell in exchange for H^+ and HCO_3^-. Additional transport mechanisms have been identified for potassium (K^+), which may be absorbed in exchange for H^+, and for calcium (Ca^{2+}), the absorption of which is regulated by vitamin D and 1,25-dihydroxyvitamin D_3, parathyroid hormone, calcitonin, and a number of calcium-binding proteins.

In addition to its absorptive function, the intestine has a secretory function. Cl^- can be secreted by intestinal crypt cells via an electrogenic mechanism, with Na^+, K^+, and water following passively through tight junctions. HCO_3^- is secreted in the duodenum, other parts of the small intestine, and into the bile and pancreatic ducts. Because of the large acid load from the stomach, secreted HCO_3^- is diluted and present in relatively low concentrations. However, in the distal gut, HCO_3^- gradually becomes the predominant anion, permitting conservation of Cl^- presumably via a Cl^--HCO_3^- exchange mechanism at the apical membrane of the epithelial cells. Intracellular cyclic nucleotides and ionized calcium (Ca^{2+}) initiate and regulate active Cl^- secretion (Fig. 39-2).

COLONIC FUNCTION As in the small intestine, an Na^+ absorptive mechanism exists in the colon. Na^+ absorption is predominantly electrogenic in that the absorbed Na^+ ion is unaccompanied by cation exchange or anion cotransport. Na^+ enters colonic epithelial cells through channels in the apical membrane and is pumped out across the basolateral membrane by Na^+, K^+-ATPase.

A variety of neural and nonneural mediators regulate colonic ion transport and motility, but the precise mechanisms are not well understood. The colon and rectum are innervated by nerve fibers that

FIGURE 39-1 Sodium, chloride, and glucose transport by intestinal epithelial cells. Passive and active transport mechanisms for sodium (Na$^+$), chloride (Cl$^-$), and sodium-glucose coupled uptake are shown. Na$^+$ is pumped out at basolateral border by the active ATPase pump; Cl$^-$ in part accompanies Na$^+$ but also is actively extruded by cyclic AMP. TJ, tight junction.

release norepinephrine, acetylcholine, and other neurotransmitters. Parasympathetic nerves stimulate peristaltic contraction and electrolyte secretion, whereas adrenergic tone inhibits cholinergic stimulation and increases electrolyte absorption. Additional regulation is provided by local reflex arcs within the autonomous enteric nervous system and intrinsic contractile responses of the colonic smooth muscle.

Differences in basal motor activity of the various segments of the colon correlate with specific function. In the ascending colon, where most fluid absorption occurs, rhythmic retrograde contractions prolong fecal contact time. In the midcolon, segmental contractions continue the process of absorption, while feces is gradually advanced to the left colon. The distal colon, including the sigmoid colon and rectum, is under the greatest neurogenic control and propels feces caudally in preparation for defecation. Additionally, throughout the colon, massive peristalsis (mass movement) occurs several times a day.

DEFECATION   The defecatory reflex is initiated by acute distention of the rectum, which results in partial and transient relaxation of the internal anal sphincter via parasympathetic innervation. As sigmoid and rectal contractions increase the pressure within the rectum, the rectosigmoid angle created by tonic contraction of the puborectalis muscle, which forms a sling around the anorectal junction, is obliterated. Contraction of the external anal sphincter, which consists of at least three bundles of striated muscle surrounding the anal canal and innervated by the pudendal nerve, can delay defecation until a socially acceptable time. Concomitant relaxation of the internal and external anal sphincters then permits the evacuation of feces, which can be augmented by an increase in intraabdominal pressure created by the Valsalva maneuver.

DIARRHEA

DEFINITION   In developed countries, normal stool weight of an adult human is less than 200 g/d; stool water accounts for 60 to 85 percent of the weight. Normal bowel frequency ranges from three times a week to three times a day. Factors that influence stool weight, consistency, and frequency include the fiber content of the diet, gender (the average daily weight of stool in women is less than that of men), ingested medications, and possibly exercise and stress. *Diarrhea* is formally defined as an increase in daily stool weight above 200 g. Typically, the patient also may describe an abnormal increase in stool liquidity and frequency.

Diarrhea must be distinguished from *pseudodiarrhea* or *hyperdefecation*, which is an increased frequency of defecation without an increase in stool weight above normal, as occurs in patients with irritable bowel syndrome, proctitis, or hyperthyroidism. Diarrhea also must be distinguished from fecal *incontinence*, which is the involuntary release of rectal contents. Incontinence is more common when stool is liquid than solid and reflects abnormal function of the anorectum or pelvic muscles. Diarrhea is considered *acute* when lasting less than 7 to 14 days and *chronic* when lasting more than 2 to 3 weeks.

ACUTE DIARRHEA   The most common causes of acute diarrhea are infectious agents. Acute diarrhea also may be caused by ingested drugs or toxins, the administration of chemotherapy, resumption of enteral feeding following a prolonged fast, fecal impaction (overflow diarrhea), or particular situations, such as marathon running. Additionally, acute diarrhea may represent the onset of a chronic diarrheal illness.

Infectious diarrhea (see Chaps. 87, 102, 115, and 117 to 120) Worldwide, acute infectious diarrhea accounts for more than 4 million deaths each year in children less than age 5, especially in developing nations, where acute infectious diarrhea is a major cause of protein-calorie malnutrition and dehydration. Contributing factors include inadequate sewage disposal and water supplies, lack of refrigeration, overcrowding and lack of personal hygiene, poverty, lack of access to health care, and lack of education. Even in the United States, significant economic loss results from acute infectious diarrhea, which accounts for 250,000 hospital admissions and nearly 8 million office visits to physicians each year.

Most infectious diarrheas are acquired by fecal-oral transmission by way of water or food contaminated by human waste as a result of poor sewage systems or by wild or domestic animal feces in inadequately purified water. Beef, pork, or poultry may be the source of infection when improperly cooked. Food-preparing surfaces may be contaminated by organisms that are spread to uncooked food. Person-to-person transmission also may occur through aerosolization (Norwalk agent, rotavirus), contamination of hands (*Clostridium difficile*) or surfaces, or sexual activity.

In the United States, groups at particularly high risk of acute infectious diarrhea include travelers to or recently from developing nations, persons who ingest shellfish, male homosexuals (gay bowel syndrome), prostitutes, and intravenous drug users. Persons with AIDS in particular are at risk for a remarkable array of serious enteric infections (Table 39-1). Among children attending day-care centers, acute infectious diarrhea commonly results from person-to-person

FIGURE 39-2 Effect of increased mucosal cyclic AMP on stimulation of ion (chloride) secretion from intestinal crypt cells and inhibition of coupled Na$^+$ and Cl$^-$ absorption by intestinal villus cells.

TABLE 39-1 **Possible causes of diarrhea in patients with AIDS**

Nonopportunistic pathogens
  Shigella
  Salmonella
  Campylobacter
  Entamoeba histolytica
  Chlamydia
  Neisseria gonorrhoeae
  Treponema pallidum and other spirochetes
  Giardia lamblia
Opportunistic infections
  Protozoa
    Cryptosporidium
    Isospora belli
    Microsporidia
    Blastocystis hominis
  Viruses
    Cytomegalovirus
    Herpes simplex
    Adenovirus
    Human immunodeficiency virus
  Bacteria
    Mycobacterium avium-intracellulare

transmission. The most common organisms involved in day-care outbreaks of diarrhea are *Shigella*, *Giardia lamblia*, and *Cryptosporidium*. Secondary attack rates ranging between 10 and 20 percent represent an important source of infection for parents and siblings. Additional high-risk institutions for outbreaks of acute infectious diarrhea include residential homes for the mentally and developmentally handicapped, nursing homes, and hospitals.

Clinical features   Patients with acute infectious diarrhea typically present with nausea, vomiting, abdominal pain, fever, and diarrhea, which may be watery, malabsorptive, or bloody, depending on the cause. Patients ingesting *toxins* or those with *toxigenic infection* typically have nausea and vomiting as prominent symptoms but rarely a high fever. Abdominal pain is mild, diffuse, and crampy and results from the high volumes of secreted fluid that stimulate peristalsis and cause watery diarrhea. Vomiting that begins within several hours of ingesting a food should suggest food poisoning due to a preformed toxin. Parasites that do not invade the intestinal mucosa such as *Giardia lamblia* and *Cryptosporidium* usually cause only mild abdominal discomfort. *Giardia* also may be associated with mild steatorrhea, gaseousness, and bloating. *Invasive bacteria* such as *Campylobacter*, *Salmonella*, and *Shigella* and organisms that produce cytotoxins such as *C. difficile* and enterohemorrhagic *Escherichia coli* cause severe intestinal inflammation, abdominal pain, and often a high fever; occasionally, peritoneal signs may suggest a surgical abdomen. *Yersinia* often infects the terminal ileum and cecum and presents with right lower quadrant pain and tenderness suggestive of acute appendicitis. Watery diarrhea is typical of organisms that invade the intestinal epithelium with *minimal inflammation*, such as enteric viruses, or organisms that *adhere* to but do not destroy the epithelium, such as enteropathogenic or enteroadherent *E. coli*, protozoa, and helminths. Some organisms such as *Campylobacter*, *Aeromonas*, *Shigella*, and *Vibrio* species both produce enterotoxins and invade the intestinal mucosa, and patients therefore often present with watery diarrhea followed within hours or days by bloody diarrhea.

The presence of systemic symptoms may provide additional clues to the underlying cause of diarrhea. Both shigellosis and infection with enterohemorrhagic *E. coli* may be accompanied by the hemolytic-uremic syndrome, particularly in persons who are very young or very old. *Yersinia* infection and occasionally other enteric bacterial infections may be accompanied by Reiter's syndrome (arthritis, urethritis, and conjunctivitis), thyroiditis, pericarditis, or glomerulonephritis.

Differential diagnosis   Virtually any *medication* can cause diarrhea, and a careful drug history should be obtained in any patient with acute diarrhea (Table 39-2). Other ingested toxins also must

be considered, including organophosphate insecticides, mushrooms, arsenic, and even caffeine. *Acute diverticulitis* may present with diarrhea accompanied by fever and abdominal pain. In patients with acute bloody diarrhea, diagnostic considerations may include *superior mesenteric arterial* or *venous thrombosis*, *ischemic* or *drug-induced colitis*, or *idiopathic inflammatory bowel disease* (ulcerative colitis or Crohn's disease). In the elderly patient with acute colitis, differentiating an ischemic cause from enterohemorrhagic *E. coli* may be difficult because both diseases may be associated with submucosal hemorrhage that presents as "thumbprinting" on a plain abdominal radiograph. While colonoscopic and radiographic findings may be indistinguishable in infectious colitis and idiopathic inflammatory bowel disease, histologic findings may be helpful in suggesting one diagnosis or the other, since the inflammatory infiltrate in acute infectious diarrhea consists mainly of polymorphonuclear leukocytes rather than the chronic inflammatory infiltrate with crypt distortion typical of idiopathic inflammatory bowel disease. The presence of pseudomembranes on colonoscopy points to *C. difficile* as the cause.

Laboratory diagnosis   Acute infectious diarrhea is usually self-limited, often resolving by the time the patient seeks medical attention. Because of the expense of stool cultures and other diagnostic tests, considerable judgment is required in deciding which patients with acute diarrhea should be evaluated and treated with antibiotics. For the patient presenting without high fever, bloody diarrhea, or dehydration, symptomatic therapy with oral fluids in the absence of specific diagnostic testing may suffice. On the other hand, a high fever, systemic toxicity, bloody diarrhea, and dehydration favor diagnostic testing, as do a known outbreak of food poisoning, recent overseas travel, immunocomprise, male homosexuality, or recent antibiotic use. In these situations, freshly collected stool should be examined for *occult blood* and *white blood cells*. The finding of primarily polymorphonuclear leukocytes on a Wright's or methylene blue stain suggests *Salmonella*, *Shigella*, invasive *E. coli*, *Yersinia*, or *Entamoeba histolytica*. Although it is common practice to obtain a qualitative fecal fat determination in patients with acute diarrhea, the presence of a small amount of fat in the stool is not uncommon in patients with acute diarrhea of any cause and provides no particular diagnostic information. The cornerstone of diagnosis in patients with severe and especially bloody diarrhea or a suggestive epidemiologic history is *bacterial culture* and *microscopic examination* of the stool for ova and parasites. Most laboratories routinely examine stool specimens sent for culture for *Salmonella*, *Shigella*, *Yersinia*, and *Campylobacter*, but special requests must be made to identify other organisms, including *C. difficile* (culture and toxin) and enterohemorrhagic *E. coli*. Special cultivation or staining techniques also may be required to identify organisms that cause watery diarrhea, including *Aeromonas*, *Cryptosporidium*, and *Vibrio* species. Certain organisms

TABLE 39-2 **Drugs that commonly cause diarrhea**

Gastrointestinal drugs	**Hypolipidemic agents**
Magnesium-containing antacids	Clofibrate
Laxatives	Gemfibrozil
Misoprostol	Lovastatin
Olsalazine	Probucol
Cardiac drugs	**Neuropsychiatric drugs**
Digitalis	Lithium
Quinidine	Fluoxetine (Prozac)
Procainamide	Alprazolam (Xanax)
Hydralazine	Valproic acid
Beta blockers	Ethosuximide
Angiotensin-converting enzyme	L-Dopa
inhibitors	**Others**
Diuretics	Theophylline
Antibiotics	Thyroid hormones
Clindamycin	Colchicine
Ampicillin	Nonsteroidal anti-
Cephalosporins	inflammatory drugs
Erythromycin	
Chemotherapeutic agents	

such as *Giardia* and *Strongyloides* as well as *Cryptosporidium* and *Isospora belli* may be difficult to detect in stool and are better diagnosed by *duodenal aspiration* or intestinal biopsy. In patients with AIDS, electron microscopic examination of small intestinal biopsy specimens may facilitate detection of Microsporidia. *Sigmoidoscopy* and occasionally *colonoscopy* are generally reserved for patients with bloody diarrhea that does not improve within 10 days. As discussed above, mucosal changes may be nonspecific, although in some cases characteristic findings may be observed, such as pseudomembranes in *C. difficile*–induced colitis. *Barium radiographs* are also best deferred until the initial course of illness has been observed and appropriate stool specimens obtained. Even with the application of all available laboratory studies, between 20 and 40 percent of all acute infectious diarrheas remain undiagnosed.

Treatment   General and nonspecific treatment of acute infectious diarrhea includes rest and fluid replacement. Because death in most instances of acute diarrhea results from dehydration, careful attention must be paid to correction of fluid and electrolyte deficits. Intravenous fluid therapy may be necessary in severely dehydrated individuals, especially infants and the elderly. The use of oral sugar-electrolyte solutions, which has proved successful in the treatment of patients with cholera, also can be considered in patients with acute diarrhea due to other enterotoxin-producing bacteria. The use of antibiotic therapy in bacterial diarrheas is controversial and generally not necessary in patients with mild or resolving disease but should be considered in patients with shigellosis, traveler's diarrhea, pseudomembranous enterocolitis, cholera, and parasitic diseases. Regardless of the cause of infectious diarrhea, patients should be treated if they are immunocompromised, have a malignancy, have an abnormal heart valve or vascular or orthopedic prosthesis, have hemolytic anemia, or are extremely young or old. Anticholinergic drugs and opiates to control diarrhea should generally be avoided when an enteroinvasive organism is suspected because of the risk of prolonging colonization or causing an ileus. However, loperamide and bismuth subsalicylate have been shown to be safe in patients with traveler's diarrhea who have neither a high fever nor blood or pus in the stool.

CHRONIC DIARRHEA   Diarrhea that persists for weeks or months, whether constant or intermittent, requires evaluation. Although in the majority of cases the cause will prove to be irritable bowel syndrome, diarrhea may represent a manifestation of an underlying serious illness, and a careful search for organic disease must be undertaken. Chronic diarrhea can be categorized pathophysiologically as inflammatory diarrhea, osmotic diarrhea (malabsorption), secretory diarrhea, intestinal dysmotility, and factitious diarrhea (Table 39-3).

Inflammatory diarrhea   Inflammatory diarrheas are characterized generally by the presence of fever, abdominal tenderness, blood or leukocytes in the stool, and inflammatory lesions evident on intestinal mucosal biopsy. In some cases, hypoalbuminemia, hypoglobulinemia, and protein-losing enteropathy may be present. In addition to inflammation, the mechanism of diarrhea may include malabsorption or intestinal secretion.

In a patient who is not systemically ill, a liquid stool containing overt or occult blood raises the possibility of a *colonic neoplasm*. Patients with *ulcerative proctitis* also may present in this manner. In a patient who is systemically ill with chronic bloody diarrhea, the diagnosis of *inflammatory bowel disease* (either *ulcerative colitis* or *Crohn's disease*) is suggested. These diagnoses also should be suspected when chronic diarrhea is associated with prominent extraintestinal manifestations, including arthritis, skin lesions such as erythema nodosum or pyoderma gangrenosum, uveitis, or vasculitis. Diarrhea in inflammatory bowel disease may result from damage to absorptive surface epithelium as well as the release into the circulation of secretagogues such as leukotrienes, prostaglandins, histamine, and other cytokines which stimulate intestinal secretion or the enteric nervous system.

Inflammatory diarrhea is seen in patients with *chronic radiation enterocolitis* as a result of pelvic irradiation for malignancies of the

TABLE 39-3   Classification of chronic diarrhea

Mechanism	Clinical features	Examples
INFLAMMATORY		
Mucosal and submucosal inflammation Damaged epithelium In some cases impaired intestinal absorption and excessive secretion	Fever, abdominal pain, blood and/or leukocytes in stool	Ulcerative colitis Crohn's disease Radiation enterocolitis Eosinophilic gastroenteritis Infections associated with AIDS
OSMOTIC		
Nonabsorbed or nondigested intraluminal solute	Improvement of diarrhea with fasting Bulky, greasy, foul-smelling stools; weight loss Nutrient deficiencies Osmotic gap in fecal water	Pancreatic insufficiency Bacterial overgrowth Celiac disease Lactase deficiency Whipple's disease Abetalipoproteinemia Short bowel syndrome
SECRETORY		
Excessive secretion of electrolytes	Watery diarrhea, persists with fasting Dehydration Other systemic effects of hormones Absence of osmotic gap in fecal water	Carcinoid syndrome Zollinger-Ellison syndrome Vasoactive intestinal peptide-secreting pancreatic adenomas Medullary carcinoma of thyroid Villous adenoma of rectum Microscopic colitis Cholerrheic diarrhea
ALTERED INTESTINAL MOTILITY		
Rapid transit In some cases associated bacterial overgrowth	Alternating diarrhea and constipation Neurologic symptoms; bladder involvement	Irritable bowel syndrome Fecal impaction Neurologic diseases
FACTITIOUS		
Self-induced	Usually women Watery diarrhea with hypokalemia, weakness, edema	Laxative abuse

female urogenital tract or the male prostate. The segments usually involved are the terminal ileum, cecum, and rectosigmoid because they are fixed in the pelvis. The risk of radiation enterocolitis correlates with the radiation dose; the frequency is 1 to 5 percent with doses of 4500 to 5500 rad and 35 percent with higher doses. Chronic radiation injury is characterized by progressive swelling of the endothelial cells in small arterioles of the submucosa leading to obliterative endarteritis and vascular thrombosis and resulting in ischemia with fibrosis, bowel wall thickening, ulceration, and fissuring of the mucosa. Colonoscopy may show luminal narrowing, ulceration, diffuse inflammatory changes, and characteristic mucosal telangiectases which may bleed severely. Diarrhea also may result from bile acid malabsorption because of ileal inflammation or bacterial overgrowth resulting from intestinal strictures or stasis.

Eosinophilic gastroenteritis is characterized by infiltration of any portion of the gastrointestinal tract with eosinophils. In addition to diarrhea, patients present with abdominal pain, nausea, vomiting, weight loss, and, in 75 percent of cases, peripheral eosinophilia; some patients may develop steatorrhea and protein-losing enteropathy. Severe *protein-losing enteropathy* is manifested by peripheral edema, ascites, and occasionally anasarca. It may occur in a variety of disease states, including infections (viral gastroenteritis, bacterial overgrowth, parasitic infestation, *C. difficile* enterocolitis, or Whipple's disease), inflammatory bowel disease, lymphoma, or other conditions associated with lymphatic obstruction, such as congenital intestinal lymphangiectasia, Menetrier's disease, systemic lupus erythematosus, or milk allergy. Recently, an increasing number of infectious causes of chronic diarrhea have been associated with infection caused by the *human immunodeficiency virus* (HIV) or with AIDS (see Table 39-1). In many patients with AIDS and diarrhea, multiple potential pathogens may be present in the stool, although the exact cause of diarrhea may be uncertain because such pathogens may also be found in the stool of AIDS patients without diarrhea. HIV itself is also thought to cause diarrhea in some cases (AIDS enteropathy), but the mechanism is not understood.

Other miscellaneous diseases associated with inflammatory diarrhea include *Behçet's syndrome* and *graft-versus-host disease* following allogeneic bone marrow transplantation.

Osmotic diarrhea (see Chap. 254) Osmotic diarrhea occurs when an orally ingested solute is not fully absorbed in the small intestine and thereby exerts an osmotic force that draws fluid into the intestinal lumen. The increased luminal fluid volume overwhelms the capacity of the colon for reabsorption. The nonabsorbed solute can be a maldigested or malabsorbed nutrient or drug. Clinical symptoms are usually recognized because of the malabsorption of *fat (steatorrhea)* or *carbohydrates*. *Protein* or *amino acid* malabsorption (*azotorrhea*) is generally not recognized clinically unless it is severe enough to cause malnutrition or the consequences of a specific deficiency in an amino acid. The various disorders associated with malabsorption and maldigestion are discussed in more detail in other chapters, specifically, mucosal malabsorptive disorders in Chap. 254 and pancreatic exocrine deficiency and related disorders in Chap. 274.

Intraluminal maldigestion may result from *pancreatic exocrine insufficiency*, which occurs when at least 90 percent of the secretory capacity of the pancreas is lost in patients with *chronic pancreatitis* or occasionally *pancreatic ductal obstruction*. Maldigestion and weight loss occur despite preserved appetite. In children, *cystic fibrosis* may cause chronic pancreatic insufficiency. *Somatostatinoma* is a rare pancreatic islet tumor that leads to gallstones, diabetes, and steatorrhea thought to be caused by inhibition of pancreatic secretion. Intraluminal maldigestion also may result from *bile duct obstruction* as a result of cancer of the head of the pancreas or from severe liver disease with *cholestasis*. Deficiency of intraluminal bile salts usually results in only mild fat malabsorption. *Bacterial overgrowth* in a blind loop of intestine or a segment of stasis may result in steatorrhea due to deconjugation of the bile salts and impaired micelle formation; additional factors leading to diarrhea include brush border enzyme injury, mucosal inflammation, hydroxylation of fat causing fatty acid diarrhea, and altered intestinal motility.

Osmotic diarrhea may result from the chronic ingestion of certain fruits or candy, gum, dietetic foods, and medications sweetened with unabsorbed carbohydrates such as sorbitol or fructose. Congenital absence of specific brush border carbohydrate hydrolases and transport proteins also may lead to chronic diarrhea; the most common of these is lactase deficiency resulting in lactose intolerance.

The classic example of *mucosal malabsorption* is *celiac sprue*, or gluten-sensitive enteropathy (see Chap. 254). In addition to presenting with typical symptoms and signs of malabsorption, patients with celiac sprue may have atypical presentations, including failure to thrive, muscle wasting, abdominal distention, and irritability in young children, and unexplained iron deficiency anemia, growth retardation, and anorexia in adolescents or young adults. Later in life, patients may present with insidious nutritional deficiencies, infertility, and neuromuscular disease. Like celiac sprue, *tropical sprue* is characterized by malabsorption and histologic changes in the small bowel of villus atrophy, crypt hyperplasia, damaged surface epithelium, and a mononuclear infiltrate in the lamina propria. A disease affecting residents in certain tropical parts of the world, tropical sprue can occur even in visitors residing for as little as 1 to 3 months in an endemic area. The onset may be acute, suggesting an infectious etiology.

Intestinal malabsorption is typical of *Whipple's disease* due to *T. whippelii*, which usually affects middle-aged men but may present at any age and in patients of either sex. Additional manifestations include arthralgias, fever and chills, hypotension, lymphadenopathy, and involvement of the central nervous system (see Chap. 254). *Abetalipoproteinemia* is caused by the absence of Apo B resulting in defective chylomicron formation. Children with this disorder present with steatorrhea, acanthocytic red blood cells, ataxia, and retinitis pigmentosa (see Chap. 254). Steatorrhea also may result from infections with *Giardia, Isospora, Strongyloides*, and *Mycobacterium avium-intracellulare*. Ingestion of certain *drugs* may result in steatorrhea because of damage to enterocytes; examples include colchicine, neomycin, and *para*-aminosalicylic acid.

Intestinal lymphangiectasia (Chap. 254) causes protein-losing enteropathy with steatorrhea but preserved absorption of carbohydrates and is thus an example of *postmucosal obstruction of lymphatic channels*. The disease may be congenital or acquired as a result of trauma, lymphoma, carcinoma, or Whipple's disease.

Finally, extensive intestinal resection may result in the *short bowel syndrome*, in which steatorrhea results from an inadequate absorptive surface, decreased transit time, and a decreased bile salt pool. Other factors that may contribute to diarrhea in short bowel syndrome include the osmotic effect of nonabsorbed solutes, gastric hypersecretion, and in some cases bacterial overgrowth.

Secretory diarrhea Secretory diarrhea is characterized by a large volume of fecal output caused by abnormal fluid and electrolyte transport not necessarily related to the ingestion of food. Therefore, diarrhea usually persists with fasting. The term *watery diarrhea* is often used synonymously with secretory diarrhea. Because there is no malabsorbed solute, fecal osmolality in secretory diarrheas can be accounted for by normal ionic constituents with no fecal osmotic gap.

The classic examples of secretory diarrhea are those mediated by hormones (see Chaps. 252 and 276). Patients with metastatic *carcinoid tumors* of the gastrointestinal tract may have watery diarrhea as part of the carcinoid syndrome that includes episodic flushing, telangiectatic skin lesions, cyanosis, pellagra-like skin lesions, bronchospasm, and cardiac murmurs due to right-sided valvular lesions. The carcinoid syndrome results from secretion of a variety of vasoactive substances which are potent intestinal secretagogues, including serotonin, histamine, catecholamines, prostaglandin, and kinins. The *Zollinger-Ellison syndrome* is characterized by recurrent, refractory, and unusually located peptic ulcers due to a gastrinoma; diarrhea occurs in up to one-third of patients and may be the presenting symptom in 10 percent of cases. The diarrhea is not strictly secretory but is due in part to the high volumes of secreted hydrochloric acid in addition to maldigestion of fat caused by inactivation of pancreatic lipase and precipitation of bile acids at low pH. *Non-beta cell pancreatic adenomas* may secrete a variety of peptides, including vasoactive intestinal polypeptide (VIP), pancreatic polypeptide (PP), secretin, neurotensin, calcitonin, prostaglandins, and others. Those which secrete VIP may be associated with the *watery diarrhea hypokalemia achlorhydria* (WDHA) *syndrome*, characterized by often massive secretory diarrhea, achlorhydria, hypokalemia, hypomagnesemia, hypercalcemia without hyperparathyroidism, and in some cases flushing, myopathy, or nephropathy. Not all patients with WDHA syndrome have a *vipoma*, and in such cases, alternative mediators of intestinal secretion have been postulated. *Medullary carcinoma of the thyroid* (Chap. 343) may be sporadic or a feature of multiple endocrine neoplasia syndrome type IIa with pheochromocytomas and hyperparathyroidism. Watery diarrhea is thought to be mediated by calcitonin produced by the tumor, although in some cases other mediators may be found. The occurrence of diarrhea in medullary carcinoma of the thyroid is usually associated with metastases and a poor prognosis. *Systemic mastocytosis* (Chap. 254), which may be associated with the skin lesion urticaria pigmentosa, also may be associated with diarrhea that is secretory and mediated by histamine or malabsorptive and due to intestinal mucosal infiltration by mast cells.

Diarrhea associated with a *villous adenoma* (Chap. 257) of the rectum or rectosigmoid usually occurs with large tumors, often more than 3 to 4 cm in diameter. Hypokalemia due to potassium loss is common.

Microscopic or *lymphocytic colitis* and *collagenous colitis* (Chap. 255) may represent variants of the same disease. Their hallmarks are a characteristic histologic lesion despite a normal mucosal appearance on colonoscopy and diarrhea that is often secretory. In both disorders, histologic findings include infiltration of the lamina propria with inflammatory cells as well as intraepithelial lymphocytes, but only in collagenous colitis is there also a characteristic subepithelial collagen band.

Secretory diarrhea may result from *severe disease, resection,* or *bypass of the distal ileum* when less than 100 cm of the ileum is affected (Chap. 254). Presumably, diarrhea results from stimulation of colonic secretion by dihydroxy bile salts that escape absorption in the terminal ileum (cholerrheic diarrhea). By preventing gallbladder contraction and the delivery of large amounts of bile into the intestine, fasting eliminates this type of secretory diarrhea. When greater than 100 cm of terminal ileum is diseased or resected, hepatic synthesis cannot maintain an adequate intraluminal bile salt pool, and steatorrhea also ensues. Bile acid–induced diarrhea may occur following cholecystectomy because of the loss of the storage capacity of the gallbladder. Rarely, *primary (idiopathic) bile acid malabsorption* by the terminal ileum may account for otherwise unexplained secretory diarrhea. Rapid small intestinal transit resulting in increased delivery of bile acids to the colon also may account for *postvagotomy diarrhea,* which occurs in up to 30 percent of patients ungoing truncal vagotomy with a drainage procedure for peptic ulcer disease; diarrhea is much less common following selective or superselective vagotomy.

Altered intestinal motility   Diarrhea may be associated with disorders that affect intestinal motility. The most common of these is *irritable bowel syndrome* (Chap. 256), in which typically diarrhea alternates with constipation and may be associated with abdominal pain, the passage of mucus, and a sense of incomplete evacuation. However, in some patients, constipation alone with lower abdominal cramps is the predominant clinical manifestation, while others present only with painless diarrhea presumably due to disordered intestinal motility. Diarrhea may occasionally occur paradoxically as a result of *fecal impaction* or an obstructing tumor with the overflow of liquid colonic contents around the impacted stool or obstruction. A variety of *neurologic diseases* also may be associated with diarrhea because of altered autonomic control of bowel function. Profuse watery diarrhea, often with incontinence, may be seen in young patients with *diabetes* and is often associated with severe neuropathy, nephropathy, and retinopathy. Additional contributing factors may include bacterial overgrowth secondary to intestinal dysmotility, pancreatic exocrine insufficiency, or, rarely, celiac disease. Diarrhea also may occur in patients with *traumatic neuropathy,* the *Shy-Drager syndrome,* or *lesions of the cauda equina.*

Factitious diarrhea   Factitious diarrhea is self-induced by the patient and may result from intestinal infection, the addition of water or urine to the stool, or self-medication with laxatives. Patients are predominantly women with severe chronic watery diarrhea, abdominal pain, nausea and vomiting, weight loss, peripheral edema, and weakness resulting from hypokalemia. The diagnosis of factitious diarrhea should be suspected in a patient with a history of psychiatric disease or multiple previous negative evaluations for diarrhea. Additional diagnoses to consider in patients with chronic diarrhea of obscure origin are listed in Table 39-4.

History and physical examination   A thorough history and physical examination are crucial initial steps in the evaluation of the patient with chronic diarrhea. The history in particular may direct the evaluation toward a general pathophysiologic mechanism or even a specific diagnosis and serves as a useful guide to the selection of a limited number of appropriate diagnostic studies.

Inflammatory diarrheas may be suggested by the presence of fever with abdominal pain, often localized to one of the lower quadrants.

TABLE 39-4   Causes of chronic diarrhea of obscure origin

Drugs (see Table 39-2)
Laxative abuse
Microscopic or collagenous colitis
Bacterial overgrowth
Carbohydrate malabsorption
Bile acid malabsorption (including after cholecystectomy and
  ileal resection)
Diabetic diarrhea
Chronic idiopathic secretory diarrhea
Fecal incontinence

Extraintestinal manifestations such as arthritis, skin lesions, or ocular symptoms suggest idiopathic inflammatory bowel disease. The presence of peripheral edema, ascites, or anasarca is compatible with protein-losing enteropathy. Intestinal malabsorption is suggested by bulky or greasy foul-smelling stools, flatulence, and weight loss. Malabsorption of specific essential nutrients may present as anemia, a bleeding tendency, osteopenia, amenorrhea, or infertility. Steatorrhea is typically more severe in pancreatic insufficiency than in intestinal mucosal disease, whereas flatulence and bloating are more typical of intestinal mucosal disease than pancreatic insufficiency because of associated carbohydrate malabsorption. Osmotic diarrhea of any cause often improves or resolves with fasting. In watery diarrheas, weight loss is unusual except in patients with advanced neuroendocrine tumors, which also may be suggested by characteristic systemic manifestations such as flushing. Symptoms of autonomic dysfunction such as postural hypotension, impotence, or disordered sweating are often found in patients with diabetic diarrhea. Diarrhea alternating with constipation is typical of the irritable bowel syndrome.

In addition to providing clues to the underlying cause of diarrhea, the physical examination is important in assessing the presence of volume depletion, as manifested by postural hypotension, tachycardia, absence of axillary sweat, decreased skin turgor, mental lethargy, and generalized weakness.

Evaluation   Numerous laboratory studies may be employed in the evaluation of chronic diarrhea, but a ''shotgun'' approach should be avoided. The workup should be guided by the history and physical examination, and simpler investigations should be carried out before more complex diagnostic studies. In many patients it is helpful to start with routine blood studies such as a complete blood count and peripheral smear and serum electrolyte, calcium, phosphate, albumin, and quantitative immunoglobulin determinations.

Inflammatory diarrheas may be associated with leukocytosis, an elevated erythrocyte sedimentation rate, or hypoalbuminemia. The hallmark of inflammatory diarrheas is the presence of either *gross or occult blood and leukocytes* in the stool; leukocytes can be detected by a Wright's or methylene blue stain. Further evaluation usually involves *upper gastrointestinal endoscopy or colonoscopy* with diagnostic biopsies. An *upper gastrointestinal radiograph with a small bowel follow-through* also may be indicated to evaluate the small intestine. [111]*Indium-labeled white blood cell scans* may detect bowel inflammation not apparent on endoscopy or conventional barium radiography. In patients with AIDS and chronic diarrhea, multiple stool specimens for culture and examination for ova and parasites should be obtained prior to more invasive diagnostic testing.

A wide array of tests may be helpful in evaluating the patient with an osmotic diarrhea. Decreased levels of iron, folate, vitamin B_{12}, and vitamin D may suggest malabsorption. The prothrombin time may be prolonged due to vitamin K deficiency, and serum carotene, cholesterol, and albumin levels may be decreased. The cornerstone of testing for intestinal malabsorption is the measurement of *fecal fat,* which is described in detail in Chap. 254.

The capacity of the small intestine to absorb simple sugars can be assessed by the D-*xylose absorption test,* in which 25 g of this five-carbon sugar is administered orally and urine is collected for the subsequent 5 h; normally, at least 25 percent of the administered dose is excreted in the urine. The sensitivity of this test may be increased by obtaining a blood sample following the oral dose; a blood level of greater than 30 mg/dL at 2 h is normal (see Chap. 254).

The definitive test for malabsorption due to intestinal mucosal disease is the *small intestinal biopsy*, which may be performed via upper endoscopy with forceps biopsy of the distal duodenum or with a specialized small bowel biopsy instrument which reaches the jejunum. Small intestinal biopsy is generally diagnostic in diseases characterized by diffuse involvement of the small intestine such as Whipple's disease, *Mycobacterium avium-intracellulare* infection, or abetalipoproteinemia but may be falsely negative in diseases with a patchy distribution such as lymphoma, eosinophilic gastroenteritis, or amyloidosis. In celiac sprue, histologic findings may be suggestive, but the diagnosis can only be confirmed by demonstrating that the histologic lesion reverses following withdrawal of gluten from the diet.

Protein-losing enteropathy is best confirmed by assaying for α_1-antitrypsin, an endogenous protein, on an aliquot of lyophilized stool (Chap. 254). The most widely used test of *pancreatic function* is the *bentiromide test*, which depends on the ability of pancreatic chymotrypsin to cleave *para*-aminobenzoic acid (PABA) from the synthetic peptide *N*-benzoyl-L-tyrosyl *para*-aminobenzoic acid (bentiromide); the cleaved PABA is absorbed by the intestine, conjugated in the liver, and excreted in the urine. This and other tests of pancreatic function are discussed in Chap. 274.

The *Schilling test*, used in the evaluation of patients with suspected pernicious anemia, also can be used as a diagnostic test for pancreatic insufficiency, in which vitamin B_{12} absorption is impaired because gastric R-proteins are not cleaved from intrinsic factor as a result of diminished pancreatic proteolytic activity in the upper small intestine; vitamin B_{12} absorption improves when the test is repeated following oral administration of pancreatic enzymes.

Bacterial overgrowth may be detected by aspirating fluid from the upper small intestine through an endoscope or a small intestinal tube placed under fluoroscopic guidance and finding a *bacterial colony count* of greater than 10^5 per milliliter. Alternatively, the diagnosis of bacterial overgrowth is suggested by an increase in exhaled $^{14}CO_2$ within 60 minutes of the ingestion of 1 g ^{14}C-D-xylose (*^{14}C-xylose breath test*) or after the ingestion of ^{14}[C]cholylglycine (*bile acid breath test*) or the detection of increased breath H_2 within the first 2 h after ingestion of either glucose or rice flour (*breath hydrogen test*) (see Chap. 254).

Radiologic tests may play a diagnostic role in patients with suspected malabsorption. An abdominal radiograph may demonstrate pancreatic calcification in patients with chronic pancreatitis. *Abdominal ultrasonography*, *computed tomography*, or *endoscopic retrograde cholangiopancreatography* also may be useful in the evaluation of suspected pancreatic disease. Standard *barium radiographs* of the gastrointestinal tract may suggest thickening of the valvulae conniventes due to infiltrative disease such as Whipple's disease, lymphoma, or amyloidosis or dilatation of the small bowel with flocculation of the barium in celiac sprue. Additional relevant findings may include a gastrocolic fistula, blind loop, stricture, or multiple diverticula.

Fecal osmolality measurements may be helpful in distinguishing osmotic from secretory diarrhea when the diarrhea is watery. Measured osmolality can be compared with the calculated fecal osmolality, which is the sum of the measured Na^+ and K^+ concentrations multiplied by 2 (to account for anions). The osmotic gap is the measured fecal osmolality minus the calculated fecal osmolality and corresponds approximately to the concentration of poorly absorbed solutes in fecal water. Measured fecal osmolality should approximate plasma osmolality, which, in general, is 290 mosmol/kg H_2O. (In fact, a measured fecal osmolality greater than 300 mosmol/kg H_2O indicates bacterial degradation of nonabsorbed carbohydrate in the collection jar or the addition of urine to the jar.) A fecal osmotic gap greater than 50 mosmol/kg H_2O is significant and suggests osmotic diarrhea due to a poorly absorbed carbohydrate or excessive ingestion of magnesium-containing laxatives. If the fecal osmolality is much

lower than that of the plasma (290 mosmol/kg H_2O), fluid has been added to the stool.

In patients with watery diarrhea, blood levels of *serotonin*, *gastrin*, *VIP*, *calcitonin*, and other potential secretagogues should be obtained, in addition to a *urinary 5-hydroxyindole acetic acid* (5-HIAA) level. *Flexible sigmoidoscopy* or *colonoscopy* should be considered to exclude villous adenoma of the rectum or sigmoid as well as microscopic or collagenous colitis. Colonoscopy also may reveal melanosis coli due to abuse of anthraquinone laxatives. Ingestion of phenolphthalein laxatives may be detected by *alkalinizing the stool* with either NaOH or KOH, which results in a pink or purple color. When the index of suspicion for laxative abuse is high, a cautious room search may be diagnostic.

In cases of suspected ileal bile salt malabsorption, a *^{75}selenahomo-taurocholic acid* (*^{75}SeHCAT*) test may be available in some centers. ^{75}SeHCAT acid is an analogue of taurocholic acid and is thus absorbed in the terminal ileum; scanning with a gamma camera can be used to quantitate ileal absorption and increased bile acid loss. Alternatively, a therapeutic trial of the bile salt–binding resin *cholestyramine* may be administered.

Antidiarrheal therapy While every effort should be made to identify and correct the specific cause of diarrhea, in many cases a cause that is specifically treatable may not be identifiable, and symptomatic therapy alone may be indicated. Psyllium and other hydrophilic agents absorb water and thereby enhance stool consistency. Most other available antidiarrheal agents act by altering intestinal motility; some also may have mild proabsorptive or antisecretory activity. *Opiate antidiarrheal agents* such as diphenoxylate and loperamide may be helpful in secretory diarrhea of mild to moderate severity. For patients with more severe symptoms, codeine or deodorized tincture of opium may be more successful. However, such antimotility agents may be contraindicated in diarrhea due to infectious agents because stasis may enhance tissue invasion by the organisms or delay their clearance from the bowel. In patients with severe inflammatory bowel disease, such drugs may contribute to the development of toxic megacolon and are contraindicated. *Octreotide*, a long-acting synthetic analogue of somatostatin, has a significant antisecretory effect in the carcinoid syndrome and other neuroendocrine tumors because of its specific inhibition of hormone secretion; it also may have some benefit in the short bowel syndrome. *Clonidine*, and alpha$_2$-adrenergic agonist, may be useful in the diarrhea of opiate withdrawal and diabetic diarrhea. H^+,K^+-*ATPase inhibitors*, such as omeprazole, and *H-2 receptor antagonists* are useful in the diarrhea that results from gastric hypersecretion in the Zollinger-Ellison syndrome. Other drugs that may have some benefit in the treatment of neuroendocrine tumors or unexplained secretory diarrheas include *phenothiazines* and *calcium antagonists*. *Indomethacin*, an inhibitor of prostaglandin synthesis and secretion, may have benefit in the diarrhea of medullary carcinoma of the thyroid and villous adenomas. A combination of H-1 and H-2 receptor antagonists may be helpful in treating the diarrhea of systemic mastocytosis. *Cholestyramine* is the drug of choice in diarrhea caused by ileal bile salt malabsorption.

CONSTIPATION

DEFINITION Constipation is a common complaint in clinical practice. Because of the wide range of normal bowel habits, constipation is difficult to define precisely. Most persons have at least three bowel movements per week, and *constipation* has been defined as a frequency of defecation of less than three times per week. However, stool frequency alone is not a sufficient criterion to use, because many constipated patients describe a normal frequency of defecation but subjective complaints of excessive straining, hard stools, lower abdominal fullness, and a sense of incomplete evacuation. Thus a combination of objective and subjective criteria must be used to define constipation.

CAUSES Pathophysiologically, constipation generally results from *disordered colonic transit or anorectal function* as a result of a primary motility disturbance, certain drugs, or in association with a large number of systemic diseases that affect the gastrointestinal tract. Constipation of any cause may be exacerbated by chronic illnesses that lead to physical or mental impairment and result in inactivity or physical immobility. Additional contributing factors may include a lack of fiber in the diet, generalized muscle weakness, and possibly stress and anxiety.

In the patient presenting with the recent onset of constipation, an *obstructing lesion* of the colon should be sought. In addition to a *colonic neoplasm*, other causes of colonic obstruction include *strictures* due to colonic ischemia, diverticular disease, or inflammatory bowel disease; *foreign bodies*; or *anal strictures*. Anal sphincter spasm due to painful *hemorrhoids* or *fissures* also may inhibit the desire to evacuate.

In the absence of an obstructing lesion of the colon, *disturbed colonic motility* may mimic colonic obstruction. Disruption of parasympathetic innervation to the colon as a result of injury or lesions of the lumbosacral spine or sacral nerves may produce constipation with hypomotility, colonic dilatation, decreased rectal tone and sensation, and impaired defecation. In patients with *multiple sclerosis*, constipation may be associated with neurogenic dysfunction of other organs. Similarly, constipation may be associated with *lesions of the central nervous system* caused by parkinsonism or a cerebrovascular accident. In South America, the parasitic infection *Chagas disease* may result in constipation because of damage to myenteric plexus ganglion cells. *Hirschsprung's disease*, or aganglionosis, is characterized by absence of myenteric neurons in a segment of distal colon just proximal to the anal sphincter. This results in a segment of contracted bowel which produces obstruction and proximal dilatation. In addition, an absent rectosphincteric inhibitory reflex results in the failure of the internal anal sphincter to relax following rectal distention. Most patients with Hirschsprung's disease are diagnosed by 6 months of age, but in occasional cases symptoms are mild enough that the diagnosis may be delayed into adulthood.

Drugs that may lead to constipation include those with anticholinergic properties, such as antidepressants and antipsychotics, codeine and other narcotic analgesics, aluminum- or calcium-containing antacids, sucralfate, iron supplements, and calcium antagonists. In patients with certain endocrinopathies such as *hypothyroidism* and *diabetes mellitus*, constipation is generally mild and responsive to therapy. Rarely, life-threatening megacolon occurs in patients with myxedema. Constipation is common during *pregnancy*, presumably as a result of altered progesterone and estrogen levels which decrease intestinal transit. *Collagen vascular diseases* may be associated with constipation, which may be a particularly prominent feature of *progressive systemic sclerosis*, in which delayed intestinal transit results from atrophy and fibrosis of colonic smooth muscle.

In the large majority of patients with severe constipation, no obvious cause can be identified. In *idiopathic childhood constipation*, both psychological and physiologic factors are thought to play a role. Affected children often have slow colonic transit localized to the distal colon and rectum, and voluntary withholding behavior or abnormal anorectal function has been suggested to play a role in this disorder. Young to middle-aged women may present with severe constipation characterized by infrequent defecation, excessive straining when defecating, and unresponsiveness to fiber supplements or mild laxatives. In 70 percent of such cases, slow colonic transit (colonic inertia) may be demonstrated by the delayed passage of radiopaque markers through the proximal colon. In 30 percent of cases colonic transit is normal, and abnormalities of anorectal sensory and motor function may be demonstrated. The terms *outlet obstruction* and *anismus* have been used to describe this form of constipation, which appears to result from failed relaxation or inappropriate contraction of the puborectalis and external anal sphincter muscles. Because relaxation of these muscles involves cortical inhibition of the spinal reflex during defecation and may be modified by biofeedback, it is speculated that such rectosphincteric dysfunction is an acquired or learned rather than an organic or neurogenic disease. Chronic straining at defecation itself may lead to descent of the perineal floor and stretching of the pudendal nerve, thus leading to an incompetent anal sphincter and fecal incontinence. Similarly, *rectal prolapse* may impair defecation as a result of rectal intussusception or chronic pudendal nerve injury. A *rectocele* is an anterior rectal herniation that may interfere with defecation by filling with feces preferentially during attempts at defecation.

Chronic idiopathic intestinal pseudo-obstruction is a rare disorder in which episodes of intestinal obstruction are unaccompanied by evidence of mechanical blockage (see Chap. 256). This disorder may be familial as a result of a neuropathy or myopathy involving the bowel and in some cases the bladder. *Idiopathic megacolon* or *megarectum* is characterized by a dilated colon or rectum, respectively, with constipation and defecatory difficulties attributed to neurogenic dysfunction.

In young to middle-aged adults, constipation is most commonly attributable to the *irritable bowel syndrome*. Unlike some of the idiopathic constipation syndromes described above, irritable bowel syndrome is typically accompanied by abdominal pain, especially in the lower abdomen, as well as by the passage of small, hard stools with a sense of incomplete evacuation and excessive straining. Patients also may complain of flatulence, abdominal bloating, heartburn, nausea, dysphagia, back pain, and genitourinary symptoms. Colonic transit is usually normal in such patients, and the precise pathophysiologic basis for the symptoms is uncertain (see Chap. 256).

HISTORY AND PHYSICAL EXAMINATION A precise description of symptoms and their duration should be obtained. Constipation that is present from birth or early childhood is likely to be congenital in origin, whereas later onset suggests an acquired disease. A recent change in bowel habits in an adult always demands an evaluation for an obstructing neoplasm. A description of the frequency and nature of defecation should be obtained, including the presence of excessive straining, hard scybalous stools, or a sense of incomplete evacuation. The patient should be questioned about associated abdominal pain and bloating and upper gastrointestinal or genitourinary symptoms. It is especially important to obtain a history of prior laxative use and its duration. A gentle but careful assessment should be made for evidence of anxiety, emotional distress, or affective disorders and the use of mood-altering drugs.

Physical examination should be directed toward the detection of nongastrointestinal diseases that may contribute to constipation. Particular attention should be paid to the neurologic examination, including an assessment of autonomic function. The abdomen should be examined for evidence of prior surgery, bowel distention, or retained stool. A careful perineal and anorectal examination should be conducted for evidence of deformity, gluteal muscle atrophy, rectal prolapse, anal stenosis, anal fissure, rectal mass, or fecal impaction. The patient may be asked to strain to demonstrate evidence of a rectocele or rectal prolapse. The presence of an "anal wink" should be assessed by demonstrating reflex contraction of the anal canal following pinprick of the perineum. A variety of complications of constipation or its treatment also may be detected and may be the reason the patient seeks medical attention (Table 39-5).

EVALUATION Studies of colorectal anatomy are important to exclude organic disease, although they provide little information

TABLE 39-5   Complications of constipation or its treatment

Hemorrhoids	Ischemic colitis
Anal fissure	Colonic volvulus
Rectal prolapse	Colonic perforation
Stercoral ulcer	Fecal incontinence
Melanosis coli	Urinary retention
Cathartic colon	Cardiac and cerebrovascular dysfunction
Fecal impaction	(e.g., syncope, arrhythmias, angina)

about colonic and anorectal function. *Flexible sigmoidoscopy* or *colonoscopy* may demonstrate melanosis coli as a brown-black discoloration of the bowel mucosa resulting from chronic use of anthraquinone laxatives. The absence of haustrations on endoscopy or barium enema suggests a "cathartic colon" due to laxative abuse. *Barium enema* also may demonstrate obstructing lesions of the colon, megacolon, or megarectum and in Hirschsprung's disease will show the characteristic denervated bowel segment with proximal dilatation of the colon. In such cases, rectal biopsies may be obtained to demonstrate the absence of neurons.

Studies of colonic and anorectal function should be reserved for patients with severe idiopathic constipation who fail to respond to simple therapeutic measures. In patients with a complaint of infrequent defecation, *colonic transit studies* may demonstrate colonic inertia. Radiopaque markers are ingested and their transit is monitored by serial abdominal radiographs until at least 80 percent have passed or a defined period of time has elapsed. The upper limit of normal for most adults is approximately 70 h. In patients with suspected outlet obstruction, *anorectal motility studies* provide information about rectal sensation, viscoelasticity, relaxation of the internal anal sphincter, and defecation of air-filled balloons of various sizes inserted into the rectum. For example, patients with constipation due to irritable bowel syndrome often have a low rectal compliance and tolerate rectal distention poorly, whereas those with megarectum have a very high rectal compliance. The absence of internal anal sphincter relaxation suggests Hirschsprung's disease. In some centers, anorectal manometry is supplemented by *electromyogram studies* to record external anal sphincter function and *defecography*, in which thickened barium approximating the consistency of stool is introduced into the rectum and its evacuation monitored by fluoroscopy while the patient sits on a commode.

TREATMENT Treatment of constipation must be individualized, taking into account the duration and severity of constipation, potential contributing factors, the age of the patient, and the patient's expectations. Symptomatic therapy is quite empirical in that there is often little objective evidence to support a particular strategy. Initial therapy is usually dietary, with an emphasis on increasing dietary fiber intake. Although there is little evidence that constipated persons consume less dietary fiber than nonconstipated persons, many constipated persons do respond to increases in dietary fiber to between 20 and 30 g/d. Fiber supplementation may increase stool weight and the frequency of defecation and decrease gastrointestinal transit time. The bulking effect of fiber on stool may relate to both increased water retention and proliferation of colonic bacteria with the production of gases in the stool. Fiber supplementation is not appropriate for patients with obstructing lesions of the gastrointestinal tract or those with megacolon or megarectum.

Except for bulk laxatives, routine use of laxatives over long periods of time should be discouraged because of the risk of side effects such as lipid pneumonia due to mineral oil or damage to myenteric plexuses resulting in "cathartic colon" due to stimulant anthraquinone laxatives such as senna. *Bulk-forming laxatives* consist of natural (psyllium) or synthetic polysaccharides or cellulose derivatives that act in a manner similar to fiber. Fluid intake should be increased with the use of these preparations. *Emollient laxatives* include mineral oil, which when given orally or by enema penetrates and softens the stool, and docusate salts, which are anionic surfactants that lower the surface tension of stool to allow mixing of aqueous and fatty substances and thereby soften the stool. *Hyperosmolar agents* include mixed electrolyte solutions containing polyethylene glycol and nonabsorbable sugars such as lactulose and sorbitol, which act as osmotic agents and are used in bowel cleansing prior to colonoscopy. *Saline laxatives* contain nonabsorbable cations and anions that exert an osmotic effect to increase intraluminal water content. *Stimulant laxatives* include castor oil, anthraquinones such as senna, and diphenylmethanes such as phenolphthalein and bisacodyl. Castor oil is converted to ricinoleic acid, which stimulates intestinal secretion and increases intestinal motility. The anthraquinones increase

fluid and electrolyte accumulation in the distal ileum and colon. Phenolphthalein and bisacodyl stimulate colonic motor activity and inhibit glucose and sodium absorption. Recently, the experimental prokinetic agent cisapride has been shown to enhance intestinal transit through the proximal colon, but its role in the management of constipation is uncertain. A role for excessive endogenous opioids in constipation related to motility disorders has been hypothesized, and the benefit of opioid receptor antagonists in the treatment of constipation has been reported but requires further study. *Biofeedback* techniques have shown promise in the treatment of constipation resulting from inappropriate contraction of the pelvic floor muscles and external anal sphincter.

Surgical treatment for severe chronic constipation is generally controversial, except in Hirschsprung's disease, in which surgical resection of the aganglionic segment is the treatment of choice. In colonic inertia, subtotal colectomy with ileorectal anastomosis may be indicated in carefully selected patients in whom upper gastrointestinal motility is normal and anorectal dysmotility has been excluded. Surgery to reduce or resect a rectocele, intussusception, or prolapse should be undertaken with caution, because symptoms often are not alleviated.

REFERENCES

BERTOMEU A et al: Chronic diarrhea with normal stool and colonic examinations: Organic or functional? J Clin Gastroenterol 13:531, 1991

DANIELSSON A et al: Chronic diarrhoea after radiotherapy for gynaecological cancer: Occurrence and aetiology. Gut 32:1180, 1991

EHERER AJ, FORDTRAN JS: Fecal osmotic gap and pH in experimental diarrhea of various causes. Gastroenterology 103:545, 1992

FIELD M (ed): *Diarrheal Diseases*. New York: Elsevier, 1991

—— et al: Intestinal electrolyte transport and diarrheal disease. N Engl J Med 321:800, 1989

FINE KD, FORDTRAN JS: The effect of diarrhea on fecal fat excretion. Gastroenterology 102:1936, 1992

—— et al: Diarrhea, in *Gastrointestinal Disease: Pathophysiology, Diagnosis, Management*, MH Sleisenger, JS Fordtran (eds). Philadelphia, Saunders, 1989

GAZZARD BG: Diarrhea in human immunodeficiency virus antibody–positive patients. Semin Gastrointest Dis 2:3, 1991

GLEESON D: Acid-base transport systems in gastrointestinal epithelia. Gut 33:1134, 1992

HEATON KW et al: Defecation frequency and timing, and stool form in the general population: A prospective study. Gut 33:818, 1992

KAWIMBE BM et al: Outlet obstruction constipation (anismus) managed by biofeedback. Gut 32:1175, 1991

PEMBERTON JH et al: Evaluation and surgical treatment of severe chronic constipation. Ann Surg 214:403, 1991

POWELL DW: Approach to the patient with diarrhea, in *Textbook of Gastroenterology*, T Yamada et al (eds). Philadelphia, Lippincott, 1991

WALD A: Approach to the patient with constipation, in *Textbook of Gastroenterology*, T Yamada et al (eds). Philadelphia, Lippincott, 1991

WISTROM J et al: Empiric treatment of acute diarrheal disease with norfloxacin. Ann Intern Med 117:202, 1992

40 GAIN AND LOSS IN WEIGHT

DANIEL W. FOSTER

GENERAL PRINCIPLES In normal persons weight is stable because food intake is matched to energy expenditure by the coordinated activity of "feeding" and "satiety" centers in the hypothalamus. The signals that regulate the interactions of these centers are multifactorial, and both short- and long-term controls are thought to be operative. Whatever the mechanisms, the system is normally efficient over periods of months to years.

Gain or loss in tissue mass is determined by the net balance between food intake and energy expenditure. Food intake is influenced by availability and attractiveness of food and by emotional and physical factors. The bulk of energy expenditure is due to basal metabolism and physical activity. The former is defined as the energy requirement when the body is in the supine position, motionless

TABLE 40-1 Percentage composition of mean daily weight loss in 13 young men during food restriction for 24 days

Days	Mean weight loss, kg/day	Water, %	Fat, %	Protein, %	Food equiv. of weight loss, kJ/kg (kcal/kg)
1–3	0.80	70	25	5	10,900 (2600)
11–13	0.23	19	69	12	29,500 (7000)
22–24	0.17	0	85	15	36,400 (8700)

SOURCE: After Brožek et al.

except for quiet respiration; it is the energy required to maintain structural and functional integrity of the body in the absence of physical activity. About half the total daily intake is normally consumed by basal processes. Nonsedentary persons spend about 40 percent of energy in physical activity; athletes may utilize 50 percent or more of ingested energy in exercise. Persons sedentary because of habit, illness, or obesity expend far less in activity. In nonobese, nonsedentary subjects 10 percent of ingested food is released as heat associated with the absorption of food, a process called *dietary thermogenesis*. This fraction, previously designated *specific dynamic action*, is usually considered a separate component of energy costs. Heat generated during and after exercise and heat released for maintenance of body temperature (*regulatory thermogenesis*) are components of the energy costs of physical activity and basal metabolism, respectively.

Change in body weight as a consequence of voluntary alteration in diet or exercise is usually not worrisome; change in weight that is not deliberately sought, on the other hand, is a frequent reason for consultation with the physician and often indicates the presence of disease. Changes in weight may reflect alteration in either tissue mass or body fluid content. Even when tissue mass is changing, fluid loss or gain plays a major role in the measured change in weight, particularly over the short run. This point is illustrated in Table 40-1, where the composition of weight loss was estimated during a 24-day period of semistarvation in 13 normal men [daily intake, 4200 kJ (1010 kcal)]. During the first 3 days 70 percent of the decrease in weight was due to water loss, while in subsequent stages weight loss was principally due to a diminution of body protein and fat. This varying contribution of fluid explains why a fixed formula cannot be used for predicting weight loss or gain. It is frequently stated that a net change of 32,000 kJ (7700 kcal) will be accompanied by a 1-kg change in body mass. While this estimate is reasonable for long-term changes in food intake, the apparent cost per kilogram of weight lost or gained varies with the accompanying fluid shifts. In the experiment summarized in Table 40-1, for example, a negative balance of only 10,900 kJ (2600 kcal) resulted in the loss of 1 kg of weight between days 1 and 3, while between days 22 and 24, loss of 1 kg of weight required a deficit of 36,400 kJ (8700 kcal). In general, if weight loss or gain occurs over a period of weeks or months, it is safe to assume that tissue mass has changed; weight loss or gain of short duration may be due to fluid shifts alone. Occasionally, true loss of tissue mass is obscured by fluid retention as in the patient with cirrhosis of the liver who develops ascites or the patient with anorexia nervosa who has edema.

WEIGHT GAIN

The diagnosis of obesity (see Chap. 73) is usually uncomplicated. Obese subjects often deny overeating, but the true situation can be assessed either by tabulating actual food intake and determining its caloric content from standard tables, by interviewing the patient's family and friends, or by estimating metabolic rates from indirect calorimetry.

Regardless of history, excess caloric intake is the usual cause of obesity. Pathologic causes are rare. In the adult, Cushing's syndrome can result in acquired obesity, but usually the diagnosis is suggested by the pattern of fat distribution and the clinical picture. Other endocrine diseases such as hypothyroidism, hypogonadism, and insulin-secreting tumors are frequently listed in the differential diagnosis of obesity but are not significant diagnostic problems. Congenital diseases that cause obesity such as the Prader-Willi, Laurence-Moon-Biedl, and Alström syndromes are also readily recognizable and appear early in life. Rarely, hypothalamic disease, such as craniopharyngioma, may cause acquired obesity. Extensive workup of the central nervous system is not indicated in obesity, however, in the absence of suspicious symptoms (headache, visual difficulties, vomiting, or endocrine changes).

WEIGHT LOSS

Weight loss in the absence of deliberate dieting is more serious than weight gain, because there is a high chance that organic disease is present. Sustained or continued weight loss in an obese person, even if dieting is in progress, should be a signal for concern, since sustained weight loss is rare in the obese. Mechanisms of pathologic weight loss include decreased food intake, accelerated metabolism, and loss of calories in urine or stool, acting singly or in combination. Almost any serious illness can cause weight loss either through direct effects or by inducing malaise and depression. The signals that cause decreased appetite and accelerated tissue loss are not known. The negative nitrogen balance that occurs following trauma, surgery, or stressful illness is likely mediated at least partially by glucagon and other catabolic hormones. Additional candidate molecules for disease-induced weight loss are cytokines such as tumor necrosis factor (cachectin) and adipsin, but proof of their involvement is lacking.

Several categories of disease need to be considered when weight loss is prominent.

DIABETES MELLITUS Initial weight loss with the onset of diabetes is largely fluid and is due to the osmotic diuresis induced by hyperglycemia. Subsequently, loss of tissue mass occurs in insulin-dependent diabetes as a result of caloric wastage (the consequence of glycosuria) and of the hormonal abnormalities that characterize the illness. Insulin deficiency and glucagon excess result in impaired synthesis of protein and fat and simultaneously cause accelerated proteolysis and lipolysis such that the net energy state is catabolic. Weight loss in diabetes is frequently associated with increased food intake.

ENDOCRINE DISEASE Hyperthyroidism usually causes weight loss. Increased appetite and food intake are the rule, and patients often consume a high-carbohydrate diet. Energy expenditure is enormous, primarily because of an increased metabolic rate and increased motor activity. The mechanism by which thyrotoxicosis causes weight loss is not settled. In rodents, thyroid hormone increases Na-K adenosine triphosphatase (ATPase) activity in many tissues resulting in a futile cycle of ATP synthesis and breakdown with energy lost as heat. This abnormality does not appear to operate in humans. Whatever the mechanism, metabolism is "uncoupled" in thyrotoxicosis, accounting for excess generation of heat and caloric wastage.

In "apathetic" hyperthyroidism, weight loss and weakness may predominate with little evidence of nervousness or other symptoms. Another endocrine cause of weight loss is pheochromocytoma, the inducing agent being catecholamine release. Panhypopituitarism and adrenal insufficiency can cause weight loss, largely as a consequence of diminished appetite secondary to cortisol deficiency.

GASTROINTESTINAL DISEASE Overt or occult steatorrhea due to sprue, chronic pancreatitis, or cystic fibrosis may produce wasting despite major increases in food intake. A variety of other diseases of the gastrointestinal tract cause weight loss: inflammatory bowel disease, parasites, esophageal strictures, obstruction secondary to chronic peptic ulcer, pernicious anemia, and cirrhosis of the liver. Mechanisms of weight loss include anorexia, obstruction with vomiting, malabsorption, and the effects of inflammation. Intraabdominal masses (e.g., massive splenomegaly) act by compressing the stomach, while weight loss in heart failure is due to visceral congestion.

INFECTION   Hidden infection must always be sought in patients with unexplained weight loss. Tuberculosis, fungal disease, amebic abscess, and subacute bacterial endocarditis should be high on the list of suspects. Infection with human immunodeficiency virus must be considered, especially in high-risk groups (male homosexuals, intravenous drug users, recipients of multiple transfusions). Weight loss with infection is probably due to inflammatory cytokines.

MALIGNANCY   Occult malignancy is probably the most common cause of weight loss in the absence of major signs and symptoms. In the search for malignancy, particular emphasis must be placed on the gastrointestinal tract, pancreas, and liver. Lymphoma and leukemia also should be considered. While silent (except for weight loss) malignancy can occur in any organ, the gastrointestinal tract is the most common site. Mechanisms of weight loss in cancer vary, and more than one factor is often operative. Anorexia is usually present, but increased metabolism also may play a role, particularly in lymphomas and leukemias. Tumor necrosis factor and other cytokines likely play a significant role in the weight loss of cancer.

PSYCHIATRIC DISEASE   The classic psychiatric illness associated with profound weight loss is anorexia nervosa (Chap. 74). Conversion disorders, schizophrenia, and depression also may cause weight loss due to decreased food intake. In a study of weight loss in the elderly, depression was the cause as often as cancer.

RENAL DISEASE   One of the earliest manifestations of uremia is anorexia. As a consequence, all patients with unexplained weight loss should be given screening renal function tests.

SUMMARY

Weight loss is more often a diagnostic problem than weight gain and more often a sign of serious organic illness. If the weight loss is associated with increased food intake, the diagnosis is likely diabetes, thyrotoxicosis, or malabsorption; less frequently, leukemias or lymphomas cause weight loss in the presence of increased food intake. If food intake is normal or decreased, malignancy, infection, renal disease, psychiatric disease, or endocrine deficiency is more likely.

REFERENCES

BEUTLER B, CERAMI A: Cachectin: More than a tumor necrosis factor. N Engl J Med 316:379, 1987

BROŽEK J et al: Changes in body weight and body dimensions in men performing work on a low calorie carbohydrate diet. J Appl Physiol 10:412, 1957

FOSTER DW: Eating disorders: Obesity and anorexia nervosa, in *Williams Textbook of Endocrinology*, 8th ed, JD Wilson, DW Foster (eds). Philadelphia, Saunders, 1992, p 1335

GARFINKEL PE et al: Differential diagnosis of emotional disorders that cause weight loss. Can Med Assoc J 129:939, 1983

MARTON KI et al: Involuntary weight loss: Diagnostic and prognostic significance. Ann Intern Med 95:568, 1981

MORLEY JE: Neuropeptide regulation of appetite and weight. Endocrine Rev 8:256, 1987

RAVUSSIN E et al: Determinants of 24-hour energy expenditure in man: Methods and results using a respiratory chamber. J Clin Inves 78:1568, 1986

ROMIJN JA, KLEIN S: One more reason for weight loss in patients with AIDS. Gastroenterology 101:861, 1991

THOMPSON MP, MORRIS LK: Unexplained weight loss in the ambulatory elderly. J Am Geriatr Soc 39:497, 1991

WILBER F: Neuropeptides, appetite regulation, and human obesity. JAMA 266:257, 1991

41 GASTROINTESTINAL BLEEDING

JAMES M. RICHTER / KURT J. ISSELBACHER

Hematemesis is defined as the vomiting of blood, and *melena* as the passage of stools rendered black and tarry by the presence of altered blood. These symptoms of gastrointestinal hemorrhage suggest a proximal source of bleeding. The color of vomited blood depends on the concentration of hydrochloric acid in the stomach and its mixture with the blood. Thus, if vomiting occurs shortly after the onset of bleeding, the vomitus appears red, and later the appearance will be dark red, brown, or black. Precipitated blood clots in the vomitus will produce a characteristic "coffee grounds" appearance. Hematemesis usually indicates bleeding proximal to the ligament of Treitz, because blood entering the gastrointestinal tract below the duodenum rarely enters the stomach.

While bleeding sufficient to produce hematemesis usually results in melena, less than half of patients with melena have hematemesis. *Melena* usually denotes bleeding from the esophagus, stomach, or duodenum, but lesions in the jejunum, ileum, and even ascending colon may cause melena provided the gastrointestinal transit time is sufficiently prolonged. Approximately 60 mL of blood is required to produce a single black stool; acute blood loss greater than this may produce melena for up to 7 days. After the stool color returns to normal, tests for occult blood may remain positive for over a week. The black color of melena results from contact of the blood with hydrochloric acid to produce hematin. Such stools are tarry ("sticky") and have a characteristic smell. This tarry consistency is in contrast to black or dark stools occurring after the ingestion of iron, bismuth, or licorice. Similarly, red stools may result from the ingestion of beets or intravenous administration of sulfobromophthalein. Gastrointestinal bleeding, even if detected only by positive tests for occult blood, indicates potentially serious disease and must be further investigated.

Hematochezia, the passage of red blood per rectum, generally signifies bleeding from a source distal to the ligament of Treitz. However, since blood must remain in the gut for approximately 8 h to produce melena, rapid hemorrhage into the esophagus, stomach, or duodenum also may result in hematochezia.

The clinical manifestations of gastrointestinal bleeding depend on the extent and rate of hemorrhage and the presence of coincidental diseases. Blood loss of less than 500 mL is rarely associated with systemic signs; exceptions include bleeding in the elderly or in the anemic patient in whom smaller amounts of blood loss may produce hemodynamic alterations. Rapid hemorrhage of greater volume results in decreased venous return to the heart, decreased cardiac output, and increased peripheral resistance due to reflex vasoconstriction (see Chap. 34). Orthostatic hypotension greater than 10 mmHg usually indicates a 20 percent or greater reduction in blood volume. Concomitant symptoms include syncope, lightheadedness, nausea, sweating, and thirst. When blood loss approaches 40 percent of blood volume, shock frequently ensues with pronounced tachycardia and hypotension. Pallor is prominent, and the skin is cool.

In the setting of rapid hemorrhage, the hematocrit may not accurately reflect the magnitude of blood loss, since equilibration with extravascular fluid and hemodilution require over 8 h. Common laboratory findings include mild leukocytosis and thrombocytosis which develop within 6 h after the onset of bleeding. The blood urea nitrogen may be elevated out of proportion to the creatinine, particularly in upper gastrointestinal bleeding, due to breakdown of blood proteins to urea by intestinal bacteria as well as from a mild reduction in the glomerular filtration rate.

Occult bleeding, detected by card test for hemoglobin peroxidase, is an important means of finding colorectal neoplasia at earlier, potentially curable stages. Testing is advocated for patients over age 40 as a part of the yearly checkup, and test kits are available for purchase by patients. The interpretation of the test is complicated by the need for examining multiple stools (usually two samples from three stools) and if positive, requires additional studies. A positive result can be due to physiologic blood loss, dietary peroxidases, or any cause of upper or lower gastrointestinal bleeding. Vitamin C ingestion over 500 mg daily may result in a false-negative test. To limit the confounding variables, patients should be tested on a high-fiber and low-meat diet with no ingestion of nonsteroidal anti-inflammatory agents or vitamin C. Quantitative and specific tests are being developed and advocated (Hemoquant) to improve the performance of fecal occult blood screening.

ETIOLOGY OF UPPER GASTROINTESTINAL BLEEDING A careful history and physical examination of the oropharynx and nasal cavity should serve to exclude swallowed blood as a source of hematemesis or melena.

The four most common causes of upper gastrointestinal hemorrhage are (1) peptic ulceration, (2) erosive gastritis, (3) varices, and (4) esophagogastric mucosal tear. These entities account for up to 90 percent of all cases of upper gastrointestinal hemorrhage in which a definite lesion can be found.

Peptic ulcer Peptic ulcer of the stomach or duodenum is the most common cause of upper gastrointestinal bleeding. Because hemorrhage may be the initial manifestation of a peptic ulcer, this lesion should be considered seriously even when a history characteristic of ulcer disease is not obtained.

Gastritis Gastritis may be associated with recent alcohol ingestion or the use of anti-inflammatory drugs such as aspirin or ibuprofen (see Chap. 252). Gastric erosions also frequently develop in patients with major trauma, surgery, and severe systemic disease, particularly burn victims and patients with increased intracranial pressure. Because there are no characteristic physical findings, the diagnosis of gastritis must be suspected when the appropriate clinical setting is encountered.

Varices and portal hypertensive gastropathy Variceal bleeding is characteristically abrupt and massive; chronic gastrointestinal blood loss is unusual. Bleeding from esophageal or gastric varices is usually the result of portal hypertension, secondary to cirrhosis. Although alcoholic cirrhosis is the most prevalent cause of esophageal varices in the United States, any condition producing portal hypertension may result in variceal bleeding. Further, while the presence of varices usually connotes long-standing portal hypertension, acute hepatitis or severe fatty infiltration of the liver may occasionally produce varices which disappear once the hepatic abnormality resolves. Although upper gastrointestinal bleeding in a patient with cirrhosis suggests a variceal source, approximately half those patients will be bleeding from peptic ulcer or portal hypertensive gastropathy. The latter results from gastric mucosal venous engorgement. Consequently, it is essential to determine the cause of bleeding so that the appropriate treatment can be instituted.

Esophagogastric mucosal tear (Mallory-Weiss syndrome) With the advent of esophagogastroduodenoscopy, the Mallory-Weiss syndrome has been observed with increasing frequency as a cause of acute upper gastrointestinal hemorrhage (see also Chap. 38). Mucosal laceration occurs in the region of the esophagogastric junction and is often characterized historically by retching or nonbloody vomiting followed by hematemesis.

Other lesions Less common bleeding esophageal lesions include esophagitis and carcinoma; these generally cause chronic blood loss and rarely produce massive bleeding.

Gastric carcinoma, lymphoma, polyps, and other tumors of the stomach and small bowel are uncommon and infrequently cause hemorrhage. Leiomyoma and leiomyosarcoma are likewise rare, but they can lead to massive hemorrhage. Bleeding from duodenal and jejunal diverticula is relatively unusual. Vascular insufficiency of the mesenteric vessels, including occlusive and nonocclusive disease, may lead to bloody diarrhea.

Rupture of arteriosclerotic aortic aneurysms into the small intestine is almost always fatal. Rupture usually occurs following arterial reconstructive surgery with fistula formation between synthetic graft and bowel lumen. A small or herald bleed may precede a sudden massive hemorrhage from an aortoenteric fistula. Sudden bleeding also may occur after trauma resulting in hepatic laceration; this may result in blood loss into the bile ducts (i.e., hemobilia).

Primary blood dyscrasias, vasculitis, and connective tissue disorders may result in significant gastrointestinal bleeding. Uremia may produce gastrointestinal blood loss; the most common presentation is chronic, occult bleeding from diffuse involvement of the mucosa of the stomach and small bowel.

ETIOLOGY OF LOWER GASTROINTESTINAL BLEEDING **Anal and rectal lesions** Small amounts of bright red blood on the surface of the stool and toilet tissue are often caused by hemorrhoids, anal fissures, or fistulas; such bleeding is generally precipitated by the strained passage of a hard stool. Proctitis is another source of rectal bleeding. It is often an idiopathic, limited variant of ulcerative colitis. In others, particularly male homosexuals or patients infected with HIV, proctitis may be due to CMV or gonorrheal or mycoplasmal infections. Rectal trauma is a cause of hematochezia, and the placement of foreign objects in the rectal vault may precipitate perforation as well as acute rectal hemorrhage. It must be emphasized that anal pathology does not preclude other sources of blood loss, and these must be sought and excluded.

Colonic lesions Carcinoma of the colon, as well as colonic polyps, may produce chronic blood loss. Angiodysplasia, a mucosal telangiectasia usually involving the ascending colon, is a major source of acute or chronic bleeding in elderly patients. Frankly bloody diarrhea is common and may be the presenting symptom in patients with ulcerative colitis; it is less frequent in granulomatous colitis, but occult blood may be present in the stool. Bleeding also may accompany diarrhea due to infections with *Shigella*, amebae, *Campylobacter*, *C. difficile*, and rarely, *Salmonella*. In the elderly patient, ischemic colitis may be a cause of bloody diarrhea; this lesion also may be seen in younger women who use oral contraceptive agents.

Diverticula Bleeding from colonic diverticula is a cause of massive lower gastrointestinal hemorrhage. The usual presentation of a diverticular hemorrhage is that of painless passage of a maroon-colored stool. Meckel's diverticulum, a congenital anomaly of the distal ileum, is present in about 2 percent of the population and is an important cause of acute hemorrhage in children and young adults. Although only about 15 percent of these diverticula contain gastric mucosa, half the lesions which cause acute bleeding contain gastric mucosa.

APPROACH TO THE PATIENT WITH GASTROINTESTINAL BLEEDING The approach to the bleeding patient depends on the site, extent, and rate of bleeding. The primary consideration in the care of the bleeding patient is maintaining adequate intravascular volume and hemodynamic stability. Patients with hematemesis have usually bled greater amounts (often greater than 1000 mL) than those who have melena alone (usually 500 mL or less), and mortality with the former is about twice that of the latter. When first seen, the patient may be in shock. Prior to taking a history and performing a thorough physical examination, vital signs should be noted, blood sent for typing and cross-matching, and a large-bore intravenous line placed for infusion of saline or other plasma expanders.

History A history or symptoms suggestive of ulcer disease may provide a useful clue. Similarly, recent heavy use of alcohol or anti-inflammatory drugs should make erosive gastritis suspect. If such alcohol use has been long-standing, esophageal varices may be a more likely source of hemorrhage. Prior history of gastrointestinal bleeding may be helpful, as may a family history of intestinal disease or hemorrhagic diathesis. Recent retching followed by hematemesis should suggest the possibility of the Mallory-Weiss syndrome. The acute onset of bloody diarrhea may indicate the presence of inflammatory bowel disease or an infectious colitis. Associated systemic illnesses, burns, or recent trauma may lead to erosive gastritis.

Physical examination Following evaluation for orthostatic changes in pulse and blood pressure, clinical assessment of central venous pressure, and institution of volume repletion, the patient should be examined for clues to the underlying illness. A nonintestinal bleeding source should be excluded by careful examination of the oral cavity and nasopharynx. Dermatologic examination may disclose the characteristic telangiectasia of Osler-Weber-Rendu disease (although these will not be visible if severe anemia is present), the perioral pigmentation of Peutz-Jeghers syndrome, the dermal fibromas of neurofibromatosis, the sebaceous cysts and bony tumors of Gardner's syndrome, the palpable purpura frequently seen with vasculitis, or the diffuse pigmentation seen in hemochromatosis. Stigmata of chronic liver disease such as spider angiomata, gynecomastia, testicular atrophy, jaundice, ascites, and hepatosplenomegaly suggest portal hypertension resulting in bleeding from esophageal or gastric varices. Significant lymph node enlargement or abdominal masses may reflect underlying intraabdominal malignancy. Careful rectal examination is important to exclude local pathology as well as to observe the color of the stool.

Laboratory studies   Initial studies should include the hematocrit, hemoglobin, careful assessment of red blood cell morphologic features (hypochromic, microcytic red blood cells suggest that blood loss is chronic), white blood cell count, differential, and platelet count. Prothrombin time, partial thromboplastin time, and other coagulation studies are needed to exclude primary or secondary clotting defects. Radiography of the abdomen is rarely helpful in establishing a diagnosis unless a perforated or ischemic viscus is suspected. Although the initial studies are valuable and essential, repeated evaluation of the laboratory data is important as one follows the clinical course of the bleeding.

Diagnostic and therapeutic approach   The diagnostic approach to the patient with gastrointestinal hemorrhage must be individualized. When there is a history of melena or hematemesis or the suspicion of bleeding from the upper part of the gastrointestinal tract, the patient should have a nasogastric tube passed to empty the stomach and to determine whether the bleeding is proximal to the ligament of Treitz. If the initial nasogastric aspirate is clear, the tube should be left in place for several hours, since active duodenal bleeding may occur with an initially clear nasogastric aspirate. If the aspirate is negative for blood during a period of active bleeding, it is reasonable to conclude that active bleeding is not occurring in the gastroduodenal region, and the nasogastric tube can be removed. However, if there is no evidence of active bleeding at the time the nasogastric tube is placed, one cannot assume bleeding did not come from the stomach or duodenum, and endoscopy may be required.

If red blood or "coffee grounds" material is aspirated from the nasogastric tube, saline irrigation of the stomach should be initiated. Irrigation serves two purposes: It provides the clinician with an assessment of the rapidity of the bleeding, and it clears the stomach of old blood prior to possible endoscopy. Subsequent diagnostic maneuvers will depend on whether bleeding continues; this can be assessed by vital signs, transfusion requirements, and the number and consistency of stools.

If the bleeding has stopped and the patient is stable, one may proceed with esophagogastroduodenoscopy. Although studies have shown that emergency endoscopy and a vigorous diagnostic approach do not generally decrease patient morbidity or mortality, emergency endoscopy may be important in planning therapy in certain patients with previous gastric surgery, portal hypertension, or complex multisystem diseases. By identifying patients with visible vessels or varices, some patients may be treated endoscopically, and possible complications can be anticipated. Endoscopy is not required if the diagnosis and therapeutic approach are clear from clinical or other data.

Persistent upper gastrointestinal hemorrhage must be viewed differently, and most clinicians would proceed immediately to esophagogastroduodenoscopy (Fig. 41-1). Determination of the site and cause of bleeding is essential to plan for appropriate therapy. Anticipation of surgery, angiography, or the suspicion of bleeding varices are strong indications for esophagogastroduodenoscopy. Bleeding from an arteriole in a peptic ulcer may be controlled by endoscopic coagulation using Nd:YAG laser, heater probe, or electrocautery. However, esophagogastroduodenoscopy is more difficult in the evaluation of *massive* hemorrhage because large amounts of blood obscure visualization of mucosal pathology, and angiography may be required in addition to endoscopy.

Should bleeding continue and endoscopy fail to reveal the bleeding source, the site of hemorrhage may be beyond the ligament of Treitz. In this situation, angiography is frequently valuable in establishing a diagnosis. Angiographic demonstration of the bleeding site requires blood loss at a rate of at least 0.5 mL/min. Clinical correlates reflecting this degree of blood loss include postural hypotension and the necessity for blood transfusion to maintain stable vital signs. Emergency angiography may localize the site of bleeding; however, the cause of the bleeding may not be determined unless varices, vascular malformations, or aneurysms are present.

Therapeutic angiography is a helpful approach to the control of persistent hemorrhage. Continuous intraarterial infusion of vasoconstrictor agents, such as vasopressin, is often successful in controlling hemorrhage due to gastric ulcer or Mallory-Weiss tear. Additionally, embolic material may be injected directly into the artery perfusing the bleeding site.

If bleeding esophageal varices are identified on upper endoscopy, peripheral infusions of vasopressin may acutely control the bleeding. The response to such therapy depends on the general condition of the patient as assessed by clinical and laboratory parameters. It has been shown that intraarterial vasopressin is no more effective than intravenous administration in the control of variceal bleeding. Endoscopic sclerosis and banding of varices have emerged as effective

FIGURE 41-1 Endoscopic photographs from a patient with hematemesis. *A.* A gastric ulcer along the lesser curvature of the stomach is identified (*arrows*). *B.* The same ulcer is bleeding actively from a spurting artery (*arrows*).

therapies for bleeding esophageal varices. Periodic endoscopic sclerotherapy and banding also appear to limit further bleeding in patients who have bled from varices but do not prolong life. Variceal bleeding also may be controlled by balloon tamponade with a Sengstaken-Blakemore tube. Like vasopressin, this technique is generally used as a stabilizing measure and should be followed by definitive therapy within 48 h whenever possible. Because of its morbidity, portosystemic shunting is reserved for the gravest circumstances. Liver transplantation may be an option for some patients with cirrhosis and bleeding varices.

In the evaluation of *lower gastrointestinal bleeding*, the most important procedures are the digital examination, anoscopy, and sigmoidoscopy. The last of these may identify a bleeding site or document bleeding coming from above the range of the instrument. In the latter case, preparation of the colon with saline lavage solutions permits a colonoscopic evaluation of the bowel within hours. Many colonic abnormalities can be detected and treated with polypectomy or electrocoagulation. If bleeding is brisk, arteriography may serve to localize the bleeding site and allow local infusion of vasoconstrictor agents to control bleeding. Because arteriography detects actively bleeding lesions only when blood loss exceeds 0.5 mL/min and gastrointestinal bleeding tends to be intermittent, arteriography is often nondiagnostic. Radiolabeled erythrocyte scanning is more sensitive than arteriography in detecting blood loss of 0.1 mL/min and may be used to investigate less severe bleeding. However, bleeding scans are less specific than arteriography, generally localizing the lesion but seldom making a discrete diagnosis. Bleeding scans are most helpful in detecting active, low-grade, or intermittent bleeding in order to better time arteriography and obtain the maximal diagnostic yield. Finally, a barium enema has a limited role in the evaluation of acute rectal bleeding. Although it may localize potential bleeding sources, it will not define the bleeding site. Furthermore, if brisk bleeding recurs, subsequent colonoscopy or angiography will be difficult to interpret due to retained contrast material. Therefore, it is advisable to withhold barium studies of both the upper and lower bowel for at least 48 h after the cessation of active bleeding.

Patients with positive tests for fecal occult blood are evaluated principally to exclude colorectal neoplasia. Any symptoms or history of disease should be investigated as well. If there are no symptoms, evaluation focusing on the colon with either a barium enema and sigmoidoscopy or colonoscopy is sufficient. Patients with anemia are unlikely to have a physiologic or trivial basis for their test result, and the evaluation should be pursued until a full explanation is obtained.

REFERENCES

AHLQUIST DA et al: Fecal blood levels in health and disease: A study using Hemoquant. N Engl J Med 312:1422, 1985

CELLO JP et al: Endoscopic sclerotherapy versus portacaval shunt in patients with severe cirrhosis and acute variceal hemorrhage; Long-term follow-up. N Engl J Med 316:11, 1987

CHOJKIER M et al: A controlled comparison of continuous intraarterial and intravenous infusions of vasopressin in hemorrhage from esophageal varices. Gastroenterology 77:540, 1979

LAINE L: Multipolar electrocoagulation in the treatment of active upper gastrointestinal tract hemorrhage. N Engl J Med 316:1613, 1987

LEVY M et al: Major upper gastrointestinal tract bleeding: Relation to the use of aspirin and other nonnarcotic analgesics. Arch Intern Med 148:281, 1988

LICHTENSTEIN JL: Accuracy and reliability of endoscopy and x-ray in upper gastrointestinal bleeding. Dig Dis Sci 26:70s, 1981

PETERSON WL et al: Routine early endoscopy in upper gastrointestinal tract bleeding: A randomized, controlled trial. N Engl J Med 304:925, 1981

RICHTER JM et al: Angiodysplasia: Clinical presentation and colonoscopic diagnosis. Dig Dis Sci 29:481, 1984

STEER ML, SILEN W: Diagnostic procedures in gastrointestinal hemorrhage. N Engl J Med 309:646, 1983

42   JAUNDICE

LEE M. KAPLAN / KURT J. ISSELBACHER

Accumulation of bilirubin in the bloodstream causes yellow pigmentation of the plasma, leading to discoloration of heavily perfused tissues. Serum bilirubin levels accumulate when its production from heme exceeds its metabolism and excretion. Imbalance between production and clearance may result either from excess release of bilirubin precursors into the bloodstream or from physiologic processes that impair the hepatic uptake, metabolism, or excretion of this metabolite (see Table 42-1). Clinically, hyperbilirubinemia appears as *jaundice* or *icterus*, yellow pigmentation of the skin and sclerae. Jaundice can usually be detected when the serum bilirubin level exceeds 34 to 43 μmol/L (2.0 to 2.5 mg/dL), or about twice the upper limit of the normal range, but may be detectable at lower bilirubin levels in patients with fair skin and profound anemia. Conversely, jaundice is frequently obscured in individuals with dark skin or edema. Scleral tissue is rich in elastin, which has a high affinity for bilirubin, so that scleral icterus is usually a more sensitive sign of hyperbilirubinemia than generalized jaundice. A similarly early sign of hyperbilirubinemia is darkening of the urine, which results from renal excretion of bilirubin in the form of bilirubin glucuronide. With pronounced jaundice, the skin may take on a greenish hue because of oxidation of some of the circulating bilirubin to biliverdin. This effect is seen more commonly in conditions with profound or long-standing *conjugated* hyperbilirubinemia such as cirrhosis (see below). Other causes of yellowed skin include *carotenemia*, usually developing as a result of ingestion and absorption of large amounts of β-carotene and related, pigmented compounds. In contrast to hyperbilirubinemia, however, carotenemia does not cause scleral icterus.

PRODUCTION AND METABOLISM OF BILIRUBIN   Sources and chemical characterization of serum bilirubin   Normal serum bilirubin concentrations range from 5 to 17 μmol/L (0.3 to 1.0 mg/dL). More than 90 percent of serum bilirubin in normal individuals is in the unconjugated form, a nonpolar molecule circulating as an albumin-bound complex. The remainder is conjugated to a polar group (primarily glucuronide), rendering it water-soluble and thus able to be filtered and excreted by the kidney. When measured by routine clinical assays, the conjugated, or direct, fraction is frequently overestimated, leading to reported normal values of 1.7 to 8.5 μmol/L (0.1 to 0.5 mg/dL).

Approximately 80 percent of circulating bilirubin is derived from senescent red blood cells. When circulating erythrocytes reach the end of their normal life span of approximately 120 days, they are destroyed by reticuloendothelial cells (Fig. 42-1). Oxidation of the heme moiety dissociated from the hemoglobin within these cells generates biliverdin, which is metabolized in turn to bilirubin. Approximately 15 to 20 percent of circulating bilirubin is derived

TABLE 42-1   Comparative properties of conjugated and unconjugated bilirubin

Properties and reactions	Unconjugated*	Conjugated
Water solubility	0	+
Affinity for lipids	+	0
Renal excretion	0	+
van den Bergh reaction	Indirect (total minus direct)	Direct
Binding to serum albumin (reversible)	+ + +	+
Formation of bilirubin-albumin complex (irreversible)	0	+[†]

* These properties apply to the naturally occurring bilirubin IXα. Other geometric and photoisomers behave like conjugated bilirubin. See text for details.
[†] Detectable in plasma under conditions of prolonged conjugated hyperbilirubinemia (see text).

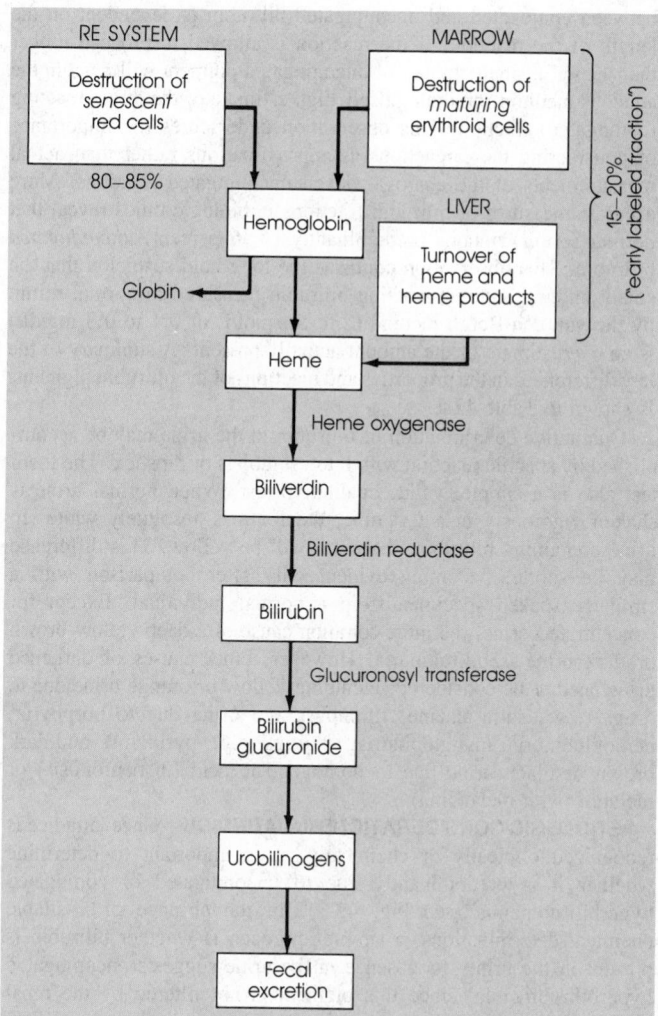

FIGURE 42-1 The sources and precursors of bilirubin and steps in its subsequent metabolism and excretion. RE, reticuloendothelial.

from sources other than senescent erythrocytes. The second major source of bilirubin is ineffective erythropoiesis resulting from destruction of maturing erythroid cells in the bone marrow. A smaller portion of circulating bilirubin derives from the metabolism of other heme-containing proteins, most notably hepatic cytochromes, muscle myoglobin, and widely distributed heme-containing enzymes.

Unconjugated bilirubin liberated into the plasma is bound tightly, but noncovalently to albumin. Certain organic anions, such as sulfonamides and salicylates, complete with bilirubin for binding sites on albumin, permitting the released pigment to enter tissues such as the central nervous system. This phenomenon may explain the neurotoxic effects of neonatal hyperbilirubinemia. Conjugated bilirubin is bound to albumin in two forms, reversible and irreversible. Reversible, noncovalent binding is similar to that of unconjugated bilirubin, although the complex is less stable. When present in serum for extended periods of time (e.g., with cholestasis, long-standing biliary obstruction, or chronic active hepatitis), conjugated bilirubin can form an irreversible, covalent complex with albumin (delta bilirubin or biliprotein). Because of the irreversibility of binding, this complex is not excreted by the kidney. This bilirubin-albumin conjugate has a serum half-life similar to that of albumin (15 to 20 days) and thus remains detectable in serum for up to several weeks after relief of biliary obstruction or during recovery from hepatocellular disease.

Bilirubin is present in body fluids (cerebrospinal fluid, joint effusions, ascites, pleural effusions, cysts, etc.) in proportion to their albumin content and is absent from true secretions such as tears,

saliva, and pancreatic juice. The appearance of jaundice is also influenced by blood flow and edema, with paralyzed extremities and edematous areas tending to remain uncolored.

Hepatic metabolism of bilirubin   The liver has a central role in the metabolism of the bile pigments. This process can be divided into three distinct phases: (1) *hepatic uptake*, (2) *conjugation*, and (3) *excretion* into bile. Of these three phases, excretion appears to be the rate-limiting step and the one most susceptible to impairment when the liver cell is damaged.

UPTAKE   Unconjugated bilirubin bound to albumin is presented to the liver cell, where the complex dissociates and the nonpolar bilirubin enters the hepatocyte by diffusion or transport across the plasma membrane. The uptake and subsequent hepatocyte storage of bilirubin involves binding of bilirubin to cytoplasmic anion-binding proteins, especially ligandin (glutathione-S-transferase B), that prevent efflux of bilirubin back into the plasma.

CONJUGATION   Unconjugated bilirubin is water-insoluble unless complexed to an amphipathic molecule such as albumin. Since albumin is absent from bile, bilirubin must be converted to a water-soluble derivative before biliary excretion. This process is accomplished predominantly by conjugation of bilirubin to glucuronic acid, generating bilirubin glucuronide. The conjugation reaction occurs in the endoplasmic reticulum of hepatocytes and is catalyzed by bilirubin glucuronosyl transferase in a two-step reaction (see Fig. 42-2).

EXCRETION   In normal circumstances, only conjugated bilirubin can be excreted into bile. Although the overall process is not well understood, bilirubin excretion appears to be an energy-dependent process limited to the canalicular membrane. Excretion is the rate-limiting step in the hepatic metabolism of this pigment. Impaired excretion leads to decreased bilirubin concentrations in the bile and concomitant "regurgitation" of *conjugated* bilirubin through the sinusoidal membrane of the hepatocyte into the bloodstream. The role of intracellular protein trafficking and membrane transport processes in normal and disordered bilirubin excretion are still poorly understood.

Intestinal phase of bilirubin metabolism   After secretion into the bile, conjugated bilirubin is transported through the biliary ducts into the duodenum. Conjugated bilirubin is not reabsorbed by the intestinal mucosa. It is either excreted unchanged in the stool or metabolized by ileal and colonic bacteria to *urobilinogen* and related products. Urobilinogen can be reabsorbed from the small intestine and colon and enters the portal circulation. Some of the portal urobilinogen is taken up by the liver and reexcreted into the bile, and the remainder bypasses the liver and is excreted by the kidney. Under normal conditions, the daily urinary excretion of urobilinogen does not exceed 4 mg. When the hepatic uptake and excretion of urobilinogen is impaired (e.g., in hepatocellular disease) or the production of bilirubin is greatly increased (e.g., with hemolysis),

FIGURE 42-2 Scheme of bilirubin uptake, conjugation, and excretion by the liver cell. The conversion of BMG to BDG is catalyzed by glucuronosyl transferase of the endoplasmic reticulum. B, bilirubin; BMG, bilirubin monoglucuronide; BDG, bilirubin diglucuronide; UDP, uridine diphosphate.

daily urinary urobilinogen excretion may increase significantly. In contrast, cholestasis or extrahepatic biliary obstruction interferes with the intestinal phase of bilirubin metabolism and leads to markedly decreased production and urinary excretion of urobilinogen. Measurement of urinary urobilinogen can thus be a useful tool in distinguishing possible causes of hyperbilirubinemia.

Renal excretion of bilirubin   The urine normally contains no detectable bilirubin by usual clinical assays, although traces may be detected by sensitive spectrophotometric procedures. Unconjugated bilirubin, being tightly bound into albumin, is not filtered by the renal glomeruli. Because there is no tubular secretory process for bilirubin, unconjugated bilirubin is not excreted in urine. In contrast, *conjugated* bilirubin is a polar molecule less tightly bound to albumin. A significant fraction circulates unbound, is filtered by the renal glomeruli, and appears in the urine. The presence of bilirubin in the urine is evidence of conjugated hyperbilirubinemia and can be a useful differentiating point early in the evaluation of jaundice. Bile salts enhance the glomerular filtration of conjugated bilirubin, and in conditions associated with increased circulating bile salts (e.g., cholestasis, extrahepatic biliary obstruction) renal bilirubin excretion is significantly enhanced. This phenomenon may explain the observation that serum conjugated bilirubin tends to plateau at levels below 510 to 680 μmol/L (30 to 40 mg/dL) in patients with *biliary tract obstruction*, while higher levels may occur in patients with severe hepatocellular injury.

For additional information about the production, metabolism, and excretion of bilirubin, please refer to Chap. 265.

PATHOPHYSIOLOGIC CONSEQUENCES OF HYPERBILIRUBINEMIA   In most cases, hyperbilirubinemia itself has little pathophysiologic effect. Unlike circulating bile salts, whose levels are also elevated in cholestasis and biliary obstruction, bilirubin does not become deposited in cutaneous tissues and does not produce pruritus. However, *unconjugated* plasma bilirubin that is not bound to albumin can cross the blood-brain barrier. In conditions such as neonatal jaundice or type I or II Crigler-Najjar syndrome (see below), extremely high concentrations (>340 μmol/L or >20 mg/dL) of unconjugated bilirubin can accumulate, and the resulting diffusion of bilirubin into the central nervous system can cause encephalopathy (kernicterus) and permanent impairment of nervous function. The risk of kernicterus is increased by conditions that favor elevated circulating levels of *unbound*, unconjugated bilirubin, such as hemolysis, hypoalbuminemia, acidosis, and increased levels of compounds that compete for albumin binding such as free fatty acids and drugs. Circulating concentrations of unconjugated bilirubin can be decreased by removing these contributory factors and by facilitating the biliary excretion of *unconjugated* bilirubin. Exposure to blue light causes conformational changes in unconjugated bilirubin, rendering it more polar and water soluble. These *photoisomers* are taken up and excreted by the liver and kidney, without need for normal conjugation. Intense treatment with blue light can provide sufficient isomerization of unconjugated bilirubin circulating through the skin to prevent kernicterus in patients with neonatal jaundice.

CHEMICAL TESTS FOR BILE PIGMENTS   The most widely employed chemical test for bile pigments in serum is the van den Bergh reaction. The bilirubin pigments are exposed to sulfanilic acid to generated diazo conjugates, and the chromogenic products are measured colorimetrically. The van den Bergh reaction can be used to distinguish between unconjugated and conjugated bilirubin because of the different solubility properties of the pigments. When the reaction is performed in an aqueous medium, the water-soluble conjugated bilirubin reacts directly with sulfanilic acid, giving a positive *direct* van den Bergh reaction. When the reaction is performed in methanol, the intramolecular hydrogen bonds of unconjugated bilirubin are broken; thus, both conjugated and unconjugated pigments react, giving a measure of the *total* bilirubin level. The *indirect* value, representative of the unconjugated bilirubin fraction, is estimated by subtracting the direct-reacting fraction from the total measured bilirubin. The ability of the *direct* van den Bergh reaction to distinguish

between conjugated and unconjugated bilirubin is dependent on the length of the reaction. If the reaction is allowed to proceed longer than 1 min, a small amount of unconjugated pigment will react in the aqueous medium, giving a falsely high estimate of the direct-reacting (conjugated) fraction. This observation underscores the importance of considering these reactions as approximations rather than actual measurements of the conjugated and unconjugated fractions. More accurate measures of bilirubin fractions in biologic fluids reveal that normal serum contains predominantly (>96 percent) *unconjugated* bilirubin. This observation confirms the long-held suspicion that the small amount of direct-reacting bilirubin measured in normal serum by the van den Bergh method (2 to 5 μmol/L or 0.1 to 0.3 mg/dL) is an overestimate of the amount actually present. A summary of the key differences in the properties and reactions of the bilirubin pigments is shown in Table 42-1.

Qualitative determination of bilirubin in the urine may be accomplished by specific reaction with Ictotest tablets or dipstick. The foam test also is a simple, valid, qualitative test. When normal urine is shaken vigorously in a test tube, the foam is absolutely white. In urine containing bilirubin, the foam will be yellow. This difference may be subtle, becoming evident only after comparison with a similarly shaken specimen from a normal individual. Except for concentrated urine, the most common cause of a deep yellow-brown or dark urine is bilirubinuria. However, other causes of darkened urine need to be considered, including yellow or orange urine due to drugs (e.g., sulfasalazine, rifampin), red urine due to porphyria, hemoglobinuria, myoglobinuria, or drugs (e.g., pyridium), and dark brown or black urine due to homogentisic acid (in ochronosis) or melanin (with melanoma).

ETIOLOGIC CONSIDERATIONS IN JAUNDICE   Once jaundice is recognized clinically or chemically, it is important to determine whether it is predominantly due to unconjugated or conjugated hyperbilirubinemia (see Fig. 42-3). In the absence of available chemical determinations, a simple approach is whether bilirubin is present in the urine. Its absence in the urine suggests unconjugated hyperbilirubinemia, since this pigment is not filtered by the renal glomeruli; its presence indicates conjugated hyperbilirubinemia. When chemical analysis (van den Bergh reaction) reveals 80 to 85 percent of the total serum bilirubin to be unconjugated, a patient is considered to have primarily *unconjugated hyperbilirubinemia*. A patient with more than 50 percent direct-reacting (conjugated) serum bilirubin is considered to have predominantly *conjugated hyperbilirubinemia*.

An approach to the classification of jaundice based on this important distinction is presented in Table 42-2. Derangements of bilirubin metabolism may occur through any of four mechanisms: (1) overproduction, (2) decreased hepatic uptake, (3) decreased hepatic conjugation, and (4) decreased excretion of bilirubin into bile (due either to intrahepatic dysfunction or extrahepatic mechanical obstruction). Jaundice may also be described on the basis of the pathogenic mechanisms or disease processes leading to increased bilirubin levels. Thus, the terms *hemolytic jaundice*, *hepatocellular jaundice*, and *obstructive* (or *cholestatic*) *jaundice* are often used. Though these classifications are helpful, in any one patient more than a single derangement in bilirubin metabolism may be operative, and more than a single "type" of jaundice may be present. For example, a patient with cirrhosis may have not only impaired liver cell function (and hence hepatocellular jaundice) but also hemolysis. Furthermore, as indicated above, obstructive jaundice or cholestasis may be due either to *mechanical* obstruction of the biliary radicles or to impaired *functional* hepatic excretion of bilirubin. This chapter presents a brief description of the major causes of jaundice. A more detailed discussion of individual diseases is found in Chap. 265.

Jaundice with predominantly unconjugated bilirubinemia   OVER-PRODUCTION OF BILIRUBIN   An increased amount of hemoglobin released from senescent or hemolyzed red blood cells leads to increased bilirubin production. Erythrocyte destruction leading to hyperbilirubinemia most commonly results from intravascular hemolysis (e.g., autoimmune, microangiopathic, or hemoglobinopathy-

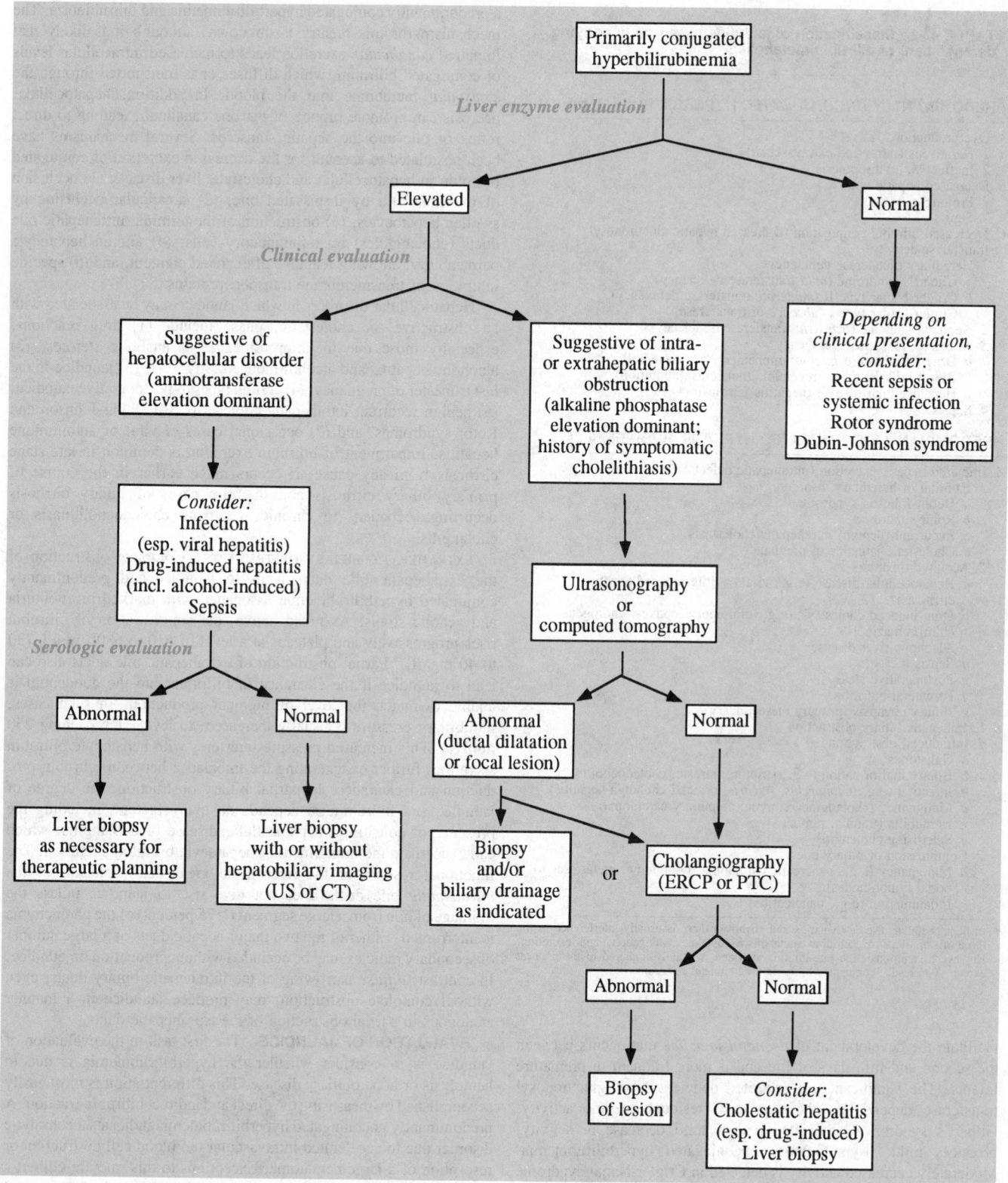

FIGURE 42-3 Algorithm for evaluation of conjugated hyperbilirubinemia. Abbreviations: CT, computed tomography, ERCP, endoscopic retrograde cholangiopancreatography; PTC, percutaneous transhepatic cholangiography; US, ultrasonography.

associated) or resorption of a large hematoma. Excess bilirubin production is reflected in increased serum bilirubin levels of up to 51 to 68 μmol/L (3 to 4 mg/dL), with a predominance of unconjugated bilirubin. For a more detailed discussion of the causes of increased bilirubin production, refer to Chap. 265.

IMPAIRED HEPATIC UPTAKE OF BILIRUBIN As indicated above, the uptake of bilirubin by hepatocytes requires dissociation of the nonpolar pigment molecule from albumin, transport across the cell

membrane, and binding to ligandin. In rare cases of drug-induced jaundice (e.g., from flavaspidic acid) and possibly in some patients with Gilbert's syndrome, there may be a disruption of this phase of bilirubin handling.

IMPAIRED GLUCURONIDE CONJUGATION Deficiency in glucuronosyl transferase activity can occur as a result of both acquired and genetic defects. In the fetus and neonate, glucuronosyl transferase activity is normally low. This deficiency, although transient, can

TABLE 42-2   Classification of jaundice based on underlying derangement of bilirubin metabolism

PREDOMINANTLY *UNCONJUGATED* HYPERBILIRUBINEMIA

A Overproduction
  1 Hemolysis (intra- and extravascular)
  2 Ineffective erythropoiesis
B Decreased hepatic uptake
  1 Prolonged fasting
  2 Sepsis
C Decreased bilrubin conjugation (decreased hepatic glucuronosyl transferase activity)
  1 Hereditary transferase deficiency
    a Gilbert's syndrome (*mild* transferase deficiency)
    b Crigler-Najjar type II (*moderate* transferase deficiency)
    c Crigler-Najjar type I (*absence* of transferase)
  2 Neonatal jaundice (*transient* transferase deficiency)
  3 Acquired transferase deficiency
    a Drug inhibition (e.g. chloramphenicol, pregnanediol)
    b Breast milk jaundice (reversible transferase inhibition)
    c Hepatocellular disease (hepatitis, cirrhosis)*
  4 Sepsis

PREDOMINANTLY *CONJUGATED* HYPERBILIRUBINEMIA

A Impaired hepatic excretion (intrahepatic defects)
  1 Familial or hereditary disorders
    a Dubin-Johnson syndrome
    b Rotor syndrome
    c Recurrent (benign) intrahepatic cholestasis
    d Cholestatic jaundice of pregnancy
  2 Acquired disorders
    a Hepatocellular disease (e.g., viral or drug-induced hepatitis, cirrhosis)*
    b Drug-induced cholestasis (e.g., oral contraceptives, androgens, chlorpromazine)
    c Alcoholic liver disease
    d Sepsis
    e Postoperative state
    f Parenteral nutrition
    g Biliary cirrhosis (primary or secondary)
B Extrahepatic biliary obstruction
  1 Intraductal obstruction
    a Gallstones
    b Biliary malformation (e.g., stricture, atresia, choledochol cyst)
    c Infection (e.g., *Clonorchis, Ascaris,* oriental cholangiohepatitis)
    d Malignancy (cholangiocarcinoma, ampullary carcinoma)
    e Hemobilia (trauma, tumor)
    f Sclerosing cholangitis
  2 Compression of biliary ducts
    a Malignancy (e.g., pancreatic carcinoma, lymphoma, metastases to portal lymph nodes)
    b Inflammation (e.g., pancreatitis)

* In hepatocellular disease (hepatitis and cirrhosis) there is usually interference in the three major steps of bilirubin metabolism—uptake, conjugation, and excretion. However, excretion is the rate-limiting step and is usually impaired to the greatest extent. As a result, conjugated bilirubin predominates in serum.

facilitate the development of *neonatal jaundice* that occurs between the second and fifth days of life and is more frequent in premature infants. The significance of inherited deficiencies of glucuronosyl transferase depends on the degree of residual enzyme activity. Gilbert's syndrome, associated with a mild decrease in activity, produces mild, asymptomatic, unconjugated hyperbilirubinemia. Moderately decreased activity is detected in Crigler-Najjar syndrome type II, and this enzyme is total absent in Crigler-Najjar syndrome type I, an autosomal recessive disorder associated with kernicterus and childhood mortality from CNS dysfunction. Acquired defects in glucuronosyl transferase activity may be induced by drugs (i.e., direct enzyme inhibition) or be associated with liver disease generally. However, in most hepatocellular disorders, bilirubin excretion is impaired to a greater extent than bilirubin conjugation, leading to a primarily *conjugated* hyperbilirubinemia.

Jaundice with predominantly conjugated bilirubinemia
IMPAIRED BILIRUBIN EXCRETION BY HEPATOCYTES   Interference with the biliary excretion of conjugated bilirubin by hepatocytes leads to "reentry" of this pigment into the systemic circulation, resulting in

a predominantly conjugated hyperbilirubinemia and bilirubinuria. The mechanism for this reentry is unknown, although it is likely that impaired *canalicular* excretion leads to increased intracellular levels of conjugated bilirubin, which diffuses or is transported through the *sinusoidal* membrane into the blood. In addition, hepatocellular necrosis can promote rupture of the bile canaliculi, leading to direct reflux of bile into the hepatic sinusoids. Several mechanisms have been postulated to account for the decreased excretion of conjugated bilirubin in hepatocellular and cholestatic liver disease: (1) occlusion of the canaliculi by inspissated bile, (2) canalicular occlusion by swollen hepatocytes, (3) obstruction of the terminal intrahepatic bile ducts (cholangioles) by inflammatory cells, (4) altered hepatocyte permeability, allowing reuptake of excreted pigment, and (5) specific inhibition of transmembrane transport proteins.

Hepatocellular disorders in which jaundice may be associated with an obstructive, or cholestatic, phase include (1) drug reactions, especially those due to chlorpromazine or anabolic steroids, (2) alcoholic hepatitis and alcohol-induced fatty liver, (3) jaundice in the last trimester of pregnancy, (4) certain types of postoperative jaundice, (5) benign recurrent intrahepatic cholestasis, (6) Dubin-Johnson and Rotor syndromes, and (7) occasional cases of viral or autoimmune hepatitis. Impairment of bilirubin excretion is common in late-stage cirrhosis from any cause. It occurs much earlier in the course of primary biliary cirrhosis and the rare cases of biliary cirrhosis occurring secondary to chronic, recurring choledocholithiasis or cholangitis.

EXTRAHEPATIC BILIARY OBSTRUCTION   Complete obstruction of the extrahepatic bile ducts leads to jaundice and predominantly conjugated hyperbilirubinemia associated with marked bilirubinuria and acholic stools. As noted above, the concentration of bilirubin rises progressively and plateaus at a level of 510 to 680 μmol/L (30 to 40 mg/dL). Partial obstruction of extrahepatic bile ducts also can lead to jaundice if the clearance of bilirubin into the duodenum is unable to match the level of pigment production. In such cases, intrabiliary pressure is usually increased (to levels approaching 250 mmHg). This increased pressure interferes with hepatocyte bilirubin secretion, further exaggerating the imbalance between bilirubin production and clearance. In partial biliary obstruction, the degree of jaundice and bilirubinuria depends on many factors, including the presence of concurrent hepatocellular disease or cholangitis, which can exacerbate the impairment of hepatocyte bilirubin excretion. The functional reserve of the liver is so great that occlusion of the *intrahepatic* bile ducts does not give rise to jaundice unless the drainage of bile from a large segment (>75 percent) of the parenchyma is interrupted. Either of the two major hepatic ducts or a large number of secondary radicles may be occluded without production of jaundice. In contrast, *diffuse* narrowing of the intrahepatic biliary ducts, even without complete obstruction, may produce jaundice in a manner analogous to partial obstruction of the extrahepatic ducts.

EVALUATION OF JAUNDICE   The first task in the evaluation of jaundice is to consider whether the hyperbilirubinemia is due to hemolysis or hepatobiliary disease. This differentiation is most easily accomplished by measuring the direct and indirect bilirubin fraction. A predominantly unconjugated hyperbilirubinemia indicates a hemolytic disorder due to accelerated intravascular red blood cell destruction or resorption of a large hematoma. Exceptions to this rule are Gilbert's syndrome, the other, rare, hereditary disorders of glucuronosyl transferase, and end-stage hepatic failure. Further evaluation of the cause of hemolysis can then proceed as described in Chap. 304, Megaloblastic Anemias, Chap. 306, Disorders of Hemoglobin, and Chap. 307, Hemolytic Anemias.

Jaundice associated with a primarily (>50 percent) *conjugated* hyperbilirubinemia usually results from one of three groups of disorders, including hepatocellular disease, intrahepatic biliary obstruction ("cholestasis") and extrahepatic biliary obstruction. An early goal is the determination of which category of disease explains the patient's jaundice. Central to this determination is a careful *clinical* evaluation, including history, physical examination, basic tests of liver function, and a complete blood count. Using these simple tools, experienced clinicians can determine the overall nature of the jaundice in the majority of cases. Most importantly, however, the results of the clinical evaluation direct the physician to a logical progression of imaging studies, serological tests, and pathological evaluation. The initial clinical evaluation should focus on features of the patient's illness that distinguish between hepatocellular disease, intrahepatic cholestasis, and extrahepatic biliary obstruction. A general algorithm for the evaluation of jaundice due to conjugated hyperbilirubinemia is shown in Fig. 42-3.

History Historical evaluation should include determination of the length of symptoms, presence and character of abdominal pain, fever or other symptoms of active inflammation, changes in appetite, weight, and bowel habits. Specific attention should be directed to a history of blood transfusions, intravenous drug use, promiscuous sexual activity, and ethanol use. A history of medication use should be sought, particularly drugs known to cause either cholestasis, such as anabolic steroids and chlorpromazine, or hepatocellular necrosis, such as acetaminophen or isoniazid. A history of arthralgias may suggest acute viral hepatitis. Viral disease should also be considered in patients with a history of travel to developing countries endemic for enterally transmitted hepatitis E or East Asian countries, where the parenterally transmitted hepatitis B and C viruses are widespread. Pruritus is most commonly associated with chronic cholestasis, developing from either extrahepatic obstruction or cholestatic liver disease such as sclerosing cholangitis or primary biliary cirrhosis. In contrast, acholic stools develop more commonly in patients with extrahepatic biliary obstruction from tumor, choledocholithiasis, or secondary to a congenital biliary abnormality such as an inflamed choledochal cyst. The presence of acholic and heme-positive stool (silver stools) should suggest a tumor of the distal biliary tract such as ampullary, periampullary, or cholangiocarcinoma. This combination may also be seen in patients with pancreatic carcinoma eroding into the biliary tract or duodenum. Jaundice, in the setting of previous biliary surgery, may suggest retained or recurrent stone disease, a biliary stricture, or recurrent obstruction from an enlarging tumor. Finally, a preexisting or underlying condition predisposing to hepatobiliary disease should be solicited. For example, inflammatory bowel disease, particularly ulcerative colitis, may be associated with sclerosing cholangitis. Pregnancy predisposes to cholestasis, steatosis, and acute liver failure. Right heart failure may result in hepatic congestion and cholestasis, and sepsis can cause selective disruption of bilirubin transport or generalized intrahepatic cholestasis.

Physical examination The examination is also important for directing the subsequent evaluation. Excoriations suggest prolonged cholestasis or high grade biliary obstruction, and a greenish hue to the jaundice is associated with particular severe or long-standing liver disease, such as biliary cirrhosis, sclerosing cholangitis, severe, chronic hepatitis, or long-standing malignant obstruction. Fever and epigastric or right upper quadrant tenderness is frequently associated with choledocholithiasis and cholangitis or cholecystitis. In contrast, malignant biliary obstruction commonly presents as painless jaundice. An enlarged, tender liver suggests acute hepatic inflammation or a rapidly enlarging hepatic tumor, while a palpable gallbladder suggests distal biliary obstruction from a malignant tumor. The presence of splenomegaly may provide a clue to the presence of portal hypertension, from chronic active hepatitis, severe alcoholic or acute viral hepatitis, or cirrhosis. Cirrhosis is also associated with a hyperestrogenic state that may be reflected in gynecomastia, testicular atrophy, or spider angiomata. Testicular atrophy may be particularly prominent in cirrhosis due to alcoholic liver disease or hemochromatosis. Palmar erythema, facial telangiectasia, and Dupuytren's contractures are also associated with cirrhosis, particularly as a result of chronic ethanol ingestion. Wasting or lymphadenopathy suggests malignancy, and in the presence of splenomegaly, these signs may direct consideration to a pancreatic tumor obstructing the splenic vein or a widely metastatic lymphoma. In patients whose history or examination

suggests malignancy, particular attention should be directed toward physical findings suggestive of a primary tumor, including heme-positive stool, abdominal or breast masses, thyroid nodules, and supraclavicular lymphadenopathy. Physical findings associated with specific liver diseases include distended neck veins and hepatojugular reflux (right heart failure), xanthomata (primary biliary cirrhosis), and Kayser-Fleischer rings (Wilson's disease).

Laboratory tests Initial laboratory evaluation should focus on serum bilirubin fractionation. Predominantly *unconjugated* (indirect) hyperbilirubinemia should prompt consideration of a hemolytic disorder, such as an autoimmune or microangiopathic hemolytic anemia, ineffective erythropoiesis, or resorption of a large hematoma. The most common cause of mild elevations in the unconjugated fraction, however, is Gilbert's syndrome, an inherited condition resulting from a mild deficiency in hepatic glucuronosyl transferase. Individuals with Gilbert's syndrome experience variable elevations in circulating unconjugated bilirubin, especially in association with physical stress, fever, intercurrent infection or surgery, fasting, or heavy ethanol ingestion. This mild metabolic abnormality produces no symptoms other than jaundice, and is *not* associated with liver enzyme abnormalities or adverse long-term effects.

Conjugated (direct) hyperbilirubinemia usually results from hepatocellular or cholestatic liver disease, or extrahepatic biliary obstruction. Because hepatic glucuronosyl transferase activity is normally present in great abundance, adequate bilirubin glucuronide formation can occur even with severe liver disease. In patients with primarily conjugated hyperbilirubinemia, the presence and nature of liver enzyme abnormalities usually provide important clues about the nature of the underlying process. Conjugated hyperbilirubinemia without liver enzyme abnormalities is relatively uncommon, but can be seen in pregnancy, sepsis, or after recent surgery. Isolated conjugated hyperbilirubinemia is the primary manifestation of two heritable disorders, Rotor and Dubin-Johnson syndromes, and can also be seen in some patients with the syndrome of recurrent benign intrahepatic cholestasis. As described more fully in Chap. 263, elevation of the aminotransferases out of proportion to other liver enzymes suggests hepatocellular damage, most commonly seen in toxic, viral, or ischemic hepatitis, while prominent elevations of the alkaline phosphatase, 5'-nucleotidase and/or gamma-glutamyl transpeptidase are more suggestive of intrahepatic cholestasis or extrahepatic obstruction. Although these patterns are not invariably diagnostic, they are helpful in directing the ensuing evaluation.

Patients with a clinical evaluation and laboratory findings suggestive of hepatocellular disease should be evaluated for evidence of viral hepatitis, drug toxicity, hepatic congestion, such as that produced by right ventricular failure or acute obstruction of the hepatic veins, or ischemic hepatitis. In the appropriate clinical setting, serological studies are extremely helpful for diagnosing, or excluding the diagnosis of, hepatitis A, acute and chronic hepatitis B, and hepatitis C and D. Common causes of toxic hepatitis include acetaminophen, isoniazid, and halogenated anesthetic agents. Patients with alcoholic liver disease are particularly susceptible to acetaminophen toxicity, which may occur after therapeutic doses in these individuals. For patients with probable hepatocellular disease, liver biopsy can provide important diagnostic and prognostic information. The results of percutaneous, transjugular, or laparoscopic biopsy may also provide important information for optimal therapy. The role of hepatobiliary imaging in these patients is less clearly defined. In some cases, identification of focal lesions by computed tomography (CT), ultrasonography (US) or magnetic resonance imaging (MRI) can increase the diagnostic accuracy of liver biopsy. These imaging techniques can also aid in diagnosis by suggesting the presence of hepatic fat deposition, cirrhosis, or the excessive hepatic iron deposition of hemochromatosis. US is an exquisitely sensitive means of detecting ascites. Combined with Doppler flow analysis, it can also determine the patency and direction of flow in the portal and hepatic veins, frequently enabling noninvasive diagnosis of portal vein thrombosis and Budd-Chiari syndrome.

Hepatobiliary imaging For patients whose clinical evaluation and liver chemistries suggest cholestasis or extrahepatic biliary obstruction, biliary imaging is an important early diagnostic tool to differentiate intrahepatic causes from extrahepatic obstruction. Both US and CT detect dilated extrahepatic biliary ducts with great sensitivity. In the absence of previous hepatobiliary surgery, the specificity of these tests for identifying dilated extrahepatic ducts is well above 90 percent. Both techniques are sensitive indicators of intrahepatic, portal, and pancreatic masses, and either can be effective in diagnosing biliary obstruction from tumors or impacted stones. In addition, US is an extremely effective means of detecting stones within the gallbladder and is somewhat more sensitive than CT. These imaging techniques are considerably less sensitive for detecting choledocholithiasis. Both fail to detect approximately 40 percent of intraductal stones, although selected studies suggest that CT is somewhat better at detecting stones within *nondilated* ducts.

In patients with clinical and radiographic evidence of extrahepatic biliary obstruction, further evaluation should be directed at determining the cause of the obstruction and providing rapid relief. Masses identified by US, CT, or MRI, are usually accessible to radiographically directed percutaneous biopsy. Further definition and relief of extrahepatic biliary obstruction can frequently be accomplished by *percutaneous* or *endoscopic cholangiography*. In the hands of experienced practitioners, dilated biliary ducts can be accessed percutaneously in more than 90 percent of patients, nondilated ducts in up to 70 percent. Percutaneous transhepatic cholangiography (PTC) may be particularly useful for imaging and drainage of patients with biliary obstruction above the bifurcation of the common bile duct and in patients whose obstruction cannot be relieved during endoscopic cholangiography. Collection of bile for cytologic analysis may also allow identification of the obstructing lesion. *Endoscopic retrograde cholangiopancreatography* (ERCP) is frequently the preferred technique for diagnosing and treating distal biliary obstructions. In addition to cholangiography, ERCP provides the opportunity for inspection and biopsy of the ampulla of Vater and surrounding duodenum (common sites of tumors obstructing the bile ducts), visualization of the pancreatic ducts to detect evidence of pancreatic ductal stones or small pancreatic tumors, and direct biopsy of the bile duct epithelium and pancreatic head. Both PTC and ERCP can afford relief of malignant obstruction and dissolution or fragmenting of ductal stones. ERCP also provides the opportunity for long-term relief of stone disease via endoscopic papillotomy and is the preferred approach to intraductal stones remaining after surgical or laparoscopic cholecystectomy.

For patients with a clinical presentation of cholestasis who have ducts of *normal* caliber, attention should focus on intrahepatic cholestasis caused by primary biliary cirrhosis, drugs or toxins (including ethanol), and extrahepatic obstruction *without* ductal dilation, which can be caused by primary sclerosing cholangitis or intrahepatic arterial chemotherapy and is occasionally seen in patients with AIDS ("vanishing duct syndrome") and cholangiocarcinoma. If the clinical picture is more suggestive of cholestasis or biliary cirrhosis, liver biopsy may provide the most direct route to diagnosis. In contrast, cholangiography with cytologic analysis of the bile and/or biopsy of the ductal epithelium is indicated in patients whose presentation suggests extrahepatic obstruction, such as patients with jaundice and nondilated ducts in the setting of weight loss, lymphadenopathy, or inflammatory bowel disease.

REFERENCES

BERLIN N, BERK P: Quantitative aspects of bilirubin metabolism for hematologists. Blood 57:983, 1981

BLANKAERT N, FEVERY J: Physiology and pathophysiology of bilirubin metabolism, in *Hepatology*, 2d ed, D Zakim, T Boyer, eds. Philadelphia, Saunders, 1989, p 254

BORSCH G et al: Clinical evaluation, ultrasound, cholescintigraphy, and endoscopic retrograde cholangiography in cholestasis: A prospective clinical study. J Clin Gastroenterol 10:185, 1988

CRONIN JJ: Ultrasound diagnosis of choledocholithiasis: A reappraisal. Radiology 161:133, 1986

FRANK BB et al: Clinical evaluation of jaundice: A guideline of the patient care committee of the American Gastroenterological Association. JAMA 262:3031, 1989

FRANSON TR et al: Frequency and characteristics of hyperbilirubinemia associated with bacteremia. Rev Infect Dis 7:1, 1985

MCDONAGH AF et al: Blue light and bilirubin excretion. Science 208:145, 1980

MURACA M et al: Analytic aspects and clinical interpretation of serum bilirubins. Semin Liver Dis 8:137, 1988

SCHARSCHMIDT BF et al: Approach to the patient with cholestatic jaundice. N Engl J Med 308:1515, 1983

SHERLOCK S, DOOLEY J (eds): *Diseases of the Liver and Biliary System*, 9th ed, Oxford, Blackwell, 1993, pp 199–213

VAN HOOTEGEM P et al: Serum bilirubins in hepatobiliary disease: Comparison with other liver function tests. Hepatology 5:112, 1985

WEISS JS et al: The clinical importance of a protein-bound fraction of serum bilirubin in patients with hyperbilirubinemia. N Engl J Med 309:147, 1983

43 ABDOMINAL SWELLING AND ASCITES

ROBERT M. GLICKMAN / KURT J. ISSELBACHER

ABDOMINAL SWELLING Abdominal swelling or distention is a common problem in clinical medicine and may be the initial manifestation of a systemic disease or of otherwise unsuspected abdominal disease. *Subjective* abdominal enlargement, often described as a sensation of fullness or bloating, is usually transient and is often related to a functional gastrointestinal disorder when it is not accompanied by objective physical findings of increased abdominal girth or local swelling. *Obesity* and lumbar lordosis, which may be associated with prominence of the abdomen, may usually be distinguished from true increases in the volume of the peritoneal cavity by history and careful physical examination.

Clinical history Abdominal swelling may first be noticed by the patient because of a progressive increase in belt or clothing size, the appearance of abdominal or inguinal hernias, or the development of a localized swelling. Often, considerable abdominal enlargement has gone unnoticed for weeks or months, either because of coexistent obesity or because the ascites formation has been insidious, without pain or localizing symptoms. Progressive abdominal distention may be associated with a sensation of "pulling" or "stretching" of the flanks or groins and vague low back pain. Localized *pain* usually results from involvement of an abdominal organ (e.g., a passively congested liver, large spleen, or colonic tumor). Pain is uncommon in cirrhosis with ascites, and when it is present, pancreatitis, hepatoma, or peritonitis should be considered. Tense ascites or abdominal tumors may produce increased intraabdominal pressure, resulting in *indigestion* and *heartburn* due to gastroesophageal reflux or *dyspnea, orthopnea,* and *tachypnea* from elevation of the diaphragm. A coexistent pleural effusion, more commonly on the right, presumably due to leakage of ascitic fluid through lymphatic channels in the diaphragm, also may contribute to respiratory embarrassment. The patient with diffuse abdominal swelling should be questioned about increased alcoholic intake, a prior episode of jaundice or hematuria, a change in bowel habits, or a past history of rheumatic heart disease. Such historical information may provide the clues that will lead one to suspect an occult cirrhosis, a colonic tumor with peritoneal seeding, congestive heart failure, or nephrosis.

Physical examination A carefully executed *general physical examination* can yield valuable clues concerning the etiology of abdominal swelling. Thus palmar erythema and spider angiomas suggest an underlying cirrhosis, while supraclavicular adenopathy (Virchow's node) should raise the question of an underlying gastrointestinal malignancy. *Inspection* of the abdomen is an important but often cursorily performed aspect of the abdominal examination. By noting the abdominal contour, one may be able to distinguish localized from generalized swelling. The tensely distended abdomen with tightly stretched skin, bulging flanks, and everted umbilicus is characteristic of ascites. A prominent abdominal venous pattern with the direction of flow away from the umbilicus often is a reflection of portal hypertension; venous collaterals with flow from the lower part of the abdomen toward the umbilicus suggest obstruction of the inferior vena cava; flow downward toward the umbilicus suggests superior vena cava obstruction. "Doming" of the abdomen with visible ridges from underlying intestinal loops is usually due to intestinal obstruction or distention. An epigastric mass, with evident peristalsis proceeding from left to right, usually indicates underlying pyloric obstruction. A liver with metastatic deposits may be visible as a nodular right upper quadrant mass moving with respiration.

Auscultation may reveal the high-pitched, rushing sounds of early intestinal obstruction or a succussion sound due to increased fluid and gas in a dilated hollow viscus. Careful auscultation over an enlarged liver occasionally reveals the harsh bruit of a vascular tumor, especially a hepatoma, or the leathery friction rub of a surface nodule. A venous hum at the umbilicus may signify portal hypertension and an increased collateral blood flow around the liver. A fluid wave and flank dullness which shifts with change in position of the patient are important signs that indicate the presence of peritoneal fluid. In obese patients, small amounts of fluid may be difficult to demonstrate; on occasion, the fluid may be detected by abdominal percussion with patients on their hands and knees. Small amounts of ascites often can only be detected by ultrasound examination of the abdomen. Careful percussion should serve to distinguish generalized abdominal enlargement from localized swelling due to an enlarged uterus, ovarian cyst, or distended bladder. Percussion also can outline an abnormally small or large liver. Loss of normal liver dullness may result from massive hepatic necrosis; it also may be a clue to free gas in the peritoneal cavity, as from perforation of a hollow viscus.

Palpation is often difficult with massive ascites, and ballottement of overlying fluid may be the only method of palpating the liver or spleen. A slightly enlarged spleen in association with ascites may be the only evidence of an occult cirrhosis. When there is evidence of portal hypertension, a soft liver suggests that obstruction to portal flow is extrahepatic; a firm liver suggests cirrhosis as the likely cause of the portal hypertension. A very hard or nodular liver is a clue that the liver is infiltrated with tumor, and when accompanied by ascites, it suggests that the latter is due to peritoneal seeding. The presence of a hard periumbilical nodule (Sister Mary Joseph's nodule) suggests metastatic disease from a pelvic or gastrointestinal primary tumor. A pulsatile liver and ascites may be found in tricuspid insufficiency.

An attempt should be made to determine whether a mass is solid or cystic, smooth or irregular, and whether it moves with respiration. The liver, spleen, and gallbladder should descend with respiration unless they are fixed by adhesions or extension of tumor beyond the organ. A fixed mass not descending with respiration may indicate that it is retroperitoneal. Tenderness, especially if localized, may indicate an inflammatory process such as an abscess; it also may be due to stretching of the visceral peritoneum or tumor necrosis. Rectal and pelvic examinations are mandatory; they may reveal otherwise undetected masses due to tumor or infection.

Radiographic and laboratory examinations are essential for confirming or extending the impressions gained on physical examination. Upright and recumbent films of the abdomen may demonstrate the dilated loops of intestine with fluid levels characteristic of intestinal obstruction or the diffuse abdominal haziness and loss of psoas margins suggestive of ascites. Ultrasonography is often of value in detecting ascites, determining the presence of a mass, or evaluating the size of the liver and spleen. CT scanning provides similar information. CT scanning is often necessary to visualize the retroperitoneum, pancreas, and lymph nodes. A plain film of the abdomen may reveal the distended colon of otherwise unsuspected ulcerative colitis and give valuable information as to the size of the liver and spleen. An irregular and elevated right side of the diaphragm may be a clue to a liver abscess or hepatoma. Studies of the gastrointestinal

tract with barium or other contrast media are usually necessary in the search for a primary tumor.

ASCITES The evaluation of a patient with ascites requires that the *cause* of the ascites be established. In most cases ascites will appear as a part of a well-recognized illness, i.e., cirrhosis, congestive heart failure, nephrosis, or disseminated carcinomatosis. In these situations, the physician should determine that the development of ascites is indeed a consequence of the basic underlying disease and not due to the presence of a separate or related disease process. This distinction is necessary even when the cause of ascites seems obvious. For example, when the patient with compensated cirrhosis and minimal ascites develops progressive ascites that is increasingly difficult to control with sodium restriction or diuretics, the obvious temptation is to attribute the worsening of the clinical picture to progressive liver disease. However, an occult hepatoma, portal vein thrombosis, spontaneous bacterial peritonitis, or even tuberculosis may be responsible for the decompensation. The disappointingly low success in diagnosing tuberculous peritonitis or hepatoma in the patient with cirrhosis and ascites reflects the too-low index of suspicion for the development of such superimposed conditions. Similarly, the patient with congestive heart failure may develop ascites from a disseminated carcinoma with peritoneal seeding. The thorough evaluation of each patient with ascites, even in the presence of an "obvious" cause, will help avoid these errors.

Diagnostic paracentesis (50 to 100 mL) should be part of the routine evaluation of the patient with ascites. The fluid should be examined for its gross appearance; and protein content, cell count, and differential cell count should be determined, and Gram's and acid-fast stains and culture performed. Cytologic and cell-block examination may disclose an otherwise unsuspected carcinoma. Table 43-1 presents some of the features of ascitic fluid typically found in various disease states. In some disorders, such as cirrhosis, the fluid has the characteristics of a transudate (<25 g protein per liter and a specific gravity of <1.016); in others, such as peritonitis, the features are those of an exudate. Rather than the total protein content of ascites, some authors prefer the use of a plasma-ascites albumin gradient to characterize ascites. If the difference between the plasma albumin and ascitic fluid albumin is greater than 1.1 g/dL, this is characteristic for uncomplicated cirrhotic ascites, while values less than 1.1 g/dL are seen in conditions characterized by exudative ascites. Although there is variability of the ascitic fluid in any given disease state, some features are sufficiently characteristic to suggest certain diagnostic possibilities. For example, blood-stained fluid with more than 25 g protein per liter is unusual in uncomplicated cirrhosis but is consistent with tuberculous peritonitis or neoplasm. Cloudy fluid with a predominance of polymorphonuclear cells and a positive Gram stain are characteristic of bacterial peritonitis; if most cells are lymphocytes, tuberculosis should be suspected. The complete examination of each fluid is most important, for occasionally only *one* finding may be abnormal. For example, if the fluid is a typical transudate but contains more than 250 white blood cells per microliter, the finding should be recognized as atypical for cirrhosis, nephrosis, or congestive heart failure and should warrant a search for tumor or infection. This is especially true in the evaluation of cirrhotic ascites where occult peritoneal infection may be present with only minor elevations in the white blood cell count of the peritoneal fluid (300 to 500 cells per microliter). Since Gram's stain of the fluid may be negative in a high proportion of such cases, careful culture of the peritoneal fluid is mandatory. Bedside innoculation of blood culture flasks with ascitic fluid results in a dramatically increased incidence of positive cultures when bacterial infection is present (90 versus 40 percent positivity with conventional cultures done by the laboratory). Direct visualization of the peritoneum (laparoscopy) may disclose peritoneal deposits of tumor, tuberculosis, or metastatic disease of the liver. Biopsies are taken under direct vision, often adding to the diagnostic accuracy of the procedure.

Chylous ascites refers to a turbid, milky, or creamy peritoneal fluid due to the presence of thoracic or intestinal lymph. Such a fluid

TABLE 43-1 Ascitic fluid characteristics in various disease states

Condition	Gross appearance	Specific gravity	Protein, g/dL	Cell count Red blood cells, >10,000/μL	White blood cells, per μL	Other tests
Cirrhosis	Straw-colored or bile-stained	<1.016 (95%)*	<25 (95%)	1%	<250 (90%);* predominantly mesothelial	
Neoplasm	Straw-colored, hemorrhagic, mucinous, or chylous	Variable, >1.016 (45%)	>25 (75%)	20%	>1000 (50%); variable cell types	Cytology, cell block, peritoneal biopsy
Tuberculous peritonitis	Clear, turbid, hemorrhagic, chylous	Variable, >1.016 (50%)	>25 (50%)	7%	>1000 (70%); usually >70% lymphocytes	Peritoneal biopsy, stain and culture for acid-fast bacilli
Pyogenic peritonitis	Turbid or purulent	If purulent, >1.016	If purulent, >2.5	Unusual	Predominantly polymorphonuclear leukocytes	+Gram's stain, culture
Congestive heart failure	Straw-colored	Variable, <1.016 (60%)	Variable, 15–53	10%	<1000 (90%); usually mesothelial, mononuclear	
Nephrosis	Straw-colored or chylous	<1.016	<25(100%)	Unusual	<250; mesothelial, mononuclear	If chylous, ether extraction, Sudan staining
Pancreatic ascites (pancreatitis, pseudocyst)	Turbid, hemorrhagic, or chylous	Variable, often >1.016	Variable, often >25	Variable, may be blood-stained	Variable	Increased amylase in ascitic fluid and serum

* Since the conditions of examining fluid and selecting patients were not identical in each series, the percentage figures (in the parentheses) should be taken as an indication of the order of magnitude rather than as the precise incidence of any abnormal finding.

shows Sudan-staining fat globules microscopically and an increased triglyceride content by chemical examination. Opaque milky fluid usually has a triglyceride concentration of more than 1000 mg/dL. A turbid fluid due to leukocytes or tumor cells may be confused with chylous fluid (pseudochylous), and it is often helpful to carry out alkalinization and ether extraction of the specimen. Alkali will tend to dissolve cellular proteins and thereby reduce turbidity; ether extraction will lead to clearing if the turbidity of the fluid is due to lipid. Chylous ascites is most often the result of lymphatic obstruction from trauma, tumor, tuberculosis, filariasis (see Chap. 182), or congenital abnormalities. It also may be seen in the nephrotic syndrome.

Rarely, ascitic fluid may be *mucinous* in character, suggesting either pseudomyxoma peritonei (Chap. 260) or rarely a colloid carcinoma of the stomach or colon with peritoneal implants.

On occasion, ascites may develop as a seemingly isolated finding in the absence of a clinically evident underlying disease. It is then that a careful analysis of ascitic fluid may indicate the direction the evaluation should take. A useful framework for the workup starts with an analysis of whether the fluid is an exudate or transudate. *Transudative ascites* of unclear etiology is most often due to occult cirrhosis, right-sided venous hypertension raising hepatic sinusoidal pressure, or hypoalbuminemic states such as nephrosis or protein-losing enteropathy. Cirrhosis with well-preserved liver function (normal albumin) resulting in ascites invariably is associated with significant portal hypertension (see Chap. 268). Evaluation should include liver function tests, liver-spleen scan, or other hepatic imaging procedure (i.e., CT or ultrasound) to detect nodular changes in the liver or a colloid shift of isotope to suggest portal hypertension. On occasion, a wedged hepatic venous pressure can be useful to document portal hypertension. Finally, if clinically indicated, a liver biopsy will confirm the diagnosis of cirrhosis and perhaps suggest its etiology. Other etiologies may result in hepatic venous congestion and resultant ascites. Right-sided cardiac valvular disease and particularly constrictive pericarditis should raise a high index of suspicion and may require cardiac imaging and cardiac catheterization for definitive diagnosis. Hepatic vein thrombosis is evaluated by visualizing the hepatic veins using imaging techniques (Doppler ultrasound, angiography, CT

scans, magnetic resonance imaging) to demonstrate obliteration, thrombosis, or obstruction by tumor. Uncommonly, transudative ascites may be associated with benign tumors of the ovary, particularly fibroma (Meigs's syndrome) with ascites and hydrothorax.

Exudative ascites should initiate an evaluation for primary peritoneal processes, most importantly infection and tumor. Routine bacteriologic culture of ascitic fluid often will yield a specific organism causing infectious peritonitis. Tuberculous peritonitis (see Table 43-1) is best diagnosed by peritoneal biopsy, either percutaneously or via laparoscopy. Histologic examination invariably shows granulomata that may contain acid-fast bacilli. Since cultures of peritoneal fluid and biopsies for tuberculosis may require 6 weeks, characteristic histology with appropriate stains allows antituberculosis therapy to be started promptly. Similarly, the diagnosis of peritoneal seeding by tumor can usually be made by cytologic analysis of peritoneal fluid or by peritoneal biopsy if cytology is negative. Appropriate diagnostic studies can then be undertaken to determine the nature and site of the primary tumor. Pancreatic ascites (see Table 43-1) is invariably associated with an extravasation of pancreatic fluid from the pancreatic ductal system, most commonly from a leaking pseudocyst. Ultrasound or CT examination of the pancreas followed by visualization of the pancreatic duct by direct cannulation (viz., endoscopic retrograde cholangiopancreatography, ERCP) will usually disclose the site of leakage and permit resective surgery to be carried out.

An analysis of the physiologic and metabolic factors involved in the production of ascites (see Chap. 268 for details), coupled with a complete evaluation of the nature of the ascitic fluid, will invariably disclose the etiology of the ascites and permit appropriate therapy to be instituted.

REFERENCES

EPSTEIN M: Treatment of refractory ascites. N Engl J Med 321:1675, 1989

GARCIA-TSAO G et al: The diagnosis of bacterial peritonitis. Hepatology 5:91, 1985

HOEFS JC: Globulin correction of the albumin gradient: Correlation with measured ascites colloid osmotic pressure gradients. Hepatology 16:396, 1992

PINTO PC et al: Large volume paracentesis in nonedematous patients with tense ascites: Its effect on intravascular volume. Hepatology 8:207, 1988

RECTOR WG JR, REYNOLDS TB: Superiority of the serum: Ascites albumin difference over the ascites total protein concentration in separation of "transudative" and "exudative" ascites. Am J Med 77:83, 1988

RUNYON BA: Ascitic fluid culture technique. Heptatology 8:893, 1988

————: Patients with deficient ascitic fluid opsonic activity are predisposed to spontaneous bacterial peritonitis. Hepatology 8:632, 1988

RUNYON BA et al: The serum-ascites albumin gradient in the differential diagnosis of ascites. Ann Int Med 117:215, 1992

section 6 Alterations in urinary function and electrolytes

44 ALTERATIONS IN URINARY FUNCTION

FREDRIC L. COE

AZOTEMIA, OLIGURIA, AND ANURIA

AZOTEMIA Urea and creatinine concentrations in serum are often measured to assess the glomerular filtration rate (GFR). Both substances are produced at a reasonably constant rate, by the liver and muscles, respectively. As discussed in Chap. 235, they undergo complete glomerular filtration and are not reabsorbed extensively by the renal tubules; hence their clearances tend to reflect the GFR. An increase in their serum concentrations, termed *azotemia* (*azo*, "containing nitrogen"), occurs as the GFR falls. Creatinine is a more reliable index of GFR than urea because of the latter's lower back-diffusion from tubule lumen to peritubular blood. The GFR may be reduced by a fall in the filtration rates of individual functioning nephrons or by a reduction in the number of functioning nephrons. (See Table 44-1.)

Reduced single-nephron GFR TUBULAR FUNCTION NORMAL An important response of the normal kidney to a severe sodium-conserving stimulus, such as extracellular fluid volume depletion, is reduction of the single-nephron glomerular filtration rate (SNGFR) and subsequent reabsorption of an increased fraction of the reduced amounts of NaCl and water that enter the tubules. The resulting azotemia is called *prerenal azotemia*, in which urinary Na concentration falls below 20 (often below 1) mmol/L (see Table 44-1). The fractional excretion of Na can be calculated (see Chap. 236) and used as an additional index of prerenal azotemia. Secretion of vasopressin is stimulated by depletion of extracellular fluid volume, and as a consequence, the distal tubules and collecting ducts become fully permeable to water. The concentrating mechanisms in the inner medulla (Chap. 235) are efficient when flow rates through the loops of Henle and the collecting ducts are low. As a result, the filtrate that escapes reabsorption in the proximal tubule undergoes maximal osmotic concentration, the urine volume becomes small, and it has a high osmolality, above 500 mmol/kg of water. Most of the filtered creatinine escapes tubular reabsorption, and consequently, the ratio of the urine-to-plasma (U/P) creatinine concentrations is high, 40 or more. Because urea can back-diffuse more completely than creatinine, the blood urea nitrogen (BUN) level rises more than the serum creatinine concentration. Normally, the ratio of BUN to serum creatinine concentration is 10:1; with depletion of the extracellular fluid volume, this ratio rises. An elevated ratio also can be produced by unrelated factors such as tetracycline administration, glucocorticoid therapy, the presence of blood in the gastrointestinal tract, and increased protein turnover due to trauma or burn.

Prerenal azotemia can occur in any edema-forming condition during the phase in which NaCl and water accumulate. Typical examples include the nephrotic syndrome and hepatic cirrhosis with ascites (Chaps. 33 and 240). When a diuretic is administered to inhibit the tubular reabsorption of NaCl, urine volume and Na concentration may be normal or elevated, even though SNGFR falls in response to the combination of the underlying edema-forming stimulus and further extracellular fluid volume depletion from the drug. Oliguria may appear upon withdrawal of the drug as the renal tubules resume intense reabsorption of NaCl and water. Prerenal azotemia also may be seen when renal blood flow is reduced by systemic hypotension, partial renal arterial or venous occlusion, or other cause (Chap. 236). Acute incomplete obstruction of the ureter and acute glomerular injury also may reduce SNGFR and leave tubule function relatively intact; *postrenal azotemia* is a term often applied when acute obstruction lowers SNGFR and causes azotemia. Whenever chronic obstruction of any portion of the urinary tract or glomerulonephritis damages nephrons extensively, the high urinary osmolality, high U/P ratios for creatinine or urea, and low urinary Na concentrations disappear, and the kidneys behave as they do when nephron number is reduced.

TUBULE FUNCTION IMPAIRED Certain acute renal diseases that produce azotemia lower SNGFR and at the same time damage the tubules sufficiently to reduce or even abolish their reabsorptive function, producing *acute renal failure*. Acute tubular necrosis, nephrotoxic agents, and acute tubulointerstitial disease are excellent examples. Azotemia and oliguria appear, but the urinary Na concentration exceeds 20 mmol and usually 40 mmol/L; the U/P ratios for urea and creatinine are below 2 and 20, respectively; and urine osmolality is below 350 mmol/kg of water. The ratio of BUN to serum creatinine is not elevated (see Chap. 236).

Reduced nephron number INCREASED SNGFR If one kidney is removed, the other grows, its nephrons enlarge, and the SNGFR increases until the total GFR becomes nearly normal for two kidneys. The tubules are overperfused with filtrate, but they appear to cope with their increased reabsorptive burdens, perhaps in part because they are longer and wider and possess more cells. If more kidney tissue is removed, the remnant nephrons enlarge further, and their SNGFR rises. Extreme overperfusion of the tubules interferes with Na conservation. At the same time, total GFR comes to depend more and more on expansion of the extracellular fluid volume, largely because the increase in SNGFR is due not only to anatomic growth of the glomeruli but also to a relatively high rate of blood flow per glomerulus. Nephron adaptations to reduced nephron number are detailed in Chap. 235.

Azotemia ensues because the total GFR, i.e., the product of the elevated SNGFR and the markedly reduced nephron number, is low. Tubular conservation of filtered H$_2$O and Na conservation are poor, so fluid and salt intake must be liberal. Clinical states that produce this picture include surgical loss of renal substance secondary to trauma, neoplasm, stone, and destruction of kidneys by bacterial infection or tuberculosis, polycystic and medullary cystic renal diseases, and all the chronic tubulointerstitial nephropathies (Chaps. 242 and 244). In each of these disorders, the nephrons that remain viable are either fully intact or behave as though the SNGFR is better preserved than tubule function.

TABLE 44-1 Pathophysiologic mechanisms of azotemia

Mechanism of reduced GFR	Clinical examples	Laboratory findings					
		Oliguria	Urine osm, mosmol/kg	Urine [Na^+], mmol/L	$\left[\dfrac{U}{P}\right]_{creat}$	$\left[\dfrac{U}{P}\right]_{urea}$	$\dfrac{BUN}{Serum\ creat}$
REDUCED SNGFR							
Tubules normal (prerenal azotemia)	Severe dehydration, edema-forming states, diuretic agents, systemic hypotension, acute glomerular disease,* acute urinary obstruction, incomplete renal vascular obstruction	Nearly always present	>500	<20	>40	>8	>10
Tubules damaged (acute renal failure)	Acute tubular necrosis, nephrotoxic agents, glomerulonephritis with tubule injury	Common	<350	>40	<20	>2	10
REDUCED NEPHRON NUMBER							
Elevated SNGFR	Chronic tubulointerstitial-renal disease Surgical loss of renal tissue	Rare†	[290	>40	3–10	3–10]	10
Normal SNGFR	Diffuse chronic glomerulonephritis Diabetic nephropathy	Rare†	[100–350‡	10–100‡	>10	>3]	>10
Reduced SNGFR	Any of the factors that can reduce SNGFR (listed above) may lower SNGFR in a patient who has a reduced number of functioning nephrons	Common	290	>20	>10	<3	>10

* Acute obstruction causing reduced SNGFR is called *postrenal azotemia*.
† Occurs only when total GFR is below 5 percent normal; urine chemistry values are helpful only when oliguria is present and are therefore enclosed in brackets.
‡ Varies with diet and with the level of GFR. When GFR is below 20 percent normal, osmotic concentration of the urine is usually impossible.
NOTE: osm = osmolality; creat = creatinine concentration; U = urine; P = plasma.

SNGFR NORMAL The SNGFR does not appear to increase despite a reduction of nephron number in diseases such as glomerulonephritis and diabetic glomerulosclerosis, where the glomerulus is the primary site of damage. In these diseases, total GFR falls directly with nephron number and is not supported by elevated SNGFR. Since the tubules are not confronted with an excessive reabsorptive burden, sodium conservation is adequate. In these disorders, superimposed conditions that lower SNGFR, such as depletion of extracellular fluid volume, can cause oliguria with low urine sodium concentration and U/P ratios for creatinine and urea above 20 and 3, respectively. The serum urea-to-creatinine ratio will rise distinctly.

SNGFR REDUCED In patients with chronic renal disease in whom total GFR is sufficient to support life only because of a very high SNGFR, inadvertent dehydration or any other factor (Table 44-1 and Chaps. 235 and 236) that lowers the SNGFR can provoke oliguria and severe azotemia. Under these circumstances, urine Na concentration falls, but not below 20 mmol/L, as in the normal person, because SNGFR, though reduced from a previously high level, may still be above normal. The U/P ratios for creatinine and urea will be low, usually below 10 and 3, respectively, despite oliguria, and urine osmolality will not rise above the plasma level. The serum urea-to-creatinine ratio may rise, but not above 20. In less extreme situations, reduction of SNGFR worsens azotemia and alters urine chemistry in the same directions but to a lesser extent.

OLIGURIA AND ANURIA *Oliguria* refers to a urine volume insufficient to sustain life, usually less than 400 mL/d in an adult of average size. Daily urine volume is difficult to measure when flow rate is low, because small absolute errors of volume measurement, in the range of 50 to 100 mL/d of urine, or of timing of collection, may represent large percentage errors.

Anuria, which is the absence of urine flow, is caused usually by urinary obstruction, which must be excluded as a first step (Chap. 246), or by total renal arterial and venous occlusion. Severe renal diseases such as cortical necrosis and rapidly progressive glomerulonephritis produce anuria in the adult so rarely that anuria should never be ascribed to a primary renal disease until patency of the urinary tract and major renal blood vessels has been established.

Approach to the patient with azotemia or oliguria A critical issue is whether azotemia has been stable and long-standing (chronic renal failure; see Chap. 234) or is recent and increasing (acute renal failure; see Chap. 236; pre- and postrenal azotemia). If azotemia is recent and oliguria is present, the most discriminating additional measurements include serum urea and creatinine concentrations and the Na, urea, and creatinine concentrations and osmolality of a concurrent urine sample. Reduction of SNGFR with well-preserved tubule function is usually present when urine osmolality exceeds 500 mmol/kg of water, Na < 20 mmol/L, the U/P ratios for urea and creatinine > 8 and 40, respectively, the urinalysis is normal, and the BUN > 10 times the serum creatinine concentration. The prognosis for recovery of adequate GFR is good if the cause of reduced SNGFR can be reversed. When urine osmolality is below 350 mmol/kg of water, Na > 40 mmol, the U/P values for urea and creatinine < 2 and 20, respectively, and the BUN exceeds the serum creatinine by only tenfold, tubule function has been lost, and some form of acute or chronic renal failure is present.

ABNORMAL URINARY CONSTITUENTS

PROTEINURIA Normal adults may excrete up to 150 mg/d protein. Of this, only 5 to 15 mg is albumin; the rest is composed of over 30 different plasma proteins and of glycoproteins that derive from the renal cells. Tamm-Horsfall mucoprotein, the most prevalent urine protein that does not arise from plasma, is produced by the cells of the ascending limb of the loop of Henle and is excreted at the rate of 50 to 75 mg/d. Daily excretion of more than 150 mg protein is properly termed *pathologic proteinuria*, but in common usage the word *proteinuria* suffices. Protein excretion above 3.5 g/24 h is termed *massive* proteinuria and usually occurs when glomeruli have been damaged enough to allow plasma proteins, especially albumin, to enter the urine. Urinary albumin loss lowers serum albumin concentration, and the consequent fall in intracapillary oncotic pressure fosters the accumulation of tissue edema (Chap. 33); serum lipids rise, for reasons detailed in Chap. 240. The combination of *massive proteinuria, hypoalbuminemia, edema*, and *hyperlipidemia* is often called the *nephrotic syndrome*, but this term is also used for massive urinary protein loss alone. Massive proteinuria causes hypoalbuminemia, elevated blood lipids, and edema only when hepatic albumin synthesis, although normal or even increased, fails to compensate for urine albumin losses; these features are not a direct result of renal disease.

Detection of proteinuria Proteinuria is usually detected by urine "dipsticks" that register a trace result in response to as little as 50 mg protein per liter and a distinct color change of the 1 + level at about 300 mg protein per liter. Since proteinuria can be missed if the urine is dilute, fasting morning samples that tend to be concentrated are usually studied. Dipsticks respond best to albumin, so a negative result can occur when large amounts of other protein, or protein fragments such as light chains, are excreted. Dipstick proteinuria requires additional documentation by the measurement of 24-h excretion rate. If total protein excretion is abnormal, it is helpful to characterize the proportions of albumin and globulins in the urine by cellulose acetate electrophoresis or other methods. Immunoelectrophoresis is required to identify immunoglobulin fragments, kappa or lambda light chains, when their presence is suggested by a monoclonal peak on routine urine electrophoresis.

Mechanisms of proteinuria TUBULAR PROTEINURIA Low-molecular-weight ($<40,000$) serum proteins, such as $beta_2$ microglobulin (11,600 mol wt), lysozyme (14,000 mol wt), or light chains (22,000 mol wt) are readily filtered by the glomeruli but are reabsorbed so efficiently that only trace amounts enter the urine. Diseases that selectively damage the tubules more than glomeruli (Chap. 242) cause excessive excretion of these small proteins with little or no increase in albumin excretion. The resulting proteinuria is usually between 1 and 3 g/24 h, and edema and lipid disorders do not occur because albumin losses are small. Bence Jones protein, which is probably a dimer of two light chains, light chains themselves, and myoglobin are examples of proteins whose plasma concentrations may increase as a consequence of disease. If the filtered load rises to exceed tubular reabsorptive capacity, "overflow" proteinuria may occur.

GLOMERULAR PROTEINURIA Normal glomeruli filter little albumin or globulin. Glomerular capillary endothelial cells form a barrier penetrated by pores of about 100 nm diameter that holds back cells and other particles but offers no impediment to most proteins. The glomerular basement membrane traps molecules about 5 nm in effective radius, above 100,000 Da molecular mass. The *foot processes (podocytes)* of the visceral epithelial cells (Fig. 44-1) cover the urinary aspect of the glomerular basement membrane and produce a series of narrow channels through which molecules traverse the basement membrane. Anionic molecules, like albumin, are filtered less freely than are neutral or positively charged molecules of the same size, so little albumin enters the filtrate. This charge selectively appears to be due to anionic glycoproteins that cover the surfaces of the foot processes and contribute to the matrix structure of the basement membrane (Chap. 235). The glycoproteins are anionic due to their content of glutamate, aspartate, and sialic acid. At the pH of blood (7.4) or urine (4.5 to 7.5) carboxylic and sialic acid residues are dissociated and, therefore, have a negative charge; albumin also carries a negative charge. The negatively charged glycoproteins repel albumin and retard albumin filtration.

Glomerular disease can disrupt any of these filtration barriers. Injury limited to the polyanion glycoproteins tends to produce selective losses of anionic proteins, such as albumin, that would be filtered more completely by the normal glomerulus but for their charge. Extensive injury that involves the entire basement membrane, not only its polyanion components, may increase losses of very large proteins as well as albumin.

The selectivity of proteinuria varies with the extent of glomerular injury. However, the clinical value of measuring selectivity has not been fully defined. The basis of such measurements is to express the excretion rate of a protein as a fraction of its theoretical maximal filtered load, which is the product of its serum concentration and the

FIGURE 44-1 *(Top).* Diagram showing normal structures separating the capillary lumen and urinary space in the glomerulus. In the process of glomerular filtration, an ultrafiltrate of plasma traverses the glomerular capillary wall through endothelial fenestrae, basement membrane, and slit diaphragms. Macromolecules in the plasma are believed to be restricted from entry into glomerular urine by each of these wall structures. In addition, circulating polyanions (e.g., albumin) are thought to be retarded by negatively charged glycosialoproteins, which, as shown by the shaded area in the upper panel, are distributed throughout the glomerular wall. *(Bottom).* A corresponding electron micrograph of the same structures. *(Drawing by NL Gahan from BM Brenner, R Beeuwkes, Hosp Prac, vol 13, no 7, 1978. Reproduced with permission.)*

GFR. This fraction must reflect the relative filtration efficiency of the protein to that of a completely filtered GFR marker, usually inulin or creatinine, provided that tubular reabsorption and renal production or catabolism are negligible. The slope of a plot of the clearance ratio against molecular weight for a variety of serum proteins is one index of filtration selectivity. A more practical version of this test is based on the ratio of the clearance fractions of two proteins of different molecular weight, such as IgG and transferrin (Chap. 240).

Approach to the patient with proteinuria If the dipstick proteinuria is 1 + or more, 24-h urine protein excretion should be measured. If it is above 150 mg, the proportions of albumin and other proteins should be determined by electrophoresis. Excretion mainly of albumin signifies a glomerular lesion. When the total daily protein excretion exceeds 3.5 g, by definition, the nephrotic syndrome is considered to be present; milder albuminuria is called an *asymptomatic urinary abnormality*. The initial steps in evaluating proteinuria are outlined in Chap. 234. Subsequent details of differential diagnosis are in Chaps. 240 and 241. Tubular proteinuria usually reflects a hereditary or acquired tubular disorder (Chap. 244) or tubulointerstitial nephropathy (Chap. 242). The presence of large amounts of Bence Jones protein suggests that multiple myeloma may be present (Chap. 280).

HEMATURIA AND CASTS **Isolated hematuria** Bleeding in the urinary tract from the urethra to the renal pelvis produces isolated hematuria, without significant proteinuria, cells, or urinary casts. Total hematuria, which occurs evenly throughout voiding, means that blood has had the opportunity to mix fully with the bladder urine. When bleeding occurs mainly at the beginning or end of micturition, a prostatic or urethral origin is more likely.

Common causes of *isolated* hematuria are urinary tract stones, benign and malignant neoplasms of the urinary tract, tuberculosis, trauma, and prostatitis; few primary renal diseases cause it. As discussed in Chaps. 234 and 240, *focal glomerulitis*, in the syndrome of benign recurrent hematuria or in Berger's disease, i.e., IgA nephropathy, is usually associated with red blood cell casts. Analgesic nephropathy and sickle cell disorders cause isolated hematuria but modest proteinuria; the coexistence of papillary necrosis or azotemia suggests a renal origin. Hemoglobin electrophoresis is appropriate whenever a sickle cell disorder is suspected.

Examination of the prostate and external urethra is the first step in the evaluation of isolated hematuria. Intravenous pyelography and renal ultrasonography are the next. If no lesion is found and no cause of bleeding such as renal stone passage is obvious, cystoscopy and retrograde pyelography may be necessary. At cystoscopy, blood may issue from only one ureter, a helpful clue which indicates a localized lesion rather than a primary renal disease. Disorders of coagulation and thrombocytopenia, as well as urinary infection, must be excluded. Because infection with tuberculosis and fungi may be difficult to detect, multiple urine samples should be cultured and examined by microscopy. Computed tomography of the kidney and sometimes renal arteriography may be needed to disclose anatomic lesions such as cysts or tumors. Urine cytology may give a clue to malignant neoplasms of the kidneys or urinary tract that otherwise escape detection.

Hematuria associated with urinary tract infection   Bacterial infection of the lower urinary tract or of the kidneys frequently causes hematuria. The presence of associated pyuria suggests the diagnosis, and the demonstration of pathogenic bacteria in concentrations above 10^5 colonies per milliliter of urine establishes it. Acute cystitis or urethritis in women is a common cause of gross hematuria; in such symptomatic patients, infection is established by documenting colony counts above 10^2 colonies per milliliter. Urinary tuberculosis can produce isolated hematuria, but pyuria often is present as well.

Hematuria with evidence of renal disease   NEPHRONAL HEMATURIA   Blood that enters the tubular fluid anywhere along the nephron can be trapped in a cylindrical mold of gelled Tamm-Horsfall protein to produce red blood cell casts. Tamm-Horsfall protein gels when concentrated at a low pH, as occurs during dehydration, or when exposed to myoglobin, hemoglobin, albumin, Bence Jones protein, or pyelographic contrast media. Degenerated red blood cells and clumps of hemoglobin can produce deeply pigmented casts that have the same significance—nephronal hematuria—as red blood cell casts.

Nephronal hematuria always connotes significant renal disease such as glomerulonephritis, tubulointerstitial injury, or a vasculitis that has damaged the circulation of the nephron. Glomerular or tubular proteinuria often accompanies renal bleeding, as a consequence of nephron injury. In general, nephronal hematuria and proteinuria alone arise from renal diseases that have a better prognosis than those in which proteinuria and hematuria occur in combination (Chap. 234).

Hematuria with proteinuria or casts   Frequently, hematuria is accompanied by proteinuria, but red blood cell and deeply pigmented granular casts are absent. The presumption is that bleeding is of nephronal origin, but a coincident independent lesion of the urinary tract must always be considered, because common renal diseases, such as diabetic glomerulosclerosis and arteriolar nephrosclerosis associated with hypertension, produce mainly proteinuria.

TYPES OF CASTS   Heavy albuminuria or dehydration can cause showers of transparent, refractile *hyaline* casts. During heavy proteinuria, tubule cells fill with cholesterol-rich lipid droplets that display a Maltese-cross appearance in polarized light. Casts that incorporate these cells are called *fatty casts* because the lipid droplets are prominent. The same lipid-rich cells free in urine are called *oval fat bodies*.

White blood cell and *epithelial cell casts* can occur in any inflammatory state that involves the nephrons. White blood cell casts are particularly common in pyelonephritis, in nephritis associated with systemic lupus erythematosus, and during transplant rejection.

When white blood or epithelial cells degenerate, they form granular nonpigmented casts that contain cellular debris and aggregated proteins. So-called *waxy* casts, with few granules and very distinct margins, arise when cell debris has broken down to a fine dispersion so that granules are no longer visible and are most common in chronic and progressive renal diseases.

Broad casts, of unusual width, are thought to arise in the dilated tubules of enlarged nephrons that have undergone compensatory hypertrophy in response to a reduction of functioning renal mass. A urine sample that contains a combination of broad and waxy casts as well as cellular or granular casts or red blood cells indicates a chronic smoldering process and has been termed a *telescoped* urine. This abnormality, first described in polyarteritis nodosa and systemic lupus erythematosus, also is found in many chronic forms of glomerulonephritis with active glomerulitis.

Approach to the patient with hematuria   Many urinalyses should be performed to determine whether the hematuria is isolated or associated with other features of primary renal disease, i.e., cells, casts, or proteinuria. The magnitude and type of associated proteinuria should be determined. Intravenous pyelography should be performed, if it can be done safely, even when the hematuria is of nephronal origin. Not only lesions of the urinary tract, but renal tumors or cysts, discrete areas of papillary necrosis, or signs of renal venous obstruction may be present. The source of isolated hematuria must always be ascertained, and this means a detailed examination of the urinary tract by cystoscopy, retrograde pyelography, and arteriography to disclose tumor, stone, cysts, or other cause. Renal ultrasonography and computed tomography are particularly helpful in detecting and evaluating renal cysts and tumors and should precede cystoscopy and arteriography. If all the studies disclose normal structures, a nephronal origin of hematuria is likely even if no red blood cell casts are present. The role of renal biopsy in such cases is detailed in Chaps. 240, 241, and 242. Hematuria with infection or overt renal disease usually requires no steps beyond intravenous pyelography. Evaluation of hematuria is detailed in Chap. 227.

POLYURIA AND NOCTURIA

POLYURIA   A reasonable definition of polyuria is a urine volume above 3 L/d, with the recognition that normal individuals who drink a large amount of fluid intake form large volumes of urine. Patients cannot always distinguish polyuria from urinary frequency, the frequent voiding of small volumes. Since voiding volumes may not be clear from the history, polyuria must be substantiated by 24-h urine collection before investigating the cause.

Causes   Polyuria can arise from inadequate secretion of vasopressin, failure of the renal tubules to respond to vasopressin, solute diuresis, or natriuresis (Table 44-2). It also may occur as a physiologic response to excessive water drinking. The physiology of urine formation and mechanisms for renal water conservation are discussed in Chap. 235.

DIABETES INSIPIDUS (See also Chap. 333)   The term *diabetes insipidus* is applied to situations in which inadequate renal water conservation causes polyuria and secondary thirst, either due to vasopressin insufficiency (central diabetes insipidus) or renal unresponsiveness to vasopressin (nephrogenic diabetes insipidus). In both, water reabsorption is reduced all along the distal nephron, because passive water movement from tubules into the hypertonic outer and inner medullary interstitium is slow. Even though the rate of water movement out of the collecting ducts is low for a given osmotic difference between the tubule lumen and interstitial fluid, however, the fluid that enters the collecting ducts is so dilute and copious in volume that more water reaches the inner medulla than normal and medullary solutes are washed into the vasa recta. Wash-out is incomplete; while vasopressin administration can lead to formation of a concentrated urine, the maximal urine osmolality attained is below normal.

TABLE 44-2 Causes of polyuria

INADEQUATE RENAL WATER CONSERVATION

A Diabetes insipidus
   1 Vasopressin-sensitive (posthypophysectomy; posttrauma; postpituitary ablation; idiopathic, supra- or intrasellar tumors or cysts; histiocystosis or granuloma; encroachment by aneurysm; Sheehan's syndrome, meningoencephalitis; Guillain-Barré syndrome; fat embolus; empty sella)
   2 Nephrogenic
       a Acquired tubulointerstitial renal disease (pyelonephritis, analgesic nephropathy, multiple myeloma, amyloidosis, obstructive uropathy, sarcoidosis, hypercalcemic or hypokalemic nephropathy, Sjögren's syndrome, sickle cell anemia, renal transplantation)
       b Drugs or toxins (lithium, demeclocycline, methoxyflurane, ethanol, diphenylhydantoin, propoxyphene, amphotericin)
       c Congenital (hereditary nephrogenic diabetes insipidus, polycystic or medullary cystic disease)
B Solute diuresis (glucosuria, high-protein tube feedings, urea or mannitol infusion, radiographic contrast media, chronic renal failure)
C Natriuretic syndromes (salt-losing nephritis, diuretic phase of acute tubular necrosis, diuretic agents)

PRIMARY POLYDIPSIA

A Psychogenic
B Hypothalamic disease
C Drugs (thioridazine, chlorpromazine, anticholinergic agents)

Vasopressin-sensitive (central) diabetes insipidus may be idiopathic or secondary to hypophysectomy or trauma or to neoplastic, inflammatory, vascular, or infectious causes (Table 44-2). Idiopathic diabetes insipidus can be inherited as an autosomal dominant trait; more commonly, it is sporadic and appears in childhood. In both forms there is selective destruction of the neurons that produce vasopressin in the supraoptic nucleus.

Rarely, nephrogenic diabetes insipidus is familial and congenital, but usually it is acquired (Table 44-2). Hypercalcemia and hypokalemic nephropathy are reversible causes of nephrogenic diabetes insipidus. Lithium carbonate, methoxyflurane anesthesia, and demeclocycline also can produce nephrogenic diabetes insipidus.

SOLUTE DIURESIS Excessive filtration of a poorly resorbed solute such as glucose, mannitol, or urea can depress reabsorption of NaCl and water in the proximal tubule and cause their loss in the urine, producing polyuria. Urine Na concentration is below that of blood, so more water than salt is lost from the body and the serum is hypertonic. Glucosuria in diabetes mellitus is a common cause of solute diuresis. Iatrogenic solute diuresis may arise from mannitol infusion, angiographic contrast media, and high-protein gavage feedings, which produce an excessive excretion of urea. Any solute diuresis can cause polyuria, so further evaluation of renal concentrating ability should be postponed until the solute diuresis is corrected.

NATRIURETIC SYNDROMES Excessive chronic Na loss may occur during the course of tubulointerstitial or cystic renal disease. Polyuria and polydipsia are accompanied by a large daily Na requirement. Examples include medullary cystic disease, Bartter's syndrome, and the diuretic phase of acute tubular necrosis, in which Na and water losses are large.

PRIMARY POLYDIPSIA Whether because of habit, predilection, psychiatric disorder, a specific lesion in the brain, or medication (Table 44-2), some people drink enough water every day to produce polyuria. The body and the kidneys rarely, if ever, are injured by chronic polydipsia, but the condition can be confused with diabetes insipidus, which it resembles closely. During deliberate polydipsia, extracellular fluid volume is normal or high, and vasopressin secretion is reduced to a basal level because serum osmolality tends to be near the lower limits of normal. Reabsorption of water from the distal convoluted tubule and collecting ducts is reduced so that all the surplus water can be excreted into the urine. The inner medulla loses its urea and NaCl gradients because of wash-out, as in diabetes insipidus. Wash-out may be more severe than in diabetes insipidus

because primary polydipsia tends to cause expansion of the extracellular fluid volume, whereas primary renal water loss does the opposite. Volume expansion raises total delivery of NaCl and water to the thick ascending limb of Henle and therefore to the inner medulla, all things being equal. It also raises renal blood flow, and increased flow through the vasa recta reduces their ability to trap solutes in the medulla.

Approach to the patient with polyuria Solute diuresis and natriuretic syndromes usually are apparent from the history, physical examination, urinalysis (glucosuria), clinical setting, blood count, blood glucose, and serum creatinine or BUN. Diagnostic problems occur mainly when stable, chronic polyuria and polydipsia of uncertain origin are present. Here one must try to distinguish between vasopressin-sensitive diabetes insipidus, nephrogenic diabetes insipidus, and primary polydipsia; the best way to make this distinction is by measuring the response of urine osmolality to water deprivation and the administration of vasopressin.

The subject should have free access to water and receive a normal diet that provides approximately 100 mmol NaCl per day for 3 days; then a total fast is instituted. During the fast, pulse and blood pressure should be measured every 30 min, and body weight should be measured every hour using an accurate balance. When 3 percent of the initial body weight has been lost or 14 h has elapsed, urine and serum osmolality are measured. In the normal subject urine volume will be below 0.5 mL/min, and urine osmolality will be above 700 mmol/kg of water. In complete diabetes insipidus, nephrogenic or vasopressin-sensitive, the urine osmolality will remain below 200 mmol/kg of water and urine flow above 0.5 mL/min, but some rise in osmolality and fall in flow occurs in incomplete diabetes insipidus. If urine osmolality is below 700 mmol/kg of water by the end of the fasting period, 5 mU/min aqueous arginine vasopressin or 1 μg desmopressin is administered by subcutaneous injection. Patients with complete or partial vasopressin-sensitive diabetes insipidus will raise their urine osmolality above the level achieved by fasting alone by more than 9 percent (see Chap. 333). No increase will occur in complete nephrogenic diabetes insipidus, although incomplete forms of nephrogenic diabetes insipidus will permit some response to vasopressin. Infusion of hypertonic saline (Chap. 333) is useful in defining defects of osmoregulator function.

Patients with primary polydipsia respond differently. During fluid restriction, the secretion of vasopressin increases, and at the completion of the test the flow rate and osmolality of the urine reflect a physiologic level of vasopressin acting on normal tubules that traverse a medullary interstitium whose urea and NaCl concentrations have been reduced by chronic wash-out. In other words, the wash-out sets the upper limit on urine osmolality, and patients with primary polydipsia thus demonstrate a submaximal concentrating ability despite intact vasopressin secretion. Exogenous vasopressin can increase urine osmolality very little (<9 percent) because medullary wash-out, not vasopressin insufficiency or insensitivity, is the main limiting factor. Usually the urine osmolality will be above 400 mmol/kg of water by the end of the fluid deprivation test, in contrast to the values of approximately 200 mmol/kg of water in patients with diabetes insipidus; in some cases it may be impossible to distinguish incomplete diabetes insipidus from primary polydipsia with the fluid deprivation test alone. Measurement of serum arginine vasopressin levels by radioimmunoassay is rarely of diagnostic help.

NOCTURIA Whether an individual sleeps through the night without urinating depends on a diurnal rhythm in which the volume of urine formed during sleep does not exceed bladder capacity, because of reduced renal osmotic concentration, high sodium excretion, solute diuresis, or low bladder capacity.

All polyuric states may cause nocturia. Urinary concentrating ability falls in most renal diseases (Chap. 235), often at an early stage. Even though overt polyuria may be absent, overnight urine volume frequently exceeds bladder capacity. Nocturia also occurs in edema-forming states. In congestive heart failure, nephrotic syndrome, and hepatic cirrhosis with ascites, fluid accumulates preferentially in dependent portions of the body during the day. At night, with recumbency, tissue capillary forces change, and some edema fluid is mobilized, producing the effect of an intravenous saline infusion. Venous insufficiency may produce dependent edema of the legs that is also mobilized at night, causing nocturia.

Reduced bladder capacity also causes nocturia. Infection, tumor, or stone can cause inflammation and increased bladder irritability. Chronic partial bladder outflow obstruction, from prostatic hyperplasia, urethral stricture, or benign or malignant neoplasm or stone, causes a stimulus to void and a thickening of the muscular wall that reduces its compliance. Frequent small voidings may be a clue to this cause of nocturia, but in its earlier phases bladder obstruction may cause only one nocturnal voiding of reasonable volume.

DYSURIA, FREQUENCY AND URGENCY, INCONTINENCE, AND ENURESIS

DYSURIA, FREQUENCY, AND URGENCY *Dysuria* refers to pain or a burning sensation during urination. *Urinary frequency* means voiding at frequent intervals, due to a sense of bladder fullness that is due not to a full bladder but to an irritable bladder that feels full even when it is not. *Urgency* is an exaggerated sense of needing to urinate, due to an irritable or inflamed bladder.

Mechanisms of dysuria REDUCED BLADDER COMPLIANCE When the ability of the bladder to expand is reduced, frequency, nocturia, and urgency result. When decreased expansion is due to inflammation of the mucosa (cystitis) from infection, radiation, chemicals, or foreign bodies (catheters, stones), a burning sensation usually is more intense than when it is due to infiltration of the muscle by tumors of the bladder or from adjacent organs (prostate, rectum, uterus).

INFECTION Acute bacterial cystitis, which occurs more frequently in women, usually causes frequent urination day and night, a burning sensation on urination, and, not infrequently, gross hematuria. Prostatitis or prostatocystitis in men can cause a picture similar to acute cystitis in women. When only the prostate is involved, milder symptoms such as vague pain or discomfort in the lower abdomen, groin, perineum, rectum, testes, or penis occur. The symptoms may be associated with urination but usually is noticed at times other than during urination or ejaculation.

PSYCHOSOMATIC CYSTITIS The *functional bladder syndrome* and *chronic glandular urethrotrigonitis* are synonyms for a very common but poorly understood affliction of middle-aged and older women, in which pain is usually vague, aching in nature, and in the lower abdomen or vagina. There is daytime frequency without nocturia; pyuria is absent. A complete urologic evaluation usually becomes necessary because symptoms are chronic and hard to eradicate. The functional bladder syndrome must be distinguished from the effects of a cystocele, which can be repaired surgically.

Approach to the patient with dysuria The medical history should focus on past as well as present urinary problems. A pelvic examination in women and prostatic examination in men are necessary components of the physical examination. A two-glass urinary sediment in all patients and the prostatic fluid in men, obtained by prostatic massage, should be examined by microscopy. When the urethra is the principal site of inflammation or infection, the first 20 mL of a voiding, if collected separately, may contain a higher concentration of leukocytes and bacteria than the remainder of the voided urine. Normal prostatic fluid, not subjected to centrifugation, contains less than 10 leukocytes per high-power field; leukocytosis in the prostatic fluid is an important clue to prostatitis and may, when prostatitis is chronic, be the only detectable abnormality. Further diagnostic studies will depend on such features as a history of chronic or recurrent episodes or associated fever, which are rare in lower urinary tract infections except in acute prostatitis; an abnormality on physical examination, such as a pelvic or rectal mass or tenderness, hematuria, or pyuria; or increased excessive leukocytes and macrophages in the prostatic fluid.

Additional evaluation of dysuria, when the cause is not evident from clinical examination, may include cultures of urine and prostatic fluid for aerobic and anaerobic bacteria, tubercle bacilli, and mycoplasmas; excretory urography; and voiding cystourethrography. If these examinations do not reveal the diagnosis but symptoms are troublesome, urologic evaluations, including cystoscopy, urethroscopy, and endoscopic biopsies of visualized abnormalities, and dynamic urinary tract studies may be useful.

INCONTINENCE *Incontinence*, the inability to retain urine in the bladder, results from neurologic or mechanical disorders of the system that controls normal micturition.

Normal bladder function The detrusor muscle, which provides the propulsive force for emptying the bladder, consists of interlacing fibers of smooth muscle that are under parasympathetic autonomic control through the pelvic nerves from sacral spinal cord segments S2, S3, and S4. The smooth muscle of the trigonal portion of the bladder, between the ureteral orifices and the posterior area of the bladder outlet, is innervated by motor fibers from thoracolumbar segments (T11 to L2) of the sympathetic nervous system, in which alpha receptor sites predominate. This layer of muscle extends into the posterior urethra and acts as an involuntary internal sphincter that helps maintain urinary continence even in the absence of voluntary control. The external urethral sphincter and perineal muscles are under voluntary control via the pudendal nerves.

Sensory tracts of pain, temperature, and distention pass from the bladder via the pelvic nerves to sacral spinal levels S2, S3, and S4, creating a spinal voiding reflex between the bladder and the sacral spinal cord. The sensory tracts from the bladder further ascend through sacrobulbar pathways to the medulla of the brain and ultimately to cortical centers, from which impulses arise, pass back down the lateral and ventral reticulospinal tracts, and normally suppress the sacral spinal reflex arc controlling bladder emptying.

The normal adult bladder can accommodate approximately 400 mL fluid without a significant increase in intravesical pressure (<20 cmH$_2$O). Above this point, sensations of fullness are transmitted to the sacral cord. If not suppressed by cortical control, the sacral cord reflexly discharges motor impulses that cause powerful sustained detrusor contraction. Urination can be prevented by cortical suppression of the reflex arc or by voluntary contraction of the external sphincter and perineal muscles. Infants and adults with spinal cord damage above S2 urinate spontaneously when the bladder fills sufficiently.

Normal urination is initiated by voluntary suppression of cortical inhibition of the reflex arc and by relaxation of the muscles of the pelvic floor and the external sphincter. The base of the bladder falls; then the trigone contracts, an action that occludes the ureters as they pass through the bladder wall and helps to prevent vesicoureteral reflux of urine during voiding. Finally, the detrusor contracts, and voiding occurs.

Causes of incontinence DETRUSOR INSTABILITY In this condition, the bladder becomes prone to uncontrollable contractions—that cause incontinence—because inhibitory neural pathways are damaged. Among the elderly, detrusor instability causes as much as 70 percent of urinary incontinence and arises from diseases of the central nervous system such as cerebrovascular accidents, Alzheimer's disease, neoplasia, and, possibly, normal-pressure hydrocephalus. Any lesion that disrupts the lateral and ventral reticulospinal tracts can reduce or abolish descending inhibiting impulses to the sacral spinal reflex and result in detrusor instability. If the descending tracts are completely destroyed, the bladder will empty automatically. Bladder or pelvic infection or tumor, fecal impaction, uterine prolapse, and prostatic hypertrophy are other causes. Whatever the cause, the usual clinical picture is of unpredictable, involuntary voiding, usually >160 mL each time. Imipramine, 25 mg at bedtime, or calcium channel blockers (such as nifedipine) reduce detrusor contractions and improve continence. Local infection, tumors, or fecal impaction are treated conventionally.

STRESS INCONTINENCE This condition is common in postmenopausal parous women. The structures of the female urethra atrophy when deprived of estrogen, and many women become unable to resist the passage of urine under the stress of increased intraabdominal pressure during coughing, sneezing, climbing stairs, and other physical activity, so small amounts of urine escape. Parturition may damage the pelvic support of the bladder so that the bladder and urethra can slip downward from their normal position above the pelvic diaphragm. As they do, the urethra shortens, and the normal urethrovesical angle, important in closing the urethral sphincter, is lost. In men, stress incontinence usually is secondary to prostatic surgery for benign prostatic hypertrophy or prostatic carcinoma. If the external sphincter is damaged during operation, total incontinence may result. Surgical elevation of the urethrovesical angle is helpful in women. Estrogen replacement therapy may prevent atrophy of the urethral mucosa.

MECHANICAL INCONTINENCE Some congenital anomalies, extrophy of the bladder, patent urachus, and ectopic ureteral openings distal to the vesical neck cause mechanical incontinence. They are correctable only by surgery. Mechanical incontinence can follow transurethral resection of the prostate that damages both the internal and external sphincter mechanisms. Pelvic surgery or irradiation of the uterus or rectum may cause incontinence because of vesicovaginal, ureterovaginal, vesicoperineal, or ureteroperineal fistulas.

OVERFLOW OR PARADOXICAL INCONTINENCE This form of incontinence arises from large residual volumes of urine secondary to obstruction at the bladder neck or the urethra (urethral stricture) or from neurologic damage. Benign prostatic hyperplasia afflicts upward of 75 percent of older men (see Chap. 323). It is manifested by nocturia, reduced size and force of the urinary stream, straining to urinate, and terminal dribbling, all due to outflow obstruction. Functional outflow obstruction can occur because of spinal cord disease; the detrusor and external sphincter contract dyssynergistically, i.e., at the same time. Hypotonic neurogenic bladders may occur in diseases that produce autonomic peripheral neuropathy, such as diabetes mellitus, uremia, hypothyroidism, chronic alcoholism, Guillain-Barré syndrome, collagen vascular diseases, and toxic neuropathies associated with some carcinomas (especially lung and kidney). It also may occur because of prolonged overdistention of the bladder. Hydronephrosis and impaired renal function can occur with chronic overflow incontinence. All causes produce a dilated, palpable bladder. Especially in diabetes, patients can control micturition but lose their sensory awareness of bladder filling. Their incontinence can be avoided by scheduled reminders. Outlet obstruction is treated surgically. If the bladder is adynamic because of prolonged overfilling, bethanechol chloride, 50 to 100 mg/d, may improve emptying.

PSYCHOGENIC AND FUNCTIONAL INCONTINENCE Children and even some young adults draw attention to themselves by feigning incontinence and thereby derive some secondary emotional satisfaction. A complete diagnostic evaluation usually is necessary to rule out organic disease even when psychogenic incontinence is strongly suspected. In elderly people, especially those with a limited ability to walk or who are confused because of central nervous system disease or drugs, incontinence may be *functional*, i.e., due simply to an inability to reach a toilet in time. Treatment depends on correcting the individual problem in each case.

ENURESIS *Enuresis* refers to the involuntary passage of urine at night or during sleep—hence the synonym *bed-wetting*. Some reserve the term enuresis for those bed-wetters who have no gross urologic abnormalities, but it is appropriate for bed-wetting in general.

The sacral spinal reflex arc alone controls urination in the infant; therefore, bed-wetting is normal under the age of 2 years. As the nervous system matures, development of cortical control over the spinal reflex arc results in the voluntary control over urination and defecation by the age of 2½ years. Even so, enuresis beyond the age of 3 years occurs to some degree in approximately 10 percent of all otherwise normal children and probably is due to a delay in maturation of bladder control, which may be familial.

Although most bed-wetting ceases by the age of puberty, organic diseases, especially infections of the urinary tract, obstructive lesions

with overflow incontinence, neurovesical dysfunction, and polyuric conditions that overload the bladder must be suspected when enuresis persists beyond the age of 3 years. Patients with organic disease usually, but not always, are incontinent during the day as well as at night. For the majority, who have no overt lesions, imipramine (75 mg at bedtime) may be useful.

REFERENCES

Azotemia, oliguria, and anuria

ABUELO JG: Proteinuria: Diagnostic principles and procedures. Ann Intern Med 98:186, 1983

BRENNER BM, LAZARUS JM (eds): *Acute Renal Failure*, 2d ed. New York, Churchill-Livingstone, 1988

GLASSOCK RJ et al: Primary glomerular diseases, in *The Kidney*, 4th ed, BM Brenner, FC Rector Jr (eds). Philadelphia, Saunders, 1991, p 1182

HILBRANDS LB et al: Cimetidine improves the reliability of creatinine as a marker of glomerular filtration. Kidney Int 40:1171, 1991

KANWAR YS: Biophysiology of glomerular filtration and proteinuria. Lab Invest 51:7, 1984

KOHLER H et al: Acanthocytosis: A characteristic marker for glomerular bleeding. Kidney Int 40:115, 1991

LEVEY AS et al: Idiopathic nephrotic syndrome. Ann Intern Med 107:697, 1987

LOON N et al: Effect of angiotensin II infusion on the human glomerular filtration barrier. Am J Physiol 257:F608, 1989

MYERS BD et al: Mechanisms of proteinuria in human glomerulonephritis. J Clin Invest 70:732, 1982

PARDO V et al: Benign primary hematuria: Clinicopathologic study of 65 patients. Am J Med 67:817, 1979

Polyuria and nocturia

BERL T (ed): Disorders of water metabolism, in *Seminars in Nephrology*, vol 4. New York, Grune & Stratton, 1984, p 285

GOLDMAN MB et al: Mechanisms of altered water metabolism in psychotic patients with polydipsia and hyponatremia. N Engl J Med 318:397, 1988

ROBERTSON GL, BERL W: Pathophysiology of water metabolism, in *The Kidney*, 4th ed, BM Brenner, FC Rector Jr (eds). Philadelphia, Saunders, 1991, p 677

SCHRIER RW, BICHET DG: Osmotic and nonosmotic control of vasopressin release and the pathogenesis of impaired water excretion in adrenal, thyroid, and edematous disorders. J Lab Clin Med 98:1, 1981

Dysuria, frequency and urgency, incontinence, and enuresis

BRADLEY WE: Diagnosis of urinary bladder dysfunction in diabetes mellitus. Ann Intern Med 92:323, 1980

——, SCOTT FB: Physiology of the urinary bladder, in *Urology*, 4th ed, JH Harrison et al (eds). Philadelphia, Saunders, 1978, vol 1, p 87

DEGROAT WC, BOOTH AM: Physiology of the urinary bladder and urethra. Ann Intern Med 92:312, 1980

HINDMARSH HR, BYRNE PO: Adult enuresis: A symptomatic and urodynamic assessment. Br J Urol 52:88, 1980

JOHNSON JR, STAMM WE: Urinary tract infections in women: Diagnosis and treatment. Ann Intern Med 111:906, 1989

LIPSKY BA: Urinary tract infections in men. Ann Intern Med 110:138, 1989

MIKKELSEN EJ, RAPOPORT JL: Enuresis: Psychopathology, sleep stage, and drug response. Urol Clin North Am 7:361, 1980

PLATT R: Quantitative definition of bacteriuria. Infectious Diseases Symposium, July 28, 1983, p 44, Supplement to Am J Med

RESNICK NM et al: The pathophysiology of urinary incontinence among institutionalized elderly persons. N Engl J Med 320:1, 1989

TURNER-WARWICK R, WHITESIDE CG (eds): *Symposium on Clinical Urodynamics: The Urologic Clinics of North America*, vol 6. Philadelphia, Saunders, 1979

WILLIAMS ME, PANNELL FC: Urinary incontinence in the elderly. Ann Intern Med 97:895, 1982

45 FLUIDS AND ELECTROLYTES

NORMAN G. LEVINSKY

SODIUM AND WATER

PHYSIOLOGIC CONSIDERATIONS (See also Chap. 235)   Both physiologically and clinically, sodium and water metabolism are closely interrelated. The sodium content of the body depends on the balance between dietary intake and renal excretion of sodium. In health, extrarenal losses of sodium are negligible. Renal sodium excretion is closely regulated to match dietary content. Within 2 to 4 days after sodium intake stops, urinary excretion decreases to 5 mmol/d or less. If dietary sodium is abruptly increased, sodium excretion promptly rises and equals intake within a few days. Thus, in normal persons, the sodium content of the body remains quite constant despite wide variations in sodium intake; over the range of 0 to 400 mmol/d, total body sodium varies only by about 10 percent.

Renal sodium excretion   This is regulated by the interplay of multiple control mechanisms. Sodium loads or deficits tend to produce corresponding changes in the central blood volume. Receptors located in the atria, central arteries, and the juxtaglomerular apparatus in the kidney respond to changes in local pressure which signal the volume/capacity relation of the central circulation (*effective blood volume*). If the effective volume is depleted, salt retention is induced, whereas expansion triggers multiple factors that favor natriuresis. With volume (salt) depletion, renal blood flow falls, due to decreased cardiac output and increased renal sympathetic nerve activity, which causes afferent arteriolar vasoconstriction.

The renin-angiotensin system is activated by autonomic stimuli and by reduced pressure in the juxtaglomerular apparatus. Angiotensin II preferentially constricts efferent arterioles and causes glomerular mesangial cell contraction. Glomerular filtration tends to fall because of reduced renal blood flow, decreased glomerular capillary pressure caused by afferent arteriolar constriction, and reduced capillary filtration area caused by mesangial contraction. In moderate to severe volume depletion, these factors outweigh the effect of angiotensin-induced efferent arteriolar constriction, which tends to maintain glomerular filtration by enhancing capillary filtration pressure. The fall in glomerular filtration reduces filtered sodium. Tubular reabsorption of sodium is enhanced. Proximal reabsorption is stimulated by changes in Starling forces in the peritubular circulation. Hydraulic pressure in peritubular capillaries is decreased by arteriolar constriction. Oncotic pressure is enhanced by concentration of plasma proteins and by increased filtration fraction (glomerular filtration tends to fall less than renal blood flow). These changes in hydraulic and oncotic Starling forces promote proximal salt and water reabsorption. Proximal reabsorption also is stimulated by angiotensin II and by sympathetic nerves which innervate proximal segments directly. Distal tubular reabsorption is enhanced by aldosterone, which is secreted at an increased rate in response to stimulation of the adrenal gland by angiotensin.

Volume expansion leads to opposite changes in renal hemodynamics and in these various regulators of tubular transport. Moreover, one or more natriuretic hormones are released in response to increased extracellular volume. Natriuretic peptides are present in the atria, the brain, and probably the kidney itself. Such peptides can augment sodium excretion both by increasing glomerular filtration and by inhibiting sodium reabsorption in the collecting ducts. There is also evidence for a ouabain-like natriuretic hormone that reduces tubular salt transport by inhibiting Na^+,K^+-adenosine triphosphatase (N^+,K^+-ATPase). Prostaglandins and kinins secreted within the kidney reduce sodium reabsorption in distal nephron segments. The exact role of these natriuretic factors in the regulation of sodium excretion is uncertain.

Undoubtedly, other regulatory mechanisms remain to be defined.

The multiplicity of control mechanisms prevents abnormalities of any single mechanism from grossly distorting the regulation of sodium excretion. For example, increased aldosterone secretion leads only to limited and transient sodium retention, because the initial accumulation of sodium tends to increase glomerular filtration and stimulates opposing natriuretic factors which decrease tubular sodium reabsorption.

Distribution of sodium   All but 2 to 5 percent of the sodium in the body is located in the extracellular fluids. (Approximately 40 percent of total body sodium is in bone, but this fraction does not participate significantly in most physiologic processes and will not be considered further.) The electrolyte compositions of plasma and interstitial fluid differ slightly because of the Gibbs-Donnan effect of anionic plasma proteins, which increases cation and decreases anion concentrations by a few percent in plasma relative to interstitial fluid. For practical purposes, plasma composition can be considered representative of the entire extracellular compartment. Total extracellular volume approximates 20 percent of body weight. Of this, 5 percent represents plasma volume and 15 percent the volume of interstitial fluids. Thus, in a 70-kg individual with plasma sodium concentration of 140 mmol/L, extracellular sodium content will approximate 2000 mmol. The volume of intracellular fluid is approximately twice as great as that of extracellular fluid, i.e., about 40 percent of body weight. However, since intracellular sodium concentration is less than 5 mmol/L, total intracellular sodium content is only about 100 to 150 mmol. The asymmetric distribution of sodium across cell membranes is maintained by expenditure of a large fraction of the energy derived from cell metabolism, which is required constantly to pump sodium out of cells against its electrochemical gradient. All the principal electrolytes are asymmetrically distributed across cell membranes. The principal electrolytes of the extracellular fluids are sodium, chloride, and bicarbonate. The major electrolytes of the intracellular fluids are potassium, magnesium, calcium, and organic anions, including proteins.

Since sodium salts account for more than 90 percent of the total osmolality of the extracellular fluids, variations in plasma sodium concentration are almost always reflected in equivalent changes in plasma osmolality. Exceptions due to accumulation of other solutes in plasma are discussed later. Although the electrolyte compositions of intracellular and extracellular fluids differ markedly, they are always in osmotic equilibrium, since water moves rapidly across cellular membranes to dissipate osmotic gradients. Therefore, although sodium is largely confined to extracellular fluids, plasma sodium concentration is an index of not only the relative proportions of sodium and water in those fluids but also the relation between total body solute and total body water. An example is the effect of shift of sodium from extracellular to intracellular fluids without a change in total body solute. Movement of sodium into cells would not cause hyponatremia, since water would shift into cells with the sodium. On the other hand, a primary decrease in the concentration of osmotically active solute within cells would decrease total body solute; although there would be no change in total body sodium or water, hyponatremia would result from the shift of intracellular water into the extracellular compartment.

Role of antidiuretic hormone   A very effective mechanism involving the *hypothalamus*, the *neurohypophysis*, and the kidney regulates plasma osmolality. Changes of 2 percent or less in plasma osmolality can be detected by osmoreceptors in the hypothalamus. Small increases in osmolality stimulate the secretion of vasopressin (the antidiuretic hormone, ADH) from the neurohypophysis, while small decreases suppress secretion of the hormone. Normal plasma osmolality is approximately 280 to 300 mosmol/kg of water; the exact level is determined by the "set" of the hypothalamic osmoreceptors in a given individual. When ADH secretion is maximal, urine volume will be about 500 mL/d, and urine osmolality will be 800 to 1400 mosmol/kg. In the absence of ADH, minimal urine osmolality is 40 to 80 mosmol/kg, and maximum water diuresis can reach 15 to 20 L/d or more. The capacity of this receptor-effector system is sufficient to maintain plasma osmolality within narrow limits despite large variations in the volume and concentration of dietary fluids. ADH secretion is also regulated by changes in extracellular volume. A reduction of 10 percent or more may trigger ADH release even in the absence of changes in plasma osmolality. If volume contraction is sufficiently severe, volume-mediated stimulation of ADH may override osmotic signals and cause water retention despite progressive dilution of body fluids. Conversely, extracellular volume expansion tends to suppress ADH release even if the body fluids are hypertonic.

The total sodium *content* of the body is determined by the renal sodium regulatory mechanisms described earlier. However, the principal determinant of plasma sodium *concentration* is water metabolism rather than total body sodium content. If excess sodium were to be ingested and retained, hypernatremia would be only transient. Water intake would increase because of thirst, and the fluid ingested would be retained because hypernatremia (hyperosmolality) would stimulate ADH secretion. Expanded extracellular volume, not hypernatremia, would be the end result. Conversely, if the osmoregulatory system is functioning normally, loss of moderate amounts of sodium without water would not result in permanent reduction of plasma sodium concentration. The initial reduction would shut off secretion of ADH, and a water diuresis would ensue. The final outcome would be contraction of extracellular volume, while plasma sodium concentration would be restored to normal. It follows that changes in total sodium content tend to cause changes in extracellular volume. In this sense, the sodium content of the extracellular fluid determines extracellular volume. On the other hand, changes in plasma sodium concentration reflect altered regulation of water excretion, not changes in total body sodium content alone. Clinically, plasma sodium concentration per se gives no information about the amount of sodium present in the body. Total body sodium content is determined by the volume of extracellular fluids as well as by the concentration of sodium in these fluids. Extracellular volume is usually the dominant factor, since changes in volume tend to be proportionately greater than changes in sodium concentration. Plasma sodium concentration reflects the relative proportions of sodium and water (or, more exactly, of total body solute and water), not the absolute amount of sodium in the body. Either hyponatremia or hypernatremia may occur when total body sodium content is decreased, normal, or increased.

CLINICAL DISORDERS Deficits and excesses of sodium and water occur in a great variety of clinical circumstances. The manifestations of the underlying illness may overshadow the clinical features of the fluid and electrolyte disorder. Theoretically, disturbances of sodium and water metabolism can be classified into four categories, reflecting a primary excess or deficit of water or sodium. Practically, such isolated disturbances are uncommon. A primary excess of sodium leads to edema; it is not ordinarily considered as an electrolyte disorder but as a feature of underlying disease, such as congestive heart failure, hepatic cirrhosis, or nephrotic syndrome. Primary sodium deficits are nearly always accompanied by water depletion, leading to the clinical syndrome of extracellular volume depletion. Pure or disproportionate water excess leads to hyponatremia, relative or absolute water depletion to hypernatremia. A practical clinical classification of the principal disorders of sodium and water metabolism is given in Table 45-1.

VOLUME DEPLETION Combined sodium and water deficits are far more frequent than isolated deficits of either constituent. Although the term *dehydration* is often used for combined deficits, this usage is confusing. Dehydration should be used to describe relatively pure water depletion leading to hypernatremia; *volume depletion* or some similar term should be used for combined deficits.

Pathogenesis As noted earlier, elimination of sodium from the diet will not by itself lead to sodium depletion in the presence of normal renal function, since urinary sodium excretion will quickly fall to very low levels. Therefore, sodium depletion is always due either to extrarenal losses or to abnormal renal losses.

TABLE 45-1   Disorders of sodium and water metabolism*

I Combined sodium and water depletion (volume depletion)
  A Extrarenal losses
    1 Gastrointestinal (vomiting, diarrhea, gastrointestinal suction, fistulas)
    2 Abdominal sequestration (peritonitis, rapid reaccumulation of ascites)
    3 Skin (sweating, burns)
  B Renal losses
    1 Renal disease (diuretic phase of acute renal failure, postobstructive diuresis, chronic renal failure, salt-wasting tubular disease)
    2 Diuretic excess
    3 Osmotic diuresis (diabetic glycosuria)
    4 Mineralocorticoid deficiency (Addison's disease, hypoaldosteronism)
II Hyponatremia
  A Associated with extracellular volume depletion (see list of causes above)
  B Associated with extracellular volume excess and edema
  C Associated with normal or modestly expanded extracellular volume (no edema)
    1 Acute and chronic renal failure
    2 Temporary impairment of water diuresis (pain, drugs, emotion)
    3 Syndrome of inappropriate secretion of antidiuretic hormone (SIADH)
    4 Endocrine (glucocorticoid deficiency, hypothyroidism)
    5 Severe polydipsia
    6 Essential ("sick-cell syndrome")
  D Without plasma hyposmolality
    1 Osmotic (hyperglycemia, mannitol)
    2 Artifactual (hyperlipemia, hyperproteinemia, laboratory error)
III Hypernatremia
  A Due solely to water loss
    1 Extrarenal
      a Skin (insensible losses)
      b Lungs
    2 Renal
      a Diabetes insipidus (central, nephrogenic)
    3 Hypothalamic dysfunction
  B Due to water loss associated with sodium loss
    1 Extrarenal
      a Sweat
    2 Renal
      a Osmotic diuresis (glycosuria, urea)
  C Due to sodium gain
    1 Excessive sodium administration
    2 Adrenal hyperfunction (hyperaldosteronism, Cushing's syndrome)

---

* For differential diagnosis, see Fig. 45-1.

GASTROINTESTINAL   The most common cause of volume depletion is loss of a significant fraction of the 8 to 10 L of gastrointestinal fluids secreted daily. As the sodium concentration of these fluids is high, their loss causes combined sodium and water deficits. Since the principal secretions contain potassium and hydrogen ion or bicarbonate in large amounts, volume depletion due to such losses is often combined with potassium depletion and acidosis or alkalosis.

Significant volume depletion may be caused by sequestration of secretions within an obstructed gastrointestinal tract or within the peritoneal cavity in peritonitis. Rapid reaccumulation of ascites after paracentesis may reduce the effective circulating blood volume.

SKIN   The sodium concentration of sweat varies from 5 to 50 mmol/L; sodium concentration increases with higher rates of sweating and in adrenal insufficiency. Because sweat is always a hypotonic solution, sweating leads to water deficits out of proportion to sodium losses. In burns, capillary damage may lead to sequestration of large amounts of sodium and water in the injured skin.

RENAL   Abnormal losses of sodium and water in the urine may occur in both acute and chronic renal diseases. Early in the recovery (diuretic) phase of *acute renal failure*, urinary sodium concentration tends to be high (50 to 100 mmol/L), and substantial deficits of both sodium and water may ensue. With rare exceptions, severe sodium and water wasting does not persist beyond the first few days. It is important to discriminate between increased excretion which eliminates excess retained during the oliguric period and true tubular sodium and water wasting which depletes normal extracellular volume. Only the latter requires replacement. Acute salt and water wasting due to tubular damage also may occur immediately after relief of prolonged *obstruction* of the urinary tract. Although such a postobstructive diuresis may be severe, it rarely persists for more than several days as a clinically important phenomenon.

Patients with *chronic renal failure* have limited ability to decrease sodium and water excretion in response to decreased intake. They will become progressively volume-depleted if their intake is restricted by the anorexia, nausea, and vomiting characteristic of uremia or because of their physician's instructions. Large deficits may develop insidiously over many days or weeks. A "self-perpetuating cycle" may result, in that volume depletion will tend further to compromise renal function. Severe sodium-wasting renal disease, i.e., negative sodium balance when dietary sodium is normal, is rare. It occurs in occasional patients with tubulointerstitial diseases of the kidney, especially medullary cystic disease.

Renal sodium wasting in the presence of normal intrinsic renal function occurs in three clinical circumstances. Perhaps the most common is sodium depletion due to continued administration of potent *diuretics* to patients after edema has been relieved or to patients whose edema is sequestered and cannot be mobilized. For example, attempted treatment of cirrhotics with ascites may result in depletion of extracellular volume rather than mobilization of ascitic fluid. An obligatory *osmotic diuresis* also may cause renal sodium and water wasting despite normal renal function. Marked glycosuria in uncontrolled diabetes mellitus is the most frequent clinical example. Volume depletion in patients receiving high-protein enteral or parenteral alimentation may be due to an osmotic diuresis of urea formed by protein metabolism. Administration of solutes such as mannitol, which act as osmotic diuretics, may cause volume depletion. Finally, renal sodium wasting despite normal intrinsic function occurs in Addison's disease and hypoaldosteronism due to a *deficiency of mineralocorticoids*.

Clinical features and diagnosis   The cause of volume depletion can usually be suspected from a history of inadequate salt and water intake together with vomiting, diarrhea, or excessive sweating; the symptoms of poorly controlled diabetes mellitus or of renal or adrenal disease may be elicited. The key findings on physical examination are those of interstitial and plasma volume depletion. Decreased interstitial volume may be recognized from reduced skin turgor, which is usually present in patients with significant volume contraction but may be difficult to evaluate in the elderly. It can be estimated clinically by noting the slow rate of return of skin to its original position when it is raised between the examiner's fingers. An area of skin normally free of wrinkles and not subject to wide variations in the thickness of subcutaneous tissue, such as that over the sternum, should be selected for this maneuver. Oral mucous membranes may be dry and axillary sweating decreased; these are less reliable diagnostic features than decreased skin turgor. Plasma volume depletion is indicated by changes in blood pressure. With moderate volume depletion, blood pressure is usually normal when the patient is recumbent, although resting tachycardia may be present. Postural hypotension, i.e., a drop of at least 5 to 10 mmHg in the sitting or standing position, is often present. With greater degrees of volume depletion, even recumbent blood pressure is reduced, and frank shock may occur. The patient with moderate or severe degrees of volume contraction is often lethargic, weak, confused, or obtunded. Such patients are usually oliguric, even when recumbent blood pressure is normal. However, an osmotic diuresis, as occurs in hyperglycemia, tends to prevent oliguria despite volume contraction.

LABORATORY FINDINGS   The hematocrit and plasma protein concentration are increased, but increases within the normal range are interpretable only if prior values are known. Plasma sodium concentration may be decreased, normal, or increased depending on the proportion between deficits of sodium and of water. Plasma creatinine and urea nitrogen are usually increased, since the glomerular filtration rate is decreased ("prerenal azotemia"). Blood urea nitrogen (BUN) tends to rise proportionately more than plasma creatinine. Urinary sodium concentration may be of value in differentiating extrarenal and renal sources of sodium loss if the probable cause is not clear from the history. With extrarenal losses, urinary sodium concentration is less than 10 mmol/L; the concentration will usually exceed 20 mmol/L if renal or adrenal disorders are at fault. However,

urinary sodium may ultimately fall below this level even in patients with renal salt wasting if sodium depletion becomes severe.

Treatment   The principal clinical manifestations of extracellular volume depletion are due to reduction of plasma and interstitial fluid volume. Since there is no convenient clinical method for quantifying these volumes, the effect of treatment must be determined by following the changes in clinical features such as blood pressure, urine output, and skin turgor. Modest deficits of sodium and water often can be corrected by increased oral intake in patients not suffering from gastrointestinal disorders. Severe depletion requires therapy with intravenous solutions. Isotonic saline (0.85%) is the infusion of choice in patients whose serum sodium concentration is approximately normal. The amount to be infused can be estimated from the history of prior losses and from the severity of the physical findings of extracellular volume contraction. Patients with moderate volume contraction usually require replacement with 2 to 3 L of saline, while patients with severe depletion may require much larger volumes. The need for correction of other concurrent electrolyte abnormalities may alter the composition of the required infusion; e.g., some of the sodium may be given as bicarbonate to patients with volume contraction and metabolic acidosis, or potassium may be added in patients with concurrent potassium depletion. In estimating the total amount to be infused, allowance for ongoing losses must be included. Since the amount to be infused cannot be calculated precisely, patients should be monitored carefully to avoid fluid overload and congestive failure.

HYPONATREMIA   Pathophysiology   Hyponatremia indicates that the body fluids are diluted by an excess of water relative to total solute. Hyponatremia is not equivalent to sodium depletion, which is only one of the clinical states in which it may occur (see Table 45-1). Most types of hyponatremia result from defective urinary dilution. The normal response to dilution of body fluids is a water diuresis, which corrects the hyposmotic state. Normal water diuresis requires three factors: (1) secretion of ADH must be suppressed; (2) sufficient sodium and water must reach the diluting sites of the nephron, in the ascending limb of Henle's loop and the distal convoluted tubule; and (3) these nephron segments must function normally, reabsorbing sodium while remaining impermeable to water.

Correspondingly, three mechanisms may cause defective water diuresis in patients with hyponatremia: (1) Secretion of ADH may continue "inappropriately" despite hypotonicity of extracellular fluid, which normally shuts off secretion of the hormone. This may be due to unregulated release of ADH by neoplasms or to nonosmotic stimuli to ADH secretion. The latter include volume depletion, neural factors such as pain and emotion, and certain drugs. (2) Insufficient sodium may reach the diluting segments to permit the formation of an adequate amount of dilute urine. Inadequate delivery of tubular fluid to distal sites may be due to reduced glomerular filtration and/or enhanced proximal tubular reabsorption. Even in the absence of ADH, distal tubular segments are not absolutely impermeable to water; small amounts of water continue to leak from the hypotonic tubular fluid into the isotonic cortical and slightly hypertonic medullary interstitial fluid. The amount of water leaking back in this manner becomes an increasingly larger fraction of the volume of dilute urine formed, since the diluting process is progressively limited by decreasing delivery. Hence urine osmolality rises progressively. In some instances, this mechanism may even result in excretion of a urine hypertonic to plasma, despite the absence of ADH. (3) Sodium transport in the diluting segments may be defective, or water permeability may be excessive at these sites even in the absence of ADH. One of these three factors can account for most types of hyponatremia, as described below.

Types of hyponatremia (See Table 45-1)   In patients with extracellular *volume depletion*, delivery of sodium and water to the diluting segments of the nephron is reduced because of decreased glomerular filtration, increased proximal tubular reabsorption, or both. ADH secretion is stimulated by the volume contraction. These changes in renal function and hormone secretion limit water diuresis during extracellular volume depletion. Hyponatremia per se is usually of little clinical significance in sodium (volume) depletion. The major features are those of extracellular volume contraction, described above. Reduction of plasma sodium concentration by more than 10 to 15 mmol/L is rare in the absence of obvious decreases in skin turgor, postural or recumbent hypotension, and some degree of azotemia. Treatment is directed to correction of the volume deficits. Restitution of extracellular volume will correct hyponatremia by reversing the pathophysiologic mechanisms which limit water diuresis. In the occasional symptomatic patient with sodium depletion whose plasma sodium concentration is less than 125 mmol/L, it may be desirable to administer some of the intravenous sodium replacement fluids as hypertonic saline (see "Treatment," below).

Multiple factors contribute to hyponatremia caused by *diuretics*. Salt loss may cause volume depletion, which limits water diuresis by mechanisms already described and stimulates thirst. Thiazides and loop diuretics (furosemide, bumetanide, and ethacrynic acid) inhibit salt reabsorption in the diluting segments of the nephron and thereby directly limit water diuresis. Thiazides are the diuretics most commonly associated with hyponatremia, because they interfere with elaboration of a hypotonic urine by inhibiting sodium reabsorption in the distal convoluted tubule but, unlike loop diuretics, do not limit urine concentration and water retention by interfering with salt transport in the loop of Henle. In addition, potassium depletion caused by many diuretics contributes to hyponatremia through uncertain mechanisms. Hyponatremia due to diuretic therapy of hypertension is frequent but usually minor in severity. However, moderate or severe hyponatremia may occur in patients who receive diuretics, usually thiazides, and who drink large quantities of water or other hypotonic fluids. Elderly women are especially prone to develop severe hyponatremia. Progressive hyponatremia is an important complication of diuretic therapy in edematous patients, in whom the underlying disease tends to cause hyponatremia (see below) and to whom large doses of diuretics may be given. The treatment of hyponatremia due to diuretics is water restriction and repletion of potassium deficits.

In *edematous states* such as congestive heart failure, cirrhosis, and the nephrotic syndrome, hyponatremia paradoxically appears to result from mechanisms similar to those which cause hyponatremia in patients with volume depletion. Although total extracellular volume is increased in edematous patients, it is believed that the "effective" volume is reduced by decreased cardiac output or sequestration of fluid outside the central circulation. The decrease in "effective" volume results in diminished delivery of sodium and water to nephron diluting segments because of reduced glomerular filtration, increased proximal tubular reabsorption, or both. Volume-mediated secretion of ADH is also triggered in these conditions. In some edematous patients, essential hyponatremia may be an additional mechanism (see below). In edematous states, the severity and frequency of hyponatremia correlate to some extent with the magnitude of the edema and the seriousness of the underlying condition. Hyponatremia is usually present in patients with advanced disease unless water intake is restricted. The hyponatremia itself is often of little clinical significance. The principal features are those of the underlying disease. However, symptomatic hyponatremia may occur, most often in connection with vigorous diuretic therapy or excessive oral or parenteral intake of dilute fluids.

Hyponatremia associated with edema responds to effective treatment of the underlying disease. Moderate nonprogressive hyponatremia in edematous patients usually does not cause symptoms. Attempts to correct such hyponatremia by restriction of fluid intake induce thirst and discomfort without improving the clinical picture or longevity. Patients with severe or progressive hyponatremia may require some restriction of water intake, especially during vigorous treatment with diuretics. However, moderate limitation to the range of 1 to 1.5 L/d will often suffice to avoid symptoms of progressive hyponatremia. More severe restriction should be instituted only if specific clinical or laboratory observations warrant. Since edematous

subjects have excess total extracellular sodium, hypertonic saline should not be administered except in rare instances in which clinical manifestations of extreme hyponatremia, such as coma or convulsions, justify emergency measures. Furosemide should be given concurrently in such cases to avoid further expansion of the extracellular space. Dialysis also can be used to correct severe hyponatremia without increasing volume in edematous patients.

Hyponatremia may result from *impaired water excretion* not associated with a substantial deficit or excess of salt. In this case, extracellular volume is only modestly expanded. Since excess water is distributed throughout both intracellular and extracellular fluids in proportion to their volumes, only one-third of a water excess will be retained in the extracellular compartment. *Oliguric* patients develop dilutional hyponatremia if the volume of oral and intravenous fluids is not restricted appropriately. The ability to excrete a normal volume of dilute urine is progressively limited in advancing *chronic renal failure*. Regulation of water intake by thirst usually prevents dilutional hyponatremia. However, hyponatremia may be precipitated by increased fluid intake (e.g., if the patient is instructed to force fluids). Since the ability to regulate salt excretion is also impaired in chronic renal failure, in many patients hyponatremia is associated with edema or salt depletion rather than normal extracellular volume. In patients with normal renal function, *water diuresis* may be *limited temporarily* by ADH secretion induced by various neural stimuli such as pain and narcotics. In the postoperative state, these factors, together with administration of large volumes of hypotonic fluids, may cause hyponatremia. The etiology of hyponatremia due to impaired water excretion is usually evident from the clinical setting and a careful review of fluid intake and output. This type of hyponatremia is treated by water restriction. Only if severe symptoms occur is hypertonic saline infusion required.

In the *syndrome* of *inappropriate antidiuretic hormone* (SIADH) secretion (see also Chap. 333), ADH is released "inappropriately" despite dilution of body fluids and increased extracellular volume. Hyponatremia in patients with SIADH is principally due to water retention, but urinary losses of sodium also may contribute to a mild negative sodium balance. Renal sodium wasting is due to water retention and consequent modest volume expansion, which increases sodium excretion by mechanisms discussed above. Clinically, SIADH is characterized by a number of features: (1) Urine osmolality is not maximally dilute even when marked hyponatremia is induced by water loading. In most cases, urine osmolality exceeds plasma osmolality. (2) Plasma creatinine and urea are normal or low, indicating that the glomerular filtration rate is normal or increased. (The elaboration of hypertonic urine is presumptive evidence of ADH secretion if the glomerular filtration rate is normal.) (3) During fluid loading (even if the fluid is saline), hyponatremia increases due to water retention and urinary sodium wasting. It should be noted that sodium wasting during volume expansion may be minimal or even absent in patients with extreme degrees of hyponatremia. (4) Since hyponatremia and salt wasting are not direct effects of vasopressin but are due to retention of ingested water, they are corrected by restriction of fluid intake. This response is helpful in occasional patients in whom it may be difficult to distinguish SIADH from mild volume depletion as the cause of hyponatremia. The plasma uric acid also may be of value in making this distinction. Since uric acid excretion tends to vary with "effective" extracellular volume, hyperuricemia is common in volume depletion, while hypouricemia is usual in SIADH.

SIADH occurs commonly in patients with oat cell carcinoma of the lung but also has been described in patients with a variety of other *neoplasms*. In some of these patients the tumor secretes ADH or a substance with analogous biologic activity (see also Chap. 333). The syndrome also has been reported in patients with various disorders of the *central nervous system*, including meningitis, encephalitis, tumors, trauma, and stroke, and in acute *porphyria*. It is assumed that ADH in these patients is secreted in response to direct stimulation of the hypothalamic osmoreceptors. *Pulmonary* diseases associated with

SIADH, in addition to tumors, include a wide variety of infections, asthma, and chronic obstructive lung disease.

Pharmacologic agents that induce SIADH include (1) the oral hypoglycemic agents chlorpropamide and tolbutamide, (2) the antineoplastic and immunosuppressive agents vincristine, vinblastine, and cyclophosphamide, and (3) psychoactive drugs such as haloperidol, thioridazine, carbamazepine, and amitriptyline. These agents exert their antidiuretic effect either by potentiating the tubular action of small amounts of ADH or by stimulating inappropriate secretion of ADH. The antipsychotic drugs also tend to stimulate fluid intake by their anticholinergic action, which dries mucous membranes.

Hyponatremia due to SIADH can be treated by limiting fluid intake; restriction to the range of 1 to 1.2 L/d is ordinarily adequate. Occasional patients who are symptomatic despite water restriction may be treated by enhancing water excretion. This can be accomplished either by increasing solute excretion (by taking a high-salt, high-protein diet or ingesting urea) or by antagonizing ADH with demeclocycline or lithium. Initial therapy with hypertonic saline infusions may be appropriate in a few symptomatic patients with marked hyponatremia. Concurrent administration of furosemide, which increases water excretion by limiting urinary concentration, may facilitate correction of hyponatremia in those patients who do not respond promptly to hypertonic saline alone.

Hyponatremia may occur in certain *endocrine* disorders, notably adrenal insufficiency and hypothyroidism. Multiple factors appear to play a role in limiting water diuresis in patients with *adrenal insufficiency*. Deficient secretion of mineralocorticoid hormones may lead to sodium depletion, with consequent reduction of glomerular filtration and enhancement of tubular sodium reabsorption. Moreover, glucocorticoid deficiency directly reduces filtration. Therefore, adrenal insufficiency will tend to decrease delivery of sodium to diluting sites. In addition, hormone deficiency prevents the maintenance of normal water impermeability in distal diluting segments of the nephron. This appears to be due in large part to inappropriate secretion of ADH, although there also may be direct effect of hormone deficiency on water permeability of distal tubular epithelium. Since patients with adrenal insufficiency may have the combination of defective dilution of the urine and sodium wasting, hyponatremia due to Addison's disease can occasionally be confused with SIADH. Usually, other clinical features of adrenal insufficiency such as hyperkalemia, pigmentation, and hypoglycemia suggest the correct diagnosis. However, specific tests of adrenal function are indicated whenever the diagnosis is in doubt. Hyponatremia due to adrenal insufficiency is corrected by appropriate hormonal therapy.

Hyponatremia may develop in moderate or severe *hypothyroidism*. Decreased delivery of tubular fluid to diluting segments and persistent release of ADH both limit water excretion in this condition. The diagnosis of this type of hyponatremia is made by recognizing the clinical features of hypothyroidism and from the response to treatment with thyroid hormone.

The normal kidney can excrete 15 to 20 L of dilute urine per day. Normal water intake, regulated by thirst and habit, is a small fraction of this maximum excretory capacity. Rarely, *psychogenic polydipsia* may be so severe that the rapid ingestion of huge quantities of fluids may overwhelm normal excretory capacity and produce symptomatic dilutional hyponatremia despite normal renal diluting mechanisms. Hyponatremia of this type is diagnosed from the history of massive fluid intake. The patients most often are women, usually with other evidence of psychiatric illness. Since water excretory capacity is normal, the urine is maximally dilute in this condition. Hyponatremia due to psychogenic polydipsia responds to water restriction. Rare patients who are symptomatic due to extreme degrees of hyponatremia may require intravenous infusion of hypertonic saline.

Low solute output will limit excretion of water. Since minimal urine osmolality is about 50 mosmol/kg, the kidney must excrete at least 50 mosmol of solute in order to excrete 1 L of water. In individuals consuming diets low in protein and electrolytes, urinary solute excretion may be reduced to less than half the usual 600 to 800 mosmol/d (mostly urea and electrolytes). Hyponatremia due to a diet which provides little urinary solute but large fluid intake has been described in beer drinkers who consume little else ("beer potomania").

Some patients may be hyponatremic in the absence of a defect in water diuresis. The terms *essential hyponatremia* and *"sick-cell" syndrome* have been applied to this category. Osmoreceptor cells in the hypothalamus are thought to be "reset" to maintain a decreased level of body fluid osmolality as though it were normal. Urine becomes dilute or concentrated, respectively, if plasma sodium falls or increases slightly from the new "normal" level for the particular patient. The genesis of such a syndrome is speculative. Changes in cellular metabolism may lead to a primary reduction in cellular osmolality. Another possibility is that essential hyponatremia is a variant of SIADH in which there is a nonosmotic stimulus to ADH secretion. When plasma osmolality is reduced sufficiently, osmotic suppression of ADH secretion overcomes the nonosmotic stimulus.

Essential hyponatremia may occur in a variety of chronic illnesses, such as pulmonary tuberculosis, congestive heart failure, and hepatic cirrhosis. This type of hyponatremia is asymptomatic; skin turgor, blood pressure, and renal function are normal, unless altered by the primary disease. Definitive diagnosis of essential hyponatremia requires the demonstration of normal urinary dilution in response to water loading, normal urinary concentration during dehydration, and normal renal sodium excretory responses to sodium loading and restriction. This type of hyponatremia does not require treatment.

Hyponatremia due to *accumulation of osmotically active solutes* in the plasma is the sole exception to the rule that hyponatremia means decreased plasma osmolality. In this type of hyponatremia, plasma osmolality is increased. Plasma sodium is diluted by movement of water out of cells along the osmotic gradient created by the addition of a solute such as glucose or mannitol. (High plasma urea levels in patients with renal failure do not cause hyponatremia because urea concentration is equal across cell membranes.) The diagnosis of hyponatremia due to increased plasma concentrations of osmotically active solutes is usually apparent from the history and clinical features of uncontrolled diabetes. Plasma sodium concentration will decrease by about 1.6 mmol/L with every elevation of 1 g/L in plasma glucose above normal. This type of hyponatremia also should be considered whenever there is a history of recent administration of mannitol, especially to oliguric patients unable to excrete it promptly. Since plasma osmolality is increased, clinical manifestations of hypotonicity are absent in this type of hyponatremia.

In patients with severe hyperlipemia or, very rarely, with extreme hyperproteinemia, *artifactual* hyponatremia may be reported by the laboratory. In severe hyperlipemia, part of any unit volume of plasma taken for analysis will be lipid, which is sodium-free. This type of hyponatremia rarely occurs unless the plasma is grossly milky. In patients with extreme hyperproteinemia, proteins occupy more than the normal 7 percent of plasma volume, thereby reducing the proportion of aqueous sodium-containing fluid per unit of plasma taken for analysis. In both cases, hyponatremia will be reported by the laboratory because the sodium concentration will be low in millimoles per liter of plasma. However, sodium concentration per liter of plasma water and plasma osmolality are normal; hence this type of hyponatremia has no clinical significance. Laboratories increasingly have adopted the sodium-selective electrode as the method for measuring plasma sodium. This technique eliminates artifactual hyponatremia because it gives accurate values regardless of plasma lipid or protein concentration.

Differential diagnosis   Although the type of hyponatremia can be defined easily in most patients, precise diagnosis may be difficult in some. In Fig. 45-1 is a flowchart that outlines the major steps in determining the cause of hyponatremia. First, assess extracellular fluid (ECF) volume. The history and physical examination are usually sufficient to determine whether the hyponatremia is associated with a decreased, increased, or normal extracellular volume. In occasional patients, moderate volume depletion may not readily be separable from

FIGURE 45-1 Flowchart for differential diagnosis of causes of hyponatremia. Categories (A, B, C, D) and types (C1–6) are keyed to Table 45-1, section II (Hyponatremia). Abbreviations: Nl = normal; ECF = extracellular fluid; creat = creatinine; CHF = congestive heart failure; BP = blood pressure; Uosm = urinary osmolality; U_{Na} = urinary Na, mmol/L; ↓ = decreased, ↑ = increased; Hx = history, PE = physical examination.

normovolemia by clinical examination. In that event, measurement of BUN and plasma creatinine may be helpful. The plasma creatinine and especially the BUN tend to be increased when hyponatremia is associated with volume depletion and normal or decreased when it is associated with a normal or expanded extracellular volume, as in SIADH. As noted above, plasma uric acid also may be helpful in making this distinction. The various types of normovolemic hyponatremia can frequently be recognized by a careful review of specific features of the history, such as associated diseases, drug therapy, and fluid intake. However, laboratory tests, such as measurement of serum cortisol, may be needed to confirm a diagnosis.

Measurements of urinary sodium concentration and osmolality are common in the workup. *Urinary sodium concentration* is low (under 10 mmol/L) if hyponatremia is associated with edema or with volume depletion due to extrarenal causes. Urine sodium concentration usually exceeds 20 mmol/L if hyponatremia is due to renal salt losses or to renal failure with water retention. In SIADH, urine sodium concentration usually exceeds 20 mmol/L unless fluid intake has been restricted. Since impaired water diuresis is the mechanism of most types of hyponatremia, measurement of *urinary osmolality* is not usually of value. A maximally dilute urine would be expected only in hyponatremia due to extreme polydipsia or during water loading in essential hyponatremia. With other causes, urinary osmolality exceeds 150 mosmol/kg of water; usually the urine is hypertonic to plasma.

Clinical manifestations   Neurologic dysfunction is the principal clinical manifestation of hyponatremia. It is due to intracellular movement of water, leading to swelling of brain cells. The severity of symptoms is related both to the degree of hyponatremia and to the rapidity with which it develops. There is some evidence that women develop more severe manifestations than men. In chronic hyponatremia, the degree of brain swelling caused by any given reduction in body fluid osmolality is reduced by cellular volume regulatory mechanisms. These transport inorganic ions, such as potassium and chloride, and organic osmolytes, such as amino acids, out of swollen brain cells. Patients may be lethargic, confused, stuporous, or comatose. If hyponatremia develops rapidly, signs of hyperexcitability such as muscular twitches, irritability, and convulsions may occur. Hyponatremia rarely causes clinical symptoms when plasma sodium is above 125 mmol/L, although symptoms may occur at higher levels if the decrease in concentration has been rapid.

Treatment   Appropriate therapy for the various types of hyponatremia has been outlined. Hyponatremia itself is often of little significance and requires no specific treatment. If severe, symptomatic hyponatremia requires intravenous treatment; the amount of sodium required to increase plasma sodium concentration is calculated by multiplying the deficit in plasma sodium concentration (millimoles per liter) by the total body water (approximately 50 to 60 percent of body weight). Although the administered sodium will remain in the extracellular compartment, the osmotic effect of hypertonic saline will cause water to shift out of cells.

The appropriate rate and extent of initial correction of hyponatremia are controversial. Severe hyponatremia can cause major neurologic dysfunction. On the other hand, rapid correction of hyponatremia also can cause serious neurologic damage [osmotic demyelination, often prominent in the pons (central pontine myelinolysis)]. Both the rate and magnitude of initial correction of hyponatremia apparently influence the likelihood of this complication. The risk of neurologic damage appears to be very low in patients whose hyponatremia has developed rapidly, e.g., patients with psychogenic polydipsia. In patients with chronic hyponatremia, osmotic demyelination is more likely, although apparently still infrequent.

Although the issue of optimal treatment has not yet been resolved, the following regimen seems reasonable in the light of current information. Only patients with severe, symptomatic hyponatremia should be treated with hypertonic saline. If hyponatremia has developed over 24 h or less, 5% saline should be administered in an amount calculated to increase plasma sodium by no more than 1 to 2 mmol/L per hour. If hyponatremia is more chronic, plasma sodium should be raised by no more than 0.5 to 1 mmol/L per hour. In either case, plasma sodium should not be increased by more than 12 mmol/L over the first 24 h. The symptoms and clinical status, especially with respect to circulatory congestion, should be assessed carefully throughout the infusion. Furosemide may be given if fluid overload is present initially or develops during the infusion. Complete correction of hyponatremia, if indicated, is usually best carried out more slowly by water restriction or oral sodium supplementation if possible.

HYPERNATREMIA   Pathophysiology   Hypernatremia is due to a deficit of body water relative to total body solute or sodium content. Without exception, hypernatremia indicates that the body fluids are hypertonic. Normally, minimal increases in tonicity stimulate both thirst and release of ADH. Although renal water retention induced by ADH helps to correct hypernatremia, thirst appears to be the principal defense mechanism. Hypernatremia is usually modest in patients with diabetes insipidus, although they lack ADH and may excrete 15 L or more of urine per day. Thirst stimulates water intake enough to balance even such large water losses. Severe persistent hypernatremia occurs only in patients who cannot respond to thirst by voluntary ingestion of fluid, e.g., infants or mentally obtunded patients, or in rare patients with disorders of thirst mechanisms. In such individuals, loss of dilute body fluids progressively elevates body fluid osmolality. Initial losses of water are from the extracellular compartment, but water deficits are rapidly equilibrated throughout total body water. The rise in extracellular fluid tonicity causes intracellular water to shift into the extracellular compartment. In effect, approximately two-thirds of pure water deficits are derived from intracellular fluid. Hence extracellular volume depletion is clinically significant in patients with relatively pure deficits of water only when such deficits are large. The principal clinical features are attributable to decreased intracellular volume, especially dehydration of cells in the central nervous system. Brain cells adapt to chronic hyperosmolality by accumulating increased intracellular solute, principally potassium and amino acids. When hyperosmolality is rapidly corrected, the increase in total intracellular solute may promote brain swelling even at normal or slightly elevated plasma osmolality. These mechanisms may account for the fact that rapid correction of hypertonicity sometimes causes deterioration of central nervous function.

Pathogenesis (See Table 45-1)   For clinical purposes it is useful to classify hypernatremia as due to water loss alone; to water deficits associated with, but proportionately in excess of, sodium deficits; or to retention of sodium. *Pure water deficits* may be due to extrarenal or renal water losses that are not replaced. Insensible losses of water from the skin or lungs may reach several liters per day, especially in patients with fever, increased respirations, or extensive burns. Renal losses may lead to hypernatremia in diabetes insipidus. Alert patients with diabetes insipidus ordinarily maintain normal or only slightly hypertonic body fluids despite massive renal water wasting by increasing fluid intake appropriately. However, diabetes insipidus may develop acutely after cerebral trauma or neurosurgical procedures. In such patients, careful attention to replacement of urinary losses is mandatory to avoid severe hypernatremia. Defective thirst and ADH regulation occurs in rare patients with hypothalamic disorders, which may be idiopathic ("essential hypernatremia") or due to specific causes such as tumors, granulomas, and cerebrovascular accidents.

Water losses leading to hypernatremia are often associated with sodium deficits. In such cases, the clinical features of extracellular volume depletion and hypernatremia may both be present, and either may predominate. Extrarenal losses of salt and water due to profuse sweating and renal losses due to osmotic diuresis are the major causes of hypernatremia in this category. Since sweat is hypotonic, hypernatremia will develop if profusely sweating patients cannot drink. In an osmotic diuresis, urinary sodium concentration is less than plasma concentration; therefore, hypernatremia tends to occur. Hypernatremia due to urea diuresis may develop when patients unable to complain of thirst are placed on high-protein feeding. Examples include patients with severe cerebrovascular accidents who are unable to swallow and postoperative neurosurgical patients. In the syndrome of hyperosmolar nonketotic diabetic coma, severe hyperosmolality of the body fluids is due to a combination of hyperglycemia and relative or absolute hypernatremia. The hypernatremia is a consequence of an intense glucose osmotic diuresis in patients who are unable to ingest fluids. Since hyperglycemia itself causes hyponatremia by inducing a shift of water from cells, the presence of hypernatremia in the face of extreme hyperglycemia indicates that total body water is severely depleted.

Infrequently, hypernatremia may result from an absolute *excess of sodium* rather than from water depletion. Examples are hypernatremia caused by accidental substitution of salt for sugar in infant feeding formulas and administration of excessive amounts of hypertonic sodium chloride or bicarbonate infusions to comatose adults unable to drink. The cause of the common mild hypernatremia in patients with adrenal hyperfunction is uncertain. Presumably, stimulation of renal tubular sodium reabsorption by adrenal steroids initiates the hypernatremia, and the hypervolemia that results resets upward the threshold for ADH release. It is not known why the thirst mechanism fails to maintain normal body fluid osmolality.

Clinical features and diagnosis   The principal manifestations of hypernatremia are observed in the central nervous system. Confusion and other evidence of altered mental state; increased neuromuscular irritability, such as twitching and seizures; and obtundation, stupor, or coma may all occur. The magnitude of symptoms depends on the severity of the hyperosmolality. The symptoms are similar whether hyperosmolality is due to hypernatremia or extreme hyperglycemia. The neurologic symptoms appear to be due to dehydration of brain cells. The clinical manifestations of acute hypernatremia are more marked than those of slowly developing hypernatremia. Severe hyperosmolality may cause irreversible neurologic sequelae, apparently due to vascular consequences such as venous sinus thrombosis and hemorrhage from vessels that rupture when the brain shrinks. High mortality rates are associated with extreme hyperosmolality, especially in children and the elderly.

In patients with pure water deficits, manifestations of extracellular volume depletion are minimal because only one-third of the deficit is derived from extracellular fluid. As noted, combined deficits are common, especially in patients who sweat or experience an osmotic diuresis; in such individuals, the signs and symptoms of volume depletion may overshadow those of hypernatremia.

The cause of hypernatremia can usually be inferred from the history when it is due to extrarenal water loss, an osmotic diuresis, or sodium excess. In these cases, the urine is hypertonic to plasma. The differential diagnosis of pituitary and nephrogenic diabetes insipidus, in which urine concentrating ability is impaired, is discussed in Chap. 333.

Treatment   Hypernatremia itself is corrected with water by mouth or by intravenous infusion of 5% dextrose in water. Calculation of water requirements must be based on total body water, since water deficits are drawn from both intracellular and extracellular fluid and both must be repleted. For example, suppose a 70-kg man has a plasma sodium of 160 mmol/L which is to be lowered to 140. Total body water is estimated as 60 percent of 70 kg, which is 42 L. To reduce plasma sodium, this volume must be increased to $(160/140) \times 42$ L, which equals 48 L. Thus a positive water balance of 6 L $(48 - 42)$ is required. Hypernatremia should be corrected slowly; no more than half the water deficit should be replaced in the first 12 to 24 h. As stated above, rapid correction of hypertonicity may cause central nervous function to deteriorate.

In patients with associated sodium deficits, saline solutions should be infused. If the predominant clinical feature is extracellular volume depletion with circulatory insufficiency, treatment should begin with 0.9% saline to replete extracellular volume promptly. If the neurologic effects of hypertonicity predominate, therapy can start with 0.45% saline. In patients with hyperosmolar diabetic coma, sodium deficits are usually large, due to prior glucose osmotic diuresis. Plasma hypertonicity is due to both hyperglycemia and hypernatremia. Treatment consists of isotonic saline (0.9%) to replete extracellular volume and insulin to lower plasma glucose and thereby partly correct hypertonicity. Later, hypotonic saline (0.45%) can replace the remaining water and salt deficits and return plasma sodium to normal.

POTASSIUM

PHYSIOLOGIC CONSIDERATIONS   Potassium is the principal intracellular cation. Active transport mediated by Na^+,K^+–stimulated

ATPase in cell membranes maintains a cellular concentration of approximately 160 mmol/L, 40 times that in extracellular fluid. All but 2 percent of the 2500 to 3000 mmol potassium in the body is within cells. Since potassium is a large fraction of total cellular solute, it is a major determinant of the volume of the cell and the osmolality of the body fluids. Moreover, potassium is an important cofactor in a number of metabolic processes. Extracellular potassium, while a small fraction of the total, greatly influences neuromuscular function. The ratio of intracellular to extracellular potassium concentration is the principal determinant of membrane potential in excitable tissues. Since extracellular potassium concentration is low, small deviations in concentration produce large variations in this ratio; conversely, only large changes in intracellular potassium influence the ratio significantly. These relationships have practical consequences. For example, toxic effects of hyperkalemia can be mitigated by inducing movement of potassium from extracellular fluid into cells.

With the exception of changes in acid-base balance (see below), in most circumstances extracellular and intracellular potassium change in the same direction. Hence alterations in plasma potassium are a useful index of alterations in total body potassium. During potassium depletion, plasma potassium initially decreases about 1 mmol/L for each 100 to 200 mmol lost. However, plasma potassium falls more slowly after it reaches 2 mmol/L. Thus a plasma potassium in the range of 2 to 3.5 mmol/L is a reasonably accurate guide to the magnitude of depletion, but plasma potassium concentrations less than 2 mmol/L may reflect a wide range of deficits, from moderate to severe. Plasma concentration increases about 1 mmol/L after acute administration of 100 to 200 mmol potassium. Assuming an extracellular volume of 15 L, 150 mmol would be expected to raise plasma potassium by about 10 mmol/L. Thus the largest fraction of administered potassium rapidly enters cells. Renal excretion also increases promptly. Chronic exposure to high-potassium diets enhances both tissue uptake and renal excretion of the ion; the mechanism of these adaptations is uncertain. Sustained hyperkalemia rarely is caused by excess intake, because these mechanisms normally function so efficiently. Impaired renal excretion and cellular transfer are the usual causes of hyperkalemia.

The relation between plasma and cellular potassium is influenced by acid-base balance and by hormones. Acidosis tends to shift potassium out of cells, and alkalosis favors movement from extracellular fluid into cells. The relation between blood pH and plasma potassium is complex and is influenced by several factors, including the type of acidosis, the duration of the altered acid-base state, and the change in plasma bicarbonate per se. In general, plasma potassium changes less with respiratory acidosis than with metabolic acidosis and less with alkalosis than with acidosis. Metabolic acidosis due to organic acids such as lactic acid or ketoacids has little or no effect on plasma potassium, while mineral acids (e.g., hyperchloremic acidosis or renal failure acidosis) increase plasma potassium by about 0.5 to 1.0 mmol/L per 0.1-unit decrease in plasma pH. While the magnitude of the change in plasma potassium cannot be predicted from changes in blood pH alone, a patient with normal total body potassium tends to be hyperkalemic if acidotic and hypokalemic if alkalotic. Hormones appear to be important parts of the mechanism for moving potassium loads out of plasma. Insulin and beta-adrenergic catecholamines promote movement of potassium into cells. Conversely, alpha-adrenergic agonists impair potassium uptake into cells.

Of the usual potassium intake of 50 to 150 mmol/d, most is excreted in the urine. Normally, stool and sweat contain only about 5 mmol/d. As noted, the kidneys respond to acute and chronic changes in potassium intake by corresponding changes in excretion. Excess potassium is excreted promptly; about half of an acute load appears in the urine within 12 h. The renal response to potassium depletion is more sluggish. Excretion does not fall to minimal levels for 7 to 14 days. During this period, a deficit of 200 mmol or more may develop in an individual on a potassium-deficient diet. Renal excretory mechanisms for potassium are complex. Potassium in the urine is derived almost entirely from potassium secreted in the distal convo-

luted tubule and collecting duct; filtered potassium is nearly quantitatively reabsorbed in more proximal segments. Potassium secretion is influenced by the potassium concentration of tubular cells, aldosterone, distal tubular fluid flow rate, acid-base balance, and factors that alter distal tubular electronegativity. Aldosterone stimulates potassium secretion. Thus hyperkalemia increases potassium excretion by two mechanisms: It stimulates adrenal secretion of aldosterone, and it directly enhances renal secretion, presumably via increased tubular cell potassium. Potassium secretion in the distal tubule is flow-dependent; increased distal delivery of tubular fluid favors potassium excretion. For example, loop diuretics, which enhance distal volume delivery, increase potassium excretion, especially in patients with edema and secondary aldosteronism. Alkalosis enhances and acidosis depresses renal potassium secretion, probably by inducing corresponding changes in tubular cell potassium. If delivery to distal segments of sodium salts of unreabsorbable anions such as excess bicarbonate or carbenicillin is augmented, tubular electronegative potential will increase as sodium is reabsorbed. The enhanced electrical gradient will promote potassium excretion.

POTASSIUM DEPLETION AND HYPOKALEMIA   Pathogenesis

The principal causes of potassium depletion are listed in Table 45-2. As noted above, renal excretion of potassium falls slowly in persons on potassium-deficient diets. During the 10 to 14 days before balance is achieved, significant deficits may occur. Thus, in contrast to sodium, moderate potassium depletion may result from *poor intake* alone. Potassium deficiency is frequent in *gastrointestinal disorders* in which vomiting, diarrhea, or loss of gastrointestinal secretions is prominent. Diarrhea may cause large potassium deficits, since the potassium concentration of liquid stool is 40 to 60 mmol/L. *Loss of gastric secretions* through vomiting or nasogastric suction is also a common cause of potassium depletion. The potassium concentration of gastric fluid is only 5 to 10 mmol/L; direct losses contribute modestly to negative potassium balance. The potassium deficit is primarily due to increased renal excretion. Potassium excretion appears to be stimulated by three mechanisms. Loss of gastric acid leads to *metabolic alkalosis*, which increases tubular cell potassium concentration. The elevated plasma bicarbonate concentration also increases delivery of bicarbonate and fluid to the distal nephron. At that site, as noted above, excess bicarbonate acts as a nonreabsorbable anion to augment potassium excretion. Finally, secondary hyperaldosteronism due to associated extracellular volume contraction may play a role in maintaining potassium excretion at high levels despite potassium depletion.

TABLE 45-2 Causes of potassium depletion and hypokalemia

I Gastrointestinal
  A Deficient dietary intake
  B Gastrointestinal disorders (vomiting, diarrhea, villous adenoma, fistulas, ureterosigmoidostomy)
II Renal
  A Metabolic alkalosis
  B Diuretics, osmotic diuresis
  C Excessive mineralocorticoid effects
    1 Primary aldosteronism
    2 Secondary aldosteronism (including malignant hypertension, Bartter's syndrome, juxtaglomerular cell tumor)
    3 Licorice ingestion
    4 Glucocorticoid excess (Cushing's syndrome, exogenous steroids, ectopic ACTH production)
  D Renal tubular diseases
    1 Renal tubular acidosis (types I and II)
    2 Leukemia
    3 Liddle's syndrome
    4 Certain antibiotics
  E Magnesium depletion
III Hypokalemia due to shift into cells (no depletion)
  A Hypokalemic periodic paralysis
  B Insulin effect
  C Alkalosis
  D Increased beta-adrenergic activity

Diuretics are among the most frequent causes of hypokalemia and potassium depletion. Thiazides, loop diuretics, and carbonic anhydrase inhibitors all increase potassium excretion. These agents augment sodium and fluid delivery to the distal potassium secretory site by inhibiting reabsorption in more proximal nephron segments. Loop diuretics also inhibit potassium reabsorption by the $Na^+-K^+-2Cl^-$ transport mechanism in the ascending limb of Henle's loop. Carbonic anhydrase inhibitors such as acetazolamide, which inhibit proximal bicarbonate reabsorption, also enhance potassium excretion by increasing distal delivery of nonreabsorbable bicarbonate. Hypokalemia and potassium depletion are frequent when diuretics are used to treat edematous patients, in whom secondary aldosteronism is the rule. Although hypokalemia also occurs in patients receiving diuretics for treatment of hypertension, potassium depletion is modest if dietary potassium is normal. Surreptitious abuse of diuretics should be considered when hypokalemic patients have renal potassium wasting of uncertain cause.

Potassium excretion is increased during an *osmotic diuresis*. This mechanism leads to potassium depletion in patients with diabetic ketoacidosis, in whom the osmotic diuresis is due to glycosuria and to increased excretion of keto acid anions. However, despite potassium depletion plasma potassium may be normal or even high due to the shift of potassium out of tissues caused principally by insulin deficiency and renal insufficiency. Failure to recognize potassium depletion may lead to serious cardiotoxicity from sudden hypokalemia when the ketoacidosis is treated with insulin or alkali. A normal plasma potassium concentration in a patient with diabetic ketoacidosis strongly suggests potassium depletion.

Urinary potassium loss is often due to *excessive mineralocorticoid activity*. Hypokalemia is characteristic of *primary aldosteronism* (Chap. 335). It may be minimal in patients with restricted sodium intake because potassium excretion is limited by decreased distal salt and fluid delivery. *Secondary aldosteronism* causes renal potassium wasting and hypokalemia in patients with malignant hypertension, Bartter's syndrome, and renin-secreting renal tumors. However, patients with congestive heart failure, hepatic cirrhosis, and nephrotic syndrome usually are not hypokalemic despite secondary aldosteronism. The decrease in effective blood volume in such patients reduces distal delivery of salt and fluid, thereby limiting potassium excretion. As noted above, treatment with diuretics, which increase distal delivery, will often provoke hypokalemia in these patients. Patients who consume huge amounts of licorice may become hypokalemic. Glycyrrhizic acid in licorice inhibits 11-β-hydroxysteroid dehydrogenase, an enzyme which normally minimizes the mineralocorticoid activity of endogenous cortisol in the kidney by converting it to an inactive metabolite. Excessive levels of *glucocorticoids* stimulate secretion of renal potassium (and hydrogen), leading to hypokalemia and alkalosis in patients with *Cushing's syndrome* (Chap. 335) and some receiving *therapeutic steroids*.

Renal tubular potassium wasting is a feature of types I and II *renal tubular acidosis* (Chap. 244). Some patients with monocytic or myelomonocytic *leukemia* develop hypokalemia. The mechanism is uncertain. Renal potassium wasting in some patients appears to correlate with lysozymuria, and the enzyme may interfere with tubular function. In *Liddle's syndrome*, a rare familial disorder (Chap. 244), renal potassium wasting is an intrinsic tubular abnormality. Certain *antibiotics* may cause hypokalemia by increasing potassium excretion. Carbenicillin and rarely other penicillin derivatives given in large amounts promote distal tubular secretion by acting as unreabsorbed anions; amphotericin B alters distal tubular permeability. Gentamicin also has been reported to cause hypokalemia by unknown mechanisms.

Magnesium depletion can cause potassium depletion, apparently due to increased renal and possibly gastrointestinal losses. Increased aldosterone secretion may play a role in stimulating potassium excretion. Hypokalemia in this condition is associated with hypocalcemia.

Hypokalemia without potassium depletion occurs in a number of conditions in which *potassium shifts into cells*. Patients with *periodic paralysis* develop repeated episodes of muscle weakness, which may be severe or even life-threatening if respiratory muscles are involved. These are due to sudden movement of potassium into cells, which causes hypokalemia. *Insulin* promotes a shift of potassium into cells. Administration of large amounts of dextrose intravenously may cause mild hypokalemia by stimulating insulin secretion. This effect may be clinically significant if dextrose solutions are used to administer potassium to hypokalemic patients. Plasma *alkalosis* tends to decrease plasma potassium modestly (less than 0.5 mmol/L per 0.1-unit increase in pH) by promoting potassium movement into cells. Treatment of acidosis with bicarbonate infusions may have a greater effect on plasma potassium because potassium entry into cells is enhanced not only by increasing plasma pH but also by a direct effect of bicarbonate ion. As discussed above, hypokalemia in alkalotic patients also may reflect loss of potassium in the urine, e.g., with vomiting, diuretic use, or excessive mineralocorticoid effects. Exogenous or endogenous *beta-adrenergic catecholamines* may cause hypokalemia by stimulating potassium shifts into cells. This phenomenon may be one factor leading to cardiac arrhythmias during stress or during treatment of asthma with beta-adrenergic agonists.

Clinical features   The most prominent features of hypokalemia and potassium depletion are neuromuscular. Moderate degrees of depletion may be asymptomatic, especially if they develop slowly. Some patients, however, complain of muscle weakness, especially in the lower extremities. With more severe or acute degrees of hypokalemia and potassium deficiency, marked and generalized weakness of skeletal muscles is prominent. Very severe or abrupt development of hypokalemia may lead to virtually total paralysis, including the respiratory muscles. Rhabdomyolysis may occur. On physical examination, in addition to decreased motor power, the patient may demonstrate decreased or absent tendon reflexes. The smooth muscle of the gastrointestinal tract may be affected, resulting in paralytic ileus.

Abnormalities in the electrocardiogram are common. The characteristic changes include flattening and inversion of the T wave, increased prominence of the U wave, and sagging of the ST segment (Fig. 189-20A). These alterations are not well correlated with the severity of the disturbance in potassium metabolism and cannot be relied on as indexes of the clinical significance of a potassium deficit. Although moderate potassium depletion rarely affects cardiac action, severe or rapid reduction in serum potassium may cause cardiac arrest. Potassium deficiency enhances the cardiac toxicity of digitalis preparations. A variety of atrial and ventricular arrhythmias may occur in hypokalemia, especially in patients receiving digitalis.

Renal tubular function is markedly impaired by potassium depletion (Chap. 242). The most prominent abnormality is decreased concentrating ability, which may cause polyuria and polydipsia. Glomerular filtration rate is normal or slightly reduced; moderate reductions may occur with chronic potassium depletion nephropathy. Renal regulation of potassium excretion remains normal. The urinalysis is benign: Protein excretion is normal or minimally increased, and the urinary sediment is normal or demonstrates only a slight increase in hyaline or granular casts.

Diagnosis   The cause of hypokalemia and potassium depletion is usually evident from the history. However, patients whose potassium deficiency is caused by chronic abuse of laxatives; psychogenic, self-induced vomiting; or surreptitious use of diuretics rarely volunteer an accurate history. Patients with villous adenomas of the rectum sometimes report that their feces are formed; careful questioning will reveal the elimination of the characteristic mucous secretion of the tumor.

In Fig. 45-2 is a flowchart that outlines the steps in differential diagnosis of hypokalemia when the cause is not evident from the history. The presence of *hypertension*, which suggests hyperaldosteronism (except Bartter's syndrome) or glucocorticoid excess, may be a clue to diagnosis. Blood pressure is normal in patients whose potassium depletion is due to the other causes listed in Table 45-2. Evaluation of *urinary potassium excretion* may be helpful in

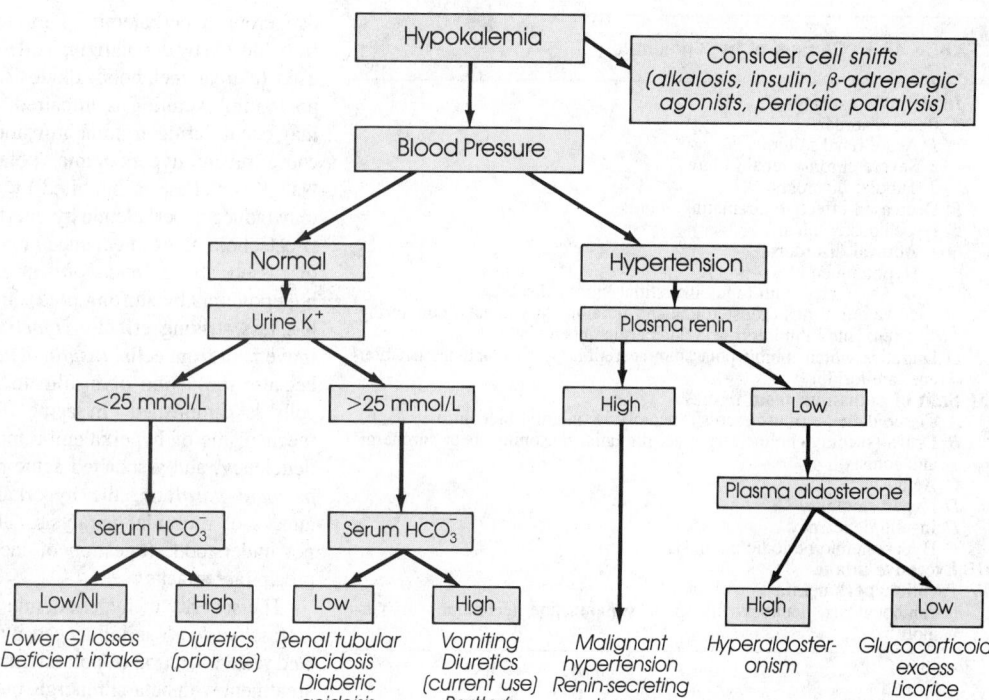

FIGURE 45-2 Flowchart for differential diagnosis of principal causes of hypokalemia. Nl = Normal.

determining the origin of the potassium deficit. If gastrointestinal losses have occurred, urinary excretion is usually less than 20 to 25 mmol/L or per day. Although renal conservation of potassium is slow, excretion falls to these levels by the time that clinically significant deficits of potassium have accumulated. On the other hand, when renal potassium wasting is the cause, urinary excretion usually exceeds 20 to 25 mmol/L or per day. However, lower concentrations and lower excretion rates may be found in severe depletion, in those patients with excessive mineralocorticoid activity while on low sodium intake, and in patients whose diuretics have been stopped at the time of examination. Evaluation of blood *acid-base status* may help in differential diagnosis. Hypokalemia is associated with metabolic acidosis in types I and II renal tubular acidosis, diarrhea, and diabetic ketoacidosis and in patients treated with carbonic anhydrase inhibitors. With other causes of hypokalemia, blood bicarbonate is normal or elevated due to associated metabolic alkalosis.

Treatment When possible, potassium depletion should be corrected by increased dietary intake or supplementation with potassium salts. Potassium chloride is the salt of choice, especially in alkalotic patients. It may be given in the form of an elixir or in tablets in which potassium chloride crystals are embedded in a wax. Enteric-coated potassium chloride tablets have been responsible for ulceration of the small bowel, due to release of high concentrations of potassium salts, and should be avoided. Organic salts such as gluconate or citrate are adequate in patients who are not severely alkalotic and often are used to treat hypokalemia due to renal tubular acidosis. In edematous patients treated with diuretics that cause hypokalemia, potassium deficits should be prevented or treated by increased dietary potassium intake, supplementation with potassium chloride, or addition of "potassium-sparing" diuretics such as spironolactone. More controversial is the need for routine dietary supplements in patients receiving diuretics for treatment of hypertension. Patients with adequate dietary potassium intake usually do not develop significant hypokalemia and probably do not require routine supplements to prevent potassium depletion. However, those who do develop hypokalemia despite adequate diets should probably receive potassium salts, since hypokalemia may be associated with an increased frequency of arrhythmias.

Intravenous treatment is required for patients with gastrointestinal disorders or when the potassium deficiency is severe. It must be emphasized that the potassium *concentration* in commonly available intravenous solutions of potassium chloride is 2000 mmol/L. Concentrations in intravenous infusions should not exceed 40 or at the most 60 mmol/L. The rate of infusion should not exceed 20 mmol/h or approximately 200 to 250 mmol/d, unless the need for more rapid infusion has been demonstrated in the individual patient by evidence of continuing losses large enough to justify more intensive therapy. The results of treatment are best monitored by repeated determinations of plasma potassium and evaluation of clinical symptoms such as muscular weakness or paralysis. Disappearance of electrocardiographic abnormalities correlates only roughly with improvement in total body potassium content. However, during rapid intravenous administration of potassium, the electrocardiogram should be monitored to avoid cardiac toxicity from inadvertent hyperkalemia.

Hypokalemia and hypocalcemia may occur together, e.g., in patients with malabsorption syndrome. The neuromuscular effect of each electrolyte abnormality is masked by the other. Treatment of either disorder alone may precipitate symptoms. Thus treatment of hypokalemia alone may precipitate tetany, and conversely, treatment of hypocalcemia without correcting the hypokalemia may exacerbate the manifestations of potassium deficiency.

HYPERKALEMIA Pathogenesis The causes of hyperkalemia are shown in Table 45-3. Inadequate renal excretion is a frequent cause (see also Chaps. 236 and 237). When oliguria or anuria is present, as in acute renal failure, progressive hyperkalemia is the rule. Plasma potassium rises by about 0.5 mmol/L per day if there are no abnormal loads. Chronic renal failure does not cause severe or progressive hyperkalemia unless oliguria supervenes. Adaptive changes increase potassium excretion per residual nephron as chronic renal failure progresses. However, patients with chronic renal failure function at the limits of their excretory capacity. Hence hyperkalemia may develop rapidly if the potassium load is increased or excretory capacity is limited, e.g., by administration of spironolactone. *Impaired tubular potassium secretion* has been described in a number of tubulointerstitial diseases. Causes include lupus erythematosus, sickle cell disease, rejection of a transplanted kidney, obstructive uropathy, and amyloidosis. Tubular H$^+$ secretion is often impaired as well, leading to the combination of hyperkalemia and hyperchloremic acidosis (type IV renal tubular acidosis). The defect in potassium secretion may result directly from a tubular disorder or may be due to hyporeninemic hypoaldosteronism (see below).

A *decrease in effective circulating volume* tends to impair potassium excretion. In conditions such as salt and water depletion or

TABLE 45-3   Causes of hyperkalemia

I Inadequate excretion
   A Renal disorders
      1 Acute renal failure
      2 Severe chronic renal failure
      3 Tubular disorders
   B Decreased effective circulating volume
   C Hypoaldosteronism
      1 Adrenal disorders
      2 Hyporeninemic
         a Associated with tubulointerstitial kidney disease
         b Due to drugs (nonsteroidal anti-inflammatory agents, converting-enzyme inhibitors, beta-adrenergic antagonists)
   D Diuretics which inhibit potassium secretion (spironolactone, triamterene, amiloride)
II Shift of potassium from tissues
   A Tissue damage (muscle crush, hemolysis, internal bleeding)
   B Drugs (succinylcholine, arginine, digitalis, poisoning, beta-adrenergic antagonists)
   C Acidosis
   D Hyperosmolality
   E Insulin deficiency
   F Hyperkalemic periodic paralysis
III Excessive intake
IV Pseudohyperkalemia
   (thrombocytosis, leukocytosis, poor venipuncture technique, in vitro hemolysis)

congestive heart failure, glomerular filtration rate is reduced and proximal fluid reabsorption is enhanced. This decreases delivery of fluid to the distal tubule, thereby limiting potassium secretion into the urine. Hyperkalemia may occur in some patients; it is usually modest and not progressive but may become severe if potassium loads are high.

Hyperkalemia is a cardinal feature of adrenal insufficiency (Addison's disease) and of certain congenital adrenal enzyme disorders, including selective *hypoaldosteronism*. Heparin inhibits aldosterone secretion; hyperkalemia may occur in patients treated with heparin who have other potentiating factors, such as volume depletion or renal insufficiency.

In adults, *hyporeninemic hypoaldosteronism* (see Chap. 335) is a frequent cause of hyperkalemia. In patients with this disorder, renin and aldosterone secretion are deficient. Hypoaldosteronism appears to be due both to the decrease in angiotensin, a major stimulus to aldosterone secretion, and to some secretory defect in the adrenal gland. Most patients have moderate renal insufficiency. In about half this is due to diabetic nephropathy, but a variety of chronic interstitial nephritides may cause this syndrome. Patients typically present with hyperkalemia, often associated with hyperchloremic acidosis (type IV renal tubular acidosis). Inhibition of the activity of the renin-angiotensin-aldosterone system by nonsteroidal anti-inflammatory drugs, converting enzyme inhibitors or beta-adrenergic blockers also may induce hyperkalemia due to hyporeninemic hypoaldosteronism. (Beta-adrenergic blockers also inhibit potassium entry into cells; see below.)

A kilogram of tissue such as muscle or erythrocytes contains about 80 mmol potassium, and damaged cells release potassium into the plasma. Hence hyperkalemia may be seen when there is muscle-crushing injury, hemolysis, or internal hemorrhage. Severe progressive hyperkalemia is not ordinarily a consequence of increased release of potassium from damaged or acidotic tissues alone. However, acidosis and tissue damage often occur together with acute renal insufficiency; under these circumstances, severe hyperkalemia may develop quickly. In contrast to the increase of 0.5 mmol/L per day typical of uncomplicated anuria, plasma potassium concentration in anuric patients with tissue damage may increase 2 to 4 mmol/L per day. Such rapidly progressive hyperkalemia may be an important cause of death in military casualties. Several *drugs* may cause hyperkalemia by altering tissue uptake of potassium. In patients with trauma, burns, or neuromuscular diseases such as paraplegia and multiple sclerosis, the muscle relaxant succinylcholine may cause

dangerous hyperkalemia. This agent apparently releases potassium from muscle by depolarizing cell membranes. Arginine hydrochloride, used to treat metabolic alkalosis, drives potassium out of cells. If potassium excretion is impaired, clinically significant hyperkalemia may occur during arginine infusions. Extreme digitalis poisoning may cause severe hyperkalemia; potassium leaks out of cells because Na^+,K^+-ATPase is inhibited by the drug. Beta-adrenergic blockers may induce hyperkalemia by interfering with the action of endogenous β-catecholamines to enhance movement of potassium into tissues. As discussed above, *metabolic acidosis* due to mineral acids causes hyperkalemia by shifting potassium out of cells. Respiratory acidosis has less striking effects. *Hyperosmolality* also enhances potassium movement from cells. *Insulin deficiency* is conducive to hyperkalemia because the action of insulin to promote potassium movement into cells is diminished. In acute diabetic ketoacidosis, the principal mechanisms of hyperkalemia appear to be hyperosmolality, insulin deficiency, and associated acute renal insufficiency. In *hyperkalemic periodic paralysis*, the hyperkalemia is associated with repeated attacks of muscular paralysis. The mechanism of this syndrome is not understood. Ingestion of increased amounts of potassium may precipitate attacks.

The severity of hyperkalemia caused by large oral or intravenous *potassium loads* is influenced by factors that modulate tissue uptake and renal excretion of potassium. For example, insulin deficiency and treatment with beta-adrenergic blockers tend to augment hyperkalemia by limiting tissue uptake. Volume depletion and administration of converting enzyme inhibitors or nonsteroidal anti-inflammatory agents enhance hyperkalemia by limiting the rate at which the kidney excretes such loads.

Patients with extreme thrombocytosis or, more rarely, extreme leukocytosis in leukemia may demonstrate the phenomenon of *pseudohyperkalemia*. Platelets or white blood cells release potassium during blood clotting in vitro. While serum potassium may be grossly abnormal, plasma potassium is not increased. Artifactual elevation of plasma potassium may occur if blood is drawn after repeated fist clenching to make veins more prominent during application of a tourniquet, due to leakage of potassium from exercising muscle. Improper technique during collection or processing of blood samples may cause hemolysis and hence hyperkalemia in vitro. Artifactual hyperkalemia may be suspected when electrocardiographic abnormalities are absent despite elevation of measured potassium levels.

Clinical features The most important toxic effects of hyperkalemia are cardiac arrhythmias. The earliest manifestation is the development of high-peaked T waves, especially prominent in precordial leads. Hyperkalemia does not prolong the QT interval, unlike other disorders which induce peaking of the T waves. Later changes include prolongation of the PR interval, complete heart block, and atrial asystole. As plasma potassium rises further, ventricular complexes may deteriorate. The QRS complex becomes progressively prolonged and finally tends to merge with the T wave in a sinewave configuration. Terminally, ventricular fibrillation and standstill may occur.

Occasionally, moderate or severe hyperkalemia has striking effects on peripheral muscles. Ascending muscular weakness can occur, progressing to flaccid quadriplegia and respiratory paralysis. Cerebral and cranial nerve function are normal, as is sensation.

Diagnosis Severe or progressive hyperkalemia is rare in the absence of renal insufficiency. Hence plasma creatinine and urine output should be determined promptly in hyperkalemic patients. Acute renal failure, especially if oliguric, will cause progressive hyperkalemia. Even in oliguric patients, an increase in plasma potassium of more than 0.5 mmol/L per day suggests the need to search for a source of potassium loads, e.g., from tissue breakdown in hematomas or muscle undergoing rhabdomyolysis. When hyperkalemia is detected in nonoliguric patients with chronic renal failure, the physician should look for sources of high dietary potassium intake or medications which interfere with potassium excretion. In the absence of such superimposed factors, hyperkalemia in these patients should suggest hyporeninemic hypoaldosteronism or a tubular disease which directly impairs tubular potassium secretion. This distinction is made by appropriate studies of renin and aldosterone levels (see Chap. 335), which are reduced in patients with hyporeninemic hypoaldosteronism but not in those with hyperkalemia due directly to tubular damage.

In all patients with hyperkalemia, the history should focus on medications that may cause elevated plasma potassium levels, such as converting enzyme inhibitors, nonsteroidal anti-inflammatory agents, beta-adrenergic blockers, and potassium-sparing diuretics. Sources of high potassium intake in the diet should be reviewed, e.g., potassium supplements or salt substitutes. Signs of extracellular volume depletion, Addison's disease, or edematous states with decreased effective extracellular volume should be sought on physical examination.

In addition to plasma creatinine, blood sugar and plasma bicarbonate levels should be determined to evaluate possible contributions of diabetes or acidosis to hyperkalemia. Urine potassium measurements are of little value in differential diagnosis. An electrocardiogram is important to evaluate the effects of hyperkalemia. In patients with no adequate explanation for hyperkalemia, especially if the electrocardiogram demonstrates no hyperkalemic features, the possibility of spurious hyperkalemia should be considered.

Treatment In considering therapy, it is helpful to classify hyperkalemia according to degree of severity. The seriousness of hyperkalemia is best estimated by considering both the plasma potassium concentration and the electrocardiogram. When the plasma potassium is less than 6 mmol/L and electrocardiographic changes are limited to peaking of T waves, hyperkalemia is mild. When the plasma potassium is 6 to 8 mmol/L and T-wave peaking is the only electrocardiographic abnormality, hyperkalemia is moderate. Severe hyperkalemia is present if the plasma potassium exceeds 8 mmol/L or if electrocardiographic abnormalities include absent P waves, widened QRS complexes, or ventricular arrhythmias.

Mild hyperkalemia can usually be treated by elimination of a cause, such as potassium-sparing diuretics, or by treatment of accompanying volume depletion or acidosis. Patients with Addison's disease require specific hormonal therapy (see Chap. 335). Those with renal tubular disorders can be treated with loop diuretics to increase potassium excretion. Patients with hyporeninemic hypoaldosteronism also respond to loop diuretics or may require mineralocorticoid therapy (see Chap. 335).

More severe or progressive hyperkalemia requires vigorous therapy. Severe cardiac toxicity responds most rapidly to infusion of calcium; 10 to 30 mL of 10% calcium gluconate may be infused intravenously within a period of 1 to 5 min under constant electrocardiographic monitoring. While calcium infusions do not alter plasma potassium, they counteract the adverse effects of potassium on neuromuscular membranes. The effect of calcium infusions, while almost immediate, is transient if the hyperkalemia is not treated directly.

In moderate or severe hyperkalemia, infusion of hypertonic glucose solutions decreases toxicity by provoking insulin release and shifting potassium into cells. In the first 30 min, 200 to 500 mL of 10% glucose may be given. An additional 500 to 1000 mL may be infused over the next several hours. Concurrently, 10 units of regular insulin is given intravenously or subcutaneously. This treatment may reduce serum potassium by 1 to 2 mmol/L within 30 to 60 min, and effects persist for a number of hours. The infusion of sodium bicarbonate also helps lower serum potassium rapidly by causing potassium to shift into cells; 50 to 150 mmol alkali (two to three ampuls) may be added to a liter of glucose. Although this agent is most valuable in acidotic patients, it also is effective in individuals with normal acid-base status. The effect occurs within 1 h and persists for a number of hours. The infusion of hypertonic sodium solutions also may be effective in reversing cardiac toxicity, especially in hyponatremic or volume-depleted patients. In part, the effect depends simply on dilution of plasma potassium, but there may be a direct effect of elevated plasma sodium to antagonize hyperkalemic neuromuscular

toxicity as well. Glucose, bicarbonate, and sodium may be combined in a "therapeutic cocktail," formulated by adding an ampul or two of sodium bicarbonate to a liter of 5% dextrose in 0.9% saline.

None of the measures just described removes potassium from the body. Cation-exchange resins such as sodium polystyrene sulfonate are useful to remove potassium in the treatment of moderate or severe hyperkalemia. Fifty grams of the resin is mixed with 100 mL of 35% sorbitol and given by retention enema. Enough potassium may be removed by a single enema to reduce potassium by 0.5 to 2 mmol/L within an hour, and repeated enemas can be given. These resins also can be given repeatedly by mouth to maintain low plasma potassium concentrations. Twenty grams is given three or four times a day together with 20 mL of a 70% sorbitol solution as required to ensure the passage of several loose stools daily. In patients with renal failure, hemodialysis and peritoneal dialysis effectively control hyperkalemia. However, they are relatively slow techniques, and patients with severe hyperkalemia should be treated first with one of the methods previously discussed.

REFERENCES

Sodium and water

DeVita MV, Michelis MF: Perturbations in sodium balance. Hyponatremia. Clin Lab Med 13:135, 1993

Kamel KS, Bear RA: Treatment of hyponatremia: A quantitative analysis. Am J Kidney Dis 21:439, 1993

Narins RG et al: Diagnostic strategies in disorders of fluid, electrolyte and acid-base homeostasis. Am J Med 72:496, 1982

Robertson GL: Thirst and vasopressin function in normal and disordered states of water balance. J Lab Clin Med 101:351, 1983

Sonnenblick, M et al: Diuretic-induced severe hyponatremia. Review and analysis of 129 reported patients. Chest 103:601, 1993

Strange K: Regulation of solute and water balance and cell volume in the central nervous system. J Am Soc Nephrol 3:12, 1992

Weisberg LS et al: Pseudohyponatremia: A reappraisal. Am J Med 86:315, 1989

Zerbe R et al: Vasopressin function in the syndrome of inappropriate diuresis. Ann Rev Med 31:315, 1980

Potassium

DeFronzo RA: Clinical disorders of hyperkalemia, in *The Kidney: Physiology and Pathophysiology*, 3d ed, DW Seldin, G Giebisch (eds). New York, Raven, 1992, p 2279

Knochel JP: The syndrome of hyporeninemic hypoaldosteronism. Ann Rev Med 30:145, 1979

———: Neuromuscular manifestations of electrolyte disorders. Am J Med 72:521, 1982

———: Hypokalemia. Adv Intern Med 30:317, 1984

Kupin WL, Narins RG: The hyperkalemia of renal failure: pathophysiology, diagnosis and therapy. Contrib Nephrol 102:1, 1993

Latta K et al: Perturbations in potassium balance. Clin Lab Med 13:149, 1993

Seldin DW, Giebisch G (eds): *The Regulation of Sodium and Chloride Balance*. New York, Raven, 1989

Sterns RH et al: Internal potassium balance and the control of the plasma potassium concentration. Medicine 60:339, 1981

Stokes JB: Potassium intoxication: Pathogenesis and Treatment, in *The Regulation of Potassium Balance*, DW Seldin, G Giebisch (eds). New York, Raven, 1989, p 269

Tannen RL: Diuretic-induced hypokalemia. Kidney Int 28:988, 1985

46 ACIDOSIS AND ALKALOSIS

NORMAN G. LEVINSKY

PHYSIOLOGIC CONSIDERATIONS Acids are produced continuously during normal metabolism. Despite the addition of some 20,000 mmol of carbonic acid and 80 mmol of nonvolatile acids to body fluids daily, the free hydrogen ion concentration of these fluids is fixed within a narrow range. The pH of extracellular fluids is normally between 7.35 and 7.45 (hydrogen ion, 45 to 35 nmol/L). The pH of intracellular fluids cannot be determined with precision, but most methods suggest a mean intracellular pH in the range of 6.9.

Intracellular hydrogen ion concentration is not uniform; it varies among intracellular organelles within individual cells. Although the free hydrogen ion concentration of body fluids is low, protons are so reactive that even minute changes in concentration influence enzymatic reactions and physiologic processes. Immediate defense against untoward changes in pH is provided by buffers that can take up or release protons instantaneously in response to changes in acidity of body fluids. Regulation of pH ultimately depends on the lungs and the kidneys.

Role of the lungs   The principal acid product of metabolism is carbon dioxide, equivalent to potential carbonic acid. The normal concentration of carbon dioxide in body fluids is fixed around 1.2 mmol/L [P_{CO_2} = 5.3 kPa (40 mmHg)] by the lungs; at this concentration, pulmonary excretion equals metabolic production. Although carbon dioxide reacts with water and body buffers during transport from cells to pulmonary alveoli, no net change in body fluid composition results, since the CO_2 excreted by the lungs is equal to the CO_2 produced by cells.

Nonvolatile acids   When a nonvolatile acid is produced by metabolism, the protons are removed instantaneously from body fluids by reaction with buffers. In extracellular fluid, bicarbonate is converted to water and carbon dioxide, which is excreted by the lungs. Although this mechanism minimizes changes in acidity, it destroys bicarbonate and uses up cell buffer capacity. The total buffer capacity of the body fluids is about 15 mmol/kg of body weight. The normal rate of production of nonvolatile acids would be sufficient to deplete the body buffers completely in 10 to 20 days, were it not for the ability of the kidney to eliminate protons from the body by secretion into the urine, thereby regenerating bicarbonate and cell buffer capacity.

The principal source of nonvolatile acid is metabolism of methionine and cystine in dietary proteins, which produces sulfuric acid. Additional sources include the incomplete combustion of carbohydrates and fats, which produces organic acids; the metabolism of nucleoproteins, which produces uric acid; and the metabolism of organic phosphorus compounds, which releases protons and inorganic phosphates. The diet does not normally contain significant amounts of preformed acid or alkali, but significant amounts of potential acid (e.g., an excess of cationic acids, such as lysine) or alkali (e.g., citrate) may be present.

Role of the kidney   The principal functions of the kidney in acid-base balance can be viewed as (1) retention of extracellular bicarbonate and (2) excretion of protons of nonvolatile acids produced by metabolic processes. Both functions are served by secretion of protons into tubular fluid, in proximal nephron segments via a sodium-proton exchanger and in distal segments by an H^+-ATPase pump. The protons secreted into tubular fluid are derived from carbon dioxide (carbonic acid); removal of protons generates bicarbonate in the tubular cell. This bicarbonate is reabsorbed with filtered sodium. When secreted protons are buffered by filtered bicarbonate, it is destroyed. The bicarbonate lost in this process is replaced by reabsorption of the bicarbonate generated in renal tubular cells, thereby conserving existing bicarbonate stores. When the secreted protons are buffered by urinary buffers other than bicarbonate, filtered bicarbonate is not destroyed; therefore, the new bicarbonate reabsorbed from tubular cells represents a net addition to extracellular bicarbonate. Normally, most protons are buffered by bicarbonate, thus reclaiming the approximately 4000 mmol/d of bicarbonate in glomerular filtrate. About 80 mmol/d is secreted onto nonbicarbonate buffers, thereby regenerating the buffer capacity used in buffering the daily production of nonvolatile acids. Of this amount, about one-third reacts with phosphate, converting HPO_4^{2-} to $H_2PO_4^-$; the remainder is titrated onto ammonia. The amount of free acid which can be excreted in the urine is negligible, even at the minimum urine pH of 4.8. However, acidification of the urine is essential for titration of protons onto phosphate and ammonia.

Changes in the pH of body fluids lead to regulatory responses by the kidney, mediated by parallel changes in renal tubular cell pH. Acidosis stimulates renal hydrogen ion secretion. Ammonia

production increases, and more protons can be excreted as ammonium, thus generating new extracellular bicarbonate. In extreme acidosis, ammonia production may increase tenfold or more above the normal rate of 40 to 50 mmol/d. Alkalosis inhibits renal proton secretion and thereby reduces reabsorption and generation of bicarbonate by renal tubules. Recent studies indicate that the kidney can secrete bicarbonate into distal tubular fluid via an HCO_3-Cl exchanger; alkalosis stimulates this process. If plasma bicarbonate rises, bicarbonate is excreted rapidly both because the increase in filtered load is not matched by a corresponding increase in tubular reabsorptive capacity and because bicarbonate is secreted. By these mechanisms, normal plasma bicarbonate is restored promptly. For example, chronic ingestion of even large amounts of sodium bicarbonate normally produces only minimal sustained elevation of plasma bicarbonate.

Renal acid-base regulatory mechanisms are influenced by a number of factors in addition to pH of body fluids, important among them the carbon dioxide tension and volume of the extracellular fluid, angiotensin, aldosterone, availability of chloride ion, and body potassium stores. Tubular bicarbonate reabsorption is directly related to the carbon dioxide concentration of body fluids, presumably because changes in CO_2 alter the pH of renal tubular acid-secreting cells. Hypercapnia, which induces intracellular acidosis, tends to stimulate renal bicarbonate reabsorption, while hypocapnia has the opposite effect. Effective extracellular volume also influences bicarbonate reabsorption. In volume-depleted states, proximal tubular bicarbonate reabsorption is increased. This effect appears to be mediated by angiotensin II, which stimulates proximal bicarbonate transport, and by a reduction in filtered load due to decreased glomerular filtration rate. Aldosterone increases proton secretion in distal tubular segments. This is due both to direct stimulation of the distal proton pump and to enhanced sodium reabsorption, which favors retention of protons in tubular fluid by increasing intraluminal electronegativity.

Chloride depletion tends to limit bicarbonate excretion. This may be due in part to reduced delivery of chloride to the collecting tubules, where it is needed for bicarbonate secretion via the HCO_3^--Cl exchanger. Moreover, sodium reabsorption is generally enhanced in chloride-depleted states owing to associated extracellular fluid volume depletion. When less chloride is available for reabsorption, a larger fraction of the sodium must be reabsorbed with bicarbonate (via increased proton secretion). In experimental animals, renal bicarbonate reabsorption is inversely related to body potassium stores. In humans, the relation is less clear, but severe potassium depletion has been associated with increased bicarbonate reabsorption and metabolic alkalosis. Hyperkalemia, on the contrary, may contribute to metabolic acidosis by suppressing renal ammonia production.

The respiratory response to changes in blood pH is almost instantaneous. Acidosis stimulates and alkalosis depresses ventilation. The respiratory center in the medulla appears to respond to a pH intermediate between those of blood and cerebrospinal fluid.

EVALUATION OF ACID-BASE BALANCE   In practice, classification of acid-base disorders is based on measurements of changes in the bicarbonate–carbonic acid system, the principal buffer of extracellular fluid. Because intracellular and extracellular buffers are functionally linked, measurement of the plasma bicarbonate system provides useful information about total body buffers. The relationship among the elements of the bicarbonate system is usually described in terms of the Henderson-Hasselbalch equation:

$$pH = pK + \log \frac{[HCO_3^-]}{[H_2CO_3]}$$

Acidosis is defined as a disturbance which tends to add acid or remove alkali from body fluids, whereas *alkalosis* is any disturbance which tends to remove acid or add base. Since compensatory processes may minimize or prevent a change in the hydrogen ion concentration of the plasma, some authors prefer to use the terms *acidemia* and *alkalemia* to indicate those situations in which the pH of the plasma is measurably altered. *Metabolic* disorders are those in which the primary disturbance is in the concentration of bicarbonate. Since bicarbonate appears in the numerator of the buffer salt/acid ratio in the Henderson-Hasselbalch equation, increased bicarbonate concentration causes increased pH (alkalemia), whereas a decrease in bicarbonate causes decreased pH (acidemia). *Respiratory* disorders are those in which the primary change is in the concentration of carbon dioxide (carbonic acid). As can be seen from the Henderson-Hasselbalch equation, a fall in carbon dioxide concentration causes alkalemia, whereas an increase in carbon dioxide concentration causes acidemia.

A major problem in the assessment of acid-base disorders results from the compensatory responses of the lungs and the kidneys. A primary change in carbon dioxide concentration induces a compensatory renal response which alters plasma bicarbonate in the same direction. Conversely, a primary alteration of plasma bicarbonate induces a compensatory respiratory response which changes plasma carbon dioxide in the same direction. Consider a patient with chronic respiratory insufficiency who has the following set of acid-base parameters: P_{CO_2} = 9.3 kPa (70 mmHg), $[HCO_3^-]$ = 31 mmol/L, pH = 7.25. The clinician needs to know whether the elevation of plasma bicarbonate is merely the appropriate renal response to the primary hypercapnia or a metabolic acid-base disorder is superimposed. No calculations or a priori reasoning will provide the answer to this key question. Such information can be derived only from in vivo observations in which the usual compensatory response to a given degree of chronic hypercapnia is determined.

Clinical and experimental observations in humans (and animals) have been made in all common primary acid-base disturbances. They are most readily visualized and used for analysis of clinical acid-base disorders by the "confidence band" technique, as shown in Fig. 46-1. Each band represents the mean ± 2 SD, that is, 95 percent

FIGURE 46-1 Nomogram showing bands for uncomplicated respiratory or metabolic acid-base disturbances in intact subjects. Each "confidence" band represents the mean ± 2 SD for the compensatory response of normal subjects or patients to a given primary disorder. Ac = acute; chr = chronic, resp = respiratory; met = metabolic; acid = acidosis; alk = alkalosis. (*Modified from Arbus.*)

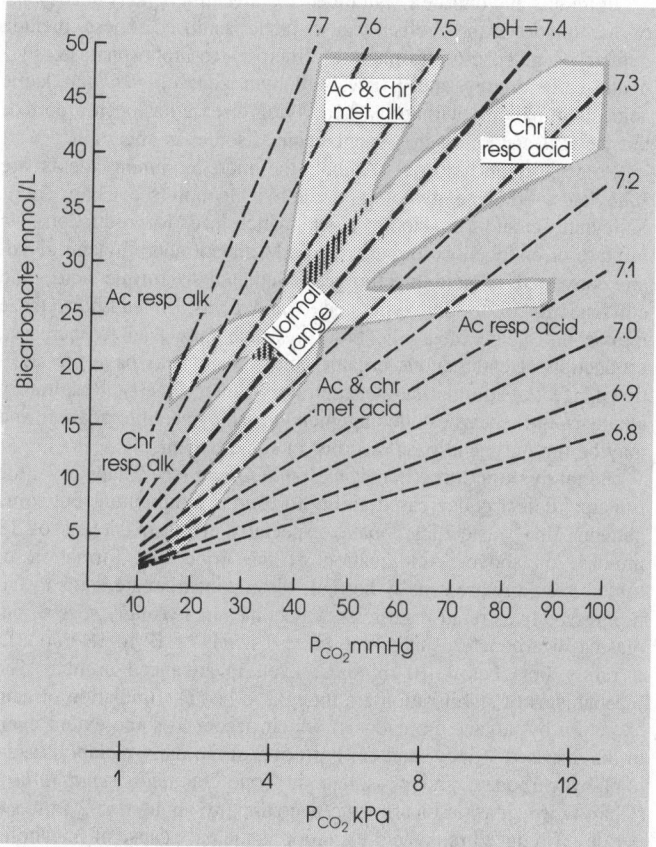

TABLE 46-1 Approximate compensatory responses to primary acid-base disorders*

Metabolic acidosis
  $P_{CO_2} \downarrow \approx 1.2\ HCO_3^- \downarrow$
Metabolic alkalosis
  $P_{CO_2} \uparrow \approx 0.7\ HCO_3^- \uparrow$
Respiratory acidosis
  A Acute: $HCO_3^- \uparrow \approx 0.1\ P_{CO_2} \uparrow$
  B Chronic: $HCO_3^- \uparrow \approx 0.35\ P_{CO_2} \uparrow$
Respiratory alkalosis
  A Acute: $HCO_3^- \downarrow \approx 0.2\ P_{CO_2} \downarrow$
  B Chronic: $HCO_3^- \downarrow \approx 0.5\ P_{CO_2} \downarrow$

* P_{CO_2} measured in mmHg, HCO_3^- in mmol/L.

---

of observations, for the compensatory response to each primary disturbance. In the example under discussion, inspection of the confidence band marked *chronic respiratory acidosis* indicates that 95 percent of individuals with chronic elevation of P_{CO_2} to 9.3 kPa (70 mmHg) would have $[HCO_3^-]$ between 34 and 44 mmol/L, due to renal compensation. Thus the $[HCO_3^-]$ of 31 mmol/L in the example cannot be interpreted as the sole result of an appropriate compensatory response to chronic hypercapnia. A second acid-base disorder, presumably metabolic acidosis, must be superimposed to account for the fact that plasma bicarbonate, although increased in response to hypercapnia, is not as high as usually observed when P_{CO_2} is 9.3 kPa (70 mmHg). Obviously, the use of this figure is no panacea, nor does it obviate the need for commonsense clinical evaluation of alternative possibilities. For example, if the patient under discussion had only recently developed hypercapnia, the $[HCO_3^-]$ of 31 mmol/L would be too high for a purely compensatory response to acute respiratory acidosis and would be interpreted as superimposed metabolic alkalosis. The difference between these two interpretations depends entirely on the clinical recognition of the chronicity of the primary respiratory disorder. The use of Fig. 46-1 in each type of acid-base disturbance is described in the appropriate sections of this chapter.* If the nomogram is unavailable, the "rules of thumb" in Table 46-1 are useful alternatives in interpreting acid-base data.

METABOLIC ACIDOSIS

PATHOPHYSIOLOGY Metabolic acidosis is caused by one of three mechanisms: (1) increased production of nonvolatile acids, (2) decreased acid excretion by the kidney, (3) loss of alkali. Extracellular bicarbonate is reduced by reaction with hydrogen ions or, in patients wasting alkali, by loss of bicarbonate in urine or stool. The decrease in pH stimulates respiration, and P_{CO_2} is lowered. Inspection of the confidence band for metabolic acidosis (Fig. 46-1) indicates that a decrease in P_{CO_2} of about 0.16 kPa (1.2 mmHg) can be expected for each decrement of 1 mmol/L in plasma bicarbonate. Complete respiratory compensation for primary metabolic acidosis does not occur. Respiratory compensation for acute acidosis tends to be somewhat greater than for chronic metabolic acidosis. The minimum level of P_{CO_2} that can be attained is approximately 1.3 kPa (10 mmHg); levels below 2 to 2.7 kPa (15 to 20 mmHg) are rarely maintained in chronic metabolic acidosis. When kidney function is normal, net acid excretion increases promptly in response to metabolic acidosis. Most of the initial rise is due to increased titration of urinary phosphate as urine pH falls below 5.2. Over several days, ammonia production by the kidney increases and becomes the most important mechanism for excreting excess protons. Net acid excretion may increase 5 to 10 times above normal, reaching a maximum of several hundred millimoles per day.

---

* Although the confidence band method does not permit automatic identification of simple or complicated acid-base disorders, it is preferable to techniques such as "buffer base" or "base excess-deficit" for reasons discussed in detail by Schwartz and Relman, N Engl J Med 268:1382, 1963. These terms are not used in this chapter.

TABLE 46-2   Causes of metabolic acidosis

INCREASED ANION GAP

I **Increased acid production**
  A Ketoacidosis
    1 Diabetic
    2 Alcoholic
    3 Starvation
  B Lactic acidosis
    1 Secondary to circulatory or respiratory failure
    2 Associated with various disorders (see text)
    3 Drugs and toxins
    4 Enzyme defects
  C Poisoning (salicylates, ethylene glycol, methanol)
II **Renal failure**

NORMAL ANION GAP (HYPERCHLOREMIC)

III **Renal tubular dysfunction**
  A Renal tubular acidosis
  B Hypoaldosteronism
  C "Potassium-sparing" diuretics
IV **Loss of alkali**
  A Diarrhea
  B Ureterosigmoidostomy
  C Carbonic anhydrase inhibitors
V **Production of HCl (ammonium chloride, cationic amino acids)**

TYPES OF ACIDOSIS   The principal causes of metabolic acidosis are listed in Table 46-2.

Ketoacidosis   In *diabetic ketoacidosis*, due to the hormonal abnormalities, acetoacetic and β-hydroxybutyric acids are produced more rapidly than they can be metabolized (see Chap. 337). Severe ketoacidosis may occur in *association* with *acute* and *chronic alcoholism*. Typically, patients give a history of prolonged abstention from food, protracted vomiting, and appreciable alcohol intake just before development of the ketoacidosis. β-Hydroxybutyrate, acetoacetate, and lactate accumulate in the plasma. The ketosis may be overlooked because the ratio of β-hydroxybutyrate to acetoacetate tends to be high; the nitroprusside test used for clinical detection of plasma ketones responds only to the latter. Blood sugar is usually normal or mildly elevated in these patients. *Starvation* may cause mild ketoacidosis; plasma bicarbonate usually falls no more than 3 to 4 mmol/L, although decreases of up to 10 mmol/L may occur with prolonged starvation. Reduced carbohydrate intake leads to low insulin and high glucagon levels in both starvation and alcoholic ketosis. These hormonal changes favor glycolysis and ketogenesis. In alcoholic ketosis, for uncertain reasons, fatty acid mobilization exceeds even that characteristic of starvation alone (see Chap. 337).

Lactic acidosis   Metabolic production and consumption of lactate are normally in balance. Under basal conditions, the liver and kidney consume lactate produced by tissues such as erythrocytes, skin, intestine, and muscle. However, if oxygen delivery is inadequate to meet energy requirements, any tissue will generate lactate. Deficient oxygen impairs electron flow through the cytochrome transport chain; ATP formation is decreased, and cell redox pairs, such as NADH/NAD, are shifted toward the reduced state. Decreases in ATP and reciprocal increases in ADP and AMP concentrations activate phosphofructokinase, the key enzyme regulating glycolysis. Accelerated glycolysis leads to increased production of pyruvate, and the increase in NADH/NAD ratio decreases its oxidation. Pyruvate and lactate are in a near-equilibrium reaction catalyzed by lactic dehydrogenase, as follows:

$$\text{Pyruvate} + \text{NADH} + \text{H}^+ \rightleftharpoons \text{lactate} + \text{NAD}$$

Thus lactate will tend to increase when pyruvate concentration increases and when the ratio of NADH to NAD rises. Since both conditions occur when tissues are oxygen-deprived, lactate formation is increased. Lactate will accumulate because it can be consumed only by conversion back to pyruvate, which is blocked so long as pyruvate concentration and the NADH/NAD ratio are elevated. Since the overall process of glycolysis generates one H^+ for each lactate molecule produced, acid production increases proportionately with lactate production.

These mechanisms, probably compounded by decreased uptake or even production of lactate by the liver, account for the development of lactic acidosis in patients with *shock* due to any cause (e.g., sepsis, myocardial infarction, hemorrhage) or with respiratory arrest. Since severe acidosis depresses myocardial and arteriolar contractility, lactic acidosis may compound the underlying cause of shock. Less commonly, lactic acidosis may be caused by *pulmonary diseases* leading to extreme hypoxia or by diminished blood oxygen–carrying capacity in severe *anemia* and *carbon monoxide* poisoning. The mortality rate is high in patients with lactic acidosis secondary to shock and tissue hypoxia. During vigorous *exercise* or convulsions, local disproportion between oxygen supply and demand in contracting muscle may lead to transient, clinically benign lactic acidosis.

Lactic acidosis also is *associated* with disorders in which tissue hypoxia does not appear to be present. It has been reported in patients with leukemia, lymphoma, and solid tumors, with poorly controlled diabetes mellitus, and with severe hepatic failure. Mechanisms causing lactic acidosis in these disorders are poorly understood. Overproduction of lactate by neoplastic tissue probably is a factor in lactic acidosis associated with tumors. Insulin deficiency, which inhibits pyruvate oxidation, presumably is an important factor in patients with poorly controlled diabetes. Decreased hepatic lactate metabolism seems a likely mechanism in severe liver disease.

A variety of *drugs* and *toxins* have been associated with lactic acidosis. *Drugs* include fructose used in parenteral alimentation, sodium nitroprusside, epinephrine and norepinephrine infusions, and, before the drug was removed from general use, the biguanide hypoglycemic agent phenformin. Lactic acidosis may contribute to the severe acidosis in *poisoning* by salicylates, ethylene glycol, or methanol. Ethanol elevates serum lactate, but clinically significant lactic acidosis does not occur in alcohol intoxication unless there are associated disorders such as hepatic or circulatory failure.

In infants and children, a number of *congenital defects in enzymes* of carbohydrate metabolism cause lactic acidosis. These include defects of glucose-6-phosphatase, fructose-1,6-biphosphatase, pyruvate carboxylase, and pyruvate dehydrogenase. *Primary* lactic acidosis in patients without an underlying disease has been reported, but the existence of such a spontaneous disorder is uncertain.

Poisoning and drugs   Among the more common agents are salicylates, ethylene glycol, and methyl alcohol (see Chap. 395). Salicylates create a metabolic block, which leads to production of a mixture of endogenous organic acids. Methanol and ethylene glycol are converted to acid metabolites, methanol to formic acid, and ethylene glycol to glyoxylic and oxalic acids. In addition, these intoxicants create metabolic blocks, which may lead to increased production of endogenous organic acids. Salicylates have the additional effect of stimulating the respiratory center directly. Respiratory alkalosis is the earliest derangement in salicylate intoxication and may be the only acid-base disorder in some patients.

Renal dysfunction   In *chronic renal failure* (see Chap. 237), the principal defect is decreased ability to excrete ammonium, but some patients also waste bicarbonate, especially at plasma levels of 18 mmol/L or above. Acidification of the urine and formation of titratable acidity are usually normal. Plasma bicarbonate tends to fall progressively as renal insufficiency becomes increasingly severe, but plasma bicarbonate usually stabilizes at levels of 12 to 18 mmol/L; it rarely falls below 10 mmol/L, even in advanced uremia. The mechanisms of stabilization are thought to be (1) stimulation of acid excretion by advancing acidosis, which occurs to some extent even in the diseased kidney, and (2) buffering of the daily metabolic acid load by carbonate and phosphate in bone. In *acute renal failure* (Chap. 236), plasma bicarbonate decreases by about 1 to 2 mmol/L per day if reduced renal acid excretion is the only cause of metabolic acidosis. Greater rates of fall suggest the presence, in addition, of some cause of increased acid production.

Chronic metabolic acidosis is the hallmark of *renal tubular acidosis* (see Chap. 244), which may be an isolated disorder of tubular acid excretion; part of a Fanconi syndrome, in which other tubular functions are also abnormal; or associated with nonrenal primary disorders (see Chap. 352). The acidosis is due to defective renal tubular acidification mechanisms, which limit renal conservation and regeneration of bicarbonate.

Aldosterone stimulates distal tubular acid and potassium secretion. In *hypoaldosteronism*, loss of this effect leads to metabolic acidosis and hyperkalemia. The acidosis is due not only to loss of the direct effect of aldosterone on acid excretion but also to the hyperkalemia, which decreases renal ammonia production. The same factors account for metabolic acidosis caused by the diuretic spironolactone, which blocks the action of aldosterone, and other "potassium-sparing" diuretics such as triamterene and amiloride, which directly inhibit distal tubular secretion of acid and potassium.

Loss of alkali   Severe *diarrhea* or intestinal malabsorption usually causes mild to moderate acidosis due to the loss of bicarbonate in liquid stool, in which concentrations of 40 to 60 mmol/L may be present. *Ureterosigmoidostomy*, i.e., transplantation of the ureters into the sigmoid colon, leads to metabolic acidosis both because of exchange of chloride for bicarbonate by intestinal epithelium and because renal disease (obstructive uropathy and pyelonephritis) often develops. However, acidosis is not a problem with the more modern technique for urinary diversion, in which a bladder is formed from a small isolated loop of ileum. *Carbonic anhydrase inhibitors*, such as acetazolamide, cause mild to moderate acidosis by increasing bicarbonate loss in the urine.

Production of HCl   Acidosis can be caused by administration of ammonium chloride and lysine or arginine hydrochloride, which form HCl during metabolism. This type of acidosis also may occur during parenteral alimentation with amino acid infusates that contain an excess of the cationic amino acids arginine, lysine, and histidine.

CLINICAL FEATURES AND DIAGNOSIS   Acute metabolic acidosis is usually caused by overproduction of a nonvolatile acid (see Table 46-2, category I). Chronic metabolic acidosis is most frequently due to renal dysfunction. Diarrhea is a common cause of either acute or chronic acidosis.

There are few specific symptoms or signs of metabolic acidosis; diagnosis depends on recognition of the clinical setting and appropriate laboratory studies. In acute metabolic acidosis, hyperventilation is usual and may be intense (Kussmaul respiration). However, it is ordinarily impossible to detect increased respiration by physical examination in patients with chronic metabolic acidosis, despite substantial reduction of P_{CO_2}. Acute, severe acidosis produces a variety of nonspecific symptoms ranging from fatigue through confusion, stupor, and coma. Cardiovascular effects include decreased cardiac contractility and vasodilatation, which may lead to heart failure or hypotension. Chronic metabolic acidosis may produce no symptoms or may be associated with fatigue and anorexia, although it is usually difficult to determine whether these symptoms reflect the acidosis per se or are related to the underlying disease.

The characteristic laboratory features are reduction of plasma bicarbonate and blood pH, together with a compensatory reduction in P_{CO_2} (see Fig. 46-1). Hyperkalemia is often present, due to shift of potassium out of cells. This phenomenon may mask significant potassium depletion (see Chap. 45). Hypokalemia is a clue to conditions in which concomitant potassium depletion is severe, e.g., diarrhea or diabetic ketoacidosis, or in which renal potassium-regulating mechanisms are affected, e.g., renal tubular acidosis or administration of carbonic anhydrase inhibitors.

When the cause of metabolic acidosis is not evident from the history or clinical setting, calculation of unmeasured anions (anion gap) may help in differential diagnosis. Unmeasured anions are calculated by subtracting the sum of plasma bicarbonate and chloride concentrations from plasma sodium concentration; the normal value

is 8 to 16 mmol/L. The negative charges on plasma proteins, principally albumin, make up most of the anion gap. Phosphate, sulfate, and organic acid anions normally contribute to unmeasured anions to a lesser degree. When metabolic acidosis is due to increased acid production or renal insufficiency (categories I and II in Table 46-2), the anion gap is usually increased. In acidosis resulting from increased acid production, the increased anion gap is due to accumulation in plasma of the anions of the various acids such as acetoacetate or lactate, which are produced faster than they can be metabolized or excreted. In renal failure, the anion gap increases because sulfate, phosphate, and organic acid anions are not excreted efficiently.

The cause of acidosis with an increased anion gap usually is easily determined from the clinical setting and simple laboratory tests. *Ketoacidosis* should be considered when acidosis occurs in patients with uncontrolled diabetes mellitus (see Chap. 337), alcoholism, or starvation. Ketonemia can be detected by testing serum dilutions with nitroprusside (Acetest) reagent. In occasional patients this test, which reacts to acetoacetate but not β-hydroxybutyrate, may be misleading. If the clinical diagnosis is uncertain, a specific assay for β-hydroxybutyrate is available. The diagnosis of *lactic acidosis* is suspected in patients with severe circulatory insufficiency when other causes of acidosis can be ruled out. A specific assay for plasma lactate is available if the diagnosis is uncertain. Plasma salicylate concentration in the toxic range [>2.9 mmol/L (>40 mg/dL)] will confirm suspected *salicylate intoxication* (see Chap. 395). Acidosis due to *poisoning* with ethylene glycol or methanol (see Chap. 395) may be suspected if measured plasma osmolality exceeds calculated plasma osmolality [$(2 \times$ plasma Na$)$ + glucose/18 + BUN/2.8 (with plasma Na in mmol/L, glucose and BUN in mg/dL)]. This "osmolal gap" reflects the plasma level of methanol or ethylene glycol, small molecules that at toxic concentrations add significantly to plasma osmolality. (Since ethanol has a similar effect, it must be measured if alcohol intoxication is suspected.) Detection of a large "osmolal gap" in a patient with severe acidosis may permit prompt treatment to be instituted while awaiting confirmation of the diagnosis with specific tests for the toxins. However, for unknown reasons, moderately elevated "osmolal gaps" (up to 10 to 15 mosmol/kg) occur in some patients with lactic acidosis or alcoholic ketoacidosis. Hence an elevated "osmolal gap" is not a specific test for methanol or ethylene glycol poisoning; clinical judgment must be used in deciding on therapeutic strategy.

In all other types of metabolic acidosis (categories III, IV, and V in Table 46-2), the anion gap is normal because there is neither increased production nor decreased excretion of organic acids, sulfate, and phosphate. Plasma chloride concentration is increased approximately as much as plasma bicarbonate is decreased (hyperchloremic acidosis). In diabetic ketoacidosis, a variety of plasma acid-base patterns may develop, depending on the balance between production and renal excretion of ketoacid anions. In most patients there is renal dysfunction, and the anions are retained, leading to an anion-gap acidosis in which the elevation in plasma unmeasured anion is about equal to the reduction in bicarbonate concentration. Patients with normal renal function may present with a component of hyperchloremic acidosis due to renal excretion of ketone anions and retention of chloride. After therapy that repairs volume depletion and hence renal dysfunction, most patients develop some degree of hyperchloremia, due to the same mechanisms.

TREATMENT   The treatment of metabolic acidosis depends on its cause and severity. In *chronic renal failure*, mild or moderate metabolic acidosis does not require treatment. When plasma bicarbonate falls below 15 mmol/L, it is reasonable to treat patients with oral alkali, such as sodium bicarbonate or sodium citrate. The dose is gradually increased until plasma bicarbonate concentration rises to about 18 to 20 mmol/L. Some patients appear to benefit symptomatically from elevation of bicarbonate to this level, and fatigue, anorexia, and malaise tend to be alleviated. Caution must be exerted to avoid excessively rapid alkalinization of the plasma, which may precipitate tetany; excess sodium given with alkali may aggravate hypertension or edema. Acidosis should be corrected as completely as possible in patients with type 1 (distal) *renal tubular acidosis;* this will avoid hypercalciuria, osteomalacia, nephrocalcinosis, and lithiasis. In type 2 (proximal) renal tubular acidosis, therapy is usually not required (see Chap. 244). Patients with *acute renal failure* also do not ordinarily require specific therapy for acidosis. Dialysis instituted for management of the renal failure should maintain an adequate plasma bicarbonate.

Diabetic *ketoacidosis* responds to insulin, and most patients do not require treatment with alkali (see Chap. 337). However, when acidosis is extreme (pH less than 7.1 or $[HCO_3^-]$ less than 6 to 8 mmol/L), intravenous bicarbonate therapy is justified. The ketoacidosis associated with alcoholism responds rapidly to infusions of glucose and saline. Insulin is not required, nor should alkali be given unless acidosis is extreme. The ketoacidosis of starvation is mild and requires no specific treatment.

In *lactic acidosis,* if the underlying disorder can be reversed, the acidosis will be corrected by metabolism of lactate, which generates bicarbonate. Since lactic acidosis is usually associated with severe circulatory or respiratory failure, the mortality rate is high. Because production of lactate and H^+ in lactic acidosis can be very rapid, it is usually resistant to treatment with alkali. Large amounts of bicarbonate may be required to raise or even to stabilize plasma bicarbonate. Some studies have suggested that alkali therapy in lactic acidosis may be counterproductive because correction of acidosis appears to increase lactate production. However, extreme acidosis may contribute to circulatory collapse (see above), thereby perpetuating the underlying cause of the lactic acidosis. Hence it seems reasonable to treat lactic acidosis with intravenous bicarbonate at a rate at least sufficient to maintain plasma bicarbonate at 8 to 10 mmol/L and pH above 7.10. If vigorous administration of sodium bicarbonate leads to circulatory overloading, diuretics should be given or dialysis with a bicarbonate-buffered fluid may be instituted. Dichloroacetate, an investigational agent that enhances pyruvate dehydrogenase activity, has shown promise for treating lactic acidosis in experimental and clinical studies.

The acidosis due to *diarrhea* or loss of alkaline upper intestinal secretions is usually associated with volume depletion and potassium deficiency. Treatment of such electrolyte disorders with intravenous infusions appropriate for the patient's specific abnormalities may be required.

Some general points about therapy with alkali deserve emphasis. Oral treatment with sodium bicarbonate usually should begin with 1 g three times daily and be increased to maintain the desired plasma bicarbonate level. Some patients find that sodium bicarbonate leads to upper gastrointestinal discomfort; a 10% sodium citrate solution may be more palatable. In the intravenous treatment of acute metabolic acidosis, sodium bicarbonate is the agent of choice. The amount of bicarbonate to be given depends on the severity of the acidosis and any associated disorders of serum sodium concentration. Typically, concentrations of bicarbonate between 50 and 150 mmol/L are achieved by adding one to three vials of sodium bicarbonate to a liter of dextrose in water. The concentration of bicarbonate in these vials is 1000 mmol/L (50 mmol in 50 mL); these bicarbonate solutions should never be given undiluted in the treatment of acidosis, since rapid infusion may induce serious or even fatal cardiac arrhythmias, especially if given as a bolus through a central venous catheter.

In metabolic acidosis, approximately equal amounts of acid appear to be buffered by extracellular bicarbonate and by intracellular buffers. (In severe acidosis, a greater fraction of the acid load may be buffered within cells.) Therefore, it is appropriate to calculate the amount of bicarbonate needed to raise plasma bicarbonate by assuming that approximately half will accept protons from intracellular buffers and be destroyed; the other half will elevate plasma bicarbonate concentration. Thus the calculation would be millimoles of bicarbonate required equals desired increment in plasma concentration (millimoles per liter) times 40 percent of body weight. The 40 percent figure represents twice the extracellular volume. It is rarely desirable to infuse enough alkali to elevate plasma bicarbonate to normal. Possible untoward effects include hypokalemic cardiac toxicity in patients who are substantially potassium-depleted, tetany in patients with renal failure or hypocalcemia, and congestive heart failure due to excess sodium. Moreover, alkalosis may supervene. Cerebrospinal fluid bicarbonate does not equilibrate rapidly with plasma. Hence the respiratory center, which responds to acidity both of blood and cerebrospinal fluid, maintains some degree of hyperventilation as plasma bicarbonate is increasing. This type of respiratory alkalosis may sometimes persist for several days after correction of metabolic acidosis. In acute acidosis due to overproduction of metabolic acids, successful treatment of the primary disorder will cause rapid metabolic conversion of lactate and ketone bodies to bicarbonate. Thus excessive administration of bicarbonate early in therapy also may lead to metabolic alkalosis at a later stage of treatment, when endogenous bicarbonate has been reconstituted by improvement in metabolism.

METABOLIC ALKALOSIS

PATHOPHYSIOLOGY Metabolic alkalosis is usually initiated by increased loss of acid from the stomach or the kidney. However, excretion of bicarbonate at high plasma concentrations is normally so rapid that alkalosis will not be sustained unless bicarbonate reabsorption is enhanced or alkali is continuously generated at a great rate. Clinically, maintenance of metabolic alkalosis is most often due to stimulation of bicarbonate reabsorption by a volume (chloride) deficit. During volume depletion, renal conservation of sodium takes precedence over other homeostatic mechanisms, such as correction of alkalosis. Since in alkalosis a large fraction of plasma sodium is paired with bicarbonate, complete reabsorption of filtered sodium requires reabsorption of bicarbonate as well. Alkalosis is sustained until volume depletion is corrected by administration of sodium chloride. This diminishes tubular avidity for sodium and provides chloride as an alternative anion for reabsorption with sodium; excess bicarbonate can then be excreted with sodium. Chloride is required for bicarbonate secretion in the collecting duct via a bicarbonate-chloride exchanger. Provision of chloride probably also facilitates bicarbonate excretion by enhancing chloride delivery to this secretory site.

The other major mechanism which can maintain metabolic alkalosis is hypermineralocorticoidism. Mineralocorticoids stimulate renal hydrogen ion secretion. In patients with excess mineralocorticoid activity, elevation of plasma bicarbonate is initiated by increased urinary loss of protons as ammonium and titratable acidity. Stimulation of tubular acid secretion also enhances bicarbonate reabsorption, thereby sustaining the metabolic alkalosis. Patients with excess mineralocorticoid activity are not volume- or chloride-deficient. Hence this type of metabolic alkalosis does not respond to sodium chloride administration.

The relation between metabolic alkalosis and potassium is incompletely understood. Alkalosis and hypokalemia often occur together. Alkalosis may cause hypokalemia and potassium depletion through mechanisms discussed in Chap. 45. Conversely, potassium depletion may help to sustain metabolic alkalosis because tubular acid secretion, and hence bicarbonate reabsorption, is stimulated. This mechanism contributes to maintenance of alkalosis in hypermineralocorticoidism. Whether potassium depletion alone can generate metabolic alkalosis is uncertain; if so, severe potassium depletion is required.

Respiratory compensation for metabolic alkalosis is limited. Alveolar ventilation decreases, and P_{CO_2} is elevated. However, since this response is limited by hypoxia, P_{CO_2} rarely rises above 7.3 to 8 kPa (55 to 60 mmHg).

PATHOGENESIS The principal causes of metabolic alkalosis are outlined in Table 46-3. *Vomiting* and *gastric drainage* usually induce only minimal or moderate alkalosis, but occasional patients, especially those with increased gastric acid secretion (e.g., with acid-peptic disease or the Zollinger-Ellison syndrome), may develop very severe

TABLE 46-3 Causes of metabolic alkalosis

I **Associated with volume (chloride) depletion**
  A Vomiting or gastric drainage
  B Diuretic therapy
  C Posthypercapnic alkalosis
II **Associated with hyperadrenocorticism**
  A Cushing's syndrome
  B Primary aldosteronism
  C Bartter's syndrome
III **Severe potassium depletion**
IV **Excessive alkali intake**
  A Acute
  B Milk-alkali syndrome

alkalosis. Loss of hydrochloric acid in the gastric fluid initiates the alkalosis. Water and sodium chloride are lost in the vomitus or gastric aspirate. Initially, sodium is lost in the urine as well, coupled with increased bicarbonate excretion (which results from elevation of plasma bicarbonate above the tubular reabsorptive threshold). These losses cause a volume (chloride) deficit, which stimulates tubular reabsorption of sodium and bicarbonate and presumably inhibits bicarbonate secretion. Thus the elevated plasma bicarbonate generated by gastric losses of hydrochloric acid is maintained.

Alkalosis may be present in patients treated with "loop" *diuretics* (furosemide, ethacrynic acid, bumetanide) or with thiazides. The diuretics cause extracellular volume contraction and inhibit sodium chloride reabsorption in the loop of Henle or distal convoluted tubule, which increases delivery of tubular fluid to more distal nephron segments. The volume deficit and consequent hyperaldosteronism, as well as concomitant hypokalemia, stimulate proton secretion in these segments, generating and maintaining the alkalosis. Alkalosis due to treatment with oral diuretics is usually mild. Acute administration of potent intravenous diuretics such as furosemide or ethacrynic acid to patients on low-sodium diets may induce more severe alkalosis due to rapid loss of sodium chloride in the urine. Sudden contraction of extracellular volume elevates plasma bicarbonate; renal excretion of excess bicarbonate is prevented by the mechanism discussed above. Diuretics that specifically inhibit bicarbonate reabsorption, such as acetazolamide, or inhibit distal cation secretion, such as spironolactone, amiloride, and triamterene, cause acidosis rather than alkalosis (see above).

Patients with chronic hypercapnia due to respiratory insufficiency maintain high plasma bicarbonate concentrations (see "Respiratory Acidosis," below). If respiration improves, P_{CO_2} falls promptly. However, urinary excretion of excess bicarbonate previously generated by renal compensatory mechanisms takes a number of days. In patients on low-salt diets or diuretics who have a volume (chloride) deficiency, *posthypercapnic* alkalosis of this type may persist indefinitely unless sodium or potassium chloride is added to the diet. The mechanism in this condition is the same as that which causes persistent alkalosis in vomiting, described earlier.

Alkalosis is variable in patients with excess mineralocorticoid activity. Minimal or moderate alkalosis is usually present in patients with *Cushing's syndrome* or *primary aldosteronism*. More marked alkalosis may be seen in patients with extreme adrenal hyperfunction associated with ACTH-secreting tumors, such as bronchogenic carcinoma. Moderate alkalosis is typical of patients with *Bartter's syndrome*.

Although alkalosis and *potassium depletion* are often associated, mild or moderate potassium depletion alone does not cause sustained metabolic alkalosis. However, extreme degrees of potassium depletion (serum potassium usually 2 mmol/L or less) may cause metabolic alkalosis. This type of alkalosis is not corrected by administration of sodium chloride but does respond to administration of potassium.

For reasons noted earlier, alkalosis due to administration of alkali cannot be sustained unless large amounts are given. When renal function is compromised, alkalosis may be sustained by small

exogenous loads. This is apparently the mechanism of alkalosis in the milk-alkali syndrome, in which hypercalcemic nephropathy and alkalosis develop in response to excessive intake of absorbable alkali. The nephropathy limits bicarbonate excretion, thus maintaining the alkalosis.

CLINICAL FEATURES AND DIAGNOSIS There are no specific clinical signs or symptoms. Severe alkalosis may cause apathy, confusion, and stupor. If serum calcium is borderline or low, rapid development of alkalosis may lead to tetany. The diagnosis of metabolic alkalosis depends on recognition of the clinical setting and appropriate laboratory studies. Plasma bicarbonate is increased. P_{CO_2} increases by about 0.01 kPa (0.7 mmHg) for each mmol/L increase in bicarbonate. Elevation of P_{CO_2} is insufficient to prevent alkalemia (see Fig. 46-1). Plasma potassium concentration is often reduced, and the electrocardiogram may reveal changes in T and U waves typical of hypokalemia (Chap. 189). These changes may be due to alkalosis itself or to associated alterations in potassium metabolism. Despite elevation of plasma bicarbonate, the urine pH is usually less than 7 in patients with sustained metabolic alkalosis. This "paradoxical aciduria" reflects the fact that bicarbonate reabsorption must be increased if metabolic alkalosis is to be sustained.

Differential diagnosis is usually made from clinical features, such as a history of vomiting or the manifestations of Cushing's syndrome. If no cause is apparent, surreptitious vomiting or use of diuretics should be considered. The urinary chloride concentration may be a helpful clue if the cause of alkalosis is not evident. When the alkalosis is associated with volume contraction (category I in Table 46-3), urinary chloride is low, usually less than 10 mmol/L. When the alkalosis is caused by hyperadrenocorticism or severe potassium depletion (categories II and III), urinary chloride is higher, usually 20 mmol/L or more.

TREATMENT Mild or moderate metabolic alkalosis rarely requires specific treatment. In patients with gastric alkalosis, infusion of saline solutions is usually sufficient to enhance renal bicarbonate excretion and to correct alkalosis by mechanisms discussed above. Administration of potassium chloride is also helpful in treating or preventing alkalosis in these patients and those with diuretic-induced alkalosis. In patients with adrenal hyperfunction, alkalosis is corrected by specific treatment of the underlying disease. In Bartter's syndrome, hypokalemia, potassium wasting, and alkalosis may be partly corrected by treatment with prostaglandin synthetase inhibitors such as indomethacin. Whenever alkalosis and potassium depletion occur together, potassium depletion should be treated with potassium chloride.

Rarely, with prolonged gastric metabolic alkalosis, losses may be severe enough to require intravenous therapy with acidifying agents. Dilute hydrochloric acid or acidifying salts such as ammonium chloride or arginine hydrochloride may be given slowly under such circumstances. In most patients the use of acidifying agents can be avoided by appropriate treatment with saline and potassium chloride. In patients who are volume-expanded or in whom volume loading is inadvisable, therapy with acetazolamide, which enhances renal bicarbonate excretion, may be helpful.

RESPIRATORY ACIDOSIS

PATHOPHYSIOLOGY Failure of ventilation promptly increases P_{CO_2} (carbonic acid) because metabolic production of carbon dioxide is so rapid. Acute respiratory acidosis is modulated to a limited degree by tissue buffers. As can be seen from the curve labeled *acute respiratory acidosis* in Fig. 46-1, immediate tissue buffering elevates plasma bicarbonate only slightly, by about 1 mmol/L for each increase of 1.3 kPa (10 mmHg) in P_{CO_2}. If hypercapnia is sustained, renal acid excretion is enhanced, and bicarbonate reabsorption is stimulated. Over a period of several days, plasma bicarbonate rises approximately 3.5 mmol/L for each increase of 1.3 kPa (10 mmHg) in P_{CO_2}, thereby minimizing the degree of acidemia. The increment in plasma bicarbonate attributable to renal activity is represented by the difference between the curves marked *chronic respiratory acidosis* and *acute respiratory acidosis.*

PATHOGENESIS *Acute* respiratory acidosis occurs whenever there is a sudden failure of ventilation. Common causes include depression of the respiratory center by cerebral disease or drugs, neuromuscular disorders, and cardiopulmonary arrest. *Chronic* respiratory acidosis occurs in pulmonary diseases such as chronic emphysema and bronchitis, in which ventilation and perfusion are mismatched and effective alveolar ventilation is decreased. Chronic hypercapnia also may result from primary alveolar hypoventilation or from alveolar hypoventilation related to extreme obesity (Pickwickian syndrome). Acute and chronic diseases characterized principally by interference with alveolar gas exchange, such as chronic pulmonary fibrosis, pneumonia, and pulmonary edema, usually cause hypocapnia rather than hypercapnia. In these conditions, hypoxia stimulates increased ventilation; since carbon dioxide is much more diffusible than oxygen, excretion of carbon dioxide is enhanced despite the barrier to gas exchange. Hypercapnia occurs only with respiratory fatigue or extremely severe disease.

CLINICAL FEATURES AND DIAGNOSIS It is often difficult to separate the manifestations of respiratory acidosis from those of associated hypoxia. Moderate hypercapnia, especially if it develops slowly, probably has no specific clinical features. When P_{CO_2} exceeds 9.3 kPa (70 mmHg), patients become progressively confused and obtunded. Asterixis may be present. Papilledema may occur, apparently because intracranial pressure is increased by the cerebral vasodilation characteristic of hypercapnia. Dilatation of conjunctival and superficial facial blood vessels may be noted.

The diagnosis of acute respiratory acidosis is usually evident from the clinical situation, especially if respiration is obviously depressed. Proof requires laboratory confirmation that P_{CO_2} is elevated. Acidemia is always present in patients with *acute* hypercapnia. Acidosis in acute cardiopulmonary arrest is usually a combination of a metabolic lactic acidosis and acute respiratory acidosis. Patients with *chronic* hypercapnia are usually acidemic. However, some individuals with minimal or moderate chronic hypercapnia may have normal or even slightly elevated plasma pH, as may be seen from Fig. 46-1. The mechanism of full compensation or of "overcompensation" in such instances is unknown. However, significant elevation of pH in patients with chronic hypercapnia is almost always due to complicating metabolic alkalosis. Diuretics, low-sodium diets, and posthypercapnic alkalosis are frequent causes of this type of superimposed acid-base disorder.

Because of the differences between plasma bicarbonate in acute hypercapnia and in chronic hypercapnia, proper interpretation of acid-base parameters in respiratory acidosis depends on clinical information.

TREATMENT The only worthwhile approach to treatment of respiratory acidosis is correction of the underlying disorder. Rapid infusion of alkali is justified in cardiopulmonary arrest. In other circumstances, infusions of alkali have no role in practical management of respiratory acidosis.

RESPIRATORY ALKALOSIS

PATHOPHYSIOLOGY Acute reduction in carbon dioxide concentration releases hydrogen ion from tissue buffers, which minimize alkalemia by reducing plasma bicarbonate. Acute alkalosis also enhances glycolysis; increased production of lactic and pyruvic acids lowers serum bicarbonate and raises plasma concentrations of the corresponding anions by a millimole or two. In chronic hypocapnia, plasma bicarbonate is further reduced because the decreased P_{CO_2} inhibits tubular reabsorption and generation of bicarbonate. As in respiratory acidosis, compensation for the chronic state is much more complete than for the acute (see Fig. 46-1). In acute hypocapnia, plasma bicarbonate falls only about 2 mmol/L for each 1.3-kPa (10-mmHg) reduction in P_{CO_2}. In chronic hypocapnia, plasma bicarbonate

TABLE 46-4 Causes of respiratory alkalosis

I Hypoxia
   A Acute (e.g., pneumonia, asthma, pulmonary edema, hypotension)
   B Chronic (e.g., pulmonary fibrosis, cyanotic heart disease, high altitude, anemia)
II Respiratory center stimulation
   A Anxiety
   B Fever
   C Gram-negative sepsis
   D Salicylate intoxication
   E Cerebral disease (tumor, encephalitis, etc.)
   F Hepatic cirrhosis
   G Pregnancy
   H After correction of metabolic acidosis
III Excessive mechanical ventilation

is reduced by 4 to 5 mmol/L for each 1.3-kPa (10-mmHg) decrease in P_{CO_2}. The decrement in plasma bicarbonate attributable to renal compensatory activity is shown by the difference between the curves labeled *acute* and *chronic respiratory alkalosis* in Fig. 46-1.

PATHOGENESIS Respiratory alkalosis is due to acute or chronic hyperventilation, which lowers P_{CO_2}. The causes of respiratory alkalosis are shown in Table 46-4.

Hypoxia from any process which reduces arterial P_{O_2} to approximately 60 mmHg or less tends to cause hyperventilation and respiratory alkalosis. Hyperventilation in lung disorders appears to be caused not only by hypoxemia but also by activation of intrapulmonary receptors which stimulate the respiratory center via neural connections. Hyperventilation may occur in patients with hypotension or severe anemia, apparently due to decreased oxygen delivery to chemoreceptors in the great vessels.

A number of disease processes and medications directly stimulate the medullary respiratory center. Persistent acidosis of the cerebrospinal fluid may stimulate hyperventilation after correction of metabolic acidosis (see "Metabolic Acidosis," above).

CLINICAL FEATURES AND DIAGNOSIS Depending on its severity and acuteness, hyperventilation may or may not be clinically apparent. In acute respiratory alkalosis, the clinical picture is rather characteristic: Patients complain of paresthesias, numbness, and tingling; of light-headedness; and if alkalosis is sufficiently severe, of manifestations of tetany. Alkalosis directly enhances neuromuscular excitability; this effect, rather than the modest decrease in ionized plasma calcium induced by alkalosis, is probably the major cause of tetany. Severe respiratory alkalosis may cause confusion or loss of consciousness, perhaps due to cerebral vasospasm induced by hypocapnia.

The diagnosis may be suspected from the clinical setting but must be confirmed by analysis of the plasma bicarbonate system. Hypocapnia together with a variable degree of alkalemia is found; plasma bicarbonate is decreased but is rarely below 15 mmol/L.

TREATMENT The only successful treatment for respiratory alkalosis is elimination of the underlying disorder. In the acute hyperventilation syndrome, sedation, reassurance, and, if symptoms are sufficiently severe, rebreathing into a bag will usually terminate the attack.

MIXED DISORDERS

In some patients, acid-base disturbances are mixed; i.e., two or occasionally even three of the primary disorders described in preceding sections may coexist. Table 46-5 lists some common causes of mixed acid-base disorders.

Metabolic acidosis and respiratory acidosis This is the typical acid-base disorder in patients with acute *cardiopulmonary arrest* or severe *pulmonary edema*. The circulatory failure causes lactic acidosis, and the respiratory failure leads to hypercapnia. Patients, often elderly, who develop *salicylate toxicity* while under treatment for a chronic disorder such as arthritis also may be receiving sedatives or

TABLE 46-5 Some common causes of mixed acid-base disorders

I **Metabolic acidosis and respiratory acidosis**
  A Cardiopulmonary arrest
  B Severe pulmonary edema
  C Salicylate plus sedative overdose
  D Pulmonary disease with superimposed renal failure or sepsis
II **Metabolic acidosis and respiratory alkalosis**
  A Salicylate overdose
  B Sepsis
  C Combined hepatic and renal insufficiency
  D Recent alcohol binge
III **Metabolic alkalosis and respiratory acidosis**
  A Chronic pulmonary disease, with superimposed
    1 Diuretic therapy
    2 Steroid therapy
    3 Vomiting
    4 Reduction of hypercapnia by ventilator
IV **Metabolic alkalosis and respiratory alkalosis**
  A Pregnancy with vomiting
  B Chronic liver disease treated with diuretics
  C Cardiopulmonary arrest treated with bicarbonate and ventilator
V **Metabolic acidosis and alkalosis**
  A Vomiting superimposed on
    1 Renal failure
    2 Diabetic acidosis
    3 Alcoholic ketoacidosis

hypnotics. These medications can depress respiration, leading to respiratory acidosis and metabolic acidosis, rather than the respiratory alkalosis and metabolic acidosis typical of salicylate toxicity alone. Mixed metabolic and respiratory acidosis also may occur in patients with *pulmonary disease* who develop *renal failure* or *sepsis*.

The mixed acidosis may be suspected from the clinical setting. Definitive diagnosis requires interpretation of blood acid-base measurements. Acidemia usually is very severe. The acid-base measurements do not fit on the confidence band for either metabolic or respiratory acidosis. If analyzed as a respiratory acidosis, the bicarbonate concentration is found to be lower than appropriate for the P_{CO_2} level. If initially interpreted as a metabolic acidosis, the P_{CO_2} is inappropriately high for the measured bicarbonate. It should be emphasized that the P_{CO_2} need not be above 5.3 kPa (40 mmHg). Even a reduced P_{CO_2} may indicate a component of respiratory acidosis if it is higher than expected for the usual compensatory response to metabolic acidosis. For example, a P_{CO_2} of 3.9 kPa (30 mmHg) represents relative hypercapnia in a patient whose bicarbonate is 7 mmol/L (see Fig. 46-1). In most cases, the acid-base parameters will fall between the bands for metabolic acidosis and acute respiratory acidosis on the nomogram. However, in patients with chronic respiratory acidosis, superimposed metabolic acidosis may reduce bicarbonate only to the area between the acute and chronic respiratory acidosis bands or even to a position on the acute respiratory acidosis band (see Fig. 46-1). In such patients, correct diagnosis of the acid-base disorder depends on analysis of the clinical history and availability of prior acid-base measurements.

Metabolic acidosis and respiratory alkalosis As discussed above, *salicylate toxicity* commonly causes this mixed (combined) disorder (see "Metabolic Acidosis," above). This mixed disorder occurs in *septic patients*; cardiovascular insufficiency causes lactic acidosis, whereas fever and endotoxemia stimulate the respiratory center and cause hypocapnia. Chronic respiratory alkalosis is often present in patients with *hepatic cirrhosis*. Acute renal failure, a frequent complication in these patients, will superimpose metabolic acidosis. Patients who recently binged on *alcohol* may develop ketoacidosis and also may hyperventilate due to delirium tremens. In patients who have vomited repeatedly, a component of metabolic alkalosis may be added, resulting in a triple disorder.

As the severity of the hypocapnia increases, acid-base values will shift to the left on the nomogram (Fig. 46-1). With mild hypocapnia, the patient's values will be in the area between the bands for metabolic acidosis and chronic respiratory alkalosis; in this case, the nature of

this disorder is relatively easily recognized. With more profound hypocapnia, the value may fall on the chronic respiratory alkalosis band or even on the area between chronic and acute respiratory alkalosis. In such patients, correct identification of the acid-base disorder depends on the clinical setting and history.

Metabolic alkalosis and respiratory acidosis In patients with chronic respiratory acidosis due to *pulmonary disease*, metabolic alkalosis is often superimposed by treatment with *diuretics*, *steroids*, or *ventilators*. The pathogenesis of metabolic alkalosis with these forms of therapy is discussed in the section of this chapter on metabolic alkalosis.

This is an important disorder to recognize in patients with chronic lung disease because the metabolic alkalosis will reduce the acidemic stimulus to ventilation. In patients with this combined disorder, blood pH is usually close to normal. The diagnosis is suggested by the clinical history and confirmed by acid-base values that are to the left of the confidence band for chronic respiratory acidosis, typically falling between that band and the one for metabolic alkalosis. Appropriate therapy for the metabolic alkalosis may improve ventilation significantly.

Metabolic alkalosis and respiratory alkalosis In *pregnant* patients, severe vomiting will superimpose metabolic alkalosis on the chronic hypocapnia characteristic of pregnancy. Diuretics or vomiting may produce a combined alkalosis in patients with the chronic respiratory alkalosis typical of *hepatic cirrhosis*. *Treatment of cardiopulmonary arrest* often leads to a combined alkalosis. Hypocapnia is caused by the ventilator setting. The blood bicarbonate level is elevated both by bicarbonate therapy and by metabolic conversion of lactate accumulated during the cardiac arrest to bicarbonate after the circulation is restored. A triple acid-base disorder also may occur during treatment of cardiopulmonary arrest. If the circulation is not adequately restored, lactic acidosis will persist, leading to the combination of metabolic acidosis (lactic acidosis), respiratory alkalosis (ventilator), and metabolic alkalosis (bicarbonate infusion).

It is important to recognize combined metabolic and respiratory alkalosis because the relatively normal blood bicarbonate concentration may conceal severe alkalemia. Most often analysis will show that acid-base parameters lie between the bands for each primary disorder on the nomogram (Fig. 46-1). During therapy of cardiac arrest, a triple disorder due to superimposed lactic acidosis is recognized from the clinical features and a persistent elevation of the anion gap (see below).

Metabolic acidosis and alkalosis Most often this disorder results when metabolic alkalosis due to vomiting is superimposed on diabetic or alcoholic ketoacidosis or on the acidosis of chronic or acute renal failure. In some patients with diabetic ketoacidosis, ingestion of large amounts of absorbable antacids for self-treatment of accompanying symptoms of gastric discomfort may be an additional cause of metabolic alkalosis. As discussed above, during therapy of cardiopulmonary arrest, either this combined disorder or a triple disturbance including ventilator-induced respiratory alkalosis may occur.

Blood pH may be normal, acidemic, or alkalemic, depending on the relative magnitude of the primary disorders. The blood acid-base pattern is not diagnostic, since it can fall on the confidence band for either metabolic alkalosis or metabolic acidosis or be in the normal range if the two disorders balance each other. Recognition depends largely on the clinical setting and history. If the acidosis is of the high-anion-gap type (see Table 46-2), recognition of the increase in unmeasured anion concentration may be a clue to a hidden metabolic acidosis (see below). If the acidosis is characterized by a normal anion gap (see Table 46-2), diagnosis is essentially dependent on analysis of the clinical features.

Diagnosis Diagnosis of combined acid-base disorders is principally dependent on evaluation of the clinical setting, especially the history, and on interpretation of blood acid-base patterns with the aid of the nomogram (Fig. 46-1). Values that do not fit on any confidence band strongly suggest a mixed disorder. However, values that do fit on the band for a single acid-base disorder do not eliminate the possibility of a mixed disorder. Even normal acid-base parameters may conceal mixed disorders.

Evaluation of the anion gap may help in interpreting complex acid-base disorders. An anion gap in excess of 25 mmol/L strongly suggests the presence of a component of metabolic acidosis even if plasma bicarbonate is normal or elevated. For example, consider a patient who has recently binged on alcohol and presents with these plasma values: [Na] = 134 mmol/L, [K] = 3.9 mmol/L, [Cl] = 81 mmol/L, [HCO_3^-] = 26 mmol/L. Although the [HCO_3^-] is normal, the anion gap is 27 mmol/L [134 − (81 + 26)]. In this clinical setting, the elevated anion gap suggests the possibility of alcoholic ketoacidosis, which can be confirmed by measurement of plasma ketones. History reveals that the patient has been vomiting. The normal [HCO_3^-] thus is probably the result of balancing metabolic alkalosis and ketoacidosis. Although helpful, an elevated anion gap is not unequivocal evidence of metabolic acidosis. It may be moderately increased and occasionally may even exceed 25 mmol/L in metabolic alkalosis.*

---

* The increase in unmeasured anions in metabolic alkalosis is due principally to increased albumin anions. Release of protons by albumin acting as a buffer increases the number of anions per molecule. Plasma albumin concentration may also be increased by associated

REFERENCES

ADROGUE HJ et al: Plasma acid-base patterns in diabetic ketoacidosis. N Engl J Med 307:1603, 1982

ARBUS GS: An in vivo acid-base nomogram for clinical use. Can Med Assoc J 109:291, 1973

EMMETT M, NARINS RG: Clinical use of the anion gap. Medicine 56:38, 1977

GENNARI FJ, MADDOX DA: Renal regulation of acid-base homeostasis: Integrated response, in The Kidney: Physiology and Pathophysiology, 3d ed, DW Seldin, G Giebisch (eds). New York, Raven, 1992, p 2695

HARRINGTON JT: Metabolic alkalosis. Kidney Int 26:88, 1984

KASSIRER JP, MADIAS NE: Respiratory acid-base disorders. Hosp Practice 15:57, 1980

MADIAS NE: Lactic acidosis. Kidney Int 29:752, 1986

NARINS RG, EMMETT M: Simple and mixed acid-base disorders: A practical approach. Medicine 59:161, 1980

PREUSS HG: Fundamentals of clinical acid-base evaluation. Clin Lab Med 13:103, 1993

ROCHER LL, TANNEN RL: The clinical spectrum of renal tubular acidosis. Ann Rev Med 37:319, 1986

STACPOOLE PW et al: Dichloroacetate in the treatment of lactic acidosis. Ann Intern Med 108:58, 1988

WRENN KD et al: The syndrome of alcoholic ketoacidosis. Am J Med 91:119, 1991

volume depletion. Small increases in plasma lactate contribute to the elevated anion gap in alkalosis.

---

section 7   Alterations in reproductive and sexual function

47   IMPOTENCE

JOHN D. MCCONNELL / JEAN D. WILSON

A variety of endocrine, vascular, neurologic, and psychiatric diseases disrupt normal sexual and reproductive function in men. Furthermore, sexual dysfunction may be the presenting symptom of systemic disease.

NORMAL SEXUAL FUNCTION   Penile erection is initiated by neuropsychological stimuli that ultimately produce vasodilation of the sinusoidal spaces and arteries within the paired corpora cavernosa. Erection is normally preceded by sexual desire (or libido), which is regulated in part by androgen-dependent psychic factors. Although nocturnal and diurnal spontaneous erections are suppressed in men with androgen deficiency, erections in response to erotic stimuli may continue. Thus continuing action of testicular androgens appears to be required for normal libido but not for the erectile mechanism itself.

The penis receives innervation from sympathetic, parasympathetic, and somatic fibers. Somatic fibers in the dorsal nerve of the penis form the afferent limb of the erectile reflex by transmitting sensory impulses from the penile skin and glans to the S2–S4 dorsal root ganglia via the pudendal nerve. Unlike the corpuscular-type endings in the penile shaft skin, the majority of afferent terminations in the glans are free nerve endings. The efferent limb begins with parasympathetic preganglionic fibers from S2–S4 which pass in the pelvic nerves to the pelvic plexus. Sympathetic fibers emerging from the intermediolateral gray areas of T11–L2 travel through the paravertebral sympathetic chain ganglia, superior hypogastric plexus, and hypogastric nerves to enter the pelvic plexus along with parasympathetic fibers. Somatic efferent fibers from S3–S4 traveling in the pudendal nerve to the ischiocavernosus and bulbocavernosus muscles and postganglionic sympathetic fibers innervating the smooth muscle

of the epididymis, vas deferens, seminal vesicle, and internal sphincter of the bladder mediate rhythmic contraction of these structures at the time of ejaculation.

Autonomic nerve impulses, integrated in the pelvic plexus, project to the penis through the cavernous nerves which course along the posterolateral aspect of the prostate before penetrating the pelvic floor muscles immediately lateral to the urethra. Distal to the membranous urethra, some fibers enter the corpus spongiosum, while the remainder enter the corpora cavernosa along with the terminal branches of the pudendal artery and exiting cavernous veins. If disruption of the cavernous nerves occurs following pelvic trauma or surgery, erectile impotence may ensue.

The brain exerts an important modulatory influence over spinal reflex pathways that control penile function. A variety of visual, auditory, olfactory, and imaginative stimuli elicit erectile responses that involve cortical, thalamic, rhinencephalic, and limbic input to the medial preoptic–anterior hypothalamic area, which is an important integrating center. Other areas of the brain, such as the amygdaloid complex, may inhibit sexual function.

Although the parasympathetic nervous system is the primary effector of erection, the transformation of the penis to an erect organ is a vascular phenomenon. In the flaccid state the arteries, arterioles, and sinusoidal spaces within the corpora cavernosa are constricted due to active sympathetic-mediated contraction of smooth muscle in the walls of these structures. The venules between the sinusoids and the dense tunica albuginea surrounding the cavernosa open freely to the emissary veins. Erection begins when relaxation of the smooth muscles leads to dilation of the sinusoids and a decrease in peripheral resistance, causing a rapid increase in arterial blood flow through internal pudendal and cavernosa arteries. Blood is trapped in the expanding sinusoidal system, which compresses the venules against the tunica albuginea, resulting in venous occlusion. The increase in intracorporeal pressure leads to tumescence and rigidity. Full rigidity, however, may in addition require stimulation of somatic fibers in the pudendal nerve and contraction of the ischiocavernosus muscle.

Erection occurs when adrenergic-induced sinusoidal tone is antagonized by sacral parasympathetic stimulation. Sinusoidal relaxation is mediated primarily by nonadrenergic-noncholinergic (NANC) neurotransmitter(s) and by the acetylcholine-dependent release of an endothelium-derived relaxing factor (EDRF). In vitro electrical stimulation of isolated corpus cavernosum strips causes release of neurotransmitters within nerve terminals which produces smooth-muscle relaxation that is resistant to adrenergic and cholinergic blockers. Both EDRF and the NANC neurotransmitter—which acts independent of the endothelium—are nitric oxide–like factors. Inhibitors of nitric oxide synthesis and cyclic guanosine monophosphate (cGMP) synthesis, as well as nitric oxide scavengers, block sinusoidal relaxation. A variety of neuropeptides found in corporal tissues, including vasoactive intestinal peptide (VIP) and calcitonin gene-related peptide, produce tumescence when injected into the penis but have uncertain physiologic roles. Norepinephrine plays an important role in the adrenergic mechanism of detumescence.

Seminal emission and ejaculation are under control of the sympathetic nervous system. Emission results from alpha-adrenergic–mediated contraction of the epididymis, vas deferens, seminal vesicles, and prostate which causes seminal fluid to enter the prostatic urethra. Concomitant closure of the bladder neck prevents retrograde flow of semen into the bladder. Antegrade ejaculation results from contraction of the muscles of the pelvic floor including the bulbocavernosus and ischiocavernosus muscles.

Orgasm is a psychosensory phenomenon in which the rhythmic contraction of the pelvic muscles is perceived as pleasurable. Orgasm can occur without either erection or ejaculation and in the presence of retrograde ejaculation.

Detumescence after orgasm and ejaculation is incompletely understood. Presumably, active tone in the vessels of the sinusoidal spaces is restored by active (probably adrenergic-mediated) contraction of smooth muscles, which decreases the inflow of blood to the penis and promotes emptying of the erectile tissue. Following orgasm, there is a refractory period that varies with age, physical condition, and psychic factors during which erection and ejaculation are inhibited.

IMPOTENCE Simply defined, *impotence* is the failure to achieve erection, ejaculation, or both. Men with sexual dysfunction present with a variety of complaints, either singly or in combination: loss of libido, inability to initiate or maintain an erection, ejaculatory failure, premature ejaculation, or inability to achieve orgasm. Sexual dysfunction can be secondary to systemic disease processes or their treatment, to specific disorders of the urogenital or endocrine systems, or to psychological disturbance. Previously, it was felt that the cause of dysfunction in the majority of men with erectile impotency was psychogenic. It is now believed that the majority of impotent men have a component of underlying organic disease. Since the selection and success of subsequent therapy depends on the specific cause, it is essential to evaluate all aspects of the erectile mechanism.

Loss of desire A decrease in sexual desire, or libido, may be due to androgen deficiency (arising from either pituitary or testicular disease), psychological disturbance, or some types of prescribed or habitually abused drugs. The possibility of androgen deficiency can be tested by measurement of plasma testosterone and gonadotropin levels. The level of testosterone required for normal erectile function remains unknown. Hypogonadism also may result in the absence of emission secondary to decreased secretion of ejaculate by the seminal vesicles and prostate.

Failure of erection The organ causes of erectile impotence can be grouped into endocrine, drug, local, neurologic, and vascular causes (Table 47-1). Decreased plasma testosterone secondary to testicular failure is an uncommon but easily recognized and treated disorder. However, hyperprolactinemia may cause impotence in some men with pituitary tumors and may not be obvious on physical examination; hyperprolactinemia suppresses luteinizing hormone–releasing hormone (LHRH) production, resulting in plasma gonadotropin and testosterone values in the low or low-normal range. Bromocrip-

TABLE 47-1 Some organic causes of erectile impotence in men

ENDOCRINE CAUSES

A Testicular failure (primary or secondary)
B Hyperprolactinemia

DRUGS

A Antiandrogens
  1 Histamine—H-2 blockers (e.g., cimetidine)
  2 Spironolactone
  3 Ketoconazole
  4 Finasteride
B Antihypertensives
  1 Central acting sympatholytics (e.g., clonidine and methyldopa)
  2 Peripheral acting sympatholytics (e.g., guanadrel)
  3 Beta blockers
  4 Thiazides
C Anticholinergics
D Antidepressants
  1 Monoamine oxidase inhibitors
  2 Tricyclic antidepressants
E Antipsychotics
F Central nervous system depressants
  1 Sedatives (e.g., barbiturates)
  2 Antianxiety drugs (e.g., diazepam)
G Drugs of habituation or addiction
  1 Alcohol
  2 Methadone
  3 Heroin
  4 Tobacco

PENILE DISEASES

A Peyronie's disease
B Previous priapism
C Penile trauma

NEUROLOGIC DISEASES

A Anterior temporal lobe lesions
B Diseases of the spinal cord
C Loss of sensory input
  1 Tabes dorsalis
  2 Disease of dorsal root ganglia
D Disease of nervi erigentes
  1 Radical prostatectomy and cystectomy
  2 Rectosigmoid operations
E Diabetic autonomic neuropathy and various polyneuropathies

VASCULAR DISEASE

A Aortic occlusion (Leriche syndrome)
B Atherosclerotic occlusion or stenosis of the pudendal and/or cavernosa arteries
C Arterial damage from pelvic radiation
D Venous leak
E Disease of the sinusoidal spaces

tine, a dopamine agonist, may lower prolactin levels and reverse impotence in such patients.

Although many drugs are associated with impotence, antihypertensive agents, cimetidine, and monoamine oxidase inhibitors are more likely to lead to erectile dysfunction. Antihypertensive drugs with peripheral and central sympatholytic action or beta-adrenergic receptor blocking activity are the most frequently implicated. Angiotensin-converting enzyme inhibitors, calcium channel blockers, and peripheral vasodilators do not cause a significant incidence of sexual dysfunction. Histamine (H-2) receptor antagonists, such as cimetidine, have antiandrogenic properties in addition to increasing prolactin secretion. The 5α-reductase inhibitor finasteride, used commonly for the treatment of benign prostate hypertrophy, produces impotence or decreased libido in 3 to 4 percent of men. Monoamine oxidase inhibitors, antipsychotic drugs, and tricyclic depressants may impair sexual function via anticholinergic and sympatholytic actions.

Penile diseases, including previous priapism, penile trauma, and Peyronie's disease, can cause impotence due to fibrosis of the sinusoidal spaces of the corpora cavernosa, corporeal artery occlusion, or neurogenic mechanisms. Peyronie's disease is not rare; patients present with a painful plaque on the dorsum of the penis and may progress to development of penile curvature and decreased rigidity.

Many types of neurologic disorders cause impotence, including lesions in the anterior temporal lobe, spinal cord disorders, insufficiency of sensory input as in tabes dorsalis, or damage to parasympathetic nerves, e.g., following surgical procedures such as radical (total) prostatectomy or cystectomy. Furthermore, the nerve supply to the penis (the nervi erigentes) runs on the posterolateral surface of the prostate, and if the nerves are preserved during radical prostate and bladder surgery, potency can be preserved in many men. If spinal cord injury is above the sacral region, reflex erections may occur, whereas diffuse injury of the sacral spinal cord results in total impotence. As many as half of men with diabetes mellitus develop impotence within 6 years of the onset of diabetes, and impotence may be the first clinical manifestation of diabetic neuropathy. Several factors contribute to neuropathic impotence, including abnormalities in afferent sensory pathways, motor neuropathy in the cavernosa nerves (which carry the efferent pathways for vasodilation in the penis), and decreased level of cavernosa neurotransmitter. Although autonomic pathways in the penis can be tested by direct recording of electrical activity in the corporal smooth muscle, the test may not be necessary because most patients demonstrate other manifestations of autonomic neuropathy on careful examination. Many of the other polyneuropathies associated with impotence have similar effects.

Men with vasculogenic impotence may present with total erectile impotence, decreased penile rigidity, or loss of erection during intercourse. Vascular insufficiency may be due to aortic occlusion (Leriche syndrome) or to more distal atherosclerotic disease in the hypogastric, pudendal, and cavernosa arteries. Significant disease in the pudendal and cavernosa arteries can occur in the absence of other clinical manifestations of peripheral vascular disease. Impotence following pelvic radiation is probably due to vasculogenic causes. Together with neuropathy, vascular insufficiency contributes to the impotence in many men with diabetes mellitus.

Premature ejaculation This disorder seldom has an organic cause. It is usually related to anxiety in the sexual situation, unreasonable expectations about performance, or emotional disorder. A variety of successful therapeutic modalities have been described by Levine.

Absence of emission This symptom may be produced by (1) retrograde ejaculation, (2) sympathetic enervation, (3) androgen deficiency, or (4) drugs. Retrograde ejaculation may occur following surgery on the bladder neck or develop spontaneously in diabetic men. Demonstration of sperm in a postcoital urine specimen establishes the diagnosis. Following sympathectomy or occasionally after extensive retroperitoneal surgery, the autonomic innervation of the prostate and seminal vesicles is lost, resulting in absence of smooth-muscle contraction at the time of ejaculation. Androgen deficiency results in a decrease in secretions of the prostate and seminal vesicles and in a diminution of the volume of ejaculate. Finally, drugs such as guanethidine, phenoxybenzamine, and phentolamine primarily impair ejaculation rather than erection or libido.

Absence of orgasm If libido and erectile function are normal, the absence of orgasm is almost always due to a psychiatric disorder.

Failure of detumescence Priapism is a persistent painful erection, often unrelated to sexual activity. Priapism can be distinguished from a normal erection by the absence of tumescence of the glans penis. Priapism may be idiopathic but can be associated with sickle cell anemia, chronic granulocytic leukemia, spinal cord injury, or, rarely, injection of vasodilator agents (such as papaverine) into the penis. The disorder may be secondary to clotting of blood within the sinusoidal spaces of the penis or to abnormalities of the adrenergic-mediated mechanism for detumescence. Failure to treat priapism promptly usually results in fibrosis and subsequent loss of erectile function. In early phases, detumescence can sometimes be achieved by aspiration, irrigation of the corpora cavernosa, and injection of

dilute vasoconstrictors. If this fails, surgical relief by shunting procedures may be necessary. In patients with priapism secondary to sickle cell anemia, conservative measures such as transfusion, oxygenation, and irrigation are generally preferred to shunting procedures.

EVALUATION OF IMPOTENCE The relative frequency of organic as opposed to psychogenic causes of erectile impotence is still debated. Nevertheless, anxiety and depressive states are common causes of impotence. Other psychological factors such as disinterest in the sexual partner, fear of sexual incompetence, martial discord, guilt about deviant sexual attitudes, worry, fatigue, and ill health often operate in various combinations to reduce sexual impulse. The central issue in the evaluation of impotence is to separate those instances due to psychological factors from those due to organic causes (see Table 47-1). Often, the separation can be made on the basis of history. With the exception of severe depression, men with psychogenic impotence usually have normal nocturnal and early morning erections. From early childhood through the eighth decade, erections occur during normal sleep. This phenomenon, termed *nocturnal penile tumescence* (NPT), occurs during rapid eye movement sleep, and the total time of NPT averages 100 min per night. Consequently, if the impotent man gives a history of rigid erections under any circumstances (often when awakening in the morning), the efferent neurologic and circulatory systems that mediate erection are intact, and dysfunction is probably due to a psychiatric disorder. In these patients the workup should be limited. (Occasional patients with early sensory neuropathy may have nocturnal erections.)

If the history of nocturnal erections is questionable, measurements of NPT can be made formally with the use of a strain gauge in a sleep laboratory or informally attached to a recorder by snap gauge or home monitor. Although false-negative and false-positive results are possible, this procedure helps to differentiate psychogenic and organic impotence. Patients with vasculogenic impotence may have some degree of penile tumescence without the development of adequate rigidity, which may result in a false-positive NPT test. An alternative to NPT testing is the visual sexual stimulation (VSS) test, which utilizes videotaped erotic material in a laboratory setting to monitor erection by strain gauge. Other features of organic impotence include a slow, insidious onset not associated with any particular psychiatric symptomatology, a previous uninterrupted period of normal erectile function, and persistent sexual desire.

Having deduced an organic cause, the fundamental problem is the differential diagnosis of the etiology (see Table 47-1). The history should be probed for diabetes mellitus, manifestations of peripheral neuropathy or bladder dysfunction, symptoms referable to the vascular system such as intermittent claudication, and symptoms of penile disease such as a history of priapism or penile curvature (Peyronie's disease). A thorough drug history should be obtained, and inquiry should be made concerning past surgery that may have produced neurologic damage. Smoking is a risk factor for atherosclerotic disease and may inhibit sinusoidal relaxation directly.

Physical examination should include a detailed genital examination to identify abnormalities of the penis, especially Peyronie's disease, which is usually easily felt as a fibrotic plaque on the dorsum of the penis. The testes should be palpated for size, symmetry, and abnormal masses; if the length is less than 3.5 cm, hypogonadism should be considered. Evidence of feminization such as gynecomastia and abnormal body hair distribution should be sought. All pulses should be palpated, and the presence of bruits should be sought. Often, the pulse in the dorsal penile artery can be felt. If there is an indication from either history or physical examination of a vascular cause, penile blood flow can be measured directly.

Pudendal arteriography provides the most accurate assessment of penile arterial disease, but it is expensive and invasive. Moreover, distal arterial lesions may not be identified unless the procedure is performed under conditions of chemical erection (e.g., papaverine injection). The penile/brachial index can be used to estimate penile blood flow by dividing the penile systolic blood pressure, as determined by Doppler technique, by the simultaneously determined supine brachial systolic pressure. An index of less than 0.6 is suggestive of vasculogenic impotence. However, the test evaluates flow only through the dorsal penile artery, which is not directly involved in the erectile process. Significant disease may be present in the cavernosa arteries despite normal flow through the dorsal artery. Pulsed Doppler analysis and high-resolution ultrasonography can be used in conjunction with intracorporeal papaverine to assess blood flow in the cavernosa arteries. Alternatively, dynamic infusion cavernosography, which measures pressure directly within the corpora, can be utilized to assess arterial inflow. Abnormalities in the venous occlusive mechanism of the penis can cause impotence due to venous leak and can be diagnosed with the use of dynamic infusion cavernosometry to demonstrate a rapid fall in corporal pressures, followed by cavernosography to document the anatomic site of leak. The incidence of venous leakage in men with normal erectile function is unknown. Moreover, venous leak is most commonly secondary to arterial inflow and sinusoidal disease. The failure rate of surgical or embolization procedures designed to obliterate the incompetent vein is high, suggesting that most patients have additional pathology.

The neurologic examination should measure anal sphincter tone, perineal sensation, and the bulbocavernosus reflex. This reflex is elicited by squeezing the glans penis and noting the degree of anal sphincter constriction. An examination for peripheral neuropathy, including assessment of distal muscle function, the tendon reflexes in the legs, and vibratory, position, tactile, and pain sensation also should be performed. In the presence of peripheral neuropathy, tests to evaluate penile neuropathy are seldom necessary. In cases with an uncertain neurogenic component, electromyographic sacral signal tracing of the bulbocavernosus reflex or direct electrical recording of the corpora cavernosa by needle or surface electrodes may be helpful. A specific test to document abnormalities in the penile autonomic efferent pathways is not available.

In the absence of hypogonadism or feminization, the serum testosterone level is usually normal. Hyperprolactinemia, however, may not be suspected on the basis of history and physical examination. Although the endocrine causes of erectile dysfunction are uncommon, serum prolactin and pooled serum testosterone and luteinizing hormone (see Chap. 339) should be measured, since abnormalities of these parameters are treatable.

TREATMENT OF IMPOTENCE Medical therapy with androgens offers little more than placebo benefit except in hypogonadal men, and empirical therapy may actually delay identification of organic causes. If a prolactin-secreting pituitary tumor is present, however, either surgical removal or treatment with bromocriptine usually results in return of potency. Yohimbine, an alpha$_2$-adrenergic antagonist, is widely prescribed but works only in psychogenic impotence by placebo effect. Surgical therapy may be useful in the treatment of decreased potency related to aortic obstruction; however, potency can be lost rather than improved after aortic surgery if the autonomic nerve supply to the penis is damaged. Penile revascularization is effective only in young men with traumatic arterial disease. Few men with venous leak impotency benefit from venous ligation.

A variety of vasoactive substances produce erection when injected into the corpora cavernosa. Self-injection with prostaglandin E and papaverine (with or without phentolamine) produces erection in patients with psychogenic, neurogenic, and mild vasculogenic impotency. Despite lack of FDA approval, occasional pain on injection, and the rare complications of priapism and penile fibrosis, use of this therapy is fairly widespread. Commercially available mechanical devices that utilize a vacuum to produce an erection and a rubber band to restrict venous return at the base of the penis provide a successful nonsurgical alternative in many patients, including some with diabetes mellitus.

Penile prostheses should only be implanted in impotent men refractory to other forms of therapy. Malleable Silastic rods inserted into the penis provide the simplest system and the lowest complication rates; however, the cosmetic and functional performance of the device

is not uniformly satisfactory. Multicomponent, hydraulically operated prostheses offer the advantage of more physiologic erection and greater increase in penile diameter. However, these devices are subject to mechanical failure.

Even in patients with organic impotence, psychotherapy is often beneficial in alleviating concomitant psychogenic factors that limit the success of medical and surgical therapy.

REFERENCES

ABRAMOWICZ M et al: Drugs that cause sexual dysfunction. Med Lett 29:65, 1987

deGROAT WC, STEERS WD: Neuroanatomy and neurophysiology of penile erection, in *Contemporary Management of Impotence and Infertility*, EA Tanagho et al (eds). Baltimore, Williams & Wilkins, 1988, pp 3–27

FISHMAN JF et al: Experience with inflatable penile prosthesis. Urology 23:86, 1984

GOLDSTEIN I: Overview of types and results of vascular procedures for impotence. Cardiovasc Intervert Radiol 11:240, 1988

———, KRANE RJ: Diagnosis and therapy of erectile dysfunction, in *Campbell's Urology*, PC Walsh et al (eds). Philadelphia, Saunders, 1992, pp 3033–3070

——— et al: Radiation-associated impotence: A clinical study of its mechanism. JAMA 251:903, 1984

KAISER FE, KORENMAN SG: Impotence in diabetic men. Am J Med 85(suppl 5A):147, 1988

KIM N et al: A nitric oxide–like factor mediates nonadrenergic-noncholinergic neurogenic relaxation of penile corpus cavernosum smooth muscle. J Clin Invest 88:112, 1991

KNISPEL HH: Penile venous surgery in impotence: Results in highly selected cases. Urol Int 47:144, 1991

KOLODNY RC et al: Sexual function in diabetic men. Diabetes 23:306, 1974

KORENMAN SG: Sexual dysfunction, in *Williams' Textbook of Endocrinology*, 7th ed, JD Wilson, DW Foster (eds). Philadelphia, Saunders, 1992, pp 1033–1048

KRANE RJ: Medical progress: Impotence. N Engl J Med 321:1648, 1989

KWAN M et al: The nature of androgen action on male sexuality: A combined laboratory–self-report study on hypogonadal men. J Clin Endocrinol Metab 57:557, 1983

LEE LM et al: Prostaglandin E, versus phentolamine/papaverine for the treatment of erectile impotence: A double-blind comparison. J Urol 141:549, 1989

LEVINE SB: Marital sexual dysfunction: Ejaculation disturbances. Ann Intern Med 84:575, 1976

LUE TF et al: Functional evaluation of penile veins by cavernosography in papaverine-induced erection. J Urol 135:479, 1986

——— et al: Vasculogenic impotence evaluated by high-resolution ultrasonography and pulsed Doppler spectrum analysis. Radiology 155:777, 1985

MEYER J: Disorders of sexual function, in *Textbook of Endocrinology*, vol 7, JD Wilson, DM Foster (eds). Philadelphia, Saunders, 1985, pp 476–491

MONTAGUE DK et al: Infusion pharmacocavernosometry and normal penile tumescence findings in men with erectile dysfunction. J Urol 145:768, 1991

RAJFER J: Nitric oxide as a mediator of relaxation in response to nonadrenergic, noncholinergic neurotransmission. N Engl J Med 326:90, 1992

SAENZ DE TEJADA I et al: Cholinergic neurotransmission in human corpus cavernosum: I. Responses of isolated tissue. Am J Physiol 254:H459, 1988

SAYPOL DC et al: Impotence: Are the newer diagnostic methods a necessity? J Urol 130:260, 1983

VIRAG R et al: Intracavernous self-injection of vasoactive drugs in the treatment of impotence: 8-year experience with 615 cases. J Urol 145:287, 1991

WABEK AJ: Bulbocavernosus reflex testing in 100 consecutive cases of erectile dysfunction. Urology 25:495, 1985

WALSH PC et al: Impotence following radical prostatectomy: Insight into etiology and prevention. J Urol 128:492, 1982

WINTER CC: Priapism. Urol Surv 28:163, 1978

WITHERINGTON R: Vacuum constriction device for management of erectile impotence. J Urol 141:320, 1989

ZORGNIOTTI AW: Autoinjection of the corpus cavernosum with a vasoactive drug combination for vasculogenic impotence. J Urol 133:39, 1985

48 DISTURBANCES OF MENSTRUATION AND SEXUAL FUNCTION IN WOMEN

BRUCE R. CARR / JEAN D. WILSON

Complaints related to the female reproductive tract can be categorized as disorders of menstruation, pelvic pain, disturbances in sexual function, or infertility. However, a single disorder, e.g., leiomyoma of the uterus, can present with symptoms referable to any one or more of these categories. Furthermore, sexual dysfunction can interdigitate with other complaints in several ways. On the one hand, in women with complaints related to other reproductive tract functions, the underlying problem may actually be severe sexual dysfunction or marital conflict. Alternatively, women with severe organic disorders of the pelvis, e.g., pelvic inflammatory disease, may present with sexual dysfunction such as dyspareunia which in fact is only a minor manifestation of the underlying disease.

Since normal reproductive function depends on the integrated action of the central nervous system, the endocrine glands, and the reproductive organs, menstrual cycle abnormalities, sexual dysfunction, and infertility may be the result of systemic and psychological disorders as well as of primary defects in the endocrine and reproductive organs. The endocrine and physiologic control—normal and abnormal—of puberty, reproductive life, and menopause are discussed in Chap. 340. The focus of this chapter is on the initial evaluation of women with disturbances of the reproductive tract.

DISTURBANCES IN MENSTRUATION　Disorders of menstruation can be divided into abnormal uterine bleeding and amenorrhea.

Abnormal uterine bleeding　The menstrual cycle is defined as the interval between the onset of one bleeding episode and the onset of the next. In normal women the cycle averages 28 ± 3 days, the mean duration of menstrual flow is 4 ± 2 days, and the average blood loss is 40 to 100 mL. Between menarche and menopause most women experience one or more episodes of abnormal uterine bleeding, here defined as any bleeding pattern outside the normal ranges of frequency, duration, and/or amount of blood loss. The decision to evaluate a patient with an abnormal bleeding pattern depends on the severity and frequency of the abnormal episodes.

When uterine bleeding is suspected, it is essential to establish first that the blood observed by the patient is derived from the uterine endometrium. Rectal, bladder, cervical, and vaginal sources of bleeding must be excluded. Once the bleeding is documented to be uterine in origin, a pregnancy-related disorder (such as threatened or incomplete abortion or ectopic pregnancy) must be excluded by physical examination and appropriate laboratory tests. Abnormal uterine bleeding also may be the initial or principal manifestation of a generalized bleeding diathesis. The remaining causes of abnormal uterine bleeding can be divided into those associated with ovulatory cycles and those associated with anovulatory cycles.

OVULATORY CYCLES　Menstrual bleeding with ovulatory cycles is spontaneous, regular in onset, predictable in duration and amount of flow, and frequently associated with discomfort. Uterine bleeding with ovulatory cycles is due to progesterone withdrawal at the end of the luteal (postovulatory) phase and requires prior estrogen priming of the endometrium during the follicular (preovulatory) phase of the cycle. When deviations from an established pattern of menstrual flow occur but the cycles are still regular, the usual cause is organic disease of the outflow tract. For example, regular, prolonged, excessive bleeding episodes unassociated with a bleeding diathesis can result from abnormalities of the uterus such as submucous leiomyomas, adenomyosis, or endometrial polyps. On the other hand, cyclic, predictable menstruation characterized by spotting or light bleeding suggests obstruction of the outflow tract as with uterine synechiae or scarring of the cervix. Intermittent bleeding between cyclic ovulatory menses is often due to cervical or endometrial lesions.

ANOVULATORY CYCLES　Uterine bleeding that is irregular in occurrence, unpredictable as to amount and duration of flow, and usually painless is called *dysfunctional uterine bleeding*. This type of bleeding is the result of a failure of normal follicular maturation with consequent anovulation and may be either transient or chronic. Transient disruption of the synchronous hypothalamic-pituitary-ovarian hormonal control necessary for ovulatory cycles occurs most often in the early menarcheal years, during the perimenopausal period, or as the consequence of a variety of stresses and intercurrent illnesses. Persistent dysfunctional uterine bleeding during the reproductive years can occur in several organic diseases that affect ovarian function and is most often due to estrogen breakthrough bleeding. Estrogen breakthrough bleeding occurs when prolonged continuous estrogen stimulation of the endometrium is not interrupted by cyclic progesterone withdrawal. For example, chronic acyclic estrogen production not associated with ovulation can occur in polycystic ovarian disease.

Amenorrhea　*Amenorrhea* is defined as failure of menarche by age 16, regardless of the presence or absence of secondary sexual characteristics, or the absence of menstruation for 6 months in a woman with previous periodic menses. Amenorrhea in a woman who has never menstruated is termed *primary*; cessation of menses is termed *secondary amenorrhea*. Because some disorders can cause both primary and secondary amenorrhea, we prefer a functional classification based on the nature of the underlying defect, namely, anatomic defects of the outflow tract (uterus, cervix, or vagina), ovarian failure, and chronic anovulation.

Anatomic defects of the outflow tract include congenital defects of the vagina, imperforate hymen, transverse vaginal septa, cervical stenosis, intrauterine adhesions (synechiae), absence of the vagina or uterus, and uterine maldevelopment. The diagnosis of an anatomic defect is usually made by physical examination and confirmed by demonstrating failure of bleeding following administration of estrogen plus a progestogen for 21 days. Pelvic ultrasonography, magnetic resonance imaging, hysterosalpingogram or hysteroscopy may be helpful in defining the defect.

Causes of *ovarian failure* include gonadal dysgenesis, deficiency of $P450_{17\alpha}$, resistant ovary syndrome, and premature ovarian failure. Ovarian failure encompasses disorders in which the ovary is deficient in germ cells and those in which the germ cells are resistant to FSH (follicle-stimulating hormone). The diagnosis of ovarian failure as the cause of amenorrhea is confirmed by a plasma FSH greater than 40 IU/L.

Women with *chronic anovulation* fail to ovulate spontaneously but have the capability of ovulating with appropriate therapy. In some women with chronic anovulation, estrogen production is adequate, but estrogen is not secreted in a cyclic fashion. In others, estrogen production is deficient.

Women who have adequate estrogen production and demonstrate withdrawal bleeding after progestogen challenge usually have polycystic ovarian disease (see Fig. 340-7). Other causes include hormone-secreting ovarian and adrenal tumors. Women with deficient or absent estrogen production, and therefore with absence of withdrawal bleeding after progestogen administration, usually have hypogonadotropic hypogonadism due to organic or functional disorders of the pituitary or central nervous system such as brain tumors, pituitary tumors (especially prolactin-secreting adenomas), primary hypopituitarism, or Sheehan's syndrome.

PELVIC PAIN　Pelvic pain may originate in the pelvis or be referred from another region of the body. A pelvic source is suggested by the history (e.g., dysmenorrhea and dyspareunia) and physical findings, but a high index of suspicion must be entertained for extrapelvic disorders that refer to the pelvis, such as appendicitis, cholecystitis, intestinal obstruction, and urinary tract infections (see Chap. 13).

"Physiologic" pelvic pain　PAIN ASSOCIATED WITH OVULATION ("MITTELSCHMERZ")　Many women experience low abdominal discomfort with ovulation, typically a dull aching pain at midcycle in one lower quadrant lasting from minutes to hours. It is rarely severe or incapacitating. The relationship of the pain to the process of ovulation is unknown. It may result from peritoneal irritation by follicular fluid released into the peritoneal cavity at ovulation. The onset at midcycle and short duration of pain are often diagnostic.

PREMENSTRUAL OR MENSTRUAL PAIN　In normal ovulatory women, somatic symptoms during the few days prior to menses may be insignificant or disabling. Such symptoms include edema, breast engorgement, and abdominal bloating or discomfort. A symptom complex of cyclic irritability, depression, and lethargy is known as the *premenstrual syndrome* (PMS). The cause of PMS is unknown, and there is no consensus about therapy.

Severe or incapacitating uterine cramping in women with ovulatory menses but no demonstrable disorders of the pelvis is termed *primary dysmenorrhea*. Primary dysmenorrhea is caused by prostaglandin-induced uterine ischemia and is treated with prostaglandin synthetase inhibitors or oral contraceptive agents.

Pelvic pain due to organic causes   Severe dysmenorrhea associated with disease of the pelvis is termed *secondary dysmenorrhea*. Organic causes of pelvic pain can be classified as (1) uterine, (2) adnexal, (3) vulvar or vaginal, and (4) pregnancy-associated.

UTERINE PAIN   Pain of uterine etiology is often chronic and continuous and increases in intensity during menstruation and intercourse. Causes include leiomyomas of the uterus (particularly submucous and degenerating leiomyomas), adenomyosis, and cervical stenosis. Infections of the uterus associated with intrauterine manipulation following dilatation and curettage or with intrauterine devices also can cause significant pelvic pain (see Chap. 340). Pelvic pain due to endometrial or cervical cancer is usually a late manifestation of disseminated disease (see Chap. 340).

ADNEXAL PAIN   The most common cause of pain in the adnexae (fallopian tubes and ovaries) is infection (see Chap. 89). Acute salpingo-oophoritis presents as low abdominal pain, fever, and chills; begins a few days after a menstrual period; and is usually due to chlamydia or gonococcal disease with or without a superimposed pyogenic infection. Chronic pelvic inflammatory disease results from either a single episode or multiple episodes of infection and may present as infertility associated with chronic pelvic pain that increases in intensity with menses and intercourse. On physical examination, the adnexae are tender, and adnexal thickening with or without masses may be present. Pelvic inflammatory disease may become a surgical emergency if peritonitis results from rupture of a tuboovarian abscess. Ovarian cysts or neoplasms may cause pelvic pain that becomes more severe with torsion or rupture of the mass, and ectopic pregnancy must be considered in the differential diagnosis (see below). Endometriosis involving fallopian tubes, ovaries, or peritoneum may cause both chronic low abdominal pain and infertility; the magnitude of tissue involvement does not always correlate with the severity of symptoms. Endometriosis pain typically increases with menstruation and, if the posterior ligaments of the uterus are involved, with intercourse.

VULVAR OR VAGINAL PAIN   Pain in these areas is most often due to infectious vaginitis caused by organisms such as *Monilia*, *Trichomonas*, or *Gardnerella* and is characteristically associated with vaginal discharge and pruritus. Herpetic vulvitis, condyloma acuminatum, and cysts or abscesses of Bartholin's glands also may cause vulvar pain.

PREGNANCY-ASSOCIATED DISORDERS   Pregnancy must be considered in the differential diagnosis of pelvic pain during the reproductive years. Threatened abortion or incomplete abortion often presents with uterine cramping, bleeding, or passage of tissue following a period of amenorrhea. Ectopic pregnancy may be insidious in presentation and result in severe intraperitoneal hemorrhage and maternal death.

Evaluation of pelvic pain   The evaluation of pelvic pain requires a careful history and pelvic examination. This often leads to the correct diagnosis and institution of appropriate treatment. If the pain is severe and the diagnosis is unclear, the workup should follow that outlined for the acute abdomen (Chap. 13). A culdocentesis is indicated if a ruptured ectopic pregnancy is suspected. If there is a question of an adnexal mass or if the patient is so obese as to preclude a thorough pelvic examination, sonography may be useful. Serial human chorionic gonadotropin (hCG) measurements may help in establishing a diagnosis of tubal pregnancy. Finally, diagnostic laparoscopy and laparotomy may be indicated with pain of undetermined etiology.

SEXUAL DYSFUNCTION   Some women with sexual dysfunction describe minor complaints related to the reproductive tract as a means of bringing sexual problems to the attention of the physician. Alternatively, sexual dysfunction may be thought to be the cause of low abdominal discomfort or dyspareunia when the actual etiology is organic. However, more and more women seek medical advice because of sexual problems that interface in provenance between medicine and sociology.

The normal sexual response begins with sexual arousal which causes genital vasocongestion that results in vaginal lubrication in preparation for intromission. The lubrication is due to the formation of a transudate in the vagina and in conjunction with genital congestion produces the so-called orgasmic platform prior to orgasm. Sexual stimuli (visual, tactile, auditory, and olfactory) as well as healthy vaginal tissue are prerequisites for genital vasocongestion and vaginal lubrication. During the second stage of the sexual response, involuntary contractions of the muscles of the pelvis result in a pleasurable cortical sensory phenomenon known as orgasm. Direct or indirect stimulation of the clitoris is important in the production of the female orgasm. In simple terms, sexual dysfunction can be due to interference with the arousal or orgasmic phases of the sexual response. Either disorder can be due to an organic or functional cause or both.

Illnesses that impair neurologic function such as diabetes mellitus or multiple sclerosis can prevent normal sexual arousal. Local pelvic diseases such as vaginitis, endometriosis, and salpingo-oophoritis may preclude normal sexual response because of resulting dyspareunia. Debilitating systemic diseases such as cancer and cardiovascular diseases may impair normal sexual response indirectly.

More commonly, failure of a normal sexual response is due to psychological factors that impair sexual arousal. Such problems include misinformation, e.g., the perception of sexual satisfaction as bad, or feelings of guilt about previous psychologically traumatic events such as incest, rape, or unwanted pregnancy. In addition, women who have had previous hysterectomy or mastectomy may perceive themselves as "incomplete." Stresses such as anxiety, depression, fatigue, and marital or interpersonal conflicts may lead to failure of the vasocongestive response and prevent normal vaginal lubrication. Women with such experiences may be unable to achieve normal sexual response unless they receive professional counseling by a family physician, psychiatrist, or sex therapist. Such problems are approached by attempting to identify and reduce the causative stresses.

Failure to achieve orgasm is a specific form of sexual dysfunction. In the absence of orgasm many women enjoy sexual encounters to variable degrees because of the pleasure derived from closeness in a cherished relationship, particularly with a loving partner. However, for other women sexual relations with rare or absent orgasms are frustrating and unsatisfying. In many instances, failure of orgasm is due to insufficient clitoral stimulation and may be rectified by appropriate counseling and patient education.

A specific entity, "vaginismus," painful, involuntary contractions of the musculature surrounding the entrance to the vagina, is a rare cause of dyspareunia. It is a conditioned response to a previous real or imagined frightening or traumatic sexual experience. Treatment is directed to elimination of the conditioned response by progressive vaginal dilation by the patient in conjunction with marital therapy.

REPRODUCTION   Problems of infertility are discussed in detail in Chap. 340. The approach to infertile couples always involves evaluation of both the man and woman. The history should elicit information as to the frequency of intercourse, the sexual responses of both, the use of contraceptives or lubricants, previous or past medical illnesses, and all medications taken.

Male-associated factors account for a third of infertility problems. Therefore, one of the first procedures in the workup of infertile couples should be a semen analysis (see Chap. 339). The initial evaluation of the woman includes documentation of normal ovulatory cycles. A history of regular, cyclic, predictable, spontaneous menses usually indicates ovulatory cycles, which may be confirmed by basal body temperature graphs, properly timed endometrial biopsies, or plasma progesterone measurements during the luteal phase of the cycle. Also, the diagnosis of luteal-phase dysfunction (low progesterone secretion during the luteal phase) can be established by these methods. If the woman is anovulatory, attempts to induce ovulation can be undertaken by a variety of methods including clomiphene, human menopausal gonadotropins, bromocriptine, luteinizing hormone–releasing hormone (LHRH) agonists, or wedge resection of the ovaries (Chap. 340).

The most common cause of infertility in women is tubal disease, usually due to infection (pelvic inflammatory disease) or endometriosis. Tubal disease can be evaluated by obtaining a hysterosalpingogram or by diagnostic laparoscopy. The treatment of tubal causes of infertility is primarily surgical.

A cervical factor as a cause of infertility is identified by a properly timed postcoital examination. During this examination, the sperm motility in cervical mucus is observed. Also, immunologic etiologies for infertility can be tested for by a variety of laboratory tests. The cause of infertility is unknown in 10 percent of couples. In many instances of infertility, it is now possible to use assisted reproductive technologies including in vitro fertilization and embryo transfer, gamete intrafallopian tube transfer, transfer of cryopreserved ova and embryos, and intrauterine insemination.

The desire for contraception is also a frequent cause for women to seek medical treatment or evaluation. The most widely used methods for fertility control include (1) rhythm and withdrawal techniques, (2) barrier methods, (3) intrauterine devices, (4) oral steroid contraceptives, (5) sterilization, and (6) abortion. These methods and their complications are discussed in Chap. 340.

REFERENCES

CUNNINGHAM FG et al: *Williams Obstetrics*, 18th ed. Norwalk, Appleton-Century-Crofts, 1989
HERBST AL et al: *Comprehensive Gynecology*, 2d ed. St. Louis, Mosby, 1992
FORDNEY DS: Dyspareunia and vaginismus. Clin Obstet Gynecol 21:205, 1978
HAMMOND DC: Screening for sexual dysfunction. Clin Obstet Gynecol 27:732, 1984
HATCHER RA et al: *Contraceptive Technology 1990–1992.* New York, Irvington, 1986
MASTERS W, JOHNSON V: *Human Sexual Response.* Boston, Little, Brown, 1966
———, ———: *Human Sexual Inadequacy.* Boston, Little, Brown, 1970
SPEROFF L et al: *Clinical Gynecologic Endocrinology and Infertility*, 4th ed. Baltimore, Williams & Wilkins, 1989

49   HIRSUTISM AND VIRILIZATION

WILLIAM J. KOVACS / JEAN D. WILSON

Hirsutism, male pattern hair growth in women, is a common and perplexing problem. The distribution and growth of hair in normal persons is under complex genetic and endocrine control so that there is considerable variability in hair growth among normal men and women. As a consequence, abnormal hair growth is difficult to define: Some patients may seek medical attention because of what the physician may consider an insignificant cosmetic defect. Others, because of personal or cultural differences, may be undisturbed by surprising degrees of hirsutism. The central issue in dealing with such patients is the separation of those infrequent instances in which hirsutism is a manifestation of a serious and remediable underlying disorder from the majority of hirsute women in whom excess hair is fundamentally a cosmetic problem.

CONTROL OF NORMAL HAIR GROWTH AND DISTRIBUTION

Endocrine control   Androgens are the major determinants of hair distribution in both sexes. There are three principal circulating androgens in women—dehydroepiandrosterone, derived from the adrenal; androstenedione, which is derived equally from adrenal and ovary; and testosterone, which is both secreted by the ovary and adrenal and formed in extraglandular tissue from circulating dehydroepiandrosterone and androstenedione. The production of adrenal androgen is regulated primarily by adrenocorticotropin while ovarian androgen secretion is regulated by luteinizing hormone (LH). These various androgens must be converted to testosterone (or dihydrotestos-

terone) before they can bind to the androgen receptor of target cells and induce an androgenic response. Thus, adrenal androgens virilize only in so far as they serve as precursors for testosterone and dihydrotestosterone.

Several types of relationships can be defined between hair growth and androgens in normal individuals. The growth of eyebrows, eyelashes, and vellus hair is not dependent on androgens, while axillary and lower pubic hair are sensitive to the small amounts of androgen secreted by the adrenal. Hair in these regions therefore grows to an approximately equal extent in men and women. Hair growth in some areas is more typical of males and appears to require the greater androgen levels normally produced by the testes; such areas include the face, upper pubic triangle, chest, and ears. Finally, scalp hair exhibits androgen-mediated regression. The reason different body regions respond differently to the same or similar androgen is unknown. Theoretically, the metabolism of androgens might differ in the various sites. The hair follicle, like some other androgen targets, requires conversion of testosterone to dihydrotestosterone for expression of androgen action, and hair follicles from all regions of the body perform this conversion. Moreover, the same receptor that is essential for androgen action in other cells (Chap. 339) mediates the effects of dihydrotestosterone in the hair follicle. Genetic disorders with normal testosterone production but absent androgen receptor have deficient or absent axillary, pubic, facial, truncal, and limb hair (Chap. 342). Regional differences in androgen responsiveness of hair in normal individuals may be the consequence of regional differences in the amount of androgen receptor in hair follicles.

Genetic factors   Despite similar hormone levels, the distribution of hair varies among individuals and among different racial groups. Dark-haired, darkly pigmented whites of either sex tend to be more hirsute than blond or fair-skinned persons. Orientals, American Indians, and blacks on average are less hirsute than whites. Orientals have scant facial and body hair except in the pubic and axillary regions, and American Indians, in addition, rarely develop baldness. Heterogeneity of hair patterns also exists within families. The inheritance of hair patterns is complex and probably polygenic in nature.

Other factors   Aging is a prerequisite for some types of hair development. For example, in men hair on the trunk and extremities frequently increases for several years after maximal levels of plasma androgens have been reached. Conversely, loss of androgen may not result in diminution of normal hair growth in men or complete reversal of hirsutism in women. The appearance of pubic hair is frequently the heralding event of puberty in females. Women in the first trimester of pregnancy commonly have increased hairiness of the face, extremities, and breasts. Menopause is often associated with the loss of hair in the pubic area, axillae, and extremities, whereas growth of hair on the face increases in postmenopausal women. These changes cannot be explained solely by changes in androgen levels.

PATHOLOGIC HAIR GROWTH AND DISTRIBUTION   A central consideration in the evaluation of women with hirsutism is whether evidence of virilization or defeminization is also present (Table 49-1) since such signs suggest androgen excess. In patients with overproduction of androgen, defeminizing signs, such as disturbances of menstruation, are more frequent than virilization. However, the

TABLE 49-1   Clinical signs of defeminization and virilization

Signs of defeminization	Signs of virilization
Amenorrhea	Frontal balding
Decrease in breast size	Increase in size of shoulder girdle
Loss of female body contours	muscles
	Clitoromegaly
	Coarsening of the voice
	Acne

After Karp L, Herrmann WL: Diagnosis and treatment of hirsutism in women. Obstet Gynecol 41:283, 1973.

presence or absence of overt virilization should be interpreted with caution for at least two reasons. First, signs of virilization (clitoromegaly, balding, coarsening of the hair, hirsutism) indicate androgen excess at some time in the patient's life but do not necessarily mean that active disease is present at the time of evaluation. It is necessary to measure plasma androgen levels and/or production rates to determine if androgen excess is ongoing. Second, severe overandrogenization may exist in the absence of marked virilization; i.e., at the same level of androgen production clitoromegaly may be present in one patient and not another.

Diagnostic considerations DRUGS Excessive hair growth can be caused by drugs that exert their effects independent of androgens and do not produce defeminization or virilization. Such drugs include phenytoin, minoxidil, diazoxide, cyclosporin, and hexachlorobenzene. Androgens produce hirsutism as well as virilization. Some synthetic progestogens have androgenic activity.

TUMORS The rapid onset of hair growth with or without accompanying signs of frank virilization suggests a neoplastic source of androgen. Such tumors include adenomas and carcinomas of the adrenal and ovarian tumors such as arrhenoblastoma, which secrete androgens directly, and Krukenberg tumors of the ovary, which stimulate the surrounding ovarian stromal tissue to produce excess androgen.

POLYCYSTIC OVARIAN DISEASE The most common cause of ovarian hyperandrogenism is polycystic ovarian disease. This disorder has a broad spectrum of manifestations that range from mild hirsutism to amenorrhea and virilization. The salient feature for the diagnosis is the pubertal onset of chronic anovulation and hirsutism; enlarged cystic ovaries, obesity, and amenorrhea (i.e., the Stein-Leventhal syndrome) are present in only half or fewer of women with this disorder and need not be present for the diagnosis (see Chap. 340). The fundamental abnormality in polycystic ovarian disease is not fully understood. Elevation of plasma LH causes enhanced androgen secretion by stromal and thecal cells of the ovary.

ATTENUATED FORMS OF ADRENAL HYPERPLASIA The adrenal can be the source of excess androgen in the absence of tumor. Heritable defects in adrenal steroidogenesis (congenital adrenal hyperplasia) such as deficiencies of 21-hydroxylase ($P450_{C21}$), 11β-hydroxylase ($P450_{C11B}$), and 3β-hydroxysteroid dehydrogenase isomerase (3β-HSD) can produce virilization, and each can occur in a "late-onset" form in which hirsutism or virilization and menstrual irregularities

appear at the time of expected puberty or in adulthood (see Chap. 342). The clinical presentation in these cases is usually indistinguishable from polycystic ovarian disease. Late-onset 21-hydroxylase deficiency is the most common of these attenuation forms of congenital adrenal hyperplasia and has been most extensively studied; its incidence in the general population of hirsute, oligomenorrheic women is probably on the order of one percent. The presence of elevated plasma levels of adrenal androgens (such as dehydroepiandrosterone sulfate) or of dexamethasone-suppressible hyperandrogenism does not necessarily imply that the overandrogenization is due to a specific adrenal steroidogenic defect, but these findings may be useful as a guide to therapy.

IDIOPATHIC HIRSUTISM In many women with hirsutism a specific diagnosis cannot be made. The term *idiopathic hirsutism* applies to those women with evidence of androgen excess but with normal menses, normal-sized ovaries, no evidence of tumors of the adrenal or ovary, and normal adrenal function. Slight elevations of plasma androstenedione and testosterone are common in such women, and testosterone production rates are increased, although to a lesser degree than in patients with polycystic ovarian disease.

Experience outside the United States with the antiandrogen cyproterone acetate indicates that this form of hirsutism is androgen-mediated, since therapy results in improvement. Women with idiopathic hirsutism could constitute the extreme end of a normal continuum of androgen production or represent a true pathologic subset. Some women with the tentative diagnosis of idiopathic hirsutism actually have mild or early polycystic ovarian disease, but in most, hirsutism is not accompanied by or followed by signs of ovarian dysfunction. If such women are merely extremes of the normal range of androgen production, then their hirsutism is fundamentally a cosmetic defect.

DIAGNOSTIC EVALUATION The decision as to when to undertake a complex diagnostic evaluation depends on several factors. Such evaluation is appropriate in all women with hirsutism accompanied by virilization; whether it should be performed in women with isolated hirsutism depends upon the severity, distribution, and rate of hair growth. An approach to the diagnostic evaluation of hirsute patients is shown in Fig. 49-1. The clinical history is taken with particular attention to drug ingestion and to the details of pubertal development and menstrual history and their relation to the onset of excessive hair growth. The physical examination is directed to the assessment of

FIGURE 49-1 Diagnostic approach to the hirsute patient. T = testosterone; DHEA-S = dehydroepiandrosterone sulfate.

sites of growth of androgen-dependent hair (pubic, axillary, facial, truncal, and extremity) and evaluation for signs of virilization, which correlate with higher levels of androgen overproduction and raise the concern of androgen-producing neoplasms. Such signs include laryngeal enlargement (deepening of the voice), temporal balding, clitoromegaly, and increased muscle mass in the limb girdles. Signs of cortisol excess (plethora, centripetal obesity, striae, and dorsocervical and supraclavicular fat pads) should also be sought. Pelvic examination should include a search for palpable ovarian masses. Appropriate laboratory tests include measurement of serum androgens and, when appropriate, radiologic imaging of ovaries and adrenal glands. Basal measurements of dehydroepiandrosterone sulfate greater than 22 μmol/L (8000 ng/mL) or of serum testosterone over 7 nmol/L (2 ng/mL) suggest neoplastic sources of androgen excess; plasma testosterone levels in the normal range are more difficult to interpret because total levels in women do not necessarily reflect the free or unbound levels of hormone under conditions when testosterone-binding globulin levels are either increased or decreased. Suspected Cushing's syndrome should be evaluated with standard dexamethasone suppression testing if a screening test (such as urinary free cortisol excretion or overnight dexamethasone suppression test) is abnormal. The diagnosis of polycystic ovarian disease is made from the history and clinical features in a woman with chronic anovulation. Women may be screened for delayed-onset adrenal hyperplasia by the short ACTH stimulation test and measurement of plasma 17-hydroxy-progesterone (see Chap. 335).

MANAGEMENT   In the case of drug-induced hirsutism and neo-plastic disease of the ovary or adrenals treatment is straightforward; administration of the drugs should be stopped, or the tumor should be removed. Adrenal steroidogenic defects are treated with glucocorticoids to suppress excess ACTH and inhibit adrenal androgen secretion. In most instances (polycystic ovarian disease as well as idiopathic hirsutism) both cosmetic treatment and suppression of androgen production or antagonism of its action at the receptor level need to be employed.

Cosmetic therapy is directed at the concealment or removal of hair from exposed skin areas. Small amounts of hair can be bleached with hydrogen peroxide. Methods for removal of hair are classified as depilatory (removal of hair from the surface of the skin) or epilatory (removal of the intact hair with the root). Depilatory techniques include shaving and chemical methods. Shaving does not have an adverse effect on hair growth rate or coarseness (although the blunt ends may feel coarse), but shaving of areas other than axillae or legs is unacceptable to most women. Chemical depilatories are effective for limited areas of hair removal and are generally safe if used properly. Most available depilatories are substituted mercaptans, such as thioglycollic acid, which reduce the disulfide bonds in the peptide chains of keratin. The hair fiber swells and softens to a consistency that can be washed from the skin. Care must be taken to avoid skin

irritation because of the alkalinity of these preparations. Temporary epilation can be achieved by plucking (useful only for isolated hairs) or wax treatment. The waxes are melted and applied to the skin. When the wax cools and sets, it is stripped off, removing hair with it. The procedure is uncomfortable, and best results can be obtained by salon treatments. Permanent epilation can be achieved only by electrolysis. The treatments are expensive and time-consuming, and success depends on the skill of the electrologist.

While cosmetic treatment is undertaken, attempts to suppress androgen overproduction may also be appropriate. Treatment with combination oral contraceptives suppresses ovarian androgen secretion when restoration of fertility is not an objective. To minimize side effects the lowest effective dosage of estrogen should be used. Women over 35 years of age, smokers, and those with hypertension, a history of thromboembolic disease, impaired liver function, or suspected estrogen-dependent neoplasm should not be treated with oral contraceptives. Suppression of adrenal androgen overproduction can be achieved with small doses of dexamethasone and is most useful in the treatment of women with late-onset 21-hydroxylase deficiency.

Antagonism of the effects of androgens at the hair follicle is the basis for the other main treatment modality, the antiandrogens. Cyproterone acetate has been used with success but is unavailable in the United States. Spironolactone has a dual action of blocking the androgen receptor and of inhibiting androgen production and is a useful alternative therapy. Cimetidine also binds to the androgen receptor and acts as an androgen antagonist but is not of general benefit in the treatment of hirsutism. The androgen antagonist flutamide has shown promise in some studies.

If pharmacologic therapy is undertaken, the patient should be prepared to make a commitment of 6 months for an adequate trial of efficacy. Even when treatment is long-term, dramatic reversal of established hair growth is unlikely to be achieved by interference with androgen synthesis or action. Such hormonal manipulations can arrest or slow the rate of hair growth, but established hair must be dealt with by use of cosmetic treatment.

REFERENCES

CUSAN L et al: Treatment of hirsutism with the pure antiandrogen flutamide. J Am Acad Dermatol 23:462, 1990

EHRMAN DA, ROSENFIELD RL: An endocrinologic approach to the patient with hirutism. J Clin Endocrinol Metab 71:1, 1990

HASSIOKOS DK et al: Late-onset congenital adrenal hyperplasia in a group of hyperandrogenic women. Arch Gynecol Obstet 249:165, 1991

KILLEEN AA et al: Prevalence of nonclassical congenital adrenal hyperplasia among women self-referred for treatment of hirsutism. Am J Med Genet 42:197, 1992

LESHIN M: Hirsutism. Am J Med Sci 294:369, 1987

O'BRIEN RC et al: Comparison of sequential cyproterone acetate/estrogen versus spironolactone/oral contraceptive in the treatment of hirsutism. J Clin Endocrinol Metab 72:1008, 1991

RITTMASTER RS, LORIAUX DL: Hirsutism. Ann Intern Med 106:95, 1987

section 8   Alterations in the skin

50   EXAMINATION OF THE SKIN

THOMAS J. LAWLEY / KIM B. YANCEY

The challenge of examining the skin lies in distinguishing normal from abnormal and significant findings from trivial ones and in integrating pertinent signs and symptoms into an appropriate differential diagnosis. The fact that the largest organ in the body is visible is both an advantage and a disadvantage to those who examine it. It

is advantageous because no special instrumentation, other than a magnifying glass, is necessary and because the skin can be biopsied with little morbidity. However, the casual observer can be overwhelmed by a variety of stimuli and overlook important, subtle signs of skin or systemic disease. For instance, the sometimes minor differences in color and shape that distinguish a malignant melanoma from a benign pigmented nevus can be difficult to recognize. To aid in the interpretation of skin lesions, a variety of descriptive terms have been developed to characterize cutaneous lesions (Tables 50-1 and 50-2 and Fig. 50-1). Mastery of this terminology is important not only for categorizing the skin lesions of a particular case but also

TABLE 50-1 Descriptions of primary skin lesions

1 **Macule:** A flat, colored lesion, <2 cm in diameter, not raised above the surface of the surrounding skin. A ''freckle,'' or ephelid, is a prototype pigmented macule.

2 **Patch:** A large (>2 cm), flat lesion with a color different from the surrounding skin. This differs from a macule only in size.

3 **Papule:** A small, solid lesion, <1 cm in diameter, raised above the surface of the surrounding skin and hence palpable (e.g., a closed comedone, or whitehead, in acne).

4 **Nodule:** A larger (1–5 cm), firm lesion raised above the surface of the surrounding skin. This differs from a papule only in size (e.g., dermal nevus).

5 **Tumor:** A solid, raised growth >5 cm in diameter.

6 **Plaque:** A large (>1 cm), flat-topped, raised lesion; edges may either be distinct (e.g., in psoriasis) or gradually blend with surrounding skin (e.g., in eczematous dermatitis).

7 **Vesicle:** A small, fluid-filled lesion, <1 cm in diameter, raised above the plane of surrounding skin. Fluid is often visible, and the lesions are often translucent [e.g., vesicles in allergic contact dermatitis caused by *Rhus* (poison ivy)].

8 **Pustule:** A vesicle filled with leukocytes. Note: The presence of pustules does not necessarily signify the existence of an infection.

9 **Bulla:** A fluid-filled, raised, often translucent lesion >1 cm in diameter.

10 **Cyst:** A soft, raised, encapsulated lesion filled with semisolid or liquid contents.

11 **Wheal:** A raised, erythematous papule or plaque, usually representing short-lived dermal edema.

12 **Telangiectasia:** Dilated, superficial blood vessels.

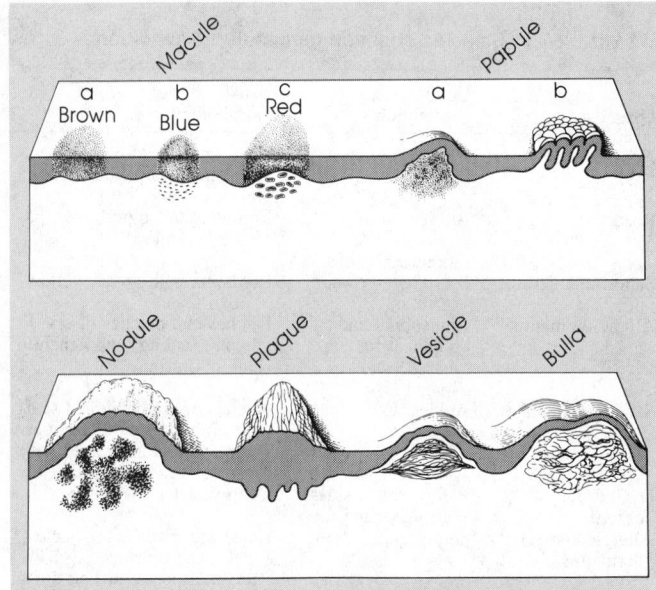

FIGURE 50-1 A schematic representation of several common primary skin lesions (see Table 50-1).

in formulating a differential diagnosis (Table 50-3). For instance, the finding of large numbers of scaling papules, usually indicative of a primary skin disease, places the patient in a different diagnostic category than would hemorrhagic papules, which may indicate vasculitis or sepsis. It is important to differentiate primary skin lesions from secondary skin changes. If the examiner focuses on linear erosions overlying an area of erythema and scaling, he or she may incorrectly assume that the erosion is the primary lesion and the redness and scale are secondary, while the correct interpretation would be that the patient has a pruritic eczematous dermatitis and the erosions have been caused by scratching.

AN APPROACH TO THE PATIENT In examining the skin it is usually advisable to assess the patient before taking a history. This way, the entire cutaneous surface is sure to be evaluated, and objective findings can be integrated with relevant historical data. Four basic features of any cutaneous lesion must be noted and considered in the examination of skin: the distribution of the eruption, the type(s) of primary lesion, the shape of individual lesions, and the arrangement of the lesions. In the initial examination it is important that the patient be disrobed as completely as possible. This will minimize chances of missing important individual skin lesions and make it possible to assess accurately the distribution of the eruption. The patient should

first be viewed from a distance of about 1.5 to 2 m (4 to 6 ft) so that the general character of the skin and the distribution of lesions can be evaluated. Indeed, distribution of lesions often correlates highly with diagnosis (Fig. 50-2). For example, a hospitalized patient with a generalized erythematous exanthem is more likely to have a drug eruption than is a patient with a similar rash limited to the sun-exposed portions of the face. The presence or absence of lesions on mucosal surfaces also should be determined. Once the distribution of the lesions has been established, the nature of the primary lesion must be determined. Thus, when lesions are distributed on elbows, knees, and scalp, the most likely possibilities based solely on distribution are psoriasis or dermatitis herpetiformis. The primary lesion in psoriasis is a scaly papule that soon forms erythematous plaques covered with a white scale, whereas that of dermatitis herpetiformis is an urticarial papule that quickly becomes a small vesicle. In this manner, identification of the primary lesion directs the examiner toward the proper diagnosis. Secondary changes in skin also can be quite helpful. For example, scale represents excessive epidermis, while crust is the result of an inadequate or inconsistent epithelial cell layer. Palpation of skin lesions also can yield insight into the character of an eruption. Thus red papules on the lower extremities that blanch with pressure can be a manifestation of many different diseases, but hemorrhagic red papules that do not blanch with pressure indicate palpable purpura characteristic of necrotizing vasculitis.

The shape of lesions is also an important feature. Flat, round, erythematous papules and plaques are common in many cutaneous diseases. However, target-shaped lesions that consist in part of erythematous plaques are specific for erythema multiforme. In the same way, the arrangement of individual lesions is important. Erythematous papules and vesicles can occur in many conditions, but their arrangement in a specific linear array suggests an external etiology such as allergic contact or primary irritant dermatitis. In contrast, lesions with a generalized arrangement are common and suggest a systemic etiology.

As in other branches of medicine, a complete history should be obtained to emphasize the following features:

1 Evolution of lesions

 a Site of onset

 b Manner in which eruption progressed or spread

 c Duration

 d Periods of resolution or improvement in chronic eruptions

TABLE 50-2 Common dermatologic terms

1 **Lichenification:** A distinctive thickening of the skin that is characterized by accentuated skin-fold markings and that feels thick and firm on palpation.

2 **Crust:** Dried exudate of body fluids that may be either yellow (serous exudate) or red (hemorrhagic exudate).

3 **Milia:** Small, firm, white papules that are filled with keratin (and may in part resemble pustules).

4 **Erosion:** Epithelial deficit resulting in a superficial disruption of skin integrity.

5 **Ulcer:** Epithelial deficit resulting in a deep surface disruption.

6 **Excoriations:** Linear, angular erosions that may be covered by crust and are caused by scratching.

7 **Atrophy:** An acquired loss of substance. In the skin, this may appear as a depression with intact epidermis (i.e., loss of dermal or subcutaneous tissue) or as sites of shiny, delicate, wrinkled lesions (i.e., epidermal atrophy).

8 **Scar:** A change in the skin secondary to trauma or inflammation. Sites may be erythematous, hypopigmented, or hypertrophic depending on their age or character. Sites on hair-bearing areas may be characterized by destruction of hair follicles.

TABLE 50-3 Selected common dermatologic conditions

Diagnosis	Common distribution	Usual morphology	Diagnosis	Common distribution	Usual morphology
Acne vulgaris	Face, upper back	Open and closed comedones, erythematous papules, pustules, cysts	Seborrheic keratosis	Trunk, face	Brown plaques with adherent, greasy scale; "stuck on" appearance
Rosacea	Blush area of cheeks, nose, forehead, chin	Erythema, telangiectasias, papules, pustules	Folliculitis	Any hair-bearing area	Follicular pustules
Seborrheic dermatitis	Scalp, eyebrows, perinasal	Erythema with greasy yellow-brown scale	Impetigo	Anywhere	Papules, vesicles, pustules, often with honey-colored crusts
Atopic dermatitis	Antecubital and popliteal fossae; may be widespread	Patches and plaques of erythema, scaling, and lichenification; pruritus	Herpes simplex	Lips, genitalia	Grouped vesicles progressing to crusted erosions
Stasis dermatitis	Ankles, lower legs	Patches of erythema and scaling on background of hyperpigmentation associated with signs of venous insufficiency	Herpes zoster	Dermatomal, usually trunk but may be anywhere	Vesicles limited to a dermatome (often painful)
Dyshidrotic eczema	Palms, soles, sides of fingers and toes	Deep vesicles	Varicella	Face, trunk, relative sparing of extremities	Lesions arise in crops and quickly progress from erythematous macules to papules to vesicles to pustules to crusts
Allergic contact dermatitis	Anywhere	Localized erythema, vesicles, scale, and pruritus, e.g., fingers, earlobes—nickel; dorsal aspect of foot—shoe dermatitis; exposed surfaces—poison ivy dermatitis; etc.	Pityriasis rosea	Trunk (Christmas tree pattern) herald patch followed by multiple smaller lesions	Symmetric erythematous patches with a collarette of trailing scale
Psoriasis	Elbows, knees, scalp, lower back, fingernails (may be generalized)	Papules and plaques covered with silvery scale; nails have pits	Tinea versicolor	Chest, back, abdomen, proximal extremities	Scaly hyper- or hypopigmented macules
Lichen planus	Wrists, ankles, mouth (may be widespread)	Violaceous flat-topped papules and plaques	Candidiasis	Groin, beneath breasts, vagina, oral cavity	Erythematous macerated areas with satellite pustules; white, friable patches on mucous membranes
Keratosis pilaris	Extensor surfaces of arms and thighs, buttocks	Keratotic follicular papules with surrounding erythema	Dermatophytosis	Feet, groin, beard, or scalp	Varies with site, e.g., tinea corporis—scaly annular patch
Melasma	Forehead, cheeks, temples, upper lip	Tan to brown patches	Scabies	Groin, axillae, between fingers and toes, beneath breasts	Excoriated papules, burrows, pruritus
Vitiligo	Periorificial, trunk, extensor surfaces of extremities, flexor wrists, axillae	Chalk-white macules	Insect bites	Anywhere	Erythematous papules with central puncta
			Cherry angioma	Trunk	Red, blood-filled papules
Actinic keratosis	Sun-exposed areas	Skin-colored or red-brown macule or papule with dry, rough, adherent scale	Keloid	Anywhere (site of previous injury)	Firm tumor, pink, purple, or brown
Basal cell carcinoma	Face	Papule with pearly, telangiectatic border on sun-damaged skin	Dermatofibroma	Anywhere	Firm red to brown nodule that shows dimpling of overlying skin with lateral compression
Squamous cell carcinoma	Face, especially lower lip, ears	Indurated and possibly hyperkaratotic lesions often showing ulceration and/or crusting	Acrochordons (skin tags)	Groin, axilla, neck	Fleshy papules
			Urticaria	Anywhere	Wheals, sometimes with surrounding flare, pruritus
			Transient acantholytic dermatosis	Trunk, especially anterior chest	Erythematous papules
			Xerosis	Extensor extremities, especially legs	Dry, erythematous, scaling patches, pruritus

2 Symptoms associated with eruption
  a Itching, burning, pain, numbness
  b What, if anything, has relieved symptoms
  c Time of day when symptoms are most severe
3 Current or recent medications (prescribed as well as over-the-counter)
4 Associated systemic symptoms (e.g., malaise, fever, arthralgias)
5 Ongoing or previous illnesses
6 History of allergies
7 Presence of photosensitivity
8 Review of systems

DIAGNOSTIC TECHNIQUES Many skin diseases can be diagnosed on gross clinical appearance, but sometimes relatively simple diagnostic procedures can yield valuable information. In most instances, they can be performed at the bedside with a minimum of equipment.

Skin biopsy A skin biopsy is a straightforward minor surgical procedure; however, it is important to biopsy the anatomic site most likely to yield diagnostic findings. This decision may require expertise in skin diseases and knowledge of superficial anatomic structures in selected areas of the body. In this procedure, a small area of skin is anesthetized with 1% lidocaine with or without epinephrine. The skin lesion in question can be excised with a scalpel or removed by punch biopsy. In the latter technique, a punch is pressed against the surface of the skin and rotated with downward pressure until it penetrates to the subcutaneous tissue. The circular biopsy is then lifted with forceps, and the bottom is cut with iris scissors. Biopsy sites may or may not need suture closure depending on size and location.

KOH preparation A potassium hydroxide (KOH) preparation is performed on scaling skin lesions when a fungal etiology is suspected. The edge of such a lesion is scraped gently with a scalpel blade, and the removed scale is collected on a glass microscope slide and treated with 1 to 2 drops of a solution of 10 to 20% KOH. KOH dissolves keratin and allows easier visualization of fungal elements. Brief heating of the slide accelerates dissolution of keratin. When the preparation is viewed under the microscope, the refractile hyphae will be seen more easily when the light intensity is reduced. This technique can be utilized to identify hyphae in dermatophyte infections, pseudohyphae and budding yeast in *Candida* infections, and frag-

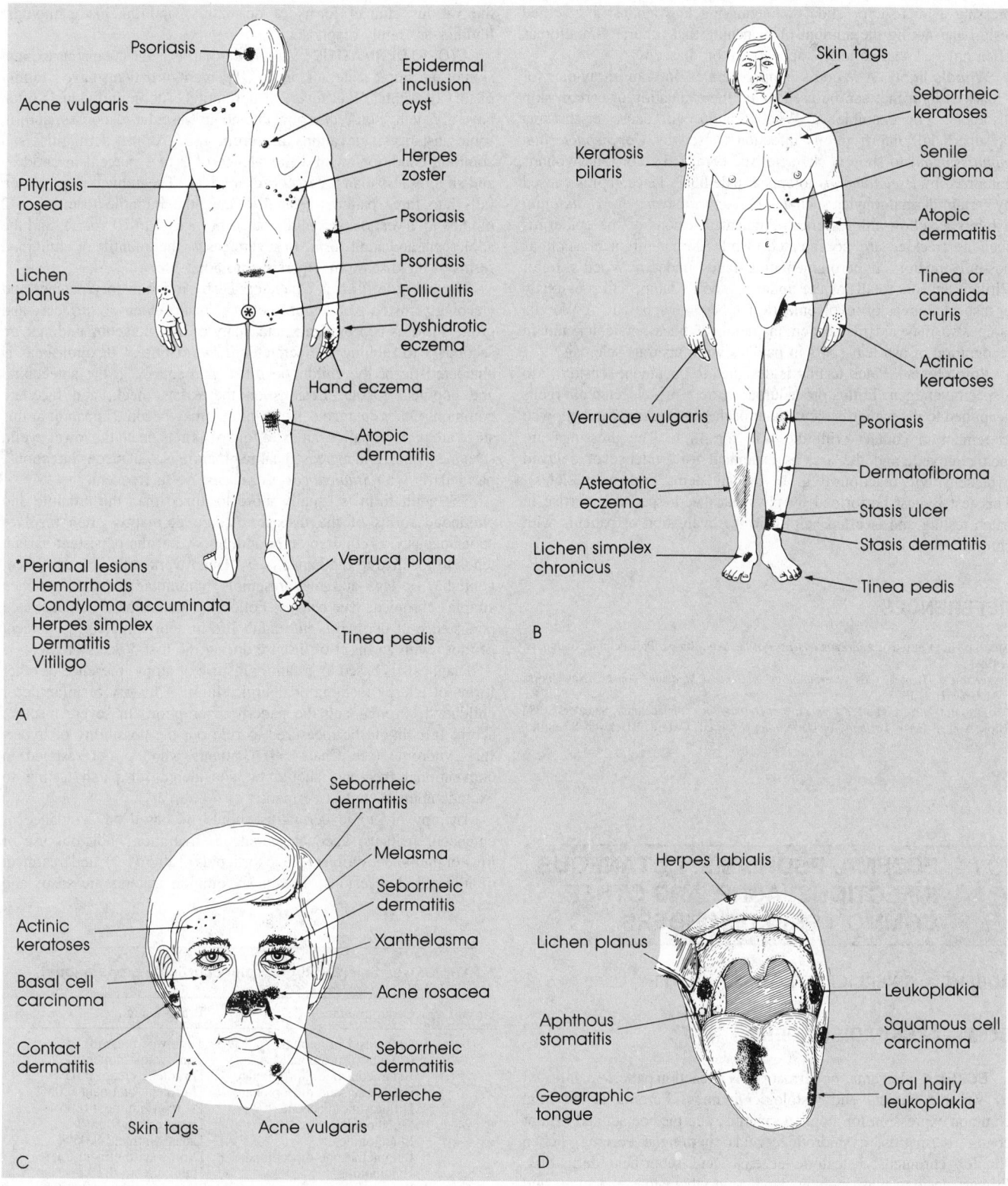

FIGURE 50-2 *A–D.* The distribution of some common dermatologic diseases and lesions.

mented hyphae and spores in tinea versicolor. The same sampling technique can be used to obtain scale for culture of selected pathogenic organisms.

Tzanck smear A Tzanck smear, named after Arnault Tzanck, is a cytologic technique most often used in the diagnosis of herpesvirus infections (simplex or varicella-zoster). An early vesicle, not a pustule or crusted lesion, is unroofed, and the base of the lesion is scraped gently with a scalpel blade. The material is then placed on a

glass slide, air-dried, and stained with Giemsa or Wright's stain. Multinucleated giant cells suggest the presence of herpes, but culture must be performed to identify the specific virus.

Diascopy Diascopy is designed to assess whether a skin lesion will blanch with pressure as, for example, in determining whether a red lesion is hemorrhagic or simply blood-filled. For instance, a hemangioma will blanch with pressure, whereas a purpuric lesion caused by necrotizing vasculitis will not. Diascopy is performed by pressing a microscope slide or magnifying lens against a specified lesion and noting the amount of blanching that occurs. Granulomas often have an ''apple jelly'' appearance on diascopy.

Wood's light   A Wood's lamp generates 360-nm ultraviolet (or ''black'') light that can be used to aid the evaluation of certain skin disorders. For example, a Wood's lamp will cause erythrasma (a superficial, intertriginous infection caused by *Corynebacterium minutissimum*) to show a characteristic coral red color, and wounds colonized by *Pseudomonas* to appear pale blue. Tinea capitis caused by certain dermatophytes such as *Microsporum canis* or *M. audouini* exhibits a yellow fluorescence. Pigmented lesions of the epidermis such as freckles are accentuated, while dermal pigment such as postinflammatory hyperpigmentation fades under a Wood's light. Vitiligo appears totally white under a Wood's lamp, and previously unsuspected areas of involvement often become apparent. A Wood's lamp also may aid in the demonstration of tinea versicolor and in recognition of ash leaf spots in patients with tuberous sclerosis.

Patch tests   Patch testing is designed to document sensitivity to a specific antigen. In this procedure, a battery of suspected allergens is applied to the patient's back under occlusive dressings and allowed to remain in contact with the skin for 48 h. The dressings are then removed, and the area is examined for evidence of delayed hypersensitivity reactions (e.g., erythema, edema, or papulovesicles). This test is best performed by physicians with special expertise in patch testing and is often helpful in the evaluation of patients with chronic dermatitis.

REFERENCES

ARNOLD HL et al (eds): *Andrew's Diseases of the Skin*, 8th ed. Philadelphia, Saunders, 1990

FITZPATRICK TB et al (eds): *Dermatology in General Medicine*, 4th ed. New York, McGraw-Hill, 1993

LOOKINGBILL DP, MARKS JG: *Principles of Dermatology*. Philadelphia, Saunders, 1986

ROOK A et al (eds): *Textbook of Dermatology*, 4th ed. Oxford, Blackwell Scientific, 1986

51   ECZEMA, PSORIASIS, CUTANEOUS INFECTIONS, ACNE, AND OTHER COMMON SKIN DISORDERS

ROBERT A. SWERLICK / THOMAS J. LAWLEY

COMMON SKIN DISORDERS

ECZEMA   Eczema, or dermatitis, is a reaction pattern manifested by variable clinical and histologic findings. Eczema is the final common expression for atopic dermatitis, allergic contact and irritant contact dermatitis, dyshidrotic eczema, nummular eczema, lichen simplex chronicus, asteatotic eczema, and seborrheic dermatitis. Primary lesions may include papules, erythematous macules, and vesicles, which can coalesce to form patches and plaques. In severe eczema, secondary lesions such as weeping and crusting may predominate. Long-standing dermatitis is often dry and is characterized by thickened, scaling skin (lichenification). The histologic changes correlate with the clinical findings. The histologic features of dermatitis have been divided into three patterns: acute, subacute, and chronic. Acute dermatitis shows a mixture of epidermal and dermal edema, epidermal vesiculation, and a mononuclear cell infiltrate. Chronic dermatitis demonstrates epidermal acanthosis, hyperkeratosis, upper dermal fibrosis, and a predominantly perivascular mononuclear cell infiltrate. Mixtures of these two histologic reaction patterns occur in subacute dermatitis. Any of these patterns may be associated with

the various clinical forms of dermatitis, and the histopathologic findings are rarely diagnostic.

ATOPIC DERMATITIS   Atopic dermatitis is the cutaneous expression of the atopic state, and up to 70 percent of patients have a family history of asthma, hay fever, or dermatitis. Atopic individuals often have dry, itchy skin, abnormal cutaneous vascular responses, and, in some instances, elevations in serum IgE. Atopic dermatitis is a common condition, with a prevalence of 2 to 3 percent in children and slightly less than 1 percent for all ages. The clinical presentation falls into three patterns related to age: the infantile form (ages 2 months to 2 years), the childhood form (ages 4 to 10 years), and the adolescent and adult form. In severe cases, the infantile or childhood forms of the disease may persist into adult life.

The infantile form is characterized by inflammatory patches and weeping, crusted plaques on the face, neck, extensor surfaces, and groin. Pruritus is prominent, and many of the cutaneous findings are secondary to rubbing and scratching. Dermatitis of flexural areas is characteristic of the childhood form, particularly in the antecubital and popliteal fossae. Lesions on the wrists, neck, and face are common. Other cutaneous stigmata that may become apparent at this stage are perioral pallor, an extra fold of skin beneath the lower eyelid (Dennie's line), and increased palmar markings. Cutaneous infections, particularly with *Staphylococcus aureus*, occur frequently.

The adult form is usually more localized than the infantile and childhood forms of the disease. Atopic dermatitis often resolves spontaneously as children enter adulthood, but the persistent variant tends to localize to the hands (see ''Hand Dermatitis''), neck, face, genitalia, or legs and may resemble nummular eczema or lichen simplex chronicus (see below). Follow-up studies have demonstrated persistence of dermatitis into adult life in approximately 60 percent of those with an onset of disease during the first 5 years of life.

Diagnosis is based on a family history of atopy, presence of other forms of allergy (asthma or allergic rhinitis), history of infantile or childhood eczema, and the pattern of eruption. In severe disease, serum IgE should be measured to rule out the possibility of hyper-IgE syndrome (see Chap. 59). Patients who do not respond to conventional therapies should be considered for patch testing to exclude allergic contact dermatitis.

Therapy of atopic dermatitis should be based on avoidance of cutaneous irritants, adequate cutaneous hydration, judicious use of low- or midpotency topical glucocorticoids (Table 51-1), and treatment of infected skin lesions. The most common irritants are soaps and

TABLE 51-1   Selected topical glucocorticoid preparations*

Group[†]	Generic name	Brand name
1	Clobetasol propionate	Temovate cream 0.05%
	Clobetasol propionate	Temovate ointment 0.05%
	Betamethasone dipropionate	Diprolene cream 0.05%
	Betamethasone dipropionate	Diprolene ointment 0.05%
	Diflorasone diacetate	Psorcon ointment 0.05%
2	Flucinonide	Lidex cream 0.05%
	Flucinonide	Lidex ointment 0.05%
	Betamethasone dipropionate	Diprosone ointment 0.05%
	Halcinonide	Halog cream 0.1%
3	Betamethasone dipropionate	Diprosone cream 0.05%
	Betamethasone valerate	Valisone ointment 0.1%
	Diflorasone diacetate	Maxiflor cream 0.05%
4	Triamcinolone acetonide	Kenalog ointment 0.1%
	Triamcinolone acetonide	Aristocort ointment 0.1%
	Flurandrenolide	Cordran ointment 0.05%
5	Triamcinolone acetonide	Kenalog cream 0.1%
	Fluocinolone acetonide	Synalar cream 0.025%
	Hydrocortisone valerate	Westcort cream 0.2%
6	Desonide	Tridesilon cream 0.05%
	Desonide	DesOwen cream 0.05%
	Alclometasone dipropionate	Alcovate cream 0.05%
7	Hydrocortisone	Many

* List not meant to be comprehensive.
† Preparations grouped according to potency: Group 1 is most potent; group 7 is least potent.

hot water. Patients should bathe using warm, but not hot, water and should limit their use of soap, particularly on extremities. Immediately after bathing, the skin should be lubricated with a low- or midpotency topical glucocorticoid in a cream or ointment base. Crusted and weeping lesions should be treated with systemic antibiotics with activity against *S. aureus* and *Streptococcus pyogenes*, since secondary infection often exacerbates eczema. Antihistamines are useful to control the pruritus that accompanies eczema, but sedation may limit their usefulness.

The role of dietary allergens in atopic dermatitis is controversial, but there is little evidence that it plays any role except in infancy. A significant number of children under age 3 who do not respond to conventional therapy have food sensitivities. Unfortunately, parental histories of food intake do not correlate with actual food allergens, and identification of the offending agents is best done with double-blind food challenges.

Treatment with systemic glucocorticoids should be limited to severe exacerbations unresponsive to topical therapy. In the patient with chronic atopic eczema, therapy with systemic glucocorticoids will generally clear the skin only briefly, but cessation of the systemic therapy will invariably be accompanied by return, if not worsening, of the dermatitis. The side effects of daily doses of systemic glucocorticoids preclude chronic use in virtually all patients with atopic dermatitis, and the efficacy of alternate-day regimens in this disease is limited.

CONTACT DERMATITIS When dermatitis is induced by contact with an external agent, it is called *contact dermatitis*. When an external agent directly damages the skin, the ensuing eruption is referred to as an *irritant contact dermatitis* (ICD). This is different from *allergic contact dermatitis* (ACD), which is caused by an immunologic reaction to an allergen which comes into contact with the skin. The exact prevalence of contact dermatitis is not known, but previous surveys suggest that a significant proportion of occupation-related disease (almost 50 percent) is due to work-related skin injury, and the most commonly involved site is the hands (see Hand eczema). Contact dermatitis represents a significant economic problem. In 1975, a survey in California demonstrated that 95 percent of all occupation-related skin disease was contact dermatitis, which, in turn, represented almost half of all occupational claims that year. The most commonly recognized form of ACD is phytodermatitis or plant dermatitis. Members of the *Rhus* family, including poison ivy, poison oak, and poison sumac, cause an allergic reaction marked by erythema, vesiculation, and severe pruritus. The eruption is often linear, corresponding to areas where plants have touched the skin. Other allergens are much more difficult to identify, especially if the exposure is chronic and the skin becomes thickened and scaly.

If ACD is suspected and an offending agent is identified and removed, the eruption resolves. Usually, treatment with high-potency fluorinated topical glucocorticoids is enough to relieve symptoms while the ACD runs its course. Patients with particularly widespread disease, or disease involving the face or genitalia, may require treatment with oral glucocorticoids. Since the natural course of ACD is 2 to 3 weeks, therapy should be continued for that length of time. Treatment of ACD with short, rapidly tapered courses of oral glucocorticoids is usually followed by recurrence of skin lesions.

Identification of a contact allergen can be a difficult and time-consuming task. Patients with a dermatitis unresponsive to conventional therapy or with an unusual and patterned distribution should be suspected of having ACD. They should be questioned carefully regarding occupational exposures, topical medications, and oral medications. Common sensitizers include preservatives in topical preparations, nickel sulfate, potassium dichromate, neomycin sulfate, fragrances, formaldehyde, and rubber curing agents. Standard patch-test trays are helpful in identifying these agents but should not be used in patients with widespread active dermatitis or in those on systemic glucocorticoids.

HAND ECZEMA Hand eczema, a common chronic skin disorder, may be associated with other cutaneous disorders such as atopic dermatitis or psoriasis or may occur by itself. Like other forms of dermatitis, both exogenous and endogenous factors play important roles in the expression of hand dermatitis. Chronic, excessive exposure to water and detergents may initiate or aggravate this disorder. It may present with dryness and cracking of the skin of the hands, as well as with variable amounts of erythema and edema. Often the dermatitis begins under rings, where water and irritants are trapped. A variant of hand dermatitis, dyshidrotic eczema, presents with multiple, intensely pruritic, small papules and vesicles on the thenar and hypothenar eminences and the sides of the fingers. Lesions tend to occur in crops, slowly crust over, and are followed by another outbreak.

The overall prevalence of hand eczema has been estimated to be approximately 2 per 1000 persons. Its prevalence is highest in the 25- to 44-year-old age group where it is two- to threefold higher. The actual prevalence of hand eczema is probably much higher, since surveys that were used to estimate the prevalence of hand eczema and occupational contact dermatitis excluded homemakers and workers in industries which failed to report work-related skin injury.

Therapy of hand dermatitis is directed toward avoidance of irritants, identification of possible contact allergens, treatment of coexistent infection, and application of topical glucocorticoids. The most common hand irritants are soap and water. Health care professionals, housewives, and food handlers are prone to hand eczema. Use of mild soap, avoidance of hot water, and compulsive use of emollients can alleviate some symptoms. Whenever possible, the hands should be protected by gloves, preferably vinyl gloves, since many patients with hand eczema may become sensitive to curing agents in rubber gloves. Predominant involvement of the dorsal surfaces of the hands with sparing of the palmar surfaces should suggest a possible contact dermatitis. Most patients can be treated by application of cool, moist compresses (dressings) to dry and debride acute inflammatory lesions and to decrease swelling, followed by a midpotency topical glucocorticoid in a cream or ointment base. If allergic contact dermatitis is suspected, ointments are preferable. Chronic use of very high potency topical glucocorticoids can lead to cutaneous atrophy and is often accompanied by loss of effectiveness. As with atopic dermatitis, treatment of secondary infection with *Staphylococcus* or *Streptococcus* is essential. All patients with hand dermatitis should be examined for dermatophyte infection by KOH preparation and culture (see "Dermatophyte Infections").

NUMMULAR ECZEMA Nummular eczema is characterized by circular or oval "coinlike" lesions. Initially, this eruption consists of small edematous papules that become crusted and scaly. The most common locations are on the trunk or the extensor surfaces of the extremities, particularly on the pretibial areas or dorsum of the hands. It occurs most frequently in middle-aged men. The etiology is unknown but appears to be related to dryness of the skin and exogenous irritants. Unlike other forms of dermatitis, nummular eczema does not respond well to hydration, topical glucocorticoids, or antihistamines. Overt infection should be treated appropriately with antibiotics; however, even in instances where infection is not apparent, treatment with oral antibiotics, such as tetracycline or erythromycin, may be useful.

LICHEN SIMPLEX CHRONICUS Lichen simplex chronicus may represent the end stage of a variety of eczematous disorders. It consists of a well-circumscribed plaque or plaques with lichenified or thickened skin due to chronic scratching or rubbing. Common areas involved include the posterior nuchal region, dorsum of the feet, or ankles. Treatment of lichen simplex chronicus centers around breaking the cycle of chronic itching and scratching. High-potency topical glucocorticoids may be helpful in alleviating pruritus, but in recalcitrant cases, application of topical glucocorticoids under occlusion or intralesional injection of glucocorticoids may be required.

ASTEATOTIC ECZEMA Asteatotic eczema, also known as xerotic eczema or "winter itch," is a mildly inflammatory variant of eczematous dermatitis that develops most commonly on the lower legs of elderly individuals during dry times of year. Fine cracks, with or without erythema, resembling cracks seen in china or porcelain, characteristically develop on the anterior surfaces of the lower extremities. Pruritus is variable. Asteatotic eczema responds well to avoidance of excessive dryness, rehydration of the skin, and application of topical emollients, particularly those containing urea or alpha-hydroxy acids (lactic acid or glycolic acid).

STASIS DERMATITIS AND STASIS ULCERATION   Stasis dermatitis develops on the lower extremities secondary to chronic edema and venous incompetence. The disorder usually begins as mild erythema and scaling associated with pruritus over the medial aspect of the ankle, often over a varicose vein. The dermatitis progresses to become pigmented as the result of extravasation of blood and hemosiderin deposition. Stasis dermatitis may become acutely inflamed, with crusting and exudation. Chronic stasis dermatitis is often associated with dermal fibrosis which results in brawny edema and may be complicated by the development of stasis ulcers.

Elevation of the legs, compression stockings, and topical emollients are the cornerstone of therapy. Patients should be instructed to elevate the affected extremity when sitting. Support stockings are a useful adjunct, particularly in individuals who stand for long periods of time. A graded compression stocking is more desirable than an antiembolism hose, which is designed for individuals confined to bed. The dermatitic component can be treated with cool dressings and the application of midpotency topical glucocorticoids. Glucocorticoids should not be applied to ulcerations, since they may retard healing. Secondarily infected lesions should be treated with appropriate oral antibiotics.

Stasis ulcerations are difficult to treat, and resolution of these lesions is slow even under the best of circumstances. The affected limb should be elevated as much as possible. External compression dressings such as an Unna boot are also helpful in aiding healing. The ulcer should be kept clear of necrotic material, and debridement may be facilitated by frequent soaks. The use of semipermeable and hydrocolloid dressings may be helpful. Some ulcerations may take months to heal and require skin grafting. Healed areas are prone to recurrent ulceration.

SEBORRHEIC DERMATITIS   Seborrheic dermatitis is a common, chronic disorder usually affecting the central face and scalp and, on occasion, the groin, axilla, submammary folds, and gluteal cleft. Rarely, it may cause a widespread generalized dermatitis. Patients commonly complain of itching or burning. It is characterized by greasy scales overlying erythematous patches or plaques. In the scalp it may be recognized as severe dandruff. On the face it affects the eyebrows, eyelids, glabella, nasolabial fold, or ears. Scaling within the external ear is often mistaken for a chronic fungal infection (otomycosis), and postauricular dermatitis often becomes macerated and tender.

Seborrheic dermatitis may be evident in infancy in the scalp ("cradle cap"), face, or groin. It is not seen in children beyond infancy but becomes evident again during adult life. Although it is frequently seen in patients with Parkinson's disease, in those who have had cerebrovascular accidents, and in those with human immunodeficiency virus (HIV-1) infection, the overwhelming majority of individuals with seborrheic dermatitis have no underlying disorder.

Treatment with low- to midpotency topical glucocorticoids in conjunction with shampoos containing coal tar and/or salicylic acid is generally sufficient to control activity of this disorder. Selenium sulfide shampoos also may be effective. Fluorinated topical glucocorticoids should not be used on the face.

PAPULOSQUAMOUS DISORDERS

PSORIASIS   Psoriasis is one of the most common dermatologic diseases, affecting 1 to 2 percent of people. It is a chronic inflammatory skin disorder characterized by erythematous, sharply demarcated papules and rounded plaques, covered by silvery micaceous scale. The lesions are variably pruritic. The most common areas of involvement are the elbows, knees, gluteal cleft, and scalp. Lesions tend to be symmetric. Traumatized areas are often involved (Koebner or isomorphic phenomenon). Most patients will have stable, slowly growing, infiltrated plaques, which remain unchanged for long periods. Eruptive psoriasis in children and young adults is notable for the development of many small lesions after upper respiratory tract infection with beta-hemolytic streptococci.

About half of patients have fingernail involvement, appearing as a punctate pitting, nail thickening, or subungual hyperkeratosis. About 5 to 10 percent of psoriatics have joint complaints, often when there is fingernail involvement. Although some have typical rheumatoid arthritis (see Chap. 285), many have joint disease specifically associated with psoriasis: (1) disease limited to a single or a few small joints (70 percent of cases), (2) a seronegative rheumatoid arthritis–like disease, (3) involvement of the distal interphalangeal joints, (4) severe destructive arthritis with the development of "arthritis mutilans," and (5) disease limited to the spine (see Chap. 298).

The histologic picture can be variable but is usually diagnostic in early lesions or at the advancing edge of a well-established plaque. The epidermis demonstrates elongation of the rete ridges, suprapapillary thinning, loss of the granular layer, parakeratotic keratin, and intraepidermal collections of neutrophils. Dilated capillaries and mononuclear cell infiltrates are common in the dermal papillae.

Treatment depends on the type, location, and extent of disease. All patients should be instructed to avoid excess drying or irritation of the skin and to maintain adequate cutaneous hydration. Most patients with localized plaque-type psoriasis can be managed with midpotency topical glucocorticoids, although their long-term use is often accompanied by loss of effectiveness. The effectiveness of topical glucocorticoids may be increased if used in conjunction with a keratolytic agent, such as salicylic acid, which removes surface scale and allows greater penetration. Crude coal tar (1 to 5% in an ointment base) is an old but useful method of treatment in conjunction with ultraviolet light therapy.

Ultraviolet light is useful for widespread psoriasis. The ultraviolet B (UV-B) spectrum is effective alone or may be combined with coal tar (Goeckerman regimen) or anthralin (Ingram regimen). Natural sunlight or an artificial light source can be used. The combination of the ultraviolet A (UV-A) spectrum and either oral or topical psoralens is also extremely effective for the treatment of psoriasis, but the photosensitizing potential of psoralens and unknown long-term toxicity may limit the use of this therapy.

Other agents can be used for widespread disease. Methotrexate is useful in patients with associated psoriatic arthritis. Long-term liver toxicity limits its use to patients with widespread disease not responsive to standard agents. The synthetic retinoid etretinate is effective in some patients with severe psoriasis, but it is a potent teratogen with an extremely long tissue half-life, thus precluding its use in women of childbearing age.

LICHEN PLANUS   Lichen planus is a papulosquamous disorder in which the primary lesions are pruritic, polygonal, flat-topped, violaceous papules. Close examination of the surface of these papules will often reveal a network of grayish lines (Wickham's striae). The skin lesions have a predilection for the wrists, shins, lower back, and genitalia. Involvement of the scalp may lead to hair loss. Lichen planus commonly involves mucous membranes, particularly the buccal mucosa, where it can present as a netlike, whitish eruption. The etiology is unknown, but cutaneous eruptions clinically resembling lichen planus can occur after administration of numerous drugs, including thiazide diuretics, gold, antimalarials, and phenothiazines, and in patients with skin lesions of chronic graft-versus-host disease. Histologic examination of lesions of lichen planus will demonstrate hyperkeratosis, irregular acanthosis, a bandlike dermal infiltrate of lymphocytes adjacent to the epidermis, and damage to the epidermal basal cells. The course is variable, but most patients have spontaneous remissions 6 months to 2 years after the onset of disease. Topical glucocorticoids are the mainstay of therapy.

PITYRIASIS ROSEA Pityriasis rosea is a papulosquamous eruption of unknown etiology that occurs more commonly in the spring and fall. Its first manifestation is the development of a 2- to 6-cm annular lesion (the herald patch). This is followed in a few days to a few weeks by many smaller annular or papular lesions with a truncal predilection. The lesions are generally oval with their long axis parallel to the skin-fold lines. The individual lesions may be red to brown in color with an erythematous border and trailing scale. Many clinical features resemble the eruption of secondary syphilis, but palm and sole lesions are rare in pityriasis rosea. The eruption tends to be moderately pruritic and lasts 3 to 8 weeks. The histologic picture is often not diagnostic, because it can resemble an acute or subacute dermatitis. Treatment is generally directed at alleviating pruritus and consists of oral antihistamines, midpotency topical glucocorticoids, and, in some cases, the use of UV-B phototherapy.

CUTANEOUS INFECTIONS

IMPETIGO AND ECTHYMA *Impetigo* is a common superficial bacterial infection caused by group A beta-hemolytic streptococci or *S. aureus*. The primary lesion is a superficial pustule that ruptures and forms a characteristic yellow-brown "honey-colored" crust. Lesions caused by *Staphylococcus* may be tense, clear bullae, and this form of the disease is called *bullous impetigo*. Lesions may occur on normal skin or in areas already affected by another skin disease. Ecthyma is a variant of impetigo on the lower extremities and causes punched-out ulcerative lesions. In addition to improving hygiene, treatment of both ecthyma and impetigo involves gentle debridement of adherent crusts, which is facilitated by the use of soaks and topical antibiotics in conjunction with appropriate oral antibiotics.

ERYSIPELAS AND CELLULITIS See Chap. 103.

DERMATOPHYTOSIS Fungi that infect skin, hair, and nails include members of the species *Trichophyton, Microsporum*, and *Epidermophyton*. Infection of the foot is most common and is referred to as *tinea pedis* (athlete's foot). Tinea pedis is often chronic and is characterized by variable erythema and edema, scaling, pruritus, and occasionally vesiculation. Involvement may be widespread or localized, but almost invariably the web space between the fourth and fifth toes is affected. Infection of the nails (tinea unguium) is characterized by opacified, thickened nails and subungual debris. The groin is the next most commonly involved area, with men affected predominantly. It presents as a scaling erythematous eruption, which spares the scrotum. Microscopic examination of scale after digestion with potassium hydroxide (KOH preparation) of either untreated tinea pedis or tinea cruris usually demonstrates hyphae. However, even short courses of topical antifungal agents may make demonstration of hyphae difficult.

Dermatophyte infection of the scalp (tinea capitis) is quite common, particularly in inner-city clinics. The predominant organism, *Trichophyton tonsurans*, can produce a relatively noninflammatory infection that may present with either well-defined or irregular, diffuse areas of mild scaling and hair loss. Close examination of the scalp may reveal many broken off hairs appearing as small black dots. Unlike infections with *Microsporum* sp., which was previously the most common cause of tinea capitis, lesions caused by *Trichophyton tonsurans* are not fluorescent under a Wood's lamp. Tinea capitis caused by *Microsporum audouini* is characterized by a sharply delineated noninflammatory area in which hairs are broken off close to the surface. Hairs infected with *M. audouini* fluoresce bright bluish green when examined with a Wood's lamp. Tinea corporis, or widespread infection on non-hair-bearing skin, may have a variable appearance, depending on the extent of the associated inflammatory reaction. It may have the typical annular appearance of "ringworm" or appear as deep inflammatory nodules (on the scalp known as *kerions*) or granulomas. KOH examination of scale or hair from patients with tinea capitis or inflammatory tinea corporis often does not reveal hyphae, and diagnosis may require culture.

Both topical and systemic therapies may be used to treat dermatophyte infection. Topical imidazoles and triazoles, including miconazole, ketaconazole, and econazole, may be effective. Haloprogin, undecylic acid, ciclopirox olamine, and tolnaftate are also effective, but nystatin is not active against dermatophytes. Griseofulvin is the drug of choice for dermatophyte infections requiring systemic therapy. While older preparations of griseofulvin required the use of as much as 1 to 2 g of drug daily, newer microsized and ultramicrosized preparations are better absorbed and allow treatment with much lower doses of drug. Generally, a daily dose of 500 mg of microsized or 350 mg of ultramicrosized griseofulvin is adequate. Unresponsive infections may respond to doubling the dose. Griseofulvin is best absorbed if administered with a fatty meal. The most common side effects of griseofulvin are gastrointestinal distress and headache. It is also rarely associated with hematologic and liver function abnormalities, and patients on long-term therapy should be carefully monitored.

The choice of treatment depends on the site involved and the type of infection. For chronic noninflammatory tinea pedis, topical imidazoles or keratolytics are useful to limit pruritus and scaling but are rarely curative. Treatment with oral griseofulvin is effective but may require months of therapy for mycologic cure and, even then, is associated with a high relapse rate, particularly if the nails are involved. The therapy of tinea corporis depends on the extent of disease. Localized infection is best treated with topical imidazoles, but widespread disease, particularly in patients with decreased cellular immunity, requires systemic antifungal therapy.

Dermatophyte infection of hair-bearing areas (such as tinea capitis) requires systemic antifungal therapy, and treatment should be continued for 6 to 8 weeks. The adjunctive use of topical antifungals in addition to systemic therapy may be useful, but topical therapy alone is not adequate. Markedly inflammatory tinea capitis may result in scarring and hair loss, and systemic or topical glucocorticoids may prevent this sequela.

TINEA VERSICOLOR Tinea versicolor is caused by a nondermatophyte dimorphic fungus which is a normal inhabitant of the skin. As the yeast form (*Pityrosporum orbiculare*), it generally does not cause disease (except for folliculitis in certain individuals). However, in some individuals, it converts to the hyphal form and causes characteristic lesions. Infection is promoted by heat and humidity. The typical lesions consist of oval scaly macules, papules, and patches concentrated on the chest, shoulders, and back and rarely on the face or distal extremities. On dark skin they often appear as hypopigmented areas, while on light skin they are slightly hyperpigmented. In some darkly pigmented individuals, they may only appear as scaling patches. A KOH preparation from scaling lesions will demonstrate a confluence of short hyphae and round spores (so-called spaghetti and meatballs). There are many effective topical treatments for tinea versicolor. Solutions containing sulfur, salicylic acid, or selenium sulfide will clear the infection if used daily for a week and then intermittently thereafter. Topical imidazoles are also effective.

CANDIDIASIS Candidiasis is caused by a related group of yeasts, whose manifestations may be localized to the skin or may be systemic and life-threatening. The causative organism is usually *Candida albicans* but also may be *C. tropicalis, C. parapsilosis*, and *C. krusei*. These organisms are normal saprophytic inhabitants of the gastrointestinal tract but can overgrow (usually due to broad-spectrum antibiotic therapy) and cause disease at cutaneous sites. Other predisposing factors include diabetes mellitus, chronic intertrigo, and cellular immune deficiency. The oral cavity is commonly involved. Lesions may occur on the tongue or buccal mucosa (thrush) and appear as white plaques. Microscopic examination of scrapings demonstrates both pseudohyphae and yeast forms. Fissured, macerated lesions at the corners of the mouth (perleche) are often seen in individuals with poorly fitting dentures and also may be associated with candidal infection. Additionally, candidal infections have an affinity for sites that are chronically wet and macerated and may occur around nails (onycholysis and paronychia) and in intertriginous areas. Intertriginous lesions are characteristically edematous, erythematous, and scaly, with scattered "satellite pustules." In men there is often involvement of the penis and scrotum as well as the inner aspect of the thighs, and in women the introitus and vagina may be infected. Diagnosis is based on the clinical pattern and demonstration of yeast on KOH preparation or on culture. Treatment involves removing any predisposing factors such as antibiotic therapy or chronic wetness, the careful control of diabetes mellitus, if present, and the use of appropriate topical or systemic antifungal agents.

WARTS   Warts are cutaneous neoplasms caused by papillomaviruses. Over 50 different human papillomaviruses (HPV) have been described. Types 1, 2, 4, and 7 cause typical verrucae vulgaris. These lesions are sessile, dome-shaped, usually about a centimeter in diameter, and have a surface made up of many small filamentous projections. These papillomaviruses also cause typical plantar warts and filiform warts in intertriginous areas. Plantar warts are endophytic and are covered by thick keratin. Paring of the wart will generally demonstrate a central core of keratinized debris and punctuate bleeding points. Filiform warts are most common on the face, neck, and skin folds and present as papillomatous lesions on a narrow base. HPV types 3 and 10 are associated with flat warts or verrucae plana. These lesions are only slightly elevated and have a velvety, nonverrucous surface. They have a propensity for the face, arms, and legs and often are spread by shaving.

HPV types 6, 11, 16, 18, 31–35, 39, 48, and 51–54 cause genital tract lesions. Types 6 and 11 are associated with typical lesions of condyloma acuminata, which generally begin as small papillomas and may grow to form large, fungating lesions. In women, they may involve either the labia, perineum, or perianal skin. Additionally, the mucosa of the vagina, urethra, and anus can be involved, as well as the cervical epithelium. In men, the lesions often occur initially in the coronal sulcus, but they may be seen on the shaft of the penis, the scrotum, perianal skin, or in the urethra. They initially appear as soft, pink, filiform lesions, which may enlarge and coalesce to form large cauliflower-like aggregates. HPV types 6 and 11 also can cause juvenile laryngeal papillomas.

HPV also plays a role in the development of neoplasia of the uterine cervix and external genitalia. A high rate of coexistence of condyloma acuminata with cervical dysplasia or carcinoma was initially reported, and HPV DNA has been found in association both with cervical carcinoma and dyplasia and with cancerous and precancerous lesions of the external genitalia. HPV types 16 and 18 have been most intensely studied; other types are also implicated. In men, these lesions may initially appear as small, flat, hyperpigmented papules on the penis or perianal skin. The surface of the lesions is generally smooth and velvety, but it may be verrucous. The detection of subtle lesions may be improved by treatment with 5% acetic acid, which makes them appear white. In women, cutaneous lesions are generally multiple and often pigmented. They can be located on the labia majora and minora of the vulva and in the perianal region. Histologic examination of biopsies from affected sites may reveal changes associated with typical warts (hyperkeratosis, papillomatosis, and vacuolated cells) and/or features typical of intraepidermal carcinoma (Bowen's disease). Features in the latter include a disordered maturational sequence of dyskeratotic keratinocytes with hyperchromatic nuclei.

Squamous cell carcinomas are also associated with papillomavirus infections in extragenital skin. This has been seen in patients immunosuppressed after renal transplantation and in patients with the disorder epidermodysplasia verruciformis. Patients in both groups tend to develop multiple cutaneous squamous cell carcinomas on sun-exposed sites associated with several HPV types, including types 5, 8, and 14.

There are many ways to treat warts, but none is universally effective. Perhaps the most useful and convenient method is cryotherapy with liquid nitrogen. Equally effective, but requiring much more patient compliance is the use of keratolytic agents such as salicylic acid plasters or combinations of lactic acid and salicylic acid in flexible collodion. Keratolytic agents are of limited use on mucous

membranes and genital lesions. For genital warts, podophyllin solution is moderately effective but may be associated with marked local reactions. Other topical agents used include trichloracetic acid or cantharidin. Electrodesiccation and curettage or carbon dioxide laser are also effective but require local anesthesia. Some caution should be exercised with electrodesiccation or carbon dioxide laser ablation because infectious viral particles may be in the vaporized tissue. Recurrence of warts appears to be common to all these modalities because viral genomic material is present in normal-appearing skin adjacent to the clinical lesions. Treatment should be tempered by recognition that most warts in normal individuals resolve spontaneously within 1 to 2 years. Also, only a fraction of warts are associated with neoplasia, and these are almost exclusively located on the genitalia or perianal skin.

HERPES SIMPLEX   See Chap. 143.
HERPES ZOSTER   See Chap. 144.

ACNE

ACNE VULGARIS   Acne vulgaris is usually a self-limited disorder of teenagers and young adults, although 10 to 20 percent of adults may experience some form of the disorder. The permissive factor for the expression of the disease is the increase in sebum release by sebaceous glands after puberty. Small cysts, called *comedones*, form in hair follicles due to blockage of the follicular orifice by retention of sebum and keratinous material. The action of lipophilic yeast (*Pityrosporum orbiculare*) and bacteria (*Proprionibacterium acnes*) within the comedones releases free fatty acids from sebum, causes inflammation within the cyst, and results in rupture of the cyst wall. An inflammatory reaction develops as a result of extrusion of oily and keratinous debris from the cyst.

The clinical hallmark of acne vulgaris is the comedo, which may be closed (whitehead) or open (blackhead). Closed comedones appear as 1- to 2-mm pebbly white papules that are accentuated when the skin is stretched. They are the precursors of inflammatory lesions, and the contents are not easily expressed. Open comedones, which rarely result in inflammatory acne lesions, have a large dilated follicular orifice and are filled with easily expressible oxidized, darkened, oily debris. Closed comedones are usually accompanied by inflammatory lesions: papules, pustules, or nodules.

The earliest lesions in adolescence are generally mildly inflamed or noninflammatory comedones on the forehead, followed by more typical inflammatory lesions on the cheeks, nose, and chin. The most common location for acne is the face, but the chest and back may be involved. Most diseases remain mild and do not lead to scarring; a subset of patients develop large inflammatory cysts and nodules, which may drain and result in significant scarring.

Exogenous and endogenous factors can alter the expression of acne vulgaris. Friction and trauma may rupture preexisting microcomedones and elicit inflammatory acne. This is commonly seen with headbands or chin straps of athletic helmets. Agents that predispose to comedone formation include topical agents in cosmetics or hair preparations such as lanolin, petrolatum, butylstearate, lauryl alcohol, and oleic acid and chronic topical exposure to certain industrial compounds that contain insoluble cutting oils (impure paraffin oil mixtures), halogenated hydrocarbons, and coal tar and its derivatives. Glucocorticoids, applied topically or administered systemically, also may elicit acne. Other systemic medications such as isoniazid, halogens, Dilantin, and phenobarbital may produce acneiform eruptions or aggravate preexisting acne.

Treatment is directed toward elimination of comedones, decreasing the population of lipophilic bacteria and yeast, and decreasing inflammation. Although areas affected with acne should be kept clean, removal of surface oils does not play an important role in therapy. Indeed, overly vigorous scrubbing may aggravate acne due to mechanical rupture of comedones. Oral tetracycline or erythromycin in doses of 250 to 1000 mg daily will decrease follicular colonization with some lipophilic organisms and may have an anti-inflammatory effect independent of antibacterial effects. Topical agents such as retinoic acid, benzoyl peroxide, or salicylic acid may alter the pattern of epidermal desquamation, prevent the formation of comedones, and aid in the resolution of preexisting cysts. Topical antibacterial agents such as benzoyl peroxide, topical erythromycin, clindamycin, or tetracycline are also useful adjuncts to therapy. Severe nodulocystic acne not responsive to oral antibiotics and topical therapy may be treated with the synthetic retinoid isotretinoin at doses of 0.5 to 1.0 mg/kg body weight per day for 15 to 20 weeks. The use of this drug is limited by its teratogenicity, and women must be screened for pregnancy prior to initiating therapy, maintain a fail-safe method of birth control during treatment, and be screened for pregnancy during treatment. Patients receiving this medication develop extremely dry skin and cheilitis and must be followed for development of hypertriglyceridemia. Patients treated with isotretinoin, particularly those on long-term therapy for disorders other than acne, are also at risk to develop calcifications of tendons and bony overgrowths of vertebrae.

ACNE ROSACEA Acne rosacea is an inflammatory disorder predominantly affecting the central face. It rarely affects patients under age 30. Rosacea is more common in women, but those most severely affected are men. It is characterized by erythema, telangiectasias, and superficial pustules and is not associated with comedones. Rosacea rarely involves the chest or back.

There is a relationship between the tendency for pronounced facial flushing and the subsequent development of acne rosacea. Initially, individuals with rosacea demonstrate a pronounced flushing reaction. This may be in response to heat, emotional stimuli, alcohol, hot drinks, or spicy foods. As the disease progresses, the flush persists longer and longer, eventually becoming permanent. Papules, pustules, and telangiectasias then become superimposed on the persistent flush.

Rosacea of long standing may lead to connective tissue overgrowth, particularly of the nose (rhinophyma), and may be complicated by inflammatory disorders of the eye, including keratitis, blepharitis, iritis, and recurrent chalazion. These ocular problems potentially threaten vision and warrant ophthalmologic evaluation.

Acne rosacea can generally be effectively treated with oral tetracycline in doses ranging from 250 to 1500 mg/d. Topical metronidazole is also effective, and low-potency, nonfluorinated topical glucocorticoids, particularly after cool soaks, may alleviate facial erythema. Fluorinated topical glucocorticoids should be avoided, since chronic use of these preparations may actually elicit rosacea. Topical therapy is not effective for ocular disease.

REFERENCES

FITZPATRICK TB et al (eds): *Dermatology in General Medicine*, 3d ed. New York, McGraw-Hill, 1987

KRANNING KK, ODLAND GF (eds): Analysis of research needs and priorities in dermatology. J Invest Dermatol 73 (Suppl 5):1, 1979

LEVER WP, LEVER GS: *Histopathology of the Skin*, 6th ed. Philadelphia, Lippincott, 1983

MOSCHELLA SL, HURLEY HH (eds): *Dermatology*, 2d ed. Philadelphia, Saunders, 1985

PETO R, ZUR HAUSEN H: *Viral Etiology of Cervical Cancer: Banbury Report*. Cold Spring Harbor, NY, Cold Spring Harbor Laboratory, 1986

PLEWIG G, KLIGMAN AM: *Acne: Morphogenesis and Treatment*. New York, Springer-Verlag, 1975

52 CUTANEOUS DRUG REACTIONS

BRUCE U. WINTROUB / ROBERT S. STERN

Cutaneous reactions are among the most frequent adverse reactions to drugs. Early in drug-induced illness, prompt therapeutic intervention may limit toxicity. This chapter focuses on adverse cutaneous reactions to drugs other than topical agents and reviews the incidence, patterns, and pathogenesis of cutaneous reactions to drugs and therapeutic agents.

USE OF PRESCRIPTION DRUGS IN THE UNITED STATES More than 1.5 billion prescriptions for 60,000 drug products, which include approximately 2000 different active agents, are dispensed each year in the United States. Hospital inpatients alone annually receive about 120 million courses of drug therapy, and half of adult Americans receive prescription drugs on a regular outpatient basis. As much as 15 percent of hospital days are devoted to treatment for drug toxicity.

INCIDENCE OF CUTANEOUS REACTIONS Although adverse drug reactions are common, it is difficult to ascertain their incidence, seriousness, and ultimate health effects. The fact that comprehensive information on these reactions is inadequate in part reflects the difficulty in establishing a system for postmarketing surveillance that is both economically feasible and capable of generating clinically useful data. Available information comes from evaluations of hospitalized patients, epidemiologic surveys, premarketing studies, and voluntary reporting.

In one study about 2 percent of medical inpatients had skin reactions consisting of rash, urticaria, or pruritus during hospitalization, and the overall reaction rate per course of drug therapy was 3:1000. Penicillins, sulfonamides, and blood products accounted for two-thirds of cutaneous reactions. Specific algorithmic estimates of drug-specific quantitative reaction rates for drugs commonly used in inpatients were calculated. Reaction rates for selected commonly used drugs are summarized in Table 52-1. This study showed that most cutaneous reactions occur within 1 week of exposure to the drug. Exceptions were semisynthetic penicillins and ampicillin; about half the reactions to these drugs occurred more than 1 week after initial administration. The risk of allergic reactions was not related to age, diagnosis, or blood level of urea nitrogen on admission. Skin reactions were more frequent among women.

The distribution of morphologic patterns of drug eruptions cared for within a Finnish hospital dermatology department with a special interest in fixed drug eruptions included exanthematous reactions (32 percent), urticaria and/or angioedema (20 percent), fixed drug eruptions (34 percent), erythema multiforme (2 percent), Stevens-Johnson syndrome (1 percent), exfoliative dermatitis (1 percent), and photosensitivity reactions (3 percent).

Documenting the risk of the most serious forms of drug eruptions associated with specific drugs remains an important challenge. Based on successful population-based retrospective case registries of toxic epidermal necrolysis and Stevens-Johnson syndrome in Germany and France, there are now prospective registries that serve as the basis

TABLE 52-1 Rates (per 1000 recipients) of skin reactions to selected medications

Drug	Reaction rate
Amoxicillin	51
Trimethoprim-sulfamethoxazole	34
Ampicillin	33
Other penicillins	20
Blood	21
Allopurinol	8
Gentamycin	5
Barbiturates	4

SOURCE: Adapted from Bigby et al.

for case-control studies in these and other countries. These data, together with data from health-maintenance organizations and Medicaid, suggest that the risk of these reactions is from 1 to 10 per million person-years. The drugs most often associated with these reactions include the sulfonamide antibiotics, the aminopenicillins, phenytoin and structurally related antiseizure medications, and some nonsteroidal anti-inflammatory drugs.

PATHOGENESIS OF DRUG REACTIONS

Untoward cutaneous responses to drugs can arise as a result of immunologic or nonimmunologic mechanisms. Immunologic reactions require activation of host immunologic pathways and are designated *drug allergy*. Drug reactions occurring through nonimmunologic mechanisms may be due to activation of effector pathways, overdosage, cumulative toxicity, side effects, ecologic disturbance, interactions between drugs, metabolic alterations, exacerbation of preexisting dermatologic conditions, or inherited protein or enzyme deficiencies. Nonimmunologic cutaneous reactions to drugs are more common, and immunologic reactions are unpredictable when they do occur. It is often not possible to specify the responsible drug or pathogenic mechanism because the skin responds to a variety of stimuli through a limited number of reaction patterns. The mechanism of many drug reactions is unknown.

IMMUNOLOGIC DRUG REACTIONS   Drugs frequently elicit an immune response, but only a small number of individuals experience clinical hypersensitivity reactions. For example, most patients exposed to penicillin develop demonstrable antibodies to penicillin but do not manifest drug reactions when exposed to penicillin. Multiple factors determine the capacity of a drug to elicit an immune response, including the *molecular characteristics* of the drug and *host effects*.

Increases in *molecular* size and complexity are associated with increased immunogenicity, and macromolecular drugs such as protein or peptide hormones are highly antigenic. Most drugs are small organic molecules less than 1000 daltons in size, and the capacity of such small molecules to elicit an immune response depends on their ability to act as haptens, i.e., to form stable, usually covalent, bonds with tissue macromolecules. Fortunately, most drugs have little or no ability to form covalent bonds with tissue components, and clinical sensitization results from minor contaminants or conversion of the drugs themselves to reactive metabolic products.

Route of administration of a drug or simple chemical can influence the nature of the *host* immune response. For example, topical application of antigens tends to induce delayed hypersensitivity, and exposure to antigens via oral or nasal cavities stimulates production of secretory immunoglobins, IgA and IgE, and occasionally IgM. Some agents, such as pentadecacatechol, sensitize readily if applied to the skin but do so poorly if ingested orally or applied to a mucosal surface. Frequency of sensitization through intravenous administration of drugs varies, but anaphylaxis is a more likely clinical consequence with this route of exposure.

The degree of drug exposure and individual variability in absorption and metabolism of a given agent may alter immunogenic load. The variable degree of in vivo acetylation of hydralazine provides a clinical example of this phenomenon. Hydralazine produces a lupus-like syndrome associated with antinuclear antibody formation more frequently in patients who acetylate the drug slowly. Frequent high-dose and interrupted courses of therapy are also important risk factors for development of drug allergy.

Pathogenesis of allergic drug reactions   IgE-dependent drug reactions are usually manifest in the skin and gastrointestinal, respiratory, and cardiovascular systems (see Chap. 282). Primary symptoms and signs include pruritus, urticaria, nausea, vomiting, cramps, bronchospasm, and laryngeal edema and, on occasion, anaphylactic shock with hypotension and death. Immediate reactions may occur within minutes of drug exposure, and accelerated reactions occur hours or days after drug administration. Accelerated reactions are usually urticarial and may include laryngeal edema. IgE-dependent reactions are usually due to penicillins; manifestations are caused by release from sensitized tissue mast cells or circulating basophilic leukocytes of chemical mediators such as histamine, adenosine, leukotrienes, prostaglandins, platelet-activating factor, enzymes, and proteoglycans. Release is triggered when polyvalent drug protein conjugates cross-link IgE molecules fixed to sensitized cells. The clinical manifestations are determined by interaction of the released chemical mediator with its target organ, i.e., skin, respiratory, gastrointestinal, and/or cardiovascular systems. Certain routes of administration favor different clinical patterns (i.e., oral route: gastrointestinal effects; intravenous route: circulating effects).

Immune-complex–dependent reactions   Serum sickness is produced by circulating immune complexes and is characterized by fever, arthritis, nephritis, neuritis, edema, and an urticarial, papular, or pruritic rash (see Chap. 283). The syndrome requires an antigen that remains in the circulation for prolonged periods so that when antibody is synthesized, circulating antigen-antibody complexes are formed. Serum sickness was first described following administration of foreign sera, but drugs are now the usual cause. Drugs that produce serum sickness include the penicillins, sulfonamides, thiouracils, cholecystographic dyes, phenytoin, aminosalicylic acid, streptomycin, heparin, and antilymphocyte globulin. Symptoms develop 6 days or more after exposure to a drug, the latent period representing the time needed to synthesize antibody. The antibodies responsible for immune-complex–dependent drug reactions are largely of the IgG or IgM class.

Cytotoxic drug–induced reactions   Immunologic reactions to drugs may damage kidneys, heart, lungs, liver, muscle, peripheral nerves, or formed elements of the blood by at least three mechanisms. First, a drug may react with the tissue and introduce haptenic groups on a cell surface that renders the tissue susceptible to antibody- or lymphocyte-mediated cytotoxicity. Second, drug-antibody complexes formed in the fluid phase may bind to the cell surface and damage the cell as an "innocent bystander." Third, drugs may induce immune responses that involve formed blood elements such as platelets and erythrocytes but do not cause cutaneous allergic drug reactions.

Cell-mediated immune responses play a role in contact drug hypersensitivity and are suspected to participate in other allergic drug reactions (i.e., pulmonary infiltration).

NONIMMUNOLOGIC DRUG REACTIONS   Nonimmunologic mechanisms are responsible for the majority of drug reactions.

Nonimmunologic activation of effector pathways   Drug reactions may result from nonimmunologic activation of effector pathways by three mechanisms: First, drugs may release mediators directly from mast cells and basophils and present as anaphylaxis or as urticaria and/or angioedema. Urticarial anaphylactic reactions induced by opiates, polymyxin B, tubocurarine, radiocontrast media, and dextrans may occur by this mechanism. Second, drugs may activate complement in the absence of antibody. This is an additional mechanism through which radiocontrast media may act. Third, drugs such as aspirin and other nonsteroidal anti-inflammatory agents may alter pathways of arachidonic acid metabolism; such drugs inhibit the cyclooxygenase that catalyzes the generation of prostaglandins from arachidonic acid in vitro.

Overdosage   The manifestations of overdosage are predictable for most drugs; symptoms are an exaggeration of the drug's pharmacologic action. Overdosage can, at times, be observed in patients given the usual doses of a drug because of differing rates of absorption, metabolism, or excretion. An example is easy bruisability caused by warfarin overdose.

Phototoxicity   Phototoxic reactions may be drug-induced or may occur in metabolic disorders in which an appropriate photosensitizing chemical is overproduced. In each case the phototoxic reaction occurs when enough chromophore (drug or metabolic product) absorbs sufficient radiation in reactive tissue. Drug-induced phototoxic reactions can occur on first exposure, and the incidence of phototoxicity is a direct function of the concentration of sensitizer and amount of light. At least three distinct photochemical mechanisms have been described: First, the reaction between the excited state of a phototoxic molecule and a biologic target may cause formation of a covalent photoaddition product. Second, the phototoxic molecule may absorb protons to form stable photoproducts that are toxic to biologic substrates. Third, radiation of a phototoxic molecule may result in transfer of energy to oxygen molecules and cause formation of toxic oxygen species, such as singlet oxygen, superoxide anion, or hydroxyl radical. Interaction of these species with biologic targets produces photooxidized molecules. Serum protein–dependent systems and circulating effector cells play a role in acute in vivo phototoxic tissue damage due to exogenous agents; normal numbers of polymorphonuclear leukocytes and an intact complement system are required for the full development of demeclocycline-induced phototoxic lesions.

Cumulative toxicity The cumulative effects of drug deposition in skin may cause disturbance in skin color. In some instances, the drug is deposited in phagocytic cells of skin or mucous membranes, as occurs after prolonged administration of silver, bismuth, mercury, or gold. In other instances, the drug or its metabolic derivatives may bind to a component of the skin (e.g., melanin), as in patients taking high doses of chlorpromazine.

Secondary or side effects Secondary effects occur uniformly as part of the normal pharmacologic action of a drug but are not the primary therapeutic objective. Examples include alopecia, gastrointestinal disturbances, or hematopoietic depression during use of chemotherapeutic agents.

Ecologic disturbances These reactions result from drug-dependent alterations of normal flora of the skin, gut, or mucous membranes, permitting overgrowth of an organism (e.g., anogenital and oral candidiasis during administration of a broad-spectrum antibiotic).

Drug interactions Drugs may interact to cause adverse reactions. First, drugs may compete for the same plasma protein binding sites. For example, warfarin may be displaced from its binding site by phenylbutazone or aspirin and result in hemorrhage. Second, a drug may inhibit or stimulate metabolic enzymes important to its degradation or to that of another agent. Third, one drug may interfere with the excretion of another; for example, probenecid reduces penicillin excretion by the kidney.

Metabolic changes Drugs may sufficiently alter nutritional or metabolic status to induce cutaneous changes. For example, drugs, such as phenytoin, that interfere with folate absorption or metabolism increase the risk of aphthous stomatitis. In addition, drugs that alter lipid metabolism, such as isotretinoin, cause xanthomas by elevation of very low-density lipoproteins.

Exacerbation of preexisting diseases A variety of agents can exacerbate preexisting diseases. For example, lithium can exacerbate acne and psoriasis in a dose-dependent manner. Beta-blocking agents may induce a psoriasiform dermatitis, and withdrawal of glucocorticoids can exacerbate psoriasis or atopic dermatitis. Exacerbations of cutaneous lupus have been noted in association with cimetidine use. Vasodilators may exacerbate rosacea.

Inherited enzyme or protein deficiencies Drug reactions may also occur as the result of inherited enzyme deficiencies. For example, patients may be deficient in an enzyme required for metabolism of the drug or clearance of a toxic drug metabolite. The phenytoin hypersensitivity syndrome occurs in patients deficient in epoxide hydrolase, an enzyme required for metabolism of a toxic epoxide derived from phenytoin. Second, patients may be deficient in an enzyme required for normal function of a biochemical pathway, and further drug-induced lowering of the factor may cause pathologic manifestations. An example is warfarin sodium (Coumadin) necrosis of skin in patients with heterozygote deficiency of protein C, a proenzyme required for normal thrombolytic function. In contrast, heparin-induced cutaneous necrosis, which has some clinical similarity to warfarin necrosis, appears to be an immune-complex reaction.

Alterations of immunologic status Alterations in patients' immunologic status also may modify the risk of cutaneous reactions. Bone marrow transplant patients often experience cutaneous reactions to drugs. These reactions may be very difficult to differentiate from acute graft-versus-host reactions even when skin biopsy is obtained.

HIV-infected persons appear to be at very high risk of developing cutaneous eruptions, and this increased risk is not accounted for merely by the higher number of drugs utilized by these patients (see Chap. 279). The risk of these reactions increases as immunologic function deteriorates. Skin reactions to trimethoprim-sulfamethoxazole are seen in about a third of HIV-infected users of this drug. Dapsone, trimethoprim alone, and amoxicillin-clavulanate are also frequent causes of drug eruptions in these patients. Some drugs result in specific problems in HIV-infected persons. For example, foscarnet causes a painful penile ulcer in a substantial fraction of users. HIV-infected persons also appear to be at higher risk of the most serious types of reactions, including toxic epidermal necrolysis and Stevens-Johnson syndrome.

CHARACTERISTIC FEATURES OF CUTANEOUS DRUG REACTIONS

Cutaneous disorders induced by drugs by known mechanisms include urticaria, photosensitivity, disturbances of pigmentation, vasculitis, phenytoin hypersensitivity syndrome, and warfarin necrosis of skin. Reactions of uncertain mechanism include morbilliform reactions, erythema multiforme, fixed drug reactions, erythema nodosum, lichenoid reactions, bullous drug reaction, and toxic epidermal necrolysis.

REACTIONS OF KNOWN CAUSE *Urticaria* *Urticaria* is a skin reaction characterized by pruritic, red wheals. Lesions may vary from a small point to a large area. Individual lesions rarely last more than 24 h. When deep dermal and subcutaneous tissues are also swollen, this reaction is known as *angioedema*. Angioedema may involve mucous membranes and may be part of a life-threatening anaphylactic reaction. Urticarial lesions, along with pruritus and morbilliform (or maculopapular) eruptions, are among the most frequent types of cutaneous reactions to drugs.

Drug-induced urticaria may be caused by three mechanisms: an IgE-dependent mechanism, circulating immune complexes (serum sickness), and nonimmunologic activation of effector pathways. IgE-dependent urticarial reactions usually occur within 36 h but can occur within minutes. Reactions occurring within minutes to hours of drug exposure are termed *immediate reactions*, whereas those which occur 12 to 36 h after drug exposure are designated *accelerated reactions*. Immune-complex–induced urticaria associated with serum sickness may occur from 4 to 12 days after challenge. In this syndrome, the urticarial eruption may be accompanied by fever, hematuria, and arthralgias, hepatic dysfunction, and neurologic symptoms.

Certain drugs, such as nonsteroidal anti-inflammatory agents, the angiotensin-converting enzyme (ACE) inhibitors, and radiographic dyes, may induce urticarial reactions, angioedema, and anaphylaxis whose time course resembles that of immediate IgE-dependent reactions. Drug-specific antibody does not play a role in such reactions, and in some cases they are thought to be induced by the action of drug on cutaneous mast cells, complement, or arachidonic acid–dependent pathways. For the ACE inhibitors, inhibition of kinin may be responsible for these reactions, which can be life-threatening. Although aspirin, penicillin, and blood products are the most frequent causes of urticarial eruptions, urticaria has been observed in association with nearly all drugs.

Drugs also may cause chronic urticaria, which lasts more than 6 weeks. The mechanisms of chronic urticaria are unclear. Aspirin frequently exacerbates this problem.

Photosensitivity eruptions Photosensitivity eruptions are usually most marked in sun-exposed areas but may extend to sun-protected areas. Phototoxic reactions are more common than photoallergic reactions. Phototoxic reactions usually resemble sunburn, can occur with the first exposure to a drug, and are dose-related. The action spectrum for phototoxicity is similar to the ultraviolet absorption spectrum of the drug. No single test system seems to be a successful predictor of the photosensitivity potential for a given compound.

The mechanism for photoallergy to systemic medications is not well defined. Drug, immune response, and light are required to produce clinical photoallergy, and photoallergic reactions may be delayed hypersensitivity responses. Eruptions range from lichenoid papules to eczematous changes.

Orally administered drugs that cause photoallergic or phototoxic reactions include chlorpromazine, tetracycline, thiazides, nalidixic acid, and two nonsteroidal anti-inflammatory agents, the quinadone antibiotics benoxaprofen and piroxicam. Based on test systems, the majority of the common photosensitizers seem to have action spectrums in the long-wave ultraviolet (UV-A) range and are usually phototoxic. This is fortunate, since phototoxic reactions will abate with removal of either the drug or ultraviolet radiation, but some photoallergic reactions may persist after the drug is withdrawn. Because UV-A and visible light which trigger these reactions are not easily absorbed by nonopaque sunscreens, these reactions may be difficult to block.

Drugs also may induce photosensitivity diseases. For example, procainamide may induce systemic lupus erythematosus.

Pigmentation changes   Drugs may cause a variety of pigmentary changes in the skin. Some drugs stimulate melanocytic activity and increase pigmentation. Drug deposition also can lead to pigmentation; this phenomenon occurs with heavy metals. Phenothiazines may be deposited in the skin and cause a slate-gray color. Antimalarial drugs may cause a slate-gray or yellow pigmentation. Inorganic arsenic, once used to treat psoriasis, is associated with diffuse macular pigmentation. Other heavy metals that cause pigmentary changes include silver, gold, bismuth, and mercury. Long-term use of phenytoin can produce a chloasma-like pigmentation in women. Certain cytostatic agents also can cause pigmentary changes. Histologic examination is often diagnostic for drug deposition diseases.

Zidovudine (AZT) is a frequent cause of pigmentation, especially of the nails. Clofazimine, an aminophenazine dye used in the treatment of leprosy, causes a red skin color that is so marked that some patients discontinue therapy. Methysergide produces a red color in the skin and an orange-peel-like texture. Nicotinic acid in large doses may cause brown pigmentation. Oral contraceptives may produce chloasma, and adrenocorticotropin may cause a hypermelanosis similar to that of primary adrenal insufficiency. In addition, amiodarone may cause violaceous hyperpigmentation which is increased in sun-exposed skin. Drugs such as heavy metals, copper, antimalarial and arsenical agents, and ACTH also may discolor oral mucosa.

Vasculitis   Cutaneous necrotizing vasculitis often presents as palpable purpuric lesions that may be generalized or limited to the lower extremities or other dependent areas (see Chap. 291). Urticarial lesions, ulcers, and hemorrhagic blisters also occur. Vasculitis may involve other organs, including the liver, kidney, brain, and joints. Drugs are only one cause of vasculitis. Immune-complex–dependent mechanisms are probably responsible for drug-induced vasculitis and/or serum sickness. Propylthiouracil induces a cutaneous vasculitis that is accompanied by leukopenia and splenomegaly. Direct immunofluorescent changes in these lesions suggest immune-complex deposition. Drugs implicated in vasculitic eruptions include allopurinol, thiazides, penicillin, and phenytoin.

Phenytoin hypersensitivity reaction   The phenytoin hypersensitivity reaction, one of many phenytoin-induced cutaneous reactions, is an erythematous eruption that eventually becomes purpuric and is accompanied by fever, facial and periorbital edema, tender generalized lymphadenopathy, leukocytosis (often with atypical lymphocytes and eosinophils), hepatitis, and sometimes nephritis. The cutaneous reaction usually begins 1 to 3 weeks after phenytoin is begun and resolves rapidly with drug cessation and treatment with systemic glucocorticoids. The eruption recurs with rechallenge, and cross-reactions with other anticonvulsants with similar structures, including carbamazepine and barbiturates, are frequent. This syndrome apparently results from an inherited deficiency of epoxide hydrolase, an enzyme required for metabolism of a toxic intermediate arene oxide that is formed during metabolism of phenytoin by the cytochrome P450 system.

Warfarin necrosis of the skin   This rare reaction occurs usually between the third and tenth days of therapy with warfarin derivatives, usually in women. Lesions are sharply demarcated, erythematous, indurated, and purpuric and may resolve or progress to formation of large, irregular, hemorrhagic bullae with eventual necrosis and slow-healing eschar formation.

Development of the syndrome is unrelated to drug dose or underlying condition. Favored sites are breasts, thighs, and buttocks. The course is not altered by discontinuation of the drug after onset of the eruption. Similar reactions have been associated with heparin. Warfarin reactions are associated with protein C deficiency. Protein C is a vitamin K–dependent protein with a shorter half-life than other clotting proteins and is in part responsible for control of fibrinolysis. Since warfarin inhibits synthesis of vitamin K–dependent coagulation factors, warfarin anticoagulation in heterozygotes for protein C deficiency causes a precipitous fall in circulating levels of protein C, permitting hypercoagulability and thrombosis in the cutaneous microvasculature, with consequent areas of necrosis.

REACTIONS OF UNCERTAIN CAUSE   **Morbilliform reactions**   *Morbilliform* or *maculopapular eruptions* may be the most common of all drug-induced reactions, often start on the trunk or areas of pressure or trauma, and consist of erythematous macules and papules that are frequently symmetric and may become confluent. Involvement of mucous membranes, palms, and soles is variable; the eruption may be associated with moderate to severe pruritus and fever.

The pathogenesis is unclear. A hypersensitivity mechanism has been suggested, although these reactions do not always recur following drug rechallenge. Diagnosis is rarely assisted by laboratory tests; differentiation from viral exanthem is the principal differential diagnostic consideration. While these reactions usually require discontinuation of drug (dechallenge), eruptions occasionally may decrease or fade with continued use of the responsible drug.

Morbilliform reactions usually develop within 1 week of initiation of therapy and last 1 to 2 weeks; however, reactions to some drugs, especially penicillin, may begin more than 2 weeks after therapy has begun and last as long as 2 weeks after therapy has ceased. These eruptions are common in patients receiving ampicillin, amoxicillin, or allopurinol; trimethoprim-sulfamethoxazole causes frequent reactions in AIDS patients.

Erythema multiforme   *Erythema multiforme* is an acute, self-limited inflammatory disorder of skin and mucous membranes characterized by distinctive iris or target lesions, often associated with sore throat and malaise. Many drugs, including sulfonamides, penicillin, phenytoin, and phenylbutazone, can cause erythema multiforme; long-acting sulfonamides are the best-studied. Erythema multiforme resulting from sulfonamides typically begins after 1 to 2 weeks of drug therapy and is accompanied by fever and mucous membrane reaction (Stevens-Johnson syndrome). An immune-complex–induced, lymphocyte-mediated mechanism may be responsible.

Fixed drug reactions   These reactions are characterized by one or more sharply demarcated, erythematous lesions in which hyperpigmentation results after resolution of the acute inflammation; with rechallenge, the lesion recurs in the same (i.e., "fixed") location. Lesions often involve the face, genitalia, and oral mucosa and cause burning. Fixed drug eruptions have been associated with phenolphthalein, sulfonamides, tetracycline, phenylbutazone, and barbiturates. Although cross-sensitivity appears to occur between different tetracycline compounds, cross-sensitivity was not elicited when different sulfonamide compounds were administered to patients as part of provocation testing.

Documentation of a characteristic papillary-dermal mononuclear cell infiltrate in close approximation to the dermoepidermal junction may confirm the clinical diagnosis. Extensive basal cell degeneration can lead to formation of bullae and pigment dispersion. Even when lesions are completely healed, melanin-laden macrophages are present in the dermis.

Erythema nodosum *Erythema nodosum* is a panniculitis characterized by tender, subcutaneous, erythematous nodules, usually on the anterior portion of the legs. Drug hypersensitivity, frequently involving oral contraceptives, is one cause of this reaction. The mechanism is unknown.

Lichenoid drug eruptions A *lichenoid cutaneous reaction*, clinically and morphologically indistinguishable from lichen planus, is associated with a variety of drugs and chemicals. Eosinophils in lichen planus are more common when the reaction is drug-induced. Gold and antimalarials are most often associated with this eruption. Antihypertensive agents, including beta blockers and captopril, also have been reported to cause a lichenoid reaction.

Bullous eruptions Blisters accompany a wide variety of cutaneous reactions, especially the severe morbilliform eruptions, and may be an integral part of erythema multiforme, toxic epidermal necrolysis, and fixed drug eruptions. Nalidixic acid and furosemide cause blistering eruptions indistinguishable from the primary bullous diseases. Other examples are a pemphigus foliaceus–like eruption seen with penicillamine and cicatricial pemphigoid that has been seen with clonidine.

Pustular eruptions Active *pustular exanthemic eruptions* also are associated with exposure to drugs, most notably antibiotics. These eruptions can be distinguished from pustular psoriasis by more rapid onset of fever and pustulation and their rapid spontaneous resolution with drug withdrawal.

Toxic epidermal necrolysis *Toxic epidermal necrolysis* is the most serious cutaneous drug reaction and may be fatal. Drugs are the most frequent cause in adults. Onset is generally acute and is characterized by epidermal necrosis with a minimal dermal inflammatory process. This reaction is often associated with sulfonamides, aminopenicillins, anticonvulsants, nonsteroidal anti-inflammatory agents, and allopurinol and has been reported with measles vaccine, fumigants, and phenytoin.

DRUGS OF SPECIAL INTEREST

PENICILLIN The incidence of reactions to penicillin is about 1 percent. Not all adverse reactions are immunologic, as illustrated by ampicillin-induced morbilliform eruptions and central nervous system reactions to procaine penicillin.

IgG, IgM, and IgE antibodies can be produced; IgG and IgM anti-penicillin antibodies play a role in the development of hemolytic anemia, whereas anaphylaxis and serum sickness appear to be due to IgE antibodies in serum.

Since penicillin reactions often occur in patients without a prior history of penicillin allergy, the utility of accurate and easily administered tests for sensitization is apparent. Current practice is to perform skin testing with a commercially available penicilloyl determinant preparation (Pre-pen, Kremers-Urban) and with fresh penicillin and, if possible, with another source of minor (nonpenicilloyl) determinants such as aged or base-treated penicillin. Antibodies to minor determinants are common in patients experiencing anaphylaxis. Testing with major determinants alone detects most patients at risk for anaphylaxis.

Twenty-seven percent (10 to 36 percent) of patients with a positive history of penicillin allergy also have a positive skin test, while 6 percent (3 to 10 percent) with a negative history demonstrate a positive skin response to penicillin. Administering penicillin to those patients with a positive skin test produces reactions in a high proportion (50 to 100 percent); conversely, only a few patients (about 0.5 percent) with negative skin tests react to the drug, and reactions tend to be mild and to occur late. Since a negative skin test may occur during or just after an acute reaction, testing should be performed either prospectively or several months after a suspected reaction. As many as 80 percent of patients lose anaphylactic sensitivity and IgE antibody after several years. Radioallergosorbent test (RAST) and other in vitro tests offer no advantage over properly performed skin testing.

Some cross-reactivity exists between penicillin and nonpenicillin β-lactam antibiotics (e.g., cephalosporins). About half of patients who react to penicillin skin testing also react to cephalosporin skin testing; anaphylaxis from cephalosporins has occurred in patients testing positive to penicillin. The benefit of skin testing with penicillin derivatives and cephalosporins in addition to penicillin is uncertain; in one study, none of 120 patients with negative results to penicillin skin tests reacted to semisynthetic penicillinase-resistant agents.

In the face of a positive clinical history of penicillin reaction, another drug should be chosen. If this is not feasible or prudent (e.g., in a pregnant patient with syphilis; with enterococcal endocarditis), skin testing with penicillin is warranted. If skin tests are negative, cautious administration of penicillin is acceptable, although some recommend desensitization of such patients. In those with positive skin tests, desensitization is mandatory if therapeutic use of β-lactam antibiotics is to be undertaken. Various protocols are available, including oral and parenteral approaches. Oral desensitization appears to carry a lesser risk of serious anaphylactic reactions during desensitization. However, desensitization carries the risk of anaphylaxis regardless of how it is performed. After desensitization, many patients experience non-life-threatening IgE-mediated untoward reactions to penicillin during their course of therapy. Desensitization is not effective in those with exfoliative dermatitis or morbilliform reactions due to penicillin.

NONSTEROIDAL ANTI-INFLAMMATORY DRUGS Nonsteroidal anti-inflammatory drugs (NSAIDs), including aspirin (but not salicylates in general) and indomethacin (indometacin), cause two broad categories of allergic-like symptoms in susceptible individuals: (1) approximately 1 percent of persons experience urticaria or angioedema, and (2) about half as many (0.5 percent) experience rhinosinusitis and asthma; however, about 10 percent of adult asthmatics and one-third of individuals with nasal polyposis and sinusitis may respond adversely to aspirin.

Urticaria/angioedema may be delayed up to 24 h and may occur at any age. The rhinosinusitis-asthma syndrome generally develops within 1 h of drug administration. In young people, the reaction pattern often begins as watery rhinorrhea, which can be complicated by nasal and sinus infection, and polyposis, bloody discharge, and nasal eosinophilia. In many individuals with this syndrome, asthma eventually ensues that can be life-threatening whenever NSAIDs are subsequently ingested, and symptoms may persist despite avoidance of these drugs. Proof of the association of symptoms and NSAID use requires either clear-cut history of symptoms following drug ingestion or an oral challenge. For the latter to be performed with relative safety, (1) asthma must be under good control, (2) the procedure must be conducted in a hospital setting by experienced personnel capable of recognizing and treating acute respiratory responses, and (3) the challenge should begin with very low doses (i.e., <30 mg) of aspirin and increase every 1 to 2 h in doubling doses as tolerated to 650 mg. In a study of 50 consecutive patients with a positive history of aspirin-induced bronchospasm, 84 percent developed pulmonary or naso-ocular symptoms with aspirin, but 16 percent did not react; moreover, when subjects who initially tested positive to a challenge were reexposed to aspirin, the clinical reaction pattern was identical in only 60 percent.

While cross-reactivity between NSAIDs is common, it is not immunologic, and patients who are sensitive to NSAIDs cannot be identified by assessment of IgE antibody to aspirin, lymphocyte sensitization, or in vitro immunologic testing. All cross-reacting drugs are cyclooxygenase inhibitors, although salicylates also inhibit cyclooxygenase but (except for aspirin) do not cause the response.

"Desensitization" to the adverse effects of NSAIDs can be accomplished by the challenge procedure above, although repeated challenge at the initial provocation dose may be required. Desensitization works by unknown mechanisms, renders the subject tolerant to all NSAIDs yet studied, persists for at least 24 and up to 96 h, and is probably universal but does not have a positive effect on the underlying disorder.

RADIOCONTRAST MEDIA   Large numbers of patients are exposed to radiocontrast agents, and 5 to 10 percent of patients receiving them develop some reaction: urticaria in 1 percent, dyspnea in 0.25 percent, and death in 0.01 percent. Reactions consisting of urticaria and angioedema, asthma, and hypotension mimicking anaphylaxis occur in less than 1 percent of radiocontrast procedures. About one-third of those with mild reactions to previous exposure rereact on reexposure.

There is no proof of an immunologic mechanism for radiocontrast media reactions. Elevations in plasma histamine occur in those with and without reaction and may be due to the hypertonicity of these media. In addition, complement activation by both classical and alternative pathways occurs in normal and reactive individuals. In short, the mechanism for these reactions is not understood, and no test identifies patients at risk for a radiocontrast medium reaction. Because repeat reactions are common, obtaining a thorough history is the best available technique for identifying those most likely to experience an adverse reaction. Several pretreatment regimens are claimed to decrease repeat reaction rate to about 10 percent. One such regimen consists of 50 mg prednisone at 13, 7, and 1 h before the procedure and 50 mg diphenhydramine 1 h before the procedure.

HYDANTOINS   Phenytoin and other hydantoins cause morbilliform eruptions, erythema multiforme, and toxic epidermal necrolysis, as well as a hypersensitivity reaction (described above) and the pseudolymphoma syndrome. In one study, 5 percent of children treated with phenytoin developed a mild dose-dependent, maculopapular eruption lasting 3 to 5 days and occurring within 2 weeks of starting treatment.

The pseudolymphoma syndrome, consisting of lymphadenopathy and histopathologic lymph node atypia, is a more chronic form of the phenytoin hypersensitivity syndrome, and the cutaneous changes are less marked in this syndrome.

Use of phenytoin is frequently associated with gingival hyperplasia and rarely with a syndrome similar to systemic lupus erythematosus, severe exfoliative dermatitis, and polyarteritis nodosa. Because many hydantoin side effects may be dose-related, drugs that interfere with its elimination (e.g., chloramphenicol) effectively prolong those effects. Sulfasalazine, other sulfonamides, and allopurinol cause reactions that are indistinguishable from the phenytoin hypersensitivity syndrome.

THIAZIDES AND SULFONAMIDES   Thiazides are among the most common causes of drug-induced urticaria and morbilliform eruptions; they also cause erythema multiforme, drug-induced cutaneous vasculitis, and lichenoid and photosensitivity eruptions. Because they are substituted sulfonamides, antibodies to these diuretics may cross-react with sulfonamide antibiotics and sulfonamide-based hypoglycemic agents. The combination of sulfamethoxazole and trimethoprim causes two distinct cutaneous reactions: (1) an urticarial eruption beginning in the first few days of treatment and (2) a morbilliform eruption often occurring more than 1 week after therapy has begun. The morbilliform reaction is frequent in patients with AIDS and is associated with pancytopenia in some patients. The eruption may have an intensely purpuric characacter, independent of the presence of vasculitis. One patient developed toxic epidermal necrolysis and pancytopenia following administration of sulfamethoxazale-trimethoprim.

AGENTS USED IN CANCER CHEMOTHERAPY   Since many agents used in cancer chemotherapy inhibit cell division, rapidly proliferating elements of the skin, including hair, mucous membranes, and appendages, are sensitive to their effects; as a result, stomatitis and alopecia are among the most frequent dose-dependent side effects of chemotherapy. Onychodystrophy (dystrophic changes in nails) is also seen with bleomycin, hydroxyurea (hydroxycarbamide), and 5-fluorouracil. Sterile cellulitis and phlebitis and ulceration of pressure areas occur with many of these agents. Urticaria, angioedema, exfoliative dermatitis, and erythema of the palms and soles also have been seen, as has local and diffuse hyperpigmentation. Diagnosis and treatment of these reactions are especially difficult because of the underlying malignancy.

TETRACYCLINES   While urticaria and morbilliform eruptions are unusual, tetracyclines sometimes cause other cutaneous side effects, including a photosensitivity reaction (as a result of drug-induced phototoxicity) and onycholysis (sometimes with no apparent cutaneous photosensitivity). These reactions occur with demeclocycline, doxycycline, minocycline, tetracycline, and oxytetracycline. Tetracyclines also cause fixed drug and lichenoid eruptions. An acne-like, gram-negative folliculitis with long-term use of tetracycline is due to overgrowth of resistant bacteria.

Several pigmentary abnormalities have been noted. If used during pregnancy or early childhood, tetracycline stains the teeth, sometimes permanently. Minocyline can cause hyperpigmentation in sun-exposed areas and in areas of previous inflammation. Histiocytes that contain iron are responsible for the pigmentary changes. Tetracycline also has been associated with a flulike syndrome (accompanied by headaches, malaise, and eosinophilia) that recurred with rechallenge. A serum sickness–like reaction to minocycline also has been reported.

GLUCOCORTICOIDS   Both systemic and topical glucocorticoids cause a variety of skin changes, including acneiform eruptions, atrophy, striae, and other stigmata of Cushing's syndrome, and in sufficiently high doses can retard wound healing. Patients using glucocorticoids are at higher risk for bacterial, yeast, and fungal skin infections that may be misinterpreted as drug eruptions but are in fact drug side effects instead.

ANTIMALARIAL AGENTS   Antimalarial agents are used as therapy for several skin diseases, including the skin manifestations of lupus and polymorphous light eruption, but they also can induce cutaneous reactions. In patients with asymptomatic porphyria cutanea tarda, chloroquine increases porphyrin levels and may exacerbate the disease.

Pigmentation disturbances, including black pigmentation of the face, mucous membranes, and pretibial and subungual areas, occur with antimalarials, and quinacrine (mepacrine) causes generalized, cutaneous yellow discoloration. Antimalarial agents may exacerbate psoriasis, and exfoliative dermatitis, fixed drug eruptions, lichenoid dermatitis, and erythema annulare centrifugum have all been reported with their use.

GOLD   Chrysotherapy has been associated with a variety of dose-related dermatologic reactions (including maculopapular eruptions) that can develop as long as 2 years after initiation of therapy and require months to resolve. Erythema nodosum, psoriasiform dermatitis, vaginal pruritus, eruptions similar to pityriasis rosea, hyperpigmentation, and lichenoid eruptions resembling those seen with antimalarial agents have been reported. After a cutaneous reaction, it is sometimes possible to reinstitute gold therapy at lower doses without recurrence of the dermatitis.

DIAGNOSIS OF DRUG REACTIONS

Possible causes of an adverse reaction can be assessed as definite, probable, possible, or unlikely based on six variables: (1) previous experience with the drug in the general population, (2) alternative etiologic candidates, (3) timing of events, (4) drug levels or evidence of overdose, (5) patient reaction to dechallenge, and (6) patient reaction to rechallenge.

PREVIOUS EXPERIENCE   Tables of relative reaction rates are available and are useful to assess the likelihood that a given drug is responsible for a given cutaneous reaction. The specific morphologic pattern of a drug reaction, however, may modify these reaction rates by increasing or decreasing the likelihood that a given drug is responsible for a given reaction. For example, since fixed eruptions due to drug are more often seen with barbiturates than with penicillin, a fixed drug reaction in a patient taking both types of agents is more likely to be due to the barbiturate, even though penicillins have a higher overall drug reaction rate.

ALTERNATIVE ETIOLOGIC CANDIDATES A cutaneous eruption may be due to exacerbation of preexisting disease or to development of new disease unrelated to drugs. For example, a patient with psoriasis may have a flare-up of disease coincidental with administration of penicillin for streptococcal infection; in this case, infection is a more likely cause for the flare-up than drug reaction.

TIMING OF EVENTS Since most drug reactions of the skin occur within 1 to 2 weeks of initiation of therapy, reactions beginning after 2 weeks are less likely to be due to drugs.

DRUG LEVELS Some cutaneous reactions are dependent on dosage or cumulative toxicity. For example, lichenoid dermatoses due to gold administration appear more often in patients taking high doses.

DECHALLENGE Most adverse cutaneous reactions to drugs remit with dechallenge (removal of the suspected agent). A reaction is unlikely to be drug-related if improvement occurs without dechallenge or if a patient fails to improve after dechallenge and appropriate therapy.

RECHALLENGE Rechallenge provides the most definitive information concerning adverse cutaneous reactions to drugs, since a reaction failing to recur on rechallenge with a drug is unlikely to be due to that agent. Rechallenge is frequently impractical, however, because the need to ensure patient safety and comfort outweighs the value of the possible information derived from rechallenge.

DIAGNOSIS OF DRUG ALLERGY

Tests for IgE responses include in vivo and in vitro methods, but such tests are available only for a limited number of drugs, including penicillins and cephalosporins, some peptide and protein drugs (insulin, xenogeneic sera), and some agents used for general anesthesia. In vivo testing is accomplished by prick puncture and/or by intradermal skin testing. A wheal-and-flare response 2×2 mm greater than that seen with a saline control within 20 min is considered indicative of IgE-mediated mast cell degranulation, provided (1) the patient is not dermographic, (2) the drug does not nonspecifically degranulate mast cells, (3) the drug concentration is not high enough to be irritating, and (4) the buffer itself does not cause wheal-and-flare responses.

Skin testing with major and minor determinants of penicillins or cephalosporins has proved useful for identifying patients at risk of anaphylactic reactions to these agents. However, skin tests themselves carry a small risk of anaphylaxis. Negative skin tests do not rule out IgE-mediated reactivity, and the risk of anaphylaxis in response to penicillin administration in patients with negative skin tests is about 1 percent; about two-thirds of patients with a positive skin test and history of a previous adverse reaction to penicillin experience an allergic response on rechallenge. Skin tests may be negative in allergic patients receiving antihistamines or in those whose allergy is to determinants not present in the test reagent. Although less well studied, similar techniques can identify patients who are sensitive to protein drugs and to agents such as gallamine and succinylcholine. Most other drugs are small molecules, and skin testing with them is unreliable.

In vitro testing for IgE may be done by assessing the ability of serum to bind to antigen and then to bind radiolabeled antibody to IgE (RAST test) or by assessing the ability of the drug to cause histamine release from basophils from drug-sensitive individuals. The RAST test is sensitive and specific but is not available for most drugs; even in the case of penicillin it is available for major determinants only. Similarly, basophil histamine release is a research technique that is not generally available.

There are no generally available and reliable tests for sensitivity

to NSAIDs, to agents that directly degranulate mast cells, or to drugs that cause manifestations via immune-complex–mediated complement activation. Although it is possible to screen for the absence of IgA antibody, the utility of this maneuver in preventing transfusion-associated anaphylaxis in IgA-deficient individuals has not been documented.

REFERENCES

ALANKO K et al: Cutaneous drug reactions: Clinical types and causative agents. Five-year survey of inpatients (1981–1985). Acta Derm Venereol (Stockh) 69:223, 1989

BAUM C et al: Prescription drug use in 1984 and changes over time. Med Care 26:105, 1988

BIELORY L et al: Human serum sickness: A prospective analysis of 35 inpatients treated with equine anti-thymocyte globulin for bone marrow failure. Medicine 67:40, 1988

BIGBY M et al: Drug-induced cutaneous reactions: A report from the Boston Collaborative Drug Surveillance Program on 15,438 consecutive inpatients, 1975–1982. JAMA 256:3358, 1986

CHAN HL et al: The incidence of erythema multiforme, Stevens-Johnson syndrome, and toxic epidermal necrolysis: A population-based study with particular reference to reactions caused by drugs among outpatients. Arch Dermatol 126:43, 1990

COOPMAN SA, STERN RS: Cutaneous drug reactions in human immunodeficiency virus infection (editorial). Arch Dermatol 127:714, 1991

LEVENSON DE et al: Cutaneous manifestations of adverse drug reactions. Immunol Allergy Clin North Am 11:493, 1991

ROUJEAU JC et al: Toxic epidermal necrolysis (Lyeel syndrome): Incidence and drug etiology in France, 1981–1985. Arch Dermatol 126:37, 1990

——— et al: Acute generalized exanthematous pustulosis: Analysis of 63 cases. Arch Dermatol 127:1333, 1991

SHEAR NH, SPIELBERG SP: Anticonvulsant hypersensitivity syndrome: In vitro assessment of risk. J Clin Invest 82:1826, 1988

53 IMMUNOLOGICALLY MEDIATED SKIN DISEASES

KIM B. YANCEY / THOMAS J. LAWLEY

A number of immunologically mediated skin diseases and the cutaneous manifestations of immunologically mediated systemic disorders are now recognized as distinct entities with relatively consistent clinical, histologic, and immunopathologic findings. Many of these disorders are due to autoimmune mechanisms. Clinically, they are characterized by morbidity (pain, pruritus, disfigurement) and in some instances by mortality (largely due to loss of epidermal barrier function and/or secondary infection). The major features of the more common immunologically mediated skin diseases are summarized in this chapter. See Table 53-1.

PEMPHIGUS VULGARIS Pemphigus vulgaris (PV) is a blistering skin disease seen predominantly in elderly patients. Patients with PV have an increased incidence of the HLA-DR4 and -DRw6 serologically defined haplotypes. This disorder is characterized by the loss of cohesion between epidermal cells (a process termed *acantholysis*) with the resultant formation of intraepidermal blisters. Clinical lesions of PV typically consist of flaccid blisters on either normal-appearing or erythematous skin. These blisters rupture easily, leaving denuded areas that may crust and enlarge peripherally. Substantial portions of the body surface may be denuded in severe cases. Manual pressure to the skin of these patients may elicit the separation of the epidermis (Nikolsky's sign). This finding, while characteristic of PV, is not specific to this disorder and is also seen in toxic epidermal necrolysis, Stevens-Johnson syndrome, and a few other skin diseases. Lesions in PV typically present on the scalp, face, neck, axilla, trunk, and oral cavity. In half or more of patients, lesions begin in the mouth; approximately 90 percent of patients have oromucosal involvement at some time during the course of their disease. Involvement of other mucosal surfaces (e.g., pharyngeal, laryngeal, esophageal, conjunctival, vulval, or rectal) can occur in severe disease. Pruritus

TABLE 53-1   Immunologically mediated blistering skin diseases

Disease	Clinical	Histology	Immunopathology
Pemphigus vulgaris	Flaccid blisters, denuded skin, oromucosal lesions	Blister formed in suprabasal layer of epidermis	Cell surface deposits of IgG on keratinocytes
Pemphigus foliaceus	Crusts and shallow erosions on scalp, central face, neck, upper chest, and back	Blister formed in superficial layers of epidermis	Cell surface deposits of IgG on keratinocytes
Bullous pemphigoid	Large tense blisters on flexor surfaces, oromucosal lesions	Blister formed in subepidermal region, usually eosinophil-rich	Linear band of IgG or C3 at BMZ*
Dermatitis herpetiformis	Extremely itchy small papules and vesicles on elbows, knees, buttocks, and posterior nuchal area	Subepidermal blister with neutrophils in dermal papillae	Granular deposits of IgA in dermal papillae
Linear IgA disease	Extremely itchy small papules and vesicles on extensor surfaces, occasionally larger arciform blisters	Subepidermal blister with neutrophils in dermal papillae	Linear band of IgA at BMZ
Epidermolysis bullosa acquisita	Blisters, scarring, and milia on dorsum of hands, elbows, knees; oromucosal lesions	Blister is subepidermal and can be inflammatory or not	Linear band of IgG or C3 at BMZ

* BMZ = basement membrane zone.

may be a feature of early pemphigus lesions; extensive denudation may be associated with severe pain. Lesions usually heal without scarring, except at sites complicated by secondary infection or mechanically induced dermal wounds. Nonetheless, postinflammatory hyperpigmentation is usually present at sites of healed lesions for some time.

Biopsies of early lesions demonstrate intraepidermal vesicle formation secondary to loss of cohesion between epidermal cells (i.e., acantholytic blisters). Blister cavities contain acantholytic epidermal cells which appear as round homogeneous cells containing hyperchromatic nuclei. Basal keratinocytes remain attached to the epidermal basement membrane, hence blister formation is within the suprabasal portion of the epidermis. Lesional skin may contain focal collections of intraepidermal eosinophils within blister cavities; dermal alterations are slight, usually limited to an eosinophil-predominant leukocytic infiltrate. Direct immunofluorescence microscopy of lesional or normal skin shows deposits of IgG on the surface of keratinocytes; in contrast, deposits of complement are typically found in lesional but not normal skin. Keratinocyte IgG deposits are derived from a circulating autoantibody directed against cell surface antigens. Circulating autoantibodies can be demonstrated in 80 to 90 percent of PV patients by indirect immunofluorescence microscopy; monkey esophagus is the optimal substrate for demonstration of these autoantibodies. In PV, autoantibodies are directed against a 130-kDa desmosomal cadherin molecule that forms a complex with plakoglobin, an 85-kDa constituent of desmosomal and adherens junctions. These autoantibodies are responsible for dysadhesion of epidermal cells. The titer of circulating autoantibody (determined by indirect immunofluorescence microscopy) correlates roughly with disease activity. These immunopathologic findings aid the diagnosis of PV and its differentiation from other blistering skin diseases.

PV can be life-threatening. Prior to the availability of glucocorticoids, the mortality ranged from 60 to 90 percent. The current mortality is approximately 5 to 15 percent. Common causes of morbidity and mortality are infection and complications of treatment with glucocorticoids. Bad prognostic factors include advanced age, widespread involvement, and the requirement for high doses of glucocorticoids (with or without other immunosuppressive agents) for control of disease. The course of PV in individual patients is variable and difficult to predict. Some patients achieve remission after variable periods of treatment (40 percent of patients in some series), but others may require long-term treatment or succumb to complications of their disease or its treatment. The mainstay of treatment is systemic glucocorticoids. Patients with moderate to severe disease are usually started on prednisone 60 to 80 mg/d. If new lesions continue to appear after 1 to 2 weeks of treatment, the dose should be increased. Many regimens have combined an immunosuppressive agent with systemic glucocorticoids for control of PV. The two frequently used are

either azathioprine (1 mg/kg per day) or cyclophosphamide (1 mg/kg per day). It is important to bring severe or progressive disease under control quickly to lessen the severity and/or duration of this disorder.

PEMPHIGUS FOLIACEUS   Pemphigus foliaceus (PF) is distinguished from PV by several features. In PF, acantholytic blisters are located high within the epidermis, usually just beneath the stratum corneum. Hence PF is a more superficial blistering disease than PV. The distribution of lesions in the two disorders is much the same, except that in PF mucous membrane lesions are rare. Patients with PF rarely demonstrate intact blisters but rather exhibit shallow erosions associated with erythema, scale, and crust formation. Mild cases of PF resemble severe seborrheic dermatitis; severe PF may cause extensive exfoliation. Sun exposure (ultraviolet irradiation) may be an aggravating factor. A blistering skin disease endemic to south central Brazil known as fogo selvagem or Brazilian pemphigus is clinically, histologically, and immunopathologically indistinguishable from PF.

Patients with PF have immunopathologic features in common with PV. Specifically, direct immunofluorescence microscopy of normal, perilesional skin demonstrates IgG on the surface of keratinocytes. As in PV, patients with PF frequently have circulating IgG autoantibodies against keratinocyte cell surface antigens. Guinea pig esophagus is the optimal substrate for indirect immunofluorescence microscopy studies of sera from patients with PF. In PF, autoantibodies are directed against desmoglein, a 160-kDa desmosomal core glycoprotein that (like PV antigen) is complexed to plakoglobin.

Although pemphigus has been associated with several autoimmune diseases, its association with thymoma and/or myasthenia gravis is particularly notable. To date, more than 30 cases of thymoma and/or myasthenia gravis have been reported in association with pemphigus, usually with PF. Patients also may develop pemphigus as a consequence of drug exposure. The most frequently implicated agent is penicillamine; other offenders include captopril, rifampin, piroxicam, penicillin, and phenobarbital. Drug-induced pemphigus usually resembles PF rather than PV; autoantibodies in these patients have the same antigenic specificity as they do in other pemphigus patients. In most patients, lesions resolve following discontinuation of the drug; however, some patients require treatment with systemic glucocorticoids and/or immunosuppressives.

PF is generally a far less severe disease than PV and carries a better prognosis. Localized disease can be treated conservatively with topical or intralesional glucocorticoids; more active cases can usually be controlled with systemic glucocorticoids.

PARANEOPLASTIC PEMPHIGUS   Paraneoplastic pemphigus is a recently described autoimmune acantholytic mucocutaneous disease associated with an occult or confirmed neoplasm. Patients with paraneoplastic pemphigus typically show painful mucosal erosive lesions in association with pruritic papulosquamous eruptions that often progress to blisters. Palm and sole involvement is common in these patients and raises the possibility that prior reports of neoplasia-associated erythema multiforme actually may have represented unrecognized cases of paraneoplastic pemphigus. Biopsies of lesional skin from these patients show varying combinations of acantholysis, keratinocyte necrosis, and vacuolar-interface dermatitis. Direct immunofluorescence microscopy of patient skin shows deposits of IgG and complement on the surface of keratinocytes as well as similar immunoreactants in the epidermal basement membrane zone. Patients with paraneoplastic pemphigus have IgG autoantibodies that react with the surface of tissues containing desmosomes (i.e., complex and simple epithelia as well as myocardium). These autoantibodies immunoprecipitate a unique complex of four polypeptides (250, 230, 210, and 190 kDa) from keratinocyte cell extracts. In sodium dodecyl sulfate–polyacrylamide gel electrophoresis, the 250-kDa antigen comigrates with the desmosomal plaque–associated protein desmoplakin I, whereas the 230-kDa antigen comigrates with bullous pemphigoid antigen (see below); the identities of the other antigens in this complex have not yet been determined. Interestingly, passive transfer of patient immunoglobulin to neonatal mice produces keratinocyte detachment, indicating that patient autoantibodies are pathogenic mediators of tissue damage. Paraneoplastic pemphigus is generally treatment-resistant, although patients may improve (or even remit) following resection of the underlying neoplasm.

BULLOUS PEMPHIGOID   Bullous pemphigoid (BP) is a subepidermal blistering skin disease usually seen in the elderly. Lesions typically consist of tense blisters on either normal-appearing or erythematous skin. The lesions are usually distributed over the lower abdomen, groin, and flexor surface of the extremities; oral mucosal lesions are found in 10 to 40 percent of patients. Pruritus may be nonexistent or severe. As lesions evolve, tense blisters tend to rupture and be replaced by flaccid lesions or erosions with or without surmounting crust. Nontraumatized blisters heal without scarring. There is no ethnic or HLA association. Despite isolated reports, several studies have shown that patients with BP do not have an increased incidence of malignancy in comparison with appropriately age- and sex-matched controls.

While biopsies of early lesional skin demonstrate subepidermal blisters, the histologic features depend on the character of the particular lesion. Lesions on normal-appearing skin generally show a sparse perivascular leukocytic infiltrate with some eosinophils. Biopsies of inflammatory lesions typically show an eosinophil-rich, leukocytic infiltrate within the papillary dermis at sites of vesicle formation and in perivascular areas. In addition to eosinophils, these cell-rich lesions also contain mononuclear cells and neutrophils. It is not always possible to distinguish BP from other subepidermal blistering skin diseases by routine histologic techniques.

Immunopathologic studies have broadened our understanding of this disease and aided its diagnosis. Direct immunofluorescence microscopy of normal-appearing perilesional skin shows linear deposits of IgG and/or C3 in the epidermal basement membrane. The sera of approximately 70 percent of these patients contain circulating IgG autoantibodies that bind the epidermal basement membrane of normal human skin in indirect immunofluorescence microscopy. No correlation exists between the titer of these autoantibodies and disease activity. In BP, autoantibodies recognize 230- and (in approximately 50 percent of BP patients) 180-kDa hemidesmosome-associated glycoproteins in basal keratinocytes. Autoantibodies are thought to develop against these antigens, deposit in situ, and activate complement that subsequently produces dermal mast cell degranulation and granulocyte-rich leukocytic infiltrates that cause tissue damage and blister formation.

BP is generally benign, but it may persist for months to years, with exacerbations or remissions. Although extensive involvement may result in widespread erosions and compromise cutaneous integrity, the mortality rate is low even in the absence of treatment. Nonetheless, deaths may occur in elderly and/or debilitated patients. The mainstay of treatment is systemic glucocorticoids. Patients with

local or minimal disease can sometimes be controlled with topical glucocorticoids alone; patients with more extensive lesions generally respond to systemic glucocorticoids either alone or in combination with immunosuppressive agents. Patients will usually respond to prednisone 40 to 60 mg/d. In some instances, azathioprine (1 mg/kg per day) or cyclophosphamide (1 mg/kg per day) are necessary adjuncts.

HERPES GESTATIONIS   Herpes gestationis (HG) is a rare, nonviral, subepidermal blistering disease of pregnancy and the puerperium. HG may begin during any trimester of pregnancy or present shortly after delivery. Lesions are usually distributed over the abdomen, trunk, and extremities; mucous membrane lesions are rare. Skin lesions in these patients may be quite polymorphic and consist of erythematous urticarial papules and plaques, vesiculopapules, and/or frank bullae. Lesions are almost always very pruritic. Severe exacerbations of HG frequently occur after delivery, typically within 24 to 48 h. HG tends to recur in subsequent pregnancies, often beginning earlier during such gestations. Brief flare-ups of disease may occur with resumption of menses and may develop in patients later exposed to oral contraceptives. Occasionally, infants of affected mothers demonstrate transient skin lesions.

Biopsies of early lesional skin show teardrop-shaped subepidermal vesicles forming in dermal papillae in association with an eosinophil-rich leukocytic infiltrate. Differentiation of HG from other subepidermal bullous diseases by light microscopy is often difficult. However, direct immunofluorescence microscopy of normal perilesional skin from HG patients reveals the immunopathologic hallmark of this disorder—linear deposits of C3 in the epidermal basement membrane zone. These deposits develop as a consequence of complement activation produced by a low titer IgG anti-basement membrane zone autoantibody. Recent studies have shown that the majority of HG sera contain autoantibodies that recognize the same 180-kDa hemidesmosome-associated glycoprotein that is targeted by autoantibodies in roughly 50 percent of patients with BP—a subepidermal bullous disease that resembles HG morphologically, histologically, and immunopathologically.

The goals of therapy in patients with HG are to prevent the development of new lesions, relieve intense pruritus, and care for erosions at sites of blister formation. Most patients require treatment with moderate doses of daily glucocorticoids (i.e., 20 to 40 mg of prednisone) at some point in their course. Mild cases (or brief flare-ups) may be controlled by vigorous use of potent topical glucocorticoids. Although HG was once thought to be associated with an increased risk of fetal morbidity and mortality, the best evidence now suggests that these infants may only be at increased risk of being slightly premature or "small for dates." Current evidence suggests that there is no difference in the incidence of uncomplicated live births in HG patients treated with systemic glucocorticoids and in those managed more conservatively. If systemic glucocorticoids are administered, newborns are at risk for development of reversible adrenal insufficiency.

DERMATITIS HERPETIFORMIS   Dermatitis herpetiformis (DH) is an intensely pruritic, chronic papulovesicular skin disease characterized by lesions symmetrically distributed over extensor surfaces (i.e., elbows, knees, buttocks, back, scalp, and posterior neck). The primary lesion in this disorder is a papule, papulovesicle, or urticarial plaque. Because pruritus is prominent, patients may present with excoriations and crusted papules but no observable primary lesions. Patients sometimes report that their pruritus has a distinctive burning or stinging component; the onset of such local symptoms reliably heralds the development of distinct clinical lesions 12 to 24 h later. Almost all DH patients have an associated, usually subclinical, gluten-sensitive enteropathy (also see Chap. 254), and more than 90 percent express the HLA-B8/DRw3 and HLA-DQw2 haplotypes. DH may present at any age, including childhood; onset in the second to fourth decades is most common. The disease is typically chronic.

Biopsy of early lesional skin reveals neutrophil-rich infiltrates within dermal papillae. Neutrophils, fibrin, edema, and microvesicle formation at these sites are characteristic of early disease. Older lesions may demonstrate nonspecific features of a subepidermal bulla or an excoriated papule. Because the clinical and histologic features of this disease can be variable and resemble other subepidermal blistering disorders, the diagnosis can be confirmed by direct immuno-fluorescence microscopy of normal-appearing perilesional skin. Such studies demonstrate granular deposits of IgA (with or without complement components) in the papillary dermis and along the epidermal basement membrane zone. IgA deposits in the skin are unaffected by control of disease with medication; however, these immunoreactants may diminish in intensity or disappear in patients maintained for long periods on a strict gluten-free diet (see below). Patients with granular deposits of IgA in their epidermal basement membrane zone do not have circulating IgA autoantibodies and should be distinguished from individuals with linear IgA deposits at this site (see below).

Although most DH patients do not report overt gastrointestinal symptoms or laboratory evidence of malabsorption, biopsies of small bowel usually reveal blunting of intestinal villi and a lymphocytic infiltrate in the lamina propria. As is true for patients with celiac disease, this gastrointestinal abnormality can be reversed by a gluten-free diet. Moreover, if maintained, this diet alone may control the skin disease and eventuate in clearance of IgA deposits from these patients' epidermal basement membrane zone. Subsequent gluten exposure in the latter patients alters the morphology of their small bowel, elicits a flare-up of their skin disease, and is associated with the reappearance of IgA in their epidermal basement membrane zone. Patients with DH also have an increased incidence of thyroid abnormalities, achlorhydria, atrophic gastritis, and antigastric parietal cell antibodies. These associations likely relate to the high frequency of the HLA-B8/DRw3 haplotype in these patients, since this marker is commonly linked to autoimmune disorders. The mainstay of treatment of DH is dapsone. Patients respond rapidly (24 to 48 h) to dapsone but require careful pretreatment evaluation and close follow-up to ensure that complications are avoided or controlled. All patients on more than 100 mg/d dapsone will have some hemolysis and methemoglobinemia. These are expected pharmacologic side effects of dapsone. It is important to employ the lowest possible maintenance dose of dapsone to control symptoms and lesions. Gluten restriction can control DH and lessen dapsone requirements, but this diet must rigidly exclude gluten to be of benefit. Moreover, many months of dietary restriction may be necessary before a beneficial result is achieved. Good dietary counselling by a trained dietitian is essential.

LINEAR IgA DISEASE   Linear IgA disease, once considered a variant form of dermatitis herpetiformis, is actually a separate and distinct entity. Clinically, these patients may resemble typical cases of DH, bullous pemphigoid, or other subepidermal blistering skin diseases. Lesions typically consist of papulovesicles, bullae, and/or urticarial plaques, predominantly on extensor (as seen in "classic" DH), central, or flexural sites. Oral mucosal involvement does occur in selected patients. Severe pruritus resembles that in patients with DH. Patients with linear IgA disease do not have an increased frequency of the HLA-B8/DRw3 haplotype or an associated enteropathy and hence are not candidates for a gluten-free diet.

The histologic alterations in early lesions may be virtually indistinguishable from those in DH. However, direct immunofluorescence microscopy of normal-appearing perilesional skin reveals linear deposits of IgA (and often C3) in the epidermal basement membrane zone. Many patients with linear IgA disease demonstrate circulating IgA autoantibodies against a 97-kDa protein in normal epidermal basement membrane. As in DH, these patients respond promptly to treatment with dapsone, 50 to 200 mg/d.

EPIDERMOLYSIS BULLOSA ACQUISITA   EBA is a rare, noninherited, polymorphic, subepidermal blistering skin disease. (The inherited form is discussed in Chap. 351.) Since lesions generally occur in sites prone to minor trauma (e.g., dorsum of the hands, elbows, knees, etc.), EBA is regarded as a mechanobullous disease. Patients with classic or noninflammatory EBA have blisters on noninflamed skin, atrophic scars, milia, nail dystrophy, and oral lesions. Other patients with EBA have widespread inflammatory, scarring, bullous lesions and oromucosal involvement that resembles severe BP. Interestingly, some patients present with an inflammatory bullous skin disease that subsequently evolves into the classic noninflammatory form of this disorder. In general, EBA is chronic; associations with multiple myeloma, amyloidosis, inflammatory bowel disease, and diabetes mellitus have been reported. The HLA-DR2 haplotype is found with increased frequency in these patients.

The histology of lesional skin varies depending on the type or character of the lesion being studied. Noninflammatory bullae show subepidermal blisters with a sparse leukocytic infiltrate and resemble those in patients with porphyria cutanea tarda. Inflammatory vesiculobullous lesions consist of a subepidermal blister and neutrophil-rich leukocytic infiltrates in the superficial dermis. EBA patients have continuous deposits of IgG (and frequently C3 as well as other complement components) in a linear pattern within the epidermal basement membrane zone. Ultrastructurally, these immunoreactants are found in the sublamina densa region in association with anchoring fibrils. Approximately 25 to 50 percent of EBA patients have circulating IgG autoantibodies directed against type VII collagen—the collagen species found in anchoring fibrils.

Treatment of EBA is generally unsatisfactory. Some patients with inflammatory EBA may respond to systemic glucocorticoids, either alone or in combination with immunosuppressive agents. Other patients (especially those with neutrophil-rich inflammatory lesions) may respond to dapsone. The chronic, noninflammatory form of this disease is largely resistant to treatment.

AUTOIMMUNE SYSTEMIC DISEASES WITH PROMINENT CUTANEOUS FEATURES

DERMATOMYOSITIS   The cutaneous manifestations of dermatomyositis (see Chap. 384) are often distinctive but at times may resemble those of systemic lupus erythematosus (SLE), scleroderma, or other overlapping connective tissue diseases. The extent and severity of cutaneous disease may or may not correlate with the extent and severity of the myositis. Patients with severe muscle involvement may have relatively minor skin changes, whereas patients with marked skin involvement may have mild muscle disease. The cutaneous manifestations of dermatomyositis are similar whether the disease appears in childhood or old age, except that calcification of subcutaneous tissue is a common late sequela in childhood dermatomyositis.

The cutaneous signs of dermatomyositis may precede or follow the development of myositis by weeks to years. Cases lacking muscle involvement (i.e., dermatomyositis sine myositis) also have been reported. The most common manifestation is a purple-red discoloration of the upper eyelids, sometimes associated with scaling ("heliotrope" erythema) and periorbital edema. Erythema on the cheeks and nose in a "butterfly" distribution may resemble the eruption in SLE. Erythematous or violaceous scaling patches are common on the upper anterior chest and the extensor surfaces of the arms, legs, and hands. Erythema and scaling may be particularly prominent over the elbows, knees, and the dorsal interphalangeal joints. Approximately one-third of patients have violaceous, flat-topped papules over the dorsal interphalangeal joints that are pathognomonic of dermatomyositis (Gottron's sign or Gottron's papules). These lesions can be contrasted with the erythema and scaling on the dorsum of the fingers in some patients with SLE which spares the skin over the interphalangeal joints. Periungual telangiectasia may be prominent, and a lacy or reticulated erythema may be associated with fine scaling on the extensor surfaces of the thighs and upper arms. Other patients, particularly those with long-standing disease, develop areas of hypopigmentation, hyperpigmentation, mild atrophy, and telangiectasia known as *poikiloderma vasculare atrophicans*. Poikiloderma is rare in both SLE and scleroderma and thus can serve as a clinical sign that distinguishes dermatomyositis from these two diseases. However, cutaneous changes may be similar in scleroderma and dermatomyositis and may include thickening and binding down of the skin of the hands (sclerodactyly) as well as Raynaud's phenomenon. However, the presence of severe muscle disease, Gottron's papules, heliotrope erythema, and poikiloderma serve to distinguish these patients as having dermatomyositis. Skin biopsy of erythematous, scaling lesions of dermatomyositis may reveal only mild nonspecific inflammation but sometimes may show changes indistinguishable from those found in SLE, including epidermal atrophy, hydropic degeneration of basal keratinocytes, edema of the upper dermis, and a mild mononuclear cell infiltrate. Direct immunofluorescence microscopy of lesional skin is usually negative. Treatment should be directed at the systemic disease. In the few instances where adjunctive cutaneous therapy is desirable, topical glucocorticoids are sometimes useful. These patients should avoid exposure to ultraviolet irradiation and use photoprotective measures such as sunscreens.

LUPUS ERYTHEMATOSUS The cutaneous manifestations of lupus erythematosus (LE) (see Chap. 284) can be divided into acute, subacute, and chronic (i.e., discoid LE) types. Acute cutaneous LE is characterized by erythema of the nose and malar eminences in a "butterfly" distribution. The erythema is often sudden in onset, accompanied by edema and fine scale, and correlated with systemic involvement. Patients may have widespread involvement of the face as well as erythema and scaling of the extensor surfaces of the extremities and upper chest. These acute lesions, while sometimes evanescent, usually last for days and are often associated with exacerbations of systemic disease. Skin biopsy of acute lesions may show only a sparse dermal infiltrate of mononuclear cells and dermal edema. In some instances, cellular infiltrates around blood vessels and hair follicles are notable, as is hydropic degeneration of basal cells of the epidermis. Direct immunofluorescence microscopy of lesional skin frequently reveals deposits of immunoglobulin(s) and complement in the epidermal basement membrane zone. Treatment is aimed at control of systemic disease; photoprotection in this, as well as in other forms of LE, is very important.

Subacute cutaneous lupus erythematosus (SCLE) is characterized by a widespread photosensitive, nonscarring eruption. About half of these patients have SLE in which severe renal and CNS involvement is uncommon. SCLE may present as a papulosquamous eruption that resembles psoriasis or annular lesions that resemble those seen in erythema multiforme. In the papulosquamous form, discrete erythematous papules arise on the back, chest, shoulders, extensor surfaces of the arms, and the dorsum of the hands but are uncommon on the face, flexor surfaces of the arms, and below the waist. The slightly scaling papules tend to merge into large plaques, some with a reticulate appearance. The annular form involves the same areas and also begins as an erythematous papule but tends to develop oval, circular, or polycyclic lesions. The lesions of SCLE are more widespread but have less tendency for scarring than do lesions of discoid LE. Skin biopsy reveals a dense mononuclear cell infiltrate around hair follicles and blood vessels in the superficial dermis, combined with hydropic degeneration of basal cells in the epidermis. Direct immunofluorescence microscopy of lesional skin reveals deposits of immunoglobulin(s) in the epidermal basement membrane zone in about half these cases. Most SCLE patients have anti-Ro antibodies. Local therapy is usually unsuccessful, and most patients require treatment with aminoquinoline antimalarials. Low-dose therapy with oral glucocorticoids is sometimes necessary; photoprotective measures against both ultraviolet B and A wavelengths are very important.

Discoid lupus erythematosus (DLE) is characterized by discrete lesions, most often on the face, scalp, or external ears. The lesions are erythematous papules or plaques with a thick, adherent scale that occludes hair follicles (follicular plugging). When the scale is removed, its underside will show small excrescences that correlate with the openings of hair follicles and is termed a "carpet tack" appearance. This finding is relatively specific for discoid LE. Long-standing lesions develop central atrophy, scarring, and hypopigmentation but frequently have erythematous, sometimes raised borders at the periphery. These lesions persist for years and tend to expand slowly. Only 5 to 10 percent of patients with DLE meet the American Rheumatism Association criteria for SLE. However, typical discoid lesions are frequently seen in patients with SLE. Biopsy of discoid LE shows hyperkeratosis, follicular plugging, and atrophy of the epidermis. The dermal-epidermal junction reveals hydropic degeneration of basal keratinocytes, and a mononuclear cell infiltrate surrounds hair follicles and blood vessels. Direct immunofluorescence microscopy demonstrates immunoglobulin(s) and complement deposits at the basement membrane zone in about 90 percent of cases. Treatment is focused on control of local cutaneous disease and consists mainly of photoprotection and topical or intralesional glucocorticoids. If local therapy is ineffective, use of aminoquinoline antimalarials may be indicated.

SCLERODERMA AND MORPHEA The skin changes of scleroderma (see Chap. 286) usually begin on the hands, feet, and face, with episodes of recurrent nonpitting edema. Sclerosis of the skin begins distally on the fingers (sclerodactyly) and spreads proximally, usually accompanied by resorption of bone of the fingertips, which may have punched out ulcers, stellate scars, or areas of hemorrhage. The fingers may actually shrink in size and become sausage-shaped, and since the fingernails are usually unaffected, the nails may curve over the end of the fingertips. Periungual telangiectasias are usually present, but periungual erythema is rare. In advanced cases, the extremities show contractures and calcinosis cutis. Face involvement includes a smooth, unwrinkled brow, taut skin over the nose, shrinkage of tissue around the mouth, and perioral radial furrowing. Matlike telangiectasias are often present, particularly on the face and hands. Involved skin feels indurated, smooth, and bound to underlying structures; hyperpigmentation and hypopigmentation are also often present. Raynaud's phenomenon, i.e., cold-induced blanching, cyanosis, and reactive hyperemia, is present in almost all patients with scleroderma and can precede development of scleroderma by many years. The combination of calcinosis cutis, Raynaud's phenomenon, esophageal dysmotility, sclerodactyly, and telangiectasia has been termed the *CREST syndrome*. Anticentromere antibodies have been reported in a very high percentage of patients with the CREST syndrome but in only a small minority of patients with scleroderma. Skin biopsy reveals thickening of the dermis and homogenization of collagen bundles. Direct immunofluorescence microscopy of lesional skin is usually negative.

Morphea, which has been called *localized scleroderma*, is characterized by localized thickening and sclerosis of skin, usually affecting young adults or children. Morphea begins as erythematous or flesh-colored plaques that become sclerotic, develop central hypopigmentation, and demonstrate an erythematous border. In most cases, patients have one or a few lesions, and the disease is termed *localized morphea*. In some patients, widespread cutaneous lesions may occur, without systemic involvement. This form is called *generalized morphea*. Most patients with morphea do not have autoantibodies. Skin biopsy of morphea is indistinguishable from that of scleroderma. Linear scleroderma is a limited form of disease which presents in a linear, bandlike distribution and tends to involve deep as well as superficial layers of skin. Scleroderma and morphea are usually quite resistant to therapy with medications. For this reason, physical therapy to prevent joint contractures and to maintain function is employed and is often helpful.

Diffuse fasciitis with eosinophilia is a clinical entity that can sometimes be confused with scleroderma. There is usually the sudden onset of swelling, induration, and erythema of the extremities frequently following significant physical exertion. The proximal portions of extremities (arms, forearms, thighs, legs) are more often involved than are the hands and feet. While the skin is indurated, it is usually not bound down as in scleroderma. These skin findings are accompanied by peripheral blood eosinophilia, increased erythrocyte sedimentation rate, and sometimes hypergammaglobulinemia. Deep biopsy of affected areas of skin reveals inflammation and thickening of the deep fascia overlying muscle. An inflammatory infiltrate composed of eosinophils and mononuclear cells is usually found. Patients with eosinophilic fasciitis appear to be at increased risk to develop bone marrow failure or other hematologic abnormalities. While the ultimate course of eosinophilic fasciitis is uncertain, many patients respond favorably to treatment with prednisone in doses ranging from 40 to 60 mg/d.

The *eosinophilia-myalgia syndrome*, a newly recognized disorder reported in epidemic numbers in 1989 and linked to ingestion of manufactured tryptophan, is a multisystem disorder characterized by debilitating myalgias and absolute eosinophilia in association with varying combinations of arthralgias, pulmonary symptoms, peripheral edema, and neuropathies (see Chap. 286). The precise cause of this syndrome, which may resemble other sclerotic skin conditions, is unknown. However, the clustering of cases suggests that an impurity or contaminant in a manufactured tryptophan preparation is likely.

REFERENCES

ANHALT GJ et al: Paraneoplastic pemphigus: An autoimmune mucocutaneous disease associated with neoplasia. N Engl J Med 323:1729, 1990

BRAVERMAN IM: Connective tissue diseases, in *Skin Signs of Systemic Disease*. Philadelphia, Saunders, 1981

GAMMON WR et al: Epidermolysis bullosa acquisita—A pemphigoid-like disease. J Am Acad Dermatol 11:820, 1984

HALL RP: The pathogenesis of dermatitis herpetiformis: Recent advances. J Am Acad Dermatol 16:1129, 1987

KATZ SI et al: Dermatitis herpetiformis: The skin and the gut. Ann Intern Med 93:857, 1980

KORMAN N: Pemphigus. J Am Acad Dermatol 18:1219, 1988

SHORNICK JK: Herpes gestationis. J Am Acad Dermatol 17:539, 1987

SHULMAN LE: Diffuse fasciitis with eosinophilia: A new syndrome. Arthritis Rheum 20(Suppl):205, 1977

STANLEY JR: Pemphigus and pemphigoid as paradigms of organ-specific, autoantibody-mediated diseases. J Clin Invest 83:1443, 1989

YANCEY KB, LAWLEY TJ: The immunology of the skin, in *Allergy: Principles and Practice*, 3d ed, E Middleton et al (eds). St. Louis, Mosby, 1988

54   SKIN MANIFESTATIONS OF INTERNAL DISEASE

JEAN BOLOGNIA / IRWIN M. BRAVERMAN

It is now a generally accepted concept in medicine that the skin can show signs of internal disease. Therefore, in textbooks of medicine one finds a chapter describing in detail the major systemic disorders that can be identified by cutaneous signs. The underlying assumption of such a chapter is that the clinician has been able to identify the disorder in the patient and needs only to read about it in the textbook. In reality, concise differential diagnoses and the identification of these disorders are actually difficult for the nondermatologist because he or she is not well versed in the recognition of cutaneous lesions or their spectrum of presentations. Therefore, the authors of this chapter have decided to cover this particular topic of cutaneous medicine not by discussing individual disorders but by describing and discussing the various presenting clinical signs and symptoms that indicate the presence of these disorders. Concise differential diagnoses will be generated in which the significant diseases will be briefly discussed and distinguished from the more common disorders that have no significance for internal diseases. The latter disorders are reviewed in table form and always need to be excluded when considering the former. For a detailed description of individual diseases, the reader should consult a dermatologic text. The categories of skin lesions that are discussed include papulosquamous lesions, erythroderma, alopecia, figurate lesions, acne, pustules, telangiectasias, hypopigmentation, hyperpigmentation, vesicles/bullae, exanthems, urticaria, papulonodular lesions, purpura, and ulcers. In an attempt to determine the appropriate category for a particular lesion, it is important to carefully examine its surface qualities, shape, and color in addition to the location and distribution (see Chap. 50).

PAPULOSQUAMOUS SKIN LESIONS (Table 54-1)   When an eruption is characterized by elevated lesions, papules (<1 cm) or plaques (>1 cm), in association with scale, it is referred to as *papulosquamous*. The most common papulosquamous diseases—*psoriasis*, *tinea*, *pityriasis rosea*, and *lichen planus*—are primary cutaneous disorders (Table 54-2). When psoriatic lesions are accompanied by arthritis, the possibility of psoriatic arthritis or *Reiter's disease* should be considered. A history of oral ulcers, conjunctivitis, uveitis, and/or urethritis points to the latter diagnosis. In *guttate psoriasis* there is an acute onset of small, widely scattered, uniform lesions, often in association with a streptococcal infection. Lithium, beta blockers, human immunodeficiency virus (HIV) infection, and a rapid taper of systemic glucocorticoids are also known to exacerbate psoriasis. Epidermal hyperproliferation and incomplete maturation are responsible for the plaque formation and scale that is characteristic of psoriasis.

Whenever the diagnosis of pityriasis rosea or lichen planus is made, it is important to review the patient's medications because the eruption can be treated by simply discontinuing the offending agent. Pityriasis rosea–like drug eruptions are seen most commonly with beta blockers, captopril, clonidine, gold, griseofulvin, isotretinoin, metronidazole, and penicillin, while the drugs that can produce a lichenoid eruption include gold, antimalarials, thiazides, quinidine, phenothiazines, sulfonylureas, furosemide, griseofulvin, beta blockers, and captopril. Lichen planus–like lesions are also observed in chronic graft-versus-host disease. *Bowen's disease* represents squamous cell carcinoma in situ, and it usually presents as a single lesion. The plaque is well demarcated, pink to red in color, and the amount of scale varies. Bowen's disease is found in both sun-exposed and sun-protected areas of the body; the possibility of arsenic exposure should be explored in these patients, and an examination of the palms and soles for arsenical keratoses should be performed.

Parapsoriasis is an intermediate disease, for it can remain solely as a primary cutaneous disease or it can progress to cutaneous T cell lymphoma (CTCL) after a latency period of as long as 40 years. There are several forms of *parapsoriasis*, including small plaque (0.5 to 5 cm), large plaque (>6 cm), and retiform. The lesions of both small plaque and large plaque parapsoriasis are thin and salmon-pink in color with fine white scale. In small plaque forms, the lesions are commonly on the trunk but can be widely scattered. In large plaque forms, the most common location is the "girdle" area, and fine wrinkling secondary to epidermal atrophy is often seen. Retiform parapsoriasis forms a netlike pattern, and the individual papules are red-brown and flat-topped. The latter two forms of parapsoriasis, large plaque and retiform, can progress to CTCL.

Cutaneous T cell lymphoma (CTCL), *secondary syphilis*, *lupus* (see "Papulonodular Skin Lesions" below), and *Bazex' syndrome* are less common papulosquamous disorders that are associated with systemic disease. A clue to the development of *CTCL* within lesions

---

TABLE 54-1   Causes of papulosquamous skin lesions

Primary cutaneous disorders
A Psoriasis
B Tinea
C Pityriasis rosea
D Lichen planus
E Parapsoriasis
F Bowen's disease
Drugs
Systemic diseases
A Lupus erythematosus
B Cutaneous T cell lymphoma
C Secondary syphilis
D Reiter's disease
E Bazex' syndrome

TABLE 54-2 Papulosquamous skin diseases (primary cutaneous disorders)

	Characteristic lesion	Location	Other findings	Diagnostic aids
Psoriasis	Pink-red, silvery scale, sharply demarcated	Elbows, knees, scalp, pre-sacral area	Nail dystrophy: pitting, ony-cholysis, yellow discoloration Arthritis: primarily small joints (hands and feet)	Skin biopsy
Tinea	Pink-red, central clearing common, active, scaling border	Inner thigh (tinea cruris), palms, soles, any area of body	Invasion of stratum corneum by dermatophytes	KOH and/or fungal culture of scale
Pityriasis rosea	Salmon-pink, oval shape, long axis follows lines of cleavage in the skin, peripheral collarette of scale	Trunk, proximal extremities	Herald patch: initial lesion and usually the largest in size Spontaneous resolution over 2–3 months	Skin biopsy, VDRL to exclude secondary syphilis
Lichen planus	Violet-colored, polygonal, flat-topped, traversed by thin white lines (Wickham's striae)	Flexor wrists, ankles, presacral area, glans penis	Oral mucosa: lacelike white plaques and/or erosions Pruritus Nail dystrophy: pterygium, longitudinal ridging	Skin biopsy

of large plaque or retiform parapsoriasis is an increase in the palpable component of the plaque (increased infiltration). In its early stages, CTCL may be confused with ezcema or psoriasis, but it often fails to respond to the appropriate therapy for those inflammatory diseases. The diagnosis of CTCL is established by skin biopsy in which collections of atypical T lymphocytes are found in the epidermis and dermis. As the disease progresses, cutaneous tumors and lymph node involvement may appear.

In *secondary syphilis* there are scattered red-brown papules with thin scale. The eruption often involves the palms and soles, and it can resemble pityriasis rosea. Associated findings are helpful in making the diagnosis, and they include annular plaques on the face, nonscarring alopecia, condyloma lata (broad-based and moist), and mucous patches, as well as lymphadenopathy, malaise, fever, headache, and myalgias. The interval between the primary chancre and the secondary stage is usually 4 to 8 weeks, and spontaneous resolution without appropriate therapy is seen. When psoriasiform lesions are seen on the nose, ears, fingers, and toes, *Bazex' syndrome* should be considered. It is a distinctive paraneoplastic eruption associated with squamous cell carcinomas of the oropharynx, tracheobronchial tree, and esophagus.

ERYTHRODERMA (Table 54-3) *Erythroderma* is the term used when the majority of the skin surface is erythematous (red in color). There may be associated scale, erosions, or pustules as well as shedding of the hair and nails. Potential systemic manifestations include fever, chills, hypothermia, reactive lymphadenopathy, peripheral edema, hypoalbuminemia, increased transepidermal water loss, and high-output cardiac failure. The major etiologies of erythroderma are (1) *cutaneous diseases* such as psoriasis and dermatitis (Table 54-4), (2) *drugs*, (3) *systemic diseases*, most commonly CTCL, and (4) *idiopathic*. In the first three groups, the location and description of the initial lesions, prior to the development of the erythroderma, aid in the diagnosis. For example, a history of red scaly plaques on the elbows and knees would point to psoriasis. It is also important to examine the skin carefully for a migration of the erythema and

associated secondary changes such as pustules or erosions. Migratory waves of erythema studded with superficial pustules are seen in *pustular psoriasis*, whereas erosive migratory erythema of the girdle area is seen in *necrolytic migratory erythema* (glucagonoma syndrome).

An erythroderma secondary to an underlying cutaneous disease is most commonly due to *psoriasis* or one of the various forms of *dermatitis* (eczema). Each type of dermatitis has its own distinguishing features, but they may be limited to the initial lesions. Uncontrolled dermatitis can evolve into an erythroderma through a process known as *autosensitization* (conditioned hyperirritability), where initially uninvolved skin becomes pruritic and eventually dermatitic.

Drug-induced erythroderma (exfoliative dermatitis) may begin as a morbilliform eruption, or it may arise as diffuse erythema. Fever and peripheral eosinophilia often accompany the eruption. There are a number of *drugs* that can produce an erythroderma, including penicillins, sulfonamides, barbiturates, phenytoin, gold, allopurinol, captopril, sulfonylureas, and furosemide. Reactions to allopurinol also may be accompanied by hepatitis and nephropathy, especially in patients with impaired renal function given full doses of allopurinol plus a diuretic.

The most common malignancy that is associated with erythroderma is *CTCL*; in some series, up to 25 percent of the cases of erythroderma were due to CTCL. The patient may progress from isolated plaques and tumors, but more commonly the erythroderma is present throughout the course of the disease (Sézary syndrome). In the Sézary syndrome, there are circulating atypical T lymphocytes, pruritus, and lymphadenopathy. Additional findings include keratoderma and leonine facies. In cases of erythroderma where there is no apparent cause (idiopathic), longitudinal follow-up is mandatory to monitor for the possible development of CTCL. Other types of *lymphoma* can be associated with erythroderma, including Hodgkin's and non-Hodgkin's lymphoma, the former being more common. There also have been isolated case reports of erythroderma secondary to some solid tumors—lung, liver, prostate, thyroid, and colon—but it is usually in a late stage of the disease.

ALOPECIA (Table 54-5) The two major forms of *alopecia* are scarring and nonscarring. In *scarring alopecia* there is associated fibrosis, inflammation, and loss of hair follicles. A smooth scalp with a decreased number of follicular openings is usually observed clinically, but in some cases the changes are seen only in biopsy specimens from the affected areas. In *nonscarring alopecia* the hair shafts are gone, but the hair follicles are preserved, explaining the reversible nature of nonscarring alopecia.

Primary cutaneous disorders are the most common causes of nonscarring alopecia and they include *telogen effluvium, androgenetic alopecia, alopecia areata, tinea capitis*, and *traumatic alopecia* (Table 54-6). In women with androgenetic alopecia, an elevation in

TABLE 54-3 Causes of erythroderma

Primary cutaneous disorders
  A Psoriasis
  B Dermatitis (atopic, stasis, contact, seborrheic)
  C Pityriasis rubra pilaris
Drugs
Systemic diseases
  A Cutaneous T cell lymphoma
  B Lymphoma
  C Necrolytic migratory erythema
Idiopathic

TABLE 54-4　Erythroderma (primary cutaneous disorders)

	Initial lesions	Location of initial lesions	Other findings	Diagnostic aids
Psoriasis	Pink-red, silvery scale, sharply demarcated	Elbows, knees, scalp, presacral area	Nail dystrophy, arthritis, pustules	Skin biopsy
Dermatitis: Atopic	Acute: Erythema, fine scale, crust, indistinct borders Chronic: Lichenification (increased skin markings)	Antecubital and popliteal fossae, neck, hands	Pruritus Family history of atopy, including asthma, allergic rhinitis or conjunctivitis, and atopic dermatitis Rule out secondary infection with *S. aureus* Rule out superimposed irritant contact dermatitis	Skin biopsy
Stasis	Erythema, crusting, excoriations	Lower extremities	Pruritus, lower extremity edema History of venous ulcers, thrombophlebitis, and/or cellulitis Rule out cellulitis Rule out superimposed contact dermatitis, e.g., topical neomycin	Skin biopsy
Contact (local)	Erythema, crusting, vesicles, and bullae	Depends on offending agent	Irritant—onset often within hours Allergic—delayed-type hypersensitivity; lag time of 48 h	Patch testing
Contact (systemic)	Erythema, fine scale, crust	Generalized	Patient has history of allergic contact dermatitis to topical agent and then receives systemic medication that is structurally related, e.g., ethylenediamine (topical) aminophylline (IV)	Patch testing
Seborrheic	Pink-red, greasy scale	Scalp, nasolabial folds, eyebrows, intertriginous zones	Flares with stress, HIV infection Associated with Parkinson's disease	Skin biopsy
Pityriasis rubra pilaris	Orange-red, perifollicular, papules	Generalized, but characteristic "skip" areas of normal skin	Wax-like keratoderma Rule out cutaneous T cell lymphoma	Skin biopsy

circulating levels of androgens may be seen as a result of ovarian or adrenal gland dysfunction. When there are signs of virilization, such as a deepened voice and enlarged clitoris, the possibility of an ovarian or adrenal gland tumor should be considered.

Exposure to various *drugs* also can cause diffuse hair loss, usually by inducing a telogen effluvium. An exception is the anagen effluvium observed with antimitotic agents such as daunorubicin. Alopecia is a side effect of the following drugs: warfarin, heparin, propylthiouracil, carbimazole, vitamin A, isotretinoin, etretinate, lithium, beta blockers, levodopa, amphetamines, and thallium. Fortunately, spontaneous regrowth usually follows discontinuation of the offending agent.

Less commonly, nonscarring alopecia is associated with *lupus erythematosus* and *secondary syphilis*. In systemic lupus there are two forms of alopecia—one is scarring secondary to discoid lesions (see below) and the other is nonscarring. The latter form may be diffuse and involve the entire scalp, or it may localized to the frontal

scalp in the form of multiple short hairs ("lupus hairs"). Scattered, poorly circumscribed patches of alopecia with a "moth-eaten" appearance are a manifestation of the secondary stage of syphilis (see "Papulosquamous Skin Lesions"). Diffuse thinning of the hair is also associated with hypothyroidism, hyperthyroidism, hypopituitarism, HIV infection, and deficiencies of protein, iron, biotin, and zinc.

Scarring alopecia is more frequently the result of a primary cutaneous disorder such as *lichen planus*, *folliculitis decalvans*, *cutaneous lupus*, or *linear scleroderma (morphea)* than it is a sign of systemic disease. Although the scarring lesions of *discoid lupus* can be seen in patients with systemic lupus, in the majority of cases the disease process is limited to the skin. Less common causes of scarring alopecia include *sarcoidosis* (see "Papulonodular Skin Lesions"), cutaneous *metastases*, and *pseudopelade*. The latter disease may be idiopathic and arise de novo, or it can represent the inactive end-stage phase of a previous inflammatory process such as lichen planus, sarcoid, or discoid lupus. The irregularly shaped areas of alopecia lack inflammation and often arise at an acute angle from the midline.

In the early phases of discoid lupus, lichen planus, and folliculitis decalvans, there are circumscribed areas of alopecia. Fibrosis and subsequent loss of follicles are observed primarily in the center of the individual lesions, while the inflammatory process is most prominent at the periphery. The areas of active inflammation in *discoid lupus* are erythematous with scale, whereas the areas of previous inflammation are often hypopigmented with a rim of hyperpigmentation. In *lichen planus* the peripheral perifollicular papules are violet-colored, and postinflammatory hyperpigmentation is a characteristic finding. Complete examination of the skin and oral mucosa combined with a biopsy and direct immunofluorescence microscopy will aid in distinguishing these two entities. The peripheral active lesions in *folliculitis decalvans* are perifollicular pustules that

TABLE 54-5　Causes of alopecia

Nonscarring alopecia	Scarring alopecia
A Primary cutaneous disorders 　1 Telogen effluvium 　2 Androgenetic alopecia 　3 Alopecia areata 　4 Tinea capitis 　5 Traumatic alopecia B Drugs C Systemic diseases 　1 Lupus erythematosus 　2 Secondary syphilis 　3 Hypothyroidism 　4 Hyperthyroidism 　5 Deficiencies of protein, 　　iron, biotin, and zinc 　6 HIV infection	A Primary cutaneous disorders 　1 Cutaneous lupus 　2 Lichen planus 　3 Folliculitis decalvans 　4 Pseudopelade 　5 Linear scleroderma 　　(morphea) B Systemic diseases 　1 Lupus erythematosus 　2 Sarcoidosis 　3 Cutaneous metastases

TABLE 54-6 Nonscarring alopecia (primary cutaneous disorders)

	Clinical characteristics	Pathogenesis
Telogen effluvium	Diffuse shedding of normal hairs Follows either major stress (high fever, severe infection) or change in hormones (post partum) Reversible without treatment	Stress causes the normally asynchronous growth cycles of individual hairs to become synchronous; therefore, large numbers of growing (anagen) hairs simultaneously enter the dying (telogen) phase
Androgenetic alopecia	Miniaturization of hairs along the midline of the scalp Recession of the anterior scalp line in men and some women	Increased sensitivity of affected hairs to the effects of testosterone Increased levels of circulating androgens (ovarian or adrenal source)
Alopecia areata	Well-circumscribed, circular areas of hair loss, 2–5 cm in diameter In extensive cases, coalescence of lesions and/or involvement of other hair-bearing surfaces of the body Pitting of the nails	The germinative zones of the hair follicles are surrounded by T lymphocytes Occasional associated diseases: hyperthyroidism, hypothyroidism, vitiligo, Down's syndrome
Tinea	Varies from scaling with minimal hair loss, to discrete patches with "black dots" (broken hairs), to boggy plaque with pustules (kerion)	Invasion of hairs by dermatophytes, most commonly *Trichophyton tonsurans*
Traumatic alopecia	Broken hairs Irregular outline	Traction with curlers, rubber bands, braiding Exposure to heat or chemicals Mechanical pulling (trichotillomania)

routinely grow *Staphylococcus aureus* or normal flora. These patients often have other forms of acne and folliculitis and can develop a reactive arthritis.

FIGURATE SKIN LESIONS (Table 54-7) In *figurate* eruptions, the lesions form rings and arcs that are usually erythematous but can be flesh-colored to brown. Most commonly, they are due to primary cutaneous diseases such as *tinea, urticaria, erythema annulare centrifugum,* and *granuloma annulare* (Table 54-8). An underlying systemic illness is found in a second, less common group of migratory annular erythemas. It includes *erythema gyratum repens, erythema migrans,* and *erythema marginatum.*

In *erythema gyratum repens,* one sees hundreds of mobile concentric arcs and wavefronts that resemble the grain in wood. A search

TABLE 54-7 Causes of figurate skin lesions

Primary cutaneous disorders
 A Tinea
 B Urticaria
 C Erythema annulare centrifugum
 D Granuloma annulare
Systemic diseases
 A Migratory
  1 Erythema migrans
  2 Erythema gyratum repens
  3 Erythema marginatum
  4 Pustular psoriasis
  5 Necrolytic migratory erythema
 B Nonmigratory
  1 Sarcoidosis
  2 Subacute lupus erythematosus
  3 Secondary syphilis
  4 Cutaneous T cell lymphoma
  5 Elastosis perforans serpiginosa

for an underlying malignancy is mandatory in a patient with this eruption. *Erythema migrans* is the cutaneous manifestation of Lyme disease, which is caused by the spirochete *Borrelia burgdorferi.* In the initial stage (3 to 30 days after tick bite), a single annular lesion is usually seen, which can expand to ≥10 cm in diameter. Within several days, approximately half the patients develop multiple smaller erythematous lesions at sites distant from the bite. Associated symptoms include fever, headache, myalgias, photophobia, arthralgias, and malar rash. *Erythema marginatum* is seen in patients with rheumatic fever, primarily on the trunk. Lesions are pink-red in color, flat to mildly elevated, and transient. If pustules are noted within a figurate eruption, consider *pustular psoriasis,* and if erosions are seen, consider *necrolytic migratory erythema.*

There are additional cutaneous diseases that present as annular eruptions, but they lack an obvious migratory component. Examples include *CTCL,* annular cutaneous *lupus,* also referred to as *subacute lupus* (see "Papulonodular Skin Lesions"), secondary *syphilis,* and *sarcoidosis* (see "Papulonodular Skin Lesions"). The most common clinical setting for the annular form of secondary lues is the face of black patients; a clue to this diagnosis is the presence of central hyperpigmentation. If keratotic plugs are noted within the annular or arciform lesions, particularly if they are localized to the neck and antecubital fossae, consider *elastosis perforans serpiginosa* (EPS). EPS is seen as a side effect of D-penicillamine and in patients with Down's syndrome and disorders of elastin and collagen. The latter include Ehlers-Danlos type IV and Marfan's syndromes, pseudoxanthoma elasticum, and osteogenesis imperfecta.

ACNE (Table 54-9) *Acne vulgaris* and *acne rosacea* are the two major forms of acne (Table 54-10). Estrogens decrease sebaceous gland activity, whereas androgens enhance sebum production. Therefore, acne vulgaris in an adult, especially if it is of recent onset, may be a reflection of increased levels of circulating *androgens.*

TABLE 54-8 Figurate eruptions (primary cutaneous disorders)

	Clinical characteristics	Pathogenesis
Tinea	Active, scaling erythematous border with central clearing Expands slowly	Invasion of stratum corneum by dermatophytes
Urticaria	Central wheal with erythematous flare Transient and/or migratory Pruritic	Release of histamine from mast cells via immunologic (IgE, type 1 hypersensitivity) or nonimmunologic mechanisms (e.g., morphine)
Erythema annulare centrifugum	Enlarges slowly Erythematous, flat or slightly raised "Trailing scale"—scale on inner aspect of expanding ring Buttock, upper thighs	Not known Usually idiopathic Sometimes associated with tinea pedis, drug hypersensitivity Rarely, paraneoplastic
Granuloma annulare	Border composed of flesh-colored to red-brown papules Extremities	Granulomatous process is limited to the skin Unknown etiology Disseminated form is associated with diabetes mellitus

---

TABLE 54-9   Causes of acneiform eruptions

Primary cutaneous disorders
  A   Acne vulgaris
  B   Acne rosacea
Drugs
Systemic diseases
  A   Increased androgen production
    1   Adrenal origin, e.g., Cushing's disease, 21-hydroxylase deficiency
    2   Ovarian origin, e.g., polycystic ovary disease
  B   Cryptococcosis, disseminated
  C   Behçet's disease

TABLE 54-11   Causes of folliculitis

Infections
  A   Bacterial
    1   *Propionibacterium acnes*
    2   *Staphylococcus aureus*
    3   Gram-negative rods, e.g., *Pseudomonas*
      a   Face and neck—in the setting of long-term antibiotic use
      b   Trunk—"hot tub" folliculitis
  B   Fungal
    1   *Pityrosporum*
      a   AIDS
    2   Dermatophytes
      a   Legs of women—*Trichophyton rubrum*
      b   Beard area of men—*Trichophyton verrucosum*
      c   Scalp—*Trichophyton tonsurans*
    3   *Candida*
      a   Occluded areas
      b   Diabetics
Inflammatory
  A   Eosinophilic folliculitis
    1   AIDS
Drugs

Dysfunction of the ovary or adrenal gland, e.g., polycystic ovary disease, Cushing's syndrome, or partial deficiency of the enzyme 21-hydroxylase, can lead to the hormonal imbalance. Examination of the patient for signs such as hirsutism, androgenetic alopecia, hypertension, and redistribution of subcutaneous fat will aid in the diagnosis. In patients with *acne conglobata*, a more severe form of acne characterized by multiple cysts and bridging scars, an associated inflammatory arthritis has been described.

Exposure to chlorinated aromatic hydrocarbons such as dioxin (TCDD) leads to a particular form of acne known as *chloracne*, which is characterized by open comedones and straw-colored cysts. Patients exposed to dioxin also can develop the signs and symptoms of porphyria cutanea tarda (see "Vesicles"). Exacerbations of acne vulgaris follow the ingestion of several *drugs*, such as iodides, bromides, glucocorticoids, and lithium, as well as the application of oil-containing compounds. Acne-like lesions can be seen in patients with Behçet's disease (see "Ulcers"), and in immunocompromised hosts, disseminated *cryptococcosis* may present as an acneiform eruption.

Patients with the carcinoid syndrome have episodes of flushing of the head, neck, and sometimes the trunk. Resultant skin changes of the face, in particular telangiectasias, mimic the clinical appearance of acne rosacea. Suffusion of the face, as is seen in polycythemia vera, also can be confused with acne rosacea.

PUSTULAR LESIONS *Acneiform eruptions* (see "Acne") and *folliculitis* represent the most common pustular dermatoses. An important consideration in the evaluation of perifollicular pustules is a determination of the associated pathogen (Table 54-11). Noninfectious forms of folliculitis include eosinophilic folliculitis and folliculitis secondary to drugs such as glucocorticoids and lithium. Eosinophilic folliculitis can be seen in HIV-infected individuals, and it is characterized by multiple pruritic lesions on the face and trunk. Administration of high dose oral glucocorticoids can result in a widespread eruption of perifollicular pustules on the trunk, characterized by lesions in the same stage of development. With regard to underlying systemic diseases, pustules are a characteristic component of pustular psoriasis and can be seen in septic emboli of bacterial or fungal origin (see "Purpura"). For example, the cutaneous lesions of disseminated gonococcemia often have a halo of erythema surrounding a central pustule.

TELANGIECTASIAS (Table 54-12) In order to distinguish the various types of telangiectasias, it is important to examine the shape and configuration of the dilated blood vessels. *Linear telangiectasias* are seen on the face of patients with *actinically damaged skin* and *acne rosacea* and are found on the legs of patients with *venous hypertension* and *essential telangiectasia* (Table 54-13). Patients with an unusual form of *mastocytosis* (telangiectasia macularis eruptiva perstans), the *carcinoid* syndrome (see "Acne"), and *ataxia-telangiectasia* also have linear telangiectasias. In ataxia-telangiectasia, linear telangiectasias appear on the bulbar conjunctiva during childhood. Eventually, there is involvement of the ears, eyelids, cheeks, and/or flexural areas such as the antecubital and popliteal fossae. Lastly, linear telangiectasias are found in areas of cutaneous inflammation. For example, lesions of discoid lupus frequently have telangiectasias within them.

TABLE 54-12   Causes of telangiectasias

Primary cutaneous disorders	Systemic diseases
A Linear	*A* Linear
1 Acne rosacea	*1* Carcinoid
2 Actinically damaged skin	*2* Ataxia-telangiectasia
3 Venous hypertension	*3* Mastocytosis
4 Essential telangiectasia	*B* Poikiloderma
B Poikiloderma	*1* Dermatomyositis
1 Ionizing radiation	*2* Xeroderma pigmentosa
2 Poikiloderma vasculare atrophicans	*C* Mat
C Spider angioma	*1* Scleroderma
1 Idiopathic	*D* Periungual
2 Pregnancy	*1* Lupus erythematosus
	2 Scleroderma
	3 Dermatomyositis
	E Papular
	1 Hereditary hemorrhagic telangiectasia
	F Spider angioma
	1 Cirrhosis

TABLE 54-10   Acne (primary cutaneous disorders)

	Clinical characteristics	Pathogenesis
Acne vulgaris	Erythematous papules, pustules, open comedones (black-heads), closed comedones (whiteheads), and cysts Areas that contain sebaceous glands: face, neck, upper trunk	Epithelial hyperproliferation within the infundibulum of the hair follicle leads to comedone formation Additional factors: sebum-derived free fatty acids, *Propionibacterium acnes*
Acne rosacea	Papules, pustules; central face Telangiectasias of nose and cheeks Facial erythema Flushing reaction to hot foods and alcohol Ocular involvement: conjunctivitis, blepharitis, keratitis	Unknown No increased reactivity of cutaneous blood vessels to vasodilators Sebum production normal

TABLE 54-13 Telangiectasias (primary cutaneous disorders)

Type	Associated disorder	Clinical characteristics	Pathogenesis
Linear: Simple red or blue line that disappears with diascopy (pressure)	Acne rosacea	Face Associated with flushing, erythema, papulopustules, and rhinophyma	Vasodilatation
	Actinically damaged skin	Face, arms, upper trunk Associated with hypopigmentation, hyperpigmentation, and keratoses	Damage to supportive connective tissue
	Essential telangiectasia	Netlike sheets Begins on lower extremities May be widespread More common in women	Unknown
Spider angioma: Central pulsating punctum with radiating legs	Idiopathic Pregnancy	Upper half of the body Halo of pallor secondary to local steal phenomenon	Proliferation of blood vessels in association with increased circulating estrogens

Poikiloderma is a term used to describe a patch of skin with (1) reticulated hypo- and hyperpigmentation, (2) wrinkling secondary to epidermal atrophy, and (3) telangiectasias. Poikiloderma does not imply a single disease entity—it is seen in skin damaged by *ionizing radiation*, in the disorders *poikiloderma vasculare atrophicans* (PVA) and *xeroderma pigmentosum*, as well as in patients with connective-tissue diseases, primarily *dermatomyositis*. PVA is a precursor lesion of CTCL, and the areas of poikiloderma usually begin in the flexural areas of the axillae and groin.

In *scleroderma*, the dilated blood vessels have a unique configuration and are known as *mat telangiectasias*. The lesions are broad macules that usually measure 2 to 7 mm in diameter; occasionally, they are larger in size. Mats have a polygonal or oval shape, and their erythematous color may be uniform or the result of delicate telangiectasias. The most common locations for mat telangiectasias are the face, oral mucosa, and hands—peripheral sites that are prone to intermittent ischemia. One theory is that the mats represent a form of neovascularization in these areas. In the CREST variant of scleroderma (see Chap. 286), which is associated with a chronic course and anticentromere antibodies, the *T* stands for telangiectasias. Mat telangiectasias are an important clue to the diagnosis of the CREST syndrome as well as systemic scleroderma, for they may be the only cutaneous finding. A minority of the patients with scleroderma will have telangiectasias indistinguishable from those found in hereditary hemorrhagic telangiectasia (see below).

Periungual telangiectasias are pathognomonic signs of the three major connective tissue diseases—*lupus erythematosus, scleroderma,* and *dermatomyositis* (DM). They are easily visualized by the naked eye, and they occur in at least two-thirds of these patients. In both DM and lupus, there is associated nailfold erythema, and in DM, the erythema is often accompanied by "ragged" cuticles and fingertip tenderness. Under 10× magnification, the blood vessels in the nailfolds of lupus patients are tortuous and resemble "glomeruli," whereas in scleroderma and DM there is a loss of capillary loops and those which remain are markedly dilated.

In *hereditary hemorrhagic telangiectasia* (Osler-Rendu-Weber disease), the lesions usually appear during adulthood and are most commonly seen on the mucous membranes, face, and distal extremities, including under the nails. They represent arteriovenous (AV) malformations of the dermal microvasculature, are dark red in color, and are usually slightly elevated. When the skin is stretched over an individual lesion, an eccentric punctum with radiating legs is seen. Although the degree of systemic involvement varies in this autosomal dominant disease, the major symptoms are recurrent epistaxis and gastrointestinal bleeding. The fact that these mucosal telangiectasias are actually AV communications helps to explain their tendency to bleed.

HYPOPIGMENTATION (Table 54-14) Disorders of hypopigmentation are classified as either diffuse or localized. The classic example of *diffuse* hypopigmentation is *oculocutaneous albinism* (OCA). The two most common forms are tyrosinase-negative OCA and tyrosinase-positive OCA; the former is characterized by a lack of enzyme

TABLE 54-14 Causes of hypopigmentation

Primary cutaneous disorders	Systemic diseases
A Diffuse	A Diffuse
1 Generalized vitiligo	*1* Oculocutaneous albinism
B Localized	B Localized
1 Vitiligo	*1* Vogt-Koyanagi-Harada
2 Chemical leukoderma	*2* Scleroderma
3 Piebaldism	*3* Melanoma-associated leukoderma
4 Nevus depigmentosus	*4* Tuberous sclerosis
5 Postinflammatory	*5* Hypomelanosis of Ito
6 Tinea versicolor	*6* Sarcoidosis
	7 Tuberculoid leprosy
	8 Cutaneous T cell lymphoma

activity. At birth, both types of OCA appear similar—white hair, gray-blue eyes, and pink-white skin. The patients with tyrosinase-negative OCA maintain this phenotype, whereas those with tyrosinase-positive OCA will acquire some pigmentation of the eyes, hair, and skin as they age. The degree of pigment formation is a function of their racial background, but a pigmentary dilution is readily apparent when they are compared to their first-degree relatives.

The ocular findings in OCA correlate with the degree of hypopigmentation, and they include decreased visual acuity, nystagmus, photophobia, and monocular vision. Patients with OCA, particularly those who reside in the tropics, develop cutaneous squamous cell carcinomas in association with severe actinic damage. The diagnosis of tyrosinase-positive OCA in a patient from Puerto Rico (Arecibo region) or southern Holland raises the possibility of the Hermansky-Pudlak syndrome. In addition to the signs and symptoms of OCA, these patients have a bleeding diathesis secondary to a platelet storage pool defect and restrictive lung disease secondary to deposits of ceroidlike material. Patients with Chédiak-Higashi syndrome also have tyrosinase-positive OCA, but their giant lysosomal granules fail to eradicate common pathogens such as *Staphylococcus aureus*. Generalized vitiligo, phenylketonuria, and homocystinuria are other unusual causes of diffuse pigmentary dilution. In generalized vitiligo, melanocytes are not found in affected skin, whereas in OCA they are present but have decreased activity. Appropriate laboratory tests exclude the other disorders of metabolism.

The differential diagnosis of *localized* hypomelanosis includes the following primary cutaneous disorders: *vitiligo, chemical leukoderma, piebaldism, nevus depigmentosus* (see below), *postinflammatory hypomelanosis,* and *tinea versicolor* (Table 54-15). In this group of diseases, the areas of involvement are macules or patches with a decrease or absence of pigmentation, and in the first four disorders, secondary changes such as scale or crust are absent. Patients with vitiligo have an increased incidence of several autoimmune disorders, including hypothyroidism, Graves' disease, pernicious anemia, Addison's disease, uveitis, alopecia areata, chronic mucocutaneous candidiasis, and the polyglandular autoimmune syndromes (types I, II, and III). Diseases of the thyroid gland are the most frequently associated disorders, occurring in up to 30 percent of patients with vitiligo.

TABLE 54-15   Hypopigmentation (primary cutaneous disorders, localized)

	Clinical characteristics	Wood's lamp examination (UV-A: peak = 365 nm)	Skin biopsy	Pathogenesis
Vitiligo	Acquired; progressive Symmetric areas of complete pigment loss Periorifical—around mouth, nose, eyes, nipples, umbilicus, anus Other areas—flexor wrists, extensor distal extremities Segmental form is less common—unilateral, dermatomal-like	More apparent Chalk-white	Absence of melanocytes Minimal inflammation	Possible autoimmune phenomenon that results in destruction of melanocytes—humoral and/or cellular Alternative hypothesis is self-destruction of melanocytes and circulating antibodies against melanocytes as a secondary phenomenon
Chemical leukoderma	Similar appearance to vitiligo Often begins on hands Satellite lesions in areas not exposed to chemicals	More apparent Chalk-white	Decreased number or absence of melanocytes	Exposure to chemicals that selectively destroy melanocytes, in particular, phenols and catechols (germicides; rubber products) Release of cellular antigens and activation of circulating lymphocytes may explain satellite phenomenon
Piebaldism	Autosomal dominant Congenital, stable White forelock Areas of hypomelanosis contain normally pigmented and hyperpigmented macules of various sizes Symmetric involvement of central forehead, ventral trunk, and mid regions of upper and lower extremities	Enhancement of leukoderma and hyperpigmented macules	Hypomelanotic areas—few to no melanocytes	Defect in migration of melanoblasts from neural crest to ventral skin or failure of melanoblasts to survive or differentiate in these areas Mutations within the *c-kit* proto-oncogene that encodes the tyrosine kinase receptor for mast/stem cell growth factor
Postinflammatory	Hypopigmentation can develop within active lesions, as in subacute lupus, or after the lesion fades, as in dermatitis	Depends on particular disease Usually less enhancement than in vitiligo	Type of inflammatory infiltrate depends on specific disease	Block in transfer of melanin from melanocytes to keratinocytes could be secondary to edema or decrease in contact time Destruction of melanocytes if inflammatory cells attack basal layer
Tinea versicolor	Common disorder Upper trunk and neck Shawl-like distribution Young adults Macules have fine white scale when scratched	Golden fluorescence	Hyphae and spores in stratum corneum	Invasion of stratum corneum by the yeast *Pityrosporum* Yeast is lipophilic and produces C_9 and C_{11} dicarboxylic acids which in vitro inhibit tyrosinase

Circulating autoantibodies are often found, and the most common ones are antithyroglobulin, antimicrosomal, and antiparietal cell antibodies.

There are three systemic diseases that should be considered in a patient with skin findings suggestive of vitiligo—*Vogt-Koyanagi-Harada syndrome*, *scleroderma*, and *melanoma-associated leukoderma*. A history of aseptic meningitis, nontraumatic uveitis, tinnitus, hearing loss, and/or dysacusis points to the diagnosis of the Vogt-Koyanagi-Harada syndrome. In these patients, the face and scalp are the most common locations of pigment loss. The vitiligo-like leukoderma seen in patients with scleroderma has a clinical resemblance to idiopathic vitiligo that has begun to repigment as a result of treatment; that is, perifollicular macules of normal pigmentation are seen within areas of depigmentation. The basis of this leukoderma is unknown; there is no evidence of inflammation in areas of involvement, but it can resolve if the underlying connective-tissue disease becomes inactive. In contrast to idiopathic vitiligo, melanoma-associated leukoderma often begins on the trunk, and its appearance should prompt a search for metastatic disease. The possibility exists that the destruction of normal melanocytes is the result of an immune response against malignant melanocytes.

There are two systemic disorders that may have the cutaneous findings of piebaldism (partial albinism) (see Table 54-15). They are *Hirschsprung's disease* and *Waardenburg's syndrome*. A possible explanation for both disorders is an abnormal embryonic migration or survival of two neural crest–derived elements, one of them being

melanocytes and the other myenteric ganglion cells (Hirschsprung's disease) or auditory nerve cells (Waardenburg's syndrome). The latter syndrome is characterized by congenital sensorineural hearing loss, dystopia canthorum (lateral displacement of the inner canthi but normal interpupillary distance), heterochromic irises, and a broad nasal root, in addition to the piebaldism.

In *tuberous sclerosis*, the earliest cutaneous sign is the ash leaf spot. These lesions are often present at birth; however, detection may require Wood's lamp examination, especially in fair-skinned individuals. The pigment within them is reduced but not absent. The average size is 1 to 3 cm, and the common shapes are oval, polygonal, and lance-ovate, whereas the less common shapes are dermatomal and confettilike. The terms *lance-ovate* and *ash leaf* are used to describe lesions with a particular shape, that is, tapered at one end and round at the other. Examination of the patient for additional cutaneous signs such as adenoma sebaceum (multiple angiofibromas of the face), ungual and gingival fibromas, fibrous plaques of the forehead, and connective-tissue nevi (shagreen patches) is recommended. It is important to remember that an ash leaf spot on the scalp will result in poliosis, which is a circumscribed patch of gray-white hair. Internal manifestations include seizures, mental retardation, central nervous system (CNS) and retinal hamartomas, renal angiomyolipomas, and cardiac rhabdomyomas. The latter can be detected in up to 60 percent of children (<18 years) with tuberous sclerosis by echocardiography.

Nevus depigmentosus is a stable, well-circumscribed hypomelanosis that is present at birth. There is usually a single circular or rectangular lesion, but occasionally, the nevus has a dermatomal or whorled pattern. It is important to distinguish this lesion from an ash leaf spot or hypomelanosis of Ito, for it is rarely associated with CNS findings. *Hypomelanosis of Ito* (incontinentia pigmenti achromians) is a neurocutaneous disorder in which swirls and streaks of hypopigmentation run parallel to one another. The pattern resembles that of a marble cake. Associated abnormalities are found in the musculoskeletal system (asymmetry), the CNS (seizures and mental retardation), and the eyes (strabismus and hypertelorism). Chromosomal mosaicism and diploid/triploid mixoploidy have been reported in these patients; this lends support to the hypothesis that the pattern is the result of the migration of two clones of primordial melanocytes, each with a different pigment potential.

Localized areas of decreased pigmentation are commonly seen as a result of cutaneous inflammation (see Table 54-15) and have been observed in the skin overlying active lesions of *sarcoidosis* (see ''Papulonodular Skin Lesions'') as well as *CTLC*. Cutaneous infections also present as disorders of hypopigmentation, and in *tuberculoid leprosy* there are a few asymmetric patches of hypomelanosis that have associated anesthesia, anhidrosis, and alopecia. Biopsy specimens of the palpable border show dermal granulomas that lack *Mycobacterium leprae* organisms.

HYPERPIGMENTATION (Table 54-16) Disorders of hyperpigmentation are also divided into two groups—localized and diffuse. The *localized* forms are due to an epidermal alteration, a proliferation of melanocytes, or an increase in pigment production. Both *seborrheic keratoses* and *acanthosis nigricans* belong to the first group (Table

---

TABLE 54-16 Causes of hyperpigmentation

Primary cutaneous disorders
A Localized
  1 Epidermal alteration
    a Seborrheic keratosis
    b Acanthosis nigricans (obesity)
    c Pigmented actinic keratosis
  2 Proliferation of melanocytes
    a Lentigo
    b Nevus
    c Melanoma
  3 Increased pigment production
    a Ephelides (freckles)
    b Café au lait spots
B Localized and diffuse
  1 Drugs
Systemic diseases
A Localized
  1 Epidermal alteration
    a Seborrheic keratoses (sign of Leser-Trélat)
    b Acanthosis nigricans (endocrine disorders, paraneoplastic)
  2 Proliferation of melanocytes
    a Lentigines (Peutz-Jeghers, LEOPARD syndromes)
    b Nevi (LAMB and NAME syndromes)
  3 Increased pigment production
    a Café au lait spots (neurofibromatosis, Albright's syndrome)
    b Urticaria pigmentosa (see ''Papulonodular Skin Lesions'')
  4 Dermal pigmentation
    a Incontinentia pigmenti
    b Dyskeratosis congenita
B Diffuse
  1 Endocrinopathies
    a Addison's disease
    b Nelson's syndrome
    c Ectopic ACTH syndrome
  2 Metabolic
    a Porphyria cutanea tarda
    b Hemochromatosis
    c Vitamin B_{12}, folate deficiency
    d Pellagra
    e Malabsorption, Whipple's disease
  3 Melanosis secondary to metastatic melanoma
  4 Autoimmune
    a Biliary cirrhosis
    b Scleroderma
    c POEMS syndrome
  5 Drugs and metals

54-17). Seborrheic keratoses are common lesions, but in one clinical setting they are a sign of systemic disease, and that setting is the sudden appearance of multiple lesions, often in association with acrochordons (skin tags) and acanthosis nigricans. This is termed the *sign of Leser-Trélat*, and it signifies an internal malignancy. *Acanthosis nigricans* also can be a reflection of an internal malignancy, most commonly of the gastrointestinal tract, and it appears as velvety hyperpigmentation (see Table 54-17). In the majority of patients, acanthosis nigricans is associated with obesity, but it may be a reflection of an endocrinopathy such as acromegaly, Cushing's syndrome, the Stein-Leventhal syndrome, or insulin-resistant diabetes mellitus (type A, type B, and lipoatrophic forms).

A proliferation of melanocytes results in the following pigmented lesions: *lentigo*, *melanocytic nevus*, and *melanoma* (see Table 54-17). In an adult, the majority of lentigines are related to sun exposure, which explains their distribution. However, in the Peutz-Jeghers and LEOPARD syndromes, lentigines do serve as a clue to systemic disease. The lentigines in patients with *Peutz-Jeghers syndrome* are located primarily around the nose and mouth, on the hands and feet, and within the oral cavity. While the pigmented macules on the face may fade with age, the oral lesions persist. However, similar intraoral lesions are also seen in Addison's disease and as a normal finding in darkly pigmented individuals. Patients with this autosomal dominant syndrome have multiple benign polyps of the gastrointestinal tract, ovarian tumors, and an approximately 6 percent risk of developing a gastrointestinal malignancy when the polyps arise in the stomach, duodenum, or colon.

In the multiple lentigines or *LEOPARD syndrome*, hundreds of lentigines develop during childhood and are scattered over the entire surface of the body. The syndrome consists of *L*, lentigines; *E*, ECG abnormalities, primarily conduction defects; *O*, ocular hypertelorism; *P*, pulmonary stenosis and subaortic valvular stenosis; *A*, abnormal genitalia (cryptorchidism, hypospadias); *R*, retardation of growth; and *D*, deafness (sensorineural). Lentigines are also seen in association with cardiac myxomas and have been described under the mnemonics *LAMB syndrome* and *NAME syndrome*. The findings in these two syndromes overlap and include *L*, lentigines; *A*, atrial myxomas; *M*, mucocutaneous myxomas; and *B*, blue nevi versus *N*, nevus; *A*, atrial myxoma; *M*, myxoid neurofibroma, and *E*, ephelides (freckles). These patients also can have evidence of endocrine overactivity in the form of Cushing's syndrome, acromegaly, or sexual precocity.

The third type of localized hyperpigmentation is due to a local increase in pigment production, and it includes *ephelides* (see Table 54-17) and café au lait spots. The latter are most commonly associated with two disorders—neurofibromatosis (NF) and Albright's syndrome. *Café au lait* (CAL) *spots* are flat, uniformly light brown in color, and can vary in size from 0.5 to 12 cm. Approximately 80 percent of the patients with *type I NF* will have six or more CAL spots measuring 1.5 cm or greater in diameter. Additional findings are discussed in the section on neurofibromas (see ''Papulonodular Skin Lesions''). In comparison with NF, the CAL spots in patients with *Albright's disease* (polyostotic fibrous dysplasia with precocious puberty in females) are usually larger, more irregular in outline, respect the midline, and rarely contain macromelanosomes. CAL spots also have been associated with pulmonary stenosis, temporal dysrhythmia, tuberous sclerosis, the LEOPARD syndrome, and ataxia telangiectasia, but a few such lesions can be found in normal individuals.

In incontinentia pigmenti, dyskeratosis congenita, and bleomycin pigmentation, the areas of localized hyperpigmentation form a pattern—swirled in the first, reticulated in the second, and flagellate in the third. Patients with the X-linked dominant disorder *incontinentia pigmenti* can have linear blisters and verrucous papules during infancy. During childhood, parallel swirls and streaks of hyperpigmentation appear on the trunk, and occasionally streaks of hypopigmentation appear on the extremities. Associated findings include seizures, mental retardation, strabismus, cataracts, and delayed or impaired dentition. Biopsy of the streaks will show pigment within dermal macrophages (''incontinent pigment''). In *dyskeratosis congenita*, atrophic reticu-

TABLE 54-17   Hyperpigmentation (primary cutaneous disorders, localized)

	Clinical characteristics	Histopathology
Seborrheic keratosis	Tan to black papule Warty and/or greasy surface "Stuck on" appearance Trunk	Epidermal hyperplasia
Acanthosis nigricans	Velvety surface Neck, axillae, groin Occasionally on dorsum of the hand, corners of mouth	Epidermal folds Increased pigment in basal layer

Pigmented actinic keratosis	Brown macule, 3–10 mm
	Rough scale
	Sun-exposed areas, in particular
	  face and dorsum of hand
		Dysplasia of keratinocytes in lower third
		  of epidermis
		Increased pigment in epidermis

Ephelides (freckles)	2–5-mm macule Tan color Sun-exposed surfaces Darkens following sun exposure	Increased pigment in epidermis
Lentigo	0.3–1.5-cm macule Tan to black Most commonly in sun-exposed areas Face, upper trunk, and extremities	Increased number of melanocytes in epidermis Increased pigment in epidermis
Nevus		
Junctional	Brown to black macule 2–6 mm	Nests of melanocytes at dermoepidermal junction
Compound	Tan to brown papule 2–6 mm	Nests of melanocytes in epidermis and dermis
Dermal	Flesh-colored Papule	Nests of melanocytes in dermis
Melanoma	Variation in color—brown, black, blue, red, white Irregular outline and surface >5 mm in diameter Asymmetric	Malignant neoplasm of melanocytes

lated hyperpigmentation is seen on the neck, thighs, and trunk, and it is accompanied by nail dystrophy, pancytopenia, and leukoplakia of the oral and anal mucosa. The latter often develops into squamous cell carcinoma. In addition to the flagellate pigmentation (linear streaks) on the trunk, patients receiving bleomycin often have hyperpigmentation on the elbows, knees, and small joints of the hand.

Localized hyperpigmentation is seen as a side effect of several other *systemic medications*, including those which produce fixed drug reactions (phenolphthalein, tetracyclines, sulfonamides, barbiturates, and analgesics) and those which can bind to melanin (antimalarials). Fixed drug eruptions recur in the same location as circular areas of erythema that can become bullous and then resolve as brown macules. The eruption usually appears within hours of administration of the offending agent, and common locations include the genitalia, extremities, and perioral region. Chloroquine and hydroxychloroquine produce gray-brown to blue-black discoloration of the shins, hard palate, and face, while blue macules are seen on the lower extremities and in sites of inflammation with prolonged minocycline administration. Estrogen in oral contraceptives can induce melasma—symmetric brown patches on the face, especially the cheeks, upper lip, and forehead. Similar changes are seen in pregnancy, in patients receiving hydantoin, and in the adult form of Gaucher's disease. In the latter group there is also hyperpigmentation of the distal lower extremities.

In the *diffuse* forms of hyperpigmentation, the darkening of the skin may be of equal intensity over the entire body, or it may be accentuated in sun-exposed areas. The causes of diffuse hyperpigmentation can be divided into four groups—endocrine, metabolic, autoimmune, and drugs. The endocrinopathies that frequently have associated hyperpigmentation include *Addison's disease, Nelson's syndrome,* and *ectopic ACTH syndrome.* In these diseases, the increased pigmentation is diffuse, but it is accentuated in the palmar creases, sites of friction, scars, and the oral mucosa. An overproduction of any or all of the pituitary hormones α-MSH (melanocyte-stimulating hormone), ACTH, and β-lipotropin can lead to an increase in melanocyte activity. All these peptides are products of the proopiomelanocortin gene, and therefore, they exhibit homology; e.g., α-MSH and ACTH share 13 amino acids. A minority of the patients with Cushing's disease or hyperthyroidism have generalized hyperpigmentation.

The metabolic causes of hyperpigmentation include *porphyria*

cutanea tarda (PCT), *hemochromatosis, vitamin B₁₂ deficiency, folic acid deficiency, pellagra, malabsorption,* and *Whipple's disease.* In patients with *PCT* (see "Vesicles/Bullae"), the skin darkening is seen in sun-exposed areas and is a reflection of the photoreactive properties of porphyrins. The increased level of iron in the skin of patients with *hemochromatosis* stimulates melanin pigment production and leads to the classic bronze color. Patients with *pellagra* have a brown discoloration of the skin, especially in sun-exposed areas, as a result of nicotinic acid (niacin) deficiency. In the areas of increased pigmentation, there is a thin varnishlike scale. These changes are also seen in patients who are vitamin B₆ deficient, have functioning carcinoid tumors (increased consumption of niacin), or take isoniazid. Approximately 50 percent of the patients with *Whipple's disease* have an associated generalized hyperpigmentation in association with diarrhea, weight loss, arthritis, and lymphadenopathy. A diffuse slate-blue color is seen in patients with melanosis secondary to *metastatic melanoma.* There is a debate as to whether the color is due to single-cell metastases in the dermis or to a widespread deposition of melanin resulting from the high concentration of circulating melanin precursors.

Of the autoimmune diseases associated with diffuse hyperpigmentation, *biliary cirrhosis* and *scleroderma* are the most common, and occasionally, both disorders are seen in the same patient. The skin is dark brown in color, especially in sun-exposed areas. In biliary cirrhosis the hyperpigmentation is accompanied by pruritus, jaundice, and xanthomas, whereas in scleroderma it is accompanied by sclerosis of the extremities, face, and, less commonly, the trunk. Additional clues to the diagnosis of scleroderma are telangiectasias, calcinosis cutis, Raynaud's phenomenon, and distal ulcerations (see "Telangiectasias"). The differential diagnosis of cutaneous sclerosis with hyperpigmentation includes the *POEMS syndrome*: P, polyneuropathy; O, organomegaly (liver, spleen, lymph nodes); E, endocrinopathies (impotence, gynecomastia); M, M-protein; and S, skin changes. The skin changes include hyperpigmentation, skin thickening, hypertrichosis, hyperhidrosis, and angiomas.

Diffuse hyperpigmentation that is due to *drugs* or *metals* can result from one of several mechanisms—induction of melanin pigment formation, complexing of the drug or its metabolites to melanin, and deposits of the drug in the dermis. Busulfan; cyclophosphamide;

long-term, high-dose ACTH; and inorganic arsenic induce pigment production. Complexes containing melanin or hemosiderin plus the drug or its metabolites are seen in patients receiving chlorpromazine and minocycline. The sun-exposed skin as well as the conjunctivae of patients on long-term, high-dose chlorpromazine can become blue-gray in color. Patients taking minocycline may develop a diffuse blue-gray, muddy appearance in sun-exposed areas in addition to pigmentation of the mucous membranes, teeth, nails, bones, and thyroid. Administration of amiodorone can result in both a phototoxic eruption (exaggerated sunburn) and/or a brown or blue-gray discoloration of sun-exposed skin. Biopsy specimens of the latter show yellow-brown granules in dermal macrophages, which represent intralysosomal accumulations of lipids, amiodarone, and its metabolites. Actual deposits of a particular drug or metal in the skin are seen with silver (argyria), where the skin appears blue-gray in color; gold (chrysiasis), where the skin has a brown to blue-gray color; and clofazimine, where the skin appears reddish brown. The associated hyperpigmentation is accentuated in sun-exposed areas, and discoloration of the eye is seen with gold (sclerae) and clofazimine (conjunctivae). Recently, an epidemic of the eosinophilia-myalgia syndrome has been described that is presumably due to contaminated L-tryptophan preparations. In addition to maculopapular eruptions and alopecia, large areas of sclerodermalike induration are observed with overlying hyperpigmentation.

VESICLES/BULLAE (Table 54-18) Depending on their size, cutaneous blisters are referred to as *vesicles* (<0.5 cm) or *bullae* (>0.5 cm). The primary blistering disorders include *pemphigus vulgaris, pemphigus foliaceus, pemphigus erythematosus, bullous pemphigoid, herpes gestationis, cicatricial pemphigoid, epidermolysis bullosa acquisita,* and *dermatitis herpetiformis* (see Chap. 53).

Vesicles and bullae are also seen in *contact dermatitis,* both allergic and irritant forms (see "Erythroderma"). When there is a linear arrangement of vesicular lesions, an exogenous cause should be suspected. Bullous disease secondary to the ingestion of drugs can take one of several forms, including phototoxic eruptions, isolated bullae, toxic epidermal necrolysis, and erythema multiforme. Clinically, phototoxic eruptions resemble an exaggerated sunburn with diffuse erythema and bullae in sun-exposed areas. The most commonly associated drugs are thiazides, tetracyclines, sulfonylureas, sulfonamides, phenothiazines, griseofulvin, and psoralens. The development of a phototoxic eruption is dependent on the doses of both the drug and UV-A irradiation.

There are several drugs, including penicillins, sulfonamides, phenobarbital, phenytoin, furosemide, and nonsteroidal anti-inflammatory agents, that cause isolated bland bullae to arise on normal skin. The characteristics of these blisters are such that they cannot

be assigned to a particular cutaneous disease. The most common location for these isolated bullae is the distal extremity. In contrast, *toxic epidermal necrolysis* (TEN) is characterized by bullae that arise on widespread areas of erythema and then slough. This results in large areas of denuded skin. The associated morbidity, such as sepsis, and mortality are relatively high, and they are a function of the extent of epidermal necrosis. In addition, these patients also may have involvement of the mucous membranes and intestinal tract. Drugs are the primary cause of TEN, and the most common offenders are phenytoin, barbiturates, sulfonamides, penicillins, allopurinol, and phenylbutazone. Severe acute graft-versus-host disease (grade 4) also can resemble TEN.

In *erythema multiforme* (EM), the primary lesions are pink-red macules and edematous papules, the centers of which may become vesicular. The clue to the diagnosis of EM rather than of a drug-induced morbilliform exanthem is the development of a "dusky" violet color or petechiae in the center of the lesions. Target or iris lesions are also characteristic of EM, and they arise as a result of active centers and borders in combination with centrifugal spread. However, iris lesions need not be present to make the diagnosis of EM. Preferred sites of involvement include the hands, extensor forearms, palms, soles, and mucous membranes (oral, nasal, ocular, and genital). Hemorrhagic crusts of the lips are characteristic of EM, as well as two other blistering disorders—pemphigus vulgaris and TEN. Fever, malaise, myalgias, sore throat, and cough may precede or accompany the eruption. The lesions of EM usually resolve over 3 to 6 weeks, but they may be recurrent.

Drugs can induce EM, in particular sulfonamides, phenytoin, barbiturates, penicillins, and carbamazepine, but they do not cause the majority of cases, especially in young adults. Infections with herpes simplex are the most common cause of EM in this age group, and the lesions appear 7 to 12 days after the viral eruption. Other infectious agents associated with EM include *Mycoplasma pneumoniae, Histoplasma capsulatum, Coccidioides immitis, Yersinia enterocolitica,* and several viruses (echovirus, coxsackievirus, Epstein-Barr, and influenza). EM also can follow vaccinations with BCG, poliomyelitis, or vaccinia viruses; radiation therapy; and exposure to environmental toxins; and it has been observed in a few patients with lupus erythematosus, Wegener's granulomatosis, and internal malignancy.

In addition to primary blistering disorders and hypersensitivity reactions, bacterial and viral infections can lead to vesicles and bullae. The most common infectious agents are herpes simplex (see Chap. 143), herpes varicella-zoster (see Chap. 144), and staphylococci (see Chap. 102).

Staphylococcal scalded-skin syndrome (SSSS) and *bullous impetigo* are two blistering disorders associated with staphylococcal (phage group II) infection. In SSSS, the initial findings are redness and tenderness of the central face, neck, trunk, and intertriginous zones. This is followed by short-lived flaccid bullae and a slough or exfoliation of the superficial epidermis. Crusted areas then develop, characteristically around the mouth. SSSS is distinguished from TEN by the following features: younger age group, more superficial site of blister formation, no oral lesions, shorter course, less morbidity and mortality, and an association with staphylococcal exfoliative toxin ("exfoliatin"), not drugs. A rapid diagnosis of SSSS versus TEN can be made by a frozen section of the blister roof or exfoliative cytology of the blister contents. In SSSS the site of staphylococcal infection is usually extracutaneous (conjunctivitis, rhinorrhea, otitis media, pharyngitis, tonsillitis), and the lesions are sterile, whereas in *bullous impetigo* the lesions are the site of infection. Impetigo is more localized than SSSS, and it usually presents with honey-colored crusts. Occasionally, superficial purulent blisters also form. *Cutaneous emboli* from gram-negative infections may present as isolated bullae, but the base of the lesion is purpuric or necrotic, and it may develop into an ulcer (see "Purpura").

Several metabolic disorders are associated with blister formation, including diabetes mellitus, renal failure, and porphyria. Local

---

TABLE 54-18 Causes of vesicles/bullae

Primary cutaneous diseases	Systemic diseases
A Primary blistering diseases	A Infections
1 Pemphigus*	*1* Cutaneous emboli†
2 Bullous pemphigoid†	B Metabolic
3 Herpes gestationis†	*1* Diabetic bullae*,†
4 Cicatricial pemphigoid†	*2* Porphyria cutanea tarda†
5 Dermatitis herpetiformis†	*3* Porphyria variegata†
6 Epidermolysis bullosa†	*4* Pseudoporphyria†
acquisita	*5* Bullous dermatosis of
B Secondary blistering diseases	hemodialysis†
1 Contact*	
2 Erythema multiforme*,†	
3 Toxic epidermal ne-	
crolysis*,†	
C Infections	
1 Varicella/zoster*,‡	
2 Herpes simplex*,‡	
3 Staphylococcal scalded-skin	
syndrome*	
4 Bullous impetigo*	

* Intraepidermal. † Subepidermal. ‡ Also systemic.

hypoxia secondary to decreased cutaneous blood flow also can produce blisters, which explains the presence of bullae over pressure points in comatose patients (coma bullae). In *diabetes mellitus*, tense bullae with clear viscous fluid arise on normal skin. The lesions can be as large as 6 cm in diameter, and they are located on the distal extremities. There are several types of porphyria, but the most common form with cutaneous findings is *porphyria cutanea tarda* (PCT). In sun-exposed areas (primarily the face and hands), the skin is very fragile, and trauma leads to erosions and tense vesicles. These lesions then heal with scarring and formation of milia; the latter are firm, 2- to 3-mm white or yellow papules that represent epidermoid inclusion cysts. Associated findings can include hypertrichosis of the lateral malar region (males) or face (females) and, in sun-exposed areas, hyperpigmentation and firm sclerotic plaques. An elevated level of urinary uroporphyrins confirms the diagnosis and is due to a decrease in uroporphyrinogen decarboxylase activity. Precipitating agents include alcohol, estrogen, iron, and chlorinated hydrocarbons.

The differential diagnosis of PCT includes (1) *porphyria variegata*—the skin signs of PCT plus the systemic findings of acute intermittent porphyria; it has a diagnostic plasma porphyrin fluorescence emission at 626 nm; (2) *drug-induced bullous photosensitivity* (pseudoporphyria)—the clinical and histologic findings are similar to PCT, but porphyrins are normal; etiologic agents are furosemide, tetracycline, nalidixic acid, dapsone, naproxen, and pyridoxine; (3) *bullous dermatosis of hemodialysis*—the same appearance as PCT, but porphyrins are usually normal or occasionally borderline elevated; patients have chronic renal failure and are on hemodialysis; (4) PCT associated with hepatomas, hepatic carcinomas, and hemodialysis; and (5) *epidermolysis bullosa acquisita* (see Chap. 53).

EXANTHEMS (Table 54-19)   Exanthems are characterized by an acute generalized eruption. The two most common presentations are erythematous macules and papules (morbilliform) and confluent blanching erythema (scarlatiniform). *Morbilliform* eruptions are usually due to either *drugs* or *viral infections*. For example, at least 5 percent of the patients receiving penicillins, sulfonamides, captopril, phenytoin, or gold will develop a maculopapular eruption. Accompanying signs may include pruritus, fever, eosinophilia, and transient lymphadenopathy. Similar maculopapular eruptions are seen in the classic childhood viral exanthems, including (1) *rubeola* (measles)— a prodrome of coryza, cough, conjunctivitis, and Koplik's spots on the buccal mucosa whose onset coincides with a second fever spike; the eruption begins behind the ears, at the hairline, and on the forehead and then spreads down the body, often becoming confluent; (2) *rubella*—it begins on the forehead and face and then spreads down the body; it resolves in the same order and is associated with retroauricular and suboccipital lymphadenopathy; and (3) *erythema infectiosum* (fifth disease)—erythema of the cheeks is followed by a reticulated pattern on extremities; it is secondary to a parvovirus infection, and an associated arthritis is seen in adults.

TABLE 54-19   Causes of exanthems

Morbilliform
 A Drugs
 B Viral
   1 Rubeola (measles)
   2 Rubella
   3 Erythema infectiosum
   4 Epstein-Barr, echovirus, coxsackievirus, and adenovirus
   5 Early HIV
 C Bacterial
   1 Typhoid fever
   2 Early secondary syphilis
   3 Early *Rickettsia*
   4 Early meningococcus
 D Acute graft-versus-host disease
Scarlatiniform
 A Scarlet fever
 B Toxic shock syndrome
 C Kawasaki's disease

Both measles and rubella are seen in unvaccinated young adults, and an atypical form of measles is seen in adults immunized with either killed measles vaccine or killed vaccine followed in time by live vaccine. In contrast to classic measles, the eruption of atypical measles begins on the palms, soles, wrists, and knuckles, and the lesions may become purpuric. The patient with atypical measles can have pulmonary involvement and be quite ill. Rubelliform and roseoliform eruptions are also associated with *Epstein-Barr virus* (5 to 15 percent of patients), *echovirus, coxsackievirus,* and *adenovirus* infections. Detection of specific IgM antibodies allows the proper diagnosis. Occasionally, a maculopapular eruption is the result of a drug-viral interaction. For example, about 95 percent of the patients with infectious mononucleosis who are given ampicillin will develop a rash.

Of note, early in the course of infections with *Rickettsia* and *meningococcus*, prior to the development of purpura, the lesions may be erythematous macules and papules. This is also the case in chickenpox prior to the development of vesicles. Maculopapular eruptions are associated with early *HIV infection*, early secondary *syphilis, typhoid fever,* and *acute graft-versus-host* disease. In the last, lesions frequently begin on the palms and soles; the macular rose spots of typhoid fever involve primarily the anterior trunk.

The prototypic *scarlatiniform* eruption is seen in *scarlet fever* and is due to an erythrotoxin produced by group A beta-hemolytic streptococcal infections, most commonly pharyngitis. There are a diffuse erythema, which begins on the neck and upper trunk, and red perifollicular puncta. Additional findings include a white strawberry tongue (white coating with red papillae) followed by a red strawberry tongue (red tongue with red papillae), petechiae of the palate, a facial flush with circumoral pallor, linear petechiae in the antecubital fossae, and desquamation of the involved skin, palms, and soles 5 to 20 days after onset of the eruption. A similar desquamation of the palms and soles is seen in toxic shock syndrome, Kawasaki's disease, and after severe febrile illnesses. Certain strains of staphylococci also produce an erythrotoxin that leads to the same clinical findings as in streptococcal scarlet fever, except that the antistreptolysin O titers are not elevated.

In *toxic shock syndrome* (TSS), staphylococcal (phage group I) infections produce an exotoxin that causes the fever and rash, as well as an enterotoxin. Initially, the majority of cases were reported in menstruating women who were using tampons. However, other sites of infection, including wounds and vaginitis, may produce TSS. The diagnosis of TSS is based on clinical criteria, and three of these involve mucocutaneous sites. The clinical criteria are (1) fever, (2) diffuse erythema of the skin, (3) desquamation of the palms and soles 1 to 2 weeks after onset of illness, (4) hypotension, and (5) involvement of three or more organ systems, including the gastrointestinal tract, muscles, kidney, liver, CNS, hematologic (thrombocytopenia), and mucous membranes. The latter is characterized as hyperemia of the vagina, oropharynx, or conjunctivae.

Although the cutaneous eruption in *Kawasaki's disease* (mucocutaneous lymph node syndrome) is polymorphous, the two common types are morbilliform and scarlatiniform. The majority of cases are seen in children less than 5 years of age, but adult cases have been reported. The diagnosis is based on a fever lasting more than 5 days plus four of the five following criteria: (1) bilateral conjunctival injection, (2) exanthem, (3) cervical lymphadenopathy, usually unilateral, (4) erythema and edema of the hands and feet followed by desquamation, and (5) diffuse erythema of the oropharynx, red strawberry tongue, and erosions with crusting on the lips. This clinical picture can resemble TSS and scarlet fever, but clues to the diagnosis of Kawasaki's disease are the cervical lymphadenopathy, lip erosions, and increased platelets. The most serious associated systemic finding in this disease is coronary aneurysm secondary to arteritis. Aneurysms may lead to sudden death, primarily within the first 30 days of the illness. Scarlatiniform eruptions are also seen in the early phase of SSSS (see "Vesicles/Bullae") and as reactions to drugs.

TABLE 54-20 Causes of urticaria

Primary cutaneous disorders
A Acute and chronic urticaria
B Physical urticaria
   1 Dermatographism
   2 Solar urticaria*
   3 Cold urticaria*
   4 Cholinergic urticaria*
C Angioedema (hereditary and acquired)*
Systemic diseases
A Urticarial vasculitis
B Hepatitis B infection
C Serum sickness
D Angioedema (acquired)

* Also systemic.

URTICARIA (Table 54-20) *Urticaria* (hives) are transient lesions that are composed of a central wheal surrounded by an erythematous halo. Individual lesions are round, oval, or figurate, and they are often pruritic. *Acute* and *chronic* urticaria have a wide variety of allergic etiologies. Less common systemic causes of urticaria are mastocytosis (urticaria pigmentosa), hyperthyroidism, malignancy, and juvenile rheumatoid arthritis (JRA). In JRA, the lesions coincide with the fever spike, and they are transient but not migratory as in erythema marginatum.

The common *physical urticarias* include *dermatographism*, *solar urticaria*, *cold urticaria*, and *cholinergic urticaria*. Patients with dermatographism exhibit linear wheals following minor pressure or scratching of the skin. It is a common disorder, affecting approximately 5 percent of the population. Solar urticaria characteristically occurs within minutes of sun exposure and is a skin sign of one systemic disease—erythropoietic protoporphyria. In addition to the urticaria, these patients have subtle pitted scarring of the nose and hands. Cold urticaria is precipitated by exposure to the cold, and therefore, exposed areas are usually affected. In some cases, the disease is associated with abnormal circulating proteins—more commonly cryoglobulins and cold hemolysins and less commonly cryofibrinogens and cold agglutinins. Additional systemic symptoms include wheezing and syncope, thus explaining the need for these patients to avoid swimming in cold water. Cholinergic urticaria is precipitated by heat, exercise, or emotion and is characterized by small wheals with relatively large flares. It is occasionally associated with wheezing.

Whereas urticaria is the result of dermal edema, subcutaneous edema leads to the clinical picture of *angioedema*. Sites of involvement include the eyelids, lips, tongue, larynx, and gastrointestinal tract as well as the subcutaneous tissue. Angioedema occurs alone or in combination with urticaria, including urticarial vasculitis and the physical urticarias. Both acquired and hereditary (autosomal dominant) forms of angioedema occur (see Chap. 282), and in the latter, urticaria is rarely seen.

Urticarial vasculitis is an immune complex disease that may be confused with simple urticaria. In contrast to simple urticaria, individual lesions tend to last longer than 24 h, and they usually develop central petechiae that can be observed even after the urticarial phase has resolved. The patient also may complain of burning rather than pruritus. On biopsy, there is a leukocytoclastic vasculitis of the small blood vessels. Although many cases of urticarial vasculitis are idiopathic in origin, it can be a reflection of an underlying systemic illness such as lupus erythematosus, Sjögren's syndrome, or hereditary complement deficiency. There is a spectrum of urticarial vasculitis that ranges from purely cutaneous to multisystem involvement. The most common systemic signs and symptoms are arthralgias and/or arthritis, nephritis, and crampy abdominal pain, with asthma and chronic obstructive lung disease seen less often. Hypocomplementemia occurs in one- to two-thirds of patients, even in the idiopathic cases. Similar cutaneous, joint, and renal findings can be seen in the prodrome of *hepatitis B infection*, *serum sickness*, and *serum sickness–like illnesses*.

PAPULONODULAR SKIN LESIONS (Table 54-21) In the *papulonodular diseases*, the lesions are elevated above the surface of the skin, and they may coalesce to form plaques. The location, consistency, and color of the lesions are the keys to their diagnosis. This section is organized on the basis of color, and the color groups are white, flesh, pink, yellow, red, red-brown, blue, violaceous, purple, and brown-black.

White lesions In *calcinosis cutis* there are firm white to white-yellow papules with an irregular surface. When the contents are discharged, a chalky white material is seen. *Dystrophic* calcification is seen at sites of previous inflammation or damage to the skin. It develops in acne scars as well as on the distal extremities of patients with scleroderma and in the subcutaneous tissue and intermuscular fascial planes in dermatomyositis. The latter is more extensive and is more commonly seen in children. An elevated calcium phosphate product, as in secondary hyperparathyroidism, can lead to nodules of *metastatic* calcinosis cutis, which tend to be subcutaneous and periarticular. This form is often accompanied by calcification of muscular arteries and subsequent ischemic necrosis.

Flesh-colored lesions There are several types of flesh-colored lesions, including epidermoid inclusion cysts, lipomas, rheumatoid nodules, neurofibromas, angiofibromas, neuromas, and adnexal tumors such as tricholemmomas. Both *epidermoid inclusion cysts* and *lipomas* are very common mobile subcutaneous nodules—the former are rubbery and compressible, and they drain cheeselike material (sebum and keratin) if incised. Lipomas are firm and somewhat lobulated on palpation. When extensive facial epidermoid inclusion cysts develop in childhood or there is a family history of such lesions, the patient should be examined for other signs of Gardner's syndrome, including osteomas and desmoid tumors (see Chap. 256). *Rheumatoid nodules* are firm, 0.5- to 4-cm nodules that tend to localize around

TABLE 54-21 Papulonodular skin lesions according to color groups

White	C Nodules
A Calcinosis cutis	1 Panniculitis
Flesh	2 Cutaneous polyarteritis
A Rheumatoid nodule	nodosa
B Neurofibromas	3 Systemic vasculitis
(von Recklinghausen's	D Primary cutaneous disorders
disease)	1 Arthropod bites
C Angiofibromas	2 Cherry hemangiomas
(tuberous sclerosis)	3 Infections, e.g., erysipelas,
D Neuromas	sporotrichosis
(multiple endocrine neoplasia	4 Polymorphous light
syndrome, type 2b)	eruption
E Adnexal tumors	5 Lymphocytoma cutis
1 Basal cell epitheliomas	(pseudolymphoma)
(basal cell nevus syndrome)	**Red-brown**
2 Tricholemmomas	A Sarcoidosis
(Cowden's disease)	B Sweet's syndrome
F Primary cutaneous disorders	C Urticaria pigmentosa
1 Epidermal inclusion cysts	D Erythema elevatum diutinum
2 Lipomas	(chronic leukocytoclastic
Pink/translucent	vasculitis)
A Amyloidosis	E Lupus vulgaris
B Papular mucinosis	**Blue**
Yellow	A Cavernous hemangiomas
A Xanthomas	(blue rubber bleb syndrome)
B Tophi	B Primary cutaneous disorders
C Necrobiosis lipoidica	1 Venous lake
D Pseudoxanthoma elasticum	2 Blue nevus
E Sebaceous adenomas	**Violaceous**
(Torre's syndrome)	A Lupus pernio (sarcoidosis)
Red	B Lymphoma cutis
A Papules	C Cutaneous lupus
1 Angiokeratomas	**Purple**
(Fabry's disease)	A Kaposi's sarcoma
2 Bacillary angiomatosis (pri-	B Angiosarcoma
marily in AIDS)	C Palpable purpura
B Papules/plaques	**Brown-black**
1 Cutaneous lupus	See "Hyperpigmentation"
2 Lymphoma cutis	**Any color**
3 Leukemia cutis	A Metastases

pressure points, especially the elbows. They are seen in approximately 20 percent of patients with rheumatoid arthritis and 6 percent of patients with Still's disease. Biopsies of the nodules show palisading granulomas. Similar lesions that are smaller and shorter-lived are seen in rheumatic fever.

Neurofibromas (benign Schwann cell tumors) are soft papules or nodules that exhibit the "button-hole" sign, that is, they invaginate into the skin with pressure in a manner similar to a hernia. Single lesions are seen in normal individuals, but multiple neurofibromas, usually in combination with six or more café au lait spots measuring >1.5 cm (see "Hyperpigmentation") and multiple Lisch nodules, are seen in von Recklinghausen's disease (NF type I). Lisch nodules are 1-mm yellow-brown spots within the iris that are best observed with slit-lamp examination. Additional manifestations include axillary freckling and peripheral and CNS tumors (see Chap. 378). In some patients the neurofibromas are localized and unilateral, whereas in others they are limited to the CNS.

Angiofibromas are firm, pink to flesh-colored papules that measure from 3 mm to several centimeters in diameter. When they are located on the central cheeks (adenoma sebaceum) or fibromas are seen around the nails, the patient has tuberous sclerosis. It is an autosomal disorder, and the associated findings are discussed in the section on ash leaf spots (see "Hypopigmentation").

Neuromas (benign proliferation of nerve fibers) are also firm, flesh-colored papules. They are more commonly found at sites of amputation and as rudimentary supernumerary digits. However, when there are multiple neuromas on the eyelids, lips, distal tongue, and/or oral mucosa, the patient should be investigated for other signs of the multiple endocrine neoplasia syndrome, type 2b. Associated findings include marfanoid habitus, protuberant lips, intestinal ganglioneuromas, and medullary thyroid carcinoma (>75 percent of patients) (see Chap. 343).

Adnexal tumors are derived from pluripotential cells of the epidermis that can differentiate toward hair, sebaceous, apocrine, or eccrine glands or remain undifferentiated. *Basal cell epitheliomas* (BCEs) are examples of adnexal tumors that have little or no evidence of differentiation. Clinically, they are translucent papules with rolled borders, telangiectasias, and central erosion. BCEs commonly arise in sun-damaged skin of the head and neck. When a patient has multiple BCEs, especially prior to age 30, the possibility of the basal cell nevus syndrome should be raised. It is inherited as an autosomal dominant trait and is associated with jaw cysts, palmar and plantar pits, frontal bossing, rib anomalies, and calcification of the falx cerebri and diaphragma sellae. *Tricholemmomas* are also flesh-colored adnexal tumors, but they differentiate toward hair follicles and can have a wartlike appearance. The presence of multiple tricholemmomas on the face and oral mucosa points to the diagnosis of Cowden's disease (multiple hamartoma syndrome). The oral tricholemmomas are found primarily on the tongue and gingiva and give these areas a cobblestone appearance. Internal organ involvement (in decreasing order of frequency) includes fibrocystic disease and carcinoma of the breast, adenomas and carcinomas of the thyroid, and gastrointestinal polyposis. Keratoses of the palms, soles, and dorsa of the hands are also seen.

Pink lesions   The cutaneous lesions associated with primary systemic *amyloidosis* are pink in color and translucent. Common locations are the face, especially the periorbital and perioral regions, and intertriginous areas. On biopsy, homogeneous deposits of amyloid are seen in the dermis and in the walls of blood vessels; the latter lead to an increase in vessel wall fragility. As a result, petechiae and purpura develop in clinically normal skin as well as in lesional skin following minor trauma, hence the term "pinch purpura." Amyloid deposits are also seen in the striated muscle of the tongue, and these result in macroglossia.

Even though specific mucocutaneous lesions are rarely seen in secondary amyloidosis and are present in only about 30 percent of the patients with primary amyloidosis, a rapid diagnosis of systemic amyloidosis can be made by an examination of abdominal subcutaneous fat. By special staining, deposits are seen around blood vessels or individual fat cells in 40 to 50 percent of patients. There are also three forms of amyloidosis that are limited to the skin and that should not be construed as cutaneous lesions of systemic amyloidosis. They are macular amyloid (upper back), lichenoid amyloidosis (usually lower extremities), and nodular amyloidosis. In macular and lichenoid amyloidosis, the deposits are composed of altered epidermal keratin. Recently, macular amyloidosis has been associated with multiple endocrine neoplasia syndrome, type 2a.

Patients with *multicentric reticulohistiocytosis* also have pink-colored papules and nodules on the face and mucous membranes as well as on the extensor surface of the hands and forearms. They have a polyarthritis that can mimic rheumatoid arthritis clinically. On histologic examination, the papules have characteristic giant cells that are not seen in biopsies of rheumatoid nodules. Pink to flesh-colored papules that are firm, 2 to 5 mm in diameter, and often in a linear arrangement are seen in patients with *papular mucinosis*. This disease is also referred to as *lichen myxedematosus* or *scleromyxedema*. The latter name comes from the brawny induration of the face and extremities that may accompany the papular eruption. Biopsy specimens of the papules show localized mucin deposition, and serum protein electrophoresis demonstrates a monoclonal spike of IgG, usually with a λ light chain.

Yellow lesions   Several systemic disorders are characterized by yellow-colored cutaneous papules or plaques—hyperlipidemia (xanthomas), gout (tophi), diabetes (necrobiosis lipoidica), pseudoxanthoma elasticum, and Torre's syndrome (sebaceous tumors). Eruptive xanthomas are the most common form of *xanthomas*, and they are associated with hypertriglyceridemia (types I, III, IV, and V). Crops of yellow papules with erythematous halos occur primarily on the extensor surfaces of the extremities and the buttocks in association with elevations of the circulating triglycerides. They spontaneously involute with a fall in serum lipids. Increased β-lipoproteins (primarily types II and III) result in one or more of the following types of xanthoma: xanthelasma, tendon xanthomas, and plane xanthomas. Xanthelasma are found on the eyelids, whereas tendon xanthomas are frequently associated with the Achilles and extensor finger tendons; plane xanthomas are flat and favor the palmar creases, face, upper trunk, and scars. Tuberous xanthomas are frequently associated with hypertriglyceridemia, but they are also seen in patients with hypercholesterolemia (type II) and are found most frequently over the large joints or hand. Biopsy specimens of xanthomas show collections of lipid-containing macrophages (foam cells).

Patients with several disorders, including biliary cirrhosis, can have a secondary form of hyperlipidemia with associated tuberous and planar xanthomas. However, patients with myeloma have *normolipemic* flat xanthomas. This latter form of xanthoma may be ≥12 cm in diameter and is most frequently seen on the upper trunk or side of the neck. It is also important to note that the most common setting for eruptive xanthomas is uncontrolled diabetes mellitus. The least specific sign for hyperlipidemia is xanthelasma because at least 50 percent of the patients with this finding have normal lipid profiles.

In *tophaceous gout* there are deposits of monosodium urate in the skin around the joints, particularly those of the hands and feet. Additional sites of *tophi* formation include the helix of the ear and the olecranon and prepatellar bursae. The lesions are firm, yellow in color, and occasionally discharge a chalky material. Their size varies from 1 mm to 7 cm, and the diagnosis can be established by polarization of the aspirated contents of a lesion. Lesions of *necrobiosis lipoidica* are found primarily on the shins (90 percent), and the majority of patients have diabetes mellitus or develop it subsequently. Characteristic findings include a central yellow color, atrophy (transparency), telangiectasias, and an erythematous border. Ulcerations also can develop within the plaques. Biopsy specimens show necrobiosis of collagen, granulomatous inflammation, and obliterative endarteritis.

In *pseudoxanthoma elasticum* (PXE) there is an abnormal deposition of calcium on the elastic fibers of the skin, eye, and blood vessels. In the skin, the flexural areas such as the neck, axillae, antecubital fossae, and inguinal area are the primary sites of involvement. Yellow papules coalesce to form reticulated plaques that have an appearance similar to that of plucked chicken skin. In severely affected skin, hanging, redundant folds develop. Some patients have a more subtle macular form of the disease, and careful inspection is required. Biopsy specimens of involved skin show swollen and irregularly clumped elastic fibers with deposits of calcium. In the eye, the calcium deposits in Bruch's membrane lead to angioid streaks and choroiditis; in the arteries of the heart, kidney, gastrointestinal tract, and extremities, the deposits lead to angina, hypertension, gastrointestinal bleeding, and claudication, respectively. Four types of PXE have been described—two with autosomal dominant and two with autosomal recessive inheritance. The extent of vessel and skin involvement varies depending on the type. Long-term administration of D-penicillamine can lead to PXE-like skin changes as well as elastic fiber alterations in internal organs.

Adnexal tumors that have differentiated toward sebaceous glands include sebaceous adenoma, sebaceous epithelioma, sebaceous carcinoma, and sebaceous hyperplasia. Except for sebaceous hyperplasia, which is commonly seen on the face, these tumors are solitary and uncommon. Patients with Torre's syndrome have *sebaceous adenomas*, and in the majority of cases there are multiple such tumors. These patients also can have sebaceous carcinomas and sebaceous hyperplasia as well as keratoacanthomas. The internal manifestations of Torre's syndrome include *multiple* carcinomas of the gastrointestinal tract (primarily colon) as well as cancers of the larynx, genitourinary tract, ovary, and endometrium. Some patients also have a strong family history of cancer.

Red lesions Cutaneous lesions that are red in color have a wide variety of etiologies, and in an attempt to simplify their identification, they will be subdivided into papules, papules/plaques, and subcutaneous nodules. Common red papules include *arthropod bites* and *cherry hemangiomas*; the latter are small, bright-red, dome-shaped papules that represent benign proliferation of capillaries. In patients with AIDS, the development of multiple red hemangioma-like lesions points to bacillary angiomatosis, and biopsy specimens show clusters of bacilli that stain positive with the Warthin-Starry stain; the pathogen has been identified as *Rochalimaea henselae*. Disseminated visceral disease is seen primarily in immunocompromised hosts, but it can occur in immunocompetent individuals.

Multiple *angiokeratomas* are seen in Fabry's disease, an X-linked recessive lysosomal storage disease that is due to a deficiency of α-galactosidase A. The lesions are red to red-blue in color and can be quite small in size (1 to 3 mm), with the most common location being the lower trunk. Associated findings include chronic renal failure, peripheral neuropathy, and corneal opacities (cornea verticillata). Electron photomicrographs of angiokeratomas and clinically normal skin demonstrate lamellar lipid deposits in fibroblasts, pericytes, and endothelial cells that are diagnostic of this disease. Widespread acute eruptions of erythematous papules are discussed in the section on exanthems.

There are several infectious diseases that present as erythematous papules or nodules in a sporotrichoid pattern, that is, in a linear arrangement along the lymphatic channels. The two most common etiologies are *Sporothrix schenckii* (*sporotrichosis*) and *Mycobacterium marinum* (atypical mycobacteria). The organisms are introduced as a result of trauma, and a primary inoculation site is often seen in addition to the lymphatic nodules. Additional causes include *Nocardia*, *Leishmania*, and other dimorphic fungi; culture of lesional tissue will aid in the diagnosis.

The diseases that are characterized by erythematous plaques with scale are reviewed in the papulosquamous section, and the various forms of dermatitis are discussed in the section on erythroderma. Additional disorders in the differential diagnosis of red papules/plaques include *erysipelas, polymorphous light eruption, lymphocytoma cutis, cutaneous lupus, lymphoma cutis,* and *leukemia cutis.*

The first three diseases represent primary cutaneous disorders. Polymorphous light eruption (PMLE) is characterized by erythematous papules and plaques in a primarily sun-exposed distribution—dorsum of the hand, extensor forearm, and face. Lesions follow exposure to both UV-B and UV-A, and in northern latitudes PMLE is most severe in the late spring and early summer. A process referred to as "hardening" occurs with continued UV exposure, and the eruption fades, but in temperate climates it will recur in the spring. PMLE must be differentiated from cutaneous lupus, and this is accomplished by histologic examination and direct immunofluorescence of the lesions. Lymphocytoma cutis (pseudolymphoma) is a *benign* proliferation of lymphocytes in the skin that presents as infiltrated pink-red to red-purple papules and plaques. It must be distinguished from cutaneous lupus and lymphoma cutis.

Several types of red plaques are seen in patients with systemic *lupus*, including (1) erythematous urticarial plaques across the cheeks and nose in the classic butterfly rash, (2) erythematous discoid lesions with fine or "carpet-tack" scale, telangiectasias, central hypopigmentation, peripheral hyperpigmentation, follicular plugging, and atrophy located on the face, scalp, external ears, arms, and upper trunk, and (3) psoriasiform or annular lesions of subacute lupus with hypopigmented centers located on the face, extensor arms, and upper trunk. Additional cutaneous findings include (1) a violaceous flush on the face and vee of the neck, (2) urticarial vasculitis (see "Urticaria"), (3) lupus panniculitis (see below), (4) diffuse alopecia, (5) alopecia secondary to discoid lesions, (6) periungual telangiectasias and erythema, (7) erythema multiforme–like lesions that may become bullous, and (8) distal ulcerations secondary to Raynaud's phenomenon, vasculitis, or livedoid vasculitis. Patients with only discoid lesions usually have the form of lupus that is limited to the skin. However, 2 to 10 percent of these patients eventually develop systemic lupus. Direct immunofluorescence of involved skin shows deposits of IgG and C3 in a granular distribution along the dermal-epidermal junction.

In *lymphoma cutis* there is a proliferation of malignant lymphocytes or histiocytes in the skin, and the clinical appearance resembles that of lymphocytoma cutis—infiltrated pink-red to red-purple papules and plaques. Lymphoma cutis can occur anywhere on the surface of the skin, whereas the sites of predilection for lymphocytomas are the malar ridge, tip of the nose, earlobes, forearms, and scrotum. Patients with non-Hodgkin's lymphomas have specific cutaneous lesions more often than those with Hodgkin's disease, and occasionally, the skin nodules precede the development of extracutaneous non-Hodgkin's lymphoma. Arcuate lesions are sometimes seen in lymphoma and lymphocytoma cutis as well as in CTLC. *Leukemia cutis* has the same appearance as lymphoma cutis, and specific lesions are seen more commonly in monocytic leukemias than in lymphocytic or granulocytic leukemias. Cutaneous chloromas (granulocytic sarcomas) may precede the appearance of circulating blasts in acute nonlymphocytic leukemia and, as such, represent a form of aleukemic leukemia cutis.

Common causes of erythematous subcutaneous nodules include inflamed epidermoid inclusion cysts, acne cysts, and furuncles. *Panniculitis*, an inflammation of the fat, also presents as subcutaneous nodules and is frequently a sign of systemic disease. There are several forms of panniculitis, including erythema nodosum, erythema induratum, lupus profundus, Weber-Christian disease, α$_1$-antitrypsin deficiency, factical, and fat necrosis secondary to pancreatic disease. In all these disorders, except for erythema nodosum, the lesions may break down and ulcerate or heal with a scar. The shin is the most common location for the nodules of erythema nodosum, whereas the calf is the most common location for lesions of erythema induratum. In erythema nodosum the nodules are initially red, but then they develop a blue color as they resolve. Patients with erythema nodosum and no underlying systemic illness can still have fever, malaise, leukocytosis, arthralgias and/or arthritis, and unilateral or bilateral hilar adenopathy. However, the possibility of an underlying illness should be excluded, and the most common associations are streptococcal infections, upper respiratory infections, sarcoidosis, and inflammatory bowel disease. The less common associations include tuberculosis, histoplasmosis, coccidioidomycosis, psittacosis, drugs (oral contraceptives, sulfonamides, aspartame, bromides, iodides), cat-scratch fever, and infections with *Yersinia*, *Salmonella*, and *Chlamydia*.

In most patients, erythema induratum/nodular vasculitis is an idiopathic disease, while in a few it may be a reflection of extracutaneous tuberculosis. The lesions of lupus profundus are found primarily on the face, upper arms, and buttocks (sites of abundant fat), and they are seen in both the cutaneous and systemic forms of lupus. The overlying skin may be normal, erythematous, or have the changes of discoid lupus. The subcutaneous fat necrosis that is associated with pancreatic disease is presumably secondary to circulating lipases and is seen in patients with pancreatic carcinoma as well as in patients with acute and chronic pancreatitis. In this disorder and in Weber-Christian disease there may be an associated arthritis, fever, and inflammation of visceral fat. Histologic examination of deep incisional biopsy specimens will aid in the diagnosis of the particular type of panniculitis.

Subcutaneous erythematous nodules are also seen in *cutaneous polyarteritis nodosa* (PAN) and as a manifestation of *systemic vasculitis*, e.g., systemic PAN, allergic granulomatosis, or Wegener's granulomatosis. Cutaneous PAN presents with painful subcutaneous nodules and ulcers within a red-purple, netlike pattern of livedo reticularis. The latter is due to slowed blood flow through the superficial horizontal venous plexus. The majority of lesions are found on the lower extremity, and while arthralgias and myalgias may accompany cutaneous PAN, there is no evidence of systemic involvement. In both the cutaneous and systemic forms of vasculitis, skin biopsy specimens of the associated nodules will show the changes characteristic of a vasculitis; the size of the vessel involved will depend on the particular disease.

Red-brown lesions   The cutaneous lesions in *sarcoidosis* are classically red to red-brown in color, and with diascopy (pressure with a glass slide) a yellow-brown residual color is observed that is secondary to the granulomatous infiltrate. The waxy papules and plaques may be found anywhere on the skin, but the face is the most common location. Usually there are no surface changes, but occasionally the lesions will have scale. Biopsy specimens of the papules show "naked" granulomas in the dermis, i.e., granulomas surrounded by a minimal number of lymphocytes. Other cutaneous findings in sarcoidosis include annular lesions with an atrophic or scaly center, papules within scars, hypopigmented macules and papules, alopecia, acquired ichthyosis, erythema nodosum, and lupus pernio (see below). Additional physical findings are peripheral lymphadenopathy and parotid and lacrimal gland enlargement. When there is cutaneous involvement of the hands, radiographs often will show lytic lesions in the underlying bone.

The differential diagnosis of sarcoidosis includes foreign-body granulomas produced by chemicals such as beryllium and zirconium, late secondary syphilis, and *lupus vulgaris*. Lupus vulgaris is a form of cutaneous tuberculosis that is seen in previously infected and sensitized individuals. There is often underlying active tuberculosis elsewhere, usually in the lungs or lymph nodes. At least 90 percent of the lesions occur in the head and neck area, and they are red-brown plaques with a yellow-brown color on diascopy. Secondary scarring and squamous cell carcinomas can develop within the plaques. Cultures of the lesions should be done because it is rare for the acid-fast stain to show bacilli within the dermal granulomas.

Sweet's syndrome is characterized by red-brown plaques and nodules that are frequently painful and occur primarily on the head, neck, and upper extremities. The patients also have fever, neutrophilia, and a dense dermal infiltrate of neutrophils in the lesions. In approximately 10 percent of the patients there is an associated malignancy, most commonly acute nonlymphocytic leukemia. Lymphoma, chronic leukemia, myeloma, myelodysplastic syndromes, and solid tumors (primarily of the genitourinary tract) also have been reported. Extracutaneous sites of involvement include joints, muscles,

eye, kidney (proteinuria, occasionally glomerulonephritis), and lung (neutrophilic infiltrates). The idiopathic form of Sweet's syndrome is seen more often in women, following a respiratory tract infection.

A generalized distribution of red-brown macules and papules is seen in the form of mastocytosis known as *urticaria pigmentosa* (see Chap. 282). Each lesion represents a collection of mast cells in the dermis, with hyperpigmentation of the overlying epidermis. Stimuli such as rubbing and heat cause these mast cells to degranulate, and this leads to the formation of localized urticaria (Darier's sign). Additional symptoms can result from mast cell degranulation, and these include headache, flushing, diarrhea, and pruritus. Mast cells also infiltrate various organs such as the liver, spleen, and gastrointestinal tract in up to 30 to 50 percent of patients with urticaria pigmentosa, and accumulations of mast cells in the bones may produce either osteosclerotic or osteolytic shadows on radiographs. In the majority of these patients, however, the internal involvement remains fairly static. A subtype of chronic leukocytoclastic vasculitis, *erythema elevatum diutinum* (EED), also presents with papules that are red-brown in color. The papules coalesce into plaques on the extensor surfaces of knees, elbows, and the small joints of the hand. Flares of EED have been associated with streptococcal infections.

Blue lesions   Lesions that are blue in color are the result of either vascular ectasias and tumors or melanin pigment in the dermis. *Venous lakes* (ectasias) are compressible dark blue lesions that are found commonly in the head and neck region. *Cavernous hemangiomas* are also compressible blue papules and nodules that can occur anywhere on the body, including the oral mucosa. When they are multiple rather than single congenital lesions, the patient may have the blue rubber bleb syndrome or Mafucci's syndrome. Patients with the blue rubber bleb syndrome also have hemangiomas of the gastrointestinal tract that may bleed, whereas patients with Mafucci's syndrome have associated dyschondroplasia and osteochondromas. In the case of single cavernous hemangiomas that are relatively large in size, there can be associated platelet consumption (Kasabach-Merritt syndrome) or musculoskeletal defects. *Blue nevi* (moles) are seen when there are collections of pigment-producing nevus cells in the dermis. These benign papular lesions are dome-shaped, and they occur most commonly on the dorsum of the hand and arm.

Violaceous lesions   Violaceous papules and plaques are seen in *lupus pernio*, *lymphoma cutis*, and *cutaneous lupus*. Lupus pernio is a particular type of sarcoidosis that involves the tip of the nose and the earlobes, with lesions that are violaceous in color rather than red-brown. This form of sarcoidosis is associated with involvement of the upper respiratory tract. The plaques of lymphoma cutis and cutaneous lupus may be red or violaceous in color and were discussed above.

Purple lesions   Purple-colored papules and plaques are seen in vascular tumors, such as *Kaposi's sarcoma* (see Chap. 279) and *angiosarcoma*, and when there is extravasation of red blood cells into the skin in association with inflammation, as in *palpable purpura* (see "Purpura"). Patients with congenital or acquired arteriovenous fistulas can develop purple papules on the lower extremities that can resemble Kaposi's sarcoma clinically and histologically, and this condition is referred to as pseudo-Kaposi sarcoma (acral angiodermatitis). *Angiosarcoma* is found most commonly on the scalp and face of elderly patients or within areas of chronic lymphedema, and it presents as purple papules and plaques. In the head and neck region the tumor often extends beyond the clinically defined borders and may be accompanied by facial edema.

Brown- and black-colored papules are reviewed in the section on hyperpigmentation.

Cutaneous metastases are discussed last because they can have a wide range of colors. Most commonly they present as either firm, flesh-colored subcutaneous nodules or firm, red to red-brown papulonodules. The lesions of lymphoma cutis range from pink-red to plum in color, whereas metastatic melanoma can be pink, blue, or black in color. Cutaneous metastases develop from hematogenous or lymphatic spread and are most often due to the following primary carcinomas: in men, lung, colon, melanoma, and oral cavity; and in women, breast, colon, and lung. These metastatic lesions may be the initial presentation of the carcinoma, especially when the primary site is the lung, kidney, or ovary.

PURPURA (Table 54-22) *Purpura* are seen when there is an extravasation of red blood cells into the dermis, and as a result, the lesions do not blanch with pressure. This is in contrast to those erythematous or violet-colored lesions that are due to localized vasodilatation—they do blanch with pressure. Purpura (≥ 3 mm) and petechiae (≤ 2 mm) are divided into two major groups, palpable and nonpalpable. The most frequent causes of *nonpalpable* petechiae and purpura are primary cutaneous disorders such as *trauma, solar purpura,* and *capillaritis.* Less common causes are *steroid purpura* and *livedoid vasculitis* (see "Ulcers"). Solar purpura are seen primarily on the extensor forearm, while glucocorticoid purpura (secondary to potent topical steroids) or endogenous or exogenous Cushing's syndrome can be more widespread. In both cases there is alteration of the supporting connective tissue that surrounds the dermal blood vessels. In contrast, the petechiae that result from capillaritis are found primarily on the lower extremities. In capillaritis there is an extravasation of erythrocytes as a result of perivascular lymphocytic inflammation. The petechiae are bright red, 1 to 2 mm in size, and scattered within annular or coin-shaped yellow-brown macules. The yellow-brown color is caused by hemosiderin deposits within the dermis.

Systemic causes of nonpalpable purpura fall into several categories, and those secondary to clotting disturbances and vascular fragility will be discussed first. The former group includes *thrombocytopenia* (see Chap. 314), *abnormal platelet function* as is seen in uremia, and *clotting factor defects.* The initial site of presentation for thrombocytopenia-induced petechiae is the distal lower extremity. Capillary fragility leads to nonpalpable purpura in patients with systemic *amyloidosis* (see "Papulonodular Skin Lesions"), disorders of collagen production such as *Ehlers-Danlos syndrome,* and *scurvy.* In scurvy there are flattened corkscrew hairs with surrounding hemorrhage on the lower extremities, in addition to gingivitis. Vitamin C is a cofactor for lysyl hydroxylase, an enzyme involved in the posttranslational modification of procollagen that is necessary for cross-link formation.

In contrast to the previous group of disorders, in which either capillary fragility or a clotting abnormality is responsible for the nonpalpable purpura, the purpura seen in the following group of diseases are associated with thrombi formation within vessels. It is important to note that these thrombi are demonstrable in skin biopsy specimens. This group of disorders includes *disseminated intravascular coagulation, monoclonal cryoglobulinemia, thrombotic thrombocytopenic purpura,* and *reactions to warfarin.* Disseminated intravascular coagulation (DIC) is triggered by several types of infection (gram-negative, gram-positive, viral, and rickettsial) as well as by tissue injury and neoplasms. Widespread purpura and hemorrhagic infarcts of the distal extremities are seen. Similar lesions are found in purpura fulminans, which is a form of DIC associated with fever and hypotension that occurs more commonly in children following an infectious illness such as varicella, scarlet fever, or an upper respiratory tract infection. In both disorders, hemorrhagic bullae can develop in involved skin.

Monoclonal cryoglobulinemia is associated with multiple myeloma, Waldenström's macroglobulinemia, lymphocytic leukemia, and lymphoma. Purpura, primarily of the lower extremities, and hemorrhagic infarcts of the fingers and toes are seen in these patients. Exacerbations of disease activity can follow cold exposure or an increase in serum viscosity. Biopsy specimens show precipitates of the cryoglobulin within dermal vessels. Similar deposits have been found in the lung, brain, and renal glomeruli. Patients with *thrombotic thrombocytopenic purpura* also can have hemorrhagic infarcts as a result of intravascular thromboses. Additional signs include thrombocytopenic purpura, fever, and microangiopathic hemolytic anemia (see Chap. 307).

Administration of *warfarin* can result in painful areas of erythema that become purpuric and then necrotic with an adherent black eschar. This reaction is seen more often in women and in areas with abundant subcutaneous fat—breasts, abdomen, buttocks, thighs, and calves. The erythema and purpura develop between the third and tenth day of therapy, most likely as a result of a transient imbalance in the levels of anticoagulant and procoagulant vitamin K–dependent factors. Continued therapy does not exacerbate preexisting lesions, and patients with an inherited or acquired deficiency of protein C are at increased risk for this particular reaction as well as for purpura fulminans.

Purpura secondary to *cholesterol emboli* are usually seen on the lower extremities of patients with atherosclerotic vascular disease. They often follow anticoagulant therapy or an invasive vascular procedure such as an arteriogram, but they also occur spontaneously from disintegration of atheromatous plaques. Associated findings include livedo reticularis, gangrene, cyanosis, subcutaneous nodules, and ischemic ulcerations. Multiple step sections of the biopsy specimen may be necessary to demonstrate the cholesterol clefts with the vessels. Petechiae are also an important sign of *fat embolism,* and they occur primarily on the upper body 2 to 3 days after a major injury. By using special fixatives, the emboli can be demonstrated in biopsy specimens of the petechiae. Emboli of tumor or thrombus are seen in patients with atrial myxomas and marantic endocarditis.

In the *Gardner-Diamond syndrome* (autoerythrocyte sensitivity), female patients develop large ecchymoses within areas of painful, warm erythema. An episode of significant trauma frequently precedes the onset of this syndrome. Intradermal injections of autologous erythrocytes or phosphatidyl serine derived from the red cell membrane can reproduce the lesions in most patients; however, there are instances where a reaction is seen at an injection site of the forearm but not in the midback region. The latter has led some observers to view Gardner-Diamond syndrome as a cutaneous manifestation of severe emotional stress. *Waldenström's hypergammaglobulinemic purpura* is a chronic disorder characterized by petechiae on the lower extremities. There are circulating complexes of IgG–anti-IgG molecules, and exacerbations are associated with prolonged standing or walking.

Palpable purpura are further subdivided into vasculitic and embolic. In the group of vasculitic disorders, *leukocytoclastic vasculitis* (LCV), also known as *allergic vasculitis,* is the one most commonly associated with palpable purpura (see Chap. 291). *Henoch-Schönlein purpura* is a subtype of acute LCV that is seen primarily in children and adolescents following an upper respiratory infection. The majority

---

TABLE 54-22 Causes of purpura

Primary cutaneous disorders
A Nonpalpable
  1 Trauma
  2 Solar purpura
  3 Steroid purpura
  4 Capillaritis
  5 Livedoid vasculitis
Systemic diseases
A Nonpalpable
  1 Clotting disturbances
    a Thrombocytopenia (including ITP)
    b Abnormal platelet function
    c Clotting factor defects
  2 Vascular fragility
    a Amyloidosis
    b Ehlers-Danlos syndrome
    c Scurvy
  3 Thrombi
    a Disseminated intravascular coagulation
    b Monoclonal cryoglobulinemia

    c Thrombotic thrombocytopenic purpura
    d Warfarin reaction
  4 Emboli
    a Cholesterol
    b Fat
  5 Possible immune complex
    a Gardner-Diamond syndrome (autoerythrocyte sensitization)
    b Waldenström's hypergammaglobulinemic purpura
B Palpable
  1 Vasculitis
    a Leukocytoclastic vasculitis
    b Polyarteritis nodosa
  2 Emboli
    a Acute meningococcemia
    b Disseminated gonococcal infection
    c Rocky mountain spotted fever
    d Ecthyma gangrenosum

of lesions are found on the lower extremities and buttocks. Systemic manifestations include fever, arthralgias (primarily of the knees and ankles), abdominal pain, gastrointestinal bleeding, and nephritis. Direct immunofluorescence examination shows deposits of IgA within dermal blood vessel walls. In *polyarteritis nodosa*, specific cutaneous lesions result from a vasculitis of arterial vessels rather than postcapillary venules as in LCV. The arteritis leads to ischemia of the skin, and this explains the irregular outline of the purpura (see below).

Several types of infectious emboli can give rise to palpable purpura. These embolic lesions are usually *irregular* in outline as opposed to the lesions of leukocytoclastic vasculitis, which are *circular* in outline. The irregular outline is indicative of a cutaneous infarct, and the size corresponds to the area of skin that received its blood supply from that particular arteriole or artery. The palpable purpura in LCV are circular because the erythrocytes simply diffuse out evenly from the postcapillary venules as a result of inflammation. Infectious emboli are most commonly due to gram-negative cocci (meningococcus, gonococcus), gram-negative rods (Enterobacteriaceae), and gram-positive cocci (staphylococcus). Additional causes include *Rickettsia* and, in immunocompromised patients, *Candida* and *Aspergillus*.

The embolic lesions in *acute meningococcemia* are found primarily on the trunk, lower extremities, and sites of pressure, and a gunmetal-gray color often develops within them. Their size varies from 1 mm to several centimeters, and the organisms can be cultured from the lesions. Associated findings include a preceding upper respiratory tract infection, fever, meningitis, disseminated intravascular coagulation, and, in some patients, a deficiency of the terminal components of complement. In *disseminated gonococcal infection* (arthritis-dermatitis syndrome), a small number of papules and vesicopustules with central purpura or hemorrhagic necrosis are found over the joints of the distal extremities. Additional symptoms include arthralgias, tenosynovitis, and fever. To establish the diagnosis, a Gram stain of these lesions should be performed. *Rocky mountain spotted fever* is a tick-borne disease that is caused by *Rickettsia rickettsii*. A several-day history of fever, chills, severe headache, and photophobia precedes the onset of the cutaneous eruption. The initial lesions are erythematous macules and papules on the wrists, ankles, palms, and soles. With time, the lesions spread centripetally and become purpuric.

Lesions of *ecthyma gangrenosum* begin as edematous, erythematous papules or plaques and then develop central purpura and necrosis. Bullae formation also occurs in these lesions, and they are frequently found in the girdle region. The organism that is classically associated with ecthyma gangrenosum is *Pseudomonas aeruginosa*, but other gram-negative rods such as *Klebsiella*, *E. coli*, and *Serratia* can produce similar lesions. In immunocompromised hosts, the list of potential pathogens is expanded to include *Candida* and *Aspergillus*.

ULCERS (Table 54-23) As an approach to the patient with a cutaneous ulcer, the etiologies are divided into two major groups: (1) primary cutaneous disorders and (2) underlying systemic diseases. Within the group of *primary cutaneous disorders*, there are three categories: vascular, tumor-associated, and infectious. The *peripheral vascular* group is the first to be discussed because it contains the most common cause of lower extremity ulcers in adults, *venous hypertension*. Stasis ulcers are characteristically painless and contain adequate granulation tissue. They are often found on the medial malleoli against a background of varicosities, stasis dermatitis, edema, and hemosiderin deposition (yellow-brown discoloration of the skin).

In contrast, lower extremity ulcers due to *arteriosclerosis obliterans* are often painful and are associated with cool, hairless, atrophic skin and dystrophic nails—all a reflection of a decrease in blood flow. The majority of patients are men, and they frequently have evidence of atherosclerosis in other large- and medium-sized arteries. *Thromboangiitis obliterans* (Buerger's disease) and *Mönckeberg's arteriosclerosis* are two less common arterial diseases that can lead to ulcers of the distal upper extremity as well as the lower extremity. The latter is found in patients with primary or secondary hyperparathyroidism, and the calcification of the tunica media of involved muscular arteries

TABLE 54-23   Causes of cutaneous ulcers
Primary cutaneous disorders
A Peripheral vascular disease
1 Venous
2 Arterial
B Livedoid vasculitis
C Squamous cell carcinoma, e.g., within scars
D Infections, e.g., ecthyma
Systemic diseases
A Legs
1 Leukocytoclastic vasculitis
2 Hemoglobinopathies
3 Cryoglobulinemia
4 Cholesterol emboli
5 Necrobiosis lipoidica
B Hands and feet
1 Raynaud's phenomenon
C Generalized
1 Pyoderma gangrenosum
D Mucosal
1 Behçet's syndrome
2 Erythema multiforme
3 Primary blistering disorders

is seen radiographically as a diffuse pipestem calcification. Buerger's disease occurs primarily in young men (ages 25 to 40) who smoke or have been smokers.

Livedoid vasculitis (atrophie blanche) represents a combination of a vasculopathy with intravascular thrombosis. Purpuric lesions and livedo reticularis are found in association with painful ulcerations of the lower extremities. These ulcers are often slow to heal, but when they do, irregularly shaped white scars are formed. The majority of cases are idiopathic in origin, but possible underlying illnesses include systemic lupus, the antiphospholipid syndrome, scleroderma, cryoglobulinemia, and cryofibrinogenemia. Patients with the antiphospholipid syndrome have anticardiolipin antibodies, biologic false-positive tests for syphilis, and prolonged activated partial thromboplastin times; the latter are due to a circulating lupus anticoagulant. These antiphospholipid antibodies are seen most commonly in patients with systemic lupus, but they are also associated with other connective tissue diseases. In addition to the lesions of livedoid vasculitis, patients with the antiphospholipid syndrome have recurrent venous thrombosis, arterial thrombosis (including cerebrovascular accidents), spontaneous abortions, and thrombocytopenia.

Several *carcinomas* can present as cutaneous ulcers, e.g., basal cell carcinoma, squamous cell carcinoma, and, less often, melanoma. When an ulcer on the lower extremity does not heal, despite appropriate treatment, it should be biopsied to rule out carcinoma, primarily squamous cell carcinoma. The same holds true for ulcers that develop within scars. Bacterial and viral *infections* also lead to cutaneous ulceration, and one of the more commonly isolated organisms is *Streptococcus*. The term *ecthyma* is used to describe the often widespread ulcerative lesions that are caused by this bacteria. Ecthyma is a primary cutaneous disorder and should not be confused with ecthyma gangrenosum, which is secondary to blood-borne emboli (see "Purpura"). In Meleney's ulcer, a gradually expanding ulcer begins at a site of trauma or surgery. The clinical appearance is similar to that of pyoderma gangrenosum, but it is due to a synergistic infection that usually includes anaerobic streptococci.

For one group of patients with cutaneous ulcers due to an underlying systemic disease, the lower extremity is the primary location for the lesions. In a young patient, ischemic cutaneous ulcers on the leg should raise the possibility of a *hemoglobinopathy* or *hereditary spherocytosis*. Intravascular thrombosis is the presumed cause of these ulcers, as well as for the ulcers seen in patients with *monoclonal cryoglobulinemia* (see "Purpura"). Primary and secondary forms of *LCV* as well as *emboli of cholesterol* can result in cutaneous ulceration, again primarily on the lower extremities (see "Purpura"). For example, lower extremity ulcers in patients with rheumatoid arthritis are often due to vasculitis. In addition, the yellow atrophic plaques of *necrobiosis lipoidica* can break down centrally into an ulcer (see "Papulonodular Skin Lesions").

Vasospasm occurs in patients with *Raynaud's phenomenon* and can lead to ulcerations of the hands as well as the feet. Raynaud's phenomenon is defined as a triphasic reaction of pallor, cyanosis, and hyperemia in response to cold or emotional stress. Vasospasm is also seen in patients who receive systemic norepinephrine, vasopressin, ergot, and bleomycin. The patient with Raynaud's phenomenon and ulcerations on the tips of the digits should be examined carefully for periungual and mat telangiectasias, the subtle signs of scleroderma. Raynaud's phenomenon is also seen in patients with dermatomyositis, systemic lupus, cryoglobulinemia, cervical rib and scalenus anticus syndromes, pneumatic hammer disease, and occupational acro-osteolysis (associated with the manufacture of polyvinyl chloride).

In *pyoderma gangrenosum*, the border of the ulcers has a characteristic appearance of an undermined necrotic bluish edge and a peripheral erythematous halo. The ulcers often begin as pustules that then expand rather rapidly to a size as large as 20 cm. Although these lesions are most commonly found on the lower extremities, they can arise anywhere on the surface of the body, including sites of trauma (pathergy). An estimated 30 to 50 percent of cases are idiopathic, and the most common associated disorders are ulcerative colitis and Crohn's disease. Less commonly, it is associated with chronic active hepatitis, seropositive rheumatoid arthritis, acute and chronic granulocytic leukemia, polycythemia vera, and myeloma. Additional findings in these patients, even those with idiopathic disease, are cutaneous anergy and a benign monoclonal gammopathy. Because the histology of pyoderma gangrenosum is nonspecific, the diagnosis is made clinically by excluding less common causes of similar-appearing ulcers such as necrotizing vasculitis, Meleney's ulcer (see above), dimorphic fungi, cutaneous amebiasis, spider bites, and factitial. In the myeloproliferative disorders, the ulcers may be more superficial with a pustulobullous border, and these lesions provide a connection between classic pyoderma gangrenosum and acute febrile neutrophilic dermatosis (Sweet's syndrome).

The clinical diagnosis of *Behçet's disease* (see Chap. 290) requires the presence of recurrent oral ulceration (at least three times in a 12-month period) in addition to two of the four following criteria: (1) recurrent genital ulcers, primarily of the vulva and scrotum, (2) eye lesions, either uveitis or retinal vasculitis, (3) skin lesions, and (4) a positive pathergy test. The oral ulcers are usually painful and well-defined with an erythematous halo, whereas the genital ulcers tend to be deeper and heal with scarring. Erythema nodosum, "pseudofolliculitis," papulopustular lesions, *or* acneiform nodules in a postadolescent patient not on glucocorticoids are the entities included under the heading of skin lesions. The test for pathergy, which is defined as a reproduction of cutaneous lesions by trauma, is performed by injecting sterile saline into the dermis. Before the diagnosis of Behçet's disease can be made, the following disorders must be excluded: recurrent erythema multiforme (see "Vesicles/Bullae"), herpes simplex, inflammatory bowel disease, systemic lupus, and primary blistering disorders.

FEVER AND RASH The major considerations in a patient with a fever and a rash are inflammatory diseases versus infectious diseases. In the hospital setting, the most common scenario is a patient who has a drug rash plus a fever secondary to an underlying infection. However, it should be emphasized that a drug reaction can lead to both a cutaneous eruption and a fever ("drug fever"). Additional inflammatory diseases that are often associated with a fever include pustular psoriasis, erythroderma, and Sweet's syndrome. Lyme disease, secondary syphilis, and viral and bacterial exanthems (see "Exanthems") are examples of infectious diseases that produce a rash and a fever. Lastly, it is important to determine whether or not the cutaneous lesions represent septic emboli (see "Purpura"). Such lesions usually have evidence of ischemia in the form of purpura, necrosis, or impending necrosis (gunmetal-gray color). In the patient with thrombocytopenia, however, purpuric lesions can be seen in inflammatory reactions such as morbilliform drug eruptions and infectious lesions.

REFERENCES

BORK K: *Cutaneous Side Effects of Drugs.* Philadelphia, Saunders, 1988

BRAVERMAN IM: *Skin Signs of Systemic Disease*, 2d ed. Philadelphia, Saunders, 1981

CALLEN JP: *Dermatology Clinics*, vol 8, no 2: *Skin Signs of Internal Disease II.* Philadelphia, Saunders, 1990

———, JORRIZZO JL: *Dermatology Clinics*, vol 7, no 3: *Skin Signs of Internal Disease.* Philadelphia, Saunders, 1989

DEVITA VT JR et al (eds): *Cancer—Principles and Practice of Oncology*, 3d ed. Philadelphia, Lippincott, 1989

JORRIZZO JL: *Dermatology Clinics*, vol 3, no 1: *Urticaria*. Philadelphia, Saunders, 1985

LEVER WF, SCHAUMBURG-LEVER G: *Histopathology of the Skin*, 7th ed. Philadelphia, Lippincott, 1990

ROOK A et al (eds): *Textbook of Dermatology*, 5th ed. Oxford, Blackwell Scientific, 1991

55 PHOTOSENSITIVITY AND OTHER REACTIONS TO LIGHT

DAVID R. BICKERS

SOLAR RADIATION Sunlight is the most visible and obvious source of comfort in the environment, and it is in the nature of humans to love light. This natural proclivity for the sun has the beneficial results of warmth and vitamin D synthesis but also can produce pathologic consequences. Few effects due to sun exposure beyond those on the skin have been identified, but cutaneous exposure to sunlight can evoke immunosuppressive responses that may be relevant to the pathogenesis of nonmelanoma skin cancer.

The sun's energy encompasses a broad range from ultrashort ionizing radiation (10^{-2} μm) to ultralong radiowaves of very low photon energy (10^7 μm). Thus the emission spectrum has a range of nine orders of magnitude, but that reaching the earth's surface is narrow and is limited to components of the ultraviolet, visible light, and portions of the infrared. The cutoff at the short end of the ultraviolet is at approximately 290 nm, because stratospheric ozone is formed by ionizing radiation of wavelengths less than 100 nm and ozone in turn absorbs solar energy between 120 and 310 nm. In effect, stratospheric ozone prevents penetration to the earth's surface of the shorter, more energetic, potentially more harmful wavelengths of solar radiation. Indeed, concern about destruction of the ozone layer by chlorofluorocarbons released into the atmosphere has led to international agreements to reduce production of these chemicals.

Measurements of solar flux indicate that there is a twentyfold regional variation in the amount of energy at 300 nm that reaches the surface of the earth. This variability is in part related to seasonal effects, the path of sunlight transmission through ozone and air, the altitude (4 percent increase for each 300 m of elevation), the latitude (increasing intensity with decreasing latitude), and the amount of cloud cover, fog, and pollution.

The major components of the photobiologic action spectrum include the ultraviolet and visible wavelengths between 290 and 700 nm. In addition, the wavelengths beyond 700 nm in the infrared primarily evoke heat, but warming of the skin may enhance the response to wavelengths in the ultraviolet and visible spectrum.

The ultraviolet (UV) spectrum is arbitrarily divided into three major segments: C, B, and A. This includes the wavelengths between 10 and 400 nm. UV-C consists of wavelengths between 10 and 290 nm and does not reach the earth because of its absorption by stratospheric ozone. These wavelengths are not a cause of photosensitivity except in occupational settings where artificial sources of this energy are employed, e.g., for germicidal effects. UV-B consists of wavelengths between 290 and 320 nm. This portion of the photobiologic action spectrum is the most efficient in producing redness or erythema in human skin, and hence it is sometimes known as the "sunburn spectrum." UV-A represents those wavelengths between 320 and 400 nm and is approximately a thousandfold less efficient in producing skin hyperemia than is UV-B.

The visible wavelengths between 400 and 700 nm include the familiar white light which when directed through a prism can be shown to consist of various colors including violet, indigo, blue, green, yellow, orange, and red. The energy possessed by photons in the visible spectrum usually is not capable of damaging human skin in the absence of a photosensitizing chemical. Photon energy levels are critical to photosensitivity, since the absorption process requires that sufficient energy be present. The absorption of a photon is an all-or-none phenomenon, and when absorbed, the photon ceases to exist. The absorption of energy is critical to the development of photosensitivity. Thus the *absorption spectrum* of a molecule is defined as the range of wavelengths absorbed by it, whereas the *action spectrum* for an effect of incident radiation is defined as the range of wavelengths that evoke the response.

Photosensitivity occurs when a photon-absorbing chemical (*chromophore*) present in the skin absorbs incident energy, becomes excited, and transfers the absorbed energy to various structures or to oxygen. The absorbed energy must subsequently be dissipated by processes including heat, fluorescence, and phosphorescence. It is important to emphasize that absorption spectra and action spectra need not be superimposable, but there must be overlap at some point to produce photosensitization.

STRUCTURE AND FUNCTION OF SKIN   The skin is accessible to incident solar radiation and has a structural heterogeneity that permits the absorption of some wavelengths and the transmission of others. Essentially, human skin is a sandwich of two distinctive compartments, the epidermis and dermis, separated by a basement membrane. The outer epidermis is a stratified squamous epithelium comprising the surface stratum corneum (a protein- and lipid-rich compact membrane), the stratum granulosum, stratum Malphigii, and the basal cell layer. The basal cell layer contains a heterogeneous population of cells, some of which migrate upward in the process of terminal differentiation that results in the expression of keratin genes and the formation of the stratum corneum. Epidermal cells include resident keratinocytes and melanocytes and immigrant cells, including the immunologically active Langerhans cells, lymphocytes, polymorphonuclear leukocytes, monocytes, and macrophages. The epidermis is a major component of the immune system. Branches of sensory nerve endings also reach into this compartment.

The second major component of skin is the dermis, which is relatively large and less densely populated with cells that include fibroblasts, endothelial cells within dermal vessels, and mast cells. Tissue macrophages and sparsely distributed inflammatory cells are also present. All these cells exist within an extracellular matrix of collagen, elastin, and glycosaminoglycans. In contrast to the epidermis, rich vascularization of the dermis allows it to play an important role in temperature regulation.

UV RADIATION (UVR) AND SKIN   The epidermis and the dermis contain several chromophores capable of interacting with incident solar energy. These interactions include reflection, refraction, absorption, and transmission. The stratum corneum is a major impediment to the transmission of UV-B, and less than 10 percent of incident wavelengths in this region penetrate the basement membrane. Approximately 3 percent of radiation below 300 nm, 20 percent of radiation below 360 nm, and 33 percent of short visible radiation reaches the basal cell layer in untanned human skin. Proteins and nucleic acids absorb intensely in the short UV-B. In contrast, UV-A penetrates the epidermis efficiently to reach the dermis, where it likely produces changes in structural and matrix proteins that contribute to the aged appearance of chronically sun-exposed skin, particularly in individuals of light complexion.

One of the consequences of UV-B absorption by DNA is the production of pyrimidine, particularly thymine dimers. These structural changes can be repaired by mechanisms that result in their recognition, excision, and the reestablishment of normal base sequences. The efficient repair of these structural aberrations is crucial, since individuals with defective DNA repair are at high risk for the development of cutaneous cancer. For example, patients with xeroderma pigmentosum, an autosomal recessive disorder, are characterized by variably decreased repair of UV-induced pyrimidine dimers and may develop the xerotic appearance of photoaging as well as basal cell and squamous cell carcinomas and melanoma in the first two decades of life.

Cutaneous optics and chromophores   Chromophores are endogenous or exogenous chemical components that can absorb physical energy. Endogenous chromophores of skin are of two types: (1) chemicals that are normally present, including nucleic acids, proteins, lipids, and cholesterol derivatives such as the precursor of vitamin D, and (2) chemicals, such as porphyrins, synthesized elsewhere in the body that circulate in the bloodstream and diffuse into the skin, where they can absorb incident radiation and evoke cutaneous photosensitivity. Normally, only trace amounts of porphyrins are present in the skin, but in the porphyrias, increased amounts of porphyrins are released into the circulation and are transported to the skin, where they absorb incident energy both in the Soret band around 400 nm (short visible) and to a lesser extent in the red portion of the visible spectrum (580–660 nm). This results in structural damage to the skin that may be manifest as erythema, edema, urticaria, or blister formation (see Chap. 346).

Acute effects of sun exposure   The immediate cutaneous consequences of sun exposure include sunburn and vitamin D synthesis.

SUNBURN   This very common affliction of human skin is caused by exposure to UV radiation. Generally speaking, the ability of an individual to tolerate sunlight is inversely proportional to melanin pigmentation. Melanin is a complex polymer of tyrosine that functions as an efficient neutral-density filter with broad absorbance within the UV portion of the solar spectrum. Melanin is synthesized in specialized epidermal dendritic cells termed *melanocytes* and is packaged into *melanosomes* that are transferred via dendritic processes into *keratinocytes*, where they provide photoprotection. A single melanocyte can provide melanin pigment for approximately 36 keratinocytes, and this group of cells is termed the *epidermal-melanin unit*. Tolerance of sun exposure is a function of the efficiency of the epidermal-melanin unit and can usually be ascertained by asking an individual two questions: (1) Do you burn after sun exposure? and (2) Do you tan after sun exposure? By the answers to these questions, it is usually possible to divide the population into six skin types varying from type I (always burn, never tan) to type VI (never burn, always tan) (see Table 55-1).

There are two general theories about the pathogenesis of the sunburn response. First, the lag phase in time between skin exposure and the development of visible redness (usually 4 to 12 h) suggests an epidermal chromophore that causes delayed production and/or release of vasoactive mediator(s) that diffuse to the dermal vasculature to evoke vasodilatation. Second, it is possible that the small amount of incident UV-B radiation (10 percent or less) that penetrates to the dermis can be absorbed by endothelial cells in the vasculature, thereby directly resulting in vasodilatation. The issue remains unresolved.

TABLE 55-1   Skin type and sunburn sensitivity

Type	Description
I	Always burn, never tan
II	Always burn, sometimes tan
III	Sometimes burn, sometimes tan
IV	Sometimes burn, always tan
V	Never burn, sometimes tan
VI	Never burn, always tan

The action spectrum for sunburn erythema includes the UV-B and the UV-A regions. Photons in the shorter UV-B are at least a thousandfold more efficient than photons in the longer UV-B and the UV-A in evoking the response. However, UV-A may contribute to sunburn erythema at midday when much more UV-A than UV-B is present.

The mechanism of injury remains poorly defined, but the action spectrum for UV-B erythema closely resembles the absorption spectrum for DNA after adjusting for the absorbance of incident energy by the stratum corneum. Damaged keratinocytes (so-called sunburn cells) are visible histologically within an hour of exposure and are maximal within 24 h. UV-A is less effective than UV-B in producing sunburn cells. Mast cells may release inflammatory mediators after exposure to UV-B and UV-A. For example, erythema doses of both UV-B and UV-A increase histamine levels in suction blisters of human skin that return to normal by 24 h (before visible erythema has subsided). Prostaglandin E_2 (PGE_2) increases to approximately 150 percent of control levels by 24 h and then diminishes. Since prostaglandins evoke both pain and redness when injected intradermally, their presence in suction blisters after UV-B exposure suggests a role in UV-B erythema. There may be an age-related decline in the amount of inflammatory mediators detectable in human skin after UV-B irradiation. UV-A erythema results in few epidermal sunburn cells, but vascular endothelial injury is greater than with UV-B. In addition, there are increased levels of arachidonic acid and of prostaglandins D_2, E_2, and I_2 that peak within 5 to 9 h and then subside before peak redness occurs. Despite the evidence for elevated prostaglandins in both UV-B– and UV-A–irradiated skin, administration of nonsteroidal anti-inflammatory drugs is more effective in reducing erythema evoked by UV-B than by UV-A.

VITAMIN D PHOTOCHEMISTRY Cutaneous exposure to UV-B causes photolysis of epidermal provitamin D_3 (7-dehydrocholesterol) to previtamin D_3, which then undergoes a temperature-dependent isomerization to form the stable hormone vitamin D_3. This compound then diffuses to the dermal vasculature and circulates to the liver and kidney, where it is converted to the functional hormone 1,25-dihydroxy vitamin D_3 [$1,25(OH)_2D_3$] (see also Chap. 356). Aging substantially decreases the ability of human skin to produce vitamin D_3. This, coupled with the widespread recommended use of sunscreens that filter out UV-B, has led to concern that vitamin D deficiency may become a significant clinical problem in the elderly. Indeed, studies have shown that the use of sunscreens can prevent the production of vitamin D_3 in human skin.

Chronic effects of sun exposure: nonmalignant The clinical features of photodamaged sun-exposed skin consist of wrinkling, blotchiness, telangiectasia, and a roughened, irregular, "weather-beaten" appearance. Whether these changes, which some refer to as *photoaging* or *dermatoheliosis*, represent accelerated chronologic aging or a separate and distinct process is not clear.

Within chronically sun-exposed epidermis there is thickening (acanthosis) and morphologic heterogeneity within the basal cell layer. Higher but irregular melanosome content may be present in some keratinocytes, indicating prolonged residence of the cells in the basal cell layer. These structural changes may help to explain the leathery texture and the blotchy discoloration of sun-damaged skin.

The dermis is the major site for sun-associated chronic damage, manifest as a massive increase in thickened irregular masses of tangled elastic fibers containing uncharacterized electron-dense material. Collagen fibers are also abnormally clumped in the deeper dermis. Fibroblasts are increased in number and show morphologic signs suggesting enhanced metabolic activity. Degraded mast cells may be present in the dermis, the relevance of which remains unclear.

These morphologic changes, both gross and microscopic, are features of chronically sun-exposed skin. The chromophore(s), the action spectra, and the specific biochemical events that result in these changes are unknown.

Chronic effects of sun exposure: malignant One of the major known consequences of chronic skin exposure to sunlight is nonmela-noma skin cancer. The two types of nonmelanoma skin cancer are basal cell and squamous cell carcinoma (see Chap. 324). There are three major steps for cancer induction: initiation, promotion, and progression. Chronic exposure of animal skin to artificial light sources that mimic solar UVR results in *initiation*, a step whereby structural (mutational) changes in DNA evoke an irreversible change in the target cell (keratinocyte) that begins the tumorigenic process. Exposure to a tumor initiator is believed to be a necessary but not sufficient step in the malignant process, since initiated skin cells not exposed to tumor promoters do not generally develop tumors. The second stage in tumor development is *promotion*, a multistep process whereby initiated cells are exposed to chemical and physical agents that evoke epigenetic changes that culminate in the clonal expansion of initiated cells and cause the development, over a period of weeks to months, of benign growths known as *papillomas*. UV-B is a *complete carcinogen*, meaning that it can function as both an initiator and a promoter, leading to tumor induction. *Incomplete carcinogens* can initiate tumorigenesis but require additional skin exposure to tumor promoters to cause the production of tumors. The prototype tumor promoter is the phorbol ester 12-*O*-tetradecanoyl phorbol-13-acetate (TPA). Tumor promotion usually requires multiple exposures over time to evoke a neoplasm.

The final step in the malignant process is the conversion of benign precursors into malignant lesions, a process thought to require additional genetic alterations in already transformed cells.

Sun exposure is believed to cause nonmelanoma and melanoma cancers of the skin, although the evidence is far more direct for its role in nonmelanoma (basal cell and squamous cell carcinoma) than in melanoma cancers. Approximately 80 percent of nonmelanoma skin cancers develop on exposed body areas, including the face, the neck, and the hands. Men of fair complexion who work outdoors are twice as likely as women to develop these types of cancers. Whites of darker complexions (e.g., Hispanics) have one-tenth the risk of developing such cancers as do light-skinned individuals. Blacks are at lowest risk for all forms of skin cancer. Between 400,000 and 500,000 individuals in the United States develop nonmelanoma skin cancer annually, and the lifetime risk for a white individual to develop such a neoplasm is estimated at approximately 15 percent. A consensus exists that the incidence of nonmelanoma skin cancer in the population is rising for reasons that are unclear.

The relationship of sun exposure to melanoma is less clear-cut, but suggestive evidence supports an association. Melanomas may develop by the teenage years, indicating that the latent period for tumor growth is less than that of nonmelanomas. Epidemiologic studies of immigrants of similar ethnic stock indicate that individuals born in one area or who migrated to the same locale before age 10 have higher age-specific melanoma rates than individuals arriving later. It is thus reasonable to conclude that life in a sunny climate from birth or early childhood increases the risk of melanoma. In general, risk does not correlate with cumulative sun exposure but may relate to sequelae of sun exposure in childhood. Thus a blistering sunburn is associated with a doubling of melanoma risk at the site of the reaction.

Immunologic effects Exposure to solar radiation influences both local and systemic immune responses. UV-B appears to be most efficient in altering immune responses, likely related to the capacity of such energy to affect antigen presentation in skin by interacting with epidermal Langerhans cells. These bone marrow–derived dendritic cells possess surface markers characteristic of monocytes and macrophages. Following skin exposure to erythema doses of UV-B, Langerhans cells undergo both morphologic and functional changes that result in decreased contact allergic responses when haptens are applied to the radiated site. This diminished capacity for sensitization is due to the induction of antigen-specific suppressor T lymphocytes. Indeed, while the immunosuppressive effect of irradiation is limited to haptens applied to the irradiated site, the net result is systemic immune suppression to that antigen because of the induction of suppressor T cells that spread throughout the body.

Higher doses of radiation evoke diminished immunologic responses to antigens introduced either epicutaneously or intracutaneously at sites distant from the irradiated site. These suppressed responses are also associated with the induction of antigen-specific suppressor T lymphocytes and may be mediated by as yet undefined factors that are released from epidermal cells at the irradiated site. The implications of this generalized immune suppression in terms of altered susceptibility to cutaneous cancer or to infection remain to be defined.

It is known that UV-induced tumors in murine skin are antigenic and are rapidly rejected when transplanted into normal syngeneic animals. If the tumors are transplanted into animals previously exposed to subcarcinogenic doses of UVR, they are not rejected and instead grow progressively in the recipients. This failure of irradiated animals to reject the transplanted tumors is due to the development of T suppressor cells that prevent the rejection response. While the mechanism of suppression of tumor rejection is unknown, such a response might be a critical determinant of cancer risk in human skin.

PHOTOSENSITIVITY DISEASES   The diagnosis of photosensitivity requires a careful history to define the duration of the signs and symptoms, the length of time between exposure to sunlight and the development of subjective complaints, and visible changes in the skin. The age of onset also can be a helpful clue; for example, the acute photosensitivity of erythropoietic protoporphyria almost always begins in childhood, whereas the chronic photosensitivity of porphyria cutanea tarda typically begins in the fourth and fifth decades. A history of exposure to topical and systemic drugs and chemicals may provide important information. Many classes of drugs can cause photosensitivity on the basis of either phototoxicity or photoallergy. Fragrances such as musk ambrette contained in numerous cosmetic products are also potent photosensitizers.

Examination of the skin also may offer important clues. Anatomic areas that are naturally protected from direct sunlight such as the hairy scalp, the upper eyelids, the retroauricular areas, the infranasal, and the submental regions may be spared, whereas exposed areas show characteristic features of the pathologic process. These anatomic localization patterns are often helpful but not infallible in making the diagnosis. For example, airborne contact sensitizers that are blown onto the skin may produce dermatitis that can be difficult to distinguish from photosensitivity, despite the fact that such material may trigger skin reactivity in areas shielded from direct sunlight.

Many dermatologic conditions may be caused or aggravated by light (Table 55-2). The role of light in evoking these responses may be dependent on genetic abnormalities ranging from the well-described defect in DNA repair that occurs in xeroderma pigmentosum to the inherited abnormalities in heme synthesis that characterize the porphyrias. In certain photosensitivity diseases, the chromophore has been identified, whereas in the majority, the energy-absorbing agent is unknown.

Polymorphous light eruption   After sunburn, the most common type of photosensitivity disease is *polymorphous light eruption*, the mechanism of which is unknown. Many affected individuals never seek medical attention because the condition is often transient, becoming manifest each spring with initial sun exposure but then subsiding spontaneously with continuing exposure, a phenomenon known as "hardening." The major manifestations of polymorphous light eruption include pruritic (often intensely so) erythematous papules that may coalesce into plaques on exposed areas of the face and arms or other areas as well, making the distribution spotty and uneven.

The diagnosis can be confirmed by skin biopsy and by performing phototest procedures in which skin is exposed to multiple erythema doses of the UV-A and UV-B. The action spectrum for polymorphous light eruption is usually within these portions of the solar spectrum.

Treatment of this disease includes the induction of "hardening" by the cautious administration of light either alone or in combination with photosensitizers such as the psoralens (see below).

Phototoxicity and photoallergy   Another photosensitivity disorder is related to the topical or systemic administration of drugs and

TABLE 55-2 Classification of photosensitivity diseases	
Type	Disease
Genetic	Erythropoietic porphyria
	Erythropoietic protoporphyria
	Albinism
	Xeroderma pigmentosum
	Rothmund-Thompson disease
	Bloom's disease
	Cockayne's disease
	Familial porphyria cutanea tarda
	Phenylketonuria
	Hepatoerythropoietic porphyria
Metabolic	Sporadic porphyria cutanea tarda
	Variegate porphyria
	Hartnup disease
	Kwashiorkor
	Pellagra
	Carcinoid
	Pseudoporphyria
Phototoxic	
Internal	Drugs
External	Drugs, plants, food
Photoallergic	
Immediate	Solar urticaria
Delayed	Drug photoallergy
	Persistent light reaction
Neoplastic and degenerative	Photoaging
	Actinic keratoses
	Basal cell carcinoma
	Squamous cell carcinoma
	Melanoma
	Dysplastic nevus syndrome
	Bowen's disease
Idiopathic	Polymorphous light eruption
	Hydroa aestivale
	Actinic reticuloid
Photoaggravated	Lupus erythematosus
	Systemic
	Subacute cutaneous
	Dermatomyositis
	Pemphigus foliaceus
	Herpes simplex
	Lichen planus actinicus
	Acne vulgaris
	Atopic dermatitis
	Transient acantholytic dermatosis

other chemicals. Photosensitivity reactions are of two broad types, phototoxicity and photoallergy, both of which require the absorption of energy by a drug or chemical resulting in the production of an excited-state photosensitizer that can transfer its absorbed energy to a bystander molecule or to molecular oxygen, thereby generating tissue-destructive chemical species.

Phototoxicity is a nonimmunologic reaction caused by drugs and chemicals, a few of which are listed in Table 55-3. The usual clinical manifestations include erythema resembling a sunburn that quickly desquamates or "peels" within several days. In addition, edema, vesicles, and bullae may occur.

Photoallergy is distinct in that the immune system participates in the pathologic process. The excited-state photosensitizer may create highly unstable haptenic free radicals that bind covalently to macromolecules to form a functional antigen capable of evoking a delayed hypersensitivity response. Some of the drugs and chemicals that produce photoallergy are listed in Table 55-4. The clinical manifestations typically differ from those of phototoxicity in that an intensely pruritic eczematous dermatitis tends to be predominant and evolves into lichenified, thickened, "leathery" changes in sun-exposed areas. A small subset (perhaps 5 to 10 percent) of patients with photoallergy may develop a persistent exquisite hypersensitivity to light even when the offending drug or chemical is identified and eliminated. Known as *persistent light reaction*, this may be incapacitating for years.

Diagnostic confirmation of phototoxicity and photoallergy often can be obtained using phototest procedures. In patients with suspected phototoxicity, determination of the minimal erythema dose (MED) while the patient is exposed to a suspected agent and then repeating

TABLE 55-3 Phototoxic drugs and chemicals

	Topical	Systemic
Coal tar derivatives		
Acridine	+	
Anthracene	+	
Phenanthrene	+	
Drugs		
Amiodarone		+
Dacarbazine		+
5-Fluorouracil	+	+
Furosemide		+
Nalidixic acid		+
Phenothiazines		+
Psoralens	+	+
Retinoids	+	+
Sulfonamides		+
Sulfonylureas		+
Tetracyclines		+
Thiazides		+
Vinblastine		+
Dyes		
Anthraquinone		+
Eosin		+
Methylene blue		+
Rose bengal		+

the MED after discontinuation of the agent may provide a clue to the causative drug or chemical. Photopatch testing can be performed to confirm the diagnosis of photoallergy. This is a simple variant of ordinary patch testing in which a series of known photoallergens is applied to the skin in duplicate and one set is irradiated with a suberythema dose of UV-A. Development of eczematous changes at sites exposed to sensitizer and light is a positive result. The characteristic abnormality in patients with persistent light reaction is a diminished threshhold to erythema evoked by UV-B.

The management of drug photosensitivity is first and foremost to eliminate exposure to the chemical agents responsible for the reaction and to minimize sun exposure. The acute symptoms of phototoxicity may be ameliorated by cool, moist compresses, topical glucocorticoids, and systemically administered nonsteroidal anti-inflammatory agents. In severely affected individuals, a rapidly tapered course of systemic glucocorticoids may be useful. Judicious use of analgesics may be necessary.

TABLE 55-4 Photoallergenic drugs and chemicals

	Topical	Systemic
Antibiotics		
Sulfonamides		+
Antifungals		
Fenticlor	+	
Jadit	+	
Multifungin	+	
Diuretics		
Thiazides		+
Fragrances		
Musk ambrette	+	
6-Methylcoumarin	+	
Plant oleoresins	+	
Halogenated salicylanilides		
Bithionol	+	
Tetrachlorosalicylanilides	+	
Tribromosalicylanilide	+	
Nonsteroidal anti-inflammatory agents		
Piroxicam	+	
Phenothiazines		
Chlorpromazine	+	
Promethazine	+	
Sulfonylureas		+
Sunscreens		
p-Aminobenzoic acid and esters	+	
Whitening agents		
Stilbenes	+	

Photoallergic reactions require similar management techniques. Furthermore, individuals suffering from persistent light reactivity must be protected against light exposure. In selected patients in whom chronic systemic high-dose glucocorticoids pose unacceptable risks, it may be necessary to employ cytotoxic agents such as azathioprine or cyclophosphamide.

Porphyria The porphyrias (see Chap. 346) are a group of diseases that have in common various derangements in the synthesis of heme. Heme is a nonchelated tetrapyrrole or porphyrin, and the porphyrins are potent photosensitizers that absorb light intensely in both the short (400–410 nm) and the long (580–650 nm) portions of the visible spectrum.

Heme cannot be reutilized and must be continuously synthesized, and the two body compartments with the largest requirement for its production are the bone marrow and the liver. Accordingly, the porphyrias originate in one or the other of these organs, with the end result of excessive endogenous production of potent photosensitizers. The porphyrins circulate in the bloodstream and diffuse into the skin, where they absorb solar energy, become photoexcited, and evoke cutaneous photosensitivity. The mechanism of porphyrin photosensitization is known to be a photodynamic or oxygen-dependent reaction that can be mediated by reactive oxygen species such as superoxide anions.

Two forms of human porphyria, porphyria cutanea tarda and erythropoietic protoporphyria, will be discussed briefly. *Porphyria cutanea tarda* is the most common type of human porphyria and is associated with decreased activity of the enzyme uroporphyrinogen decarboxylase. There are two basic types of porphyria cutanea tarda: the sporadic or acquired type, generally seen in individuals ingesting ethanol or receiving estrogens and associated with increased hepatic iron stores, and the inherited type, in which there is autosomal dominant transmission of deficient enzyme activity.

In both types of porphyria cutanea tarda, the predominant feature is a chronic photosensitivity characterized by increased fragility of sun-exposed skin, particularly areas subject to repeated trauma such as the dorsa of the hands, the forearms, the face, and the ears. The predominant skin lesions are vesicles and bullae that rupture, producing moist erosions often with a hemorrhagic base, and which heal slowly with crusting and purplish discoloration of the affected skin. Hypertrichosis, mottled pigmentary change, and scleroderma-like induration are associated features. Biochemical confirmation of the diagnosis can be obtained by measurement of urinary porphyrin excretion and by assay of uroporphyrinogen decarboxylase.

Treatment consists of repeated phlebotomies to diminish the excessive hepatic iron stores and/or intermittent low doses of the antimalarial drugs chloroquine and hydroxychloroquine. Long-term remission of the disease can be achieved if the patient eliminates exposure to porphyrinogenic agents.

Erythropoietic protoporphyria originates in the bone marrow and is due to a decrease in the enzyme ferrochelatase. The major clinical features include an acute photosensitivity characterized by subjective burning and stinging of exposed skin that often develops during or just after exposure. There may be associated skin swelling and, after repeated episodes, a waxlike scarring.

The diagnosis is confirmed by demonstration of elevated measurement of free erythrocyte protoporphyrin. Detection of increased plasma protoporphyrin helps to differentiate lead poisoning and iron-deficiency anemia, in both of which elevated erythrocyte protoporphyrin occurs in the absence of cutaneous photosensitivity and of elevated plasma protoporphyrin.

Treatment consists of reducing sun exposure and the oral administration of the carotenoid β-carotene, which is an effective scavenger of free radicals. Many affected individuals are able to tolerate sun exposure while ingesting this drug, but it has no effect on the metabolic defect in porphyrin-heme synthesis.

PHOTOPROTECTION Since photosensitivity of the skin results from exposure to sunlight, it follows that avoidance of the sun would eliminate these disorders. Unfortunately, social pressures make this

TABLE 55-5   Properties of selected sunscreens

Ingredients	Trade names	SPF* (outdoors)	Substantivity†
p-Aminobenzoic acid (PABA) (5% in ethanol)	Pre-Sun-15	10–12	Excellent
p-Aminobenzoic acid esters (3.5% padimate A + 3.0% octyldimethyl PABA)	Original Eclipse	4–6	Fair
p-Aminobenzoic acid ester combinations (7.0% padimate 0 + 2.5% oxybenzone + 5.0% dioxybenzone)	Bain de Soleil	9	Excellent
Non-p-aminobenzoic acid (3% 2-hydroxy-4-methoxy benzophenone)	Ti-Screen-15	10–12	Excellent
Physical sunscreens (5% titanium dioxide + 5% methyl anthranilate)	A-Fil	4–6	Good

* SPF = sun protective factor.
† Substantivity = ability to remain on the skin.

an impractical alternative for most individuals, and this has led to a search for better approaches to photoprotection.

Natural photoprotection is provided by structural proteins in the epidermis, particularly keratin and melanin. The amount of melanin and its distribution in cells is genetically regulated, and individuals of darker complexion (skin types IV to VI) are at decreased risk for the development of cutaneous malignancy.

Other forms of photoprotection include clothing and sunscreens. Clothing constructed of tightly woven fabrics irrespective of color affords substantial protection. Wide-brimmed hats, long sleeves, and pants all reduce direct exposure. Sunscreens are of two major types—chemical and physical. Chemical sunscreening agents are chromophores that absorb energy in the UV-B and/or UV-A regions, thereby diminishing photon absorption by the skin (Table 55-5). Sunscreens are rated for their photoprotective effect by their *sun protective factor* (SPF). The SPF is simply a ratio of the time required to produce sunburn erythema with and without sunscreen application. SPF ratings of 15 or higher provide effective protection against UV-B and, to a lesser extent, UV-A. The major categories of chemical sunscreens include p-aminobenzoic acid and its esters, benzophenones, anthranilates, cinnamates, and salicylates. Physical sunscreens are light-opaque mixtures containing zinc oxide, talc, or titanium oxide that scatter light, thereby reducing absorption by the skin.

In addition to light absorption, a critical determinant of the photoprotective effect of sunscreens is their ability to remain on the skin, a property known as *substantivity*. In general, the PABA esters formulated in moisturizing vehicles provide the greatest substantivity.

Photoprotection also can be achieved by limiting the time of exposure during the day. Since as much as half an individual's total lifetime sun exposure may occur by the age of 18, it is important to educate parents and young children about the hazards of sunlight. Simply eliminating exposure at midday will achieve substantial reduction in UV-B exposure.

PHOTOTHERAPY AND PHOTOCHEMOTHERAPY   While greatest attention has been paid to the damaging effects of sunlight in the skin, this same energy is employed in the management of selected dermatologic diseases. The administration of UV-B alone or in combination with topically applied compounds such as emollient ointments with or without crude coal tar induces remissions in psoriasis, an inflammatory disorder in which excessively rapid epidermal cell turnover is associated with thick scaling and redness of the skin.

Photochemotherapy in which UV-A radiation is administered in combination with topically applied or systemically administered psoralens (PUVA) is also effective in treating psoriasis and in the early stages of cutaneous T cell lymphoma and vitiligo. Psoralens are tricyclic furocoumarins which when intercalated into DNA and exposed to UV-A produce monofunctional adducts to pyrimidine bases and eventually form DNA cross-links. These structural changes are thought to decrease DNA synthesis and effect the improvement that occurs in psoriasis. The reason that PUVA photochemotherapy is effective in cutaneous T cell lymphoma is not clear.

In addition to its effects on DNA, PUVA photochemotherapy also stimulates melanin synthesis, and this provides the rationale for its use in the depigmenting disease vitiligo. Oral 8-methoxypsoralen and UV-A appear to be most effective in this regard, but as many as 100 treatments extending over 12 to 18 months may be required to promote satisfactory repigmentation.

The major side effects of phototherapy and PUVA photochemotherapy are due to the cumulative effects of photon absorption and include skin dryness, actinic keratoses, and an increased risk of nonmelanoma skin cancer. Despite these risks, the therapeutic index of these modalities is positive.

REFERENCES

FRAIN-BELL W: *Cutaneous Photobiology.* Oxford, Oxford University Press, 1985
HARBER LC, BICKERS DR: *Photosensitivity Diseases*, 2d ed. Toronto, Decker, 1989
HÖNIGSMANN H, STINGL G: *Therapeutic Photomedicine.* Basel, Karger, 1986
MAGNUS IA: *Dermatological Photobiology.* Oxford, Blackwell, 1976
MORISON WL et al: Photobiology. J Am Acad Dermatol 25:327, 1991
PATHAK MA et al: Preventive treatment of sunburn, dermatoheliosis, and skin cancer with sun-protective agents, in *Dermatology in General Medicine*, 4th ed, TB Fitzpatrick et al (eds). New York, McGraw-Hill, 1993

section 9 Hematologic alterations

56 ANEMIA

H. FRANKLIN BUNN

By definition, patients with anemia have a significant reduction in red cell mass and a corresponding decrease in the oxygen-carrying capacity of the blood. Normally, blood volume is maintained at a nearly constant level. Therefore, anemia entails a decrease in the concentration of red cells or hemoglobin in peripheral blood. Normal blood values for individuals of various ages are shown in the Appendix of this book. In women in the childbearing age group, these values are 10 percent lower than in men. At high altitudes, higher values are found, roughly in proportion to the elevation above sea level. Anemic patients have a reduction of more than 10 percent below the mean values for the sex. However, since the variations in normal hemoglobin values approach this limit, the documentation of mild anemia may be uncertain.

SIGNS AND SYMPTOMS OF ANEMIA   The clinical presentation of the anemic patient depends on the underlying disease as well as on the severity and chronicity of the anemia. The manifestations of anemia per se can be explained by the pathophysiologic principles outlined in this chapter and in Chap. 302. Most of these signs and symptoms represent cardiovascular and ventilatory adjustments which compensate for the decrease in red blood cell mass.

The degree to which symptoms occur in an anemic patient depends on several contributing factors. If the anemia has developed rapidly, there may not be adequate time for compensatory adjustments to take place, and the patient may have more marked symptoms than if an anemia of equivalent severity had developed insidiously. Furthermore, the patient's complaints may depend on the presence of local vascular disease. For example, angina pectoris, intermittent claudication, or transient cerebral ischemia may be unmasked by the development of anemia.

Individuals with mild anemia are often asymptomatic. They may complain of fatigue as well as dyspnea and palpitation, particularly following exercise. Severely anemic patients will often be symptomatic at rest and unable to tolerate significant exertion. When the hemoglobin concentration falls below 75 g/L (7.5 g/dL), resting cardiac output rises significantly with an increase in both heart rate and stroke volume. The patient may be aware of this hyperdynamic state and complain of palpitation or a pounding pulse. Symptoms of cardiac failure may develop if the patient's myocardial reserve is reduced.

The symptoms of severe anemia extend to other organ systems. Patients often complain of dizziness and headache and may experience syncope, tinnitus, or vertigo. Many patients are irritable and have difficulty sleeping or concentrating. Because of decreased blood flow to the skin, patients may become hypersensitive to cold. Gastrointestinal symptoms such as anorexia, indigestion, and even nausea or bowel irregularity are attributable to shunting of blood away from the splanchnic bed. Females commonly develop abnormal menstruation, both amenorrhea and increased bleeding. Males may complain of impotence or loss of libido.

Physical findings   *Pallor* is the physical finding most commonly associated with anemia. However, the usefulness of this sign is limited by other factors that affect the color of the skin. The thickness and texture of the skin vary widely among individuals. Furthermore, the blood flow to the skin can undergo wide fluctuations. The concentration of melanin in the epidermis is another important determinant of skin color. Individuals with a fair complexion may look pale even though they are not anemic. Conversely, pallor is difficult to detect in deeply pigmented individuals. Furthermore, acquired disorders of melanin pigmentation (e.g., Addison's disease, hemochromatosis) or jaundice may interfere with detection of pallor. Nevertheless, even in blacks, the presence of anemia may be suspected by the color of the palms or of noncutaneous tissues such as oral mucous membranes, nail beds, and palpebral conjunctivas. The color of the creases of the palm is a useful sign. When they are as pale as the surrounding skin, the patient usually has a hemoglobin of less than 70 g/L (7 g/dL).

Two factors contribute to the development of pallor in patients with anemia. There is, of course, a decrease in the hemoglobin concentration of blood perfusing the skin and mucous membranes. Also, blood is shunted away from the skin and other peripheral tissues, permitting enhanced blood flow to vital organs. Redistribution of blood flow is an important mode of compensation in anemia.

Other physical findings associated with anemia include tachycardia, wide pulse pressure, and a hyperdynamic precordium. A systolic ejection murmur is often heard over the precordium, particularly at the pulmonic area. In addition, a venous hum may be detected over the neck vessels. These cardiac findings disappear when the anemia is corrected. Patients with hemolytic anemia often have icterus and splenomegaly and occasionally develop superficial skin ulceration over the ankle bones.

APPROACH TO THE PATIENT WITH ANEMIA

In evaluating the anemic patient, the physician should proceed in an orderly fashion so that the correct diagnosis can be established with a minimum of laboratory tests and procedures. As in other clinical disciplines, a comprehensive history and meticulous physical examination are of paramount importance in the initial workup of the anemic patient. For example, a family history which reveals a dominant inheritance pattern provides strong support for the diagnosis of hereditary spherocytosis. The discovery of a heart murmur and splenomegaly raises the possibility that the anemic patient may have subacute bacterial endocarditis.

Under unusual circumstances, the blood values do not accurately reflect alterations in the red cell mass. For example, hemoglobin level and hematocrit are falsely elevated in patients who have sustained an acute reduction in plasma volume owing to hemorrhage, extensive burns, vigorous diuresis, or other types of severe dehydration. In contrast, the blood values may be falsely low in patients who have an expanded plasma volume, as in pregnancy or congestive heart failure.

The evaluation of the anemic patient should be based on a firm understanding of the pathophysiologic principles outlined in Chap. 302. As shown in Table 56-1, the clinician must first ask whether the anemia is due to a decreased production of red cells or to enhanced destruction. Moreover, the possibility of blood loss either as the sole cause or as a contributing factor must always be considered. The examination of the stool for occult blood is an indispensable part of the evaluation of all anemic patients.

RED CELL INDEXES   Accurate measurements of the hematocrit, hemoglobin concentration, and red blood cell count enable the

TABLE 56-1   Initial evaluation of anemia

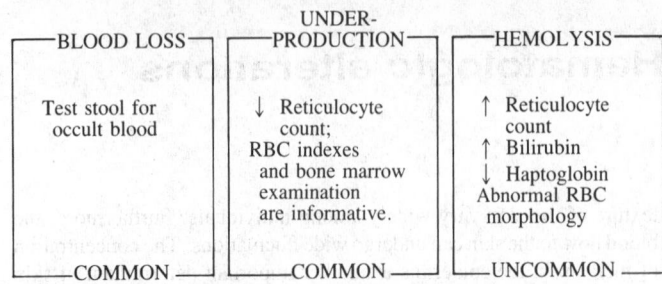

BLOOD LOSS	UNDER-PRODUCTION	HEMOLYSIS
Test stool for occult blood	↓ Reticulocyte count; RBC indexes and bone marrow examination are informative.	↑ Reticulocyte count ↑ Bilirubin ↓ Haptoglobin Abnormal RBC morphology
——— COMMON ———	——— COMMON ———	——— UNCOMMON ———

calculation of red cell indices which, as shown in Table 56-2, are very useful in the classification of anemias of underproduction. Measuring the hematocrit or PCV is the simplest and one of the most precise ways to ascertain the concentration of red cells in the blood. Generally, a small sample of anticoagulated blood is drawn into a capillary tube which is sealed at one end and centrifuged. The PCV is the ratio of the volume of packed red cells to the total volume. Alternatively, the concentration of hemoglobin can be determined spectrophotometrically from the absorbance of the cyanmethemoglobin form at a specific wavelength. With the advent of automated red blood cell counting technology, very precise measurements of red blood cell indexes are now readily available in nearly all hospitals and clinical laboratories. The electronic counter makes a direct measurement of the red cell count (RBC/μL) and the mean red cell volume (MCV):

$$MCV \text{ (fL)} = \frac{PCV \text{ (L/L)}}{(RBC/\mu L) \times 10^{-9}}$$

This instrument calculates the PCV from the direct measurement of MCV and RBC/μL. In addition, hemoglobin concentration is measured directly on a separate channel. The mean corpuscular hemoglobin concentration (MCHC) is then computed as follows:

$$MCHC \text{ (g/dL)} = \frac{Hb \text{ (g/dL)}}{PCV \text{ (L/L)}}$$

TABLE 56-2   Anemias due to decreased red cell production

RBC Indexes	Marrow	Additional lab tests	Diagnosis
Hypochromic, microcytic (↓ MCV)	0 Iron	↓ Fe, ↑ TIBC	Iron deficiency
	+ Iron Ring sideroblasts	↑ Hb A$_2$ or ↑ Hb F ↓ Hb A$_2$	β Thalassemia Sideroblastic anemia
Macrocytic (↑ MCV)	Megaloblastic	↓ Serum B$_{12}$, achlorhydria	Vitamin B$_{12}$ deficiency, pernicious anemia
		↓ Serum folate	Folic acid deficiency
Normochromic, normocytic	Normal	↓ Fe, ↓ TIBC	Anemia of chronic inflammation
		↑ Creatinine	Anemia of uremia
		Abn LFT	Anemia of liver disease
		↓ T$_4$	Anemia of myxedema
	Aplastic	Pancytopenia	Aplastic anemia
Normoblasts, teardrops	Infiltrated: tumor, lymphoma, etc.	↑ LAP	Myelophthisic
	Fibrosis		Myeloid metaplasia

NOTE: Fe, iron; TIBC, total iron-binding capacity; Hb, hemoglobin; LAP, leukocyte alkaline phosphatase; LFT, liver function tests; Abn, abnormal; MCV, mean corpuscular volume.

A third red blood cell index, the mean corpuscular hemoglobin (MCH), is determined as follows:

$$MCH \text{ (pg)} = \frac{Hb \text{ (g/dL)}}{(RBC/\mu L) \times 10^{-7}}$$

Generally, an automated system provides a printout which includes hemoglobin concentration, red cell count, packed cell volume, and the three red cell indexes (MCV, MCHC, and MCH).

As Table 56-2 shows, the MCV is particularly useful in classifying the anemias due to decreased red cell production. Microcytic anemias have low MCV values. On microscopic examination, the red cells appear small and often pale. In contrast, in the macrocytic anemias the MCV is elevated, and large, oval cells (macroovalocytes) are seen on microscopic examination. Unlike the anemias of underproduction, nearly all the hemolytic anemias are normocytic or slightly macrocytic owing to the preponderance of young red cells which are somewhat large. Exceptions include the severe forms of thalassemia in which microcytic red cells are accompanied by brisk hemolysis.

RETICULOCYTE COUNT   This is the most useful laboratory test for distinguishing anemias secondary to underproduction of red blood cells from those caused by hemolysis. When an appropriate supravital stain is applied to a sample of peripheral blood, the 1- to 2-day-old red cells exhibit a network of purple strands which are aggregates of ribosomes. Reticulocytosis is a reflection of the release of an increased number of young cells from the bone marrow. The rate of red cell production can be assessed more quantitatively by determining the reticulocyte index, which uses the hematocrit or packed cell volume (PCV) and is calculated as follows:

$$\text{Reticulocyte index} = \text{reticulocyte \%} \times \frac{\text{patient's PCV}}{\text{normal PCV}}$$

This measure fails to consider the distribution of reticulocytes between the bone marrow and the peripheral blood. When the marrow is greatly stimulated, marrow reticulocytes enter the circulation prematurely. On a routinely prepared smear, these ''shift reticulocytes'' appear larger than average and have a lavender hue, so-called polychromatophilia. Since the circulation of ''shift reticulocytes'' in the peripheral blood is prolonged, the reticulocyte index should be divided by about 2. This factor varies from 1.5 to 3 depending on the severity of the anemia and the degree of erythropoietin stimulation. This correction should always be made if normoblasts are encountered in the peripheral blood, since this finding indicates the premature release of red cell precursors into the circulation.

A failure to produce red cells is reflected in an inappropriately low reticulocyte count. In contrast, a significant elevation of reticulocytes is suggestive of hemolysis. Exceptions include (1) the brisk reticulocyte response that is seen in a patient with hemorrhage, (2) reticulocytosis encountered in patients recovering from impaired erythropoiesis (e.g., an individual with pernicious anemia who received an injection of vitamin B$_{12}$ 1 week earlier), and (3) mild to moderate elevations in reticulocytes (3 to 7 percent) encountered in myelophthisic anemia in which the orderly release of cells is affected by alterations of the marrow stroma owing to tumor, fibrosis, or granulomata. These exceptions are often readily appreciated in the initial evaluation of the patient. Furthermore, a number of ancillary laboratory tests described below are useful in determining to what extent hemolysis is occurring. The measurement of unconjugated bilirubin in the serum is a particularly useful guide to the presence of accelerated red blood cell breakdown. Once this information is obtained, the workup can be directed toward the establishment of a specific etiology.

EXAMINATION OF THE BLOOD SMEAR   In the evaluation of a patient with anemia, the physician should take the time to examine a well-stained peripheral blood film. Figures A9-1 to A9-12 show examples of abnormalities in red cell morphology encountered in various types of anemia. Many subtleties escape the attention of the technologist whose primary purpose in examining the slide is to obtain a white cell differential count. Furthermore, the clinician can approach the specimen with a prepared mind and can scrutinize it for specific abnormalities. As suggested above, the examination can confirm the size and color of red cells as estimated by RBC indexes. Furthermore, while these indexes provide mean statistical values, the microscopic examination can reveal variation in red cell size (anisocytosis) or shape (poikilocytosis), changes which are helpful in the diagnosis of specific anemias. Examination of the blood smear is particularly important in evaluating a patient with hemolysis. Most hemolytic anemias have characteristic morphologic abnormalities. Finally, this practice may yield unexpected dividends. The finding of rouleaux suggests the presence of dysproteinemia, as occurs in multiple myeloma. The examination may provide the initial clue that the patient has significant thrombocytopenia.

BONE MARROW EXAMINATION   A microscopic examination of the bone marrow is often useful and may be critical in the workup of any *unexplained* anemia. Study of the bone marrow is particularly informative in the anemias of underproduction. The more severe the anemia, the more likely it is that the procedure will be informative. An assessment of the quantity and quality of red cell precursors may determine whether there is a primary defect in cell production. A marrow biopsy is particularly useful in estimating overall cellularity. The normal differential of nucleated cells in the marrow is shown in the Appendix. The ratio of myeloid (M) to erythroid (E) precursors is normally about 2:1 but may be artifactually increased by the inclusion of circulating leukocytes. The ratio is increased in patients with infection, a leukemoid reaction, or neoplastic proliferation of myeloid cells. Rarely, a high M/E ratio is due to selective aplasia of the red cell precursors. A decreased M/E ratio indicates erythroid hyperplasia (seen in hemolysis or hemorrhage) or ineffective erythropoiesis (e.g., megaloblastic and sideroblastic anemias). The morphology of the precursors may reveal a maturation deficit such as megaloblastic anemia. The bone marrow examination is also important in demonstrating the presence of cellular infiltrates such as those found in leukemia, lymphoma, or multiple myeloma. The demonstration of tumor, fibrosis, or granulomata usually requires a biopsy. A portion of the marrow specimen should be stained with Prussian blue. In addition to providing an assessment of iron stores, this iron stain is required for the identification of sideroblasts.

VARIOUS FORMS OF ANEMIA

ANEMIA DUE TO BLOOD LOSS   This form of anemia varies considerably in its clinical presentation depending on the site, severity, and rapidity of the hemorrhage. At opposite extremes are acute fulminant bleeding producing hypovolemic shock and chronic occult blood loss leading to iron-deficiency anemia.

Patients who have sustained an acute hemorrhage generally present with signs and symptoms secondary to hypoxia and hypovolemia. Depending on the severity of the process, the patient will have weakness, fatigue, lightheadedness, stupor, or coma and will often appear pale, diaphoretic, and irritable. Vital signs are a reflection of cardiovascular compensation for the acute blood loss (Chap. 34). The patient will have hypotension and tachycardia in proportion to the degree of hemorrhage. Elicitation of postural signs is useful in the initial evaluation of patients with acute blood loss. If the pulse rises 25 percent or more or the systolic blood pressure falls 20 mmHg or more upon going from a supine to sitting position, the patient is likely to have significant hypovolemia (blood loss >1000 mL) and requires prompt replacement. Acute blood loss in excess of 1500 mL usually leads to cardiovascular collapse.

If the blood loss has been acute and recent, the peripheral blood may not reveal a significant decrease in packed cell volume or hemoglobin, since the red cell mass and plasma volume are contracted in parallel. There often is a moderate leukocytosis and a ''shift to the left'' in the white cell differential count. Thrombocytosis may be encountered in both acute and chronic blood loss, particularly when

the patient is iron-deficient. During the first few days following an acute hemorrhage there is usually an increase in reticulocytes. Occasionally, nucleated red cells may appear in the peripheral blood. Since young red cells are larger than old ones, the patient may develop slightly macrocytic red cell indexes (MCV = 95 to 105 fL). As mentioned above, sustained reticulocytosis will be seen if significant blood loss continues, or until iron stores have been exhausted. Internal bleeding may be accompanied by an increase in unconjugated bilirubin. This abnormality is a reflection of an increase in catabolism of heme from extravasated red cells. Patients with acute gastrointestinal blood loss will often have an elevation of blood urea nitrogen owing to impaired renal blood flow and perhaps to the absorption of digested blood protein.

It is of critical importance to assess these patients promptly and institute treatment without delay. A large-bore intravenous line should be placed. While blood is being typed and cross matched, saline, Ringer's lactate, or, preferably, a colloid such as 5% albumin should be infused to correct hypovolemia. Whole blood is then administered as soon as it is available. Monitoring of vital signs and central venous pressure is useful in determining the appropriate amount of volume replacement. During and following these emergency measures, diagnostic studies may reveal the site or sites of bleeding. If the bleeding is unexplained, an emergency coagulation profile should be obtained. Demonstration of bleeding from the gastrointestinal tract may require the insertion of a nasogastric tube. Appropriate radiologic studies may be indicated to determine sites of internal bleeding such as retroperitoneal hemorrhage.

Chronic blood loss is usually due to lesions in the gastrointestinal tract or the uterus. The testing of stool specimens for occult blood is an essential, though frequently overlooked, part of the evaluation of anemia. It may be necessary to examine serial specimens over a prolonged period of time, since gastrointestinal bleeding is often intermittent. The hematologic manifestations of chronic blood loss are those of iron-deficiency anemia, discussed in detail in Chap. 303.

ANEMIAS DUE TO DECREASED RBC PRODUCTION   As shown in Table 56-2, red cell indexes are useful in classifying the anemias due to underproduction of red cells. They can be conveniently grouped into three major categories: microcytic, macrocytic, and normocytic.

The *microcytic* anemias include iron-deficiency anemia (Chap. 303), sideroblastic anemias (Chap. 303), and the thalassemias (Chap. 306). Collectively, they represent a decrease in the availability or synthesis of one of the three major constituents of the hemoglobin molecule: iron, porphyrin, and globin. Since hemoglobin makes up over 90 percent of the protein within the erythrocyte, it is not surprising that these defects in hemoglobin synthesis result in the formation of small, pale red cells. These disorders involve a variable degree of ineffective erythropoiesis (Chap. 302). In addition, the anemias of chronic inflammation and malignancy may be slightly microcytic (Chap. 305). This phenomenon is due to a defect in the availability of iron. However, these disorders are more often normocytic and have been so classified in Table 56-2. Measurement of serum iron and iron-binding capacity and evaluation of marrow iron stores are particularly useful in distinguishing between these anemias.

The *macrocytic* anemias generally are associated with megaloblastic morphology in the bone marrow. In most cases, a deficiency of either vitamin B_{12} or folic acid results in an impairment of the replication of DNA, particularly in cells having a high turnover rate. Because nuclear maturation lags behind cytoplasmic development, large red cells tend to be produced in the bone marrow. Megaloblastic anemias are discussed in detail in Chap. 304. Like the microcytic anemias, these disorders are maturation defects associated with ineffective erythropoiesis. Macrocytosis, generally of a lesser degree, also may be encountered in patients with liver disease, hypothyroidism, acute blood loss, hemolytic anemia, aplastic anemia, and alcoholism. However, in these conditions, the red cell precursors in the bone marrow do not appear megaloblastic. The macrocytes in liver disease and hypothyroidism may be related to an increased deposition of lipid in the red cell membrane.

The *normocytic* anemias of underproduction comprise a diverse group of disorders. As shown in Table 56-2, this group can be conveniently subdivided into two categories: those secondary to some other underlying disease and those due to intrinsic pathology within the bone marrow.

The primary disorders of the bone marrow, such as the leukemias, myelodysplasia, aplastic anemia, and myelophthisis, are best approached by microscopic examination of a marrow aspirate and biopsy. This group of anemias is often accompanied by leukopenia and thrombocytopenia. Pancytopenia, usually to a lesser degree, also can be seen in hypersplenism and in the megaloblastic anemias. Aplastic anemia, myelodysplasia, and the myelophthisic anemias are discussed in Chap. 308.

The diagnosis of anemia secondary to some underlying disease is usually quite straightforward. Conversely, the presence of an unexplained normocytic anemia should prompt the search for an underlying disorder such as chronic renal failure, infection, or myxedema. If the presence of such an illness is established, the physician is obliged to investigate whether other factors such as blood loss or a nutritional deficiency contribute to the patient's anemia. Generally, the anemias due to liver disease, chronic inflammation, or an endocrinopathy are of only moderate severity. Unlike the other "secondary" anemias, that due to chronic renal failure is often severe. All these anemias are discussed in more detail in Chap. 305.

HEMOLYTIC ANEMIAS Hemolytic anemias (Table 56-3) are encountered much less frequently than the anemias due to decreased red cell production. Although they are a diverse group, the hemolytic anemias have a number of clinical features in common. Signs and symptoms of patients with hemolysis are briefly mentioned above.

A number of laboratory tests are available to establish the presence of accelerated breakdown of red cells. The reticulocyte count is the single most useful test. Patients with hemolysis nearly always have an elevated reticulocyte count. A variety of serum and urine tests are useful in confirming the presence of hemolysis and assessing its magnitude. Serum unconjugated bilirubin and haptoglobin are particularly useful (see Table 56-1). Others are described in detail in Chap. 307 and are summarized in Table 307-2.

Classification of hemolytic anemias Once the presence of hemolysis is established, a large battery of laboratory tests is available for determining the specific diagnosis. Some of these tests are listed in Table 56-3. No other area of internal medicine is better suited to detailed and fruitful diagnostic probing. In the interest of time and money, the clinician should use the available tests in an orderly fashion. This complex group of disorders is easier to approach diagnostically if a concise and workable classification is used. The hemolytic anemias can be grouped in several ways: congenital versus acquired, intracorpuscular versus extracorpuscular, or by anatomic site of the erythrocyte defect. The various kinds of hemolytic anemia are discussed in Chap. 307.

APPROACH TO THE TREATMENT OF ANEMIA

The effective treatment of anemia, like other disorders, is predicated on a thorough diagnostic evaluation. There is no reason to administer hematinics such as iron, vitamin B_{12}, or folic acid unless a specific deficiency of these substances has been demonstrated or is anticipated. Although the indiscriminate administration of vitamin B_{12} is not deleterious per se, it lulls both the patient and the physician into a sense of false security. In contrast, the inappropriate use of iron preparations over a prolonged period of time can be directly harmful, leading to a state of iron overload. Pyridoxine is indicated only in the treatment of sideroblastic anemias.

Many kinds of anemias can be corrected if a precipitating cause can be uncovered and reversed. If a drug or toxin can be incriminated, its withdrawal may allow full recovery. The outcome of the "secondary" anemias is dependent on whether the underlying condition can be corrected. Anemias due to an endocrinopathy or infection should respond favorably to appropriate treatment. Occasionally, the anemia of malignancy is corrected by removal of the primary tumor. One of the most dramatic sequelae of a successful renal transplant is the prompt correction of the "anemia of uremia." Moreover, the anemia associated with renal failure can be corrected by the administration of recombinant human erythropoietin. This agent also may prove to be effective in the treatment of anemia associated with other chronic disorders such as malignancies, rheumatoid arthritis, or AIDS.

Primary disorders of bone marrow such as aplastic anemia or myelophthisic anemia are often irreversible and are treated with supportive measures such as transfusions of red cells and platelets. *Androgens* are sometimes employed in this group of anemias, but their efficacy is marginal. The availability of recombinant hematopoietic growth factors may provide more specific and effective treatment. Because prognosis is so bleak in these disorders, a radical approach to treatment is justified. As described in Chaps. 308 and 313, bone marrow transplantation is a reasonable therapeutic alternative in selected cases of severe aplastic anemia and acute leukemia.

Several factors should be weighed in determining whether an anemic patient should be transfused. The risks and complications of the administration of blood products are discussed in Chap. 312. Patients with chronic or long-standing anemias are able to compensate in several ways, discussed earlier in this chapter. A considerable reduction in red cell mass can be surprisingly well tolerated, especially if the patient is young or sedentary. Transfusion is seldom indicated in a patient with a chronic anemia whose hemoglobin is 90 g/L (9 g/dL) or greater. Those who are expected to respond to the administration of a specific agent such as iron, folic acid, or vitamin B_{12} can usually be spared transfusions. If the anemia has precipitated an episode of congestive heart failure or myocardial ischemia, prompt but cautious administration of packed red cells is indicated. In general, whole blood should be given only if the patient is hypovolemic.

Glucocorticoids have only a limited role in the treatment of anemia. These agents are not effective in stimulating erythropoiesis. High doses of a glucocorticoid are indicated in the treatment of immunohemolytic anemia and pure red cell anemia. Otherwise, steroids should be prescribed sparingly unless some coexisting condition dictates their use.

Splenectomy is indicated in the treatment of certain hemolytic anemias. The efficacy of splenectomy correlates with the degree to which the abnormal or defective red cells are sequestered. Splenectomy

---

TABLE 56-3   Hemolytic anemias

Blood smear	Additional lab tests	Diagnosis
Schistocytes, helmet cells		Traumatic hemolytic anemia
Spherocytes	+ Coombs' test	Immunohemolytic anemia
	↑ Osmotic fragility	Hereditary spherocytosis
Spur cells	Abnormal LFT	Spur cell anemia
	+ Sucrose lysis	Paroxysmal nocturnal hemoglobinuria
Sickle cells	+ Sickle prep	Sickle cell syndromes
Target cells	Abn Hb electrophoresis	Hb C, D, etc.
Heinz bodies	Abn Hb electrophoresis	Congenital Heinz body hemolytic anemia
	↓ G6PD	G6PD deficiency

NOTE: Hb, hemoglobin; G6PD, glucose-6-phosphate dehydrogenase; LFT, liver function tests; Abn, abnormal.

is virtually curative in hereditary spherocytosis. The operation may be beneficial in selected patients with immunohemolytic anemia, congestive splenomegaly, spur cell anemia, and certain hemoglobinopathies and enzymopathies. The operative morbidity and mortality from elective splenectomy are very low. Occasional patients develop a left subphrenic abscess. Following splenectomy, young children are at risk of developing overwhelming septicemia. This complication is much rarer in adults. Thrombocytosis generally develops promptly following splenectomy. However, in most cases, it is transient. In patients with continued hemolysis or a myeloproliferative disorder (Chap. 309), the thrombocytosis usually persists and may occasionally be associated with thromboembolic phenomena.

REFERENCES

Babior BM, Stossel TP: *Hematology, A Pathophysiological Approach*, 2d ed. New York, Churchill Livingstone, 1990
Beck WS (ed): *Hematology*, 5th ed. Boston, MIT Press, 1991
Crosby WH: Red cell mass: Its precursors and perturbations. Hosp Prac 15:2, 71, 1980
Jandl JH: *Blood Pathophysiology*. Boston, Blackwell, 1991

57 BLEEDING AND THROMBOSIS

ROBERT I. HANDIN

Hemorrhage, intravascular thrombosis, and embolism are common clinical manifestations of many diseases. The normal hemostatic system limits blood loss by precisely regulated interactions between components of the vessel wall, circulating blood platelets, and plasma proteins. However, when disease or trauma damage large arteries and veins, excessive bleeding may occur, despite a normal hemostatic system. Less frequently, hemorrhage is caused by an inherited or acquired disorder of the hemostatic machinery itself. A large number of such bleeding disorders have now been identified.

In addition, unregulated activation of the hemostatic system may cause thrombosis and embolism, which can reduce blood flow to critical organs like the brain and myocardium. Although we understand less about the pathophysiology of thrombosis than of hemostatic failure, certain patient groups have been identified that are particularly prone to thrombosis and embolism. These include patients (1) immobilized after surgery, (2) with chronic congestive heart failure, (3) with atherosclerotic vascular disease, (4) with malignancy, or (5) who are pregnant. Most of these "thrombosis-prone" patients have no identifiable hemostatic disorder. However, there are certain patient groups who have inherited or acquired a "hypercoagulable" or "prethrombotic" state which predisposes them to recurrent thrombosis.

The cardinal manifestations of disordered hemostasis which cause bleeding or thrombosis are discussed below, along with the clinical approach to diagnosis and evaluation of these patients. Certain information in the patient's history, such as the mode of onset and sites of bleeding, a family bleeding tendency, and a record of drug ingestion help establish the correct diagnosis. Physical examination can identify bleeding in the skin or joint deformities due to previous hemarthroses. Ultimately, however, bleeding disorders are diagnosed by laboratory tests. General screening tests are utilized first, to document a systemic disorder, and are then supplemented by specific tests of coagulation protein or platelet function to arrive at an accurate diagnosis.

The hypercoagulable or prethrombotic patient can also be identified by a careful history. There are three important clues to this diagnosis: (1) repeated episodes of thromboembolism without an obvious predisposing condition; (2) a family history of thrombosis; and (3) well-documented thromboembolism in adolescents and young adults. There are, as yet, no clinically useful screening tests for the prethrombotic state. However, several of the prethrombotic disorders can be diagnosed with specific immunologic and functional assays.

NORMAL HEMOSTASIS

Accurate diagnosis and treatment of patients with either bleeding or thrombosis requires some knowledge of the pathophysiology of hemostasis. The process can be divided into primary and secondary components and is initiated when trauma, surgery, or disease disrupt the vascular endothelial lining and blood is exposed to subendothelial connective tissue. *Primary hemostasis* is the name given to the process of platelet plug formation at sites of injury. It occurs within seconds of injury and is of prime importance in stopping blood loss from capillaries, small arterioles, and venules (see Fig. 57-1). *Secondary hemostasis* describes the reactions of the plasma coagulation system which result in fibrin formation. It requires several minutes for completion. The fibrin strands which are produced strengthen the primary hemostatic plug. This reaction is particularly important in larger vessels and prevents recurrent bleeding hours or days after the initial injury. Although presented here as separate events, primary and secondary hemostasis are closely linked. For example, activated platelets accelerate plasma coagulation, and products of the plasma coagulation reaction, such as thrombin, stimulate platelet aggregation.

Effective primary hemostasis requires three critical events— platelet adhesion, granule release, and platelet aggregation. Within a few seconds of injury, platelets adhere to collagen fibrils in vascular subendothelium via a specific platelet collagen receptor, glycoprotein Ia/IIa, which is a member of the integrin family. As shown in Fig. 57-2, this interaction is stabilized by the von Willebrand factor, an adhesive glycoprotein which allows platelets to remain attached to the vessel wall despite the high shear forces generated within the vascular lumen. The von Willebrand factor accomplishes this task by forming a link between a platelet receptor site on glycoprotein Ib/IX and subendothelial collagen fibrils. The adherent platelets then release preformed granule constituents and generate de novo mediators like those depicted in Fig. 57-1.

As in other cells, platelet activation and secretion are regulated by changes in the level of cyclic nucleotides, the influx of calcium,

FIGURE 57-1 Schematic presentation of the major events in primary hemostasis. The first event is platelet adhesion, the interaction of platelets with a nonplatelet surface such as vascular subendothelium. This is followed by platelet activation and secretion. Some of the products secreted by platelets are depicted. Abbreviations—ADP, adenosine diphosphate; PDGF, platelet-derived growth factor, vWF, von Willebrand's factor. The final event is the binding of activated platelets to the adherent monolayer in the process of platelet aggregation.

Activation/Secretion

FIGURE 57-4 The biochemical basis of platelet activation and secretion. Binding of agonists such as thrombin, epinephrine, or collagen sets in motion a chain of events which hydrolyzes membrane phospholipids, inhibits adenylate cyclase, mobilizes intracellular calcium, and phosphorylates critical intracellular proteins. The net result is shape change, movement of granules to the canalicular system, generation of mediators like thromboxane A_2, and granule secretion. Abbreviations—A.C., adenylate cyclase; G, guanine nucleotide–binding protein; PIP_2, phosphatidylinositol-4,5-bisphosphate; PLC, phospholipase C; DAG, diacylglycerol; PLA_2, phospholipase A_2; PC, phosphatidylcholine; AA, arachidonic acid; CO, cyclooxygenase; O_2, oxygen; IP_3, inositol triphosphate; cAMP, cyclic AMP; Ca-CM, calcium calmodulin complex; MLCK, myosin light chain kinase.

FIGURE 57-2 The molecular basis of platelet adhesion and aggregation. Adhesion of platelets to vascular subendothelium is facilitated by von Willebrand's factor, which forms a bridge between collagen fibrils in the vessel wall and receptors on platelet glycoprotein Ib/IX (GpIb–IX). In a similar manner, platelet aggregation is mediated by fibrinogen which links adjacent platelets via receptors on the platelet glycoprotein IIb and IIIa complex (GpIIb–IIIa).

hydrolysis of membrane phospholipids, and phosphorylation of critical intracellular proteins. The relevant pathways are depicted in Figs. 57-3 and 57-4. The binding of agonists such as epinephrine, collagen, or thrombin to platelet surface receptors activates two membrane enzymes—phospholipase C and phospholipase A_2. These enzymes catalyze the release of arachidonic acid from two of the major

FIGURE 57-3 Generation of thromboxane A_2 in platelets and prostacyclin (PGI_2) in endothelial cells.

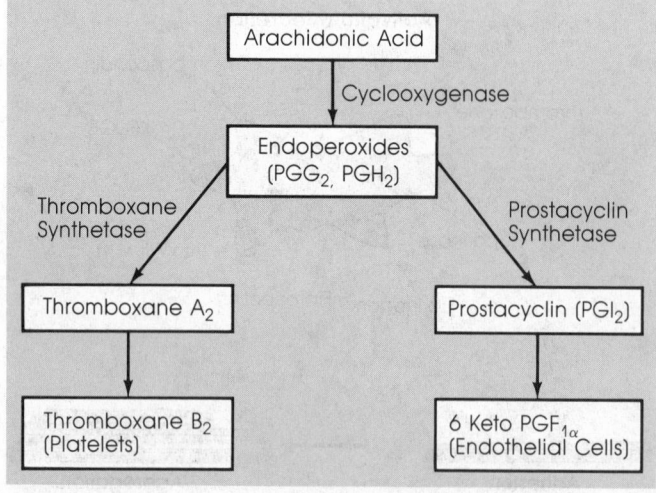

membrane phospholipids, phosphatidylinositol and phosphatidylcholine. Initially, a small quantity of the released arachidonic acid is converted to thromboxane A_2 (TXA_2), which, in turn, can activate phospholipase C. The formation of TXA_2 from arachidonic acid is mediated by the enzyme cyclooxygenase (see Fig. 57-3). This enzyme is inhibited by aspirin and nonsteroidal anti-inflammatory drugs. Inhibition of TXA_2 synthesis is a cause of mild bleeding in some patients, as well as the basis for the action of some antithrombotic drugs.

Hydrolysis of the membrane phospholipid, phosphatidylinositol 4,5-bisphosphate (PIP_2), produces diacylglycerol (DAG) and inositol triphosphate (IP_3), both of which play critical roles in platelet metabolism. IP_3 mediates the movement of calcium into the platelet cytosol and stimulates the phosphorylation of myosin light chains. The latter interact with actin to facilitate granule movement and platelet shape change. DAG activates protein kinase C which, in turn, phosphorylates several substrates including myosin light chain kinase and a 47,000-Da protein (plekstrin). Phosphorylation of these or other proteins may regulate platelet granule secretion.

A finely balanced mechanism controls the rate and extent of platelet activation, which is illustrated in Fig. 57-3. TXA_2, a platelet product of arachidonic acid, stimulates platelet activation and secretion. In contrast, prostacyclin (PGI_2), an endothelial cell product of arachidonic acid, inhibits platelet activation by raising intraplatelet cyclic AMP levels. Similar pathways to regulate activation and secretion occur in other cells.

Following activation, platelets secrete their granule contents into plasma. Endoglycosidases and a heparin-cleaving enzyme are released from lysosomes; calcium, serotonin, and adenosine diphosphate (ADP) are released from the dense granules; and several proteins including the von Willebrand factor, fibronectin, thrombospondin, the platelet-derived growth factor (PDGF), and a heparin-neutralizing protein (platelet factor 4) are released from alpha granules. Released ADP binds to a specific purinergic receptor which, when activated, changes the conformation of the glycoprotein IIb/IIIa complex so that

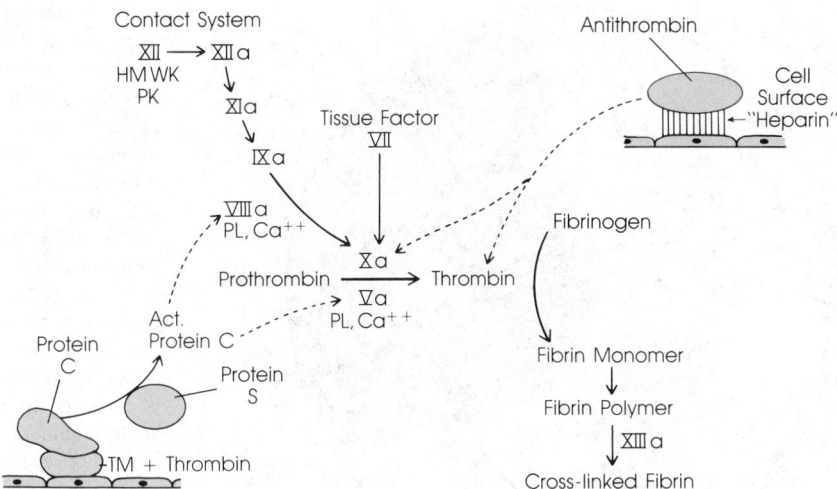

FIGURE 57-5 A schematic diagram of some of the clinically important coagulation reactions. The unactivated or precursor proteins are indicated by roman numerals, and the active form by the addition of a lowercase "a"—a standard convention. Other abbreviations are HMWK, high-molecular-weight kininogen; PK, prekallikrein; PL, phospholipid; TM, thrombomodulin; Ca^{2+}, calcium. There are two independent activation pathways, the contact system and the tissue factor–mediated or extrinsic system. They both merge at the point of factor X activation and lead to the generation of thrombin, which converts fibrinogen into fibrin. These reactions are regulated by antithrombin, which forms complexes with all of the coagulation protein serine proteases except factor VII, and the protein C–protein S system which inactivates factors V and VIII.

it binds fibrinogen, linking adjacent platelets into a hemostatic plug (Fig. 57-2). Released PDGF, stimulates the growth and migration of fibroblasts and smooth muscle cells within the vessel wall, which is an important part of the repair process.

As the primary hemostatic plug is being formed, plasma coagulation proteins are activated to initiate secondary hemostasis. An overall picture of the coagulation scheme, including the role of various inhibitors, is shown in Fig. 57-5. The coagulation pathway can be broken down into a series of reactions (outlined in Fig. 57-6) which culminate in the production of sufficient thrombin to convert a small portion of plasma fibrinogen to fibrin. Each of the reactions requires the formation of a surface-bound complex, the conversion of inactive precursor proteins into active proteases by limited proteolysis, and each is regulated by both plasma and cellular cofactors and calcium.

In *reaction 1*, the intrinsic or contact phase of coagulation, three plasma proteins, Hageman factor (factor XII), high-molecular-weight kininogen (HMWK), and prekallikrein (PK) form a complex on vascular subendothelial collagen. After binding to HMWK, factor XII is slowly converted to an active protease (XIIa), which then converts both PK to kallikrein and factor XI to its active form (XIa). Kallikrein (K) in turn accelerates XII conversion to XIIa, while XIa participates in subsequent coagulation reactions. Although these interactions are well-characterized in vitro, an alternative mechanism for the activation of factor XI may exist, as patients who are deficient in either factor XII, HMWK, or PK have apparently normal hemostasis and no clinical bleeding.

Reaction 2 provides a second pathway to initiate coagulation by converting factor VII to an active protease. In this extrinsic or tissue-factor-dependent pathway, a complex is formed between factor VII, calcium, and tissue factor, a ubiquitous lipoprotein present in cellular membranes which is exposed following cellular injury. There is increasing evidence that the tissue factor–VII pathway is continuously active and makes a major contribution to basal coagulation. Factor VII and three other coagulation proteins—factors II (prothrombin), IX, and X—require calcium and vitamin K for biologic activity. These proteins are synthesized in the liver, where a vitamin K–dependent carboxylase catalyzes a unique posttranslational modification which adds a second carboxyl group to certain glutamic acid residues. Pairs of these di-γ-carboxyglutamic acid (Gla) residues bind calcium, which anchors these proteins to negatively charged phospholipid surfaces and confers biologic activity. Inhibition of this posttranslational modification by vitamin K antagonists (e.g., warfarin) is the basis of one of the most common forms of anticoagulant therapy.

In *reaction 3*, factor X is activated by the proteases generated in the two previous reactions. In one reaction, a calcium- and lipid-dependent complex is formed between factors VIII, IX, and X. Within this complex, factor IX is first converted to IXa by factor XIa that was generated within the intrinsic pathway (reaction 1). Factor X is then activated by factor IXa in concert with factor VIII. Alternatively, both factors IX and X can be activated more directly by factor VIIa, which has been generated via the extrinsic pathway (reaction 2).

FIGURE 57-6 The major coagulation reactions are subdivided and depicted in schematic form to emphasize their similarity. They all rely on the formation of surface bound enzyme-cofactor complexes. Abbreviations are PK, prekallikrein; K, kallikrein; HMWK, high-molecular-weight kininogen; TF, tissue factor; Ca^{2+}, calcium; PT, prothrombin; Thr, thrombin. By convention other coagulation factors are indicated by roman numerals, with a lowercase "a" appended to indicate their active form. The $\wedge\wedge\wedge$ is used to indicate the Gla (di-γ-carboxyglutamic acid)–containing domains of factors VII, IX, X, Xa, and PT which bind calcium and phospholipid. Hatching is used to indicate proteins that adhere to surfaces by hydrophobic interaction.

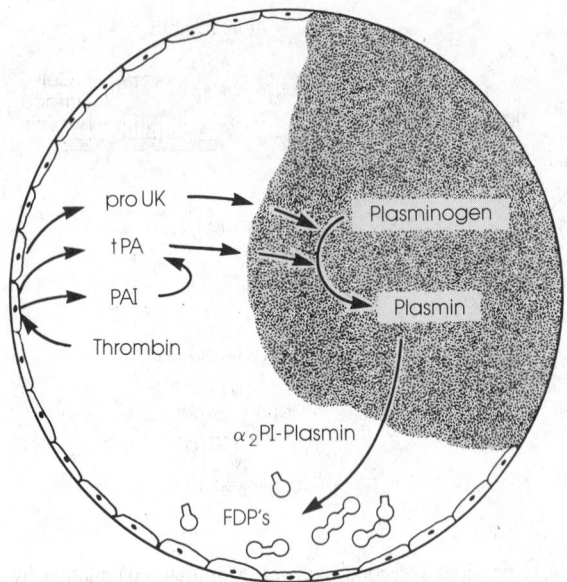

FIGURE 57-7   A schematic diagram of the fibrinolytic pathway. tPA (tissue plasminogen activator) is released from endothelial cells, enters the fibrin clot, and activates plasminogen to plasmin. Any free plasmin is complexed with α_2 PI (alpha$_2$ plasmin inhibitor). Fibrin is degraded to low-molecular-weight fragments, abbreviated as FDPs, fibrin degradation products.

Activation of factors IX and X provides an important link between the intrinsic and extrinsic coagulation pathways (see Fig. 57-5).

Reaction 4, the final step, converts prothrombin to thrombin in the presence of factor V, calcium, and phospholipid. Although prothrombin conversion can take place on various natural and artificial phospholipid-rich surfaces, it accelerates several-thousand-fold on the surface of activated platelets. Thrombin, the product of this reaction, has multiple functions in hemostasis. Although its principal role in hemostasis is the conversion of fibrinogen to fibrin, it also activates factors V, VIII, and XIII and stimulates platelet aggregation and secretion. Following the release of fibrinopeptides A and B from the alpha and beta chains of fibrinogen, the modified molecule, now called fibrin monomer, polymerizes into an insoluble gel. The fibrin polymer is then stabilized by the cross-linking of individual chains by factor XIIIa, a plasma transglutaminase (Fig. 57-5).

Clot lysis and vessel repair begin immediately after the formation of the definitive hemostatic plug. There are three major activators of the fibrinolytic system, Hageman factor fragments, urokinase (UK), and tissue plasminogen activator (tPA). The principal physiologic activator, tPA, diffuses from endothelial cells and converts plasminogen, adsorbed to the fibrin clot, into plasmin (see Fig. 57-7). Plasmin then degrades fibrin polymer into small fragments which are cleared by the monocyte-macrophage scavenger system. Although plasmin can also degrade fibrinogen, the reaction remains localized because (1) tPA activates plasminogen more effectively when it is adsorbed to fibrin clots, (2) any plasmin that enters the circulation is rapidly bound and neutralized by the alpha$_2$ plasmin inhibitor. The importance of this inhibitor is underscored by the fact that patients who lack it have unchecked fibrinolysis and bleed and (3) endothelial cells release a plasminogen activator inhibitor (PAI-1) which blocks the action of tPA.

As noted above, the plasma coagulation system is tightly regulated so that only a small quantity of each coagulation enzyme is converted to its active form. As a consequence, the hemostatic plug does not propagate beyond the site of injury. Precise regulation is important, since there is enough clotting potential in a single milliliter of blood to clot all the fibrinogen in the body in 10 to 15 s. Blood fluidity is maintained by the flow of blood itself, which reduces the concentration of reactants, the adsorption of coagulation factors to surfaces, and the presence of multiple inhibitors in plasma. Antithrombin, proteins C and S and the tissue factor pathway inhibitor (TFPI) are the most important inhibitors which collectively maintain blood fluidity.

These inhibitors have distinct modes of action. Antithrombin forms complexes with all the serine protease coagulation factors except factor VII (see Fig. 57-5). Rates of complex formation are accelerated by heparin and heparin-like molecules on the surface of the endothelial cells. This ability of heparin to accelerate the activity of antithrombin is the basis for heparin's action as a potent anticoagulant. Protein C is converted to an active protease by thrombin after it is bound to an endothelial cell protein called thrombomodulin. Activated protein C then inactivates the two plasma cofactors V and VIII by limited proteolysis which slows down two critical coagulation reactions. Protein C may also stimulate the release of tissue plasminogen activator from endothelial cells. The inhibitory function of protein C is enhanced by protein S. As one might predict, reduced levels of antithrombin or proteins C and S, or dysfunctional forms of the molecule, result in a hypercoagulable or prethrombotic state.

The preceding description of blood coagulation implies that the process is uniform throughout the body. In fact, the process is not uniform and composition of the blood clot varies with the site of injury. Hemostatic plugs or thrombi that form in veins where blood flow is slow are richly endowed with fibrin and trapped red blood cells and contain relatively few platelets. They are often called red thrombi due to their appearance in surgical and pathologic specimens. The friable ends of these red thrombi, which often form in leg veins, can break off and embolize to the pulmonary circulation. Conversely, clots that form in arteries under conditions of high flow are predominantly composed of platelets and have little fibrin. These white thrombi may readily dislodge from the arterial wall and embolize to distant sites to cause temporary or permanent ischemia. This is particularly common in the cerebral and retinal circulation and may lead to transient neurologic dysfunction (transient ischemic attacks) including temporary monocular blindness (amaurosis fugax) or strokes. In addition, most episodes of myocardial infarction are due to thrombi which form after the rupture of atherosclerotic plaques within diseased coronary arteries. It is important to remember that there is little difference between hemostatic plugs, which are a physiologic response to injury, and pathologic thrombi. To underscore the similarity, thrombosis has been described as coagulation occurring in the wrong place or at the wrong time.

CLINICAL EVALUATION

HISTORY   Certain elements of the history are particularly useful in determining whether bleeding is caused by an underlying hemostatic disorder rather than a local anatomic defect. One clue is a history of bleeding following common hemostatic stresses such as dental extraction, childbirth, or minor surgery. Bleeding that is sufficiently severe to require a blood transfusion merits special attention. A family history of bleeding and bleeding from multiple sites that cannot be linked to trauma or surgery also suggest a systemic disorder. Since bleeding can be mild, lack of a family history of bleeding does not exclude an inherited hemostatic disorder.

It may be possible to localize the defect to the platelet or plasma coagulation system (Table 57-1). Bleeding from a platelet disorder is usually localized to superficial sites such as the skin and mucous membranes, comes on immediately after trauma or surgery, and is readily controlled by local measures. In contrast, bleeding from secondary hemostatic or plasma coagulation defects occurs hours or days after injury and is unaffected by local therapy. Such bleeding most often occurs in deep subcutaneous tissues, muscles, joints, or body cavities. A careful and thorough history is probably the most important step in establishing the presence of a hemostatic disorder and in guiding initial laboratory testing.

PHYSICAL EXAMINATION   In conjunction with a careful history, physical examination can also be of help in evaluating patients with hemostatic disorders. The most common site to observe bleeding is

TABLE 57-1 Differences in the clinical manifestations of disorders of primary and secondary hemostasis

	Primary hemostasis (platelet defect)	Secondary hemostasis (plasma proteins)
Onset of bleeding after trauma	Immediate	Delayed—hours or days
Sites of bleeding	Superficial—skin; mucous membranes; nose; gastrointestinal, genitourinary tracts	Deep—joints, muscle, retroperitoneum
Physical findings	Petechiae, ecchymoses	Hematomas, hemarthroses
Family history	Autosomal dominant	Autosomal or X-linked recessive
Response to therapy	Immediate; local measures effective	Requires sustained systemic therapy

TABLE 57-2 Causes of thrombocytopenia

Decreased marrow production of megakaryocytes
  A Marrow infiltration with tumor, fibrosis
  B Marrow failure—aplastic, hypoplastic anemias
Splenic sequestration of circulating platelets
  A Splenic hypertrophy—tumor, portal hypertension
Increased destruction of circulating platelets
  A Nonimmune destruction
    1 Vascular prostheses, cardiac valves
    2 Disseminated intravascular coagulation
    3 Sepsis
    4 Vasculitis
  B Immune destruction
    1 Autoantibodies to platelet antigens
    2 Drug-associated antibodies
    3 Circulating immune complexes—systemic lupus erythematosus, viral agents, bacterial sepsis

in the skin and mucous membranes. Collections of blood in the skin are called *purpura* and may be subdivided on the basis of the site of bleeding in the skin. Small pinpoint hemorrhages into the dermis due to the leakage of red cells through capillaries are called *petechiae* and are characteristic of platelet disorders—in particular, severe thrombocytopenia. Larger subcutaneous collections of blood due to leakage of blood from small arterioles and venules are *ecchymoses* (common bruises) or, if somewhat deeper and palpable, *hematomas*. They are also common in patients with platelet defects and result from minor trauma. There are other skin and mucous membrane lesions like dilated capillaries or *telangiectasia* that may cause bleeding without any hemostatic defect. In addition, the loss of connective tissue support for capillaries and small veins that accompanies aging increases the fragility of superficial vessels, such as those on the dorsum of the hand, leading to extravasation of blood into subcutaneous tissue—*senile purpura*. Menorrhagia is sometimes a serious problem in women with severe thrombocytopenia or platelet dysfunction. In addition, some patients with primary hemostatic defects, especially von Willebrand's disease, may have recurrent gastrointestinal hemorrhage.

As mentioned previously, bleeding into body cavities, retroperitoneum, or joints is a common manifestation of plasma coagulation defects. Repeated joint bleeding may cause synovial thickening, chronic inflammation, and fluid collections and may erode articular cartilage and lead to chronic joint deformity and limited mobility. Such deformities are particularly common in factors VIII and IX deficiency, the two sex-linked coagulation disorders referred to as the *hemophilias*. For unclear reasons, hemarthroses are much less common in other plasma coagulation defects. Blood collections in various body cavities or soft tissues can cause secondary necrosis of tissues or nerve compression. Retroperitoneal hematomas can cause femoral nerve compression, and large collections of poorly coagulated blood in soft tissues may occasionally mimic malignant growths—the pseudotumor syndrome. Two of the most life-threatening sites of bleeding are in the oropharynx, where bleeding can compromise the airway, and in the central nervous system. Intracerebral hemorrhage is one of the leading causes of death in patients with severe coagulation disorders.

LABORATORY TESTS The most important screening tests of the primary hemostatic system are (1) a *bleeding time* (a sensitive measure of platelet function) and (2) a *platelet count*. The latter is particularly useful as it is readily available and correlates well with the propensity to bleed. The normal platelet count is 150,000 to 450,000 platelets per cubic millimeter of blood. As long as the count is above 100,000 per cubic millimeter, however, patients are not symptomatic and the bleeding time remains normal. Platelet counts of 50,000 to 100,000 per cubic millimeter cause mild prolongation of the bleeding time so that bleeding occurs only after severe trauma or other stress. Patients with platelet counts less than 50,000 per cubic millimeter have easy bruising, which is manifested by skin purpura with minor trauma and bleeding after mucous membrane

surgery. Patients with a platelet count below 20,000 per cubic millimeter have an appreciable incidence of spontaneous bleeding, usually have petechiae, and may have intracranial or other spontaneous internal bleeding. The major causes of thrombocytopenia are outlined in Table 57-2.

Patients with qualitative platelet abnormalities have a normal platelet count and a prolonged bleeding time (Table 57-3). The bleeding time is ascertained by making a small, superficial skin incision and timing the duration of blood flow from the wounded area. Although this is a rather crude "bioassay," by careful standardization it has become a reliable and sensitive test of platelet function. The most widely used technique uses a template or an automated scalpel to control the length and depth of the incision (usually 1 mm deep by 9 mm long) and a sphygmomanometer inflated to 40 mmHg to distend the capillary bed of the forearm uniformly. In order to be useful the bleeding time must be performed by an experienced technician as small differences in techniques have a big effect on the outcome of the test. Although any patient with a bleeding time over 10 min has a slightly increased risk of bleeding, the risk does not become great until the bleeding time exceeds 15 or 20 min. As shown in Fig. 57-8, there is a roughly linear relationship between the platelet count and the bleeding time. When a defect in primary hemostasis is uncovered, specialized testing is needed to determine the cause of the platelet dysfunction (Table 57-3). A precise diagnosis is important since patients with bleeding due to a primary hemostatic disorder may need therapy with platelets, one of several hormones (desmopressin, estrogen, glucocorticoids), or plasma fractions, depending on the nature of the disorder. Occasional patients with a strong history of bleeding, particularly those with mild von Willebrand's disease, may have a normal bleeding time when initially tested due to cyclical variations in the level of the von Willebrand factor. They may need repeated testing to establish an accurate diagnosis.

Plasma coagulation function is readily assessed with a few simple

TABLE 57-3 Primary hemostatic (platelet) disorders

Platelet adhesion defects:
  Von Willebrand's disease
  Bernard-Soulier syndrome (absence, dysfunction of GpIb/IX)
Platelet aggregation defects
  Glanzmann's thrombasthenia (absence, dysfunction of GpIIb/IIIa)
Platelet release defects
  1 Decreased cyclooxygenase activity
    Drugs—aspirin, nonsteroidal anti-inflammatory agents
    Congenital
  2 Granule storage pool defects
    Congenital
    Acquired
  3 Uremia
  4 Platelet coating (e.g., penicillin or paraproteins)
Platelet coagulant defect
  Scott's syndrome

ABBREVIATION: Gp = glycoprotein.

FIGURE 57-8   The relationship between the platelet count and the bleeding time. (*From Harker LA, Hemostasis Manual, 2d ed. Philadelphia, FA Davis Company, 1974.*)

laboratory tests—the partial thromboplastin time (PTT), prothrombin time (PT), thrombin time (TT), or a quantitative fibrinogen determination (Fig. 57-5, Table 57-4). The PTT screens the intrinsic limb of the coagulation system and tests for the adequacy of factors XII, HMWK, PK, XI, IX, and VIII. The PT screens the extrinsic or tissue factor–dependent pathway. Both tests also evaluate the common coagulation pathway involving all the reactions that occur after the activation of factor X. Prolongation of the PT and PTT that does not correct after the addition of normal plasma suggests a specific or nonspecific coagulation inhibitor. A specific test for fibrinogen conversion to fibrin is needed when both the PTT and PT are prolonged—either a TT or a clottable fibrinogen level can be employed. When abnormalities are noted in any of the screening tests, more specific coagulation factor assays can be ordered to determine the nature of the defect.

There are three rare coagulation abnormalities that may be missed as they do not perturb the screening tests just discussed. They are factor XIII deficiency, alpha₂ plasmin inhibitor deficiency, and Scott's syndrome, a platelet coagulant defect. A test for factor XIII–dependent fibrin cross-linking, such as clot solubility in 5 *M* urea, should be ordered when the PT and PTT are both normal but there is a strong

history of bleeding. The fibrinolytic system can be assessed by measuring the rate of clot lysis with the euglobulin lysis or whole blood clot lysis tests and by measuring the level of alpha₂ plasmin inhibitor. Scott's syndrome can be detected by ordering a serum prothrombin time, which assesses the amount of residual prothrombin.

There are no clinical tests to screen patients suspected of having hypercoagulable or prethrombotic disorders, although tests are being developed in research laboratories which measure small peptides or enzyme-inhibitor complexes generated during coagulation. For example, radioimmunoassays have been developed for fibrinopeptides A and B, for the thrombin-antithrombin complex, and for prothrombin cleavage fragments. Elevated levels of these products have been reported in patients with prethrombotic disorders and in patients with thromboembolism. At present, patients suspected of having a hypercoagulable state on the basis of clinical information, should have specific assays to screen for the small number of known defects. Currently available tests can identify 10 to 20 percent of the cases of familial thrombosis and represent only a small fraction of the many patients who present to physicians with thromboembolism.

Inhibitor syndromes or circulating anticoagulants are usually due to antibodies which impair coagulation factor activity. They are an infrequent cause of bleeding which require specialized diagnostic testing. Inhibitors are likely when screening test abnormalities cannot be reversed by adding normal plasma to patient plasma. Antibodies against specific coagulation factors may develop in (1) postpartum females; (2) patients with autoimmune disorders such as systemic lupus erythematosus; (3) patients taking drugs like penicillin and streptomycin; and (4) otherwise healthy elderly individuals. In addition, between 10 and 20 percent of patients with severe hemophilia who have received multiple plasma infusions develop inhibitor antibodies. Some patients, especially those with systemic lupus erythematosus, may also have a nonspecific form of anticoagulant antibody which interferes with phospholipid binding of coagulation factors and prolongs the PT and PTT but does not cause clinical bleeding. The presence of the lupus anticoagulant may increase the risk of thromboembolism and may cause placental infarction and recurrent midtrimester abortion. Occasionally, patients develop inhibitors that are not antibodies. For example, several patients with circulating mucopolysaccharides that have heparin-like activity have been described with clinical bleeding.

REFERENCES

BROZE GJ: The role of tissue factor pathway inhibitor in a revised coagulation cascade. Blood 29:159, 1992

COLMAN RW et al (eds): *Hemostasis and Thrombosis: Basic Principles and Clinical Practice*, 3d ed. Philadelphia, Lippincott, 1993

HANDIN RI et al (eds): *Blood: Principles and Practice of Hematology and Hematologic Oncology*, 4th ed. Philadelphia, Lippincott, 1993

HAWIGER J, HANDIN RI: Structure and function of platelets, in *Hematology of Infancy and Childhood*, 4th ed., DG Nathan et al (eds). Philadelphia, Saunders, 1992, pp 1512–1533

LIND SE: The bleeding time does not predict surgical bleeding. Blood 77: 2547, 1991

ROBERTS HR, LOZIER JN: New perspectives on the coagulation cascade. Hosp Prac Jan 1992, 97–112

ROSENBERG RD, SOFF G: Physiology of hemostasis: The fluid phase, in *Hematology of Infancy and Childhood*, 4th ed., DG Nathan et al (eds). Philadelphia, Saunders, 1992, pp 1534–1560

TABLE 57-4   Relationship between secondary hemostatic disorders and coagulation test abnormalities

Prolonged partial thromboplastin time (PTT)
No clinical bleeding—factors XII, HMWK, PK
Mild or rare bleeding—factor XI
Frequent, severe bleeding—factors VIII and IX
Prolonged prothrombin time (PT)
Factor VII deficiency
Vitamin K deficiency—early
Warfarin anticoagulant ingestion
Prolonged PTT and PT
Factor II, V, or X deficiency
Vitamin K deficiency—late
Warfarin anticoagulant ingestion
Prolonged thrombin time (TT)
Mild or rare bleeding—afibrinogenemia
Frequent, severe bleeding—dysfibrinogenemia
Heparin-like inhibitors or heparin administration
Prolonged PT and/or PTT not corrected with normal plasma
Specific or nonspecific inhibitor syndromes
Clot solubility in 5 *M* urea
Factor XIII deficiency
Inhibitors or defective cross-linking
Rapid clot lysis
Alpha₂ plasmin inhibitor

ABBREVIATIONS: HMWK = high-molecular-weight kininogen; PK = prekallikrein.

58 ENLARGEMENT OF LYMPH NODES AND SPLEEN

BARTON F. HAYNES

Lymph nodes and spleen constitute a major portion of the peripheral immune system and become enlarged in a wide spectrum of infectious, malignant, autoimmune, and metabolic diseases. Enlargements of lymph nodes (lymphadenopathy) and spleen (splenomegaly) are common clinical findings that can lead to a wide range of diagnostic and therapeutic procedures. The goal of this chapter is to serve as an introduction to these two components of the immune system and to highlight clinical features and diagnostic evaluation of some of the diseases in which lymphadenopathy and splenomegaly occur.

LYMPH NODES

LYMPH NODE STRUCTURE AND FUNCTION   Lymph nodes are peripheral lymphoid organs that are connected to the circulation by afferent and efferent lymphatic vessels (Fig. 58-1) and by postcapillary high-endothelial venules. A number of cell types make up the lymph node supportive framework and stroma. Fibroblasts are the predominant cell type in the lymph node capsule and trabeculae. Fibroblast-derived reticular cells are supporting cells found frequently in the follicles and germinal centers, i.e., the B cell areas of lymph nodes. Tissue macrophages derived from circulating monocytes are present throughout the normal node. Within cortical areas are interdigitating reticular cells (also called *dendritic cells*) and Langerhans cells, both of which are specialized nonphagocytic, Ia-bearing cells of bone marrow origin that along with macrophages participate in antigen presentation to thymus-derived (T) and B cells (Chap. 277). The outer lymph node cortex contains lymphoid follicles with germinal centers that are the B cell areas of lymph node (see Fig. 58-1). Primary lymphoid follicles are aggregates of IgM- and IgD-bearing B cells and CD4 + helper/inducer T cells prior to antigenic challenge. Secondary lymphoid follicles are the result of antigen stimulation and contain an outer or mantle layer of IgM- and IgD-bearing B cells and an inner zone (germinal center) of activated B cells, macrophages, reticular cells, and scattered CD4 + helper T cells. Between primary and secondary follicle areas (interfollicular zones) and inner lymph node medullary regions are T cell (paracortical) areas. The majority of T cells in lymph nodes are CD4 + helper T cells (approximately 80 percent), while the minority are CD8 + suppressor/cytotoxic T cells (approximately 20 percent).

FIGURE 58-1   Schematic lymph node structure. Lymph flows into nodes via afferent lymphatics (A) and leaves nodes via efferent lymphatics (E). B cell areas are primary and secondary follicles in lymph node cortex while T cells are concentrated in paracortical areas.

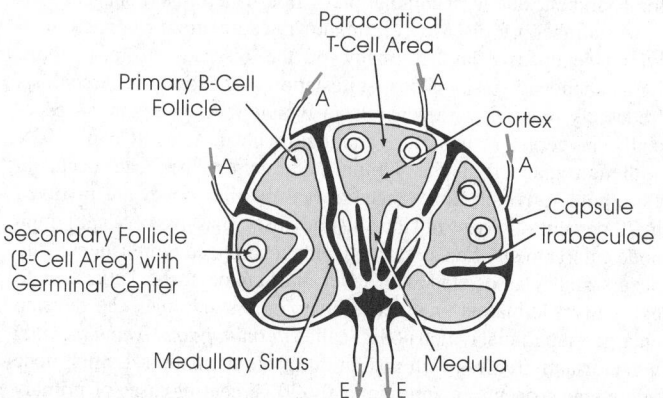

The two most important factors contributing to the composition and distribution of lymphoid cells within lymph node are (1) generation of memory B and T cells de novo from proliferation of antigen-stimulated precursors within lymph nodes and (2) selective recirculation to and homing of specific types of lymphoid cells to lymph nodes from the circulation. Traffic through lymph nodes is via two general routes (see Fig. 58-1). Afferent lymph, containing lymphocytes, macrophages, and antigens, enters the lymph node via the subcapsular space and drains through paracortical and medullary areas into medullary sinuses that converge to form efferent lymphatic vessels through which lymph exits. B cells from bone marrow and T cells from the thymus enter lymph nodes from the circulation by binding to specific receptors on cells of postcapillary high-endothelial venules. After activation by antigen and clonal expansion, sensitized T and B cells and antibody-secreting plasma cells leave the node in efferent lymph and rejoin the peripheral blood circulation via the thoracic duct.

Lymph nodes function as sites of antigen presenting cell, T cell, and B cell contact with antigen, with a specialized structure that gives rise to optimal T cell, B cell, and antigen presenting cell interactions. Under normal conditions, such interactions result in efficient recognition of antigen, activation of the cellular and humoral arms of the immune response, and ultimate elimination of antigen (see Chap. 277).

In normal immune responses, antigen stimulation of macrophages and lymphocytes in lymph nodes exerts profound influences on lymphocyte traffic. One of the earliest effects of antigen is to increase blood flow through the affected node, which during antigen stimulation may reach 10 to 25 times normal levels. Lymphocytes accumulate in antigen-stimulated nodes by increase in traffic through the node, decreased egress of lymphocytes from antigen-stimulated nodes, and proliferation of responding T and B cells. A lymph node may thus reach 15 times its normal size 5 to 10 days after antigenic stimulation.

DISEASES ASSOCIATED WITH LYMPHADENOPATHY   Lymph node enlargement can be due to (1) an increase in the number of benign lymphocytes and macrophages during response to antigens, (2) infiltration by inflammatory cells in infections involving lymph nodes (lymphadenitis), (3) in situ proliferation of malignant lymphocytes or macrophages, (4) infiltration of nodes by metastatic malignant cells, or (5) infiltration of lymph nodes by metabolite-laden macrophages in lipid storage diseases. Under normal conditions in adults, the inguinal lymph nodes may be palpable and are generally 0.5 to 2 cm in size. Elsewhere in the body, smaller lymph nodes due to past infections may be present normally. Enlargement of lymph nodes requires investigation when there are one or more new nodes present equal to or greater than 1 cm in diameter and not known to arise from a previously recognized cause. However, this is not a rigid criterion, and under certain circumstances, new multiple or single smaller lymph nodes may warrant investigation as well. Important factors in assessing the significance of enlarged lymph nodes are (1) the patient's age, (2) the physical characteristics of the lymph node, (3) node locations, and (4) the clinical setting associated with lymphadenopathy. Lymphadenopathy reflects significant disease more often in adults than in children because children are more likely to respond to minor stimuli with lymphoid hyperplasia. Lymphadenopathy in patients under 30 years of age is due to benign causes in approximately 80 percent of cases, whereas in patients greater than 50 years of age lymphadenopathy is due to benign causes in only 40 percent of cases.

The physical characteristics of peripheral nodes are important. Nodes of lymphomas tend to be rubbery, firm, matted together, and nontender. Nodes involved with metastatic carcinomas are usually hard and fixed to underlying tissue. In acute infections, nodes are tender, asymmetrically enlarged, and matted together, and the overlying skin may be erythematous.

The clinical setting is important in assessing lymphadenopathy. In a young college student with fever and recent onset of lymph node enlargement, infectious mononucleosis syndromes are important to consider. In homosexuals, hemophiliacs, and intravenous drug users with systemic lymphadenopathy, AIDS an AIDS-related complex syndrome should be considered (see Chap. 279).

The location of enlarged lymph nodes may suggest important clues to the diagnosis. Enlarged posterior cervical nodes are frequently present in scalp infections, toxoplasmosis, and rubella, whereas anterior auricular nodes suggest infections of the eyelids and conjunctiva. Lymphomas commonly involve cervical lymph nodes and can occasionally involve posterior auricular and occipital nodes as well. Enlarged suppurative cervical nodes are seen in mycobacterial lymphadenitis (scrofula). Unilateral jugular or mandibular lymph node enlargement suggests lymphoma or nonlymphoid head and neck malignancy. Supraclavicular and scalene lymph node enlargement is always significant and frequently results from metastasis from intrathoracic or gastrointestinal malignancies or from lymphomas. Virchow's node is an enlarged left supraclavicular lymph node infiltrated with metastatic tumor usually from the gastrointestinal tract. Unilateral epitrochlear node enlargement is usually due to hand infections; bilateral epitrochlear node enlargement is seen in sarcoidosis, tularemia, and secondary syphilis.

Unilateral axillary adenopathy can be seen with breast carcinoma, lymphomas, infections of the upper extremities, cat-scratch disease, and brucellosis.

Bilateral inguinal adenopathy can be seen in a variety of venereal infections; however, lymphogranuloma venereum and syphilis are associated with unilateral inguinal adenopathy. Progressive inguinal lymph node enlargement without obvious infection suggests malignant disease. Femoral node involvement has been reported to occur in *Pasteurella pestis* infections and lymphomas.

Symptoms that should raise the suspicion of hilar or mediastinal node enlargement are cough or wheezing due to airway compression, recurrent laryngeal nerve compression with hoarseness, paralysis of the diaphragm, dysphagia with esophageal compression, and swelling of the neck, face, or arms due to superior vena cava or subclavian vein compression. Bilateral mediastinal adenopathy is frequently seen in lymphomas, especially the nodular sclerosing type of Hodgkin's disease. Unilateral hilar adenopathy indicates a high likelihood of metastatic carcinoma (usually lung), while bilateral hilar adenopathy is more often benign and is seen in sarcoidosis, tuberculosis, and systemic fungal infections. Bilateral hilar adenopathy in asymptomatic patients or in association with erythema nodosum or uveitis is almost always due to sarcoidosis (Chap. 292). The association of bilateral hilar adenopathy with an anterior mediastinal mass, pleural effusion, or pulmonary mass suggests neoplastic disease.

Enlarged retroperitoneal and intraabdominal nodes are not usually inflammatory in origin but are frequently due to lymphomas or other neoplastic diseases. Tuberculosis can cause mesenteric lymphadenitis with large matted and sometimes calcified nodes.

Some of the diseases associated with lymph node enlargement are listed in Table 58-1 and fall into six general categories: infectious diseases, immunologic diseases, malignant diseases, endocrine diseases, lipid storage diseases, and miscellaneous.

The manifestations of infectious diseases are protean and are best considered according to the type of infectious agent. The most common viral infection associated with systemic lymphadenopathy is Epstein-Barr (EB) virus–associated infectious mononucleosis (see Chap. 145). A variety of other viral diseases, including viral hepatitis, cytomegalovirus, rubella, and influenza, can cause clinical syndromes similar to those induced by the EB virus. AIDS is caused by a retrovirus, human immunodeficiency virus (HIV). In the HIV-associated lymphadenopathy syndrome, cervical, axillary, and occipital nodes are the most commonly involved (see Chap. 279).

Chronic bacterial infections as well as fungal infections may produce considerable lymph node enlargement without signs of local inflammation. Cat-scratch disease is a regional lymphadenitis occurring approximately 2 weeks following a cat scratch or bite. The nodes involved relate to lymph drainage of the wound site, with upper extremity adenopathy being the most common, occurring in 50 percent of cases. Fungi associated with primary pulmonary infections

TABLE 58-1 Diseases associated with lymph node enlargement

Infectious diseases
A Viral infections: infectious hepatitis, infectious mononucleosis syndromes (cytomegalovirus, EB virus), AIDS, rubella, varicella–herpes zoster, vaccinia
B Bacterial infections: streptococci, staphylococci, salmonella, brucella, Francisella tularensis, *Listeria monocytogenes, Pasteurella pestis, Haemophilus ducreyi*, cat-scratch disease, *Yersinia pseudotuberculosis, Y. enterocolitica*
C Fungal infections: coccidioidomycosis, histoplasmosis
D Chlamydial infections: Lymphogranuloma venereum, trachoma
E Mycobacterial infections: tuberculosis, leprosy
F Parasitic infections: trypanosomiasis, microfilariasis, toxoplasmosis
G Spirochetal diseases: syphilis, yaws, endemic syphilis (bejel), leptospirosis
Immunologic diseases
A Rheumatoid arthritis
B Systemic lupus erythematosus
C Dermatomyositis
D Serum sickness
E Drug reactions: phenytoin, hydralazine, allopurinol, silicone implants
F Angioimmunoblastic lymphadenopathy
G Sjögren's syndrome
H Primary biliary cirrhosis and other forms of chronic hepatitis
Malignant diseases
A Hematologic: Hodgkin's lymphoma, acute and chronic T, B, myeloid, and monocytoid cell leukemias and lymphomas, malignant histiocytosis
B Metastatic tumors to lymph nodes: melanoma, Kaposi's sarcoma, neuroblastoma, seminoma, tumors of lung, breast, prostate, kidney, head and neck, gastrointestinal tract
Endocrine diseases: hyperthyroidism
Lipid storage diseases: Gaucher's and Niemann-Pick diseases
Miscellaneous diseases and diseases of unknown cause
A Giant follicular lymph node hyperplasia (Castleman's disease)
B Sinus histiocytosis
C Dermatopathic lymphadenitis
D Sarcoidosis
E Amyloidosis
F Mucocutaneous lymph node syndrome
G Lymphomatoid granulomatosis
H Multifocal Langerhans cell (eosinophilic) granulomatosis
I Familial Mediterranean fever
J Kikuchi's histiocytic necrotizing lymphadenitis

(coccidioidomycosis, histoplasmosis) can cause hilar adenopathy. Acute and chronic mycobacterial, parasitic, and spirochetal diseases against which there is a profound cellular and humoral immune response all can result in either systemic or regional enlarged lymph nodes depending on the clinical syndrome in question. Virtually any disease characterized by immune cell activation (systemic lupus erythematosus, rheumatoid arthritis, serum sickness, reactions due to drugs such as diphenylhydantoin, angioimmunoblastic lymphadenopathy) can be associated with regional or systemic adenopathy. Lymph node enlargement associated with malignant disease may be due to direct node involvement by tumor, lymphoid hyperplasia in response to tumor, or both. Generalized lymphoid hyperplasia may occur with hyperthyroidism. Patients with lipid storage diseases such as Gaucher's and Niemann-Pick can have enlarged lymph nodes, particularly in the abdomen, due to accumulation of lipid-laden macrophages.

A number of diseases of unknown cause are associated with lymphadenopathy, and in many of the diseases in this group, lymphadenopathy is a major manifestation of the disease. Sarcoidosis frequently presents with generalized lymph node enlargement, especially in cervical, inguinal, and epitrochlear areas (Chap. 292). Although giant follicular lymph node hyperplasia can occur in extrathoracic lymph nodes, mediastinal or hilar nodes are involved in 70 percent of cases. In sinus histiocytosis, massive cervical lymph node enlargement often associated with generalized lymphadenopathy occurs and is associated with fever and leukocytosis. Patients with exfoliative dermatitis or other dermatologic syndromes can develop enlarged superficial lymph nodes (called *dermatopathic lymphadenitis*) which usually regress with resolution of the dermatitis. Lymph node involvement occurs in approximately 30 percent of cases of primary and secondary amyloidosis; only rarely is amyloid lymphadenopathy the major or only organ involvement. The mechanism of node enlargement in amyloidosis is the accumulation of extracellular masses of amyloid fibrils that compress and eventually obliterate normal lymph node architecture (Chap. 281).

Mucocutaneous lymph node syndrome (Kawasaki's disease) is a systemic lymphadenopathy syndrome, the hallmarks of which are fever, conjunctivitis, erythema of the tongue with protrusion of papillae (strawberry tongue), a truncal exanthem with desquamation of palms and soles, and acute nonsuppurative enlargement of cervical lymph nodes (see Chap. 291).

Lymphomatoid granulomatosis is a disease characterized by infiltration of various organs (lungs, skin, central nervous system) with an angiocentric and angioinvasive polymorphic cellular infiltrate consisting of atypical lymphocytes and macrophages. The disease has characteristics of both an inflammatory granulomatous process and a lymphoproliferative disease, with progression to frank lymphoma in up to 50 percent of cases. Lymphadenopathy in the prelymphoma state of lymphomatoid granulomatosis occurs in 40 percent of cases affecting primarily intrathoracic nodes while peripheral adenopathy occurs only rarely (10 percent) (see Chap. 291).

Angioimmunoblastic lymphadenopathy is a disease characterized by fever, generalized lymphadenopathy, hepatosplenomegaly, polyclonal hypergammaglobulinemia, and Coombs-positive hemolytic anemia. Although it is not thought to be a malignant disease, it evolves into B cell lymphoma in 35 percent of patients (see Chap. 311).

Diseases characterized by benign and malignant proliferation of tissue macrophages (histiocytes) or of specialized bone marrow–derived cells called *Langerhans cells* have been termed *histiocytoses* or *histiocytosis X*. In the past, these terms encompassed a number of diseases, including unifocal and multifocal eosinophilic granuloma, Hand-Schüller-Christian syndrome, Letterer-Siwe disease, and frank neoplasms of undifferentiated histiocytes. However, the identification of the Langerhans cell as the predominant cell in forms of eosinophilic granuloma has prompted reevaluation of these syndromes.

One term currently in use for eosinophilic granuloma syndromes is *Langerhans cell (eosinophilic) granulomatosis*, and this term will be used here. The term *histiocytosis X* is an outmoded term that refers to a spectrum of diseases encompassing both the benign disorder of Langerhans cell (eosinophilic) granulomatosis and malignant lymphomatous disease.

The classic triad of the *Hand-Schüller-Christian syndrome* (exophthalmus, diabetes insipidus, and destructive bone lesions) occurs with 25 percent of cases of multifocal eosinophilic granuloma but also may occur in malignant lymphoma and carcinoma. *Letterer-Siwe disease* is an acute clinical syndrome of unknown cause in infants that consists of hepatosplenomegaly, lymphadenopathy, hemorrhagic diathesis, anemia, no familial occurrence, and generalized hyperplasia of tissue macrophages in a variety of organs. It is currently felt that Letterer-Siwe disease represents an unusual form of malignant lymphoma and is distinct from forms of eosinophilic granuloma.

Histologically, Langerhans cell granulomatosis consists of aggregates of mature eosinophils and Langerhans cells. Langerhans cells are bone marrow–derived cells normally found among epidermal cells of skin and rarely in B cell areas of lymph node and the medulla of thymus. Langerhans cells contain distinct cytoplasmic granules (Birbeck granules) and adenosine triphosphatase and alpha naphthyl acetate esterase. Surface markers of Langerhans cells include class II major histocompatibility complex antigens (Ia-like) and the CD1 antigen that is also expressed by the cortical (immature) thymocytes (see Chap. 277).

Unifocal Langerhans cell (eosinophilic) granulomatosis is a benign disease of children and young adults, predominantly in males. Occasionally, it occurs as late as 60 to 70 years of age and presents as a solitary osteolytic lesion in the femur, skull, vertebrae, ribs, or occasionally the pelvis. Since there are no consistent accompanying laboratory abnormalities, the diagnosis of unifocal Langerhans cell

granulomatosis requires biopsy of the lytic bone lesion. Treatment of choice of this condition is excision or curettage of the lesion. Rarely, lesions in inaccessible sites such as cervical vertebrae require moderate doses of irradiation [3 to 6 Gy (300 to 600 rad)]. After initial bone scan and radiographic survey to assess extent of disease, follow-up studies should be performed at 6-month intervals for 3 years. If no additional lesions are present 12 months after diagnosis, development of subsequent lesions is unlikely.

Multifocal Langerhans cell (eosinophilic) granulomatosis also usually presents in childhood and is characterized by the development of multiple bony lesions at virtually any site—though less commonly in the feet and hands.

Transient or permanent diabetes insipidus due to granulomatous involvement of the hypothalamus occurs in one-third of patients; 20 percent develop hepatomegaly, 30 percent splenomegaly, and 50 percent have focal or generalized lymph node involvement. Lesions also may involve the skin, vulva, gingiva, lung, and thymus. Laboratory studies are rarely helpful in the diagnosis of multifocal Langerhans cell granulomatosis, necessitating biopsy of lesions. While generally a benign disease, multifocal Langerhans cell granulomatosis is best treated with low to moderate doses of methotrexate, prednisone, or vinblastine, usually with regression of lesions.

Kikuchi's histiocytic necrotizing lymphadenitis was originally described in Japan in 1972 but also has been seen in the United States and Europe. This syndrome occurs most often in young adults and frequently presents with viral upper respiratory tract symptoms and fever. Lymphadenopathy occurs in most cases, with cervical adenopathy the most common site. Histologically, involved nodes show localized proliferation of histiocytes and immunoblasts associated with abundant nuclear debris and tissue necrosis. An increase in CD8 + TCRγδT cells has been reported in necrotizing lymphadenitis lymph nodes. Splenomegaly is also rarely seen in this condition. Although suspected to be caused by an infectious agent, no viral or bacterial etiologic agent has been identified.

EVALUATION OF THE PATIENT WITH LYMPHADENOPATHY

Good physical examination techniques for palpation and assessment of lymph nodes are essential for providing useful information on which diagnostic and therapeutic decisions can be based. For serial evaluation of nodes, the documentation of each node with regard to size, location, consistency, and mobility at each examination is critical. For cervical nodes, the examiner may stand behind or in front of the seated patient to palpate the neck and to examine in sequence the sites of various groups of nodes. Submental nodes are under the chin in the midline and on either side; submandibular nodes are under the jaw near its angle; jugular nodes are along the anterior border of the sternocleidomastoid muscle; supraclavicular nodes are found behind the midportion of the clavicle. Suboccipital nodes are found in the apex of the posterior cervical triangle, and pre- and postauricular nodes are found in front of and behind the ear pinnae, respectively. Central axillary nodes occur near the middle of the thoracic wall of the axilla; lateral axillary nodes are located near the upper part of the humerus along the axillary vein and are best felt by having the patient's arm elevated. Subscapular nodes can be felt under the anterior edge of the latissimus dorsi muscle, and pectoral nodes are beneath the lateral edge of the pectoralis major muscle. Infraclavicular nodes can be felt under the distal end of the clavicle. Epitrochlear nodes are located approximately 3 cm proximal to the medial humeral epicondyle. Palpation of epitrochlear nodes is best accomplished by palpation across the epitrochlear node area in an anterior to posterior direction. Enlarged abdominal lymph nodes can be difficult to palpate and may only be felt if the patient has a shallow abdominal cavity. Pelvic nodes are best evaluated with deep palpation of the lower abdomen by rolling the extended fingers over the pelvic brim.

The investigation of lymphadenopathy can be organized according to where nodes occur and the type of clinical symptoms present. Enlarged supraclavicular nodes most often result from lymphoma or gastrointestinal or intrathoracic tumors and should be biopsied. Acute onset of cervical adenopathy in young adults in the absence of head and neck infections suggests the diagnosis of infectious mononucleosis syndromes. If localized cervical node enlargement persists and serologic evaluation for EB virus, cytomegalovirus, and toxoplasmosis infections as well as chest x-ray and intermediate-strength PPD skin test are negative, then lymph node biopsy is indicated to seek lymphoma, sarcoidosis, carcinoma, and other diseases listed in Table 58-1.

Unilateral cervical adenopathy warrants a careful ear, nose, and throat examination for malignancy. In the asymptomatic patient with persistent new axillary and/or inguinal adenopathy, a biopsy specimen should be obtained. If fever and constitutional symptoms are present, the cause of infectious mononucleosis–like syndromes should be sought prior to node biopsy.

Generalized lymph node enlargement can be caused by systemic infections, drug reactions, malignancy, or one of the systemic lymphadenopathy syndromes (see Table 58-1). History and physical examination can yield clues regarding the possibility of these diagnoses and direct further evaluation (e.g., complete blood count, blood cultures, chest x-ray, serologies, skin tests). If systemic adenopathy persists without an obvious cause being identified, lymph node biopsy is warranted. Once the decision to perform lymph node biopsy has been made, tissue should be processed for culture of appropriate organisms, frozen in liquid nitrogen for lymphocyte typing or other special diagnostic studies for malignant cell types (such as Southern blot analysis of DNA for T cell receptor or immunoglobulin gene clonal rearrangements), and processed for routine pathologic evaluation. One can expect information that will lead to a diagnosis in 50 to 60 percent of lymph node biopsies. About 25 percent of patients with nondiagnostic lymph node biopsies will subsequently develop within a year a disease (usually a lymphoma) related to the indication for biopsy. Therefore, there should be little hesitation to repeat a nondiagnostic biopsy, especially if enlarged lymph nodes and symptoms persist.

The term *atypical hyperplasia of lymph nodes* refers to neither a clinical nor a pathologic entity but designates cases in which the pathologist expresses concern about neoplasia and is unable to unequivocally diagnose lymphoma. Since 30 percent of patients whose lymph node biopsies are read as atypical hyperplasia subsequently develop lymphoma, a repeat biopsy is recommended at a later date if node enlargement persists. Needle aspiration biopsy is a safe technique for initial evaluation of superficial adenopathy. While lymph node aspiration can aid in the diagnosis of metastatic tumor and infections, it is rarely helpful in the diagnosis of lymphomas and other hematologic malignancies.

SPLEEN

SPLEEN STRUCTURE AND FUNCTION   The spleen is a lymphoreticular organ that serves at least four major physiologic functions. First, it is an organ of the immune system and a major site of clearance of microorganisms and particulate antigens from the bloodstream and of generation of humoral or cellular responses to foreign antigens. Second, the spleen is instrumental in sequestration and removal of normal and abnormal blood cells. Third, the vasculature of the spleen plays a role in regulation of portal blood flow. Fourth, while hematopoiesis in the normal adult takes place primarily in the bone marrow, under pathologic conditions when the marrow is replaced or overstimulated to respond, the spleen may become a major site of extramedullary hematopoiesis.

The spleen is arranged into units of areas called *red* and *white pulp* (Fig. 58-2). Red pulp contains blood-filled sinuses and pulp cords lined by reticuloendothelial cells. White pulp contains centrally located arterioles, surrounded by densely packed small lymphocytes, which are primarily CD4+ helper T lymphocytes. Adjacent to the T cell periarteriolar lymphocyte sheath is the follicular zone of B lymphocytes which also contains germinal centers made up of B cells

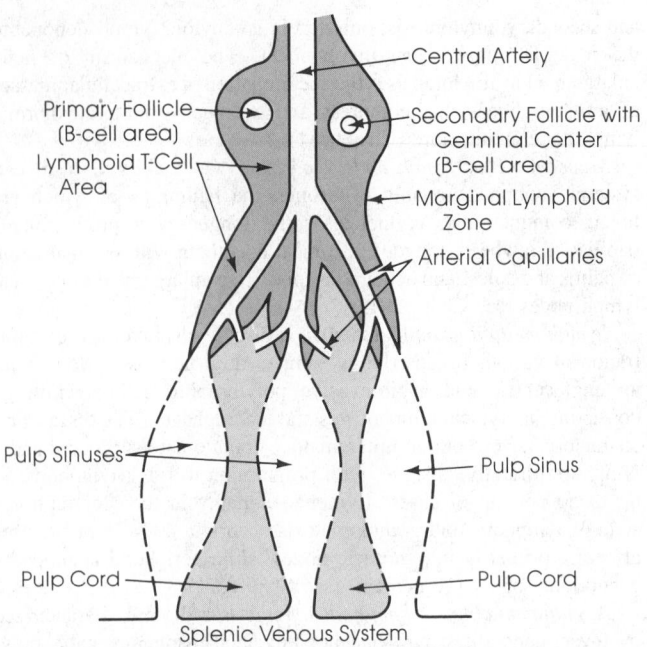

FIGURE 58-2   Schematic spleen structure. The spleen is made up of multiple units of red and white pulp centered around small branches of the splenic artery called central arteries. White pulp areas of spleen are lymphoid areas while red pulp areas include pulp sinuses and pulp cords. In white pulp, B cell areas are primary and secondary follicles and the marginal lymphoid zone, while T cell areas are lymphoid cells around follicles and arterial capillaries. (*Redrawn with permission from Videbaek et al.*)

and macrophages. The outermost portion of white pulp is another B cell layer called the *marginal zone* which blends into red pulp areas.

The blood supply and the route of blood flow are unique in the spleen, and splenic anatomy can best be defined in terms of route of blood flow (see Fig. 58-2). Blood enters the spleen by the splenic artery. The splenic artery divides into branches which penetrate into the spleen via connective tissue projections called *trabeculae* and from the trabeculae branch into smaller arteries called *central arteries*. From central arteries the bloodstream reaches the arterial capillaries. The periarteriolar lymphoid sheaths of T cells surrounding B cell follicles persist around the arterial vessels until they become small arterioles. Blood in central arterioles empties partly through arterial capillaries directly into splenic venules and then into splenic veins. The central arterioles also empty into macrophage-lined sinuses of red pulp and into the fibrous network of reticuloendothelial cells and tissue macrophages called *pulp cords*. Blood in red pulp sinuses and pulp cords empties directly into the splenic venous system. During red blood cell passage from central arteries to pulp cords, and finally to spleen sinuses, red cells are concentrated in the macrophage-rich pulp cords. Normally circulating red cells accumulate in pulp cords with subsequent passage through critical small openings of sinus endothelium into red pulp sinuses and on to the splenic venous system. Packing of red cells in pulp cords with subsequent passage through small slits into sinuses is termed *erythrocyte conditioning*. Upon senescence, red cells become less deformable and are unable to pass into sinuses; they are retained in pulp cords and phagocytosed by macrophages—a process termed *culling*. Erythrocyte particulate matter such as nuclear material (Howell-Jolly bodies), denatured hemoglobin (Heinz bodies), or malaria parasites can be pinched off during passage of red cells from pulp cords into sinuses and retained in the spleen while the rest of the red cell passes back into the circulation—a process termed *pitting*.

Many of the mechanisms of spleen enlargement are exaggerated forms of normal spleen function. While a wide variety of diseases are associated with enlargement of the spleen, there are six basic pathophysiologic mechanisms of splenic enlargement. (1) Splenic enlargement occurs from reticuloendothelial or immune system hyperplasia in infectious diseases such as bacterial endocarditis or in immune diseases such as Felty's syndrome. Reticuloendothelial hyperplasia also occurs in diseases associated with destruction of abnormal red blood cells such as hereditary spherocytosis, thalassemia, or early in the course of sickle cell disease. (2) Splenic enlargement occurs due to altered splenic blood flow in hepatic cirrhosis or splenic, hepatic, or portal vein thrombosis. (3) Malignant neoplasms can involve the spleen either primarily, as with lymphomas or angiosarcomas, or secondarily, as with leukemias or metastatic solid tumors. (4) Splenic enlargement can occur in situations leading to extramedullary hematopoiesis in the spleen, such as in myeloid metaplasia or other myelophthisic syndromes. (5) Infiltration of the spleen with abnormal material in amyloidosis and Gaucher's disease can result in splenomegaly. (6) Splenomegaly also can result from space-occupying lesions such as hemangiomas and cysts.

DISEASES ASSOCIATED WITH SPLENIC ENLARGEMENT   A wide variety of diseases lead to an increase in cellularity and vascularity of the spleen (Table 58-2). Increase in cellularity in infections is due to lymphocyte and macrophage proliferation in both red and white pulp areas. Splenomegaly is often present in acute systemic bacterial infections. Infectious granulomas due to mycobacterial and fungal infections occur in both red and white pulp. In diseases associated with disordered immunoregulation such as rheumatoid arthritis and systemic lupus erythematosus, splenic enlargement is often due to lymphoid hyperplasia, with enlarged lymphoid follicles present in white pulp areas and increased numbers of plasma cells and macrophages around red pulp arterioles and pulp cords. Splenic enlargement associated with abnormal splenic blood flow is most commonly due to chronic passive congestion from increased portal vein pressure or from portal vein obstruction. *Banti's syndrome* is *congestive splenomegaly* with hypersplenism associated with cirrhosis and portal hypertension and is manifested histologically by red pulp congestion with accumulation and concentration of erythrocytes in widened pulp cords and sinuses. In congestive splenomegaly, reticuloendothelial hyperplasia occurs with proliferation of cells lining red pulp cords and sinuses. In splenic enlargement in conditions associated with abnormal erythrocytes such as hereditary spherocytosis, there is pooling of abnormal red cells in sinuses and pulp cords because of increased red cell rigidity and therefore decreased ability to traverse the red pulp sinusoidal endothelium.

Myelosclerosis with myeloid metaplasia is characterized by splenic intrasinusoidal extramedullary hematopoiesis involving all three myeloid cell lines associated with dilated and distended pulp sinuses. In cases of secondary extramedullary hematopoiesis such as in myelophthisic syndromes, extramedullary hematopoiesis may only involve one or two cell lineages, particularly red cells. Infiltrative malignant disease can cause focal or generalized increases in white pulp lymphoid cells, as in the case of Hodgkin's disease and lymphocytic lymphoma, or infiltration of red pulp areas with malignant cells, as in chronic granulocytic leukemia, acute leukemia syndromes, systemic mast cell disease, and metastatic carcinoma. Infiltrative diseases of the spleen such as Gaucher's and Niemann-Pick produce splenic enlargement by increasing the number of splenic red pulp histiocytes. Thyrotoxicosis can be associated with splenomegaly and is due to thyroid hormone–induced lymphoid hyperplasia. Sarcoidosis causes splenic enlargement by the development of areas of granulomatous inflammation in white pulp lymphoid tissue. A splenic artery aneurysm may cause unexplained splenomegaly, cramping, and left upper abdominal pain; a calcified ring in the splenic area may be seen on x-ray.

The degree of splenomegaly varies with the disease entity. Slight or mild enlargement occurs in chronic passive congestion of the liver due to congestive heart failure, acute malaria, typhoid fever, bacterial endocarditis, systemic lupus erythematosus, rheumatoid arthritis, and thalassemia minor. Moderate splenic enlargement occurs in hepatitis, cirrhosis, lymphomas, infectious mononucleosis, hemolytic anemias, splenic abscesses and infarcts, and amyloidosis. Massive enlargement of the spleen occurs in chronic myelocytic leukemia, agnogenic myeloid metaplasia with myelofibrosis, hairy cell leukemia, Gaucher's and Niemann-Pick diseases, sarcoidosis, thalassemia major, chronic malaria, congenital syphilis, leishmaniasis, and in some cases of portal vein obstruction.

DIAGNOSTIC EVALUATION OF THE PATIENT WITH SPLENIC ENLARGEMENT   When normal in size and position, the spleen is generally inaccessible to abdominal palpation. A normal-sized spleen is about 12 cm long, 7 cm wide, and 250 cm³. Because of the oblique orientation of the spleen to the abdominal cavity, its long axis lies behind and parallel to the tenth rib in the midaxillary line, with splenic width located between the ninth and eleventh ribs. Palpation of the left upper quadrant is performed with the patient supine or on the right side by the examiner's right hand; the examiner's left hand is placed under the lower thorax, grasping the lower ribs posteriorly. Palpation for spleen enlargement is performed with the patient taking deep breaths to permit the examiner to feel the inferior tip of an enlarged spleen. To avoid missing a massively enlarged spleen, palpation of the left upper quadrant should begin in the lower abdominal cavity with gradual movement up to the left upper quadrant.

Demonstration of mild to moderate splenic enlargement by physical examination may be difficult, particularly in obese patients. Other techniques for assessment of spleen size include ⁹⁹Tc-colloid liver-spleen scan, computed tomography, and ultrasound scanning of the left upper quadrant. These three techniques can be useful in defining

---

TABLE 58-2   Diseases associated with enlargement of the spleen

Infections
- A Infectious mononucleosis
- B Bacterial septicemias
- C Bacterial endocarditis
- D Tuberculosis
- E Malaria
- F Leishmaniasis
- G Trypanosomiasis
- H AIDS
- I Viral hepatitis
- J Congenital syphilis
- K Splenic abscess
- L Disseminated histoplasmosis

Diseases of disordered immunoregulation
- A Rheumatoid arthritis (Felty's syndrome)
- B Systemic lupus erythematosus
- C Immune hemolytic anemias
- D Angioimmunoblastic lymphadenopathy
- E Drug reactions with serum sickness syndromes
- F Immune thrombocytopenias and neutropenias

Diseases of disordered splenic blood flow
- A Laennec's and postnecrotic cirrhosis
- B Hepatic vein obstruction
- C Hepatic schistosomiasis
- D Portal vein obstruction or cavernous sinus transformation
- E Splenic vein obstruction
- F Chronic congestive heart failure
- G Splenic artery aneurysm

Diseases associated with abnormal erythrocytes
- A Spherocytosis
- B Sickle cell disease
- C Ovalocytosis
- D Thalassemia

Infiltrative diseases of the spleen
- A Benign—amyloidosis, Gaucher's disease, Niemann-Pick disease, Hurler's syndrome, Tangier disease, multifocal Langerhans cell (eosinophilic) granulomatosis, extramedullary hematopoiesis, hamartomas, fibromas, hemangiomas, lymphangiomas, splenic cysts
- B Malignant—leukemias, lymphomas, Hodgkin's lymphoma, primary splenic tumors, angiosarcomas, metastatic tumors, myeloproliferative syndromes

Miscellaneous diseases or diseases of unknown cause
- A Idiopathic splenomegaly
- B Thyrotoxicosis
- C Iron-deficiency anemia
- D Sarcoidosis
- E Berylliosis
- F Kikuchi's histiocytic necrotizing lymphadenitis

splenic defects such as cysts, infarct, or tumors or in defining accessory splenic tissue that may be due to congenital accessory spleens or residual foci of splenic tissue following splenic rupture (splenosis). One study has documented palpable spleens in 3 percent of entering college freshmen and no increased risk of any disease during the ensuing 6 years.

In evaluation of the patient with splenomegaly, it is helpful to consider splenomegaly with acute or subacute illnesses separately from splenomegaly with chronic illness. Acute left upper quadrant pain with an enlarged tender spleen suggests subcapsular hematoma, splenic rupture, or splenic infarcts. Rupture of the spleen with splenic hematoma most often follows direct or remote trauma but can occur as well in the setting of infectious diseases such as malaria, typhoid fever, and EB virus–induced infectious mononucleosis. Splenic infarcts due either to in situ red cell sickling (in sickle cell disease) or to emboli (from mural thrombus, atrial myxoma, or cardiac valve vegetation) can usually be detected by spleen scan or arteriogram. More unusual disorders presenting acutely are diffuse splenic metastatic disease and hemorrhage into a splenic cyst.

An acute febrile illness associated with splenomegaly may be due to bacterial endocarditis, infectious mononucleosis syndromes, tuberculosis, and histoplasmosis. Fever, peripheral adenopathy, and splenomegaly, with or without a rash or arthralgias, should suggest (in addition to infectious mononucleosis) sarcoidosis, Hodgkin's lymphoma, a collagen vascular disease such as systemic lupus erythematosus, or a serum sickness syndrome.

An acute illness with splenomegaly associated with the signs and symptoms of anemia, with or without bleeding, suggests autoimmune hemolytic anemia, myeloproliferative syndromes, or acute leukemia.

Splenomegaly with signs and symptoms of chronic illness suggests a wide range of disorders, many of which are listed in Table 58-2. Liver disease with portal hypertension is a common etiology of splenomegaly in this setting. Patients with congestive splenomegaly from liver disease or portal or splenic vein thrombosis are often asymptomatic. With clinical features of rheumatoid arthritis and leukopenia, Felty's syndrome should be considered. The presence of lymphadenopathy should suggest chronic lymphocytic leukemia or lymphoma. Plethora and an elevated hematocrit suggest polycythemia vera or chronic lung disease, with right-sided heart failure and congestive splenomegaly. Weight loss or other signs of chronic illness suggest leukemia or other myeloproliferative syndromes, as well as a variety of hemoglobinopathies. Bone marrow aspiration and biopsy can aid in the diagnosis of leukemia and lymphoma, lipid storage diseases, disseminated fungal or mycobacterial diseases, metastatic malignant diseases, and amyloidosis.

Occasionally, laparotomy and splenectomy are indicated in the evaluation of splenomegaly. The decision to perform diagnostic laparotomy in a patient with unexplained splenomegaly is difficult and must take into account the patient's age and clinical signs, symptoms, and laboratory abnormalities present. Palpation of moderately enlarged spleens (750 to 800 cm^3) has been reported to miss up to 44 percent of spleens shown to be enlarged on radionuclide scan. In contrast, 97 percent of spleens are palpable when they reach three times normal size (900 cm^3). In a study of older subjects (average age 49) who had undergone splenectomy for undiagnosed splenomegaly and had signs and symptoms of chronic illness, a diagnosis of an underlying disorder was obtained in the majority of patients by splenectomy.

HYPERSPLENISM   The term *hypersplenism* applies to any clinical situation in which the spleen removes excessive quantities of erythrocytes, granulocytes, or platelets from the circulation. General mechanisms of removal of formed blood elements include increased sequestration of cells due to hemodynamic abnormalities of splenic blood flow or production of anti–red cell, granulocyte, or platelet antibodies, making the cells vulnerable to clearance by splenic macrophages. Situations in which passive congestion of the spleen occurs produce abnormal sludging of blood in sinuses and red pulp cords. Under these conditions, there is plasma pooling, producing

marked intrasplenic hemoconcentration and hypoxia and making blood cells more vulnerable to the phagocytic action of pulp cord macrophages. Criteria for diagnosis of hypersplenism include (1) splenomegaly, (2) splenic destruction of one or more cell lines in the peripheral blood, (3) normal or hyperplastic cellularity of bone marrow with normal representation of the cell line deficient in the circulation, and (4) variably, evidence of increased cell turnover in the cell lines affected (i.e., reticulocytosis), increased band forms of neutrophils, or circulating immature platelet forms.

Therapy for hypersplenism relates in large part to the underlying disease or the underlying pathophysiologic process. If the underlying disorder responsible for hypersplenism cannot be corrected, splenectomy is an option for cases in which a severe deficit is present (see below for indications for splenectomy).

HYPOSPLENISM   The terms *hyposplenia* and *asplenia* are used to indicate diminished or absent splenic function, respectively. The usual causes of hyposplenism are splenectomy, congenital absence of the spleen, sickle cell anemia in patients older than 5 years (with autosplenectomy due to repeated infarcts), and splenic irradiation (Table 58-3). In sickle cell anemia, persistence of a palpable spleen after age 5 suggests coexisting α thalassemia. Findings in the peripheral blood that indicate diminished splenic function include the presence of nucleated red cells, erythrocyte Howell-Jolly bodies, erythrocyte Heinz bodies, basophilic stippling, as well as target and burr forms of red cells, and rarely, circulating nucleated red blood cells.

Splenectomized patients or patients with functional asplenia (such as in sickle cell disease) are prone to bacterial infections, which are frequently overwhelming and life-threatening, particularly with encapsulated organisms such as *Streptococcus pneumoniae, Neisseria meningitidis, Escherichia coli,* and *Haemophilus influenzae.* The overall risk of bacterial sepsis in splenectomized patients has been estimated to be approximately 7 percent over a 10-year period. In addition, patients with hyposplenia are susceptible to infections with the parasite *Babesia,* which causes the parasitic disease *babesiosis.* This is due to a reduction or absence of the filtration function of the spleen for clearance of antibody-coated bacteria as well as to decreased production of IgG and IgM antibodies (opsonins) needed to bind bacteria. Immunization with 23-valent pneumococcal vaccine is recommended in patients older than 2 years with hyposplenism and prior to elective splenectomy. The presence of peripheral blood manifestations of hyposplenism in a normal-sized or enlarged spleen suggests splenic infiltrative disease such as a primary splenic angiosarcoma.

TABLE 58-3 Causes of functional and anatomical hyposplenism

1 Congenital hyposplenism—Fanconi's syndrome
2 Surgical splenectomy
3 Hyposplenism of old age
4 Hyposplenism due to splenic congestion—sickle hemoglobinopathies, myeloproliferative disorders such as essential thrombocytosis and myelofibrosis
5 Hyposplenism due to impaired vascular supply to the spleen
6 Immunologic or autoimmune disorders—systemic lupus erythematosus, rheumatoid arthritis, systemic necrotizing vasculitis syndromes, sarcoidosis, bone marrow transplantation complicated by graft-versus-host disease, IgA deficiency, thyroiditis, and thyrotoxicosis
7 Gastrointestinal diseases—celiac disease, dermatitis herpetiformis, ulcerative colitis, regional enteritis, intestinal lymphangiectasia, chronic active hepatitis
8 Malignancies—Sézary syndrome, multiple myeloma, gastric carcinoma, breast carcinoma, primary splenic angiosarcoma, non-Hodgkins lymphoma, splenic irradiation, Thorotrast therapy
9 Miscellaneous—systemic amyloidosis, drug-induced (IV gamma globulin, methyldopa, glucocorticoids), nephrotic syndrome, splenosis following splenectomy or splenic trauma, malignant mastocytosis, disseminated varicella

SOURCE: *C Pochedly et al (eds).*

INDICATIONS FOR SPLENECTOMY   Splenic trauma, whether accidental blunt trauma or intraoperative iatrogenic injury, is the most common indication for splenectomy. En bloc removal of the spleen may be indicated either because of tumor involvement or for a splenorenal shunt. Staging laparotomy with splenectomy remains a major diagnostic procedure for many early stage Hodgkin's disease patients being considered for radiation therapy alone. Splenectomy for selected patients with idiopathic splenomegaly is often necessary when other investigations fail to produce a diagnosis; however, the spleen should not be removed simply because it is palpable. Hypersplenism in lymphomas can cause persistent cytopenias and in select cases responds to splenectomy. B cell hairy cell leukemia frequently presents with hypersplenism, and in those patients who fail medical treatments, splenectomy is beneficial.

Felty's syndrome (rheumatoid arthritis and hypersplenism) and Gaucher's disease both require splenectomy when splenomegaly leads to symptomatic neutropenia or other complications of hypersplenism. Immune thrombocytopenic purpura which persists after trials of medical therapy may benefit from splenectomy (see Chap. 314). Of the hemolytic anemias, hereditary spherocytosis, hereditary elliptocytosis, immune hemolytic anemia with warm-reacting IgG antibody, and pyruvate kinase deficiency have been improved by splenectomy. Splenectomy is usually necessary late in the course of thalassemia major when neutropenia or thrombocytopenia develops or when transfusion requirements double. Chronic lymphocytic leukemia (CLL), chronic granulocytic leukemia, and agnogenic myeloid metaplasia may be complicated by symptomatic hypersplenism or, in the case of CLL, immune hemolytic anemia and thrombocytopenia, often necessitating splenectomy (Chaps. 309 and 310.)

REFERENCES

Lymph node enlargement

BUTCHER E, WEISSMAN I: Lymphoid tissues and organs in *Fundamental Immunology*, WE Paul (ed). New York, Raven, 1984, pp 109–127

GREENFIELD S, JORDAN MC: The clinical investigation of lymphadenopathy, in primary care practice. JAMA 240:1388, 1978

IOACHIM HL: *Lymph Node Biopsy*. Philadelphia, Lippincott, 1982

LENNERT K, STEIN H: The germinal center, in *Morphology, Histochemistry, and Immunohistology in Lymphoproliferative Diseases of Skin*, M Goos, E Christopher (eds). Berlin, Heidelberg, New York, Springer-Verlag, 1982

LIEBERMAN PH et al: A reappraisal of eosinophilic granuloma of bone, Hand-Schüller-Christian syndrome, and Letterer-Siwe syndrome. Medicine 48:375, 1969

NATHWANI BN et al: Malignant lymphoma arising in angioimmunoblastic lymphadenopathy. Cancer 41:578, 1978

POPPEMA S et al: Distribution of T cell subsets in human lymph nodes. J Exp Med 153:30, 1981

SCHROER KR, FRANSSILA KO: Atypical hyperplasia of lymph nodes: A follow-up study. Cancer 44:1155, 1979

SINCLAIR S et al: Biopsy of enlarged, superficial lymph nodes. JAMA 228:602, 1974

THOMAS JA et al: Combined immunological and histochemical analysis of skin and lymph node lesions in histiocytosis X. J Clin Pathol 35:327, 1982

WINTERBAUER RH et al: A clinical interpretation of bilateral hilar adenopathy. Ann Intern Med 78:65, 1973

YEN-TSU N et al: Lymph node biopsy for diagnosis: A statistical study. J Surg Oncol 14:53, 1980

Splenic enlargement

BUTLER JJ: Pathology of the spleen in benign and malignant conditions. Histopathology 7:453, 1983

EICHNER ER, WHITFIELD CL: Splenomegaly: An algorithmic approach to diagnosis. JAMA 246:2858, 1981

ENRIQUEZ E, NEIMAN RS (eds): *The Pathology of the Spleen: A Functional Approach*. Chicago, American Society of Clinical Pathologists, 1976

HERMANN RE et al: Splenectomy for the diagnosis of splenomegaly. Ann Surg 168:896, 1964

LEWIS SM (ed): *Clinics in Haematology*, vol 12: *The Spleen*. London, Saunders, 1983, pp 361–608

McINTYRE OR, EBAUGH FG: Palpable spleens in college freshmen. Ann Intern Med 66:301, 1967

POCHEDLY C et al (eds): *Disorders of the Spleen: Pathophysiology and Management*. New York, Marcel Dekker, 1989

STEINBERG MH et al: Evidence of hyposplenism in the presence of splenomegaly. Scand J Haematol 31:437, 1983

VIDEBAEK A et al: *The Spleen in Health and Disease*. Chicago, Yearbook, 1982

ZHANGE B, LEWIS SM: A study of the reliability of clinical palpation of the spleen. Clin Lab Haematol 11:7, 1989

59   QUANTITATIVE AND QUALITATIVE DISORDERS OF PHAGOCYTES

JOHN I. GALLIN

Leukocytes are the major cellular components of inflammatory and immune responses and include neutrophils, T and B lymphocytes, monocytes, eosinophils, and basophils. These cells have been assigned specific functions, such as antibody production by B lymphocytes or destruction of bacteria by neutrophils, but in no single infectious disease is the exact role of each of the cell types completely established. Thus, whereas neutrophils are classically thought to be critical to host defense against bacteria, there is increasing evidence that neutrophils play important roles in viral infections.

The blood is the most readily obtainable source of leukocytes and serves as the vehicle for their delivery to the various tissues from the bone marrow, where they are produced. Normal blood leukocyte counts for adults are given in Table 59-1 and those for different ages in the Appendix. The various leukocytes are thought to derive from a common stem cell in the bone marrow. Three-fourths of the nucleated cells of bone marrow are committed to the production of leukocytes. Leukocyte maturation in the marrow is under the regulatory control of a number of different factors, known as colony stimulating factors and interleukins. Because an alteration in the number and type of leukocytes is a frequent association with disease processes, a total white blood count (WBC) (cells per microliter) and differential counts are obtained frequently. The lymphocytes and basophils are discussed elsewhere. This chapter focuses on the neutrophils, monocytes, and eosinophils.

NEUTROPHILS

MATURATION   Important events in the neutrophil life are summarized in Fig. 59-1. In normal humans, neutrophils are only produced in the bone marrow. Best estimates indicate that the appropriate number of stem cells necessary to support hematopoiesis is between 400 and 500. There is convincing evidence that human blood monocytes and tissue macrophages produce colony stimulating factors, hormones required for the growth of monocytes and neutrophils in the bone marrow. The hematopoietic system not only produces enough neutrophils (approximately 1.3×10^{11} cells per 80-kg person per day) to carry out physiologic functions but also has a large reserve stored in the marrow which can be mobilized in response to inflammation or infection. An increase in the number of blood neutrophils is called *neutrophilia*, and the presence of immature cells is termed a ''shift to the left.'' A diminution in the number of blood neutrophils is referred to as *neutropenia*.

Neutrophils evolve from pluripotent stem cells (Fig. 59-2). Proliferation of the earliest pluripotent stem cells appears to be augmented

TABLE 59-1   Normal values for concentration of blood leukocytes*

Cell type	Mean, cells per microliter	95% Confidence limits, cells per microliter
Neutrophil	3650	1830–7250
Lymphocyte	2500	1500–4000
Monocyte	430	200–950
Eosinophil	150	0–700
Basophil	30	0–150

* Total leukocyte counts from venous blood samples were done in a Coulter counter, and 200 leukocytes were differentiated on Wright-stained blood smears made on coverglass. (From DC Dale, in JD Wilson et al, eds, *Harrison's Principles of Internal Medicine*, 12th ed, Chap 64.)

FIGURE 59-1 Events in inflammation. The four basic symptoms of inflammation are indicated by bold print.

by a multipotent growth factor (mgf). Interleukin 6 (IL-6) has no effect alone at this stage but synergistically augments the effect of mgf. As a consequence, the pluripotent stem cell is driven toward lymphocyte progenitors and toward granulocytes, erythrocytes, monocytes, megakaryocytes (GEMM), and mast cells. A multipotential colony stimulating factor known as interleukin 3 (IL-3) enhances proliferation toward erythrocytes, megakaryocytes, and mast cells, and interleukin 1 (IL-1) enhances proliferation at a later stage. Granulocyte-macrophage colony stimulating factor (GM-CSF) appears to act only on monomyeloid precursors. Granulocyte colony stimulating factor (G-CSF) is highly specific and influences neutrophil precursors only. By the myeloblast stage, cells under the influence of G-CSF enter the committed differentiation phase of development. The final stages of neutrophil development are characterized by the appearance of cells with distinct morphologic features. The myeloblast is the first recognizable precursor cell and is followed by the *promyelocyte* (see Fig. A9-15). The promyelocyte evolves when the classic lysosomal granules, called the *primary* or *azurophil granules*, are produced. The primary granules contain hydrolases, elastase, myeloperoxidase, cationic proteins, and bactericidal/permeability-increasing protein (BPI) important for killing gram-negative bacteria. Azurophil granules also contain *defensins*, a family of cystine-rich polypeptides with broad antimicrobial activity against bacteria, fungi, and certain enveloped viruses. The promyelocyte divides to produce the *myelocyte*, a cell responsible for the synthesis of the *specific* or *secondary granules* which contain unique (specific) constituents such as lactoferrin, vitamin B_{12}–binding proteins, membrane components of the NADPH oxidase required for hydrogen peroxide production, histaminase, and receptors for certain chemoattractants and adherence-promoting factors (CR3) as well as receptors for the connective tissue element laminin. The secondary granules do not contain acid hydrolases and therefore are not classic lysosomes. They are readily released extracellularly, and their mobilization is probably important in modulating inflammation. During the final stages of maturation there is no cell division, and the cell passes through the *metamyelocyte* stage and then to the *band* neutrophil with a sausage-shaped nucleus (see Fig. A9-17). As the band cell matures, the nucleus assumes a lobulated configuration. The nucleus of neutrophils normally contains

up to four segments. Excessive segmentation (greater than five nuclear lobes) may be a manifestation of folate or vitamin B_{12} deficiency. The Pelger-Hüet anomaly (see Fig. A9-19*B*), an infrequent dominant benign inherited trait, results in neutrophils with distinctive bilobed nuclei that must be distinguished from band forms. The physiologic role of the multilobed nucleus of neutrophils is unknown, but it may allow great deformation of neutrophils during migration into tissues at sites of inflammation.

In settings of severe acute bacterial infection, prominent neutrophil cytoplasmic granules called *toxic granulations* are occasionally seen (see Fig. A9-16). Toxic granulations are thought to be immature or abnormally staining azurophil granules. Cytoplasmic inclusions, also called *Doehle bodies* (see Fig. A9-17), can be seen during infection and probably represent fragments of ribosome-rich endoplasmic reticulum. Large neutrophil vacuoles are often present in acute bacterial infection and probably represent pinocytosed (internalized) membrane.

Neutrophils have long been thought to be a homogeneous population of cells. However, studies of neutrophil function have suggested that they are heterogeneous. Recently, monoclonal antibodies have been developed that recognize only a subset of mature neutrophils. The meaning of neutrophil heterogeneity is not known.

MARROW RELEASE AND CIRCULATING COMPARTMENTS

Specific signals, including interleukin 1, tumor necrosis factor-α, the colony stimulating factors, the complement fragment C3e, and perhaps other cytokines mobilize leukocytes from the bone marrow and deliver them to the blood in an unstimulated state. Under normal conditions, about 90 percent of the neutrophil pool is in the bone marrow, 2 to 3 percent in the circulation, and the remainder in the tissues. The blood pool exists as two compartments. The marginated pool is adherent to endothelial cells in capillary beds (especially in lung and spleen) and comprises about 50 percent of blood leukocytes. The freely flowing circulating pool makes up the remainder of blood leukocytes. In response to chemotactic stimuli from tissues (e.g., the complement product C5a, the arachidonic acid derivative leukotriene B_4, the cytokine interleukin 8, or the bacterial product *N*-formylmethionylleucylphenylalanine), neutrophil adhesiveness increases, and the circulating cells aggregate to each other and adhere to the endothelium.

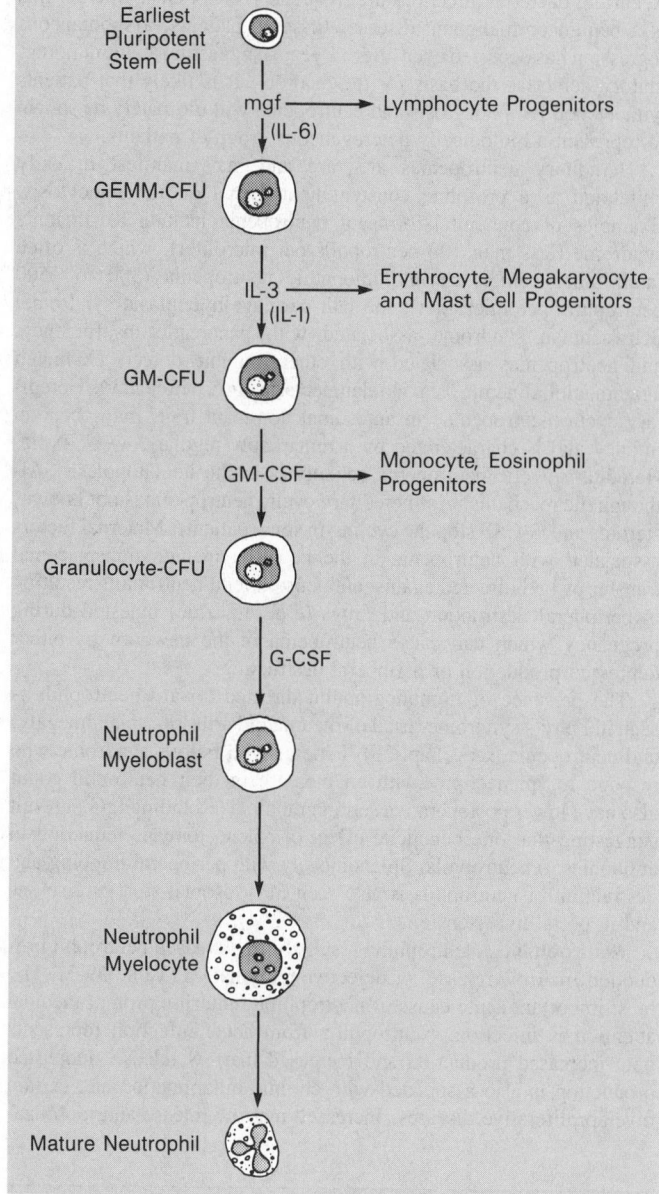

FIGURE 59-2 Regulation of myelopoiesis by growth factors (mgf, multipotent growth factor; IL, interleukin; GEMM, granulocyte, erythrocyte, monocyte, megakaryocyte; CFU, colony forming unit; CSF, colony stimulating factor; GM, granulocyte-macrophage; G, granulocyte).

An increased expression of the adhesion glycoprotein receptors called *integrins* [i.e., C3bi (also called CR3), LFA-1] on phagocytes is intimately involved with the increased adhesion. In addition, a novel family of adhesion molecules, called *selectins*, utilizes protein-carbohydrate interactions for specific cell-cell binding between leukocytes and endothelial cells. Receptors for chemoattractants and opsonins are also mobilized; the phagocytes orient toward the chemoattractant source in the extravascular space, increase their motile activity (chemokinesis), and migrate with direction (chemotaxis) into tissues. The biochemistry and cell biology of these processes are rapidly unfolding (see "References"). The process of migration into tissues is called *diapedesis* and involves the crawling of neutrophils between postcapillary endothelial cells which open junctions between adjacent cells to permit leukocyte passage. The endothelial responses (increased blood flow secondary to increased vasodilation and permeability) are mediated by anaphylatoxins (e.g., complement products C3a and C5a) as well as vasodilators such as histamine, bradykinin, serotonin, and prostaglandins E and I. In the healthy adult, most

neutrophils leave the body by migration through the mucous membrane of the gastrointestinal tract. Normally, neutrophils spend a relatively short time in the circulation, with a half-life of 6 to 7 h. Senescent neutrophils are cleared from the circulation by macrophages in the lung and spleen. Once in the tissues, neutrophils release enzymes such as collagenase and elastase, which may help establish abscess cavities. Neutrophils ingest (phagocytose) pathogenic materials that have been properly altered (opsonized) by substances such as immunoglobulin G (IgG) and the complement product C3b. Fibronectin and the tetrapeptide tuftsin facilitate the phagocytic process.

Concomitant with phagocytosis there is a burst of oxygen consumption and activation of the hexose-monophosphate shunt. A membrane-associated nicotinamide-adenine dinucleotide phosphate (NADPH) oxidase, consisting of membrane and cytosolic components, is assembled and catalyzes the reduction of oxygen to superoxide anion, which is then converted to hydrogen peroxide and other toxic oxygen products (e.g., hydrogen peroxide and hydroxyl radical). Hydrogen peroxide + chloride + neutrophil myeloperoxidase provide a particularly toxic system that generates hypochlorous acid, hypochlorite, and chlorine. These products oxidize and halogenate microorganisms and tumor cells and, when uncontrolled, can damage host tissue. Strongly cationic proteins and defensins also participate in microbial killing. Other enzymes, such as lysozyme and acid proteases, help digest microbial debris. After 1 to 4 days in tissues neutrophils die. Under certain conditions, such as in delayed-type hypersensitivity immunity, monocyte accumulation occurs within 6 to 12 h of initiation of inflammation. Neutrophils, monocytes, microorganisms in various states of digestion, and altered local tissue cells make up pus, which derives its characteristic green color from myeloperoxidase. Myeloperoxidase and other factors may be important in turning off the inflammatory process by inactivating chemoattractants and immobilizing phagocytic cells.

NEUTROPHIL DYSFUNCTION A defect anywhere in the neutrophil life cycle (summarized in Fig. 59-1) can lead to dysfunction and compromised host defenses. Inflammation is often depressed, and the clinical result is often recurrent and severe bacterial and fungal infections creating novel and often difficult management problems. Diagnosis of phagocytic cell disorders is suggested by clinical evaluation. Aphthous ulcers of mucous membranes (gray ulcers without pus) and gingivitis and periodontal disease are common. Patients with congenital phagocyte defects can have infections within the first few days of life. Skin, ear, upper and lower respiratory tract, and bone infections are common. Sepsis and meningitis are rare. In some disorders the frequency of infection is variable, and patients can go for months or even years without major infection. In the past it was unusual for persons with congenital defects to live beyond the age of 30 years. However, aggressive management of these diseases has extended the life span of patients.

Neutropenia The consequences of absent neutrophils are a dramatic demonstration of their importance in host defense. A large body of clinical data indicates that susceptibility to infectious diseases increases sharply when neutrophil levels fall below 1000 cells per microliter; when there are fewer than 200 cells per microliter, the inflammatory process is absent. The causes of neutropenia are multiple and are related to depressed production, peripheral destruction, and peripheral pooling. A falling neutrophil count or a significant decrease in neutrophils below steady state levels, together with a failure to increase neutrophil counts in the setting of infection or other challenge to the bone marrow reserve, requires investigation. Such acute neutropenia is more likely to be associated with increased risk of infection than neutropenia of long duration (months to years) that has a reversal in response to infection or carefully controlled administration of endotoxin (see "Laboratory Diagnosis," below).

Some causes of inherited and acquired neutropenia are listed in Table 59-2. The most common neutropenias are iatrogenic, resulting from the widespread use of cytotoxic or immunosuppressive therapies for malignancy or control of autoimmune disorders. These drugs cause neutropenia because they are toxic and result in decreased

TABLE 59-2　Causes of neutropenia

DECREASED PRODUCTION

Drug-induced—alkylating agents (nitrogen mustard, busulfan, chlorambucil, cyclophosphamide); antimetabolites (methotrexate, 6-mercaptopurine, 5-flurocytosine); noncytotoxic agents [antibiotics (chloramphenicol, penicillins, sulfonamides), phenothiazines, tranquilizers (meprobamate), certain diuretics, anti-inflammatory agents, antithyroid drugs, many others]
Hematologic diseases—idiopathic, cyclic neutropenia, Chédiak-Higashi syndrome, aplastic anemia, infantile genetic disorders (see text)
Tumor invasion, myelofibrosis
Nutritional deficiency—vitamin B_{12}, folate (especially alcoholics)
Infection—tuberculosis, typhoid fever, brucellosis, tularemia, measles, infectious mononucleosis, malaria, viral hepatitis, leishmaniasis, AIDS

PERIPHERAL DESTRUCTION

Antineutrophil antibodies and/or splenic or lung (alveolar macrophage) trapping
Autoimmune disorders—Felty's syndrome, rheumatoid arthritis, lupus erythematosus
Drugs as haptens—aminopyrine, α-methyl dopa, phenylbutazone, mercurial diuretics, some phenothiazines
Wegener's granulomatosis

PERIPHERAL POOLING (TRANSIENT NEUTROPENIA)

Overwhelming bacterial infection (acute endotoxemia)
Hemodialysis
Cardiopulmonary bypass

production of rapidly growing progenitor (stem) cells of the marrow. Cytotoxic chemotherapeutic agents fall into this category, but certain antibiotics such as chloramphenicol, trimethoprim-sulfamethoxazole, 5-flurocytosine, adenine arabinoside, and the antiretroviral drug zidovudine may cause neutropenia by inhibiting proliferation of myeloid precursors. The marrow suppression is generally dose-related and dependent on continued administration of the drug. Recombinant human G-CSF is an important drug for reversing this form of neutropenia and is particularly useful in cancer chemotherapy.

Another important mechanism for iatrogenically induced neutropenia is the effect of drugs that serve as immune haptens and sensitize neutrophils or neutrophil precursors to immune-mediated peripheral destruction. This form of drug-induced neutropenia can be seen within 7 days of exposure to the drug; with previous drug exposure, neutropenia may occur a few hours after administration of the drug. Although any drug can cause this form of neutropenia, the most frequent causes are commonly used antibiotics, such as sulfa-containing compounds, penicillins, and cephalosporins. Fever and eosinophilia also may be associated drug reactions, but often these signs are not present. Drug-induced neutropenia can be severe, but discontinuation of the sensitizing drug is sufficient for recovery, which is usually seen within 5 to 7 days and is complete by 10 days. Readministration of the sensitizing drug should be avoided, since abrupt neutropenia often will result. For this reason, diagnostic challenge, even with a brief exposure, should be avoided in most situations.

Autoimmune neutropenias caused by circulating antineutrophil antibodies are another form of acquired neutropenia that results in increased destruction of neutrophils. Acquired neutropenia also may be seen with viral infections, including those with the human immunodeficiency virus. Rarely, acquired neutropenia may be cyclic in nature, occurring at intervals of several weeks. Acquired cyclic neutropenia may be associated with increased natural killer (NK) cells and may be responsive to steroids.

Syndromes have been described in which clonal expansion of T8 cells is associated with neutropenia. T8 cells are granulated T lymphocytes, and patients with T8 cell lymphocytosis have moderate blood and bone marrow lymphocytosis, neutropenia, polyclonal hypergammaglobulinemia, splenomegaly, and absence of lymphadenopathy. Such patients have a chronic and relatively stable course.

Recurrent bacterial infections are frequent. It is not clear whether this is a benign or malignant disease. In some patients, a spontaneous regression has occurred even after 11 years, suggesting an immunoregulatory defect as the basis for the disorder. It is likely that patients with T8 cell lymphocytosis and neutropenia will ultimately be shown to represent a biologically heterogeneous group of patients.

Hereditary neutropenias are rare and may manifest in early childhood as a profound constant neutropenia or agranulocytosis. Examples of congenital forms of neutropenia include Kostmann's syndrome (less than 100 neutrophils per microliter), which is often fatal; more benign chronic idiopathic neutropenia (300 to 1500 neutrophils per microliter); the hair-cartilage-hypoplasia syndrome; Schwachman syndrome associated with pancreatic insufficiency; and neutropenias associated with other immune defects (X-linked agammaglobulinemia, ataxia telangiectasia, IgA deficiency). Hereditary cyclic neutropenia, an autosomal dominant trait, may occur in infancy and is characterized by a remarkably regular 3-week cycle. Hereditary cyclic neutropenia actually is cyclic hematopoiesis. Although the mechanism for hereditary cyclic neutropenia is not known, steroids and G-CSF stop the cycling in some patients. Maternal factors associated with neutropenia in the newborn include transplacental transfer of IgG directed against antigens on fetal neutrophils resulting in peripheral destruction and drugs (e.g., thiazide) ingested during pregnancy which can cause neutropenia in the newborn by either depressed production or peripheral destruction.

The presence of immunoglobulin directed toward neutrophils is seen in Felty's syndrome (triad of rheumatoid arthritis, splenomegaly, and neutropenia; see Chap. 58). Patients with Felty's syndrome who respond to splenectomy with an increase in their neutrophil count also have lower postoperative serum granulocyte-binding IgG, a result suggesting that one beneficial effect of splenectomy is reduction in antibodies to neutrophils. Splenomegaly with peripheral trapping and destruction of neutrophils is also seen in lysosomal storage diseases and in portal hypertension.

Neutrophilia　Neutrophilia results from increased neutrophil production, marrow release, or defective margination (Table 59-3). The most important acute cause of neutrophilia requiring prompt medical attention is infection. Neutrophilia from acute infection represents both increased production and increased marrow release. Increased production is also associated with chronic inflammation and certain myeloproliferative diseases. Increased marrow release and mobiliza-

TABLE 59-3　Causes of neutrophilia

INCREASED PRODUCTION

Idiopathic
Drug-induced—corticosteroids
Infection—bacterial, fungal, rarely viral
Inflammation—thermal injury, tissue necrosis, myocardial and pulmonary infarction, hypersensitivity states, collagen vascular diseases
Myeloproliferative diseases—myelocytic leukemia, myeloid metaplasia, polycythemia vera

INCREASED MARROW MOBILIZATION

Corticosteroids
Acute infection (endotoxin)
Inflammation—thermal injury

DEFECTIVE MARGINATION

Drugs—epinephrine, corticosteroids, nonsteroidal anti-inflammatory agents
Stress, excitement, vigorous exercise
Leukocyte adhesion protein [C3bi (CR3) receptor] deficiency

MISCELLANEOUS

Metabolic disorders—ketoacidosis, acute renal failure, eclampsia, acute poisoning
Drugs—lithium
Other—metastatic carcinoma, acute hemorrhage or hemolysis

tion of the marginated leukocyte pool are induced by corticosteroids. Release of epinephrine, as with vigorous exercise, excitement, or stress, will demarginate neutrophils in the spleen and lungs and double the neutrophil count. Administration of exogenous epinephrine is a useful test to distinguish neutrophilia due to decreased margination, as seen in leukocyte adhesion deficiency, from that due to increased marrow production or release. Leukocytosis with counts of 10,000 to 25,000 cells per microliter occurs in response to infection and other forms of acute inflammation and results from both release of the marginated pool and mobilization of marrow reserves. Persistent neutrophilia of 30,000 to 50,000 cells per microliter or greater is called a *leukemoid reaction*, a term often used to distinguish this degree of neutrophilia from leukemia. In a leukemoid reaction, the circulating neutrophils are usually mature.

ABNORMAL NEUTROPHIL FUNCTION The types of inherited and acquired abnormalities of phagocyte function are described in Table 59-4. The resulting diseases are best considered in terms of the functional defects of adherence, chemotaxis, and microbicidal activity. The distinguishing features of the important inherited disorders of phagocyte function are shown in Table 59-5, several of which are discussed below.

Patients with inherited (autosomal recessive) abnormal phagocyte adherence, *leukocyte adhesion protein deficiency*, lack the plasma membrane receptor for the fragment of the third complement component called C3bi (CR3 by other terminology). The mutation is in the gene of the beta subunit of the leukocyte adhesion molecules LFA-1, Mac-1, and gp150,95. The gene is located on the most distal portion of the long arm of chromosome 21. Variable expression of the defect determines the magnitude of clinical disease. Complete lack of expression of the leukocyte adhesion proteins by resting neutrophils results in the severe phenotype in which inflammatory cytokines do not increase the expression of leukocyte adhesion proteins on neutrophils or activated T and B cells. The functional abnormalities are predictable because of the role these molecules play in normal leukocyte function. Neutrophils (and monocytes) from patients with leukocyte adhesion protein deficiency adhere poorly to endothelial cells and protein-coated surfaces and exhibit defective spreading, aggregation, and chemotaxis. Patients with this syndrome have recurrent bacterial and fungal infections involving skin, oral and genital mucosa, and respiratory and intestinal tracts, persistent leukocytosis (15,000 to 20,000 neutrophils per microliter) because cells do not marginate, and usually a history of delayed separation of

the umbilical stump. Infections, especially of the skin, tend to become necrotic with progressively enlarging borders, slow healing, and the development of dysplastic scars. The most common bacteria are *Staphylococcus aureus* and enteric gram-negative bacteria.

Abnormal neutrophil and monocyte chemotaxis occurs in the *hyperimmunoglobulin E–recurrent infection (Job's) syndrome*. The molecular basis for the syndrome is not known. For many years the cold abscesses were thought to be a reflection of impaired chemotaxis with too few phagocytes arriving too late, perhaps secondary to a lymphocyte factor inhibiting chemotaxis. However, it is now clear that the chemotactic defect in these patients is variable and the fundamental basis for the impaired defenses is complex and inadequately delineated.

The most common neutrophil defect is *myeloperoxidase deficiency*, which is inherited as an autosomal recessive trait and may have an incidence as high as about 1 in 2000 persons. Isolated myeloperoxidase deficiency is not associated with severely compromised defenses, because other defense systems such as hydrogen peroxide generation are accelerated. Microbicidal activity of neutrophils is delayed but not absent. However, if another underlying defect in host defense, such as poorly controlled diabetes mellitus, accompanies myeloperoxidase deficiency, then host defenses are likely to be significantly compromised. An acquired form of myeloperoxidase deficiency occurs in myelomonocytic leukemia and acute myeloblastic leukemia (also referred to as *myelogenous leukemia*). Dapsone and sulfones also inhibit myeloperoxidase-mediated hypochlorous acid (bleach) production by neutrophils.

Chédiak-Higashi syndrome (CHS) is a rare disease with autosomal recessive inheritance. Neutrophils and all cells containing lysosomes from patients with CHS characteristically have large granules (see Fig. A9-19A). CHS patients have increased infections due to a multitude of infectious agents. CHS neutrophils and monocytes have impaired chemotaxis and abnormal rates of microbial killing due to slow rates of fusion of the lysosomal granules with phagosomes. Natural killer cell function is also impaired.

Chronic granulomatous disease (CGD) represents a group of patients with disorders of neutrophil and monocyte oxidative metabolism. Although CGD is rare, occurring about once in 1 million individuals, it is an important model of defective neutrophil oxidative metabolism. Most often CGD is inherited as an X-linked recessive pattern, although in 35 percent of patients the disease is inherited with an autosomal recessive pattern. Mutations of four genes corre-

---

TABLE 59-4 Types of phagocyte dysfunction

Function	Cause of indicated dysfunction		
	Drug-induced	Acquired	Inherited
Adherence-aggregation	Aspirin, colchicine, alcohol, glucocorticoids, ibuprofen, piroxicam	Neonatal state, hemodialysis	Leukoctye adhesion protein deficiency
Deformability		Leukemia, neonatal state, diabetes mellitus, immature neutrophils	
Chemokinesis-chemotaxis	Glucocorticoids (high dose), auranofin, colchicine (weak effect), phenylbutazone, naproxen, indomethacin, interleukin 2	Thermal injury, malignancy, malnutrition, periodontal disease, neonatal state, systemic lupus erythematosus, rheumatoid arthritis, diabetes mellitus, sepsis, influenza virus infection, herpes simplex virus infection, acrodermatitis enteropathica, Down syndrome, α-mannosidase deficiency, severe combined immunodeficiency, Wiskott-Aldrich syndrome, AIDS	Chédiak-Higashi syndrome, neutrophil specific granule deficiency, hyper IgE–recurrent infection (Job's) syndrome (in some patients)
Microbicidal activity	Colchicine, cyclophosphamide, glucocorticoids (high dose)	Leukemia, aplastic anemia, certain neutropenias, tuftsin deficiency, thermal injury, sepsis, neonatal state, diabetes mellitus, malnutrition, AIDS	Chédiak-Higashi syndrome, neutrophil specific granule deficiency, chronic granulomatous disease

TABLE 59-5   Inherited disorders of phagocyte function: Differential features

Clinical manifestations	Cellular or molecular defects	Diagnosis
CHRONIC GRANULOMATOUS DISEASES OF CHILDHOOD (60% X-LINKED, 30% AUTOSOMAL RECESSIVE)		
Severe infections of skin, ears, lungs, liver, and bone with catalase-positive microorganisms such as *S. aureus*, *Pseudomonas cepacia*, *Aspergillus* sp., *Chromobacterium violaceum*; often hard to culture organism; excessive inflammation with granulomas, frequent lymph node suppuration; granulomas can obstruct GI or GU tracts; gingivitis, aphthous ulcers, seborrheic dermatitis	Absent respiratory burst due to the lack of one of four NADPH oxidase subunits in neutrophils, monocytes, and eosinophils	NBT test; absent superoxide and H_2O_2 production by neutrophils
CHEDIAK-HIGASHI SYNDROME (AUTOSOMAL RECESSIVE)		
Recurrent pyogenic infections, especially with *S. aureus*; many patients get lymphomatous-like illness during adolescence; periodontal disease; partial oculocutaneous albinism, nystagmus, progressive peripheral neuropathy, mental retardation in some patients	Reduced chemotaxis and phagolysosome fusion, increased respiratory burst activity, defective egress from marrow, abnormal skin window	Clinical features, giant lysosomal granules in granule-bearing cells (Wright stain)
SPECIFIC GRANULE DEFICIENCY (AUTOSOMAL RECESSIVE?)		
Recurrent infections of skin, ears, and sinopulmonary tract; delayed wound healing; decreased inflammation; bleeding diathesis	Abnormal chemotaxis, impaired respiratory burst and bacterial killing, failure to upregulate chemotactic and adhesion receptors with stimulation, defect in transcription of granule proteins	Lack of Wright-stained secondary (specific) granules in neutrophils, absent neutrophil-specific granule contents (i.e. lactoferrin), and absent eosin-staining granulocytes due to abnormal eosinophil-specific granules, platelet alpha granule abnormality
MYELOPEROXIDASE DEFICIENCY (AUTOSOMAL RECESSIVE)		
Clinically normal except in patients with underlying disease such as diabetes mellitus; then candidiasis or other fungal infections	Absent myeloperoxidase due to pre- and posttranslational defects	Absent peroxidase in neutrophils
LEUKOCYTE ADHESION PROTEIN DEFICIENCY* (AUTOSOMAL RECESSIVE)		
Delayed separation of umbilical cord, sustained granulocytosis, recurrent infections of skin and mucosa, gingivitis, periodontal disease	Impaired phagocyte adherence, aggregation, spreading, chemotaxis, phagocytosis of iC3b coated particles; leukemoid reaction; defective production of beta subunit common to leukocyte adhesion proteins	Reduced phagocyte surface expression of leukocyte adhesion receptors using a monoclonal antibody against Mac-1
HYPER IgE–RECURRENT INFECTION SYNDROME† (NON-X-LINKED)		
Eczematoid or pruritic dermatitis, "cold" skin abscesses, recurrent pneumonias with *S. aureus* with bronchopleural fistulas and cyst formation, mild eosinophilia, mucocutaneous candidiasis, atopy, coarse facies, restrictive lung disease, scoliosis	Reduced chemotaxis in some patients, reduced suppressor T cell activity	Clinical features, serum IgE > 2000 IU/mL, high serum anti-*S. aureus* IgE, low or absent serum and salivary anti-*S. aureus* IgA

* C3bi (CR3) receptor, Mac-1,LFA-1, gpl50,95 deficiency.
† Job's syndrome.

sponding to four proteins that assemble at the plasma membrane account for all patients with CGD. Two proteins (a 91-kDa protein, abnormal in X-linked CGD, and a 22-kDa protein, absent in autosomal recessive CGD) form the heterodimer cytochrome b-558 in the plasma membrane, and two other proteins (47 and 67 kDa, abnormal in autosomal recessive forms of CGD) are cytoplasmic in origin and interact with the cytochrome following cell activation to form NADPH oxidase, required for hydrogen peroxide production. Leukocytes from patients with CGD have severely diminished hydrogen peroxide production. The genes involved in each of the defects have been cloned and sequenced and the chromosome location identified. Patients with CGD characteristically have increased infection with catalase-positive microorganisms (organisms which destroy their own hydrogen peroxide). When patients with CGD become infected, they often have extensive inflammatory reactions, and lymph node suppuration is common despite the administration of appropriate antibiotics. Aphthous ulcers and chronic inflammation of the nares are usually present. Granulomas are frequent and can obstruct the gastrointestinal or genitourinary tracts. The excessive inflammatory reactions probably reflect abnormal turnoff of inflammation by failure to degrade chemoattractants and antigens which cause persistent neutrophil accumulation. Impaired killing of intracellular microorganisms by macrophages may lead to persistent cell-mediated immunity and granuloma formation.

MONONUCLEAR PHAGOCYTES

The mononuclear phagocyte system is defined as a continuum linking monoblasts, promonocytes, and monocytes with the structurally diverse tissue macrophages which make up what was previously referred to as the reticuloendothelial system. Macrophages are long-lived phagocytic cells capable of many of the functions of neutrophils. In addition, they are important secretory cells that, through their receptors and secretory products, participate in many complex immunologic and inflammatory processes not attributed to neutrophils. Monocytes leave the circulation by diapedesis more slowly than neutrophils and have a half-life in the blood of 12 to 24 h.

After blood monocytes arrive in the tissues, they differentiate into macrophages ("big eaters") with specialized functions suited for specific anatomic locations. Macrophages are particularly abundant in capillary walls of the lung, spleen, liver, and bone marrow, where they function to remove microorganisms and other noxious elements from the blood. Alveolar macrophages, liver Kupffer cells, splenic macrophages, peritoneal macrophages, bone marrow macrophages, lymphatic macrophages, brain microglial cells, and dendritic macrophages all have specialized functions. Macrophage-secreted products include lysozyme, neutral proteases, acid hydrolases, arginase, numerous complement components, enzyme inhibitors (plasmin, alpha$_2$ macroglobulin), binding proteins (transferrin, fibronectin, transcobalamin II), nucleosides, cachectin, and interleukin 1 (pyrogen). Interleukin 1 (see Chaps. 16 and 277) has many important functions, including stimulating the hypothalamus to initiate fever, mobilizing leukocytes from the bone marrow, as well as activating lymphocytes and neutrophils. Tumor necrosis factor (also called *cachectin*) is a pyrogen that duplicates many of the actions of interleukin 1 and plays an important role in the pathogenesis of gram-negative shock (see Chap. 83). It can stimulate vigorous production of hydrogen peroxide and related toxic oxygen species by macrophages and neutrophils. In addition, tumor necrosis factor induces catabolic responses of chronic inflammation which contribute to the profound wasting (cachexia) associated with many chronic diseases.

Other macrophage-secreted products include reactive oxygen metabolites, bioactive lipids (arachidonate metabolites and platelet-activating factors), a neutrophil chemoattractant, factors regulating synthesis of proteins by other cells, bone marrow colony stimulating factors, factors stimulating fibroblast and microvasculature proliferation, as well as factors inhibiting replication of lymphocytes, tumors, viruses, and certain bacteria (*Mycobacterium tuberculosis* and *Listeria monocytogenes*). Macrophages are key effector cells in the elimination of intracellular microorganisms. Their ability to fuse to form giant cells which coalesce into granulomas in response to some inflammatory stimuli is important in the elimination of intracellular microbes and may be under the control of interferon-γ.

Macrophages play an important role in the immune response (see Chap. 277). They process antigen for presentation to lymphocytes, their secreted products modulate lymphocyte function, and macrophages participate in autoimmune phenomena by removing immune complexes and other immunologically active substances from the circulation. Furthermore, they play a role in wound healing, in the disposal of senescent cells, and in the development of atheromas.

DISORDERS OF THE MONONUCLEAR PHAGOCYTE SYSTEM
Many disorders of neutrophils extend to mononuclear phagocytes. Thus drugs which suppress neutrophil production in the bone marrow usually lead to monocytopenia. Transient monocytopenia also can be seen after stress or glucocorticoid administration. Monocytosis is associated with certain infections such as tuberculosis, brucellosis, subacute bacterial endocarditis, Rocky Mountain spotted fever, and malaria. Monocytosis is also seen in kala azar, malignancies, leukemias, myeloproliferative syndromes, hemolytic anemias, chronic idiopathic neutropenias, granulomatous diseases such as sarcoidosis, regional enteritis, and some collagen vascular diseases. Patients with leukocyte adhesion protein deficiency, the hyperimmunoglobulin E–recurrent infection (Job's) syndrome, Chédiak-Higashi syndrome, and chronic granulomatous diseases all have defects in the mononuclear phagocyte system.

Certain viral infections impair mononuclear phagocyte function. For example, influenza virus infection is associated with abnormal monocyte chemotaxis. Mononuclear phagocytes can be infected by the human immunodeficiency virus (HIV), and abnormal monocyte chemotaxis and abnormal clearance of IgG-coated erythrocytes (discussed below) by macrophages is also seen in AIDS (see Chap. 279). It is likely that these defects of the monocyte-macrophage system in AIDS contribute to the disordered immunoregulation and increased susceptibility to opportunistic infection due to intracellular microorganisms such as *Pneumocystis carinii* and *Mycobacterium avium-intracellulare*. T lymphocytes produce interferon-γ, which induces Fc-receptor expression and phagocytosis and stimulates hydrogen

peroxide production by mononuclear phagocytes. In certain diseases, such as AIDS, interferon-γ production may be deficient, while in other diseases, such as T cell lymphomas, excessive release of interferon-γ is thought to cause erythrophagocytosis by splenic macrophages.

Specific defects of the mononuclear phagocytes have been described in certain autoimmune diseases. Removal of IgG-coated radiolabeled autologous erythrocytes, presumably via the Fc receptor of splenic macrophages, is profoundly abnormal in patients with active systemic lupus erythematosus. Patients with other autoimmune diseases characterized by tissue deposition of immune complexes, as seen in Sjögren's syndrome, mixed cryoglobulinemia, dermatitis herpetiformis, and chronic progressive multiple sclerosis, also have defects in Fc-receptor function as judged by clearance of IgG-coated erythrocytes (see Chap. 283). Clinically, normal subjects with genetic haplotypes commonly associated with autoimmune disease (i.e., HLA-B8/DRw3) also have an increased incidence of defective Fc-receptor–specific functional activity, suggesting that this defect may predispose individuals with this genetic profile to immune-complex disease.

Monocytopenia occurs with acute infections, with stress, and following administration of glucocorticoids. Monocytopenia also occurs in aplastic anemia and acute myelogenous leukemia and as a direct result of myelotoxic and immunosuppressive drugs.

EOSINOPHILS

Eosinophils and neutrophils share similar morphology, many lysosomal constituents, most chemotactic responses, phagocytic capacity, and oxidative metabolism. However, there are major differences between the two cell types, and little is known about the natural function of eosinophils. Eosinophils are much longer lived than neutrophils, and unlike neutrophils, tissue eosinophils can recirculate. During most infections, eosinophils do not appear to have any important function. However, in invasive parasite infections, such as hookworm, schistosomiasis, strongyloidiasis, toxocariasis, trichinosis, filariasis, echinococcosis, and cysticercosis, the eosinophil likely plays a central role in host defense. Eosinophils are also associated with bronchial asthma, cutaneous allergic reactions, and other hypersensitivity states.

The characteristic red-staining eosinophil granules (Wright's stain) contain a number of unique constituents. The distinctive feature of the eosinophil granule is its crystalline core consisting of an arginine-rich protein (major basic protein) with histaminase activity, which is probably important in host defense against parasites. Eosinophil granules also contain a unique eosinophil peroxidase which catalyzes the oxidation of many substances by hydrogen peroxide and may facilitate killing of microorganisms.

Eosinophil peroxidase, in the presence of hydrogen peroxide and halide, initiates mast cell secretion in vitro and thereby may contribute to inflammation. Other substances found in eosinophils include cationic proteins, some of which bind to heparin and reduce its anticoagulant activity. Eosinophil cytoplasm contains Charcot-Leyden crystal protein, a hexagonal bipyramidal crystal first described in leukemia and then in sputum from asthma patients, which is lysophospholipase and may function to restrict the toxicity of certain lysophospholipids. Eosinophils also contain a powerful neurotoxin. Because patients with hypereosinophilic syndrome and cerebral spinal fluid eosinophilia exhibit varied neurologic abnormalities, eosinophil-derived neurotoxin may play an important role in central nervous system disease.

Several factors enhance the eosinophil's function in host defense. For example, T cell–derived eosinophil stimulation promoter enhances the ability of eosinophils to kill parasites. Mast cell–derived eosinophil chemotactic factor of anaphylaxis (ECFa) increases the number of eosinophil complement receptors and enhances eosinophil killing of parasites. In addition, eosinophil colony stimulating factors produced by macrophages may not only increase eosinophil production in the bone marrow but also may activate eosinophils to kill parasites.

EOSINOPHILIA   Eosinophilia is the presence of more than 500 eosinophils per microliter of blood and is common in many settings besides parasite infection. Significant tissue eosinophilia can occur without an elevated blood count. The most common cause of eosinophilia is probably allergic reactions to drugs such as iodides, aspirin, sulfonamides, nitrofurantoin, penicillins, and cephalosporins. Allergies such as hay fever, asthma, eczema, serum sickness, allergic vasculitis, and pemphigus commonly are associated with eosinophilia. Eosinophilia is also seen in collagen vascular diseases (e.g., rheumatoid arthritis, eosinophilic fasciitis, allergic angiitis, periarteritis nodosa, and granulomatosis) and malignancies (e.g., Hodgkin's disease, mycosis fungoides, chronic myelogenous leukemia, and cancer of the lung stomach, pancreas, ovary, or uterus), as well as rare diseases such as Job's syndrome and the chronic granulomatous diseases; the mechanisms for the eosinophilia in these diseases are not known. Eosinophilia is commonly seen in helminthic infections, such as hookworm, strongyloidiasis, toxocariasis, trichuriasis, trichinosis, filariasis, schistosomiasis, echinococcosis, and cysticercosis. The most dramatic increases in eosinophils occur in hypereosinophilic syndromes, including Loeffler's syndrome, Loeffler's endocarditis, eosinophilic leukemia, and idiopathic hypereosinophilic syndrome (with counts as high as 50,000 to 100,000 per microliter).

The idiopathic hypereosinophilic syndrome represents a heterogeneous group of disorders with the common feature of prolonged eosinophilia of unknown cause and associated organ system dysfunction, including the heart, central nervous system, kidneys, lungs, gastrointestinal tract, and skin. The bone marrow is involved in all subjects, but the most severe complications involve the heart and central nervous system. Eosinophils are found in the involved tissues and are thought to cause tissue damage by local deposition of toxic eosinophil proteins such as eosinophil cationic protein and eosinophil major basic protein. In the heart, the pathologic changes lead to thrombosis, which may result in endocardial fibrosis and restrictive endomyocardiopathy. Similar pathologic changes are thought to contribute to the damage of tissues in other organ systems. Although the mechanism for the hypereosinophilia is not known, it has been shown that chemotherapy with glucocorticoids usually induces remission. In patients unresponsive to glucocorticoids, a cytotoxic agent such as hydroxyurea has been used successfully to lower the peripheral blood eosinophil counts and to improve markedly the prognosis. Aggressive medical and surgical approaches are also employed for management of patients with cardiovascular complications.

The *eosinophilia-myalgia syndrome* is a multisystem disease with prominent cutaneous, hematologic, and visceral manifestations that frequently evolves into a chronic course and can occasionally be fatal. The syndrome is characterized by blood eosinophilia (greater than 10^9 eosinophils per liter) and generalized disabling myalgias without other recognized causes. Eosinophil fasciitis, pneumonitis and myocarditis, neuropathy culminating in respiratory failure, and encephalopathy have been described. The association of the disease with ingestion of L-tryptophan–containing products originating from a single source has led to the identification and characterization of a putative etiologic agent present as a contaminant in these preparations. Although the accumulation of eosinophils, lymphocytes, macrophages, and fibroblasts in the affected tissues suggests that these cells play important roles in the pathogenesis of the eosinophilia-myalgia syndrome, the precise mechanism of their involvement has not been established. Several studies have demonstrated the activation of eosinophils and the deposition of eosinophil-derived toxic proteins in affected tissues. Fibroblast activation and increased expression of genes coding for various connective tissue macromolecules have been demonstrated with use of in situ hybridization with complementary DNAs. Furthermore, interleukin 5 and transforming growth factor-β have been implicated as potential mediators. Treatment has included withdrawal of L-tryptophan–containing products and the administra-

tion of corticosteroids. Most patients recover fully, remain stable, or show slow recovery, but in some patients (up to 5 percent) the disease can be fatal. This disease emphasizes the importance of chemical and environmental factors in the development of systemic disorders characterized by chronic inflammation and fibrosis.

EOSINOPENIA   This occurs with stress, such as acute bacterial infection, and following administration of glucocorticoids. The mechanism of eosinopenia of acute bacterial infection is unknown but is independent of endogenous glucocorticoids, since it occurs in animals following total adrenalectomy. There is no known adverse effect of eosinopenia.

LABORATORY DIAGNOSIS AND MANAGEMENT OF PHAGOCYTE DYSFUNCTION

Initial studies of white blood count and differential and often a bone marrow examination are followed by assessment of bone marrow reserves (steroid challenge test), marginated circulating pool of cells (epinephrine challenge test), and marginating ability (endotoxin challenge test). In vivo assessment of inflammation is possible with a Rebuck skin window test or an in vivo blister assay, which measures the ability of leukocytes and inflammatory mediators to accumulate locally within the skin. In vivo clearance of IgG-coated erythrocytes provides a useful way to monitor the mononuclear phagocyte system. In vitro tests of phagocyte aggregation, adherence, chemotaxis, phagocytosis, degranulation, and microbicidal activity (for *Staphylococcus aureus*) help pinpoint cellular or humoral lesions which can then be further characterized at the molecular level. Deficiencies of oxidative metabolism are screened with the nitroblue tetrazolium dye (NBT) test, which is based on the ability of products of oxidative metabolism to reduce yellow, soluble NBT to blue-black formazan, an insoluble material which precipitates intracellularly and can be seen microscopically. Further aspects of neutrophil oxidative metabolism are defined by studies of superoxide and hydrogen peroxide production.

The most important aspect of patient management is to appreciate that patients with leukopenias or leukocyte dysfunction often have delayed inflammatory responses. Therefore, clinical manifestations may be minimal despite overwhelming infection, and unusual infections must always be suspected in some patients. Early signs of infection demand prompt, aggressive culturing for microorganisms and use of antibiotics and surgical drainage of abscesses. Prolonged antibiotics are often required, and in life-threatening infections, daily white blood cell transfusions (enriched for neutrophils) are probably beneficial, although their use is still controversial. In patients with the chronic granulomatous diseases of childhood (CGD), prophylactic antibiotics (trimethoprim-sulfamethoxazole) probably diminish the frequency of life-threatening infections. Surgery is required for thorough drainage of abscesses in lung, liver, and bones. Short courses of glucocorticoids have had dramatic effects in the management of the granulomas of CGD. For example, obstruction of the gastrointestinal or genitourinary tract in CGD can be diminished with a short course of steroids followed by a long one of a nonsteroidal anti-inflammatory agent. Recent studies indicate that recombinant human interferon-γ, which nonspecifically stimulates phagocytic cell function, reduces the frequency of infections in CGD patients by 70 percent and reduces the severity of infection (hospital days for infection) as well. This effect of interferon-γ in CGD is additive to the effect of prophylactic antibiotics. Interferon-γ has been approved by the U.S. Food and Drug Administration for use in CGD at a recommended dose of 50 μg/m² of body surface area.

Rigorous oral hygiene reduces but does not eliminate the discomfort of gingivitis, periodontal disease, and aphthous ulcers; chlorhexidine mouth wash and tooth brushing with a hydrogen peroxide–sodium bicarbonate paste helps many patients. Ketoconazole has caused dramatic improvement of mucocutaneous candidiasis in patients with Job's syndrome. Treatment to restore myelopoiesis in patients with neutropenia due to impaired production has included use of androgens, glucocorticoids, lithium, and immunosuppressive therapy. Recombinant G-CSF is useful in the management of certain forms of neutropenia due to depressed production, especially that related to chemotherapy for cancer. Patients with chronic neutropenia with evidence of a good bone marrow reserve should not receive prophylactic antibiotics.

Patients with constant or cyclic neutrophil counts below 500 cells per microliter may benefit from prophylactic antibiotics. Oral trimethoprim-sulfamethoxazole (160/800 mg) twice daily is commonly used to prevent infection, although concerns about its predisposing to fungal infections have been raised. Increased fungal infection is not seen in CGD patients on this regimen. Oral quinolones such as norfloxacin and ciprofloxacin have been suggested alternatives.

In the setting of cytotoxic chemotherapy with severe, persistent neutropenia, the proven effectiveness of trimethoprim-sulfamethoxazole in preventing *Pneumocystis carinii* pneumonia may offer another incentive to use this form of prophylaxis. These patients, and patients with phagocytic cell dysfunction, should avoid heavy exposure to airborne soil, dust, or decaying matter (mulch, manure) which could be rich in spores of *Aspergillus* or other fungi. Restriction of activities or social contact probably makes little difference in risk of infection.

Cure of some congenital phagocyte defects is theoretically possible by bone marrow transplantation (see Chap. 313). However, complications of bone marrow transplantation are still great, and with rigorous medical care many patients with phagocytic disorders can go for years without a life-threatening infection. The identification of specific gene defects in patients with leukocyte adhesion protein deficiency and chronic granulomatous disease of childhood and the successful correction of B cells from these patients by gene transfection make gene therapy a likely and exciting future possibility.

REFERENCES

ANDERSON DC, SPRINGER TA: Leukocyte adhesion deficiency: An inherited defect in the Mac-1, LFA-1, and p150,95 glycoproteins. Annu Rev Med 38:175, 1987

BEUTLER B (ed): Tumor necrosis factors, in *The Molecules and Their Emerging Role in Medicine*. New York, Raven Press, 1992

CURNUTTE JT (ed): Phagocyte defects: Abnormalities outside the respiratory burst. Hematol Clin North Am 2, 1988

GALLIN JI: Interferon-γ in the management of chronic granulomatous disease. Rev Infect Dis 13:1973, 1991

——— et al: Delineation of the phagocyte NADPH oxidase through studies of chronic granulomatous diseases of childhood. Curr Opin Immunol 4:53, 1991

——— et al (eds): *Inflammation: Basic Principles and Clinical Correlates*, 2d ed. New York, Raven Press, 1992

GEHA RS, LEUNG DY: Hyper-immunoglobulin-E syndrome. Immunodefic Rev 1:155, 1989

GLEICH GJ, ADOLPHSON C: The eosinophil leukocyte: Structure and function. Adv Immunol 39:177, 1986

JOHNSTON RB: Monocytes and macrophages. N Engl J Med 318:747, 1988

KLEMPNER MS, MALECH HL: Phagocytes: Normal and abnormal neutrophil host defenses, in *Infectious Diseases*, SL Gorbach et al (eds). Philadelphia, Saunders, 1992

KUHNS DB et al: Dynamics of the cellular and humoral components of the inflammatory response elicited in skin blisters in humans. J Clin Invest 89:1734, 1992

LAWRENCE MB, SPRINGER TA: Leukocytes roll on a selectin at physiologic flow rates: Distinction from and a prerequisite for adhesion through integrins. Cell 65:859, 1991

LIESCHKE GJ, BURGESS AW: Granulocyte colony-stimulating factor and granulocyte-macrophage colony-stimulating factor. N Engl J Med 327:28, 99, 1992

LOMAX KJ et al: The molecular biology of selected phagocyte defects. Blood Rev 3:94, 1989

MALECH HL, GALLIN JI: Neutrophils in human diseases. N Engl J Med 317:687, 1987

METCALFE DM: Control of granulocytes and macrophages: Molecular, cellular and clinical aspects. Science 254:529, 1991

MOORE MAS: The clinical use of colony stimulating factors. Annu Rev Immunol 9:159, 1991

NAUSEEF WM: Myeloperoxidase deficiency. Hematol Pathol 4:165, 1990

SAMTER M (ed): *Immunological Diseases*, 4th ed. Boston, Little, Brown, 1988

VARGA J et al: The cause and pathogenesis of the eosinophil-myalgia syndrome. Ann Intern Med 116:140, 1992

WEISS SJ: Tissue destruction by neutrophils. N Engl J Med 320:365, 1989

60   GENETIC ASPECTS OF DISEASE

JOSEPH L. GOLDSTEIN / MICHAEL S. BROWN

GENETIC PRINCIPLES

More than one-fifth of the proteins (and hence genes) in each human being exist in a form that differs from the one present in the majority of the population. This remarkable genetic variability, or polymorphism, among "normal" people accounts for much of the normal variation in body traits such as height, intelligence, and blood pressure. These genetic differences also determine the ability of each individual to meet environmental challenges, including those which produce disease. All human diseases can be considered to result from an interaction between an individual's unique genetic makeup and the environment. In certain diseases, the genetic component is so overwhelming that it expresses itself in a predictable manner without a requirement for extraordinary environmental challenges. Such diseases are termed *genetic disorders*.

MOLECULAR BASIS OF GENE EXPRESSION   All hereditary information is transmitted from parent to offspring through the inheritance of deoxyribonucleic acid (DNA). DNA is a linear polymer composed of purine and pyrimidine bases whose sequence ultimately determines the sequence of amino acids in every protein made by the body. The four types of bases in DNA are arranged in groups of three, each triplet forming a code word, or codon, that signifies a particular amino acid. A *gene* represents the total sequence of bases in DNA that specifies the amino acid sequence of a single polypeptide chain of a protein molecule.

Genetic information encoded in the DNA of the chromosomes is first transcribed into a *ribonucleic acid* (RNA) copy. During transcription, the ribose nucleotides align themselves along the DNA according to base-pairing rules. Thus adenine of DNA pairs with uridine of RNA, cytosine pairs with guanine, thymine pairs with adenine, and guanine pairs with cytosine. The ribose bases are joined together by RNA polymerase. The resulting *RNA transcript* forms the template for translation into the amino acid sequence of a protein. The DNA and mRNA code words for each of the amino acids in protein are shown in Fig. 60-1.

A schematic diagram of the genetic control of protein synthesis in higher organisms is illustrated in Fig. 60-2. The DNA of most genes is fragmented into discrete coding regions (exons) separated by noncoding regions (introns or intervening sequences). The *coding regions* contain the bases that specify the sequence of amino acids in the polypeptide chain. The *intervening sequences* are composed of bases that act as spacers between the coding regions; they are not translated into protein. The transcription of DNA produces a faithful copy of the entire gene sequence; thus the RNA transcript contains alternating coding and intervening sequences. The RNA transcript is edited in the nucleus before it passes into the cytoplasm. In the editing process, the intervening sequences are excised, and the coding regions are spliced together to form one continuous RNA (Fig. 60-2).

FIGURE 60-1   The genetic code.

		A or U		G or C		T or A		C or G		
A or **U**	**AAA** **AAG** *UUU* *UUC* } Phe	**AGA** **AGG** *UCU* *UCC* } Ser	**ATA** **ATG** *UAU* *UAC* } Tyr	**ACA** **ACG** *UGU* *UGC* } Cys	**A** or **U**
	AAT **AAC** *UUA* *UUG* } Leu	**AGT** **AGC** *UCA* *UCG*	**ATT** **ATC** *UAA* *UAG* } Stop	**ACT** **ACC** *UGA* *UGG* Stop / Trp	**G** or **C** / **T** or **A** / **C** or **G**
G or **C**	**GAA** **GAG** **GAT** **GAC** *CUU* *CUC* *CUA* *CUG* } Leu	**GGA** **GGG** **GGT** **GGC** *CCU* *CCC* *CCA* *CCG* } Pro	**GTA** **GTG** *CAU* *CAC* } His; **GTT** **GTC** *CAA* *CAG* } Gln	**GCA** **GCG** **GCT** **GCC** *CGU* *CGC* *CGA* *CGG* } Arg	**A** or **U** / **G** or **C** / **T** or **A** / **C** or **G**
T or **A**	**TAA** **TAG** **TAT** *AUU* *AUC* *AUA* } Ile; **TAC** *AUG* Met	**TGA** **TGG** **TGT** **TGC** *ACU* *ACC* *ACA* *ACG* } Thr	**TTA** **TTG** *AAU* *AAC* } Asn; **TTT** **TTC** *AAA* *AAG* } Lys	**TCA** **TCG** *AGU* *AGC* } Ser; **TCT** **TCC** *AGA* *AGG* } Arg	**A** or **U** / **G** or **C** / **T** or **A** / **C** or **G**
C or **G**	**CAA** **CAG** **CAT** **CAC** *GUU* *GUC* *GUA* *GUG* } Val	**CGA** **CGG** **CGT** **CGC** *GCU* *GCC* *GCA* *GCG* } Ala	**CTA** **CTG** *GAU* *GAC* } Asp; **CTT** **CTC** *GAA* *GAG* } Glu	**CCA** **CCG** **CCT** **CCC** *GGU* *GGC* *GGA* *GGG* } Gly	**A** or **U** / **G** or **C** / **T** or **A** / **C** or **G**

Second nucleotide

First nucleotide (left side label)   *Third nucleotide* (right side label)

Note: The DNA codons appear in boldface type; the complementary RNA codons are in italics. A = adenine, C = cytosine, G = guanine, T = thymine, U = uridine (replaces thymine in RNA). In RNA, adenine is complementary to thymine of DNA; uridine is complementary to adenine of DNA; cytosine is complementary to guanine, and vice versa. "Stop" = termination. The amino acids are abbreviated as follows:

Ala = alanine	Cys = cysteine	His = histidine	Met = methionine	Thr = threonine
Arg = arginine	Gln = glutamine	Ile = isoleucine	Phe = phenylalanine	Trp = tryptophan
Asn = asparagine	Glu = glutamic acid	Leu = leucine	Pro = proline	Tyr = tyrosine
Asp = aspartic acid	Gly = glycine	Lys = lysine	Ser = serine	Val = valine

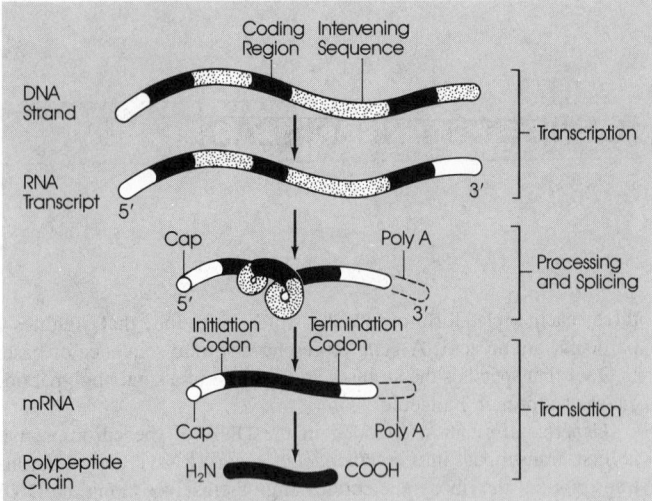

FIGURE 60-2 A schematic diagram of the genetic control of protein synthesis, illustrating the flow of genetic information from the base sequence of DNA to the RNA transcript (transcription) to mRNA (processing) to the polypeptide chain of a protein molecule (translation). Although DNA exists in a double-stranded form, only one of the two strands is used as a template for transcribing the RNA transcript. Solid sections represent coding regions in DNA, RNA transcript, mRNA, and amino acid sequence in polypeptide chain; dotted sections represent intervening sequences in DNA and RNA transcript.

After processing, the edited RNA, called *messenger RNA* (mRNA), leaves the nucleus and enters the cytoplasm, where it becomes associated with *ribosomes* and thereby serves as a template for the ribosomal synthesis of proteins. Each of the 20 amino acids is attached in the cell cytoplasm to a specific molecule called *transfer RNA* (tRNA). Each tRNA contains a triplet sequence of purine and pyrimidine bases that is "complementary" to a specific codon in the mRNA. These tRNA molecules with their attached amino acids line up along the mRNA molecule in the precise order dictated by the genetic code. Under the action of cytoplasmic enzymes (initiation factors, elongation factors, and termination factors), peptide bonds are formed between the various amino acids, and the completed protein is released from the ribosome. For a more detailed account of the molecular basis of gene expression, see Chap. 61.

MAINTENANCE OF GENETIC DIVERSITY THROUGH TRANSMISSION AND SEGREGATION OF GENES The amount of DNA in the nucleus of each human cell is sufficient to code for more than 50,000 genes and hence to specify more than 50,000 polypeptide chains. The genes are arranged in a linear sequence of DNA that together with certain histone proteins form rod-shaped bodies called *chromosomes*. Each somatic cell contains 46 chromosomes, arranged in 23 pairs, one of each pair derived from each parent. Thus each individual inherits two copies of each chromosome and hence two copies of each gene. The chromosomal location of the two copies of each gene is termed the *genetic locus*. When a gene occupying a genetic locus exists in two or more different forms, these alternate forms of the gene are referred to as *alleles*.

In humans, a given gene always resides at a specified genetic locus on one particular chromosome. For example, the genetic locus for the Rh blood group is on the short arm of chromosome 1; at this site there are two Rh genes, one on chromosome 1 derived from the mother and the other on chromosome 1 derived from the father. When two genes at the same genetic locus are identical, the individual is a *homozygote*. When the two genes differ (i.e., two different alleles are present at the locus), the individual is a *heterozygote*. Each normal human is heterozygous at approximately 20 percent of genetic loci and homozygous at 80 percent. A map of human chromosome 1,

shown in Fig. 60-3, illustrates the location of a representative sample of genes that have been assigned loci on this chromosome.

The genetic information carried on chromosomes is transmitted to daughter cells under two different sets of circumstances. One of these occurs whenever a somatic cell (i.e., a nongerm cell) divides. This process, called *mitosis*, transmits identical copies of each gene to each daughter cell, thus maintaining a uniform genetic makeup in all cells of a single individual. The other set of circumstances prevails when genetic information must be transmitted from one individual to an offspring. This process, called *meiosis*, produces germ cells (i.e., ova or spermatozoa) that possess only one copy of each parental chromosome, thus allowing for new combinations of chromosomes to occur when ovum and sperm cell fuse during fertilization.

During meiosis, the 46 chromosomes of an immature germ cell arrange themselves in 23 pairs at the center of the nucleus, each pair being composed of one chromosome derived from the mother and its homologous chromosome derived from the father. At a specified point in the meiotic process, the two partner chromosomes separate, only one of each pair going into each daughter cell, or gamete. Thus meiosis produces gametes with a reduction in the number of chromosomes from 46 to 23, each gamete having received one chromosome from each of the 23 pairs. The assortment of the chromosomes within each pair is random so that each germ cell receives a different combination of maternal and paternal chromosomes. During the process of fertilization, the fusion of ovum and sperm cell, each of which has 23 chromosomes, produces an individual with 46 chromosomes.

The independent assortment of chromosomes into gametes during meiosis produces an enormous diversity among the possible genotypes

FIGURE 60-3 Gene map of human chromosome 1, illustrating a representative sample of the more than 250 genes that have been localized to this chromosome. The black bands represent those genetic regions of the chromosome which stain brightly by a fluorescent dye such as quinacrine; the white bands are the negatively staining regions; the hatched area is a variable region that stains differently (i.e., either brightly or negatively) in the chromosomes of different individuals. Each gene is listed opposite its genetic locus on the right. (*Data provided by VA McKusick.*)

of the progeny. For each 23 pairs of chromosomes, there are 2^{23} different combinations of chromosomes that could occur in a gamete, and the likelihood that one set of parents will produce two offspring with the identical complement of chromosomes is 1 in 2^{23} or 1 in 8.4 million (assuming no monozygotic, or identical, twins).

RECOMBINATION Adding to the genetic diversity in humans is the phenomenon of *genetic recombination*. During meiosis, when homologous chromosomes are paired, bridges frequently form between corresponding regions of the chromosome pair. These bridges, or *chiasmata*, are regions in which the two chromosomes break at identical points along their length and subsequently rejoin, the distal segments having been switched from one homologous chromosome to another. This process is designated *crossing-over*. Although no net change in the amount of genetic material occurs during crossing-over, a recombination of genes does occur. For example, consider a chromosome with two loci, A and B, located at opposite ends of the same chromosome. On this particular chromosome, the A locus has a rare allele *x*, and the B locus also has a rare allele *y*. Without the phenomenon of recombination, every offspring that inherited the *x* allele at the A locus also would inherit the *y* allele at the B locus. However, if recombination occurs, the A locus with the *x* allele would then be on the opposite chromosome from the B locus with the *y* allele. In this case, any offspring that inherited the *x* allele at the A locus could not inherit the *y* allele at the B locus.

Crossing-over occurs with great frequency in every meiosis in humans, and the resultant recombination of genes may occur at any point on a chromosome. The farther apart two genes are on the same chromosome, the greater is the likelihood that a crossing-over will occur in the space between them. When two genes are on the opposite ends of a long chromosome, the probability of recombination is so great that their respective alleles are transmitted to offspring almost independently of one another, just as if the two gene loci were on different chromosomes. On the other hand, gene loci that are close together on the same chromosome are said to be *linked* so that there is a great likelihood that offspring will inherit the same combination of alleles that are present on the parental chromosome.

Several examples of *gene linkage* can be seen from the map of human chromosome 1 (Fig. 60-3). For example, the locus for the gene specifying the Rh blood group factor and the locus for the gene producing one form of the dominant trait hereditary elliptocytosis occur in close proximity on this chromosome. Thus, if a subject with hereditary elliptocytosis transmits the disease to an offspring, the offspring will usually inherit the allele that is present at the Rh locus on this chromosome. If the Rh allele happens to be a rare one in the population (such as *r'*), one can assume that whichever offspring inherits the *r'* allele at the Rh locus also will inherit the abnormal allele at the elliptocytosis locus. On the other hand, if an offspring does not exhibit the *r'* allele, he or she will not usually have elliptocytosis. The concept of linkage does not imply an association between any particular set of Rh alleles and the disease state elliptocytosis, rather between the two genetic loci. Thus in different families the abnormal elliptocytosis allele may be linked to the R^1, R^0, r_2, or any other allele at the Rh locus depending on the allele that happened to be at that locus when the elliptocytosis mutation occurred. Stated another way, the elliptocytosis locus is linked to the Rh locus in every family, but the particular Rh allele with which it is associated differs from family to family.

MUTATION Broadly defined, a *mutation* is a stable, heritable alteration in DNA. Although the causes of mutation in humans are largely unknown, a variety of environmental agents, such as radiation, viruses, and chemicals, are among the factors that are implicated. Mutations can involve a visible alteration in the structure of a chromosome, such as a deletion or translocation of a portion of a chromosome, or they can involve a minute change in one of the purine or pyrimidine bases of a single gene. Most commonly, such "point" mutations consist of the substitution of one base for another, changing the meaning of the codon containing that base, hence their

designation as *missense mutations*. For example, in the gene coding for the β chain of hemoglobin, the sixth position normally contains the nucleotide triplet CTC, which codes for the amino acid glutamic acid (Fig. 60-1). The mutation that gives rise to hemoglobin C produces a change of the first base of this triplet from cytosine to thymine, changing the triplet to TTC, which codes for lysine. On the other hand, the mutation that gives rise to hemoglobin S produces a change in the second base of the same triplet (from thymine to adenine), producing CAC, which codes for valine. Thus, in the sixth position of the β chain of hemoglobin, the normally occurring glutamic acid may be replaced with either lysine (producing hemoglobin C) or valine (producing hemoglobin S). More than 100 such single-base mutations in the hemoglobin β chain have been identified, and many of these mutations produce distinct clinical syndromes. Of the mutations so far elucidated in humans, most involve such single-base changes.

Besides producing an amino acid substitution, a single-base substitution also can cause another abnormality in protein synthesis— premature chain termination. Three mRNA code words (UAA, UAG, and UGA) normally do not specify an amino acid but constitute the signal that the message has ended and that the protein chain should be released from the ribosome (Fig. 60-1). If a change occurs in DNA that produces one of these mRNA code words [e.g., a switch in an mRNA triplet from UAU (tyrosine) to UAA (termination)], the polypeptide chain would be terminated prematurely when translation had reached that point. Such mutations, called *non-sense mutations*, produce short fragments of proteins that have reduced function.

CELLULAR MECHANISM BY WHICH MUTANT GENES PRODUCE DISEASES Critical to the understanding of heredity is the concept that the only information transmitted from generation to generation is the sequence of bases in DNA and that these sequences in turn specify only the primary structure of RNA and protein molecules. All other chemical reactions—such as the synthesis of complex lipids and carbohydrates, the formation of membranes and other cellular organelles, and the accumulation and partitioning of inorganic ions—occur as a secondary consequence of the action of specific proteins. Many of these proteins are enzymes that catalyze the biochemical conversion of one molecule into another. Others are structural proteins such as collagen and elastin, and still others are regulatory proteins that dictate how much of each enzyme and each structural protein is made.

Since proteins are the cellular molecules whose structures are encoded by genes, mutations in genes exert their deleterious effects by altering the structure of enzymes, structural proteins, or regulatory proteins. For example, in a disease such as glycogen storage disease, type I (von Gierke's disease), massive accumulation of glycogen in the liver is due not to a primary structural abnormality in the polysaccharide glycogen but to a structural abnormality in a protein, glucose-6-phosphatase, an enzyme that is required to liberate glucose so as to permit glycogen breakdown. Other examples of the biochemical mechanisms by which mutant genes alter cellular metabolism are discussed below under "Simply Inherited Disorders."

GENETIC HETEROGENEITY When two or more mutations can produce a similar clinical syndrome, *genetic heterogeneity* is said to exist. Hemophilia is an example of a genetically heterogeneous syndrome. A clinically similar bleeding disorder can be caused by mutations at either of two loci on the X chromosome, one leading to a deficiency of factor VIII (classic hemophilia) and the other causing a deficiency of factor IX (Christmas disease). Most, if not all, hereditary diseases, when carefully analyzed, will probably prove to be genetically heterogeneous.

Genetic heterogeneity may result from the existence of a series of different mutations at a single genetic locus (allelic mutations) or from mutations at different genetic loci (nonallelic mutations). For example, drug-induced hemolysis of red blood cells can occur in patients with several different types of allelic mutations at the glucose-6-phosphate dehydrogenase locus. On the other hand, hemophilia is an example of a syndrome in which nonallelic mutations can produce a similar clinical picture (see above).

In some cases of heterogeneity, both the genetic locus and the mode of inheritance differ. Diseases such as spastic paraplegia, Charcot-Marie-Tooth peroneal muscular atrophy, and retinitis pigmentosa are inherited as autosomal dominant traits in some families, as autosomal recessives in others, and as X-linked recessives in still others. The identification of such genetic heterogeneity in these disorders is of obvious importance for correct genetic counseling.

TAKING THE FAMILY HISTORY

The investigation of a patient with a possible genetic disorder begins with the *family history*. The first step is to obtain certain information on the *proband* or *index case* (i.e., the clinically affected person who has brought the family to attention) and on each of the *first-degree relatives* (i.e., the parents, siblings, and offspring of the proband). This information includes the given name, surname, maiden name, birth date or current age, age at death, cause of death, and name or description of any disease or defect.

The second step is to ask questions designed to survey the family for the presence of disease or defect. (1) Has any relative an identical or similar trait? (2) Has any relative a trait that is absent in the proband but is known to occur in some patients with the same disease? This question requires that the physician have some knowledge about the manifestations of the disease in question. For example, when obtaining the family history from a proband with dissecting aneurysm caused possibly by Marfan's syndrome, one should ask about the occurrence of eye abnormalities, cardiac abnormalities, and skeletal abnormalities in the relatives. (3) Has any relative a trait that is recognized to be genetically determined? The purpose of this question is to ascertain the occurrence of hereditary disease in the family even though the particular patient may not be involved. (4) Has any relative an unusual disease, or has any relative died of a rare condition? The purpose of this question is to identify a condition that might be genetically determined though not recognized as such by the informant. In addition, this question may help to identify conditions in relatives that might be etiologically related to the patient's problem. For example, a patient with pheochromocytoma should be suspected of having von Recklinghausen's disease if he or she has a brother with scoliosis and mental retardation, both of which can be manifestations of the neurofibromatosis (von Recklinghausen's) gene. (5) Is there any consanguinity in the family? This inquiry should be made directly. In addition, one should ask whether common last names appear in the families of husband-wife pairs. Consanguineous marriage may be the source of a rare autosomal recessive syndrome, and sometimes its presence in the family may not be known by the proband. (6) What is the ethnic origin of the family? Persons of various ethnic origins, such as blacks, Jews, and Greeks, have increased chances of specific genetic diseases. Table 60-1 lists examples of simply inherited disorders that are found with increased frequency in various ethnic groups.

CATEGORIES OF GENETIC DISORDERS

Genetic diseases generally fall into one of three categories: (1) *Chromosomal disorders* involve the lack, excess, or abnormal arrangement of one or more chromosomes, producing excessive or deficient genetic material. (2) *Mendelian*, or *simply inherited*, *disorders* are determined primarily by a single mutant gene. These disorders display inheritance patterns which can be classified into autosomal dominant, autosomal recessive, or X-linked types. (3) *Multifactorial disorders* are caused by an interaction of multiple genes and multiple exogenous or environmental factors. Although many of these multifactorial disorders, such as essential hypertension and cleft lip and palate, are said to run in families, the inheritance pattern is complex and the risk

TABLE 60-1   Examples of simply inherited disorders that occur with increased frequency in specific ethnic groups

Ethnic group	Simply inherited disorder
African blacks	Hemoglobinopathies, especially Hb S, Hb C, persistent Hb F, α and β thalassemias Glucose-6-phosphate dehydrogenase deficiency
Armenians	Familial Mediterranean fever
Ashkenazi Jews	Abetalipoproteinemia Bloom's syndrome Dystonia musculorum deformans (recessive form) Factor XI (PTA) deficiency Familial dysautonomia (Riley-Day syndrome) Gaucher's disease (adult form) Neimann-Pick disease Pentosuria Tay-Sachs disease
Chinese	α Thalassemia Glucose-6-phosphate dehydrogenase deficiency Adult lactase deficiency
Eskimos	Pseudocholinesterase deficiency Adrenogenital syndrome
Finns	Congenital nephrosis Mulibrey nanism
French Canadians	Tyrosinemia Homozygous familial hypercholesterolemia
Japanese	Acatalasemia
Lebanese	Homozygous familial hypercholesterolemia
Mediterranean peoples (Italians, Greeks, Sephardic Jews)	β Thalassemia Glucose-6-phosphate dehydrogenase deficiency Familial Mediterranean fever Glycogen storage disease, type III
Northern Europeans	Cystic fibrosis
Scandinavians	Alpha₁-antitrypsin deficiency LCAT (lecithin:cholesterol acyltransferase) deficiency
South African whites	Porphyria variegata Homozygous familial hypercholesterolemia

to relatives is less than in the single-gene (mendelian) disorders. Each of these categories presents different problems with respect to causation, prevention, diagnosis, genetic counseling, and treatment.

CHROMOSOMAL DISORDERS   The karyotype of an individual (i.e., the number and structure of the chromosomes) can be ascertained from readily accessible body tissues, such as peripheral blood lymphocytes or skin, by growing them in tissue culture until active cell proliferation occurs and then preparing single cells for examination of chromosomes by microscopy. Each individual chromosome can be identified by special staining of DNA sequences, e.g., by the affinity of fluorescent dyes (such as quinacrine hydrochloride) for certain chromosomal segments that can be visualized by fluorescence microscopy or by treatment with special dyes (Giemsa) and proteolytic enzymes (trypsin). These techniques produce characteristic *banding patterns* for each chromosome (Fig. 60-4).

The number of chromosomes in normal individuals is 46, of which 44 are the 22 pairs of *autosomes* and the other 2 are the *sex chromosomes*. Women have two X chromosomes (XX), and men have one X chromosome and one Y chromosome (XY). Each of the 22 pairs of autosomes and the 2 sex chromosomes can be distinguished on the basis of size, location of the centromere (which divides the chromosome into arms of equal or unequal length), and the unique banding pattern (Fig. 60-4). The relative length of the arms and the position of the centromere are used as further criteria to divide the human chromosomes into seven groups (designated A to G) (Fig. 60-4).

F
((

FIGURE 60-4 The karyotype of a normal woman showing the chromosomes of a single somatic cell in the metaphase stage of cell division. The photographic images of the chromosomes have been cut out and arranged according to descending length and varying arm ratio. The chromosomes have been stained by the Giemsa technique, which allows each chromosome pair to be identified by its unique banding pattern. Chromosomes 1 to 22 are the autosomes. The sex chromosomes in this normal female are both X. The normal male has an identical karyotype except for the absence of one X chromosome and the presence instead of one Y chromosome. (*Courtesy of David H. Ledbetter.*)

For a complete discussion of the etiology and clinical features of chromosomal abnormalities affecting humans, the reader is referred to Chap. 62.

SIMPLY INHERITED DISORDERS Disorders caused by the transmission of a single mutant gene show one of three simple (or mendelian) patterns of inheritance: (1) autosomal dominant, (2) autosomal recessive, or (3) X-linked. The distinction between "dominant" and "recessive" is one of convenience in pedigree analysis and does not imply a fundamental difference in genetic mechanism. The term *dominant* means that a mutation is clinically manifest when an individual has a single dose of this mutation (or is *heterozygous* for it), while *recessive* implies that a double dose (or *homozygosity*) is required for clinical detection. Genes are never dominant or recessive; their effects, however, produce clinical patterns that are classified as dominant or recessive. Despite their overall clinical "normality," individuals who are heterozygous for "recessive" genes often have biochemical abnormalities that are demonstrable in the laboratory; on the other hand, those who are homozygous for "dominant" genes are usually more severely affected than are the heterozygotes.

With few exceptions, each of the approximately 2500 mendelian diseases is rare. However, as a group, these disorders constitute an important cause of morbidity and death, accounting directly for more than 5 percent of all hospital admissions.

The genes for more than 450 simply inherited diseases have been assigned to specific chromosomes. Disease-producing genes assigned to the X chromosome outnumber those so far assigned to any single autosome. This is so because assignment to the X chromosome requires only pedigree studies showing X-linked inheritance (see below). Assignment to an autosome is more complicated, requiring sophisticated techniques of somatic cell hybridization or pedigree studies showing linkage between a disease-producing gene and a "marker" gene that is known to be on a certain chromosome.

Several hundred disease-producing genes have been cloned and analyzed at the molecular level. The vast majority of these genes, such as those responsible for the hemoglobinopathies, familial hypercholesterolemia, and glucose-6-phosphate dehydrogenase deficiency, have been identified after the protein product was characterized biochemically and functionally. In the past few years, a new strategy for cloning disease genes has emerged. This approach depends on first mapping the responsible gene to its correct chromosomal location

by means of linkage analysis or deletion mapping in affected patients. The relevant segment of DNA is then cloned, and the gene is identified by strategies designed to localize transcribed regions within the DNA segment. The sequence of the gene is thus obtained even before the protein has been identified. Inferences about the protein's function are drawn from the predicted protein sequence. This approach, originally referred to as *reverse genetics*, is more accurately called *positional cloning*. The first 13 disease genes that have been cloned and characterized by positional cloning are shown in Table 60-2.

The demonstration that a particular disease or syndrome shows one of the three mendelian patterns of inheritance implies that its pathogenesis, no matter how complex, is due to an abnormality in a single protein molecule. For example, in sickle cell anemia, the entire clinical syndrome, including such seemingly unrelated disturbances as anemia, pain crises, nephropathy, and predisposition to pneumococcal infections, is the consequence of having thymine instead of adenine at a specific site in the gene that codes for the β chain of hemoglobin, producing a substitution of a valine for a glutamic acid in the sixth amino acid position in the protein sequence.

In many mendelian disorders, especially in those with dominant inheritance, it is not possible to demonstrate directly the protein that is primarily altered by the mutation. In such cases (e.g., adult polycystic kidney disease and tuberous sclerosis), only the distal physiologic effects of the mutation are recognizable. Nevertheless, it is safe to assume that a single primary defect exists whenever a disease is transmitted by a single-gene mechanism and that the various manifestations of the disease all can be related to the mutational event by a more or less complicated "pedigree of causes." Table 60-3 lists the most commonly encountered mendelian disorders affecting adults.

Autosomal dominant disorders Dominant diseases are those manifest in the heterozygous state, i.e., when only one abnormal gene (*mutant allele*) is present and the corresponding partner allele on the homologous chromosome is normal. The gene responsible for an autosomal dominant disorder is located on one of the 22 autosomes, and both males and females can be affected. Since alleles segregate independently at meiosis, there is a 1 in 2 chance that the offspring of an affected heterozygote will inherit the mutant allele and, similarly, a 1 in 2 chance of the offspring inheriting the normal allele.

A typical pedigree involving an autosomal dominant trait is shown in Fig. 60-5. The following features are characteristic: (1) Each affected individual has an affected parent (unless the condition arose by a new mutation or is mildly expressed in the affected parent); (2) an affected individual will bear, on average, both normal and affected offspring in equal proportions; (3) normal children of an affected individual will have only normal offspring; (4) males and females are affected in equal proportions; (5) each sex is equally likely to transmit the condition to male and female offspring, with male-to-male transmission occurring; and (6) vertical transmission of the condition through successive generations occurs, especially when the trait does not impair reproductive capacity.

TABLE 60-2 Some disease genes identified by positional cloning

Disease locus	Chromosomal location	Date of identification
Chronic granulomatous disease	X	1986
Duchenne's muscular dystrophy	X	1986
Retinoblastoma	13	1986
Cystic fibrosis	7	1989
Wilm's tumor	11	1990
Sex determining gene	Y	1990
Choroideremia	X	1990
Fragile-X syndrome (mental retardation)	X	1991
Familial polyposis coli	5	1991
Kallman syndrome	X	1991
Aniridia	11	1991
Myotonic dystrophy	19	1991

TABLE 60-3 Some relatively frequent mendelian disorders affecting adults

AUTOSOMAL DOMINANT DISORDERS

Familial hypercholesterolemia
Hereditary hemorrhagic telangiectasia
Marfan's syndrome
Hereditary spherocytosis
Adult polycystic kidney disease
Huntington's chorea
Acute intermittent porphyria
Osteogenesis imperfecta tarda
von Willebrand's disease
Myotonic dystrophy
Idiopathic hypertrophic subaortic stenosis (IHSS)
Noonan's syndrome
Neurofibromatosis
Tuberous sclerosis

AUTOSOMAL RECESSIVE DISORDERS

Deafness
Albinism
Wilson's disease
Hemochromatosis
Sickle cell anemia
β Thalassemia
Cystic fibrosis
Hereditary emphysema (alpha$_1$-antitrypsin deficiency)
Homocystinuria
Familial Mediterranean fever
Friedreich's ataxia
Phenylketonuria

X-LINKED DISORDERS

Hemophilia A
Glucose-6-phosphate dehydrogenase deficiency
Fabry's disease
Ocular albinism
Testicular feminization
Chronic granulomatous disease
Hypophosphatemic rickets
Fragile-X syndrome (mental retardation)
Color blindness

TABLE 60-4 Approximate percentage of patients affected by new mutations in some autosomal dominant disorders

Disorder	Percentage
Achondroplasia	80
Tuberous sclerosis	80
Neurofibromatosis	40
Marfan's syndrome	30
Myotonic dystrophy	25
Huntington's chorea	4
Adult polycystic kidney disease	1
Familial hypercholesterolemia	Very low

however, cause a defective gene product that gives rise to a dominant trait. The parent in whose germ cells the mutation arose is clinically normal. Likewise, the siblings of the affected individual are normal, since the mutation affects only a single germ cell. However, the affected individual transmits the disease to half of his or her children.

The proportion of patients with dominant disorders who represent new mutations is inversely proportional to the effect of the disease in question on biologic fitness. The term *biologic fitness* refers to the ability of an affected individual to produce children who survive to adult life and reproduce. In the extreme case, if a dominant mutation produced absolute infertility, then all observed cases would, of necessity, represent new mutations, and it would be impossible to prove the genetic transmission of the trait. In less severe disorders, as in tuberous sclerosis, the severe mental retardation reduces biologic fitness to about 20 percent of normal, and the proportion of cases due to new mutations is about 80 percent. Other examples of the relation between biologic fitness and the proportion of new mutations in dominant disorders are shown in Table 60-4.

Many new mutations appear to occur in the germ cells of fathers who are of relatively advanced age. Such a "paternal age effect" is seen, for example, in Marfan's syndrome, in which the average age of fathers of sporadic or "new mutation" cases (37 years) is in excess of the mean age of fathers generally (30 years) and also in excess of the age of fathers who transmit Marfan's disease due to an inherited mutation (30 years).

Before one concludes that a dominant disorder in a given patient with unaffected parents is the result of a new mutation, it is important to consider two other possibilities: (1) that the gene may be carried by one parent in whom the disease is of low expressivity (discussed below) and (2) that extramarital paternity may have occurred. The latter is found in about 3 to 5 percent of randomly studied children in the United States.

Most autosomal dominant disorders show two characteristic features that are not usually seen in recessive syndromes: (1) *delayed age of onset* and (2) *variability in clinical expression.* Delayed age of onset is seen in disorders such as Huntington's chorea and adult polycystic kidney disease. These disorders do not manifest clinically until adult life, even though the mutant gene is present from the time of conception. Variability in clinical expression is illustrated dramatically by the multiple endocrine neoplasia syndrome. Patients in the same family inheriting the same abnormal gene may have hyperplasia or neoplasia of one or more endocrine glands (including the pancreas, parathyroid glands, and pituitary gland) as well as of adipose tissue. The resulting clinical manifestations are diverse; different members of the same family may develop peptic ulcers, hypoglycemia, kidney stones, multiple lipomas of the skin, or bitemporal hemianopsia. The recognition that each family member suffers from the same genetic abnormality can be difficult, as illustrated by the family pedigree in Fig. 60-6.

Dominant mutations involve a type of gene product that produces clinical symptoms when only 50 percent of the gene product is defective. The defective genes usually do not encode enzymes, since a 50 percent deficiency of most enzymes produces no symptoms (see "Recessive Disorders" below). Rather, dominant diseases are likely

While half the offspring of an individual with an autosomal dominant condition will inherit the disease, it is not necessarily true that each affected person must have an affected parent. In every autosomal dominant disease a certain proportion of affected persons owe their disorder to a new mutation rather than to an inherited mutation. Since the estimated frequency of mutation is 5×10^{-6} mutations per gene per generation, and since a dominant trait, by definition, requires a mutation in only one of a pair of alleles, one would expect that about 1 in 100,000 newborn persons would possess a new mutation at any given genetic locus. Many of these mutations either do not impair the function of the gene product or involve a recessive function so that the mutation is clinically silent. Others,

FIGURE 60-5 Pedigree pattern of an autosomal dominant trait. Note the *vertical* pattern of inheritance.

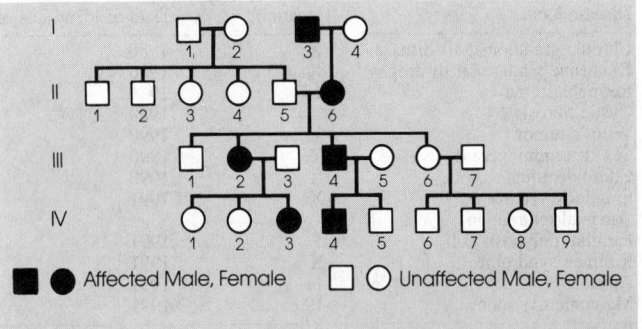

■ ● Affected Male, Female   □ ○ Unaffected Male, Female

FIGURE 60-6 Pedigree of a family affected with the multiple endocrine neoplasia, type 1 (MEN-1) syndrome, a disorder inherited as an autosomal dominant trait. Circles denote females; squares, males. Open circles and squares denote unaffected relatives; closed circles and squares denote affected relatives. Deceased relatives are indicated by the oblique line. The age of each relative is indicated below his or her symbol. Note the marked variation in clinical expression among living affected heterozygotes.

to involve abnormalities in two classes of proteins: (1) those which regulate complex metabolic pathways, such as membrane receptors and rate-limiting enzymes in pathways under feedback control, and (2) key structural proteins, such as hemoglobin or collagen.

The basic biochemical defects have been identified in only a handful of the approximately 600 autosomal dominant disorders. These include familial hypercholesterolemia (abnormal cell surface receptor that binds plasma low-density lipoprotein and thereby regulates cholesterol metabolism); Marfan's syndrome (abnormal fibrillin molecule); osteogenesis imperfecta (abnormal collagen molecule); hereditary methemoglobinemia and several hemolytic anemias due to unstable forms of hemoglobin (abnormal hemoglobin molecule); hereditary angioedema (abnormal protein inhibitor of an enzyme involved in the serum complement system); acute intermittent porphyria (abnormal enzyme that catalyzes a rate-limiting step in the heme biosynthetic pathway); and pseudohypoparathyroidism, type 1 (abnormal guanine nucleotide-binding regulatory component or G-protein of the adenylate cyclase system).

Autosomal recessive disorders   Autosomal recessive conditions are clinically apparent only in the homozygous state, i.e., when both alleles at a particular genetic locus are mutant. By definition, the gene responsible for an autosomal recessive disorder must be on one of the 22 autosomes; thus both males and females can be affected.

A pedigree in which an autosomal recessive trait is present in the family is shown in Fig. 60-7. The following features are characteristic: (1) The parents are clinically normal; (2) only siblings are affected and vertical transmission does not occur; and (3) males and females are affected in equal proportions.

FIGURE 60-7 Pedigree pattern of an autosomal recessive trait. Note the *horizontal* pattern of inheritance.

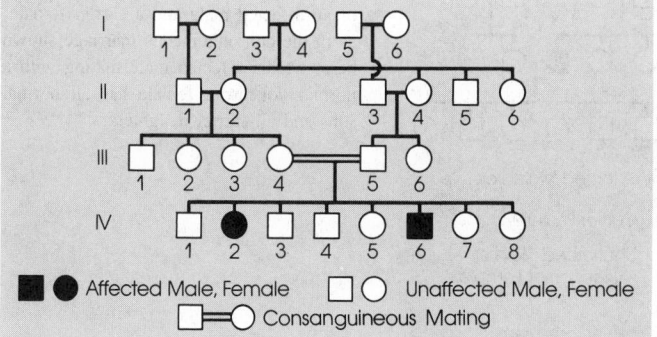

The relative infrequency of recessive genes in the population and the requirement for two abnormal genes for clinical expression combine to create special conditions for autosomal recessive inheritance: (1) The more infrequent the mutant gene in the population, the stronger is the likelihood that affected individuals are the product of consanguineous matings (see below); (2) if a husband and a wife are both carriers for the same autosomal recessive gene, 25 percent of the children will be normal, 50 percent will be heterozygous carriers, and 25 percent will be homozygous and affected with the disease; (3) if an affected individual marries a heterozygote (as may occur with consanguineous marriage), half the children will be affected, and a pedigree simulating dominant inheritance will result; and (4) if two individuals with the same recessive disease marry, all their children will be affected.

The clinical picture in autosomal recessive disorders tends to be more uniform than that of dominant diseases, and the age of onset is often early in life. As a general rule, recessive disorders are more commonly diagnosed in children, while dominant diseases are more frequently encountered in adults.

Since with recessive inheritance only one of four children in a sibship is expected to be affected, multiple cases in a family may not occur. This is especially true in a society in which small families are common. Consider, for example, 16 families in which both parents are heterozygous for the same recessive disorder. If each family has two children, 9 of the families will have no affected children, 6 will have one affected and one normal child, and only 1 of the 16 families will have two affected children. In the United States, physicians usually see sporadic or isolated cases of a recessive disorder without an affected sibling to alert them to the possibility of a genetic disorder. Fortunately, because of the relatively uniform clinical picture of recessive disorders, and because most can be diagnosed directly by biochemical tests, the correct diagnosis usually can be made even when no other members of a family are clinically affected.

The basic biochemical lesions underlying many autosomal recessive disorders have been identified. Of the three types of proteins in which mutations could occur (i.e., enzymes, structural proteins, and regulatory proteins), the enzymes have been the easiest to study. A mutation that destroys the catalytic activity of an enzyme generally does not impair the health of a heterozygote (i.e., an individual who has one mutant allele specifying a functionless enzyme and one normal allele on the partner chromosome specifying a normal enzyme). In this situation, each cell in the body usually produces about 50 percent of the normal number of active enzyme molecules. However, normal regulatory mechanisms function to avert any clinical consequences of this 50 percent deficiency, and so heterozygotes usually are clinically normal. On the other hand, when an individual inherits functionless alleles at both loci specifying an enzyme, the reduction in enzyme activity is too great for a compensatory mechanism to overcome, and a disease results. For example, heterozygotes for phenylketonuria have half the normal activity of phenylalanine hydroxylase, but they are clinically asymptomatic because the body compensates for the half-normal level of the enzyme by raising the substrate concentration approximately twofold. Under these conditions, a normal amount of phenylalanine can be metabolized with no symptoms. On the other hand, the homozygote for phenylketonuria has such a severe reduction in phenylalanine hydroxylase activity that enormous levels of phenylalanine and its derivatives accumulate, causing detrimental brain development. As in the case of phenylketonuria, the majority of enzyme deficiency states produce *simultaneously* both a simple accumulation of one or more metabolites preceding the enzymatic block and a deficient production of other metabolites distal to the block in the metabolic pathway.

Most of the genetic enzyme deficiencies that have been elucidated are not only inherited as recessive traits but also tend to involve enzymes that participate in catabolic pathways. Frequently these enzymes degrade organic molecules that are ingested in the diet, such as galactose (galactosemia), phenylalanine (phenylketonuria), and phytanic acid (Refsum's syndrome). A special class of such catabolic diseases is that in which the deficiency affects an acid hydrolase that occurs within lysosomes. In these *lysosomal storage disorders* the substrate, usually a complex lipid or polysaccharide, accumulates within swollen lysosomes in specific organs, giving the cells a foamy appearance. Examples of such lysosomal diseases include the mucopolysaccharidoses such as Hurler's syndrome (α-iduronidase deficiency) and the lipid storage diseases such as Gaucher's disease (glucocerebrosidase deficiency) (see Chap. 349).

In general, recessive diseases are rare because the reduced biologic fitness of homozygotes acts to remove the mutant gene from the population. However, a few recessive disorders, such as cystic fibrosis and sickle cell anemia, are common. To explain this paradox, it has been postulated that the biologic fitness of heterozygotes is greater than that of noncarriers for these genes. In such a case, the frequency of the gene in the population depends on the balance between the increased fitness of the relatively numerous heterozygotes and the reduced fitness of the less common homozygotes. A small selective advantage of the heterozygote over the normal results in a high gene frequency and hence a high birth frequency of homozygotes even when the disease is lethal. Thus about 1 in 22 Caucasians is a heterozygous carrier for the genetically lethal disease cystic fibrosis, and the disease occurs in about 1 in 2000 Caucasian births. To maintain such a high gene frequency, heterozygotes for cystic fibrosis must have a definite reproductive advantage over noncarriers, but the nature of this advantage is unknown. In sickle cell anemia, another recessive disorder with high frequency among certain populations, heterozygotes appear to have increased resistance to malaria.

Inasmuch as recessive diseases require the inheritance of a mutation at the same genetic locus from each parent, when the genes are rare, the likelihood of any two parents being carriers for the same defect becomes small. However, if the parents have a common ancestor and if that ancestor was a carrier for the recessive gene, then the likelihood that two of the descendants have inherited the gene becomes relatively great. The rarer the recessive gene, the stronger is the likelihood that an affected individual will have resulted from such a consanguineous mating. On the other hand, certain recessive genes are so common in the population that the likelihood of two random parents being carriers is great enough to eliminate the need for consanguinity. For common traits such as sickle cell anemia, phenylketonuria, cystic fibrosis, and Tay-Sachs disease, all of which have a high carrier frequency in certain populations, consanguinity in the parents is unusual.

In general, consanguinity is infrequent in families with recessive diseases in the United States. This is so because the rate of consanguinity in the general population is low. In most of the United States (as opposed to areas with relative geographic isolation such as northern Norway and Switzerland), a disorder must indeed be rare before it is associated with a high frequency of consanguinity. For example, consanguinity is expected in a large proportion of families

having children with very rare disorders, such as the Laurence-Moon-Biedl syndrome and abetalipoproteinemia.

Compound heterozygotes represent a special type of recessively inherited disorder in which the affected individual's two mutant genes, although located at the same genetic locus, are not identical. The mutations in the paternal and maternal alleles presumably involve different alterations in the DNA of the same gene. SC hemoglobinopathy is an example of such a *heteroallelic* compound state in which individuals have a gene for sickle cell hemoglobin on one chromosome and a gene for hemoglobin C on the homologous chromosome.

X-linked disorders The genes responsible for X-linked disorders are located on the X chromosome; therefore, the clinical risk and severity of the disease are different for the two sexes. Since a female has two X chromosomes, she may be either heterozygous or homozygous for a mutant gene, and the trait may therefore demonstrate either recessive or dominant expression. Males, on the other hand, have only one X chromosome, so they can be expected to display the full syndrome whenever they inherit the gene regardless of whether the gene behaves as a recessive or as a dominant trait in the female. Thus the terms *X-linked dominant* or *X-linked recessive* refer only to the expression of the gene in women.

An important feature of all X-linked inheritance is the absence of male-to-male (i.e., father-to-son) transmission of the trait. This follows because a male must always contribute his Y chromosome to his sons; hence he can never contribute his X chromosome. On the other hand, a male contributes his one X chromosome to all his daughters.

The pedigree in Fig. 60-8 illustrates the characteristic features of X-linked recessive inheritance. (1) In contrast to the vertical transmission in dominant traits (parents and children affected) and the horizontal transmission in autosomal recessive traits (siblings affected), the pedigree pattern in X-linked recessive traits tends to be oblique because of the occurrence of the trait in the sons of normal carrier sisters of affected males (uncles and nephews affected) (Fig. 60-8A); (2) male offspring of carrier women have a 50 percent chance of being affected; (3) all female offspring of affected males are carriers, and affected males do not transmit the disease to their sons (Fig. 60-8C); (4) unaffected males do not transmit the trait to any offspring; and (5) affected homozygous females occur only when an affected male fathers the child of a carrier female (Fig. 60-8B).

Examples of X-linked recessive disorders in humans include hemophilia A, nephrogenic diabetes insipidus, the Lesch-Nyhan syndrome, Duchenne's muscular dystrophy, glucose-6-phosphate dehydrogenase deficiency, testicular feminization, and Fabry's disease. Color blindness is also inherited as an X-linked recessive trait, but it is so frequent (occurring in about 8 percent of white males) that the occurrence of homozygous color-blind females is no rarity.

X-linked dominant inheritance is illustrated by the pedigree in Fig. 60-9. Its characteristic features are as follows: (1) Females are

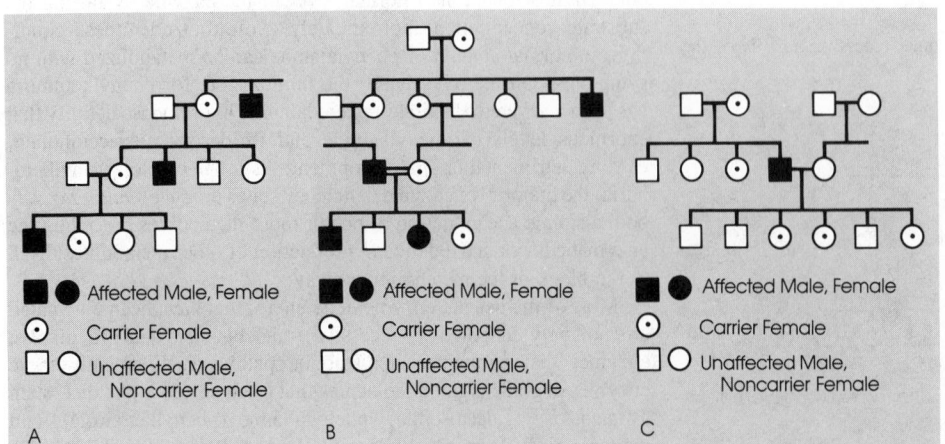

FIGURE 60-8 Pedigree patterns of an X-linked recessive trait. *A*. Note the oblique pattern of inheritance. *B*. An affected female can result from the mating of an affected male and a carrier female, as in the consanguineous marriage shown here. *C*. An affected male mating with a normal noncarrier female has all normal sons and all carrier daughters.

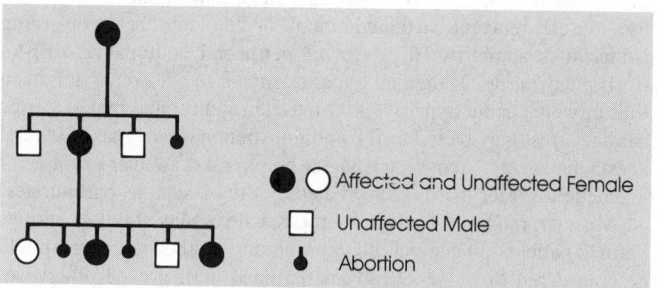

FIGURE 60-9 Pedigree pattern of an X-linked dominant trait.

affected about twice as often as males; (2) an affected female transmits the disorder to half her sons and half her daughters; (3) an affected male transmits the disorder to all his daughters and to none of his sons; and (4) the syndrome is more variable and less severe in heterozygous affected females than in hemizygous affected males. One common trait, the Xg(a +) blood group, is inherited as an X-linked dominant trait, as is hypophosphatemic rickets.

Some rare conditions may be inherited as X-linked dominant traits in which there is lethality in the hemizygous male. The characteristics of this form of inheritance are illustrated by the pedigree in Fig. 60-10: (1) The disorder occurs only in females who are heterozygous for the mutant gene; (2) an affected mother transmits the trait to half her daughters; and (3) an increased frequency of abortions occurs in affected women, the abortions representing affected male fetuses. Conditions that appear to be transmitted by this mode of inheritance include incontinentia pigmenti, focal dermal hypoplasia, orofaciodigital syndrome, and hyperammonemia due to ornithine transcarbamylase deficiency.

Expression of X-linked traits in females tends to be variable because of the phenomenon of X-chromosome inactivation. Early in embryonic development one of the two X chromosomes in each somatic cell of a female is inactivated. The inactivation process is random, so for each cell there is an equal probability that the paternally or maternally derived X chromosome will be inactivated. The inactivated X chromosome is rendered permanently nonfunctional, so all progeny of the initial cell inherit the same active and inactive X chromosomes. Thus each female is a mosaic; on average, half her cells express the X chromosome of the father, and half express the X chromosome of the mother. If a mutation in a gene is carried on one of the X chromosomes, about one-half of the cells in each tissue will be normal and the other half will manifest the mutant phenotype. However, chance or selection of one or the other set of clones of cells may disturb these proportions in any given individual. Depending on the proportions of mutant and normal X chromosomes in each tissue, a genetically heterozygous female may either be clinically

FIGURE 60-10 Pedigree pattern of an X-linked dominant trait lethal in the hemizygous male.

normal or have mild or severe manifestations of the disease. To illustrate, mothers of boys with the X-linked recessive Duchenne muscular dystrophy may occasionally show mild manifestations of the disease, such as limb girdle weakness or hypertrophied calves.

In each female cell the nonfunctional X chromosome can be visualized by several techniques. By ordinary staining, the inactivated X chromosome in metaphase appears heteropyknotic (condensed in appearance), and it replicates late in the mitotic cycle ("late-labeling" with tritiated thymidine). In nondividing cells the inactivated X chromosome can be observed as a clump of chromatin at the periphery of the nucleus—the so-called X chromatin or Barr body. In abnormal states with more than two X chromosomes such as 47,XXX, all but one of the X chromosomes are inactivated, so female cells may have multiple X chromatin bodies (see Chap. 62).

Since a single mutant allele is sufficient for the expression of X-linked recessive disorders, consanguinity does not increase the likelihood of expression in males, unlike the case in the rare autosomal recessive disorders. On the other hand, just as in the dominantly inherited disorders, new mutations can be a factor. In general, if an X-linked recessive condition reduces biologic fitness to zero, one-third of affected males will be a result of new mutations, and an additional one-third will be born to mothers who themselves are carriers as a result of a new mutation. Thus only one-third will come from a classic pedigree manifesting oblique transmission. An example of such a disease is Duchenne's muscular dystrophy in which affected hemizygous males are so severely disabled that they never reproduce. In hemophilia A, in which the biologic fitness is greater than zero, about 20 percent of affected males represent new mutations.

In families in which only one male is affected with an X-linked recessive disease and there is no other family history of the trait, it is essential for proper genetic counseling that the mother undergo biochemical tests or other relevant studies to determine whether she is a carrier. If she is a carrier, half her daughters will be carriers and half her sons will be affected. On the other hand, if her affected son represents a new mutation, only his daughters will inherit the gene. At present, biochemical tests can identify female carriers for several X-linked diseases, including the Lesch-Nyhan syndrome, Fabry's disease, Hunter's syndrome, hemophilia, testicular feminization, fragile X syndrome, and Duchenne's muscular dystrophy.

The distinction between X-linked inheritance and *sex-influenced autosomal dominant inheritance* is important. Baldness is probably inherited as an autosomal dominant trait, yet it is manifested mainly in men and rarely in women. Heterozygous females express the baldness gene only when a source of testosterone becomes available, as occurs with a virilizing tumor of the ovary.

MULTIFACTORIAL GENETIC DISEASES The common chronic diseases of adults (such as essential hypertension, coronary heart disease, diabetes mellitus, peptic ulcer disease, and schizophrenia) as well as the common birth defects (such as cleft lip and palate, spina bifida, and congenital heart disease) have been long known to "run in families." They fit best into the category of *multifactorial genetic diseases*. The genetic element in these disorders rarely manifests itself in an all-or-none fashion as it does in the simply inherited (mendelian) disorders and in chromosomal aberrations. Instead, it is the interaction of multiple genes with multiple environmental factors that produces the familial aggregation.

In the multifactorial genetic diseases, there is a *polygenic component* consisting of a series of genes that interact in a cumulative fashion. An individual who inherits the right combination of these genes passes beyond a "threshold of risk," at which point an *environmental component* determines whether and to what extent that person is clinically affected. In order for another individual in the same family to express the same syndrome, the same or a similar combination of genes must be inherited. Since the first-degree relatives of an affected individual (i.e., parents, siblings, and offspring) each share half that person's genes, they are all at increased risk of exhibiting the same polygenic syndrome. Second-degree relatives (uncles, aunts, and grandparents) share, on average, one-fourth of an individual's genes, that is, $(\frac{1}{2})^2$, and third-degree relatives (cousins) share one-eighth, that is, $(\frac{1}{2})^3$. Thus, as the degree of relation becomes more distant, the likelihood of a relative inheriting the same combination of genes becomes less. Moreover, the chances of any relative inheriting the right combination of risk genes decrease as the number of genes required for the expression of a given trait increases.

Since the precise number of genes responsible for polygenic traits is unknown, the risk of inheritance for a relative of an affected individual is difficult to calculate, and the standard is based on empiric risk figures (i.e., a direct tally of the proportion of affected relatives in previously reported families). In contrast to the simply inherited disorders, in which 25 or 50 percent of the first-degree relatives of an affected proband are at genetic risk, multifactorial genetic disorders are generally observed empirically to affect no more than 5 to 10 percent of first-degree relatives. Moreover, in contrast to mendelian traits, the recurrence risk of multifactorial conditions varies from family to family, and its estimation is significantly influenced by two factors: (1) the number of affected persons already present in the family and (2) the severity of the disorder in the index case. The greater the number of affected relatives and the more severe their disease, the higher is the risk to other relatives. For example, the risk of cleft lip in the siblings of a child with unilateral cleft lip is about 2.5 percent, but if the lesion in the index case is bilateral, the risk in the siblings rises to 6 percent. Table 60-5 lists the empiric risk figures for the familial recurrence of a number of multifactorial genetic diseases.

The hypothesis of a polygenic component in the inheritance of multifactorial diseases has been given a sound basis by the demonstration that at least one-third of all gene loci harbor polymorphic alleles that vary among individuals. Such a large degree of variation in normal genes undoubtedly provides the substrate for variations in genetic predisposition with which environmental factors can interact. So far, the genetic loci most strikingly associated with predisposition to specific diseases are those which constitute the HLA system (also called the *major histocompatibility gene complex*) (see Chap. 64). The HLA gene complex is located on the short arm of chromosome 6. It consists of four closely linked but distinct loci (A, B, C, and D). The products of these genes are proteins that are found on the surfaces of body cells and that enable an individual's immune system to distinguish its own cells from those of someone else. Each HLA locus in the population consists of multiple alleles, each of which produces an immunologically distinct protein. For example, an individual may inherit any 2 of 20 alleles at the HLA-B locus.

An important observation of recent years has been the finding that certain alleles at the HLA loci predispose individuals to certain specific diseases. For example, if the B27 allele at the HLA-B locus is inherited by an individual, that person has a 121-fold greater chance of developing ankylosing spondylitis than an individual who lacks this allele (Table 60-6). Ankylosing spondylitis remains a multifactorial disease, however, because its development clearly requires one or

TABLE 60-6 Alleles at the HLA loci associated with multifactorial genetic diseases

Disease	HLA locus	Specific allele	Relative risk*
Ankylosing spondylitis	B	B27	121
Reiter's syndrome	B	B27	40
Psoriasis with arthritis	B	B27	5
Celiac disease	B	B8	10
Chronic active hepatitis	B	B8	4
Myasthenia gravis	B	B8	4
Diabetes mellitus (insulin-dependent)	DR	DR3/DR4	33
Hyperthyroidism	DR	DR3	4
Addison's disease	B	B8	7
	DR	DR4	10
Multiple sclerosis	DR	DR2	7

* *Relative risk* is the probability of the disease developing in an individual with the specific allele, divided by the probability of its development in an individual who does not possess this specific allele.

more other factors in addition to the B27 allele. Thus less than 15 percent of people who inherit this allele develop this disease. Table 60-6 lists some of the diseases associated with alleles at the HLA loci. Several of them are suspected to be of viral etiology, suggesting that the HLA loci may dictate the mode of expression of certain viral diseases. A more detailed discussion of the HLA system is presented in Chap. 64.

Multifactorial disorders are heterogeneous in the sense that the relative contribution of the polygenic factors ("risk genes") and environmental factors to the etiology vary greatly from patient to patient. However, it is important to remember that among common phenotypes which are largely multifactorial, often a small proportion will be created by major mutant genes. For example, although coronary heart disease is usually of multifactorial etiology, about 5 percent of subjects with premature myocardial infarctions are heterozygotes for familial hypercholesterolemia, a single-gene disorder that produces atherosclerosis in the absence of any other predisposing factor. Similarly, in a small proportion of patients with other common diseases such as peptic ulcer disease or "essential" hypertension, the condition is not multifactorial but determined by a single gene, as in the multiple endocrine adenoma–peptic ulcer syndrome or the medullary thyroid carcinoma–pheochromocytoma syndrome, respectively.

INTERACTION BETWEEN SINGLE GENETIC AND ENVIRONMENTAL FACTORS

Many diseases result from an interaction between a specific genotype and a specific environmental factor. In particular, inherited single-gene mutations may produce clinically significant and often life-threatening idiosyncratic responses to certain drugs.

Table 60-7 lists the most important of these *pharmacogenetic disorders*, which encompass all the mendelian modes of inheritance. Perhaps the most common is glucose-6-phosphate dehydrogenase deficiency, an X-linked recessive trait in which a variety of drugs may precipitate a hemolytic anemia. Plasma pseudocholinesterase deficiency and hepatic transacetylase deficiency are examples of autosomal recessive traits which alter drug catabolism so that when the muscle relaxant suxamethonium or the antituberculous drug isoniazid is administered, apnea or peripheral neuropathy, respectively, may ensue. Malignant hyperthermia is an autosomal dominant trait in which acute hyperpyrexia, muscle rigidity, and hyperkalemic cardiac arrest may be induced by administration of any one of several anesthetic agents. Acute intermittent porphyria is another example of a genetic disorder that is exacerbated by drugs, such as barbiturates.

Misinterpretation of adverse drug reactions may result in serious harm to patients. In general, all unusual idiosyncratic reactions should be considered to be genetically determined until proved otherwise. Fortunately, the pharmacogenetic disorders are a group of diseases

TABLE 60-5 Empiric risks for some common multifactorial genetic diseases affecting adults

Disorder in index case	Estimated absolute risk for first-degree relatives, %
Cleft lip and/or palate	3
Congenital heart disease	4
Coronary heart disease	8 for male relatives
	3 for female relatives
Diabetes mellitus	5–10
Epilepsy	5–10
Hypertension	10
Manic-depressive psychosis	10–15
Psoriasis	10–15
Schizophrenia	15
Thyroid disease (autoimmune disorders including hyperthyroidism, thyroiditis, primary myxedema, simple goiter)	10

TABLE 60-7 Examples of inherited disorders involving an abnormal response to drugs

Disorder	Molecular abnormality	Mode of inheritance	Frequency	Clinical effect	Drugs producing abnormal response
Slow inactivation of isoniazid	Isoniazid acetylase in liver	Autosomal recessive	50% of U.S. population	Polyneuritis	Isoniazid, sulfamethazine, sulfamaprine, phenelzine, dapsone, hydralazine
Suxamethonium sensitivity	Pseudocholinesterase in plasma	Autosomal recessive	Several mutant alleles; most common affects 1 in 2500	Apnea	Suxamethonium, succinylcholine
Warfarin insensitivity	? Altered receptor or enzyme in liver with increased affinity for vitamin K	Autosomal dominant	Rare	Inability to achieve anticoagulation with usual doses of drug	Warfarin
Glaucoma	Unknown	? Autosomal dominant	Common	Increased intraocular pressure	Glucocorticoids
Malignant hyperthermia	Ryanodine receptor	Autosomal dominant	1 in 20,000 anesthetized patients	Severe hyperpyrexia, muscle rigidity, death	Such anesthetics as halothane, succinylcholine, methoxyflurane, ether, cyclopropane
Unstable hemoglobins: Hemoglobin Zurich	Arginine substitution for histidine at sixty-third position of β chain of hemoglobin	Autosomal dominant	Rare	Hemolysis	Sulfonamides
Hemoglobin H	Hemoglobin composed of four β chains	Autosomal dominant	Rare	Hemolysis	Sulfisoxazole
Glucose-6-phosphate dehydrogenase deficiency	Glucose-6-phosphate dehydrogenase in erythrocytes	X-linked recessive	~1 × 10⁸ affected persons in world; common in persons of African, Mediterranean, Asiatic origin; multiple mutant alleles	Hemolysis	Analgesics, sulfonamides, antimalarials, nitrofurantoin, other drugs

SOURCE: Modified from ES Vesell, N Engl J Med 287:904, 1972.

for which therapy is straightforward: avoidance of the noxious drug by patient and relatives.

In addition to drugs, other factors in the environment may aggravate specific genetic traits. Cigarette smoke may have deleterious effects on persons homozygous and possibly heterozygous for alpha₁-antitrypsin deficiency, who are predisposed to the development of emphysema. Patients with xeroderma pigmentosa and anhydrotic ectodermal dysplasia are unusually sensitive to sunlight and high temperatures, respectively. Avoidance of milk at an early age prevents many of the complications ordinarily seen in persons with galactosemia.

Genetic-environmental interactions are particularly important in pregnancy. Women who are affected with phenylketonuria may develop high plasma phenylalanine levels during pregnancy, and thus their offspring may suffer from a variety of phenylalanine-induced birth defects even though the offspring may not themselves have phenylketonuria. Other examples of diseases resulting from an adverse genetic relation between the mother and fetus include erythroblastosis caused by Rh incompatibility and *diabetic embryopathy*, a term that refers to a series of major birth defects occurring in about 5 percent of the offspring of women who are clinically diabetic during pregnancy.

REFERENCES

GELEHRTER TD, COLLINS FS: *Principles of Medical Genetics.* Baltimore, Williams & Wilkins, 1990

LEWIN B: *Genes,* 4th ed. New York, Wiley, 1990

MCKUSICK VA: *Mendelian Inheritance in Man: Catalogs of Autosomal Dominant, Autosomal Recessive and X-Linked Phenotypes,* 11th ed. Baltimore, Johns Hopkins University Press, 1992

SCRIVER CR et al: *The Molecular and Metabolic Basis of Inherited Disease,* 7th ed. New York, McGraw-Hill, in press

THOMPSON MW et al: *Genetics in Medicine,* 5th ed. Philadelphia, Saunders, 1991

VOGEL F, MOTULSKY AG: *Human Genetics: Problems and Approaches,* 2d ed. Berlin, Springer-Verlag, 1986

WEATHERALL DJ: *The New Genetics and Clinical Practice,* 3d ed. Oxford, Oxford University Press, 1991

61 MOLECULAR GENETICS AND MEDICINE

ARTHUR L. BEAUDET / ANDREA BALLABIO

The haploid human genome is comprised of approximately 3×10^9 (3 billion) base pairs of DNA and is estimated to contain 30,000 to 100,000 genes encoding a large number of protein products. Each individual inherits one copy of the genome from each parent. In the cell, the genomic DNA is packaged as 23 pairs of chromosomes, each containing a single linear duplex DNA molecule. Most of the DNA sequences that encode proteins occur as unique (single copy) sequences in the genome. These protein coding genes are usually divided into coding exons and intervening introns in the genomic DNA. The messenger RNA (mRNA) is formed by splicing the RNA to link the exon and eliminate the introns. Many genes and their products show similarities in nucleotide and amino acid sequence and can be viewed as members of large gene families, e.g., the globin gene family, the immunoglobulin superfamily, or the serine protease family. Many proteins contain domains that are functionally distinct and show sequence homology to related domains in other proteins. Complex genes are believed to have commonly arisen by reassortment of preexisting protein domains through a protein of "exon shuffling." A large amount of DNA in the genome *appears* not to be functional, and hundreds, if not thousands, of repetitive DNA sequences of unknown function are present; some are dispersed, and some are clustered. The length of DNA frequently is quantitated in thousands of bases (kilobases, kb) or in millions of bases (megabases, Mb) so that the genome comprises 3 million kb or 3000 Mb.

If one were to print *one copy* of *one strand* of the haploid human genome, it would fill a text 170 times the size of *Harrison's.* The analogy of the human genome to a large text can be carried further. The text can be envisioned as being bound into 23 separate volumes of various sizes, each the equivalent of one chromosome. Individuals would inherit one paternal set of 23 volumes and one maternal set of 23 volumes. The mutation causing sickle cell anemia would be the equivalent of changing a single letter on one page of one volume, while deletion of the α-globin gene cluster in α-thalassemia might represent the equivalent of the loss of one or two pages of text in each set. The text can also be envisioned as having been copied over and over again for thousands of generations with frequent errors or alterations (mutations) being introduced and then passed to the progeny copies. Finally, to carry this analogy to the concept of crossing-over and linkage, one can envision a parent with two sets of 23 volumes needing to pass one set to an offspring. Each volume of each set will exchange parts with its corresponding partner at one to six sites per volume so that a unique 23 volume text comprised of mixed portions of the two available sets will be passed to the next generation. This results in the unique genotype that is the basis of genetic individuality.

The human genome is extraordinarily polymorphic so that the DNA of each individual (except identical twins) varies in millions of ways from the DNA of another. A polymorphic site or locus is any site in the genome that varies so much that more than 1 percent of the chromosomes have a sequence different from the most common sequence. Much of this variation involves single base substitutions (e.g., a C:G base pair versus a T:A base pair at a position). About 1 in 200 to 1 in 500 of the 3 billion base pairs in the genome is polymorphic, i.e., varies beyond the 1 percent criterion. Genetic variation or polymorphism includes the presence or absence of base pairs or longer segments. Genetic variation arises through single base mutation, deletion, insertion, unequal crossing-over, and other rearrangements of the DNA. This genetic variation gives rise to different alleles; an allele is defined as one of a series of possible alternative forms of a given gene, e.g., the sickle allele at the β-globin locus. The term allele is now commonly used to refer to differing DNA sequences for a DNA marker without regard to whether this occurs in a gene or not, as will be discussed below.

What are the phenotypic effects of this extensive variation in DNA? There is a tendency to think of the common variations in DNA and protein (i.e., the polymorphisms) as benign and without phenotypic effect, and this belief is justified to some extent. DNA sequence is more conserved in protein coding regions and more variable in introns and intergenic regions. The vast majority of variations in DNA presumably have little or no phenotypic effect, although they provide DNA markers of clinical utility as discussed below. Another class of genetic variation contributes to racial, ethnic, and individual differences but not in a way that affects health or susceptibility to disease. Of greater medical relevance are those genetic variations that affect disease susceptibility, often through the interaction of genes with nongenetic factors, giving rise to conditions of multifactorial etiology. This type of genetic variability contributes to the etiology and pathogenesis of most of the disease processes described in this textbook. Approximately 60 percent of individuals experience genetically influenced diseases during their lifetime, if multifactorial diseases of late onset are included. The separation between benign individuality and variation with subtle medical implications is often unclear, as exemplified by the variations in HLA loci and blood groups. Finally, in some instances a change (mutation) in the DNA of a single gene has a major phenotypic effect and causes a single gene defect or Mendelian disorder, since such disorders segregate in families according to simple Mendelian rules (see Chap. 60). Even for these "single gene" disorders, the phenotype is often influenced by genes at other loci and by nongenetic factors. Mutations causing single gene disorders can be common and exceed the 1 percent criterion for polymorphism (e.g., cystic fibrosis, sickle cell disease, and G6PD deficiency) so that polymorphism does not uniformly imply a benign circumstance. Although single gene disorders are the most obvious example of the role of genetic variation in disease processes, the genetic contribution to common multifactorial diseases is quantitatively more important, although more complex to unravel.

The molecular heterogeneity of individuals has an important implication for medical practice. Physicians should constantly be aware in their diagnostic and therapeutic activities that patients are as unique in biochemistry, physiology, pharmacologic responses, laboratory results, and disease processes as in their physiognomy and personality; everyone is different.

METHODS FOR ANALYSIS OF HUMAN DNA

Molecular analyses of clinical relevance rely on multiple features and strategies, including: (1) the ability to clone genes and DNA fragments using recombinant methods, (2) determination of the sequence of DNA fragments, (3) the specificity of nucleic acid hybridization, (4) the specificity of recognition sites of restriction endonucleases, and (5) the power of DNA amplification using the polymerase chain reaction. Various combinations of these capabilities are used for diverse diagnostic procedures.

MOLECULAR CLONING AND SEQUENCING　The size, the complexity, and the variability of the human genome constitute barriers to the analysis of individual traits and genes. The feasibility for such analysis was greatly enhanced by the development of recombinant DNA technology, which allows for isolation of small DNA fragments and production of unlimited amounts of the cloned material. The methodology for gene cloning is now well established. Hundreds of human genes have been cloned, and progress in this regard has been extraordinary as the genes for cystic fibrosis, Marfan syndrome, polyposis of the colon, neurofibromatosis, myotonic dystrophy, fragile X mental retardation, Huntington's disease, and many other diseases have been cloned since the last edition of this text. Once cloned, the various genes and gene products can be utilized for studies of gene structure and function in normal and disease states with diagnostic, therapeutic, and research implications.

The cloning of DNA involves isolation of DNA fragments and their insertion into the nucleic acid from another biologic source (vector) for manipulation and propagation. The most widely used vectors are maintained in bacterial host cells and are based on bacterial plasmids or bacteriophage such as phage λ or M13, some variations of which (cosmids) can accommodate DNA fragments up to 45 kb in size. In addition, vectors designed to function as yeast artificial chromosomes are maintained in yeast host cells and can be utilized for cloning DNA fragments up to hundreds of kilobases in size. Space does not allow presentation of the various methods for DNA cloning, but these are well described in Watson et al.

Most genes encode proteins and are divided into coding exons and intervening introns in the genomic DNA. The messenger RNA (mRNA) from a gene is spliced to link the coding segments, and it is often useful to copy mRNA in vitro to synthesize cDNA (DNA complementary to mRNA) for analysis and cloning. Genomic DNA and cDNA clones have been isolated for hundreds of human genes. In addition, many hundreds of *anonymous* genomic DNA clones are in widespread use. These anonymous DNA clones are generally of interest because they represent a unique site in the genome and often are associated with polymorphic markers that map to that site, as will be discussed below. Radioactive, biotinylated, or otherwise modified copies of DNA can be prepared from any cloned fragment and can serve as specific molecular *probes*. Radioactive probes can be detected by autoradiography, and biotinylated probes can be detected with avidin and secondary detection methods. Sequencing of DNA is readily accomplished using manual or semiautomated methods. The amino acid sequence of a protein can be deduced from the cDNA sequence and frequently provides insight into the function of a gene. If a gene is cloned, it is relatively straightforward to analyze the DNA from a patient to determine if the sequence deviates from the normal. The availability of sequence data allows for the use of the polymerase chain reaction for DNA amplification. Thus, some of the fruits of molecular cloning are the availability of probes for analytical procedures, the availability of DNA sequence data both to deduce protein sequence and to allow for DNA amplification (see below), and the ability to analyze for disease mutations.

NUCLEIC ACID HYBRIDIZATION Many of the steps in recombinant DNA analysis take advantage of the complementary nature of nucleic acid interaction which is so essential for the synthesis of DNA and RNA (see Chap. 60). Linear pieces of double-stranded (native) DNA can be treated with heat or alkali to dissociate the two strands to yield single-stranded (denatured) DNA. When a strand is incubated under conditions that allow for nucleic acid hybridization, bases of the denatured DNA recognize complementary bases, and reformation of double-stranded molecules by base pairing takes place. Nucleic acid hybridization is so sensitive that a single-stranded DNA molecule can be hybridized specifically to a complementary strand of RNA or DNA present at about 1 part in 10,000. Many recombinant DNA studies involve the preparation of one radioactive or biotinylated strand of nucleic acid that is then used as a "probe" in the analysis. It is possible to identify and distinguish both fully homologous and partially homologous sequences. The specificity of nucleic acid hybridization, often in combination with fractionation or amplification procedures, allows detection of a single gene among tens of thousands or of a sequence from an infectious organism that may be present at a frequency of less than one copy per human cell.

A variation of nucleic acid hybridization involves the use of allele-specific oligonucleotides (ASO). The ASO probe is a synthetic, single-stranded oligonucleotide, usually 15 to 20 bases in length. Two probes are synthesized, usually differing at a mutation site by a single base, one perfectly matching the normal sequence and one perfectly matching the mutant sequence, with the variable nucleotide in the midportion of the oligonucleotide. Hybridization conditions are adjusted so that the oligonucleotide detects a perfectly matched sequence but fails to hybridize if there is a single base mismatch. Allele-specific oligonucleotides can be used in combination with Southern blotting or in combination with DNA amplification, as described below.

RESTRICTION ENDONUCLEASES The discovery in microorganisms of restriction endonucleases, commonly known as *restriction enzymes,* facilitated recombinant DNA manipulations. These enzymes recognize a specific short sequence in double-stranded DNA, typically 4 to 8 base pairs, and cleave the DNA at this site. Hundreds of enzymes are known, each recognizing a unique DNA sequence (Fig. 61-1). An example of an enzyme that recognizes sequences only four base pairs in length is *Hae*III, which cleaves the sequence 5'-GGCC-3'. By convention, only one strand of DNA is printed as the recognition site, but the enzymes recognize double-stranded DNA. The sequence specificity of restriction enzymes is a powerful tool in dissection of large genomes. When human DNA is digested with a particular restriction enzyme, hundreds of thousands of DNA fragments are generated with remarkable reproducibility. Such fragments can vary from a few base pairs to several thousand base pairs in length, depending on the enzyme used. Restriction enzymes that recognize a sequence only four base pairs long cleave the DNA into smaller fragments than enzymes that recognize longer sequences, since recognition sites of the former enzymes occur more often in a relatively random sequence. With the use of multiple restriction enzymes to analyze a particular segment of DNA, it is possible to construct a detailed map of restriction endonuclease cleavage sites for the region. Such a map can span a region of from hundreds to thousands of base pairs of DNA. Enzymes that cut DNA infrequently can be used to prepare DNA maps over megabase distances. As

FIGURE 61-2 Southern blotting analysis of genomic DNA.

described below, variations in the sequences of cleavage sites can be analyzed as polymorphisms or mutations in the genome.

SOUTHERN BLOTTING Many analyses of the human genome utilize the blotting procedure developed by E. M. Southern, which involves hybridizing DNA in solution to DNA transferred to a membrane support. For clinical analysis, *Southern blotting* (Fig. 61-2) begins with the isolation of genomic DNA from any source but frequently from peripheral leukocytes or fetal cells. The high-molecular-weight genomic DNA is digested with a restriction enzyme to yield a series of reproducible fragments. These DNA fragments are separated by electrophoresis in agarose gels, and the DNA is transferred from the gel through the capillary action of a blotting procedure to a membrane that binds the DNA tightly. The membrane is treated to denature the DNA and is soaked in a solution containing a radioactive or otherwise labelled single-stranded nucleic acid probe. The probe will form a double-stranded nucleic acid complex at sites on the membrane where homologous DNA is present. The membrane

FIGURE 61-1 DNA sequence specificity and nuclease activity for three restriction endonucleases. Hae*III* leaves a blunt end while the other enzymes leave single-stranded ends.

| *Hae* III | 5'-G-G\|C-C-3'
3'-C-C\|G-G-5' | *Hind* III | 5'-A\|A-G-C-T-T-3'
3'-T-T-C-G-A\|A-5' | *Mst* II | 5'-C-C\|T-N-A-G-G-3'
3'-G-G-A-N-T\|C-C-5' |

is washed to remove unbound radioactivity, and regions on the membrane where homologous DNA sequences are bound are detected using x-ray film. The sensitivity of Southern blotting is enhanced by splitting the DNA into small segments, fractionating the fragments, and applying sensitive detection methods to identify specific fragments (nucleic acid hybridization). Overall, this method can detect unique genomic DNA fragments that typically represent about 1 part in 1 million in the genome. The clinical power of Southern blotting resides in the capacity to analyze a tiny portion of the primary structure of human genomic DNA taken from an individual. The procedure is ideal for detecting gross rearrangements in DNA and for distinguishing some point mutations, but the majority of point mutations are not detected by routine Southern blotting.

An analogous procedure starting with RNA has been termed *northern* (in contrast to Southern) *blotting*. In this procedure, the presence or absence and the approximate size of a particular mRNA can be determined. The term *immunoblotting* or *western blotting* describes a derivative procedure designed to analyze protein antigens. Proteins are separated by electrophoresis and transferred to a solid membrane through a blotting procedure. The membrane is analyzed by incubation with antibodies followed by a second step for enzymatic or radioactive detection of bound antibody. Thus, Southern blotting, northern blotting, and immunoblotting or western blotting each combines fractionation and a detection method to provide a sensitive technique for the analysis of DNA, RNA, and protein, respectively (Table 61-1).

POLYMERASE CHAIN REACTION (PCR) FOR DNA AMPLIFICATION   The PCR technique for DNA amplification has had a revolutionary impact on molecular diagnosis. The technique is based on knowing the nucleic acid sequence for a region, which, for diagnostic purposes, is to be analyzed repeatedly from different individuals. Oligonucleotide primers are prepared that are complementary to opposite strands of the DNA and are separated by up to a few hundred base pairs (Fig. 61-3). The oligonucleotide primers are incubated with the target DNA to be amplified and with a DNA polymerase that synthesizes a complementary strand in a 5′-to-3′ direction. Specificity is provided by the requirement that primers must lead to convergent synthesis for amplification to be effective. The reaction is subjected to a sequence of temperature variations including a denaturing temperature where double-stranded DNA is dissociated to single-stranded DNA, an annealing temperature where oligonucleotide primers hybridize to target DNA, and a polymerization temperature for the synthetic step. The reaction is usually carried out using a thermostable polymerase so that the polymerase remains active during the temperature cycles (usually ranging from 50 to 95°C). After a number of such cycles, typically 20 to 30 or more, hundreds of thousands of copies of the original target sequence are synthesized as depicted in Fig. 61-3. The bulk of the product is a double-stranded DNA fragment of specific length. The technique is so sensitive that it can be used to amplify and analyze DNA from a single human sperm which contains one duplex target DNA molecule. PCR is easily performed with minimal preparation of crude and even degraded samples allowing analysis from whole blood, dried blood filters, mouthwash, old tissue sections, and other sources. Molecular diagnosis with PCR can include: (1) determining the presence or the absence of an amplified product, (2) digesting the amplified product with a

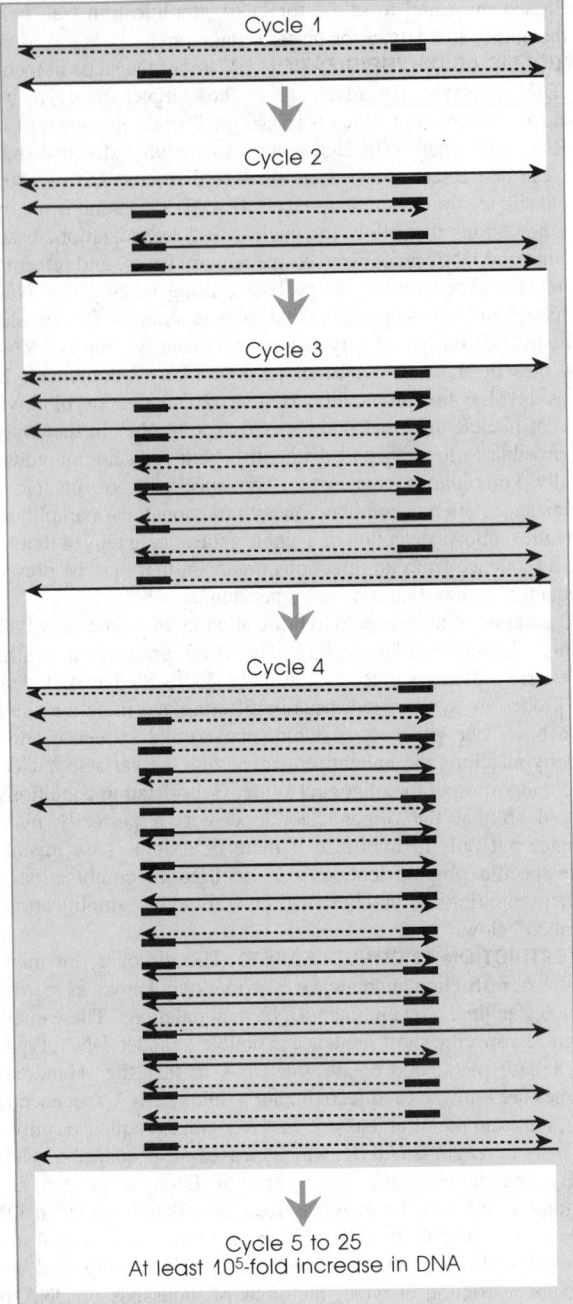

FIGURE 61-3 Polymerase chain reaction for amplification of DNA. The target DNA is shown as a solid line in cycle 1. Newly synthesized DNA is indicated by dotted lines in each cycle. Primer oligonucleotides are indicated by solid rectangles. Each DNA strand is marked with an arrow indicating 5′-to-3′ orientation.

restriction enzyme, (3) hybridizing the PCR product with allele-specific oligonucleotides, and (4) direct sequencing of the PCR product. Many variations have been devised to take advantage of the PCR concept. These include synthesis of cDNA from mRNA using reverse transcriptase followed by amplification of the cDNA. Single-stranded DNA can be synthesized by altering the ratio of the oligonucleotide primers. Other applications include preparation of recombinant DNA constructs, mutagenesis of cloned DNA, detection of rare nucleotide sequences, and detection of nucleotide sequences of infectious agents. The PCR method provides rapid analysis (single day), ease of automation, relative economy, and extraordinary specificity.

LIGASE CHAIN REACTION (LCR)   The LCR method is based on the ability of DNA ligase to covalently link two immediate adjacent

TABLE 61-1   Analytical blotting procedures

Blot method	Material analyzed	Fractionation	Detection
Southern	DNA	Electrophoresis	Nucleic acid hybridization
Northern	RNA	Electrophoresis	Nucleic acid hybridization
Western or immunoblot	Protein	Electrophoresis	Immunologic

oligonucleotides hybridized to a longer template that can bind both oligonucleotides. For example, if four 20-mer oligonucleotides forming two complementary, adjacent pairs are incubated with a heat stable ligase and the reaction is subjected to temperature cycles similar to PCR, oligonucleotides will be ligated to yield two longer complementary 40-mer oligonucleotides dependent on the presence or absence of a longer DNA template in the reaction. One useful feature of LCR is the ability to distinguish templates with single base differences at the ligation site. By placing six oligonucleotides in the reaction (two common and complementary on one side of a mutation, plus two matching the normal sequence and two matching the mutant sequence on the opposite side with the mutation site at the end adjacent to the common oligonucleotides to be ligated), a genotype analysis for a single base mutation is easily determined by the presence or absence of products that reflect the normal and/or mutant template. LCR has the potential advantage over most forms of PCR that the presence or absence of a distinct product is diagnostic, and the product does not need further characterization, although PCR offers greater versatility for many procedures. LCR is particularly useful in screening for known mutations in any given population.

ANALYZING THE HUMAN GENOME

The human genome map is the topographical description of human genomic DNA. Traditionally, the map is divided into regions corresponding to the chromosomal bands of the 24 chromosomes (22 autosomes and X and Y).

As of early 1993, over 2500 loci have been assigned to specific positions on the human genetic map. The main information contained in the map is the relative order and distance of genetic markers and their positions within a defined region. Two types of maps containing this kind of information have been developed, the genetic and the physical maps. There is a major conceptual difference between the two; the first is an indirect statistical analysis based on genetic recombination, whereas the second hinges on direct measurement of the length of DNA.

THE GENETIC MAP AND THE PRINCIPLE OF GENETIC LINKAGE

Genetic linkage is essential for preparation of the map of the human genome, and it is used routinely for molecular diagnosis in the clinical setting. Genetic distance, which is expressed in centimorgans (cM), is a measure of the likelihood of crossover between two loci. Two loci are 1 cM apart if there is a 1 percent probability of a crossover between them at meiosis. There are on average 30 to 35 crossovers per cell during meiosis in males and perhaps twice as many during meiosis in females. The frequency of meiotic crossing-over is not uniform along the length of the chromosomes.

One essential requirement for linkage analysis is the availability of DNA markers; the feasibility of human linkage analysis was revolutionized in 1978 when Kan and Dozy demonstrated genetic variation in the size of fragments generated after digestion of normal human DNA with restriction endonucleases. These restriction fragment length polymorphisms (RFLPs) are the consequence of the DNA sequence polymorphisms discussed above and are inherited according to Mendelian principles. Restriction enzyme digestion and Southern blotting made it possible to identify these polymorphisms and utilize them as genetic markers for sites within the genome. If one of the base pairs in the recognition sequence for a restriction enzyme is variable between individual copies of the genome or if there is a length variation in the DNA, there will be variation in the size of DNA fragments generated by the restriction enzyme digestion. The inheritance of an RFLP is depicted in Fig. 61-4.

A particularly informative subset of RFLPs occurs at variable number tandem repeat (VNTR) sites. These are sites of length variation in the genome in which a DNA sequence is tandemly repeated a different number of times on different chromosomes. The result is that there are many different sizes of DNA fragments, which can be regarded as different alleles at a VNTR site. The repeat unit

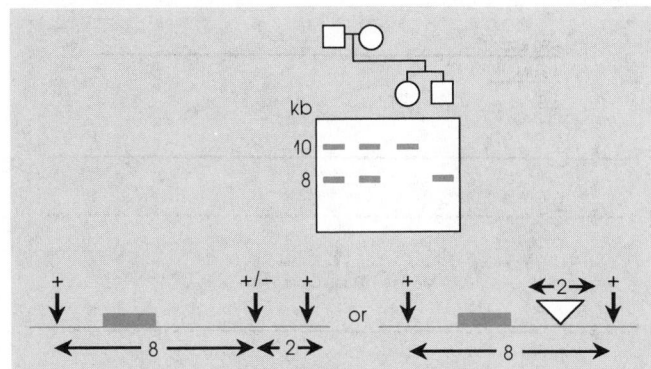

FIGURE 61-4 Example of restriction fragment length polymorphism (RFLP) in human DNA using Southern blotting. The solid blocks indicate segments of DNA used as probe. Parents are heterozygous and children are homozygous for the RFLP. Symbols above the arrows indicate cutting (+) or noncutting (−) by the restriction endonuclease. Numbers indicate DNA length in kilobases.

in VNTRs can be tens or hundreds of bases in length with variation arising through unequal crossing-over. In the case of the apolipoprotein for Lp(a), a VNTR repeat unit includes two exons giving rise to polymorphism in both the length of the gene and the protein. Another important group of polymorphic DNA markers is the short tandem repeats (STRs) which are repeats of tetra-, tri-, di-, and mononucleotides in the genome; variation arises through "slippage" of the DNA polymerase at replication to increase or decrease the number of repeat units on a chromosome. STRs are highly polymorphic, easily analyzed, and widely distributed in the genome. Dinucleotide repeats, of $(GT)_n$ on one strand and $(CA)_n$ on the other strand, with 10 to 40 repeat units, are the most common as depicted in Fig. 61-5. An

FIGURE 61-5 Depiction of a short tandem repeat (STR) polymorphism for a dinucleotide $(GT)_n$ repeat. Each repeat is separated by a vertical line. Sites for two primers for PCR are indicated by arrows. Four alleles of 24, 21, 18, and 15 GT repeats are indicated. Inheritance of the alleles in a family as detected by PCR is shown below.

FIGURE 61-6 Depiction of meiotic crossing over and linkage analysis. Panel A shows two copies of one chromosome (one in solid line and one in dashed line) from an individual before (above) and after (below) meiotic crossing over. The individual is heterozygous for a disease locus with a normal allele (open rectangle) and a disease allele (hatched rectangle) and is heterozygous for four DNA markers with alleles A/B, F/G, K/L, and R/S at 0, 1, 10, and >50 centimorgans (cM) from the disease locus, respectively. Panel B depicts analysis in a family for an autosomal dominant disorder. The DNA marker with K/L alleles at 10 cM from the disease locus on chromosome 4 and another DNA marker with Y/Z alleles on chromosome 7 are depicted. The chromosomes 4 and 7 for each parent are shown and the genotypes given for each family member. The disease phenotype is inherited from the father with the L allele for the DNA marker except for the last child who represents a crossover of the type shown in the upper panel. See text for discussion.

essential issue for linkage analysis, whether for construction of the human gene map or for clinical diagnosis, is that DNA markers in any individual have two different alleles at the marker locus of interest so that the two chromosomes of the individual can be distinguished.

Genetic linkage can be assessed between any group of markers, one of which may represent a mutation causing a disease phenotype (Fig. 61-6). For autosomal genes, each new individual inherits one copy of each chromosome from each parent. Panel A of Fig. 61-6 depicts one pair of chromosomes ready to enter meiosis with one normal copy of a gene (open rectangle) and one defective copy of the same gene (hatched rectangle). Four DNA markers, typically dinucleotide repeat polymorphisms, with A/B, F/G, K/L, and R/S alleles are depicted at 0, 1, 10, and >50 centimorgans from the disease gene. After meiosis and three crossover events, gametes are formed containing one chromosome with various segments of the original chromosomes. The A and F alleles of the DNA markers are within the gene of interest (A) or very close to it (F) and remain on the chromosome with the normal copy of the gene. DNA markers further away have a greater probability to undergo crossing-over, and the L allele of one DNA marker is now on the chromosome with the

normal copy of the gene, although it was previously on the chromosome with the defective copy of the gene. The greater the distance between markers and genes, the greater the probability of crossovers. Alleles for a gene and a marker on different chromosomes are inherited independently.

Panel B of Fig. 61-6 depicts the analysis of DNA markers in a family with an autosomal dominant disease such as Huntington's chorea. Data are shown for the K/L DNA marker which is 10 cM from the disease gene and for a Y/Z DNA marker which resides on a different chromosome. A researcher trying to map a disease gene is likely to study many DNA markers like the Y/Z markers which show no correlation between which allele of the marker is inherited and whether or not the disease phenotype is inherited. Eventually a marker such as the K/L marker is discovered where there is significant linkage to the disease gene. Analysis of additional families can provide conclusive statistical evidence that a polymorphic DNA marker is near a disease gene. Identification of a genetic linkage allows for immediate application of the marker for predictive diagnosis within a family such as that shown in Fig. 61-6 (see "Diagnosis by Linkage Analysis," below) and opens the way for positional cloning of the disease gene (see "Cloning and Identifying Human Disease Genes," below). The frequency of crossovers as shown for the last offspring in Fig. 61-6 is a measure of the genetic distance between the DNA marker and the disease gene. Once a linked DNA marker is found, the gene is mapped to a specific site on a chromosome, and closer DNA markers can be identified rapidly.

With the availability of an unlimited number of polymorphic DNA markers, there is already a relatively detailed linkage map for the entire human genome. In one recent study, 814 polymorphic markers (dinucleotide repeats) were placed into 23 linkage groups corresponding to the 22 autosomes and the X chromosome and spanning 90 percent of the estimated length of the genome.

THE PHYSICAL MAP   The physical map provides different information than the genetic map since it is based on direct DNA analysis and is not influenced by regional differences in recombination frequency. A physical map facilitates both the isolation of abundant DNA markers and the identification and cloning of all the genes in a region.

Four major strategies are used for physical mapping of the human genome: *in situ* hybridization, deletion mapping, long range restriction mapping, and isolation of yeast artificial chromosome clones. With *in situ* hybridization the direct hybridization of a DNA marker to a chromosome allows the assignment of the marker to a specific chromosomal band. With the advent of FISH (fluorescent *in situ* hybridization), the use of different colors for different probes makes it possible to map simultaneously more than one DNA marker. Hybridization to interphase nuclei allows determination of the order of markers within a particular chromosomal region. This technique is also useful for identification of chromosomal abnormalities, as described in Chap. 62.

Deletion mapping is based on the presence or absence of a particular region or locus in the DNA from patients with chromosomal abnormalities or from human/rodent somatic cell hybrids that retain known segments of the human chromosomes. Deletion mapping is particularly useful for mapping the X chromosome because of the large number of X chromosome abnormalities identified. Deletions of the X chromosome frequently result in a disease phenotype in males, and the deleted region can be identified without having to separate the abnormal chromosome from any normal homologue in somatic cell hybrids. Deletion mapping is also useful in establishing relative orders of sets of markers in the genome, although it does not provide precise information on the distance involved.

Information about physical distance is provided by long range restriction mapping. In this technique, high-molecular-weight DNA is cut into large fragments (from 100 kb up to 4 Mb) using restriction enzymes. These fragments are separated by pulsed field gel electrophoresis (PFGE) and then can be hybridized to DNA markers using conventional Southern blotting procedures. If two DNA probes hybridize, for example, to the same 200-kb restriction fragment, it can be concluded that the maximum distance between the two loci is 200 kb.

A particularly useful strategy in physical mapping utilizes yeast artificial chromosome (YAC) clones. The YAC cloning vectors are capable of carrying large-size fragments of genomic DNA (from 50 kb to 1 or 2 Mb). These vectors contain yeast telomeres and centromeres, and the clones are actually propagated as separate chromosomes in a yeast host. The human genome project will attempt the cloning of the entire human genome in overlapping YAC clones, and this has been accomplished for chromosomes 21 and Y. When this goal is achieved, physical mapping will be largely completed at one level of resolution, and further molecular analysis of the human genome will be facilitated because it will be possible to assign all genes and DNA markers to specific locations in the genome as defined by YAC clones.

THE HUMAN GENOME PROJECT The human genome project is an international effort, started in the mid 1980s, aimed at the characterization of human genomic DNA. Specific goals of the human genome project are: (1) the development of detailed physical and genetic maps, (2) the cloning of the entire genome in overlapping YACs, (3) the identification and characterization of all genes, (4) the sequencing of all the 3×10^9 bp forming the haploid human genome, and finally (5) the biological interpretation of the information hidden in the nucleotide sequence. Although technology is now adequate to carry out the first two objectives and to identify a large fraction of all genes in a reasonable length of time (2 to 5 years), new methods of sequence determination and analysis will be needed for the last two goals. The human genome project will foster a tremendous advancement in basic biology and in medicine. In the latter field, the identification of genes involved in genetic predisposition to cancer and to common multifactorial disorders, such as hypertension and atherosclerosis, is among the most important goals.

CLONING AND IDENTIFYING HUMAN DISEASE GENES Cloning of human disease genes can be categorized according to four general strategies: (1) knowledge and availability of the protein; (2) the ability to select for function of the gene; (3) knowledge of its genetic location (positional cloning); and (4) some combination of information regarding the phenotype, the genetic map location of the disease, and the genetic map location of biologically relevant genes (a regional candidate gene approach). Much of gene cloning relies on purification of a protein, determination of partial amino acid sequence, preparation of antibodies, and development of enzymatic or other assays. Using this information, cDNA clones can be isolated using approaches such as mRNA purification, hybridization screening with oligonucleotides based on available amino acid sequence, PCR amplification based on similar oligonucleotides, immunological screening of expression cDNA libraries, and other related approaches. In some instances, it has been possible to clone genes based on a functional property without knowing the protein or the genetic map location. For example, various genes involved in DNA repair disorders have been isolated using selection in tissue culture to identify clones that correct the cellular phenotype of defective DNA repair.

Positional cloning, often in the past, termed reverse genetics, is the isolation of a disease gene based on its location in the genome with no knowledge of its function. This strategy depends on the identification in samples from affected families of a DNA marker that is located close to the disease locus, as discussed above and depicted for an autosomal dominant disorder in Fig. 61-6B. Analogous efforts can be applied to autosomal recessive and X-linked diseases. Having localized the disease gene in a general way, it is possible to isolate the DNA of the relevant region in overlapping clones, identify genes in the region, and eventually prove which is the disease gene, often by identifying small mutations within one of the genes (Fig. 61-7). This strategy is facilitated if chromosomal translocations are available to assist in mapping and identifying the disease gene. This approach is labor intensive but has yielded landmark success in the case of genes for Duchenne's muscular dystrophy, cystic fibrosis, retinoblastoma, polyposis of the colon, neurofibromatosis, and Huntington's disease.

FIGURE 61-7 A positional cloning strategy. DNA markers at sites A and B are found to flank a disease gene. Overlapping DNA clones are isolated for the region, and the disease gene is identified within the region.

As human gene mapping becomes easier and as more genes are identified from human and other species, the regional candidate gene approach will be facilitated. A pure candidate gene strategy might involve simply guessing the disease gene from among known proteins based on the disease phenotype, but this is rarely possible. More often the candidate gene approach requires a limited amount of genetic mapping information for a disease, much less than would be adequate for a strictly positional cloning effort. Based on the limited mapping information, on information about relevant genes mapping to the general region, and perhaps taking into account information from other species such as the mouse, one can formulate and test the hypothesis that a particular gene is mutated in a specific genetic disease. Such testing is usually done by amplification and/or cloning of the gene in question from affected patients to search for mutations. A regional candidate gene approach led to the identification of mutations in the cardiac myosin heavy chain genes as the cause of familial hypertrophic cardiomyopathy. Use of information from the mouse led to the recognition that the *PAX3* gene is mutated in Waardenburg syndrome based on very limited mapping information and relevant information from the mouse. Many genes have been and will be cloned according to some combination of positional genetic information and candidate gene hypothesis, as exemplified by Marfan's syndrome, where mapping information and characterization of a candidate protein both contributed to the identification of the disease gene. One variation on the candidate gene approach would depend on the production of mice with targeted mutations and identification of candidate genes by phenotypes in humans that might resemble a phenotype observed in the mouse.

TRANSGENIC AND MUTANT MICE Gene structure and function are usually similar in mouse and human, and studies in the mouse can provide insight into human disease. The germline DNA of mice can be manipulated in a variety of ways (Fig. 61-8). The creation of transgenic mice typically involves microinjection of cloned DNA sequences into the male pronucleus of fertilized mouse eggs. The injected DNA becomes integrated into the mouse chromosomal DNA in a fraction of the injected cells. The transgenic DNA can be expressed in the resulting animals and transmitted in the germ cells so that a series of transgenic descendant animals can be obtained. Each site of integration of foreign DNA behaves as a single Mendelian trait, and heterozygous and homozygous animals can be obtained.

Transgenic animals have been particularly useful for the evaluation of *cis*-acting regulatory DNA sequences that control tissue-specific and temporal aspects of gene expression. Putative regulatory sequences are linked to a reporter gene, which produces an easily detectable product. Using this strategy, short DNA sequences have been identified that provide exquisite tissue specificity for genes such as insulin and elastase, and more complex and distant regulatory sequences have been shown to control the expression of globin genes. The transgenic method has also been utilized to introduce viral or cellular oncogenes that induce tumors in animals, opening new approaches for the study of tumor biology. A tissue-specific regulatory sequence can be linked to the SV40 T antigen to produce tumors in specific cell types. Another transgenic mouse strategy involves linking of regulatory sequences to a toxin that will selectively kill cells that express the sequence. As an example, linking of insulin regulatory

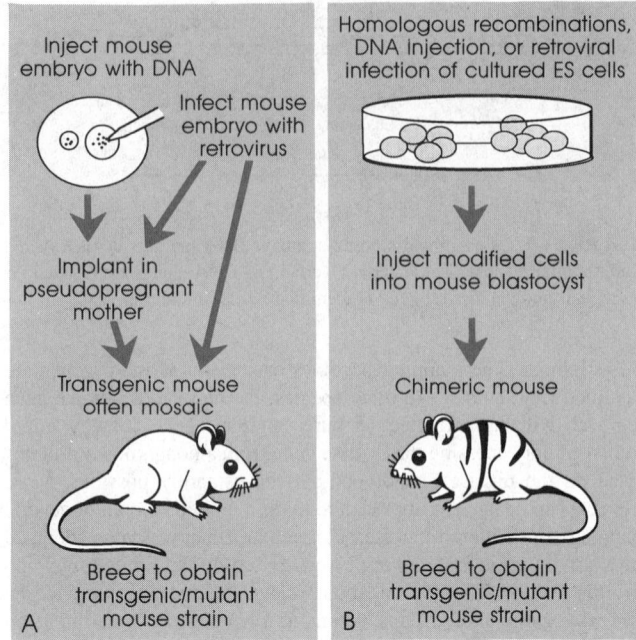

FIGURE 61-8 Various strategies for producing transgenic and mutant mice. DNA can be injected into the male pronucleus of fertilized mouse eggs followed by implantation in pseudopregnant mothers. Mouse embryos can be infected with retroviruses in vivo or in vitro. Transgenic mice may be mosaic, but the transgene can be recovered in nonmosaic form in the offspring of these mice. These strategies are depicted on the left. On the right, cultured embryonic stem (ES) cells can be modified by homologous or nonhomologous recombination or by retroviral infection. The modified cells can be selected and injected into a mouse blastocyst to produce a chimeric mouse with subsequent recovery of the mutation in the germline of the offspring of the chimeric mouse.

sequences to diphtheria toxin can generate mice with selective absence of pancreatic β cells. In yet another application, larger transgenic animals can be used for production of pharmaceuticals to be harvested from milk or blood.

Since integration of transgenic DNA is relatively random, it results in interruption of normal mouse genes in a certain percentage of cases. Retroviruses can also be used to infect mouse embryonic cells with the goal of relatively random insertional mutagenesis in the mouse. Mutant phenotypes can then be sought in the resulting heterozygous or homozygous offspring, including the identification of defects that are benign in heterozygotes but lethal in the homozygous state. Because the cloned DNA inserts at the site of the affected gene, it is possible to clone the gene associated with the mutant phenotype. Thus, it is possible to identify many new mutations and to clone the relevant genes.

The ability to carry out homologous recombination with mouse embryonic stem (ES) cells provides additional exciting opportunities. ES cells are totipotent cells that can be manipulated in culture and then reintroduced into mouse embryos. Using homologous recombination in ES cells, it is possible to target one specific gene for inactivation ("knockout") or subtle mutation. The injection of altered ES cells into recipient blastocysts results in chimeric animals composed partially of mutant cells derived from the ES cell culture. The genetically altered cells are often represented in the germ cells of the resulting chimeric animals, and mutant mice can be obtained and bred to study heterozygotes and homozygotes. The technique has allowed for the production of mouse models of many human genetic diseases including retinoblastoma, p53 oncogene deficiency (Li Fraumeni familial cancer syndrome), cystic fibrosis, Lesch-Nyhan syndrome, Gaucher's disease, apolipoprotein E deficiency, and others. In some instances there are major phenotypic differences for the same mutation in mouse and human, and delineation of the basis of these

differences will provide major insights into pathophysiology. In other cases, the phenotypes in mice and humans are similar, and the animals will be valuable for therapeutic trials. It is likely that mutant mice of these types will be particularly useful for unraveling the genetic factors in multifactorial disease processes such as atherosclerosis and for analysis of complex neurological functions. The ability to obtain mouse mutants for virtually any cloned gene provides an opportunity to analyze the function of cloned genes whose biologic roles are not delineated.

MOLECULAR DIAGNOSIS OF GENETIC DISEASE

NATURE AND ORIGIN OF MUTATIONS Typical genes which encode proteins are composed of promoters, exons, introns, and polyadenylation signals (see Fig. 60-2) and are subject to a wide variety of mutations. These include deletions, expanding triplet repeats, other gross rearrangements, and smaller mutations which can be characterized as missense, nonsense, frameshift, splicing, promoter, or other type. Some mutations are ancient in origin, and individuals in the population will carry the same mutation which originated from a rare event (a founder effect) as in the case of the common mutations for cystic fibrosis, sickle cell anemia, thalassemias, α_1-antitrypsin deficiency, Tay-Sachs disease, and other disorders. In the case of mutations that impair reproductive fitness and are eliminated from the population relatively quickly, disease mutations are more recent and tend to be different in each family, as in the case of X-linked lethal disorders and many dominant disorders including neurofibromatosis, Marfan's syndrome, and others. This consideration impacts on whether it is practical to search for known common mutations or to anticipate the need to search for an unpredictable mutation that is unique to a given family. In any consideration of molecular diagnosis, it is necessary to distinguish when one is dealing with the disease causing mutation as opposed to a variation in a DNA marker which is within or near the disease gene but is not the cause of the disease. Failure to distinguish the disease-causing mutation from variation in a DNA marker is a frequent source of misunderstanding in mutation analysis and linkage analysis.

Some mutations occur in stepwise fashion, progressing from premutation to mild mutation to severe mutation as exemplified by expanding triplet repeats in genes (see Caskey et al.). In addition, some genes are imprinted, in that only the paternal or maternal copy is expressed. This complicates the pattern of transmission of the phenotype within the family, since the appearance of the disease depends both on whether the disease gene was inherited or not and also on whether it was inherited from the mother or the father (see Hall). Imprinting is exemplified by the Prader-Willi syndrome where only the paternal copy of the gene appears to be active and the Angelman syndrome where only the maternal copy of the gene seems functional. The genes for Prader-Willi and Angelman syndromes appear to be distinct but close to each other on chromosome 15.

STRATEGIES FOR DIAGNOSIS OF MENDELIAN DISORDERS As for all clinical diagnosis, a detailed workup including family history and clinical examination, is the appropriate starting point. In some cases, the phenotype may be characteristic of a specific genetic disease, and the diagnostic information may be supplemented by family history or by specific biochemical laboratory tests. A general scheme for utilization of molecular methods for clinical diagnosis is depicted in Fig. 61-9.

Definite clinical and/or biochemical genetic diagnosis In many cases, a definite clinical genetic diagnosis is established before undertaking DNA analysis. The goals in such cases may include genotype/phenotype correlation, i.e., predicting the severity of the disease based on the mutations present. For example, some mutations cause nonneuronopathic Gaucher's disease, and others cause neuronopathic disease. Analysis may further confirm a diagnosis that is already considered to be established. Genotype/phenotype correlation and confirmation of diagnosis rely on mutation analysis and generally

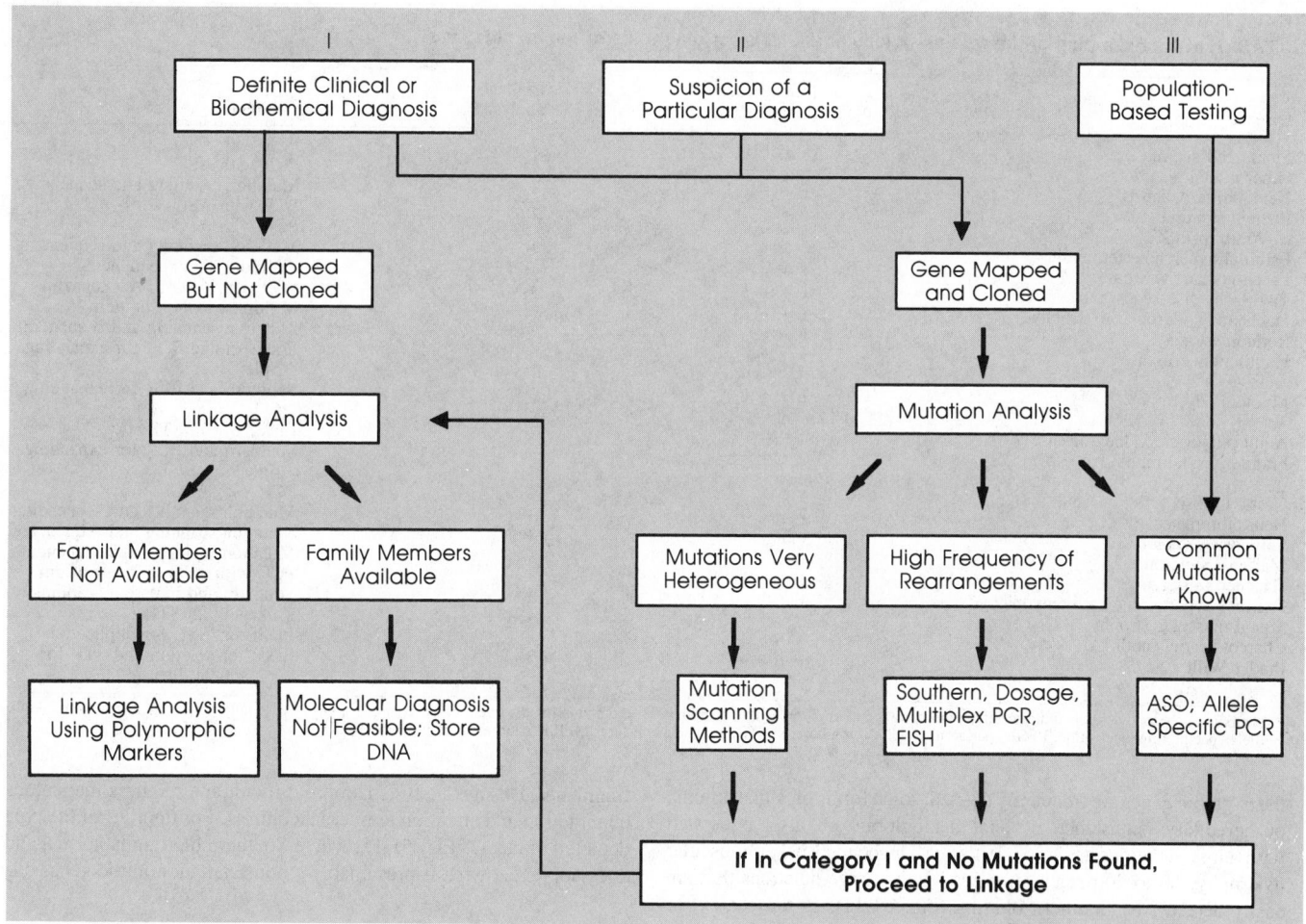

FIGURE 61-9 A scheme for utilization of DNA analysis for genetic diagnosis.

cannot be based on linkage analysis. Another application is studies of various family members for purposes of heterozygote detection, presymptomatic diagnosis, or prenatal diagnosis. Family studies should be performed using mutation analysis if possible and linkage analysis, where necessary, if suitable family members are available.

Clarification of a possible genetic diagnosis   In some cases, there may be a suspicion of a particular genetic disease, but the findings may be inconclusive, the patient may be early in the clinical course, or the case may be atypical. This frequently occurs in a circumstance where it is possible to detect some fraction of the disease mutations but not to search the entire coding and flanking regions to exclude an undetected mutation. In the case of dominant disorders or X-linked diseases in males, a diagnosis may be established by demonstration of a single copy of a definitive deleterious change in the DNA such as a deletion, frameshift, or nonsense mutation. Failure to find a mutation usually does not rule out the diagnosis but in some diseases makes it less likely. For autosomal recessive disorders, the situation is more complex: Identification of pathologic mutations in both copies of the gene establishes a diagnosis; identification of one pathologic mutation increases the probability that the suspect phenotype is related to mutation at this locus but does not prove a diagnosis; and failure to identify any pathologic mutations lessens the likelihood that the disease is related to mutation at this locus, but does not eliminate that possibility. For example, failure to detect a mutation may mean that the mutation is outside the region analyzed or that the patient has a separate but similar disease. Linkage analysis is usually not a practical way of resolving diagnostic problems of this type.

Population based DNA testing   Utilization of DNA testing for population-based screening offers the potential for many applications, similar to nonmolecular methods of population screening such as

newborn screening; cholesterol measurements; mammography; measurement of prostate specific antigen; carrier screening for Tay-Sachs, sickle-cell, or thalassemia; and maternal serum α-fetoprotein screening. DNA testing may be useful for (1) presymptomatic detection of disease susceptibility with plans for intervention, (2) carrier screening and reproductive counseling, or (3) prenatal testing. Many forms of genotypic analysis based on protein methods (e.g., sickle cell, α_1-antitrypsin and Tay-Sachs testing) might be more specific and more economic using DNA methods. The question of whether DNA testing for carrier detection for cystic fibrosis should be offered routinely has been controversial but is likely to become widespread in time. With DNA variation of known or likely disease significance occurring in the genes for apolipoprotein E, apolipoprotein Lp(a), angiotensinogen, angiotensin-converting enzyme, α_1-antitrypsin, and many others, it is likely that population-based DNA testing might become a powerful preventive approach with pharmacologic and lifestyle interventions for individuals with high-risk genotypes. Such strategies might well apply to familial cancer risks, such as breast cancer. Novel technologies such as ASO analysis using DNA fixed on electronic chips to allow multiple determinations at very low cost offers the promise of both economical and preventive strategies.

EXAMPLES OF MUTATION DETECTION   As indicated in Fig. 61-9, different methods of analysis are employed for molecular diagnosis depending on the most common type of mutation for a particular disorder, whether the mutations are usually large rearrangements or point mutations, and whether the mutations are usually of predictable type from ancient origins or are more heterogeneous and recent in origin. Examples of common genetic disorders are listed in Table 61-2 with the type of analysis that is most applicable for a disorder.

Examples of large defects in genes include α-thalassemia, where

TABLE 61-2   Examples of the role of molecular analysis for diagnosis of genetic disease

Disease	Detection of mutation*	Linkage analysis*	Comments
Sickle cell anemia	+ + + +		PCR with ASO
Other globin disorders	+ + + +	+	PCR with ASO
Hemophilia A and B	+ + +	+ +	Mutation scanning and sequencing
Phenylketonuria	+ +	+ +	PCR with ASO
α₁-Antitrypsin ZZ	+ + + +		PCR with ASO
Familial hypercholesterolemia	+ +	+ +	Mutation scanning and sequencing
Lesch-Nyhan syndrome	+ + + +	+	PCR and direct sequencing
Tay-Sachs disease	+ + +	+	PCR with ASO in Ashkenazim
Duchenne's muscular dystrophy	+ + +	+ +	Multiplex PCR, Southern
Retinoblastoma	+ + +	+	Mutation scanning and sequencing
Huntington's disease	+ + +		Southern and PCR for expanding triplet
Myotonic dystrophy	+ + + +		Southern and PCR for expanding triplet
Adult polycystic kidney disease		+ + + +	Linkage with STR
Fragile X syndrome	+ + + +		Southern and PCR for expanding triplet
Cystic fibrosis	+ + +	+	PCR with ASOs
Neurofibromatosis I	+ +	+ +	Mutation scanning and sequencing
Polyposis of colon	+ +	+ +	Mutation scanning and sequencing
Marfan's syndrome	+ +	+ +	Mutation scanning and sequencing
Gaucher's disease	+ + + +	+	PCR with ASO in Ashkenazim
Familial hypertrophic cardiomyopathy	+ + +	+	Southern and mutation scanning
Spinal muscular atrophy		+ + + +	Linkage with STR
Charcot-Marie-Tooth IA	+ + + +	+	PFGE or FISH for duplication
Prader-Willi	+ + + +		FISH for deletion and STR for uniparental disomy

* Symbols of + to + + + + indicate relative importance of an approach as of mid 1993; the status for disorders could change rapidly. PCR, polymerase chain reactions; ASO, allele specific oligonucleotide; PFGE, pulsed field gel electrophoresis; STR, short tandem repeat; FISH, fluorescence in situ hybridization.

the α-globin genes are frequently deleted; some forms of β-thalassemia or hereditary persistence of fetal hemoglobin are also associated with large deletions (Fig. 61-10). For Duchenne/Becker muscular dystrophy, 60 to 70 percent of cases involve large deletions that are easily detected by Southern blotting (Fig. 61-11). In the context of carrier detection for family members, a case such as lane 1 in Fig. 61-11 with a novel, junctional DNA fragment is optimal since the presence of this fragment will be absolutely diagnostic for carrier status for females in this family. For cases such as lane 3, heterozygote detection would depend on dosage analysis with one copy of the deleted fragments in carrier females, and two copies of the nondeleted

fragments. Dosage analysis is more difficult and requires meticulous quantitation and attention to internal controls. For families of the type depicted in lane 2, Fig. 61-11, where Southern blotting is normal and does not detect what is presumably a point mutation in the gene, this

FIGURE 61-11 Detection of deletions in the DNA isolated from Duchenne's muscular dystrophy patients using a dystrophin cDNA probe. Southern blot analysis detects deletions (absence of fragments) in five of eight patients (arrows). A junction fragment is clearly demonstrated in patients 1 and 6. *(From M Koenig et al, Cell 50:509, 1987.)*

FIGURE 61-10 Depiction of Southern blot analysis of human globin genes. Above, DNA was isolated from a normal individual and from patients with homozygous hereditary persistence of fetal hemoglobin (HPFH) or homozygous α-thalassemia. DNA was digested with the enzyme *Eco*RI. A mixed DNA probe was prepared by reverse transcription of reticulocyte globin mRNA. Below, arrows indicate *Eco*RI cut sites in the α- and β-globin regions, and numbers indicate DNA fragment sizes in kilobases. *(Adapted from YW Kan, AM Dozy, Proc Natl Acad Sci USA 75:5631, 1978.)*

FIGURE 61-12 Multiple amplification of DNA using PCR to detect deletions in the dystrophin gene. Nine amplifications detecting fragments of nine different exons are performed in a single tube and analyzed on an agarose gel. Deletions can be seen as missing fragments for the Duchenne dystrophy patients shown in lanes b, d, e, g, and h, while no deletion is detected in lanes a, c, f, and i. φX indicates DNA markers. *(Used by permission, Multicenter Study Group: JAMA 267:2609, 1992.)*

analysis would not be useful for carrier detection. Deletions such as those seen in Duchenne/Becker dystrophy can also be detected using PCR to test for the presence or absence of various sites in the gene (Fig. 61-12). Deleted segments are identified by the absence of particular PCR products in a multiplex reaction testing for the presence of various sites along the length of the gene.

Expanding triplet repeat mutations have been described as the cause of myotonic dystrophy, fragile X mental retardation, Huntington's and Kennedy's syndrome, a form of spinomuscular atrophy associated with this type of mutation in the androgen receptor. In the case of fragile X mental retardation and myotonic dystrophy, there is increasing severity of the disease as permutation progresses to mild mutation and mild mutation progresses to severe mutation, a genetic phenomenon called anticipation (see Caskey et al). Depending on the size of the expanding triple repeat, these mutations can be detected by Southern blotting and/or PCR analysis. An example of an expanding triplet repeat mutation with anticipation and more severe disease in later generations is depicted in Fig. 61-13.

For many disorders, including all autosomal recessive disorders and autosomal dominant or X-linked disorders with minimal effect on reproduction, known mutations of ancient origin may be present in thousands or even millions of people in the population. Despite the fact that there may be ancient common mutations, there may still be extensive molecular heterogeneity as is depicted for β-thalassemia in Fig. 61-14. The situation is similar for cystic fibrosis where the

FIGURE 61-13 Diagramatic representation of Southern blot analysis revealing an expanding triplet mutation in a myotonic dystrophy family. A grandmother and mother with the adult form of the disease and a child with the infantile form of the disease are shown. The normal size genomic DNA fragment (lowest band) is present in homozygous form in the unaffected individuals and in heterozygous form in the affected family members. The larger mutant fragment is present in all affected individuals with increasing size from grandmother, to mother, to child.

common mutation (designated ΔF508 for deletion of phenylalanine, F at position 508) accounts for about 70 percent of all mutations in most populations, but over 200 different mutations have been identified among the remaining 30 percent of mutant chromosomes. Common mutations of this type are usually best tested using some allele-specific method such as hybridization with ASOs. Typically, ASO analysis for a single disease may require testing for only a few alleles as in α_1-antitrypsin deficiency or for 10, 20, or more mutations as in the case of β-thalassemia or cystic fibrosis. A simple example of a traditional or "forward" ASO analysis is shown in Fig. 61-15 for S and C hemoglobin. In this case, PCR product is fixed on a filter, and the filter is hybridized to labeled oligonucleotide probes. In the reverse ASO or dot blot procedure, oligonucleotides are fixed on a membrane,

FIGURE 61-14 Point mutations in β-globin gene is shown with numbered hatched areas representing the coding regions of exons. Boxed open areas between the exons are introns, and boxed open areas at the 5' and 3' ends of

the gene are untranslated regions that appear in the messenger RNA. The various types of mutations are depicted by different symbols. *(From HH Kazazian, Jr., CD Boehm, Blood 72:1107, 1988.)*

FIGURE 61-15 Genotype analysis of PCR amplified genomic DNA using allele-specific oligonucleotides (ASO) probes. DNA was extracted from the blood of individuals of β-globin genotypes AA, AS, SS, SC, CC, and AC and homozygous deletion (XX). The DNA was applied to replicate filters for hybridization with ASO as follows: β^A probe (19A), β^S probe (19S) or β^C probe (19C). *(From K Mullis et al, Cold Spring Harbor Symp Quant Biol 51:263, 1986.)*

and labeled PCR product is hybridized to the membrane. Forward and reverse ASO procedures yield similar information and are in widespread use today. An example of a reverse ASO analysis for cystic fibrosis mutations is shown in Fig. 61-16.

The data from mutation analysis is generally relatively straightforward to interpret, although it is important to determine which mutations are present in affected family members in some cases as depicted in Fig. 61-17. It is currently recommended that carrier testing be offered to all reproductive aged individuals with a positive family history of cystic fibrosis. In the case shown in Fig. 61-17, two uncles and an aunt undergo testing. Consider first the circumstance where the mutation analysis is not available on the index case and his parents, i.e., missing the shaded information in Fig. 61-17. One uncle is found to have the ΔF508 mutation and is a definite carrier without regard to other family information. The other uncle and the aunt have negative mutation studies, and the probability that they are carriers is substantially reduced from the approximate prior risk of 1 chance in 2, particularly for the male, since the ΔF508 mutation is present on his side of the family. Once DNA analysis is performed on the propositus and his parents, and it is determined that the father carries the common ΔF508 mutation and the mother carries an unidentified mutation, the carrier risk for the uncle with negative mutation studies remains at a very low level while that for the aunt rises substantially to the original 1 in 2 risk. This example demonstrates the importance of obtaining mutation analysis on appropriate family members and the significant impact of such information on risk calculations.

In some cases, mutation analysis is quite difficult because the majority of patients carry point mutations, and the point mutations are heterogeneous. This typically includes autosomal dominant disorders with some impairment of reproductive capacity and X-linked disorders that limit reproduction in males. The factors influencing the proportion of cases of autosomal dominant disorders due to new mutation are discussed in Chap. 60. In these cases of heterogeneous mutations,

FIGURE 61-16 Reverse dot ASO analysis for various point mutations causing cystic fibrosis. For each mutation, the PCR product is hybridized to an ASO dot on the left for the normal allele and on the right for the mutant allele. The positions for each ASO are indicated as follows: F and Δ for the ΔF508 mutation, G and X for the G542X mutation, G and D for the G551D mutation, R and X for the R553X mutation, N and K for the N1303K mutation, and 10 or 11 or 21 under control for the ASO to detect the amplification of exons of those numbers. Mutations are designated by single letter amino acid code (X = non-sense) with the normal amino acid followed by the position number followed by the substituted amino acid. Thus G551D is substitution of aspartic acid (D) for glycine (G) at position 551. ΔF508 is described in the text. Letters at the right margin identify individuals of the following genotypes: A = no mutation, B = ΔF508/G542X compound heterozygote, C = ΔF508/R553X compound heterozygote; D = G542X heterozygote, E = G551D heterozygote, F = R553X heterozygote, and G = N1303K heterozygote. *(Modified from H. Erlich, Cetus Corporation.)*

508		542		551		553		1303		Control			
F ● Δ		G ○ X		G ● D		R ● X		N ● K		10 ○	11 ●	21 ○	A
F ● Δ		G ○ X		G ● D		R ● X		N ● K		10 ○	11 ●	21 ○	B
F ○ Δ		G ○ X		G ● D		R ○ X		N ● K		10 ○	11 ○	21 ○	C
F ● Δ		G ○ X		G ● D		R ○ X		N ● K		10 ○	11 ○	21 ○	D
F ● Δ		G ○ X		G ● D		R ● X		N ● K		10 ○	11 ○	21 ○	E
F ○ Δ		G ● X		G ● D		R ● X		N ● K		10 ○	11 ●	21 ○	F
F ○ Δ		G ○ X		G ● D		R ○ X		N ● K		10 ○	11 ●	21 ○	G

FIGURE 61-17 Mutational analysis in a cystic fibrosis family. Designations are as follows: ΔF = ΔF508 mutation, UK = unknown mutation, NL = normal allele, and NEG = negative mutation studies. See text for discussion.

some method of analyzing the entire gene is needed. Sequencing all of the exons of a gene is feasible in a few cases if the coding region of the gene is small, and this has been utilized for Lesch-Nyhan syndrome and to some extent for hemophilias A and B. However, this is impractical using current technology in most cases, and identification of mutations depends on a variety of procedures designed to detect single base differences in DNA sequences. In many cases, this remains an activity for research laboratories and is beyond the level of routine clinical service, although it would be extremely desirable to develop more powerful methods for detection of disease mutations in all families of this type.

DIAGNOSIS BY LINKAGE ANALYSIS If it is not possible to identify the mutation or mutations in the disease gene in a given family, then molecular diagnosis must be based on linkage analysis. In other cases, the disease gene may not be cloned but DNA markers

so close as to show negligible recombination with the disease phenotype may be available. In these cases, linkage diagnosis can be performed with a negligible possibility of crossovers. The general concepts for genetic recombination and linkage are discussed earlier in this chapter and in Chap. 60. For clinical linkage analysis, some genetic marker near the disease locus (or near the mutation if the locus is very large) must be *informative*. The genetic marker is informative if an individual has two different alleles at the marker locus. Linkage analysis often is appropriate when an individual carries one mutant gene and one normal gene and the goal is to determine which has been transmitted to the next generation. Most analyses can be made informative since highly polymorphic dinucleotide repeat polymorphisms are easily identified within and near genes causing diseases.

A second requirement for linkage analysis is that of *phase* information between the marker locus and the disease locus for genetic analysis. If an individual is heterozygous for a marker (genotype 1/2) that is tightly linked to a mutation, it must be determined whether allele 1 for the marker is on the chromosome with the disease allele or on the homologous chromosome with the normal allele, assuming that allele 2 for the marker would be on the chromosome with the alternate allele. When the genetic marker is informative and the phase is known, genetic diagnosis can be made for purposes of heterozygote detection, presymptomatic diagnosis, detection of failure of penetrance, and prenatal diagnosis. When the DNA probe or marker is within the gene that is mutated, crossing-over between the genetic marker and the disease-causing mutation is usually negligible. Duchenne's muscular dystrophy is an exception because it is an extremely large gene within which crossing-over occurs at a detectable frequency.

Examples of molecular diagnosis by linkage, when recombination between the loci is negligible, are presented in Fig. 61-18. Genetic marker data are presented as letters that might represent simple marker alleles or haplotypes of markers. A *haplotype* is a cluster of tightly

FIGURE 61-18 Examples of molecular diagnosis by genetic linkage with negligible recombination between the DNA probe and the disease locus. Letters below pedigree symbols indicate alleles for a DNA marker. Families *A* and *B* depict autosomal recessive disorders; *C* through *E* depict autosomal dominant disorders; and *F* through *I* depict X-linked disorders. Complete penetrance is assumed. See text for discussion.

linked specific alleles on a chromosome. Phase can usually be determined from a single index case for autosomal recessive disorders (Fig. 61-18*A*). Fetuses of AC genotype are predicted to be affected in Fig. 61-18*A* while fetuses of AA or BC genotype are predicted to be carriers and those of AB genotype to be noncarriers. In Fig. 61-18*B*, carrier detection is sought for the aunt and uncle of the affected. The data on the maternal side require analysis of the grandparents and predict that the aunt is a noncarrier. Although the paternal grandparents are deceased, it is still possible to conclude that the uncle is a noncarrier since he does not inherit the C haplotype which is linked to disease allele on the paternal side. For autosomal dominant disorders, linkage phase usually cannot be determined from a single affected individual (Fig. 61-18*C*). Exceptions include retinoblastoma, when analysis of tumor DNA may distinguish the allele on the abnormal chromosome (often retained in the tumor) from the allele on the normal chromosome (often lost in the tumor). Linkage phase for autosomal dominant disorders can be determined from two appropriate individuals; it is not essential that both be affected if penetrance is complete (Fig. 61-18*D* and *E*). Fetuses of AA or AC genotype in Fig. 61-18*D* and fetuses of AB or BC genotype in Fig. 61-18*E* are predicted to be affected. For X-linked disorders, phase information is most readily obtained from a single affected male (Fig. 61-18*F*). In general, linkage information can be used to determine the genotype in children of individuals of known genotype. Linkage information generally cannot be used consistently to determine the genotype of antecedents because of the possibility of new mutation from one generation to the next. This is exemplified by an X-linked disorder, where linkage information will not clarify whether the mother of an isolated affected male is a heterozygote or whether there is a new mutation in the propositus (Fig. 61-18*G*). This represents an important difference between direct detection of a mutation and linkage analysis. Occasionally, linkage analysis can suggest the genotype of an antecedent. Note in Fig. 61-18*G* that the mutation arose on the chromosome that was inherited from the unaffected maternal grandfather; the maternal grandmother and maternal aunt of the index case do not carry the mutation, and the new mutation occurred either in the mother or the index case. The situation is similar in Fig. 61-18*H* except that the mutation is on the chromosome from the maternal grandmother, and the site of the new mutation is unknown and could be from the mother, from the grandmother, or from further back in the family. Still by linkage analysis, the maternal aunt is not a carrier of the mutation. The genotype of an antecedent also can be inferred when a woman has two sons with the same DNA marker, one son being affected and one son being unaffected with the X-linked disorder (Fig. 61-18*I*). In this instance, the mother is not a heterozygote for the X-linked disorder, although the possibility of gonadal mosaicism (i.e., some of the maternal germ cells have the new mutation) is not eliminated. An example of the use of a dinucleotide repeat polymorphism for presymptomatic and prenatal diagnosis in a family with an autosomal dominant disease is depicted in Fig. 61-19.

LINKAGE WITH DETECTABLE RECOMBINATION Linkage analysis using a genetic marker that shows detectable recombination with a disease mutation has the same requirements for informativeness and phase as discussed above but is further complicated by the possibility of recombination at each meiosis in the family. The result is that predictions of genotype are given as probabilities (e.g., a 0.95 probability a fetus is affected and a 0.05 probability that it is not). These calculations are best performed using a computer program designed for linkage analysis. With the continued improvement of the human gene map and the ability to identify highly polymorphic markers, the use of markers that show significant recombination with a disease locus will decrease.

LINKAGE DISEQUILIBRIUM Linkage disequilibrium refers to the fact that certain alleles at two or more nearby loci may be found together more often than would be predicted from their frequency in the general population. Although linkage disequilibrium occurs routinely between multiple polymorphic sites, for purposes of genetic

FIGURE 61-19 Linkage analysis in an autosomal dominant disorder with variable age of onset or incomplete penetrance. A dinucleotide repeat polymorphism is analyzed by PCR to detect alleles A–D. Solid symbols are affected and open symbols are asymptomatic. The brother of the affected in the second generation is predicted to carry the normal allele while the pregnant sister has received the disease allele. The fetus received the normal allele (with the D marker) from the mother. Thus presymptomatic diagnosis indicates an affected genotype for the pregnant sister and an unaffected genotype for the brother and fetus.

diagnosis this is most readily discussed in terms of a genetic marker and a disease mutation. In Fig. 61-20 is depicted the occurrence of a disease susceptibility mutation (Z) at a locus where the normal allele is represented as Y. The mutation arises on a chromosome carrying the A allele for a nearby polymorphic DNA marker. With the passage of time, chromosomes carrying the A allele for the DNA marker and the Z allele for the disease locus grow to represent 10 percent of the chromosomes in the population. Not all chromosomes carrying the A form of the marker carry the disease susceptibility allele, but the disease allele is carried only on chromosomes bearing

FIGURE 61-20 Depiction of the development of linkage disequilibrium within a population of chromosomes. *A* and *B* indicate alleles for a DNA polymorphism. *Y* represents a normal allele and *Z* a disease susceptibility allele at a locus. See text for discussion.

the A form of the marker. This model also implies that it might be possible at a future date to identify and detect directly the Z mutation to provide a more accurate prediction of disease susceptibility. For linkage disequilibrium to be present, the two genetic markers must be tightly linked. In addition there must be one or only a few origins for the disease mutations, or the mutations will be found randomly with different alleles for the marker site. Linkage disequilibrium can often be found using a group of close genetic markers to form a haplotype.

Linkage disequilibrium is extensive within the HLA complex, and numerous diseases are found in association with various HLA haplotypes (see Chap. 60 in this text and Chap. 9 in Scriver et al.). For example, insulin-dependent diabetes mellitus is associated with HLA-DR3 and HLA-DR4, and susceptibility to this disease may be attributable to the presence of an aspartic acid residue in position 57 of the HLA-DQβ locus. The genotype at this position can be directly determined using PCR and allele-specific oligonucleotides. By comparison to Fig. 6-20, the HLA-DR data for diabetes could be equivalent to the A/B marker, while the aspartic acid residue could be the equivalent of the Z mutation. By analogy, DNA polymorphisms near any gene might detect linkage disequilibrium with a disease susceptibility. Using this rationale, attempts have been made to determine if certain DNA markers adjacent to the apolipoprotein genes are associated with increased risk of atherosclerosis. If such associations are proven, they would imply that some genetic variation in the coding or regulatory portions of an apolipoprotein gene itself is responsible for the altered disease susceptibility. Ultimately these genetic variations could be used directly for assessment of disease risks.

MOLECULAR CYTOGENETICS Recombinant DNA techniques provide a bridge between single-gene disorders and cytogenetics (see Chap. 62 in this text and Chaps. 16 to 20 in Scriver et al.). Genetic alterations range in size from single-base changes to gain or loss of an entire chromosome. As an example, some patients with Duchenne's muscular dystrophy have gross cytogenetic abnormalities, some patients have large deletions of DNA detectable by molecular but not by conventional cytogenetic analysis, and presumably others have single-base changes. In some cases, large deletions may involve multiple adjacent disease genes giving rise to complex phenotypes (contiguous gene syndromes). Samples from patients with detectable constitutional cytogenetic abnormalities or with acquired abnormalities in tumors have facilitated the cloning of numerous X-linked and autosomal genes. Reciprocally, molecular probes have been used to define cytogenetic translocations, deletions, and insertions. DNA probes are used to detect Y chromosome–specific sequences including the testes-determining factor in 46,XX males and to demonstrate the absence of regions of the Y chromosome in 46,XY females.

The technique of FISH (fluorescence in situ hybridization) is a major breakthrough in diagnostic molecular genetics and cytogenetics (Chap. 62). In addition to its use in disorders traditionally considered as cytogenetic conditions, FISH makes possible diagnosis of deletions in Prader-Willi syndrome, DiGeorge's syndrome, and other conditions and detection of the typical duplications of chromosome 17 that cause Charcot-Marie-Tooth disease.

MOLECULAR ONCOLOGY Just as these diagnostic techniques can be used to detect mutations in the constitutional DNA of all cells, they can also detect somatic mutations in malignant cells. Southern blotting and/or PCR can be used to detect alterations affecting both dominant and recessive oncogenes. Single-base changes in dominant oncogenes such as substitutions in codon 12 of H-*ras*, have been demonstrated in human colon and pancreatic cancer among others. Oncogenes can be shown to be amplified in numerous human tumors. Loss of heterozygosity at loci for recessive oncogenes can be demonstrated, using polymorphisms linked to these loci, e.g., loss of heterozygosity on chromosomes 5, 17, and 18 in human colon cancer. Chromosomal translocations such as those between immunoglobin loci and oncogenes can be demonstrated by Southern blotting. Molecular techniques are invaluable in the analysis of the basic

alterations in tumor cells, in the classification and staging of tumors, and in the monitoring of therapeutic strategies (see Chap. 63 in this text and Chaps. 10 to 15 in Scriver et al.).

DIAGNOSTIC VIROLOGY AND MICROBIOLOGY Virtually all microorganisms have DNA or RNA sequences that can be detected by nucleic acid hybridization techniques. As discussed above, nucleic acid hybridization is sensitive and specific and can be combined with PCR to detect a low abundance of foreign nucleic acid sequences. Other diagnostic procedures such as detection of infectious antigens with monoclonal antibodies and detection of human immune responses with immunoblotting can also provide rapid, sensitive, and specific diagnostic procedures. Each strategy offers special advantages. Some advantages of the detection of foreign nucleic acid sequences are as follows: (1) sequences can be detected without the delay required for the host to mount immune responses, (2) sequences can be detected without regard to passive acquisition of antibody whether by maternal transfer or by transfusion, (3) sequences can be detected even if the host fails to mount an immune response, (4) sequences can be detected even if no foreign proteins are being synthesized, and (5) the extraordinary ability of PCR to detect even a single molecule in a sample may make it the most sensitive technique in many circumstances. These techniques have been used for a broad range of viral diagnoses including cytomegalovirus, rotavirus, Epstein-Barr virus, and others. PCR has been used to detect hepatitis B sequences in serum and to detect HIV-1 sequences in peripheral blood mononuclear cells. In one study using PCR, HIV-1 sequences were detected in all specimens from seropositive, virus culture-positive subjects and in 64 percent of specimens from seropositive, virus culture-negative subjects. DNA amplification required 3 days rather than the 3 to 4 weeks required for virus isolation. PCR can also be used to detect nucleic acids from infectious organisms.

IDENTITY TESTING Analysis for only a few highly polymorphic tandem repeat sites, often tetra-, tri-, or dinucleotide repeats, provides the ability to distinguish the genotype of virtually all individuals except identical twins. This powerful method of identification is useful in paternity testing, in settling immigration disputes, in criminal investigations, and in monitoring bone marrow transplantation. The use of PCR for analysis of short tandem repeats is particularly powerful for forensic analysis, since identification can be made from minuscule samples of semen, blood, hair root, skin, or other tissue. Tissue typing at the HLA loci is also feasible using molecular analysis of polymorphisms.

PROSPECTS FOR SOMATIC GENE THERAPY (See also Chap. 65)

The general visions regarding both the significance of the role for somatic gene therapy and mechanisms for implementation have evolved dramatically. One change involves the breadth of disorders which might be considered amenable to therapy. Thinking has expanded from treatment of single-gene disorders to include treatment of cancer, AIDS, and atherosclerosis; in addition, a recombinant protein therapy (e.g., insulin, erythropoietin, clotting factor) could be converted to in vivo production via somatic gene therapy. The repertoire of delivery systems has expanded from retroviral vectors to include vectors based on adenovirus, herpes virus, vaccinia, and other viruses. Nonviral systems such as liposomes, DNA-protein conjugates, and DNA-protein–defective virus conjugates are also promising. Emphasis has shifted from ex vivo modification of cells to in vivo delivery, although ex vivo manipulation of bone marrow cells, tumor cells, and cultured fibroblasts and epithelium remains attractive. In general, retroviral vectors provide integration of the foreign DNA and permanent alteration of the recipient cell, but they require dividing cells as a target and allow only low titers of virus to be generated and are therefore relatively impractical for most in vivo approaches. Adenoviral vectors, in contrast, offer high titer and easier ability to infect large numbers of cells in vivo, but there is concern about toxic effects on infected cells and about the transient nature of their expression. Vaccinia vectors and nonviral systems also cause only transient expression, since they are not integrated into DNA. There is little information as yet as to whether repeated administration of agents that provide transient expression is feasible. Transient expression may be acceptable for applications such as eliciting an altered immune response to malignant cells or treatment of acute disease. There is need for new delivery systems or vectors that can be delivered efficiently in vivo preferably by intravenous injection, targeted to specific cell types, alter resting or dividing cells, and persist indefinitely whether by integration into the chromosome or by an extrachromosomal (episomal) mechanism.

At least three strategies may be useful for integration of the expressed DNA for somatic gene therapy. In one, a cDNA might be inserted under the control of a foreign promoter so that the product is synthesized without proper regulation. In a second strategy, genomic DNA could include the sequences necessary for proper regulation of the level and tissue specificity of expression. Artificial "minigene" constructions that link genomic regulatory regions with cDNA may provide constructions that are of manageable size and that show proper regulation. These strategies would typically involve random insertion of DNA sequences into the chromosome, although expression of extrachromosomal sequences is also a possibility. A third strategy would utilize site-specific recombination so that the mutant region would be replaced by normal DNA sequence. This approach is theoretically optimal and, although challenging, is more feasible since homologous recombination has been achieved in various cultured cells. In the case of enzyme or other protein deficiencies, any of these three approaches might suffice. For hemoglobin disorders, the relative accessibility of bone marrow stem cells and the advantages of maintaining all the normal regulatory mechanisms make homologous recombination a desirable goal.

Retroviral vectors provide viral particles that encode foreign nucleic acid and contain mechanisms for chromosomal integration. One current strategy (Fig. 61-21) involves insertion of cDNA or minigene DNA constructions between two viral long terminal repeats (LTRs) in a plasmid vector. These constructions can be introduced into cultured cell lines that provide the viral proteins necessary to package pseudovirus particles that include the gene sequence of interest. For example, bone marrow cells could be removed from a patient with a specific defect, purified bone marrow stem cells could be infected with these viral particles, and the patient's bone marrow could be repopulated with the altered cells. Retroviral infection of hepatocytes ex vivo has also been tried for homozygous familial hypercholesterolemia, but in vivo alteration of hepatocytes is likely to be more useful.

Adenovirus vectors typically are deleted for an essential viral gene and are then produced in cultured cells which complement this defect to yield a vector that can infect target cells but not produce further virus. Human trials to deliver adenovirus encoding the cystic fibrosis cDNA to the airway of patients are being initiated, and adenoviral delivery to hepatocytes is feasible, although expression is expected to be transient in these cases. Various in vivo strategies for gene therapy are being explored (Fig. 61-21).

Several single-gene disorders are candidates for gene therapy, and many protocols are being developed (Table 61-3). Life-threatening, recessive diseases involving bone marrow–derived cells would be excellent choices (e.g., adenosine deaminase deficiency, chronic granulomatous disease, and leukocyte adhesion deficiency), as are disorders in which extracellular products such as hormones or clotting factors might be produced in altered bone marrow cells. Dominant, neurologic disorders such as Huntington's disease appear to be the least approachable. If proper regulation of globin genes could be achieved, sickle cell anemia and thalassemia would constitute important opportunities because of the accessibility of bone marrow for in vitro treatment.

FIGURE 61-21   Comparison of ex vivo and in vivo strategies for somatic gene therapy. A procedure for ex vivo retroviral infection of bone marrow stem cells is shown on the left. On the right, this is compared to delivery by inhalation of aerosol for a disease such as cystic fibrosis or parenteral injection for targeting to organs such as liver or muscle using a variety of vectors or delivery systems.

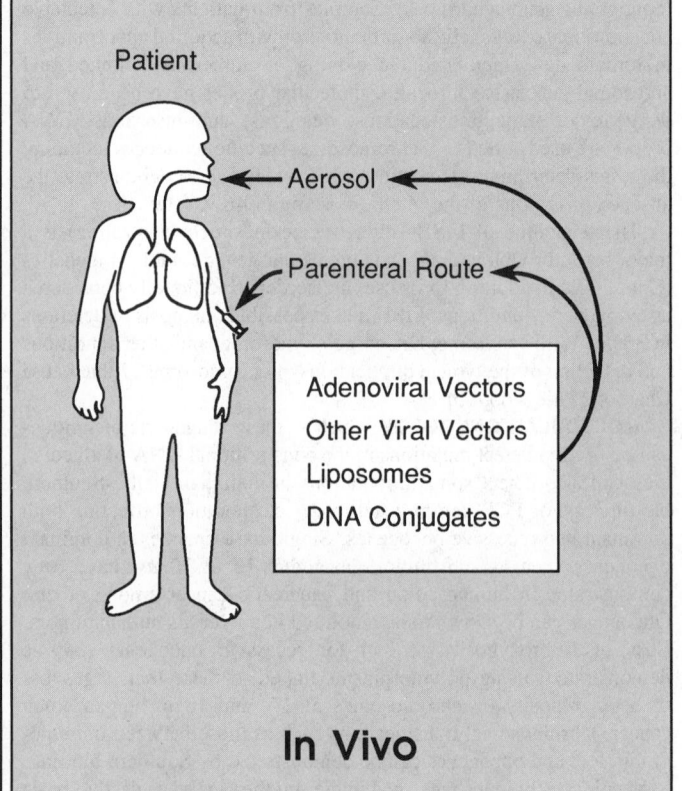

TABLE 61-3 Human diseases as candidates for gene replacement therapy*

Disorder	Burden of disease	Alternative treatment	Disease frequency	Requirement for tissue specificity	Regulation	Relative feasibility[†]
Hemoglobinopathies	Great	Transfusion, fair to poor	1 in 600 in ethnic groups	Erythroid	Required	+ + +
Lesch-Nyhan syndrome	Great	Poor	Rare	Brain, ?other	?Not essential	+ +
Adenosine deaminase and nucleoside phosphorylase deficiency	Great	Transplant, enzyme replacement, fair to good	Very rare	Bone marrow	?Not essential	+ + +
Leukocyte adhesion deficiency	Great	Transplant, fair to poor	Very rare	Bone marrow	?Not essential	+ + + +
Phenylketonuria	Small to moderate	Diet, good	1 in 11,000	Liver, ?other	?Not essential	+ +
Urea cycle disorders	Moderate to great	Diet, drug, good to poor	1 in 30,000 for all types	Liver, ?other	?Not essential	+ + +
α_1-Antitrypsin	Moderate	Poor, ?recombinant drug	1 in 3500	Liver, ?other	?Not essential	+ + +
Hemophilia A and B	Moderate to great	Replacement, fair	1 in 10,000 males	?Any organ,	?Not essential	+ + + +
Lysosomal storage diseases	Great	Poor	1 in 1500 for all types	Brain for many	?Not essential	+ +
Familial hypercholesterolemia	Great	Diet, drug, fair	1 in 500 heterozygotes	Liver, ?other	Some importance	+ +
Cystic fibrosis	Great	Supportive, fair/poor	1 in 2500 whites	Lung	?	+ + +
Duchenne's muscular dystrophy	Great	Poor	1 in 10,000 males	Muscle	?	+ +
Huntington's disease	Great	Poor	1 in 20,000	?Brain	?	?Poor
Various cancers	Great	Often poor	Very high	?Tumor cells	?	+ +
AIDS	Great	Poor	High	?Bone marrow	?	+ +
Atherosclerosis	Great	Fair	Very high	?Intravascular	?	+ +

* See Anderson for clinical protocols as of 1992.
† Attempts to take into account requirements for regulation, accessibility of target organs, alternative treatment, and risk vs benefit.

GENE THERAPY FOR CANCER, AIDS, ATHEROSCLEROSIS, AND PHARMACOTHERAPY The concept of somatic gene therapy has expanded beyond replacement strategies for genetic deficiencies (see Anderson). Many protocols for treatment of cancer are under evaluation, particularly for otherwise untreatable conditions. Strategies include (1) alteration of cancer cells or other host cells to produce cytokines or other molecules to alter the host response to the malignancy, (2) expression of antigens (e.g., allogeneic HLA proteins) on cancer cells to induce a host immune response, (3) insertion of tumor suppressor gene sequences or other sequences to slow cell growth, and (4) introduction of drug resistance genes into normal cells (e.g., bone marrow) to facilitate more aggressive chemotherapy. The first two "immunomodulatory" approaches are the basis of numerous research protocols.

A variety of strategies for gene therapy of bone marrow stem cells to introduce resistance to HIV or otherwise blunt expression of its effects are being proposed. In transgenic mice overexpression of apolipoprotein A-I can protect against atherosclerosis, and various strategies are being proposed for prevention and reversal of atherosclerosis whether of single-gene or multifactorial origin. As mentioned above, recombinant proteins could be produced in vivo rather than ex vivo with repeated injection. Transient and rapid expression of therapeutic proteins after injection of a viral or nonviral vector could greatly expand current therapeutic avenues.

ETHICAL CONSIDERATIONS Molecular genetic diagnosis provides an increasing capacity for presymptomatic and prenatal diagnosis of disease and disease susceptibility. It is possible to diagnose a newborn infant with familial polyposis of the colon, Huntington's disease, or dominant polycystic kidney disease decades before the onset of symptoms. What might be the impact of such diagnosis on the psychological development, career opportunities, and insurability of such individuals? Diagnosis of major increased susceptibility to coronary disease, diabetes mellitus, colon cancer, breast cancer, and other disorders is also likely to bring both the potential for therapeutic intervention and the risk of anxiety and discrimination. Prenatal diagnosis is now possible for diseases with a wide range of burden, such as α_1-antitrypsin deficiency, phenylketonuria, sickle cell anemia, muscular dystrophy, and familial hypercholesterolemia. Societies and individuals are divided regarding the option of abortion under such circumstances. Development of somatic gene therapy and other means

of treating presently untreatable genetic diseases may ultimately result in a reduced utilization of abortion.

Gene therapy raises other ethical considerations. Somatic gene replacement therapy requires conventional risk-benefit analyses for individual patients. So long as there is no modification of the germline DNA, few people have serious ethical concerns other than the question of whether such treatment is in the best interest of an individual patient. Experience with cancer chemotherapy suggests that some low level of damage to germline DNA might be an acceptable risk of such therapy if the patient received great benefit. In the future, it is conceivable that methods for site-specific recombination would allow replacement of mutant DNA in the germline with normal material. If one could permanently correct the cystic fibrosis mutation, the Huntington's disease mutation, or the sickle cell mutation in the germline of an individual and if such treatment were safe and effective, would society consider such therapeutic intervention? If introduction of an extra copy of a tumor suppressor gene into the germline of mice greatly protected against carcinogen-induced tumors without harmful effects, would this be relevant to humans?

REFERENCES

ANDERSON WF: Human gene therapy. Science 256:808, 1992

CASKEY CT et al: Triplet repeat mutations in human disease. Science 256:784, 1992

COOPER DN, SCHMIDTKE J: Diagnosis of genetic disease using recombinant DNA. Third edition. Hum Genet 87:519, 1991

ERLICH H et al (eds): *Polymerase Chain Reaction.* Cold Spring Harbor, Cold Spring Harbor Laboratory, 1989

HALL JG: Genomic imprinting: Review and relevance to human diseases. Am J Hum Genet 46:857, 1990

MULTICENTER STUDY GROUP: Diagnosis of Duchenne and Becker muscular dystrophies by polymerase chain reaction. JAMA 267:2609, 1992

PALMITER RD, BRINSTER RL: Germ-line transformation of mice. Annu Rev Genet 20:465, 1986

SAMBROOK J et al: *Molecular Cloning, A Laboratory Manual,* 2d ed. Cold Spring Harbor, Cold Spring Harbor Laboratory, 1989

SCRIVER CR et al (eds): *The Molecular and Metabolic Basis of Inherited Disease,* 7th ed. New York, McGraw-Hill, in press

WATSON JD et al: *Recombinant DNA,* 2d ed. New York, Scientific American Books, distributed by Freeman, 1992

WEISSENBACH J et al: A second-generation linkage map of the human genome. Nature 359:794, 1992

62 CYTOGENETIC ASPECTS OF HUMAN DISEASE

JAMES GERMAN

The chromosome complement is guarded carefully against change; most chromosome mutations, either structural or numerical, are deleterious. Only rarely is a structural rearrangement introduced into the population and transmitted from generation to generation, i.e., a chromosome mutation, that results in neither deficiency nor duplication of significant chromosome segments. As a rule an abnormal number of autosomes results in early death, except for trisomy of the shortest chromosome. In contrast, an abnormal number of sex chromosomes is often tolerated reasonably well although infertility or subfertility usually is present. Nevertheless, among human embryos abnormalities in chromosome structure and number are the major known cause of embryonic and early fetal wastage. However, not every fetus with an abnormal chromosome complement is aborted, and those that survive become the material of medical cytogenetics. Chromosome imbalance causes varying features including abnormal anatomic development, mental deficiency, behavioral disorders, and disturbances in growth and sexual development. Sometimes persons with abnormal chromosome complements whose own general development is normal present with infertility, repeated abortion, or the birth of malformed children.

The disorders just referred to are due to chromosome imbalance that affects tissues throughout the body. In addition, change can occur in the chromosome complement in a single cell of some somatic tissue. Such a mutant cell may have a proliferative advantage over normal cells if the mutation affects certain growth-controlling loci and is of a specific type, in which case a clone bearing the abnormal chromosome complement can develop among otherwise normal cells. Although such mutant clones are in many cases clinically insignificant, some are of importance in the etiology of cancer and possibly in other conditions that can be referred to as somatic mutational disease.

This chapter is addressed to those aspects of normal chromosome structure and function that constitute the basis for understanding the important chromosome alterations that have been or will be discovered. A selected number of those alterations and their consequences are mentioned as examples.

CHROMOSOME STRUCTURE AND FUNCTION The human autosomes are numbered 1 through 22, and the sex chromosomes are denoted X and Y. (The normal human chromosome complement is shown in Fig. 62-1. In the legend of the figure several terms used in human cytogenetics are defined.) Only seven of the chromosomes can be identified microscopically by their relative lengths and centromere positions, but unique staining characteristics—banding patterns—make possible the identification of all.

A mammalian chromosome consists of one double-stranded helix of DNA that extends from one end through the centromere to the other end. The paternally and the maternally derived autosomes that compose a pair and the pair of X chromosomes in females are genetically homologous, their differences being qualitative, i.e., dependent on the alleles received from each parent at polymorphic loci. In contrast, the X and Y chromosomes in males are almost completely different with the exception of their *pseudoautosomal regions*, short homologous segments at the ends of the short arms. The two homologues of each autosomal pair synapse and exchange chromatid segments at meiosis, as do the pseudoautosomal regions, which in effect constitute a 24th autosomal pair. With respect to the sex chromosomes, in germ line cells in the ovary, the two Xs pair at meiosis and undergo *recombination* just as the autosomes do; in the male, pairing and recombination of the X and Y chromosomes normally is limited to the pseudoautosomal regions. In somatic cells of the female, except in early embryonic life, one X is extensively inactivated, thereby giving the male and female approximately equivalent numbers of active X-linked genes. Inactivation of an X originates at a single active locus, *XIST*, on the long arm (band Xq13) of the inactivated X and affects most loci on that X, excluding the pseudoautosomal region. Similarly, one locus on the Y, *SRY* (*Sex-determining Region on the Y* chromosome), is pivotal in testis determination.

Cell-division cycle Chromosomes must duplicate before cell division can occur. This duplication occurs prior to the onset of mitosis or meiosis in a phase of the cell cycle termed *S*, for synthesis of DNA (Fig. 62-2). Thus, from the completion of S to the completion of metaphase, each chromosome contains two identical double-stranded helices of DNA, and the nucleus contains four times as much DNA as a spermatozoon or ovum. During mitosis chromosomes are condensed, and the two sister chromatids can be visualized by late prophase or early metaphase (Fig. 62-1). (Metaphase is the stage in the cell-division cycle ordinarily employed for cytogenetic analysis.)

At the onset of anaphase the centromeric regions of each chromosome separate, and the two chromatids move quickly to opposite poles of the mitotic spindle. When the poles receive their full complements of chromatids (now called chromosomes), nuclear membranes assemble about each cluster to form the nuclei of the two sister cells that will emerge from mitosis. (The nuclear membrane had been disassembled late in prophase.) The sister cells emerge in what is called the G_1 phase of the cell cycle where they remain unreplicated unless another division is to be prepared for, in which case they enter S. Cells engaged in some differentiated function ordinarily remain unreplicated.

Most normal cells in the human body are diploid; i.e., they have twice the haploid number of chromosomes, the number in a gamete (haploid = 23, diploid = 46). In the germ line, the lineage of cells devoted to gamete formation, cells destined eventually to differentiate into spermatozoa or ova, undergo mitotic cell cycling until they enter *meiosis*, two specialized divisions unique to this lineage. In meiosis, pairing of homologous chromosomes takes place (the paternally derived chromosome 1 with the maternally derived chromosome 1, the paternal 2 with the maternal 2, and so on), and genetic recombination occurs by a process called *crossing-over*, an exchange of entire segments between paternal and maternal chromosomes whereby the genetic constitution of each is altered qualitatively (see Chap. 60). At the first meiotic division homologous chromosomes are segregated, and the diploid chromosome number is reduced to the haploid; i.e., each cell then contains one of each of the 22 (duplicated) autosomes plus one (duplicated) sex chromosome. No S phase takes place between the first and second meiotic divisions (depicted in Fig. 62-2, right), so that at the second division, in which sister chromatids separate, emerging cells maintain the haploid number of chromosomes but are reduced in their content of DNA to half the amount of diploid G_1 cells of somatic tissues. With fertilization, both the chromosome constitution and the DNA content of the zygote are restored to that of a G_1 somatic cell. An S period in the zygote then permits reinstitution of regular cell-division cycles characteristic of somatic cells.

Chromosome differentiation A chromosome is differentiated along its length, and some aspects of this differentiation are resolvable microscopically. The DNA is complexed with a number of proteins in a highly specific way. The DNA-protein complex together with some associated RNA is referred to as *chromatin*. The fine structure, the manner in which the DNA is compacted and interacts with proteins, and the organization of chromatin in the interphase nucleus are thought to pertain to the control of RNA production and DNA replication and perhaps to cellular differentiation as well.

The sequences of nucleotide bases in DNA that constitute the genes and that can be transcribed into messenger RNA are distributed throughout the length of the various chromosomes. (These sequences are too short to be resolved microscopically.) Over 1500 genes have been assigned to specific chromosomes, in many cases to specific bands of a chromosome, where the order in which they are *linked* also has been determined.

Certain visible segments of at least 12 chromosomes vary in

FIGURE 62-1 Normal human lymphocyte chromosomes arrested in metaphase and stained for G bands (G standing for Giemsa). The inset shows the arrangement of chromosomes in an intact cell, and the remainder of the figure shows their ordered arrangement into a karyotype. By the time mitosis begins, each chromosome consists of two identical parts called sister chromatids and is identified by its relative length, the location of its centromere, and a distinctive sequence of bands of varying lengths and depth of staining. The number of bands visible microscopically varies from cell to cell, depending on the degree of chromosome condensation. The 300 to 400 bands seen in this particular cell can be increased to several times that number if cells with longer chromosomes are chosen for analysis, i.e., many of the bands seen here will resolve into subbands. Normally, the band patterns of the two chromosomes of a pair are alike, with the exception of certain polymorphic regions, examples of which are shown in Fig. 62-3.

The centromere of a chromosome divides it into a short arm (p) and a

long arm (q). Numbers 13 to 15, 21, 22, and Y are called acrocentric because of the nearly terminal positions of their centromeres; the minute p of each acrocentric autosome bears a nucleolus-organizing region which often causes a secondary constriction in the metaphase chromosome (the constriction at the centromere being the primary constriction).

By standard nomenclature, this karyotype is described as 46,XY, indicating that its chromosome number is 46, its sex chromosomes are an X and a Y, and the autosomes (those besides the X and Y) number 44. The following examples show the general use of this nomenclature: A normal female karyotype is described as 46,XX. A female cell with an extra chromosome 18 (trisomic for 18) would be described as 47,XX, + 18. A cell with only one sex chromosome, an X, and with deletion in the short arm of chromosome 5 would be described as 45,X,5p − . A male cell with a translocation between chromosomes 2 and 3, with breakpoints in band 13 of 2p and band 22 of 3p, would be described as 46,XY,t(2;3)(p13;p22). (See also Table 62-2 footnote.)

length among individuals. These can be delineated by their staining characteristics (e.g., Fig. 62-3). The variable segments consist of nontranscribed, highly repetitive nucleotide sequences of DNA and are transmitted from parent to child in a straightforward mendelian fashion. The techniques of molecular genetics make possible the identification and molecular definition of innumerable heritable polymorphic segments of DNA, segments that, like genes themselves, are submicroscopic. These noncoding segments are referred to as *restriction fragment length polymorphisms* (RFLPs) or *variable number of tandem repeats* (VNTRs). Variations in both microscopically visible and invisible segments are usually unassociated with detectable phenotypic effect. However, they serve as useful genetic markers in prenatal diagnosis when they are tightly linked to disease-

associated loci (e.g., in Duchenne's muscular dystrophy) and in the determination of zygosity of twins, paternity, and survival of transplants. Also, these DNA markers, especially those VNTRs composed of short oligonucleotide repeats that are highly polymorphic and are widely dispersed throughout the genome, are invaluable in the effort to map the human genome. In this undertaking, loci of importance in normal development and differentiated cell function, including those that when mutant result in human disease, are being assigned their correct order and relationship to one another along each of the chromosomes.

Microscopically recognizable segments in the short arms of the acrocentric autosomes (mentioned in the legend to Fig. 62-1) are devoted to the production of ribosomal RNA and nucleoli. As

FIGURE 62-2 Schematic representation of the mitotic and meiotic cell-division cycles, as described in the text. G_1 and G_2 = time gaps before and after S, the period in which DNA replicates. Each of these intervals is several hours in duration; together they constitute interphase. M = mitosis; I and II = the two divisions of meiosis. The DNA content of the cycling cells is indicated on the vertical axis: 1c = the content in a gamete; 2c = that in either an egg immediately postfertilization or a somatic cell emerging from mitosis; 4c = the amount in a cell which has completed chromosome duplication and is ready to enter mitosis or meiosis.

mitosis progresses, these nucleolus-organizer regions remain relatively uncondensed. Consequently, at metaphase they appear understained and demarcate condensed segments of chromatin distal to them on the chromosome arms—*satellites*. (The DNA of satellites contains no genes; satellites are examples of the polymorphic segments just mentioned.) Several other regions that remain relatively uncondensed at metaphase are recognizable in a low percentage of cells and are called *fragile sites* because they may undergo outright disruption (''breakage'') in metaphase preparations. The only such region known to be of significance in relation to a human trait, the clinical condition called the *fragile-X syndrome*, is one located near the distal end (the

FIGURE 62-3 Metaphase chromosomes stained for C bands (C standing for centromeric or constitutive heterochromatin), showing inherited variation in lengths of C bands in chromosome 1 (arrows).

end away from the centromere) of the long arm of the X chromosome (see below, under ''Sex Chromosome Imbalance''). Other examples of segmental specialization along the chromosome include *telomeres* and *centromeres*. Telomeres, the distal termini of each arm, have some relationship to the nuclear membrane and probably are important in the maintenance of order in the interphase nucleus and of accurate pairing of homologues in meiosis; centromeric regions are sites of microtubule attachment at metaphase.

A further example of chromosome differentiation is the sequence by which various segments replicate during S; certain segments replicate early, others late. In general, late replication of a chromosome segment correlates with genetic inertness. This correlation is exemplified by one of the two X chromosomes in female cells; the X in which the entire chromosome, except for the terminal pseudoautosomal region and a few additional loci that are inactivated by a phenomenon referred to as the *Lyon effect* (see Chap. 60), is almost entirely late-replicating.

A little-understood type of chromatin is referred to as *heterochromatin*. It is tightly condensed, not just at metaphase but throughout interphase. Such condensation of chromatin correlates with genetic inactivity and also with late replication. Some regions are condensed and inactive in all cells (constitutive heterochromatin), while others, e.g., the X chromosome, may be either condensed and inactive or decondensed and active (facultative heterochromatin). Many chromosome imbalances that permit viability beyond intrauterine life involve chromosome segments that are rich in this apparently inactive, or inactivatable, type of chromatin, e.g., chromosomes that can be trisomic in live-born individuals or, in the case of the X, monosomic. The activity of genes can sometimes be affected, even inactivated, if they are positioned aberrantly near regions of heterochromatin, as can occur in chromosome breakage and rearrangement.

Therefore, in chromosome imbalance both the specific genetic loci and the particular types of chromatin deleted or duplicated are important. Also, the significance of a chromosome rearrangement probably depends on the new and abnormal positioning of structural and regulatory genes in relation to each other and to heterochromatin.

Fortunately for the cytogeneticist, several differentiated features of the chromosome correlate with cytologic artifacts that can be produced and visualized in the laboratory. A number of techniques are now in use to display the constant pattern of bands of various lengths and staining characteristics already mentioned (Figs. 62-1 and 62-3). These patterns are identical in each chromosome 1, each chromosome 2, etc., varying only in the inert polymorphic regions mentioned above, so that they can be used in clinical cytogenetics to identify chromosomes and to detect and define structural rearrangements.

Sources of error   A large number of genetic loci must be active to produce the enzymes and structural proteins required to initiate and complete a cell-division cycle. Remarkable precision and accuracy are demanded over and over in matters such as the passage of a cell from G_1 into S, orderly progression of replication, assembly of the mitotic spindle, and the spindle action that segregates chromatids at mitosis. In the germ line additional loci are activated to permit a cell of the germ line to pass successfully through meiotic prophase including pairing of homologous chromosomes, genetic recombination, and then disjoining of recombined homologous chromosomes at anaphase of the first division. These mechanisms and processes are subject to errors, some spontaneous, others promoted by unfavorable environmental influences (e.g., Fig. 62-4) or the consequence of inherited or new mutations that affect one of the many steps in the cell cycle. Furthermore, the genetic material itself is subject to damage, and certain types of unrepaired or erroneously repaired lesions in DNA predispose to mutation, including chromosome rearrangement. Errors at many of these steps or errors introduced during the repair of damaged DNA lie behind chromosome imbalance. Mutations that arise in germ cells, during fertilization, or in early postfertilization divisions are important causes of embryonic maldevel-

FIGURE 62-4 Breaks and rearrangements (arrows) in metaphase chromosomes of a blood lymphocyte that received ionizing irradiation before being stimulated by phytohemagglutinin to enter S and divide.

opment and infertility; mutations in somatic cells are important in causes of somatic mutational disease, particularly neoplasia.

CHROMOSOME ABNORMALITIES Mutations of a single base in a gene and deletions and duplications of chromosome segments involving even hundreds of base pairs are not visible microscopically. In fact, for the normal chromosome banding pattern to be detectably disturbed, a lengthy segment of DNA must be deleted, duplicated, or transposed. This means that a chromosome mutation that is microscopically detectable must involve large amounts of DNA. However, the same environmental agents that produce point mutations (mutagens in the usual sense) are also chromosome-breaking agents, and vice versa. Thus, it seems safe to assume the existence of a spectrum extending all the way from mutations visible to the cytogeneticist to those that must be defined by nucleotide sequencing. Visible mutations ordinarily exert a more widespread effect on development than do point mutations; ordinary genes—often many of them—as well as other specialized types of chromatin whose function or significance is unknown are involved in cytologically visible mutations.

If an entire chromosome is affected in an imbalance, the genome is said to be either *trisomic* or *monosomic* for the chromosome (thus, trisomy 13, monosomy X). Genes and chromatin carried on the affected chromosome then are present in triple or single dose, respectively, rather than the normal double—*disomic*—dose. Abnormal dosage affecting less than an entire chromosome, the result of chromosome breakage and rearrangement, is often termed *partial trisomy* or *partial monosomy*, to indicate that segments rather than entire chromosomes are involved (thus, partial trisomy 13q, partial monosomy 4p). Some of the recurring chromosome imbalances, both numerical and structural, are listed in Table 62-1.

Uniparental disomy refers to the situation in which both chromosomes of a pair, or perhaps just a segment of both, are erroneously inherited from a single parent. In such cases the presence of a homozygous chromosome segment can have unfavorable effects on development, presumably because of homozygosity of some recessive gene or genes that by chance were carried on that segment in the (heterozygous and therefore healthy) parent from whom the segment was inherited in double dose or possibly from an inappropriate balance of imprintable genes (see discussion of genomic imprinting under "Structural Abnormalities" below).

Incidence The frequency with which chromosome imbalance is detectable depends on the population investigated. It is estimated that a minimum of 1 in 10 human conceptions has a chromosome abnormality. In spontaneously aborted human embryos and fetuses, the incidence of chromosome imbalance is higher the earlier in pregnancy the sampling is made. The contribution of imbalance to late abortion and stillbirth, though not well studied, probably also is significant. From surveys of more than 65,000 live-born babies examined in different laboratories, approximately 1 in 200 has a significant chromosome abnormality, either numerical or structural. In such studies, at least 1 in 700 newborns is trisomic for one of the autosomes 21, 18, or 13; about 1 in 350 newborn males has the complement 47,XXY or 47,XYY. One in every several thousand newborns has monosomy X. One in 500 has some structural rearrangement, most of which are genetically balanced. Samplings of the general adult population reveal an occasional inherited balanced structural rearrangement as well as the expected number of XXY, XYY, and XXX complements; the inherited, apparently innocuous segmental polymorphisms (e.g., Fig. 62-3) and minor structural rearrangements demonstrable by banding techniques are found in abundance.

In individuals with mental deficiency, 10 to 15 percent have a significant chromosome abnormality, the proportion being greater if anatomic malformations are also present. In some groups of men with behavioral disorders or infertility, an increased incidence of individuals with an extra X or Y chromosome is found. Infertile women also include many individuals with extra or missing sex chromosomes and an appreciable number with structural chromosome rearrangement; approximately one-fourth of women with primary amenorrhea have some abnormality of the X chromosome. Among infertile men and women, individuals may have inherited mutations that interfere with meiosis, so-called meiotic mutants.

Numerical abnormalities Trisomy (47 chromosomes) is the most common chromosome imbalance in early spontaneous abortuses, followed by monosomy (45 chromosomes) and triploidy (69 chromosomes). The extra or missing chromosomes can be either paternal or maternal in origin, and the error in segregation of chromosomes can occur in the germ line, fertilized egg (zygote), or early embryo. Trisomy of every chromosome except the no. 1 has been observed in spontaneous abortions, trisomy 16 being the most frequent.

Sex chromosome trisomy (XXY, XYY, and XXX) is compatible with intrauterine survival; in contrast, autosomal trisomy rarely permits survival to term. However, a small proportion of autosomal trisomics are born alive. For practical purposes these are trisomy 21, 18, or 13, in decreasing frequency. Trisomies 18 and 13 cause death during infancy. Therefore, trisomies of significance in adults are only trisomy 21, XXY, XXX, and XYY. A few other autosomal trisomies, such as trisomy 8, occur rarely, usually in mosaicism with a normal cellular component. (*Mosaicism* is the coexistence in one individual of multiple, genetically different populations of cells, all derived originally, however, from a single zygote.)

Autosomal monosomy is rare even in abortion material. In contrast, monosomy X (45,X) occurs in approximately 1.5 percent of recognized conceptions. It is common among spontaneously aborted human embryos (approximately 10 percent) and is present in one in every several thousand live-born babies. The reason for the failure of 45,X embryos and fetuses to survive is unknown, although anatomic abnormalities probably contribute; cardiovascular and renal anomalies are common in the few that do survive. The genetic basis for the lethality may be hemizygosity for some vital locus or loci in the portions of the Y and in the portions of the second X in 46,XX individuals that fail to be inactivated by the Lyon effect, including the pseudoautosomal region. A possible explanation for the survival of an occasional 45,X individual is occult mosaicism, the nonmonosomic cells, perhaps limited just to a few tissues, going undetected. In monosomy X, the missing sex chromosome can have been either a Y or an X and either paternal or maternal in origin. Often the second

TABLE 62-1   **Some recurring chromosome imbalances that result in distinct syndromes***

Class of imbalance	Chromosome affected	Karyotypes[†]	Clinical features[‡]
Monosomy	X	45,X	Turner syndrome
Segmental deficiency ''partial monosomy''	X	46,XX,p−; 46,XX,q−; 46,X,r(X); 46,X,iso(Xp); 46,X,iso(Xq)	Turner syndrome or some features of it
	Y	46,XY,p−; 46,XY,q−; 46,X,r(Y); 46,X,iso(Yp); 46,X,iso(Yq)	Turner syndrome, or some features of it, sometimes with ''mixed gonadal dysgenesis'' when a 45,X cell line coexists
	4	46,XY,4p−	Gr, Cf, Mi, Ey, Sk, Ge, Ht, Co, Me
	5	46,XY,5p−	5p− syndrome: Cr, Mi, Cf, Me
	8	46,XY,8q−	Langer-Gideon syndrome
	11	46,XY,11p−	WT, Ge, Me
	13	46,XY,13q−	RB, Cf, Me
	15	46,XY,15q−	Prader-Willi (or Angelman) syndrome
	17	46,XY,17p−	Miller-Dieker syndrome
	18	46,XY,18p−	Gr, Cf, Ea, Te, Po, Sk, Ht, Me
	18	46,XY,18q−	Cf, Hy, Sk, Ey
	21	46,XY,r(21)	Cf, Hp, Ea, Me
Trisomy	X	47,XXX	Se, Me (mild), Ps
	X	47,XXY	Klinefelter syndrome
	Y	47,XYY	Ta, Ac, Su, B; but often normal
	8	46,XY/47,XY, +8	Cf, Sk, Me (moderate)
	13	47,XY, +13	Trisomy 13 syndrome: Cp, Ey, Pd, Po, Ht, D, V, Sc, F, Ar, Me
	18	47,XY, +18	Trisomy 18 syndrome: Cf, Ea, V, F, Gr, D, He, Me
	21	47,XY, +21	Trisomy 21 (Down syndrome)
Segmental duplication ''partial trisomy''	Y	46,X,t(X;Y)[§]	XX male
	9	9p+[†]	Cf
	21	21q+(distal q)	Trisomy 21 syndrome
	22	22q+[¶]	Gr, Cf, Ea, Cp, Hy, Co
Chimerism	Entire complement	46,XY/46,XX	Pseudo- or true hermaphroditism; dimorphism of blood-cell-surface antigens
Triploidy	Entire complement	69,XXY	Hc, Me, Sy, Ht, Ge, D

* For complete listing, consult DeGrouchy and Turleau.

[†] The sex chromosome constitution might be either XY or XX, but in the example karyotypes given, XY arbitrarily is used in most.

[‡] The clinical features given include only some of the more constant ones. Deficiency of one segment often is accompanied by duplication of another, and the phenotypic effect is the consequence of the combined imbalance. Abbreviations are defined below.

[§] Translocation onto an X of a segment of the Y bearing the locus responsible for testicular differentiation.

[¶] Brought about through any of several rearrangements.

Abbreviations: Ac, acne; Ar, arrhinencephaly; B, behavior disorder; Cr, characteristically abnormal cry; Cf, characteristic craniofacial dysmorphism; Co, convulsions; Cp, cleft lip–palate; D, early death; Ea, characteristically abnormal ears; Ey, eye anomaly; F, characteristically flared, overlapping fingers; Ge, abnormality of external genitalia; Gr, severe growth deficiency; Hc, hydrocephaly; Hp, hypertonia; Ht, cardiac malformation; Hy, infantile hypotonia; Me, intellectual deficit; Mi, microcephaly; Om, omphalocele; Po, characteristically abnormal posture; Pd, polydactyly; Ps, psychotic predisposition; RB, retinoblastoma; Sc, scalp defect; Se, secondary amenorrhea; Sk, skeletal anomalies; Su, subfertility; Sy, syndactyly; Ta, tallness; Te, characteristically abnormal ears; V, visceral anomalies; WT, Wilms's tumor with aniridia.

sex chromosome is not completely absent but is replaced by a structurally rearranged Y or X. Mosaicism is often demonstrable in live-borns with monosomy X; here, tissues are populated not only by cells with a 45,X complement but by other cells, perhaps with a normal complement, 46,XY or 46,XX, or with a complement in which the second sex chromosome is rearranged in some way.

The phenotypic effects of the autosomal trisomies, of 47,XXY, and of monosomy X (45,X) are characteristic and well defined so that their diagnosis usually is not difficult (see Chap. 342). The effects of the 47,XYY and 47,XXX constitutions are less striking, and therefore these complements are underdiagnosed. In mosaicism with coexistence of abnormal and normal populations of cells, the phenotype may approach the normal.

The mechanisms responsible for the numerical abnormalities are undefined and may be multiple. In trisomy 21 the extra chromosome is maternal in 95 percent of cases, and it usually results from nonsegregation of the no. 21 chromosomes at the first meiotic division. A maternal age effect exists in trisomies 21, 18, 13, XXY, and XXX. Over a third of babies with trisomy 21 are born to women over 35, whereas only about a tenth of all births occur in this group. The frequency of trisomy 21 rises from 0.5 to 0.7 per 1000 live births between ages 21 and 23 to 3 per 1000 at age 35, 10 per 1000 at age 40, and 34 per 1000 at age 45. After a child with trisomy 21 is born, the risk of recurrence in future pregnancies is approximately 1 percent. As to the cause of monosomy X, the frequent association of the 45,X complement in mosaicism with normal complements and with structural rearrangements of the X and Y suggests that the zygote or the preimplantation embryo is often the target of a chromosome-breaking event, rather than a nondisjunctional event during meiosis as in the trisomies.

Structural abnormalities Some structural chromosome rearrangements are inherited, and others represent new mutations. The cause of the new rearrangements is unknown, although they are assumed to be partly spontaneous and partly the effect of environmental agents such as mutagenic chemicals or ionizing radiation (Fig. 62-4) acting on the germ line, zygote, or early embryo. The majority of de novo rearrangements are in paternally derived chromosomes.

Many chromosome rearrangements have been detected only once or a few times. Others are detected repeatedly, the same one recurring in unrelated individuals and families. For example, the commonest translocation, one that can occur either as result of de novo mutation or by inheritance, affects one chromosome 13 and one 14 at or near their centromeres. In this translocation only inert chromatin or functional chromatin that is represented elsewhere in the genome—

the nucleolus-organizing regions and satellites referred to earlier—is lost from the tiny short arms. A similar recurring translocation affects chromosomes 14 and 21.

Chromosome complements bearing rearrangements can be genetically balanced or effectively so, thus imparting no unfavorable effect to their bearers; about two-thirds of rearrangements detected during surveys of live-born babies are balanced. Or, the complement can be unbalanced and impair development, the usual case when rearrangements are detected during surveys of spontaneous abortuses or of individuals with multiple anomalies and mental deficiency.

A phenomenon that can influence the developmental consequence of chromosome abnormalities is *genomic imprinting*. Certain genetic loci are subject to functional modulation, presumably during passage through the germ line. The modulation differs, depending on whether the genome passed through spermatogenesis or oogenesis. The parental source of a chromosome mutation that affects an imprintable locus/loci can determine whether a developmental defect will arise and the nature of the defect. An example of imprinting concerns deletion of chromosome band 15q11 (fifteen-q-one-one): If the affected (deleted) chromosome 15 is the one inherited from the father, the Prader-Willi syndrome is the consequence; if from the mother, the Angelman syndrome (Table 62-1).

Some balanced chromosome rearrangements are transmitted from generation to generation without producing clinical effects. In other cases, they are responsible for the conception of embryos with unbalanced genomes. For example, inherited translocations involving chromosome 21 predispose to the trisomy 21 syndrome. Approximately 5 percent of live-borns with that syndrome have a translocation, and in about a fifth of those it is detectable in one of the parents. Because most babies with the trisomy 21 syndrome due to translocation are born to women under 30, a search for a translocation can be important when a child with this clinical syndrome is born to young parents. Different translocations bestow on their carriers different risks of having offspring with unbalanced rearrangements, i.e., partial trisomies or partial monosomies. These risks frequently cannot be predicted on theoretical grounds. Useful empiric risk figures have been accumulated for the common translocations; e.g., the 14;21 translocation bestows a 2 percent risk on a balanced male carrier and more than a 10 percent risk on a female carrier of having a child with the trisomy 21 syndrome. In contrast, the balanced carrier of a 21;21 translocation can expect unbalanced offspring almost exclusively. Information of this type is indispensable for counseling in relation to chromosome disorders.

DISEASE ASSOCIATIONS Various combinations of abnormalities in malformed and mentally defective individuals correlate with variations in the chromosome complement. (Many of the conditions are of little significance in adult medicine because of their lethality in infancy or early childhood.)

Autosome imbalance Of the three autosomal trisomies found in live-born babies, only trisomy 21 is compatible with survival past infancy. The phenotype produced by an extra chromosome 21, formerly known as *mongolism* but now called the *Down syndrome* or *trisomy 21 syndrome*, is characteristic and easily diagnosed. Cardiac malformations lead to death in infancy in a third of individuals with trisomy 21, and other malformations and infections may also cause early death. However, subjects who survive infancy often reach adulthood, and some old age. Affected females occasionally become pregnant, and, as expected, approximately half their children have trisomy 21.

Mosaicism of trisomy 21 with normal cells (46/47, +21) may occur in individuals with modified features of the trisomy 21 syndrome, or even in normal persons. The risk that a person with such mosaicism will have trisomic children is increased, but unfortunately the abnormal cell population usually is detected only after the birth of an affected child.

Partial trisomy, partial monosomy, or a combination of the two affecting any of many chromosomal segments throughout the genome explains many instances of multiple developmental defects combined with mental deficiency. Sometimes a balanced autosomal translocation is detected in normally developed adults who have repeated spontaneous abortion or subnormal fertility, with or without abnormal liveborn children.

Although the phenotypic effects of many segmental chromosome imbalances are varied and nonspecific, the anomalies sometimes compose recognizable clinical syndromes. Two examples are the following: (1) If a rearrangement causes partial trisomy of just the distal band of 21q, the long arm of chromosome 21, the clinical features of the full Down syndrome associated with an extra entire 21 develop. (A triple dose of other segments of the long arm of chromosome 21 also produces adverse effects but not the Down syndrome.) (2) Partial monosomy of a short segment within the short arm of chromosome 5 causes mental deficiency, a characteristic facies, and a characteristic cry during infancy. This group of signs is known as the *5p* − (five-p-minus), or cri-du-chat, syndrome.

Additional recognizable syndromes produced by imbalance of many different chromosome segments now are known (Table 62-1), e.g., the *4p* −, 9p partial trisomy, 13q −, and 18q − syndromes, to name a few. Furthermore, the application of high-resolution banding techniques and fluorescence in situ hybridization (FISH) (described below under "Technical Considerations") make possible identification of the exact band(s) deficient or duplicated. Rearrangements not previously described and their corresponding clinical syndromes still are being recognized. These syndromes may appear as the result either of de novo chromosome rearrangement or through formation of a genetically unbalanced gamete in a person carrying in balanced state a rearrangement affecting the segment involved.

In many individuals with chromosome imbalance, regardless of which segments are affected a degree of phenotypic similarity is present. These recurring and nonspecific features include mental deficiency, growth deficiency, dysmorphic ears, nose, and mouth, cardiac malformations of standard types, abnormalities of dermal ridges and creases, and dysmorphic digits. (As a rule, autosomal imbalance need not be considered in the etiology of anatomic defects unaccompanied by mental deficiency.) Why similar abnormalities occur with so many different segmental imbalances is unknown, but when several such features are observed in a single individual, they can be a valuable clinical indication for cytogenetic analysis. Imbalance affecting certain segments also causes specific phenotypic changes, examples being the 5p − syndrome, retinoblastoma [mutation of a particular band of chromosome 13 (band 13q14.2)], the WAGR syndrome (Wilms's tumor, aniridia, genital anomalies, and mental deficiency) caused by deletion of band 11p13, and the Prader-Willi syndrome, which is often the consequence of deletion of a specific band near the centromere of chromosome 15 (band 15q11). Whereas the nonspecific changes serve to call attention to the possibility of some chromosome imbalance, the specific features or constellation of features can suggest the exact segment of the genome affected. These conditions are sometimes referred to as contiguous gene-deletion syndromes, the case, for example, in the WAGR syndrome (above) and in deletions of segments of Xp that may result in loss of contiguous loci that individually are responsible for Duchenne's muscular dystrophy, chronic granulomatous disease, retinitis pigmentosa, and the MacLeod phenotype.

Sex chromosome imbalance (See also Chap. 342) In contrast to autosome imbalance, sex chromosome imbalance causes relatively mild phenotypic effects. This is because X chromosomes beyond one in the complement of somatic cells are usually almost totally inactivated, because the pseudoautosomal region is much shorter than any of the autosomes, and because the strictly sex-linked portions of the Y bears few genes. X-linked loci (in contrast to autosomal loci) function normally in single dose: the female is functionally hemizygous for most loci on the X through the Lyon effect; the male, with only one X chromosome, is hemizygous for X-linked genes with the exception of loci clustered in the pseudoautosomal segment and a few scattered in the proximal Yp and Yq. The addition of an extra sex chromosome has a phenotypic effect but insufficient to interfere with intrauterine survival. Since major anatomic defects are usually absent, men with the complements 47,XXY and 47,XYY and 47,XXX females often go unrecognized.

The *Klinefelter syndrome* (Chap. 342), which in classic form consists of small testes, infertility, gynecomastia, and variable degrees of underandrogenization, sometimes with mild mental deficiency, antisocial behavior, or both, is the consequence of the addition of an extra X to the male complement: 47,XXY. The extra X interferes with the survival of germ cells, and atrophy of the spermatogenic tubules and azoospermia are the consequence. Sometimes the phenotypic effects are mild, the testicular atrophy being the only noteworthy feature in otherwise healthy and socially well-adjusted men. The mosaicism 46,XY/47,XXY sometimes occurs and may ameliorate the phenotypic effect of the extra X. More extreme phenotypic effects and mental deficiency result when more than one extra X chromosome is added to the normal male complement: 48,XXXY or 49,XXXXY.

The phenotypic effect of 47,XYY is less well defined; although increased height, behavioral difficulties, and infertility are common, the extra Y is sometimes found in otherwise normal men. The rare complement 48,XXYY results in infertility. The phenotype associated with 47,XXX is also poorly defined; although women with mild mental deficiency, psychosis, and menstrual abnormalities sometimes have this complement, it is also detected in normal, healthy women. Further clarification is needed concerning the effects on personality and behavior of all three of the complements 47,XXY, 47,XYY, and 47,XXX.

Loss of the Y or of the second X has drastic effects on development. If it does not cause abortion (as already discussed), it may or may not be recognizable at birth. Loose nuchal skin folds and edema of the hands and feet in a newborn girl, with or without renal or cardiovascular anomalies, may point to the diagnosis of the 45,X complement. The *Turner syndrome* is the manifestation in subsequent life (Chap. 342): short stature, infantilism of otherwise normal female external and internal genitalia, germ-cell-free gonads referred to as gonadal streaks, and variable renal, cardiovascular, skeletal, and ectodermal anomalies.

The Turner syndrome may be the developmental consequence of several chromosome constitutions besides 45,X. Mosaicism as well as structural abnormalities affecting certain segments of a second sex chromosome, either a Y or an X, cause a spectrum of disorders at both the clinical and cytogenetic levels. A normal male or normal female cellular component may be present along with the 45,X cellular component, or one component may bear a structurally abnormal chromosome. Common abnormalities of the Y and X are isochromosome formation (one arm deleted and the other duplicated) or deletion of part or all of one arm. In some affected individuals all cells have 46 chromosomes, with one normal X plus an abnormal Y or X, for example, 46,XXp−, deletion of a segment of the short arm of one of the X chromosomes. In others a second or third cellular component may be present as well, for example, 45,X/46,XX/46,XXp−. Typical Turner syndrome may be found in association with various combinations of these karyotypes if one of them is either monosomic or partially monosomic for X. However, when Y-bearing cells coexist with the 45,X cells, for example, 45,X/46,XY, genital ambiguity often develops, and gonadal morphology ranges from streaks to functional testes (the syndrome of *mixed gonadal dysgenesis*); in mosaicism that includes 45,X cells and other cells with a Y the risk of gonadal neoplasia is significant. When 46,XX cells coexist with 45,X, varying degrees of ovarian function may be maintained, including ovulation. Although the phenotype may approach that of a normal male or female when normal and abnormal cells coexist, the effects of mosaicism are unpredictable. Thus, the phenotype associated with monosomy X and structurally abnormal Ys or Xs ranges from male through the Turner syndrome to female.

Two other rare disturbances of sexual development deserve mention here—*true hermaphroditism* and the *46,XX male* (see also Chap. 342). True hermaphroditism is present when testicular and ovarian tissue coexist in the same individual. In most cases the chromosome complement is 46,XX, and it appears normal by banding. Exceptionally, true hermaphrodites have the complement 46,XY, and sometimes *chimerism* 46,XY/46,XX is demonstrable, the two cellular components having been derived from different zygotes. Second, males occasionally have complement that appears by banding to be 46,XX. As in 47,XXY men, the second X interferes with meiosis and azoospermia results. In both the 46,XX true hermaphrodite and the 46,XX male, the rule that a Y is required for testicular differentiation appears to break down. The explanation in some XX males is that the testis-determining locus actually is present, having been erroneously translocated from Yp to Xp, demonstrable not by microscopy but by molecular cytogenetics.

In the general population more males than females are mentally deficient, and familial mental deficiency affects males preferentially. In some such kindreds, mental deficiency segregates as an X-linked trait, and several such syndromes are now recognized.

The commonest of these, the *fragile-X syndrome*, is characterized by mental retardation, a characteristic facies, and macroorchia. The condition can be recognized by cytogenetic techniques. In a variable but usually small proportion of metaphases from affected persons and in an even smaller number from the mothers, the abnormal X chromosome exhibits a so-called fragile site near the distal end of Xq. This site is responsible for the decondensed appearance of the region at metaphase, and its fragility is due to excess amplification of the trinucleotide sequence CGG. This base sequence is normally repeated 2 to 50 times at the fragile-X locus, whereas in the fragile-X syndrome the number of repeats expands to more than 160. This amplification is believed to affect the normal functioning of neighboring genetic determinants and thereby to cause the abnormal phenotype. Other examples of this mode of inheritance, heritable selective amplification of an oligonucleotide, are known, e.g., amplification of the trinucleotide CTG within a specific locus on chromosome 19 can cause familial myotonic dystrophy, though in this instance unassociated with a microscopically visible chromosome lesion.

Chromosome change in cancer The theory that chromosomal abnormalities may cause cancer was advanced many years ago, and with improved cytogenetic techniques and the advent of recombinant DNA technology firm evidence supporting the theory has become available. Indeed, most human cancers have chromosome complements that are altered in a microscopically detectable way.

Table 62-2 lists some of those found with regularity. In the leukemias, lymphomas, and certain myeloproliferative disorders the alterations are less extensive than in solid tumors and, therefore, easier to define. As examples, chromosome 14 is often found to have undergone structural rearrangement in certain lymphomas, with the breakpoint near or in the immunoglobulin heavy chain locus; the rearrangement translocates the *myc* locus from its normal position on chromosome 8 to chromosome 14. Also, in over 95 percent of cases of chronic granulocytic leukemia a translocation affecting chromosomes 9 and 22 (already mentioned) is detected, resulting in the Philadelphia, or Ph, chromosome, an abnormally short no. 22. (The abnormality in chromosome 9 is difficult to detect microscopically.) If the leukemia progresses into a "blastic" phase, the already mutated karyotype evolves; certain new chromosome changes are added stepwise in a nonrandom sequence. In this and certain other leukemias, the chromosome changes, demonstrable either by conventional cytogenetics techniques and microscopy or by microscopy supplemented by molecular techniques, may have diagnostic utility as well as some value in prognosis and choice of therapy. Common carcinomas such as of the lung, breast, and colon, although more difficult to study by conventional cytogenetics techniques, also have specific chromosome mutations, often analyzed more readily by molecular techniques.

The microscopically visible chromosome mutations that are found with regularity in human neoplasms often affect loci that play growth regulatory roles in normal cells. In some cases the chromosome breakpoints affect already known cellular oncogenes, but analysis of

TABLE 62-2 Some recurring chromosome abnormalities encountered in human neoplasms*

Neoplasm	Aberration	Chromosome region affected
Leukemia		
Chronic granulocytic	Translocation	9q34 and 22q11
Acute nonlymphocytic		
M1	Translocation	9q34 and 22q11
M2	Translocation	8q22 and 21q22
M3	Translocation	15q22 and 17q11
Chronic lymphocytic	Trisomy	12
Acute lymphocytic		
L1–L2	Translocation	9q34 and 22q11
L3	Translocation	4q21 and 11q23
	Translocation	8q24 and 14q32
Lymphoma		
Burkitt's	Translocation	8q24 and 14q32
Follicular	Translocation	14q32 and 18q21
Solid tumors		
Benign		
Meningioma	Deletion or monosomy	22q
Leiomyoma, uterus	Translocation	2q13–15 and 14q23–24
Adenomas, salivary gland	Translocation	3p25 and 8q12
Malignant		
Ewing's sarcoma	Translocation	11q24 and 22q12
Rhabdomyosarcoma, alveolar	Translocation	2q35–37 and 13q14
Germ cell tumors, testis	Isochromosome	12p
Lung, small cell carcinoma	Deletion	3p13–23
Liposarcoma, myxoid	Translocation	12q13 and 16p11
Sarcoma, synovial	Translocation	Xp11 and 18q11
Neuroblastoma	Deletion	1p31 to 3p36
Ovary, cystadenocarcinoma	Translocation	6q21 and 14q24
Retinoblastoma	Deletion	13q14
Wilms's tumor	Deletion	11p13

* For more complete listing see Solomon.
NOTE: The FAB (French-American-British) classification of leukemias is employed above. The chromosome breakpoint and band nomenclature is that of the Paris Conference (Birth Defects: Original Articles Series VIII (7):1–46, 1971). The chromosome and chromosome-arm designation (e.g., 9q means the long arm of chromosome no. 9) appears first and is followed by the chromosome region and band on that arm (e.g., 9q34 means the fourth band in the third region of the long arm of chromosome no. 9).

the breakpoints in the acute leukemias has resulted in identification of previously unrecognized genetic determinants in basic cell biology, e.g., transcription regulatory factors and loci concerned with the regulation of normal development. In the lymphoma examples given, *myc* in its new position on chromosome 14 is abnormally regulated, brought now under the influence of the activating elements of the transcribing immunoglobulin locus in cells differentiated to synthesize antibodies. In the Ph chromosome, the cellular-oncogene *abl* is translocated from its normal position on chromosome 9 into a specific region called *bcr* on chromosome 22, thereby creating what is referred to as a *fusion gene*; in myeloid cells, this mutant locus is transcribed, and the mRNA is translated into a novel protein that presumably plays a causative role in the autonomous growth of the neoplastic cell lineage that is recognized clinically as chronic granulocytic leukemia.

Another process that appears to be important in progression of some tumors is *gene amplification*. One particular chromosome segment is replicated selectively, sometimes to such a degree that the normal banding pattern at the chromosome region affected is visibly disturbed, a *homogeneously staining region* (HSR) being the result. Sometimes the region amplified rather than producing an HSR is released from the chromosome, and multiple tiny centromereless bodies of DNA, known as *double minutes* (DMs), accumulate in the nucleus and can be seen at metaphase. Presumably, in both HSRs and DMs, amplification of the DNA of some particular locus is of selective value to the neoplastic cell, thus enhancing the neoplastic clone's progression or perhaps resistance to chemotherapeutic agents.

Another chromosome mechanism in human neoplasia is *somatic crossing-over*. Through somatic crossing-over, a recessive mutation at a genetic locus concerned with growth regulation—a mutation that

preexisted in a cell but that had remained occult because of the presence of a normal locus on the homologous chromosome—can become homozygous. The recessive mutation may either have been inherited or arisen de novo in somatic cells. The consequence then of homozygosity at such a mutant locus is loss of normal growth control, i.e., acquisition of autonomous growth by the affected cell and its progeny. Such mutations were first recognized in the rare neoplasms retinoblastoma and Wilms's tumor, where the loci affected were on chromosomes 13 and 11, respectively. In some cases of retinoblastoma the original (recessive) mutation consisted of outright deletion of the locus; then, when somatic crossing-over occurred, homozygosity of the affected chromosome arm distal to the point of exchange was the consequence, and a cell and its progeny became *nullisomic* for the retinoblastoma locus. Transmission through the germ line of such occult recessive mutations at growth- or tumor-suppressor loci explains familial instances of those neoplasms.

Thus, chromosome mutations of at least four types constitute crucial steps in the initiation and progression of malignant neoplasia: (1) translocations that disturb the regulation of loci concerned with growth or that produce novel genes that affect growth; (2) deletion-mutation of recessive growth-controlling loci (e.g., the retinoblastoma locus just referred to), mutations that can either be inherited through the germ line or occur de novo in a somatic cell; (3) recombination yielding homozygosity for preexisting mutations affecting this last-mentioned type of locus; and (4) amplification of some locus that facilitates expansion of the neoplastic population. These mutations and their oncogenic consequences are the subject of intense investigation, both basic and clinical. In turn, the breakpoints in neoplasms are helping identify genetic determinants that together orchestrate normal cellular proliferation and tissue growth; thus the cytogenetics of human cancer is contributing not only to clinical medicine but also to the understanding of normal cell biology.

The cytogenetic findings in leukemias and solid tumors were some of the first evidence of the clonal nature of human cancer.

TECHNICAL CONSIDERATIONS Human metaphase chromosomes can be examined by light microscopy in any tissue in which sufficient cells are cycling. Preparations can therefore be made directly from almost any embryonic tissue and from adult bone marrow, lymphoid tissue, and selected malignant tissues. In searches for mosaicism and chimerism, the study of multiple tissues is often required. Some tissues unlikely to contain cells in metaphase can be placed in culture, and chromosome preparations can be made from cells that reach mitosis in vitro. Blood T lymphocytes stimulated to enter cell-division cycles by phytohemagglutinin are the standard material for diagnosing constitutional chromosome imbalance. In some myeloproliferative disorders and leukemias, unstimulated circulating blood cells will divide spontaneously after a few hours in culture. Long-term cultures of fibroblasts can be derived from minute skin biopsies or from fragments of many other types of tissue, although more elaborate laboratory facilities and a longer period of time are required before cytogenetic preparations can be made. Amniotic fluid is among the sources of cells suitable for culture, and the cells, which are fetal in origin, are widely used in the prenatal diagnosis of chromosome imbalance. Metaphase preparations also can be made from chorionic villi biopsied in the first trimester of pregnancy or from aborted fetal tissue.

Meiotic chromosome preparations from testicular biopsies are sometimes useful in obscure cases of infertility. Translocations and genetically determined disturbances of meiotic pairing may be identified there.

The combination of conventional techniques with those of recombinant DNA technology and fluorescence microscopy makes it possible to detect promptly abnormalities such as trisomy, translocation, and segmental duplication or deficiency and to characterize the abnormalities in some detail. The availability of molecular probes for many specific loci whose map position is known and that blanket the genome makes it possible to identify rearrangements not detectable by banding techniques alone. By FISH, molecular probes specific for each chromosome can be used to "paint" a chromosome differentially throughout its length, determining, for example, whether part of one chromosome might be translocated aberrantly to another, or whether some specific chromosome or chromosome segment might be trisomic. FISH also permits the exact chromosome localization of known DNA sequences including specific genes, even determining their order. For answering certain questions, study of interphase nuclei using either painting (chromosome-specific) probes or cloned gene sequences obviates the ordinary requirement of bringing cells into metaphase for identification of numerical or structural mutation. Often the use of FISH along with microscopy, Southern blotting, and polymerase chain reaction can provide minute definition of chromosome rearrangements, both constitutional ones and those in clones of neoplastic cell lineages.

Sometimes, metaphase or anaphase chromosomes are analyzed to determine whether damage to the genetic material has been induced by some environmental agent (radiation, chemical, virus), or whether constitutional genomic instability is present. Cells that have proliferated in vivo and then been incubated only briefly in vitro may be used in search of microscopically visible evidence of damage to the genetic material of a given person or of a population (e.g., Fig. 62-4). The number of chromatid gaps, breaks, and rearrangements can be estimated directly in cells reaching their first mitosis in vitro.

REFERENCES

CHAGANTI RSK, GERMAN J (eds): *Genetics in Clinical Oncology*. New York, Oxford, 1985

DE GROUCHY J, TURLEAU C: *Clinical Atlas of Human Chromosomes*, 2d ed. New York, Wiley, 1984

GERMAN JL: Studying human chromosomes today. Am Sci 58:182, 1970

GRUMBACH MM, CONTE FA: Disorders of sex differentiation, in *Williams Textbook of Endocrinology*, 8th ed, JD Wilson, DW Foster (eds). Philadelphia, Saunders, 1992, pp 853–951

SCHINZEL A: *Catalogue of Unbalanced Chromosome Aberrations*. Berlin and New York, W de Gruyter, 1983

SOLOMON E et al: Chromosome aberrations and cancer. Science 254:1153, 1991

63   GENES AND NEOPLASIA

STANLEY J. KORSMEYER

The past decade has witnessed enormous progress in understanding the genetic basis of human cancer. Cancer is nearly always of clonal origin, having originated from a single cell. Multiple genetic mutations are required for such a cell to result in a malignant tumor. Mutations that result in cancer can either be inherited in the germ line or acquired in somatic tissues. Cellular proto-oncogenes have emerged as the common targets for endogenous or exogenous events. Not infrequently, the same genes that are altered by carcinogens, radiation, or viruses also may be deregulated by translocation, amplification, or deletion.

Distinct aberrations of oncogenes are being defined for specific tumors at a rapid pace. This chapter will not attempt to provide a complete catalogue of mutations associated with human cancers. Instead, it will illustrate examples of genetic mechanisms to provide a framework for understanding developments in this field.

RNA TUMOR VIRUSES REVEAL ONCOGENES   Many malignancies of animals are transmissible. Extracts from chicken sarcomas were able to transmit the neoplasia to healthy recipients. The agent was proven to be the Rous sarcoma virus. A number of animal leukemias and carcinomas are induced within a matter of weeks by such acute transforming retroviruses. Retroviruses possess a single-stranded RNA genome. They are novel among viruses in that they

convert to a double-stranded DNA copy during their life cycle. After entry into the host cell via a cell surface receptor, the RNA template is copied into DNA by an RNA-dependent DNA polymerase known as *reverse transcriptase*. This viral DNA is efficiently integrated into the host cell's chromosomal DNA via specialized ends known as *long terminal repeats* (LTRs). LTRs are multifunctional, possessing promoter and enhancer elements as well as providing a signal for polyadenylation. The integrated DNA form of the virus is known as the *provirus*. The retroviral genome possesses genes which encode the core proteins of the viral capsid (gag), the reverse transcriptase (pol), and the viral envelope glycoproteins (env) (Fig. 63-1).

Retroviruses possessing only the gag, pol, and env genes may induce tumors but only after a long latency period. This results from *insertional activation*, whereby the integrated provirus activates a neighboring cellular gene which promotes transformation. In contrast the acute transforming retroviruses all carry a viral oncogene (v-*onc*). Often the v-*onc* gene interrupts one of the viral genes, necessitating a coinfection with a "helper virus" to provide the missing replicative machinery.

Insight into cancer pathogenesis was revolutionized by the discovery that v-*onc* genes represented copies of genes obtained from mammalian cells. The transforming element in Rous sarcoma virus, v-*src*, was shown to have originated from a normal cellular homologue in the chicken, c-*src*. v-*onc* genes lack introns, arguably because they were generated through an RNA intermediate. Moreover v-*onc* genes have been altered compared with their normal cellular counterparts in order to become transforming. They are often truncated, fused with viral proteins, or mutated. In contrast, the cellular homologues, c-*onc* genes, are correctly regulated in normal cells, where they frequently play pivotal roles in the control of cell growth and differentiation. However, it is these same c-*onc* genes that are often the sites of genetic alteration within human tumors.

THE SEARCH FOR HUMAN RETROVIRUSES   The observation that retroviruses were responsible for a number of malignancies in animals prompted an extensive search for retroviral counterparts in humans. However, only rarely have retroviruses been implicated in human tumorigenesis. The most notable exception is human T cell lymphotropic virus type I (HTLV-I), which causes adult T cell lymphoma/leukemia (ATL), an aggressive malignancy. ATL is characterized by leukemia, skin involvement, bone marrow infiltration, and hypercalcemia. A related virus, HTLV-II, was isolated from a patient with hairy cell leukemia. While the HTLVs do not possess a classic oncogene, an additional region, pX, was noted between env and the 3' LTR. This region encodes the 40-kDa tax protein that serves as a transcription factor capable of upregulating the IL-2 and IL-2 receptor genes. This may establish an autocrine loop important in the early stages of leukemogenesis. HTLV is endemic in southern Japan and the Caribbean, where the disease is more prevalent.

DNA TUMOR VIRUSES   Many DNA viruses can transform cells in culture or induce tumors in animal models. It has been more difficult to prove a causative role in humans because tumors arise during latent or persistent infection. Simian virus 40 (SV40) is a highly oncogenic virus isolated from monkeys that has proven highly instructive. SV40 encodes a transforming "early" gene product, large T antigen. Importantly large T antigen has been shown to bind to both the p53 and *Rb* tumor suppressor gene products of cellular origin. This finding has influenced the thinking concerning the pathogenic mechanism of DNA viruses implicated in human malignancies.

Epidemiologic studies have implicated papilloma virus, Epstein-Barr virus, and hepatitis B virus in human tumors. Human papilloma virus (HPV) induces condylomas and papillomas. Moreover, HPV has been implicated in cervical carcinoma in which invasive cervical cancers often contain HPV16 and 18. The *E6/E7* early genes of HPV have been mapped as the region responsible for transformation. Of interest, *E7* has been shown to interact with *Rb*, while E6 binds to p53.

Epstein-Barr virus (EBV) is a herpesvirus consistently detected in

FIGURE 63-1 Structure of a retrovirus as it would be integrated into genomic DNA as a provirus. LTR, long terminal repeats containing R, U5, U3 regulatory regions; gag, viral capsid; pol, reverse transcriptase; and env, envelope glycoproteins.

endemic Burkitt's lymphoma of Africa but in only 10 percent of sporadic cases. EBV infects B cells and is the etiologic agent of infectious mononucleosis. The virus has the ability to immortalize normal B cells in culture. EBV genome is also found in nasopharyngeal carcinomas, which are common in Southeast Asia.

Hepatitis B virus (HBV) has clearly been implicated in hepatocellular carcinoma. The acquisition of chronic infection by HBV in the Orient results in a several hundred–fold increased risk of hepatocellular carcinoma. Recent transgenic mouse models have indicated that overexpression of HBsAg results in progression to hepatocellular carcinoma.

TRANSFECTION OF TUMOR DNA IDENTIFIES ACTIVATED PRO-TO-ONCOGENES A valuable approach to detect activated oncogenes utilizes tumor DNA in a DNA-mediated gene transfer. Nonmalignant NIH3T3 mouse fibroblasts will take up exogenous DNA and incorporate portions into their own genome. DNA from chemically induced sarcomas was shown to transform NIH3T3 cells. Moreover, DNA from many human tumors also was capable of transforming these fibroblasts. Serial transfection of DNA from transformed foci enabled the isolation of a single human gene responsible for transformation. The transforming gene was often a member of the *ras* gene family. This includes the cellular homologues of viral Harvey ras (c-H-*ras*) and Kirsten ras (c-K-*ras*) as well as c-N-*ras*, which has no viral counterpart. Comparison of the DNA sequence of the transforming *ras* genes from tumors with their normal counterparts revealed an additional mechanism of tumorigenesis, somatic point mutations. Remarkably, single-base changes were noted to cluster in codons 12, 13, 59, or 61, resulting in amino acid substitutions responsible for the activation. The *ras* genes encode highly related p21^{ras} proteins that bind guanine nucleotides (GTP and GDP) and possess intrinsic GTPase activity (Fig. 63-2). Mutations which replaced gly^{12} with val^{12} or asp^{12} still retain the capacity to bind GTP but demonstrate less GTPase activity. The intrinsic GTPase activity of p21 is markedly accelerated by a GTPase-activating protein (GAP) which catalyzes the conversion of p21-GTP to p21-GDP. Oncogenic p21 molecules with mutations at position 12, 59, or 61 are resistant

to the effects of GAP. This locks the mutated ras protein in the GTP-ras activated form. While the precise role of mammalian ras proteins is under intensive scrutiny, it is known that they are located on the inner surface of the cell membrane and are similar to G proteins. This argues that ras proteins, which have been noted in some receptor complexes, may be intimately involved in the early phase of signal transduction. A wide variety of hematologic and solid tumors possess *ras* gene mutations. Mutated K-*ras* and H-*ras* are more common in cancers of epithelial origin, whereas N-*ras* mutations are noted in neural and hematologic malignancies. Mutations of *ras* genes are not a universal prerequisite for tumorigenesis. However, when present, the same alteration is found in all cells of the tumor, indicating a selective advantage. Moreover, activated *ras* genes have been noted in premalignant diseases, including myelodysplastic syndromes and adenomas of the colon, indicating that they can be an early event. In addition, the gene responsible for neurofibromatosis type 1 (NF-1) has substantial homology to the catalytic domains of GAP, suggesting an expanded role for this family in tumorigenesis.

GENE AMPLIFICATIONS IDENTIFY ONCOGENIC EVENTS Karyotypic analysis of neuroblastomas often reveals extrachromosomal double minute chromosomes or homogeneous staining regions (HSRs) within chromosomes. These regions were initially examined to determine if they bore genes involved in drug resistance. However, a survey of oncogenes indicated that the N-*myc* gene from chromosome 2 was uniformly amplified in these HSRs and double minutes. The sequence of events in amplification is felt to be an excision of a small chromosomal piece containing N-*myc* which is propagated as an extrachromosomal double minute. Later this can be randomly integrated into chromosomes resulting in HSRs.

Studies of primary tumors have indicated an important clinical correlation. Benign ganglioneuromas never have N-*myc* amplification. Low-stage neuroblastomas, generally associated with a good prognosis, have a low incidence of N-*myc* amplification (5 to 10 percent). However, those cases identified with N-*myc* amplification were destined to have rapid tumor progression similar to advanced-stage patients. *Over 30 percent of advanced-stage tumors have N-myc amplification* (Table 63-1). N-*myc* amplification appears to be an intrinsic biologic property of certain neuroblastomas, generally being present at the time of diagnosis rather than demonstrating acquisition over time.

CHROMOSOMAL TRANSLOCATIONS REVEAL NOVEL PROTO-ONCOGENES At the beginning of this century, it was proposed that chromosomal abnormalities would be the basis for malignant transformation. Since then, careful observations by cancer cytogeneticists have revealed over 125 recurrent cytogenetic abnormalities in a wide range of neoplasms. Specific interchromosomal translocations are found repeatedly within distinct types of malignancies but not their normal cellular counterparts. These sites of chromosomal breakage have proven an extremely rich source of novel proto-

FIGURE 63-2 Schematic of *ras* activation pathway and abnormalities induced by *ras* point mutation. GAP, GTPase-activating protein.

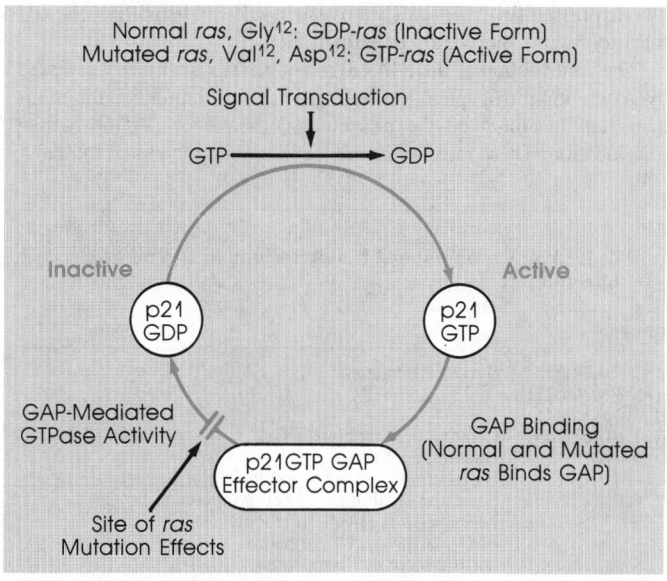

TABLE 63-1 N-*myc* copy number and stage in neuroblastoma

Stage at diagnosis	Frequency of N-*myc* amplification, %
Benign ganglioneuromas	0
Low stages (A, B; I, II)	3
Stage D-S or IVS	7
Advanced stages (C, D; II, IV)	31

SOURCE: Modified from Brodeur GM, Fong CT: Cancer Genet Cytogenet 41:153, 1989.

oncogenes integral to normal development as well as neoplasia. Of these, the best understood are the abnormalities in hematopoietic neoplasms.

The first generation of interchromosomal translocations to be characterized at a molecular level juxtaposed a known cellular oncogene, c-*myc*, with the immunoglobulin (Ig) locus in Burkitt's lymphoma (Table 63-2). A second generation of interchromosomal translocations introduces new putative proto-oncogenes into known loci. In B cell tumors this was often the immunoglobulin loci and in T cell malignancies the T cell receptor genes. The t(9;22), which generated the Philadelphia chromosome found in chronic myelogenous leukemia, serves as a prototype (see Table 63-2). This breakpoint revealed the *bcr* gene from chromosome segment 22q11 juxtaposed with the known c-*abl* gene on 9q34. Most translocations and deletions represent a third generation, and that presents the greatest challenge. The majority of chromosomal aberrations possess no certain candidate genes at either chromosomal site. Conquering these abnormalities requires new strategies that bridge the resolution gap between cytogenetics (≈5000 to 10,000 kb per band) and cosmid clones (50 kb). Yeast artificial chromosome (YAC) libraries of the human genome have permitted the isolation of large fragments containing over 1000 kb of human DNA. YACs have allowed the isolation of candidate oncogenes from the t(4;11) abnormality found in extremely aggressive mixed-lineage leukemias. Thus the technology now exists to address all these signatures of human cancer cells.

BURKITT'S LYMPHOMA JUXTAPOSES C-*MYC* WITH IMMUNO-GLOBULIN HEAVY OR LIGHT CHAIN LOCI
The most common chromosomal aberration in the B cell lymphoma of childhood, Burkitt's lymphoma, is a t(8;14) reciprocal translocation that introduces the c-*myc* proto-oncogene from 8q24 into the immunoglobulin heavy chain locus at 14q32 (Fig. 63-3). This correlation between Burkitt's translocations and immunoglobulin gene loci was substantially strengthened when variant forms of Burkitt's translocations were shown to involve the home of the κ gene locus at 2p11 or the λ genes at 22q11 (see Table 63-3).

The repositioning of c-myc next to an immunoglobulin gene markedly altered its regulatory control. Immunoglobulin genes are actively transcribed at this stage of differentiation, and the c-*myc* gene may be influenced by mechanisms that augment antibody expression.

THE t(14;18) OF FOLLICULAR LYMPHOMA REVEALS THE *bcl*-2 PROTO-ONCOGENE
The t(14;18) (q32;q21) is the most common translocation in hematologic malignancies (Table 63-3). Approximately 85 percent of follicular and 20 percent of diffuse B cell lymphomas possess this translocation. Molecular cloning of the

FIGURE 63-3 A schematic representation of the normal and reciprocally translocated chromosomes in Burkitt's lymphoma t(8;14). A normal chromosome 14 possesses an effective $V_H D_H J_H$ and $C\mu$ responsible for the IgM produced. The normal chromosome 8 retains a nonexpressed copy of c-*myc*. The 14q+ chromosome has received a portion of chromosome 8 bearing the c-*myc* gene. The 8q− chromosome breaks at 8q24 and receives part of chromosome 14, often including some V_H genes.

t(14;18) breakpoint revealed a putative proto-oncogene, *bcl*-2, at 18q21. Despite the mature B cell phenotype of lymphomas bearing t(14;18), the translocation appears to occur earlier in development at a pre-B cell stage. Immunoglobulin recombinase initiates the first attempt at rearrangement in pre-B development by cleaving at a D and J immunoglobulin segment (Fig. 63-4). Instead of completing that recombination, however, progenitor cells of follicular lymphoma introduce a broken *bcl*-2 gene from 18q21 into these sites.

The cloning of this second-generation breakpoint provided a new gene, *bcl*-2, which demonstrates the novel function of blocking programmed cell death (apoptosis) rather than promoting proliferation. Overexpressed *bcl*-2 prevents apoptosis in selected hematopoietic cell lines following deprivation of growth factors.

The contribution of the t(14;18) to neoplasia was directly assessed by generating transgenic mice bearing a *bcl*-2–immunoglobulin mini-gene that recapitulated the molecular consequences of the human translocation. These mice uniformly developed a polyclonal follicular

---

TABLE 63-2 Chromosomal translocations in lymphomas and leukemias

Candidate genes on both sides of breakpoint

	14q32	8q24
Burkitt's lymphoma t(8;14)	Ig H chain	c-*myc*

Candidate gene on one side, new gene on the other

	14q32	18q21
Follicular lymphoma t(14;18)	Ig H chain	*bcl*-2

	14q11	11p15, 11p13, 10q24
T acute lymphoblastic leukemia	α/δTCR	*ttg*-1, *ttg*-2, *Hox11*
Chronic myelogenous leukemia	9q34	22q11
Ph acute lymphoblastic leukemia	c-*abl*	*bcr*

No certain candidate gene on either side of breakpoint

	11q23	4q21
Mixed lineage leukemia t(4;11)	MLL	AF4

TABLE 63-3 Chromosomal translocations in B lymphoid neoplasms

Chromosomes	Neoplasm	Gene
t(8;14)(q24;q32) t(8;22)(q24;q11) t(2;8)(p11;q24)	Burkitt's lymphoma	*myc*
t(11;14)(q13;q32)	Centrocytic lymphoma (Kiel classification) B cell chronic lymphocytic leukemia	*bcl*-1 (*PRAD*-1)
t(14;18)(q32;q21)	Follicular small cleaved cell lymphoma Follicular mixed cell lymphoma Follicular large cell lymphoma Diffuse large cell lymphoma	*bcl*-2

FIGURE 63-4 Mechanisms of the t(14;18) recombination. Der(14) chromosomes have breakpoints at J segments, while der(18) breakpoints involve D segments. This indicates that the translocation occurs at a pre-B cell stage following endonucleolytic cleavage at a D and J segment by immunoglobulin recombinase. Such ends illegitimately recombine with a double-stranded DNA break in the major breakpoint region (MBR) of *bcl-2* exon III at 18q21.

lymphoproliferation that selectively expanded small resting B cells. These recirculating B cells accumulate as a result of extended survival rather than increased proliferation. Like patients with follicular lymphoma, these mice progress from indolent follicular hyperplasia to diffuse large cell lymphoma. This satisfies a molecular Koch's postulate for the t(14;18) in B cell lymphoma. Moreover, they also indicate that prolonged cell survival is oncogenic. Thus *bcl-2* represents the first member of a new category of oncogenes, regulators of programmed cell death. Extended cell survival may prove to be a key event in carcinogenesis that enables the acquisition of further genetic changes (Fig. 63-5).

CLL, CENTROCYTIC LYMPHOMA, AND THE *bcl-1* GENE, CYCLIN D1. One of the first interchromosomal breakpoints to be cloned was t(11;14) (q13;q32), first noted in a handful of B cell type chronic lymphocytic leukemias (CLLs). Once again, the immunoglobulin locus at 14q32 had recombined with a region on chromosome segment 11q13 entitled the *bcl-1* locus. However certain intermediate-grade lymphomas, especially the centrocytic B cell lymphomas of the Kiel classification, have a much higher incidence (30 to 50 percent) of *bcl-1* rearrangement. In parallel, a number of parathyroid adenomas bear clonal rearrangements of their phenotypic landmark gene, parathyroid hormone (PTH). This proved to be a translocation with 11q13 that overexpressed a newly identified gene located there, *PRAD-1* (parathyroid adenomatosis). *PRAD-1* encodes a novel cyclin that is expressed in the G_1 phase of the cell cycle and has been named *cyclin D1*. Cyclins regulate cell cycle transitions, and D cyclins appear to interact with a kinase protein (cdk) as well as Rb, the retinoblastoma gene product (Fig. 63-6). Cyclin D1 appears to be the *bcl-1* gene, since it is also deregulated in B cell tumors t(11;14). This

FIGURE 63-5 Alternative pathways to neoplasia. Normal tissue homeostasis represents a balanced equation between input (cell proliferation) and output (cell death). Considerable evidence indicates that an increase in proliferation can lead to neoplasia. Studies of *bcl-2* indicate that a decrease in the rate of cell death is also tumorigenic.

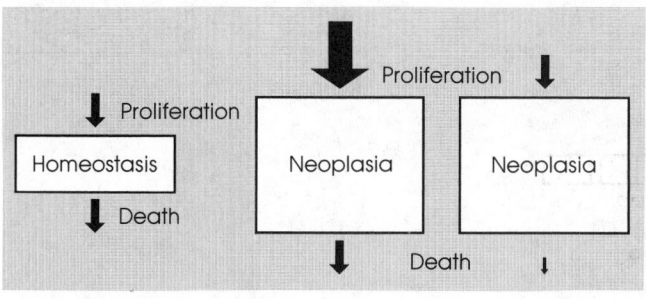

gene provides an avenue to determine how a cyclin which appears to act at the G_1–S boundary influences cell growth and neoplasia.

TWO MOLECULAR FORMS OF THE PHILADELPHIA CHROMO-SOME IN CML AND ALL (See also Chaps. 309 and 310) The description in 1960 of the Philadelphia chromosome in chronic but not acute myelogenous leukemia initiated the field of cancer cytogenetics. The Philadelphia chromosome, Ph, is present in virtually all patients with chronic myelogenous leukemia (CML) and in approximately 25 percent of adults and 5 percent of children with acute lymphoblastic leukemia (ALL). CML is a disease of a multipotential hematopoietic stem cell in which multiple lineages including myeloid, erythroid, lymphoid, and megakaryocytic are affected. ALLs with Ph are of pre-B cell type. The t(9;22) (q34;q11) was found to involve c-*abl* on 9q34 and a limited region on 22q11 designated the *breakpoint cluster region* (bcr). Later this was shown to be part of a gene that spans over 90 kilobases. The molecular consequence of the t(9;22) is to generate a fusion gene between 5' *bcr* sequences and 3' *abl* sequences on the Ph chromosome. This results in a chimeric peptide that is part *bcr* and part *abl* (Fig. 63-7).

The breakpoints within the *bcr* gene at 22q11 are focused in two areas. The original breakpoint cluster region is within the heart of the *bcr* gene. This is where nearly all cases of CML break and results in a 8.5-kb *bcr-abl* fusion RNA and a fusion protein of p210 (210 kDa) size. In contrast, many ALLs break far upstream within the first intron of the *bcr* gene. This creates a smaller 7.0-kb fusion RNA and p190 fusion protein. Clinical studies indicate that Ph-positive ALL has a much worse prognosis than the Ph-negative ALL. Moreover, Ph-positive adult ALL can possess either the p210 form ($\approx$40 percent of cases) or the p190 form ($\approx$60 percent). The capacity of the p210 and p190 forms of the hybrid *bcr-abl* proteins to transform cells correlates with their augmented tyrosine kinase activity. Moreover, animal models bearing the p210 or p190 forms of *bcr-abl* develop leukemia. As the human disease first suggested, the molecular forms of *bcr-abl* may predetermine the type of disease. While it is not absolute, the p190 form appears to favor acute pre-B cell leukemia, whereas the p210 form favors a chronic stem cell leukemia.

T CELL TRANSLOCATIONS REDIRECT TRANSCRIPTION FAC-TORS The most frequent interchromosomal translocations within T cell neoplasms also involve their antigen receptor genes. Chromosome segment 14q11, the home of the α/δ TCR, is most frequently involved, but translocations into the β TCR locus at 7q34 are also noted. Analysis of transcripts from the other participating chromosome has proven rewarding. While TCR loci are involved on one side, a large number of different chromosomal partners participate on the far side. Characterization of six separate proto-oncogene candidates indicates that they belong to classic transcription factor families principally intended for lineages other than T cells. This includes *ttg-1*, *ttg-2*,

FIGURE 63-6 Schematic presentation of the role of the retinoblastoma protein Rb in the regulation of cell cycle. Rb is progressively phosphorylated during cell cycle progression. Underphosphorylated Rb is active in inhibiting proliferation and interacts with the E2F transcription factor, which is displaced by the viral oncogene products E1A, T antigen (TAg), and E7. Rb also may complex with the highly regulated cyclin proteins and cyclin-dependent kinases (cdks). Inactive Rb is hyperphosphorylated, which appears to displace a number of these interacting proteins.

scl, *tal*-2, and *lyl*-1. *HOX11* completes this group. Redirected expression of these transcription factors to the thymus results in T cell lymphoblastic lymphoma/leukemia. These aberrantly expressed products may substitute for homologues in T cells or inappropriately activate a gene program intended for another cell type.

EWING'S SARCOMA: SOLID TUMORS ALSO POSSESS RECIPROCAL TRANSLOCATIONS Highly recurrent interchromosomal translocations are not restricted to hematopoietic neoplasms. Ewing's sarcoma and related subsets of primitive neuroectodermal tumors bear a reciprocal translocation t(11;22) (q24;q12). Molecular cloning of the breakpoint has revealed the generation of a chimeric protein with the *fli*-1 proto-oncogene, a member of the *ets* family of oncogenes, located at 11q24.

TUMOR SUPPRESSOR GENES: THE RETINOBLASTOMA MODEL A class of cancer-related genes exists which suppresses tumorigenesis and contributes to neoplasia in a recessive manner. It has been noted that transfer of a single normal chromosome into certain tumor cells can suppress their tumorigenicity. For example,

a normal chromosome 11 will suppress the malignant behavior of a Wilms' tumor cell. These observations prompted the thesis that the absence or functional loss of such chromosomes would result in unchecked growth. Definitive data that indicated the existence of tumor suppressor genes were provided by several inherited forms of cancer, retinoblastoma and Wilms' tumor. Knudson advanced the "two hit" hypothesis to explain such pediatric tumors that occurred in families. In familial retinoblastoma he proposed that one mutation is present in the germ line while the second allele is altered in somatic development. In sporadic cases of retinoblastoma, both mutational events would occur in the retinal lineage cells. This accounts for the fact that familial retinoblastoma occurs at an earlier age and is typically bilateral.

Evidence for a recessive mechanism in retinoblastoma was first provided by cytogenetics in which deletions of the long arm of chromosome 13, 13q14, were noted in normal as well as tumor cells of some patients. This prompted the use of polymorphic genetic markers mapped to 13q14 to search for more refined losses in other

FIGURE 63-7 *c-abl* and *bcr* genes in CML and ALL. Normal genomic *c-abl* gene at 9q24; sites of breakpoints noted. Normal genomic *bcr* gene at 22q11; sites of ALL versus CML breakpoints noted. Two species of fusion RNAs, CML (8.5 kb) versus ALL (7.0 kb).

FIGURE 63-8 Schematic of the genetic mechanisms observed for the loss of heterozygosity in the *Rb* gene in familial retinoblastoma. *(Adapted from Cavenee et al, Nature 305, 780, 1983.)*

cases. These studies revealed a loss of heterozygosity for polymorphic DNA markers at 13q14 in tumor cells versus normal cells of patients. Loss of heterozygosity can occur by a number of genetic mechanisms (Fig. 63-8). While the second allele may be altered by a spontaneous mutation, other events are more common, including chromosomal nondisjunction, nondisjunction with duplication, mitotic recombination, and gene conversion. The loss of heterozygosity for a genetic marker has become the hallmark of a potential tumor suppressor gene.

The mapping of the locus to 13q24 soon led to the isolation of the retinoblastoma (*Rb*) gene. *Rb* encodes a 105-kDa nuclear phosphoprotein that has protein-protein interaction properties (see Fig. 63-6). The underphosphorylated form of *Rb* predominates in the G_1 phase of the cell cycle, whereas *Rb* is progressively phosphorylated toward the S phase. The underphosphorylated active form of Rb complexes with the E2F transcription factor, whereas the heavy phosphorylated inactive form of Rb releases E2F. Of note, the DNA viral oncoproteins T antigen of SV40, E1A of adenovirus, and E7 of the human papilloma virus all bind Rb and displace E2F. The loss of *Rb* protein results in neoplastic transformation and unregulated cell growth. Proof that the *Rb* gene was the responsible tumor suppressor gene was obtained when normal *Rb* was reintroduced into tumor cells and cell growth was arrested at the G_1 stage of the cell cycle.

WILMS' TUMOR AND THE INACTIVATION OF TUMOR SUPPRESSOR GENES Wilms' tumor is an embryonal malignancy of the kidney that represents the most common abdominal malignancy of childhood. Documented familial transmission is rare (≈ 10 percent), but 10 percent of Wilms' tumors present with bilateral disease. The mapping of genes involved in Wilms' tumor was advanced by the analysis of patients with associated congenital anomalies. Children with the WAGR syndrome (Wilms' tumor, aniridia, genitourinary abnormalities, and mental retardation) had overlapping deletions of chromosome segment 11p13. Molecular dissection of this common region of deletion yielded the *WT1* gene. *WT1* is a zinc finger containing transcription factor that interacts with a specific DNA motif. This DNA sequence is also recognized by other transcription factors involved in early growth response. This observation suggests how *WT1* might compete for target genes and function as a tumor suppressor. Initial studies had shown loss of heterozygosity for polymorphic DNA markers on 11p in sporadic cases of Wilms' tumor. Mutations have been documented for the *WT1* gene within sporadic Wilms' tumor. Moreover, germ-line mutations have been noted in cases with bilateral tumors.

The genetics of Wilms' tumor is complex, and loci beyond *WT1* are also implicated. The Beckwith-Wiedeman syndrome is characterized by congenital anomalies of macroglossia, hemihypertro-

phy, organomegaly, and an increased incidence of Wilms' tumor, adrenocortical carcinoma, and hepatoblastoma. Genetic linkage and cytogenetics have mapped the Beckwith-Wiedeman locus to 11p15. Moreover, some sporadic cases of Wilms' tumor demonstrate loss of heterozygosity of 11p15. In addition, evidence exists for differential imprinting of the parental genes at 11p15 in both Beckwith-Wiedeman syndrome and Wilms' tumor. It is believed that only the maternal or paternal copy is expressed, a phenomenon known as *parental imprinting*. Studies of Wilms' tumors suggest that mutations may be selective for the paternal chromosome, while the maternal allele may be prone to loss. Details of this differential regulation await the isolation of a putative *WT* gene at 11p15.

Familial cases of Wilms' tumor further emphasize the genetic complexity of this single disease. Genetic linkage analysis of several large pedigrees with multiple cases of Wilms' tumor excluded 11p13 and 11p15 as the sites of inherited susceptibility. Thus evidence exists that at least three genes can participate in the genesis of Wilms' tumor.

LI-FRAUMENI SYNDROME AND THE p53 GENE IN CANCER Mutation or loss of the p53 gene is the most common genetic alteration found in human cancer. p53 was first noted as a cellular origin protein that associated with T antigen in SV40-transformed cells. Reminiscent of the *Rb* tumor suppressor gene, p53 is also inactivated by the E1B product of adenovirus and the E6 oncoprotein of human papilloma virus. Indeed p53 was often found at much higher levels in tumor cells. This was demonstrated to reflect a marked prolongation of its normally short protein half-life. In fact, p53 was initially classified as a dominant-acting oncogene since an isolated p53 cDNA would cooperate with other oncogenes to transform cells. However, the transforming clones of p53 proved to be mutants. Subsequently, the wild-type form of p53 has been shown to suppress the transformation of cells. Reintroduction of wild-type p53 into tumor cells that had lost the gene arrested their growth by blocking the cell cycle at the G_1–S transition. p53 also had been shown to interact with other endogenous cellular proteins and to bind DNA. Those proteins include the heat shock protein Hsc70 as well as *mdm*2, a probable oncogene that is amplified in certain tumors. Thus p53 has emerged as a most important DNA-binding protein that regulates cell cycle progression at the G_1–S boundary.

Perhaps 5 to 10 percent of common cancers, including breast, ovarian, and colon cancer, cluster in families, reflecting an underlying genetic susceptibility. One of the best detailed familial cancer syndromes is the rare autosomal dominant Li-Fraumeni syndrome (LFS). Affected families have a high incidence of very diverse childhood and adult tumors. The spectrum includes breast carcinoma, soft tissue sarcomas, brain tumors, osteosarcomas, leukemia, and adrenocortical carcinoma. Germ-line p53 mutations have been found in at least five such Li-Fraumeni families studied. Inherited mutations are found in the heterozygous state in normal cells which predispose them to the development of cancer.

Mutations in the regions of p53 conserved by evolution are exceptionally common in a wide variety of sporadic human tumors. Loss of heterozygosity for markers on 17p or loss of p53 itself is common in cancer cells. In colon cancer studies have revealed loss of wild-type p53 alleles by either deletion or point mutation in 75 to 80 percent of cases. Missense point mutations are the most frequent p53 gene mutation. Of interest, these mutations are clustered in four limited regions of the protein that constitute functional domains. Experimental studies indicate that such mutated p53 alleles can function as dominant negatives that outcompete any wild-type p53 protein. p53 alterations are widespread in cancer of the colon, lung, esophagus, breast, liver, brain, and hematopoietic lineages. Thus p53 has emerged as a rather global regulator of cell growth with a prominent role in a wide spectrum of human cancers.

MULTISTEP BASIS OF CANCER While individual oncogenes have distinct effects on tumorigenesis, multiple events are usually required before a single cell is fully transformed. Transformation of embryonic fibroblasts requires the cooperation of two oncogenes. Epidemiologic studies of human cancer indicate an age-dependent tumor incidence that argues for multiple independent steps. Cytogenetic data indicate that many tumors acquire further chromosomal alterations with progression of the disease. This reflects a clonal evolution in which the most malignant cells are selected.

Detailed analysis of the molecular aberrations in colorectal carcinoma has provided the clearest evidence for the multistep progression of human cancer. Colon tumorigenesis represents a progression from benign adenomas to highly metastatic carcinoma (see Chap. 257). Approximately 10 percent of small adenomas and roughly half of

large adenomas possess a mutated *ras* gene, usually K-*ras*. Overall, alteration of at least four to five genes may often be required for the generation of malignant colon tumor. These reflect mutational activation of oncogenes together with the inactivation of tumor suppressor genes (Fig. 63-9). The chromosomes that are most frequently deleted include 5q, 17p, and 18q. Proven or candidate tumor suppressor genes have been isolated from each site. This includes the familial adenomatous polyposis (FAP) gene at 5q responsible for the hyperproliferative epithelium in these predisposed patients and also noted to be altered in sporadic examples of colon carcinoma. p53 appears to be the principal gene participating on 17p. The deleted in colon carcinoma (DCC) gene that resembles an adhesion molecule is the candidate recessive oncogene from 18q. Losses of 17p and 18q often occur in later stages of tumorigenesis. However, there is no strict order, and the accumulation of defects appears more critical than the order of events. Recently, a predisposition to colon cancer has been shown to be linked to a gene on chromosome 2. Most familial (nonpolyposis) colon cancers and 13 percent of sporadic colon cancers have mutations in this gene. These mutations are associated with widespread alterations in short (dinucleotide) repeat sequences throughout the genome, suggesting that numerous replication errors occurred during tumor development. Thus these cancers develop by a mechanism of genetic instability rather than by classic tumor suppressor genes.

The enormous progress in defining the sequential genetic events in carcinogenesis holds great promise and challenge for the future. Understanding changes that are inherited or acquired may enable the identification of environmental contributions and lead to preventive steps. Pinpointing the precise biochemical effect of each of these genetic changes should ultimately refine therapeutic approaches as well.

REFERENCES

Bishop JM: Viral oncogenes. Cell 42:23, 1985
Fearon ER, Vogelstein B: A genetic model for colorectal tumorigenesis. Cell 61:759, 1990
Levine AJ et al: The p53 tumour suppressor gene. Nature 351:453, 1991
McCormick F: GTPase-activating protein: Signal transmitter and signal terminator. Cell 56:5, 1989
Mitelman F: *Cancer Cytogenetics.* New York, Liss, 1987
Rabbitts TH: Translocations, master genes, and differences between the origins of acute and chronic leukemias. Cell 67:644, 1991
Rowley JD: Identification of the constant chromosome regions involved in human hematologic malignant disease. Science 216:749, 1982
Weinberg RA: Tumor suppressor genes. Science 254:1138, 1991

FIGURE 63-9 Genetic changes depicted for stages of progression in colorectal tumorigenesis. Not shown are gene mutations on chromosome 2 that lead to colon cancer by causing replication errors throughout the genome. *(After Fearon and Vogelstein.)*

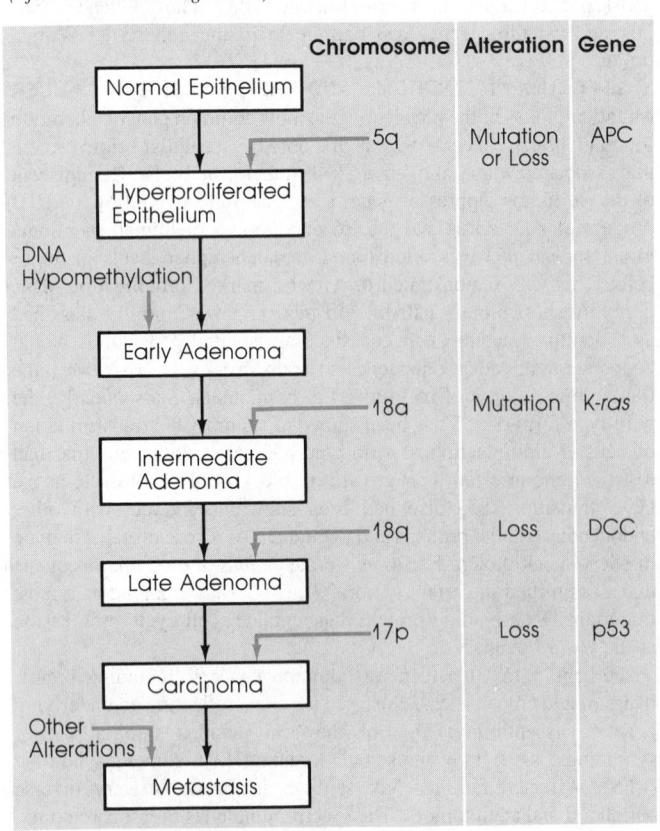

	Chromosome	Alteration	Gene
Normal Epithelium			
	5q	Mutation or Loss	APC
Hyperproliferated Epithelium			
DNA Hypomethylation			
Early Adenoma			
	18a	Mutation	K-ras
Intermediate Adenoma			
	18q	Loss	DCC
Late Adenoma			
	17p	Loss	p53
Carcinoma			
Other Alterations			
Metastasis			

64 THE MAJOR HISTOCOMPATIBILITY GENE COMPLEX

CHARLES B. CARPENTER

Antigenic differences between members of a species are called *alloantigens*, and when these play a determining role in the rejection of allogeneic tissue grafts, they are called *histocompatibility antigens*. Evolution has conserved a single closely linked region of histocompatibility genes, the products of which are prominently displayed on cell surfaces and provide a strong barrier to allotransplantation. The terms *major histocompatibility antigens* and *major histocompatibility gene complex* (MHC) refer to the gene products and genes of this chromosomal region. Their principal function is to bind peptide fragments so that they are optimally presented to T lymphocytes for recognition. Many minor histocompatibility antigens, in contrast, are encoded throughout the genome. They represent weaker allotypic differences on molecules that serve a variety of functions. Structures

FIGURE 64-1   Schematic representation of human chromosome 6 showing the location of the HLA region in the 21 region of the short arm. The HLA-A, HLA-B, and HLA-C loci encode class I heavy chains (44,000 Da), while the beta$_2$-microglobulin light chain (11,500 Da) of the class I molecule is encoded by genes of chromosome 15. HLA-D region (class II) is centromeric to the A, B, and C loci, with genes for closely linked complement components C4A, C4B, Bf, and C2 in the B–D region. Two genes for tumor necrosis factor (TNFα,β) also lie between HLA-B and the complement genes. The order of the complement genes is uncertain. Additional loci shown are P for the proteosome (LMP) and T for the peptide transporter (TAP) genes and the Hsp$_{70}$ heat-shock protein gene. Each D region class II molecule is made up

of an α and β chain (their genes are written as A and B). They appear on the cell surface in distinct heterodimers, DP, DQ, and DR. The numbers following A or B indicate that there are different genes for the chains of a given set; e.g., for DR, there are 9 β-chain genes (three are shown). The expressed molecule may be β1α(B1A) or β3α(B3A), for example. The β2 gene is not expressed (pseudogene). The antigens DR51, DR52, and DR53 are on the expressed B5, B3, and B4 chains, respectively, while the other DR antigens are on B1. DRA is not polymorphic, while the molecules bearing the DQ antigens have polymorphism in both A1 and B1 chains. DQA2 and DQB2 are pseudogenes. Polymorphism in DP is greater for B1 than for A1. The overall length of the HLA region is about 3 cM (3400 kilobases).

bearing MHC antigens play a major role in immunity and in self-recognition in the differentiation of cells and tissues. Much of the evidence for MHC control of the immune response comes from work in animal models in which immune-response genes have been mapped within the mouse (H-2), rat (RT1), and guinea pig (GPLA) MHC. In humans, the MHC is called *HLA*. The individual letters of HLA have various meanings, and by international agreement HLA is the logo for the human MHC.

Several generalizations can be made about the MHCs. *First*, three classes of gene products are encoded within the 4-kilobase region of the MHC. Class I molecules, expressed on virtually all cell surfaces, consist of one heavy and one light polypeptide chain and are the products of three reduplicated loci: HLA-A, HLA-B, and HLA-C. Class II molecules, restricted in expression to B lymphocytes, some monocytes, and activated T lymphocytes, consist of two polypeptide chains (α and β) of unequal length and are the products of several closely linked genes, collectively termed the HLA-D region. Class III molecules are the C4, C2, and Bf components of complement. *Second*, class I and class II molecules form complexes with immunogenic peptides (e.g., from bacteria or viruses), and they are conjointly recognized by T lymphocytes having appropriate antigen receptors. Selection of the T cell receptor repertoire occurs during development in the thymus, where various self-peptide + MHC combinations promote survival or elimination of T cell clones. Self versus nonself discrimination in the initiation and effector phase of the immune response is thereby intimately directed by class I and II molecules. *Third*, genes for enzyme systems having no apparent relationship to immunity are located in the region of the MHC, as are genes of importance in skeletal growth and development. *Fourth*, genes for tumor necrosis factors TNFα and TNFβ, heat-shock protein (Hsp$_{70}$), and peptide processing and transport lie also within the MHC. Loci of the HLA region on the short arm of chromosome 6 are shown in Fig. 64-1.

LOCI OF THE HLA SYSTEM   Class I antigens   HLA antigens of the class I type are defined serologically by human sera, principally from multiparous females, and to a limited extent by monoclonal antibodies. They are present in varying densities in most body tissues, including B cells, T cells, and platelets, but not in mature red blood cells. The number of serologically defined specificities is large, and the HLA system is the most polymorphic genetic system known in humans. Three clearly defined loci are recognized within the HLA complex for class I, serologically defined (SD), HLA antigens. Each class I antigen consists of an 11,500-Da beta$_2$-microglobulin subunit and a 44,000-Da heavy chain that carries the antigenic specificities

(Fig. 64-2). There are over 80 clearly defined A and B specificities, and 10 C-locus specificities are known. Antigens of the major complex are prefixed by HLA, but this may be omitted when the context is clear. The number following the locus designation is the name of the antigen. HLA antigens of African, Asian, and Oceanic peoples include many of the antigens commonly found in people of western European ancestry. However, the distribution of HLA antigens is distinctive for certain racial groups and can serve as anthropologic markers in the study of migration patterns and diseases.

Since chromosomes are paired, each individual has six serologically defined HLA-A, HLA-B, and HLA-C antigens, three from each parent. Each of these chromosomal sets is termed a *haplotype*, and

FIGURE 64-2   Schematic representation of class I and class II molecules on the cell surface. Class I molecules are composed of two polypeptide chains. The 44,000-Da heavy chain passes through the plasma membrane. Its external portion consists of three domains (α$_1$, α$_2$, α$_3$) formed by disulfide bonding. The beta$_2$-microglobulin (β$_{2μ}$) light chain (11,500 Da) encoded by chromosome 15 is noncovalently bound to the heavy chain. Amino acid sequence homology among class I molecules is 80 to 85 percent, falling to 50 percent or less in portions of α$_1$ and α$_2$ which represent the sites of alloantigenic polymorphism. Class II molecules consist of two noncovalently associated polypeptide chains, a 34,000-Da α and a 29,000-Da β. Each chain has two domains formed by disulfide bridging (the α$_1$ domain lacks a sulfide bridge). (*From Carpenter and Strom.*)

Haplotypes:
a = A1, Cw3, B8, Dw3
b = A29, Cw4, B35, Dw1
a_r = A1, Cw3, B8, Dw1
b_r = A29, Cw4, B35, Dw3

Inheritance:

ab x cd

ac   ad   bc   bd

FIGURE 64-3 HLA region, chromosome 6: inheritance of HLA haplotypes. Each chromosomal segment of linked genes is termed a *haplotype*, and each individual inherits one haplotype from each parent. The A, B, C, and D antigens of haplotypes a and b are shown for this hypothetical individual in chromosomal order on the diagram and also below as they would be written in text. If individual ab were to marry cd, their offspring would be of four types only, as far as HLA is concerned. Occasionally (*dashed cross*) recombination occurs in the germ line (meiosis) of a parent, resulting in an altered haplotype. The frequency of recombinant children is a measure of the map distance (1 percent recombination frequency = 1 cM; see Fig. 64-1). (*From CB Carpenter, Kidney Int, 14:283, 1978.*)

by simple Mendelian inheritance, one-fourth of siblings have identical haplotypes, one-half share a haplotype, and the remaining one-fourth are completely incompatible (Fig. 64-3). Evidence that this gene complex plays the major role in the transplantation response comes from the fact that haplotype-matched sibling donor-recipient combinations show excellent results in kidney transplantation, in the vicinity of 85 to 90 percent long-term survival (see Chap. 238).

Class II antigens The HLA-D region is separated from the class I loci on the short arm of chromosome 6 by 1000 kilobases (see Fig. 64-1). This region encodes a series of class II molecules, each consisting of a 29,000-Da β chain and a 34,000-Da α chain (see Fig. 64-2). Incompatibility for this region, particularly concerning the DR antigens, determines the in vitro proliferative response of lymphocytes to mismatched haplotypes. This mixed lymphocyte response (MLR) is assessed by the degree of proliferation of a *mixed lymphocyte culture* (MLC) and is positive even when HLA-A, HLA-B, and HLA-C antigens are identical (see Fig. 64-3). When parental recombination has occurred between HLA-B and -DR, for example, a new haplotype appears in the child, who will be identical for class I but different for class II (a versus a_r in Fig. 64-3). HLA-D antigens are defined by reference-stimulating lymphocytes that are homozygous for HLA-D and are inactivated by x-irradiation or mitomycin C to make the reaction unidirectional. There are 26 such antigens recognized by homozygous typing cells.

Attempts to define HLA-D by serology first established a series of D-related (DR) antigens expressed on class II molecules of B lymphocytes, monocytes, and activated T lymphocytes. Macrophages, dendritic cells, and skin Langerhans cells are also class II–positive. Other closely related antigen systems were soon discovered and given various local names (MB, MT, DC, SB), which have been replaced by subregion names DR, DQ, and DP. The separate identity of these sets of class II molecules is now established, and the genes for their respective α and β chains have been isolated and sequenced. There are 24 DR, 9 DQ, and 6 DP antigens recognized by serology. The class II gene map shown in Fig. 64-1 describes a minimal number of genes and molecular sets. Although a class II molecule may be composed of a DQα (DQA1 gene) from one parental haplotype and a DQβ (DQB1 gene) from the other parent (transcomplementation), α and β combinations outside each DP, DQ, DR set rarely, if ever, occur. DR, and to some extent DQ, molecules provide the stimuli for the primary mixed lymphocyte response. The secondary MLR is called the *primed lymphocyte test* (PLT) and occurs rapidly over 24 to 36 h instead of 6 to 7 days. DP alloantigens were discovered from their ability to provide PLT stimulation, although they do not

contribute much to a primary MLR. DQ and DP molecules also can be identified serologically. While B lymphocytes and activated T lymphocytes express all three sets of class II molecules, DQ antigens are not expressed on 60 to 90 percent of monocytes, which are virtually all DP- and DR-positive.

Three-dimensional structure of HLA X-ray diffraction studies of HLA class I molecules show a groove or cleft on the surface facing away from the cell membrane with dimensions sufficient to bind a peptide fragment 8 to 15 amino acids long. In fact, class I molecules usually bind sequences of 9 amino acids. The margins of the binding site are formed by α helices, and the base is floored by eight antiparallel β strands, with the α1 and α2 domains contributing equally to each side of the structure (Fig. 64-4). The HLA variable regions which are recognized by alloantibodies or cytotoxic T cells lie along the α helices that form the margins of the groove. When the bound materials released by acidification of redissolved HLA class I crystals were analyzed by HPLC, hundreds of different peptides were found. Of those analyzed further, a 9 amino acid length and a binding consensus motif at positions 2 and 9 were characteristic. Although class II molecules have yet to be studied to the same resolution, preliminary results suggest a similar groove formed by the α1 and β1 domains, and the known sequence polymorphisms also lie along the presumed location of the groove. It is likely that virtually all MHC molecules come to the surface of the cell with a peptide in place. In the case of class I, the pathway is primarily one of selection of peptides endogenous to the cell (e.g., from intracellular viral infection), and for class II, the pathway is primarily an exogenous one which processes endocytosed or pinocytosed polypeptides. The latter function is classically performed by macrophages, but any cell which expresses class II MHC (e.g., B lymphocytes, epithelial cells) can serve as an antigen-presenting cell (APC). The phenomenon of MHC restriction, which requires the T cell to recognize both self-MHC and antigen, can now be viewed as the function of a single T cell receptor that binds to the surface formed by both α-helical sides of the HLA groove and peptide lying within it. Some of the MHC polymorphisms, those on the inner surfaces of the helices and on the floor of the groove, are not accessible in the presence of bound peptide; hence the polymorphisms serve to bind the peptide fragments having a certain sequence motif.

Molecular genetics Each polypeptide chain of class I and class II molecules bears several polymorphic sites in addition to the "private" antigen defined by alloantisera. In the *cell-mediated lympholysis* (CML) test, the specificity of killer T cells (T_c), which arise during the proliferative events in MLR, is determined by testing on target cells from donors other than those providing the MLR stimulus. Antigen systems defined by this method show a close but imperfect correlation with class I private antigens. Cloning of cytotoxic cells has revealed the presence of a variety of polymorphic target determinants on HLA molecules, some of which are identifiable by alloantisera or monoclonal antibodies derived from immunization of mice with human cells. Some of these reagents can be used to identify private determinants of HLA, while others are directed to more "public" (sometimes called *supertypic*) determinants. One such system of public HLA-B antigens has two alleles, Bw4 and Bw6. Most HLA-B private antigens are associated with either Bw4 or Bw6. Other systems are restricted to subsets of HLA antigen groups. For example, HLA-B–bearing heavy chains carry additional sites that are common to B7, B27, B22, and B40 or to B5, B15, B18, and B35. Other types of shared antigenic determinants exist, as exemplified by a monoclonal antibody which reacts with a site shared between HLA-A and HLA-B heavy chains.

The amino acid sequence and peptide maps of several HLA molecules show that the class I hypervariable regions are clustered in the peptide-binding region of the outer α1 domain (see Fig. 64-2) and the adjacent portion of α2. Variability in the sequences of class II molecules also differs in a similar manner. Remarkably, the class I α3 domain, the class II α2 and β2 domains, and the portions of the CD8 (T8, Leu 2) cell surface molecule that function in T cell

FIGURE 64-4 Structure of the HLA class I molecule as determined by x-ray crystallography. *A.* Shown is the face of the HLA-A2 molecule that points away from the cell surface. This ribbon diagram shows the groove that is formed by two α helices and is supported by a floor of eight β strands. N is the amino terminal of the α_1 domain; the two small circles represent a disulfide bond. (*From PA Bjorkman et al.*) *B.* Composite display of polymorphic sites from several human and mouse class I alleles using the HLA-A2 structure as the model. The symbols show a composite of the polymorphisms along the groove. Localization of variable amino acids and/or sites for alloantibody and/or cytotoxic T cell recognition is shown to be along the α helices (*circles*). Polymorphic sites exist also in the β strands (*squares*). The numbers indicate the amino acid sequence. (*After PA Bjorkman et al.*)

interactions, as well as the T cell receptor (TCR) itself, are all considered members of the immunoglobulin supergene family because of significant amino acid sequence homologies with immunoglobulin constant regions (see Chap. 277). These findings suggest evolutionary elaboration within a family of gene products that have immune recognition functions. When genomic DNA for HLA is examined, typical exon-intron sequences of DNA have been found for class I and class II, exons having been identified for signal peptides (5′), each of the domains, a transmembrane hydrophobic segment, and a cytoplasmic segment (3′). cDNA probes are available for most of the HLA chains, and enzymatic digests have been used to study patterns of *restriction fragment length polymorphisms* (RFLP), many of which correlate with class II serologic and MLR patterns. There are 20 to 30 class I genes, however, making assessment of polymorphism by RFLP difficult. Many of these genes are not expressed (pseudogenes), while some could represent additional class I loci that are expressed only on activated T cells and are of uncertain function. Tissue typing by the detection of variable nucleotide sequences begins with the polymerase chain reaction (PCR) technique to amplify specific segments of DNA, as defined by oligonucleotide primers, from genomic DNA obtained from a small sample of blood or tissue. The primers are usually locus-specific (e.g., the β1 chain of HLA-DR) or may be allele-specific (e.g., amplifying only genes having a particular polymorphic sequence). The products are then analyzed by hybridization with sequence-specific labeled probes or by RFLP analysis of the amplified DNA. The technique has already demonstrated ability to identify sequences in the human population in a more accurate fashion than with the established serologic technique. The official HLA nomenclature has been changed to reflect the definition of distinct sequences and to document the presence of polymorphisms not clearly understood from the definitions of classical serology (e.g., an HLA-DQ molecule is made up of both α and β chains, each of which is polymorphic). To illustrate, HLA-DR1 is written as DRB1*0101. DRB1 indicates the β chain of the DR locus, and *0101 indicates that it is antigen 1, first variant. In similar fashion, DQA1*0302 indicates the α chain of the DQ locus, antigen 3, variant 2. Many recent observations of disease associations wih HLA antigens use this more precise nomenclature in order to define the molecular

basis for peptide binding, as well as to provide better genetic markers for ethnic and population diversity.

Complement (class III) Structural genes for three complement components, C4, C2, and Bf (factor B), are present in the HLA-BD region (see Fig. 64-1). There are two loci for C4, coding for C4A and C4B, formerly recognized as the Rodgers and Chido red blood cell antigens, respectively. These antigens are, in fact, adsorbed plasma C4 molecules. Other complement components are not closely linked to HLA. No crossovers have been found between the C2, Bf, and C4 loci. They are all encoded within a 100-kilobase segment between HLA-B and HLA-DR. There are two alleles of C2, four of Bf, seven of C4A, and three of C4B, plus blanks (null genes) for each locus (QO). The extensive polymorphism of complement types (complotypes) makes them useful for genetic studies. The four most common extended haplotypes found in people of western European ancestry are shown in Table 64-1. MLRs between unrelated individuals who are matched for these extended haplotypes are nonreactive, whereas reactivity is common if unrelated individuals are matched for only HLA-DR and -DQ. Such identical extended haplotypes may be conserved from a common ancestor.

Other sixth-chromosome genes Deficiency of steroid 21-hydroxylase, an autosomal recessive trait, results in the syndrome of congenital adrenal hyperplasia (see Chaps. 335 and 342). The genes for the enzyme are also localized in the HLA-B-D region. The 21-hydroxylase gene adjacent to C4A is deleted in affected individuals along with C4A (C4AQO), and the HLA-B locus gene may have been altered to convert B13 to the rare B47 found only in affected

TABLE 64-1 Comnmon extended HLA haplotypes

HLA-B	HLA-DR	Bf	C2	C4A	C4B
8	3	S	C	QO	1
7	2	S	C	3	1
57	7	S	C	6	1
44	7	F	C	3	1

TABLE 64-2　Linkage of genetic defects to HLA

	Gene location	Common haplotype found
C2 deficiency	HLA-B-D	A25, B18, BfS, DR2
21-OH deficiency	HLA-B-D	A3, B47, BfF, DR7
21-OH deficiency (late onset)	HLA-B-D	B14, BfS, DR1
Idiopathic hemochromatosis	HLA-A	A3, B14
Paget's disease	HLA-A-D	
Spinocerebellar ataxia	HLA-A-D	
Hodgkin's disease	HLA-A-D	

haplotypes. A late-onset variant of 21-hydroxylase deficiency is also linked to HLA. Congenital adrenal hyperplasia due to 11β-hydroxylase deficiency is not HLA-linked. Idiopathic hemochromatosis, an autosomal recessive disorder, is linked to HLA, as has been shown in several family studies (see Chap. 345). Although the pathogenesis of this disease is unknown, the gene that modulates gastrointestinal iron absorption is near HLA-A (Table 64-2).

Immune-response genes　As originally defined in the guinea pig and the mouse, high and low immune responsiveness to haptens or synthetic peptide motifs was shown to be determined by genes in the region of the MHC. It is now clear that these genes encode the class II molecules and that the ability to bind the relevant antigen is the major determinant of a strong T cell–dependent response initiated by CD4+ T cells. Class I genes are also important in the effector phases of a response, especially with regard to recognition by CD8+ T cells of foreign peptide bound to class I molecules. For example, human cell lines infected with the influenza virus are lysed by immune cytotoxic T cells (T_c) only if a class I (HLA-A or HLA-B) antigen is shared between the attacking and target cells. Class I and II molecules are said to be the *restriction elements* in immune responsiveness because they must be able to bind and present peptide fragments properly to T cells. In the allogeneic response, there is evidence that recognition may be of either the amino acid differences on the external face of the intact MHC molecule or of an MHC peptide fragment presented by a responder strain MHC molecule. In this special case, instead of restricting the response, the MHC antigenic differences become the stimulus. In transplantation, the induction and effector phases of a rejection response follow the general rules of CD4+ T_H and CD8+ T_c interacting with MHC class II and I, respectively (Fig.

64-5). Although B lymphocytes can be directly activated via their surface immunoglobulin receptors, they also express high concentrations of class I and II molecules and can process antigens for presentation on the cell surface. It is the response of the T cell to such antigen presentation which provides the "help" required for a mature IgG secretory response by the B cells.

DISEASE ASSOCIATIONS　Not all genes involved in regulating the immune response are in the MHC region. It is nevertheless a fact that most human inflammatory diseases thought to have some autoimmune basis are in some way promoted by genes of the HLA region. In most cases, these are *associations* of particular HLA antigens in populations of individuals with certain diseases. Since it is becoming apparent that the extensive polymorphism of the MHC is directly related to the ability of a given molecule to bind a particular peptide sequence, the critical biologic function of MHC polymorphism may be to ensure survival of the species in relation to the large numbers of microbiologic agents present in the environment. Self-tolerance which happens to crossreact with microbiologic agents would produce a high degree of susceptibility, resulting in lethal infection, whereas the polymorphism of the HLA system ensures that segments of the human population will recognize offending agents as foreign and initiate the appropriate response. The importance of the MHC for species survival could be of the highest order, since there is need for local mechanisms, not entirely understood, to prevent allorecognition in the special case of pregnancy. The extent to which the MHC plays a role in immune surveillance against neoplasia and whether such a role contributes to survival in an evolutionary sense are not established.

Table 64-3 summarizes the most significant HLA and disease associations. It should be noted that such associations do not in themselves prove that variations in antigen presentation to T cells is necessarily at the root of autoimmunity. It also can be that HLA genes are markers for haplotypes in which mutations have occurred in other linked genes.

Most striking is the increased frequency of HLA-B27 in certain rheumatic diseases, particularly ankylosing spondylitis, a condition with a strong familial tendency. B27 is present in about 7 percent of people of western European ancestry, while it appears in 80 to 90 percent of patients with ankylosing spondylitis. Expressed as a relative risk, the antigen B27 confers a susceptibility to the development of ankylosing spondylitis that is 87 times that in the general population. Similarly, acute anterior uveitis, Reiter's syndrome, and reactive arthritis to at least three bacterial infections (*Yersinia*, *Salmonella*,

FIGURE 64-5　Schema of the relative roles of HLA-A, HLA-B, HLA-C, and HLA-D antigens in initiation of the alloimmune response and in the development of effector cells and antibodies. Two main classes of T lymphocytes recognize antigens: T_c, the precursors to the cytotoxic "killer" cells, and T_H, the helper cells for amplification of the cytotoxic response. T_H also provide help to B lymphocytes for production of a fully mature IgG response. Note that T_c generally recognize class I antigens, while the T_H signal is provided by antigens of the HLA-D region (class II). (*From CB Carpenter, Kidney Int, 14:283, 1978.*)

TABLE 64-3 HLA antigens and disease, showing the most highly associated antigens

Disease	Antigen	Relative risk*	Disease	Antigen	Relative risk*
RHEUMATIC			**ENDOCRINE**		
Ankylosing spondylitis	B27	69.1	Type 1 diabetes mellitus	DR4	3.6
Reiter's syndrome	B27	37.0		DR3	4.8
Acute anterior uveitis	B27	8.2		DR2	0.2
Reactive arthritis (*Yersinia, Salmo-nella,* gonococcus)	B27	18.0		BfF1	15.0
Psoriatic arthritis, central	B27	10.7	Hyperthyroidism (Graves')	B8	2.5
	B38	9.1		DR3	3.7
Psoriatic arthritis, peripheral	B27	2.0	Hyperthyroidism (Japanese)	B35	4.4
	B38	6.5		A2	2.2
Juvenile rheumatoid arthritis	B27	3.9		DP5	4.4
	DR8	3.6		A2 + DP5	10.5
Juvenile arthritis, pauciarticular	DR5	3.3	Adrenal insufficiency	Dw3	10.5
Rheumatoid arthritis	Dw4/DR4	3.8	Subacute thyroiditis (de Quervain)	B35	13.7
Sjögren's syndrome	Dw3	5.7	Hashimoto's thyroiditis	DR5	3.2
Systemic lupus erythematosus			Congenital adrenal hyperplasia	B47	15.4
Causasian	DR3	2.6			
Japanese	DR2	5.3	**NEUROLOGIC**		
Chinese	DQ3	11.5	Myasthenia gravis	B8	2.7
Systemic lupus erythematosus (hy-dralazine)	DR4	5.6		DR3	2.5
			Multiple sclerosis	DR2	6.0
GASTROINTESTINAL			Manic-depressive disorder	B16	2.3
Gluten-sensitive enteropathy	DR3	11.6	Narcolepsy	DR2	130.0
Chronic active hepatitis	DR3	6.8	Schizophrenia	A28	2.3
Ulcerative colitis	B5	3.8			
			RENAL		
HEMATOLOGIC			Idiopathic membranous glomerulone-phritis	DR3	5.7
Idiopathic hemochromatosis	A3	6.7	Goodpasture's syndrome (anti-GBM)	DR2	15.9
	B14	26.7	Minimal change disease (steroid re-sponse)	B12	4.2
	A3, B14	90.0	Polycystic kidney disease	B5	2.6
Pernicious anemia	DR5	5.4	IgA nephropathy (Caucasians)	DR2	0.6
Hodgkin's disease			Gold nephropathy	DR3	14.0
Caucasian	DP3	2.0		DR4	0.3
Japanese	DP4	0.2			
			INFECTIOUS		
SKIN			Tuberculoid leprosy (Asians)	B8	6.8
Dermatitis herpetiformis	Dw3	17.3	Paralytic polio	B16	4.3
Psoriasis vulgaris	Cw6	7.5	Low vs. high response to vaccinia virus	Cw3	12.7
Psoriasis vulgaris (Japanese)	Cw6	8.5			
Pemphigus vulgaris (Jews)	DR4	14.6	**IMMUNODEFICIENCY**		
	A10	4.8	IgA deficiency (blood donors)	DR3	13.0
Behçet's disease					
Caucasian	B5	3.8			
Japanese	B51	12.4			
Chinese	B51	5.5			

* Relative risk = $\dfrac{(\%\ \text{antigen-positive patients})(\%\ \text{antigen-negative controls})}{(\%\ \text{antigen-negative patients})(\%\ \text{antigen-positive controls})}$.

and gonococcus) show a high degree of association with B27. Although the ordinary form of juvenile rheumatoid arthritis (JRA) also shows a similar association with B27, the pauciarticular form of JRA with iritis is DR5-associated. The increased incidence of B27 in psoriatic arthritis is also significant for the central type (axial skeleton) of the disorder, while B38 is associated with both the central and peripheral types. Psoriasis is associated with Cw6. Patients with degenerative arthritis or gout show no alteration in antigen frequencies.

Most other disease associations are with HLA-D region antigens. The rheumatoid arthritis associations with DR4 involve 3 of the 12 DR4 variants (DRB1*0401, *0404, and *0405), as well as DRB1*0101 and DRB1*1402 in some ethnic groups. Narcolepsy is virtually 100 percent associated with DR2 in both Japanese and Caucasians. Affected individuals need inherit only a single gene dose of DR2. Although there is no apparent autoimmune component to this condition, there is speculation that an abnormality in a neurotransmitter or its receptor may be influenced by the DR2 gene or another closely linked gene. Gluten-sensitive enteropathy (celiac disease, nontropical sprue) in children and adults is associated with DR3 (relative risk = 12). Recent DNA typing shows a higher relative risk of 52 with DQA1*0501 and DQB1*0201. The actual percentage of such patients having DR3 ranges from 63 to 96 percent compared with 22 to 27 percent of controls. The same antigen is also present

in increased frequency in patients with chronic active hepatitis and in patients with dermatitis herpetiformis who also have gluten-sensitive enteropathy. Juvenile-onset insulin-dependent diabetes mellitus (type I) is associated with DR4 and DR3 and is negatively associated with DR2. Resistance to type I diabetes is strongly associated with the inheritance of aspartate at position 57 of the β chain of HLA-DQ, in linkage disequilibrium with HLA-DR2. Other amino acids at position 57, especially when HLA-DR3 or -DR4 are on the same haplotype, are associated with an increased risk of disease. Recent studies show that having nonaspartate at position 57 of DQB1 of both haplotypes confers a relative risk for type 1 diabetes of 7.4, whereas a single or double dose of aspartate at position 57, as with DQB1*0601 or *0602, provides protection (relative risk of 0.2). Maturity-onset diabetes is not HLA-associated. A rare allele of Bf (F1) is also found in 17 to 25 percent of patients with type I diabetes. Hyperthyroidism in Caucasians is associated with B8,DR3, while in Japanese populations the association is with B35, A2, and DP5. This is an example of a disease in which racial differences display different HLA associations in contrast with rheumatoid arthritis and type I diabetes, in which the DR4 associations are more universal. Sometimes an HLA marker is clearly associated only with a subgroup within a syndrome. For example, myasthenia gravis without thymoma is more strongly B8,DR3-associated, and the association of DR2 with multiple sclerosis is stronger in patients with rapidly progressive deterioration. The common DR2 and DQ haplotype found in normal individuals (DRB1*1501, DQA1*0102, DQB1*0602) is also most commonly increased in multiple sclerosis. Renal diseases strongly HLA-DR–associated are Goodpasture's syndrome due to an autoantibody to glomerular basement membrane (DR2), idiopathic membranous glomerulonephritis (DR3 in Caucasians, DR2 in Japanese) which may be an autoimmune process involving antibodies to an antigen of the glomerulus, and gold-induced nephritis (DR3). Studies of HLA associations with AIDS suggest that HLA-B35 is a risk factor for more rapid progression of the disease (see Chap. 279).

LINKAGE DISEQUILIBRIUM   Although the distribution of HLA alleles varies in racial and ethnic populations, the most salient feature of population genetics of HLA antigens is the presence of linkage disequilibria among certain antigens of the A and B, B and C, and B, D, and complement loci. *Linkage disequilibrium* means that antigens of closely linked loci appear together more frequently than predicted by random association. The classic example is the linkage disequilibrium present between the A-locus antigen HLA-A1 and the B-locus antigen HLA-B8 in people of western European ancestry. The coincidence of A1 and B8 should be the product of their individual gene frequencies ($0.17 \times 0.11 \cong 0.02$). The observed frequency of A1 and B8 is 0.08, four times that expected, an increase of 0.06. The latter value is termed Δ (delta) and is a measure of the disequilibrium. Other A- and B-locus haplotype disequilibria have been recognized and include (A3, B7), (A2, B12), (A29, B12), and (A11, B35). Furthermore, some D-region determinants are in linkage disequilibrium with B-locus antigens (e.g., DR3 and B8), as are some B- and C-locus antigens. Serologically defined HLA antigens can serve as markers for the genes of an entire haplotype within a family and as markers for specific genes within a population, but only where a linkage disequilibrium exists.

Linkage disequilibrium is of importance because such gene associations may have some bearing on their function. For example, selective pressures during the course of evolution may have been the major factor in the survival of certain gene combinations in a haplotype. Such a theory suggests, for example, that A1 and B8, along with certain D-region and other determinants, conferred a selective advantage in the face of epidemics such as the plague or smallpox. It also would follow that the descendants of the survivors may display susceptibility to certain diseases because their unique gene complex happens to confer an abnormal response to other environmental agents. The major difficulty with this hypothesis is the assumption that selection must work on several genes simultaneously to account for the observed Δ's; however, the need for complex interactions among the products of the several loci of the major histocompatibility complex is only beginning to be appreciated, and selection might force multiple linkage disequilibria. The conservation of certain extended haplotypes, mentioned above, supports this view.

On the other hand, the selection hypothesis is not necessary to explain linkage disequilibrium. When a population lacking certain antigens is crossed with one in which a high frequency of antigens is in equilibrium, a Δ can develop within a few generations. For example, the increasing Δ value for A1,B8 found in populations from east to west, from India to western Europe, can be explained on the basis of migration and fusion. In smaller groups, consanguinity, founder effects, and gene drift may account for disequilibria. Finally, certain linkage disequilibria could occur as a result of nonrandom crossing over during gametic meiosis because of chromosomal segments which are either more or less likely to break. Unless there are selective pressures or restrictions in crossing over, linkage disequilibria disappear over a period of several generations. A large number of nonrandom associations occur throughout the HLA gene complex, and elucidation of the reasons for their existence may provide insight into the mechanism underlying certain disease susceptibilities.

LINKAGE AND ASSOCIATION   The diseases listed in Table 64-2 are examples of HLA linkage wherein the inherited conditions are marked within families by the relevant HLA haplotypes. For C2

deficiency, 21-hydroxylase deficiency, and idiopathic hemochromatosis, the mode of inheritance is recessive, with heterozygotes showing partial deficiencies. These genetic defects are also HLA-associated, with an excess of certain HLA alleles in affected unrelated individuals. Also, C2 deficiency is commonly linked to the HLA-A25, B18, BfS, Dw/DR2 haplotype, and idiopathic hemochromatosis exhibits both linkage and strong association with HLA-A3 and -B14. The high degree of linkage disequilibria in these HLA-linked diseases may result from mutations in a single founder, and a sufficient period of time may not have passed to bring the gene pool back into equilibrium. In this view, the HLA antigens are simple markers for the linked gene. Alternatively, expression of the defect may require interaction with specific HLA alleles. This latter hypothesis would require a higher mutation rate, with defective gene expression occurring only when linked with certain HLA genes.

Paget's disease and spinocerebellar ataxia are HLA-linked autosomal dominant traits in families having multiple affected members, and Hodgkin's disease shows an HLA-linked recessive pattern of inheritance. Except for a weak association of HLA-DP3 with Hodgkin's disease, no HLA associations have been discerned for these disorders, suggesting that there were multiple founders with mutations of as yet undefined genes in linkage with different HLA alleles.

HLA linkage is readily recognized when recessive or dominant inheritance patterns are clear-cut, i.e., when expressivity is high and the process is mostly, if not entirely, determined by a single gene defect. In most of the associations, HLA markers represent risk factors involving the operation and modulation of the immune response under the influence of multiple genes. An example of a polygenic immunologic disease is atopic allergy, in which the association to HLA may be evident only in individuals whose genetically controlled (non-HLA) levels of IgE production are low. Another is IgA deficiency (see Table 64-3), which is HLA-DR3–associated.

CLINICAL APPLICATIONS   The clinical value of HLA typing for diagnosis of disease is limited to B27 and ankylosing spondylitis, where nevertheless there are 10 percent false-positive and false-negative rates. HLA studies are also of value in genetic counseling and early recognition of disease in families with idiopathic hemochromatosis or congenital adrenal hyperplasia due to steroid 21-hydroxylase deficiency, particularly since HLA typing can be performed on cells obtained by amniocentesis. The high degree of polymorphism of the HLA system also makes it a powerful tool for paternity testing and other medicolegal applications. The implications for diseases such as type I diabetes mellitus and the other diseases showing HLA associations require further study of the components of the HLA system and their role in the pathogenesis of disease. Matching for HLA antigens in allogeneic transplantation is reviewed in Chap. 238.

REFERENCES

Bjorkman PA et al: Structure of the human class I histocompatibility antigen, HLA-A2. Nature 329:506, 1987

———— et al: The foreign antigen binding site and T cell recognition regions of class I histocompatibility antigens. Nature 329:512, 1987

Bodmer JG et al: Nomenclature for factors of the HLA system, 1991. Tissue Antigens, 39:161, 1992

Brown MG et al: Structural and serological similarity of MHC-linked LMP and proteosome (multicatalytic proteinase) complexes. Nature 353:355, 1991

Carpenter CB, Strom TB: Immunobiology of renal transplantation, in *Contemporary Issues in Nephrology*, vol 19: *Renal Transplantation*, EL Milford et al (eds). New York, Churchill Livingstone, 1989

Duquesnoy RJ, Trucco M: Genetic basis of cell surface polymorphism encoded by the major histocompatibility complex in humans. CRC Crit Rev Immunol 8:103, 1988

Ehrlich HA, Gyllensten UB: Shared epitopes among HLA class II alleles: Gene conversion, common ancestry and balancing selection. Immunol Today 12:411, 1991

Glynne R et al: A proteosome-related gene between the two ABC transporter loci in the class II region of the human MHC. Nature 353:357, 1991

Itescu S et al: HLA-B35 is associated with accelerated progression to AIDS. J Acquired Immune Deficiency Syndrome 5:37, 1992

Nelson JL, Hansen JA: Autoimmune disease and HLA. CRC Crit Rev Immunol 10:307, 1990

Rotzsche O, Falk K: Naturally occurring peptide antigens derived from the MHC class I-restricted processing pathway. Immunol Today 12:447, 1991

Trowsdale J et al: Map of the human MHC. Immunol Today 12:443, 1991

65   TREATMENT AND PREVENTION OF GENETIC DISEASE

DAVID VALLE

Normal development and physiologic homeostasis depend on the coordinated interactions of the products of many genes working together in metabolic systems. These systems are adaptable within limits, allowing normal homeostasis to occur over a range of environmental conditions. For instance, the products of some 30 to 40 genes participate in blood glucose regulation; in concert they maintain a relatively constant blood glucose concentration despite intermittent and highly variable ingestion of glucose precursors. On a larger scale, developmental and homeostatic interactions of 10,000 or so gene products are believed to be necessary for normal development and function of the central nervous system. Mutations that reduce the adaptive capacity of these systems result in abnormalities that we recognize as genetic disease. The mutant gene may so compromise a particular developmental or homeostatic system that the system functions poorly or not at all under all circumstances, thereby producing a monogenic disorder. Alternatively, the mutant gene may have modest effects under ordinary conditions but in certain environments cause maldevelopment or dyshomeostasis that we recognize as a multifactorial disorder. Thus the role of the genes in health and disease is both central and complex. Consequently, treatment of genetic disease is both difficult and frequently less than completely effective.

TREATMENT

Effective treatment of genetic disorders requires accurate diagnosis, early intervention prior to development of irreversible tissue damage, and an understanding of the abnormal biochemistry or metabolic pathophysiology. Progress in delineating the molecular basis of genetic disease has improved our capability for accurate diagnosis of monogenic disorders. Understanding of the metabolic pathophysiology is increasing at a slower rate mainly because progress in this area often requires elucidation of integrative physiology by study of the intact organism. The development of noninvasive metabolic monitoring techniques such as positron emission tomography and topical magnetic resonance spectrometry, as well as new genetic technologies for the production of animal models of human genetic disease, offers promise for progress in this area.

Approaches to treatment of genetic disease can be organized proceeding from the clinical phenotype through the abnormal metabolites and dysfunctional protein to the level of the defective gene (Table 65-1).

TREATMENT OF THE CLINICAL PHENOTYPE   Treatment of the clinical phenotype includes conventional medical practices such as patient education, pharmacologic interventions, and surgical procedures. It depends on a thorough understanding of the natural history of the particular disorder so that potential complications can be avoided or addressed early in the course to minimize the consequences. Although therapy at this level is not aimed at correcting the primary defect, it can markedly improve the quality of life. Examples include instruction to patients with albinism or xeroderma to limit sun exposure or to patients with glucose-6-phosphate dehydrogenase deficiency to avoid the offending drugs; administration of beta blockers to Marfan's syndrome patients to prevent or slow dilatation of the aortic root, anticonvulsants to patients with neurogenic disorders, or antihypertensive agents to patients with secondary hypertension; and a host of surgical interventions for patients with genetic malformations, skeletal dysplasias, and malignancies.

TREATMENT OF THE METABOLIC PHENOTYPE   Treatment at the metabolite level involves nutritional or pharmacologic approaches

TABLE 65-1   Some treatments for monogenic disorders

Level of treatment and method	Disorder(s)
CLINICAL PHENOTYPE	
Patient education	
Avoidance of aggravating agents (high carbohydrate diet, exposure to cold)	Periodic paralysis syndromes
Avoidance of certain drugs	Pharmacogenetic disorders, acute intermittent porphyria
Avoidance of sun exposure	Xeroderma pigmentosa, albinism
Avoidance of certain physical activity	Chondrodystrophies
Notify physician for rapid increase in size of mass or tinnitus	Neurofibromatosis
Pharmacologic	
Beta blockers	Marfan's syndrome
Anticonvulsants	Neurodegenerative disorders
Surgical	
Orthopedic reconstruction	Chondrodystrophies
Colectomy	Familial polyposis coli
Plastic reconstruction of facial malformations	Treacher-Collins syndrome, several monogenic cleft lip and/or palate syndromes
METABOLIC PHENOTYPE	
Metabolite alteration	
Substrate restriction	
Phenylalanine	Phenylketonuria
Branch-chain amino acids	Maple syrup urine disease
Galactose	Galactosemia
Fructose	Hereditary fructose intolerance
Lactose	Lactase deficiency
Phytanic acid	Refsum's disease
Alternative pathway utilization	
Benzoate and phenylacetate	Urea cycle disorders
Glycine	Isovaleric acidemia
Carnitine	Organic acidosis
Cysteamine	Cystinosis
Penicillamine	Wilson's disease
Metabolic inhibition	
Allopurinol	Gout
Mevinolin	Familial hypercholesterolemia
Replacement of deficient products	
Glucose polymers (cornstarch)	Glycogen storage disease, types I and III
Uridine	Hereditary orotic aciduria
Glucocorticoids	Congenital adrenal hyperplasia
Thyroxine	Familial goiter
Biotin	Biotinidase deficiency
Protein alteration	
Activation of the mutant protein	
Pyridoxine (vitamin B_6)	Homocystinuria
Thiamine	Maple syrup urine disease
Hydroxycobalamin (vitamin B_{12})	Some forms of methylmalonic acidemia
Replacement of the mutant protein	
Growth hormone	Growth hormone deficiency
Factor VIII	Classic hemophilia
α_1-Antitrypsin	α_1-Antitrypsin deficiency
Polyethylene glycol-adenosine deaminase	Adenosine deaminase deficiency
Mannose-terminated glucocerebrosidase	Gaucher disease
Organ transplantation	
As a source for a specific protein	
Allogeneic bone marrow	Lysosomal storage diseases, β thalassemia
Liver	Glycogen storage disease, type I, familial hypercholesterolemia, ornithine transcarbamylase deficiency
As a protein source and replacement of damaged organ	
Liver	α_1-Antitrypsin deficiency, hepatorenal tyrosinemia
Kidney	Cystinosis

and is dependent on understanding the biochemical pathophysiology (Fig. 65-1). Deficient function of a mutant protein may result in a disease phenotype because a substrate accumulates to toxic levels (precursor toxicity), because the product of an alternative pathway is produced in excessive amounts (alternative pathway overflow), be-

FIGURE 65-1 Pathophysiologic consequences of a genetic defect in a metabolic pathway. Substrate A is converted via a series of intermediates to a final product, D. The enzymes catalyzing these reactions are indicated by the horizontal arrows. A also is converted to F in an alternative pathway. Genetic deficiency of the enzyme converting A to B (indicated by the hatched rectangle) may have pathophysiologic consequences related to accumulation of A (precursor toxicity), overflow to F (alternative pathway overflow), reduced formation of D (product deficiency), or some combination of these possibilities.

cause of reduced formation of the reaction product or some downstream metabolite (product deficiency), or because of some combination of these possibilities. Although this paradigm is most easily visualized for enzymes in a metabolic pathway, it holds for virtually all proteins. The pathophysiology may be *local* within the cell or tissue normally expressing the mutant protein, or it may involve *distant* biochemical effects as a consequence of perturbations of metabolite concentrations in the extracellular fluid. For example, the neurologic phenotype of Tay Sachs disease results from destruction of neurons caused by deficiency of hexosaminidase A, whereas the mental retardation of untreated phenylketonuria due to deficiency of phenylalanine hydroxylase is mediated by the systemic accumulation of phenylalanine.

Precursor toxicity Correction of precursor toxicity frequently involves dietary restriction of a substrate whose major source is nutritional. Inborn errors of amino acid and carbohydrate metabolism are examples of this approach. A diet restricted in the branch-chain amino acids (leucine, isoleucine, valine) is effective in preventing the mental retardation associated with maple syrup urine disease caused by deficiency of branch-chain ketoacid decarboxylase (see Chap. 352). Such diets should be started soon after birth, continued for life, and monitored so that intake of these essential amino acids is just sufficient for normal growth. Illnesses that cause protein catabolism (e.g., those associated with intercurrent infections or trauma) periodically complicate this therapy by releasing large amounts of the offending amino acids from the breakdown of endogenous protein. These episodes may require hospitalization for administration of intravenous fluids or dialysis. Similarly, lifetime restriction of dietary galactose in patients with galactosemia due to deficiency of galactose-1-phosphate uridyl transferase corrects growth failure, prevents cataracts, and improves intellectual outcome (see Chap. 354).

Alternative pathway utilization For some disorders, alternative metabolic pathways may be utilized to remove toxic metabolites. The effectiveness of this approach is limited by the capacity of the alternative pathway and often must be combined with dietary restriction of the offending substrate. Administration of benzoate and phenylacetate to patients with inborn errors of urea metabolism is a good example of this approach. These compounds are conjugated with endogenous glycine and glutamine, forming hippurate and phenylacetylglutamine, respectively. When used in conjunction with restriction of dietary protein, this therapy reduces the accumulation of ammonia in patients with inborn errors of the urea cycle and organic acid metabolism. Similar approaches include the administration of carnitine, which conjugates with a variety of accumulated CoA esters, to patients with defects of organic acid metabolism; cysteamine, which helps to eliminate excess cystine in cystinosis; and penicillamine to reduce excessive stores of copper in Wilson's disease and iron in hemochromatosis.

Inhibition of an overactive pathway For other disorders, particularly those in which alternative pathway overflow produces a toxic

level of a particular metabolite, it may be possible to prevent the accumulation by inhibiting an enzyme in the affected pathway. This approach may lead to accumulation of upstream substrates that must be well tolerated if the treatment is to be successful. For instance, in gout and other disorders in which excessive purine degradation leads to uric acid accumulation, inhibition of xanthine oxidase by allopurinol reduces uric acid production and lowers the incidence of uric acid nephropathy and gouty arthritis. Xanthine, which accumulates as a consequence, has greater aqueous solubility than uric acid and usually is well tolerated. In a similar fashion, hypercholesterolemic patients heterozygous for mutations of the low-density lipoprotein receptor exhibit significant reductions in plasma cholesterol when treated with lovastatin, a drug that acts in part to inhibit hydroxymethylglutaryl coenzyme A reductase that catalyzes an early, rate-limiting step in the synthesis of cholesterol (see Chap. 344).

Product deficit For disorders in which the pathophysiology involves product deficit, nutritional or pharmacologic approaches to replenishing the product can be effective if the administered material reaches the appropriate physiologic compartment. For example, many of the inborn errors in hormone biosynthesis such as the various forms of congenital adrenal hyperplasia and hereditary defects in thyroid hormone biosynthesis respond well to pharmacologic replacement of the deficient hormones. By contrast, the administration of melanin to albinos would not correct the pigment deficit in melanocytes.

TREATMENT DIRECTED TO THE PROTEIN PHENOTYPE Therapy at the level of dysfunctional protein involves either activation or replacement of the mutant protein.

Activation of the mutant protein Activation may be possible if the protein requires a vitamin cofactor and the vitamin is one that is well tolerated in pharmacologic doses. Obviously, not all mutations of a gene encoding a vitamin-dependent protein will respond. Those that do are likely to be missense mutations that either decrease the affinity of an enzyme for its cofactor or destabilize a protein in a way that can be partially overcome by substantial increments in cofactor concentration. About one-third of the cases of homocystinuria due to deficiency of the pyridoxal phosphate–requiring enzyme cystathione-β-synthase exhibit a significant increment in the activity when treated with pharmacologic doses (50 to 500 mg/d) of pyridoxine (vitamin B_6). The actual increase in enzyme activity may be small, but it suffices to improve metabolic flux in the impaired pathway. Since activation of residual activity both reduces precursor accumulation and increases product formation, knowledge of the pathophysiologic mechanism is less critical for this form of treatment.

Protein replacement therapies An alternative approach involves replacement with an exogenous supply of the protein. To be efficacious, the protein must be administered directly into or reach the appropriate physiologic compartment. Thus blood proteins or proteins that traverse the vascular compartment (e.g., peptide hormones) are candidates for this approach. Other considerations include the availability, stability, and immunogenicity of the protein. In some instances, the administered protein may be modified to enhance stability and/or targeting to the appropriate cell or tissue. For example, linkage of adenosine deaminase to polyethylene glycol increases stability, and partial deglycolsylation of glucocerebrosidase exposes mannose residues on the surface of the protein that target it to macrophages via the mannose receptor. Recombinant DNA technology can sometimes be utilized to supply sufficient amounts of the pure protein (e.g., human growth hormone and α_1-antitrypsin). Other proteins (e.g., clotting factor VIII) are available from natural sources but may eventually be produced by recombinant technology. This advance ensures an adequate supply and avoids the risk of transmission of pathologic viruses contaminating the protein purified from natural sources.

ORGAN TRANSPLANTATION Organ transplantation is on the borderline between therapy at the level of the dysfunctional protein and gene therapy. On the one hand, a transplanted organ supplies a deficient protein; on the other, the transplant tissue also brings new genetic information which, in contrast to standard models of gene therapy, is not integrated into the recipient's genome. Kidney, liver, and bone marrow transplantation are utilized for a variety of genetic diseases. The development of more effective and specific immunosuppressants (cyclosporine and FK5061) and the inadequacy of many less invasive therapies account, in part, for the increased utilization of this form of treatment. In some instances, the goal of transplantation is to supply a tissue that can replace a mutant protein (e.g., liver transplant for deficiency of low-density lipoprotein receptor or one of the urea cycle enzymes). For other disorders (e.g., α_1-antitrypsin deficiency or hepatorenal tyrosinemia), the transplant both provides the protein and replaces a damaged organ. The pathophysiologic mechanism of the disease is relevant; the physician must consider if the newly supplied protein will only be used locally or, if not, will gain access to the involved tissue(s). The long-term efficacy and consequences of organ transplantation as treatment for genetic disorders remain to be determined.

PROSPECTS FOR GENE THERAPY Several methods are now available to introduce new genetic material into mammalian cells. These methods allow consideration of a more direct approach to treatment of genetic disease, namely, gene therapy or introduction of a functional gene to replace or supplement the activity of a resident defective gene. Typically, two strategies have been considered, germline and somatic cell gene therapy, which differ in the nature of the recipient cells. In the germline model, foreign DNA is introduced into the zygote or early embryo with the expectation that the newly introduced material will contribute to the germline of the recipient, i.e., be passed on to the next generation. By contrast, in somatic gene therapy models, genetic material is introduced only into somatic cells and is not transmitted to the germ cells. A third approach to gene therapy involves activation of endogenous genes to augment or circumvent a defective gene.

Much of the technology for germline gene therapy has been developed in transgenic mice. Fertilized mouse eggs are harvested from a superovulated female, microinjected with DNA molecules, and reimplanted in a pseudopregnant female. Several murine genetic diseases, including deficiency of growth hormone, myelin basic protein, and β-globin, have been "treated" in this fashion with the general result that the disease phenotype is markedly ameliorated. These experiments have provided considerable information on the regulation of gene expression and the pathogenesis of genetic disease. However, the method is inefficient: Only 15 to 20 percent of injected eggs produce transgenic animals, and of these, only 20 to 30 percent actually express the introduced gene. Furthermore, there are appreciable risks, including damage to a resident gene by the random insertion of the foreign DNA (insertional mutagenesis). For human disorders, availability of the molecular reagents for this approach makes prenatal diagnosis possible. The certainty of having an unaffected child as established by prenatal diagnosis is preferable to the uncertainty and risks of the transgenic approach. Thus germline gene therapy is not applicable to human genetic disease.

Conversely, somatic gene therapy experiments for human genetic disease are beginning (Fig. 65-2). The methods for introducing the genetic material and the recipient cells vary, depending, in part, on the disease to be treated. Currently, modified retroviral vectors that allow high-efficiency introduction of foreign DNA into dividing cells are favored. Other viral vectors that do not require the recipient cell to be dividing (e.g., replication-deficient recombinant adenovirus vectors) may also be useful. Bone marrow stem cells, hepatocytes, endothelial cells, fibroblasts, myoblasts, and epithelial cells are all candidates for recipient cells. Difficulties with long-term, high-level expression of the introduced gene and with reintroduction of the recipient cells into the organism are obstacles to progress in this area. Developments in directing the introduced gene to its normal location in the genome (homologous recombination) offer promise for achieving normal regulation of the introduced gene and elimination of possible detrimental effects of the endogenous mutant gene. The lessons learned from conventional therapies will apply to somatic gene therapy. The importance of early intervention, consideration of

pathophysiologic mechanism(s), and the need for regulated interactions of the product of the introduced gene with other members of the involved homeostatic system are all relevant. Each disorder will have its own therapeutic requirements and problems. These considerations suggest that many genetic disease will remain resistant to treatment despite advances in the ability to perform somatic gene therapy.

Activation of the expression of endogenous genes is another form of therapy that is being attempted for human genetic disease. Interferon γ, a potent transcriptional regulator of several genes, including those involved in X-linked chronic granulomatous disease (X-CGD), improves neutrophil function in that subset of X-CGD patients with mutations that impair a cytochrome involved in superoxide metabolism. Likewise, hydroxyurea increases the expression of the fetal globin genes in some patients with sickle cell disease, providing an alternative, nonsickling hemoglobin. The long-term efficacy and the possible detrimental effects of administering agents that affect the expression of many genes are unknown.

EVALUATION OF THERAPY FOR GENETIC DISEASE

Two general questions should be posed in an evaluation of therapy for a genetic disease. First, does the treatment provide therapeutic benefit? Second, does the treatment restore the patient to normality? These questions can be asked of any disease treatment but have special significance for genetic disorders that are predictable and preventable. Studies by Costa, Scriver, and Childs evaluated the effectiveness of therapy of 351 representative monogenic disorders on three basic variables: life span, reproductive capability, and social adaptation; in their study, available therapies returned life span to normal in 15 percent, allowed reproductive capability in 11 percent, and improved social adaptation in 6 percent of the disorders. Only slightly better outcomes were found with a subset of 65 diseases in which the basic defect is known. Because severe diseases are more quickly recognized, this sample may be skewed toward diseases most difficult to treat. Nevertheless, the results of therapy are worse than

FIGURE 65-2 One model for somatic gene therapy involving retroviral-mediated gene transfer into hepatocytes.

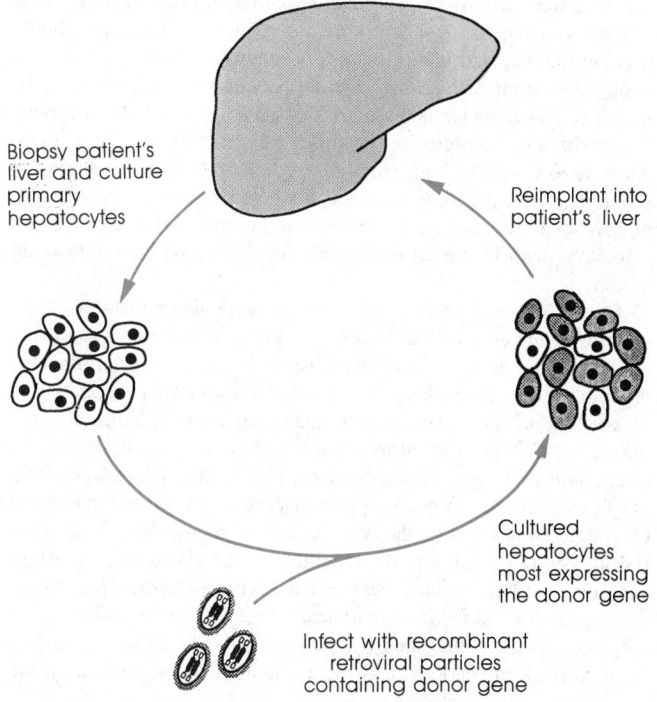

Biopsy patient's liver and culture primary hepatocytes

Reimplant into patient's liver

Cultured hepatocytes most expressing the donor gene

Infect with recombinant retroviral particles containing donor gene expected, emphasize the difficulty in developing effective therapies for genetic diseases, and highlight the need for continued work in this area. The results also underscore the value of preventive measures as therapy for genetic disease.

PREVENTION OF GENETIC DISEASE

Recognition of the limitation of therapy in genetic disease plus the predictability of the pattern of transmission of genes from one generation to the next has focused attention on prevention as the most reliable and effective means of dealing with hereditary disorders. The preventive approach includes genetic screening, counseling, and prenatal diagnosis.

GENETIC SCREENING   There are two types of genetic screening programs for autosomal recessive disorders: Homozygote screening programs search for individuals who have the disorder; by contrast, heterozygote screening programs search for individuals who are carriers of a mutant gene and thus are at risk of having offspring with a particular disorder. Successful homozygote screening programs require an inexpensive and reliable test, the recognition of some benefit (treatment, counseling) of early diagnosis, and education of the individuals and/or families screened so that they understand the significance of the results. The best example of such programs are the newborn screening programs. The diseases screened vary from state to state but include phenylketonuria, homocystinuria, maple syrup urine disease, galactosemia, cystic fibrosis, hypothyroidism, and sickle cell disease. In each instance, the screening test allows early detection and the opportunity to initiate appropriate therapy prior to the onset of irreversible damage. Also, the parents of an affected individual are made aware of the risk to future offspring and have the option of prenatal diagnosis. Heterozygote screening programs are best exemplified by the program to detect carriers of Tay Sachs disease, a fatal autosomal recessive lysosomal storage disease for which there is no effective treatment. Heterozygote screening of defined subpopulations with an increased carrier frequency (e.g., Ashkenazi Jews, in whom the carrier frequency is approximately 1/25 as compared with approximately 1/300 in Anglo Saxons) identifies couples at risk in which both potential parents are carriers with a 25 percent chance of having an affected child. Prenatal diagnosis is possible, and the procedure provides a means for the couple to have unaffected children.

GENETIC COUNSELING   Prospective parents who seek information regarding the risk of genetic disease in their offspring may come to the physician for genetic counseling. Thus all physicians should become familiar with the principles of medical genetics and use this knowledge to understand and counsel patients. The couples may be identified as having an increased risk for having a child with a genetic disease because of a previously affected child or other near relative. Alternatively, one or both parents may belong to a known high-risk group (e.g., identified as a carrier in a heterozygote screening test), or advanced maternal age (>35 years at the time of delivery) may be associated with increased risk of having a baby with an autosomal trisomy.

One aspect of genetic counseling involves determination of the risk for having an affected child so that prospective parents can make informed reproductive decisions. The first step is to determine the reliability of the diagnosis. This usually requires critical examination of existing medical data and/or additional evaluation of affected family member(s). The information is then assembled in the format of the family pedigree to determine the pattern of transmission within the family and to compare it with that expected for the diagnosed condition. Depending on the type of disease (monogenic, multifactorial, or chromosomal) and the reliability of the diagnosis, the risk to subsequent offspring may be predicted with a degree of certainty ranging from a rough estimate to nearly perfect. The reliability of the diagnosis will be influenced by the existence of multiple etiologies for a particular phenotype and the availability of specific diagnostic tests. Molecular tests that directly and unambiguously determine the parental genotype are sometimes available and allow precise prediction of the risk of recurrence and prenatal diagnosis for some monogenic disorders (see Chap. 62). For autosomal recessive and X-linked disorders in which a primary biochemical defect is known, reliable diagnosis is possible by a functional test of the gene product (e.g., assay of enzyme activity). For most autosomal dominant disorders, the primary biochemical defect is not known, and identification of parental genotype is subject to error resulting from heterogeneity of manifestations. Availability of linked molecular markers, e.g., RFLPs, and identification of the involved genes will greatly improve the reliability and precision of counseling for some of these conditions.

Counseling for many common multifactorial disorders (e.g., diabetes mellitus, hypertension, atherosclerosis, congenital malformations, and psychiatric disorders) is imperfect and will be so until we have a better understanding of the interactions of the various genes and environmental factors that produce these diseases. In some families the etiology may involve a major contribution of a single gene, and in others a mix of multiple genes and environmental factors is the cause. In the former the risk may be predicted by a monogenic model, while in the latter no simple model suffices. In these instances, the physician must resort to empiric risk estimates derived from retrospectively assembled data based on the average outcome in many different families.

In addition to determining risk, other information should be obtained prior to counseling. The prognosis and treatment of the disorder should be reviewed, and the availability of prenatal diagnosis and carrier testing should be determined. Finally, the counselor must be sensitive to the emotional impact this information may have on those counseled.

During the counseling session, effective communication of the information depends on expressing the essentials in language understandable to those being counseled. Written notes and diagrams frequently are helpful and can be given to them at the end of the session. Finally, review at subsequent visits helps correct misconceptions and increase retention of the information. In this regard, the physician who has an established relationship with the family may have an advantage over a trained counselor who meets with the subjects on only one or two occasions.

PRENATAL DIAGNOSIS   Following genetic counseling, the couple at risk for having a child with a genetic disease has several options depending, in part, on the type of disorder. They may be reassured and proceed despite the risk without any subsequent monitoring. Or they may view the risks as too high and choose to have no additional children or to adopt. Alternatively, when both parents are heterozygous for an autosomal recessive disorder, they may choose to reduce the risk by utilizing artificial insemination by donor. The magnitude of the decrease in the risk provided by this option will depend on the carrier frequency for the particular disorder in the general population. For a couple with a 1 in 4, or 25 percent, chance of having a child with phenylketonuria, the risk with donor insemination will drop to 1 in 130 ($\frac{1}{2} \times \frac{1}{65}$), or less than 1 percent, because the carrier frequency in the general population is 1 in 65. When mutant alleles for the gene in question are preferentially associated with particular linked markers (linkage dysequilibrium), it may be possible to reduce the risk further by avoiding donors with the mutant-associated markers.

Finally, if the disorder can be detected antenatally, the couple may decide to proceed with reproduction and utilize prenatal diagnosis with elective abortion of affected fetuses. Because the risk of having an affected fetus ranges from a maximum of 50 percent for heterozygotes with autosomal dominant disorders to less than 10 percent for nearly all chromosomal and multifactorial disorders, the majority of pregnancies monitored by prenatal diagnosis have an unaffected fetus. This relatively low frequency of affected fetuses, together with an increase in reproductive activity which often results from the reassurance provided by the availability of prenatal diagnosis, leads to significant increases in the family size of at-risk couples. Thus, in contrast to some public misconceptions, availability of

TABLE 65-2   Major indications for prenatal diagnosis

Indication	Risk for affected fetus, %	Method of detection
CHROMOSOMAL DISORDERS		
Advanced maternal age (>35 y)	1–10 depending on maternal age	
Parent with a balanced translocation	3–20 depending on the translocation	Chromosomal analysis of cells obtained by CVS* or amniocentesis
Previous child with chromosomal abnormality	~1	
MONOGENIC DISORDERS		
Couple at risk for having a child with an autosomal recessive inborn error of metabolism	25	Biochemical and/or molecular analysis of cells obtained by CVS or amniocentesis
Couple at risk for having a child with a monogenic disorder for which molecular markers are available	25–50	Molecular analysis of DNA obtained from cells obtained by CVS or by amniocentesis
Couple at risk for having a child with a monogenic malformation syndrome without biochemical or molecular markers	25–50	Fetal imaging by ultrasound
MALFORMATION DISORDERS		
Couples at risk for having a child with a neural tube defect (anencephaly or meningomyelocele) or other multifactorial malformation syndrome	1–10	Fetal imaging by ultrasound and, for neural tube defects, measurement of alpha fetoprotein and other fetal markers in amniotic fluid obtained by amniocentesis

* CVS, chorionic villus sampling

prenatal diagnosis actually results in increased numbers of offspring. The indications for prenatal diagnosis are based on a comparison of the risk of the procedures with the risk of having an affected child (Table 65-2).

Several methods for prenatal diagnosis are available (Table 65-3). Choice of a method depends on the disorder in question and on family preferences. Measurement of alpha fetoprotein (AFP) and other fetal proteins in maternal serum is noninvasive and can be used to screen for pregnancies at risk for neural tube defects (increased maternal serum AFP) and for fetal aneuploidies (decreased maternal serum AFP). It is possible by ultrasonography to visualize many fetal malformations and growth abnormalities and to monitor more invasive fetal sampling techniques with attendant reductions in the risks of the procedures. Although second-trimester (15 to 16 weeks of gestation) fetal sampling by amniocentesis is widely used for obtaining fetal cells, the techniques of transcervical and transabdominal chorionic villus sampling (CVS) also provide fetal cells and can be performed at 9 to 12 weeks of gestation. CVS has the advantage of allowing the diagnosis to be made earlier, and if an abortion is chosen, it will take place at a stage of pregnancy when maternal-fetal bonding is less. Finally, elective abortion at 12 weeks of gestation is a 2- to 3-h outpatient procedure, whereas a second-trimester elective abortion requires a 1- to 3-day hospitalization. The risks of CVS in experienced hands appear to compare well with those of amniocentesis. The tissue obtained at CVS is fetal trophoblastic tissue, expresses nearly all enzymes found in amniocytes, and provides an excellent source of fetal DNA.

REFERENCES

ANDERSON WF: Human gene therapy. Science 256:808, 1992

COSTA T, SCRIVER CR, CHILDS B: The effect of mendelian disease on human health: A measurement. Am J Med Genet 21:231, 1985

HARRISON MR et al: *The Unborn Patient: Prenatal Diagnosis and Treatment*, 2d ed. Philadelphia, Saunders, 1991

SCRIVER CR et al (eds): *The Molecular and Metabolic Basis of Inherited Disease*, 7th ed. New York, McGraw Hill, in press

TABLE 65-3   Methods of prenatal diagnosis

Method	Stage of gestation, weeks	Sample	Fetal disorders	Risks
Maternal serum sampling	15–18	Alpha fetoprotein and other fetal proteins	Neural tube defects, aneuploidies	Negligible
Fetal ultrasonography	6–40	Image	Fetal dating, morphologic abnormalities, skeletal dysplasis	Negligible
Fetal sampling				
Chorionic villus sampling	9–12	Fetal trophoblastic tissue	Cytogenetic, biochemical, molecular	1–2% fetal loss
Amniocentesis	15–18	Amniotic fluid and cells	Cytogenetic, biochemical, molecular, neural tube defects	0.2–0.5% fetal loss
Fetal biopsy	18–20	Fetal skin	Dermatologic	~2% fetal loss
		Fetal liver	Liver-specific, enzyme deficiencies	2–5% fetal loss
		Umbilical cord, blood	Blood disorders	~2% fetal loss

PART FOUR

66 PRINCIPLES OF DRUG THERAPY

JOHN A. OATES / GRANT R. WILKINSON

QUANTITATIVE DETERMINANTS OF DRUG ACTION

Safe and effective therapy with drugs requires their delivery to target tissues in concentrations within the narrow range that yields efficacy without toxicity. Optimal precision in achieving concentrations of drug within this therapeutic ''window'' can be achieved with regimens that are based on the kinetics of the drug's availability to target sites. This chapter deals with the principles of drug elimination and distribution that form the basis for loading and maintenance regimens for the average patient and considers instances in which elimination of the drug is impaired (e.g., renal failure). The basis for optimal utilization of plasma level data is also discussed.

PLASMA LEVELS AFTER A SINGLE DOSE The levels of lidocaine in plasma following intravenous administration decline in two phases, as illustrated in Fig. 66-1; such a biphasic decline is typical for many drugs. Immediately following rapid injection, essentially all of the drug is in the plasma compartment, and the high initial plasma level reflects its confinement to this small volume. Subsequently, the drug is transferred into the extravascular compartment, and the period of time during which this occurs is referred to as the *distribution phase*. For lidocaine the distribution phase is virtually complete within 30 min; then a slower rate of fall ensues, referred to as the *equilibrium phase* or *elimination phase*. During this latter phase, the drug levels in plasma and those in the tissues change in parallel.

Distribution phase Pharmacologic events during the distribution phase depend on whether the level of drug at the receptor site is similar to that in the plasma. If this is the case, the pharmacologic effects, whether favorable or adverse, may be inordinately great during this period because of the high initial levels in plasma. For example, following a small bolus dose (50 mg) of lidocaine, antiarrhythmic effects may be evident during the early distribution phase but disappear as levels fall below those which are minimally effective and even before equilibrium between plasma and tissue is reached. Thus larger single doses or multiple small doses must be administered to achieve an effect that is sustained into the equilibrium phase. Toxicity resulting from high levels of some drugs during the distribution phase precludes administration of a single intravenous loading dose that will achieve therapeutic levels during the equilibrium phase. For example, the administration of a loading dose of phenytoin as a single intravenous bolus can cause cardiovascular collapse due to the high levels during the distribution phase. If a loading dose of phenytoin is administered intravenously, it must be given in fractions at intervals sufficient to permit substantial distribution of the prior dose before the next is given (e.g., 100 mg every 3 to 5 min). For similar reasons, the loading dose of many potent drugs that rapidly equilibrate with their receptors is divided into fractional doses for intravenous administration.

After an oral dose that delivers an equivalent amount of drug into the systemic circulation, plasma levels during the initial period after administration are not as high as after an intravenous bolus dose.

Because the drug is not absorbed instantly after oral administration and is delivered into the systemic circulation more slowly, much of the drug is distributed by the time absorption is complete. Thus procainamide, which is almost totally absorbed after oral administration, can be given as a single 750-mg loading dose with little risk of hypotension; in contrast, loading of the drug by the intravenous route is more safely accomplished by giving the dose in fractions of about 100 mg at 5-min intervals to avoid the hypotension that might ensue during the distribution phase if the entire loading dose were given as a single bolus.

In contrast, other drugs are distributed slowly to their sites of action during the distribution phase. For example, levels of digoxin at the receptor site (and its pharmacologic effect) do not reflect plasma levels during the distribution phase. Digoxin is transported (or bound) to its cardiac receptors more slowly by a process that proceeds throughout distribution. Thus plasma levels fall during a distribution phase of several hours, while levels at the site of action and pharmacologic effect increase. Only at the end of the distribution phase, when the drug has reached equilibrium with the receptor, does the concentration of digoxin in plasma reflect pharmacologic effect. For this reason, there should be a 6- to 8-h wait after administration before plasma levels of digoxin are obtained for a guide to therapy.

Equilibrium phase After distribution has proceeded to the point where the concentration of drug in plasma is in dynamic equilibrium with that in the tissues outside the vascular compartment, the levels in plasma and tissues fall in parallel as the drug is eliminated from the body. Thus the *equilibrium phase* is sometimes also referred to as the *elimination phase*. Measurement of drug concentration in plasma provides the best reflection of drug level in tissues during this phase.

Most drugs are eliminated as a first-order process. During the equilibrium phase, a characteristic of the first-order process is that the time required for the level of drug in plasma to fall to one-half the original value (the half-life, $t_{1/2}$) is the same regardless of which

FIGURE 66-1 Concentrations of lidocaine in plasma following the administration of 50 mg intravenously. The half-life of 108 min is computed as the time required for levels to fall from any given value during the equilibrium phase ($Cp_{initial}$) to one-half that level. Cp_0 is the hypothetical concentration of lidocaine in plasma at time zero if equilibrium had been achieved instantly.

point on the plasma level curve is chosen as a starting point for the measurement. Another characteristic of the first-order process is that a semilogarithmic plot of the concentrations in plasma versus time during the equilibrium phase is linear. From such a plot (Fig. 66-1) it can be seen that the half-life of lidocaine is 108 min.

One can calculate what amount of the administered dose remains in the body at any multiple of the half-life interval following administration:

Number of half-lives	Amount of dose remaining in the body, %	Amount of dose eliminated, %
1	50	50
2	25	75
3	12.5	87.5
4	6.25	93.75
5	3.125	96.875

In principle, the elimination process never reaches completion. From a clinical standpoint, however, elimination is essentially complete when it has reached 90 percent. Therefore, for practical purposes, *a first-order elimination process reaches completion after 3 to 4 half-lives.*

DRUG ACCUMULATION—LOADING AND MAINTENANCE DOSES With repeated administration of a drug, the amount in the body accumulates if the elimination of the first dose is incomplete when the second dose is given, and both the amount of drug in the body and its pharmacologic effect increase with continuing administration until they reach a plateau. The accumulation of digoxin administered in repeated maintenance doses (without a loading dose) is illustrated in Fig. 66-2. Since digoxin's half-life is about 1.6 days in a patient with normal renal function, 65 percent of digoxin remains in the body at the end of 1 day. Thus the second dose will raise the amount of digoxin in the body (and average plasma level) to 165 percent of that following the first dose. Each subsequent dose will result in greater amounts in the body until a *steady state* is achieved. At this point, drug intake per unit of time is the same as the rate of elimination, with the fluctuation between peak and trough plasma levels remaining constant. If the rate of drug delivery is subsequently altered, a different and new steady state will be attained. Continuing infusion of a drug at constant rate also will result in progressive accumulation to a predictable steady state (Fig. 66-3). In this case, a constant plasma level (Cp_{ss}) is achieved which is between the peak and trough values attained when the same rate of drug delivery is administered in an intermittent fashion. For *all* drugs with first-order kinetics, the time required to achieve steady state levels can be predicted from the half-life because accumulation also is a first-order process with a half-life identical to that for elimination. Hence

FIGURE 66-2 The time course of digoxin accumulation when a single daily maintenance dose is given without a loading dose. Note that accumulation is more than 90 percent complete by the end of 4 half-lives.

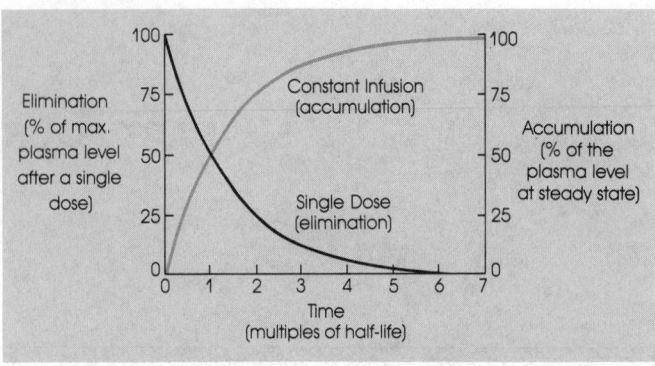

FIGURE 66-3 The time course of plasma levels of a drug following a single intravenous dose compared with those during a constant intravenous infusion. This relationship applies to all drugs that rapidly achieve equilibrium between plasma and tissues.

accumulation reaches 90 percent of steady state levels at the end of 3 to 4 half-lives. For digoxin, with a half-life of 1.6 days (with normal renal function), accumulation will be practically complete in 5 days. Continuous infusion of a drug at a constant rate also will result in progressive accumulation to a steady state with a time course predictable from the elimination curve for that drug (Fig. 66-3).

When the time required to reach steady state is longer than one wishes to wait, desired plasma levels may be achieved more rapidly by the administration of a *loading dose*. Loading entails the administration of an amount that will bring the concentration in plasma (at equilibrium) to the level present during steady state. If the desired plasma level (Cp_{ss}) is known, the loading dose can be estimated with knowledge of the extent of the drug's extravascular distribution at equilibrium, the apparent volume of distribution, or V_d:

$$\text{Loading dose} = \text{desired plasma level} \times \text{volume of distribution at steady state}$$

$$= Cp_{ss} \times V_d$$

Loading may be accomplished by the administration of the loading amount as a single dose, or in the case of drugs for which there is risk of toxicity if all the drug is introduced into the plasma compartment rapidly, the loading amount is administered in a series of fractions of the total loading amount. Since the accumulation of procainamide to 90 percent of steady state by infusion would require approximately 10 h (the $t_{1/2}$ is 3 h), a loading regimen is almost always desirable. The load required to suppress an arrhythmia, however, varies among individuals from 300 to 1000 mg, and rapid intravenous administration of the *average loading dose* causes hypotension during the distribution phase in some patients. Therefore, the intravenous loading dose of procainamide is given in fractions (e.g., 100 mg every 5 min) until the arrhythmia is controlled or adverse effects such as hypotension indicate that no further drug should be given. Dividing the loading dose into fractions is appropriate for most drugs that have a low therapeutic index (the *therapeutic index* is the ratio of toxic dose to the therapeutic dose). This permits better individualization of the loading amount and minimizes adverse effects.

The size of the loading dose required to achieve the plasma levels at steady state also can be determined from the fraction of drug eliminated during the dosage interval and the maintenance dose (in the case of intermittent drug administration). For example, if the fraction of digoxin eliminated daily is 35 percent and the planned maintenance dose is to be 0.25 mg daily, then the loading dose to achieve steady state levels should be 100/35 times the maintenance dose, or approximately 0.75 mg. Thus

$$\frac{\text{Loading}}{\text{dose}} = \frac{100}{\% \text{ of drug eliminated per dosage interval}} \times \text{maintenance dose}$$

The fraction of drug eliminated during any dosage interval can be determined from a semilogarithmic graph in which the total amount in the body at time zero is set at 100 percent and the fraction remaining at the end of one half-life is 50 percent.[1] Conversely, if the loading dose is known, the maintenance dose can be similarly calculated.

To calculate a loading dose designed to achieve the plasma concentration of a known infusion rate at steady state,

$$\text{Loading dose} = \frac{\text{infusion rate}}{k}$$

where k is the fractional elimination constant that describes the rate of drug elimination.[1]

Regardless of the size of the loading dose, *after maintenance therapy has been given for 3 to 4 half-lives, the amount of drug in the body is determined by the maintenance dose.* The independence of the plasma levels at steady state from the load is illustrated in Fig. 66-3, which indicates that the elimination of the loading dose would be practically complete after three to four half-lives.

DETERMINANTS OF PLASMA LEVELS DURING THE EQUILIB-RIUM PHASE An important determinant of the level of drug in plasma during the equilibrium phase after a single dose is the extent to which the drug is distributed outside the plasma compartment. For example, if the distribution of a 3-mg dose of a large macromolecule is confined to a plasma volume of 3 L, then the concentration in plasma will be 1 mg/L. However, if a different drug is distributed so that 90 percent of it leaves the plasma compartment, then only 0.3 mg will remain in the 3-L plasma volume and the concentration in plasma will be only 0.1 mg/L. The *apparent volume of distribution*, or V_d, expresses the relationship between the amount of drug in the body and the plasma concentration at equilibrium:

$$V_d = \frac{\text{amount of drug in body}}{\text{plasma concentration}}$$

The amount of drug in the body is expressed as mass (e.g., milligrams), and the plasma concentration is expressed as mass per volume (e.g., milligrams per liter). Thus V_d is a hypothetical volume into which a quantity of drug would distribute if its concentration in the entire volume were the same as that in plasma. Although it is not a real volume, it is an important concept because it determines the fraction of total drug in the plasma and therefore the fraction available to the organs of elimination. An approximation of V_d in the equilibrium phase can be obtained by estimating the concentration of drug in plasma at time zero (Cp_0) by back-extrapolation of the equilibrium-phase plot to zero time, as illustrated in Fig. 66-1. Then, after intravenous administration when the amount in the body at time zero is the dose, we have

$$V_d = \frac{\text{dose}}{Cp_0}$$

For the administration of the large macromolecule mentioned above, the measured Cp_0 of 1 mg/L after a 3-mg dose indicates a V_d that is a real volume, the plasma volume. This is the exception, however, for the V_d of most drugs is larger than plasma volume; many drugs are so extensively taken up by cells that tissue levels exceed those in plasma. For such drugs, the hypothetical V_d is large, even greater than the volume of body water. For example, Fig. 66-1 indicates that the Cp_0 obtained by extrapolation after administration of 50 mg lidocaine is 0.42 mg/L, yielding a V_d of 119 L.

Since elimination is performed largely by the kidneys and liver, it is useful to consider the elimination of drugs according to the *clearance* concept. For example, in the kidney, regardless of the

extent to which removal of drug is determined by filtration, secretion, or reabsorption, the net result is a reduction of the concentration of drug in plasma as it passes through the organ. The extent to which the concentration is reduced is expressed as the *extraction ratio*, or E, which is constant as long as first-order elimination occurs.

$$E = \frac{C_a - C_v}{C_a}$$

where C_a = arterial plasma concentration
C_v = venous plasma concentration

If the extraction is complete, $E = 1$. If the total plasma flow to the kidneys is Q (mL/min), the total volume of plasma from which drug is completely removed in a unit time (clearance from the body, Cl) is determined as

$$\text{Cl}_{renal} = QE$$

If the renal extraction ratio of penicillin is 0.5 and renal plasma flow is 680 mL/min, then penicillin's renal clearance is 340 mL/min. If the extraction ratio is high, as is the case for renal extraction of aminohippurate or hepatic extraction of propranolol, then clearance is a function of organ blood flow.[2]

Clearance from the body is the sum of clearance from all organs of elimination and is the best measure of the efficiency of the elimination processes. If a drug is removed by both the kidney and liver, then

$$\text{Cl} = \text{Cl}_{renal} + \text{Cl}_{hepatic}$$

Thus, if penicillin is eliminated by both renal clearance (340 mL/min) and hepatic clearance (36 mL/min) in a normal individual, total clearance is 376 mL/min. If renal clearance is reduced to half, total clearance is 170 + 36 or 206 mL/min. In anuria, total clearance equals hepatic clearance.

Only the drug in the vascular compartment can be cleared during each passage through an organ. To ascertain the effect of a given plasma clearance by one or more organs on the rate of removal of drug from the body, the clearance must be related to the volume of "plasma equivalents" to be cleared, that is, the volume of distribution. If the volume of distribution is 10 L and clearance is 1 L/min, then one-tenth of the drug in the body is eliminated per minute. This fraction, Cl/V_d, is known as a *fractional elimination constant* and is designated as k:

$$k = \frac{\text{Cl}}{V_d}$$

If the fraction k is multiplied by the total amount of drug in the body, the actual rate of elimination at any given time can be determined:

$$\text{Rate of elimination} = k \times \text{amount in body} = \text{Cl}Cp$$

This is the general equation for all first-order processes and expresses the fact that rate is proportional to the declining quantity in a first-order process.

Since half-life is a temporal expression of the exponential first-order process, half-life ($t_{1/2}$) can be related to k as follows:

$$t_{1/2} = \frac{0.693}{k}$$

$$\text{Because} \quad k = \frac{\text{Cl}}{V_d}$$

$$\text{then} \quad t_{1/2} = \frac{0.693 V_d}{\text{Cl}}$$

As shown in the section on drug dosage in renal failure, the linear relationship of k to creatinine clearance makes k a useful parameter

---

[1] Alternatively, the fraction of drug lost from the body during a dosage interval can be determined nongraphically from this equation:

$$\text{Fraction of drug lost from body} = 1 - e^{-kt}$$

Values for e^{-kt} can be obtained from a table of natural exponential functions or by a calculator, where $k = (0.693/t_{1/2})$ is the fractional elimination constant (described in the next section) and t is the time interval after drug administration.

[2] When drug is present in the formed elements of blood, then calculation of extraction and clearance from blood is more physiologically meaningful than from the plasma.

upon which to estimate changes in drug elimination with reduction in creatinine clearance in renal insufficiency. Half-life is not linearly related to clearance.

The important relationship

$$t_{1/2} = \frac{0.693 V_d}{Cl}$$

indicates clearly the dependency of half-life, a measure of rate of elimination, on the two physiologically independent variables of volume of distribution and clearance, which expresses the efficiency of elimination. Thus half-life is shortened when phenobarbital induces the enzymes responsible for hepatic clearance of a drug, and half-life is lengthened when a drug's renal clearance is attenuated in renal failure. Also, the half-life of some drugs is shortened when their volume of distribution is reduced. If, as in the case of cardiac failure, the volume of distribution is reduced at the same time that clearance is reduced, there may be little change in drug half-life to reflect the impaired clearance, but steady state plasma levels will be increased, as is the case with lidocaine. In treating patients after an overdose, the effects of hemodialysis on a drug's elimination are dependent on its volume of distribution. When the volume of distribution is large, as with tricyclic antidepressants (V_d of desipramine equals more than 2000 L), the removal of drug, even with a high-clearance dialyzer, proceeds slowly.

The extent to which a drug is bound to plasma protein also determines the fraction extracted by the organ(s) of elimination. Altered binding changes the extraction ratio significantly, however, only when elimination is limited to the unbound (free) drug in plasma. The extent to which binding influences elimination depends on the relative affinity of the plasma binding versus the affinity of the drug for the extraction process. The high affinity of the renal tubular anion transport system for many drugs leads to extraction of bound and unbound drug, and the efficient process by which the liver removes propranolol extracts most of this highly bound drug from blood. However, in the case of drugs with low organ extraction ratios, only unbound drug is available for elimination.

STEADY STATE   With a constant infusion of drug, the infusion rate equals elimination rate at steady state. Therefore,

| Infusion rate | = | Cp_{ss} | × | Cl |
| (amt/unit time) | | (amt/vol) | | (vol/unit time) |

when the units for amount, volume, and time are consistent.

Thus, if clearance (Cl) is known, the infusion rate to achieve a given steady state plasma level can be calculated. Estimation of drug clearance is discussed in the section on renal disease.

When the dose is given intermittently instead of by infusion, the above relationship between plasma concentration and the dose administered at each dosage interval can be expressed as

$$\text{Dose} = Cp_{av} \times Cl \times \text{dosage interval}$$

The average plasma concentration (Cp_{av}) implies, as seen in Fig. 66-2, that levels can be higher and lower than the average during the dosage interval.

When a drug is given orally, the fraction (F) of the administered dose that reaches the systemic circulation is an expression of the drug's *bioavailability*. A reduction in bioavailability may reflect a poorly formulated dosage form that fails to disintegrate or dissolve in the gastrointestinal fluids. Regulatory standards have reduced the extent of this problem. Drug interactions also can impair absorption after oral dosing. Bioavailability also may be reduced due to drug metabolism in the gastrointestinal tract and/or the liver during the absorption process, the *first-pass effect*. This is a particular problem for drugs that are extensively extracted by these organs, and considerable interpatient variability often exists in bioavailability. Lidocaine for the control of arrhythmias is not administered orally because of the first-pass effect. Drugs that are injected intramuscularly also may have low bioavailability, e.g., phenytoin. An unexpected drug response should lead to consideration of bioavailability as a possible factor. Calculation of a dosage regimen should be corrected for bioavailability:

$$\text{Oral dose} = \frac{Cp_{av} \times Cl \times \text{dosage interval}}{F}$$

DRUG ELIMINATION THAT IS NOT FIRST-ORDER   The elimination of some drugs such as phenytoin, salicylate, and theophylline does not follow first-order kinetics when amounts of drug in the body are in the therapeutic range. For these drugs, the clearance changes as levels in the body fall during elimination or after alterations in dose. This pattern of elimination is said to be *dose-dependent*. Accordingly, the time for the concentration to fall to one-half becomes less as plasma levels fall; this halving time is not truly a half-life, because the term *half-life* applies to first-order kinetics and is a constant. The elimination of phenytoin is dose-dependent, and when very high levels are present (in the toxic range), the halving time may be longer than 72 h, whereas as the concentration in plasma declines, the clearance increases and the concentration in plasma will halve in 20 to 30 h. When a drug is eliminated by first-order kinetics, the plasma level at steady state is directly related to the amount of the maintenance dose, and a doubling of the dose should lead to doubling of the steady state plasma level. However, for drugs with dose-dependent kinetics, increases in the dose may be accompanied by disproportionate increases in plasma level. Thus, if the daily dose of phenytoin is increased from 300 to 400 mg, plasma levels rise by more than 33 percent. The extent of increase is not predictable because of the interpatient variability in the extent to which clearance deviates from first order. Theophylline and salicylates also are eliminated by dose-dependent kinetics, and in children particular caution must be taken with the administration of salicylates in high doses. Changes in dosage regimens for such drugs should always be accompanied by surveillance for adverse effects and by measurement of the concentration of the drug in plasma after sufficient time to establish a new steady state. Ethanol metabolism also is dose-dependent, with obvious implications. The mechanisms involved in dose-dependent kinetics may include the saturation of the rate-limiting step in metabolism or a feedback inhibition of the rate-limiting enzyme by a product of the reaction.

INDIVIDUALIZATION OF DRUG THERAPY

Optimal drug therapy requires administration of just the right amount of drug for the particular patient—too little and efficacy is not likely, whereas too large a dose increases the risk of undesirable effects. When the desired response is a readily determined clinical effect, such as altered blood pressure or coagulation time, then an optimal dosage requirement can be achieved in an empirical fashion. Dosage alterations should, however, involve modest changes in amount (50 percent) and no more frequently than every two to three half-lives. In most cases, however, drug therapy must be guided by the concept of a "therapeutic window" within which drug concentrations must be achieved and maintained. If this therapeutic window is large, i.e., little dose-related toxicity, then maximal efficacy, should this be desired and achievable, may be obtained by administering a supraeffective dose. Such a strategy is often used for penicillins and many beta-adrenoceptor blocking agents. It is also possible under these circumstances to usefully extend the duration of action of the drug, especially when it is rapidly eliminated from the body. Thus 75 mg of captopril will result in reduced blood pressure for up to 12 h, even though the elimination half-life of the ACE-inhibitor is about 2 h. The therapeutic window for most drugs, however, is much narrower, and in certain instances (see Table 66-4), as little as a twofold difference distinguishes the dose (concentration) of drug producing the desired response from that eliciting an adverse effect. In these cases, the application of pharmacokinetic principles is critical to achieving the defined therapeutic objective.

During long-term therapy, the most important pharmacokinetic factor is the drug's clearance, since this determines the steady state plasma concentration. Thus, after an oral dose, and assuming that clearance is constant regardless of the dose,

$$Cp_{av} = \frac{\text{dosage rate}}{\text{clearance}} = \frac{F \times \text{oral dose}}{Cl \times \text{dosage interval}}$$

Accordingly, steady state drug levels and, therefore, the intensity of response can be adjusted by changing the dosing rate. In most cases this is best achieved by changing the drug dose and maintaining the same dosage interval, e.g., 250 mg every 8 h versus 200 mg every 8 h—drug levels will change in a proportional fashion, but the relative fluctuation between the maximum and minimum values will remain the same. On the other hand, the steady state level may be changed by altering the frequency of intermittent dosing while maintaining the amount of administered drug the same. This strategy, however, will result in changes in the relative fluctuations around the average steady state concentration. If a drug is administered every half-life, the trough concentration at the end of the dosing interval will be about one-half that of the peak level, assuming that absorption is rapid. At shorter intervals the fluctuations will be smaller, with the ultimate smooth curve when the drug is continuously given by infusion. By contrast, reaching a given steady state using a longer dosage interval and a proportionally large dose leads to wider fluctuations between the maximum and minimum levels (Fig. 66-4). Only if very high concentrations are nontoxic and it is acceptable that drug concentrations are below the minimum effective concentration for a considerable period of time during the longer dosage interval can larger doses be given to achieve a desired average steady state level.

With drugs that have a long elimination half-life and in which, therefore, steady state is only achieved after a considerable period of time, the previously described loading-dose strategy may be appropriate. Also, knowledge of a drug's rate of elimination is important in predicting when the full effects of any dosage change made to alter a steady state will be expected, since this takes three to four times the elimination half-life.

RENAL DISEASE Where urinary excretion is an important route of elimination, renal failure results in decreased drug clearance and therefore slower removal of the drug from the body, so administration of the usual dosage leads to greater accumulation and an increased likelihood of toxicity. The goal in such cases is to modify the dosage schedule so that a similar drug concentration–time profile is achieved in the plasma of the patient with renal insufficiency and the steady

state is reached after a similar time interval as in the patient with normal renal function. This is particularly appropriate for drugs with long half-lives and narrow therapeutic indexes (e.g., digoxin). Since

$$Cp_{av} = \frac{\text{dose}}{\text{dose interval}} \times \frac{F}{Cl}$$
$$= \frac{\text{dose}}{\text{dose interval}} \times \frac{F}{k\,V_d}$$

the Cp_{av} achieved with normal renal function can be obtained in patients with renal impairment, i.e., decreased Cl, by either decreasing the dose while maintaining the normal dosing interval, administering the usual dose but less frequently, or a combination of the two. Moreover, the modification factor for the dosage regimen is dependent on the ratio of the drug's clearance or rate of elimination in renal failure to that in uncompromised patients. Although such pharmacokinetic strategies in renal failure result in the same Cp_{av} during the dosage interval, the peak-to-trough fluctuations differ considerably from those seen in patients with normal renal function. Selection of the most appropriate modifications, therefore, depends on the levels associated with efficacy or toxicity, e.g., peak, Cp_{av}, or trough, and the drug's therapeutic index.

One approach is to calculate the *fraction of the normal dose* that is to be given at the usual dosage interval. This fraction can be determined from either drug clearance (Cl) or the fractional rate constant (k) based on the fact that both renal clearance and k are proportional to creatinine clearance (Cl_{cr}). Creatinine clearance is best determined directly. However, serum creatinine (C_{cr}) may be used to estimate the value by the following equation which is applicable to men:

$$Cl_{cr} = \frac{(140 - \text{age}) \times \text{weight (kg)}}{72 \times C_{cr}\,(\text{mg/dL})}\,(\text{mL/min})$$

For women, the value should be reduced to 85 percent of that estimated by this equation. This approach to estimation of Cl_{cr} is invalid in severe renal insufficiency ($C_{cr} > 5$ mg/dL) or with rapidly changing renal function.

The clearance approach Calculation of drug dosage is most accurately based on the clearance of a drug. From data on the clearance of a drug, the dose in renal insufficiency ($Dose_{ri}$) may be calculated as follows:

$$Dose_{ri} = \text{dose} \times \frac{Cl_{ri}}{Cl}$$

where ri = renal insufficiency

    Cl = clearance from the whole body with normal renal function

    Cl_{ri} = clearance from the whole body with renal insufficiency

    Dose = maintenance dose with normal renal function ($Cl_{cr} \approx$ 100 mL/min)

The normal clearance and that in renal impairment can be obtained by employing the data in Table 66-1 in the following equations:

$$Cl = Cl_{renal} + Cl_{nonrenal}$$

$$Cl_{ri} = Cl_{renal} \times \frac{\text{measured } Cl_{cr}}{100\,\text{mL/min}} + Cl_{nonrenal}$$

The Cl_{renal} values in Table 66-1 are those found with $Cl_{cr} = 100$ mL/min, and the renal clearance of drug in renal insufficiency is obtained by multiplying Cl_{renal} by the ratio of measured Cl_{cr} (in milliliters per minute) to 100 mL/min.

For gentamicin, with a normal Cl_{renal} of 78 mL/min and $Cl_{nonrenal}$ of 3 mL/min, Cl = 81 mL/min. Therefore, with a Cl_{cr} of 12 mL/min, $Cl_{ri} = 78 \times (12/100) + 3 = 12.4$ mL/min. If the dose of gentamicin for a given infection should be 1.5 mg/kg per 8 h in the presence of normal renal function, then

$$Dose_{ri} = \frac{1.5\,\text{mg/kg}}{8\,\text{h}} \times \frac{12.4\,\text{mL/min}}{81\,\text{mL/min}} = \frac{0.23\,\text{mg/kg}}{8\,\text{h}}$$

FIGURE 66-4 Plasma concentrations of a drug with an elimination half-life of 12 h during chronic therapy using different dosage regimens for a period sufficient to reach steady state. Proportionally reducing or increasing both the size of the maintenance dose and the interval between dosage changes the magnitude of the fluctuations in plasma levels but has no effect on the average steady state (Cp_{av}) value, since this depends on the ratio between D and τ.

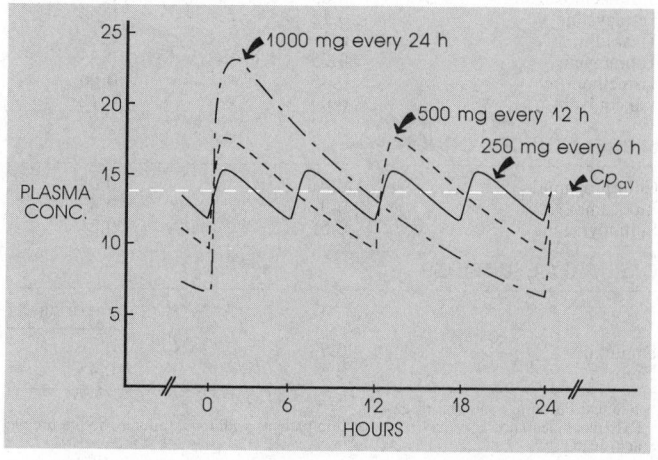

TABLE 66-1   Clearance of drugs

Drug	Renal clearance,* mL/min	Nonrenal clearance, mL/min
Ampicillin[†]	340	12
Carbenicillin	68	10
Digoxin[†]	110	36
Gentamicin	78	3
Kanamycin	60	0
Penicillin G[‡]	340	36

* The "normal" renal clearances are those associated with a clearance of creatinine of 100 mL/min.
† The fraction of digoxin absorbed after an oral dose (F) is approximately 0.75, and F for ampicillin is 0.5.
‡ One microgram of penicillin G = 1.6 units.

In the patient with renal insufficiency, this computation provides an average plasma level during a dosage interval that is the same as the average plasma level during the dosage interval with normal renal function; the fluctuations between peaks and troughs, however, will be less pronounced, but the peak value could be below the therapeutic level. Alternatively, the normal (1.5 mg/kg) dose of gentamicin could be administered but the dosage interval prolonged by the modification factor based on the change in clearance

$$8 \text{ h} \times \frac{81 \text{ mL/min}}{12.4 \text{ mL/min}} = 52 \text{ h}$$

In this case, the plasma levels may be subtherapeutic for a deleterious length of time during the dosage interval.

In some instances it may be desirable to calculate a dose that will yield a certain plasma level at steady state. This approach is most appropriate for constant intravenous infusions where 100 percent of the dose is delivered to the systemic circulation. When clearance of a drug in a patient with renal insufficiency is calculated as above, then

$$\underset{\text{(amt/unit time)}}{\text{Dose}_{ri}} = \underset{\text{(vol/unit time)}}{\text{Cl}_{ri}} \times \underset{\text{(amt/vol)}}{Cp}$$

where the time, amount, and volume terms are uniform.

If a plasma concentration of carbenicillin of 100 μg/mL is the therapeutic objective in a patient with a creatinine clearance of 25 mL/min, the infusion rate is calculated as follows. Carbenicillin clearance is

$$\text{Cl}_{ri} = \left(68 \times \frac{25}{100}\right) + 10 = 27 \text{ mL/min}$$

Therefore, carbenicillin should be infused at a rate of 2700 μg/min.

Should the method of calculating dose based on the desired plasma level be applied to intermittent-dose therapy, particular attention should be given to the fact that the calculation is based on an *average* plasma level and that peak plasma levels will be higher. In addition, if an oral drug is not completely absorbed, the computed dose must be divided by the fraction (F) that reaches the systemic circulation (see "Steady State" above).

The fractional rate constant (k) approach   For many drugs, clearance data in renal failure are not available. In these cases, the fraction of the normal dose that is required in a patient with renal failure can be approximated from the ratio of the fractional rate constant for elimination from the body in renal failure (k_{ri}) to that with normal renal function (k). This approach requires the assumption that the distribution of the drug (V_d) is not affected by renal disease. The approach is the same as that employed with clearance data:

$$\text{Dose}_{ri} = \text{dose} \times \frac{k_{ri}}{k}$$

Since the ratio k_{ri}/k is the fraction of the usual dose employed in a given degree of renal insufficiency, it is termed the *dose fraction* and

may be estimated from the information in Table 66-2 and the nomogram (Fig. 66-5). Table 66-2 gives the fraction of the usual dose of a drug required at a creatinine clearance of zero (dose fraction$_0$). The nomogram presents the dose fraction as a linear function of creatinine clearance.

To calculate the dose fraction$_{ri}$, the dose fraction$_0$ is obtained from Table 66-2, plotted on the left ordinate of the nomogram, and connected by a straight line to the upper right-hand corner of the nomogram. This line describes the dose fraction over a range of creatinine clearances from 0 to 100 mL/min. The point of intersection between the measured creatinine clearance (on the lower abscissa) and this dose-fraction line is a coordinate with the dose fraction (on the left ordinate) corresponding to that particular creatinine clearance. For example, if a patient with a creatinine clearance of 20 mL/min

TABLE 66-2   Estimated fraction of usual dose of drug required for a patient with a creatinine clearance of zero (dose fraction$_0$) and average overall fractional elimination rate constant for a patient with normal renal function (k)

Drug	Dose fraction$_0$	k (per hour)
ANTIBIOTICS		
Amikacin	0.05	0.4
Amoxicillin	0.15	0.7
Ampicillin	0.1	0.6
Aztreonam	0.25	0.4
Carbenicillin	0.1	0.6
Cefazolin	0.06	0.35
Cefotaxime*	0.3	0.7
Cefoxitin	0.1	0.8
Ceftazidime	0.1	0.4
Ceftriaxone[†]	0.5	0.09
Cephalexin	0.04	0.7
Cephalothin	0.02	1.4
Chloramphenicol	0.8	0.3
Ciprofloxacin	0.33	0.2
Clindamycin	0.8	0.2
Cloxacillin	0.25	1.2
Dicloxacillin	0.5	1.2
Doxycycline	0.8	0.03
Erythromycin	0.7	0.5
Gentamicin	0.05	0.3
Imipenem	0.25	0.7
Isoniazid:		
Fast inactivators	0.8	0.5
Slow inactivators	0.5	0.25
Methicillin	0.12	1.4
Minocycline	0.9	0.06
Nafcillin	0.4	1.2
Norfloxacin	0.5	0.2
Oxacillin	0.25	1.4
Penicillin G	0.1	1.4
Piperacillin	0.33	0.5
Rifampin	1.0	0.25
Streptomycin	0.05	0.25
Sulfadiazine	0.45	0.7
Sulfamethoxazole	0.85	0.07
Tetracycline	0.12	0.08
Ticarcillin	0.1	0.6
Tobramycin	0.05	0.35
Trimethoprim	0.45	0.06
Vancomycin	0.03	0.12
MISCELLANEOUS DRUGS		
Chlorpropamide	0.4	0.02
Lidocaine	0.9	0.4
Sulfinpyrazone	0.55	0.3
CARDIAC GLYCOSIDES		k (per day)
Digitoxin	0.7	0.1
Digoxin	0.3	0.45

* See text on dosage in renal disease.
† Extrarenal clearance also may be reduced in patients with renal failure who are uremic and/or ill.

FIGURE 66-5 Nomogram for estimation of the dose fraction in patients with renal insufficiency. Cr = creatinine; Cl_{cr} = creatinine clearance. (*From Dettli L, Clin Pharmacokin 1:126, 1976.*).

However, the plasma concentration of one of its metabolites, normeperidine, is increased when its renal elimination is impaired. Since normeperidine has more convulsant activity than meperidine, its accumulation in patients with renal failure probably accounts for the signs of central nervous system excitation such as irritability, twitching, and seizures that result from the administration of multiple doses of meperidine to patients in renal insufficiency.

The metabolite of procainamide, N-acetylprocainamide, also has cardiac effects. Since N-acetylprocainamide is eliminated almost entirely by the kidney, its concentration in plasma is increased by renal failure. Thus the potential of procainamide to produce toxicity in renal insufficiency cannot be assessed by measuring the plasma concentration of procainamide alone. Cefotaxime is metabolized predominantly to desacetylcefotaxime, which also has antimicrobial activity. Desacetylcefotaxime accumulates in renal failure to an even greater degree than does the parent drug, but no adverse effects are known to accrue to the accumulation of this metabolite.

LIVER DISEASE In contrast to the predictable decline in renal clearance of drugs when glomerular filtration is reduced, it is not possible to make a general prediction of the effect of liver disease on hepatic biotransformation of drugs (Chap. 261). Rather, in hepatitis and cirrhosis, changes may range from impaired to increased drug clearance. Even in advanced hepatocellular disease, the magnitude of impairment in drug clearance usually is only about two- to fivefold. The extent of such changes, however, cannot be predicted by the common tests of liver function. Consequently, even when it is suspected that drug elimination is altered in liver disease, there is no quantitative base on which to adjust the dosage regimen other than assessment of clinical response and concentration of drug in plasma.

Portacaval shunting creates a special condition because the effective hepatic blood flow is reduced. This situation has its greatest effect on drugs that normally have a high hepatic extraction ratio so that their clearance is largely a function of blood flow; thus the clearance of such drugs (e.g., propranolol and lidocaine) is remarkably reduced by portacaval shunting. In addition, the fraction of an administered oral dose reaching the systemic circulation is increased, because drug that is shunted around the liver during the absorption process escapes the first-pass metabolism by this organ (e.g., meperidine, pentazocine).

CIRCULATORY INSUFFICIENCY—CARDIAC FAILURE AND SHOCK Under conditions of decreased tissue perfusion, redistribution of the cardiac output occurs to preserve blood flow to the heart and brain at the expense of other tissues (Chap. 34). As a result, the drug is distributed into a smaller volume of distribution, higher drug concentrations are present in the plasma, and the tissues that are best perfused are exposed to these higher concentrations. If either the brain or heart is sensitive to the drug, an alteration in response will occur.

Furthermore, the decreased perfusion of the kidney and liver may impair drug clearance by these organs directly or indirectly. Thus, in severe congestive heart failure, in hemorrhagic shock, and in cardiogenic shock, the response to the usual dose of drug may be excessive, and dosage modification may be necessary. For example, the clearance of lidocaine is reduced by about 50 percent in cardiac failure, and therapeutic plasma levels are achieved at infusion rates of only about half those usually required. In cardiac failure there also is a significant reduction in lidocaine's volume of distribution, which results in the requirement of a smaller loading dose. Similar situations are thought to exist for procainamide, theophylline, and possibly quinidine. Unfortunately, predictors of these types of pharmacokinetic alterations are unavailable. Therefore, loading doses should be conservative, and continued therapy should be monitored closely, following clinical indicators of toxicity and plasma levels.

DISEASE-INDUCED CHANGES IN PLASMA BINDING Many drugs circulate in the plasma partly bound to the plasma proteins. Since only the unbound or free drug can distribute to the site of pharmacologic action, the therapeutic response should be related to the free rather than the total circulating plasma drug concentration.

requires penicillin G for an infection that would be treated with 10 million units daily in patients with normal renal function, then an appropriate dose would be 2.8 million units daily. This dose is estimated by plotting the dose fraction$_0$ for penicillin G (0.1) on the left-hand ordinate and connecting it to the top right-hand corner of the nomogram (Fig. 66-5). On this dose-fraction line for penicillin G, the coordinate for a creatinine clearance of 20 mL/min corresponds on the left ordinate to a dose fraction of 0.28. Hence the dose is 0.28 × 10 million units daily.

The loading dose In addition to adjusting the maintenance dose in renal failure, consideration also must be given to the loading dose. Since this dose is designed to bring the plasma concentration, or more particularly, the amount of drug in the body, rapidly to the level at steady state, there is no need to modify the usual loading dose if one is normally used. The elimination of many drugs is sufficiently rapid in patients with normal renal function that the time required to reach steady state is not significant, and no loading dose is usually used. On the other hand, in renal failure, where the half-life may be significantly prolonged, this accumulation period may become unacceptably long. In such a case, a loading dose may be indicated; it would be the same amount of drug administered with normal renal function as described in "Drug Accumulation" above.

General considerations for determining dosage in renal insufficiency Because of the differences in volumes of distribution and rates of metabolism, calculations of drug dose in renal failure must be viewed as valuable approximations which prevent the use of doses that are grossly excessive or inadequate for most patients. However, *maintenance dosages are most accurate when plasma-level data are employed to enable adjustment of the dose where necessary.*

In all the above calculations, it is assumed that the nonrenal clearance and nonrenal k are constant in renal failure. In fact, when cardiac failure accompanies renal failure, metabolic clearance for many drugs is reduced. Accordingly, when a drug with a narrow therapeutic index, such as digoxin, is used in cardiac failure, an appropriate precaution would be to reduce the value for nonrenal clearance (or k) to about one-half.

Active or toxic metabolites of drugs also may accumulate in renal failure. Meperidine, for example, is cleared largely by metabolism, and its concentration in plasma is little altered by renal insufficiency.

In most cases the degree of binding is fairly constant across the therapeutic concentration range so that significant error is not caused by individualizing therapy on the basis of total drug levels in plasma. However, states such as hypoalbuminemia, liver disease, and renal disease can decrease the extent of drug binding, particularly of acidic and neutral drugs, so that at any total plasma level there is a greater concentration of free drug and a risk of increased response and toxicity. Other conditions, e.g., myocardial infarction, surgery, neoplastic disease, rheumatoid arthritis, and burns, that lead to an increased plasma concentration of the acute-phase reactant alpha$_1$-acid glycoprotein have the opposite effect on the basic drugs that are bound to this macromolecule. The drugs for which changes in binding are important are those which are normally highly bound in the plasma (>90 percent) because a small alteration in the extent of binding produces a large change in the amount of drug in the unbound form.

The consequences of these binding changes, particularly with respect to total drug levels, depend on whether the clearance and distribution are dependent on the unbound or total drug. For many drugs, elimination and distribution are largely restricted to the unbound fraction, and therefore, a decrease in binding leads to an increase in the clearance and distribution of the drug. The relative magnitudes of these changes are such that the net effect is to shorten the half-life. The appropriate modification of the dosage regimen in conditions with reduced drug binding, as is the case of phenytoin in renal failure, is simply to administer the usual daily dose of the drug but in divided doses at more frequent intervals. Individualization of therapy can then be based on either the clinical response or the plasma concentration of unbound drug. It is critical that the patient not be titrated into the usual therapeutic range for concentration of *total* drug in plasma, since this will lead to excessive response and toxicity.

In the case of drugs bound to alpha$_1$-acid glycoprotein, the disease-induced increase in binding has the opposite effects of reducing the clearance and distribution of total drug. Accordingly, constant rate infusion of lidocaine to control arrhythmias after myocardial infarction leads to an accumulation of total drug. However, the clearance of unbound and pharmacologically active drug remains essentially unchanged. Again, it is critical that the patient not be dosed on the basis of total drug concentrations in the plasma, since this will be associated with subtherapeutic levels of unbound drug.

VARIABLE ACTIONS OF DRUGS CAUSED BY GENETIC DIFFERENCES IN THEIR METABOLISM

ACETYLATION Isoniazid, hydralazine, procainamide, and a number of other drugs are metabolized by acetylation of a hydrazino or amino group. This reaction is catalyzed by *N*-acetyl transferase-2, an enzyme in the liver cytosol that transfers an acetyl group from acetyl coenzyme A to the drug. Individuals differ markedly in the rate at which drugs are acetylated, and there is a bimodal distribution of the population into "rapid acetylators" and "slow acetylators." The rate of acetylation is under genetic control; slow acetylation is an autosomal recessive trait.

Responses to hydralazine therapy are dependent on the acetylation phenotype. The hypotensive effect of hydralazine is greater in patients who acetylate the drug slowly, and the lupus erythematosus–like syndrome produced by hydralazine occurs almost exclusively in those with slow acetylation. Thus it may be of value to know the acetylation phenotype as a predictor of which patients with hypertension might benefit from an increase in the dose of hydralazine above the 200 mg daily that can be safely employed in the population at large.

Acetylation phenotype can be determined by measuring the ratio of acetylated to nonacetylated dapsone or sulfamethazine in plasma or urine following administration of a test dose of these acetylation substrates. The ratio of monoacetyldapsone to dapsone in plasma at 6 h after dapsone administration is less than 0.30 for slow acetylators and greater than 0.35 for rapid acetylators. At 6 h following the administration of sulfamethazine, less than 25 percent of the drug in

the plasma is in the acetylated form in slow acetylators (in rapid acetylators, more than 25 percent); in the urine collected in the 5- to 6-h interval after administration, less than 70 percent of the drug is in the acetylated form in slow acetylators (in rapid acetylators, more than 70 percent). More recently, the acetylation of a metabolite of caffeine, possibly the most widely consumed drug worldwide because of its presence in a variety of foodstuffs, has been used as an indicator of phenotypic status. In this procedure, the urinary molar ratio of 5-acetylamino-6-amino-3-methyluracil to methylxanthine after ingestion of a drink of coffee or cola is determined. Antimodes of about 1.8 and 6.6 separate slow, intermediate, and rapid acetylators; moreover, these three groups appear to correspond to the expected genotypes.

METABOLISM BY MIXED-FUNCTION OXIDASES In healthy individuals taking no other medications, the major determinant of the rate of metabolism of drugs by the hepatic mixed-function oxidases is genetic. Hepatic endoplasmic reticulum contains a family of cytochrome P450 isoenzymes with different substrate specificities. Many drugs undergo oxidative metabolism by more than one iso-enzyme, and the steady state concentrations of such drugs in the plasma is a function of the sum of the activities of these and other metabolizing enzymes. When a drug is metabolized by multiple pathways, the catalytic activities of the participating enzymes are regulated by a number of genes so that the frequency of clearance rates and steady state concentrations of the drug tend to distribute unimodally within the population. The range of activity may differ markedly (tenfold or more) between different individuals, as is the case for chlorpromazine, and there is no way to make a prior prediction of the rate.

For certain metabolic pathways, bimodally distributed activity suggests control by a single gene, and several polymorphisms have been identified. As a result, two phenotypic populations are usually present analogous to the situation with *N*-acetylation (see above). A majority of the population are extensive metabolizers (EM), and a smaller group of individuals of the poor metabolizer (PM) phenotype have an impaired, if not an absent, ability to metabolize the drug. For example, about 8 to 10 percent of whites are unable to form the 4-hydroxy metabolite of the test drug debrisoquin, and this trait is inherited in an autosomal recessive fashion. Importantly, the putatively involved cytochrome P450 isoenzyme 2D6 is also at work in the biotransformation of other drugs whose metabolic fate, therefore, cosegregates with the debrisoquin trait. These other drugs include antiarrhythmic agents (propafenone, flecainide), beta-adrenoceptor blockers (alprenolol, metoprolol, timolol), tricylic antidepressants (nortriptyline, desipramine, imipramine, clomipramine), neuroleptic drugs (perphenazine, thioridazine, and possibly fluoxetine), and certain opiates such as codeine. Thus a much reduced analgesic effect of codeine is obtained in PM patients because of impaired production of the active metabolite morphine. A similar situation occurs with the oxidative polymorphism that involves the metabolism of mephenytoin. The situation is further complicated by interethnic differences in the frequency of the polymorphisms. For example, impaired hydroxylation of mephenytoin is present in only 3 to 5 percent of whites, but the incidence is about 20 percent in individuals of Japanese descent; likewise, the frequency of the PM phenotype for debrisoquin hydroxylation appears to decrease as one moves from western (8 to 10 percent) to eastern (0 to 1 percent) population groups.

Polymorphisms in drug-metabolizing ability may be associated with large differences in the disposition of the drug among individuals, especially when the involved pathway is a major contribution to the overall elimination of the drug. For example, the oral clearance of mephenytoin differs 100- to 200-fold between individuals of the EM and PM phenotypes. As a result, peak plasma concentrations and bioavailability after oral administration may be profoundly increased and the rate of drug elimination decreased in PM individuals. This in turn results in drug accumulation and exaggerated pharmacologic responses, including toxicity, when usual drug dosages are administered to patients with the PM phenotype. Drug interactions between compounds that are metabolized by cytochrome P450 2D6 or which inhibit its activity noncompetitively, e.g., quinidine, may be of considerable clinical importance in patients with the EM phenotype, since such concomitant administration often leads to impaired drug handling similar to that in the PM phenotype. Effective individualization of drug therapy is even more critical when using drugs exhibiting polymorphic drug metabolism.

DRUG USE IN THE ELDERLY (See also Chap. 8)

The elderly (>65 years) constitute about 12 percent of the U.S. population, and will increase to about 20 percent, or 50 to 60 million individuals, over the next 20 years. These patients use a disproportionate amount of prescription medications (30 percent), and in addition, 70 percent of the elderly regularly use over-the-counter drugs, compared with only 10 percent in the general adult population. Aging results in changes in organ function, especially in those organs involved in drug disposition, as well as alterations in body size and composition. Not surprisingly, therefore, pharmacokinetic differences are often present in elderly individuals compared with younger cohorts. Unfortunately, few generalizations appear to exist with respect to the type, magnitude, or clinical importance of any age-related changes or their extent in an individual patient. Multiple diseases are also common in geriatric patients, and it is not unusual, therefore, that a large number of drugs are required, which may result in drug interactions that, along with increased vulnerability to morbidity and mortality, contribute to the higher incidence of adverse drug reactions in elderly patients. Increased sensitivity of target organs and impaired physiologic control systems, such as those involved in the regulation of the circulation, also may be a factor. Accordingly, optimization of drug therapy in the elderly, particularly frail patients, is often difficult, since a variety of factors that are frequently poorly defined accentuate the usual interindividual variability in drug response.

Although many individuals preserve good renal function into old age, as a group, elderly patients have an increased and predictable likelihood of impaired renal excretion of drugs. Even in the absence of kidney disease, renal clearance is generally reduced by about 35 to 50 percent in elderly patients. Dosage adjustments analogous to those in patients with kidney dysfunction (see above) are therefore necessary for drugs that are predominantly eliminated from the body by the renal route, e.g., digoxin, aminoglycosides, lithium, and other drugs listed in Table 66-2. In this regard, it is important to recognize that the reduced muscle mass present in older individuals results in a reduction in the rate of creatinine production; thus a normal serum creatinine concentration can be present even though creatinine clearance is impaired.

Aging also results in a decrease in liver size and blood flow, and possibly reduced activity of hepatic drug-metabolizing enzymes; accordingly, the hepatic clearance of some drugs is impaired in the elderly. Unfortunately, no consistent pattern of clinical application appears to be present. Moreover, changes that may exist are often modest relative to the interindividual variability within the patient population. However, even small reductions in hepatic extraction may result in a significant increase in oral bioavailability of drugs with a high first-pass effect, such as propranolol and labetalol.

As a consequence of impaired clearance and/or increased distribution, the elimination half-lives of drugs may increase with aging. Thus, if a dosage modification in an elderly patient is required, it is often possible to accomplish this by decreasing the frequency of drug administration, possibly along with a reduction in dose.

Even if the pharmacokinetics of a drug are not altered, elderly patients may require a smaller drug dosage because of an increase in pharmacodynamic sensitivity. Examples include increased analgesic effects of opioids, increased sedation from benzodiazepines and other central nervous system depressants, and increased risk of bleeding while receiving anticoagulant therapy, even when clotting parameters are well controlled. Exaggerated responses to cardiovascular drugs

are also common because of the impaired responsiveness of normal homeostatic mechanisms. Such age-related changes require close monitoring of the patient's clinical response and appropriate dosage titration.

In general, drug therapy for the elderly should be attended by increased alertness to the possibility of moderate reductions in the clearance of drugs and instances of exaggerated pharmacodynamic responsiveness.

INTERACTIONS BETWEEN DRUGS

The effect of some drugs can be altered markedly by the administration of other agents. Such interactions can sabotage therapeutic intent by producing excessive drug action (with adverse effects) or decreasing the action of a drug, rendering it ineffective. Drug interactions must be considered in the differential diagnosis of unexpected responses to drugs, recognizing that patients often come to the physician with a legacy of drugs acquired during previous medical experiences. A meticulous drug history will minimize the unknown elements in the therapeutic milieu; it should include examination of the patient's medications and calls to the pharmacist to identify prescriptions, if necessary.

There are two principal types of interactions between drugs. *Pharmacokinetic interactions* result from alteration in the delivery of drugs to their sites of action. *Pharmacodynamic interactions* are those in which the responsiveness of the target organ or system is modified by other agents.

An index of the drug interactions discussed in this chapter is provided in Table 66-3. Included are interactions which have verified significance in patients and a few of such potential danger that cognizance should be taken of experimental data or case reports suggesting their likely occurrence.

I PHARMACOKINETIC INTERACTIONS CAUSING DIMINISHED DRUG DELIVERY

A Impaired gastrointestinal absorption Cholestyramine, an ionic exchange resin, binds thyroxine, triiodothyronine, and the cardiac glycosides with sufficiently high affinity to impair their absorption from the gastrointestinal tract. This resin probably also interferes with the absorption of other drugs, and it is safest not to give it within 2 h of their administration. Aluminum ions, present in antacids, form insoluble chelates with the tetracyclines, thereby preventing absorption of these drugs. Ferrous ions similarly block tetracycline absorption. Kaolin-pectin suspensions bind digoxin, and when the drugs are administered together, digoxin absorption is reduced by about one-half. However, when kaolin-pectin is administered 2 h after digoxin, there is no effect on absorption of digoxin.

Ketoconazole is a weak base that dissolves well only at acidic pH. Thus histamine-2 antagonists such as cimetidine, by neutralizing gastric pH, impair the dissolution and subsequent absorption of ketoconazole. By contrast, absorption of fluconazole is not impaired by increasing gastric pH. Oral administration of aminosalicylate interferes with the absorption of rifampin by an unknown mechanism.

Impaired absorption results in reduction in the total amount of drug absorbed, i.e., decreased bioavailability, F, with reduced area under the plasma level curve, reduced peak plasma levels, and lower steady state concentrations of the drug involved.

B Induction of hepatic drug-metabolizing enzymes When the elimination of the drug is largely by metabolism, an increase in the rate of metabolism reduces its availability to sites of action. The metabolism of most drugs occurs largely in the liver because of its mass, high blood flow, and concentration of enzymes that metabolize drugs. The initial step in metabolism of many drugs is mediated by a group of mixed-function oxidase isoenzymes in the endoplasmic reticulum. These enzyme systems containing cytochrome P450 oxidize drug molecules by a variety of reactions including aromatic hydroxylations, N-demethylations, O-demethylations, and sulfoxidations. The

TABLE 66-3 Drug interaction index

Drug	Section of chapter describing interaction
Acetohexamide	IIB
Allopurinol	IIA
p-Aminosalicylate	IA
Amiodarone	IIA, IIC
Amphetamine	IC
Antidepressants, tricyclic (desipramine, nortriptyline, imipramine, doxepin, protriptyline, amitriptyline)	IC
Aspirin	IIB, III
Azathioprine	IIA
Barbiturates (class)	IB
Bethanidine	IC
Carbamazepine	IB, IIA
Chlorpromazine	IC, IIA
Cholestyramine	IA
Cimetidine	IA, IIA, IIB
Clofibrate	IIA
Clonidine	IC
Codeine	IIA
Cyclosporin A	IB, IIA
Dexamethasone	IB
Digitoxin	IA, IB, IIC
Digoxin	IA, IIC
Diltiazem	IIA
Diuretics	III
Erythromycin	IIA
Ephedrine	IC
Ethanol	IIA
Famotidine	IIA
Guanadrel	IC
Guanethidine	IC
Haloperidol	IIA
Indomethacin	III
Isoniazid	IIA
Kaolin-pectin	IA
Ketoconazole	IA, IB, IIA
Lidocaine	IIA
Lovastatin	IIA
6-Mercaptopurine	IB
Methadone	IIB
Methotrexate	IIB
Methylprednisolone	IB, IIA
Metronidazole	IB, IIA
Metyrapone	IB
Mexiletine	IB
Nicardipine	IIA
Nifedipine	IIA
Nonsteroidal anti-inflammatory drugs	III
Oral contraceptive steroids	IB
Phenobarbital	IB
Phenylbutazone	IIA, IIB
Phenytoin (diphenylhydantoin)	IB, IIA
Piroxicam	III
Potassium	III
Prednisone	IB
Probenicid	IIB
Procainamide	IIB
Propranolol	III
Quinidine	IB, IIA, IIC, III
Ranitidine	IA, IIA
Rifampin	IA, IB
Salicylate	IIB
Spironolactone	III
Terfenadine	IIA
Tetracycline	IA
Theophylline	IIA
Thiazide diuretics	III
Tolbutamide	IIA
Triamterene	III
Triazolam	IIA
Verapamil	IB, IIA, IIC
Warfarin	IB, IIA, III

products of these reactions are usually more polar (and more readily excreted by the kidney).

The biosynthesis of some of the mixed-function oxidase isoenzymes is under regulatory control, and their content in the liver can be induced by a number of drugs. Phenobarbital is the prototype of these inducers, and all barbiturates in clinical use increase mixed-function oxidase isoenzymes. Induction with phenobarbital can occur with doses of as little as 60 mg daily. Mixed-function oxidases also are induced by rifampin, carbamazepine, phenytoin, and glutethimide, by smoking and exposure to chlorinated insecticides such as DDT, and by chronic alcohol ingestion.

Phenobarbital, rifampin, and other inducers lower plasma levels of many drugs, including warfarin, digitoxin, quinidine, mexiletine, verapamil, ketoconazole, cyclosporin A, dexamethasone, methylprednisolone, prednisolone (the active metabolite of prednisone), oral contraceptive steroids, methadone, metronidazole, and metyrapone. These interactions all have obvious clinical significance. With the coumarin anticoagulants, the patient is placed at major risk when an appropriate level of anticoagulation is achieved while the coumarin drug is coadministered with an inducing agent. Should the inducer then be discontinued, e.g., following discharge from the hospital, plasma levels of the coumarin anticoagulant will rise as the induction effect wears off, leading to excessive anticoagulation.

There is considerable variation among individuals in the extent to which drug metabolism can be induced. In some patients, phenobarbital leads to marked acceleration in the rate of drug metabolism, whereas little induction is seen in others.

In addition to inducing certain of the mixed-function oxidase isoenzymes, phenobarbital has other effects on hepatic function. It increases liver blood flow, bile flow, and the hepatocellular transport of organic anions. The conjugation of drugs and bilirubin also may be enhanced by inducing agents.

C Inhibition of cellular uptake or binding The guanidinium antihypertensives guanethidine, guanadrel, and bethanidine are transported to their site of action in adrenergic neurons by an energy-requiring membrane transport system for biogenic monoamines. Although the physiologic function of the transport system is reuptake of the adrenergic neurotransmitter, it also transports a variety of ring-substituted bases, including guanethidine and related guanidiniums, into the adrenergic neuron against a concentration gradient. Inhibitors of norepinephrine uptake prevent the uptake of the guanidinium antihypertensives into adrenergic neurons and thereby block their pharmacologic effects. The tricyclic antidepressants are potent inhibitors of norepinephrine uptake. Consequently, concomitant administration of clinical doses of tricyclic antidepressants, including desipramine, protriptyline, nortriptyline, and amitriptyline, almost totally abolishes the antihypertensive effects of guanethidine, guanadrel, and bethanidine. Although they are less potent inhibitors of norepinephrine uptake, doxepin and chlorpromazine produce dose-related antagonism of the action of the guanidinium antihypertensives. Ephedrine, a component of many drug combinations used in asthma, also antagonizes the effect of guanethidine. In patients with severe hypertension, the loss of control of blood pressure from these drug interactions can lead to stroke and malignant hypertension.

The antihypertensive effect of clonidine is partially antagonized by tricyclic antidepressants. Clonidine lowers arterial pressure by reducing sympathetic outflow from the blood pressure–regulating centers in the hindbrain (Chap. 209). This central hypotensive action is antagonized by the tricyclic antidepressants.

II PHARMACOKINETIC INTERACTIONS CAUSING INCREASED DRUG DELIVERY

A Inhibition of drug metabolism If the active form of a drug is eliminated largely by biotransformation, inhibition of its metabolism leads to a reduced clearance, prolonged half-life, and accumulation of the drug during maintenance therapy. Excessive accumulation due to inhibited metabolism can lead to adverse effects.

Cimetidine is a potent inhibitor of the oxidative metabolism of many drugs, including warfarin, quinidine, nifedipine, lidocaine, theophylline and phenytoin. Adverse reactions, many of them severe, have resulted from the administration of these drugs in conjunction with cimetidine. Cimetidine is a more potent inhibitor of mixed-function oxidases than ranitidine, whereas ranitidine is more potent as a histamine-2 antagonist. Thus ranitidine, when administered in doses of 150 mg twice daily, does not inhibit the oxidative metabolism of most drugs; where reduced drug elimination has been observed, the effects of ranitidine have been less than those of cimetidine and devoid of appreciable pharmacodynamic consequence. Doses of ranitidine higher than 150 mg, however, may produce greater inhibition of drug oxidation. Famotidine and nizatidine are not known to produce clinically appreciable inhibition of drug metabolism.

Knowledge of the P450 isoenzyme that catalyzes the predominant pathway of metabolism of a drug provides a basis for predicting and understanding drug interactions. For example, the P450 3A family of isoenzymes catalyzes the metabolism of many drugs that produce toxicity when their metabolism is blocked. Drugs that depend on P450 3A as a major route of metabolism include cyclosporin A, quinidine, lovastatin, warfarin, nifedipine, lidocaine, terfenadine, erythromycin, methylprednisolone, carbamazepine, midazolam, and triazolam.

Erythromycin and ketoconazole are potent inhibitors of enzymes in the P450 3A family. Some of the calcium antagonists, diltiazem, nicardipine, and verapamil also can inhibit P450 3A, as can some of its other substrates such as cyclosporin A. Thus serious toxicity from cyclosporin A can result from inhibition of its metabolism by erythromycin, ketoconazole, diltiazem, nicardipine, and verapamil. Lovastatin causes severe myopathy with rhabdomyolysis when administered together with erythromycin or cyclosporin A, and it is highly probable that other of the known inhibitors of P450 3A also can inhibit the disposition of lovastatin. Terfenadine-induced polymorphic ventricular tachycardia can occur when the metabolism of this antihistamine is blocked by ketoconazole and erythromycin.

Whenever erythromycin or ketoconazole are administered to patients, there should be a high level of alert regarding the potential for serious interactions with drugs that are metabolized by P450 3A.

The P450 2D6 isoenzyme that catalyzes the polymorphic metabolism of debrisoquin is markedly inhibited by quinidine and also is blocked by a number of neuroleptic drugs such as chlorpromazine, fluoxetine, and haloperidol. The analgesic effect of codeine depends on its metabolism to morphine via P450 2D6 in individuals with the extensive metabolizer phenotype. Thus quinidine abrogates the analgesic efficacy of codeine in extensive metabolizers. Since desipramine is cleared largely by metabolism via P450 2D6 in extensive metabolizers, its levels are increased substantially by concurrent administration of quinidine or the neuroleptic drugs that block P450 2D6.

Some drugs are inactivated by mechanisms other than the hepatic drug-metabolizing enzymes. Azathioprine is converted in the body to an active metabolite, 6-mercaptopurine, which in turn is oxidized by xanthine oxidase to 6-thiouric acid. When allopurinol, a potent inhibitor of xanthine oxidase, is administered concurrently with standard doses of azathioprine or 6-mercaptopurine, life-threatening toxicity (bone marrow suppression) can result.

Other drugs that inhibit biotransformation of pharmacologic compounds (with examples of drugs that have their metabolism blocked by the inhibitor listed in parenthesis) include:

Amiodarone (warfarin, quinidine)
Clofibrate (phenytoin, tolbutamide)
Excessive ingestion of ethanol (warfarin)
Isoniazid (phenytoin)
Metronidazole (warfarin)
Phenylbutazone (warfarin, phenytoin, tolbutamide)

B Inhibition of renal elimination A number of drugs are secreted by the renal tubular transport systems for organic anions. Inhibition of this tubular transport system can cause excessive accumulation of a drug. Phenylbutazone, probenecid, and salicylates competitively inhibit this transport system. Salicylate, for example, reduces the renal clearance of methotrexate, an interaction that may lead to methotrexate toxicity. Renal tubular secretion contributes

substantially to the elimination of penicillin, which can be inhibited by probenecid.

Inhibition of the tubular cation transport system by cimetidine impedes the renal clearance of procainamide and its active metabolite N-acetylprocainamide.

C Inhibition of clearance by multiple mechanisms The concentrations of digoxin and digitoxin in plasma are elevated by quinidine, due largely to inhibition of renal elimination and in part to inhibition of nonrenal clearance as well. An increase in cardiac arrhythmia may occur when quinidine is given in conjunction with a cardiac glycoside.

Amiodarone, cyclosporin A, and verapamil also inhibit the clearance of digoxin and increase the concentration of digoxin in plasma.

III PHARMACODYNAMIC AND OTHER INTERACTIONS BETWEEN DRUGS Therapeutically useful interactions occur in which the combined effect of two drugs is greater than that of either drug alone. These favorable drug combinations are described in specific therapeutic sections in this text, and the following is directed toward those interactions which create unwanted effects. Two drugs may act on separate components of a common process and yield effects greater than either alone. For example, small doses of aspirin (less than 1 g daily) do not alter the prothrombin time appreciably in patients who are on warfarin therapy. However, the addition of aspirin to patients anticoagulated with warfarin increases the risk of bleeding because aspirin inhibits platelet aggregation. Thus the combination of impaired functions of platelets and the clotting system increases the potential for hemorrhagic complications in patients receiving warfarin therapy.

Indomethacin, piroxicam, and probably other nonsteroidal anti-inflammatory drugs antagonize the antihypertensive effects of beta-adrenergic receptor blockers, diuretics, converting enzyme inhibitors, and other drugs. The resultant elevation in blood pressure ranges from trivial to severe. Aspirin and sulindac, however, do not elevate the blood pressure in treated hypertensive patients.

Polymorphic ventricular tachycardia (torsades de pointes) during quinidine administration occurs much more frequently in patients receiving diuretics, probably as a consequence of potassium and/or magnesium depletion.

The administration of supplemental potassium leads to more frequent and more severe hyperkalemia when potassium elimination is reduced by concurrent treatment with angiotensin-converting enzyme inhibitors, spironolactone, or triamterene.

CONCENTRATION OF DRUGS IN PLASMA AS A GUIDE TO THERAPY

Optimal individualization of therapy is assisted by measuring the concentration of certain drugs in plasma. Genetic variation in elimination rates, interactions with other drugs, disease-induced alterations in elimination and distribution, and other factors combine to yield a wide range of plasma levels in patients given the same dose. Furthermore, the problem of noncompliance with prescribed regimens during continuing therapy is an endemic and elusive cause of therapeutic failure (see below). Clinical indicators assist the titration of some drugs into the desired range, and no chemical determination is a substitute for careful observations of the response to treatment. However, the therapeutic and adverse effects are not precisely quantifiable for all drugs, and in complex clinical situations, estimates of the action of a drug may be misleading. For example, previously existing neurologic disease may obscure the neurologic consequences of intoxication with phenytoin. Because clearance, half-life, accumulation, and steady state plasma levels are difficult to predict, the measurement of plasma levels is often useful as a guide to the optimal dose. This is particularly so when there is a narrow range between the plasma levels yielding therapeutic and adverse effects. For drugs having such characteristics, e.g., digoxin, theophylline, lidocaine, aminoglycosides, and anticonvulsants, dose optimization should involve modification of the standard dose based on the pharmacokinetic principles described above. In certain instances, predictive nomograms and algorithms have been developed to facilitate the necessary modifications. However, the most flexible and accurate method for individualizing drug dosage appears to be a feedback approach using a small number of previously obtained plasma levels and Bayesian forecasting. In controlled studies, this type of computer-assisted dosing has been shown to improve patient care. However, the overall cost/benefit ratio of such methods in routine management still remains to be conclusively demonstrated.

For those drugs with a narrow therapeutic window that exhibit first-order elimination, then, dosage adjustments may be made on the basis that the average, maximal, minimum steady state concentrations are linearly related to the dosing rate. Accordingly, the dose may be adjusted on the basis of the ratio between the desired and measured concentrations:

$$\frac{Cp_{SS} \text{ (desired)}}{Cp_{SS} \text{ (measured)}} = \frac{\text{dose (new)}}{\text{dose (previous)}}$$

In instances where dose-dependent kinetics are present (e.g., phenytoin and theophylline), plasma concentrations change disproportionately more than the alteration in the dosing rate. Not only should changes in dose be small to minimize the degree of unpredictability, but plasma concentration monitoring also is critical to ensure appropriateness of the modification.

The variability among individual responses to given plasma levels must be recognized. This is illustrated by a hypothetical population concentration-response curve (Fig. 66-6) and its relationship to the therapeutic range or therapeutic window of desired plasma levels. The defined therapeutic window should include the levels at which the majority of patients achieve the intended pharmacologic effect. However, a few people, sensitive to the therapeutic effects, respond to lower levels, whereas others are sufficiently refractory as to require levels that impose the likelihood of adverse effects as a price for therapeutic benefit. For example, a few patients with strong seizure foci require plasma levels of phenytoin exceeding 20 μg/mL to control seizures. Dosages to achieve this effect may be appropriate.

As also illustrated in Fig. 66-6, some patients are prone to adverse effects at levels that are tolerated by most of the population, and therefore, elevation of levels to those with a high probability of therapeutic effect may bring on unwanted actions in the exceptional patient. Table 66-4 presents the concentrations of a number of drugs

FIGURE 66-6 The cumulative percentage of patients responding to increasing levels of drug in plasma with both therapeutic and adverse effects. The therapeutic window defines the range of concentrations of drug that will achieve therapeutic effects in most patients with adverse effects in only a small percentage.

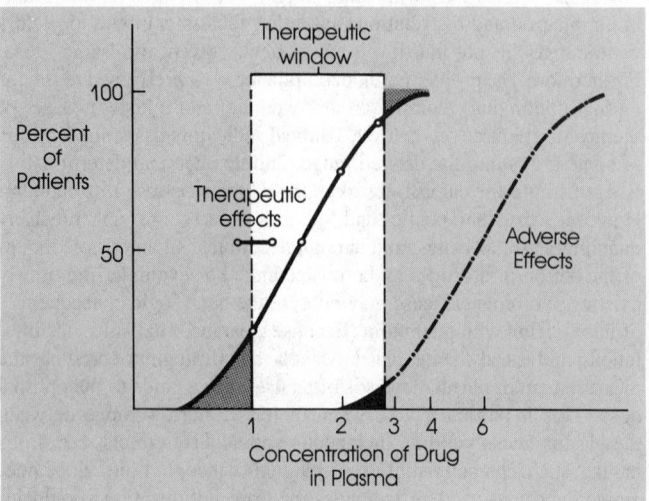

TABLE 66-4   Concentrations of drugs in plasma: Relation to efficacy and adverse effects

Drug	Efficacy*	Adverse effects[†]
Amikacin (peak)	20 μg/mL	40 μg/mL
Carbenicillin	100 μg/mL[‡]	300 μg/mL
Carbamazepine	3 μg/mL	10 μg/mL
Digitoxin	12 ng/mL	25–30 ng/mL
Digoxin	0.8 ng/mL	2.0 ng/mL
Ethosuximide	40 μg/mL	100 μg/mL
Gentamicin (peak)	5 μg/mL	10 μg/mL
Gentamicin (predose)		2.5 μg/mL
Lidocaine	1.5 μg/mL	5 μg/mL
Lithium	0.5 mEq/L	1.3 mEq/L
Penicillin G	1–25 μg/mL[¶]	
Phenytoin (diphenylhydantoin)	10 μg/mL	20 μg/mL
Procainamide	4 μg/mL	10 μg/mL
Quinidine	2.5 μg/mL	6 μg/mL
Theophylline	8 μg/mL	20 μg/mL

* The therapeutic effect is infrequent or slight at levels below these.
[†] The frequency of adverse effects increases sharply when these levels are exceeded.
[‡] Minimal inhibitory concentration (MIC) for most strains of *Pseudomonas aeruginosa*. MIC for other, more sensitive, organisms is less.
[¶] There is a wide range of MIC of penicillin for various organisms, and the MIC of all those for which penicillin is used is < 20. "Massive" penicillin therapy with 20 million units daily achieves levels of 20 to 25 μg/mL in patients with clearance of creatinine of 100 mL/min.

in plasma that are associated with adverse and therapeutic effects in most patients. Its use within the guidelines discussed should permit more effective and safer therapy for those patients who are not "average."

EFFECTIVE PARTICIPATION OF THE PATIENT IN THERAPEUTIC PROGRAMS   Measurement of the concentration of a drug in plasma is the most effective approach to determine when patients have failed to take the drug. Such "noncompliance" is a frequent problem in the long-term treatment of diseases such as hypertension and epilepsy, occurring in 25 percent or more of patients in therapeutic environments that lack special efforts to involve patients in the responsibility for their own health. Occasionally, noncompliance can be uncovered by sympathetic, nonincriminating questioning, but more often it is recognized only after determining that the concentration of drug in plasma is nil or is recurrently low. Because other factors can cause plasma levels to be lower than expected, comparison with levels obtained during inpatient treatment may be required to confirm that noncompliance did, in fact, occur. Once the physician is certain of noncompliance, a nonaccusatory discussion of the problem with the patient may elucidate a reason for the noncompliance and serve as a basis for more effective cooperation of the patient. Many approaches have been tried to enhance patients' exercise of responsibility for their own treatment, most based on improved communication regarding the nature of the disease and the expectations of treatment success and treatment failure. This communication includes an opportunity for the patient to relate problems associated with treatment, and it may be improved by involving nurses and other paramedical personnel in the process. Minimizing the complexity of the regimen is helpful in terms of both the number of drugs and the frequency of administration. Educating patients to assume the principal role in their own health care requires a blend of the art and science of medicine.

REFERENCES

BENET LZ, WILLIAMS RL: Design and optimization of dosage regimens: Pharmacokinetic data, in *Goodman and Gilman's The Pharmacological Basis of Therapeutics*, 8th ed, AG Gilman et al (eds). New York, Macmillan, 1990, p 1650, Appendix II

BENNETT WM et al: *Drug Prescribing in Renal Failure: Dosing Guidelines for Adults*. Philadelphia, American College of Physicians, 1987

BROWN GR et al: Drug concentration monitoring. An approach to rational use. Clin Pharmacokinet 24:187, 1993

MEYER UA: Drugs in special patient groups: Clinical importance of genetics in drug effects, in *Clinical Pharmacology: Basic Principles in Therapeutics*, 3rd ed, KL Melmon et al (eds). New York, McGraw-Hill, 1992, p 875

NEBERT DW et al: The P450 superfamily: Update on new sequences, gene mapping and recommended nomenclature. DNA Cell Biol 10:1, 1992

REYNOLDS DJ, ARONSON JK: ABCs of monitoring drug therapy. Making the most of plasma drug concentration measurements. BMJ 306:48, 1993

TUKEY RH, JOHNSON EF: Molecular aspects of regulation and structure of drug metabolizing enzymes, in *Principles of Drug Action: The Basis of Pharmacology*, 3d ed, WB Pratt, P Taylor (eds). New York, Churchill Livingstone, 1990, p 423

67 ADVERSE REACTIONS TO DRUGS

ALASTAIR J. J. WOOD*

The beneficial effects of drugs are coupled with the inescapable risk of untoward effects. The morbidity and mortality from these untoward effects often present diagnostic problems because they can involve every organ and system of the body and are frequently mistaken for signs of underlying disease.

Major advances in the investigation, development, and regulation of drugs ensure in most instances their uniformity, effectiveness, and relative safety, as well as identify their recognized hazards. However, the large number and variety of drugs available over the counter (OTC) or by prescription make it impossible for patient or physician to obtain or retain the knowledge necessary to use all drugs well. It is understandable, therefore, that many OTC drugs are used unwisely by the public and that restricted drugs may be prescribed incorrectly by physicians.

Most physicians use no more than 50 drug products in their practice, gaining familiarity with their effectiveness and safety. Most patients probably use only a limited number of OTC drugs. Nevertheless, many patients receive care and drug prescriptions from more than one physician, and in any 30-day period many patients consume more than three different OTC drug products containing nine or more different chemical agents.

Twenty-five to fifty percent of patients may make errors in self-administration of prescribed medicines, and this can be responsible for adverse drug effects. Elderly patients are most likely to commit such errors, perhaps reflecting their consumption of increased numbers of medicines. One-third or more of patients also may not take their prescribed medications. Similarly, patients commit errors in taking OTC drugs by not reading or following the directions for use of the medicines on the containers. Physicians must recognize that providing directions with prescriptions does not always guarantee compliance.

Every drug can produce untoward consequences, even when used according to standard or recommended methods of administration. When used incorrectly, the effectiveness may be reduced, and adverse reactions can be expected to occur more frequently. The administration of several drugs during the same period of time also may result in adverse interactions between drugs (see Chap. 66).

In the hospital, all drugs a patient is given should be under the control of a physician, and patient compliance is, in general, ensured. Errors may occur nevertheless, in that the wrong drug or dose may be given or the drug may be given to the wrong patient, although improved drug distribution and administration systems have reduced this problem. On the other hand, there are no means for controlling how ambulatory patients take prescription or OTC drugs.

EPIDEMIOLOGY Epidemiologic studies of adverse drug reactions have been helpful in evaluating the magnitude of the overall problem, in calculating the rate of reactions to individual drugs, and in characterizing some of the determinants of adverse drug effects.

Patients receive, on average, 10 different drugs during each hospitalization. The sicker the patient, the more drugs are given, and there is a corresponding increase in the likelihood of adverse drug reactions. When fewer than 6 different drugs are given to hospitalized patients, the probability of an adverse reaction is about 5 percent, but if more than 15 drugs are given, the probability is over 40 percent. Retrospective analyses of ambulatory patients have revealed adverse drug effects in 20 percent.

Thus the magnitude of drug-induced disease is large. Two to five percent of patients are admitted to the medical and pediatric services of general hospitals because of illnesses attributed to drugs. The case/fatality ratio from drug-induced disease in hospitalized patients varies from 2 to 12 percent. Furthermore, some fetal or neonatal abnormalities are due to medicines taken by the mother during pregnancy or parturition.

A small group of widely used drugs accounts for a disproportionate number of reactions; aspirin, digoxin, anticoagulants, diuretics, antimicrobials, steroids, antineoplastics, and hypoglycemic agents account for 90 percent of reactions.

ADVERSE DRUG REACTIONS IN THE ELDERLY (See also Chap. 8) The elderly as a group have a greater burden of disease and receive a greater number of medications. Thus it is not surprising that adverse drug reactions occur frequently in elderly patients. The issue of whether an elderly individual is more likely to develop an adverse drug reaction than a young person with a similar number of concurrent diseases and other therapy has not been unequivocally demonstrated. Although it is widely believed that the elderly are more sensitive to drugs than the young, this is not true for all drugs. For example, a consistent decrease in sensitivity to drugs acting at the beta-adrenergic receptor has been demonstrated in the elderly. The consequences of adverse drug effects may differ in the elderly because of their greater likelihood of other disease. For example, long half-life benzodiazepine use is linked to the occurrence of hip fractures in elderly patients, perhaps reflecting both a risk of falls from these drugs and the increased incidence of osteoporosis in elderly patients. Even when a drug impairs function similarly in different age groups the poorer baseline function in the elderly may put them at greater risk for an adverse drug reaction. When prescribing for an individual elderly patient the possibility that drug excretion, either by hepatic metabolism or renal excretion, may be impaired should be taken into account by the prescribing physician. Adverse drug effects in the elderly may be subtle and, as in all populations, the physician must be alert to the possibility that a patient's signs and symptoms may reflect an adverse effect of medication.

ETIOLOGY Most adverse reactions can be classified into two groups. The most frequent result from the exaggerated but predicted pharmacologic action of the drug. Other adverse reactions ensue from toxic effects unrelated to the intended pharmacologic actions. These therefore are often unpredictable, are frequently severe, and result from recognized as well as undiscovered mechanisms. Some mechanisms of extrapharmacologic toxicity include direct cytotoxicity, initiation of abnormal immune responses, and perturbation of metabolic processes in individuals with genetic enzymatic defects.

EXAGGERATION OF THE INTENDED PHARMACOLOGIC EFFECT By prior consideration of the known factors that modify drug action, these adverse reactions often are preventable.

Abnormally high drug concentration at the receptor site (site of action) due to the pharmacokinetic variability is the usual cause (see Chap. 66). For example, reduction in the volume of distribution, in the rate of metabolism, or in the rate of excretion all result in higher than expected concentration of drug at the receptor site with consequent increase in pharmacologic effect.

Recently, the specific cytochrome P450s involved in drug metabolism have been identified. Recognition of the polymorphic distribution of some of these enzyme activities within the population provides both an explanation for the interindividual variability in drug clearance and the expectation that as simple tests are developed to characterize an individual's specific cytochrome P450 activity it will be possible to identify, in advance, individuals at particular risk for concentration-related adverse effects. For enzymes whose activity is polymorphically distributed, a proportion of the population has low or absent enzyme activity. In these individuals, the concentration of drugs achieved will

* John A. Oates was coauthor in the 12th edition and this chapter represents a revision of that work.

be higher than normal and may produce toxicity. Conversely, where toxicity or efficacy is produced by a metabolite, the inability of poor metabolizers to produce that metabolite will limit toxicity or efficacy in such individuals. The polymorphic distribution of drug-metabolizing enzymes may explain some adverse drug effects previously labeled as idiosyncratic.

Alteration in the dose-response curve due to increased receptor sensitivity results in an increase in drug effect at the same concentration. An example of this is seen in the excessive response to the anticoagulant warfarin at normal or lower than normal blood levels in the elderly.

The shape of the dose-response curve itself also determines the likelihood of the development of adverse drug reactions. Drugs with a steep dose-response curve are more likely to be associated with dose-related toxicity because of the small increase in dose required to produce a large change in pharmacologic effect. An increase in the dose of drugs which exhibit nonlinear kinetics, such as phenytoin (see Chap. 66), may produce a proportionately greater increase in the blood level, resulting in toxicity.

Concomitant drug therapy may affect the pharmacokinetics or pharmacodynamics of other drugs. Pharmacokinetics may be affected by alterations in bioavailability, protein binding, or the rate of metabolism or excretion. Pharmacodynamics may be altered by competition for receptor sites, by preventing the drug from reaching its site of action, or by antagonism or enhancement of the drug's pharmacologic effect. Inhibition of the metabolism of one drug by another may occur when both drugs bind to the same cytochrome P450. Therefore, with increased identification of the specific cytochrome P450 responsible for metabolism of individual drugs, prediction of drug interactions is now on a more rational scientific basis (see Chap. 66).

TOXICITY UNRELATED TO A DRUG'S PRIMARY PHARMACO-LOGIC ACTIVITY Cytotoxic reactions The understanding of so-called idiosyncratic reactions has greatly improved with the recognition that many of these reactions are due to irreversible binding of drug or metabolites to tissue macromolecules by shared electron (covalent) bonds. Some chemical carcinogens such as the alkylating agents combine directly with DNA. Usually, it is only after metabolic activation to reactive metabolites that covalent binding occurs. This activation usually occurs in the microsomal mixed-function oxidase system, the hepatic enzyme system responsible for the metabolism of many drugs (Chap. 66). During the course of drug metabolism, reactive metabolites may covalently bind to tissue macromolecules, causing tissue damage. Because of the reactive nature of these metabolites, covalent binding often occurs close to the site of production, such as the liver, but the mixed-function oxidase system is found in other tissues as well.

An example of this type of adverse drug reaction is the hepatotoxicity associated with isoniazid, which is metabolized principally by acetylation to acetylisoniazid, which is then hydrolyzed to acetylhydrazine. The further metabolism of acetylhydrazine by the mixed-function oxidase system liberates reactive metabolites that covalently bind to hepatic macromolecules, causing hepatic necrosis. The administration of drugs known to increase the activity of the mixed-function oxidase system, such as phenobarbital or rifampin, together with isoniazid is associated with the production of increased amounts of reactive metabolites, increased covalent binding, and hepatic damage.

The hepatic necrosis produced by overdosage of acetaminophen is also caused by reactive metabolites. Normally these metabolites are detoxified by combining with hepatic glutathione. When glutathione becomes exhausted, the metabolites bind instead to hepatic protein, with resultant hepatocyte damage. The hepatic necrosis produced by the ingestion of acetaminophen can be prevented, or at least attenuated, by the administration of substances such as *N*-acetylcysteine, which reduce the binding of electrophilic metabolites to hepatic proteins. The risks of hepatic necrosis are increased in patients receiving drugs such as phenobarbital that increase the rate of drug metabolism and rate of production of toxic metabolite(s).

It is likely, though as yet not proven, that other idiosyncratic reactions are caused by the covalent binding of reactive metabolites to tissue macromolecules, with either direct cytotoxicity or via the initiation of an immunologic response.

Immunologic mechanisms Most pharmacologic agents are poor immunogens because they consist of small molecules with molecular weights less than 2000. Stimulation of antibody synthesis or sensitization of lymphocytes by a drug or one of its metabolites usually requires in vivo activation and covalent linkage to protein, carbohydrate, or nucleic acid.

Drug stimulation of antibody production may mediate tissue injury by one of several mechanisms. The antibody may attack the drug affixed to a cell by covalent linkage and thereby destroy the cell, as occurs in penicillin-induced hemolytic anemia. Complexes of antibody-drug-antigen may be passively adsorbed by a bystander cell which is destroyed by activation of complement; this occurs in quinine- and quinidine-induced thrombocytopenia. Drugs or their reactive metabolites may alter host tissue, rendering it antigenic, and stimulate autoantibodies; for example, hydralazine and procainamide can chemically alter nuclear material, stimulate formation of antinuclear antibodies, and occasionally cause lupus erythematosus. Autoantibodies may be stimulated by drugs which neither interact with the host antigen nor have any chemical similarity to the host tissue; e.g., alpha methyldopa frequently stimulates formation of antibodies to host erythrocytes, yet the drug does not itself attach to the erythrocyte or share any chemical similarities with the antigenic determinants on the erythrocyte.

Drug-induced *pure red cell aplasia* (Chap. 308) is due to an immunologic-based drug reaction. Red cell formation in bone marrow cultures can be inhibited by phenytoin and purified IgG obtained from a patient with pure red cell aplasia associated with phenytoin.

Serum sickness (Chap. 282) results from deposition of circulating drug-antibody complexes on endothelial surfaces. Complement activation occurs, chemotactic factors are generated locally, and an inflammatory response appears at the site of complex entrapment. Arthralgias, urticaria, lymphadenopathy, glomerulonephritis, or cerebritis may result. Penicillin is the most common cause of serum sickness today. Many drugs, particularly the antimicrobial agents, induce production of IgE, which affixes to mast cell membranes. Contact with a drug antigen initiates a series of biochemical events within the mast cell and results in the release of mediators that may produce urticaria, wheezing, flushing, rhinorrhea, and occasionally hypotension characteristic of anaphylaxis.

Drugs also may excite cell-mediated immune responses. Topically administered substances may interact with sulfhydryl or amino groups in the skin and react with sensitized lymphocytes to produce the rash characteristic of contact dermatitis. Other types of rashes also may appear from the interaction of serum factors, drugs, and sensitized lymphocytes. The role of drug-activated lymphocytes in the immune mechanisms governing destruction of visceral tissue is unknown.

Toxicity associated with genetically determined enzymatic defects In the porphyrias, drugs that increase the activity of enzymes proximal to the deficient enzyme in the biosynthetic pathway of porphyrins can increase the quantity of porphyrin precursors that accumulate proximal to the deficient enzyme (Chap. 346). These drugs are listed in Table 67-1.

Patients with a deficiency of glucose-6-phosphate dehydrogenase (G6PD) develop hemolytic anemia on primaquine and a number of other drugs (Table 67-1) that do not cause hemolysis in patients with adequate quantities of this enzyme (Chap. 307).

Diagnosis The manifestations of drug-induced diseases frequently resemble those of other diseases and may be produced by different and dissimilar drugs. Recognition of the role of a drug or drugs responsible for illness is dependent on appreciation of the possible adverse reactions to drugs in any disease, identification of a temporal relationship between drug administration and development of illness, and familiarity with the manifestations most often caused by particular drugs. Although specific reactions have been described

TABLE 67-1   Clinical manifestations of adverse reactions to drugs

I MULTISYSTEM MANIFESTATIONS

Anaphylaxis
  ACE inhibitors and dialysis
  Cephalosporins
  Demeclocycline
  Dextran
  Insulin
  Iodinated drugs or contrast
    media
  Iron dextran
  Lidocaine
  Penicillins
  Procaine
  Streptomycin
  Sulfobromophthalein

Angioedema
  ACE inhibitors

Drug-induced lupus
    erythematosus
  Acebutolol
  Asparaginase
  Barbiturates
  Bleomycin
  Cephalosporins
  Hydralazine
  Iodides
  Isoniazid
  Methyldopa
  Phenolphthalein
  Phenytoin
  Procainamide
  Quinidine
  Sulfonamides
  Thiouracil

Fever
  Aminosalicylic acid
  Amphotericin B
  Antihistamines
  Novobiocin
  Penicillins
Hyperpyrexia
  Antipsychotics
Serum sickness
  Aspirin
  Penicillins
  Propylthiouracil
  Streptomycin
  Sulfonamides

II ENDOCRINE MANIFESTATIONS

Addisonian-like syndrome
  Busulfan
  Etomidate
  Ketoconazole
Galactorrhea (may also
    cause amenorrhea)
  Methyldopa
  Phenothiazines
  Reserpine
  Tricyclic antidepressants
Gynecomastia
  Calcium channel
    antagonists
  Digitalis
  Estrogens
  Ethionamide
  Griseofulvin
  Isoniazid
  Methyldopa
  Phenytoin
  Reserpine
  Spironolactone
  Testosterone

Sexual dysfunction
  Impaired ejaculation:
    Bethanidine
    Debrisoquin
    Guanethidine
    Thioridazine
  Decreased libido and impotence:
    Beta blockers
    Clonidine
    Diuretics
    Lithium
    Major tranquilizers
    Methyldopa
    Oral contraceptives
    Sedatives
  Impairment of spermatogenesis
    or oogenesis:
    Cytotoxics
  Priapism:
    Trazodone

Thyroid function tests,
    disorders of
  Acetazolamide
  Amiodarone
  Bromsulfophthalein
  Chlorpropamide
  Clofibrate
  Colestipol and
    nicotinic acid
  Dimercaprol
  Gold salts
  Iodides
  Lithium
  Oral contraceptives
  Phenindione
  Phenothiazines (long-term)
  Phenylbutazone
  Phenytoin
  Sulfonamides
  Tolbutamide

Vaginal carcinoma
  Diethylstilbestrol (given to
    mother)

III METABOLIC MANIFESTATIONS

Hyperbilirubinemia
  Novobiocin
  Rifampin
Hypercalcemia
  Antacids with absorbable
    alkali
  Thiazides
  Vitamin D
Hyperglycemia
  Chlorthalidone
  Diazoxide
  Encainide
  Ethacrynic acid
  Furosemide
  Glucocorticoids
  Growth hormone
  Oral contraceptives
  Thiazides
Hypoglycemia
  Insulin
  Octreotide
  Oral hypoglycemics
  Pentamidine
  Quinine

Hyperkalemia
  ACE inhibitors
  Amiloride
  Cytotoxics
  Digitalis overdose
  Heparin
  Lithium
  Pentamidine
  Potassium preparations
    including salt substitute
  Potassium salts of drugs
  Spironolactone
  Succinylcholine
  Triamterene
Hypokalemia
  Alkali-induced alkalosis
  Amphotericin B
  Carbenoxolone
  Corticosteroids
  Diuretics
  Gentamicin
  Insulin
  Laxative abuse
  Mineralocorticoids,
    some glucocorticoids
  Osmotic diuretics
  Sympathomimetics
  Tetracycline (degraded)
  Theophylline
  Vitamin B_{12}

Hyperuricemia
  Aspirin
  Chlorthalidone
  Cytotoxics
  Ethacrynic acid
  Fructose (IV)
  Furosemide
  Hyperalimentation
  Thiazides
Hyponatremia
  Dilutional:
    Antipsychotics
    Carbamazepine
    Chlorpropamide
    Cyclophosphamide
    Desmopressin
    Diuretics
    Octreotide
    Vincristine
  Salt wasting:
    Diuretics
    Enemas
    Mannitol

Metabolic acidosis
  Acetazolamide
  Paraldehyde (degraded)
  Phenformin
  Salicylates
  Spironolactone
Porphyria exacerbation
  Barbiturates
  Chlordiazepoxide
  Chlorpropamide
  Estrogens
  Glutethimide
  Griseofulvin
  Meprobamate
  Oral contraceptives
  Phenytoin
  Rifampin
  Sulfonamides

(continued)

TABLE 67-1   Clinical manifestations of adverse reactions to drugs *(continued)*

IV DERMATOLOGIC MANIFESTATIONS

Acne
  Anabolic and androgenic
    steroids
  Bromides
  Glucocorticoids
  Iodides
  Isoniazid
  Oral contraceptives
  Troxidone
Alopecia
  Beta blockers
  Cytotoxics
  Ethionamide
  Heparin
  Oral contraceptives (withdrawal)
Eczema
  Captopril
  Cream and lotion
    preservatives
  Lanolin
  Topical antihistamines
  Topical antimicrobials
  Topical local anesthetics

Erythema multiforme or
  Steven-Johnson
  syndrome
  Barbiturates
  Chlorpropamide
  Codeine
  Ethosuximide
  Penicillins
  Phenylbutazone
  Phenytoin
  Salicylates
  Sulfonamides
  Sulfones
  Tetracyclines
  Thiazides
  Tocainide
Erythema nodosum
  Oral contraceptives
  Penicillins
  Sulfonamides
Exfoliative dermatitis
  Barbiturates
  Gold salts
  Penicillins
  Phenylbutazone
  Phenytoin
  Quinidine
  Sulfonamides
Fixed drug eruptions
  Barbiturates
  Captopril
  Foscarnet (penile ulceration)
  Phenolphthalein
  Phenylbutazone
  Quinine
  Salicylates
  Sulfonamides

Hyperpigmentation
  Bleomycin
  Busulfan
  Chloroquine and other
    antimalarials
  Corticotropin
  Cyclophosphamide
  Gold salts
  Hypervitaminosis A
  Oral contraceptives
  Phenothiazines
Lichenoid eruptions
  Aminosalicylic acid
  Antimalarials
  Chlorpropamide
  Gold salts
  Methyldopa
  Phenothiazines
Photodermatitis
  Captopril
  Chlordiazepoxide
  Furosemide
  Griseofulvin
  Nalidixic acid
  Oral contraceptives
  Phenothiazines
  Sulfonamides
  Sulfonylureas
  Tetracyclines, particularly
    demeclocycline
  Thiazides

Purpura (see also
    thrombocytopenia)
  Aspirin
  Glucocorticoids
  Rashes (nonspecific)
  Allopurinol
  Ampicillin
  Barbiturates
  Indapamide
  Methyldopa
  Phenytoin
Skin necrosis
  Warfarin
Toxic epidermal necrolysis
    (bullous)
  Allopurinol
  Barbiturates
  Bromides
  Iodides
  Nalidixic acid
  Penicillins
  Phenolphthalein
  Phenylbutazone
  Phenytoin
  Sulfonamides
Urticaria
  Aspirin
  Barbiturates
  Captopril
  Enalapril
  Penicillins
  Sulfonamides

V HEMATOLOGIC MANIFESTATIONS

Agranulocytosis (see also
    pancytopenia)
  Aprindine
  Captopril
  Carbimazole
  Chloramphenicol
  Cotrimoxazole
  Cytotoxics
  Gold salts
  Indomethacin
  Methimazole
  Oxyphenbutazone
  Phenothiazines
  Phenylbutazone
  Propylthiouracil
  Sulfonamides
  Tolbutamide
  Tricyclic antidepressants
Clotting abnormalities/
    Hypothrombinemia
  Cefamandole
  Cefoperazone
  Moxalactam
  Valproic acid
Eosinophilia
  Aminosalicylic acid
  Chlorpropamide
  Erythromycin estolate
  Imipramine
  L-Tryptophan
  Methotrexate
  Nitrofurantoin
  Procarbazine
  Sulfonamides

Hemolytic anemia
  Aminosalicylic acid
  Cephalosporins
  Chlorpromazine
  Dapsone
  Insulin
  Isoniazid
  Levodopa
  Mefenamic acid
  Melphalan
  Methyldopa
  Penicillins
  Phenacetin
  Procainamide
  Quinidine
  Rifampin
  Sulfonamides
Hemolytic anemia (in G6PD
    deficiency)
  Aminosalicylic acid
  Antimalarials, e.g.,
    primaquine
  Aspirin
  Chloramphenicol
  Cotrimoxazole
  Dapsone
  Nalidixic acid
  Nitrofurantoin
  Phenacetin
  Probenecid
  Procainamide
  Quinidine
  Sulfonamides
  Vitamin C
  Vitamin K

Leukocytosis
  Glucocorticoids
  Lithium
Lymphadenopathy
  Phenytoin
  Primidone
Megaloblastic anemia
  Cotrimoxazole
  Folate antagonists
  Nitrous oxide (repeated or
    prolonged exposure)
  Oral contraceptives
  Phenobarbital
  Phenytoin
  Primidone
  Triamterene
  Trimethoprim
Pancytopenia (aplastic anemia)
  Carbamazepine
  Chloramphenicol
  Cytotoxics
  Gold salts
  Mepacrine
  Mephenytoin
  Oxyphenbutazone
  Phenylbutazone
  Phenytoin
  Potassium perchlorate
  Quinacrine
  Sulfonamides
  Trimethadione
  Zidovudine (AZT)

Pure red cell aplasia
  Azathioprine
  Chlorpropamide
  Isoniazid
  Phenytoin
Thrombocytopenia
    (see also pancytopenia)
  Acetazolamine
  Aspirin
  Carbamazepine
  Carbenicillin
  Chlorpropamide
  Chlorthalidone
  Cotrimoxazole
  Digitoxin
  Furosemide
  Gold salts
  Heparin
  Indomethacin
  Isoniazid
  Methyldopa
  Moxalactam
  Novobiocin
  Oxyphenbutazone
  Phenylbutazone
  Phenytoin and other
    hydantoins
  Quinidine
  Quinine
  Thiazides
  Ticarcillin

(continued)

TABLE 67-1   Clinical manifestations of adverse reactions to drugs (continued)

VI CARDIOVASCULAR MANIFESTATIONS

Acute chest pain (nonischemic)
  Bleomycin
Angina exacerbation
  Alpha blockers
  Beta-blocker withdrawal
  Ergotamine
  Excessive thyroxine
  Hydralazine
  Methysergide
  Minoxidil
  Nifedipine
  Oxytocin
  Vasopressin
	Arrhythmias
	  Adriamycin
	  Antiarrhythmic drugs
	  Astemizole
	  Atropine
	  Anticholinesterases
	  Beta blockers
	  Daunorubicin
	  Digitalis
	  Emetine
	  Erythromycin
	  Guanethidine
	  Lithium
	  Papaverine
	  Phenothiazines, particularly thioridazine
	  Sympathomimetics
	  Terfenadine
	  Theophylline
	  Thyroid hormone
	  Tricyclic antidepressants
	  Verapamil
	AV block
	  Clonidine
	  Methyldopa
	  Verapamil
	Cardiomyopathy
	  Adriamycin
	  Daunorubicin
	  Emetine
	  Lithium
	  Phenothiazines
	  Sulfonamides
	  Sympathomimetics
		Fluid retention/congestive heart failure/edema
		  Beta blockers
		  Calcium blockers
		  Carbenoxolone
		  Diazoxide
		  Estrogens
		  Indomethacin
		  Mannitol
		  Minoxidil
		  Phenylbutazone
		  Steroids
		  Verapamil
		Hypotension (see also arrhythmias)
		  Amiodarone (perioperative)
		  Calcium channel blockers, e.g., nifedipine
		  Citrated blood
		  Diuretics
		  Interleukin 2
		  Levodopa
		  Morphine
		  Nitroglycerin
		  Phenothiazines
		  Protamine
		  Quinidine
			Hypertension
			  Clonidine withdrawal
			  Corticotropin
			  Cyclosporine
			  Glucocorticoids
			  Monoamine oxidase inhibitors with sympathomimetics
			  NSAIDs (some)
			  Oral contraceptives
			  Sympathomimetics
			  Tricyclic antidepressants with sympathomimetics
			Pericarditis
			  Emetine
			  Hydralazine
			  Methysergide
			  Procainamide
			Pericardial effusion
			  Minoxidil
			Thromboembolism
			  Oral contraceptives

VII RESPIRATORY MANIFESTATIONS

Airway obstruction (bronchospasm, asthma; see also anaphylaxis)
  Beta blockers
  Cephalosporins
  Cholinergic drugs
  NSAIDs, e.g., aspirin, indomethacin
  Penicillins
  Pentazocine
  Streptomycin
  Tartrazine (drugs with yellow dye)
	Cough
	  ACE inhibitors
	Nasal congestion
	  Decongestant abuse
	  Guanethidine
	  Isoproterenol
	  Oral contraceptives
	  Reserpine
	Pulmonary edema
	  Contrast media
	  Heroin
	  Hydrochlorthiazide
	  Interleukin 2
	  Methadone
	  Propoxyphene
		Pulmonary infiltrates
		  Acyclovir
		  Amiodarone
		  Azothioprine
		  Bleomycin
		  Busulfan
		  Carmustine (BCNU)
		  Chlorambucil
		  Cyclophosphamide
		  Melphalan
		  Methotrexate
		  Methysergide
		  Mitomycin C
		  Nitrofurantoin
		  Procarbazine
		  Sulfonamides
			Respiratory depression
			  Aminoglycosides
			  Hypnotics
			  Opiates
			  Polymyxins
			  Sedatives
			  Trimethaphan

(continued)

as resulting from the use of particular drugs, there is always a "first," and any drug should be suspected of causing an adverse effect if the clinical setting is appropriate.

Illness related to a drug's pharmacologic action may be more easily recognized than illness attributable to immunologic or other mechanisms. For example, side effects such as cardiac arrhythmias in patients receiving digitalis, hypoglycemia in patients given insulin, and bleeding in patients receiving anticoagulants are more easily related to the drug than are symptoms such as fever or rash, which may be caused by many drugs or by other factors.

Once an adverse reaction is suspected, discontinuance of the suspected drug followed by disappearance of the reaction is presumptive evidence of a drug-induced illness. Reappearance of the reaction upon cautious readministration of the drug may provide confirmatory evidence of the relationship if such confirmation adds useful information to the future management of the patient without entailing undue risk. With concentration-dependent adverse reactions, lowering the dosage also may be followed by disappearance of the reaction, and increasing the dose may cause it to reappear. When the reaction is thought to be allergic, however, readministration of the drug may be hazardous, since anaphylactic shock may develop. Readministration is unwise under these conditions unless alternative drugs are not available and treatment is mandatory.

If the patient is receiving many different drugs when an adverse reaction is suspected, the drugs most likely to be incriminated can usually be identified. All drugs may be discontinued at once, or if this is not practical, then drugs should be discontinued one at a time, starting with the drug under greatest suspicion, and the patient observed for signs of improvement. The time needed for a concentration-dependent adverse effect to disappear depends on the time required for the concentration to fall below the range associated with the adverse effect, and this, in turn, depends on the initial blood level and on the rate of elimination or metabolism of the drug. Adverse effects of drugs with long half-lives, such as phenobarbital, take a considerable time to disappear.

Drugs recognized as producing a number of reactions are listed in

TABLE 67-1　Clinical manifestations of adverse reactions to drugs (continued)

VIII GASTROINTESTINAL MANIFESTATIONS

Cholestatic hepatitis
  Acetohexamide
  Anabolic steroids
  Androgens
  Chlorpropamide
  Clavulanic acid/amoxicillin
  Cyclosporine
  Erythromycin estolate
  Flucloxacillin
  Gold salts
  Methimazole
  Nitrofurantoin
  Oral contraceptives
  Phenothiazines
Constipation or ileus
  Aluminum hydroxide
  Barium sulfate
  Calcium carbonate
  Ferrous sulfate
  Ganglionic blockers
  Ion exchange resins
  Opiates
  Phenothiazines
  Tricyclic antidepressants
  Verapamil
Diarrhea or colitis
  Antibiotics (broad-
    spectrum)
  Clindamycin
  Colchicine
  Digitalis
  Guanethidine
  Lactose excipients
  Lincomycin
  Magnesium in antacids
  Methyldopa
  Purgatives
  Reserpine
  Ticlopidine

Diffuse hepatocellular damage
  Acetaminophen
    (paracetamol)
  Acebutolol
  Allopurinol
  Aminosalicylic acid
  Amiodarone
  Aprindine
  Cyclophosphamide
  Dapsone
  Diclofenac
  Erythromycin estolate
  Ethionamide
  Glyburide
  Halothane
  Isoniazid
  Ketoconazole
  Labetalol
  Lovastatin
  Methimazole
  Methotrexate
  Methoxyflurane
  Methyldopa
  Monoamine oxidase
    inhibitors
  Niacin
  Nifedipine
  Nitrofurantoin
  Oxyphenisatin
  Phenytoin and other
    hydantoins
  Propoxyphene
  Propylthiouracil
  Pyridium
  Rifampin
  Salicylates
  Sodium valproate
  Sulfonamides
  Tetracyclines
  Verapamil
  Zidovudine (AZT)

Gallstones/biliary pseudolithiasis
  Ceftriaxone
Intestinal ulceration
  Solid KCl preparations
Malabsorption
  Aminosalicylic acid
  Antibiotics (broad spectrum)
  Cholestyramine
  Colchicine
  Colestipol
  Cytotoxics
  Neomycin
  Phenobarbital
  Phenytoin
  Primidone
Nausea or vomiting
  Digitalis
  Estrogens
  Ferrous sulfate
  Levodopa
  Opiates
  Potassium chloride
  Tetracyclines
  Theophylline
Oral conditions
  Dental discoloration:
    Tetracycline
  Dry mouth:
    Anticholinergics
    Clonidine
    Levodopa
    Methyldopa
    Tricyclic antidepressants
  Gingival hyperplasia:
    Calcium antagonists
    Cyclosporine
    Phenytoin

Salivary gland swelling:
  Bethanidine
  Bretylium
  Clonidine
  Guanethidine
  Iodides
  Phenylbutazone
Taste disturbances:
  Acetazolamide
  Biguanides
  Captopril
  Griseofulvin
  Lithium
  Metronidazole
  Penicillamine
  Rifampin
Ulceration:
  Aspirin
  Cytotoxics
  Gentian violet
  Isoproterenol (sublingual)
  Pancreatin
Pancreatitis
  Azathioprine
  Ethacrynic acid
  Furosemide
  Glucocorticoids
  Opiates
  Oral contraceptives
  Sulfonamides
  Thiazides
Peptic ulceration or
  hemorrhage
  Aspirin
  Ethacrynic acid
  Glucocorticoids
  NSAIDs
  Reserpine (large doses)

IX RENAL MANIFESTATIONS

Bladder dysfunction
  Anticholinergics
  Disopyramide
  Monoamine oxidase
    inhibitors
  Tricyclic antidepressants
Calculi
  Acetazolamide
  Vitamin D
Concentrating defect with
  polyuria (or
  nephrogenic diabetes
  insipidus)
  Demeclocycline
  Lithium
  Methoxyflurane
  Vitamin D

Hemorrhage cystitis
  Cyclophosphamide
Interstitial nephritis
  Ciprofloxacin
  Allopurinol
  Furosemide
  NSAIDs
  Penicillins, esp.
    methicillin
  Phenindione
  Sulfonamides
  Thiazides
Nephropathies
  Due to analgesics
    (e.g., phenacetin)

Nephrotic syndrome
  Captopril
  Gold salts
  Penicillamine
  Phenindione
  Probenecid
Obstructive uropathy
  Extrarenal: methysergide
  Intrarenal: cytotoxics
Renal dysfunction
  Cyclosporin
  NSAIDs
  Pentamidine
  Triamterene
Renal tubular acidosis
  Acetazolamide
  Amphotericin B
  Degraded tetracycline

Tubular necrosis
  Aminoglycosides
  Amphotericin B
  Cephaloridine
  Colistin
  Cyclosporin
  Methoxyflurane
  Polymyxins
  Radioiodinated contrast
    medium
  Sulfonamides
  Tetracyclines

(continued)

Table 67-1. This table includes well-documented and some less well-documented reactions that are sufficiently devastating as to require consideration. It should be used to suggest the likely causative drug, but the absence of a drug from the table does not mean that it is not responsible for the reaction.

Serum antibody has been demonstrated in some persons with drug allergy involving cellular blood elements, as in agranulocytosis, hemolytic anemia, and thrombocytopenia. For example, both quinine and quinidine can produce platelet agglutination in vitro in the presence of complement and the serum from a patient who has developed thrombocytopenia following this drug.

Eliciting a drug history from patients is important for diagnosis.

Attention must be directed to nonprescription, or OTC, as well as to prescription drugs. Each type can be responsible for adverse drug effects, and adverse interactions may occur between OTC drugs and prescribed drugs. In addition, it is common for patients to be cared for by several physicians, and duplicative, additive, counteractive, or synergistic drugs may therefore be taken if the physicians are not aware of the patients' drug histories. Every physician should determine what drugs a patient has been taking, at least during the preceding 30 days, before prescribing any medications. A frequently overlooked source of additional drug exposure is topical therapy; for example, the patient complaining of bronchospasm who is using an ophthalmic beta blocker may not volunteer such drug use to the physician unless

TABLE 67-1   Clinical manifestations of adverse reactions to drugs (continued)

X NEUROLOGIC MANIFESTATIONS

Exacerbation of myasthenia
  Aminoglycosides
  Polymyxins
Extrapyramidal effects
  Butyrophenones,
    e.g., haloperidol
  Levodopa
  Methyldopa
  Metoclopramide
  Oral contraceptives
  Phenothiazines
  Reserpine
  Tricyclic antidepressants
Headache
  Bromides
  Ergotamine (withdrawal)
  Glyceryl trinitrate
  Hydralazine
  Indomethacin

Peripheral neuropathy
  Amiodarone
  Chloramphenicol
  Chloroquine
  Chlorpropamide
  Cisplatin
  Clioquinol
  Clofibrate
  Demeclocycline
  Disopyramide
  Ethambutol
  Ethionamide
  Glutethimide
  Hydralazine
  Isoniazid
  Methysergide
  Metronidazole
  Mustine
  Nalidixic acid
  Nitrofurantoin

  Perhexiline
  Phenelzine
  Phenytoin
  Polymyxin, colistin
  Procarbazine
  Streptomycin
  Tolbutamide
  Tricyclic antidepressants
  Vincristine
Pseudotumor cerebri (or
    intracranial hypertension)
  Amiodarone
  Glucocorticoids,
    mineralocorticoids
  Hypervitaminosis A
  Oral contraceptives
  Tetracyclines

Seizures
  Amphetamines
  Analeptics
  Imipenem
  Isoniazid
  Lidocaine
  Lithium
  Nalidixic acid
  Penicillins
  Phenothiazines
  Physostigmine
  Theophylline
  Tricyclic antidepressants
  Vincristine
Sleep disorders
  Lovastatin
Stroke
  Oral contraceptives
Tremor
  Beta-adrenergic agonists

XI OCULAR MANIFESTATIONS

Cataracts
  Busulfan
  Chlorambucil
  Glucocorticoids
  Phenothiazines
Color vision alteration
  Barbiturates
  Digitalis
  Methaqualone
  Streptomycin
  Sulfonamides
  Thiazides
  Troxidone

Corneal edema
  Oral contraceptives
Corneal opacities
  Chloroquine
  Indomethacin
  Mepacrine
  Vitamin D
Eye pain
  Nifedipine
Glaucoma
  Ipratropium bromide
  Mydriatics
  Sympathomimetics

Optic neuritis
  Aminosalicylic acid
  Chloramphenicol
  Clioquinol
  Ethambutol
  Isoniazid
  Penicillamine
  Phenothiazines
  Phenylbutazone
  Quinine
  Streptomycin

Retinopathy
  Chloroquine
  Phenothiazines

XII EAR MANIFESTATIONS

Deafness
  Aminoglycosides
  Aspirin
  Bleomycin
  Chloroquine
  Cisplatin
  Deferoxamine
  Erythromycin
  Ethacrynic acid
  Furosemide
  Mustine
  Nortriptyline
  Quinine

Vestibular disorders
  Aminoglycosides
  Mustine
  Quinine

XIII MUSCULOSKELETAL MANIFESTATIONS

Bone disorders
  Osteoporosis:
    Glucocorticoids
    Heparin
  Osteomalacia:
    Aluminum hydroxide
    Anticonvulsants
    Glutethimide

Myopathy or myalgia
  Amphotericin B
  Carbenoxolone
  Chloroquine
  Clofibrate
  Glucocorticoids
  Oral contraceptives
Rhabdomyolysis
  Gemfibrozil
  Lovastatin

XIV PSYCHIATRIC MANIFESTATIONS

Delirious or confusional states
  Amantadine
  Aminophylline
  Anticholinergics
  Antidepressants
  Bromides
  Cimetidine
  Digitalis
  Glucocorticoids
  Isoniazid
  Levodopa
  Methyldopa
  Penicillins
  Phenothiazines
  Sedatives and hypnotics

Depression
  Amphetamine withdrawal
  Beta blockers
  Centrally acting
    antihypertensives
    (reserpine, methyldopa,
    clonidine)
  Glucocorticoids
  Levodopa
Drowsiness
  Antihistamines
  Anxiolytic drugs
  Clonidine
  Major tranquilizers
  Methyldopa
  Reserpine
  Tricyclic antidepressants

Hallucinatory states
  Amantadine
  Beta blockers
  Levodopa
  Meperidine
  Narcotics
  Pentazocine
  Tricyclic antidepressants
Hypomania, mania, or excited
  reactions
  Glucocorticoids
  Levodopa
  MAO inhibitors
  Sympathomimetics
  Tricyclic antidepressants
Hypersexuality
  Antiparkinsonians

Schizophrenic-like or
  paranoid reactions
  Amphetamines
  Bromides
  Glucocorticoids
  Levodopa
  Lysergic acid
  Monoamine oxidase
    inhibitors
  Tricyclic antidepressants
Sleep disturbances
  Anorexiants
  Levodopa
  Monoamine oxidase
    inhibitors
  Sympathomimetics

specifically asked. A history of previous adverse drug effects in patients is common. Since these patients have a predisposition to other drug-induced illnesses, eliciting such a history should dictate added caution in prescribing drugs.

Patients with biochemical abnormalities such as erythrocyte G6PD deficiency can be identified; patients with the defect are usually blacks or of Mediterranean descent. Drug-induced hemolytic crisis can be avoided by testing for the enzyme defect before administering these drugs. Similarly, persons with an abnormal serum pseudocholinesterase may have abnormally prolonged apnea when given succinylcholine.

General comments No drug is completely without side effects, and a side effect in one patient may be the desired pharmacologic effect in another. Current drug regulations allow physicians to prescribe drugs with considerable confidence in their purity, bioavailability, and effectiveness. However, physicians have to weigh the potential toxicity against the possible benefits. Thus toxicity that would be acceptable for an effective antineoplastic agent would not be permitted in an oral contraceptive. Because of the necessarily small number of patients treated in premarketing studies, rare adverse reactions cannot be identified, so the first responsibility for identifying and reporting these effects must rest with the practicing clinician through the use of the various national adverse reaction reporting systems, such as those operated by the Food and Drug Administration in the United States and the Committee on Safety of Medicines in Great Britain. The publication of a newly recognized adverse reaction can in a short time stimulate many similar such reports of reactions that previously had gone unrecognized.

The prevention of adverse drug reactions first involves a high index of suspicion that the development of a new symptom or sign may be drug-related. Reduction of the dose or discontinuation of the suspected agent usually clarifies the position in concentration-dependent toxic reactions. Physicians should be familiar with the common adverse effects of the drugs they use and, if they are in doubt, should consult the literature.

REFERENCES

BRENNAN TA et al: Incidence of adverse events and negligence in hospitalized patients: Results of the Harvard Medical Practice Study I. N Engl J Med 324:370, 1991

DAVIES DM: *Textbook of Adverse Drug Reactions*, 4th ed. New York, Oxford University Press, 1991

FELDMANN U: Design and analysis of drug safety studies, with special reference to sporadic drug use and acute adverse reactions. J Clin Epidemiol 46:237, 1993

HOIGNÉ R et al: Risk factors for adverse drug reactions: Epidemiological approaches. Eur J Clin Pharmacol 39:321, 1990

LEAPE LL et al: The nature of adverse events in hospitalized patients. Results of the Harvard Medical Practice Study II. N Engl J Med 324:377, 1991

Reactions Annual 89. Auckland, New Zealand, Adis Press, 1989

Reactions Annual 90. Auckland, New Zealand, Adis Press, 1990

RIEDER MJ: Immunopharmacology and adverse drug reactions. J Clin Pharmacol 33:316, 1993

STOUKIDES CA et al: Adverse drug reaction surveillance in an emergency room. Am J Hosp Pharm 50:712, 1993

WALLER PC: Measuring the frequency of adverse drug reactions. Br J Clin Pharmacol 33:249, 1992

68   PHYSIOLOGY AND PHARMACOLOGY OF THE AUTONOMIC NERVOUS SYSTEM

LEWIS LANDSBERG / JAMES B. YOUNG

FUNCTIONAL ORGANIZATION OF THE AUTONOMIC NERVOUS SYSTEM

The autonomic nervous system innervates vascular and visceral smooth muscle, exocrine and endocrine glands, and parenchymal cells throughout the various organ systems. Functioning below the conscious level, the autonomic nervous system responds rapidly and continuously to perturbations that threaten the constancy of the internal environment. The many functions governed by this system include the distribution of blood flow and the maintenance of tissue perfusion, the regulation of blood pressure, the regulation of the volume and composition of the extracellular fluid, the expenditure of metabolic

energy and supply of substrate, and the control of visceral smooth muscle and glands.

Autonomic responses, like those of the somatic nervous system, are induced promptly and dissipated quickly, in contrast to the slower, more prolonged effects of circulating hormones. The autonomic nervous system, like the endocrine system, regulates the rate of processes that have intrinsic activities of their own, while the somatic nervous system initiates responses de novo. Although certain autonomic responses are discriminating, many are generalized and influence a variety of effectors in different organs. The interface between the autonomic nervous system and the endocrine system is exemplified by the adrenal medulla. This gland, homologous in many respects with the postganglionic sympathetic neuron, secretes a hormone (epinephrine) into the circulation to interact with adrenergic receptors throughout the body.

ANATOMIC ORGANIZATION The autonomic neurons, located in ganglia outside the central nervous system, give rise to the postganglionic autonomic nerves that innervate organs and tissues throughout the body (Fig. 68-1). The activity of autonomic nerves is regulated by central neurons responsive to diverse afferent inputs. After central integration of afferent information, autonomic outflow

FIGURE 68-1 Schematic representation of the autonomic nervous system. (*From Moskowitz M: Diseases of the autonomic nervous system. Clin Endocrinol Metab 6:77, 1977.*)

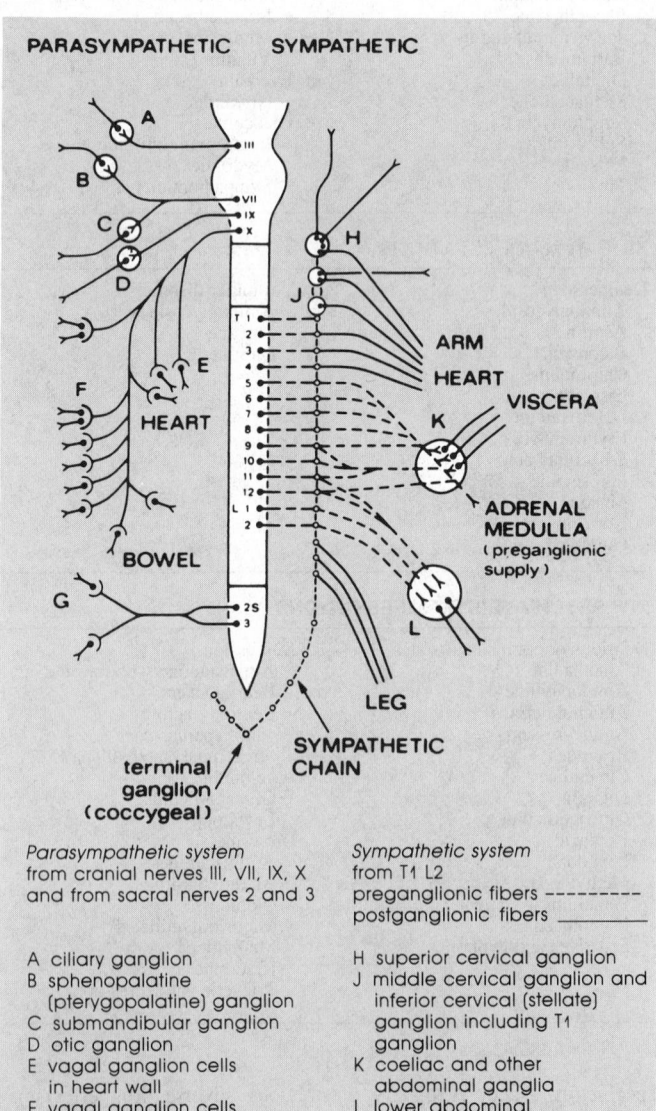

PARASYMPATHETIC   SYMPATHETIC

ARM
HEART
VISCERA
ADRENAL MEDULLA (preganglionic supply)
HEART
HEART
BOWEL
LEG
SYMPATHETIC CHAIN
terminal ganglion (coccygeal)

Parasympathetic system from cranial nerves III, VII, IX, X and from sacral nerves 2 and 3

Sympathetic system from T1 L2
preganglionic fibers - - - - - - - -
postganglionic fibers _____

A   ciliary ganglion
B   sphenopalatine (pterygopalatine) ganglion
C   submandibular ganglion
D   otic ganglion
E   vagal ganglion cells in heart wall
F   vagal ganglion cells in bowel wall
G   pelvic ganglia

H   superior cervical ganglion
J   middle cervical ganglion and inferior cervical (stellate) ganglion including T1 ganglion
K   coeliac and other abdominal ganglia
L   lower abdominal sympathetic ganglia

is adjusted to permit the functioning of the major organ systems in accordance with the needs of the organism as a whole. Connections between the cerebral cortex and the autonomic centers in the brainstem coordinate autonomic outflow with higher mental functions.

The sympathetic and parasympathetic divisions The preganglionic neurons of the parasympathetic nervous system leave the central nervous system in the third, seventh, ninth, and tenth cranial nerves and in the second and third sacral nerves, while the preganglionic neurons of the sympathetic nervous system exit the spinal cord between the first thoracic and the second lumbar segments (Fig. 68-1). Responses to sympathetic and parasympathetic stimulation are frequently antagonistic, as exemplified by their opposing effects on heart rate and gut motility. This antagonism reflects highly coordinated interactions within the central nervous system; the resultant changes in parasympathetic and sympathetic activity, often reciprocal, provide more precise control of autonomic responses than could be achieved by the modulation of a single system.

Neurotransmitters *Acetylcholine* (ACh) is the preganglionic neurotransmitter for both divisions of the autonomic nervous system, as well as the postganglionic neurotransmitter of the parasympathetic neurons. Nerves that release ACh are said to be cholinergic. *Norepinephrine* (NE) is the neurotransmitter of the postganglionic sympathetic neurons; these nerves are said to be adrenergic. Within the sympathetic outflow, postganglionic neurons innervating the eccrine sweat glands (and perhaps some blood vessels supplying skeletal muscle) are of the cholinergic type.

THE SYMPATHETIC NERVOUS SYSTEM AND THE ADRENAL MEDULLA

CATECHOLAMINES All three of the naturally occurring catecholamines, NE, *epinephrine* (E), and *dopamine*, function as neurotransmitters within the central nervous system. NE, the neurotransmitter of postganglionic sympathetic nerve endings, exerts its effects locally, in the immediate vicinity of its release. E, the circulating hormone of the adrenal medulla, influences processes throughout the body. A peripheral dopaminergic system also exists but has not been characterized in detail.

Biosynthesis (Fig. 68-2) Catecholamines are synthesized from the amino acid tyrosine, which is sequentially hydroxylated to form dihydroxyphenylalanine (dopa), decarboxylated to form dopamine, and hydroxylated on the beta position of the side chain to form NE. The initial step, the hydroxylation of tyrosine, is rate-limiting and is regulated so that synthesis of dopa is coupled to norepinephrine release. This regulation is achieved by alterations in both the activity and the amount of tyrosine hydroxylase. In the adrenal medulla and in those central neurons utilizing E as neurotransmitter, NE is *N*-methylated to E by the enzyme phenylethanolamine-*N*-methyltransferase (PNMT).

Catecholamine metabolism (Fig. 68-2) The major metabolic transformations of catecholamines involve *O*-methylation at the metahydroxyl group and oxidative deamination. *O*-Methylation is catalyzed by the enzyme catechol-*O*-methyltransferase (COMT), and oxidative deamination is promoted by monoamine oxidase (MAO). COMT in liver and kidney is important in the metabolism of circulating catecholamines. MAO, a mitochondrial enzyme present in most tissues, including nerve endings, has a lesser role in the metabolism of circulating catecholamines but is important in regulating the catecholamine stores within the peripheral sympathetic nerve endings. The metanephrines and 4-hydroxy-3-methoxymandelic acid (VMA) are the major end products of N and NE metabolism. Homovanillic acid (HVA) is the end product of dopamine metabolism.

STORAGE AND RELEASE OF CATECHOLAMINES In both the adrenal medulla and sympathetic nerve endings catecholamines are stored in subcellular granules and released by exocytosis. The large stores of catecholamines in these tissues provide an important physiologic reserve that maintains an adequate supply of catechol-

amines in the face of intense stimulation. A variety of substances may be stored along with catecholamines in sympathetic nerve endings and adrenal medulla and released with catecholamines during exocytosis. These substances, which may function as cotransmitters or neuromodulators, include peptides such as neuropeptide Y, substance P, and enkephalins; purines such as ATP and adenosine; and other amines such as serotonin. At the neuroeffector junction, coreleased neuromodulators modify the response to NE, while cotransmitters exert physiologic effects independent of those induced by NE.

Adrenal medulla The adrenal medullary chromaffin tissue in a pair of normal human adrenal glands weighs about 1 g and contains approximately 6 mg catecholamines, 85 percent of which is E. Catecholamines are maintained in high concentration within the storage (chromaffin) granule by several complex processes including (1) an inwardly directed H^+-transporting ATPase in the chromaffin granule membrane which maintains a steep hydrogen ion concentration and an acidic (pH 5.5) internal milieu, (2) an amine carrier that is saturable, stereospecific, favors the naturally occurring substrate (dopamine), and is inhibited by the reserpine class of agents, and (3) an intragranular storage complex that involves ATP and acidic glycoproteins called *chromagranins*. The high internal H^+ concentration tends to trap catecholamines in their protonated form and provides the driving force for the amine pump; H^+ egress down its electrochemical gradient is coupled to carrier-mediated amine uptake from the cytoplasm. These mechanisms permit very high concentrations of catecholamines to be stored within the granules. Both the inwardly directed H^+-ATPase and chromagranins have a widespread distribution in the neurosecretory granules of other parts of the endocrine system, including the anterior pituitary, pancreatic islets, and parathyroids.

Catecholamine secretion, stimulated by ACh from the preganglionic sympathetic nerves, occurs after calcium influx triggers fusion of the chromaffin granule membrane and cell membrane; obliteration of the cell membrane at the point of fusion and extrusion of the entire soluble contents of the granule into the extracellular space complete the process of exocytosis (Fig. 68-2). Although the molecular mechanisms involved in the exocytotic process are only partially understood, evidence has accumulated that a specific calcium-binding protein is involved. Once bound, calcium induces a conformational change in this protein which forms a hydrophobic rod that penetrates chromaffin granule membranes favoring fusion of granules and docking of granules at the cell membrane. Approximately 2 to 10 percent of the total adrenal medullary catecholamine store is turned over each day.

Peripheral sympathetic nerve endings The peripheral sympathetic nerve endings form a reticulum or ground plexus that brings the terminal fibers into close contact with effector cells. All the NE in peripheral tissues is in the sympathetic nerve endings, and heavily innervated tissues contain as much as 1 to 2 μg/g of tissue. NE stored in the nerve endings is in discrete subcellular particles analogous to the adrenal medullary chromaffin granules. MAO in the mitochondria of the nerve endings plays an important role in regulating the local concentration of NE (Fig. 68-2). Amines in storage vesicles are protected from oxidative deamination; amines within the cytoplasm, however, are deaminated to inactive metabolites. Release from the nerve ending occurs in response to action potentials propagated in terminal sympathetic fibers (Fig. 68-2).

THE PERIPHERAL ADRENERGIC NEUROEFFECTOR JUNCTION Neuronal uptake The peripheral sympathetic nerve endings possess an amine transport system that actively takes up amines from the extracellular fluid. A variety of synthetic and naturally occurring amines are substrates for this process. Neuronal uptake or recapture of locally released NE terminates the action of the transmitter and contributes to the constancy of the NE stores (Fig. 68-2). An NE transporter from human cells has been cloned and the amino acid sequence deduced. The structure of the protein inferred from the nucleotide sequence is remarkably similar to the transporter for gamma aminobutyric acid (GABA) as well as to recently cloned transporters

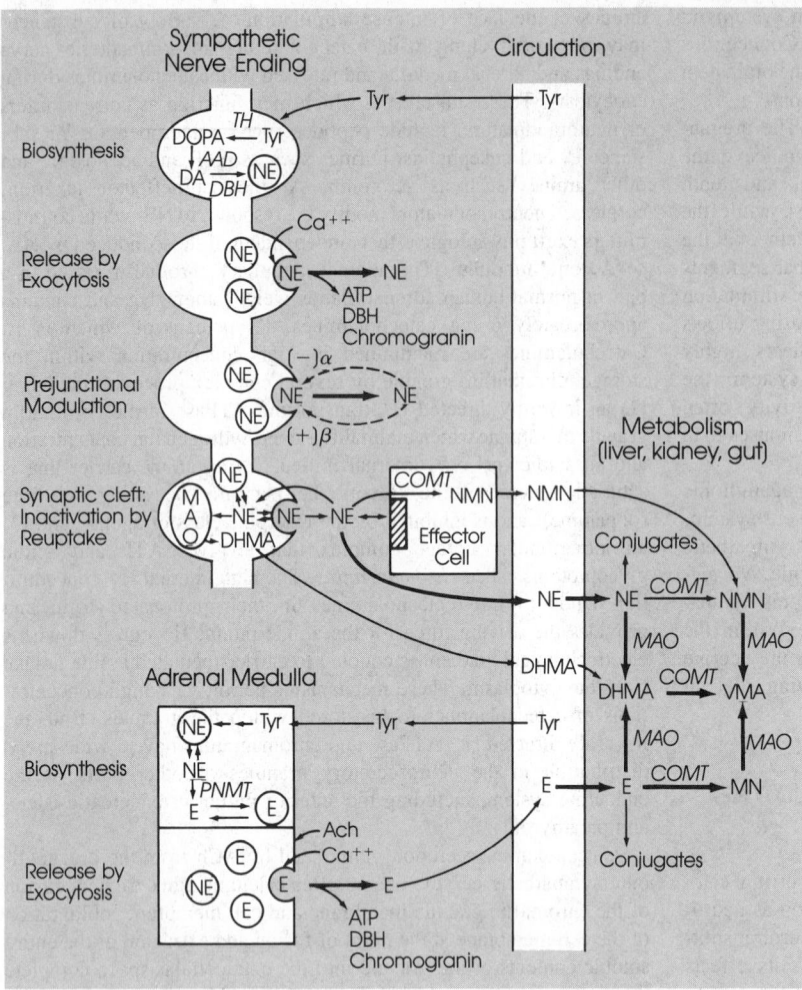

FIGURE 68-2 Catecholamine biosynthesis, release, and metabolism. Schematic representation of a peripheral sympathetic nerve ending is shown at the top; the bulbous areas on the terminal fiber represent varicosities identified by histochemical fluorescence techniques as areas of high neurotransmitter concentration. The processes of biosynthesis, release, modulation, and reuptake are shown sequentially for demonstration purposes only; in vivo they proceed concurrently. Adrenal medullary chromaffin cells are shown at the bottom of the diagram. (TH = tyrosine hydroxylase, AAD = aromatic-l-amino acid decarboxylase, DA = dopamine, DBH = dopamine-β-hydroxylase, NE = norepinephrine, PNMT = phenylethanolamine-N-methyltransferase, E = epinephrine, COMT = catechol-O-methyltransferase, NMN = normetanephrine, MAO = monoamine oxidase, DHMA = 3,4-dihydroxymandelic acid, VMA = 3-methoxy-4-hydroxymandelic acid.)

for dopamine and serotonin, suggesting the existence of a superfamily of neurotransmitter transporter genes.

Prejunctional modulation A variety of factors alter the relationship between neuronal impulse traffic and NE release. Diminished temperature and acidosis, for example, both decrease the amount of NE released in response to sympathetic impulses. Several chemical mediators operate at the peripheral sympathetic nerve ending (referred to as prejunctional or presynaptic sites) to modify sympathetic neurotransmission by influencing the amount of NE released in response to nerve impulses. Prejunctional modulation may be either inhibitory or facilitatory. Certain modulators, such as catecholamines and ACh, may either inhibit or facilitate NE release, antagonistic effects that are mediated by different adrenergic or cholinergic receptors, respectively. Those compounds exerting an *inhibitory* effect on NE release at the prejunctional nerve ending include the following: catecholamines (alpha$_2$ receptor), ACh (muscarinic receptor), dopamine (D-2 receptor), histamine (H-2 receptor), serotonin, adenosine, enkephalins, and prostaglandins. *Facilitatory* prejunctional modulators include catecholamines (beta$_2$ receptor), ACh (nicotinic receptor), and angiotensin II. The overall significance of prejunctional modulation, as well as the relative importance of the various mediators, has yet to be established, although increasing evidence indicates that many of these compounds exert a significant modulatory role in vivo. Antagonizing the facilitatory actions of angiotensin II at the neuroeffector junction may contribute to the antiadrenergic effects of angiotensin-converting enzyme inhibitors.

PREJUNCTIONAL ADRENERGIC RECEPTORS Catecholamines reduce NE release via prejunctional alpha receptors in a classic negative feedback system. Feedback regulation is complicated by the fact that beta-receptor activation facilitates NE release. This may be explained by the finding that prejunctional beta receptors (beta$_2$, see below) are

more sensitive to E than NE; this differential sensitivity could result in facilitation of NE release by circulating E. Infused E in fact augments NE release in humans. Release of E from sympathetic nerve endings (under conditions of intense adrenal medullary stimulation) also has been demonstrated, implying that E taken up in sympathetic nerve endings from the circulation and released as a cotransmitter may influence NE release as well.

PREJUNCTIONAL CHOLINERGIC RECEPTORS Though both inhibitory and facilitatory effects of ACh on NE release have been described, the inhibitory effect of ACh, mediated by the muscarinic cholinergic receptor, occurs at lower ACh concentrations and is probably of greater physiologic significance. This peripheral inhibitory effect of ACh on adrenergic neurotransmission may reinforce the reciprocal changes in central parasympathetic and sympathetic outflow that occur in the regulation of numerous physiologic responses.

CENTRAL REGULATION OF SYMPATHOADRENAL OUTFLOW

Brainstem sympathetic centers Sympathetic outflow is initiated from the reticular formation of the medulla oblongata and pons and from centers in the hypothalamus. The rostral ventral portion of the medulla, particularly the area designated the rostral ventrolateral medulla (RVLM), appears to contain especially important sympathoexcitatory areas. Descending fibers originating from these centers synapse in the intermediolateral cell column of the spinal cord with the preganglionic sympathetic neurons. The brainstem sympathetic centers, which have an intrinsic activity of their own, are regulated by many stimuli, including impulses from more rostral areas of the central nervous system (cortex, limbic lobe, hypothalamus), neural afferents that interact at the level of the brainstem centers and at the higher centers, and changes in the physical and chemical properties of the extracellular fluid, including the circulating levels of hormones and substrates. The area postrema, in the floor of the fourth ventricle, lies outside the blood-brain barrier and may play an important role in this regard. The higher centers, which have connections with the brainstem, coordinate sympathetic outflow with higher mental functions, emotional reactions, and the homeostatic needs of the internal environment. Although the hallmark of intense sympatho-adrenal stimulation is a global response (the fight-or-flight reaction of Cannon), discrete changes in sympathetic outflow to different organ systems continuously regulate many autonomic functions.

RELATIONSHIP BETWEEN THE SYMPATHETIC NERVOUS SYSTEM AND THE ADRENAL MEDULLA   Sympathetic nervous system activity and adrenal medullary secretion are coordinated but not always congruent. During periods of intense sympathetic stimulation, such as cold exposure and exhaustive exercise, the adrenal medulla is progressively recruited, and circulating E reinforces the physiologic effects of sympathetic stimulation. In other situations, the sympathetic nervous system and the adrenal medulla are stimulated independently. The response to upright posture, for example, involves predominantly the sympathetic nervous system, while hypoglycemia stimulates only the adrenal medulla. An important role for the adrenal medulla may be to provide circulating catecholamines to support vital functions when the sympathetic nervous system is suppressed.

Sympathetic regulation of the cardiovascular system   Stretch receptors in the systemic and pulmonary arteries and veins continuously monitor intravascular pressures; the resulting afferent impulses, after relay and integration in the brainstem, alter sympathetic activity in defense of blood pressure and blood flow to critical areas (Fig. 68-3).

ARTERIAL BARORECEPTORS   An increase in blood pressure stimulates receptors in the carotid sinus and aortic arch. The ensuing afferent impulses, after relay within the nucleus of the solitary tract (NTS) in the brainstem, suppress the brainstem sympathetic centers (Fig. 68-3). This baroreceptor reflex arc forms a negative-feedback loop in which a rise in arterial pressure results in the inhibition of central sympathetic outflow. A brainstem noradrenergic pathway interacts with the NTS to participate in suppression of sympathetic outflow. This noradrenergic inhibitory pathway is stimulated by centrally acting alpha-adrenergic agonists and may be involved in the action of certain antihypertensive drugs, such as clonidine, that

potentiate the baroreceptor-mediated vasodepressor response (Chap. 209). In the opposite manner, when the blood pressure falls, decreased afferent impulses diminish central inhibition, resulting in an increase in sympathetic outflow and a rise in arterial pressure.

CENTRAL VENOUS PRESSURE   Receptors in the walls of the great veins and within the atria are also involved in the regulation of sympathetic outflow. Stimulation of these receptors by high venous pressure suppresses the brainstem sympathetic centers; when central venous pressure is low, sympathetic outflow increases. The central connections are poorly understood, but the afferent impulses are carried in the vagus (Fig. 68-3).

ASSESSMENT OF SYMPATHOADRENAL ACTIVITY   The clinical assessment of sympathoadrenal activity involves the measurement of catecholamines in plasma and of catecholamines and catecholamine metabolites in urine. Quantitation of urinary catecholamines and metabolites is useful in the diagnosis of pheochromocytoma (Chap. 336).

Plasma catecholamines   Catecholamines in human plasma may be measured by radioenzymatic isotope derivative techniques or by high-performance liquid chromatography in conjunction with electrochemical detection. Plasma catecholamine measurements provide an index of sympathetic nervous system and adrenal medullary activity and have been widely used to assess sympathoadrenal activity in clinical investigation in human subjects. The usefulness of plasma catecholamine measurements is, however, compromised by factors that alter the relationship between the plasma concentration of catecholamines and the functional state of the sympathoadrenal system, and also by important regional differences in sympathetic outflow. Techniques utilizing tracer infusions of tritiated NE, which correct for changes in NE clearance when applied across a particular anatomic region, estimate regional sympathetic outflow with some precision and have helped to define differentiated sympathetic nervous system activity in the investigational setting. The clinical usefulness of plasma catecholamine levels remains limited to the evaluation of patients with autonomic insufficiency and, on occasion, patients with suspected pheochromocytoma (Chap. 336).

Basal plasma NE concentrations are in the range of 0.09 to 1.8 nmol/L (150 to 350 pg/mL); basal E levels are about 135 to 270 pmol/L (25 to 50 pg/mL). The half-time of disappearance of NE from the circulation is approximately 2 min. The plasma NE level is markedly affected by a variety of factors, including posture; accordingly, the conditions under which blood is obtained for assay must be controlled. By convention, basal plasma NE levels are those obtained through an indwelling intravenous line after the patient has rested supine in a relaxed environment for 30 min.

PLASMA NE RESPONSE TO UPRIGHT POSTURE   The predictable increase in circulating NE concentration during upright posture provides a convenient test of sympathetic nervous system function. Five minutes of quiet standing results in a two- to threefold increase in plasma NE level. A normal response requires an intact afferent system, appropriate central nervous system relays, and an intact peripheral sympathetic nervous system; a defect of any of these components reduces the increment in circulating NE.

Plasma E levels are also dependent on the physical and mental state of the subject. Change in plasma E with upright posture is usually small. Hypoglycemia, strenuous exercise, and various types of mental stress, however, can cause large increments in the plasma E level.

PERIPHERAL DOPAMINERGIC SYSTEM

In addition to its role as neurotransmitter in the central nervous system, dopamine functions as an inhibitory transmitter in the carotid body and the sympathetic ganglia. A distinct peripheral dopaminergic system is also believed to exist. Dopamine elicits a variety of responses not attributable to stimulation of classic adrenergic receptors; it relaxes the lower esophageal sphincter, delays gastric emptying,

FIGURE 68-3   Sympathetic regulation of the circulation. Receptors in the venous and arterial circulations are stimulated by stretch, caused by an increase in pressure; afferent impulses from these receptors are carried to the central nervous system by the ninth (IX) and tenth (X) cranial nerves. The net result of these afferent impulses, after relay in the brainstem, is to inhibit central sympathetic outflow. The arterial baroreceptor reflex involves a relay in the nucleus of the tractus solitarius. (+ = stimulation; − = inhibition.)

causes vasodilation in the renal and mesenteric arterial circulation, suppresses aldosterone secretion, directly stimulates renal sodium excretion, and suppresses NE release at sympathetic nerve terminals by a presynaptic inhibitory mechanism. The mediation of these dopaminergic effects in vivo is poorly understood. Dopamine does not appear to be a circulating hormone. Unequivocal evidence of peripheral autonomic dopaminergic nerves has not been produced, although such nerves may be present in the kidney. The kidney, furthermore, produces much of the dopamine in the urine, since the amount excreted each day (approximately 200 µg per 24 h) cannot be accounted for by clearance of plasma dopamine. Decarboxylation of circulating dopa, which is present in high concentration in the plasma [9 nmol/L (1500 pg/mL)] may contribute to urinary dopamine production. Dopamine generated from the decarboxylation of circulating dopa also might be involved in the mediation of dopaminergic effects in the kidney and other sites. Thus the nature of the peripheral dopaminergic system is obscure, but the existence of a dopaminergic system in those tissues that respond uniquely to dopamine seems likely.

ADRENERGIC RECEPTORS

Catecholamines influence effector cells by interacting with specific *receptors* on the cell surface. When stimulated by catecholamines, the adrenergic receptor initiates a series of membrane changes followed by a cascade of intracellular events that culminates in a measurable response. Compounds that elicit the response are referred to as *agonists;* those that block the interaction of the agonist with the receptor are referred to as *adrenergic receptor blocking agents* or *antagonists.*

Two major categories of response to catecholamines reflect the activation of two populations of adrenergic receptors, designated *alpha* and *beta*. Selective agonists and antagonists are available, enabling pharmacologic stimulation or blockade of the physiologic effects mediated by one receptor without influencing those mediated by the other. Both alpha and beta receptors have been further divided into subtypes that serve different functions and are susceptible to differential stimulation and blockade.

ALPHA-ADRENERGIC RECEPTORS The alpha-adrenergic receptor mediates vasoconstriction, intestinal relaxation, and pupillary dilatation. E and NE are approximately equipotent as alpha-receptor agonists. Distinct alpha$_1$- and alpha$_2$-receptor subtypes are also recognized. Originally the postsynaptic or postjunctional alpha-adrenergic receptors on effector cells were designated alpha$_1$, while the prejunctional alpha-adrenergic receptors on the sympathetic nerve endings were designated alpha$_2$. It is now recognized that nonneuronal (postsynaptic) processes are mediated by the alpha$_2$ receptor as well. The alpha$_1$ receptor mediates the classic alpha effects, including vasoconstriction; phenylephrine and methoxamine are selective alpha$_1$ agonists, and prazosin is a selective alpha$_1$ antagonist. The alpha$_2$ receptor mediates presynaptic inhibition of NE release from adrenergic nerves and other responses, including inhibition of ACh release from cholinergic nerves, inhibition of lipolysis in adipocytes, inhibition of insulin secretion, stimulation of platelet aggregation, and vasoconstriction in some vascular beds. Specific alpha$_2$ agonists include clonidine and α-methylnorepinephrine; these agents, the latter derived from α-methyldopa in vivo, exert an antihypertensive effect by interacting with alpha$_2$ receptors within the brainstem sympathetic centers that regulate blood pressure. Yohimbine is a specific alpha$_2$ antagonist. Molecular biologic techniques support the further subdivision of both the alpha$_1$ and alpha$_2$ receptors into more or less distinct subtypes, suggesting the eventual potential for differential stimulation and blockade.

BETA-ADRENERGIC RECEPTORS Physiologic events associated with beta-adrenergic receptor responses include stimulation of heart rate and contractility, vasodilation, bronchodilation, and lipolysis. Beta-receptor responses also can be divided into two types.

The beta$_1$ receptor responds equally to E and NE and mediates cardiac stimulation and lipolysis. The beta$_2$ receptor is more responsive to E than to NE and mediates responses such as vasodilation and bronchodilation. Isoproterenol stimulates and propranolol blocks both beta$_1$ and beta$_2$ receptors. Other agonists and antagonists that have partial selectivity for the beta$_1$ or beta$_2$ receptors have been used therapeutically where the desired response involves predominantly one of the two subtypes. Both pharmacologic and molecular genetic studies have suggested the possibility of an additional distinct beta$_3$-adrenergic receptor that subserves so-called atypical beta-adrenergic responses. Stimulation of heat production in brown adipose tissue has been suggested as a potentially important process mediated by this receptor. The full significance of this receptor remains to be elucidated.

DOPAMINERGIC RECEPTORS Specific dopaminergic receptors, distinct from the classic alpha- and beta-adrenergic receptors, are present in the central and peripheral nervous system and in several nonneural tissues. Two types of dopaminergic receptors serve different functions and have different second messengers. Dopamine is a potent agonist of both types of receptors; the action of dopamine is antagonized by phenothiazines and thioxanthenes. The dopamine 1 receptor mediates vasodilation in the renal, mesenteric, coronary, and cerebral vascular beds. Fenoldopam is an investigational agonist selective for the dopamine 1 receptor. The dopamine 2 receptor inhibits transmission in the sympathetic ganglia, inhibits NE release from sympathetic nerve endings by an effect on the presynaptic membrane (Fig. 68-2), inhibits prolactin release from the pituitary, and causes vomiting. Selective agonists of the dopamine 2 receptor include bromocriptine, lergotrile, and apomorphine, while butyrophenones such as haloperidol (active within the central nervous system), domperidone (does not cross blood-brain barrier readily), and the benzamide sulpiride are relatively selective dopamine 2 antagonists.

STRUCTURE AND FUNCTION OF ADRENERGIC RECEPTORS
The utilization of recombinant DNA technology has substantially increased current understanding of the structure and function of adrenergic receptors. cDNAs of the four major adrenergic receptor subtypes have been cloned and their primary amino acid sequences deduced. It is clear from these studies that the adrenergic receptors belong to a superfamily of related membrane proteins that includes the visual protein rhodopsin and the muscarinic acetylcholine receptors. These proteins share significant sequence homologies and, as deduced from the properties of the constituent amino acids, a similar topographic structure in the cell membrane. The postulated structure of this family of receptor proteins is shown schematically in Fig. 68-4. The characteristic features include seven membrane-spanning hydrophobic domains containing 20 to 28 amino acids each (possibly arranged as alpha helices), a hydrophilic extracellular *N* terminus and three extracellular connecting loops, and a hydrophilic intracellular *C* terminus with three cytoplasmic connecting loops.

Specificity for agonist binding and effector response is apparently conferred by differences in the tertiary structure of the various domains. Beta receptors, for example, have short third cytoplasmic loops (C-III) and long *C*-terminal chains, while the alpha$_2$ receptor has a long C-III and a short *C* terminus. The C-III loop appears to influence binding to the appropriate regulatory protein within the cell membrane (see below). The membrane-spanning domains, particularly M-7 (Fig. 68-4), appear to be important in determining the characteristic agonist binding.

Coupling of receptor occupancy with cellular response The major mediators of adrenergic (as well as many other) cellular responses are a family of regulatory proteins termed G (or N) proteins that, when activated, bind the nucleotide guanosine triphosphate (GTP). The best-characterized G proteins are those that stimulate or inhibit adenylyl cyclase, designated G$_s$ or G$_i$, respectively (Fig. 68-5) (see Chap 69). The beta$_1$, beta$_2$, and dopamine 1 receptors are coupled to G$_s$; receptor occupancy is therefore associated with stimulation of adenylyl cyclase and results in an increase in intracellular cyclic adenosine monophosphate (cAMP), which in turn results in activation of protein kinase A and other cAMP-dependent protein kinases. The

FIGURE 68-4 Proposed structure of adrenergic receptors as deduced from primary amino acid sequences. The single protein chain contains a hydrophilic *N* terminus (extracellular) and *C* terminus (intracellular) connected by seven lipophilic membrane-spanning regions (M-1 to M-7) which are interconnected by three extracellular loops (E-I to E-III) and three cytoplasmic loops (C-I to C-III). The beta$_1$, beta$_2$, alpha$_1$, and alpha$_2$ adrenergic receptors have appreciable sequence homologies and are believed to fit the general structural model represented. Specificity of agonist binding may be conferred by the tertiary structure of several of the membrane-spanning domains while specificity of intracellular response may be related to the length and tertiary structure of the cytoplasmic loops and *C* terminus. The top portion of the figure is a longitudinal representation of the receptor protein in the cell membrane; shown below is a hypothetical, more compact arrangement seen from the membrane surface. ECF = extracellular fluid; ICF = intracellular fluid. (*From Landsberg and JB Young, 1992.*)

resultant protein phosphorylation alters the activity of enzymes and the function of other proteins, culminating in a cellular response that is characteristic of the tissue being stimulated. The alpha$_2$, M-2 subtype of the muscarinic acetylcholine receptor and the dopamine 2 receptor are coupled to G$_i$, resulting in diminished adenylyl cyclase activity and a fall in cAMP. The subsequent alterations in enzyme activity and function of other proteins produce an alternate, frequently opposite, series of cellular responses. Although many alpha$_2$ responses can be explained by inhibition of adenylyl cyclase, other mechanisms may be involved as well.

The alpha$_1$-adrenergic receptor (as well as the M-1 subtype of the acetylcholine receptor) appears to be coupled to a different G protein that activates phospholipase C; this G protein has not been well characterized but is sometimes tentatively designated G$_p$. Receptor occupancy in this system stimulates phospholipase C, which catalyzes the breakdown of membrane-bound phospholipids, particularly phosphatidylinositol-4,5-bisphosphate (PIP$_2$) with the production of inositol-1,4,5-trisphosphate (IP$_3$) and 1,2-diacylglycerol (DAG), both of which act as second messengers (Fig. 68-5). IP$_3$ rapidly mobilizes calcium from intracellular stores within the endoplasmic reticulum, producing an increase in free cytoplasmic calcium which by itself and via calcium-calmodulin–dependent protein kinases influences cellular processes appropriate to the stimulated cell. The transient rise in calcium induced by IP$_3$ from the intracellular stores is reinforced in the presence of continued agonist stimulation by alterations in membrane calcium flux that result eventually in net calcium uptake from the extracellular fluid by mechanisms that have been incompletely defined.

DAG, the other second messenger produced by the action of phospholipase C on PIP$_2$ (as well as other membrane phospholipids), remains associated with the cell membrane and activates protein kinase C, which has different substrates than the calcium-calmodulin kinases stimulated by IP$_3$. Protein phosphorylation stimulated by protein kinase C contributes to the tissue-specific response in ways that remain poorly understood. Increases in intracellular calcium also potentiate the activation of protein kinase C (Fig. 68-5).

REGULATION OF ADRENERGIC RECEPTORS Radiolabeled adrenergic-receptor agonists and antagonists have been utilized as ligands to study adrenergic receptors. In combination with studies of peripheral tissue sensitivity, these studies demonstrated that changes

FIGURE 68-5 Interaction of autonomic agonists with membrane-bound regulatory proteins and cellular effectors systems. The designations α and β refer to adrenergic receptors, DA refers to dopaminergic receptors, and M, to muscarinic receptors. G designates the GTP-associated regulatory protein which may have a stimulatory (s) or inhibitory (i) effect on adenylyl cyclase or may stimulate phospholipase C (p). (+) designates stimulation; (−) designates inhibition. PIP$_2$ = phosphatidylinositol-4,5-bisphosphate; DAG = 1,2-diacylglycerol; IP$_3$ = inositol-1,4,5-trisphosphate. See text for details.

in adrenergic receptors occur under a variety of physiologic conditions. Prolonged exposure to alpha- or beta-adrenergic agonists decreases the number of corresponding adrenergic receptors on effector cells. Although the biochemical mechanisms involved are obscure, internalization of the beta-adrenergic receptor within the cell occurs during agonist exposure in some systems, suggesting that internal translocation contributes to the decrease in receptor number under these circumstances.

Alteration in agonist concentration also may affect the affinity of the receptor for the agonist. Adrenergic receptors that utilize adenylyl cyclase for the second messenger (beta receptors, alpha$_2$ receptors) exist in high and low affinity states; exposure to agonist diminishes the proportion of receptors in the high-affinity state. Such alterations in adrenergic receptors induced by adrenergic agonists are termed *homologous regulation*. Agonist-induced alterations in adrenergic-receptor density and affinity are believed to contribute to the diminished physiologic response that occurs after prolonged exposure of an effector tissue to adrenergic agonist, a phenomenon known as *tachyphylaxis* or *desensitization*. Recent evidence suggests that phosphorylation of the beta receptor by a specific beta-receptor kinase is involved in the desensitization phenomenon.

Adrenergic receptors are also influenced by factors other than adrenergic agonists, so-called *heterologous regulation*. Enhanced alpha-adrenergic-receptor affinity, for example, may underlie the potentiation of alpha-adrenergic responses that occur in response to lowered environmental temperatures. Thyroid hormones potentiate beta-receptor responses by alterations in beta-receptor number and in the efficiency of coupling receptor occupancy with physiologic response. Estrogen and progesterone alter the sensitivity of the myometrium to catecholamines by effects on alpha-adrenergic receptors. Glucocorticoids may influence adrenergic function by antagonizing agonist-induced decreases in adrenergic receptors, thereby counteracting tachyphylaxis in response to intense adrenergic stimulation. Some forms of heterologous desensitization may involve modifications in the membrane regulatory proteins or in adenylyl cyclase itself.

Alterations in sensitivity to catecholamines also occur as a consequence of postreceptor changes, although the latter remain poorly characterized.

PHYSIOLOGY OF THE SYMPATHOADRENAL SYSTEM

Catecholamines influence all the major organ systems. The effects take place in seconds as compared with the minutes, hours, or days that characterize the actions of the endocrine system and most other control systems that regulate bodily processes. The sympathoadrenal system, moreover, may respond in anticipation of physiologic requirement. An increase in sympathoadrenal activity prior to strenuous exercise, for example, lessens the impact of exercise on the internal environment.

DIRECT EFFECTS OF CATECHOLAMINES Cardiovascular system   Catecholamines stimulate vasoconstriction in the subcutaneous, mucosal, splanchnic, and renal vascular beds by alpha-receptor–mediated mechanisms. Although vasoconstriction was originally considered an alpha$_1$-receptor response, vascular tone appears to be more complexly regulated and, in many areas, involves alpha$_2$-mediated responses as well. The venous portion of the circulation, in particular, is endowed with alpha$_2$ receptors. Differential regulation of the two types of alpha receptors, under certain circumstances, contributes to an integrated physiologic response, as described below under "Cold Exposure." Since vasoconstriction in the coronary and cerebral circulations is minimal, flow to these areas is maintained during sympathetic stimulation. The adaptive significance of this priority given the heart and brain is clear; in both these organs the metabolic requirements relative to blood flow are high, and continuous perfusion is essential for life. Skeletal muscle vasculature contains beta receptors sensitive to low circulating levels of E so that skeletal muscle blood flow is augmented during adrenal medullary activation.

The effects of catecholamines on the heart are mediated by beta$_1$ receptors and include increase in heart rate, enhancement of cardiac contractility, and increase in conduction velocity. The increase in myocardial contractility is illustrated by a leftward and upward shift of the ventricular function curve (Fig. 194-5) that relates cardiac work to ventricular diastolic fiber length; at any initial fiber length, catecholamines increase cardiac work. Catecholamines also enhance cardiac output by stimulating venoconstriction, enhancing venous return, and increasing the force of atrial contraction, thereby augmenting diastolic volume and hence fiber length. The acceleration of conduction in the junctional tissues results in a more synchronous, and hence more effective, ventricular contraction. Cardiac stimulation increases myocardial oxygen consumption, a major factor in the pathogenesis and treatment of myocardial ischemia.

Metabolism   Catecholamines increase metabolic rate. In small mammals, mitochondrial respiration in brown adipose tissue is functionally uncoupled by NE. In a reaction unique to brown adipose tissue, NE activates a specific mitochondrial uncoupling protein that dissipates the proton gradient between the inner mitochondrial matrix and the cytoplasm, thereby uncoupling substrate utilization and ATP synthesis. In humans, a functional role for brown adipose tissue has not been established with certainty, but increasing evidence suggests a potential role for this tissue in catecholamine-stimulated heat production in human beings.

SUBSTRATE MOBILIZATION   In a variety of tissues, catecholamines stimulate the breakdown of stored fuel with the production of substrate for local consumption; glycogenolysis in the heart, for example, provides substrate for immediate metabolism by the myocardium. Catecholamines also accelerate fuel mobilization in liver, adipose tissue, and skeletal muscle, liberating substrates (glucose, free fatty acids, lactate) into the circulation for use throughout the body. Activation of enzymes involved in fuel breakdown occurs by a beta-receptor (beta$_1$) mechanism for adipose tissue lipolysis and by alpha- and beta-receptor (beta$_2$) mechanisms for hepatic glycogenolysis and gluconeogenesis. In skeletal muscle, catecholamines stimulate glycogenolysis (beta receptor), thereby increasing lactate efflux.

Fluids and electrolytes   Catecholamines contribute to regulation of the volume and composition of extracellular fluid. By a direct action on the renal tubule, NE stimulates sodium reabsorption, thereby defending extracellular fluid volume. Dopamine, in contrast, promotes sodium excretion. NE and E also promote cellular uptake of potassium, thereby defending against the development of hyperkalemia. Effects of catecholamines on calcium, magnesium, and phosphate metabolism are complex and depend on a variety of factors.

Viscera   Catecholamines affect visceral function by actions on smooth muscle and glandular epithelium. Urinary bladder and intestinal smooth muscle are relaxed while the corresponding sphincters are stimulated. Gallbladder emptying also involves sympathetic mechanisms. Catecholamine-mediated smooth-muscle contraction in the female aids ovulation and ovum transport along the fallopian tubes, and in the male provides propulsive force for the seminal fluid during ejaculation. Inhibitory alpha$_2$ receptors on cholinergic neurons within the gut contribute to intestinal relaxation. Catecholamines induce bronchodilation by a beta$_2$-receptor mechanism.

INDIRECT EFFECTS OF CATECHOLAMINES   The ultimate physiologic response induced by catecholamines involves changes in hormone secretion and in blood flow distribution, both of which support and amplify the direct effects of catecholamines.

Endocrine system   Catecholamines influence the secretion of renin, insulin, glucagon, calcitonin, parathormone, thyroxine, gastrin, erythropoietin, progesterone, and, possibly, testosterone. Secretion of each of these hormones is governed by complex feedback loops. With the exception of thyroxine and the gonadal steroids, each is a polypeptide not under the direct control of the pituitary gland. Sympathoadrenal input into the secretion of these hormones provides a mechanism for regulation by the central nervous system and ensures a coordinated hormonal response in accord with the homeostatic needs of the organism.

RENIN (See also Chap. 209) The juxtaglomerular apparatus of the kidney is heavily innervated. Sympathetic stimulation increases renin release by a direct beta-receptor effect independent of vascular changes within the kidney. The renin response to volume depletion is sympathetically mediated and is initiated by a fall in central venous pressure. Since renin secretion activates the angiotensin-aldosterone system, angiotensin-induced vasoconstriction supports the direct effects of catecholamines on blood vessels, while aldosterone-mediated sodium reabsorption complements the direct increase in sodium reabsorption induced by sympathetic stimulation. Beta-receptor blocking agents suppress renin secretion.

INSULIN AND GLUCAGON The pancreatic islets also receive an extensive sympathetic innervation. Stimulation of pancreatic sympathetic nerves or an elevation in circulating catecholamines suppresses insulin and increases glucagon release. Inhibition of insulin secretion is mediated by the alpha$_2$ receptor, and stimulation of glucagon is mediated by the beta receptor. This combination of effects supports substrate mobilization, reinforcing the direct effects of catecholamines on hepatic glucose output and lipolysis. Although alpha-receptor–mediated suppression of insulin release usually predominates, a beta-receptor mechanism may augment insulin secretion under some circumstances.

SYMPATHOADRENAL FUNCTION IN SELECTED PHYSIOLOGIC AND PATHOPHYSIOLOGIC STATES Support of the circulation

The sympathetic nervous system functions to maintain an adequate circulation. During upright posture and volume depletion, reduction of afferent venous and arterial baroreceptor impulse traffic diminishes an inhibitory input to the vasomotor center, thereby increasing sympathetic activity (Fig. 68-3) and reducing efferent vagal tone. As a result, heart rate is increased, and cardiac output is diverted from the skin, subcutaneous tissues, mucosa, and viscera. Sympathetic stimulation of the kidney increases sodium reabsorption, and sympathetically mediated venoconstriction enhances venous return. With pronounced hypotension, the adrenal medulla is recruited and E reinforces the effects of the sympathetic nervous system. A similar pattern of sympathetic activation occurs in the postprandial state when blood and extracellular fluid are sequestered in the splanchnic circulation and in the lumen of the gut, respectively.

The intense sympathoadrenal stimulation that accompanies severe volume depletion may contribute to the development of ketoacidosis in alcoholics as well as to the ketoacidosis sometimes seen in association with hyperemesis gravidarum. Under these circumstances, catecholamine-mediated suppression of insulin and stimulation of glucagon markedly potentiate ketogenesis. Volume resuscitation and provision of adequate glucose promptly reverse the ketoacidosis in most cases.

CONGESTIVE HEART FAILURE The sympathetic nervous system also provides circulatory support during congestive heart failure (Chap. 195). Venoconstriction and sympathetic stimulation of the heart increase cardiac output while peripheral vasoconstriction directs blood flow to the heart and brain. The afferent signals are less clear than in simple volume depletion because the venous pressure is usually elevated. In severe heart failure, depletion of cardiac NE may impair the effectiveness of sympathetic circulatory support.

TRAUMA AND SHOCK In acute traumatic injury or shock, adrenal catecholamines support the circulation and mobilize substrates. It is presumed, but unproved, that the sympathetic nervous system is activated as well, although some evidence suggests that suppression of the sympathetic nervous system may contribute to the hypotension that occurs in association with trauma. In the chronic, reparative phase following injury, catecholamines contribute to substrate mobilization and to the elevation in metabolic rate.

EXERCISE Sympathetic activation during exercise increases cardiac output, maintains blood flow, and ensures sufficient substrate to meet the increased needs. Central neural factors, such as anticipation, and circulatory factors, such as fall in venous pressure, trigger the sympathetic response. Mild degrees of exercise stimulate the sympathetic nervous system alone; during more severe exertion the

adrenal medulla is activated as well. Conditioning is associated with a decrease in sympathetic nervous system activity both at rest and during exercise, in comparison with the untrained state.

Hypoglycemia (See also Chap. 338) Hypoglycemia causes a marked increase in adrenal medullary E secretion. When glucose concentrations fall below overnight fasting levels, regulatory glucose-sensitive neurons in the central nervous system initiate a prompt increase in adrenal medullary secretion. The increase is especially intense at plasma glucose levels below 2.8 mmol/L (50 mg/dL), when plasma E levels increase 25 to 50 times above baseline, thereby increasing hepatic glucose output, providing alternative substrate in the form of free fatty acids, suppressing endogenous insulin release, and inhibiting insulin-mediated glucose utilization in muscle. Many clinical manifestations of hypoglycemia, such as tachycardia, palpitations, nervousness, tremor, and widened pulse pressure, are secondary to increased E secretion. These manifestations of E secretion constitute an "early warning" system in insulin-requiring diabetics. In patients with long-standing diabetes mellitus, however, the E response to hypoglycemia may be diminished or absent, leaving affected patients at greater risk to develop severe hypoglycemia.

Cold exposure The sympathetic nervous system plays a critical role in the maintenance of normal body temperature during exposure to a cold environment. Receptors in the skin and central nervous system respond to a fall in temperature by activating hypothalamic and brainstem centers that increase sympathetic activity. Sympathetic stimulation leads to vasoconstriction in the superficial vascular beds, thereby diminishing heat loss. The sympathetic response involves a complex interaction between lowered environmental temperatures and alpha$_2$-adrenergic receptors. The superficial veins of the extremities are prominently endowed with alpha$_2$ receptors. Cold directly increases the vasoconstrictor response mediated by the alpha$_2$ receptor. The deep venous system, in contrast, is endowed with alpha$_1$ receptors which, in nonspecific fashion, diminish the constrictor response during environmental cooling. The net result is a shunting of blood from the superficial to the deep venous system. Since the deep veins run in close proximity to the major arteries supplying the limb, heat is efficiently returned to the central venous pool by a countercurrent exchange mechanism. Heat production is simultaneously increased by shivering, generation of metabolic heat, and substrate mobilization. Acclimatization during chronic cold exposure increases the capacity for metabolic heat production in response to sympathetic stimulation.

Dietary intake Fasting suppresses and overfeeding stimulates the sympathetic nervous system. The reduction in sympathetic activity during fasting or starvation contributes to the decrease in metabolic rate, bradycardia, and hypotension in these states. Enhanced sympathetic activity during periods of increased caloric intake contributes to the elevation in metabolic rate associated with a chronic increase in dietary intake.

Hypoxia Chronic hypoxia is associated with stimulation of the sympathoadrenal system, and some of the cardiovascular changes attendant to hypoxia are dependent on catecholamines.

THE SYMPATHETIC NERVOUS SYSTEM IN PATHOGENESIS OF SELECTED DISEASE STATES

HYPERTENSION (See also Chap. 209) As shown in Fig. 68-6, regulation of arterial pressure by the sympathetic nervous system involves blood vessels, the heart, and the kidneys. The sympathetic nervous system increases peripheral resistance by direct stimulation of the resistance vessels and by activation of the renin-angiotensin system. Increased cardiac output is the result of enhanced cardiac contractility and augmented venous return, the latter a result of venoconstriction and increased renal sodium reabsorption. Stimulation of sodium retention alters the pressure natriuresis relationship, thereby diminishing the capacity of the kidney to compensate for the increase in blood pressure. Antiadrenergic agents lower blood pressure by interacting at many of the sites shown in Fig. 68-6.

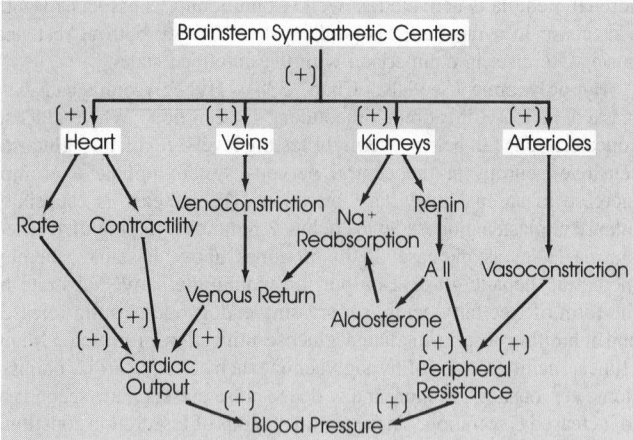

FIGURE 68-6 Sympathetic nervous system effects on blood pressure. Sympathetic stimulation (+) increases blood pressure by effects on the heart, the veins, the kidneys, and the arterioles. The net result of sympathetic stimulation is an increase in both cardiac output and peripheral resistance. AII = angiotensin II. *[From JB Young, L Landsberg, in P Sleight et al (eds), Scientific Foundations of Cardiology, London, Heinemann, 1981.]*

Whether primary sympathetic overactivity plays a role in the pathogenesis of essential hypertension is uncertain owing to the insensitivity of currently available methods of assessing regional sympathetic activity in humans. It is well established, however, that the sympathetic nervous system plays at least a permissive role in hypertension. Despite the elevated blood pressure, sympathetic nervous system activity is not suppressed in hypertensive patients, and reflex control of the circulation is retained, due in part to upward resetting of the baroreceptors. In addition, peripheral sensitivity of the vasculature to NE is either normal or enhanced. The maintenance of sympathetic nervous system activity in patients with hypertension accounts for the hypotensive effects of antiadrenergic agents.

During antihypertensive treatment with vasodilators or diuretics, the sympathetic nervous system may be activated in response to decreased pressure in either the venous or arterial circulation (Fig. 68-3). The heightened sympathetic activity that results, in addition to causing tachycardia, may oppose the antihypertensive therapy by activating the various effector systems shown in Fig. 68-6. Agents with antiadrenergic effects, therefore, have a fundamental role in the therapy of most hypertensive patients.

ANGINA PECTORIS (See also Chap. 203) Sympathetic stimulation of the cardiovascular system increases myocardial oxygen consumption as a consequence of elevated heart rate, enhanced myocardial contractility, and increased myocardial wall tension. Attacks of angina, therefore, are often precipitated by situations associated with sympathetic activation such as exercise, eating, and cold exposure. Beta blockade is beneficial in the treatment of angina because of reduction in sympathetic stimulation of the heart. Alpha-adrenergically mediated coronary vasoconstriction also may contribute to coronary spasm.

HYPERTHYROIDISM (See also Chap. 334) Many of the peripheral manifestations of hyperthyroidism suggest a hyperadrenergic state. Enhancement of beta-receptor responses in hyperthyroidism is due in part to effects on the beta receptor. Thyroid hormone, in some tissues and in some species, increases receptor number; in other tissues, even when beta-receptor number is not increased, coupling of receptor occupancy to the adenylate cyclase cyclic-AMP system is augmented to amplify catecholamine-induced responses. Since thyroid hormone excess does not suppress sympathetic nervous system activity (plasma NE levels are normal in thyrotoxic patients), a "normal" level of sympathetic activity may evoke an exaggerated physiologic response. Many of the adrenergic manifestations of hyperthyroidism are diminished by treatment with beta-receptor blocking agents.

ORTHOSTATIC HYPOTENSION The maintenance of arterial pressure during upright posture depends on an adequate blood volume, an unimpaired venous return, and an intact sympathetic nervous system. Significant postural hypotension, therefore, often reflects extracellular fluid volume depletion or dysfunction of the circulatory reflexes. Diseases of the nervous system, such as tabes dorsalis, syringomyelia, or diabetes mellitus, may disrupt these sympathetic reflexes with resultant orthostatic hypotension. Although any antiadrenergic agent may impair the postural sympathetic response, orthostatic hypotension is most prominent with drugs that block neurotransmission within the ganglia or adrenergic neurons.

The term *idiopathic orthostatic hypotension* refers to a group of degenerative diseases involving either the pre- or postganglionic sympathetic neurons. Involvement of the postganglionic sympathetic nervous system is characterized by low basal NE levels, while involvement at the level of the central nervous system or preganglionic sympathetic neurons is associated with normal basal plasma NE levels. In both cases, the plasma NE response to upright posture is deficient. Orthostatic hypotension caused by disruption of the preganglionic autonomic neurons within the intermediolateral cell column of the spinal cord often occurs in association with degenerative changes of basal ganglia and other portions of the central nervous system. In the latter situation, known as *multiple-systems atrophy*, or the *Shy-Drager syndrome*, orthostatic hypotension occurs along with a variety of neurologic disturbances, including Parkinson's disease.

Treatment of orthostatic hypotension is usually unsatisfactory except in the mildest cases. There is no way of reestablishing the normal relationship between fall in venous return and sympathetic neuronal activation. Volume expansion with fludrocortisone and a liberal salt diet in conjunction with fitted stockings to the waist, as well as elevation of the head of the bed to avoid recumbency, will maintain plasma volume and venous return and frequently provide symptomatic improvement. Rarely a beneficial response may be obtained from treatment with sympathomimetic amines (including clonidine).

PHARMACOLOGY OF THE SYMPATHOADRENAL SYSTEM

A variety of therapeutic agents affect sympathetic nervous system function or interact with adrenergic receptors, making it possible to stimulate or suppress effects mediated by catecholamines with some degree of specificity (Table 68-1).

SYMPATHOMIMETIC AMINES Sympathomimetic amines may directly activate adrenergic receptors (direct acting) or release NE from the sympathetic nerve endings (indirect acting). Many agents have both direct and indirect effects.

Epinephrine and norepinephrine The naturally occurring catecholamines act predominantly by the direct stimulation of adrenergic receptors. NE is employed to support the circulation and elevate the blood pressure in hypotensive states (Chap. 34). Peripheral vasoconstriction is the major effect, although cardiac stimulation occurs as well. E, also employed as a pressor, has special usefulness in the treatment of allergic reactions, especially those associated with anaphylaxis. E antagonizes the effects of histamine and other mediators on vascular and visceral smooth muscle and is useful in the treatment of bronchospasm.

Dopamine *Dopamine* is used in treating hypotension, shock (Chap. 34), and certain forms of heart failure (Chap. 195). At low infusion rates it exerts a positive inotropic effect both by a direct action on the cardiac beta$_1$ receptors and by the indirect release of NE from sympathetic nerve endings in the heart. At low doses direct stimulation of dopaminergic receptors in the renal and mesenteric vasculature also results in vasodilation in the gut and kidney and facilitates sodium excretion. At higher infusion rates interaction with alpha-adrenergic receptors results in vasoconstriction, an increase in peripheral resistance, and an elevation of blood pressure.

Beta-receptor agonists *Isoproterenol*, a direct-acting beta-receptor agonist, stimulates the heart, decreases peripheral resistance, and relaxes bronchial smooth muscle. It raises the cardiac output and accelerates atrioventricular conduction while increasing the automaticity of ventricular pacemakers. Isoproterenol is used in the treatment of heart block and bronchoconstriction. *Dobutamine*, a congener of dopamine with relative selectivity for the beta$_1$ receptor and with a greater effect on myocardial contractility than on heart rate, is also used in the treatment of congestive heart failure, often in combination with vasodilators (Chap. 195). In conjunction with radionuclide imaging or echocardiographic assessment of wall motion, dobutamine, as well as other investigational congeners that have a relatively greater effect on heart rate, is used in the diagnosis of demand-induced myocardial ischemia.

SELECTIVE BETA$_2$-RECEPTOR AGONISTS The cardiac stimulation caused by nonselective beta agonists, such as isoproterenol or epinephrine, is occasionally dangerous when these agents are used in the treatment of bronchoconstriction (see Chap. 217). Selective beta$_2$ agonists (*metaproterenol, albuterol, terbutaline, pirbuterol,* and *isoetharine*) improve the therapeutic ratio by achieving bronchial dilatation with less activation of the cardiovascular system (see Chaps. 217 and 223); selectivity is relative, and cardiac stimulation does occur with these agents, particularly at the higher dose levels. *Ritodrine*, another selective beta$_2$ agonist, is used as a tocolytic agent (as is *terbutaline*) to relax the uterus and antagonize premature labor.

Alpha-adrenergic agonists *Phenylephrine* and *methoxamine* are direct-acting alpha agonists that elevate blood pressure by increasing peripheral vasoconstriction. They are used primarily in the treatment of hypotension and paroxysmal supraventricular tachycardia (Chap. 198), in the latter case by increasing cardiac vagal tone through reflex baroreceptor stimulation. Phenylephrine and a related proprietary compound, *phenylpropanolamine*, are common constituents of decongestant medications (often combined with antihistamines) for the treatment of allergic rhinitis and upper respiratory infections.

Miscellaneous sympathomimetic amines with mixed actions *Ephedrine* has both direct beta-receptor agonist properties and an indirect effect on sympathetic nerve endings, from which it releases NE, and is used primarily as a bronchodilator. *Sudephedrine*, a congener of ephedrine, is less potent at dilating bronchi and serves as a nasal decongestant. *Metaraminol* has both direct and indirect effects on sympathetic nerve endings and is employed in the treatment of hypotensive states.

Dopaminergic agonists The dopamine 2–receptor agonist *bromocriptine* is used to suppress prolactin secretion (Chap. 331). *Apomorphine*, another dopamine 2–receptor agonist, is used to induce emesis.

ANTIADRENERGIC OR SYMPATHOLYTIC AGENTS (See also Chap. 209) **Agents inhibiting central sympathetic outflow** The antihypertensive agents *methyldopa, clonidine, guanabenz,* and *guanfacine* diminish central sympathetic outflow by stimulating a central alpha-adrenergic pathway (alpha$_2$ receptor) that diminishes vasomotor outflow. Central nervous system side effects such as sedation are common. When administration of clonidine is stopped abruptly, a withdrawal syndrome characterized by rebound hyperactivity of the sympathetic nervous system can produce a state resembling the crises of patients with pheochromocytoma. *Opiates* also may exert a central sympatholytic effect; the sympathetic excitation of morphine withdrawal responds to clonidine and vice versa. *Propranolol* and *reserpine* may exert some sympatholytic effects at the level of the central nervous system.

Ganglionic blocking agents Ganglionic transmission may be antagonized by drugs that block the (nicotinic) cholinergic synapse between the preganglionic and postganglionic autonomic nerves. These agents inhibit the parasympathetic as well as the sympathetic nervous system. Only *trimethaphan* is in general clinical use; its major application is in the treatment of hypertensive crises, particularly aortic dissection, when controlled hypotension and decreased myocardial contractility are desirable (Chap. 210).

Agents acting at the peripheral sympathetic nerve endings Adrenergic neuron-blocking agents depress the function of the peripheral sympathetic nerves by decreasing the amount of neurotransmitter released. *Guanethidine*, the prototype of this class of drugs, is concentrated in the sympathetic nerve endings by the amine-uptake mechanism. Within the terminal it blocks the release of NE in response to nerve impulses and eventually depletes the nerve of NE by displacing it from the intraneuronal storage granules. The drug is occasionally useful in the management of severe hypertension, although orthostatic hypotension is a limiting side effect. *Bretylium*, an agent whose effects are similar to those of guanethidine, is employed in the treatment of ventricular fibrillation (Chap. 198). Both guanethidine and bretylium are antagonized by agents that affect the amine-uptake transport process such as sympathomimetic amines, tricyclic antidepressants, phenoxybenzamine, and phenothiazines. The antihypertensive action of guanethidine may be rapidly reversed by these drugs.

Reserpine depletes catecholamines from the peripheral sympathetic nerve endings, the brain, and the adrenal medulla. Its antihypertensive effect in humans is usually attributed to depletion of peripheral NE stores within sympathetic nerve endings. The sedation and occasionally morbid depression attending its use result from NE depletion within the central nervous system.

Adrenergic-receptor blocking agents Adrenergic blocking agents antagonize the effects of catecholamines at the level of the peripheral tissue.

ALPHA-ADRENERGIC-RECEPTOR BLOCKING AGENTS *Phenoxybenzamine* and *phentolamine* are utilized principally in treating pheochromocytoma (Chap. 336). Phenoxybenzamine produces prolonged, noncompetitive alpha blockade, while phentolamine leads to reversible, competitive blockade. Because of its rapid action and short duration, phentolamine is commonly used in the treatment of acute hypertensive paroxysms secondary to catecholamine excess, such as occur with pheochromocytoma, with pressor reactions in patients receiving monoamine oxidase inhibitors, and in clonidine withdrawal. Both phentolamine and phenoxybenzamine antagonize alpha$_1$ and alpha$_2$ receptors, although phenoxybenzamine is more potent at the alpha$_1$ receptor site. *Prazosin*, an alpha-adrenergic blocking agent with selectivity for the alpha$_1$ receptor, possesses properties that resemble those of primary vasodilators and is used in the treatment of essential hypertension and as an afterload-reducing agent in congestive heart failure. Doxazosin and terazosin, long-acting selective alpha$_1$ blockers, are used in the treatment of essential hypertension. Selective alpha$_1$ blockers are potentially useful in the symptomatic treatment of urinary outflow track obstruction because they antagonize contraction of the sphincter at the bladder trigone.

BETA-ADRENERGIC-RECEPTOR BLOCKING AGENTS These drugs antagonize the cardiovascular effects of catecholamines in angina pectoris, hypertension, and cardiac arrhythmias. The benefit of beta blockade in angina derives from the decrease in myocardial oxygen consumption following reduction in heart rate and myocardial contractility (Chap. 203). The hypotensive effect of beta blockade is not clearly understood (Chap. 209). Diminished cardiac output, decreased NE release at postganglionic sympathetic nerve endings, reduced renin secretion, and suppressed central sympathetic outflow are possible mechanisms. The efficacy of beta blocking agents in the treatment of arrhythmias depends on reduction of the rate of spontaneous depolarization of pacemaker cells in the sinus node and junctional pacemakers and on slowing conduction within the atria and atrioventricular node. Beta blockade is also effective in the symptomatic management of hyperthyroidism and the control of tachycardia and arrhythmias in patients with pheochromocytoma. Beta-adrenergic blocking agents are also useful in the treatment of migraine, essential tremor, idiopathic hypertrophic subaortic stenosis, and aortic dissection. Several trials have demonstrated that beta-receptor blocking agents, administered long-term, diminish mortality following acute myocardial infarction. The mechanism of this cardioprotective effect may involve antiarrhythmic action, prevention of reinfarction, and reduction in infarct size (Chap. 202).

TABLE 68-1 Some commonly used autonomic drugs[a,b,c]

Agent	Indication	Dose and Route	Comment
ADRENERGIC AGONISTS[d]			
Epinephrine	Anaphylaxis	100–500 μg SC or IM (0.1–0.5 mL of 1/1000 solution of hydrochloride salt); 25–50 μg IV (slowly) every 5–15 min; titrate as needed	Nonselective alpha and beta agonist; increases BP, heart rate Bronchodilation
Norepinephrine	Shock Hypotension	2–4 μg of NE base/min IV; titrate as needed	Alpha and beta$_1$ agonist Vasoconstriction predominates Extravasation causes tissue necrosis; infuse through IV cannula
Isoproterenol	Cardiogenic shock Bradyarrhythmias AV block	0.5–5.0 μg/min IV; titrate as needed	Nonselective beta agonist Increases cardiac rate and contractility (beta$_1$) Tachycardia limits usefulness
	Asthma	Inhalation	Dilates bronchi (beta$_2$); cardiac stimulation also occurs
Dobutamine	Refractory CHF Cardiogenic shock	2.5–25 (μg/kg)/min IV	Selective beta$_1$ agonist with greater effect on contractility than heart rate; a congener of dopamine but not a dopaminergic agonist
Phenylephrine	Hypotension	40–180 μg/min IV	Selective alpha$_1$ agonist; useful in antagonizing hypotension of spinal anesthesia
	Supraventricular tachycardia	150–800 μg slow IV push	Pressor effect induces vagotonic response; do not exceed 160 mmH systolic BP
Terbutaline	Asthma	2.5–5.0 mg PO tid; 0.25–0.5 mg SC; inhalation every 4–5 h	Selective beta$_2$ agonist; beta$_1$ (cardiac) effects at higher doses
Albuterol	Asthma	2.0–4.0 mg PO tid or qid; inhalation every 4–6 h	Selective beta$_2$ agonist; beta$_1$ effects (cardiac) at higher doses
Isoetharine	Asthma	Inhalation every 2–4 h	Selective beta$_2$ agonist; some beta$_1$ effects
Metaproterenol	Asthma	10–20 mg PO tid or qid; inhalation every 3–4 h	Selective beta$_2$ agonist; some beta$_1$ effects
Pirbuteral	Asthma	Inhalation every 4–6 h	Selective beta$_2$ agonist; some beta$_1$ effects
Ritodrine	Premature labor	100–350 μg/min IV; 10–20 mg every 4–6 h PO	Selective beta$_2$ agonist; hypokalemia. hyperglycemia, hypotension, cardiac stimulation may occur Neonatal hypoglycemia, hypocalcemia reported
DOPAMINERGIC AGONISTS			
Dopamine	Shock	2–5 (μg/kg)/min IV (dopaminergic range) 5–10 (μg/kg)/min IV (dopaminergic and beta range) 10–20 (μg/kg)min IV (beta range) 20–50 (μg/kg)/min IV (alpha range)	Pharmacologic effects are dose dependent: renal and mesenteric vasodilation predominate at lower doses; cardiac stimulation and vasoconstriction develop as the dose is increased
Bromocriptine	Amenorrhea-galactorrhea	2.5 mg PO bid or tid	Selective agonist of dopamine-2 receptor; inhibits prolactin secretion
	Acromegaly	5–15 mg PO tid or qid	Lowers growth hormone in a minority of patients with acromegaly
INHIBITORS OF CENTRAL SYMPATHETIC OUTFLOW			
Clonidine	Hypertension	0.1–0.6 mg PO bid	Selective alpha$_2$ agonist; potentiates central baroreceptor depressor reflex Abrupt discontinuation may result in withdrawal syndrome with rebound hypertension
Methyldopa	Hypertension	250–500 mg PO every 6–8 h	Metabolized by decarboxylation and beta hydroxylation to α-methyl-norepinephrine, a centrally active selective alpha$_2$ agonist
ADRENERGIC NEURON BLOCKING AGENTS			
Guanethidine	Hypertension	10–100 mg PO qd	Concentrated in sympathetic nerve endings; blocks release of NE in response to nerve impulses and depletes NE stores; prominent orthostatic hypotension
Bretylium	Ventricular fibrillation and tachycardia	5 mg/kg IV	In addition to blocking NE release, has direct effect on electrical properties of cardiac muscle
BETA BLOCKING AGENTS[e]			
Propranolol	Hypertension	40–160 mg PO bid (or higher)	Lipophilic, nonselective Dosage highly variable
	Angina	10–40 mg PO tid or qid	
	Myocardial infarction	60–80 mg PO tid	Prolongs survival post MI
	Arrhythmias	10–30 mg PO tid or qid; 1–3 mg IV	
	Hypertrophic cardiomyopathy	20–40 mg PO tid or qid	
	Pheochromocytoma	10–20 mg PO tid or qid; 0.5–2.0 mg IV	After alpha blockade initiated
	Essential tremor	20–80 mg PO tid	
	Migraine	20–80 mg PO bid or tid	
	Hyperthyroidism	10–60 mg PO tid or qid	
Metoprolol	Hypertension	50–200 mg PO bid	Selective beta$_1$ (cardiac), lipophilic
	Myocardial infarction	100 mg PO bid	Prolongs survival post MI

TABLE 68-1 Some commonly used autonomic drugs[a,b,c] (continued)

Agent	Indication	Dose and Route	Comment
BETA BLOCKING AGENTS[e] (continued)			
Nadolol	Hypertension Angina	80–320 mg PO qd 80–240 mg PO qd	Hydrophilic, nonselective; lengthen dosage interval with renal failure
Timolol	Hypertension Myocardial infarction	10–30 mg PO bid 10 mg PO bid	Lipophilic, nonselective Prolongs survival post MI
Atenolol	Hypertension	50–100 mg PO qd	Selective beta$_1$, hydrophilic; lengthen dosage interval with renal failure
Pindolol	Hypertension Angina	5–30 mg PO bid 10 mg PO qid	Nonselective, lipophilic with partial agonist activity
Acebutolol	Hypertension Arrhythmias	200–800 mg qid 200–600 mg bid	Selective beta$_1$, hydrophilic, partial agonist activity
Penbutolol	Hypertension	20–40 mg PO qd	Nonselective
Betaxolol	Hypertension	15–20 mg PO qd	Selective β_1, hydrophilic
Carteolol	Hypertension	2.5–10 mg PO qd	Nonselective, partial agonist activity, hydrophilic; lengthen dosage interval with renal failure
Esmolol	Supraventricular tachycardia	50–200 (μg/kg)/min IV after loading dose of 500 μg/kg/min for 1 min	Selective beta$_1$, very short duration of action
ALPHA BLOCKING AGENTS			
Phenoxybenzamine	Pheochromocytoma	10–60 mg PO bid; titrate as needed	Noncompetitive, nonselective alpha blockade
Phentolamine	Pheochromocytoma	5 mg IV (after test dose of 0.5 mg)	Competitive, nonselective alpha blockade
Prazosin	Hypertension CHF	1–5 mg PO bid or tid 2–7 mg PO qid	Competitive, selective alpha$_1$ blockade
Doxazosin	Hypertension	1–16 mg PO qd	Competitive selective alpha$_1$ blockade, long duration of action
Terazosin	Hypertension	1–5 mg PO qd	Competitive, selective alpha$_1$ blockade, long duration of action
COMBINED ALPHA-BETA BLOCKING AGENT			
Labetalol	Hypertension	100–1200 mg PO bid; titrate slowly as needed; 20–80 mg IV (by increments up to 300 mg); 2 mg/min by IV infusion	Competitive alpha and beta antagonist with relatively more activity against beta receptors
DOPAMINERGIC ANTAGONIST[f]			
Metoclopramide	Diabetic gastroparesis	10 mg PO qid	Competitive dopaminergic antagonist with prominent cholinergic agonist activity
	Gastroesophageal reflex Antiemetic (cancer chemotherapy)	10–15 mg PO qid 10 mg IV	
GANGLIONIC BLOCKING AGENT			
Trimethaphan	Hypertensive crisis (aortic dissection)	1–3 mg/min IV	Competitive ganglionic blocker; some direct vasodilating effects; inhibits parasympathetic as well as sympathetic nervous system
CHOLINERGIC AGENT			
Bethanechol	Urinary retention (nonobstructive)	10–100 mg PO tid or qid; 5 mg SC	M-2 receptor agonist
ANTICHOLINESTERASE AGENTS[g]			
Physostigmine	Central cholinergic blockade	1–2 mg IV (slow)	Tertiary amine; penetrates CNS well; may cause seizures; used to reverse central anticholinergic effects produced by overdose of atropine or tricyclic antidepressants
Edrophonium	Paroxysmal supraventricular tachycardia	5 mg IV (after 1.0-mg test dose)	Induces vagotonic response; rapid onset, short duration of action; effects reversed by atropine
CHOLINERGIC BLOCKING AGENTS[h]			
Atropine	Bradycardia and hypotension	0.4–1.0 mg IV every 1–2 h	Competitive inhibition of M-1 and M-2 receptor; blocks hemodynamic changes associated with increased vagal tone

[a] Consult complete prescribing information. [b] Doses for children are not given. [c] Only the more common indications and routes of administration are listed.
[d] Dopaminergic agonists are listed separately although dopamine, at high doses, is an adrenergic agonist as well.
[e] Clinical efficacy of most beta blockers appears similar for major indications. Not all beta blockers are FDA approved for all indications listed in the table. When beta blocking agents are discontinued, gradual dosage reduction is recommended. Both beta$_1$ selective and nonselective agents have cardioprotective effects after myocardial infarction.
[f] Neuroleptic and antipsychotic agents are also dopaminergic antagonists; these are not included in the table.
[g] A major use of cholinesterase inhibitors is in myasthenia gravis (Chap 386). These agents, quaternary amines that do not penetrate the CNS, are not included here.
[h] A wide variety of synthetic atropine derivatives are available for the purpose of (1) diminishing GI tract motility and secretion and (2) increasing urinary bladder capacity. Their usefulness is limited by anticholinergic side effects. Some may be useful as adjuncts in the treatment of peptic ulcer disease.

PHARMACOLOGIC PROPERTIES OF BETA-RECEPTOR BLOCKING AGENTS   Eleven beta blocking agents (atenolol, acebutolol, betaxolol, carteolol, esmolol, metoprolol, nadolol, pindolol, penbutolol, propranolol, and timolol) are available for use in the United States. Other agents (alprenolol, bevantolol, oxprenolol, sotalol, etc.) are in use in other countries and investigational within the United States. The utility of these agents is derived predominantly from blockade of beta-adrenergic receptors. In general, the various agents have similar clinical efficacy.

Although much has been written about other pharmacologic properties, including cardioselectivity, membrane stabilizing (local anesthetic) effects, intrinsic sympathomimetic (partial-agonist) activity, and lipid solubility, the clinical significance of these additional properties is small. Local anesthetic properties are most prominent with propranolol; however, membrane stabilization probably does not contribute substantially to the clinical utility. The various beta blockers do differ in their water and lipid solubility. The lipophilic agents (propranolol, metoprolol, oxprenolol) are readily absorbed from the gastrointestinal tract, metabolized by the liver, have large volumes of distribution, and penetrate the central nervous system well; the hydrophilic agents (acebutolol, atenolol, betaxolol, carteolol, nadolol, sotalol) are less readily absorbed, not extensively metabolized, and have relatively long plasma half-lives. As a consequence, the hydrophilic agents may be administered once per day. Hepatic failure may prolong the plasma half-life of the lipophilic agents, whereas renal failure may prolong the action of the hydrophilic group. The degree of lipid solubility, therefore, provides a basis for choice of a particular agent in patients with hepatic or renal insufficiency. Although the hydrophilic agents penetrate the central nervous system less well, central nervous system side effects (sedation, depression, hallucinations) are well described with the hydrophilic as well as with the lipophilic agents.

Some beta-adrenergic blocking agents possess beta-agonist activity. This has been referred to as "intrinsic sympathomimetic activity" (or ISA). Agents with partial agonist activity (pindolol, alprenolol, acebutolol, carteolol, oxprenolol) cause little or no depression of resting heart rate (partial agonist effect) while blocking the increase in heart rate that occurs in response to exercise or the administration of a beta agonist such as isoproterenol. The presence of partial agonist activity may be useful when bradycardia limits treatment in patients with slow resting heart rates. Although theoretically attractive in patients with depressed left ventricular function and reactive airways, no decisive advantage of these agents over beta blockers without partial agonist activity has been demonstrated under these circumstances. Pindolol also produces mild vasodilation, perhaps in part related to peripheral beta$_2$ stimulation. Agents with partial agonist activity appear to cause less change in blood lipid levels than agents without agonist properties. On theoretical grounds, intrinsic sympathomimetic activity would be undesirable in the treatment of thyrotoxicosis, idiopathic hypertrophic subaortic stenosis, aortic dissection, and tachyarrhythmias.

CARDIOSELECTIVE (BETA$_1$) ADRENERGIC RECEPTOR BLOCKING AGENTS   Propranolol, the prototype of the nonselective beta-adrenergic blocking agent, induces a competitive blockade of both beta$_1$ and beta$_2$ receptors. Other nonselective beta blocking agents include alprenolol, carteolol, nadolol, oxprenolol, penbutolol, pindolol, sotalol, and timolol. Metoprolol, acebutolol, atenolol, and betaxolol possess relative selectivity for the beta$_1$ receptor. Although beta$_1$-selective agents have the theoretical advantage of producing less bronchoconstriction and less peripheral vasoconstriction, a clear-cut clinical advantage of the cardioselective agents has not been demonstrated, since the beta$_1$ selectivity is only relative. Bronchoconstriction may occur when beta$_1$-selective agents are administered in full therapeutic doses.

ADVERSE EFFECTS OF BETA-RECEPTOR BLOCKING AGENTS   Aside from the effects on the central nervous system, most adverse reactions to beta blocking agents are consequences of beta-adrenergic blockade. These include the precipitation of heart failure in patients in whom cardiac compensation depends on enhanced sympathetic drive; the aggravation of bronchospasm in patients with asthma; predisposition to the development of hypoglycemia in insulin-requiring diabetics (blockade of catecholamine-mediated counterregulation and antagonism of the adrenergic warning signs of hypoglycemia); the development of hyperkalemia in diabetic or uremic patients with impaired potassium tolerance; the enhancement of coronary or peripheral arterial vasospasm; and elevation in triglycerides and depression of high-density lipoprotein (HDL) levels. The lipid effects are less (or absent) in agents with partial agonist activity.

MISCELLANEOUS ADRENERGIC BLOCKING AGENTS   *Labetalol*, approved for use in the United States as an antihypertensive agent, is a competitive antagonist of both alpha- and beta-adrenergic receptors. Although labetalol induces relatively more beta- than alpha-receptor blockade, fall in peripheral resistance may be marked following acute administration of the drug. Vasodilation may be mediated in part by a partial agonist effect on the beta$_2$-adrenergic receptor; labetalol does not possess partial agonist activity for the beta$_1$ (cardiac) receptor.

Metoclopramide is a dopaminergic antagonist with cholinergic agonist properties. It enhances gastric emptying, increases the tone of the lower esophageal sphincter, increases prolactin and aldosterone secretion, and antagonizes emesis induced by apomorphine. It is useful clinically in enhancing gastric emptying (in the absence of organic obstruction such as in diabetic gastroparesis), in antagonizing gastroesophageal reflux, and as an antiemetic during cancer chemotherapy.

THE PARASYMPATHETIC NERVOUS SYSTEM

ACETYLCHOLINE   Acetylcholine (ACh) serves as the neurotransmitter at all autonomic ganglia, at the postganglionic parasympathetic nerve endings, at the postganglionic sympathetic nerve endings innervating the eccrine sweat glands, and at the skeletal muscle end plate (neuromuscular junction). The enzyme choline acetyltransferase catalyzes the synthesis of ACh from acetyl CoA produced within the nerve ending and from choline, actively taken up from the extracellular fluid. Within the cholinergic nerve endings ACh is stored in discrete synaptic vesicles and released in response to nerve impulses that depolarize the nerve terminals and increase calcium influx.

Cholinergic receptors   Different receptors for ACh exist on the postganglionic neurons within the autonomic ganglia and at the postjunctional autonomic effector sites. Those within the autonomic ganglia and adrenal medulla are stimulated predominantly by nicotine (*nicotinic receptors*) and those on autonomic effector cells by the alkaloid muscarine (*muscarinic receptors*). Ganglionic blocking agents antagonize the nicotinic receptors, while atropine blocks the muscarinic receptors. The muscarinic (M) receptor, furthermore, has been recently subdivided into additional types. The M-1 receptor is localized to the central nervous system and perhaps parasympathetic ganglia; the M-2 receptor is the nonneuronal muscarinic receptor on smooth muscle, cardiac muscle, and glandular epithelium. Bethanechol is a selective agonist of the M-2 receptor; pirenzepine, an investigational agent, is a selective antagonist of the M-1 receptor. This agent markedly reduces gastric acid secretion. The M-2 receptor inhibits adenylyl cyclase and utilizes the regulatory G_i protein; the M-1 receptor interacts with G_p and stimulates phospholipase C (Fig. 68-5). The M-3 receptor, present on smooth muscle and secretory glands, is antagonized by atropine and utilizes phospholipase C, IP_3, and DAG as second messengers. Other subtypes have been identified by molecular biologic techniques but have not yet been fully characterized.

Acetylcholinesterase   Hydrolysis of ACh by acetylcholinesterase inactivates the neurotransmitter at cholinergic synapses. This enzyme (also known as specific or true cholinesterase) is present within neurons and is distinct from butyrocholinesterase (serum cholinesterase or pseudocholinesterase). The latter enzyme is present in plasma and nonneuronal tissues and is not primarily involved in the termination of the effects of ACh at autonomic effector sites. The pharmacologic effects of anticholinesterase agents are due to inhibition of neuronal (true) acetylcholinesterase.

PHYSIOLOGY OF THE PARASYMPATHETIC NERVOUS SYSTEM

The parasympathetic nervous system participates in the regulation of the cardiovascular system, the gastrointestinal tract, and the genitourinary system. Tissues such as liver, kidney, pancreas, and thyroid also receive parasympathetic innervation, suggesting a role for the parasympathetic nervous system in metabolic regulation as well, although cholinergic effects on metabolism are not well characterized.

Cardiovascular system   Parasympathetic effects on the heart are mediated by the vagus nerve. ACh reduces the rate of spontaneous depolarization of the sinoatrial node and decreases heart rate. The heart rate in different physiologic states is the result of coordinated interaction between sympathetic stimulation, parasympathetic inhibition, and the intrinsic activity of the sinoatrial pacemaker. ACh also delays impulse conduction within the atrial musculature while shortening the effective refractory period, a combination of factors which may initiate or perpetuate atrial arrhythmias. At the atrioventricular node, ACh reduces conduction velocity, increases the effective refractory period, and thus diminishes the ventricular response during atrial flutter or fibrillation (Chap. 198). The decrease in inotropy induced by ACh is related to a prejunctional inhibitory effect on sympathetic nerve endings as well as to a direct inhibitory effect on the atrial myocardium. The ventricular myocardium is not much affected since innervation by cholinergic fibers is minimal. A direct cholinergic contribution to the regulation of peripheral resistance appears unlikely since parasympathetic innervation of the vasculature is not extensive. The parasympathetic nervous system, however, may influence peripheral resistance indirectly by inhibiting NE release from sympathetic nerves.

Gastrointestinal tract   Parasympathetic innervation of the gut is via the vagus nerve and the pelvic sacral nerves. The parasympathetic nervous system increases the tone of gastrointestinal smooth muscle, enhances peristaltic activity, and relaxes the gastrointestinal sphincters. ACh stimulates exocrine secretion from the glandular epithelium and enhances the secretion of gastrin, secretin, and insulin.

Genitourinary and respiratory systems   Sacral parasympathetic nerves supply the urinary bladder and genitalia. ACh increases ureteral peristalsis, contracts the urinary detrusor muscle, and relaxes the trigone and sphincter, thereby playing a critical role in the coordination of urination. The respiratory tract is innervated with parasympathetic fibers derived from the vagus nerve. ACh increases tracheobronchial secretions and stimulates bronchial constriction.

PHARMACOLOGY OF THE PARASYMPATHETIC NERVOUS SYSTEM   Cholinergic agonists

ACh itself has no therapeutic role because of its widespread effects and short duration of action. Congeners of ACh are less susceptible to hydrolysis by cholinesterase and have a narrower range of physiologic effects. Bethanechol, the only systemic cholinergic agonist in general use, stimulates gastrointestinal and genitourinary smooth muscle with minimal effect on the cardiovascular system. It is used in the treatment of urinary retention in the absence of outflow tract obstruction and, less commonly, in gastrointestinal disorders such as postvagotomy gastric atony. Pilocarpine and carbachol are topical cholinergic agonists used in the treatment of glaucoma.

Acetylcholinesterase inhibitors   Cholinesterase inhibitors enhance the effects of parasympathetic stimulation by diminishing the inactivation of ACh. The therapeutic application of reversible cholinesterase inhibitors depends on the role of ACh as neurotransmitter at the skeletal muscle neuroeffector junction and within the central nervous system and includes the treatment of myasthenia gravis (Chap. 386), the termination of neuromuscular blockade following general anesthesia, and the reversal of intoxication by agents with a central anticholinergic action. Physostigmine, a tertiary amine, penetrates the central nervous system well, while related quaternary amines (neostigmine, pyridostigmine, ambenonium, and edropho-

nium) do not. Organophosphorous cholinesterase inhibitors produce irreversible cholinesterase blockade; these agents are used principally as insecticides and are primarily of toxicologic interest. With regard to the autonomic nervous system, cholinesterase inhibitors are of limited use in the treatment of intestinal and bladder smooth-muscle dysfunction such as occurs in paralytic ileus and atonic urinary bladder. Cholinesterase inhibitors induce a vagotonic response in the heart and may be useful in terminating attacks of paroxysmal supraventricular tachycardia (Chap. 198).

Cholinergic-receptor blocking agents   Atropine blocks muscarinic cholinergic receptors, with little effect on cholinergic transmission at the autonomic ganglia and the neuromuscular junctions. Many of the central nervous system actions of atropine and atropine-like drugs are attributable to blockade of central muscarinic synapses. The related alkaloid, *scopolamine*, is similar to atropine but causes drowsiness, euphoria, and amnesia, effects that make it suitable as a preanesthetic medication.

Atropine increases heart rate and enhances atrioventricular conduction, actions that may be useful in combating the bradycardia or heart block associated with heightened vagal tone. In addition, atropine reverses cholinergically mediated bronchoconstriction and diminishes respiratory tract secretions. These effects contribute to its utility as a preanesthetic medication.

Atropine also decreases gastrointestinal tract motility and secretion. Although various derivatives and congeners of atropine (such as *propantheline, isopropamide,* and *glycopyrrolate*) have been advocated in patients with peptic ulcer or with diarrheal syndromes, the chronic use of such agents is limited by other manifestations of parasympathetic inhibition such as dry mouth and urinary retention. The investigational selective M-1 inhibitor pirenzepine inhibits gastric secretion at doses that have minimal anticholinergic effects at other sites; this agent may be useful in the treatment of peptic ulcer. Atropine and its congener *ipratropium*, when given by inhalation, cause bronchodilation and have been used experimentally in the treatment of asthma.

REFERENCES

CARON MG, LEFKOWITZ RJ: Catecholamine receptors: Structure, function and regulation. Recent Prog Horm Res 48:277, 1993

CHALMERS J, PILOWSKY P: Brainstem and bulbospinal neurotransmitter systems in the control of blood pressure. J Hypertens 9:675, 1991

ESLER M et al: Overflow of catecholamine neurotransmitters to the circulation: Source, fate, and functions. Physiol Rev 70:963, 1990

HADCOCK JR, MALBON CC: Agonist regulation of gene expression of adrenergic receptors and G proteins. J Neurochem 60:1, 1993

HOLLENBERG MD: Structure-activity relationships for transmembrane signaling: The receptor's turn. FASEB J 5:178, 1991

KUPFERMANN I: Functional studies of cotransmission. Physiol Rev 71(3):683, 1991

LANDSBERG L, YOUNG JB: Catecholamines and the adrenal medulla, in *Williams' Textbook of Endocrinology*, 8th ed, DW Foster, JD Wilson (eds). Philadelphia, Saunders, 1992, p 621

————, ————: The influence of diet on the sympathetic nervous system, in *Neuroendocrine Perspective*, vol 4, EE Muller et al (eds). Amsterdam, Elsevier, 1985, p 191

LOKHANDWALA MF, AMENTA F: Anatomical distribution and function of dopamine receptors in the kidney. FASEB J 5:3023, 1991

LOW PA: Autonomic nervous system function. J Clin Neurophysiol 10:14, 1993

MEISTER B, APERIA A: Molecular mechanisms involved in catecholamine regulation of sodium transport. Semin Nephrol 13:41, 1993

PACHOLCZYK T et al: Expression cloning of a cocaine- and antidepressant-sensitive human noradrenaline transporter. Nature 350:350, 1991

RUFFOLO RR et al: Structure and function of α-adrenoceptors. *Pharmacol Rev* 43:475, 1991

SCHONDORF R: New investigations of autonomic nervous system function. J Clin Neurophysiol 10:28, 1993

WILLIAMS JL et al: Area postrema: A unique regulator of cardiovascular function. NIPS 7:30, 1992

69 G PROTEINS AND THE REGULATION OF SECOND MESSENGER SYSTEMS

MICHAEL FREISSMUTH / ALFRED G. GILMAN

Hormones, neurotransmitters, growth factors, and autacoids (local regulators such as histamine and adenosine) interact with specific receptors to produce biologic effects. These receptors are classified into distinct categories, based on structural homologies and on similarities in their mechanism of action. For example, the receptors for insulin and certain growth factors (e.g., platelet-derived growth factor) are membrane-bound tyrosine protein kinases, and this enzymatic activity is essential for their function (see Chap. 337). The binding site for ANF (atrial natriuretic factor; see Chap. 187) is in the extracellular domain of a guanylate cyclase that spans the plasma membrane; the intracellular portion of this protein synthesizes a second messenger, guanosine-3′,5′-monophosphate (cyclic GMP). Steroid hormones and triiodothyronine form hormone-receptor complexes that act as regulators of gene transcription (see Chap. 329). Yet another class of receptors, exemplified by the nicotinic cholinergic receptor, acts as ligand-gated ion channels. Lastly, a large family of plasma membrane–bound receptors (the known number exceeds 100) activates heterotrimeric guanosine triphosphate–binding (GTP-binding) regulatory proteins, or *G proteins*, in the plasma membranes of cells. Each G protein, in turn, controls the activity of one or more membrane-bound effectors, such as adenylate cyclase, ion channels, and phospholipases (Table 69-1).

G PROTEIN–LINKED RECEPTORS A diverse group of ligands interacts with G protein–linked receptors. These include peptide hormones (e.g., glucagon, ACTH), lipids (prostaglandins), nucleosides and nucleotides (adenosine, ATP), and amines (epinephrine, histamine). Nevertheless, almost all such receptors possess common structural features—including the topology of the proteins with respect to the plasma membrane (Fig. 69-1). The amino terminus of each receptor is outside the cell and is modified with *N*-linked oligosaccharides. The carboxyl terminus is intracellular and contains sites that can be phosphorylated and that play a crucial role in desensitization to hormone actions. The central portion of the receptor molecule is believed to fold into seven α helices that span the membrane bilayer and form the hydrophobic core of the receptor. The ligand-binding site lies within this hydrophobic core and is formed by reactive side chains that are contributed by more than one transmembrane helix. Portions of the intracellular loops that connect the individual membrane-spanning α helices form the sites of interaction between the ligand-bound receptor and the appropriate G protein.

G PROTEINS AND THEIR EFFECTORS G proteins are composed of three different subunits designated α, β, and γ in order of decreasing mass. A few of the distinctive properties of individual G protein subunits are summarized in Table 69-1.

G protein α subunit G proteins are classified on the basis of the α subunit. The hormone-sensitive adenylate cyclase system and the retinal cyclic GMP phosphodiesterase that participates in vision have served as models for the elucidation of the mechanisms of G protein–mediated transmembrane signaling. In both cases, the α subunit of the G protein interacts with and regulates the effector. The α subunits bind Mg^{2+} and guanine nucleotide (GTP or GDP) with high affinity and also possess GTPase activity that is essential for deactivation of the pathway. In addition, many G protein α subunits are substrates for bacterial toxins that catalyze the incorporation of an ADP-ribosyl moiety into the polypeptide at specific amino acid residues. G_s (the G protein that activates adenylate cyclase) and G_t (the major retinal G protein that activates the cyclic GMP phosphodiesterase) are substrates for cholera toxin; G_s in intestinal cells is the natural target for the toxin, since cholera is an intraluminal infection. The

incorporation of ADP-ribose into G_s causes its persistent activation, and this is the crucial reaction in the pathogenesis of cholera. The various isoforms of G_i, G_o, and G_t are ADP-ribosylated by pertussis toxin, and this modification blocks the ability of the G protein to interact with receptors. The precise role of ADP-ribosylation in the pathogenesis of whooping cough is not clear.

G_s ALPHA SUBUNIT Apparently all molecular species of $G_{s\alpha}$ can activate each of the several isoforms of adenylate cyclase. $G_{s\alpha}$ also activates dihydropyridine-sensitive (L-type) Ca^{2+} channels in skeletal and cardiac muscle and inhibits cardiac Na^+ channels. The fact that a single G protein α subunit can interact with more than one effector is an important general point. Not only can G proteins integrate the input from several receptors, they also represent a branch point for regulation of multiple effectors in response to a single signal. In the olfactory neuroepithelium, G_{olf}, a specialized form of G_s, couples receptors for odorants to activation of adenylate cyclase.

G_i AND G_o ALPHA SUBUNITS The G_i family consists of oligomers with at least three closely related α subunits, designated $G_{i\alpha1}$, $G_{i\alpha2}$, and $G_{i\alpha3}$; they are products of distinct genes and are broadly expressed in many cell types. Two splice variants of $G_{o\alpha}$ are closely related to the $G_{i\alpha}$ proteins and are expressed in neurons and neuroendocrine cells. The G_i proteins were discovered as mediators of hormonal inhibition of adenylate cyclase, although the mechanism of this effect is still not clear (see "Mechanism," below). The G_i proteins can

TABLE 69-1 Properties of G protein subunits

Families of subunits	Subunit	Toxin	Role
$G_{s\alpha}$ ($M_r \approx 45,000$)	α_s ($\times 4$)	Cholera toxin	Activates adenylate cyclase and L-type calcium channels; inhibit cardiac Na^+ channels
	$\alpha_{s,olf}$	Cholera toxin	Activates olfactory adenylate cyclase
$G_{i\alpha}/G_{o\alpha}$ ($M_r \approx 40,000$)	α_i ($\times 3$)	Pertussis toxin	Inhibit adenylate cyclase (indirectly?); stimulate K^+ channels; inhibit neuronal Ca^{2+} channels
	α_o ($\times 2$)	Pertussis toxin	Regulates neuronal Ca^{2+} and K^+ channels; implicated in pertussis toxin–sensitive activation of phospholipase C
	α_z	None known	Unknown; structurally related to $G_{i\alpha}/G_{o\alpha}$
Transducins ($G_{t\alpha}$'s) ($M_r \approx 40,000$)	$\alpha_{t,r}$	Pertussis toxin, cholera toxin	Activate cyclic GMP phosphodiesterase in retinal rods
	$\alpha_{t,c}$	Pertussis toxin, cholera toxin	Activate cyclic GMP phosphodiesterase in retinal cones
	α_g	Pertussis toxin (?), cholera toxin (?)	Hypothesized to activate cyclic AMP phosphodiesterase in taste buds (gustducin)
$G_{q\alpha}$ ($M_r \approx 42,000$)	α_q, α_{11}	None known	Activate phospholipase C
	α_{14}, α_{15}, α_{16}	None known	
$G_{\alpha12}$ ($M_r \approx 42,000$)	α_{12}, α_{13}	None known	Unknown
βγ-complex (β: $M_r \approx 37,000$); γ: $M_r \approx 8000$–10,000):	β ($\times 5$) γ ($> \times 7$?)	— —	βγ required for interaction with receptor; direct regulation of effectors; modulation of effector response to G_α

FIGURE 69-1 Schematic representation of the topology of a G protein–coupled receptor. The barrels represent membrane-spanning α helices. The ligand-binding site of the receptor is located within the core formed by these membrane-spanning segments.

activate K$^+$ channels in atrial myocardial cells. Stimulation of this pathway by muscarinic cholinergic agonists hyperpolarizes the cell and results in both negative chronotropic and inotropic responses. In the central nervous system, G$_o$ and the G$_i$ family apparently couple a variety of receptors to Ca^{2+} channels; G$_o$ also can modulate K$^+$ currents in brain cells. The resulting ion fluxes mediate the actions of myriad neurotransmitters. Regulation of ion channels by G proteins results largely from direct interaction between the G protein α subunit and the channel-forming protein(s). Thus the structure of adenylate cyclase resembles that of an ion channel, and some adenylate cyclases serve a dual role, as both channel and enzyme.

G$_t$ AND G$_g$ ALPHA SUBUNITS   The retinal G proteins, G$_t$'s or *transducins*, play a pivotal role in vision. The photon receptor, *rhodopsin*, is localized in membranous disks in the outer segments of retinal rod cells; analogous color receptors are present in the cones. These molecules resemble the other G protein–linked receptors. Upon activation by light, rhodopsin interacts with and activates G$_t$; G$_t$ in turn activates a cyclic GMP–specific phosphodiesterase. Intracellular concentrations of cyclic GMP fall rapidly, resulting in the closing of Na$^+$ channels and hyperpolarization of the rod cells. This represents the initial electrical signal that is eventually transmitted to the visual cortex. Retinal rods and cones differ not only in their individual photon receptors; they also have distinct G$_t$ molecules (G$_{t,r}$ and G$_{t,c}$) and distinct cyclic GMP phosphodiesterases.

G$_g$, or *gusducin*, the gustatory homologue of the transducins, is expressed exclusively in taste buds. Because of its close structural relationship to the transducins, it too is presumed to regulate a cyclic nucleotide phosphodiesterase.

G$_q$ ALPHA SUBUNIT   The G$_q$ α subunit and its homologues (α$_{11}$, α$_{14}$, α$_{15}$, and α$_{16}$) constitute a related group of proteins that are not substrates for pertussis toxin and are candidates for regulation of signaling pathways that cannot be disrupted by this toxin. In most cells, agonist-mediated, GTP-dependent activation of phospholipase C is not blocked by pertussis toxin, and, indeed, G$_q$ and at least some of its homologues interact with and activate the β1-isoform of phospholipase C.

G protein βγ-subunit complex   The β and γ subunits form a tightly associated complex, and the proteins have not been resolved in their active forms. The βγ-subunit complex contributes to the receptor recognition site on the G protein oligomer and facilitates the attachment of the oligomer to the inner face of the plasma membrane (with the help of a lipid modification—a C-20 prenyl group—attached to γ). The βγ complex is believed to deactivate the α subunit by

formation of the intact G protein. In addition, free βγ also can interact with and regulate the activity of effectors such as adenylate cyclase or phospholipase C, either by itself or in concert with regulators such as G protein α subunits or calmodulin.

At least five genes encode closely related but distinct β subunits, while the number of different forms of γ is at least seven. The functional implications of this heterogeneity are discussed below.

MECHANISM OF G PROTEIN–MEDIATED SIGNAL TRANSDUCTION   A widely accepted model of the mechanism of G protein–mediated signal transduction is shown schematically in Fig. 69-2. The central thesis is that the G protein α subunit cycles between an inactive, GDP-liganded oligomeric form and an active, GTP-liganded monomeric state. *These two forms of the α subunit represent the "off" and "on" positions of a molecular switch.* The dissociation of GDP from α is the rate-limiting step. That is, the slow rate of spontaneous dissociation of GDP from α holds the switch in the off position. Interaction of the G protein with an agonist-receptor complex (H·R) facilitates dissociation of GDP. Binding of GTP to this ternary complex of hormone, receptor, and G protein has two consequences. First, the affinity of the receptor for the agonist is lowered, resulting in dissociation of the ternary complex. The receptor is thus free to recycle and activate additional G protein molecules, as long as agonist is present. As a result, considerable amplification occurs at this step. Second, the α subunit is activated by its dissociation from the βγ complex. The switch is now on, and the activated α subunit interacts with the appropriate effector and modulates its activity. The G protein switch is programmed to turn itself off automatically, since deactivation results from hydrolysis of bound GTP by the α subunit. However, the lifetime of the activated α subunit is relatively long (several seconds), since the intrinsic rate of hydrolysis of GTP is slow; this kinetic feature permits additional signal amplification. To complete the cycle, the GDP-bound α subunit associates with βγ, and the system relaxes to its basal state. As mentioned above, the free βγ subunit may itself regulate effectors directly.

Inhibition of adenylate cyclase may be due in part to the capacity of the βγ subunit, released on activation of G$_i$, to interact with and deactivate G$_s$; βγ can thus inhibit adenylate cyclase indirectly. This subunit exchange hypothesis predicts that the activation of one pathway can cause inhibition of effectors that are controlled by other G protein α subunits if the concentration of appropriate forms of βγ in the membrane is raised sufficiently.

Molecular heterogeneity   As the number of identified G protein subunits increases, the task of unraveling the complexity of the G protein–regulated cellular switchboard also expands. The known number of α, β, and γ subunits indicates roughly 1000 possible combinations; this number may get much larger. Furthermore, an individual cell must sort through a vast number of choices to complete its own customized G protein–controlled regulatory network. Additional complexity at each step in the signal transduction cascade compounds the problem. There is divergence and convergence of protein-protein interactions at both the receptor G protein level and the G protein effector level, and α and βγ subunits presumably interact to dictate the specificities of these choices and to control, synergistically or in opposition, the activities of effectors. Thus activation of a given receptor in different cells can produce a varied constellation of activated G proteins and effectors, and cellular responses will change with development or with exposure to regulatory signals. Such enormous "combinatorial power" endows cells and organisms with extraordinary capacity for fine-tuning both the magnitude and the nature of their responses to the environment.

SECOND MESSENGER SYSTEMS UNDER THE CONTROL OF G PROTEINS (Fig. 69-3)   **Cyclic AMP**   The conversion of ATP to cyclic AMP is accomplished by various isoforms of the enzyme adenylate cyclase. These membrane-bound proteins are believed to span the plasma membrane several times; their topology resembles that usually found in transporters and channels.

Cyclic AMP acts as a second messenger for a number of hormones. The primary mechanism of action of the cyclic nucleotide is to cause

1. Basal State

2. Receptor Activation

5. GTPase

3. Subunit Dissociation

4. Effector Activation

FIGURE 69-2 G protein–mediated transmembrane signaling. In the basal state **(step 1)**, G proteins exist as heterotrimers with GDP bound tightly to the α subunit; the hormone receptor (R) is unoccupied, and the effector (E) is inactive. Upon hormone binding and receptor activation **(step 2)**, receptor interacts with the heterotrimer to promote a conformational change and dissociation of GDP from the guanine nucleotide binding site; at normal cellular concentrations of guanine nucleotides, GTP fills the site immediately. Binding of GTP to α induces a conformational change with two consequences **(step 3)**. The G protein dissociates from the H·R complex, reducing the affinity of hormone for receptor and, in turn, freeing the receptor for another liaison with a neighboring quiescent G protein. GTP binding also reduces the affinity of α for βγ, and subunit dissociation occurs. This frees α·GTP to fulfill its primary role as a regulator of effectors **(step 4)**. At least in some systems, the free βγ subunit complex may also interact directly with an effector (E_1) and modulate the activity of the active complex, or it may act independently at a distinct effector (E_2). α subunits possess an intrinsic GTPase activity **(step 5)**. The rate of this GTPase determines the lifetime of the active species and the associated physiologic response. α-catalyzed hydrolysis of GTP leaves GDP in the binding site and causes dissociation and deactivation of the active complex. The GTPase activity of α is, in essence, an internal clock that controls an on/off switch. The GDP bound form of α has high affinity for βγ; subsequent reassociation of α·GDP with βγ returns the system to the basal state **(step 1)**.

dissociation of a dimer of cyclic AMP–binding regulatory subunits from the catalytic subunits of a protein kinase. The free catalytic subunits of the protein kinase are enzymatically active, and they transfer the γ phosphate from ATP to serine and threonine residues in target proteins. Such phosphorylation can either increase the activity (e.g., glycogen phosphorylase kinase, triacylglycerol lipase, protein phosphatase inhibitor 1) or decrease the activity (e.g., glycogen synthase, myosin light chain kinase) of the various substrates.

Termination of cyclic AMP action is accomplished by several mechanisms that are themselves subject to regulation by cyclic AMP and Ca^{2+}-calmodulin, a molecule with related second messenger functions (see below). Cyclic AMP is degraded to 5′-AMP by cyclic nucleotide phosphodiesterases. Some of these isoenzymes are activated by Ca^{2+}-calmodulin; they are inhibited by several drugs, including the methylxanthines (caffeine and theophylline) and milrinone. In addition, most cells possess a mechanism for the facilitated extrusion of cyclic AMP.

The regulatory effects of protein kinases are reversed by phosphoprotein phosphatases, which hydrolytically cleave the phosphate ester bond. These enzymes differ in their substrate specificities and in their regulation. For example, in the presence of elevated concentrations of cyclic AMP, protein phosphatase inhibitor 1 is phosphorylated by the cyclic AMP–dependent protein kinases; in this phosphorylated form, the inhibitor suppresses the activity of protein phosphatase 1. By contrast, protein phosphatase 2B is activated by Ca^{2+}-calmodulin. This network of stimulatory and inhibitory mechanisms integrates input from additional second messenger systems, which is necessary for efficient fine-tuning of cellular activities. All intracellular effects of cyclic AMP were initially believed to result from activation of protein phosphorylation, but ionic (Na^+) channels in olfactory neuroepithelial cells can be regulated (gated) directly by cyclic AMP.

Inositol trisphosphate, diacylglycerol, and calcium Inositol-1,4,5-trisphosphate (IP_3) and diacylglycerol are second messengers generated by activation of a family of phosphoinositidases, commonly

termed *phospholipase C*. These enzymes use phosphatidylinositol-4,5-bisphosphate, a minor phospholipid component of the plasma membrane, as substrate. A large number of hormones and related molecules are known to activate phospholipase. Whereas the γ-isoform of phospholipase C is phosphorylated and activated by receptors belonging to the tyrosine kinase family, the β1-isoform is stimulated by G_q and related G protein α subunits in most cells. However, in certain cells (e.g., granulocytes and mast cells) agonist-mediated, GTP-dependent activation of phospholipase C is blocked by pertussis toxin, presumably indicating a role for G_i or G_o (either their α or βγ subunits).

Inositol trisphosphate releases Ca^{2+} from intracellular stores (endoplasmic/sarcoplasmic reticulum) and promotes Ca^{2+} influx from the extracellular fluid. Additional mechanisms for entry of Ca^{2+} into the cytosolic compartment include voltage-gated Ca^{2+} channels and exchange mechanisms activated by other ions. G proteins regulate the activity of some of these channels and exchangers.

Ca^{2+} both regulates the activity of target enzymes directly and, more important, exerts its second messenger functions by interactions with Ca^{2+}-binding proteins such as troponin C and calmodulin. Calmodulin is a ubiquitous intracellular protein that binds four molecules of Ca^{2+}. This Ca^{2+}-calmodulin complex regulates several enzymes of the cyclic AMP system, including at least one type of adenylate cyclase, certain cyclic nucleotide phosphodiesterases, and protein phosphatase 2B (calcineurin). Several protein kinases are also activated by Ca^{2+}-calmodulin; the resulting effect can be either synergistic with (e.g., activation of phosphorylase kinase) or antagonistic to (e.g., activation of myosin light chain kinase) the cyclic AMP–mediated action. The effects of Ca^{2+}-calmodulin on its target enzymes can be blocked by certain phenothiazine drugs. The relationship between this effect and the therapeutic efficacy or toxicity of these drugs is unknown.

Deactivation of the pathway is achieved by active transport of Ca^{2+} into intracellular compartments and extrusion of the ion by

FIGURE 69-3   The role of G proteins in transmembrane signaling. The top panel shows G protein–regulated channels and adenylate cyclase. The bottom panel depicts pathways that involve activation of phospholipases.

AA = arachidonic acid
AC = adenylate cyclase
Ca²⁺/Cam PKC = calcium-calmodulin-dependent protein kinase
Cam = calmodulin
CH = channel
DG = diacylglycerol
E.R./S.R. = endoplasmic/sarcoplasmic reticulum
G = G protein
12-HETE = 12-hydroxyeicosatetraenoic acid
15-HETE = 15-hydroxyeicosatetraenoic acid
IP₃ = inositol trisphosphate
LL = lysophospholipid
LT = leukotriene
PDE = cyclic nucleotide phosphodiesterase
PG = prostaglandin
PIP₂ = phosphatidylinositol trisphosphate
PLC = phospholipase C
PKA = cyclic AMP–dependent protein kinase
PKC = protein kinase C
R = receptor for hormone or agonist

plasma membrane–bound Ca^{2+}-pumping ATPases. Inositol trisphosphate is degraded by sequential dephosphorylation. The phosphatase that catalyzes the removal of phosphate from inositol-1-phosphate is inhibited by Li^+. This effect of Li^+ may be related to its efficacy in psychiatric disorders.

The second product of the phospholipase C reaction is diacylglycerol, which acts as a second messenger by activating a family of isoenzymes referred to as *protein kinase C*. Upon binding of diacylglycerol, the requirement of these enzymes for Ca^{2+} decreases into the range of free Ca^{2+} concentrations found in cytosol. Activated

protein kinase C phosphorylates many intracellular proteins, including some substrates of cyclic AMP–dependent protein kinase. The phorbol esters, which act as tumor promoters, are structurally related to diacylglycerol and also bind to and activate protein kinase C. This action is believed to explain their carcinogenicity.

The effect of diacylglycerol is terminated by enzymatic recycling to form phosphatidylinositol. Alternatively, diacylglycerol is broken down by a diacylglycerol lipase. Of interest, one of the fatty acids in the diacylglycerol molecule is usually arachidonate, the precursor of prostaglandins, leukotrienes, and other eicosanoids.

Stimulation of phospholipase A₂ and release of arachidonic acid
Release of arachidonate from membrane phospholipids is the rate-limiting step in the biosynthesis of prostaglandins, leukotrienes, and other eicosanoids (see Chap. 70). Free arachidonate can arise by two distinct mechanisms. First, a family of enzymes, termed *phospholipase A₂*, cleaves the ester bond at the 2 position of the glycerol moiety of membrane phospholipids, giving rise to equimolar amounts of arachidonate and lysophospholipids. The enzymes require Ca^{2+} for activity. Second, as mentioned above, free arachidonate can be produced by the sequential action of phospholipase C and diacylglycerol lipase. Thus hormones that stimulate the hydrolysis of phosphatidylinositol-4,5-bisphosphate also cause the release of arachidonate and the subsequent synthesis of eicosanoids. In addition, these hormones increase intracellular concentrations of free Ca^{2+} and stimulate protein kinase C through inositol trisphosphate and diacylglycerol, respectively. Both these effects also may contribute to the generation of free arachidonate via activation of phospholipase A₂. Phospholipase A₂ is activated by Ca^{2+}, and direct stimulation of protein kinase C by phorbol esters promotes release of arachidonate.

In view of the interdigitation of the regulatory mechanisms that control these pathways, it is not surprising that the regulation of phospholipase A₂ by G proteins is poorly understood. However, phospholipase A₂ can be activated independently of concomitant stimulation of phospholipase C.

Most eicosanoids are not second messengers as defined originally, since they produce their biologic effects by interacting with specific cell surface receptors coupled to G proteins. However, some metabolites of the 12-lipoxygenase pathway, in particular HEPETE (8-hydroxy-11,12-epoxy-5,9,14-icosotrienoic acid), may affect neuronal K^+ channels through a direct intracellular mechanism and thus act as typical second messengers.

Stimulation of phospholipase D   Phospholipase D utilizes phosphatidylcholine, another phospholipid component of the plasma membrane, as its preferred substrate and generates choline and phosphatidic acid. Phosphatidic acid may function directly as a second messenger or serve as an alternative source of diacylglycerol. This signaling pathway appears to be under the direct control of unidentified G proteins, both pertussis toxin–insensitive and –sensitive. Phospholipase D is also stimulated by Ca^{2+} and protein kinase C.

REGULATION OF RECEPTOR-EFFECTOR COUPLING   Desensitization   Prolonged exposure of cells to a hormonal stimulus leads to a gradual attenuation of the biologic response, despite the continuing presence of the stimulus; this phenomenon is termed *desensitization*, *refractoriness*, or *tolerance*. Such adaptation is a general biologic mechanism, as exemplified by pharmacodynamic tolerance to massive concentrations of opioids. Desensitization is traditionally divided into two categories. *Homologous* or *receptor-specific desensitization* refers to the refractoriness that develops only to agonists that act on the same receptor as the desensitizing stimulus. In addition, stimulation of a particular receptor by an agonist can lead to the subsequent attenuation of the response to multiple hormones that influence the same pathway through distinct receptors. This phenomenon is termed *heterologous desensitization*.

Beta-adrenergic-receptor–mediated stimulation of adenylate cyclase has served as a model system for elucidation of the molecular events that underlie desensitization, and both homologous and heterologous desensitization appear to result from phosphorylation of the receptor on its carboxyl-terminal domain.

Desensitization is a multistep process which can be considered in three phases: uncoupling (seconds to minutes), sequestration (minutes), and down-regulation (hours). Initially, receptors are uncoupled from G_s, as judged in part by their inability to stimulate adenylate cyclase. This process is reversible upon removal of agonist. Homologous desensitization is mediated by a novel protein kinase termed *beta-adrenergic-receptor kinase* (βARK), which specifically phosphorylates the agonist-bound receptor. Unliganded and antagonist-bound receptors do not serve as substrates. However, βARK also phosphorylates other agonist-bound receptors, including those that mediate inhibition of adenylate cyclase, such as the alpha$_2$-adrenergic and M$_2$-muscarinic receptors.

Heterologous desensitization of receptors that stimulate adenylate cyclase is probably mediated predominantly by a classic negative feedback loop. Activation of cyclic AMP–dependent protein kinase leads to phosphorylation of the receptors in a largely agonist-independent manner, and this modification also interferes with their ability to interact with G_s.

An analogous mechanism of desensitization is observed with receptors that mediate stimulation of phospholipase C (e.g., the alpha$_1$-adrenergic receptor). As a result of release of diacylglycerol, protein kinase C phosphorylates the receptors near the carboxyl terminus and is thereby presumed to interfere with the receptor–G protein interaction.

The mechanisms responsible for sequestration of beta-adrenergic receptors (the rapid removal of receptor into an ill-defined cellular compartment) are not well understood. The sequestered receptors may return to the functionally active pool upon hydrolytic cleavage of the incorporated phosphate by a phosphatase. Long-term exposure of cells to agonists leads to a decline in the number of receptors in the plasma membrane. This down-regulation is not readily reversible, and protein synthesis is required to replenish the receptors on the surface. Down-regulation results from both degradation of phosphorylated receptors and a cyclic AMP–dependent reduction in the steady state level of the mRNA that encodes the protein.

Additional forms of regulation   The steady state concentration of receptors in the plasma membrane represents the balance between synthesis and insertion into the bilayer versus internalization and degradation. As mentioned, the continuous presence of agonist tilts this balance in favor of degradation. Conversely, removal of agonist by pharmacologic blockade of the receptor, denervation of tissue, or extirpation of the source of the agonist favors accumulation of receptors on the cell surface and sensitization of target tissues to the appropriate agonist. Such sensitization may underlie the clinical syndrome associated with abrupt withdrawal of beta-adrenergic blocking agents.

Several other regulatory mechanisms influence signal transduction and thus the sensitivity of target cells to agonists. Since these events are not promoted by the receptor agonist, they are referred to as *heterologous regulation*. The most remarkable examples of heterologous regulation at the clinical level are the alterations in adrenergic receptor-effector coupling produced by thyroid and steroid hormones. Both triiodothyronine and glucocorticoids appear to be necessary to maintain normal coupling between beta-adrenergic receptors and G_s. In addition, thyroid hormones and glucocorticoids can increase transcription of mRNA for beta-adrenergic receptors. As one example, symptoms of increased sympathetic activity in the absence of elevated concentrations of plasma catecholamines are characteristic of hyperthyroidism. Similarly, heterologous regulation may underlie the permissive role of glucocorticoids in neurohormonal control of blood pressure.

ROLE OF G PROTEIN SYSTEMS IN DISEASE   The pivotal role of G proteins in regulatory biology is understood in considerable detail. Comparatively little is known about the degree to which perturbations of these pathways participate in pathophysiology. However, a link to alterations in a G protein–regulated second messenger system has been established in several entities.

Cholera (See also Chap. 120)   Pathogenic strains of *Vibrio cholerae* produce an exotoxin that transfers an ADP-ribosyl moiety to the α subunit of G_s, using intracellular nicotinamide adenine dinucleotide (NAD) as the donor. This reaction can occur in virtually all cells. However, the bacteria remain confined to the intestinal lumen, and the toxin binds to the intestinal epithelium but is not absorbed into the systemic circulation. Cell-surface binding of cholera toxin is dependent on the interaction between the B subunits of the toxin and gangliosides (GM$_1$) on the cell surface. Following such binding, the catalytically active A subunit of the toxin penetrates the cell. The ensuing modification of $G_{s\alpha}$ leads to its persistent activation, and the resultant high intracellular concentrations of cyclic AMP trigger the secretion of water and electrolytes into the intestinal lumen. The resulting watery diarrhea is the hallmark of cholera. Enteropathogenic strains of *Escherichia coli* produce a heat-labile toxin that is quite similar to cholera toxin and causes diarrhea by an identical mechanism (see Chap. 87). By contrast, other strains of *E. coli* cause diarrhea by elaboration of a low-molecular-weight, heat-stable toxin that activates guanylate cyclase. Enzymes capable of removing mono-ADP-ribosyl moieties from cellular proteins have not been detected. Upon removal of the toxin, its effects fade slowly as ADP-ribosylated $G_{s\alpha}$ is gradually replaced by newly synthesized protein. This explains why the symptoms of cholera persist after eradication of the bacteria.

Pertussis (See also Chap. 114)   The molecular pathogenesis of whooping cough and cholera are similar. *Bordetella pertussis* remains confined to the bronchi and produces two exotoxins. The first is commonly referred to as *pertussis toxin* or *islet-activating protein*. Like cholera toxin, this protein is an enzyme that catalyzes the NAD-dependent ADP-ribosylation of proteins; the targets for pertussis toxin are members of the $G_{i\alpha}$ family and $G_{o\alpha}$ (see above). This modification interferes with the ability of these G proteins to interact with receptors; among other effects, cyclic AMP concentrations are thus elevated. Again, restoration of normal G protein function depends on de novo synthesis of the α subunits, explaining in part why the symptoms of pertussis can persist for weeks after eradication of the microorganisms. In contrast to cholera, the sequence of events that links ADP-ribosylation of G protein α subunits to clinical symptoms is not understood. However, *B. pertussis* also interferes with cellular regulation of cyclic AMP concentrations by another mechanism, since the second exotoxin is itself an invasive calmodulin-dependent adenylate cyclase. Elevated concentrations of cyclic AMP in neutrophils impair their ability to kill ingested bacteria. In addition, ADP-ribosylation of G protein α_i subunits (presumably $G_{i\alpha1}$ and $G_{i\alpha2}$) uncouples the neutrophil chemotactic receptor from the pathway that controls superoxide generation and bactericidal activity. This may contribute to the increased susceptibility to pulmonary infection by other pathogens—a frequent complication of whooping cough.

Anthrax (See also Chap. 104)   Cutaneous infection with *Bacillus anthracis* produces a lesion characterized by central necrosis and prominent subcutaneous edema. The edema is due to the presence of a bacterial exotoxin, referred to as *edema factor*. Edema factor is an adenylate cyclase that shares many characteristics with the *B. pertussis* enzyme, including host cell penetration and dependence on calmodulin. Rare patients who ingest *Bacillus* organisms can develop a watery diarrhea indistinguishable from cholera. This syndrome may result from penetration of edema factor into cells of the intestinal mucosa.

Pseudohypoparathyroidism/Albright's hereditary osteodystrophy (See also Chap. 357)   Pseudohypoparathyroidism type I is an inherited disorder characterized by target-organ resistance to parathyroid hormone. In addition, many patients exhibit partial resistance to other hormones that act by stimulation of adenylate cyclase (e.g., thyroid-stimulating hormone, vasopressin, glucagon). In one variant of the disorder (termed *pseudohypoparathyroidism type Ia*), the molecular defect results in reduced cellular concentrations of $G_{s\alpha}$, and this partial deficiency is apparently due to lower cellular levels of the mRNAs that encode the polypeptide. The underlying genetic defect is heterogeneous. Several point mutations in one allele of the $G_{s\alpha}$ gene have been identified in affected kindreds. These result in aberrant splicing of the pre-mRNA, frame shifts, or loss of the codon for the initiating methionine residue. Pseudohypoparathyroidism type Ib is a similar syndrome in which cellular concentrations of $G_{s\alpha}$ are normal.

G proteins as products of oncogenes   G proteins control pathways that are linked to cellular proliferation. Cyclic AMP is a trophic stimulus for endocrine target tissues (pituitary, thyroid, adrenals, gonads); stimulation of G_i-coupled receptors is mitogenic for many cells; tumor-promoting phorbol esters are believed to act via persistent stimulation of protein kinase C, and ectopic expression of receptors coupled to G_q and phospholipase C results in tumor formation. Certain point mutations within the genes that encode G protein α subunits interfere with the GTPase activity of the proteins. Such mutations cause constitutive activation of the pathways that they regulate and act in a dominant fashion. Activating point mutations have been identified in the genes encoding $G_{s\alpha}$ and $G_{i\alpha2}$. About 50 percent of growth hormone–producing pituitary adenomas contain a mutated $G_{s\alpha}$ allele (see Chap. 331); these mutations also occur in thyroid carcinomas and in the neoplastic lesions found in the McCune-Albright syndrome (see Chap. 362). A mutation in the $G_{i\alpha2}$ gene has been found in tumors derived from the adrenal cortex and the ovary. In addition, constitutively active mutant alpha$_2$-adrenergic (G_i-coupled) and alpha$_1$-adrenergic (G_q-coupled) receptors can be produced experimentally; expression of these mutated receptors causes transformation of the transfected cells. Thus alterations at any of several levels of the transmembrane signaling cascade that abolish the abnormal regulatory cycle of activation and deactivation may participate in carcinogenesis.

REFERENCES

DOHLMAN HG et al: Model systems for the study of seven-transmembrane-segment receptors. Annu Rev Biochem 60:653, 1991

GILMAN AG: G proteins and regulation of adenylyl cyclase. JAMA 262:1819, 1989

LYONS J et al: Two G protein oncogenes in human endocrine tumours. Science 249:655, 1990

PATTEN JL et al: Mutations in the gene encoding the stimulatory G protein of adenylate cyclase in Albright's hereditary osteodystrophy. N Engl J Med 322:1412, 1990

SIMON MI et al: Diversity of G proteins in signal transduction. Science 252:802, 1991

WATSON S, ABBOTT A: TIPS receptor nomenclature supplement. Trends Pharmacol Sci 12:S1, 1991

WEINSTEIN LS et al: Activating point mutations of the stimulatory G protein in the McCune-Albright syndrome. N Engl J Med 325:1688, 1991

70   EICOSANOIDS AND HUMAN DISEASE

R. PAUL ROBERTSON

This chapter focuses on the formation and mechanism of action of the physiologically active metabolites of arachidonic acid and on the biologic phenomena in which these compounds may be involved.

FORMATION OF THE EICOSANOIDS   Prostaglandins, the first arachidonic acid metabolites to be recognized, were so named because they were originally identified in seminal fluid and thought to be secreted by the prostate. Subsequently, two major pathways relevant to human disease—the cyclooxygenase and the lipoxygenase pathways—were characterized. These synthetic pathways are summarized schematically in Fig. 70-1, and structures of representative metabolites are shown in Fig. 70-2. All products of both the cyclooxygenase and the lipoxygenase pathways are called *eicosanoids*. The products of the cyclooxygenase pathway—the prostaglandins and the thromboxanes—are termed *prostanoids*.

The initial synthetic step for both pathways involves the cleavage of arachidonic acid from phospholipid in the plasma membrane of cells. Phospholipase A_2 cleaves arachidonic acid from phospholipid. A phospholipase-activating protein termed *PLAP* is present in some cells. Free arachidonic acid also can be derived by phospholipase C cleavage of diacylglycerol from phospholipids and subsequent cleavage of arachidonic acid from diacylglycerol. Free arachidonic acid can then be oxygenated by the cyclooxygenase or lipoxygenase pathway. The first product of the cyclooxygenase pathway is the cyclic endoperoxide prostaglandin G_2 (PGG_2), which is converted to prostaglandin H_2 (PGH_2). PGG_2 and PGH_2 are the key intermediates in the formation of physiologically active prostaglandins (PGD_2, PGE_2, $PGF_{2\alpha}$, and PGI_2) and thromboxane A_2 (TXA_2). Several lipoxygenase pathways, including 5-lipoxygenase and 12-lipoxygenase, are important to human physiology. The first product of the 5-lipoxygenase pathway is 5-hydroperoxyeicosatetraenoic acid (5-HPETE), which is an intermediate in the formation of 5-hydroxyeicosatetraenoic acid (5-HETE), and the leukotrienes (LTA_4, LTB_4, LTC_4, LTD_4, and LTE_4). 5-Lipoxygenase is activated by a membrane protein termed *FLAP*. The subscripts designate the number of double bonds between carbon atoms in the side chains. Arachidonic acid forms prostaglandin products with subscript 2 and leukotrienes with subscript 4. Two fatty acids other than arachidonic acid [3,11,14-eicosatrienoic acid (dihomo-γ-linolenic acid) and 5,8,11,14,17-eicosapentaenoic acid] can be converted to metabolites closely related to these eicosanoids. Prostanoid products of the former substrate carry the subscript 1; the leukotriene subscript is 3. Prostanoid products of the latter substrate have the subscript 3 while leukotrienes have the subscript 5. Omega-3 fatty acids found in fish oils can decrease production of some arachidonate metabolites and increase levels of prostanoids with the subscript 3. Feeding of these fatty acids has been used as a therapeutic strategy to diminish platelet aggregation by decreasing TXA_2 and increasing TXA_3 synthesis by platelets.

Virtually all cells have the necessary substrates and enzymes to form some of the metabolites of arachidonic acid, but tissues differ in enzyme profile and consequently in the products they form. Eicosanoids are synthesized in response to immediate need and are not stored in significant amounts for later release.

The cyclooxygenase products   Prostaglandins D_2, E_2, $F_{2\alpha}$, and I_2 are formed from the cyclic endoperoxides PGG_2 and PGH_2. Of these, PGE_2 and PGI_2 exert the broadest physiologic effects. PGE_2 is synthesized by many tissues. PGI_2 (also called *prostacyclin*) is a dominant product in the endothelial and smooth muscle cells of vessel walls and in some nonvascular tissues. PGI_2 is a vasodilator, a bronchodilator, and an inhibitor of platelet aggregation. PGD_2 is also believed to play a role in platelet aggregation and brain function. $PGF_{2\alpha}$ plays a role in uterine and ovarian function. Both PGD_2 and $PGF_{2\alpha}$ are bronchoconstrictors.

Thromboxane synthetase catalyzes the incorporation of an oxygen atom into the ring of the endoperoxide PGH_2 to form the thromboxanes. TXA_2, which is synthesized by platelets, enhances platelet aggregation, and causes vasoconstriction and bronchodilation.

The lipoxygenase products   The leukotrienes and HETE are the end products of the lipoxygenase pathway. The leukotrienes have histamine-like actions, including enhancement of vascular permeability and induction of bronchospasm, and appear to have mediator activities for leukocytes. On a molar basis, leukotrienes are more potent brochoconstrictors than histamine. LTC_4, LTD_4, and LTE_4 together have been identified as slow-reacting substance of anaphylaxis (SRS-A). (The pathophysiology of the leukotrienes is discussed in detail in Chap. 217.)

EFFECTS OF DRUGS ON THE SYNTHESIS OF EICOSANOIDS
Many drugs block the synthesis of eicosanoids by inhibiting one or more enzymes in the biosynthetic pathways. Glucocorticoids and antimalarial drugs such as mepacrine interfere with the cleavage of arachidonic acid from phospholipids in some cells (Fig. 70-1). Cyclooxygenase is directly inhibited by nonsteroidal anti-inflammatory drugs including salicylates, indomethacin, and ibuprofen. Drugs under development inhibit more distal steps in the cyclooxygenase and lipoxygenase pathways. However, the fact that a drug inhibits

FIGURE 70-1 The overall scheme of arachidonic acid metabolism. The various drugs act at the various enzymatic steps to inhibit the reactions. The major pathways are the cyclooxygenase and the lipoxygenase pathways. PLAP and FLAP are proteins that activate, respectively, cyclooxygenase and 5-lipoxygenase. Phospholipase A_2 is inhibited by glucocorticoids and mepacrine, and cyclooxygenase is inhibited by certain salicylates, indomethacin, and ibuprofen. 5-Lipoxygenase is inhibited by zileuton.

the synthesis of a certain eicosanoid does not necessarily mean that a given effect of the drug is the direct result of a deficiency of that eicosanoid. Most currently available drugs inhibit early reactions in the synthetic pathways and therefore block the formation of more than one product. Additionally, some of the drugs have other effects. For example, indomethacin not only inhibits formation of cyclic endoperoxides by cyclooxygenase but also disrupts calcium flux across membranes, inhibits cyclic adenosine monophosphate (cyclic AMP)–dependent protein kinase and phosphodiesterase, and inhibits one of the enzymes responsible for degradation of PGE_2.

Truly specific synthesis inhibitors and receptor antagonists for individual arachidonic acid metabolites are needed for human use. The lack of such drugs has been a major barrier to elucidating the pathophysiologic roles of these metabolites.

METABOLISM AND ASSAY OF EICOSANOIDS Arachidonic acid metabolites are catabolized rapidly in vivo. Prostaglandins of the E and F series, although chemically stable, are almost completely degraded during a single passage through the liver or the lung. Thus essentially all nonmetabolized PGE_2 measurable in urine is derived from renal and seminal vesicle secretion, whereas PGE_2 metabolites in urine represent total-body PGE_2 synthesis. PGI_2 and TXA_2 are both chemically unstable and also rapidly catabolized. Because PGE_2, PGI_2, and TXA_2 are short-lived in vivo, measurement of their inactive metabolites is commonly used as an index of the rates of their formation. As examples, PGE_2 is converted to 15-keto-13,14,-dihydro-PGE_2, PGI_2 is converted to 6-keto-$PGF_{1\alpha}$, and TXA_2 is converted to TXB_2, and these metabolites can be reliably measured. Six methods are generally available to measure arachidonic acid metabolites in physiologic fluids: bioassay, radioimmunoassay, enzyme immunoassay (ELISA), chromatography, receptor assay, and mass spectrometry. Bioassay provides direct physiologic data but is not very sensitive. Radioimmunoassay is the most convenient and sensitive but, as with bioassay and receptor assay, should be preceded by extraction and chromatography of samples to ensure specificity. ELISA is sensitive and eliminates the need for radioisotopes. Mass spectrometry preceded by chromatography is accurate but laborious. With each method precautions must be taken in handling samples because prostaglandin synthesis may be enhanced during the collection of biologic samples. For example, if blood is allowed to clot or if platelets are not carefully separated from plasma, the generation of large amounts of PGE_2 and TXA_2 during processing can lead to erroneous results. Use of an inhibitor of prostaglandin synthesis in the collection tube diminishes this problem.

PHYSIOLOGY Prostaglandins and leukotrienes have specific receptor sites on the plasma membranes of cells such as liver, corpus luteum, adrenal gland, adipocytes, thymocytes, uterus, pancreatic islets, platelets, and red blood cells. Most of the binding sites exhibit specificity for eicosanoids of a given type. For example, the liver plasma membrane PGE receptor binds PGE_1 and PGE_2 with high affinity but not prostaglandins of the A, F, and I configurations. The postreceptor mechanisms by which the binding of the prostaglandins alters cell function are poorly understood. Some involve modulation of cyclic AMP production through interactions with two G proteins, the stimulatory (G_s) and inhibitory (G_i) subunits of adenylate cyclase (see Chap. 69). The physiologic actions of eicosanoids are not mediated as circulating hormones. Instead, eicosanoids act as local, intercellular, and/or intracellular modulators of biochemical activity in the tissues in which they are formed (e.g., a paracrine function). They are autacoids, not hormones. Most are short-lived in the circulation because of chemical instability and/or rapid degradation.

FIGURE 70-2 Structures of representative biologically active eicosanoids.

Lipolysis PGE_2 and PGI_2 are synthesized by adipose tissue and are potent endogenous regulators of lipolysis. Since the formation of cyclic AMP is necessary in the action of hormones that stimulate lipolysis, the interactions between PGE and adenylate cyclase have been examined in considerable detail. PGE inhibits lipolysis by decreasing the formation of cyclic AMP in response to epinephrine, adrenocorticotropic hormone (ACTH), glucagon, and thyroid-stimulating hormone (TSH). Thus PGE may act as an endogenous antilipolytic substance by interfering with the stimulation of cyclic AMP formation by hormones. During catecholamine-induced lipolysis, coordinate modulation is provided by the antilipolytic action of PGE_2 and the lipolytic action of PGI_2.

Insulin and PGE may act independently during their antilipolytic actions on the adipocyte. For example, insulin but not PGE inhibits the stimulation of lipolysis by exogenous cyclic AMP in isolated adipocytes, but both agents inhibit hormone-stimulated generation of cyclic AMP. This suggests a site of action of insulin distal to the stimulation of adenylate cyclase. In some animals, PGE inhibits glucagon-induced lipolysis whereas insulin does not.

Sodium and water balance The renin-angiotensin-aldosterone system is a major regulator of sodium homeostasis, and vasopressin exerts the principal control over water balance. Arachidonic acid metabolites influence both systems. PGE_2 and PGI_2 stimulate renin secretion, and inhibitors of prostaglandin synthesis have the opposite effect. PGI_2 and PGE_2 decrease renal vascular resistance and increase blood flow. Conversely, inhibitors of prostaglandin synthesis, such as indomethacin and meclofenamate, decrease total renal blood flow, which can lead to acute renal venoconstriction and decreased renal function in circumstances such as volume depletion and edematous states. PGE_2 is natriuretic, whereas cyclooxygenase inhibitors cause sodium and water retention.

Indomethacin also increases sensitivity to exogenous vasopressin in dogs. Conversely, PGE_2 decreases vasopressin-stimulated water transport. Since this effect of PGE_2 is circumvented by the administration of dibutyryl–cyclic AMP, PGE_2 most likely interferes with the stimulation of adenylate cyclase by vasopressin.

Platelet aggregation Platelets synthesize PGE_2 and PGD_2, but TXA_2 is the dominant eicosanoid produced. TXA_2 is a potent stimulator of platelet aggregation; in contrast PGI_2, formed by the endothelial cells of blood vessel walls, is an antagonist of platelet aggregation. TXA_2 and PGI_2 may exert their opposing effects by decreasing and increasing, respectively, platelet generation of cyclic AMP.

Inhibitors of endogenous prostaglandin synthesis interfere with platelet aggregation. For example, a single dose of aspirin can suppress normal platelet aggregation for 48 h and longer, presumably by suppressing cyclooxygenase-mediated TXA_2 synthesis. Cyclooxygenase inhibition by a single dose of aspirin is of longer duration in platelets than in other tissues, because the platelet, in contrast to nucleated cells that can synthesize new proteins, does not have the machinery to form new enzyme. Consequently, the effect of aspirin persists until newly formed platelets are released. Endothelial cells, on the other hand, rapidly recover cyclooxygenase activity following discontinuation of aspirin, and PGI_2 production is thus restored. This is one reason that aspirin therapy does not predispose to formation of excessive platelet thrombi. In addition, the platelet is more sensitive than the endothelial cell to aspirin.

Endothelial damage may lead to platelet aggregation along the blood vessel wall by causing a local decrease in PGI_2 synthesis, thereby allowing unbridled platelet aggregation at the site of vessel wall damage.

Vascular effects The vasoactive properties of arachidonic acid metabolites are among their most impressive actions. PGE_2 and PGI_2 are vasodilators, whereas $PGF_{2\alpha}$, TXA_2, and LTC_4-LTD_4-LTE_4 are vasoconstrictors in most vascular beds. These effects appear to be the result of direct action on the smooth muscle of the vessel wall. Provided that systemic blood pressure is maintained, the vasodilatory arachidonic acid metabolites act to increase blood flow. If blood

pressure falls, however, blood flow decreases because with systemic hypotension catecholamine-induced vasoconstriction offsets the vasodilatory effect of the prostaglandins. Thus significant alterations in systemic blood pressure must be excluded when evaluating the effects of arachidonic acid metabolites on organ blood flow.

Gastrointestinal effects Prostaglandins of the E series influence gastrointestinal function. Infusion of either PGI_2 or PGE_2 into the gastric artery of dogs causes increases in blood flow and inhibition of acid output, and several PGE analogues both inhibit gastric acid output and directly protect the gastrointestinal mucosa when taken orally. In in vitro experiments prostaglandins stimulate gastrointestinal smooth muscle and thereby increase motility, but it is not clear whether these actions are physiologically important. Therapeutically, PGE analogues prevent damage to the stomach and duodenum by aspirin and other NSAIDs.

Neurotransmission PGE inhibits egress of norepinephrine from sympathetic nerve terminals. The effect of PGE on norepinephrine secretion appears to be prejunctional, i.e., at a site on the nerve terminal proximal to the synaptic cleft, and can be reversed by increases in calcium concentration in the perfusing medium. Therefore, PGE_2 may inhibit norepinephrine release by blocking calcium influx.

Catecholamines can release PGE_2 from a variety of tissues, probably by an alpha-adrenergic–mediated mechanism. For example, in innervated tissues such as the spleen, nerve stimulation or injection of norepinephrine causes release of PGE_2. This release is blocked after denervation or administration of alpha-adrenergic blockers. Thus a stimulus that activates the nerve causes release of norepinephrine, which in turn stimulates synthesis and release of PGE_2; PGE_2 then feeds back at the prejunctional level of the nerve terminal to decrease the amount of norepinephrine released.

Pancreatic endocrine function PGE_2 has primarily inhibitory effects on insulin secretion by the pancreatic beta cell in vitro and on insulin response to intravenous glucose. This effect is mediated by G proteins, since it is associated with decreased production of cyclic AMP and is preventable by pertussis toxin, an agent that inhibits G_i and G_o activity. This inhibitory effect appears to be specific for glucose because the insulin responses to other secretagogues are not influenced by PGE_2. Studies with inhibitors of prostaglandin synthesis support the concept that endogenous PGE_2 acts in vivo to inhibit insulin secretion. In general, such drugs augment insulin secretion and improve carbohydrate tolerance. An exception is indomethacin, which inhibits glucose-induced insulin secretion and can cause hyperglycemia. The discordant results with indomethacin are likely due to some action other than inhibition of cyclooxygenase. Aracidonic acid stimulates insulin secretion in vitro, and the lipoxygenase pathway appears to play a role in potentiating insulin secretion by participating in stimulus-secretion coupling. In this case a likely active arachidonic acid product may be 12-HPETE.

Luteolysis In the sheep, hysterectomy during the luteal phase of the ovarian cycle results in maintenance of the corpus luteum, suggesting that the uterus normally produces a luteolytic substance. A candidate for this substance is $PGF_{2\alpha}$, since it can cause luteal regression.

PATHOPHYSIOLOGY Most postulated roles for arachidonic acid metabolites in disease involve excessive production, but a few disorders may be the result of decreased production. The latter could result from dietary deficiency of arachidonic acid (an essential fatty acid), from damage to a tissue where prostaglandin synthesis takes place, or from therapy with drugs that inhibit enzymes in the synthetic pathway.

Bone resorption: Hypercalcemia of malignancy (See also Chaps. 327 and 357) Hypercalcemia occurs in association with nonparathyroid malignancies of many different types. Parathyroid hormone excess, as the result either of autonomous production by parathyroid tissue or ectopic formation by the tumor itself, is a rare cause. Most patients with hypercalcemia of malignancy do not have elevated plasma levels of parathyroid hormone, and secretion of parathyroid hormone–related peptide by tumors is the usual cause (see Chap. 357).

Prostaglandin E_2 is a potent inducer of bone resorption and of calcium release from bone, and PGE_2 production is elevated in certain hypercalcemic animals with transplantable tumors. Treatment of these animals with inhibitors of PGE_2 synthesis causes reduction of PGE_2 levels and a concomitant decrease in hypercalcemia. Likewise, rare patients with hypercalcemia and malignancy have excessive amounts of PGE_2 metabolites in urine. Drugs that inhibit prostaglandin synthesis may decrease circulating calcium levels in such patients. Thus a subset of approximately 5 percent of patients with hypercalcemia of malignancy have elevated PGE production and can be treated with drugs that inhibit prostaglandin synthesis.

The source of the excess PGE_2 in these patients has not been identified. Increased liver and lung degradation of PGE would be expected to compensate if large amounts of PGE were present in the circulation. It is possible, of course, that such large amounts of PGE_2 are released by a tumor into the circulation that liver and lung degradation cannot handle the load. Alternatively, if lung metastases are present, the venous drainage from the tumors could be delivered into the systemic circulation without passing through lung tissue. A third possible mechanism involves metastatic seeding of bone. Tumor cells synthesize PGE in culture, and metastatic tumor cells in bone could synthesize PGE that acts locally to cause bone resorption. Part of this hypothetical mechanism may involve PGE_2 production by circulating white cells which congregate at metastatic sites. Bone-resorbing effects of cytokines (particularly IL-1 and TNF) are mediated in part by local prostaglandin production in bone. Hypercalcemia of malignancy can occur in the absence of demonstrable bone metastases, but the clinical tools for excluding such metastases, such as radioisotope scans and computed tomography, may not be sensitive enough to detect many small lesions.

Bone resorption: Rheumatoid arthritis and dental cysts (See Chap. 285) Overproduction of PGE_2 has been postulated as a cause of the juxtaarticular osteoporosis and bony erosions in some patients with rheumatoid arthritis. Rheumatoid synovia synthesize PGE_2 in tissue culture, and media from these cultures promote bone resorption; moreover, the inclusion of indomethacin in the culture medium blocks this resorptive capacity.

Cells from benign dental cysts also cause bone resorption and synthesize PGE_2 in tissue culture. Again, bone resorption caused by the culture medium from such cells is decreased if indomethacin is added prior to the incubation. A related problem is that of alveolar bone resorption in patients with periodontal disease, a common inflammatory disease of the gums. PGE_2 levels in inflamed gingiva are greater than in healthy gingival tissue. Thus it is possible that alveolar resorption might be due, in part at least, to local overproduction of these metabolites.

Bartter's syndrome (See Chap. 244) Bartter's syndrome is characterized by elevated levels of plasma renin, aldosterone, and bradykinin; resistance to the pressor effect of angiotensin; hypokalemic alkalosis; and renal potassium wasting in the presence of normal blood pressure. A role for prostaglandins has been postulated since PGE_2 and PGI_2 stimulate the release of renin and since the pressor response to infused angiotensin is blunted by the vasodilator effects of PGE_2 and PGI_2. The increase in renin release leads to increased aldosterone secretion, which in turn can increase urinary kallikrein activity.

In keeping with this postulate, elevated levels of PGE_2 and 6-keto-$PGF_{1\alpha}$ are present in urine. Hyperplasia of renal medullary interstitial cells (which synthesize PGE in culture) also occurs. These findings led to therapeutic trials of inhibitors of prostaglandin synthesis in the disorder. Indomethacin (and other inhibitors) reverse virtually all the abnormalities except hypokalemia. Thus a prostaglandin, probably PGE_2 and/or PGI_2, probably mediates some of the manifestations of Bartter's syndrome.

Diabetes mellitus (See Chap. 337) Intravenous administration of glucose to normal individuals causes a sudden (first-phase) increase in secretion of insulin into plasma followed by a slower, more prolonged response termed *second-phase insulin secretion*. Patients with type II (non-insulin-dependent, adult-onset) diabetes mellitus have absent first-phase insulin release in response to glucose and a variable decrease in second-phase insulin secretion. Insulin response to other secretagogues, such as arginine, isoproterenol, glucagon, and secretin, is preserved. Thus diabetics appear to have a specific defect that interferes with normal recognition of glucose signals. Since PGE_2 inhibits glucose-induced insulin secretion in normal individuals, inhibitors of endogenous prostaglandin synthesis have been given to patients with type II diabetes to ascertain whether insulin secretion can be improved. Both sodium salicylate and aspirin elevate basal plasma insulin levels, partially restore the first-phase insulin response, increase second-phase insulin secretion, and improve glucose tolerance. This suggests that the defect in glucose-induced insulin secretion in patients with type II diabetes mellitus may be associated with excessive local production of, or hypersensitivity to, endogenous PGE_2.

Patients with diabetic ketoacidosis have elevated levels of PGE_2 metabolites, and diabetic animals have elevated levels of PGI_2 metabolites. PGE_2 production may be increased to inhibit lipolysis, and both PGE_2 and PGI_2 may play roles in the decreased vascular resistance and hypotension in diabetic ketoacidosis.

Patent ductus arteriosus (See Chap. 199) The ductus arteriosus in sheep is sensitive to the vasodilatory properties of PGE_2, and PGE-like material is present in the ductal wall. Thus enhanced endogenous PGE_2 might maintain prenatal patency of the ductus. Since inhibitors of prostaglandin synthesis cause constriction of the ductus of fetal lambs, trials with indomethacin were undertaken in premature human infants with isolated patent ductus arteriosus. Such treatment for several days is followed by closure of the vessel in the majority, although some require a second course of therapy, and a minority require surgical ligation. Infants under 35 weeks of gestational age are most likely to respond.

Patients with certain types of congenital heart disease require a patent ductus arteriosus to survive. Ductus-dependent pulmonary blood flow is essential under circumstances in which the ductus is the major channel by which nonoxygenated blood reaches the lungs from the aortic arch, e.g., in pulmonary atresia and tricuspid atresia. Since PGE relaxes the smooth muscle in the lamb ductus arteriosus, intravenous PGE has been administered to such patients to attempt to maintain patency of the ductus. Short-term PGE infusions cause a temporary increase in blood flow to the lungs and improve arterial oxygen saturation until the necessary corrective heart surgery can be performed. The large right-to-left shunt in these cardiac malformations allows the intravenously infused PGE_2 to escape pulmonary degradation before arriving at the ductus. In this instance, the disease process itself facilitates delivery of the therapeutic agent.

Peptic ulcer disease (See Chap. 252) Gastric acid secretion in patients with peptic ulcer disease is increased. Various analogues of PGE_2 inhibit gastric acid secretion and are also inherently cytoprotective. These agents are more effective than placebo in relieving pain and decreasing gastric acid secretion in patients with ulcer disease. Moreover, the healing of ulcer craters as assessed by endoscopic criteria is accelerated in patients receiving PGE analogues.

Dysmenorrhea (See Chap. 340) Dysmenorrhea is usually associated with increased uterine contractions. The fact that some analgesics used to treat this disorder also inhibit prostaglandin synthesis suggests that arachidonic acid metabolites may play a role in the pathogenesis of dysmenorrhea. Prostaglandins of the E and F series are present in human endometrium. Intravenous infusion of either produces uterine contractions, and PGF and PGE levels in menstrual blood are decreased by administration of prostaglandin synthesis inhibitors. Controlled trials in women with dysmenorrhea suggest that symptomatic improvement is greater following therapy with inhibitors of prostaglandin synthesis.

Asthma (See Chap. 217)

Inflammatory response and immune response (See Chaps. 277 and 282) Drugs such as aspirin have antipyretic, anti-inflammatory, and analgesic effects. Several arguments support a relation between inflammation and the arachidonic acid metabolites: (1) Inflammatory stimuli such as histamine and bradykinin release endogenous prostaglandins in parallel. (2) Leukotriene C_4-D_4-E_4 is more potent than histamine in causing bronchoconstriction. (3) Several arachidonic acid metabolites cause vasodilatation and hyperalgesia. (4) PGE_2 and LTB_4 are present in areas of inflammation. Polymorphonuclear cells release these products during phagocytosis, and they are chemotactic for leukocytes. (5) Some eicosanoids (PGD_2, PGE_2, LTC_4, LTD_4, LTE_4) cause increased vascular permeability, a feature of the inflammatory response that gives rise to local edema. (6) Vasodilation induced by PGE is not abolished by atropine, propranolol, methysergide, or antihistamines, known antagonists of other possible mediators of the inflammatory response. Thus PGE may have a direct inflammatory effect, and some mediators of inflammation may act by influencing PGE release. (7) Some arachidonic acid metabolites can cause pain in animal models and hyperalgesia or an increased sensitivity to pain in humans. (8) PGE can cause fever after injection into the cerebral ventricles or into the hypothalamus of animals. (9) Pyrogens cause increased concentrations of prostaglandins in cerebrospinal fluid, whereas prostaglandin synthesis inhibitors decrease fever and decrease release of prostaglandins into cerebrospinal fluid.

PGD_2 is believed to play a major role in the manifestations of systemic mastocytosis and other disorders of mast cell activation. These symptoms include flushing, tachycardia, hypotension, abdominal cramping, diarrhea, chest pain, headache, dyspnea, and pruritus. NSAIDs in combination with antihistamines are effective therapy, but a subset of patients have attacks provoked by aspirin.

Arachidonic acid metabolites also may play a role in the immune response. Small amounts of PGE_2 can suppress stimulation of human lymphocytes by mitogens such as phytohemagglutinin, and the inflammatory response is associated with the local release of arachidonic acid metabolites; thus these substances may act as negative modulators of lymphocyte function. The release of PGE by mitogen-stimulated mononuclear cells may play a role in the negative feedback control mechanism by which lymphocyte activity is regulated. Sensitivity of lymphocytes to the inhibiting effects of PGE_2 increases with age, and indomethacin augments lymphocyte responsiveness to mitogens to a greater degree in the elderly. Mononuclear cells from patients with Hodgkin's disease release more PGE_2 after the addition of phytohemagglutinin, and lymphocyte responsiveness is enhanced by indomethacin. When suppressor T cells are removed from the cultures, the amount of PGE_2 synthesized is diminished, and the responsiveness of the lymphocytes from the Hodgkin's patients and controls is no longer different. Depressed cellular immunity in patients with Hodgkin's disease may be the result of PGE inhibition of lymphocyte function.

REFERENCES

ADVANCES IN PROSTAGLANDINS AND GASTROENTEROLOGY. Symposium. Am J Med 83(1A): 1, 1987

HENDERSON WR: Eicosanoids and platelet-activating factor in allergic respiratory diseases. Am Rev Respir Dis 143:S86, 1991

HEYMAN MA: Prostaglandins and leukotrienes in the perinatal period. Clin Perinatol 14:857, 1987

NEEDLEMAN P et al: Arachidonic acid metabolism. Annu Rev Biochem 55:69, 1986

OATES JA et al: Clinical implications of prostaglandin and thromboxane A_2 formation. N Engl J Med 319(11):689, 1988 and 319(12):761, 1988

ROBERTSON RP (ed): Symposium on prostaglandins in health and disease. Med Clin North Am 65:711, 1981

———: Eicosanoids as pluripotential modulators of pancreatic islet function. Diabetes 37:367, 1988

SCHARSCHMIDT L et al: Glomerular prostaglandins, angiotensin II, and nonsteroidal anti-inflammatory drugs. Am J Med 81(2B):30, 1986

PART FIVE

NUTRITION

71 NUTRITION AND NUTRITIONAL REQUIREMENTS

IRWIN H. ROSENBERG

Maintenance of nutrition is essential for both the management and the prevention of disease. Many complications can be prevented or modified by attention to nutritional status and prevention of nutritional deficits. The effective management of the sick patient, therefore, requires detailed evaluation of diet and nutritional status and a projection of the interaction of diet and nutritional status on the clinical course. Only then can proper goals and techniques of nutritional management be selected and nutritional guidance be provided for disease prevention and health promotion.

The purpose of this section is to summarize some of the basic considerations for the estimation of nutritional needs and the setting of goals for treatment. Determination of the nutritional needs of the individual patient must take into account both the physiologic responses to normal dietary intake and the nutritional impairments induced by disease.

EATING BEHAVIOR AND NUTRITIONAL NEEDS Eating behavior is by nature intermittent, yet energy needs are continuous. This feature of mammalian biology has resulted in the evolution of metabolic controls that promote the ebb and flow of nutrients after feeding and during the postabsorptive period and, in addition, provide for the maintenance of near-normal function during fasting.

In a nutritional perspective, the mechanisms that control appetite and eating behavior are directed to maintain energy intake adequate for the needs of the healthy adult, for growth in the child, and for the requirements of pregnancy and lactation. Under conditions of disease or trauma, the increased requirements must be met through appropriate modifications in eating behavior or caloric supplementation.

The usual remarkable stability of body weight and body composition requires that energy intake and expenditure be balanced over time. The nature of the internal signals that relay the information that caloric intake is appropriate for energy needs during the preceding days is not known. Such signals do not adjust eating behavior on a meal-to-meal time scale. With an individual meal, volume and chemoreceptors in the stomach and small bowel initiate neural and hormonal responses that contribute to satiety. The nutrient density of the food eaten, in terms of the protein or calorie content per unit volume, is not sensitively perceived, and therefore total energy or protein intake can fluctuate substantially over the short run. The neurophysiologic mechanisms that control eating behavior recognize calorie deficiencies on roughly a 24-h time scale and make compensatory changes in the volume of food eaten over periods of 1 to 2 days. That these controls work is attested to by the stability of body weight and general nutritional health of most people who have access to adequate food intake. Aberrations in these control factors can produce serious and even life-threatening imbalance, as evidenced by obesity and syndromes of anorexia and depletion.

METABOLIC RESPONSES TO CALORIC INTAKE When dietary or energy intake is adequate, several metabolic controls act to maintain essential body functions. One essential function is the maintenance of a steady fuel supply to the brain. Under the usual conditions the brain uses glucose for energy at a rate of about 5 g/h during both the fasted and fed states. The brain is also capable of utilizing ketones as an energy source and will do so in preference to glucose if the ketones are present in high concentration. In contrast to tissues such as skeletal muscle, the brain uses energy at a fairly constant rate, whether awake, sleeping, thinking, or dreaming.

During the influx of nutrients into blood after feeding and absorption, the energy and amino acid needs of the body are readily met by the supply entering from the gastrointestinal tract. When this flow of nutrients subsides, however, the body's needs are met by release of energy from stores. In the period immediately after feeding, these stores are generated under hormonal control, particularly insulin. The excess amino acids, fatty acids, and glucose not required immediately for energy are stored as proteins, triglycerides, and glycogen. This storage process also serves to mitigate the large extracellular osmotic shifts that might occur between the fed and the fasting states by depositing excess nutrients in intracellular depots.

NUTRITIONAL REQUIREMENTS To formulate a plan for nutritional management, one must consider the nutritional requirements of the patient and the impact of disease on these requirements. Energy balance means energy intake that maintains a steady body weight. Energy insufficiency is reflected in weight loss, and energy overabundance causes weight gain. Conditions that can modify nutritional requirements include infection, trauma, surgery, alcohol abuse, and malabsorption.

ESTIMATION OF ENERGY REQUIREMENT Although malnutrition, literally abnormal nutrition, could result from either excessive or inadequate energy balance, in general the term refers to undernutrition. Undernutrition can be due to inadequate intake or absorption or to increased metabolic requirements imposed by disease, including excessive loss of nutrients and drug-nutrient antagonisms.

The components of energy requirements in humans are summarized in Table 71-1. Total daily energy requirement consists of basal metabolic rate plus energy of activity and the thermic effect of food. Basal metabolic rate (BMR) or, more appropriately, resting metabolic rate (RMR) is a measure of the amount of energy expended at rest and without food; energy of activity is a measure of the energy

---

TABLE 71-1 Example of estimation of daily energy requirement

The information presented above can be utilized as in the following example: A 45-year-old, 70-kg male office worker presents with rheumatoid arthritis of mild severity. Calorie intake is good, but recent activity has been limited.

Resting energy expenditure*	7500 kJ (1800 kcal)
Activity-related expenditure	1700 kJ (400 kcal)
Illness-related expenditure (10 percent of 1800 kcal)	750 kJ (180 kcal)
Diet-induced thermogenesis (10 percent of 2380 kcal)	955 kJ (238 kcal)
Total	10,945 kJ (2618 kcal)

* Resting energy expenditure (RMR) is calculated as in Table 71-2.

TABLE 71-2   Estimation of resting metabolic rate (RMR)

Age (years)	Male kJ (a)	Male kcal (b)	Female kJ (a)	Female kcal (b)
3–10	Wt* × 95 + 2110	Wt* × 22.7 + 505	Wt* × 85 + 2033	Wt* × 20.3 + 486
10–18	Wt × 74 + 2754	Wt × 17.7 + 659	Wt × 56 + 2898	Wt × 13.4 + 693
18–30	Wt × 63 + 2896	Wt × 15.1 + 693	Wt × 62 + 2036	Wt × 14.8 + 487
30–60	Wt × 48 + 4653	Wt × 11.5 + 1113	Wt × 34 + 3538	Wt × 8.1 + 846
>60	Wt × 59 + 2459	Wt × 11.7 + 588	Wt × 38 + 2755	Wt × 9.1 + 659

*Body weight in kilograms
(a) To convert the RMR from kJ to kcal multiply kJ by 0.239.
(b) To convert the RMR from kcal to kJ multiply the kcal by 4.186.
SOURCE: Modified from WN Schofield.

expended to support a variety of physical activities; diet-induced thermogenesis (DIT) (also called *thermic effect of food* and previously termed *specific dynamic action*) is the increase in energy expenditure above basal values associated with consuming food. RMR accounts for about two-thirds of the total energy requirements and is affected by body size (height and weight), age, sex, and habitus (Table 71-2). Several methods are available for estimating resting energy expenditure. The most accurate technique for measuring total energy expenditure is the doubly labeled water technique, which utilizes the different distribution of ^{18}O and deuterium in CO_2 and body H_2O.

Estimation of resting metabolic rate (RMR)   Most methods are based on calorimetry, a measurement of oxygen consumption under carefully controlled conditions, e.g., during fasting, in the morning, and for one hour. A more meaningful metabolic rate would reflect the rate at which energy is consumed in a normal life situation at rest throughout the day, including the period of food assimilation. Clinical estimates of RMR, based on indirect assessments rather than true measurements, are frequently very useful.

The estimations of Harris and Benedict for calculating BMR (in kcal/d) are as follows:

$$BMR_{women} = 655 + (9.5 \times W) + (1.8 \times H) - (4.7 \times A)$$
$$BMR_{men} = 66 + (13.7 \times W) + (5 \times H) - (6.8 \times A)$$

where W is actual or usual weight (kg), H is height (cm), and A is age (years).

The equations for RMR are simpler and are based on more comprehensive data. Because people of the same weight but of different heights have similar RMRs, the formulas are based only on weight, age, and sex (Table 71-2). It should be remembered that predicted RMR (or BMR) may over- or underestimate the measured values by 20 or even 30 percent for any individual.

Diet-induced thermogenesis (DIT)   The ingestion of nutrients in food causes heat or energy production in excess of basal metabolic rates. A mixed diet causes approximately a 6 to 10 percent increase above basal in calories expended as heat. DIT can be divided into two components, *obligatory thermogenesis* and *facultative thermogenesis*. The former is the component of DIT that is expended in digestion, transport, and processing of food. The remainder is energy that may dissipate surplus energy and thus participate in weight maintenance and prevention of obesity. The thermogenic effect of protein is greatest, that of carbohydrate is next, and fat is least effective. The calorigenic effect of food seems to be closely related to the energy required for ATP formation, in which protein (via amino acid breakdown) is the oxidative substrate. Most of the effect is generated in the muscle and liver and occurs whether intake is enteral or parenteral. In hypermetabolic patients, diet-induced thermogenesis is less marked because heat production is already elevated. In calculating additional energy requirements for hypermetabolic patients, the DIT should be estimated at no more than 5 percent of total energy requirements.

Estimates of energy for activity   The energy expenditure of physical activity accounts for about one-third of total energy expenditures under most conditions and can vary from 6 to 36 kJ (1.5 to 8.5

kcal) per kilogram body weight per hour (Table 71-3). This factor is obviously more important in calculating energy requirements for active, ambulatory patients. Some types of work (e.g., gardening) can cause fatigue without using a large number of calories. Usually, exercise that results in lifting the body from the ground (e.g., running) uses the most calories. Although precise measurements can be made for a wide range of activities, it is easiest to use an approximation when estimating energy needs.

Additional energy requirements of illness   Heat production increases with fever and inflammation. However, as oxygen consumption increases, DIT decreases, and the energy of activity often declines owing to immobility. For these reasons, the daily energy requirement in ill persons is usually only slightly greater than the requirement when well. Indeed, the energy requirement for most patients, even during severe illness, rarely exceeds 12,500 kJ (3000 kcal) per day. (The earlier estimates of massively increased calorie requirements in patients with sepsis have not been substantiated.) Approximately 20 percent should be added to resting energy estimates for a patient confined to bed, and 30 percent should be added for ambulatory patients. Severe illness requires additional caloric supplementation, namely, addition of 10 percent of estimated RMR for mild illness, 25 percent for moderate illness, and 50 percent for severe illness.

Malabsorption is a special cause of increased energy requirement. The most accurate but impractical way to assess calorie loss would be calorimetry of the feces. However, fat excretion (in g/d) (as determined in a 72-h fecal fat assay) × 38 kJ (9 kcal) per gram equals the daily energy loss due to fat malabsorption. To estimate total fecal energy loss from all sources, the fecal energy loss from fat (in kJ or kcal) is multiplied by 2.5. This estimate assumes an average dietary composition and equivalent malabsorption of fat, carbohydrate, and protein.

ESTIMATION OF PROTEIN REQUIREMENT   Protein balance, like energy balance, is a function of intake relative to utilization and loss. Normally, nitrogen derived from amino acids is lost in urine and feces and from skin. Unlike the energy stored in triglycerides and glycogen, no proteins (or amino acids) are stored in the body solely for subsequent utilization. Every protein serves either a structural or metabolic function; when excess protein is ingested the amino acids are transaminated, and the nonnitrogenous portion of the

TABLE 71-3   Estimation of additional energy expenditure by activity

Type of work	Calories added to BMR kJ/d	kcal/d
Sedentary	1670–3350	400–800
Light: office, professional and clerical	3350–5000	800–1200
Moderate: walking, lifting	5000–7500	1200–1800
Heavy: construction, athletic	7500–19,000	1800–4500

SOURCE: Modified from DW Wilmore, *The Metabolic Management of the Critically Ill.* New York, Plenum Press, 1977.

molecule serves as a source of calories for storage as glycogen and/or fat.

Obligatory nitrogen losses Urea accounts for over 80 percent of urinary nitrogen. The remaining nitrogen is excreted as creatinine, porphyrins, and other nitrogen-containing compounds. Thus total urine loss of nitrogen = urinary urea nitrogen (mg/dL) × daily volume (dL) ÷ 0.8. Urinary nitrogen is related to the RMR. The larger the body muscle mass, the more transamination of amino acids occurs to fulfill energy needs. Each kilocalorie needed for basal metabolism leads to the excretion of 1 to 1.3 mg of urinary nitrogen. For the same reason, nitrogen excretion increases during exercise and heavy work.

Fecal and skin losses account for a large proportion of nitrogen loss from the body (about 40 percent) in normal circumstances, but the magnitude of these losses varies in disease states. Thus, measurement of urinary nitrogen often provides a useful index of daily nitrogen requirement.

Minimal nitrogen loss (in g/d) from a 70-kg person on a diet that is nitrogen free but energy adequate approximates 1.9 to 3.1 in urine, 0.7 to 2.5 in stool, and 0.3 from skin for a mean total loss of 4.4 g/d. Equivalent protein loss can be calculated by multiplying nitrogen loss by 6.25 so that total loss by metabolism of protein is 4.4 × 6.25 or 27.5 g/d or about 0.4 g/kg body weight for a 70-kg person. The recommended protein allowance for adults varies from 0.6 to 0.9 g/kg to allow for a margin of safety. Vigorous exercise may increase protein requirements to 1 g/kg body weight or higher.

Protein requirements are highest during the growth spurts of infancy and adolescence. During infancy, total body protein reserve is lowest, and obligatory losses are greatest. Thus, protein deficiency is most likely to occur during infancy. Protein requirements decline slightly during childhood and again increase with adolescence. Minimal requirements for these stages of life are about 1.5 g/kg body weight per day. The recommended allowance (2 g/kg body weight per day) allows a margin of safety for children who have increased needs or who ingest proteins of low biologic value. Low-quality proteins include certain vegetable proteins that do not support growth as well as protein from milk, eggs, or meat. The differences in the nutritional value of protein are largely due to the higher content of essential amino acids in animal proteins and to differences in digestibility. Protein (and energy) requirements also increase during pregnancy and lactation.

CALORIC REQUIREMENTS FOR PROTEIN UTILIZATION

Amino acids ingested without other energy sources are not efficiently incorporated into protein partly because of the energy lost during amino acid metabolism. Moreover, incorporation of each amino acid molecule into peptides requires three high-energy phosphate bonds. Consequently, excess of dietary energy over basal needs improves the efficiency of nitrogen utilization. During the period of intense growth in children, about 300 kJ (76 kcal) of nonprotein energy are required for each gram of protein. In ambulatory adults about 200 kJ (50 kcal) from nonprotein sources are needed per gram of protein. This high ratio usually cannot be achieved with parenteral feeding, since energy intake is limited by the volume needed to be infused. Acceptable figures for parenteral nutrition are about 100 to 125 kJ (25 to 30 kcal) from nonprotein sources per gram of protein or 600 to 750 kJ (150 to 180 kcal) per gram of nitrogen.

RECOMMENDED DIETARY ALLOWANCES OF PROTEIN AND MICRONUTRIENTS

Guidelines of nutritional requirements in health have been formulated in the reports, updated periodically, of the Food and Nutrition Board of the National Research Council of the United States. These Recommended Dietary Allowances, expressed for age and sex and modified for such conditions as pregnancy and lactation, are designed to cover the requirements of virtually all healthy individuals. With the exception of energy, the allowances are not average requirements but rather a recommended intake sufficient to meet the needs of all healthy individuals.

The recommended allowances for protein (nitrogen), iron, and calcium are based upon experiments in which normal requirement is

TABLE 71-4 Recommended dietary allowances for healthy adults

	Range of allowance	
	Men	Women
Protein, g	45–63	44–50
Vitamin A, μg retinol equivalents	1000	800
Vitamin D, μg	5–10	5–10
Vitamin E, mg α-tocopherol equivalents	10	8
Vitamin K, μg	45–80	45–65
Vitamin C, mg	50–60	50–60
Thiamine, mg	1.2–1.5	1–1.1
Riboflavin, mg	1.4–1.8	1.2–1.3
Niacin, mg niacin equivalents	15–20	13–15
Vitamin B$_6$, mg	1.4–2.0	1.4–1.6
Folate, μg	150–200	150–180[†]
Vitamin B$_{12}$, μg	2.0	2.0
Biotin, μg*	30–100	50–100
Pantothenic Acid, mg*	4–10	4–7
Calcium, mg	800–1200	800–1200
Phosphorus, mg	800–1200	800–1200
Magnesium, mg	270–400	280–300
Iron, mg	10–12	10–15
Zinc, mg	15	12
Iodine, μg	150	150
Selenium, μg	40–70	45–55
Copper, mg*	1.5–3	1.5–3
Manganese, mg*	2–5	2–5
Fluoride, mg*	1.5–4	1.5–4
Chromium, μg*	50–200	50–200
Molybdenum, μg*	75–250	75–250

* Estimated safe and adequate daily dietary intakes. From the National Research Council: *Recommended Dietary Allowances*, 10th ed. Washington, D.C., National Academy of Sciences, 1989.
† The allowance increases to 400–800 in women of childbearing age and for pregnancy.

defined as the intake necessary to achieve zero balance between intake versus output. For most vitamins the recommended allowance is the daily intake required to maintain full function and safe levels of body stores. Most estimates assume normal digestion and absorption and normal metabolism. In some cases, estimates of daily turnover are used to determine the amount of nutrient required to maintain body stores. It follows, therefore, that diseases that influence efficiency of absorption or that change the metabolism or nutritional requirements will change the safe allowance for that individual. It further follows that the recommended dietary allowances are at best a rough guide for requirements for enteral nutrient intake by any individual. Such allowances may be an overestimation of parenteral requirements, particularly in the case of micronutrients, since in that case no allowance need be made for the inefficiency of extraction from food and absorption. A listing of these essential nutrients and an estimation of the ranges of required intake for healthy adults are presented in Table 71-4.

The 1989 Recommended Dietary Allowances make little provision for changes in nutrient requirements for the elderly. Energy requirements decline progressively beyond age 50 or 60 as the lean (muscle) mass declines and as resting metabolic energy expenditure decreases. Energy needs for activity also decline as aging often leads to more sedentary lifestyle. At present, it is prudent to recommend full adult levels of protein, vitamins, and minerals even in the face of declining energy intake. For many elderly people, especially women, this may require careful dietary planning and dietary supplements. Increased physical activity at all ages promotes the retention of lean muscle mass and increases appetite and food intake.

REFERENCES

ALPERS DH et al: *Manual of Nutritional Therapeutics.* Boston, Little, Brown, 1987, chap 3

HAVEL RJ: Caloric homeostasis and disorders of fuel transport. N Engl J Med 1987:1186, 1972

Kissileff HR, Van Itallie TB: Physiology of the control of food intake. Ann Rev Nutr 2:271, 1982

National Research Council: *Recommended Dietary Allowances*, 10th ed. Washington, DC, National Academy of Sciences, 1989

Schofield WN: Predicting basal metabolic rate, new standards and review of previous work. Human Nutr Clin Nutr 39C(Suppl 1), 1985

Woo R et al: Regulation of energy balance. Ann Rev Nutr 5:411, 1985

72 PROTEIN-ENERGY MALNUTRITION

JOEL B. MASON / IRWIN H. ROSENBERG

Protein-energy malnutrition (PEM), also called protein-calorie malnutrition (PCM), is present when insufficient energy or protein is available to meet metabolic demands, thereby leading to impairments in normal physiologic processes. Inadequate dietary intake is only one of several mechanisms by which this may occur. Increased metabolic demands due to disease and increased nutrient losses are two other common mechanisms by which the body's protein and energy economy may become disrupted enough to cause PEM. Protein deficiency may also arise in the face of adequate protein intake if the dietary protein is of poor quality (i.e., the content of one or more essential amino acids is inadequate and thus becomes the limiting factor in protein utilization); such is the case when the entire protein intake is derived from a single vegetable source. Protein nutrition is also influenced by the intake of energy relative to the intake of protein because the efficient utilization of dietary protein requires energy from nonprotein calories.

Adaptive responses function over the short term when protein and energy sources are limited. As a consequence, the pathologic effects of undernutrition require a sustained inadequacy of protein or energy sources. The adaptive mechanisms that respond to protein and calorie deprivation are finite, particularly because protein has no storage form in the body.

The rapidity with which PEM develops and its severity depend on a number of factors, including the nutritional state when the nutritional deprivation begins, the underlying illness, and the developmental stage. Some of these factors are outlined in Table 72-1.

PROTEIN-ENERGY MALNUTRITION AS A GLOBAL PROBLEM

Recognition of PEM emerged from studies in the tropics that were focused primarily on the problem in children. Preschool children, particularly those between the ages of 1 and 2 are more susceptible to PEM. They are dependent on others for determining the quantity and quality of food intake; their protein and energy requirements are substantially higher per unit weight; and unhygienic habits and immaturity of the immune system heighten susceptibility to infections.

Gastrointestinal infections, in particular, constitute a major precipitant of PEM in infants and children because such illnesses result in altered feeding habits, vomiting, decreased intestinal absorption, increased metabolic needs, and increased metabolic losses. The magnitude of the problem is immense; the World Health Organization estimated in 1983 that 300 million children have growth retardation secondary to malnutrition. Increased mortality and impaired cognitive, social, and economic development are additional features but are difficult to quantitate.

PROTEIN-ENERGY MALNUTRITION IN DEVELOPED NATIONS

PEM is confined neither to children nor to the less-developed countries. Although the overall prevalence of PEM is low, specific sectors of the U.S. population, such as the institutionalized elderly and children of the poor, have a significant prevalence. For example, the Ten State Survey, which focused on low income areas in the United States, found that 22 to 35 percent of the children aged 2, 4, and 6 were below the 15th percentile for weight. In this survey income level and minority status were predictors of growth retardation among children. In a 1987 survey 11 percent of low income children had height for age below the 5th percentile standard. Moreover, in large urban teaching hospitals as well as smaller community hospitals 30 to 70 percent of general medical and surgical patients have anthropometric and/or biochemical evidence of PEM. Similar statistics have been noted in surveys of pediatric inpatients. It is perhaps more disturbing that the nutritional status of the majority of hospitalized patients *declines* during the course of hospitalization. Positive associations between the degree of PEM and the incidence of postoperative infections, impaired healing of surgical wounds, and prolongation of hospitalization indicate that more attention needs to be paid to the maintenance of adequate nutrition in individual patients. There are tangible benefits from such nutritional diligence. For example, aggressive preoperative nutritional restitution of malnourished patients can decrease perioperative morbidity such as infection.

Most modern-day hospital malnutrition is compounded by insufficient attention by medical personnel to nutrition (Table 72-2). Indeed, most factors contributing to the high prevalence of malnutrition in hospitalized patients are reversible or preventable.

PROTEIN-ENERGY METABOLISM DURING STRESS
Physiological adaptation to starvation During periods of protein and/or energy deficit, compensatory mechanisms serve to lessen the pathologic impact of these deficiencies. To understand how malnutrition develops, it is important to understand the responses to such inadequate intake. During the first 24 h of fasting, circulating glucose, fatty acids, and triglycerides and liver and muscle glycogen are used as fuel sources. However, the sum of these stores in a 70-kg man is only about 5000 kJ (1200 kcal) and provides less fuel than is needed for basal metabolism for a single day. Triglycerides, derived primarily from adipose tissue, can be catabolized to fatty acids and ketone

---

TABLE 72-1 Factors that condition the response to inadequate nutrient intake

A Nutritional factors
  1 Underlying adequacy of reserves/depot of that nutrient
  2 Severity of the inadequate intake; duration of deprivation
  3 Concurrent deficiencies of other nutrients
B Underlying illnesses
  1 Fever, infection, trauma, and other conditions associated with increased requirements and catabolic losses
  2 Malabsorptive, maldigestive states
  3 Illnesses associated with excessive loss of nutrients (e.g., protein-losing enteropathy, nephrotic syndrome, enteric fistulas)
  4 Conditions associated with altered metabolism of nutrients (e.g., diabetes mellitus, hyperthyroidism)
C Physiologic states in which increased requirements are present
  1 Pregnancy, lactation
  2 Growth and development during infancy, childhood, and adolescence

---

TABLE 72-2 Undesirable practices that affect the nutritional health of hospital patients

1 Failure to record height and weight in the hospital chart
2 Diffusion of responsibility for patient care
3 Prolonged use of glucose and saline intravenous feedings
4 Failure to observe and record patients' dietary intake
5 Withholding meals because of diagnostic tests
6 Use of enteral or parenteral feedings of uncertain composition and in inadequate amounts
7 Ignorance of the composition of nutritional products
8 Failure to recognize increased nutritional needs due to injury or illness
9 Lack of communication and interaction between physician, nurse, and dietician
10 Delay of nutritional support until the patient is in a state of severe depletion
11 Limited availability of laboratory tests to assess nutritional status; failure to use those that are available
12 Limited emphasis on nutrition education in medical schools

SOURCE: Butterworth CE: The skeleton in the hospital closet. Nutr Today 9:4, 1974 bodies by most tissues. However, over the short run tissues such as the brain can only use glycolytic pathways to obtain energy. Since fatty acids are not converted to carbohydrate, these glycolytic tissues must utilize either glucose or substrates that can be converted to glucose. Amino acids derived primarily from skeletal muscle constitute the major endogenous substrate for glucose production for this purpose. Since there is no storage form of protein in the body, a fasting individual sustains a daily loss of functionally significant protein.

The provision of adequate fuel substrate to critical tissues, particularly the brain, has homeostatic priority during protein/energy deprivation. Brief starvation leads to acute adaptive responses that sustain the supply of glucose to tissues that require it and minimize the amount of protein breakdown to meet this need. To accomplish this end, certain tissues, such as the heart, kidney, and skeletal muscle, change their primary fuel substrate from glucose to fatty acids and ketone bodies. Other tissues, such as the bone marrow, renal medulla, and peripheral nerves, switch from the full oxidation of glucose to anaerobic glycolysis, resulting in the production of lactate and pyruvate. These compounds can be converted to glucose in the liver with energy derived from fat oxidation and then released for systemic consumption. This shuttle, the Cori cycle, enables energy stored as fat to be utilized for glucose synthesis and thus conserves protein energy that would otherwise be necessary for the de novo synthesis of glucose.

With more extended starvation other adaptations appear. A decrease in physical exertion decreases energy consumption, and the resting metabolic rate generally declines by about 10 percent. The brain, which ordinarily obtains energy only by glucose oxidation, acquires the ability to use keto acids for its fuel requirements, and this contributes further to protein conservation. Animal studies and, less definitively, human studies suggest that protein that is consumed during relative protein starvation is utilized more efficiently. Moreover, chronic protein deprivation leads to a reduced rate of protein turnover, and amino acids are reutilized more efficiently for the synthesis of new proteins, contributing to savings in both energy and amino acid requirements.

During relative or total caloric starvation, such adaptations allow the body to provide the energy necessary for metabolism and to minimize the obligatory loss of protein, which appears primarily as nitrogen-containing compounds in the urine. After several weeks of starvation, nitrogen loss in the urine may decrease by more than 65 percent. However, these homeostatic mechanisms do not compensate entirely for the imposed deficits, and eventually the negative caloric and/or protein balance lead to pathologic consequences.

Effects of physical stress Infection, trauma, and other physical stress cause inflammatory responses. In such situations, protein and energy metabolism change in ways that increase both energy demands and nitrogen losses and thereby predispose to the development of PEM.

Resting metabolic rate (RMR) increases dramatically during critical illness in a fashion that is roughly proportional to the severity of the stress. Patients with burns over more than 40 percent of the body have a RMR approximately twice normal, patients with sepsis have a RMR that is about one and a half times normal, and patients with a single bone fracture or a localized infection have RMRs that are about 1.3 times normal. Factors that contribute to the increased energy consumption include increases in circulating catecholamines, the increase in energy expenditure required for gluconeogenesis, and the hypermetabolism associated with fever.

Nitrogen loss during critical illness is also increased proportional to the severity of the stress, but the magnitude of the increase is generally larger than the increase in energy consumption. A healthy adult loses approximately 12 g of nitrogen in urine per day in the fasting state; sepsis and trauma commonly increase that value by 50 to 100 percent. Since 1 g of urinary nitrogen represents approximately 30 g of lean body mass, critical illness induces a daily loss of 0.6 kg of lean body mass. Most of this loss comes from the skeletal muscle,

and the efflux of amino acids from skeletal muscle increases two- to sixfold in critically ill patients. Increased efflux from skeletal muscle is probably due to increased protein catabolism rather than decreased protein synthesis.

The mobilization of amino acids from skeletal muscle is an adaptive response. The liberated amino acids are in part used as fuel. They are also taken up by the liver and other visceral organs (the "visceral protein compartment"). The proteolysis of muscle under physical stress thus enables the body to shift protein substrate from skeletal muscle (the "somatic protein compartment") to visceral organs whose function is more critical for immediate survival. Hormonal factors play a significant role in this shift; circulating levels of cortisol, glucagon, epinephrine, and growth hormone are increased in physically stressed individuals. Increased local or circulating levels of interleukin 1 and tumor necrosis factor alpha (TNF-α) in patients with a systemic inflammatory process probably play a major role in sparing the visceral protein compartment at the expense of the skeletal muscle. Eventually, continued deficits in protein and energy, particularly when superimposed on sustained physical stress, lead to a contraction of the visceral protein compartment and its associated functions.

CLASSIFICATION AND ASSESSMENT OF PROTEIN-ENERGY MALNUTRITION Protein-energy malnutrition may be *primary*, due to an inadequate intake of protein and/or energy source, or *secondary*, due to illness that impairs intake or utilization of nutrients or that increases nutrient requirements or metabolic losses. Malignancy, intestinal malabsorption, inflammatory bowel disease, AIDS, and chronic renal failure are a few of the illnesses commonly associated with secondary PEM.

There are no universally accepted criteria for defining the severity of PEM although it is often categorized as mild, moderate, or severe. An effective nutritional assessment requires the synthesis of information provided by a dietary history, physical examination, biochemical data, and functional and/or anthropometric measurements of nutritional status. No single piece of evidence is sufficient to indicate the nutritional status. A corollary is that each parameter used to assess nutritional status can be, and often is, influenced by factors that have little to do with the nutritional state.

In adults, the most commonly used indication of caloric status is body weight. Standard tables of desirable or ideal body weight are available, but individual variation is so great that comparison with the pre-morbid weight of the individual is more informative. It therefore follows that an obese individual who has ongoing deficits in protein or caloric balance, although considerably above ideal body weight, can have PEM with its associated pathologic consequences.

The degree of unintentional weight loss in an ill individual correlates with the extent of total body protein depletion, the integrity of many physiologic functions, and clinical endpoints such as the rate of in-hospital infections and the duration of hospitalization. Consequently, an unintentional decrease of more than 20 percent of the usual body weight, which is almost always associated with a 25 to 35 percent decrease in lean body mass, significant impairment in many physiologic functions, a higher rate of in-hospital morbidity, and extended hospitalization, is the most accessible indicator of *severe* PEM. Patients whose weight loss is >10 and ≤20 percent (*moderate* PEM) have significant losses of body protein, impairments in physiologic functions, increased rates of in-hospital morbidity, and hospitalization stays that are intermediate between individuals with severe PEM and individuals whose weight loss is less than or equal to 10 percent. Unintentional weight loss of ≤10 percent is not associated with physiologic impairments or increased morbidity.

Fat stores are the major energy reserve in the body and, as such, also can be used to assess energy status. The reduction in subcutaneous fat is often evident by inspecting the extremities or face, although a significant reduction in fat mass is frequently overlooked unless more objective criteria than visual inspection are used. Skin-fold measurements or more sophisticated indicators of body consumption can be used to quantify the reduction in body mass that is composed

TABLE 72-3 Normative values for triceps skin-fold thickness

Age group, years	Mean, mm	Percentile						
		5	10	25	50	75	90	95
MEN								
18–74	12.0	4.5	6.0	8.0	11.0	15.0	20.0	23.0
18–24	11.2	4.0	5.0	7.0	9.5	14.0	20.0	23.0
25–34	12.6	4.5	5.5	8.0	12.0	16.0	21.5	24.0
35–44	12.4	5.0	6.0	8.5	12.0	15.5	20.0	23.0
45–54	12.4	5.0	6.0	8.0	11.0	15.0	20.0	25.0
55–64	11.6	5.0	6.0	8.0	11.0	14.0	18.0	21.5
65–74	11.8	4.5	5.5	8.0	11.0	15.0	19.0	22.0
WOMEN								
18–74	23.0	11.0	13.0	17.0	22.0	28.0	34.0	37.5
18–24	19.4	9.4	11.0	14.0	18.0	24.0	30.0	34.0
25–34	21.9	10.5	12.0	16.0	21.0	26.5	33.5	37.0
35–44	24.0	12.0	14.0	18.0	23.0	29.5	35.5	39.0
45–54	25.4	13.0	15.0	20.0	25.0	30.0	36.0	40.0
55–65	24.9	11.0	14.0	19.0	25.0	30.5	35.0	39.0
65–74	23.3	11.5	14.0	18.0	23.0	28.0	33.0	36.0

SOURCE: Heymsfield and Williams.

of fat. The triceps fat fold, when compared to standard values, provides an indication of the adequacy of body fat since more than half of total body fat is subcutaneous (Table 72-3). A triceps fat fold measurement that is less than the 10th percentile is indicative of a substantial deficit of fat stores.

Protein status can be assessed in several different ways. Separate assessments of the somatic and visceral protein compartments are useful and physiologically meaningful since these two protein depots are handled differently by the body. The somatic protein compartment can be objectively assessed by determining the mid-arm muscle area and comparing it to normative values such as in Table 72-4. Estimation of the creatinine-height index performs a similar function (Table 72-5). Physical examination also can provide evidence of decreased

muscle mass but tends to be an insensitive means of assessment. The visceral protein compartment can be estimated by several methods. The total lymphocyte count in the peripheral blood and the presence of delayed cutaneous hypersensitivity are effective in this respect. A total lymphocyte count less than 1500 cells per microliter or the absence of cutaneous hypersensitivity to common antigens suggests a deficit in the visceral protein compartment. The concentrations of certain serum proteins, albumin being the most common, are also useful parameters. However, the accuracy of serum albumin to reflect the status of the visceral protein compartment or the general state of nutrition is poor in the setting of acute or critical illness: the long half-life of albumin (20 days), the fact that it is distributed extensively in the extravascular and intravascular compartments, and the fact that its synthesis is influenced by circulating inflammatory mediators and by liver disease all contribute to its inaccuracy as a measure of nutrition. Other serum proteins with shorter half-lives such as transferrin, transthyretin (prealbumin) and retinol-binding protein are better in this regard (Table 72-6).

Alterations in body habitus and composition frequently occur in

TABLE 72-4 Normative values for midarm muscle area*

Age group	Arm muscle area percentiles, mm^2						
	5	10	25	50	75	90	95
MEN							
16–16.9	3625	4044	4352	4951	5753	6576	6980
17–17.9	3998	4252	4777	5286	5950	6886	7726
18–18.9	4070	4481	5066	5552	6374	7067	8355
19–24.9	4508	4777	5274	5913	6660	7606	8200
25–34.9	4694	4963	5541	6214	7067	7847	8436
35–44.9	4844	5181	5740	6490	7265	8034	8488
45–54.9	4546	4946	5589	6297	7142	7918	8458
55–64.9	4422	4783	5381	6144	6919	7670	8149
65–74.9	3973	4411	5031	5716	6432	7074	7453
WOMEN							
16–16.9	2308	2567	2865	3248	3718	4353	4946
17–17.9	2442	2674	2996	3336	3883	4552	5251
18–18.9	2398	2538	2917	3243	3694	4461	4767
19–24.9	2538	2728	3026	3406	3877	4439	4940
25–34.9	2661	2826	3148	3573	4138	4806	5541
35–44.9	2750	2948	3359	3783	4428	5240	5877
45–54.9	2784	2956	3378	3858	4520	5375	5964
55–64.9	2784	3063	3477	4045	4750	5632	6247
65–74.9	2737	3018	3444	4019	4739	5566	6214

* Estimates based on data from the U.S. Health and Nutrition Examination Survey, 1971–1974 (HANES I). Mid-arm muscle area (MAMA) =

$$\frac{[\text{mid-arm circumference} - \pi(\text{triceps skin fold, mm})]^2}{4(\pi)}$$

SOURCE: AJ Frisancho, Am J Clin Nutr 34:2540, 1981.

TABLE 72-5 Normative values for creatinine excretion based on height

Men*		Women†	
Height, cm	Ideal creatinine, mg	Height, cm	Ideal creatinine, mg
157.5	1288	147.3	830
160.0	1325	149.9	851
162.6	1359	152.4	875
165.1	1386	154.9	900
167.6	1426	157.5	925
170.2	1467	160.0	949
172.7	1513	162.6	977
175.3	1555	165.1	1006
177.8	1596	167.6	1044
180.3	1642	170.2	1076
182.9	1691	172.7	1109
185.4	1739	175.3	1141
188.0	1785	177.8	1174
190.5	1831	180.3	1206
193.0	1891	182.9	1240

* Creatinine coefficient (men) = 23 mg/kg of ideal body weight.
† Creatinine coefficient (women) = 18 mg/kg of ideal body weight.

Creatinine-Height Index = $\dfrac{\text{Actual 24-h urinary creatinine excretion}}{\text{normative value for height and sex}}$

SOURCE: GL Blackburn et al., J Parent Ent Nutr 1:11, 1977.

TABLE 72-6 Serum proteins used in nutritional assessment

Serum protein	Approximate molecular mass, Da	Biosynthetic site	Normal value $\overline{X} \pm$ SD or (range)*	Half-life, days	Function	Comment[†]
Albumin	66,000	Hepatocyte	45 (35–50)	14–20	Maintain plasma oncotic pressure; carrier for small molecules	Serum levels are determined by many different processes
Transferrin	77,000	Hepatocyte	2.3 (2.0–3.2)	8–9	Binds Fe^{2+} in plasma and transports to bone	Iron nutriture influences plasma level; increased during pregnancy, estrogen therapy, and acute hepatitis; reduced in protein-losing enteropathy and nephropathy, chronic infections, uremia, and acute catabolic states; often measured indirectly as total iron-binding capacity
Transthyretin (Prealbumin)	61,000	Hepatocyte	0.30 (0.2–0.5)	2–3	Binds T_3 and to a lesser extent T_4. Carrier for retinol-binding protein	Increased in patients with chronic renal failure on dialysis; reduced in acute catabolic states, after surgery, in hyperthyroidism; serum level determined by overall energy and nitrogen balance
Retinol-binding protein (RBP)	21,000	Hepatocyte	0.0372 ± 0.0073[‡]	0.5	Transports vitamin A in plasma; binds noncovalently to prealbumin	Catabolized in renal proximal tubular cell; with renal disease RBP increases and $t_{1/2}$ is prolonged; low in vitamin A deficiency, acute catabolic states, after surgery, and in hyperthyroidism

* Units are g/L. Normal range varies between centers; check local values.
† All of the listed proteins are influenced by hydration and the presence of hepatocellular dysfunction.
‡ Normal values are age- and sex-dependent. Table value is for pooled subjects.
SOURCE: Heymsfield and Williams.

acute illness: fluid retention, for example, may dilute the apparent concentration of serum proteins, alter anthropometric measurements of edematous body structures, and increase body weight. Because all the traditional measures of protein-energy status may fall prey to such artifacts in acutely ill individuals there is increasing reliance on functional measures of protein-calorie status. Measures of skeletal muscle strength correlate very highly with more conventional measures of somatic and visceral protein status, with total body protein, and with clinical outcomes. A handgrip dynamometer is a simple and highly effective tool in this regard (Fig. 72-1). Table 72-7 outlines parameters to classify an individual as either moderately or severely malnourished.

CLINICAL FEATURES Weight loss and a reduction in subcutaneous fat are the most consistent physical features of mild to moderate PEM in adults. Children with PEM exhibit additional features related to retarded physical development such as a stunted (low height for age) or wasted (low weight for height) body habitus and delayed puberty. PEM also causes retardation of cognitive and psychosocial development in children.

Mild to moderate PEM The reduction in lean body mass in mild to moderate PEM is usually not as great as the reduction in fat but can be identified by measurement of the mid-arm muscle area or the creatinine-height index. The decrease in urinary urea nitrogen, in contrast, is more a reflection of the physiologic adjustments made by the body in response to inadequate protein and/or calories. A contraction of the visceral protein compartment may be reflected in decreased levels of serum albumin, transferrin, retinol-binding protein, and thyroxine-binding prealbumin, a reduction in the total lymphocyte count, or a loss of delayed cutaneous hypersensitivity. Functionally, there may be a decrease in handgrip strength; impairments in work capacity are usually evident only in individuals whose daily activities are particularly high in energy demands. Pregnant women with mild

FIGURE 72-1 Handgrip strength, expressed as percent predicted (*A*) correlates with visceral protein status (*B* and *C*), somatic protein status (data not shown), and total body protein (data not shown). Protein index = measured total body protein/predicted total body protein. Physiologic impairments are common when the protein index is <0.8. (*From Hill.*)

TABLE 72-7 Assessment of protein-energy status

Method of assessment	Moderate PEM	Severe PEM
Percent of premorbid weight	80–90	<80
Percent of ideal weight	60–80	<60
Creatinine-height index (see Table 72-5)	60–80	<60
Grip strength, % predicted	60–70	<60
Serum albumin, g/L	21–30	<21
Serum transferrin, g/L	1.0–1.5	<1
Total lymphocyte count, μL	800–1200	<800
Delayed hypersensitivity index*	1	0
Prognostic Nutritional Index, %†	40–50	>50

* Delayed hypersensitivity Index quantitates the amount of induration elicited by skin testing with a common antigen such as *Candida*, trichophyton, or mumps. Grading: 0 = <0.5 cm induration, 1 = 0.5 cm, 2 = 1.0 cm

† Prognostic Nutritional Index is a weighted combination of four measures (see Table 72-8): PNI % = 158 − [1.66 × albumin (g/L)] − [0.78 × triceps skin fold (mm)] − [2.0 × transferrin (g/L)] − [5.8 × delayed hypersensitivity index].

to moderate PEM are at risk of delivering an infant with low weight or length for gestational age. The volume of breast milk in such women is decreased as is its fat and energy content.

Severe PEM More severe PEM is characterized by more severe alterations in the body habitus and in laboratory parameters. Deficiency states of specific micronutrients are common in conjunction with severe PEM although the latter usually has the most impact on health. There is further loss of subcutaneous fat and decrease in the somatic protein compartment as evidenced by muscle wasting in the extremities. The decrease in muscle mass can be identified by examining for atrophy of the interosseous muscles in the hand or the temporalis muscle on the sides of the head or by estimating the mid-arm muscle area. The loss of subcutaneous fat and muscle mass, in conjunction with a decrease in the elasticity of the skin, results in loose fitting, wrinkled skin with reduplicated folds. Skin lesions are common in advanced PEM, particularly over edematous areas. They may appear as shiny, erythematous, atrophic areas or as hyperkeratotic, hyperpigmented regions ("flaky paint" dermatitis). Decubitus ulcers are also common. The hair becomes sparse and dry, loses its usual sheen, and can be pulled out with little effort. The color of the hair may change to reddish or dull brown, and alternating periods of nutritional depletion and repletion may give rise to bands of color changes in the hair.

Lethargy is common. Alterations in gastrointestinal function include constipation and difficulty ingesting normal-sized meals due to early satiety and vomiting. The heart rate, blood pressure, and core body temperature may be subnormal. Infections may not be accompanied by appropriate hyperthermic and tachycardic responses.

When severe PEM arises from an inadequate intake of both protein and calories the diminution in the somatic protein compartment is disproportionately large compared to the decrease in the visceral protein compartment (*marasmic* PEM). Individuals with this form of PEM demonstrate marked muscle wasting in the extremities and trunk while maintaining relative normality of the visceral protein compartment. Weakness accompanies the loss in muscle mass and can be profound. The decrease in subcutaneous fat throughout the body, combined with the loss in muscle mass, results in a "skin-and-bones" appearance. Edema is not present in these individuals and constitutes a major feature distinguishing marasmic PEM from pure protein malnutrition.

When the inadequacy of protein intake outweighs the extent of caloric deprivation, and particularly when there is a superimposed inflammatory stress, the subcutaneous fat and somatic protein compartments are spared relative to the reduction in the visceral protein compartment. The interpretation of the anthropometric measurements of the fat and somatic protein compartments are complicated by the presence of edemas but are relatively normal in the face of substantial decreases in the concentrations of serum proteins. This is "hypoproteinemic PEM" (called *kwashiorkor* in the original descriptions of

children in under-developed nations). It is rare in its pure form among malnourished hospitalized patients but may occur in a mixed form with features of both hypoproteinemic and marasmic PEM. Such individuals have subnormal fat and somatic protein compartments, as indicated by anthropometric measurements, as well as depressed levels of serum proteins and the accompanying edema. The edema in hypoproteinemic PEM is usually dependent but may extend more cephalad and even be generalized. Individuals with hypoproteinemic PEM are particularly misleading because they do not have the marked fat and muscle wasting characteristic of marasmic protein-energy malnutrition. This does not imply that this type of PEM is associated with less morbidity. Indeed, hospitalized patients with hypoproteinemic PEM may have a worse prognosis than those with marasmic PEM, and there is a greater susceptibility for development of superimposed infections.

In hypoproteinemic PEM the liver may be enlarged and tender to palpation as a result of fatty infiltration: fat droplets initially appear in the periportal hepatocytes and, with increasing severity, spread to the pericentral regions of the hepatic lobule. Fatty liver is thought to be due to the inadequate transport of lipids out of the hepatic parenchyma due to the decreased availability of lipoproteins. Serum concentrations of VLDL and LDL are subnormal in hypoproteinemic PEM, and the severity of the fatty infiltration correlates with the degree of depression of these lipoproteins.

Several factors determine whether a malnourished individual develops a hypoproteinemic, marasmic, or combined form of PEM including the relative degree of protein versus energy deprivation, the presence of superimposed inflammatory processes, and individual host responses to the same type of nutritional deprivation and inflammatory insult. Children with marasmic PEM have higher glucocorticoid levels than those with hypoproteinemic PEM, and this hormonal difference may be responsible for maintaining the visceral protein compartment at the expense of the skeletal muscle.

PHYSIOLOGIC IMPAIRMENTS ASSOCIATED WITH PROTEIN-ENERGY MALNUTRITION PEM impairs the function of all organs. Most, if not all, of the impairments are reversible with nutritional restitution.

Gastrointestinal tract Alterations in gastrointestinal structure and function with PEM arise partially from undernutrition and partially from decreased stimulation of the gut by ingested nutrients. The sustained absence of nutrients in the intestine of nutritionally replete, parenterally fed individuals results in structural and functional atrophy of the intestine. The changes have been best described in children and are presumed to occur also in adult PEM and include both histologic and functional abnormalities. Marked blunting, or total absence, of the intestinal villi is associated with decreased levels of disaccharidases and aminopeptidases in the mucosa. Gastric and pancreatic secretions are reduced in volume and contain decreased concentrations of acid and digestive enzymes. The volume of bile and the concentration of conjugated bile acids in bile are reduced. Substantial populations of facultative and strict anaerobic bacteria are frequently present in the upper small bowel, probably explaining the increase in free bile acids. Malabsorption of carbohydrates, fat- and water-soluble vitamins, and fat may occur, the degree of steatorrhea being proportional to the severity of PEM. These alterations in absorption impair the ability to assimilate an adequate quantity of nutrients.

Immunologic functions PEM impairs both the cell-mediated and humoral immune systems. The functional integrity of T lymphocytes, polymorphonuclear leukocytes, and the complement system is uniformly blunted, and B lymphocyte function may be impaired.

A cycle is established whereby malnutrition impairs host defenses and thereby enhances the susceptibility to infection which, in turn, worsens the malnourished state. Atrophy, and thereby impairment, of epithelial integrity and decreased gastric acid and lysozyme secretion contribute to the propensity toward infection. Infection worsens malnutrition through a series of events that includes: anorexia, which decreases the intake of nutrients; a shift in the balance of protein metabolism to the catabolic state, thereby promoting loss of lean body mass; and enhancement of the metabolic rate which increases about 13 percent for every 1°C elevation of body temperature. Interleukin 1, interleukin 6, and TNF-α appear to play roles in these processes. Tumor necrosis factor (sometimes called cachectin) also inhibits several enzymes of lipid metabolism and therefore impairs utilization of fat stores as an energy source.

The total lymphocyte count, delayed skin hypersensitivity, and some nutritional indices that incorporate these parameters (see below) correlate with the visceral protein compartment and can be used to predict the risk of postoperative infections and, in some cases, postoperative mortality. Additional factors other than nutritional status also influence lymphocytes, and nutritional status is therefore not the sole determinant of the predictive utility of these tests.

Endocrine system Hormonal alterations are common in PEM; most appear to be physiologic adaptations to the undernourished state. The inadequate intake of food leads to a decrease in the availability of circulating glucose and amino acids, low circulating levels of insulin, and increased levels of growth hormone. These alterations, in conjunction with the decreased levels of somatomedins and increased levels of cortisol in PEM, promote muscle protein catabolism and at the same time enhance incorporation of the liberated amino acids into visceral organs. Urea synthesis is inhibited, decreasing nitrogen loss and enhancing the reutilization of amino acids. The enhancement of lipolysis and gluconeogenesis provides substrate for energy.

The serum levels of triiodothyronine (T_3) and thyroxine (T_4) are commonly decreased in association with increased concentrations of reverse T_3 (3,5,5'-triiodothyronine), resembling the pattern observed in the *euthyroid sick syndrome*. The decreased concentrations of T_3 may play a role in the decrease in metabolic rate and decrease in protein catabolism in PEM.

Primary gonadal dysfunction is common in adults with moderate to severe PEM, including decreased levels of circulating testosterone and estrogen and impairment in reproductive potential. Amenorrhea is common. Fertility is further reduced in women by an increased risk of resorption of an implanted embryo. Impaired secretion of the hypothalamic hormone luteinizing hormone releasing hormone (LH-RH) may also play a role in the impaired reproduction. In prepubertal children with PEM the basal level of FSH and the response of this gonadatropin to LHRH are variously reported to be low or normal. Delay of puberty appears to be due to a decrease below a critical lean body mass. These changes in the pituitary-gonadal axis can be viewed as an adaptation, since the availability of energy and protein substrate is more critical for immediate survival than is the need for sexual maturation in children or reproduction in adults.

Cardiovascular system Moderate to severe PEM produces both quantitative and qualitative alterations in the heart. Myocardial mass is decreased, although proportionately less than the loss in body weight. Microscopic analysis of the myocardium reveals myofibrillar atrophy, edema, and, less commonly, patchy necrosis and infiltration with chronic inflammatory cells. Involvement of the myocardial conduction system may explain the conduction abnormalities in the PEM associated with anorexia nervosa and total starvation.

These structural changes are associated with alterations in myocardial performance, most evident under conditions of increased demand, as a decrease in cardiac output, stroke volume, and maximal work capacity. The cardiac alterations associated with PEM are reversible: both left ventricular mass and cardiac output increase with several weeks of nutritional repletion.

Respiratory system All muscles, including the diaphragm and the other respiratory muscles, undergo structural and functional atrophy, causing decreases in the inspiratory and expiratory pressures and in the vital capacity. Decreased respiratory muscle strength and a blunted ventilatory drive impair the ability to sustain ventilation in the severely malnourished individual. In tracheostomy patients, adherence of bacteria to tracheal epithelial cells correlates with the degree of malnutrition. Thus the immunologic integrity of the respiratory tract, as previously discussed, appears to be compromised by malnutrition.

Nutritional repletion leads to improvements in impaired pulmonary physiology and in the probability of weaning from a ventilator.

Wound healing Well-nourished individuals lay down more collagen at the site of a surgical wound than do those individuals with even mild malnutrition. Repletion of the malnourished surgical patient before surgery leads to better wound healing than if nutritional needs are only addressed postoperatively. Nevertheless, the provision of adequate nutrition after surgery enhances the deposition of collagen at the wound. Furthermore, intestinal anastomoses in well-nourished animals have a higher bursting strength than those in malnourished animals, and collagen deposition, tensile strength, and resistance to complications at the site of intestinal anastomses are greater in nutritionally replete animals.

Influence of malnutrition on the hospital course Numerous studies have demonstrated a correlation between protein-energy status and the outcome of hospitalization. For example, a depressed serum albumin or transferrin level, recent unintentional weight loss of >10 percent, a moderately depressed grip strength, a decreased total lymphocyte count (<1200 per microliter), or an anergic skin response to foreign antigens are all predictive of an increased incidence of morbid events within the hospital. Moreover, several of these parameters are predictors of the duration of postoperative hospitalization, in-hospital mortality, and the risk of morbidity following discharge.

Several nutritional indices, each of which incorporates various combinations of these parameters, have been utilized to assess the nutritional status of hospitalized patients (Table 72-8). However, every parameter used for the clinical assessment of nutritional status

TABLE 72-8 Prognostic indices in hospitalized patients

Index	Incorporated parameters	Correlates with	Reference
Likelihood of malnutrition	Serum folate, serum vitamin C, serum albumin, lymphocyte count, hematocrit, triceps skinfold, arm muscle circumference, weight	Duration of hospitalization	Am J Clin Nutr 32:418, 1979
Prognostic nutritional index	Serum albumin, serum transferrin, delayed hypersensitivity, triceps skinfold	Incidence of postoperative complications and mortality	Cancer 47:2375, 1981
Instant nutritional index	Serum albumin, lymphocyte count	Incidence of postoperative infection	J Parent Ent Nutr 12:195, 1988
Hospital prognostic index	Serum albumin, delayed hypersensitivity, presence of sepsis or cancer	Hospital mortality	Am J Clin Nutr 34:2013, 1981

and the indices that integrate several parameters, are influenced by disease as well as by nutritional status. Such indices are more properly considered assessments of the severity of illness and the "likelihood" of malnutrition rather than as indicators of nutritional status alone. Nevertheless, aggressive attention to nutritional restitution can mitigate the morbidity associated with PEM, confirming both the predictive and practical value of these nutritional measures. Furthermore, the response to nutritional intervention emphasizes the importance of attending to both nutritional assessment and therapy in hospitalized patients.

REFERENCES

BARACOS V et al: Stimulation of degradation of muscle proteins during fever. A mechanism for the increased degradation of muscle proteins during fever. New Engl J Med 308:553, 1983
BECKER DJ: The endocrine responses to protein calorie malnutrition. Ann Rev Nutr 3:187, 1983
BEUTLER B, CERAMI A: Cachectin: more than a tumor necrosis factor. New Engl J Med 316:379, 1987
BISTRIAN BR et al: Protein status of general surgical patients. JAMA 230:858, 1974
——— et al: Prevalence of malnutrition in general medical patients. JAMA 235:1567, 1976
BISTRIAN BR et al: Cytokines, muscle proteolysis, and the catabolic response to infection and inflammation. Proc Soc Exp Biol Med 200:220, 1992
CAHILL GF: Starvation in man. New Engl J Med 282:668, 1970
HEYMSFIELD SB, WILLIAMS PJ: Nutritional assessment by clinical and biochemical methods, in Modern Nutrition in Health and Disease, 7th ed, ME Shils, VR Young (eds). Philadelphia, Lea & Febiger, 1988
HILL GL: Body composition research: Implications for the practice of clinical nutrition. J Parent Ent Nutr 16:197, 1992
KEUSCH GT, FARTHING MJG: Nutrition and infection. Ann Rev Nutr 6:131, 1986
LONG CL, LOWRY SF: Hormonal regulation of protein metabolism. J Parent Ent Nutr 14:555, 1990
ROSENBLATT S et al: Exchange of amino acids by muscle and liver in sepsis. Arch Surg 118:167, 1983

73 OBESITY

JERROLD M. OLEFSKY

The ability to store food energy as fat provides survival value when the food supply is scarce or sporadic. Unlike glycogen or protein, triglyceride does not require water or electrolytes for storage purposes and can be retained essentially as pure fat; 1 g adipose tissue yields close to the full theoretical equivalent of 38 kJ (9 kcal). Because of the efficient storage of energy in adipose tissue, an individual of normal weight can survive up to 2 months of total starvation. However, western society is generally not characterized by periodic or insufficient food supply but rather by constant and abundant food. As a consequence, the ability to store fat frequently is of negative survival value because of overconsumption and resulting obesity.

DEFINITION AND INCIDENCE Obesity can most easily be assessed in terms of height and weight. One way is to relate weight to an average range for height and age. This measure of *relative weight* can lead to an underestimation of the incidence of obesity, since in the United States the "average" individual is somewhat obese. Tables of *ideal* and *desirable* weight are based on actuarial estimates of what is consistent with longest life expectancy. Such tables are more useful if adjusted for differences in body build. An alternative method of estimating obesity is the *body mass index* or *BMI* [body weight (in kilograms) divided by height^2 (in meters)]. For adults ages 20 to 29, the 85th percentile for BMI is 27.8 for males and 27.3 for females. Although relative weight and BMI correlate with the degree of adiposity, excess weight can be either lean or fat tissue. For example, heavily muscled individuals would be considered obese using these measurements. Nevertheless, such assessments correlate fairly well

with the risk of adverse effects on health and longevity. More precise assessment of obesity can be made with measurements of body density or with isotopic dilution methods, but these are unsuitable for routine use. Alternatively, anthropometry can be utilized for assessing the degree of adiposity. Assessment of skin-fold thickness over various areas of the body together with height, weight, and age can be used to assess the degree of adiposity. Triceps and subscapular skin folds are most commonly employed (see Chap. 72). From a health standpoint, certain patterns of obesity may be less desirable than others. Fat deposition about the waist and flank, as evidenced by a high ratio of waist to hip circumference, is associated with a greater health risk than fat deposition at the hips.

The term *obesity* implies an excess of adipose tissue, but the meaning of *excess* is hard to define. Aesthetic considerations aside, obesity is best defined as any degree of excess adiposity that imparts a health risk. This cutoff between normal and obese can only be approximated, and the health risk imparted by obesity is probably a continuum with increasing adiposity. The Framingham Study demonstrated that a 20 percent excess over desirable weight clearly imparted a health risk. A National Institutes of Health consensus panel on obesity agreed with this definition and concluded that a 20 percent increase in relative weight or a BMI above the 85th percentile for young adults constitutes a health risk; by use of these criteria, 20 to 30 percent of adult men and 30 to 40 percent of adult women are obese, with the highest rates among the poor and minority groups. Significant health risks at lower levels of obesity can occur in the presence of diabetes mellitus, hypertension, heart disease, or other associated risk factors.

The Surgeon General's 1988 report on obesity notes that even mild obesity increases the risk for premature death, diabetes mellitus, hypertension, atherosclerosis, gallbladder disease, and certain types of cancer. In the United States the prevalence of obesity has increased in the past few decades. Because of the frequency of obesity and its health consequences, its prevention and treatment should be a high public health priority.

ETIOLOGY When energy intake exceeds expenditure, the excess calories are stored in adipose tissue, and if this net positive balance is prolonged, obesity results; i.e., there are two components to weight balance, and an abnormality on either side (intake or expenditure) can lead to obesity.

The regulation of eating behavior is incompletely understood. To some extent, appetite is controlled by discrete areas in the hypothalamus: a feeding center in the ventrolateral nucleus of the hypothalamus (VLH) and a satiety center in the ventromedial hypothalamus (VMH). The cerebral cortex receives positive signals from the feeding center that stimulate eating (Fig. 73-1), and the satiety center modulates this process by sending inhibitory impulses to the feeding center. In animals, destruction of the feeding center results in decreased food intake, and destruction of the satiety center leads to overeating and obesity. Several regulatory processes may influence these hypothalamic centers. The satiety center may be activated by the increases in plasma glucose and/or insulin that follow a meal. It is of interest in this regard that the VMH contains insulin receptors and is insulin-sensitive. Meal-induced gastric distention is another possible inhibitory factor. The total adipose tissue mass also may influence the activity of the hypothalamic centers; i.e., there is a relatively fixed "set point" for body adiposity. An elevated set point may account for the frequent recidivism in obese patients who have lost weight. How the "set point" is established and how the hypothalamus senses total fat stores are unknown. Glycerol release from fat cells, ascending neural impulses, and/or circulation of adipocyte-derived peptides such as adipsin may be signals of adipose tissue size. Additionally, the hypothalamic centers are sensitive to catecholamines, and beta-adrenergic stimulation inhibits eating behavior. This provides at least one rationale for the anorexiant effects of amphetamines.

Ultimately, the cerebral cortex controls eating behavior, and impulses from the feeding center to the cerebral cortex are only one

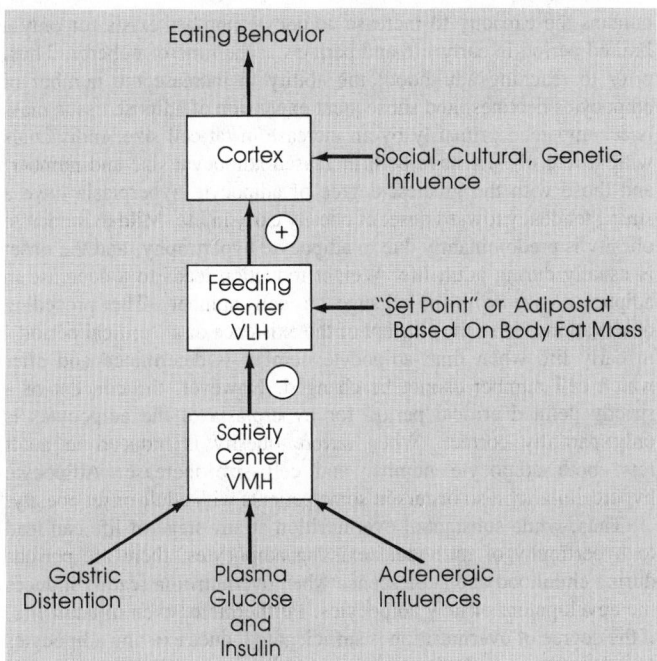

FIGURE 73-1 The regulation of eating. The ventromedial satiety center is considered to be inhibitory, and the ventrolateral feeding center stimulatory. See text for discussion.

input. Psychological, social, and genetic factors also influence food intake. In many obese subjects these influences are overriding; indeed, obese subjects usually respond to external signals such as time of day, social setting, and smell or taste of food to a greater extent than do persons of normal weight.

Although overeating is the usual cause of obesity, other factors may participate. Daily caloric needs normally range between 110 to 130 kJ (27 to 32 kcal) per kilogram of body weight; this figure is higher in active and lower in sedentary individuals. Physical activity clearly modulates overall caloric balance, and obese individuals tend to be less active. This can be a contributory factor in the maintenance of excess weight, but decreased physical activity is unlikely to be an important cause of major weight gain in most obese subjects. Rather, obesity leads to inactivity. The modest increase in weight that often accompanies the middle years may be related more directly to diminished physical activity. Injury or illness may lead to chronic restricted activity and predispose to weight gain unless caloric intake is appropriately curtailed. Perhaps the greatest factor tending to diminish energy output is simply a sedentary life-style.

Decreased caloric expenditure and a metabolic abnormality associated with overefficient caloric utilization also have been postulated as involved in the pathogenesis of obesity. With rare exceptions, major metabolic abnormalities have not been detected in obese individuals, although subtle defects may be undetected. There are three major components to overall energy expenditure: resting metabolic rate, exercise-induced thermogenesis, and the thermic response to food.

The resting metabolic rate accounts for 60 to 75 percent of daily energy expenditure and is measured in a thermoneutral environment while the subject is at rest following an overnight fast and several hours after any significant physical activity. An average resting metabolic rate in a 70-kg man is 6300 kJ (1500 kcal)/d. The resting metabolic rate should be expressed as a function of fat-free body weight (by subtracting the subject's total adipose mass from body weight), since triglyceride mass is metabolically inert in that negligible energy is expended to maintain triglyceride depots. When expressed in this way, the resting metabolic rate is normal in most obese subjects. However, a distinction must be made between static obesity

and the actual process of gaining weight. When normal subjects consume hypercaloric diets, less weight is gained than would be predicted on the basis of the excess calories ingested. This effect is most marked when carbohydrate is consumed and disappears when the excess calories consist of fat. Thus humans can apparently partially adapt to chronic excessive carbohydrate and protein intake, and this protective effect attenuates the weight gain. Part of this adaptive response is related to an increase in thermogenesis manifested as an increase in the resting metabolic rate. The mechanism of adaptive thermogenesis is unknown, but overeating of carbohydrate or mixed nutrients leads to increased plasma levels of triiodothyronine (T_3) and decreased levels of reverse T_3 (rT_3). A converse effect is seen in starvation, with decreased T_3 and increased rT_3 levels. The conversion of thyroxine to T_3 occurs largely in the liver; excess food may induce adaptive thermogenesis by increasing the concentration of T_3 relative to that of T_4 and rT_3. Increased central or peripheral sympathetic outflow leading to increased catecholamine-induced caloric utilization and increased heat production also may play a role in the thermogenic response to overnutrition. Adaptive thermogenesis can lead to a 10 to 15 percent increase in resting metabolic rate, and this effect is seen after a 2- to 3-week period of hypercaloric intake. The rate of onset and the degree of adaptive thermogenesis is the same in obese and nonobese individuals when expressed on the basis of fat-free body mass. Specifically, the increase in resting metabolic rate, changes in thyroid hormone metabolism, and thermic responses to infused catecholamines are similar in normal and obese subjects during periods of overnutrition.

Work performance, or energy expenditure per standard physical work load, can be normal or increased in obesity depending on the kind of work performed. The energy expenditure of exercise is increased in obese compared with lean subjects due to the extra effort involved in moving or supporting an increased body mass. When this effect of increased body mass is taken into account, work performance is normal in obesity. Clearly, normal or increased energy expenditure during physical work cannot contribute to the development of obesity. On the other hand, the total daily energy expenditure due to exercise is less in many sedentary obese subjects simply because they engage in less daily physical activity than their lean counterparts.

The third important aspect of caloric balance is the thermic response to food, so-called dietary thermogenesis. This consists of the heat, or energy, expended above the resting metabolic rate for several hours after the ingestion of a meal. About 75 percent of the thermic response to food is due to the energy cost of digestion, absorption, metabolism, and storage of foodstuffs; the remainder is probably due to activation of the sympathetic nervous system. The heat produced following nutrient ingestion is a form of caloric expenditure and is greater for protein and less for carbohydrate and fat. The thermic response to mixed meals can equal 10 to 15 percent of the calories ingested, and decreased thermic responses have been described in some studies of human obesity. This difference may be due to altered flux rates through different pathways of intermediary metabolism, with more energy-efficient pathways being favored in obesity. As an example, the higher the rate of glucose utilization, the greater the thermic response to carbohydrate-containing meals, and small decreases in the thermic response to food may be due to insulin resistance and decreased glucose disposal in obese subjects. It is clear that small differences in caloric utilization maintained over years can lead to a significant net positive caloric balance. However, while it is tempting to postulate that this decreased thermic response may contribute to obesity, most of the published comparisons have been made between normal persons and subjects who are already obese. Thus the obesity-associated changes in thermic response to food may be secondary to the obese state rather than a primary abnormality. More important, differences in the thermic response to meals between the obese and nonobese are at most in the range of 125 to 210 kJ (30 to 50 kcal) per day. Such minor differences can easily be counterbalanced by minor decreases in food intake and/or increases in exercise-induced thermogenesis. Since such compensation does not occur, it seems more probable that obesity is the result of impaired coupling between caloric intake and expenditure.

Another potential regulatory process in the control of adipose tissue mass involves adipose tissue lipoprotein lipase (ATLPL). This enzyme is synthesized within adipocytes, secreted into the extracellular space, and attaches to the luminal surface of nearby endothelial cells. At this location, ATLPL hydrolyzes fatty acids from the triglycerides of circulating triglyceride-rich lipoproteins. The released fatty acids are taken up by adipocytes, converted to triglycerides, and stored. Thus ATLPL participates in the storage of excess fat calories in adipose tissue. The *lipoprotein lipase hypothesis* holds that in some obese states excessive levels of this enzyme induce obesity by causing preferential deposition of fat calories in adipose tissue. In support of this hypothesis, ATLPL levels are increased in obese rodents and humans. More important, levels of this enzyme do not return to normal following weight reduction. This latter finding is of particular interest because it is one of the few characteristics of the obese state that is not corrected by weight reduction and could explain the propensity of obese patients to regain lost weight.

Environmental, cultural, and genetic influences all contribute to obesity, and in population studies it is impossible to quantitate the separate impact of these factors. Nevertheless, the role of genetics has been demonstrated in studies of twins and adopted siblings. The BMI of adopted individuals correlates better with that of the biologic rather than the adoptive parents. Among biologic and adoptive siblings, there is a genetic influence on the amount and distribution of fat, and similarities are not as close among adopted siblings. Most likely, both nature and nurture contribute to obesity.

SECONDARY OBESITY **Hypothyroidism** Obesity can result from hypothyroidism because of decreased caloric needs. However, only a minority of hypothyroid patients are truly obese, and an even smaller proportion of obese patients are hypothyroid. Indiscriminate use of thyroid hormone in the treatment of obesity is to be deplored and should never be instituted in the absence of decreased thyroid function.

Cushing's disease Cushing's disease is a rare cause of obesity. Hyperadrenocorticism elicits a typical pattern of obesity with predominantly centripetal fat stores, characteristic rounded or moon facies, and cervical or supraclavicular fat deposits.

Insulinoma Hyperinsulinemia, secondary to an insulinoma, can occasionally cause obesity, presumably because of increased caloric intake secondary to recurrent hypoglycemia. Most patients with islet cell tumors and hypoglycemia are not obese.

Hypothalamic disorders Froehlich's syndrome in boys is characterized by obesity and hypogonadotrophic hypogonadism with other variable features such as diabetes insipidus, visual impairment, and mental retardation. The anterior pituitary is usually normal, and the syndrome is thought to be the result of hypothalamic dysfunction. This syndrome likely includes a number of overlapping disorders having in common a hypothalamic lesion that leads to overeating and to hypogonadotrophism. Occasionally, pituitary tumors (as in Froehlich's original case) may physically impair the hypothalamus.

Other rare causes of obesity include the Laurence-Moon-Biedl syndrome, characterized by retinitis pigmentosa, mental retardation, skull deformities, polydactyly, and syndactyly and the Prader-Willi syndrome, which is associated with hypotonia, mental retardation, and a predilection for diabetes mellitus. In both these disorders obesity and hypogonadism are thought to be hypothalamic in origin.

PATHOLOGIC SEQUELAE Increased adipose tissue stores are deposited subcutaneously, around internal organs, throughout the omentum, and in the intramuscular spaces. Obese individuals also have an expansion of lean body mass, as evidenced by increased size of the kidneys, heart, liver, and skeletal muscle mass. Fatty livers are common in extreme obesity.

Adipocyte size and number Attempts have been made to classify obesity on the basis of the relative degree of adipocyte hypertrophy versus hyperplasia. This classification was generated as the result of experimental data indicating that in several rodent species and in humans the capacity to increase adipocyte number exists for only a limited period in early life and perhaps at the time of puberty. Thus, prior to reaching adulthood, the ability to increase the number of adipocytes declines, and subsequent expansion of adipose tissue mass is accompanied primarily by an increase in fat cell size. Individuals with severe obesity have both increased adipocyte size and number, and those with the greatest degree of adipocyte hyperplasia have a strong tendency toward onset of obesity early in life. Mild to moderate obesity is predominantly due to adipocyte hypertrophy, and the onset is usually during adult life. Weight reduction leads to a decrease in adipocyte size with no change in cell number. The preceding observations led to the concept of the existence of a "critical period" in early life when final adipocyte number is determined and after which cell number cannot be changed. However, the concept of a strictly defined critical period for hyperplasia of the adipocytes is only partially correct. When severe obesity is induced in adult rats, both adipocyte number and cell size increase. Adipocyte hypercellularity also occurs in some patients with adult-onset obesity.

Thus, while substantial overnutrition at any stage of life can lead to hypertrophy of individual existing adipocytes, there are periods during childhood and adolescence when overnutrition readily induces the development of new adipocytes. Furthermore, even in adult life, if the degree of overnutrition is sufficient to induce existing adipocytes to enlarge to some limiting size, new adipocytes will form. Whether this latter population of cells represents new cell formation or simply the filling with lipid of previously undetectable preadipocytes formed earlier in life is not known. Regardless of the cause or time of development of increased adiposity (adipocyte hypertrophy with or without hyperplasia), subsequent weight reduction only leads to a decrease in the size of existing adipocytes and not a decrease in adipocyte number. Thus, once a given complement of adipocytes is attained, this number is fixed and cannot be reduced.

METABOLIC SEQUELAE Obesity has a profound impact on diabetes mellitus and on various hyperlipoproteinemic states primarily through its influences on insulin secretion and insulin sensitivity.

Hyperinsulinemia: Insulin resistance Increased insulin secretion is a common feature of obesity. It occurs in the basal state and in response to a wide variety of insulinogenic agents. A correlation exists between the degree of obesity and the magnitude of the hyperinsulinemia—particularly the basal insulin levels. Some obese patients exhibit hyperglycemia or frank diabetes in the face of hyperinsulinemia. The combination of hyper- or euglycemia and hyperinsulinemia indicates an insulin-resistant state, and decreased hypoglycemic responses to insulin are common in obese humans and animals. Insulin resistance could be due to an abnormal beta cell product, circulating insulin antagonists, or tissue insulin insensitivity. Since abnormal islet secretory products or circulating antagonists have not been identified, it is thought that the insulin resistance of obesity is due primarily to tissue insensitivity. The initial step in insulin action involves binding to cell surface receptors in target tissues. Cells from obese animals and humans contain decreased numbers of insulin receptors, and this decrease doubtless plays a role in the insulin resistance. Binding of insulin to the receptor activates the tyrosine kinase activity of the cytoplasmic domain of the receptor, and this kinase activity is important for many, if not all, of insulin actions. While defects in insulin receptor tyrosine kinase activity have been found in several insulin-resistant states, including type II diabetes mellitus, receptor kinase activity is normal in obesity. Thus defects in insulin action distal to the insulin receptor participate in the insulin resistance of obesity. The enlarged adipocytes of obese rats have both a decrease in insulin receptors and an even greater defect in the capacity to metabolize glucose, suggesting a major biochemical abnormality downstream of the receptor mechanism. A similar postreceptor defect presumably exists in other insulin target tissues such as muscle and liver. In the obese human, insulin resistance is due to a combination of receptor and postreceptor defects in insulin action. In those obese patients with the mildest degree of hyperinsulinemia and insulin resistance, the decrease in insulin action is predominantly due to a decreased number of insulin receptors. As the insulin-resistant state worsens, a postreceptor defect emerges, and in obese subjects with the most severe degree of insulin resistance, the postreceptor defect is the predominant abnormality.

Diabetes mellitus (See also Chap. 337) Although only a minority of obese patients are diabetic, the converse is not the case. Non-insulin-dependent, or type II, diabetes comprises about 90 percent of the diabetic population in the United States, and 80 to 90 percent of type II diabetics are obese. Obesity is an important contributory factor to the diabetes in these patients, predominantly through its influences on insulin resistance. Obesity exacerbates the diabetic state, and in many cases diabetes can be ameliorated by weight reduction.

Hyperlipoproteinemia (See also Chap. 344) Most plasma cholesterol circulates in the low-density lipoprotein (LDL) fraction, and in the fasting state, very low density lipoproteins (VLDL) contain most of the circulating triglyceride. The association between obesity and elevated LDL levels is modest at best, especially when the relationship is corrected for factors such as age. Total-body cholesterol is increased in obesity, but this is mainly accounted for by adipose tissue cholesterol stores. Cholesterol turnover may be increased, leading to increased biliary excretion of cholesterol. This may contribute to the increased incidence of gallstone formation. Obesity has a more pronounced effect on VLDL metabolism. Hypertriglyceridemia is frequent, and the degree of obesity correlates with the level of hypertriglyceridemia. The increased triglyceride levels are due to increased hepatic VLDL production with no defect in the removal of VLDL from plasma. As discussed earlier, plasma insulin levels are elevated, particularly in the portal venous blood. Hyperinsulinemia can promote increased hepatic VLDL synthesis and secretion. In addition, increased plasma free fatty acid (FFA) turnover exists in obesity, and FFA extraction by the liver provides an important precursor for hepatic triglyceride synthesis. Thus the hypertriglyceridemia in obesity may be secondary to increased hepatic VLDL secretion due to hyperinsulinemia and augmented FFA availability.

MANIFESTATIONS AND COMPLICATIONS Gross obesity produces mechanical and physical stresses that aggravate or cause a number of disorders, including osteoarthritis (especially of the hips) and sciatica. Varicose veins, thromboembolism, ventral and hiatal hernias, and cholelithiasis are more common.

Hypertension In significantly obese persons, use of the standard size blood pressure cuff leads to erroneously high readings; an oversize cuff should always be used. A strong association between hypertension and obesity is observed even when accurate measurements are obtained. The mechanism by which obesity causes hypertension is uncertain, but peripheral vascular resistance is usually normal while blood volume is increased. Weight loss leads to reductions in systemic blood pressure independent of changes in sodium balance.

Hypoventilation syndrome (pickwickian syndrome) The obesi-ty-hypoventilation syndrome is a heterogeneous group of disorders with differing clinical manifestations. The hypersomnolence that can occur in obesity is a manifestation of nighttime sleep apnea. In these individuals, once sleep begins, upper airway obstruction leads to hypoxemia and hypercapnia, causing arousal with return of normal respiration. Many such episodes occur each night, leading to chronic sleep deprivation and daytime somnolence. The combination of the obese habitus plus sleep-induced relaxation of the pharyngeal musculature is believed to be the cause of the intermittent upper airway obstruction. Occasionally, such episodes are life-threatening (causing serious cardiac arrhythmias) and require long-term tracheos-tomy. Chronic daytime hypoventilation is usually not as severe as that during sleep and may be due to abnormalities of the respiratory control centers. Patients with hypoventilation display blunted ventila-tory responses to hypercapnia and hypoxia and often develop hypercap-nia and hypoxemia due to decreased basal ventilation; in addition, ventilation-perfusion mismatch may result from mechanical factors. In severe cases, polycythemia, pulmonary hypertension, and cor pulmonale can result. Weight reduction will reverse these abnormali-ties if instituted before permanent cardiac damage develops. Some

obese patients with sleep apnea and hypersomnolence do not have daytime hypoventilation and have normal ventilatory responses to hypoxia and hypercapnia. Progestational agents have been used therapeutically in the obesity-hypoventilation syndrome because they stimulate the ventilatory response to hypercapnia and hypoxia in normal subjects. Medroxyprogesterone increases ventilation and im-proves heart failure and erythrocytosis in these patients, although obstructive sleep apnea continues.

Adrenal function Although Cushing's disease can usually be distinguished from simple obesity on clinical grounds, laboratory testing is occasionally necessary. This can lead to confusion, since 24-h urinary 17-hydroxycorticoid excretion is often elevated in obesity. Less commonly, plasma cortisol levels are also increased. Glucocorticoid levels are usually suppressible with dexamethasone in obesity, but occasionally suppression is incomplete, rendering the diagnosis difficult (also see Chap. 335).

Growth hormone Secretory responses of growth hormone to a variety of stimuli such as hypoglycemia, exercise, and arginine infusion are reduced, and the starvation-induced rise in plasma growth hormone levels is attenuated.

Atherosclerosis Obesity is a risk factor for the development of coronary artery disease and stroke. Most of the risk is mediated through the associated hypertension, hyperlipoproteinemia, and diabetes. Nevertheless, even when these abnormalities are factored out, an additional, smaller risk can be ascribed to obesity per se.

TREATMENT Amelioration of hyperinsulinemia, insulin resist-ance, diabetes, hypertension, and hyperlipidemia can occur following weight loss. These changes are significant and enduring provided the weight loss is maintained. During weight loss, all adipose tissue depots diminish proportionately. Sometimes generalized loss does not produce the attractive cosmetic effects desired for those individuals wishing to achieve adipose tissue mass reduction in particular anatomic regions. Many techniques have been proposed to effect selective regional adipose tissue reduction, but none is effective.

Methods of weight reduction When obesity is secondary, the therapy is to treat the underlying disease. Most of the time, primary weight reduction must be undertaken.

Diet Caloric restriction is the cornerstone of weight reduction. For the patient and physician this is a frustrating and demanding undertaking. The basic principles are simple. If food intake is less than energy expenditure, stored calories, predominantly in the form of fat, will be consumed. In general, a deficit of 32,000 kJ (7700 kcal) leads to loss of about 1 kg fat. By estimating the patient's daily caloric needs [approximately 125 to 150 kJ (30 to 35 kcal) per kilogram of body weight], one can calculate the daily deficit necessary to achieve a given rate of weight loss.

Dietary restriction can range from total starvation to mild caloric deprivation, and these approaches will be discussed separately. Dietary recommendations are most effective when they are specific and geared to the patient's life-style. A dietitian or a similarly trained health professional should interview each patient and estimate average daily caloric intake, identify food preferences, and characterize the eating patterns. The amount of calories to be consumed on the restricted diet should be carefully explained in terms of amounts of specific foodstuffs. Frequently, the therapist must balance the degree of restriction against potential noncompliance. The more restrictive the diet, the more rapid is the weight loss, but this often leads to a greater rate of nonadherence. It is preferable to take the individual's needs and motivation into account and design a diet containing a degree of caloric restriction tailored to the patient's ability to comply. Such a diet should produce a consistent and relatively steady rate of weight loss.

Schemes for weight reduction have become a profitable business in the United States, and there are almost as many diets as there are therapists. Each proponent claims that the presence or absence of certain foodstuffs is desirable for more effective weight loss. However, little evidence exists that calorie for calorie one hypocaloric diet leads to greater weight loss than another. The relationship between the patient and the therapist, plus patient education and encouragement, is more important to success than the specific dietary constituents. The major virtue of "fad" diets is that patients are usually motivated to try them, at least initially, and patient cooperation is often better. Provided a particular diet is not harmful, the best course for the therapist is to maintain flexibility in the treatment program. Nevertheless, diets markedly deficient in any major class of foodstuff are to be avoided. For example, whole-food diets that are exceedingly low in carbohydrate are by nature high in fat and, depending on the type and quantity of fat ingested, may lead to hypercholesterolemia. The major virtue of a low-carbohydrate diet is the attendant ketosis (ketone bodies have a central anorexiant effect). This feature provided part of the rationale for the widely touted liquid or powdered protein diets that were previously popular. These diets have been dubbed "protein-sparing modified fasts" and were said to allow drastic long-term caloric restriction without inducing negative nitrogen balance. These claims have not been substantiated, nor has it been shown that the diets lead to a greater degree of true weight loss than mixed diets of equal caloric value. Basically, a calorie is a calorie whether it comes from protein, carbohydrate, or fat. Furthermore, deaths have been reported in otherwise healthy individuals participating in such long-term dietary programs, even under medical supervision. This has been attributed to the fact that some of these early diets contained mostly collagen-derived protein of low biologic value. The newer very low calorie diets involve formula preparations containing 500 to 800 kcal/d, with 50 to 80 g of high-quality protein. The remaining calories consist of carbohydrate and fat. Vitamin and micronutrient supplements are incorporated in the formula or provided as an added supplement. Such high-quality low-calorie diet formulas lead to relatively rapid weight loss but should not be taken continuously as the sole caloric source for more than 6 weeks. In the absence of coexisting diseases such as gout, renal insufficiency, cardiac arrhythmias, etc., such diets are safe when taken under medical supervision. As a general guideline, caloric intake below 800 kcal/d has been taken as the definition of a very low calorie diet (VLCD). Diets providing adequate high-quality protein and greater than 800 kcal/d are referred to as low-calorie diets (LCDs) and are safe in otherwise healthy obese individuals. While very low or low-calorie diets are often effective in achieving rapid and substantial amounts of weight loss, long-term maintenance of weight loss usually requires additive approaches (see below). There are several categories of subjects in whom VLCDs and LCDs are absolutely or relatively contraindicated; these include pregnant women, adolescents, growing children, and patients with significant liver, kidney, and cardiac diseases. In addition, there are conditions in which VLCDs and LCDs should only be used under medical supervision. Examples in this category are gout, diabetic patients taking insulin or oral hypoglycemic agents, preexisting gallbladder disease, and hypertensive patients on antihypertensive drugs.

Prior to therapy it is wise to warn patients that there is usually a marked initial weight loss when caloric restriction is started, in large part due to fluid loss, but such rapid rates of loss will not persist. Likewise, positive shifts in fluid balance can sometimes mask loss of adipose mass, a fact that can sometimes be demonstrated to the patient's satisfaction by recording skin-fold thickness at periodic intervals.

Total-starvation diets have been advocated for the treatment of obesity; provided gout, renal insufficiency, and ketosis-prone diabetes are not present, short-term (2- to 3-day) fasts are usually well tolerated. Ketonemia and hyperuricemia regularly develop during starvation but rarely lead to acidosis or gout. Because of these potential complications, total fasting should be carried out only under medical supervision. Probably the major usefulness of total fasting is as a motivational aid at the beginning of a dietary program or when weight loss has stopped. Even though much of the weight loss during short-term fasting represents fluid, this weight loss can be encouraging to frustrated patients and motivate them to improve compliance with the long-term weight reduction program.

The major problem in the treatment of obesity is not weight reduction but maintenance of the reduced weight. Provided the therapist works hard and long enough, most motivated patients can eventually lose weight. Unfortunately, only the rare patient maintains the weight loss permanently. Obesity is an eating disorder, and the underlying mechanisms are not reversed by limiting food intake.

Behavior modification   In recognition of the problems involved, the techniques of behavior modification have been applied to treat abnormal patterns of eating behavior. Many studies demonstrate that obese individuals respond less well than normal individuals to internal cues that regulate eating behavior such as gastric contractions, fear, and previous food ingestion. Conversely, obese subjects overrespond to external cues such as taste, smell, food attractiveness, food abundance, and the ease of obtaining food. Given the fact that the obese individual is unusually susceptible to external stimuli, food intake may be altered by changing the pattern and nature of these external cues, and this is the major premise underlying the behavior modification approach to weight reduction.

Behavior modification begins with a detailed individual history of the patient's eating patterns with respect to time of day, length of eating period, place of ingestion (restaurant, dining table, standing in front of open refrigerator), simultaneous activities (watching television, reading, idleness), emotional state, companions (relatives, friends, or alone), and finally the kinds and quantities of foods ingested. Once this detailed record is obtained, the therapist and patient can design specific behavioral changes aimed at disrupting or aborting recurring behavior patterns which initiate or prolong abnormal eating activity. As examples: if a patient eats in response to certain emotional states, then other activities can be substituted when the patient perceives such a state; if the patient snacks frequently from readily available food storage areas (refrigerators, cookie jars, etc.), then he or she is encouraged to eat only while sitting down at a table with a fixed place setting; if eating frequently occurs while watching television alone, then efforts to avoid this activity can be initiated. Results with behavior modification techniques indicate that many patients can maintain long-term weight reduction providing the new behavior patterns are truly "learned."

Exercise   Exercise has a place in any weight reduction program. However, the importance of exercise in terms of caloric balance must be clearly understood. Even moderate daily exercise would not lead to a large enough increase in energy expenditure to alter significantly the initial rate of weight reduction (Table 73-1). This does not mean that exercise is unimportant in weight reduction, since even modest increases in caloric expenditure can lead to large long-term differences in caloric balance, provided exercise is performed on a regular basis. For example, a daily increase in caloric expenditure of 1250 kJ (300 kcal) over a period of 4 months could lead to a 4.5-kg weight loss. More important, incorporation of regular exercise into the overall weight reduction program improves the chances that the weight loss will be maintained.

Drugs   Two classes of drugs are frequently used in the treatment of obesity: anorexiants and thyroid hormone. The addition of levothyroxine or liothyronine to a weight reduction program is ineffective in promoting adipose tissue loss and, if anything, accentuates lean tissue loss and causes negative nitrogen balance. Cardiotoxicity may occur. Thus, unless hypothyroidism is clear-cut, thyroid supplementation has no role in the treatment of obesity.

The major anorexiants are amphetamine-like agents that presumably exert their effect at the level of the hypothalamus. They probably have a modest effect in promoting short-term weight loss in some individuals. However, they are effective only for short periods, and problems of habituation, addiction, and drug abuse limit their usefulness. Two anorexiants, diethylpropion and fenfluramine, may be less addictive and, therefore, somewhat more useful. However, none of these agents treats the underlying eating disorder, and they are of little use in maintenance of weight reduction.

Injections of human chorionic gonadotropin (hCG) have been tried as an adjunct to weight reduction, but no evidence exists to indicate

TABLE 73-1 Energy equivalents of food calories expressed in minutes of activity

Food	Energy value, kJ (kcal)	Walking*	Riding bicycle†	Swimming‡	Running§	Reclining¶
Apple, large	422 (101)	19	12	9	5	78
Bacon, 2 strips	401 (96)	18	12	9	5	74
Beer, 1 glass	477 (114)	22	14	10	6	88
Bread and butter	326 (78)	15	10	7	4	60
Carbonated beverage, 1 glass	444 (106)	20	13	9	5	82
Carrot, raw	176 (42)	8	5	4	2	32
Cheese, cottage, 1 tbsp	113 (27)	5	3	2	1	21
Chicken, fried, ½ breast	971 (232)	45	28	21	12	178
Cookie, chocolate chip	213 (51)	10	6	5	3	39
Egg, fried	460 (110)	21	13	10	6	85
Ham, 2 slices	699 (167)	32	20	15	9	128
Ice cream, ⅛ qt	808 (193)	37	24	17	10	148
Mayonnaise, 1 tbsp	385 (92)	18	11	8	5	71
Milk, skim, 1 glass	339 (81)	16	10	7	4	62
Milk shake	1762 (421)	81	51	38	22	324
Orange, medium	285 (68)	13	8	6	4	52
Pancake with syrup	519 (124)	24	15	11	6	95
Peas, green, ½ cup	234 (56)	11	7	5	3	43
Pizza, cheese, ¼	753 (180)	35	22	16	9	138
Potato chips, 1 serving	462 (108)	21	13	10	6	83
Sandwiches:						
Hamburger	1456 (350)	67	43	31	18	269
Tuna fish salad	1163 (278)	53	34	25	14	214
Sherbet, ⅛ qt	741 (177)	34	22	16	9	136

* Energy cost of walking for 70-kg individual = 22 kJ (5.2 kcal)/min.
† Energy cost of riding bicycle = 34 kJ (8.2 kcal)/min.
‡ Energy cost of swimming = 47 kJ (11.2 kcal)/min.
§ Energy cost of running = 81 kJ (19.4 kcal)/min.
¶ Energy cost of reclining = 5 kJ (1.3 kcal)/min.

a beneficial effect. The primary effectiveness of the hCG-diet program is due to the caloric restriction, frequent physician contact, and placebo effects. Comparable weight loss is achieved if saline injections are substituted for hCG, suggesting a placebo effect of parenteral injection.

Jejunoileal shunt Small-bowel bypass is an effective means of achieving weight reduction in morbidly obese patients. However, it is an experimental procedure and should be attempted only in institutions where a trained team is committed to regular, systematic, and long-term follow-up. Because of accompanying morbidity and mortality, most such institutions have abandoned this form of surgery in favor of the more benign and effective gastric plication or bypass approach described below.

The most common operative procedures for the jejunoileal bypass involve end-to-end or end-to-side anastomosis of about 38 cm of proximal jejunum to 10 cm of terminal ileum. Weight loss is initially rapid, reaching a plateau at 18 to 24 months. The mean weight loss is about 30 to 50 percent of initial excess weight, leaving patients still about 50 percent overweight once a steady state is reached. Although some malabsorption occurs, the major portion of the weight loss is due to decreased food intake.

Teams still performing this surgery select patients who are at least 50 kg overweight and in whom adequate attempts at medical management have failed repeatedly. Because of postoperative morbidity, older (>50 years) and psychologically unstable individuals are usually excluded.

The overall surgical mortality ranges from 0.5 to 7.8 percent, with an average of around 4 percent. Mortality is inversely related to the experience of the surgical team. The major postoperative morbidity is related to wound infection and thromboembolism. The common serious complications are cirrhosis and hepatic failure, nephrolithiasis, electrolyte imbalances, cholelithiasis, and arthritis (Table 73-2). Severe liver disease probably occurs in 5 percent of patients, and mild hepatic dysfunction is more common. The long-range implications of mild hepatic abnormalities are unknown. Possible causes of liver damage following small-bowel bypass include (1) protein and particularly essential amino acid deficiency, (2) accumula-

tion of hepatotoxic secondary bile salts, and (3) release of unknown toxic substances from the excluded bowel. Hypokalemia is likely secondary to diarrhea. Persistent deficiency of calcium and magnesium can result from malabsorption and must be treated with appropriate replacement. Transient depression of plasma 25-hydroxyvitamin D

TABLE 73-2 Complications of ileal bypass surgery

Complication	Percentage
EARLY	
Perioperative mortality	2–6
Thromboembolic disease	1–5
Wound infection	2–5
Renal failure	3
Severe nausea, vomiting	3
Wound dehiscence	1–3
LATE	
Urinary calculi	3–10
Severe electrolyte imbalance	5–8
Acute cholecystitis	0–5
Progressive liver disease	2–4
Intestinal obstruction	2
Peptic ulcer	1–2
Osteoporosis	?
Tuberculosis	1
MINOR	
Diarrhea	100
Weakness	80
Hypokalemia	80
Hypoproteinemia	50
Vomiting	50
Thirst	50
Hypocalcemia	30
Arthralgias	15
Incisional hernias	3
Hyperuricemia	<10
Anemias	<10

levels also may contribute to abnormal mineral metabolism. Nephrolithiasis occurs in up to 30 percent of patients and is due to hyperoxaluria secondary to calcium malabsorption. It can be treated by calcium supplements and a low oxalate intake. Migratory polyarthritis occurs in up to 6 percent of patients and may be due to circulating immune complexes. This operation is now rarely performed, in part due to the decision of many insurance companies not to pay for the procedure.

Gastric surgery   Gastroplasty establishes a small upper gastric remnant connected to a larger lower gastric pouch by a narrow 1- to 1.5-cm channel. Gastric bypass excludes the lower 90 percent of the stomach pouch and maintains intestinal continuity of the upper 10 percent via a retrocolic gastrojejunostomy. Both these procedures cause patients to limit food intake by delaying gastric emptying and providing a small gastric reservoir so that fullness is experienced after a small meal. Weight loss with these procedures is comparable with that achieved with small-bowel bypass operations but without malabsorption, diarrhea, and hepatic dysfunction. The procedure can be reversed if a decision to restore normal anatomy is made at a later time. At institutions with a large experience with this procedure, operative mortality and morbidity are low, the efficacy is good, and weight loss is relatively long lasting. This surgical approach should only be considered in morbidly obese individuals who have failed repeated attempts at weight management through other means.

SUMMARY   For most patients, obesity is an eating disorder, and a major hope for effective long-term treatment of this disease lies in understanding the causes of overeating. No single etiology explains all cases, and different causes exist for different individuals. At present, a variety of techniques are available to effect initial weight loss. Unfortunately, initial weight loss is not the real therapeutic goal. Rather, the problem is that most obese patients eventually regain their weight. Once obesity occurs, it is a lifelong, chronic illness requiring continuous treatment, even if successful weight loss has occurred. An effective means to sustain weight loss is the major challenge in the treatment of obesity today. The technique of behavioral modification, when professionally and rigorously applied and coupled with an appropriate exercise regimen, is the best tool for this task. As information develops concerning the hypothalamic "set point," or *adipostat*, and the factors that regulate it, other therapies may emerge that will effect long-term correction of abnormal eating patterns.

REFERENCES

BRAY GA: Obesity: An endocrine perspective, in *Endocrinology*, 2d ed, LJ DeGroot et al (eds). Philadelphia, Saunders, 1989, p 2303
———: Obesity: Basic aspects and clinical implications. Med Clin North Am 73:1, 1989
——— et al: Treatment of obesity. Diabetes Metab Rev 4:653, 1988
CARO JF: Clinical review 26: Insulin resistance in obese and nonobese man. J Clin Endocrinol Metab 73:691, 1991
FOSTER DW: Eating disorders: Obesity and anorexia nervosa, in *Williams' Textbook of Endocrinology*, 8th ed, JD Wilson, DW Foster (eds). Philadelphia, Saunders, 1992, p 1335
HENRY RR et al: Metabolic consequences of very low calorie diet therapy in obese non-insulin-dependent diabetic and non-diabetic subjects. Diabetes 35:155, 1986
HIRSCH J et al: Clinical review 28: A biological basis for human obesity. J Clin Endocrinol Metab 73:1153, 1991
KOLTERMAN OG et al: Mechanisms of insulin resistance in human obesity: Evidence for receptor and postreceptor defects. J Clin Invest 65:1272, 1980
NATIONAL INSTITUTES OF HEALTH CONSENSUS DEVELOPMENT PANEL: Gastrointestinal surgery for severe obesity. Ann Intern Med 115:956, 1991
NATIONAL INSTITUTES OF HEALTH CONSENSUS DEVELOPMENT PANEL: Health implications of obesity. Ann Intern Med 103:147, 1985
RAVUSSIN E et al: A brief overview of human energy metabolism and its relationship to essential obesity. Am J Clin Nutr 55:242S, 1992
STUNKARD AJ et al: An adoption study of human obesity. N Engl J Med 314:193, 1984
The Surgeon General's Report on Nutrition and Health, US Department of Health and Human Services Public Health Service (DHHS PHS) Publication 88-50210, 1988
WADDEN TA et al: Treatment of obesity by very low calorie diet, behavior therapy and their combination: A five-year perspective. Int J Obesity 13:39, 1989
WOO R et al: Regulation of energy balance, in *Annual Review of Nutrition*, vol. 5. Palo Alto, Calif., Annual Reviews, Inc, 1985, pp 411–433

74   ANOREXIA NERVOSA AND BULIMIA

DANIEL W. FOSTER

Anorexia nervosa and bulimia are eating disorders in young, previously healthy women who develop a paralyzing fear of becoming fat. The population at risk consists largely of white women from middle-class backgrounds. The disorders rarely occur in black or oriental women, in the poor, or in men. The driving force is the pursuit of thinness, all other aspects of life being secondary. In anorexia nervosa this aim is achieved primarily by radical restriction of caloric intake, the end result being emaciation. In bulimia massive binge eating is followed by vomiting and excessive use of laxatives. Weight loss in bulimic subjects is not great despite the obsession with food. Some authors consider anorexia nervosa and bulimia to be distinct illnesses, while others classify bulimia as a variant of anorexia nervosa. Overlap syndromes exist since emaciated patients fulfilling the criteria of true anorexia nervosa may exhibit bulimic behavior, subjects with bulimia often pass through a phase of anorexia. In this chapter it is assumed that the two disorders are different expressions of a psychologic obsession with body weight.

PREVALENCE   Estimates of prevalence for anorexia nervosa range from 0.4 to 1.5 per 100,000 population. In adolescent white girls from middle- or upper-class families rates as high as 1 per 100 have been reported. Prevalence is believed to be increasing. Subclinical variants may occur in up to 5 percent of the group at highest risk. The incidence of bulimia is less certain. Vomiting after eating may occur in as many as 18 percent of women college students. The frequency of self-induced vomiting is probably 1 to 2 percent, but full-blown bulimia is less frequent.

DIAGNOSIS   The diagnosis of both anorexia nervosa and bulimia is made on clinical grounds. No specific diagnostic tests exist. For many years the criteria of Feighner et al. were standard (Table 74-1). These criteria included both psychological and clinical/physical components. Revised criteria in the American Psychiatric Association's *Diagnostic and Statistical Manual of Mental Disorders, Third Edition, Revised* (DSM-IIIR) focus on the psychological components of the illnesses. "Softening" of the criteria allows inclusion of subjects that do not yet have a full blown eating disorder but who clearly have abnormal eating patterns.

In the revised criteria the weight loss required for diagnosis was decreased from 25 to 15 percent of expected or ideal weight. Three other features include intense fear of gaining weight or becoming fat even when underweight; disturbance in the way body weight, size, or shape is experienced such that the individual "feels fat"; and, in women, either primary amenorrhea or secondary amenorrhea for at least three consecutive periods. The Feighner criteria remain useful, although it seems reasonable to substitute the 15 percent figure for weight loss. Since the spectrum of restricted eating ranges from a mild disorder of little consequence to life-threatening starvation, neither set of criteria is definitive.

The diagnostic value of the disturbance in body image in patients with eating disorders has been questioned, and some authorities have recommended its omission on the grounds that many normal young women demonstrate the same perceptual distortion. In practice a presumptive diagnosis of anorexia nervosa is justified if the following elements are elicited: (1) a history of major weight loss; (2) absence of organic disease to account for weight loss; (3) absence of severe primary psychiatric illness that might account for failure to eat; (4) extreme restriction of food intake with or without intermittent induction of vomiting; (5) ritualized exercise; and (6) denial of hunger, fatigue, or emaciation. While there is an emphasis on the absence of organic disease to cause weight loss, anorexia nervosa may coexist with other disease that can cause loss of weight, for example, insulin-dependent diabetes mellitus. Late-onset disease is also now recognized although usually symptoms begin in the teen years or early adulthood.

TABLE 74-1   Diagnostic criteria for anorexia nervosa and bulimia nervosa

Anorexia nervosa		Bulimia nervosa
Feighner et al.	DSM-IIIR	DSM-IIIR

1 Onset prior to age 25.
 2 Anorexia with weight loss of at least 25% of original body weight.
 3 Distorted attitude toward eating, food, or weight that overrides hunger, admonitions, reassurances, and threats.
 4 No known medical illness that could account for the weight loss.
 5 No other known psychiatric disorder.
 6 At least two of the following manifestations:
   a Amenorrhea
   b Lanugo hair
   c Bradycardia (persistent resting pulse of 60 beats per minute or less)
   d Periods of overactivity
   e Episodes of bulimia
   f Vomiting (may be self-induced)
	1 Refusal to maintain body weight over a minimal normal weight for age and height, e.g., weight loss leading to maintenance of body weight 15% below that expected; or failure to make expected weight gain during period of growth, leading to body weight 15% below that expected.
	 2 Intense fear of gaining weight or becoming fat, even though underweight.
	 3 Disturbance in the way in which one's body weight, size, or shape is experienced, e.g. the person claims to "feel fat" even when emaciated, believes that one area of the body is "too fat" even when obviously underweight.
	 4 In women, absence of at least three consecutive menstrual cycles when otherwise expected to occur (primary or secondary amenorrhea). A woman is considered to have amenorrhea if periods occur only following hormone, e.g. estrogen, administration.
		1 Recurrent episodes of binge eating (rapid consumption of a large amount of food in a discrete period of time).
		 2 A feeling of lack of control over eating behavior during the eating binges.
		 3 The person regularly engages in either self-induced vomiting, use of laxatives or diuretics, strict dieting or fasting, or vigorous exercise to prevent weight gain.
		 4 At least two binge-eating episodes a week for at least 3 months.
		 5 Persistent overconcern with body shape and weight.

SOURCE: JP Feighner et al: American Psychiatric Association: Diagnostic and Statistical Manual of Mental Disorders, Third Edition, Revised. American Psychiatric Association, Washington D.C. 1987

The criteria for the diagnosis of bulimia in DSM-IIIR are also given in Table 74-1. The picture is that of a normal- or near-normal-weight subject whose life is dominated by gorging and regurgitation in the absence of profound weight loss.

ETIOLOGY   The cause is unknown. Although primary dysfunction of the hypothalamus has been postulated, the associated hypothalamic abnormalities revert to normal with weight gain and thus are secondary rather than causal.

Most investigators favor a psychiatric etiology, but there is disagreement about its nature. One view holds that the disorders begin in response to inadequate or destructive interpersonal relationships in families that are goal-oriented and highly achieving. Despite an outward appearance of normality, interpersonal communication within the family tends to be inadequate, frequently following a pattern in which the father seeks success in his work while the mother turns to her children for fulfillment and in the process becomes overdirective. It is often stated that the families are "enmeshed," meaning that generational boundaries are blurred and that parents and children are constantly involved in each other's problems. Psychoanalytic interpretation tends to focus on anorexia as a mechanism whereby the patient reestablishes control of her own life independent of parental direction. It is not clear how this sequence might cause the intense fear of being fat that is the central feature of both anorexia and bulimia.

Although the absence of serious psychiatric disease is a common criterion for diagnosis (Table 74-1), it is now widely held that depression plays a significant role in the eating disorders, especially in bulimia. Abnormalities of neurotransmitter concentrations have been reported in blood and cerebrospinal fluid, but such changes are inconsistent and are likely secondary rather than primary.

Cultural issues are also important in anorexia nervosa. The quest for health and slimness is a powerful force in modern western society and may reinforce the fear of fatness in patients with established anorexia or tip the borderline case into full-blown disease. Occupation may play a role; dancers, for example, have a prevalence of anorexia nervosa 10 times that of the general population. Likewise athletes, particularly runners, often seek to decrease body fat to very low levels (5 to 7 percent). Thus far no genetic component has been identified. Whatever the mechanism(s) involved, the behavioral response is obsessive and is difficult to treat.

CLINICAL PICTURE   While anorexia nervosa and bulimia may coexist in the same patient, the clinical pictures are ordinarily distinct (Table 74-2).

Anorexia nervosa   The anorexia nervosa syndrome usually begins before or shortly after puberty but may appear later (usually by the middle twenties). Many patients were overweight in childhood. Emaciation is equivalent to that seen in the concentration camp victims of World War II. Despite profound weight loss patients deny hunger, thinness, or fatigue. They are often physically active, and ritualized exercise is common. Frenzied calisthenics or running may follow food intake. There is a preoccupation with food, and elaborate meals may be prepared for others. If social circumstances require them to eat more than usual, vomiting is induced as soon as possible, often in a public restroom. As noted, episodic binge eating may occur and is also followed by emesis. Amenorrhea usually accompanies or follows weight loss but may appear prior to any physical change. Constipation and cold intolerance are common. The latter is presumably due to a defect in regulatory thermogenesis secondary to hypothalamic dysfunction.

In advanced cases bradycardia, hypothermia, and hypotension are present. Body fat is undetectable, and the bones protrude through the

TABLE 74-2   The eating disorders

	Anorexia nervosa	Bulimia
Predominant sex	Female	Female
Method of weight control	Restriction of intake	Vomiting
Binge eating	Uncommon	Invariant
Weight at diagnosis	Markedly decreased	Near normal
Ritualized exercise	Usual	Rare
Amenorrhea	100%	50%
Antisocial behavior	Rare	Frequent
Cardiovascular changes (bradycardia, hypotension)	Common	Uncommon
Skin changes (hirsutism, dryness, carotenemia)	Usual	Rare
Hypothermia	Usual	Rare
Edema	+/−	+/−
Medical complications	Hypokalemia, cardiac arrhythmias	Hypokalemia, cardiac arrhythmias, aspiration of gastric contents, esophageal or gastric rupture

NOTE: These features are characteristic of pure anorexia nervosa and pure bulimia. Overlap syndromes occur, and anorexia may evolve to bulimia (the bulimia → anorexia transformation is rare).

skin. Interestingly, breast tissue is often preserved. The skin may be dry and scaly and is often yellow due to carotenemia (particularly visible in the palms). Body hair is often increased; it is usually of fine, lanugo quality, but frank hirsutism may occur. Parotid glands may be enlarged as in other forms of starvation. Mitral valve prolapse is due to valve–ventricular volume mismatch secondary to starvation-induced decrease in left ventricular volume. Edema in the absence of hypoalbuminemia is thought to be due to failure of extracellular fluid volume to diminish proportionately with body mass during weight loss. Because of edema in the legs and parotid enlargement, which gives a fullness to the face, the true state of emaciation may be masked when the patient is fully dressed.

Laboratory abnormalities include anemia and leukopenia (with hypocellularity of the bone marrow), hypokalemia, and hypoalbuminemia. Serum β-carotene levels tend to be elevated. Prerenal azotemia may occur if vomiting or laxative use are prominent. The blood urea nitrogen may be as high as 21 to 25 mmol/L (60 to 70 mg/dL). Renal concentrating ability is impaired, possibly due to blunted responsiveness to vasopressin. Release of vasopressin in response to an osmotic stimulus is also abnormal. Plasma cholesterol is occasionally high, but triglyceride levels are not increased despite low activities of hepatic and lipoprotein lipases. Glucose tolerance is abnormal as in other forms of starvation.

Miscellaneous abnormalities include low levels of IgG, IgM, and a variety of complement proteins. Despite these findings immune function is generally preserved, and serious infections are rare. Plasma iron and ceruloplasmin are normal, but iron binding capacity is decreased. Serum zinc and copper are decreased, but concentrations of these metals are normal in hair. Serum amylase may be increased in the absence of pancreatitis.

Basal levels of luteinizing hormone (LH) and follicle-stimulating hormone (FSH) are low when weight loss is severe, and the LH response to luteinizing hormone–releasing hormone (LHRH) is impaired. FSH response to LHRH is normal, although time to peak increase may be delayed. Studies of the 24-h circadian pattern of LH secretion show regression of the mature stage to the pattern characteristic of prepubertal or early pubertal girls; i.e., episodic LH release is missing or occurs only during sleep. These findings presumably account, at least in part, for the amenorrhea. Menses return with weight gain, although the weight required for reinitiation of menstruation may be somewhat higher (about 10 percent) than that needed for the original induction of menarche. Ovulatory menses may be induced in subjects with anorexia nervosa by prolonged treatment with LHRH agonists, suggesting that pituitary gonadotropin release is impaired because of hypothalamic dysfunction. Prolactin levels are normal. Plasma estradiol levels are low, but plasma testosterone is in the normal female range. Testosterone levels are low in men with anorexia nervosa.

Growth hormone (GH) in the basal state may be normal or elevated. A rise in GH occurs after injection of thyrotropin-releasing hormone (TRH), as in other states with elevated basal levels of GH such as acromegaly, uremia, and protein-calorie malnutrition. Insulin-like growth factor I (somatomedin C) concentrations are low and may contribute to growth hormone elevation via diminished negative feedback. Plasma cortisol levels are high due to increased secretion of corticotropin-releasing hormone from the hypothalamus. The cortisol negative feedback mechanism in the hypothalamus is believed to be impaired. Dexamethasone suppression tests may be abnormal. Norepinephrine concentrations in plasma are depressed.

Thyroxine (T_4) levels are in the low-normal range; free T_4 is normal. Triiodothyronine (T_3) concentrations are reduced, while reverse T_3 (rT_3) levels are increased. Basal levels of thyroid-stimulating hormone (TSH) are usually normal, and TSH response to TRH is intact. The primary defect in thyroid hormone metabolism is decreased activity of the 5′-deiodinase that converts T_4 to T_3 and rT_3 to diiodothyronine in nonthyroidal tissues. These changes are characteristic of starvation and wasting diseases and are not specific for anorexia nervosa.

Bone density is decreased in women with anorexia nervosa. The mechanism is thought to be estrogen deficiency. Cortisol excess may contribute.

Bulimia Bulimia, which means "ox-hunger," refers to the episodic ingestion of large amounts of food in a compulsive fashion, coupled with awareness that the eating pattern is abnormal, a fear that eating cannot be stopped voluntarily, and feelings of depression at completion of the act. Bulimics have a morbid fear of becoming fat. While binge eating may occur in several types of emotional disorders, many patients give a history of overt or cryptic anorexia nervosa, suggesting that bulimia is a variant of anorexia nervosa. Episodes of binge eating are followed by induced vomiting, with or without the subsequent ingestion of laxatives. Initially vomiting is induced by placing a toothbrush or fingers in the throat, but eventually most patients learn to vomit reflexly.

Binge eating generally occurs daily in the active phase; in 40 patients the mean number of episodes per week was 12, ranging from 1 to 46. The duration of the eating period averaged 1.2 h but could last as long as 8 h. The amount of food ingested may be enormous, up to 200,000 kJ (50,000 kcal). High-carbohydrate foods are favored, and more than one food is usually eaten. The order of frequency in one report was: ice cream→bread→candy→doughnuts→soft drinks. The term "dietary chaos" describes the eating pattern. Because of the high sugar content of the diet, dental caries are frequent.

Other behavioral abnormalities are common. Secrecy about the eating-vomiting sequence is characteristic so that family and friends are often unaware. Stealing is common, and food is the item most often taken. There is a high rate of alcohol and drug abuse. Depression tends to be more severe than in anorexia nervosa, making suicide a definite risk. Hysterical behavior may occur. Families of patients with bulimia have a higher incidence of affective disorders, alcoholism, and illicit drug use than in families of patients with anorexia nervosa.

Despite the close relationship with anorexia nervosa, a number of differences are noted. While many patients with bulimia are thin, emaciation is not seen; generally weight is within 15 percent of the normal range as defined by life insurance tables of ideal weight. Fluctuating weight is common, with cyclical gains and losses. Some patients are modestly overweight. In contrast to anorexia nervosa, many patients continue to menstruate and may become pregnant. Persistent menstruation probably reflects the absence of extreme weight loss. Sexual activity is greater in bulimic subjects than in those with anorexia.

The physical findings are usually minimal, although more extensive weight loss may cause some of the changes seen with anorexia nervosa.

The most common laboratory abnormality is hypokalemia with metabolic alkalosis secondary to vomiting and laxative use. Endocrine abnormalities are similar to those in anorexia nervosa. One study suggested that LH response to LHRH is exaggerated in bulimic patients. It has been reported that peptide YY, a putative stimulant of feeding behavior in animals, is elevated in the cerebrospinal fluid of bulimic patients. Some also have deficient secretion of serotonin and cholecystokinin, thought to be satiety signals. The significance of these findings is not known. Dexamethasone suppression is frequently abnormal. Unlike patients with anorexia nervosa, some women with bulimia have low basal prolactin levels and an exaggerated prolactin response to TRH. Serum amylase may be elevated in the absence of pancreatitis in both anorexia and bulimia.

COMPLICATIONS Patients with anorexia nervosa are vulnerable to sudden death from ventricular tachyarrhythmias. Electrocardiograms show prolonged QT intervals. The risk of death becomes high when weight loss reaches 35 percent below ideal, probably because of protein deficiency. (Since there is no reserve store of protein, critical enzymes and cellular structures are affected by starvation-induced decreases in lean body mass; see Chap. 72.) Major complications include aspiration, esophageal or gastric rupture, pneumomediastinum, hypokalemia with cardiac arrhythmias, pancreatitis, and ipecac-induced myopathy and/or cardiomyopathy.

PROGNOSIS The course of anorexia nervosa is variable. In long-term follow-up about half of patients achieve normal weight, 20 percent improve but remain underweight, 20 percent continue anorexic, 5 percent become obese, and 6 percent die. Even when weight gain occurs, signs of persistent illness remain since intermittent dieting, binge eating, vomiting, and laxative use persist in up to two-thirds of patients. Death is usually due to starvation (cardiac arrhythmias primarily) or suicide. Poor prognostic signs include older age of onset, longer duration of illness, history of bulimia or vomiting, extreme weight loss, and presence of significant depression. Fewer reports of long-term follow-up are available for bulimia. Because the psychiatric disturbance tends to be more severe (suicide occurs at higher rates) and because the medical dangers of gorging are greater, prognosis is believed to be worse in bulimia than in anorexia. One report indicates that 40 percent of treated patients remained bulimic after 18 months of treatment and that relapse occurred in 65 percent after 1 year of recovery.

TREATMENT There is no specific treatment for anorexia nervosa or bulimia. The intense fear of becoming fat coupled with a perceptual disturbance that causes overestimation of body size results in powerful resistance to therapy. The benefits of psychiatric intervention are marginal. The same can be said of behavior modification techniques and for group and family therapy. Supportive care by an understanding physician may accomplish as much as formal psychotherapy. The patient should be seen regularly for a review of weight change, diet, and exercise patterns. It is often useful to establish a mutually agreeable explicit contract; e.g., if the patient weighs 65 pounds and ideal body weight determined from life insurance tables is 115 pounds, a goal of 90 pounds might be set as a first stage. At every visit the patient should be reassured by the physician that "we will not let you get fat." A calm but realistic review of the dangers of starvation, including sudden death, should be given, coupled with statements like "my job is to help you deal with this illness so that you can have a normal life expectancy with reasonable happiness." The physician must be perceived not as an enemy or a parental surrogate but an advisor and partner in the struggle.

A similar approach should also be used with bulimic patients. Even if the gorging-regurgitation cycle cannot be stopped, the lesser goal of limiting the load of food ingested (to minimize the chance of aspiration or gastric rupture) and decreasing the frequency of events may be achieved. Because depression and antisocial behavior are more common in bulimia, psychiatric therapy is usually required. Drug therapy appears to be of little use in anorexia nervosa although fluoxetine may help in preventing relapse in patients responding to behavior modification strategies. Antidepressant therapy appears to be superior to placebo in the treatment of bulemia nervosa. Potassium supplementation may be required for vomiters.

Hospitalization may be a lifesaving measure with severe anorexia nervosa. As noted above, sudden death may occur at weights more than 35 percent below ideal, particularly if weight loss has been rapid. Hypokalemia, hypotension, and prerenal azotemia due to volume depletion are other indications for hospitalization. A nasogastric tube may be required, but it is better to persuade the patient to eat. Supervision of every meal is initially required, ideally by the same person. During hospitalization the patient should never be allowed to eat alone. Total parenteral nutrition is rarely indicated. Instruction about nutrition, occupational therapy, group work with the family, and individual psychotherapy should be included in the treatment plan. The "safety" of eating and assurances that obesity will not result should be emphasized repetitively. Some specialists feel that all seriously affected anorexia patients benefit from initial hospitalization, but this is not a universal view. Hospitalization for bulimic subjects is normally only required for medical complications (e.g., aspiration).

Treatment of the anorexia-bulimia syndrome is a long-term proposition, rife with failure, and requires perseverance by the subject, family, and physician.

REFERENCES

FEIGHNER JP et al: Diagnostic criteria for use in psychiatric research. Arch Gen Psychiatry 26:57, 1972

FOSTER DW: Eating disorders: Obesity, anorexia nervosa and bulimia nervosa in *Williams Textbook of Endocrinology*, 8th ed, JD Wilson, DW Foster (eds). Philadelphia, Saunders, 1992, pp 1335–1365

HERZOG DB, COPELAND PM: Eating disorders. N Engl J Med 313:295, 1985

HERZOG DB et al: The course and outcome of bulimia nervosa. J Clin Psychiatry supp. 52:4, 1991

ISNER JM et al: Anorexia nervosa and sudden death. Ann Intern Med 102:49, 1985

KAYE WH, WELTZIN TE: Neurochemistry of bulimia nervosa. J Clin Psychiatry supp. 52:21, 1991

LEVY AB: Neuroendocrine profile in bulimia nervosa. Biol Psychiatry 25:98, 1989

———— et al: How are depression and bulimia related? Am J Psychiatry 146:162, 1989

LOVE L, GOLD PW: The hypothalamic-pituitary-adrenal axis in anorexia nervosa and bulimia nervosa: Pathophysiologic implications. Adv Pediatr 38:287, 1991

LUCAS AR et al: Anorexia nervosa in Rochester, Minnesota: A 45-year study. Mayo Clin Proc 63:433, 1988

MITCHELL JE et al: Medical complications and medical management of bulimia. Ann Intern Med 107:71, 1987

NEWMAN MM, HALMI KA: The endocrinology of anorexia nervosa and bulimia nervosa. Endocrin Metab Clin North Am 17:195, 1988

WALSH BT, DEVLIN MJ: The pharmacological treatment of eating disorders. Psychiatr Clin N Amer 15:149, 1992

75 DIET THERAPY

JOHANNA T. DWYER / JODI ROY

The primary aims of diet therapy are to prevent or treat malnutrition, control diet-related manifestations of disease, delay progression of chronic disease, and provide support for other medical or surgical treatments. Diet therapy also plays an important role in rehabilitation and in palliation, e.g., maintaining or enhancing the quality of life in the terminally ill. Dietary advice is useful for health promotion, disease prevention, nutritional support, and rehabilitation. Nutrition therapy may involve slight modifications of usual food intakes, use of special purpose oral supplements, or feeding by enteral or parenteral routes.

Four principles guide sound diet therapy. First a nutrition-related problem must be present for which an accepted dietary therapy exists. Second, the diet therapy must be based on a solid scientific rationale. Ideally, documentation of the effectiveness of the therapeutic diet in ameliorating symptoms, slowing progression, lessening secondary problems or offering other positive effects on function should be available. Anecdotal evidence alone is insufficient to warrant diet therapy. Third, the patient must be able and willing to eat and must have a functional gastrointestinal tract. (For patients who require parenteral or enteral nutrition therapy, see Chap. 76.) Finally, the patient must adhere to the diet. Little effort is required for a patient to consume a diet in the hospital since appropriate meals are served and no other food choice may be available, but a great deal of motivation is needed to prepare and eat therapeutic diets after discharge.

PLANNING DIET THERAPY

ASSESSMENT Dietary assessment attempts to discover what is eaten. It requires cataloguing what the individual usually eats and the nutritional quality and adequacy of that pattern. It also helps determine nutritional status, establishes or refines differential diagnoses, and furnishes the background information on food intakes and preferences that are needed for implementing diet therapy. Nutritional status assessment (Chap. 72) measures the interaction of diet, disease, and nutrition requirements by integrating information on food intake and clinical, biochemical and anthropometric measurements. Both dietary assessment and nutritional status assessment are needed to identify nutrition-related problems and plan therapeutic diets.

Dietary assessment can be performed at qualitative or quantitative levels. Qualitative assessment involves determining (1) whether the patient is currently eating and following a specific diet, and if so, the number of meals per day, any use of nutritional supplements (e.g., amounts and types of vitamin or mineral supplements), special dietary preferences or dietary practices (e.g., consumption of only one or a few foods), or medications that may influence nutritional status; (2) whether there has been recent weight loss or gain; (3) the physical state (e.g., chewing problems, dysphagia, diarrhea, ability to shop, cook and feed oneself); and (4) social circumstances that may influence intake (e.g., economic resources, social isolation, social support systems). If the qualitative assessment suggests that nutritional problems may exist, more quantitative approaches may be in order. For example, a complete record of all food intake (less uneaten food) and its ability to meet nutrient needs can be ordered if the patient is hospitalized. For outpatients, current dietary intake (e.g., the past day) can be catalogued using 24-h recalls. The patient is asked to describe what was consumed over the past 24 h, starting with the last meal eaten. Intake is then assessed by comparing it to a food grouping system or by calculating the nutrient contributions of each food from a table of food composition, and comparing the adequacy of nutrients with the Recommended Dietary Allowances or some other criteria of desirable food intake. Computer programs are now available for performing these analyses. This method is easy to administer, places little burden on the patient, and provides some estimate of intakes. However, one day may not be long enough to provide a truly representative intake, so habitual diet may not be assessed. If assessment of nutritional status is to be meaningful, dietary intake data must reflect a period of weeks or months. If changes in intake have occurred, it may also be helpful to probe previous intakes before the illness or other events that might have caused dietary alteration.

The habitual diet is assessed with either semiquantitative food frequency questionnaires, using a standardized list of foods and portion sizes, or the periodic collection of food records for several days at a time. Semiquantitative food frequency questionnaires can be analyzed on a computer. Food records are better for identifying the intake of unusual foods not included on food frequency questionnaires, but records are more difficult to obtain and analyze. Other methods for dietary assessment include the dietary history, in which the patient provides information on usual intakes in an interview with a dietitian. In skilled hands this can reveal dietary patterns quickly and is less burdensome to the patient than keeping food records, but training and time are required to interview in a reproducible manner.

PRESCRIPTION A diet prescription or diet order that specifies the dietary modifications needed for nutritional therapy is the first step in nutritional intervention. It is usually brief, stated in terms of the additional assessment needed, the disease to be treated, and the modifications to deal with the disease. The physician is also responsible for making appropriate changes in diet orders. Failure to make changes can result in such unfortunate events as keeping patients indefinitely on nutritionally inadequate "clear liquid" diets with resulting debilitation and/or delayed healing.

The rendering of nutrition care requires knowledge about food composition, dietary assessment, diet planning, and diet counseling techniques. In acute care and inpatient settings, the diet order is translated by dietitians into actual foods, menus, or eating plans acceptable to the patient. In outpatient settings, the physician may counsel patients directly, or they may be referred to dietitians.

CARE PLAN A nutrition care plan is then formulated for the implementation of the diet. The individual who undertakes diet therapy must record the nutritional care plan in the medical record and supervise its implementation. The care plan should include a summary of the needs uncovered during the assessment and an implementation plan for achieving nutritional objectives including additional resources needed, such as assistance in purchasing food, help with eating (if necessary) and any follow up plans for counseling

TABLE 75-1 Modifications in diet consistency

Consistency	Purpose	Use	Nutritional adequacy	Comments
Clear liquid: clear broth, gelatin, popsicles, ices; sugar, honey, hard candy; clear fruit juices; clear coffee, tea, and carbonated beverages (as tolerated); low-residue, high-protein, high-calorie clear oral supplements.	Short term (1–2 days preferably): to supply fluid and some energy [2500 kJ/d (600 kcal/d)] in a form that requires minimal digestion after surgery, trauma, or in acute illness.	Initial feeding after surgery or IV feeding to relieve thirst and hydrate, while minimizing the need to chew and GI-tract stimulation.	Falls seriously short of nutrient needs in energy, protein, vitamins, and minerals; if this diet is to continue beyond 3–5 days, nutritional support is necessary.	Produces few or no feces; greatly different from usual diets.
Full liquid: clear liquids plus: all milk and milk drinks, yogurt; vegetable and fruit juices; refined cooked cereals; butter, margarine; custard, ice cream, pudding; high-protein, high-calorie oral supplements.	Supply fluid and meet energy and other nutrient needs more completely with foods that are liquid at body temperature; usually higher in calories than clear liquid diet.	Transition between clear liquid and solid foods after surgery and in acute illness; in esophageal or stomach disorders with strictures or anatomical irregularity; and for inability to chew or swallow solid foods.	May be inadequate in niacin, folacin, and iron due to lack of meat, whole grain, and vegetable intake; adequacy may be improved using high-protein, high-calorie supplements or the addition of a multivitamin supplement.	More complete diet than clear liquid; beneficial as a transitional feeding for weak patients who cannot adequately chew food; greatly different from usual diets.
Soft	Provide foods that can be swallowed with little or no chewing.	For patients who are alert or acutely ill with difficulty in chewing/swallowing, or who are too ill or weak to tolerate a usual diet; for head and neck surgical patients; those with esophageal strictures or poor dentition. Also useful for those with inflammatory ulceration, neurologic changes, or anatomic alterations.	Can be adequate in all nutrients based on menu selection. Oral nutritional supplements may be helpful as well.	Textures can range from pureed (blenderized, strained, or smooth foods) to ground, chopped, or soft solids.

and nutrition education. Special attention should be directed to easing the transition from special routes of feeding back to usual oral routes. Plans for review, follow-up, and evaluation of progress should also be specified.

IMPLEMENTING DIET THERAPY

USUAL INTAKE The starting point for planning therapeutic diets is the patient's usual intake. The fewer the changes from usual intake, the greater the likelihood that individual preferences will be met and that the new eating plan will be followed. If the usual intake is not nutritionally adequate, the therapeutic plan includes modifications to ensure nutritional sufficiency.

MODIFICATIONS Therapeutic diets can involve three basic alterations: modifications in food constituents, consistency, and route of feeding (see Chap. 76). The appropriate diet for a given condition depends on the stage or severity of disease, characteristics of the patient (age, sex, educational level, ethnicity), the treatment environment (e.g., inpatient, outpatient), and the social situation. For example, there are many diets for patients with diabetes mellitus, depending on individual needs such as whether the patient is on insulin, whether there is a need for weight reduction, and coexisting medical complications (such as hyperlipidemia, hypertension, or renal disease).

Additional considerations must be taken into account. The first is to meet the recommended dietary allowances (RDAs) for nutrients (see Table 71-4). The second is to deal with relevant medical concerns (such as ease of swallowing in a stroke patient or the timing of feeding in a patient with insulin-dependent diabetes mellitus), patient food preferences, and drug-nutrient interactions. Diet manuals in individual hospitals specify the diets available.

CONSISTENCY (See Table 75-1) Variations in consistency usually involve two factors. The first is liquidity; major categories are clear liquid, full liquid, and soft. The form and nature of the ingredients constitute the second factor. Options include common foods that have been chopped and blenderized, commercial nutritional supplements formulated with ingredients not usually available in the home, and "elemental diets" using nutrients in simple forms such as protein hydrolysates or amino acids. In general, the commercial products are more appetizing because they use stabilizers and other means to keep particles in suspension and because they are more palatable.

Nutritional adequacy and palatability must be considered in plans that alter consistency. Clear liquid diets are nutritionally inadequate and include only a few foods that most people eat regularly, but they may be necessary immediately after surgery or during severe medical emergencies. Full liquid diets include more foods and may be nutritionally adequate but are limited in choice compared to normal diets. Soft diets are also limited in terms of palatability. For these reasons, modifications in consistency should only be used when necessary and for as limited a time as feasible.

CONSTITUENTS (See Table 75-2) Modifications in the composition of diets may include energy level, type and amount of nutrients (e.g., lactose-free; low fat, low saturated fat), or type and amount of other constituents (e.g., 30-g soluble fiber, 300-mg cholesterol; low oxalate). Other therapeutic regimens are described in standard textbooks.

Several points need emphasis in planning alterations in dietary composition: First, the supporting evidence and documentation of

TABLE 75-2 Dietary modifications in various diseases

Therapeutic diet modification	Disease	Known benefit(s)	Possible benefit(s)
ENERGY			
Energy controlled	Diabetes mellitus	Increased glucose tolerance, decreased acute side effects	Decreased long-term complications (large vessel atherosclerosis, nephropathy, hypertension)
Low energy	Obesity	Weight loss	
	Hypertension	Decreased systolic and diastolic blood pressure	
	Non-insulin dependent diabetes mellitus	Increased glucose tolerance, decreased short-term symptoms	Decreased long-term complications
High energy	Anorexia, emaciation	Increased weight, lean body mass, and fat; promotes normal fat and lean tissue	
Small feedings	Gastroesophageal reflux	Decreased gastric volume, decreased likelihood of reflux (small feedings in an upright position)	
ENERGY-YIELDING NUTRIENTS			
Carbohydrate			
Low simple sugar	Postgastrectomy to prevent dumping syndrome (with low liquids) and to control symptoms due to lactose intolerance, sucrase or lactase deficiency, or other inborn errors of sugar absorption	Controls symptoms	
High carbohydrate (65–70% kcal)	When undertaken a week or so before event, increases muscle glycogen stores and energy reserves for endurance activities	May increase athletic performance by increasing energy reserves in muscle during long sustained activity in athletic events	
Protein			
Low protein	Chronic renal failure (end stage renal disease)	Control of blood urea nitrogen, electrolytes, and phosphorus levels (amino acid supplements are used)	
	Hepatic encephalopathy	Prevention of hepatic encephalopathy	
	Early chronic progressive renal insufficiency Nephrotic syndrome		Decreased decline in glomerular filtration rate Decreased protein wasting

(continued)

TABLE 75-2 Dietary modifications in various diseases *(continued)*

Therapeutic diet modification	Disease	Known benefit(s)	Possible benefit(s)
ENERGY-YIELDING NUTRIENTS			
Fat			
Low fat	Steatorrhea, radiation enteritis, Gastroesophageal reflux	Decreased malabsorption Increased lower esophageal sphincter pressure	
	Acute hepatic, pancreatic, and gall bladder disease	Decreased need for bile salts	
	Crohn's disease	Decreased malabsorption in patients with functional lactase deficiency	
	Postgastrostomy dumping	Decreased malabsorption in patients with functional lactase deficiency	
	Colon, prostate, and breast cancers		Reduced risks in promotion stage via hormone actions
	Hyperlipidemia	Reduced serum lipids	
Low fat, low saturated fat, low cholesterol	Coronary heart disease	Reduced serum lipids	Some arterial plaques regress (if diet is extreme and long continued)
OTHER DIETARY ALTERATIONS			
Low sodium	Hypertension	Decreased blood-pressure in salt-sensitive persons	
	Congestive heart failure	Decreased sodium retention, reducing hypertension	
	Chronic renal failure	Decreased sodium retention, reducing hypertension	
	Ascites	Decreased sodium retention	
Low potassium	Hyperkalemia	Decreased serum potassium	
	Chronic renal failure	Decreased serum potassium	
High potassium	Hypokalemia	Increased serum potassium	
High calcium	Osteoporosis		Risk reduction in postmenopausal women
Low phosphorus	Hyperphosphatemia	Decreased serum phosphorus	
	Renal failure	Decreased serum phosphorus	
Low oxalate	Oxalate kidney stones	Decreased concentration of oxalate in the urine	
	Crohn's disease	Decreased malabsorption in patients with steatorrhea	
High fiber	Hyperlipidemia	Decreased serum cholesterol (if high water-soluble fiber or oat gum)	
Low fiber	Crohn's disease, inflammatory bowel disease, regional enteritis, ulcerative colitis (active phase)	Reduced diarrhea and pain	
	Crohn's disease (inactive phase)		Symptom control
Low fiber, low residue	Postoperative transition poststomy, diverticulitis, active inflammatory bowel disease, or other conditions with narrowed or stenosed colon	Symptom control and reduces total post-digestive luminal contents, decrease in fecal output	Unproved if diet improves gut healing
Sulfite restricted	Prevents adverse reactions such as asthma, hives, and anaphylaxis in sulfite sensitive persons	Decreases symptoms	
Phenylalanine restricted	Prevents adverse metabolic effects among persons with phenylketonuria or hyperphenylalaninemia	Decreases symptoms and reduces ill effects on mental function in children, and reduces fetal levels in utero of affected mothers	
Tyramine controlled	Prevents reactions from consumption of foods with tyramine and other amines while receiving monoamine oxidase inhibitor therapy	Reduces symptoms	
Purine restricted diet	Decreases elevated blood and urinary uric acid levels in patients with gout, urinary calculi, etc. when used in conjunction with other drug and diet therapy.	Other measures, such as drug therapy, weight reduction, limited alcohol intake, and control of hypertriglyceridemia also recommended if this is used	Not always required but may help to reduce drug doses
Gluten-free, gliadin free	Celiac disease	Decreased malabsorption and gut damage due to improved absorption	

benefits for therapeutic diets vary in their completeness (Table 75-2). For some diseases, such as the hyperlipidemias, the role of diet modification in decreasing serum cholesterol and risk of coronary artery disease is well documented. For other diseases, such as diabetes mellitus, diet can control acute and short-term complications, but the efficacy for long term sequelae, such as retinopathy and kidney disease, is not established. Patients need to be informed as to what can be expected from the diet instituted.

Second, changes both in consistency and in composition may be required. For example, simultaneous modifications in a number of constituents are mandatory in patients with diabetes mellitus and renal failure. Such a patient may require an eating plan that controls energy intake, type and amount of carbohydrate, timing of carbohydrate intake, amount of dietary fiber, and the content of fat, protein, and sodium. In some cases, there are so many constraints that priority ranking must be given to the important alterations. With other

TABLE 75-3 Recommendations of American Heart Association/National Cholesterol Education Program: step 1 (with PBR*) and step 2 diets for hypercholesterolemia

Indications
 LDL cholesterol >4.1 mmol/L (>160 mg/dL)
 LDL cholesterol >3.4 mmol/L (>130 mg/dL) with definite coronary disease or two other risk factors[†]

Minimal goals
 Without coronary disease or two risk factors: Lower LDL cholesterol below 4.1 mmol/L (150 mg/dL)
 With coronary disease or two risk factors: Lower LDL cholesterol below 3.4 mmol/L (130 mg/dL)

Recommended intake	% of total kilocalories	
	Step 1 diet and PBR* for persons of age >2 y	Step 2 diet (if serum lipid goal not reached)
Total fat	<30%	<25%
Saturated fatty acids	<10%	< 7%
Polyunsaturated fatty acids	<10%	<10%
Monounsaturated fatty acids	10–15%	10–15%
Carbohydrates	50–60%	50–60%
Protein	10–20%	10–20%
Cholesterol	<300 mg/d	<200 mg/d
Total energy intake	To achieve and maintain desirable weight	To achieve and maintain desirable weight

* Population Based Recommendations.
† Risk factors include male sex, family history of premature coronary distress, cigarette smoking, hypertension, low HDL cholesterol level, diabetes mellitus, history of definite cerebrovascular or occlusive peripheral vascular disease, severe obesity.
NOTE: LDL = low-density lipoprotein; HDL = high-density lipoprotein.
SOURCE: Adapted from National Cholesterol Education Program: Arch Intern Med 148:36, 1988; and National Cholesterol Education Program: *Report of the Expert Panel on Population Strategies for Blood Cholesterol Reduction*, U.S. Department of Health and Human Services, Public Health Service, National Institutes of Health, Bethesda MD, 1990.

TABLE 75-4 Nutritional goals for patients with diabetes mellitus

Energy intake: achieve and maintain a reasonable body weight
Carbohydrate: (1) up to 55–60% of total energy; (2) substitute unrefined complex carbohydrates high in fiber for highly refined carbohydrates; (3) modest amounts of sucrose and other refined sugars are acceptable depending on metabolic control; (4) individualization is important
Protein: no lower than the RDA for adults of 0.8 g/kg of ideal body weight, or approximately 12–20% of total calories, but further modifications and individualization may be needed for pregnancy, lactation, in aging, and in presence of renal complications.
Total fat: ideally <30% total calories from fat, with no more than 10% saturates, up to 10% polyunsaturated, and remainder from monounsaturated fatty acids
Dietary cholesterol: <300 mg/d
Fiber: up to 40 g/d recommended, with 25g/4200 kJ (100 kcal) calories if individual is on a low calorie diet
Sodium intake: <3000 mg/d, but may need further restrictions in presence of renal or other medical complications
Alcohol use: limit to 1–2 alcohol equivalents once or twice a week
Vitamins and minerals: at levels specified in Recommended Dietary Allowances
Alcohol: if at all, in moderation
Alternative sweeteners: nutritive and nonnutritive sweeteners both acceptable in moderation
Meal timing: in insulin-dependent diabetes, meal timing and size may need to be adjusted depending on type of insulin used, physical activity, sick days, and other factors
Other: presence of nephropathy, atherosclerosis, or high blood pressure may require further modifications

SOURCE: Modified and adapted from American Diabetes Association, Position statement: Nutritional recommendations and principles for individuals with diabetes mellitus. Diabetes Care 10:126, 1987; and Beebe CA: Kilocalorie and nutrient controlled diet for diabetes, in *Handbook of Clinical Dietetics*, 2d ed, American Dietetic Association 1992, pp 405–427.

modifications, less precision is acceptable. Otherwise, it may be impractical to implement diet therapy.

Third, modifications in nutrient composition may be necessary to meet physiologic needs (infancy, puberty, pregnancy, lactation, aging). Factors to be taken into account include inadequacies in recent intake, the timing of nutrient intake (as in insulin-dependent diabetes mellitus), and the presence of specific food allergies or intolerances (e.g., patients on monoamine oxidase inhibitors). Other problems, include inability to feed oneself, vegetarianism, religious beliefs that prohibit certain foods, alcoholism, and specific likes and dislikes.

Fourth, elaborate diet prescriptions place a burden on patients. Complicated diets may cause only minor problems in the hospitalized patients but create major compliance problems for outpatients. When

TABLE 75-5 Exchange list for meal planning for diabetics

Exchange list food group	Carbohydrate, grams	Protein, grams	Fat, grams	Energy intake, kilojoules (kilocalories)
Starch/bread 120 mL (½ cup) cereal, grain, or pasta 30 g (1 oz) of a bread product	15	3	Trace	335 (80)
Meat 30 g (1 oz) cooked				
Lean	—	7	3	230 (55)
Medium-fat	—	7	5	315 (75)
High-fat	—	7	8	415 (100)
Vegetable 120 mL (½ cup) cooked or juice 240 mL (1 cup) raw	5	2	—	105 (25)
Fruit 120 mL (½ cup) fresh or juice 60 mL (¼ cup) dried	15	—	—	250 (60)
Milk 240 mL (1 cup)				375 (90)
Skim	12	8	Trace	500 (120)
Low-fat	12	8	5	625 (150)
Whole	12	8	8	
Fat 5 mL butter, margarine, oil, mayonnaise (1 tsp.) 15 mL salad dressing (1 Tbsp.)	—	—	5	190 (45)

NOTE: Saturated fat, fiber and sodium intakes are controlled by choices within food groups
SOURCE: American Diabetes Association and the American Dietetic Association: *Exchange Lists for Meal Planning*, 1986.

the continuation of such diets is necessary, diet counseling prior to discharge should be supplemented by frequent outpatient visits.

Even within a given disease category, the role of dietary therapy may vary, and there may be no single "therapeutic diet" for a given disease. Rather, the appropriate dietary measures depend on symptoms and other manifestations of the disease.

Modifications for hypercholesterolemia   The associations between diet and levels of serum cholesterol are well documented and, at least in men, predictable, and the association between lowering of serum cholesterol and decreases in the complications of coronary artery disease is clear-cut. Hence, diet therapy is the first step in the treatment of most hyperlipidemic states. Table 75-3 summarizes the current recommendations for diet therapy of those adults at high risk [(e.g., total serum cholesterol >6.2 mmol/L (<240 mg/dL)] jointly endorsed by the National Cholesterol Education Program (NCEP) and the American Heart Association and includes the indications for diet therapy in terms of the individual's serum lipid values (see also Chaps. 208 and 344).

The NCEP recommends a "step-care" approach in dealing with hyperlipidemia. Patients at risk are first placed on the step 1 diet (unless they are at very high risk), which is modified in total fat, saturated fat, cholesterol, and energy intake. After a period of 2 months the serum cholesterol is evaluated. Those who, despite adherence, do not achieve the goals of therapy on the step 1 diet are asked to continue the diet trial and are provided with additional assistance. Patients whose serum cholesterol is still not within acceptable levels are moved to the step 2 diet, which is even lower in saturated fat and cholesterol. If serum cholesterol levels are still not reduced sufficiently, drug therapy is added. Hyperlipidemic patients may also have hypertension, diabetes mellitus, chronic renal insufficiency, or other diseases that require additional dietary modifications.

Modifications for diabetes mellitus   Table 75-4 outlines the nutritional recommendations for individuals with diabetes mellitus, and Table 75-5 summarizes a widely used tool—the exchange list. Exchange lists describe the serving size of various foods in groups that are similar in nutrient value. Exchange lists vary depending on the disease and the desired dietary modifications. Such lists provide an overall meal plan that allows selection of different foods and menus. However, the type and amount of dietary carbohydrate and fat and the energy intake ingested throughout the day need to be considered in planning the diet, drug administration schedule, and physical activity patterns. Diet therapy in diabetes is helpful in controlling the acute manifestations (excessive thirst, frequent urination, blurred vision, etc.) of hyperglycemia and may reduce the risk of accelerated atherosclerosis.

Alterations in dietary fiber   Modifications in the type and amount of dietary fiber can sometimes ameliorate functional constipation or diarrhea. Increased dietary fiber intakes, particularly of water-insoluble fibers like wheat bran, also provide symptomatic relief in diverticulosis of the colon. Some water-soluble fibers in large doses may decrease serum cholesterol levels; these include fiber derived from oat bran, beans, and psyllium seeds.

Lactose-free diets   Many adults, especially Orientals, blacks, and Ashkenazic Jews, have hereditary lactase deficiency. Lactose intolerance may also be secondary, either acquired or as a result of

TABLE 75-6   Rich food sources of vitamins

Vitamin	Alternative names	Richest sources
Vitamin A (plus carotenoids)	Retinol (vitamin A alcohol)	Liver, egg yolk, chicken meat; whole milk, butter; breakfast cereals and margarines fortified with vitamin A
Carotenoids	β-Carotene (most plentiful)	Dark-green leafy vegetables like spinach, chard; deep-yellow vegetables like carrots, squash; yellow fruits like mango, cantaloupe
Vitamin D	D_3 (cholecalciferol) D_2 (ergocalciferol)	Fatty fish like salmon and fish oils; eggs; butter; liver; milk fortified with vitamin D
Vitamin E	Alpha tocopherol	Oils from soybean, sunflower, corn, and cottonseed; germ of whole grains; fish liver oils; nuts
Thiamine	Vitamin B_1	Whole grains, dried legumes; pork muscle, liver; products made with enriched flour
Riboflavin	Vitamin B_2	Milk and milk products; eggs; whole- and enriched-grain products; lean meat, liver, poultry, fish; dark-green vegetables like spinach, asparagus
Niacin	Nicotinic Acid	Meats, poultry, fish; yeast; whole- and enriched-grain products; legumes; nuts; in addition, some of the tryptophan present in meats, poultry, fish, cheese, legumes, and seeds can be converted in the body to niacin
Vitamin B_6	Pyridoxine Pyridoxal Pyridoxamine	Meat, poultry, fish; bananas; yeast; bran; nuts
Vitamin B_{12}	Cobalamin	Only in foods of animal origin: liver, muscle meat, fish, eggs, and milk and milk products
Folacin	Folic Acid Folate	Liver; dark-green leafy vegetables like spinach, romaine lettuce; dried beans, peanuts, wheat germ, whole grains; yeast
Vitamin C	Ascorbic Acid	Citrus fruits like oranges, lemons, grapefruit; dark-green leafy vegetables like broccoli, asparagus

SOURCE: National Academy of Sciences Committee on Diet and Health: *Diet and Health: Recommendations to Reduce Chronic Disease Risk*, National Academy Press, Washington, 1989.

TABLE 75-7   Rich food sources of minerals

Mineral	Sources
Calcium	Milk, cheese, broccoli, dark-green leafy vegetables such as collard, turnip, and mustard greens
Phosphorus	Meat, milk products, grains, phosphate, food additives
Magnesium	Green vegetables, nuts, seeds, dried beans, whole grains, and meat
Iron	Liver, red meat, whole-grain and enriched-grain products, beans, nuts, and dark-green leafy vegetables
Zinc	Shellfish, meat, poultry, cheese, whole grains, dried beans, nuts
Copper	Crab meat, fresh vegetables and fruits, nuts, seeds, legumes
Sodium	Salt (sodium chloride); cured meats (ham, bacon, sausage, frankfurters, luncheon meats); cheeses; olives; pickles; condiment sauces; frozen and canned meat and fish entrees and dinners; canned and dried soups; commercial pasta, noodle, and potato dishes; salted snacks; commercial mixes for waffles, muffins, and cakes; canned vegetables with sauces; baking powder; baking soda; certain emulsifiers and other food additives; drinking water; drugs such as some antacids
Potassium	Milk, fruits (especially oranges, prunes, apples, pears, peaches, bananas, and grapefruit), vegetables (especially fresh broccoli, carrots, tomatoes, and potatoes), fish, shellfish, turkey, chicken, and cooked oatmeal

SOURCE: National Academy of Sciences Committee on Diet and Health: *Diet and Health: Recommendations to Reduce Chronic Disease Risk*, National Academy Press, Washington, 1989.

gastrointestinal disease. Elimination of lactose from the diet reduces the diarrhea due to the osmotic action of unabsorbed lactose in the gut lumen (see Chap. 254).

Gluten-free diets Gluten, a protein found primarily in wheat products, produces a toxic reaction causing villous atrophy in patients with sprue or celiac disease. Elimination of gluten from diet requires substitution of gluten-poor foods, e.g., rice or potato (Chap. 254).

Caffeine restriction Caffeine can cause untoward behavioral effects in large doses (e.g., 1000 mg or more, the equivalent of 10 cups of coffee a day, and in some individuals at lower doses). Some patients with reflux esophagitis, hypermotility syndrome, and peptic ulcer disease may also benefit from reducing or eliminating caffeine from the diet.

Questionable dietary remedies Many legitimate therapeutic diets exist in addition to those mentioned in Table 75-2. However, not all popular dietary remedies are documented to be useful. For example, there is no evidence that special diets have any role in alleviating or treating premenstrual syndrome, hyperactivity, fibrocystic disease of the breast, or acne; that a polyunsaturated fat diet is beneficial for multiple sclerosis; or that a macrobiotic diet is useful in patients with cancer.

HOW DIETARY CHANGES ARE ACHIEVED Dietary change is achieved by altering the amount and frequency of food consumption. Nutrients are not equally distributed throughout all foods. Tables 75-6 and 75-7 list food sources rich in selected vitamins and minerals.

Substitutions within food groups can alter diet composition. For example, using skimmed milk instead of whole milk lowers the amount of fat but does not alter its contribution of other nutrients (protein, calcium, and phosphorus). Lean cuts of meat, skinned chicken, and lean fish contain less fat than fried meats but have the same content of protein, vitamins, and minerals.

When many simultaneous reductions must be made in nutrient intakes, development of a reasonable eating plan can be time-consuming and difficult. Computerized menu planning systems or use of simplified exchanges' and menu-planning guides may be helpful in some circumstances. However, for most physicians the best first step is to consult a dietitian.

ORAL NUTRITIONAL SUPPLEMENTS WITH SPECIAL CHARACTERISTICS Diets to meet therapeutic needs may utilize readily available foods, but flexibility is enhanced by the use of specially formulated dietary products (Table 75-8). These products can be of great help in planning menus that are palatable and that permit some

TABLE 75-8 Nutrient composition of oral nutritional supplements

	Manufacturer	kJ/mL	kcal/mL	Percent of energy Protein	Fat	Carbohydrate	Comments
CLEAR LIQUID FORMULAS							
Citrotein	Sandoz Nutrition	2.8	0.66	25	2	73	
Ross SLD (surgical liquid diet)	Ross	2.9	0.70	21	1	78	
FULL LIQUID FORMULAS							
Milk-based formulas							
Carnation Instant Breakfast	Carnation Company	4.4	1.06	21	27	52	
Meritene Liquid	Sandoz Nutrition	4.0	0.96	24	30	46	
Meritene Powder	Sandoz Nutrition	4.4	1.06	26	29	45	
Sustacal Nutritional Powder	Mead Johnson	5.4	1.30	23	23	54	
Sustagen	Mead Johnson	7.7	1.85	24	8	68	
Blenderized formulas							
Compleat Modified Formula	Sandoz Nutrition	4.5	1.07	16	31	53	Lactose-free; gluten-free
Compleat Regular Formula	Sandoz Nutrition	4.5	1.07	16	36	48	
Vitaneed	Sherwood Medical	4.2	1.00	16	35	49	Lactose-free
Formulas with fiber							
Enrich	Ross	4.6	1.10	14	29	57	Lactose-free; 14 g fiber per L
Sustacal with Fiber	Mead Johnson	4.4	1.06	17	29	54	Lactose-free; 5 g fiber per L
Jevity	Ross	4.4	1.06	16	30	54	Isotonic,* lactose-free; 14 g fiber per L
Nutren 1.0 with Fiber	Clinitec Nutrition Co.	4.2	1.0	16	33	51	Lactose free, 14 g fiber per L
Ultracal	Mead Johnson	4.2	1.06	17	37	46	Lactose free, 14 g fiber per L
Fibersource	Sandoz	4.4	1.20	14	30	56	Lactose free, 10 g fiber per L
Fibersource HN	Sandoz	5.0	1.20	18	30	52	Lactose free, 7 g fiber per L
Profiber	Sherwood	4.2	1.0	16	36	48	Lactose free, 12 g fiber per L
Newtrition Isofiber	OBrien/KMI	5.0	1.20	17	30	53	Lactose free, 14 g fiber per L
Lactose-free formulas							
Ensure	Ross	4.4	1.06	14	31	55	Low-residue*
Resource Plus Liquid	Sandoz Nutrition	6.2	1.50	15	32	53	Gluten-free; low-residue
Sustacal Liquid	Mead Johnson	4.2	1.01	24	20	56	Low-residue
Travasorb MCT Diet	Clinitec Nutrition Co.	6.7	1.60	20	30	50	
Resource Instant Crystals	Sandoz Nutrition	4.4	1.06	14	31	55	Low-residue
Resource Liquid	Sandoz Nutrition	4.4	1.06	14	31	55	Gluten-free; low-residue
Comply	Sherwood Medical	6.2	1.50	16	36	48	
Ensure Plus	Ross	6.2	1.50	15	32	53	Low-residue
Sustacal HC	Mead Johnson	6.4	1.52	16	34	50	Low-residue
Ensure Plus HN	Ross	6.2	1.50	17	30	53	Low-residue
Isocal HCN	Mead Johnson	8.4	2.00	15	45	40	
Magnacal	Sherwood Medical	8.4	2.00	14	36	50	Low-residue
Two Cal HN	Ross	8.4	2.00	17	40	43	

(continued)

TABLE 75-8   Nutrient composition of oral nutritional supplements (continued)

	Manufacturer	kJ/mL	kcal/mL	Percent of energy			Comments
				Protein	Fat	Carbohydrate	

FULL LIQUID FORMULAS (continued)

Isotonic formulas*

Attain	Sherwood Medical	4.2	1.00	16	30	54	Lactose-free; low-residue
Osmolite	Ross	4.4	1.06	14	32	54	Lactose-free; low-residue
Precision Isotonic Diet	Sandoz Nutrition	4.0	0.96	12	28	60	Lactose-free; gluten-free
Isocal	Mead Johnson	4.4	1.06	13	37	50	Lactose-free; low-residue; gluten-free
Isosource	Sandoz Nutrition	5.2	1.20	14	30	56	Lactose-free; low-residue
Isotein HN	Sandoz Nutrition	5.0	1.20	23	25	52	Lactose-free; low-residue; gluten-free
Isosource HN	Sandoz Nutrition	5.4	1.20	18	30	52	High-nitrogen; isotonic; lactose-free; gluten-free; low-residue
Nutren 1.0	Clinitec Nutrition Co.	4.2	1.0	16	33	51	
Nutren 1.5	Clinitec Nutrition Co.	6.2	1.5	16	39	45	
Nutren 2.0	Clinitec Nutrition Co.	8.4	2.0	16	45	39	
Replete	Clinitec Nutrition Co.	4.2	1.0	25	30	45	
NEntrition	Clinitec Nutrition Co.	4.2	1.0	14	31	55	
Newtrition	O'Brien/KMI	4.4	1.06	15	32	54	
Osmolite HN	Ross	4.4	1.06	14	31	55	Lactose-free; low-residue

Specialized use formulas

Amin-Aid Instant Drink	Kendall McGraw	8.2	1.90	4	21	75	Requires vitamin, mineral, and electrolyte supplementation
Attain L.S.	Kendall McGraw	8.2	1.90	16	36	48	Lactose-free; low-residue
Pre-Attain	Sherwood Medical	2.1	0.50	16	36	48	Lactose-free
Hepatic Aid II Instant Drink	Kendall McGraw	4.9	1.18				Requires vitamin, mineral, and electrolyte supplementation
Lonalac	Mead Johnson	4.2	1.00	21	49	30	
Portagen	Mead Johnson	4.2	1.01	14	40	46	Lactose-free
Precision High Nitrogen Diet	Sandoz Nutrition	4.4	1.05	9	1	90	Lactose-free; low-residue; gluten-free
Precision LR Diet	Sandoz Nutrition	4.2	1.10				Lactose-free; low-residue; gluten-free
Pulmocare	Ross	6.3	1.50	17	55	28	Lactose-free
Stresstein	Sandoz Nutrition	5.0	1.20	23	21	56	Lactose-free; no residue
Traum-Aid HBC	Kendall McGraw	4.2	1.00	24	6	70	Lactose-free; low-residue
TraumaCal	Mead Johnson	6.3	1.50	22	40	38	Lactose-free
Travasorb Hepatic	Clinitec Nutrition Co.	4.6	1.10	7	12	77	Low aromatic amino acids
Travasorb Renal	Clinitec Nutrition Co.	5.7	1.35	7	12	81	Requires vitamin, mineral, and electrolyte supplementation

Hydrolyzed protein-elemental formulas*

Accept HPF	Sherwood Medical	4.2	1.0	16	76	9	Lactose-free
Carnation Peptamen Liquid, Isotonic, Complete, Elemental Diet	Clinitec Nutrition Co.	4.2	1.00	16	33	51	
Criticare HN	Mead Johnson	4.4	1.06	16	33	83	Lactose-free; low resid.
Pepti 2000	Sherwood Medical	4.2	1.00	18	12	70	Lactose-free; low-residue
Reabilan	Clinitec Nutrition Co.	4.2	1.0	13	35	54	
Tolerex	Norwich Eaton	4.2	1.0	15	3	73	
Travasorb HN	Clinitec Nutrition Co.	4.2	1.00	12	12	76	Lactose-free; low-residue
Travasorb STD	Clinitec Nutrition Co.	4.2	1.00	17	10	73	Lactose-free; low-residue
Vital High Nitrogen	Ross	4.2	1.00	17	1	82	Lactose-free; low-residue
Vivonex HN	Norwich Eaton	4.2	1.00	17	1	82	Lactose-free; no residue
Vivonex Standard	Norwich Eaton	4.2	1.00	9	1	90	Lactose-free; no residue
Vivonex T.E.N.	Norwich Eaton	4.2	1.00	15	3	82	Lactose-free; low-residue

HIGH CALORIE SOFT SUPPLEMENTS

		kJ/g	kcal/g				

Puddings

Ensure Pudding	Ross	7.5	1.8	11	35	54	Gluten-free
Sustacal Pudding	Mead Johnson	7.5	1.7	11	36	53	
Forta Pudding	Ross	7.5	1.6	11	35	54	Lactose-free

TABLE 75-8 Nutrient composition of oral nutritional supplements (*continued*)

	Manufacturer	kJ/mL	kcal/mL	Percent of energy			Comments
				Protein	Fat	Carbohydrate	
MODULAR SYSTEMS (SINGLE NUTRIENT SOURCES)		kJ/g or /mL	kcal/g or /mL				
Protein modules							
Casec	Mead Johnson	15.5	3.7	96	4	<1	Powder
Nutrisource Amino Acids	Sandoz Nutrition	16.3	3.9	100	0	0	Powder
Nutrisource Amino Acids -High BCAA	Sandoz Nutrition	15.9	3.8	100	0	0	Powder
Nutrisource Protein	Sandoz Nutrition	16.7	4.0	75	10	6	Powder
Pro Mod	Ross	17.6	4.2	72	19	9	Powder
Propac	Sherwood Medical	16.7	4.0	77	18	5	Powder
RDP	Corpak, Inc.	15.1	3.6	84	10	6	Powder
Fat modules							
High Fat Supplement	Corpak, Inc.	25.5	6.12	3	70	27	Powder
MCT Oil	Mead Johnson	32.3	7.7	0	100	0	Liquid
Nutrisource Lipid—Long-Chain Triglycerides	Sandoz Nutrition	9.2	2.2	0	100	0	Liquid
Nutrisource Lipid—Medium-Chain Triglycerides	Sandoz Nutrition	8.4	2.0	0	100	0	Liquid
Microlipid	Sherwood Medical	18.8	4.5	0	100	0	Liquid
Carbohydrate modules							
Liquid Carbohydrate Supplement	Corpak, Inc.	10.5	2.5	0	0	100	Liquid
Modical	Mead Johnson	15.9	3.8	0	0	100	Powder
Nutrisource Carbohydrate	Sandoz Nutrition	13.4	3.2	0	0	100	Liquid
Polycose Powder	Ross	15.9	3.8	0	0	100	Powder
Polycose Liquid	Ross	8.4	2.0	0	0	100	Liquid
Pure Carbohydrate Supplement	Corpak, Inc.	16.7	4.0	0	0	100	Powder
Sumacal	Sherwood Medical	15.9	3.8	0	0	100	Powder
LOW-PROTEIN PRODUCTS		kJ/20 g	kcal/20 g				
WelPlan low-protein pasta	Dietary Specialties Dist.	282	67	.006	2.4	97	Corn and potato starch
Aproten low-protein rusks	Dietary Specialties Dist.	353	84	.01	19	81	Melba toast-like product with wheat, rice, starch
WelPlan low protein brown bread	Dietary Specialties Dist.	180	43	.02	8.5	91	
Prono low protein gelled dessert	Dietary Specialties Dist.	328	78	.001	0	99	
DP low protein chocolate chip cookies	Dietary Specialties Dist.	420	100	.004	45	54	Wheat starch
Low Pro rice starch loaf	Med-Diet	265	63	.003	23	76	Rice starch
Poi Bread	Ener-G	282	67	.04	41	51	Gluten free rice flour and tapioca flour
Alterna Low Protein Milk Substitute	Ross	30.5	7.25	11	38	51	Comes in powder form (values are for prepared version, which compares to 2% milk)
Low protein cookies	Kingsmill	1046	250	<1	41	59	
FIBER SUPPLEMENTS		kJ/20 g	kcal/20 g				
Fiber Med	Purdue Frederick Co.	243	70	11	26	63	
Fiberall	Ciba-Geigy Corp.	331	79	5	46	49	
OTHER SPECIAL FORMULAS		kJ/g	kcal/mL				
Alitraq	Ross	4.2	1.0	21	13	66	Elemental nutrition with glutamine
Fibrael	Ross	29 kJ/9 g serving	5 kcal/9g serving				7 g dietary fiber per serving (9 g); concentrated dietary fiber supplement
Glucerna	Ross	4.2	1.0	17	50	33	Diabetic product
Impact	Sandoz	4.2	1.0	22	25	53	Critical care
Introlite	Ross	2.2	.53	17	30	54	Fortified .5 Calorie liquid nutrition
Lipisorb	Mead Johnson	4.2	1.0	14	40	46	MCT oil and corn oil mixture
Nepro	Ross	8.4	2.0	16	43	43	For dialysis patients
Replena	Ross	8.4	2.0	6	43	51	For predialysis patients

* Definitions: Low-residue = producing little or no stool; isotonic = having the tonicity of plasma (308 mosmol/L); hydrolyzed protein-elemental formula = nutrients partially or completely digested.

SOURCE: Modified from the American Dietetic Association: *Manual of Clinical Dietetics*, 1988.

latitude on the part of the patients. Some of the products are particularly useful for complex diets.

SPECIAL PROBLEMS IN DIET THERAPY

TRANSITIONS FROM ONE ROUTE OF FEEDING TO ANOTHER
Transitional feeding refers to the process of return to the usual feeding pattern after total parenteral nutrition, peripheral hyperalimentation, or enteral feeding by gastrotomy, jejunostomy, esophagostomy, or nasogastric tube. After extended periods of disuse, the gut may not function normally, and unless the transition process is carefully monitored, ad libitum oral intake and/or food absorption may be inadequate.

ADHERENCE TO DIET   Compliance with therapeutic dietary recommendations is relatively easy to monitor in the hospitalized patient. A menu that conforms to the diet orders is offered, and choices and made in line with the therapeutic prescription (and if choices are not appropriate, substitutions are made). However, the patient may refuse or be unable to eat or may miss meals because of diagnostic tests. Therefore, nutritional status and patient adherence should be monitored carefully even in the hospital.

To implement therapeutic diets in outpatients, the patient must be motivated and must understand the diet instructions and the changes in what is to be eaten. New food buying, food preparation, and eating habits may be required. Selections when dining out are also altered. These changes are difficult to make and even more difficult to sustain.

Psychological support; assistance in learning new food preparation, buying, and management skills; help with eating (in disabilities such as stroke); help in obtaining financial assistance to buy special foods; and general education about the importance of diet are as important as nutritional advice.

ASSURING THE CONTINUITY OF NUTRITIONAL CARE: THE TEAM CONCEPT   Nutrition is too important to be the sole responsibility of a single member of the health team. Nutritional counseling can and does change dietary habits, and each health-care provider has a critical role in assuring that nutrition is adequate. However, physicians rarely obtain thorough diet histories, address potential barriers to change in eating habits, or offer special guidance on food selection. The major role of physicians is to expand the content of the nutritional information they provide, to emphasize the health benefits of good nutrition to refer those requiring help to dietitians or other specialized providers.

REFERENCES

AMERICAN DIABETES ASSOCIATION, INC. AND THE AMERICAN DIETETIC ASSOCIATION: *Exchange Lists for Meal Planning*, Revised 1989. Alexandria, Va., American Diabetes Association, 1989

CHICAGO DIETETIC ASSOCIATION AND SOUTH SUBURBAN DIETETIC ASSOCIATION: *Manual of Clinical Dietetics*, 3rd ed. Chicago, The American Dietetic Association, 1992

COMMITTEE ON DIET AND HEALTH: *Diet and Health; Modifications to Reduce Chronic Disease Risk*. Washington, National Academy Press, 1993

Handbook of Clinical Dietetics, 2d ed. Chicago, American Dietetic Association, 1992

JOINT NATIONAL COMMITTEE V: *The Fifth Report of the Joint National Committee on Detection Evaluation and Treatment of High Blood Pressure* (JNCV), National High Blood Pressure Education Program. Bethesda, National Heart, Lung and Blood Institute, National Institutes of Health, 1992

NATIONAL RESEARCH COUNCIL: *Recommended Dietary Allowances*, 10th ed. Washington DC, National Academy of Sciences, 1989

Nutrition Interventions Manual for Professionals Caring for Older Americans. Washington DC, Nutrition Screening Initiative

Nutrition Screening Manual for Professionals Caring for Older Americans. Washington DC, Nutrition Screening Initiative

REPORT OF THE US PREVENTIVE SERVICES TASK FORCE: *Guide to Clinical Preventive Services: An Assessment of the Effectiveness of 169 Interventions*. Philadelphia, Williams & Wilkins, 1989

SHILS ME (ED): *Modern Nutrition in Health and Disease*. Philadelphia, Lea and Febiger, 1993

ZEMAN FJ: *Clinical Nutrition and Dietetics*. New York, Macmillan, 1983

76   PARENTERAL AND ENTERAL NUTRITION THERAPY

LYN HOWARD

Parenteral and enteral nutrition provide life-sustaining therapy for patients who cannot take adequate nutrition by mouth and who consequently are at risk for the debilitating effects of malnutrition. These effects include susceptibility to infection and the consequences of immobility, such as pulmonary embolism, aspiration pneumonia, and pressure sores, all of which delay recovery from illness and result in an increased mortality.

The term *enteral* refers to feeding via the gut and hence includes normal eating, but in the present context it implies the infusion of formulas via a tube inserted into the upper gastrointestinal tract. *Parenteral* refers to the infusion of nutrient solutions into the bloodstream. While these approaches to nutritional support are different, their goals are by and large the same. Where feasible, enteral nutrition is the preferred route because it sustains gastrointestinal function both from a digestive and an absorptive standpoint and as an immunologic barrier. Enteral feeding costs about one-tenth as much as parenteral feeding.

Enteral tube feeding initially involved large-bore rubber tubes placed via the nose or through an ostomy into the stomach or jejunum; these tubes have largely been replaced by small-bore pliable tubes that remain soft with exposure to digestive juices. Feeding tubes can now be placed directly (percutaneously) into the stomach or jejunum by endoscopic or radiologic techniques and seldom require surgical placement except when the gastrostomy is part of a larger operation. These advances have enhanced the acceptance of the technique by patients, and tube feedings are now used in medical conditions where malnutrition is due to impaired oral intake or defective nutrient assimilation as well as for swallowing or esophageal dysfunction.

Parenteral nutrition is more recent. After Gamble demonstrated in the 1940s that glucose (100 g/d) spares protein breakdown in fasting subjects, intravenous glucose infusions became routine therapy for hospitalized patients unable to eat. In the 1960s, Dudrick and colleagues showed that total nutrition (calories, amino acids, minerals, and vitamins) can be delivered on a long-term basis through infusion into a high-flow central vein. Such therapy results in positive nitrogen balance and promotes wound healing in adults and normal growth and development in children. Total parenteral nutrition is now available in all large hospitals and for certain patients at home. The development of high-energy, isotonic intravenous fat solutions also makes it possible to deliver adequate calories and other essential nutrients via a peripheral vein. However, peripheral veins usually cannot sustain nutrient infusions indefinitely, and long-term support requires central venous access.

THE DECISION PROCESS FOR USING PARENTERAL OR ENTERAL NUTRITION   The decision to use specialized nutrition support should be based on the likelihood that averting or redressing malnutrition will improve the quality of life or the ability to recover from a life-threatening condition. At least 15 to 20 percent of hospitalized patients have evidence of malnutrition. Some of these patients will benefit from specialized nutrition support, but for others wasting is an inevitable component of a terminal disease. Distinguishing between these possibilities requires critical clinical judgment: (1) knowledge of the potential benefits and risks of nutritional support, (2) the ability to communicate the benefits and risks to the patient and the family, and (3) awareness of the legal requirements pertinent to this issue. Figure 76-1 is a flow diagram of the steps involved in making this decision.

The first step requires the physician to formulate the nutritional implications of the disease process. Since it is easier to prevent than to treat malnutrition, this first step must be part of the initial workup. Clinicians can categorize a patient as severely, moderately, or

FIGURE 76-1   Should specialized nutrition support (SNS) be undertaken? An algorithm.

minimally malnourished by careful attention to the history and physical examination. The history must encompass recent weight change, the functional status of the patient, and the effects of the primary disease on food intake and assimilation. The physical examination must assess muscle wasting, fat stores, edema, anemia, and other signs of nutrient deficiencies (see Chap. 72). Table 76-1 summarizes some of the criteria for documenting protein-energy malnutrition. Except for delayed hypersensitivity testing, these criteria rely mainly on changes in body composition. In the future, more emphasis may be placed on functional tests of nutritional status, such as muscle strength, pulmonary reserve, and wound healing. Once it is recognized that the patient is at risk for or has developed

malnutrition, the question of whether artificially supplied nutrition is appropriate involves ethical and risk-versus-benefit considerations.

While the provision of food and water is a basic element of medical care, nutrition support delivered by enteral or parenteral means is associated with discomfort and should only be recommended if the benefits exceed the risks and only after obtaining the consent of the patient or the legal surrogate. In many situations the dividing line between comfort and medical therapy is not clear, especially in the incompetent patient. Physicians should advise all patients to address this issue by preparing advance directions such as a "living will" and designating a health care proxy. Without such preplanning, nutritional support may distressingly protract a terminal illness.

TABLE 76-1 Means for assessment of protein-energy malnutrition (PEM)

Method of assessment	Moderate PEM	Severe PEM
Weight loss, %	15–25	>25
Fat depletion*	<16 ± 6	<12 ± 5
Albumin, g/L	25–30	<25
Transferrin, g/L	1–2.0	<1
Total lymphocyte count, 10^6/L	0.8–1.2	<0.8
Delayed hypersensitivity index†	1	0

* Fat depletion assessed from triceps skin fold in millimeters.
† Delayed hypersensitivity index quantitates the centimeters of induration with common antigens such as *Candida*, trichophytin, or mumps: 0 = <0.5, 1 = 0.5, 2 = 1.0.

If it is determined that preventing or treating malnutrition with specialized nutrition support would improve the prognosis and quality of life, the nutritional requirements must be determined, and the route of nutrient delivery must be selected.

RISKS AND BENEFITS OF NUTRITION SUPPORT The risks are chiefly determined by the route required to deliver effective nutrition support. If nutrient requirements can be met by special attention to oral intake, by use of liquid supplements (if necessary), and by monitoring food intake with frequent calorie counts, this is the best approach. Normal nutrient assimilation starts with the cephalic phase of digestion, and tube-fed infants grow better if the cephalic stimulus is provided by having the infant suck on a pacifier.

Anorexia, impairment of swallowing, or more distal bowel disease may limit oral intake, in which case tube enteral nutrition is the next option. Enteral feeding maintains the digestive and absorptive functions of the gastrointestinal tract and also sustains the immunologic barrier which the gut provides, preventing enteric organisms from invading the body. The nutrient and immunologic functions of the gut are supported by luminal nutrients and by the normal gastrointestinal hormones, blood flow, and neural stimulation, all of which are activated by enteral feeding. Certain nutrients, including glutamine, nucleotides, and short-chain fatty acids, may be particularly important for the maintenance of gut mucosal integrity. Specific growth factors such as epidermal growth factor or human growth hormone also may promote bowel adaptation and positive nitrogen balance even in the presence of hypocaloric feeding.

To support the barrier functions of the gut, some enteral nutrition should be provided whenever possible, even if parenteral nutrition is also required. This is particularly important in debilitated, immunosuppressed patients. In the past, bowel rest, through total parenteral nutrition, was thought to be the cornerstone for the treatment of several severe gastrointestinal disorders. The value of some enteral nutrition is now established, and strict bowel rest is rarely advocated. Parenteral nutrition alone is still the mainstay of treatment in the early phase of extreme short bowel syndrome, severe hemorrhagic pancreatitis, necrotizing enterocolitis, and prolonged ileus.

Since parenteral nutrition is more costly and more hazardous than enteral nutrition, most risk-versus-benefit studies to date have focused on parenteral nutrition. Increasingly, the end points required of such studies involve evidence that the therapy improves outcome, such as decreased mortality rates, a reduced incidence of major complications, or shorter duration of hospital stay. End points such as better nitrogen balance, increased levels of serum albumin, and improved delayed hypersensitivity are no longer acceptable.

Perioperative nutrition While there is a clear-cut association between preoperative malnutrition and poor surgical outcome, it has been difficult to demonstrate a beneficial impact of preoperative parenteral nutrition on the outcome of surgery in malnourished patients. However, a meta-analysis of 18 small studies and a large cooperative Veterans Administration study suggests that preoperative parenteral nutrition does provide a net benefit for severely malnourished surgical patients. In treated patients, noninfectious complications (e.g., pulmonary emboli and delayed wound healing) were reduced in the postoperative period. In surgical patients with mild or moderate malnutrition, the risks of infection from preoperative therapy outweigh the benefits. These risks include sepsis and infectious complications not directly related to the central line, such as pneumonia and wound infection. Effective preoperative parenteral nutrition requires at least 7 to 14 days.

Preoperative enteral nutrition has not been studied extensively but is a safe and economical option where feasible. A randomized, controlled trial of postoperative enteral nutrition (needle catheter jejunostomy) versus parenteral nutrition showed equal benefit, with the enteral approach being less expensive. Postoperative parenteral nutrition should be considered in the nutritionally impaired patient if enteral nutrition cannot be resumed for 7 days or longer.

Cancer cachexia Early nonrandomized studies suggested that cachectic cancer patients benefit from parenteral nutrition support, but randomized trials have shown more risk than benefit for such patients receiving chemotherapy or radiation. Where enteral feeding is not tolerated, parenteral nutrition should be provided only if clinical improvement can be expected.

Severely malnourished cancer patients undergoing surgery appear to benefit from preoperative parenteral nutrition, as do other malnourished patients. In two randomized, prospective trials, bone marrow transplantation patients supported by parenteral or enteral nutrition in the cytoreduction phase showed better long-term survival. The nutrition support did not influence the frequency of initial infectious complications, nor was graft rejection or graft-versus-host disease reduced.

Liver failure Since malnutrition is common in advanced liver disease, the effects of nutritional intervention have been investigated extensively. Patients with acute or chronic liver failure have decreased levels of branched chain amino acids (BCAA) and elevated levels of aromatic amino acids (AAA) in plasma and brain. Randomized, prospective trials with parenteral and enteral formulas high in BCAA and low in AAA have demonstrated better nitrogen balance and less risk of encephalopathy. One large multicenter study reported improved nitrogen balance and improved survival. The BCAA-enriched formulas are expensive and should only be used in liver failure patients who have encephalopathy or who cannot tolerate a standard protein formula without developing encephalopathy.

Critical illness In randomized, controlled trials, BCAA-enriched formulas improved nitrogen balance in severely ill patients but did not alter clinical outcome. However, in both burn and head injury patients, initiation of parenteral or enteral nutrition support within the first 12 hours decreased weight loss and reduced length of hospital stay.

Renal failure Since renal failure is associated with impaired nitrogen excretion, there has been a long-standing belief that outcome in renal failure would be improved if protein intake were restricted. An early controlled trial showed improved survival of acute renal failure patients receiving parenteral essential amino acids and glucose compared with those receiving glucose alone. Subsequent trials demonstrated similar benefit with standard solutions supplying equal amounts of essential and nonessential amino acids; thus the superiority of costly formulas rich in essential amino acids or their keto analogues is not established.

Pancreatitis Parenteral nutrition does not improve the medical outcome of patients with mild or moderate pancreatitis. However, severe pancreatitis is associated with impaired nutrition, and survival decreases as malnutrition increases. These observations provide indirect evidence for the use of parenteral nutrition in severe pancreatitis. In the absence of severe hyperlipidemia or thrombocytopenia complicating pancreatitis, intravenous lipids are safe and are especially useful if glucose intolerance is present.

Inflammatory bowel disease (IBD) Evidence of nutritional deficiencies such as weight loss, growth failure, anemia, and hypoalbuminia are common in IBD, more so in Crohn's disease than in ulcerative colitis (see Chap. 255). Nutrition support plays a role in redressing these nutritional deficiencies, particularly prior to elective surgery. Since IBD often improves with diversion of the fecal stream, the question has been raised as to whether bowel rest and parenteral nutrition might have a role as primary treatment. However, randomized, prospective studies have shown no special benefit from bowel rest. Elemental diets can be used in place of glucocorticoids for inducing remission in acute Crohn's disease, but relapse is common when a normal diet is resumed.

Because of the possibility that specific dietary fats may have a beneficial effect in several immune disorders, probably by altering prostaglandin pathways, diets high in omega 3 fatty acids are under investigation in IBD. While some studies suggest a benefit to IBD patients from high-fiber diets, this may cause problems in patients with strictures. In controlled studies, remissions may be longer in Crohn's disease if wheat and dairy products are eliminated.

Short bowel syndrome   Before the advent of parenteral nutrition, patients with severe short bowel syndrome, as from mesenteric vascular infarction or surgical resection, seldom survived. Parenteral nutrition has allowed many patients with only a foot or two of small intestine to survive indefinitely. In some the short bowel eventually adapts so that only parenteral fluid and electrolyte support is required or they can graduate to enteral nutrition alone.

Acquired immunodeficiency syndrome   Parenteral nutrition is frequently used in AIDS patients with severe gastrointestinal disease, weight loss, and intolerance for enteral feeding. There have been anecdotal reports of temporary clinical benefit, but there have been no randomized, controlled studies of parenteral support in these patients.

Pulmonary disease   Weight loss in patients with advanced pulmonary disease is due to increased work of breathing and poor food intake. In cystic fibrosis, malnutrition may hasten pulmonary deterioration, and enteral feeding via gastrostomy tubes enhances growth and stabilizes or improves pulmonary function, particularly in young children. The criteria for selection of patients and the psychological costs of such treatment have not been defined. The use of a low-carbohydrate formula is beneficial in the weaning of patients from ventilators, but the superiority of such formulas in ambulatory patients with chronic lung disease is not established.

Pregnancy   Severe hyperemesis gravidarum can make any oral or tube enteral nutrition impossible, and profound weight loss and ketosis may be harmful to the fetus. Hyperemesis is relieved by abortion or delivery, but the underlying mechanism is not understood. There are numerous reports of successful otucome of pregnancy following temporary support of the pregnant woman by parenteral nutrition, but nausea and vomiting tend to persist despite bowel rest.

THE DESIGN OF INDIVIDUAL REGIMENS   Fluid requirements These can be estimated by adding the normal daily requirement (120 mL/kg of body weight for infants, 35 mL/kg of body weight for adults) to any abnormal loss. If the patient is on parenteral therapy, any enteral intake should be subtracted from the abnormal loss. For examples, see Table 76-2. Since abnormal loss of enteric fluid implies significant mineral losses, extra amounts of these nutrients (Table 76-3) also must be added to any standard parenteral or enteral formula.

Energy requirements   These can be estimated as outlined in Chap. 71. Measurements of energy expenditure in ill patients have shown that the Harris-Benedict formula tends to overestimate expenditures. Direct measurements, using a bedside metabolic cart and calculation of energy requirements from gas exchange, are also difficult to interpret, since energy expenditure fluctuates throughout the day and calorimetry assessments are confounded by starvation or any ongoing nutritional support. A reasonable approach is to provide 100 kJ/kg (25 kcal/kg) per day for an unstressed patient and 125, 145, and 165 kJ/kg (30, 35, and 40 kcal/kg) per day, respectively, for mildly, moderately, and severely stressed patients.

The most desirable balance of carbohydrate to fat in parenteral and enteral solutions is unsettled. Wound healing, white blood cells, the brain, and the renal cortex depend on glucose metabolism. The majority of energy is usually supplied as glucose in parenteral solutions and as oligosaccharides and disaccharides in enteral solutions. Parenteral lipid solutions are available as 10% or 20% emulsions of vegetable oils (soybean or safflower oils emulsified into artificial lipoproteins with egg phospholipid and made isotonic with glycerin). Parenteral lipids can be infused separately or as a "three in one" nutrient solution with amino acids and glucose. "Three in one" solutions are well tolerated and can obviate the need for an extra infusion pump for the separate solution. However, such solutions are not as stable as the more traditional glucose and amino acid mix, and destabilized fat particles have the potential of coalescing into larger droplets and becoming fat emboli. To be safe "three in one" solutions must be mixed by a pharmacist knowledgeable about the necessary mixing sequence of the separate ingredients and the amounts of divalent cations and trace elements that can be added. Patients who require parenteral iron or generous amounts of zinc must alternate between "three in one" and non-lipid-containing parenteral solutions.

Polyunsaturated vegetable oils are used in most enteral formulas because they are better absorbed by the compromised gastrointestinal tract. The fat in parenteral and enteral formulas must supply the

---

TABLE 76-2   Estimation of daily fluid requirements

NORMAL 70-KG MAN

Intake	Output
Normal requirement: 35 × 70 = ~2500 mL/d (derived from oral liquids of 1200 mL, or 5 glasses/cups per day, and solid food providing 1300 mL, 1000 mL from water in food, 300 mL from water generated by metabolism of foods)	Urine: 1600 mL/d Insensible loss: 800 mL/d Stool: 100 mL/d [sweat loss can be up to 2 L/d. Each degree of fever (C) = 200 mL/d]

TUBE ENTERAL PATIENT

A 58-kg woman recovering from total gastrectomy for gastric cancer and supported by jejunostomy feedings, taking nothing by mouth or intravenously, but experiencing 600 mL of diarrheal losses per day:
Normal requirement 35 × 58 = ~2000 mL/d
Abnormal loss (600 − 100) = 500 mL/d
Total requirement = 2500 mL/d

PARENTERAL PATIENT

A 66-kg man with a high jejunostomy following massive bowel resection for Crohn's disease with oral intake of 2000 mL/d and jejunostomy loss of 4000 mL/d:
Normal requirement 35 × 66 = 2300 mL/d
Abnormal loss (4000 − 100) minus oral intake (2000) = 1900 mL/d
Total requirement = 4200 mL/d

TABLE 76-3   Enteric fluid volumes and their sodium, potassium, chloride, and bicarbonate content*

	L/d†	Na mmol/L	K‡ mmol/L	Cl mmol/L	HCO$_3$§ mmol/L
Oral intake	2–3				
Enteric secretions					
Saliva	1–2	10	30	10	30
Gastric juice	2	60	9	90	0
Bile	2–3	150	10	90	70
Small bowel	1	100	5	100	20
Colon	Variable	40	100	15	60

* Enteric secretions are also rich in divalent cations (Ca, Mg, Zn, Cu), and their loss is increased by steatorrhea, a high bowel fistula, or prolonged suction.
† Of the 9 L/d of oral and enteric fluid presented to the upper small bowel, normally 50 percent is absorbed in the jejunum, 40 percent in the ileum, and 10 percent in the colon. In short bowel patients, the colon can absorb greater amounts, up to 3 L/d.
‡ Potassium losses are small except in secretions distal to the ileocecal valve. The colon ion exchange is partly controlled by aldosterone, and therefore, Na$^+$ depletion increases K$^+$ loss in the stool.
§ Bicarbonate losses must be replaced in parenteral solutions as acetate or lactate because of potential precipitation of bicarbonate with ingredients such as calcium.

essential fatty acid requirement (1 to 2 percent of energy from linoleic and linolenic acid). The provision of 30 percent of energy as fat may reduce the problems that arise from providing excess carbohydrate calories (e.g., hepatic steatosis). Substitution of ordinary polyunsaturated vegetable fats by omega 3 polyunsaturated fish oils may reduce the inflammatory response to burn injury, trauma, and radiation by reducing the synthesis of prostaglandins that enhance gut mucosal permeability to enteric toxins.

Protein or amino acid requirements　The recommended dietary protein allowance of 0.8 g/kg per day is adequate for nonstressed patients (e.g., a patient with a high-grade esophageal stricture or anorexia nervosa). Catabolic patients may require up to 1.5 g/kg per day of protein to induce positive nitrogen balance and reconstitute normal body mass. In a stable patient the adequacy of protein and energy support can be assessed by a balance study:

$$\text{Protein balance} = \text{protein intake} - \text{protein loss}$$

where protein loss = [24-h urine urea nitrogen (g) + 4] × 6.25, and by documenting wound healing, restoration of normal body composition, or resumption of longitudinal growth.

In states of disturbed protein utilization (e.g., renal and hepatic failure), azotemia and abnormal plasma amino acid patterns develop. The benefit of special enteral and parenteral solutions that correct these aberrations is not established.

Certain amino acids and peptides that are not essential nutrients (because they can be synthesized endogenously) may become essential in severely ill patients when endogenous production or salvage pathways are impaired. This is true of glutamine, arginine, and the products of methionine metabolism. Glutamine is an important fuel, particularly for the enterocyte. The oxidation of one molecule of glutamine produces 30 mmol ATP, which makes this amino acid almost as rich an energy source as glucose. The free amino acid pool of the enterocyte is glutamine-rich. Glutamine is fairly insoluble and is absent from many parenteral formulas and present only in low concentrations in most enteral formulas. Soluble glutamine-containing dipeptides are under investigation.

Parenteral amino acids are infused systemically rather than via the more physiologic portal route. Under these circumstances, methionine,

the only sulfur-containing amino acid in parenteral solutions, tends to be transaminated rather than transulfurated. As a result, downstream products such as carnitine, taurine, and glutathione become relatively deficient. Preliminary studies suggest the addition of S-adenosyl methionine to parenteral solutions results in less cholestasis.

Mineral and vitamin requirements　(See Table 76-4)　Parenteral requirements of some minerals and vitamins may be higher than the enteral requirements for several reasons: First, the micronutrients are delivered into the systemic rather than the portal circulation, thereby potentially bypassing the liver and being rapidly excreted into the urine. Second, many patients who require parenteral support have enteric losses that can result in sodium, potassium, chloride, and bicarbonate wasting (see Table 76-3) and in loss of divalent cations and vitamins that normally have an enterohepatic circulation, including folate, cobalamin, vitamin D, and other fat-soluble vitamins. The tubing and delivery bags and exposure to oxygen and light also can destroy vitamins (particularly vitamin A).

PARENTERAL NUTRITION　Infusion technique and patient monitoring　Partial and short-term parenteral nutrition can be provided via a peripheral vein if the majority of the energy intake is supplied by isotonic fat solutions, but long-term total parenteral support should be administered via a central vein catheter because the solutions contain hypertonic glucose that must be rapidly diluted in a high-flow system. The preferred sites for central vein access and the catheter choices available are summarized in Table 76-5, and typical nutrient content of a standard daily parenteral formula is given

---

TABLE 76-4　Daily enteral (EN) and parenteral (PN) requirements of essential fatty acids, minerals, and vitamins

Nutrient	Daily requirement, adult range	
	EN	PN
Essential fatty acids, % kcal	1–2	2–4
Calcium, g	0.8–1.2	0.4
Phosphorus, g	0.8–1.2	0.8
Potassium, g	2–5	3–4
Sodium, g	1–3	1–2
Chloride, g	2–5	2
Magnesium, g	0.3	0.3
Iron, mg	10	1–2
Zinc, mg	15	3–12
Copper, mg	2–3	0.3–0.5
Iodine, mg	0.15	0.15
Manganese, mg	2–5	2–5
Chromium, mg	0.05–0.2	0.015
Molybdenum, mg	0.15–0.3	0.01–0.5
Selenium, mg	0.05–0.02	0.05–0.1
Ascorbic acid, mg	60	100
Thiamine, mg	1.4	3.0
Riboflavin, mg	1–6	3.6
Niacin, mg	18	40
Biotin, μg	60	60
Pantothenic acid, mg	5	15
Pyridoxine, mg	2.0	4.0
Folic acid, μg	400	400
Cobalamin, μg	3.0	5
Vitamin A, μg	1000	1300
Vitamin D, μg	10	5
Vitamin E, mg	8–10	10–15
Vitamin K, μg	70–140	200

TABLE 76-5　Central vein parenteral nutrition catheters

SITES OF VENOUS ACCESS

A　Distal tip of catheter best placed in midportion of superior vena cava
B　Enters venous system via
　1　Percutaneous stick into the subclavian, external or internal jugular, or antecubital vein
　2　Cutdown site on external jugular (via common facial vein), femoral, axillary, or intercostal vein
C　All catheters can be tunneled subcutaneously to a distal site, which
　1　May provide a barrier to skin organisms infecting the line
　2　Places exit site at convenient place for self-care in patients at home

TYPES OF CATHETERS

A　Externalized
　1　Single, double, or triple lumen
　　a　Second and third channels used for IV medications or drawing of blood
　　b　Higher incidence of infectious complications with multiple-lumen catheters
　2　In home patients, avoids the need for a nightly needle stick but requires constant aseptic dressing
　3　Repair kits available if a leak or tear develops in the externalized portion
B　Subcutaneous port
　1　Involves a small reservoir with an overlying rubber diaphragm that is self-sealing
　2　Port must be entered by a J-shaped needle
　3　Not all patients like the daily needle stick
　4　If line is not in use, the buried port makes taking showers and swimming less hazardous

CATHETER MATERIAL

A　Polyvinylchloride, polyethylene, polyurethane, or polytetrafluoroethylene
　1　Advantage:
　　a　Inherent stiffness may allow easy threading into the vein
　2　Disadvantages:
　　a　Stiffness allows catheter to be in direct contact with vessel wall, causing phlebitis and thrombosis
　　b　Stiffness increases with time, causing kinks or fractures
B　Silicone rubber
　1　Advantages:
　　a　Very pliable, less kinking
　　b　Less traumatic to vessel wall
　　c　Inert, inducing little reaction or adherence
　2　Disadvantages:
　　a　Difficult to thread into vein
　　b　Falls out more easily owing to nonadherence
　　c　Potential for tearing

TABLE 76-6   Standard total parenteral nutrition solution (24 h) for a 70-kg adult

Fluid	3 L
Protein (amino acids)	0.2–0.3 g nitrogen/kg
Energy value*	100–165 kJ/kg (25–40 kcal/kg)
Essential fatty acids (lipids)	2% of total calories
Electrolytes	
Sodium	100 mmol
Potassium†	100 mmol
Chloride	130 mmol
Acetate/gluconate	90 mmol
Calcium	7.5 mmol
Magnesium	10 mmol
Phosphorous†	600 mg
Trace elements	
Zinc	5 mg
Copper	1.5 mg
Iodine	120 μg
Selenium	100 μg
Chromium	15 μg
Maganese	2 mg
Vitamins	
Ascorbic acid	100 mg
Thiamine	3 mg
Riboflavin	3.6 mg
Niacin	40 mg
Panthothenic acid	15 mg
Pyridoxine	4 mg
Biotin	60 μg
Folic acid	400 μg
Cobalamin	5 μg
Vitamin A	1300 μg
Vitamin D	10 μg
Vitamin E	15 mg
Vitamin K	200 μg

* Provided principally as dextrose.
† More potassium and phosphorus may be needed in the repletion phase after severe cachexia. Chronic starvation results in total-body potassium and phosphorus depletion.

TABLE 76-8   Complications of total parenteral nutrition (TPN)

First 48 h	First 2 weeks	3 months onward
MECHANICAL		
Complications from catheter insertion: Cephalad displacement Pneumothorax Hemothorax Detachment of line at catheter hub with blood loss or air embolism	Catheter coming out of vein, more common if Silastic Detachment of line at catheter hub with blood loss or air embolism	Detachment of line at catheter hub with blood loss or air embolism Fractures or tears in catheter
METABOLIC		
Fluid overload Hyperglycemia Hypophosphatemia Hypokalemia	Cardiopulmonary failure Hyperosmolar nonketotic hyperglycemic coma Acid-base imbalance Electrolyte imbalance	Essentially fatty acid deficiency Zinc, copper, chromium, selenium, molybdenum, deficiency Iron deficiency Vitamin deficiencies Refeeding edema TPN metabolic bone disease TPN liver disease
INFECTIOUS		
	Catheter-induced sepsis	Catheter-induced sepsis Tunnel infections

in Table 76-6. The glucose content is increased gradually as the patient demonstrates tolerance of the high glucose load. Appropriate clinical and laboratory monitoring for patients on parenteral nutrition is summarized in Table 76-7.

Complications (See Table 76-8)   MECHANICAL   The insertion of a central venous catheter should only be done by trained personnel

TABLE 76-7   Monitoring the patient on total parenteral nutrition

CLINICAL DATA MONITORED DAILY

Sense of well-being: symptoms suggesting fluid overload, high or low blood glucose, electrolyte imbalance, etc.
Strength as judged by graded activity: getting out of bed, walking, stair climbing.
Vital signs: temperature, blood pressure, pulse rate and respiratory rate.
Fluid balance: weight; fluid input (intravenous +/− enteral) versus fluid output (urine, stool, gastric suction, etc.).
Delivery equipment for parenteral nutrition: composition of nutrient solution, tubing, pump, filter, catheter, dressing (skin checked for local infection at time of dressing change).

LABORATORY DATA

Plasma glucose	Four times daily until patient stable
Blood glucose Na$^+$, K$^+$, Cl$^-$, HCO$_3^-$ Blood urea nitrogen	Daily until glucose infusion load and patient stable, then twice weekly
Serum albumin, transferrin (or TIBC) Liver function studies Serum creatinine Ca^{2+}, PO$_4^{2-}$, Mg^{2+} Hb/Hct, WBC	Baseline, then twice weekly
Prothrombin time, partial thromboplastin time Micronutrient tests as indicated	Baseline, then weekly

under stringent aseptic techniques. Major mechanical complications include pneumothorax, hemothorax from laceration of the subclavian artery or vein, brachial plexus injury, and malpositioning of the catheter in a cerebral vein, the azygos vein, or the right ventricle. The correct catheter position must be confirmed by x-ray before hypertonic nutrient solution is infused. Catheters can subsequently back out of the vein, develop leaks, or become detached from the hub and embolize into the heart or pulmonary artery. Catheter thrombosis may occur, especially if the catheter is used for withdrawing blood samples. Thrombosis of the catheter with involvement of the central vein is frequently coincident with infection. Thrombosed catheters can sometimes be unblocked by urokinase treatment. The addition of low-dose heparin (1000 units per liter) to limit thrombosis in parenteral catheters is controversial; no randomized, controlled studies demonstrate benefit, and heparin can contribute to loss of bone mineral, which is a particular problem in long-term parenteral nutrition.

METABOLIC   Fluid overload produces congestive heart failure especially in elderly and debilitated patients. Glucose overload can lead to osmotic diuresis and, via the stimulation of insulin, result in massive extracellular to intracellular shifts of phosphorous and potassium. Such shifts are most likely in cachectic patients with total-body phosphorus and potassium depletion; the reduction in plasma potassium and phosphorus levels can result in arrhythmias, cardiopulmonary dysfunction, and neurologic symptoms. To avoid these problems, parenteral nutrition should be started slowly and monitored carefully.

Late metabolic complications include cholestatic liver disease with bile sludging and gallstone formation. The exact cause of the liver disease is not understood, but defective sulfur amino acid metabolism may play a role. Cholestasis appears to be associated with the lack of enteral stimulation and is less likely to occur if some enteral feeding is maintained. Parenteral nutrition induces hypercalcuria, which can result in negative calcium balance and osteopenia. The hypercalcuria appears to be due to several factors, including effects of infused amino acid and the high fixed acid load of the bisulfite preservative. With earlier protein hydrolysate solutions aluminum contamination occurred which blocked bone mineralization; aluminum may still be a contaminant of some parenteral solution additives. Once patients on long-term parenteral nutrition move from catabolic breakdown to sustained anabolism, deficiencies of micronutrients such as essential fatty acids, trace minerals, and vitamins may develop unless they are provided in the parenteral nutrient solution (see Table 76-4).

INFECTIOUS Infection of the access line rarely occurs in the first 72 h, and early fever is usually due to infection elsewhere or some other cause. Infection of the access line is likely if the patient defervesces when the infusion rate of the parenteral formula is tapered. Positive central line cultures suggest catheter sepsis, especially if no other infectious source is identified and if the organism is *Staphylococcus* or *Candida*. While removal of the central catheter may allow the patient to clear fungemia spontaneously, antibiotic therapy is usually necessary for bacterial infections. Catheter sepsis is less likely if central vein parenteral nutrition is provided via a single-lumen catheter; triple-lumen catheters, even if frequently replaced over a guidewire, are associated with a greater incidence of sepsis. Recurrent catheter sepsis may be avoided if small amounts of an antibiotic solution are left in the line along with a heparin lock.

ENTERAL NUTRITION Tube placement and patient monitoring The types, techniques of insertion, uses, and potential problems of enteral tubes are outlined in Table 76-9. Some of the available enteral formulas and their nutrient compositions are listed in Table 75-8 and in a more generic form in Table 76-10. Patients on enteral feeding are at risk for some of the same metabolic complications as parenterally fed patients and should receive the same clinical and laboratory monitoring (Table 76-10). Since small-bore tubes are easily displaced, tube position should be tested by aspirating and measuring the pH of the gut fluid (<4 in stomach, >6 in jejunum).

Complications ASPIRATION The debilitated patient with poor gastric emptying and an impaired swallow and cough mechanism is at risk for aspiration. In patients on respirators, effective tracheal suctioning induces coughing and provokes gastric regurgitation, and the cuff on the endotracheal tube or tracheostomy seldom provides adequate protection against aspiration. Under these circumstances, it may be safer to use a large-bore rubber feeding tube to allow for an accurate check of residual gastric contents and, if necessary, removal of gastric contents prior to tracheal suction.

Although normal gastric motility provides a churning and fragmenting activity with intermittent propulsion of liquid and small food fragments into the duodenum, constant gastric infusion of an enteral formula is better tolerated in sick patients than is intermittent bolus feeding. A continuous infusion is best achieved with an enteral feeding pump, especially with fine-bore feeding tubes that have a greater potential to clog. If long-term gastric feeding is anticipated, endoscopic, radiologic, or surgical placement of a gastric tube is

---

TABLE 76-9 Enteral feeding tubes

Placement technique	Clinical uses	Potential problems	Placement technique	Clinical uses	Potential problems
NASOGASTRIC TUBE			**GASTROSTOMY TUBE**		
External measurement: nostril, ear to xiphisternum; placed by professional or, with instruction, by family member or patient; tube stiffened by ice water or a stylet; position tested by injecting air and auscultating air bubble passing through fluid, by aspirating acid gastric contents, or by checking an x-ray.	Short-term clinical situations (a few weeks); placement can be intermittent; normal gastric emptying required; bolus feeds or continuous drip.	Aspiration pneumonia from regurgitated stomach contents; irritation of nasopharynx or esophagogastric junction with bleeding and/or stricture.	Tube placed through the abdominal wall into the stomach, either by a percutaneous radiologic or endoscopic technique using local anesthetic or surgically via an abdominal incision using a spinal or general anesthetic; can be converted to gastric "button" for long-term ambulatory patients.	Long-term access; once tract is established, tubes can be replaced; used when swallowing is impaired because of either mechanical obstruction or neurologic discoordination.	Irritation around tube site; aspiration of stomach contents; displacement of tube into peritoneal cavity or, if held in situ by balloon, migration and obstruction of the pylorus.
NASODUODENAL OR NASOJEJUNAL TUBE			**JEJUNOSTOMY TUBE**		
External measurement: nostril, ear to anterosuperior iliac spine in adults; to the medial malleolus in infants; weighted tube may pass spontaneously through pylorus if patient lies on right side; or tube is placed in jejunum with stiffening stylet under fluoroscopy; position tested by aspirating alkaline duodenal contents or by checking an x-ray.	Short-term clinical situations; used if gastric emptying is impaired or to infuse beyond a high bowel fistula such as an esophageal tear or gastric or duodenal fistula.	Passing tube through pylorus; preventing the spontaneous pulling back into stomach; continuous drip required and tends to cause diarrhea; tubes stiffen with time; can lacerate pylorus or gastroesophageal junction if pulled out rapidly.	Tube placed radiologically or surgically through abdominal wall into proximal loop of jejunum and tethered to anterior wall by suture; fine-bore tube inserted by diagonal tract into bowel lumen or large bore secured with an anchoring suture.	Long-term access; used for defective gastric emptying; fine-bore tube recommended as postoperative backup when prolonged gastric atony might occur.	Irritation at tube exit site, especially with large-bore tube; clogging or displacement of tube; continuous drip usually required; diarrhea
PHARYNGOSTOMY/ESOPHAGOSTOMY TUBE			**COMBINED GASTROJEJUNOSTOMY TUBE**		
Tube placed surgically through side of neck into pharynx.	Long-term access; no nasopharyngeal irritation; once tract is established, tubes can be replaced.	Aspiration; pharyngeal scarring causes distortion of normal anatomy.	Tube placed intragastrically with jejunal arm threaded beyond the pylorus.	Allows for simultaneous gastric suction and jejunal infusion; used in patient particularly at risk for aspiration of gastric contents.	Not yet widely available.

TABLE 76-10 Types of enteral feeding formulas

Description	Clinical indications	Delivery method	Comments on cost, amount needed to meet RDAs*
BLENDERIZED FORMULA			
Mixture of pureed meat, fruit, vegetables, sometimes added nonfat milk, fiber, vitamins, and minerals; highly viscous.	Normal digestion and absorption required; can be fed into esophagus, stomach, duodenum, or jejunum.	By sipping or via a large-bore tube (12–18 French); bolus or drip with pump.	Lowest cost; 2 L or more daily†
POLYMERIC FORMULA			
Mixture of whole proteins, polysaccharides, and triglycerides; seldom contain fiber; lower viscosity than blenderized formulas.	Normal digestion and absorption required; can be fed into esophagus, stomach, duodenum, or jejunum.	By sipping or via a small-bore tube (8–12 french); bolus or drip with pump.	2 L or more needed daily.
MONOMERIC FORMULA			
Mixture of predigested protein, carbohydrate (CHO), and a small amount of trigylceride; enough to provide essential fatty acids; contains no fiber; lowest viscosity of all formulas.	Used for inflammatory bowel disease, chronic pancreatitis, GI fistula, enteritis from radiation or chemotherapy, pan-malabsorption, or as a transition feeding from parenteral to enteral therapy.	Small-bore tube (5–8 French) drip with pump	Higher cost than polymeric formulas; 1.5–3 L needed daily.
DISEASE-RELATED FORMULA			
Devised to meet the nutritional needs of specific disease states; varying amounts of protein, amino acid ratios, CHO, electrolytes, and caloric density; low viscosity.	Used for fluid restricted, heart failure, renal failure, hepatic encephalopathy, high protein requirement, trauma, burn.	Small-bore tube (5–8 French) drip with pump	Highest cost; 1–2 L needed daily.
MODULAR FORMULA			
Made-to-order feedings of individual constitutents; viscosity depends on quantities of protein, CHO, and fat.	Used for specific metabolic abnormalities, such as glycogen storage disease.	Varies, depending on viscosity.	Higher cost than monomeric formula; 1.5 L or more needed daily.

* RDA = recommended daily allowance of nutrient.
† Commercially made blenderized formulas are now available which can be delivered through small-bore tubes (8 French); relatively expensive.

preferred by most patients. For long-term ambulatory patients, a gastrostomy tube can be converted to a gastric "button," an access device that is flush with the skin.

A nasojejunal tube reduces the risk of aspirations. However, placement of such tubes through the pylorus is time-consuming, and such tubes frequently pull back into the stomach. Radiologic placement of a percutaneous gastric-jejunal tube is more reliable. If a debilitated patient with poor gastric emptying goes to surgery, it is appropriate to ask the surgeon to place a jejunostomy tube for feeding. This can involve a traditional (10 to 14 French) or a fine-bore (5 to 8 French) tube inserted through an oblique needle track that seals rapidly when the jejunostomy tube is removed.

DIARRHEA Enteral feeding often causes diarrhea, especially if absorption is compromised by bowel disease or drugs such as antibiotics. The diarrhea may be controlled by the use of continuous drip feeding or the addition of enteral bulking agents, such as psyllium hydrophilic mucilogs, or an anticholinergic medication, in the formula. Diarrhea, stimulated by enteral feeding, does not necessarily imply inadequate absorption of nutrients other than water and electrolytes. Furthermore, since luminal nutrients induce trophic effects on the gut mucosa and stimulate the enteric immunologic barrier, it may be appropriate to persist despite the diarrhea, even when this necessitates temporary supplemental parenteral fluid support.

THE COST OF NUTRITION SUPPORT Specialized nutrition support accounts for 1 percent of health care costs or approximately $6 billion per year in the United States. Most nutrition support is provided to hospitalized patients. Characteristically, such patients are among the most sick and have an above-average length of hospital stay, and many are high users of other life-sustaining therapies. Such patients are typically referred from smaller hospitals to tertiary-

care centers. With pressure mounting to contain health care costs, randomized, control trials such as those described above are important to determine the appropriate use of this treatment. The costs and complications of parenteral nutrition can be reduced if patient management is supervised by a nutrition support service. In one study, catheter sepsis decreased from 29 to 5 percent after such a service was instituted, and in another study, routine consultations with a nutrition support service resulted in a 20 percent reduction in average hospital stay and a 26 percent average reduction in costs per patient.

In patients with benign forms of extreme short bowel syndrome such as extensive surgical resection for Crohn's disease or mesenteric bowel infarction, home parenteral nutrition is associated with low morbidity and high rates of rehabilitation. Longitudinal data from a national registry for home parenteral nutrition patients show that 97 percent of Crohn's patients experience partial or complete rehabilitation. Home parenteral nutrition costs about half as much as in-hospital treatment. Enteral feeding is now common for many other debilitated patients both in nursing homes and at home. The clinical outcome for such patients has not been well studied.

REFERENCES

ALEXANDER WJ et al: The importance of lipid type in the diet after burn injury. Ann Surg 240:1, 1986

ALUN JONES V: Comparison of total parenteral nutrition and elemental diet in induction of remission of Crohn's disease. Dig Dis Sci 332:100S, 1987

ANDERSON GF, STEINBERG EP: DRGs and specialized nutritional support: The need for reform. J Parenter Enter Nutr 10:3, 1986

AMERICAN COLLEGE OF PHYSICIANS: Position paper: Parenteral nutrition in patients receiving cancer chemotherapy: A meta-analysis. Ann Intern Med 110:734, 1989

BOWER RH et al: Branched chain amino acid–enriched solutions in the septic patient: A randomized, prospective trial. Ann Surg 203:13, 1986

CERRA FB et al: Disease-specific amino acid infusion (FO80) in hepatic encephalopathy: A prospective, randomized, double blind, controlled trial. J Parenter Enter Nutr 9:288, 1985

CHIARELLI A et al: Very early nutrition supplementation in burned patients. Am J Clin Nutr 51:1035, 1990

DETSKY AS et al: Perioperative parenteral nutrition: A Meta-analysis. Ann Intern Med 107:195, 1987

Evaluating total parenteral nutrition: Assessment and practice guidelines forum, Georgetown University School of Medicine. Dig Dis Sci 34:489, 1989

FOX AD et al: Effect of glutamine-supplemented enteral diet on methotrexate-induced enterocolitis. J Parenter Enter Nutr 12:325, 1988

GIAFFER MH et al: Controlled trial of polymeric versus elemental diet in treatment of active Crohn's disease. Lancet 335:816, 1990

GREENBERG GR et al: Controlled trial of bowel rest and nutritional support in the management of Crohn's disease. Gut 29:1309, 1988

HILL A: Body composition research: Implications for the practice of clinical nutrition. J Parenter Enter Nutr 16:197, 1992

HOWARD L et al: Medical effectiveness of home parenteral nutrition support as judged by four years of North American Registry data. J Parenter Enter Nutr 15:384, 1991

KIRBY DF, CRAIG RM: The value of intensive nutritional support in pancreatitis. J Parenter Enter Nutr 9:353, 1985

———— et al: Intravenous nutritional support during pregnancy. J Parenter Enter Nutr 12:72, 1988

KOPPLE JD: Dietary considerations in patients with advance chronic renal failure, acute renal failure, and transplantation, in Diseases of the Kidney, vol 3, 4th ed, RW Schrier, CW Gohschalk (eds). Philadelphia, Saunders, 1988

LOCHS H et al: Comparison of enteral nutrition and drug treatment in active Crohn's disease. Gastroenterology 101:881, 1991

NAYLOR CD et al: Parenteral nutrition with branched-chain amino acids in heptic encephalopathy: A meta-analysis. Gastroenterology 97:1033, 1989

Perioperative total parenteral nutrition in surgical patients: Veterans Administration total parenteral nutrition cooperative study. N Engl J Med 325:525, 1991

RAPP RP et al: The favorable effect of early parenteral feeding on survival in head injured patients. J Neurosurg 58:90, 1983

RIGAUD D et al: Controlled trial comparing two types of enteral nutrition in treatment of active Crohn's disease: Elemental v. polymeric diet. Gut 32:1492, 1991

SAX HC et al: Early total parenteral nutrition in acute pancreatitis: Lack of beneficial effects. Am J Surg 153:117, 1987

SEIDMAN E: Nutritional management of inflammatory bowel disease. Gastroenterol Clin North Am 17:129, 1989

SITZMANN JV et al: Statement on guidelines for total parenteral nutrition. Dig Dis Sci 34:489, 1989

SZELUGA DJ et al: Nutritional support of bone marrow transplant recipients: A prospective, randomized clinical trial comparing total parenteral nutrition to an enteral feeding program. Cancer Res 47:3309, 1987

WEINSIER RL et al: Cost containment: A contribution of aggressive nutrition support in burn patients. J Burn Care Rehabil 6:436, 1985

WEISDORF S et al: Influence of prophylactic total parenteral nutrition on long-term outcome of bone marrow transplantation. Transplantation 43:833, 1987

77   VITAMIN DEFICIENCY AND EXCESS*

JEAN D. WILSON

Vitamins play several roles in human disease. Deficiencies of single vitamins are now rarely endemic, even in developing nations, and are more likely to occur either as a portion of states of general malnutrition, as a result of food faddism, as a complication of another disease such as malabsorption, as a consequence of complex therapy such as hemodialysis or total parenteral nutrition, or as the result of an inborn error of metabolism. Indeed, disorders of vitamin excess may now be more common than vitamin deficiency.

In considering the pathophysiology of vitamins, several points are worth emphasis: (1) The fact that organic compounds cannot be synthesized within the body and are required constituents of the diet is the result of mutations, and the provision of vitamins in the diet is a form of therapy for an inborn error of metabolism. In some instances, such as the limited ability to synthesize thiamine, the requirement is common to many, if not all, animals, and the mutation must have occurred early in evolution; in others, such as the single-gene defect that prevents ascorbic acid synthesis, humans share the defect with

only a few species, such as the guinea pig. (2) The feature that separates vitamins from other necessary organic constituents in the diet is that small amounts are required in contrast to the relatively large amounts of essential amino acids and essential fatty acids. This is a consequence of the fact that vitamins function not as building blocks of tissue mass or as substrates for energy production but as prosthetic groups for quantitatively minor tissue constituents or as catalytic cofactors for biologic reactions; like most catalysts, they are required only in small amounts. (3) Deficiency of some vitamins (e.g., pantothenic acid) has never been described in humans, implying that these vitamins either are so ubiquitous in food sources or are conserved so efficiently by the body that deficiency can become manifest, if at all, only in the context of a mixed nutritional and vitamin deficiency. (4) Alcoholism is the background upon which many vitamin deficiencies develop. This is the consequence of several interlocking factors, including diminished intake, impairment of absorption and storage of vitamins, and, in some cases, predisposing genetic factors. (5) Biochemical means of proving vitamin deficiency, once suspected, are limited, and the role of vitamin deficiency in disease states is frequently not recognized because nonspecific vitamin therapy is a common part of standard supportive care. As a consequence, knowledge of the manifestations of vitamin deficiency and a high index of suspicion in the appropriate setting are essential for considering the diagnosis, and demonstration of a response to replacement therapy may be the most accurate way to confirm a diagnosis. (6) The consumption of excessive amounts of vitamins can occur either as the indirect consequence of dietary practice or, more commonly, as the result of deliberate ingestion. Syndromes of excess for the fat-soluble vitamins A and D are well characterized, whereas the toxicity syndromes produced by the water-soluble vitamins are inconsistent and less well understood.

DEFICIENCY STATES

NIACIN (PELLAGRA)   **Biochemistry**   *Niacin* is the generic term for nicotinic acid (pyridine-3-carboxylic acid) and derivatives that exhibit the nutritional activity of nicotinic acid (Fig. 77-1). In one sense, niacin is not a vitamin, since it can be formed from the essential amino acid tryptophan. In the human, an average of about 1 mg of niacin is formed from 60 mg of dietary tryptophan. Accordingly, estimates of the adequacy of dietary intake must take into account the tryptophan content of the diet as well as the content of niacin. Many foodstuffs, especially cereals, contain bound forms of niacin from which the vitamin is not nutritionally available.

The vitamin is absorbed rapidly from the intestine by both active and passive transport mechanisms. The capacity to absorb niacin is approximately 3 to 4 g/d in the human. Approximately one-fifth of the vitamin is decarboxylated to nicotinuric acid, and the remainder is excreted in the urine as methylated products, largely *N*-methylnicotinamide (NMN) and *N*-methyl-2-pyridone-5-carboxamide.

Mechanism of action   Niacin is an essential component of nicotinamide adenine dinucleotide (NAD) and nicotinamide adenine dinucleotide phosphate (NADP), coenzymes for many oxidation-reduction reactions.

Requirements   The requirements and recommended daily allowances for niacin and tryptophan are listed in Table 71-4. In contrast to most vitamins, the requirement for niacin does not appear to be increased during pregnancy. Requirement is determined primarily by the amino acid composition of the diet.

Experimental depletion   After the institution of a diet deficient in niacin and tryptophan, the urinary excretion of niacin metabolites reaches minimal values (<1.5 mg/d) after 1 to 2 months. Clinical deficiency develops shortly thereafter and consists of dermatitis, glossitis, stomatitis, diarrhea, proctitis, mental depression, abdominal pain, vaginitis, dysphagia, and amenorrhea, findings similar to those in pellagra.

* For vitamin D, see Chap. 358, and for the hematologic vitamins, see Chap. 304.

Vitamin	Active Derivative or Cofactor Form	Principal Function
Niacin	Nicotinamide Adenine Dinucleotide Phosphate (NADP) and Nicotine Adenine Dinucleotide (NAD)	Coenzymes for Oxidations and Reductions
Thiamine	Thiamine Diphosphate	Coenzyme for Cleavage of Carbon-Carbon Bonds
Pyridoxine	Pyridoxal Phosphate	Cofactor for Enzymes of Amino Acid Metabolism
Riboflavin	Flavin Mononucleotide (FMN) and Flavin Adenine Dinucleotide (FAD)	Cofactor for Oxidation-Reduction Reactions and Covalently Attached Prosthetic Groups for Some Enzymes
Ascorbic Acid	Ascorbic Acid and Dehydroascorbic Acid	Participation as a Redox Ion in Many Biological Oxidation Reactions
Biotin	Biotin	Apoenzyme for Carboxylase Enzymes
Vitamin A	Retinol, Retinal, and Retinoic Acid	Formation of Carotenoid Proteins (Vision) and Glycoproteins (Epithelial Cell Function)
Vitamin E	Tocopherol	Antioxidant
Vitamin K	Menaquinone	Cofactor for Post-Translational Carboxylation of Many Proteins Including Essential Clotting Factors

FIGURE 77-1 The structure and principal functions of some of the vitamins associated with human disorders.

Clinical deficiency Pellagra was previously an endemic disease in the American South and in many other parts of the world. The endemic disease is usually associated with a high intake of maize (American corn) or of millet (sorghum, jowar) and can be cured by the administration of niacin; nevertheless, the fact that large populations of people exist on a diet in which maize is the major source of protein but are free of endemic pellagra implies that the relation between maize intake and the development of the disease is not straightforward. The niacin equivalent (available niacin and tryptophan) of maize, although low, is no lower than that of some cereals that are unassociated with endemic pellagra. As a consequence, the concept of the pathogenesis of pellagra has evolved from that of a pure vitamin deficiency or a mixed deficiency of tryptophan and available niacin in the diet to a more complicated etiology. The disorder may be due to an imbalance in dietary amino acids or to a complex deficiency state. Alternatively, the milling of maize influences the bioavailability of the niacin in the cereal. Treatment of maize with alkali in the preparation of foods in Latin America may serve to hydrolyze bound nicotinic acid and inactivate toxins that accumulate in stored grain contaminated with molds. Alternatively, degermination of the cereal during the common milling process in the United States may inhibit the liberation of bound niacin. The effect of these treatments, respectively, would be to prevent or to predispose to the development of pellagra when maize is a major element of the diet.

Whatever the cause, endemic pellagra disappeared coincident with the improvement of nutritional education and the widespread supplementation of grain cereals with niacin. Pellagra is a rare manifestation of two disorders of tryptophan metabolism, the carcinoid syndrome, in which up to 60 percent of tryptophan is catabolized by what is ordinarily a minor pathway (see Chap. 276), and Hartnup disease (see Chap. 352), an inherited disorder in which several amino acids including tryptophan are absorbed poorly from the diet. In both conditions, pellagra is due to diminished availability of effective niacin equivalents and can be cured by the administration of large amounts of the vitamin.

Pellagra is a chronic wasting disease typically associated with dermatitis, dementia, and diarrhea. The dermatitis is bilateral, symmetric, and present in sites exposed to sunlight and is due to photosensitivity. The mental changes are less discrete; fatigue, insomnia, and apathy may precede the development of an encephalopathy characterized by confusion, disorientation, hallucination, loss of memory, and eventually, organic psychosis. Paresthesias and polyneuritis may be the result of coexisting deficiencies of other vitamins. Diarrhea, when present, results from widespread inflammation of the mucous surfaces; other mucosal abnormalities include achlorhydria, glossitis, stomatitis, and vaginitis. The skin lesions are characterized by hyperkeratosis, hyperpigmentation, and desquamation. The course is progressive over a several-year period, and death is usually due to secondary complications.

The relation between the coenzyme functions of NAD and NADP and the symptoms has not been defined. Levels of NAD and NADP in erythrocytes are low in patients with pellagra, but the coenzymes are essential to so many reactions in intermediary metabolism that profound deficiency of NAD and NADP is incompatible with life. The mental changes in pellagra may be due to diminished conversion of tryptophan to serotonin.

No biochemical test is of diagnostic value, and diagnosis must be based on suspicion and response to replacement therapy. As predicted, urinary excretion of the metabolites of nicotinic acid and tryptophan is low but not lower than in patients with generalized malnutrition. Plasma tryptophan and erythrocyte NAD and NADP levels are also low.

The administration of small amounts of niacin (10 mg/d) in the face of adequate amounts of dietary tryptophan is sufficient to cure endemic pellagra. Large amounts of niacin (40 to 200 mg/d) may be required in Hartnup disease and in the carcinoid syndrome.

THIAMINE (BERIBERI) **Biochemistry** Thiamine contains pyrimidine and thiazole moieties linked by a methylene bridge (see Fig. 77-1). The vitamin is synthesized by a variety of plants and microorganisms but not ordinarily by animals. However, rats and pigeons fed a thiamine-free diet can be protected from deficiency by large quantities of the pyrimidine and thiazole moieties, suggesting a small capacity to couple the subunits together. Small amounts may be synthesized by microorganisms in the gastrointestinal tract. Thiamine is absorbed both by an active-transport process and by passive diffusion. The capacity to absorb the vitamin in the human intestine is about 5 mg/d. Approximately 25 to 30 mg is stored in the body, 80 percent as thiamine diphosphate (pyrophosphate), 10 percent as thiamine triphosphate, and the remainder as thiamine monophosphate. Large amounts are present in skeletal muscles, heart, liver, kidneys, and brain. A number of thiaminase enzymes inactivate thiamine by splitting the vitamin into its two component parts. Several metabolites are excreted in the urine, principally thiamine itself (which is secreted by the renal tubules), an acetylated derivative, and derivatives of thiazole acetate and pyrimidine carboxylate.

Mechanism of action Thiamine diphosphate acts as a coenzyme for several reactions that cleave carbon-carbon bonds—the oxidative decarboxylation of α-keto acids (pyruvate and α-ketoglutarate) and keto analogues of leucine, isoleucine, and valine and the transketolase reaction in the pentose phosphate pathway. Many features of thiamine deficiency are the result of inhibition of these enzymatic reactions and/or the accumulation of the proximal metabolites. Thiamine also may have a specific role in neurons independent of its function in general metabolism; thiamine and its esters are present in axonal membranes, and electrical stimulation of nerves effects the hydrolysis and release of thiamine diphosphate and triphosphate.

Requirements The recommended daily allowances for thiamine are given in Table 71-4. The vitamin has a widespread distribution in food and is absent only from oils, fats, cassava, and refined sugar. In vegetable products, the vitamin is largely in the form of thiamine. The outer layers of cereal grains are especially rich in the vitamin; hence machine-milled rice is a poor source. In animal tissues, thiamine is present largely in the form of phosphate esters. The esters are dephosphorylated by phosphatases in the intestine, and only the free vitamin is absorbed. A substantial loss of the vitamin takes place during cooking above 100°C.

Several factors influence the absorption and metabolism of the vitamin (and hence alter daily requirements). One is the presence of thiaminases in foods such as fresh fish, clams, shrimp, mussels, and some raw animal tissues and in microorganisms in the colon. Two, daily needs decrease when fat forms a large part of the diet and increase as carbohydrate intake increases. Requirements are increased by pregnancy, lactation, thyrotoxicosis, and fever. Accelerated loss of thiamine may occur with diuretic therapy, hemodialysis, peritoneal dialysis, and diarrhea. Defective absorption can occur in malabsorption states, alcoholism, chronic malnutrition, and folate deficiency.

Experimental depletion Following the institution of a thiamine-free diet in control subjects, urinary thiamine excretion decreases to 5 percent of the control value after a week and is undetectable after 2 weeks. However, the excretion of the pyrimidine and thiazole catabolites remains unchanged for as long as a month, indicating that the body pool is slowly utilized when intake is low.

Within a week after the institution of a deficient diet, subjects develop a resting tachycardia, followed by the onset of weakness, decreased deep tendon reflexes, and (in some) sensory neuropathy. Symptoms include generalized malaise, headache, nausea, and aching of the muscles. Appearance of these symptoms is paralleled by a fall in red blood cell transketolase activity. Within a week of thiamine repletion (2 mg/d), all abnormal physical findings disappear, and the subjective symptoms clear after 2 weeks. (Experimental depletion in humans has not been carried to the point of development of severe manifestations.)

Clinical deficiency In developed nations, thiamine deficiency occurs in alcoholics or food faddists or in the context of special clinical situations, such as chronic peritoneal dialysis, hemodialysis, refeeding after starvation, or after the administration of glucose to asymptomatic but thiamine-depleted patients. In developing countries, the disorder is commonly due to the consumption of milled rice or foods containing thiaminases or (possibly) other antithiamine factors.

Development of thiamine deficiency in chronic alcoholics is due to low thiamine intake, impaired thiamine absorption and storage, accelerated destruction of thiamine diphosphate, and varying degrees of energy expenditure. However, clinical manifestations develop in only a fraction of alcoholics and other chronically malnourished persons. Genetic factors may be involved in susceptibility.

The two major manifestations of thiamine deficiency involve the cardiovascular (wet beriberi) and nervous systems (dry beriberi and the Wernicke-Korsakoff syndrome). The typical patient has mixed symptoms involving both the cardiovascular and nervous systems, but pure cardiovascular, neuropathic, and cerebral forms also occur. The relative preponderance of these manifestations is related in part to the duration and severity of deficiency, the degree of physical exertion, and the caloric intake. Severe physical exertion, high carbohydrate intake, and a moderate degree of chronic deficiency favor wet beriberi with little or no peripheral neuritis, whereas an equal deficiency with caloric restriction and relative inactivity favors the development of dry beriberi.

Beriberi heart disease comprises three major physiologic derangements: (1) peripheral vasodilatation leading to a high-output state, (2) retention of sodium and water leading to edema, and (3) biventricular myocardial failure. In the chronic form, peripheral vasodilatation leads to increased arteriovenous shunting of blood, rapid circulation time, tachycardia, increased cardiac output, and a venous congestive state characterized by elevated peripheral venous pressure, elevated right ventricular end-diastolic pressure, decreased arteriovenous extraction of oxygen, sodium retention, and edema. Decreased cerebral and renal blood flow and increased flow to muscles are common. Cardiac output increases so that notwithstanding the lowered peripheral vascular resistance, ventricular work, arterial blood pressure, and pulmonary wedge pressure tend to be elevated. Temporary appearance or worsening of hypertension may occur during thiamine repletion, presumably due to closing of arteriovenous shunts and temporary volume overload.

In acute fulminant cardiovascular (shoshin) beriberi, the myocardial lesion is the central feature of a course in which dyspnea, restlessness, and anxiety eventuate in acute cardiovascular collapse and death within hours to days. Physical findings include stocking-glove cyanosis, tachycardia, marked cardiomegaly, hepatomegaly, arterial bruits, and neck vein distention. The venous pressure is high, and the circulation time is rapid. Because of the fulminant course, edema may be minimal or absent. Administration of thiamine rapidly restores peripheral vascular resistance, but improvement in the myocardial abnormality may be delayed so that low-output failure supervenes during treatment.

Three types of nervous system involvement occur: peripheral neuropathy, Wernicke's encephalopathy (cerebral beriberi), and the Korsakoff syndrome. The neuropathy may or may not be painful and is characterized by a symmetric impairment of sensory, motor, and reflex function that affects predominately the distal segments of limbs. The histologic lesion is a noninflammatory degeneration of myelin sheaths. No meaningful distinction can be made between this disorder and so-called alcoholic neuropathy on the basis of clinical criteria.

Wernicke's encephalopathy ordinarily develops in an orderly sequence and consists of vomiting, nystagmus (horizontal more commonly than vertical), palsies of the rectus muscles leading to unilateral or bilateral ophthalmoplegia (and decrease in the nystagmus), fever, ataxia, and progressive mental deterioration that eventuates in a global confusional state and may progress to coma and death. Improvement occurs after thiamine replacement, although Korsakoff's syndrome may supervene. Thus the eye palsies are corrected, the nystagmus improves in one-half, the ataxia improves or disappears in two-thirds, and the global confusional state disappears to be replaced by Korsakoff's syndrome. The latter consists of retrograde amnesia, impaired ability to learn, and (usually) confabulation. The patient is typically alert and responsive and exhibits no serious defect in behavior. Recovery (complete or partial) from Korsakoff's syndrome occurs only in one-half.

In summary, Wernicke's encephalopathy and the amnesic psychosis of Korsakoff's syndrome are not separate clinical events; instead, the changing ocular and ataxic signs, the transformation of the global confusional state into the amnesic-confabulatory syndrome, and the development of a nonconfabulatory amnesic state are successive stages in the recovery from a single process. The clinical features, differential diagnosis, course, and pathology of cerebral beriberi are discussed in detail in Chap. 377.

Various biochemical tests to detect thiamine deficiency include the measurement of blood thiamine, pyruvate, α-ketoglutarate, lactate, and glyoxylate; measurement of the urinary excretion of thiamine and thiamine metabolites; the thiamine-loading test; and measurement of urinary methylglyoxal. The most reliable is the measurement of whole-blood or erythrocyte transketolase activity. Any enhancement in enzymatic activity resulting from added thiamine diphosphate (TPP) is referred to as the *TPP effect* (expressed in percent). If the activity of the enzyme is increased more than 15 percent by the added thiamine diphosphate, then a deficiency state is probably present. Due to variability in activity, measurement of isolated transketolase levels is not useful, but demonstration of an increase in activity after treatment coupled with a positive TPP test prior to treatment suggests thiamine deficiency.

Another criterion for the diagnosis is the assessment of clinical response to thiamine administration. Clinical improvement may be dramatic in cardiovascular beriberi, with an increase in blood pressure and a decrease in heart rate within 12 h after start of therapy and diuresis and reduction in heart size within 1 to 2 days.

Prompt administration of thiamine is indicated when beriberi is diagnosed or suspected. Fifty milligrams per day should be given intramuscularly for several days, after which 2.5 to 5 mg/d can be administered by mouth. Larger amounts are usually not absorbed. All patients also should receive other water-soluble vitamins in therapeutic quantities.

Thiamine-responsive inborn errors of metabolism Thiamine-responsive inborn errors of metabolism, in which patients respond to pharmacologic doses of thiamine, include thiamine-responsive megaloblastic anemia, for which the mechanism is unknown; thiamine-responsive lactic acidosis, which is due to low activity of pyruvate carboxylase in liver; thiamine-responsive branched-chain ketoaciduria, which is due to low activity of a ketoacid dehydrogenase; and intermittent cerebellar ataxia, which may result from an abnormal pyruvate dehydrogenase. In addition, the autosomal recessive disorder subacute necrotizing encephalomyelopathy (Leigh's disease) may be related to a diminished amount of thiamine triphosphate in neural tissue; a factor has been isolated from the urine of such patients that inhibits the enzyme that synthesizes thiamine triphosphate. The response of patients with Leigh's disease to pharmacologic doses appears to be minor, however.

PYRIDOXINE (VITAMIN B$_6$)   Biochemistry The biologic activity of the vitamin B$_6$ group is displayed by pyridoxine, pyridoxal, and pyridoxamine and their 5-phosphate esters (see Fig. 77-1). The coenzyme form is pyridoxal-5-phosphate, and the other compounds owe their activity to conversion to pyridoxal-5-phosphate. The vitamin is widely and uniformly distributed in all foods; muscle meats, liver, vegetables, and whole-grain cereals are among the best sources.

Mechanism of action Pyridoxal phosphate acts as a cofactor for many enzymes involved in amino acid metabolism, including transaminases, synthetases, and hydroxylases. In humans, the vitamin is of particular importance in the metabolism of tryptophan, glycine, serine, glutamate, and the sulfur-containing amino acids. Pyridoxal phosphate is also required for the synthesis of the heme precursor δ-aminolevulinic acid. A large portion of body stores is in muscle phosphorylase, where it functions to stabilize the enzyme rather than as a catalyst. It also plays a poorly understood role in neuronal excitability, possibly as a result of its function in transsulfuration reactions or in γ-aminobutyric acid metabolism.

Requirements The recommended daily allowances are given in Table 71-4. Even more than for most vitamins, the requirement is increased in pregnancy and by the administration of estrogens. Estrogens appear to inhibit the role of pyridoxal phosphate in tryptophan metabolism. Pyridoxine requirement also may be increased by high protein intake and by either chronic hemodialysis or peritoneal dialysis. The ethanol metabolite acetaldehyde displaces pyridoxal phosphate from proteins and thus enhances its degradation.

Experimental depletion The feeding of pyridoxine-deficient diets leads to chemical evidence of deficiency (increased xanthurenic acid and decreased pyridoxine in urine) within a week. Electroencephalographic abnormalities occur within 3 weeks, and some subjects have grand mal seizures. Deficiency induced with the pyridoxine antagonist deoxypyridoxine causes, in addition, seborrheic dermatitis, cheilosis, glossitis, nausea, vomiting, weakness, and dizziness.

Clinical deficiency The widespread occurrence of the vitamin in food is probably the reason that pure pyridoxine deficiency is rare except when the pyridoxine content of food is either destroyed or converted to less available protein-bound forms during processing, as has happened in some infant formulas. It is a paradox, therefore, that pyridoxine deficiency is now common because many drugs act as pyridoxine antagonists. Isoniazid, cycloserine, penicillamine, and carbonyl reagents in general form complexes with the aldehyde moiety of the vitamin and prevent normal function of the coenzyme. In each case abnormal tryptophan metabolism and convulsions can be prevented by supplementation with the vitamin.

Estimates of vitamin deficiency have been based on the correction of clinical signs of deficiency following administration of the vitamin, measurement of the excretion of tryptophan metabolites after tryptophan-loading tests, measurement of various amino acid transferase activities in blood, and measurement of the excretion of pyridoxine or its metabolites or of oxalate in urine. One index is the measurement of urinary tryptophan metabolites, particularly xanthurenic acid, following tryptophan loading. Alternatively, cystathionine can be assayed after administration of a methionine load. In vitro measurement of red blood cell glutamic pyruvic transaminase in the presence and absence of pyridoxal phosphate may be a better indicator of pyridoxine status than either loading test.

The appropriate management is prevention of deficiency. Supplementation of the diet with 30 mg pyridoxine returns tryptophan metabolism to normal in pregnancy, in users of oral contraceptives, and in patients taking isoniazid. Doses as high as 100 mg/d may be required in subjects taking penicillamine.

Pyridoxine-responsive diseases Several genetic disorders cause abnormalities in vitamin B_6 metabolism. In one group, infants develop convulsions and brain damage and die if not provided with large daily supplements of pyridoxine; these children have an apoenzyme for glutamic acid decarboxylase that has a decreased binding affinity for pyridoxal phosphate. Consequently, they do not form normal amounts of γ-aminobutyric acid, a physiologic inhibitor of neurotransmission. Another group has pyridoxine-responsive chronic anemia; pyridoxine supplementation results in prompt hematologic improvement but does not correct the morphologic abnormality in the erythrocytes.

The synthesis of cystathionine from homocystine and serine and its cleavage to cysteine and homoserine are catalyzed by two pyridoxal phosphate enzymes. The changes that occur with deficiency of these two enzymes and in xanthurenic aciduria due to kynureninase deficiency have been reviewed by Mudd. Some patients with vitamin B_6-responsive xanthurenic aciduria or cystathioninuria have a mutant apoenzyme that interacts abnormally with pyridoxal phosphate, a defect that can be largely corrected by elevated concentrations of the cofactor. In contrast, the vitamin B_6 response in patients with homocystinuria due to cystathionine synthetase deficiency results from enhancement of the activity of the residual amount of normal enzyme present rather than from a restoration of the affected enzyme levels to normal.

RIBOFLAVIN Riboflavin in the form of the coenzymes flavin mononucleotide (FMN) and flavin adenine dinucleotide (FAD) (see Fig. 77-1) participates in a variety of oxidation-reduction reactions. In addition, covalently attached flavins are essential to the structure of such enzymes as succinate dehydrogenase and monoamine oxidase. The vitamin is absorbed from the gastrointestinal tract either as free riboflavin or the 5'-phosphate by an active transport process. The recommended daily allowance is listed in Table 71-4. Covalently linked vitamin accounts for less than one-tenth of the tissue pool. The vitamin is excreted in urine predominantly in the free form, although a small fraction of the daily turnover is the result of catabolism by microorganisms in the gastrointestinal tract.

Riboflavin deficiency can be induced by feeding a riboflavin-deficient diet or by the administration of riboflavin antagonists such as galactoflavin. Deficiency is characterized by sore throat, hyperemia and edema of the oral mucous membranes, cheilosis, angular stomatitis, glossitis, seborrheic dermatitis, and normochromic, normocytic anemia due to red cell hypoplasia of the bone marrow. These features can be reversed by riboflavin administration. Thyroid hormones and adrenal steroids enhance FMN and FAD synthesis; phenothiazines and tricyclic antidepressants competitively inhibit flavin coenzyme biosynthesis, but these agents alone do not induce deficiency. Instead, riboflavin deficiency almost invariably occurs in combination with deficiencies of other water-soluble vitamins. Riboflavin requirements are increased in subjects on chronic hemodialysis or peritoneal dialysis.

VITAMIN C (SCURVY) Biochemistry In most animals, ascorbic acid (vitamin C) can be synthesized from glucose. However, humans, other primates, and the guinea pig are unable to synthesize L-ascorbic acid and require vitamin C in the diet. These species can perform the various reactions required for the biosynthesis of the vitamin from D-glucose except for one step, the conversion of L-gluconogammalactone to L-abscorbic acid. The enzyme that catalyzes this reaction (L-gluconolactone oxidase) is missing because of a mutation; thus the need for vitamin C in the diet is the result of an inborn error in carbohydrate metabolism.

Mechanism of action L-Ascorbic acid readily undergoes reversible oxidation and reduction as follows:

$$\text{L-ascorbic acid} \rightleftharpoons \text{dehydro-L-ascorbic acid} + 2H^+ + 2e$$

This property of the vitamin is the key to understanding its role as a redox agent for biologic oxidation. However, ascorbic acid does not act as a conventional cofactor because its requirement can usually be replaced by other compounds with similar redox properties. The vitamin reduces the prosthetic metal ions in many enzymes to the required forms and performs other antioxidant functions by removing free radicals. The best understood function is in the synthesis of collagen; absence of the vitamin leads to impairment of peptidyl hydroxylation of procollagen and a reduction in collagen formation and secretion by connective tissue. Nonhydroxylated collagen cannot form the triple helix required for normal tissue structure. Many features of scurvy result from this defect in collagen synthesis, including the capillary fragility that underlies the hemorrhagic features, the poor healing of wounds, and (in part) the bony abnormalities of children. Collagens with the highest content of hydroxyproline are most severely affected, accounting for the early disruption of the adventitia, media, and basal laminae of blood vessels. Ascorbic acid also prevents oxidation of tetrahydrofolate and thus protects the active folic acid pool and regulates iron distribution and storage, probably by influencing the valence of stored iron and maintaining a normal ratio of ferritin to hemosiderin. Scorbutic patients excrete incompletely oxidized products of tyrosine metabolism, but the significance is not clear.

Requirements The recommended daily allowance for vitamin C is described in Table 71-4. The vitamin is present in milk and some meats (kidney, liver, fish) and is widely distributed in fruits and vegetables. A portion is lost after prolonged storage of unprocessed fruits and vegetables (e.g., potatoes), but it is partially preserved (half or greater) by most means of food processing (boiling, steaming, pressure cooking, preserving jams and jellies, freezing, dehydration, and canning). As a consequence, the recommended daily allowances can be met with even a modest intake of fruits and vegetables. Utilization of the vitamin is increased during pregnancy and lactation and in thyrotoxicosis, and absorption is decreased in diarrheal states and in achlorhydria.

Experimental depletion The total-body pool of vitamin C varies from 1.5 to 3 g. When a deficient diet is instituted, the pool is depleted at a rate that approximates 4 percent per day. In monkeys, the major catabolic pathway involves oxidation of the alcohol at carbon 6 to an aldehyde and then to an acid. Because of differences in initial pool size and rates of turnover, differences in the completeness of deficiency in various experimental diets, and variation among normal subjects at the cellular or enzymatic level, the time required for development of symptoms ranges from 1 to 3 months in different studies. Manifestations of deficiency correlate better with the total pool size than with plasma or blood levels. The first symptoms (petechial hemorrhages and ecchymoses) develop when the pool size is less than 0.5 g; with further depletion (pool size 0.1 to 0.5 g), manifestations include gum involvement, hyperkeratosis, congested hair follicles, arthralgias, Sjögren's syndrome, coiled hairs, and joint effusions. When depletion is extreme (pool size <0.1 g), dyspnea, edema, oliguria, and neuropathy supervene. Progress of the disease may then be rapid.

Symptoms do not improve until the pool is repleted, and the larger the therapeutic dose, the more rapid is the repletion. However, with doses as small as 6.5 mg/d the body pool eventually returns to normal, and amelioration of symptoms follows.

Clinical deficiency   Scurvy now occurs for the most part in areas of urban poverty. An increased incidence occurs at 6 to 12 months of age in infants whose processed milk formulas are unsupplemented with citrus fruit or vegetables as a result of maternal error or neglect. Another peak occurs in middle and old age; edentulous men who live alone and cook for themselves are particularly prone. Clinical scurvy is more severe than the experimental disease, doubtlessly because affected individuals usually have deficiencies of other dietary constituents as well and because the groups at risk (infants and the elderly) are especially vulnerable.

In adults, the features include perifollicular hyperkeratotic papules in which hairs become fragmented and buried; perifollicular hemorrhages; purpura beginning on the backs of the lower extremities coalescing to become ecchymoses (Fig. 77-2); hemorrhage into the muscles of the arms and legs with secondary phlebothromboses; hemorrhages into joints; splinter hemorrhages in the nail beds; gum involvement (only in people with teeth) that includes swelling, friability, bleeding, secondary infection, and loosening of the teeth; poor wound healing and breakdown of recently healed wounds; petechial hemorrhages in the viscera; and emotional changes. Symptoms resembling those of Sjögren's syndrome may occur. Terminally, icterus, edema, and fever are common, and convulsions, hypotension, and death may occur abruptly.

In infancy and childhood, hemorrhage into the periosteum of long bones causes painful swellings and may result in epiphyseal separation. The sternum may sink inward, leaving a sharp elevation at the rib margins (scorbutic rosary). Purpura and ecchymoses may develop in the skin, and gum lesions occur if the teeth have erupted. Retrobulbar, subarachnoid, and intracerebral hemorrhages rapidly culminate in death if treatment is delayed.

FIGURE 77-2   Hemorrhages and ecchymoses in a patient with scurvy. (*Photograph courtesy of Leonard L. Madison.*)

Normochromic, normocytic anemia is common and is due to bleeding into tissues. Anemia also may be macrocytic and/or megaloblastic (one-fifth of patients in one series). Many foods that contain vitamin C also contain folate, and diets that cause scurvy also may cause folate deficiency. However, ascorbic acid deficiency also results in an increased oxidation of formyl tetrahydrofolic acid to inactive folate metabolites and may cause a decrease in the active folate pool. Whether changes in iron distribution and storage are involved in the pathogenesis of the anemia is unclear. The anemia is corrected with replenishment of vitamin C and institution of a balanced diet.

In some hospitals, platelet ascorbic acid levels are useful in diagnosing scurvy and are usually less than one-fourth of the normal value. Plasma levels of the vitamin correlate less well with the clinical state. In infants, x-ray changes of the bones may be diagnostic. Bilirubin is frequently elevated. Capillary fragility is abnormal.

Scurvy is potentially fatal; if the diagnosis is suspected, blood should be obtained, and ascorbic acid therapy should be instituted promptly. The usual dose in adults is 100 mg three to five times a day by mouth until 4 g has been administered, then 100 mg/d. In infants and children, administration of 10 to 25 mg three times a day is adequate. A diet rich in vitamin C should be initiated simultaneously. Spontaneous bleeding usually ceases within 24 h, muscle and bone pains subside quickly, and the gums begin to heal within 2 to 3 days. Even large ecchymoses and hematomas resolve in 10 to 12 days, although pigmentary changes in areas of hemorrhage may persist for months. Serum bilirubin becomes normal within 3 to 5 days, and the anemia is ordinarily corrected within 2 to 4 weeks.

BIOTIN   Biotin (see Fig. 77-1) functions as a cofactor in mammalian carboxylases. The vitamin is largely ingested in a form bound to protein, hydrolyzed by pancreatic biotinidase, and absorbed by what is probably an active transport process. The recommended daily allowance is given in Table 71-4. In cells, biotin is covalently attached to apocarboxylases to form four haloenzymes that catalyze the incorporation of biocarbonate into substrate, acetyl-CoA carboxylase, pyruvate carboxylase, methylcrotonyl CoA carboxylase, and propionyl CoA carboxylase. Biotin deficiency in the human occurs under at least three conditions: following the prolonged consumption of raw egg white (which binds biotin in the gut and prevents its absorption), after parenteral nutrition without biotin supplementation in patients with malabsorption, and in subjects with biotinidase deficiency. In all three conditions the common manifestations of biotin deficiency resemble those of essential fatty acid deficiency and include perioral dermatitis, conjunctivitis, alopecia, ataxia, and, in children, developmental delay. In addition, biotinidase deficiency may cause serious neurologic defects.

The diagnosis can be established by documenting reduced urinary excretion of biotin or by demonstrating resolution of the deficiency in response to supplementation with 100 μg/d.

VITAMIN A   **Biochemistry**   Vitamin A (retinol) can either be ingested or synthesized within the body from plant carotenes (see Fig. 77-1). The best sources of preformed vitamin A are liver, milk, and kidney, where it occurs largely in the form of fatty acid esters. The esters are hydrolyzed during digestion, absorbed in the free form, reesterified with fatty acids within the intestinal mucosa, and enter the circulation with lymph chylomicrons. The carotene substrates for synthesis of vitamin A, mainly β-carotenes, are widely distributed in plants. β-Carotene can either be absorbed intact or cleaved in the intestinal tract to form two molecules of retinaldehyde. Retinaldehyde is subsequently reduced by an aldehyde reductase to retinol. Retinol from whatever source is stored as retinyl esters in the liver. The normal body pool is 300 to 900 mg.

Prior to release from the liver, retinyl esters are hydrolyzed, and the free alcohol is bound to a specific transport protein, retinol-binding protein (RBP), for transport to peripheral tissues. In vitamin A deficiency, the release of RBP from the liver is inhibited, and the protein accumulates in liver; with repletion, RBP is rapidly released from preformed stores. Approximately equal amounts of retinol are excreted in the bile and urine.

Mechanism of action   The best-defined function of vitamin A is its role in vision; in the retina vitamin A constitutes the prosthetic group of carotenoid proteins that provide the molecular basis for visual excitation. In addition, vitamin A is required for growth, reproduction, and the maintenance of life. Retinol-phosphate-mannose glycolipid is present in a variety of cell membranes, and the vitamin plays a primary role in the synthesis of glycoproteins. The importance of glycoprotein to every cell implies that this is an equally important function of the vitamin. In all its functions, the vitamin is believed to act by binding to a transcription regulatory protein that controls gene expression (see Chap. 329).

Requirements   The recommended daily allowance for vitamin A is listed in Table 71-4. The assumed utilization efficiency for the conversion of β-carotene to vitamin A in the human is one-sixth (0.167). Other carotenoids with provitamin A activity have, on average, about half the activity of β-carotene. Pregnancy and disease states with impaired absorption or storage, excessive utilization, or increased excretion of vitamin A may lead to increased requirements.

Experimental depletion   When experimental subjects are fed a diet deficient in both retinol and carotene, plasma levels fall, and the body pool shrinks to less than half the control value. Deficiency is manifested by follicular hyperkeratosis, impaired dark adaptation, and abnormalities of the electroretinogram. These changes are corrected after supplementation with 150 μg retinol or 300 μg β-carotene per day.

Clinical deficiency   Endemic deficiency results from inadequate amounts of the vitamin and the provitamins in the diet and occurs in conjunction with deficiency of other nutrients or complicating diseases. In some developing countries, vitamin A deficiency is a major cause of blindness in the young as a consequence of failure to incorporate green leafy vegetables or other sources of the provitamin or vitamin into the diet. Such children appear to be particularly susceptible to the complications of measles. Vitamin A deficiency also may contribute to protein-calorie malnutrition, and here the deficiency is due in part to a defective release mechanism from the liver secondary to inadequate retinol-binding protein. In developed nations, vitamin A deficiency is usually due either to intestinal malabsorption (as in sprue or after intestinal bypass surgery), abnormal storage (liver disease), or enhanced destruction or excretion of the vitamin (proteinuria). Vitamin A deficiency also has occurred in patients receiving total parenteral nutrition because of loss of vitamin A after prolonged storage of intravenous fluid.

Night blindness is the earliest symptom of deficiency, followed by degenerative changes in the retina. The bulbar conjunctiva becomes dry (xerosis), and small gray plaques with foamy surfaces develop (Bitôt's spots). These early lesions are reversible with vitamin A. The more serious effects of deficiency are ulceration and necrosis of the cornea (keratomalacia), leading to perforation, endophthalmitis, and blindness. Dryness and hyperkeratosis of the skin may be present.

Vitamin A levels in plasma are not reliable for the assessment of stores in individual cases. Measurements of dark adaptation, rod scotometry, and electroretinography are useful indicators of vitamin A stores but require trained personnel and expensive equipment; consequently, the diagnosis is usually based on a high index of suspicion in malnourished children or in patients with predisposing factors for its development.

Night blindness and the milder conjunctival changes respond well to 30,000 IU vitamin A daily for a week. Corneal damage constitutes a therapeutic emergency, and the usual treatment is 20,000 IU/kg of body weight per day for 5 days. Children who are at risk for vitamin A deficiency and who develop measles should be given 200,000 IU orally each day for 2 days.

VITAMIN E   Biochemistry   Eight naturally occurring tocopherols possess vitamin E activity. The structure of alpha tocopherol, the most widely distributed and most active of the tocopherols, is shown in Fig. 77-1. The vitamin is absorbed from the gastrointestinal tract by a mechanism similar to that for other fat-soluble vitamins and enters the bloodstream via the lymph, associated first with chylomicrons and

then with plasma β-lipoproteins. Indeed, plasma levels correlate with plasma lipid levels. The vitamin is stored in all tissues, and the tissue stores can protect against vitamin deficiency for long periods. Approximately three-fourths of the vitamin is excreted in bile, and the balance is excreted as glucuronides in urine. Metabolites with quinone structures (including one similar to ubiquinone) are present in tissues.

Mechanism of action   The vitamin probably acts as an antioxidant rather than as a specific cofactor. In so acting it presumably inhibits oxidation of essential cellular constituents and prevents the formation of toxic oxidation products. Other antioxidants such as selenium, sulfur-containing amino acids, and the ubiquinone group can reverse the symptoms of vitamin E deficiency in animals.

Requirements   The recommended daily requirement is 10 to 30 mg/d (see Table 71-4). Diets containing large amounts of polyunsaturated fatty acids increase and diets containing antioxidants decrease the requirement. The vitamin is widely distributed in food, so a primary deficiency state has never been recognized in otherwise healthy children or adults. Newborn infants have plasma concentrations about one-fifth that of maternal levels, implying poor placental transfer, but human milk (in contrast to cow's milk) has sufficient levels to meet the requirements in infants.

Experimental depletion   In long-term studies, vitamin E concentrations in plasma declined significantly only after months on a deficient diet. No manifestations of the depletion were detected in normal volunteers, making it difficult to establish that tocopherol is a human vitamin.

Clinical deficiency   In the appropriate clinical setting, vitamin E deficiency is associated with a discrete syndrome. Rarely, deficiency is due to a selective malabsorption of the vitamin. More commonly, intestinal fat malabsorption can cause deficiency of all fat-soluble vitamins including vitamin E, and children with abetalipoproteinemia or chronic cholestatic liver disease appear to be particularly susceptible. Measurement of the ratio of serum vitamin E to total-serum lipid is the preferred index for assessing vitamin E status. The manifestations of deficiency include areflexia, gait disturbance, decreased proprioceptive and vibratory sensation, and paresis of gaze and are associated with degeneration of the posterior columns of the spinal cord, selective loss of large-caliber, myelinated axons in peripheral nerves, and appearance of spheroids in the gracile and cuneate nuclei of the brain. Treatment (50 to 100 IU/d by mouth) is most effective when initiated early in the course of the disease.

VITAMIN K   Vitamin K consists of a quinone ring attached to a side chain (labeled R in Fig. 77-1) that varies depending on the source of the vitamin. Vitamin K_1 (phylloquinone) is present in most edible vegetables, particularly in green leaves, and vitamin K_2 is produced by intestinal bacteria. The many compounds with vitamin K activity are structurally related to the simpler compound, 2-methyl-1,4-naphthoquinone (menadione). Menadione is formed in the gut by the removal of the side chain from the vitamin by intestinal bacteria. After absorption, menadione is converted in the body to the active menaquinone. The vitamin is a component of a specialized microsomal enzyme system that effects the posttranslational γ carboxylation of glutamic acid in proteins of the plasma, bone, kidney, and urine, including the precursor proteins for the clotting factors VII, IX, X, and possibly V. Death from hemorrhage in deficiency states ensues before deficiency of the other carboxylated proteins becomes manifest. The warfarin anticoagulant drugs induce hypoprothrombinemia by inhibiting the γ carboxylation of the precursor protein.

Under ordinary circumstances, about 80 percent of vitamin K is absorbed from the small bowel into the intestinal lymph. Deficiency can occur in association with diseases that interfere with fat absorption. In addition, long-term treatment with oral antibiotics may temporarily eliminate intestinal bacteria as a source for vitamin K and promote deficiency when the diet is marginal or deficient.

Newborn infants tend to be deficient in vitamin K and have low plasma levels of several coagulation factors in the prothrombin complex. Such deficiencies result from minimal stores of vitamin K at birth, lack of an established intestinal flora, and a limited dietary intake of the vitamin.

Routine determination of prothrombin should be performed prior to surgical procedures or delivery. Subjects with levels below 70 percent of normal should receive therapy with vitamin K. Vitamin K deficiency can be separated from hypoprothrombinemia of liver disease by demonstration of the noncarboxylated prothrombin precursor that accumulates in plasma in the vitamin deficiency.

VITAMIN EXCESS

According to the National Health Interview Survey, more than 50 percent of adults in the United States use vitamin and/or mineral supplements, and in many instances ingestion is within a potentially toxic range. Multivitamins are the most common type ingested by children, whereas single vitamins are consumed commonly among adults. Supplement use is higher with the level of education and income and in those whose health is good.

Fat-soluble vitamins are stored to a variable extent in the body and hence are more likely to cause adverse effects when taken in excess; excess states for vitamins D (see Chap. 358) and A are well characterized. Water-soluble vitamins are readily excreted in the urine and stored only to a limited extent. Consequently, toxicity states for these vitamins only occur when large amounts are taken for prolonged periods.

VITAMIN A AND CAROTENES **Carotenemia** Carotenemia results from excessive intake of vitamin A precursors in foods, principally carrots. Excess carotene is not injurious apart from the cosmetic effect; the fact that carotenemia does not cause hypervitaminosis A indicates that the conversion of carotene to vitamin A must be regulated. Carotenemia is manifested by yellowing of the skin with greatest intensity on the palms and soles and by a corresponding yellowness of serum. The yellowing of the skin differs from jaundice in that the sclerae remain white. Hypothyroid patients are particularly susceptible. The omission of carrots from the diet leads to the rapid disappearance of the pigmentation. Discoloration of the skin also can result from the consumption of large amounts of other colored fruits and vegetables.

Vitamin A toxicity Hypervitaminosis A can result from accidental overingestion by hunters or explorers (polar bear liver), as the result of food faddism (usually caused by overly solicitous parents), or as a side effect of inappropriate therapy. Acute toxicity from a single massive dose consists of abdominal pain, nausea, vomiting, headache, dizziness, sluggishness, papilledema, and in infants a bulging fontanel followed within a few days by generalized desquamation of the skin and recovery. Chronic toxicity occurs after ingestion of 25,000 units or more daily for protracted periods and is characterized by bone and joint pain, hyperostoses, hair loss, dryness and fissures of the lips, anorexia, benign intracranial hypertension, low-grade fever, pruritus, weight loss, and hepatosplenomegaly. The only diagnostic laboratory finding is elevation of the vitamin in serum, chiefly in the form of retinyl esters. The concentration of retinol-binding protein is normal, and the excess vitamin A circulates in association with lipoprotein. Relief is prompt on discontinuation of the vitamin.

VITAMIN E Relatively large doses of vitamin E have been taken by some for extended periods without apparent harm. In others, malaise, gastrointestinal complaint, headaches, and possibly hypertension have occurred. However, true toxicity appears to occur in two situations—in subjects receiving oral anticoagulants and in premature infants. In large amounts, vitamin E can antagonize vitamin K and prolong the prothrombin time; this phenomenon results in a potentiation of oral anticoagulants. Premature infants given parenteral vitamin E have developed ascites associated with hepatosplenomegaly, cholestatic jaundice, azotemia, and thrombocytopenia.

VITAMIN K Large amounts of vitamin K can block the effects of oral anticoagulants and when given to pregnant women can cause jaundice in the newborn.

PYRIDOXINE Most adults can consume up to 10 times the recommended daily allowance of 2 mg pyridoxine per day without adverse effects. However, severe peripheral neuropathies have developed after ingestion of several grams per day for prolonged periods; symptoms include ataxia, perioral numbness, and clumsiness of the hands and feet, and the findings include loss of position and vibration sense without impairment of reflexes or sensory function. Recovery is slow after ingestion ceases. Lower doses (25 mg/d) can antagonize the effects of levodopa in Parkinson's disease and decrease the anticonvulsant effects of phenytoin and barbiturates.

VITAMIN C Vitamin C is consumed by 85 percent of all vitamin users because of the claim that large amounts of the vitamin (a gram or greater per day) prevent or minimize the symptoms of the common cold. However, in controlled studies, no significant differences in occurrence, severity, or duration of colds have been demonstrated in subjects treated with the vitamin. Use of the vitamin in this way is unwarranted and probably unwise. The long-term use of ascorbic acid in these doses can interfere with the absorption of vitamin B_{12}, enhance blood levels of estrogens in women on exogenous estrogens, cause uricosuria, and predispose to formation of oxalate kidney stones. In addition, large doses enhance the development of metabolizing enzymes in the fetus and may cause rebound scurvy in the offspring of mothers who have ingested large amounts of the vitamin during pregnancy. However, pharmacologic doses (200 mg daily) may correct leukocyte abnormalities in patients with the Chédiak-Higashi syndrome (see Chap. 59).

NIACIN Large doses of niacin are used for treatment of hypercholesterolemia and occasionally for other purposes. The vitamin causes release of histamine, which in turn can cause severe flushing, pruritus, and gastrointestinal disturbances and may aggravate asthma. Acanthosis nigricans may occur. In doses of 3 g/d niacin can cause elevation of serum uric acid and of fasting glucose. Large doses can also cause hepatic toxicity including cholestatic jaundice.

In women who consume vitamin supplements, the median dose of pyridoxine approaches the level of 120 mg/d found to cause paresthesia and muscle weakness in all 103 volunteers who consumed the vitamin for 6 months or greater.

REFERENCES

General

BROWN ML: *Present Knowledge in Nutrition*. Washington, International Life Science Institute, 1990

COMBS GF JR: *The Vitamins*. San Diego, Academic, 1992

ELSAS LJ, MCCORMICK DB: Genetic defects in vitamin utilization. Part I: General aspects and fat-soluble vitamins. Vitam Horm 43:103, 1986

GOODHART RS, SHILS ME (eds): *Modern Nutrition in Health and Disease*, 6th ed. Philadelphia, Lea & Febiger, 1980

HOYUMPA AM: Mechanisms of vitamin deficiencies in alcoholism. Alcoholism (NY) 10:573, 1986

LINDEN MC: *Nutritional Biochemistry and Metabolism*. New York, Elsevier, 1991

MUDD SH: Inborn errors of metabolism. Vitamin-responsive genetic disease. J Clin Pathol 27(Suppl) 8:38, 1974

RUDMAN D, WILLIAMS PJ: Nutrient deficiencies during total parenteral nutrition. Nutr Rev 43:1, 1984

Niacin deficiency

CARPENTER KJ: The relationship of pellagra to corn and the low availability of niacin in cereals. Experientia(Suppl) 44:197, 1983

———, LEWIN WJ: A reexamination of the composition of diets associated with pellagra. J Nutr 115:543, 1985

CASTIELLO RJ, LYNCH PJ: Pellagra and the carcinoid syndrome. Arch Dermatol 105:574, 1972

FU CS et al: Biochemical markers for assessment of niacin status in young men. J Nutr 119:1949, 1989

GOLDSMITH GA: Experimental niacin deficiency. J Am Dietetic Assoc 32:312, 1956

HENDERSON LM: Niacin. Ann Rev Nutr 3:289, 1983

JUKES TH et al: The conquest of pellagra. Fed Proc 40:1519, 1980

LEVY HL: Hartnup disorder, in *The Metabolic Basis of Inherited Disease*, 6th ed, CR Scriver et al (eds). New York, McGraw-Hill, 1989, p 2515

Thiamine deficiency

BROWN GM: Biogenesis and metabolism of thiamine, in *Metabolic Pathways*, 3d ed, DM Greenberg (ed). New York, Academic, 1970, p 369

DURAN M, WADMAN SK: Thiamine-responsive inborn errors of metabolism. J Inherited Metab Dis 8(Suppl 1):70, 1985

DYCKNER T et al: Aggravation of thiamine deficiency by magnesium depletion. Acta Med Scand 218:129, 1985

HAAS RH: Thiamin and the brain. Annu Rev Nutr 8:483, 1988

HARPER CG et al: Clinical signs in the Wernicke-Korsakoff complex: A retrospective analysis of 131 cases diagnosed at necropsy. J Neurol Neurosurg Psychiatry 49:341, 1986

HOYUMPA AM: Mechanisms of thiamine deficiency in chronic alcoholism. Am J Clin Nutr 33:2750, 1980

KAWAI C et al: Reappearance of beriberi heart disease in Japan. Am J Med 69:383, 1980

KOZAM RL et al: Cardiovascular beriberi. Am J Cardiol 30:418, 1972

KURIYAMA M et al: Blood vitamin B_1, transketolase, and thiamine pyrophosphate (TPP) effect in beriberi patients. Clin Chim Acta 108:159, 1980

VICTOR M et al: *The Wernicke-Korsakoff Syndrome*. Philadelphia, Davis, 1971

ZIPORIN ZZ et al: Excretion of thiamine and its metabolites in the urine of young adult males receiving restricted intakes of the vitamin. J Nutr 85:287, 1965

Pyridoxine deficiency

BASSIER KH: Megavitamin therapy with pyridoxine. Int J Vitam Nutr Res 58:105, 1988

BHAGAVAN HN, BRIN M: Drug–vitamin B_6 interaction. Curr Concepts Nutr 12:1, 1983

GERSHOFF SN: Vitamin B_6, in *Nutrition Reviews' Present Knowledge in Nutrition*, 4th ed, DM Hegsted et al (eds). Washington, The Nutrition Foundation, 1976, p 149

HARRIS JW, HORRIGAN DL: Pyridoxine-responsive anemia-prototype and variations on the theme, in *Vitamins and Hormones*, vol 22, RS Harris et al (eds). New York, Academic, 1964, p 721

LUHBY AL et al: Vitamin B_6 metabolism in users of oral contraceptive agents: I. Abnormal urinary xanthurenic acid excretion and its correction by pyridoxine. Am J Clin Nutr 24:684, 1971

ROSS EA et al: Vitamin B_6 requirements of patients on chronic peritoneal dialysis. Kidney Int 36:702, 1989

SAUERLICH HE et al: Biochemical assessment of the nutritional status of vitamin B_6 in the human. Am J Clin Nutr 25:629, 1972

YOUNG RC, BASS JP: Iatrogenic nutritional deficiencies. Annu Rev Nutr 2:201, 1982

Riboflavin deficiency

BATES CJ: Human riboflavin requirements, and metabolic consequences of deficiency in man and animals. World Rev Nutr Diet 50:215, 1987

MERRILL AH JR et al: Formation and mode of action of flavoproteins. Annu Rev Nutr 1:281, 1981

PINTO JT, RIVLIN RS: Drugs that promote renal excretion of riboflavin. Drug Nutr Interact 5:143, 1987

———— et al: Mechanisms underlying the differential effects of ethanol on the bioavailability of riboflavin and flavin adenine dinucleotide. J Clin Invest 79:1343, 1987

Ascorbic acid deficiency

BARNESS LA: Nutritional aspects of vegetarianism, health foods, and fad diets. Nutr Rev 59:153, 1977

BOXER LA et al: Correction of leucocyte function in Chédiak-Higashi syndrome by ascorbate. N Engl J Med 295:1041, 1971

BURNS JJ et al: Third conference on vitamin C. Ann NY Acad Sci 498, 1987

ENGLAND S, SEIFTER S: The biochemical functions of ascorbic acid. Annu Rev Nutr 6:365, 1986

FRANCESCHI RT: The role of ascorbic acid in mesenchymal differentiation. Nutr Rev 50:65, 1992

HODGES RE et al: Clinical manifestations of ascorbic acid deficiency in man. Am J Clin Nutr 24:432, 1971

LEVINE M: New concepts in the biology and biochemistry of ascorbic acid. N Engl J Med 314:892, 1986

PADH H: Vitamin C: Newer insights into its biochemical functions. Nutr Rev 49:65, 1991

REID GM: Scurvy: Old disease—New insight. Med Hypotheses 12:167, 1983

REULER JB et al: Adult scurvy. JAMA 253:805, 1985

SATO D, UNDENFRIEND S: Studies on ascorbic acid related to the genetic basis of scurvy, in *Vitamins and Hormones*, vol 36, P Munson et al (eds). New York, Academic, 1978, p 33

TOLBERT BM et al: New information on synthesis and metabolism of ascorbic acid. Nutr Rev 35:22, 1977

VILTER RW: Effects of ascorbic acid deficiency in man, in *The Vitamins*, WH Sebrell Jr et al (eds). New York, Academic, 1967, vol 1, p 457

WALLERSTEIN RO, WALLERSTEIN RO JR: Scurvy. Sem Hematol 13:211, 1976

Biotin

MARSHALL MM: The nutritional importance of biotin—An update. Nutr Today 22:26, 1987

MOCK DM et al: Effects of biotin deficiency on serum fatty acid composition: Evidence for abnormalities in humans. J Nutr 188:342, 1988

SWEETMAN L, NYHAN WL: Inheritable biotin-treatable disorders and associated phenomena. Annu Rev Nutr 6:317, 1986

WOLF B et al: Biotinidase deficiency: Initial clinical features and rapid diagnosis. Ann Neurol 18:614, 1985

Vitamin A deficiency

BARCLAY AJG et al: Vitamin A supplements and mortality related to measles: A randomised clinical trial. Br Med J 294:294, 1987

DELUCA LM: The direct involvement of vitamin A in glycosyl transfer reactions of mammalian membranes, in *Vitamins and Hormones*, vol 35, PL Munson et al (eds). New York, Academic, 1977, p 1

GIGUERE V et al: Identification of a receptor for the morphogen retinoic acid. Nature 330:624, 1987

GOODMAN DS: Vitamin A and retinoids in health and disease. N Engl J Med 310:1023, 1984

HOWARD L et al: Vitamin A deficiency from long-term parenteral nutrition. Ann Intern Med 93:576, 1980

SAUERLICH HE et al: Vitamin A metabolism and requirements in the human studied with the use of labeled retinol, in *Vitamins and Hormones*, vol 32, RS Harris et al (eds). New York, Academic, 1974

SMITH FR, GOODMAN DS: Vitamin A transport in human vitamin A toxicity. N Engl J Med 294:805, 1976

SOMMER A: New imperatives for an old vitamin (A). J Nutr 119:96, 1989

TIELSCH JM, SOMMER A: The epidemiology of vitamin A deficiency and xerophthalmia. Annu Rev Nutr 4:183, 1974

VAHLQUIST A: Clinical use of vitamin A and its derivatives—Physiological and pharmacological aspects. Clin Exp Dermatol 10:133, 1985

Vitamin A for measles. Lancet 1:1067, 1987

WALD G: Molecular basis of visual excitation. Science 162:230, 1968

Vitamin E deficiency

BIERI JG et al: Medical uses of vitamin E. N Engl J Med 308:1063, 1983

HORWITT MK: Interrelations between vitamin E and polyunsaturated fatty acids in adult men, in *Vitamins and Hormones*, vol 20, GF Marrian, KV Thimann (eds). New York, Academic, 1962, p 541

LLOYD JK: The importance of vitamin E in human nutrition. Acta Paediatr Scand 79:6, 1990

PERLMUTTER DH et al: Intramuscular vitamin E repletion in children with chronic cholestasis. Am J Dis Child 141:170, 1987

SITRIN MD et al: Vitamin E deficiency and neurologic disease in adults with cystic fibrosis. Ann Intern Med 107:51, 1987

SOKOL RJ et al: Vitamin E deficiency with normal serum vitamin E concentrations in children with chronic cholestasis. N Engl J Med 310:1209, 1984

———— et al: Isolated vitamin E deficiency in the absence of fat malabsorption—familial and sporadic cases: Characterization and investigation of causes. J Lab Clin Med 111:548, 1988

———— et al: Intestinal malabsorption of vitamin E in primary biliary cirrhosis. Gastroenterology 96:479, 1989

TRABER MG et al: Lack of tocopherol in peripheral nerves of vitamin E–deficient patients with peripheral neuropathy. N Engl J Med 317:262, 1987

Vitamin K deficiency

BERTINA RM et al: New method for the rapid detection of vitamin K deficiency. Clin Chim Acta 105:93, 1980

DOISY EA JR, MATSCHINER JT: Biochemistry of vitamin K, in *Fat-Soluble Vitamins*, vol 9, RA Morton (ed). Elmsford, NY, Pergamon, 1970, p 293

IBER FL et al: Vitamin K deficiency in chronic alcoholic males. Alcoholism (NY) 10:679, 1986

OLSON RE, SUTTIE JW: Vitamin K and α-carboxyglutamate biosynthesis, in *Vitamins and Hormones*, vol 35, PL Munson et al (eds). New York, Academic, 1977, p 59

SHEARER MJ et al: Studies on the absorption and metabolism of phylloquinone (vitamin K) in man, in *Vitamins and Hormones*, vol 32, RS Harris et al (eds). New York, Academic, 1974, p 513

SUTTIE JW: *Vitamin K Metabolism and Vitamin K-Dependent Proteins*. Baltimore, University Park Press, 1988

SUTTIE JW et al: Vitamin K deficiency from dietary vitamin K restriction in humans. Am J Clin Nutr 47:475, 1988

Vitamin excess

ALHADEFF L: Toxic effects of water-soluble vitamins. Nutr Rev 42:33, 1984

CHALMERS TC: Effects of ascorbic acid on the common cold. Am J Med 58:532, 1975

CORRIGAN JJ JR: The effect of vitamin E on warfarin-induced vitamin K deficiency. Ann NY Acad Sci 82:361, 1982

DALTON K, DALTON MJT: Characteristics of pyridoxine overdose neuropathy syndrome. Acta Neurol Scand 76:8, 1987

LEMONS JA, MAISELS MJ: Vitamin E—How much is too much? Pediatrics 76:625, 1985

LOMBAERT A, CARTON H: Benign intracranial hypertension due to A-hypervitaminosis in adults and adolescents. Eur Neurol 14:340, 1976

LORCH V et al: Unusual syndrome with fatalities among premature infants: Association with a new intravenous vitamin E product. Morb Mort Week Rep 33:198, 1984

MOSS AJ et al: Use of vitamin and mineral supplements in the United States. Advance Data No. 174. Hyattsville, Md: National Center for Health Statistics, 1989

SCHAUMBURG H et al: Sensory neuropathy from pyridoxine abuse: A new megavitamin syndrome. N Engl J Med 309:445, 1983

SHIN HB et al: Ascorbic acid–induced uricosuria: A consequence of megavitamin therapy. Ann Intern Med 84:385, 1976

Toxic effects of vitamin overdosage. Med Lett Drugs Ther 26:73, 1984

WOOLLISCROFT JO: Megavitamins: Fact and fancy. Dis-A-Month 24:1, 1983

78 DISTURBANCES IN TRACE ELEMENT METABOLISM

KENNETH H. FALCHUK

CLASSIFICATION AND FUNCTIONS The "trace elements" comprise metals in biologic fluids at concentrations <1 μg/g wet weight. Most are essential nutrients for humans (Table 78-1). Others (As, Ni, Sn, V, Si) are essential for some species and may be required by humans. The functions of trace elements and of more abundant metals (Na, K, Ca, Mg) are determined, in part, by their charges, mobilities, and binding constants to biologic ligands. Elements in one group (Na, K) bind weakly to negatively charged ligands and can cross cellular membranes without major impediment. They are used by living systems as charge carriers to conduct electric impulses along nerves, etc. Those in a second group (Mg, Ca) form moderately stable complexes with enzymes, nucleic acids, and other ligands. They act as biochemical "triggers," altering and/or controlling the functions of these molecules, e.g., Ca affects muscle contraction and relaxation (Chap. 385). Those in a third group (Fe, Zn, Cu, and others) form strong, static complexes with and become integral functional components of enzymes (Table 78-1).

METAL DEFICIENCY OR TOXICITY Metals can cause disease through deficiency, imbalance, or toxicity. Deficiency usually results when dietary intake is inadequate or when intake is adequate but other conditioning factors come into play. Deficiencies can be caused by metal malabsorption in chronic diarrheal diseases, surgical resection of the small intestine, or formation of metal complexes with dietary components that are not readily absorbed, e.g., between phytates and Zn. Deficiency states also can result from increased losses through urine, pancreatic juice, or other exocrine secretions or from metabolic imbalances produced by antagonistic or synergistic interactions between metals. Large amounts of Ca, for example, decrease the absorption and induce deficiency of Zn. Zinc supplements in excess of 10 times the recommended daily allowance cause a conditioned deficiency of copper including anemia. Similarly, Mo and Cu compete with each other; excessive Mo in cattle leads to Cu deficiency characterized by diarrhea and wasting. Trace element deficiencies in humans, except for iron, were previously thought to be rare but have been recognized more frequently with the use of total parenteral nutrition (TPN) (Chap. 76). Criteria for the recognition of deficiency states include decreases in metal content of whole blood, serum, hair and/or other accessible fluids and tissues, changes in the activities of metalloenzymes, and characteristic signs and symptoms (Table 78-2).

Toxic effects are dependent on the chemical form, the amount ingested, the route of entry into the body, the biologic ligands bound by the metal, the tissue distribution, the concentration achieved, and the excretion rate. Mechanisms of toxicity include inhibition of enzyme activity by binding to essential amino acid residues, alterations in nucleic acid function and structure, impairment in protein synthesis, effects on membrane permeability, and inhibition of phosphorylation, among others. Metal toxicity in patients undergoing chronic renal dialysis is important because of the frequency and severity of the resulting problems and because of the number of metals involved, e.g., Al, Zn, Cu, Ni, and Sn (Chap. 238). For example, even when present only in trace amounts in dialysis fluids, Al is readily absorbed into blood and accumulates in brain, bone, and erythroid tissues, causing disabling neurologic, skeletal, and hematologic disorders. These include malaise, memory loss, asterixis, dementia, twitches, and other manifestations of metabolic encephalopathy, including seizures and death. Osteomalacia unresponsive to vitamin D, fractures, muscular pain, weakness, and anemia may occur. Documentation of increase in plasma Al concentration following deferoxamine administration is diagnostic.

DISORDERS OF METABOLISM OF SPECIFIC METALS **Zinc** Absorption of Zn in the small intestine is decreased by fibers, phytate, phosphate, Ca, and Cu and increased by amino acids, peptides, iodoquinol and other chelating agents. Excretion of Zn occurs principally through secretions of the pancreas and intestine. Nearly 99 percent of total-body Zn is inside cells, the remainder in plasma

TABLE 78-1 Requirements and functions of trace elements in humans

Element	Requirements, mg/d*	Amount† Total, g/70 kg body weight	Serum μmol/L	Serum μg/dL	Selected biochemical functions	Enzymes Class	Examples
Fe	10–20	4.0	18	100	Oxygen transport	Oxidoreductases	Cytochrome oxidase
Zn	15–20	3.0	15	100	Nucleic acid and protein synthesis and degradation, alcohol metabolism	Transferases, hydrolases, lyases, isomerases, ligases, oxidoreductases, transcription factors	RNA polymerases, alcohol dehydrogenases, glucocorticoid receptor
Cu	2–6	0.25	16	100	Hemoglobin synthesis, connective tissue metabolism, bone development	Oxidoreductases	Superoxide dismutase, ferroxidase (ceruloplasmin)
Co	0.0001	1.1	0.0001	0.0007	Methionine metabolism	Transferases	Homocysteine methyltransferase
Mn	2–5	0.02	0.001	0.06	Oxidative phosphorylation; fatty acid, mucopolysaccharide, and cholesterol metabolism	Oxidoreductases, hydrolases, ligases	Diamine oxidase, pyruvate carboxylase
Mo	0.15–0.5	0.07	0.007	0.07	Xanthine metabolism	Oxidoreductases	Xanthine oxidase
Se	0.05–0.2	(−)	1.6	13	Antioxidant	Oxidoreductases, transferases	Glutathione peroxidase
Ni	(−)	(−)	0.02	0.01	?Stabilizing RNA structure	Oxidoreductases, hydrolases	Urease
Cr	0.005–0.2	0.0006	0.004	0.02	?Binding of insulin to cells, glucose metabolism		

* Requirements may differ for different age groups and physiologic states, e.g., pregnancy.
† Reported normal values vary owing to differences in sample preparation, analytical instruments, and small quantities present in biologic materials.
(−), Reported values variable or not available.

TABLE 78-2 Disorders of metal metabolism in humans

Element	Deficiency	Toxicity*
Fe	Anemia	Hepatic failure, diabetes, testicular atrophy, arthritis, cardiomyopathy, peripheral neuropathy, hyperpigmentation
Zn	Growth retardation, alopecia, dermatitis, diarrhea, immunologic dysfunction, failure to thrive, psychological disturbances, gonadal atrophy, impaired spermatogenesis, congenital malformations	Gastric ulcer, pancreatitis, lethargy, anemia, fever, nausea, vomiting, respiratory distress, pulmonary fibrosis
Cu	Anemia, growth retardation, defective keratinization and pigmentation of hair, hypothermia, degenerative changes in aortic elastin, mental deterioration, scurvy-like changes in skeleton	Hepatitis, cirrhosis, tremor, mental deterioration, Kayser-Fleischer rings, hemolytic anemia, renal dysfunction (Fanconi-like syndrome)
Mn	Bleeding disorder (increased prothrombin time)	Encephalitis-like syndrome, Parkinson-like syndrome, psychosis, pneumoconiosis
Co	Anemia (B_{12} deficiency)	Cardiomyopathy, goiter
Mo	?Esophageal cancer	?Hyperuricemia
Cr	? Impairment of glucose tolerance	Renal failure, dermatitis (occupational), pulmonary cancer
Se	Cardiomyopathy, congestive heart failure, striated muscle degeneration	Alopecia, abnormal nails, emotional lability, lassitude, garlic odor to breath
Ni	?	Dermatitis (occupational), lung and nasal carcinomas, liver necrosis, pulmonary inflammation
Si	? Impaired early bone development	Pulmonary inflammation, granuloma, fibrosis
F	? Impaired bone and dental structure	Mottled dental enamel, nausea, abdominal pain, vomiting, diarrhea, tetany, cardiovascular collapse

* Symptoms are dependent on route of entry and tissue distribution (see text).

and extracellular fluids. Serum Zn, approximately 70 percent of which is bound to albumin and other proteins, is the source of metal for cellular needs. Serum Zn content is fairly constant, but small diurnal variations may occur. It decreases when intake or absorption is reduced (e.g., in regional enteritis) or when urinary losses are increased (e.g., in nephrotic syndrome, in cirrhosis of the liver or other hypoalbuminemic states, during the administration of penicillamine or other chelating agents, in high catabolic states as after trauma, burns, or surgery, and in hemolytic anemias and sickle cell disease). Plasma Zn also decreases with acute myocardial infarction, infections, malignancies, hepatitis, and other diseases. The decreases may be due to redistribution from plasma to tissues and are probably mediated by ACTH, cortisol, and/or cytokines (interleukins 2 and 6). Clinical deficiency may follow these decreases in serum content. The Zn requirement of the developing fetus, pregnant woman, and growing child or adolescent is higher than that of adult men or nonpregnant women. Therefore, the former groups are more susceptible to Zn depletion. Zn deficiency in pregnant animals can lead to fetal Zn deficiency, manifested by high mortality rates or congenital malformations of nearly all organ systems. Zinc deficiency has not been described in pregnant women but has been reported in adolescents who eat dirt, in patients who receive TPN without supplemental Zn

(see Chap. 76), and in patients with the autosomal recessive defect acrodermatitis enteropathica. In the latter disease, Zn deficiency may be the consequence of a defect in Zn absorption. The onset of symptoms often occurs when an affected infant is weaned from human to cow's milk. Zn also may play a role in the maintenance of normal taste and in wound healing.

Tissues with a high cellular turnover, including skin, gastrointestinal mucosa, chondrocytes, spermatogonia, and thymocytes are characteristically affected (Table 78-2). The dermatologic manifestations (hyperkeratosis, parakeratosis, acrodermatitis, and alopecia) call attention to the possibility of Zn deficiency. The usual distribution of the keratotic lesions is in areas that are readily traumatized (elbows, knees), but the lesions can develop in other areas as well. The keratotic lesions can become pustular or crusting, red, scaly plaques. Immunologic defects of T cell function are typical. The ability to mount an immunologic response to parasites is reduced. Superinfections are common with either fungi or bacteria.

Toxicity follows inhalation of Zn fumes (by welders), oral ingestion, or intravenous administration. Inhalation of high concentrations of zinc oxide fumes leads to an acute illness called *metal-fume fever* or *brass chills*, manifested by fever, chills, excessive salivation, headaches, cough, and leukocytosis. Dialysis fluids can be contaminated with Zn from the adhesive plaster used on the dialysis coils or from galvanized pipes. The toxic syndrome associated with hemodialysis is characterized by anemia, fever, and central nervous system disturbances (Table 78-2). Toxic amounts of Zn decrease chemotaxis, phagocytosis, pinocytosis, and platelet aggregation.

Copper The liver, kidney, heart, and brain contain the highest amounts of Cu. Over 90 percent of plasma Cu is associated with ceruloplasmin, and 60 percent of that in red blood cells is bound to superoxide dismutase. The major excretory pathway is through the bile. The serum Cu concentration is normally constant. Increases occur in patients with acute myocardial infarction, leukemia, solid tumors, infections, cirrhosis of the liver, hemochromatosis, thyrotoxicosis, and connective tissue disorders. The consequences of the increases are unknown. Decreases occur in the nephrotic syndrome, kwashiorkor, the hepatolenticular degeneration of Wilson's disease (see Chap. 348), severe diarrheal diseases with malabsorption, and other conditions associated with increased excretion or decreased synthesis of ceruloplasmin. Premature infants who are fed diets deficient in Cu develop decreased serum ceruloplasmin and Cu levels, anemia, osteopenia, skin and hair depigmentation, and psychomotor retardation. Cu deficiency in subjects receiving TPN causes anemia and neutropenia.

A more complex disorder of Cu metabolism occurs in Menkes' disease, an X-linked recessive disorder (see also Chap. 353). Intestinal Cu uptake is normal, and tissue Cu content varies; that of intestinal, kidney, and skin (fibroblast) cells is normal or high, while that of serum, liver, brain, and (likely) vascular cells is low. Ceruloplasmin content and the activities of some Cu enzymes (e.g., connective tissue amine oxidases) are decreased. The clinical picture is similar to that of Cu deficiency in animals except that anemia does not occur (Table 78-2). The patients have kinky hair, and decreased amounts of mature collagen and elastin cause dissecting aneurysms, sudden cardiac rupture, emphysema, and osteoporosis. Death usually occurs in the first 5 years of life.

Excessive oral intake of Cu or hemodialysis with water contaminated with Cu is toxic. The acute symptoms include hemolytic anemia, nausea, vomiting, and diarrhea. The renal and hepatic failure and the central nervous system disorders that eventually develop (Table 78-2) are typical of the Cu toxicity syndrome in Wilson's disease (see Chap. 348).

Cobalt Co is a component of vitamin B_{12}, and deficiency syndromes are those associated with deficiency of the vitamin (see Chap. 304). Pharmacologic amounts of Co induce erythropoiesis. Chronic administration blocks iodine uptake by the thyroid, resulting in development of goiter.

Cardiomyopathy, congestive heart failure with pericardial effusions, polycythemia, thyroid enlargement, and neurologic abnormalities have been reported as manifestations of Co toxicity in drinkers of beer to which the metal had been added as a foam stabilizer. Co accumulates in the heart, forms a complex with lipoic acid, and interferes with decarboxylation reactions critical to both pyruvate and fatty acid metabolism.

Manganese Mn acts both as an activator of enzymes and as a component of metalloenzymes (Table 78-1). Defects of the skeletal, central nervous, and gonadal systems occur in Mn deficiency in animals. Humans obtain sufficient Mn from normal dietary intake so that a deficiency syndrome is rare. Increase in prothrombin time, unresponsive to vitamin K, has been noted. In serum, Mn is bound to transmanganin. Mn is excreted primarily in bile and pancreatic secretions.

Serum Mn increases following myocardial infarction and decreases in children with convulsive disorders. Miners who inhale large quantities of Mn dust over long periods of time develop asthenia, anorexia, apathy, headache, impotence, leg cramps, speech disturbances, and occasionally even more severe symptoms (Table 78-2).

Selenium As a component of glutathione peroxidase, Se plays a critical role in the control of oxygen metabolism, particularly in catalyzing the breakdown of H_2O_2. The metal is required for the growth of human fibroblasts and other cells in tissue culture. Furthermore, Se cures or prevents Keshan disease, a syndrome endemic to Keshan Province in China, where the soil may be deficient in the metal. Keshan disease is characterized by multifocal myocardial necrosis and reduced serum Se content. The clinical severity varies from severe arrhythmias and cardiogenic shock to a mild form with cardiac enlargement as the only significant finding. Peripheral myopathies may develop as a consequence of muscle degeneration (Table 78-2). Children and women of childbearing age are particularly susceptible. Se protects animals from a number of carcinogenic chemicals and viruses; a role in human cancer prevention is not established. Se binds Cd, Hg, and other metals and mitigates their toxic effects, even though tissue levels of the metals remain elevated. Se poisoning has been reported due to ingestion of water containing large amounts of the metal.

Other trace elements *Silicon* is present in bone and skin and may play a role in the cross-linkage of collagen. Deficiency in animals results in decreased growth, abnormal bone development, and decreased hexosamine content of epiphyses and epiphyseal plates. Deficiency in humans has not been described. Inhalation of fine particles of SiO_2 causes granuloma formation and fibrosis (silicosis) of the lungs (see Chap. 219).

Fluoride is a constituent of teeth and bone. It prevents dental caries, and its use in patients with osteoporosis may result in increased mineralized bone (see Chap. 362). Complications of long-term ingestion by such patients include calcification of bony ligaments and tendons. Chronic intake of fluorides also causes fluorosis, a syndrome characterized by weakness, weight loss, anemia, brittle bones, and mottling of teeth (if taken during stages of enamel formation). Acute ingestion of toxic amounts, as found in some insect poisons, causes severe abdominal pain, nausea, vomiting, diarrhea, and hypocalcemia. Eventually, tetany and cardiorespiratory arrest occur.

Deficiencies of *arsenic, nickel, tin,* or *vanadium* cause pathologic manifestations in plants and some vertebrates. Their roles in human health are undefined.

REFERENCES

FALCHUK KH: Effect of acute disease and ACTH on serum zinc proteins. N Engl J Med 296:1129, 1977

KARCIOULU ZA, SARPER RM: *Zinc and Copper in Medicine*, Springfield, Ill., Charles C Thomas, 1980

Metabolic and physiological consequences of trace element deficiency in animals and man. Philos Trans R Soc Lond [Biol] 294:1, 1981

MILLINER DS et al: Use of the deferoxamine infusion test in the diagnosis of aluminum-related osteodystrophy. Ann Intern Med 101:775, 1984

PRASAD AS: *Trace Elements in Human Health and Disease*, vol 2. New York, Academic, 1976

REINHOLD JG: Trace elements—A selective survey. Clin Chem 21:476, 1975

TING-KAI L, VALLEE BL: The biochemical and nutritional roles of other trace elements, in *Modern Nutrition in Health and Disease*, 6th ed, RS Goodhart and ME Shils (eds). Philadelphia, Lea and Febiger, 1980

UNDERWOOD EJ: *Trace Elements in Human and Animal Nutrition*, 3d ed. New York, Academic, 1971

WILLIAMS RJP: The Tilden lecture. Q Rev Chem Soc (Lond) 24:331, 1970

section 1 Basic considerations in infectious disease

79 INTRODUCTION TO INFECTIOUS DISEASE: HOST-PARASITE INTERACTION

LAWRENCE C. MADOFF / DENNIS L. KASPER

Despite decades of dramatic progress in their treatment and prevention, infectious diseases remain a major cause of death and debility and are responsible for worsening the living conditions of many millions of people around the world. Infections, which must be considered in the differential diagnosis of syndromes affecting every organ system, frequently challenge the physician's diagnostic skill by involving a multitude of organ systems.

With the advent of antimicrobial agents, many people believed that infectious diseases would be relegated to medical history. Indeed, the years since World War II have seen the development of hundreds of chemotherapeutic agents, many of which are potent, safe, and effective not only against bacteria but also against viruses, fungi, and parasites. Yet we now realize that as antimicrobial agents developed, so did the ability of the microbes to elude our best strategies and to counterattack with their own strategies for survival. Antibiotic resistance occurs at an alarming rate among all classes of mammalian pathogens. Diseases once thought to have been nearly eradicated from the developed world—tuberculosis and rheumatic fever, for example—have rebounded with a new ferocity. Recently discovered and emerging infectious agents—the Lyme disease spirochete, the AIDS retrovirus, the hepatitis C virus, and the rickettsia causing ehrlichiosis—humble us even as our understanding of pathogenesis at the most basic, molecular level deepens. The role of infectious agents in the etiology of diseases once believed to be noninfectious is being increasingly recognized. For example, *Helicobacter pylori* has recently been shown to play a role in the development of gastrointestinal ulcers and perhaps malignancy. The possibility certainly exists that other diseases of unknown cause, such as rheumatoid arthritis, sarcoidosis, or inflammatory bowel disease, may in fact be infectious.

Medical advances over infectious diseases have been hindered by changes in the patient population. Immunocompromised hosts now constitute a significant proportion of the population who are being treated for infectious diseases. Physicians immunosuppress their patients to prevent the rejection of transplants and to treat neoplastic and inflammatory diseases. Some infections, most notably that caused by human immunodeficiency virus (HIV), immunocompromise the host. Lesser degrees of immunosuppression are associated with other infections, such as influenza and syphilis. Aging of and malnutrition in the host tip the survival balance toward the infecting pathogen. Implantable devices such as heart valves, automatic defibrillators,

pacemakers, prosthetic joints, indwelling intravenous catheters, and ventriculoperitoneal shunts all provide foci predisposed to infection; many infections associated with implantable devices are difficult or impossible to cure without removal of the foreign hardware. Infectious agents that coexist peacefully with the immunocompetent hosts wreak havoc in those who lack a complete immune system. AIDS has brought to prominence once-obscure organisms such as *Pneumocystis carinii*, *Cryptosporidium parvum*, and *Mycobacterium avium*. Thus the understanding of infectious diseases remains crucial and ever-changing.

For any infectious process to occur, the parasite and the host must first encounter each other. Factors such as geography, environment, and behavior thus influence the likelihood of infection. Some organisms can be harbored in the host for years before disease becomes clinically evident. A detailed history, including information on travel, behavioral factors, exposures to animals or potentially contaminated environments, and living and occupational conditions, must be elicited and considered in the evaluation of a patient in whom infection is suspected. For example, the likelihood of infection by *Plasmodium falciparum* can be significantly affected by altitude, climate, terrain, season, and even time of day. Certain antibiotic-resistant strains are localized to specific geographic regions, and a seemingly minor alteration in a travel itinerary can dramatically influence the likelihood of acquiring chloroquine-resistant malaria. If such important details in the history are overlooked, inappropriate treatment may result in the death of the patient. Likewise, the chance of acquiring a sexually transmitted disease can be dramatically affected by relatively minor variation in sexual practices, such as the method used for birth control. Knowledge of the relationship between specific risk factors and disease allows the physician to influence a patient's health even before the development of infection by modifying these factors and administering appropriate vaccines.

Many specific host factors influence the likelihood of acquiring an infectious disease. Age, immunization history, prior illnesses, level of nutrition, pregnancy status, coexisting illness, and perhaps emotional state all have some impact on the risk of infection after exposure to a potential pathogen. The importance of individual host defense mechanisms, either specific or nonspecific, becomes apparent in their absence, and our understanding of these immune mechanisms is enhanced by studies of clinical syndromes developing in immunodeficient patients. For example, the frequent occurrence of meningococcal disease in people with deficiencies in specific complement proteins of the "membrane attack complex" underscores the importance of an intact complement system for preventing meningococcal infection.

Medical care itself increases the risk of acquiring an infection in several ways: (1) through contact with pathogens during hospitalization; (2) through breaching the skin (with intravenous devices or surgical incisions) or mucosal surfaces (with endotracheal tubes or bladder catheters); (3) through introduction of foreign bodies; (4)

through alteration of the natural flora with antibiotics; and (5) through treatment with immunosuppressive drugs.

Infection involves complicated interactions of parasite and host, inevitably affecting both. In most cases, several steps in the pathogenic process are required for the development of infection. Since the competent host has a complex series of barricades in place to prevent infection, the successful parasite must utilize specific strategies at each of these steps. The specific strategies used by bacteria (see Chap. 99), viruses (see Chap. 141), and parasites (see Chap. 170) have some remarkable conceptual similarities, but the strategic details are unique for each organism.

SURFACE CONTACT   Most often, the first contact between host and parasite is at a mucosal or cutaneous surface. In order to prevent the initiation of the infectious process during such contact, the host has developed highly effective defense mechanisms operating at the body's interface with the outside world. Many of these initial mechanisms of host defense are not specifically directed at individual species of organisms. Mechanical barriers, for example, including the tough cornified epithelium of the skin and the flow of secretions from glands tend to prevent infection by any potential pathogen. Chemical barriers, such as the acidic environment of the stomach and urinary bladder, represent hostile environments for most microorganisms. The normal microflora, composed of nonpathogenic organisms that inhabit mucosal surfaces, make colonization by pathogens more difficult by competing for environmental resources. Behavioral and neurologic mechanisms, such as gagging and coughing, help prevent infection of the lower respiratory tract.

We recognize the importance of these mechanisms when we observe the diseases that arise when they are impaired. Patients with suppressed coughing (for example, due to pain associated with a fractured rib) are very susceptible to pneumonia. Achlorhydric individuals are particularly likely to develop salmonellosis after the ingestion of contaminated food or drink because a lower inoculum is required. The abnormal bronchial secretions in cystic fibrosis usually lead to chronic pulmonary infection with *Pseudomonas aeruginosa.* A break in the skin resulting from an animal or insect bite, a burn, a scratch, trauma, or surgery allows the entry of pathogenic or opportunistic agents. The eradication of the normal bowel flora by antibiotics may render organisms such as *Clostridium difficile* pathogenic.

The host has also evolved an organism-specific immune system that functions at mucosal surfaces. Specialized macrophages and lymphocytes, which play a role in the specific defense system, reside in the epithelium of the gut, in the nasal mucosa, and at other sites that interface with the environment. This mucosa-associated lymphoid tissue appears to play a role in trapping antigens and allowing them to be presented to lymphocytes at the mucosal barrier. In certain areas, these tissues become recognizable anatomically; examples include the oropharyngeal tonsils, and—in the gastrointestinal tract—Peyer's patches and the appendix. Central to this defense system is the elaboration of surface immunoglobulins, particularly secretory IgA, which prevents adherence and penetration of organisms.

Pathogens have evolved an array of methods for breaching this well-developed boundary between the host and the outside world. In order to invade, most pathogens must first attach. Many microorganisms have developed a highly specialized apparatus for binding to the surface of the host. For example, pili of uropathogenic *Escherichia coli* recognize certain host glycoproteins that serve as sites for attachment to epithelial cells. The binding of Epstein-Barr virus to a specific complement receptor (CR2) on B lymphocytes allows the subsequent internalization of the virus. HIV binds to the CD4 complex present in certain human T lymphocytes. Many bacterial pathogens produce enzymes or surface components that bind to or inactivate secretory IgA. Others impair ciliary motility thus hindering their own clearance by this mechanism.

Some potentially pathogenic organisms are capable of living symbiotically with the host, colonizing but not infecting for extended periods. It is important for the astute clinician to distinguish coloniza-

tion from infection. *E. coli* are normally present in large numbers in the colon. At this site, these organisms are certainly harmless and may even be beneficial to the normal healthy host, contributing to the synthesis of vitamin K and inducing natural immunity to other gram-negative bacteria. It is only when *E. coli* penetrate the normal mucosal barriers and enter another site that they become opportunists and cause disease. The penetration of *E. coli* into the peritoneum through a mechanical breach in the bowel wall, their entry into the urinary bladder, and their invasion of the bloodstream are events associated with infection and disease. Some virulent pathogens, such as group A streptococci and *Neisseria meningitidis,* are able to colonize most individuals for prolonged intervals without untoward effects. In these cases the colonized individuals may already have developed specific immunity to the organism, or invasion may be prevented by nonspecific host defenses while specific immunity is being stimulated. Certain viruses (e.g., herpesviruses) inhabit tissue for the life of the host, causing little harm as long as the host's immune system is intact but inducing severe symptomatic disease if the immune status is altered.

INVASION   Microorganisms attached to a mucosal surface use specific mechanisms to invade deeper host structures. Meningococci and gonococci penetrate the mucosal barrier after engulfment by mucosal epithelial cells. *Haemophilus influenzae* penetrate by squeezing through the junction between epithelial cells. Salmonellae induce the host's gastrointestinal macrophages (i.e., in Peyer's patches) to engulf and phagocytose them; these bacteria then resist killing by the phagolysosome of the unactivated macrophage and subsequently proliferate, spilling into the bloodstream. Schistosomal cercariae enter the epidermis of hosts exposed to contaminated fresh water; in the presence of a specific host, they are able to uncoat, mature, and enter the circulation. Other pathogens, including bacteria (e.g., *Rickettsia rickettsii* and *Yersinia pestis*), viruses (e.g., dengue and eastern equine encephalitis virus), and parasites (e.g., *Plasmodium* and *Trypanosoma*), may enlist the aid of an insect vector to breach the protective skin and enter the circulation.

Infection has a major impact on the microorganism as well as the host. It is increasingly recognized that the invading microbe senses and adapts to changes in its environment through complex regulatory mechanisms, "turning on" the virulence factors necessary for invasion and survival in the host. For example, *Yersinia* sp., *Shigella* sp., and *Bordetella pertussis* all express virulence factors in response to exposure to the 37°C temperature likely to be encountered at the time of infection. Other virulence determinants—the Shiga-like toxin of enterohemorrhagic *E. coli,* for example—are expressed in response to the low-free-iron conditions existing in the host, where iron is tightly bound by transferrin and other proteins. Many such bacterial virulence factors are controlled by two-component regulatory systems: one protein component senses environmental changes and signals (often by phosphorylation) a second protein which coordinately regulates the expression of a group of genes whose products facilitate survival in the host milieu.

Once in the bloodstream or a normally sterile body site, the microorganism faces the host's tightly integrated cellular and humoral immune systems. Cellular immunity (Chap. 277), comprising T lymphocytes, macrophages, and NK cells, primarily recognizes and combats pathogens that proliferate intracellularly. Cellular immune mechanisms are important in immunity to all classes of infectious agents, including most viruses and many bacteria (e.g., *Mycoplasma, Chlamydia, Listeria, Salmonella, Mycobacterium*), parasites (e.g., *Trypanosoma, Toxoplasma, Leishmania*), and fungi (e.g., *Histoplasma, Cryptococcus,* and *Coccidioides*). Usually, T lymphocytes are activated by macrophages and B lymphocytes, which present foreign antigens along with the host's own major histocompatibility complex antigen. Activated T cells may then act in several ways to fight infection. They may directly attack and lyse host cells that express foreign antigens. Some act as helper T cells to stimulate the proliferation of B cells and the production of immunoglobulins. They may elaborate cytokines (interferon, for example) which directly inhibit the growth of pathogens or stimulate killing by host macrophages and cytotoxic cells. Cytokines also augment host immunity by stimulating the inflammatory response (fever, the production of acute-phase serum components, and the proliferation of leukocytes). Cytokine stimulation does not always result in a favorable response in the host; septic shock (see Chap. 83) and toxic shock syndrome (see Chap. 102) are among the conditions that are mediated by these inflammatory substances.

Extracellular pathogens, including most encapsulated bacteria (e.g., streptococci, staphylococci, and pathogenic *E. coli*), are attacked by the humoral immune system, comprising primarily the complement cascade, antibodies, and phagocytic cells. Polymorphonuclear leukocytes (PMNs) are short-lived blood cells that engulf and kill invading microbes; these migratory cells are capable of finding sites of inflammation via chemotaxis and exiting the circulation into infected tissue. In order to efficiently localize at the site of inflammation, PMNs make use of cellular adhesion molecules elaborated by endothelial cells in response to inflammation. For example, endothelial cells respond to inflammatory cytokines by transiently expressing the selectin molecules CD62 and ELAM-1. The binding of these molecules to specific receptors on PMNs results in the adherence of the latter to the endothelium. Other adhesion molecules, such as ICAM-1, may then bind to β_2 integrins on the PMN and facilitate diapedesis into the extravascular compartment. Although PMNs are capable of killing microorganisms without help, they function much more efficiently when pathogens are first "opsonized" (from the Greek for "to prepare for eating") by components of the complement system and/or by antibodies.

Antibodies are complex glycoproteins, also called immunoglobulins (Ig), that are produced by mature B lymphocytes and circulate in body fluids. They specifically recognize and bind to foreign antigens. One of the most impressive features of the immune system is the ability to generate an incredible diversity of antibodies capable of recognizing virtually every foreign antigen yet not reacting with self. In addition to their antigen specificity, antibodies of different structural and functional classes exist: IgG predominates in the circulation and persists for many years after exposure; IgM is the earliest specific antibody to appear in response to infection; IgA is important in immunity at mucosal surfaces; and IgE is important in allergic and parasitic diseases. Antibodies may act by directly impeding the function of an invading organism, by neutralizing secreted toxins and enzymes, or by facilitating the removal of the parasite by phagocytic cells. Immunoglobulins participate in cell-mediated immunity by promoting antibody-dependent cellular cytotoxicity functions of certain T lymphocytes. Antibodies also promote the deposition of complement components on the surface of the invader.

The complement system consists of a group of serum proteins that function as a cooperative, self-regulating cascade of enzymes that adhere to—and in some cases disrupt—the surface of invading organisms. Some of these surface-adherent proteins (e.g., C3b) can then act as opsonins for destruction of microbes by phagocytes. The later, "terminal" components (C7, C8, and C9) can directly kill some bacterial invaders (notably, many of the neisseriae) by forming a "membrane attack complex" and spoiling the integrity of the bacterial membrane. Other complement components, such as C5a, act as chemoattractants for PMNs. Complement activation and deposition occurs by either or both of two pathways: the classic pathway is primarily activated by immune complexes (i.e., antibody bound to antigen), and the alternative pathway is activated by microbial components, frequently in the absence of antibody. PMNs have receptors for both antibody and C3b, and antibody and complement function together to aid in the clearance of infectious agents.

Microbes have developed a variety of strategies for overcoming host immunity. Many bacteria are encapsulated with polysaccharides that allow them to evade host defense mechanisms and proliferate freely until the host is able to generate capsule-specific antibodies. Group B *Streptococcus* and serogroups B and C meningococci have capsules containing the sugar sialic acid, whose presence on the bacterial surface gives the organism an advantage in evading nonspecific (nonantibody-dependent) clearance by the alternative pathway of complement. The sialic acid residue increases the affinity of binding of the complement regulatory protein factor H to C3b on the bacterial surface; C3b bound to factor H is susceptible to degradation by another complement regulatory protein, factor I. Therefore, surface sialic acid prevents the accumulation of quantities of C3b on the bacterial surface that are sufficient to initiate the killing of organisms in the absence of specific antibody. Several gram-positive bacteria possess surface proteins that bind immunoglobulins, perhaps interfering with immune recognition. Other organisms even employ the host immune response as a survival strategy. *Schistosoma mansoni* recognizes the host lymphokine tumor necrosis factor (TNF) and responds to it by depositing eggs.

TOXINS AND ENZYMES   Some pathogenic organisms elaborate toxins and enzymes that facilitate invasion of the host and are often responsible for the disease state. Pathogenic strains of *Vibrio cholerae* elaborate a potent and well-characterized toxin that enters host enterocytes via a specific receptor (the monosialyl GM_1 ganglioside) and then enzymatically activates the host cell adenylate cyclase system. This event in turn leads to the copious electrolyte and fluid secretion by the enterocyte and the voluminous watery diarrhea that is characteristic of cholera. *Staphylococcus aureus* expresses a large number of extracellular proteins that contribute to the variety of disease states associated with this bacterium. Enterotoxins cause staphylococcal food poisoning even though viable organisms may never enter the host. Toxic shock syndrome toxin 1 is responsible for the many systemic effects of toxic shock syndrome even though host tissue barriers may remain intact. Damage to mucosal surfaces, mediated by toxins, may permit a pathogen to proliferate at a mucosal site whether or not the organism invades. Pertussis toxin impairs the ability of ciliated epithelium to clear the pathogen from the host bronchial tree. Enteropathogenic *E. coli* and *V. cholerae* are examples of toxin-producing bacteria that normally do not invade. In contrast, other toxins are clearly capable of promoting invasion and spread. The extracellular enzymes of *Streptococcus pyogenes*, such as hyaluronidase, facilitate movement through tissue planes, and streptolysins O and S disrupt leukocyte membranes and thus impair host defense.

Integral components of pathogens are often responsible for much of the disease process that results from infection. Lipopolysaccharides of gram-negative bacteria act as a potent endotoxin ("endo" in this case referring to the fact that they are part of the bacterial membrane, not a secreted product) that is the proximate cause of the syndrome of sepsis. The cell walls of gram-positive bacteria appear to elicit a similar host inflammatory response. The anaerobic pathogen *Bacteroides fragilis* possesses a capsular polysaccharide that promotes abscess formation by the host.

TROPISM   In order to successfully infect a host, many pathogens occupy highly specific niches within the host and thus are tropic to a particular body site or cell type. This type of tropism has many implications for the life cycle of the pathogen, for the immune system of the host, and for the disease process. Malaria sporozoites, for example, are rapidly cleared from the blood into hepatocytes, where they undergo maturation and release into the circulation; trophozoites, in turn, can infect only the erythrocyte. The bacterial pathogen *Helicobacter pylori* produces the enzyme urease, which, by cleaving urea to form ammonium ion, may allow the organism to inhabit a neutral microenvironment within the highly acidic gastric epithelium. Many viruses are tropic for specific tissues; for example, the hepatitis viruses are tropic for hepatocytes, HIV for CD4-bearing T lymphocytes, herpesviruses for neural tissues, and rhinoviruses for the nasal epithelium.

The central nervous system is uniquely protected from perturbations in the environment by a blood-brain barrier—a system of tight junctions at capillaries within the CNS that resists the entry of inflammatory cells, pathogens, and even macromolecules into the subarachnoid space. Yet certain pathogens have devised highly specialized, and as yet poorly understood, mechanisms for breaching this barricade. One strategy employed by organisms such as rabies and herpes simplex viruses in humans and by reovirus in experimental animals is to travel within peripheral nerves into the CNS. Other organisms, such as certain highly encapsulated bacteria and fungi, enter from the bloodstream and possess surface components that allow them to traverse the capillary tight junctions. The degree of specialization required for this mechanism is demonstrated by the predilection of certain serotypes of organisms within a species to cause meningitis. The type III strains account for the vast majority of cases of meningitis caused by group B *Streptococcus,* even though other serotypes cause much of the invasive disease outside the CNS. This disparity appears to be due solely to the arrangement of the component sugars of the capsular polysaccharide: other serotypes of group B *Streptococcus* rarely cause meningitis even though their capsules possess the same four component sugars in different structural arrangements.

CLINICAL MANIFESTATIONS OF INFECTION   The clinical manifestations of infectious diseases at presentation are myriad, varying from fulminant, life-threatening processes to brief and self-limited conditions to indolent, chronic maladies. The clinician must use all of the skills of medicine to diagnose and prescribe appropriate treatment. First, a careful history is essential and must include details on underlying chronic diseases, medications, occupation, travel, risk factors for exposure to certain types of pathogens, such as those associated with sexual contacts, illicit drug use, particular animals, or bites of insect vectors. Since infectious diseases may involve many organ systems, the review of systems may elicit important clues as to the disease process. The physical examination must be thorough, and attention must be paid to seemingly minor details: a soft heart murmur that might indicate bacterial endocarditis; an evanescent skin rash that suggests rheumatic fever; a retinal lesion that suggests disseminated candidiasis.

LABORATORY INVESTIGATIONS   Laboratory studies must be carefully considered and directed toward establishing an etiologic diagnosis in the shortest possible time, at the lowest possible cost, and with the least possible discomfort to the patient. Cultures must be performed in a manner that minimizes the likelihood of contamination while maximizing the yield. A sputum sample is far more likely to be valuable when elicited with careful coaching by the clinician than when collected in a container simply left at the bedside with cursory instruction. Gram stains of specimens should be interpreted carefully and the quality of the specimen assessed. The findings on gram staining should correspond to the results of culture. A discrepancy may suggest diagnostic possibilities such as infection due to fastidious or anaerobic bacteria.

The microbiology laboratory must be an ally in the diagnostic endeavor (see Chap. 80). Astute laboratory personnel will suggest optimal culture and transport conditions or alternative tests to facilitate diagnosis. If informed about specific potential pathogens, an alert laboratory staff will allow sufficient time for these organisms to become evident in culture, even when present in small numbers or when slow-growing. The parasitology technician who is attuned to the specific diagnostic considerations relevant to a particular case may be able to detect the rare, otherwise-elusive egg or cyst in a stool specimen. In cases where a diagnosis appears difficult, serum should be stored during the early acute phase of the illness so that a diagnostic rise in titer of antibody to a specific pathogen can be detected later. Bacterial and fungal antigens can sometimes be detected in body fluids, even when cultures are negative or are rendered sterile by antibiotic therapy. Newer techniques such as the polymerase chain reaction allow the amplification of specific DNA sequences so that minute quantities of foreign nucleic acids can be recognized in host specimens.

THERAPY   Optimal therapy for infectious diseases requires a broad knowledge of medicine and careful clinical judgment. Life-threatening infections such as bacterial meningitis or sepsis, viral encephalitis, or falciparum malaria must be treated immediately, often before a specific causative organism is identified. Antimicrobial agents must be chosen empirically and must be active against the range of potential infectious agents consistent with the clinical scenario. Good clinical judgment is necessary in making decisions to withhold antimicrobials in a self-limited process or until a specific diagnosis is made. The dictum *primum non nocere* should be adhered to, and it should be remembered that all antimicrobials carry a risk (and a cost) to the patient. Direct toxicity may be encountered, e.g., ototoxicity due to aminoglycosides, bone marrow toxicity of zidovudine, and hepatotoxicity of antituberculous agents such as isoniazid and rifampin. Allergic reactions are common and can be serious. Since superinfection may follow eradication of the normal flora and colonization by resistant organism, one invariant principle is that infectious disease therapy should be directed toward as narrow a spectrum of infectious agents as possible. Treatment specific for the pathogen should result in as little perturbation as possible of the host's microflora. With few exceptions, abscesses require surgical or percutaneous drainage for cure. Likewise, infected foreign bodies, including medical devices, must generally be removed in order to eliminate an infection of the device or adjacent tissue. Other infections, such as necrotizing fasciitis, peritonitis due to a perforated organ, gas gangrene, and chronic osteomyelitis, require surgery as their primary means of cure, with antibiotics serving only an adjunctive role.

Recently, the role of immunomodulators in the management of infectious diseases has received increasing attention. Glucocorticoids have been shown to be of benefit in the treatment of *H. influenzae* meningitis in children and in therapy for *P. carinii* pneumonia in patients with AIDS. Their use in other infectious processes remains less clear, and in some cases (in cerebral malaria and septic shock, for example) is detrimental. Other agents that modulate the immune response include prostaglandin inhibitors, specific lymphokines, and TNF inhibitors. Specific antibody therapy has been shown to play a role in the treatment and prevention of many diseases. Specific immunoglobulins have long been known to prevent the development of symptomatic rabies and tetanus. More recently, cytomegalovirus (CMV) immune globulin has been recognized as important not only in preventing transmission of CMV during organ transplantation but also in treating CMV pneumonia in the bone marrow transplant recipient. There is a strong need for well-designed clinical trials to evaluate each new interventional modality.

PERSPECTIVE   The genetic simplicity of many infectious agents allows them to undergo rapid evolution and to develop selective advantages that result in constant variation in the clinical manifestations of infection. Moreover, changes in the environment and the host can predispose new populations to infection. An epidemic of lethal respiratory failure on a Navajo reservation in the southwestern United States in 1993, which caused nationwide alarm, exemplifies the fear that new plagues induce in the human psyche. In this outbreak, patients presented with fever, myalgias, headache, and cough, which were followed by the rapid development of respiratory failure with unexplained noncardiogenic pulmonary edema. Among the etiologic agents potentially responsible for the clinical syndrome were the hantaviruses, which had never been described as human pathogens in the Western Hemisphere. Although patients had respiratory involvement, they lacked the renal failure and hemorrhagic manifestations previously described with hantavirus infection. Nonetheless, most of these patients demonstrated rises in antibody titer to the hantaviruses. This cluster of fatal illness emphasizes the propensity of new infectious diseases to arise in new populations. The potential for infectious agents to emerge in novel and unexpected ways requires that physicians and public health officials be knowledgeable, vigilant, and open-minded in their approach to the consideration of unexplained illness.

There has existed a perception that infectious diseases no longer represented as serious a concern to world health as they once did. The progress that science, medicine, and society as a whole have made in combatting these maladies is impressive, and it is ironic that, as we stand on the threshold of understanding the most basic biology of the microbe, infectious diseases are posing renewed problems. We are threatened by new diseases such as AIDS, hepatitis C, and Lyme disease and by the reemergence of old foes like tuberculosis, cholera, and rheumatic fever. True students of infectious diseases were, perhaps, the least surprised by these developments. Those who know pathogens are aware of their incredible adaptability and diversity. As ingenious and successful as therapeutic approaches may be, our ability to develop methods to counter infectious agents so far has not matched the myriad strategies employed by the sea of microbes that surrounds us. Their sheer numbers and the rate at which they can evolve are daunting. Though new vaccines, new antibiotics, and new modalities for treating and preventing infection will be developed, pathogenic microbes will continue to develop new strategies of their own, presenting us with an unending and dynamic challenge.

REFERENCES

DiRita VJ, Mekalanos JJ: Genetic regulation of bacterial virulence. Annu Rev Genet 23:455, 1989

Fields BN: Pathogenesis of viral infections, in Virology, BN Fields (ed). New York, Raven, 1990, pp 191–239

Gorbach SL et al (eds): Infectious Diseases. Philadelphia, Saunders, 1992

Kasper DL: Introduction to bacterial diseases, in Principles and Practice of Infectious Diseases, 3d ed, GL Mandell et al (eds). New York, Wiley, 1990, pp 1484–1489

Mahmoud A: Parasitic protozoa and helminths. Science 246:1015, 1989

Quagliarello V, Scheld MW: Bacterial meningitis: Pathogenesis, pathophysiology, and progress. New Engl J Med 327:864, 1992

Report of the Task Force on Microbiology and Infectious Diseases. NIAID. NIH Publication No. 92-3320, April 1992

80 LABORATORY DIAGNOSIS OF INFECTIOUS DISEASES

ANDREW B. ONDERDONK

The laboratory diagnosis of infection requires the demonstration, either directly or indirectly, of viral, bacterial, mycotic, or parasitic agents in tissues, fluids, or excreta of the host. Clinical microbiology laboratories are responsible for processing these specimens and also for determining antibiotic susceptibility for bacterial pathogens. Traditionally, the detection of pathogenic agents largely relies on either the microscopic visualization of pathogens in clinical material or growth of microorganisms in the laboratory. Identification is generally based on phenotypic characteristics, such as fermentation profiles for bacteria, cytopathic effects produced by viral agents in tissue culture, and microscopic morphology for fungi and parasites. These techniques are reliable but are often time-consuming.

DETECTION METHODS Reappraisal of the methods employed in the clinical microbiology laboratory has led to development of strategies for detecting pathogenic agents through nonvisual biologic signal-detection systems. Much of this methodology is based on computerization of detection systems with relatively inexpensive, but sophisticated, computers. In this chapter, both the methods currently available and those under development will be discussed. Detection of parasitic agents is the subject of a separate chapter.

Biologic signals A biologic signal is a material that can be reproducibly differentiated from other substances present in the same physical environment. The issue for biologic (and electronic) signals is distinguishing the signal from background "noise" and translating the signal into meaningful information. Examples of biologic signals as applicable to clinical microbiology include structural components of bacteria, fungi, and viruses; specific antigens; metabolic end products; unique DNA or RNA base sequences; enzymes; toxins or other proteins; and surface polysaccharides.

Detection systems A detector is used to sense (or detect) a signal to allow discrimination between the signal and background noise. Detection systems range from morphologic variations that are detected by the trained eyes of a technologist to sensitive electronic instruments, such as gas-liquid chromatographs coupled to computer systems for signal analysis. The sensitivity with which signals can be detected varies widely. It is essential to utilize a detection system that discerns small amounts of signal (sensitivity) even when biologic background noise is present (specificity). Some common detection systems used in microbiology are immunofluorescence, substrate utilization reactions or end-product formation detected as color changes, enzyme activity detected as change in light absorbance, flame ionization detection of short- or long-chain fatty acids, turbidity changes, cytopathic effects in cell lines, and agglutination of particles.

Amplification Amplification of weak signals enhances the sensitivity with which signals can be detected. The most common microbiologic amplification technique is growth of a single bacterium into a discrete colony on an agar plate or into a suspension containing many identical organisms. The advantage of growth as an amplification method is that it does not require anything but an appropriate medium; the disadvantage is the amount of time required for amplification to occur. More rapid, specific amplification of biologic signals can be achieved with techniques such as polymerase (ligase) chain reactions (for DNA/RNA), enzyme immunoassays (for antigens and antibodies), electronic amplification (for gas-liquid-chromatography assays), antibody capture methods for concentration and/or separation, and selective filtration or centrifugation.

Although a variety of methods are available for the amplification and detection of biologic signals on a research basis, thorough testing is required before they are validated as diagnostic assays.

DIRECT DETECTION Microscopy The field of microbiology has been defined largely by the development and use of the microscope. The examination of specimens by microscopic methods often provides rapid and useful diagnostic information. Staining techniques permit organisms to be seen more clearly. Some examples of common microbiologic stains are listed in Table 80-1.

The simplest method for microscopic evaluation is the wet mount, which is used for the examination of samples such as cerebrospinal fluid (CSF) for the presence of Cryptococcus neoformans, with India ink as a background against which to visualize yeasts with large capsules. Wet mounts with dark-field illumination are also used to detect spirochetes from genital lesions. Skin scrapings and hair samples can be examined with use of either 10% KOH wet mount preparations or the calcofluor white method and ultraviolet (UV) illumination to detect fungal elements as fluorescing structures. Stained wet mounts, such as the lactophenol cotton blue stain for fungal elements, are often used for morphologic identification. These techniques enhance signal detection and decrease the background by making it easier to identify specific fungal structures.

Staining GRAM'S STAIN Without staining, bacteria are difficult to see at the magnification (400 to 1000 ×) required for their detection. Although simple, one-step stains can be used, differential stains are more common. Gram's stain differentiates between those organisms with thick peptidoglycan cell walls (gram-positive) and those in which outer membranes can be dissolved with alcohol or acetone (gram-negative).

Gram's stain is particularly useful for examining sputum for the presence of polymorphonuclear cells (PMNs) and bacteria. Sputum specimens with 25 or more PMNs and fewer than 10 epithelial cells per low-power field often provide clinically useful information. However, "sputum" samples with more than 10 epithelial cells per low-power field and multiple bacterial types suggest contamination with oral microflora. Despite the difficulty in discriminating between normal microflora and pathogens, Gram's stain may prove useful for specimens from areas with a large resident microflora if a useful biologic marker (signal) is available. Gram's stain of vaginal swab specimens is useful for detecting epithelial cells covered with gram-positive bacteria, which are regarded as a sign of bacterial vaginitis. Similarly, examination of stool specimens for the presence of leukocytes is useful as a screening procedure before testing for Clostridium difficile toxin or other enteric pathogens.

TABLE 80-1   Selected microbiologic stains

Stain	Use	Expected result
Acridine orange (uses UV light)	Visualization of bacteria, yeast, and leukocytes	Bacteria and yeast are red-orange, and leukocytes are pale green.
Auramine/rhodamine (uses UV light)	Visualization of *Mycobacterium* spp.	Yellow fluorescing bacteria indicate *Mycobacterium*.
Calcofluor white (uses UV light)	Visualization of fungal elements	Fungal elements appear as green fluorescing structures.
Gram's	Visualization and differentiation of bacteria into two groups	Gram-positive bacteria appear purple, and gram-negative bacteria are red.
Kinyoun acid-fast	Detection of *Mycobacterium* spp.	Acid-fast bacteria are pink against a blue background.
Modified acid-fast	Detection of weakly acid-fast organisms, such as *Nocardia*	Weakly acid-fast organisms are pink against a blue background.
Giemsa	Varied, used for visualization of chlamydiae and malarial and other intracellular parasites	Varied, depending on agent.
Methenamine-silver	Detection of *Pneumocystis carinii*	Cell wall of *P. carinii* appears black against a light green background.
Spore	Visualization of spores and cellular location	Spores are light green against a pink/red background, and bacteria stain red.
Toluidine blue	Detection of *P. carinii*	*P. carinii* cysts appear light purple/lavender against a blue background.
Wet mount India ink	Detection of *Cryptococcus neoformans*	*Cryptococcus* mucoid capsules appear as clear halos around a yeast cell against a dark background.
Lactophenol cotton blue	Visualization of fungal structures	Fungal elements stain a more intense blue against a light blue background.

SOURCE: After Eisenberg et al.

The examination of CSF and joint, pleural, or peritoneal fluid using Gram's stain is useful for determining whether bacteria and/or PMNs are present. The sensitivity is such that $>10^4$ bacteria per liter should be detected. Centrifugation is often performed before staining to concentrate specimens suspected of containing low numbers of organisms. The pellet is then examined after staining. This simple method is particularly useful for examination of CSF for bacteria and white blood cells or sputum for acid-fast bacilli.

ACID-FAST STAIN   The acid-fast stain differentiates organisms capable of retaining carbol fuchsin dye after acid/organic solvent disruption (*Mycobacterium* spp.). Modifications of this procedure also allow differentiation between *Actinomyces* and *Nocardia* or other weakly acid-fast organisms. The acid-fast stain is employed for sputum, gastric aspirates, tissue samples, or other fluids when acid-fast bacilli (*Mycobacterium* spp.) are suspected. The identification of the pink/red acid-fast bacilli (AFB) against the blue background of the counterstain requires a trained eye, since few AFB may be detected in an entire smear, even when the signal is amplified by centrifugation. An alternative is the auramine-rhodomine combination fluorescent dye technique.

FLUOROCHROME STAINS   Fluorochrome stains, such as acridine orange, are used to identify white blood cells, yeast, and bacteria in body fluids.

Other specialized stains, such as Dappe's stain, may be used for detecting *Mycoplasma* in cell cultures designated for this purpose.

Capsular, flagellar, and spore stains are also used for identification or demonstration of characteristic structure.

IMMUNOFLUORESCENT STAINS   Direct immunofluorescence staining (DFA) uses antibody coupled to a fluorescing compound, such as fluorescein, directed at a specific antigenic target to visualize organisms or subcellular structures. When samples are examined under appropriate conditions, the fluorescing compound absorbs the UV light and reemits light at a higher (visible) wavelength that can be detected by the human eye. In the indirect immunofluorescent antibody (IFA) technique, an unlabeled (target) antibody binds a specific antigen. The specimen is then stained with labeled polyclonal antibody directed at the target antibody. Because each unlabeled target antibody attached to the appropriate antigen has multiple sites for attachment of the second antibody, the visual signal can be intensified (amplification). This form of staining is called *indirect* because a two-antibody system is used to generate the signal for detection of the antigen. Both direct and indirect fluorescence methods can be used to detect cultured cells infected with viruses such as cytomegalovirus and herpes simplex and many difficult-to-grow bacterial agents such as *Legionella pneumophila*.

Macroscopic antigen detection   Latex agglutination assays and enzyme immunoassays (EIAs) are rapid and inexpensive methods for identifying organisms or extracellular toxins and viral agents using protein and polysaccharide antigens. Such assays may be performed directly on clinical samples or after growth on agar plates or in viral cell cultures. The biologic signal in each case is the antigen to be detected; such methods utilize monoclonal or polyclonal antibodies.

Techniques such as direct agglutination of bacterial cells with specific antibody are simple but relatively insensitive, while latex agglutination procedures and enzyme immunoassays are more sensitive. Some cell-associated antigens, such as capsular polysaccharides, lipopolysaccharides, and other surface-expressed antigens, can be detected by agglutination of a suspension of bacterial cells when antibody is added, a method useful for typing the somatic antigens of *Shigella* and *Salmonella*. Systems such as EIA employ monoclonal antibodies coupled to an enzyme in which antigen is detected by development of a color when colorless substrate is converted to a colored product after an antigen-antibody reaction has occurred. Because the coupling of an enzyme to the monoclonal antibody can amplify a weak biologic signal, the sensitivity of such assays is often high. In each instance, the basis for detection is antigen-antibody binding, with the detection system changed to accommodate the biologic signal. Most such assays provide information as to whether antigen is present but do not quantify the amount.

DETECTION OF PATHOGENIC AGENTS BY CULTURE   Specimen collection and transport   To culture bacterial, mycotic, or viral pathogens, an appropriate sample must be placed into the proper medium for growth (amplification). The success or failure of identification of a specific microbial pathogen often relies on the collection and transport process. Table 80-2 lists procedures for collection and transport of commonly obtained specimens. Because there are many pathogen-specific paradigms for these procedures, it is important to seek advice from the microbiology laboratory when in doubt about a particular situation.

Isolation of bacterial pathogens   The isolation of the suspect pathogen(s) from clinical material relies on the use of artificial media designed to support the growth of bacteria in vitro. Such media are composed of agar, which is not metabolized by bacteria, and nutrients to support the growth of the microbial species of interest, often in combination with substances to inhibit the growth of other bacteria. Broth for growth (amplification) of organisms is employed for specimens with low numbers of bacteria, such as peritoneal dialysis fluids, CSF, or samples in which anaerobes may be present. Two basic strategies are used to isolate pathogenic bacteria. The first uses enriched media to allow the growth of any bacteria that may be present in a sample such as blood or CSF. Since bacteria are not present in such fluids under normal conditions, the finding of organisms is usually significant. Broths that allow for the growth of

TABLE 80-2 Culture collection and transport

Body fluids
Specimen: Aseptically aspirated body fluids
Minimum volume: 1 mL
Container: Sterile tubes with a tight-fitting cap. The specimen may be left in the syringe used for collection if the needle is removed and a rubber cap placed over the barrel of the syringe before transport to the laboratory.
Other considerations: For some body fluids, such as peritoneal lavage samples, increased volumes are helpful for isolation of low numbers of bacteria.

Bronchial aspirates
Specimen: Transtracheal aspirate (TTA) or bronchoscopy specimen
Minimum volume: 1 mL of aspirate or brush in transport medium
Container: Sterile TTA or bronchoscopy tube, bronchoscopy brush in other sterile container

Cerebrospinal fluid (CSF or lumbar puncture)
Specimen: Spinal fluid
Minimum volume: 1 mL for routine cultures, 5 mL or greater for detection of *Mycobacterium*
Container: Sterile tube with tight-fitting cap

Genital sites
Specimen: Vaginal or urethral secretions, cervical swabs, uterine fluid, prostatic fluid, etc.
Minimum volume: 1 swab or 0.5 mL of fluid
Container: Transwab containing Amies transport medium or similar system containing holding medium for *Neisseria gonorrhoeae*
Other considerations: Vaginal swab samples for "routine culture" should be discouraged whenever possible, unless the presence of a particular pathogen is suspected. If detection of multiple organisms, such as group B *Streptococcus, Trichomonas, Chlamydia,* or *Candida* species is being requested, one swab per test should be sent.

Miscellaneous sterile sites
Specimen: Tissue removed at surgery, bone, anticoagulated bone marrow, biopsy samples, or other specimens from areas that are normally sterile sites
Minimum volume: 1 mL of fluid or a 1-g piece of tissue
Container: Sterile "culturette" type swab or similar transport system containing a holding medium. A sterile bottle or jar should be used for tissue specimens.
Other considerations: Accurate identification of the specimen and source is important for processing purposes. Enough tissue should be collected for both microbiologic and histopathologic evaluations.

Nares
Specimen: Swab from the nares
Minimum volume: 1 swab
Container: Sterile "culturette" or similar transport system containing holding medium
Other considerations: Swabs made of calcium alginate may be used.

Wounds
Specimen: Purulent material or abscess contents obtained from a wound or abscess without contamination by normal microflora
Minimum volume: Two swabs or 0.5 mL of aspirated pus
Container: "Culturette" swab or similar transport system or a sterile tube with a tight-fitting screw cap. If anaerobic cultures are to be ordered at the same time, send specimen in anaerobic transport device or closed syringe.
Collection: Abscess contents or other fluids should be collected in a syringe (see above) when possible to provide adequate sample volume and an anaerobic environment.

Sputum
Specimen: Fresh sputum (not saliva)
Minimum volume: 2 mL
Container: Commercially available sputum collection system or similar sterile container with a screw top
Cause for rejection: Care must be taken to ensure that the specimen is sputum and not saliva. Results of Gram's stain noting the number of epithelial cells and PMNs can serve as an important part of the evaluation process.

Stool for enteric pathogens
Synonyms: Stool for routine culture, stool for *Salmonella, Shigella,* and *Campylobacter*
Specimen: Rectal swab or a fresh, randomly collected stool (preferable)
Minimum volume: At least 1 g of stool or two rectal swabs
Container: Plastic-coated cardboard cup or plastic cup with a tight-fitting lid. Other leak-proof containers are also acceptable.
Other considerations: If *Vibrio* species are suspected, the laboratory must be notified, and appropriate collection and transport methods must be used.

Stool for *Yersinia*
Specimen: A fresh, randomly collected stool
Minimum volume: At least 1 g of stool
Container: Plastic-coated cardboard cup or plastic cup with a tight-fitting lid
Limitations: Procedure requires enrichment techniques.

Stool for *Aeromonas* and *Plesiomonas*
Specimen: A fresh, randomly collected stool
Minimum volume: At least 1 g of stool
Container: Plastic-coated cardboard cup or plastic cup with a tight-fitting lid
Limitations: Stool should not be cultured for *Aeromonas* or *Plesiomonas* unless culture for other enteric pathogens is also performed.

Throat
Specimen: Swab of posterior pharynx, ulcerations, or areas of suspected purulence
Minimum volume: 1 swab
Container: Sterile "culturette" or other sterile swab specimen collection system containing holding medium
Note: Normal microflora includes alpha-hemolytic streptococci, saprophytic *Neisseria* spp., diphtheroids, and nonhemolytic *Staphylococcus* spp. Aerobic culture of a throat ("routine") includes screening for and identification of beta-hemolytic *Streptococcus* species and any potentially pathogenic organism. Although considered normal microflora, organisms such as *Staphylococcus aureus, Haemophilus influenzae, Haemophilus parainfluenzae,* and *Streptococcus pneumoniae* will be identified by most laboratories, if requested. When *N. gonorrhoeae* or *Corynebacterium diptheriae* is suspected, a special culture request is recommended.

Urine
Specimen: Clear voided urine specimen or urine collected by catheter
Minimum volume: 0.5 mL
Container: Sterile, leak-proof container with a screw cap
Limitations: Isolates should be identified under the following circumstances:
  1 Clear voided specimen, midvoid specimen, and Foley or indwelling catheter-specimens that yield 50,000 organisms per milliliter or more and from which no more than three species are isolated.
  2 Straight catheterized, bladder tap, and similar urine specimens should have complete workup (identification and susceptibility test) for all potentially pathogenic organisms, regardless of colony count.
  3 Certain clinical problems (e.g., acute dysuria in women) may warrant identification and susceptibility testing of isolates present at concentrations lower than 50,000 organisms per milliliter.

Blood culture, routine
Synonyms: Blood culture for aerobes, anaerobes, and yeast
Specimen: Whole blood
Minimum volume: 10 mL, in each of two bottles for adults and children; 5 mL, if possible, in each of two bottles for infants, less for neonates
Containers: For adults, two bottles (smaller sizes are available for pediatric patients), one with dextrose phosphate, tryptic soy, or other appropriate broth and the other with thioglycollate or other broth containing reducing agents appropriate for isolation of obligate anaerobes. For special situations, e.g., suspected fungal identification, culture-negative endocarditis, or mycobacteremia, different blood collection systems may be used (Isolator systems, see below).
Collection: An appropriate disinfecting technique should be used on both the bottle septum and the patient. Do not allow air bubbles to get into anaerobic broth bottles.
Special considerations: There is no more important clinical microbiology test than the detection of blood-borne pathogens. The rapid identification of bacterial and fungal agents is a major determinant of patient survival. Bacteria may be present either continuously in blood, as is the case for endocarditis, overwhelming sepsis, and the early stages of salmonellosis and brucellosis, or intermittently, as is the case for most other bacterial infections in which bacteria are shed into the blood on a sporadic basis. Most blood culture systems employ two separate bottles containing broth medium, one that is vented in the laboratory for the growth of facultative and aerobic organisms and a second bottle that is maintained under anaerobic conditions. For suspected continuous bacteremia/fungemia, two to three samples should be drawn before the start of therapy, with additional sets obtained if fastidious organisms are suspected. For intermittent bacteremia, two to three sets should be obtained at least 1 h apart during the first 24 h.

Blood culture, fungus/*Mycobacterium* species
Volume of specimen: 10 mL in each bottle, as with routine blood cultures, or alternatively, request Isolator tube from the laboratory
Container: See Blood culture, routine.
Special instruction: Be sure to specify "hold for extended incubation," since many fungal agents require 7 to 14 days to grow in standard blood culture bottles.

Blood culture, Isolator (lysis centrifugation)
Specimen: Blood
Container: Isolator tubes
Note: Used mainly for the isolation of fungi, *Mycobacterium,* or other fastidious aerobes and for elimination of antibiotics from cultured blood in which organisms are concentrated by centrifugation.

TABLE 80-2 Culture collection and transport (continued)

Cultures: Fungus

Specimen: Specimen types listed in the aerobic culture section may be cultured for fungi. When urine or sputum are to be cultured for fungi, a first morning specimen is usually preferred.
Minimum volume: 1 mL or as specified for aerobic cultures under individual listing of specimens
Container: A sterile, nonleaking container with a tight-fitting cap
Collection: The specimen should be transported to the microbiology laboratory within 1 h of collection. Contamination with normal flora from the skin, rectum, vaginal tract, or other body surfaces should be avoided as much as possible.

Cultures: Mycobacterium

Synonyms: AFB culture, culture for acid-fast bacilli
Specimen: Sputum, tissue, urine, body fluids
Minimum volume: 10 mL of fluids or small piece of tissue. Swabs should not be used.
Container: A sterile container with a tight-fitting cap
Other considerations: The detection of *Mycobacterium* spp. is improved by the use of concentration techniques. Smears and cultures of pleural, peritoneal, and pericardial fluids often have low yields. Multiple cultures from the same patient are encouraged.

Cultures: Legionella

Specimen: Pleural fluid, lung tissue (biopsy), bronchial lavage (BAL), bronchial biopsy, transbronchial biopsy. Rapid transport to the laboratory is required.
Minimum volume: 1 mL of fluids; any size piece of tissue, although it is preferable to submit a 0.5-g sample when possible.

Cultures: Anaerobes

Specimen: Aspirated specimens in capped syringes or other transport devices designed to limit oxygen exposure are suitable for the cultivation of obligate anaerobes. A variety of commercially available transport devices may be used. Contamination of specimens with normal microflora from the skin, rectum, vaginal vault, or other body site should be avoided. Specimens cultured for obligate anaerobes should be cultured for facultative bacterial species as well.
Minimum volume: At least 1 mL of aspirated fluid or two swabs and an appropriate anaerobic transport device are required. Collection containers for aerobic culture, such as dry swabs, and inappropriate specimens, such as refrigerated samples, expectorated sputum, stool, gastric aspirates, vaginal, and throat, nose, and rectal swabs, should be rejected as unsuitable for culture.

Cultures: Viral agents

Specimen: Respiratory secretions, wash aspirates from the respiratory tract, nasal swabs, blood samples (including buffy coats), vaginal and rectal swabs, and swab specimens from suspect skin lesions. Stool samples may be employed for detection of some agents. Laboratories generally employ diverse methods for detecting viral agents, and the specific requirements for each specimen should be checked before sending a sample. In general, fluid samples or stool in sterile containers or swab samples in viral "culturette" devices kept on ice, but not frozen, are suitable. Plasma specimens and buffy coats in sterile collection tubes are adequate but should be kept at 4 to 8°C. If specimens are to be shipped or kept for extended periods of time, freezing at -80°C usually preserves viable replicating units.
Minimum volume: 1 mL of fluid, one swab, or 1 g of stool in each appropriate transport medium
Other considerations: Most samples for culture are transported to the laboratory in a holding medium containing antibiotics to prevent bacterial overgrowth and to provide an environment in which viral particles will not be inactivated. Many specimens should be kept cool but not frozen. Procedures and transport media vary depending on viral agent to be cultured and the length of time for transport.

TABLE 80-3 Examples of primary plating media

Medium	Incubation	Purpose
Blood agar(s), 5% defibrinated sheep blood in an enrichment agar base, chocolate agar with additives	CO_2 or anaerobic	Growth and amplification of many medically significant bacteria, including obligate anaerobes
MacConkey agar, deoxycholate agar, eosin–methylene blue agar	O_2	Select for Enterobacteriaceae and other gram-negative rods; inhibits growth of most gram-positive organisms; differentiate Lac-positive and Lac-negative organisms
Phenylethyl alcohol agar, Columbia CNA agar	CO_2	Select for gram-positive species, particularly *Staphylococcus* and *Streptococcus*; inhibits many gram-negative organisms
Hektoen enteric agar, deoxycholate-citrate, *Salmonella-Shigella* agar	O_2	Select for enteric pathogens; characteristics vary, depending on medium
GN broth, selenite broth, tetrathionate broth	O_2	Selective amplification for certain enteric pathogens
Thayer-Martin agar, Martin-Lewis agar, New York City agar	CO_2	Selective amplification for *Neisseria* spp.
Brain-heart infusion, tryptic digest, thioglycollate, chopped-meat glucose	O_2, CO_2, anaerobic	General-purpose amplification broths

SOURCE: After Eisenburg et al.

identification of specific isolates. Phenotypic characteristics include readily detectable traits (colony size, color, hemolytic reactions, odor) after growth on agar media, use of specific substrates and carbon sources (such as carbohydrates), the formation of specific end products during growth, and the microscopic appearance of the organisms themselves. Broth tubes containing specific substrates are commonly employed for such characterization procedures.

Classical phenotyping Automated systems allow identification of bacterial pathogens on the basis of phenotypic characteristics within a matter of hours. Most such systems are based on biotyping techniques, in which isolates are grown in multiple substrates and the pattern of reactions is compared with known patterns for various bacterial species. This procedure is relatively fast, and commercially available systems include a coding system to simplify recording of results, probability calculations for likely identification, and miniaturized biotyping methods. By automating the biotyping approach and coupling the reading process to computer-based data analysis, rapidly growing organisms, such as the Enterobacteriaceae, can be identified within hours of detection on agar plates.

To speed identification, several systems use preformed enzymes for 2- to 3-h identification methods. Such systems do not rely on bacterial growth per se to determine whether a substrate has been used or not. They employ a heavy inoculum in which enzymes are present in sufficient quantity to convert substrate to product rapidly. In addition, some systems use fluorogenic substrate/end-product detection methods to increase sensitivity (through signal amplification).

Gas-liquid chromatography Gas-liquid chromatography (GLC) is used for the detection of metabolic end products of bacterial fermentations. A common application of this technique is identification of the short-chain fatty acid products produced by obligate anaerobes during the fermentation of glucose. Because the types of volatile acids and relative concentrations differ among the various genera and

small numbers of organisms may be subcultured to solid media when growth is detected. The second is to isolate (amplify) specific bacterial species from stool, genital tract secretions, or sputum, which contain large numbers of bacteria under normal conditions. For this purpose, antimicrobial agents or other inhibitory substances are incorporated into the agar medium to inhibit growth of all but the bacteria of interest. Following incubation, organisms that grow on such media are further characterized to determine whether they are pathogens. Selection for organisms that may be pathogens from normal microflora shortens the time required to make the diagnosis. Some of the more common types of primary plating media and their uses for specific specimen types are listed in Tables 80-3 and 80-4.

IDENTIFICATION METHODS Once organisms are isolated, traditional methods of phenotypic characterization are used for the

TABLE 80-4 Examples of commonly employed media by specimen type

Specimen	Medium	Time required for isolation and identification
Abscess or pus, deep wounds	Blood, chocolate, and MacConkey agar; anaerobic agar(s); enrichment broth	24–48 h for facultative species; 72–96 h for most anaerobes
Body fluids (other than blood, CSF, and urine)	Blood, chocolate agar enrichment broth; anaerobic agar(s), or MacConkey as indicated by site	Same as above
Blood	Enrichment broth for facultative and aerobic organisms; second enrichment broth for anaerobes	6 h to 14 days depending on organism; most facultative and anaerobic species detected in 7 days or less
CSF	Blood, chocolate, anaerobic agar(s), and enrichment broth; fungal agar as necessary	24–48 h for facultative species and dimorphic fungi; 72–96 h for most anaerobes
Intestinal tract (feces, rectal swabs, and ileostomy or colostomy contents)	MacConkey, Hektoenenteric, and other selective agar for *Salmonella* and *Shigella*; special agar(s) for *Campylobacter*, *Yersinia*, and *Vibrio*	18–24 h for *Salmonella* and *Shigella*; longer for other agents
Respiratory tract (bronchial lavage, sputum, tracheal aspirates)	Blood, chocolate, and MacConkey agars; medium for *Legionella*; medium for *Mycobacterium* if indicated	24–48 h for most facultative species; up to 14 days for *Legionella*; up to 2 months for *Mycobacterium* cultures
Throat swab for group A *Streptococcus*	Blood agar	18–24 h
Tissue (biopsy or surgical)	Blood, chocolate, MacConkey, and anaerobic agar; selective agar for gram-positives; fungal agar as required	24–48 h for most facultative species; longer for obligate anaerobes and fungal agents
Urine (clean voided or catheterized)	Blood and MacConkey agar; quantitative culture required	24–48 h

species that make up this group of organisms, such information serves as a metabolic "fingerprint" for identification of a particular isolate.

GLC also can be coupled to a sophisticated signal-analysis computer software system for identification and quantitation of long-chain fatty acids (LCFA) in the outer membranes and cell walls of bacteria and fungi. For any given species, the types and relative concentrations of LCFA are different enough to allow identification of even closely related species. Definitive identification may be obtained within a few hours after growth of the organism on appropriate media. LCFA analysis is one of the most advanced procedures currently available for phenotypic characterization.

Nucleic acid probes Organisms can be identified with absolute specificity by analysis of the unique DNA or RNA base sequences for that species. Probes have been developed for identification of a wide variety of pathogens from Epstein-Barr virus to *Mycoplasma* and *Cryptococcus*, and some of these are available for use in the clinical laboratory. The routine use of this methodology for direct detection from clinical specimens is limited at present because the sensitivity of this method without amplification is often less than that of other techniques. The use of ribosomal RNA as the target for oligonucleotide probes helps increase sensitivity, since there are many

more rRNA molecules in a single bacterial cell than DNA molecules. Readily available probe technology can be used for the direct detection of *Chlamydia*, *Neisseria gonorrhoeae*, *Gardnerella*, and *Trichomonas* from vaginal/cervical swabs and for identification of bacterial agents such as *Salmonella* and *Mycobacterium*. Much work remains to be done with regard to signal amplification to provide adequate sensitivity for direct detection of pathogens such as *Mycobacterium* spp. in clinical material. An important application for probe technology, either directly on clinical specimens or by in situ hybridization, is the detection of viral agents such as HIV, human papilloma virus, hepatitis A, B, and C, cytomegalovirus, parvovirus, varicella zoster, and herpes simplex virus. In some cases, these techniques are more sensitive for direct detection of viral agents than are conventional culture or serologic methods. Many viral probes are now available only for research purposes, but DNA/RNA probes will probably become the method of choice for identification of hard-to-detect viral agents in the future.

One unresolved issue with regard to use of probes on a routine basis is how best to amplify weak biologic signals. The polymerase chain reaction requires repeated heating of the DNA or RNA to separate the two complementary strands of the double helix, hybridization of a primer sequence to the appropriate base sequence, target amplification via complementary strand extension, and signal detection via a labeled probe. At the present time, the complexity of this procedure often makes other methods for detection, including growth of organisms, easier and less expensive. One of the interesting advantages of probe technology is that live organisms need not be present to detect a positive biologic signal. The impact of detecting dead organisms and the inability to perform susceptibility testing remain to be elucidated.

SUSCEPTIBILITY TESTING One of the principal responsibilities of the clinical laboratory is to determine which antimicrobial agents are inhibitory for a specific bacterial isolate. Two approaches are useful for this purpose. The first is to use a qualitative assessment of susceptibility to categorize responses as susceptible, resistant, or intermediate. This qualitative approach can be accomplished either by placing paper disks containing antibiotics onto an agar surface inoculated with the bacterial strain to be tested (Kirby-Bauer or disk/agar-diffusion method) or by using broth tubes containing a set concentration of antibiotic (breakpoint method). These methods have been carefully calibrated against quantitative methods and clinical experience with each antibiotic.

The second is to inoculate the test strain of bacteria in a series of broth tubes (or agar plates) with increasing concentrations of antibiotic. The lowest concentration of antibiotic that inhibits microbial growth in this test system is known as the *minimum inhibitory concentration* (MIC). If tubes in which no growth occurs are subcultured, the minimum concentration of antibiotic required to kill the starting inoculum also can be determined. This measurement is called the *minimum bactericidal concentration* (MBC). A miniaturized version of the macrobroth dilution technique in microwell plates is called the *microbroth dilution method*. Quantitative susceptibility testing using the microbroth dilution technique lends itself to automation and is used commonly in larger clinical laboratories.

A novel version of the disk/agar-diffusion method employing a quantitative diffusion gradient uses an absorbent strip with a known gradient of antibiotic concentrations along its length. When the strip is placed on the surface of an agar plate seeded with a bacterial strain to be tested, antibiotic diffuses into the medium, and bacterial growth is inhibited. Quantitative measures of the MIC are estimated by determining the lowest point on the gradient strip that inhibits microbial growth.

AUTOMATION OF MICROBIAL DETECTION IN BLOOD The detection of microbial growth in blood is difficult because the numbers of organisms present in the sample are often low and because the integrity of the organisms and their ability to replicate may be damaged by humoral defense mechanisms or antimicrobial agents. Over the years, automated systems that relied on the detection of CO_2

produced by the organisms present in blood culture bottles have allowed for the automation of this procedure. The most common system involves inserting a sampling device into each bottle at periodic intervals and drawing off the head-space gas of the bottle. An infrared monitor is used to determine the CO_2 level. The system interprets levels exceeding a set concentration as indicative of microbial growth. Such methods are not any more sensitive than the human eye in detecting a positive culture, but because the bottles in an automated system are generally monitored more frequently, a positive culture is often detected more rapidly than by manual techniques, and consequently, important information, including Gram's stain and preliminary susceptibility assays, can be obtained sooner.

One technique for automated blood culture monitoring uses reflectance optics consisting of a photodiode and a light-emitting diode to monitor the amount of CO_2 produced in each blood culture bottle every 10 min through a self-contained sensor that is part of each bottle. Each reflectance measurement is then stored in computer memory, and when an appropriate change in reflectance occurs, the system alerts the clinical laboratory to the presence of a positive culture via audible and visible alarms. The continuous scanning of bottles used in this system provides shortened detection times with the concomitant advantage of early reporting for positive cultures, and the noninvasive monitoring procedure decreases the likelihood of laboratory contamination.

Automated systems also have been applied for detection of microbial growth from specimens other than blood, such as peritoneal and other normally sterile fluids. *Mycobacterium* spp. also can be detected in certain automated systems if appropriate media are used for culture.

DETECTION OF VIRAL AGENTS **Serologic methods** Measurement of antibodies provides an indirect marker for past or current infection with a specific viral agent. The biologic signal is usually either IgM or IgG antibody directed at viral antigen(s). The detection systems include those used for bacterial antigens (agglutination reactions, immunofluorescence, and EIA) and unique detection systems such as hemolysis inhibition and complement fixation. Serologic methods generally fall into two categories: tests to determine protective antibody levels or measurements of changing antibody titers as a method for detecting current infection. Documentation of an antibody response as a measure of current immunity is important for viral agents such as rubella or varicella zoster; assays for this purpose normally use one or two dilutions of serum for a qualitative determination of protective antibody levels. Quantitative serologic assays to detect increases in antibody titers most often employ paired serum samples obtained 10 to 14 days apart (acute and convalescent phase). Since the incubation period before symptoms are noted may be long enough for an antibody response to occur, the demonstration of acute phase antibody alone is often not enough to establish the diagnosis of active infection as opposed to past exposure. In such circumstances, the finding of IgM may be useful as a measure of an early, acute antibody response. A fourfold increase in total antibody titer or in EIA activity between the acute and convalescent samples is also regarded as evidence for active infection.

For certain viral agents, such as Epstein-Barr virus, the antibodies produced may be directed at different antigens during different phases of the infection. For this reason, most laboratories test for antibody directed at both viral capsid antigens and antigens associated with recently infected host cells to determine the stage of infection.

Culture methods Pathogenic viral agents are often cultured when the presence of antibody is not a criterion of active infection or when an increase in serum antibody may not be detected during infection. The biologic signal, virus, is thus amplified to a level at which detection can occur. Although a number of techniques are available, the essential elements include a monolayer of cultured mammalian cells sensitive to infection with the suspect viral pathogen. These cells serve as the amplification system by allowing for the proliferation of viral particles. Virus may be detected by direct observation of the cultured cells for cytopathic effects or by immuno-

fluorescent detection of viral antigens following incubation. Culture methods are particularly useful for detection of rapidly propagated agents, such as cytomegalovirus or herpes simplex virus.

REFERENCES

EISENBERG HD et al: Specimen collection and handling, in *Manual of Clinical Microbiology*, 5th ed, A Ballows et al (eds). Washington, American Society for Microbiology, 1991

FUCCILLO DA et al: Rapid viral diagnosis, in *Manual of Clinical Laboratory Immunology*, 3d ed, Rose, NR et al (eds). Washington, American Society for Microbiology, 1986

HOPKIN JM et al: DNA hybridization for the diagnosis of microbial disease. Q J Med 75:415, 1990

LENNETTE DA: Preparation of specimens for virological examination, in *Manual of Clinical Microbiology*, 5th ed, A Ballows et al (eds). Washington, American Society for Microbiology, 1991

MURRAY PR: Comparison of the lysis-centrifugation and agitated biphasic blood culture systems for detection of fungemia. J Clin Microbiol 29:96, 1991

NOWINSKI RC et al: Monoclonal antibodies for diagnosis of infectious diseases in humans. Science 219:637, 1983

SCHOCHETMAN G et al: Polymerase chain reaction. J Infect Dis 158:1154, 1988

YOLKEN RH: Enzyme immunoassays for the detection of infectious antigens in body fluids: Current limitations and future prospects. Rev Infect Dis 4:35, 1982

81　INFECTIONS IN PATIENTS WITH INFLAMMATORY AND IMMUNOLOGIC DEFECTS

HENRY MASUR / ANTHONY S. FAUCI

DEFINITION Qualitative or quantitative defects in inflammatory or immunologic host defenses are caused by a wide variety of processes, including primary congenital syndromes, cancer, trauma, malnutrition, retroviral infection, and drug therapy. When these defects—or those in other host protective mechanisms—are diminished significantly, patients develop increased susceptibility to infection and are considered ''compromised hosts.'' Microbial processes are increasingly important causes of morbidity and mortality in compromised hosts because progressively more potent suppressive regimens are being used to manage conditions such as cancer and organ transplants and because patients are living longer as a result of improvements in the management of noninfectious complications.

HOST DEFENSE MECHANISMS

Antimicrobial defense mechanisms (Table 81-1) consist of complex, interacting systems that protect the host from endogenous and exogenous microbes (Chap. 79). The degree to which a patient becomes abnormally susceptible to infection by these microbes depends on the mechanism(s) compromised, the severity of the derangements, and their interactions. For instance, as isolated abnormalities, total absence of serum IgA or complement component C9 would probably have minor, if any, impact on host susceptibility to infection. In contrast, isolated abnormalities such as total absence of circulating neutrophils, serum IgG, or complement component C3 would lead to recurrent and life-threatening infections. Simultaneous damage to multiple host defenses may lead to especially ominous vulnerability. For instance, a combination of absent neutrophils and extensive disruption of the skin or mucous membranes would together constitute a particularly dangerous compromise that would likely be much worse than the sum of the risks posed by the individual abnormalities.

Recognition of which specific and nonspecific host defenses are compromised is important in order to develop effective clinical

TABLE 81-1   Mechanisms of host defense

Physical and chemical barriers
    Morphologic integrity of skin, mucous membranes
    Sphincters
    Epiglottis
    Normal secretory and excretory flow
    Endogenous microbial flora
    Gastric acidity
Inflammatory response
    Circulating phagocytes
    Complement
    Other humoral mediators (bradykinins, fibrinolytic systems, arachidonic acid cascade)
Reticuloendothelial system
    Tissue phagocytes
Immune response
    T lymphocytes and their soluble products
    B lymphocytes and immunoglobulins

strategies for predicting the probable timing of onset of infection and the most likely causative organisms, for formulating the appropriate diagnostic approach, and for developing the optimal therapeutic and preventive plan. However, based on an understanding of the mechanisms of host defenses, such an approach must be supplemented by clinical experience with specific patient populations. Because there are complexities of various host defense mechanisms that are not easily measured or fully understood, it cannot be assumed that all patient populations with the same measured deficiency in antimicrobial defense (as assessed by current laboratory techniques) will behave identically. For example, certain patients with AIDS and certain patients with hematologic malignancies will have neutrophil counts below 500 cells per microliter, but only the latter will have greatly increased frequency of infections due to gram-positive and gram-negative bacteria.

PHYSICAL AND CHEMICAL BARRIERS   Physical and chemical barriers (Table 81-1) are part of a complex and interacting system of nonspecific host defense mechanisms that are essential for preventing the introduction and spread of endogenous and exogenous microbial organisms, including both those which normally colonize various anatomic sites and those which are highly pathogenic and whose presence is abnormal. These barriers utilize a wide variety of properties to protect the host, including the morphologic and functional integrity of skin or mucous membranes, the epiglottis, or sphincters; chemical processes (e.g., gastric acidity, pancreatic enzymes, cutaneous fatty acids or lysozyme); physical removal of organisms (e.g., peristalsis, sloughing of squamous cells, urine flow); and competition from less virulent flora. Interference with any of these mechanisms, e.g., by tumors, procedures, devices, infarcts, or drugs, can increase the host's susceptibility to infection. Common causes of disruption of physical and chemical barriers include intravenous catheters, which breach the skin; antacids, which remove the gastric barrier; and cytotoxic chemotherapy, which disrupts the gastrointestinal mucosa.

INFLAMMATORY RESPONSES   Circulating phagocytes (neutrophils, monocytes, eosinophils, and basophils) arise from the bone marrow and upon appropriate signals enter the peripheral circulation and are distributed to local tissues, where they form the cornerstone of the inflammatory response. Recruitment of phagocytes from the bloodstream is a complicated process which involves the phagocytes' aggregation, adherence to the vascular endothelium, passage through endothelial spaces, and migration to local tissue sites (Chap. 59). An effective inflammatory response depends on the ability of the phagocyte to adhere, deform, have random locomotion, and respond to a chemical signal with directed movement. Humoral mediators influence local structures in ways that affect the phagocyte's ability to reach various loci; an example is the influence the complement cascade (especially C3a and C5a) has on the potential spaces between endothelial cells. Humoral mediators, including the complement system, the arachidonic acid cascade, kinin-generating systems, and cellular products such as interleukin 1 and tumor necrosis factor,

microbial peptides, or endotoxins, also promote directed locomotion of the phagocytes. Once the phagocyte arrives at a focus of infection, it may be able to adhere to the microorganism, ingest it, and digest it, particularly if the organism has been opsonized by antibodies or complement products. A wide variety of bacteria as well as fungi are killed by neutrophils in this manner.

RETICULOENDOTHELIAL SYSTEM   Circulating microorganisms are cleared from the bloodstream by tissue phagocytes that are derived from circulating monocytes. These phagocytes include macrophages in the liver (Kupffer cells), spleen, lymph nodes, lung (alveolar macrophages), kidney (mesangial cells), and brain (microglial cells). The antimicrobial activities of these monocytes and macrophages are strongly influenced by opsonins such as IgG or C3b, which enhance the rate of particle ingestion, and by a large variety of soluble mediators produced primarily by mononuclear leukocytes (see Chap. 59). The efficacy of the reticuloendothelial system is also influenced by characteristics of specific organisms which allow the microbes to resist phagocytosis, lysosome-phagosome fusion (*Toxoplasma*), or intraphagosomal inactivation (*Leishmania*).

Immune response   The major cellular components of the immune response are T lymphocytes and B lymphocytes (Chap. 277). These cells are distributed throughout the body in the bloodstream and at tissue sites. They interact in a highly complex fashion among themselves and with monocytes, macrophages, immunoglobulins, and the complement cascade. T lymphocytes are major components of the cell-mediated immune system. They secrete a multitude of cytokines which influence the functional status of other T lymphocytes, B lymphocytes, monocytes, and macrophages to eradicate infection and participate directly in cytotoxic reactions against tumor cells, HLA-incompatible cells, and certain virus-infected host cells. B lymphocytes and plasma cells secrete specific antibodies which have important roles in eradicating certain infections. The ability of the monocytes and macrophages to ingest and kill a wide variety of bacteria, fungi, and protozoa is augmented by lymphokines released by T lymphocytes, in particular, γ-interferon. Production of opsonizing, neutralizing, or microbicidal antibodies can also be profoundly influenced by the regulatory effect of T lymphocytes on B lymphocytes (Chap. 277).

ETIOLOGY AND PATHOGENESIS OF INFECTION

In compromised hosts, the development of infections reflects the interaction of impaired immunologic and nonimmunologic host defense mechanisms with the host's endogenous and exogenous microbial environment. Factors which change the microbial flora have an important impact on the organisms that are likely to cause disease. Such factors include antimicrobial therapy, invasive procedures or trauma, ingestion or inhalation of infected material, and hospitalization itself. The type of infections which develop are usually the consequence of specific alterations in host defenses, however.

Numerous processes can predispose to serious infection by compromising the anatomic and physical barriers of host defense. For example, the skin and mucous membranes can be breached by tumor invasion, tumor necrosis, or vascular insufficiency induced by arteritis or atherosclerosis; by injuries such as burns, pressure, or trauma; by radiation or cytotoxic chemotherapy; by a drug-induced cutaneous slough; and by procedures such as venipuncture or surgery. The respiratory tract can become the site of infection when its anatomic barriers are disrupted: the epiglottis may fail to protect the lower tract when the patient's consciousness is impaired or during intubation or bronchoscopy. The patient's ability to expel organisms may be adversely affected by infection, tumors, or drugs that alter the state of consciousness or prevent coughing; by disruption of mucociliary transport by a congenital disorder of ciliary subunits (such as Kartagener's syndrome) or by smoke or other inhaled toxins, anesthetic agents, or cytotoxic therapy; or by airway obstruction as a result of tumor, a foreign body, or lymph node enlargement.

The gastrointestinal tract can become a less effective barrier against entry of organisms if gastric acidity is abolished by a surgical procedure or antacid therapy (infections with *Salmonella* and other gram-negative rods are a typical consequence) or if its mucosa is eroded by tumor or cytotoxic therapy, especially in neutropenic patients. Obstruction of the intestinal or biliary tract by tumor, a stricture, or a stone allows endogenous or introduced flora to gain access to the involved tissues and often the bloodstream.

The genitourinary tract can become a portal of entry for infections if its mucosa is eroded by tumor, irradiation, or cytotoxic therapy or there is urinary obstruction. Renal failure associated with oliguria or anuria deprives the genitourinary system of the ability to flush out microorganisms and obviates the antimicrobial effects of urine itself. The insertion of foreign bodies into the urethra during catheterization or cystoscopy allows exogenous organisms to be introduced into the urinary tract.

Any locus in the body can become the site of infection if devitalized tissue or foreign bodies are seeded by bacteria or become infected by direct penetration. Hematomas, necrotic tissue, infarcts, calcified heart valves, and prosthetic devices (joints, heart valves, or central nervous system appliances) are particularly prone to bacterial infection.

Defects in inflammatory and immune function may permit infections that would normally be promptly eradicated to progress and cause clinically important disease. These quantitative or qualitative defects may be due to a congenital disorder, an underlying acquired disease, or drug therapy. Several specific types of defects are associated with particularly frequent or severe infectious complications.

LEUKOCYTE DISORDERS   The clinical consequences of leukocyte disorders depend on which subpopulations of leukocytes are numerically or functionally affected and the duration of the dysfunction (Table 81-2) (Chap. 59). Neutropenia (less than 1800 neutrophils per microliter) is the most commonly encountered defect in inflammatory host defense mechanisms (Chap. 59). When the neutrophil count falls below 1000 cells per microliter, there is a progressive increase in susceptibility to bacterial and fungal infections and a progressive decrease in the localizing signs and symptoms of inflammation. Susceptibility to infection increases dramatically when the peripheral neutrophil count falls below 500 cells per microliter, particularly when the count falls below 100 cells per microliter. The rate of decline and the duration of neutropenia are also important parameters which influence the development of infection. Neutropenia can occur because of bone marrow failure, peripheral destruction, or pooling or sequestration of cells. The most common causes of neutropenia are cytotoxic chemotherapy, neoplastic invasion of the bone marrow, aplastic anemia, and idiosyncratic drug reactions.

Neutrophil dysfunction also can result in a substantial predisposition to serious infection. Dysfunction may be a manifestation of a congenital disorder such as chronic granulomatous disease or Chédiak-Higashi syndrome (Chap. 59). Glucocorticoids and some multiple-drug chemotherapeutic regimens may alter both the number and the function of circulating neutrophils.

Lymphopenia in adults is defined as less than 1000 lymphocytes per microliter. The clinical consequences of lymphopenia depend on the subset(s) affected. Regardless of the total lymphocyte count, severe infections may occur if profound deficiencies of either B lymphocytes or T lymphocytes are present. Substantial reductions in helper T lymphocytes (CD4-positive lymphocytes) (<200 per microliter) can have particularly important infectious consequences, especially when caused by human immunodeficiency virus (HIV). The most common causes of lymphopenia are hematologic malignancies, glucocorticoid therapy, antilymphocyte globulins, cytotoxic drugs, and infection with certain viruses such as cytomegalovirus (Chap. 146) and HIV (Chap. 279). Congenital lymphopenias also can have severe consequences (Chap. 278).

Lymphocyte dysfunction can predispose to life-threatening infection even if the lymphocyte number is normal. Lymphocyte dysfunc-

tion is most often a consequence of therapy with glucocorticoids or cytotoxic drugs.

IMMUNOGLOBULIN DISORDERS   Decreased production of functional immunoglobulins, particularly IgG, can cause a marked increase in susceptibility to microbial disease (Chap. 278). Patients with significant reductions in IgG (usually less than 200 to 300 mg/dL) characteristically have recurrent infections due to encapsulated bacteria, particularly *Streptococcus pneumoniae*, *Haemophilus influenzae*, and *Neisseria meningitidis*, and to other organisms (*Pneumocystis carinii* and *Giardia lamblia*). Selective IgA deficiency can lead to respiratory or systemic bacterial infections (particularly when accompanied by IgG$_2$ deficiency) as well as intestinal giardiasis or severe viral hepatitis. The few documented cases of selective IgM deficiency also have been associated with severe infections, in particular with gram-negative organisms such as *Neisseria meningitidis*. Clinically important causes of immunoglobulin deficiency or dysfunction include congenital and acquired disorders, such as malignancies (multiple myeloma, chronic lymphocytic leukemia), sickle cell disease, and splenectomy (Table 81-2) (Chap. 278).

COMPLEMENT DISORDERS   The consequences of total absence of functional complement proteins depend on which of the specific components are deficient (Table 81-2) (Chap. 277). Deficiencies of C1 or C3 have been associated with pneumococcal infections, while deficiencies of C5, C6, C7, or C8 may lead to relapsing *Neisseria meningitidis* or *Neisseria gonorrhoeae* infections. Most severe deficiencies are due to inherited disorders, although there are reports of significant deficiencies in patients with systemic lupus erythematosus, cirrhosis, or splenectomy.

SPLENECTOMY   The spleen contains large numbers of B lymphocytes, monocytes, and macrophages and is a major site for T cell–independent immune responses such as the production of antibodies to polysaccharide antigens. The spleen has an important role in the phagocytosis of circulating opsonized organisms. Following splenectomy, young children are at high risk for fulminant infections due to *Streptococcus pneumoniae*, *Haemophilus influenzae*, *Neisseria meningitidis*, and the fastidious gram-negative bacterium DF-2. Adults who undergo splenectomy are also at increased risk for these infections, especially during the first 3 years after surgery. Splenectomized patients may develop fulminant infection with intraerythrocytic protozoa such as *Plasmodium malariae* and *Babesia*.

DIAGNOSIS

Clinicians managing compromised patients must recognize that the diagnosis of infectious processes requires special attention, persistence, and expertise. Compromised patients often present initially with manifestations that may be subtle or atypical. All infections can become life-threatening in extremely short time periods in many of these patients, so the diagnostic evaluation needs to begin promptly when the first signs or symptoms or laboratory abnormalities become apparent. These evaluations should proceed in rapid sequence, with use of tests that have the shortest feasible processing times. A thorough approach is necessary to make certain that the true etiologic agent is being treated and to minimize the likelihood that unnecessary drugs with toxic effects will be employed. The spectrum of potential etiologic agents is usually wide, so the diagnostic tests must often be broad-gauged as well. On the basis of a knowledge of the factors that render the patient compromised, the organisms associated with particular defects in host defense, and the patient's individual history and presentation, the clinician in concert with the laboratory must consider whether special testing should be done for unusual bacteria, fungi, viruses, helminths, protozoa, or other microorganisms. It is usually desirable to have a standard protocol for evaluating common clinical syndromes (e.g., pneumonia, fever, meningitis) in compromised patients, with modifications being made in the protocol as warranted by the individual patient's circumstances. For instance, when an HIV-infected patient has a helper T lymphocyte (T4-positive

TABLE 81-2 Infections associated with common defects in inflammatory or immunologic response

Host defect	Examples of diseases or therapies associated with defects	Common etiologic agents of infections
INFLAMMATORY RESPONSE		
Neutropenia	Hematologic malignancies, cytotoxic chemotherapy, aplastic anemia	Gram-negative enteric bacilli, *Pseudomonas* species, *Staphylococcus* species, *Candida* species, *Aspergillus* species
Chemotaxis	Chédiak-Higashi syndrome	*Staphylococcus aureus*, *Streptococcus pyogenes*
	Job's syndrome, protein-calorie malnutrition	*Staphylococcus aureus*, *Haemophilus influenzae*, gram-negative bacilli
Phagocytosis (cellular)	Systemic lupus erythematosus, chronic myelogenous leukemia, megaloblastic anemia	*Streptococcus pneumoniae*, *Haemophilus influenzae*
Splenectomy		*Haemophilus influenzae*, *Streptococcus pneumoniae*, other streptococci, DF-2, *Babesia microti*, *Salmonella* species
Microbicidal defect	Chronic granulomatous disease	Catalase-positive bacteria and fungi: staphylococci, *Escherichia coli*, *Klebsiella* species, *Pseudomonas aeruginosa*, *Aspergillus* species, *Nocardia* species
	Chédiak-Higashi syndrome	*Staphylococcus aureus*, *Streptococcus pyogenes*
COMPLEMENT SYSTEM		
C3	Congenital liver disease, systemic lupus erythematosus	*Staphylococcus aureus*, *Streptococcus pneumoniae*, *Pseudomonas* species, *Proteus* species
C5	Congenital	*Neisseria* species, gram-negative rods
C6, C7, C8	Congenital, systemic lupus erythematosus	*Neisseria meningitidis*, *Neisseria gonorrhoeae*
Alternate pathway	Sickle cell disease	*Streptococcus pneumoniae*, *Salmonella* species
IMMUNE RESPONSE		
T lymphocyte deficiency/dysfunction	Thymic aplasia, thymic hypoplasia, Hodgkin's disease, sarcoidosis, lepromatous leprosy	*Listeria monocytogenes*, *Mycobacterium* species, *Candida* species, *Aspergillus* species, *Cryptococcus neoformans*, herpes simplex virus, varicella-zoster virus
	Acquired immunodeficiency syndrome	*Pneumocystis carinii*, cytomegalovirus, herpes simplex, *Mycobacterium avium-intracellulare*, *Cryptococcus neoformans*, *Candida* species
	Mucocutaneous candidiasis	*Candida* species
	Purine nucleoside phosphorylase deficiency	Fungi, viruses
B cell deficiency/dysfunction	Bruton's X-linked agammaglobulinemia, agammaglobulinemia, chronic lymphocytic leukemia, multiple myeloma, dysglobulinemia	*Streptococcus pneumoniae*, other streptococci, *Haemophilus influenzae*, *Neisseria meningitidis*, *Staphylococcus aureus*, *Klebsiella pneumoniae*, *Escherichia coli*, *Giardia lamblia*, *Pneumocystis carinii*, enteroviruses
	Selective IgM deficiency	*Streptococcus pneumoniae*, *Haemophilus influenzae*, *Escherichia coli*
	Selective IgA deficiency	*Giardia lamblia*, hepatitis virus, *Streptococcus pneumoniae*, *Haemophilus influenzae*
Mixed T and B cell deficiency/dysfunction	Common variable hypogammaglobulinemia	*Pneumocystis carinii*, cytomegalovirus, *Streptococcus pneumoniae*, *Haemophilus influenzae*, various other bacteria
	Ataxia-telangiectasia	*Streptococcus pneumoniae*, *Haemophilus influenzae*, *Staphylococcus aureus*, rubella virus, *Giardia lamblia*
	Severe combined immunodeficiency	*Staphylococcus aureus*, *Streptococcus pneumoniae*, *Haemophilus influenzae*, *Candida albicans*, *Pneumocystis carinii*, varicella-zoster virus, rubella virus, cytomegalovirus
	Wiskott-Aldrich	Agents of infections seen in T and B cell abnormalities

or CD4-positive) count below 200 to 300 per microliter, and especially when the count falls below 100 per microliter, mild cough with fever must be evaluated promptly and aggressively because pneumocystis or cytomegalovirus pneumonia are much more likely than in HIV-positive patients with normal T4 counts. Kidney transplant recipients are known to be at very high risk for bacterial wound and urinary tract infections during the first postoperative month, while opportunistic viral, fungal, and protozoan diseases are more common during the second through sixth months. The development of fever during the first postoperative month should prompt an evaluation that focuses initially on the wound and urinary tract, while similar symptoms occurring several months after surgery should direct studies for protozoan, fungal, or viral infections.

Patients with leukemias and lymphomas need particular scrutiny for complicating bacterial or fungal infections when their neutrophil counts fall below 100 cells per microliter (a time that is usually predictable from the pharmacokinetics of the chemotherapeutic regimen).

THERAPY

In compromised patients the therapy of infectious complications should include drainage of localized collections of infected material, specific antimicrobials, and, if possible, reconstitution of deficient antimicrobial defenses. Examples of the last include the infusion of fresh frozen plasma to augment complement components, the administration of immune serum globulin to restore IgG levels, and the tapering of immunosuppressive drugs (such as glucocorticoids or cytotoxic agents) to restore cell-mediated immune mechanisms or neutrophil production. In certain neutropenic patients, augmentation or restoration of neutrophils can be achieved by the use of colony-stimulating factors (see Chap. 59) or white blood cell transfusions or permanently by bone marrow transplantation. Patients must be carefully selected for which of these procedures is likely to be effective.

Empiric antimicrobial therapy is clearly appropriate for some patient populations. For example, newly developing fever in severely neutropenic patients is frequently due to infection with bacteria, and therapy with a broad-spectrum regimen directed against potential major gram-positive and gram-negative pathogens before culture results are available can be lifesaving. The use of antibiotic combinations that are synergistic against infecting bacteria has been more successful in reducing morbidity and mortality from bacterial infection in neutropenic patients than single agents or nonsynergistic combinations. Examples of such combinations are vancomycin, ticarcillin, and amikacin or ceftazidime and amikacin (see Chap. 100). Empiric use of amphotericin B in the febrile neutropenic patient unresponsive after several days of antibacterial treatment is a common practice and may reduce morbidity from fungal superinfection.

PREVENTION OF INFECTION

In compromised patients, certain types of infections can be prevented by avoiding damage to physical barriers, bolstering host defenses, reducing acquisition of new potential pathogens, and suppressing colonizing flora. The use of invasive procedures, including repeated venipuncture, indwelling peripheral venous catheterization, and urinary catheterization, should be minimized or avoided completely. Surgical procedures should be chosen only when absolutely essential and should be performed with meticulous care. Bolstering host defenses can be accomplished directly in some patient groups. For example, immune serum globulin can be given prophylactically to hypogammaglobulinemic patients (see Chap. 278); hyperimmune varicella-zoster immunoglobulin can prevent or reduce the severity of varicella-zoster virus disease after acute exposure; immunization with vaccines against pneumococci, *Haemophilus*, and meningococci may be helpful for patients with conditions of particular susceptibility, such as those needing splenectomy (see Chap. 59).

Maintaining an optimal nutritional status will improve cellular immune mechanisms and aid wound repair. Most other methods to enhance depressed cell-mediated immunity have been clinically ineffective. Colony-stimulating factors offer promise in restoring neutrophil numbers and preventing infection in neutropenic subjects but require further investigation (see Chap. 59). Reducing the acquisition of potential pathogens can be facilitated by simple techniques, such as having hospital personnel wash their hands before patient contact, and by appropriate isolation from specific potentially contagious organisms, such as varicella-zoster virus, *Mycobacterium tuberculosis*, or multiply antibiotic-resistant gram-negative bacilli (see Chap. 98). More stringent measures, such as laminar flow isolation or control of sterility of food and water, have not proved to be useful or cost-effective for ultimate survival, although these measures will decrease the rate of infection for patients with prolonged and profound granulocytopenia. Selective or total suppression of endogenous bacteria or fungi is an important concept, since they cause more than 80 percent of infections in neutropenic cancer patients. Gut sterilization or prophylactic systemic antibiotics may have proved useful as temporary measures in certain neutropenic patients but cannot be practically sustained for more than a few weeks. Prolonged antimicrobial prophylaxis of certain specific infections that have exceedingly high attack rates in certain defined populations can be quite effective. The impressive protection provided by trimethoprim-sulfamethoxazole or aerosolized pentamidine against *Pneumocystis carinii* pneumonia in certain patients with AIDS or acute lymphocytic leukemia is a striking example.

REFERENCES

BODEY GP et al: Quantitative relationships between circulating leukocytes and infection in patients with acute leukemia. Ann Intern Med 64:328, 1966

BUCKLEY RH, SCHIFF RI: The use of intravenous immune globulin in immunodeficiency diseases. N Engl J Med 325:110, 1991

DWYER JM: Manipulating the immune system with immune globulin. N Engl J Med 326:107, 1992

FIGUEROA JE, DENSEN P: Infectious diseases associated with complement deficiencies. Clin Microbiol Rev 4:359, 1991

HUGHES WT et al: Successful chemoprophylaxis for *Pneumocystis carinii* pneumonitis. N Engl J Med 297:1419, 1977

——— et al: Guidelines for the use of antimicrobial agents in neutropenic patients with unexplained fever. J Infect Dis 161:381, 1990

INTERNATIONAL CHRONIC GRANULOMATOUS DISEASE COOPERATIVE STUDY GROUP: A controlled trial of interferon gamma to prevent infection in chronic granulomatous disease. N Engl J Med 324:509, 1991

MASUR H et al: CD4 counts as predictors of pneumonias in human immunodeficiency virus–infected individuals. Ann Intern Med 111:223, 1989

SANDE MA, VOLBERDING PA: *The Medical Management of AIDS*, 2d ed. Philadelphia, Saunders, 1990

SHELHAMER J et al (eds): *Respiratory Disease in the Immunosuppressed Host*. Philadelphia, Lippincott, 1991

WINSTON DJ et al: Beta-lactam antibiotic therapy in febrile granulocytopenic patients. Ann Intern Med 115:849, 1991

82 IMMUNIZATION PRINCIPLES AND VACCINE USE

GERALD T. KEUSCH / KENNETH J. BART

Most humans live their lives ignoring the certainty of their own mortality. Perhaps this explains why the adage "an ounce of prevention is worth a pound of cure" weighs so little in our everyday behavior. This is certainly true among adults, but even when it comes to acting to protect their young, humans are capable of either ignoring the potential mortality of their children in the developed world or accepting the certainty of childhood deaths in the developing world. In both settings, they all too often fail to seek out and demand the best preventive measures available. Unless mandated by the law in the former or provided by benevolent organizations or governments in the latter setting, universal immunization will invariably fall far short of the goal. Compulsion and benevolence, it seems, are two essential components of public health.

However, the integration of immunization practices (a major component of primary disease prevention) into routine health care services has provided caregivers with control over a substantial proportion of the disease and mortality that plagued the United States during the first half of the twentieth century (Table 82-1). For society today, immunization represents one of the most cost-effective means of preventing serious infectious disease. Presently, more than 50 biologic products are licensed in the United States and 11 antigens are used for routine immunization in the young, including diphtheria-tetanus-pertussis (DTP), trivalent polio, measles-mumps-rubella (MMR), *Haemophilus influenzae* type b (Hib), and hepatitis B vaccines. Five vaccines are designed for routine use in adults, including adult tetanus-diphtheria (Td) toxoids, hepatitis B virus, influenza virus, and polyvalent pneumococcal polysaccharides. The epidemiologically appropriate use of vaccines has resulted in the global eradication of smallpox, the virtual eradication of poliomyelitis in the Americas, and the near elimination of congenital rubella syndrome, tetanus, and diphtheria and a dramatic reduction in pertussis, rubella, measles, and mumps in the United States. Figure 82-1 shows the effect of vaccines on the incidence of *H. influenzae* type b meningitis. The Hib conjugate vaccines in particular have exerted a remarkable influence on invasive *Haemophilus* infections, presumably because they reduce nasopharyngeal carriage of *H.*

TABLE 82-1   Changes in vaccine-preventable disease incidence in the United States

		Cases reported		
	Peak year		1992*	Decreases, %
Diphtheria	1921	206,939	4	99.99
Measles	1941	894,134	2200	99.75
Mumps	1968	152,209	2460	98.38
Pertussis	1934	265,269	3359	98.73
Poliomyelitis (paralytic)	1952	21,269	0†	100.00
Rubella	1969	57,686	148	99.74
Congenital rubella syndrome	1964–5	20,000	9	99.96
Tetanus	1923	1,560	42	97.31

* Provisional.
† Projected to be 5 to 10 vaccine-associated cases.
SOURCE: Centers for Disease Control and Prevention, National Program for Immunization.

influenzae and induce protection before the period of greatest vulnerability in infancy.

Vaccine development depends on the systematic application of a four-phase strategy: (1) identify a protective antigen, (2) determine how to effectively present it to the immune system, (3) define the safety of the preparation, and (4) evaluate its efficacy in the target population. Each of these steps is simple in concept but difficult in execution, not the least so for the clinical trials necessary to assess safety and efficacy; failure at any level stops the development process. Progress in immunology has taught us much about the organization and function of the immune system (see Chap. 277); it also has taught us that the immune system is complicated and that details of antigen composition and presentation are critical for stimulating desired immune responses.

The development of vaccines goes beyond the technology and proof of principle to issues of development costs, manufacturers' liability and indemnity, perceived public health needs, and the likelihood of the product being used or sold. Given the complex science required, the costs of vaccine development are high and success is uncertain, adding risk to the development decision. It is unfortunate that the one certain implication of uncertainty in vaccine development is increased cost. In addition, a rational assignment of costs between public and private sectors in the United States has never been achieved. Under the National Vaccine Injury Compensation Program, the potential of associated or attributed adverse reactions following the use of vaccines adds to the risk and capitalization needs for vaccine development.

DEFINITIONS   *Vaccination* and *immunization* are often used as interchangeable terms; however, the former denotes only the administration of a vaccine or toxoid, whereas the latter describes the process of inducing or providing immunity by any means, whether by active or passive measures. Thus vaccination does not guarantee

immunization. *Active immunization* refers to the induction of immune defenses by the administration of vaccines or toxoids, whereas *passive immunization* involves the provision of temporary protection by administration of exogenously produced immune substances. Immunizing agents thus include vaccines, toxoids, and antibody-containing immunoglobulin (Ig) preparations from human or animal donors (Table 82-2) and in the future may include immunocompetent cells, whether derived from the host himself or herself or from cell lines maintained in vitro or even DNA designed to express specific antigens which in turn induce protective antibodies or cell-mediated immunity.

PRINCIPLES OF IMMUNIZATION   Artificial induction of immunity closely follows two well-tested principles of nature. The first, active immunization, can be traced at least as far back as Thucydides, who noted that people surviving epidemics of plague in Athens were spared during later outbreaks of the same disease. Having symptomatic disease is an uncomfortable way of acquiring immunity, however, and some diseases do not provide subsequent resistance. The second, passive immunization, is a natural process as well, e.g., transplacental transmission of maternal antibodies to the fetus, which provides protection against several diseases during the first months of life. When practiced by clinicians, the two measures are complementary and only rarely mutually exclusive. Depending on whether there are multiple species or serotypes of an organism and whether there are common, cross-reactive, protective antigens, a specific vaccine may induce protection against all representative forms of an infectious agent or just the immunizing strain.

However, because the immune response to specific antigens is controlled genetically, individuals cannot be expected to respond equally to the same vaccine. One of the intrinsic virtues of whole-organism vaccines is that they potentially might contain all protective antigens of the organism. This is also an inherent problem of such vaccines: the possibility of adverse reactions to unnecessary materials present in the mix.

Approaches to active immunization   The principal approaches to active immunization are (1) the use of live, generally attenuated infectious agents (e.g., measles) and (2) the use of inactivated agents, detoxified extracts or toxins from them, or specific antigens obtained

FIGURE 82-1   *H. influenzae* vaccine doses sold or distributed and meningitis incidence in children more than 5 years old. (*From Centers for Disease Control and Prevention.*)

TABLE 82-2   Definitions

Vaccine: A suspension of attenuated live or killed microorganisms or antigenic portions of these agents presented to a potential host to induce immunity and prevent disease.

Toxoid: A modified bacterial toxin that has been made nontoxic but retains the capacity to stimulate the formation of antitoxin.

Immune globulin: An antibody-containing solution derived from human blood obtained by cold ethanol fractionation of large pools of plasma and used primarily for the maintenance of immunity of immunodeficient persons or for passive immunization. Intramuscular and intravenous preparations are available.

Antitoxin: An antibody derived from the serum of animals after stimulation with specific antigens used to provide passive immunity.

by genetic recombination (e.g., hepatitis B virus). For many diseases (e.g., poliomyelitis, influenza), both approaches have been employed. Live, attenuated vaccines are believed to induce an immunologic response more nearly like that resulting from natural infection than the response induced by killed vaccines. Currently available inactivated or killed vaccines and those being developed consist of inactivated whole organisms (e.g., standard pertussis vaccine), detoxified protein exotoxins (e.g., tetanus toxoid), recombinant protein antigens (e.g., hepatitis B vaccine), fusion proteins with other antigens or carrier peptides or as conjugates with lipopolysaccharides, or in the case of carbohydrate antigens either as soluble purified capsular material (e.g., *Streptococcus pneumoniae* polysaccharides) or conjugated to a protein carrier (e.g., *H. influenzae* type b or group B streptococcal polysaccharides conjugated to diphtheria or tetanus toxoids).

Since the organisms in live vaccines multiply in the recipient host, antigen production generally increases logarithmically until checked by the onset of the immune response it is intended to induce. In those who respond, live, attenuated virus vaccines (e.g., measles, rubella, mumps) are believed to confer lifelong protection with one dose, although it is already clear that in some individuals immunity wanes and requires subsequent boosting for long-term protection. By contrast, except for purified polysaccharide antigens, killed vaccines generally do not induce permanent immunity with one dose, making both a series of multiple initial inoculations and subsequent periodic boosters necessary to develop and maintain high levels of antibody (e.g., diphtheria, rabies). Although the amount of antigen initially introduced is greater with inactivated vaccines, the multiplication of organisms in the host given live vaccines results in a cumulatively greater antigenic input.

Approaches to passive immunization Passive immunization is generally used to provide temporary immunity in an unimmunized subject exposed to an infectious disease when active immunization is either unavailable (e.g., hepatitis A) or has not been given prior to exposure (e.g., rabies). Passive immunization is used in the treatment of certain disorders associated with toxins (e.g., diphtheria), in certain bites (e.g., snake and spider), and as a specific [e.g., Rho(D) immune globulin] or nonspecific (e.g., antilymphocyte globulin) immunosuppressant.

Three types of preparations are used in passive immunization: (1) standard human immune serum globulin for general use (e.g., gamma globulin) and for intramuscular or intravenous administration, (2) special immune serum globulins with a known antibody content for specific agents (e.g., hepatitis B or varicella-zoster immune globulin), and (3) animal serums and antitoxins.

Determinants of the immune response The nature and extent of the response to vaccines or toxoids are determined by the chemical and physical states of the antigen, the mode of administration, the rate of antigen degradation, the genetic characteristics of the recipient, and various other host factors, some known and many unknown. The relationship between antigen dose and peak response describes a dose-response curve with a threshold at the low end and a plateau at the high end.

Route of administration The route of administration in part determines the rapidity and nature of the immune responses to vaccines. Parenterally administered vaccine may not induce mucosal secretory IgA, and mucosal immunization may or may not induce good systemic responses.

Age The age of the individual influences the response to vaccines, and therefore, recommended schedules for immunization are based on age-dependent responses and empirical data from clinical trials. The presence of high levels of maternal antibody and/or the immaturity of the immune system in the early months of life impairs the initial immune response to some antigens. In the elderly, vaccine responses may be diminished because of natural waning of the immune system. Hence larger amounts of an antigen may be required to produce the desired response (e.g., influenza).

Adjuvant potentiation The immune response to some antigens is potentiated by the addition of adjuvants such as aluminum salts or, in the case of polysaccharides (e.g., the polyribose phosphate polysaccharide of *H. influenzae* type b), by covalent conjugation to a peptide. Adjuvants, nonspecific boosters of immune responses, are used with inactivated products such as diphtheria and tetanus toxoids, acellular pertussis (aP), and hepatitis B vaccines. The mechanism for adjuvant enhancement of antigenicity is not well defined but may relate to the rendering of soluble antigens into a particulate form, the ability to mobilize phagocytes to the site of antigen deposition, and slower release of antigens, which prolongs stimulation of the immune response. Although many constituents of infectious microorganisms and their products, such as exotoxins, are or can be made to be antigenic, only a limited number stimulate a protective immune response.

Mucosal immunity Many pathogens replicate only at musocal surfaces (e.g., *Vibrio cholerae*), while other pathogens replicate at the mucosa before host invasion (e.g., poliovirus, rubella, or influenza). At the mucosal site, these organisms induce secretory IgA. Induction of secretory IgA by vaccines may be an efficient way to block the essential steps in pathogenesis, whether the organism is restricted to mucosal surfaces or systemically invades the host across mucosal surfaces.

Measurement of the immune response Immune responses to vaccines are often gauged by the concentration of specific antibody in serum. While seroconversion serves as a dependable indicator of an immune response, it measures only one immunologic parameter and does not necessarily indicate protection. The development of circulating antibodies after immunization often correlates directly with clinical protection (e.g., measles or rubella). Some responses may not in themselves reflect immunity but may be sufficiently associated with protection that they remain useful proxy measures (e.g., vibriocidal serum antibodies in cholera). At the same time, the absence of measurable antibody in a previously immunized individual does not mean that he or she is unprotected if a secondary protective IgG antibody response occurs rapidly enough after challenge. In some instances, the titer of antibody is critical, and for certain vaccines (e.g., tetanus), protection is predictable by the level of circulating antitoxin antibody.

Herd immunity It is not necessary to immunize every person to stop transmission of an infectious agent through a population. For those organisms dependent on person-to-person transmission, there may be a definable prevalence of immunity in the population above which it becomes difficult for the organism to circulate and reach new susceptibles. This prevalence is called *herd immunity*, and it permits the goals of immunization to be converted from the need to immunize every person in the community to a population goal, in which the target is to immunize a specified minimum percentage of the persons at risk. Herd immunity may be lost when individuals refuse to be immunized (as happened with pertussis in the United Kingdom in the 1970s because of the concerns about severe vaccine reactions, which exceeded the fear of the disease itself) or when immunity wanes (as in diphtheria). In both settings, loss of immunity has led to reacquisition of susceptibility with later encounters with the organism, resulting in transmission of infection in the community and significant illness.

Target populations and timing of immunization For the common and highly contagious childhood diseases, such as measles, the target population is the whole universe of susceptibles, and the time to immunize is as early in life as feasible. Epidemiologic differences in measles in different settings, however, dictate different strategies of immunization. In the industrialized world, immunization with live virus vaccine at 15 months has been the norm because the vaccine protects over 95 percent of those immunized at this age and there is little measles morbidity/mortality among very young infants. In contrast, in the developing world, measles fatalities are a significant proportion of young infant deaths. This has driven the desire to immunize in the first few months of life in order to close the window of vulnerability between the rapid decline of maternal antibody after 4 to 6 months and the subsequent vaccine-induced active immunity.

Problems have cropped up in measles immunization programs in both the developed and the developing world. In the United States, recent outbreaks of measles have occurred among unvaccinated infants younger than 15 months and preschoolers from underserved inner-city populations, as well as among previously vaccinated college students. These outbreaks represent both vaccine failure and program failure. Among the former, most are *primary* failures, i.e., no initial response to the vaccine. However, some are due to secondary loss of immunity with time after immunization, especially after the unstabilized pre-1980 vaccines, or when vaccines were given along with gamma globulin. Program failures represent an inability to reach and immunize the target population, often because no systematic program of immunization exists.

H. influenzae type b causes severe invasive disease and is the leading cause of meningitis, epiglotitis, and pneumonia in early childhood. Similar to measles, the majority of severe disease occurs in early childhood, rising sharply after the disappearance of maternally derived antibody. In contrast to measles vaccine, however, primary failure of Hib vaccine during infancy is due more to the age-related inability to respond to polysaccharide antigens. To overcome this innate deficit, the protective polysaccharide has been coupled with protein to convert it to a T cell–dependent antigen to which young infants respond.

In some diseases, such as rubella, infection is primarily a threat to the fetus, since young infants and children are not at risk of serious illness. While it is not clinically necessary to immunize early in life, the goal is to ensure immunity before females enter the reproductive age group. Theoretically, immunization of all reproductive-age women prior to pregnancy would be an ideal strategy. Because of the difficulties in systematically reaching all adolescents and young females and in ensuring the protection of as many women as possible, it was recognized that universal childhood immunization both to reach susceptibles and to interrupt transmission was necessary.

Some vaccines are now used primarily for adults, e.g., influenza virus and polyvalent pneumococcal polysaccharide vaccines to prevent pneumonia deaths in the elderly. They are, unfortunately, underused in large part because physicians and patients in the target group ignore the indication in otherwise healthy older adults and partly because there is a tendency to think about prevention with vaccines as a strategy for children. In addition, pneumococcal polysaccharide vaccine is recommended for children over 2 years who are at risk of severe, life-threatening pneumococcal infection, such as those with sickle cell disease, asplenia (whether functional or anatomic), renal failure and nephrotic syndrome, cerebrospinal fluid leak, and human immunodeficiency virus (HIV) infection or other immunosuppressive disease states. Because infection with *S. pneumoniae* is a major cause of otitis media, lung, and central nervous system infections in young children, however, the vaccine (which is immunogenic in infancy) may at some future time be considered for routine use in all children.

Biologic impediments   Each of the vaccines mentioned below illustrates major technical problems to be overcome in vaccine development. Thus influenza virus, characterized biologically by its antigenic drift, periodically emerges in a new antigenic version capable of causing a global pandemic for which a new vaccine must be rapidly devised, produced, and distributed. In contrast to the circulation of one major antigenic type of influenza A at any one time, many prevalent pneumococcal polysaccharide serotypes are in circulation at all times. Because immunity is serotype-specific, however, an individual is susceptible to all serotypes for which he or she lacks antibody. The reality of serotype-specific protection is one reason why it was more difficult to develop an effective pneumococcal vaccine than it was to develop a vaccine for *H. influenzae,* where almost all severe disease is related to one capsular serotype, type b. To overcome this problem, pneumococcal vaccine includes 23

polysaccharides which represent approximately 80 percent of the commonly encountered virulent serotypes. Unfortunately, some serotype polysaccharides are poorly immunogenic, and immunized individuals will remain susceptible to the serotypes excluded from the vaccine. Improved immunization awaits either a safe, effective conjugate vaccine to break the polysaccharide-response barrier in early childhood or the development of a common protective protein antigen vaccine that protects against all pneumococcal serotypes.

The use of hepatitis B virus (HBV) vaccine illustrates another technical issue. Because hepatitis B is of low endemicity in the general population in the United States, the high cost of the original serum-derived vaccine led to its being targeted to populations at high risk of acquiring HBV infection and its sequelae, chronic active hepatitis, including medical personnel handling blood and blood products, injection drug users, and homosexuals. In contrast, the most important sequela of HBV in Africa and Asia is neither acute nor chronic hepatitis but rather the long-term effect of chronic infection acquired in infancy on the later induction of liver cancer in young adults. The need for immunization in the developing world was therefore different from in the United States, first to prevent liver cancer in adult life and only second to prevent acute and chronic hepatitis. To accomplish the first goal, it would be necessary to immunize as close to birth as possible. The advent of recombinant HBV vaccines and reductions in cost have permitted a change in strategy. HBV vaccine is now recommended for universal use in infants in the United States as well as in unimmunized older children and adults at high risk of infection, including household members exposed to HBV surface (HBVs) antigen–positive adopted or foster immigrant children from HBV-endemic countries. Universal immunization at birth has been adopted in a few African and Asian countries, but proof of its efficacy to prevent liver cancer will require decades of surveillance, and ambitious studies are now in progress.

Testing of vaccines   In the development of vaccines, initial studies are typically carried out in animal models, if available, to demonstrate the production of immune responses, their ability to protect the host, and their relative safety. Ultimately, vaccines for humans must be tested in humans. There are three questions to be answered: (1) Is the vaccine immunogenic and safe? (2) Is the vaccine efficacious under controlled conditions? And (3) is the vaccine effective in reducing disease prevalence in a population? Thus, when initial in vitro and animal data look promising, graded doses of vaccine are given to small numbers of humans to assess immune responses and safety. Human clinical trials are then performed in larger numbers to demonstrate vaccine efficacy often by challenge of a group of informed volunteers with a virulent strain. After clinical trials in the community, typically involving 1000 to 10,000 vaccinees, licensure may be sought. Because of their limited size, however, these trials cannot be expected to detect rare but serious adverse effects. Thus licensing does not guarantee that a new vaccine is completely safe, and postlicensing monitoring of safety and efficacy is needed to ensure effectiveness and determine the occurrence of adverse effects of low frequency.

Vaccine formulations   The development of the science of immunology has led to the understanding that living and dead antigens do not necessarily induce the same immune responses and that the requirements for protective immunity differ with the organism. These insights, together with the refinement of epidemiologic concepts surrounding immunization, have changed the strategy of vaccine development. Now the goal is not only to select the correct antigens but also to ensure that the vaccines will result in the type of immune response needed for protection, whether T cell–mediated macrophage activation or generation of cytotoxic T cells or B cell–mediated secretory IgA or a particular IgG subtype response to a specific polysaccharide epitope.

Living vaccines are selected or genetically altered to be avirulent or dramatically attenuated yet still remain immunogenic. In effect, these agents are expected to cause a subclinical illness that mimics natural infection except for the lack of clinical disease. They have the advantage of replication in vivo, which increases the antigenic load presented to the host immune system; they present a diversity of antigens to overcome immunogenetic restrictions in some hosts; they may reach the local sites most appropriate for inducing protective immunity; and they also may produce important protective antigens in vivo that are not efficiently expressed in vitro.

In contrast, with nonviable vaccines, in essence, what you give is what you get vis-à-vis antigen load and the specific antigenic determinants presented. In addition, these preparations often fail to elicit mucosal IgA-mediated immunity, since they lack a delivery system to the local antigen-processing cells as effective as a living organism, and, except for pure polysaccharide antigens, they almost always require multiple exposures to induce effective responses. However, killed vaccines can be extremely effective. For example, for hepatitis A, a nonviable vaccine formulation close to being licensed appears to be nearly 100 percent effective in inducing protective immunity.

Despite these characteristics, living vaccines are not always the preferred type. For example, there are populations in whom live oral polio vaccine (OPV) is less than ideally effective. Thus, in India, it requires up to 9 to 10 doses of Sabin vaccine to fully immunize the majority of subjects, whereas the usual series of the highly immunogenic enhanced-potency inactivated polio vaccine (IPV-e) will protect nearly all. There is a tradeoff, however, since the new killed vaccine does not immunize the gut and can neither reduce the circulation of wild-type poliovirus nor immunize contacts of vaccine recipients. There is also no risk of vaccine-strain poliomyelitis occurring. In some settings, a combination schedule of killed and living polio vaccine may make the most sense, and this strategy is currently being evaluated.

To create a deliverable vaccine, constituents other than the antigens are required (Table 82-3). These constituents can affect immunogenicity, efficacy, and safety of a vaccine, and they determine the success of one formulation over another.

Production of vaccines As products to be given to healthy individuals to prevent disease, there is a special requirement for vaccines to be not only efficacious but also without the capacity to cause harm. In the United States, this quality assurance is the responsibility of the manufacturers. Standards of manufacture of biologicals (quality control) are regulated and supervised by the Food and Drug Administration. Proof of both safety and efficacy is required, and sterility and purity of products are monitored. On rare occasions, either good manufacturing practice or quality assurance have broken down, e.g., the release of incompletely killed Salk polio vaccine in 1955, which caused an outbreak of poliomyelitis in nearly 200 vaccine recipients and their contacts. Unregulated and uncontrolled manufacture of vaccines in developing countries has sometimes led to the release and use of inactive products that fail to provide the expected protective immunity. These episodes are ordinarily not detected and their clinical consequences remain unmeasured.

Another problem in production of vaccines has cropped up unexpectedly in the past decade in violation of the basic law of supply and demand. For multiple reasons, including the high costs of vaccine development and testing, liability of pharmaceutical companies to claims of vaccine-related injury, and the prospect of much higher profitability from investing in other products, the number of vaccine manufacturers in the United States has declined and the costs of some basic childhood vaccines have increased. There is, therefore, legitimate concern about the future availability of these essential biologicals for national use. In addition, pricing decisions made within the private-sector pharmaceutical industry can have a major impact on vaccine use. This has stimulated an initiative toward increasing public oversight and price negotiations with industry. The recent increase in the UNICEF contract price of polio vaccine from 4 to 8 cents per dose has had no effect on the use of this vaccine in the United States but has severely stressed the ability of UNICEF to meet its vaccine procurement obligations for immunization in developing countries.

Administration of vaccines The number of vaccines that can be given at one time without interfering with response or increasing side effects—and the cost of buying and administering them—affect the ability to deliver vaccines. There is clearly as much art to the programming of vaccine administration as there is to the development and testing of protective antigens. Wherever effective primary health care systems ensure access to medical services for the majority and the population is educated about the need for and efficacy of vaccines, high coverage rates for basic immunization should be achieved, regardless of the route of administration of a vaccine or the number of doses necessary. However, without attention to the infrastructure needed for follow-up on multiple-dose vaccine schedules, coverage rates for second, third, and booster doses of vaccines may drop off significantly. The simple act of providing "road to health" cards to mothers in developing countries on which immunizations, growth, and major illnesses are recorded has increased the rates of complete basic immunization of infants because the mothers can more effectively participate in the process.

VACCINE USE Recommendations for vaccine use in the United States are developed by several different groups, including the Advisory Committee on Immunization Practices (ACIP) of the Centers for Disease Control and Prevention (CDC), the Committee on Infectious Diseases of the American Academy of Pediatrics (AAP, The Red Book), the American College of Physicians (ACP), the American Academy of Family Practice (AAFP), and the American College of Obstetrics and Gynecology (ACOG).

Vaccines recommended in 1993 for routine use for infants, children, and adults and vaccines for special use are shown in Tables 82-4 and 82-5, respectively. Intervals between doses longer than those recommended do not diminish the ultimate protective response but merely delay it. It is not necessary to restart an interrupted schedule from the beginning or to add an extra dose. In contrast, giving vaccines at shorter than recommended intervals may result in poor responses.

Recording and reporting requirements Certain aspects of vaccine use are directed by the National Childhood Vaccine Injury Act (NCVIA) of 1986. The act requires that all mandated childhood vaccinations be recorded by health care providers in the child's permanent medical record, including date of administration, the manufacturer and lot number, and the name of the provider administering the vaccine. Parents also should keep an up-to-date immunization record on their children. The act also requires that the benefits to the child and possible reactions be explained to parents. Educational materials providing the required information are available from the CDC or the AAP.

VACCINES FOR ROUTINE USE   Infants and children Recommended schedules for administration of vaccines to infants and children are shown in Table 82-6. It is current practice that all children in the United States should receive DTP, polio, measles, mumps, rubella, *H. influenzae* type b, and HBV vaccines unless contraindicated (Table 82-7). Four doses of DTP and three doses of OPV constitute the primary series. A fifth dose of DTP is given at 4 to 6 years of age. Adult formulation tetanus-diphtheria (Td) boosters are recommended every 10 years thereafter. A fourth dose of OPV is also recommended

---

TABLE 82-3 Constituents of vaccines

Preservatives, stabilizers, antibiotics
  Used to inhibit or prevent bacterial growth or to stabilize the antigen. Materials such as mercurials or antibiotics are used. Allergic reactions to any of the additives may occur.

Adjuvants
  An aluminum salt is used in some vaccines to enhance the immune response (e.g., toxoids, hepatitis B).

Suspending fluid
  Sterile water, saline, buffer, or more complex fluids derived from the growth medium or biologic system in which the agent is produced (e.g., egg antigens, cell culture ingredients, serum proteins).

TABLE 82-4   Routinely recommended vaccines for infants, children, and adults

Vaccine	Type of immunizing agent	Recommended route of administration	Efficacy	Adverse events
Diphtheria and tetanus toxoids and pertussis vaccine	Toxoids and inactivated whole bacteria	IM	D = 95%	Frequent local reactions; seizures, hypotonic hyporesponsive episodes, acute encephalopathy (DTP)
Diphtheria and tetanus toxoids, pediatric			P = 80%	
Tetanus, diphtheria toxoids, adult			T = 95%	Arthus-like reaction in persons who have received multiple boosters (Td)
Acellular pertussis	Inactivated bacterial antigen	IM	?	Reduce local reactions; no serious reactions reported
Haemophilus influenzae type b	Bacterial polysaccharide conjugated to protein	IM	90%	Local reactions, 10%; no serious reactions
Hepatitis B	Inactivated viral antigen	IM	80–95%	Mild local reaction; Guillain-Barré syndrome, rare
Influenza	Inactivated virus or viral components	IM	40–70%	Mild local reaction; Guillain-Barré syndrome with swine flu; rare allergic reaction in those allergic to eggs
Measles, mumps, rubella virus vaccine combined	Live viruses	SQ	M = 95% Mu = 95% R = 95%	Acute encephalopathy (measles) Parotitis and orchitis reported rarely (mumps) Arthralgia (40%); arthritis (<2%); rare arthropathy; 5–15% fever 5–21 days after vaccinations; 5% rash
Pneumococcal polysaccharide	Bacterial polysaccharide of 23 types	IM or SQ	60–80%	Local reactions—50% (pain); rare anaphylaxis; arthus-like reaction with booster doses
Poliomyelitis Oral polio virus	Live virus of three serotypes	Oral	95%	Vaccine-associated poliomyelitis, rare
Inactivated polio virus– enhanced (IPV-e)	Inactivated virus of three serotypes	SQ	95%	None significant

SOURCE: Recommendations of the Advisory Committee on Immunization Practices, the American Academy of Pediatrics, and the American College of Physicians.

TABLE 82-5   Special-use vaccines

Vaccine	Year licensed	Type of immunizing agent	Route of administration	Indications	Efficacy	Adverse events
Adenovirus types 4 and 7	1980	Unattenuated live viruses	Oral	Used solely for military recruits	>90%	Essentially non-existent
Anthrax	1970	Inactivated avirulent bacteria	SQ (6 doses primary; annual booster)	For high risk of exposure, i.e., persons in contact with or manufacture of animal hides, furs, bone meal, wool, goat hair	90% antibody response but efficacy uncertain	No serious adverse effects are known
Tuberculosis (BCG)	1950	Living bacteria	ID	PPD-negative individuals in prolonged contact with active TB patient	Controversial, reduces disseminated disease in children	Regional adenitis, disseminated BCG, osteitis
Cholera	1914	Inactivated bacteria	SC or ID	Not recommended for public health use	50% (short-lived)	Frequent fever, local pain, swelling
Meningococcal A, C, Y, W135	1981	Bacterial polysaccharide of four serotypes	SC	Military; principally travelers to epidemic areas	90% for 2–3-year-olds Annually for <4-year-olds	Rare
Plague	1911	Inactivated bacteria	IM	Laboratory workers; foresters in endemic areas; travelers	90% antibody response but efficacy uncertain	10% local reactions; rare sterile abscesses and hypersensitivity
Rabies (human diploid)	1980	Inactivated virus	IM or ID	Travelers; laboratory workers; veterinarians	Virtually 100%	25% local reactions; 6% arthropathy, arthritis, angioedema
Yellow fever	1953	Live virus	SC	Laboratory workers; travelers	High	Encephalitis; encephalopathy
Japanese encephalitis	1993	Inactivated virus	SC	Travelers	80–90%	Anaphylactic/severe delayed allergic reactions common; observe for 10 days
Typhoid				Not routinely recommended in United States		
Phenol and heat killed	1952	Killed whole bacteria	IM	Travelers, contact with carrier	50–70% (short-lived)	Frequent fever, local swelling, pain
Ty$_{21a}$	1992	Live mutant bacteria	Oral	Travelers, contact with carrier	50–70%	None

SOURCE: Recommendations of the Advisory Committee on Immunization Practices, the American Academy of Pediatrics, and the American College of Physicians.

TABLE 82-6 Recommended schedule of vaccinations for all children

Vaccine	2 Months	4 Months	6 Months	12 Months	15 Months	4–6 Years (before school entry)
DTP	√	√	√		√*	√
Polio	√	√			√*	√‡
MMR					√†	√‡
Hib						
Option 1§	√	√	√		√	
Option 2§	√	√		√		

	Birth	1–2 Months		6–18 Months		
HBV						
Option 1	√	√¶		√¶		
Option 2		√¶	√¶	√¶		

NOTE: DTP: diphtheria, tetanus, and pertussis vaccine (combined); polio: live oral polio drops (OPV) or killed (inactivated) polio vaccine shots (IPV); MMR: measles, mumps, and rubella vaccine (combined); Hib: *Haemophilus* b conjugate vaccine; HBV: hepatitis B vaccine.

* Many experts recommend these vaccines at 18 months.
† In some areas this dose of MMR vaccine may be given at 12 months.
‡ Many experts recommend this dose of MMR vaccine be given at entry to middle school or junior high school.
§ HIB vaccine is given in either a four-dose schedule (1) or a three-dose schedule (2) depending on the type of vaccine used.
¶ Hepatitis B vaccine can be given simultaneously with DTP, polio, MMR, and *Haemophilus* b conjugate vaccine at the same visit.
SOURCE: ACIP: General recommendations on immunization. Morb Mort Week Rep 38:205, 1989.

TABLE 82-7 Vaccination contraindications and precautions[1]

Vaccine	Valid	Invalid
General for all vaccines (DTP/DTaP, OPV, IPV, MMR, Hib, HBV)	Anaphylactic reaction to a vaccine contraindicates further doses of that vaccine Anaphylactic reaction to a vaccine constituent contraindicates the use of vaccines containing that substance Moderate or severe illnesses with or without a fever	Mild to moderate local reaction (soreness, redness, swelling) following a dose of an injectable antigen Mild acute illness with or without low-grade fever Current antimicrobial therapy Convalescent phase of illnesses Prematurity (use same dosage and indications as for normal, full-term infants) Recent exposure to an infectious disease History of penicillin or other nonspecific allergies or fact that relatives have such allergies
DTP/DTaP	Encephalopathy within 7 days of administration of previous dose of DTP Fever of ≥40.5°C (105°F) within 48 h after vaccination with a prior dose of DTP[2] Collapse or shocklike state (hypotonic-hyporesponsive episode) within 48 h of receiving a prior dose of DTP[2] Seizures within 3 days of receiving a prior dose of DTP (see note 3 regarding management of children with a personal history of seizures at any time)[2] Persistent, inconsolable crying lasting ≥3 h within 48 h of receiving a prior dose of DTP[2]	Temperature of >40.5°C (105°F) following a previous dose of DTP Family history of convulsions[3] Family history of an adverse event following DTP administration Family history of sudden infant death syndrome
OPV[4]	Infection with HIV or a household contact with HIV Known immunodeficiency (hematologic and solid tumors; congenital immunodeficiency syndrome; and long term immunosuppressive therapy) Immunodeficient household contact Pregnancy[2]	Breast feeding Current antimicrobial therapy Diarrhea
IPV	Anaphylactic reactions to neomycin or streptomycin Pregnancy[2]	
MMR[4]	Anaphylactic reactions to eggs or to neomycin[5] Pregnancy Known immunodeficiency (hematologic and solid tumors; congenital immunodeficiency syndrome; and long term immunosuppressive therapy) Recent (within 3 months) IG administration[2]	Tuberculosis or positive PPD Simultaneous TB skin testing[6] Breast feeding Pregnancy of mother of recipient Immunodeficient family member or household contact Infection with HIV Nonanaphylactic reactions to eggs or neomycin
Hib	None identified	
HBV		Pregnancy
Influenza	Avoid during 1st trimester of pregnancy on theoretical grounds Anaphylactic reactions to eggs	
Pneumococcus	Has not been evaluated in pregnancy	

[1] Based on the recommendations of the Advisory Committee on Immunization Practices (ACIP) and those of the Committee on the Infectious Diseases (Red Book Committee) of the American Academy of Pediatrics (AAP) as of October 1992. Sometimes these recommendations vary from those contained in the manufacturers' package inserts. For more detailed information, providers should consult the current published recommendations of the ACIP, the AAP, the AAFP, and the manufacturers' package inserts.
[2] The events or conditions listed as precautions, although not contraindications, should be carefully reviewed. The benefits and risks of administering a specific vaccine to an individual under the circumstances should be considered. If the risks are believed to outweigh the benefits, the immunization should be withheld; if the benefits are believed to outweigh the risks (e.g., during an outbreak or foreign travel), the immunization should be given. Whether and when to administer DTP to children with proven or suspected underlying neurologic disorders should be decided on an individual basis. It is prudent on theoretical grounds to avoid vaccinating pregnant women. However, if immediate protection against poliomyelitis is needed, OPV, not IPV, is recommended.
[3] Acetaminophen given prior to administering DTP and thereafter every 4 h for 24 h should be considered for children with a personal or with a family history of convulsions in siblings or parents.
[4] There is a theoretical risk that the administration of multiple live virus vaccines (OPV and MMR) within 30 days of one another if not given on the same day will result in a suboptimal immune response. There are no data to substantiate this.
[5] Persons with a history of anaphylactic reactions following egg ingestion should be vaccinated only with extreme caution. Protocols have been developed for vaccinating such persons and should be consulted (J Pediatr 1983; 102:196–9, J Pediatr 1988; 113:504–6).
[6] Measles vaccination may temporarily suppress tuberculin reactivity. If testing can not be done the day of MMR vaccination, the test should be postponed for 4–6 weeks.
SOURCES: Standards for Pediatric Immunization Practices, Centers for Disease Control and Prevention; ACIP: Pneumococcal polysaccharide vaccine. Morb Mort Week Rep 38:64, 1989; ACIP: Prevention and control of influenza. Morb Mort Week Rep 40:73, 1991.

at 4 to 6 years of age. One dose of a combined measles, mumps, and rubella vaccine is recommended at 15 months and again at school entry or in middle school. DTP, MMR, OPV, and Hib vaccines may be given simultaneously at 15 months of age without increasing adverse reaction rates or impairing the immune response.

Adults All adults should be immune to diphtheria and tetanus. If not previously immunized, adults require a primary immunizing course of three doses of Td, with the second dose 4 to 8 weeks after the first and the third dose at 12 months, plus boosters administered every 10 years thereafter. Many individuals remain immune to tetanus into adulthood because they have received tetanus toxoid rather than Td after injuries, but they are commonly at risk of diphtheria. Routine immunization against polio is not recommended for adults unless they are at particular risk of exposure, as with travel to endemic regions of the world (see "Travel," below). Adults should be protected from measles, mumps, and rubella and should be vaccinated unless they are known to have either received vaccine on or after their first birthday or had physician-diagnosed disease. Rubella vaccine should be given to all women of childbearing age unless they have documentary proof of immunization after their first birthday or laboratory evidence of immunity. A history of prior rubella disease is unreliable and should not be accepted.

Current recommendations also include influenza vaccine for routine annual administration to adults 65 years of age and older and to individuals at any age with chronic illness. Polyvalent pneumococcal polysaccharide vaccine is similarly recommended for the elderly or chronically ill. Hepatitis B is recommended for individuals at high risk of exposure, including health care workers exposed to potentially infected blood, homosexuals, injection drug users, individuals living and working in institutions for the mentally retarded, and household contacts of known carriers of hepatitis B surface antigen.

Adverse events following vaccination Modern vaccines, while safe and effective, are associated with adverse effects which range from the very mild to the life-threatening. Because no vaccine can be expected to be 100 percent effective, some persons who have received a full course of vaccine or toxoid may develop disease upon exposure. The decision to use a vaccine involves assessment of the risks of disease, the benefits of vaccination, and the risks associated with vaccination. These factors may change over time, and consequently, continued assessment of vaccines is essential. Table 82-7 presents a guide to contraindications to immunization and appropriate precautions in the use of specific vaccines.

All detected adverse events temporally related to vaccination are expected to be reported to both the local health department and the vaccine manufacturer. The NCVIA requires health care providers to report certain suspected adverse events after a mandated vaccine to the FDA's Vaccine Adverse Events Reporting System (VAERS) (Table 82-8). Although a temporal relationship does not establish cause and effect, surveillance is essential to collect data needed to form conclusions and make decisions.

Vaccine components, including the protective antigens, animal proteins introduced during vaccine production, and antibiotics or other preservatives or stabilizers, can cause allergic reactions in some recipients. These may be local or systemic, including serious anaphylaxis and urticaria. The most common extraneous allergen is egg protein introduced when vaccines are prepared in embryonated eggs, such as occurs with measles, mumps, influenza, and yellow fever vaccines. Local or systemic reactions can result from the too frequent administration of some vaccines, such as Td, DT, or rabies, and are probably due to antigen-antibody complexes.

In addition, live virus vaccines can interfere with tuberculin test responses. When a tuberculin skin test is indicated, it may be done either on the day of immunization or 6 weeks later.

USE OF VACCINES IN SPECIAL CIRCUMSTANCES Pregnancy Because of theoretical risks to the fetus and the risk of litigation to the practitioner, immunization of pregnant women is usually avoided. Notwithstanding, it is essential to ensure that pregnant women are immune to tetanus, since transfer of maternal antitoxin antibodies is

TABLE 82-8 Reportable events following vaccination, as required by the National Vaccine Injury Act of 1986

Vaccine/toxoid	Event	Interval from vaccination
DTP; P; DTP/polio combined	Anaphylaxis or anaphylactic shock	24 h
	Encephalopathy (or encephalitis)*	3 days
	Shock-collapse or hypotonic-hyporesponsive collapse*	3 days
	Residual seizure disorder*	(See Aids to Interpretation)
	Any acute complication or sequela (including death) of above events	No limit
	Events in vaccinees described in manufacturer's package insert as contraindications to additional doses of vaccine† (such as convulsions)	(See package insert)
Measles, mumps, and rubella, DT, Td, tetanus toxoid (TT)	Anaphylaxis or anaphylactic shock	24 h
	Encephalopathy (or encephalitis)*	15 days for measles, mumps and rubella; 3 days for DT, Td, TT
	Residual seizure disorder*	(See Aids to Interpretation)
	Any acute complication or sequela (including death) of above events	No limit
	Events in vaccinees described in manufacturer's package insert as contraindications to additional doses of vaccine†	(See package insert)
Oral polio vaccine (OPV)	Paralytic polio in a nonimmunodeficient recipient	30 days
	Paralytic polio in an immunodeficient recipient or vaccine-associated community case	6 months
	Any acute complication or sequela (including death) of the above	No limit
	Events in vaccinees described in manufacturer's package insert as contraindications to additional doses of vaccine†	(See package insert)
Inactivated polio vaccine–enhanced (IPV-e)	Anaphylaxis or anaphylactic shock	24 h
	Any acute complication or sequela (including death) of above events	No limit
	Events in vaccines described in manufacturer's package insert as contraindications to additional doses of vaccine†	(See package insert)

* Aids to Interpretation: Shock-collapse or hypotonic-hyporesponsive collapse may be evidenced by signs or symptoms such as decrease in or loss of muscle tone, paralysis (partial or complete), hemiplegia, hemiparesis, loss of color or turning pale white or blue, unresponsiveness to environmental stimuli, depression of or loss of consciousness, prolonged sleeping with difficult arousing, or cardiovascular or respiratory arrest. Residual seizure disorder may be considered to have occurred if no other seizure or convulsion unaccompanied by fevers or accompanied by a fever of less than 102°F occurred before the first seizure or convulsion after the administration of the vaccine involved; if in the case of measles, mumps, or rubella-containing vaccines, the first seizure or convulsion occurred within 15 days after vaccination; or in the case of any other vaccine, the first seizure or convulsion occurred within three days after vaccination, and, if two or more seizures or convulsions unaccompanied by fever or accompanied by a fever of less than 102°F occurred within 1 year after vaccination. The terms *seizure* and *convulsion* include grand mal, petit mal, absence, myoclonia, tonic-clonic, and focal motor seizures and signs. *Encephalopathy* means any significant acquired abnormality of, injury to, or impairment of function of the brain. Among the frequent manifestations of encephalopathy are focal and diffuse neurologic signs, increased intracranial pressure, or changes in level of consciousness lasting at least 6 h with or without convulsions. The neurologic signs and symptoms of encephalopathy may be temporary with complete recovery, or they may result in various degrees of permanent impairment. Signs and symptoms such as high-pitched and unusual screaming, persistent inconsolable crying, and bulging fontanel are compatible with an encephalopathy, but in and of themselves are not conclusive evidence of encephalopathy. Encephalopathy usually can be documented by slow wave activity on an electroencephalogram.
† The health-care provider must refer to contraindication section of the manufacturer's package insert for each vaccine.
SOURCE: National Childhood Vaccine Injury Act of 1986.

an important means of prevention of neonatal tetanus and pregnant women can safely receive tetanus as well as diphtheria toxoids. Although live virus vaccines, in general, should be withheld during pregnancy, polio and yellow fever vaccines are exceptions and may be administered if the risk of exposure to disease is great. If indicated, some inactivated virus vaccines, e.g., influenza, are safe to give to pregnant women.

Breast feeding Breast-fed infants can be immunized on a normal schedule. Breast feeding does not adversely affect the immune response and is not a contraindication for any vaccine. Breast-feeding women also may be vaccinated without problem. Although live vaccines multiply within the mother's body, most are not excreted in breast milk. Mothers may therefore receive oral polio or yellow fever vaccines without interrupting breast feeding.

Occupational exposure Immunization recommendations for most occupational groups remain to be developed. Specific requirements for immunization of health care workers against hepatitis B in the United States are now mandated by the Occupational Safety and Health Administration (OSHA). Those at particular risk of exposure to hepatitis B, such as health workers dealing with blood products or surgeons, must be immunized. Many medical institutions now give HBV vaccine to all health care workers and medical, dental, and nursing students. Transmission of rubella in medical facilities to and from health care workers, particularly in pediatrics, occurs as well. Health care workers who might transmit rubella to pregnant patients should therefore be immune to rubella, and it is prudent to screen them for antibodies to rubella and immunize susceptibles. Health care workers are also at greater risk from measles than the general public, and those likely to come in contact with measles patients should be immune. Health care workers caring for patients with chronic diseases can transmit influenza; such workers should be vaccinated annually. Unfortunately, these recommendations often are not fully implemented, even in academic institutions.

HIV infection and other immunocompromised states Limited studies in HIV-infected individuals have not shown an increased risk of adverse events from live or inactivated vaccines. However, immune responses in immunocompromised individuals may not be as vigorous as in subjects with a normal immune system. Except for polio, persons known to be HIV infected should be immunized with recommended vaccines as early in the course of their disease as possible in the same manner as individuals without immunocompromise, before significant impairment in immune function occurs. This includes the use of live, attenuated MMR vaccine (Table 82-9), although IPV-e should be used when vaccination against polio is indicated because the risk of vaccine-associated poliomyelitis is too great. Care should be taken to ensure that household contacts to be immunized against polio receive IPV-e and not OPV. However, it is not necessary to test for HIV before making immunization decisions for asymptomatic individuals from known HIV risk groups.

Live, attenuated vaccines are normally contraindicated in other immunocompromised patients such as the congenital immunodeficiency syndromes and in patients receiving immunosuppressive therapy. Passive immunization with immunoglobulin preparations or antitoxins can be considered in individual cases, either as postexposure prophylaxis or as part of the therapy of established infection.

Postexposure immunization For certain infections, active or passive immunization soon after exposure prevents or attenuates disease expression. The immune globulins and antitoxins currently available in the United States are listed in Table 82-10, and the recommended postexposure immunization regimens are compiled in Table 82-11. Measles immune globulins given within 6 days of exposure may prevent or modify infection, and administration of measles vaccine within the first few days after exposure may prevent symptomatic infection. Although clinical manifestations of rubella are minimized by postexposure passive immunization, this may not prevent viremia, fetal infection, and congenital rubella syndrome. Therefore, the administration of immune globulin is recommended only for women developing rubella during pregnancy who will not consider abortion under any circumstances. Tetanus immune globulin can be used in patients with tetanus; however, survivors with no history of tetanus immunization should receive a primary series of toxoid. Administration of rabies immune globulin plus rabies vaccine in the immediate postexposure period is highly effective in preventing disease. Similarly, the use of immune globulin within 2 weeks of exposure to hepatitis A is likely to prevent clinical illness. There are also good data indicating the efficacy of special human HBV immune globulin in preventing disease after exposure. While there is no high-titer preparation for postexposure protection against non-A, non-B hepatitis, standard human immune serum globulin is efficacious.

Simultaneous administration of vaccines The simultaneous administration of the most widely used live and inactivated vaccines has not resulted in impaired antibody responses or increased rates of adverse reactions. Simultaneous administration of vaccines is important to increase the probability that a child will ultimately be fully immunized and when there is imminent exposure to multiple infectious diseases in any age group in preparation for travel to endemic countries. Inactivated vaccines often can be given in a single injection or at separate sites at the same time. Vaccines that result in frequent local or systemic side effects, such as killed typhoid or plague vaccines, may result in accentuated reactions when given together.

Prior or simultaneous DTP or DT may be necessary to elicit an optimal response to certain *H. influenzae* conjugate vaccines (i.e., tetanus or diphtheria toxoid conjugates) but not others (conjugates with meningococcal outer membrane proteins). Administration of the

---

TABLE 82-9 Recommendations for routine immunization of HIV-infected persons in the United States

| Vaccine | HIV clinical status | | Comments |
	Asymptomatic	Symptomatic	
DTP/Td	Yes	Yes	No change in usual immunization schedule
OPV	NO	NO	Increased risk of vaccine virus proliferation and paralytic polio IPV-e should be used for household contacts of HIV-infected persons
IPV-e	Yes	Yes	Antibody response may be impaired in symptomatic patients
MMR	Yes	Yes	No change in usual immunization schedule If high risk of exposure to measles, immunize at 6–11 months of age, with second dose at >12 months of age; with documented infection, measles immune globulin may be administered (see Table 82-10)
HIB conjugate	Yes	Yes	No change in usual immunization schedule
HBV	Yes	Yes	Antibody response may be impaired; a higher-dose vaccine is available, but there are no data addressing the optimal dose; it may be wise to check the antibody titer after immunization and give additional doses if inadequate
Pneumococcus	Yes	Yes	Should be given to all 2 years and older
Influenza	Yes	Yes	Antibody response may be impaired in symptomatic patients

SOURCE: Recommendations of the Advisory Committee on Immunization Practices (ACIP): Use of vaccines and immunoglobulins in persons with altered immunocompetence. Morb Mort Week Rep 42(No.RR-4):1, 1993.

TABLE 82-10 Preparations available for passive immunity*

Immunobiological	Indication(s)
STANDARD HUMAN IMMUNE GLOBULIN	
Intravenous immune globulin (IVIG)	Replacement therapy for antibody deficiency disorders; immune thrombocytopenic purpura (ITP); hypogammaglobulinemia in chronic lymphocytic leukemia; Kawasaki disease
Intramuscular immune globulin (IMIG)	Antibody immunodeficiency; hepatitis A pre- and postexposure prophylaxis; hepatitis B prophylaxis; hepatitis non-A, non-B prophylaxis; measles postexposure prophylaxis; chickenpox postexposure prophylaxis
SPECIAL HUMAN IMMUNE SERUM GLOBULIN	
Hepatitis B immune globulin (HBIG)	Perinatally exposed newborn infants; hepatitis B postexposure prophylaxis
Varicella-zoster immune globulin (VZIG)	Postexposure prophylaxis of susceptible immunocompromised persons, certain susceptible pregnant women, and perinatally exposed newborn infants
Rabies immune globulin† (RIG)	Rabies postexposure management of persons not previously immunized with HDCV
Tetanus immune globulin (TIG)	Tetanus treatment; postexposure prophylaxis of persons not adequately immunized with tetanus toxoid
Cytomegalovirus immune globulin, intravenous (CMV-IGIV)	Prophylaxis for bone marrow and kidney transplant recipients
Rho(D) immune globulin	Prevention of Rh hemolytic disease of the newborn
ANIMAL SERUM AND GLOBULINS	
Diphtheria antitoxin (equine)	Prevention or treatment of respiratory diphtheria
Botulinum antitoxin (equine)	Treatment of botulism

* Immune globulins and antitoxins are administered intramuscularly unless indicated otherwise.
† Rabies immune globulin is administered around wound in addition to the intramuscular injection.
SOURCE: Center for Biologics Evaluation and Research, Food and Drug Administration.

TABLE 82-11 Recommended postexposure immunization with immunoglobulin preparations in the United States

Disease	Indicated	Comments.
Measles	Yes	Standard human immune globulin recommended for exposed infants and adults with normal immunocompetence but contraindication to measles vaccine and for immunocompromised patients exposed to measles regardless of immunization status Patients should be immunized 3–6 months after immunoglobulin Recommended dose 0.25–0.5 mL/kg IM; maximum 15 mL
Rubella	No	Efficacy unreliable; therefore, standard human immune globulin is recommended for use only for antibody-negative pregnant women in the first trimester with a documented rubella exposure and who will not consider terminating pregnancy Recommended dose 0.55 mL/kg IM
Tetanus	Yes	Special human tetanus immune globulin (TIG) has replaced equine tetanus antitoxin because of the risk of serum sickness with equine serum Recommended dose for postexposure prophylaxis 250–500 units of TIG Recommended dose for treatment of tetanus 500–3000 units of TIG
Rabies	Yes	Special human rabies immune globulin (RIG) is preferred over equine rabies antiserum because of the risk of serum sickness, but RIG is not always available RIG or antiserum is recommended in nonimmunized individuals for all animal bites in which rabies cannot be ruled out and for other exposures to rabid animals Recommended dose of RIG 20 IU/kg; recommended dose of antiserum 40 IU/kg Rabies vaccine is given as well at 0, 3, 7, 14, and 28 days
Hepatitis A	Yes	Standard immune serum globulin is given in a single dose of 0.02–0.04 mL/kg or up to 0.06 mL/kg every 5 months for continuous exposure
Hepatitis B	Yes	Standard immune serum globulin is not reliably effective; special human hepatitis B immune globulin (HBIG) is useful and recommended for neonates born to an infected mother and after mucous membrane or parenteral contact with infected persons or infected blood or serum Recommended dose for neonates 0.5 mL IM within 12 h of birth; recommended dose for percutaneous or mucosal exposure is 0.06–0.12 mL/kg IM
Non-A, non-B hepatitis	Yes	Standard immune serum globulin may be valuable Recommended dose 0.12 mL/kg up to 10 mL

SOURCES: Recommendations of the Advisory Committee on Immunization Practices (ACIP): Use of vaccines and immunoglobulins in persons with altered immunocompetence. Morb Mort Week Rep 42(RR-4):1, 1993; Update on adult immunization: recommendations of the Immunization Practices Advisory Committee (ACIP). Morb Mort Week Rep 40(RR-12):1, 1991; Rabies prevention—United States, 1991: Recommendations of the Immunization Practices Advisory Committee (ACIP). Morb Mort Week Rep 40(RR-3):1, 1991; Hepatitis B virus: A comprehensive strategy for eliminating transmission in the United States through universal childhood immunization: Recommendations of the Immunization Practices Advisory Committee (ACIP). Morb Mort Week Rep 40(RR-13):1, 1991; Rubella prevention: Recommendations of the Immunization Practices Advisory Committee (ACIP). Morb Mort Week Rep 39(RR-15):1, 1990.

combined measles, mumps, and rubella vaccine (MMR) yields results comparable with administration of the individual vaccines given at different sites and has greatly increased the ease of achieving effective immunization for the three infections at little increase in cost. Although recent OPV is not a contraindication to use of MMR, in general, other live virus vaccines not given together on the same day should be given at least 30 days apart.

Neither OPV nor yellow fever vaccine responses are altered by administration of immune globulins. High doses of immune globulin may inhibit the efficacy of measles and rubella vaccines, and an interval of at least 3 months following administration of immune globulin is recommended. Postpartum vaccination of rubella-susceptible women should not be delayed because of the administration of anti-Rho(D) immune globulin or any other blood product during the last trimester or at delivery. If administration of an immune globulin preparation becomes necessary after vaccination, it should be postponed if possible for at least 14 days to allow time for vaccine virus replication and development of immunity to occur. In general, there is little interaction between immune globulin and inactivated vaccines, and postexposure passive prophylaxis can be given together with HBV vaccine or tetanus toxoid, resulting in both immediate and long-standing protection.

Travel The International Sanitary Regulations allow countries to impose requirements for yellow fever and cholera vaccines as a condition for admission, even though the currently available killed parenteral cholera vaccine is not an effective public health tool. Travelers should know whether these vaccines are required for entry into the countries on their itinerary to avoid being turned back or,

perhaps worse, immunized on the spot. Infants, children, and adults should be up to date with all routine immunizations before traveling, with particular attention to polio, measles, and DTP or Td. Pooled human gamma globulin for hepatitis A, at least until the vaccine is widely available, may be advisable for travelers to some locales. Use of rabies, meningococcal A and C polysaccharide, typhoid (oral live or Vi polysaccharide when available), Japanese encephalitis, and plague vaccines should be considered for those individuals who expect to go beyond the usual tourist routes or to spend extended time in rural areas in disease-endemic regions. In most U.S. cities, there are one or more travel clinics which maintain up-to-date epidemiologic monitoring, have supplies of the more uncommon vaccines available, and are prepared to provide general health information, including precautions for travelers' diarrhea and malaria prophylaxis.

DELIVERY OF VACCINES   Over the past 20 years, considerable progress has been made to ensure that every child in the United States is fully immunized by the time of school entry. All 50 states now require immunization for school entry, and most have laws addressing attendance at preschool and day-care centers. As a result, up to 98 percent* of all children are immunized against nine vaccine-preventable diseases by the time they enter school. The impact of immunization, and other improvements in the health of the American population, on the incidence of vaccine-preventable illness is shown in Table 82-1 and Fig. 82-1.

Despite these successes, large numbers of preschool children are not fully immunized by 15 months of age. Only 37 to 56 percent of preschoolers in the United States have been completely immunized,† and this rate is as low as 10 percent in some communities. The failure to vaccinate preschool children was largely responsible for the resurgence of measles between 1989 and 1991, which included 55,467 cases and over 11,200 admissions to the hospital, with more than 44,100 hospital days and over 130 measles-related deaths. Congenital rubella syndrome also increased from 6 cases in 1988 to 47 in 1991. Outbreaks of pertussis and mumps have been on the rise for the same reason—low immunization rates among preschool children.

Standards for immunization practices   National standards for immunization for pediatric and adult practice have been established which define common policies and practices for public health clinics and in physicians private offices (Table 82-12). These guidelines highlight the need to distinguish between true contraindications and conditions which often, but needlessly, preclude immunization. Among the true contraindications applicable to all vaccines are a history of anaphylaxis or allergic reaction to a vaccine or vaccine component and the presence of a moderate or severe illness with or without fever. Diarrhea, minor respiratory illness with or without fever, mild to moderate local reactions to a previous dose of vaccine, the concurrent or recent use of antimicrobials, mild to moderate malnutrition, and the convalescent phase of an acute illness are not valid contraindications to routine immunization. Failure to vaccinate children with these conditions is increasingly being viewed as a missed opportunity for immunization. Infants who develop an encephalopathy within 7 days of a dose of DTP should not receive further doses of DTP. Because of theoretical risks to the fetus, pregnant women should not receive MMR vaccine.

Access to immunization   There are four major barriers to successful infant and childhood immunization within the health care system: (1) low public awareness and lack of public demand for immunization, (2) inadequate access to immunization services, (3) missed opportunities to administer vaccines, and (4) inadequate resources for public health and preventive programs. These problems are current public concerns and are a priority for national health policy in the United States.

In contrast, there has been little progress and virtually no publicity about the goals for adult immunization in the United States promulgated under *Healthy People 2000,* a set of national health promotion and disease prevention objectives for the year 2000 (Table 82-13). These objectives were established by the U.S. Department of Health and Human Services in consultation with the Institute of Medicine, the National Academy of Sciences, and after extensive public review and comment. Adult immunization goals are important, for as many as 60,000 adults are estimated to die each year from vaccine-

TABLE 82-12   Standards for immunization practices

PEDIATRIC PRACTICE

Standard 1: Immunization services are *readily available.*
Standard 2: There are *no barriers* or *unnecessary prerequisites* to the receipt of vaccines.
Standard 3: Immunization services are available *free* or for a *minimal fee.*
Standard 4: Providers utilize all clinical encounters to *screen* and, when indicated, *immunize* children.
Standard 5: Providers *educate* parents and guardians about immunization in general terms.
Standard 6: Providers *question* parents or guardians about *contraindications* and, before immunizing a child, *inform* them in specific terms about the risks and benefits of the immunizations their child is to receive.
Standard 7: Providers follow only true *contraindications.*
Standard 8: Providers administer *simultaneously* all vaccine doses for which a child is eligible at the time of each visit.
Standard 9: Providers use accurate and complete *recording procedures.*
Standard 10: Providers *co-schedule* immunization appointments in conjunction with appointments for other child health services.
Standard 11: Providers *report adverse events* following immunization promptly, accurately, and completely.
Standard 12: Providers operate a *tracking system.*
Standard 13: Providers adhere to appropriate procedures for *vaccine management.*
Standard 14: Providers conduct semiannual *audits* to assess immunization coverage levels and to review immunization records in the patient populations they serve.
Standard 15: Providers maintain up-to-date, easily retrievable *medical protocols* at all locations where vaccines are administered.
Standard 16: Providers operate with *patient-oriented* and *community-based approaches.*
Standard 17: Vaccines are administered by *properly trained individuals.*
Standard 18: Providers receive *ongoing education* and *training* on current immunization recommendations.

ADULT PRACTICE

Standard 1: Promote appropriate vaccine use through information campaigns for health-care practitioners and trainees, employers, and the public about the benefits of immunizations
Standard 2: Providers are completely immunized to protect themselves and prevent transmission to patients
Standard 3: Providers routinely determine the immunization status of their adult patients, offer vaccines for those for whom they are indicated, and maintain complete immunization records
Standard 4: Providers identify high-risk patients in need of influenze vaccine and develop a system to recall them for annual immunization
Standard 5: Providers and institutions identify high-risk adult patients in hospitals and other treatment centers and assure that appropriate vaccination is considered either prior to discharge or as part of discharge planning
Standard 6: Licensing/accreditation agencies support the development by health-care institutions of comprehensive immunization programs for staff, trainees, volunteer workers, inpatients, and outpatients
Standard 7: States establish preenrollment immunization requirements for colleges and other institutions of higher education
Standard 8: Institutions that train health-care professions, deliver health care, or provide laboratory or other medical support services require appropriate immunizations for persons at risk of contracting or transmitting vaccine-preventable illnesses
Standard 9: Health-care benefit programs, third part payers and government healt-care programs provide coverage for adult immunization services
Standard 10: Adopt a standard personal and institutional immunization record as a means of verifying the immunization status of patients and staff

SOURCE: Ad Hoc Working Group for the Development of Standards for Pediatric Immunization Practices. JAMA 269:1817, 1993
The National Coalition for Adult Immunization

preventable diseases for which effective vaccines are not being optimally used. As few as 40 percent of persons aged 65 and older receive influenza vaccine each year, and less than 15 percent have ever received pneumococcal vaccine (Table 82-14). Health care providers as often miss opportunities to vaccinate adults as they do infants and children. Between 60 and 90 percent of adults hospitalized for, or dying of, influenza-associated respiratory disease received medical care during the previous year during which they *could have* been immunized.

Financing immunization   Many private health insurance policies do not provide adequate coverage for immunization, and physicians and other health care providers pass these costs directly on to patients.

---

* These data do not include HBV vaccine and *H. influenzae* type b conjugate vaccine.
† By the second birthday, a fully immunized child will have received four doses of diphtheria and tetanus toxoids combined with pertussis vaccine (DTP), three doses of oral polio vaccine (OPV), one dose of measles, mumps, and rubella (MMR) vaccine, three doses of HBV vaccine, and three to four doses of a suitable *H. influenzae* type b conjugate vaccine (HibCV).

TABLE 82-13 Vaccine-preventable disease targets

Vaccine-preventable diseases	1987 baseline	2000 target
Diphtheria among people aged 25 and younger	1	0
Tetanus among people aged 25 and younger	3	0
Polio (wild-type virus)	0	0
Measles	3058	0
Rubella	225	0
Congenital rubella syndrome	6	0
Mumps	4866	<500
Pertussis	3450	<1000

SOURCE: *Healthy People 2000: National Health Promotion and Disease Prevention Objectives*. Washington, U.S. Department of Health and Human Services, Public Health Service, 1990.

A major impediment to the delivery of vaccines under public-sector programs is the low reimbursement rates to providers of these services, which in 1990 served 5.3 million children under age 6 under Medicaid. Since states may reimburse Medicaid providers at less than the cost of the vaccines, let alone the cost of administration, there is little incentive for private providers to offer and promote immunizations for Medicaid-enrolled children. The result is that all too often children are referred to overburdened public clinics, thereby contributing to fragmentation of care and lower coverage rates against vaccine-preventable diseases. At the same time, 40 to 91 percent of unvaccinated preschool children who developed measles during the epidemic of 1989–1990 were enrolled in one or more public assistance programs which *could have* served as a referral source for children in need of immunization.

Similar gaps for immunization of adults exist under Medicare. While Medicare coverage includes the cost of influenza and pneumococcal vaccines and their administration to all enrolled individuals and HBV vaccine for those at high risk of exposure (i.e., renal dialysis patients), reimbursement is not adequate to encourage vaccine use among providers, and the program does not cover inexpensive vaccines such as tetanus-diphtheria toxoid (Td).

The role of industry With the exception of the states of Michigan and Massachusetts, which manufacture certain vaccines and immune globulin preparations, the American public is entirely dependent on the willingness of the commercial sector to make and market vaccines. This willingness has been in decline over the last two decades, and many manufacturers no longer produce vaccines. There are currently just one or two United States–based commercial sources for most childhood vaccines.

The National Vaccine Injury Compensation Program The use of mandated vaccines benefits society as a whole by reducing morbidity and the cost of care for preventable diseases and by reducing childhood mortality. For these reasons, and because the vaccines are sometimes associated with severe adverse reactions or sequelae, in the United States, society has assumed the obligation to care for those injured by the administration of mandated vaccines. The National

TABLE 82-14 Estimates of vaccine coverage or immunity among adults, 1993

Vaccine	Percent
Influenza (age 65+)	40
Pneumococcal (age 65+)	14
Hepatitis B (age 65+)	1–60*
Tetanus	16–59[†]
Diphtheria	34–51[†]
Measles	85–95[†]
Rubella	80–90[†]

* Varies by risk group.
[†] Varies by study.
SOURCE: Centers for Disease Control and Prevention: National Program on Immunization.

Childhood Vaccine Injury Compensation Act of 1986 is the instrument in use to ensure fairness to injured persons and protection for federal, state, and local immunization programs, private immunization providers, and vaccine manufacturers. The act was designed to carry out two vital public policies: (1) to provide prompt and fair compensation to the families of children who have died or have been injured as a result of routine mandated immunization and (2) to reduce the adverse impact of the tort system on vaccine supply, cost, and innovation and development. The intent is to encourage predictable, speedy, and equitable compensation for persons injured by vaccines. The success of immunization programs in the United States depends on the continued viability of the NVICP.

CONTROL OF VACCINE-PREVENTABLE DISEASE A continuing task of public health practice is to maintain individual and herd immunity. The job is not over once a population is fully vaccinated, since it is imperative to immunize each subsequent generation as long as the threat of the disease persists. Ongoing surveillance and prompt reporting of disease to local or state health departments are essential to this goal by ensuring a continuing awareness of the possibility of vaccine-preventable illness. Nearly all vaccine-preventable diseases are now notifiable and individual case data are routinely forwarded to the CDC. These data are used to detect outbreaks or other unusual events in need of investigation and to evaluate prevention and control policies, practices, and strategies.

A similar informations system for immunization coverage levels needs to be developed to determine if infants, children, and adults are actually receiving vaccines according to recommended schedules. This information could be used to ensure complete immunization of individuals, as well as to assess vaccine effectiveness and adverse events, to evaluate the performance of immunization programs, and to promote the efficient use of scarce resources.

Influencing acceptance of vaccines As a direct consequence of the success of immunization, vaccine-preventable disease has become less visible, and parents and health care providers can become complacent about immunization of children. Even among the affluent and educated, low levels of immunization may prevail, reflecting a gross misunderstanding of the continuing threat of disease with which parents and health care providers have limited experience and/or an inappropriately greater fear of vaccine adverse reactions than with the illness and death caused by vaccine-preventable diseases. Health care workers play an essential role in influencing the attitudes of patients regarding appropriate immunization, and therefore, it is essential for health care workers to continually update their own knowledge about vaccines and the epidemiology of vaccine-preventable illnesses.

VACCINE AND IMMUNIZATION RESEARCH To accomplish the preventive goals of *Healthy People 2000,* current immunization recommendations in the United States call for every child to receive nine different vaccines (many in combination and all requiring more than one dose) between birth and entry into kindergarten. This requires at least five visits to a health care provider by age 2, with an additional visit before starting school. This is a formidable task, particularly for those with limited access to health care, and compliance can be expected to become more difficult as new vaccines are licensed.

The Children's Vaccine Initiative The potential to eradicate selected diseases and build sustainable immunization programs that reach every child is not being achieved with existing vaccines and delivery technology. New vaccines or new formulations are required that will not only improve protective responses but also will simplify the immunization schedule. The Children's Vaccine Initiative (CVI) is an international effort to accomplish this goal. The ultimate ideal is to develop vaccines which may be administered orally early in life, provide lifelong protection to multiple infections, require one or a few doses, and be less reactive and more heat stable than current vaccines. Reaching these ambitious goals may take years or decades, but rapid progress is being made right now in developing new combinations of current vaccines to increase the feasibility of complete immunization. Thus DTP plus inactivated polio vaccine, Hib-conju-

TABLE 82-15   Examples of directed scientific research to improve the immunization delivery system

Delivery system change desired	Scientific input	Products in process
Decrease number of visits required for full immunization	Developing new combination vaccines	MMRV, DTP-HIB-HBV, DTP-HIB
	Research on recombinant live multiantigen vaccines	Canarypox-measles, Canarypox-RSV, *Vaccinia*-rabies, *Vaccinia*-influenza, *Salmonella*, BCG
Decrease number of doses	Development of time-release products	Microencapsulated tetanus toxoid Microencapsulated hepatitis B Microencapsulated pertussis Microencapsulated influenza
Decrease number of injections	Reseach on oral vaccines	Pertussis
	Understanding mucosal immunity	Cholera
	Research in antigen presentation	Influenza
Immunization as early in life as possible	Research on maternal immunization	*Haemophilus* type B; *Meningococcus*
	Research on neonatal immunity	Group B streptococcus, *Pneumococcus*, influenza
Decrease in adverse events	Research on the mechanisms of adverse events	Acellular pertussis
		OPV neurovirulence, genetic determinants
Increase protection	Research on more immunogenic antigens	Group B streptococcus
	Development of conjugated vaccines	*Meningococcus, Pneumococcus*, influenza group B streptococcus
	Research on adjuvants	Typhoid
Increase thermal stability	Research on stabilizers	Polio, chemical stabilizer, freeze drying

SOURCE: National Vaccine Program Office, Office of the Assistant Secretary for Health, Department of Health and Human Services.

gate plus DTP, and HBV plus DTP vaccines are being evaluated, and a six-valent vaccine is a likely next step. Strategies of directed scientific research to improve vaccine delivery are listed in Table 82-15. The results will be applicable to both developed and developing country immunization programs.

Reemergence of controlled disease and emergence of new disease   The emergence of new pathogens is fostered by the genetic potential of microbes to evolve as well as by rapid changes in demographics and human behavior and in global ecology that create new or more hospitable hosts. The emergence of new infectious diseases such as HIV, Lyme borreliosis, and hepatitis C and the increase in global incidence and in drug resistance of familiar diseases such as tuberculosis and malaria, once considered under control, are proof of the need for continuing vaccine research. In addition, some common illnesses without a known etiology, such as peptic ulcer disease and cervical and nasopharyngeal cancer, are now epidemiologically linked to specific infection and thus may be vaccine-preventable.

Development of new vaccines   Many serious, life-threatening infectious diseases cannot be controlled because there are no effective vaccines. Many new vaccines are in development (Table 82-16); however, the task is proving to be very complex. Priority efforts for the United States are currently targeted toward HIV, acellular pertussis vaccine, group B streptococcus, respiratory syncytial virus, rotavirus, varicella, tuberculosis, hepatitis C, and two virus-associated tumors, human papilloma virus (cervical cancer) and Epstein-Barr virus (nasopharyngeal cancer).

INTERNATIONAL CONSIDERATIONS   Since the establishment of the World Health Organization's Expanded Programme on Immunization (EPI), immunization levels for the six basic children's vaccines have risen from 5 percent in the early 1980s to approximately 80 percent worldwide today. Each year, at least 2.7 million deaths from measles, neonatal tetanus, and pertussis and 200,000 cases of paralysis due to polio are prevented. Despite the successes of the EPI, many vaccine-preventable diseases remain prevalent in the developing world. Measles, for example, continues to kill an estimated 1.5 million children each year, and cases of diphtheria, whooping cough, polio, and neonatal tetanus still occur at unacceptably high levels. It is estimated that between 20 and 35 percent of all deaths in children under age 5 are associated with vaccine-preventable diseases.

Global targets   Eight antigens are recommended for routine use in the developing world by the EPI, including BCG, DTP, trivalent polio, and measles vaccines for children and tetanus toxoid for pregnant women. Others (Hib, Japanese B encephalitis, yellow fever, HBV, group A meningococcus, mumps, and rubella) are used

regionally, depending on disease epidemiology and resources. Polio has been targeted for eradication by the year 2000, and great progress has been achieved in the Americas by the Pan American Health Organization.

Because infectious diseases know no geographic or political boundaries, uncontrolled disease anywhere in the world poses a threat to the United States. Vaccines offer the opportunity to control and even eradicate some diseases, and successful eradication means that vaccines are no longer needed. The experience with smallpox has shown that the eradication of disease is a remarkably good economic investment. The entire sum that the United States spent for the global smallpox eradication campaign has been recouped, in 1968 dollars, every $2\frac{1}{2}$ months since 1971. A similar achievement with polio would save the United States over $300 million a year in vaccine and associated delivery costs, and the goal is feasible.

TABLE 82-16   Vaccines in human trial, 1993

Bacterial
Vibrio cholerae
Mycobacterium leprae
Salmonella typhi
Bordetella pertussis
Neisseria meningitidis
Streptococcus pneumoniae
Group B streptococcus
Shigella spp.
Enterotoxigenic *E. coli*
Lyme disease
Fungal
Cryptococcus neoformans
Parasitic
Plasmodium spp.
Viral
Hepatitis A
Dengue
Rotavirus
Japanese B encephalitis
Influenza A and B
Varicella
Measles
Cytomegalovirus
Rabies
Junin
Chikungunya
Rift Valley fever
Respiratory syncytial virus
Parainfluenza virus

SOURCE: National Vaccine Program Office, Office of the Assistant Secretary for Health, Department of Health and Human Services.

REFERENCES

AMERICAN ACADEMY OF PEDIATRICS: *Report of the Committee on Infectious Diseases* ("Red Book"), 22d ed, G. Peter et al (eds). Elk Grove Village, Ill., 1991

AMERICAN COLLEGE OF PHYSICIANS: *Guide for Adult Immunization*, 2d ed. Philadelphia, American College of Physicians, 1990

AMERICAN PUBLIC HEALTH ASSOCIATION: *Control of Communicable Diseases in Man*, 15th ed, AS Benenson (ed). Washington, D.C., American Public Health Association, 1990

CENTERS FOR DISEASE CONTROL AND PREVENTION: Recommendations of the Advisory Committee on Immunization Practices (ACIP): Use of vaccines and immune globulins in persons with altered immunocompetence. Morb Mort Week Rep 42(RR-4):1, 1993

————: Standards for pediatric immunization practices. Morb Mort Week Rep 42(RR-5):1, 1993

————: Update on adult immunization. Recommendations of the Immunization Practices Advisory Committee (ACIP). Morb Mort Week Rep 40(RR-12):1, 1991

———— : *Health Information for International Travel* (published yearly) and *Advisory Memoranda on Travel* (published periodically)

section 2 Clinical syndromes— community acquired

83 SEPSIS AND SEPTIC SHOCK

ROBERT S. MUNFORD

DEFINITIONS The host reaction to invading microbes involves a rapidly amplifying polyphony of signals and responses that may spread beyond the invaded tissue. Fever or hypothermia, chills, tachypnea, and tachycardia often herald the onset of the systemic inflammatory response to microbial invasion, also called *sepsis*. Sepsis is usually limited by counterregulatory mechanisms. When these mechanisms are overwhelmed, often as the microbe moves from a local site to invade the bloodstream, homeostasis may fail, and dysfunction of major organs can supervene *(severe sepsis)*. Further failure of counterregulatory control leads to *septic shock*, characterized by hypotension as well as organ dysfunction. As sepsis progresses to septic shock, the risk of dying increases substantially. Early sepsis is usually reversible, whereas many patients with septic shock succumb despite aggressive therapy.

ETIOLOGY Sepsis can be a response to infection caused by any class of microorganism. Although gram-negative and gram-positive bacteria account for most cases, sepsis may occur with diseases caused by fungi, mycobacteria, rickettsiae, viruses, or protozoans. Microbial bloodstream invasion, with positive blood cultures, is not essential to the development of sepsis, since systemic spread of microbial signal molecules or toxins also can elicit the response. Approximately 30 to 60 percent of patients with sepsis and 60 to 80 percent of patients with septic shock have blood cultures that yield bacteria or fungi, and gram-negative bacteria account for approximately two-thirds of these isolates. The remaining cases are caused by gram-positive cocci (10 to 20 percent) or fungi (2 to 5 percent) or a mixture of microorganisms. In patients whose blood cultures are negative, the etiologic agent may often be established by culture or microscopical examination of infected material from a local site. Occasional patients with established bacteremia do not mount a septic response.

EPIDEMIOLOGY Sepsis now contributes to more than 100,000 deaths per year in the United States. The incidence is probably between 300,000 and 500,000 cases per year. Approximately two-thirds of the cases occur in hospitalized patients. Factors that predispose to gram-negative rod bacteremia include diabetes mellitus, lymphoproliferative diseases, cirrhosis of the liver, burns, invasive procedures or devices, and drugs that cause neutropenia. Major risk factors for gram-positive bacteremia include vascular catheters, indwelling mechanical devices, burns, and intravenous drug injection. Fungemia occurs most often in immunosuppressed patients with neutropenia, often after broad-spectrum antimicrobial therapy. The increasing incidence of sepsis in the United States is attributable to the aging of the population, the increasing longevity of patients with chronic diseases, and the relatively high frequency of sepsis in AIDS. The widespread use of antimicrobial agents, glucocorticoids, indwelling catheters and mechanical devices, and mechanical ventilation also contributes.

PATHOPHYSIOLOGY The septic response is usually triggered when commensal microorganisms spread from the gastrointestinal tract or skin into contiguous tissues. Localized infection in the genitourinary tract, biliary tract, lungs, or gastrointestinal tract may then lead to bloodstream infection. Microorganisms also may be introduced directly into the bloodstream (e.g., via intravenous catheters). In a minority of cases, no primary site of infection is apparent.

Microbial signals Animals recognize certain microbial molecules as signals that microorganisms have invaded. Lipopolysaccharide (LPS, also called *endotoxin*) is the most potent and best-studied gram-negative bacterial signal molecule. LPS binds to CD14 (and perhaps to other receptors) on monocytes, macrophages, and neutrophils. Plasma proteins, such as LPS-binding protein, facilitate the binding of LPS to CD14, thereby augmenting and accelerating the LPS-cell interaction. Cellular responses to LPS include the production and release of mediators that amplify and transmit the microbial signal to other cells and tissues. The peptidoglycan and lipoteichoic acids of gram-positive bacteria, certain polysaccharides, extracellular enzymes, and toxins elicit responses in animals that are similar to those induced by LPS. The molecular basis for the stimulatory potency of these molecules is less well understood than that for LPS.

Host responses Sepsis results from complex interactions among microbial signal molecules, leukocytes, humoral factors, and the vascular endothelium.

CYTOKINES The inflammatory cytokines may have endocrine, paracrine, and autocrine actions (see Chap. 277). Tumor necrosis factor alpha (TNFα) stimulates leukocytes and vascular endothelial cells to release other cytokines (as well as additional TNFα), to express cell-surface adhesion molecules, and to increase arachidonic acid turnover. Blood levels of TNFα are high in most patients with severe sepsis; in patients with fulminant meningococcemia, TNFα levels correlate with levels of circulating endotoxin and with clinical outcome. Moreover, intravenous infusion of TNFα can elicit many of the characteristic abnormalities of sepsis, including fever, tachycardia, tachypnea, leukocytosis, myalgias, and somnolence. In animals, larger doses of TNFα induce shock, disseminated intravascular coagulation (DIC), and death. Monoclonal antibodies to TNFα can abrogate the septic response and prevent the deaths of experimental animals from endotoxin challenge.

Although TNFα is a central mediator of sepsis, it is only one of many cytokines that contribute to the septic response. Interleukin 1β (IL-1β) is also present in the blood of patients with septic shock; this cytokine can elicit many of the same responses as TNFα when injected intravenously. Recombinant IL-1 receptor antagonist and monoclonal antibodies to IL-1β can protect animals from endotoxic death. Antibodies to IL-6 also may be protective. TNFα, IL-1β, IL-6, interferon-γ, and other cytokines probably interact synergistically with each other and with additional mediators. In addition, some mediators (such as IL-1 and TNFα) may enhance their own rates of synthesis by positive feedback. In animal models, the septic response can be interrupted by interventions that neutralize one or another of its many mediators; this observation testifies to the importance of mediator interactions for the overall result.

PHOSPHOLIPID-DERIVED MEDIATORS Arachidonic acid, released from membrane phospholipids by phospholipase A_2, is converted by the cyclooxygenase pathway into prostaglandins and thromboxanes. Prostaglandin E_2 and prostacyclin cause peripheral vasodilatation, whereas thromboxane is a vasoconstrictor and promotes platelet aggregation. Leukotrienes, products of the lipoxygenase pathway of arachidonate metabolism, are potent mediators of ischemia and shock; the principal arachidonate metabolite in human neutrophils is leukotriene B_4, which promotes leukocyte activation and may contribute to local vascular injury and thrombosis.

Another important phospholipid-derived mediator is platelet-activating factor (PAF), 1-O-alkyl-2-acetyl-sn-glycero-3-phosphocholine. Its precursor, lyso-PAF, is produced by the degradation of membrane choline phosphoglycerides by phospholipase A_2. PAF is a potent stimulus for neutrophil aggregation and degranulation, promotes platelet aggregation, and may contribute to tissue injury.

COAGULATION FACTORS   Intravascular deposition of fibrin, thrombosis, and DIC are important features of the septic response. Although LPS can activate the intrinsic clotting cascade in vitro, and although factor XII levels are low in patients with severe sepsis, LPS and TNFα probably promote intravascular coagulation initially by inducing blood monocytes to express tissue factor, by increasing the release of plasminogen activator inhibitor 1 (PAI-1), and by inhibiting the expression of thrombomodulin and plasminogen activator by vascular endothelial cells. Tissue factor is the high-affinity receptor and cofactor for factor VIIa. When tissue factor is expressed on monocytes, it complexes with factor VIIa to form an active complex that can convert factors X and IX to enzymatically active forms. The result is the activation of both extrinsic and intrinsic clotting pathways, culminating in the generation of thrombin. Decreased levels of antithrombin III and tissue plasminogen activator and increased concentrations of PAI-1 also promote clotting. Contact system activation may occur with severe sepsis, when denuded vascular basement membrane provides an appropriate activating surface.

COMPLEMENT   C5a and other products of complement activation may promote neutrophil chemotaxis, leukotriene synthesis, aggregation, degranulation, and oxygen radical production. When administered to animals, C5a induces hypotension, pulmonary vasoconstriction, neutropenia, and vascular leakiness due, in part, to endothelial damage. C5a-induced hypotension can be blocked by cyclooxygenase inhibitors.

ACTIVATION OF THE VASCULAR ENDOTHELIUM   Many tissues may be damaged by sepsis. The probable underlying mechanism is widespread vascular endothelial injury, with fluid extravasation and microthrombosis that decrease oxygen and substrate utilization by the affected tissues. Leukocyte-derived mediators and platelet-leukocyte-fibrin thrombi contribute to this injury, but the vascular endothelium itself also plays an active role. Stimuli such as LPS and TNFα induce vascular endothelial cells to produce and release cytokines, procoagulant molecules, PAF, endothelium-derived relaxation factor (nitric oxide), and other mediators. In addition, regulated cell adhesion molecules promote the adherence of neutrophils to endothelial cells. While these responses may attract phagocytes to infected sites and activate their antimicrobial arsenals, endothelial cell activation also can promote increased vascular permeability, microvascular thrombosis, DIC, and hypotension. Moreover, vascular integrity may be damaged by neutrophil enzymes (such as elastase) and toxic oxygen metabolites so that local hemorrhage ensues. Blocking the adhesion of leukocytes to endothelial cell surfaces, as with monoclonal antibodies to ICAM-1, can prevent tissue necrosis in response to endotoxin administration in animals.

SEPTIC SHOCK   The actual mediators of septic shock are not known. TNFα and IL-1β probably cause hypotension by triggering the release of additional mediators. Among the prominent hypotensive agents are β-endorphin, bradykinin, PAF, endothelium-derived relaxation factor (nitric oxide), leukotrienes, and prostacyclin. Agents that inhibit the synthesis or action of each of these mediators can prevent or reverse endotoxic shock in animals.

The sepsis cascade: Clues to the early events   Septic shock is associated with derangements of the proteolytic cascades that control clotting, kinin metabolism, and complement activation. Activation of the intrinsic (contact) clotting pathway, activation of kallikrein,

proteolytic inactivation of C1 inhibitor, and generation of C5a and other active complement components have been reported. In contrast, useful clues to the early changes during sepsis have come from studies of the effects of the intravenous administration of endotoxin. After injection of an endotoxin bolus, blood levels of TNFα, IL-6, and IL-8 increase (Fig. 83-1). Concentrations of TNFα typically increase by 30 min and peak at 90 min, whereas levels of IL-6 and IL-8 increase more slowly and peak around 2 to 4 h after infusion. Blood levels of tissue plasminogen activator and plasmin also increase transiently, and these rises are followed by a longer-lasting increase in PAI-1. An early fibrinolytic phase is thus followed by a period of hypercoagulability. Similar changes occur after infusion of TNFα. Activation of complement or of the intrinsic clotting pathway has not been detected in these studies; these derangements may occur only with more severe sepsis and may not be induced directly by endotoxin.

Ibuprofen, a cyclooxygenase inhibitor, blocks many of the responses to endotoxin infusion, including most symptoms (fever, myalgia, nausea, headache) and endotoxin-induced increases in adrenocorticotropin (ACTH), cortisol, epinephrine, and norepinephrine. On the other hand, ibuprofen does not prevent endotoxin-induced leukocytosis or hypoferremia, and blood levels of TNFα and IL-8 are actually higher after administration of ibuprofen and endotoxin than after endotoxin infusion alone. Prostanoids therefore mediate many of the effects of TNFα and IL-1β; some prostaglandins, such as prostaglandin E_2, appear to mediate certain cytokine actions (such as the production of fever and muscle proteolysis), yet they inhibit the production of TNFα and IL-8. They thus may provide an autoregulatory mechanism for limiting the inflammatory response.

Control mechanisms   Elaborate counterregulatory mechanisms limit the inflammatory response. Elevated plasma concentrations of ACTH occur within 1 h of intravenous endotoxin administration, and plasma cortisol levels peak shortly thereafter. Glucocorticoids inhibit cytokine synthesis by monocytes in vitro, and when administered with or shortly after the inflammatory stimulus, they may protect animals from septic shock. Presumably, endogenous glucocorticoids play a similar role in damping inflammatory responses. Certain cytokine antagonists also may dampen or control the septic response.

FIGURE 83-1   Typical time course and levels (relative to baseline) of cytokines (TNFα, IL-6, IL-8), tissue plasminogen activator (tPA), and plasminogen activator inhibitor-1 (PAI-1) in the plasma of volunteers receiving a bolus infusion of endotoxin. Data are taken from articles by Martich, van Deventer, and Suffredini. In patients with sepsis, multiple microbial signal molecules are probably produced and released intermittently at various tissue sites and in different doses. The host response is therefore much more complex than is shown here.

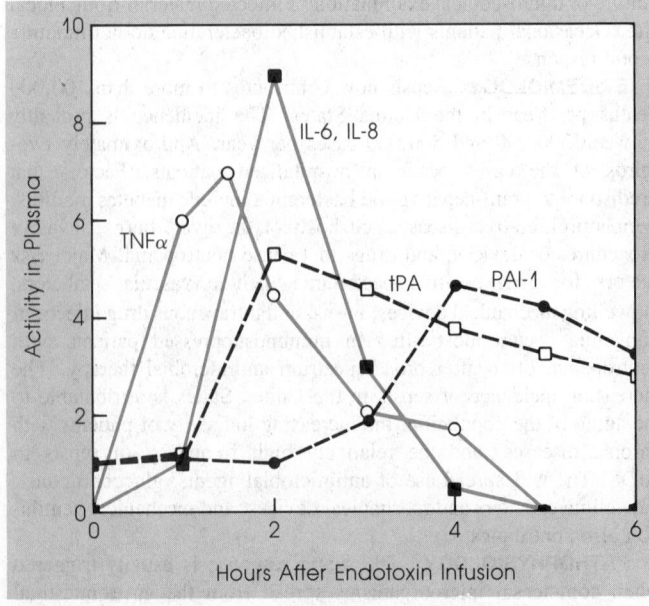

After endotoxin infusion into human subjects, for example, IL-1β rapidly appears in the blood, yet blood levels of IL-1 receptor antagonist rapidly exceed those of circulating IL-1β and may inhibit IL-1β binding to its receptors. IL-4, IL-6, IL-8, and IL-10 also can inhibit LPS-induced responses by human monocytes in vitro. Along with prostaglandin E$_2$, α-melanocyte-stimulating hormone, IL-1 receptor antagonist, and soluble TNF receptors, these molecules probably act to prevent the progression of most instances of sepsis to death. Much less is known about these control processes than about the activation arm of the septic response, however.

CLINICAL MANIFESTATIONS Sepsis is easily suspected in the patient with localized infection who abruptly develops fever, chills, tachycardia, tachypnea, altered mental status, and hypotension. However, the septic response may develop more slowly and have more subtle manifestations. For example, some septic patients have normal temperature or may even be hypothermic; the absence of fever is most common in neonates, in elderly patients, and in persons with uremia or alcoholism.

Hyperventilation is often a useful clue to the diagnosis, although its cause is poorly understood. Disorientation, confusion, and other manifestations of encephalopathy also may be early signs, particularly in the elderly and in individuals with preexisting neurologic impairment. Focal neurologic signs are uncommon, although preexisting focal deficits may become more prominent.

Hypotension and DIC predispose to acrocyanosis and ischemic necrosis of peripheral tissues, most commonly the digits. Cellulitis, pustules, bullae, or hemorrhagic lesions may develop when bacteria or fungi seed the skin or underlying soft tissues by hematogenous spread. Bacterial toxins also may be distributed hematogenously to elicit diffuse cutaneous reactions. On occasion, skin lesions may suggest specific pathogens. When sepsis is accompanied by cutaneous petechiae or purpura, infection with *Neisseria meningitidis* (or, less commonly, *Haemophilus influenzae*) should be suspected; in a patient who has been bitten by a tick while in an endemic area, petechial lesions also should suggest Rocky Mountain spotted fever. A cutaneous lesion seen almost exclusively in neutropenic patients is ecthyma gangrenosum, usually caused by *Pseudomonas aeruginosa* or *Aeromonas hydrophila*; a bullous lesion, surrounded by edema, undergoes central hemorrhage and necrosis. Histopathologic examination shows bacteria in and around the wall of a small vessel, with little or no neutrophilic response. Hemorrhagic or bullous lesions in a septic patient who has recently eaten raw oysters should suggest *Vibrio vulnificus* bacteremia, while in a patient who has recently suffered a dog bite, such lesions may indicate bacteremia due to *Capnocytophaga canimorsus* or *C. cynodegmi* (DF2). Generalized erythroderma in a septic patient should suggest the toxic shock syndrome due to *Staphylococcus aureus* or *Streptococcus pyogenes*.

Gastrointestinal manifestations such as nausea, vomiting, diarrhea, and ileus may suggest acute gastroenteritis. Stress ulceration can lead to upper gastrointestinal bleeding. Cholestatic jaundice, with elevated levels of serum bilirubin (mostly conjugated) and alkaline phosphatase, may precede other signs of sepsis. Hepatocellular or canicular dysfunction appears to underlie most cases, and hepatic function tests return to normal with resolution of the infection. Prolonged or severe hypotension may induce acute hepatic injury or ischemic bowel necrosis.

Blood lactate levels rise early, in part because of increased glycolysis in peripheral tissues with incomplete hepatic clearance of the resulting lactate and pyruvate. As hypoperfusion develops, tissue hypoxia generates more lactic acid, worsening the metabolic acidosis. The blood glucose concentration often increases, particularly in diabetics, although impaired gluconeogenesis and excessive insulin release may on occasion produce hypoglycemia. Hypertriglyceridemia reflects, at least in part, the inhibitory action of TNFα on lipoprotein lipase. The cytokine (IL-6, IL-1β, TNFα)–mediated acute-phase response inhibits albumin synthesis while enhancing the production of C-reactive protein, fibrinogen, complement components, and transferrin.

COMPLICATIONS Cardiopulmonary complications Ventilation-perfusion mismatching produces a fall in arterial P$_{O_2}$ early in the course. Increasing alveolar capillary permeability results in increased lung water, which decreases pulmonary compliance and interferes with oxygen exchange. Progressive, diffuse pulmonary infiltrates, decreasing compliance, and arterial hypoxemia (often refractory to supplemental oxygen therapy, indicating right-to-left shunting) indicate development of the acute respiratory distress syndrome (ARDS). ARDS (or "shock lung") develops in 20 to 50 percent of patients with sepsis, and sepsis is the leading cause of ARDS. Leukocyte-induced pulmonary microvascular injury, with damage to pulmonary capillary endothelial cells, contributes to its pathogenesis. Respiratory muscle failure can worsen hypoxemia and hypercapnia. An elevated pulmonary capillary wedge pressure (>18 mmHg) suggests fluid volume overload or cardiac failure rather than ARDS. Pneumonia due to viruses or severe *Pneumocystis carinii* infection may be clinically indistinguishable from ARDS.

Septic shock usually results from a severe decrease in systemic vascular resistance, a generalized maldistribution of blood flow, and functional hypovolemia that is due, at least in part, to diffuse capillary leakage of intravascular constituents. Cardiac output is initially normal or elevated. Indeed, the normal or increased cardiac output and decreased systemic vascular resistance distinguish septic shock from cardiogenic, extracardiac obstructive, and hypovolemic shock; other processes that can produce this combination include anaphylaxis, beriberi, cirrhosis of the liver, and overdoses of nitroprusside or narcotics.

Depression of myocardial function, manifested as increased end-diastolic and systolic ventricular volumes with decreased ejection fraction, occurs within 24 h in most patients with severe sepsis. Cardiac output is maintained despite the low ejection fraction because ventricular dilatation permits a normal stroke volume. In survivors, myocardial function returns to normal over several days. While myocardial dysfunction may contribute to hypotension, refractory hypotension is usually due to a low systemic vascular resistance, and death results from refractory shock or the failure of multiple organs rather than from cardiac dysfunction per se.

Renal complications Oliguria, azotemia, proteinuria, and nonspecific urinary casts are frequent. Most renal failure is due to acute tubular necrosis induced by hypotension or capillary injury, although some patients also have glomerulonephritis, renal cortical necrosis, or interstitial nephritis. Drug-induced renal damage also may complicate therapy, particularly when hypotensive patients are given aminoglycoside antibiotics.

Coagulation abnormalities Although thrombocytopenia occurs in 10 to 30 percent of patients, the underlying mechanism(s) are not understood. Very low platelet counts (below 50,000 per microliter) are usually found in patients with DIC, typically reflecting diffuse endothelial injury (see Chap. 315).

Multiple organ dysfunction syndrome Dysfunction or failure of multiple organs, usually reflecting widespread vascular endothelial injury, is associated with high fatality rates. The severity of the insult and the risk of dying correlate with the number of organs affected.

LABORATORY FINDINGS In early sepsis, abnormalities often include leukocytosis with a left shift, thrombocytopenia, hyperbilirubinemia, and proteinuria. Leukopenia may occur. The neutrophils may contain toxic granulations, Döhle bodies, or cytoplasmic vacuoles. As the septic response becomes more severe, thrombocytopenia worsens (often with prolongation of the thrombin time, decreased fibrinogen, and the presence of D-dimers, suggesting DIC), azotemia and hyperbilirubinemia become more prominent, and levels of aminotransferases become elevated. Active hemolysis suggests clostridial bacteremia, malaria, a drug reaction, or DIC; in the case of DIC, microangiopathic changes may be seen on blood smear.

During early sepsis, hyperventilation induces respiratory alkalosis. With respiratory muscle fatigue and the accumulation of lactate, metabolic acidosis (with increased anion gap) typically supervenes. Arterial blood gases also reveal hypoxemia, initially correctable with supplemental oxygen but later refractory to 100% oxygen inhalation, indicating right-to-left shunting. The chest radiograph may be normal or may show an underlying pneumonia, volume overload, or diffuse infiltrates of ARDS. The electrocardiogram may show only sinus tachycardia or nonspecific ST-T wave abnormalities.

Most diabetics with sepsis develop hyperglycemia. Severe infection may precipitate diabetic ketoacidosis, which may worsen hypotension (see Chap. 337). Hypoglycemia occurs rarely. The serum albumin level, initially within the normal range, declines as sepsis continues. Serum lipid concentrations are often elevated. Hypocalcemia is rare.

DIAGNOSIS There is no reliable laboratory test. Suggestive findings include tachypnea, tachycardia, altered mental status, leukocytosis or leukopenia, and thrombocytopenia. The septic response can be quite variable, however. In one study, 36 percent of patients with sepsis had a normal temperature, 44 percent had a normal mental status, 60 percent had a normal respiratory rate, 10 percent had a normal pulse rate, and 78 percent had normal platelet counts. The typical symptoms and signs of sepsis are also not specific, since similar systemic responses (recently named the *systemic inflammatory response syndrome,* or SIRS) may occur in uninfected patients with other conditions. Strictly speaking, the diagnosis of *sepsis* requires confirmation that SIRS has a microbial cause. Conditions that may mimic sepsis include pancreatitis, burns, trauma, adrenal insufficiency, pulmonary embolism, dissecting or ruptured aortic aneurysm, myocardial infarction, occult hemorrhage, cardiac tamponade, anaphylaxis, and drug overdose.

Definitive diagnosis requires isolation of the microorganism from blood or a local site of infection. At least two blood samples (10 mL each) should be obtained, from different venipuncture sites, for culture. Gram-negative bacteremia is typically low grade (fewer than 10 organisms per milliliter of blood), so multiple blood cultures or prolonged culture incubation may be necessary for the diagnosis; *S. aureus* grows more readily, and most blood cultures will be positive within 48 h. In approximately one-third of cases, blood cultures are negative; this result can reflect prior antibiotic administration, the presence of slowly growing or fastidious organisms, or the absence of microbial invasion of the bloodstream. In these cases, Gram's stain and culture of the primary site of infection—or of infected cutaneous lesions—are necessary to establish the microbial cause. The skin and mucosae should be examined carefully and repeatedly for lesions that might yield diagnostic information. In patients with the staphylococcal toxic shock syndrome, for example, the clinical diagnosis is often supported by isolating *S. aureus* from a cutaneous lesion or mucosal site. With overwhelming bacteremia (e.g., pneumococcal sepsis in splenectomized individuals, fulminant meningococcemia), microorganisms are sometimes seen on buffy coat smears of peripheral blood.

TREATMENT Sepsis can kill quickly. Successful management requires urgent measures to treat the local site of infection, to provide hemodynamic and respiratory support, and to eliminate the offending microorganism. The outcome is also influenced by the patient's underlying disease, which should be aggressively treated.

Antimicrobial agents Antimicrobial chemotherapy should be initiated as soon as samples of blood and other relevant sites have been cultured. The choice of initial therapy can be based on knowledge of the likely pathogens at specific sites of local infection. Available information about antimicrobial susceptibility patterns in bacterial isolates from the community, the hospital, and the patient also should be taken into account. It is also important to recall that the signs and symptoms of sepsis can be elicited by many different microorganisms. Consequently, pending culture results, empirical antimicrobial therapy usually should be effective against both gram-positive and gram-negative bacteria. Maximal recommended doses of antimicrobial drugs should be given intravenously, with adjustment for impaired renal function when necessary. Cefotaxime (3 g IV every 6 h) or ceftazidime (2 g IV every 8 h) plus gentamicin or tobramycin (1.5 mg/kg every 8 h) is an appropriate initial empirical regimen in patients with no apparent site of primary infection. (If infection with *P. aeruginosa* is suspected, ceftazidime and tobramycin should be used.)

Nafcillin (3 g IV every 6 h) or vancomycin (15 mg/kg IV every 12 h) should be added if the patient has injected drugs intravenously or has an indwelling vascular catheter, and clindamycin (600 mg IV every 6 h) or metronidazole (500 mg IV every 6 h) should be added if an intraabdominal source is suspected. When culture results become known, the regimen often can be simplified, since a single antimicrobial agent is frequently adequate for the treatment of infection with a known pathogen. On the other hand, a combination of bactericidal antimicrobial agents (typically a β-lactam and an aminoglycoside) may be indicated for definitive treatment of sepsis in neutropenic patients and for the treatment of sepsis due to bacteria such as *P. aeruginosa* and enterococci, against which antimicrobial synergy has been documented.

Removal of the source of infection Removal or drainage of a focal source of sepsis is essential. Sites of occult infection should be sought carefully. Indwelling intravenous catheters should be removed, the tip should be rolled over a blood agar plate for quantitative culture, and a new catheter should be inserted at a different site. Foley and drainage catheters should be replaced if obstructed. Paranasal sinusitis (often caused by hospital-acquired gram-negative bacteria) should be considered in any patient who has undergone nasal intubation. In the neutropenic patient, cutaneous sites of tenderness and erythema should be sought, particularly in the perianal region. The possibility of pelvic or other soft tissue pus collections should be excluded (with use of computed tomography, if necessary) in patients with sacral or ischial decubitus ulcers. Ureteral obstruction, perinephric abscess, and renal abscess should be excluded by sonography or computed tomography in patients with urosepsis.

Hemodynamic support Here, the goal is to restore adequate oxygen and substrate delivery to the tissues. Effective intravascular volume depletion is common in septic patients, and initial management of the hypotensive septic patient should include the administration of intravenous fluids, typically 1 to 2 L of normal saline over 1 to 2 h. Larger volumes may be needed. Monitoring of the pulmonary capillary wedge pressure or central venous pressure is essential in patients with refractory shock or underlying cardiac or renal disease. To avoid pulmonary edema, the pulmonary capillary wedge pressure should be maintained between 12 and 15 mmHg or the central venous pressure between 10 and 12 cmH$_2$O. The urine output should be kept above 30 mL/h by continuing fluid administration; a diuretic such as furosemide may be used if needed. In about one-third of patients, hypotension responds to fluid resuscitation; a reasonable goal is to maintain a mean arterial blood pressure of >60 mmHg (systolic pressure > 90 mmHg). Dopamine is the most widely used pressor agent. When given in low doses [5 to 10 (μg/kg)/min] it has beta$_1$-adrenergic effects, increasing cardiac output and dilating tissue arterioles by stimulating dopaminergic receptors. Caution is necessary, however, since higher doses [>20 (μg/kg)/min] stimulate alpha-adrenergic receptors and can cause peripheral vasoconstriction, with ischemia and gangrene. Because of its alpha$_1$ stimulatory effect, norepinephrine should be carefully titrated to achieve a mean blood pressure of at least 60 mmHg; this agent is often reserved for patients who remain hypotensive despite dopamine therapy. Low-dose dopamine [1 to 4 (μg/kg)/min] may be combined with norepinephrine to maintain adequate renal and intestinal perfusion and achieve maximal pressor support.

Adrenal insufficiency, an uncommon complication of sepsis, should be considered in septic patients with refractory hypotension, fulminant *N. meningitidis* bacteremia, prior glucocorticoid use, disseminated tuberculosis, or AIDS. The cosyntropin ($α^{1-24}$-ACTH) stimulation test (see Chap. 335) may suggest absolute or partial adrenal insufficiency. Supplemental hydrocortisone (50 mg IV every 6 h) may be given while awaiting the results of the cosyntropin test.

Ventilator therapy is indicated for progressive hypoxemia, hypercapnia, neurologic deterioration, or respiratory muscle failure. Intubation is often undertaken to ensure adequate oxygenation, divert blood from the muscles of respiration, and reduce the cardiac afterload.

Blood or erythrocyte transfusion is indicated if oxygen delivery is compromised by a low hemoglobin concentration.

Therapy of acidosis and DIC Bicarbonate is sometimes administered for severe metabolic acidosis (arterial pH <7.2); efficacy is not established. DIC, if complicated by major bleeding, should be treated with transfusion of fresh frozen plasma and platelets. Successful treatment of the underlying infection is essential to reverse both acidosis and DIC.

Other measures Despite early diagnosis, surgical drainage of infected sites, prompt administration of appropriate antimicrobial therapy, and careful fluid and pressor resuscitation, many patients with sepsis die. Two kinds of agents are under investigation to prevent these deaths: drugs that neutralize bacterial endotoxin, thereby benefiting patients with gram-negative bacterial sepsis, and drugs that interfere with one or more mediators of the inflammatory response, thereby potentially benefiting patients with sepsis of all etiologies.

ANTIENDOTOXIN AGENTS The toxic moiety of endotoxin, called *lipid A,* is structurally conserved in the LPS of pathogenic gram-negative bacteria. Much effort has been devoted to developing antibodies to lipid A—or to a conserved core oligosaccharide moiety—that would neutralize endotoxin in vivo and protect patients from endotoxic shock. Studies with polyclonal antisera to endotoxin core structures seemed very promising, but in placebo-controlled trials, two monoclonal antibodies to lipid A did not prevent death among patients with gram-negative bacterial sepsis. These and other antibodies to endotoxin are being evaluated further. Other investigational agents include a human neutrophil protein that neutralizes endotoxin (bactericidal permeability-increasing protein) and nontoxic lipid A analogues that inhibit host responses to endotoxins.

ANTIMEDIATOR AGENTS Other adjunctive therapies for sepsis are designed to control the inflammatory response, regardless of the microbial stimulus. Of these agents, glucocorticoids have received most attention. However, two large-scale, randomized clinical trials of high-dose methylprednisolone therapy in patients with sepsis indicated that the regimens used did not prevent death or reverse septic shock. High-dose glucocorticoid therapy therefore is not currently recommended. Agents that directly interfere with cytokine actions, including recombinant IL-1 receptor antagonist, genetically engineered soluble receptors for TNFα, and monoclonal antibodies to TNFα, are now under evaluation. Since TNFα and IL-1β probably play some beneficial role in the host response to microbial invasion, anticytokine drugs could have both beneficial and detrimental consequences in patients with sepsis. Other investigational compounds include PAF antagonists, nitric oxide synthase inhibitors, pentoxifylline, soluble complement receptors (CR1), and anticoagulants such as recombinant α_1-antitrypsin Pittsburgh, antithrombin III, and protein C.

PROGNOSIS Overall, more than 25 percent of septic patients die. Although one-third of the deaths occur within the first 48 h after the onset of symptoms, mortality can occur 14 or more days later. Late deaths are often due to poorly controlled infection, complications of intensive care, or failure of multiple organs.

The risk of dying is influenced by the prior clinical condition of the patient and the rate at which complications develop. Patients with rapidly fatal diseases such as leukemia have higher case-fatality rates from sepsis than do patients with less severe underlying diseases. Analyses using prognostic stratification systems (such as the APACHE scoring system) indicate that factoring in the patient's age and certain physiologic variables results in more accurate estimates of the risk of dying. Variables associated with high case-fatality rates include ARDS, DIC, renal insufficiency, severe acidosis, hypothermia, altered mental status, and multiple organ dysfunction. Microbial variables are less important than host- and treatment-related factors, although high case-fatality rates have been observed for patients with sepsis due to *P. aeruginosa* and for patients with polymicrobial infection.

PREVENTION Prevention offers the best opportunity to reduce morbidity and mortality from sepsis. Most episodes of severe sepsis and septic shock are nosocomial complications; these cases might be prevented by reducing the number of invasive procedures, by limiting the use (and duration) of indwelling vascular and bladder catheters, by reducing the incidence and duration of profound neutropenia (<500 neutrophils per microliter), and by more aggressive treatment of localized nosocomial infections. Indiscriminate use of antimicrobial agents and glucocorticoids should be avoided, and optimal infection control measures (see Chap. 98) should be used. In addition, prompt and aggressive management of patients with early sepsis is imperative. Investigational approaches to preventing or damping the septic response include active and passive immunization to enhance antibody titers to key bacterial cell wall molecules, including endotoxin.

REFERENCES

AMERICAN COLLEGE OF CHEST PHYSICIANS/SOCIETY OF CRITICAL CARE MEDICINE CONSENSUS CONFERENCE COMMITTEE: Definitions for sepsis and organ failure and guidelines for the use of innovative therapies in sepsis. Crit Care Med 20:864, 1992

DANNER RL et al: Endotoxemia in human septic shock. Chest 99:169, 1991

GRANOWITZ EV et al: Production of interleukin-1-receptor antagonist during experimental endotoxaemia. Lancet 338:1423, 1991

HARRIS RL et al: Manifestations of sepsis. Arch Intern Med 147:1895, 1987

Increase in national hospital discharge survey rates for septicemia, United States, 1979–1987. Morb Mort Week Rep 39:31, 1990

KNAUS WA et al: The APACHE III prognostic system: Risk prediction of hospital mortality for critically ill hospitalized adults. Chest 100:1619, 1991

KREGER BE et al: Gram-negative bacteremia: IV. Re-evaluation of clinical features and treatment in 612 patients. Am J Med 68:344, 1980

MARTICH GD et al: Detection of interleukin 8 and tumor necrosis factor in normal humans after intravenous endotoxin: The effect of antiinflammatory agents. J Exp Med 173:1021, 1991

MARTIN MA et al: Gram-negative sepsis and the adult respiratory distress syndrome. Clin Infect Dis 14:1213, 1992

PARILLO JE: Septic shock in humans: Advances in the understanding of pathogenesis, cardiovascular dysfunction, and therapy. Ann Intern Med 113:227, 1990

SPRUNG CL et al: Impact of encephalopathy on mortality in the sepsis syndrome. Crit Care Med 18:801, 1990

SUFFREDINI AF et al: Promotion and subsequent inhibition of plasminogen activation after administration of intravenous endotoxin to normal subjects. N Engl J Med 320:1165, 1989

VAN DEVENTER SJH et al: Experimental endotoxemia in humans: Analysis of cytokine release and coagulation, fibrinolytic, and complement pathways. Blood 76:2520, 1990

VETERANS ADMINISTRATION SYSTEMIC SEPSIS COOPERATIVE STUDY GROUP: Effect of high-dose glucocorticoid therapy on mortality in patients with clinical signs of systemic sepsis. N Engl J Med 317:659, 1987

84 INFECTIOUS DISEASES OF THE UPPER RESPIRATORY TRACT

ROBERT LEBOVICS / ANN SULLIVAN BAKER

The head and neck form an anatomically complex region that includes the nose, paranasal sinuses, ears and mastoids, oral cavity, pharynx, and larynx. The functions of this region include the exchange and filtering of air, the intake and separation of food and liquids from the air stream entering the tracheobronchial tree, the expression of speech, and the senses of taste, smell, and hearing. Respiratory ciliated epithelium lines those portions involved in air exchange and filtration; squamous cells line the oral cavity, tongue, and oropharynx. The senses are controlled by a complex neural network, and local immunity is provided by a collection of lymphoid tissues. The proximity of these structures to the brain and mediastinum and the potential for airway obstruction require prompt recognition and treatment of head and neck infections.

NOSE AND FACE

EXTERNAL DISORDERS Any bacterial skin infection can affect the nose and face. Furunculosis commonly occurs around the nasal vestibule, in the region of the hair follicles. *Staphylococcus aureus* is the most commonly isolated pathogen. Infection in the nasal vestibule can spread to the cavernous sinus via facial veins that communicate with the central nervous system. Treatment of furunculosis should be prompt and consist of local heat and oral antibiotics with antistaphylococcal activity (see Chap. 102). Marked local edema, fever, or signs of generalized sepsis necessitate hospitalization and parenteral antibiotic therapy with careful evaluation for sinus or intracranial extension. Diabetic and immunocompromised patients are at especially high risk for rapid spread of infection. Incision and drainage of large lesions are usually necessary.

Staphylococcus aureus and group A beta-hemolytic *Streptococcus (e.g., S. pyogenes)* are the foremost agents of impetigo and erysipelas of the nose and face. Impetigo features skin pustules overlaid with yellow crusts. Erysipelas is a form of cellulitis, commonly in a malar distribution, with an advancing border raised above the surrounding skin. The area is red-hot, erythematous, and tender. Intravenous antibiotics with coverage of gram-positive pathogens are required (see Chaps. 102, and 103).

Lupus vulgaris is a form of tuberculosis involving the external nose and adjacent facial structures. The lesions appear as brown gelatinous nodules. Confirmatory histology and positive mycobacterial cultures are usually required for diagnosis; the therapy is the same as for tuberculosis (see Chap. 130). Syphilis (see Chap. 133) of the nose and face is rare and usually presents with a painless ulcerative lesion or chancre at the mucocutaneous junction of the nose or within the nasal septum several weeks after infection. Widespread secondary lesions, which usually progress as the primary lesion disappears, appear as erythematous papulosquamous eruptions, annular lesions, or condylomata. Tertiary syphilis presents with a nasal gumma and circumscribed swellings covering the inflamed mucosa; the nasal septum is usually involved, and destruction of the septal cartilage may ultimately lead to a cosmetic deformity known as "saddle-nose."

INTERNAL NASAL INFECTIONS Infection with *Mycobacterium tuberculosis* (see Chap. 130) in the nasal cavity is uncommon in the United States. Symptoms may include pain, nasal obstruction, rhinorrhea, and epistaxis. The septum and inferior turbinate are most commonly affected. Septal perforations are common, and the gross appearance of the lesion varies from ulceration to a papillomatous growth. Diagnosis is made by smear, culture, and deep submucosal biopsies that demonstrate tissue invasion by mycobacteria. *M. leprae* (see Chap. 131), the pathogen of leprosy, causes a chronic granulomatous inflammation of the superficial tissues of the nose and may extend to the face to involve either skin or peripheral nerves. Symptoms include epistaxis, nasal obstruction, crusting, and generalized signs of atrophic rhinitis. Nasal septal perforations and saddle-nose deformity are common.

Pseudomonas mallei causes glanders, which is a nasal infection transmitted to humans from horses (see Chap. 116). It produces an extensive ulcerative granulomatous disease of the nasal mucosa that causes pain, with mucopurulent discharge. Diagnosis is confirmed by both culture and histology, and treatment is with appropriate antibiotics. Rhinoscleroma is a granulomatous infection caused by *Klebsiella rhinoscleromatis* (see Chap. 115), prevalent mainly in Central America, Central Europe, and the Middle East. Clinical presentation includes atrophic rhinitis with foul-smelling rhinorrhea and crusting. The granulomatous inflammation progresses to severe fibrosis and stenosis of the nasal cavity. Culture of *K. rhinoscleromatis* from infected tissue is diagnostic, and histologically the McKulicz cell (or foamy histiocyte) is characteristic. Tetracycline is the drug of choice. Rhinosporidiosis is caused by *Rhinosporidium seeberi*, a fungus-like organism. The lesion usually presents with either sessile or pedunculated nasal growths; epistaxis, foul odor, and nasal obstruction are common. Surgical excision is followed by administration of dapsone.

Mucormycosis (see Chap. 168) is a life-threatening illness that classically presents in patients with diabetic ketoacidosis or severe neutropenia. Rapid diagnosis and treatment are essential as the infection quickly spreads to the paranasal sinuses, orbits, and central nervous system. Black crusts overlying necrotic tissues within the nasal cavity should heighten suspicion of mucormycosis. Histologic sections of deep tissue biopsies are required to confirm the diagnosis.

Actinomyces israelii (see Chap. 127) can cause a purulent abscess in the nasal cavity. Sulfur granules are a distinguishing histologic feature, and long-term parenteral penicillin treatment is indicated.

Histoplasmosis (see Chap. 162) usually involves the lungs, larynx, and tongue. Nodules and ulcers are frequently visualized; a classic epithelioid or histiocytic granuloma is seen in addition to the organisms within the granuloma.

Cryptococcus neoformans (see Chap. 165) frequently infects the central nervous system but can be localized in the nasal cavity. *Cryptococcus* classically produces granulomatous lesions without acute inflammation. *Blastomyces hominis* (see Chap. 164) also causes granulomatous and suppurative inflammation that involves the respiratory tract and extends from the nose to the face and paranasal sinuses.

PARANASAL SINUSES

ANATOMY AND DEVELOPMENT The paranasal sinuses are cavities within the facial skeleton that are lined by ciliated respiratory epithelium and drain into the nose. The maxillary and ethmoid sinuses are present at birth; the ethmoid labyrinth grows and expands with age, so that the anterior ethmoid cells usually project above the orbital rim to develop into the frontal sinuses. Unilateral agenesis of the frontal sinuses is common. The anterior table of the frontal sinus is composed of marrow-containing bone. The sphenoid sinuses are the last to develop and often do not mature until individuals reach their early twenties. The cavernous sinus lies laterally and proximal to the sphenoid sinus and is traversed by cranial nerves II, III, IV, V_1, and VI.

SINUSITIS In the immunocompetent host acute sinusitis is usually a bacterial infection that often follows a viral infection of the upper respiratory tract. Rhinovirus, adenovirus, and influenza and parainfluenza viruses may be recovered along with bacteria in about one-fifth of cases. It is estimated that 1 to 3 percent of upper respiratory infections are complicated by sinusitis. Adults have approximately two to three episodes of upper respiratory infection and children six to eight per year.

The major factor leading to sinusitis is obstruction of the ostia of the anterior ethmoid and middle meatal complex. The ethmoid ostia are very small, ranging from 1 to 2 mm in size. A viral upper respiratory infection leads to retained secretions secondary to mucosal edema, with obstruction of the sinus ostia and impaired drainage and precipitation of acute purulent sinusitis. Obstruction may also be due to allergy with swelling of the mucosa or secondary to polyps. The maxillary sinuses are the most common site of infections, followed by the ethmoids, frontal, and sphenoid sinuses.

Sinusitis has been recognized as a frequent nosocomial infection in the intensive care unit. The single greatest risk factor for the development of nosocomial sinusitis is prolonged (more than 48 h) intubation with a nasal tracheal or nasal gastric tube. In one study, purulent sinusitis occurred in one (1.9 percent) of 53 patients with oral tracheal tubes and in 25 (43 percent) of 58 patients with nasal tracheal tubes.

Barotrauma from deep sea diving and airplane travel are recognized precipitating factors for sinusitis. Other predisposing conditions include quantitative and qualitative ciliary transport abnormalities (e.g., ciliary syndromes, cystic fibrosis, Young's syndrome), excessive production of secretions, chronic granulomatous disease (e.g., Wegener's granulomatosis, sarcoid), and midline granuloma. Chemical irritants such as chlorine may impair secretion clearance and foster microbial proliferation.

Symptoms of acute sinusitis depend on the site of involvement. Patients with maxillary sinusitis have pain over the malar area and upper teeth. The infraorbital nerve runs through the maxillary route and the first and second molars often project into the sinus floor. Patients with anterior ethmoid sinusitis may complain of headache in the temporal or retroorbital area or the upper nose. Patients with posterior ethmoid sinusitis present with pain over the distribution of the trigeminal nerve, particularly around the mastoid area. With sphenoid sinusitis, the patient may complain of pain in the frontal, retroorbital, or facial area. Facial complaints are found in one-third of the patients. Nasal congestion and discharge frequently occur.

Evaluation of acute sinusitis requires good clinical judgment. Radiographs are not necessarily required for the first episode of sinusitis. If one chooses to evaluate the patient by radiograph, sinus films that include a lateral view are optimal. CT scanning is useful for evaluating the orbital areas, the sphenoid sinus, and the possibility of osteomyelitis. MRI should be limited to evaluation for fungal concretions or tumor. The bacteriology in acute sinusitis has been incompletely defined. The most common organisms include *S. pneumoniae*, *Haemophilus influenzae*, streptococci, and *Moraxella*, and in the intensive care unit, gram-negative organisms. *Staphylococcus aureus* is more common in sphenoid sinusitis. Rhinovirus, adenovirus, and influenza and parainfluenza viruses may be recovered in one-fifth of cases.

Symptoms of chronic sinusitis include nasal congestion and discharge. Pain may be intermittent; fever is uncommon. Patients may have a chronic cough due to a postnasal drip. CT scan is most useful for revealing bony erosion, mucopyoceles, or sclerosis. In addition to the organisms isolated in acute sinusitis, anaerobic bacteria and *S. aureus* are frequently found in chronic sinusitis. Patients with chronic sinusitis should be evaluated for granulomatous disease, ciliary dysfunction, and hypogammaglobulinemia.

Therapy of sinusitis Treatment must be directed at promoting adequate drainage. Patients should be instructed to decrease nasal swelling with vasoconstricting local agents such as oxymetazolin nasal spray. In addition to obstruction, the quality of mucus secretions is important. In patients with cystic fibrosis, for example, adequate hydration is often implemented to decrease mucus viscosity. Patients with sinusitis should inhale steam from a basin or hot shower to loosen secretions. Oral antihistamines thicken rather than liquify the material trapped within the sinuses and are not useful.

Antibiotic therapy is indicated in the setting of purulent discharge, fever, and leukocytosis. Amoxicillin-clavulanic acid, trimethoprim-sulfamethoxazole, or a second generation cephalosporin (such as cefuroxime-axetil) for 2 to 4 weeks are reasonable agents, assuming resolution of symptoms. Acute sinusitis that fails to clear completely after this time should be reevaluated and referred to the otolaryngologist for further medical and surgical attention.

Sinusitis is treated in the intensive care unit with removal of all nasal tubes and administration of appropriate antibiotics, including either oxacillin or vancomycin along with a third-generation cephalosporin or sulbactam-ampicillin. Sinus puncture by the otolaryngologist may be useful for obtaining aerobic and anaerobic material. Pus from the ostium is suboptimal culture material as the nasopharynx is colonized. Patients with sinusitis that has not resolved may be evaluated by endoscopy to investigate possible anatomic cause and obtain adequate specimens for culture. If symptoms persist in chronic sinusitis, endoscopic sinus surgery may be required to obtain a histologic diagnosis, remove polyps, and establish proper ventilation of the infected sinuses.

Complications of sinusitis Infection of the frontal sinus mucosal wall may spread to the bone directly or by thrombophlebitis of the veins from sinus mucosa to diploic veins of the frontal bone. The infection may spread externally to the outer table and result in cortical breakthrough and periosteal abscess (Potts' puffy tumor). Inferior extension results in involvement of upper ethmoid cells and the roof of the orbit or in a periosteal abscess; posterior extension results in epidural abscess. Clinical presentation of frontal bone osteomyelitis includes a local soft doughy swelling. Evaluation should be by CT or MRI. Bacterial pathogens include *S. aureus*, streptococci,

anaerobes, and gram-negative organisms. Antibiotic therapy should be given intravenously for 4 weeks with a combination of agents such as (1) oxacillin, metronidazole, and a second- or third-generation cephalosporin or (2) ampicillin-sulbactam. Surgical drainage of the infected sinus is necessary should medical therapy fail.

Intracranial complications of sinusitis include cerebral epidural abscess, subdural empyema, cerebral abscess, and thrombosis of the large dural sinuses (cortical thrombophlebitis) (see Chap. 374). The most common intracranial complications of sphenoid sinusitis are meningitis and cavernous vein thrombophlebitis. The wall of the cavernous sinus surrounds the sphenoid sinus, thereby allowing easy access to the cavernous sinus and central nervous system. The patient with cavernous sinus thrombophlebitis presents with evidence of nerve palsies in cranial nerves III, IV, V_1, and VI. Patients should be evaluated with CT or MRI. Intravenous antibiotics are required, and drainage of the sphenoid sinus is important if the patient does not improve on antibiotics alone.

The most frequent extracranial complication is spread of infection to the orbit from an infected ethmoid sinus. The medial border of the orbit is also the lateral border of the ethmoid labyrinth. Acute ethmoid sinusitis can result in infection traversing the thin plate separating the bone to cause an orbital cellulitis. Orbital cellulitis is accompanied by pain, lid edema, and conjunctival chemosis (erythema, swelling). Orbital cellulitis requires hospitalization, broad spectrum intravenous antibiotics, and drainage of the sinus if no improvement is seen in 48 h.

FUNGAL SINUSITIS This condition may be divided into (1) allergic, e.g., secondary to *Aspergillus* (see Chap. 167) or *Dreschlera* infection; (2) invasive sinusitis caused by organisms such as *Aspergillus, Curvularia,* and *Alternaria;* (3) rhinocerebral phycomycosis caused by genera of the class Zygomycetes. The patient with allergic fungal sinusitis may be treated symptomatically and may benefit from glucocorticoid therapy. Some patients may also have accompanying bronchopulmonary aspergillosis and a hypersensitivity type of allergic infection in the sinuses. Bronchospasm occurs, and Charcot-Leyden crystals (proteins originating in the cytoplasm of eosinophils) may be found in the discharge. Consultation with an allergist is advisable to coordinate possible glucocorticoid therapy. Patients with chronic invasive sinusitis should be treated with intravenous amphotericin or another antifungal agent appropriate for the specific organism (see Chap. 161). Patients with phycomycosis are often diabetic, leukemic, or otherwise immunocompromised. These patients need rapid, wide debridement of the infected area and intravenous amphotericin.

Candidiasis also can present as chronic sinusitis (see Chap. 166).

EAR

ACUTE OTITIS MEDIA Viral upper respiratory tract infection is most commonly associated with acute otitis media. The hallmark of middle ear infection is pain. A sense of fullness, purulent otorrhea, hearing loss, vertigo or tinnitus, fever, and leukocytosis may be present. Otoscopic examination will confirm the diagnosis of acute otitis media by demonstrating a red, dull, and bulging or perforated tympanic membrane. *S. pneumoniae* (approximately 35 percent) and *H. influenzae* (approximately 20 percent) are the bacteria most frequently isolated from middle ear effusions in acute otitis media. The majority of *H. influenzae* isolates are nontypable strains. In children, infection by *H. influenzae* type b can cause severe systemic toxicity and may be associated with meningitis. Other commonly isolated bacteria include *Branhamella catarrhalis,* group A, *Streptococcus,* and *S. aureus.* Mixed anaerobic bacteria can occasionally cause acute otitis media. Respiratory viruses such as respiratory syncytial and influenza viruses are implicated in the pathogenesis but are rarely cultured.

Treatment of acute otitis media includes the use of antibiotics such as amoxicillin-clavulanic acid, trimethoprim-sulfamethoxazole, and cefuroxime-axetil. Antihistamines have not proven effective. Occasionally, in refractory cases, tympanocentesis is required for bacteriologic diagnosis. In persistent infection, a myringotomy with or without the insertion of a ventilating tube may be necessary. Severe pain, infection in immunologically compromised patients, and failure of antibiotic therapy are indications for surgical drainage of the middle ear space. Bullous myringitis may be associated with mycoplasma infection, while multiple perforations of the tympanic membrane suggest tuberculosis.

SEROUS OTITIS MEDIA   Serous otitis media with chronic effusion is a leading cause of hearing loss in children and occasionally in adults. Otoscopic examination will show a retracted tympanic membrane associated with fluid in the middle ear cavity. Pure tone audiometry and tympanometry can reveal a conductive hearing loss and a flat tympanogram consistent with restrictive disease in the middle ear space.

Therapy can be divided into conservative and surgical approaches. Decongestants, antihistamines, and glucocorticoids have been advocated in the treatment of serous effusions, although their usefulness is unproven. Antibiotics have been used as well as mechanical insufflation via the eustachian tube (politerization). Control of predisposing factors may include the treatment of allergy, nasal infection, or chronic sinus infection. Occasionally the use of ventilating tubes is required for management of a chronic effusion in the middle ear with or without infection. This provides drainage for an infected middle ear and will improve a conductive hearing loss caused by the accumulation of serous fluid in the middle ear. Unilateral serous otitis media in an adult should raise suspicion of a noninfectious process, e.g., tumor.

Mastoiditis   The mastoid air cells are patent with the middle ear unless blocked by an intervening mass. Because of the direct communication between the two cavities, every case of otitis media is in the truest sense a mastoiditis. The organisms causing mastoid infections are generally those that cause acute middle ear infections. Radiographs of the mastoid air cells frequently demonstrate fluid or mucosal thickening within the honeycomb labyrinth of the mastoid suggesting chronic infection. Treatment is similar to that of acute otitis media.

Intravenous antibiotics and emergency mastoidectomy are indicated when there are high fever and leukocytosis with radiographic evidence of destruction of trabeculae and the honeycombing of the mastoid air cells. Signs of acute otitis media are usually evident. A subperiosteal abscess may be present, in which case examination will reveal an ear that is displaced inferiorly and laterally, with a red fluctuant mass behind the pinna. When abscess is suspected clinically, CT scanning will usually confirm the diagnosis.

Chronic otitis media with otorrhea is defined as a chronic draining ear resulting from untreated acute or recurrent otitis media. The bacterial flora are variable. *Pseudomonas aeruginosa* and *S. aureus* are the most commonly isolated aerobic organisms, followed by *Escherichia coli* and *Proteus* species. Chronic, foul-smelling otorrhea may indicate anaerobic infection (one-third of patients). Chronic suppuration of the middle ear is associated with perforation of the tympanic membrane and may be associated with cholesteatoma (involuted squamous epithelium and keratin debris) formation. Imaging by conventional radiography or CT will show mucosal thickening in the middle ear space as well as in the mastoid cavity. Cholesteatoma may erode the temporal bone and rarely enters the cranial cavity. Treatment is directed at eradicating infection with a combination of local care, antibacterial ear drops, and systemic antibiotics selected according to antibiotic sensitivities defined by cultures. Cholesteatomas must be excised.

COMPLICATIONS OF OTITIS MEDIA AND MASTOIDITIS   Extracranial complications of otitis media and mastoiditis include conductive, sensorineural, and mixed hearing loss. Other complications include labyrinthitis manifested by vertigo as well as weakness or complete paralysis of the ipsilateral facial nerve. Gradenigo's syndrome consists of otalgia, a draining middle ear, and paralysis of the ipsilateral sixth cranial nerve, reflecting infection of the petrous

apex of the temporal bone. Cultures of draining material should be obtained. Therapy requires antibiotics directed at organisms that cause otitis media and they should be adjusted based on culture results. Surgical intervention should be reserved for refractory cases. Intracranial complications of otitis media include meningitis, brain abscess, epidural abscess, lateral sinus thrombophlebitis, and otitic hydrocephalus.

EXTERNAL OTITIS   The external auditory canals are lined by skin and are subject to the same diseases of skin as the rest of the body. Psoriasis may be the cause of an external otitis. Glands within the external auditory canal secrete cerumen, which acidifies the external auditory canal and minimizes the overgrowth of bacteria. Otitis externa ("swimmer's ear") is most common in the summer months and is thought to arise from a change in the milieu of the external auditory canal by increased alkalinization, which leads to the overgrowth of bacteria, most commonly *Staphylococcus*, *Streptococcus*, and *Pseudomonas* species. Treatment includes topical antibacterial ear drops, although occasionally systemic antibiotics (choice based on antibiotic sensitivities) are required. Mycotic infections causing otitis externa are diagnosed by smears and culture and are treated with topical antifungal ear drops. *Herpes zoster* in the external auditory canal can cause an associated loss of the sensory and motor functions of the facial nerve (Ramsay-Hunt syndrome); acyclovir is helpful in treating severe otalgia.

Necrotizing (malignant) otitis externa   This progressive necrotizing infection results in osteomyelitis of the temporal bone and is almost always caused by *P. aeruginosa*. The soft tissues and cartilage of the pinna may also be involved. The disorder occurs most commonly in patients with insulin-dependent diabetes mellitus. The diagnosis should be suspected in patients with swelling of the external canal and severe pain. Physical examination will often reveal granulation tissue in the posterior ear canal wall that is eroding into the temporal bone. The auricle and surrounding scalp may be swollen, tender, and necrotic. CT and bone scans are useful for making the diagnosis. Treatment consists of local care including debridement and antibacterial ear drops combined with intravenous antibiotics directed against *P. aeruginosa* (see Chap. 116). Good control of coexisting diabetes mellitus may hasten recovery. Occasionally radical surgical debridement of the temporal bone is required. Gallium scanning is helpful in monitoring recovery.

Perichondritis   Perichondritis is an infection or inflammation of the cartilage of the pinna usually arising after trauma. The most common organism isolated in infectious perichondritis is *P. aeruginosa*. The lobule is spared infection because it contains no cartilage. Relapsing polychondritis is an inflammatory disease of the external ear that initially may mimic infection and needs to be distinguished from perichondritis.

PHARYNX

ORAL CAVITY   The oral cavity begins at the vermilion border of the lips and extends posteriorly to the circumvallate papillae of the tongue. *Gingivitis* is inflammation of the gums covering the maxilla and mandible. Anaerobic bacteria are the usual cause of gingivitis. Poor oral and dental hygiene, tobacco use, and excessive alcohol are the main predisposing factors. Vincent's angina (also known as trench mouth or acute necrotizing ulcerative gingivitis) is usually caused by *Borrelia vincenti*, a fusiform bacillus. Patients will present with malodorous breath, excessive salivation, and frequent perigingival bleeding. Treatment is a combination of oral penicillin and hygiene.

Herpes viruses (see Chap. 143) infect the lip, causing common cold sores and lesions on the buccal mucosa, tongue, and pharyngeal wall. Patients complain of severe pain and odynophagia. Characteristic pustular eruptions are visible over the mucosa. Diagnosis is confirmed by viral culture or immunofluorescence staining. Herpes zoster can present similarly, and the treatment is a combination of local care, acyclovir, and analgesia. Herpangina, caused by group A coxsackievirus, can present with pain, dysphagia, odynophagia, and fever. Thrush, caused by *Candida albicans,* usually affects immunocompromised patients. Oral antifungals will control the overgrowth. Cancrum oris may occur in severely debilitated patients. Noma is a mixed bacterial infection of the oral cavity caused by fusospirochetal bacteria and/or streptococci. In developing countries with poor sanitation and hygiene, noma is associated with high rates of mortality. Treatment requires a combination of debridement, local care, and parenteral antibiotics directed at oral bacteria (see Chap. 128).

Ludwig's angina (see Chap. 128) is a rapidly progressing life-threatening infection that frequently follows a lower molar tooth infection with spread to the submandibular or sublingual space. Patients present with pain, dysphagia, drooling, fever, and leukocytosis. The floor of the mouth is red, inflamed, and swollen. The tongue is pushed posteriorly and superiorly and ultimately causes airway obstruction. Prompt hospitalization to control the airway, followed by possible incision and drainage and parenteral antibiotics (directed at oral bacteria) is the treatment of choice. The bacteriology is mixed, with anaerobic streptococci predominating.

OROPHARYNX   The cause of acute pharyngitis is almost always infection, although pharyngeal inflammation and ulceration may be caused by agranulocytosis, trauma, or injury by chemicals or radiation. The major symptom of acute pharyngitis regardless of etiology is sore throat, with or without associated dysphagia. Examination may reveal exudate, erythema, and mucosal congestion with hypertrophy of the lymphoid tissue, particularly the palatine tonsils. The presence of exudate suggests bacterial infection, particularly by group A beta-hemolytic streptococci (see Chap. 103). *Neisseria gonorrhoeae* (see Chap. 110) can cause pharyngeal exudate but special culture technique is required to confirm its presence. *Corynebacterium diphtheriae* (see Chap. 104) pharyngitis can become life-threatening. A pseudomembrane over the mucosa can enlarge to the point of airway obstruction. Examination reveals a dark gray mucosa. *Mycoplasma pneumoniae* (see Chap. 139) and the TWAR strains of *Chlamydia* (see Chap. 140) can cause exudative pharyngitis. Exudate may be seen with a variety of viral infections, in particular those caused by Epstein-Barr virus, herpes simplex virus, or adenovirus. Infection with respiratory syncytial, parainfluenza, and influenza viruses may also cause pharyngitis without exudate; in rhinovirus infections a "scratchy" throat may be a prominent feature.

Pus that accumulates between the middle pharyngeal constrictor and the tonsillar capsule constitutes a peritonsillar abscess. Patients complain of fever, pain, dysphagia, and odynophagia and speak with a "hot potato" voice. Physical examination reveals trismus, unilateral swelling, and deviation of the uvula. Incision and drainage provides prompt relief.

LARYNX

SIGNS AND SYMPTOMS OF LARYNGEAL DISEASE   Persistent, unexplained change in the voice, e.g., hoarseness or weakness, is pathognomonic of laryngeal disorders. Other symptoms include cough that may be dry or associated with the production of clear, purulent, or blood-streaked sputum; pain that may refer to other branches of the vagus nerve, manifested by otalgia; and upper respiratory obstruction causing stridor. Dysphagia and odynophagia may develop with either infectious or neoplastic lesions of the larynx. Besides evaluation of the neck, oropharynx, and gag and swallowing reflexes, physical examination should include an indirect mirror examination and, if available, flexible fiberoptic endoscopy. Vocal cord dysfunction, mass lesions, mucosal ulceration, infection of the larynx, structural abnormalities, and occasionally subglottic lesions will be evident on these inspections. Definitive diagnosis requires biopsy, usually under anesthesia, and culture, if possible.

LARYNGEAL INFECTIONS   Acute epiglottitis (supraglottitis)
This is a rapidly progressive cellulitis of the epiglottis and surrounding tissues in the supraglottic airway. It can cause acute airway obstruction. In infants and children the causative agent is most commonly *H. influenzae* type b, and bacteremia is frequent.

In adolescents and adults with acute bacterial epiglottitis, the clinical presentation may be less fulminant and other organisms have been implicated in some cases *(S. pneumoniae, S. aureus).* Frequently, the patient complains of dysphagia, odynophagia, and fever that has progressed over 1 to 2 days. Depending on the degree of respiratory obstruction, stridor may or may not be present, but hoarseness and loss of voice power are almost universal findings. As in children, the adult with epiglottitis usually leans forward, drooling oral secretions. Because the caliber of the airway is larger in the adult, intubation or tracheotomy may not be necessary, but the possibility of complete airway obstruction dictates management. Edematous, cherry-red epiglottis and surrounding pharyngeal mucosa are characteristic findings on fiberoptic examination, which in adults is the best way to confirm the diagnosis (see below). In infants and children this approach is contraindicated because of the threat of acute airway obstruction. A lateral radiograph of the neck may reveal an enlarged epiglottis—the so-called "thumb sign."

Until the possibility of airway obstruction has passed, the patient is best managed by admission to an intensive care unit where adequate monitoring is available. In adults, fiberoptic examination with a nasopharyngoscope should be performed only after preparations have been made to secure the airway by endotracheal intubation or, if necessary, tracheotomy. After blood is obtained for culture, appropriate intravenous antibiotic treatment is initiated with cefuroxime or a third-generation cephalosporin such as cefotaxime. Oxygen should be administered as dictated by O_2 saturations on pulse oximetry or arterial blood gas determination. Humidified air by face tent is advisable. If respiratory obstruction worsens, endotracheal intubation is required. Glucocorticoids have been administered as part of the treatment but with unproven benefit. Resolution of clinical manifestations usually occurs over 36 to 48 h. A child should not be extubated nor a patient removed from an intensive care setting unless the acute cellulitis has resolved, as confirmed by endoscopy.

Croup (laryngotracheobronchitis)   Croup is a syndrome produced by acute infection of the lower air passages and is most commonly seen in children below age 3. The most common pathogen is the parainfluenza virus, but a variety of respiratory viruses and *Mycoplasma pneumoniae* can produce acute laryngotracheobronchitis and the croup syndrome. The pathophysiology is primarily one of circumferential mucosal inflammation in the subglottic larynx and trachea, with variable involvement and spasm of the vocal cords; the epiglottis is not involved. The clinical hallmark is a barking or brassy cough with or without stridor and hoarseness. Croup can be readily distinguished from epiglottitis by lateral films of the neck, which show no epiglottal edema, or by careful direct examination. Management of severe croup requires hospitalization, close observation, humidification, oxygenation as dictated by pulse oximetry, and rarely intubation. Glucocorticoid administration has been advocated by some, but the benefits are questionable.

Tuberculous laryngitis   Tuberculous laryngitis is usually associated with active pulmonary tuberculosis. Characteristic manifestations include hoarseness, cough, and blood-tinged sputum; because of the large number of organisms in the sputum, it is usually highly contagious. The most common site of laryngeal disease is the interarytenoid fold (in the posterior portion of the larynx). Because granulomas tend to be subepithelial, deep submucosal biopsies may be essential for diagnosis. Treatment is the same as for pulmonary tuberculosis (see Chap. 130), and symptomatic measures include voice rest and analgesics for pain. Occasionally tracheostomy is needed to protect the airway.

Fungal infections   The most commonly found fungal infections, usually in immunocompromised patients, are histoplasmosis (Chap. 162); candidiasis (Chap. 166); and blastomycosis (Chap. 164). Symptoms can include hoarseness, cough, dyspnea, dysphagia, and odynophagia. Examination may reveal oral and esophageal thrush (candidiasis) or nodules on the vocal cords with or without ulceration (histoplasmosis or blastomycosis). With the latter, diagnosis is confirmed by biopsy showing microabscesses in an epithelium infiltrated with giant cells, mononuclear cells, and yeast. Treatment with systemic antifungal agents is necessary.

Other laryngeal infections These include tertiary syphilis, lepromatous leprosy, diphtheria, glanders, and actinomycosis. Biopsy is usually required for the diagnosis of syphilis and leprosy, both of which may produce infiltrating nodular lesions.

PERICHONDRITIS Perichondritis in the larynx due to pyogenic bacterial infection or an inflammatory process may be difficult to distinguish from traumatic injury, certain neoplasms, or injury induced by radiation. The thyroid cartilage is the most common cartilage affected, and an abscess may form beneath the mucoperichondrium. Symptoms and signs include pain, tenderness, and swelling that are usually slowly progressive but occasionally acute. Hoarseness, airway compromise, dysphagia, and odynophagia require prompt radiographic evaluation to exclude the possibility of a foreign body. The airway should then be secured in the operating room. Treatment may require antibiotics directed at the causative agent or glucocorticoids and debridement of laryngeal granulations.

DEEP NECK INFECTIONS

Deep neck infections are often difficult to diagnose clinically, and the potential for rapid spread and death should not be underestimated. Detailed knowledge of neck spaces and fascial planes facilitates the understanding of etiology, symptoms, complications, and treatment of these infections. Infections of the submandibular, lateral pharyngeal (parapharyngeal), and retropharyngeal spaces are particularly onerous, because pus in these locations can cause airway obstruction or spread contiguously to such structures as the mediastinum or carotid sheath.

The lateral pharyngeal space (also called the parapharyngeal or pharyngomaxillary space) can become infected from a variety of sources, including the palatine tonsils, pharynx, parotid gland, and infected lymph nodes that drain the pharynx and nose. Dental infections, particularly those originating from the third mandibular molar can spread to either the submandibular or the lateral pharyngeal spaces. Diabetics are particularly susceptible to such infections. The mode of spread includes direct dissection through the fascial spaces or direct extension from other communicating spaces within the neck. Lymphatic spread or septic thrombosis of peritonsillar veins can also precede lateral pharyngeal space infection. Clinical manifestations include fever, leukocytosis, and deep neck pain. Dysphagia and/or odynophagia may be present. On physical examination, one may see edema over the parotid gland; on intraoral examination, there may be medial bulging and displacement of the pharyngeal wall. Trismus may also be present. CT scanning with contrast can help to define the location of infection. Treatment consists of securing the airway, following external drainage in the operating room. The most common complication is a septic thrombosis of the internal jugular vein; clinical features include shaking chills with fever spikes, and tenderness at the mandibular angle. The diagnosis is confirmed by MRI. Intravenous antibiotic treatment should be directed against *Fusobacterium, Peptostreptococcus, Porphyromonas,* and *Prevotella* (see Chap. 128) for several weeks. Surgical removal of the thrombosed vein is reserved for special circumstances. Anticoagulation therapy is controversial. Complications of the thrombosed internal jugular vein include septic pulmonary emboli, lateral sinus thrombosis, cavernous sinus thrombosis, and brain abscess. Carotid artery "blowouts" are a rare but possibly fatal complication of lateral pharyngeal space infections. Clinical features include sentinel bleeding from the nose, mouth, or ear. Ipsilateral Horner's syndrome and cranial neuropathy (IX to XII) can be associated with an impending blowout. Sentinel bleeding is an acute surgical emergency that necessitates major vessel ligation. Inferior spread of infection along the carotid sheath may progress into the chest causing mediastinitis. Mortality rates approach 50 percent when mediastinitis is present.

SUBMANDIBULAR SPACE INFECTIONS See Ludwig's angina above under "Oral Cavity."

RETROPHARYNGEAL SPACE INFECTION The retropharyngeal space extends from the base of the skull superiorly to the level of the tracheal bifurcation inferiorly. It contains lymph nodes and connective tissue. The source of infection is usually located cephalad from the nose, sinuses, adenoids, and nasopharynx. Infection may extend from the lateral pharyngeal space to the retropharyngeal space directly or secondary to lymphatic spread. The greatest number of retropharyngeal lymph nodes are found in children under the age of 5 years, which accounts for the greater incidence of retropharyngeal space abscesses in this age group. These lymph nodes, including the adenoidal lymphoid pad, involute over time and are thus less likely to cause infection in older children.

Retropharyngeal space infections in young children are primarily complications of acute upper respiratory tract infections. Dysphagia and odynophagia are common and, in advanced cases, drooling is present. There is cervical rigidity and a hot-potato voice. Advanced infections present with dyspnea and/or stridor. Treatment includes securing of an airway, emergency surgical drainage, and intravenous antibiotics. In some cases, intraoral drainage may be accomplished; advanced cases, however, may require an external approach. Complications include intraoral rupture of the abscess, with secondary aspiration and pneumonia. Mediastinitis and airway obstruction are potentially life-threatening complications.

The microbiology of the various deep neck infections is similar. The most common organisms are *Streptococcus pyogenes, Peptostreptococcus, Prevotella, Porphyramonas,* and *Fusobacterium.* Many deep neck infections have mixed flora, with the majority of bacteria sensitive to a combination of penicillin G and metrinidazole or ampicillin-sulbactam.

REFERENCES

ALLAN BP et al: Orbital abscess of odontogenic origin. Case report and review of the literature. Int J Oral Maxillofac Surg 20:268, 1991

BROOK I: Diagnosis and management of anaerobic infections of the head and neck. Ann Otol Rhinol Laryngol Suppl 155:9, 1992

CHOW AW: Life threatening infections of the head and neck. Clin Infect Dis 14:991, 1992

DE FOER et al: Sinus aspergillosis. J Craniomaxillofac Surg 18:33, 1990

DUDLEY JP: *Branhamella catarrhalis* and croup: Toxicity in the upper respiratory tract. Am J Otolaryngol 12:113, 1991

ENGLISH GM (ed): *Otolaryngology,* revised edition. New York, Harper & Row, 1993

EVANS et al: Sinusitis of the maxillary antrum. N Engl J Med 293:735, 1975

GOYCOOLES MV et al: Otitis media. Otolaryngol Clin Am 24:757, 1991

LEW D et al: Sphenoid sinusitis: A review of 30 cases. N Engl J Med 309:1149, 1983

PARADISE JL: Etiology and management of pharyngitis and pharyngotonsillitis in children: A current review. Ann Otol Rhinol Laryngol Suppl 155:51, 1992

RANDALL DA et al: Indications for tonsillectomy and adenoidectomy. Am Fam Physician 44:1639, 1991

RUBEN RJ et al: Recent advances in otitis media. Complications and sequelae. Ann Otol Rhinol Laryngol Suppl 139:46, 1989

SALORD E et al: Nosocomial maxillary sinusitis during mechanical ventilation: A prospective comparison of orotracheal versus the nasotracheal route for intubation. Intens Care Med 16:390, 1990

SINAVE CP et al: The Lemierre syndrome: Suppurative thrombophlebitis of the internal jugular vein secondary to oropharyngeal infection. Medicine 68:85, 1989

---

85 INFECTIVE ENDOCARDITIS

DONALD KAYE

DEFINITION Infective endocarditis is an infection which produces vegetations on the endocardium. It is virtually always fatal if untreated. A heart valve is usually involved, but infection may be on a septal defect or mural endocardium. Infection of an arteriovenous shunt or coarctation of the aorta is more properly called *endarteritis* and produces a similar clinical syndrome. The subsequent discussion of endocarditis also applies to endarteritis.

CLASSIFICATION

Endocarditis can be divided into native valve endocarditis, endocarditis in intravenous drug abusers, and prosthetic valve endocarditis, each with different infecting microorganisms and courses. Endocarditis also can be classified as acute or subacute. Acute endocarditis most frequently is caused by *Staphylococcus aureus*, occurs on a normal heart valve, is rapidly destructive, produces metastatic foci, and, if untreated, is fatal in less than 6 weeks. Subacute endocarditis usually is caused by viridans streptococci, occurs on damaged valves, does not produce metastatic foci, and, if untreated, takes more than 6 weeks or even a year to be fatal. Correlations between organism and course are not perfect. Viridans streptococci can be associated with an acute course and *S. aureus* with a subacute course. Most important is classification by infecting organisms (e.g., *S. aureus* endocarditis), because the organism has implications for therapy as well as course.

NATIVE VALVE ENDOCARDITIS Etiology Although almost any bacteria can produce endocarditis, streptococci, enterococci, and staphylococci account for the vast majority of cases.

STREPTOCOCCI Streptococci cause about 55 percent of cases of native valve endocarditis in patients who do not abuse intravenous drugs. Viridans streptococci (most commonly *S. sanguis*, *S. mutans*, or *S. milleri*) account for about 75 percent of these; *S. bovis* and other streptococci cause 20 and 5 percent, respectively. Viridans streptococci are normal inhabitants of the oropharynx and generally are highly susceptible to penicillin. Two group D streptococci, *S. bovis* and *S. equinus*, are also highly susceptible to penicillin G. *S. bovis* endocarditis occurs in elderly individuals; 80 percent of cases are in persons over 60 years of age. More than a third of these individuals have a malignant or premalignant gastrointestinal lesion, most often colonic cancer or a villous adenoma or polyp of the colon.

Group A beta-hemolytic streptococci attack normal or damaged heart valves and may cause their rapid destruction. Group B streptococci, which have been reported as an increasing cause of endocarditis in recent years, also attack normal valves and result in large friable vegetations and large emboli. Other streptococci are much more likely to infect damaged valves and rarely cause rapid valve destruction. *S. milleri* can cause metastatic abscesses, which are uncommon with other streptococci.

ENTEROCOCCI Enterococci cause about 6 percent of cases of native valve endocarditis. Enterococci are alpha-, beta-, or gamma-hemolytic and are normal inhabitants of the gastrointestinal tract, the anterior urethra, and occasionally the mouth. All enterococci are in Lancefield's group D and may be distinguished from streptococci by biochemical tests. They are relatively resistant to penicillin G, and an aminoglycoside must be added to achieve a bactericidal effect. Enterococcal endocarditis is most common in males, who develop infection at an average age of 60, while the average age of women with enterococcal endocarditis is under 40. Many patients give a recent history of genitourinary tract manipulation, trauma, or disease (e.g., cystoscopy, urethral catheterization, prostatectomy, abortion, pregnancy, or cesarean section), which occur mainly in older men and younger women.

STAPHYLOCOCCI Staphylococci cause about 30 percent of cases of native valve endocarditis (with *S. aureus* 5 to 10 times more frequent than *S. epidermidis*). *S. aureus* attacks normal or damaged heart valves, often causing rapid destruction. The course is often fulminant, with death from bacteremia within days or heart failure within weeks. Abscesses are common at multiple sites (e.g., kidneys, lungs, and brain). *S. epidermidis* infects abnormal valves without causing rapid destruction.

HACEK ORGANISMS The HACEK group of bacteria (*Haemophilus*, *Actinobacillus*, *Cardiobacterium*, *Eikenella*, and *Kingella*) are part of the oropharyngeal flora. They produce endocarditis with a subacute presentation and very large vegetations. They are difficult to isolate from blood.

OTHER BACTERIA Almost all species of bacteria are occasional causes of endocarditis, including *Strep. pneumoniae*, *Neisseria gonorrhoeae*, enteric gram-negative bacilli, *Pseudomonas*, *Salmonella*, *Streptobacillus*, *Serratia marcescens*, *Bacteroides*, *Brucella*, *Mycobacterium*, *N. meningitidis*, *Listeria*, *Legionella*, and diphtheroids, and can result in an acute or chronic course.

FUNGI Fungi rarely cause native valve endocarditis in persons who do not abuse intravenous drugs. However, *Candida* and *Aspergillus* endocarditis can occur in patients with intravascular catheters who frequently have received glucocorticoids, broad-spectrum antimicrobial drugs, or cytotoxic agents. The course is usually subacute. Large friable vegetations are common and give rise to large emboli, often to the lower extremities. The prognosis is grave, partly because of the relatively poor activity of available antifungal agents.

OTHER MICROORGANISMS Spirochetes (e.g., *Spirillum minor*), cell wall–deficient bacteria, rickettsiae (*Coxiella burnetii*), and chlamydiae (*C. psittaci*, *C. pneumoniae*, and *C. trachomatis*) are rare causes of endocarditis.

Epidemiology In native valve endocarditis, the proportion of males is higher than females, and most patients are over age 50. Endocarditis is uncommon in children.

Between 60 and 80 percent of patients have an identifiable predisposing cardiac lesion. *Rheumatic valvular disease* accounts for about 30 percent of cases. The mitral valve is most commonly involved, followed by the aortic. Right-sided endocarditis usually affects the tricuspid valve but is rare on rheumatic valves.

Congenital heart disease other than mitral valve prolapse is the underlying lesion in about 10 to 20 percent of patients with endocarditis. Predisposing lesions include patent ductus arteriosus, ventricular septal defect, tetralogy of Fallot, coarctation of the aorta, pulmonary stenosis, and bicuspid aortic valve but not uncomplicated atrial septal defect. *Mitral valve prolapse* is the underlying lesion in about 10 to 33 percent of cases.

Degenerative heart disease predisposes to endocarditis. *Calcific aortic stenosis* (from degenerative disease or bicuspid valve) is an important lesion in the elderly. Other predisposing but unusual lesions are *asymmetric septal hypertrophy*, *Marfan's syndrome*, and *syphilitic aortic valve*. Arterioarterial or *arteriovenous fistulas* also can be underlying lesions. In 20 to 40 percent of patients with infective endocarditis, *no underlying heart disease* can be recognized.

ENDOCARDITIS IN INTRAVENOUS DRUG ABUSERS Drug abusers with endocarditis are frequently young males. The skin is the most frequent source of microorganisms responsible for endocarditis; contamination of drugs is less common. *S. aureus* causes over 50 percent of cases, streptococci and enterococci about 15 percent, and fungi (mainly *Candida*) and gram-negative bacilli (usually *Pseudomonas* species) about 10 percent each. Infection with multiple organisms is common. The onset is usually acute. Only about 20 percent of addicts with their first episode of endocarditis have previously damaged heart valves. The tricuspid valve is infected in over 50 percent of cases, the aortic in 25 percent, and the mitral in about 20 percent. Over 75 percent with *S. aureus* infection and a much lower percent with other organisms have tricuspid valve endocarditis. Pulmonary emboli or pneumonia consequent to septic pulmonary emboli is common in tricuspid valve endocarditis, and murmurs are frequently absent.

PROSTHETIC VALVE ENDOCARDITIS Any intravascular prosthesis predisposes to endocarditis and makes cure difficult. Infections of prosthetic valves now account for 10 to 20 percent of cases of endocarditis. Intravascular sutures, pacemaker wires, and Teflon-Silastic tubes also can be foci of infection. Patients with prosthetic valve endocarditis are mainly males over age 60. Endocarditis occurs in 1 to 2 percent of these patients during the first year after operation and in 1 percent per year thereafter. Aortic valve prostheses are much more likely to be involved than mitral valve prostheses. The infection is usually on the suture line.

Early-onset endocarditis (onset of symptoms within 60 days of surgery) is usually a consequence of valve contamination during the procedure or bacteremia perioperatively. *Late-onset endocarditis* (onset of symptoms after 60 days) may have the same pathogenesis as early endocarditis (especially during the first year) but with a long incubation period or may result from transient bacteremia.

About half the episodes of early and one-third of late endocarditis are caused by staphylococci, and *S. epidermidis* is more frequent than *S. aureus*. Gram-negative bacilli cause up to 15 percent and fungi (most commonly *Candida*) up to 10 percent of early cases and are less common in late endocarditis. A prosthetic valve may malfunction because of large vegetations (often fungal). Streptococci are the most frequent single cause of late endocarditis (about 40 percent of cases) but are uncommon in early endocarditis.

Early prosthetic valve endocarditis is often associated with valve dysfunction or dehiscence and a fulminant course. Although late endocarditis may be similarly fulminant, the course is commonly indistinguishable from that of patients without prosthetic valves, especially when the organism is a streptococcus.

PATHOGENESIS AND PATHOLOGY

The characteristic lesions of infective endocarditis are vegetations on valves or elsewhere on endocardium. The disease usually arises secondary to localization of microorganisms on sterile vegetations composed of platelets and fibrin. Sterile vegetations, termed *nonbacterial thrombotic endocarditis*, form over areas of trauma to the endothelium (e.g., from intracardiac foreign bodies), in areas of turbulence (as on deformed valves), over scars, or in patients with wasting disease, particularly malignancy (marantic endocarditis).

Infection of a sterile vegetation is most likely when bacteremia occurs with bacteria that adhere well to platelets, fibrin, and fibronectin. The vegetation of infective endocarditis then results from deposition of platelets and fibrin over the bacteria, forming a "protected site" into which phagocytic cells penetrate poorly.

Endocarditis tends to occur in high-pressure areas (left side of heart) and downstream from where blood flows through a narrow orifice at a high velocity from a high- to low-pressure chamber (e.g., distal to the constriction in coarctation of the aorta). Endocarditis is unusual in sites with a small pressure gradient, as in atrial septal defects. Endocarditis occurs more frequently in valvular incompetence than in pure stenosis and is characteristically on the atrial side of the regurgitant mitral valve and the ventricular surface of the regurgitant aortic valve. A high-velocity stream of blood can produce satellite-infected lesions at distant points of impact.

Microorganisms that possess little pathogenicity in other situations, e.g., viridans streptococci, usually implant only on deformed heart valves with nonbacterial thrombotic endocarditis, but more virulent microorganisms, e.g., *S. aureus* and *Strep. pneumoniae*, can infect apparently normal valves.

Transient bacteremia is common in various infections and during traumatic procedures involving epithelial surfaces that are colonized by a bacterial flora (oropharynx, genitourinary and gastrointestinal tracts, and skin). For example, after trauma to tissues of the mouth, viridans streptococci are the most common bacteria isolated from blood, alone or more often mixed with other bacteria. The frequency and magnitude of bacteremia are related to the severity of periodontal disease and the severity of trauma. The portal of entry for the initiating episode of bacteremia is usually not apparent in viridans streptococcal endocarditis. Dental procedures, the most common apparent portals of entry, precede viridans streptococcal endocarditis in only 15 to 20 percent of cases.

Bacteremia also is common with prostatic surgery, cystoscopy, urethral dilation or catheterization, and procedures on the female reproductive tract. The organisms are usually enterococci and gram-negative bacilli. About 50 percent of patients with enterococcal endocarditis have had a recent operation or instrumentation on the genitourinary or gastrointestinal tract. About 35 percent with staphylococcal endocarditis have had a preceding staphylococcal infection at a remote site.

The clinical features of endocarditis result from the vegetations and an immune reaction to the infection. Extensive vegetations, especially in fungal endocarditis, may occlude the valve orifice. Rapid destruction with consequent valvular regurgitation may occur, especially with *S. aureus*. Healing may cause scar formation with subsequent valvular stenosis or regurgitation. Infection may extend into the myocardium, producing burrowing abscesses. Conduction abnormalities, fistulas (between chambers of the heart and the pericardium or major vessels), or rupture of the chordae, a papillary muscle, or the ventricular septum may result.

Pieces of vegetation break off and embolize to the heart, brain, kidney, spleen, liver, extremities, and lung (in right-sided endocarditis). Infarcts and occasionally abscesses result. Septic embolization to the vasa vasorum or direct bacterial invasion of the arterial wall may result in formation of mycotic aneurysms, which may rupture. Mycotic aneurysms most often develop in the cerebral arteries, aorta, sinuses of Valsalva, ligated ductus arteriosus, and the superior mesenteric, splenic, coronary, and pulmonary arteries.

Patients with endocarditis usually have high antibody titers against the infecting microorganism. This contributes to formation of circulating immune complexes that may result in glomerulonephritis (focal, membranoproliferative, or diffuse), arthritis, or various mucocutaneous manifestations of vasculitis.

Myocarditis may be due to small coronary artery emboli, myocardial abscesses, or immune complex vasculitis.

MANIFESTATIONS

Symptoms of endocarditis generally start within 2 weeks of the precipitating event. With organisms of low pathogenicity (e.g., viridans streptococci), the *onset* is usually gradual, with mild fever and malaise. With organisms of high pathogenicity (e.g., *S. aureus*), the onset is often acute with high fever. *Fever* is present in almost all patients with endocarditis (except occasionally in the elderly or those with renal failure, congestive heart failure, or severe debility). The fever is usually low grade (less than 39.4°C) except with acute disease. Arthralgias are common, and arthritis occurs occasionally.

Cardiac murmurs are almost always present except early in acute endocarditis or in intravenous drug abusers with tricuspid valve infection. True changes in murmurs or the appearance of a new murmur is uncommon except in acute endocarditis, where a new murmur (particularly aortic regurgitation) is frequent. Changes in intensities of murmurs are often due to changes in heart rate and/or cardiac output (e.g., from anemia) and not necessarily to progressive valvular damage.

Splenomegaly and *petechiae* each tend to occur in about 30 percent of cases, mainly in disease of long duration. Petechiae are most frequently found on the conjunctivae, palate, buccal mucosa, and upper extremities. *Splinter hemorrhages* are subungual, linear, dark-red streaks that may appear in endocarditis but also commonly result from trauma. *Roth spots* (oval, retinal hemorrhages with a clear pale center) are seen in less than 5 percent of patients and also may occur in connective tissue disease and severe anemia. *Osler nodes* (small tender nodules, usually on the finger or toe pads, which persist for hours to days) occur in 10 to 25 percent of patients but also in other diseases. *Janeway lesions* are small hemorrhages with a slightly nodular character on the palms and soles and are most commonly seen in acute endocarditis. *Clubbing* of the fingers is present in some patients with long-standing disease. *Embolic episodes* are recognized in about one-third of patients and may occur during or after therapy. Emboli to large arteries (e.g., femoral arteries) are often the result of fungal endocarditis with its large friable vegetations. Pulmonary emboli are common in drug abusers with right-sided endocarditis and may be seen in left-sided endocarditis with left-to-right cardiac shunts.

Mycotic aneurysms occur in about 10 percent of patients. Symptoms are usually lacking but may be those of an expanding mass. The aneurysms can rupture during or even years after therapy. *Neurologic manifestations* are present in about one-third of patients with endocarditis and are more common with left-sided endocarditis than with right-sided disease and with *S. aureus* infection than with viridans streptococcal infection. Clinically apparent cerebral emboli occur in about 20 percent of patients, encephalopathy (from microemboli with or without microabscess formation) in 10 percent, leakage from mycotic aneurysm in less than 5 percent, and meningitis or macroscopic brain abscess in less than 5 percent. Major cerebral emboli as well as mycotic aneurysms usually involve the middle cerebral artery system. The majority of patients with brain abscess or purulent meningitis have *S. aureus* endocarditis. *Heart failure* may occur during the course of the disease or long after cure. Contributing factors are valve destruction, myocarditis, coronary artery emboli with infarction, and myocardial abscesses. *Myocardial abscess* most commonly occurs with acute endocarditis (most commonly *S. aureus*) or with a prosthesis. Conduction defects may result from ventricular septal invasion secondary to extension from a valve (most frequently the aortic valve). A valve ring abscess or less commonly a myocardial abscess may extend into the epicardium and cause pericarditis. Echocardiography may be helpful in the diagnosis of myocardial abscess, and surgery is often indicated, especially with a prosthesis. *Renal disease* is present in most patients with endocarditis and is due to renal emboli or glomerulonephritis. Renal insufficiency may result.

LABORATORY FEATURES

A normocytic normochromic anemia is usual in infective endocarditis. The white blood cell and differential counts are often normal. However, in acute disease, leukocytosis without anemia may be present. Proteinuria and/or microscopic hematuria is found in most patients, and the serum creatinine level may be elevated. The erythrocyte sedimentation rate is almost always elevated except when heart failure is present.

About 50 percent of patients with endocarditis of at least 6 weeks' duration have a positive serum test for rheumatoid factor, and virtually all have circulating immune complexes. These tend to disappear with cure. The serum complement level may be decreased, especially with diffuse glomerulonephritis. Bacteria can be seen inside leukocytes in buffy coat preparations of blood in about 50 percent of patients with endocarditis.

The critical diagnostic finding in endocarditis is bacteremia or fungemia. Blood cultures are positive in over 95 percent of patients. The bacteremia is continuous; if any cultures are positive, all are likely to be positive. There is no advantage to obtaining cultures at any particular time or body temperature. Arterial blood or bone marrow offers no advantage over antecubital vein blood.

In subacute disease, in the absence of previous therapy, three cultures should be obtained over 3 to 6 h and therapy initiated. With previous therapy, treatment may be expeditiously delayed in an attempt to obtain positive blood cultures. In general, in acute disease, therapy should not be delayed for more than 2 to 3 h while obtaining cultures. Only one culture should be obtained from each venipuncture; anaerobic as well as aerobic techniques should be used. Cultures should be spaced at least 30 to 60 min apart to demonstrate continuous bacteremia. The rate of positive cultures is increased by observing them over 3 weeks with periodic sampling for Gram stain and subculture even in the absence of turbidity. Addition of pyridoxal hydrochloride to the media will improve the chances of isolating nutritionally deficient variant streptococci.

Blood cultures may be negative in infections with fastidious organisms such as *Haemophilus parainfluenzae*. Fifty percent of patients with *Candida* endocarditis and almost all with *Aspergillus*, *Histoplasma*, and *Coxiella burnetii* endocarditis have negative blood cultures. With fungi, large peripheral emboli are common, necessitat-

ing embolectomy. Histologic examination and culture of the embolus may be diagnostic. Serologic tests for *C. burnetii* and *C. psittaci* are positive in endocarditis caused by these organisms.

Although not diagnostic, transthoracic echocardiograms will demonstrate the vegetation in 50 to 80 percent of patients with native valve endocarditis. Transesophageal echocardiograms are much more sensitive (positive in over 90 percent of cases) and are much more likely to demonstrate intracardiac abscesses. Serial phonocardiography and cineradiography are useful in evaluating infection on prosthetic valves. Disappearance of an opening click or sound produced by a closing valve suggests the presence of a vegetation. With dehiscence, cineradiography of the valve will show abnormal motion.

DIAGNOSIS

Endocarditis should be suspected either when a heart murmur and unexplained fever are present for at least 1 week or in febrile intravenous drug abusers, even in the absence of a murmur. However, a definitive clinical diagnosis requires positive blood cultures.

Atrial myxoma, nonbacterial thrombotic endocarditis, acute rheumatic fever, lupus erythematosus, and sickle cell disease can duplicate the syndrome of infective endocarditis. Any patient with an existing heart murmur can develop fever related to another occult illness or to drugs. Therefore, in the absence of positive blood cultures, a search must be made for other causes of fever.

Following cardiac surgery, fever may be related to infection at other sites, to the postcardiotomy syndrome, or to a "postpump syndrome" (e.g., cytomegalovirus infection).

TREATMENT

PRINCIPLES OF THERAPY Cure of endocarditis requires eradication of all microorganisms from the vegetation. Therefore, microbicidal drug regimens must be used in high enough concentrations and for a long enough duration to sterilize the vegetation. Regimens including penicillins, cephalosporins, and vancomycin give far better results than when these drugs cannot be used because of resistant organisms or drug reactions.

The minimal inhibitory and bactericidal concentrations (MIC and MBC) should be determined. To follow efficacy of therapy for a drug regimen, it may be useful to measure the bactericidal activity of the patient's serum against his or her isolate. A bactericidal titer of $\geq 1:8$ in serum drawn 30 min after drug infusion probably indicates adequate therapy. While this determination is not necessary in most cases, it may be useful when infection is caused by organisms other than gram-positive cocci, treatment has failed, or regimens do not include penicillins, cephalosporins, or vancomycin. Except for unusual circumstances, antibiotic administration should be parenteral to guarantee adequate absorption of drugs. The infecting microorganism should be saved for future testing (e.g., serum antibacterial activity, evaluation of different antibiotics, or comparison with a relapse strain).

SPECIFIC ANTIMICROBIAL REGIMENS Therapy before culture results are known The treatment of subacute infective endocarditis on a native valve while awaiting culture results should be for enterococci, which are more resistant to antibiotics than streptococci.

With an acute course, therapy should be directed against *S. aureus*. In intravenous drug abusers, initial therapy should be directed against *S. aureus*, and gentamicin should be included for the possibility of gram-negative bacilli. In many cities, most *S. aureus* isolated from drug abusers are methicillin-resistant, and vancomycin must be used. With prosthetic valves, vancomycin plus gentamicin should be used because of the high incidence of methicillin-resistant *S. epidermidis* and the need to cover enterococci.

Once the organism is isolated, the regimen should be altered appropriately. If cultures remain sterile and culture-negative endocarditis is likely, treatment is continued provided that the response is adequate.

Streptococci with MIC of ≤0.1 µg/mL penicillin G   Most streptococci are inhibited by serum concentrations of 0.1 µg/mL penicillin
G. Three regimens including penicillin G (Table 85-1) can be used
for these highly penicillin-susceptible strains. Penicillin G alone for
4 weeks (regimen A) gives cure rates of 99 percent. Addition of
gentamicin or streptomycin (regimen B) results in a more rapid
bactericidal effect and gives equivalent cure rates in 2 weeks. Regimen
B should be standard for uncomplicated infection, but regimen A is
preferred in patients likely to have side effects with aminoglycosides
(i.e., those with renal insufficiency or eighth nerve disease or older
than 65 years). Penicillin for 4 weeks with an aminoglycoside for the
first 2 weeks (regimen C) is used for nutritionally deficient variant
strains, a relapse, or complications (e.g., metastatic abscesses).
Regimen D can be substituted with a history of a delayed rash to
penicillin. Regimen E should be used with a history of anaphylaxis
to penicillin.

**Streptococci with MIC of > 0.1 µg/mL but < 0.5 µg/mL penicil-
lin G**   Endocarditis caused by streptococci with MIC of >0.1 but
<0.5 µg/mL penicillin G is managed with regimen F, a compromise
between the regimens for highly susceptible (MIC ≤ 0.1 µg/mL) and
relatively resistant (MIC ≥ 0.5 µg/mL) streptococci.

**Enterococci or streptococci with MIC of ≥ 0.5 µg/mL penicil-
lin G**   Penicillin, ampicillin, and vancomycin are not bactericidal for
most enterococci. With the addition of an aminoglycoside, a synergistic bactericidal effect occurs. Enterococcal endocarditis requires
penicillin, ampicillin, or vancomycin plus an aminoglycoside for cure
of most patients (regimens G and H, with H used for hypersensitivity
to penicillin G). An alternative to regimen H consists of skin testing
with major and minor determinants of penicillin, followed by attempts
at desensitization to penicillin. This process involves a scratch test
through a drop of penicillin G (100 units per mL), followed in 30
min by graded amounts of penicillin intradermally, begun at 0.01

unit in 0.1 mL of saline solution and continued in tenfold increments
every 30 min; with increasing amounts, administration is changed
to the subcutaneous, intramuscular, and finally intravenous route.
Epinephrine and diphenhydramine should be on hand for emergency
use during the procedure in case of anaphylaxis, and preferably the
procedure should be carried out in an intensive care unit. If a reaction
occurs, alternative therapy should be initiated.

Therapy is usually given for 4 weeks but is prolonged to 6 weeks
when symptoms have been present for longer than 3 months or the
course is complicated. Cephalosporins cannot be used in enterococcal
endocarditis because the organisms are highly resistant.

A synergistic bactericidal effect against enterococci occurs with
penicillin and aminoglycosides only when growth is inhibited by
2000 µg/mL of the aminoglycoside. Synergism is most likely
with gentamicin. However, enterococci resistant to 2000 µg/mL of
gentamicin are now common. Some of these gentamicin-resistant
strains are inhibited by 2000 µg/mL of streptomycin, but most are
resistant to 2000 µg/mL of all aminoglycosides. With aminoglycoside-
resistant strains, it may be best to exclude aminoglycosides from the
regimen and treat for 6 to 8 weeks. However, relapses may occur.
Isolates of enterococci have been observed that are highly resistant
to penicillin (either by production of penicillinase or other mechanisms) or vancomycin. Therefore, in vitro susceptibility testing of
enterococci is required to choose appropriate therapy.

Endocarditis caused by streptococci with MIC ≥ 0.5 µg/mL is
managed in the same way as enterococcal endocarditis.

Staphylococci   Methicillin-susceptible *S. aureus* and *S. epidermidis* are treated with regimen I or J. Methicillin-resistant staphylococci are resistant to all penicillins and cephalosporins. In these cases,
or in patients who cannot tolerate penicillins or cephalosporins,
vancomycin as in regimens K and L must be used. Some experts
advocate addition of gentamicin for the first 3 to 5 days because of

---

TABLE 85-1   Therapy of infective endocarditis caused by gram-positive cocci*

STREPTOCOCCI† WITH MIC ≤ 0.1 µg/mL PENICILLIN G

Regimen A	Penicillin G, 10–20 million units/d IV in divided doses every 4 h × 4 weeks *or*
Regimen B	Penicillin as in regimen A plus streptomycin, 7.5 mg/kg IM every 12 h or gentamicin, 1 mg/kg IV every 8 h, both × 2 weeks *or*
Regimen C	Penicillin plus streptomycin or gentamicin × 2 weeks as in regimen B with penicillin continued 2 weeks longer *or*
Regimen D	Cefazolin, 1–2 g IV or IM every 6–8 h × 4 weeks *or*
Regimen E	Vancomycin, 15 mg/kg IV every 12 h × 4 weeks

STREPTOCOCCI WITH MIC > 0.1 BUT < 0.5 µg/mL PENICILLIN G

Regimen F	Use regimen C *or* regimen E if penicillin allergic

ENTEROCOCCI OR STREPTOCOCCI WITH MIC ≥ 0.5 µg/mL PENICILLIN G

Regimen G	Penicillin G, 20–30 million units/d or ampicillin, 12 g/d IV in divided doses every 4 h plus gentamicin, 1 mg/kg IV every 8 h or streptomycin, 7.5 mg/kg IM every 12 h, both × 4–6 weeks *or*
Regimen H	Vancomycin, 15 mg/kg IV every 12 h plus gentamicin or streptomycin as in regimen G, both × 4–6 weeks

METHICILLIN-SUSCEPTIBLE *S. AUREUS* OR *S. EPIDERMIDIS*

Regimen I	Nafcillin, 2 g IV every 4 h × 4–6 weeks with or without gentamicin, 1 mg/kg IV every 8 h × the first 3–5 d *or*
Regimen J	Cefazolin, 2 g IV every 6 h × 4–6 weeks with or without gentamicin as in regimen I *or*
Regimen K	Vancomycin, 15 mg/kg IV every 12 h × 4–6 weeks with or without gentamicin as in regimen I

METHICILLIN-RESISTANT STAPHYLOCOCCI OR *CORYNEBACTERIUM SP.*

Regimen L	Vancomycin with or without gentamicin as in regimen K

ENDOCARDITIS CAUSED BY THE ABOVE ORGANISMS ON A PROSTHETIC VALVE

Regimen C but with 20 million units of penicillin each day and a longer duration of penicillin (a total of 6 weeks)
Regimen D × 6 weeks with gentamicin or streptomycin × the first 2 weeks
Regimen E × 6 weeks with gentamicin or streptomycin × the first 2 weeks
Regimen F, but continue penicillin × 6 weeks
Regimen G or H × 6 weeks
Regimen I, J, or K × 6–8 weeks with gentamicin × the first 2 weeks
Regimen L × 6–8 weeks with gentamicin × the first 2 weeks
In the presence of *S. epidermidis* also add rifampin, 300 mg orally every 8 h × 6–8 weeks. The use of rifampin with *S. aureus* is controversial.

* Peak serum concentrations of gentamicin should be about 3 µg/mL. Streptomycin peaks should be about 20 µg/mL. The maximum dose of vancomycin is 1 g every 12 h.
† For Group A streptococci or *S. pneumoniae* use regimen A.
NOTE: MIC = minimal inhibitory concentration.

an increase in the rate of bactericidal activity. However, clinical evidence of improved outcome is lacking and routine use of the drug is not recommended. Four weeks' therapy is standard, but with metastatic or intracardiac abscess (or other complications) therapy should be extended to 6 weeks or even longer.

Streptococci, enterococci, and staphylococci in prosthetic valve endocarditis Prolonged therapy (Table 85-1) and combinations with an aminoglycoside are usual. When a methicillin-resistant *S. epidermidis* is involved, addition of rifampin improves outcomes.

In vitro testing with added rifampin has shown a synergistic bactericidal effect with some staphylococci and an antagonistic one with others. Except for the case of *S. epidermidis*, addition of rifampin is controversial and therefore should be based on poor clinical response and in vitro evidence of synergism.

HACEK organisms Therapy for the HACEK group consists of ampicillin (2 g every 4 h IV) or a third-generation cephalosporin (e.g., ceftriaxone 1 g every 12 h IV or IM) plus gentamicin (1.7 mg/kg every 8 h IV) for 4 weeks.

Other organisms In endocarditis caused by other organisms, bactericidal antibiotics, preferably a penicillin, cephalosporin, or vancomycin with or without an aminoglycoside, should be given and therapy continued for 4 to 6 weeks. With gram-negative bacilli, the penicillin or cephalosporin which has the greatest potency against the infecting bacteria in vitro should be administered in large doses intravenously along with an aminoglycoside to which the bacterium is susceptible (e.g., ampicillin, 2 g every 4 h; piperacillin, 3 g every 4 h; cefotaxime, 2 g every 4 to 6 h; or ceftazidime, 2 g every 8 h; plus gentamicin, 1.7 mg/kg every 8 h). A quinolone such as ciprofloxacin alone, which is bactericidal for gram-negative bacilli, also should be useful.

With *Corynebacterium* species, which are often resistant to all penicillins and cephalosporins, regimen L in Table 85-1 is most likely to be effective.

When the organisms are resistant to penicillins, cephalosporins, quinolones, and vancomycin, therapy will probably be unsuccessful. Under these circumstances, treatment should be with the bactericidal drug grouping that demonstrates the best activity in vitro. If the response is poor or relapse occurs, antimicrobial therapy plus valve replacement will probably be necessary.

HOME THERAPY Home therapy is very cost effective and has been used successfully with stable, non-IV drug users who are highly motivated, able to administer the therapy, and living with someone else. Ceftriaxone, 2 g IV once daily, for streptococcal endocarditis, and vancomycin, 1 g IV every 12 h, for streptococcal and staphylococcal endocarditis, have been used most frequently.

SURGERY IN THE MANAGEMENT OF ENDOCARDITIS When appropriate microbicidal therapy is not available (as in fungal endocarditis) or positive blood cultures persist on therapy or relapse occurs after appropriate therapy, replacement of the valve should be considered. Ideally, surgery should be performed after several days of the best available antimicrobial therapy. With organisms that tend to produce metastatic foci, therapy should then be continued long enough to eradicate these foci. Persistence of infection with the same organism following valve replacement has been uncommon. Immediate replacement (even after only hours of therapy) is essential in patients developing heart failure secondary to severe valvular regurgitation. Surgery is necessary to drain myocardial or valve ring abscesses and should be considered with recurrent emboli despite adequate antimicrobial therapy. It also should be considered in patients with aortic valve endocarditis who develop first- and second-degree atrioventricular block. In some centers, the presence of a large vegetation on echocardiography may be an indication for surgery.

Replacement of a prosthesis is often necessary for infections with organisms other than streptococci, for valve dysfunction or dehiscence, or for myocardial invasion. Myocardial invasion is common with prosthetic valves and is suggested by continued fever after 10 days of therapy, a new regurgitant murmur, and/or atrioventricular conduction disturbance.

COURSE

Defervescence usually occurs after 3 to 7 days of antimicrobial therapy. Blood cultures should be obtained periodically during treatment and generally become negative after several days of therapy. Lack of response of fever and bacteremia may be associated with myocardial or metastatic abscess formation (especially associated with *S. aureus*).

The most common cause of persistent or recurrent fever during therapy is a drug reaction; less commonly, emboli are responsible. If a rash develops, therapy can be continued and antihistamines or even glucocorticoids given to suppress the reaction. If the rash is severe, therapy should be altered.

Weight gain and a rise in hemoglobin may not be seen until weeks after therapy has been completed. Petechiae, Osler nodes, and emboli may occur during and for weeks after successful antimicrobial therapy. Mycotic aneurysms may regress on drug therapy or may rupture weeks to years later. Heart failure may occur during or after therapy and is the principal cause of death.

Anticoagulants should be used only with a pressing indication (such as certain prosthetic valves, but not including infected emboli) because of increased risk of hemorrhage (especially intracranial). Warfarin is preferable to heparin. Blood cultures 2 and 4 weeks after discontinuation of the therapy detect the vast majority of relapses.

PROGNOSIS

Factors that predispose to a poor prognosis are (1) nonstreptococcal disease, (2) development of heart failure, (3) aortic valve involvement, (4) infection on a prosthetic valve, (5) older age, and (6) valve ring or myocardial abscess. The cure rate in streptococcal endocarditis is about 90 percent. Failures are not due to uncontrolled infection but to death from heart failure, embolus, rupture of mycotic aneurysm, or renal failure. The mortality rate in nonaddicts with *S. aureus* endocarditis is at least 40 percent, and most deaths are due to overwhelming infection or heart failure. In drug addicts with *S. aureus* infection on the tricuspid valve, cure rates are over 90 percent, and in the absence of infected emboli, therapy has been successful with 2 weeks of nafcillin plus an aminoglycoside. Results are poor in endocarditis caused by fungi and gram-negative bacilli resistant to penicillins and cephalosporins. The presence of large vegetations on echocardiogram may indicate a poorer prognosis than small or absent vegetations. About 10 percent of patients will have additional episodes of endocarditis, months or years later. The prognosis in early prosthetic valve endocarditis is much worse than in late disease, with mortality rates of 40 to 80 percent versus 20 to 40 percent.

ANTIMICROBIAL PROPHYLAXIS OF ENDOCARDITIS

Although the risk of endocarditis is small and there is no proof of efficacy, prophylaxis is recommended for patients with predisposing cardiac lesions undergoing procedures known to cause bacteremia. The conditions for which prophylaxis is recommended are valvular or congenital heart disease (except uncomplicated atrial septal defect), intracardiac prostheses, asymmetric septal hypertrophy, and previous episode of endocarditis. Mitral valve prolapse increases the risk of endocarditis to a low to moderate extent. However, it is so common that it is neither risk- nor cost-effective to give prophylaxis to all patients with prolapse for all procedures. It is, however, reasonable to use prophylaxis in individuals with mitral valve prolapse who have holosystolic murmurs and who presumably are at greatest risk. The finding of thickened redundant mitral valve leaflets on echocardiography apparently also selects a subset of patients at greater risk.

Oral hygiene should be optimal in patients with cardiac lesions that predispose to endocarditis, especially those who are to have prosthetic cardiac valves implanted.

For dental and other procedures in the mouth, nose, or throat likely to cause bleeding or significant trauma, prophylaxis is aimed at viridans streptococci. The regimen recommended by the American Heart Association is amoxicillin, 3 g orally 1 h before the procedure followed by 1.5 g 6 h later. With penicillin allergy, the recommendation is 800 mg oral erythromycin ethylsuccinate or 1.0 g erythromycin stearate 2 h before the procedure or 300 mg oral clindamycin 1 h before, in each case followed by half the dose 6 h later. In high-risk patients (e.g., those with prosthetic valves), an alternative but optional more stringent regimen is ampicillin, 2 g intramuscularly or intravenously, plus gentamicin, 1.5 mg/kg intramuscularly or intravenously, both 30 min before the procedure, and amoxicillin, 1.5 g orally, 6 h later or, with penicillin allergy, vancomycin, 1 g intravenously over 1 h starting 1 h before the procedure.

For genitourinary and gastrointestinal tract procedures likely to cause significant trauma (e.g., cystoscopy, prostatic surgery, and colonic or gallbladder surgery), prophylaxis is directed against enterococci. The regimen is ampicillin plus gentamicin as above. With penicillin allergy, the vancomycin regimen above is given, but 1.5 mg/kg gentamicin, given intravenously or intramuscularly, is added 1 h before the procedure. For low-risk patients, amoxicillin may be used, 3 g orally 1 h before the procedure, followed by 1.5 g 6 h later. Fiberoptic endoscopy, even with biopsy, is so low risk for endocarditis that prophylaxis is difficult to justify. If used, it should be only in high-risk patients.

Prophylaxis for cardiac surgery with placement of intracardiac prostheses, patches, or sutures is directed against staphylococci and has usually consisted of 2 g cefazolin intravenously plus 1.5 mg/kg gentamicin intravenously starting immediately preoperatively, followed by repeated doses 8 and 16 h later. However, since strains of *S. epidermidis* may be methicillin-resistant, substitution of vancomycin for cefazolin in a dose of 15 mg/kg intravenously over 1 h starting 1 h before the procedure, 10 mg/kg after completion of bypass, and then 7.5 mg/kg every 6 h for 3 doses is reasonable. Vancomycin also can be used when patients have hypersensitivity to penicillins and cephalosporins.

Patients with coronary artery bypass grafts or transvenous pacemakers in place do not require prophylaxis for endocarditis, nor is it indicated for patients undergoing cardiac catheterization.

REFERENCES

ABRUTYN E, KAYE D: Prevention of bacterial endocarditis: 1991. Ann Intern Med 114:803, 1991

BISNO AL et al: Antimicrobial treatment of infective endocarditis due to viridans streptococci, enterococci and staphylococci. JAMA 261(10):1471, 1989

CHAMBERS HF et al: Right-sided *Staphylococcus aureus* endocarditis in intravenous drug abusers: Two-week combination therapy. Ann Intern Med 109:619, 1988

DAJANI AS et al: Prevention of bacterial endocarditis: Recommendation by the American Heart Association. JAMA 264:2919, 1990

DANIEL WG et al: Improvement in diagnosis of abscesses associated with endocarditis by transesophageal echocardiography. N Engl J Med 324:795, 1991

DURACK D: Prophylaxis of infective endocarditis, in *Principles and Practice of Infectious Diseases*, 3d ed, GL Mandell et al (eds). New York, Churchill Livingstone, 1990

KANTER MC, HART RG: Neurologic complications of infective endocarditis. Neurology 41:1015, 1991

KAYE D (ed): *Infective Endocarditis*, 2d ed. New York, Raven Press, 1992

KORZENIOWSKI O, KAYE D: Infective endocarditis, in *Heart Disease*, 4th ed, E Braunwald (ed). Philadelphia, Saunders, 1992

MARKS AR et al: Identification of high-risk and low-risk subgroups of patients with mitral-valve prolapse. N Engl J Med 320:1031, 1989

SCHELD M, SANDE M: Endocarditis and intravascular infections, in *Principles and Practice of Infectious Diseases*, 3d ed, GL Mandell et al (eds). New York, Churchill Livingstone, 1990

SHIVELY BK et al: Diagnostic value of transesophageal compared with transthoracic echocardiography in infective endocarditis. J Am Coll Cardiol 18:391, 1991

STECKELBERG JM et al: Emboli in infective endocarditis: The prognostic value of echocardiography. Ann Intern Med 114:635, 1991

THRELKELD M, COBBS G: Infections of prosthetic valves and intravascular devices, in *Principles and Practice of Infectious Diseases*, 3d ed, GL Mandell et al (eds). New York, Churchill-Livingstone, 1990

86   INTRAABDOMINAL INFECTIONS AND ABSCESSES

DORI F. ZALEZNIK / DENNIS L. KASPER

Intraperitoneal infections generally arise because a normal anatomic barrier is disrupted. This disruption may occur when the appendix, a diverticulum, or an ulcer ruptures; when the bowel wall is weakened by ischemia, tumor, or inflammation (e.g., in inflammatory bowel disease); or with adjacent inflammatory processes, such as pancreatitis or pelvic inflammatory disease, in which enzymes (in the former case) or organisms (in the latter) may leak into the peritoneal cavity. Whatever the inciting event, once inflammation develops and organisms usually contained within the bowel or another organ enter the normally sterile peritoneal space, a predictable series of events takes place. Intraabdominal infections occur in two stages: peritonitis and—if it goes untreated—abscess formation. The types of microorganisms predominating in each stage of infection are responsible for the pathogenesis of disease.

PERITONITIS

The peritoneal cavity is large but divided into compartments. The upper and lower peritoneal cavities are divided by the transverse mesocolon; the greater omentum extends from the transverse mesocolon and from the lower pole of the stomach to line the lower peritoneal cavity. The pancreas, duodenum, and ascending and descending colons are located in the anterior retroperitoneal space; the kidneys, ureters, and adrenals are found in the posterior retroperitoneal space. The other organs, including liver, stomach, gallbladder, spleen, jejunum, ileum, transverse and sigmoid colon, cecum, and appendix, are found within the peritoneal cavity itself. Normally the cavity is lined with a serous membrane that can serve as a conduit for fluids—a property utilized in peritoneal dialysis. A small amount of fluid sufficient to allow movement of organs is normally present in the peritoneal space. This fluid is serous, with a protein content (consisting mainly of albumin) of <30 g/L and fewer than 300 white blood cells (WBCs, generally mononuclear cells) per microliter. Certain of the compartments in the peritoneal cavity more commonly than others collect fluid or pus in the presence of infection. These include the pelvis (the most dependent portion), the subphrenic spaces on both the right and left, and Morrison's pouch, which is a posterior, superior extension of the subhepatic spaces and is the most dependent area of the paravertebral groove when a patient is recumbent. The falciform ligament separating the right and left subphrenic spaces appears to act as a barrier to the spread of infection; consequently, it is unusual to find bilateral subphrenic collections.

SPONTANEOUS BACTERIAL PERITONITIS   Peritonitis is either primary (without apparent inciting event) or secondary. The types of organisms found and the clinical presentation of these two processes are different. In adults primary or spontaneous bacterial peritonitis (SBP) occurs most commonly in conjunction with cirrhosis of the liver (frequently the result of alcoholism). It virtually always develops in patients with ascites. Nevertheless, it is not a common event, occurring in no more than 10 percent of cirrhotic patients. The cause of SBP has not been established definitively but is believed to involve hematogenous spread of organisms with the diseased liver and altered portal circulation resulting in a defect in the usual filtration function. Organisms are able to multiply in ascites, a good medium for growth. The proteins of the complement cascade have been found in peritoneal fluid, with lower levels in cirrhotic patients than in patients with other causes of ascites. The opsonic and phagocytic properties of neutrophils are also decreased in patients with advanced liver disease.

The presentation of SBP differs from that of secondary peritonitis. The most common manifestation is fever, which is documented in as many as 80 percent of patients. Ascites is found but virtually always predates infection. Abdominal pain, an acute onset of symptoms, and peritoneal irritation detected during physical examination can be helpful diagnostically, but the absence of any of these findings does not exclude this often subtle diagnosis. It is vital to sample the peritoneal fluid of any cirrhotic patient with ascites and fever. The finding of more than 300 polymorphonuclear leukocytes (PMNs) per microliter is diagnostic for SBP, according to Conn. The microbiology of SBP also is distinctive. While enteric gram-negative bacilli such as *Escherichia coli* are the most common organisms encountered, gram-positive organisms such as streptococci, enterococci, or even pneumococci are sometimes found. The characteristic microbiologic features of SBP are that generally only a single organism is recovered and anaerobes are rarely found. This microbiologic picture contrasts with that of secondary peritonitis, in which a mixed flora, including anaerobes, is the rule. In fact, if SBP is suspected and multiple organisms, including anaerobes, are recovered from the peritoneal fluid, the diagnosis must be reconsidered and a source of secondary peritonitis sought.

The diagnosis of SBP is not easy. The level of suspicion needs to be high. It may be difficult to recover organisms from cultures of peritoneal fluid, presumably because the burden of organisms is low. The yield can be improved if 10 mL of peritoneal fluid is placed directly into a blood culture bottle. Bacteremia may accompany SBP; therefore, blood should be cultured simultaneously. No specific radiographic studies are helpful in the diagnosis of SBP. A plain film of the abdomen would be expected to show ascites. Chest and abdominal radiography should be performed in cases with abdominal pain to exclude free air, which signals a perforation. Treatment for SBP is directed at the isolate from blood or peritoneal fluid. Until culture results become available, empirical therapy should cover gram-negative aerobic bacilli and gram-positive cocci. Empirical coverage for anaerobes is not necessary.

SECONDARY PERITONITIS Secondary peritonitis develops when bacteria contaminate the peritoneum as a result of spillage from an intraabdominal process. The organisms found almost always constitute a mixed flora in which aerobic gram-negative bacilli and anaerobes predominate, especially when the source is colonic. Early in the course of infection, free-flowing exudate with PMNs is found. Early mortality is attributable to gram-negative bacillary sepsis and potent endotoxins circulating in the bloodstream (see Chap. 83). Gram-negative bacilli, particularly *E. coli,* are common bloodstream isolates, but *Bacteroides fragilis* bacteremia is common as well. The severity of abdominal pain and the clinical course depend on the inciting process. The types of organisms isolated from the peritoneum also vary with the initial process and the normal flora present. There also are differences in peritonitis that primarily results from chemical irritation and that resulting primarily from bacterial contamination. For example, as long as the patient is not achlorhydric, a ruptured gastric ulcer will release low pH gastric contents that will serve as a chemical irritant. The normal flora of the stomach comprises the same organisms found in the oropharynx (see Chap. 128) but in numbers at least two logs lower. The surfaces of teeth contain approximately 10^7 aerobic and 10^7 anaerobic organisms per milliliter of saliva; the normally acidic stomach contains an equal ratio of aerobic and anaerobic species, but in concentrations more in the range of 10^5 per milliliter. After meals, when gastric acidity is highest, this number may fall to 10^3. The bacterial burden, then, in a ruptured gastric ulcer—or even duodenal ulcer—is negligible compared with that in a ruptured appendix. The normal flora of the colon below the ligament of Treitz contains about 10^{11} anaerobic organisms per gram of feces but only 10^8 aerobes per gram; therefore, anaerobic species account for 99 percent of the bacteria. There is not a significant chemical peritonitis from leakage of colonic contents (pH 7 to 8), but infection from the heavy bacterial load is severe.

Depending on the inciting event, local symptoms may initially be found in secondary peritonitis—for example, epigastric pain from a ruptured gastric ulcer. In appendicitis the initial presenting symptoms often are vague, with periumbilical discomfort and nausea followed in a number of hours by pain more localized to the right lower quadrant. Variable locations of the appendix (including a retrocecal position) can complicate this presentation further. Once infection has spread to the peritoneal cavity, however, pain increases, particularly with infection involving the parietal peritoneum, which is innervated extensively. Patients usually lie motionless, often with knees drawn up to avoid stretching the nerve fibers of the peritoneal cavity. Coughing and sneezing, which increase pressure within the peritoneal cavity, are associated with sharp pain. There may or may not be pain localized to the infected or diseased organ from which secondary peritonitis has arisen. Patients with secondary peritonitis generally have abnormal abdominal examinations with marked voluntary and involuntary guarding of anterior abdominal musculature. Later findings include tenderness, especially rebound tenderness. In addition, there may be localized findings in the area of the inciting event. In general, patients are febrile, with marked leukocytosis and a left shift of the WBCs to earlier granulocyte forms.

While recovery of organisms from peritoneal fluid is easier in secondary than in primary peritonitis, a tap of the abdomen is rarely the procedure of choice in secondary peritonitis. An exception is in cases involving trauma, where the possibility of a hemoperitoneum may need to be excluded early. Treatment for secondary peritonitis includes administration of early antibiotics targeted particularly at aerobic gram-negative bacilli and anaerobes as well as etiologic studies. Most secondary peritonitis requires both surgical intervention to address the inciting process and antibiotic administration to treat early bacteremia, to decrease the incidence of abscess formation and wound infection, and to avoid more distant spread of infection. In SBP in adults, surgery is rarely indicated. In secondary peritonitis, surgery may be life-saving.

INTRAPERITONEAL ABSCESSES

Abscess formation is common in untreated peritonitis if overt gram-negative sepsis either does not occur or does occur but is not fatal. In experimental models of abscess formation, mixed aerobic and anaerobic organisms have been implanted intraperitoneally. Without therapy directed at anaerobes, animals develop intraabdominal abscesses. As in patients, these experimental abscesses may stud the peritoneal cavity, lie within the omentum or mesentery, or even develop on the surface of or within viscera such as the liver.

ROLE OF BACTERIAL VIRULENCE FACTORS *B. fragilis,* although accounting for only 0.5 percent of the normal colonic contents, is found in 65 percent of intraabdominal infections and is the most common anaerobic bloodstream isolate. Therefore, it appears to be uniquely virulent on clinical grounds. Moreover, *B. fragilis* causes abscesses in the animal model of intraabdominal infection, whereas most other *Bacteroides* species must be implanted with a facultative organism in order for abscesses to form.

Several virulence factors have been identified in *B. fragilis* and some are critical to abscess formation. The most important virulence factor is the capsular polysaccharide complex (CP) found on the surface of this organism. Two distinct surface polysaccharides comprise the CP of most, if not all, *B. fragilis* strains. The CP by itself can provoke abscesses. Structural analysis of each polysaccharide in the CP shows unusual features thought to be responsible for abscess formation. In addition, immunization of animals with CP leads to immunity from abscess formation. Other virulence properties of *B. fragilis* CP include the ability to adhere to peritoneal mesothelial cells and antiphagocytic activity.

B. fragilis also contains a surface lipopolysaccharide that lacks the potency of the endotoxins produced by aerobic gram-negative bacilli. In addition, *B. fragilis* elaborates an important enzyme, superoxide dismutase, which facilitates bacterial survival in the presence of oxygen by counteracting the toxic effects of superoxide radicals. One reason that anaerobic species thrive in intraabdominal infections is the reduced oxidation-reduction potential associated with necrotic tissue. The oxidation-reduction potential in the center of an abscess also is low, but, before an abscess becomes established, some oxygen is present. Anaerobic species such as *B. fragilis*, which display a degree of oxygen tolerance, have an enhanced ability to survive.

PATHOGENESIS AND IMMUNITY   There is often disagreement about whether an abscess represents a disease state or a host response. In a sense, it represents both: while an abscess is an infection in which viable organisms and PMNs are contained within a fibrous capsule, it is also a process by which the host confines microbes to a limited space, thereby preventing further spread of infection. Experimental work has helped to define both the host cells involved in abscess formation and the bacterial virulence factors responsible— most notably those of the most common gram-negative anaerobic isolate, *B. fragilis*. Several host factors have been found experimentally to participate in abscess formation, including the alternative pathway of complement and fibrinogen. T cells also are important; nude mice can form small abscesses, but animals depleted of CD4+/CD8+ T cells cannot. Although most organisms involved in abscess induction are extracellular pathogens and would be expected to elicit an immune response that is primarily humoral, in intraabdominal abscess the immune response to *B. fragilis* is T cell dependent and directed to the CP. Two different CD8+, non-H_2–restricted T cells are responsible for immunity to experimental intraabdominal abscesses. While antibodies to CP are not critical in immunity to abscesses, they enhance bloodstream clearance of *B. fragilis*.

CLINICAL PRESENTATION   Most intraperitoneal abscesses result from secondary bacterial peritonitis due to fecal spillage from a colonic source, such as an inflamed appendix. Seventy-four percent of intraabdominal abscesses are intraperitoneal or retroperitoneal and are not associated with a specific organ. Abscesses arise from a number of different processes as well. They usually form within weeks of the development of peritonitis and may be found in a variety of locations from omentum to mesentery, pelvis to psoas muscles, and subphrenic space to the surface of (or deeper in) viscera such as the liver. Infections of the female genital tract and pancreatitis are among the more common causative events. When abscesses occur in the female genital tract—either as a primary infection (e.g., tuboovarian abscess) or as an infection extending into the pelvic cavity or peritoneum—*B. fragilis* figures prominently among the organisms isolated. *B. fragilis* is not found in large numbers in the normal vaginal flora. It is encountered less commonly in pelvic inflammatory disease and endometritis, for example, without an associated abscess. In pancreatitis with leakage of damaging pancreatic enzymes, inflammation is prominent. Therefore, clinical findings such as fever, leukocytosis, and even abdominal pain do not distinguish pancreatitis itself from complications such as pancreatic pseudocyst, pancreatic abscess, or intraabdominal collections of pus. Some authors have advocated early needle aspiration of pancreatic collections under computed tomographic (CT) guidance as a means of distinguishing pseudocyst from abscess, but this procedure is associated with some hazard, and the recovery of organisms is not of clear significance.

The psoas muscle of the anterior back is another location in which abscesses are encountered. These abscesses may arise from a presumed hematogenous source, from contiguous spread from an intraabdominal or pelvic process, or from contiguous spread from nearby bony structures such as vertebral bodies. Associated osteomyelitis due to spread from bone to muscle or from muscle to bone is common in psoas abscess. When Pott's disease was common, *Mycobacterium tuberculosis* was a frequent cause of psoas abscess. Currently in the United States, the usual isolates from psoas abscesses are either *Staphylococcus aureus* or a mixture of enteric organisms including aerobic gram-negative bacilli. *S. aureus* is most likely to be isolated when a psoas abscess arises from hematogenous spread or a contiguous focus of osteomyelitis; a mixed enteric flora is most likely when the abscess has an intraabdominal or pelvic source.

DIAGNOSIS   A variety of scanning procedures have facilitated considerably the diagnosis of intraabdominal abscesses. Abdominal CT scans probably have the highest yield, although ultrasonography is particularly useful for the right upper quadrant, kidneys, and pelvis. Both gallium- and indium-labeled WBCs tend to localize in abscesses and may be useful in finding a collection. Since gallium is taken up in the bowel, indium-labeled WBCs may have a slightly greater yield for abscesses near the bowel. Neither gallium- nor indium-labeled WBC scans serve as a basis for a definitive diagnosis, however; both need to be followed by other, more specific studies, such as CT, if an area of possible abnormality is identified. Abscesses contiguous with or contained within outpouchings of bowel are particularly difficult to diagnose with scanning procedures. Occasionally, a barium enema may detect a diverticular abscess not diagnosed by other procedures, although barium should not be injected if a free perforation is suspected. If one study is negative, a second study sometimes reveals a collection. On occasion, exploratory laparotomy still must be undertaken if an abscess is strongly suspected on clinical grounds, although this procedure has been less commonly used since the advent of CT.

TREATMENT   The treatment of intraabdominal infections involves the establishment of the initial focus of infection, the administration of broad-spectrum antibiotics targeted at organisms involved in the associated infection, and the performance of a drainage procedure if one or more definitive abscesses have formed already. It cannot be overemphasized that antimicrobial therapy, in general, is adjunctive to drainage and/or surgical correction of an underlying lesion or process in intraabdominal abscesses. Unlike the intraabdominal abscesses precipitated by most infections, for which drainage of some kind generally is required, abscesses associated with diverticulitis usually wall off locally after rupture of a diverticulum, so that surgical intervention is not routinely required.

A number of antimicrobial agents exhibit excellent activity against aerobic gram-negative bacilli. Since mortality in intraabdominal sepsis is linked to gram-negative bacteremia and endotoxin release, empirical therapy for intraabdominal infection always needs to include adequate coverage of these organisms. Aminoglycosides and second- and third-generation cephalosporins are the agents most widely tested and used in intraabdominal processes. Newer antibiotics such as aztreonam, imipenem, ticarcillin/clavulanic acid, and quinolones (e.g., ciprofloxacin) cover these organisms as well, although at a higher cost. Second-generation cephalosporins such as cefoxitin or cefotetan are not as uniformly active as the other agents against all of the aerobic gram-negative species. Aztreonam, ciprofloxacin, aminoglycosides, and most of the third-generation cephalosporins are not active against anaerobes and therefore need to be used in combination with another antibiotic. There are conflicting studies in the literature about the anaerobic activity of ceftizoxime, a third-generation cephalosporin. There may be a discrepancy between in vitro sensitivities and in vivo activity. Since a number of antibiotics highly effective against anaerobes are available, third-generation cephalosporins should generally not be considered for treatment of anaerobes.

The most active and cost-effective antibiotic for anaerobic coverage currently is metronidazole. Although rare isolates of *B. fragilis* have been reported to be resistant to this drug, the clinical significance of resistance in anaerobic species is not known. Other first-line agents include cefoxitin and clindamycin. Neither metronidazole nor clindamycin covers aerobic gram-negative bacilli; thus these drugs must be combined with other agents. Cefotetan has a spectrum of activity similar to that of cefoxitin and including *B. fragilis,* but its lesser activity against other *Bacteroides* species limits its utility. The rate of resistance to cefoxitin or clindamycin among *B. fragilis* isolates has ranged from 6 to 30 percent in certain areas, although, again, the clinical significance of this finding is unclear. Among newer agents, imipenem, ticarcillin/clavulanic acid, and ampicillin/sulbactam are highly active against anaerobes. Chloramphenicol, which exhibits strong activity against *B. fragilis* in vitro, nevertheless should probably not be considered a first-line drug for anaerobes since failures of treatment have been documented in both experimental and clinical intraabdominal infections. The emerging surgical literature on scoring systems and stratification by diagnosis, severity of disease, and outcome measures should permit more accurate clinical trials of antibiotic regimens for the treatment of intraabdominal infections.

VISCERAL ABSCESSES Liver abscesses The liver is the organ most commonly subject to the development of abscesses. Altemeier and associates studied 540 intraabdominal abscesses over a 12-year period. Visceral abscesses accounted for 26 percent of these abscesses; moreover, liver abscesses made up 13 percent of the total number, or 48 percent of all visceral abscesses. Liver abscesses may be solitary or multiple; they may arise from hematogenous spread of bacteria or from local spread from contiguous infections within the peritoneal cavity. In the past, appendicitis with rupture and subsequent spread of infection was the most common route for the development of a liver abscess. Currently, associated disease of the biliary tract is the most common etiology. Suppurative pylephlebitis, usually arising from infection in the pelvis but also from infection elsewhere in the peritoneal cavity, is another common source for bacterial seeding of the liver.

Fever is the most common presenting sign of liver abscess. Some patients, particularly those with active associated disease of the biliary tract, have symptoms and signs localized to the right upper quadrant, including pain, guarding, punch tenderness, and even rebound tenderness. Nonspecific symptoms such as chills, anorexia, weight loss, nausea, and vomiting also may develop. Only 50 percent of patients with liver abscesses, however, have hepatomegaly, right upper quadrant tenderness, or jaundice; thus half of patients have no symptoms or signs that would direct attention to the liver. Fever of unknown origin (FUO) may be the only presenting manifestation of liver abscess, especially in the elderly. Diagnostic studies of the abdomen, especially the right upper quadrant, should be a part of any FUO workup. The single most reliable laboratory finding is an elevated serum concentration of alkaline phosphatase, which is documented in 90 percent of patients with liver abscesses. Other tests of liver function may yield normal results, but 50 percent of patients have elevated serum levels of bilirubin and 48 percent have elevated concentrations of aspartate aminotransferase. Other associated laboratory findings include leukocytosis in 77 percent of patients, anemia (usually normochromic, normocytic) in 50 percent, and hypoalbuminemia in 33 percent. Concomitant bacteremia is found in one-third of patients. A liver abscess is sometimes suggested by chest radiography, especially if a new elevation of the right hemidiaphragm is seen; other suggestive findings include a right basilar infiltrate and a right pleural effusion.

Imaging studies are the most reliable methods for diagnosing liver abscesses. These studies include ultrasonography, CT scan, gallium- or indium-labeled WBC scans, and even magnetic resonance imaging. In an occasional case, more than one such study may be required. Organisms recovered from liver abscesses vary with the etiology. In liver infection arising from the biliary tree, enteric gram-negative aerobic bacilli and enterococci are common isolates. Unless previous surgery has been performed, anaerobes are not generally involved in liver abscesses arising from biliary infections. In contrast, in liver abscesses arising from pelvic and other intraperitoneal sources, a mixed flora including aerobic and anaerobic species (especially *B. fragilis*) is common. With hematogenous spread of infection, usually only a single organism is encountered; this species may be *S. aureus* or a streptococcal species such as *Streptococcus milleri*.

Liver abscesses also may be caused by *Candida* species; such abscesses usually follow fungemia in patients receiving chemotherapy for cancer and often present as a return of neutrophils after a period of neutropenia. Treatment of candidal liver abscesses usually entails lengthy administration of amphotericin B, although recent reports have described successful maintenance therapy with fluconazole after an initial course of amphotericin (see Chaps. 96 and 166).

Amebic liver abscesses are not an uncommon problem (see Chap. 173). Amebic serology gives positive results in more than 95 percent of cases; thus a negative result assists in excluding this diagnosis.

While drainage—either percutaneous with a pigtail catheter kept in place or surgical—remains the mainstay of therapy for intraabdominal abscesses (including liver abscesses), there is growing interest in medical management alone for pyogenic liver abscesses. Cases treated without definitive drainage generally require longer courses of antibiotic therapy. When percutaneous drainage was compared with open surgical drainage, the average length of hospital stay for the former was almost double that for the latter, although both the time required for fever to resolve and mortality were the same for the two procedures. Mortality was appreciable despite treatment, averaging 15 percent. Several factors may predict the failure of percutaneous drainage and therefore may favor primary surgical intervention. These include the presence of multiple, sizable abscesses; viscous abscess contents which tend to plug the catheter; associated disease (e.g., of the biliary tract) that requires surgery; or the lack of a clinical response to percutaneous drainage in 4 to 7 days.

Splenic abscesses Splenic abscesses are much less common than liver abscesses. In fact, no splenic abscesses were observed in Altemeier's series of 540 intraabdominal abscesses. The incidence of splenic abscesses has ranged from 0.7 to 0.22 percent in various autopsy series. The clinical setting and the organisms isolated usually differ from the corresponding findings for liver abscesses. The degree of clinical suspicion for splenic abscess needs to be high as this condition frequently is fatal if left untreated. Even in the most recently published series, diagnosis was made only at autopsy in 37 percent of cases. While splenic abscesses may arise occasionally from contiguous spread of infection or from direct trauma to the spleen, hematogenous spread of infection is the usual mode of development. Bacterial endocarditis is the most common associated infection. Splenic abscesses also are seen in patients who have received extensive immunosuppressive therapy (particularly those who have malignancy involving the spleen) and in patients with hemoglobinopathies or other hematologic disorders (especially sickle cell anemia).

While approximately 50 percent of patients with splenic abscesses have abdominal pain, the pain is localized to the left upper quadrant in only half of these cases. Splenomegaly is found in approximately 50 percent of patients. Fever and leukocytosis generally are present; the development of fever preceded diagnosis by an average of 20 days in a recent series. Left-sided chest findings may include abnormalities to auscultation, and chest radiographic findings may include an infiltrate or a left-sided pleural effusion. When splenic abscesses are being considered in a differential diagnosis, CT scan of the abdomen has been the most sensitive diagnostic tool. Ultrasonography can yield the diagnosis, but cases have been missed with this modality. Liver-spleen scan or gallium scan also may be useful. Streptococcal species are the most common bacterial isolates from splenic abscesses and *S. aureus* is the next most common organism; presumably these prevalences reflect the bacterial cause of the associated endocarditis. An increase in the frequency of isolation of gram-negative aerobic organisms from splenic abscesses has been reported; these organisms often derive from a urinary tract focus, with associated bacteremia, or another intraabdominal source. *Salmonella* species are seen fairly commonly, especially in patients with sickle cell hemoglobinopathy. Anaerobic species accounted for only 5 percent of isolates in the largest collected series, but the reporting of a number of "sterile abscesses" may indicate that optimal techniques for the isolation of anaerobes were not employed. Because of the high mortality figures reported for splenic abscesses, the treatment of choice is splenectomy with adjunctive antibiotics. However, percutaneous drainage was recently successful in one group of patients. The most important factor in successful treatment of splenic abscesses is early consideration of the diagnosis.

Perinephric and renal abscesses Perinephric and renal abscesses are not common: the former accounted for only about 0.02

percent of hospital admissions and the latter for about 0.2 percent in Altemeier's series of 540 intraabdominal abscesses. While liver abscesses generally arise from contiguous foci of infection or track from other intraabdominal sources and splenic abscesses usually arise from hematogenous spread (e.g., bacterial endocarditis), perinephric and renal abscesses have a different pathogenesis. Before antibiotics became available, the majority of renal and perinephric abscesses were hematogenous in origin, with *S. aureus* most commonly recovered. In contrast, at the present time, more than 75 percent of perinephric and renal abscesses arise from an initial urinary tract infection. Infection ascends from the bladder to the kidney, with pyelonephritis occurring first. Bacteria may directly invade the renal parenchyma from medulla to cortex. Local vascular channels within the kidney may also facilitate the transport of organisms. Areas of abscess developing within the parenchyma may rupture into the perinephric space. The kidneys and adrenal glands are surrounded by a layer of perirenal fat that, in turn, is surrounded by Gerota's fascia, which extends superiorly to the diaphragm and inferiorly to the pelvic fat. When abscesses extend into the perinephric space, tracking may occur through Gerota's fascia into the psoas or transversalis muscles, into the anterior peritoneal cavity, superiorly to the subdiaphragmatic space, or inferiorly to the pelvis. Of the several risk factors that have been associated with the development of perinephric abscesses, the most important is the presence of concomitant nephrolithiasis producing local obstruction to urinary flow. Twenty to sixty percent of patients with perinephric abscess have renal stones. In addition, other structural abnormalities of the urinary tract, a prior history of urologic surgery, trauma, and diabetes mellitus all have been identified as risk factors.

The organisms most frequently encountered in perinephric and renal abscesses are *E. coli*, *Proteus* sp., and *Klebsiella* sp. *E. coli*, the aerobic species most commonly found in colonic flora, seems to have unique virulence properties in the urinary tract, including factors promoting adherence to uroepithelial cells. The urease of *Proteus* sp. splits urea, thereby creating a more alkaline and hospitable environment for bacterial proliferation. *Proteus* sp. frequently are found in association with large struvite stones caused by the precipitation of magnesium ammonium sulfate in an alkaline environment. These stones serve as a nidus for recurrent urinary tract infection. While a single bacterial species usually is recovered from a perinephric or renal abscess, multiple species also may be found. If a urine culture is not contaminated with periurethral flora and is found to contain more than one organism, a perinephric abscess or renal abscess should be considered in the differential diagnosis. Urine cultures also may be polymicrobial in cases of bladder diverticulum.

Candida sp. is another organism to consider in the etiology of renal abscesses. This fungus may spread to the kidney via the hematogenous route or by ascension from the bladder. The hallmark of the latter route of infection is ureteral obstruction with large fungal balls.

The presentation of perinephric and renal abscesses is quite nonspecific. Flank pain and abdominal pain are common. At least 50 percent of patients are febrile. Pain may be referred to the groin or leg, particularly with extension of infection. The diagnosis of perinephric abscess, like that of splenic abscess, is frequently delayed, and mortality in some series is appreciable although lower than in the past. Perinephric or renal abscess should be most seriously considered when a patient presents with symptoms and signs of pyelonephritis and remains febrile after 4 or 5 days, by which time the fever should have resolved. Moreover, when a urine culture yields a polymicrobial flora, when a patient has known renal stone disease, or when fever and pyuria coexist with a sterile urine culture, the diagnosis of perinephric or renal abscess should be entertained.

Renal ultrasonography and abdominal CT scan are the most useful diagnostic modalities. If a renal abscess or perinephric abscess is diagnosed, nephrolithiasis should be excluded, especially when a high urinary pH suggests the presence of a urea-splitting organism. Treatment for perinephric or renal abscesses, like that for other

intraabdominal abscesses, includes drainage of pus and antibiotic therapy directed at the organism(s) recovered. For perinephric abscesses, percutaneous drainage usually is successful.

REFERENCES

Altemeier WA et al: Intra-abdominal abscesses. Am J Surg 125:70, 1973

Chun CH et al: Splenic abscess. Medicine 59:50, 1980

Hutchison FN, Kaysen GA: Perinephric abscess: The missed diagnosis. Med Clin North Am 72:993, 1988

Levison ME, Bush LM: Peritonitis and other intra-abdominal infections, in *Principles and Practice of Infectious Diseases*, 3d ed, GL Mandell et al (eds). New York, Churchill Livingstone, 1990

Maher JA et al: Successful medical treatment of pyogenic liver abscess. Gastroenterology 77:618, 1979

Nystrom P-O et al: Proposed definitions for diagnosis, severity scoring, stratification, and outcome for trials on intraabdominal infection. World J Surg 14:148, 1990

Tzianabos AO et al: The capsular polysaccharide of *Bacteroides fragilis* comprises two ionically linked polysaccharides. J Biol Chem 267:18230, 1992

Zaleznik DF, Kasper DL: *Bacteroides* species, in *Principles and Practice of Infectious Diseases*, 3d ed, GL Mandell et al (eds). New York, Churchill Livingstone, 1990

87 ACUTE INFECTIOUS DIARRHEAL DISEASES AND BACTERIAL FOOD POISONING

JOAN R. BUTTERTON / STEPHEN B. CALDERWOOD

Ranging from mild annoyances during vacations to devastating dehydrating illnesses that can kill within hours, acute gastrointestinal illnesses rank second only to acute upper respiratory illnesses as the most common diseases worldwide. In children less than 5 years old, attack rates range from 2 to 3 illnesses per child per year in developed countries to as high as 10 to 18 illnesses per child per year in developing countries. In Asia, Africa, and Latin America, acute diarrheal illnesses are not only a leading cause of morbidity in children—producing an estimated 1 billion cases per year—but also the major cause of mortality, being responsible for 4 to 6 million deaths per year, or a sobering total of 12,600 deaths per day. In some areas, more than 50 percent of deaths of children are directly attributable to acute diarrheal illnesses. In addition, by contributing to malnutrition and thereby reducing resistance to other infectious agents, gastrointestinal illnesses may be indirect factors in a far greater burden of disease.

The wide range of clinical manifestations observed in acute gastrointestinal illnesses is matched by the wide variety of infectious agents, which include viruses, bacteria, and parasitic pathogens, that can cause these diseases (Table 87-1). This chapter will discuss factors that enable gastrointestinal pathogens to cause disease, review host defense mechanisms, and present an approach to the evaluation and treatment of patients presenting with acute diarrhea. Detailed discussions of individual organisms are presented in subsequent chapters.

PATHOGENIC MECHANISMS Enteric pathogens have developed a variety of tactics to overcome host defenses and ultimately cause disease by a number of mechanisms. Understanding the virulence factors employed by these organisms is important in the diagnosis and treatment of clinical disease.

Inoculum size The number of microorganisms that must be ingested to cause disease varies considerably from species to species. For *Escherichia coli*, *Salmonella*, and *Vibrio cholerae*, for example, 10^5 to 10^8 organisms must be ingested orally to cause disease, whereas for *Shigella*, *Giardia lamblia*, and *Entamoeba* as few as 10 to 100 bacteria or cysts can produce infection. The ability of organisms to overcome host defenses has important implications for transmission;

TABLE 87-1 Gastrointestinal pathogens causing acute diarrhea

Mechanism	Location	Illness	Stool findings	Examples of pathogens involved
Noninflammatory (enterotoxin)	Proximal small bowel	Watery diarrhea	No fecal leukocytes	*Vibrio cholerae* Enterotoxigenic *Escherichia coli* (LT and/or ST) *Clostridium perfringens* *Bacillus cereus* *Staphylococcus aureus* *Aeromonas hydrophila* *Plesiomonas shigelloides* Rotavirus Norwalk-like viruses Enteric adenoviruses *Giardia lamblia* *Cryptosporidium*
Inflammatory (invasion or cytotoxin)	Colon	Dysentery	Fecal polymorphonuclear leukocytes	*Shigella* sp. *Salmonella enteritidis* *Campylobacter jejuni* Enterohemorrhagic *Escherichia coli* Enteroinvasive *E. coli* *Vibrio parahemolyticus* *Clostridium difficile* ?*Aeromonas hydrophila* ?*Plesiomonas shigelloides* *Entamoeba histolytica*
Penetrating	Distal small bowel	Enteric fever	Fecal mononuclear leukocytes	*Salmonella typhi* *Yersinia enterocolitica*

SOURCE: After Guerrant, in Mandell et al.

Shigella, *Entamoeba*, and *Giardia* can spread by person-to-person contact, whereas bacteria such as *Salmonella* may have to grow in food for several hours before reaching an effective infectious dose.

Adherence Many organisms must adhere to the gastrointestinal mucosa as an initial step in the pathogenic process; thus organisms that can compete with the normal bowel flora and colonize the mucosa have an important advantage in causing disease. Specific cell-surface proteins involved in attachment of bacteria to intestinal cells are important virulence determinants. *V. cholerae*, for example, adheres to the brush border of small intestinal enterocytes via specific surface adhesins, including the toxin-coregulated pilus (Tcp) and other accessory colonization factors. Enterotoxigenic *E. coli* produces an adherence protein, called *colonization factor antigen* (CFA), that is necessary for colonization of the upper small intestine by the organism prior to its production of enterotoxin. Enteropathogenic strains of *E. coli* produce virulence determinants that allow these organisms to attach to and efface the brush border of the intestinal epithelium, while enterohemorrhagic strains of *E. coli* produce fimbriae that mediate attachment of bacteria to cells in culture.

Toxin production The production of one or more exotoxins is important in the pathogenesis of numerous enteric organisms. Such toxins include *enterotoxins,* which cause watery diarrhea by acting directly on secretory mechanisms in the intestinal mucosa; *cytotoxins,* which cause destruction of mucosal cells and associated inflammatory diarrhea; and *neurotoxins,* which act directly on the central or peripheral nervous system. Some exotoxins act by more than one mechanism; *S. dysenteriae* type 1, for example, produces an exotoxin that has neurotoxic, enterotoxic, and cytotoxic activities.

The prototypical enterotoxin is cholera toxin, a heterodimeric protein composed of one A and five B subunits. The A subunit contains the enzymatic activity of the toxin, while the B subunit pentamer binds holotoxin to the enterocyte surface receptor, the ganglioside G_{M1}. After the binding of holotoxin, a fragment of the A subunit is translocated across the eukaryotic cell membrane into the cytoplasm, where it catalyzes the ADP-ribosylation of a GTP-binding protein and causes persistent activation of adenylate cyclase. The end result is an increase of cAMP in the intestinal mucosa, which increases Cl^- secretion and decreases Na^+ absorption, leading to loss of fluid and the production of diarrhea.

Enterotoxigenic strains of *E. coli* may produce a protein, called *heat-labile enterotoxin* (LT), that is similar to cholera toxin and

causes secretory diarrhea by the same mechanism. Alternatively, enterotoxigenic strains of *E. coli* may produce *heat-stable enterotoxin* (ST), which causes diarrhea by activation of guanylate cyclase and elevation of intracellular cGMP. Some enterotoxigenic *E. coli* produce both LT and ST.

Bacterial cytotoxins, in contrast, destroy intestinal mucosal cells and produce the syndrome of dysentery, with bloody stools containing inflammatory cells. Enteric pathogens that produce such cytotoxins include *S. dysenteriae, V. parahemolyticus,* and *Clostridium difficile.* Enterohemorrhagic strains of *E. coli,* most commonly serotype 0157:H7, also produce potent cytotoxins that are highly related to Shiga toxin from *S. dysenteriae* and have been termed *Shiga-like toxins* (SLTs). Such strains of *E. coli* have been associated with outbreaks of hemorrhagic colitis and hemolytic-uremic syndrome.

Neurotoxins usually are produced by the responsible organism outside the host and therefore produce symptoms soon after ingestion. These include the staphylococcal and *Bacillus cereus* toxins, which act on the central nervous system to produce vomiting.

Invasion Dysentery may result not only from the production of cytotoxins but also from bacterial invasion and destruction of intestinal mucosal cells. Infections due to *Shigella* and enteroinvasive *E. coli,* for example, are characterized by invasion of mucosal epithelial cells, intraepithelial multiplication, and subsequent spread to adjacent cells. *Salmonella,* on the other hand, causes inflammatory diarrhea by invasion of the bowel mucosa but is generally not associated with destruction of enterocytes or the full clinical syndrome of dysentery. *S. typhi* and *Yersinia enterocolitica* can penetrate intact intestinal mucosa, multiply intracellularly in Peyer's patches and intestinal lymph nodes, and then disseminate through the bloodstream to cause enteric fever, a syndrome characterized by fever, headache, relative bradycardia, abdominal pain, splenomegaly, and leukopenia.

HOST DEFENSES Given the enormous number of microorganisms ingested with every meal, it is evident that the normal host must possess effective defense mechanisms to combat a constant influx of potential enteric pathogens. Observations of infections in patients with alterations in these defenses has led to a greater understanding of the variety of ways in which the normal host can protect itself against disease.

Normal flora The large numbers of bacteria that normally inhabit the intestine act as an important host defense by preventing colonization by potential enteric pathogens. Persons with fewer intestinal bacteria, such as infants who have not yet developed normal enteric colonization or patients receiving antibiotics, are at significantly greater risk of developing infections with enteric pathogens. The composition of the intestinal flora is as important as the number of organisms present. More than 99 percent of the normal colonic flora is anaerobic bacteria, and the acidic pH and volatile fatty acids produced by these organisms appear to be critical elements in the colonization resistance offered by the normal enteric flora.

Gastric acid   The acidic pH of the stomach is an important barrier to enteric pathogens, and an increased frequency of *Salmonella*, *Shigella*, *G. lamblia*, and a variety of helminthic infections has been observed in patients who have undergone gastric surgery or are otherwise achlorhydric. Neutralization of gastric acid with antacids or with H-2 blockers, as commonly occurs in hospitalized patients, similarly increases the risk of enteric colonization. Some microorganisms, however, can survive the extreme acidity of the gastric environment; rotavirus, for example, is highly stable to acid.

Intestinal motility   Normal peristalsis is the major mechanism for clearance of bacteria from the proximal small intestine, although gastric acidity and secreted immunoglobulins also play a role in limiting the number of organisms present. When intestinal motility is impaired, as by treatment with opiates or other antimotility drugs, anatomic abnormalities (diverticulas, fistulas, or afferent-loop stasis following surgery), or hypomotility states (as in diabetes mellitus or scleroderma), the frequency of bacterial overgrowth and infection of the small bowel with enteric pathogens is much increased. Some patients with *Shigella* infection treated with diphenoxylate hydrochloride with atropine (Lomotil) demonstrate prolonged fever and shedding of organisms, while patients treated with opiates for mild *Salmonella* gastroenteritis have a higher frequency of bacteremia.

Immunity   Both cellular immune responses and antibody production play important roles in protecting susceptible hosts from enteric infections. The wide spectrum of gastrointestinal viral, bacterial, parasitic, and fungal infections in patients with AIDS highlights the importance of cell-mediated immunity in protecting the normal host from these pathogens. Humoral intestinal immunity is also important and consists both of systemic IgG and IgM and secretory IgA. Growing evidence supports the concept of a common mucosal immune system for secretory IgA in which binding of bacterial antigens to the luminal surface of M cells in the distal small bowel and subsequent presentation to subepithelial lymphoid tissue leads to the proliferation of sensitized lymphocytes that circulate and populate all of the mucosal tissues of the body as IgA-secreting plasma cells.

CLINICAL EVALUATION   History   The answers to questions with high discriminating value can quickly narrow the potential cause of diarrhea and help determine if treatment is needed: (1) What is the *duration* of symptoms? Is the diarrhea acute or chronic? Diarrhea lasting more than 2 weeks generally is defined as chronic; in such cases, many of the causes of acute diarrhea are much less likely, and a new spectrum of causes needs to be considered. (2) Is there *fever*? Fever often implies invasive disease, although fever and diarrhea also may result from infection outside the gastrointestinal tract, as with malaria and a variety of febrile illnesses in children. (3) What is the *appearance of the stool*? Stools that contain blood or mucus indicate ulceration of the large bowel. Bulky, white stools suggest a small-intestinal process that is causing malabsorption. Profuse, "rice-water" stools suggest cholera or a similar toxigenic process. (4) What is the *frequency* of bowel movements? The number of stools over a given period can be the first warning of impending dehydration. (5) Does the patient have *abdominal pain*? Abdominal pain may be most severe in inflammatory processes, such as with *Shigella*, *Campylobacter*, and necrotizing toxins. Painful abdominal muscle cramps, caused by electrolyte loss, can be seen in severe cases of cholera. Bloating is common in giardiasis. (6) Is there *tenesmus* (cramps in the rectum felt after a bowel movement)? Tenesmus may be present when there is inflammation of the rectum, as is seen with shigellosis. (7) Has the patient been *vomiting*? Vomiting implies an acute infection, such as with a toxin-mediated illness or food

poisoning, but also can be prominent in a variety of systemic illnesses (e.g., malaria) and in intestinal obstruction. (8) Is there evidence of a *common source* of infection? Asking patients if anyone else is sick is a more efficient means of identifying a common source than is constructing a list of recently eaten foods. If a common source seems likely, specific foods can then be investigated.

Epidemiology   TRAVEL HISTORY   Of the 12 to 20 million people who travel from temperate industrialized countries to tropical regions of Asia, Africa, and Central and South America each year, 20 to 50 percent will experience a sudden onset of abdominal cramps, anorexia, and watery diarrhea, making *traveler's diarrhea* the most common travel-related illness. The onset is usually 3 days to 2 weeks after the traveler's arrival in a tropical area, with most cases beginning within the first 3 to 5 days. The illness is generally self-limited, lasting 1 to 5 days. The high rate of diarrhea in travelers to underdeveloped areas is related to the ingestion of contaminated food or water.

The organisms that cause traveler's diarrhea vary considerably with location. In all areas, enterotoxigenic *E. coli* is the organism most commonly isolated in cases of the classical secretory traveler's diarrhea syndrome, ranging from a high of approximately 50 percent in Latin America to a low of 15 percent in Asia. *Shigella*, *Salmonella*, and *Campylobacter* spp. are classically considered to cause more invasive, dysenteric disease than enterotoxigenic *E. coli*, but clinical differentiation can be difficult. *Shigella*, *Salmonella*, and *Campylobacter* are isolated in 1 to 15 percent of cases, with different organisms being more common in different locations. *Vibrio* species are most common in Asia, although *V. cholerae* disease reached epidemic proportions in parts of Central and South America in 1991 and has become a significant concern to travelers to these regions. Less common bacteria are *Aeromonas hydrophila* and *Plesiomonas shigelloides*, which have been isolated in travelers to Thailand. Parasitic causes of traveler's diarrhea include *Entamoeba histolytica*, which is responsible for up to 5 percent of cases in Mexico and Thailand, and *G. lamblia*, which has been associated with contaminated freshwater supplies in many areas of the world. *Giardia* is found in association with zoonotic reservoirs in the northern United States and poses a risk for hikers and campers who drink from freshwater streams. A striking association also has been noted with contaminated water supplies in St. Petersburg. *Cryptosporidium* has been recognized as a problem in travelers to the Commonwealth of Independent States, Mexico, and Africa. Viruses, such as rotavirus and Norwalk-like viruses, have been isolated in up to 12 percent of visitors to Latin America, Asia, and Africa.

LOCATION   Day-care centers are sites of particularly high attack rates of enteric infections. Rotavirus is most common in children less than 2 years old, with attack rates of 75 to 100 percent among those exposed. *G. lamblia* is more common in older children, with somewhat lower attack rates. Other common organisms, often spread by fecal-oral contact, are *Shigella*, *C. jejuni*, and *Cryptosporidium*. A characteristic feature of infection in day-care centers is the high rate of secondary cases among family members.

Similarly, hospitals are sites for concentrations of enteric infections. In medical intensive-care units and pediatric wards, diarrhea is among the most common nosocomial infections. *C. difficile* and *Salmonella* species are predominant causes of nosocomial diarrhea in the United States; viral pathogens, especially rotavirus, can spread rapidly in pediatric wards. Enteropathogenic *E. coli* has been associated with outbreaks of diarrhea in newborn nurseries. One-third of elderly patients in chronic-care institutions develop a significant diarrheal illness each year. Surveillance stool cultures suggest that 25 percent of these residents harbor cytotoxin-producing *C. difficile*, which causes more than one-half the cases of diarrhea in this population. Antimicrobial therapy can predispose to pseudomembranous colitis by altering normal colonic flora and allowing multiplication of *C. difficile*.

AGE   The majority of the morbidity and mortality from enteric pathogens is in children less than 5 years of age. Breast-fed infants are protected from contaminated food and water and derive some protection from maternal antibodies, but their risk of infection rises dramatically when they begin to eat solid foods. Infants and younger children are more likely than adults to develop rotaviral disease, while older children and adults are more commonly infected with Norwalk-like viruses. Other organisms that produce disease with higher attack rates in children than in adults include enterotoxigenic and enteropathogenic *E. coli*, *C. jejuni*, and *G. lamblia*. In children, the incidence of *Salmonella* infections is highest in infants under 1 year of age, while the attack rate for *Shigella* infections is greatest in children aged 6 months to 4 years.

Physical examination   The examination of patients for signs of dehydration provides essential information about the severity of the diarrheal illness and the need for rapid therapy. Mild dehydration is indicated by thirst, dry mouth, decreased axillary sweat, decreased urine output, and slight weight loss. Signs of moderate dehydration include an orthostatic fall in blood pressure, skin tenting, and sunken eyes or, in infants, a sunken fontanelle. Signs of severe dehydration range from hypotension and tachycardia to confusion and frank shock.

Diagnostic approach   The most important distinction that the clinician must make is between *inflammatory* and *noninflammatory* disease. By using the history and epidemiology as guides to this distinction, the clinician can rapidly assess the need for further efforts to define a specific etiology and the need for therapeutic intervention. Examination of a stool sample is an important addition to the narrative history. Grossly bloody or mucoid stool suggests an inflammatory process, but all stools should be examined for fecal leukocytes by making a thin smear of the stool on a glass slide, adding a drop of methylene blue, and examining the wet mount. Causes of acute infectious diarrhea, divided into inflammatory and noninflammatory etiologies, are listed in Table 87-1.

BACTERIAL FOOD POISONING   If the history and stool examination indicate a noninflammatory etiology of diarrhea and there is evidence of a common-source outbreak, questions concerning the ingestion of specific foods and the time of onset of the diarrhea after a meal can provide clues to the bacterial cause of the illness. Potential etiologies of bacterial food poisoning are shown in Table 87-2. Bacteria that cause disease by an enterotoxin elaborated outside the host, such as *Staphylococcus aureus* and *Bacillus cereus*, have the shortest incubation periods, averaging 1 to 6 h, and illness generally lasts less than 12 h. The majority of cases of staphylococcal food poisoning are

caused by contamination from infected human carriers. Staphylococci can multiply at a wide range of temperatures, so if food is left to cool slowly and remains at room temperature after cooking, the organisms will have the opportunity to form enterotoxin. Outbreaks following picnics where potato salad, mayonnaise, and cream pastries were served are classic examples of staphylococcal food poisoning. Diarrhea, nausea, vomiting, and abdominal cramping are common, while fever is less so. *B. cereus* produces both a syndrome with a short incubation period, the *emetic* form, mediated by a staphylococcal type of enterotoxin, and one with a longer incubation period (8 to 16 h), the *diarrheal* form, caused by an *E. coli* LT type of enterotoxin in which diarrhea and abdominal cramps are characteristic but vomiting is uncommon. The emetic form of *B. cereus* food poisoning is associated with contaminated fried rice; the organism is common in uncooked rice, and its heat-resistant spores survive boiling. If cooked rice is not refrigerated, the spores can germinate and produce toxin. Frying before serving may not destroy the preformed, heat-stable toxin. Food poisoning due to *C. perfringens* also has a slightly longer incubation period (8 to 14 h) and results from the survival of heat-resistant spores in inadequately cooked meat, poultry, or legumes. Toxin is produced after ingestion in the intestinal tract, causing moderately severe abdominal cramps and diarrhea; vomiting is rare, as is fever. The illness is self-limited, rarely lasting for more than 24 h.

Not all food poisoning has a bacterial cause; diagnostic confusion can result from diarrhea caused by nonbacterial causes of short-incubation food poisoning. These include the chemical effects of capsaicin, which is found in hot peppers, and of a variety of toxins found in fish and shellfish.

LABORATORY EVALUATION   Many cases of noninflammatory diarrhea are self-limited or can be treated empirically, and for these, the clinician may not need to determine a specific etiology. Potentially pathogenic *E. coli* cannot be distinguished from normal fecal flora by routine culture. Special tests to detect LT and ST are not available in most clinical laboratories. In situations in which cholera is a concern, stool should be cultured on thiosulfate citrate bile salt sucrose agar (TCBS). A latex agglutination test has made the rapid detection of rotavirus in stool practical for many laboratories, but electron microscopy or measurement of serologic response with a radioimmunoassay is still necessary for identification of Norwalk-like viruses. At least three stool specimens should be examined for *Giardia* cysts or stained for *Cryptosporidium* if clinical suspicion for these organisms is high.

All patients with fever and evidence of inflammatory disease should have stool cultured for *Salmonella*, *Shigella*, and *Campylobacter*. *Salmonella* and *Shigella* can be selected on MacConkey's agar as non-lactose-fermenting (colorless) colonies or grown on *Salmonella-Shigella* agar or in selenite enrichment broth, both of which inhibit most organisms except these pathogens. Isolation of *Campylobacter* requires inoculation of fresh stool on selective growth media and incubation at 42°C in a microaerophilic atmosphere. Enterohemorrhagic *E. coli* strains of serotype 0157:H7 can be identified in specialized laboratories by serotyping but also can be identified presumptively as lactose-fermenting, indole-positive colonies that are nonsorbitol fermenters (white colonies) on sorbitol MacConkey plates. Fresh stools should be examined for amebic cysts and trophozoites. Pathogenic strains of *C. difficile* generally produce two toxins, A and B. Toxin B can be detected with a cytotoxin assay; if the toxin is present, a monolayer culture of fibroblasts will show cytopathic effects within 6 to 24 h. Rapid enzyme immunoassays and latex agglutination tests for both toxin A and toxin B are a recent development.

TREATMENT   In many cases, a specific diagnosis is not necessary or available to guide treatment; the clinician can proceed with the information available from the history, stool examination, and evaluation of the severity of dehydration of the patient.

Nonspecific therapy   Most causes of noninflammatory diarrhea can be treated effectively with nonspecific therapy. The mainstay of

TABLE 87-2   Bacterial food poisoning

Organisms	Symptoms	Common food sources
1 TO 6 H INCUBATION		
Staphylococcus aureus	Nausea, vomiting, diarrhea	Ham, poultry, potato and egg salad, mayonnaise, cream pastries
Bacillus cereus	Nausea, vomiting, diarrhea	Fried rice
8 TO 16 H INCUBATION		
Clostridium perfringens	Abdominal cramps, diarrhea (vomiting rare)	Beef, poultry, legumes, gravies
Bacillus cereus	Abdominal cramps, diarrhea (vomiting rare)	Meats, vegetables, dried beans, cereals
>16 H INCUBATION		
Vibrio cholerae	Watery diarrhea	Shellfish
Enterotoxigenic *Escherichia coli*	Watery diarrhea	Salads, cheese, meats, water
Salmonella sp.	Inflammatory diarrhea	Beef, poultry, eggs, dairy products
Shigella sp.	Dysentery	Potato and egg salad, lettuce, raw vegetables
Vibrio parahemolyticus	Dysentery	Mollusks, crustaceans

treatment is adequate rehydration. The treatment of cholera and other dehydrating diarrheal diseases was revolutionized by the promotion of oral rehydration solutions, which depend on the fact that glucose-facilitated sodium and water absorption in the small intestine remains intact in the presence of cholera toxin. The availability of oral rehydration solutions has reduced the mortality from cholera from greater than 50 percent in untreated cases to less than 1 percent. The World Health Organization recommends a solution containing 3.5 g sodium chloride, 2.5 g sodium bicarbonate, 1.5 g potassium chloride, and 20 g glucose (or 40 g sucrose) per liter of water. Patients who are severely dehydrated or in whom vomiting precludes the use of oral therapy should be treated with intravenous solutions such as Ringer's lactate.

Bismuth subsalicylate, marketed in the United States as Pepto-Bismol since 1918, is hydrolyzed in the stomach to salicylic acid and insoluble bismuth salts. It has been demonstrated to be an active antimicrobial compound in vitro and to have antisecretory and anti-inflammatory properties, yet it does not significantly affect normal bowel flora. It effectively treats traveler's diarrhea when given at a dosage of 2 tablets (525 mg) every 30 to 60 min for up to 8 doses following the onset of symptoms. It should not be taken with other salicylate-containing drugs.

Antiperistaltic agents such as codeine, diphenoxylate hydrochloride with atropine (Lomotil), or loperamide (Imodium) also can reduce the frequency of stools and hasten the relief of symptoms in traveler's diarrhea. Loperamide, at a dose of 4 mg at the onset of symptoms followed by 2 mg after each loose stool (not to exceed 16 mg/d), is effective more rapidly than bismuth subsalicylate. Antiperistaltic agents should be avoided in patients with inflammatory disease, since they may prolong diarrhea in patients with infection due to *Shigella* and other invasive organisms.

Antibiotics Although most secretory forms of traveler's diarrhea, most commonly due to enterotoxigenic *E. coli,* can be treated effectively with nonspecific therapy, antimicrobial agents can shorten the duration of illness from 3 to 4 days to 24 to 36 h. Trimethoprim-sulfamethoxazole, doxycycline, and ciprofloxacin, each given in a 3-day course, have all been found to be effective. Patients with dysenteric disease should receive empirical therapy tailored to the most likely infectious agent. Ampicillin, trimethoprim-sulfamethoxazole, and ciprofloxacin are effective in treating shigellosis, depending on the local antimicrobial resistance pattern of the organism. *C. jejuni* infections can be treated with erythromycin (see Chap. 119). Treatment of *Salmonella* gastroenteritis (see Chap. 117) with ciprofloxacin may reduce fecal shedding and the duration of illness, but other oral antibiotics have not been shown to be efficacious and may prolong fecal shedding of bacteria. Therapy should be directed toward other organisms if they are likely on epidemiologic grounds. *V. cholerae* infections (see Chap. 120.), for example, can be shortened by treatment with tetracycline or a fluoroquinolone. *C. difficile* colitis (see Chap. 108) may be treated by discontinuing any implicated antibiotics and, if necessary, with oral metronidazole or vancomycin.

Prophylaxis Improvements in hygiene to reduce fecal-oral spread of enteric pathogens will be necessary before significant reductions in the prevalence of diarrheal diseases will be seen in developing countries. Travelers can reduce their risk of diarrhea by eating only hot, freshly cooked food; by avoiding raw vegetables, salads, and unpeeled fruit; and by drinking only boiled or treated water and avoiding ice.

Bismuth subsalicylate is an inexpensive method of prophylaxis against traveler's diarrhea, when taken at a dosage of 2 tablets (525 mg) four times a day. Treatment appears to be effective and safe for up to 3 weeks. Prophylactic antimicrobial agents, although effective, are not generally recommended for the prevention of traveler's diarrhea. The risk of side effects from antibiotic therapy and the possibility of developing an infection with a drug-resistant organism or with more serious, invasive bacteria make a short course of therapy once symptoms have developed a more reasonable therapeutic approach.

The possibility of exerting a major impact on the worldwide morbidity and mortality of diarrheal diseases has led to intense research activity in the development of effective vaccines against the common bacterial and viral enteric pathogens. The currently available vaccines for cholera and typhoid fever are not highly effective. Recent research has shown promising advances in the development of vaccines against these organisms as well as against rotavirus, *Shigella*, and enterotoxigenic *E. coli*.

REFERENCES

BELL DR: *Lecture Notes on Tropical Medicine,* 2d ed. Oxford, Blackwell, 1987, chap. 15

BLACK RE: Epidemiology of travelers' diarrhea and relative importance of various pathogens. Rev Infect Dis 12(suppl 1):S73, 1990

GUERRANT RL: Principles and syndromes of enteric infection, in *Principles and Practice of Infectious Diseases,* 3d ed, GL Mandell et al (eds). New York, Churchill Livingstone, 1990, chap 81

——— et al: Diarrhea in developed and developing countries: Magnitude, special settings, and etiologies. Rev Infect Dis 12(suppl 1):S41, 1990

LEVINE MM: *Escherichia coli* that cause diarrhea: Enterotoxigenic, enteropathogenic, enteroinvasive, enterohemorrhagic, and enteroadherent. J Infect Dis 155:377, 1987

LUND BM: Foodborne disease due to *Bacillus* and *Clostridium* species. Lancet 336:982, 1990

PETRUCCELLI BP: Treatment of traveler's diarrhea with ciprofloxacin and loperamide. J Infect Dis 165:557, 1992

TRANTER HS: Foodborne staphylococcal illness. Lancet 336:1044, 1990

88 SEXUALLY TRANSMITTED DISEASES

KING K. HOLMES / H. HUNTER HANDSFIELD

In all societies, sexually transmitted diseases (STDs) are among the most common of all infections. In the developing countries, three bacterial STDs—gonorrhea, chlamydial infections, and syphilis—rank among the top 10 to 20 diseases causing the loss of years of healthy, productive life due to major complications such as salpingitis, infertility, ectopic pregnancy, and perinatal morbidity. Among the viral STDs, infection with human immunodeficiency virus (HIV) has become the leading cause of death in some developing countries within the past decade, while two of the most common sexually transmitted viruses—human papillomavirus (HPV) and hepatitis B virus (HBV)—are important causes of cervical carcinoma and hepatocellular carcinoma. There is also a growing awareness of the sexual transmission of human T lymphotropic virus type I (HTLV-I) in many developing countries of Latin America, Africa, and the Caribbean. Although the bacterial STDs remain extremely common in all parts of the world, their incidence is rapidly declining in virtually all the industrialized countries except some parts of the United States. The Centers for Disease Control and Prevention in Atlanta estimates that at least 12 million U.S. residents acquire an STD each year, and some authorities estimate that half or more of all Americans acquire an STD by age 35. In industrialized countries, the unexpectedly high prevalence of certain incurable viral STDs [e.g., HPV infection, genital herpes, and cytomegalovirus (CMV) infection] is being increasingly recognized. The marked enhancement of the efficiency of transmission of HIV by both the genital ulcerative and the genital mucosal STDs adds to the urgency of STD prevention and control.

CLASSIFICATION OF AND GENERAL APPROACH

STDs can be classified on the basis of either cause or clinical manifestations. Table 88-1 summarizes the etiologic classification of STDs. Several of the pathogens listed are also transmitted nonsexually,

TABLE 88-1 Sexually transmitted pathogens

Bacteria	Viruses	Other*
TRANSMITTED IN ADULTS PREDOMINANTLY BY SEXUAL INTERCOURSE		
Neisseria gonorrhoeae	Human immunodeficiency viruses (HIV-1 and -2)	*Trichomonas vaginalis*
Chlamydia trachomatis	Human T lymphotropic virus type I (HTLV-I)	*Phthirus pubis*
Treponema pallidum	Herpes simplex virus type 2 (HSV-2)	
Calymmatobacterium	Human papillomavirus (multiple types)	
granulomatis	Hepatitis B virus[†]	
Ureaplasma urealyticum	Cytomegalovirus	
	Molluscum contagiosum virus	
SEXUAL TRANSMISSION REPEATEDLY DESCRIBED BUT NOT WELL DEFINED OR NOT THE PREDOMINANT MODE		
Mycoplasma hominis	Human T lymphotrophic virus type II (HTLV-II)	*Candida albicans*
Gardnerella vaginalis and	(?) Hepatitis C, D viruses	*Sarcoptes scabiei*
other vaginal bacteria	Herpes simplex virus type 1 (HSV-1)	
Group B streptococcus	(?) Epstein-Barr virus (EBV)	
TRANSMITTED BY SEXUAL CONTACT INVOLVING ORAL-FECAL EXPOSURE; OF DECLINING IMPORTANCE IN HOMOSEXUAL MEN		
Shigella spp.	Hepatitis A virus	*Giardia lamblia*
Campylobacter spp.		*Entamoeba histolytica*

* Includes protozoa, ectoparasites, and fungi.
[†] Among U.S. patients for whom a risk factor can be ascertained, most hepatitis B virus infections are sexually transmitted.

but in each instance sexual transmission is clinically and epidemiologically important.

No single STD can be regarded as an isolated problem because multiple infections are common and because the presence of one STD denotes high-risk sexual behavior that is often associated with other, more serious infections. STDs are not endogenous, and rarely if ever are they transmitted by fomites, food, flies, or casual contact. *At least one sexual partner is always infected*; the apparent exceptions usually can be attributed to prolonged subclinical infection in one or both partners. The elicitation of a sexual history and the management of sexual partners are therefore of paramount importance. The failure to identify and to examine or refer the infected partner represents a failure in management, both at the community level (since sources of spread of infection are not identified) and at the individual patient level (since reinfection is not prevented).

Most persons with overt genital discharge, lesions, or pain cease sexual activity and seek medical care. Accordingly, those who transmit infection usually are among the minority who are infected but asymptomatic or who do not understand the implications of their symptoms and thus do not seek medical attention spontaneously. Physicians must see that such partners are examined and treated or referred. In the United States, local health departments will usually help to identify and treat contacts of patients with some of the curable diseases [e.g., syphilis, gonococcal pelvic inflammatory disease (PID)] and will help notify partners of persons with HIV infection, but for most STDs this responsibility is shared by the patient and the clinician.

In general, persons with a new-onset STD have a *source contact* from whom it was acquired; in addition, they may have a *secondary contact* (also known as a *spread contact* or *exposed contact*). The identification and treatment of both types of contacts are important but generally for different reasons. Identification and treatment of the source contract (often a casual contact who, by definition, is spreading infection) are of greatest importance from the public health/community standpoint, since these measures will prevent further transmission. Identification and treatment of the recently exposed secondary contact (more often a spouse or steady sexual partner) will help prevent the development of serious complications, such as PID.

The increasing importance of the viral STDs, most of which are incurable and lifelong, underscores the central role of primary prevention. Whereas early detection and treatment can curtail the spread of the bacterial STDs, control of the viral STDs depends entirely on the avoidance of unprotected exposure to infected persons; the sole exception is vaccination against HBV infection.

Because STDs disproportionately affect women and newborn children, the prevention of these diseases is an important women's health issue. Many STDs are transmitted more efficiently from men to women than from women to men. Early in the course of infection, women are more likely than men to have subclinical infections or minor, nonspecific symptoms—a situation than can result in delayed diagnosis. The lesser specificity of clinical findings and the lesser sensitivity of several microbiologic tests make the diagnosis of STDs more difficult in women than in men. Most important, women and newborn children are at far greater risk than are men for long-lasting or permanent sequelae.

STDs are propagated most efficiently in populations with frequent changes of sexual partners and with poor access to or low motivation in obtaining early treatment. In most of the United States, these groups consist predominantly of young individuals of low socioeconomic status. These individuals often reside within circumscribed, deteriorating, crowded urban neighborhoods, although rates of STDs are also high in rural areas (in the southeastern United States, for example). The treatable bacterial STDs, such as syphilis, gonorrhea, and chancroid, are increasingly concentrated in "core populations" and increasingly involve prostitutes and their sexual partners and persons involved in the use of illicit drugs, particularly "crack" cocaine in the United States. Members of these core populations have been difficult to reach for the purposes of education and contact tracing and may continue to be sexually active despite STD symptoms. Other STDs are more evenly distributed in society. For example, chlamydial infection and the incurable viral STDs persist (often asymptomatically) and are propagated widely in populations that do not share the characteristics of STD core groups.

Various STDs differ in the extent to which their spread and persistence in the population depend on high rates of sexual partner change. In general, the initial rate of spread of an STD pathogen within a population depends on the product of three factors: the average rate of partner change in the population, the average duration of infectiousness of the pathogen, and the average efficiency of transmission per exposure of a susceptible person to an infected person. For diseases with a high efficiency of transmission and/or a long duration of infectiousness, rates of partner change need not be very high to sustain an epidemic. For STDs with a low efficiency of transmission (e.g., HIV infection) or a short duration of infectiousness (e.g., chancroid), high rates of partner change may be necessary to sustain an epidemic. Efforts to prevent and control STDs involve attempts to decrease the duration of infectiousness (through early diagnosis and treatment), to decrease the efficiency of transmission (through promotion of condom use), and to decrease the rate of partner change (through provision of information, health education, and counseling and efforts to change the norms of sexual behavior).

MANAGEMENT OF COMMON STD SYNDROMES

Table 88-2 lists some of the most common clinical STD syndromes and their associated complications. Strategies for the management of some of the common STD syndromes are outlined below. AIDS is discussed in Chap. 279.

An overall approach to the management of a patient with an STD begins with risk assessment (of sexual behaviors, specific exposures, and sociodemographic and other markers for high risk) and clinical assessment (elicitation of specific symptoms and signs of STDs). In light of the results of these assessments, confirmatory diagnostic tests or screening tests (e.g., culture, antigen detection test, most serologic tests) may be ordered. In developing countries and in office practices in most industrialized countries, treatment is usually given on a syndromic basis (i.e., it is selected to cover the most likely causes) while the results of confirmatory tests are pending. For certain syndromes in industrialized countries, rapid tests may be used to narrow the spectrum of this initial therapy (e.g., wet mount for women with vaginal discharge, Gram's stain for men with urethral discharge). After the institution of syndromic treatment (or of specific treatment when rapid tests have been diagnostic), it is essential to complete the first phase of STD management with what has been termed "the three C's": contact notification and treatment; condom promotion, where appropriate; and counseling regarding the reduction of future risk.

The following approach to the management of common STD syndromes is geared toward clinicians in industrialized countries, where rapid tests and confirmatory tests are widely available but less widely used then they should be.

URETHRITIS IN MEN   Urethritis is the most commonly recognized STD syndrome in men. During the past decade, the incidence of gonococcal urethritis has fallen precipitously in nearly all industrialized countries, while that of nongonococcal urethritis (NGU) remains high—a pattern suggesting that current measures for control of NGU are relatively ineffective. In general, gonorrhea and NGU occur with similar frequencies among men seen in STD clinics in the United States, whereas NGU is several times more common than gonorrhea among men seen by physicians in most other settings.

About 30 to 40 percent of NGU cases are caused by *Chlamydia trachomatis*, although the proportion may have declined in populations where chlamydial control programs have been implemented. Herpes simplex virus (HSV) and *Trichomonas vaginalis* each cause a small proportion of NGU cases in the United States. However, most cases cannot be attributed to any of these three pathogens. *Ureaplasma urealyticum* has been implicated in case-control studies as a probable cause of many of the *Chlamydia*-negative cases. A few cases are caused by coliform bacteria in men who are the insertive partners in unprotected anal intercourse. The diagnosis of male urethritis usually does not include specific tests for pathogens aside from *Neisseria gonorrhoeae* and *C. trachomatis*. However, diagnostic testing for *C. trachomatis* is now widely available; the agent can be isolated from tissue cell culture, or its antigens or genetic material can be detected. The following steps should be taken in evaluating sexually active men with symptoms of urethral discharge and/or dysuria.

1 Establish the presence of urethritis. The first step is examination for purulent or mucopurulent urethral discharge. Sometimes the urethra must be milked after the patient has not voided for several hours, preferably overnight. Whether or not an abnormal discharge is evident, inflammation should be evaluated by examination of a Gram-stained smear after passage of a small swab 2 to 3 cm into the urethra; the presence of 5 or more neutrophils per 1000× field in areas containing cells suggests urethritis. Alternatively, the centrifuged sediment of the first 20 to 30 mL of voided urine can be examined for inflammatory cells, either by microscopy or by the leukocyte esterase test. Patients with symptoms who lack objective evidence of urethritis on two occasions 1 week apart may have functional rather than organic problems and generally do not benefit from repeated courses of antibiotics.

2 Evaluate for complications or alternative diagnoses. Epididymitis and systemic complications, such as the gonococcal arthritis-dermatitis syndrome and Reiter's syndrome, should be excluded by a brief history and examination. Bacterial prostatitis and cystitis should be excluded by appropriate testing of men with dysuria who lack evidence of urethritis and of sexually inactive men with urethritis. Digital examination of the prostate gland is seldom informative in the evaluation of sexually active young men with urethritis.

3 Evaluate for gonococcal and chlamydial infection. Gonorrhea is diagnosed by the demonstration of typical gram-negative diplococci within neutrophils, and a preliminary diagnosis of NGU is warranted if gram-negative diplococci are not found. Confirmation of gonococcal urethritis by culture is optional if the Gram's stain is interpreted by an experienced reader as positive; culture is recommended if the Gram's stain is equivocal. Diagnostic testing for *C. trachomatis* is also recommended, even if empirical treatment for chlamydial infection is planned, because the results predict the patient's prognosis and guide the counseling given to the patient and the management of the patient's sexual partner(s).

TABLE 88-2   Common STD syndromes and etiologic agents

Syndrome	Primary sexually transmitted (ST) agents
Urethritis: males	*N. gonorrhoeae, C. trachomatis, U. urealyticum,* HSV
Epididymitis	*C. trachomatis, N. gonorrhoeae;* **non-ST agents:** urinary tract pathogens
Lower genital tract infections: females	
Cystitis/urethritis	*C. trachomatis, N. gonorrhoeae,* HSV; **non-ST agents:** urinary tract pathogens
Mucopurulent cervicitis	*C. trachomatis, N. gonorrhoeae*
Vulvovaginitis	*C. albicans, T. vaginalis;* **non-ST agents:** chemical irritants, allergens
Bacterial vaginosis (BV)	BV-associated bacteria (see text)
Acute pelvic inflammatory disease	*N. gonorrhoeae, C. trachomatis,* BV-associated bacteria; **non-ST agents:** coliform bacteria
Ulcerative lesions of the genitalia	HSV-1, *T. pallidum, H. ducreyi, C. trachomatis* (LGV strains), *C. granulomatis;* **non-ST agents:** *C. albicans,* pyogenic bacteria
Proctitis	*C. trachomatis, N. gonorrhoeae,* HSV, *T. pallidum*
Enteritis, enterocolitis, proctocolitis	*G. lamblia, Campylobacter* spp., *Shigella* spp., *E. histolytica,* other enteric pathogens
Acute arthritis	*N. gonorrhoeae* (e.g., DGI), *C. trachomatis* (e.g., Reiter's syndrome), HBV, HIV
Genital and anal warts	Human papillomavirus (genital types)
AIDS	HIV-1, HIV-2; also many opportunistic pathogens
Mononucleosis syndrome	Cytomegalovirus, HIV, EBV
Viral hepatitis	HBV; **non-ST agents:** HAV, HCV, HDV
Neoplasias	
Squamous cell cancer of the cervix, anus, vulva, or penis	Human papillomavirus (especially types 16, 18, 31)
Kaposi's sarcoma	HIV; other (?)
Lymphoid neoplasia	HIV, HTLV-I
Hepatocellular carcinoma	HBV
Tropical spastic paraparesis	HTLV-I
Scabies	*S. scabiei*
Pubic lice	*P. pubis*

Abbreviations: HSV = herpes simplex virus; DGI = disseminated gonococcal infection; EBV = Epstein-Barr virus; HAV, HBV, HCV, HDV = hepatitis A, B, C viruses and "delta" agent.

4 Treat the urethritis. In practice, urethritis is treated with a regimen effective for NGU if gonorrhea is excluded by Gram's stain; for example, doxycycline (100 mg orally, twice daily) or tetracycline (500 mg orally, four times daily) for 7 days may be administered. If gonococci are demonstrated by Gram's stain or if no diagnostic tests are performed, treatment should include one of the single-dose regimens for gonorrhea (see Chap. 110) plus a 7-day course of doxycycline or tetracycline for possible chlamydial infection. Sexual partners should be tested for gonorrhea and chlamydial infection and should receive the regimen given to the male index case.

EPIDIDYMITIS Acute epididymitis is almost always unilateral and must be differentiated from testicular torsion, tumor, and trauma. Torsion, a surgical emergency, usually occurs in the second or third decade of life and is suggested by sudden onset of pain, elevation of the testicle within the scrotal sac, rotation of the epididymis from a posterior to an anterior position, and absence of blood flow on Doppler examination or ^{99m}Tc scan. Testicular tumor is suggested by persistence of symptoms after a course of therapy. In sexually active men under age 35, acute epididymitis is caused most frequently by *C. trachomatis* and less commonly by *N. gonorrhoeae* and is usually associated with overt or subclinical urethritis. Antimicrobial agents are the mainstays of therapy; the optimal syndromic treatment for epididymitis due to *C. trachomatis* or *N. gonorrhoeae* is ceftriaxone (250 mg intramuscularly) followed by doxycycline (100 mg orally, twice daily for 10 days). Alternatively, ofloxacin (300 mg orally, twice daily for 10 days) is effective against both *N. gonorrhoeae* and *C. trachomatis* as well as against Enterobacteriaceae.

Acute epididymitis in older men or following urinary tract instrumentation is usually caused by gram-negative bacilli or other urinary pathogens. Similarly, epididymitis in young homosexual men is often caused by Enterobacteriaceae. Urethritis is usually absent in these cases, but bacteriuria is present.

LOWER GU TRACT INFECTION IN WOMEN Infections of the female lower urinary tract, cervix, vulva, and vagina produce various combinations of dysuria, vulvar irritation, dyspareunia, and increased or altered vaginal discharge. Diagnostic confusion may be attributable to the nonspecific symptomatology, to the tendency of specific pathogens to produce inflammation and symptoms at multiple contiguous sites (e.g., genital herpes can cause dysuria, vulvar pain, and vaginal discharge), and to the lack of consistent application of available laboratory tests. Two steps are required in the evaluation of symptoms of the lower genitourinary tract in women: (1) differentiation among cystitis, urethritis, vulvovaginitis, and cervicitis and (2) exclusion of associated upper tract disease (e.g., pyelonephritis, salpingitis).

Urethritis and the urethral syndrome *C. trachomatis, N. gonorrhoeae*, and occasionally HSV are causes of symptomatic urethritis— with or without cervicitis— in women. Sexually acquired urethritis in women often presents as the *urethral syndrome*, characterized by "internal" dysuria (usually without urinary urgency or frequency) and pyuria, with $\geq 10^2$ *Escherichia coli* or other uropathogens per milliliter of urine. The urethral syndrome in the absence of pyuria usually is idiopathic, associated with neither uropathogens nor STD pathogens. Although dysuria occurs more frequently in bacterial urinary tract infection (UTI) or urethral syndrome than in vulvar or vaginal infection, this symptom is often attributable to vulvovaginitis because in many settings the latter are more common than UTI. The dysuria associated with vulvar herpes or vulvovaginal candidiasis (and perhaps with trichomoniasis) is often described as "external," being caused by painful contact of urine with the inflamed labia or introitus.

Among women with acute dysuria and frequency, the first step in diagnosis is to exclude the possiblity of acute pyelonephritis (e.g., costovertebral pain and tenderness and fever). The management of bacterial UTI is discussed in Chap. 90. The next step in diagnosing cases in sexually active women is the differentiation of cystitis from urethritis or vaginal infection. Among women without signs of vulvovaginitis, bacterial UTI must then be differentiated from the urethral syndrome by assessment of risks, evaluation of the pattern of symptoms and signs, and specific microbiologic testing. An STD etiology is suggested by young age, more than one current sexual partner or a new partner within the past month, or coexisting mucopurulent cervicitis (see below). Bacterial cystitis is suggested by acute onset, hematuria, or suprapubic bladder tenderness. The finding of a single conventional urinary pathogen, such as *E. coli* or *Staphylococcus saprophyticus*, in a concentratoin of $\geq 10^2$ per milliliter in a properly collected specimen of midstream urine from a symptomatic woman with pyuria indicates probable bacterial UTI, whereas pyuria with $< 10^2$ conventional uropathogens per milliliter of urine ("sterile" pyuria) suggests acute urethral syndrome due to *C. trachomatis* or *N. gonorrhoeae*. Gonorrhea should be evaluated by Gram's staining and culture of specimens from the cervix and urethra. Chlamydial infection should be evaluated by culture or other specific tests for chlamydial antigen in urethral and cervical specimens. Treatment with a tetracycline (e.g., doxycycline, 100 mg twice daily for 7 days) alleviates dysuria in women with sterile pyuria but not in women without pyuria or isolation of a uropathogen.

Vulvovaginal infections Vulvovaginal symptoms are among the most common reasons for visits to physicians by young women. Further, vulvovaginal infections may have serious sequelae and may increase sexual transmission of HIV; rarely, vulvovaginal symptoms may represent serious upper genital tract or systemic disease. A recent multicenter study (sponsored by the National Institutes of Health) of vaginal infections in pregnancy found that vaginal trichomoniasis and bacterial vaginosis early in pregnancy were independent predictors of premature onset of labor. Bacterial vaginosis also appears to be a risk factor for PID and may be involved in the pathogenesis of anaerobic bacterial infection of the upper genital tract. Trichomoniasis has been associated with about a twofold increase in the risk of acquiring HIV infection in one study of prostitutes in Zaire. Vaginitis may be an early and prominent feature of toxic shock syndrome, and recurrent or chronic vulvovaginal candidiasis develops with increased frequency among women with systemic illnesses, such as diabetes mellitus or HIV infection with impaired immunity (although only a very small proportion of women with recurrent vulvovaginal candidiasis in the United States actually have a serious predisposing illness). Vaginal discharge may be the presenting manifestation of mucopurulent cervicitis caused by gonorrhea or chlamydial infection and may reflect the presence of PID.

Thus vulvovaginal symptoms or signs warrant careful evaluation and appropriate therapy that is specific for the anatomic site and type of infection. A careful pelvic examination is, in fact, within the purview of general medicine and should usually precede more invasive or expensive tests in the evaluation of women with vulvovaginal, pelvic, or abdominal symptoms—and even in the evaluation of some systemic illnesses.

Bacterial vaginosis is the most common cause of vulvovaginal symptoms in most clinical settings; next most common are candidiasis, then trichomoniasis. Vaginal infection may be characterized by one or more of the following: increased volume of discharge; abnormal yellow color of discharge caused by increased concentration of polymorphonuclear leukocytes; vulvar pruritus, irritation, or burning, often with external dysuria; vulvar dyspareunia; and vaginal malodor. An important component of the clinical evaluation of vaginal discharge is ascertaining by speculum examination whether this discharge emanates from the vagina or the cervix and whether it is, in fact, abnormal. Occasionally, increased discharge or other vaginal signs and symptoms are not associated with objective signs of vaginitis or cervicitis. The diagnosis and treatment of the three types of vaginal infection are summarized in Table 88-3.

VAGINAL TRICHOMONIASIS (See also Chap. 179) Sexual transmission of *T. vaginalis* is well documented. Routine culture indicates that many infected women and most infected men are asymptomatic. However, treatment of asymptomatic as well as symptomatic cases

TABLE 88-3   Diagnostic features and management of vaginal infection

Feature	Normal vaginal examination	Vulvovaginal candidasis	Trichomonal vaginitis	Bacterial vaginosis (BV)
Etiology	Uninfected; *Lactobacillus* predominant	*Candida albicans* and yeasts	*Trichomonas vaginalis*	Associated with *G. vaginalis*, various anaerobic bacteria, and mycoplasmas
Typical symptoms	None	Vulvar itching and/or irritation, increased discharge	Profuse purulent discharge; vulvar itching	Malodorous, slightly increased discharge
Discharge				
Amount	Variable; usually scant	Scant to moderate	Profuse	Scant to moderate
Color*	Clear or white	White	Yellow	White or gray
Consistency	Nonhomogeneous, floccular	Clumped; adherent plaques	Homogeneous	Homogeneous, low viscosity; uniformly coats vaginal walls
Inflammation of vulvar or vaginal epithelium	None	Erythema of vaginal epithelium, introitus; vulvar dermatitis common	Erythema of vaginal and vulvar epithelium; colpitis macularis	None
pH of vaginal fluid†	Usually ≤4.5	Usually ≤4.5	Usually ≥5.0	Usually >4.5
Amine ("fishy") odor with 10% KOH	None	None	May be present	Present
Microscopy‡	Normal epithelial cells; lactobacilli predominant	Leukocytes, epithelial cells; yeast, mycelia, or pseudomycelia in up to 80%	Leukocytes; motile trichomonads seen in 80% to 90% of symptomatic patients, less often in the absence of symptoms	Clue cells; few leukocytes; lactobacilli outnumbered by profuse mixed flora, nearly always including *G. vaginalis* plus anaerobic species on Gram's stain
Usual treatment	None	Miconazole or clotrimazole intravaginally, each 100 mg nightly for 3 to 7 nights Fluconazole, 150 mg orally (single dose)	Metronidazole, 2 g orally (single dose) Metronidazole, 500 mg orally, twice daily for 7 days	Clindamycin, 2% vaginal cream, twice daily for 7 days Metronidazole, 0.75% vaginal gel, twice daily for 5 days Metronidazole, 500 mg orally, twice daily for 7 days
Usual management of sexual partner	None	None; topical treatment if candidal dermatitis of penis is present	Examination for STD; treatment with metronidazole, 2 g orally (single dose)	Examination for STD; no treatment if normal

* Color of discharge is best determined by examination against the white background of a swab.
† pH determination is not useful if blood is present.
‡ To detect fungal elements, vaginal fluid is digested with 10% KOH prior to microscopic examination; to examine for other features, fluid is mixed (1:1) with physiologic saline. Gram's stain is also excellent for detecting yeasts and pseudomycelia and for distinguishing normal flora from the mixed flora seen in bacterial vaginosis, but it is less sensitive than the saline preparation for detection of *T. vaginalis*.
SOURCE: From KK Holmes et al.

is recommended to reduce the reservoir of infection and the risk of transmission and to prevent the later development of symptoms.

Symptomatic trichomoniasis characteristically produces a profuse, yellow, purulent, homogeneous vaginal discharge and vulvar itching. The vaginal and vulvar epithelium are often visibly inflamed, and petechial lesions are seen by colposcopy on the cervix ("strawberry cervix") in about 50 percent of cases. The pH of vaginal fluid is usually 5.0 or greater. In women with typical symptoms and signs of trichomoniasis, the diagnosis usually can be confirmed by the demonstration of motile trichomonads and polymorphonuclear leukocytes in vaginal secretions mixed with normal saline and promptly examined microscopically. In such cases, wet-mount examination is at least 80 percent as sensitive as culture. However, in women without symptoms or signs, culture is often required for detection of the organism. The diagnosis of *T. vaginalis* infection in men is more difficult and requires culture of early-morning first-voided urine sediment or of a urethral swab specimen obtained before voiding. New methods of identifying *T. vaginalis* by immunofluorescence or by use of oligonucleotide probes are under investigation and may prove diagnostically helpful for cases in both men and women.

Nitroimidazoles are the only drugs that are consistently effective for the treatment of trichomoniasis. Several studies show that a single 2.0-g oral dose of metronidazole is at least 90 percent as effective as more prolonged dosage schedules. Other nitroimidazoles such as tinidazole and ornidazole have longer half-lives than metronidazole but have not been shown clearly to give better results in trichomoniasis. Routine treatment of sexual partners is recommended to reduce both the risk of reinfection and the reservoir of infection. Vaginal treatment with 0.75% metronidazole gel, although effective for bacterial

vaginosis (see below), is not highly effective for vaginal trichomoniasis. Metronidazole is not recommended during the first trimester of pregnancy. Alcohol must be avoided for 24 h after its use because of occasional disulfiram-like effects. When practical, the partners of patients with trichomoniasis (or with any sexually transmitted infection, for that matter) should be seen in person rather than treated without examination and counseling.

BACTERIAL VAGINOSIS   Vaginal discharge not associated with *T. vaginalis*, yeast, or cervical infection is usually due to bacterial vaginosis. This syndrome (formerly termed *nonspecific vaginitis*, *anaerobic vaginitis*, or *Gardnerella-associated vaginal discharge*) is characterized by vaginal malodor and a slightly to moderately increased white discharge that is homogeneous, low in viscosity, and smoothly coats the vaginal mucosa. It is unclear whether bacterial vaginosis is a sexually transmitted infection. The syndrome is associated with STD risk factors, such as multiple sexual partners and recent intercourse with a new partner, but no single sexually transmitted pathogen has been clearly implicated as the cause. Antibiotic treatment of male partners does not seem to influence the rate of recurrence among affected women. Formerly considered a benign condition, bacterial vaginosis has been implicated as a risk factor for acute salpingitis, premature labor, and related neonatal and perinatal complications.

The increased prevalence and concentrations of *G. vaginalis*, *Mycoplasma hominis*, and several anaerobic bacteria [e.g., *Mobiluncus* spp., *Prevotella* spp. (formerly *Bacteroides* spp.), and some *Peptostreptococcus* spp.] in vaginal fluid of women with bacterial vaginosis probably contribute to its pathogenesis. Of the various microorganisms associated with bacterial vaginosis, *Prevotella* spp.

and *M. hominis* have been most strongly correlated with premature delivery. However, none of these organisms is found only among women with this syndrome, and *G. vaginalis* has been isolated from the vagina of up to 50 percent of healthy women. The hydrogen peroxide–producing *Lactobacillus* spp., which constitute most of the normal vaginal flora (with *L. acidophilus* and *L. jensenii* most commonly found), are usually absent from the vagina in bacterial vaginosis. Hydrogen peroxide–producing lactobacilli may protect against a variety of vaginal and cervical pathogens, and it has been hypothesized that selective depletion of these organisms facilitates the overgrowth of the vagina by anaerobic bacteria, *M. hominis*, and *G. vaginalis*.

In a patient with symptoms of abnormal vaginal discharge and malodor or with objective signs of increased white homogeneous vaginal discharge, bacterial vaginosis can be diagnosed with reasonable certainty by the following:

1 *Exclusion of candidal and trichomonal vaginitis and mucopurulent cervicitis.* This process must include the collection of endocervical specimens to be tested for *C. trachomatis* and *N. gonorrhoeae.*
2 *Liberation of a distinct fishy odor immediately after mixing of vaginal secretions with a 10% solution of KOH.* This odor is attributable to volatile amines (e.g., trimethylamine, putrescine, and cadaverine) in the vaginal fluid, presumably resulting from anaerobic bacterial metabolism.
3 *Demonstration of a pH of vaginal secretions of > 4.5.* The elevated pH may be partly due to the presence of amines as well as to decreased production of lactate.
4 *Microscopic demonstration of "clue cells" and characteristic alterations of the vaginal microflora.* Clue cells are vaginal epithelial cells coated with coccobacillary organisms. On wet mount, prepared by mixing of vaginal secretions with normal saline in a ratio of approximately 1:1, clue cells have a granular appearance and indistinct borders (Fig. 88-1). Clue cells also can be detected on a Gram-stained smear. The Gram-stained smear permits assessment of the vaginal flora; the normally predominant lactobacilli (large, gram-positive rods) are mostly or completely replaced by a profusion of bacterial morphotypes consistent with *G. vaginalis* and anaerobic organisms. The demonstration of many clue cells by wet mount microscopy and the documentation of characteristically altered vaginal flora by Gram's stain represent the most sensitive, specific, and objective criteria for the diagnosis of bacterial vaginosis in women with symptoms and/or signs of this condition.

Attempts to isolate *G. vaginalis*, genital mycoplasmas, or anaerobic bacteria are of little utility in the diagnosis of bacterial vaginosis because these organisms are components of the vaginal flora in many women without the syndrome. However, semiquantitative techniques that detect high concentrations of *G. vaginalis* (equivalent to $\geq 10^6$ organisms per milliliter) are being evaluated.

The standard regimen for bacterial vaginosis has been metronidazole (500 mg orally, twice daily for 7 days). Clindamycin (300 mg orally, twice daily for 7 days) is also effective. Recent data suggest that intravaginal treatment with 2% clindamycin cream (5 g each night for 7 nights) or 0.75% metronidazole gel (5 g twice daily for 5 days) is comparable to oral therapy in efficacy but produces fewer adverse reactions. Intravaginal clindamycin cream is likely to become the treatment of choice for pregnant women with bacterial vaginosis. Oral amoxicillin formerly was considered a therapeutic option, but is much less effective than metronidazole or clindamycin (perhaps because it is active against *Lactobacillus* spp., preventing reestablishment of a protective *Lactobacillus* flora) and is no longer recommended. Sulfonamide-containing vaginal creams are usually ineffective, probably because sulfonamides are inactive against both *G. vaginalis* and many vaginal anaerobes, and there is no rationale for their use. Tetracycline therapy also is ineffective. No controlled data support the use of vaginal or oral preparations of *Lactobacillus* spp. in the treatment of bacterial vaginosis. However, few if any of the commercial preparations of lactobacilli used so far have contained

A

B

FIGURE 88-1 *A.* Vaginal epithelial "clue cells." Note granular appearance due to adherent *G. vaginalis* and indistinct cell margins (400×). *B.* Normal vaginal epithelial cells. The cell margins are distinct and lack granularity.

hydrogen peroxide–producing vaginal strains, and studies with such isolates will be of interest.

Treatment of male partners of women with bacterial vaginosis does not seem to prevent recurrence in these women and therefore is not indicated.

VULVOVAGINAL CANDIDIASIS The predominant symptom in vulvovaginal candidiasis is vulvar pruritus. There is usually no distinct odor. Vulvar erythema is common. The vaginal discharge typically is white and scanty and sometimes takes the form of thrushlike plaques or cottage cheese–like curds adhering loosely to the vaginal mucosa. *Candida albicans* accounts for about 80 percent of yeasts isolated from the vagina, while *Torulopsis glabrata* and other less commonly encountered *Candida* spp. are found in the remainder. Most cases of vulvovaginal candidiasis probably result from increased growth of yeasts that previously colonized the vagina or the intestinal tract. However, occasional cases of recurrent vulvovaginal candidiasis may be due to sexual transmission from a colonized male, and some men whose partners have vulvovaginal candidiasis develop symptomatic yeast dermatitis of the penis.

The diagnosis of vulvovaginal candidiasis involves the demonstration of fungi by microscopic examination of vaginal fluid in saline or 10% KOH or by Gram's stain. Demonstration of pseudohyphae strengthens the diagnosis of vaginitis due to *C. albicans*. Polymorphonuclear leukocytes often are present. Microscopic examination is less sensitive than culture, but correlates better with symptoms. Culture commonly detects coincidental colonization in women who may not require therapy. The pH of vaginal secretions is usually less than 4.5, and no amine odor is produced when vaginal secretions are mixed with 10% KOH. Vulvitis often accompanies vaginitis and may result in superficial erosions or fissures that must be differentiated from genital herpes and other causes of genital ulcer.

In most circumstances, therapy for candidal vaginal infection is indicated only if the patient is symptomatic, if she has signs of vulvovaginitis, or if inflammatory cells or pseudohyphae are evident. The usual treatment is intravaginal administration of any of several imidazole antibiotics (e.g., miconazole or clotrimazole) for 3 to 7 days. The recent over-the-counter marketing of such preparations undoubtedly has reduced the cost of care and made treatment more convenient for many women with yeast vulvovaginitis. However, the symptoms of vulvovaginitis are nonspecific, and self-treatment of presumed yeast infections may delay the detection and treatment of other, more serious infections. Therefore, self-treatment should be strictly limited to women with classic symptoms in whom previous episodes of yeast vulvovaginitis have been documented by an experienced clinician. Single-dose oral treatment with fluconazole (150 mg) is also effective and is preferred by many patients. Prolonged or periodic oral therapy with fluconazole or ketoconazole may be indicated for especially severe or frequently recurrent cases or for those which do not respond to intravaginal or single-dose oral therapy. Such patients probably should be evaluated for diabetes or HIV infection, although such systemic illnesses are uncommon explanations for recurrent vulvovaginal candidiasis. Treatment of sexual partners is not routinely indicated, although its value has not been studied rigorously.

Mucopurulent cervicitis Mucopurulent cervicitis refers to inflammation of the columnar epithelium and subepithelium of the endocervix and of any contiguous columnar epithelium that lies exposed in an ectopic position on the exocervix. Mucopurulent cervicitis in women can be regarded as the "silent partner" of urethritis in men, being equally common and caused by the same agents but more difficult to recognize. It is the most common major STD syndrome in women, can be a harbinger or sign of PID, and—in pregnant women—can lead to obstetrical complications. Improved recognition and treatment of this syndrome would greatly facilitate the control of STDs. Mucopurulent cervicitis is caused most commonly by C. trachomatis and sometimes by N. gonorrhoeae; the relative proportions of cases due to these two organisms depend on their prevalence in the community. However, up to one-half of cases are associated with neither of these organisms and currently must be considered idiopathic. The syndrome usually can be differentiated clinically from cervicitis caused by HSV, which produces lesions on the stratified squamous epithelium of the exocervix as well as on the columnar epithelium.

The diagnosis is made by the demonstration of mucopurulent discharge from the cervical os or of increased numbers of polymorphonuclear leukocytes in Gram-stained or Papanicolaou smears of endocervical mucus. Edematous cervical ectopy (see below) and endocervical bleeding induced by gentle swabbing are common signs of mucopurulent cervicitis due to C. trachomatis. The color of cervical mucus on a white swab removed from the endocervix should be noted; a yellow color indicates the presence of polymorphonuclear leukocytes. The mucus should be rolled *thinly* on a slide for Gram's staining. An area of the slide should be identified that contains strands of cervical mucus not contaminated by vaginal squamous epithelial cells or vaginal bacteria. The presence of 30 or more polymorphonuclear cells per 1000× microscopic field within strands of cervical mucus suggests cervicitis. A characteristic pattern of inflammatory cells on endocervical Papanicolaou smears is sometimes considered by cytopathologists to suggest chlamydial infection. However, such findings are not sufficiently specific to warrant a diagnosis of chlamydial infection; they signify only a need for specific confirmatory testing.

Mucopurulent cervicitis requires antimicrobial therapy. An etiologic diagnosis should always be established to guide the management of sexual partners, but therapy for these men should be initiated against the most likely causes of this syndrome while results of diagnostic tests are pending.

In settings where both gonorrhea and chlamydial infection are common, therapy should include a single-dose regimen effective for gonorrhea, such as ceftriaxone (125 mg intramuscularly), followed by doxycycline (100 mg orally, twice daily for 1 week). When doxycycline is contraindicated, erythromycin base or stearate (500 mg four times daily for 7 days) can be substituted. Ofloxacin (300 mg orally, twice daily for 7 days) is an alternative regimen that is effective for both gonorrhea and chlamydial infection. In settings where gonorrhea is much less common than chlamydial infection, initial therapy for mucopurulent cervicitis may be designed to cover chlamydial infection only (e.g., a regimen of doxycycline, erythromycin or azithromycin). Azithromycin in a single dose of 1.0 g orally can be substituted for a 7-day course of doxycycline or erythromycin but is not reliable for the treatment of gonorrhea. The sexual partner(s) of a woman with mucopurulent cervicitis should be examined and given a regimen similar to that chosen for the woman unless results of tests for gonorrhea or chlamydial infection in either partner warrant a change in therapy. Gonococcal cervicitis is diagnosed by culture of an endocervical specimen. When carefully collected endocervical specimens are examined by experienced personnel, Gram's stain is an insensitive but fairly specific test, and the observation of intracellular gram-negative diplococci indicates gonococcal infection even if the culture is negative. The sensitivity of a single endocervical culture for N. gonorrhoeae is 80 to 90 percent (see Chap. 110). Chlamydial infection of the cervix can be confirmed by culture, antigen detection, or DNA probe or DNA amplification tests (see Chap. 140).

Cervical ectopy Cervicitis must be differentiated from *cervical ectopy*, which is often mislabeled "cervical erosion." Ectopy represents the presence of the one-cell-thick columnar epithelium extending from the endocervix out onto the visible ectocervix. In ectopy, the cervical os may contain clear or slightly cloudy mucus but usually does not include yellow mucopus. Colposcopy shows that the epithelium is intact and not ulcerated. Ectopy is normally found during early adolescence and gradually recedes as squamous metaplasia replaces the ectopic columnar epithelium. Oral contraceptive use favors the persistence or reappearance of ectopy. Cauterization for the elimination of ectopy is not warranted. Ectopy may make the cervix more susceptible to infection with N. gonorrhoeae or C. trachomatis by exposing a larger area of susceptible columnar epithelium. Moreover, ectopy may increase susceptibility to HIV infection. If mucopurulent cervicitis supervenes, the area of ectopy may become edematous and fragile, with bleeding induced by gentle swabbing. In addition, edema of the cervix may result in eversion of the os, with enlargement of the apparent area of ectopy.

PELVIC INFLAMMATORY DISEASE PID is a syndrome that comprises various combinations of endometritis, salpingitis, and pelvic peritonitis resulting from ascending genital infection, which usually arises from gonococcal or chlamydial mucopurulent cervicitis and/or from bacterial vaginosis (see Chap. 89). PID and its sequelae predominantly affect sexually active adolescents and young women, in whom at least 90 percent of cases are sexually acquired. Although sometimes clinically severe, with tuboovarian abscess or overt peritonitis, most cases of acute PID are relatively mild or even subclinical; however, such cases can nevertheless result in significant tubal damage, as evidenced by the frequent lack of history of PID or pelvic pain in *Chlamydia*-seropositive women with tubal scarring and infertility or ectopic pregnancy. Accordingly, the clinician must have a low threshold for considering PID in the differential diagnosis of mild or even trivial abdominal pain in young women. The approach represents a shift in thinking from the days when PID was considered likely only in women with severe adnexal tenderness plus an elevation in temperature, white blood cell count, or erythrocyte sedimentation rate.

The proportion of cases caused by N. gonorrhoeae recently has declined in most industrialized countries, a trend reflecting the declining incidence of gonococcal infections in general. C. trachomatis remains a common cause of PID in many countries. Numerous other pathogens contribute to PID, including M. hominis and various anaerobic members of the vaginal flora found in bacterial vaginosis.

Recent data also suggest that vaginal douching is an important risk factor for ascending pelvic infection. PID is discussed in detail in Chap. 89.

ULCERATIVE LESIONS OF THE GENITALIA The incidence and etiology of ulcerative lesions of the genitalia vary greatly in different areas of the world (Table 88-4). In Asia and Africa, genital ulcers are seen as frequently as gonorrhea in some STD clinics; chancroid is the most common cause, while genital herpes is relatively uncommon. In the industrialized western countries, genital ulcers are considerably less common than urethritis, mucopurulent cervicitis, and vaginitis; genital herpes is the most common cause, and chancroid is relatively uncommon. Syphilis is the second most common form of genital ulcer in almost all areas of the world, and the possiblity of its presence must always be excluded. Lymphogranuloma venereum (LGV) and donovanosis (granuloma inguinale) are very rare in North America and Europe. Other causes of genital ulcer include candidiasis and traumatized genital warts, both of which are usually readily recognized, and various non-sexually transmitted dermatoses.

Trauma is an uncommon cause of genital ulcer unless there is clear history of definite injury accompanied by bleeding. Chancroid, syphilis, genital herpes, and probably all causes of genital ulcer enhance the efficiency of sexual transmission and acquisition of HIV. Moreover, genital ulcers, especially chancroid and syphilis, are most common in inner-city populations with low socioeconomic status and high rates of prostitution and illicit drug use—independent risk factors for HIV infection. In the late 1980s in the United States, chancroid and syphilis spread at epidemic rates in such populations, although these rates began to decline in the early 1990s.

In industrialized countries, the differential diagnosis of genital ulceration usually includes genital herpes, syphilis, and chancroid. The clinical findings are occasionally definitive (e.g., the presence of herpetic vesicles), and clinical findings plus epidemiologic considerations can usually guide initial therapy pending the results of further studies. Nevertheless, most genital ulcerations cannot be diagnosed confidently on clinical grounds. It is axiomatic to exclude syphilis by appropriate serologic studies in all cases. All lesions except those highly characteristic of infection with HSV should be subjected to dark-field examination or a direct immunofluorescence test for *Treponema pallidum*. Selective enrichment media are available for isolation of *Haemophilus ducreyi*.

The following general guidelines are recommended for management of ulcerative genital lesions:

Lesions typical of genital herpes In industrialized countries, where the probability of prior herpes is high, a clinical diagnosis of genital herpes is warranted if typical vesicles or pustules are evident or if there is a cluster of painful ulcers that was preceded by vesiculopustular lesions. These clinical presentations are sufficiently typical that confirmation of the diagnosis by isolation of HSV, immunochemical detection of the virus, or type-specific serology is optional. A serologic test for syphilis should be performed not primarily for diagnostic purposes, but because screening is indicated in all patients with a newly diagnosed STD.

All other acute genital ulcers The appearance of genital herpetic lesions is highly variable, and—except in the relatively clear-cut cases described above—a specific test for HSV is indicated whenever feasible. Isolation of HSV by culture or immunochemical identification of HSV antigens or genetic material should be attempted. Type-specific serologic tests may be useful in some cases, but commercially available serologic tests do not distinguish between antibodies to the two types of HSV and are of little use (see Chap. 143). Cytologic methods (Tzanck preparation with Wright-Giemsa or Papanicolaou staining) for the detection of HSV-infected multinucleated cells are very insensitive except in the presence of intact vesicles and are seldom useful in diagnosing genital ulcer disease. An attempt should be made to isolate *H. ducreyi* if the genital ulcer is painful and inguinal lymphadenopathy with fluctuance or overlying erythema is noted; if chancroid is prevalent in the community; if the patient is at high risk for chancroid (e.g., through the use of injection drugs or "crack" cocaine or through prostitution); or if the patient has recently had a sexual exposure in a chancroid-endemic area (e.g., a developing country or certain North American cities). Enlarged, fluctuant lymph nodes should be aspirated for culture and Gram's staining to detect *H. ducreyi* and pyogenic bacteria. Syphilis should be excluded by dark-field examination and serologic testing, and the latter should be repeated 1 to 2 weeks later if the results are initially negative and if another diagnosis cannot be established.

Lesions typical of syphilis If lesions are at all suggestive of syphilis (e.g., painless, nontender, indurated) or there are epidemiologic reasons to suspect syphilis (e.g., recent exposure), dark-field examination and a rapid serologic test for syphilis should be performed. If the results are negative and the patient is reliable in terms of follow-up and sexual abstinence, there should be two more dark-field examinations on successive days before treatment is attempted, and the serologic test should be repeated 1, 2, and 6 weeks later. Direct immunofluorescence staining of *T. pallidum* is quite reliable and should be used if dark-field examination by experienced examiners is impossible.

Chronic genital ulceration When genital ulcers persist beyond the usual course of herpes (2 to 3 weeks) or chancroid or syphilis (up to 6 weeks) and do not resolve with syndromic antimicrobial therapy, then—in addition to the usual tests for herpes, syphilis, and chancroid—biopsy is indicated to exclude donovanosis, carcinoma, and other nonvenereal dermatoses. A test for HIV infection should be done, since chronic, persistent genital herpes is common in HIV infection with reduced concentrations of CD4 cells.

Ideally, treatment for genital ulceration should be withheld until the diagnosis is secure. However, immediate syndromic treatment for acute genital ulcerations (after collection of all necessary diagnostic specimens) is sometimes necessary, e.g., when it is believed that a patient may not return for follow-up. Initial treatment in such cases should generally include 2.4 million units of benzathine penicillin G for possible primary syphilis. Immediate empirical therapy for chancroid also is indicated if the patient has been exposed in an area where chancroid is endemic and especially if regional lymph node suppuration is evident or appears imminent (see Chap. 112). Prompt systemic therapy with acyclovir is indicated for patients with initial episodes of genital or anorectal herpes (see Chap. 143). Finally, empirical antimicrobial therapy may be indicated if ulcers persist and the diagnosis remains unclear after 1 to 2 weeks of observation and repeated attempts to diagnose herpes, syphilis, and chancroid.

PROCTITIS, PROCTOCOLITIS, ENTEROCOLITIS, AND ENTERITIS Sexually acquired proctitis, or inflammation limited to the rectal mucosa, results from direct rectal inoculation of typical STD pathogens. In contrast, inflammation that extends from the rectum to the colon (proctocolitis), that involves both the small and the large bowel (enterocolitis), or that involves the small bowel alone (enteritis) can result from ingestion of typical intestinal pathogens through sexual contact involving oral-fecal exposure. Anorectal pain and

TABLE 88-4 Etiologies of genital ulcer disease in industrialized and tropical developing countries

Diagnosis	Percent of cases	
	Industrialized countries	Tropical developing countries
Genital herpes	50–70	0–10*
Syphilis	10–20	10–20
Chancroid	0–10†	50–60
Donovanosis	<1	<1‡
Other/unknown	10–20	10–30

* The proportion of genital ulcers caused by HSV appears to be increasing as the prevalence of HIV infection increases in developing countries.
† Highly variable; may account for >25% of cases in selected U.S. cities during chancroid outbreaks.
‡ Donovanosis accounts for higher proportions of cases in some geographic areas (e.g., southern Africa, western Australia, Papua New Guinea, and the Indian subcontinent).

mucopurulent or bloody rectal discharge suggest proctitis or proctocolitis. Proctitis is commonly associated with tenesmus (causing frequent attempts to defecate, but not true diarrhea) and constipation, whereas proctocolitis and enterocolitis are more often associated with true diarrhea. In all three conditions anoscopy usually shows the presence of mucosal inflammation with exudate and easily induced mucosal bleeding (i.e., a positive "wipe test"). Petechiae or mucosal ulcers also may be observed. Exudate should be sampled for microbiologic studies and Gram's staining. Sigmoidoscopy or colonoscopy—which should be performed, if possible, without an enema—shows inflammation limited to the rectum (in proctitis) or disease extending at least into the sigmoid colon (in proctocolitis).

Most cases of sexually transmitted intestinal infection in the past have involved homosexual men. During the AIDS era, there has been an extraordinary shift in the clinical and etiologic spectrum of intestinal infections among homosexual men. The number of opportunistic intestinal infections (see Chap. 279) has risen rapidly among persons with AIDS. At the same time, the number of sexually transmitted intestinal infections (as described below) has fallen rapidly as high-risk sexual behaviors have become less common in this group.

Most cases of infectious proctitis are due to *N. gonorrhoeae*, HSV, or *C. trachomatis;* these are acquired via receptive anorectal intercourse. Primary and secondary syphilis also can produce anal or anorectal lesions, with or without symptoms. Proctitis due to *N. gonorrhoeae* or to common strains of *C. trachomatis* typically involves the most distal rectal mucosa and the anal crypts and is clinically mild, without systemic manifestations. In contrast, primary proctitis due to HSV and proctocolitis due to the strains of *C. trachomatis* that cause LGV usually produce severe anorectal pain and often cause fever. Perianal ulcers and inguinal lymphadenopathy, most commonly due to HSV, also can occur in LGV or syphilis. Sacral nerve root radiculopathies, usually presenting as urinary retention, laxity of the anal sphincter, or constipation, are common in primary herpetic proctitis. Sigmoidoscopy most commonly shows ulcerative proctitis in either herpes or LGV but may reveal intact vesicopustular lesions in anorectal herpes. In herpes, biopsy of the rectal mucosa shows microulcerations and may show intranuclear inclusions or perivascular lymphocytic cuffing. In LGV, biopsy typically shows crypt abscesses, granulomas, and giant cells—findings that may be indistinguishable from those of Crohn's disease. Syphilis also can produce rectal granulomas, usually in association with infiltration by plasma cells or other mononuclear cells.

The occurrence of diarrhea and abdominal bloating or cramping pain without anorectal symptoms and in association with normal anoscopy and sigmoidoscopy is consistent with inflammation of the small intestine (enteritis) or with proximal colitis. In homosexual men without HIV infection, enteritis limited to the small intestine is often attributable to *G. lamblia*. Sexually acquired proctocolitis is most often due to *Campylobacter* spp., *Shigella* spp., or *E. histolytica*.

HUMAN PAPILLOMAVIRUS INFECTION AND GENITAL WARTS
Genital warts and infection with HPV were long considered inconvenient but benign conditions. However, evolving evidence indicates that some strains of HPV—e.g., types 16, 18, and 31—are closely linked with (and probably a direct cause of) moderate to severe squamous dysplasia and overt cancer of the cervix, anus, vulva, vagina, and penis; thus infection with this virus is now recognized as one of the most important STDs. The number of visits to clinicians because of genital warts has been estimated at more than 1.2 million each year in the United States. However, most HPV infections are subclinical, and increasingly sensitive tools for the detection of HPV (e.g., the polymerase chain reaction) show that most sexually active young men and women seen at STD clinics have genital HPV infection, usually without visible clinical abnormalities. Treatment of HPV infection yields largely unsatisfactory results; destruction of visible condylomata with cryotherapy, other chemical or physical cytotoxic agents, or surgery does not cure subclinical infection of adjacent tissues. Accordingly, the primary goal of treatment of genital warts is cosmetic, and therapy should be conservative. Although genital warts are no more predictive than other STDs of severe cervical dysplasia (since the types of HPV that commonly cause genital warts are not the types that cause severe dysplasia or invasive cancer), women with any STD should undergo routine cervical cytologic screening. These conditions are addressed in detail in Chap. 149.

ACUTE ARTHRITIS The gonococcal arthritis-dermatitis syndrome and Reiter's syndrome are among the most common forms of acute arthritis in sexually active young adults. These two syndromes must be differentiated from each other, from other forms of infective arthritis, from various diseases associated with immune-complex deposition, from crystal-induced arthritis, from acute rheumatoid arthritis, and from other, less common rheumatic disorders, such as systemic lupus erythematosus. Meningococcemia, infection with *Yersinia*, sarcoidosis, and syphilis are other occasional causes of acute arthritis in young adults.

Demonstration of *N. gonorrhoeae* by culture or by a specific immunochemical method in synovial fluid, blood, skin lesions, or cerebrospinal fluid is diagnostic of disseminated gonococcal infection (DGI). Gonococcal arthritis is highly probable if such tests fail to detect the organism, if it is recovered from a mucosal site of infection or from the patient's sexual partner, and if there are typical pustular or hemorrhagic skin lesions distributed primarily on the extremities. Suspected and confirmed cases of DGI should be treated promptly with an antibiotic effective against antibiotic-sensitive and antibiotic-resistant gonococci, such as ceftriaxone (see Chap. 110).

Reiter's syndrome occurs in a sporadic (apparently sexually transmitted) form that usually follows chlamydial infection and in a postdysenteric form that usually follows infection with *Yersinia, Campylobacter,* or *Shigella* spp. Discrete epidemics of the latter form are sometimes documented (see Chap. 289).

HEPATITIS B VIRUS, CYTOMEGALOVIRUS, AND HUMAN T LYMPHOTROPIC VIRUSES HBV and CMV are carried in the blood, are shed in genital secretions, and can be transmitted through sexual and perinatal exposure as well as through contact with blood. Sexual transmission and perinatal transmission predominate with HTLV-I, whereas transmission by injection drug users predominates with HTLV-II. HTLV-II also is endemic among some Native American tribes. All these agents cause primary infections that usually are asymptomatic, with subsequent chronic or latent infection and a potential for complications or transmission for many years—perhaps indefinitely.

Sexually transmitted HBV infection was an extremely common problem among homosexual and bisexual men until the mid-1980s, and sexual contact among men continues to account for 5 to 10 percent of adult HBV infections in the United States. About 25 percent of cases of hepatitis B in adults currently are attributed to heterosexual transmission and 30 percent to sharing of injection equipment by illicit drug users. The route of acquisition is unknown in 35 to 40 percent of cases, many of which are probably acquired sexually. Hepatitis B is the only STD for which an effective vaccine is available, and current recommendations in the United States include universal vaccination of infants and targeted vaccination of adolescents in high-risk communities, people with multiple sexual partners or other STDs, sexual partners of individuals with acute hepatitis B, and seronegative sexual partners of chronic carriers of the hepatitis B surface antigen.

Sexual contact is the most important mode of transmission of CMV in some settings. Among initially seronegative women attending STD clinics, the annual incidence of seroconversion is 8 to 30 percent. CMV is among the most common causes of congenital neurodevelopmental abnormalities and of life-threatening morbidity in patients with advanced cellular immunodeficiency due to HIV, malignancy, or chemotherapy. Until an effective vaccine is developed, the prevention of sexually transmitted CMV infection will be problematic.

HTLV-I is endemic as a sexually transmitted virus in parts of the Caribbean, Latin America, Asia, and Africa and is associated with

T cell leukemia and tropical spastic paresis (HTLV-I–associated myelopathy). HTLV-II is found in up to 15 to 20 percent of injection drug users in the United States. The clinical consequences of infection with this virus have yet to be defined.

PREVENTION AND CONTROL OF STDs

The control of bacterial STDs has traditionally depended on early diagnosis and treatment. The emergence of the incurable viral STDs has required increasing emphasis on health education and health promotion as a means of discouraging casual sex and high-risk sexual practices and encouraging the use of condoms. Medical students and physicians require training in eliciting a sexual history, determining the extent to which their patients (especially adolescents and young adults) are at risk for STDs, and counseling these patients appropriately. Public education and personal counseling should begin in early adolescence and should emphasize responsible sexual behavior (abstinence, maintenance of monogamous relationships); the use of condoms for nonmonogamous sexual encounters; the avoidance of traumatic sexual practices, such as anal intercourse; the recognition of early symptoms and signs of STDs; and the importance of early health care for such symptoms and signs.

Maintenance of clinical skills in the recognition, diagnosis, and treatment of STDs is essential to the prevention of STD transmission and STD complications. Screening tests for gonorrhea, chlamydial infection, syphilis, and HIV infection as well as cervical cytology should be made widely available and should be used by physicians serving populations at risk. In region X (the Northwest) of the United States, a federally funded program for selective chlamydial diagnostic screening in more than 150 family planning clinics was associated with a decline in chlamydial prevalence from 10 to 5 percent during a 5-year period from 1987 to 1992. It is appalling that, as of early 1993, other regions still had not implemented similar programs for this preventable STD. Health departments should provide high-quality STD clinical services and screening for high-risk populations; these departments are also responsible for STD surveillance and for the coordination of targeted control measures—efforts that require the cooperation of physicians in reporting cases. Notification of the sexual partners of infected persons is the joint responsibility of the patient and the physician. In most communities, the local health department will assist in this effort for cases of syphilis, for some cases of gonorrhea, and increasingly, for cases of HIV infection.

REFERENCES
General

ADIMORA A et al: *Sexually Transmitted Diseases, 2d ed, Companion Handbook*. New York, McGraw-Hill, 1993

ARAL SO, HOLMES KK: Sexually transmitted diseases in the AIDS era. Sci Am 264:62, 1991

BRANDT AM: *No Magic Bullet: A Social History of Venereal Disease in the United States Since 1890*, 2d ed. New York, Oxford Univ Press, 1989

CENTERS FOR DISEASE CONTROL: 1989 sexually transmitted diseases treatment guideline. Morb Mort Week Rep 38(suppl 8):1, 1989

HOLMES KK et al (eds): *Sexually Transmitted Diseases*, 2d ed. New York, McGraw-Hill, 1990

HANDSFIELD HH: *Color Atlas and Synopsis of Sexually Transmitted Diseases*. New York, McGraw-Hill, 1992

Urethritis in males

BOWIE WR: Urethritis in males, in *Sexually Transmitted Diseases*, 2d ed, KK Holmes et al (eds). New York, McGraw-Hill, 1990, chap 52
——— et al: Etiology of nongonococcal urethritis: Evidence for *Chlamydia trachomatis* and *Ureaplasma urealyticum*. J Clin Invest 59:735, 1977

KREIGER J et al: Clinical manifestations of trichomoniasis in men. Ann Intern Med 118:844, 1993

SHAFER MD et al: Urinary leukocyte esterase screening test for asymptomatic chlamydial and gonococcal infection in males. JAMA 262:2562, 1989

Epididymitis

BERGER RE et al: Etiology and manifestations of epididymitis in young men: Correlation with sexual orientation. J Infect Dis 155:1341, 1987

Urethral syndrome

STAMM WE et al: Urinary tract infection: From pathogenesis to treatment. J Infect Dis 159:400, 1989

Vaginal infections

ESCHENBACH DA et al: Diagnosis and clinical manifestations of bacterial vaginosis. Am J Obstet Gynecol 158:819, 1988

HILLIER SL et al: The relationship of hydrogen peroxide–producing lactobacilli to bacterial vaginosis and genital microflora in pregnant women. Obstet Gynecol 79:369, 1992

SOBEL J: Genital candidiasis, in *Sexually Transmitted Diseases*, 2d ed, KK Holmes et al (eds). New York, McGraw-Hill, 1990

WØLNER-HANSSEN P et al: Clinical manifestations of vaginal trichomoniasis. JAMA 261:571, 1989

Mucopurulent cervicitis

BRUNHAM RC et al: Mucopurulent cervicitis—The ignored counterpart in women of urethritis in men. N Engl J Med 311:1, 1984

Genital ulcers

KOUTSKY LA et al: Underdiagnosis of genital herpes by current clinical and viral isolation procedures. N Engl J Med 326:1533, 1992

SIMONSEN JN et al: Human immunodeficiency virus infection among men with sexually transmitted diseases. N Engl J Med 319:274, 1988

Proctitis, proctocolitis, enterocolitis, and enteritis

QUINN TC et al: The polymicrobial etiology of intestinal infections in homosexual men. N Engl J Med 309:576, 1983

Arthritis

HANDSFIELD HH, POLLOCK PS: Arthropathies associated with sexually transmitted diseases, in *Sexually Transmitted Diseases*, 2d ed, KK Holmes et al (eds). New York, McGraw-Hill, 1990

Pelvic inflammatory disease

SOPER DE: Diagnosis and laparoscopic grading of acute salpingitis. Am J Obstet Gynecol 164:1370, 1991

WØLNER-HANSSEN P et al: Association between vaginal douching and acute pelvic inflammatory disease. JAMA 263:1936, 1990

HPV/warts

KOUTSKY LA et al: A cohort study of the risk of cervical intraepithelial neoplasia grade 2 or 3 in relation to papillomavirus infection. N Engl J Med 327:1272, 1992

HBV, CMV, HTLV-I, and HTLV-II

ALTER MJ et al: The changing epidemiology of hepatitis B in the United States: Need for alternative vaccination strategies. JAMA 263:1218, 1990

COLLIER AC et al: Cytomegalovirus infection in women attending a sexually transmitted disease clinic. J Infect Dis 162:46, 1990

89 PELVIC INFLAMMATORY DISEASE

KING K. HOLMES

DEFINITION The term *pelvic inflammatory disease* (PID) usually refers to ascending infection of the endometrium and/or fallopian tubes. Intrauterine infection can be primary (spontaneously occurring and usually sexually transmitted) or secondary to invasive intrauterine surgical procedures (e.g., dilatation and curettage, termination of pregnancy, insertion of an intrauterine device, or hysterosalpingography) or to parturition. Endometritis or endomyometritis is particularly common following delivery by cesarean section.

PID is uncommon during pregnancy itself. The uterotubal junction is closed as early as the seventh week of pregnancy, and the chorioamnion becomes approximated to the endocervical os, sealing off the intrauterine cavity, at the twelfth to fifteenth week of gestation. As a consequence, ascending intrauterine infection prior to the twelfth week of gestation may be associated (as either cause or effect) with endometritis and spontaneous abortion, while ascending infection after the twelfth week may be associated with chorioamnionitis. Rarely, infection may extend secondarily to the pelvic organs from adjacent foci of inflammation, such as appendicitis, regional ileitis, or diverticulitis; as a result of hematogenous dissemination, such as tuberculosis; or as a rare complication of certain tropical diseases, such as schistosomiasis.

Spontaneously occurring PID can be divided into chronic and acute types. Chronic PID due to tuberculosis has become uncommon in industrialized countries. However, subacute or chronic PID caused by chronic infection with *Chlamydia trachomatis* is thought to be common.

PID is the term most often used today to refer to cases of acute spontaneously occurring infection ascending from the cervix or vagina. The clinical diagnosis of PID is imprecise. Use of endometrial biopsy together with laparoscopy provides evidence of a continuum, progressing from cervicitis alone to endometritis, to salpingitis, to pelvic peritonitis, to generalized peritonitis, perihepatitis, or pelvic abscess. In this chapter, PID is used to refer to the clinical syndrome which includes each of these conditions, and the term *salpingitis* is restricted to patients with visually or histopathologically confirmed inflammation of the fallopian tubes. The distribution between endometritis and salpingitis may be important, because long-term sequelae are common after salpingitis. These sequelae include infertility due to bilateral tubal occlusion, peritubal adhesions, ectopic pregnancy due to tubal damage without occlusion, chronic pelvic pain, and recurrent PID.

ETIOLOGY   The etiology of PID has seemed to vary greatly in several studies for reasons related to patient selection as well as methodology. As is summarized in Table 89-1, the agents most often implicated in acute PID include those which are primary causes of cervicitis (*Neisseria gonorrhoeae* and *C. trachomatis*) and those which can be regarded as abnormal components of the vaginal flora.

In the United States, gonococci were isolated from 44 percent of women with acute PID in a multicity cooperative study during the 1970s. From 1980 through 1990 in Seattle, *N. gonorrhoeae* or *C. trachomatis* were found in 85 percent of patients with proven salpingitis and endometritis, with gonorrhea being nearly twice as common as chlamydial infection and dual infection being common. However, in Scandinavian countries, where gonococcal infection is under much better control, endocervical gonococcal infection has been found in a declining proportion of women with PID during the past decade, while chlamydial infection remains more common in this group. In general, PID is most often associated with gonorrhea where there is a high incidence of gonorrhea, e.g., in developing countries and in indigent, inner-city populations in developed countries. In several studies of women with PID, up to two-thirds with positive endocervical cultures for *N. gonorrhoeae* have had positive endometrial, peritoneal, or tubal cultures for this organism. Similarly, studies of women with proven PID have shown that *C. trachomatis* can be demonstrated by culture or immunofluorescent staining in the endometrium or tubes of the majority of those who have endocervical chlamydial infection.

Anaerobic and facultative anaerobic organisms (especially *Prevotella* spp., peptostreptococci, *Escherichia coli*, and group B streptococci) and genital mycoplasmas have been isolated from specimens obtained at laparoscopy from the peritoneal fluid or fallopian tubes in a varying proportion—typically one-fourth to one-third—of women with PID studied in the United States. These vaginal organisms can be found in association with chlamydial or gonococcal infection, as well as in women without them. The importance of vaginal organisms in salpingitis has probably been overestimated in studies based on culture of specimens obtained by culdocentesis or endometrial aspiration, procedures in which contamination of the aspirated specimen by vaginal flora could occur. However, specimens obtained by laparoscopy also have contained anaerobic and facultative species in some patients with PID. It is extremely difficult to determine the exact microbial etiology in the individual patient with PID because of the frequency of mixed infection, the difficulty in sampling the fallopian tube itself, and the complexity of microbiologic techniques required to detect the various fastidious pathogens involved.

In general, first episodes of acute PID are particularly likely to be caused by *N. gonorrhoeae* and/or *C. trachomatis*. These sexually transmitted pathogens are somewhat less often implicated in recurrent bouts of acute PID, episodes occurring in IUD users, and episodes precipitated by invasive intrauterine diagnostic or therapeutic procedures, which are often associated with ascending infection caused by certain components of the endogenous vaginal flora.

EPIDEMIOLOGY   It has been estimated that the annual incidence of PID in the United States during the mid-1970s was about 850,000 cases per year. PID is not a reportable disease in the United States; surveillance of physicians in private practice and of hospital discharges suggests that the incidence of PID increased from the mid-1960s through the mid-1970s and may then have decreased. Hospitalization for acute PID declined from 1982 through 1990, but visits to physicians' offices remained steady during that period. The 1988 National Survey of Family Growth indicated that 11 percent of women have been treated for PID.

Acute PID is almost exclusively a disease of sexually active women. The risk may be greater in sexually active teenagers than among older women. Important risk factors other than young age include a history of salpingitis, recent history of vaginal douching, and use of an intrauterine device, particularly the Dalkon shield. In most studies, the relative risk of PID among IUD users was higher in nulliparous than in parous women, and was greatest during the first few months after insertion. The increased risk of PID among IUD users appears mainly among those with multiple sex partners. On the other hand, women using oral contraceptives appear to be at decreased risk of PID. Barrier methods of contraception also prevent PID by reducing the risk of chlamydial and gonococcal infection. Tubal sterilization reduces (but does not completely eliminate) the risk of salpingitis by preventing intraluminal spread of infection into the tubes.

PATHOGENESIS   Factors cited as possibly contributing to intracanalicular upward spread of gonococci and *Chlamydia* from the endocervix to the endometrium and endosalpinx include estrogen-dominated (thin) cervical mucus, attachment to sperm which migrate upward into the tubes, use of an intrauterine device, vaginal douching, and menstruation. The onset of symptoms of gonorrhea-associated PID and of *Chlamydia*-associated PID often occurs during or soon after the menstrual period. In fallopian tube organ cultures in vitro, gonococci attach to the surface of the secretory columnar cells (but not the ciliated cells) of the endosalpinx. Gonococcal pili and perhaps other surface proteins are important in this attachment. Gonococci then are taken into the secretory cells by endocytosis. They pass through the cells, and perhaps between cells, and are extruded through the base of the cell into the submucosal connective tissue. Ciliary motion ceases, and then ciliated cells, although not directly invaded by gonococci, are sloughed from the mucosa during this process—a factor which may render the tubes more susceptible to superinfection by other organisms. It is uncertain whether this loss of ciliated cells is irreversible in vivo. Gonococcal endotoxin and peptidoglycan and certain cytokines appear responsible for these cytotoxic effects.

TABLE 89-1   Cervical and vaginal organisms most often implicated in acute PID

Cervical pathogens	Vaginal flora

N. gonorrhoeae
C. trachomatis
	Anaerobic bacteria
	   Prevotella spp., Peptostreptococci, *Mobiluncus* spp., *Actinomyces* spp.
	Facultative bacteria
	   Enterobacteriaceae, *H. influenzae*, *G. vaginalis*, Group B, streptococcus
	Mycoplasmas
	   M. hominis,
	   U. urealyticum

Gonococci associated with PID have been significantly more resistant to penicillin and less likely to belong to the Arg-Hyx-Ura auxotype than are strains causing uncomplicated gonorrhea.

C. trachomatis also infects the columnar cells of the fallopian tube but produces little damage in tubal organ cultures, perhaps because the host response is more important than directly toxic effects of bacterial products in the pathogenesis of chlamydial salpingitis. In chlamydial mucopurulent cervicitis (MPC), cervical biopsies show inclusions containing *Chlamydia* within columnar cells; columnar epithelial infiltration by neutrophils; submucosal and stromal infiltration by plasma cells, lymphocytes, histiocytes, and neutrophils; and lymphoid aggregates containing transformed lymphocytes. Routine endometrial biopsies from consecutive women with chlamydial MPC show endometritis in approximately one-half. Although endometritis detected in this way is sometimes associated with uterine tenderness, abnormal menstrual bleeding, and leukocytosis, symptoms of abdominal pain and fever, as well as signs of adnexal tenderness, are usually lacking, underscoring the subclinical nature of many cases of upper genital tract chlamydial infection. It is not known what proportion of those with endometritis also have salpingitis, since laparoscopy has not been performed in the absence of more suggestive symptoms and signs of salpingitis. However, among women with chlamydial MPC who do have such symptoms and signs, the great majority who undergo endometrial biopsy and laparoscopy have both endometritis and salpingitis. Chlamydial inclusions are demonstrable by direct immunofluorescence in columnar epithelial cells of the endometrium and endosalpinx. The endometrial biopsies usually show neutrophils infiltrating the epithelium and plasma cells infiltrating the stroma, findings also seen in gonococcal endometritis but not in the uninfected endometrium. Other inflammatory changes analogous to those seen in the cervix are also found in the endometrium with chlamydial infection. Experimental inoculation of the fallopian tubes of lower primates produces mild acute salpingitis and ciliary sloughing, which is transient and reversible. However, if experimental tubal inoculation is preceded by repeated inoculation of the fallopian tubes or cervix, a more intense salpingitis results and progresses to peritubular scarring. This suggests that in the female genital tract, as in the eye, repeated exposure to *C. trachomatis* leads to the greatest degree of tissue inflammation and damage.

The pathogenesis of PID attributable to mycoplasmas or other vaginal anaerobic or facultative organisms is less well studied. It is possible that other vaginal organisms implicated in PID often cause tubal infection in women whose tubes have already been damaged by a primary sexually transmitted pathogen (i.e., *N. gonorrhoeae* or *C. trachomatis*). The organisms and mycoplasmas implicated in PID are found in the vagina most often and in greatest concentration in bacterial vaginosis (nonspecific vaginitis), and there is epidemiologic evidence that bacterial vaginosis itself is a predisposing factor for PID (just as poor oral hygiene is a risk factor in aspiration pneumonia).

Certain other iatrogenic factors, such as dilatation and curettage or cesarean section, are known to increase the risk of PID in women with endocervical gonococcal or chlamydial infection. Recent evidence indicates that among women undergoing cesarean section, the presence of bacterial vaginosis increases the risk of postpartum endometritis.

CLINICAL MANIFESTATIONS **Tuberculous salpingitis** Unlike nontuberculous salpingitis, genital tuberculosis often occurs in older women, about half of whom are postmenopausal. In a large review of cases in Sweden, 38 percent had had previously diagnosed tuberculosis. The most common presenting symptoms were abnormal vaginal bleeding, pain (including dysmenorrhea), and infertility. Most had normal bimanual pelvic examinations, though about one-quarter had adnexal masses. The most common method of diagnosis was endometrial biopsy, showing tuberculous granulomas, often associated with a positive culture.

Nontuberculous salpingitis The evolution of symptoms classically proceeds from a mucopurulent vaginal discharge caused by

cervicitis—possibly associated with dysuria and frequency due to urethritis or with anorectal pain, tenesmus, rectal discharge, and bleeding due to proctitis—to midline abdominal pain and abnormal vaginal bleeding caused by endometritis, followed by bilateral lower abdominal and pelvic pain caused by salpingitis, with nausea and vomiting and increased abdominal tenderness caused by peritonitis. Some patients have diffuse abdominal pain caused by generalized peritonitis or pleuritic right upper quadrant pain caused by perihepatitis. The pattern in which symptoms evolve varies from patient to patient and is also related to the etiology of the PID.

The onset of IUD-associated PID is typically gradual and may be preceded by typical malodorous vaginal discharge characteristic of bacterial vaginosis. The onset of gonococcal PID has been more acute than that of chlamydial PID in some, but not all studies, and both are often associated with menses.

The abdominal pain is usually described as dull or aching. In some cases, pain is lacking or is atypical, and active inflammatory changes can be found in the course of an unrelated evaluation or procedure such as a tubal ligation or laparoscopic evaluation for infertility. Abnormal uterine bleeding precedes or coincides with the onset of pain in about 40 percent of women with PID, symptoms of urethritis occur in 20 percent, and symptoms of proctitis occasionally are seen in those with gonococcal or chlamydial infection.

Speculum examination shows evidence of mucopurulent cervicitis in the majority of women with gonococcal or chlamydial PID. Cervical motion tenderness is produced by stretching of the adnexal attachments on the side toward which the cervix is pushed. Bimanual examination reveals uterine fundal tenderness due to endometritis and abnormal adnexal tenderness due to salpingitis which is usually, but not necessarily, bilateral. Adnexal swelling is palpable in about one-half of women with acute salpingitis, but evaluation of the adnexae in a patient with marked tenderness is not reliable, even by an experienced examiner. An initial temperature >38°C is found in only about one-third of patients with acute salpingitis, and fever is not required for the diagnosis.

Laboratory findings include elevation of the erythrocyte sedimentation rate (ESR) in 75 percent and elevation of the peripheral white blood cell count in up to 60 percent of patients with acute salpingitis. Microscopic examination of a saline wet-mount preparation of vaginal fluid has revealed more than one polymorphonuclear leukocyte per vaginal epithelial cell, or findings consistent with bacterial vaginosis, in nearly all patients with laparoscopically confirmed salpingitis in Swedish studies. However, exceptions have not been uncommon in U.S. studies.

Certain clinical manifestations of acute PID have been correlated with etiologic findings. For example, the onset of salpingitis is related to menses in women with gonorrhea or chlamydial infection. Women with gonorrhea or *Chlamydia*-associated salpingitis are significantly younger than women with other forms of salpingitis. In a Swedish study, women with *Chlamydia*-associated salpingitis had a more indolent disease with mild symptoms of significantly longer duration and with less fever than women who had gonorrhea-associated salpingitis. It is suspected that for all recognized cases of symptomatic *Chlamydia* salpingitis, there is a comparable number of unrecognized cases of indolent subclinical *Chlamydia* salpingitis, and that subclinical chronic or recurrent *Chlamydia* salpingitis may be a major cause of infertility in women.

IUD-associated PID has been much less common since withdrawal of the Dalkon shield from the market. It tends to be indolent and is associated less often with fever, but more often with adnexal masses, than is PID not associated with IUD use.

Perihepatitis and periappendicitis Symptoms of perihepatitis, including pleuritic upper abdominal pain and tenderness, usually localized to the right upper quadrant, occur in 3 to 10 percent of women with acute PID. The onset of symptoms of perihepatitis occurs during or after onset of symptoms of PID and may overshadow the lower abdominal symptoms, leading to a mistaken diagnosis of cholecystitis. In perhaps 5 percent of cases of acute salpingitis, laparoscopy performed early reveals inflammation ranging from edema and erythema of the liver capsule to exudate with fibrinous adhesions between the visceral and parietal peritoneum. When treatment is delayed and laparoscopy is performed late, dense "violin-string" adhesions are seen over the liver; these cause chronic exertional or positional right upper quadrant pain when traction is placed on the adhesions. Although perihepatitis, also known as the *Fitz-Hugh–Curtis syndrome,* was for many years attributed to gonococcal PID, in recent studies most cases of perihepatitis have been associated with chlamydial salpingitis. In patients with chlamydial salpingitis, serum microimmunofluorescent antibody titers against *C. trachomatis* are typically much higher when perihepatitis is present than when it is absent, and it has been suggested that repeated chlamydial infections are responsible for perihepatitis.

Physical findings include right upper quadrant tenderness and usually include adnexal tenderness and cervicitis, even in patients whose symptoms are not suggestive of salpingitis.

Liver function tests are nearly always normal, since inflammation is largely limited to the liver capsule, usually sparing the parenchyma. Oral cholecystogram may show nonfunction of the gallbladder, but ultrasonography of the right upper quadrant is normal. The presence of mucopurulent cervicitis and pelvic tenderness in a young woman with subacute pleuritic right upper quadrant pain with normal ultrasonography of the gallbladder points to a diagnosis of perihepatitis.

Periappendicitis (appendiceal serositis without involvement of the intestinal mucosa) has been found in approximately 5 percent of patients undergoing appendectomy for suspected appendicitis and can occur as a complication of gonococcal or chlamydial salpingitis.

DIAGNOSIS Early diagnosis and initiation of therapy are essential to minimize tubal scarring. Appropriate treatment must not be withheld from patients who have an equivocal diagnosis. Since delay in therapy may lead to progression of tubal scarring, it is better to err on the side of overdiagnosis and overtreatment. On the other hand, it is essential to differentiate between salpingitis and other pelvic pathology, particularly surgical emergencies such as appendicitis and ectopic pregnancy.

No clinical or laboratory finding short of laparoscopy is pathognomonic for salpingitis, and there is reluctance to perform laparoscopy in all cases of suspected salpingitis. Most patients with acute PID have lower abdominal pain of less than 3 weeks' duration, pelvic tenderness on bimanual pelvic examination, and evidence of lower genital tract infection (e.g., white blood cells outnumber all other cells in the vaginal fluid). Approximately 60 percent of such patients have salpingitis at laparoscopy. Among the patients with these findings, a rectal temperature above 38°C, a palpable adnexal mass, and elevation of the ESR over 15 mm/h also raise the probability of salpingitis, which has been found at laparoscopy in 68 percent of patients with one of these additional findings, 90 percent of patients with two or more, and 96 percent of patients with three or more additional findings. However, only 17 percent of all patients with laparoscopy-confirmed salpingitis had all three additional findings.

Mucopurulent cervicitis is probably responsible for the presence of neutrophils in vaginal fluid in PID. In a woman with pelvic pain and tenderness, demonstration of an increased number of neutrophils (≥30 per 1000× microscopic field in strands of cervical mucus) increases the predictive value of a clinical diagnosis of acute PID.

Several clinical features other than the presence of cervicitis also favor the diagnosis of acute PID. These include onset with menses, history of recent menstrual bleeding, presence of an IUD, history of previous salpingitis, and exposure to a male with urethritis. Detection of polymorphonuclear leukocytes in fluid aspirated by culdocentesis supports a diagnosis of suspected salpingitis. Urethritis or proctitis may occur in chlamydial or gonococcal infection but also may represent a urinary tract infection or an intestinal source for the patient's symptoms. Early onset of nausea and vomiting favors appendicitis or other disorders of the gut. A missed menstrual period dictates evaluation for ectopic pregnancy. The more sensitive assays

for human beta-chorionic gonadotropin are usually positive. Ultrasonography is sometimes useful to identify tuboovarian abscess or pelvic abscess, and intravaginal ultrasound assessment of the tubes has recently been reported to show increased tubal diameter, intratubal fluid, or tubal wall thickening in salpingitis (confirmatory experience is needed).

Laparoscopy is the most specific method for diagnosis of acute salpingitis. Although laparoscopy may be normal if inflammation is limited to the endosalpinx or endometrium, patients with suspected PID who have normal laparoscopy have a better prognosis, with few, if any, sequelae, than patients who have abnormal laparoscopic findings. The primary and uncontested value of laparoscopy in women with lower abdominal pain is exclusion of other surgical problems. Table 89-2 clearly shows that the most common and serious problems that may be confused with salpingitis are usually unilateral. Unilateral pain or pelvic mass, though not incompatible with PID, is a strong indication for laparoscopy unless the clinical picture warrants laparotomy instead. Atypical clinical findings such as the absence of lower genital tract infection, a missed menstrual period, or failure to respond to appropriate therapy are other frequent indications for laparoscopy.

Laparoscopic criteria used for the diagnosis of salpingitis include (1) erythema of the fallopian tube, (2) edema of the fallopian tube, and (3) seropurulent exudate or fresh, easily lysed adhesions at the fimbriated end or on the serosal surface of a fallopian tube.

Endometrial biopsy is relatively sensitive and specific for the diagnosis of endometritis when the endometrial changes described above are found, and the presence of endometritis correlates well with the presence of salpingitis. Endometritis is found in at least three-fourths of women with laparoscopically confirmed salpingitis and is absent in women without PID.

The etiologic diagnosis of PID can be further studied by cultures or other tests on specimens obtained by endocervical swab, endometrial aspiration, or culdocentesis or by laparoscopy or laparotomy. Endocervical swab specimens should be examined by Gram's stain for neutrophils and gram-negative diplococci and by culture for *N. gonorrhoeae.* The sensitivity of Gram's stain is about 60 percent, and specificity is more than 95 percent, compared with culture. The endocervical swab specimen also should be tested for *C. trachomatis* by culture, immunofluorescence, or assays for chlamydial DNA or RNA. Although isolation of either *N. gonorrhoeae* or *C. trachomatis* from the cervix does not prove that either agent is also present in the upper genital tract, this finding strongly supports the diagnosis of PID. The clinical diagnosis of PID made by expert gynecologists is confirmed by laparoscopy or endometrial biopsy in only about 60 percent of all consecutive patients but in about 90 percent of those who also have positive cultures for *N. gonorrhoeae* or *C. trachomatis.* There is no evidence that isolation of anaerobes or facultative aerobes from the cervix or vagina correlates with the presence of these organisms in the upper genital tract in acute PID, but this has not been well studied. The value of culture of culdocentesis and endometrial aspirate specimens is disputed because of the risk of contamination

TABLE 89-2　Laparoscopic findings in patients with false-positive or false-negative clinical diagnoses of acute PID

False-positive clinical diagnosis		False-negative clinical diagnosis, unexpected PID at laparoscopy	
Laparoscopic diagnosis	Percent	Clinical diagnosis	Percent
Acute appendicitis	24	Ovarian tumor	20
Endometriosis	16	Acute appendicitis	18
Corpus luteum bleeding	12	Ectopic pregnancy	16
Ectopic pregnancy	11	Chronic salpingitis	6
Pelvic adhesions only	7	Acute peritonitis	6
Benign ovarian tumor	7	Endometriosis	5
Chronic salpingitis	6	Uterine myoma	5
Miscellaneous	15	Atypical pelvic pain	6
		Miscellaneous	6

SOURCE: L Jacobsen and L Weström, Am J Obstet Gynecol 105:1088, 1969.

of the specimen with vaginal flora. When laparoscopy is performed, material can be obtained directly from the cul-de-sac or the fimbriated opening of the tube or by tubal aspiration if pyosalpinx is present. Such specimens should be cultured for anaeorbic and facultative pathogens, as well as for *N. gonorrhoeae* and *C. trachomatis.*

TREATMENT Hospitalization should be considered in all women with PID and is strongly recommended when (1) the diagnosis is uncertain, (2) surgical emergencies such as appendicitis and ectopic pregnancy must be excluded, (3) a pelvic abscess is suspected, (4) severe illness precludes outpatient management, (5) the patient is pregnant, (6) the patient is an adolescent (among adolescents, compliance is less predictable), (7) the patient is assessed as unable to follow or tolerate an outpatient regimen, (8) the patient has failed to respond to outpatient therapy, or (9) clinical follow-up after 48 to 72 h of instituting antibiotic treatment cannot be arranged. Treatment should cover *N. gonorrhoeae, C. trachomatis,* gram-negative facultative bacteria (especially *E. coli*), vaginal anaerobes, and group B streptococcus. No single agent is active against the entire spectrum of pathogens (Table 89-3). Several antimicrobial combinations do provide a broad spectrum of activity against the major pathogens in vitro, but many have not been adequately evaluated for clinical efficacy in PID.

A recent survey showed that physician antibiotic prescribing for PID improved from 1979 (when only 32 percent of patients received an antichlamydial drug) to 1989 (when 74 percent received such treatment). However, in 1989, only 21 percent of patients received a two-drug regimen that included an antichlamydial agent.

Examples of combination regimens with broad activity against major pathogens in PID Clinicians have had extensive experience with the following two inpatient regimens:

1 Doxycycline 100 mg, twice a day, IV, plus cefoxitin 2.0 g, four times a day, IV, or cefotetan 2.0 g, every 12 h, IV. These drugs should be continued IV for at least 48 h after the patient improves. Doxycycline should be continued in a dose of 100 mg by mouth, twice a day, after discharge from the hospital to complete 14 days of therapy. This regimen provides excellent coverage for *N. gonorrhoeae*, including penicillinase-producing *N. gonorrhoeae* (PPNG), and *C. trachomatis.*

2 Clindamycin 900 mg, every 8 h, IV, plus gentamicin 2.0 mg/kg, IV, followed by 1.5 mg/kg, every 8 h, IV, in patients with normal renal function. These drugs should be continued for at least 48 h after the patient improves. After discharge from the hospital, doxycycline 100 mg orally, twice a day, should be given to complete 14 days of therapy. This regimen provides good activity against anaerobes and facultative gram-negative rods and is active against *C. trachomatis* and *N. gonorrhoeae.* Doxycycline provides definitive therapy for chlamydial infection.

Patients who are not hospitalized also should receive a combined regimen with broad activity, such as ceftriaxone 250 mg, IM, followed by doxycycline, 100 mg, by mouth, twice a day for 14 days. Cefoxitin, 2.0 g, IM, given concurrently with probenecid 1.0 g, orally, can be used in place of ceftriaxone. Tetracycline also can be used in a dose of 500 mg, four times·a day, in place of doxycycline but requires more frequent dosing, which is a major drawback in the treatment of PID. An alternative outpatient regimen, which requires more evaluation but which provides good coverage of the major pathogens, is ofloxacin, 400 mg, twice daily, plus either metronidazole, 500 mg, twice daily, or clindamycin, 450 mg, four times daily, for 14 days.

Management of sexual partners All persons who are sexual partners of patients with PID should be examined for STD and promptly treated with a regimen effective against uncomplicated gonococcal and chlamydial infection. Treatment of PID should be considered inadequate until sexual partners have been properly evaluated and treated.

Follow-up All patients who are treated as outpatients should be clinically reevaluated in 48 to 72 h. Those not responding favorably should be hospitalized. A culture for *N. gonorrhoeae* or *C. trachomatis* to test whether cure has been achieved should be performed as needed.

Removal of an intrauterine device Although possible benefit of IUD removal on the response of acute salpingitis to antimicrobial therapy and on the risk of recurrent salpingitis has not been proven, removal of the IUD soon after antimicrobial therapy has been initiated seems reasonable. When an IUD is removed, contraceptive counseling is necessary.

Surgery Surgery is necessary only rarely for treatment of salpingitis, except in the face of life-threatening infection such as rupture or threatened rupture of a tuboovarian abscess or for drainage of an abscess. Ultrasonography is useful for diagnosing and following pelvic abscesses. When surgery is performed, conservative procedures are usually sufficient. Pelvic abscesses often can be drained by posterior colpotomy, and peritoneal lavage can be used if there is generalized peritonitis.

PROGNOSIS In a cooperative trial in the United States, nearly 20 percent of women treated for PID on an ambulatory basis with IM penicillin followed by a 10-day course of ampicillin or with a 10-day course of tetracycline alone were judged to be clinical failures.

Among 900 women who underwent long-term follow-up for a mean period of 8 years after successful treatment of the acute episode with various regimens in Sweden, late sequelae included infertility due to bilateral tubal occlusion, ectopic pregnancy due to tubal scarring without occlusion, chronic pelvic pain, and recurrent salpingitis. Chronic pain lasting longer than 6 months was seen in 18 percent of patients and infertility due to tubal occlusion in 17 percent; 4 percent of pregnancies that did occur were ectopic, representing approximately a sixfold increase over the expected rate of ectopic pregnancies. The rate of infertility after salpingitis was found to be related to age of the patient, duration of symptoms when treatment was started, severity of salpingitis by laparoscopy at the time of

TABLE 89-3   Relative activities of the antimicrobial agents most commonly used to treat PID

	N. gonorrhoeae	C. trachomatis	Vaginal anaerobes GPC*	GNR†	Facultative GNR	M. hominis
Ampicillin/amoxicillin	2+	2+	4+	2+	2+	0
Tetracycline HCl	2+	4+	4+	2+	2+	2+
Doxycycline	2+	4+	4+	3+	2+	2+
Cefoxitin, cefotetan	3+	0	4+	3+	4+	0
Ceftriaxone	4+	0	3+	2+	4+	0
Gentamicin/tobramycin	2+	0	1+	0	4+	2+?
Ofloxacin	4+	3+	1+	1+	4+	1+
Clindamycin	1+	3+	4+	4+	0	3+
Metronidazole	0	0	4+	4+	0	0

* GPC = Gram-positive cocci (peptostreptococci).
† GNR = Gram-negative rods (anaerobic GNR include *Prevotella;* facultative GNR include Enterobacteriaceae, *H. influenzae*).
NOTE: No single antimicrobial agent offers optimal activity against all of these pathogens, but certain combinations (e.g., cefoxitin plus doxycycline, gentamicin plus clindamycin) or ofloxacin plus metronidazole have complementary activity. Relative activity is indicated on a 0→4+ scale.

diagnosis, and number of episodes of salpingitis. The rate of infertility due to tubal occlusion among women exposed to a chance of pregnancy was 14 percent for women 15 to 24 years of age and 26 percent for women 25 to 34 years of age; the risk for women of all ages combined was 11 percent after one episode of salpingitis, 23 percent after two episodes, and 54 percent after three or more episodes. The risk of infertility after gonococcal salpingitis was comparable with the risk after chlamydial salpingitis in one small prospective study. A study of outcomes of PID at the University of Washington found a sevenfold increase in risk of ectopic pregnancy and an eightfold increase in hysterectomies after PID.

A striking relationship also has been shown in several countries between infertility due to tubal occlusion and the prevalence and titer of antibody to *C. trachomatis*. Recurrent salpingitis has been seen in approximately 15 to 25 percent of women treated for salpingitis in various studies.

PREVENTION Prevention of PID depends first on the effective control of gonococcal and chlamydial infection. Effective methods include promotion of changes in sexual behavior and use of barrier contraceptives while providing ready access to modern methods of diagnosis and effective treatment of sex partners to control further spread. The decline in popularity of the intrauterine device, particularly in nulliparous women, has undoubtedly helped to reduce the incidence of PID. It is also possible, but not proven, that use of oral contraceptives and avoidance of vaginal douching may reduce the risk of PID.

The complications of salpingitis can be minimized by early diagnosis and prompt treatment. It seems logical, but is unproven, that broad-spectrum therapy effective against all of the common causes of PID would offer the best outcome. Similarly, hospitalization to ensure rest and adequate compliance may improve the rather dismal long-term prognosis for tubal function. One placebo-controlled study showed that concurrent anti-inflammatory therapy with prednisolone hastened the reduction of acute inflammatory changes but did not improve the end results as measured by fertility, hysterosalpingographic findings, or chronic pain. However, the potential value of anti-inflammatory therapy remains to be evaluated adequately.

REFERENCES

CATES WJ et al: Worldwide patterns of infertility: Is Africa different? Lancet 2:596, 1985

CENTERS FOR DISEASE CONTROL: Policy guidelines for the prevention and management of pelvic inflammatory disease. Morb Mort Week Rep 40RR-5:1, 1992

ESCHENBACH DA et al: Polymicrobial etiology of acute pelvic inflammatory disease. N. Engl J Med 293:166, 1975

FALK V et al: Genital tuberculosis in women. Am J Obstet Gynecol 138:974, 1980

GERMAINE A et al: *Reproductive Tract Infections: Global Impact and Priorities for Women's Reproductive Health.* New York, Plenum, 1992

KIVIAT N et al: Endometrial histopathology in patients with culture-proven upper genital tract infection and laparoscopically diagnosed acute salpingitis. Am J Surg Pathol 14:167, 1990

LANDERS DV et al: Combination antimicrobial therapy in the treatment of acute pelvic inflammatory disease. Am J Obstet Gynecol 164:849, 1991

MÅRDH PA et al: *Chlamydia trachomatis* infection in patients with acute salpingitis. N Engl J Med 296:1377, 1977

PLUMMER FA et al: Postpartum upper genital tract infections in Nairobi, Kenya: Epidemiology, etiology, and risk factors. J Infect Dis 156:92, 1987

REED SD et al: Antibiotic treatment of tuboovarian abscess: Comparison of broad-spectrum beta-lactam agents versus clindamycin-containing regimens. Am J Obstet Gynecol 164:1556, 1991

SOPER DE et al: Microbial etiology of urban emergency department acute salpingitis: Treatment with ofloxacin. Am J Obstet Gynecol 167:653, 1992

ST JOHN RK, BROWN ST (eds): International symposium on pelvic inflammatory disease. Am J Obstet Gynecol 138:845, 1980

SVENSSON L et al: Differences in some clinical and laboratory parameters in acute salpingitis related to culture and serologic findings. Am J Obstet Gynecol 138:1017, 1980

—— et al: Infertility after acute salpingitis—With special reference to *Chlamydia trachomatis*–associated infections. Fertil Steril 40:322, 1983

WASHINGTON AE, KATZ P: Cost of and payment source for pelvic inflammatory disease: Trends and projections, 1983 through 2000. JAMA 266:2565, 1991

WASSERHEIT JN et al: Microbial causes of proven pelvic inflammatory disease and efficacy of clindamycin with tobramycin. Ann Intern Med 104:187, 1986

WØLNER-HANSSEN P et al: Atypical pelvic inflammatory disease: Subacute, chronic, or subclinical upper genital tract infections in women, in *Sexually Transmitted Diseases*, 2d ed, KK Holmes et al (eds). New York, McGraw-Hill 1990, pp 615–620

90 URINARY TRACT INFECTIONS AND PYELONEPHRITIS

WALTER E. STAMM

DEFINITIONS Acute infections of the urinary tract can be subdivided into two general anatomic categories: lower tract infection (urethritis, cystitis, and prostatitis) and upper tract infection (acute pyelonephritis and intrarenal and perinephric abscesses). Infections at these various sites may occur together or independently and may be asymptomatic or present as the clinical syndromes outlined below. Infections of the urethra and bladder are often considered superficial (or mucosal) infections, while prostatitis, pyelonephritis, and renal suppuration signify tissue invasion.

Microbiologically, urinary tract infection exists when pathogenic microorganisms are detected in the urine, urethra, bladder, kidney, or prostate. In most instances, growth of more than 10^5 organisms per milliliter from a properly collected midstream "clean catch" urine sample indicates infection. However, significant bacteriuria may be absent in some circumstances when true urinary infection exists. Especially in symptomatic patients, a smaller number of bacteria (10^2 to 10^4 per milliliter of midstream urine) may accompany infection. In urine specimens obtained by suprapubic aspiration or "in and out" catheterization, or from a patient with an indwelling catheter, colony counts of 10^2 to 10^4 per milliliter generally indicate infection. Conversely, colony counts in excess of 10^5 per milliliter of midstream urine are occasionally due to specimen contamination, especially when multiple species are present.

Recurrent infections after antibiotic therapy can be due to persistence of the originally infecting strain, as judged by species identification, serotype, and antibiogram, or to reinfection with a new strain. "Same strain" recurrent infections that occur within 2 weeks of cessation of therapy can result from unresolved renal or prostatic infection (termed *relapse*) or from persistent vaginal colonization that leads to rapid reinfection of the bladder.

Symptoms of dysuria, urgency, and frequency unaccompanied by significant bacteriuria have been termed the *acute urethral syndrome*. Although widely used, this term lacks anatomic precision because many cases of urethral syndrome are actually bladder infections. Moreover, since the causative agent can usually be identified in these patients, the term *syndrome*, implying unknown causation, is inappropriate.

Chronic pyelonephritis refers to chronic interstitial nephritis believed to result from bacterial infection of the kidney (see Chap. 242). Many noninfectious diseases also cause an interstitial nephritis indistinguishable pathologically from chronic pyelonephritis.

ACUTE INFECTIONS OF THE URINARY TRACT: URETHRITIS, CYSTITIS, AND PYELONEPHRITIS

EPIDEMIOLOGY Epidemiologically, urinary tract infections should be subdivided into catheter-associated (or nosocomial) infections and non-catheter-associated (or community-acquired) infections. In either category, infections may be symptomatic or asymptomatic. Acute infections in noncatheterized patients are very common, especially in women, and account for over 6 million office visits annually in the United States. These infections occur in 1 to 3 percent of schoolgirls and then increase markedly in incidence with the onset of sexual activity in adolescence. The vast majority of acute symptomatic infections occur in young women. Acute symptomatic urinary infections are unusual in men under the age of 50. The occurrence of asymptomatic bacteriuria parallels that of symptomatic infection and is rare in men under 50 but is common in women between the ages of 20 and 50. Asymptomatic bacteriuria is very common in elderly men and women, being identified in up to 40 to 50 percent of patients in some studies.

ETIOLOGY   Many different microorganisms can infect the urinary tract, but by far the most common agents are the gram-negative bacilli. *Escherichia coli* causes approximately 80 percent of acute infections in patients without catheters, urologic abnormalities, or calculi. Other gram-negative rods, especially *Proteus* and *Klebsiella* and occasionally *Enterobacter*, account for a smaller proportion of uncomplicated infections. These organisms, plus *Serratia* and *Pseudomonas*, assume increasing importance in recurrent infections and infections associated with urologic manipulation, calculi, or obstruction. They play a major role in nosocomial, catheter-associated infections (see below). *Proteus* species, by virtue of urease production, and *Klebsiella* species, through production of extracellular slime and polysaccharides, predispose to stone formation and are isolated more frequently from patients with calculi.

Gram-positive cocci play a lesser role in urinary tract infections. However, *Staphylococcus saprophyticus*, a novobiocin-resistant, coagulase-negative staphylococcus, accounts for 10 to 15 percent of acute symptomatic urinary tract infections in young females. Enterococci and *Staphylococcus aureus* cause infections in patients with renal stones or previous instrumentation. Isolation of *S. aureus* from the urine should arouse suspicion of bacteremic infection of the kidney.

About one-third of women with dysuria and frequency have either a nonsignificant number of bacteria in midstream urine cultures or completely sterile cultures and have been previously defined as having the urethral syndrome. About three-quarters of these women have pyuria, while one-quarter have no pyuria and little objective evidence of infection. In the women with pyuria, two groups of pathogens account for the majority of infections. Low quantities (10^2 to 10^4 bacteria per milliliter) of typical bacterial uropathogens such as *E. coli*, *S. saprophyticus*, *Klebsiella*, or *Proteus* in midstream urine specimens are found in the majority of these women. They are probably the causative agents in these women because they can usually be isolated from a suprapubic aspirate, are associated with pyuria, and respond to appropriate antimicrobial therapy. In other women with acute urinary symptoms, pyuria, and sterile urine (even on suprapubic aspiration), sexually transmitted urethritis-producing agents such as *Chlamydia trachomatis, Neisseria gonorrhoeae*, and herpes simplex virus are important etiologic agents. These sexually transmitted agents are most frequently found in young, sexually active women with new sexual partners.

The causative role of nonbacterial pathogens in urinary tract infections remains poorly defined. *Ureaplasma urealyticum* has frequently been isolated from the urethra and urine of patients with acute dysuria and frequency but is also found in many patients without urinary symptoms. Thus ureaplasmas probably account for some cases of urethritis and cystitis. *U. urealyticum*, as well as *Mycoplasma hominis*, has also been isolated from prostatic and renal tissues in patients with acute prostatitis and pyelonephritis and probably accounts for some of these infections. Adenoviruses cause acute hemorrhagic cystitis in children and in some young adults, often in epidemics. Although many other viruses can be isolated from urine (cytomegalovirus, Jakob-Creutzfeldt virus, and others), they are not thought to cause urinary infection. *Candida* and other fungal species often colonize the urine of catheterized patients or diabetics and in some patients progress to symptomatic invasive infection (see Chap. 166). Mycobacterial infection of the genitourinary tract is discussed in Chap. 130.

PATHOGENESIS AND SOURCES OF INFECTION   The urinary tract should be viewed as a single anatomic unit connected by a continuous column of urine that extends from the urethra to the kidney. In the vast majority of infections, bacteria gain access to the bladder via the urethra. Ascent of bacteria from the bladder may then follow and is probably the usual pathway for most renal parenchymal infections.

The vaginal introitus and distal urethra are normally colonized with diphtheroids, streptococcal species, lactobacilli, and staphylococcal species but not with the enteric gram-negative bacilli that commonly cause urinary tract infections. In females prone to development of cystitis, however, enteric gram-negative organisms residing in the bowel colonize the introitus, the periurethral skin, and the distal urethra prior to and during episodes of bacteriuria. Factors predisposing to periurethral colonization with gram-negative bacilli remain poorly understood but probably involve alteration of the normal perineal flora by antibiotics, other genital infections, or contraceptives, especially diaphragms and spermicide. Small numbers of periurethral bacteria probably gain entry to the bladder frequently, facilitated in some women by urethral massage during intercourse. Whether bladder infection ensues then depends on interaction between the pathogenicity of the strain, the inoculum size, and local and systemic host defense mechanisms.

Under normal circumstances, bacteria placed in the bladder are rapidly cleared. This results partly from the flushing and dilutional effects of voiding but also from direct antibacterial properties of urine and the bladder mucosa. Due mostly to high urea concentration and high osmolarity, the bladder urine of many normal persons inhibits or kills bacteria. Prostatic secretions possess antibacterial properties as well. Polymorphonuclear leukocytes in the bladder wall also appear to play a role in clearing bacteriuria. The role of locally produced antibody remains unclear.

Hematogenous pyelonephritis occurs most often in debilitated patients who either have chronic illnesses or are receiving immunosuppressive therapy. Staphylococcal pyelonephritis may follow bacteremia from distant foci of infection in the bone, skin, endothelium, or elsewhere.

CONDITIONS AFFECTING PATHOGENESIS   Gender and sexual activity   The female urethra appears particularly prone to colonization with colonic gram-negative bacilli, owing to its proximity to the anus, its short length (about 4 cm), and its termination beneath the labia. Urethral massage, as occurs during sexual intercourse, causes introduction of bacteria into the bladder and appears to be important in the pathogenesis of urinary infections in younger women. (Voiding after intercourse has been shown to reduce the risk of cystitis, probably because it promotes eradication of bacteria introduced during intercourse.) In addition, diaphragm and spermicide use dramatically alter the normal introital bacterial flora and have been associated with a marked increase in vaginal colonization with *E. coli* and risk of urinary infection. In males, prostatitis or urethral obstruction due to prostatic hypertrophy are important factors predisposing to bacteriuria. Homosexuality also predisposes to an increased risk of cystitis, probably associated with rectal intercourse. HIV-infected men with CD-4-positive T cell counts less than 200 cells per microliter have recently been shown to have an increased risk of both bacteriuria and symptomatic urinary tract infection. Finally, lack of circumcision has been identified as a risk factor for urinary tract infection in both neonates and young men.

Pregnancy   Depending on socioeconomic status, urinary infections are detected in 2 to 8 percent of pregnant women. In particular, symptomatic upper tract infections occur more commonly during pregnancy; fully 20 to 30 percent of pregnant women with asymptomatic bacteriuria subsequently develop pyelonephritis. This predisposition to upper tract infection during pregnancy results from the decreased ureteral tone, decreased ureteral peristalsis, and temporary incompetence of the vesicoureteral valves seen in pregnancy. Bladder catheterization during or after delivery causes additional infections. Cystitis and pyelonephritis are no more common in women with toxemia of pregnancy than in other pregnant women. An increased prevalence of prematurity and newborn mortality may result from urinary infections during pregnancy, particularly those involving the upper urinary tract.

Obstruction   Any impediment to the free flow of urine—tumor, stricture, stone, or prostatic hypertrophy—results in hydronephrosis and a greatly increased frequency of urinary tract infection. Infection superimposed on urinary tract obstruction may lead to rapid destruction of renal tissue. It is of utmost importance, therefore, when infection is present, to repair obstructive lesions. On the other hand, with minor degrees of obstruction that are not progressive or associated with infection, great caution should be exercised in attempting surgical correction. The introduction of infection in such patients may be more damaging than uncorrected minor obstructions that do not significantly impair renal function.

Neurogenic bladder dysfunction   Interference with the nerve supply to the bladder, as in spinal cord injury, tabes dorsalis, multiple sclerosis, diabetes, or other diseases, may be associated with urinary tract infection. The infection may be initiated by the use of catheters for bladder drainage and is favored by the prolonged stasis of urine in the bladder. An additional factor often present in these patients is bone demineralization due to immobilization, which causes hypercalciuria, calculus formation, and obstructive uropathy.

Vesicoureteral reflux   This condition is defined as reflux of urine from the bladder cavity up into the ureters and sometimes into the renal pelvis. It occurs during voiding or with elevation of pressure in the bladder. In practice, vesicoureteral reflux exists when retrograde movement of radiopaque or radioactive material can be demonstrated during a voiding cystourethrogram. An anatomically impaired vesicoureteral junction facilitates reflux of bacteria and thus upper tract infection. However, since a fluid connection between the bladder and kidney always exists even in the normal urinary system, some retrograde movement of bacteria probably occurs during infection but is not detected by radiologic techniques.

Vesicoureteral reflux is common in children with anatomic abnormalities of the urinary tract and in children with anatomically normal but infected urinary tracts. In the latter group, reflux disappears with advancing age and probably results from causes other than urinary infection. Long-term follow-up of children with urinary tract infection who were found to have reflux establishes that renal damage correlates with marked reflux, not with infection.

The routine search for reflux would be aided by development of noninvasive tests applicable to young children, where the need is greatest. In the meantime, it appears reasonable to search for reflux in anyone with unexplained failure of renal growth or renal scarring, because urinary tract infection per se is an insufficient explanation for these abnormalities. On the other hand, it is doubtful that all children with recurrent urinary tract infections but normal urinary tracts on pyelography should be subjected to voiding cystoureterography merely to detect the rare patient with marked reflux that did not reveal itself on the intravenous pyelogram.

Bacterial virulence factors   Bacterial virulence factors influence the likelihood that a given strain, once introduced into the bladder, will cause urinary tract infection. Not all *E. coli* are equally able to infect the intact urinary tract. The majority of strains that cause symptomatic urinary tract infections in noncatheterized patients belong to a small number of specific O, K, and H serogroups, produce hemolysin, and share certain other "uropathogenic" properties. Adherence of bacteria to uroepithelial cells is a critical first step in the initiation of infection. For both *E. coli* and *Proteus*, fimbriae (hairlike surface proteinaceous appendages) mediate bacterial attachment to specific receptors on epithelial cells. Nearly all *E. coli* strains that cause pyelonephritis in patients with anatomically normal urinary tracts possess a particular pilus (the P pilus or gal-gal pilus) that mediates attachment to the digalactoside portion of glycosphingolipids present on uroepithelium. Strains that produce pyelonephritis are also usually hemolysin producers, have aerobactin (a siderophore for scavenging iron), and are resistant to the bactericidal action of human serum. Since most strains that produce acute pyelonephritis in the intact host possess all or nearly all these virulence factors, the concept has arisen that a small number of uropathogenic clones cause most such cases of infection. In patients with structural or functional abnormalities of the urinary tract, infections are frequently caused by bacterial strains that lack these uropathogenic properties, implying that these properties are not needed for infection of the compromised urinary tract.

Genetic factors   Increasing evidence suggests that host genetic factors influence susceptibility to urinary infection. The number and type of receptors on uroepithelial cells to which bacteria may attach are at least in part genetically determined. Many of these structures to which uropathogenic bacteria bind are components of blood group antigens and are present on erythrocytes and uroepithelial cells. For example, P fimbriae mediate attachment of *E. coli* to P-positive erythrocytes and are present on nearly all strains causing acute uncomplicated pyelonephritis. Conversely, P blood group–negative individuals, who lack these receptors, have a decreased likelihood of pyelonephritis. It also has been demonstrated that nonsecretors of blood group antigens may have an increased risk of recurrent urinary infection, which may relate to a different profile of genetically determined glycolipids that are present on the uroepithelial cells of nonsecretors.

LOCALIZATION OF INFECTION   Infections involving the upper urinary tract usually cause a significant rise in serum antibodies directed against the O antigen of the infecting strain. They also produce a temporary defect in renal concentrating ability in many patients and may be associated with formation of leukocyte casts. Lower tract infections rarely result in increased antibody titers, concentrating defects, or white cell casts. Unfortunately, these methods of distinguishing renal parenchymal infection from cystitis are neither reliable nor convenient enough for routine clinical use. More sensitive tests for distinguishing pyelonephritis from cystitis (bilateral ureteral catheterization and the bladder wash-out technique originated by Fairley) are inherently invasive and too complex for routine clinical practice. A simpler, noninvasive test to separate upper and lower tract infections based on antibody coating of bacteria in the urine does not have sufficient sensitivity and specificity to be of value in the routine clinical management of patients. An elevated C-reactive protein often accompanies acute pyelonephritis and rarely is seen in cystitis, but this acute-phase reactant is nonspecific and occurs in infections other than pyelonephritis as well.

CLINICAL PRESENTATION   Clinical signs and symptoms cannot be relied on to diagnose urinary tract infection accurately or to localize the site of infection. Many patients with significant bacteriuria (including some with upper tract infection) have no symptoms at all. Of those with significant bacteriuria and symptoms of cystitis, about two-thirds have lower tract infection and about one-third have clinically silent upper tract infection that is evident only upon performing localization studies. Clinical symptoms and signs of pyelonephritis, though usually suggestive, do not always indicate upper tract infection. Finally, among women presenting with acute dysuria and frequency, only 60 to 70 percent have significant bacteriuria, but the majority of those without significant bacteriuria also have urinary tract or urethral infections.

Enumeration of the number and type of bacteria in the urine is an extremely important diagnostic procedure. In symptomatic infections of the urinary tract, uropathogenic bacteria are usually demonstrable in the urine in large numbers. Quantitative estimation of the number of bacteria in voided urine specimens as a rule makes it possible to distinguish contaminants from true bacteriuria, and 10^5 or more bacteria per milliliter has been the criterion traditionally used for this purpose. However, in symptomatic women with pyuria, bacterial colony counts of 10^2 to 10^4 *E. coli, Klebsiella, Proteus,* or *S. saprophyticus* per milliliter of midstream urine usually indicate infection, not contamination, and should not be disregarded. In asymptomatic patients, two or three consecutive urine specimens should be examined bacteriologically before instituting therapy, and 10^5 or more per milliliter of a single species should be demonstrable in the repeated specimens. Since the large number of bacteria in the bladder urine is due in part to bacterial multiplication during residence in the bladder cavity, samples of urine from the ureters or renal pelvis may contain fewer than 10^5 bacteria per milliliter and yet indicate infection. Similarly, the presence of bacteriuria of any degree in suprapubic aspirates or of 10^2 or more bacteria per milliliter of urine obtained by catheterization usually indicates infection. In some circumstances (antibiotics, high urea concentration, high osmolarity, low pH), urine will inhibit bacterial multiplication, resulting in a lower number of bacteria in the presence of infection. For this reason, antiseptic solutions should not be used in washing the periurethral area prior to collection of the urine specimen. Water diuresis or recent voiding also reduces the bacterial counts in urine.

Rapid methods of detection of bacteriuria have been developed as alternatives to standard culture methods. They detect bacterial growth using photometry, bioluminescence, or other means and provide results rapidly, usually in 1 to 2 h. These methods generally achieve a sensitivity of 95 to 98 percent and >99 percent negative predictive value as compared with urine cultures when bacteriuria is defined as 10^5 colony forming units per milliliter. However, the sensitivity of these tests falls to 60 to 80 percent when bacteriuria of 10^2 to 10^4 colony forming units per milliliter is the standard of comparison.

Microscopy of urine from symptomatic patients can be of great diagnostic value. Microscopic bacteriuria, which is best assessed using Gram-stained, uncentrifuged urine, is found in over 90 percent of specimens from patients whose infections have colony counts of 10^5 per milliliter and is a very specific finding. However, bacteria cannot usually be detected microscopically in lower colony count infections (10^2 to 10^4 per milliliter). The presence of bacteria on urinary microscopy is firm evidence of infection, but its absence does not exclude the diagnosis. When carefully sought using a chamber count microscopy method, pyuria is a highly sensitive indicator of urinary tract infection in symptomatic patients. Pyuria is present in nearly all patients with acute bacterial urinary tract infection, and its absence should cause the diagnosis to be questioned. The leukocyte esterase "dipstick" method is less sensitive than microscopy in identifying pyuria but is a useful alternative where microscopy is not available.

Cystitis Patients with dysuria, frequency, urgency, and suprapubic pain usually have cystitis. The urine often becomes grossly cloudy, malodorous, and, in about 30 percent of cases, bloody. White cells and bacteria should be present on examination of the unspun urine in most patients. However, some women with cystitis have only 10^2 to 10^4 bacteria per milliliter of urine, which cannot be seen on a Gram stain of unspun urine. Physical examination generally reveals only a tender urethra or suprapubic tenderness. If a genital lesion or a vaginal discharge is present, especially with fewer than 10^5 bacteria per milliliter on culture, causes of urethritis, vaginitis, or cervicitis such as *C. trachomatis*, gonorrhea, *Trichomonas, Candida*, and herpes simplex virus should be considered. Prominent systemic manifestations such as temperature >38.3°C (101°F), nausea, vomiting, and costovertebral angle tenderness usually indicate concomitant renal infection. However, the absence of these findings does not ensure that infection is limited to the bladder and urethra.

Acute pyelonephritis Symptoms generally develop rapidly over a few hours or a day and include temperature ≥39.4°C (103°F), shaking chills, nausea, vomiting, and diarrhea. Symptoms of cystitis may or may not be present. Besides fever, tachycardia, and generalized muscle tenderness, physical examination reveals marked tenderness on deep pressure in one or both costovertebral areas or on deep abdominal palpation. In some patients, signs and symptoms of gram-negative sepsis predominate. Most patients have significant leukocytosis, pyuria with leukocyte casts in the urine, and bacteria on a Gram stain of unspun urine. Hematuria may be present during the acute phase of the disease, but if it persists after acute manifestations of infection have subsided, a stone, tumor, or tuberculosis should be considered.

Except in individuals with papillary necrosis or urinary obstruction, the manifestations of acute pyelonephritis usually subside within a few days, even without specific antibacterial therapy. However, despite the absence of symptoms, bacteriuria or pyuria may persist. With severe pyelonephritis, fever subsides more slowly and may not disappear for several days, even after appropriate antibiotic treatment has been instituted.

Urethritis Approximately 30 percent of women with acute dysuria, frequency, and pyuria have midstream urine cultures that show either no growth or nonsignificant bacterial growth. Clinically, these women cannot be readily distinguished from those with cystitis. In these women, distinction should be made between those with sexually transmitted pathogens such as *C. trachomatis, Neisseria gonorrhoeae*, or herpes simplex virus, and those with low-count *E. coli* or staphylococcal infection of the urethra and bladder. Women with a gradual onset of illness, no hematuria, no suprapubic pain, and a history of more than 7 days of symptoms should be suspected of having chlamydial or gonococcal infection. The additional history of a recent sex partner change, especially if the patient's partner has recently had chlamydial or gonococcal urethritis, should heighten the suspicion of a sexually transmitted infection, as would the finding of mucopurulent cervicitis. Gross hematuria, suprapubic pain, abrupt onset of illness, a duration of illness of less than 3 days, and a history of previous urinary tract infections favor *E. coli* or staphylococcal infection.

Catheter-associated urinary tract infections Bacteriuria occurs in at least 10 to 15 percent of hospitalized patients with indwelling urethral catheters. The risk of infection is about 3 to 5 percent per day of catheterization. *Proteus, Pseudomonas, Klebsiella*, and *Serratia*, in addition to *E. coli*, usually cause these infections. Many infecting strains show marked antimicrobial resistance compared with organisms that cause community-acquired urinary infections. Factors associated with an increased risk of infection include female sex, lengthy period of catheterization, severe underlying illness, disconnection of the catheter and drainage tube, other types of faulty catheter care, and absence of systemic antimicrobials.

Infection occurs when bacteria reach the bladder by one of two routes: by migrating through the column of urine in the catheter lumen (intraluminal route) or by moving up the mucous sheath outside the catheter (periurethral route). Hospital-acquired pathogens reach the patient's catheter or urine-collecting system on the hands of hospital personnel, in contaminated solutions or irrigants, and via contaminated instruments or disinfectants. Entry of bacteria into the catheter system usually occurs at the catheter–collecting tube junction or at the drainage bag portal. Bacteria then ascend intraluminally into the bladder within 24 to 72 h. Alternatively, the patient's own bowel flora colonize the perineal skin and periurethral area and reach the bladder via the external surface of the catheter. This route is particularly common in women. Recent studies have demonstrated the important role of attachment and growth of bacteria on the inner surface of the catheter in the pathogenesis of catheter-associated urinary tract infection. Such bacteria growing in biofilms on the inner surface of the catheter eventually produce encrustations consisting of bacteria, bacterial glycocalyxes, host urinary proteins, and urinary salts. Encrustations provide a refuge for bacteria and may protect them from antimicrobials and phagocytes.

Clinically, most catheter-associated infections cause minimal symptoms and no fever and often resolve after withdrawal of the catheter. The frequency of upper tract infection associated with catheter-induced bacteriuria is unknown. Gram-negative bacteremia, which follows 1 to 2 percent of cases of catheter-associated bacteriuria, is the most significant recognized complication of catheter-induced urinary infections. The catheterized urinary tract has repeatedly been demonstrated to be the most common source of gram-negative bacteremia in hospitalized patients. It also has been suggested that bacteriuria in hospitalized catheterized patients is associated with an adjusted increased relative risk of death of approximately threefold compared with similar patients without bacteriuria.

Catheter-associated urinary tract infections can be partially prevented in patients catheterized less than 2 weeks by use of a sterile closed collecting system, by attention to aseptic technique during insertion and care of the catheter, and by measures to minimize cross-infection. Other preventive approaches, including short courses of systemic antimicrobials, topically applied periurethral antimicrobial ointments, preconnected catheter–drainage tube units, and antimicrobials added to the drainage bag, have all been protective in one or more controlled trials but are not recommended for general use. Despite precautions, the majority of patients catheterized longer than

2 weeks eventually develop bacteriuria. The need for treatment and, if given, the optimal type and duration of treatment for such patients with asymptomatic bacteriuria have not been established. Removal of the catheter and a short course of antibiotics to which the organism is susceptible are probably the best course of action and nearly always eradicate the bacteriuria. Treatment of asymptomatic catheter-associated bacteriuria may be of greatest benefit in elderly women, who more often develop symptoms if left untreated. If the catheter cannot be removed, antibiotic therapy usually proves to be unsuccessful and may result in infection with a more resistant strain. In this situation, the bacteriuria should be ignored unless the patient develops symptoms or is at high risk of developing bacteremia. In these cases, systemic antibiotics or urinary bladder antiseptics may reduce the degree of bacteriuria and the likelihood of bacteremia. Because of spinal cord injury, incontinence, or other factors, some patients in hospitals or nursing homes require long-term or semipermanent bladder catheterization. Preventive measures have been largely unsuccessful, and essentially all such chronically catheterized patients develop bacteriuria. If feasible, intermittent catheterization by a nurse or by the patient appears to reduce the occurrence of bacteriuria and associated complications in such patients. Treatment should be provided when symptomatic infections arise, but treatment of asymptomatic bacteriuria in such patients has no apparent benefit.

DIAGNOSTIC TESTING   Although many authorities have recommended that urine culture and antimicrobial susceptibility testing be performed in any patient with a suspected urinary tract infection, it may be more practical and cost-effective to manage women who have symptoms and urinalysis findings characteristic of acute uncomplicated cystitis without an initial urine culture. Thus women with symptoms and signs of acute cystitis in whom no complicating factors are present can be managed with urinary microscopy (or alternatively, a leukocyte esterase test). If positive for pyuria, hematuria, and/or bacteriuria, these tests provide sufficient documentation of infection such that urine culture and susceptibility testing can be omitted and the patient treated empirically. Urine culture should be obtained, however, in women in whom symptoms and urine examination findings leave the diagnosis of cystitis in question. Pretherapy cultures and susceptibility testing are also essential in the management of all patients with suspected upper tract infections and those in whom complicating factors are present, since in these situations a variety of pathogens may be present and antibiotic therapy is best tailored to the individual organism.

TREATMENT   Several therapeutic principles should underlie treatment of urinary tract infections:

1 In most circumstances, a quantitative urine culture, a positive Gram stain, or an alternative rapid diagnostic test should be obtained to confirm infection before starting treatment. When cultures are obtained, antimicrobial sensitivity testing should be used to direct therapy.
2 Factors predisposing to infection, such as obstruction, neurogenic bladder, calculi, etc., should be identified and corrected if possible.
3 Relief of clinical symptoms does not always indicate bacteriologic cure.
4 After completion of therapy, each treatment episode should be classified as a failure (symptoms and/or bacteriuria not eradicated during therapy or in the immediate posttreatment culture) or a cure (resolution of symptoms and elimination of bacteriuria). Recurrent infections should be classified as same strain or different strain and early (within 2 weeks of stopping therapy) or late.
5 In general, uncomplicated infections confined to the lower urinary tract respond to low doses and short courses of therapy, while upper tract infections require longer periods of treatment. After therapy, early recurrences with the same strain may result from an unresolved upper tract focus of infection but often (especially after short-course therapy for cystitis) result from persistent vaginal colonization rather than from recurrent bladder infection. Recurrences more than 2 weeks after the cessation of therapy are nearly

always reinfections, even though some may be with the same strain.
6 Community-acquired infections, especially initial infections, are usually due to antibiotic-sensitive strains.
7 Patients with repeated infections, instrumentation, or recent hospitalization should be suspected of harboring resistant strains.

The anatomic location of a urinary tract infection greatly influences success or failure of a therapeutic agent. Bladder bacteriuria (cystitis) can usually be eliminated with nearly any antimicrobial to which the infecting strain is sensitive; in the past, it was demonstrated that as little as a single dose of 500 mg of intramuscular kanamycin eliminated bladder bacteriuria in most patients. Currently, a 7-day course of therapy with oral drugs appears more than adequate. With upper tract infections, however, single-dose therapy fails in the majority of cases, and even a 7-day course will be unsuccessful in many patients. Longer periods of treatment (2 to 6 weeks) aimed at eradicating a persistent focus of infection may be necessary in some cases.

In *acute uncomplicated cystitis*, more than 80 percent of infections are due to E. coli, and although resistance patterns vary geographically, most strains are sensitive to many antibiotics. Single doses of trimethoprim-sulfamethoxazole (4 single-strength tablets), trimethoprim (400 mg), sulfa alone (2.0 g), and most fluoroquinolones (norfloxacin, ciprofloxacin, ofloxacin) have been used successfully to treat acute uncomplicated episodes of cystitis. A single 3-g dose of amoxicillin (amoxicilline) appears to result in lower cure rates than these other agents, especially in women infected with amoxicillin-resistant strains. In most areas, about one-third of E. coli strains causing acute cystitis are amoxicillin-resistant. The advantages of single-dose therapy include less expense, ensured compliance, fewer side effects, and perhaps less intense selective pressure for emergence of resistant organisms in the gut or vaginal or perineal flora. However, several studies now suggest that more recurrences with the same strain occur shortly after single-dose therapy than after 3 to 7 days of treatment and that single-dose therapy does not effectively eradicate vaginal colonization with E. coli. Nevertheless, single-dose therapy does appear safe and efficacious for women presenting with *acute uncomplicated cystitis*. Single-dose therapy should be used only in reliable patients, in whom posttreatment follow-up can be ensured, and in patients in whom symptoms have been present for less than 7 days. Three days of therapy with trimethoprim-sulfamethoxazole, norfloxacin, ciprofloxacin, or ofloxacin appears to preserve the lower side-effects rate of single-dose therapy but improves efficacy. Neither single-dose nor 3-day therapy should be used in women with symptoms or signs of pyelonephritis, in women with urologic abnormalities or stones, or in women with previous infections due to antibiotic-resistant organisms. Males with urinary tract infection often have urologic abnormalities or prostatic involvement and hence are not candidates for single-dose or 3-day therapy.

Treatment of women with acute urethritis depends on the etiologic agent involved. In chlamydial infection, doxycycline (100 mg orally bid for 7 days) should be used. Women with acute dysuria and frequency, negative urine cultures, and no pyuria do not usually respond to antimicrobial agents.

Acute uncomplicated pyelonephritis in women without accompanying clinical evidence of calculi or urologic disease is due to E. coli in most cases. Although the optimal route and duration of therapy have not been established, a 14-day course of trimethoprim-sulfamethoxazole, trimethoprim alone, a fluoroquinolone, an aminoglycoside, or a cephalosporin usually provides adequate therapy. Ampicillin or amoxicillin should not be used as initial therapy because 20 to 30 percent of E. coli are now resistant in vitro. Intravenous antibiotics, at least for the first few days of treatment, should probably be given to most patients, but mildly symptomatic patients can be treated with 2 weeks of oral antibiotics (usually trimethoprim-sulfamethoxazole, ciprofloxacin, or ofloxacin). Patients who relapse following therapy should be investigated to determine whether unrecognized suppurative foci, calculi, or urologic disease is present. If not, treatment should be extended to 2 to 6 weeks to eliminate a presumed upper tract focus causing recurrent bacteriuria.

Complicated urinary tract infections (those arising in the setting of catheterization, instrumentation, urologic anatomic or functional abnormalities, stones, obstruction, immunosuppression, renal disease, or diabetes) are typically due to hospital-acquired bacteria, including *E. coli*, *Klebsiella*, *Proteus*, *Serratia*, *Pseudomonas*, enterococci, or staphylococci. Many of these strains are antibiotic-resistant. Thus initial empiric antibiotic therapy for complicated urinary tract infections ideally should provide broad-spectrum coverage against these pathogens. In patients with minimal symptoms, oral therapy with a fluoroquinolone such as ciprofloxacin or ofloxacin can be utilized until culture results and antibiotic sensitivities are known. In patients with more severe illness attributable to complicated urinary tract infection, including acute pyelonephritis or suspected urosepsis, hospitalization and parenteral therapy should be provided. Commonly used empiric regimens include imipenem alone, a penicillin or cephalosporin plus an aminoglycoside, ceftriaxone, and ceftazadime (when enterococci are unlikely). When the antimicrobial sensitivity pattern of the infecting strain becomes available, a more specific antimicrobial regimen can be selected. Therapy should generally be provided for 7 to 21 days, depending on the severity of the infection. Follow-up cultures 2 to 4 weeks after cessation of therapy should be obtained to demonstrate cure.

In *pregnancy*, acute cystitis can be managed with 3 to 7 days of amoxicillin, nitrofurantoin, or a cephalosporin. All pregnant women should be screened for asymptomatic bacteriuria during the first trimester, and if bacteriuric, they should be treated with one of the regimens just outlined. After treatment, a culture should be obtained to ensure cure and repeated monthly thereafter. Acute pyelonephritis in pregnancy should be managed with hospitalization and parenteral antibiotics, generally a cephalosporin or an extended-spectrum penicillin. Continuous low-dose prophylaxis with nitrofurantoin should be given to women who have recurrent infections during pregnancy.

Asymptomatic bacteriuria should be documented with at least two positive cultures before treatment is given. Seven days of an oral agent to which the organism is sensitive should be given initially. If bacteriuria persists, it can be followed without further treatment in most patients. High-risk patients with neutropenia, renal transplants, or other complicating conditions may require longer periods of treatment.

UROLOGIC EVALUATION   Very few women with recurrent urinary tract infections have correctable lesions discovered at cystoscopy or upon intravenous pyelography, and these procedures should not be performed routinely in such patients. In selected women, namely those with relapsing infection, those with a history of childhood infections, those with stones or painless hematuria, and those with recurrent pyelonephritis, urologic evaluation should be performed. Most males with urinary infection should be considered to have complicated infection and thus be evaluated urologically. Exceptions may include young men who have sexually associated cystitis, are uncircumcised, or have AIDS. Men or women presenting with acute infection and signs or symptoms suggestive of an obstruction or stones should undergo urologic evaluation, generally by means of ultrasound.

PROGNOSIS   In patients with uncomplicated cystitis or pyelonephritis, treatment ordinarily results in complete resolution of symptoms. In fact, symptoms usually remit even without specific therapy. Lower tract infections in adult women are of concern mainly because they cause discomfort, minor morbidity, and time lost from work. Cystitis also may result in upper tract infection or in bacteremia (especially during instrumentation), but there is little evidence to suggest that renal impairment follows. When repeated episodes of cystitis occur, they are nearly always reinfections, not relapses.

Uncomplicated acute pyelonephritis in adults rarely progresses to functional impairment and chronic renal disease. Repeated upper tract infections often indicate relapse rather than reinfection, and a vigorous search for renal calculi or an underlying urologic abnormality should be undertaken. If neither is found, 6 weeks of chemotherapy may be useful in eradicating an unresolved focus of infection.

Repeated symptomatic urinary tract infections in children, and in adults with obstructive uropathy, neurogenic bladder, structural renal disease, or diabetes, more often progress to chronic renal disease. Asymptomatic bacteriuria in these groups, as well as in adults without urologic disease or obstruction, predisposes to increased episodes of symptomatic infection but does not result in renal impairment in most instances.

PREVENTION   Patients with frequent symptomatic infections may benefit from long-term low-dose antibiotics directed at preventing recurrences. A single dose of trimethoprim-sulfamethoxazole (80 mg trimethoprim and 400 mg sulfamethoxazole), trimethoprim alone (100 mg), or nitrofurantoin (50 mg) given daily or thrice weekly has been particularly effective. Prophylaxis should be initiated only after bacteriuria has been eradicated with a full-dose treatment regimen. Women having more than two infections every 6 months should be considered for such preventive antibiotics. These same regimens can be used after sexual intercourse to prevent episodes of symptomatic infections in women whose infectious episodes are temporally related to intercourse. Other patients for whom prophylaxis appears to have some merit include men with chronic prostatitis; patients undergoing prostatectomy, both during the operation and in the postoperative period; and pregnant women with asymptomatic bacteriuria. All pregnant women should be screened for bacteriuria in the first trimester and should be treated if bacteriuria is found.

PAPILLARY NECROSIS

When infection of the renal pyramids develops in association with vascular diseases of the kidney or with urinary tract obstruction, renal papillary necrosis is likely to result. Patients with diabetes, sickle cell disease, chronic alcoholism, and vascular disease seem peculiarly susceptible to this complication. Hematuria, pain in the flank or abdomen, and chills and fever are the most common presenting symptoms. Acute renal failure with oliguria or anuria sometimes occurs. Rarely, sloughing of a pyramid may take place without symptoms in a patient with chronic urinary infection, and the diagnosis is made when the necrotic tissue is passed in the urine or identified as a "ring shadow" on pyelography. If renal function deteriorates suddenly in a diabetic or a patient with chronic obstruction, the diagnosis of renal papillary necrosis should be entertained, even in the absence of fever or pain. Although renal papillary necrosis is often bilateral, when it is unilateral, nephrectomy may be lifesaving in the management of overwhelming infection.

RENAL AND PERINEPHRIC ABSCESS

See p. 529.

PROSTATITIS

The term *prostatitis* has been used for various inflammatory conditions affecting the prostate, including acute and chronic infections with specific bacteria and, more commonly, instances in which signs and symptoms of prostatic inflammation are present but no specific organisms can be detected. Patients with acute bacterial prostatitis can usually be identified on the basis of typical symptoms and signs, pyuria, and bacteriuria. To classify patients with suspected chronic prostatitis correctly, each patient should be evaluated using first-void and midstream urine specimens, a prostatic expressate, and a postmassage urine specimen. All specimens should be quantitatively cultured and evaluated for numbers of leukocytes. Based on the results of these studies, patients can be classified as having chronic bacterial prostatitis, chronic nonbacterial prostatitis, or prostatodynia. Patients with suspected chronic prostatitis usually have low back pain, perineal or testicular discomfort, mild dysuria, and lower urinary obstructive symptoms. Microscopic pyuria may be the only objective manifestation of prostatic disease.

ACUTE BACTERIAL PROSTATITIS This disease generally affects young male adults when it occurs spontaneously, but it also may be associated with an indwelling urethral catheter. It is characterized by fever, chills, dysuria, and a tense or boggy, extremely tender prostate on examination. Although prostatic massage usually produces purulent secretions with a large number of bacteria on culture, bacteremia may result from manipulation of the inflamed gland. For this reason, and because the etiologic agent can usually be identified on urine Gram stain and culture, vigorous prostatic massage should be avoided. In non-catheter-associated cases, the infection is generally due to common gram-negative urinary tract pathogens (*E. coli* or *Klebsiella*). Initially, intravenous trimethoprim-sulfamethoxazole, a cephalosporin, a fluoroquinolone, or an aminoglycoside can be utilized if gram-negative rods are seen in the urine Gram stain, and a cephalosporin or nafcillin if gram-positive cocci are seen. Although many of these drugs do not readily diffuse into the noninflamed prostate gland, the response to antibiotics in acute bacterial prostatitis is usually prompt, perhaps because drugs penetrate more readily into the acutely inflamed prostate. In catheter-associated cases, a broader spectrum of etiologic agents is seen, including hospital-acquired gram-negative rods and enterococci. In such cases, an aminoglycoside, a fluoroquinolone, or a third-generation cephalosporin should be used for initial therapy until the organism has been isolated and susceptibilities determined. The long-term prognosis is good, although in some instances acute infection may result in abscess formation, epididymoorchitis, seminal vesiculitis, septicemia, and residual chronic bacterial prostatitis. Since the advent of antibiotics, the frequency of acute bacterial prostatitis has diminished markedly. Many so-called cases of acute prostatitis are probably posterior urethritis.

CHRONIC BACTERIAL PROSTATITIS This entity is now infrequent but should be considered in men with a history of recurrent bacteriuria. Symptoms are usually absent, and the prostate usually feels normal on palpation. Obstructive symptoms or perineal pain occurs in some patients. Intermittently, infection spreads to the bladder, producing frequency, urgency, and dysuria. A pattern of relapsing infection in a middle-aged man strongly suggests chronic bacterial prostatitis. Classically, the diagnosis is established by culturing *E. coli*, *Klebsiella*, *Proteus*, or other uropathogenic bacteria in higher quantities from the expressed prostatic secretion or postmassage urine than are found in first-void or midstream urine. Antibiotics promptly relieve the symptoms associated with acute exacerbations but have been less effective in eradicating the focus of chronic infection in the prostate. The relative ineffectiveness of antimicrobials, in terms of long-term cure, in part results from the poor penetration of most antibiotics into the prostate because the low pH which prevails in this organ precludes solubility of most drugs. Sulfonamide-trimethoprim, ciprofloxacin, and ofloxacin have been employed successfully in some cases, but they must be given for at least 12 weeks to be effective. Patients with frequent episodes of acute cystitis can be managed with prolonged courses of antimicrobials (usually sulfonamide, trimethoprim, or nitrofurantoin), with a view toward suppressing symptoms and keeping the bladder urine sterile. Total prostatectomy produces cure of chronic prostatitis but is associated with considerable morbidity. Transurethral prostatectomy is safer but cures only one-third of patients.

NONBACTERIAL PROSTATITIS Patients who present with symptoms and signs of prostatitis, increased leukocytes in their expressed prostatic secretions and postmassage urine, and no bacterial growth in cultures are classified as having nonbacterial prostatitis. In addition, such patients do not have a history of recurrent episodes of bacterial cystitis. Prostatic inflammation can be considered present when the expressed prostatic secretion and postmassage urine contain at least tenfold more leukocytes than the first-void and midstream specimens or when the expressed prostatic secretion contains ≥1000 leukocytes per microliter. The presumed infectious etiology of this condition remains unidentified. Evidence for the causative role of both *Ureaplasma urealyticum* and *Chlamydia trachomatis* has been presented but is not conclusive. Since most cases of nonbacterial prostatitis occur in young, sexually active men, and since many cases arise following an episode of nonspecific urethritis, the causative agent may well be sexually transmitted. The effectiveness of antimicrobial agents in this condition remains uncertain. Some patients benefit from a 4- to 6-week course of erythromycin, doxycycline, trimethoprim-sulfamethoxazole, or a fluoroquinolone, but controlled trials are lacking.

PROSTATODYNIA Patients who have symptoms and signs of prostatitis but no evidence of prostatic inflammation (normal leukocyte counts) and negative urine cultures are classified as having prostatodynia. Despite their symptoms, these patients most likely do not have prostatic infection and should not be given antimicrobial agents.

REFERENCES

HOOTON TM et al: *Escherichia coli* bacteriuria and contraceptive method. JAMA 265:64, 1991

————, STAMM WE: Management of acute uncomplicated urinary tract infection in adults. Med Clin North Am 75:339, 1991

JOHNSON JR, STAMM WE: Diagnosis and treatment of urinary tract infections. Infect Dis Clin North Am 1:773, 1987

KRIEGER JN: Complications and treatment of urinary tract infections during pregnancy. Urol Clin North Am 13:685, 1986

KUNIN CM: *Detection, Prevention and Management of Urinary Tract Infections*, 4th ed. Philadelphia, Lea & Febiger, 1987

LIPSKY BA: Urinary tract infections in men. Ann Intern Med 110:138, 1989

MEARES EM JR: Acute and chronic prostatitis: Diagnosis and treatment. Infect Dis Clin North Am 1:855, 1987

PEZZLO M: Detection of urinary tract infections by rapid methods. Clin Microbiol Rev 1:268, 1988

STAMM WE et al: Causes of the acute urethral syndrome in women. N Engl J Med 303:409, 1980

———— et al: Diagnosis of coliform infection in acutely dysuric women. N Engl J Med 307:463, 1982

———— et al: Urinary tract infections: From pathogenesis to treatment. J Infect Dis 159:400, 1989

————: Catheter-associated urinary tract infections: Epidemiology, pathogenesis, prevention. Am J Med 91(suppl 3B):B655, 1991

SVANBORG-EDEN C et al: Host-parasite relationship in urinary tract infection. J Infect Dis 157:421, 1988

WARREN JW: Catheter-associated urinary tract infections. Infect Dis Clin North Am 1:823, 1987

91 INFECTIOUS ARTHRITIS

DANIEL ROTROSEN

NONGONOCOCCAL SEPTIC ARTHRITIS Acute bacterial arthritis is a common medical problem affecting individuals of all ages. Prompt recognition and treatment are important to avoid permanent articular disability.

Etiology, pathogenesis, and predisposing factors Approximately 75 percent of nongonococcal pyoarthroses are due to gram-positive cocci, with *Staphylococcus aureus* isolated particularly often. Pneumococci and group A beta-hemolytic and viridans streptococci collectively account for fewer than half of isolates. Among immunocompromised individuals, group G streptococci are an infrequent cause of septic arthritis; among neonates, group B streptococci are an important cause of arthritis. *Staphylococcus epidermidis* is the leading cause of prosthetic joint infection.

Gram-negative bacilli account for approximately 20 percent of cases, typically in patients with obvious risk factors for gram-negative bacteremia. *Pseudomonas aeruginosa* is an important cause of septic arthritis in intravenous drug addicts and neonates. *Haemophilus influenzae* type b is a prominent cause of pyoarthrosis among children under age 5.

Septic arthritis usually results from direct hematogenous seeding of the synovium. Factors that predispose to septic arthritis include infancy, immunosuppressive therapy, alcoholism, drug abuse, some chronic systemic illnesses, hemoglobinopathies, complement and immunoglobulin deficiencies, phagocytic cell dysfunction, chronic arthritis, and previous joint damage. Infection may occur as a complication of arthroscopy, intraarticular glucocorticoid injection, or prosthetic joint surgery. A history of minor joint trauma is a common but often-overlooked feature in patients with suppurative arthritis. An extraarticular focus of infection (e.g., cutaneous abscesses) can be identified in about 25 percent of patients and can be helpful in establishing a cause and choosing antibiotics before results of joint fluid cultures become available.

The synovium is well vascularized and lacks a limiting basement membrane, allowing relatively free access of bloodborne microorganisms to the joint space once extravasation has occurred. In experimentally induced arthritis, microorganisms are found scattered throughout the synovium 1 to 2 h after inoculation. Within 1 to 2 days, vascular congestion, leukocyte infiltration, and hyperplasia of the synovial lining cells are prominent. The host response may be sufficient to eradicate infection, but early changes usually progress to purulent effusion and microabscess formation within the synovium and subchondral bone. Increased intraarticular pressure causes ischemia and impairs cartilage biomechanics and nutrition. The formation of granulation tissue and release of chondrolytic enzymes contribute to the destruction of articular cartilage, subchondral bone, and the joint capsule.

Clinical and experimental observations suggest that host immune mechanisms play a critical role in the development and maintenance of synovial inflammation. For example, sterile bacterial products, including endotoxins, exotoxins, and cell wall peptidoglycan, induce acute and chronic arthritis in laboratory animals. Deposition of immune complexes in the synovium and periarticular tissues may be followed by a sterile synovitis during the convalescent phase of certain bacterial and viral infections. In addition, individuals who develop postinfectious arthritis or Reiter's syndrome following *Shigella, Salmonella, Yersinia*, and *Campylobacter* infection of the gastrointestinal tract are more likely than matched controls to have the specific histocompatibility antigen HLA-B27.

Manifestations Nongonococcal septic arthritis presents as a monarticular synovitis with a predilection for large weight-bearing joints. The knee is the most frequently involved joint in children and adults, followed by the hip. The ankle, wrist, elbow, shoulder, sternoclavicular, and sacroiliac joints are involved less often. The interphalangeal joints are rarely affected in bacterial arthritis, except in patients with gonococccal synovitis or mycobacterial infection. Gram-positive coccal arthritis usually presents as an acute illness with severe constitutional symptoms accompanied by swelling, pain, warmth, and restricted motion of the involved joint. In septic arthritis of the hip, effusion may not be readily appreciated, and pain may be minimal or referred to the groin, buttock, lateral thigh, or anterior knee. Patients with suppurative arthritis usually seek medical attention within 3 to 4 days of the onset of symptoms. Signs of inflammation may be masked in patients taking glucocorticoids or other immunosuppressive medications and in those with chronic debilitating illnesses. Individuals with coexistent rheumatoid or gouty arthritis often attribute their symptoms to a flare-up of the underlying disease and consequently delay medical evaluation. In this setting a high degree of suspicion is warranted, and studies to exclude infection are important when articular symptoms fail to respond to anti-inflammatory agents.

If medical attention is sought early in the illness, a source of bacteremia is usually identified, and the responsible pathogen can be isolated from the blood in about 50 percent of cases. In contrast to the gram-positive arthritides, gram-negative bacillary arthritis follows a more indolent course with less prominent articular manifestations.

These differences contribute to the more prolonged time to diagnosis in gram-negative bacillary arthritis (typically 3 weeks from the onset of symptoms) and to the high incidence of coexistent osteomyelitis at the time of diagnosis.

Prosthetic joint infection is associated with mild symptoms and an indolent course resulting in a mean diagnostic delay of 2 to 8 months. *S. epidermidis* and *S. aureus* account for most of these infections, but polymicrobial infections or infections due to gram-negative bacilli or anaerobes are not uncommon. Infection occurs in 1 to 4 percent of prostheses followed for 10 years and is more frequent after revision of a previous total joint replacement. It invariably is accompanied by osteomyelitis at the site of implantation. Eradication of the infection usually requires removal of the prosthesis.

Certain pathogens are likely to cause infection at unusual sites. Spinal arthritis is often associated with osteomyelitis of adjacent vertebral bodies. It is usually due to *S. aureus*, but *Brucella, Salmonella*, and *Mycobacterium tuberculosis* also preferentially involve the spine. Among intravenous drug addicts, *P. aeruginosa* infection can occur in the sternoclavicular and sacroiliac joints.

Laboratory findings and diagnosis Analysis of synovial fluid is essential in the evaluation of suspected bacterial arthritis. Fluid sufficient for complete analysis usually can be obtained by percutaneous arthrocentesis. Care should be taken not to contaminate the joint space by inserting the needle through an area of overlying cellulitis or through an infected bursa. Fluoroscopic guidance may facilitate aspiration of the hip, shoulder, spinal, or sacroiliac joints. When joints are difficult to aspirate, arthrotomy may be required to obtain fluid or synovial tissue. Synovial fluid in septic arthritis is usually turbid or grossly purulent. The synovial fluid leukocyte count is greater than 100,000 per microliter (range < 10,000 to > 300,000 per microliter, usually > 90 percent polymorphonuclear neutrophils) in one-third to one-half of patients. In patients with unexpectedly low leukocyte counts on initial evaluation, repeat joint aspiration 12 to 24 h later almost always demonstrates leukocytosis. The synovial fluid leukocyte count and differential are of limited value in establishing an infectious cause because of overlap with other acute inflammatory arthritides. However, serial counts are important in monitoring response to therapy.

Gram's stain of synovial fluid is important in establishing the cause of septic arthritis. Stains are positive in 75 to 95 percent of gram-positive coccal and in approximately 50 percent of gram-negative bacillary infections. Regardless of the results of Gram's stain, synovial fluid should be cultured aerobically and anaerobically to identify specific pathogens and to provide data on antimicrobial sensitivity. Joint fluid cultures are positive in most patients with nongonococcal bacterial arthritis. If the patient has taken oral antibiotics prior to arthrocentesis, the microbiology laboratory should be notified, because growth of the organism may be delayed and cultures may require special handling. Blood cultures should be obtained, and a diligent search should be made for occult sources of bacteremia. Bacterial antigen detection by counterimmunoelectrophoresis has been advocated as a rapid diagnostic test for certain etiologic agents (e.g., *Streptococcus pneumoniae* and *H. influenzae*) but is not widely used.

In septic arthritis the synovial fluid glucose level may be low and lactate elevated compared with the corresponding levels in serum, but neither test is sufficiently sensitive or specific to be generally used. Elevated synovial fluid protein and poor mucin clot are nonspecific.

Unless arthritis arises by extension of adjacent osteomyelitis, distention of the joint capsule and periarticular soft tissue swelling are the only radiographic findings expected on initial evaluation. Nonetheless, early films are useful to establish a baseline. Destructive changes are rarely noted before the second to third week of untreated infection. At that time, periosteal elevation, juxtaarticular osteoporosis, bony erosions on the articular surface, and joint space narrowing may be apparent. In prosthetic joint infection radiographic evidence of implant loosening and osteomyelitis is usually seen.

In the setting of staphylococcal or gram-negative bacillary arthritis, computed tomography (CT) or magnetic resonance imaging (MRI) is helpful, particularly when the sternoclavicular joint or the hip is involved. These joints are poorly visualized by conventional techniques, and CT or MRI may reveal extensive bony involvement and parasynovial abscesses when conventional x-ray films are negative. Such findings have important implications for surgical intervention and for the duration of antimicrobial therapy. Radioisotope scans lack diagnostic specificity and may be positive in noninfectious inflammatory joint disease. However, scans are useful to identify inapparent foci of osteomyelitis and to substantiate suspicions of low-grade infection in the hip, shoulder, spine, and sacroiliac joints.

Other conditions to be considered in the differential diagnosis of oligoarticular arthritis include septic bursitis (usually olecranon or prepatellar), adult or juvenile rheumatoid arthritis, psoriatic arthritis, acute rheumatic fever, Reiter's syndrome, sarcoid arthropathy, trauma, villonodular synovitis, aseptic necrosis, and intermittent hydroarthrosis. Lyme disease and infections caused by mycobacteria and fungi typically present as oligoarticular arthritis.

Management and outcome Optimal management of suppurative arthritis includes parenteral antimicrobial therapy, drainage, and articular rest. Most antibiotics achieve therapeutic levels in the infected joint following parenteral administration. There is no rationale for intraarticular administration of antibiotics, and direct injection of antibiotics can induce chemical synovitis. The initial choice of antibiotics should be guided by Gram's stain of synovial fluid and revised as dictated by culture results. Antibiotic regimens for specific organisms are provided in the chapters dealing with these organisms and in Chap. 100. When no organisms are seen on Gram's stain, the antimicrobial regimen should be tailored to cover the likely pathogens based on the patient's age and the clinical setting. Infants under 1 month of age should be treated with a semisynthetic penicillin and an aminoglycoside to provide coverage against *S. aureus*, gram-negative bacilli, and group B streptococci. In children under 5 years of age, therapy should be targeted against *S. aureus* and ampicillin-resistant *H. influenzae*. Children over 5 years and adults should receive a semisynthetic penicillin and an aminoglycoside until culture results are available. Vancomycin is the drug of choice in patients with serious penicillin allergy, renal failure, or prosthetic joint infection. The results of single-drug therapy of gram-negative bacillary arthritis have been disappointing, despite in vitro sensitivity to the agents used. Because of the high rates of failure and relapse in this setting, combination chemotherapy is generally advised. After an initial clinical response, substitution of a newer β-lactam or quinolone antibiotic may avoid the toxicities of prolonged aminoglycoside therapy.

Most cases of streptococcal arthritis are cured by a 10- to 14-day course of antibiotics, whereas staphylococcal and gram-negative bacillary infections require longer treatment, usually 3 to 6 weeks. Drainage of purulent joint fluid is essential to relieve pain, to diminish the risk of loculation and pressure necrosis, and to remove chondrolytic products that promote destructive changes within the joint. Drainage of acidic, purulent fluid improves the bactericidal activity of neutrophils and certain antibiotics. Percutaneous needle aspiration and joint irrigation can be performed daily or twice daily for the first 5 to 7 days. The development of loculations, continued culture positivity, and persistence of a purulent effusion are indications that arthroscopy or open drainage may be required. When the hip is involved, surgical intervention is usually warranted from the outset, especially in children, because of the difficulty of repeated percutaneous aspiration and the risk of vascular compromise from elevated intracapsular pressure. Exploratory arthrotomy and open drainage have been beneficial in septic arthritis of the shoulder and sternoclavicular joints. Persistence of culture positivity despite adequate drainage is an indication for repeat studies to look for the emergence of antibiotic-resistant strains.

During the acute phase the joint should be immobilized in a position that minimizes capsular tension, usually midway between full extension and flexion. Passive range-of-motion exercises should be started as the synovitis improves, but weight bearing should be avoided until pain and signs of inflammation are gone.

Most cases of streptococcal arthritis resolve without sequelae, whereas in staphylococcal and gram-negative bacillary arthritis the response is generally less salutary. In this setting healing may be delayed by a sterile, postinfectious synovitis. Such patients may be left with limitation of motion and persistence of pain. Other major determinants of a poor outcome are failure to recognize and treat the infection within 7 days of onset and involvement of the hip joint. In children with hip or ankle arthritis, impaired ambulation and shortening of the extremity are not uncommon.

GONOCOCCAL ARTHRITIS (See Chap. 110) Gonococcal infection is the leading cause of bacterial arthritis in young adults and the most common form of infectious arthritis seen at urban medical centers. It may be a complication of sexual abuse in young children. In disseminated gonococcal infection, an early arthritis-dermatitis syndrome is typically followed by a joint-localization stage. The early phase is characterized by constitutional symptoms, migratory tenosynovitis and arthralgias, vesiculopustular skin lesions, and minimal joint effusion. The knee, shoulder, wrist, and interphalangeal joints of the hands are commonly involved. Cultures of blood and skin lesions may be positive at this stage of the illness, whereas culture and Gram's stain of synovial fluid are usually negative. A presumptive diagnosis can be made if the gonococcus is isolated from a silent primary focus (e.g., urogenital tract, pharynx, or rectum). Without treatment, constitutional symptoms and dermatitis usually abate, but joint involvement progresses to a purulent mon- or polyarticular arthritis. Synovial fluid cultures may be positive at this stage, whereas blood cultures are almost always negative. In 30 to 40 percent of patients a biphasic pattern of illness is not observed, and some patients present with a monarticular purulent arthritis and few systemic manifestations. Terminal complement component deficiencies, menstruation, and pregnancy predispose to gonococcal dissemination.

The differential diagnosis of disseminated gonococcal infection includes acute rheumatic fever, Reiter's syndrome, chronic meningococcemia, and *Streptobacillus moniliformis* infection. In Reiter's syndrome, constitutional toxicity is usually less pronounced, there is often a history of symptomatic urethritis and conjunctivitis, and distinct but subtle mucocutaneous lesions are usually present. Sacroiliitis and Achilles tendonitis are more common in Reiter's syndrome, and involvement of the upper extremity, especially the wrist, is unusual. A clinical response to antibiotics (in gonococcal disease) or to salicylates (in rheumatic fever) may help to differentiate among these syndromes.

In the United States most gonococcal isolates causing disseminated infection are penicillin-sensitive. However, penicillin resistance is increasingly common in some urban areas and in the Philippines, Southeast Asia, and Africa. Ceftriaxone or spectinomycin is effective. After an initial response, therapy can be continued with cefuroxime or amoxicillin plus clavulanic acid. Hospitalization and administration of parenteral antibiotics are warranted for unreliable patients and for those with purulent monarticular arthritis or uncertain diagnoses.

CHRONIC MONARTICULAR ARTHRITIS Certain mycobacteria and fungi cause chronic oligoarticular arthritis that is clinically and histologically distinct from other forms of septic arthritis.

Tuberculous arthritis (See Chap. 130) *Mycobacterium tuberculosis* causes a slowly progressive arthritis that is monarticular in up to 90 percent of cases. With the decline in primary tuberculosis in developed countries, spinal arthritis is rare, and involvement of the knee, hip, wrist, ankle, or small joints of the hand is more common. These sites become infected by reactivation of long-dormant lymphohematogenous foci. Rupture of such a focus (often in the epiphyseal region of long bones) into the joint space causes effusion and a progressive granulomatous reaction of synovial membranes, articular cartilage, and tendons. Localized pain may precede other signs of inflammation or x-ray changes by weeks or even months. The insidious nature of the infection usually delays diagnosis by weeks or months (the average time elapsed was 19 weeks from onset in one series). The granulomatous process eventually imparts a boggy, doughy feeling to the joint and periarticular structures. Cold abscesses and draining sinuses may develop. Constitutional symptoms are not prominent, and active pulmonary tuberculosis is unusual. Most patients are tuberculin-positive. Radiographs initially show subchondral osteoporosis and periarticular bone destruction with overlying periosteal thickening. Eventually, destructive changes are noted within the joint. The synovial fluid leukocyte count ranges from about 1000 to >100,000 per microliter (average about 15,000 per microliter), with a preponderance of polymorphonuclear neutrophils when counts are high, but frankly purulent fluid is uncommon. Acid-fast bacilli are not often seen on smears of synovial fluid (approximately 20 percent yield), but cultures of synovial fluid or tissue are positive in 80 to 90 percent of cases. Granulomatous changes in synovium are indications for antituberculous therapy while awaiting culture results. Infection due to atypical mycobacteria (e.g., *M. kansasii, M. marinum, M. avium-intracellulare*) may produce a chronic granulomatous arthritis with similar clinical and histopathologic features. These organisms are highly resistant to antimicrobial agents. The correct diagnosis and choice of an appropriate regimen depend on isolation of the organism (Chaps. 130 and 132). In spinal tuberculosis, surgery is usually reserved for drainage of abscesses or stabilization of the spine and is rarely required for treatment of other joints. Arthritis due to *Brucella* sp., *Nocardia asteroides*, and fungi may resemble mycobacterial infection.

Fungal arthritis Any of the invasive mycoses may involve bone and articular structures (see Chaps. 161–169). With the exception of acute arthritis due to *Candida* sp. or blastomycosis, the fungal arthritides tend to be slowly progressive and may elude accurate diagnosis for months or years. All show a predilection for involvement of large weight-bearing joints, especially the knee, and joint infection usually occurs without extraarticular dissemination. A history of serious underlying illness is common in blastomycotic arthritis but not in other fungal arthritides.

In acute pulmonary *coccidioidomycosis* (see Chap. 163), self-limited sterile synovitis is a component of the acute hypersensitivity syndrome known as "desert fever." Persistent coccidioidal synovitis may arise via direct hematogenous seeding of the synovium or via extension from an adjacent osteomyelitic focus. In the former case the disease tends to follow an indolent course with recurrent effusion, maintenance of joint space integrity, no evidence of osteomyelitis, and only late progression to a destructive villonodular arthritis with pannus formation. With extension from an adjacent bony focus, effusion is less prominent, and destructive changes tend to occur earlier. Diagnosis depends on culture and histology of synovial tissue; joint fluid cultures are positive in < 5 percent of cases.

Sporotrichotic arthritis (see Chap. 169) usually occurs in the absence of the more familiar lymphocutaneous syndrome. There is a predilection for involvement of the small joints of the hand and wrist in addition to the knee. Articular disability is uncommon until late in the disease. The etiologic agent, *Sporothrix schenckii*, is easily cultured from synovial fluid. As opposed to cutaneous sporotrichosis, articular disease is relatively refractory to iodide therapy, and response to amphotericin B may be slow.

Isolated articular involvement is unusual in *blastomycosis* (see Chap. 164), and patients usually present with a rapidly progressive "pulmonary-cutaneous-arthritic" syndrome. Involvement of multiple joints is the rule. In contrast to other granulomatous arthritides, articular blastomycosis is characterized by frankly purulent joint fluid, and the organism is easily visualized on wet-mount microscopy of synovial aspirates.

Candida arthritis usually follows direct hematogenous seeding of synovium in patients with risk factors for disseminated candidiasis (see Chap. 166). The acute articular infection may spread to adjacent bone.

In *histoplasmosis* (see Chap. 162), a migratory polyarthritis

accompanied by erythema nodosum may be analogous to the acute hypersensitivity syndrome of coccidioidomycosis; osseous and articular infection is exceedingly rare.

In disseminated *cryptococcal* infection, bone involvement is common, but synovitis is unusual.

Successful management of fungal arthritis usually requires prolonged administration of amphotericin B; surgical debridement is helpful in cases with extensive pannus formation.

VIRAL ARTHRITIS Self-limited polyarthritis is a common manifestation of rubella, type B hepatitis, human immunodeficiency virus infection, and arboviral diseases not found in the Western Hemisphere (chikungunya and O'nyong-nyong in Africa and Ross River arthritis in Australia). Synovitis is less common in mumps, varicella, adenoviral infection, and parvoviral infection. Destructive joint changes are uncommon in viral arthritis, even with recurrent disease.

Arthritis occurs in natural *rubella* infection and following immunization with live, attenuated rubella virus. Approximately 15 percent of postpubertal women develop frank arthritis in the course of natural rubella infection. Large and small joints may be involved; the small joints of the hand and wrist are most severely affected. Occasional involvement of the distal interphalangeal joints helps to differentiate this syndrome from the onset of rheumatoid arthritis. The onset of arthritis in rubella usually occurs at the same time as—or within a few days of—the rash in natural infection and within 2 to 10 weeks after immunization. Rubella arthritis usually abates spontaneously within 1 to 2 weeks; recalcitrant cases respond to salicylates. Joint symptoms may recur for a year or more in natural rubella, but rarely recur after rubella immunization.

The synovitis that accompanies *type B hepatitis* resembles serum sickness, with abrupt onset of fever and articular symptoms. Symmetric polyarthritis of the small joints of the hand may be associated with rheumatoid arthritis–like morning stiffness. The knee, shoulder, ankle, elbow, and wrist are also involved, but the joints of the feet are typically spared. Synovitis is usually accompanied by an urticarial rash, but the rash may be erythematous, maculopapular, or petechial. The possibility of hepatitis-associated arthritis is rarely entertained at the onset of the illness because synovitis usually occurs in the anicteric/prodromal phase. Over a third of patients never become jaundiced, but liver function tests show evidence of hepatitis. Immune complexes containing hepatitis B antigens are present in serum and synovium during the prodromal stage of hepatitis, lending support to the concept that this form of synovitis is immunologically mediated.

In contrast to that of rubella, the arthritis of *mumps* has a predilection for men. It usually occurs after parotitis has subsided, may be accompanied by high fever, and does not respond to salicylates. In children and adults, *coxsackieviral* and *adenoviral* infections have been associated with recurrent fever, polyarthritis, and a polyserositis resembling Still's disease. *Parvoviruses* cause a self-limited acute polyarthritis, predominately in women.

SPIROCHETAL ARTHRITIS Articular disease occurs in congenital, secondary, and tertiary *syphilis* (see Chap. 133). Congenital syphilis is associated with metaphyseal osteochondritis of the long bones that abates spontaneously after 6 months of age. Periostitis continues after that age, and at puberty a painless bilateral synovitis of the knees and elbows (Clutton's joints) may develop. Synovial fluid shows a lymphocytic pleocytosis. Arthralgias, arthritis, and tenosynovitis may accompany the classic signs of secondary syphilis. Gummatous synovitis of the large joints occurs in tertiary syphilis. Neurogenic joint degeneration (Charcot's joint) occurs in neurosyphilis. Articular manifestations also may occur in the nonvenereal treponematoses.

Lyme disease (see also Chap. 137) is a multisystem disorder caused by a spirochete, *Borrelia burgdorferi*, that is transmitted by the bite of *Ixodes dammini* or related ticks. The hallmark of the disease is a characteristic rash, erythema chronicum migrans, during the early phase of infection. Weeks to months later, neurologic and cardiac abnormalities occur, accompanied by polyarthralgias and tenosynovitis. Joint manifestations may evolve to frank arthritis, particularly of the large joints, and recur for years. Prompt oral therapy with tetracycline or amoxicillin eradicates the rash and generally prevents late manifestations, whereas erythromycin does not reliably prevent sequelae. Less than 5 percent of patients are seronegative but develop late manifestations, possibly related to a spirochetal ''persister'' state induced by suboptimal antibiotic therapy. Established late manifestations are cured by parenteral penicillin or ceftriaxone; response to therapy may take several months, and repeated treatment may be necessary.

REFERENCES

BAYER AS, GUZE LB: Fungal arthritis. II. Coccidioidal synovitis; Clinical, diagnostic, therapeutic, and prognostic considerations. Semin Arthritis Rheum 8:200, 1979

GOLDENBERG DL, REED JI: Bacterial arthritis. N Engl J Med 312:764, 1985

HOFFMAN GS: Mycobacterial and fungal infections of bones and joints, in *Textbook of Rheumatology*, 2d ed, WN Kelley, ED Harris, Jr, S Ruddy (eds). Philadelphia, Saunders, 1985

STEIGBIGEL NH: Diagnosis and management of septic arthritis, in *Current Clinical Topics in Infectious Diseases*, JS Remington, MN Swartz (eds). New York, McGraw-Hill, 1983, vol 4, pp 1–29

92   OSTEOMYELITIS AND INFECTIONS OF PROSTHETIC JOINTS

JAMES H. MAGUIRE

Osteomyelitis, an infection of bone, is caused most commonly by pyogenic bacteria and mycobacteria. Case classification on the basis of the causative agent and the route and duration of infection provides a useful framework for evaluating the patient and planning treatment.

PATHOGENESIS AND PATHOLOGY   Microorganisms enter bone by the hematogenous route, by direct introduction from a contiguous focus of infection, or by a penetrating wound. Trauma, ischemia, and foreign bodies enhance the susceptibility of bone to microbial invasion. Phagocytes attempt to contain the infections and, in the process, release enzymes that lyse bone. Pus spreads into vascular channels, raising intraosseous pressure and impairing the flow of blood; as the untreated infection becomes chronic, ischemic necrosis of bone results in the separation of large devascularized fragments (*sequestra*). When pus breaks through the cortex, subperiosteal or soft tissue abscesses form, and the elevated periosteum deposits new bone (the *involucrum*) around the sequestrum. Bacteria escape host defenses by adhering tightly to damaged bone and by coating themselves and underlying surfaces with a protective biofilm.

Microorganisms, infiltrates of neutrophils, and congested or thrombosed blood vessels are the principal histologic findings of acute osteomyelitis. The distinguishing feature of chronic osteomyelitis is necrotic bone, which is recognized by the absence of living osteocytes. Mononuclear cells predominate in chronic infections, and granulation and fibrous tissues replace bone that has been resorbed by osteoclasts. In the chronic stage, organisms may be too few to be seen.

HEMATOGENOUS OSTEOMYELITIS   Hematogenous infection accounts for approximately 20 percent of cases of osteomyelitis and primarily affects children, in whom the long bones are infected, and older adults and intravenous drug users, in whom the spine is the usual site of infection.

Acute hematogenous osteomyelitis   Infection usually involves a single bone, most commonly the tibia, femur, or humerus. Bacteria settle in the well-perfused metaphysis, where functioning phagocytes are scarce and a network of venous sinusoids slows the flow of blood. Because of a different vascular anatomy in children and adults, hematogenous infection of long bones is uncommon during adulthood and, when it occurs, usually involves the diaphysis.

In children, the source of bacteremia is often inapparent, although there may have been recent blunt trauma to the extremity. On presentation, the child usually appears acutely ill, with high fever, chills, localized pain and tenderness, and leukocytosis. Cutaneous erythema and swelling indicate extension of pus through the cortex. During infancy and after puberty, infection may spread through the epiphysis into the joint space.

Plain radiographs initially show soft tissue swelling, but the first change in bone—a periosteal reaction—is not evident until at least 10 days after the onset of infection. Lytic changes can be detected after 2 to 6 weeks, when 50 to 75 percent of bone density has been lost. Rarely, a well-circumscribed lytic lesion, or *Brodie's abscess*, is seen in a child who has had pain for several months but no fever.

Chronic hematogenous osteomyelitis   With prompt treatment, fewer than 5 percent of cases of acute hematogenous osteomyelitis progress to chronic osteomyelitis. On average, 10 days are required for the formation of necrotic bone, but plain radiographs are unable to detect sequestra or sclerotic new bone for many weeks.

A protracted clinical course, long periods of quiescence, and recurrent exacerbations are characteristic of chronic osteomyelitis. Sinus tracts between bone and skin may drain purulent material and occasionally pieces of necrotic bone. An increase in drainage, pain, or the erythrocyte sedimentation rate (ESR) signals an exacerbation. Fever is unusual except when obstruction of a sinus tract leads to soft tissue infection. Rare late complications include pathologic fractures, squamous cell carcinoma of the sinus tract, and amyloidosis.

Vertebral osteomyelitis   Organisms reach the well-perfused vertebral body of adults via spinal arteries and quickly spread from the end plate into the disk space and then to the adjacent vertebral body. The infection may originate in the urinary tract and reach the spine via the prostatic venous (Baston's) plexus; such cases develop particularly often among elderly men. Other sources of the bacteremia include endocarditis, soft tissue infection, and a contaminated intravenous line; these sources usually are obvious. Penetrating injuries and surgical procedures to the vertebrae may cause nonhematogenous vertebral osteomyelitis.

Most patients with vertebral osteomyelitis complain of neck or back pain, although 15 percent describe atypical pain in the chest, abdomen, or an extremity that is due to irritation of nerve roots. Symptoms are localized to the lumbar spine (over 50 percent) more often than the thoracic (35 percent) or cervical spine in pyogenic infections, but the thoracic spine is involved most commonly in tuberculous spondylitis (Pott's disease). Percussion over the involved vertebra elicits tenderness, and physical examination may reveal spasm of the paraspinal muscles and a limitation of motion. Approximately 50 percent of patients experience a subacute illness in which a vague, dull pain gradually intensifies over the course of 2 to 3 months; fever is low grade or absent, and the white blood cell count is normal. An acute presentation with high fever and toxicity is less common and suggests an ongoing bacteremia.

Usually, by the time the patient seeks medical attention, the ESR is elevated, and plain radiographs show irregular erosions in the end plates of adjacent vertebral bodies and narrowing of the intervening disk space. This radiographic pattern is virtually diagnostic of bacterial infection because tumors and other diseases of the spine rarely cross the disk space. Computed tomography (CT) or magnetic resonance imaging (MRI) may demonstrate epidural, paraspinal, retropharyngeal, mediastinal, retroperitoneal, or psoas abscesses that originate in the spine. An epidural abscess may evolve suddenly or over the course of several weeks; irreversible paralysis may be the consequence of failure to recognize the classic clinical presentation of a spinal epidural abscess, consisting of spinal pain progressing to radicular pain and weakness.

Microbiology   Over 95 percent of cases of hematogenous osteomyelitis are caused by a single organism. *Staphylococcus aureus* accounts for 50 percent of isolates. Vertebral osteomyelitis is due to *Escherichia coli* and other enteric bacilli in approximately 25 percent of cases. *Pseudomonas aeruginosa* and *Serratia* infections are associated with intravenous drug use in some parts of the United States and may involve the sacroiliac, sternoclavicular, or pubic joints as well as the spine. *Salmonella* spp. and *S. aureus* are the major causes of long bone osteomyelitis complicating sickle cell anemia and other hemoglobinopathies. Tuberculosis and brucellosis affect the spine more often than other bones.

Unusual causes of hematogenous osteomyelitis include disseminated histoplasmosis, coccidioidomycosis, and blastomycosis in endemic areas. Immunocompromised persons on rare occasions develop osteomyelitis due to species of *Candida, Cryptococcus, Aspergillus,* or *Pneumocystis.* Syphilis, yaws, varicella, and vaccinia may involve bone. The etiology of chronic relapsing multifocal osteomyelitis, an inflammatory condition of children characterized by recurrent episodes of painful lytic lesions in multiple bones, has not yet been identified.

OSTEOMYELITIS SECONDARY TO A CONTIGUOUS FOCUS OF INFECTION   Clinical features   This broad category includes infections introduced by penetrating injuries and surgical procedures and direct extension of infection from adjacent soft tissues. It accounts for the greatest number of cases of osteomyelitis and occurs most commonly in adults.

Frequently the diagnosis is not made until the infection has already become chronic. The pain, fever, and inflammatory signs due to acute osteomyelitis may be attributed to the original injury or soft tissue infection. An indolent infection may become apparent only weeks or months later when a sinus tract develops, a surgical wound breaks down, or a fracture fails to heal. It may be impossible to distinguish the radiographic abnormalities due to osteomyelitis from those due to the precipitating condition.

A special category of contiguous focus osteomyelitis occurs in the setting of peripheral vascular disease and nearly always involves the small bones of the feet of adult diabetics. Diabetic neuropathy exposes the foot to frequent trauma and pressure sores, and the patient may be unaware of infection as it spreads into bone. Poor tissue perfusion impairs normal inflammatory responses and wound healing and creates a milieu that is conducive to anaerobic infections. It is often during the evaluation of a nonhealing ulcer or acute cellulitis that a radiograph provides the first evidence of osteomyelitis.

Microbiology   *S. aureus* is a pathogen in more than half of cases, but in contrast to hematogenous osteomyelitis, these infections often are polymicrobial and more likely to involve gram-negative and anaerobic bacteria. Hence a mixture of staphylococci, streptococci, enteric organisms, and anaerobic bacteria may be isolated from a diabetic foot infection or pelvic osteomyelitis underlying a decubitus ulcer. Aerobic and anaerobic bacteria cause osteomyelitis following surgery or soft tissue infection of the oropharynx, paranasal sinuses, gastrointestinal tract, or female genital tract. *S. aureus* is the principal cause of postoperative infections; coagulase-negative staphylococci are common pathogens following implantation of orthopedic appliances; and these organisms as well as gram-negative enteric bacilli, atypical mycobacteria, and *Mycoplasma* may cause sternal osteomyelitis after cardiac surgery. Infection with *P. aeruginosa* is frequently associated with puncture wounds of the foot or thermal burns, and *Pasteurella multocida* infection commonly follows cat bites (see Chap. 95).

DIAGNOSIS   Early diagnosis of acute osteomyelitis is critical because prompt antibiotic therapy may prevent the necrosis of bone. The evaluation usually begins with plain radiographs because of their ready availability, although they frequently show no abnormalities during early infection. The ESR is elevated in most cases of active osteomyelitis, including those in which constitutional symptoms and leukocytosis are missing. It is not a specific test for osteomyelitis, however, and occasionally is normal in early infections. In 95 percent of cases the technetium radionuclide scan using ^{99m}Tc diphosphonate is positive within 24 h of onset of symptoms. Falsely negative scans usually indicate obstruction of blood flow to the bone. Because the uptake of technetium reflects osteoblastic activity and skeletal vascularity, the bone scan cannot differentiate osteomyelitis from fractures, tumors, infarction, or neuropathic osteopathy. ^{67}Ga citrate–

and ^{111}In-labeled leukocyte or immunoglobulin scans, which have greater specificity for inflammation, may help distinguish infectious from noninfectious processes and indicate inflammatory changes within bones that are already abnormal by radiography and the technetium scan for other reasons.

MRI is as sensitive as the bone scan for the diagnosis of acute osteomyelitis because it is able to demonstrate changes in the water content of marrow. MRI gives better anatomic resolution of epidural abscesses and other soft tissue processes than CT and is currently the imaging technique of choice for vertebral osteomyelitis.

The role of diagnostic imaging in chronic osteomyelitis is to determine the presence of active infection and delineate the extent of debridement necessary to remove necrotic bone and abnormal soft tissues. Although plain films accurately reflect chronic changes, the CT scan is more sensitive for detecting sequestra, sinus tracts, and soft tissue abscesses. Sequential technetium and gallium or indium scans may help determine whether infection is active and may distinguish infection from noninflammatory bone changes; they do not, however, provide good anatomic detail. MRI gives detailed information about the activity and the anatomic extent of infection but does not always distinguish osteomyelitis from healing fractures and tumors. MRI is particularly useful in distinguishing cellulitis from osteomyelitis in the diabetic foot; however, no imaging modality consistently distinguishes infection from neuropathic osteopathy.

Appropriate samples for microbiologic studies should be obtained in all cases of suspected osteomyelitis before initiation of antimicrobial therapy. Blood cultures are indicated in acute cases and are positive in over one-third of children with hematogenous osteomyelitis and 25 percent of adults with vertebral osteomyelitis. If the clinical picture demands immediate antibiotic therapy or if blood cultures are negative, samples from needle aspiration of pus in bone or soft tissues or a bone biopsy should be obtained for culture.

The results of culture of specimens obtained by swabbing a sinus tract or the base of an ulcer correlate poorly with the organisms infecting the bone. For this reason, in cases of chronic osteomyelitis and contiguous focus osteomyelitis, samples for aerobic and anaerobic culture should be obtained by percutaneous needle aspiration, percutaneous biopsy, or intraoperative biopsy at the time of debridement. Isolates of coagulase-negative staphylococci and other organisms of low virulence should not be automatically disregarded as contaminants, especially in the presence of prosthetic materials. Special culture media may be necessary to isolate mycobacteria, fungi, and other less common pathogens. In some cases, histopathologic examination of biopsy specimens may be the only way to make a diagnosis.

TREATMENT   Antibiotic therapy   Antibiotics are administered only after appropriate specimens have been obtained for culture. The antibiotics selected should be bactericidal for the organism(s) isolated from bone or blood and in most cases should be given intravenously in the same high doses used to treat endocarditis. When necessary, empirical therapy is guided by the findings of a Gram-stained specimen from the bone or abscess or is chosen to cover the most likely pathogens. Empirical therapy in most cases should include an agent active against *S. aureus,* such as oxacillin, nafcillin, a cephalosporin, or vancomycin and, if gram-negative organisms are likely to be involved, a third-generation cephalosporin, an aminoglycoside, or a fluoroquinolone.

The duration of therapy is typically 4 to 6 weeks; in some cases, at-home intravenous administration of antibiotics or oral therapy is appropriate. Children with acute hematogenous osteomyelitis routinely receive oral antibiotics after 5 to 10 days of parenteral therapy if signs of active infection have resolved; such treatment has been as successful as the standard parenteral therapy. The doses of oral penicillins or cephalosporins required for treating osteomyelitis are several times higher than the doses of these drugs given for common infections. Adults do not tolerate these high doses as well as children, and except in case of the fluoroquinolones, there are few data to support the use of oral antibiotics by adults. Oral administration of an agent such as ciprofloxacin (750 mg every 12 h) has been as successful as the intravenous administration of β-lactam antibiotics. Caution should be exercised in the use of these agents as the sole treatment of infection due to *S. aureus* or *P. aeruginosa* because resistance may develop during therapy.

Serum minimal bactericidal concentrations (MBC) against isolates of the responsible pathogen should be measured to document compliance and adequate serum levels in patients who receive an oral antibiotic. Otherwise, there are few data to support the routine use of the MBC to monitor therapy of osteomyelitis.

Acute osteomyelitis Early treatment of acute hematogenous osteomyelitis of childhood with 4 to 6 weeks of an appropriate antibiotic is usually successful; treatment for less than 3 weeks has resulted in a 10-fold greater rate of failure. Surgical intervention in childhood cases is indicated for intraosseous or subperiosteal abscesses, concomitant septic arthritis, and failure of the acute signs of infection to improve in 24 to 48 h. Acute hematogenous osteomyelitis of bones other than the spine in adults often requires surgical debridement.

Four to 6 weeks of an appropriate antibiotic are usually sufficient to cure vertebral osteomyelitis. Failure of the ESR to drop to at least two-thirds of pretreatment levels is an indication for longer treatment. Surgery is seldom necessary, even in cases of many months' duration, except in the case of spinal instability, new or progressive neurologic deficits, large soft tissue abscesses, or a failure of medical treatment. Patients should maintain bed rest until back pain has declined to the point at which ambulation is possible. Body casts are no longer used.

Contiguous focus osteomyelitis usually requires surgery in addition to 4 to 6 weeks of appropriate antibiotics, even when diagnosed early, because of underlying soft tissue infection or damage to bone from an injury or surgery.

Chronic ostemyelitis The risks and benefits of aggressive therapy of chronic osteomyelitis should be weighed before any attempt to eradicate the infection is undertaken. Some patients with extensive disease prefer to live with their infections rather than undergo multiple surgical procedures, take prolonged courses of antimicrobial therapy, and face the risk of loss of an extremity. Such persons often benefit from intermittent courses of oral antibiotics to suppress acute exacerbations.

Once the decision has been made to treat chronic osteomyelitis aggressively, antibiotics should be started several days before surgery to reduce inflammation if the etiology of the infection is known preoperatively. If not, antibiotic therapy should be withheld until surgical debridement. An empirical antibiotic regimen is started intraoperatively after culture specimens are obtained. Four to 6 weeks of appropriate antibiotic therapy are given postoperatively on the basis of the susceptibility pattern of organisms isolated from the bone. The benefit of prolonged oral antibiotic therapy following 4 to 6 weeks of parenteral therapy remains unproven. There currently is insufficient information to recommend the routine use of hyperbaric oxygen to enhance the killing of microorganisms by phagocytes or instillation pumps and antibiotic-impregnated methacrylate beads to deliver high levels of antibiotics to the bone.

Success in treating chronic osteomyelitis rests largely on the complete surgical removal of necrotic bone and abnormal soft tissues. Modern imaging techniques allow accurate preoperative delineation of tissues to be debrided, but it remains difficult for the surgeon to determine intraoperatively whether all necrotic and infected tissue has been removed. In the past, the inability to restore large defects in bone and soft tissue limited the extent of debridement. Muscle flaps and skin grafts are now used routinely to cover large soft tissue defects and fill dead space, and bone grafts and vascularized bone transfer may restore a seriously compromised bone to a functional state.

In infections of recent fractures, internal fixators are often left in place, and the infection is controlled by limited debridement and suppressive antibiotic therapy. Definitive surgical antimicrobial therapies are delayed until after bony union of the fracture is achieved. If there is nonunion of the fracture or loosening of the fixator, the appliance should be removed and an external fixator applied.

Osteomyelitis of the small bones of the feet in persons with vascular disease also requries surgery for successful treatment. The effectiveness of the surgery is limited by the blood supply to the site and the patient's ability to heal the wound. Revascularization of the extremity is indicated if the vascular disease involves large arteries. In cases of decreased perfusion due to small-vessel disease, treatment is likely to fail, and the best option is suppressive therapy or amputation. The duration of antibiotic therapy depends on the surgical procedure performed. When the infected bone is removed entirely but residual infection of soft tissues remains, 2 weeks of antibiotics should be given; if amputation eliminates infected bone and soft tissue, standard surgical prophylaxis is given; otherwise 4 to 6 weeks of postoperative antibiotics are required.

INFECTIONS OF PROSTHETIC JOINTS Infection complicates 1 to 4 percent of total joint replacements. The majority of infections are acquired intraoperatively or in the immediate postoperative period due to wound breakdown or infection and, less commonly, at any time after joint replacement by the hematogenous route or by direct inoculation. The presentation may be acute with fever, pain, and local signs of inflammation, especially in infections due to *S. aureus*, pyogenic streptococci, and enteric bacilli, or infection may persist for months or years without causing constitutional symptoms when less virulent organisms such as coagulase-negative staphylococci or diphtheroids are involved. Such indolent infections are usually acquired during joint implantation and are discovered during evaluation of chronic unexplained pain or after a radiograph shows loosening of the prothesis; the ESR is usually elevated in such cases.

The diagnosis is best made by needle aspiration of the joint; accidental introduction of organisms during aspiration must be meticulously avoided. Synovial fluid pleocytosis with a predominance of polymorphonuclear leukocytes is highly suggestive of infection, since other inflammatory processes uncommonly affect prosthetic joints. Culture and Gram's stain usually yield the responsible pathogen. Special media for unusual pathogens such as fungi, atypical mycobacteria, and *Mycoplasma* may be necessary if routine and anaerobic cultures are negative.

Treatment includes surgery and high doses of parenteral antibiotics, which are given for 4 to 6 weeks because bone is usually involved. In most cases, the prosthesis must be replaced in order to cure the infection. Implantation of a new prosthesis is best delayed for several weeks or months because relapses of infection occur most commonly within this time frame. In some cases, reimplantation is not possible, and the patient must manage without a joint, with a fused joint, or, at times, with amputation. Cure of infection without removal of the prosthesis occasionally is possible in cases of infection due to streptococci or pneumococci and without radiologic evidence of loosening of the prosthesis. In these cases, antibiotic therapy must begin within several days of the onset of infection, and the joint should be vigorously drained either by open arthrotomy or arthroscopically.

To avoid the disastrous consequences of infection, candidates for joint replacement should be selected with care. Rates of infection are particularly high in patients with rheumatoid arthritis, persons who have undergone previous surgery on the joint, and persons with medical conditions requiring immunosuppressive therapy. Perioperative antibiotic prophylaxis, usually cefazolin, and measures to decrease intraoperative contamination, such as laminar flow, have decreased the rates of perioperative infection to less than 1 percent in many centers. Following implantation, measures should be taken to prevent and rapidly treat extraarticular infections that might give rise to hematogenous spread of infection to the prosthesis. The effectiveness of prophylactic antibiotics for prevention of hematogenous infection following dental procedures has not been demonstrated, and in fact, viridans streptococci and other components of the oral flora are extremely unusual causes of prosthetic joint infection.

REFERENCES

ESOLEN LM et al: *Pneumocystis carinii* osteomyelitis in a patient with common variable immunodeficiency. N Engl J Med 326:999, 1992

ESTERHAI JL JR (ed): Orthopedic infection. Orthop Clin North Am 22:363, 1991

MADER JT et al: Evaluation of new anti-infective drugs for the treatment of osteomyelitis in adults. Clin Infect Dis 15(suppl 1):S155, 1992

MAY JW JR et al: Treatment of chronic traumatic bone wounds. Microvascular free tissue transfer: A 13-year experience in 96 patients. Ann Surg 214:241, 1991

NORDEN CW (ed): Osteomyelitis. Infect Dis Clin North Am 4:361, 1990

WALDVOGEL FA et al: Osteomyelitis: A review of clinical features, therapeutic considerations, and unusual aspects. N Engl J Med 282:198, 1970

93 INFECTIONS OF THE SKIN, MUSCLE, AND SOFT TISSUES

DENNIS L. STEVENS

ANATOMICAL RELATIONSHIPS: CLUES TO THE DIAGNOSIS OF SOFT TISSUE INFECTIONS   Protection against infection of the epidermis is dependent upon the mechanical barrier afforded by the stratum corneum, since the epidermis itself is devoid of blood vessels (Fig. 93-1). Disruption of this layer by burns, bites, abrasion, or foreign body allows penetration of bacteria to the deeper structures. Similarly, the hair follicle can serve as a portal for either normal flora (*Staphylococcus*) or for extrinsic bacteria (*Pseudomonas*—hot tub folliculitis). Intracellular infection of the squamous epithelium with vesicle formation may arise from cutaneous inoculation with viruses such as herpes simplex 1, from the dermal capillary plexus with viruses associated with viremia (varicella), or from cutaneous nerve roots (herpes zoster). Bacteria infecting the epidermis such as *Streptococcus pyogenes* may be translocated laterally to deeper structures via lymphatics, thus resulting in the rapid superficial spread of erysipelas. Later, engorgement or obstruction of lymphatics causes flaccid edema of the epidermis, another characteristic of erysipelas.

The rich plexus of capillaries beneath the dermal papillae provides nutrition to the stratum germinativum, and physiologic responses of this plexus provide important clinical signs and symptoms. For example, infective vasculitis of the plexus results in petechiae, Osler's nodes, Janeway lesions, and palpable purpura, which are important clues for the existence of endocarditis (Chap. 85). In addition, metastatic infection within this plexus can also result in cutaneous manifestations of disseminated fungal infection (Chap. 166), gonococcal infection (Chap. 110), salmonella infections (Chap. 117), pseudomonas infection, i.e. ecthyma gangrenosa (Chap. 116), meningococcemia (Chap. 109), and staphylococcal infection (Chap. 102). This plexus also provides access for bacteria to the circulation, thereby facilitating local spread or bacteremia. Postcapillary venules of this plexus are a major site of polymorphonuclear leukocyte sequestration, diapedesis, and chemotaxis to the site of cutaneous infection. Exaggeration of these physiologic mechanisms by excessive cytokines or bacterial toxins causes leukostasis, venous occlusion, and pitting edema. Edema with purple bullae and ecchymosis suggests loss of vascular integrity and requires exploration of the deeper structures for evidence of necrotizing fasciitis or myonecrosis. To make an earlier diagnosis requires a high level of suspicion in patients with unexplained fever and pain and tenderness in the soft tissue, even in the absence of acute cutaneous inflammation.

INFECTIONS ASSOCIATED WITH VESICLES (Table 93-1)   Vesicle formation due to infection is caused by viral proliferation within the epidermis. In variola, viremia precedes the onset of a diffuse centrifugal rash that progresses from macules to vesicles, then pustules, and finally scabs over the course of 1 to 2 weeks. Vesicles of varicella have a "dew drop" appearance and occur in crops randomly about the trunk, extremities, and face over the course of 3 to 4 days. Herpes zoster occurs in a single dermatome and is preceded by pain for several days before the appearance of vesicles. Zoster occurs predominately in elderly patients and AIDS victims, whereas most varicella occurs in young children. Vesicles due to herpes simplex (HSV) are found on or around the lips (HSV-1) or genitals (HSV-2) but may appear on the head and neck in young wrestlers (herpes gladitorum) or on the digits (herpetic whitlow) in health care workers. Coxsackie A-16 characteristically causes vesicles on the

FIGURE 93-1   Structural components of the skin and soft tissue are identified at the left. Superficial infections are depicted along the top of the figure and infections of the deeper structures of the soft tissue at the right edge. The rich capillary network beneath the dermal papillae plays a key role in localizing infection and in the development of the acute inflammatory reaction.

TABLE 93-1 Skin and soft-tissue infections

Lesion	Agent/ Clinical syndrome	Chapter Reference
Vesicles	Variola (smallpox)	147
	Varicella (chickenpox)	144
	Herpes zoster (shingles)	144
	Herpes simplex types I and II	143
	Coxsackie A-16 (hand, foot, and mouth disease)	154
	Orf	147
Bullae	Staphylococcal scalded-skin syndrome	102
	Necrotizing fasciitis	128
	Gas gangrene	108
	Halophilic vibrio	120
Crusted lesions	Impetigo	103
	Superficial dermatophytes	169
	Systemic dimorphic fungi	162
	Cutaneous leishmaniasis	175
	Mucocutaneous candidiasis	166
	Cutaneous tuberculosis	130
	Nocardiosis	126
Folliculitis	*Staphylococcus aureus*	102
	Pseudomonas aeruginosa (hot tub folliculitis)	116
	Schistosomiasis (swimmer's itch)	183
	Acne vulgaris	51
Ulcers with or without eschars	Anthrax	104
	Cutaneous diptheria	104
	Ulceroglandular tularemia	122
	Bubonic plague	123
	Mycobacterium ulcerans	132
	Mycobacterium leprae	131
	Mycobacterium tuberculosis	130
Erysipelas	*Streptococcus pyogenes*	103
Necrotizing fasciitis	*Streptococcus pyogenes*	103
	Mixed aerobic/anaerobic infection	128
Myositis	Pyomyositis	102
	Streptococcal necrotizing myositis	103
	Gas gangrene	108
	Nonclostridial (crepitant) myositis	128
	Synergistic nonclostridial anaerobic myonecrosis	128

hands, feet, and mouth in children. Orf is caused by a DNA virus related to smallpox and infects the fingers of individuals who work around goats and sheep.

INFECTIONS ASSOCIATED WITH BULLAE (Table 93-1) Staphylococcal scalded-skin syndrome (SSSS) in neonates is caused by a toxin from phage group II *Staph. aureus*. SSSS must be distinguished from toxic epidermal necrolysis (TEN) which occurs primarily in adults, is drug induced, and has a higher mortality. Punch biopsy with frozen section is useful since the cleavage plane in SSSS is the stratum corneum (Fig. 93-1), and in TEN is the stratum germinativum. Necrotizing fasciitis and gas gangrene also induce bullae formation (see Necrotizing Fasciitis, below). Halophilic vibrio infection can be as aggressive and fulminant as necrotizing fasciitis, and a helpful clue would be a history of exposure to waters of the Gulf of Mexico or Atlantic seaboard, or a patient with cirrhosis who has ingested raw seafood.

INFECTIONS ASSOCIATED WITH CRUSTED LESIONS (Table 93-1) Impetigo contagiosa is caused by *Streptococcus pyogenes*, and bullous impetigo is due to *Staph. aureus*. Both skin lesions may have an early bullous stage but then appear as thick crusts with a golden brown color. Streptococcal lesions are most common in children 2 to 5 years of age, and epidemics may occur in settings of poor hygiene, particularly in children of lower socioeconomic status in tropical climates. It is important to recognize impetigo contagiosa because of its relationship to poststreptococcal glomerulonephritis. Superficial dermatophyte infections (ringworm) can occur on any skin surface, and skin scrapings with KOH staining are diagnostic. Primary dimorphic fungal infections such as *Blastomyces* (Chap. 164) and

Sporothrix schenkii (Chap. 169) can initially present as crusted skin lesions resembling ringworm. Disseminated *Coccidioides immitis* (Chap. 163) also can involve skin, and biopsy and culture should be performed on crusted lesions in patients from endemic areas.

FOLLICULITIS (Table 93-1) Hair follicles serve as a portal of entry for a number of bacteria, though *Staph. aureus* is the most common cause of localized folliculitis. Sebaceous glands empty into hair follicles and ducts, which if blocked (sebaceous cyst), may resemble staphylococcal abscess or may become secondarily infected. Infection of sweat glands (hidradenitis suppurativa) can also mimic infected hair follicles particularly in the axillae. Chronic folliculitis is uncommon except in acne vulgaris where normal flora, e.g., *Propionibacterium acnes*, may play a role.

Diffuse folliculitis occurs in two settings. "Hot-tub folliculitis" is caused by *Pseudomonas aeruginosa* in waters that are insufficiently chlorinated and maintained at temperatures between 37 and 40°C. Infection is usually self-limited, though bacteremia and shock have been reported. Swimmer's itch occurs when a skin surface is exposed to water infested with freshwater avian schistosomes. Warm water temperatures and alkaline pH are suitable for molluscs that serve as intermediate hosts between bird and human. Free-swimming schistosomal cercariae (see Chap. 183) readily penetrate human hair follicles or pores but quickly die and elicit a brisk allergic reaction causing intense itching and erythema.

ULCERS WITH OR WITHOUT ESCHARS (Table 93-1) Cutaneous anthrax begins as a pruritic papule which develops within days to an ulcer with surrounding vesicles and edema and then to an enlarging ulcer with black eschar. Cutaneous diphtheria may cause chronic nonhealing ulcers with an overlying dirty-gray membrane, though lesions may also mimic psoriasis, eczema, or impetigo. Ulceroglandular tularemia may have associated ulcerated skin lesions with painful regional adenopathy. Although bubos are the major cutaneous manifestation of plague (see Chap. 123), cutaneous lesions in 25 percent of cases include ulcers with eschars, papules, or pustules.

Mycobacterium ulcerans typically causes chronic skin ulcers on the extremities of individuals living in the tropics. *M. leprae* may be associated with cutaneous ulcerations in patients with lepromatous leprosy associated with the Lucio phenomenon or during reversal reactions. *M. tuberculosis* may also cause ulcerations, papules, or erythematous macular lesions of the skin in both normal and immunocompromised patients.

Decubitus ulcers are due to tissue hypoxia secondary to vascular insufficiency caused by pressure and may become secondarily infected with skin and gastrointestinal flora including anaerobes. Ulcerative lesions on the anterior shins may be due to pyoderma gangrenosa, which must be distinguished from infectious etiology by means of histological evaluation of biopsy sites.

ERYSIPELAS (Table 93-1) Erysipelas is due to *S. pyogenes* and is characterized by an abrupt onset of fiery, red swelling of the face or extremities. Distinctive features are its well-defined margins, particularly along the nasolabial fold, rapid progression, and intense pain. Flaccid bullae may develop during the second or third day of illness, but extension to deeper soft tissues is rare. Treatment with penicillin is effective; swelling may progress despite appropriate treatment, though fever, pain, and the intense red color diminish. Desquamation of the involved skin occurs 5 to 10 days into the illness. Infants and elderly adults are most commonly afflicted, and the severity of systemic toxicity may vary.

CELLULITIS Cellulitis is an acute inflammatory condition of skin characterized by localized pain, erythema, swelling, and heat. Small breaks in the skin are associated with streptococcal infection, whereas staphylococcal cellulitis is commonly associated with larger wounds, ulcers, or abscesses. Fever suggests streptococcal infection. Cellulitis of the lower extremity is more common with chronic lymphedema, chronic venous stasis, and saphenous vein donor sites. Infection is usually due to group A streptococci, though group C and G streptococci may cause saphenous donor site infections. *S.*

agalactiae infection may occur in diabetes mellitus or peripheral vascular disease. *Haemophilus influenzae* causes periorbital cellulitis in children in association with sinusitis, otitis media, or epiglottitis.

Exogenous bacteria may be introduced into the skin by a variety of means: *Pasteurella multocida*—cat bites; *Staph. intermedius*—dog bites; *Aeromonas hydrophila*—cuts in fresh water; *P. aeruginosa*—sweaty tennis shoe syndrome; *Erysipelothrix rhusiopathiae*—fish monger's cellulitis; *Mycobacterium marinum*—fish tank exposure; and gram-negative rod cellulitis—compromised hosts.

Bacterial diagnosis is difficult in acute cellulitis, and needle aspiration or even punch biopsy yields positive cultures in only about 20 percent of cases. The low number of bacteria identified suggests that toxins or host response to infection may be largely responsible for the signs and symptoms of cellulitis.

NECROTIZING FASCIITIS (Table 93-1) Necrotizing fasciitis, formerly called streptococcal gangrene, may be associated with group A streptococcus, mixed aerobic-anaerobic bacteria, or as part of gas gangrene caused by *Clostridium perfringens*. Early diagnosis may be difficult when pain or unexplained fever are the only presenting symptoms and signs. Swelling then occurs and is followed by brawny edema and tenderness. With progression, dark red induration of the epidermis appears along with bullae filled with blue or purple fluid. Later skin becomes friable and takes on a bluish, maroon, or black color. By this stage, extensive thrombosis of blood vessels occur in the dermal papilla (see Fig. 93-1). Extension of infection to the level of the deep fascia causes a brownish-gray appearance. Rapid spreading occurs along fascial planes, through venous channels and lymphatics. Patients in the later stages are toxic and frequently manifest shock and multiorgan failure.

Necrotizing fasciitis caused by mixed aerobic-anaerobic bacteria begins with a breach in integrity of a mucous membrane barrier such as the mucosa of the gastrointestinal or genitourinary tract. The portal can be a malignancy, diverticulum, hemorrhoid, anal fissure, or urethral tear. Other predisposing factors include peripheral vascular disease, diabetes mellitus, surgery, or penetrating injury to the abdomen. Leakage into the perineal area results in a syndrome called *Fournier's gangrene*, characterized by massive swelling of the scrotum and penis with extension into the perineum, or abdominal wall, and legs.

Necrotizing fasciitis caused by *S. pyogenes* has increased in frequency and severity since 1985. It frequently begins deep at the site of nonpenetrating minor trauma such as a bruise or muscle strain. Seeding of the site by transient bacteremia is likely, though most patients deny antecedent streptococcal infection. Necrotizing fasciitis due to mixed aerobic-anaerobic bacteria may be associated with gas in the deep tissue, but gas is not usually present when the cause is *S. pyogenes*. Toxicity is severe, and renal impairment may precede the development of shock. In 20 to 40 percent of cases, myositis occurs concomitantly, and, as in gas gangrene (see below), serum creatinine phosphokinase values may be markedly elevated. Prompt surgical exploration down to the deep fascia and muscle is essential. Necrotic tissue must be surgically removed, and Gram's stain of material will be useful to establish whether group A streptococci, mixed aerobic-anaerobic bacteria, or *Clostridium* species are present. (See "Treatment," below.)

MYOSITIS (Table 93-1) Muscle involvement can occur with virus infection [influenza, dengue, coxsackievirus B (pleurodynia)]; or parasitic invasion [*Trichinella spiralis* (trichinosis), *Taenia solium* (cysticercosis), *Toxoplasma gondii* (toxoplasmosis)]. Although myalgia can occur in most of these infections, severe muscle pain is the hallmark of pleurodynia, trichinosis, and bacterial infection. Acute rhabdomyolysis predictably occurs with clostridial and streptococcal myositis but may also be associated with influenza, echovirus, coxsackievirus, Epstein-Barr virus, and *Legionella* infection.

Pyomyositis is usually due to *Staph. aureus*, is common in tropical areas, and commonly has no known portal of entry. Infection remains localized and unless organisms produce toxic shock syndrome toxin

1 or certain enterotoxins, shock does not occur. In contrast, *S. pyogenes* may induce a primary myositis referred to as *streptococcal necrotizing myositis*, which is associated with severe systemic toxicity. Such infections occur as part of the streptococcal toxic shock syndrome.

Gas gangrene usually occurs following severe penetrating injuries that result in interruption of blood supply and introduction of soil into wounds. Such cases of traumatic gangrene are usually caused by *C. perfringens*, *C. septicum*, or *C. histolyticum*. Rarely, latent or recurrent gangrene can occur years after penetrating trauma, most likely due to dormant spores that reside at the previous site of injury. Spontaneous nontraumatic gangrene among patients with neutropenia, gastrointestinal malignancy, diverticulosis, or recent radiation therapy to the abdomen is caused by *C. septicum*. Tolerance of this anaerobe to oxygen probably explains why *C. septicum* can initiate infection spontaneously in normal tissue anywhere in the body.

Synergistic nonclostridial anaerobic myonecrosis, also known as necrotizing cutaneous myositis and synergistic necrotizing cellulitis, is a variant of necrotizing fasciitis caused by mixed aerobic and anaerobic bacteria with the exclusion of clostridial organisms (see "Necrotizing Fasciitis," above).

TREATMENT OF DEEP-SEATED SOFT TISSUE INFECTIONS
Early and aggressive surgical exploration is essential in patients with suspected necrotizing fasciitis, myositis, or gangrene in order to (1) visualize the deep structures, (2) remove necrotic tissue, (3) reduce compartment pressure, and (4) obtain suitable material for Gram's stain and aerobic and anaerobic cultures. Appropriate empirical antibiotic treatment pending culture results could be either A or B below:

A 1 Clindamycin 600–800 mg IV every 8 h or metronidazole 750 mg every 6 h
    plus
  2 Ampicillin or ampicillin/sulbactam 2–3 grams IV every 6 h
    plus
  3 Gentamicin 1.0–1.5 mg/kg every 8 h
or
B Ampicillin/sulbactam or cefoxitin alone

For Group A streptococcal and clostridial infection of the fascia and/or muscle, mortality of 20 to 50 percent occurs with penicillin treatment. In experimental models of streptococcal and clostridial necrotizing fasciitis/myositis, clindamycin has superior efficacy, but no comparative trials have been performed in humans. Hyperbaric oxygen treatment may also be useful in gas gangrene due to clostridia species. Antibiotic treatment should be continued until all signs of systemic toxicity have resolved, all devitalized tissue has been removed, and granulation tissue has developed (Chaps. 103, 108, 128).

In summary, infections of the skin and soft tissues are diverse in presentation and severity and offer a great challenge to the clinician. This chapter is meant to provide an approach to diagnosis and understanding of the pathophysiologic mechanisms. More in-depth information may be found in individual chapters.

REFERENCES

Hook EW et al: Microbiologic evaluation of cutaneous cellulitis in adults. Arch Intern Med 146:295, 1986
Simmons RL, Ahrenholz DH: Infections of the skin and soft tissue, in *Surgical Infectious Diseases*, 2d ed, RJ Howard, RL Simmons (eds). Norwalk, Appleton & Lange, 1988, pp 377–441
Stevens DL: Invasive group A Streptococcus infections. Clin Infect Dis 14:2, 1992
Stevens DL et al: Spontaneous, nontraumatic gangrene due to *Clostridium septicum*. Rev Infect Dis 12(2):286, 1990

94 INFECTIONS (EXCLUDING AIDS) IN INJECTION DRUG USERS

GERALD H. FRIEDLAND / PETER A. SELWYN

The injection of illicit drugs is a widespread practice whose prevalence has increased dramatically since the 1950s in association with successive epidemics of heroin and cocaine use. Injection drug users are a hidden population, engaging in an illegal and societally disapproved activity. It is impossible to determine their precise number and, therefore, the true incidence of infectious complications in this population. In the 1980s, the total number of heroin addicts in the United States was estimated yearly at 500,000, with heavy concentrations in urban areas, particularly but not exclusively in the Northeast. The number of injection drug users may be almost three times this figure when users of cocaine and occasional injection users are included. In addition, there are large numbers of injection drug users in Europe and increasing numbers in developing countries, often at sites of drug production and along routes of drug trade and distribution.

Markedly higher age-specific mortality among injection drug users than in the general population was documented even before the epidemic of infection with human immunodeficiency virus (HIV) and AIDS (see Chap. 279). For example, in New York City between 1965 and 1972, the death rate among young (20- to 54-year-old) adult heroin addicts not involved in drug treatment programs was estimated to be five times greater than that among age-matched, non-heroin-addicted adults (28.2 per 1000 versus 5.6 per 1000). A substantial portion of this excess mortality was the result of infectious complications of injection drug use. Data from the New York City Medical Examiner during the 1960s indicated that 27 percent of narcotic-related deaths were associated with infections. During this period, a wide array of infectious complications of injection drug use was described. More recently, as a consequence of the HIV epidemic, overall mortality and cause-specific mortality secondary to both AIDS and bacterial infections have dramatically increased in this population. Mortality rates of 3.41 per 100 person-years from AIDS and 1.08 per 100 person-years from bacterial infection preceding AIDS have been reported in HIV-infected injection drug users.

Most infectious complications in injection drug users reflect the events surrounding drug injection and associated life-style issues rather than the direct effects of the illicit drugs themselves. Drugs are purchased in powdered form and often contain adulterants such as quinine, talc, and dextrose. The drugs are dissolved in water (obtained from any available source) or occasionally in saliva in bottle caps or "cookers," filtered through cotton wool or gauze, aspirated into tuberculin or diabetic syringes, and injected intravenously or subcutaneously. Skin preparation is usually minimal and may consist of rubbing saliva on the injection site. A small amount of blood may remain in the needle and syringe after use and may be diluted by rinsing in tap water or bleach. Needles and syringes are often shared among injection drug users, either by a few friends or relatives or by larger numbers of users sequentially and anonymously in "shooting galleries." These clandestine locations where injection drug users gather to rent injection equipment and administer drugs are ideal sites for the transmission of bloodborne infectious agents.

Within this setting, the characteristics of injection drug users that increase the risk of infection are (1) increased rates of skin, mucous membrane, and nasopharyngeal carriage of pathogenic organisms, particularly staphylococci, (2) unsterile injection technique resulting in the introduction of components of the skin or nasopharyngeal flora into soft tissues or the bloodstream, (3) contamination of injection equipment or drugs with viral, bacterial, and parasitic microorganisms, which may be present in residual blood in shared injection equipment or in contaminated water used to dissolve drugs before injection or to rinse equipment afterward, (4) humoral, cell-mediated, and phagocytic defects induced by HIV infection and/or drug use (even before the HIV/AIDS epidemic, injection drug users were known to have abnormal immunologic parameters, including high levels of globulins, false-positive serologic reactions to multiple antigens, and abnormalities in phagocytosis, and these defects have been markedly exacerbated by HIV-induced B and T cell dysfunction), (5) poor dental hygiene and drug-induced impairment of gag and cough reflexes, (6) alteration of the normal microbial flora by intermittent antibiotic use, (7) low socioeconomic status, with increased prevalence of exposure to certain pathogens (notably *Mycobacterium tuberculosis*), (8) behaviors associated with injection drug use, such as cigarette smoking, alcohol use, or exchange of sex for drugs or money, and (9) decreased access to and/or lack of appropriate use of preventive and primary health care services, resulting in low levels of immunization and prophylaxis and delay in the diagnosis and treatment of minor infectious complications.

SPECIFIC INFECTIONS OCCURRING AMONG INJECTION DRUG USERS

SKIN AND SOFT TISSUE INFECTIONS (See also Chap. 93) Infections of the skin and soft tissues represent the most common bacterial infectious complication of injection drug use and, before the AIDS epidemic, were the most common cause of hospital admissions of injection drug users. The clinical spectrum of infection is broad, ranging from simple cellulitis and abscess to life-threatening necrotizing fasciitis and septic thrombophlebitis. The high frequency of skin and soft tissue infections is attributable to several factors: the practice of injecting drugs subcutaneously ("skin popping"), the extravasation of drugs into soft tissue during intravenous injection, the presence in injected material of adulterants that may cause tissue necrosis, and the increased skin carriage of pathogenic organisms.

Most skin and soft tissue infections occur on the upper and lower extremities, but occasionally atypical sites (e.g., the abdomen or back, groin, scrotum, and neck) may be involved as a result of injection into the jugular or femoral veins. Cellulitis may extend from a fresh injection site or may result from superinfection of an open wound sustained earlier. The clinical appearance is often atypical because of chronic damage to the skin and to venous and lymphatic systems in both the upper and the lower extremities, with resultant underlying lymphedema, hyperpigmentation, scarring, and regional lymphadenopathy. Nevertheless, careful examination often reveals characteristic redness, warmth, and tenderness, with tender inguinal or axillary lymph nodes. Fever is variable and bacteremia infrequent.

Uncomplicated cellulitis is most frequently due to group A streptococci, other streptococci, or *Staphylococcus aureus*. Unless an associated open, draining wound is present or bacteremia develops, the precise microbial etiology is difficult to determine. For localized abscesses presenting either as draining lesions or as fluctuant subcutaneous masses, Gram's staining and culture of pus or aspirated material are required. Although these abscesses are usually staphylococcal in etiology, they are sometimes due to a more complex mixture of anaerobic and aerobic bacteria. A foul odor and Gram's staining of pus suggest the presence of mixed organisms.

Treatment consists of hospitalization in most cases, incision and drainage in instances of abscess formation, and administration of intravenous antistaphylococcal β-lactam antibiotics such as oxacillin or nafcillin. Cefazolin may be an alternative choice. In areas where methicillin-resistant *S. aureus* is highly prevalent, vancomycin should be used empirically pending the results of susceptibility tests. The total duration of therapy should be 10 to 14 days; for the latter part of this course, oral agents may or may not be used, depending on the individual's clinical response. For injection drug users who have an established realtionship with a health care provider, mild infections may be treated with oral agents on an outpatient basis; therapy should be followed by frequent visits at which the response is assessed.

Indolent skin ulcers are common. These lesions are shallow and indurated and may become superinfected. Their etiology is unclear, but they are likely the result of foreign-body inflammatory changes, necrosis, and low-grade infection. They usually respond to local wound care and oral or topical antibiotic treatment. Occasionally, these ulcers are extensive enough to require skin grafting. When lesions heal, they leave depressed, hyperpigmented scars.

Necrotizing fasciitis and myositis and septic thrombophlebitis are life-threatening local complications of injection drug use. Although infrequent, they should always be considered when skin or soft tissue infection develops in injection drug users. The presence of fasciitis and myositis is associated with exquisite pain and tenderness at the injection site and with toxicity and hemodynamic instability out of proportion to the local lesion. Crepitus may be noted, and soft tissue radiographs may reveal gas in tissues. Immediate surgical exploration, with extensive drainage and debridement of infected and nonviable tissue, is required. These infections often have a polymicrobial etiology that includes *S. aureus*, aerobic and anaerobic streptococci, enteric gram-negative bacilli, and other anaerobes. Parenteral antibiotic therapy aimed at gram-positive and gram-negative organisms, with anaerobic coverage, is essential. Several regimens, including vancomyicin or nafcillin, plus metronidazole or clindamycin, plus an aminoglycoside, a third-generation cephalosporin, or an expanded-spectrum penicillin, are indicated.

Septic thrombophlebitis of extremity, jugular, or femoral veins often appears as septic pulmonary emboli. Bacteremia is invariably found, and pus may be expressed from injection sites of infected vessels. Parenteral antibiotic therapy as well as ligation and excision of infected thrombosed veins (if technically feasible) is advocated. The value of heparin remains unproved, and it is generally not recommended.

Other, infrequent complications of injection drug use under unsterile circumstances include wound botulism, tetanus, malaria, and disseminated candidiasis. The first two have been sporadically reported, usually in long-term users and often in "skin poppers," whereas outbreaks of malaria have resulted from the sharing of needles contaminated with infected blood. Botulism should be considered in patients with unusual, progressive cranial nerve palsies; wounds should be cultured for *Clostridium botulinum*. Tetanus should be suspected in drug users with seizures, muscle rigidity, and autonomic hyperactivity.

ENDOCARDITIS (See Chap. 85) Although bacterial endocarditis is less frequent than skin and pulmonary infections among injection drug users, its potential life-threatening complications and the usual need for prolonged intravenous antibiotic therapy in the hospital make it a disease of great consequence in this population. In several studies of consecutive hospital admissions of injection drug users before the AIDS epidemic, endocarditis accounted for 5 to 16 percent of admissions and for 2 to 8 percent of all deaths.

Microbiology The predominant organism causing endocarditis in injection drug users is *S. aureus*. In various published series, this organism has accounted for 60 percent to more than 90 percent of cases. In many geographic locations, a substantial and increasing proportion of *S. aureus* isolates are resistant to methicillin. Although this organism was originally believed to be a contaminant of drugs and injection paraphernalia, it is now clear that *S. aureus* is part of the patient's own flora, carried in the nares and oropharynx and on the skin and subsequently introduced into the bloodstream by unsterile injection. In the published studies, 60 to 100 percent of injection drug users with *S. aureus* endocarditis on admission to the hospital had an identical organism in the blood and at one or more of these sites, while cultures of heroin and injection equipment were negative for *S. aureus*.

Certain bacteria are encountered more frequently in right-sided rather than in left-sided endocarditis. Right-sided endocarditis is caused by *S. aureus* in more than 80 percent of cases, whereas the organisms isolated in aortic or mitral valve endocarditis are more similar to those found in other patients. Streptococci and enterococci, including α-hemolytic viridans streptococci and *Enterococcus fae-*

calis, are the second most common organisms but account for only 5 to 10 percent of cases of endocarditis in various series. Geographic and temporal clustering of more unusual infecting organisms has occasionally been reported. These organisms include *Pseudomonas aeruginosa*, which was isolated from injection drug users in Chicago and Detroit in the 1970s and early 1980s in relation to pentazocine and tripelennamine abuse; *Pseudomonas cepacia*, isolated in New York; *Serratia marcescens*, isolated in San Francisco; enterococci, isolated in Cleveland; and recently, methicillin-resistant *S. aureus*, isolated in Detroit. Infrequent cases of endocarditis due to *Candida* spp., *Bacillus* spp., diphtheroids, and fastidious gram-negative or anaerobic components of the oral flora have been described as well. *Bacillus* spp. have been the most frequent contaminants of drugs and injection paraphernalia. Polymicrobial endocarditis due to both gram-positive and gram-negative organisms has been documented.

Pathogenesis and clinical presentation Longer duration and increased frequency of the use of drugs are associated with a cumulative increase in the risk of endocarditis. Most cases of endocarditis in this populatoin involve the right side of the heart and the tricuspid valve. In one series, 76 percent of cases of endocarditis in injection drug users were right-sided, while the corresponding figure was only 9 percent among non-drug-using patients.

The frequency of involvement of the tricuspid valve may be a function of its proximity to the injection site and its consequent bombardment with injected particulate matter, including talc and cotton. Microscopic examination of uninfected tricuspid valve surfaces in injection drug users reveals pitting and disruption of the smooth endothelial lining—changes that may facilitate the attachment of pathogenic organisms. Left-sided endocarditis may occur with or without right-sided involvement and usually develops in the setting of underlying valvular heart disease.

The various characteristic clinical presentations depend on the site of valvular involvement. In tricuspid valve endocarditis, the predominant picture is one of an abrupt illness with persistent high fever, pulmonary involvement, and an absence of systemic embolic or microvascular phenomena. Approximately 50 percent of patients present with cough and pleuritic chest pain, and some exhibit hemoptysis; these signs and symptoms are the result of multiple septic pulmonary emboli and infarctions. The characteristic murmur of tricuspid regurgitation may be heard in 50 percent of patients: a midsystolic medium-pticxhed murmur at the lower left sternal border that increases in intensity with inspiration.

Characteristically, the chest x-ray shows multiple patchy or nodular infiltrates which progress to cavitation during therapy and eventually resolve. Endocarditis involving the mitral and aortic valves also has an acute onset, with high fever, toxicity, and signs and symptoms resulting from multiple systemic emboli (including arterial emboli and septic infarcts of the skin, liver, spleen, kidneys, and central nervous system). Toxic encephalopathy, focal neurologic abnormalities (the result of mycotic aneurysm or brain abscess), and bacterial meningitis may ensue. Petechiae and splenomegaly occur in approximately 50 percent of patients, and aortic and mitral regurgitant murmurs are reported in almost all cases.

Diagnosis The diagnosis of endocarditis in injection drug users can be problematic, even in the emergency room setting, where most febrile drug users are evaluated and this diagnosis is often suspected. Right-sided endocarditis may be particularly difficult to diagnose because systemic emboli and a regurgitant murmur are usually absent. The diagnosis rests on a composite of clinical, microbiologic, radiologic, and imaging data.

The clinical criteria used include sustained bacteremia involving an organism likely to cause endocarditis and the presence of compatible pulmonary, systemic, or cardiac findings. A clinically useful case definition employed by Marantz et al. divides cases into definite (pathologic confirmation), probable (several positive blood cultures, new regurgitant murmur, or peripheral or pulmonary embolic phenomena), and presumed (several positive blood cultures and no other source found). However, the diagnostic accuracy of emergency room evaluation to predict endocarditis in febrile injection drug users was quite low. Of 87 consecutive febrile injection drug users, 13 percent ultimately met the case definition for definite or probable endocarditis. Only 4 of 12 suspected of having endocarditis in the emergency room proved to have this diagnosis, while 8 of 30 admitted with other diagnoses ultimately proved to have endocarditis. In this series, bacterial pneumonia and minor illnesses were more frequent. The authors conclude that the emergency room diagnostic accuracy is insufficient to distinguish between endocarditis and nonendocarditis and that febrile injection drug users in emergency rooms should be admitted for observation and/or therapy.

Injection drug users may self-medicate with oral antibiotics. Although, unfortunately, this behavior is not always disclosed when the patient's medical history is taken, it may be critically important in the evaluation of patients with suspected endocarditis because blood cultures may be falsely negative. In addition, a large-scale study from Detroit suggested that use of nonprescribed antibiotics before admission to the hospital was an important factor predicting endocarditis due to methicillin-resistant *S. aureus* among drug injectors.

As the above comments indicate, all febrile injection drug users should have a careful history taken, with an emphasis on the frequency and type of drug injection and on antibiotic use. The physical examination should focus attention on the presence of septic emboli in the skin and on mucosal surfaces and of regurgitant murmurs. Chest radiography should be used to detect the characteristic radiologic findings of septic emboli or focal infections that may result in bacteremia. Typically, the radiograph shows multiple patchy or nodular infiltrates that progress to cavitation during therapy and eventually resolve. Ideally, three sets of blood cultures—spaced over several hours, as clinical exigency permits—should be obtained. Gram's staining of peripheral lesions and buffy coat smear of blood may provide a more rapid diagnosis in some cases of bacterial infection. Cardiac imaging studies are a valuable adjunct to diagnosis, although they cannot usually be undertaken at the time of initial presentation and are of variable sensitivity and specificity; false-negative results are frequent in right-sided involvement, and false-positive results also have been documented. Echocardiography may be invaluable in following patients with potentially unstable lesions (i.e., valve incompetence or intramyocardial abscess).

Therapy   After blood cultures are obtained, empirical antibiotic therapy should be instituted if patients are acutely ill, if left-sided endocarditis is highly suspected, and/or if septic pulmonary emboli are seen on radiographs. However, it is not necessary to institute therapy for endocarditis in all injection drug users with fever. In fact, it is often reasonable to withhold antibiotics and to observe the patient carefully until the results of blood cultures are known. Some patients will be found to have a minor transient illness or a pyrogenic or hypersensitivity reaction to injected drugs and will defervesce within 24 h. In others, an alternative diagnosis will become apparent.

Appropriate empirical antibiotic therapy should be given parenterally and should always include an antistaphylococcal agent. Depending on local susceptibility patterns and the severity of the patient's illness, the agent selected is usually either a β-lactam antibiotic, such as oxacillin or nafcillin or—if infection with methicillin-resistant *S. aureus* is suspected—vancomycin. If local patterns warrant, gram-negative coverage with an added aminoglycoside may be appropriate. For endocarditis due to methicillin-susceptible staphylococci, conventional therapy consists of 4 weeks of oxacillin or nafcillin at a dose of 1.5 to 2 g every 4 hours. In severe endocarditis, some clinicians add an aminoglycoside, usually gentamicin (1.5 mg/kg every 8 h) for the first 2 weeks of therapy; this addition may result in more rapid resolution of bacteremia, although an improved outcome has never been shown. In cases of allergy to penicillin or infection with methicillin-resistant *S. aureus*, vancomycin (1 g every 12 h) is given. Therapy targeting other organisms should be selected on the basis of antimicrobial susceptibility patterns. There is no evidence that treatment for 6 weeks instead of 4 weeks improves outcome. A few

studies have reported successful treatment of uncomplicated right-sided endocarditis with a 2-week course of a β-lactam antibiotic plus an aminoglycoside. Given the difficulty of obtaining long-term secure intravenous access, this alternative regimen may prove valuable in selected cases. Its value in HIV-infected injection drug users with endocarditis remains to be determined. Most experts advocate parenteral therapy for the duration of the course, although this decision often necessitates the placement of an indwelling central line.

The prognosis of right-sided staphylococcal endocarditis in this population is excellent, with only rare deaths and infrequent lack of response to medical therapy. Endocarditis caused by other organisms and left-sided involvement carries a more serious prognosis with higher complication and fatality rates. These are largely determined by valve destruction and site and severity of peripheral arterial emboli. The role of surgery remains controversial in this as in other populations with endocarditis (see Chap. 85). The same criteria for surgical intervention should apply: intractable heart failure, undrained myocardial abscess, and failure of medical therapy, particularly in candidal or fungal endocarditis. The surgical approach varies with the cardiac valve(s) involved. Valve excision alone appears to be sufficient for severe tricuspid endocarditis. In mitral and aortic valve endocarditis, valve replacement is required and usually can be accomplished safely. Concerns about subsequent reinfection in the setting of continued injection drug use engender heated debates and require medical, surgical, and patient joint decisions.

PNEUMONIA (See also Chap. 220)   Community-acquired bacterial pneumonia, most often caused by *Streptococcus pneumoniae* and *Haemophilus influenzae*, was commonly described among drug injectors in the 1960s and 1970s. Although population-based epidemiologic data were lacking, these infections were thought to be more frequent among drug users than among the general population. The putative risk factors in drug users included pulmonary aspiration resulting from intermittent overdose, deleterious effects of opiates on lung defenses and cough reflex, hypoventilation due to respiratory depression, and smoking. These factors have all been outweighed by HIV infection, which has dramatically increased the risk of bacterial pneumonia in drug injectors. Beginning in the mid-1980s, epidemiologic surveillance data from New York City showed rising mortality from bacterial pneumonia and other bacterial infections among drug injectors—a phenomenon linked to HIV infection. In some cases, HIV-infected drug users died from pyogenic bacterial infections even before the diagnosis of AIDS. Prospective studies demonstrated that even when they were not actively injecting drugs, HIV-infected drug users had a four- to fivefold greater risk of bacterial pneumonia and sepsis (up to 10 cases per 100 person-years) than their HIV-seronegative counterparts. Among febrile drug users presenting to an emergency room, pneumonia was the single largest diagnostic category, accounting for 38 percent of admissions. The 1993 Revised AIDS Case Definition of the Centers for Disease Control and Prevention includes recurrent bacterial pneumonia in persons with HIV infection as an AIDS-defining condition; the inclusion of this criterion is expected to increase the proportion of AIDS cases reported among injection drug users. The organisms involved in HIV-related pneumonia among drug injectors are predominantly those reported in the earlier literature on community-acquired pneumonia in this group, i.e., *S. pneumoniae* and *H. influenzae*.

The clinical presentation of bacterial pneumonia and the strategies for its diagnosis and therapy are similar in injection drug users and in other populations, despite an expanded array of differential diagnostic possibilities. The typical presentation includes fever, productive cough, pleuritic chest pain, and findings of consolidation and segmental or lobar infiltrate on chest radiography. Specific etiologic diagnosis requires cultures of sputum and/or blood. Therapy aimed at *S. pneumoniae* and/or *H. influenzae*, given parenterally for 10 days to 2 weeks, is recommended, with modifications based on Gram's stain and culture results and on clinical course.

Among other infectious entities to be considered in the differential diagnosis of pulmonary infiltrates in this population of patients are septic pulmonary emboli, tuberculosis, and *Pneumocystis carinii* pneumonia (in patients infected with HIV). Noninfectious pulmonary complications of injection drug use also should be considered. Heroin-induced pulmonary edema, the most common of these complications, occurs most often in drug-use neophytes but also develops in experienced users exposed to particularly potent opiates and results rapidly in death by asphyxiation unless treated promptly with a narcotic antagonist (e.g., naloxone) and respiratory support. Heroin users who relapse and return to drug injection after a period of abstinence appear to be at especially high risk for the complication. Other noninfectious pulmonary complications of drug injection include (1) pulmonary vascular or talc granulomatosis, which develops in fewer than 5 percent of injectors and is caused by repeated intravenous injection of crushed oral medications or by injection of cotton or other particulate material that may contaminate injected drugs (a syndrome characterized by a diffuse reticulonodular pattern on chest radiography and often by disabling symptoms of pulmonary hypertension), (2) bullous disease, which often involves the peripheral upper lobe areas and which is of uncertain etiology but may be another complication of particulate matter injection, (3) reactive airway disease, which may be exacerbated by heroin use or by "crack" cocaine inhalation, and (4) mechanical complications, such as pneumothorax resulting from attempted venous injection into the deep veins of the neck ("pocket shot") or (as has been described more recently in cocaine smokers) pulmonary barotrauma with pneumothorax or pneumomediastinum resulting from intense Valsalva's or other maneuvers used in the inhalation of drugs.

Finally, the virtual universality of heavy cigarette smoking among drug injectors may not only predispose them to the usual sequelae of this behavior but also complicate the differential diagnosis of pulmonary symptoms (e.g., cough, shortness of breath, sputum production).

TUBERCULOSIS (See also Chap. 130)   The other important pulmonary infection described in drug injectors is tuberculosis. Infections due to *M. tuberculosis* were well documented in drug users before the AIDS epidemic, accounting for greater morbidity and mortality in this population than in the non-drug-using population. Although some authors attributed this greater impact to poverty, poor housing, and the social and demographic factors associated with both drug use and tuberculosis, others found an elevated risk of tuberculosis among drug users even after attempting to control for these other factors. AIDS has now overwhelmed all other potential risk factors and has resulted in a new epidemic of resurgent tuberculosis among HIV-infected drug users and their contacts (see Chaps. 130 and 279). Among persons with HIV infection, tuberculosis has disproportionately affected injection drug users. This observation may reflect higher levels of latent infection with *M. tuberculosis* in drug-using populations, associated environmental factors, or a combination of factors. In parts of the urban northeastern United States, where 20 percent of drug injectors have evidence of latent *M. tuberculosis* infection and 40 percent are infected with HIV, the overlap of these two endemic infections has resulted in an unprecedented increase in the incidence of tuberculosis since 1985. This finding highlights the importance of aggressive chemoprophylaxis with isoniazid in this population.

Pulmonary tuberculosis should always be suspected and included in the differential diagnosis in injection drug users with pneumonia. Particularly among those with HIV infection, extrapulmonary tuberculosis has greatly increased in frequency. The therapy administered to injection drug users is similar to that given to other populations, but special efforts must be made to ensure long-term adherence to the regimen.

SKELETAL INFECTIONS (See Chap. 92)   Skeletal infections in injection drug users result both from hematogenous dissemination and, less commonly, from contiguous spread from chronically infected skin and soft tissue sites to underlying bone. In one series, skeletal infections represented 9 percent of admissions of injection drug users to a large urban hospital. Septic arthritis of large synovial joints may be seen during the course of staphylococcal endocarditis or of

bacteremia arising from other infected sites and may appear as a complication of disseminated gonococcal disease. The joints most frequently involved are the knees, hips, shoulders, and elbows, but there is predilection for involvement of unusual joints as well—e.g., the vertebral column, the symphysis pubis, and the sternoclavicular, sternochondral, and sacroiliac joints. These infections are usually unilateral and subacute, with an indolent, progressive course characterized by pain, limitation of motion, and absence of fever. The diagnosis may be easily missed or overlooked. Point tenderness over the affected joint is usually elicited. Sternoarticular infections are often associated with soft tissue swelling of the chest wall and bacteremia. Vertebral osteomyelitis may be associated with paraspinal soft tissue masses and (in cases of posterior extension) with the formation of spinal epidural abscesses. Radiologic and imaging studies may suggest the diagnosis by findings which are most characteristic of vertebral osteomyelitis, where the disk space is lost, contiguous bone erosion and new bone formation are evident, and several vertebrae are involved. Infection of the sacroiliac joints and symphysis pubis results in joint space separation and erosion of the articular surfaces.

S. aureus is the pathogen most commonly isolated from sites of skeletal infection, but gram-negative organisms—notably *P. aeruginosa*, *Serratia marcescens*, and fungi—also have been well documented. *M. tuberculosis* should be included in the differential diagnosis, particularly in cases of vertebral osteomyelitis. Because etiologic agents and their antimicrobial susceptibilities vary, efforts should be made to obtain a specific microbiologic diagnosis. This process may involve diagnostic aspiration or closed or open biopsy, with fluid or material sent for staining and culture for bacterial, mycobacterial, and fungal pathogens.

Treatment consists of a combination of drainage of the synovial joints and the contiguous soft tissue collections and prolonged administration of appropriate antimicrobial agents.

CENTRAL NERVOUS SYSTEM COMPLICATIONS   The nervous system, especially the CNS, is another important site for adverse sequelae of drug injection. Drug injectors are at increased risk for certain noninfectious complications, including intracerebral hemorrhage and other stroke syndromes (especially in cocaine and amphetamine users), particulate emboli to the brain and spinal cord, vasculitis, and the consequences of head trauma. Among the infectious complications, the most common is systemic embolization to the brain as a result of bacterial endocarditis or bacteremia, which frequently involves multiple small septic emboli, from either aortic or mitral valve vegetations or, even more commonly given the more frequent occurrence of right-sided endocarditis in drug users, from pulmonary arteriovenous shunting or bacteremic seeding of the meninges and brain. Patients may present with focal neurologic deficits, seizures, altered mental status, and/or meningismus. *S. aureus* and other bacteria that cause endocarditis in drug injectors are most commonly involved in these manifestations. Cerebral mycotic aneurysms and spinal and epidural abscesses also have been described as complications of endocarditis in this population. Less commonly, drug users have been reported to be at risk for focal brain abscesses, not related to endocarditis, caused by organisms such as *Aspergillus*, *Mucor*, other fungi, and *Nocardia*. There is also evidence that tuberculous meningitis and focal tuberculomas of the brain may be more common in drug users than in other patients with tuberculosis, with and without HIV infection. Finally, ocular infections, including episcleritis, chorioretinitis, and endophthalmitis have been well described in drug injectors, involving such organisms as *B. cereus*, *Aspergillus*, and *C. albicans* (the last often in conjunction with the syndrome of systemic candidiasis, described in several populations of European drug injectors in the early 1980s, associated with "brown" heroin and the use of lemon juice as a medium for dissolving the drug).

HEPATITIS (See also Chaps. 266 and 267)   Injection drug users have long been known to be at high risk for hepatitis, primarily through parenteral transmission of bloodborne infectious agents. The incidence of hepatitis B has risen over the past decade in the United States, and the proportion of all cases occurring among injection drug users has increased from 15 percent to close to 30 percent since the mid-1980s. The acquisition of hepatitis B is a relatively early event for most drug injectors, occurring within the first several years of illicit drug use. Since the 1970s, seroprevalence studies in a wide range of drug-using populations have indicated that 75 to 90 percent of long-term drug injectors have serologic evidence of past exposure to hepatitis B. Approximately 5 to 10 percent of these individuals will remain chronic carriers of hepatitis B surface antigen; the remainder will develop immunity to hepatitis, producing antibody to hepatitis B core antigen and/or that to hepatitis B surface antigen. While most hepatitis B–infected drug users do not progress to chronic forms of clinically significant hepatitis or cirrhosis, at least 40 percent of most series of entrants in drug-treatment programs exhibit abnormalities of liver function. In addition to infectious causes, the toxic effects of adulterants used in the production of illicit drugs and the hepatotoxic effects of alcohol are responsible in part for these abnormalities. Indeed, while chronic active and chronic persistent hepatitis have been linked to infection with hepatitis B virus and ongoing injection of illicit drugs, hepatic cirrhosis in drug users is most often associated with coexisting alcohol abuse.

Another infectious agent commonly found in drug injectors is hepatitis D virus, previously referred to as the *delta agent*. This defective hepatotropic RNA virus depends on coexisting infection with hepatitis B virus for expression and replication. First detected in Italy in the mid-1970s, hepatitis D virus has since been documented in numerous seroprevalence studies among drug users in the United States, Europe, and Southeast Asia. In most such surveys, antibody to hepatitis D virus has been found in 10 to 15 percent of patients with antibody to hepatitis B surface or core antigen and in as many as 50 to 70 percent of patients with chronic carriage of hepatitis B surface antigen. Fulminant hepatitis B may show a characteristic biphasic pattern in the setting of hepatitis D coinfection. Moreover, hepatitis D has been associated among drug users with chronic active hepatitis and persistent abnormalities of liver function. Among persons with hepatitis B in the United States, coexisting hepatitis D infection has shown a greater predilection for injection drug users and hemophiliacs than for homosexual men; thus the parenteral route may be important in the transmission of hepatitis D virus.

The third significant bloodborne agent of hepatitis in injection drug users is hepatitis C virus. This virus, which has been identified in recent years as the cause of a large proportion of cases of what had previously been termed non-A, non-B hepatitis, is highly prevalent in many different populations of drug users. In seroprevalence studies in the United States and Europe, antibody to hepatitis C virus has been detected in up to 70 percent of drug injectors—a rate reflecting a level of infection comparable with that for hepatitis B. Like hepatitis B, hepatitis C appears to be acquired relatively soon after the start of illicit drug injection. While hepatitis C has been associated with chronic active hepatitis, persistent abnormalities of liver function, and cirrhosis, further studies must fully elucidate the natural history of this infection in drug users. Preliminary data suggest that interferon-α may be of benefit in patients with progressive hepatitis B or hepatitis C. This treatment has not yet been widely administered to drug users, however, and its requisite duration is unknown. Preliminiary follow-up studies suggest that disease quickly recrudesces after cessation of therapy.

Although not considered to be a bloodborne infection, hepatitis A has been associated with injection drug use. In 1970, 60 percent of more than 1000 entrants in a drug-treatment program at the Federal Addiction Treatment Center in Lexington, Kentucky, showed serologic evidence of exposure to hepatitis A. While the high rate of seropositivity in this study cannot be compared with the background rate in the general population at the time, several surveillance-based investigations since then have indicated that injection drug users may have up to a 50-fold higher risk of acquiring hepatitis A than non-injection drug users. In addition, recent outbreaks of hepatitis A have been linked to groups of injection drug users in both the United States and Europe. While the exact mechanism of spread has not been

determined, investigation of these outbreaks has suggested that fecal-oral contamination, close personal contact, and poor hygiene are the most likely factors; viral contamination of drugs or injection equipment was considered less likely but could not be ruled out.

These observations suggest that in long-term drug injectors with known past exposure to hepatitis B and/or hepatitis C, hepatitis A (and—for chronic carriers of hepatitis B—hepatitis D) should be strongly considered in the differential diagnosis of new-onset acute hepatitis syndromes. The acquisition of bloodborne hepatitis soon after the start of illicit injection drug use suggests the importance of developing public health strategies for reaching adolescent and young-adult drug users with information about preventive interventions (such as hepatitis B vaccine) and risk-reducing behaviors.

HTLV-I/II   Injection drug users are at relatively high risk not only for infection with HIV but also for that with human T lymphotropic retrovirus types I and II (see Chap. 151). In the United States, injection drug use has been the most important behavioral factor associated with the presence of antibody to HTLV-I/II in blood donors screened for retroviral infection. Seroprevalence studies in the United States have documented HTLV-I/II infection in more than 10 percent of certain populations of drug users; in some areas the rate of HTLV infection has exceeded that of HIV infection. HTLV infection has often been associated with black race, older age, and a history of heroin injection. Rates of infection have shown wide geographic variation. Molecular genetic techniques have recently indicated that more than three-fourths of the HTLV infections in drug injectors are due to HTLV-II; this observation may account for the relatively low rate of clinical disease reported to date in patients with such infections. Two studies have suggested, however, that coinfection with HTLV-I/II and HIV may be associated with more rapid progression of HIV infection and early mortality; if corroborated, this observation might make serologic testing for HTLV-I/II an important prognostic tool for HIV-infected drug users.

HARM REDUCTION FOR INJECTION DRUG USERS

The myriad infectious consequences of injection drug use mandate the development of preventive harm-reduction strategies which are based on the underlying principle that if people are going to inject drugs, they should do so in a way that minimizes harm to themselves and others. Prevention of the infectious complications of injection and education about more hygienic injection practices are primary goals. Needle- and syringe-exchange programs are the most obvious example of the harm-reduction approach. In addition to the distribution or exchange of injection equipment, these programs typically include AIDS education, condom distribution, and enrollment in a variety of medical and social services.

Provision of primary medical care services linked to drug-abuse treatment is a way to promote preventive regimens to enhance harm reduction. In this and all other clinical settings, injection drug users should be routinely screened for hepatitis B, latent *M. tuberculosis* infection, and syphilis and other sexually transmitted diseases. They should be offered pneumococcal, influenza, tetanus, and hepatitis B immunization and (when appropriate) prophylaxis for tuberculosis and complications of HIV disease.

Clearly, the ultimate goal of harm-reduction strategies should be the reduction or prevention of illicit drug use itself. A high priority must be assigned to the development of strategies that will minimize the serious medical consequences of drug abuse as well as to those that will eliminate drug abuse and its root causes.

REFERENCES

CHAMBERS HF et al: *Staphylococcus aureus* endocarditis: Clinical manifestations in addicts and non-addicts. Medicine 62:170, 1983

——— et al: Right-sided *Staphylococcus aureus* endocarditis in intravenous drug users: Two-week combination therapy. Ann Intern Med 109:619, 1988

CHANDRASEKAR PH, NARULA AP: Bone and joint infections in intravenous drug abusers. Rev Infect Dis 8:904, 1986

DONAHUE JG et al: Antibody to hepatitis C virus among cardiac surgery patients, homosexual men and intravenous drug users in Baltimore, Maryland. Am J Epidemiol 134:1206, 1991

FELTON CP: Pulmonary infections in the addict, in *Medical Aspects of Drug Abuse*, RW Richter (ed). Hagerstown, MD, Harper & Row, 1975

HAVERKOS HW, LANGE WR: Serious infections other than human immunodeficiency virus among intravenous drug users. J Infect Dis 161:894, 1990

HIND CRK: Pulmonary complications of intravenous drug users: I. Epidemiology and noninfective complications. Thorax 45:891, 1990; II. Infective and HIV-related complications. Thorax 45:957, 1990

KHABBAZ RA et al: Seroprevalence of HTLV-I and HTLV-II among intravenous drug users and persons in clinics for sexually transmitted diseases. N Engl J Med 326:375, 1992

LANGE WR et al: The Lexington addicts, 1971–72: Demographic characteristics, drug use patterns, and selected infectious disease experience. Int J Addict 24:609, 1989

LETTAU LA et al: Outbreak of severe hepatitis due to delta and hepatitis B viruses in parenteral drug abusers and their contacts. N Engl J Med 317:1256, 1987

LEVINE DP, SOBEL JD (eds): *Infections in Intravenous Drug Abusers*. New York, Oxford University Press, 1991

MARANTZ PR et al: Inability to predict diagnosis in febrile intravenous drug abusers. Ann Intern Med 106:823, 1987

NOVICK DM et al: Hepatitis D virus antibody in HBsAg-positive and HBsAg-negative substance abusers with chronic liver disease. J Med Virol 15:351, 1985

SANDE MA et al: Endocarditis in intravenous drug users, in *Infective Endocarditis*, 2d ed, D Kaye (ed). New York, Raven, 1992, pp 345–359

SELWYN PA et al: Clinical manifestations and predictors of disease progression in drug users with human immunodeficiency virus infection. N Engl J Med 327:1697, 1992

SHEAGREN JN: Endocarditis complicating parenteral drug abuse, in *Current Clinical Topics in Infectious Diseases*, 2d ed, JS Remington, MN Schwartz (eds). New York, McGraw-Hill, 1981, pp 211–233

STIMSON GV: Editorial review: Syringe exchange programs for injection drug users. AIDS 3:253, 1989

STONEBURNER RL et al: A larger spectrum of severe HIV-1 related disease in intravenous drug users in New York City. Science 242:916, 1988

VON HAASTRECHT HJA et al: The course of the HIV epidemic in Amsterdam, The Netherlands. Am J Public Health 81:59, 1991

95 INFECTIONS FROM BITES AND SCRATCHES, BURNS, AND ENVIRONMENTAL ORGANISMS

JAMES L. BREELING / LOUIS WEINSTEIN

ANIMAL BITES AND SCRATCHES

Infections following animal bites are caused by deep inoculation of bacteria into the skin or soft tissues. Early culture of the wound often discloses small numbers of organisms representative of a particular animal's oral flora; many bites never become overtly infected. Patients with infected wounds usually present 12 to 24 h after the injury with inflammation caused by invasion by common organisms.

EPIDEMIOLOGY Most domestic animal bites are inflicted by pets. There are more than 100 million dogs and cats in the United States. Dogs inflict 80 to 90 percent of the bites and cats about 6 percent. (Other animals that inflict bites are monkeys, rodents, livestock, and reptiles.) However, 20 to 50 percent of the bites by cats and about 5 percent by dogs become infected. Most of the 2 to 4 million bite wounds each year result in minor injury: 10 percent may require suturing, and an estimated 1 to 2 percent require hospitalization. Children are bitten more often than adults. Occupational groups at high risk include animal breeders, veterinary surgeons, zookeepers, wild animal trainers, laboratory workers, and postal carriers. The hands and arms are the most common sites of bites. Wounds of the hands tend to become infected most often. Because of the structure of the hand and the ease with which infection spreads along tissue planes, every bite on the hand must be considered potentially serious.

ETIOLOGY The oropharynx of an animal is the most important source of organisms involved in infections following a bite. However, the microflora of the skin, soil, and excreta also may be involved in the development of infection. The average dog or cat harbors a wide range of pathogens, such as *Pasteurella, Staphylococcus aureus*, streptococci, and mixed oral anaerobic organisms. The oral microfloras of other animal species have been less well studied. Infections caused by *Actinobacillus* may occur following bites by horses or sheep. Bites by dolphins may lead to infection by halophilic and waterborne organisms such as *Mycobacterium marinum*. An unidentified agent that responds to tetracycline is responsible for infection following a bite by a seal ("seal finger"). Bites by monkeys may lead to the development of fatal encephalomyelitis caused by herpesvirus simiae. Leptospirosis, brucellosis, and tularemia have been attributed to animal bites, although documentation of actual transmission has been scanty. Rabies is transmitted by the bite of some animals (see Chap. 158).

Bites by animals may lead to damage of soft tissues and loss of skin, acute cellulitis, chronic localized infection of deep tissues (septic arthritis, osteomyelitis), or septicemia with or without disseminated intravascular coagulation.

SPECIFIC ORGANISMS Pasteurella multocida *P. multocida* is a small gram-negative coccobacillus present in the naso-oropharynx and gastrointestinal tract of mammals and birds. Cats have the highest carriage rate (70 to 90 percent), but dogs, great cats (lions and tigers), swine, sheep, cattle, rabbits, and rats may harbor the organism. The most common human infection is cellulitis surrounding the wound, but localized abscess, osteomyelitis, septic arthritis, peritonitis, mycotic aneurysm, meningitis, acute epiglottis, pneumonia, and chorioamnionitis may occur. *P. multocida* infections may follow nonbite exposure to animals, including scratches and respiratory spread of droplets from carrier animals to the respiratory tract of patients with chronic pulmonary disease. Patients with cirrhosis who come into contact with animal saliva are at risk of developing primary bacteremia.

Pasteurella infections following animal bites are characterized by the rapid development in <24 h of intense inflammation and purulent drainage. Because bites are often small but penetrate deeply, the possibility of septic arthritis, tendon sheath involvement, or osteomyelitis is great, even when the puncture wounds are trivial.

The preferred oral treatment of wounds infected by *Pasteurella* is penicillin VK (500 mg orally every 6 h) or, in the penicillin-allergic patient, tetracycline (500 mg orally every 6 h). Erythromycin, cephalosporins, clindamycin, and dicloxacillin are ineffective and should not be used.

Capnocytophaga canimorsus (CDC group DF-2) Formerly an unclassified microorganism (CDC group DF-2 for dysgonic fermenter), *C. canimorsus* is a gram-negative rod associated with septicemia following dog bites, particularly in immunocompromised alcoholics or splenectomized subjects (see Chap. 112).

Fever is the most common presenting symptom. The illness is usually mild in patients with an intact spleen, but systemic meningitis and endocarditis can cause an overall mortality rate approaching 30 percent. In splenectomized patients, disseminated intravascular coagulation (DIC), gangrene of the extremities, adrenal hemorrhage, hemorrhagic pulmonary edema, and fulminant sepsis may occur. The organism can be seen on microscopic examination of the buffy coat (with use of Wright's or Gram's stain) in splenectomized patients. *Capnocytophaga* is generally sensitive to penicillin, tetracycline, clindamycin, and erythromycin.

CLINICAL MANIFESTATIONS The likelihood of infection depends on the location and nature of the wound. Signs of infection almost always appear 1 to 3 days after injury; disease produced by *Pasteurella* usually presents in 12 to 24 h. Redness, swelling, and tenderness are accompanied by drainage that may be scant or purulent. Localization of infection in the hand usually occurs, but the process can spread through the tendon sheath to distant sites. In patients with systemic signs and symptoms out of proportion to the degree of local injury, sepsis with *Pasteurella* or *Capnocytophaga* should be suspected. Persistence of local inflammation after treatment of an infected wound warrants a search for deeper infection in joints, bones, or subcutaneous spaces.

DIAGNOSIS AND TREATMENT After infection is established, Gram's stain and culture of a wound swab or exudate may be helpful in the evaluation of its etiology. However, interpretation of the frequently complex results of early culture (within 8 h of injury) may be misleading. Thorough cleansing of the lesion (high-pressure irrigation and careful debridement) followed by closure in low-risk injuries (e.g., dog bites, bites not involving the hand) is often sufficient for healing. For wounds first seen 24 h after injury and those clearly infected at presentation, specimens for culture should be labeled as "bite wound" to alert the microbiology laboratory to the possibility of anaerobes and unusual organisms. Primary closure of older wounds is rarely advisable; provision should be made for observation of such wounds over the next few days. Prophylaxis for tetanus (see Chap. 106) and rabies (see Chap. 158) and administration of antimicrobial prophylaxis should be considered (1) at the time of debridement and/or closure of wounds seen later than 24 h after injury, (2) for puncture wounds from cats, (3) for deep wounds (especially of the hand) involving tendons or bone, and (4) for facial wounds. In addition, splenectomized patients with dog bites are at extra risk of *C. canimorsus* sepsis and should receive penicillin prophylaxis. *Pasteurella* spp. are generally sensitive to penicillin, but most *S. aureus* strains require penicillinase-resistant penicillins. Treatment with penicillin VK and dicloxacillin, cephalexin, or amoxicillin/clavulanic acid offers coverage for most potential pathogens. Established wound infections are usually treated for 10 to 14 days. Prophylaxis for apparently noninfected but high-risk wounds should be given for 3 to 5 days. Tetracycline offers some degree of coverage for the penicillin-allergic patient. Erythromycin may be considered in the pregnant woman or the child with severe allergy. Response to treatment should be monitored carefully; surgical intervention and parenteral antibiotics may be required.

RAT-BITE FEVER Fever and arthralgias following a rat bite may be caused by two microorganisms: *Streptobacillus moniliformis* and *Spirillum minus*. Infection becomes manifest after the wound heals, distinguishing rat-bite fever from the animal bites described above.

Both *S. moniliformis* and *S. minus* normally reside in the rodent oral cavity. Rat-bite fever may be transmitted by rats, laboratory animals, and domestic and wild rodents. Also, outbreaks of rat-bite fever have been associated with the ingestion of contaminated milk or drinking water (Haverhill fever).

S. moniliformis is a pleomorphic gram-negative rod. The incubation period is usually 3 to 10 days, sufficient time for the original rodent bite wound to heal. High-grade fever, rigors, headache, vomiting, and myalgias followed by regional lymphadenopathy, arthralgias, and arthritis constitute the clinical syndrome. A maculopapular rash on the palms and soles may progress to petechial hemorrhages. If the patient is not treated, fever persists, and the patient may die.

S. minus is a spirochete that causes febrile illness approximately 1 to 3 weeks after a bite. A healed initial wound may break down at the onset of systemic illness. High-grade fever, rigors, and myalgias develop, but joint involvement is rare. Unlike streptobacillary rat-bite fever, there is no rash. Transmission by contaminated food or water has not been reported, but other spirochetes present in animals (*Leptospira* spp. and *Anaerobiospirillum succiniciproducens*) may be transmitted in this fashion. Spirillar rat-bite fever is more common in Asia than in the United States and should be considered in travelers from Asia who develop cryptic fever.

The diagnosis of streptobacillary rat-bite fever is established by culture of the organism from blood or infected tissues, which may require the use of special media. The diagnosis of spirillar rat-bite fever is made only by dark-field examination of blood, examination of infected tissues, or animal inoculation. *S. minor* infection may cause the serologic test for syphilis to be falsely positive.

Treatment of either form of rat-bite fever with procaine penicillin G (600,000 units IM twice daily for 14 days) is curative. Alternative therapy for penicillin-allergic patients is tetracycline (500 mg orally four times daily for 14 days).

CAT-SCRATCH DISEASE **Definition and etiology** Tender regional lymphadenopathy persisting for 3 weeks or longer, frequently preceded by a primary skin lesion after contact with cats, has been called *benign inoculation lymphoreticulosis*, *nonbacterial regional lymphadenitis*, *cat-scratch fever*, and *cat-scratch disease*. Cat-scratch disease appears to be caused primarily by *Rochalimaea hensleae*, a small, pleomorphic gram-negative bacillus that has been identified in the excised lymph nodes of patients (see Chap. 124). Another organism, *Afipia felis*, appears to be responsible for some cases. *A. felis* belongs to the alpha-1 subgroup of the class Proteobacteria. This class contains other pathogens such as *Bartonella* and *Brucella*. Cats acquire the organism from the soil and carry it orally and/or on their paws. Inoculation of a human occurs with a scratch or bite.

Epidemiology Cat-scratch disease occurs throughout the world and most often in children. Exposure to an immature cat is the most common means of transmission, although older cats and dogs may transmit the disease. Scratches are the most common mode of infection, but transmission may occur by licks, bites, and handling of objects with which a cat has recently made contact or by inoculation of organisms into mucous membranes (e.g., conjunctivae). Organisms are usually introduced into the skin and multiply at the local site. Most cases occur from July to October.

Clinical manifestations Three to five days after a bite, scratch, or lick by a cat, the patient may develop a papule that progresses to a pustule which crusts over. Within 1 to 2 weeks, tender regional lymphadenopathy develops. Since the hands are most often involved, epitrochlear, axillary, pectoral, and cervical lymph node involvement is common. There does not appear to be lymphangitis from the site of primary inoculation to the enlarged regional lymph nodes. Mild generalized aching, malaise, and/or anorexia is rarely accompanied by fever unless secondary bacterial infection produces suppuration of the lymph node. Conjunctival inoculation may lead to Parinaud's oculoglandular syndrome with conjunctivitis and preauricular lymphadenopathy. The lymphadenopathy usually persists for 3 to 6 weeks but may be protracted. Other manifestations not limited to immunocompromised hosts include encephalitis, meningitis, transverse myelitis, granulomatous hepatitis, osteomyelitis, and disseminated infection. In patients with AIDS, two additional manifestations, bacillary (epithelioid) angiomatosis and bacillary peliosis hepatis, have been described and appear also to be related to *R. hensleae* (see Chap. 124).

Diagnosis Cat-scratch disease should be suspected if the patient has lymphadenopathy, exposure to a cat, and a skin lesion at the site of inoculation. Other causes of regional or generalized lymphadenopathy should be excluded (see Chap. 58). The diagnosis may be confirmed by pathologic examination of the involved nodes. Concern about transmission of viral illness has lessened the utility of a skin test with cat-scratch antigen because the antigen is prepared from material aspirated from human lymph nodes. Typical pathology includes granulomas, central necrosis of the germinal centers, and infiltration by neutrophils.

Treatment Cat-scratch disease is generally benign and self-limited and does not require treatment with antibiotics for resolution. Antipyretics and analgesics may be used as needed. Immunocompromised patients and those with severe or long-lasting illness have been treated with a variety of agents, including aminoglycosides, erythromycin, doxycycline, and ciprofloxacin. Since no comparative antibiotic trials have been carried out, firm recommendations for therapy cannot be made at this time.

HUMAN BITE INFECTIONS

Human bites may occur in adults during fights or child abuse, in hospital personnel bitten while caring for patients, in partners during sexual play, and in persons sustaining "clenched fist" injuries involving the metacarpophalangeal joint.

ETIOLOGY Human bites (occlusional and clenched-fist) are thought to be more prone to infection than animal bites because the human oropharyngeal flora contains a large number of species of microorganisms, including anaerobic bacteria (see Chap. 128). Anaerobes are present in 39 percent of animal bites, in 50 percent of human bites, and in 56 percent of clenched-fist injuries. Anaerobes, including the oral *Bacteroides* spp. (now called *Prevotella* and *Porphyromonas*), and aerobic organisms, such as *S. aureus, Eikenella corrodens,* and non-beta-hemolytic streptococci, are commonly involved.

Clenched-fist injuries inflicted by humans have a worse prognosis than other bites, perhaps because the injury occurs with the fingers flexed, and when the fingers are extended, bacteria are sealed beneath the skin. Infection of clenched-fist injuries also may appear to be more common because many patients report the injury only after infection has developed, usually 24 or 48 h later. The rates of infection following human bites of the face or lip are much lower, possibly because patients with these injuries are likely to seek more immediate medical attention.

CLINICAL MANIFESTATIONS Clenched-fist injuries are produced by piercing of the thin skin over the flexed metacarpophalangeal joint, the teeth often penetrating the joint. There is often delayed development of pain and a proximally spreading swelling of the hand, with or without discharge. Suppurative arthritis, ankylosis, and osteomyelitis may develop. Radiographs must be examined for the presence of foreign bodies, fractures, or air in the joints. Plain films may show early osteomyelitis.

Occlusional bites on any body surface may lead to the development of cellulitis, tenosynovitis, osteomyelitis, or septic arthritis. In addition to organisms of the normal oral flora that cause infection, hepatitis B, syphillis, and tuberculosis have been transmitted by human bite.

TREATMENT Clenched-fist injuries must be treated aggressively. Patients presenting more than 24 h after injury or those with obviously infected wounds should be considered for admission, surgical exploration, irrigation, and parenteral antibiotic therapy. Aerobic and anaerobic cultures are required. Empirical antimicrobial therapy must be effective against *Bacteroides, S. aureus,* and *E. corrodens.* Organisms expressing β-lactamases *(Bacteroides, S. aureus)* and pathogens usually resistant to clindamycin but sensitive to penicillin *(Eikenella)* make monotherapy difficult. Among the drugs thought to provide adequate coverage are clindamycin, amoxicillin and clavulanic acid in combination and cefoxitin or cefotetan alone. The duration of therapy is usually 10 to 14 days when the infection appears to be responding. When osteomyelitis is present, antibiotics should be given intravenously for 4 to 6 weeks. Some patients require a second surgical debridement and may suffer residual disability.

Although HIV-1 may be present in saliva, human bites have not been documented to transmit the virus. The issue of counseling victims of human bites to be tested for HIV is unclear, but testing is probably advisable.

BURN-WOUND INFECTION

Each year 130,000 persons in the United States are hospitalized for thermal burns. About 70,000 require intensive care. Infection is the major cause of death in nearly 10,000 patients. Thermal burns to the skin are often complicated by smoke injury to the lungs.

ETIOLOGY During the first or second week after thermal injury, host immunity becomes depressed: concentrations of immunoglobulins, complement, and fibronectin fall; clearance of particulates by the reticuloendothelial system is impeded; phagocytic function is depressed and there is a decline in cell-mediated immunity, as evidenced by the impairment of cutaneous hypersensitivity, rejection of skin allografts, decreased activity of natural killer cells, lessened

mitogen responses, and decreased numbers of helper T cells. Suppressor T cells become activated. The magnitude of burn-induced changes in humoral and cellular immunity is related to the extent of the burn. The relation between the magnitude of injury and the risk of infection is linear. Mortality due to infection increases when burns cover more than 40 percent of the body surface area.

The combination of destruction of the skin barrier to bacteria and immunodeficiency permits colonizing bacteria to multiply and invade adjacent viable tissue or even to enter the systemic circulation (burn-wound sepsis). Thermal injury, hypermetabolism, and the catabolic state caused by a burn and endotoxemia from infected wounds also appear to promote "translocation" of intestinal bacteria into the portal and systemic circulations by causing a breakdown in the mucosal barriers and immune defenses of the normal gut. Intensive resuscitation and surgical intervention, including intubation and mechanical ventilation (especially in patients with adult respiratory distress syndrome or smoke inhalation), predispose to pneumonia, the third major route of systemic infection in burn patients.

CLINICAL MANIFESTATIONS Burned skin is initially free of major bacterial contamination. However, because of the exudation of body fluid, necrosis of tissues, and contamination from environmental sources, the surface area of the burn wound rapidly becomes colonized with the microbial flora of the hospital unit. Early use of topical antimicrobial agents (sodium mafenide, silver sulfadiazine, nystatin) serves to delay but not prevent infection of a burn wound. If bacterial counts reach a level of 10^5 organisms per gram of tissue, invasion of viable subcutaneous tissue with bloodstream dissemination is likely. Gram-negative, gram-positive, fungal, and even viral (herpes simplex) pathogens may cause sepsis. Suppurative thrombophlebitis and suppurative chondritis may develop.

DIAGNOSIS Quantitative bacterial cultures of biopsy specimens of a burn wound at 48-h intervals provide adequate monitoring of the wound. High densities of organisms in the area of a burn increase the risk of sepsis and interfere with the ability of skin allografts to "take," thus delaying closure of open areas.

TREATMENT Current surgical approaches to early excision of a wound and closure with autografts or skin substitutes within the first week of a burn have improved survival. Removal of the necrotic eschar appears to reverse many of the immunologic defects that occur. Debridement also promotes drainage of seromas and hematomas and improves the delivery of host resistance factors and antibiotics to the sites of injury and inflammation. Topical and appropriate systemic antimicrobial therapy and early enteral nutrition also improve survival. Selective decontamination of the intestine with antibacterial and antifungal agents may be helpful.

Systemic antimicrobial therapy must be directed toward the microorganism responsible for clinical sepsis. Since no single agent or combination of agents destroys all organisms, and because multidrug therapy may promote development of resistance, parsimonious use of antibiotics administered long enough to reverse sepsis but not long enough to permit secondary infection must be the rule.

MISCELLANEOUS ENVIRONMENTAL ORGANISMS

AEROMONAS HYDROPHILA *A. hydrophila,* a gram-negative, facultative anaerobe of the family Vibrionaceae, may cause a variety of infections in persons who have had contact with flowing or stagnant fresh water, aquaria, tap water, or freshwater fish. If ingested, *A. hydrophila* may cause gastroenteritis. When inoculated into the skin via puncture or contamination of simple wounds, it may cause rapid-onset cellulitis and even septicemia in immunocompromised or cirrhotic individuals. The skin is characteristically necrotic; formation of bullae is common. Involvement of muscle may occur early, especially in cases of wounds contaminated by water. Metastatic complications include osteomyelitis, peritonitis, meningitis, and endocarditis. Inoculation into the eye may cause conjunctivitis. A closely related species, *Plesiomonas shigelloides,* may produce rapid-onset wound infections and sepsis after marine contact. Antibiotic sensitivity patterns suggest the use of trimethoprim-sulfamethoxazole, aminoglycosides, quinolones, or third-generation cephalosporins.

PSEUDOMONAS   Many species of *Pseudomonas*, including *P. aeruginosa,* are present in fresh and salt water and may cause cutaneous infection via inoculation (see Chap. 116). *Pseudomonas* folliculitis is associated with contaminated heated indoor whirlpool hot tubs, and saunas. It is treated with topical agents such as chlorhexidine and povidone-iodine; antibiotics are reserved for patients with cellulitis. Otitis externa, "swimmer's ear," is produced by *Pseudomonas* as well as other aquatic species in individuals with exposure to pools for long periods of time during the summer months. Puncture wounds of the foot by nails may lead to the development of osteomyelitis, septic arthritis, and infection of soft tissues by soil or aquatic microorganisms. The risk is especially high for infection by *Pseudomonas,* perhaps because the organism can survive and proliferate in the moist, humid environment of the inside of a shoe. Treatment usually involves surgical debridement and long courses of antipseudomonal agents.

ERYSIPELOID (ERYSIPELOTHRIX RHUSIOPATHIAE)   *E. rhusiopathiae* is a small, slender, gram-positive rod found in many mammals, birds, and fish. Human infection follows a scratch or a puncture of the skin, usually the fingers, while handling fish, shellfish, or organic matter containing the organism. The infection is an occupational hazard for fish handlers, farmers, and veterinarians. A purplish, painful pruritic area appears at the site of inoculation after 1 to 4 days and is followed by a slowly spreading erythematous rash, pruritic vesicles, and papules. Fever and regional lymphadenopathy are uncommon. Rare cases of disseminated infection or endocarditis have been reported. The disease may be self-limited and run a course of several weeks. Erysipeloid responds to treatment with penicillin or erythromycin. Persons at risk of inoculation are advised to wear puncture-proof gloves and wash their hands frequently.

REFERENCES

BRENNER DJ et al: Proposal of *Afipia* gen. nov., with *Afipia felis* sp. nov. (formerly the cat scratch disease bacillus), *Afipia clevelandensis* sp. nov. (formerly the Cleveland Clinic Foundation strain), *Afipia broomeae* sp. nov., and three unnamed genospecies. J Clin Microbiol 29:2450, 1991

GOLDSTEIN EJC: Bite wounds and infection. Clin Infect Dis 14:633, 1992

────── et al: Role of anaerobic bacteremia in bite-wound infections. Rev Infect Dis 6(suppl):S177, 1984

HICKLIN H et al: Dysgonic fermenter-2 septicemia. Rev Infect Dis 9:884, 1987

JACOBS RF et al: *Pseudomonas* osteochondritis complicating puncture wounds of the foot in children: A 10-year evaluation. J Infect Dis 160:657, 1989

KULLBERG BJ et al: Purpura fulminans and symmetrical peripheral gangrene caused by *Capnocytophaga canimor sus* (formerly DF-2) septicemia: A complication of dog bite. Medicine 70:287, 1991

MARGILETH AM et al: Systemic cat-scratch disease: Report of 23 patients with prolonged or recurrent severe bacterial infection. J Infect Dis 155:390, 1987

McEVOY M et al: Outbreak of fever caused by *Streptobacillus moniliformis.* Lancet 2:1361, 1987

PITLIK S et al: Nonenteric infections acquired through contact with water. Rev Infect Dis 9:54, 1987

ROBERGE RJ: Cat-scratch disease. Emerg Med Clin North Am 9:327, 1991

SCHLOSSBERG D et al: Culture-proved disseminated cat-scratch disease in acquired immunodeficiency syndrome. Arch Intern Med 149:1437, 1989

SCHWARTSMAN WA: Infections due to Rochalimaea: The expanding clinical spectrum. Clin Infect Dis 15:893, 1992

WEBER DJ et al: *Pasteurella multocida* infections: Report of 34 cases and review of literature. Medicine 63:133, 1984

section 3   Clinical syndromes—nosocomial infections

96   INFECTIONS IN THE IMMUNOCOMPROMISED HOST

ROBERT FINBERG

In dealing with infections in immunocompromised patients, the type of defect and the anticipated infection should guide therapy (Tables 96-1 and 96-2). This chapter will discuss the approach to diagnosis and treatment of infections in patients who are immunocompromised by virtue of chemotherapy-induced granulocytopenia and immunosuppression related to organ or bone marrow transplantation. Many defects in host response are covered in other areas of this book.

INFECTIONS IN NEUTROPENIC PATIENTS

INITIAL MANAGEMENT   The neutropenic patient is unusually susceptible to bacterial infection, so antibiotic therapy should be initiated promptly to cover likely pathogens if infection is suspected. Indeed, early initiation of antibacterial agents is mandatory to prevent fatal events. These patients are susceptible to common gram-positive and gram-negative organisms found on the skin and in the bowel (Table 96-3). Treatment with narrow-spectrum agents leads to infection with organisms not covered by the antibiotics used, and for this reason, the initial regimen should be designed to treat pathogens likely to be initial causes of bacterial infection in neutropenic hosts (see Table 96-3).

Selection of antibiotics   Hundreds of antibiotic regimens have been tested for use in this setting. Many of these studies involved small populations in which the outcomes were generally good, and most did not have the statistical power to detect differences among the regimens studied. Each febrile neutropenic patient should be approached as a unique problem, with particular attention to previous infections and recent exposures to antibiotics. Several general guidelines are useful in the initial therapy of neutropenic patients with fever (Fig. 96-1):

1 It is necessary to treat with antibiotics active against both gram-negative and gram-positive pathogens (see Table 96-3) in the initial regimen.
2 An aminoglycoside or ciprofloxacin alone is not adequate therapy in this setting.
3 The agents used should reflect both the epidemiology and the antibiotic resistance pattern of the hospital [e.g., in hospitals where there is gentamicin resistance, amikacin-containing regimens should be considered, and in hospitals with frequent *Pseudomonas aeruginosa* infections, a regimen with the highest activity against this pathogen (such as tobramycin plus a semisynthetic penicillin) would be a reasonable initial regimen].
4 A single third-generation cephalosporin is an appropriate initial regimen for many hospitals (if the pattern of resistance justifies its use).
5 Most standard regimens are designed for patients who have not been treated previously with prophylactic antibiotics. The development of fever in a patient receiving antibiotics affects the choice of subsequent therapy (which should be tailored to treat resistant organisms or organisms known to cause infections in patients being treated with the antibiotics used at the time).

TABLE 96-1 Normal barriers to infections

Type of defense	Specific lesion	Cells involved	Organism	Disease
Physical barrier	Breaks in skin	Epithelial cells	Staphylococci, streptococci	Cellulitis, extensive skin infection
Phagocytosis	Splenectomy	Reticuloendothelial cells	S. pneumoniae, H. influenzae, N. meningitidis	Rapid overwhelming bacteremia
Phagocytosis	Lack of granulocytes	Granulocytes (neutrophils)	Staphylococci, streptococci, enteric organisms	Bacteremia
Humoral immunity	Lack of antibody	B cells	S. pneumoniae, H. influenzae, N. meningitidis	Infections with encapsulated organisms, sinusitis, pneumonia
Cellular immunity	Lack of T cells	T cells and macrophages	M. tuberculosis, Listeria, herpes viruses, fungi, other intracellular parasites	Infections with intracellular bacteria, fungi, parasites

The initial regimen should be refined on the basis of culture results (see Fig. 96-1). Blood cultures are the most relevant culture on which to base therapy; surface cultures of skin and mucous membranes may be misleading. In the case of bacteremia or other gram-positive infections, it is important that the antibiotic is optimal for the organism isolated. If the infection is caused by certain gram-negative pathogens (especially *P. aeruginosa*), a synergistic combination of antibiotics, usually a semisynthetic penicillin (such as mezlocillin) plus an aminoglycoside (such as tobramycin), may be appropriate. Although it is not desirable to leave the patient unprotected, adding more and more antimicrobials is not appropriate unless there is a clinical or microbiologic reason to do so. *Planned progressive therapy* (the serial, empirical addition of one drug after another without culture data) is not efficacious in most settings and may have unfortunate consequences. Cephalosporins can cause bone marrow suppression, and vancomycin is associated with neutropenia in some normal people. Furthermore, the addition of multiple cephalosporins may induce β-lactamase production in some organisms (cephalosporins and particularly double β-lactam combinations probably should be avoided altogether in the case of *Enterobacter* infections).

Antifungal therapy Most clinicians add amphotericin B to antibiotic regimens after a patient has been febrile on antibacterial agents for 4 to 7 days. The rationale for the "empirical" addition of amphotericin B is based on the difficulty in culturing fungi prior to their causing disseminated disease and the high fatality rate of disseminated fungal infections in granulocytopenic patients. The imidazoles (especially fluconazole) may have prophylactic efficacy in this regard, but the spectrum of the imidazoles is less broad than that of amphotericin B. Amphotericin B is the mainstay of therapy for disseminated *Candida* or *Aspergillus* infection in the neutropenic patient. The use of the combination of an imidazole and amphotericin B is controversial because of the theoretical antagonistic effects of these agents.

Other therapeutic modalities Another way to address the problems of the febrile neutropenic patient is to replace the neutrophils. Although granulocyte transfusions may be efficacious in refractory gram-negative bacteremia, they do not have a documented role in prophylaxis. Because of the expense, the risk of leukoagglutinin reactions (although this risk is probably decreased because of improved cell separation procedures), and the risk of transmitting cytomegalovirus (CMV) in unscreened donors, granulocyte transfusion is reserved for patients unresponsive to antibiotics. This modality may be efficacious for documented gram-negative bacteremia refractory to antibiotics, particularly in situations where the granulocytes will be depressed for only a short period. A variety of cytokines, including granulocyte colony stimulating factor (G-CSF) and granulocyte macro-

TABLE 96-2 Infections and cancer

Cancer	Underlying immune abnormality	Organisms causing infection
Multiple myeloma	Hypogammaglobulinemia	S. pneumoniae, H. influenzae, N. meningitidis
CLL	Hypogammaglobulinemia	S. pneumoniae, H. influenzae, N. meningitidis
AML, ALL	Granulocytopenia, skin and mucous membrane lesions	Extracellular gram-positive and gram-negative organisms, fungi
Hodgkin's disease	Abnormal T cell function	Intracellular pathogens (M. tuberculosis, Listeria, Salmonella, Cryptococcus, M. avium-intracellulare)
Non-Hodgkin's lymphoma and ALL	Steroid chemotherapy, T and B cell dysfunction	P. carinii
Colon and rectal tumors	Local abnormalities*	S. bovis bacteremia
Hairy cell leukemia	Abnormal T cell function	Intracellular pathogens (M. tuberculosis, Listeria, Cryptococcus, M. avium-intracellulare)

* The reason for this association is not well defined.

TABLE 96-3 Organisms likely to cause infections in granulocytopenic patients

GRAM-POSITIVE COCCI

Staphylococcus epidermidis
Staphylococcus aureus
Streptococcus viridans
Streptococcus fecalis (enterococcus)
Streptococcus pneumoniae

GRAM-NEGATIVE RODS

E. coli
Klebsiella
Pseudomonas aeruginosa
Pseudomonas nonaeruginosa (often IV catheter-associated)
Enterobacter
Serratia
Acinetobacter (ofter IV catheter-associated)
Citrobacter

GRAM-POSITIVE RODS

Diphtheroids
JK bacillus (often associated with IV catheters)

FUNGI

Candida species
Aspergillus species

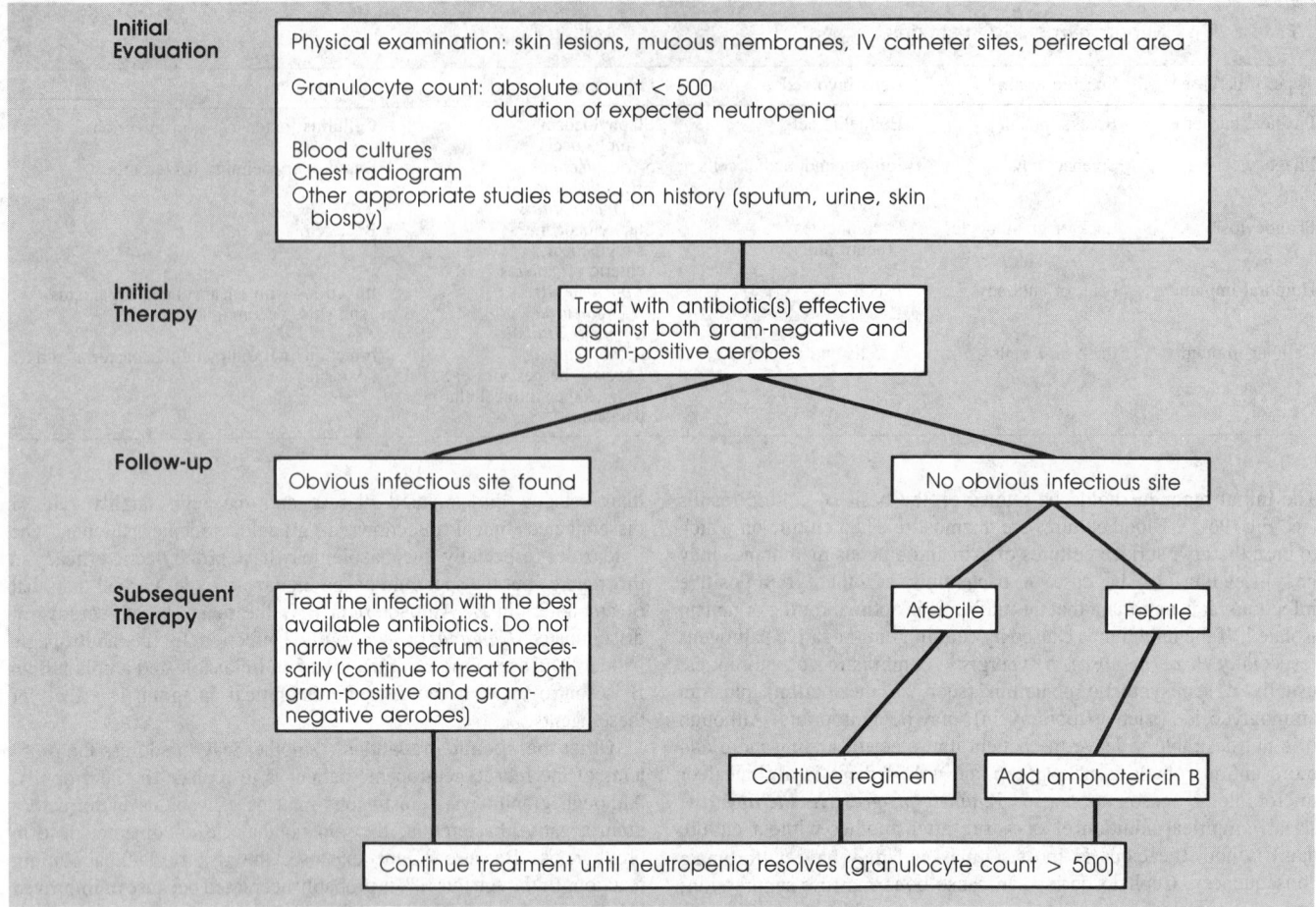

Initial Evaluation

Physical examination: skin lesions, mucous membranes, IV catheter sites, perirectal area

Granulocyte count: absolute count < 500
                duration of expected neutropenia

Blood cultures
Chest radiogram
Other appropriate studies based on history (sputum, urine, skin biospy)

Initial Therapy

Treat with antibiotic(s) effective against both gram-negative and gram-positive aerobes

Follow-up

Obvious infectious site found   No obvious infectious site

Subsequent Therapy

Treat the infection with the best available antibiotics. Do not narrow the spectrum unnecessarily (continue to treat for both gram-positive and gram-negative aerobes)

Afebrile   Febrile

Continue regimen   Add amphotericin B

Continue treatment until neutropenia resolves (granulocyte count > 500)

FIGURE 96-1   Diagnosis and treatment of febrile neutropenic patients: an algorithm.

phage colony stimulating factor (GM-CSF), enhance granulocyte recovery after chemotherapy and consequently shorten the period of maximal vulnerability to fatal infections. The role of other cytokines, such as macrophage colony stimulating factor (M-CSF) for monocytes or interferon (IFN-γ), in preventing or treating infections in granulocytopenic patients is under investigation.

Catheter infections   Infections of catheters in the neutropenic patient can be caused by both bacteria and fungi. The decision to remove the line should be based on the necessity of its remaining (it is always easier to treat the infection if the line can be removed). In general, an infection that involves the tunnel (the area where the catheter runs underneath the skin) mandates removal of the catheter. Infections at the exit site can be treated without removing the catheter with variable success depending on the organism causing the infection. Most coagulase-negative staphylococcal infections can be treated even with the line in place. Treatment of coagulase-positive staphylococcal or fungal infections has a high rate of failure and complication. Treatment of catheter infections due to JK bacilli or *Pseudomonas* species with antibiotics alone also is often associated with failure, and removal of the catheter may be required to achieve a cure.

Duration of therapy   In general, therapy should be continued until the granulocytopenia resolves in an infected (or febrile) neutropenic patient. If there is no evidence of focal infection and the fever resolves with resolution of granulocytopenia, antibiotics can be discontinued after the neutrophil count rises.

DISORDERS UNIQUE TO NEUTROPENIC HOSTS   **Skin lesions**
The appearance of skin lesions in a neutropenic patient merits careful attention, since these lesions are often an important clue to serious infection. While most lesions (whether due to bacteria or fungi) begin as innocent-looking macules or papules, in the neutropenic host they may progress rapidly to ulceration with a necrotic center (ecthyma gangrenosum) (Fig. 96-2). Ecthyma gangrenosum, which is usually

painless, is often associated with *Pseudomonas* bacteremia but can be caused by other gram-negative rods (e.g., *Escherichia coli*) or fungi. The use of occlusive dressings is associated with the development of infection with *Rhizopus* and *Aspergillus* species. Biopsy should be considered when a skin nodule develops in a neutropenic patient, since histologic identification and positive bacterial or fungal cultures may precede the development of blood cultures positive for the infecting agent. Such lesions may evolve rapidly (even with the patient on appropriate antibiotics), and surgical debridement may be required (see Fig. 96-2A–E).

Sweet's syndrome   Sweet's syndrome, acute febrile neutrophilic dermatosis, usually presents as fever and multiple painful cutaneous plaques or tender nodules (and sometimes as pustules, vesicles, or bullae) on the face and upper extremities (see Fig. 96-2F) or at intravenous sites (Koebner phenomenon) and is characterized by a dermal infiltrate of neutrophils, often with edema, and elevated erythrocyte sedimentation rates. The syndrome was originally described in middle-aged women with elevated neutrophil counts unassociated with malignancy. In the last two decades it has been recognized increasingly as a cancer-associated syndrome [particularly associated with acute myelogenous leukemia (AML)] and, paradoxically, may occur in the setting of profound neutropenia. Cultures and stains of biopsy specimens for microorganisms are negative. Patients respond dramatically to prednisone, with lysis of fever within hours and resolution of skin lesion in days.

Typhlitis   Typhlitis (cecitis) is an inflammatory process of the cecum in granulocytopenic patients, particularly children with acute lymphocytic leukemia (ALL), that presents like appendicitis, with fever and right lower quadrant pain and tenderness. Pathologically, the involved bowel has ulcerations, necrotic tissue, and dilated blood vessels. Masses of organisms are often found, and the disease is associated with gram-negative bacteremia (particularly with *Pseudo-*

FIGURE 96-2 Skin lesions of neutropenic patients. *A.* Papules related to *E. coli* bacteremia in a neutropenic patient with acute lymphocytic leukemia. *B.* The same papule 2 h later. *C.* The same patient the following day. *D.* Ecthyma gangrenosum in a neutropenic patient with *P. aeruginosa* bacteremia. *E.* Papule in a neutropenic patient with *C. tropicalis* fungemia. *F.* Plaques of Sweet's syndrome in a patient with acute myelocytic leukemia.

Perirectal infections Leukemic patients (especially those with myelomonocytic leukemias) frequently develop perirectal infections. These infections, which like other infections in neutropenic patients often present with a minimum of physical findings, are usually caused by aerobic gram-negative organisms, and do not necessarily mandate the use of agents active against intestinal anaerobes such as *Bacteroides fragilis*. In the presence of deep infection or intestinal fistulas, antibiotics should be changed to include agents with activity against *B. fragilis* (e.g., metronidazole) (see Chap. 128).

Clostridium difficile–induced diarrhea Neutropenic patients, because of exposure to multiple antibiotics, commonly develop *C. difficile*–induced diarrhea. While this diarrhea must be distinguished from chemotherapy-induced diarrhea, patients with *C. difficile* toxin–positive stools respond to therapy with oral vancomycin. The intravenous vancomycin preparation can be given as an elixir at low dose (125 mg PO qid). Therapy with metronidazole is an alternative (see Chap. 108).

Pneumonias in neutropenic patients Pneumonias in immunocompromised patients may be difficult to diagnose because conventional methods of diagnosis depend on the presence of neutrophils. Bacterial pneumonias in neutropenic patients may present without purulent sputum or without any sputum and may not produce physical findings suggestive of chest consolidation (rales or egophony).

Chest x-rays are needed in the situation of persistent or recurrent fever in granulocytopenic patients. The x-ray pattern may provide localizing information which is helpful in further defining which investigative tests and procedures and in narrowing therapeutic options (Table 96-4). The difficulties in management of pulmonary infiltrates relates in part to the difficulties in performing diagnostic procedures on these patients. When platelet counts can be increased to adequate levels with transfusion, microscopic and microbiologic evaluation of the fluid obtained by endoscopic bronchial lavage is often diagnostic. Lavage fluid should be cultured for *Mycoplasma, Chlamydia, Legionella, Nocardia*, fungi, and the usual bacterial pathogens. In addition, *Pneumocystis carinii* pneumonia should be considered, especially in ALL and lymphoma patients who have not had prophylactic trimethoprim-sulfamethoxazole. The characteristics of the infiltrate may be helpful in determining further diagnostic and therapeutic maneuvers. Nodular infiltrates suggest fungal pneumonia (e.g., *Aspergillus* or *Mucor*). Diffuse interstitial infiltrates suggest a viral or parasitic pneumonia. If the patient has a diffuse interstitial pattern on chest x-ray, it may be reasonable to treat empirically with trimethoprim-sulfamethoxazole (for *Pneumocystis*) and erythromycin (for *Chlamydia, Mycoplasma*, and *Legionella*) while considering invasive diagnostic procedures. Noninvasive procedures such as staining of sputum smears for *Pneumocystis* and serum *Cryptococcus* antigen tests may be helpful on occasion. In transplant recipients who are CMV-seropositive, culturing CMV from another site may be worthwhile.

While bleomycin is the most common cause of chemotherapy-induced lung disease, other causes include alkylating agents (such

monas). It is difficult to diagnose the disease without surgical intervention or postmortem examination. Surgery in neutropenic patients can be difficult, because healing is likely to be impaired and the risk of infectious complications is high. Therapy of typhlitis is controversial. Surgical resection has been successful in some patients. On the other hand, in many neutropenic patients, right lower quadrant pain and fever resolve with antibiotics alone, making it hard to define the role of surgery. In general, if the underlying problem can wait until the neutropenia has resolved, surgery is likely to be less complicated. If surgery is absolutely required during the neutropenic period, the patient should be treated with appropriate antibiotics and the necessary procedure should be performed, assuming adequate platelet support can be given.

TABLE 96-4 Differential diagnosis of chest infiltrates in immunocompromised patients

	Cause of pneumonia	
Infiltrate	Infectious	Noninfectious
Localized	Bacteria, *Legionella,* Mycobacteria	Local hemorrhage or embolism, tumor
Nodular	Fungi (e.g., *Aspergillus* or *Mucor*), *Nocardia*	Recurrent tumor
Diffuse	Viruses (especially CMV), *Chlamydia, P. carinii, T. gondii*, mycobacteria	Congestive heart failure, radiation pneumonitis, drug-induced lung injury, diffuse alveolar hemorrhage (described after BMT)

as cyclophosphamide, chlorambucil, and melphalan), nitrosoureas (BCNU, CCNU, methyl-CCNU), busulfan, procarbazine, methotrexate, procarbazine, and hydroxyurea. Both infectious and drug- and/or radiation-induced pneumonitis can cause fever and chest x-ray abnormalities, so the differential diagnosis of an infiltrate in a patient receiving chemotherapy is broad (see Table 96-4). Since the treatment of radiation pneumonitis (which may respond dramatically to glucocorticoid) or drug-induced pneumonitis is different than that of infectious pneumonia, a biopsy may be important in the diagnosis. Unfortunately, a definitive diagnosis is not made in approximately 30 percent of cases even after bronchoscopy.

Open lung biopsy is the standard of diagnostic techniques. Biopsy via a visualized thoracostomy may replace an open procedure in many cases. When a biopsy cannot be performed, empirical treatment may be undertaken with erythromycin and trimethoprim-sulfamethoxazole in the case of diffuse infiltrates or amphotericin B in the case of nodular infiltrates. The risks should be weighed carefully in these cases. Empirical treatment may result in drug toxicity from administration of inappropriate drugs or in a failure to administer appropriate therapy, either of which may be more harmful than biopsy.

FUNGAL INFECTIONS IN NEUTROPENIC PATIENTS Neutropenic patients are predisposed to the development of invasive fungal infections, most commonly including *Candida* species and *Aspergillus* and, on occasion, *Fusarium, Trichosporon,* and *Dreschlera.* *Cryptococcus* infection, which is common in patients on immunosuppressive agents, is uncommon in neutropenic patients receiving chemotherapy for AML. Invasive candidal disease is usually caused by *C. albicans* or *C. tropicalis* but can be caused by *C. krusei, C. parapsilosis,* and *C. glabrata.*

Candida infections in other settings include superficial candidiasis, candidal sepsis, and hepatic (or hepatosplenic) candidiasis.

Superficial or mucous membrane infection with *Candida* As with any patients who receive antibiotics for prolonged periods, superficial colonization with *Candida* is likely to occur in the skin, mouth, and anal and genital areas. Such colonization is usually unassociated with evidence of tissue invasion. Local care and treatment of the area may be all that is required. Prophylactic oral nystatin, as commonly employed to prevent these mucocutaneous "superinfections," is probably of little or no efficacy. Treatment with fluconazole is effective against *C. albicans* but may be associated with an increased risk of *C. kruseii* or *Aspergillus* infection. Colonization of mouth, skin, and stool with *C. tropicalis* but not with *C. albicans* may be predictive of invasive disease in neutropenic patients. *Candida* esophagitis, often a complication of antibiotic treatment, may respond to low doses of amphotericin or imidazole and may be accompanied by invasive disease.

Candida sepsis Early in neutropenia, *Candida* may cause acute sepsis with fungemia, skin nodules, and hypotension—manifestations similar to those of gram-negative bacteremia. *Candida* may seed almost any organ; joint disease and thyroid disease have been reported, and the organism appears to have a predilection for the kidney and for retinal embolization. The presence of a maculopapular rash and subcutaneous nodules is suggestive of *C. tropicalis* infection. If the candidemia results from colonization of an indwelling catheter, the catheter should be removed as soon as possible. Although transient candidemia may not always require therapy in the noncompromised patient, documentation of candidemia in the neutropenic host should lead to immediate administration of amphotericin B.

Hepatic candidiasis Hepatic candidiasis in neutropenic patients usually develops around the time of resolution of the neutropenia. The characteristic picture is that of persistent fever unresponsive to antibiotics, abdominal symptoms, and elevated serum alkaline phosphatase levels in a patient with hematologic malignancy who has recently recovered from neutropenia. The diagnosis of this disease (which may present in an indolent manner and persist for several months) is based on the finding of yeasts or pseudohyphae in granulomatous lesions. Hepatic ultrasound or computed tomographic (CT) scans may reveal bull's eye lesions. In some cases, magnetic

resonance imaging (MRI) scans may reveal small lesions not seen by other imaging modalities. The pathology (revealing a granulomatous response) and the timing (with resolution of neutropenia and higher granulocyte counts) suggest that the host response is important in the manifestations. In many cases, although organisms may be visualized, cultures of biopsied material may be negative. The designation *hepatosplenic candidiasis* or *hepatic candidiasis* is a misnomer because the disease often involves the kidneys and other tissues, and the term *chronic disseminated candidiasis* might be more appropriate. Because of the risk of bleeding with liver biopsy, diagnosis is often made on the basis of radiographic abnormalities. Although the traditional therapy is with amphotericin B (often for several months until all manifestations of disease have disappeared), fluconazole may be useful for outpatient therapy.

***Aspergillus* infection** As with *Candida, Aspergillus* species can colonize the skin and respiratory tract or cause fatal systemic illness. Although *Aspergillus* may cause invasive aspergillosis, aspergilloma in a previously existing cavity, or allergic bronchopulmonary aspergillosis, the major problem of neutropenic patients is with invasive disease due to *A. fumigatus* or *flavus.* Entry is often through colonization of the respiratory tract with subsequent invasion of the blood vessels. The disease is likely to present with a thrombotic or embolic event because of the ability of the organisms to invade blood vessels. The risk of infection with *Aspergillus* correlates with the duration of neutropenia. In prolonged neutropenia, surveillance cultures for colonization of the nasopharynx with *Aspergillus* may be predictive of the development of disease.

Patients with *Aspergillus* infection often present with pleuritic chest pain and fever sometimes accompanied by cough. Hemoptysis may be an ominous sign. Chest x-rays may reveal new focal infiltrates or nodules (see Table 96-4). Chest CT scans may reveal a characteristic "halo" consisting of a masslike infiltrate surrounded by an area of low attenuation. The presence of a "crescent sign" on chest x-ray or chest CT, in which the mass progresses to central cavitation, is characteristic of invasive *Aspergillus* but may occur only with resolution of the lesions.

In addition to pulmonary presentations, *Aspergillus* may invade through the nose or palate, with deep sinus penetration. The appearance of a discolored area in the nasal passages or on the hard palate should prompt investigation for invasive *Aspergillus.* These cases are likely to require surgical debridement. Treatment with high doses of amphotericin B has been successful in curing granulocytopenic patients of invasive *Aspergillus* following return of the granulocytes. Catheter infections with *Aspergillus* usually require both removal of the catheter and antifungal therapy.

PREVENTION OF INFECTIONS IN NEUTROPENIC PATIENTS
Air handling Outbreaks of fatal *Aspergillus* infections have been associated with construction and construction materials in several hospitals. The association between spore counts and risk of infection suggests the need for a high-efficiency air handling system in hospitals that care for large numbers of neutropenic patients. The use of laminar flow rooms and prophylactic antibiotics has decreased the number of infectious episodes in severely neutropenic patients. But because of the expense of such a program and the failure to show any dramatic effects on mortality, most centers do not routinely use laminar flow to care for neutropenic patients. Some centers use "reverse isolation," in which health care providers and visitors to a patient who is neutropenic are dressed in gowns and gloves. Since most of the infections the patients develop are due to organisms that colonize the patients' own skin and bowel, the validity of such schemes is dubious, and limited clinical data do not support their use. Hand washing may prevent spread of resistant organisms.

Food The presence of large numbers of bacteria (particularly *P. aeruginosa*) in certain foods (particularly fresh vegetables) has led some to recommend a special low-bacteria diet. A diet consisting of cooked and canned food is satisfactory to most neutropenic patients and does not involve elaborate disinfection or sterilization protocols. Some spices (such as black pepper) are likely to be contaminated with fungal spores, and these, like fresh flowers and live plants, probably should be avoided during the period of severe neutropenia.

Antibiotic prophylaxis   There is no consensus on the use of prophylactic antibiotics in neutropenic patients. The incidence of infection is decreased in patients treated prophylactically with broad-spectrum antibiotics, and trimethoprim-sulfamethoxazole appeared to prevent infections in some series. Because of a prolongation of neutropenia which may be associated with use of trimethoprim-sulfamethoxazole, some clinicians have used such broad-spectrum agents as the quinolones (e.g., ciprofloxacin). Either regimen can be given orally, and both have the theoretical advantage that the antibiotics are not active against anaerobic organisms and are thus less likely to disrupt the bowel flora and permit colonization with new aerobes or *Candida*. However, both have adverse effects and can lead to resistance in a hospital. For this reason, many clinicians reserve their use for patients with the longest periods of neutropenia (e.g., bone marrow transplant recipients; see below). The same issues exist concerning the use of antifungal agents; again, the administration of antifungals such as fluconazole may prevent infections with susceptible organisms (e.g., *C. albicans*) but cause a concomitant increase in infections due to resistant fungi (e.g., *C. krusei*). Thus the decision to use antifungal prophylaxis may vary depending on what fungi are endemic in a given hospital.

Treatment after resolution of the neutropenic episode   Once neutropenia has resolved, the patient is not at high risk of infection. However, patients who continue on chemotherapeutic protocols, depending on what drugs they receive, continue to be at high risk for certain diseases. Any patient on more than a maintenance level of glucocorticoids (including many diffuse lymphoma treatment regimens) should have prophylactic trimethoprim-sulfamethoxazole because of the risk of *P. carinii* infection; those with ALL should be maintained on trimethoprim-sulfamethoxazole prophylaxis for as long as they are receiving chemotherapy.

INFECTIONS IN BONE MARROW TRANSPLANT (BMT) RECIPIENTS

Bone marrow transplantation for either immune deficiency or cancer results in a transient state of complete immune incompetence. Immediately following transplantation, both phagocytes and immune cells (T cells and B cells) are absent, and the host is susceptible to infection. The reconstitution that occurs following transplantation has been likened to maturation of the immune system in neonates. The analogy does not entirely predict infections seen in these patients, however, because the new marrow is usually expressed in an old host who has several latent infections already (Table 96-5).

TIMETABLE OF COMMON INFECTIONS (See also Fig. 96-3)   In the first month after transplantation, infectious complications are similar to those in granulocytopenic patients receiving chemotherapy for AML or ALL (see above). Because of the anticipated 3- to 4-week duration of neutropenia in this population, many centers give prophylactic antibiotics to patients with the initiation of chemotherapy.

TABLE 96-5   Herpes group virus syndromes in transplant recipients

Virus	Reactivation disease
Herpes simplex type 1	Oral lesions, sometimes with spread (pneumonia described in BMT patients)
Herpes simplex type 2	Severe and/or persistent anogenital lesions
Varicella zoster	Zoster (dissemination may occur)
Cytomegalovirus	Associated with graft rejection, fever
Epstein-Barr virus	B cell lymphoproliferative disease
Human herpes virus 6	Fever, rash,* pneumonitis
Human herpes virus 7	Undefined

* A characteristic rash (seen in primary infection) has not been well defined.

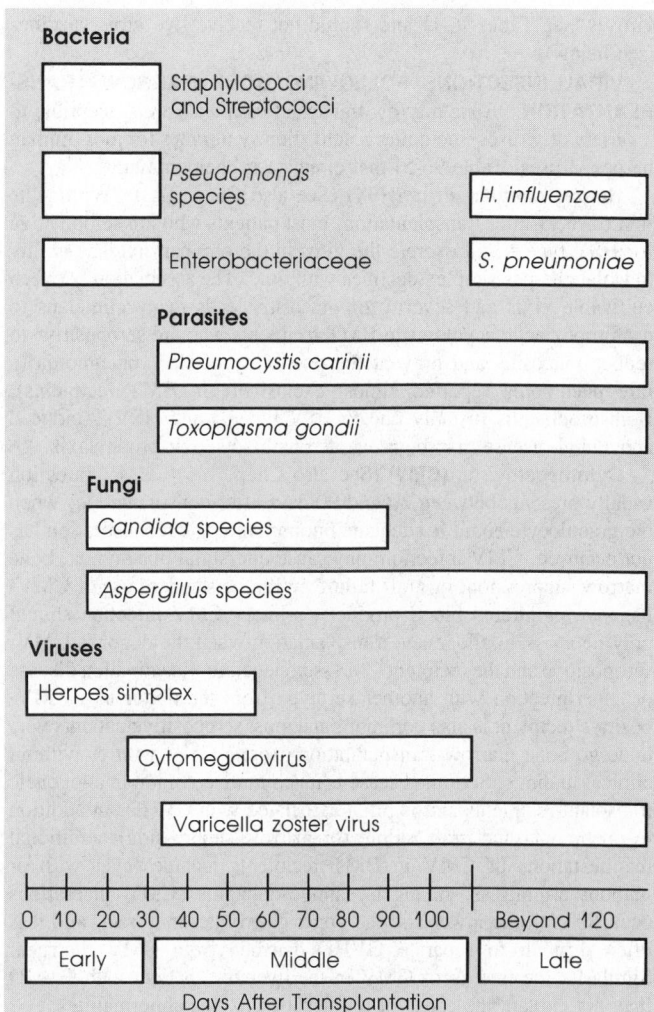

FIGURE 96-3   Infections after bone marrow transplantation.

Prophylactic trimethoprim-sulfamethoxazole or ciprofloxacin decreases the incidence of gram-negative bacteremia in these patients.

In the second month after transplantation, a major concern (particularly in allogeneic transplant recipients) is CMV disease. The diagnosis of pneumonia in these patients presents some special problems (see Table 96-4). Because they have been treated with multiple chemotherapeutic agents and radiation, the differential diagnosis of pneumonitis in this group should include CMV pneumonitis, diffuse alveolar hemorrhage (DAH), viral and fungal causes of pneumonia, and parasites. Because of the high risk of *P. carinii* pneumonia (especially in patients being treated for hematologic malignancies), most patients should be maintained on prophylactic doses of trimethoprim-sulfamethoxazole. Trimethoprim-sulfamethoxazole also may provide protection for patients seropositive for *Toxoplasma gondii,* which may cause a pneumonia in the early weeks after transplantation or central nervous system (CNS) lesions later.

The late posttransplantation period (6 months following bone marrow reconstitution) is marked by bacteremias due to encapsulated organisms and reactivation of varicella zoster virus (Fig. 96-3). The advantages of maintaining patients on trimethoprim-sulfamethoxazole for 1 year after transplantation include protection against late bacterial infections with pneumococci and *Haemophilus influenzae* which are a consequence of the inability of the immature bone marrow to respond to polysaccharide antigens (see Fig. 96-3). After recovery from transplantation and full restoration of immune function, patients should be revaccinated with all recommended vaccines (based on the age of the patient). Patients who continue to take immunosuppressive drugs for graft-versus-host disease (GVHD) are susceptible to intracellular pathogens such as *Listeria, Nocardia,* fungi, *Pneumocystis,* and viruses (see Table 96-1) and should not receive live virus vaccines (see below).

VIRAL INFECTIONS FOLLOWING BONE MARROW TRANS-PLANTATION   Bone marrow transplant recipients are susceptible to a variety of viruses, including reactivation syndromes for most human herpes viruses (Table 96-5) that circulate in the community.

Herpes simplex virus (HSV) (See also Chap. 143)   Within the first 6 weeks after transplantation, most patients who are seropositive for HSV type 1 will excrete the virus in the oropharynx. The ability to isolate herpes simplex declines with time. The association between cultivable virus and severity of mucositis leads many clinicians to use prophylactic acyclovir in BMT recipients who are seropositive to reduce mucositis and prevent the possibility of HSV pneumonia (a rare pneumonia reported almost exclusively in BMT recipients). Both esophagitis (usually due to HSV type 1) and HSV-2–induced anogenital disease may be prevented with acyclovir prophylaxis.

Cytomegalovirus (CMV) (See also Chap. 146)   CMV infection usually presents between 30 and 90 days after transplantation, when the granulocyte count is adequate but immunologic reconstitution has not occurred. CMV infection may cause interstitial pneumonia, bone marrow suppression, or graft failure. With the standard use of CMV-negative or filtered blood products, primary CMV infection should only be a risk in allogeneic transplantation when the donor is CMV-seropositive and the recipient CMV-seronegative. Reactivation disease or superinfection with another serotype from the donor in a CMV-positive recipient is also common, and most seropositive patients who undergo bone marrow transplantation excrete CMV with or without clinical findings. Serious disease is much more common in allogeneic transplant recipients and is often associated with GVHD. In addition to pneumonia and graft failure (or marrow suppression), additional manifestations of CMV in BMT recipients include fever with or without arthralgias, myalgias, and esophagitis. CMV ulcerations occur in both the lower and the upper gastrointestinal tract, and it is often difficult to separate GVHD diarrhea from CMV diarrhea. Similarly, the finding of CMV in the liver of a patient with GVHD may not explain the cause of the hepatic enzyme abnormalities.

Because of the high fatality rate of CMV pneumonia in bone marrow transplantation and the difficulty in diagnosing infection early, prophylactic ganciclovir is given in some centers during the period of maximum vulnerability (from engraftment to day 120 after transplant). The major problem with its administration relates to adverse effects that include a dose-related neutrophil suppression. Because the frequency of CMV pneumonia is lower in autologous transplant recipients (2 to 7 percent versus 10 to 40 percent for allogeneics), prophylactic therapy in this group will not become the rule unless a less toxic antiviral agent is available. A common practice among many centers treating allogeneic transplant patients is to culture blood and urine (and bronchial secretions in some) and treat those patients who have positive CMV cultures with ganciclovir as prophylaxis against the development of CMV pneumonia. The development of improved antigen testing methods should make surveillance of those at high risk for CMV disease more reliable. Treatment of CMV pneumonia in BMT recipients requires both IVIG and ganciclovir, although ganciclovir alone is effective prophylactically.

Varicella zoster (VZV) (See also Chap. 144)   Reactivation of herpes zoster may occur as early as 1 month but more commonly occurs several months after transplantation. Attack rates are approximately 40 percent for allogeneic and 25 percent for autologous transplant recipients. Localized zoster can spread in the face of immunosuppressives. Fortunately, disseminated disease usually can be controlled with high doses of acyclovir (Fig. 96-4; see also Chap. 142). Because of the high incidence of dissemination of herpes zoster in patients with skin lesions, acyclovir is given prophylactically in some centers to prevent severe disease. Low doses of acyclovir (400 mg PO tid) appear to be effective prophylaxis for preventing reactivation of varicella zoster virus. However, administration of acyclovir inhibits development of VZV-specific immunity. Thus, administration for only 6 months following transplantation does not prevent zoster

A

B

FIGURE 96-4   Spread of herpes zoster with chemotherapy. *A.* The patient complained of external ear pain. A vesicular rash on the concha and antihelix suggested Ramsey-Hunt syndrome. *B.* Following chemotherapy for prostate cancer, the patient developed disseminated zoster which was eventually controlled with acyclovir.

infection from occurring when acyclovir is stopped. Some data suggest that administration of low doses of acyclovir for an entire year following transplantation is effective and may eliminate most post-transplantation zoster.

Epstein-Barr virus (See also Chap. 145)   Primary Epstein Barr virus (EBV) infection can be fatal in transplant recipients, and EBV reactivation can cause a B cell lymphoproliferative disease (EBV lymphoproliferative syndrome), which also may be fatal in patients taking immunosuppressive drugs. The localization of EBV to B cells leads to several interesting phenomena in marrow transplants. The marrow ablation that occurs as part of the bone marrow transplantation procedure eliminates latent EBV from the host. The disease can then be reacquired following transplantation when a susceptible pool of B cells is regenerated.

The EBV lymphoproliferative syndrome can develop in the recipient's B cells (if any should survive marrow ablation) but is more likely to be a consequence of reactivation in the donor cells. Reactivation of EBV is more likely during immunosuppression (e.g., it is associated with GVHD and the use of anti-T cell antibodies). Although less likely in the autologous transplant recipient, it can occur in the case of T cell–depleted autologous recipients (e.g., patients being treated for a T cell lymphoma with marrow depletion using anti-T cell antibodies). The EBV lymphoproliferative syndrome usually presents 1 to 3 months after engraftment and can cause high fevers and cervical adenopathy, similar to those in infectious mononucleosis, but more commonly resembles disseminated lymphoma. An incidence of 0.6 percent has been found among allogeneic bone marrow transplants recipients, in contrast to the figures of approximately 5 percent for renal transplant recipients and 20 percent after cardiac transplantation. In all cases, EBV lymphoproliferative syndrome is more likely to occur with continued immunosuppression (especially with the use of anti-T cell antibodies and cyclosporin).

Other (nonherpes) viruses Both respiratory syncytial virus (RSV) and parainfluenza virus type 3 can cause severe and sometimes fatal pneumonias in BMT recipients. Infections with both these agents can occur as disastrous nosocomial epidemics. Therapy with ribavirin has been reported to ameliorate disease. Influenza is also seen in BMT recipients and generally mirrors the presence of infection in the community. In addition, adenovirus can be isolated at rates varying from 5 to 18 percent of BMT recipients. Although hemorrhagic cystitis, pneumonia, and fatal disseminated infection have been reported, adenovirus infection, which usually occurs in the first or second month after transplantation (similar to CMV), is often asymptomatic. No treatment has proven efficacy. Infections with B19 parvovirus (presenting with anemia) and enteroviruses (with fatalities) can occur, rotaviruses are a common cause of gastroenteritis in BMT recipients, and BK and JC virus can be found in the urine of some transplant recipients.

VACCINATION OF BMT RECIPIENTS Because of their lack of immunologic memory, BMT recipients should be vaccinated against organisms they are likely to encounter. Vaccines against pneumococci and *H. influenzae* should be administered (see Table 96-9), particularly if the patient is splenectomized. In addition patients should be inoculated against poliovirus with an inactivated vaccine. Because of the risk of spread, household contacts of marrow transplant recipients (or patients immunosuppressed by virtue of chemotherapy) should receive the inactivated polio vaccine as well. It is safe to give live measles, mumps, and rubella vaccine to allogeneic transplant recipients 2 years after transplantation if they are free of overt GVHD. This vaccine also has a lower risk of spreading to a household contact than the polio vaccine. In patients who have active GVHD and/or are maintained on high doses of glucocorticoids, it may be prudent to avoid all live virus vaccines.

INFECTIONS IN SOLID ORGAN TRANSPLANT RECIPIENTS

The most important cause of death among early kidney transplant recipients was infection with organisms not susceptible to conventional antibiotic therapy. These infections occurred in patients requiring prolonged courses of glucocorticoids and other immunosuppressive drugs. Morbidity and mortality in solid organ transplantation have been reduced with the use of better antibiotics.

The organisms that cause infections in these patients are different from those in BMT recipients because solid organ recipients do not go through a period of neutropenia. On the other hand, since organ transplant patients are immunosuppressed for more prolonged periods (usually permanently), they are susceptible to the same organisms as cancer patients with impaired T cell immunity (see Table 96-1). In addition, since the transplantation procedure involves surgery, the recipients are subject to wound infections.

TIMETABLE OF INFECTIONS (See also Table 96-6) During the early period (less than 1 month after transplantation), infections are most often caused by extracellular bacteria (staphylococci, streptococci, *E. coli,* other gram-negative organisms) which often originate in surgical wound or anastomotic sites. Thus the infections are largely determined by the type of transplant.

In subsequent weeks, the consequences of the administration of agents that suppress cell-mediated immunity and of the acquisition (from the transplanted organ) or reactivation of parasites and viruses become apparent. CMV is often a problem at this time and may present as severe systemic disease or as an infection of the transplanted organ. CMV is associated not only with generalized immunosuppression but also (in some series) with organ-specific, rejection-related syndromes. CMV is associated with glomerulopathy in kidney transplant recipients, bronchiolitis obliterans in lung transplant recipients, premature atherosclerosis in heart transplant recipients, and the vanishing bile duct syndrome in liver transplant recipients. Whether these syndromes are actually caused by CMV, which itself is an opportunistic invader, or are merely associated has not been established. It is clear that the presence of CMV and CMV disease is associated with a poor outcome after transplantation. For this reason, considerable attention has focused on the diagnosis, treatment, and prophylaxis of CMV in organ transplant recipients.

During the period beyond 6 months after transplantation, infections characteristic of patients with defects in cell-mediated immunity develop. Thus infections with *Listeria monocytogenes, Nocardia,* various fungi, and other intracellular parasites may be a problem. Elimination of these late infections will not be possible until specific tolerance to the transplanted organ can be achieved without the administration of drugs that lead to generalized immunosuppression. Meanwhile vigilance, prophylaxis (when indicated), and rapid diagnosis and therapy of infections can be lifesaving in the solid organ transplant recipient who, unlike most BMT recipients, continues to be immunosuppressed.

Solid organ transplant recipients are susceptible to EBV lymphoproliferative disease from as early as 2 months to many years after transplantation. The prevalence of this complication is increased by potent immunosuppressive drugs and may be reversed (in some cases) by decreasing the immunosuppression. The proliferation of B cells, which is the pathologic problem in this disease, occurs with increased frequency in renal and liver transplantation. Among organ transplant

---

TABLE 96-6 Infections after renal transplantation

	Period after transplantation		
	Early (<1 month posttransplant)	Middle (1–4 months posttransplant)	Late (>6 months posttransplant)
Urinary tract	Bacteria (*E. coli, Klebsiella,* Enterobacteriaceae, *Pseudomonas,* enterococcus), associated with bacteremias and pyelonephritis, *Candida*	Cytomegalovirus (fever alone is common)	Bacteria, late UTIs usually not associated with bacteremia
Lungs	Bacteria (including *Legionella* in endemic settings)	CMV diffuse interstitial pneumonitis, *P. carinii, Aspergillis, Legionella*	*Nocardia, Aspergillis, Mucor*
CNS		*Listeria monocytogenes,* bacteremia and meningitis, CMV encephalitis, toxoplasmosis	CMV retinitis, listerial meningitis, cryptococcal meningitis, *Aspergillis, Nocardia*

patients, lung and heart transplants are most likely to present with EBV-induced B cell proliferation in the lungs. Whether the tendency of EBV lymphoproliferation to present in the transplanted organ relates to local factors (e.g., lack of access of host T cells to the transplanted organs because of disturbed lymphatics) or to the differences in major histocompatibility loci between the host T cells and the organ (which may lead to lack of cell migration or lack of effective T cell–macrophage cooperation) has not been established.

INFECTIOUS COMPLICATIONS OF KIDNEY TRANSPLANTATION

Early infections Early infections following kidney transplantation are often caused by bacteria associated with skin or wound infections. Some data indicate a role for perioperative antibiotic prophylaxis, and many centers give cephalosporins or a penicillin with an aminoglycoside to decrease the risk of postoperative complications. Immediately after transplantation, urinary tract infections are usually related to anatomic alterations due to surgery (see Table 96-6). Such early infections may require prolonged treatment as for pyelonephritis (6 weeks of antibiotics). Urinary tract infections that occur more than 6 months after transplantation do not seem to be associated with the high rate of pyelonephritis or relapse seen with infections that occur in the first 3 months and may be treated for shorter time periods.

Prophylaxis with trimethoprim-sulfamethoxazole, i.e., 1 double-strength tablet (800 mg sulfamethoxazole and 160 mg trimethoprim) per day, for the first 4 months following transplantation decreases the incidence of early and middle period infections (see below and Table 96-7).

Middle-period infections Because of continuing immunosuppression, renal transplant recipients are predisposed to lung infections characteristic of patients with T cell deficiencies (i.e., *Listeria*, *Mycobacteria*, *Nocardia*, fungi, viruses, and parasites). The high mortality associated with *Legionella pneumophila* infection led to the closing of renal transplant units in hospitals with endemic *Legionella*. Fifty percent of all renal transplant recipients presenting with fever in the period 1 to 4 months after transplantation have evidence of CMV disease, and CMV itself accounts for over two-thirds of the fevers, making it the predominant pathogen during this period. CMV infection also may present as arthralgias or myalgias. CMV can cause primary disease (in the case of a seronegative recipient who receives a kidney from a seropositive donor) or may present as either reactivation disease or superinfection during this period. Patients may have an atypical lymphocytosis, but unlike nonimmunosuppressed patients, they often do not have lymphadenopathy or splenomegaly, thereby making clinical suspicion (and laboratory confirmation) necessary for diagnosis. The clinical syndrome may be accompanied by bone marrow suppression (particularly leukopenia). CMV is associated with an increased incidence of other opportunistic infections (e.g., fungal infections) and glomerulopathy. Because of the frequency and severity of CMV disease, a considerable effort has been addressed to its prevention and treatment in renal transplant recipients. Administration of an immune globulin preparation enriched for antibodies to cytomegalovirus (CMV-Ig) decreases the incidence in the group at highest risk for severe infections (seronegative recipients of seropositive kidneys). Ganciclovir is useful for the treatment of serious CMV disease.

The other herpes group viruses may present within 6 months of the transplant or later. Early after transplantation, herpes simplex may cause either oral or anogenital lesions that are usually responsive to acyclovir. Large ulcerating lesions in the anogenital area may lead to bladder and rectal dysfunction as well as predisposing to bacterial infection. VZV may cause a fatal disseminated infection in nonimmune renal transplant recipients, but immune patients usually do not have dissemination of reactivation zoster outside the dermatome; thus it is a less fearsome complication in renal than in bone marrow transplantation.

EBV reactivation disease is more serious; it often presents as a polyclonal proliferation of B cells that invade the CNS, nasopharynx, liver, small bowel, heart, and transplanted kidney. The disease is diagnosed by the finding of a proliferation of EBV-positive B cells. The incidence of the syndrome is higher in patients on high doses of cyclosporin. Fortunately, the B cells usually regress with withdrawal of immunosuppression with or without antiviral therapy (acyclovir). Human herpes virus type 6 infection and reactivation also occur after renal transplantation.

The papovaviruses BK and JC have been cultured from the urine of renal transplant recipients (as they have from BMT recipients). BK virus excretion is associated with ureteral strictures, and JC virus with progressive multifocal leukoencephalopathy. Adenoviruses also may persist in patients with continued immunosuppression.

Renal transplant recipients are also subject to infections with other intracellular organisms. These patients are likely to have pulmonary infections with *Nocardia*, *Aspergillus*, and *Mucor* and infections with other pathogens in which the T cell–macrophage axis plays an important role. In patients without intravenous catheters, *L. monocytogenes* is the most common cause of bacteremia 1 month or more after transplantation. Renal transplant recipients also may have *Salmonella* bacteremia, which can lead to endovascular infections and require prolonged therapy. Pulmonary infections with *P. carinii* are common unless the patient is maintained on trimethoprim-sulfamethoxazole prophylaxis. The addition of cyclosporine to azathioprine and prednisone is probably associated with an increased risk of *P. carinii* pneumonia. *Nocardia* infection may present in the skin, bones, lungs, or CNS (usually single or multiple brain abscesses). *Nocardia* infection usually occurs 1 month or more after transplantation and may follow treatment (increased immunosuppression) for an episode of rejection. Pulmonary findings are nonspecific; localized disease with or without cavities is most common, but the disease may disseminate. The diagnosis is made by culture of the organism from sputum or from the involved nodule. Most patients are now cured with prolonged sulfonamide therapy. Prophylaxis with trimethoprim-sulfamethoxazole also appears to be efficacious in the prevention of disease. *Nocardia* infections can occur more than 2 years after transplantation, suggesting that long-term prophylaxis is justified.

Toxoplasmosis occurs in seropositive patients, usually in the first few months after transplantation. In endemic areas, histoplasmosis, coccidioidomycosis, and blastomycosis may cause pulmonary infiltrates or disseminated disease.

Late infections Late infections (more than 6 months after transplantation) include CMV retinitis and a variety of CNS complica-

---

TABLE 96-7 Prophylaxis against infections in transplant recipients

Risk factors	Organism	Prophylactic antibiotics	Examinations
Travel or residency in area with known risk of fungal infection	Coccidiodomycosis, histoplasmosis, blastomycosis	? Imidazoles* or amphotericin B	Chest radiogram
Latent viruses	Herpes simplex, varicella zoster, EBV, CMV	Acyclovir after BMT for HSV and VZV; ganciclovir in some settings	Serology—test for HSV, VZV, CMV, EBV
Latent parasites	*P. carinii, T. gondii*	Trimethoprim-sulfamethoxazole or dapsone plus pyrimethamine	Serology for *Toxoplasma*
History of exposure to tuberculosis	*M. tuberculosis*	Isoniazid, if recent conversion for positive chest x-ray and no previous treatment	PPD and chest radiogram

* The use of imidazoles in this setting is under study.

tions. Patients (and particularly those in whom immunosuppression has been increased) are also at risk for subacute meningitis due to *Cryptococcus* as well as aspergillomas (usually originating from a lung source) and for cryptococcal disease, which may present in an insidious manner (sometimes as a skin infection before the development of clear CNS findings). *Listeria* meningitis may present acutely and requires prompt therapy to avoid a fatal outcome.

In addition, patients who remain on glucocorticoid therapy are predisposed to infection. "Transplant elbow" is a recurrent bacterial infection in and around the elbow that is said to result from a combination of poor tensile strength of the skin of steroid-treated patients and steroid-induced proximal myopathy that requires patients to push themselves up with their elbows to get out of chairs. Recurrent bouts of cellulitis (usually caused by *Staphylococcus aureus*) occur until patients are provided with elbow protection.

These patients are susceptible to other fungal infections with *Aspergillus* and *Rhizopus,* for example, which may present as superficial lesions before dissemination disease. Mycobacteria (particularly *M. marinum*) can be diagnosed by skin examination. *Prototheca wickerhamii* (an achlorophyllic alga) has been diagnosed by skin biopsy. Warts caused by human papillomaviruses are a late consequence of persistent immunosuppression. Local therapy is usually satisfactory treatment.

INFECTIONS IN HEART TRANSPLANT RECIPIENTS   Early infections   Mediastinitis is an early complication of heart transplantation. An indolent course is common, with fever or a mildly elevated white blood cell count preceding the development of site tenderness or drainage. Clinical suspicion based on evidence of sternal instability and failure to heal may lead to the diagnosis. Although common skin organisms such as *S. aureus* and *S. epidermidis* are common pathogens, mediastinitis in these patients also can be due to *Mycoplasma hominis*. Since these organisms require an anaerobic environment for growth and may be difficult to see on conventional medium, the laboratory should be alerted that *M. hominis* is suspected. *M. hominis* mediastinitis has been cured with a combination of surgical debridement (sometimes requiring muscle flap placement) and clindamycin and tetracycline. Other organisms, including *P. aeruginosa* and *Candida,* can cause mediastinitis. The organisms may be cultured from accompanying pericarditis fluid.

Middle-period infections   *Toxoplasma gondii* may be transmitted to a seronegative recipient in the heart of a seropositive donor, thus making serologic screening for *T. gondii* infection important in the months after transplantation. The incidence of disease is so high in this setting that some centers have advocated prophylaxis with pyrimethamine. CMV and HIV also have been transmitted by heart transplantation. CNS infections can be due to *Toxoplasma, Nocardia,* and *Aspergillus,* and *L. monocytogenes* meningitis should be considered in heart transplant recipients with fever and headache.

CMV infection is associated with poor outcomes after heart transplantation. The virus is usually cultivable 1 to 2 months after transplantation, causes manifestations (usually fever and atypical lymphocytosis, often associated with leukopenia and thrombocytopenia) in 2 to 3 months, and develops into severe disease such as pneumonia 3 to 4 months after transplantation. Seropositive recipients usually develop cultivable virus faster than patients whose primary CMV infection is a consequence of the transplant. Between 40 and 70 percent of patients develop symptomatic CMV disease: (1) CMV pneumonia, the most likely to be fatal, (2) CMV esophagitis and gastritis, sometimes accompanied by abdominal pain with or without ulcerations and bleeding, and (3) the CMV syndrome, comprising CMV in the blood, fever, leukopenia, thrombocytopenia, and hepatic enzyme abnormalities. Ganciclovir is efficacious in the treatment of CMV infection; prophylaxis with ganciclovir may reduce the incidence of CMV-related disease.

Late infections   EBV infection usually presents as a lymphoma-like proliferation of B cells as a late complication, particularly with increased immunosuppression. A subset of heart-lung transplant recipients may develop early (within 2 months of transplantation)

fulminant EBV lymphoproliferative disease, often in the transplanted lung. Prophylaxis against *P. carinii* infection is required for these patients (see below and Table 96-8).

LUNG TRANSPLANTATION   Early infections   It is not surprising that lung transplants are predisposed to the development of pneumonia. The combination of ischemia and the resulting mucosal damage together with accompanying denervation and lack of lymph drainage probably contribute to the high rate (66 percent in one series) of pneumonia. The prophylactic use of high doses of broad-spectrum antibiotics for the first 3 to 4 days after surgery decreases the incidence of pneumonia. Gram-negative pathogens (Enterobacteriaceae and *Pseudomonas* species) are troublesome in the first 2 weeks after surgery (the period of maximum vulnerability). Pneumonia also can be caused by *Candida* (possibly as result of colonization of the donor lung), *Aspergillus,* and *Cryptococcus.*

Mediastinitis   Mediastinitis may occur at an even higher rate than in heart transplant recipients. *Staphylococcus, M. hominis,* and *C. albicans* are common causes of mediastinitis that occurs within 2 weeks of surgery. Mediastinitis due to CMV (which may be transmitted as a consequence of the transplant) usually presents between 2 weeks and 3 months after surgery, with primary disease occurring later than reactivation disease. The incidence of CMV infection, either reactivation or primary, is between 75 and 100 percent if either the donor or the recipient is seropositive for CMV. CMV-induced disease appears to be more severe in recipients of lung and heart-lung transplants. Whether this relates to the mismatch in lung antigen-presenting and host immune cells or occurs for other (nonimmune) reasons is not known. Over half of lung transplant recipients with symptomatic CMV disease have pneumonia, and it may be difficult to distinguish the radiographic picture of CMV from organ rejection, thereby further complicating therapy. CMV also can be associated with bronchiolitis obliterans in lung transplants. The development of pneumonitis related to herpes simplex has led to use of acyclovir for the prevention of herpes simplex pneumonia. Acyclovir prophylaxis also may affect CMV isolation. Ganciclovir is probably more efficacious than acyclovir in lung transplant recipients.

EBV lymphoproliferative syndrome   As in other transplant recipients, infection with EBV may cause either a mononucleosis-like syndrome or lymphoproliferative disease. The tendency of the B cell blasts to present in the lung appears to be greater after lung than in other organ transplantation. Reduction of cyclosporine dosage causes remission in most cases, but lymph node compression can cause fatalities.

Late posttransplantation infections   The incidence of *P. carinii* infection (which may present with a paucity of findings) is high in lung or heart-lung transplants. Some form of prophylaxis against *P. carinii* pneumonia (PCP) is indicated in all organ transplant situations (see Table 96-7 and Table 96-8). Trimethoprim-sulfamethoxazole prophylaxis for 12 months after transplantation may be sufficient to prevent disease in patients whose immunosuppression is not increased.

LIVER TRANSPLANTATION   Early complications   As in the case of other transplantation, early bacterial infections are a major problem following liver transplantation. Many centers administer systemic broad-spectrum antibiotics for the first 5 days following

TABLE 96-8   Prophylactic antibiotics or vaccination for immunocompromised patients

Underlying problem	Therapy
Splenectomy	Vaccination for pneumococci, *H. influenzae,* meningococci*
T cell defects (e.g., solid organ transplantation)	Prophylaxis for *P. carinii* while patient is immunosuppressed
Antibody defects (e.g., BMT, CLL, or multiple melanoma)	Vaccination for *Pneumococcus, H. influenzae, N. meningitidis*

* Patients should be advised of the importance of seeking immediate medical attention for suspected infections [it may be advisable for patients to have antibiotics (e.g., amoxicillin or amoxicillin/clavulanate) at home].

surgery, even in the absence of documented infection. However, despite prophylaxis, infectious complications are still common and are correlated with duration of surgical procedure and the type of biliary drainage. An operation of greater than 12 h is associated with an increased likelihood of infection. Patients with a choledochojejunostomy with drainage of the biliary duct to a roux en Y jejunal bowel loop have more fungal infections than those whose bile is drained via a choledochocholedochostomy (with anastomosis of the donor common bile duct to the recipient common bile duct).

Cholangitis The development of postoperative biliary stricture predisposes to cholangitis. These patients may lack the characteristic signs and symptoms of cholangitis: fever, abdominal pain, and jaundice. In fact, even if present, these findings may suggest graft rejection. The diagnosis of cholangitis in liver transplant recipients therefore requires documentation of bacteremia or demonstration of aggregated neutrophils in bile duct biopsy specimens. Unfortunately, invasive studies of the biliary tract (either T-tube cholangiograms or endoscopic retrograde cholangiopancreatography) may lead to cholangitis. For this reason, many clinicians recommend prophylactic antibiotics covering gram-negative organisms and anaerobes when these procedures are performed in liver transplant recipients.

Peritonitis Peritonitis and intraabdominal abscesses are common complications. Bacterial peritonitis may result from biliary leaks and primary or secondary infection following leakage of bile. Peritonitis in liver transplant recipients is often polymicrobial, commonly due to enterococci, aerobic gram-negative organisms, staphylococci, anaerobes, or *Candida*. Only one-third of patients with intraabdominal abscesses have bacteremia. Abscesses within the first postoperative month may occur not only over the liver but also in the spleen, pericolic area, and pelvis. Treatment includes antibiotics and drainage as necessary.

As is true of other transplant recipients, liver transplant patients have a high incidence of fungal infections, and the occurrence of fungal infection (often candidiasis) correlates with preoperative use of glucocorticoids, duration of treatment with antibacterial agents, and posttransplant use of immunosuppressive agents.

Viral infections Viral hepatitis is a common complication of liver transplantation (see Chap. 266). As in other transplant settings, reactivation disease with herpes group viruses is common (see Table 96-5). Herpes simplex, human herpes virus 6, and CMV can be transmitted in donor organs. Although CMV hepatitis occurs in about 4 percent of liver transplant recipients, it is usually not so severe as to require retransplantation. While CMV disease develops in the majority of seronegative recipients who receive organs from CMV-positive donors, fatality rates are lower than in lung or heart-lung transplant recipients. CMV disease is associated with the vanishing bile duct syndrome after liver transplantation. While patients respond

to treatment with ganciclovir, prophylaxis with CMV-Ig and acyclovir may modify disease. EBV lymphoproliferative disease after liver transplantation shows a propensity for involvement of the liver.

PANCREAS TRANSPLANTATION Transplantation of the pancreas is complicated by early abdominal infection in approximately 20 percent of cases. To prevent contamination of the allograft with enteric bacteria and yeasts, some surgeons, instead of draining the pancreas through the bowel, drain secretions into the urinary tract or bladder. A cuff of duodenum if often utilized in the anastomosis between the pancreas graft and the bladder. In addition to the attendant bicarbonate loss, this technique causes a high rate of urinary tract infections (30 to 40 percent), possibly related to the retention of the duodenum. An alternative method, the transplantation of only the islet cells, may eliminate the problems of wound and urinary tract sepsis which are characteristic of pancreas transplant recipients.

Issues related to the development of CMV infection, EBV lymphoproliferative disease, and infection with opportunistic pathogens are similar in patients receiving pancreas as in other solid organ transplant recipients.

VACCINATION OF TRANSPLANT RECIPIENTS

In addition to antibiotic prophylaxis (Table 96-8), transplant recipients should be vaccinated against likely pathogens (Table 96-9). In the case of BMT recipients, optimal responses cannot be achieved until after reconstitution; allogeneic transplant BMT recipients require reimmunization to be protected against pathogens, despite previous immunization of the donor and recipient. The situation is complex in the case of autologous transplants. T and B cells in the peripheral blood may reconstitute the response if they are transferred in adequate numbers. However, cancer patients (particularly those with Hodgkin's disease, in whom it has been extensively studied) on chemotherapy do not respond normally to immunization, and titers to infectious agents fall more rapidly than in normal hosts. Therefore, even immunosuppressed patients who have not had marrow transplants may need booster vaccine injections. If memory cells are specifically eliminated as part of a marrow "cleanup" procedure, it will be necessary to reimmunize the recipient with a new primary series. Optimal times for immunization for different transplant populations are currently being evaluated.

In the absence of compelling data as to the best time to immunize BMT recipients, it is reasonable to vaccinate both autologous and allogeneic transplant recipients with pneumococcal vaccine at 12 months after transplantation followed by another injection 12 months later (since the response to the initial vaccine is weak in the early posttransplantation period). The *H. influenzae* conjugate vaccine, *N. meningitidis* polysaccharide vaccine, and diphtheria, tetanus, and inactivated polio vaccines can all be given at these same intervals (12 and 24 months after transplantation). Some authorities recommend instead a new primary series for tetanus/diphtheria and inactivated polio vaccine (vaccination at 12, 14, and 16 months after transplantation). The live-virus measles/mumps/rubella vaccine can be given to autologous transplant recipients 24 months after transplantation and to most allogeneic bone transplant recipients if they are not maintained on immunosuppressive drugs and do not have ongoing GVHD.

In the case of solid organ transplant recipients, vaccination with all usual vaccines and the indicated booster shots should be given prior to immunosuppression, if possible, since responses will be improved. For patients on immunosuppressive agents, administration of the pneumococcal vaccine should be repeated every 6 years. No data are available for the meningococcal polysaccharide vaccine, but it is probably reasonable to administer it along with the pneumococcal vaccine. The *H. influenzae* conjugate vaccine is safe and should have efficacy in this population; therefore, administration is recommended prior to transplantation. Booster doses of this vaccine are not recommended in adults. Solid organ transplant recipients who remain on immunosuppressive drugs (glucocorticoids, cyclosporine) should

---

TABLE 96-9 Vaccination for bone marrow or solid organ transplant recipients

Vaccine	Bone marrow	Solid organ
Pneumococcus, H. influenzae, Meningococcus	After transplantation (optimal timing not established) preimmunization*	Immunize prior to transplant and every 6 years for Pneumovax (others not established)
Seasonal influenza	Yes	Before transplantation if possible
Poliomyelitis	Inactivated vaccine	Inactivated vaccine; live vaccine may be given prior to immunosuppression
Measles/ mumps/ rubella	Immunize 24 months after transplantation if no graft-versus-host disease	Prior to transplant
Tetanus, diptheria	Reimmunize after transplantation	Before transplantation; boosters at 10 years or as required; does not require new primary series

* Some studies suggest that it may be helpful to "immunize the graft" prior to transplant.

not receive live-virus vaccines. Thus a person in this group exposed to measles should be given immune globulin. Similarly, an immunocompromised patient who is seronegative for varicella and who comes in contact with a person who has chickenpox should be given varicella zoster immune globulin (VZIG) as soon as possible (and certainly within 96 h).

Immunocompromised patients who travel benefit from some but not all vaccines. If patients travel to areas where *N. meningitidis* meningitis or polio is common, they should be protected against these diseases. The current typhoid vaccines are not recommended for use in most immunocompromised patients because the inactivated preparation has too many adverse effects and the live vaccine is contraindicated. The yellow fever live vaccine also should not be administered. Phenol-inactivated cholera vaccine is probably of little use in this setting. On the other hand, immunization with the purified protein hepatitis B vaccine is reasonable if patients are likely to be exposed. The inactivated hepatitis A vaccine has not been licensed at this time but may have efficacy in this population as well. In the absence of an approved vaccine for hepatitis A, travelers should consider receiving passive protection with immune globulin (the dose depends on the length of travel in the high-risk area).

REFERENCES

ANAISSIE E et al: Fluconazole therapy for chronic disseminated candidiasis in patients with leukemia and prior amphotericin B therapy. Am J Med 91:142, 1991

DAUBER JH et al: Infectious complications in pulmonary allograft recipients. Clin Chest Med 11(2):291, 1990

DENNING DW, STEVENS DA: Antifungal and surgical treatment of invasive aspergillosis: Review of 2,121 published cases. Rev Infect Dis 12(6):1147, 1990

EMANUEL D et al: Cytomegalovirus pneumonia after bone marrow transplantation successfully treated with the combination of ganciclovir and intravenous immune globulin. Ann Intern Med 109:777, 1988

EORTC INTERNATIONAL ANTIMICROBIAL THERAPY COOPERATIVE GROUP: Empiric antifungal therapy in febrile granulocytopenic patients. Am J Med 86:668, 1989

ETTINGER NA, TRULOCK EP: Pulmonary considerations of organ transplantation (parts 1, 2, and 3). Am Rev Respir Dis 144:1386, 144:213, 144:433, 1991

GOODRICH JM et al: Early treatment with ganciclovir to prevent cytomegalovirus disease after allogeneic bone marrow transplantation. N Engl J Med 325:1601, 1991

HUGHES WT et al: Guidelines for use of antimicrobial agents in neutropenic patients with unexplained fever. J Infect Dis 161:381, 1990

KRAMER MR et al: Trimethoprim-sulfamethoxazole prophylaxis for *Pneumocystis carinii* infections in heart-lung and lung transplantation: How effective and for how long? Transplantation 53:586, 1992

KUSNE S et al: Infections after liver transplantation: An analysis of 101 consecutive cases. Medicine 67(2):132, 1988

RAAD II, BODEY GP: Infectious complications of indwelling vascular catheters. Clin Infect Dis 15:197, 1992

RUBIN RH, YOUNG LS (eds): *Clinical Approach to Infection in the Compromised Host.* New York, Plenum, 1988

———— et al: Infection in the renal transplant recipient. Am J Med 70:405, 1981

SHAH G et al: Incidence, prevalence and clinical course of hepatitis C following liver transplantation. Gastroenterology 103:323, 1992

SNYDMAN DR et al: Use of cytomegalovirus immune globulin to prevent cytomegalovirus disease in renal-transplant recipients. N Engl J Med 317:1049, 1987

STRATTA RJ et al: Successful prophylaxis of cytomegalovirus disease after primary CMV exposure in liver transplant recipients. Transplantation 51:90, 1991

THALER M et al: Hepatic candidiasis in cancer patients: The evolving picture of the syndrome. Ann Intern Med 108:88, 1988

TSEVAT J et al: Which renal transplant patients should receive cytomegalovirus immune globulin? Transplantation 52:259, 1991

WINGARD JR et al: Cytomegalovirus infection after autologous bone marrow transplantation with comparison to infection after allogeneic bone marrow transplantation. Blood 71:1432, 1988

WOLFSON JS et al: Dermatologic manifestations in immunocompromised patients. Medicine 64:115, 1985

WRIGHT TL et al: Recurrent and acquired hepatitis C viral infection in liver transplant recipients. Gastroenterology 103:317, 1992

ZUTTER MM et al: Epstein-Barr virus lymphoproliferation after bone marrow transplantation. Blood 72:520, 1988

97 EVALUATION AND MANAGEMENT OF PATIENTS WITH HOSPITAL-ACQUIRED INFECTIONS

DORI F. ZALEZNIK

Nosocomial infections are defined as infections acquired during or as a result of hospitalization. Generally, a patient who has been in the hospital for less than 48 h and develops an infection is considered to have been incubating the infection prior to hospital admission. Most infections manifested after 48 h are considered to be *nosocomial*. Patients may still develop a nosocomial infection after hospital discharge if the organism presumably was acquired in the hospital. Surgical wound infection developing in the weeks after hospital discharge is an example of nosocomial infection.

INCIDENCE AND COSTS Nosocomial infections contribute significantly to morbidity and even mortality, as well as to excess costs, for hospitalized patients. It is estimated that 3 to 5 percent of patients admitted to an acute care hospital in the United States acquire a new infection, which accounts for about 2 million nosocomial infections per year and an annual cost in excess of 2 billion dollars. Some estimate that the odds of death double in patients who develop a nosocomial infection, although clearly such factors as underlying disease and severity of illness also play an important role.

Although immunosuppressed hosts are especially vulnerable to infections acquired in a hospital, there are common nosocomial infections that occur even in normal hosts. The most common hospital-acquired infection is a urinary tract infection, accounting for about 40 to 45 percent of all nosocomial infections. Pneumonia accounts for 15 to 20 percent, surgical wound infection 25 to 30 percent, and bacteremia, mainly associated with intravascular devices, 5 to 7 percent.

The potential impact of nosocomial infections is considerable when assessed in terms of incidence, morbidity, mortality, and increased financial burden. These types of analyses examine nosocomial infections as medical and economic issues. The clinical problem for the physician is a patient in the hospital developing a new fever. In the evaluation of such a patient, information about the most common categories of infection may not be helpful. The clinician must use clinical clues from the patient's presentation and hospitalization as well as information about common hospital-acquired infections to diagnose a nosocomial infection.

The evaluation of a hospitalized patient with new fever should include a careful history. Particular attention should be paid to symptoms of headache, cough, abdominal pain, diarrhea, flank pain, dysuria, urinary frequency, and leg pain. Other features related to the hospitalization also are important, such as presence and type of intravenous devices, history or current use of a urinary catheter, surgical procedure if any was performed, and new medications administered, including those for surgical prophylaxis. The physical examination should be directed at possible sources of infection and should pay particular attention to the skin to look for rash or possible embolic lesions; lungs; abdomen, especially the right upper quadrant; costovertebral angles; surgical wounds, if present; and calves and current and old intravenous sites for signs of phlebitis. The laboratory evaluation of all hospitalized patients with new fever should include a complete blood count with differential, chest radiograph, and blood and urine cultures. Other diagnostic tests to consider, depending on the patient, include liver function tests, plain film or other study of the abdomen, routine aerobic cultures of sputum, stool, or other relevant body fluids, and testing of stool for *Clostridium difficile* toxin in cases of diarrhea.

CATEGORIES OF INFECTION   Pneumonia Although the astute clinician will question the patient thoroughly and perform a rapid, comprehensive physical examination, one way to approach the development of fever in a hospitalized patient is to consider potential infectious sites which may be life-threatening. One important infection to consider is pneumonia. Patients most at risk for developing nosocomial pneumonia are those in an intensive care unit (ICU), especially intubated patients; patients with altered levels of consciousness, especially those with nasogastric tubes; elderly patients; patients with chronic lung disease; postoperative patients; and any of the above patients taking H-2 blockers or antacids. Nosocomial pneumonia in the National Nosocomial Infections Surveillance (NNIS) Registry is diagnosed 0.6 to 1.0 times per 100 hospitalizations and is common in postoperative patients. In patients on ventilators, the occurrence of pneumonia may be 10 to 20 times higher. Mortality figures for nosocomial pneumonia are as high as 33 percent.

Oropharyngeal and gastric colonization play a critical role in the pathogenesis of pneumonia in the hospitalized patient. The oropharynx of hospitalized patients can become colonized by many species of aerobic gram-negative organisms within 48 h of hospitalization. Aspiration occurs commonly during sleep and is increased by such factors as a nasogastric tube, altered consciousness, decreased gag reflex, or delayed gastric emptying. In recent years, the role of gastric colonization in nosocomial pneumonia has been recognized. Bacterial counts in the stomach rise in the presence of medications that raise gastric pH, such as H-2 blockers and antacids, as well as in malnourished, achlorhydric, or some elderly patients. The prevalence of pneumonia in intubated patients is reportedly two to three times higher in patients receiving H-2 blockers or antacids for stress ulcer prophylaxis than in those receiving sucralfate, a medication that heals ulcers without altering gastric pH.

Gastric colonization is believed to influence development of pneumonia by retrograde colonization of the oropharynx. Ventilated patients are also at risk of developing pneumonia by leakage of bacteria around the cuff of the endotracheal tube and by nebulized bacteria from nebulizers, condensate within ventilator circuits, and humidifiers.

In patients outside intensive care, pneumonia should be suspected when a patient develops a new cough, fever, leukocytosis, sputum production, and a new infiltrate on chest x-ray. Diagnosis can be complicated in patients with congestive heart failure, in whom concomitant chest x-ray abnormalities are present, or in patients with chronic sputum production. Some organisms, such as *Legionella* spp., may not be associated with peripheral leukocytosis.

The signs of pneumonia are more subtle, and therefore, diagnosis of pneumonia often is more complex in ICU patients, especially those who are intubated. In particular, chest x-ray films are much more difficult to interpret, since fluid overload, congestive heart failure, and adult respiratory distress syndrome (ARDS) are all common findings in intubated patients. Polymorphonuclear leukocytes (PMNs) often are present on Gram's stains of the purulent secretions common in intubated patients. An important clue to pneumonia is a change in output or character of these secretions. If increased quantity or thickness or change in color of secretions is noted, a sputum Gram's stain should be performed and pneumonia seriously considered in the differential diagnosis. Serial Gram's stains are useful, since the number of PMNs may increase substantially, and the type(s) of organisms may shift. For example, the baseline sputum from an intubated patient may contain about 25 PMNs per high-power field and have mixed gram-positive and gram-negative organisms of several morphologic types in moderate amounts. On the day of a new fever, the same patient may have copious amounts of more tenacious sputum with more PMNs and a predominance of enteric-appearing gram-negative rods. Even without distinct changes in chest x-ray, this patient would be considered to have developed pneumonia. Another subtle sign of pneumonia in the intubated patient is a requirement for change in ventilator settings in the absence of (1) fluid overload, (2) a mechanical alteration such as a shift in endotracheal tube placement, or (3) the presence of a pneumothorax.

The major organisms of concern in nosocomial pneumonia are gram-negative aerobic organisms. In the NNIS survey, *Pseudomonas aeruginosa* was the leading pathogen causing nosocomial pneumonia in 1984, followed by *Staphylococcus aureus, Klebsiella pneumoniae,* and *Enterobacter* spp. While surveys of this kind are useful, it is essential to know which pathogens are common in a particular institution, since there are differences among hospitals in resident flora, particularly in ICUs. In some institutions, methicillin-resistant *S. aureus, Xanthomonas* spp., *Flavobacterium* spp., and even *Legionella* spp. may be of particular concern. Viruses such as respiratory syncytial virus and adenovirus as etiologic agents in nosocomial pneumonia in the adult and the pediatric population are receiving more attention. Viruses have been underrepresented as agents of nosocomial pneumonia because diagnosis is more difficult, and many microbiology laboratories do not have the capability to isolate viruses.

Antibiotic resistance is another important issue to address in the hospitalized patient. In addition to knowing the sensitivity patterns of the hospital flora, one must consider whether a patient has been on continuous or multiple courses of antibiotic therapy. To reduce the likelihood of altering the sensitivity patterns of the patient's flora, antibiotic courses for pneumonia should be kept as short as possible, with coverage as narrow as possible for the organism(s) involved.

Bacteremia   Another potentially life-threatening nosocomial infection to consider in the evaluation of the patient with a new fever is bacteremia, which is usually related to the presence of an intravascular device. While many common nosocomial infections such as pneumonia or urinary tract infection can be accompanied by bacteremia, a primary bacteremia is defined by isolation of a recognized pathogen from the blood without an infection at another site. The NNIS survey from 1989 reported bloodstream infection rates at 1.3 to 6.5 per 1000 patient discharges, with large teaching hospitals having the highest rates. In one study, bacteremia led to 14-fold higher in-hospital mortality, with length of stay increased by at least 2 weeks.

One difficulty in assessing the significance of bacteremia is to distinguish true pathogens from contaminating skin flora. This problem is especially important in establishing an infection of an indwelling intravascular catheter because organisms that inhabit the skin, such as coagulase-negative staphylococci, also commonly cause infection. The most common entry site for infection related to intravascular devices is at the insertion site, with spread of infection along the outside of the device initially. Other sources of entry, however, include contaminated infusates and tubing, introduction of organisms through ports or leaking connections, and hematogenous seeding of a catheter during bacteremia. While gram-negative aerobic bacilli are probably the most feared nosocomial bloodstream pathogens, the NNIS survey from 1980–1989 showed that these organisms had not increased in frequency of isolation over the decade. The bacteremia-associated group of organisms that increased the most in frequency was the coagulase-negative staphylococci, followed by *Candida* spp. Other leading causes of line-related bacteremia were *S. aureus* and enterococci.

For practical purposes, establishing an infection of an intravascular device or primary bacteremia as the cause of fever in a hospitalized patient is a diagnosis of exclusion. If a patient has a fever and signs of cutaneous involvement (erythema, induration, tenderness, or purulent drainage) at the insertion site of a catheter, full cultures should be obtained, the vascular access line removed, and the catheter tip sent for quantitative culture. Studies have correlated growth of 15 colonies or more from a catheter tip with infection of the line. More commonly, the exit site does not show signs of infection, and there is considerable debate about the necessity of removing a line at that point in a febrile patient. Unless another site of infection is obvious, it is generally advisable to remove a line when a patient develops a new fever. While central line changes over a guidewire have been shown to be safe, it is not clear that maintaining the same insertion site with possible line infection is wise. In general, when a line is removed for possible infection, the site should be changed. If vascular access is a problem and one wishes to continue intravascular therapy despite the intravascular device infection, it is probably not necessary to change the line over a guidewire. Traditional teaching suggested automatic removal of an infected intravenous device. In current practice, however, especially with surgically implanted intravenous catheters, a decision may be made to attempt treatment with antibiotics leaving the catheter in place. This practice often is successful when the infecting organism is a coagulase-negative *Staphylococcus* and less so with other organisms, particularly *Candida* spp.

Another controversial management issue is whether to draw blood for culture through a line. While some studies document correlation of cultures drawn through vascular access lines in the 90 percent range with peripheral blood cultures, there are both false-positive and false-negative cultures of blood obtained through a line. If the culture is positive and no peripheral blood has been drawn, it is impossible to determine whether the patient has a true bacteremia or the culture merely reflects bacteria associated with the line. In turn, if multiple peripheral blood cultures are positive, it is reasonable to assume that the line is at least infected secondarily. Whether a bacteremia is high grade or sustained may influence duration of antibiotic therapy and cannot be determined from cultures of specimens obtained through a line.

Surgical wound infection   Evaluation of fever in the postoperative patient must include careful evaluation of the surgical wound. Although surgical wound infection accounts for 25 to 30 percent of nosocomial infections, the true incidence of postoperative wound infection is difficult to assess, particularly at a time when patients are hospitalized for shorter periods. In a number of studies, careful follow-up for the development of wound infections after discharge, especially observation of the wound by a trained observer such as a nurse, has shown the actual rates of wound infections in all categories of surgery to be greater than reported rates. Surgical procedures have long been classified as clean, clean-contaminated, contaminated, and dirty-infected. The risk of wound infection varies from 2.9 percent for clean procedures to 12.6 percent for already infected sites. In 1985, a more sophisticated system was proposed for assessing risk of wound infection. This index uses abdominal operation, surgery lasting >2 h, contaminated or dirty-infected surgery by the classic wound classification system, and the presence of three or more diagnoses in the patient and predicts wound infection rates between 1 and 27 percent.

Other risk factors for the development of postoperative wound infection include the presence of a drain; preoperative length of stay, with the rates doubling for each week of extra preoperative hospitalization; preoperative shaving of the field, especially 24 h or more before the procedure; length of surgery; presence of an untreated remote infection; and surgeon. Perioperative antibiotic prophylaxis has been shown to decrease wound infection rates in a number of careful studies, including those of clean surgical procedures. Antibiotic coverage after the surgical wound is closed has not been shown to provide additional benefit.

A surgical wound should be examined for erythema extending more than 2 cm beyond the margin of the wound, localized tenderness and induration, fluctuance, drainage of purulent material, or dehiscence of sutures. Mechanical factors, as well as infection, can cause wound dehiscence. Sternal wounds following cardiac surgery are of special concern, since the consequence of infection can be great. The surface of the wound may not present an obvious cause for concern, but in some patients ongoing fevers and especially development of rocking or instability of the sternum may be sufficient cause for surgical exploration of the wound. Mediastinitis or sternal osteomyelitis is a severe complication of cardiac surgery. Wounds associated with the placement of prosthetic devices such as mechanical joints also are of special concern. Infection of these wounds can lead to infection of the prosthesis, which generally requires surgical removal to clear the infection.

Urinary tract infection   Urinary tract infections (UTIs) are the most common nosocomial infection and generally the easiest to treat with the least severe sequelae. In a study that controlled for potential confounding factors such as severity of illness, length of hospitaliza-

tion, and duration of catheterization, the overall case-fatality rate was 2.8 times higher in bacteriuric patients than in patients without bacteriuria. A follow-up study of sealed catheter junctions showed a decrease in this mortality rate associated with a decrease in UTIs. Four principal risk factors have been associated repeatedly with the development of UTI in hospitalized patients: female sex, duration of urinary catheterization, absence of systemic antibiotics, and breach of appropriate catheter care. Administration of systemic antibiotics in patients with urinary catheters in place for 1 to 5 days has been associated with a decrease in rates of bacteriuria. For patients with catheters in place for 6 or more days, however, this benefit is no longer observed.

The pathogenesis of catheter-associated UTI appears to differ in men and women. In women, periurethral colonization with fecal flora, with tracking of organisms up the catheter to the bladder, resembles the pathogenesis of UTI in noncatheterized female patients, in whom bacteria track up the short female urethra. In contrast, periurethral colonization often cannot be demonstrated in men; the majority of infections seem to arise from intraluminal spread of organisms to the bladder. Some organisms such as *Proteus* and *Pseudomonas* spp. appear to facilitate growth of a biofilm along the inside of the urinary catheter which encrusts and obstructs the flow of urine.

Although UTI is an extremely common nosocomial infection, it is important to define infection precisely. Especially in evaluating a febrile hospitalized patient, it is crucial to think carefully about all possible sources of infection and not to assume UTI is the probable cause. In patients who have had urinary catheters in place for a number of days, fever, dysuria, frequency, leukocytosis, and especially flank pain or costovertebral angle tenderness are highly suggestive of bladder infection or pyelonephritis. In patients with fever but no other symptoms or signs referable to the urinary tract, one should look for ancillary findings suggestive of urinary tract involvement, such as white blood cells without epithelial cells in the urine sediment or leukocyte esterase or nitrite on urinalysis. A urine culture positive for a single organism should not be accepted as definitive evidence of UTI in an asymptomatic patient. While one might treat the febrile patient with a positive urine culture with antibiotics, it is prudent to repeat the culture before the institution of therapy. Inability to recover an organism or the same organism on repeat culture, particularly if the patient does not respond to antibiotics, should raise questions about the validity of the diagnosis of UTI. In addition, isolation of two or more bacteria in a single specimen is most likely due to contamination unless there is reason to suspect a bladder diverticulum or a perinephric abscess.

Other infectious sources of fever   Several other types of infections may cause fever in the hospitalized patient and should be considered in the differential diagnosis of new fever. In patients who have received antibiotics, even a single dose as surgical prophylaxis, antibiotic-associated diarrhea may develop. This is caused usually by the spore-forming organism *C. difficile,* which produces toxins that cause diarrhea. Some patients may appear quite toxic with this infection, with high fevers, leukocytosis, and profuse diarrhea. The organism is quite hardy and is difficult to eradicate from the hospital environment. The hands of hospital personnel have been implicated as a mode of transmission of this organism, as have electronic rectal thermometers despite use of individual covering sheaths for each patient. The colon may become colonized with *C. difficile* while the patient is in the hospital, but particularly for patients still on antibiotics when sent home, diarrhea may not present until after discharge. Other infections to consider in the hospitalized patient include decubitus ulcers, particularly in patients on chronic care wards or confined to bed rest for prolonged periods, and sinusitis, especially in patients with nasotracheal tubes.

NONINFECTIOUS SOURCES OF FEVER   Several common noninfectious causes of fever in hospitalized patients also are part of a thorough evaluation of new fever. Drugs are the major noninfectious cause of fever. Drug fever may occur with or without an accompanying rash or eosinophilia and can be caused by new medication or by medications the patient has been receiving for some time. Particular agents associated with drug fever include phenytoin, H-2 blockers, procainamide, and antibiotics, most notably sulfonamides. Fevers, even drug-associated, can be quite high in some patients and may take up to 5 days to resolve after removal of the offending agent. Other noninfectious causes of fever include phlebitis, often at the site of an old intravenous line and sometimes followed by suppurative thrombophlebitis with clots or septic emboli, and pulmonary emboli, especially in patients on prolonged bed rest, although prophylactic heparin or mechanical boots often are used to reduce the risk of pulmonary embolism in these patients.

The range of possibilities for the etiology of a new fever in a hospitalized patient is quite broad. Attention to detail, a careful history and physical examination and knowledge of infections and organisms likely to cause nosocomial problems usually lead to an accurate diagnosis.

REFERENCES

HALEY RW et al: Identifying patients at high risk of surgical wound infection: A simple multivariate index of patient susceptibility and wound contamination. Am J Epidemiol 121:206, 1985

HOLTZ TH, WENZEL RP: Postdischarge surveillance for nosocomial wound infection: A brief review and commentary. Am J Infect Control 20:206, 1992

MARTONE WJ, GARNER JS (eds): Proceedings of the Third Decennial International Conference on Nosocomial Infections. Am J Med 91(suppl 3B), 1991

PLATT R et al: Epidemiology of nosocomial infections, in Infectious Diseases, SL Gorbach et al (eds). Philadelphia, Saunders, 1992, p 96

——— et al: Mortality associated with nosocomial urinary tract infection. N Engl J Med 307:637, 1982

WEBER DJ et al: Relative frequency of nosocomial pathogens at a university hospital during the decade 1980 to 1989. Am J Infect Control 20:192, 1992

98 INFECTION CONTROL IN THE HOSPITAL

ROBERT A. WEINSTEIN

The costs of nosocomial (hospital-acquired) infections are great, whether measured in dollars or in morbidity and mortality (see Chap. 97). Although infection control and hospital epidemiology activities have been the subjects of increasing scientific study over the past 20 years, efforts to lower infection risks have been continually challenged by the growing numbers of immunocompromised patients, of antibiotic-resistant bacteria, of fungal and viral superinfections, and of new invasive devices and procedures. Three international decennial conferences on infection control, organized by the Centers for Disease Control and Prevention (CDC), have clearly documented these formidable trends. This chapter reviews the basic surveillance and prevention activities that have been developed to deal with these problems and that form the foundation for current hospital epidemiology programs.

ORGANIZATION AND RESPONSIBILITIES OF INFECTION-CONTROL PROGRAMS The standards of the Joint Commission on Accreditation of Healthcare Organizations require all accredited hospitals to have an active program for surveillance, prevention, and control of nosocomial infections and a multidisciplinary infection control committee that meets not less than quarterly to oversee the program. The agents of the committee are the chairperson, preferably an infectious disease physician, and the infection control practioner(s), who are usually trained in nursing or medical technology and in epidemiology and public health.

In the 1970s, the CDC's extensive Study on the Efficacy of Nosocomial Infection Control found that hospitals that established programs with organized surveillance and control activities, a trained, effectual infection-control physician, and 1 infection-control practitioner per 250 beds experienced a 32 percent reduction in nosocomial infection rates, while rates in hospitals without effective programs increased by 18 percent. Since that study, however, the responsibilities and roles of hospital epidemiology programs have expanded in several ways. Diagnosis-related reimbursement has led hospital administrators to place increased emphasis on cost containment and on documenting that infection control is cost-effective. The quality-improvement movements and the Joint Commission's Agenda for Change have redirected infection-control attention, in part, beyond just writing policies and procedures to improving the actual processes and optimizing the outcomes. In a few hospitals, epidemiology programs have even taken on additional pharmacoepidemiologic and antibiotic utilization review reponsibilities. Finally, all programs must now respond to increasing governmental regulation of hospital waste and to Occupational Safety and Health Administration (OSHA)–mandated standards for protecting health care workers from occupational exposure to bloodborne pathogens and tuberculosis.

SURVEILLANCE Traditionally, infection-control practitioners survey inpatients for the occurrence of nosocomial infections (defined as those neither present nor incubating at the time of admission). Surveillance involves review of microbiology laboratory results, "shoe leather" epidemiology on the nursing wards, standardized definitions of infection, ongoing dialogue with hospital workers, and common sense. Some innovative infection-control programs have taken advantage of the increased use of computerized pharmacy, microbiology, and other data bases in hospitals to create algorithm-driven surveillance activities.

Because total hospital surveillance leaves little time for data analysis and education, most hospitals now aim surveillance at infections that have high morbidity (e.g., ICU-related infections and nosocomial pneumonia), are costly (e.g., cardiac surgery wound infections) or difficult to treat (e.g., those due to antibiotic-resistant bacteria), present recurring epidemic problems (e.g., Clostridium difficile–related diarrhea), and are potentially preventable (e.g., vascular access–related infections). Quality assurance activities in infection control have led to increased surveillance of personnel compliance with policies (e.g., monitoring actual use of universal precautions).

The results of surveillance are expressed as rates; e.g., 5 to 10 percent of patients develop nosocomial infections. Although such overall statistics are often requested of hospitals by administrators or surveyors, they have little value unless qualified by site of infection, by patient population, and by exposure to risk factors. Meaningful denominators for infection rates include the number of patients exposed to a specific risk (e.g., rates of pneumonia in patients on mechanical ventilators) and the number of intervention days (e.g., pneumonias per patient-days on a ventilator).

Temporal trends in rates should be reviewed, and ideally, rates should be compared with regional and national norms. However, even comparison rates generated by the CDC's ongoing National Nosocomial Infection Surveillance (NNIS) system, which collects data from over 100 hospitals that use standardized definitions of nosocomial infections, have not been validated independently and represent a nonrandom sample of hospitals. Interhospital comparisons are easily confounded by the wide range in risk factors and severity of underlying illnesses—unless rates are adjusted for these factors, comparisons may be misleading. Unfortunately, systems for making such adjustments either are rudimentary or have not been well validated.

The ongoing analysis of an individual hospital's infection rates helps to determine whether ongoing control efforts are succeeding and where increased education and control measures should be focused. Knowledge of infection rates also helps in discussions with the hospital administration regarding areas to which additional resources should be directed.

PREVENTION AND CONTROL MEASURES **Epidemiologic basis and general measures** Nosocomial infections follow basic epidemiologic patterns that help to direct prevention and control measures. Nosocomial pathogens have reservoirs, follow predictable modes of transmission, and require susceptible hosts. Reservoirs and sources exist in the inanimate environment (e.g., tap water contaminated with *Legionella*) and in the animate environment (e.g., infected or colonized health care workers, patients, and visitors). The modes of transmission most often are either cross-infection (e.g., indirect spread of pathogens from one patient to another on the inadequately washed hands of hospital personnel) or autoinoculation (e.g., aspiration of oropharyngeal flora into the lung along an endotracheal tube). Occasionally, pathogens (e.g., group A streptococci and many respiratory viruses) are spread indirectly from person-to-person by infectious droplets released by coughing or sneezing. Much less common, but often devastating in epidemic risk, is true airborne spread of droplet nuclei (e.g., as in nosocomial chickenpox) or common-source spread by contaminated materials (e.g., iodophors contaminated with *Pseudomonas*). Factors that increase host susceptibility include underlying conditions discussed elsewhere in this text and the many medical-surgical interventions and procedures that bypass normal host defenses.

The hospital's infection-control committee, through its infection control program, must determine the general and specific measures used to control infections and must review and recommend the specific antiseptics and disinfectants for hospital use. Given the prominence of cross-infection, handwashing is the single most important preventive measure in hospitals. There have been many studies of the antimicrobial activity of a large variety of antiseptic-containing handwashing agents. Such agents are important for handwashing before invasive procedures and possibly in intensive care unit (ICU) settings; however, given the poor general compliance with handwashing recommendations, the importance of handwashing with any hand cleanser between patient contacts cannot be overemphasized.

The fact that 25 to 50 percent of nosocomial infections are due to the combined effect of the patient's own flora and invasive devices highlights the importance of improvements in use and design of devices. Intensive educational programs can be associated with at least temporary reduction in infection rates through improved asepsis in handling and earlier removal of invasive devices, but sustaining such gains is often difficult. Nevertheless, it is encouraging to note that epidemiologic studies have been used increasingly to assess the value of newer devices and site-specific control measures, which are discussed below, and to debunk some traditional yet ineffective and costly measures, such as routine culturing of the environment and personnel for "pathogens."

Urinary tract infections Although urinary tract infections (UTIs) cause 40 to 45 percent of nosocomial infections, they contribute only 10 to 15 percent to prolongation of hospital stay and to extra costs. Almost all nosocomial UTIs are associated with preceding instrumentation or indwelling bladder catheters, which increase the risk of UTI by about 7 percent per day. As discussed in Chap. 97, UTI is caused by pathogens that spread up the periurethral space from the patient's perineum or gastrointestinal tract and by cross-infection via caregivers who are irrigating catheters or emptying drainage bags. Occasionally, pathogens come from inadequately disinfected urologic equipment and rarely from contaminated supplies (e.g., dilute aqueous benzalkonium chloride, an ineffective disinfectant).

Attempts at prevention have included the use of topical meatal antimicrobials, drainage bag disinfectants, antimicrobial-coated catheters, and sealed catheter–drainage tube junctions to eliminate inadvertent breaks in the system. Because of conflicting study results, none of these measures is considered routine. Systemic antimicrobials given for other purposes decrease the risk of UTI during the first 4 days of catheterization, after which resistant bacteria or yeasts emerge

as pathogens. Selective decontamination of the gut also is associated with a reduced risk; however, neither approach is routine. Moreover, irrigation of catheters, with or without antimicrobials, may actually increase the risk of infection.

Pneumonia Pneumonia causes 15 to 20 percent of nosocomial infections but is responsible for 24 percent of extra hospital days and 39 percent of extra costs. Almost all bacterial nosocomial pneumonias are caused by aspiration of endogenous or hospital-acquired oropharyngeal and gastric flora (viral pneumonias, which are particularly important in pediatric and immunocompromised patients, are discussed in Chaps. 96 and 220). Nosocomial pneumonia is associated with mortality rates up to 50 percent in ICUs; however, prevention of pneumonia often does not reduce overall ICU mortality, thereby suggesting that this infection is a marker for patients with otherwise heightened mortality risk. Surveillance and accurate diagnosis of pneumonia are often problematic because many ICU patients have abnormal chest roentgenograms, fever, and leukocytosis attributable to multiple causes.

Control measures are aimed at remediable risk factors in general patient care (e.g., minimizing supine aspiration-prone positioning and possibly avoiding prophylactic gastric alkalization because of increased risk of colonization with gram-negative rods when gastric pH is over 4) and at meticulous aseptic care of respirator equipment (e.g., disinfecting or sterilizing all in-line reusable components such as nebulizers, replacing tubing circuits at ≥48-h intervals rather than more frequently to lessen the number of breaks into the system, and teaching aseptic technique for suctioning). Two additional, more controversial issues have been the infection-control benefits of sucralfate, which provides stress ulcer prophylaxis without altering gastric pH, and of selective decontamination of the oropharynx and gut with nonabsorbable antimicrobials. Each approach warrants further investigation.

Surgical wound infections Wound infections cause approximately 25 to 30 percent of nosocomial infections but contribute up to 57 percent of extra hospital days and 42 percent of extra costs. They are usually caused by the patient's endogenous or hospital-acquired skin and mucosal flora and occasionally by airborne spread of skin squames that may be shed into the wound from members of the operating room team. True airborne spread of infection due to droplet nuclei is rare in operating rooms unless there is a "disseminator" (e.g., of group A streptococci or of staphylococci) among the staff. Because the average wound infection incubation period is 5 to 7 days, which is now longer than many postoperative stays, and because many procedures now are performed on an outpatient basis, over 50 percent of wound infections may not be detected unless postdischarge surveillance is performed.

The most important risk factors are the surgeon's judgment and operative technique, the patient's general health (e.g., presence of diabetes), and the specific operative procedure and its duration. The most important control measures include use of antimicrobial prophylaxis at the start of high-risk procedures, attention to technical surgical issues and operating room asepsis (e.g., not shaving the preoperative site until surgery and avoiding open or prophylactic drains), and preoperative therapy of any active infection. Reporting of surveillance results to surgeons also has been associated with reductions in infection rates. Interest in reporting results to surgeons, and the growing review of infection rates by regulatory agencies and payor sources, emphasizes the importance of stratifying rates by patient risk factors and of developing meaningful systems for interhospital comparisons.

Infections related to vascular access and monitoring Infection rates for peripheral intravenous (IV) catheters are very low (approximately 0.2 to 0.5 percent), but infections of central venous and arterial catheters are at least 20-fold more frequent, depending primarily on duration of use. Control measures include moving peripheral or arterial catheters to a new site at specified intervals (e.g., every 72 h for peripheral IVs), which may be facilitated by use of an IV team; using disposable transducers and aseptic technique when accessing transducers or other vascular ports; and removing "idle" catheters. Unresolved issues include the frequency for rotating central venous catheter sites (guidewire-assisted catheter changes at the same site do not lessen infection risk); the best antiseptics for site preparation and for catheter dressing; the appropriate role for mupirocin ointment, a topical antibiotic with excellent antistaphylococcal activity, for site care; whether newer designs—tunneled, totally implanted, or peripherally inserted central catheters (PICC lines)—offer a lessened infection risk than percutaneous central catheters; and the role of other costly catheter innovations, such as impregnating catheters with antimicrobials or attaching subcutaneous cuffs that contain bactericidal silver. In several studies, the use of semitransparent polyurethane dressings has increased infection rates, although these dressings have potential nursing benefits (ease of bathing and site inspection and protection of site from secretions).

Isolation techniques Written policies for isolation of infectious patients are a standard component of infection-control programs. The CDC recommends that hospitals use either category-specific (based on suspected infection) or disease-specific (based on likely mode of transmission) isolation. The category-specific system includes *strict* (e.g., for chickenpox), *contact* (e.g., for staphylococcal wound infections), *respiratory* (e.g., for untreated bacterial meningitis), *acid-fast bacillus*, or AFB (for *M. tuberculosis* infection, which has specific ventilation requirements, described below), *isolation and enteric* (e.g., for bacterial diarrhea), and *drainage/secretion* (e.g., for minor wound infections) precautions. Some hospitals also use blood and body fluid precautions, although universal precautions have largely supplanted them. For each of the six category-specific modes, a door sign lists the necessary protective measures (e.g., gown, gloves, and mask for strict isolation). In the disease-specific system, the caregiver checks off the appropriate measures on a generic isolation sign, on the basis of an understanding of the patient's infection and its specific mode(s) of transmission.

In body substance isolation, the preceding systems are abandoned in favor of instructing personnel to wear gloves for contact with any body substance or mucous membrane. Other barriers, such as gowns, are required if soiling or splashing is anticipated. For patients with airborne pathogens such as tuberculosis, additional isolation precautions are required (see below).

In addition to these three alternative systems, all hospitals are mandated by OSHA to provide annual in-service training in and to monitor compliance with universal precautions to protect health care workers from bloodborne pathogens, including HIV and hepatitis B and C viruses. In essence, these precautions are similar to body substance isolation and require gloves, gown, mask, and/or eye protection depending on the likelihood of contact or splash with *any* blood or potentially contaminated body fluids. Some hospitals use additional guidelines for handling infected mothers and their newborns and antibiotic resistance precautions for patients colonized or infected with problematic strains.

EPIDEMIC PROBLEMS Outbreaks are always big news but probably account for less than 5 percent of nosocomial infections. The investigation and control of epidemics in hospitals require that infection-control personnel develop a case definition, confirm that an outbreak really exists (since many apparent epidemics are actually pseudo-outbreaks due to surveillance or laboratory artifacts), review aseptic practices and disinfectant use, determine the extent of the outbreak, perform an epidemiologic investigation to determine modes of transmission, work closely with microbiology personnel to culture for common sources or personnel carriers as appropriate and to type epidemiologically important isolates, and heighten surveillance to judge the effect of control measures. Control measures generally include early reinforcement of routine aseptic practices while seeking compliance problems that may have fostered the outbreak, ensuring appropriate isolation of cases (and instituting cohort isolation and nursing if needed), and implementing further controls on the basis of the findings of the investigation. Examples of some potential epidemic problems follow.

Chickenpox When health care workers are exposed to chickenpox in the community or by patients with initially unrecognized infections or work during the 24 h before developing chickenpox, infection-control practitioners institute a varicella exposure investigation and control plan, which includes obtaining names of exposed workers and patients, reviewing medical histories and (if needed) obtaining serologic tests for immunity, notifying physicians of susceptible exposed patients, administering prophylactic varicella-zoster immune globulin and/or instituting early acyclovir treatment where appropriate, and furloughing susceptible exposed employees during the at-risk period for disease. The varicella vaccine, if approved by the FDA, could be used to decrease risk for susceptible employees.

Tuberculosis The resurgence of pulmonary tuberculosis in the United States since 1987 and a series of nosocomial outbreaks of multiply drug-resistant strains primarily involving patients with AIDS and caregivers have led to a reevaluation of tuberculosis control. Important control measures include prompt recognition, isolation, and treatment of cases; recognition of atypical presentations (e.g., lower-lobe infiltrates without cavitation); use of negative pressure, 100 percent exhaust, private isolation rooms with closed doors, and six air changes per hour; use of particulate respirator face masks by caregivers entering isolation rooms; possible use of HEPA (high-efficiency particulate arrest) filter units and/or ultraviolet lights for disinfecting air when other engineering controls are not feasible or reliable; and follow-up skin-testing of susceptible personnel who have been exposed to infectious patients before isolation.

Group A streptococci The potential for a group A streptococcal outbreak should be suspected when even a single nosocomial case occurs. Most outbreaks involve surgical wounds and are due to the presence of an asymptomatic carrier in the operating room. Investigation can be confounded by extrapharyngeal sites of carriage, such as the rectum and vagina. Carriers who have been linked to nosocomial transmission of group A streptococci are removed from patient care and are not returned until carriage has been eliminated by antimicrobial therapy.

Aspergillus *Aspergillus* spores are common in the environment, particularly on dusty surfaces. When hospital ceiling tiles are removed for access to electrical wiring or plumbing or when dusty areas are disturbed during hospital renovation, the spores become airborne. Inhalation of spores by immunosuppressed, particularly neutropenic, patients creates a risk of pulmonary and/or paranasal sinus infection and disseminated aspergillosis. Routine surveillance among neutropenic patients for infections with filamentous fungi, such as *Aspergillus* and *Fusarium*, helps hospitals to determine whether they have undue environmental loads. To lower the risk, hospitals should inspect and clean air-handling equipment on a routine schedule, review all planned hospital renovations with infection-control personnel and construct appropriate barriers, remove immunosuppressed patients from renovation sites, and consider use of HEPA filters for air supplied to rooms housing immunosuppressed patients.

Legionella Sporadic and epidemic cases of nosocomial *Legionella* pneumonia are most often due to contaminated potable water or to contamination of air-handling systems and predominantly affect immunosuppressed patients, particularly those receiving glucocorticoid medication. The nosocomial risk varies greatly by geographic region and within an area depending on the extent of hospital hot-water contamination, on the presence of high-risk patient populations, and on specific hospital practices (e.g., use of nonsterile water in respiratory therapy equipment.) Laboratory-based surveillance for nosocomial *Legionella* should be performed, and a diagnosis of legionellosis should probably be considered more often than it is. If cases are detected, environmental cultures (e.g., hot-water tank sediment, faucets, and showerheads) should be obtained. If cultures grow *Legionella* and typing of clinical and environmental isolates correlate, eradication measures should be pursued (see Chap. 113).

An alternative approach is to periodically culture water tanks and water on wards housing high-risk patients. If *Legionella* is found, a concerted effort should be made to culture for *Legionella* in all patients with nosocomial pneumonia.

Antibiotic-resistant bacteria   Outbreaks of antibiotic resistance reflect Darwinian selection of bacterial chromosomal mutations, spread of plasmid- and/or transposon-borne resistance among bacterial species, and/or (re)admission of patients chronically infected with resistant bacteria—all further complicated by clonal dissemination of resistant strains by cross-infections and occasionally by personnel carriers and/or environmental contamination. Outbreak control depends on close laboratory surveillance to allow early detection of problems, on reinforcing routine asepsis (e.g., handwashing), on barrier precautions for all colonized and/or infected patients, on use of patient surveillance culture surveys to more fully ascertain extent of patient colonization, on use of antibiotic control policies, and on timely epidemiologic investigation when rates increase. Colonized personnel who are implicated in nosocomial transmission and problematic patients may be decontaminated; e.g., methicillin-resistant *Staphylococcus aureus* colonization may be controlled by use of oral antibiotics, such as trimethoprim-sulfamethoxazole and rifampin, and topical agents, including hexachloraphene or chlorhexidine and mupirocin. In a few ICUs, selective decontamination has been used successfully as an emergency control measure for outbreaks of infection due to gram-negative bacilli.

EMPLOYEE HEALTH SERVICE ISSUES   Employee health services (EHSs) are a critical component of infection control. New employees should be processed through the EHS where a contagious disease history can be taken; evidence of immunity to a variety of diseases, such as hepatitis B, chickenpox, measles, and rubella can be determined; immunizations for hepatitis B, measles, and rubella can be given as needed and a reminder about need for yearly influenza immunization can be imparted; a baseline PPD skin test can be performed; and education about personal responsibility for infection control can begin. Evaluations of employees should be codified to meet the requirements of accrediting and regulatory agencies; e.g., the CDC recommends at least annual PPD skin testing of susceptible caregivers, and OSHA requires that employees who have potential exposure to blood or blood-containing fluids must receive free hepatitis B vaccination or sign a specific declination form.

The EHS must have protocols for dealing with employees who have been exposed to contagious diseases. The newest problem is counseling, treating, and following personnel after percutaneous or mucosal exposure to blood of HIV-infected patients. Protocols are also needed for dealing with caregivers who have common contagious diseases, such as chickenpox, group A streptococcal infections, respiratory infections, and infectious diarrheas, and for caregivers who have less common but very high visibility public health problems, such as chronic hepatitis B or HIV—for which exposure-control guidelines have been published recently by the CDC.

REFERENCES

BENNETT JV, BRACHMAN PS (eds): *Hospital Infections*, 3d ed. Boston, Little, Brown, 1992

CENTERS FOR DISEASE CONTROL: Report of the Nosocomial Infections Surveillance (NNIS) System: Nosocomial infection rates for interhospital comparison: Limitations and possible solutions. Infect Control Hosp Epidemiol 12:609, 1991

HALEY RW et al: The efficacy of infection surveillance and control programs in preventing nosocomial infections in U.S. hospitals. Am J Epidemiol 121:182, 1985

MARTONE WJ, GARNER JS (eds): Proceedings of the Third Decennial International Conference on Nosocomial Infections. Am J Med 91(suppl 3B):1S, 1991

section 4   Bacterial disease: general considerations

99   MOLECULAR MECHANISMS OF BACTERIAL PATHOGENESIS

GERALD B. PIER

The past decade has seen an explosion of information about the bacterial and host molecules that contribute to the infectious and disease processes, which are thought by many to consist of three stages: (1) bacterial entry and colonization of the host; (2) bacterial invasion and growth in host tissues along with elaboration of toxic substances; and (3) the host response. These three stages reflect the more traditional concepts of *infection* (presence of bacteria in a host) and *disease* (reaction to the infection)—terms that are often used interchangeably. Bacterial pathogenesis is the measure of an organism's capacity to cause disease and is a function of the myriad pathogenic or virulence factors elaborated by bacteria. These virulence factors may be classified in two groups: those that promote bacterial colonization and infection (usually surface molecules) and those that cause disease (often, but not exclusively, secreted toxins or toxic metabolites). In addition, the host's inflammatory response to infection can contribute greatly to the observed disease and its attendant clinical signs and symptoms. Knowledge of the molecular architecture of the bacterial surface (Fig. 99-1), its interaction with the host, and the host response are critical to an understanding of the basic process of infection and disease.

CELL WALL STRUCTURE OF GRAM-POSITIVE AND GRAM-NEGATIVE BACTERIA

GRAM-POSITIVE BACTERIA   Gram-positive bacteria have a typical lipid bilayer cytoplasmic membrane surrounded by a rigid cell wall that gives the organisms their characteristic shape, differentiates them from eukaryotic cells, and allows them to survive in osmotically unfavorable environments. The cell wall is composed mainly of peptidoglycan, a polymer of *N*-acetylglucosamine and its lactyl ether, *N*-acetylmuramic acid, with peptide side chains covalently bound to the lactyl group. The peptide chains consist of alternating D and L amino acids and are usually linked to each other by a pentaglycine bridge binding a terminal D-alanine on one peptide substituent to the penultimate L-lysine on a neighboring peptide. Variations in this basic structure have been described for a number of bacterial genera.

In addition, the cell walls of gram-positive bacteria contain teichoic acids, phosphate-linked polymers of ribitol or glycerol that can have additional compounds linked to available side groups. Lipid tails anchor these acids to the cytoplasmic membrane, giving rise to lipoteichoic acids. Some organisms have cell wall teichoic acids wherein the glycerol or ribitol phosphate polymer is directly linked to *N*-acetylmuramic acid in the peptidoglycan. The various substituents on teichoic acids are often responsible for the biologic and immunologic properties associated with disease due to pathogenic gram-positive bacteria.

Most pathogenic gram-positive bacteria have additional extracellular structures. These include surface polysaccharides (such as the

FIGURE 99-1 Schematic representations of bacterial surface structures. *A.* Cytoplasmic membrane and cell wall typical of gram-positive bacteria. *B.* Outer structure of a gram-negative organism (*OM* = outer membrane). *C.* Detailed structure of peptidoglycan showing backbone of *N*-acetylmuramic acid (*MurNac*) and *N*-acetylglucosamine (*GlcNac*); tetrapeptide bridges composed of L-alanine (L-*ala*), D-glutamate (D-*Glu-N*), L-lysine (L-*Lys*), and D-alanine (D-*ala*); and pentaglycine [*Gly(5)*] cross-bridges. *D.* Teichoic acid backbone. *E.* Detailed structure of lipopolysaccharide typical of *Salmonella* spp., including the lipid A sugars glucosamine (*GlcN*) and 4-amino arabinose (*AraN*) and the core sugars 2-keto-3-deoxyoctonate (*KDO*), heptose (*Hep*), glucose (*Glc*), galactose (*Gal*), and *N*-acetylglucosamine (*GlcNAc*). Hexagons depicting the O-specific chain represent variable monosaccharide residues that comprise this structure. (*Drawing courtesy of T.J. DiCesare.*)

group antigens of streptococci), capsular polysaccharides, and surface proteins and polypeptide capsules needed for survival in blood or useful for epidemiologic classification.

GRAM-NEGATIVE BACTERIA   In addition to having a cytoplasmic membrane and a peptidoglycan layer similar to but reduced from that found in gram-positive organisms, gram-negative bacteria are characterized by an outer membrane that is covalently linked to the tetrapeptides of the peptidoglycan layer by a lipoprotein; this protein also contains a special lipid substituent on the terminal cysteine that embeds the lipoprotein in the outer membrane. The outer layer of the outer membrane contains the lipopolysaccharide (LPS) constituent, and embedded in this membrane are special proteins with important functions, including maintaining the outer membrane's integrity, acting as a selective barrier for diffusion of molecules into the cell, serving as receptors for bacteriophages, and binding siderophores that scavenge iron for transport into the bacterial cell.

Lipopolysaccharide   The LPS is made up of a relatively conserved di-*N*-acetylglucosamine backbone linked β 1→6, containing phosphate groups on the reducing 1 and nonreducing 4′ carbons. The hydroxyl and amino groups on carbons 2, 3, 2′, and 3′ are esterified with 2-hydroxy fatty acids of varying length, and these fatty acids also can be derivatized on their 2-hydroxy residue with additional fatty acids. This structure is termed *lipid A* and likely possesses most

of the important biologic properties associated with LPS or endotoxin. Attached to carbon 6′ is the inner polysaccharide core, which is usually, but not always, composed of a di- or trisaccharide of 2-keto-3-deoxyoctonate (KDO). Some pathogens, such as *Vibrio cholerae*, do not use KDO here. Additional sugar substituents are linked to the inner core, forming a complete core that is somewhat conserved among related gram-negative pathogens. Attached to the complete core are the O polysaccharide side chains, which, when present, confer serologic variability on different strains within a species and provide protection for the cell against host proteins such as lytic complement components. O polysaccharides can be composed of a variety of monosaccharides, ranging from the common pentoses and hexoses to more complex and often unique structures such as pseudaminic acid (5,7- diamino-3,5,7,9-tetradeoxynonulosonic acid), which is found in LPS from some strains of *Pseudomonas aeruginosa* and *Shigella boydii* type 7. These sugars can be substituted by a variety of components, such as formyl, acetyl, and hydroxy-butyryl side chains; amino acids or peptides; and phosphate groups. This high level of chemical variability is thought to be key to bacterial pathogenesis in that it allows various strains of pathogenic organisms to avoid host defenses.

Pili   Pili or fimbriae extend through the outer membrane into the external environment. They are seen in electron micrographs as hairlike projections that may be confined to one end of the organism (polar pili) or distributed more evenly over the surface, with up to several hundred per cell. An individual cell may make multiple pili with different functions. Most pili comprise a major pilin protein subunit with a molecular weight of 17,000 to 30,000 that polymerizes to form the pilus. Some pili, such as the gal-gal binding pili of *Escherichia coli,* have additional proteins located at their tips that are functionally critical. The major function attributed to pili to date is mediation of the binding of bacteria to host tissues.

Flagella Flagella are long appendages attached to either one or both ends of the bacterial cell (polar flagella) or distributed over the entire cell surface (peritrichous flagella). Flagella, like pili, are composed of a polymerized or aggregated basic protein. In flagella, the protein subunits form a tight helical structure and show serologic variability among different species. Spirochetes such as *Treponema pallidum* and *Borrelia burgdorferi* have axial filaments similar to flagella running down the long axis of the center of the cell and swim by rotation around these filaments. Some bacteria can glide over a surface in the absence of obvious motility structures.

INITIAL STAGE OF BACTERIAL INFECTION: COLONIZATION OF HOST SURFACES

Most bacterial pathogens initially enter the host through a mucosal surface of the respiratory, ocular, gastrointestinal, or genitourinary tract. The skin can be an important site of bacterial colonization (particularly for staphylococci), and direct inoculation of pathogens into the host is always a risk factor for subsequent disease. Successful colonization usually requires bacterial adherence to the mucosal surface. The ability to adhere is most often attributed to the pili, capsular polysaccharides, and lipoteichoic acids exposed on the cell surface, although any surface structure is capable of mediating adherence to host tissues. Host targets for bacterial adherence are either the epithelial cells lining mucosal tracts or the mucous layer itself. In the latter case, the bacteria must circumvent the host's normal ability to clear mucus-embedded cells. Such circumvention is thought to occur in states like ciliary dyskinesis in the respiratory tract or chronic *P. aeruginosa* colonization of the respiratory tract of individuals with cystic fibrosis.

It now appears that an individual bacterial cell expresses multiple, often serologically variable adhesins and that the cell uses different adhesins during different stages of colonization. For example, most strains of *E. coli* express type 1 pili, whose binding to host tissues is inhibited by D-mannose. These pili appear to help these organisms bind to mucus. Strains of *E. coli* causing pyelonephritis express a different adhesin, the Pap or P pilus, that mediates binding to digalactose residues on globosides of the human P blood groups. Adherence here is due to minor components of the pilus proteins that are found only on the tip. *E. coli* cells causing diarrheal disease express receptors for enterocytes on the small bowel, along with other receptors termed *colonization factors.*

A common type of pilus found in *Neisseria* spp., *Moraxella* spp., *V. cholerae,* and *P. aeruginosa* appears to be involved in adherence of these organisms to target surfaces. These pili tend to have a relatively conserved amino-terminal region and a more variable carboxy-terminal region. For some species such as *N. gonorrhoeae* and *N. meningitidis,* the pili are critical for attachment to mucosal epithelial cells. For others, such as *P. aeruginosa,* the pili mediate only some of the epithelial cell adherence. *V. cholerae* cells appear to use two different types of pili for intestinal colonization. While interference with this stage of colonization would appear to be an effective antibacterial strategy, attempts to develop pilus-based vaccines for human diseases have not been highly successful to date. In some instances, diarrhea due to *E. coli* in pigs, calves, and lambs has been prevented by pilus immunization, but a recent trial of a gonococcal pilus vaccine in humans failed to demonstrate efficacy. The serologic variability among pili is one barrier to this approach.

Other bacterial structures involved in adherence to host tissues include specific proteins found among staphylococci that bind to human proteins such as fibrin, fibronectin, laminin, and collagen. These bacterial structures probably promote the normal colonization of the nares and skin. Fibronectin appears to be a commonly used receptor for various pathogens; a particular sequence, Arg-Gly-Asp or RGD, is critical to binding. Surface lipoteichoic acids promote adherence of streptococci to mucosal surfaces. The mucoid exopolysaccharide or alginate capsule of *P. aeruginosa* promotes binding of mucoid strains to respiratory mucins. Coagulase-negative staphylococci have emerged as important pathogens through their ability to colonize prosthetic devices and catheters commonly used in medical care; the surface capsular polysaccharide of these organisms promotes binding to the prosthetic material.

TISSUE INVASION AND TISSUE TROPISM

TISSUE INVASION Bacteria may invade deeper layers of mucosal tissue via intracellular uptake by epithelial cells or via traversal of epithelial cell junctions. Among virulent *Shigella* strains and invasive *E. coli,* outer membrane proteins are critical to epithelial cell invasion and bacterial multiplication. *Neisseria* and *Haemophilus* penetrate mucosal cells by poorly understood mechanisms before dissemination into the bloodstream. Staphylococci and streptococci elaborate a variety of extracellular enzymes, such as hyaluronidase, lipases, nucleases, and hemolysins, that are probably important in breaking down cellular and matrix structures and allowing the bacteria access to deeper tissues and blood. Organisms that colonize the gastrointestinal tract can often translocate through the mucosa into the blood and, under circumstances in which host defenses are inadequate, cause bacteremia. *Yersinia enterocolitica* can invade the mucosa through the activity of the invasin protein. Some bacteria (e.g., *Brucella*) can be carried from a mucosal site to a disant site by phagocytic cells (e.g., polymorphonulcear leukocytes, or PMNs) that ingest but fail to kill the bacteria.

A number of major pathogens cause disease without further invasion of host tissues; these include *Bordetella pertussis,* *V. cholerae, Clostridium tetani, Clostridium botulinum, Corynebacterium diphtheriae, Mycobacterium tuberculosis,* and *Mycobacterium leprae.* Some pathogens can cause both local disease (such as pharyngitis and epiglottitis, skin ulcerations, or diarrhea) and disease due to tissue invasion. Some pathogens require a breach in host tissues to cause deeper infections; an example of this situation is peritonitis due to *Bacteroides fragilis* or other intestinal organisms after bursting of the appendix or intestinal trauma. In such cases, bacterial factors are not critical for invasion.

TISSUE TROPISM The propensity of certain bacteria to cause disease by infecting specific tissues has been known since the early days of bacteriology, yet the molecular basis for this propensity is much less well understood than is viral tissue tropism. By analogy, receptor-ligand interactions may be expected to underlie bacterial tissue tropism, and some good evidence from studies of gastrointestinal infection supports this possibility. However, there is no well-accepted explanation of why *N. gonorrhoeae* colonizes and infects the human genital tract, while the closely related species *N. meningitidis* principally colonizes the human oropharynx. *N. meningitidis* expresses a capsular polysaccharide, while *N. gonorrhoeae* does not; however, there is no indication that this property plays a role in the different tissue tropisms displayed by these two bacterial species. *N. gonorrhoeae* can use the enzyme sialytransferase from host tissues to add *N*-acetyl neuraminic acid (sialic acid) to its LPS O side chain, and this alteration appears to make the organism resistant to host defenses. Whether this enzyme is present in a special form or amount in the genital tract of humans is not known. Bacteria with sialic acid sugars in their capsules, such as *N. meningitidis, E. coli* K1, and group B streptococci, have a propensity to cause meningitis, but this generalization has many exceptions. For example, all six recognized serotypes of group B streptococci contain sialic acid in their capsules, but only one of these serotypes (type III) is responsible for most cases of meningitis due to infection by these organisms. In addition, both *H. influenzae* and the pneumococcus can readily cause meningitis, and these organisms do not have sialic acid in their capsules.

DISEASE

Disease is a complex phenomenon resulting from bacterial colonization, invasion, toxin elaboration, and host response. Toxin elaboration is one of the best-characterized molecular mechanisms of bacterial pathogenesis, while host factors such as interleukin 1 (IL-1) and IL-6, tumor necrosis factor α (TNFα), kinins, inflammatory proteins and products of complement activation, and mediators derived from arachidonic acid metabolites (leukotrienes) and cellular degranulation (histamines) readily contribute to the severity of disease.

TOXINS Among the first diseases emanating from bacterial infection to be understood were those due to toxin-elaborating organisms. Diphtheria, botulism, and tetanus toxins are responsible for the disease associated with local infections due to *C. diphtheriae*, *C. botulinum*, and *C. tetani*, respectively. Enterotoxins produced by *E. coli*, *Salmonella*, *Shigella*, *Staphylococcus*, and *V. cholerae* contribute to diarrheal disease caused by these organisms. Staphylococci, streptococci, *P. aeruginosa*, and *Bordetella* elaborate a variety of toxins that cause or contribute to disease, including toxic shock syndrome toxin 1 (TSST-1), erythrogenic toxin, exotoxin A, and pertussis toxin. A number of these toxins (e.g., cholera toxin, diphtheria toxin, pertussis toxin, *E. coli* heat-labile toxin, and *P. aeruginosa* exotoxin) have adenosine diphosphate (ADP)–ribosyltransferase activity, wherein the toxins enzymatically catalyze the transfer of the ADP-ribosyl portion of nicotinamide adenine diphosphate to target proteins and inactivate them. The staphylococcal enterotoxins, TSST-1, and streptococcal pyogenic exotoxins have been shown recently to behave as "superantigens," stimulating certain T cells to proliferate without processing of the protein toxin by antigen-presenting cells. Part of this process involves stimulation of the antigen-presenting cells to produce IL-1 and TNFα, which have been implicated in many of the clinical features of diseases such as toxic shock syndrome and scarlet fever.

ENDOTOXIN The lipid A portion of gram-negative LPS has potent biologic activities that are thought to cause many of the clinical features seen in gram-negative bacterial sepsis. These include fever, muscle proteolysis, uncontrolled intravascular coagulation, and shock. This effect appears to be mediated by production from mononuclear cells of IL-1, TNFα, and perhaps IL-6. These molecules exhibit potent hypothermic activity via effects in the hypothalamus, increase vascular permeability, alter the activity of endothelial cells, and induce these cells to procoagulant activity. Numerous therapeutic strategies aimed at neutralizing the effects of endotoxin are under study, including the use of antibodies to lipid A and to TNF and the administration of the IL-1 receptor antagonist (IL-1RA), which blocks the binding of IL-1 to its cellular receptor. Unfortunately, the clinical trial of one human monoclonal antibody to endotoxin, HA-1A, was halted in January 1993 because of excess mortality in the treated group, and disappointing results with the IL-1RA clinical trial reported in February 1993 have raised some doubts about the efficacy of this drug. Whether future clinical trials of these reagents will show efficacy is unclear at this time.

BACTERIAL INVASION Some diseases are likely caused primarily by the presence of bacteria in tissue sites that are normally sterile. Invasion of the bloodstream by gram-negative rods gives rise to sepsis and bacteremia without obvious exotoxin involvement, although endotoxin is very important in this situation. Pneumococcal pneumonia is mostly attributed to the growth of *Streptococcus pneumoniae* in the lung and the attendant host inflammatory response; there is little evidence that bacterial toxins are important in this disease. Disease following bacteremia and invasion of the meninges by meningitis-producing bacteria such as *N. meningitidis*, *H. influenzae*, *E. coli* K1, and group B streptococci appears to be due solely to the ability of these organisms to get into these tissues and multiply. Most of the tissue destruction here results from bacterial growth and host inflammation.

If organisms are to effectively invade host tissues (particularly the blood), they must avoid the major host defenses of complement and phagocytic cells. This avoidance is most often accomplished through the presence of cell surface polysaccharides—either capsular polysaccharides or long O side chain antigens characteristic of the smooth LPS of gram-negative bacteria. These molecules appear to function by preventing activation and/or deposition of complement opsonins or by limiting access of phagocytic cells with receptors for complement opsonins to these molecules when they are deposited on the bacterial surface below the capsular layer. Another potential mechanism of microbial virulence is the ability of some organisms to present the capsule as an apparent self-antigen via molecular mimicry. For example, the polysialic acid capsule of group B *N. meningitidis* is chemically identical to an oligosaccharide found on human brain cells. The M proteins of group A streptococci appear to convey resistance to phagocytic activity in blood. Some bacteria such as *Brucella*, *Yersinia*, *Listeria*, *Francisella*, and *Mycobacterium* resist destruction inside phagocytic cells. Even in the absence of an obvious bacteremic phase, such as that seen in shigellosis, production of a smooth LPS is critical for bacterial pathogenesis and disease.

Immunochemical studies of capsular polysaccharides have led to an appreciation of the tremendous chemical diversity that can result from the linking of a few monosaccharides. For example, three different hexoses can link up in more than 300 different, potentially serologically distinct ways, while three different amino acids have only six different possible peptide combinations. This immunochemical diversity may be the reason why many pathogenic bacteria use capsular polysaccharides to avoid host defenses. Capsular polysaccharides have been employed as effective vaccines against meningococcal meningitis as well as pneumococcal and *H. influenzae* infections and are currently under development as vaccines against infections due to group B streptococci, *P. aeruginosa*, *Klebsiella*, *S. aureus*, and *S. epidermidis*. In fact, capsular polysaccharides can function as a vaccine against any organism expressing a nontoxic, immunogenic capsular polysaccharide. In addition, most encapsulated pathogens become virtually avirulent when capsule production is interrupted via genetic manipulation; this observation emphasizes the importance of this structure in bacterial pathogenesis. Some encapsulated bacteria may alter their expression of capsular antigens during pathogenesis, producing a capsule when avoiding host defenses (such as during bloodstream dissemination) but not when adhering to and invading an epithelial cell during mucosal colonization.

HOST RESPONSE The inflammatory response of the host is critical for interruption and resolution of the infectious process but also is often responsible for the signs and symptoms of disease. Bacterial infection promotes a complex series of host responses involving the complement, kinin, and coagulation pathways. Most likely, the initial recognition of a foreign pathogen involves the activation of complement, and the generation of molecules such as C3a and C5a initiate inflammation. Consequently, changes take place in endothelial membranes; receptors for inflammatory cells are produced on the luminal side of the blood vessel, causing these cells to adhere to the endothelium and migrate through the vessel wall to the site of infection. The subsequent production of factors such as IL-1, IL-6, and TNF leads to fever, muscle proteolysis, and other effects noted above. An inability to kill or contain the microbe usually results in further damage due to the progression of inflammation and infection. For example, in many chronic infections, degranulation of host inflammatory cells can lead to release of host proteases, elastases, histamines, and other toxic substances that can degrade host tissues. Chronic inflammation in any tissue will eventually lead to the destruction of that tissue and to clinical disease associated with loss of organ function, such as sterility from pelvic inflammatory disease caused by chronic infection with *N. gonorrhoeae*.

The nature of the host response is often a critical factor in the type of pathology associated with a particular infection. Most bacterial pathogens provoke either local or systemic inflammation or the formation of a granuloma or an abscess. Local inflammation, as noted above, produces local tissue damage, while systemic inflammation, such as that seen during sepsis, can result in the signs and symptoms of septic shock. The latter can occur with either gram-negative or gram-positive infections, and its severity is associated with the degree of production of host effectors such as IL-1 and TNFα. Disease due to intracellular parasitism arising from infection with bacteria that cause tuberculosis, leprosy, or brucellosis results from the formation of granulomas, wherein the host attempts to wall off the parasite inside a fibrotic lesion surrounded by fused epithelial cells that make up so-called multinucleated giant cells. A number of pathogens, particularly anaerobic bacteria, staphylococci, and streptococci, provoke the formation of an abscess. It has been suggested that a network of T cells is involved in abscess formation following inoculation of *B. fragilis* into the peritoneum of experimental animals to mimic human peritonitis. IL-8 may play a role in recruiting and activating PMNs during abscess formation. The outcome of a bacterial infection will depend on the balance between an effective host response that eliminates a pathogen and an excessive inflammatory response that is associated with an inability to eliminate a pathogen and with the resultant tissue damage that leads to disease.

REFERENCES

BITTERSUERMANN D: Influence of bacterial polysialic capsules on host defense: Masquerade and mimicry, in *Polysialic Acid,* J Roth et al (eds). Basel, Birkhauser-Verlag, 1993, p 11

BOSLEGO JW et al: Efficacy trial of a parenteral gonococcal pilus vaccine in men. Vaccine 9:154, 1991

CRABB JH et al: T cell regulation of *Bacteroides fragilis*–induced intraabdominal abscesses. Rev Infect Dis 12:S178, 1990

DAVIS BD: Bacterial architecture, in *Microbiology,* BD Davis et al (eds). Philadelphia, Lippincott, 1990, p 21

DENICH K et al: Frequency and organization of *papA* homologous DNA sequences among uropathogenic digalactoside-binding *Escherichia coli* strains. Infect Immun 59:2089, 1991

DINARELLO CA, THOMPSON RC: Blocking IL-1: Interleukin-1 receptor antagonist in vivo and in vitro. Immunol Today 12:404, 1991

GREENMAN RL et al: A controlled clinical trial of E5 murine monoclonal IgM antibody to endotoxin in the treatment of gram negative sepsis. JAMA 266:1097, 1991

ISBERG RR: Discrimination between intracellular uptake and surface adhesion of bacterial pathogens. Science 252:934, 1991

MARRACK P, KAPPLER J: The staphylococcal enterotoxins and their relatives. Science 248:705, 1990

MEKALANOS JJ: Environmental signals controlling expression of virulence determinants in bacteria. J Bacteriol 174:1, 1992

PIER GB et al: Complement deposition by antibodies to *Pseudomonas aeruginosa* mucoid exopolysaccharide (MEP) and by non-MEP specific opsonins. J Immunol 147:1869, 1991

ZIEGLER EJ et al: Treatment of gram-negative bacteremia and septic shock with HA-1A human monoclonal antibody against endotoxin: A randomized, double-blind, placebo-controlled trial. N Engl J Med 324:429, 1991

100 TREATMENT AND PROPHYLAXIS OF BACTERIAL INFECTIONS

GORDON L. ARCHER / RONALD E. POLK

The discovery and development of drugs able to prevent and cure bacterial infections have represented one of this century's major contributions toward improving human longevity and quality of life. Antibacterial agents are among the most commonly prescribed drugs of any kind worldwide. Used properly and appropriately, these drugs are lifesaving. However, their indiscriminate use drives up the cost of health care, leads to a plethora of side effects and drug interactions, and fosters the emergence of bacterial resistance, rendering valuable drugs useless. The rational use of antibacterial agents is dependent on an understanding of their mechanisms of action; their pharmacokinetics, toxicities, and interactions; bacterial strategies for resistance; and testing in vitro for susceptibility of bacteria to antibacterial activity. In addition, patient-associated parameters, such as the site of infection and both the immune and the excretory status of the host, are critically important to appropriate therapeutic decisions.

This chapter provides specific data required for making an informed choice of antibacterial agent. Throughout the chapter the term *antibacterial agent* is used to refer to all natural, synthetic, and semisynthetic compounds that kill bacteria or inhibit their growth. The term *antibiotic* is reserved for those compounds produced by living organisms.

MECHANISMS OF ACTION

Antibacterial agents, like all antimicrobial drugs, are directed against unique targets not present in mammalian cells. The goal is to limit toxicity to the host and maximize chemotherapeutic activity affecting invading microbes only. The mechanisms of action of the antibacterial agents to be discussed in this section are summarized in Table 100-1.

INHIBITION OF CELL WALL SYNTHESIS One major difference between bacterial and mammalian cells is the presence in bacteria of a rigid wall external to the cell membrane. The wall protects bacterial cells from osmotic rupture because of the difference between the markedly hyperosmolar (up to 20 atm) cell interior and the usually isosmolar or hyposmolar host environment. The structure conferring cell wall rigidity and resistance to osmotic lysis in both gram-positive and gram-negative bacteria is peptidoglycan, a large, covalently linked sacculus that surrounds the bacterium. In gram-positive bacteria, peptidoglycan is the only layer external to the cell membrane and is large (20 to 80 nm); in gram-negative bacteria, there is an outer membrane external to a very thin (1-nm) peptidoglycan layer.

Chemotherapeutic agents directed at any stage of the synthesis, export, assembly, or cross-linking of peptidoglycan lead to inhibition of bacterial cell growth and, in most cases, to cell death. Peptidoglycan is composed of a backbone of two alternating sugars, N-acetylglucosamine and N-acetylmuramic acid; a chain of four amino acids that extend down from the backbone (stem peptides); and a peptide bridge that cross-links the peptide chains. Peptidoglycan is formed by the addition of subunits (a sugar with its five attached amino acids) that are assembled in the cytoplasm and transported through the cytoplasmic membrane to the cell surface. Subsequent cross-linking is driven by cleavage of the terminal stem peptide amino acid. Antibacterial agents act to inhibit cell wall synthesis in the following ways.

Bacitracin, a cyclic peptide antibiotic, inhibits the conversion to its active form of the lipid carrier that moves the water-soluble cytoplasmic peptidoglycan subunits through the cell membrane to the cell exterior. Cell wall subunits accumulate in the cytoplasm and cannot be added to the growing peptidoglycan chain.

Glycopeptides (vancomycin and teichoplanin) are high-molecular-weight antibiotics that bind to the terminal D-alanine–D-alanine component of the stem peptide when the subunits are external to the cell membrane and still linked to the lipid carrier. This binding sterically inhibits the addition of subunits to the peptidoglycan backbone.

β-*Lactam* antibiotics (penicillins, cephalosporins, carbapenems, and monobactams; see Table 100-2), characterized by a four-membered β-lactam ring, prevent the cross-linking reaction called *transpeptidation.* Energy for attaching a peptide cross-bridge from the stem peptide of one peptidoglycan subunit to another is derived from the cleavage of a terminal D-alanine residue from the subunit stem peptide. The cross-bridge amino acid is then attached to the penultimate D-alanine by transpeptidase enzymes. The β-lactam ring of the antibiotic forms an irreversible covalent acyl bond with the

TABLE 100-1 Mechanisms of action and resistance for major classes of antibacterial agents

Antibacterial agent*	Major cellular target	Mechanism of action	Major mechanisms of resistance
β-Lactams (penicillins and cephalosporins)	Cell wall	Inhibits cell wall cross-linking	1 Drug inactivation (β-lactamase) 2 Insensitive target (altered penicillin-binding protein) 3 Decreased permeability (altered gram-negative outer-membrane porins)
Vancomycin	Cell wall	Interferes with the addition of new cell wall subunits (muramyl pentapeptides)	Alteration of target (substitution of terminal amino acid of peptidoglycan subunit)
Bacitracin	Cell wall	Prevents addition of cell wall subunits by inhibiting recycling of membrane lipid carrier	Not defined
Macrolides (erythromycin)	Protein synthesis	Binds to 50 S ribosomal subunit	Alteration of target (ribosomal methylation)
Lincosamides (clindamycin)	Protein synthesis	Binds to 50 S ribosomal subunit	Alteration of target (ribosomal methylation)
Chloramphenicol	Protein synthesis	Binds to 50 S ribosomal subunit	Drug inactivation (chloramphenicol acetyltransferase)
Tetracycline	Protein synthesis	Binds to 30 S ribosomal subunit	1 Decreased intracellular drug accumulation (active efflux) 2 Insensitive target
Aminoglycosides (gentamicin)	Protein synthesis	Binds to 30 S ribosomal subunit	Drug inactivation (aminoglycoside-modifying enzyme)
Mupirocin	Protein synthesis	Inhibits isoleucine t-RNA synthetase	Insensitive target (mutation of target gene or acquisition of gene for new, insensitive enzyme)
Sulfonamides and trimethoprim	Cell metabolism	Competitively inhibits enzymes involved in two steps of folic acid biosynthesis	Production of insensitive targets [dihydropteroic acid (sulfonamides) and dihydrofolic acid (trimethoprim)] that bypass metabolic block
Rifampin	DNA synthesis	Inhibits DNA-dependent RNA polymerase	Insensitive target (mutation of polymerase gene)
Metronidazole	DNA synthesis	Intracellularly generates short-lived reactive intermediates by electron transfer system	Not defined
Quinolones (ciprofloxacin)	DNA synthesis	Inhibition of DNA gyrase (A subunit)	1 Insensitive target (mutation of gyrase genes) 2 Decreased intracellular accumulation (active efflux)
Novobiocin	DNA synthesis	Inhibition of DNA gyrase (B subunit)	Not defined
Polymixins (polymyxin B)	Cell membrane	Disrupts membrane permeability by charge alteration	Not defined
Gramicidin	Cell membrane	Forms pores	Not defined

* Compounds in parentheses are major representatives for the class.

transpeptidase enzyme (probably because of the antibiotic's steric similarity to the enzyme's D-alanine–D-alanine target), preventing the cross-linking reaction. Transpeptidases and similar enzymes involved in cross-linking are called *penicillin-binding proteins* (PBPs) because they all have active sites that bind β-lactam antibiotics.

Virtually all the antibiotics that inhibit bacterial cell wall synthesis are bactericidal. That is, they eventually result in the cell's death due to osmotic lysis. However, much of the loss of cell wall integrity following treatment with cell wall–active agents is due to the bacteria's own cell wall–remodeling enzymes (autolysins) that cleave peptidoglycan bonds in the normal course of cell growth. In the presence of antibacterial agents that inhibit cell wall growth, autolysis proceeds without normal cell wall repair; weakness and eventual cellular lysis occur.

TABLE 100-2 β-Lactam antibiotics

Class	Route of administration	
	Parenteral	Oral
Penicillins		
β-Lactamase susceptible		
Narrow spectrum	Penicillin G	Penicillin V
Enteric active	Ampicillin	Amoxicillin, ampicillin
Enteric active and antipseudomonal	Carbenicillin, ticarcillin, mezlocillin, azlocillin, piperacillin	Indanyl carbenicillin
β-Lactamase resistant		
Antistaphylococcal	Methicillin, oxacillin, nafcillin	Cloxacillin, dicloxacillin
Combinations with β-lactamase inhibitors	Ticarcillin plus clavulanic acid, ampicillin plus sulbactam	Amoxicillin plus clavulanic acid
Cephalosporins		
First generation	Cefazolin, cephalothin, cephapirin	Cephalexin, cephradine, cefadroxil
Second generation		
Haemophilus active	Cefamandole, cefuroxime, cefonicid, ceforanide	Cefaclor, cefuroxime axetil, cefixime,* cefprozil, cefpodoxime,* loracarbef
Bacteroides active	Cefoxitin, cefotetan, cefmetazole	None
Third-generation		
Extended-spectrum	Ceftriaxone, cefotaxime, ceftizoxime	None
Extended-spectrum and antipseudomonal	Ceftazidime, cefoperazone	
Carbapenems	Imipenem-cilastatin	None
Monobactams	Aztreonam	None

* Some sources classify cefixime and cefpodoxime as a third-generation oral agents because of a marginally broader spectrum.

INHIBITION OF PROTEIN SYNTHESIS Most of the antibacterial agents that inhibit protein synthesis interact with the bacterial ribosome. The difference between the composition of bacterial and mammalian ribosomes gives these compounds their selectivity.

Aminoglycosides (gentamicin, kanamycin, tobramycin, streptomycin, netilmicin, neomycin, and amikacin) are a group of structurally related compounds containing three linked hexose sugars. They exert a bactericidal effect by binding irreversibly to the 30 S subunit of the bacterial ribosome and blocking initiation of protein synthesis. The reason for the lethal effect of aminoglycosides—as opposed to the largely bacteriostatic effect of other protein synthesis–inhibiting antibacterial drugs (macrolides, lincosamides, chloramphenicol, and tetracycline)—is not completely understood. Uptake of aminoglycosides and their penetration through the cell membrane constitute an aerobic, energy-dependent process. Thus aminoglycoside activity is markedly reduced in an anaerobic environment. *Spectinomycin*, an aminocyclitol antibiotic, also acts on the 30 S ribosomal subunit but has a different mechanism of action from the aminoglycosides and is bacteriostatic rather than bactericidal.

Macrolides (erythromycin, clarithromycin, and azithromycin) are antibiotics that consist of a large lactone ring to which sugars are attached. They bind specifically to the 50 S portion of the bacterial ribosome. After attachment of mRNA to the initiation site of the 30 S ribosomal subunit (the process blocked by aminoglycosides), the 50 S subunit becomes bound to the 30 S component to form the 70 S ribosomal complex, and protein chain elongation proceeds. Binding of macrolides to the 50 S ribosomal subunit inhibits protein chain elongation.

Lincosamides (clindamycin and lincomycin), although structurally unrelated to macrolides, bind to a site on the 50 S ribosome nearly identical to the binding site for macrolides. Although the mechanism and site of action of macrolides and lincosamides are similar, the number and type of bacteria against which these two groups of agents are active differ.

Chloramphenicol, a small antibiotic with a single aromatic ring and short side chain, binds reversibly to the 50 S portion of the bacterial ribosome at a site close but not identical to the sites binding the macrolides and lincosamides. The ribosomal binding of chloramphenicol inhibits peptide bond formation.

Tetracyclines (tetracycline, doxycycline, and minocycline) consist of four aromatic rings with various substituent groups. They interact reversibly with the bacterial 30 S ribosomal subunit, blocking the binding of aminoacyl tRNA to the mRNA-ribosome complex. This mechanism is markedly different from that of the aminoglycosides, which also bind to the 30 S subunit. The specificity of tetracyclines for bacteria depends both on their selectivity for bacterial (as opposed to mammalian) ribosomes and on their requirement for active, energy-dependent transport into the bacterial cell by a system not found in mammalian cell membranes.

Mupirocin (pseudomonic acid) is produced by the bacterium *Pseudomonas fluorescens*. Its mechanism of action is unique in that it inhibits the enzyme isoleucine tRNA synthetase by competing with bacterial isoleucine for its binding site on the enzyme. Inhibition of this enzyme depletes cellular stores of isoleucine-charged tRNA and therefore leads to a cessation of protein synthesis. The antibiotic is selective for bacteria because of the lack of affinity of mammalian isoleucine tRNA synthetase for the compound.

INHIBITION OF BACTERIAL METABOLISM The antimetabolites are all synthetic compounds that interfere with bacterial synthesis of folic acid. Products of the folic acid synthesis pathway function as coenzymes for the one-carbon transfer reactions that are essential for the synthesis of thymidine, all purines, and several amino acids. Inhibition of folate synthesis leads to cessation of cell growth and, in some cases, to bacterial cell death. The principal antibacterial antimetabolites are sulfonamides (sulfisoxazole, sulfadiazine, and sulfamethoxazole) and trimethoprim.

Sulfonamides are structural analogues of *p*-aminobenzoic acid (PABA), one of the three structural components of folic acid (the

other two being pteridine and glutamate). The first step in the synthesis of folic acid is the addition of PABA to pteridine by the enzyme dihydropteroic acid synthetase. Sulfonamides compete with PABA as substrates for the enzyme. The selective effect of sulfonamides is due to the fact that bacteria synthesize folic acid while mammalian cells cannot synthesize the cofactor and must have exogenous supplies. However, the activity of sulfonamides can be greatly reduced in the presence of excess PABA or by the exogenous addition of end products of one-carbon transfer reactions (e.g., thymidine and purines). High concentrations of the latter substances may be present in some infections as a result of tissue and white cell breakdown, compromising sulfonamide activity.

Trimethoprim is a diaminopyrimidine, a structural analogue of the pteridine moiety of folic acid. It is a competitive inhibitor of dihydrofolate reductase, the enzyme responsible for reduction of dihydrofolic acid to tetrahydrofolic acid, the essential final component in the folic acid synthesis pathway, necessary for all one-carbon transfer reactions. Like the sulfonamides, trimethoprim is bactericidal in the absence of thymine but is only bacteriostatic when this pyrimidine is present in high concentration. The selective antibacterial activity of trimethoprim is based on the extreme sensitivity of bacterial dihydrofolate reductase to inhibition by this drug in comparison with the mammalian enzyme. The bacterial enzyme is approximately 50,000 times more sensitive to such inhibition.

INHIBITION OF NUCLEIC ACID SYNTHESIS OR ACTIVITY Numerous antibacterial compounds have disparate effects on nucleic acids. The *quinolones*, including nalidixic acid and its fluorinated derivatives (norfloxacin, ciprofloxacin, ofloxacin, and lomefloxacin), are synthetic compounds that inhibit the activity of one of the subunits (the A subunit) of the bacterial enzyme DNA gyrase. DNA gyrase is responsible for negative supercoiling of DNA, an essential conformation for DNA replication in the intact cell. Inhibition of the activity of DNA gyrase is lethal to bacterial cells. The antibiotic *novobiocin* also interferes with the activity of DNA gyrase, but it interferes with the B subunit.

Rifampin, used primarily as an antituberculous agent, is an antibiotic that is also active against a variety of bacteria other than *Mycobacterium tuberculosis*. Rifampin binds tightly to bacterial DNA–dependent RNA polymerase, thus inhibiting transcription of DNA into RNA. Mammalian cell RNA polymerase is not sensitive to the compound.

Nitrofurantoin, a synthetic compound, causes DNA damage. The nitrofurans, compounds containing a single five-membered ring, are reduced by a bacterial enzyme to highly reactive, short-lived intermediates that are thought to cause DNA strand breakage, either directly or indirectly.

Metronidazole, a synthetic compound, is an imidazole that has activity against a wide range of anaerobic bacteria and protozoa. This activity is totally dependent on the organism's system for anaerobic energy production. In the presence of the anaerobic electron transport system, the nitro group of metronidazole is reduced to a series of transiently produced, reactive intermediates that are thought to cause DNA damage. Although the unique redox system of anaerobes accounts for the selective antibacterial activity of metronidazole, this compound is also a mutagen and a radiosensitizer of hypoxic mammalian cells.

ALTERATION OF CELL MEMBRANE PERMEABILITY The *polymyxins* (polymyxin B and colistin, or polymyxin E) are cyclic, basic polypeptides. They behave as cationic, surface-active compounds that disrupt the permeability of both the outer and the cytoplasmic membranes of gram-negative bacteria.

Gramicidin A is a polypeptide of 15 amino acids that acts as an ionophore, forming pores or channels in lipid bilayers.

MECHANISMS OF RESISTANCE

Some bacteria are *intrinsically resistant* to certain classes of antibacterial agents (e.g., obligate anaerobic bacteria to aminoglycosides and gram-negative bacteria to vancomycin). Clearly these agents can never be used alone in the treatment of infections caused by resistant bacteria. However, bacteria that are ordinarily susceptible to antibacterial agents can acquire resistance. *Acquired resistance* is one of the major limitations to effective antibacterial chemotherapy. Resistance can develop by mutation of resident genes or by acquisition of new genes. New genes mediating resistance are usually spread from cell to cell by way of mobile genetic elements such as plasmids, transposons, and bacteriophages. The resistant bacterial populations flourish in areas of high antimicrobial use, where they enjoy a selective advantage over susceptible populations.

The major mechanisms used by bacteria to resist the action of antimicrobial agents are destruction of the compound, alteration or overproduction of the antibacterial target, decreased permeability of the cell envelope to the agent, and active elimination of the compound from the interior of the cell. Specific mechanisms of bacterial resistance to the major antibacterial agents are outlined below and are summarized in Table 100-1.

β-LACTAMS Bacteria develop resistance to β-lactam antibiotics by a variety of mechanisms. Most common is the destruction of the drug by β-lactamases. These enzymes have a higher affinity for the antibiotic than the antibiotic has for its target. Binding results in hydrolysis of the β-lactam ring. Genes encoding β-lactamases have been found in both chromosomal and extrachromosomal locations and in both gram-positive and gram-negative bacteria; these genes are often on mobile genetic elements. One strategy that has been devised for circumventing resistance mediated by β-lactamases is to combine the susceptible β-lactam with an inhibitor that avidly binds the inactivating enzyme, preventing its attack on the antibiotic. Unfortunately, the inhibitors (e.g., clavulanic acid and sulbactam) do not bind all classes of β-lactamase and cannot be depended on to prevent the inactivation of β-lactam antibiotics by all β-lactamases. No β-lactam antibiotic or inhibitor has been produced that can resist all of the many β-lactamases that have been identified.

A second mechanism of bacterial resistance to β-lactam antibiotics is an alteration in PBP targets so that the PBPs have a markedly reduced affinity for the drug. While this alteration may occur by mutation of existing genes, the acquisition of new PBP genes (as in staphylococcal resistance to methicillin) or of new pieces of PBP genes (as in pneumococcal, gonococcal, and meningococcal resistance to penicillin) is more important.

A final resistance mechanism is the alteration by gram-negative bacteria of their outer membrane so that it is no longer permeable to the antibiotic. Mutations of genes encoding the outer membrane proteins called *porins* mediate this alteration in permeability. The resistance of Enterobacteriaceae to some cephalosporins and that of *Pseudomonas* spp. to ureidopenicillins are the best examples of this mechanism. More than one of these resistance mechanisms commonly coexist in the same bacterial cell.

VANCOMYCIN Clinically important resistance to vancomycin was first described among enterococci in France in 1988. Vancomycin-resistant enterococci have subsequently become disseminated worldwide. The genes encoding resistance are carried on plasmids that can transfer themselves from cell to cell. Resistance is mediated by enzymes that alter the terminal amino acid on the peptidoglycan stem peptide so that there is no longer an appropriate target for vancomycin binding. This alteration does not appear to affect cell wall integrity, however. Vancomycin resistance is so far confined to enterococci and one species of coagulase-negative staphylococci (*Staphylococcus haemolyticus*); *S. aureus* and *S. epidermidis* remain susceptible.

AMINOGLYCOSIDES The most common resistance mechanism is inactivation of the antibiotic. Aminoglycoside-modifying enzymes, usually encoded on plasmids, transfer phosphate, adenyl, or acetyl residues from intracellular molecules to hydroxyl or amino side groups on the antibiotic. The modified antibiotic is less active because of decreased transport across the cytoplasmic membrane and diminished binding to its ribosomal target. Modifying enzymes that can inactivate

any of the available aminoglycosides have been found in both gram-positive and gram-negative bacteria.

A second resistance mechanism that is uncommon but has been identified in clinical isolates of *P. aeruginosa* is decreased antibiotic uptake, presumably due to alterations in the outer membrane.

MACROLIDES AND LINCOSAMIDES Resistance in gram-positive bacteria, the usual target organisms for macrolides and lincosamides, is due to the production of an enzyme—most commonly plasmid-encoded—that methylates ribosomal RNA, interfering with binding of the antibiotics to their target. Methylation mediates resistance to erythromycin, newer macrolides, and clindamycin. However, the enzyme usually needs to be induced by exposure to low concentrations of macrolides before resistance is fully expressed; clindamycin is a poor inducer. The need for induction can lead to false reports of susceptibility when bacterial isolates are tested in vitro.

CHLORAMPHENICOL Most bacteria resistant to this antibiotic produce a plasmid-encoded enzyme, chloramphenicol acetyltransferase, that inactivates the compound by acetylation. Occasionally, gram-negative bacteria acquire a mutation affecting the permeability of the outer membrane to this antibiotic.

TETRACYCLINE The most common mechanism of resistance in gram-negative bacteria is a plasmid-encoded active-efflux pump that is inserted into the cytoplasmic membrane and extrudes antibiotic from the cell. Resistance in gram-positive bacteria is due either to active efflux or to ribosomal alterations that diminish binding of the antibiotic to its target. Genes involved in ribosomal protection are found on mobile genetic elements.

MUPIROCIN Although this topical compound was only recently introduced into clinical use, resistance is already becoming widespread in some areas. The mechanisms appear to be mutation of the target isoleucine tRNA synthetase so that it is no longer inhibited by the antibiotic or plasmid-encoded production of a form of the target enzyme that binds mupirocin poorly.

TRIMETHOPRIM AND SULFONAMIDES The most prevalent resistance mechanism in both gram-positive and gram-negative bacteria is the acquisition of plasmid-encoded genes that produce a new, drug-insensitive target. Bacteria produce an insensitive dihydrofolate reductase for trimethoprim and an altered dihydropteroate synthetase for sulfonamides.

QUINOLONES Resistance to the newer fluoroquinolones emerged rapidly among *Staphylococcus* and *Pseudomonas* spp. after the introduction of these agents. The most common mechanism is the development of one or more mutations in the target DNA gyrase so that the antibacterial agent no longer interferes with the activity of the enzyme. Some gram-negative bacteria also acquire mutations in their outer-membrane porins so that cells are no longer permeable to the drugs; some gram-positive bacteria develop a mutation that allows them to actively pump the antibacterial agents from the cell.

RIFAMPIN Bacteria rapidly become resistant to rifampin by developing mutations in RNA polymerase that render the enzyme unable to bind the antibiotic. The rapid selection of resistant mutants is the major limitation to the use of this antibiotic against otherwise susceptible staphylococci and requires that it be used in combination with another antistaphylococcal agent.

MULTIPLE ANTIBIOTIC RESISTANCE Acquired resistance of one bacterium to multiple antibacterial agents is becoming increasingly common. The two major mechanisms are the acquisition of multiple unrelated resistance genes and the development of mutations in a single gene or gene complex that mediate resistance to a series of unrelated compounds. The construction of multiresistant strains by acquisition of multiple genes occurs by sequential steps of gene transfer and environmental selection in areas of high antimicrobial use. In contrast, mutations in a single gene can conceivably be selected in a single step. Bacteria that are multiresistant by virtue of the acquisition of new genes include hospital-associated gram-negative bacteria, enterococci and staphylococci, and community-acquired strains of salmonellae, gonococci, and pneumococci. Most of the latter bacterial isolates originated in other countries but have become established in some areas of the United States. Mutations that confer resistance to multiple unrelated antimicrobial agents occur in the outer-membrane proteins (porins) of gram-negative bacteria. These mutations affect the permeability of these bacteria to β-lactams, quinolones, tetracycline, chloramphenicol, and trimethoprim. Multi-resistant bacterial isolates pose increasing problems in U.S. hospitals; strains resistant to all available antibacterial chemotherapy have already been identified.

PHARMACOKINETICS

The *pharmacokinetic profile* of an antibacterial agent refers to concentrations in serum and tissue versus time after administration of the drug and reflects the processes of absorption, distribution, metabolism, and excretion. Important characteristics include peak and trough serum concentrations and mathematically derived parameters such as half-life, clearance, and distribution volume. Pharmacokinetic information is useful for estimating the appropriate antibacterial dose and frequency of administration, for adjusting dosages in patients with impaired excretory capacity, and for comparing one drug with another.

ABSORPTION Data on absorption can refer to oral, intramuscular (IM), or intravenous (IV) administration.

Oral administration Most patients with infection are treated with oral antibacterial agents in the outpatient setting. Advantages of oral therapy over parenteral therapy include lower costs, generally fewer adverse effects (including complications of indwelling lines), and greater acceptance by patients. The percentage of an orally administered antibacterial agent that is absorbed (i.e., the agent's *bioavailability*) ranges from as little as 10 to 20 percent (erythromycin and penicillin G) to nearly 100 percent (clindamycin, metronidazole, doxycycline, and trimethoprim-sulfamethoxazole). These differences in bioavailability are not clinically important as long as concentrations at the site of infection are sufficient to inhibit or kill the pathogen. However, therapeutic efficacy may be compromised when absorption is reduced as a result of physiologic or pathologic conditions (such as the presence of food for some drugs or the shunting of blood away from the gastrointestinal tract in the patient with hypotension), drug interactions (such as that of quinolones and metal cations), or noncompliance. The oral route is usually used for patients with relatively mild infections in whom absorption is not thought to be compromised by the preceding conditions.

Intramuscular administration Although the IM route of administration usually results in 100 percent bioavailability, it is not as widely used in the United States as the oral and IV routes, in part because of the pain often associated with IM injections and the relative ease of IV access in the hospitalized patient. Intramuscular injection may be suitable for specific indications requiring an "immediate" and reliable effect (e.g., with long-acting forms of penicillin, including benzathine and procaine, and with single doses of ceftriaxone for uncomplicated gonococcal infection).

Intravenous administration The IV route is appropriate when oral antibacterial agents are not effective against a particular pathogen, when bioavailability is uncertain, or when larger doses are required than are feasible with the oral route. After IV administration, bioavailability is 100 percent, and peak serum concentrations occur at the end of the infusion. For many patients requiring long-term therapy, outpatient IV administration using convenient portable pumps may be cost-effective and safe when oral therapy is not feasible. Alternatively, some newer oral antibacterial drugs are sufficiently active against some organisms to rival parenteral therapy; their use may allow the patient to return home earlier or to avoid hospitalization entirely.

DISTRIBUTION After absorption, the resulting serum concentrations of most antibacterial agents must exceed the minimum concentration required to inhibit bacterial growth (MIC; see Chap. 80) to be effective. Since most infections are extravascular, an antibiotic also must *distribute* to the site of infection. Concentrations of most antibacterials in interstitial fluid are similar to free drug concentrations in serum. However, when the infection is located in a "protected" site where penetration is poor, such as cerebrospinal fluid, the eye, the prostate, or infected cardiac vegetations, high parenteral doses or local administration for prolonged periods may be required for cure. In addition, even though an antibacterial agent may penetrate to the site of infection, its activity may be antagonized by local factors, such as an unfavorable pH or inactivation by cellular degradation products. For example, since the activity of aminoglycosides is reduced at acidic pH, the acidic environment in many infected tissues may be partly responsible for the relatively poor efficacy of aminoglycoside monotherapy. In addition, the abscess milieu reduces the activity of many antibacterial compounds so that surgical drainage is required for cure.

Most bacteria causing human infections are located extracellularly. Intracellular pathogens such as *Legionella, Chlamydia, Brucella,* and *Salmonella* may persist or cause relapse if the antibacterial agent does not enter the cell. In general, β-lactams, vancomycin, and aminoglycosides penetrate cells poorly, whereas macrolides, tetracyclines, metronidazole, chloramphenicol, rifampin, trimethoprim-sulfamethoxazole, and quinolones penetrate cells well.

METABOLISM AND ELIMINATION Like other drugs, antibacterial agents are disposed of by hepatic elimination (metabolism or biliary elimination), by renal excretion in unchanged or metabolized form, or by a combination of the two processes. For most antibacterial drugs, metabolism leads to loss of in vitro activity, although some agents such as cefotaxime, rifampin, and clarithromycin have bioactive metabolites that may contribute to their overall efficacy.

The most practical consequence of the mode of excretion of an antibacterial agent is the need to adjust the dosage when elimination capability is impaired. Direct, nonidiosyncratic toxicity from antibacterial drugs most often results from failure to reduce the dosage appropriately in a patient with impaired elimination. For agents that are primarily cleared intact by glomerular filtration, drug clearance is linearly correlated with creatinine clearance. Commonly used antibacterial drugs that require dosage adjustment in patients with renal impairment are listed in Table 100-3. Unfortunately, for drugs whose elimination is primarily hepatic, no simple marker (such as serum creatinine) is useful for dosage adjustment in subjects with liver disease. Even in patients with severe hepatic disease, residual metabolic capability is usually sufficient for the avoidance of accumulation and toxic adverse effects. However, for drugs that undergo hepatic metabolism and have a narrow therapeutic index (such as chloramphenicol), alternative therapy may be warranted in patients with liver disease, since the technology for the monitoring of serum levels is not widely available.

PRINCIPLES OF ANTIBACTERIAL CHEMOTHERAPY

The choice of an antibacterial compound for a particular patient and a specific infection involves more than just a knowledge of the agent's mechanism of action and pharmacokinetic profile. The basic tenets of chemotherapy, to be elaborated on below, include the following: First, whenever possible, material containing the infecting organism(s) should be obtained so that presumptive identification can be made by microscopic examination of stained specimens and the organism can be grown for definitive identification and susceptibility testing. Second, once the organism is identified and its susceptibility to antibacterial agents is determined, the regimen with the narrowest effective spectrum should be chosen. Third, the choice of antibacterial agent is guided by the pharmacokinetic and adverse-reaction profile of active compounds, the site of infection, the immune status of the host, and evidence of efficacy from well-performed clinical trials.

TABLE 100-3 Pharmacokinetics of selected antibacterial agents

Drug	Dose, route	Peak serum concentration, μg/mL	Breakpoint,* μg/mL	Half-life, h	Dose alteration in renal disease
Penicillin G	2×10^6 U, IV	60	0.1[†]	0.5	Yes
Ampicillin	1000 mg, IV	40	8[‡]	1	Yes
Dicloxacillin	500 mg, PO	15	2	1	No
Nafcillin	1000 mg, IV	40	2	1	No
Ticarcillin	3000 mg, IV	160	16[‡]	1	Yes
Cefazolin	1000 mg, IV	188	8	2	Yes
Cefaclor	500 mg, PO	15	8	1	Yes
Cephalexin	500 mg, PO	15	8	1	Yes
Cefoxitin	1000 mg, IV	110	8	1	Yes
Cefuroxime	1000 mg, IV	100	8	1.5	Yes
Ceftriaxone	1000 mg, IV	150	8	8	Slight
Ceftazidime	2000 mg, IV	170	8	2	Yes
Aztreonam	2000 mg, IV	200	8	2	Yes
Imipenem	500 mg, IV	43	4	1	Yes
Gentamicin	1.5 mg/kg, IV	8	4	2	Yes
Amikacin	7.5 mg/kg, IV	35	16	2	Yes
Doxycycline	100 mg, PO	2.5	4	18	Yes
Tetracycline	500 mg, PO	4	4	8	§
Erythromycin	500 mg, PO	1	0.5	0.5–2.0	No
Clindamycin	600 mg, IV	10	0.5	2.4	No
Metronidazole	500 mg, PO	10	NA[¶]	6	No
Vancomycin	1000 mg, IV	30	4	6	Yes
Trimethoprim-sulfamethoxazole	160/800 mg, PO	2/40	2/38	11/9	Yes
Ciprofloxacin	500 mg, PO	3	1	4	Yes
Ofloxacin	400 mg, PO	6	2	6	Yes

* For fully susceptible organisms.
† For most gram-positive organisms.
‡ For Enterobacteriaceae.
§ Contraindicated in renal impairment.
¶ NA = not applicable.

Finally, if all other factors are equal, the antibacterial regimen that is the least expensive should be chosen.

SUSCEPTIBILITY OF BACTERIA TO ANTIBACTERIAL DRUGS IN VITRO (See also Chap. 80) The determination of the susceptibility of the patient's infecting organism to a panel of appropriate antibacterial agents is an essential first step in devising a chemotherapeutic regimen. The details of susceptibility testing are discussed elsewhere (Chap. 80). However, susceptibility testing is designed to estimate the susceptibility of a bacterial isolate to an antibacterial drug under standardized conditions that favor rapidly growing aerobic or facultative organisms. Under certain circumstances, specialized testing is required. (1) Strict anaerobes require testing under anaerobic conditions. Problems with poor growth of the inoculum or unstable activity of some antibacterial agents (i.e., metronidazole) in testing media have led to significant interlaboratory variation. (2) Production of β-lactamase by such fastidious organisms as *Haemophilus influenzae* and *Neisseria gonorrhoeae* has a major effect on therapy. Therefore, production of this enzyme must be measured directly; β-lactam susceptibility testing cannot be relied on. (3) Resistance genes that require induction for expression may require longer incubation (e.g., erythromycin resistance in staphylococci) or detection of inducible enzymes (e.g., β-lactamase production by staphylococci). (4) Methicillin resistance in staphylococci requires specialized testing with larger inocula, longer incubation, and the addition of salt to the medium because of the variable expression of resistance under standardized testing conditions. (5) Resistance of enterococci to aminoglycosides needs to be assessed with use of very high levels of antibiotics in testing media because of intrinsic resistance. Resistance of enterococci to greater than 2000 μg/mL of an aminoglycoside such as gentamicin suggests that the isolate will be resistant to the bactericidal synergy of a β-lactam plus an aminoglycoside. (6) The minimum bactericidal concentration (MBC) of an antibacterial agent for a particular bacterial isolate may need to be determined rather than the minimal inhibitory concentration (MIC) that is the result of routine susceptibility testing. It must be performed manually by broth dilution with a carefully standardized protocol that defines the endpoint

for growth after subculture to agar. It is generally only indicated for certain patients with endocarditis or osteomyelitis.

RELATIONSHIP OF PHARMACOKINETICS AND IN VITRO SUSCEPTIBILITY TO RESPONSE The relationship between the report of susceptibility in vitro and the clinical pharmacokinetics of the antibacterial agent helps predict clinical response. Bacteria are usually considered to be *susceptible* to a drug if the achievable peak serum concentration exceeds the MIC by at least fourfold. The *breakpoint* is the concentration of the antibiotic that separates susceptible from resistant bacteria. When a majority of the isolates of a given bacterial species are inhibited at concentrations below the breakpoint, the species is within the spectrum of the drug (see "Choice of Antibacterial Therapy," below). Antibacterial agents are frequently administered every 3 to 4 half-lives, since serum concentrations will by then be below the breakpoint and may be below the MIC for the organism. These relationships are illustrated in Fig. 100-1. *Pharmacodynamics* refers to the relationship between drug concentrations in serum and tissues, in vitro susceptibility, and microbial response at the site of infection. Pharmacodynamic parameters that appear to correlate with reduction in the number of bacteria at the site of infection include the ratio of the peak antibacterial concentration to the MIC (especially for aminoglycosides and quinolones), the length of time that concentrations exceed the MIC (especially for β-lactams), and the postantibiotic effect (or length of time that bacterial growth is inhibited after concentrations fall below the MIC). For some drugs, such as the aminoglycosides, it is not necessary to maintain serum concentrations above the MIC for the entire dose interval. Many microbiology laboratories report quantitative susceptibilities (MIC); Table 100-3 lists peak serum concentrations and breakpoints for some common antibacterial agents.

STATUS OF THE HOST Various host factors must be considered when devising antibacterial chemotherapy. The host's antibacterial *immune function* is of importance, particularly as it relates to opsonophagocytic function. Since the major host defense against acute, overwhelming bacterial infection is the polymorphonuclear leukocyte, patients with neutropenia must be treated aggressively and

FIGURE 100-1 Relationship between pharmacokinetics of an antibiotic and susceptibility. Organism A is resistant, organism B is moderately susceptible, and organism C is very susceptible.

empirically with bactericidal drugs for suspected infection (see Chap. 96). Likewise, patients who have deficient humoral immunity (e.g., those with chronic lymphocytic leukemia and multiple myeloma) and individuals with surgical or functional asplenia (e.g., those with sickle cell disease) should be treated empirically for infections with encapsulated organisms, especially the pneumococcus.

Genetic factors may determine the type of infection, the pathogen, and susceptibility to antibacterial side effects. For example, in patients with chronic granulomatous disease, the survival of catalase-positive microorganisms (e.g., *S. aureus*) inside phagocytes is enhanced, and therapy not only must be directed against these bacteria but also must include agents that are taken up by phagocytes and are active intracellularly.

Pregnancy increases the risk of toxicity of certain antibacterial drugs for the mother (e.g., the hepatic toxicity of tetracycline), affects drug disposition and pharmacokinetics, and—because of the risk of fetal toxicity—severely limits the choice of agents for treating infections. Certain antibacterials are contraindicated in pregnancy either because safety has not been established or because of known toxicity. These include all fluoroquinolones, clarithromycin, erythromycin estolate (but not erythromycin base), and tetracyclines. Data on the safety of many other antibacterial drugs are limited, but they may be used cautiously when there is no suitable alternative and the perceived benefit outweighs the risk. These include aminoglycosides, azithromycin, clindamycin, imipenem, metronidazole, trimethoprim, and vancomycin. The following drugs are contraindicated in the third trimester but can be used cautiously in the first two trimesters: chloramphenicol, nitrofurantoin, and sulfonamides.

In patients with *concomitant viral infections*, the incidence of adverse reactions to antibacterial drugs may be unusually high. For example, persons with infectious mononucleosis and those infected with HIV may react more often to ampicillin and folic acid synthesis inhibitors, respectively.

In addition, the patient's age, sex, racial heritage, and excretory status all determine the incidence and type of side effects that can be expected with certain antibacterial agents.

SITE OF INFECTION The location of the infected site may play a major role in the choice and dose of antimicrobial drug. Patients with suspected *meningitis* should receive drugs that can cross the blood–cerebrospinal fluid (CSF) barrier; in addition, because of the relative paucity of phagocytes and opsonins at the site of infection, the agents should be bactericidal. Chloramphenicol, one of the standard drugs for therapy, is bactericidal for common organisms causing meningitis (i.e., meningococcus, pneumococcus, and *H. influenzae, not* enteric gram-negative bacilli), is highly lipid-soluble, and enters the CSF well. However, β-lactams, the mainstay of therapy for most of these infections, do not normally reach high levels in

CSF. Their efficacy is based on the increased permeability of the blood-brain and blood-CSF barriers to hydrophilic molecules during inflammation and the extreme susceptibility of most infectious organisms to even small amounts of β-lactam drug.

The vegetation that is the major site of infection in *bacterial endocarditis* is also a focus that is protected from normal host defense mechanisms. Antibacterial therapy needs to be bactericidal, administered at a dose that produces serum levels at least eight times higher than the MBC for the infecting organism, and given parenterally for a prolonged period. Likewise, *osteomyelitis* involves a site that is somewhat resistant to opsonophagocytic removal of infecting bacteria; furthermore, avascular bone (sequestrum) represents a foreign body that thwarts normal host defense mechanisms. *Chronic prostatitis* is exceedingly difficult to cure because most antibiotics do not penetrate nonfenestrated capillaries serving the prostate, especially when acute inflammation is absent. Drugs that are "ion trapped" after entering prostatic tissue, such as trimethoprim and fluoroquinolones, may be uniquely effective because of this mechanism. *Intraocular infections*, especially endophthalmitis, are difficult to treat because drug penetration into the vitreous from blood is hindered by retinal capillaries lacking fenestration. Inflammation does little to disrupt this barrier. Thus direct injection into the vitreous is necessary in many cases. *Abscesses* also represent infections where antibiotic penetration is usually poor. In addition, even when an antibiotic does penetrate into the abscess, local conditions, such as low pH or the presence of enzymes that hydrolyze the drug, may antagonize activity. In contrast, *urinary tract infections*, when confined to the bladder, are relatively easy infections to cure, in part because of the higher concentration of most antibiotics in the urine than in blood. Since blood is the usual reference fluid in defining susceptibility, even organisms found to be "resistant" to achievable serum concentrations may be susceptible to achievable urine concentrations. For drugs that are used only for the treatment of urinary tract infections, such as nitrofurantoin and methenamine salts, achievable urine concentrations are used to determine susceptibility.

COMBINATION CHEMOTHERAPY One of the tenets of antibacterial chemotherapy is that if the infecting bacterium has been identified, the most specific chemotherapy possible should be used. The use of a single agent with a narrow spectrum of activity against the pathogen diminishes the alteration of normal flora and thus limits overgrowth of resistant nosocomial organisms (e.g., *Candida albicans*, enterococci, *C. difficile*, or methicillin-resistant staphylococci), limits the potential toxicity of multiple drug regimens, and reduces cost. However, certain circumstances call for the use of more than one antibacterial agent. These are summarized below.

1 *Prevention of the emergence of resistant mutants.* Spontaneous mutations occur at a detectable frequency in certain genes encoding the target proteins for some antibacterial agents. The use of these agents can eliminate the susceptible population, select out resistant mutants at the site of infection, and result in the failure of chemotherapy. Resistant mutants are usually selected when the MIC of the antibacterial agent for the infecting bacterium is close to achievable levels in serum or tissues and/or when the site of infection limits the access or activity of the agent. The most common examples are rifampin for staphylococci, imipenem for *Pseudomonas*, and ciprofloxacin for staphylococci and *Pseudomonas*. Small-colony variants of staphylococci resistant to aminoglycosides also emerge during monotherapy with these antibiotics. A second antibacterial agent with a mechanism of action different from that of the first is added to prevent the emergence of these resistant mutants (e.g., imipenem plus an aminoglycoside for systemic *Pseudomonas* infections). However, since resistant mutants have emerged following combination chemotherapy, this approach is not uniformly successful.

2 *Synergistic or additive activity.* Against some bacteria, two antibacterial agents are clearly more active than one; whether or not this is the case is usually judged on the basis of testing in vitro.

Synergistic or *additive activity* is defined as a lowering of the MIC or MBC of *each* of two drugs tested in combination against a specific bacterium. Thus *each* agent is more active when combined with a second drug than it would be alone. The best examples of a synergistic or additive effect, confirmed both in vitro and by animal studies, are the enhanced bactericidal activities of certain β-lactam–aminoglycoside combinations against enterococci, viridans streptococci, and *P. aeruginosa*. The synergistic or additive activity of these combinations also has been demonstrated for selected isolates of enteric gram-negative bacteria and staphylococci. The combination of trimethoprim and sulfamethoxazole also has synergistic or additive activity against many enteric gram-negative bacteria. Most other antimicrobial combinations show indifferent activity (i.e., the combination is *no better* than the more active of the two agents alone), and some combinations (e.g., penicillin plus tetracycline against pneumococci) may be antagonistic (i.e., the combination is *worse* than either drug alone).

3 *Therapy directed against multiple potential pathogens.* For certain infections, either a mixture of pathogens is documented or the patient is desperately ill; in these situations, the most important infecting bacteria need to be covered by therapy until culture and susceptibility results become available. Examples of the former infections are intraabdominal or brain abscesses and infected limbs in diabetic patients with microvascular disease. The latter situations include fevers in neutropenic patients, acute pneumonia from aspiration of oral flora by hospitalized patients, and septic shock or sepsis syndrome. However, in circumstances where presumptive therapy with more than one agent is begun, monotherapy should always be given subsequently if a single infecting bacterium that can be treated effectively with one agent is identified.

CHOICE OF ANTIBACTERIAL THERAPY

The antibacterial spectrum of specific agents and the infections for which they represent the treatment of choice are detailed below. No attempt has been made to include all the potential situations in which antibacterial agents may be used. A more detailed discussion of specific bacteria and infections that they cause can be found elsewhere in this volume.

β-LACTAMS (See also Table 100-2)   All *penicillins* (except for the semisynthetic, penicillinase-resistant, antistaphylococcal agents) are hydrolyzed by β-lactamases and are ineffective against isolates that produce these enzymes. Penicillin G has a spectrum that includes spirochetes (*Treponema pallidum, Borrelia,* and *Leptospira*), streptococci (groups A and B, viridans, and *Streptococcus pneumoniae*), enterococci, most *Neisseria* spp., a few staphylococci, many fastidious oral bacteria [*Bacteroides* (*Porphyromonas* and *Prevotella*), streptococci, *Actinomyces,* and *Fusobacterium*], *Clostridium* spp. (except *C. difficile*), *Pasteurella multocida, Erysipelothrix rhusiopathiae,* and *Streptobacillus moniliformis*. However, resistance is widespread among staphylococci, is increasing among gonococci and enterococci, and is emerging among pneumococci, oral strains of *Bacteroides* (*Porphyromonas* and *Prevotella*), and meningococci. Penicillin G is the drug of choice for syphilis, yaws, leptospirosis, group A and B streptococcal infections, pneumococcal infections (in the United States), actinomycosis, oral and periodontal infections, meningococcal meningitis and meningococcemia, viridans streptococcal endocarditis, clostridial myonecrosis, tetanus, anthrax, rat-bite fever, *P. multocida* infections, and erysipeloid (*E. rhusiopathiae*).

Ampicillin extends the spectrum of penicillin G to some gram-negative rods. It is active against some isolates of *Escherichia coli, Proteus mirabilis, Salmonella, Shigella,* and *H. influenzae* and is one of the drugs of choice for susceptible organisms causing urinary tract infections, salmonellosis, *H. influenzae* meningitis and epiglottitis, and *Listeria monocytogenes* meningitis. High rates of resistance have lessened its value as empirical therapy in some situations. For example, more than 80 percent of isolates of *E. coli* and *P. mirabilis*

are resistant in some hospitals, as are 10 to 30 percent of isolates of *H. influenzae*; moreover, in some outbreaks of infection due to salmonellae, all isolates are ampicillin-resistant.

The *penicillinase-resistant penicillins* are used solely for the treatment of staphylococcal infections and are the drugs of choice for systemic or deep staphylococcal infections caused by susceptible organisms. Unfortunately, on average, approximately 20 percent of *S. aureus* isolates and more than 60 percent of coagulase-negative staphylococcal isolates acquired in U.S. hospitals are resistant to these agents (i.e., methicillin-resistant). While the spectrum of these agents also includes most of the same gram-positive bacteria that are susceptible to penicillin G, the MIC values of penicillinase-resistant penicillins for these organisms are higher than those of penicillin G, and the latter remains the drug of choice.

The spectrum of the *antipseudomonal penicillins* includes the bacteria covered by ampicillin as well as some additional nonpseudomonal enteric gram-negative bacilli. For example, piperacillin is active against many indole-positive *Proteus, Enterobacter, Klebsiella, Providencia,* and *Serratia* spp. However, the susceptibility of these penicillins to β-lactamase markedly limits their utility as empirical therapy when infections caused by gram-negative enteric organisms are suspected. The major use of these compounds is in the treatment of proven or suspected infections with *P. aeruginosa* and *Acinetobacter,* for which they are among the drugs of choice. Their relative antipseudomonal activities can be ranked as follows: piperacillin > mezlocillin, ticarcillin > carbenicillin.

The addition of β-*lactamase inhibitors* (clavulanic acid or sulbactam) to ampicillin, amoxicillin, or ticarcillin extends the spectrum of these agents to include many organisms that are resistant by virtue of β-lactamase production. These species include *E. coli, Klebsiella,* all *Proteus* spp., *H. influenzae, Moraxella* (formerly *Branhamella*) *catarrhalis, Providencia,* and *B. fragilis*. Such combinations are also active against staphylococci that produce β-lactamase but are not methicillin-resistant. However, the efficacy of these combinations in serious staphylococcal infections has not been adequately proven. Furthermore, *Enterobacter, Pseudomonas, Acinetobacter,* and various enteric gram-negative isolates either produce β-lactamases not inhibited by these compounds or develop resistance attributable to non-β-lactamase-mediated mechanisms.

The *first-generation cephalosporins* have a spectrum that includes penicillinase-producing, methicillin-susceptible staphylococci and streptococci. While these drugs may be used when infections with gram-positive bacteria are suspected, they are *not* the drugs of choice for such infections. They have excellent activity against many isolates of *E. coli, K. pneumoniae,* and *P. mirabilis* and are among the drugs of choice in presumptive therapy for non-hospital-acquired urinary tract infections. They have no activity against *B. fragilis,* enterococci, methicillin-resistant staphylococci, *Pseudomonas, Acinetobacter, Enterobacter,* indole-positive *Proteus,* and *Serratia* and poor activity against *H. influenzae*.

The *parenteral second-generation cephalosporins* extend the gram-negative spectrum of first-generation compounds. The various second-generation agents have differing activities. Cefuroxime and cefamandole retain activity against gram-positive cocci and are also active against *H. influenzae, Neisseria,* some *Enterobacter* isolates, and indole-positive *Proteus* but exhibit poor activity against *B. fragilis*. Cefoxitin and cefotetan have reasonably good activity against *B. fragilis,* but cefotetan is less effective against some other *Bacteriodes* spp. (see Chaps. 86 and 128). However, they display poor activity against gram-positive cocci and *Enterobacter*. No second-generation cephalosporin is active against *Pseudomonas* or *Acinetobacter*.

Oral second-generation cephalosporins have fair activity against gram-positive cocci and *H. influenzae* and are widely used in outpatient therapy for otitis media, sinusitis, and lower respiratory tract infections, although cheaper agents that are equally effective are preferable. Cefixime is one of the drugs of choice for single-dose treatment of gonococcal urethritis.

Third-generation cephalosporins all have a broad spectrum of activity against enteric gram-negative rods and are especially useful for treating hospital-acquired infections caused by multiresistant organisms. In addition, ceftazidime has excellent antipseudomonal activity. Cefoperazone has modest antipseudomonal activity, and the other third-generation cephalosporins have poor antipseudomonal activity. Since resistance to third-generation cephalosporins is increasing among all nosocomial gram-negative rods, the use of these agents should be guided by susceptibility testing. The gram-positive spectrum of the third-generation cephalosporins is variable, the relative rank being cefotaxime, ceftizoxime, ceftriaxone > cefoperazone > ceftazidime. Because of its excellent gram-negative spectrum, its activity against *Haemophilus*, *S. pneumoniae*, and penicillin-resistant *Neisseria*, its long serum half-life, and its high serum and CSF levels, ceftriaxone has become one of the drugs of choice for presumptive therapy for bacterial meningitis (except that caused by *Listeria*), all gonococcal infections, salmonellosis, and typhoid fever and is one of the drugs of choice for nonpseudomonal, hospital-acquired pneumonia. Third-generation cephalosporins have poor activity against *B. fragilis* and no activity against methicillin-resistant staphylococci, *Enterococcus, Acinetobacter*, or *Xanthomonas*.

The only *carbapenem* currently available in the United States is imipenem, marketed in combination with the renal dipeptidase inhibitor cilastatin, which enables imipenem to escape renal inactivation, thus increasing urinary levels of the drug. Imipenem has a spectrum that provides excellent activity in vitro against virtually all bacterial pathogens except *Xanthomonas*, methicillin-resistant staphylococci, and *E. faecium*. Limitations to its use are its relatively low blood levels, short serum half-life, central nervous system side effects, and cost. Resistance to imipenem is a problem only among nosocomial isolates of *P. aeruginosa*, approximately 20 percent of which are resistant. Imipenem is *not* the drug of choice for any bacterial infection, but because of its broad spectrum, it can be used as presumptive therapy for serious nosocomial infections thought to be caused by multiple bacterial species or multiresistant organisms. This antibiotic is often held in reserve as therapy for nosocomial infections due to gram-negative pathogens resistant to third-generation cephalosporins.

The only *monobactam* currently available is aztreonam. This antibiotic has a spectrum limited to facultative, gram-negative enteric bacilli. It has no activity against any gram-positive or anaerobic bacterium. Its gram-negative spectrum is similar to that of ceftazidime, with equally good activity against *Pseudomonas*. Its primary advantages are its theoretical ability to preserve the normal gram-positive and anaerobic flora and the lack of cross-reactive immediate hypersensitivity reactions in patients with histories of these reactions to other β-lactam antibiotics.

VANCOMYCIN The spectrum of vancomycin is limited to gram-positive cocci, especially streptococci and staphylococci. It is second-line therapy for most gram-positive bacterial infections but is the drug of choice for infections caused by methicillin-resistant staphylococci or the JK group of *Corynebacterium* and for serious infections in penicillin-allergic patients. Given orally (a route by which it is not absorbed), it is one of the drugs of choice for antibiotic-associated pseudomembranous colitis caused by *C. difficile*.

AMINOGLYCOSIDES The aminoglycosides are rapidly bactericidal in vitro at low concentrations, with activity limited to facultative gram-negative bacteria and staphylococci. They have no activity against anaerobic bacteria and are not effective in environments that are acidic or have a low oxygen tension. However, their spectrum includes virtually all gram-negative bacteria that are not strict anaerobes, and they are among the drugs of choice for any suspected gram-negative bacteremic infection, particularly in neutropenic patients. Aminoglycosides are synergistically bactericidal in combination with a penicillin for treating staphylococcal, enterococcal, or viridans streptococcal endocarditis and are usually combined with a β-lactam antibiotic for treating gram-negative bacteremia. Aminoglycosides are also among the drugs of choice for severe infections of the upper urinary tract. The major limitations to aminoglycoside use are their renal and otic toxicity, their diminished activity at certain sites of infection (e.g., abscesses and the central nervous system), the resistance of target bacteria, and the need to monitor serum levels to minimize the risk of toxicity and to ensure adequate concentrations. Among the available agents, gentamicin is generally preferred because of its low cost, but tobramycin has slightly greater activity against *P. aeruginosa*, and amikacin retains activity against many tobramycin- and gentamicin-resistant gram-negative bacteria because it is inactivated by fewer aminoglycoside-modifying enzymes. Streptomycin is still one of the drugs of choice in initial therapy for tularemia, plague, glanders, and brucellosis and is a second-line agent for treating tuberculosis.

MACROLIDES Erythromycin has broad spectrum activity against gram-positive bacteria, with additional activity against *Legionella, Mycoplasma, Campylobacter*, and some *Chlamydia* isolates. It is the drug of choice for infections due to *Legionella, Campylobacter*, and *Mycoplasma* and is one of the drugs of choice for pneumococcal pneumonia and pharyngitis and for skin and soft tissue infections due to group A streptococci in penicillin-allergic patients. However, resistance to erythromycin among group A streptococci and pneumococci is increasing in some countries. Erythromycin also appears to be one of the drugs of choice for infections caused in immunocompromised patients by the newly identified agent of bacillary angiomatosis (*Rochalimaea henselae*). The newer macrolides clarithromycin and azithromycin have an antibacterial spectrum similar to that of erythromycin in vitro. However, azithromycin has greater activity against *Chlamydia*. Both are active against nontuberculous mycobacteria, and both appear to have fewer gastrointestinal side effects than does erythromycin.

LINCOSAMIDES The only lincosamide used in the United States is clindamycin. It shares the gram-positive coccal spectrum of erythromycin but is more active, in some cases showing bactericidal activity, against susceptible staphylococci. However, resistance among staphylococci and many streptococci, mediated by the same genes responsible for macrolide resistance, limits clindamycin's usefulness against gram-positive cocci. In general, all gram-positive cocci resistant to erythromycin should be considered resistant to clindamycin regardless of the results of in vitro susceptibility testing. Clindamycin is one of the drugs of choice for anaerobic infections because of its broad spectrum of activity against both gram-positive and gram-negative strict anaerobes. In contrast, clindamycin, like erythromycin, has no clinically significant activity against facultative gram-negative enteric bacilli. Appropriate use is limited only by resistance or the development of pseudomembranous colitis, the major serious side effect of this drug.

CHLORAMPHENICOL Chloramphenicol has a broad spectrum of activity against gram-positive and gram-negative bacteria, although plasmid-mediated resistance has diminished its effective spectrum. However, this antibiotic is rarely used in adult infections because of the rare idiosyncratic side effect of irreversible bone marrow aplasia and the availability of other agents with similar activity. It remains one of the drugs of choice for typhoid fever and plague and is still useful for the treatment of brucellosis and both pneumococcal and meningococcal meningitis in penicillin-allergic patients.

TETRACYCLINES Tetracyclines have a broad spectrum of bacteriostatic activity against gram-positive and gram-negative bacteria and are widely used in a variety of non-hospital-acquired infections. These agents are among the drugs of choice for chronic bronchitis, granuloma inguinale, brucellosis (with streptomycin), tularemia, glanders, melioidosis, spirochetal infections caused by *Borrelia* (Lyme disease and relapsing fever; doxycycline), infections caused by *Vibrio vulnificus*, some *Aeromonas* infections, infections caused by *Xanthomonas* (minocycline), and plague. The tetracyclines are also used in penicillin-allergic patients for treating leptospirosis, syphilis, actinomycosis, and skin and soft tissue infections caused by gram-positive cocci. They are among the drugs of choice for infections due to chlamydiae (doxycycline) and rickettsiae and for granulomatous skin infection due to *M. marinum* (minocycline).

SULFONAMIDES AND TRIMETHOPRIM The folic acid synthesis inhibitors have a broad spectrum of bacteriostatic activity individually; in combination, they can be bactericidal against facultative gram-negative bacteria and staphylococci. The fixed combination of sulfamethoxazole and trimethoprim, the major folic acid synthesis inhibitors used in therapy for bacterial infections, has only modest activity against some streptococci and no activity against strict anaerobes. The individual sulfonamides are rarely used in the treatment of bacterial infections but are among the drugs of choice for treating nocardial infections, leprosy (dapsone, a sulfone), and toxoplasmosis (sulfadiazine). Trimethoprim-sulfamethoxazole is the drug of choice for the treatment of uncomplicated urinary tract infections (except for those caused by enterococococci) and is widely used in the treatment of otitis media. It can be used in therapy for upper respiratory tract infections in which *H. influenzae* and *M. catarrhalis* are suspected, gonococcal and meningococcal infections, chancroid, and infections thought to be caused by *Aeromonas, Xanthomonas, P. cepacia, Acinetobacter*, and *Yersinia enterocolitica*. For nosocomial infections due to *Xanthomonas*, trimethoprim-sulfamethoxazole is the drug of choice.

FLUOROQUINOLONES The fluoroquinolones have excellent activity against most facultative gram-negative rods, fair activity against staphylococci, variable to poor activity against streptococci, and no activity against obligate anaerobes. They are the oral agents with greatest activity against *P. aeruginosa*; ciprofloxacin is the most active against this species. All the quinolones have good to excellent oral absorption, while ciprofloxacin and ofloxacin are also administered as intravenous formulations. Treatment with norfloxacin can be used for urinary tract infections, and it has been recommended for infectious diarrhea. However, it should not be used for systemic gram-negative infections; the other quinolones should be used for this purpose. The quinolones are among the drugs of choice for complicated urinary tract infections, bacterial gastroenteritis, and enteric fever and may be useful in therapy for chronic infections caused by gram-negative organisms, such as osteomyelitis and chronic otitis externa in adults. The use of quinolones is limited by the development of resistance among staphylococci and *P. aeruginosa* and by interactions with other drugs.

RIFAMPIN Rifampin has been used in combinations for the treatment of serious infections due to methicillin-resistant staphylococci (e.g., coagulase-negative staphylococcal foreign-body infections). Because the spontaneous selection of rifampin-resistant mutants occurs rapidly, rifampin should never be used alone in treating staphylococcal infections. Rifampin is also used in the chemoprophylaxis of persons at risk for developing meningococcal meningitis and in the therapy of *Legionella* pneumonia.

METRONIDAZOLE Metronidazole has a spectrum limited to anaerobic bacteria. It is one of the drugs of choice for the treatment of any abscess in which the involvement of obligate anaerobes is suspected (e.g., lung, brain, or intraabdominal abscesses) because of its spectrum and its ability to penetrate into the area of infection. Other antibacterial agents should be used in combination with metronidazole if additional facultative and aerobic pathogens are suspected. Metronidazole is also one of the drugs of choice for treating bacterial vaginosis and antibiotic-associated pseudomembranous colitis.

URINARY TRACT ANTISEPTICS Urinary tract antiseptics are active only in the lower urinary tract and cannot be used for treating upper urinary tract or systemic infections. Their activity is limited to susceptible gram-negative enteric bacteria. The available agents in this category include nitrofurantoin and methenamine salts.

TOPICAL ANTIBACTERIAL AGENTS Mupirocin is available only as a topical preparation for use against staphylococci and streptococci. Its major applications are for impetigo and eradication of the staphylococcal carrier state. It is the drug of choice for the elimination of nasal carriage of both methicillin-susceptible and methicillin-resistant staphylococci. Unfortunately, the emergence of resistance is limiting its usefulness in some hospitals.

Although their efficacy has never been well documented, topical preparations that include sulfonamides, polymyxin B, neomycin, bacitracin, gramicidin, and novobiocin in a variety of combinations are widely used as eye drops, irrigation solutions, and ointments for superficial skin infections.

ADVERSE REACTIONS

Adverse drug reactions are frequently classified by mechanism as either dose-related ("toxic") effects or unpredictable reactions. Unpredictable reactions are further categorized as either idiosyncratic or allergic. Dose-related reactions include aminoglycoside nephrotoxicity, penicillin-induced seizures, and vancomycin anaphylactoid reactions. Many of these reactions can be avoided by reducing dosage, limiting the duration of therapy, or reducing the frequency or rate of administration. Adverse reactions to antibacterial agents are a common cause of morbidity, requiring alteration in therapy and additional expense, and they occasionally result in death. The elderly, often those with the more severe infections, may be especially prone to certain adverse reactions. These reactions to antibacterial agents are summarized below.

β-LACTAMS The therapeutic index for β-lactam antibiotics is large, and dose-related adverse reactions are uncommon and largely preventable. The greatest concern is allergic reactions. All types can occur, including anaphylaxis (type 1, hypersensitivity reactions), nephritis and Coombs-positive hemolytic anemia (type 2, cytotoxic reactions), drug fever and serum sickness (type 3, immune-complex formation), contact dermatitis (type 4, cell-mediated effects), and maculopapular eruption (type 5, idiopathic reactions). Approximately 1 to 4 percent of treatment courses result in an allergic reaction, and approximately 0.004 to 0.015 percent of treatment courses result in anaphylaxis. Fewer than half the patients who claim an allergy to penicillin react to skin testing with the major and minor determinants (penicilloyl polylysine and benzylpenicillin degradation products, respectively); those with negative skin tests only rarely react adversely to subsequent therapeutic doses. However, a careful history for allergy is still required before any β-lactam is administered, since the consequences may be life-threatening. Generally, a suitable alternative to β-lactams is available for patients who have a severe allergy, and penicillin desensitization can be carefully undertaken if there is no suitable alternative. A small number of persons (<2 percent) who are allergic to penicillin react similarly when a cephalosporin is administered; thus the latter drugs are contraindicated in patients with a history of an immediate reaction to penicillin (although they are often used in patients with a history of mild reactions). The same precaution applies to imipenem, but aztreonam is antigenically distinct and can be administered safely to the penicillin-allergic patient.

Other reactions thought to have an allergic basis include nephritis (associated with methicillin), hepatitis (related to oxacillin), leukopenia (following high doses of most β-lactams administered for prolonged periods), and severe skin rashes (toxic epidermal necrolysis and Stevens-Johnson syndrome). These reactions are not IgE-mediated, and skin testing is not predictive of their occurrence. For unclear reasons, most patients who have infectious mononucleosis develop a rash when given ampicillin.

Miscellaneous reactions to β-lactams include gastrointestinal side effects ranging in severity from mild diarrhea (5 to 10 percent) to pseudomembranous colitis (<1 percent). Drugs excreted to a large extent through the bile, such as ampicillin, ceftriaxone, and cefoperazone, may be especially prone to cause diarrhea. The addition of clavulanic acid to amoxicillin further increases the frequencey of diarrhea. Ceftriaxone, because of extremely high concentrations in bile, can cause "sludging" in the gall bladder and occasionally cause symptoms compatible with acute cholecystitis.

In high doses—and most often in patients with renal impairment who receive an excessive dose—penicillins (especially carbenicillin, ticarcillin, and penicillin G) can cause bleeding from impaired platelet aggregation. In addition, bleeding also is occasionally associated with use of cephalosporins containing a methylthiotetrazole group at the 3′ position (most commonly, cefamandole and cefoperazone); this reaction may result from impairment of prothrombin formation. These same cephalosporins can cause a disulfiram-like reaction if ethanol is administered. Carbenicillin and ticarcillin are disodium salts and in high doses can cause hypokalemia and fluid overload.

Seizures are occasionally observed with β-lactams, especially penicillin G and imipenem. This reaction is most common when excessive doses relative to renal function are administered or in patients with a history of seizures.

VANCOMYCIN When vancomycin was first used clinically in 1956, local intolerance at the infusion site was common, as were systemic reactions, including ototoxicity and nephrotoxicity. Current formulations are of higher purity and, with proper dosage guidelines, are very safe, although phlebitis can still be troublesome. The most common adverse reaction is called *red man syndrome* and is characterized by pruritus, flushing, and erythema of the head and upper torso. This anaphylactoid reaction usually follows the first dose, is dependent on dose and infusion time, and results from vancomycin-induced release of histamine. The reaction is usually mild in adult patients who receive 1 g over 60 min and diminishes with repeated doses. If vancomycin is mistakenly given as a bolus, severe hypotension may result. In unusually sensitive patients, extending the infusion time or administering H-1 receptor antagonists is usually effective in preventing this reaction or reducing its severity. Patients with this reaction must not be mislabeled as having an allergy to vancomycin, since vancomycin may be the only effective treatment for certain infections, such as those due to methicillin-resistant staphylococci.

Nephrotoxicity from vancomycin is mild and occurs in fewer than 5 percent of patients. Although some data suggest that aminoglycosides and vancomycin are synergistically nephrotoxic, this is difficult to prove, and the simultaneous use of these agents should not be avoided if clinically indicated, as in the treatment of enterococcal endocarditis in penicillin-allergic patients.

Ototoxicity from vancomycin is rare as long as doses are appropriately reduced in patients with renal insufficiency. Other uncommon adverse reactions include leukopenia, skin rashes, and true allergy.

AMINOGLYCOSIDES Aminoglycoside antibiotics have a narrow therapeutic index. The two most common adverse reactions are nephrotoxicity and ototoxicity. Rarely, respiratory depression is observed. Nephrotoxicity results from accumulation of the aminoglycoside in the peritubular space, with damage to the proximal tubule and a corresponding reduction in the glomerular filtration rate. The incidence of nephrotoxicity, defined as a greater than 0.5 percent increase over baseline in serum creatinine, is approximately 5 to 10 percent among adult patients who receive a therapeutic course for 10 to 14 days. However, many cofactors also influence the frequency of toxicity, such as extremes of age (toxicity is uncommon among children, more common among the elderly), concomitant drug therapy, hydration status, and magnitude of serum concentrations. Toxicity is manifested clinically by a gradual rise in serum creatinine after a few days of therapy and is reversible if the dosage is reduced or discontinued. Serum creatinine levels should be monitored every 3 to 5 days or more often if changes are seen. There is not an important difference in the frequency of nephrotoxicity among the most useful agents (gentamicin, tobramycin, and amikacin); streptomycin is a rare cause of nephrotoxicity.

Ototoxicity from aminoglycoside therapy presents as either auditory or vestibular damage. Since the aminoglycosides can destroy hair cells within the inner ear, this ototoxicity may be permanent. The risk of ototoxicity increases with prolonged therapy, higher serum concentrations (especially in patients with renal impairment), hypovolemia, and concurrent treatment with other ototoxins, especially ethacrynic acid. Clinically apparent ototoxicity, manifested by diminished acuity or vestibular imbalance, is uncommon (probably occurring in <1 percent of cases) when serum concentrations are monitored and the duration of therapy is kept to a minimum. With

more sensitive monitoring, e.g., audiograms, asymptomatic high-tone hearing loss is more commonly noted. There are no clinically important differences in the overall frequency of ototoxicity among the aminoglycosides.

Neuromuscular depression from aminoglycosides is caused by reduced acetylcholine activity at postsynaptic membranes and can result in rare but severe respiratory depression. Risk factors include hypocalcemia, peritoneal administration, use of neuromuscular blockers, and preexisting respiratory depression. It is largely avoided by administering the aminoglycoside IV over 30 min or by IM injection; if respiratory depression occurs, it is antagonized by the administration of calcium.

Fear of toxicity should not prevent the use of aminoglycosides when there is a legitimate indication, since toxicity is usually mild and reversible. Serum concentrations are monitored both to minimize the risk of toxicity and to ensure that sufficient drug is administered to treat targeted infections.

MACROLIDES Serious adverse reactions to the macrolide antibiotics are very rare. Gastrointestinal effects, such as burning, nausea, and vomiting, are the most common adverse reactions to the macrolides; depending on dosage, these reactions may occur in up to 50 percent of patients, occasionally requiring early discontinuation of therapy. The mechanism is thought to be the binding of erythromycin to motilin receptors, with a consequent increase in gastrointestinal motility. Gastrointestinal side effects appear equally common for all the oral formulations and also occur with IV administration. Clarithromycin and possibly azithromycin may be better tolerated than erythromycin, although gastrointestinal distress is still their most common adverse effect.

Less common reactions include hepatotoxicity and ototoxicity. Hepatotoxicity is a rare, nonfatal complication of treatment with erythromycin estolate and appears as an allergic cholestatic jaundice. Ototoxicity is rare after oral administration but may occur in a dose-dependent pattern in up to 20 percent of adults who receive IV erythromycin (4 g/d) and have audiograms performed. Ototoxicity is usually reversible and mild. Allergic cutaneous reactions are observed in rare cases.

LINCOSAMIDES The most common adverse effect of clindamycin is gastrointestinal distress. Diarrhea has been reported in up to 20 percent of patients and pseudomembranous colitis in 0.01 to 10 percent. The mechanism of pseudomembranous colitis is production of a toxin by *C. difficile* (see Chap. 108). *C. difficile* colonizes the gastrointestinal tract, and may produce a toxin when normal flora is suppressed by clindamycin. This toxin causes mucosal damage that results in cramps, pain, and diarrhea that may be bloody. Pseudomembranous colitis may follow both IV and oral administration and may not become manifest until after completion of therapy. Oral metronidazole or vancomycin is effective in treating symptomatic patients with toxin-positive stools, but some spores may survive and relapse is frequent. Although diarrhea and pseudomembranous colitis can be caused by most antibacterial agents, the incidence in relation to the amount used appears to be highest for clindamycin. Allergic reactions (such as rashes and fever), hepatotoxicity, and neutropenia are observed only rarely.

CHLORAMPHENICOL Chloramphenicol causes two types of bone marrow suppression; a dose-related, reversible suppression of all elements, which occurs commonly during therapy at the maximal recommended doses (4 g/d in adults), and an idiosyncratic, irreversible aplastic anemia, which occurs in approximately 1 in every 25,000 to 40,000 exposures. The irreversible form has been reported to follow all types of chloramphenicol treatment, including ocular administration, and often develops months after therapy is discontinued.

In premature neonates and infants, chloramphenicol can cause a dose-related "gray syndrome" characterized by cyanosis, hypotension, and death resulting from an inability of the newborn to metabolize chloramphenicol. These potentially serious toxicities and the availability of newer drugs have substantially reduced the indications for chloramphenicol.

TETRACYCLINES Gastrointestinal effects are the most common adverse reactions to the tetracyclines. These problems may be related to a direct irritant effect, since tetracyclines also can cause esophageal ulceration when they dissolve before reaching the stomach. Concurrent food intake may improve tolerance, but absorption of tetracycline HCl is impaired when it is taken with food.

Hepatotoxicity has been reported after administration of more than 2 g of tetracycline IV and at lower doses during pregnancy. There are currently no indications for IV tetracycline treatment in pregnancy. All tetracyclines can cause phototoxic skin reactions, although they are most common with doxycycline. Other dermal reactions, including rash, are uncommon. Tetracyclines are contraindicated in children less than 8 years of age because of mottling of the permanent teeth, although doxycycline may be less likely to cause this problem. Worsening of renal function in patients with preexisting renal dysfunction has been reported with use of tetracycline, although some of the increased azotemia may be due to amino acid catabolism. Doxycycline and perhaps minocycline appear to be free from these renal side effects. Alternative effective agents are nearly always available for use in such patients. Minocycline can cause vertigo in up to 70 percent of women receiving therapeutic doses, with a lower frequency in men.

SULFONAMIDES AND TRIMETHOPRIM The sulfonamides are generally safe, but the list of possible adverse reactions is very long. These compounds occasionally cause a number of allergic reactions, from relatively minor skin rashes (including maculopapular rashes and urticarial reactions typically appearing after a week of therapy) to severe, life-threatening reactions such as erythema multiforme, Stevens-Johnson syndrome, and toxic epidermal necrolysis. The severe hypersensitivity reactions have occurred most commonly after treatment with the "long-acting" sulfonamides, such as sulfamethoxypyridazine, which are no longer used. Fansidar (pyrimethamine plus sulfadoxine), used for malaria prophylaxis, may cause severe allergic reactions, including hepatic and hematologic toxicities, in addition to dermatologic toxicity. Photosensitivity reactions are also relatively common with sulfonamides.

For reasons that are not clear, many patients infected with human immunodeficiency virus (HIV) who receive trimethoprim-sulfamethoxazole have adverse dermatologic reactions. These are usually not life-threatening and appear to regress in many cases despite continuation of therapy.

Sulfonamides and trimethoprim also may cause severe hematologic complications, including agranulocytosis, hemolytic and megaloblastic anemia, and thrombocytopenia. These dose-related side effects may be greater in patients with renal insufficiency. Hemolytic anemia is most common in patients with glucose-6-phosphate dehydrogenase (G6PD) deficiency who take long-acting compounds; trimethoprim-sulfamethoxazole rarely causes hemolysis in such subjects. Granulocytopenia from trimethoprim-sulfamethoxazole is especially common in HIV-infected patients, occurring in 10 to 50 percent of subjects.

Renal insufficiency, caused by crystals of the relatively insoluble acetyl metabolite, is observed primarily with the long-acting sulfonamides. A number of cases of crystalluria in HIV-infected patients taking sulfadiazine for toxoplasmosis have been reported. A high level of fluid intake and urinary alkalization may prevent this complication.

It is recommended that sulfonamides not be administered to the newborn because of concerns that bilirubin may be displaced from protein binding sites, with subsequent jaundice and kernicterus.

In addition to the preceding problems, sulfonamides may occasionally cause drug fever with serum sickness, hepatic toxicity (including necrosis), systemic lupus erythematosus, and central nervous system symptoms such as drowsiness, fatigue, and insomnia.

FLUOROQUINOLONES Fluoroquinolones are relatively safe; adverse reactions rarely require discontinuation of therapy. The most common reactions include gastrointestinal distress, such as nausea or diarrhea (<5 percent), and central nervous system effects, including insomnia and dizziness (<5 percent). Rarely, hepatic and renal dysfunction and anaphylactoid and allergic reactions are observed. The use of these drugs is contraindicated in children less than 18 years of age because of evidence in animals of cartilage damage in developing joints. In carefully selected situations, in which the perceived benefits outweigh the risks, such as in adolescent patients with cystic fibrosis who have pulmonary exacerbations, fluoroquinolones may be useful for short-term therapy. They are contraindicated in pregnancy because of concern for the developing fetus. Temafloxacin was withdrawn after a few months on the world market because it occasionally caused hypoglycemia in the elderly and hemolysis with renal failure.

RIFAMPIN Rifampin is generally well tolerated but has several important side effects. Some patients have transient rises in hepatic transaminases, but these levels usually return to normal without discontinuation of the drug. Although hepatitis from rifampin itself develops only rarely, the drug is thought by some investigators to potentiate the hepatic toxicity of concomitantly administered isoniazid. Intermittent administration of rifampin, usually less than three times per week, has been associated with symptoms that seem to have an immunologic basis. These include flulike symptoms and (rarely) hemolysis, thrombocytopenia, shock, and renal failure. Minor gastrointestinal side effects, skin rashes, and interstitial nephritis also have been reported. Patients should be warned that rifampin and its metabolites cause secretions such as urine, tears, sweat, and saliva to turn orange and that contact lenses may be stained.

METRONIDAZOLE Serious adverse reactions to metronidazole are uncommon. Gastrointestinal side effects such as nausea are most frequent but rarely necessitate discontinuation of therapy. Pseudomembranous colitis in association with metronidazole has been reported but appears to be very rare. A metallic taste is relatively common, and stomatitis and glossitis are occasionally reported. Disulfiram-like reactions can occur if ethanol is administered. Peripheral neuropathy occurs in some patients, and seizures and encephalopathy have been reported after high doses or in patients with hepatic failure.

Concerns about mutagenicity and carcinogenicity from metronidazole have led to recommendations that it not be used in pregnancy (especially during the first trimester) when alternative agents are available. Although retrospective studies have found no association between metronidazole and carcinogenesis, long-term administration of high doses should be avoided when therapeutic alternatives are available.

DRUG INTERACTIONS

Historically, clinically important interactions involving antibacterial drugs were generally of little concern, since β-lactams were the most widely used agents and rarely interacted with other drugs in a manner that affected the patient adversely. However, fluoroquinolones, macrolides, and rifampin are more widely used, and interactions are of increasing concern. Table 100-4 lists the most common and best documented interactions and their clinical relevance. Coadministration of two of the drugs paired in Table 100-4 does not necessarily result in clinically important adverse consequences. The result also depends on timing of administration, dose and duration of therapy, baseline serum concentration of the non-antibacterial drug administered, the patient's susceptibility to the pharmacologic effect of the non-antibacterial drug, and other less well described cofactors. Recognition of the potential for an interaction before the administration of an antibacterial agent is crucial to the rational use of these drugs, since adverse consequences often can be prevented if the interaction is anticipated. Table 100-4 is intended only to heighten awareness of the potential for an interaction. Additional sources should be consulted to identify appropriate options.

MACROLIDES Erythromycin can inhibit the hepatic metabolism of many concurrently administered drugs, such as theophylline, carbamazepine, terfenadine, warfarin, and ergot alkaloids—an effect

TABLE 100-4 Interactions of antibacterial agents with other drugs

Antibacterial agent (A)	Drug (B)	Effect	Clinical relevance*
Erythromycin	Theophylline	Increased levels of B	1
	Carbamazepine	Increased levels of B	1
	Digoxin	Increased levels of B	3
	Triazolam	Increased levels of B	2
	Ergotamine	Increased levels of B	1
	Warfarin	Increased levels of B	2
	Cyclosporine	Increased levels of B	1
	Terfenadine/astemazole	Increased levels of B	1
	Valproate	Increased levels of B	2
Fluoroquinolones	Theophylline	Increased levels of B[†]	2
	Divalent/trivalent cations (Al, Fe, Mg, etc.)	Decreased levels of A	1
Tetracyclines	Divalent/trivalent cations	Decreased levels of A	1
	Digoxin	Increased levels of B	3
Sulfonamides	Oral hypoglycemic agent	Increased levels of B	2
	Phenytoin	Increased levels of B	2
	Warfarin	Increased levels of B	2
Metronidazole	Ethanol	Disulfiram-like reaction	2
	Warfarin	Increased levels of B	2
Rifampin	Warfarin	Decreased levels of B	1
	Oral contraceptive	Decreased levels of B	1
	Cyclosporine	Decreased levels of B	1
	Oral hypoglycemic	Decreased levels of B	1
	Glucocortoids	Decreased levels of B	1
	Methadone	Decreased levels of B	1
	Digoxin/digitoxin	Decreased levels of B	1
	Quinidine	Decreased levels of B	1
	Azole antifungal agent	Decreased levels of B	2
	Phenytoin	Decreased levels of B	2
	Zidovudine	Decreased levels of B	1
	Diltiazem	Decreased levels of B	1
	Verapamil	Decreased levels of B	1

* 1 = a well-documented interaction with clinically important consequences; 2 = an interaction of uncertain frequency but possible clinical importance; 3 = an unusual interaction of possible clinical importance in some patients.
[†] Enoxacin > ciprofloxacin > norfloxacin/ofloxacin > lomefloxacin.

leading to increased serum concentrations and toxicity. The magnitude of the theophylline interaction is highly variable and proportional to the dose and duration of erythromycin treatment. In contrast, cyclosporine levels predictably increase when erythromycin is administered, since erythromycin inhibits the specific enzyme responsible for cyclosporine metabolism. Decreased metabolism of terfenadine and probably astemazole has been reported to cause severe cardiac dysfunction. Clarithromycin appears to be similar to erythromycin in its inhibitory potential, although azithromycin may have little effect on the metabolism of other drugs. In approximately 10 percent of patients receiving digoxin, concentrations will increase when erythromycin is also given; the mechanism is increased absorption of digoxin because of the killing of digoxin-metabolizing bacteria by erythromycin.

TETRACYCLINES Drug interactions with tetracyclines are relatively uncommon. The most important interaction is the reduction in absorption when tetracyclines are coadministered with di- and trivalent cations, such as antacids, iron compounds, or dairy products. A similar interaction is seen with quinolones (see below). Food also adversely affects absorption of most tetracyclines. Inducers of hepatic isoenzymes, such as phenytoin and barbiturates, increase the clearance of doxycycline; although the clinical significance of this effect is unknown, use of an alternative antibiotic may be appropriate.

SULFONAMIDES Sulfonamides may increase the hypoprothrombinemic effect of warfarin by inhibition of metabolism of the more potent isomer of warfarin and possibly by protein-binding displacement. Sulfonamides also may potentiate the effects of oral hypoglycemic agents and phenytoin through reduction in metabolism or displacement from serum protein.

FLUOROQUINOLONES There are two clinically important drug interactions with fluoroquinolones. First, as with tetracyclines, divalent and trivalent cations chelate all fluoroquinolones and prevent most of the dose from being absorbed. Second, certain fluoroquinolones (enoxacin, ciprofloxacin, and, to a lesser extent, norfloxacin and ofloxacin, but not lomefloxacin) can inhibit hepatic enzymes which metabolize theophylline, with resultant theophylline toxicity. The same mechanism accounts for increases in serum caffeine concentrations, but the clinical significance of this interaction is unknown. Scattered reports indicate that quinolones also can potentiate the nephrotoxicity of cyclosporine, exaggerate the effects of warfarin, and increase neurotoxicity when coadministered with nonsteroidal anti-inflammatory agents. However, these interactions have not been confirmed by controlled trials.

RIFAMPIN Rifampin is an excellent inducer of many cytochrome P450 enzymes and increases the hepatic clearance of a number of drugs, including the following (with the indicated predictable outcomes): oral contraceptives (pregnancy), warfarin (decreased prothrombin times), cyclosporine and prednisone (organ rejection or exacerbations of any underlying inflammatory condition), and verapamil and diltiazem (increased dosage requirements).

METRONIDAZOLE Metronidazole can cause a disulfiram-like syndrome when alcohol is ingested, and patients should be instructed to avoid alcohol. Inhibition of the metabolism of warfarin by metronidazole leads to significant rises in prothrombin times.

PROPHYLAXIS OF BACTERIAL INFECTIONS

INDICATIONS FOR PROPHYLAXIS Antibacterial agents are occasionally indicated for use in patients who have no evidence of infection but who have been or are expected to be exposed to bacterial pathogens under circumstances that constitute a major risk of infection. The basic tenets of antimicrobial prophylaxis are as follows: First, the risk or potential severity of infection should be greater than the risk of side effects from the antibacterial agent. Second, the antibacterial agent should be given for the shortest period necessary to prevent target infections. Third, the antibacterial agent should be given before the expected period of risk (e.g., surgical prophylaxis) or as soon as

TABLE 100-5   Prophylaxis of bacterial infections in adults

Condition	Antibacterial agent	Duration of prophylaxis
Nonsurgical		
Cardiac lesions susceptible to bacterial endocarditis	Amoxicillin*	Before and after procedures causing bacteremia
Recurrent *S. aureus* infections	Mupirocin	Intranasally for 5 days
Contact with patient with meningococcal meningitis	Rifampin	2 days
Bite wounds[†]	Penicillin V or amoxicillin–clavulanic acid	3–5 days
Recurrent cystitis	Trimethoprim-sulfamethoxazole	3 times per week for up to 1 year or after sexual intercourse
Surgical		
Clean (cardiac, vascular, neurologic, orthopedic)	Cefazolin (vancomycin)[‡]	Before and during procedure
Ocular	Topical combinations and subconjunctival cefazolin	During and at end of procedure
Clean-contaminated (head and neck, high-risk gastroduodenal, biliary tract, cesarean section, hysterectomy)	Cefazolin (or clindamycin for head and neck)	Before and during procedure
Clean-contaminated (colorectal, appendectomy)	Cefoxitin or cefotetan (add oral neomycin + erythromycin for colorectal)	Before and during procedure
Dirty[†] (ruptured viscus)	Cefoxitin or cefotetan ± gentamicin (clindamycin + gentamicin) or another appropriate regimen directed at anaerobes and gram-negative aerobes	Before and for 3–5 days after procedure
Dirty[†] (traumatic wound)	Cefazolin	Before and for 3–5 days after trauma

* Gentamicin should be added to amoxicillin for high-risk gastrointestinal and gentourinary procedures.
† In these cases, use of antibacterial agents is actually treatment of infection rather than prophylaxis.
‡ Vancomycin is recommended only in those institutions which have a high incidence of infection with methicillin-resistant staphylococci.

possible after contact with an infected individual (e.g., prophylaxis for meningococcal meningitis).

Table 100-5 lists the major indications for antibacterial prophylaxis in adults. (The use of antibacterial agents in children to prevent rheumatic fever and otitis media under certain circumstances is also common practice.) The table includes only those indications which are widely accepted, supported by well-designed studies, or recommended by expert panels. Those conditions for which prophylaxis is also used but is less widely accepted include administration of antibacterials to prevent recurrent cellulitis in conjunction with lymphedema, recurrent pneumococcal meningitis in patients with deficiencies in humoral immunity or CSF leaks, traveller's diarrhea, gram-negative sepsis in neutropenic patients, and spontaneous bacterial peritonitis in patients with ascites.

The major use of antibacterial prophylaxis in the United States is for infections following surgical procedures. Antibacterial agents are administered just before and, for long operations, during the surgical procedure in order to ensure high levels in serum and tissues during surgery. The objective is to eradicate bacteria originating from the air of the operating suite, the skin of the surgical team, or the patient's own flora that may contaminate the wound. In all but colorectal surgical procedures, prophylaxis is predominantly directed against staphylococci. Prophylaxis is intended to prevent wound infection or infection of implanted devices, not all infections that may occur during the postoperative period (e.g., urinary tract infections or pneumonia). Prolonged prophylaxis merely alters normal flora and favors infections with organisms resistant to the antibacterial agents used.

ANTIBACTERIAL COSTS AND INAPPROPRIATE USE   Use of antibacterial agents in hospitals in the United States accounts for 20 to 50 percent of all drug costs and represents the largest expenditure for any pharmacologic class. In the outpatient setting, costs of antibacterial drugs are second only to those of cardiovascular agents. It is not unusual for the purchase cost (in 1993 dollars) of a newer parenteral antibiotic to be $1000 to $2000 for a 10- to 14-day course of treatment. Therapy with a new oral antibiotic can easily cost $50 to $60. Administration costs, monitoring costs, and pharmacy charges must be added to these figures. While some newer antibacterial agents

undeniably represent important advances in therapy, many newer drugs offer no advantage over older, less expensive agents.

Clinicians are understandably confused by the bewildering array of available drugs. Numerous surveys have reported that approximately 50 percent of antibiotic use is in some way "inappropriate." Aside from the monetary cost of unnecessary antibiotics, there are the costs of excess morbidity from adverse effects and drug interactions and the eventual costs of treating more resistant organisms. The following suggestions are intended to provide guidance through the antibiotic maze. First, objective evidence regarding the merits of newer drugs is available through publications such as *The Medical Letter*, including the annual update of *Drugs of Choice*. Second, clinicians should become comfortable using a few drugs recommended by independent experts and should resist the temptation to use a new drug unless the merits are clear. A new antibacterial agent with a "broader spectrum and greater potency" or a "longer half-life and higher tissue levels" does not necessarily mean greater clinical efficacy. Third, the clinician must become familiar with local bacterial susceptibility profiles. It may not be necessary to use a new drug with "improved activity against *P. aeruginosa*" if that pathogen is rarely encountered or if it retains full susceptibility to older drugs. Finally, with regard to inpatient use of antibacterial drugs, appropriate empirical treatment with one or more broad-spectrum agents may often be simplified with use of a narrower-spectrum agent or even an oral drug once the results of cultures and susceptibility tests become available. While there is an understandable temptation to not alter effective therapy, no data suggest that switching to a more specific agent, once the patient has improved clinically, alters efficacy. If these guidelines are followed, the care of patients will not be compromised, many unnecessary complications and expenses can be avoided, and the useful life of valuable drugs will be extended.

REFERENCES

Antimicrobial prophylaxis in surgery. Med Lett Drugs Ther 34:5, 1992
DONOWITZ GR, MANDELL GL: Beta-lactam antibiotics. N Engl J Med 319:419, 1988
EBERT SC, CRAIG WA: Pharmacodynamic properties of antibiotics: Application of drug monitoring and dosage regimen design. Infect Control Hosp Epidemiol 11:319, 1990

Handbook of Adverse Drug Interactions: New Rochelle, The Medical Letter, 1991

HOOPER DC, WOLFSON JS: Fluoroquinolone antimicrobial agents. N Engl J Med 324:384, 1991

JACOBY GA, ARCHER GL: Mechanisms of disease: New mechanisms of bacterial resistance to antimicrobial agents. N Engl J Med 324:601, 1991

KUNIN CM: Problems in antibiotic usage, in *Principles and Practice of Infectious Disease,* GL Mandell et al (eds). New York, Churchill Livingstone, 1990, pp 427–434

O'HANLEY P et al: Infectious disorders, in *Basic Principles in Therapeutics,* KL Melmon et al (eds). New York, McGraw-Hill, 1992, pp 642–720

PRATT WB, FEKETY R (eds): *The Antimicrobial Drugs.* New York. Oxford University Press, 1986

The choice of antibacterial drugs: Med Lett Drugs Ther 34:49, 1992

section 5 Diseases caused by gram-positive bacteria

101 PNEUMOCOCCAL INFECTIONS

ROBERT AUSTRIAN

ETIOLOGY The pneumococcus (*Streptococcus pneumoniae*) is a gram-positive encapsulated coccus that usually grows in pairs or short chains. In the diplococcal form, the adjacent margins are rounded and the opposite ends slightly pointed, giving the organisms a lancet shape. In stained preparations of exudate, gram-negative forms are sometimes present. Pneumococcal colonies are surrounded by greenish discoloration on or in blood agar and are confused at times with other alpha-hemolytic streptococci to which they are closely related. Their isolation from respiratory secretions may be facilitated by inclusion of 5 μg gentamicin per milliliter in the medium. Pneumococci can be distinguished by their bile solubility and mouse virulence or by serologic typing. Another method with approximately 90 percent specificity, utilizing inhibition of pneumococci by Optochin-impregnated paper disks, is less cumbersome.

The capsular substances are complex polysaccharides and are the basis for dividing pneumococci into serotypes. Organisms exposed to type-specific antiserum show a positive capsular precipitin reaction, the Neufeld quellung reaction; by this means, 84 serotypes have been identified. All are pathogenic for human beings, but types or groups 3, 4, 6, 7, 9, 12, 14, 18, 19, and 23 are encountered currently most often in clinical practice. Types or groups 6, 9, 14, 19, and 23 frequently cause pneumonia and otitis media in children.

Specific typing of pneumococci remains of great clinical importance if pneumococcus is to be identified with regularity, and recognition of pneumococcus has decreased significantly since the abandonment of capsular typing by most clinical laboratories. The detection of pneumococcal capsular polysaccharides in sputum and other body fluids by immunologic methods such as counter-immuno-electrophoresis (CIE) or latex agglutination provides an alternative to bacteriologic techniques for the presumptive diagnosis of pneumococcal infection. Because of cross reactions between the polysaccharides of pneumococci and of other bacterial species, immunologic diagnosis is less specific than bacteriologic diagnosis.

PATHOGENESIS The mechanism by which pneumococci damage the mammalian host is obscure, and no toxin elaborated by the organism has been shown to play a major pathogenic role in pneumococcal infection, although the teichoic acid component of the cell wall may cause inflammation. The capsular polysaccharides, although nontoxic, are known to be necessary factors in virulence and to offer some protection of the organism from phagocytosis.

Although "pneumococcal pharyngitis" is a doubtful clinical entity, invasion of nasopharyngeal tissue may occur in the infant and occasionally in the nonimmune adult and be followed by spread to the circulation via the cervical lymphatics. At times, secondary infection of serous cavities in the absence of demonstrable focal infection of the upper or lower respiratory tract may occur. The organisms multiply readily in vivo and may produce acute inflammation of the lungs, serous cavities, and endocardium.

The normal human respiratory tract is provided with a variety of mechanisms which guard the lungs from infection. The lower respiratory tract is protected by the glottis and larynx, and material passing these barriers stimulates the expulsive cough reflex. Removal of small particles impinging on the walls of the trachea and bronchi is facilitated by their mucociliary lining (see Chap. 220), and growth of bacteria reaching normal alveoli is inhibited by their relative dryness and by the phagocytic activity of alveolar macrophages. Any anatomic or physiologic derangement of these coordinated defenses tends to augment the susceptibility of the lungs to infection. Anesthesia, alcoholic intoxication, convulsions, and disturbed innervation of the larynx depress the cough reflex and may permit aspiration of infected material. Alterations in the tracheobronchial tree leading to anatomic changes in the epithelial lining or to localized obstruction increase the vulnerability of the lungs to infection. Pulmonary edema, local or generalized, resulting from viral infection, inhalation of irritant gases, cardiac failure, or contusion of the chest wall provides a fluid menstruum in the alveoli for the growth of bacteria and their spread to adjacent areas of the lung. Viral infection of the respiratory epithelium with concomitant disruption of its component cells interferes significantly with the clearance of bacteria from the lungs, an observation in accord with the high incidence of pneumococcal pneumonia during epidemics of viral influenza and its frequent clinical association with sporadic viral respiratory infections.

Pneumonia usually begins in the right lower, right middle, or left lower lobe, those areas to which gravity is most likely to carry upper respiratory secretions aspirated during sleep. Bronchial embolization with infected mucinous secretions during the course of an upper respiratory infection appears to be the initiating factor in many cases of pneumococcal pneumonia. Protected initially from phagocytosis by mucinous material, the bacteria multiply and, in infected alveoli, evoke the outpouring of proteinaceous fluid which serves both as a nutrient and as a vehicle for spread to adjacent alveoli. Soon thereafter, polymorphonuclear leukocytes migrate from the pulmonary capillaries to phagocytize a part of the pneumococcal population before the appearance of detectable antibody. Delay in the polymorphonuclear leukocytic response occurs during alcoholic intoxication and certain forms of anesthesia, permitting spread of infection. Glucocorticoids also may interfere with leukocyte migration. Later, as the pneumonic lesion evolves, macrophages appear in the exudate and remove the debris of fibrin and cells. It is probable that antibody to the capsular polysaccharide of the invading pneumococcus makes its appearance locally in the lung before being detectable in the circulation. Such antibody increases the efficiency of phagocytosis approximately twofold and causes agglutination of the organisms and their adherence to alveolar walls, thereby slowing their dissemination in the lung. The outcome of infection depends, therefore, on the rate at which bacteria can multiply in the edema fluid and spread and on the host's ability to immobilize and destroy them by phagocytosis. Individuals with deficiencies of the early components of complement or hypogammaglobulinemia and patients with multiple myeloma (see Chap. 81) incapable of producing anticapsular antibody are prone to recurrent attacks of pneumococcal pneumonia. Repeated infection with the same pneumococcal type should always prompt a search for dysgammaglobulinemia.

The attack rates of bacterial pneumonia and of pneumococcal bacteremia are markedly increased in individuals infected with HIV both before and after the development of AIDS. Neither the clinical manifestations of pneumococcal infection nor the distribution of capsular types causing infection differ significantly from those of the general population.

Failure of local defense mechanisms in the lung results in lymphatic spread of pneumococci to the hilar lymph nodes. In the sinusoids of these organs, a sequence of events not unlike that in the lung ensues. If infection is not checked in this secondary line of defense, organisms find their way into the thoracic duct and then into the circulation. Although transient bacteremia may occur at the onset of many cases of pneumococcal pneumonia, it is detectable in only 20 to 30 percent of cases. Bacteremia, which reflects the body's inability to localize the pulmonary infection, is a poor prognostic sign and carries with it the danger of metastatic infection. The mortality of treated or untreated bacteremic pneumococcal pneumonia is four times that resulting from comparably managed nonbacteremic infections. Metastatic infection secondary to bacteremia may occur in the meninges, joints, or peritoneum or on the endocardium. Direct spread from the infected lung may give rise to empyema or to pericarditis.

Natural recovery from pneumococcal infection coincides usually, but not invariably, with the appearance of detectable type-specific antibody in the circulation and is often accompanied by a dramatic and abrupt fall in temperature, the so-called crisis. Antibody aids recovery by increasing the efficiency of phagocytosis and by limiting dissemination of the organisms. Bacteriostatic drugs, such as sulfonamides, facilitate control of the infection by limiting the size of the pneumococcal population, but the host's defense mechanisms are still required for the elimination of the bacteria. Bactericidal agents, such as penicillin, cause the death of pneumococci in the lung and are effective when some of the host's defense mechanisms are compromised. With the arrest of infection, the alveolar exudate undergoes liquefaction, the inflammatory debris is removed by expectoration and via the lymphatic channels, and the lung is restored to its normal state. Necrosis of pulmonary tissue as a result of pneumococcal infection is distinctly uncommon. Primary pneumococcal lung abscess is a rare clinical entity, although the diagnosis is mistakenly made at times when pneumococcal infection complicates lung abscess of other origins.

In addition to causing pneumonia and its metastatic sequelae, pneumococcus can extend from the nasopharynx to its adjacent structures, giving rise to otitis media, mastoiditis, paranasal sinusitis, or conjunctivitis. Soft tissue abscesses are rare but may occur, notably in patients with systemic lupus erythematosus and complement deficiency.

PNEUMOCOCCAL PNEUMONIA

Pneumococcal pneumonia is a disease of considerable uniformity, in contrast to other infections such as typhoid fever and tuberculosis. The diseases produced by different pneumococcal serotypes show little variation in severity or in clinical manifestations. The prognosis in type 3 pneumococcal pneumonia is usually regarded as poor, probably because type 3 infections occur frequently in the aged and in patients with other debilitating diseases, such as diabetes and congestive heart failure. The usual lesion in adults is segmental or lobar in distribution, but in children and the aged, bronchopneumonia, characterized by patchy involvement, is frequent.

MANIFESTATIONS   Pneumonia is often preceded for a few days by coryza or some other form of common respiratory disease. The onset is frequently so abrupt that the patient can state the exact hour that illness began. There is a sudden *shaking chill* in more than 80 percent of the cases and a rapid rise in temperature, with corresponding tachycardia and an increase in respiratory rate (tachypnea). Most patients with pneumococcal pneumonia have a single rigor unless antipyretic drugs are administered, and repeated chills should suggest another etiologic agent.

About 75 percent of patients develop severe *pleuritic pain* and *cough*, productive of pinkish or "rusty" mucoid sputum, within a few hours. The chest pain is agonizing, and respirations become rapid, shallow, and grunting as the patient tries to splint the affected side. Many patients are mildly cyanotic as a result of hypoxia caused by $\dot{V}/\dot{Q}$ (ventilation-perfusion ratio) abnormality or shunt, which accompanies altered respiration, and show dilatation of the alae nasi when first seen. Patients appear acutely ill, but nausea, headache, and malaise are not prominent, and most individuals are alert. Pleuritic pain and dyspnea are the dominant complaints.

In the untreated disease, there are sustained fever of 39.2 to 40.5°C (103 to 105°F) and continued pleuritic pain, cough, and expectoration; and *abdominal distention* is frequent. *Herpes labialis* is a common complication. After 7 to 10 days, there are diaphoresis, abrupt defervescence, and dramatic improvement in well-being, the "crisis."

In cases which terminate fatally, there is usually extensive pulmonary involvement, and dyspnea, cyanosis, and tachycardia are prominent. Circulatory collapse or a picture resembling adult respiratory distress syndrome has been observed. Death in a few patients is associated with empyema or some other suppurative complication such as meningitis or endocarditis.

Physical examination reveals restricted motion of the affected hemithorax. Tactile fremitus may be decreased during the initial day of illness but is usually increased when consolidation is fully established. Deviation of the trachea away from the affected lung suggests pleural effusion or empyema. The percussion note is dull, and if the lesion is in an upper lobe, impaired motion of the diaphragm can be detected on the affected side. Very early in the course of infection, breath sounds are diminished, but as the lesion evolves, they become tubular or bronchial in quality, and bronchophony and whispered pectoriloquy can be elicited. These findings are accompanied by fine crepitant rales.

EFFECT OF SPECIFIC CHEMOTHERAPY   Pneumococcal pneumonia usually improves promptly when an appropriate antimicrobial drug is given. Within 12 to 36 h after initiation of treatment with penicillin, temperature, pulse, and respiration begin to fall and may reach normal values, pleuritic pain subsides, and the spread of the inflammatory process is halted. The temperature of approximately half the patients, however, requires 4 days or longer to become normal, and failure of the patient's temperature to reach normal in 24 to 48 h should not prompt a change in antibacterial therapy in the absence of other indications.

COMPLICATIONS   The typical course of pneumococcal pneumonia can be modified by the development of one or more local or distant complications:

In the lung   ATELECTASIS   Atelectasis of all or part of a lobe may occur during the active stage of pneumonia or after treatment has been instituted. The patient may complain of sudden recurrence of pleuritic pain and show rapid respirations. Small areas of atelectasis are often detected by x-ray in the absence of symptoms. These areas usually clear with coughing and deep breathing, but bronchoscopic aspiration is occasionally necessary. If atelectasis is allowed to persist, the affected area becomes fibrotic and functionless.

DELAYED RESOLUTION   Return of physical findings in the lung to normal after pneumococcal pneumonia is usually complete within 2 to 4 weeks. X-ray evidence of residual pulmonary consolidation, however, may persist as long as 8 weeks, and other radiologic manifestations of the infection (volume loss, stranding, and pleural disease) may persist for up to 18 weeks. The process of resolution may require a longer time in those over 50 years of age and in those with chronic obstructive airway disease or alcoholism.

ABSCESS   Lung abscess is a rare sequel to pneumococcal infection, although pneumococcal pneumonia is a not uncommon complication of lung abscess of other origins. It is manifested by continued fever and profuse expectoration of purulent sputum. X-ray shows one or more cavities. This complication is exceedingly rare in patients who receive penicillin therapy and is most likely to follow infection with pneumococcus type 3.

In adjacent structures   PLEURAL EFFUSION   Pleural effusion detectable in lateral decubitus x-rays of the chest occurs in approximately half of patients with pneumococcal pneumonia and is associated with delay in the initiation of therapy and with bacteremia. Usually the effusion is sterile and is absorbed spontaneously within a week or two. At times, however, the effusion is large and requires aspiration or drainage.

EMPYEMA   Before the introduction of effective chemotherapy, empyema occurred in 5 to 8 percent of patients with pneumococcal pneumonia; it is now observed in less than 1 percent of treated cases. It is manifested by persistent fever or pleuritic pain, together with signs of pleural effusion. In the early stages, the gross appearance of infected fluid may not differ from that of a sterile pleural effusion; later, there is a profuse outpouring of polymorphonuclear leukocytes and fibrin, resulting in an exudate of thick greenish pus containing large clots of fibrin. The quantity of exudate may become large enough to displace mediastinal structures. In neglected cases, this process leads to extensive pleural scarring, with limitation of thoracic movement. Rupture and drainage through the chest wall *(empyema necessitatis)* occur but are rare. Metastatic *brain abscess* is an occasional complication of chronic empyema.

PERICARDITIS   A particularly serious complication is spread of infection to the pericardial sac. This lesion is characterized by pain in the precordial region, a friction rub synchronous with the heartbeat, and distention of cervical veins, although one or all of these findings may be absent. The possibility of coexisting purulent pericarditis should be considered whenever a very ill patient with pneumonia develops empyema.

Metastatic infections   *Arthritis* occurs more often in children than in adults. The affected joint is swollen, red, and painful, with a purulent effusion. It usually subsides promptly with systemic administration of penicillin, although aspiration and intraarticular injection of penicillin may be necessary in adults.

Acute bacterial endocarditis and *meningitis,* complications of pneumococcal pneumonia, are discussed subsequently.

Paralytic ileus   Gaseous abdominal distention is commonly present and in severely ill patients may assume such serious proportions that the term *paralytic ileus* is justified. This complication further impairs respiratory movement by elevation of the diaphragm and constitutes a difficult problem in management. A rarer and more serious gastrointestinal complication is acute gastric dilatation.

Impaired liver function   Alterations in hepatic function are common during the course of pneumococcal pneumonia, and mild jaundice is not at all rare. The pathogenesis of the jaundice is not entirely clear, although in some patients it appears to be related to glucose-6-phosphate dehydrogenase deficiency.

LABORATORY FINDINGS   *Sputum* should be obtained in the physician's presence before the administration of antimicrobial drugs to ensure its quality. Although resort to transtracheal aspiration or lung puncture may be necessary on occasion to establish the cause of pneumonia, routine use of these invasive techniques is not recommended because of their attendant, albeit infrequent, complications. When stained by Gram's method, the sputum shows polymorphonuclear leukocytes and variable numbers of gram-positive cocci, singly and in pairs. These can be typed directly by the Neufeld quellung technique, and this procedure should be used to facilitate diagnosis whenever possible. The *blood culture* is positive for pneumococci during the first days of untreated illness in 20 to 30 percent of cases. The white blood cell count usually shows a polymorphonuclear *leukocytosis* ranging from 12×10^9 to 25×10^9 cells per liter (12,000 to 25,000 cells per microliter). A normal white count or

leukopenia is sometimes observed in patients with overwhelming infection and bacteremia. Occasionally, pneumococci may be seen directly in granulocytes of patients with bacteremia by examining the buffy coat after staining with Wright's stain. These patients often have asplenia. *X-ray of the chest* usually reveals a homogeneous density in the affected area of the lung. In well-established cases, the density may occupy one or more entire lobes. Atypical patterns of consolidation may be seen in patients with underlying chronic pulmonary disease.

EXTRAPULMONARY PNEUMOCOCCAL INFECTION

PNEUMOCOCCAL MENINGITIS   The pneumococcus is second only to the meningococcus as a cause of purulent meningitis in adults; in children, meningitis caused by *Haemophilus influenzae* is also more frequent than pneumococcal infection.

Pneumococcal meningitis can develop as a "primary" disease without preceding signs of infection elsewhere; as a complication of pneumococcal pneumonia; by extension from otitis, mastoiditis, or sinusitis; or following a skull fracture which creates an opening between the subarachnoid space and the nasal cavity or paranasal sinuses. Patients with pneumococcal endocarditis frequently develop meningeal infection. Patients with multiple myeloma and with sickle cell disease seem to be prone to pneumococcal infection of the meninges, just as they are to pneumonia.

The *manifestations* are those of any acute pyogenic meningitis (see Chap. 374) and include chills, fever, headache, nuchal rigidity, Kernig's and Brudzinski's signs, delirium, and cranial nerve palsies. Evidence of otitis, sinusitis, or pneumonia should be carefully sought by physical and roentgenographic examination in all patients.

The *spinal fluid* is under increased pressure, appears cloudy, often with a greenish tint, and shows a high protein and low glucose content. Stained smears usually reveal gram-positive diplococci and polymorphonuclear leukocytes; in some patients, the number of cells in the spinal fluid is surprisingly small, and much of the cloudiness is produced by the bacterial content. The diagnosis can be established rapidly by identification of pneumococci in the spinal fluid by Gram's stain or by the Neufeld quellung reaction. Immunologic tests (CIE or latex agglutination) are positive in approximately 80 percent of culture-positive cases and may provide a presumptive bacterial cause of infection in some patients from whose spinal fluid no organism is recovered.

With appropriate chemotherapy, recovery can be expected in 70 percent of cases; the prognosis is better in children than in infants or adults, and limited but inconclusive data suggest that anti-inflammatory therapy may be of benefit. Relapse may occur but is unusual if adequate treatment is carried out. Subarachnoid block, the result of accumulation of large amounts of thick exudate in the meningeal space and at the base of the brain, is an infrequent complication.

PNEUMOCOCCAL ENDOCARDITIS   Endocarditis is a rare complication of pneumonia or meningitis. The clinical picture is that of acute bacterial endocarditis (see Chap. 85), with remittent fever, splenomegaly, and metastatic infection of the lungs, meninges, joints, eye, and other tissues. Petechiae are uncommon. The infection can attack normal valves and is particularly likely to occur on the aortic valve. The valvular infection is destructive, and loud murmurs and heart failure develop rapidly. Rupture or perforation of cusps or even rupture of the aorta may occur. The blood culture is consistently positive for the pneumococcus in the absence of treatment with antimicrobial drugs, yet at the same time antibodies to the infecting organism may be demonstrable in the blood, a combination of findings seldom observed except in endocarditis or brucellosis. Although the infection is relatively easy to cure with penicillin, damage to valve leaflets, especially to the cusps of the aortic valve, may be followed by rapidly progressive heart failure. Surgical repair or replacement of damaged valvular structures should be carried out early, before heart failure becomes intractable.

PNEUMOCOCCAL PERITONITIS Pneumococcal peritonitis is a rare disease and is probably the sequel to transient pneumococcal bacteremia, although, because of its somewhat greater frequency in young girls, it has been hypothesized that the organism may gain entry to the peritoneum via the vagina and fallopian tubes. Peritonitis was formerly a common complication of the nephrotic syndrome, particularly in children, but it occurs now with a frequency of less than 2 percent. In adults, the disease is seen in association with cirrhosis or with carcinoma of the liver. The diagnosis is made by examination of the ascitic fluid; blood cultures are often positive, and a polymorphonuclear leukocytosis is the rule.

TREATMENT

SPECIFIC ANTIMICROBIAL THERAPY Although resistance of pneumococci to antimicrobial drugs was long regarded as an insignificant problem, increasing numbers of strains from widely separated geographic areas throughout the world have been found in the last decade to be resistant to one or to all of the following agents: penicillins, cephalosporins, tetracyclines, chloramphenicol, erythromycin, clindamycin, cotrimoxazole, and aminoglycosides. For this reason, sensitivity of the infecting organism to the drug(s) to be used should be determined, particularly in treating extrapulmonary infection. In the absence of resistance or of hypersensitivity to it, penicillin G (benzylpenicillin) is the drug of choice for all manifestations of pneumococcal infection. Strains of pneumococcus manifesting increased resistance to penicillin are being recovered with increasing frequency from humans in a number of areas throughout the world. Although the level of such resistance rarely precludes treatment with this antibiotic when infection is confined to the lung, awareness of the phenomenon is necessary. A dose of 600,000 units daily provides a good margin of safety in treating adults with bacteremic or nonbacteremic infection in the absence of an extrapulmonary focus when caused by pneumococci lacking increased resistance to the drug, but the occurrence of pneumococci showing increased resistance to penicillin makes the initiation of therapy with larger amounts desirable. Treatment may be started with doses of 600,000 units of aqueous crystalline penicillin G or procaine penicillin administered at 6-h intervals to be continued until the patient has been afebrile for 48 to 72 h. Pneumococcal pneumonia can be treated with an oral penicillin, preferably one resistant to gastric acid (see Chap. 100), in dosage equivalent to 2.4 to 4.8 million units of penicillin G. *Peritonitis* caused by sensitive strains responds usually within 36 to 48 h to 2 to 4 million units of penicillin daily.

Pneumococcal meningitis in adults should be treated with 18 to 24 million units of penicillin G daily intravenously. Larger amounts should not be used, to avoid neurotoxicity from excessive dosage. Intrathecal administration of penicillin is unnecessary, and supplementation of penicillin with broad-spectrum bacteriostatic drugs such as tetracyclines may exert a deleterious effect. All pneumococcal isolates from cerebrospinal fluid should be tested promptly for their sensitivity to antibacterial drugs, including ceftriaxone, resistance to which has been demonstrated. Vancomycin is the drug of choice for treatment of meningitis caused by pneumococci resistant to multiple antimicrobial agents.

Moderate doses of penicillin G are used to treat pneumococcal endocarditis—8 to 12 million units daily by intravenous infusion. Rapidly developing heart failure as a result of valvular injury and a tendency to form myocardial abscess, however, often lead to a fatal outcome despite the use of antibiotics. Prompt surgical repair or replacement of damaged heart valves should be considered when cardiac failure develops.

Cephalosporins in parenteral doses of 1 to 2 g daily are effective in pneumococcal pneumonia but must be administered with caution to those hypersensitive to penicillin. Many members of this class of β-lactam drugs cannot be used to treat meningitis because of their poor ability to penetrate the blood–cerebrospinal fluid barrier. Several of the newer cephalosporins, including cefotaxime and ceftriaxone, show promise of efficacy in treating pneumococcal meningitis, although experience with each is limited. The tetracyclines in doses of 1 to 2 g daily, erythromycin in doses of 1.6 g daily, or clindamycin in doses of 1.2 g daily are effective treatment for pneumococcal pneumonia if it is caused by a sensitive strain, but they are recommended only for patients who have had untoward reactions to penicillins or cephalosporins. Despite its efficacy, chloramphenicol should not be used to treat pneumococcal infections other than meningitis in patients hypersensitive to penicillin who are infected with a drug-sensitive strain. For patients with illness caused by multiply drug-resistant pneumococci, vancomycin in doses of 2 g daily is the drug of choice. Sulfonamides have little place in the present-day treatment of pneumococcal pneumonia and are useless in endocarditis and meningitis. Aminoglycosides, such as gentamicin, tobramycin, and amikacin, should not be employed to treat pneumococcal infection.

Pneumococcal arthritis responds to systemic penicillin, but aspiration and intraarticular instillation of the drug may be necessary.

Empyema should be detected and treated as early as possible. When an effusion is found, fluid should be removed and examined for bacteria, leukocytes, glucose concentration, and pH. The presence of bacteria or pus, a pH below 7.0, and/or a pleural fluid glucose level below 2.2 mmol/L (40 mg/dL) are indications for institution of closed chest tube drainage. Failure to cure empyema early may be followed by pleural fibrosis and may necessitate subsequent surgical decortication of the lung to restore pulmonary function.

OTHER MEASURES Oxygen administered through a face mask should be used to treat significant cyanosis, cardiac failure, and delirium. In the presence of adult respiratory distress syndrome, positive end-expiratory pressure may be indicated. Codeine, 32 to 64 mg every 4 h, will usually control pleuritic pain. When pain is severe, it may require intercostal nerve block with 1% to 2% procaine for relief.

PROGNOSIS AND PREVENTION

Although the mortality from pneumococcal pneumonia has diminished significantly since the advent of antimicrobial drugs, available evidence indicates that the incidence of the disease has changed little, if at all. The fatality rate in patients over the age of 12 years with bacteremic pneumococcal pneumonia treated with an antibiotic is 18 percent, and in patients over the age of 50 and in those with underlying systemic illness, it is significantly higher.

Signs of poor prognosis in pneumonia include leukopenia, bacteremia, multilobar involvement, any extrapulmonary focus of pneumococcal infection, presence of preexisting systemic disease, asplenia, circulatory collapse, and occurrence of the infection in the first year of life or after the age of 55. Infection with pneumococcus type 3 has a higher mortality rate than that caused by other pneumococcal types. Death is most likely to occur in individuals sustaining irreversible physiologic damage early in the course which is unaltered by antimicrobial therapy. Until the nature of the injury produced by pneumococcus is understood and ways are devised to repair it, vaccination will remain the principal means of protecting those at high risk of a fatal outcome.

A 23-valent vaccine containing the capsular polysaccharides of pneumococcal types 1, 2, 3, 4, 5, 6B, 7F, 8, 9N, 9V, 10A, 11A, 12F, 14, 15B, 17F, 18C, 19F, 19A, 20, 22F, 23F, and 33F, which include the serotypes or groups responsible for 90 percent of bacteremic infections in the United States, is recommended for prevention of pneumococcal infection caused by these serotypes in individuals at high risk of a fatal outcome. In immunocompetent subjects, the vaccine has an aggregate efficacy of 61 percent in preventing infection with any of the pneumococcal types represented in it. Those at higher-than-average risk are individuals over the age of 55 and patients with a variety of chronic systemic illnesses, including heart disease, chronic bronchopulmonary disease, hepatic disease, renal insufficiency, diabetes, and a variety of malignancies. Persons of all ages with sickle cell disease have an increased risk of developing pneumococcal infection, and the vaccine is recommended for those with this disorder over the age of 2 years. Since anatomic or functional asplenia is associated with fulminant overwhelming pneumococcal septicemia with disseminated intravascular coagulation, giving rise to a clinical picture resembling that of the Waterhouse-Friderichsen syndrome, such individuals also should be immunized. However, the vaccine does not contain the antigens of all pneumococcal types, and infection caused by nonincluded types may occur occasionally in immunized subjects. Reactions to the vaccine are usually absent or mild, although in the occasional individual they may resemble those following immunization with typhoid vaccine: local pain, erythema, and elevation of temperature. Recent evidence suggests gradual waning of immunity induced by pneumococcal vaccine over a period of several years, especially in individuals over age 65. Reimmunization of such individuals at intervals of 5 years may be beneficial, although evidence to support such a practice is lacking currently. The aggregate efficacy of vaccine in preventing bacteremic infection is 60 to 70 percent in immunocompetent adults. It may afford little, if any, protection, however, to those with agamma- or dysgammaglobulinemia or to patients who have been subjected recently to intensive antitumor chemotherapy and radiation. Although the efficacy of polyvalent pneumococcal vaccine in those infected with HIV has not been quantified, and although the immunologic responses of small numbers of infected individuals are less than those in their uninfected counterparts, administration of the vaccine to the former should be considered in view of the potential benefit it may confer to those at greatly increased risk and its lack of harmful side effects. In children, immunologic responsiveness to different capsular antigens develops at different times prior to puberty as a result of maturational characteristics of the human immune system and, in infancy, may be manifested only by antibodies of the IgM class. Currently, vaccines of capsular polysaccharide conjugated to proteins such as diphtheria toxoid, which are antigenic in infancy, are under development for pediatric populations. If circumstances dictate, pneumococcal vaccine may be administered concomitantly with influenza viral vaccine, provided each vaccine is injected from a separate syringe at a separate site.

REFERENCES

AUSTRIAN R: *Life with the Pneumococcus.* Philadelphia, University of Pennsylvania Press, 1985
———: Untreated pneumococcal bacteraemia of cryptic origin in the human adult with spontaneous recovery. S Afr Med J 70(suppl):46, 1986
BRADLEY JS, CONNOR JD: Ceftriaxone failure in meningitis caused by *Streptococcus pneumoniae* with reduced susceptibility to beta-lactam antibiotics. Pediatr Infect Dis J 10:871, 1991
DiNUBILE MJ et al: Pneumococcal soft-tissue infections: Possible association with connective tissue diseases. J Infect Dis 163:897, 1991
FRUCHTMAN SM et al: Adult respiratory distress syndrome as a cause of death in pneumococcal pneumonia. Chest 83:598, 1983
HEFFRON R: *Pneumonia with Special Reference to Pneumococcus Lobar Pneumonia.* Cambridge, Mass, Harvard University Press, 1979
KLUGMAN KP: Pneumococcal resistance to antibiotics. Clin Microbiol Rev 3:171, 1990
LEE BL et al: Infectious complications with respiratory pathogens despite ciprofloxacin therapy. N Engl J Med 325:520, 1991
REDD SC et al: The role of human immunodeficiency virus infection in pneumococcal bacteremia in San Francisco residents. J Infect Dis 162:1012, 1990
RESEARCH COMMITTEE, BRITISH THORACIC SOCIETY: Community acquired pneumonia in adults in British hospitals in 1982–83: A study of aetiology, mortality, prognostic factors and outcome. Q J Med 62:195, 1987
ROSS JC, DENSEN P: Complement deficiency states and infection: Epidemiology, pathogenesis and consequences of neisserial and other infections in an immune deficiency. Medicine 63:243, 1984
SHAPIRO ED et al: The protective efficacy of polyvalent pneumococcal polysaccharide vaccine. N Engl J Med 325:1453, 1991
STEPHAN JJ et al: The radiographic resolution of *Streptococcus pneumoniae* pneumonia. N Engl J Med 293:798, 1975
TUOMANEN E et al: Induction of pulmonary inflammation by components of the pneumococcal cell surface. Am Rev Respir Dis 135:869, 1987
VILADRICH PF et al: Evaluation of vancomycin for therapy of adult pneumococcal meningitis. Antimicrob Agents Chemother 35:2467, 1991

102 STAPHYLOCOCCAL INFECTIONS

RICHARD M. LOCKSLEY

The staphylococci, of which *Staphylococcus aureus* is the most important human pathogen, are hardy, gram-positive bacteria that colonize the skin of most human beings. If the skin or mucous membranes are disrupted by surgery or trauma, staphylococci may gain access to and proliferate in the underlying tissues, giving rise to a typically localized, superficial abscess. Although these cutaneous infections are most commonly harmless and self-limited, the multiplying organisms may invade the lymphatics and the blood, leading to the potentially serious complications of staphylococcal bacteremia. These complications include septic shock, which may be indistinguishable from that caused by gram-negative bacteria, and serious metastatic infections, including endocarditis (see Chap. 85), arthritis (see Chap. 91), osteomyelitis (see Chap. 92), pneumonia (see Chap. 220), and abscesses (see Chap. 86) in virtually any organ. Certain strains of *S. aureus* produce toxins that cause skin rashes or that mediate multisystem dysfunction, as in toxic shock syndrome. Coagulase-negative staphylococci, particularly *S. epidermidis*, are important nosocomial pathogens, with a predilection for infecting vascular catheters and prosthetic devices. *S. saprophyticus* is a common cause of urinary tract infection.

ETIOLOGY AND MICROBIOLOGY Staphylococci are gram-positive, nonmotile, aerobic or facultatively anaerobic, catalase-positive cocci within the family Micrococcaceae. The name derives from the typical clustering of organisms (the Greek *staphyle*, "bunch of grapes") observed microscopically in stained specimens taken from colonies grown on solid media. Pathogenic staphylococci are distinguished from nonpathogenic micrococci by the ability of staphylococci to ferment glucose anaerobically and by their sensitivity to lysostaphin endopeptidase. *S. aureus*, the most important human pathogen in the genus, is named for the golden color of colonies grown aerobically on solid media. Staphylococcal strains producing coagulase are designated *S. aureus*. In contrast to coagulase-negative staphylococci, *S. aureus* ferments mannitol, produces DNase, and displays greater susceptibility to lysostaphin. *S. aureus* strains are generally hemolytic when cultured on blood agar and exhibit greater expression of biochemical activity (production of coagulase, toxins, hemolysis) than coagulase-negative staphylococci.

There are 21 recognized species of coagulase-negative staphylococci. Twelve are part of the normal human flora, of which *S. epidermidis* and *S. saprophyticus* are the most important clinically.

Differentiation among strains of *S. aureus* or *S. epidermidis* has been used to identify a common source during epidemics or intrahospital outbreaks of staphylococcal disease. Strains may be distinguished by antimicrobial susceptibility profiles, patterns of lysis by staphylococcal bacteriophages (phage typing), biochemical testing (biotyping), and molecular analysis of plasmids or of plasmid or chromosomal DNA. Of these tests, antibiotic susceptibility testing has the least, and molecular analysis the most, discriminatory ability.

EPIDEMIOLOGY The coagulase-negative staphylococci are part of the normal flora of the skin, mucous membranes, and lower bowel; *S. epidermidis* is the most common species isolated. *S. aureus* transiently colonizes the anterior nares in 70 to 90 percent of persons and may be recovered for relatively prolonged periods of time in 20 to 30 percent of them. Nasal carriage is often accompanied by secondary colonization of the skin. Independent colonization of the perineal area occurs in 5 to 20 percent of persons, and vaginal carriage has been demonstrated in 10 percent of menstruating females. Higher carriage rates of *S. aureus* have been documented in hospital employees (including physicians and nurses), hospitalized patients, persons with atopic dermatitis, and patients whose care requires frequent puncture of the skin, e.g., with insulin-dependent diabetes, dialysis-dependent renal failure, or frequent desensitization injections for allergies. Drug abusers who use needles also have enhanced *S. aureus* carriage rates. Presumably, disturbances in the local cutaneous barrier allow *S. aureus* to establish and maintain colonization successfully.

S. saprophyticus demonstrates greater adherence to urothelial cells than *S. epidermidis*. Approximately 5 percent of healthy males and females have low colony counts of *S. saprophyticus* in the urethral or periurethral areas (see Chap. 90).

Although staphylococci can survive in the environment for prolonged periods of time and airborne spread of organisms can be demonstrated, person-to-person transfer via contaminated hands is the most important mechanism for transmission of these organisms. Hospitalized patients with active staphylococcal infection or those who become heavily colonized, particularly at cutaneous sites (surgical wounds, burns, decubitus ulcers), constitute the greatest reservoir for nosocomially acquired infection. Such patients shed an enormous number of organisms, and the hands of hospital personnel caring for these patients are readily colonized. Failure to use aseptic technique and neglect of hand washing allow transmission of the organisms to the skin of other patients. Strains of both *S. aureus* and *S. epidermidis* may become endemic in areas of the hospital housing patients with large integumental defects, particularly when widespread antimicrobial use favors the acquisition of multiply resistant strains (burn units, intensive care units, bone marrow transplant units). Less frequently, otherwise healthy hospital employees who are nasal carriers have been implicated in nosocomial outbreaks. Upon careful examination, most of these carriers will have active dermatologic infections during the time that effective transmission of staphylococci is documented.

If infections arising from the urinary tract are excluded, *S. aureus* and *S. epidermidis* together have become the most common cause of nosocomial infection in U.S. hospitals. They are the most frequently isolated pathogens in both primary and secondary bacteremias and in cutaneous and surgical wound infections.

PATHOGENESIS Infection by staphylococci usually results from a combination of bacterial virulence factors and diminution in host defense. Important microbial factors include the ability of the staphylococcus to survive under harsh conditions, its cell wall constituents, the production of enzymes and toxins that promote tissue invasion, its capacity to persist intracellularly in certain phagocytes, and its potential to acquire resistance to antimicrobials. Important host factors include an intact mucocutaneous barrier, an adequate number of functional neutrophils, and removal of foreign bodies or devitalized tissues.

Microbial factors Cell wall components of *S. aureus* include a large peptidoglycan complex that confers rigidity on the organism and enables it to survive under unfavorable osmotic conditions, a unique teichoic acid linked to peptidoglycan, and protein A, found both attached to peptidoglycan over the outermost parts of the cell and released in soluble form. Most isolates of *S. aureus* are coated by serologically distinct, thin, polysaccharide capsules. Serotypes 5 and 8 are most prevalent. Both peptidoglycan and teichoic acid are capable of activating the complement cascade via the alternative pathway. Although important for opsonization of organisms for ingestion by phagocytes, complement activation also may play a role in the pathogenesis of shock and disseminated intravascular coagulation. Protein A binds in the Fc portion of certain classes of IgG as well as to the Fc receptor on phagocytes and may serve as a blocking factor preventing neutrophil ingestion of the organism. Specific receptors for laminin and fibronectin may mediate the widespread metastatic potential of *S. aureus*. Activation of tissue factor (procoagulant activity) occurs when endothelial cells and monocytes are incubated with *S. aureus*. The cell wall of certain strains of *S. epidermidis* is also capable of activating complement; shock and disseminated intravascular coagulation during infections by these organisms have been described, although less frequently than with *S. aureus*. The capacity of *S. epidermidis* to adhere to intravascular cannulas and prosthetic devices may explain the propensity of these organisms to cause foreign-body infections. These

organisms bind fibronectin and other matrix proteins that coat catheters and secrete an exopolysaccharide slime that forms a protective biofilm over the colonizing organisms.

Certain enzymes produced by *S. aureus* may play a role in virulence. Catalase degrades hydrogen peroxide and may protect the organism during phagocytosis, when it must withstand the phagocyte's respiratory burst. Coagulase is present in both soluble and cell-bound forms and causes plasma to clot by formation of thrombin-like material. The high correlation between coagulase production and virulence suggests that this substance is important in the pathogenesis of staphylococcal infections, but its precise role as a determinant of pathogenicity has not been determined. Many strains also produce hyaluronidase, an enzyme that degrades hyaluronic acid in the connective tissue matrix and that may promote spreading of infection. A trypsin-like protease from some strains enhances influenza virus infection by proteolytic cleavage of the viral precursor hemagglutinin into its active fragments and may contribute to the morbidity of such coinfections. *S. saprophyticus* produces urease, an enzyme capable of breaking down urea to ammonium, alkalinizing the urine and favoring the formation of struvite stones.

S. aureus may produce numerous extracellular toxins. The expression of multiple toxins, as in gram-negative bacilli, is coordinately regulated by an accessory gene regulator protein, presumably in response to physicochemical environmental stimuli. Toxins may be encoded by chromosomal or plasmid DNA. Four different red cell hemolysins—designated alpha, beta, gamma, and delta toxins—have been identified. Alpha toxin is also dermonecrotic when injected subcutaneously into animals. Delta toxin inhibits water absorption by elevating cyclic AMP in guinea pig ileum and may play a role in the acute watery diarrhea seen in some cases of staphylococcal infection. Leukocidin lyses granulocyte and macrophage membranes by producing membrane pores permeable to cations.

While the role of the above factors in virulence is incompletely understood, the exfoliatin toxins A and B, the staphylococcal enterotoxins, and the toxic shock syndrome toxin—TSST-1—have been implicated in disease. These exotoxins belong to the enlarging family of microbial superantigens. Superantigens bind to regions that lie outside of the normal peptide recognition domains on both MHC class II molecules and certain families of T cell antigen receptors, thus bridging antigen-presenting cells and T cells, resulting in activation. A number of cytokines are produced that subsequently mediate local or systemic effects depending on the amount of toxin formed, the immune status of the host, and the access of the toxin to the circulation.

The exfoliatin toxins mediate the dermatologic manifestations of the staphylococcal scalded-skin syndrome and bullous impetigo. These toxins cause intraepidermal cleavage of the skin at the stratum granulosum, leading to bullae formation and denudation. Antibodies to the toxins are protective in both humans and animals. Seven distinct enterotoxins (A, B, C1, C2, C3, D, and E) have been implicated in food poisoning due to *S. aureus*. The toxins enhance intestinal peristalsis and seem to induce vomiting by a direct effect on the central nervous system. Enterotoxins B and C1 also may mediate toxic shock syndrome (TSS), although this is more frequently due to TSST-1. TSST-1 is produced by over 90 percent of *S. aureus* recovered from women with menstrual TSS and over 60 percent of nonmenstrual cases. Most TSST-1–negative strains produce enterotoxin B and, rarely, enterotoxin C1. These superantigens activate large numbers of T cells and monocyte/macrophages, resulting in release of a number of cytokines, including tumor necrosis factor (TNF), that mediate most of the symptoms of TSS (see Chaps. 16 and 83). The *tst* gene encoding TSST-1 is present in 5 to 25 percent of clinical isolates of *S. aureus* as part of a large, mobile, transposon-like element. Similar elements encode the enterotoxin B and C genes.

Antimicrobial resistance by staphylococci favors their persistence in the hospital environment. Over 90 percent of both hospital and community strains of *S. aureus* causing infection are resistant to penicillin. Resistance is due to the production of β-lactamases; the genes for these enzymes are usually carried by plasmids. A subgroup of *S. aureus* hyperproduce β-lactamase in vitro and show borderline in vitro susceptibility to oxacillin that disappears when clavulanic acid (β-lactamase inhibitor) is added. Infections due to these organisms with "acquired resistance to oxacillin" can be treated safely with penicillinase-resistant β-lactam antimicrobial agents. The true penicillinase-resistant *S. aureus* organisms, called methicillin-resistant *S. aureus* (MRSA), are resistant to all the β-lactam antimicrobials, as well as to the cephalosporins, despite the fact that standard disk susceptibility testing may indicate sensitivity to cephalosporin drugs. Resistance of MRSA is chromosomally mediated and involves production of an altered penicillin-binding protein (PBP 2a or PBP 2′) with a low binding affinity for β-lactams. Not uncommonly, MRSA has acquired R plasmids mediating resistance to some combination of erythromycin, tetracycline, chloramphenicol, clindamycin, and aminoglycosides. MRSA has become increasingly common worldwide, particularly in tertiary-care referral hospitals. In the United States, approximately 5 percent of hospital isolates of *S. aureus* are MRSA; one-third of hospitals surveyed have experienced bacteremias due to MRSA. The isolation of these organisms has remained relatively constant since 1980. Outbreaks continue to occur periodically in the form of intrahospital epidemics. The community carriage rate of MRSA is low, although selected patient populations, such as parenteral drug abusers, may have MRSA at the time of admission to the hospital. These isolates remain susceptible to vancomycin.

Tolerance of staphylococci to β-lactams is an in vitro phenomenon characterized by resistance to the lethal action of normally cidal antimicrobials. It is characterized by a marked discrepancy between the minimal inhibitory and the minimal bactericidal concentrations of the drug. The mechanism may relate to a defect in the normal activation of autolytic enzymes of the bacteria by cell wall–active antimicrobials. Demonstration of the trait is influenced markedly by physicochemical conditions. Although tolerance has been reported to influence the outcome of severe staphylococcal infection adversely, it has been difficult to incriminate tolerance to β-lactams as a significant cause of antibiotic failure because of the in vitro observation that continued treatment with β-lactams will kill tolerant *S. aureus*, although killing proceeds more slowly.

Most cases of *S. epidermidis* infection are nosocomially acquired, and the infecting strains typically express greater variability and degrees of antimicrobial resistance than those of *S. aureus*. Virtually all isolates contain R plasmids that produce β-lactamase and are resistant to penicillin. Approximately one-third are resistant to aminoglycosides and two-thirds are resistant to tetracycline, erythromycin, clindamycin, and chloramphenicol. Hospital isolates of *S. epidermidis* containing multiple antimicrobial-resistant plasmids can serve as important reservoirs for the acquisition of resistance by *S. aureus* and *Enterococcus* species.

Methicillin resistance is common among *S. epidermidis* strains; over 80 percent of isolates from cases with prosthetic valve endocarditis in one study were methicillin-resistant. Conditions of temperature, pH, osmolality, and the presence of chelating agents and heavy metals all may influence the demonstration of resistance. Methicillin-resistant isolates may appear susceptible by routine susceptibility testing. The most reliable identification of these organisms is by their growth from a large inoculum (10^7 cells) spread on agar containing 6 µg/mL oxacillin. Cross-resistance to the other β-lactam antimicrobials and to the cephalosporins is always present, although, as with MRSA, these bacteria may appear susceptible to cephalosporins by conventional disk testing. As with *S. aureus*, *S. epidermidis* strains remain susceptible to vancomycin, although resistance has occurred in strains of *S. haemolyticus*. Although the quinolone antibiotics may be active against methicillin-resistant staphylococci, resistance is widespread due to rapid, single-step mutations in the DNA gyrase or expression of an active efflux transporter.

HOST FACTORS The importance of host factors in resisting staphylococcal infections is demonstrated by the observation that enormous numbers of bacteria are required to establish experimental infections in humans and animals. Areas where skin or mucosal continuity is broken provide portals of entry for staphylococci. More than 50 percent of serious staphylococcal infections of deep tissues arise from cutaneous foci; a smaller number originate from the respiratory, gastrointestinal, or less frequently, the genitourinary tract. Direct inoculation of organisms into the blood is an important route of infection in hospitalized patients with intravenous catheters and in drug abusers.

Staphylococci often invade the integument via plugged hair follicles and sebaceous glands or areas involved by burns, wounds, abrasions, insect bites, or dermatitis. Colonization and invasion of the lungs may occur when the normal mucociliary clearance mechanisms are either bypassed, as occurs with endotracheal intubation, or depressed, as occurs following viral infections of the lung (influenza) or in patients with cystic fibrosis. Mucosal damage to the gastrointestinal tract following cytotoxic chemotherapy or radiotherapy predisposes to invasion from that site.

Once the integument has been breached, local bacterial multiplication is accompanied by inflammation and tissue necrosis at the site of infection. Neutrophils rapidly enter the area and ingest large numbers of staphylococci. Thrombosis of surrounding capillaries occurs; fibrin is deposited about the periphery; later, fibroblasts create a relatively avascular wall about the area. The fully developed staphylococcal abscess consists of a central core of dead and dying leukocytes and bacteria which gradually liquefies to form characteristic thick, creamy pus, surrounded by a fibroblastic wall. When host mechanisms fail to contain the cutaneous or submucosal infection, staphylococci may enter the lymphatics and the bloodstream. Common sites of metastatic seeding include the diaphyseal ends of long bones in children and the lungs, kidneys, cardiac valves, myocardium, liver, spleen, and brain.

Polymorphonuclear leukocytes appear to be the major protective mechanism against staphylococcal disease. Persons with neutropenia or inherited or acquired defects of neutrophil chemotaxis, ingestion, or killing are particularly susceptible to staphylococcal infections. A low number of staphylococci are capable of surviving within phagocytes, which may account for the relatively slow response of staphylococcal infections to antimicrobials and the potential for relapse.

Although infections may occur in all age groups, serious staphylococcal infections most commonly afflict the young and old—particularly those with underlying debilitating disease. Primary staphylococcal pneumonia is common in infants but rare in adults. Superficial staphylococcal pyoderma is more frequent in infants, whereas actual abscess formation occurs more often in adults. While these examples suggest some role for immunity in resistance against staphylococci, there has been no satisfactory demonstration that human staphylococcal disease is followed by effective immunity or that infection can be modified significantly by vaccination. Virtually 100 percent of adults possess antistaphylococcal antibodies in their serum. Except for the efficacy of neutralizing antibodies to toxins in staphylococcal toxin–mediated diseases, the role of humoral immunity in modifying or protecting against staphylococcal infection is unclear.

The presence of a foreign body such as a suture or a prosthetic device markedly decreases the inoculum of staphylococci required to produce experimental infection. Once established, such infections are very difficult to cure without removal of the foreign body. Strains of *S. epidermidis* are capable of adhering firmly to and invading plastic catheters and of secreting a protective glycocalyx covering the adherent colonies. Neutrophil function is also altered in the presence of a foreign body; phagocytosis and killing of *S. aureus* are diminished.

DIAGNOSIS The diagnosis of all staphylococcal infections is made by Gram stain and culture of purulent material, either aspirated pus or involved tissue, or by culture of normally sterile body fluids. Typical clustering of organisms may not be seen in clinical specimens; individual cocci and even short chains of three or four organisms may be present. Bacteria in the static phase or within leukocytes may appear gram-negative. Abundant neutrophils, many containing intracellular organisms, are usually present, except in severely neutropenic patients.

SPECIFIC DISEASES   Superficial infections   Infection of hair follicles manifested as a collection of minute erythematous papules without involvement of the surrounding skin or deeper tissues is termed *folliculitis*. A more extensive and invasive follicular or sebaceous gland infection with some involvement of subcutaneous tissues is termed a *furuncle*, or *boil*. Itching and mild pain are followed by progressive local swelling and erythema, and the overlying skin becomes exquisitely painful on pressure or motion. Relief of pain occurs promptly after spontaneous or surgical drainage.

Furuncles occur most commonly in areas subject to maceration or friction and poor personal hygiene or involved by acne or dermatitis. The face, neck, axillae, buttocks, and thighs are common sites. Staphylococcal infection may involve the apocrine sweat glands in the axilla or groin (hidradenitis suppurativa). These infections may be deep-seated and slow to localize and drain and are prone to recurrence and scarring.

Staphylococcal infections within the thick, fibrous, inelastic skin of the back of the neck and upper part of the back lead to formation of a *carbuncle*. The relative thickness and impermeability of the overlying skin lead to lateral extension and loculation, and a large, indurated, painful lesion with multiple ineffective drainage sites results. Carbuncles produce fever, leukocytosis, extreme pain, and prostration. Bacteremia is common.

Staphylococci frequently colonize impetiginous lesions, but most impetigo is due to group A streptococci. However, staphylococcal impetigo does occur, and while it cannot be clearly differentiated on the basis of its clinical features from streptococcal impetigo, it tends to produce multiple superficial, localized lesions at different stages of development, has a grayish rather than golden-yellow crust, and less often produces high fever. Staphylococcal bullous lesions are caused by exfoliatin-producing strains.

Treatment of most superficial infections does not require the use of antibiotics. Local moist heat, attention to personal hygiene, and washing with germicidal soaps that leave an inhibitory residue on the skin (hexachlorophene, chlorhexidine, triclosan) are usually sufficient. For more severe or recurrent disease, oral antibiotic therapy with dicloxacillin or cloxacillin (2 g/d in four divided doses) for 7 to 10 days may be effective. Incision and drainage should be utilized selectively. Disease presenting with prominent constitutional symptoms or facial or periorbital infection should be treated with intravenous doses of appropriate antimicrobials as outlined in the section on bacteremic disease.

Toxin-mediated staphylococcal diseases   STAPHYLOCOCCAL SCALDED-SKIN SYNDROME (SSSS)   SSSS is a generalized exfoliative dermatitis complicating infection by toxin (exfoliatin)–producing strains of *S. aureus*. The disease typically occurs in newborns (Ritter's disease) and in children under the age of 5; it is rare in adults. Strains of *S. aureus* causing SSSS in the United States are frequently phage group II. The disease begins with a localized cutaneous infection often accompanied by a nonspecific virus-like prodrome. Fever and leukocytosis are mild. A scarlatiniform rash begins in the perioral area, becomes generalized over the trunk and extremities, and finally desquamates. The disease may consist of rash alone (staphylococcal scarlet fever), or large, flaccid bullae develop that may be localized (more common in adults) or generalized. The bullae burst, resulting in red, denuded skin resembling a burn. Friction applied to healthy areas of skin causes the epidermis to wrinkle and separate (Nikolsky's sign). *S. aureus* can usually be recovered from the skin and nasopharynx. Most adults with SSSS are immunosuppressed or have renal insufficiency. Blood cultures are frequently positive, and mortality is significant. Therapy includes antistaphylococcal antibiotics and local skin care. Recovery usually occurs in infants and children.

In adults, SSSS has been grouped with other severe scalding syndromes such as toxic epidermal necrolysis (Lyell's disease). Drug reactions are the most frequent cause of toxic epidermal necrolysis in adults, and the syndrome may be differentiated from SSSS by skin biopsy. Cleavage of the skin in drug-induced toxic epidermal necrolysis occurs at the basal cell layer, resulting in full-thickness denudation, with a greater potential for superinfection and significant fluid and electrolyte loss. In SSSS, cleavage occurs within the epidermis. Kawasaki's disease and toxic shock syndrome also should be considered in the differential diagnosis of SSSS.

TOXIC SHOCK SYNDROME   Toxic shock syndrome (TSS) was described in 1978 as a multisystem disease presenting with high fever, a "sunburn" rash that subsequently desquamated, and hypotension in children who had group I *S. aureus* isolated from mucosal or sequestered sites. In 1980, TSS became epidemic among young, primarily white, women, with onset during menstruation. A strong correlation was found between TSS and recovery of *S. aureus* from vaginal or cervical cultures of affected patients. Subsequently, a marker toxin, TSST-1, that mediates most cases of this syndrome was identified. Staphylococcal enterotoxins B or C1 also may mediate TSS. The pathogenesis involves establishment of a toxin-producing strain in a nonimmune individual under conditions favoring toxin formation, i.e., an aerobic, nutrient environment favoring late log to stationary phase growth of the organism. The attack rate of TSS among the 10 percent of persons lacking sufficient levels of antitoxin antibodies approaches 25 percent in those infected with toxin-positive strains.

Epidemiologically, TSS was associated with the introduction of certain brands of hyperabsorbent tampons. Public education and removal of hyperabsorbent tampons from the market have resulted in a marked decrease in the number of reported cases of TSS. Although the majority of cases continue to occur among menstruating females, nonmenstrual TSS now accounts for up to 45 percent of TSS cases in the United States.

The diagnosis of TSS is based on clinical criteria that include high fever, a diffuse rash that desquamates on the palms and soles over the subsequent 1 to 2 weeks, hypotension that may be orthostatic, and evidence of involvement in three or more organ systems. Such involvement commonly includes gastrointestinal dysfunction (vomiting or diarrhea), renal or hepatic insufficiency, mucous membrane hyperemia, thrombocytopenia, myalgias with elevated creatine phosphokinase (CK) levels, and disorientation with a normal cerebrospinal fluid examination. Hypocalcemia is common. Milder forms of the syndrome have been reported.

The onset is acute and typically occurs around the start of menses in a young woman using tampons or barrier contraception methods. The vaginal mucosa is hyperemic, and *S. aureus* can be cultured from the vaginal discharge. Blood cultures are usually negative. Clinical findings are the same in nonmenstrual-associated TSS. Cutaneous infections, postpartum vaginal and cesarean section wound infections, focal tissue infections (abscesses, empyema, osteomyelitis), postinfluenza pneumonia, and rarely, primary staphylococcal bacteremia have been associated with TSS. Signs of infection may be minimal among patients with postoperative wound infections where the onset typically occurs on the second day after surgery. Nosocomial transmission has been described. The mortality rate of TSS is 3 percent and is most often due to refractory hypotension and the development of the adult respiratory distress syndrome (ARDS) with or without disseminated intravascular coagulation.

Treatment is directed at correcting shock and treating renal failure, pulmonary insufficiency, and disseminated intravascular coagulation when present. Antistaphylococcal antibiotics should be administered parenterally. Focal collections of *S. aureus* must be drained. Because neutralizing antibodies are widespread, the use of intravenous pooled gamma globulin is being investigated. Up to 30 percent of menstruating women with TSS may have recurrences with subsequent menses, although these are generally milder. The use of antistaphylococcal antibiotics to treat TSS and discontinuation of tampon use significantly decrease the likelihood of recurrences.

The differential diagnosis of TSS includes Rocky Mountain spotted fever, meningococcemia, streptococcal scarlet fever, toxic epidermal necrolysis, and Kawasaki's syndrome. A similar syndrome has been described following group A streptococcal infection.

Staphylococcal food poisoning See Chap. 87.

Invasive staphylococcal infections BACTEREMIA AND ENDO-CARDITIS Bacteremia due to *S. aureus* may arise from any local infection, at either extravascular (cutaneous infections, burns, cellulitis, osteomyelitis, arthritis) or intravascular foci (intravenous catheters, dialysis access sites, intravenous drug abuse). Up to one-third of patients do not have an identifiable focus.

Rarely, patients with bacteremia die within 12 to 24 h with high fever, tachycardia, cyanosis, and vascular collapse. Disseminated intravascular coagulation may produce a disease mimicking meningococcemia. Commonly, the disease progresses more slowly, with hectic fever and metastatic abscess formation in the bones, kidneys, lungs, myocardium, spleen, brain, or other tissues.

A major complication of *S. aureus* bacteremia is endocarditis (see Chap. 85). *S. aureus* is the second most common cause of endocarditis and the most common cause among drug addicts. Among nonaddicts, normal valves are involved in 30 to 60 percent of cases, and older, frequently hospitalized, patients with underlying medical disease are most often infected. The mitral, aortic, or both valves may be involved. The disease typically pursues an acute course with high fever, progressive anemia, and frequent embolic and extracardiac septic complications. Progressive valvular insufficiency leads to significant murmurs in 90 percent of patients. Valve ring and myocardial abscesses are common. The mortality rate is 20 to 30 percent. Infection of the aortic valve, the development of uncontrolled congestive heart failure, or evidence of central nervous system involvement are poor prognostic signs; these patients frequently require surgical intervention.

Among addicts, *S. aureus* frequently involves the tricuspid valve. Evidence for septic pulmonary emboli (chest pain, hemoptysis, nodular infiltrates) is common. Audible murmurs and peripheral stigmata of endocarditis are less common than in nonaddicts. Myalgias and back pain may be the major presenting symptoms and obfuscate the diagnosis. The mortality rate is 2 to 10 percent.

Differentiation of bacteremia from endocarditis may be difficult. Patients with normal heart valves with an identifiable, easily managed or removable primary focus of infection, who receive and respond promptly to appropriate antibiotic therapy, and who do not develop evidence of metastatic complications during the subsequent 2 weeks on therapy usually can be treated for bacteremia alone. Patients with underlying valvular disorders, with murmurs of valvular regurgitation, with community-acquired disease and no obvious focus, with infection secondary to drug abuse, with evidence for embolic events, or with echocardiographic evidence for vegetations should be treated for endocarditis. The presence of antibodies to the teichoic acid cell wall component of *S. aureus* after 2 weeks of illness does not distinguish reliably between endocarditis or bacteremia with metastatic foci and uncomplicated bacteremia.

Three carefully collected blood cultures are adequate for the diagnosis in most instances; usually all are positive for *S. aureus*. More cultures may be required if the patient has previously received antibiotics. Purulent skin lesions and urine also should be cultured before instituting antibiotic therapy. The urine may be positive in up to a third of cases of staphylococcal bacteremia (with colony counts typically lower than 10^5 per milliliter); staphylococcal bacteriuria in this setting does not indicate metastatic renal infection.

Intravenous therapy should be initiated with a penicillinase-resistant agent. Nafcillin (1.5 g every 4 h) and oxacillin (2.0 g every 4 h) are preferred to methicillin because of the high incidence of interstitial nephritis with methicillin. Gentamicin (1 mg/kg every 8 h, adjusted for renal function) may be added for the first 48 to 72 h because of evidence for synergy with β-lactam antimicrobials against *S. aureus* and the tendency for patients treated with both drugs to

defervesce more rapidly and to achieve earlier sterilization of the bloodstream. Rare isolates that do not produce β-lactamase should be treated with intravenous penicillin G (4×10^6 units every 4 h). First-generation cephalosporins (cephalothin, cefazolin) also have been used successfully in infections with both penicillinase-positive and -negative strains of *S. aureus*. Patients with serious penicillin allergy or with infections due to methicillin-resistant *S. aureus* should be treated with vancomycin 30 mg/kg per day in two or three divided doses, adjusted for renal function.

Cases of uncomplicated *S. aureus* bacteremia can be treated for 2 weeks. These patients should be followed carefully; relapses should be treated as endocarditis. Uncomplicated right-sided endocarditis in drug addicts has been treated successfully with 2 weeks of intravenous nafcillin plus tobramycin or gentamicin. All other cases of endocarditis should receive 4 to 6 weeks of parenteral antimicrobials. Prosthetic valve endocarditis should be treated with an appropriate penicillin or vancomycin plus gentamicin, with or without rifampin, for 6 weeks. Most cases will require surgery as well.

The response to antimicrobials in staphylococcal endocarditis may be slow, particularly when MRSA is treated with vancomycin. The fever may not disappear until the second week of therapy. Persistent fever or signs of sepsis should prompt a search for metastatic abscesses that require drainage.

S. epidermidis is the most common isolate in primary nosocomial bacteremias and the most frequent organism infecting intravenous access devices. It has been recognized as a major cause of bacteremia among neutropenic cancer patients, arising either from long-term indwelling central catheters or from the gastrointestinal tract, and among high-risk neonates receiving intravenous lipid emulsions. Continued fever, progressive sepsis, multiple pulmonary abscesses, and death may result if this complication is left untreated.

Although an uncommon cause of native valve endocarditis, *S. epidermidis* is the most common cause of prosthetic valve endocarditis (40 percent of cases). Most cases are due to inoculation of organisms at the time of surgery but may not become clinically apparent until 1 year later. Infections frequently involve the valve ring and require surgical intervention. Over 50 percent of patients die.

Because coagulase-negative staphylococci are frequent blood culture contaminants, distinguishing infection from contamination can be difficult. Positive blood cultures demand careful inspection of catheter sites and repeat blood cultures, even in the absence of symptoms, in patients with indwelling catheters or with prosthetic heart valves or vascular grafts. Speciation of multiple isolates may be useful if isolates can be demonstrated to be the same; plasmid analysis may be required. Catheters should be removed and cultured, although antibiotic therapy alone has been successful for treatment of bacteremic catheter-related infections.

Hospital-acquired *S. epidermidis* infections are usually multiply antibiotic-resistant. Methicillin resistance is heterotypic and difficult to exclude. For these reasons, all serious *S. epidermidis* infections should be treated with vancomycin in doses used for *S. aureus*. Prosthetic valve endocarditis should be treated for 6 weeks with vancomycin plus gentamicin, with or without rifampin. Monitoring of renal function and ototoxicity is required.

OSTEOMYELITIS *S. aureus* is responsible for the majority of cases of acute osteomyelitis (see Chap. 92). Although most common in persons under the age of 20, adults over 50 make up an increasingly prevalent group, particularly with involvement of the spine. A primary portal of entry is frequently not identified. In children, the frequent localization in the diaphyseal end of the long bones is thought to be due to the endarterial circulation of the diaphysis. Many patients give a history of preceding trauma to the involved area. Clavicular osteomyelitis has complicated septic thrombosis of a catheterized subclavian vein.

Once established, infection spreads through the newly formed juxtaepiphyseal bone to the periosteum or along the marrow cavity. If the infection reaches the subperiosteal space, the periosteum is lifted, a subperiosteal abscess forms, and rupture with infection of the subcutaneous tissues may occur. Rarely, the joint capsule is penetrated, producing pyogenic arthritis. There is death of bone, producing a sequestrum, followed by new bone formation, the involucrum. Occasionally, indolent staphylococcal infections of bone may persist for years within dense granulation tissue about a central necrotic cavity, a so-called Brodie's abscess.

Osteomyelitis in children may present as an acute process beginning abruptly with chills, high fever, nausea, vomiting, and progressive pain at the site of bony involvement. Muscle spasm about the affected bone is a common early sign, and the child may refuse to move the affected limb. Leukocytosis is common. Blood cultures are positive for *S. aureus* in 50 to 60 percent of cases early in disease. The tissues overlying the involved bone become edematous and warm, and the skin becomes erythematous. Anemia develops during the course of untreated disease.

Staphylococcal vertebral osteomyelitis in the adult differs considerably from acute osteomyelitis in the child. The onset is less abrupt, and there is a greater tendency for bony fusion with obliteration of the disk space. The lumbar spine is most frequently affected.

Osteomyelitis should be suspected in any child with fever, limb pain, and leukocytosis. Similarly, back or neck pain in an adult, when accompanied by fever, should raise the possibility of vertebral osteomyelitis. A history of a preceding cutaneous infection, local tenderness over the bone, and culture of *S. aureus* from the blood are confirmatory. Roentgenograms are usually normal during the first week, but radionuclide and MRI scans are generally abnormal. Bony rarefaction, local periosteal elevation, and new bone formation can frequently be seen during the second week. Needle aspiration or bone biopsy should be performed if necessary to obtain a specific etiologic diagnosis prior to institution of chemotherapy. In chronic osteomyelitis, sinus tracts are often present, but cultures of the sinus tracts are not reliable in the diagnosis.

Therapy should be initiated parenterally using a penicillinase-resistant semisynthetic penicillin as outlined for bacteremia and endocarditis and continued for 4 to 6 weeks. Cephalosporins and clindamycin also have been used. Uncomplicated osteomyelitis in children has been managed with 2 weeks of intravenous therapy followed by 2 to 4 weeks of oral therapy. Vancomycin can be used in penicillin-allergic patients and in infections due to methicillin-resistant organisms. Surgery may be required to remove devitalized bone and to drain soft tissue and periosteal abscesses. Neurologic findings due to epidural abscess and cord compression complicating vertebral osteomyelitis demand early surgical intervention. Aggressive treatment of acute osteomyelitis has decreased the incidence of chronic osteomyelitis, with its penchant for recurrent flare-ups and sinus formation. The cure rate for acute staphylococcal osteomyelitis is approximately 90 percent, and death is rare.

PNEUMONIA   (See Chap. 207) *S. aureus* causes approximately 3 percent of community-acquired bacterial pneumonias. This disease occurs sporadically except during influenza outbreaks, when staphylococcal pneumonia is relatively more common, although still less frequent than pneumococcal pneumonia.

Primary staphylococcal pneumonia in infants and children frequently presents with high fever and cough. Multiple thin-walled abscesses, or pneumatoceles, are present on the chest roentgenogram. Empyema formation is common. Cough may be nonproductive, and blood cultures are usually negative, frequently necessitating empiric antistaphylococcal therapy. In older children and healthy adults, staphylococcal pneumonia is generally preceded by an influenza-like respiratory infection (influenza, measles, or other viruses). Onset of staphylococcal involvement is abrupt, with chills, high fever, progressive dyspnea, cyanosis, cough, and pleural pain. The sputum may be bloody or frankly purulent.

Staphylococci frequently colonize the bronchiectatic airways in children with cystic fibrosis and may cause recurrent episodes of bronchopneumonia. Nosocomial staphylococcal pneumonia typically occurs in intubated patients in intensive care units and in debilitated

patients who are prone to aspiration. Residents of nursing homes may have an increased incidence of staphylococcal pneumonia. Infections distal to an obstructing bronchogenic carcinoma also may be caused by *S. aureus*. These infections can begin insidiously, with increasing fever, tachycardia, and tachypnea the only indications of infection. The disease also may be less abrupt when pulmonary involvement occurs during the course of staphylococcal bacteremia, as in patients with right-sided endocarditis or septic thrombophlebitis. Cavitation and pleural effusions are common, but empyema is unusual.

The course of staphylococcal pneumonia may be stormy despite adequate antimicrobial therapy. Gradual defervescence starting 48 to 72 h after the initiation of therapy is typical.

Staphylococcal pneumonia must be differentiated from other pneumonias. The preceding influenza-like illness, rapid onset of pleural pain, cyanosis, and prostration out of proportion to physical findings should suggest primary staphylococcal pneumonia. Sputum Gram stain showing masses of neutrophils and gram-positive intraleukocytic cocci provides supportive evidence. Leukocytosis is generally present. Blood cultures are positive in 20 to 30 percent of cases. When pneumonia develops suddenly or insidiously in debilitated hospital patients, staphylococci should be considered.

Parenteral therapy should be initiated with antistaphylococcal antimicrobials as outlined for serious bacteremia and endocarditis. Two weeks of intravenous therapy is usually adequate if complications do not develop. Empyema usually necessitates chest tube drainage and may be complicated by the formation of loculations or bronchopleural fistulas. Ultrasound or computed tomography (CT) scan may be required to identify loculated collections of pus for drainage.

CNS INFECTION   *S. aureus* causes 1 to 9 percent of cases of bacterial meningitis and 10 to 15 percent of brain abscesses. Most commonly, spread from a focus outside the CNS, typically from infective endocarditis or by extension from a paraspinal or parameningeal abscess, or nosocomial infection following neurosurgical procedures have been involved. Blood cultures are usually positive. Over 50 percent of epidural abscesses are due to *S. aureus*; up to half these cases may be associated with vertebral osteomyelitis. The thoracic spine and lumbar spine are most frequently involved. Patients present with either acute (<2 weeks) or chronic back pain, usually with low-grade fever and malaise. The onset of radicular pain is an ominous sign that portends progression to frank neurologic dysfunction and ultimate paralysis. The diagnosis is most reliably established using magnetic resonance imaging, although CT scanning and myelography have been useful. Surgical drainage, often with decompression laminectomy, and parenteral antibiotics are required. The duration of therapy is dependent on the adequacy of drainage and the presence or absence of coexisting osteomyelitis.

URINARY TRACT INFECTION   *S. saprophyticus* is, after *Escherichia coli*, the most common cause of primary, nonobstructive urinary tract infection in sexually active young women (see Chap. 90). It is responsible for 10 to 20 percent of infections in healthy outpatients. Symptoms of urgency, frequency, and burning are indistinguishable from urinary infections due to other agents. Fever is absent or low-grade. Although lower tract infection is most common, pyelonephritis has been reported.

The diagnosis is established by examination of the urinary sediment, which characteristically reveals pyuria, microscopic hematuria, and cocci in clumps. The organism may be identified by its resistance to novobiocin and nalidixic acid. *S. saprophyticus* grows readily on blood agar but less well on MacConkey agar and may be missed by currently available rapid diagnostic methods that depend on nitrate reduction or glucose utilization. The criterion for greater than 10^5 bacteria per milliliter developed for gram-negative urinary tract infection is unreliable.

The organism is susceptible to most antimicrobials used for urinary tract infection, including ampicillin, trimethoprim, sulfonamides, and nitrofurantoin. Relapses after appropriate therapy should raise the consideration of infected renal calculi, which may be formed because of the organism's capacity to produce urease.

Isolation of *S. aureus* from a well-collected urine specimen should prompt consideration of staphylococcal bacteremia, which may have been complicated by renal, perinephric, or prostatic abscesses.

Other infections   Infection of the vascular access site with *S. aureus* is a major cause of morbidity and death among patients on hemodialysis. Chronic nasal carriage is the source of most infections. The use of 5-day courses of oral rifampin and topical bacitracin every 3 months significantly decreases the incidence of infection and should be considered in hemodialysis centers where such infections are endemic. *S. epidermidis* and *S. aureus* rank first and second among pathogens infecting prosthetic devices and intravascular grafts and are particularly problematic in AIDS patients with indwelling catheters. Acute *S. aureus* pyomyositis also may complicate the course of HIV infection. *S. epidermidis* infections tend to be more insidious and frequently pursue a prolonged course with high morbidity due in part to the temptation to regard positive cultures as contaminants. *S. epidermidis* is a common cause of endophthalmitis complicating ocular surgery. *S. aureus* is a frequent cause of mastitis among nursing mothers.

CONTROL OF HOSPITAL OUTBREAKS   (See Chap. 98)   Hospital outbreaks of staphylococcal disease may develop rapidly in burn units, intensive care units, or neonatal care units—areas housing debilitated patients under continuous antibiotic pressure. The index case is frequently a patient recently discharged or transferred from another hospital where the organism is endemic. The implicated strains of *S. aureus* are frequently methicillin-resistant (MRSA).

Control demands the rapid identification of the patient reservoir in the affected care units by cultures of wounds, nares, and perineum; urine cultures should be performed for patients with indwelling urinary catheters. Isolation of culture-positive patients together with reinforcement of the need for proper aseptic technique and hand washing by hospital personnel decreases transmission. Housekeeping antisepsis using phenolic cleaning agents should be carried out in the rooms of colonized patients. Early discharge of colonized patients should be encouraged. Charts should be labeled and the patient returned to strict isolation upon readmission to the hospital until shown to be culture-negative.

Although nasal carriers among hospital personnel may transmit the organism, efficient dissemination is by cutaneous diseases (eczema, atopic dermatitis) that have become colonized with *S. aureus*. Such personnel should be removed from clinical duties until they become culture-negative either spontaneously or following therapy.

Decolonization of the skin and nares in patients and personnel has been accomplished by whole-body washing with antiseptic soaps that leave an inhibitory residue on the skin—hexachlorophene, chlorhexidine, or triclosan. Topical antibiotics are generally ineffective. Although intranasal application of mupirocin has eradicated carriage, resistance can develop. Oral antibiotics may be required to abolish the carrier state. Rifampin (600 mg every day for 5 days) has been used successfully alone or, depending on the sensitivity of the staphylococcal isolate, combined with trimethoprim-sulfamethoxazole, doxycycline, or dicloxacillin to prevent the emergence of rifampin resistance.

REFERENCES

BOHACH GA et al: Staphylococcal and streptococcal pyrogenic toxins involved in toxic shock syndrome and related illnesses. Crit Rev Microbiol 17:251, 1990

BRUMFITT W, HAMILTON-MILLER J: Methicillin-resistant *Staphylococcus aureus*. N Engl J Med 320:1188, 1989

ESPERSEN F et al: Changing pattern of bone and joint infections due to *Staphylococcus aureus*: Study of cases of bacteremia in Denmark, 1959–1988. Rev Infect Dis 13:347, 1991

MARTIN MA et al: Coagulase-negative staphylococcal bacteremia: Mortality and hospital stay. Ann Intern Med 110:9, 1989

RAAD II, SABBAGH MF: Optimal duration of therapy for catheter-related *Staphylococcus aureus* bacteremia: A study of 55 cases and review. Clin Infect Dis 14:75, 1992

SCHWARTZMAN WA et al: Staphylococcal pyomyositis in patients infected by the human immunodeficiency virus. Am J Med 90:595, 1991

TRUCKIS M et al: Emerging resistance to fluoroquinolones in staphylococci: An alert. Ann Intern Med 114:424, 1991

103   STREPTOCOCCAL INFECTIONS

MICHAEL R. WESSELS

Many varieties of streptococci are found as part of the normal human flora colonizing the respiratory, gastrointestinal, and genitourinary tracts. Several species are important causes of human disease. Group A streptococcus, or *Streptococcus pyogenes,* is the organism responsible for streptococcal pharyngitis, one of the most common bacterial infections of school-age children, and for the postinfectious syndromes of acute rheumatic fever and poststreptococcal glomerulonephritis. Group B streptococcus, or *S. agalactiae,* is the leading cause of bacterial sepsis and meningitis in newborns and a major cause of endometritis and fever in parturient women. Enterococci are important causes of urinary tract infection, intraabdominal infections, and endocarditis. Viridans streptococci are the most common cause of bacterial endocarditis.

Streptococci are gram-positive bacteria of spherical to ovoid shape that characteristically form chains when grown in liquid media. Most streptococci that cause human infections are facultative anaerobes, although some are strict anaerobes. Streptococci are relatively fastidious organisms, requiring enriched media for growth in the laboratory. No single scheme for classification of streptococci is entirely satisfactory. Consequently, clinicians and clinical microbiologists commonly identify streptococci by any of several classification systems, including hemolytic pattern, Lancefield group, species name, or a common or trivial name. Many of the streptococci associated with human infection produce a zone of complete hemolysis around the bacterial colony when cultured on blood agar, a pattern known as *beta hemolysis.* The beta-hemolytic streptococci can be classified by the Lancefield system, a serologic grouping based on the reaction of specific antisera with cell wall carbohydrate antigens of the bacteria. With rare exceptions, organisms belonging to Lancefield groups A, B, C, and G are all beta-hemolytic streptococci, and each is associated with characteristic patterns of human infections. Other streptococci produce a zone of partial, or alpha, hemolysis, often imparting a greenish appearance to the agar. These alpha-hemolytic streptococci are further identified by biochemical testing and include *S. pneumoniae,* an important cause of pneumonia, meningitis, and other infections (discussed in Chap. 101), and several species of streptococci referred to collectively as the *viridans streptococci,* part of normal oral flora and important as agents of subacute bacterial endocarditis. Finally, some streptococci are nonhemolytic, a pattern sometimes called *gamma hemolysis.* Classification of the major groups of streptococci responsible for human infections is outlined in Table 103-1. Among the group D streptococci, the species previously designated as *S. faecalis* and *S. faecium* have recently been renamed *Enterococcus faecalis* and *E. faecium,* respectively, on the basis of DNA homology studies. Although, technically, these organisms now fall into a separate genus from true streptococci, they will be discussed in this chapter, since clinical syndromes associated with the enterococci are generally considered within the context of other streptococcal infections from which they must be distinguished.

GROUP A STREPTOCOCCUS

Lancefield's group A consists of a single species, *S. pyogenes.* As its species name implies, this organism is associated with a variety of suppurative infections. In addition, group A streptococci are unique among known bacterial pathogens in their capacity to trigger the postinfectious syndromes of acute rheumatic fever (see Chap. 200) and poststreptococcal glomerulonephritis (see Chap. 240).

Group A streptococci elaborate a number of cell surface components and extracellular products important both in the pathogenesis of infection and in the immune response of the human host. The cell

TABLE 103-1   Classification of streptococci

Lancefield group	Representative species	Hemolytic pattern	Typical infections
A	S. pyogenes	Beta	Pharyngitis, impetigo, cellulitis, scarlet fever
B	S. agalactiae	Beta	Neonatal sepsis and meningitis, puerperal infections, urinary tract infection, diabetic ulcer infection, endocarditis
C	S. equi	Beta	Cellulitis, bacteremia, endocarditis
D	Enterococci E. faecalis E. faecium	Usually nonhemolytic	Urinary tract infection, wound infection, endocarditis
	Nonenterococci S. bovis	Usually nonhemolytic	Bacteremia, endocarditis
G	S. canis	Beta	Cellulitis, bacteremia, endocarditis
Variable or nongroupable	Viridans streptococci S. mutans S. sanguis	Alpha	Endocarditis, dental abscess, brain abscess
	Intermedius or milleri group S. milleri	Beta	Brain abscess, visceral abscess
	Anaerobic streptococci Peptostreptococcus magnus	Usually nonhemolytic	Sinusitis, pneumonia, empyema, brain abscess, liver abscess

wall contains a carbohydrate antigen that may be released from the bacterial cells by treatment with acid. The reaction of such acid extracts with group A–specific antiserum is the basis for the definitive identification of a streptococcal strain as *S. pyogenes*. The major surface protein of group A streptococci is M protein, which occurs in more than 80 antigenically distinct types and is the basis for serotyping strains with specific antisera. The M protein molecules are fibrillar structures anchored in the cell wall of the organism and extending as hairlike projections away from the cell surface. The amino acid sequence of the distal or amino-terminal portion of the M protein molecule is quite variable, accounting for the antigenic variation of the different M types, while more proximal regions of the protein are relatively conserved. The presence of M protein correlates with the capacity of a strain to resist phagocytic killing in fresh human blood, a phenomenon that appears to be due, at least in part, to binding of plasma fibrinogen to M protein molecules on the streptococcal surface, thereby interfering with complement activation and deposition of opsonic complement fragments on the bacterial cell. This resistance to phagocytosis may be overcome by M protein–specific antibodies, accounting for the observation that individuals with antibodies to a given M type acquired as a result of prior infection are protected against subsequent infection with organisms of the same, but not different, M types. Group A streptococci also elaborate, to varying degrees, a polysaccharide capsule composed of hyaluronic acid. Certain strains produce large amounts of hyaluronic acid capsule, resulting in a characteristic mucoid appearance to the bacterial colonies. The capsular polysaccharide also plays an important role in protecting the organisms from ingestion and killing by phagocytes. In contrast to M protein, the hyaluronic acid capsule is a weak immunogen, and antihyaluronate antibodies have not been shown to be important in protective immunity, presumably because of the apparent structural identity between streptococcal hyaluronic acid and the hyaluronic acid of mammalian connective tissues.

Group A streptococci produce a large number of extracellular products that may be important in local and systemic toxicity and in facilitating the spread of infection through tissues. These products include streptolysins S and O, toxins that damage cell membranes and account for the hemolysis produced by the organisms; streptokinase; DNAses; protease; and pyrogenic exotoxins A, B, and C. The pyrogenic exotoxins, previously known as *erythrogenic toxins*, cause the rash of scarlet fever. More recently, exotoxin A–producing strains of group A streptococcus have been linked to unusually severe, invasive infections, including necrotizing fasciitis and a systemic syndrome termed the *streptococcal toxic shock–like syndrome*. Several extracellular products stimulate specific antibody responses useful in serodiagnosis of recent streptococcal infection. These antibody tests are used primarily as evidence of preceding streptococcal infection in cases of suspected acute rheumatic fever or poststreptococcal glomerulonephritis.

PHARYNGITIS   Group A streptococcal pharyngitis is one of the most common bacterial infections of childhood, accounting for 20 to 40 percent of cases of exudative pharyngitis. Streptococcal pharyngitis is seen in patients of all ages; it is most common in children but is rare in children under the age of 3. Younger children may manifest streptococcal infection with a syndrome of fever, malaise, and lymphadenopathy without exudative pharyngitis. Infection is acquired through contact with another individual carrying the organism. Respiratory droplets are the usual mechanism of spread, although other routes are well described, including food-borne outbreaks.

Clinical features   The incubation period is 1 to 4 days. Symptoms include sore throat, fever and chills, malaise, and sometimes abdominal complaints and vomiting, particularly in children. Both symptoms and signs are quite variable, ranging from mild throat discomfort with minimal physical findings to high fever and severe sore throat associated with intense erythema and swelling of the pharyngeal mucosa and the presence of purulent exudate over the posterior pharyngeal wall and tonsillar pillars. Enlarged, tender anterior cervical lymph nodes are commonly found accompanying exudative pharyngitis.

The differential diagnosis of streptococcal pharyngitis includes the many other bacterial and viral causes of pharyngitis. Other infections commonly producing exudative pharyngitis include infectious mononucleosis and adenovirus infection. Now rare in the United States, the pseudomembrane of diphtheria also may give a similar appearance. *Corynebacterium (Arcanobacterium) hemolyticum* may cause pharyngitis, often in association with a scarlet fever–like rash. Other causes of pharyngitis, usually without a purulent exudate, include coxsackievirus, influenza, *Mycoplasma*, *Neisseria gonorrhoeae*, and acute infection with HIV. Because of the range of clinical presentations of streptococcal pharyngitis and the large number of other agents that can produce the same clinical picture, diagnosis of streptococcal pharyngitis on clinical grounds alone is not reliable.

The throat culture remains the gold standard for diagnosis of streptococcal pharyngitis. When properly collected (a sterile swab rubbed vigorously over both tonsillar pillars) and processed, the throat culture is the most sensitive and specific means available to make a definitive diagnosis. Rapid diagnostic kits using latex agglutination or enzyme immunoassay of swab specimens are now widely available and can serve as a useful adjunct to the throat culture. While precise figures on sensitivity and specificity vary among studies, in general, the rapid diagnostic kits are highly specific (greater than 95 percent), so a positive result can be relied on for definitive diagnosis and precludes the need for a throat culture. However, the rapid diagnostic tests are less sensitive than throat culture, with a relative sensitivity ranging from 55 to 90 percent in comparative studies, so a negative rapid diagnostic test should be confirmed with a throat culture.

The usual course of uncomplicated streptococcal pharyngitis is resolution of symptoms after 3 to 5 days. The course is shortened little by treatment, which is given primarily to prevent suppurative complications and rheumatic fever. Prevention of rheumatic fever depends on eradication of the organism from the pharynx, not simply on resolution of symptoms, and requires 10 days of penicillin treatment, either as a single intramuscular dose of benzathine penicillin G or as a 10-day course of oral penicillin (Table 103-2). Erythromycin may be substituted for individuals allergic to penicillin. Follow-up culture after treatment is no longer routinely recommended, though it may be warranted in selected cases, such as patients or families with frequent streptococcal infections or situations in which the risk of rheumatic fever is thought to be high, e.g., when cases have occurred recently in the community.

Suppurative complications of streptococcal pharyngitis have become uncommon with the widespread use of antibiotics for most cases of symptomatic streptococcal infection. These complications arise as a result of spread of infection from the pharyngeal mucosa to deeper tissues, either by direct extension or via hematogenous or lymphatic spread, and may include cervical lymphadenitis, peritonsillar or retropharyngeal abscess, sinusitis, otitis media, meningitis, bacteremia, endocarditis, and pneumonia. Local complications such as abscess formation in the peritonsillar or parapharyngeal space should be considered in a patient with unusually severe or prolonged symptoms or localized pain associated with high fever and toxic appearance.

ASYMPTOMATIC CARRIER STATE Surveillance cultures have shown that up to 20 percent of individuals, in certain populations, may have asymptomatic pharyngeal colonization with group A streptococci. There are no definitive guidelines for management of these asymptomatic carriers or of asymptomatic individuals with a positive throat culture after a full course of treatment for symptomatic pharyngitis. A reasonable course of action is to give a single 10-day course of penicillin for symptomatic pharyngitis but not to retreat if positive cultures persist unless symptoms recur. Studies of the natural history of streptococcal carriage and infection have shown that the risk both of developing rheumatic fever and of transmitting infection to others is substantially less in asymptomatic carriers than in individuals with symptomatic pharyngitis, so overly aggressive attempts at eradicating carriage are probably not justified under most circumstances. An exception to this general statement is the situation in which an asymptomatic carrier is a source of infection to others. Outbreaks of food-borne infection and nosocomial puerperal infections have been traced to asymptomatic carriers who may harbor the organisms in the throat, on the skin, or in the vagina or anus. In cases in which a carrier is transmitting infection to others, attempts to eradicate carriage are warranted, although data are limited on the best regimen to clear the organism after penicillin alone has failed. The combination of penicillin and rifampin has been used to eliminate pharyngeal carriage, and addition of oral vancomycin has been successful in eradicating rectal colonization, although there is not extensive experience with any regimen.

SCARLET FEVER Scarlet fever is streptococcal infection, usually pharyngitis, accompanied by a characteristic rash. The rash arises from the effects of one of three toxins, currently designated streptococcal pyrogenic exotoxins A, B, and C and known previously as erythrogenic or scarlet fever toxins. Scarlet fever was thought to reflect infection of an individual lacking toxin-specific immunity with a toxin-producing strain of group A streptococcus. Susceptibility to scarlet fever was correlated with results of the Dick test: A small amount of erythrogenic toxin injected intradermally produced local erythema in susceptible individuals but no reaction in those with specific immunity. Subsequent studies have suggested that development of the scarlet fever rash may reflect a hypersensitivity reaction requiring prior exposure to the toxin. For reasons that are not clear, scarlet fever has become less common in recent years, although strains of group A streptococci that produce exotoxins B or C continue to be prevalent in the population. The symptoms of scarlet fever are the same as for pharyngitis alone. The rash typically begins on the first or second day of illness over the upper trunk, spreading to involve the extremities but sparing the palms and soles. The rash is made up of minute papules, giving a characteristic "sandpaper" feel to the skin. Associated findings include circumoral pallor, "strawberry tongue" (enlarged papillae on a coated tongue which may later become denuded), and accentuation of the rash in the skin folds (Pastia's lines). The rash subsides after 6 to 9 days and is followed after several days by desquamation of the palms and soles. The differential diagnosis of scarlet fever includes other causes of fever and generalized rash, such as measles and other viral exanthems, Kawasaki's disease, toxic shock syndrome, and systemic allergic reactions such as drug eruptions.

SKIN AND SOFT TISSUE INFECTIONS Group A streptococci, and occasionally other streptococcal species, cause a variety of infections involving the skin, subcutaneous tissues, muscles, and fascia. While several clinical syndromes, recognized according to the tissues involved, are a useful means for classification of skin and soft tissue infections, not all cases fit exactly into a single category. The classic syndromes should be considered as general guides to predicting the level of tissue involvement in a particular patient, the likely clinical course, and the likelihood that surgical intervention or aggressive life support will be required.

Impetigo (pyoderma) Impetigo is a superficial infection of the skin caused primarily by group A streptococci, occasionally by other streptococci or by *Staphylococcus aureus*. Impetigo is seen most often in young children, tends to occur during the warmer months, and is more common in semitropical or tropical climates than in cooler regions. Infection is more common among children living under conditions of poor hygiene. Prospective studies have shown that colonization of unbroken skin with group A streptococci precedes the development of clinical infection. Minor trauma, such as a scratch or insect bite, may then serve to inoculate organisms into the skin. Impetigo is best prevented, therefore, by attention to adequate hygiene. The usual sites of involvement are the face, particularly around the nose and mouth, and the legs, although lesions may occur at other locations. Individual lesions begin as red papules that evolve quickly to vesicular and then pustular lesions which break down and coalesce to form characteristic honey-like crusts. Lesions are generally not painful, and patients do not appear ill. Fever is not a feature of impetigo and, if present, should suggest infection extending to deeper tissues or another diagnosis.

The classic presentation of impetigo usually is not difficult to diagnose. Cultures of impetiginous lesions often show *S. aureus* as well as group A streptococci, but longitudinal studies have shown that, in almost all cases, streptococci can be isolated initially, with staphylococci appearing later, presumably as secondary colonizing flora. Penicillin is nearly always effective in these infections, although most staphylococcal strains are resistant, further supporting the primary role of streptococci in the infection. An exception to this general rule is bullous impetigo due to *S. aureus*, distinguished from streptococcal infection by the presence of more extensive, bullous

---

TABLE 103-2 **Treatment of group A streptococcal infections**

Infection	Treatment
Pharyngitis	Benzathine penicillin G, 1.2 million units IM or penicillin V, 250 mg PO qid x 10 days (Children <27 kg: Benzathine penicillin G, 600,000 units IM or penicillin V, 125 mg PO qid x 10 days)
Impetigo	Same as pharyngitis
Erysipelas/cellulitis	Severe: Penicillin G, 1 to 2 million units IV q4h Mild to moderate: Procaine penicillin, 1.2 million units IM bid
Necrotizing fasciitis/ myositis	Surgical debridement plus penicillin G, 2 to 4 million units IV q4h
Pneumonia/empyema	Penicillin G, 2 to 4 million units IV q4h plus drainage of empyema

* Penicillin allergy: Erythromycin (10 mg/kg PO qid up to maximum of 250 mg per dose) may be substituted for oral penicillin. Alternative agents for parenteral therapy include first-generation cephalosporins if the nature of the allergy is not an immediate hypersensitivity reaction (anaphylaxis or urticaria) or other potentially life-threatening manifestation (e.g., severe rash and fever) or vancomycin.

lesions that break down and leave thin, paper-like crusts, in contrast to the thick, amber crusts of streptococcal impetigo. Other skin lesions which may be confused with impetigo include herpetic lesions, either of orolabial herpes simplex or of chicken pox or zoster. Herpetic lesions can generally be distinguished by their appearance as more discrete, grouped vesicles and by a positive Tzanck test. In difficult cases, cultures of vesicle fluid should yield group A streptococci in the case of impetigo and the responsible virus in herpesvirus infections.

Treatment of impetigo is the same as for streptococcal pharyngitis. Rheumatic fever is not a sequel to streptococcal skin infections, in contrast to pharyngitis, although poststreptococcal glomerulonephritis may follow either skin or throat infection. The reason for this difference is not known. One hypothesis is that the immune response necessary for development of rheumatic fever only occurs following infection of the pharyngeal mucosa. In addition, the strains of group A streptococci that cause pharyngitis are generally of different M-protein types from those associated with skin infections, suggesting that the strains that cause pharyngitis may have rheumatogenic potential, while the skin strains do not.

Cellulitis Inoculation of organisms into the skin may lead to infection involving the skin and subcutaneous tissues, or cellulitis. The portal of entry may be a traumatic or surgical wound, an insect bite, or any break in skin integrity. Often, no entry site is apparent.

A particular form of streptococcal cellulitis is known as *erysipelas*. Erysipelas is characterized by a bright red appearance of the involved skin which forms a plateau, sharply demarcated from surrounding normal skin. The lesion is warm to touch, may be tender, and appears shiny and swollen. The skin often has a *peau d'orange* texture, thought to reflect involvement of superficial lymphatics; superficial blebs or bullae may form, usually 2 or 3 days after onset. The lesion typically develops over a few hours and is associated with fever and chills. Erysipelas tends to occur in certain characteristic locations; the malar area of the face, often with extension over the bridge of the nose to the contralateral malar region, and the lower extremities are the usual sites. After one episode, recurrence at the same site, sometimes years later, is not uncommon.

Classic cases of erysipelas, with the typical features described above, are almost always due to group A streptococci. Often, however, the appearance of streptococcal cellulitis is not sufficiently distinctive to permit a specific diagnosis on clinical grounds; the area of involvement may be other than one of the typical sites for erysipelas, the lesion may be less intensely red and may fade into surrounding skin, and patients may appear only mildly ill. In such cases, it is prudent to broaden empirical antimicrobial therapy to include other potential pathogens, particularly *S. aureus*, that can produce cellulitis with the same appearance.

Streptococcal cellulitis tends to occur at anatomic sites in which the normal lymphatic drainage has been disrupted, such as sites of prior episodes of cellulitis, the arm ipsilateral to a mastectomy and axillary lymph node dissection, a lower extremity previously involved with deep venous thrombosis or chronic lymphedema, and the leg from which a saphenous vein has been harvested for coronary artery bypass grafting. The organism may enter via a breach in the dermal barrier at a location some distance from the eventual site of clinical cellulitis. For example, some patients with recurrent episodes of leg cellulitis following saphenous vein removal have stopped having recurrent episodes only after treatment of tinea pedis on the foot of the affected extremity, fissures in the skin presumably having served as a portal of entry for streptococci which then produced infection more proximally in the leg at the site of previous injury. Another setting in which streptococcal cellulitis may occur is recent surgical wounds. Group A streptococci are among the few bacterial pathogens that typically produce signs of wound infection and surrounding cellulitis within the first 24 h after surgery. These wound infections are usually associated with a thin exudate and may spread rapidly, either as cellulitis in the skin and subcutaneous tissue or as a deeper tissue infection (see below). Streptococcal wound infection or

localized cellulitis also may be associated with *lymphangitis*, manifested by red streaks extending proximally along superficial lymphatics from the site of infection.

Deep soft tissue infections *Necrotizing fasciitis*, also referred to as *hemolytic streptococcal gangrene*, is an infection involving the superficial and/or deep fascia investing the muscles of an extremity or the trunk. The source of the infection is either organisms on the skin, introduced into the tissue as a result of trauma that may be trivial, or bowel flora released during abdominal surgery or from an occult enteric source such as a diverticular or appendiceal abscess. The site of inoculation in both forms of necrotizing fasciitis may be inapparent and often is some distance from the site of clinical involvement, e.g., minor trauma to the hand associated with clinical infection of the tissues overlying the shoulder or chest. In cases of necrotizing fasciitis associated with bowel flora, the infection is usually polymicrobial, involving a mixture of anaerobic bacteria, such as *Bacteroides fragilis* or anaerobic streptococci, and facultative organisms, usually gram-negative bacilli. Cases unrelated to contamination from bowel organisms are most commonly caused by group A streptococci, either alone or in combination with other organisms, most often *S. aureus*. Overall, group A streptococci are implicated in about 60 percent of cases of necrotizing fasciitis. The onset of symptoms is usually quite acute and is marked by severe pain at the site of involvement, malaise, fever, chills, and a toxic appearance. The physical findings, particularly early in the illness, may not be striking, with only minimal erythema of the overlying skin. Pain and tenderness are usually severe, in contrast to more superficial cellulitis in which the skin appearance is more abnormal, but pain and tenderness are only mild or moderate. As the infection progresses, often in a matter of several hours, the severity and extent of symptoms worsen, and skin changes become more apparent, with the appearance of dusky or mottled erythema and edema. The marked tenderness of the involved area may evolve to anesthesia, as the spreading inflammatory process produces infarction of cutaneous nerves. Once the diagnosis is suspected, early surgical exploration is indicated, both to confirm the diagnosis and for treatment. The findings at operation are necrosis and inflammatory fluid tracking along the fascial planes above and between muscle groups, without involvement of the muscles themselves. The process usually is found to extend beyond the area of clinical involvement, and extensive debridement is required. Drainage and debridement are central to the management of necrotizing fasciitis; antibiotic treatment is useful as adjunctive therapy (see Table 103-2), but surgery is lifesaving.

Group A streptococci may produce abscesses in skeletal muscles (*streptococcal myositis*) with little or no involvement of surrounding fascia or overlying skin. This syndrome is more commonly due to *S. aureus* infection but is occasionally caused by group A streptococci. Presentation is usually subacute, but a fulminant form of streptococcal myositis has been described, associated with severe systemic toxicity, bacteremia, and a high mortality. The fulminant form may reflect the same basic disease process as that seen in necrotizing fasciitis, but with extension of the necrotizing inflammatory process into the muscles themselves, rather than remaining limited to fascial layers. Treatment for streptococcal myositis is surgical drainage, usually by an open procedure, to evaluate the extent of the infection and ensure adequate debridement of involved tissues and high-dose penicillin (see Table 103-2).

PNEUMONIA AND EMPYEMA Group A streptococci are an occasional cause of pneumonia, generally in previously healthy individuals. Onset of symptoms may be abrupt or gradual. Pleuritic chest pain, fever, chills, and dyspnea are the usual symptoms. Cough is usually present but may not be prominent. Approximately one-half of patients with group A streptococcal pneumonia have an accompanying pleural effusion. In contrast to the sterile parapneumonic effusions typically seen with pneumococcal pneumonia, those complicating streptococcal pneumonia are almost always infected. The empyema fluid is usually visible by chest x-ray on initial presentation and may enlarge rapidly. These pleural collections should be drained early because they tend to become loculated rapidly, resulting in a chronic fibrotic reaction that may require thoracotomy for removal.

BACTEREMIA, PUERPERAL SEPSIS, AND STREPTOCOCCAL TOXIC SHOCK–LIKE SYNDROME Bacteremia with group A streptococcus is usually associated with an identifiable local infection. Bacteremia occurs rarely with otherwise uncomplicated pharyngitis, somewhat more frequently with cellulitis or pneumonia, and relatively frequently in patients with necrotizing fasciitis. Occasionally, there is no apparent source for the bacteremia. Bacteremia without an identified source should raise suspicion of endocarditis, an occult abscess, or osteomyelitis. A variety of focal infections may arise secondarily from streptococcal bacteremia, including endocarditis, meningitis, septic arthritis, osteomyelitis, peritonitis, and visceral abscesses.

Group A streptococci are occasionally implicated in infectious complications of childbirth, usually endometritis and associated bacteremia. In the preantibiotic era, puerperal sepsis was commonly caused by group A streptococci, but currently it is more often caused by group B streptococci. Several nosocomial outbreaks of puerperal infections due to group A streptococci have been traced to an asymptomatic carrier, usually an individual present at the time of delivery of the infant. The site of carriage may be the skin, throat, anus, or vagina.

In 1987, Cone and associates described a series of patients with group A streptococcal infections associated with shock and multisystem disease. Several subsequent reports have described the same syndrome, which has been called the *streptococcal toxic shock–like syndrome* because it shares certain features with staphylococcal toxic shock syndrome. While a formal case definition has not been established, the general features of the illness include fever, hypotension, renal impairment, and respiratory distress syndrome. Various types of rashes have been described, but rash is usually absent. Laboratory abnormalities include a marked shift to the left in the white blood cell differential, with many immature granulocytes, hypocalcemia, hypoalbuminemia, and thrombocytopenia, which usually becomes more pronounced on the second or third day of illness. In contrast to those with staphylococcal toxic shock, the majority of patients with the streptococcal syndrome are bacteremic. The most common associated infection is a soft tissue infection—necrotizing fasciitis, myositis, or cellulitis—although a variety of other local infections have been described in association with the syndrome, including pneumonia, peritonitis, osteomyelitis, and myometritis. Streptococcal toxic shock–like syndrome is associated with a 30 percent mortality, with most deaths secondary to shock and respiratory failure. Because of the rapidly progressive and lethal course of the illness, early recognition of the syndrome is essential. Patients should be given aggressive supportive care in the form of fluid resuscitation, pressors, and mechanical ventilation, in addition to antimicrobial therapy and, in cases associated with necrotizing fasciitis, surgical debridement. Exactly why certain patients develop this fulminant syndrome is not known; however, studies of the streptococcal strains isolated from patients with streptococcal toxic shock–like syndrome have shown a strong association with production of pyrogenic exotoxin A. While exotoxin A–producing strains currently are rare among clinical isolates from other types of infections, 80 to 90 percent of the strains associated with streptococcal toxic shock–like syndrome have been exotoxin A producers, suggesting that the toxin may play a role in pathogenesis of the syndrome. In light of the possible role of this or other streptococcal toxins in streptococcal toxic shock–like syndrome, treatment of these patients with clindamycin has been advocated by some authorities, who argue that, through its direct action on protein synthesis, clindamycin is more effective than penicillin, a cell wall agent, in rapidly terminating toxin production. Support for this view comes from studies of an experimental model of streptococcal myositis, in which mice treated with clindamycin

had improved survival over those that received penicillin. Comparable data for treatment of human infections are not available.

GROUP C AND G STREPTOCOCCAL INFECTIONS

Group C and group G streptococci are beta-hemolytic streptococci that occasionally cause infections in humans similar to those caused by group A streptococci, including pharyngitis, pneumonia, cellulitis and soft tissue infections, bacteremia, septic arthritis, and endocarditis. Bacteremia due to group C or G streptococci occurs most commonly in patients who are elderly or chronically ill and, in the absence of an obvious local infection, is likely to reflect endocarditis. Septic arthritis, sometimes involving multiple joints, may complicate endocarditis or occur in the absence of endocarditis. Response to treatment is slow, and patients with joint infections often require repeated aspiration or open drainage and debridement for cure. Penicillin is the drug of choice for therapy of infections due to group C or G streptococci; because of poor clinical response in some patients treated with penicillin alone, the addition of gentamicin (1 mg/kg every 8 h for patients with normal renal function) is recommended for treatment of endocarditis or septic arthritis.

GROUP B STREPTOCOCCUS

Identified first as a cause of mastitis in cows, streptococci belonging to Lancefield's group B have since been recognized as a major cause of sepsis and meningitis in human neonates. Group B streptococci are also a frequent cause of peripartum fever in women and an occasional cause of serious infection in nonpregnant adults. Lancefield group B consists of a single species, *S. agalactiae*. Definitive identification of the organism is made serologically using antiserum specific for the group B cell wall–associated carbohydrate antigen. Presumptive identification of a streptococcal isolate as belonging to group B may be made on the basis of biochemical testing, including hydrolysis of sodium hippurate (99 percent are positive), hydrolysis of bile esculin agar (99 to 100 percent are negative), bacitracin susceptibility (92 percent are resistant), and production of so-called CAMP factor (98 to 100 percent are positive). CAMP factor is a phospholipase produced by group B streptococci that results in synergistic hemolysis with β-lysin produced by certain strains of *S. aureus*. Its presence can be demonstrated by cross-streaking the test isolate and staphylococcal strain on a blood agar plate. Most group B streptococci causing human infections are encapsulated by one of six antigenically distinct polysaccharides. The capsular polysaccharide has been shown experimentally to be important in virulence of the organism. Antibodies to the capsular polysaccharide afford protection against group B streptococci of the same, but not of different, capsular type.

INFECTION IN NEONATES Two general types of infections in infants are defined by the age of the patient at presentation. Early-onset infections occur within the first week of life, with a median age at onset of illness of 20 h. Approximately half these infants have signs of group B streptococcal disease at birth. The infection is acquired during or shortly before birth from organisms colonizing the maternal genital tract. Surveillance studies have shown 5 to 40 percent of women are vaginal or rectal carriers of group B streptococci. Approximately 50 percent of infants vaginally delivered from carrier mothers become colonized, although only 1 to 2 percent of those colonized develop clinically evident infection. Prematurity and maternal risk factors of prolonged labor, obstetric complications, and maternal fever are often present. The presentation of early-onset infection is the same as that of other forms of neonatal sepsis. Typical findings include respiratory distress, lethargy, and hypotension. Essentially all infants with early-onset disease are bacteremic, one-third to one-half have pneumonia and/or respiratory distress syndrome, and one-third have meningitis. Late-onset infections occur in infants between 1 week and 3 months of age, with a mean age of 3 to 4 weeks. Acquisition of the infecting organism may occur during birth, as in early-onset cases, or later from contact with a colonized mother, nursery personnel, or other sources. Meningitis is the most common manifestation of late-onset infection and in 80 to 90 percent of cases is associated with infection by a strain of capsular type III. Infants present with fever, lethargy or irritability, poor feeding, and seizures. Poor prognostic signs include presentation with hypotension, coma, status epilepticus, and the presence of neutropenia. Up to 50 percent of survivors have some degree of long-term neurologic impairment ranging from mild language delay or hearing loss to profound mental retardation, blindness, and uncontrolled seizures. A variety of other types of late-onset infections occur, including bacteremia without an identified source, osteomyelitis, septic arthritis, and facial cellulitis associated with submandibular or preauricular adenitis.

Penicillin is the treatment of choice for all group B streptococcal infections. Neonates with suspected bacterial sepsis are generally begun on empirical broad-spectrum therapy with ampicillin and gentamicin until culture results are known. If cultures return positive for group B streptococci, many pediatricians will continue gentamicin, along with ampicillin or penicillin, for a few days, until clinical improvement is evident. The basis for this practice is in vitro studies showing synergistic killing of group B streptococci by the two agents in combination. Certainly for infants with group B streptococcal meningitis, combined therapy for the first few days is recommended, although rigorous clinical data to support this view are lacking. Therapy with penicillin alone should be continued for 10 days for bacteremia and local infections and for a minimum of 14 days for meningitis because of the risk of relapse in patients treated with shorter courses.

Because the usual source of the organism in infected neonates is the mother's birth canal, efforts have been made to prevent group B streptococcal infections by identification and treatment of high-risk carrier mothers with various forms of antibiotic or immunoprophylaxis. This approach has been hampered by the logistical difficulties of identifying colonized women before delivery, since vaginal cultures early in pregnancy are poor predictors of carrier status at the time of delivery. Rapid diagnostic tests are available, using latex agglutination or enzyme immunoassay, for testing vaginal swab specimens directly; however, these tests currently are less sensitive than cultures, with a false-negative rate of approximately 10 to 30 percent. The incidence of group B streptococcal infection is increased in infants of women with risk factors: preterm delivery, prolonged rupture of membranes (>24 h), prolonged labor, fever, or chorioamnionitis. While prophylactic administration of ampicillin to such patients during delivery has been shown to prevent infection of the newborn, it should be emphasized that indiscriminate antibiotic treatment of colonized women is likely to do more harm than good, since the risk of adverse reactions to the antibiotic outweighs the risk of infection in the absence of maternal risk factors. Prophylaxis should be reserved for women with vaginal or rectal colonization *and* one or more of the risk factors noted above or a history of having delivered an infant with group B streptococcal infection. Because transplacental passage of maternal antibodies produces protective levels in the newborn, efforts are underway to develop a vaccine against group B streptococci that could be given to childbearing women before or during pregnancy.

INFECTION IN ADULTS The majority of group B streptococcal infections in adults are related to pregnancy and parturition. Peripartum fever is the most common manifestation, sometimes accompanied by symptoms and signs of endometritis or chorioamnionitis (abdominal distention and uterine or adnexal tenderness). Blood cultures are often positive, as are cultures of vaginal swabs. Bacteremia is usually transitory but occasionally results in meningitis or endocarditis. Infections in adults not associated with the peripartum period generally occur in individuals who are elderly or have some underlying chronic illness, particularly diabetes mellitus or a malignancy. Infections that occur with some frequency include cellulitis and soft tissue infections

(including infected diabetic skin ulcers), urinary tract infections, pneumonia, endocarditis, and septic arthritis. Other reported infections include meningitis, osteomyelitis, and intraabdominal or pelvic abscesses.

Group B streptococci are less sensitive to penicillin than group A, requiring 10- to 100-fold higher concentrations for inhibition of growth in vitro. Therefore, somewhat higher doses of penicillin are needed for treatment of group B infections. Adults with serious localized infections (pneumonia, pyelonephritis, abscess) should receive doses in the range of 12 million units of penicillin G daily, while patients with endocarditis or meningitis should receive 18 to 24 million units per day, in divided doses. Vancomycin is an acceptable alternative for patients allergic to penicillin.

GROUP D STREPTOCOCCAL INFECTIONS

Group D includes the enterococci, organisms now classified in a separate genus from other streptococci, and nonenterococcal group D streptococci. Enterococci are distinguished from nonenterococcal group D streptococci by their ability to grow in the presence of 6.5% sodium chloride and other biochemical tests. The enterococcal species that are significant pathogens for humans are E. faecalis and E. faecium. They tend to produce infection in patients who are elderly or debilitated or who have had disruption of mucosal or epithelial barriers or alterations in the balance of normal flora through antibiotic treatment. Urinary tract infections due to enterococci are quite common, particularly in patients who have had antibiotic treatment or instrumentation of the urinary tract. These organisms account for 10 to 20 percent of cases of bacterial endocarditis on both native and prosthetic valves. The presentation of enterococcal endocarditis is usually subacute but may be acute with rapidly progressive valve destruction. Enterococci are frequently cultured from bile and are commonly involved in infectious complications of biliary surgery and in liver abscesses. Enterococci are often isolated from mixed infections arising from bowel flora, such as intraabdominal abscesses. Similarly, enterococci are often found in polymicrobial infections arising from abdominal surgical wounds and in diabetic foot ulcers. While such mixed infections are often cured by antimicrobials not active against enterococci, specific therapy directed against enterococci is warranted in circumstances in which these organisms are the predominant species or in which enterococci are isolated from blood cultures.

Unlike other streptococci, enterococci are not reliably killed by penicillin or ampicillin alone at concentrations of antibiotic achieved clinically in the blood or tissues. Because in vitro testing has shown evidence of synergistic killing by the combination of penicillin or ampicillin with an aminoglycoside for most enterococcal strains, combined therapy is recommended for serious enterococcal infections. Ampicillin reaches sufficiently high urinary concentrations to be adequate as single-drug therapy for uncomplicated urinary tract infections. For other types of enterococcal infections, however, addition of gentamicin at moderate doses (e.g., 1 mg/kg every 8 h for patients with normal renal function) is recommended. Vancomycin, in combination with gentamicin, may be substituted for penicillin in allergic patients. Enterococci are resistant to all cephalosporins, and this class of antibiotics should not be used for treatment of enterococcal infections.

Antimicrobial susceptibility testing should be performed routinely on enterococcal isolates from patients with serious infections. Most enterococci are resistant to streptomycin, and this drug should not be used for treatment of enterococcal infection unless in vitro testing of the strain indicates susceptibility. Though less widespread than streptomycin resistance, high-level resistance to gentamicin (minimum inhibitory concentration greater than 2000 μg/mL) has become common. Gentamicin-resistant enterococci should be tested for susceptibility to other aminoglycosides. If the isolate is resistant to all aminoglycosides, treatment with penicillin or ampicillin alone may be successful. Prolonged (at least 6 weeks), high-dose (e.g., 12 g/d ampicillin) therapy is recommended for endocarditis due to these highly resistant enterococci. β-Lactamase production (mediating resistance to penicillin and ampicillin) has been reported but currently appears to be rare among clinical isolates. β-Lactamase–producing strains may be treated with vancomycin plus gentamicin or with ampicillin combined with a β-lactamase inhibitor such as sulbactam in combination with gentamicin.

The main nonenterococcal group D streptococcal species that causes human infections is *S. bovis*. *S. bovis* endocarditis is often associated with neoplasms of the gastrointestinal tract, most often a colon carcinoma or polyp, but is also reported in association with other bowel lesions. When occult gastrointestinal lesions are carefully sought, abnormalities have been found in 60 percent or more of patients with *S. bovis* endocarditis. In contrast to the enterococci, nonenterococcal group D streptococci such as *S. bovis* are reliably killed by penicillin as a single agent, and penicillin is the treatment of choice for *S. bovis* infections.

VIRIDANS AND OTHER STREPTOCOCCI

Consisting of multiple species of alpha-hemolytic streptococci, the viridans streptococci are a heterogeneous group of organisms important as agents of bacterial endocarditis. Several species of viridans streptococci, including *S. salivarius*, *S. mutans*, *S. sanguis*, and *S. mitis*, are part of the normal mouth flora, where they live in close association with the teeth and gingiva. Some contribute to development of dental caries. Transient bacteremia induced by eating, tooth brushing and flossing, and other minor trauma, together with the ability of these organisms to adhere to biologic surfaces, is thought to account for their predilection for causing endocarditis. Viridans streptococci are also isolated, often as part of a mixed infection, in sinusitis, brain abscess, and liver abscess. A group of organisms referred to variously as *S. milleri*, *S. intermedius*, and *S. anginosus* are often considered as viridans streptococci, although they differ somewhat from other viridans streptococci in both hemolytic pattern (usually beta-hemolytic) and disease syndromes. These organisms often cause suppurative infections, particularly abscesses of brain and abdominal viscera.

Most viridans streptococci are sensitive to penicillin. Occasional isolates from blood cultures of patients with endocarditis fail to grow when subcultured on solid media. These *nutritionally variant streptococci* require supplemental thiol compounds or active forms of vitamin B_6 (pyridoxal or pyridoxamine) for growth in the laboratory. Because treatment failure and relapse appear to be more common for cases of endocarditis due to nutritionally variant streptococci than for usual viridans streptococci, the addition of gentamicin (1 mg/kg every 8 h for patients with normal renal function) to penicillin is recommended for therapy of endocarditis due to these organisms.

S. suis is an important pathogen in swine and has been reported to cause meningitis in humans, usually in individuals with occupational exposure to pigs. Strains of *S. suis* associated with human infections have generally reacted with Lancefield group R typing serum and sometimes with group D as well. Isolates may be alpha- or beta-hemolytic and have been sensitive to penicillin. *Anaerobic streptococci* are part of the normal flora of the oral cavity, bowel, and vagina. They are involved, usually in mixed infections, in brain abscess, sinusitis, dental abscess, and other odontogenic infections (Ludwig's angina, abscesses of the retropharyngeal or lateral pharyngeal space); in aspiration pneumonia, lung abscess, and empyema; and in intraabdominal and pelvic abscesses. Anaerobic and microaerophilic streptococci, together with facultative bacteria, also may play a role in invasive soft tissue infections, generally related to trauma or surgical wounds. Management of these infections involves debridement of infected tissues and treatment with high-dose penicillin (12 to 18 million units per day for serious infections).

REFERENCES

BASILIERE JL et al: Streptococcal pneumonia. Am J Med 44:580, 1968

BISNO AL: Group A streptococcal infections and acute rheumatic fever. N Engl J Med 325:783, 1991

CONE LA et al: Clinical and bacteriologic observations of a toxic shock–like syndrome due to *Streptococcus pyogenes*. N Engl J Med 317:146, 1987

EDWARDS MS, BAKER CJ: *Streptococcus agalactiae* (group B streptococci), in *Principles and Practice of Infectious Diseases*, 3d ed, GL Mandell et al (eds). New York, Churchill Livingstone, 1990, p 1554

KLEIN RS et al: Association of *Streptococcus bovis* with carcinoma of the colon. N Engl J Med 297:800, 1977

LANCEFIELD RC: A serological differentiation of human and other groups of hemolytic streptococci. J Exp Med 57:571, 1933

MOELLERING RC JR.: Emergence of *Enterococcus* as a significant pathogen. Clin Infect Dis 14:1173, 1992

STEVENS DL et al: Severe group A streptococcal infections associated with a toxic shock–like syndrome and scarlet fever toxin A. N Engl J Med 321:1, 1989

VARTIAN C et al: Infections due to Lancefield group G streptococci. Medicine 6:75, 1985

VIGLIONESE A et al: Recurrent group A streptococcal carriage in a health care worker associated with widely separated nosocomial outbreaks. Am J Med 91(suppl 3B):329S, 1991

WANNAMAKER LW: Differences between streptococcal infections of the throat and of the skin. N Engl J Med 282:23, 78, 1970

WELLS VD et al: Infections due to beta-lactamase–producing, high-level gentamicin-resistant *Enterococcus faecalis*. Ann Intern Med 116:285, 1992

YODER EL et al: Spontaneous gangrenous myositis induced by *Streptococcus pyogenes*: Case report and review of the literature. Rev Infect Dis 9:382, 1987

104 DIPHTHERIA, OTHER CORYNEBACTERIAL INFECTIONS, AND ANTHRAX

RANDALL K. HOLMES

DIPHTHERIA

DEFINITION Diphtheria is a localized infection of mucous membranes or skin caused by *Corynebacterium diphtheriae*. A characteristic pseudomembrane may be present at the site of infection. Some strains of *C. diphtheriae* produce diphtheria toxin, a protein that can cause myocarditis, polyneuritis, and other systemic toxic effects. Respiratory diphtheria is usually caused by toxinogenic (tox$^+$) *C. diphtheriae*, but cutaneous diphtheria is frequently caused by nontoxinogenic (tox$^-$) strains.

ETIOLOGY *C. diphtheriae* is an aerobic, nonmotile, nonsporulating, irregularly staining, gram-positive rod. The bacteria are 2 to 6 μm long, 0.5 to 1 μm wide, club shaped, and often arranged in clusters (Chinese letters) or parallel arrays (palisades). *C. diphtheriae* forms gray to black colonies on selective media containing potassium tellurite. Three biotypes, designated *gravis*, *mitis*, and *intermedius*, are distinguished on the basis of colonial morphology, hemolytic activity, sugar fermentation reactions, and other biochemical tests. Both tox$^+$ and tox$^-$ strains cause infections, and tox$^+$ strains of all three biotypes can cause severe disease. Individual strains of *C. diphtheriae* within a biotype can be identified by phage typing, analysis of bacterial polypeptides or DNA restriction patterns, DNA hybridization tests or polymerase chain reactions with specific probes, ribotyping, or other methods.

The gene for diphtheria toxin is present in specific corynephages. Nontoxinogenic *C. diphtheriae* acquires the ability to produce diphtheria toxin by infection with tox$^+$ phages, a process termed *phage conversion*. Growth of *C. diphtheriae* under low-iron conditions mimicking the environment of host tissues induces the synthesis of diphtheria toxin and the expression of a siderophore-dependent, high-affinity iron uptake system.

IMMUNOLOGY Treatment of diphtheria toxin with formaldehyde converts it to a nontoxic product called *diphtheria toxoid*. Immunization with the toxoid elicits antibodies (antitoxin) that neutralize the toxin and prevent diphtheria. Antitoxin does not prevent colonization by *C. diphtheriae* or eradicate the carrier state. If most individuals in a population have antitoxic immunity, the carriage of tox$^+$ strains of *C. diphtheriae* decreases to a low level. Thus herd immunity reduces the risk that nonimmune individuals in the population will be exposed to tox$^+$ *C. diphtheriae*. Nonimmune individuals may contract diphtheria if they travel to regions where the disease is present or if tox$^+$ strains of *C. diphtheriae* are introduced into their community.

No specific amount of antitoxin provides absolute protection against diphtheria, but the attack rate and the mortality rate for diphtheria are much lower among individuals with more than 0.01 unit of antitoxin per milliliter. This antitoxin level is often used, therefore, as an index of immunity for epidemiologic studies. Antitoxic immunity is also demonstrated by the Schick test, in which standardized doses of diphtheria toxin and toxoid are injected intracutaneously at separate sites on the volar surface of the forearm. A tender, swollen, erythematous lesion reaching maximal intensity in 4 to 5 days at the site of the toxin injection only (a positive reaction) is caused by the direct action of diphtheria toxin and indicates that the individual is not immune. The absence of a lesion at either site (a negative reaction) indicates that the toxin has been neutralized by circulating antitoxin and that the individual is immune. Tuberculin-like reactions at both sites that reach a maximum in 2 to 3 days and then fade (pseudoreaction) indicate delayed hypersensitivity to toxin/toxoid in an immune individual. Delayed hypersensitivity reactions at both sites combined with a subsequent positive reaction at the site of toxin administration only (a combined reaction) indicate delayed hypersensitivity in an individual who does not have a protective level of antitoxin.

EPIDEMIOLOGY AND IMMUNITY   Humans are the reservoir for *C. diphtheriae*. The organism is transmitted primarily by close contact of diphtheria patients or carriers with susceptible individuals, but the risk of transmission from patients appears to be substantially greater than that of transmission from asymptomatic carriers. Transmission involving fomites and indirect routes is less common, although *C. diphtheriae* can survive for weeks to months in the environment. The incubation period for respiratory diphtheria is typically 2 to 5 days and rarely up to 8 days. Cutaneous diphtheria is usually a secondary infection whose signs develop an average of 7 days (range 1 to >21 days) after the appearance of primary skin lesions.

In populations in temperate climates, diphtheria primarily involves the respiratory tract, occurs throughout the year with a peak incidence in colder months, and is usually caused by tox$^+$ *C. diphtheriae*. Before the introduction of active immunization, diphtheria was usually a disease of children, affected up to 10 percent of this group, and sometimes occurred in devastating epidemics. Most infants were immune because of transplacental transfer of maternal IgG antitoxin, but children became susceptible by 6 to 12 months of age. Approximately 75 percent of individuals became immune by age 10 as a result of clinical or subclinical infection with *C. diphtheriae*. Mortality rates of 30 to 40 percent were common in untreated disease and sometimes exceeded 50 percent in epidemics. Treatment with antitoxin reduced the case mortality rate to 5 to 10 percent.

Routine immunization of children in the United States resulted in a progressively decreasing incidence of diphtheria and a shift of cases to older age groups, but the case mortality rate remained at 5 to 10 percent. More than 206,000 cases of diphtheria occurred in 1921. Only 22 cases were reported in 1980–1987, and 5 cases were reported in 1991. Forty-eight percent of cases in 1971–1981 were in persons over 15 years of age. Rates of immunization by school entry are high (96 percent), but rates for younger children are substantially lower. Many older adults (25 to 50 percent) are susceptible to diphtheria.

Large local outbreaks of diphtheria occurred in San Antonio, Texas (1969–1970, 201 cases), and Seattle, Washington (1972–1982, 1100 cases). Alcoholism, low socioeconomic status, crowded living conditions, and Native American ethnic background were significant risk factors in these and other recent diphtheria outbreaks. A recent report from England documented pharyngeal infections by tox$^-$ *C. diphtheriae* developing predominantly among homosexual men, often causing symptomatic pharyngitis and sometimes resulting in a tonsillar exudate.

In the tropics, cutaneous diphtheria is more common than respiratory diphtheria, occurs throughout the year, and often develops as a secondary infection complicating other dermatoses. Isolates of *C. diphtheriae* from skin lesions are more often tox$^-$ than tox$^+$. A study in Rangoon, Burma, demonstrated *C. diphtheriae* (18.5 percent tox$^+$ strains) in more than 60 percent of bacterially infected skin lesions in patients under 12 years of age. Eighty percent of isolates were from impetiginous scabies, with most of the remainder from impetiginous eczema or impetigo. Cutaneous diphtheria also has been increasingly recognized in temperate climates during the past two decades and accounted for 86 percent of the 1100 cases in Seattle.

Molecular epidemiologic studies demonstrated that the Seattle epidemic actually consisted of three discrete but overlapping outbreaks involving intermedius, gravis, and mitis strains, respectively. The intermedius strains (433 tox$^+$ isolates in 1972–1977) and gravis strains (8 tox$^+$ and 8 tox$^-$ isolates in 1973–1976; 3 tox$^+$ and 173 tox$^-$ isolates in 1978–1982) were shown to be distinct clones of *C. diphtheriae*, with tox$^-$ variants of the gravis clone predominating late in the epidemic. The mitis strains isolated throughout the epidemic, all but 4 of which were tox$^-$, were heterogeneous and represented multiple clones. In Sweden, a recent outbreak (1984–1986) with high mortality (>20 percent) was found to be caused by a single tox$^+$ mitis strain that differed from *C. diphtheriae* strains isolated concurrently from carriers. These observations suggest that traits of *C. diphtheriae* in addition to toxinogenicity contribute to virulence. In England, evidence was found for the initiation of an epidemic by phage conversion of tox$^-$ to tox$^+$ strains in vivo in one individual, with subsequent dissemination over other susceptible subjects.

PATHOLOGY AND PATHOGENESIS   *C. diphtheriae* infects mucous membranes, most commonly in the respiratory tract, and also invades open skin lesions resulting from insect bites or trauma. In infections caused by tox$^+$ *C. diphtheriae*, initial edema and hyperemia are often followed by epithelial necrosis and acute inflammation. Coagulation of the dense fibrinopurulent exudate produces a pseudomembrane, and the inflammatory reaction accompanied by vascular congestion extends into the underlying tissues. The pseudomembrane contains large numbers of *C. diphtheriae* cells, but the bacteria are rarely isolated from the blood or internal organs.

Diphtheria toxin acts both locally and systemically. Very small amounts cause dermonecrosis (as in the Schick test), and toxin presumably contributes to pseudomembrane formation. The lethal dose of diphtheria toxin for nonimmune humans and highly susceptible animals is about 0.1 μg/kg of body weight. Absorbed toxin can cause myocarditis, neuritis, and focal necrosis in various organs, including the kidneys, liver, and adrenal glands. Early changes in diphtheritic myocarditis include cloudy swelling of muscle fibers and interstitial edema. These are followed within weeks by hyaline and granular degeneration of muscle fibers (sometimes with fatty degeneration of the myocardium) progressing to myolysis and finally to the replacement of lost muscle by fibrosis. Thus diphtheria can cause permanent cardiac damage. In diphtheritic polyneuritis, pathologic changes include patchy breakdown of myelin sheaths in peripheral and autonomic nerves, but recovery of damaged nerves is the rule if the patient survives.

Diphtheria toxin is produced by *C. diphtheriae* as an extracellular polypeptide. It is cleaved by proteases to form nicked toxin consisting of fragments A and B, which remain linked by a disulfide bond. Fragment B binds to a plasma membrane receptor (an integral membrane protein corresponding to the precursor of a heparin-binding growth factor resembling epidermal growth factor) on cells from humans or susceptible animals, and the bound toxin is internalized by receptor-mediated endocytosis. Fragment A is translocated across the endosomal membrane and released into the cytoplasm, where it catalyzes the transfer of the adenosine diphosphate ribose moiety from nicotinamide adenine dinucleotide (NAD) to a modified histidine residue (diphthamide) on elongation factor 2, thereby inactivating this factor and inhibiting protein synthesis. One molecule of fragment A in the cytoplasm can kill a cell. Other metabolic alterations in intoxicated cells are secondary to inhibition of protein synthesis. The depletion of carnitine noted in the intoxicated heart may contribute to the pathogenesis of diphtheritic myocarditis. Diphtheria toxin and exotoxin A of *Pseudomonas aeruginosa* have the same enzymatic activity, and their catalytic domains are structurally homologous. Nevertheless, their biologic effects differ because they bind to different cell-surface receptors and exhibit different cellular tropisms.

CLINICAL MANIFESTATIONS Patients with *C. diphtheriae* in the respiratory tract are classified as diphtheria cases if they have symptoms consistent with local infection and as diphtheria carriers if they are asymptomatic. Signs and symptoms vary with the site and severity of the local infection, the patient's age, and the presence or absence of preexisting nasopharyngeal disease or concomitant systemic disease. Onset is often gradual, but most patients seek medical care within a few days of becoming ill. Sore throat is the most common symptom, but children are less likely than adults to complain of sore throat and are more likely to have nausea and vomiting. Fever of 37.8 to 38.9°C (100 to 102°F) and dysphagia are documented in about half of patients, but cough, hoarseness, chills, and rhinorrhea are less common. Systemic manifestations are primarily due to the effects of diphtheria toxin. Patients without toxicity exhibit discomfort and malaise associated with local infection, whereas severely toxic patients may have listlessness, pallor, and tachycardia that can progress rapidly to vascular collapse.

Primary infection in the respiratory tract is most often tonsillopharyngeal (one-half to two-thirds of cases) but also may be (in decreasing order of frequency) laryngeal, nasal, and tracheobronchial. Multiple sites are frequently involved, and secondary spread of pharyngeal infection upward to the nasal mucosa or downward to the larynx and tracheobronchial tree is much more common than primary infection at those sites. Systemic toxicity is usually less severe in nasal diphtheria than in tonsillopharyngeal diphtheria and is most severe when extensive pseudomembrane extends from the tonsils and pharynx into contiguous regions. A small percentage of patients present with malignant, or "bull neck," diphtheria, with abrupt onset, extensive pseudomembrane formation, foul breath, massive swelling of the tonsils and uvula, thick speech, cervical lymphadenopathy, striking edematous swelling of the submandibular region and anterior neck, and severe toxicity.

In tonsillopharyngeal diphtheria, only erythema may be noted initially, but isolated spots of gray or white exudate are common. These often extend and coalesce within a day to form a confluent, sharply demarcated pseudomembrane that becomes progressively thicker, more tightly adherent to the underlying tissue, and darker gray. Unlike the exudate in streptococcal pharyngitis, the diphtheritic pseudomembrane often extends beyond the margin of the tonsils onto the tonsillar pillars, palate, or uvula. Dislodging the membrane is likely to cause bleeding. Estimates of the proportion of patients with pharyngeal diphtheria who develop typical pseudomembranes vary widely, from as few as one-third to almost all. The higher estimates may be biased by failure to consider and confirm the diagnosis of diphtheria in patients who do not develop pseudomembranes. Patients with nasal diphtheria often present with serosanguineous nasal discharge, which may be unilateral or bilateral, and may cause irritation of the nares or lip. Laryngeal diphtheria often presents with hoarseness and cough. Demonstration of laryngeal pseudomembrane by laryngoscopy is helpful for distinguishing diphtheria from other infectious forms of laryngitis. Primary or secondary diphtheritic infection occasionally involves other mucous membranes, including the conjunctiva and the membranes of the genitourinary and gastrointestinal tracts.

Cutaneous diphtheria usually presents as an infection by *C. diphtheriae* of preexisting dermatoses involving (in decreasing order of frequency) the lower extremities, upper extremities, head, or trunk.

The clinical features are similar to those of other secondary cutaneous bacterial infections. In the tropics, the presentation of cutaneous diphtheria occasionally includes morphologically distinct "punched-out" ulcers that are covered by necrotic slough or membrane and have well-demarcated edges.

COMPLICATIONS Obstruction of the respiratory tract, presenting as tachypnea, dyspnea, stridor, cyanosis, and use of accessory muscles of respiration, can be caused by extensive pseudomembrane formation and swelling during the first few days of the disease or by sloughed pseudomembrane that becomes lodged in the airways at a later stage. The risk of respiratory obstruction is greater when infection involves the larynx or the tracheobronchial tree and is higher in children because of the small size of the airways.

Myocarditis and polyneuritis are the most prominent toxic manifestations of diphtheria. The risk of developing these manifestations is proportional to the severity of local disease, and the two can occur together in the same patient. Myocarditis may present during the acute phase of illness, develop as local disease is resolving, or begin insidiously after several weeks. One-half to two-thirds of patients with typical diphtheria have subtle evidence of cardiac dysfunction, including electrocardiographic abnormalities, but clinically apparent myocarditis develops in 10 to 25 percent of patients and is usually more severe when the onset is early. Electrocardiographic abnormalities include ST-T-wave changes, varying degrees of heart block, and arrhythmias, including atrial fibrillation, ventricular premature beats, ventricular tachycardia, or ventricular fibrillation. Clinical signs include diminished heart sounds, gallop rhythm, systolic murmurs, and (less commonly) acute or insidiously progressive congestive heart failure. Serum levels of aspartate aminotransferase reflect the intensity of myocardial damage and can be used to monitor its course.

Polyneuritis is uncommon in mild diphtheria but occurs in approximately 10 percent of cases of average severity and in up to 75 percent of severe cases. Bulbar dysfunction typically develops during the first 2 weeks. Palatal and pharyngeal paralysis usually develops first. Swallowing is difficult, the voice sounds nasal, and ingested fluids may be regurgitated through the nose. With unilateral pharyngeal infection, ipsilateral palatal paralysis is more common than contralateral or bilateral paralysis. Additional bulbar signs may develop over several weeks, with oculomotor and ciliary paralysis occurring more often than facial or laryngeal paralysis. Peripheral polyneuritis typically begins from 1 to 3 months after the onset of diphtheria with proximal weakness of the extremities that spreads distally. The severity of the disease varies from mild weakness of the pelvic muscles with unsteady gait to total paralysis, including failure of respiration. Paresthesias may develop, most often in a glove-and-stocking distribution. Approximately one-half of patients with diphtheritic neuropathy have evidence of cardiac vagal denervation, and a smaller proportion of this group has abnormal baroreceptor function. Polyneuritis usually resolves completely, with the time needed for improvement approximately equal to that elapsing from exposure to the development of symptoms. Severe muscular weakness may develop 1 to 2 weeks before maximal abnormalities in the peripheral nerve conduction velocity are demonstrated, the result being a striking dissociation between clinical and electrophysiologic findings. Cerebrospinal fluid (CSF) most often contains moderately increased levels of albumin, occasionally with pleocytosis, but the abnormalities in CSF do not determine prognosis.

Pneumonia occurs in more than half of fatal cases of diphtheria. Less common complications include renal failure, encephalitis, cerebral infarction, pulmonary embolism, and bacteremia or endocarditis due to invasive infection by *C. diphtheriae*. Serum sickness may result from antitoxin therapy.

COURSE AND PROGNOSIS Most cases of diphtheria occur in nonimmunized patients. The attack rate, severity of disease, and risk of complications are much lower in immunized patients. The pseudomembrane may continue to increase in size during the first day after administration of antitoxin. During the next several days to a week, it becomes softer, less adherent, and nonconfluent and eventually disappears as the normal mucosa is regenerated. In the preantibiotic era, *C. diphtheriae* persisted in the throat for about 2 weeks in one-half of patients and for 1 month or more in about one-fifth. Mortality increases with the severity of local disease, the extent of pseudomembrane formation, and the delay between onset of local disease and administration of antitoxin. The death rate is highest during the first week of illness; among patients with "bull neck" diphtheria; among patients with myocarditis who develop ventricular tachycardia, atrial fibrillation, or complete heart block; among patients with laryngeal or tracheobronchial involvement; among infants and patients over 60 years of age; and among alcoholics. In cutaneous diphtheria both mortality and the risk of myocarditis or peripheral neuropathy are significantly lower than in respiratory diphtheria.

DIAGNOSIS A characteristic pseudomembrane on the mucosa of the oropharynx, palate, nasopharynx, nose, or larynx suggests diphtheria but is not uniformly present. Diphtheritic pseudomembrane must be distinguished from other pharyngeal exudates, including those of group A beta-hemolytic streptococcal infections, infectious mononucleosis, viral pharyngitides, fusospirochetal infection, and candidiasis. Diphtheria should be considered in patients with sore throat, cervical adenopathy or swelling, and low-grade fever, especially when these manifestations are accompanied by systemic toxicity, hoarseness, stridor, palatal paralysis, and/or serosanguineous nasal discharge with or without demonstrable pseudomembrane. Treatment with diphtheria antitoxin should be begun as soon as the clinical diagnosis of diphtheria is made.

Definitive diagnosis of diphtheria depends on the isolation of *C. diphtheriae* from local lesions. The laboratory should be notified that diphtheria is suspected so that use of selective tellurite medium appropriate for the isolation of *C. diphtheriae* is ensured. All isolates of *C. diphtheriae* should be subjected to toxicity testing. Primary isolates can be rapidly screened for toxinogenicity by the polymerase chain reaction, although occasional strains of *C. diphtheriae* that carry an inactive toxin gene may give false-positive results. The biochemical tests needed to differentiate *C. diphtheriae* from corynebacteria of the normal flora (diphtheroids) require several days. Group A beta-hemolytic streptococci and *Staphylococcus aureus* are also isolated frequently from patients with diphtheria.

Although, as has been mentioned, cutaneous diphtheria may present as a characteristic "punched-out" ulcer with a membrane, it is more often indistinguishable from other inflammatory dermatoses. Diagnosis depends on a high degree of suspicion and on culture of cutaneous lesions on laboratory media appropriate for the isolation of *C. diphtheriae*. Throat samples from all patients with cutaneous diphtheria should be cultured for *C. diphtheriae*.

TREATMENT The decision to administer diphtheria antitoxin must be based on the clinical diagnosis of diphtheria without definitive laboratory confirmation, since each day of delay is associated with increased mortality. Because diphtheria antitoxin is produced in horses, it is necessary to inquire about possible allergy to horse serum and to perform a conjunctival or intracutaneous test with diluted antitoxin for immediate hypersensitivity. Epinephrine must be available for immediate administration to patients with severe allergic reactions. Patients with immediate hypersensitivity should be desensitized before a full therapeutic dose of antitoxin is given. The dose of diphtheria antitoxin currently recommended by the Committee on Infectious Diseases of the American Academy of Pediatrics is based on the site of the primary infection and the duration and severity of disease: 20,000 to 40,000 units for disease present for 48 h or less and involving the pharynx or larynx, 40,000 to 60,000 units for nasopharyngeal infections, and 80,000 to 100,000 units for disease that is extensive, has been present for 3 or more days, or is accompanied by brawny anterior cervical edema. Antitoxin is administered intravenously by infusion in saline over 60 min to neutralize unbound toxin rapidly. The approximately 10 percent risk of serum sickness is acceptable because of the established therapeutic value of antitoxin in decreasing mortality from respiratory diphtheria. During the early phase of the Seattle epidemic, all patients with cutaneous

diphtheria received 20,000 units of antitoxin. Later, when most isolates were tox$^-$, antitoxin was withheld initially and administered only to patients from whom tox$^+$ strains of *C. diphtheriae* were isolated. The potential systemic complications of cutaneous diptheria must be weighed against the potential adverse effects of antitoxin treatment; authorities are not unanimous in recommending antitoxin therapy for cutaneous diphtheria.

Antibiotics have little demonstrated effect on healing of the local infection in diphtheria patients treated with antitoxin. The primary goal of antibiotic therapy for patients or carriers is therefore to eradicate *C. diphtheriae* and prevent its transmission from the patient to susceptible contacts. Erythromycin, penicillin G, rifampin, or clindamycin is recommended by most authorities. Commonly recommended regimens for the treatment of adults with respiratory diphtheria are erythromycin (500 mg four times daily, parenterally or orally) or intramuscular procaine penicillin G (600,000 units at 12-h intervals) for 14 days. Patients with cutaneous diphtheria and carriers can be treated orally with erythromycin (500 mg four times daily) or rifampin (600 mg once daily) for 7 days. If compliance is in question, a single dose of benzathine penicillin G (1.2 to 2.4 million units intramuscularly) can be administered. Eradication of *C. diphtheriae* should be documented by negative cultures of samples taken on two or three successive days, beginning at least 24 h after the completion of antibiotic therapy. Some authorities also recommend a repeat throat culture 2 weeks later. The small percentage of patients who continue to be infected with *C. diphtheriae* after treatment should receive an additional 10-day course of oral erythromycin or rifampin. Plasmid-mediated erythromycin resistance of the MLS type emerged transiently in *C. diphtheriae* during the Seattle epidemic, but its frequency declined dramatically after the routine use of erythromycin was discontinued.

Patients with respiratory or cutaneous diphtheria caused by tox$^+$ *C. diphtheriae* or strains of unknown toxinogenicity should be hospitalized, kept in bed initially, handled with isolation procedures appropriate for the site of infection, and given supportive care as needed. Respiratory and cardiac function must be monitored closely. Early intubation or tracheostomy is recommended when the larynx is involved or signs of impending airway obstruction are present. Tracheobronchial membrane can sometimes be mechanically removed via the endotracheal tube or tracheostomy. Primary or secondary pneumonia should be diagnosed and treated promptly. Sedative or hypnotic drugs that may mask respiratory symptoms are contraindicated. Close electrocardiographic monitoring, treatment of arrhythmias, and electrical pacing for heart block are essential. Congestive heart failure should be treated as described in Chap. 195. Glucocorticoids do not reduce the risk of diphtheritic myocarditis or polyneuritis. Oral therapy with DL-carnitine (100 mg/kg per day, given in twice-daily doses for 4 days) may be beneficial in diphtheritic myocarditis, but such therapy should be considered experimental until additional data becomes available. Ulcerative or ecthymatous cutaneous lesions should be treated with Burow's solution applied on wet compresses after debridement of necrotic areas, and treatment for associated conditions such as pediculosis, scabies, or underlying dermatoses should be instituted.

PREVENTION Vaccines available in the United States for immunization against diphtheria include diphtheria and tetanus toxoids and pertussis vaccine adsorbed (DTP), diphtheria and tetanus toxoids adsorbed (DT) (for pediatric use), and tetanus and diphtheria toxoids adsorbed (Td) (for adult use). Each vaccine contains one dose in 0.5 mL and is administered intramuscularly. The adsorbent is alum, which functions as an adjuvant and enhances immunogenicity of the vaccines. Td contains less diphtheria toxoid than DTP or DT and causes fewer adverse reactions in adults.

Initial immunization against diphtheria requires completion of a primary series. Booster doses are required periodically throughout life for the maintenance of immunity. The recommended primary series for immunization of children up to the seventh birthday consists of four doses of DTP: the first at 6 weeks of age or older, the second and third doses after successive intervals of 4 to 8 weeks, and the fourth 6 to 12 months after the third. DT is substituted for DTP if pertussis vaccine is contraindicated (see Chap. 114). If primary immunization is delayed until after the seventh birthday, the primary series consists of three doses of Td, with the second dose given 4 to 8 weeks after the first and the third dose given 6 to 12 months after the second. If primary immunization is interrupted, the series should simply be completed; there is no need to start a new series. Children who complete a primary series should receive a booster dose of DTP before entering kindergarten unless the final dose of the primary series was given after the fourth birthday. Adults with an uncertain history of immunization should receive a primary series. Patients with diphtheria should be actively immunized after recovery. Booster doses of Td should be given at intervals of 10 years throughout life, preferably at the middecade ages (15 years, 25 years, etc).

Close contacts of patients with diphtheria should be cultured for *C. diphtheriae*, kept under surveillance for 1 week, and treated with appropriate antibiotics if cultures are positive. Previously immunized close contacts should receive an appropriate booster containing diphtheria toxoid if their last booster was given more than 5 years earlier. If the immunization status is uncertain, close contacts should receive an antibiotic regimen appropriate for carriers and a primary immunization series appropriate for their age.

OTHER CORYNEBACTERIAL INFECTIONS

DEFINITION Medically important *coryneform bacteria* (formerly called *diphtheroids*) include members of the normal flora that cause opportunistic infections, human pathogens of relatively low virulence, and animal pathogens that cause occasional zoonotic infections. Reported infections caused by coryneform bacteria have increased substantially in number over the last two decades. Isolates of *C. jeikeium* and group D-2 coryneform bacteria are often resistant to multiple antibiotics.

ETIOLOGY AND LABORATORY FEATURES Because coryneform bacteria are potential pathogens, it is important not to dismiss them as constituents of the normal flora or contaminants when they are found in clinical specimens. Laboratory differentiation of coryneform bacteria is important when they are isolated repeatedly, when they are recovered in pure culture or in large numbers, or when they form pigmented or hemolytic colonies.

The coryneform bacteria are a large, taxonomically heterogeneous, poorly classified group of gram-positive, pleomorphic, irregularly staining bacilli or coccobacilli that superficially resemble *C. diphtheriae*. The scheme recommended by the Centers for Disease Control and Prevention (CDC) for the classification of coryneform bacteria assigns them to several genera, including *Actinomyces, Arcanobacterium, Corynebacterium, Oerskovia,* and *Rhodococcus,* as well as to several groups that have not yet been categorized at the genus and species level.

ECOLOGY AND EPIDEMIOLOGY Humans are the probable natural habitat for *C. xerosis, C. pseudodiphtheriticum* (formerly *C. hofmanii*), *C. striatum, C. minutissimum, C. jeikeium* (fomerly CDC group JK), *Arcanobacterium haemolyticum* (formerly *C. haemolyticum*), and members of CDC coryneform groups A-4, D-2, G, I, 1, and 2. Animals are the probable natural habitat for *Actinomyces pyogenes* (formerly *C. pyogenes*; cows, sheep, pigs), *C. ulcerans* (cows, horses), and *C. pseudotuberculosis* (sheep, goats, horses). The natural habitat for *Rhodococcus equi* (formerly *C. equi*) is soil. The ecologic niches for most other coryneform bacteria of medical importance are not well defined.

The coryneform bacteria found most frequently as components of the normal flora include *C. pseudodiphtheriticum* (pharynx, skin), *C. xerosis* (conjunctival sac, nasopharynx, skin), and *C. striatum* (anterior nares, skin). Those which often colonize the skin of hospitalized patients include *C. jeikeium* (axilla, groin, perineum) and CDC group D-2. *C. jeikeium* most frequently colonizes patients with malignancies

or severe immunodeficiency; it also can be isolated from environmental sources (surfaces, air) in hospitals and from the hands of ward staff. *C. ulcerans* infections are acquired by consumption of raw milk. *C. pseudotuberculosis* infections are acquired by contact with animals or animal products or by consumption of raw milk.

PATHOGENESIS AND CLINICAL MANIFESTATIONS *C. jeikeium* was recognized in 1976 as a cause of infections in immunocompromised hosts. It also causes infections in immunocompetent hosts, but severe infections continue to be most frequent in patients with hematologic malignancies and neutropenia. Colonization of the skin precedes clinical infection. Additional risk factors for nosocomial *C. jeikeium* sepsis include prolonged hospitalization, breaks in the integument, chronic intravascular catheterization, and prior treatment with broad-spectrum antibiotics. Other presentations of *C. jeikeium* infection include endocarditis, device-related infections, pulmonary infiltrates, cutaneous septic emboli, soft tissue infections, and skin rashes. Endocarditis due to *C. jeikeium* occurs primarily in patients with prosthetic heart valves. *C. jeikeium* is a rare cause of infections of the central nervous system in patients with ventricular shunts.

Group D-2 coryneform bacteria were identified in 1985 as a significant cause of nosocomial urinary tract infections, including acute and chronic cystitis and pyelonephritis. These organisms closely resemble *C. jeikeium* but differ by producing urease and failing to convert glucose to acidic metabolites. Hydrolysis of urea by urease causes alkalinization of the urine and formation of ammonium magnesium phosphate (struvite) stones. Group D-2 coryneform bacteria cause alkaline-encrusted cystitis in patients with preexisting bladder lesions that serve as foci for precipitation of struvite crystals. Risk factors associated with symptomatic urinary tract infections include preexisting immunosuppression, recent urologic procedures (including renal transplantation), underlying disorders of the genitourinary tract, and a history of urinary tract infections.

A. haemolyticum causes pharyngitis, with 90 percent of cases occurring in patients between 10 and 30 years old. In this age group, *A. haemolyticum* pharyngitis is 5 to 13 percent as frequent as *Streptococcus pyogenes* pharyngitis. An erythematous rash is present in 30 to 67 percent of cases. The rash is usually scarlatiniform and most pronounced on the extremities, but it sometimes resembles urticaria or erythema multiforme. Because rash is more common in *A. haemolyticum* infections than in *S. pyogenes* infections, older children and adults presenting with the scarlet fever syndrome are as likely to have *A. haemolyticum* as *S. pyogenes* infection. Infection due to *A. haemolyticum* also can present with extensive pharyngeal exudate and can mimic diphtheria. *A. haemolyticum* occasionally causes peritonsillar abscess, sepsis, endocarditis, or meningitis.

C. minutissimum is frequently isolated from the lesions of erythrasma, a common superficial skin infection characterized by the presence in intertriginous areas of reddish brown, scaly, pruritic, macular patches that exhibit coral-red fluorescence under a Wood's light. The etiology of erythrasma has not been definitively established; infection of the skin by *C. minutissimum* has been shown to develop after the onset of maceration and scaling. Deep infections caused by *C. minutissimum* are rare and include abscesses, bacteremia, and endocarditis.

Among coryneform bacteria that cause disease in animals and occasionally in humans, *R. equi* is emerging as a potentially important intracellular opportunistic pathogen in immunocompromised patients. Most reported cases are pulmonary infections that resemble tuberculosis in patients with severely defective cell-mediated immunity. Several cases of *R. equi* infection have recently been documented in patients with AIDS. *A. pyogenes* causes bovine mastitis, a disease transmitted by flies. Yearly epidemics of leg ulcers infected with *A. pyogenes* occurred among schoolchildren in Thailand between 1979 and 1984 and were postulated to have resulted from introduction of the organism into traumatic skin lesions by flies. Reported *A. pyogenes* infections among adults in Denmark have included abscesses, cystitis, intraabdominal infections, and mastoiditis with bacteremia. Infections due to *C. ulcerans* in humans usually present as pharyngitis and can mimic respiratory diphtheria, whereas infections caused by *C. pseudotuberculosis* typically present as suppurative granulomatous lymphadenitis. *C. ulcerans* and *C. pseudotuberculosis* can be lysogenized by tox$^+$ phages and can produce diphtheria toxin. Human infections by tox$^+$ strains of *C. ulcerans*—but not by tox$^+$ strains of *C. pseudotuberculosis*—have been reported.

C. pseudodiphtheriticum, a commensal of low virulence, is an uncommon cause of pneumonia in men with AIDS and of endocarditis, necrotizing tracheitis, tracheobronchitis, and urinary tract infection in patients without known immune deficiencies. Likewise, *C. xerosis* and *C. striatum* occasionally cause infections in humans.

DIAGNOSIS The clinical features of *C. jeikeium* infections are not pathognomonic. Thus the diagnosis of *C. jeikeium* infections is based on a high index of suspicion, identification of the organism by culture from appropriate clinical specimens, and exclusion of other likely causes of infection.

Group D-2 coryneform bacteria often are not detected by routine urine cultures; rather, it is necessary to incubate the cultures for 24 to 48 h on blood agar or special media. Cultivation should be prolonged in selected cases—i.e., those involving patients (especially elderly men who have preexisting genitourinary abnormalities) with alkaline urine, ammonium magnesium phosphate stones, gram-positive bacilli in the urine, or negative standard urine cultures despite clinical evidence of bacteriuria. Other microbes that can cause urinary tract infections with alkaline urine include *Proteus, Ureaplasma,* and some *staphylococci* and *streptococci.* Alkaline-encrusted cystitis is an anatomic diagnosis made by cystoscopy.

The differential diagnosis of *A. haemolyticum* pharyngitis with rash includes scarlet fever; rubella; staphylococcal and streptococcal toxic shock syndromes; infections caused by Epstein-Barr virus, cytomegalovirus, and enteroviruses (especially coxsackieviruses); disseminated gonococcal infection; secondary syphilis; and drug allergy. Routine diagnostic methods of throat culture are not ideal for the detection of *A. haemolyticum,* nor is this organism detected by rapid tests for *S. pyogenes* that are sometimes substituted for throat cultures. Pharyngitis caused by *A. haemolyticum* in adolescents and adults is likely to be underdiagnosed until improved tests for the organism are used by diagnostic laboratories.

Erythrasma is diagnosed clinically. Because of uncertainty about the etiologic role of *C. minutissimum,* culture of erythrasma lesions is not currently recommended. Pharyngitis caused by tox$^+$ strains of *C. ulcerans* may be clinically indistinguishable from diphtheria. The presentations of infections caused by other coryneform bacteria are not usually diagnostic; cultures are required for identification of the causal organisms.

TREATMENT AND PREVENTION Strains of *C. jeikeium* are typically resistant to most antibiotics except vancomycin, which is the drug of choice. Some recent isolates of *C. jeikeium* are susceptible or only moderately resistant to β-lactam antibiotics. Infections due to fully susceptible strains can be treated with β-lactam antibiotics alone, and those due to moderately resistant strains can be treated with β-lactam antibiotics plus an aminoglycoside. Quinolones, especially ciprofloxacin, exhibit excellent in vitro activity against *C. jeikeium,* but clinical data on their therapeutic effectiveness are not yet available. For device-related *C. jeikeium* infections, removal of the infected device is usually required in addition to appropriate antibiotic therapy.

Group D-2 coryneform bacteria are often resistant to the antibiotics used commonly for the treatment of urinary tract infections. Early isolates were uniformly susceptible to vancomycin and quinolones, but recent isolates have exhibited increasing resistance to norfloxacin and ciprofloxacin. Isolates are often susceptible to erythromycin, rifampin, novobiocin, and tetracyclines. Treatment of urinary tract infections due to group D-2 strains is often difficult; several courses of antibiotic may be necessary for bacteriologic cure. Patients with alkaline-encrusted cystitis require resection of the encrusted lesions in addition to antibiotic therapy.

Controlled trials of treatment for infections caused by *A. haemolyticum* have not been performed. In vitro tests have demonstrated susceptibility to erythromycin but tolerance or relative resistance to penicillin. Limited data suggest that the clinical course of *A. haemolyticum* pharyngitis may be shortened by treatment with erythromycin.

Infections caused by *C. ulcerans* that present like diphtheria or that are known to be caused by tox$^+$ strains should be treated like diphtheria. Oral erythromycin is usually effective for the treatment of erythrasma. Initial treatment of infections caused by other coryneform bacteria should be based on the identity of the organism and on published data regarding antibiotic susceptibility. Therapy should be modified, when necessary, in light of the results of antibiotic susceptibility tests. All isolates of *Corynebacterium* and of coryneform bacteria reported to date have been susceptible to vancomycin.

ANTHRAX

DEFINITION Anthrax is an acute bacterial infection caused by *Bacillus anthracis* that occurs most frequently in herbivorous animals. Humans become infected when spores of *B. anthracis* are introduced into the body by contact with infected animals or contaminated animal products, insect bites, inhalation, or ingestion. In humans, the most common form is cutaneous anthrax, which is characterized by a localized skin lesion with a central eschar surrounded by marked nonpitting edema. Inhalation anthrax (woolsorters' disease) typically involves hemorrhagic mediastinitis, rapidly progressive systemic infection, and very high mortality. Gastrointestinal anthrax is rare and is associated with high mortality.

ETIOLOGY *B. anthracis* is a large (1 to 1.5 μm by 4 to 10 μm), nonmotile, encapsulated, chain-forming, aerobic, gram-positive rod that forms centrally located, oval spores. Oxygen is required for sporulation but not for germination of spores, and sporulation does not take place in living animals. The rectangular shape of the individual bacteria gives chains of *B. anthracis* a boxcar-like appearance. On blood agar, virulent *B. anthracis* usually forms nonhemolytic or weakly hemolytic, grayish white, rough colonies that have irregular, comma-shaped projections and are said to resemble a medusa's head; however, if the medium contains bicarbonate and incubation is carried out in the presence of excess CO_2, the colonies are smooth and mucoid. Virulent strains of *B. anthracis* are pathogenic for animals, including mice and guinea pigs. Known virulence factors include three proteins collectively called *anthrax toxin* (see below) and an antiphagocytic capsular polypeptide composed of D-glutamic acid residues linked by peptide bonds involving the gamma carboxyl group. The genes that determine the production of anthrax toxin and of capsular polypeptide are on separate plasmids of *B. anthracis.* Determination of susceptibility to bacillus phage gamma and demonstration of species-specific antigens by direct fluorescent antibody tests or by hemagglutination tests are helpful in laboratory identification of *B. anthracis.* Spores of *B. anthracis* can survive for years in dry earth but are destroyed by boiling for about 10 min, by treatment with oxidizing agents such as potassium permanganate or hydrogen peroxide, or by dilute formaldehyde. Most strains of *B. anthracis* are susceptible to penicillin.

EPIDEMIOLOGY The distribution of anthrax is worldwide. All animals are susceptible to varying degrees, but the disease is most prevalent among domestic herbivores (including cattle, sheep, horses, and goats) and wild herbivores.

Grazing animals become infected when they are foraging for food in areas contaminated with spores of *B. anthracis* under appropriate climatic conditions. Anthrax in herbivores tends to be severe, with high mortality. Terminally ill animals have overwhelming bacteremia and often bleed from the nose, mouth, and bowel, thereby contaminating soil or watering places with vegetative *B. anthracis* that can subsequently sporulate and persist in the environment. The carcasses of infected animals provide additional potential foci of contamination. Whether or not *B. anthracis* multiplies to any significant extent in the soil is controversial, and environmental factors affecting the probability that animals grazing in contaminated areas will become infected have not been fully defined. Epidemics among animals may spread from an initial focus to contiguous geographic areas in a pattern consistent with the movement of infected animals. Biting flies also have been implicated as vectors for the spread of anthrax, and vultures that feed on infected carcasses are believed to be involved in the occasional spread of anthrax from a contaminated area to noncontiguous areas, probably by contamination of surface water pools. A striking example of the impact of anthrax in animals is provided by an outbreak on a pig farm in northern Wales in 1989 that necessitated the slaughter and incineration of 4492 pigs; decontamination of excrement, farm buildings, equipment, paths, roadways, and farmland with formalin; and disposal of the decontaminated excrement as toxic waste–all at public expense.

The natural resistance of humans to anthrax is greater than that of herbivorous animals. It is difficult to determine the annual worldwide incidence of human anthrax because many cases do not receive medical attention and are not reported; estimates of 20,000 to 100,000 cases per year have been made. Human cases are classified as agricultural or industrial on the basis of the epidemiologic setting in which they occur. Agricultural cases result most often from contact with animals that have anthrax (during skinning, butchering, dissecting, etc.), from bites of contaminated or infected flies, and, in rare instances, from consumption of contaminated meat. Industrial cases are associated with exposure to contaminated hides, goat's hair, wool, or bones. Anthrax in animals has been a long-standing problem in Iran, Turkey, Pakistan, and Sudan, and the probability is high that animal products (especially goat's hair) originating from these areas will be contaminated with anthrax spores.

Only 4 cases of human anthrax were documented in the United States from 1984 through 1988, and gastrointestinal anthrax has never been documented in this country. Large epidemics of anthrax occurred in the former Soviet Union at Sverdlovsk in 1979 and in Zimbabwe between 1978 and the early 1980s. Initially, the cases in Sverdlovsk were reported to be cutaneous and gastrointestinal anthrax and were attributed to exposure to meat from infected animals. Intense international interest was stimulated by the suspicion that the release of B. anthracis from a nearby military facility was responsible for the outbreak. A recent analysis of 42 necropsies from the Sverdlovsk outbreak, including most of the fatal cases, describes the pathologic findings and documents that the disease was, in fact, inhalation anthrax. The outbreak in Zimbabwe involved more than 9700 cases of agricultural anthrax in humans. This massive outbreak occurred during wartime and was associated with disruption of the veterinary and medical infrastructure and cessation of veterinary anthrax vaccination programs (see below).

PATHOGENESIS B. anthracis is an extracellular pathogen that can evade phagocytosis, invade the bloodstream, multiply rapidly to a high population density in vivo, and kill quickly. Capsular polypeptide and anthrax toxin are recognized as the principal virulence factors of B. anthracis. The capsule of B. anthracis consists of poly-D-glutamic acid and confers resistance to phagocytosis. Anthrax toxin consists of three proteins called *protective antigen* (PA), *edema factor* (EF), and *lethal factor* (LF). The toxin was discovered by the demonstration that the transfer of sterile blood from guinea pigs dying of anthrax to uninfected guinea pigs killed the recipients.

PA, EF, and LF have been purified and characterized and their structural genes cloned and sequenced. PA binds to plasma membranes of target cells and is cleaved by a cellular protease into two fragments. The larger fragment remains on the cell surface and displays a binding site for a domain that is present in both EF and LF, but the smaller fragment is released. The larger PA fragment on the cell surface serves as a specific receptor that mediates entry of either EF or LF into the target cells by receptor-mediated endocytosis. Recent studies have demonstrated that PA also can be cleaved in the blood of infected animals and that the larger PA fragment can interact with LF to form circulating complexes. EF is a calmodulin-dependent adenylate cyclase, and EF activity is expressed within human or animal cells

that provide both the calmodulin activator and the ATP substrate for EF. The biologic effects of EF, which include formation of edema in anthrax lesions and inhibition of polymorphonuclear leukocyte functions, are mediated by the cyclic AMP that is formed intracellularly from ATP by the enzymatic action of EF. PA-mediated entry of LF into susceptible cells leads to cell death, but the mechanism of action of LF has not yet been determined.

Cutaneous anthrax is initiated by the introduction of spores of B. anthracis into the skin through cuts or abrasions or by biting flies. The spores germinate within hours, and the vegetative cells multiply and produce anthrax toxin. Histologically, the lesion in cutaneous anthrax is characterized by necrosis, vascular congestion, hemorrhage, and gelatinous edema. The number of leukocytes is disproportionately small in comparison with the amount of tissue damage. The clinical description of this lesion as a "malignant pustule" is not in concordance with the pathologic findings.

In inhalation anthrax, B. anthracis spores in airborne particles less than 5 μm in diameter are deposited directly into the alveoli or alveolar ducts. The spores are phagocytized by alveolar macrophages, and some are carried to and germinate in mediastinal nodes. Hemorrhagic necrosis of the nodes, in association with hemorrhagic mediastinitis and overwhelming B. anthracis bacteremia, may develop rapidly. Secondary pneumonia sometimes occurs.

Gastrointestinal anthrax usually results from ingestion of inadequately cooked meat from animals with anthrax. Primary infection can be initiated in the intestine by organisms that survive passage through the stomach, but an oropharyngeal form of the disease also has been described. Lesions in the throat or intestine are usually accompanied by hemorrhagic lymphadenitis.

B. anthracis bacteremia can develop in any form of anthrax and is documented in almost all fatal cases. Autopsies reveal large numbers of bacteria in blood vessels, lymph nodes, and many organs.

CLINICAL MANIFESTATIONS Approximately 95 percent of human cases of anthrax are the cutaneous form and about 5 percent the inhalation form. Gastrointestinal anthrax is rare. Anthrax meningitis occurs in a small percentage of all cases and is a frequent complication of overwhelming B. anthracis bacteremia.

Cutaneous anthrax The cutaneous lesion in anthrax is most often found on exposed areas of skin. In the Zimbabwe outbreak, lesions in children under 5 years old were significantly more likely to be on the head, neck, or face and less likely to be on the upper limbs than in adults. This distribution correlates with the fact that children have less contact than adults with carcasses of infected animals and are more likely to acquire infection through fly bites.

Within days after inoculation of B. anthracis spores into the skin, a small red macule appears. During the next week the lesion typically progresses through papular and vesicular or pustular stages to the formation of an ulcer with a blackened necrotic eschar surrounded by a highly characteristic, expanding zone of brawny edema. The early lesion may be pruritic, and the fully developed lesion is painless. Small satellite vesicles may surround the original lesion, and painful nonspecific regional lymphadenitis is common. Most patients are afebrile, with mild or no constitutional symptoms; in severe cases, however, edema may be extensive and associated with shock. Spontaneous healing occurs in 80 to 90 percent of untreated cases, but edema may persist for weeks. In the 10 to 20 percent of untreated patients who have progressive infection, bacteremia develops and is often associated with high fever and rapid death. The differential diagnosis includes staphylococcal skin infections, tularemia, plague, and orf. Cutaneous anthrax should be considered when patients have painless ulcers associated with vesicles and edema and have had contact with animals or animal products.

Inhalation anthrax The frequent similarity of the presenting symptoms of inhalation anthrax (woolsorters' disease) to those of severe viral respiratory diseases makes early diagnosis difficult. After 1 to 3 days an acute phase supervenes, with increasing fever, dyspnea, stridor, hypoxia, and hypotension usually leading to death within 24 h. Occasionally, patients present with fulminant disease. A characteristic radiologic finding associated with hemorrhagic mediastinitis is symmetrical mediastinal widening.

Gastrointestinal anthrax   Symptoms of gastrointestinal anthrax are variable and include fever, nausea and vomiting, abdominal pain, bloody diarrhea, and sometimes rapidly developing ascites. Diarrhea is occasionally massive, causing hemoconcentration and severe contraction of intravascular volume. The major features of oropharyngeal anthrax are fever, sore throat, dysphagia, painful regional lymphadenopathy, and toxemia; respiratory distress may be evident. The primary lesion is most often on the tonsils.

LABORATORY DIAGNOSIS   *B. anthracis* is present in large numbers in cutaneous lesions of anthrax and can be demonstrated by Gram's stain, direct fluorescent antibody staining, or culture unless the patient has been treated with antibiotics. A small proportion of patients with anthrax have bacteremia, but the disease may progress to death before blood cultures become positive. Patients with anthrax meningitis have bloody spinal fluid containing large numbers of *B. anthracis* cells demonstrable by staining or culture. The virulence of suspected isolates of *B. anthracis* can be demonstrated by the inoculation of guinea pigs; death results within 24 h with positive cultures of heart blood. Patients with mild disease usually have normal leukocyte counts, but patients with disseminated disease typically have polymorphonuclear leukocytosis. Tests for antibody to *B. anthracis* are useful in confirming the diagnosis of anthrax. A sensitive and specific polymerase chain reaction method developed for the detection of spores of *B. anthracis* may be useful for rapid testing of potentially contaminated animal or agricultural products.

TREATMENT   Viable *B. anthracis* disappears from the lesions of cutaneous anthrax within 5 h of the initiation of treatment with parenteral penicillin G. Recommended therapy for adults is 2 million units of penicillin G at intervals of 6 h until edema subsides, with the subsequent administration of oral penicillin to complete a 7- to 10-day course. For penicillin-sensitive adults, erythromycin or tetracycline (500 mg every 6 h) can be substituted. Chloramphenicol also has been used successfully. Antibiotics decrease local edema and systemic toxicity in patients with cutaneous anthrax but do not prevent eschar formation. Cutaneous lesions should be cleaned and covered, and used dressings should be decontaminated. For inhalation anthrax, high-dose penicillin therapy (2 million units at 2-h intervals) is recommended; for gastrointestinal anthrax or anthrax meningitis, the recommended regimen is similar. A rational case can be made for passive immunization with anthrax antitoxin in addition to antibiotic therapy in severely ill patients with anthrax, but an appropriate antitoxin is not commercially available.

PREVENTION   Inhalation anthrax was essentially eliminated in England before 1940 through the development of methods to decontaminate wool and goat's hair and the improvement of working conditions for handlers of animal products.

Nonliving vaccines consisting of alum-precipitated or aluminum hydroxide–adsorbed extracellular components of unencapsulated *B. anthracis* are used in the United Kingdom and the United States for agricultural workers, veterinary personnel, and others at risk of exposure to anthrax. The major active component of these vaccines is PA. Live attenuated vaccines containing spores of *B. anthracis* are used in both developed and developing countries for the immunization of domestic herbivores; these preparations are also used for the immunization of humans in Russia but not in the United States. The probable basis for attenuation of the original Pasteur spore vaccine is partial loss of the plasmid that encodes anthrax toxin during prolonged incubation of *B. anthracis* cultures at 42°C. The basis for attenuation of the current Sterne spore vaccine is loss of the plasmid that encodes capsular polypeptide.

Improved anthrax vaccines for humans are needed because the current vaccines are impure and chemically complex, elicit only slow-onset protective immunity, provide incomplete protection, and cause significant adverse reactions. In addition to agricultural and industrial anthrax, the possible use of *B. anthracis* as an agent of biological warfare is stimulus to the development of an improved vaccine.

Current strategies for vaccine development include purification of candidate protective antigens, expression of protective antigens in recombinant microbial vaccines, and construction of improved live attenuated strains of *B. anthracis*. A mutant form of PA that lacks the protease-sensitive sequence and that cannot be processed to interact with EF or LF to mediate toxicity has been produced by genetic engineering as one candidate vaccine against anthrax.

Carcasses of animals that succumb to anthrax should be buried intact or cremated. Necropsies or butchering of infected animals should be avoided because sporulation of *B. anthracis* occurs only in the presence of oxygen.

PROGNOSIS   The mortality rate is 10 to 20 percent for untreated cutaneous anthrax but is very low with appropriate antibiotic therapy. In contrast, the mortality rate for inhalation anthrax approaches 100 percent, and therapy is usually unsuccessful. The mortality rate for treated gastrointestinal anthrax is approximately 50 percent. Meningitis as a complication of anthrax is usually fatal.

The opinions expressed herein are those of the author and do not necessarily represent the views of the Department of Defense or the Uniformed Services University of the Health Sciences.

REFERENCES

ABRAMOVA FA et al: Pathology of inhalational anthrax in 42 cases from the Sverdlovsk outbreak of 1979. Proc Natl Acad Sci USA 90:2291, 1993

AKSARAY N et al: Cutaneous anthrax. Trop Geogr Med 42:168, 1990

CENTERS FOR DISEASE CONTROL: Diphtheria, tetanus, and pertussis: Recommendations for vaccine use and other preventive measures: Recommendations of the Immunization Practices Advisory Committee (ACIP). Morb Mort Week Rep 40(No. RR-10):1, 1991

COHEN Y et al: *Corynebacterium pseudodiphtheriticum* pulmonary infection in AIDS patients. Lancet 340:114, 1992

COMMITTEE ON INFECTIOUS DISEASES: Diphtheria, in *Report of the Committee on Infectious Diseases*, 22d ed. Elk Grove Village, IL, American Academy of Pediatrics, 1991, p 91

COYLE MB et al: The molecular epidemiology of three biotypes of *Corynebacterium diphtheriae* in the Seattle outbreak from 1972–1982. J Infect Dis 159:670, 1989

COYLE MB, LIPSKY BA: Coryneform bacteria in infectious diseases: Clinical and laboratory aspects. Clin Microbiol Rev 3:227, 1990

FARIZO KM et al: Fatal respiratory disease due to *Corynebacterium diphtheriae*: Case report and review of guidelines for management, investigation, and control. Clin Infect Dis 16:59, 1993

HARNISH JP et al: Diphtheria among alcoholic urban adults. A decade of experience in Seattle. Ann Intern Med 111:71, 1989

HEDLUND KW: Anthrax toxin: History and recent advances and perspectives. J Toxicol Toxin Rev 11:41, 1992

HÖFLER W: Cutaneous diphtheria. Int J Dermatol 30:845, 1991

KAIN KC et al: *Arcanobacterium hemolyticum* infection: Confused with scarlet fever and diphtheria. J Emerg Med 9:33, 1991

LAFORCE FM: Bacillus anthracis (anthrax), in *Principles and Practice of Infectious Diseases*, 3d ed, GL Mandell et al (eds). New York, Churchill Livingstone, 1990, p 1593

MORRIS A, GUILD I: Endocarditis due to *Corynebacterium pseudodiphtheriticum*: Five case reports, review, and antibiotic susceptibilities of nine strains. Rev Infect Dis 13:887, 1991

RAPPUOLI R et al: Molecular epidemiology of the 1984–1986 outbreak of diphtheria in Sweden. N Engl J Med 318:12, 1988

ROZDZINSKI E et al: *Corynebacterium jeikeium* bacteremia at a tertiary care center. Infection 19:201, 1991

SORIANO F et al: Urinary tract infection caused by *Corynebacterium* group D2: Report of 82 cases and review. Rev Infect Dis 12:1019, 1990

TURNBULL PCB: Anthrax vaccines: Past, present and future. Vaccine 9:533, 1991

WILSON APR et al: Unusual nontoxigenic *Corynebacterium diphtheriae* in homosexual men. Lancet 339:998, 1992

105 INFECTIONS CAUSED BY *LISTERIA MONOCYTOGENES*

ANNE SCHUCHAT / CLAIRE V. BROOME

Listeria monocytogenes is a gram-positive rod which can be isolated from soil, vegetation, and many animal reservoirs. Human disease due to *L. monocytogenes* generally occurs in the setting of pregnancy or immunosuppression due to illness or medication. A substantial portion of human listeriosis occurs through food-borne transmission of *L. monocytogenes*. Unlike the majority of food-borne pathogens which primarily cause gastrointestinal illness, *L. monocytogenes* causes invasive syndromes such as meningitis, sepsis, chorioamnionitis, and stillbirth.

ETIOLOGY *Listeria* are aerobic or facultatively anaerobic non-sporulating bacilli that grow well at temperatures between 1 and 45°C and have a characteristic tumbling motility when cultured at 20 to 25°C. Characteristics which help distinguish *L. monocytogenes* from other *Listeria* species include formation of a narrow zone of beta hemolysis on sheep blood agar and production of acid from glucose, maltose, and rhamnose but not from xylose or mannitol. Determination of serotype of *L. monocytogenes* is based on somatic (O) and flagellar (H) antigens. Most cases of human disease are caused by serotypes 1/2a, 1/2b, and 4b. Molecular subtyping techniques, including multilocus enzyme electrophoresis, phage typing, and ribosomal DNA analysis, have improved the ability to discriminate among strains of *Listeria*, thus complementing efforts to link environmental or food isolates with clinical infections.

PATHOGENESIS *L. monocytogenes* is an intracellular pathogen with a predilection to cause illness in persons with deficient cell-mediated immunity. The organism is present in normal gastrointestinal flora in healthy individuals. Lack of gastric acidity and abnormal gastrointestinal function may increase the risk of invasive disease following exposure to the organism in the gastrointestinal tract. Invasion, intracellular multiplication, and cell-to-cell spread of the organism appear to be mediated through proteins such as internalin, the hemolysin listeriolysin O, and phospholipase C. Local immunosuppression at the maternal-fetal interface of the placenta may facilitate intrauterine infection following transient maternal bacteremia.

EPIDEMIOLOGY Long recognized as a veterinary pathogen, *L. monocytogenes* causes basilar meningitis ("circling disease") and stillbirth in sheep and cattle. The occurrence of listeriosis among humans has received increasing attention as a result of recognition of the role of contaminated foods in the pathogenesis of epidemic listeriosis and the increased reports of disease associated with the expanding immunosuppressed population.

Invasive listeriosis confirmed by culture of blood or cerebrospinal fluid occurs in approximately 7.4 per million population annually in the United States, or an estimated 1850 cases per year. Perinatal listeriosis complicates 16 of every 100,000 births. These are minimal estimates of the real disease burden, which includes milder or unrecognized illness. Recent multistate surveillance suggests that 23 percent of infections are fatal or result in stillbirth, although higher case-fatality rates have been observed during listeriosis epidemics and in earlier series. Although the majority of disease due to *L. monocytogenes* occurs sporadically, investigation of several listeriosis outbreaks during the 1980s demonstrated that common-source food-borne transmission caused human illness and that the incubation period for disease following consumption of contaminated food may be 2 to 6 weeks. The largest North American outbreak, in Los Angeles in 1985, involved over 100 cases and resulted in 48 deaths or stillbirths. Foods implicated in outbreaks include contaminated cole slaw, pasteurized milk, soft cheeses, paté, and pork tongue. Epidemiologic studies also have implicated consumption of undercooked chicken, uncooked hot dogs, soft cheeses, and food from store delicatessen counters as risk factors for sporadic listeriosis. *Listeria*

contamination of foods is relatively common. Among foods contaminated with the organism, those which are ready-to-eat, contaminated with serotype 4b, and contaminated at a relatively high level may be the most likely to cause illness. The long incubation period associated with listeriosis contributes to the difficulty of implicating specific foods as the cause of both common-source outbreaks and sporadic cases.

Although food-borne transmission appears to be the major cause of epidemic and sporadic disease, several clusters of late-onset neonatal infection suggest that nosocomial transmission of *L. monocytogenes* can occur. Contaminated multiuse materials and equipment have been suggested as causes for some nosocomial clusters. Listeriosis has been reported in veterinarians and others with close contact with infected animals.

CLINICAL PRESENTATION *Pregnancy-associated listeriosis* may occur during any stage of pregnancy, although the majority of infections are detected during the third trimester, possibly because of failure to obtain bacterial cultures in abortions and stillbirths occurring earlier in gestation. One-half to two-thirds of pregnant women with perinatal listeriosis experience a mild illness characterized by fever, myalgias, malaise, and backache, sometimes accompanied by diarrhea, abdominal pain, nausea, and/or vomiting during the bacteremic phase of illness. Blood cultures should be used for diagnosis, since isolation of the organism from rectal or vaginal culture is not diagnostic. Transplacental spread of the organism results in intrauterine infection, which can lead to chorioamnionitis, premature labor, intrauterine fetal demise, or early-onset infection (<7 days of age) of the newborn. Women with listeriosis diagnosed during pregnancy have a favorable clinical outcome following antibiotic therapy or delivery. Although often included in the differential diagnosis of recurrent abortion, infection with *L. monocytogenes* appears to cause fewer than 2 percent of stillbirths.

Neonatal listeriosis can be classified by the same categories used in group B streptococcal infection (see Chap. 103), with early-onset infection evident during the first week of life and late-onset disease occurring thereafter. Infants may be symptomatic at birth; most infants with early-onset infection are symptomatic by the second day of life. Aspiration of infected amniotic fluid contributes to pathogenesis. Early-onset disease may include sepsis, respiratory distress, skin lesions, and the syndrome *granulomatosis infantisepticum*, which is characterized by disseminated abscesses involving the liver, spleen, adrenal glands, lung, and other sites. Infants with late-onset neonatal disease (≥7 days of age) are more likely than those with early-onset disease to develop meningitis. While early-onset disease often occurs in association with obstetrical complications such as premature delivery and chorioamnionitis, late-onset disease typically affects infants born at term by uncomplicated deliveries. Infants may acquire the organism during passage through the birth canal, but with the exception of several clusters of late-onset neonatal infection linked to nosocomial transmission, the pathogenesis of late-onset disease is not well understood.

Listeriosis not associated with pregnancy usually occurs in persons with immunosuppressive conditions, although invasive disease also can occur in immunocompetent adults, particularly the elderly. Data from a multistate study of listeriosis revealed that the most common underlying conditions seen in nonpregnant adults with listeriosis were the chronic use of glucocorticoid medications and the presence of solid or hematologic malignancies, diabetes mellitus, renal disease, liver disease, or AIDS. Although the incidence of listeriosis in AIDS patients is much higher than the incidence in the general population, listeriosis is a relatively uncommon opportunistic infection in AIDS. Bacteremic and central nervous system (CNS) disease are the most common presentations of listeriosis in nonpregnant adults.

Sepsis Recent clinical series have shown that bacteremic infection without evident focus is the most common clinical manifestation of listeriosis, followed by CNS infection. Listerial sepsis cannot be distinguished clinically from bacteremia due to other organisms. Patients are usually febrile, often appear extremely ill, and may have prodromal symptoms including myalgia, nausea, vomiting, and diarrhea. Immunocompromised patients with listeriosis are less likely than other adults to present with CNS infection. Immunocompromised patients may be more likely to have blood cultured during febrile episodes, while in other adults transient bacteremia due to *L. monocytogenes* may go unrecognized.

Central nervous system infection The majority of CNS infections due to *L. monocytogenes* are meningitic. Meningitis due to *L. monocytogenes* is not distinguishable clinically from other types of bacterial meningitis, and presenting symptoms include fever, headache, and altered level of consciousness. Typically, examination of cerebrospinal fluid (CSF) reveals pleocytosis, increased protein, and normal glucose, although other patterns (including low CSF sugar) can occur. As is the case in other forms of bacterial meningitis, Gram's stain is often unrevealing; the diagnosis is made when *L. monocytogenes* is identified on culture. Despite its name, *L. monocytogenes* infection is rarely associated with monocytosis of either the CSF or blood. Other syndromes seen with CNS infection include encephalitis, cerebritis, and brainstem, spinal cord, or intracranial abscesses. Symptoms may include fever, ataxia, seizures, personality changes, and coma. Nuchal rigidity is rare. CSF cultures may be sterile, and blood cultures are usually diagnostic.

Endocarditis Like most forms of bacterial endocarditis, endocarditis due to *L. monocytogenes* typically occurs in patients with prosthetic or previously damaged valves. The organism has a predilection for the left side of the heart, and endocarditis due to *L. monocytogenes* is often associated with systemic embolization.

Focal infections Other focal infections that can occur following unrecognized bacteremia include endophthalmitis, peritonitis, osteomyelitis, visceral abscess, pleuropulmonary infection, and cholecystitis. Cutaneous lesions may occur without systemic involvement and have been reported in veterinarians and poultry workers.

Recurrent infection with *L. monocytogenes* has been reported but is rare. Many recurrences are due to the subtype responsible for the initial infection, suggesting that recurrences result either from insufficient treatment of a focus of primary infection or from repeated exposure to a persistently contaminated source.

DIAGNOSIS Listeriosis is diagnosed when the organism is cultured from usually sterile sites such as blood, CSF, or amniotic fluid. The organism will grow readily within 36 h on routine culture media, but there are morphologic similarities between *Listeria* and both diphtheroids and streptococci; biochemical tests are needed to identify the species. Serologic assays have not been useful in diagnosing listeriosis, because exposure to the organism may be common and infected individuals may not show elevated antibody titers following infection. Culture of the organism from nonsterile sites such as vaginal and rectal specimens is not useful for diagnosis because the organism may be carried in approximately 5 percent of healthy individuals.

Differential diagnosis of prematurity, spontaneous abortion, or stillbirth includes infectious diseases such as group B streptococcal infection, congenital syphilis, and toxoplasmosis; pathogens such as group B streptococci and *Escherichia coli* are more common than *L. monocytogenes* as causes of meningitis and sepsis in the newborn period. Because *L. monocytogenes* is not sensitive to cephalosporins, these agents should not be used as a single agent in empirical therapy of neonatal sepsis and meningitis. Listerial infection should always be considered in the differential diagnosis of meningitis in immunosuppressed persons, particularly in transplant recipients and others receiving glucocorticoid treatment, as well as in patients with hematologic malignancy or HIV infection. Among healthy adults, meningitis is much more likely to be caused by *Neisseria meningitidis*, *Streptococcus pneumoniae*, or viral pathogens than by *L. monocytogenes*.

TREATMENT The treatment of choice for listeriosis is intravenous therapy with either ampicillin or penicillin, often in combination with an aminoglycoside. Trimethoprim-sulfamethoxazole has been used successfully in patients with penicillin allergy, although clinical experience with this regimen is limited. *L. monocytogenes* is suscepti-

---

TABLE 105-1 Dietary recommendations for the prevention of food-borne listeriosis

Recommendations to all individuals
1 Thoroughly cook raw food from animal sources such as beef, pork, and poultry.
2 Wash raw vegetables thoroughly before eating.
3 Keep uncooked meats separate from vegetables and from cooked foods and ready-to-eat foods.
4 Avoid raw (unpasteurized) milk or foods made from raw milk.
5 Wash hands, knives, and cutting board after handling uncooked foods.

Additional recommendations to high-risk individuals*
1 Avoid soft cheeses such as Mexican-style, feta, Brie, Camembert, and blue-veined cheese. There is no need to avoid hard cheeses, cream cheese, cottage cheese, or yogurt.
2 Left-over foods or ready-to-eat foods such as hot dogs should be reheated until steaming hot before eating.
3 Although the risk of listeriosis associated with foods from delicatessen counters is relatively low and poorly characterized, pregnant women and immunosuppressed persons may choose to avoid these foods or to thoroughly reheat cold cuts before eating.

* Persons immunocompromised by illness or medications and pregnant women.

---

ble in vitro to penicillin G, ampicillin, erythromycin, trimethoprim-sulfamethoxazole, chloramphenicol, rifampin, tetracyclines, aminoglycosides, and imipenem. However, chloramphenicol and rifampin may antagonize the bactericidal effect of penicillins. Cephalosporins are not recommended.

Dosages and duration of therapy have not been subjected to controlled trials. For treatment of neonatal listeriosis and listeriosis in pregnancy, a 2-week course of either penicillin G (240,000 to 320,000 units per kilogram per day) or ampicillin (150 to 200 mg/kg per day) in six divided doses is recommended. Addition of an aminoglycoside (gentamicin, 6 mg/kg per day in four divided doses) should be considered for neonatal infection. Higher dosage may be appropriate for CNS disease (penicillin G, 320,000 to 480,000 units per kilogram per day, or ampicillin, 200 to 300 mg/kg per day, in six divided doses). Penicillin-allergic patients may be treated with trimethoprim-sulfamethoxazole, as 15/75 mg/kg per day, intravenously, in three equal doses every 8 h. Meningitis in a patient without immunosuppression may require 2 to 3 weeks of antibiotic therapy following defervescence. Bacteremia, endocarditis, and nonmeningitic listeriosis in immunosuppressed patients should be treated longer, probably 4 to 6 weeks.

PROGNOSIS Treatment of maternal bacteremia during pregnancy can prevent neonatal infection. Antibiotic therapy for the newborn can limit sequelae, although the widely disseminated disease characteristic of granulomatosis infantisepticum is frequently fatal regardless of treatment. Early-onset disease carries a higher mortality rate than late-onset infection, and immunocompromised hosts have a worse prognosis than do otherwise healthy adults with listeriosis.

PREVENTION *L. monocytogenes* is frequently isolated from foods; the U.S. Food and Drug Administration, U.S. Department of Agriculture, and manufacturers are actively pursuing further measures to reduce *L. monocytogenes* contamination of foods that have been subjected to listericidal processing. Prevention of listeriosis requires dietary counseling of persons at increased risk of disease (Table 105-1). There is no role for prophylaxis of contacts of patients with listeriosis. Clinicians are encouraged to report cases of listeriosis to local or state health departments to facilitate early recognition of listeriosis outbreaks and prevention of subsequent cases.

REFERENCES

NIEMAN RE, LORBER B: Listeriosis in adults: A changing pattern. Report of eight cases and review of the literature, 1968–1978. Rev Infect Dis 2:207, 1980

PINNER RW et al: Role of foods in sporadic listeriosis: II. Microbiologic and epidemiologic investigation. JAMA 267:2046, 1992

SCHLECH WF et al: Epidemic listeriosis—Evidence for transmission by food. N Engl J Med 308:203, 1983

SCHUCHAT A et al: Role of foods in sporadic listeriosis: I. Case-control study of dietary risk factors. JAMA 267:2041, 1992

——— et al: Epidemiology of human listeriosis. Clin Microbiol Rev 4:169, 1991

SEELIGER HPR: *Listeriosis*. Basel, Karger, 1961

106   TETANUS

ELIAS ABRUTYN

DEFINITION   Tetanus is a neurologic disorder, characterized by increased muscle tone and spasms, that is caused by tetanospasmin, a powerful protein toxin elaborated by *Clostridium tetani*. Tetanus occurs in several clinical forms, including generalized, neonatal, and localized disease.

MICROBIOLOGY   The organism is an anaerobic, motile gram-positive rod that forms an oval, colorless, terminal spore creating a shape that resembles a tennis racket or drumstick. It is found worldwide in soil, in the inanimate environment, in animal feces, and occasionally in human feces. Spores may survive for years in some environments and are resistant to various disinfectants and boiling for 20 min. Vegetative cells, however, are easily inactivated and are susceptible to several antibiotics (penicillin and others).

Tetanospasmin is formed in vegetative cells under plasmid control. It is a single-polypeptide chain. With autolysis, the single-chain toxin is released and cleaved to form a heterodimer consisting of a heavy chain (100,000 mol wt) and a light chain (50,000 mol wt) joined by a disulfide bond. The amino acid structures of the two most powerful toxins known, botulinum and tetanus toxin, are partially homologous.

EPIDEMIOLOGY   Tetanus occurs sporadically and almost always affects nonimmunized or partially immunized persons, or fully immunized individuals who fail to maintain adequate immunity with booster doses of vaccine. Although entirely preventable by immunization, worldwide the burden of disease is large. The disease is common where soil is cultivated, in rural areas, in warm climates, during summer months, and in males. In countries without a major immunization program, neonatal tetanus and tetanus in the young predominate; worldwide an estimated 800,000 neonates die each year. In the United States and other nations with successful immunization programs, neonatal tetanus rarely occurs, and the disease affects other age groups and those in groups inadequately reached by immunization such as nonwhites. The elderly, in particular, are prominently involved. Under 100 cases have been reported to the Centers for Disease Control annually: 94 percent of cases occurred in persons over 20 years of age and 68 percent in individuals over 50. The burden of illness, however, is greater because reporting is incomplete.

In the United States, most tetanus occurs after an acute injury, such as a puncture wound, laceration, or abrasion, and is often acquired indoors, during farming or gardening, or in other outdoor settings. The injury may be major but often is trivial, so medical attention is not sought. The disease may complicate chronic conditions such as skin ulcers, abscesses, and gangrene. Tetanus is also associated with burns, frostbite, ear infection, surgery, abortion, childbirth, and drug abuse, notably skin "popping." In some patients no portal of entry can be identified.

PATHOGENESIS   Contamination of wounds with spores is probably frequent. Germination and toxin production, however, only occur in wounds with low oxidation-reduction potential such as those containing devitalized tissue, foreign bodies, or active infection. *Clostridium tetani* does not itself evoke inflammation, and the portal of entry appears benign unless infection from other organisms is present.

Toxin released in the wound binds to peripheral alpha motor neuron terminals, enters the axon, and is transported to the nerve cell body in the brainstem and spinal cord by retrograde intraneuronal transport. Toxin then migrates across the synapse to presynaptic terminals, where it blocks release of the inhibitory neurotransmitters glycine and gamma-aminobutyric acid (GABA). With diminished inhibition, the resting firing rate of the alpha motor neuron increases, producing rigidity. With lessened activity of reflexes, which limits polysynaptic spread of impulses (a glycinergic activity), agonists and antagonists may be recruited rather than inhibited, thereby producing spasms. Loss of inhibition also may affect preganglionic sympathetic neurons in the lateral gray matter of the spinal cord and produce sympathetic hyperactivity and high circulating catecholamine levels. Tetanospasmin, like botulinum toxin, also may block neurotransmitter release at the neuromuscular junction and produce weakness or paralysis; recovery requires sprouting of new nerve terminals.

In local tetanus, only the nerves supplying the affected muscles are involved. Generalized tetanus occurs when toxin released in the wound enters the bloodstream and is spread to other nerve terminals; the blood-brain barrier blocks direct entry into the central nervous sytem. Assuming equal intraneuronal transport times for all nerves, short nerves are affected before long nerves; this fact explains the sequential involvement of nerves of the head, trunk, and extremities in generalized tetanus.

CLINICAL MANIFESTATIONS   Generalized tetanus, the most common form, is characterized by increased muscle tone and generalized spasms. The median onset after injury is 7 days; 15 percent of cases occur within 3 days and 10 percent after 14 days.

Typically, the patient first notices increased tone in the masseter muscles (trismus or lockjaw). Dysphagia or stiffness or pain in the neck, shoulder, and back muscles occurs concurrently or appears soon thereafter. Then other muscles are involved, producing a rigid abdomen and stiff proximal limb muscles; the hands and feet are relatively spared. Sustained contraction of the facial muscles produces a grimace or sneer (risus sardonicus), and contraction of the back muscles produces an arched back (opisthotonos). Some patients develop paroxysmal, violent, painful, generalized muscle spasms that may cause cyanosis and threaten ventilation. They occur repetitively and may be spontaneous or provoked by even the slightest stimulation. A constant threat during generalized spasms is reduced ventilation or apnea or laryngospasm. The severity of illness may be mild (muscle rigidity and few or no spasms), moderate (trismus, dysphagia, rigidity, and spasms), or severe (frequent explosive paroxysms). The patient may be febrile, although many have no fever; mentation is unimpaired. Deep tendon reflexes may be increased. Dysphagia or ileus may preclude oral feeding.

Autonomic dysfunction commonly complicates severe cases and is characterized by labile or sustained hypertension, tachycardia, arrhythmias, hyperpyrexia, profuse sweating, peripheral vasoconstriction, and increased plasma and urinary catecholamine levels. Periods of bradycardia and hypotension also may occur and are usually easily reversed by physical stimulation such as suctioning; however, pacemaker insertion is occasionally required. Sudden cardiac arrest occurs, but the basis for it is unknown.

Complications include pneumonia, fractures, muscle rupture, deep vein thrombophlebitis, pulmonary emboli, decubitus ulcer, and rhabdomyolysis.

Neonatal tetanus usually occurs as generalized tetanus and untreated is usually fatal. It develops in children born to inadequately immunized mothers, frequently after unsterile treatment of the umbilical cord stump. The onset generally occurs during the first 2 weeks of life. Poor feeding, rigidity, and spasms occur.

Local tetanus is an uncommon form in which manifestations are restricted to muscles near the wound. The prognosis is excellent.

Cephalic tetanus, a rare form of local tetanus, follows head injury or ear infection. Trismus and dysfunction of one or more cranial nerves, often the seventh nerve, are found. The incubation period is a few days and the mortality is high.

DIAGNOSIS   The diagnosis of tetanus is made entirely on the basis of clinical findings. Tetanus is unlikely if a reliable history indicates completion of a primary vaccination series and receipt of appropriate booster doses. Wound cultures should be done. However, *C. tetani* can be isolated from wounds of patients without tetanus, and frequently the organism cannot be recovered from the wounds of those with tetanus. The leukocyte count may be elevated. The cerebrospinal fluid examination is normal. Electromyograms may show continuous discharge of motor units and shortening or absence of the silent interval normally seen after an action potential. Nonspecific changes may be seen on the electrocardiogram. Muscle enzyme levels may be raised. Serum antitoxin levels of 0.01 units/mL or higher are considered protective and would make tetanus unlikely.

The differential diagnosis includes local conditions also producing trismus such as alveolar abscess, strychnine poisoning, dystonic drug reactions (e.g., phenothiazines and metoclopramide), and hypocalcemic tetany. Other conditions possibly confused with tetanus include meningitis/encephalitis, rabies, and an acute intraabdominal process (because of the rigid abdomen). The marked increased tone in central muscles (face, neck, chest, back, and abdomen) with superimposed generalized spasms and relative sparing of the hands and feet strongly suggests tetanus.

TREATMENT   General measures   The goals of therapy are to eliminate the source of toxin, neutralize unbound toxin, prevent muscle spasms, and provide support, especially respiratory support, until recovery. Patients should be admitted to a quiet room in an intensive care unit where observation and cardiopulmonary monitoring can be maintained continuously, but stimulation can be minimized. Protection of the airway is vital. Wounds should be explored, carefully cleansed, and thoroughly debrided.

Antibiotic therapy   Although it is of questionable benefit, parenteral penicillin (10 to 12 million units daily for 10 days) is administered to eradicate vegetative cells, the source of the toxin. Clindamycin, erythromycin, or metronidazol may be given as a substitute to patients with penicillin allergy. Specific therapy should be given for active infection caused by other organisms.

Antitoxin   Given to neutralize circulating toxin and unbound toxin in the wound, antitoxin effectively lowers mortality; toxin already bound to neural tissue is unaffected. Tetanus immune globulin (human) (TIG) is the preparation of choice and should be given promptly. The dose is 3000 to 6000 units intramuscularly, usually in divided doses, because the volume is large. The optimal dose is not known, however, and results from one study indicated that 500 units was as effective as higher doses. It may be best to administer antitoxin before manipulating the wound; the value of injecting a dose proximal to the wound or infiltrating the wound is unclear. Additional doses are unnecessary because the half-life of the antitoxin is long. Antibody does not penetrate the blood-brain barrier. Intrathecal administration should be considered experimental. Equine tetanus antitoxin (TAT) is also available. It is cheaper, but the half-life is shorter and hypersensitivity and serum sickness are common; doses up to 100,000 units are given, part intramuscularly and part intravenously, but 10,000 units may suffice.

Control of muscle spasms   Many agents, alone and in combination, have been used to treat the muscle spasms, which are painful and can threaten ventilation by causing laryngospasm or sustained contraction of ventilatory muscles. Ideal therapy would abolish spasmodic activity without causing oversedation and hypoventilation. Diazepam, a benzodiazepine and GABA agonist, is in wide use. The dose is titrated, and large doses (250 mg/d or more) may be required. Lorazepam, with a longer duration of action, and midazolam, whose short half-life necessitates administration by continuous intravenous infusions, are other options. Barbiturates and chlorpromazine are also used. Neuromuscular blockade (with vecuronium or equivalent agent) with mechanical ventilation is highly effective for treating severe spasms unresponsive to medication or spasms that threaten ventilation. Dantrolene and baclofen are being investigated as treatment to shorten the period of therapeutic paralysis.

Respiratory care   Intubation or tracheostomy, with or without mechanical ventilation, may be required for hypoventilation from oversedation or laryngospasm or to avert aspiration in patients with trismus, disordered swallowing, or dysphagia. The need should be anticipated, and the procedure performed electively and early.

Autonomic dysfunction   The optimal therapy for sympathetic overactivity has not been defined. Considerations include labetalol (an alpha- and beta-adrenergic blocking agent that is recommended by some experts, but sudden death has been reported), esmolol by continuous infusion (a beta blocker whose short half-life may be advantageous in the event of hypotension or bradycardia), clonidine (a centrally acting antiadrenergic drug), and morphine sulfate. Parenteral magnesium sulfate and continuous spinal anesthesia have been used but may be more difficult to administer and monitor. The relative efficacy of these modalities is yet to be determined.

Vaccine   Active immunization should be initiated because immunity is not induced by the small amount of toxin that produces disease.

Additional measures   These include hydration to control insensible and other fluid losses, which may be high; increased nutritional requirements, which can be met by enteral or parenteral means; physiotherapy to prevent contractures; and heparin to prevent pulmonary emboli. Bowel, bladder, and renal function must be monitored. Gastrointestinal bleeding and decubitus ulcers must be prevented, and intercurrent infection should be treated.

PREVENTION   Active immunization   All partially immunized and unimmunized adults should receive vaccine, as should those recovering from tetanus. The primary series for adults consists of three doses: the first and second doses are given 4 to 8 weeks apart, and the third dose is given 6 to 12 months after the second. A booster dose is required every 10 years and may be given at middecade ages, 35, 45, and so on. Combined tetanus and diphtheria toxoid adsorbed (for adult use) (Td) rather than single-antigen tetanus toxoid is preferred for persons over 7 years of age.

Wound management   Proper wound management requires consideration of the need for (1) passive immunization with TIG and (2) active immunization with vaccine, preferably Td in those over age 7. For clean, minor wounds, Td is administered to persons who have (1) unknown tetanus immunization histories, (2) received less than three doses of adsorbed tetanus toxoid, (3) received three or more doses of adsorbed vaccine but more than 10 years have elapsed since the last dose, and (4) received three doses of *fluid* (nonadsorbed) vaccine. The recommendations for contaminated or severe wounds are identical, except that vaccine should be given to those who received three or more doses of adsorbed tetanus toxoid if more than 5 years have elapsed since the last dose. TIG is not recommended for clean, minor wounds but is given for all other wounds if the vaccination history indicates unknown or partial immunization. The dose of TIG for passive immunization of wounds of average severity is 250 units intramuscularly, which produces a protective antibody level in the serum for at least 4 to 6 weeks; the dose of equine antitoxin is 3000 to 6000 units. Vaccine and tetanus antitoxin should be administered at separate sites in separate syringes.

Neonatal tetanus   Preventive efforts include maternal vaccination, even during pregnancy, measures to increase the number of in-hospital births, and training for nonmedical birth attendants.

PROGNOSIS   The application of methods to support respiration has markedly improved the prognosis in tetanus; mortality rates as low as 10 percent have been reported from units accustomed to handling such cases. In the United States, the overall mortality for the years 1987 to 1988 was 2 percent. The outcome is poor in neonatal tetanus and the elderly and in those with a short incubation period, a short interval from the onset of symptoms to admission, or a short period from onset of symptoms to the first spasm (period of onset).

The course of tetanus extends over 4 to 6 weeks, and patients may require ventilatory support for 3 weeks during this period. Increased tone and minor spasms can last for months, but recovery is usually complete.

REFERENCES

ABRUTYN E, BERLIN JA: Intrathecal therapy of tetanus: A meta-analysis. JAMA 266:2262, 1991

BLECK TP: Tetanus, in *Infections of the Central Nervous System*, WM Scheld et al (eds). New York, Raven, 1991

CENTERS FOR DISEASE CONTROL: Diphtheria, tetanus, and pertussis: Recommendations for vaccine use and other preventive measures. Recommendations of the Immunization Practices Advisory Committee. Morb Mort Week Rep 40(RR-10):1, 1991

———: Tetanus—United States, 1987 and 1988. Morb Mort Week Rep 39:37, 1990

KING WW, CAVE DR: Use of esmolol to control autonomic instability of tetanus. Am J Med 91:425, 1991

ROOS KL: Tetanus. Semin Neurol 11:206, 1991

SUTTON DN et al: Management of autonomic dysfunction in severe tetanus: The use of magnesium sulphate and clonidine. Intensive Care Med 16:75, 1990

TRAVERSON HP et al: A reassessment of risk factors for neonatal tetanus. Bull WHO 69:573, 1991

WRIGHT KD et al: Autonomic nervous system dysfunction in severe tetanus: Current perspectives. Crit Care Med 17:371, 1989

WESLEY AG, PATHER M: Tetanus in children: An 11-year review. Ann Trop Pediatr 7:32, 1987

107 BOTULISM

ELIAS ABRUTYN

DEFINITION Botulism is a paralytic disease that begins with cranial nerve involvement and progresses caudally to involve the extremities. It is caused by potent protein neurotoxins elaborated by *Clostridium botulinum*. Cases may be classified as (1) *food-borne botulism*, from ingestion of preformed toxin in food contaminated with *C. botulinum*, (2) *wound botulism*, from toxin produced in wounds contaminated with the organism, (3) *infant botulism*, from ingestion of spores and production of toxin in the intestine of infants, (4) *adult infant botulism*, for older children and adults whose mechanism for disease resembles that found in infant botulism, or (5) *indeterminate*.

ETIOLOGY *C. botulinum*, a heterogeneous group of anaerobic gram-positive organisms that form subterminal spores, is found in soil and marine environments throughout the world and elaborates the most potent bacterial toxin known. Types A through G have been distinguished by the antigenic specificities of their toxins. Rare strains of other clostridial species—*C. butyricum* and *C. baratii*— also have been found to produce toxin. Types of *C. botulinum* with proteolytic activity can digest food and produce a spoiled appearance; nonproteolytic types leave the appearance of food unchanged.

Eight distinct toxin types (A, B, C_1, C_2, D, E, F, and G) have been described. All are neurotoxins, except for C_2, which is a cytotoxin of unknown significance that has vascular permeability and lethal, but not paralytic, activities. Botulinum neurotoxin, whether ingested or produced in the intestine or a wound, enters the vascular system and is transported to peripheral cholinergic nerve terminals, including neuromuscular junctions, postganglionic parasympathetic nerve endings, and peripheral ganglia. The central nervous system is not involved. Active neurotoxin (150,000 Da) is composed of a heavy chain (100,000 Da) and a light chain (50,000 Da). The heavy chain attaches to a receptor and enables translocation of the light chain into the nerve cell. Once intracellular, the light chain irreversibly blocks release of the neurotransmitter acetylcholine by an undefined mechanism(s) that may involve depression of calcium-mediated release reactions. Cure follows sprouting of new nerve terminals. The toxin resists degradation by acid and proteolytic enzymes but is inactivated by heat at 100°C for 10 min, as during routine home cooking. Spores, in contrast, are highly heat resistant, requiring exposure to 120°C for inactivation, as in steam sterilizers or pressure cookers.

Toxin types A, B, E, and rarely F cause human disease; type G has been associated with sudden death in a few patients in Switzerland; and types C and D cause animal disease.

EPIDEMIOLOGY Human botulism occurs worldwide. In the United States, the geographic distribution of cases by toxin type parallels the distribution of organism types found in the environment. Type A predominates west of the Rocky Mountains; type B is generally distributed but is more common in the East; and type E is found in the Pacific Northwest, Alaska, and the Great Lakes area. In the United States, food-borne botulism has been associated primarily with home-canned food, particularly vegetables, fruit, and condiments, and less commonly with meat and fish. Type E outbreaks are frequently associated with fish products. Commercial products occasionally cause outbreaks, but some of these have resulted from improper handling after purchase. Outbreaks in restaurants, schools, and private homes have been traced to uncommon sources (commercial pot pies, beef stew, turkey loaf, sauteed onions, baked potatoes, and chopped garlic in oil). Food-borne botulism can occur when (1) a food to be preserved is contaminated with spores, (2) preservation does not inactivate the spores but kills other putrefactive bacteria that might inhibit growth of *C. botulinum* and also provides anaerobic conditions at a pH and temperature that allow germination and toxin production, and (3) food is not heated to a temperature that destroys toxin before being eaten.

CLINICAL MANIFESTATIONS **Food-borne botulism** Following ingestion of food containing toxin, illness varies from a mild one for which no medical advice is sought to very severe disease which may result in death in 24 h. The incubation period is usually 18 to 36 h but depending on toxin dose ranges from a few hours to several days. A symmetric descending paralysis is characteristic and can lead to respiratory failure and death. Cranial nerve involvement, which almost always marks the onset of symptoms, usually produces diplopia, dysarthria, and/or dysphagia; weakness progresses, often rapidly, from the head to involve the neck, arms, thorax, and legs. Nausea, vomiting, and abdominal pain may occur before or after onset of paralysis. Dizziness, blurred vision, dry mouth, and very dry, occasionally sore throat are common. Occasionally, the weakness is asymmetric. Patients are generally alert and oriented, but they may be drowsy, agitated, and anxious. Typically, fever is absent. Ptosis is frequent; the pupillary reflexes may be depressed, and fixed or dilated pupils are seen in half the patients. The gag reflex may be suppressed, and deep tendon reflexes may be normal or decreased. Paralytic ileus, severe constipation, and urinary retention are common.

Wound botulism When wounds are contaminated with *C. botulinum* spores, the spores may germinate to vegetative organisms that produce toxin. This rare condition resembles food-borne illness except that the incubation period is longer, averaging about 10 days, and gastrointestinal symptoms are absent. Wound botulism has been noted after traumatic wounds contaminated with soil, in chronic drug abusers, and after cesarean delivery. The illness has occurred even when antibiotics were given to prevent wound infection. When present, fever is probably from concurrent infection with other bacteria. The wound may appear benign.

Infant botulism In infant botulism, the most common form of disease, toxin is produced in and absorbed from the intestine following germination of ingested spores. The severity ranges from mild illness with failure to thrive to fulminant, severe paralysis with respiratory failure and may be one cause of sudden infant death, but this is controversial. Ingestion of contaminated honey has been defined as one source of spores, leading to the recommendation that honey not be fed to children less than 12 months of age. Most cases cannot be attributed to a particular food source. The factors permitting intestinal colonization with *C. botulinum* are not fully defined, but cases usually occur in infants under 6 months of age; susceptibility may decrease as normal intestinal flora develop.

Adult infant botulism Also called *adult enteric infectious botulism* or *adult infectious botulism of unknown source*, this disorder resembles infant botulism in that toxin is produced in the intestine of persons colonized with the organism. Toxin and organisms may be found in the stool over prolonged periods, and spores, but not toxin, may be found in the suspect food. Gastrointestinal disease or surgery may predispose to illness. Previously, such cases would have been classified as *indeterminate*.

DIAGNOSIS Botulism must be considered in afebrile, mentally intact patients who have a symmetric descending paralysis without sensory findings. Conditions often confused with botulism include myasthenia gravis, which may be excluded by electromyography and appropriate antibody studies, and the Guillain-Barré syndrome, which is characterized by ascending paralysis, sensory abnormalities, and elevation in cerebrospinal fluid protein. The Miller-Fisher variant of Guillain-Barré—a descending paralysis—can be difficult to differentiate. Other conditions that may mimic botulism include poliomyelitis, tick paralysis, acute abdomen, pharyngitis, cerebrovascular accidents, and intoxications from mushrooms, medications, or chemicals.

The demonstration of toxin in serum by bioassay in mice is definitive, but the test may be negative, particularly in wound and infant botulism. It is only performed by specific laboratories, which can be identified by contacting regional public health authorities. The demonstration of toxin or the organism in vomitus, gastric fluid, or stool is strongly suggestive, because intestinal carriage is rare. Isolation of the organism from food without toxin is insufficient for diagnosis. Wound cultures showing the organism are suggestive. The edrophonium chloride (Tensilon) test for myasthenia gravis may be falsely positive in botulism but is usually less dramatic. Nerve conduction velocity is normal, but on routine electromyography, action potentials are decreased with a supramaximal stimulus and facilitation is found after repetitive stimulation at high frequency. Single-fiber electromyography may be helpful. The white blood cell count and sedimentation rate are normal.

TREATMENT Patients should be hospitalized and monitored closely both clinically and by spirometry, pulse oximetry, and measurement of arterial blood gases for incipient respiratory failure. Intubation and mechanical ventilation should be strongly considered when the vital capacity is less than 30 percent of predicted, especially when paralysis is progressing rapidly and hypoxemia with absolute or relative hypercarbia is present (see Chap. 231). Serial measurement of the maximal static inspiratory pressure may be useful in predicting respiratory failure.

In food-borne illness, trivalent (types A, B, and E) equine antitoxin should be administered as soon as possible after obtaining specimens for laboratory analysis. Laboratory confirmation, which may take days, is unnecessary before initiating treatment. After testing for hypersensitivity to horse serum, two vials are given, either both intravenously or one intravenously and one intramuscularly; the dose may be repeated in 2 to 4 h. Anaphylaxis and serum sickness are risks inherent in use of the equine product, and in allergic patients desensitization may be necessary. If there is no ileus, cathartics and enemas may be given to purge the gut of toxin; emetics or gastric lavage is used also if the time since ingestion is brief, e.g., only a few hours. Antibiotics to eliminate an intestinal source for possible continued toxin production and guanidine hydrochloride and other drugs used to reverse paralysis are of unproven value. In the United States, antitoxin and help in clinical management and laboratory confirmation are available at *any* time by calling the state health department or the Centers for Disease Control.

Treatment of infant botulism requires supportive care. Neither equine antitoxin nor antibiotics have been shown to be beneficial, and the value of human botulism immune globulin, an experimental preparation, is under evaluation. In wound botulism, equine antitoxin is administered. The wound should be thoroughly explored and debrided, and an antibiotic such as penicillin should be given to eradicate *C. botulinum* from the wound, although the benefit of this therapy is unproven; results of wound cultures should guide the use of other antibiotics.

PROGNOSIS Type A disease is generally more severe than type B, and mortality is higher above age 60. With improved respiratory and intensive care, the case-fatality rate in food-borne illness has fallen to about 7.5 percent and is low in infant botulism as well. Artificial respiratory support may be required for months in severe cases. Some patients experience residual weakness and autonomic dysfunction for as long as a year after disease onset.

BOTULINUM TOXIN THERAPY Botulinum toxin is being used as therapy for strabismus, blepharospasm, and other dystonias and appears safe and effective.

REFERENCES

ELSTON HR et al: Arm abscesses caused by *Clostridium botulinum*. J Clin Microbiol 29:2678, 1991

HAMBLETON P: *Clostridium botulinium* toxins: A general review of involvement in disease, structure, mode of action and preparation for clinical use. J Neurol 239:16, 1992

HATHEWAY CL: Toxigenic clostridia. Clin Microbiol Rev 3:66, 1990

JANKOVIC J, BRIN MF: Therapeutic uses of botulinum toxin. N Engl J Med 324:1186, 1991

MCCARTHY JD et al: Fever, dyspnea, and slurred speech following lower extremity trauma. Rev Infect Dis 13:172, 1991

MCCROSKEY LM, HATHEWAY CL: The large intestine as the site of *Clostridium botulinum* colonization in human infant botulism. J Clin Microbiol 26:1052, 1988

MORSE DL et al: Garlic-in-oil associated botulism: Episode leads to product modification. Am J Public Health 80:1372, 1990

SCHREINER MS et al: Infant botulism: A review of 12 years' experience at the Children's Hospital of Philadelphia. Pediatrics 87:159, 1991

SCHWARZ PJ, ARNON SS: Botulism immune globulin for infant botulism arrives—one year and a Gulf War later. West J Med 156:197, 1991

SMITH LDS, SUGIYAMA H: *Botulism: The Organism, Its Toxins, the Disease*, 2d ed. Springfield, Ill., Thomas, 1988

WILCOX PG et al: Recovery of the ventilatory and upper airway muscles and exercise performance after type A botulism. Chest 98:620, 1990

108 GAS GANGRENE AND OTHER CLOSTRIDIAL INFECTIONS

DENNIS L. KASPER / DORI F. ZALEZNIK

DEFINITION Bacteria of the genus *Clostridium* are gram-positive, spore-forming, obligate anaerobes that are ubiquitous in nature. There are over 60 recognized species of clostridia, many of which generally are considered saprophytic. Some of these species are pathogenic for humans and animals, particularly under conditions of lowered oxidation-reduction potential. Infections associated with these organisms range from localized wound contamination to overwhelming systemic disease. The four major disease categories for which clostridia are responsible include intestinal disorders, deep tissue suppurative infections, skin and soft tissue infections, and bacteremias (see Table 108-1). Toxins play a major role in some of these syndromes.

ETIOLOGY In humans, clostridia normally reside in the gastrointestinal tract and in the female genital tract, although they occasionally can be isolated from the skin or the mouth. As with other pathogenic anaerobic bacteria, clostridia are quite aerotolerant. Of the known species of the genus *Clostridium*, at least 30 have been isolated from human infections. Clostridia characteristically produce abundant gas

---

TABLE 108-1　Classification of diseases caused by other clostridia

Intestinal syndromes
- A　Food poisoning
- B　Enteritis necroticans
- C　Antibiotic-associated colitis

Suppurative deep tissue infections
- A　Mixed bacterial infections
- B　Only microorganism isolated

Skin and soft tissue infections
- A　Simple contamination
- B　Local infection without systemic signs
- C　Spreading cellulitis and fasciitis
- D　Myonecrosis

Bacteremia
- A　Transient bacteremia
- B　Sepsis

in artificial media and form subterminal endospores. *C. perfringens*, one of the most important of the species, is encapsulated, nonmotile, and rarely sporulates in artificial media; the spores usually can be destroyed by boiling. *C. tetani* and *C. botulinum* are discussed in Chaps. 106 and 107, respectively.

Clostridia are present in the normal colonic flora in concentrations of 10^9 to 10^{10} per gram. Of the 30 or more species that normally colonize humans, *C. ramosum* is the most common, followed by *C. perfringens*. These organisms are universally present in soil in concentrations of up to 10^4 per gram. Clostridia are gram-positive organisms, but in clinical specimens or stationary phase cultures, many species may appear to be gram-negative. Therefore, Gram's stains of cultures or clinical material should be interpreted with great care.

C. perfringens is the most common of the clostridial species isolated from tissue infections and bacteremias, followed in frequency by *C. novyi* and *C. septicum*. In the category of enteric infections, *C. difficile* is an important cause of antibiotic-associated colitis, and *C. perfringens* is associated with food poisoning and enteritis necroticans.

PATHOGENESIS Despite the isolation of clostridial species in many severe, traumatic wounds, the incidence of severe infections due to these organisms is low. Essential to the development of severe disease appears to be the presence of tissue necrosis and a low oxidation-reduction potential. *C. perfringens* requires about 14 amino acids and 6 or 7 additional growth factors for optimal growth. These nutrients are not found in appreciable concentrations in normal body fluids but are present in necrotic tissue. When *C. perfringens* grows in necrotic tissue, a zone of tissue damage due to the toxins elaborated by the organism allows for progressive growth. In contrast, when only a few bacteria leak into the bloodstream from a small defect in the intestinal wall, the organisms do not have the opportunity to multiply rapidly because blood as medium for growth is relatively deficient in certain amino acids and growth factors. Therefore, in a patient without tissue necrosis, bacteremia is usually benign.

C. perfringens possesses 17 possible virulence factors, including 12 active tissue toxins and enterotoxins. *C. perfringens* has been divided into five types (A through E) on the basis of four major toxins: alpha, beta, epsilon, and iota. The alpha toxin is a phospholipase C (lecithinase) that splits lecithin into phosphorylcholine and diglyceride. This alpha toxin has been associated with gas gangrene and is known to be hemolytic, destroy platelets and polymorphonuclear leukocytes, and cause widespread capillary damage. When injected intravenously, it causes massive intravascular hemolysis and damages liver mitochondria. Alpha toxin may be important in the initiation of muscle infections that may progress to gas gangrene. Experimentally, the higher the concentration of alpha toxin present in the culture fluid, the smaller the infecting dose of *C. perfringens* required to produce infection. The protective effect of antiserum is directly proportional to its content of alpha antitoxin. Beta, epsilon, and iota toxins are also known to increase capillary permeability.

C. difficile produces two major toxins, designated A and B. Toxin B is a cytotoxin and is the toxin measured in the sensitive tissue culture assay system employed in many clinical laboratories as the gold standard for diagnosing antibiotic-associated diarrhea. Toxin A is an enterotoxin which is believed to play an important role in causing diarrhea but is not reliably measured in assays currently in widespread use. Diarrheal disease due to *C. difficile* is toxin-mediated. Teaching about pathogenesis of this disease has centered on overgrowth of *C. difficile* when antibiotics suppress normal bowel flora. The mechanism is probably more complex, since many of the antibiotics that cause this disease are active against *C. difficile* as well as other bowel flora, and many patients who become colonized with *C. difficile* do not develop diarrhea. Critical features in the pathogenesis of this disease include mechanisms of toxin production and the interaction of *C. difficile* with other bowel flora. Some antibiotics may actually trigger toxin production by the organism. In turn, other bowel flora may

suppress or inhibit toxin production. *C. sordellii*, for example, neutralizes cytotoxin B in vitro. In addition, when antibiotics eliminate more sensitive bowel flora, more resistant organisms may produce enzymes such as β-lactamases that can inactivate antibiotics and thereby facilitate growth of *C. difficile*.

CLINICAL MANIFESTATIONS **Intestinal disorders** FOOD POISONING *C. perfringens* is the second or third most common cause of food poisoning in the United States (see Chap. 87). Outbreaks generally have resulted from problems in the cooling and storage of foods cooked in bulk. The food sources primarily involved are meat, meat products, and poultry. Generally, the implicated meats have been cooked, allowed to cool, and then recooked the following day, often in a stew or hash. Strains of *C. perfringens* that contaminate meat manage to survive initial cooking. During reheating, the organisms sporulate and germinate. The disease is associated with an attack rate often as high as 70 percent. Symptoms of food poisoning from type A strains develop 8 to 24 h after ingestion of foods heavily contaminated with the organism. The primary symptoms include epigastric pain, nausea, and watery diarrhea lasting 12 to 24 h. Fever and vomiting are uncommon. Symptoms usually last less than 24 h. Diarrhea appears to be caused by a heat-labile protein enterotoxin. The enterotoxin inhibits glucose transport, damages the intestinal epithelium, and causes protein loss into the intestinal lumen.

ENTERITIS NECROTICANS Enteritis necroticans (*pigbel*), caused by type C strains of *C. perfringens*, has been the cause of necrotizing enteritis and death, occurring after a feast, in children and adults in New Guinea. A similar disease, *darmbrand*, was epidemic in Germany after World War II and also was reported from an evacuation site on the Thai-Kampuchean border. Clinical features include acute abdominal pain, bloody diarrhea, vomiting, shock, and peritonitis; death occurs in 40 percent of patients. Pathologically, there is an acute ulcerative process of the bowel restricted to the small intestine. The mucosa is lifted off the submucosa, forming large denuded areas. Pseudomembranes composed of sloughed epithelium are common, and gas may dissect into the submucosa. The source of the organisms may be the patient's own intestinal flora, because cultures of ingested pork have failed to yield the organism. Antitoxin against the beta toxin of *C. perfringens* has been of considerable benefit in changing the course of established disease, and in a large-scale trial, children immunized with *C. perfringens* beta toxoid were protected.

ANTIBIOTIC-ASSOCIATED COLITIS Strains of *C. difficile* that produce toxins detectable in the stool have been identified as the major cause of colitis in patients with antibiotic-associated diarrhea. In order to diagnose this type of colitis, there should be no other identifiable cause of diarrhea and the onset of symptoms must occur either during antimicrobial administration or within 4 weeks after the implicated agent has been discontinued. Essentially any antibiotic can cause this syndrome, and even metronidazole and vancomycin, which treat the disease, have been implicated as etiologic agents in some cases. On a per-use basis, clindamycin, which was the first antibiotic described to cause this entity, is the most commonly implicated antibiotic. But since other antibiotics are prescribed more often than clindamycin in the United States, currently cephalosporins are the antibiotics which most commonly cause *C. difficile* enterocolitis, followed by penicillins.

Antimicrobial-associated diarrhea can be divided into four categories based on the appearance of the colon: (1) normal colonic mucosa, (2) mild erythema with some edema, (3) granular, friable, or hemorrhagic mucosa, and (4) pseudomembrane formation. Most patients with antibiotic-associated diarrhea have a normal, minimally erythematous colonic mucosa with some edema. Occasionally, colitis is more severe and is characterized by granular, friable, or hemorrhagic mucosa. Stool examination in these patients may reveal large numbers of red blood cells and some leukocytes. Biopsy shows subepithelial edema with round cell infiltration of the lamina propria and focal extravasation of erythrocytes. *C. difficile* cytotoxin B has been found in 15 to 46 percent of stools from patients in these first three categories, suggesting that either toxin A or other factors exist in the pathogenesis of antibiotic-associated diarrhea. The most characteristic form of antibiotic-associated colitis caused by *C. difficile* is pseudomembranous colitis (PMC). More than 95 percent of patients with documented PMC have positive stool toxin assays. Close inspection of pseudomembranes reveals exudative, punctate, raised plaques with skip areas or edematous hyperemic mucosa. These plaques can enlarge and coalesce over large segments of intestine in the later stages of disease. The clinical spectrum of antibiotic-associated PMC is diverse. Diarrhea is the common feature and is usually watery, voluminous, and without gross blood or mucus. Most patients have abdominal cramps and tenderness, fever, and leukocytosis. However, the symptoms may vary considerably. At one end of the spectrum are patients with annoying diarrhea but no systemic signs or symptoms, while at the other end there is severe systemic toxicity, fever to 40 or 40.6°C (104 or 105°F), and peripheral white blood cell counts of up to 50,000 per microliter. Fecal examination frequently reveals leukocytes. Without specific therapy, the course is highly variable. Some patients have prompt resolution of symptoms with discontinuation of the drug, while others have protracted diarrhea with large stool volumes for up to 8 weeks, with resultant hypoalbuminemia and electrolyte imbalance. Severely ill patients with toxic megacolon and colonic perforation have been reported. In those who are severely ill, mortality rates may be as high as 30 percent, while most patients with minimal symptoms have resolution of disease with discontinuation of antibiotics alone. In the majority of patients, symptoms begin 4 to 10 days after antibiotic therapy is initiated. However, about 25 percent of patients do not have symptoms until the implicated antimicrobial has been discontinued, in some cases as long as 4 weeks afterward. Some cases have been reported within hours after initiation of antibiotic therapy or after a single dose of antibiotic administered for surgical prophylaxis.

Diagnostic evaluation of patients with PMC should include examination of the stool for the presence of *C. difficile* cytotoxin. Although several assays are available, the tissue culture assay is the most practical and sensitive. The assay is performed by incubating stool filtrates with tissue culture cells and monitoring for a cytopathic effect which can be neutralized by antitoxin to either *C. sordellii* (which is cross-reactive with *C. difficile* but does not cause PMC) or *C. difficile*. Endoscopy, although useful in establishing the presence of PMC, does not establish the etiology and should be reserved for more serious disease manifestations to exclude alternative diagnoses. Isolation of *C. difficile* from stool cultures is difficult, and *C. difficile* may be present as part of the "normal" flora in asymptomatic patients, particularly infants.

Suppurative deep tissue infection   Clostridia are recovered frequently from various suppurative conditions in conjunction with other anaerobic and aerobic bacteria but also can be the only organisms isolated. These conditions exist with severe local inflammation but usually without systemic signs induced by clostridial toxins. These infections include intraabdominal sepsis, empyema, pelvic abscess, subcutaneous abscess, frostbite with gas gangrene, infected stumps in amputees, brain abscess, prostatic abscess, perianal abscess, conjunctivitis, infection of a renal cell carcinoma, and infected aortic grafts.

Clostridia are isolated in approximately two-thirds of patients with intraabdominal infections resulting from intestinal perforation. *C. ramosum*, *C. perfringens*, and *C. bifermentans* are the most commonly isolated species. The presence of clostridial species does not affect the clinical presentation or outcome of these infections (see Chap. 128).

An association has been made between malignancy and the isolation of *C. septicum* in the absence of grossly contaminated deep traumatic wounds. A major site for these malignancies is the gastrointestinal tract, particularly the colon. An association with leukemia or with other solid tumors also has been noted. Some of these patients present with *C. septicum* bacteremia and have a fulminant clinical course (discussed below). Others develop localized

suppurative infection in the abdomen or the abdominal wall without bacteremia. Presumably this infection arises from a silent perforation that leads to intraabdominal abscess formation.

Clostridia have been isolated from suppurative infections of the female genital tract, particularly tuboovarian and pelvic abscess. The major species involved has been *C. perfringens*. Most of these are mild suppurative infections without evidence of uterine gangrene. Isolation of *C. perfringens* has been reported in as many as 20 percent of diseased gallbladders at surgery. One clinical syndrome, emphysematous cholecystitis, is caused by clostridial species at least 50 percent of the time. In this syndrome there is gas formation in the biliary radicles and the wall of the gallbladder. It is seen most often in diabetic patients. Although the mortality rate in this entity is higher than in more common forms of cholecystitis, there is no evidence of myonecrosis.

Clostridia are among the many organisms found in empyema fluid or isolated by transtracheal aspiration from patients with lung abscesses. There is no clinical clue to the presence of clostridia (as opposed to other organisms) in these infections. *C. perfringens* has been reported as a cause of empyema arising from aspiration pneumonia, pulmonary emboli, and infarction. However, the majority of cases of clostridial empyema are secondary to trauma.

Skin and soft tissue infections   Various categories of traumatic wound infections due to clostridia have been described: simple contamination, anaerobic cellulitis, fasciitis with or without systemic manifestations, and anaerobic myonecrosis.

SIMPLE CONTAMINATION   Clostridia are cultured most often from wounds in the absence of clinical signs of sepsis. As many as 30 percent of battle wounds can be contaminated by clostridia without signs of suppuration, and 16 percent of penetrating abdominal wounds yield clostridia on culture despite treatment with cephalothin and kanamycin. In cases of trauma, clostridia are isolated with equal frequency from suppurative and well-healing wounds. Based on these findings, the diagnosis of clostridial infection should be clinical rather than bacteriologic.

LOCALIZED INFECTION OF THE SKIN AND SOFT TISSUE WITHOUT SYSTEMIC SIGNS   This condition was originally referred to as *anaerobic cellulitis*. It is a localized infection involving the skin and soft tissue due to clostridia in pure or mixed culture. There are no systemic signs of toxicity, although the infection may invade locally, producing necrosis. These infections tend to be relatively indolent, spreading slowly to contiguous areas. Localized infections tend to be relatively free of pain and edema. Perhaps because of the lack of edema, gas that is limited to the wound and the immediately surrounding tissue may be more evident than in gas gangrene. In these localized infections, gas is never found intramuscularly. Cellulitis, perirectal abscesses, and diabetic foot ulcers are typical infections from which clostridial species can be isolated. If inadequately treated, these localized infections advance by extension through subcutaneous tissue and fascial planes into muscle and may produce severe systemic disease with signs of toxemia.

A localized form of suppurative myositis has been described in heroin addicts. These patients develop local pain and tenderness in discrete areas (particularly the thigh and forearm) with the subsequent appearance of fluctuance and crepitance that require surgical drainage. The unusual aspect of these infections is that they remain localized without systemic signs of toxicity. Moreover these local areas are not necessarily sites of trauma or heroin injection. Pathologically, there are subcutaneous abscesses, purulent myositis, and fasciitis from which clostridia are recovered in pure culture; on occasion, mixed infections involving aerobes and anaerobes are found.

SPREADING CELLULITIS AND FASCIITIS WITH SYSTEMIC TOXICITY   This is diffuse spreading cellulitis and fasciitis, but myonecrosis is absent, and only mild inflammation is seen in muscle. These patients present with the abrupt onset of a syndrome which progresses rapidly through the fascial planes within hours. When suppuration and gas in soft tissues as well as overwhelming toxemia are present, the infection is rapidly fatal. On physical examination there is subcutaneous crepitance but little localized pain. Surgery is of no proven value because there are no discretely involved tissues amenable to resection, as may be the case in myonecrosis. However, incision of the affected area should be performed, because in rapidly advancing fasciitis, it is still the cornerstone of therapy. The initial local lesion may be quite innocuous and arises from an area involved by tumor or other infection and not from injury. The systemic toxic effects include hemolysis and injury of capillary membranes. Usually, this infection is uniformly fatal within 48 h, despite intensive therapy involving antitoxin and exchange transfusion. This syndrome is seen most commonly in patients with carcinoma, especially of the sigmoid or the cecum. Presumably, the tumor invades the fascia, and colonic contents leak into the abdominal wall. These patients present with extreme toxicity and occasionally with total-body crepitance. The syndrome differs from necrotizing fasciitis caused by other organisms in three respects: (1) rapid mortality, (2) rapid tissue invasion, and (3) the systemic effects of the toxin typified by massive hemolysis.

CLOSTRIDIAL MYONECROSIS (GAS GANGRENE)   Clostridial myonecrosis occurs when bacteria invade healthy muscle from adjacent traumatized muscle or soft tissue. The infection originates in a wound contaminated with clostridia. Despite the fact that more than 30 percent of deep wounds are infected with clostridia, the incidence of clostridial myonecrosis is quite low. These infections occur in military or civilian settings. An essential factor in the genesis of gas gangrene appears to be trauma, particularly involving deep lacerated muscle wounds. The entity of clostridial myonecrosis is relatively uncommon after simple, through-and-through bullet wounds without shattering of bone and relatively common following shrapnel fragmentation wounds, particularly when deep muscle is involved. In civilian cases, gas gangrene can occur after trauma, surgery, or intramuscular injection. The trauma need not be severe; however, the wound must be deep, necrotic, and without communication to the surface.

The incubation period of gas gangrene is usually short: almost always less than 3 days and frequently less than 24 h. Eighty percent of cases are caused by *C. perfringens*, while *C. novyi*, *C. septicum*, and *C. histolyticum* cause most of the other cases. Typically, gas gangrene begins with the sudden appearance of pain in the region of the wound, which helps to differentiate it from spreading cellulitis. Once established, the pain increases steadily in severity but remains localized to the infected area and only spreads if the infection spreads. Soon after pain develops, local swelling and edema, accompanied by a thin, often hemorrhagic exudate, appear. These patients frequently develop marked tachycardia, but elevation in temperature may be only minimal. Gas usually is not obvious at this early stage and may be completely absent. Frothiness of the wound exudate may be noted. The skin is tense, white, often marbled with blue and cooler than normal. The symptoms progress rapidly; swelling, edema, and toxemia increase, and a profuse serous discharge, which may have a peculiar sweetish smell, appears. Gram's stain of the wound exudate shows many gram-positive rods with relatively few inflammatory cells.

At surgery, muscle may appear pale because of the amount of edema, but it does not contract when probed with a scalpel. When dissected, the muscle is beefy red and nonviable and can progress to become black, friable, and gangrenous. It is important to establish a diagnosis early, preferably by frozen section biopsy of muscle.

Despite hypotension, renal failure, and often body crepitance, patients with myonecrosis often have a heightened awareness of their surroundings until just before death, when they lapse into toxic delirium and coma. In untreated cases, as the local wounds progress, the skin becomes bronzed; bullae appear, become filled with dark red fluid, and are accompanied by dark patches of cutaneous gangrene. Gas appears in later phases but may not be as obvious as in anaerobic cellulitis. Jaundice is rarely seen in wound gas gangrene (in contrast to uterine infections) and, when it does appear, is almost invariably associated with hemoglobinuria, hemoglobinemia, and septicemia. There have been reports of cases of clostridial myonecrosis without a history of trauma. These patients have bullous lesions and crepitance

of the skin; they present with a rapidly worsening course which includes myonecrosis, especially of the extremities.

Bacteremia and clostridial septicemia   The relatively common entity of transient bacteremia due to clostridia can arise in any hospitalized patient but is most common with a predisposing focus in the gastrointestinal tract, biliary tract, or uterus. Fever frequently resolves within 24 to 48 h without therapy. Despite the finding of clostridial bacteremia following septic abortions and the frequent isolation of clostridia from the lochia, most of these patients do not have evidence of septicemia. In one series of 60 patients with clostridial bacteremia, half the cases could be associated with an infected site, while the other half had a totally unrelated illness, such as tuberculous pneumonia, meningitis, or benign gastroenteritis. Frequently, by the time the blood culture reports return, the patients are completely well and sometimes have been discharged. Therefore, when a blood culture report is positive for clostridia, the patient must be assessed clinically rather than simply treated for the positive blood culture.

Clostridial septicemia is an uncommon but almost invariably fatal illness occurring after clostridial infection primarily of the uterus, colon, or biliary tract. This entity must be differentiated from transient clostridial bacteremia, which is much more common than septicemia. *C. perfringens* causes the majority of septicemic infections, as well as the majority of cases of transient bacteremia. *C. septicum*, *C. sordellii*, and *C. novyi* account for most of the remainder of cases. Clostridia account for 1 to 2.5 percent of all positive blood cultures in major hospital centers.

The majority of cases of clostridial septicemia originate from the female genital tract following septic abortion. Introduction of a foreign body is a common antecedent event. In the uterus there may be residual necrotic fetal and placental tissues and traumatized endometrium that allow the growth of clostridia. Only a small fraction of cases of septic abortion (1 percent) are followed by serious septicemic illness.

In these patients, sepsis, fever, and chills begin from 1 to 3 days after the attempted abortion. The initial signs are malaise, headache, severe myalgias, abdominal pain, nausea, vomiting, and occasionally diarrhea. Frequently a bloody or brown vaginal discharge is noted. Patients may rapidly develop oliguria, hypotension, jaundice, and hemoglobinuria. The hemolysis, which is secondary to *C. perfringens* alpha toxin, causes a characteristic bronzing of the skin. As in myonecrosis, the mental status of severely ill patients is characterized by increased alertness and apprehension. Local examination of the pelvis reveals foul cervical discharge, occasionally with gas. Frequently, laceration marks around the cervix or perforation of the cervical segment are evident. If the infection involves the myometrium or has spread to the adnexa, extreme tenderness, guarding, and an adnexal mass may be found.

Laboratory studies in septicemic patients reveal an elevated white count and may show pink, hemoglobin-tinged plasma. Anemia is proportional to the degree of hemolysis, and the hematocrit may be extremely low. Platelets may be reduced, and there is often evidence of disseminated intravascular coagulation. Oliguria or anuria, increasingly refractory hypotension, and hemorrhage and bruising may develop.

Clostridia may enter the bloodstream from the gastrointestinal or biliary tract. This occurrence is associated with ulcerative lesions or obstruction of the small or large intestine, necrotic or infiltrating malignancy, bowel surgery, or various abdominal catastrophes. The patient may present with an acute febrile illness with chills and fever but no other signs of localized infection. Intravascular hemolysis occurs in as many as half the cases. Biliary or gastrointestinal symptoms, if present, may be the only clue to the etiology. Positive blood cultures provide the definitive clue for the diagnosis.

Patients with malignant disease also can develop rapidly fatal clostridial sepsis, particularly from a gastrointestinal focus. The most common species in this setting is *C. septicum*. Characteristic signs and symptoms include fever, tachycardia, hypotension, abdominal pain or tenderness, nausea, vomiting, and, preterminally, coma. The tachycardia may be out of proportion to the fever. Only about 20 to 30 percent of patients develop hemolysis. A striking feature of this syndrome is the rapidity of death, which frequently occurs in less than 12 h.

DIAGNOSIS The diagnosis of clostridial disease must be based primarily on clinical findings. Because of the presence of clostridia in many wounds, their mere isolation from any site, including the blood, does not necessarily indicate severe disease. Smears of wound exudates, uterine scrapings, or cervical discharge may show abundant large gram-positive rods as well as other organisms. Cultures should be placed in selective media and incubated anaerobically for identification of clostridia.

The urine of patients with severe clostridial sepsis may contain protein and casts, and some patients may develop severe uremia. Profound alterations of circulating erythrocytes are seen in severely toxemic patients. Patients have a hemolytic anemia, which develops extremely rapidly, along with hemoglobinemia, hemoglobinuria, and elevated levels of serum bilirubin. Spherocytosis, increased osmotic and mechanical red blood cell fragility, erythrophagocytosis, and methemoglobinemia have been described. Disseminated intravascular coagulation may be seen in patients with severe infection. In patients with severe septicemia, a Wright's or Gram's stain smear of peripheral blood or buffy coat may demonstrate clostridia.

X-ray examination sometimes provides an important clue to the diagnosis by revealing gas in muscles, subcutaneous tissue, or the uterus. However, the finding of gas is not pathognomonic for clostridial infection. Other bacteria, particularly anaerobes, mixed with aerobic organisms may produce gas.

The diagnosis of clostridial myonecrosis can be established by frozen section biopsy of muscle. The diagnosis of *C. difficile*–associated colitis is made by the identification of *C. difficile* toxin in stool.

TREATMENT The treatment of choice for clostridial infection is penicillin G, 20 million units a day in adults. In cases of penicillin sensitivity or allergy, other antibiotics should be considered, but all should be tested for in vitro efficacy because of the occasional isolation of resistant strains. Chloramphenicol, 4 g/d, usually is an effective alternative. Clostridia are frequently, but not universally, susceptible in vitro to cefoxitin, carbenicillin, clindamycin, metronidazole, doxycycline, minocycline, tetracycline, third-generation cephalosporins, and vancomycin. For severe clostridial infections, sensitivity testing should be done before using an antimicrobial with unpredictable susceptibility. Simple contamination of a wound with clostridia should not be treated with antibiotics. Localized skin and soft tissue infection can be managed by debridement rather than with systemic antibiotics. Drugs are required when the process extends into adjacent tissue, or when fever and systemic signs of sepsis are present. Surgery is an important mainstay of therapy in clostridial myonecrosis or gas gangrene. Amputation may be required for rapidly spreading infection involving a limb. Hysterectomy is required for uterine myonecrosis. Repeated surgical debridement of all involved muscle is necessary for abdominal wall myonecrosis where ongoing myonecrosis usually occurs despite initial aggressive surgery and antibiotics.

Suppurative infections should be treated with antibiotics. Frequently, broad-spectrum antibiotics must be used because of mixed flora in these infections. Aminoglycosides can be used for the aerobic gram-negative bacteria in mixed infections.

The use of a polyvalent gas gangrene antitoxin is still recommended by some authorities. At present, the antitoxin is not produced in the United States, and most centers have discontinued its use in management of patients with suspected gas gangrene or clostridial postabortion sepsis because of questionable efficacy and the substantial risk of hypersensitivity to horse serum.

The use of hyperbaric oxygen in the treatment of gas gangrene is also controversial. Studies in humans are not well designed to answer questions on efficacy, but several knowledgeable authors believe that hyperbaric oxygen therapy has contributed to dramatic clinical improvement. It may, however, be associated with untoward effects due to oxygen toxicity and high atmospheric pressure. Some centers without hyperbaric chambers have reported acceptable mortality rates, indicating that expert surgical and medical management and control of complications are probably the most important factors in treating gas gangrene.

Treatment of *C. difficile* enterocolitis The treatment of *C. difficile*–associated colitis requires discontinuation of the offending antimicrobial agent. In some patients, symptoms will resolve over a period of 2 weeks. However, specific therapy shortens the duration of symptoms. The most widely used agent in the treatment of antibiotic-associated diarrhea ascribed to *C. difficile* is oral vancomycin. Most strains of *C. difficile* are susceptible to achievable concentrations of oral vancomycin. This antibiotic is poorly absorbed after oral administration and high levels appear in the stool. Dosing should begin with 125 mg orally four times a day for 7 to 10 days, but the dose may be increased to 500 mg orally four times a day. A randomized trial comparing vancomycin with metronidazole demonstrated equal efficacy between the two regimens. The dose of metronidazole used was 250 mg four times a day, although 500 mg three times a day should be equally effective. Relapse rates were 8 to 9 percent for both regimens. Because metronidazole is considerably less costly than vancomycin, initial treatment should begin with this agent. If diarrhea persists, therapy should be changed to vancomycin. In patients with refractory symptoms and fever unresponsive to either regimen, the addition of rifampin to vancomycin has helped in some cases. Since resistance can develop to rifampin, it should not be used alone. A number of patients who respond to initial therapy present with relapse of symptoms and a repeat positive toxin assay. A number of options are available. Some patients have been shown to acquire a different strain of *C. difficile* despite the appearance of relapsing disease. These patients respond to a second trial of the same agent used to treat the first episode. Alternatively, patients who receive vancomycin and relapse can be treated with metronidazole, and vice versa. Some authors report success with tapering regimens of vancomycin given daily or every other day for 2 weeks to avoid relapse. The resin cholestyramine binds the cytotoxin of *C. difficile* and has been used with some success to treat severe cases. Since cholestyramine also binds vancomycin, the two agents should not be used in combination. Efforts to repopulate the normal colonic flora also have been tried in relapsing disease. Ingestion of capsules of the yeast *Saccharomyces boulardii* showed some promise in one trial.

REFERENCES

BARTLETT JG: Antibiotic-associated diarrhea. Clin Infect Dis 15:573, 1992

———: Gas gangrene (other clostridium-associated diseases), in *Principles and Practice of Infectious Diseases*, 3d ed, GL Mandell et al (eds). New York, Churchill Livingstone, 1990

——— et al: Antibiotic-associated pseudomembranous colitis due to toxin-producing clostridia. N Engl J Med 298:531, 1978

BORNSTEIN DL: Clostridial myonecrosis, in *Medical Microbiology and Infectious Diseases*, A Braude (ed). Philadelphia, Saunders, 1981, chap 239

BUGGY BP et al: Therapy of relapsing *Clostridium difficile*–associated diarrhea and colitis with the combination of vancomycin and rifampin. J Clin Gastroenterol 9:155, 1987

FINEGOLD SM: *Anaerobic Bacteria in Human Disease*. New York, Academic, 1977

———: Anaerobic infections and *Clostridium difficile* colitis emerging during antibacterial therapy. Scand J Infect Dis (Suppl)49:160, 1986

GORBACH SL, THADEPALLI H: Isolation of *Clostridium* in human infections: Evaluation of 114 cases. J Infect Dis 131:S81, 1975

JENDRZEJEWSKI JW et al: Nontraumatic clostridial myonecrosis. Am J Med 65:542, 1978

JOHNSON S et al: Enteritis necroticans among Khmer children at an evacuation site in Thailand. Lancet 2:496, 1987

KORANSKY JR et al: *Clostridium septicum* bacteremia. Am J Med 66:63, 1979

PETERSON LR et al: Detection of *Clostridium difficile* toxin A (enterotoxin) and B (cytotoxin) in clinical specimens. Am J Clin Pathol 86:208, 1986

PRITCHARD JA, WHALLEY PJ: Abortion complicated by *Clostridium perfringens* infection. Am J Gynecol 111:484, 1971

SMITH LDS: Virulence factors of *Clostridium perfringens*. Rev Infect Dis 1:254, 1979

TEASLEY DG et al: Prospective, randomized trial of metronidazole versus vancomycin for *Clostridium difficile*–associated diarrhea and colitis. Lancet 2:1043, 1983

section 6 Diseases caused by gram-negative bacteria

109 MENINGOCOCCAL INFECTIONS

J. McLEOD GRIFFISS

DEFINITION *Neisseria meningitidis* is an ordinary commensal of the human oropharynx that can cause a variety of diseases, most notably bacteremia and meningitis. Its pathogenic potential can be expressed as epidemic disease or as sporadic cases and focal outbreaks.

ETIOLOGY Meningococci are gram-negative single cocci or diplococci with flattened adjacent sides. They grow well on media containing blood at temperatures between 35 and 37°C in a moist atmosphere reduced in oxygen and containing 5 to 10 percent CO_2. The organism is recovered readily when fresh specimens are inoculated on warm chocolate agar and incubated 18 to 24 h in a candle jar or other apparatus that provides a suitable environment.

Neisseria make cytochrome oxidase, which is responsible for the positive "oxidase" test; species are differentiated by their ability to use simple and compound sugars as sources of energy. Typically, meningococci use both glucose and maltose. Meningococci differ from other *Neisseria* in that they are surrounded by a polysaccharide "capsule."

Meningococci are divided into serologic groups on the basis of antigenic differences among their capsular polysaccharides. Groups A, B, C, W, and Y cause most serious disease; other groups frequently colonize the oropharynx but only very rarely disseminate. The serogroups are further divided into serotypes and subtypes based on independent antigenic differences among outer membrane protein and glycolipid constituents.

EPIDEMIOLOGY The natural habitat of meningococci is the human throat. Transmission from person to person is through inhalation of droplets of infected oropharyngeal secretions. Colonization only rarely proceeds to disease, because specific antibodies and complement lyse the organisms as they enter the bloodstream and thereby provide an effective barrier to dissemination. The incidence of disseminated infection varies cyclically, with peaks of increased frequency occurring every 10 to 15 years and lasting 4 to 6 years. Each cycle spreads slowly and is called a *hyperendemic wave* to distinguish it from the truly endemic disease that occurs between waves. Hyperendemic waves are often punctuated by focal outbreaks. Widespread epidemics have been rare in developed areas of the world since the end of World War II; hyperendemic waves continue to occur. The between-waves endemic incidence in temperate climates is a fairly constant 1 reported case per 100,000 population per year. The prevalence of meningococcal infection is also subject to seasonal influences; the lowest attack rate occurs in midsummer and the highest in winter and early spring.

Epidemic disease receives the greatest public attention. An epidemic begins as a focal outbreak in a demographically discrete population in which a strain of a single serotype, the *epidemic strain*, emerges from among the endemic strains. In less developed areas the outbreak quickly spreads, develops high attack rates, and involves large segments of the community. It remains either multicentric or evolves in the same pattern as a hyperendemic wave. Each focal outbreak in multicentric epidemics lasts 1 to 3 years, while the epidemic as a whole may last 5 or more years. In developed areas foci usually involve economically deprived segments of the population and do not spread or develop into generalized epidemics.

Group A strains caused most epidemics in the United States in the first half of this century; since World War II, groups B and C meningococci have caused outbreaks in both military and civilian populations. Hyperendemic waves are caused by group B, C, or W organisms that share a limited set of serotypes. Group A strains do not share serotypes with other groups and do not cause hyperendemic waves. Group W strains have been associated with endemic and hyperendemic disease only. Group Y organisms only cause sporadic disease in older children and teenagers. Endemic disease predominantly is caused by group B organisms of diverse serotypes.

The attack rate of endemic meningococcal disease is highest for children between 6 and 36 months of age. The age distribution of epidemic cases is always shifted to proportionately older individuals, and those of any age may be involved. The attack rate in household contacts of sporadic cases is up to 1000 times the overall endemic rate and may be as much as 15,000 times that of the general population in epidemic periods.

Carriers Between epidemics, 2 to 30 percent of individuals, depending on age, carry meningococci on their throats. When sporadic disease occurs, the carrier rate in close contacts may rise to 40 percent, and in closed populations or during epidemics, it may approach 100 percent. However, the prevalence of meningococcal disease cannot be attributed to the prevailing carrier rate. Only a small proportion of the meningococci carried on the throats of those who share a patient's environment are of the same clonotype as the patient's, and individual levels of immunity to it will vary. Case-to-case transmission of infection is rare; carriers, not patients, are the foci from which disease is spread. Although some individuals harbor meningococci for years, oropharyngeal infection is usually transient, and in 75 percent of carriers the organism disappears within a few weeks to a few months.

Immunity The occurrence of clinical disease is most dependent on the immunologic status of the host. Natural immunity is usually type-specific and develops in most individuals within the first two decades of life. Natural immunization may result from pharyngeal colonization during the first few years of life by a closely related bacterium, *Neisseria lactamica*. *N. lactamica* strains are genetically diverse but many share important outer-membrane protein and lipooligosaccharide antigens with virulent strains of *N. meningitidis*. They are not encapsulated and therefore do not survive in the bloodstream to cause disseminated disease. *N. lactamica* colonizes the throat earlier in life than does *N. meningitidis;* colonized infants develop bactericidal antibodies that initiate complement-mediated lysis of a broad range of potentially pathogenic meningococci.

Colonization with *N. meningitidis* gradually replaces that with *N. lactamica* as the child grows older, and *N. lactamica* carriage is only rarely encountered in teenagers, in whom meningococcal carrier rates of 15 to 25 percent are the rule, regardless of season. Meningococcal carriage induces antibodies to the infecting strain as well as to other strains, thereby reinforcing and broadening naturally acquired immunity. Many enteric bacteria make capsules that are chemically similar to those of meningococci. Asymptomatic colonization with them can induce group-specific antibody. Second episodes of meningococcal disease are encountered. Deficiency of properdin or one of the terminal complement components, C5, C6, C7, C8, or C9, is a risk factor for repeated episodes of bacteremia with pathogenic *Neisseria* and should always be sought in patients with second episodes.

PATHOGENESIS   Meningococcal infection begins in the oropharynx. In most instances, this infection is subclinical, but occasionally mild symptoms develop. Dissemination from the pharynx is via the bloodstream and generally is followed by clinical manifestations. Purulent meningitis, the most common manifestation, may predominate, or it may be associated with signs and symptoms of meningococcemia. Rarely, extensive inflammation may cause an acute diffuse encephalitis.

There is a correlation between susceptibility to meningococcal disease and the absence of complement-mediated bactericidal activity in serum. The pathogenetic mechanisms that account for the different epidemiologic forms of meningococcal disease all interfere with the generation of bactericidal activity by the membrane attack complex of complement (C5–9) (see Chap. 277). Hypogammaglobulinemia, deficiencies of complement components, and interference by the organism's capsular polysaccharides with the effective deposition of the attack complex into its outer membrane account for endemic disease. Primary isolated IgM deficiency is a rare cause of susceptibility that is disproportionately reported. Deficiencies of complement components are seen more frequently in patients than in the general population. They may be either primary or secondary and should always be sought in patients infected with the less common W, X, Y, Z, and 29E serogroups or in those with recurrent disseminated meningococcal or gonococcal infections. Inheritance of properdin deficiency and ineffective alternative pathway complement activity is sex-linked. Males in these pedigrees are at extremely high risk of fulminant meningococcal disease. Several systemic diseases, notably systemic lupus erythematosus and membranoproliferative glomerulonephritis, can result in secondary deficiencies of complement components and sporadic meningococcal disease. People with functional asplenia are also at increased risk of sporadic meningococcal disease, although pneumococcal infection is a more common complication.

The generation of hyperendemic waves remains incompletely understood. An "out-of-phase" response to fluctuations in antibody levels in the population is a possible mechanism. Focal outbreaks during hyperendemic waves can be correlated with the presence of elevated levels of circulating strain-specific IgA which blocks initiation of complement-mediated lysis by IgM or IgG, but the precise contribution of IgA-mediated susceptibility to hyperendemic waves remains unclear. When a sufficiently large part of the population has developed blocking serum IgA, conditions are established for an epidemic to occur. The environmental events that cause IgA levels to be elevated within the epidemic focus are not known with certainty, but epidemic disease has been correlated with prevalent enteric colonization with cross-reacting organisms. The extent of induction of blocking IgA in the epidemic focus may explain the extent and intensity of the epidemic as well as the failure of focal outbreaks to develop into generalized ones. Asplenia and coincidental diseases that interfere with the normal hepatic clearance of IgA, such as alcoholism, biliary tract disease, hemoglobinopathies, and hemosiderosis, increase susceptibility within the epidemic focus.

The meningococcal outer membrane contains lipooligosaccharides (LOS) that are chemically and biologically similar to the lipopolysaccharide endotoxins of enteric bacilli. They induce tumor necrosis factor (TNF-α) and interleukins 1 (IL-1) and 6 (IL-6), which seem to be responsible for the hypotension and vascular collapse observed in fulminant meningococcemia, the purpura and visceral hemorrhages associated with meningococcal bacteremia, and the influx of leukocytes into the cerebrospinal fluid during meningitis. Release of cytokines is associated with a fatal outcome (see Chap. 83). The presence of LOS sialic acid and release of redundant outer-membrane blebs into the circulation have been correlated with "virulence" and a poor prognosis, respectively.

CLINICAL MANIFESTATIONS   Of patients with meningococcal disease, 90 to 95 percent have meningococcemia and/or meningitis.

Meningococcemia   Thirty to fifty percent of patients who develop overt disease have meningococcemia without meningitis. The onset of clinical illness may be abrupt, but patients usually have nonspecific prodromal symptoms of cough, headache, and sore throat followed by the sudden development of spiking fever, chills, arthralgias, and myalgias. Patients usually appear acutely ill with an inordinate degree of prostration. In addition to high fever, tachycardia, and tachypnea, mild hypotension may be present. However, clinical shock does not occur unless fulminant meningococcemia supervenes. In the course of meningococcal bacteremia, about three-fourths of the patients develop a characteristic petechial rash. Lesions are frequently sparse, and the axillae, flanks, wrists, and ankles are most commonly involved. Often petechiae are located in the center of lighter-colored macules, and they may become nodular as the disease progresses. The diagnosis of meningococcemia occasionally can be established by demonstrating gram-negative diplococci in scrapings from these nodular lesions. In severe cases, purpuric spots or large ecchymoses develop, and a widespread petechial or purpuric eruption suggests fulminating disease. However, the absence of rash does not necessarily indicate that the illness will be mild. The levels of circulating endotoxin, or of the cytokines it induces, are sensitive markers for the development of fulminant disease and a poor prognosis. Patients with terminal complement-component deficiencies have a more favorable prognosis; those with properdin deficiency usually do not survive.

Fulminant meningococcemia, or the Waterhouse-Friderichsen syndrome, is meningococcemia associated with vasomotor collapse and shock. It occurs in the 10 to 20 percent of patients in whom high levels of endotoxin circulate. The onset is abrupt, and profound prostration frequently occurs within a few hours. Petechiae and purpuric lesions enlarge rapidly, and hemorrhage into the skin may be extensive. Early in the preshock stage, there is generalized vasoconstriction; patients are alert and pale, with circumoral cyanosis and cold extremities. In the early shock stage, however, the cardiac output decreases, and the blood pressure falls; mentation decreases, and coma may develop. Despite appropriate therapy, 40 to 60 percent of patients die from cardiac and/or respiratory failure. Patients who recover may have extensive sloughing of skin lesions or loss of digits because of gangrene.

Occult meningococcemia is an uncommon form of meningococcal infection that affects children between the ages of 3 and 24 months. It is characterized by fever and bacteremia without an obvious source. Infection usually resolves without treatment but may lead to the development of meningitis or other metastatic infection.

Chronic meningococcemia is a very rare form of meningococcal infection that may be associated with terminal complement component deficiencies, lasts for weeks or months, and is characterized by fever, rash, and arthritis or arthralgia. Typically, the fever is intermittent, and during afebrile periods, which may last several days, patients appear remarkably well. The usual maculopapular or polymorphous rash waxes and wanes with the fever. Petechial and nodular lesions are occasionally seen. Joint involvement is present in two-thirds of the patients, and splenomegaly is detected in about 20 percent. If treatment is delayed, meningitis, carditis, or nephritis may occur.

Meningitis   Meningitis is a common form of meningococcal disease that occurs primarily in children from 6 months to 10 years of age. Fever, vomiting, headache, and confusion or lethargy are the most common symptoms; in about one-fourth of patients, symptoms begin abruptly and rapidly increase in severity. The more typical patient, however, has symptoms of an upper respiratory tract infection followed by an illness that progresses over several days. Twenty to forty percent of patients have meningitis without clinical evidence of meningococcemia, and the diagnosis depends on bacteriologic examination of the cerebrospinal fluid. However, when meningitis occurs in association with a petechial or purpuric rash, a presumptive diagnosis of meningococcal disease is warranted because this pattern of illness is seen only rarely in other infections.

Rarer manifestations   The meningococcus may cause purulent conjunctivitis or sinusitis. Primary pneumonia occurs rarely, but secondary pneumonia not infrequently follows viral respiratory infections, particularly influenza. Bacterial endocarditis, primary pericarditis, arthritis, and osteomyelitis also have been reported. Meningococci also can produce genital infections clinically indistinguishable from gonococcal disease, including urethritis and endometritis.

LABORATORY FINDINGS Aside from bacteriologic data, laboratory studies are of little value in establishing a specific diagnosis of meningococcal infection. Polymorphonuclear leukocyte counts usually are elevated but may be normal or low in meningococcemia; a left shift usually is present. Patients with hemorrhagic manifestations may have low platelet counts and decreased levels of circulating clotting factors as a result of disseminated intravascular coagulation (see Chap. 57). In meningitis, the cerebrospinal fluid (CSF) pressure is increased; the fluid usually contains from 1000 to 40,000 polymorphonuclear leukocytes per microliter; the protein content is increased, and the concentration of glucose is low (see Chap. 374).

Meningococci usually can be recovered from cultures of blood or spinal fluid and, on occasion, of material aspirated from skin lesions or joints. In addition, gram-negative diplococci may be seen in stains of nodular petechiae or the buffy coat of blood from patients with meningococcemia. In meningococcal meningitis, a smear of the spinal fluid is diagnostic in about half the patients but often shows only a few intracellular bacteria, which are located with difficulty, particularly early in the course of the infection, when organisms may be present in the absence of CSF abnormalities. The infecting organisms shed their capsular polysaccharide, which usually can be detected in CSF, joint fluid, serum, or urine with use of highly specific antibodies in counterimmunoelectrophoresis (CIE) or latex agglutination (LA) assays. The sensitivity of these assays is dependent on the antibodies used and is least for group B; LA is somewhat more sensitive and easier to perform. In general, the immunoassays are more sensitive than culture alone and in combination with Gram's stain will provide a diagnosis in over 98 percent of cases. They are particularly helpful early in infection and when the patient has been treated with antibiotics, causing negative cultures.

COMPLICATIONS Herpes labialis occurs in 5 to 20 percent of patients with meningococcal disease. Other complications, which result from neurologic damage or secondary foci of infection, are uncommon following appropriate treatment and are often transient. Seizures or deafness occur in 10 to 20 percent of patients during the acute stages of meningitis, but postmeningitic epilepsy is rare, and the frequency of permanent nerve damage is probably less than 5 percent. A number of patients complain of recurrent headache, emotional lability, insomnia, backache, memory loss, and difficulty in concentrating for months after an episode of meningitis. These symptoms usually disappear a year or two after the infection.

Septic arthritis is a not uncommon complication of meningococcemia that may accompany meningitis or occur as the only metastatic manifestation. The joint fluid usually contains many granulocytes (see Chap. 91), but meningococci are recovered infrequently. It can be diagnosed by Gram's stain, CIE, or LA or by recovery of the organism on culture. It is treated in the same way as meningitis; recovery without sequelae is to be expected.

Immune-complex arthritis occurs in about 10 percent of patients during convalescence. As a rule, multiple joints are involved, primarily the larger ones. Inflammation appears between days 7 and 15 of treatment when newly produced antibodies form insoluble complexes with the infecting organism's capsular polysaccharide. No specific therapy is indicated; permanent joint changes are rare.

Other pyogenic complications have become extremely uncommon since antibiotics have been used routinely. Bacterial endocarditis is quite rare, but a high proportion of patients who die of meningococcal infection have myocarditis. A pericardial friction rub or electrocardiographic changes of pericarditis are seen in about 5 percent of patients; rarely, purulent pericarditis may develop.

DIAGNOSIS The diagnosis of meningococcal disease depends on recovering *N. meningitidis* or detecting antigens in blood, spinal fluid, joint fluid, urine, or petechial scrapings from patients with a typical clinical picture. Capsular polysaccharides of serogroups A, B, C, Y, and W can be detected in fluids by LA or CIE. Recovery of meningococci from the pharynx does not establish the diagnosis of meningococcal disease; throat cultures are not indicated.

Few diseases need to be considered seriously in the differential diagnosis of meningococcal disease. If meningococcal meningitis is not accompanied by rash or other manifestations of bacteremia, it is indistinguishable from meningitis caused by other common pathogens (see Chap. 374). Occasionally, the common viral exanthems, *Mycoplasma* infection, Rocky Mountain spotted fever (see Chap. 138), and vascular purpuras (see Chaps. 53 and 291) may be confused with meningococcemia.

TREATMENT In the absence of fulminant meningococcemia, the treatment of meningococcal disease is not difficult, and the mortality rate should not exceed 5 percent. Therapy should be instituted as early as possible. Penicillin G remains the drug of choice, although low-level penicillin resistance has been reported in Europe, and should be administered intravenously. The usual dosage for treatment of meningitis in adults with normal renal function is 12 to 24 million units per day (2 to 4 million units intravenously every 4 h), and in the pediatric age group, 200,000 to 300,000 units per kilogram per day, intravenously every 4 h in divided doses. When treatment is continued for a minimum of 7 days, or 4 to 5 days after the patient becomes afebrile, relapse is extremely rare. Chloramphenicol is just as effective as penicillin and may be the drug of choice in less-developed countries. It should be used when a patient is allergic to penicillin in a dosage of 75 to 100 mg/kg per day or, in adults, 2.0 to 4.0 g/d in divided doses every 6 h given intravenously until the patient is able to take oral medication. Cefotaxime, ceftriaxone, and cefuroxime (see Chaps. 100 and 374), are also effective and are often used to initiate therapy when the etiology of meningitis is uncertain. A significant proportion of meningococci are resistant to sulfonamides, so these should not be used routinely unless the infecting organism is shown to be susceptible. Sulfadiazine (2 to 3 g initially followed by 1 g every 6 h thereafter given intravenously until the patient can take oral medication) or trimethoprim-sulfamethoxazole (160/800 mg intravenously every 6 h) is effective treatment for susceptible strains. The dosages must be reduced in renal failure and in children, depending on age (see Chap. 100).

Patients with meningococcal infections require supportive treatment as well as antimicrobial therapy. Maintenance of fluid and electrolyte balance and prevention of respiratory complications in comatose patients are of primary concern. When shock occurs, visceral perfusion must be improved. Vasoactive drugs should be employed according to the pathophysiologic derangement (see Chaps. 34 and 83). When disseminated intravascular coagulation is recognized, treatment with heparin, whole blood, or fibrinogen can be tried, but these are not certain to be effective.

PROGNOSIS Before the introduction of antibiotics, meningococcal meningitis and meningococcemia were almost invariably fatal. With prompt and appropriate chemotherapy, the mortality rate of meningitis without fulminant meningococcemia has dropped to less than 10 percent in the United States, and neurologic sequelae are rare. The mortality of fulminant infection remains high primarily because patients are often in irreversible shock when treatment is instituted. Most deaths occur within 24 to 48 h of admission, and the capacity of the meningococcus to kill a previously healthy individual within a few hours remains one of the most awesome characteristics of this disease.

PREVENTION The capsular polysaccharides from organisms of serogroups A, C, Y, and W induce group-specific bactericidal antibody responses after subcutaneous injection. A tetravalent vaccine containing these antigens is available for use to prevent or control outbreaks. Routine immunization of recruits has eliminated nearly all disease among military personnel, but in the United States, immunization is recommended routinely only for travelers to areas where epidemic disease is occurring and for individuals with complement deficiencies or splenic dysfunction. An effective group B vaccine has not been developed. Chemoprophylaxis should be administered to intimate household, day-care center, and nursery school contacts of sporadic cases. If the organism isolated from the patient is sensitive to sulfonamides, 2 days of prophylaxis with one of these drugs is recommended. When sensitivities are not known or the organism is resistant to sulfonamides, rifampin in a dosage of 10 mg/kg, up to 600 mg, every 12 h for 2 days for children and adults and 5 mg/kg every 12 h for infants can be expected to eradicate the carrier state temporarily and minimize spread of meningococci. Resistance to rifampin has been reported, however. Vaccination is over 99 percent effective in preventing secondary cases (as compared with approximately 89 percent effectiveness for rifampin chemoprophylaxis), and vaccination of household or other intimate contacts should be encouraged.

REFERENCES

COUNTS GW et al: Group A meningococcal disease in the U.S. Pacific Northwest: Epidemiology, clinical features, and effect of a vaccination control program. Rev Infect Dis 6:640, 1984

DENSEN P et al: Familial properdin deficiency and fatal meningococcemia: Correction of the bactericidal defect by vaccination. N Engl J Med 316:922, 1987

FIJEN CA et al: Complement deficiencies in patients over ten years old with meningococcal disease due to uncommon serogroups. Lancet 2:585, 1989

GRIFFISS J McL: Epidemic meningococcal disease: Synthesis of a hypothetical immunoepidemiologic model. Rev Infect Dis 4:159, 1982

JARVIS GA et al: Sialic acid of group B Neisseria meningitidis regulates alternative complement pathway activation. Infect Immun 55:174, 1987

KIM JJ et al: Neisseria lactamica and Neisseria meningitidis share lipooligosaccharide epitopes but lack common capsular and class 1, 2, and 3 protein epitopes. Infect Immun 57:602, 1989

MOORE PS et al: Intercontinental spread of an epidemic group A Neisseria meningitidis strain. Lancet 2:260, 1989

WAAGE A et al: The complex pattern of cytokines in serum from patients with meningococcal septic shock: Association between interleukin 6, interleukin 1, and fatal outcome. J Exp Med 169:333, 1989

WOLF RE, BIRBARA CA: Meningococcal infections at an army training center. Am J Med 44:243, 1968

110 GONOCOCCAL INFECTIONS

KING K. HOLMES / STEPHEN A. MORSE

DEFINITION Gonorrhea, an infection of columnar and transitional epithelium caused by Neisseria gonorrhoeae, is the most common reportable communicable disease in the United States. Anatomic sites which can be infected directly by the gonococcus include the urethra, rectum, conjunctivas, pharynx, and endocervix. Local complications include endometritis, salpingitis, peritonitis, and bartholinitis in the female and periurethral abscess and epididymitis in the male. Systemic manifestations of gonococcemia include arthritis, dermatitis, endocarditis, and meningitis as well as myopericarditis and hepatitis.

ETIOLOGY Neisseria gonorrhoeae is a gram-negative coccus usually found in pairs with flattened adjacent sides. It forms oxidase-positive colonies and is differentiated from other Neisseria by its ability to utilize glucose but not maltose, sucrose, or lactose; by nucleic acid probes; and by specific immunologic reactions.

Organisms present in colonies examined within 20 h of inoculation from clinical specimens are covered by fimbriae (pili). Pili mediate attachment to various epithelial cells and interfere with neutrophil phagocytosis. Each pilus is composed of repeating peptide subunits (pilin) which have a molecular weight of about 20,000. The pilin subunits consist of conserved and variable regions. Pili undergo both antigenic and phase variation. Chromosomal rearrangements, leading to expression of any one of a large number of incomplete (silent) pilin genes, lead to antigenic variation in pili. If the rearrangement involves a defective pilin gene, piliated gonococci (pil+) produce nonpiliated variants (pil-), a process known as phase variation. Piliated organisms cause infection and urethritis after inoculation into the urethras of male volunteers, whereas nonpiliated organisms do not. Antigenic variation of pilin may allow gonococci to attach to different types of epithelial surfaces and to evade the host's antibody response to pilin. Phase variation from pil+ to pil- may permit detachment and facilitate spread.

The trilaminar outer membrane of the gonococcus contains several classes of proteins, including proteins I, II, and III, and lipopolysaccharide (Fig. 110-1). Like pili, protein II (now referred to as opacity-associated outer membrane proteins, or OPAs) also is thought to function as a ligand, mediating the attachment of gonococci to various types of human cells. An individual gonococcus can possess about a dozen OPA genes and can express zero to three or more OPAs at a time. Gonococci possessing certain OPAs adhere to and are phagocytosed by human neutrophils in the absence of serum. Certain OPAs may be responsible for the clumping of gonococci that is so evident on Gram-stained smears of urethral exudate.

Opaque colonies contain organisms that express OPAs and predominate in isolates from the male urethra and in cervical isolates obtained from women in midcycle. Transparent colonies often lack OPAs and predominate in isolates from women during menses and in isolates from blood, synovial fluid, or fallopian tubes.

Protein I is quantitatively the major outer membrane protein; it exhibits intrastrain differences in molecular mass that vary between 34,600 and 37,700 Da. Protein I molecules associate in a trimeric structure, forming anion-selective transmembrane channels (porins) that permit the exchange of hydrophilic molecules through the outer membrane. Protein I also interacts with other outer membrane components, such as protein III and lipopolysaccharide (LPS), to form complex outer membrane structures. Protein I molecules have been shown to move rapidly from gonococcal outer membranes to the more fluid cytoplasmic membrane of human cells, where they form pores. This process may initiate endocytosis of the gonococcus, the first step in gonococcal invasion of the epithelium.

The LPS of the gonococcus contains lipid A and an oligosaccharide. Features that distinguish gonococcal LPS from enteric LPS are the highly branched oligosaccharide structure and the absence of repeating O-antigen subunits. For these reasons, gonococcal LPS is often referred to as lipooligosaccharide (LOS). Gonococci produce several discrete LOS components. The type of LOS produced can be altered by a mechanism that is not well understood. Host-derived cytidine monophospho-N-acetylneuraminic acid can be used by gonococci to sialylate the oligosaccharide component of one of its LOSs. This sialylation results in the conversion of a serum-sensitive organism into one that is serum-resistant and markedly reduces nonopsonic interactions of OPA-expressing gonococci with human neutrophils. Gonococci observed in urethral exudate are sialylated, thereby indicating that sialylation occurs in vivo. Recent structural and immunochemical analyses of gonococcal LOS revealed that the antigenicity and immunogenicity of the LOS is complex due in part to the structural similarity of the oligosaccharide to host glycosphingolipids. No capsular polysaccharide has been isolated, but high-molecular-weight surface polyphosphates have been demonstrated that may have functions similar to those of capsular polysaccharides in other organisms.

Gonococcal typing Gonococcal strains can be typed on the basis of nutritional requirements (auxotyping) or antigenic differences of protein I (serotyping). Unlike pili and protein II, the protein I expressed by any single strain of gonococcus is antigenically stable, although there is considerable antigenic heterogeneity of protein I between strains. There are two structurally related forms of protein I, known as IA and IB, and individual strains contain either but not both. Protein IA and IB genes are alleles of the same gene. Monoclonal antibodies against different epitopes of protein IA and protein IB can be used to classify gonococci into a large number of serovariants, known as serovars IA1 to IA24 and IB1 to IB32.

FIGURE 110-1 Diagram of the envelope of *N. gonorrhoeae*, showing structures thought to influence pathogenesis, antimicrobial susceptibility, and antigenicity.

EPIDEMIOLOGY The only natural hosts for *N. gonorrhoeae* are humans. In the United States, the annual age-specific incidence rates tripled from 1963 to 1975, when over 1 million cases were reported and an equal number probably went unreported. During this period of epidemic gonorrhea, the incidence increased fastest in young white females. The incidence of gonorrhea has decreased from a peak of 473 cases per 100,000 in 1975 to about 277 per 100,000 in 1990.

Gonorrhea incidence and prevalence rates are known to be related to age, sex, sex preference, race, socioeconomic status, marital status, urban residence, and level of education—risk factors which influence sexual behavior, illness behavior, and accessibility of health care. Among sexually active individuals, the highest rates occur in teenagers, in nonwhites, in the poor and poorly educated, in large cities, and in unmarried persons—particularly those who live alone. Such individuals comprise a "core group" of "efficient transmitters" who play a disproportionate role in the spread of gonorrhea. Since 1985, the incidence of gonorrhea has continued to fall among white and Hispanic men and women but has leveled off among black men and women. There is some evidence that the spread of gonorrhea, like that of syphilis and chancroid, is associated with the "crack" cocaine epidemic and with exchange of sex by women for illegal drugs such as cocaine. The incidence of gonorrhea is highest in men, while the prevalence is highest in women. The prevalence rate remains so high among women in the United States that routine endocervical cultures have been advocated for gonorrhea case detection in asymptomatic women age 30 or under who are considered to be at high risk because of sexual behavior or demographic factors cited above. However, greater reliance should be placed on partner notification (contact tracing), which is far more efficient for control of gonorrhea, than on routine endocervical culturing, which is expensive and does not focus on those most likely to transmit the infection. The single most important axiom about the epidemiology of this disease is that *gonorrhea is usually spread by carriers who have no symptoms or have ignored symptoms.* Symptomatic patients, male or female, have usually been recently infected by such carriers, who must in turn be traced and treated to prevent reinfection. *Men and women with symptomatic gonorrhea should always be interviewed to identify their recent sex contacts, who should be examined and treated if infected.* The growing association of gonorrhea, syphilis, and chancroid with the exchange of sex for drugs such as "crack" cocaine presents a new and unique challenge for sexually transmitted disease (STD) control and calls for intensified and innovative control efforts.

There are interesting regional differences in the antibiotic resistance of *N. gonorrhoeae*. In 1976, penicillinase-producing strains of *N. gonorrhoeae* (PPNG), completely resistant to penicillin and ampicillin, appeared almost simultaneously in two areas of the world: in England, where they had probably been imported from West Africa, and in the United States, where they had been imported from the Philippines. PPNG first became established and then spread in areas of the world where prostitution is exceptionally common and where access to subcurative antimicrobial therapy is unrestricted. PPNG now comprise 50 percent or more of all gonococci in many areas of Africa and Asia and have by now become well established in many regions of the United States and Europe. Plasmid-borne penicillin resistance results from the presence of a TEM-type β-lactamase gene on one of six small R factors which make up a very closely related family of plasmids. Plasmid-borne, tetracycline resistance (TRNG) resulted from introduction of the streptococcal resistance determinant *tetM* into *N. gonorrhoeae*, where it resides on a plasmid derived in part from a gonococcal conjugative plasmid. This new plasmid is self-transmissible and retains the capacity to mobilize some of the β-lactamase plasmids. TRNG are clinically resistant to tetracycline, minocycline, and doxycycline. Strains possessing both penicillin and tetracycline resistance plasmids are increasing in prevalence in some parts of the country, and one or the other type of plasmid was present in about one-fifth of gonococcal isolates in the United States by 1992. Of equal importance has been the spread of gonococci with chromosomally mediated resistance to penicillin and tetracycline. These strains are referred to as chromosomally mediated resistant *N. gonorrhoeae* (CMRNG). Auxotyping and monoclonal antibody serotyping have shown that in a midsized metropolitan city, as many as 60 to 100 different gonococcal strains are circulating, and new strains are being continuously introduced. Against this background, local outbreaks of PPNG, TRNG, or CMRNG belonging to a single auxotype-serovar class have been identified, and public health efforts have at times been successfully focused on the control of such strains.

Recent epidemiologic studies have shown interesting relationships between gonorrhea and HIV infection. Gonorrhea in female prostitutes has been associated with increased susceptibility to acquiring HIV infection; gonococcal urethritis has been associated with shedding of HIV in urethral exudate in HIV-seropositive men; and HIV infection in prostitutes has been associated with both increased risk of gonococcal reinfection and increased risk of clinical signs of salpingitis when gonococcal infection occurs.

IMMUNOLOGY AND PATHOGENESIS Epidemiologic data suggest that only about one-third of men become infected after a single exposure to *N. gonorrhoeae*, and under experimental conditions an inoculum of 10^3 organisms appears necessary to establish urethral infection in 50 percent of male volunteers. Factors that may confer resistance to infection are undefined. However, components of the urethral or vaginal flora, such as *Candida albicans, Staphylococcus epidermidis*, and certain types of lactobacilli, can inhibit *N. gonorrhoeae* in vitro and may provide some natural resistance in vivo.

In humans, most extracellular iron is bound by the major iron-binding proteins transferrin and lactoferrin. The resulting concentration of free iron ($10^{-18} M$) is far too low to support gonococcal growth. Under these iron-limiting conditions, gonococci produce iron-repressible proteins (FeRPs) that function in the removal of iron from transferrin and lactoferrin. Gonococci will only bind human transferrin and lactoferrin. This specificity has been used to explain why gonococci are obligate human pathogens. Gonococci presumably compete with the lactoferrin present at mucosal surfaces for iron, which is required for growth of the organism. Strains of gonococci requiring arginine, hypoxanthine, and uracil (AHU) for growth are generally unable to remove iron from lactoferrin, which could explain the tendency of such strains to cause asymptomatic mucosal infections.

Gonococci infect mucus-secreting epithelial surfaces, and mucus could be a physical barrier or competitive inhibitor. Attachment of gonococci to mucosal cells is mediated in part by pili and by protein II. Local antibody to pili or protein II can partially block attachment. Pili also impede phagocytosis of gonococci by neutrophils, and antibody to pili (as well as antibody to protein II) is opsonic. An enzyme produced by the pathogenic *Neisseria*, IgA1 protease, which inactivates sIgA1, may interfere with IgA-mediated antiadherence activity, resulting in increased attachment.

Following attachment to columnar or transitional epithelium, gonococci penetrate through or between cells to reach the subepithelial connective tissue. Transfer of gonococcal protein I into the host cell may initiate endocytosis by the epithelial cell. Gonococcal LOS produces mucosal damage in fallopian tube organ cultures. Recent evidence suggests that gonococcal LOS stimulates the production of tumor necrosis factor (TNF) in fallopian tube organ cultures; inhibition of TNF with specific antiserum prevents tissue damage. Peptidoglycan fragments are also toxic for fallopian tube mucosa and may contribute to the intense inflammatory reactions characteristic of gonococcal disease. Gonococci also produce several proteases, peptidases, and phospholipases which may play a role in pathogenesis. In subepithelial tissue, as well as in blood, gonococci presumably interact with serum antibody, including natural IgM antibody directed against LOS antigens, with generation of the chemotactic factor C5a and formation of the bactericidal C5b-C9 attack complex. Insertion of the attack complex into the outer membrane of serum-sensitive gonococci results in gonococcal cell lysis, making antibody to LOS (like antibody to protein I) bactericidal. Although an attack complex is also formed when serum interacts with gonococci characterized by stable serum resistance, insertion of the complex into the outer membrane of the organism has an abnormal configuration which does not result in rapid cell lysis. Furthermore, human serum also appears to contain complement-fixing IgG antibody directed against epitopes on protein III which blocks the bactericidal antibodies directed against other antigens. Protein III has extensive homology to the enterobacterial Omp A protein and the meningococcal class 4 protein. Since Enterobacteriaceae and *N. meningitidis* are both common commensal microorganisms, it is possible that the protein III–blocking antibodies result from prior exposure to cross-reacting proteins from other microbial species.

Oxygen-independent antimicrobial mechanisms contribute significantly to intraleukocytic killing of gonococci following their phagocytosis by neutrophils. Despite effective intraleukocytic killing of gonococci in in vitro assay systems, a small but reproducible number survive. Whether gonococci survive within neutrophils in vivo remains a subject of controversy.

Spread of gonococci from the cervix to the endometrium and salpinges may be enhanced in women using an intrauterine device.

Menstruation further increases the risk of intraluminal ascent from the cervix and also predisposes to gonococcal bacteremia.

CLINICAL MANIFESTATIONS   The clinical spectrum of gonococcal infection depends on the site of inoculation, the duration of infection, the virulence of the infecting strain, and the presence or absence of local or systemic spread of the organism. The influence of inoculum size, variations in host susceptibility, and coinfection with *C. trachomatis* or other genital pathogens on clinical manifestations has not been well-defined.

Gonorrhea in the male   The usual incubation period of gonococcal urethritis ("clap") in the male is 2 to 7 days following exposure, although longer intervals are not infrequent, and some men never develop symptoms. In one study, one auxotype with distinctive nutritional requirements was associated with 96 percent of asymptomatic infections and only 40 percent of symptomatic infections. Symptoms of urethritis include a purulent urethral discharge, usually associated with dysuria, and meatal erythema. Approximately 90 to 95 percent of men who acquire urethral gonococcal infection develop urethral discharge, and most symptomatic men seek treatment and are removed from the infectious pool. The remaining men who never develop symptoms or who ignore their symptoms constitute about two-thirds of the infected men at any point in time, and they serve as the main source of spread of infection to women. Before antibiotic treatment became available, symptoms of urethritis persisted for an average of 8 weeks, and unilateral epididymitis occurred in 5 to 10 percent of untreated men. Epididymitis is now an uncommon complication (see below), and gonococcal prostatitis occurs rarely, if at all. Other local complications of gonococcal urethritis which are now unusual include inguinal lymphadenitis, edema of the penis due to dorsal lymphangitis or thrombophlebitis, submucous inflammatory "soft" infiltration of the urethral wall, periurethral abscess or fistula, unilateral inflammation or abscess of Cowper's gland (which lies between the thumb and forefinger when the forefinger is in the anal canal and the thumb is positioned anteriorly on the perineum), and, rarely, seminal vesiculitis.

In homosexual men, the frequency of gonococcal infection fell by 90 percent or more throughout the United States during the early AIDS era of the 1980s, but a disturbing resurgence of gonorrhea in young homosexual men has been seen in a few cities during the early 1990s. Gonococcal isolates from homosexual men tend to be more resistant to antimicrobials than are isolates from heterosexuals. This may be due to the fact that certain highly susceptible strains are rapidly killed by bile salts and fatty acids in feces and rarely occur in homosexual men, while gonococci possessing a gene for multidrug resistance (*mtr*) are more resistant to bile salts and fatty acids and occur with increased frequency in homosexual men. Rectal infection may be asymptomatic from the outset or may produce anorectal pain, pruritus, tenesmus, and a bloody, mucopurulent rectal discharge. Proctoscopy and appropriate laboratory studies are essential to exclude several other conditions which cause similar symptoms (see Chap. 88). These symptoms may subside without treatment, leaving a chronic asymptomatic carrier state. Pharyngeal gonococcal infection occurs in approximately 20 percent of homosexual men or heterosexual women who engage in fellatio with men who have urethral infection and in a smaller proportion of heterosexual men who engage in cunnilingus. Pharyngeal infection may produce exudative tonsillitis but frequently is asymptomatic; asymptomatic pharyngeal gonococcal infection usually clears spontaneously over several weeks, even without therapy.

Gonorrhea in the female   Acute uncomplicated gonorrhea in the female often causes dysuria, increased vaginal discharge due to exudative endocervicitis, abnormal menstrual bleeding due to endometritis, and anorectal discomfort. While dysuria in young men arouses the suspicion of gonococcal urethritis, the same symptom in a young woman is often automatically attributed to "cystitis." Actually, some of those without bacteriuria have gonococcal or chlamydial infection of the urethra. Young women with dysuria should have a thorough pelvic examination. Compression of the urethra through the anterior vaginal wall against the symphysis pubis may express urethral exudate which can be examined by Gram's stain and culture. Symptomatic young women with "sterile pyuria" (i.e., ≥10 neutrophils per 100× microscopic field in the centrifuged sediment of clean-catch midstream urine; no uropathogens isolated from the urine) should be evaluated for gonococcal and chlamydial infection. Acute symptoms of gonococcal urethritis in the female may subside spontaneously or following subcurative therapy with sulfonamides or urinary antiseptics. The proportion of women with gonorrhea who never develop symptoms is undefined.

Asymptomatic gonococcal infection in the female involves the endocervix, urethra, anal canal, and pharynx, in decreasing order of frequency. Extension of infection from the endocervix to the fallopian tubes occurs in at least 15 percent of women with gonorrhea. This tends to occur soon after acquisition of infection or during menstruation and results in acute endometritis, with abnormal menstrual bleeding and midline low abdominal pain and tenderness, followed by *acute salpingitis*, the major complication of gonorrhea. Coexisting *C. trachomatis* infection may increase the rate of pelvic inflammatory disease (PID). Extension of infection to the pelvis may produce signs of pelvic peritonitis, accompanied by nausea and vomiting, and may lead to pelvic abscess. Early antibiotic treatment, before development of adnexal masses, restores normal tubal function and fertility in nearly all cases of gonococcal salpingitis. However, if prominent adnexal swelling has occurred before treatment is begun, bilateral tubal damage occurs in 15 to 25 percent.

Spread of gonococci or chlamydiae into the upper abdomen may cause *perihepatitis* (Fitz-Hugh–Curtis syndrome), manifested by right upper quadrant or bilateral upper abdominal pain and tenderness and occasionally by a hepatic friction rub.

Acute inflammation of Bartholin's gland is usually unilateral and frequently is due to gonococcal infection. The acutely infected duct is surrounded by a red halo and exudes pus at the posterior third of the labium majus. Occlusion of the duct results in formation of a Bartholin's abscess. Chronic Bartholin cysts are rarely caused by active gonococcal infection.

There is evidence that peripartum endocervical gonococcal infection is associated with premature rupture of membranes, preterm delivery, and postpartum endometritis.

Gonorrhea in children During childbirth, the gonococcus may infect the conjunctivas, pharynx, respiratory tract, or anal canal of the newborn. The risk of infection increases with prolonged rupture of membranes. Prevention of gonococcal ophthalmia by prophylactic use of 1% silver nitrate eyedrops or ophthalmic preparations containing erythromycin or tetracycline is a cost-effective measure in most areas of the world, including the United States. However, with the emergence of TRNG, it is not certain whether ophthalmic tetracycline prophylaxis is effective in preventing neonatal conjunctivitis caused by such strains of *N. gonorrhoeae*. Since neonates and young infants lack bactericidal IgM antibody against *N. gonorrhoeae*, they may be at increased risk for gonococcal bacteremia. During the first year of life, infection of the infant usually results from accidental contamination of the eye or vagina by an adult. Between 1 year of age and puberty, many cases of gonorrhea involve vulvovaginitis in females who have been molested, and medicolegal considerations necessitate a complete bacteriologic diagnosis and child welfare consultation. Auxotyping and serotyping of isolates from the sexual assault victim and accused assailant have been used as evidence in court.

Disseminated gonococcal infection The incidence of disseminated gonococcal infection (DGI) varies with time and place in relation to the local incidence of infection with strains of gonococci that have a propensity to produce bacteremia. Approximately two-thirds of patients with DGI are women, and symptoms of bacteremia often begin during menses. The majority of men and women with gonococcemia do not have symptoms of urogenital, anorectal, or pharyngeal gonococcal infection.

Patients typically present either with symptoms and signs of gonococcemia or with purulent arthritis affecting one or two joints.

The onset of gonococcemia is characterized by fever, polyarthralgias, and papular, petechial, pustular, hemorrhagic, or necrotic skin lesions. Approximately 3 to 20 such lesions appear, usually on the distal extremities. Gonococci are demonstrable by immunofluorescent staining in about two-thirds of gonococcal skin lesions. The initial joint involvement is characteristically limited to tenosynovitis involving several joints asymmetrically. The wrists, fingers, knees, and ankles are most often involved. Circulating immune complexes have been demonstrated at this stage of infection in some studies. Serum complement levels are normal (except in those with complement deficiency), and the role of immune complexes, if any, is uncertain. Without treatment, the duration of gonococcemia is variable; the systemic manifestations of bacteremia may subside spontaneously within a week. Alternatively, septic arthritis ensues, often without prior symptoms of fever, polyarthralgias, or skin lesions. Pain and swelling then increase in one or, very occasionally, more joints, with accumulation of purulent synovial fluid, leading to progressive destruction of the joint if treatment is delayed.

IgM antibody to gonococcal LOS, present in normal human serum, is bactericidal for most strains of gonococci in the presence of complement. Gonococci isolated from patients with DGI have stable resistance to normal human serum. These strains usually contain outer membrane protein IA and are highly susceptible to penicillin. They often require arginine, hypoxanthine, and uracil for growth, and belong to the AHU auxotype. The decline in incidence of such strains in the United States during the past two decades has been associated with a sharp decline in incidences of DGI as well. Patients deficient in complement components C5, C6, C7, and C8 are uniquely susceptible to gonococcemia and meningococcemia because they cannot mount a serum bactericidal response to gonococci or meningococci. Although perhaps 5 percent of patients with a first episode of gonococcemia or meningococcemia are complement-deficient, the porportion is higher among those with recurrent gonococcemia or meningococcemia. Strains isolated from these patients may not be resistant to normal human serum. However, gonococci isolated from DGI patients without complement deficiency are resistant to pooled normal human serum. Isolates from patients with tenosynovitis and skin lesions are even more serum-resistant than are isolates from patients with purulent arthritis, suggesting that the two different DGI syndromes may be determined by characteristics of the causative organism.

The probability of positive blood cultures decreases after 48 h of illness, and the probability of recovery of gonococci from synovial fluid increases with increasing duration of illness. Gonococci are infrequently recovered from early effusions containing less than 20,000 leukocytes per microliter but are usually recovered from effusions containing more than 80,000 leukocytes per microliter. In the individual patient, gonococci are seldom recovered from blood and synovial fluid simultaneously.

Other common manifestations of disseminated gonococcal infection include mild myopericarditis and "toxic" hepatitis. Endocarditis and meningitis are infrequent but severe complications. Endocarditis is suggested by pathologic or changing heart murmurs, major embolic phenomena, severe myocarditis, deterioration of renal function, or an unusually large number of skin lesions.

DIFFERENTIAL DIAGNOSIS Gonococcal infection produces several common clinical syndromes which have multiple etiologies or which mimic other conditions. In particular, the epidemiology and clinical manifestations of *Chlamydia trachomatis* infections closely resemble those of gonococcal infections. The differential diagnosis of urethritis, epididymitis, and proctitis in men; vaginitis and cervicitis in women; and acute arthritis in young adults is discussed in Chap. 88. The differential diagnosis of pelvic inflammatory disease is discussed in Chap. 89.

LABORATORY DIAGNOSIS A presumptive diagnosis of gonorrhea may be made if intracellular gram-negative diplococci are observed in leukocytes on Gram-stained smears of urethral or endocervical exudate. A diagnosis is equivocal if only extracellular or atypical gram-negative diplococci are seen and is negative if no gram-negative diplococci are seen. When these criteria are employed by experienced microbiologists, the sensitivity and specificity of Gram's stain of the urethral exudate approach 100 percent. Presumptive diagnosis of gonorrhea cannot be made on the basis of gram-negative diplococci in pharyngeal smears because other *Neisseria* spp. are normal flora at this site. In areas where resistant gonococci are seen, culture should be performed to allow testing of isolates for antimicrobial resistance. The specificity of Gram's stain of purulent cervical exudate also is high, but the sensitivity is only about 50 percent. Selective media, i.e., Thayer-Martin (TM) medium, modified TM medium, and Martin-Lewis medium, which contain antibiotics to selectively inhibit most other organisms, are most useful for recovering the gonococcus from the urethra, endocervix, and pharynx. Rectal specimens are plated on modified TM medium or equivalent media containing trimethoprim lactate, which suppresses swarming organisms such as *Proteus* spp. The concentration of vancomycin in the selective medium should not exceed 3 μg/mL, and even this concentration may inhibit a small proportion of gonococci. After inoculation, the medium should be placed in a chamber with 70 percent humidity and an atmosphere containing 3 to 10 percent carbon dioxide to permit growth of the gonococcus. This can be accomplished in a candle jar, by generation of carbon dioxide chemically within packets that are sealed after inoculation, or within special CO_2 incubators. Inoculated media should be incubated at 35 to 37°C for 24 to 48 h, and putative gonococcal colonies should be confirmed by oxidase reaction, Gram's stain, and either sugar utilization tests, rapid enzyme tests, nucleic acid probes, or agglutination reactions using antibodies that are specific for *N. gonorrhoeae*. The last four tests are especially important for isolates from the pharynx and rectum, for cultures obtained from populations which have a low prevalence of gonorrhea, such as prenatal patients, and for isolates from victims of rape or sexual child abuse.

In men with incubating or chronic asymptomatic urethral infection without exudate or as a test of cure following treatment, a very thin swab should be inserted 2 cm into the anterior urethra and used to inoculate TM or other selective medium. Cultures of the pharynx and rectum should be obtained from homosexual men with suspected gonorrhea.

The most efficient test for gonorrhea in women is the endocervical culture, which is positive on a single examination in approximately 80 to 90 percent of those with gonorrhea. This diagnostic yield can be increased by performing a second endocervical culture and by performing cultures of the rectum, urethra, and pharynx.

Standard blood culture broth medium (tryptic soy, Columbia, brain-heart infusion) should be used in culturing blood and is also recommended for culturing synovial fluid. The broth should be vented and incubated under increased CO_2 tension. Synovial fluid also can be plated onto chocolate agar rather than a selective medium because it is not likely to be contaminated with commensal bacteria. In pus from skin lesions, *N. gonorrhoeae* is demonstrable by immunofluorescent staining, but this test is seldom performed. Techniques designed to detect gonococcal infection by testing of a single serum for antibody to *N. gonorrhoeae* have been limited by an inability to differentiate antibody due to past gonorrhea from antibody due to current infection and by false-positive tests caused by cross-reactive antibody to *N. meningitidis*. For these reasons, serologic tests for gonorrhea have had a very low predictive value and are not used in clinical practice.

Another diagnostic approach is the detection of gonococcal antigen in urethral or cervical secretion by enzyme-linked immunosorbent assay (ELISA). In men with urethritis, the Gram's stain is just as accurate, quicker, and cheaper. In women, such tests may be an acceptable alternative to culture for diagnosis of endocervical gonococcal infection in settings where culture is not feasible. However, the positive predictive value of antigen detection tests requires careful study, particularly in populations with a low prevalence of gonorrhea. Nucleic acid probes also have been used to detect gonococci in urethral and cervical specimens. However, additional

evaluations are required. The medicolegal and psychosocial implications of a false-positive diagnosis of gonorrhea can be troublesome for both the physician and patient.

TREATMENT Until 1986, the preferred drugs for gonococcal infection were penicillin G, ampicillin or amoxicillin, tetracycline hydrochloride, and spectinomycin. Although long-acting forms of penicillin (such as benzathine penicillin G) are effective in syphilotherapy, they have *no place* in the treatment of gonorrhea. Penicillin V and the isoxazolyl penicillins are not recommended for the treatment of gonococcal infection. Similarly, first-generation cephalosporins are not used for gonorrhea. In 1986, the Centers for Disease Control published new guidelines for treatment of gonorrhea. These 1986 guidelines, which are presented in this chapter but modified by the authors to include newer, single-dose oral regimens which appear to be highly effective alternatives, are based on several observations: the importance of single-dose efficacy; the increasing proportion of infections due to antibiotic-resistant strains of *N. gonorrhoeae*, including PPNG, TRNG, and strains with chromosomally mediated resistance to multiple antimicrobials; the high frequency of coexisting chlamydial infections in persons with gonorrhea; the absence of a cheap, rapid test for chlamydial infection; and the severity of complications of gonococcal and chlamydial infections. The guidelines do not represent a comprehensive list of all possible treatment regimens. As is shown in Table 110-1, a regimen combining a single intramuscular 125-mg dose of ceftriaxone, together with a 7-day course of tetracycline or doxycycline, is recommended for uncomplicated urethral, endocervical, rectal, or pharyngeal gonococcal infections in heterosexual adults. This combination regimen can be expected to provide adequate therapy for gonorrhea at any site and

TABLE 110-1   Recommended treatment for gonococcal infection

Diagnosis	Treatment of choice
Uncomplicated urethral, endocervical, rectal, or pharyngeal infection	Ceftriaxone, 125 mg single IM dose *plus* Doxycycline, 100 mg PO twice daily for 7 days.
Treatment failure	True treatment failure with the above regimen has so far occurred rarely, if ever. Evaluate for reinfection, alternative diagnosis.
Alternative regimens (all given with 7 days of doxycycline)	Cefixime, 400 mg single oral dose Ofloxacin, 400 mg single oral dose Spectinomycin, 2 g single IM dose Ciprofloxacin, 500 mg single oral dose
Gonorrhea in pregnancy	Ceftriaxone, 125 mg single IM dose *plus* Erythromycin base 500 mg PO four times daily for 7 days. Equivalent dose of erythromycin stearate (500 mg) or ethylsuccinate (800 mg) can be used.
Disseminated gonococcal infection (DGI)	Hospitalization is recommended. Ceftriaxone, 1 g IM or IV every 24 h *or* Ceftizoxime, 1 g IV every 8 h *or* Cefotaxime, 1 g IV every 8 h (see text for duration of inpatient and subsequent ambulatory therapy).
Gonococcal PID	Hospitalization is recommended. See Chap. 89 for recommended therapy.
Gonococcal epididymitis	See Chap. 88.
Pediatric gonococcal infections Infants	Ceftriaxone, 25–50 mg/kg once daily *or* Cefotaxime, 25 mg/kg twice daily. Usual duration of therapy is 7 days (longer for meningitis or endocarditis).
Children	Children who weigh 100 lb (45 kg) should receive adult doses; for those weighing less, see text.

will eliminate coexisting *C. trachomatis* infections. Tetracycline hydrochloride, 500 mg orally four times daily, can be substituted for doxycycline. Pregnant women and those unable to tolerate doxycycline or tetracycline can instead be given erythromycin base or stearate, 500 mg by mouth four times daily for 7 days, or erythromycin ethylsuccinate, 800 mg by mouth four times daily for 7 days, to accompany the ceftriaxone. All tetracyclines are ineffective as single-dose therapy for gonorrhea, and even a 7-day course of tetracycline has been ineffective in a growing proportion of patients owing to the spread of TRNG and the high proportion of strains with chromosomal resistance to tetracycline. Ceftriaxone can be prepared in 1% lidocaine as diluent (for intramuscular injection only) to reduce discomfort due to the injection. Other intramuscular β-lactam antibiotics (cefotaxime, cefuroxime, ceftizoxime) are also very effective for resistant gonorrhea, but the long half-life of ceftriaxone, together with its in vitro activity, makes it the optimal drug for single-dose therapy of gonorrhea. For patients who cannot take ceftriaxone, the preferred alternative is spectinomycin, 2 g intramuscularly as a single dose. Although spectinomycin resistance has emerged where that drug was used commonly for gonorrhea (e.g., in England and Korea), it has been rare in the United States. Other convenient alternatives to ceftriaxone for uncomplicated urethral, endocervical, or rectal gonorrhea include cefixime, given as a single 400-mg oral dose, ofloxacin, as a 400-mg single oral dose, or ciprofloxacin, in a 500-mg single oral dose. Although the fluoroquinolones ofloxacin and ciprofloxacin remain highly effective for gonorrhea, lessened gonococcal susceptibility to these drugs has been seen in Asia and recently in England, Canada, and the United States.

All patients with gonorrhea should have a serologic test for syphilis at the time of diagnosis and should be offered confidential testing for human immunodeficiency virus (HIV). Patients with incubating seronegative syphilis, without clinical signs of syphilis, are likely to be cured of syphilis by the recommended ceftriaxone-doxycycline regimen. However, patients with gonorrhea who also have syphilis or who are established contacts of someone with syphilis should be given additional treatment appropriate to the stage of syphilis (see Chap. 133).

Follow-up and treatment failure Treatment failure following combined ceftriaxone-doxycycline therapy is exceedingly rare; therefore, a follow-up culture is not essential. Patients should be advised to return for reexamination if any symptoms persist or recur after completion of treatment. Persistent or recurrent symptoms or signs after treatment for gonorrhea should be evaluated by culture for *N. gonorrhoeae* and a specific test for chlamydial infection. Any gonococcal isolate should be tested for antibiotic susceptibility. Additional treatment for persistent or recurrent gonorrhea should be with ceftriaxone, 250 mg intramuscularly, or with spectinomycin, 2.0 g intramuscularly (except in areas where spectinomycin resistance is a problem). Recurrent gonococcal infections after treatment with the recommended schedule are almost certainly due to reinfection, and indicate a need for improved sex partner referral and patient education.

Postgonococcal urethritis (PGU) usually becomes apparent about 2 to 3 weeks after treatment of gonorrhea with a penicillin or a cephalosporin. PGU often is caused by *C. trachomatis* which may have been acquired at the same time as gonorrhea but did not become clinically apparent until later because of the longer incubation period of chlamydial infection. When PGU occurs, it can be managed, like nongonococcal urethritis, with doxycycline, 100 mg orally twice daily, or tetracycline, 0.5 g four times a day, for 7 days. Similarly, mucopurulent cervicitis in women which often persists or appears after treatment of gonorrhea with cephalosporin, penicillin, or spectinomycin is often caused by *C. trachomatis* and can be treated like PGU. Men and women exposed to gonorrhea should be examined, cultured, and treated with one of the recommended treatment schedules.

All pregnant women should be cultured for *N. gonorrhoeae* (and tested for *C. trachomatis* infection and syphilis) at the time of the first visit as an integral part of the prenatal care. A second culture late in the third trimester (as well as tests for chlamydial infection and syphilis) should be obtained from women at high risk of sexually transmitted disease.

The regimen of choice for gonorrhea in pregnancy is ceftriaxone, in a single 125-mg intramuscular dose, plus erythromycin for a possible coexisting chlamydial infection. Pregnant women allergic to β-lactams can be treated with a single dose of spectinomycin, 2.0 g intramuscularly, plus erythromycin. Doxycycline and tetracycline should not be used in pregnant women because of potential toxic effects for mother and fetus.

The management of pelvic inflammatory disease is discussed in Chap. 89.

Treatment of gonococcal arthritis can be accomplished satisfactorily with several regimens. Gonococci recovered from patients with gonococcal arthritis have been significantly less resistant to penicillin or tetracycline than isolates from patients with uncomplicated gonorrhea. However, several cases of DGI caused by PPNG have been reported. Because of the threat of endocarditis, meningitis, and joint sepsis, all patients with disseminated infection should be hospitalized and treated with ceftriaxone intravenously, 1 g once a day, or with the alternatives listed in Table 110-1. Reliable patients without endocarditis or meningitis can be discharged 24 to 48 h after symptoms resolve, to complete a total of 7 to 10 days' therapy with an oral regimen of cefixime, 400 mg twice a day. If the infecting gonococcus is shown to be penicillin-sensitive, treatment can be completed with oral amoxicillin, 500 mg three times a day, without clavulanic acid. Failure to improve with appropriate antimicrobial regimens as listed above strongly suggests a diagnosis other than disseminated gonococcal infection. Repeated joint aspiration or closed irrigation of the joint with sterile saline may be required to reduce inflammation in patients with high synovial fluid leukocyte counts. Open drainage is seldom, if ever, required for gonococcal arthritis, except in infants with hip infection. Temporary immobilization of the joint may reduce discomfort and may be useful during initial ambulation in patients with persistent effusions of the knee or ankle. Antibiotics should not be injected directly into the joint. Once the diagnosis of gonococcal arthritis is proven, then occasional patients may benefit from use of anti-inflammatory agents along with antimicrobial therapy. However, if the diagnosis is suspected, but not proven, then early use of anti-inflammatory drugs will prevent monitoring the response to antimicrobial therapy, which is usually rapid and often of diagnostic importance in gonococcal arthritis.

Meningitis and endocarditis caused by the gonococcus require high-dose intravenous therapy with an agent effective against the strain causing the disease: ceftriaxone, 1 g intravenously every 12 h, for 10 to 14 days for meningitis and for 1 month for endocarditis. Patients with gonococcal endocarditis or meningitis, and perhaps all patients with DGI, should be evaluated for complement deficiency.

Gonococcal conjunctivitis in the adult or in children over 20 kg should be managed as a medical emergency by irrigation of the conjunctiva with saline, together with ceftriaxone, 1 g in a single intramuscular dose. All patients must have careful ophthalmologic evaluation, including slit-lamp examination.

Pediatric gonococcal infection The infant born to a mother with gonorrhea is at high risk of infection and requires prophylactic treatment with a single injection of ceftriaxone, 50 mg/kg intravenously or intramuscularly, not to exceed 125 mg. Ceftriaxone should be given with caution to hyperbilirubinemic infants, especially premature babies. Topical prophylaxis for neonatal ophthalmia is not adequate treatment for infections at other sites. Infants with gonococcal infection at any site (e.g., eye) should be evaluated for DGI by examination and culture of blood and CSF. They should be treated for 7 days with ceftriaxone, 25 to 50 mg/kg in a single daily intravenous or intramuscular dose. Alternatively, cefotaxime can be used in a dose of 25 mg/kg twice daily intravenously. Limited data suggest that uncomplicated gonococcal ophthalmia in the infant can be cured with a single injection of ceftriaxone, 50 mg/kg, up to a dose of 125 mg. Irrigation of the eyes with saline or buffered ophthalmic solutions should be performed immediately and then repeated as often as necessary to eliminate discharge. Topical antibiotic preparations alone are not sufficient or required when appropriate systemic antibiotic therapy is given. Both the parents of a newborn with gonococcal ophthalmia must be treated for gonorrhea. The parents and infant also should be tested for chlamydial infection.

Children who weigh 45 kg or more should be treated with adult regimens. Children who weigh less than 45 kg should be treated as follows: For uncomplicated vulvovaginitis, cervicitis, urethritis, proctitis, and pharyngitis, the recommended treatment is ceftriaxone, a single 125-mg intramuscular dose. The alternative regimen is spectinomycin, a single 40-mg/kg intramuscular dose. Children 8 years of age or older can, in addition, be given doxycycline, 100 mg twice a day for 7 days. Children with gonorrhea should be evaluated for coexisting syphilis and chlamydial infection.

Topical and/or systemic estrogen therapy is of no benefit in gonococcal vulvovaginitis. All children should have follow-up cultures, and the source of infection should be identified, examined, and treated. Child abuse should be carefully considered and evaluated. For treatment of complicated disease, the alternative regimens recommended for adults may be used in appropriate pediatric dosages.

Treatment of gonorrhea in developing countries The proportion of gonococcal infections caused by PPNG, TRNG, or CMRNG is highest in developing countries, which can least afford ceftriaxone, spectinomycin, or other new antimicrobials effective against these strains. Inexpensive alternatives to penicillin G and tetracycline, the traditional mainstays of gonorrhea therapy, have been disappointing. For example, a sulfonamide-trimethoprim combination which initially cured over 95 percent of cases of gonorrhea in African countries fell to less than 75 percent efficacy within 2 years after it became a popular regimen in Kenya. One approach has been the use of 4.8 million units of procaine penicillin G intramuscularly plus 1.0 g probenecid orally (a standard regimen for non-PPNG infections) together with 125 mg of clavulanic acid (in the form of one capsule of amoxicillin-clavulanate) to inhibit gonococcal β-lactamase. This inexpensive regimen has been effective in small trials in Kenya, even against PPNG infections. Gentamicin, in a single 280-mg intramuscular dose, also has been used effectively in this setting. Newer cephalosporins in lower than recommended doses, to reduce cost, should be discouraged. Norfloxacin, ciprofloxacin, and ofloxacin are increasingly prescribed or dispensed without prescription for urethritis in developing countries. None of these drugs is effective as a single-dose regimen for chlamydial urethritis, and the impact of increased fluoroquinolone use on gonococcal resistance to the quinolones remains to be assessed. There is a growing need for clinical trials with less expensive regimens and for ongoing surveillance of in vitro sensitivity of *N. gonorrhoeae*.

PREVENTION AND CONTROL There is probably no more striking illustration than gonorrhea of the failure of a specific treatment alone to eradicate a communicable disease. Vaccination is not available. A field trial of a purified gonococcal pili vaccine in U.S. soldiers in Korea showed that the vaccine was not effective. Use of the condom can prevent transmission, and the extensive use of condoms for contraception may be responsible for the low rates of gonorrhea in some countries (e.g., Japan). Spermicidal preparations used with a diaphragm or cervical sponges impregnated with nonoxynol-9 probably offer some protection against gonorrhea and chlamydial infection. Prophylactic antibiotics (e.g., 200 mg minocycline or doxycycline taken soon after sexual exposure) reduce the risk of infection but are not recommended for general use or for individuals with known exposure to gonorrhea, who should receive one of the regimens recommended for established gonorrhea.

To contain the increasing spread of antimicrobial-resistant gonococci, several measures are important: (1) routine use of diagnosis by cultures and testing of isolates for antimicrobial resistance or β-lactamase production, (2) routine use of highly effective antibiotics, such as ceftriaxone, to prevent gonorrhea treatment failures, and (3)

rapid identification and treatment of sexual partners of patients with gonorrhea, particularly partners of those with recurrent infection and those known to be infected with resistant gonococci. One of the most effective public health measures now available for control of gonorrhea is treatment of sexual partners of infected patients. In addition, public health education and individual patient counseling are essential to promote fewer sexual partners, condom use during casual sexual encounters, and early health care for symptoms of urethritis or unusual vaginal discharge, with or without lower abdominal pain.

REFERENCES

Boslego JW et al: Effect of spectinomycin use on the prevalence of spectinomycin resistant and of penicillinase-producing *Neisseria gonorrhoeae*. N Engl J Med 317:272, 1987

Britigan BE, Sparling PF: Gonococcal infection: A model of molecular pathogenesis. N Engl J Med 312:1683, 1985

Centers for Disease Control: 1989 Sexually transmitted diseases treatment guidelines. Morb Mort Week Rep 38(Suppl 8):1, 1989

———: Policy guidelines for the detection, management, and control of antibiotic resistant strains of *Neisseria gonorrhoeae*. Morb Mort Week Rep 36(5S):1, 1987

Cohen MS, Sparling PF: Mucosal infection with *Neisseria gonorrhoeae*. Bacterial adaptation and mucosal defenses. J Clin Invest 89:1699, 1992

Handsfield HH et al: Localized outbreak of penicillinase-producing *Neisseria gonorrhoeae:* Paradigm for introduction and spread of gonorrhea in a community. JAMA 261:2357, 1989

——— et al: A comparison of single-dose cefixime with ceftriaxone as treatment for uncomplicated gonorrhea. N Engl J Med 325:1337, 1991

Knapp JS et al: Serologic classification of *Neisseria gonorrhoeae* using monoclonal antibodies directed against outer membrane protein I. J Infect Dis 150:44, 1985

Mandrell RE et al: In vitro and in vivo modification of *Neisseria gonorrhoeae* lipooligosaccharide epitope structure by sialylation. J Exp Med 171:1649, 1990

Morse SA et al: High-level tetracycline resistance in *Neisseria gonorrhoeae* is result of acquisition of streptococcal *tetM* determinant. Antimicrob Agents Chemother 30:664, 1986

——— (eds): Perspectives on pathogenic *Neisseria* spp. Clin Microb Rev 2:1S, 1989

Rice PA et al: Immunoglobulin G antibodies directed against protein III block killing of serum-resistant *Neisseria gonorrhoeae* by immune serum. J Exp Med 164:1735, 1986

Rice R et al: Sociodemographic distribution of gonorrhea incidence: Implications for prevention and behavioral research. Am J Public Health, 81:1252, 1991

Schwarcz SK et al: National surveillance of antimicrobial resistance in *Neisseria gonorrhoeae*: The Gonococcal Isolate Surveillance Project. JAMA 264:1413, 1990

Sparling PF: Biology of *Neisseria gonorrhoeae*, in *Sexually Transmitted Diseases*, 2d ed, KK Holmes et al (eds). New York, McGraw-Hill, 1990, pp 131–147

van Putten JPM: Iron acquisition and the pathogenesis of meningococcal and gonococcal disease. Med Microbiol Immunol 179:289, 1990

111 MORAXELLA (BRANHAMELLA) CATARRHALIS, OTHER MORAXELLA SPECIES, AND KINGELLA

DANIEL M. MUSHER

MORAXELLA (BRANHAMELLA) CATARRHALIS

This gram-negative coccus has undergone three changes of name in as many decades. Originally called *Micrococcus catarrhalis*, it was renamed *Neisseria catarrhalis* in the 1960s because of its morphologic similarity to *Neisseria* species, and then, in 1970, it was given status as a distinct genus, *Branhamella*, on the basis of DNA homology. In 1979 this organism was placed into the genus *Moraxella*, although many authorities continue to call it *Moraxella (Branhamella) catarrhalis*. A component of normal bacterial flora of the upper airways, *M. catarrhalis* has been increasingly recognized as a cause of otitis media, sinusitis, and bronchopulmonary infection.

BACTERIOLOGY AND IMMUNITY On Gram's stain, *M. catarrhalis* appears as large round cocci that tend to retain crystal violet during the decolorizing step and occasionally are confused with *Staphylococcus aureus*. Colonies grow well on blood or chocolate agar and are readily distinguishable from *Neisseria* species by biochemical tests.

Unlike many other pathogenic bacteria, *M. catarrhalis* shows a surprising degree of homogeneity of outer-membrane proteins. Antibody to certain of these proteins is generally present in serum of children over the age of 4 years; however, isolates that cause disease are generally serum resistant; i.e., they survive in serum despite this naturally present antibody and complement. Bactericidal antibody emerges following natural infection and may be directed against one or more conserved outer-membrane proteins, a property of potential value in vaccine development.

EPIDEMIOLOGY With use of selective media, *M. catarrhalis* can be isolated from the upper respiratory tract or saliva of 50 percent of healthy school children and from the nasopharynx of up to 7 percent of healthy adults. The rate of nasopharyngeal colonization increases to 86 percent in children who have otitis media. Investigators in both the Northern and Southern Hemispheres have reported a striking seasonal variation in the isolation of this organism from clinical specimens, with a peak in late winter/early spring and a nadir in late summer/early fall. Direct contact has not been shown to contribute to community-acquired infection, but nosocomial spread of infection has rarely been documented.

OTITIS MEDIA, SINUSITIS *M. catarrhalis* has repeatedly been shown to be the third most common bacterial isolate from middle ear fluid of children who have otitis media, following *Streptococcus penumoniae* and nontypable *Haemophilus influenzae*. Recent studies also show this organism to be a prominent isolate from sinus cavities in acute and chronic sinusitis.

PURULENT TRACHEOBRONCHITIS, PNEUMONIA *M. catarrhalis* causes acute exacerbations of chronic bronchitis (increased production and/or purulence of sputum), purulent tracheobronchitis (above, plus fever and leukocytosis), and pneumonia. The great majority of infected persons are greater than 50 years of age with a long history of cigarette smoking and underlying chronic obstructive pulmonary disease (COPD); lung cancer is often present as well. In one recent study, 76 percent of affected persons had COPD (often severe), together with lung cancer in one-third of cases; most patients also had clinical evidence of malnutrition. In one extensive series of cases, *Branhamella* pneumonia was not discovered in an otherwise healthy host.

Symptoms of patients with *M. catarrhalis* pneumonia have been regarded as modest in severity, perhaps due more to a diminished febrile response because of the advanced age of the affected individuals than to any lack of pathogenic capacity of this organism. Cough usually is increased, as are the amount and purulence of the sputum, but these symptoms may not be noticeably increased above baseline. Chills are present in one-quarter of patients, pleuritic pain in one-third, and malaise in 40 percent. The majority of patients have peak temperatures < 101°F (38.3°C), and peripheral white blood cell counts are < 10,000 per cubic millimeter in nearly one-quarter of cases. Microscopic examination of a good sputum specimen following Gram's stain regularly reveals profuse numbers of organisms (approximately 2×10^8 colony forming units per milliliter). A variable radiologic appearance is seen; in one study, 43 percent of subjects had segmental or lobar infiltrates, and the remainder had a mixed pattern of subsegmental, segmental, interstitial, and diffuse involvement. These clinical, laboratory, and radiographic findings do not differ from those of pneumococcal pneumonia in an older patient population. By comparison with pneumococcal infection, however, a far lesser degree of bloodstream invasion is apparent; in one series, none of 25 patients with *M. catarrhalis* pneumonia had bacteremia. Nevertheless, *Branhamella* pneumonia is a marker for severe underlying disease in that nearly one-half of patients die within 3 months of onset.

OTHER SYNDROMES Local extension causing empyema is very uncommon, and as might be inferred from the low rate of bacteremia,

metastatic complications of *Branhamella* pneumonia such as septic arthritis are exceedingly rare. As of 1990, 27 cases of bacteremic infection due to *M. catarrhalis* had been reported, mainly in children less than 10 years or adults more than 60 years of age; most occurred in immunocompromised patients. Syndromes have included bacteremia with no apparent focus, endocarditis, and meningitis. A petechial or purpuric rash, reminiscent of that observed in meningococcal sepsis and associated with disseminated intravascular coagulation, has been described in a few cases, nearly all in children.

TREATMENT Treatment of presumed *M. catarrhalis* infection with a penicillin–clavulanic acid combination seems highly appropriate. Penicillin resistance first appeared in *Branhamella* isolates in the mid-1970s but is now found in 85 percent of clinical isolates. Resistance is mediated by two closely related β-lactamases, BRO-1 and BRO-2 (acronyms derived from *Branhamella* and *Moraxella*) that are present in 90 and 10 percent, respectively, of resistant isolates. These enzymes are active against penicillin, ampicillin, and amoxicillin but less so against cephalosporins, especially third-generation cephalosporins, and they bind avidly to clavulanic acid and sulbactam.

Cephalosporins, especially of the second and third generations, are effective alternatives. A 5-day course of therapy has been shown to cure respiratory infection, although a slightly longer course may be required in sinusitis. Isolates in the United States are nearly uniformly susceptible to tetracycline, erythromycin, and chloramphenicol, although tetracycline resistance, perhaps due to Tet B determinants, is increasing in Europe and Asia and has been documented in two isolates in the United States. *M. catarrhalis* is also susceptible to trimethoprim-sulfamethoxazole and to quinolones.

After the identification of gram-negative cocci in a Gram-stained specimen and pending final identification by culture, the severity of the condition and the potential presence of other infecting organisms should dictate antibiotic selection. For example, an exacerbation of bronchitis caused by *Branhamella* might be treated with tetracycline or trimethoprim-sulfamethoxazole, but in a patient with pneumonia, the possibility that pneumococci resistant to these agents also might be present dictates the choice of ampicillin sulbactam, at least until results of culture are available.

MORAXELLA

Moraxella species cause a wide range of infections, including bronchitis, pneumonia, empyema, endocarditis, meningitis, conjunctivitis, urinary infection, septic arthritis, and wound infection. In a report of all *Moraxella* isolates submitted to the Centers for Disease Control (CDC) between 1953 to 1980, certain clinical associations were apparent (Table 111-1). *M. osloensis* and *M. nonliquefaciens* were the most commonly isolated species, emanating from a wide range of body sites including blood, cerebrospinal fluid, and joints. *M. osloensis* was the *Moraxella* species most commonly isolated from blood; *M. nonliquefaciens* tended to be isolated from the ears, nose, or throat (47 percent) or sputum (8 percent). *Moraxella* M-5 (an as yet unnamed group) had a striking association with infected wounds from dog bites (72 percent of all isolates), whereas *M. lacunata* was associated with conjunctivitis and keratitis (70 percent of isolates). *M. urethralis* was isolated most often from urine and the genital tract and is probably the *Moraxella* species that had previously been implicated in urethritis. More than one-half of isolates of *M. phenylpyruvica* and *M. atlantis* were obtained from normally sterile sites. The clinical features of such infections and the nature of the hosts in which they occur are not fully characterized.

KINGELLA

Kingella kingae was originally *Moraxella* new species 1 (M-1) and was subsequently named in honor of Dr. Elizabeth King of the CDC,

TABLE 111-1   *Moraxella* species and *Kingella*

Species	Number of isolates	Common sites/ clinical association	Number (percent) for each site
M. osloensis	199	Blood	44 (22)
		CSF	18 (9)
		Urine	17 (9)
		Respiratory tract	24 (12)
M. nonliquefaciens	356	Blood	27 (8)
		CSF	6 (2)
		Respiratory tract	196 (55)
M-5	74	Dog bite wound	53 (72)
M-6	47	Blood, bone	15 (32)
M. lacunata	33	Conjunctivitis, keratitis	23 (70)
M. urethralis	28	Urine	16 (57)
		Genital tract	3 (11)
M. phenylpyruvica	73	Blood	19 (26)
		CSF	8 (11)
		Urine	12 (16)
M. atlantis	44	Blood	20 (45)
		CSF	5 (11)
Kingella kingae	79	Blood	38 (48)
		Joint	10 (13)
		Bone	11 (14)

SOURCE: Taken from a summary of CDC experience (Graham et al, Rev Infect Dis 12:423, 1990).

who first described it. A fastidious organism, *K. kingae* has been found to cause endocarditis, arthritis, and osteomyelitis (see Table 111-1); isolated instances of other infections have been recorded. Most bone and joint infections occur in young children. The failure to implicate this organism more frequently as a cause of pneumonia may indicate true tissue tropism for heart valve, bones, and joints, or it may reflect the difficulty in separating *Kingella* from normal respiratory flora on sputum culture.

Most moraxellae and kingellae remain susceptible to penicillins, cephalosporins, tetracyclines, and chloramphenicol, but some strains of *Moraxella* produce BRO β-lactamases, and clinical specimens must be tested for lactamase production and antibiotic susceptibility. Initial therapy with a penicillin or cephalosporin is reasonable pending susceptibility testing.

REFERENCES

CATLIN BW: *Branhamella catarrhalis:* An organism gaining respect as a pathogen. Clin Microbiol Rev 3:293, 1990

DEGROOT R et al: Bone and joint infections caused by *Kingella kingae:* Six cases and review of the literature. Rev Infect Dis 10:998, 1988

GRAHAM D et al: Infections caused by *Moraxella, Moraxella urethralis, Moraxella*-like groups M-5 and M-6, and *Kingella kingae* in the United States, 1953–1980. Rev Infect Dis 12:423, 1990

HAGER H et al: *Branhamella catarrhalis* respiratory infections. Rev Infect Dis 9:1140, 1987

MORRISON VA, WAGNER KF: Clinical manifestations of *Kingella kingae* infections: Case report and review. Rev Infect Dis 11:776, 1989

NASH DR et al: Comparison of the activity of cefixime and activities of other oral antibiotics against adult clinical isolates of *Moraxella (Branhamella) catarrhalis* containing BRO-1 and BRO-2 and *Haemophilus influenzae.* Antimicrob Agents Chemother 35:192, 1991

VERGHESE A, BERK SL: *Moraxella (Branhamella) catarrhalis.* Infect Dis Clin North Am 5:523, 1991

WALLACE RJ JR et al: Antibiotic susceptibiolities and drug resistance in *Moraxella (Branhamella) catarrhalis.* Am J Med 88(suppl 5A), 1990

WRIGHT PW et al: A descriptive study of 42 cases of *Branhamella catarrhalis* pneumonia. Am J Med 88(suppl 5A):5A, 1990

112   INFECTIONS DUE TO *HAEMOPHILUS INFLUENZAE,* HACEK GROUP, *CAPNOCYTOPHAGA,* AND *H. DUCREYI*

MICHAEL A. APICELLA

HAEMOPHILUS INFLUENZAE INFECTIONS   The species *H. influenzae* encompasses a group of pleomorphic gram-negative human pathogens whose sole ecologic niche is the human environment. When visualized by Gram's stain directly from biologic specimens (CSF or sputum), these organisms can appear coccobacillary with deeply staining polar bodies that cause misidentification as gram-positive cocci. *H. influenzae* is not a fastidious species and can be recovered readily from clinical specimens. However, it has an absolute growth requirement for hemin (factor X) and/or nicotinamide adenine dinucleotide (factor V). These factors can be supplied by direct addition to the medium. Factor V is heat labile and must be added to the media after autoclaving. Hemin can be supplied from the autoclaved hemoglobin of lysed erythrocytes as in chocolate media. Factor V is produced by certain bacteria such as *Staphylococcus aureus. H. influenzae* will grow around a staphylococcal streak on routine blood agar. This is a useful means of identifying factor V– requiring *Haemophilus* organisms. Species of *Haemophilus* that do not require factor X are designated by the *para* prefix (*H. parainfluenzae*).

There are six capsular serotypes of *H. influenzae*, a to f. *H. influenzae* serotype b (Hib) is the capsular serotype most frequently involved in human disease. Encapsulation is best detected by counter-immunoelectrophoresis of extracts prepared from organisms. Alternatively, agglutination can be used to determine capsular type. Genetic analyses indicate that Hib strains are clonally related. Unencapsulated *H. influenzae* strains are termed *nontypable H. influenzae* (NTHi). Unlike Hib strains, NTHi strains have wide genetic and antigenic diversity.

Pathogenesis   *H. influenzae* is part of the normal flora of the upper respiratory tract. The mechanism by which it invades the mucosal surface has been studied in human adenoidal organ culture models. Some mucosal pathogens such as *Neisseria gonorrhoeae, N. meningitidis,* and strains of *H. influenzae* biogroup *aegyptius* cross the mucosal barrier through nonciliated epithelial cells. In contrast, most *H. influenzae* move across by passing between rather than through cells.

The capsular polysaccharide of Hib strains, which is a polymer of ribosyl-ribitol phosphate, acts as an antiphagocytic barrier and is an important virulence factor. *H. influenzae* has a potent endotoxin (LPS) that can act systemically to induce CSF inflammation and signs associated with sepsis. Locally LPS can damage mucosal cells in the respiratory tract during middle ear infection and acute bronchitis. *H. influenzae* strains express pili which are probably important because of their ability to colonize the respiratory mucosal surface. The outer membrane proteins have been well defined, and antibodies to several (P2, P4, and P6) have been shown to be protective in experimental animals, suggesting that they may be useful as future human vaccines.

NTHi strains primarily cause disease by damaging the respiratory mucosal epithelial cell surface. The factors associated with invasiveness of *H. influenzae* biogroup *aegyptius* have not been identified. Its members are not encapsulated but contain LPS and outer membrane proteins similar to other NTHi strains.

Epidemiology   Vaccines composed of Hib polyribosyl-ribitol phosphate (PRP) capsule, chemically conjugated to modified diphtheria toxoid, tetanus toxoid, or proteosomes, have greatly reduced the incidence of Hib infections in infants below the age of 6 months since their use in the United States beginning in 1991. Before introduction of these vaccines, approximately 10,000 cases of Hib meningitis occurred per year in the United States in children below the age of 2. In regions of the world where this vaccine is not being utilized, the yearly incidence of Hib meningitis still ranges between 20 and 50 cases per 100,000 children between 6 months and 2 years of age.

H. influenzae infections also cause morbidity and mortality in adults. In one study in Atlanta, invasive *H. influenzae* infections in adults had an annual incidence of 5.6 cases per 100,000 population. Over 75 percent of the patients (representing 70 percent of the cases) were women with bacteremic pneumonia and most of them had underlying conditions, such as chronic lung disease. Other risk factors include pregnancy, HIV infection, and malignancy. Overall the mortality in adults was 28 percent, and more than half of the pregnancy-related infections resulted in fetal death. Approximately one half of the strains isolated from invasive *H. influenzae* infections in adults were nontypable.

Clinical aspects PNEUMONIA AND TRACHEOBRONCHITIS *H. influenzae* is an important cause of community-acquired bacterial pneumonia in adults. NTHi strains account for over 80 percent of these infections. The patients are generally elderly and have chronic lung disease or a long smoking history. Patients with HIV infection are also susceptible to serious respiratory infection by Hib and NTHi and appear to have an increased incidence of bacteremia. The clinical features of pneumonia caused by *H. influenzae* are indistinguishable from those of other bacterial pneumonias; fever, cough, and purulent sputum, usually of several days' duration. Chest radiographs show either lobar or patchy infiltrate and are not specific.

NTHi may play a role in acute exacerbations of chronic bronchitis in patients with obstructive lung disease. However, the organism can be found in serial cultures of sputum in the majority of patients with chronic bronchitis during quiescent periods so that the mere presence of the organism does not imply a pathogenic role in this setting. Nevertheless, the isolation of NTHi from sputum during exacerbations, the development of serum antibodies to NTHi after exacerbations, and the response of patients to antibiotics suggest that NTHi is the etiologic agent in many acute exacerbations of chronic bronchitis.

MENINGITIS AND SEPSIS *H. influenzae* is the most common cause of meningitis in children between the ages of 2 months and 2 years, with 95 percent of these cases attributable to Hib. As mentioned above, the introduction of the PRP Hib capsule vaccine in 1991 has reduced the incidence of Hib meningitis. In adults, *H. influenzae* is a relatively uncommon cause of meningitis, and approximately 50 percent of the isolates are NTHi. In children, spread to the meninges is hematogenous after invasion of the organism across the nasopharyngeal barrier. In young children, Hib is the leading cause of septic arthritis which is frequently associated with sepsis. Hib cellulitis with sepsis is also a cause of serious morbidity and mortality in this age group. In adults, infection commonly spreads to the meninges from a contiguous site, an infected sinus, CNS trauma with a CSF leak, or a middle ear infection. Since the upper respiratory tract is frequently colonized, NTHi is the second most common cause (after *Pneumococcus*) of recurrent meningitis. The clinical presentation of meningitis due to Hib and NTHi is otherwise no different from that due to other bacterial pathogens.

H. influenzae biogroup *aegyptius* is the cause of Brazilian purpuric fever, a serious systemic illness of children that begins with purulent conjunctivitis and is characterized by fever, petechiae, purpura, and shock.

OTITIS MEDIA AND SINUSITIS NTHi strains are responsible for 20 to 40 percent of bacteriologically confirmed cases of otitis media in children. It is the most common illness during early childhood; some 60 to 70 percent of children experience one to three ear infections before the age of 2 years.

OBSTETRIC AND NEONATAL INFECTIONS Obstetric infections due to *H. influenzae* are a serious complication of pregnancy as both the mother and the child become infected and there appears to be maternal-fetal transmission of the organism. The isolates are almost invariably NTHi. Symptoms in mother and child occur within 24 h of birth, and there is a high frequency of prematurity. Infant mortality is high.

ADULT EPIGLOTTITIS *H. influenzae* is an important cause of adult epiglottitis. In one large review, the incidence of acute epiglottitis in adults was 9.7 cases per million population. The average age was 44 years with an equal sex distribution. Patients presented with an elevated temperature, sore throat (90 percent), dysphagia (80 percent), respiratory difficulty (45 percent), and hoarseness or drooling. Visualization by indirect laryngoscopy of an inflamed epiglottis has proven to be more reliable in making the diagnosis (positive in 86 percent of cases) than by soft-tissue x-rays of the neck. Laryngoscopy can induce laryngospasm, particularly in children, and clinicians should be prepared to maintain the airway with tracheostomy when this procedure is performed. Mortality is 7 percent, with all deaths related to airway obstruction. It has been suggested that an airway should be established at the time of presentation rather than waiting for a worsening clinical picture. Antibiotic therapy of epiglottitis in adults is primarily directed against *H. influenzae*, group A streptococci, and pneumococci.

OTHER INFECTIONS Less common manifestations of *H. influenzae* infection in adults include empyema, pericarditis, osteomyelitis, endocarditis, cholecystitis, intraabdominal infections, urinary tract infections, mastoiditis, and aortic graft infection.

Management of *H. influenzae* infections Resistance has become more prevalent among isolates. It varies, but overall 10 to 20 percent of *H. influenzae* strains exhibit β-lactamase-mediated resistance and approximately 3 percent of strains exhibit nonenzymatic resistance secondary to modified penicillin-binding proteins or outer membrane proteins. Antibiotic resistance is approximately twice as frequent among Hib strains as among NTHi strains. Chloramphenicol resistance is a significant problem in less-developed countries and in the United States. Fortunately, there are a number of effective therapeutic choices. All isolates from seriously ill patients should be assumed resistant to ampicillin until proven otherwise, and initial therapy should be based on this assumption. Once the sensitivity of the organism is known, therapy should be adjusted to minimize cost and risk of superinfection. For serious systemic infection, combined therapy with ampicillin and chloramphenicol is recommended. In addition, several third-generation cephalosporins (including ceftriaxone and cefotaxime) penetrate the CSF to therapeutic levels and are effective in management of serious *H. influenzae* infection. The early administration of glucocorticoids may reduce the incidence of hearing loss in children with type b meningitis. Preschool contacts of children with the infection should receive prophylaxis with rifampin (20 mg/kg per day) for 4 days. This has been shown to reduce the risk of secondary cases significantly.

Less serious infections, such as otitis, sinusitis, and acute bronchitis due to ampicillin-sensitive strains, can be treated with ampicillin or amoxicillin. Infections due to ampicillin-resistant strains can be managed with ampicillin/β-lactamase inhibitors, trimethoprim-sulfamethoxazole, cefadroxil, or quinolones. Penicillin-allergic patients can be treated with trimethoprim-sulfamethoxazole, cefadroxil, or quinolones.

HACEK GROUP INFECTIONS The group of organisms including *Haemophilus aphrophilis*, *H. paraphrophilis*, *H. parainfluenzae*, *Actinobacillus actinomycetemcomitans*, *Cardiobacterium hominis*, *Eikenella corrodens*, and *Kingella kingae* is known as *HACEK*. Culture of these fastidious organisms requires incubation in an atmosphere containing carbon dioxide. They require longer incubation for isolation in blood than *H. influenzae* organisms. When HACEK organisms are suspected, blood cultures should be observed for at least 7 days. The improved ability to isolate these fastidious organisms may be the reason for the reported increased incidence. The pathogenicity of these species is lower than that of *H. influenzae*.

Haemophilus species cause about 5 percent of infective endocarditis. The course of the endocarditis is similar to that due to viridans streptococci. Underlying valvular disease, intravenous drug abuse, and prosthetic valves are predisposing factors. Vegetations tend to be large. Embolization, a frequent complication (up to 60 percent of cases), may be due in part to delay in diagnosis as a result of the difficulty in isolation of these species.

Therapy should ultimately be based on antibiotic sensitivity. Initial treatment with ampicillin and aminoglycosides, which are synergistic against some *Haemophilus* species, is recommended. Even in effectively managed cases, the mortality in *Haemophilus* endocarditis is between 10 and 15 percent.

Actinobacillus actinomycetemcomitans is part of the endogenous flora of the mouth. It is often recovered from the sites of lesions associated with juvenile periodontitis. It can cause endocarditis (especially on damaged or prosthetic valves) and has been isolated from infections of the meninges, bone, urinary tract, and pericardium. It is susceptible to the newer cephalosporins, rifampin, trimethoprim-sulfamethoxazole, quinolones, and chloramphenicol.

Cardiobacterium hominis is a small gram-negative rod. Almost all clinical isolates of *C. hominis* have been associated with endocarditis, usually of abnormal or prosthetic valves. The valvular infection tends to be insidious, and patients present with splenomegaly, anemia, and hematuria indicative of a long-standing infection before diagnosis. It is frequently difficult to determine antibiotic susceptibility because the organisms are slow-growing. *C. hominis* is usually susceptible to penicillin, chloramphenicol, and tetracycline. Penicillin alone or combined with aminoglycosides is the most common therapy. Complications caused by embolization, mycotic aneurysm, or heart failure have necessitated valvular replacement in a number of cases.

Eikenella corrodens is a gram-negative facultative anaerobic bacillus and a part of the normal oral and respiratory mucosal flora. The most common clinical types of infection are human bites, head and neck infections, and respiratory tract infections. Gynecologic infections may be associated with intrauterine devices. Other sites of *Eikenella* infection include synovial fluid, bone, and brain abscess. As with other organisms in the HACEK group, *Eikenella corrodens* has been associated with endocarditis. *Eikenella* species are resistant to clindamycin. Ampicillin, penicillin, second- and third-generation cephalosporins have been reported effective in management of such infections.

The *Kingella* genus contains three species, *K. kingae*, *K. indologenes*, and *K. denitrificans*. *Kingella* have been associated with mucous membrane, joint, bone, and valvular infections. *Kingella* infections have been treated successfully with β-lactam–aminoglycoside combinations.

Capnocytophaga infections *Capnocytophaga* are gram-negative facultative anaerobic bacilli that grow optimally under anaerobic conditions in the presence of 5 to 10 percent carbon dioxide on blood or chocolate media. *Capnocytophaga* are motile on agar but lack flagellae. They are commonly isolated from the gingival sulcus and can cause gingival ulcers in neutropenic patients. *Capnocytophaga* cause serious infections predominantly in immunocompromised patients, but bacteremia and endocarditis can occur in patients with normal immune function. *Capnocytophaga* species are sensitive to a wide range of antibiotics including penicillin, clindamycin, erythromycin, quinolones, third-generation cephalosporins, metronidazole, chloramphenicol, and imipenem.

HAEMOPHILUS DUCREYI INFECTIONS The etiologic agent associated with soft genital ulcers (the chancroid ulcer) is a short, compact, rodlike organism that initially could not be cultured. Its role in soft ulcer disease was established by documenting its ability to cause ulcers by autoinoculation. The chancroid bacillus was designated *Haemophilus ducreyi* because of the requirement for factors X and V, but genetic studies suggest that *H. ducreyi* does not belong within this genus. An enriched chocolate medium is necessary for reliable cultivation of the organisms from ulcers, and vancomycin can be added to the medium to reduce contamination with gram-positive bacteria. Samples for culture are usually taken from the base and sides of the ulcers. Aspiration of inguinal buboes is a less-common source of positive cultures.

Epidemiology of chancroid ulcer disease Genital ulcers from *H. ducreyi* occur on a world-wide basis but are more common in less-developed tropical countries. In Africa, chancroid ulcers are implicated as a cofactor in the transmission of HIV. In the United States before 1960 there were approximately 10,000 cases reported per year. This number dropped to an average of 1000 cases per year during the 1960s and 1970s and increased during the 1980s. In 1991, 3476 cases were reported to the Centers for Disease Control and Prevention. Outbreaks in several major cities occurred among heterosexual blacks and Hispanics, mostly men, a fact suggesting that a small number of females was infecting a large number of males. The failure to identify an asymptomatic carrier state for *H. ducreyi* suggests that female prostitution is the mechanism of transmission.

Pathogenesis and clinical features *H. ducreyi* invades via a break in the integrity of the epithelium and causes, over 4 to 7 days, an ingress of polymorphonuclear leukocytes, with edema and disruption of epithelial cells. A small papule surrounded by an erythematous halo ruptures within 2 to 4 days to form a sharply defined ulcer with ragged edges and minimal induration. The base of the ulcer contains grey or yellow friable granulomatous material and bleeds easily. While the papular stage may go unnoticed by the patient, chancroid ulcers are always painful. The most common sites of involvement in men are the distal prepuce, the mucosal surface of the prepuce on the frenulum, and the coronal sulcus. Local extension can occur to other regions in the genital area. In women most lesions are at the entrance to the vagina including the fourchette, labia, vestibule, and clitoris. Painful unilateral inguinal lymphadenopathy occurs in over half of patients. Buboes can form and rupture with the formation of inguinal ulcers. Despite the development of large ulcers, systemic invasion by *H. ducreyi* is rare.

Management Oral erythromycin (500 mg four times a day) for 7 days is effective therapy. Other drugs used include ceftriaxone as a single dose agent (250 mg intramuscularly) and trimethoprim-sulfamethoxazole for 5 to 7 days; considerably less clinical experience is available for the latter therapies.

REFERENCES

FARLEY MM et al: Invasive *Haemophilus influenzae* disease in adults: A prospective population based surveillance. Ann Intern Med 116:806, 1992

MAYOSMITH MF et al: Acute epiglottis in adults. An eight-year experience in the state of Rhode Island. N Engl J Med 314:1133, 1986

MEYER DJ, GERDING DN: Favorable prognosis of patients with prosthetic valve endocarditis caused by gram-negative bacilli of the HACEK group. Am J Med 85:104, 1988

MORSE FS: Chancroid and *Haemophilus ducreyi*. Clin Microbiol Rev 2:137, 1989

MURPHY TF, APICELLA MA: Nontypable *Haemophilus influenzae*: A review of clinical aspects, surface antigens and the human immune response to infection. Rev Infect Dis 9:1, 1987

PARKER SW et al: *Haemophilus* endocarditis in two patients with complications. Arch Intern Med 143:48, 1983

SCHLAMM HT, YANCOVITZ SR: *Haemophilus influenzae* pneumonia in young adults with AIDS, ARC or risk of AIDS. Am J Med 86:11, 1989

WESTERINK MAJ et al: Septicemia due to DF-2; cause of a false-positive cryptococcal latex agglutination test. Am J Med 83:155, 1987

113 LEGIONELLA INFECTIONS

MICHAEL S. BERNSTEIN / RICHARD M. LOCKSLEY

DEFINITION The family Legionellaceae consists of over 30 species of fastidious gram-negative, aerobic bacilli. The organisms are ubiquitous in the environment and cause disease when a sufficient environmental inoculum is aerosolized and inhaled by a human host. The course of the subsequent disease is determined both by virulence factors of the bacterium and by the immune competence of the host. The organism in humans behaves as a facultative intracellular bacterium. Legionnaires' disease, a fulminant pneumonia caused by *Legionella pneumophila*, is the prototypic illness caused by these organisms. Pontiac fever is a self-limited, flulike syndrome that occurs in immunocompetent individuals. The spectrum of disease caused by these organisms is designated *legionellosis*.

HISTORY *Legionnaires' disease* refers to an epidemic of pneumonia that affected 221 people and caused 34 deaths during the American Legion Convention at the Bellevue-Stratford Hotel in Philadelphia during July and August 1976. Initially referred to as the *Legionnaires' disease agent*, the organism was shown to be a new species of bacterium and subsequently designated *L. pneumophila*. Serotyping revealed that this organism had been responsible for previous epidemics of pneumonia, including 20 cases of severe pneumonia among attendees at a convention in Philadelphia at the same hotel in 1974. Furthermore, in July 1968, 144 employees and visitors in a health department building in Pontiac, Michigan, developed a self-limited illness consisting of fever, myalgias, headache, and malaise, subsequently termed *Pontiac fever*. Exposure of guinea pigs to aerosols of water from the building's air conditioning system led to isolation of the organism, eventually identified as *L. pneumophila*.

The discovery of *L. pneumophila* led rapidly to the isolation of related organisms within the family Legionellaceae (Table 113-1). There are more than 50 species (33 named) and over 60 distinct serogroups. Many isolates cause pneumonia indistinguishable from that caused by the initial strain, designated *Legionella pneumophila* serotype 1. This isolate accounts for 50 percent of human infection, followed in frequency by serotype 6 (10 percent). *L. micdadei* (Pittsburgh pneumonia agent) accounts for 7 percent of cases. The serologically unrelated, unnamed legionellae are designated *Legionella*-like organisms (LLOs).

ETIOLOGY The legionellae are classified in a single genus, *Legionella*, within the family Legionellaceae. The legionellae are gram-negative, aerobic, nonencapsulated bacilli measuring 0.3 to 0.9 μm in width and 2 to 5 μm in length. They are non-spore-forming, and most are motile due to polar or subpolar flagellae. Electron microscopy reveals multiple fimbriae (pili) extending from the surface. Legionellae have complex growth requirements and do not grow on standard bacteriologic media. All species require supplementation of growth media with L-cysteine and ferric salts and grow best at pH 6.8 to 7.0. Legionellae display an unusual dependence on amino acids, as opposed to carbohydrates, for energy and carbon sources. The fatty acids of legionellae contain an unusually high proportion of branched-chain acids, permitting identification by gas-liquid chromatography.

In most clinical laboratories, legionellae are recognized by their growth on selective media. Identification is confirmed by serologic reactivity with defined antisera. A commercially available slide agglutination test identifies 22 *Legionella* species and 33 serogroups. Further identification of a *Legionella* isolate may require analysis in a reference laboratory. Biochemical analysis, autofluorescence, immunofluorescence staining, and gas-liquid chromatography are used to characterize different species and strains. Less widely available techniques include restriction endonuclease analysis, alloenzyme typing, and plasmid DNA profiling.

ECOLOGY AND TRANSMISSION Legionellae are ubiquitous in aquatic environments. Diverse natural *reservoirs* harbor these organisms, including mud, frozen streams, hot springs, and stagnant lakes. Certain algae provide all the nutritional and growth requirements for *L. pneumophila*. Some amebas and ciliated protozoa ingest legionellae and support their intracellular multiplication, protecting the bacteria from disinfectants and other adverse conditions. Legionellaceae have no animal or human reservoir.

Amplifiers are man-made water supplies that favor the growth of legionellae. Growth is enhanced by elevated temperatures (36 to 70°C), a source of iron and simple nutrients, and low levels of other competing bacteria. Hot water systems and heat exchange units are frequently contaminated due to stagnation, infrequent decontamination, and the presence of sediment or decayed plumbing, all of which contribute to suboptimal levels of chlorine. Decomposing rubber gaskets and sealing washers are capable of supporting the growth of these organisms. Legionellae have been isolated from such diverse man-made aqueous environments as potable water systems, ice machines, hot tubs, and humidifiers.

Disseminators facilitate transmission to the human respiratory tract by generating infectious aerosols. Airborne transmission by environmentally generated aerosols was suggested by epidemiologic evidence and has been reproduced in experimental animals. Aerosolized *L. pneumophila* can survive for more than 2 h and have been isolated nearly 1 mile downwind of cooling towers. Infectious aerosol particles are less than 5 μm in diameter and can be inhaled directly into the alveoli. A variety of sources have been identified in outbreaks of Legionnaires' disease, including cooling towers, air-conditioning systems, humidifiers, whirlpool baths, respiratory nebulizers, showers, and vegetable misters used in grocery stores. Aerosolized legionellae have been traced to contaminated soil disturbed by excavation and to industrial lubricants used to cool machinery.

Other routes of transmission may exist. Microaspiration of drinking water may be a mechanism of infection, particularly in sporadic, community-acquired disease. Postoperative wound infections have developed following exposure to contaminated tap water and whirlpool baths. There is no evidence of person-to-person transmission.

EPIDEMIOLOGY *Legionella* infections account for up to 7 percent of community-acquired pneumonias and, in some studies, up to one-fourth of "atypical" community-acquired pneumonias. *L. pneumophila* may be responsible for 10 percent of nosocomial pneumonias and as much as 30 percent during endemic hospital outbreaks. About half of adults show evidence of prior exposure to at least one *Legionella* species.

Legionella infections occur in epidemic outbreaks, sporadic cases,

TABLE 113-1 Identified *Legionella*

Species (serogroups)	Pneumonia	Pontiac fever	DFA*
L. pneumophila (15)	X	1,6[†]	1–10
L. micdadei	X	X	X
L. bozemanii (2)	X		1
L. dumoffii	X	?	X
L. gormanii	X		X
L. longbeachae (2)	X		1,2
L. jordanis	X		X
L. oakridgensis	X		
L. wadsworthii	X		
L. feeleii (2)	X	X	
L. sainthelensi (2)	X	?	
L. anisa	X		
L. maceachernii	X		
L. jamestownensis			
L. rubrilucens			
L. erythra			
L. hackeliae (2)	X		
L. spiritensis		?	
L. parisiensis			
L. cherrii	X		
L. steigerwaltii			
L. santicrucis			
L. israelensis			
L. cincinnatiensis	X		
L. quinlivanii			
L. birminghamensis	X		
L. moravica			
L. brunensis			
L. tucsonensis	X		
L. gratiana			
L. fairfieldensis			
L. adelaidensis			
L. shakespearei			
L. lansingensis	X		

* Direct fluorescent antibody reagents available.
[†] Numbers refer to serogroups.

or highly endemic clusters related to sustained nosocomial outbreaks. Both pneumonic and nonpneumonic legionelloses exist in epidemic form but differ in their attack rates and incubation periods. *Legionella* pneumonia has an attack rate of 1 to 7 percent, whereas Pontiac fever affects 95 to 100 percent of those exposed. The incubation period for pneumonia is 2 to 12 days, while that for nonpneumonic outbreaks is 24 to 48 h. There is a higher incidence of legionellosis during summer, presumably due to warmer water temperatures and increased use of water-cooling systems that transmit the organism.

Pneumonic legionellosis affects men three times as often as women and is uncommon in children. Other risk factors for pneumonic disease include cigarette smoking, heavy alcohol use, advanced age, chronic illness, and use of immunosuppressive medication. Organ transplant patients appear to be at particular risk. *Legionella* infection remains uncommon among patients infected with HIV. Nonpneumonic legionellosis has no demonstrable risk factors.

PATHOGENESIS AND PATHOLOGY   Direct alveolar deposition of infectious aerosols containing legionellae is the predominant form of inoculation in *Legionella* infections. The short incubation period and the association with environmental aerosols are consistent with this mechanism. The inoculum of aerosolized bacteria and variability in virulence among strains may be important in determining the outcome of infection. Common-source exposures can result in non-pneumonic illness or severe pneumonia in different individuals, depending on the extent of exposure to infectious aerosols.

Legionellae appear to be susceptible to clearance by the mucociliary apparatus. Asymptomatic colonization does not occur, and during disease, pathologic findings are limited to the lower respiratory tract. Alveolar deposition via aerosol and factors, such as smoking, that impair mucociliary clearance permit the organism to establish infection within resident alveolar macrophages. In the human host, legionellae are facultative intracellular pathogens of monocytes and macrophages. The organisms activate complement by the classic pathway but are resistant to lysis. Mononuclear phagocytes ingest *L. pneumophila* by a mechanism termed *coiling phagocytosis* that is mediated by complement receptors CR1 and CR3 following C3 deposition on the major outer membrane protein of the bacterium. A surface protein designated *macrophage infectivity potentiator*, or mip, has been shown to enhance infectivity and virulence in experimental systems. Proteins for mip-related proteins are present in all *Legionella* species. Interestingly, the sequence of mip reveals significant homology to mammalian isomerases that bind the immunosuppressive drug FK506. Ingested organisms inhibit fusion of the phagosome to primary and secondary lysosomes, blocking the transfer of microbicidal substances into the phagosome and interfering with acidification of the vacuole. The sequestered organisms divide by binary fission within unusual vacuoles studded by host ribosomes and surrounded by glycogen granules and mitochondria. Continued replication results in lysis of the mononuclear cell and spread to adjacent cells. Both neutrophils and monocytes are recruited to the developing inflammatory lesion but are unable to inhibit bacterial growth efficiently. Specific antibody is produced, but the organisms remain resistant to antibody-mediated complement lysis. Phagocytosis is enhanced by specific antibody, thus further targeting the bacteria to the intracellular environment.

From the initial site, infection spreads by endobronchial, hematogenous, and lymphatic routes or by contiguous invasion. Bacteremia occurs in as many as one-third of patients with legionellosis and is the most common source of extrapulmonary infection.

As with infections due to other intracellular pathogens, *Legionella* infection is contained as cell-mediated immunity appears. Sensitized T lymphocytes secrete macrophage activating factors, primarily interferon-γ, that enable the cell to inhibit intracellular replication. Interleukin 2–activated natural killer cells are also capable of destroying *Legionella*-infected monocytes in vitro. The importance of cell-mediated immunity is supported by the increased incidence and severity of legionellosis among immunosuppressed patients, particularly transplant recipients.

Macroscopically, bronchopneumonia ranges from a patchy lobular process to more extensive multilobar consolidation. Round, nodular lesions are sometimes present. Abscesses with central necrosis occur in 25 percent of fatal cases. Pleuritis and small serosanguinous pleural effusions are common, but empyema is rare. Microscopically, infection is characterized by intense alveolitis and bronchiolitis. Alveolar spaces are filled with polymorphonuclear leukocytes, macrophages, fibrin, and proteinaceous exudate. Many inflammatory cells have undergone leukocytoclasis, leaving only nuclear debris and fibrin. Organisms can be visualized using the Gimenez stain, Dieterle silver impregnation stain, or direct fluorescent antibody and are predominantly located within phagocytes. Alveolar septae and interstitial spaces are thickened by edema and inflammatory cells. More severe disease, including diffuse alveolar damage with hyaline membrane formation, occurs in immunocompromised patients. Pathologic changes do not extend proximal to terminal bronchioles, a finding consistent with inoculation by aerosol. Pathologic changes are usually limited to the lungs. Brain tissue is normal even in cases with neurologic abnormalities.

CLINICAL MANIFESTATIONS   Legionnaires' disease and Pontiac fever are the two well-described syndromes. The complete spectrum of infection by Legionellaceae remains undefined, however, and probably includes asymptomatic seroconversion, mild self-resolving illness, and isolated extrapulmonary manifestations.

Pneumonic illness typically begins with an abrupt prodrome of malaise, headache, myalgia, and weakness. Fever and intermittent rigors appear 24 h later, with temperatures exceeding 40°C in more than half of patients. Nonproductive cough is common. About half of patients eventually produce thin or minimally purulent sputum, and one-third may have scant hemoptysis. Pleuritic chest pain and dyspnea can raise the suspicion of pulmonary embolism. Gastrointestinal symptoms include diarrhea, nausea, vomiting, and abdominal pain. Altered mental status suggesting toxic encephalopathy may include confusion, disorientation, lethargy, hallucinations, depression, delirium, obtundation, or coma. Seizures are rare, but cranial or peripheral neuropathy and cerebellar dysfunction are not uncommon. Physical examination usually shows a toxic appearance and high fever. Relative bradycardia is common. Lung examination reveals rales and consolidation, but the physical findings are mild when compared to radiographic findings. Complications and systemic manifestations include lung abscess, empyema, respiratory failure, hypotension, shock, rhabdomyolysis, disseminated intravascular coagulation (DIC), thrombotic thrombocytopenic purpura (TTP), and renal failure.

Pontiac fever is an acute, self-limited illness lasting 2 to 5 days. A prodrome of malaise, myalgia, and headache is followed rapidly by fever, chills, and, variably, cough, coryza, and sore throat. Diarrhea, nausea, and mild neurologic symptoms such as dizziness or photophobia may be present.

Legionellae also may cause extrapulmonary infections related to bacteremia at the time of pneumonia or local exposure to contaminated water. Pericarditis, myocarditis, pyelonephritis, pancreatitis, sinusitis, peritonitis, and hemodialysis fistula infections; abscesses in liver, skin, and the perirectal area; and postoperative wound infections have been reported. *L. pneumophila* and *L. dumoffii* can cause subacute and chronic prosthetic valve endocarditis with annular and myocardial abscesses. The organisms are nosocomially acquired during the perioperative period when the primary infection may cause a postpericardiotomy-like syndrome. Emboli are rare.

LABORATORY FINDINGS   *Legionella* pneumonia is usually accompanied by leukocytosis with an increase in early granulocyte forms; the total leukocyte count exceeds 20,000 cells per microliter in 10 to 20 percent of cases. None of the laboratory abnormalities associated with pneumonic legionellosis is specific, although hyponatremia occurs in 50 to 70 percent, more commonly than in other forms of pneumonia. Other laboratory findings may include hypophosphatemia, azotemia, microhematuria, proteinuria, and abnormal tests of liver function. Hematologic findings are typically normal unless the illness is complicated by DIC or TTP. Cerebrospinal fluid examination is usually normal, although pleocytosis and elevated protein have been reported. Gram stain of the sputum may show inflammatory cells, but legionellae stain poorly or not at all in clinical specimens. *L. micdadei* is acid-fast by Kinyoun and modified Ziehl-Neelsen stains.

Early roentgenographic patterns include diffuse patchy infiltrates or ill-defined nodular densities. Pneumonia progresses to bilateral infiltrates in 50 percent of patients; a lobar-segmental pattern predominates. Small pleural effusions are present in 20 to 50 percent. Cavitation is uncommon but may occasionally be seen, particularly in immunosuppressed patients.

Leukocytosis is frequently the only laboratory abnormality in Pontiac fever.

DIAGNOSIS The diagnosis of *Legionella* infection may be made by culturing the organism, identifying its antigens or nucleic acids in tissue or secretions, or demonstrating a serologic response in the host (Table 113-2). A positive culture is diagnostic, since no carrier state occurs. Cultures are performed on buffered charcoal yeast extract agar with α-ketoglutarate (BCYE-α agar), but 2 to 5 days may be required to identify the organism. BCYE-α agar is not selective, and supplementation with antibiotics or acidification is required for sputum samples to inhibit the growth of other bacteria. Typical results of the culture of clinical specimens are listed in Table 113-2. Blood cultures must be subcultured on BCYE-α agar after 24 h of aerobic incubation.

Legionellae may be visualized in clinical specimens by direct fluorescent antibody (DFA) staining. Clinical specimens are treated with fluorescein-conjugated rabbit antibody and examined by fluorescence microscopy. The test requires only 2 to 4 h. Commercially available DFA reagents detect over 90 percent of strains responsible for clinical disease (see Table 113-1). However, the relatively low sensitivity (50 percent) and the need for an experienced technician are disadvantages. DFA may be less sensitive after a patient has received appropriate antibiotics.

Available tests for *Legionella* antigens in urine include an enzyme-linked immunosorbent assay, radioimmunoassay, and latex agglutination. The relative ease of specimen collection and assay performance may make urinary diagnosis an attractive rapid test. However, antigenuria may persist for months, obscuring the distinction between acute and past infection. A radiolabeled nucleic acid hybridization kit is moderately sensitive and detects all *Legionella* species, although false-positive results have been reported. The radioactive isotope limits the shelf life of the assay.

Serum antibody is most commonly measured by the indirect fluorescent antibody (IFA) assay. Routinely available reagents detect antibody directed only against *L. pneumophila* serogroup 1, believed to account for half of human disease. A diagnosis of legionellosis is made by a fourfold rise in titer between acute and convalescent sera to at least 1:128 or by a single titer of 1:256 or greater. Serum samples should be obtained acutely and after 3 weeks, although as many as one-fourth of patients may seroconvert within the first week of illness. Seroconversion develops in 80 percent of patients by 10 weeks.

While no clinical features of *Legionella* pneumonia are unique, the diagnosis should be suspected in a patient with severe pneumonia, high fever, nonproductive cough, hyponatremia, and altered mental

status, particularly in the setting of immunosuppression. Each of the tests employed to diagnose legionellosis has its limitations. Combined approaches are recommended. No diagnostic test may be used to exclude the disease absolutely. Thus clinical judgment must often prevail in decisions regarding therapy.

The diagnosis of Pontiac fever requires a compatible clinical illness, evidence of serologic conversion, and, preferably, isolation of the organism from the environment. Viable legionellae have never been isolated from a case of Pontiac fever, raising the possibility that the pathogenesis involves hypersensitivity to bacterial antigens rather than true infection.

TREATMENT Erythromycin is the antibiotic of choice for pneumonic legionellosis. For serious infection, patients should receive 4 g/d intravenously. Dosage reduction may be necessary in renal or hepatic failure to avoid ototoxicity. Immunocompromised patients and those with severe disease should receive rifampin (rifampicin) concurrently in a dose of 600 mg twice daily. Immunosuppressive medications should be tapered when possible. Response to therapy occurs in 24 to 48 h, although fever may persist for up to a week. With improvement, erythromycin may be reduced to 2 g/d orally. Therapy should continue for 3 weeks; shorter courses have been associated with relapse. Doxycycline, trimethoprim-sulfamethoxazole, ciprofloxacin, and other quinolones are potential alternatives when erythromycin is not tolerated or in the rare patients failing to respond to erythromycin. Clarithromycin also has been effective in treating severe legionellosis. Effective antibiotics are those which diffuse readily into phagocytic cells, suggesting that their role may be to arrest intracellular multiplication until effective cellular immunity develops.

Legionella prosthetic valve endocarditis usually requires valve replacement and prolonged antibiotic therapy (3 to 12 months). Pontiac fever is a self-limited illness requiring no therapy.

PROGNOSIS AND IMMUNITY Overall case fatality rates for *Legionella* pneumonia are approximately 15 percent. Mortality is 80 percent among untreated immunosuppressed patients and is reduced to 25 percent with appropriate antibiotic treatment. Untreated immunocompetent hosts have a 25 percent mortality rate; with proper therapy, only 7 percent succumb.

Patients who survive usually have no permanent sequelae. Full recovery of pulmonary function is usual, although pulmonary fibrosis with respiratory disability has been reported. Immunocompetent individuals who recover from infection are immune to reinfection with the same strain. Reinfection with an identical serotype has been reported in an immunocompromised patient.

PREVENTION AND CONTROL Understanding the chain of transmission of legionellae from natural reservoirs to man-made amplifiers and disseminators is important in devising control strategies. Surveillance efforts should concentrate on documenting human infection, rather than routinely screening the environment. During epidemic or endemic outbreaks, sentinel cases occur among immunosuppressed patients. Once detected, a careful search for the environmental source should be conducted. Multiple legionellae may be recovered from environmental cultures, many of which are not associated with human disease. Therefore, clinical isolates should be characterized so that control measures can focus on the source of pathogenic strains. Legionellosis is a reportable infection, and local health departments can provide assistance in the isolation and characterization of environmental strains.

Sources of environmental aerosols (disseminators), such as shower heads and air-conditioning systems, must be identified so that transmission can be interrupted. Contaminated water systems (amplifiers) can be sterilized. Legionellae may be present in low titer in potable water systems and may thus require culture of large volumes on selective media or pretreatment with heat or acid to enhance recovery. Rusted plumbing and decayed rubber gaskets should be replaced. Sites of stagnation and sediment in water tanks may require elimination. Decontamination of potable water systems is accomplished by hyperchlorination (2 to 3 ppm) and/or intermittent

TABLE 113-2 Laboratory tests in Legionnaires' disease

Test	Sensitivity, %	Specificity, %
Culture		
Sputum	60	100
Transtracheal	80	100
Lung biopsy	90	100
Blood	38	100
DFA	50	95
Urine antigen*	80	99
DNA probe	70	99
Serology (IFA)*	80	99

* *L. pneumophila* serogroup 1 only.

heating to 60°C with flushing of distal outlets. During nosocomial outbreaks, prophylactic treatment of high-risk patients with oral erythromycin has been effective. Periodic monitoring of hospital water may be necessary to detect reemergence of the organism.

REFERENCES

CIANCIOTTO NP et al: A mutation in the *mip* gene results in attenuation of *Legionella pneumophila* virulence. J Infect Dis 162:121, 1990

FANG GD et al: Disease due to the Legionellaceae (other than *Legionella pneumophila*): Historical, microbiological, clinical, and epidemiologic review. Medicine 68:116, 1989

FRASER DW et al: Legionnaire's disease: Description of an epidemic of pneumonia. N Engl J Med 297:1189, 1977

LOWRY PW et al: A cluster of *Legionella* sternal-wound infections due to postoperative topical exposure to contaminated tap water. N Engl J Med 324:109, 1991

MASTRO TD et al: Nosocomial Legionnaires' disease and use of medication nebulizers. J Infect Dis 163:667, 1991

NGUYEN MH et al: Legionellosis. Infect Dis Clin North Am 5:561, 1991

SNYDER MB et al: Reduction in *Legionella pneumophila* through heat flushing followed by continuous supplemental chlorination of hospital hot water. J Infect Dis 162:127, 1990

STOUT JE et al: Potable water as a cause of sporadic cases of community-acquired Legionnaires' disease. N Engl J Med 326:151, 1992

114 PERTUSSIS

GEORGE R. SIBER / MATTHEW H. SAMORE

DEFINITION Pertussis, or whooping cough, is an acute infection of the respiratory tract caused by *Bordetella pertussis*. The name *pertussis*, coined by Sydenham in 1679, means "violent cough" and describes the most characteristic feature of this disease. The Chinese call this illness "the cough of 100 days" because of its chronic nature. A dramatic inspiratory whoop following a paroxysmal cough is a hallmark of severe pertussis in children but is frequently absent, particularly in infants and adults. Thus the term *whooping cough* may mislead clinicians by implying that whoops are an essential feature of the disease.

The clinical features that should suggest pertussis are a chronic cough lasting 2 weeks or longer and coughing spells that are typically sudden in onset and paroxysmal in nature. The episodes may, in severe cases, be followed by a whoop or vomiting. Fever is absent or low, unless a superinfection has occurred. An absolute lymphocytosis may provide an additional clue to the diagnosis, particularly in unimmunized children.

MICROBIOLOGY The etiologic agent of pertussis, *B. pertussis*, was first isolated by Bordet and Gengou in 1900 using the medium that bears their names. Humans are the only known host of *B. pertussis*. Other species in the genus include *B. parapertussis*, which is associated with a milder, less chronic respiratory illness in humans, and *B. bronchiseptica*, an animal pathogen that on rare occasions causes respiratory or opportunistic infections in humans.

B. pertussis is a small, nonmotile, gram-negative coccobacillus that is slow growing and fastidious in its growth requirements. After 3 to 6 days of growth at 36°C on special medium such as Bordet-Gengou agar, glistening pinpoint colonies with surrounding zones of hemolysis appear. Preliminary identification is accomplished by direct fluorescent antibody staining or by agglutination with antiserum to *B. pertussis*. *B. pertussis* is distinguished from *B. bronchiseptica* and *B. parapertussis* by further tests such as motility and nitrate reduction. *B. pertussis*, *B. parapertussis*, and *B. bronchiseptica* show extensive DNA homology and share many non-virulence-related enzymes and some virulence factors. However, only *B. pertussis* expresses pertussis toxin.

Like many other bacterial pathogens, *B. pertussis* possesses a precise mechanism for coordinated regulation of its virulence factors that is under control of a central genetic locus. This process is typically mediated by a two-component system consisting of a sensory protein and a regulatory protein which transmits specific environmental signals to regulatory genes. In *B. pertussis*, the central regulatory locus is called the *Bordetella* virulence gene (*bvg*). Reversible down-regulation of virulence factors (i.e., pertussis toxin, filamentous hemagglutinin, pertactin, fimbriae, adenyl cyclase, dermonecrotic toxin) and up-regulation of other proteins occur in response to environmental stimuli such as high sulfate, high nicotinic acid, or low temperature. This process, called *antigenic modulation*, is mediated by transmembrane sensory protein (BvgS) and a gene regulatory factor (BvgA). In addition, mutations in the *bvg* locus that occur at a frequency of 10^{-3} to 10^{-6} organisms may abolish expression of virulence factors. This process is called *phase variation*.

Both antigenic modulation and phase variation occur in vitro and in vivo. It is likely that these processes play a critical role in the ecology of the organism and its adaptation to the environment. It has been suggested that phase variation or antigenic modulation may facilitate expulsion of the organism from the respiratory tract by lowering adherence, enable it to survive hostile environmental conditions during transmission, or enable it to survive intracellularly in a quiescent state protected from attack by immune mechanisms directed toward its virulence factors.

PATHOGENESIS *B. pertussis* initiates colonization of the respiratory tract by adhering to ciliated epithelial cells, grows to high numbers producing local mucosal damage, and induces the paroxysmal cough which enhances its expulsion and transmission to contacts. A number of virulence factors that enable the organism to produce this cycle of events have been described. Fimbriae or pili, hairlike appendages on the surface of the organism, may play a role in the initial stages of adherence to ciliated cells. The fimbriae induce serotype-specific agglutinating antibodies (agglutinins) and are therefore called *agglutinogens*. Filamentous hemagglutinin, a large 220-kDa rodlike surface protein, and pertactin, a 69-kDa protein residing in the outer membrane, enable the organism to adhere closely to ciliated and other mammalian cells. Both these adherence factors have arginine, glycine, aspartic acid repeat sequences (RGD) typical of eukaryotic adhesins that stick to the integrin family of mammalian cell surface proteins.

A variety of toxins then impair local defenses (tracheal cytotoxin by inducing ciliostasis and adenyl cyclase by inhibiting phagocytes) and cause local tissue damage (tracheal cytotoxin and dermonecrotic toxin), thereby enhancing the supply of nutrients and perhaps facilitating systemic absorption of pertussis toxin. Pertussis toxin conforms to the general A/B model of enzymatic bacterial exotoxins. It contains an enzymatic moiety, the A subunit, consisting of a single peptide (S1), and a binding moiety, the B-oligomer, consisting of four peptides (S2, S3, S4, and S5) in a molar ratio of 1:1:2:1. The B-oligomer adheres to mammalian cells and delivers the A subunit to its targets. The B-oligomer exerts some biologic functions directly (e.g., mitogenesis of T cells) and may contribute to adherence of the whole organism to mammalian cells. The A subunit transfers ADP-ribose from NAD to certain members of a family of guanine nucleotide–binding regulatory membrane proteins (G proteins) in target cells. By this mechanism pertussis toxin produces a variety of biologic effects, including the inhibition of normal lymphocyte migration, which results in lymphocytosis (lymphocytosis-promoting factor), the sensitization of mice to histamine and serotonin (histamine-sensitizing factor), the enhancement of insulin secretion in response to regulatory signals such as beta-adrenergic stimulation (islet-activating protein), and the enhancement of certain immune functions such as the production of IgG and IgE class antibodies.

The mechanisms whereby the organism produces the paroxysmal cough typical of pertussis have not been elucidated. The best evidence that pertussis toxin plays a critical role in producing the pertussis syndrome was provided by studies in which infants immunized only with pertussis toxoid had an 80 to 90 percent lower rate of severe pertussis than did controls.

EPIDEMIOLOGY Pertussis is a highly communicable disease, with attack rates of 90 to 100 percent in nonimmune household contacts. Transmission of the organism is mediated via exposure to respiratory droplets expelled in large numbers by symptomatic individuals.

Before the introduction of pertussis vaccine in the late 1940s, 115,000 to 270,000 cases of pertussis were reported annually in the United States (average incidence 150 per 100,000 population per year). Epidemics of pertussis recurred at 3- to 4-year intervals without significant seasonality. Incidence was highest in children aged 1 to 5 years and was 10 to 20 percent higher in females than in males. In infants, attack rates were lower than in older children, perhaps due to maternally derived antibodies. However, case fatality rates were highest in infants. During the years 1940–1948, pertussis caused more infant deaths than did diphtheria, polio, measles, meningitis, and scarlet fever combined. Most adults were immune due to long-lasting protection induced by natural disease and perhaps boosting by frequent reexposure.

The incidence of pertussis declined 100- to 150-fold after adoption of universal whole-cell pertussis vaccination. Discontinuation or curtailment of pertussis vaccine use was associated with a rapid resurgence of pertussis in countries such as Great Britain, Sweden, and Japan. In the United States, the incidence of pertussis has been increasing gradually after reaching a low point in the mid-1970s; an average of 2783 cases were reported per year from 1980 to 1989. The reported incidence of pertussis is highest in young infants and declines with age. Approximately two-thirds of children with pertussis in the United States have not received the appropriate number of immunizations for their age group. In developed countries, mortality from pertussis has declined markedly. In the United States, the case-fatality rate is 0.4 percent overall but 1.3 percent in infants less than 2 months of age. From 1980 to 1989, infants less than 1 year of age accounted for 50 percent of reported pertussis cases and 79 percent of pertussis deaths.

Epidemiologic studies suggest that the actual incidence of pertussis is much higher than estimates based on passively reported cases. Only one-third of patients hospitalized with pertussis and an even smaller proportion of patients with less severely symptomatic pertussis are reported to the Centers for Disease Control and Prevention. Furthermore, pertussis rates continue to peak cyclically at 3- to 4-year intervals, indicating that widespread transmission still occurs in the population despite childhood immunization.

Persons aged 15 years or older comprised 13 percent of pertussis cases reported from 1980 to 1989 in the United States. The proportion of all cases that were within this age group rose during this period. In some states with active surveillance and serologic investigation of outbreaks, the proportion of pertussis in adolescents and adults is much higher. Data from pertussis outbreaks indicate that vaccine-induced protective immunity wanes after about 12 years, in contrast to natural pertussis, which usually induces life-long immunity. Consequently, a progressively larger proportion of adolescents and adults are susceptible to pertussis. Large outbreaks of pertussis that have occurred in schools, nursing homes, hospitals, and residential facilities indicate the high transmissibility of this organism in susceptible adolescent and adult populations.

Careful studies of household contacts show that while 40 to 80 percent of family members have serologic evidence of infection, only one-third to one-half of them were ever clinically symptomatic. Symptomatic undiagnosed pertussis in adults is believed to be an important source of transmission to infants and children and a mechanism of perpetuating the disease in the population. There is no evidence that asymptomatic individuals transmit *B. pertussis* to others. Chronic carriers of pertussis have not been identified.

CLINICAL MANIFESTATIONS Pertussis is typically a prolonged illness, with an average duration of 6 to 8 weeks. The incubation period ranges from 5 to 14 days but is usually 7 to 10 days. The symptoms of pertussis generally evolve through three stages: the catarrhal, the paroxysmal, and the convalescent. The catarrhal stage lasts 1 to 2 weeks and is characterized by nonspecific symptoms of coryza, mild cough, lacrimation, malaise, and low-grade fever. The paroxysmal stage, which usually lasts 2 to 4 weeks, is characterized by the paroxysmal cough, defined as sudden, forceful, repetitive coughing. The number of coughs per spasm is variable, ranging from 10 to 30; the paroxysms of pertussis characteristically occur during a single exhalation, a feature useful in distinguishing it from the repetitive cough caused by other pathogens in which there are inspirations between coughs. In severe cases, the physical effort associated with each spasm may be extreme, and there may be neck vein distention, bulging of the eyes, and cyanosis. The distinctive whoop is heard in 40 to 60 percent of pediatric cases and is due to sudden inspiration against a closed glottis at the end of the paroxysm. The paroxysm, which often results in the expectoration of viscous respiratory secretions, may be triggered by external stimuli, such as loud noises or physical contact. Typically, 10 to 25 paroxysms occur per 24-h period, with disruption of nocturnal sleep. Posttussive vomiting is common and should be considered suggestive of pertussis. Fever is generally absent during the paroxysmal stage, unless there is bacterial superinfection. Most complications of pertussis occur during the paroxysmal stage. The convalescent stage is defined by the gradual waning in intensity of the cough. Complete resolution of the cough may require several months, and superimposed viral or bacterial respiratory infections may lead to severe clinical exacerbations with recurrence of paroxysmal coughing.

An absolute lymphocytosis is a characteristic but not universal laboratory finding in children with pertussis. Typically, the total white blood cell count ranges between 10,000 and 30,000 cells per microliter, with 50 to 75 percent lymphocytes. Lymphocytosis is much less common in teenagers and adults.

The most common presentation of pertussis in adolescents and adults is cough, with or without paroxysms, persisting for 2 weeks or more. Other useful clinical clues are shortness of breath during coughing spells, nocturnal cough, a tingling sensation in the back of the throat, posttussive vomiting, and a history of exposure to other patients with prolonged coughing illness. Whooping and lymphocytosis are infrequently present. Thus, as the pool of susceptible adults increases, this nonclassical presentation of pertussis has become more common than the classical presentation seen in preschool children.

B. pertussis has been isolated from human immunodeficiency virus–infected patients with chronic respiratory symptoms. It is not known whether the incidence of pertussis is increased in these patients.

COMPLICATIONS Minor complications of pertussis secondary to increased intrathoracic pressure include subconjunctival hemorrhage and upper torso petechiae. Episodes of cyanosis and apnea are common in infants and small children (prevalence 20 to 50 percent). Malnutrition and weight loss may occur because of inadequate caloric intake. The major respiratory complication of pertussis is pneumonia, usually a secondary infection due to encapsulated bacterial pathogens such as *Streptococcus pneumoniae* and *Haemophilus influenzae*. Pneumonia is more common in infants (incidence 21 percent) than in children aged 1 to 2 (12 percent) or in adults (3 percent). Nonimmune infants may develop a severe primary pneumonia due to *B. pertussis*. Neurologic complications are infrequent and include encephalopathy (0.7 percent) and seizures (2 percent). The mechanisms of pertussis-associated encephalopathy, though unknown, are postulated to include hypoxia, hypoglycemia due to pertussis toxin, hemorrhages secondary to increased venous pressure, effects of neurotoxins, and co-infection by neurotoxic viruses.

DIAGNOSIS Laboratory confirmation should be attempted in all cases of suspected pertussis. The standard diagnostic test is isolation of *B. pertussis* on nasopharyngeal swab culture. A calcium alginate swab is inserted into the nares and maintained in contact with the nasopharynx for 10 s to permit moistening. The swab should be placed immediately into transport medium (such as Regan-Lowe charcoal medium) or plated directly onto fresh Bordet-Gengou agar or other suitable agar. A nasopharyngeal aspirate collected with a syringe attached to a fine plastic catheter is a suitable alternative specimen and should be handled in the same fashion. Growth typically requires 3 to 5 days of incubation at 36°C. Suspicious colonies may be presumptively identified by direct fluorescent antibody staining or agglutination. The fluorescein-labeled antibody also may be used to detect organisms directly in nasopharyngeal secretions but with less sensitivity and specificity than culture. Nasopharyngeal cultures are positive in 70 to 80 percent of cases when obtained within 2 weeks of the onset of symptoms (during the catarrhal and early paroxysmal stage). The diagnostic yield declines rapidly thereafter. By 4 weeks, cultures are rarely positive. Newer diagnostic tests, such as detection of B. pertussis–specific DNA from nasopharyngeal swabs by polymerase chain reaction, promise to enhance the detection of this organism.

Serologic tests for pertussis have been used more frequently in outbreak and contact investigation than for routine clinical diagnosis. Typically, ELISA is used to measure IgG and IgA antibodies to filamentous hemagglutinin and to pertussis toxin in acute and convalescent sera. High titers of one or more of these antibodies on a single specimen (e.g., >3 SD above the mean of appropriately matched controls) or a significant rise in at least one of the antibody titers is considered diagnostic evidence of pertussis. However, antibody levels increase early in the disease course, particularly in previously immunized individuals, so that in practice the rise in titer is frequently missed. Serologic assays are particularly useful in evaluating adults in whom the disease was not suspected until more than 2 weeks after onset, when cultures are no longer sensitive. Adequately standardized serologic assays for pertussis are not yet available in most areas of the United States.

DIFFERENTIAL DIAGNOSIS   A variety of respiratory pathogens may cause paroxysmal cough. However, the constellation of prolonged (>2 weeks) paroxysmal cough accompanied by whoops and lymphocytosis is highly specific for B. pertussis. B. parapertussis typically causes a milder respiratory illness. Although the organisms are distinct species, B. parapertussis and B. pertussis are occasionally associated epidemiologically. They have been isolated from the same patients simultaneously or sequentially.

Viruses such as respiratory syncytial virus and adenovirus have been isolated from patients with clinical pertussis (with or without isolation of B. pertussis). However, there is no convincing evidence that these viruses alone can cause the full pertussis syndrome with whooping and lymphocytosis.

TREATMENT   Antibiotics   The major aim of antibiotics is to eradicate B. pertussis from the respiratory tract. Erythromycin, preferably the estolate form, at a dose of 50 mg/kg per day (maximum 2 g/d) in two to four divided doses, reliably eradicates the organism from nasopharyngeal cultures within 5 days. Treatment should be continued for a full 14 days to prevent bacteriologic relapse. Patients unable to tolerate erythromycin may be treated with trimethoprim-sulfamethoxazole (8/40 mg/kg per day in two divided doses), but its efficacy is unproven.

Erythromycin ameliorates the clinical illness when begun during the catarrhal phase. According to classic teaching, antibiotics have little effect once paroxysmal cough occurs, but recent studies indicate some reduction in whooping when erythromycin is begun within 2 weeks of onset of paryoxysmal cough.

Supportive care   Infants have the highest rates of complications and death due to pertussis. Accordingly, most infants and those older patients with severe pertussis should be hospitalized. Supportive care includes monitoring for apnea and cyanosis, gentle nasotracheal suctioning, oxygen, hydration, and nutritional support. Glucocorticoids and the beta-adrenergic stimulant salbutamol have been advocated but not proven to be effective. Cough suppressants are ineffective.

Isolation of hospitalized patients   Patients should be placed on respiratory isolation for 5 days after initiation of erythromycin or for 3 weeks if unable to tolerate appropriate antimicrobial therapy.

PREVENTION   Management of contacts   All household and other close contacts, whether children or adults and irrespective of immunization status, should receive chemoprophylaxis with erythromycin (preferably the estolate) at 40 to 50 mg/kg per day in four divided doses (maximum 2 g/d) for 14 days. Prompt use of erythromycin is effective in limiting secondary transmission. Children younger than 7 years should have pertussis immunization initiated or continued according to the recommended schedule.

Vaccines   The vaccine currently used for primary immunization of infants consists of killed whole-cell pertussis organisms combined with diphtheria and tetanus toxoids (DTP) adsorbed to aluminum phosphate adjuvant. The standard schedule involves three primary doses at 2-month intervals initiated at 6 to 8 weeks of age, followed by booster doses at 15 to 18 months and 4 to 6 years of age. The vaccine is not recommended for anyone above the age of 6 but has been used in special circumstances for control of nosocomial outbreaks.

The whole-cell vaccine is believed to be 80 to 95 percent efficacious in preventing pertussis during 3 years following immunization. Thereafter, protective immunity wanes, with attack rates reaching 95 percent in household contacts exposed more than 12 years after immunization. Fortunately, the disease in previously immunized individuals is usually mild.

Injection of DTP containing a whole-cell pertussis component is associated with a variety of adverse effects. Local reactions and fever occur after one-third to one-half of injections and are maximal during the first 24 h. Fever of 40.5°C (105°F) or greater occurs after 1 in 300 doses, persistent crying (>3 h) after 1 in 100 doses, and high-pitched, unusual crying after 1 in 1000 doses. More severe reactions include seizures, which are usually febrile (1 in 1750 doses), and collapse or shocklike state (1 in 1750 doses).

There appears to be an excess incidence of acute neurologic illness during the 7 days after DTP administration, but the rate is extremely low, and a causal relationship with the vaccine has not been shown. There is no evidence for a causal relation between DTP administration and chronic neurologic illnesses, infantile spasms, or sudden infant death syndrome. Anaphylaxis is estimated to occur 1 in 50,000 DTP doses.

Two acellular pertussis vaccines formulated with diphtheria and tetanus toxoids (DTaP) have been licensed in the United States for use as booster doses at 15 to 18 months and 4 to 6 years of age in children previously immunized with three primary doses of whole-cell DTP. Both DTaP vaccines contain acellular pertussis components developed and manufactured by Japanese manufacturers. The Biken-type vaccine contains purified formalin-treated pertussis toxin and filamentous hemagglutinin. The Takeda-type vaccine contains a mixture of formalinized antigens including filamentous hemagglutinin, the predominant component, as well as smaller amounts of pertussis toxin, pertactin, and agglutinogen 2. Both acellular pertussis vaccines have shown epidemiologic evidence of efficacy in children 2 years of age or older in Japan, and both induce booster antibody responses to their constituent antigens similar to those of whole-cell pertussis vaccine. Both DTaP vaccines produce significantly fewer local reactions, fever, and other systemic symptoms than does whole-cell DTP and are therefore preferred for booster immunization in children. Whether rare severe reactions are less frequent after DTaP administration is unknown.

Licensure of DTaP vaccines for primary immunization of infants awaits the outcome of clinical efficacy studies currently underway comparing DTaP vaccines containing from 1 to 5 purified pertussis antigens and whole-cell DTP vaccine.

Neither DTaP nor whole-cell DTP vaccine is currently approved for use in adults. Whole-cell DTP has been used rarely in the control of hospital outbreaks of pertussis but is associated with high rates of adverse reactions. Routine use of DTaP vaccines in adults may offer a means for reducing symptomatic pertussis in older children and adults, thereby enhancing herd immunity and reducing transmission to incompletely immunized infants and children. However, further studies are needed before this approach can be recommended routinely.

REFERENCES

Addiss DG et al: A pertussis outbreak in a Wisconsin nursing home. J Infect Dis 164:704, 1991

Ad Hoc Group for the Study of Pertussis Vaccines: Placebo-controlled trial of two acellular pertussis vaccines in Sweden: Protective efficacy and adverse events. Lancet 1:955, 1988

Aoyama T et al: Pertussis in adults. Am J Dis Child 146:163, 1992

Coote JG: Antigenic switching and pathogenicity: Enviromental effects on virulence gene expression in *Bordetella pertussis*. J Gen Microbiol 137:2493, 1991

Farizo KM et al: Epidemiological features of pertussis in the United States, 1980–1989. Clin Infect Dis 14:708, 1992

Herwaldt LA: Pertussis in adults: What physicians need to know. Arch Intern Med 151:1510, 1991

Keller MA et al: Etiology of pertussis syndrome. Pediatrics 66:50, 1980

Long SS et al: Widespread silent transmission of pertussis in families: Antibody correlates of infection and symptomatology. J Infect Dis 161:480, 1990

Mink CAM et al: A search for *Bordetella pertussis* infection in university students. Clin Infect Dis 14:464, 1992

Pertussis outbreaks: Massachusetts and Maryland, 1992. Morb Mort Week Rep 11:197, 1993

Olson LC: Pertussis. Medicine 54:427, 1975

Pittman M: The concept of pertussis as a toxin-mediated disease. Pediatr Infect Dis J 3:467, 1984

Steketee RW et al: Evidence for a high attack rate and efficacy of erythromycin prophylaxis in a pertussis outbreak in a facility for the developmentally disabled. J Infect Dis 157:434, 1988

Sutter RW, Cochi SL: Pertussis hospitalizations and mortality in the United States, 1985–1988. JAMA 267:386, 1992

115   DISEASES CAUSED BY GRAM-NEGATIVE ENTERIC BACILLI
(*Escherichia coli, Klebsiella, Enterobacter, Serratia, Proteus, Morganella, Providencia,* and *Acinetobacter*)

BARRY I. EISENSTEIN

The gram-negative enteric bacilli frequently reside in the human colon without causing disease. They also normally colonize other environmental niches with which hospitalized patients come in contact. Because of their ubiquity within and outside the body, they often cause opportunistic infections, such as pneumonia, in debilitated patients. As a group, the enteric bacteria account for approximately one-third of the septicemia isolates, two-thirds of the bacterial gastroenteritis isolates, and three-quarters of the urinary tract isolates in all infected patients. One of the organisms, *Escherichia coli*, is also the most frequent cause of urinary tract infection and of bacterial gastroenteritis in otherwise healthy individuals.

GENERAL PROPERTIES

CLASSIFICATION AND PHYSIOLOGY   These organisms belong to the family Enterobacteriaceae, which includes other pathogens (*Shigella, Edwardsiella, Salmonella, Citrobacter, Yersinia*) discussed elsewhere. Some characteristics of members of this family are the lack of spore formation, the ability to grow both aerobically and anaerobically (i.e., facultative anaerobes), the ability to ferment glucose to acid, lack of oxidase production, and variable motility (depending on the presence of flagella).

STRUCTURE   Enterobacteriaceae share with all bacteria a peptidoglycan-containing cell wall, a single circular chromosome consisting of double-stranded DNA located throughout the cytoplasm, and prokaryote-type ribosomes (see Chap. 99). These structures are different enough from those of eukaryotes to make them ideal targets

for antimicrobial chemotherapy (see Chap. 100). For example, β-lactam antibiotics, the most frequently used agents for these organisms, bind to the bacterial cytoplasmic membrane and inhibit the cross-linking of the peptidoglycan. Gram-negative bacteria possess a unique multilayered cell envelope consisting of the typical inner (cytoplasmic) membrane, a surrounding polymeric peptidoglycan, and a complex outer membrane. The outer layer contains lipopolysaccharide (LPS or endotoxin), porins (multimeric proteins that are important channels for the penetration of antimicrobials and nutrients), and the polysaccharide capsule, which generally serves an antiphagocytic function. Many bacterial strains with intrinsic or acquired drug resistance contain porins that are impermeable to at least some antimicrobial agents.

Three classes of surface antigens have been used for serotyping for the clonal identification of *E. coli* and *Salmonella* strains: (1) the O or somatic antigens, (2) the H or flagellar antigens, and (3) the K or capsular antigens. (At present, genetically based methods are the preferred way of identifying bacteria both for taxonomy and epidemiology.) All gram-negative bacteria have the core part of LPS, which includes the toxic moiety, lipid A, responsible for the endotoxic shock seen in many episodes of bacteremia. Most pathogenic strains (at least in *E. coli*) also contain O antigens, which are repeating polysaccharide side chains attached to the core LPS. The O antigenic types are widely shared among all the Enterobacteriaceae, but in some cases cross-reactivity is particularly pronounced, even extending to cell-surface antigens from mammalian tissue. These O antigens are found on "smooth" strains and distinguish them from "rough" strains (terms that refer to differences in colonial morphology) and, along with other surface factors, mediate bacterial resistance to the killing effect of normal serum. Serum-resistant isolates, by surviving longer in the bloodstream, typically cause more severe disease.

A number of the O, H, and K serogroupings of *E. coli* act as markers for strains capable of causing a particular infectious disease; these strains also possess additional virulence factors required for pathogenesis. Thus certain O serogroups possess adhesive/colonization factors needed for urinary tract infection, other O serogroups have colonization factors and toxins that cause gastroenteritis, and another O serogroup is associated with the hemolytic-uremic syndrome. H antigens, which are proteins found on bacterial flagella, are also linked to the hemolytic-uremic syndrome (i.e., serogroup O157:H7), and the K1 capsular antigen is associated with neonatal meningitis, bacteremia, and urinary tract infection.

THE HOST-PARASITE INTERACTION   Many enteric bacteria, like relatively nonpathogenic strains of *E. coli*, colonize the gastrointestinal tract without causing symptoms. Significant disease requires either an exceptionally virulent organism, debilitated host (or one with broached defenses), or some combination of the two. A particularly pathogenic bacterium, such as *Shigella dysenteriae*, can produce dysentery even in normal hosts. A normally colonizing bacterium, such as a commensal strain of *E. coli*, can produce peritonitis or bacteremia in an otherwise healthy individual with a ruptured appendix or in a granulocytopenic individual receiving chemotherapy for cancer. A moderately pathogenic bacterium, such as K1-encapsulated strains of *E. coli*, can cause meningitis in newborns, who are particularly susceptible to this illness.

Regardless of the initial state of the host defenses, disease due to enteric bacteria consists of several sequential stages, beginning with the entry into and colonization of the gastrointestinal tract, nasopharynx, or oropharynx. Those bacteria which colonize the gastrointestinal tract, whether they are pathogenic or merely commensal, must survive the acidity of the stomach, the alkalinity and high concentrations of detergent (bile salts) and digestive enzymes in the small intestine, the immune system, and phagocytic cells. The cell wall of the gram-negative organism is well suited for coping with these challenges. Moreover, these bacteria, to avoid dislodgment by the passing intestinal contents, must attach to epithelial cell receptors or to the cell-associated mucus. This attachment is a function of hairlike proteinaceous organelles, known as *fimbriae* or *pili*, which cover the entire surface of the bacterial cell and contain lectin-like molecules that bind to specific mucosal receptors. The fimbriae of strains of *E. coli* that cause gastroenteritis have binding specificities appropriate to the gastrointestinal tract, and strains of *E. coli* associated with urinary tract infections contain P fimbriae (so-called because of affinity for the P blood group antigen found on uroepithelial cells), also called *pyelonephritis-associated pili* (PAP).

Normal host defenses limit the majority of bacterial interactions to benign commensalism. Therefore, to produce disease in healthy hosts, these organisms need additional attributes, known as *virulence factors*. For localized diseases (e.g., diarrhea, dysentery), the bacteria use secretory and cytologic toxins and, occasionally, cellular invasive factors. For successful penetration into the bloodstream, capsules inhibit opsonization, and other factors (such as smooth LPS and outer-membrane proteins) inhibit the bactericidal effect of serum.

In contrast, infections in debilitated individuals can occur with relatively avirulent organisms (see Chap. 96). Such organisms are typically robust enough to survive in various hospital environments (e.g., water supplies, the hands of caregivers) and sufficiently drug resistant to be part of the flora of an antibiotic-treated host. A debilitated host recovering from surgery or trauma or suffering from organ failure or immunodeficiency can become ill merely from the inadvertent relocation of a commensal strain to a site either normally sterile or normally not colonized with enteric bacteria. Examples include colonization of the upper airways, which with aspiration can lead to gram-negative pneumonia, and contamination of surgical wounds or intravascular or urinary catheters. The resultant "opportunistic" infections can be particularly severe because of the inability of the host to mount a normal immune response. Moreover, because the setting is most often the antimicrobial-laden hospital environment, the bacteria, preselected for drug resistance, are particularly difficult to treat.

Whether the pathogen is a virulent invader or an opportunistic commensal, the host response and appropriate antimicrobial therapy are the major determinants of recovery. Some bacteria, by possessing such antiopsonic and anticomplementary shields as K1 capsule and smooth LPS, are able to withstand the immune response of the host and can produce severe and complicated infections. Paradoxically, the normal immune response also can potentiate the disease by eliciting inflammatory responses beyond those needed for bacterial containment. Complement activation, the liberation of cytokines (e.g., tumor necrosis factor, the numerous interleukins), leukocyte mobilization and degranulation, and platelet and coagulation pathway activation can mediate the lethal manifestations of endotoxemia, including excessive fluid extravasation and circulatory collapse, renal tubular necrosis, adult respiratory distress syndrome, and damage to the central nervous system in cases of meningitis. Therapy of severe gram-negative infection is directed not only toward eliminating the invading microbe but also toward attenuating the immune response.

DRUG RESISTANCE AND VIRULENCE FACTORS   Successful therapy for bacterial infection depends on the use of antimicrobial agents to which the infecting microbe is susceptible. Unfortunately, bacteria have enormous ability to evade the effects of these drugs (see Chap. 100). Most drug resistance occurs from the acquisition of new genes, usually in the form of transposons. Transposons (a segment of DNA which can migrate between plasmids and between chromosomes) are more typically found on R-plasmids, which are self-replicating, nonchromosomal units of DNA that are frequently capable of being transferred from one bacterial cell to another, even of a different species, by conjugation.

The genetic organization of genes involved in drug resistance promotes their spread through the Enterobacteriaceae. Since R-plasmids move across bacterial populations readily, the presence of several antimicrobials in the environment readily selects those bacteria which contain multiple-drug-resistance elements. With time and the continued use of many drugs in the hospital and in agriculture, R-plasmids have become larger; each now consists of many different transposons strung together like pearls on a necklace. Many individual

virulence factors, including colonization factors, enterotoxins, and hemolysin, are found on plasmids, occasionally R-plasmids, which promote their spread. Also, some virulence factors can be carried together and need to be present together to cause disease, as is seen with genes for enterotoxin production and colonization factor antigens in some strains of enterotoxigenic *E. coli*.

ESCHERICHIA COLI INFECTIONS

ETIOLOGY, EPIDEMIOLOGY, AND MANIFESTATIONS   *E. coli*, primarily a commensal in the gastrointestinal tract, can be associated with disease in a number of settings. Normal individuals, if exposed to certain pathogenic strains, will develop gastroenteritis or other enteric infections. Debilitated individuals can develop pneumonia, sepsis, or urinary tract infection from otherwise avirulent strains, particularly with the placement of foreign bodies (such as endotracheal, endovascular, or endovesicular catheters). Previously healthy individuals are subject to contiguous infection from normal contents of a ruptured intestine, as may occur with appendicitis or abdominal trauma. Some otherwise healthy individuals, particularly sexually active females, are subject to repeated urinary tract infections from contiguous spread of uropathogenic strains from the gastrointestinal tract.

Enteric infections   First recognized as an agent of infantile diarrhea in the 1920s, *E. coli* is also the major cause of bacterial gastroenteritis in individuals traveling abroad. As discussed in Chap. 87, this organism comes in multiple pathogenic varieties. The most important are enterotoxigenic *E. coli* (ETEC), a cause of travelers' diarrhea; enteropathogenic (enteroadherent) *E. coli* (EPEC), a cause of childhood diarrhea; enteroinvasive *E. coli* (EIEC), which causes a dysentery-like disease; and enterohemorrhagic *E. coli* (EHEC), which causes hemorrhagic colitis and the hemolytic-uremic syndrome in children.

In industrialized countries, travelers' diarrhea typically occurs in otherwise healthy individuals visiting tropical or subtropical regions that lack advanced hygienic conditions. The organism is passed by the fecal-oral route, usually through contamination of unbottled water and salad vegetables. The inoculum of organisms must be high enough to resist the normal defensive barriers of the acid pH of the stomach. (Individuals with achlorhydria are more susceptible.) In most cases, the patient, within 1 to 2 days of exposure, develops symptoms of abdominal cramps and frequent explosive bowel movements lasting 3 to 4 days. The major manifestations are a consequence of the copious outpouring of fluid from the gastrointestinal tract due to the action of enterotoxin(s) on the gastrointestinal mucosa. The clinical presentation is similar whether the enterotoxin is of the heat-stable (ST) or heat-labile (LT) variety. Gastroenteritis in travelers also can be caused by other bacteria (e.g., *Shigella, Salmonella, Campylobacter*), viruses (e.g., rotavirus, Norwalk agent), and parasites (e.g., *Giardia, Entamoeba*). Cholera, which is caused by *Vibrio cholerae*, develops into a much more severe, life-theatening disease.

EPEC strains cause childhood diarrhea, especially in underdeveloped countries and in nursery outbreaks. These bacteria bind to the membranous cells of Peyer's patches and disrupt the overlying mucous gel of the host cell. In contrast to ETEC and EPEC, the EIEC strains, rare in the United States, invade the host cell and provoke a significant inflammatory response. Manifestations are those of bacterial dysentery with fever and bloody diarrheal stool containing polymorphonuclear leukocytes.

EHEC strains, which all belong to the serotype O157:H7, cause hemorrhagic colitis. These strains produce shiga-like toxins that kill certain cells in tissue culture. Although the typical patient is afebrile, the sequelae can be severe. In the elderly the disease is often confused with ischemic colitis and can lead to death. Children and occasionally adults with EHEC infection can develop the hemolytic-uremic syndrome (HUS), which also can lead to death. HUS is seen occasionally with bacteria other than O157:H7, including other *E. coli* serotypes and *Shigella*.

Urinary tract infections (See also Chap. 90)   Unlike the gastrointestinal tract, the urinary tract is normally sterile. Most uncomplicated urinary tract infections (i.e., those lacking foreign bodies, anatomic defects, prior surgery, pregnancy, stones, or prostate or other obstructions) are due to *E. coli*. The typical acute infection occurs in a sexually active woman following bacterial colonization of the periurethral region and ascension up the urethra. Disease can include asymptomatic bacteriuria, urethritis, cystitis, and pyelonephritis. Patients with the predisposing problems listed above also become infected with other Enterobacteriaceae and strains of *Pseudomonas* and are more likely to develop chronic or relapsing infection.

Intraabdominal infections (See also Chap. 86)   *E. coli* represents a small part of the normal bowel flora—over 99 percent of the bacteria are strict anaerobes—but is a significant pathogen in those infections resulting from spillage of normal bowel contents into previously sterile environments. Studies in animals indicate that the aerobic flora (including *E. coli*) of normal bowel contents are primarily responsible for the early septicemia associated with bowel spillage, whereas the anaerobic species are required for abscess formation. Thus *E. coli* is usually cultured from peritonitis resulting from a perforated appendix, diverticulum, or peptic ulcer and is often found in the bloodstream of patients with more severe cases. It is also associated with intraabdominal abscesses and cholecystitis and ascending cholangitis. Severe intraabdominal infections can occur with ischemia of the bowel or other organs, as frequently occurs in patients with diabetes mellitus and atherosclerotic vascular disease. Such individuals are at risk for developing acute emphysematous cholecystitis, characterized by gangrene and perforation, and septic thrombophlebitis of the portal vein (pylephlebitis), leading to liver abscesses. *E. coli* is a prominent pathogen in each of these processes.

Bacteremia (See also Chap. 83)   Bloodstream invasion by *E. coli* is most likely to lead to severe sequelae including death. Septic shock, which can be caused by the bloodstream invasion of virtually any bacterial species, is mediated by the inflammatory response of the host to the invading pathogen or to circulating constituents of the pathogen (e.g., the lipopolysaccharide, or endotoxin, of gram-negative organisms). By definition, septic shock includes hypotension, which often occurs 12 to 16 h after bacteremia but may be present from the onset. Bacteremia also can give rise to a milder "sepsis syndrome" not associated with hypotension and characterized by the sudden onset of fever and chills, tachycardia, tachypnea, and mental confusion. (The sepsis syndrome also can occur with bacterial infection in the absence of demonstrated bacteremia.) Septic shock also can occur with only one or two signs predominating, so bacteremia should be considered in any patient with unexplained confusion or hypotension. Hypothermia, rather than fever, occurs in 5 to 10 percent of patients. Combinations of uremia, hepatic failure, respiratory failure [adult respiratory distress syndrome (ARDS)], stupor, and coma can develop. The most common antecedent diseases are urinary tract, biliary, and intraperitoneal infections, and the most typical patient is the elderly man with prostatic obstruction and a history of urethral instrumentation and catheterization. Patients with persistent bacteremia despite adequate therapy often have undrained abscesses, most typically intraabdominally. Some patients, especially those with poor filtering capacity in the liver (i.e., those with cirrhosis or portosystemic shunts), diminished reticuloendothelial function, or diminished numbers of circulating phagocytic cells, may have no obvious portal of entry. In most of these the gastrointestinal tract is the source.

Other manifestations   *E. coli* can produce abscesses anywhere in the body as a consequence of bacteremia or contiguous spread. Individuals with vascular disease, especially common in diabetics, are prone to infections of the distal extremities and of surgical wounds, whereas those with diminished numbers of circulating phagocytes are prone to perirectal abscesses. Many of these subcutaneous infections are polymicrobial, with anaerobic as well as aerobic organisms, and, particularly in diabetics, gas may be demonstrable in the tissues by crepitation or by x-ray. *E. coli* may cause septic arthritis, perinephric

abscess, endophthalmitis, suppurative thyroiditis, brain abscess, endocarditis, osteomyelitis, sinusitis, pneumonia, and other infections. Neonates, most notably premature infants, are especially susceptible to bacteremia and meningitis with K1-encapsulated *E. coli*.

E. coli and other gram-negative bacteria are frequently cultured from endotracheal tubes and chronic indwelling Foley catheters, particularly in individuals on antimicrobial therapy. Whether such infestations reflect true infection requiring specific therapy or instead indicate mere colonization requires broader assessment of the patient's condition.

DIAGNOSIS   The diagnosis of *E. coli* infection depends on the combination of clinical findings (e.g., signs and symptoms of urinary tract infection) and isolation of *E. coli* by the clinical microbiology laboratory. In general, infections by *E. coli* either are due to a single organism in a previously sterile (e.g., urinary tract infections, meningitis) or nonsterile background (e.g., gastroenteritis) or are part of a polymicrobial process (e.g., ruptured appendix, infected foot in a diabetic). These distinctions are important in the interpretation of laboratory results. Thus the genital tract flora in women will contaminate urine during culturing unless assiduous attempts at obtaining and processing a clean-catch specimen are made. Urine samples from which other microbes grow along with *E. coli* should be considered contaminated. Because of the normal presence of *E. coli* in the stool, diagnosis of *E. coli* gastroenteritis is problematic but can be attempted with techniques that screen for specific strains of *E. coli* (e.g., sorbitol positivity in EHEC). Recovery of *E. coli* from tracheal aspirates in intubated patients must be analyzed in the context of the patient's clinical state to distinguish between colonization and infection (either tracheitis or pneumonia). In contrast, any growth of *E. coli* in the normally sterile environs of the bloodstream, cerebrospinal fluid, biliary tract, pleural fluid, or peritoneal cavity (the latter often in the context of polymicrobial growth) should be assumed to be diagnostic of *E. coli* infection at the site of recovery of the organism.

Rapid identification of gram-negative organisms at the site of infection is possible with Gram's stain, but this technique is unable to distinguish well among the other gram-negative bacteria that often cause similar infectious diseases. Techniques that involve amplification of nucleic acid show promise in identifying virulence genes and drug-resistance genes associated with specific microbes. One great advantage of the culture method, although it is slow, is the opportunity for antimicrobial susceptibility testing, which is particularly important with the emergence of drug-resistant pathogens.

TREATMENT   As for any infectious process, the mainstay of treatment is appropriate antimicrobial therapy and elimination of suppuration, necrotic tissue, and foreign bodies. Duration and breadth of antimicrobial therapy depend on the site and severity of the infection. For example, uncomplicated cystitis in otherwise healthy women often can be managed with a single dose of drug, whereas septicemia typically requires 2 weeks of therapy, and prostatitis or deep-seated renal infection requires as much as 6 weeks of treatment; a ruptured appendix requires coverage of anaerobic bacteria in addition. When a microorganism(s) can be recovered, antimicrobial susceptibility testing is indicated and should direct subsequent therapy of each of these conditions. Until test results are available, empirical therapy should be based on the severity and site of the infection, the status of the host, and the known drug resistance patterns in the treatment setting. For more detailed recommendations, the reader is referred to the chapters dealing with specific sites of infections.

KLEBSIELLA, ENTEROBACTER, AND SERRATIA INFECTIONS

The genera *Klebsiella, Enterobacter,* and *Serratia* belong to the tribe Klebsielleae and are typically differentiated only by certain amino acid decarboxylase tests and the fact that strains of *Klebsiella* are usually nonmotile and form large mucoid colonies on solid media. Like *E. coli,* all are colonizers of the human gastrointestinal tract and are rarely associated with disease in the normal host; however, they are a major cause of nosocomial and opportunistic infection. In many hospitals, strains of *Klebsiella* are among the most antimicrobial-resistant microbes isolated, with their ready acquisition of R-plasmids carrying aminoglycoside-inactivating enzymes, a wide variety of β-lactamases, and other drug resistance genes.

K. pneumoniae (the Friedlander bacillus) can cause community-acquired lobar pneumonia, found typically in alcoholic men over 40 with diabetes mellitus or chronic obstructive pulmonary disease. The disease is clinically indistinguishable from pneumococcal pneumonia, except for the greater tendency for disease due to *K. pneumoniae* to progress to lung abscess and empyema. Occasionally, this type of pneumonia causes the radiographic features of bulging fissures and loss of lung volume, findings that can be seen in any severe bacterial pneumonia. Gram's stain of the sputum reveals a predominance of short, plump, gram-negative bacilli, often surrounded by a capsule, which appears as a clear space. Because of the severity of the infection and to delay the emergence of resistance, acceptable antibiotic regimens should include a combination of a cephalosporin and an aminoglycoside, depending on susceptibility results.

In the hospital, *K. pneumoniae* and its tribal relatives are major causes of infections (in order of frequency) of the urinary tract, lower respiratory tract, biliary tract, and surgical wounds. Many of these infections are associated with bacteremia and life-threatening septic shock. Less common conditions caused by strains closely related to *K. pneumoniae* include rhinoscleroma, a chronic granulomatous disease involving the mucosa of the upper respiratory system leading occasionally to bony invasion and airway obstruction, associated with *K. rhinoscleromatis,* and ozena, a chronic severe rhinitis associated with turbinate atrophy and progressive anosmia, associated with *K. ozenae.* These strains actually belong to the species *K. pneumoniae,* and indole-positive strains of *K. pneumoniae* have been assigned to a new species, *K. oxytoca.*

The genus *Enterobacter* consists of *E. aerogenes, E. cloacae, E. agglomerans* (formerly called *erwinia*), and several other species. These organisms were originally lumped into the classification, *Klebsiella-Aerobacter. Enterobacter* strains are opportunistic pathogens clinically indistinguishable from *Klebsiella* but may produce cephalosporinases that inactivate even third-generation cephalosporins. *E. cloacae* accounts for the majority of hospital-acquired infections with this genus.

Like the genus *Enterobacter, Serratia* is an opportunist that has been recognized as a human pathogen only since the 1960s. Only *S. marcescens* and *S. liquifaciens* have been associated with human disease. The epidemiology of *S. marcescens* is somewhat different from that of other Enterobacteriaceae in that *S. marcescens* is less likely to colonize the gastrointestinal tract but more likely to colonize the respiratory and urinary tracts of hospitalized adults. Serious infections due either to *Enterobacter* or *Serratia* should be treated with a combination of antibiotics to which the organisms are susceptible. Two-drug combinations typically include an aminoglycoside and a cephalosporin (assuming susceptibility).

PROTEUS, MORGANELLA, AND *PROVIDENCIA* INFECTIONS

Proteeae are actively motile bacteria that do not ferment lactose. This tribe consists of at least three genera, *Proteus, Morganella,* and *Providencia,* and seven species, *Proteus vulgaris, Proteus mirabilis, Proteus myxofaciens, Morganella morganii* (previously *Proteus morganii*), *Providencia alcalifaciens, Providencia stuartii,* and *Providencia rettgeri* (previously *Proteus rettgeri*). Virtually all *P. mirabilis* strains, which cause the majority of *Proteus* infections, are indole-negative, whereas most strains in the tribe are indole-positive. *Proteus* strains are unique in their ability to swarm on moist agar media. These organisms are normally found in soil, water, and sewage

and are part of the normal fecal flora. Except for urinary tract infections, *Proteus* rarely causes primary disease in otherwise healthy individuals but is a common opportunistic invader in debilitated individuals on broad-spectrum antimicrobial therapy. Like other gram-negative bacteria, *Proteus* can contaminate burns, decubitus ulcers, and surgical wounds and is associated with destructive chronic infections of the middle ear and mastoid that occasionally lead to deafness or extension to the central nervous system with lateral sinus thrombosis, meningitis, brain abscess, and death. Although not as important as *Pseudomonas* in this regard, following trauma to the eye, *Proteus* can cause corneal ulcers, leading to panophthalmitis. *Proteus* is also an important cause of chronic urinary tract infections, in part by possession of the enzyme urease, which produces ammonium hydroxide by splitting urea and raises urinary pH to levels that promote struvite stone formation. These stones act as foreign bodies that obstruct urinary flow, serve as a nidus for persistence of infection, and promote destruction of renal parenchyma.

As with other gram-negative bacteria that cause focal infections, a serious complication of *Proteus* infection is bloodstream invasion. Clinical manifestations are typical of gram-negative sepsis, even including shock. The urinary tract serves as the portal of entry in the majority of cases, followed by the biliary tree, gastrointestinal tract, and other foci. A surgical procedure often precedes bloodstream invasion. Like *Proteus* infections, those due to *Providencia rettgeri* and *stuartii* may cause nosocomial urinary tract infections and are often resistant to multiple antimicrobials.

Treatment of these infections is similar to that of the other gram-negative bacteria, with two differences. Most strains of *P. mirabilis* are sensitive to most β-lactam and aminoglycoside antibiotics and are less difficult to treat. Nevertheless, the occurrence of struvite stones in these infections poses a challenge; by providing a nidus of bacterial persistence, untreated obstruction can lead to rapid renal destruction and sepsis. Contaminated stones often require surgical intervention for eradication of the infection.

ACINETOBACTER INFECTIONS

Acinetobacter organisms are ubiquitous water and soil saprophytes, which, along with the genera *Moraxella, Neisseria,* and *Kingella,* belong to the family Neisseriaceae. The two well-characterized pathogens are *Acinetobacter calcoaceticus* var. *lwoffi,* formerly called *Mima polymorpha,* and *Acinetobacter calcoaceticus* var. *anitratis,* formerly called *Herellea vaginicola.* Like other family members, they are gram-negative diplococci when grown on agar but differ by typically negative oxidase reactions, simple growth requirements, and bacillary appearance in broth. Unlike Enterobacteriaceae, they give a negative nitrate reaction.

The infections caused by members of this genus are similar in many respects to those of the Enterobacteriaceae, particularly nosocomial and community-acquired infections of the urinary tract, meninges, and lower respiratory tract. Likewise, *Acinetobacter* strains can cause bacteremia and both subacute and acute endocarditis. With their low innate virulence but high prevalence on the skin of normal individuals, these bacteria demonstrate a predilection for bloodstream invasion in individuals with intravenous catheters, surgical wounds, or burns. Occasionally, a bacteremic episode can be fulminant and suggestive of meningococcemia, with high fever, shock, and petechiae. Many of the bacteremias are polymicrobial.

Given the ubiquity of these organisms, disease due to *Acinetobacter* must be distinguished from mere colonization. True infection may be difficult to treat because it frequently occurs in debilitated patients and because these bacteria are frequently resistant to standard antimicrobials. Until susceptibility test results are available, the infection should be treated with the combination of an extended-spectrum β-lactam agent plus an aminoglycoside, any foreign body should be removed, and necrotic tissue, if present, should be debrided.

REFERENCES

Enterobacteriaceae: General

BONE RC: The pathogenesis of sepsis. Ann Intern Med 115:457, 1991

EISENSTEIN BI: Enterobacteriaceae, in *Principles and Practice of Infectious Diseases*, 3d ed, GL Mandell, RG Douglas, JE Bennett (eds). New York, Churchill Livingstone, 1990

————: New molecular techniques for microbial epidemiology and the diagnosis of infectious diseases. J Infect Dis 161:595, 1990

MURRAY BE: New aspects of antimicrobial resistance and the resulting therapeutic dilemmas. J Infect Dis 163:1184, 1991

SCHABERG DR et al: Major trends in the microbial etiology of nosocomial infection. Am J Med 91(suppl 3B):72S, 1991

Escherichia coli infections

GRANSDEN WR et al: Bacteremia due to *Escherichia coli:* A study of 861 episodes. Rev Infect Dis 12:1008, 1990

JOHNSON JR: Virulence factors in *Escherichia coli* urinary tract infection. Clin Microbiol Rev 4:80, 1991

OSTROFF SM et al: Infections with *Escherichia coli* O157:H7 in Washington State. JAMA 262:355, 1989

RUBINOFF MJ, FIELD M: Infectious diarrhea. Annu Rev Med 42:403, 1991

Klebsiella, Enterobacter, and *Serratia* infections

BODEY GP et al: Bacteremia caused by *Enterobacter:* 15 years of experience in a cancer hospital. Rev Infect Dis 13:550, 1991

CARPENTER JL: *Klebsiella* pulmonary infections: Occurrence at one medical center and review. Rev Infect Dis 12:672, 1990

CHOW JW et al: *Enterobacter* bacteremia: Clinical features and emergence of antibiotic resistance during therapy. Ann Intern Med 115:585, 1991

SCHWIMMBECK PL, OLDSTONE MB: Molecular mimicry between human leukocyte antigen B27 and *Klebsiella:* Consequences for spondyloarthropathies. Am J Med 85:51, 1988

Proteus infections

RAIMONDI A et al: Imipenem- and meropenem-resistant mutants of *Enterobacter cloacae* and *Proteus rettgeri* lack porins. Antimicrob Agents Chemother 35:1174, 1991

Acinetobacter infections

HARTSTEIN AI et al: Multiple intensive care unit outbreak of *Acinetobacter calcoaceticus* subspecies *antitratus* respiratory infection and colonization associated with contaminated, reusable ventilator circuits and resuscitation bags. Am J Med 85:624, 1988

116 PSEUDOMONAS INFECTIONS

MATTHEW POLLACK

Pseudomonas species are ubiquitous, free-living, opportunistic gram-negative pathogens. *P. aeruginosa*, the most common human pathogen among this group, is the primary subject of this chapter. Also discussed are *P. cepacia*, primarily an opportunistic pathogen; *Xanthomonas maltophilia*, which primarily infects hospitalized patients; *P. pseudomallei*, an organism that inhabits soil and water (primarily in the tropics) and that causes melioidosis—a systemic disease with acute or chronic manifestations—in nonimmunocompromised patients; and *P. mallei*, a pathogen of animal origin that occasionally produces glanders in humans.

P. AERUGINOSA INFECTIONS

P. aeruginosa is a small, aerobic gram-negative rod belonging to the family Pseudomonadaceae. It is motile by virtue of its single polar flagellum. More than half of clinical isolates produce the blue-green pigment pyocyanin; this pigment is helpful in the identification of the organism and accounts for the species name *aeruginosa*, which refers to the distinctive color of copper oxide. *P. aeruginosa* is readily identified in the clinical laboratory. It is a straight or slightly curved, nonsporulating, motile gram-negative rod that grows aerobically on most common media.

EPIDEMIOLOGY *P. aeruginosa* is widespread in nature, inhabiting soil, water, plants, and animals, including humans. It has a predilection for moist environments. This organism occasionally colonizes the skin, external ear, upper respiratory tract, or large bowel of healthy humans. Rates of carriage are relatively low, however, except in patients who have serious underlying disease, whose host defenses have been naturally or iatrogenically compromised, who have received prior antibiotic therapy, and/or who have been exposed to the hospital environment. Under these circumstances, colonization with *P. aeruginosa* frequently precedes infection, and factors that predispose to the former also increase the likelihood of the latter.

Most *P. aeruginosa* infections are hospital acquired. Many potential reservoirs of infection have been identified, including respiratory equipment, cleaning solutions, disinfectants, sinks, vegetables, flowers, endoscopes, and physiotherapy pools. Most reservoirs are associated with moisture. It is assumed that the organism is transmitted to patients via the hands of hospital personnel or via fomites.

While some infecting strains of *P. aeruginosa* appear to be endemic within the hospital environment, others are traced to a common source associated with a specific outbreak or epidemic. Epidemiologic investigation is facilitated by serotyping (immunotyping) of strains on the basis of differences in lipopolysaccharide structure or by the use of DNA probes.

PATHOGENESIS The pathogenesis of infections due to *P. aeruginosa* is complex, as is evidenced by the clinical diversity of the diseases related to this organism and by the multiplicity of virulence factors it produces. *P. aeruginosa* rarely causes disease in the healthy host. It may undergo a "malignant" transformation, however, when normal cutaneous or mucosal barriers have been breached or bypassed (e.g., by burn injury, penetrating trauma, surgery, endotracheal intubation, urinary bladder catheterization, or intravenous drug abuse); when immunologic defense mechanisms have been compromised (e.g., by chemotherapy-induced neutropenia, hypogammaglobulinemia, extremes of age, diabetes mellitus, cystic fibrosis, cancer, or AIDS); when the protective function of the normal bacterial flora has been disrupted by broad-spectrum antibiotic therapy; and/or when the patient has been exposed to reservoirs associated with a hospital environment. The ubiquity of the organism, its flexible nutritional and metabolic requirements, its environmental resiliency, and its relative resistance to antibiotics help account for the frequency and success with which it acts as an opportunistic pathogen.

Infections caused by *P. aeruginosa* usually begin with bacterial attachment and superficial colonization of cutaneous or mucosal surfaces and progress to localized bacterial invasion and damage to underlying tissues. This process may continue with bloodstream invasion, dissemination, sepsis syndrome, and ultimately death. Alternatively, the infection may remain anatomically localized or may spread by direct extension to contiguous structures. The organism and its products may cause tissue injury at primary and secondary sites of infection, while the release of systemically acting toxins may contribute directly or indirectly to the sepsis syndrome.

The initial attachment of *P. aeruginosa* to the respiratory epithelium and other epithelial surfaces appears to be mediated by bacterial organelles called *pili* or *fimbriae* and by the mucoid exopolysaccharide termed *alginate*, which is produced by mucoid strains. Receptors for these adhesins are found, for example, on tracheal epithelial cells and tracheobronchial mucin and are composed, at least in part, of *N*-acetylneuraminic acid (sialic acid) and *N*-acetylglucosamine, respectively.

Surface moieties of *P. aeruginosa*, including exopolysaccharide and lipopolysaccharide, may protect the organism from direct antibody- and complement-mediated bactericidal mechanisms and from opsonophagocytosis. Meanwhile, the organism produces a number of extracellular enzymes, including alkaline protease, elastase, phospholipase, cytotoxin, and exoenzymes (or exotoxins) A and S. The breakdown of host tissues by these extracellular bacterial products creates conditions conducive to enhanced bacterial proliferation, invasion, and tissue injury.

The preceding process is particularly likely to culminate in bloodstream invasion and dissemination in the face of immune compromise such as that resulting from profound neutropenia. Septicemia or sepsis syndrome due to *P. aeruginosa* shares many of the features of gram-negative sepsis caused by other bacteria, and the lipopolysaccharide or endotoxin produced by this organism, like that produced by other bacterial species, is thought to play a pivotal role in the pathogenesis of this syndrome.

In addition to lipopolysaccharide, which is a structural component of the bacterial outer membrane, the extracellular enzyme exotoxin A, diphtheria-like toxin, is produced by most clinical isolates of *P. aeruginosa*. Exotoxin A inhibits mammalian protein synthesis by transferring the adenosine diphosphate (ADP) ribose moiety of the nicotinamide adenine dinucleotide into covalent linkage with elongation factor 2, an enzyme that catalyzes the elongation step in polypeptide assembly but is inactivated by exotoxin-mediated ADP ribosylation. Exotoxin A appears to cause both local and systemic disease. It is cytotoxic in vitro and necrotizing in vivo and produces fatal shock in experimental animals, including nonhuman primates. Toxinogenic clinical isolates are more virulent than nontoxinogenic strains. Moreover, the rate of survival is higher among patients with *P. aeruginosa* bacteremia in the presence of adequate preexisting levels of exotoxin A–specific serum antibodies.

CLINICAL MANIFESTATIONS AND DIAGNOSIS Respiratory infections Lower respiratory tract infections due to *P. aeruginosa* occur mainly in immunocompromised patients. Primary or nonbacteremic pneumonia results from aspiration of upper respiratory tract secretions, often develops in patients with chronic lung disease or congestive heart failure, and is most common in an intensive care setting. Bacteremic pneumonia, in contrast, complicates hematopoietic malignancies, especially after chemotherapy that induces severe neutropenia. Chronic infection of the lower respiratory tract with *P. aeruginosa* is prevalent among patients with cystic fibrosis. It occurs typically in older children or young adults and is caused almost exclusively by mucoid strains.

Primary or nonbacteremic pneumonia caused by *P. aeruginosa* may present as an acute, life-threatening infection characterized by fever, chills, severe dyspnea, cyanosis, productive cough, apprehension, confusion, and other signs of severe systemic toxicity. Chest roentgenograms typically show bilateral bronchopneumonia with nodular infiltrates and small areas of radiolucency; pleural effusions are common; empyema is rare; and lobar consolidation is occasionally seen. Pathologic lesions include alveolar necrosis, focal hemorrhages, and microabscesses.

Bacteremic pneumonia due to *P. aeruginosa*, typically associated with neutropenia, begins as a respiratory infection, but subsequent bloodstream invasion and resulting metastatic spread produce characteristic lesions in the lung and other viscera. Alveolar hemorrhage and necrosis are common. The signs and symptoms of this fulminant disease include those described for nonbacteremic pneumonia caused by this organism as well as those associated with gram-negative sepsis. Chest roentgenograms characteristically demonstrate a rapid progression from pulmonary vascular congestion to interstitial edema, to pulmonary edema, to diffuse necrotizing bronchopneumonia with cavity formation. The patient typically dies 3 to 4 days after initial presentation.

Mucoid strains of *P. aeruginosa* infect the lower respiratory tract of patients with cystic fibrosis, contributing to the acute exacerbations and chronic progression that characterize pulmonary disease in these individuals. Colonization with *P. aeruginosa* correlates with bronchial airway disease in cystic fibrosis patients. It is unclear whether mucus plugging precedes infection or vice versa. This uncertainty notwithstanding, airway obstruction appears to begin with bronchiolitis, which causes mucus plugging and predisposes to *P. aeruginosa* infection. The latter produces more mucus plugging, chronic suppuration, bronchiectasis, atelectasis, and ultimately fibrosis. This process progresses to pulmonary insufficiency, hypoxemia, and alterations in cardiopulmonary dynamics resulting in pulmonary hypertension and cor pulmonale.

Clinical manifestations of lower respiratory tract infections due to *P. aeruginosa* in cystic fibrosis vary with the severity and duration of underlying lung disease and with the frequency and intensity of acute episodes. Early in the disease, patients may experience recurrent upper respiratory symptoms followed by a lingering cough. Episodes of pneumonia develop later, with persistent cough between acute episodes. Eventually, patients exhibit a chronic productive cough, diminished appetite, weight loss, and decreased activity. Other symptoms may include wheezing, tachypnea, and irritability. Acute exacerbations are typically accompanied by low-grade fever and heightened respiratory symptoms. Physical signs include evidence of malnutrition, increase in anteroposterior diameter, intercostal retractions, cyanosis, inspiratory and expiratory wheezing, rhonchi, moist rales, abdominal distention, and clubbing of the fingers and toes. Laboratory abnormalities include leukocytosis with a left shift and hypoxemia with or without hypercarbia. Tests of pulmonary function demonstrate obstructive and restrictive defects. Chest roentgenograms reveal overaeration, patchy atelectasis, peribronchial fibrosis, and patchy infiltrates associated with pneumonia. In more advanced disease, there may be evidence of severe overaeration, depressed diaphragms, increased anteroposterior diameter, extensive peribronchial infiltration, generalized bronchiectasis, and cyst formation.

Bacteremia *P. aeruginosa* causes one of the most common and life-threatening forms of gram-negative bacteremia in immunocompromised patients. *P. aeruginosa* bacteremia is usually associated with nosocomial infections and is frequently iatrogenic. It is either primary (no identifiable source) or secondary to a discrete extravascular focus. *P. aeruginosa* bacteremia is associated with underlying abnormalities such as hematologic malignancies, neutropenia, immunoglobulin deficiencies, severe burns, dermatitis, diabetes mellitus, AIDS, and prematurity. Predisposing iatrogenic factors include cancer chemotherapy resulting in neutropenia or mucosal ulceration, genitourinary instrumentation or catheterization, placement of intravascular hardware, recent surgery, steroid therapy, and antibiotic administration.

The clinical features of *P. aeruginosa* bacteremia are similar to those of other forms of bacteremia. Common primary sites of infection include the urinary tract, gastrointestinal tract, lungs, intravascular foci, skin, and soft tissues. Fever, tachypnea, tachycardia, and prostration are common. Disorientation, confusion, or obtundation may be evident. Hypotension can progress to refractory shock. Renal failure, adult respiratory distress syndrome, or disseminated intravascular coagulation may occur as complications. Jaundice is seen more commonly in *P. aeruginosa* bacteremia than in other forms of gram-negative sepsis.

Pathognomonic skin lesions termed *ecthyma gangrenosum* develop in a relatively small minority of patients with *P. aeruginosa* bacteremia. The lesions begin as small, hemorrhagic vesicles surrounded by a rim of erythema and undergo central necrosis with subsequent ulceration. They occur singly or in small numbers on the perineum, buttocks, and extremities; in the axillae; or elsewhere. Ecthyma-like lesions are occasionally noted on the mucous membranes of the mouth or gingiva. Histologic study shows that these lesions contain numerous bacteria invading blood vessels but few inflammatory cells. Bacteria are readily visible on Gram's stain and may be cultured from aspirated material.

Endocarditis *P. aeruginosa* infects native heart valves in intravenous drug users as well as prosthetic heart valves. The source of *P. aeruginosa* strains infecting drug users appears to be standing water contaminating drug paraphernalia. Moreover, foreign materials that are mixed with heroin may cause injury to valve leaflets or mural endocardium leading to fibrosis. These factors, combined with the apparent high affinity of the organism for human endocardium, may explain the association between *P. aeruginosa* endocarditis and intravenous drug use. The particularly frequent exposure of the tricuspid valve to both trauma and bacteria apparently accounts for the high incidence of tricuspid involvement in association with intravenous drug use.

The pulmonic, mitral, or aortic valve or the mural endocardium of either atrium also may be affected in *P. aeruginosa* endocarditis. Multiple-valve infections are common. Tricuspid or right-sided involvement is often associated with septic pulmonary emboli. Right-sided *P. aeruginosa* endocarditis usually presents subacutely, while the appearance of left-sided disease is likely to be more acute or even fulminant. Fever is almost invariable, and murmurs are usually detectable at initial presentation or shortly thereafter. Septic pulmonary emboli associated with right-sided disease result in cough, pleuritic chest pain, sputum production, pulmonary infiltrates (with or without abscess formation), and pleural effusions. Left-sided infections may present as intractable heart failure or large systemic emboli. Mycotic aneurysms, cerebritis, or brain abscess may occur; septic infarcts are occasionally found in the spleen, but skin and soft tissue manifestations, including Janeway lesions, Osler's nodes, and ecthyma gangrenosum, are relatively uncommon.

The diagnosis of *P. aeruginosa* endocarditis is based on a positive blood culture in the absence of an extracardiac source; an indication of valvular dysfunction or vegetation on an echocardiogram; evidence of septic pulmonary lesions on a chest roentgenogram (in right-sided disease); and the actual demonstration of infected heart valves at the time of surgery.

Central nervous system infections *P. aeruginosa* infections of the central nervous system include meningitis and brain abscess. These infections follow extension from a contiguous, parameningeal structure such as the ear, mastoid, or paranasal sinus; direct inoculation into the subarachnoid space or brain through head trauma, surgery, or diagnostic procedures; or bacteremic spread from a distant site such as the urinary tract, lung, or heart valve. Like *P. aeruginosa* infections at other anatomic sites, central nervous system infections are documented almost exclusively in patients with compromised local or systemic immune defense mechanisms. Predisposing factors include recent neurosurgical procedures, penetrating head trauma, lumbar puncture or spinal anesthesia, cancer of the head and neck, parameningeal infection, and *P. aeruginosa* infections occurring at distant sites and associated with bloodstream invasion.

The clinical signs of *P. aeruginosa* meningitis, like those of other forms of acute bacterial meningitis, include fever, headache, stiff neck, confusion, and obtundation. The onset of illness may be acute or even fulminant, particularly in bacteremic patients, with a precipitous downhill course, shock, coma, and early death. In nonbacteremic patients, *P. aeruginosa* meningitis or brain abscess may present more insidiously, with a paucity of systemic symptoms. This presentation is especially common in infections resulting from recent neurosurgery, cancer of the head and neck, or direct extension from a parameningeal focus of chronic infection. Occasionally, *P. aeruginosa* meningitis runs a subacute or relapsing course that is thought to be related to the intermittent release of bacteria from a loculated site of infection. Chronic or recurrent meningitis may result from altered cranial anatomy associated with central nervous system tumors, traumatic injury, neurosurgical procedures, indwelling hardware, or cerebrospinal fluid leaks.

Ear infections *P. aeruginosa* is often found in the external auditory canal, particularly under moist conditions and in the presence of inflammation or maceration (as in "swimmer's ear"). Moreover, this organism is the predominant pathogen associated with external otitis, a usually benign inflammatory process affecting the external auditory canal. This self-limited condition provides a local environment conducive to the growth of *P. aeruginosa*, which, in turn, appears to contribute to the inflammatory process. The ear is painful or merely itchy, there is a purulent discharge, and pain is elicited by pulling on the pinna. The external canal appears edematous and is filled with detritus that often prevents visualization of the tympanic membrane.

P. aeruginosa occasionally penetrates the epithelium overlying the floor of the external auditory canal at the junction between bone and cartilage and invades underlying soft tissue. The ensuing invasive process, which involves soft tissue, cartilage, and cortical bone, is typically slow but destructive. Termed *malignant external otitis*, this condition occurs predominantly in elderly diabetics but is reported occasionally in young infants with other underlying diseases and rarely in elderly nondiabetic patients. Virtually all cases of malignant external otitis are caused by *P. aeruginosa*. From the external ear, the infection advances to the retromandibular area or parotid space and enters the mastoid air cells and temporal bone. Advancing osteomyelitis at the base of the skull often involves the seventh, ninth, tenth, and eleventh cranial nerves. The cavernous sinus can become involved, as can the contralateral petrous apex. The middle ear is commonly spared; meningitis and brain abscess are relatively rare complications.

Otalgia and otorrhea are common presenting symptoms of malignant external otitis. Facial nerve paralysis tends to occur early, while other cranial nerve palsies appear later. There may be a loss of hearing, the pinna of the ear is typically tender, and trismus indicates temporomandibular involvement. Constitutional symptoms such as fever and weight loss are relatively uncommon. Physical examination almost always reveals abnormalities of the external auditory canal, including swelling, erythema, purulent discharge, debris, and granulation tissue in the canal wall. The tympanic membrane is often hidden from view and is sometimes perforated. Inflammation may involve the pinna as well as the periauricular, retromandibular, and mastoid areas. Bilateral disease is unusual but does occur.

Peripheral leukocytosis is relatively infrequent in malignant external otitis, while the erythrocyte sedimentation rate usually is markedly elevated. Cerebrospinal fluid occasionally exhibits pleocytosis and an elevated protein level. Computed tomographic (CT) scans or polytomograms of the mastoid or temporal bone typically reveal bony erosions and new bone formation, while the floor of the skull may have soft tissue densities associated with areas of cellulitis. Magnetic resonance imaging (MRI) may delineate soft tissue involvement with greater sensitivity and accuracy than CT scans. Technetium 99m bone scans and gallium 67 scans also are frequently positive. Cultures of samples from the external auditory canal and surgical specimens are almost always positive for *P. aeruginosa*.

P. aeruginosa is commonly implicated in chronic suppurative otitis media in children and adults. It is either the sole bacterial isolate or among the organisms isolated from the middle or external ear in a majority of cases and is thought to play a central pathogenic role.

Eye infections *P. aeruginosa* causes bacterial keratitis or corneal ulcer and endophthalmitis in the human eye. Keratitis due to *P. aeruginosa* may result from even minor corneal injury, which interrupts the integrity of the superficial epithelial surface and permits bacterial access to the underlying stroma. Corneal ulcer may complicate contact lens use, particularly when extended-wear soft contact lens are involved. Contact lens solutions or the lens themselves may be the source of the organism, which is probably inoculated into the eye at sites of minor lens-induced corneal damage. Patients who have sustained serious burns, have undergone ocular irradiation or tracheostromy, have been exposed to the intensive care environment, and/or are in a coma are also susceptible to *P. aeruginosa*–associated corneal ulcers. *P. aeruginosa* keratitis usually starts as a small central ulcer; spreads concentrically to involve a large portion of the cornea, sclera, and underlying stroma; and in some cases progresses to posterior corneal perforation.

The clinical manifestations of *P. aeruginosa* keratitis include a rapidly expanding, necrotic stromal infiltrate in the bed of an epithelial injury; surrounding epithelial edema; an anterior chamber reaction; and mucopurulent discharge adherent to the ulcer's surface. Corneal ulcer due to *P. aeruginosa* may advance rapidly to involve the entire cornea in 2 days or less or may evolve subacutely over several days. Systemic symptoms are uncommon. Complications include corneal perforation, anterior chamber involvement, and endophthalmitis.

P. aeruginosa endophthalmitis may complicate penetrating injuries of the eye, intraocular surgery, hematogenous spread from other sites of *Pseudomonas* infection, or posterior perforation of corneal ulcers. It is typically a rapidly progressive, sight-threatening condition that demands immediate therapeutic intervention. Clinical manifestations may include eye pain, conjunctival hyperemia, chemosis, lid edema, decreased visual acuity, hypopyon, severe anterior uveitis, and signs of possible vitreous involvement. Panophthalmitis may result from this intraocular infection.

Bone and joint infections Vertebral osteomyelitis due to *P. aeruginosa* is associated with complicated urinary tract infection, genitourinary instrumentation or surgery, and intravenous drug abuse. Vertebral infections associated with a urinary tract source most often develop in the elderly and usually affect the lumbosacral spine. Drug use–related infections typically occur in younger patients and may affect the cervical or lumbosacral spine. *P. aeruginosa* vertebral osteomyelitis is usually an indolent disease. Accordingly, the duration of symptoms before diagnosis may be weeks or even months. Back or neck pain is generally reported, while fever and systemic symptoms are relatively uncommon. Local tenderness and decreased range of motion of the affected spine are typical. Neurologic deficits are documented in a minority of patients. Leukocytosis may be noted, the erythrocyte sedimentation rate is almost always markedly elevated, and blood cultures are sometimes positive. Roentgenograms reveal loss of bone density, narrowed intervertebral space, destruction of vertebral end plates, lytic lesions of vertebral bodies, sclerosis, and possible osteophyte formation. CT or MRI may be the most sensitive means of defining the lesions. Technetium bone scans and gallium scans are usually positive, while myelograms are revealing only if granulation tissue impinges on the epidural space. An etiologic diagnosis requires culture of material obtained by needle aspiration or biopsy of the affected spine under fluoroscopic guidance, while open biopsy is occasionally needed.

Sternoclavicular pyarthrosis caused by *P. aeruginosa* is another complication of intravenous drug abuse; in some cases it is associated with *P. aeruginosa* endocarditis, but more often it is not. Joint involvement is usually monoarticular, with the sternoclavicular joint more often affected than sternochondral joints. Localized pain in the anterior chest wall is the usual presenting complaint, movement of the homolateral shoulder may be restricted by discomfort, associated fever is common, and symptoms typically last for months (although some cases do have more acute presentations). Physical examination reveals tenderness, erythema, and swelling over the affected joint. Leukocytosis is common, and an elevated erythrocyte sedimentation rate is almost invariable. Roentgenograms show soft tissue edema, bone demineralization, lytic lesions, and periosteal elevation of the clavicular head, rib, or sternum. Material obtained by arthrocentesis or synovial biopsy yields *P. aeruginosa* in culture.

P. aeruginosa infections of the symphysis pubis are associated with pelvic surgery and intravenous drug use. The symphysis pubis, like other fibrocartilaginous joints, exhibits a peculiar susceptibility to bloodborne infection with *P. aeruginosa*. Affected patients report pain in the groin, hip, thigh, and/or lower abdomen that is made worse by walking. Fever is variable, and the duration of symptoms before diagnosis ranges from days to months. As in other bone and joint infections caused by *P. aeruginosa*, leukocytosis is variable, while the erythrocyte sedimentation rate is markedly elevated. Roentgenograms show irregularities of the pubic margins, separation of the symphysis pubis, and osteomyelitic abnormalities of the pubic rami that may be extensive. Bone scans are usually positive. Needle aspiration or biopsy is necessary to obtain material for culture. A positive culture is particularly important for the discrimination of *P. aeruginosa* infections and other pyogenic infections from osteitis pubis, which is thought to be a noninfectious condition complicating pelvic surgery, childbirth, or trauma.

P. aeruginosa osteochondritis of the foot follows puncture wounds of the foot, primarily in children. The organism infects the small joints and bones of the foot, including the proximal phalanges, metatarsals, metatarsophalangeal joints, tarsal bones, and calcaneus. *P. aeruginosa* shows a particular predilection for cartilage. Systemic symptoms are usually lacking. On average, symptoms last for several weeks. There may be plantar cellulitis over the involved area or tenderness upon deep palpation. Roentgenograms and bone scans are generally positive. Aspiration of the affected joint usually yields purulent material in which *P. aeruginosa* can be demonstrated by Gram's stain and by culture.

P. aeruginosa is one of the most common causative agents in a variety of other, less specific syndromes involving nonhematogenous infections of bones and joints and collectively referred to as *chronic contiguous osteomyelitis*. These infections may result, for example, from compound fractures, contamination associated with open reduction and fixation of closed fractures, sternotomy performed in conjunction with cardiac surgery, contiguous spread from infected ischemic ulcers related to peripheral vascular disease or diabetes mellitus, and cellulitis in general. The chronicity, indolence, and heterogeneity of these infections explain their varied clinical manifestations and the frequent need for complicated long-term management.

Gastrointestinal infections *P. aeruginosa* infections involving virtually every portion of the human gastrointestinal tract—from oropharynx to rectum—have been documented. *P. aeruginosa*–associated gastrointestinal disease is most common in young infants and in adults with hematologic malignancies and neutropenia. Moreover, asymptomatic large-bowel colonization resulting from prolonged exposure to the hospital environment and the selective pressure of antibiotics may be a silent source of organisms that subsequently invade the bloodstream during severe chemotherapy-induced neutropenia or other forms of immunosuppression.

P. aeruginosa causes necrotizing enterocolitis in young infants and a similar disease in neutropenic patients with cancer. The most common sites of involvement are the distal ileum, cecum, and colon. The pathologic lesions are hemorrhagic and necrotic ulcers that begin in the bowel mucosa and extend into the submucosa. Vascular invasion by bacteria may be documented in the submucosa, with associated bacteremia, local spread to the muscularis and serosa, and subsequent perforation leading to peritonitis. Necrotic ulcers are also documented occasionally in the oropharynx, esophagus, stomach, or proximal small bowel. Typhlitis, a disease developing most frequently in patients with leukemia, involves localized lesions of the cecum that are associated with necrosis and gangrene and sometimes result in perforation, bacterial peritonitis, and early death; *P. aeruginosa* is the agent most commonly identified in this condition. This organism is also among the pathogens most frequently isolated from rectal abscesses in neutropenic patients with cancer. These lesions, which may be associated with few signs and symptoms, must be carefully sought in susceptible patients because they may give rise to life-threatening sepsis if not surgically drained.

P. aeruginosa has been implicated in epidemics of moderate to severe diarrhea in children, a form of enteric fever sometimes referred to as *Shanghai fever*, and a cholera-like illness attributed to a putative but still-unidentified *Pseudomonas* enterotoxin.

Urinary tract infections *P. aeruginosa* is one of the most common causes of complicated and nosocomial infections of the urinary tract. These infections may result from urinary tract catheterization, instrumentation, surgery, or obstruction; they may arise from persistent foci (e.g., the prostate or stones) and may be chronic or recurrent. The urinary tract may be a target for bloodborne infection in patients with *P. aeruginosa* bacteremia but more often is the source of bacteremia. Chronic *P. aeruginosa* infections of the urinary tract are relatively common in patients with indwelling Foley catheters, altered urinary tract anatomy secondary to diversionary procedures, and paraplegia.

The clinical features of urinary tract infections due to *P. aeruginosa* are usually indistinguishable from those of other bacterial infections. However, *P. aeruginosa* infections exhibit a propensity for persistence, chronicity, resistance to antibiotic therapy, and recurrence. More unusual forms of urinary tract involvement peculiar to *P. aeruginosa* include ulcerative lesions of the renal pelvis, ureters, and bladder that cause sloughing of vesical membrane in the urine and bacterial invasion of renal blood vessels that produces ecthyma-like lesions in association with *Pseudomonas* sepsis.

Skin and soft tissue infections As indicated above, *P. aeruginosa* bacteremia may be associated with ecthyma gangrenosum. These disseminated skin lesions, which frequently begin as small vesicles, are characterized by hemorrhage, necrosis, surrounding erythema, and histologic evidence of blood vessel invasion by bacteria. *P. aeruginosa* can almost always be cultured from the lesions. Other, less common skin manifestations of *P. aeruginosa* sepsis include vesicular or pustular lesions, bullae, subcutaneous nodules, deep abscesses, and cellulitis. Metastatic lesions of the skin or mucous membranes complicate *Pseudomonas* sepsis and occasionally produce massive necrosis or gangrene of the extremities, perineum, face, or oropharynx.

Primary *P. aeruginosa* pyoderma occurs when the skin breaks down secondary to trauma, burn injury, dermatitis, or ulcers related to peripheral vascular disease or pressure sores. Moist conditions, such as those in the perineum or diaper area of infants, contribute to the development of *P. aeruginosa* pyoderma. Neutropenia also may predispose to this condition. The clinical appearance of primary *P. aeruginosa* pyoderma, which frequently includes hemorrhage and necrosis, resembles that of metastatic *P. aeruginosa* skin lesions. Histologic studies document vascular invasion by bacteria in both diseases. A rare distinguishing feature of *P. aeruginosa* pyoderma is its association with a blue-green exudate and a characteristic fruity odor.

P. aeruginosa wound sepsis complicating extensive third-degree burn injuries results from colonization of the burn site or burn eschar, invasion of the subeschar space and underlying dermis, vascular invasion, and systemic spread. The development and progression of *P. aeruginosa* burn wound sepsis are facilitated by the injury-associated breakdown of normal skin, antibiotic selection, and burn-related immune defects. Local manifestations include black, dark brown, or violaceous discoloration of the burn eschar; degeneration of underlying granulation tissue, hemorrhage, and premature eschar separation; edema, hemorrhage, and necrosis of skin adjacent to the burn site; erythematous nodular lesions in unburned skin; and formation of brown or black neoeschars. Systemic manifestations include fever or hypothermia, confusion or obtundation, oliguria, hypotension, ileus, and sometimes respiratory failure or pneumonia. The diagnosis of *P. aeruginosa* burn sepsis is based on these local and systemic clinical manifestations and a burn wound biopsy that reveals $> 10^5$ colony-forming units of *P. aeruginosa* per gram of tissue and histologic evidence of bacterial invasion of unburned tissue, vasculitis, or intense inflammation at the burn margin.

P. aeruginosa causes diffuse pruritic maculopapular and vesiculopustular rashes associated with exposure to contaminated hot tubs, spas, whirlpools, and swimming pools. Most cases of *P. aeruginosa* dermatitis have occurred as part of a common-source outbreak. At least two nosocomial common-source outbreaks—one related to a physiotherapy pool—have been reported. Skin rashes may be limited to areas covered by swimsuits or may be more diffuse, sparing only the head and neck. Associated symptoms may include dizziness, headache, earache, sore eyes, sore nose, sore throat, swollen breasts, or abdominal cramps. Low-grade fever is uncommon. The illness is usually self-limited, and the rash resolves without specific therapy after cessation of exposure. One nosocomial outbreak involving immunocompromised patients, however, resulted in *P. aeruginosa* folliculitis evolving into full-blown ecthyma gangrenosum.

TREATMENT AND PROGNOSIS Most types of *P. aeruginosa* disease are treated with one or more antibiotics to which the infecting organism is sensitive. Exceptions are external otitis (nonmalignant) and dermatitis associated with exposure to contaminated water. Both these infections are self-limited and usually require no specific antimicrobial therapy.

In general, the choice of antibiotics with antipseudomonal activity includes the aminoglycosides (e.g., gentamicin, tobramycin, netilmicin, amikacin), selected third-generation cephalosporins (e.g., ceftazidime, cefoperazone), selected extended-spectrum penicillins (e.g., carbenicillin, ticarcillin, ticarcillin/clavulanate, piperacillin, mezlocillin, azlocillin), carbapenem (imipenem), monobactams (e.g., aztreonam), and fluoroquinolones (e.g., ciprofloxacin, ofloxacin). All these agents are available in parenteral form; ciprofloxacin and ofloxacin are also available in oral form. Local patterns of antimicrobial susceptibility should influence the initial choice of antibiotic agents, while the susceptibility profile of the isolate from a particular case should dictate definitive antibiotic therapy.

In most severe or life-threatening infections due to *P. aeruginosa*, two antibiotics to which the infecting strain is (or is likely to be) sensitive should be administered together. The combination of an aminoglycoside and a β-lactam antibiotic is usually appropriate. The goals of combined therapy are to achieve additive or synergistic killing, to exploit the pharmacologic strengths and offset the pharmacologic limitations of each agent, and to prevent the emergence of antibiotic resistance. Particularly in acute or fulminant infections, antibiotics should be employed at the maximal doses consistent with safety. Likewise, when sites of infection are relatively inaccessible (e.g., the central nervous system or the heart), maximal or even supramaximal antibiotic doses may be required for the attainment of therapeutic concentrations in infected tissues.

The appropriate duration of antibiotic therapy for disease caused by *P. aeruginosa* depends on the type, location, and severity of infection. Precise, prospectively defined treatment guidelines are sometimes problematic; it may be more appropriate to tailor the duration of therapy to the specific circumstances of a case, including the initial response to treatment. In general, chronic infections associated with extensive tissue injury, disruption of normal anatomy, foreign or prosthetic material, or suboptimal antibiotic accessibility require therapy for weeks or even months rather than days. More acute infections may be treated aggressively but for shorter periods.

Infections of the lower respiratory tract in patients with cystic fibrosis pose a special challenge because they represent long-standing, chronic conditions complicated by acute exacerbations and a downhill course. Antibiotic therapy for acute exacerbations clearly results in clinical improvement. A more aggressive approach featuring periodic, expectant courses of antimicrobial therapy may limit disease progression. Frequent pulmonary toilet is important in the management of this disease, while periodic bronchial lavage has been employed to good effect to relieve symptoms associated with mucus plugging. Aerosolized antibiotics also have been used successfully in some instances.

Optimal management of infections due to *P. aeruginosa* often requires surgical intervention as well as antimicrobial therapy. The presence of necrotic tissue or of prosthetic or foreign material necessitates surgical debridement (e.g., in malignant external otitis and some cases of chronic osteomyelitis or osteochondritis); loculated pus demands drainage (e.g., in sternoclavicular pyarthrosis, brain abscess, and endophthalmitis); left-sided endocarditis is an indication for early valve replacement; perforated bowel requires laparotomy and bowel resection (e.g., in necrotizing enterocolitis); and urinary tract obstruction may necessitate appropriate surgery.

All infections caused by *P. aeruginosa* are treatable and—with the possible exception of lung infections in patients with cystic fibrosis—potentially curable. The heterogeneity of these infections, however, accounts for major differences in short- and long-term prognosis. At one end of the spectrum are acute fulminant infections such as bacteremic pneumonia, septicemia, burn wound sepsis, and meningitis, which are associated with extremely high mortality despite appropriate therapy. At the other end of the spectrum are more chronic, indolent infections, including certain cases of chronic contiguous osteomyelitis, malignant external otitis, and lower respiratory tract infections in patients with cystic fibrosis. Although the latter infections may not be imminently life-threatening, they are often difficult to eradicate and (as in the case of cystic fibrosis lung disease) may end fatally in the longer term.

INFECTIONS CAUSED BY OTHER *PSEUDOMONAS* SPECIES

P. cepacia, like *P. aeruginosa*, is primarily an opportunistic pathogen that is implicated in both endemic infections and occasional nosocomial outbreaks. Hospital epidemics are most frequently associated with a liquid reservoir or a moist environmental surface. Under these circumstances, the organism may colonize various body sites, with the subsequent development of invasive disease. The distinction between colonization and true infection is often difficult and may hinge on the presence of clinical signs of infection as well as a positive culture. *P. cepacia* has been reported to cause pneumonia, urinary tract infections, meningitis, peritonitis, surgical and burn wound infections, bacteremia, and endocarditis related to injection drug use. In addition, *P. cepacia* has been implicated, either alone or together with *P. aeruginosa*, in chronic infections of the lower respiratory tract in patients with cystic fibrosis. In some of these patients, the appearance of *P. cepacia* has been associated with fulminant necrotizing pneumonia, bacteremia, and a rapid downhill course.

The treatment of *P. cepacia* infections is complicated by the resistance of the organism to aminoglycosides and many β-lactam agents. Although trimethoprim-sulfamethoxazole and chloramphenicol have been used successfully in the treatment of *P. cepacia* infections, resistance to these two antimicrobial agents has been reported. Third-generation cephalosporins and fluoroquinolones have variable activity against *P. cepacia*. However, ciprofloxacin and ampicillin-sulbactam may be considered as alternative agents for use against sensitive strains. While in vitro synergy has been demonstrated for certain antibiotic combinations, such as ciprofloxacin, imipenem, and rifampin, the clinical efficacy of such combinations has not been fully documented.

Xanthomonas (formerly *Pseudomonas*) *maltophilia* is a ubiquitous, free-living opportunistic pathogen that colonizes and occasionally infects hospitalized patients, particularly in an intensive care setting. This organism has been associated with pneumonia, urinary tract infection, wound infection, peritonitis, cholangitis, meningitis, bacteremia, and endocarditis. *X. maltophilia*, like other *Pseudomonas* species, has been implicated in pseudoinfections, particularly pseudobacteremia related to contaminated blood-drawing materials. It is thus essential to consider clinical signs and symptoms in distinguishing exogenous contamination or simple colonization from genuine infection. Urinary tract infection is usually associated with a chronic indwelling urinary catheter or with urinary tract instrumentation; line-related sepsis complicates intravenous therapy; peritonitis has occurred in patients undergoing chronic ambulatory peritoneal dialysis; native valve endocarditis has been described in intravenous drug users; and prosthetic valve endocarditis also has been reported. Acute *X. maltophilia* pneumonia is being seen increasingly often in debilitated patients on intensive care units; it can be a devastating disease and is frequently associated with bacteremia.

Antibiotic resistance in *X. maltophilia*, based on both low outer-membrane permeability and inducible β-lactamases, is at least partly responsible for the emergence of this organism as a nosocomial pathogen under the selective pressure of antibiotic treatment. Trimethoprim-sulfamethoxazole is often useful for the treatment of infections due to drug-resistant strains. Alternative agents include ticarcillin-clavulanate, ciprofloxacin, and minocycline or doxycycline. The third-generation cephalosporins cefoperazone and ceftazidime may be active against *X. maltophilia* in some instances, but in vitro susceptibilities should be tested in each case. The aminoglycosides and imipenem are usually inactive.

P. fluorescens occasionally causes human disease; it is implicated particularly often in infections related to the administration of contaminated (stored) blood products and other pseudoinfections. Additional *Pseudomonas* spp. that are associated only rarely with human infections include *P. putida*, *P. stutzeri*, *P. alcaligenes*, *P. pseudoalcaligenes*, *P. pickettii*, *P. acidovorans*, *P. testosteroni*, *P. diminuta*, and *P. vesicularis*.

MELIOIDOSIS

Infections caused by *P. pseudomallei* constitute a broad spectrum of acute and chronic, local and systemic, clinical and subclinical disease processes collectively called *melioidosis*. *P. pseudomallei* and the infections it causes are found mainly in the tropics and are endemic in Southeast Asia and surrounding areas. *P. pseudomallei* is a free-living, small, motile, aerobic gram-negative rod belonging to rRNA homology group II of *Pseudomonas* and related species. The organism is a saprophyte that is normally found in soil, ponds, and rice paddies and on produce from endemic areas. It is occasionally a pathogen for animals. Humans contract the disease through soil contamination of abrasions, ingestion, nasal instillation, or inhalation. Person-to-person transmission is apparently rare.

Acute infections most often involve the lungs, although lesions sometimes develop in other organs. Pulmonary lesions tend to be more extensive and dissemination to other organs tends to be more widespread in subacute melioidosis. Acute abscesses exhibit necrosis, polymorphonuclear leukocyte infiltration, and surrounding hemorrhage; multinucleated histiocytes are observed in areas of necrosis. Subacute lesions, in contrast, are characterized by caseation necrosis, with mononuclear and plasma cell infiltration.

Melioidosis presents in different forms. High rates of seropositivity in endemic areas such as Vietnam, Thailand, and Malaysia suggest that many infections are clinically inapparent. The occasional diagnosis based solely on abnormal routine chest roentgenograms represents asymptomatic pulmonary infection. Acute, localized, suppurative skin infections associated with nodular lymphangitis and regional lymphadenitis result from direct inoculation at sites of minor skin trauma. Acute pulmonary infections may originate in the respiratory tract or result from hematogenous spread, their severity varying from mild bronchitis to extensive necrotizing pneumonia. Onset may be sudden or gradual. Fever, productive cough, and marked tachypnea are frequent. Chest roentgenograms typically reveal upper lobe consolidation or thin-walled cavities. Progressive upper lobe disease mimics tuberculosis.

Acute suppurative infections or pulmonary disease may give rise to hematogenous dissemination and the acute septicemic form of melioidosis. This progression is more likely in chronically debilitated patients, such as those with diabetes mellitus or alcoholism. Patients with pulmonary infections in particular may present with severe tachypnea, confusion, headache, pharyngitis, diarrhea, and pustular lesions of the head, trunk, and extremities. The skin may be flushed or cyanotic; signs of meningitis or arthritis may be apparent; the liver and spleen may be enlarged; and muscle tenderness may be striking. Chest roentgenograms show diffuse nodular densities that may expand, coalesce, and finally cavitate. The acute septicemic form of melioidosis usually follows a rapid downhill course ending in early death unless arrested by early and aggressive therapy.

Chronic suppurative melioidosis is characterized by acute or chronic abscesses of the skin and various organs. Recrudescent disease arising from inactive sites of infection and perhaps triggered by intercurrent illness or other events may present in any acute or chronic form.

The diagnosis of melioidosis should be entertained when a febrile patient who has been in an endemic area presents with an acute lower respiratory tract illness associated with tachypnea, exhibits unusual skin or subcutaneous lesions, or has a chest roentgenogram suggesting tuberculosis in the absence of sputum-associated tubercle bacilli. An etiologic diagnosis may be made by microscopic demonstration of small, irregularly staining, gram-negative rods in exudate material; by characteristic bipolar ("safety-pin") staining of organisms with methylene blue; and by a culture positive for *P. pseudomallei* and/or a fourfold or greater rise in the titer of serum antibody to the organism.

The mainstay of treatment for melioidosis is antibiotic administration combined with appropriate surgical drainage of abscesses and aggressive support for patients with septicemic forms of the disease. The guidelines for antibiotic therapy are somewhat imprecise. Subclinical infection or mere seropositivity does not usually require specific therapy. Ceftazidime may be the agent of choice for clinical disease, while trimethoprim-sulfamethoxazole, cefotaxime, imipenem, and amoxicillin/clavulanate are possible alternatives. Therapy with a combination such as ceftazidime plus trimethoprim-sulfamethoxazole is indicated in severe forms of melioidosis. However, the resistance of many strains of *P. pseudomallei* to trimethoprim-sulfamethoxazole, particularly in Southeast Asia, necessitates other antibiotic choices. Acute septicemic infections probably should be treated with combinations of multiple agents administered parenterally. Patients with acute pulmonary infections should receive antibiotics for 60 to 150 days, while chronic disease associated with persistently positive sputum cultures may require longer treatment. Extrapulmonary suppurative disease is appropriately treated for 6 months to 1 year. When initial therapy for acute infections involves a third-generation cephalosporin such as ceftazidime, a switch can often be made after 30 days to an oral agent such as trimethoprim-sulfamethoxazole or amoxicillin-clavulanate.

Most cases of melioidosis are curable if appropriately treated. However, septicemic infections are still associated with very high mortality despite optimal therapy, while all forms of melioidosis are subject to possible early or very late recrudescence.

GLANDERS

Glanders is primarily a systemic equine disease that is caused by *P. mallei* and is associated with pulmonary involvement, subcutaneous ulcerative lesions, and lymphangitis. Once widespread, glanders still occurs in Africa, Asia, and South America but not in the United States or western Europe. The infection may be communicated to humans during close contact with horses, mules, or donkeys, probably by cutaneous inoculation or nasal exposure to contaminated discharges. Glanders assumes the following forms in humans: acute localized suppurative infection, acute pulmonary infection, acute septicemic infection, and chronic suppurative infection. Inoculation of *P. mallei* into the skin usually produces a nodule with an area of lymphangitis. Fever, malaise, and prostration are common. Mucous membrane infection results in the production of a mucopurulent discharge from the eye, nose, or lips, with the subsequent development of granulomatous ulcers. Pulmonary infection secondary to inhalation of the organism is accompanied by typical local and systemic signs and symptoms of pneumonia. Lymphadenopathy and splenomegaly may be documented. Chest roentgenograms reveal circumscribed densities suggesting early lung abscesses; bronchopneumonia or lobar consolidation also may be evident. Chronic suppurative infection presents as multiple subcutaneous and intramuscular abscesses, particularly often involving the extremities; visceral lesions are documented in some patients. The acute septicemic form of glanders may be associated with a diffuse papular or pustular eruption, severe systemic symptoms, and early death.

The diagnosis of glanders may be suggested by the clinical setting (including a history of close contact with equines) and confirmed by culture of the causative agent from clinical material and by demonstration of *P. mallei*–specific seroconversion.

Optimal antimicrobial therapy for glanders has not been adequately defined. Sulfadiazine has proven effective historically both in animals and in humans. It has been suggested, however, that rational therapy consists of the same antibiotics recommended for the treatment of melioidosis, with the specific agent chosen on the basis of in vitro susceptibility testing. Antibiotics are administered for at least 30

days in uncomplicated infections and longer in complicated cases. Abscesses may require surgical drainage, and appropriate supportive measures are necessary in acute septicemic forms of the disease.

REFERENCES

Pseudomonas aeruginosa infections

BARKER LF: The clinical symptoms, bacteriologic findings and postmortem appearances in cases of infection of human beings with the *Bacillus pyocyaneus*. JAMA 29:213, 1897

BODEY GP et al: *Pseudomonas* bacteremia: Retrospective analysis of 410 episodes. Arch Intern Med 145:1621, 1985

FICK RB (ed): *Pseudomonas aeruginosa: The Opportunist, Pathogenesis and Disease.* Boca Raton, CRC, 1992

KORVICK JA, YU VL: Antimicrobial agent therapy for *Pseudomonas aeruginosa.* Antimicrob Agents Chemother 35:2167, 1991

MORRISON AF, WENZEL RP: Epidemiology of infections due to *Pseudomonas aeruginosa.* Rev Infect Dis 6(suppl):S267, 1984

POLLACK M: The virulence of *Pseudomonas aeruginosa.* Rev Infect Dis 6(suppl):S617, 1984

————: *Pseudomonas aeruginosa,* in *Principles and Practice of Infectious Diseases,* 3d ed, GL Mandell et al (eds). New York, Churchill Livingstone, 1990, pp 1673–1691

Infections caused by other *Pseudomonas* species

ELTING LS, BODEY GP: Septicemia due to *Xanthomonas* species and non-aeruginosa *Pseudomonas* species: Increasing incidence of catheter-related infections. Medicine 69:296, 1990

GOLDMANN DA, KLINGER JD: *Pseudomonas cepacia:* Biology, mechanisms of virulence, epidemiology. J Pediatr 108:806, 1986

MURRAY AE et al: Blood transfusion-associated *Pseudomonas fluorescens* septicemia: Is this an increasing problem? J Hosp Infect 9:243, 1987

POLLACK M: *Pseudomonas,* in *Infectious Diseases,* SL Gorbach et al (eds). Philadelphia, Saunders, 1992, pp 1502–1513

TOMASHEFSKI JF et al: *Pseudomonas cepacia*–associated pneumonia in cystic fibrosis. Arch Pathol Lab Med 112:166, 1988

Melioidosis

LEELARASAMEE A, BOVORNKITTI S: Melioidosis: Review and update. Rev Infect Dis 11:413, 1989

SANFORD JP: *Pseudomonas* species (including melioidosis and glanders), in *Principles and Practice of Infectious Diseases,* 3d ed, GL Mandell et al (eds). New York, Churchill Livingstone, 1990, pp 1692–1696

117 SALMONELLOSIS

GERALD T. KEUSCH

Organisms of the genus *Salmonella* are capable of causing a large variety of infections in humans, including typhoid (or enteric) fevers, focal systemic infections, septicemias, and gastroenteritis varying clinically from watery diarrhea to dysentery. *Nontyphoidal salmonellosis* usually refers to enteric disease caused by many members of the genus except *S. typhi.* Convalescent carriage of gastroenteritis strains is usually transient. A few subjects, generally young children under 5 years of age, may become long-term (longer than 1 year) asymptomatic carriers, although they are not important in the spread of infection. Patients with *S. typhi* are more likely to become long-term carriers, for years or possibly for life, and they serve as reservoirs for the spread of infection.

ETIOLOGY The salmonellae are nonencapsulated gram-negative bacilli, almost always motile by means of peritrichous flagella, expressing two or more forms of H antigens. They are generally lactose nonfermenters, and this property is used for initial selection in the clinical microbiology laboratory. The salmonellae ferment glucose, resulting in a typical acid butt and alkaline slant on triple sugar iron agar (TSI). They generally produce H_2S, which is detectable as a black reaction product and serves initially to distinguish isolates from *Shigella,* which also give an alkaline/acid TSI reaction. There are a very large number of *Salmonella* O and H antigens, allowing the separation of over 2200 different organisms on the basis of the patterns of the O and H antigens. Since these isolates have often been named after the place they were first detected, *Salmonella* classification more closely resembles geography. On the basis of major somatic antigens, a limited number of serogroups have been defined, and most human pathogens are members of groups A to D.

More rational classification schemes have been introduced that divide the genus into three species. One scheme includes *S. cholerasuis*, the prototype species; *S. typhi*, the major cause of typhoid (enteric) fever; and *S. enteritidis*, a catchall designation for all the remaining serotypes only some of which are pathogenic for humans. These serotypes do not have the taxonomic rank of species and should not be italicized, but for clinical and epidemiologic ease the convention is to use only the serotype name. Thus *S. enteritidis* serotype typhimurium becomes *S. typhimurium*, and *S. enteritidis* serotype enteritidis becomes *S. enteritidis*.

Some salmonellae are highly host-adapted to humans (e.g., *S. typhi*, *S. paratyphi A*, and *S. paratyphi B*), while most animal-adapted species cause no human disease. Others infect both humans and lower animals causing gastroenteritis or, less commonly, localized or septicemic infections.

TYPHOID FEVER

Typhoid fever is a distinctive acute systemic febrile infection of the mononuclear phagocytes and deserves separate consideration. Since it may be caused by several *species* (*S. typhi*, *S. paratyphi A* and *paratyphi B*, and occasionally *S. typhimurium*), many clinicians prefer the term *enteric fever*. But because typhoid is fundamentally not an enteric disease, this term is also inappropriate. On balance, *typhoid fever* is still the best term, for it is understood by nearly all clinicians to describe a particular syndrome that is, in fact, due primarily to *S. typhi*.

EPIDEMIOLOGY Because the cause of clinical typhoid fever is almost always a human-adapted *Salmonella*, most cases can be traced to a human carrier. The proximate cause may be water (the most common route) or food contaminated by a human carrier. Chronic carriers are generally over 50 years old, are more commonly women, and often have gallstones. *S. typhi* reside in the bile, even within the interiors of stones, and intermittently reach the lumen of the bowel and are excreted in the stool, thereby contaminating water or food.

With improvements in environmental sanitation in the United States, the incidence of typhoid has gradually dropped. Compared with 1920 when almost 36,000 cases were detected, the annual number now is approximately 500. Over 80 percent of these are active typhoid cases, and the others are convalescent carriers. The median age of patients is around 24 years, while the median age of carriers is over 60 years. Data gathered by the Centers for Disease Control and Prevention (CDC) show that the incidence in the United States dropped fivefold from 1955 to 1966, from 1 per 100,000 to 0.2 per 100,000 population, and has remained steady since then. At the same time, the proportion of infections acquired abroad increased from 33 percent in the 1960s to over 60 percent in the 1980s and continues to increase. Mexico is the leading source for Americans, accounting for 39 percent of cases from 1975 to 1984, although the risk to travelers to Peru, Chile, India, and Pakistan is significantly greater. Students are most at risk. In England, the majority of cases are also acquired abroad, usually in India or Pakistan. Known hot spots for typhoid include Alexandria, Egypt; Jakarta, Indonesia; and Santiago, Chile.

Typhoid contracted in the United States is primarily due to association with known or newly diagnosed carriers (30 percent) or from food-borne outbreaks (28 percent). The highest rates occur in states bordering Mexico. Other than travelers, the groups most likely to be at risk are bacteriology laboratory workers and household contacts of known carriers. The number of patients in the United

States is clearly underestimated, and an unknown proportion of patients escape detection because appropriate cultures are not done or the patients have already taken antibiotics.

In *S. typhi*–endemic regions, the rate of clinical typhoid is approximately 25-fold greater in HIV-positive than in HIV-negative individuals in the 15- to 35-year-old age group and as much as 60-fold greater than in the general population. Asymptomatic HIV-positive patients have a typical clinical presentation and response to therapy; AIDS patients can present with fulminant diarrhea and/or colitis and are far more likely to relapse. While this fact has little practical significance for AIDS patients in low-typhoid countries, it may become a problem for those who travel to highly endemic countries.

PATHOGENESIS Following ingestion of a suitable inoculum, *S. typhi* pass the gastric barrier to reach the small bowel. Experimental human infections with the Quailes strain have revealed that 10^3 organisms will not cause symptomatic disease but that 10^5 bacteria cause symptoms in 27 percent of volunteers. Higher doses result in more frequent illness, especially if the organisms produce the Vi capsular polysaccharide antigen. Animal studies suggest that *S. typhi* invade the host in the upper small bowel and produce a transient and asymptomatic bacteremia. The organisms are ingested by mononuclear phagocytes and must survive and multiply intracellularly to cause illness.

Persistent bacteremia initiates the clinical phase of infection. The ability of the inoculum to invade mononuclear cells and multiply intracellularly determines whether or not this secondary bacteremia occurs. The absence of bactericidal antibodies allows organisms to be phagocytized in a viable state. Intracellular survival is dependent on microbial factors that promote resistance to killing and on specific host T lymphocyte–activated cell-mediated immunity, which is under genetic control. Dose dependence of clinical disease appears to be governed by the balance between bacterial multiplication and acquired host extracellular and intracellular defenses. When the number of intracellular bacteria surpasses a critical threshold, secondary bacteremia occurs and results in the invasion of the gallbladder and Peyer's patches of the intestine. The sustained bacteremia is responsible for the persistent fever of clinical typhoid, while inflammatory responses to tissue invasion determine the pattern of clinical expression (cholecystitis, intestinal hemorrhage, or perforation). With invasion of the gallbladder and Peyer's patches, bacteria regain entry to the bowel lumen, and may be recovered in stool cultures beginning in the second week of clinical disease. Seeding of the kidney leads to positive urine cultures but in a much lower percentage of patients than those with positive blood cultures. The lipopolysaccharide endotoxin of *S. typhi* may contribute to causing fever, leukopenia, and other systemic symptoms, but the occurrence of such symptoms in subjects made tolerant to endotoxin supports a role for other factors, such as cytokines released from infected mononuclear phagocytes, that can mediate inflammation (see Chap. 16).

CLINICAL MANIFESTATIONS The incubation period is variable and depends on both the inoculum size and the state of host defenses. A range of 3 to 60 days has been reported. The disease classically presents with a steplike daily increase in temperature to 40 to 41°C, associated with headache, malaise, and chills. The hallmark of typhoid fever is prolonged, persistent fever (4 to 8 weeks in untreated patients). Mild and brief illness may occur, but in some patients acute, severe infection with disseminated intravascular coagulation and central nervous system involvement rapidly results in death. In other patients, necrotizing cholecystitis or intestinal bleeding and perforation can occur in the third or fourth week of illness, when the patient is otherwise improving. In most, the onset of these complications is dramatic and clinically obvious. Intestinal perforation appears to be less common in children under 5 years of age.

Early intestinal manifestations include constipation, especially in adults, or mild diarrhea in children, associated with abdominal tenderness. Mild hepatosplenomegaly is detectable in the majority of patients. Bradycardia relative to the height of the fever may be a clinical clue to typhoid but is present in a minority of patients. Epistaxis may occur in the early stages of illness. "Rose spots," appearing as small, pale red, blanching, slightly raised macules, are occasionally seen on the chest and abdomen during the first week. They also can evolve into nonblanching small hemorrhages that are difficult to see in dark-skinned patients. The major characteristics of untreated typhoid are persistent high fever, severe anorexia, weight loss, and changes in sensorium, but a variety of other complications may develop, including hepatitis, meningitis, nephritis, myocarditis, bronchitis, pneumonia, arthritis, osteomyelitis, parotitis, and orchitis. Excepting relapse, the frequency of all these complications, including hemorrhage and perforation, is reduced by prompt use of appropriate antibiotics.

Multidrug-resistant *S. typhi* is becoming more prevalent in many endemic countries. These patients present with more severe illness, they look "toxic," and they have a higher incidence of disseminated intravascular coagulation and hepatomegaly and a threefold increased mortality rate thought to be related to the longer duration of disease and prior ineffective oral antibiotic therapy.

Around 3 to 5 percent of patients become long-term asymptomatic carriers, some for life unless treated. Many carriers give no history of typhoid fever and probably had an undiagnosed mild infection.

LABORATORY FINDINGS In around 25 percent of patients, leukopenia and neutropenia are present. In most patients, the white blood cell count is normal, albeit low in relation to the degree of fever, which may be a clue to the diagnosis. Rarely, severe leukopenia (<2000 cells per microliter) can occur. In the event of intestinal perforation or pyogenic complications, secondary leukocytosis develops. The anemia of blood loss may be superimposed on the anemia of chronic infection.

Definitive diagnosis depends on isolation of the organism. The recovery of organisms from blood is highest in the first week of illness, when it approaches 90 percent. Bacteremia is detectable in 50 percent in the third week and at a progressively lower frequency later on. Early in the illness culture of bone marrow aspirates will yield the organism in the majority of patients with negative blood cultures, even after brief prior antimicrobial treatment. Stool cultures are frequently negative in the first week but become positive in 75 percent of patients during the third week. By the eighth week, stools are positive in only 10 percent of patients but in approximately 3 to 5 percent of patients will remain so for at least 1 year. The frequency of positive urine cultures parallels the yield from stools and may represent, in some patients, contamination with feces.

Serologic diagnosis is less reliable than culture. Most, but not all, patients will develop agglutinating antibodies to O, H, and Vi antigens (the Widal test). In the absence of recent immunization, a high titer of antibody to O antigen (>1:640) is suggestive but not specific because other serogroup D salmonellae share the antigen used in the Widal test, as do some organisms in groups A and B. H antibodies may be found in even higher titer but because of their broad cross-reactivity are difficult to interpret. A fourfold rise in antibody in paired samples is a good criterion but is of little use in the acutely ill patient and may be blunted by early effective antimicrobial therapy. The earlier the baseline sample is obtained, the more likely a significant rise will be detected. Vi antibodies typically rise later, after 3 to 4 weeks of illness, and are of less use in the early diagnosis of infection.

DIFFERENTIAL DIAGNOSIS When all the classic clinical manifestations are present, including rose spots, prolonged fever, relative bradycardia, and leukopenia, the diagnosis of typhoid will be strongly suggested. However, most cases do not fit this "typical" profile. Differential diagnosis includes infections associated with prolonged fever such as the rickettsioses, brucellosis, tularemia, leptospirosis, miliary tuberculosis, viral hepatitis, infectious mononucleosis, cytomegalovirus infections, and malaria, as well as noninfectious causes such as lymphoma (see Chap. 16). In the United States, typhoid should be considered in any patient with prolonged, unexplained fever, especially after recent travel to places with endemic typhoid fever.

TREATMENT Since its introduction, chloramphenicol has been the antimicrobial gold standard for treatment. No drug has been better in promoting a favorable clinical response, which usually becomes apparent within 24 to 48 h of the start of treatment in the appropriate dosages (3 to 4 g/d in adults or 50 to 75 mg/kg of body weight per day in young children). The drug is given orally for 2 weeks, and the dose may be reduced to 2 g/d or 30 mg/kg per day when the patient becomes afebrile, which usually is not before day 5 of treatment. However, because of the specter of aplastic anemia associated with chloramphenicol, the drug is little used in the United States. Other effective oral regimens include amoxicillin (4 to 6 g/d in four divided doses in adults or 100 mg/kg per day in children), trimethoprim-sulfamethoxazole (640 and 3200 mg, respectively, in two divided doses daily in adults or 185 mg/m^2 of body surface area per day of the trimethoprim component for children), or in those over 17 years of age a 4-fluoroquinolone such as ciprofloxacin or ofloxacin.

A variety of intravenous drugs are also effective, and both chloramphenicol and trimethoprim-sulfamethoxazole can be given intravenously in those unable to take oral medications. Other effective parenteral antimicrobials include high-dose ampicillin, cefotaxime, aztreonam, and the 4-fluoroquinolones. However, none has been as rapidly acting or as effective as ceftriaxone, which rivals or betters chloramphenicol in rapidity of defervescence. Initial recommendations for a 7-day course of ceftriaxone have since been pared down to 3 days of 3 to 4 g once daily in adults or 80 mg/kg once daily for 5 days in children without apparent loss of efficacy. In addition, compared with that associated with other drugs, the relapse rate appears lower in adults or children given ceftriaxone; however, the number of patients reported is still small.

Prevalence of multidrug resistance of *S. typhi* to first-line oral drugs has been rising in developing countries, sometimes strikingly, due to acquisition of plasmids encoding inactivating β-lactamase and chloramphenicol acetyl transferase enzymes. In regions where this multidrug resistance is a problem, ceftriaxone or a 4-fluoroquinolone should be used initially for adults over 17 years of age, with ceftriaxone as the best choice for children, at least until the new quinolones are proven safe for young children. The higher cost of ceftriaxone is somewhat offset by the efficacy of a short course and the economy of once-daily dosing.

Studies in Indonesia of patients with severe typhoid who present with central nervous system manifestations and/or evidence of disseminated intravenous coagulation suggest that intravenous dexamethasone, 3 mg/kg as a loading dose over 30 min followed by 1 mg/kg every 6 h for 24 to 48 h, in addition to parenteral antimicrobials, reduces mortality. Salicylates should be avoided to diminish the danger of intestinal hemorrhage. Prompt surgical management of bleeding and bowel perforation reduces mortality, which is associated primarily with peritonitis. Bowel perforations should be closed in two layers for best results. Antibiotics should be selected to treat not only *S. typhi* but also the facultative and anaerobic bowel flora. Selective angiography, radioisotopic scanning methods, or sometimes endoscopy (see Chap. 46) to localize the bleeding site can facilitate operative repair. In developing countries, however, patients often present late after perforation, they may be severely malnourished and poor surgical risks, and only limited surgical and postoperative care may be available. Supportive medical care and antibiotics alone have been recommended in this setting, although limited surgery to close the perforation site without bowel resection is increasingly favored. With the use of double-layer closure of the lesion and an inexpensive broad antibiotic regimen including chloramphenicol, gentamicin, and metronidazole, mortality rates have been reduced from 25 to 30 percent to well under 10 percent.

The early use of effective antimicrobials is associated with a relatively high rate of relapse; relapse rates of 20 percent can be expected, compared with 5 to 10 percent in untreated patients. This is presumably because prompt therapy inhibits the development of an adequate immune response. Relapses are usually milder than the initial attack and will respond to the same antimicrobial used initially.

Eradication of the chronic carrier state, especially in the presence of gallstones, is notoriously difficult. Traditional regimens have used 100 mg/kg per day of ampicillin or amoxicillin plus probenecid (30 mg/kg per day) or trimethoprim-sulfamethoxazole (160/800 mg) twice daily plus rifampin (600 mg) once daily for at least 6 weeks. Recent studies suggest that a 4-week course of a 4-fluoroquinolone is at least as good and probably much better because the organism is exquisitely sensitive in vitro and the drugs reach the gut lumen, liver, gallbladder, and bile in active form. The new quinolones provide the best chance of eradicating *S. typhi* in the presence of gallstones, and because of simplicity and safety, they should be the first choice in patients without stones as well. The optimal dose and duration of treatment have yet to be defined. These drugs would be the best choice for chronic suppression of typhoid relapse in AIDS patients as well.

PREVENTION AND CONTROL   Worldwide experience has shown that improvement of environmental sanitation, including sewage disposal and water supplies, will sharply reduce the incidence of typhoid fever. Where this approach is not yet possible, and for travelers, immunization has been used. The protective efficacy of multiple doses of traditional heat-killed phenol-extracted whole typhoid vaccine is, at best, 65 percent and lasts just a few months, at a cost of certain local pain and fever. It has been largely replaced in the United States by three doses of a first-generation live oral vaccine (Ty21a). While this strain is invasive, because it is also metabolically defective, it dies after a few cycles of replication and therefore is avirulent. Nonetheless, it provides protection equivalent to the killed vaccine and lasts for at least several years. In Europe, one dose of purified Vi polysaccharide vaccine has proven as effective and long lasting as multiple doses of Ty21a, yet this product is inexplicably not available in the United States. New genetically engineered live typhoid vaccines are actively being developed by mutation of aromatic biosynthesis pathway genes, the adenylate cyclase and cAMP regulatory genes, or other virulence genes or by combination of several genetic changes in the same candidate strain. These strains are being pursued not only for immunization against typhoid but also for development of live vectors into which extraneous genes can be cloned for oral delivery of protective antigens from unrelated species. In addition, Vi-protein conjugates are being made and evaluated as immunogens suitable for infants, especially in endemic regions where infantile typhoid is prevalent and remains a dangerous disease.

Typhoid is a reportable disease in the United States. Patients should be monitored for prolonged carriage and treated for it if necessary. Precautions in food handling by carriers and in disposal of their stools are obvious and important (see Chap. 98).

PROGNOSIS   Appropriate therapy of typhoid fever, especially if patients present for medical care in the early stage of disease, is highly successful. The mortality rate should be under 1 percent, and few complications should occur.

NONTYPHOIDAL SALMONELLOSIS

Infections caused by any *Salmonella* other than *S. typhi* are termed *nontyphoidal salmonellosis*. These infections can present as acute diarrhea, a septicemic syndrome, focal abscesses, meningitis, osteomyelitis, endocarditis, or mycotic aneurysm or can be asymptomatic.

EPIDEMIOLOGY   The species *S. cholerasuis* and *S. enteritidis* include a diverse group of organisms with both host-adapted and non-host-adapted serotypes. Two human-adapted serotypes, *S. paratyphi* A and *S. schottmuelleri* (more often called *S. paratyphi B*) mimic *S. typhi* and cause a milder form of typhoid fever. Of the more than 2200 known *S. enteritidis* serotypes, just 10 account for 75 percent of all human disease isolates in the United States, and 4 serotypes (*S. typhimurium, enteritidis, heidelberg,* and *newport)* cause about two-thirds of all disease. *S. typhimurium* has previously been the most frequent isolate, representing around 35 percent of all strains

reported to the CDC. In past surveillance studies, periodic increases in recovery of certain serotypes have represented either the introduction of a new transmission source or the occurrence of a large outbreak. For example, a fivefold increase in *S. enteritidis* isolates between 1976 and 1986 was due to ingestion of contaminated grade A eggs primarily in the northeastern United States. Infections from this source have continued to increase in North and South America, Europe, and probably Africa as well. By 1992, *S. enteritidis* overtook *S. typhimurium* as the most frequently isolated *Salmonella* in the United States and at least eight countries in Europe, suggesting a new global pandemic related primarily to infected poultry eggs.

Careful analysis of surveillance data in the United States has shown that not only is the number of nontyphoidal *Salmonella* isolates increasing, but the incidence appears to be increasing as well, from 8 per 100,000 of the general population in 1965 to 12 per 100,000 in 1975, peaking at around 18 per 100,000 in 1985, and dropping slightly to approximately 16 per 100,000 in 1991. While the incidence of disease in young children is five times higher than in older subjects, the rate is also somewhat higher in adults over 70 years. Between 1970 and 1986, the median age of infected individuals rose from 6 years to 20 years and has remained as high since then. The greatest increase has been in the 20- to 39-year-old population, suggesting that foods consumed by young adults are becoming important vehicles or that they are traveling more to endemic areas. For example, the emergence of serious systemic infections in southern California due to *S. dublin* carrying a large virulence plasmid has been associated with the ingestion of unpasteurized dairy products or nontraditional nutritional treatments using raw calf-liver extracts contaminated with this serotype. A reasonable estimate of the total incidence of symptomatic *Salmonella* infection in the United States is around 2 million cases per year. This degree of morbidity implies a significant economic impact in lost productivity and medical costs and, by extension, a serious and underestimated cause of mortality.

Because nontyphoidal *Salmonella* are so often non-host-adapted, many kinds of domestic animals can harbor the organism and serve as the source for human infection. From 50 to 75 percent of broiler and layer chicken flocks in Canada are infected with a large variety of *Salmonella* serotypes, many of which are virulent for humans. In one experimental setting, 10 percent of the intact eggs of a naturally infected layer flock were positive for a human virulent *S. enteritidis* phage type 4. Although the number of organisms per egg was less than 10 at laying, growth to large numbers quickly occurs if eggs are not kept at 4°C; after 2 days at room temperature, over 10^8 organisms per gram of yolk can be isolated. At this level of contamination, viable organisms will survive cooking by any method. The source of the *Salmonella* can be the surface of the shell if the egg rests for a short time on infected hen feces or even the dry bedding of an infected hen, since the bacteria can penetrate the intact egg through microscopic pores normally present in the shell. Because the epidemic is so profound and so unlike past problems of *Salmonella* associated with cracked eggs, and because it has involved free-range as well as commercial henhouse eggs, a transovarian route is more likely and presents a rather major problem for infection control. Conditions of raising, shipping, slaughtering, and marketing contribute to the spread of *Salmonella* in the food supply. Introduction of the organism into processed foods can result in widespread dissemination, and contamination of such common foods as eggs or milk leads to large-scale outbreaks, including nosocomial hospital epidemics. Dried or frozen foods preserve viable salmonellae. For these reasons, salmonellosis is more a disease of the industrialized world than of the developing world. Additional sources of human infection are animals sold as pets, including baby chicks or ducks and turtles, and medical products of animal origin, such as carmine dye (from insects), pancreatin, bile salts, or tissue extracts from thyroids, adrenals, stomaches, or rattlesnakes.

A potentially serious problem is the selection of antibiotic-resistant strains of salmonellae by unregulated drug use in animal husbandry.

There are a number of instances where transmission to humans has occurred. Persistent and severe salmonellosis also has been recognized as a problem among patients with AIDS (see Chap. 279).

PATHOGENESIS As with *S. typhi*, the events following ingestion of the organism are determined by environmental factors (dose), microbial factors (the ability to invade epithelial cells and multiply within mononuclear phagocytes and to resist intestinal peptide antibiotic defensins), and host resistance factors (gastric acid and the ability to rapidly mobilize phagocytic cells and to activate and expand clones of T cells involved in protection, such as V gamma 9–bearing gamma-delta T cells). As few as 10^3 virulent organisms may cause disease, especially in patients with achlorhydria or having recent antimicrobial therapy. Systemic invasion is more likely in patients with "reticuloendothelial blockade" due to hemolysis (malaria, bartonellosis, leptospirosis, sickle cell anemia) or intracellular infections (histoplasmosis). The incidence of documented bacteremia varies from 5 to 45 percent but is assumed to occur early in the course of many, and possibly all, *Salmonella* infections. Bacteremia is quickly cleared in patients infected with most *S. enteritidis* serotypes. Certain serotypes, such as *dublin, infantis, virchow, panama,* and *newport,* may be more invasive; this property is associated with an 80-kilobase virulence plasmid in *S. dublin. S. typhimurium* isolated from the bloodstream are significantly more likely (76 percent) to hybridize with a probe from the highly conserved EcoR1 fragment of the *S. dublin* plasmid than are fecal isolates (42 percent). *S. typhimurium* is the most frequent blood isolate, but the rate of isolation is no more than the average for all nontyphoidal *Salmonella.* Systemic and focal tissue infections are secondary to bacteremia. *S. cholerasuis* is a highly invasive serotype that usually causes a septicemia syndrome and is commonly isolated from blood but not from stool. Microbial factors, which determine the invasiveness of salmonellae, include motility and the presence of chromosomal and plasmid genes needed to invade and replicate within mononuclear phagocytes. Many of these genes are turned on by contact of the organism with host cells and are regulated by a two-component system, *PhoP/PhoQ.* Invasion is also associated with visible ruffling of the surface membrane and a major rearrangement of actin filaments, alpha-actinin, and tropomyosin to generate the force necessary for entry and appears to require host cell tyrosine kinase and phospholipase C activity, which results in a flux of inositol phosphate and release of intracellular calcium.

The pathogenesis of *Salmonella* enteritis is not clear. Virulent strains are invasive and able to induce inflammatory responses in the gut mucosa. Some strains produce a heat-labile enterotoxin which is structurally, functionally, and immunologically related to the cholera and *E. coli* LT toxins and/or heat-labile cytotoxins that act like Shiga toxins to inhibit intestinal protein synthesis.

CLINICAL MANIFESTATIONS Gastroenteritis The incubation period of *Salmonella* gastroenteritis is generally short, 24 to 48 h. Sporadic illness is likely to go undiagnosed because culture specimens are not taken. Large outbreaks, often considered as "food poisoning" and characterized by self-limited fever and diarrhea, are more likely to be investigated and diagnosed. Diarrhea may be associated with nausea, vomiting, and abdominal cramps and occasionally becomes bloody or even dysenteric when the colon becomes involved. Direct microscopic examination of stool shows many leukocytes, which are a clue to the invasive nature of the infection. The illness is generally mild and resolves without use of specific therapy, but it may cause severe dehydration or disseminate and lead to death in debilitated elderly patients or neonates. Blood cultures often become positive as the patient is improving. Treatment may be discontinued after identification of the organism unless there is an underlying immunosuppressive disease (e.g., sickle cell disease, AIDS, malignancy such as a lymphoma) or the patient is receiving glucocorticoid or immunosuppressive drug therapy. In these conditions, an appropriate antibiotic should be administered for 7 to 10 days. Carriage of salmonellae in the stool lasts several weeks after symptomatic disease but rarely exceeds 2 months.

Localization of systemic infections Bloodborne salmonellae can invade any tissue or organ. The most common isolates are *S. typhimurium, S. enteritidis, S. virchow,* and *S. cholerasuis.* Localized infections usually follow intestinal infection, although there may be no prior diarrhea. Endocarditis is rare, but when it occurs, there may be destructive cardiac lesions, including valve perforations or ring or septal abscesses. Therapy may require both appropriate antimicrobials and surgery (see Chap. 85).

Arterial infection generally occurs in preexisting arteriosclerotic infrarenal aortic aneurysms, especially in men older than 50. *S. cholerasius,* which accounts for about 20 percent of these infections, is isolated in fewer than 1 percent of patients with *Salmonella* diarrhea, thus reflecting its capacity to cause systemic invasive disease. *S. typhimurium* accounts for approximately 25 percent of isolates in arterial infections, consistent with its high prevalence in gastrointestinal salmonellosis. In addition to treatment with antimicrobials, eradication usually requires prompt excision and drainage with bypass through uninvolved tissue. The disease should be suspected when elderly men develop prolonged fever following gastroenteritis, accompanied by back, abdomen, or chest pain; when bacteremia is present or recurrent after therapy for the initial illness; or when bacteremia occurs in patients with vertebral osteomyelitis or in those with prosthetic valves.

Cholecystitis, other *hepatobiliary infection,* and *splenic abscess* are the most common intraabdominal localized infections due to *Salmonella.* In addition to *S. typhimurium* and *S. enteritidis, S. typhi* is an important cause.

Urinary tract infections due to *Salmonella* sometimes occur, especially in patients with urolithiasis, structural abnormalities, or immunosuppressive diseases or therapy, and can coexist with renal tuberculosis or *Schistosoma haematobium* infection.

Pneumonia or *empyema* caused by *Salmonella* is rare and usually seen in patients with preexisting abnormalities of the lungs or pleura or with conditions that predispose to infection, including malignancy, diabetes, glucocorticoid use, sickle cell disease, or alcohol abuse.

Meningitis caused by *Salmonella* is also rare and is most prevalent in infants and young children. Gram's stains of cerebrospinal fluid are usually positive. Mortality rates of 40 to 60 percent are reported in children and adults, respectively. In survivors, residua include seizures, hydrocephalus, subdural empyemas, and permanent disabilities such as retardation, paresis, athetosis, and visual disturbances.

Septic arthritis due to *Salmonella* is associated with positive joint fluid cultures and should not be confused with reactive arthritis (a culture-negative inflammatory joint disease occurring after invasive diarrheas, especially in HLA-B2– or -B7–positive patients). Underlying conditions that are often present include glucocorticoid or immunosuppressive drug therapy, sickle cell disease, prosthetic joints, or aseptic necrosis. Drainage may be needed in addition to appropriate antibiotics.

Salmonella osteomyelitis is predictably associated with sickle cell disease, sickle-C disease, and sickle thalassemia. It generally affects long bones and occurs primarily in young patients; blood cultures are often positive (the most common isolate is *S. typhimurium*).

Bacteremia Sepsis, with prolonged fever and positive blood cultures but generally without prior diarrhea, occurs most commonly with *S. cholerasuis* or *S. dublin* infection. While this presentation is "typhoidal," typical manifestations of typhoid (rose spots, relative bradycardia, leukopenia) are absent, and the illness is more acute in onset. *S. cholerasuis* or *S. dublin* sepsis is a severe disease, associated with high mortality.

Intermittent symptomatic *Salmonella* bacteremia is seen in patients with hepatosplenic or urinary schistosomiasis. Clinically severe *Salmonella* sepsis due to *S. typhimurium* also occurs in AIDS patients (see Chap. 279), is often recurrent, and may develop before the diagnosis of AIDS is made. The infection may be refractory to treatment or recurrent despite appropriate therapy. The incidence of salmonellosis in AIDS patients in the United States is now estimated to be between 46 and 384 per 100,000, which is 100- to 1000-fold greater than the incidence in the general population (0.3 per 100,000).

DIAGNOSIS Specific diagnosis depends on the isolation of the organisms from stool, blood, or tissue fluids. All clinical laboratories should be able to make the initial isolation and identify common serotypes. Uncommon serotypes usually must be sent to reference laboratories for identification.

TREATMENT Treatment for focal systemic infections requires selection of the most appropriate antibiotic and, at times, drainage or resection of infected tissue. Bactericidal antibiotics by the parenteral route are the usual choice and may include ampicillin in a dose of 6 to 12 g/d in adults or 100 mg/kg in young children in divided doses or appropriate doses of third-generation cephalosporins such as ceftriaxone. Chloramphenicol in a dose of 2 to 4 g/d in adults or 50 mg/kg in children in divided doses or a 4-fluoroquinolone such as ciprofloxacin or ofloxacin in patients older than 17 is also effective.

The proper treatment of *Salmonella* gastroenteritis is not clear; antibiotics do not shorten illness but do increase the duration of convalescent carriage. For this reason it is generally recommended that no treatment other than supportive care and fluid replacement be administered. Results suggest that 4-fluoroquinolones reduce the duration of illness and rapidly eradicate the organism from stool, although contradictory data have been published as well. Positive blood cultures in the setting of otherwise uncomplicated gastroenteritis do not require antibiotic therapy; treatment is usually reserved for patients with underlying immunosuppressive disease. In an infant under 3 months of age with diarrhea, the stool should be cultured, a workup to localize the septic process initiated, and presumptive treatment begun with a third-generation cephalosporin until culture results are available. Fever is often absent in very young infants and is not a reliable indicator of systemic infection. Asymptomatic patients with salmonellae other than *S. typhi* in the stool should *not* receive antimicrobial treatment, since active disease may be provoked and the carriage state prolonged.

PREVENTION AND CONTROL It is probably not possible to eradicate nontyphoidal salmonellosis because the organisms are so widespread in nature. Reduction in the use in animal feed of antimicrobials employed for human infection and improved animal rearing and marketing practices would be useful. Vigilance in food preparation and in quality testing of the known and commonly contaminated foods should help as well. It is recommended that eggs not be eaten raw or partially cooked, especially in those at high risk, but even fully cooked eggs can harbor viable *Salmonella*. If universal body substance precautions are not routinely utilized, hospital staff caring for patients with salmonellosis should be placed on "enteric precautions," with gowning and gloving when handling stool and urine and careful handwashing after patient contact (see Chap. 98).

During outbreaks, food handlers may be responsible for transmission. Much effort is given to the identification by stool culture of asymptomatic food handlers who are carriers during food-borne outbreaks, and they are usually kept from work until they become culture-negative. However, it is more important that standards are maintained to ensure the environmental and personal hygiene of food handlers to prevent the problem in the first place, since carriage may be intermittent and is often not uniform within a single stool sample and foods contaminated with the organism require improper handling to permit the growth of a sufficient inoculum to cause disease. It may be truly justifiable to restrict carriers from the workplace only in the course of a hospital outbreak or when there are workers who refuse to improve their personal hygiene.

The development of effective vaccines may be difficult because of the great number of serotypes involved in infection. Some progress has been made with galactose epimerase and aroA vaccine mutants of *S. typhimurium* for use in animals, and these may ultimately be tested in humans. Of all the nontyphoidal salmonellae, it would be most useful to have vaccines for *S. cholerasuis*, *S. typhimurium*, and *S. enteritidis*. *S. dublin* and *S. virchow*, while quite virulent, are still uncommon causes of human disease.

REFERENCES

ASPERGILLA MO et al: Quinolone antibiotics in the treatment of *Salmonella* infections. Rev Infect Dis 12:873, 1990

BHUTTA ZA: Multidrug-resistant typhoid in children: Presentation and clinical features. Rev Infect Dis 13:832, 1991

COHEN JI et al: Extra-intestinal manifestations of *Salmonella* infections. Medicine 66:349, 1987

FANG FC, FIERER J: Human infection with *Salmonella dublin*. Medicine 70:198, 1991

FINLEY BB, FALKOW S: *Salmonella* as an intracellular parasite. Mol Microbiol 3:1833, 1989

GOTUZZO E et al: Association between the acquired immunodeficiency syndrome and infection with *Salmonella typhi* or *Salmonella paratyphi* in an endemic typhoid area. Arch Intern Med 151:381, 1991

HUMPHREY TJ et al: *Salmonella enteritidis* phage type 4 from the contents of intact eggs: A study involving naturally infected hens. Epidemiol Infect 103:415, 1989

LASSERRE R et al: Three-day treatment of typhoid fever with two different doses of ceftriaxone, compared to 14-day therapy with chloramphenicol: A randomized trial. J Antimicrob Chemother 28:765, 1991

LEVINE WC et al: Epidemiology of nontyphoidal *Salmonella* bacteremia during the human immunodeficiency virus epidemic. J Infect Dis 164:81, 1991

MOCK CN et al: Improvement in survival from typhoid ileal perforation: Results of 221 operative cases. Ann Surg 215:244, 1992

NAQVI SH et al: Therapy of multidrug resistant typhoid in 58 children. Scand J Invest Dis 24:175, 1992

PAVIA AT et al: Epidemiologic evidence that prior antimicrobial exposure decreases resistance to infection by antimicrobial-sensitive *Salmonella*. J Infect Dis 161:255, 1990

PUNJABI NH et al: Treatment of severe typhoid fever in children with high-dose dexamethasone. Pediatr Infect Dis J 7:598, 1988

RODRIGUE DC et al: International increase in *Salmonella enteritidis:* A new pandemic? Epidemiol Infect 105:21, 1990

RODRIQUES-NORIEGA E et al: Quinolones in the treatment of *Salmonella* carriers. Rev Infect Dis 11(suppl 5):S1179, 1989

RYAN CA et al: *Salmonella typhi* infections in the United States, 1975–1984: Increasing role of foreign travel. Rev Infect Dis 11:1, 1989

ST. LOUIS ME et al: The emergence of grade A eggs as a major source of *Salmonella enteritidis* infections: New implications for the control of salmonellosis. JAMA 259:2103, 1988

WOODRUFF BA et al: A new look at typhoid vaccination. Information for the practicing physician. JAMA 265:756, 1991

118 SHIGELLOSIS

GERALD T. KEUSCH

DEFINITION *Shigellosis* is an acute infectious inflammatory colitis due to one of the members of the genus *Shigella*. Although the disease is often referred to as "bacillary dysentery," many patients have only mild watery diarrhea and never develop dysenteric symptoms. The less severe illness predominates in industrialized countries such as the United States, whereas more severe, often fatal dysentery occurs in patients in developing countries.

ETIOLOGY *Shigella* are slender, gram-negative, nonmotile bacilli and are members of the family Enterobacteriaceae and tribe Escherichae. They are so closely related to *Escherichia coli* that the two genera cannot be distinguished by DNA hybridization methods. There are four *Shigella* species (*dysenteriae, flexneri, boydii,* and *sonnei*), defined on the basis of surface somatic O antigens and carbohydrate fermentation patterns. Most are lactose-negative (*S. sonnei* are late lactose fermenters) and produce acid but not gas from glucose, resulting in a typical acid butt and alkaline slant in triple sugar iron agar (TSI), without H_2S production, in contrast to *Salmonella*. The genus is characterized by its ability to invade intestinal epithelial cells and to produce highly potent protein toxins that irreversibly inhibit eukaryotic cell protein synthesis by a specific enzymatic action.

EPIDEMIOLOGY It is estimated that at least 140 million cases and almost 600,000 deaths due to shigellosis occur annually in young children under the age of 5 years, primarily in developing countries. The organism is found everywhere in the world but is most common where poor environmental sanitation and crowding facilitate transmission from person to person. The reported incidence in the United States is around 15,000 cases each year. This is no doubt a gross underestimate, since organisms from most patients are neither cultured nor identified. In industrialized countries and developing countries alike, most patients are young children. In the United States from 1974 to 1980, 93,516 cases were identified by means of a nationwide passive surveillance system. While the overall isolation rate was 4.7 per 100,000 population per year, among children aged 1 to 4 the rate was 22.3 per 100,000 children per year. In the United States, the disease is most common in the urban poor, in infants in day-care centers, and in retarded children institutionalized for custodial care. One high-risk group has also been identified: male homosexuals, who transmit infection by anal-oral sexual practices.

Since the description of the genus, major global shifts in prevalence of the four species have been noted. Until World War I, *S. dysenteriae* type 1 was the predominant isolate, frequently occurring in devastating epidemics with high mortality until it was replaced by *S. flexneri*. Since World War II, however, *S. flexneri* has been steadily replaced by *S. sonnei* in the industrialized countries. The reasons for these shifts are not clear. *S. boydii*, the fourth species, has remained largely confined to the Indian subcontinent and is uncommon elsewhere.

The genus is highly host-adapted and is a natural pathogen of only humans and a few subhuman primates. Transmission is fecal-oral from person to person and is generally via direct contact, although contaminated food, water, flies, and fomites may serve as vectors. Direct contact is efficient, and only a few hundred organisms suffice to transmit disease so that even recreational water sports in contaminated pools or lakes are sufficient to transmit infection. Also for this reason, rapid spread can occur among confined populations kept in close contact, for example, in day-care centers, in institutions for the mentally retarded, on cruise ships, or among military personnel. *Shigella* is also one of several pathogens associated with *gay bowel syndrome*. These cases are almost always due to *S. flexneri,* and homosexual young men may be a major reservoir for these organisms in the United States (see Chap. 279).

Shigellosis is associated with a high secondary household transmission rate. As many as 40 percent of children and 20 percent of adult household contacts of a case (generally a preschool child) will develop *Shigella* infection, often symptomatic in children but asymptomatic in adults, who seem to have an acquired immunity. In contrast, epidemic disease affects all ages, with a clustering of severe and fatal cases in the very young and very old. Since 1969, epidemic *S. dysenteriae* type 1 has reappeared in Latin America, in the Indian subcontinent and elsewhere in Asia, and in central Africa and was accompanied by relatively high mortality rates until the cause was recognized and effective therapy initiated. Prolonged asymptomatic carriage is uncommon, and unless there is underlying malnutrition which is associated with prolonged fecal excretion, organisms are cleared in a few weeks.

PATHOGENESIS AND PATHOLOGY *Shigella* are orally ingested, and because they survive low pH better than other enteric pathogens (a genetically regulated property), they seem to have little difficulty in passing the gastric acid barrier. An essential step in pathogenesis is invasion of colonic epithelial cells and cell-to-cell spread of infection. Invasion and cell-to-cell spread involve the initial attachment of the organism to colonic cells, entry by an endocytic mechanism in which organisms are initially encased in and then escape from plasma membrane–enclosed vesicles, and a jet propulsion–like movement to the epithelial cell surface that is powered by bacteria-induced actin polymerization at the trailing end of the bacterium. This not only provides the organism with a means to evade host defenses but also allows effective local spread. Although invasion is initially innocuous, with subsequent intracellular multiplication, cell damage and death occur, resulting in characteristic mucosal ulcerations.

These processes are extremely complicated and require the functions of multiple genes and regulatory elements encoded on both chromosomal and plasmid DNA. Early studies on the genetics of *Shigella* virulence demonstrated that conjugal transfer of *E. coli* chromosomal DNA from the *xyl-rha, his,* or *pur*E loci to virulent *S. flexneri* 2a recipients yielded hybrids able to invade but not survive within cells. The *xyl-rha* region is known to code for aerobactin and iron-regulated outer membrane proteins (OMPs), while the *his* region controls specific side chains of lipopolysaccharide, which respectively may help the organism compete for iron with the host and protect it from host defenses. However, transfer of these regions from *S. flexneri* to *E. coli* K12 does not confer virulence until other genes present on the large 120- to 140-MDa plasmids in all clinical *Shigella* isolates are transferred as well. These plasmids contain certain highly conserved regions common to all *Shigella* and invasive *E. coli* that encode a group of antigenic OMPs called *invasion plasmid antigens* (IPAs) and an operon called *mxi*, which controls insertion of the IPA proteins into the outer membrane of the organism. Mutation of some, but not all, IPAs inhibits invasiveness.

Invasion of epithelial cells by *Shigella* has been likened to the process of neutrophil phagocytosis. Internalization of *Shigella* by cells in culture or intestinal cells occurs within membrane-bounded vesicles associated with the polymerization of actin filaments. By use of transposon mutagenesis, a plasmid-encoded, acid pH–activated contact hemolysin has been found to mediate the rapid lysis of the phagocytic vacuole that allows the organisms to gain entry into the cytoplasm. While the basis for intracytoplasmic multiplication of *Shigella* is uncertain, another plasmid gene, *ics*A (for intraintercellular spread and formerly called *vir*G), encodes a 120-kDa antigenic OMP that governs the ability of the organism to spread within the cytoplasm or to form plaques in HeLa cell monolayers indicative of cell-to-cell extension of infection. These intra- and intercellular migrations of *Shigella* occur along a network of actin stress fibers within the cells and are powered by actin polymerization induced by the organism after invasion and are blocked by the addition of cytochalasins.

Several plasmid and chromosomal genes regulate these virulence properties. A plasmid locus, *vir*F, codes for a 30-kDa protein that activates the IPA genes and *ics*A. Another chromosomal locus, *vir*R, is a temperature-dependent repressor of the plasmid invasion genes at 30°C but not at 37°C, while *kcp*A, originally defined as a locus essential for keratoconjunctivitis in guinea pigs, also controls the expression of *ics*A.

A second property of apparent importance in virulence, at least for *S. dysenteriae* type 1, is the ability to produce cytotoxic proteins. Shiga toxin, encoded by an iron-regulated chromosomal gene, *stx,* is composed of two distinct peptide subunits, each with highly conserved active regions. The first, located on the larger A subunit, is an *N*-glycosidase enzyme which hydrolyzes adenine from specific sites of ribosomal RNA of the mammalian 60-S ribosomal subunit, resulting in the irreversible inhibition of protein synthesis. The second common region is a binding site on the B subunit that recognizes glycolipids of target cell membranes that terminate in a galactose $\alpha 1 \rightarrow 4$-galactose disaccharide. The glycolipid Gb3, containing a gal-gal trisaccharide, is a specific receptor present on toxin-sensitive rabbit intestinal villus cells but not crypt cells, and toxin action is specific for the former.

In shigellosis, the epithelial surface of the human colon shows extensive ulcerations, with an exudate consisting of desquamated colonic cells, polymorphonuclear leukocytes, and erythrocytes; the ulcerations may resemble a pseudomembrane in severely affected areas. Marked mucus depletion and increased mitotic activity are seen in the crypt regions, presumably as a response to the loss of surface colonic cells. The lamina propria is edematous and hemorrhagic and infiltrated with neutrophils and plasma cells. There is also swelling of capillary and venular endothelial cells, with margination of neutrophils. The tropism of toxin for endothelial cells can explain this pathology, which may contribute to fluid losses and underlie the systemic complications of *S. dysenteriae* type 1 infection such as glomerular damage and microangiopathic hemolysis (hemolytic-uremic syndrome). At the ultrastructural level, bacteria can be seen within vesicles as well as free in the cytoplasm.

Epidemiologic evidence indicates that immunity develops and is serotype specific. The precise nature of this immunity, however, is not known. Common surface OMPs involved in invasion are known to elicit serum antibodies; however, these are cross-reactive among *Shigella* species and serotypes and do not seem to be protective. The serotype-specific determinants are likely to be somatic antigens, as serum antibody to O antigens predicts resistance to infection, and there is evidence of IgA-mediated mucosal anti-O antigen responses during convalescence from shigellosis. Cellular mechanisms also have been proposed that involve antibody-dependent cellular cytotoxicity responses by Fc receptor–positive lymphocytes and phagocytic cells.

CLINICAL MANIFESTATIONS The spectrum of clinical shigellosis was shown in a study in which human volunteers ingested 10,000 *S. flexneri* type 2a. While approximately one-quarter of the volunteers never became ill, over the first 24 to 48 h approximately 25 percent of volunteers developed a transient fever, another 25 percent had fever and a self-limited watery diarrhea, and the remaining 25 percent had fever and watery diarrhea that progressed to bloody diarrhea and dysentery. In young children, in particular, the temperature can rapidly rise to 40 to 41°C and sometimes result in generalized seizures. These rarely recur or result in serious sequelae. Dysentery is characterized by frequent (usually 10 to 30 times per day) small-volume stools consisting of blood, mucus, and pus, plus abdominal cramps and tenesmus, the painful straining with stooling that may lead to rectal prolapse, especially in young children. The likelihood of severe dysentery is greatest in *S. dysenteriae* type 1 and *S. flexneri* infection and least likely in *S. sonnei*. With mild disease, patients generally recover without specific therapy in a few days to a week. Severe shigellosis can progress to toxic dilatation and colonic perforation, which may be fatal.

Endoscopy shows the mucosa to be hemorrhagic with mucous discharge and focal ulcerations, sometimes with overlying exudate. The majority of the lesions are in the distal colon and progressively diminish in the more proximal segments of large bowel. Mild dehydration is common in patients with watery diarrhea; severe dehydration is very rare. With extensive colonic involvement, protein-losing enteropathy occurs and can have very important adverse nutritional consequences for the already poorly nourished child.

A variety of *extraintestinal complications* of shigellosis have been described. The majority of these occur in patients in developing countries and are related to both the prevalence of *S. dysenteriae* type 1 and *S. flexneri* infection as well as to the poor nutritional state of the patients. For example, bacteremia, thought to be relatively infrequent in the United States, occurs in up to 8 percent of patients hospitalized for shigellosis in Dacca, Bangladesh. The causative *Shigella* species is isolated in half the patients; other Enterobacteriaceae are found in the remainder. Bacteremia is associated with higher than usual mortality and is more common in infants under 1 year of age and in those with protein-energy malnutrition. Persistent and clinically severe *Shigella* bacteremia has been encountered in the United States in patients with AIDS (see Chap. 279).

Hemolytic-uremic syndrome (HUS) may occur with *S. dysenteriae* type 1 infection. In the United States, the more likely cause of HUS is a hemorrhagic colitis–causing strain of *E. coli* producing high levels of Shiga-family toxins, such as *E. coli* O157:H7. HUS usually develops toward the end of the first week of shigellosis, when the dysentery is already resolving. Oliguria and a marked drop in hematocrit (as much as a 10 percent decrease within 24 h) are the first signs and may progress to anuria and renal failure or severe anemia with congestive heart failure, respectively. With HUS, leukemoid reactions with leukocyte counts over 50,000 per microliter may occur; thrombocytopenia (30,000 to 100,000 platelets per microliter) is common. Profound hyponatremia and severe hypoglycemia may be present. Central nervous system abnormalities include encephalopathic symptoms, seizures, altered consciousness, and bizarre posturing.

Other less common extraintestinal manifestations include seizures in some patients and reactive arthritis in others, both usually due to infection with *S. flexneri* strains. In patients expressing histocompatibility antigen HLA-B27, the full triad of Reiter's syndrome sometimes develops (see Chap. 289). Pneumonia, meningitis, vaginitis in prepubertal girls, keratoconjunctivitis, and "rose spot" rashes are rare events.

DIAGNOSIS AND LABORATORY FINDINGS Shigellosis is the principal bacterial cause of dysentery and should be considered in every patient presenting with bloody diarrhea. However, in the United States, because *S. sonnei* is the most common species, most patients will present with fever and a nonbloody watery diarrhea, indistinguishable from other bacterial or viral causes of mild to moderate diarrhea, while many patients with bloody diarrhea will have enterohemorrhagic *E. coli* as the cause. The specific diagnosis is made by culturing *Shigella* from the stool; however, polymerase chain reaction (PCR) diagnosis is possible. The yield of *Shigella* is increased by only culturing stool from patients with fecal leukocytes or bloody diarrhea. The organism is very labile and must be quickly transferred to plates or holding media (such as buffered glycerol saline) or it will not survive. Stool samples are preferable to swabs; when the latter are used, a rectal sample should be obtained. For culturing, more than one selective medium should be used, including MacConkey and one other, such as Hektoen enteric or xylose-lysine-deoxycholate.

Serology can be performed, since antibodies to somatic antigens develop early in the acute phase of disease; however, such tests are not generally available and are usually used only for epidemiologic studies.

The differential diagnosis includes other microbial causes of inflammatory colitis: enterohemorrhagic and enteroinvasive *E. coli*, *Campylobacter jejuni*, *Salmonella enteriditis* serotypes, *Yersinia enterocolitica*, *Clostridium difficile*, and the protozoan *Entamoeba histolytica*. Ulcerative colitis or Crohn's colitis are among the "noninfectious" causes (see Chap. 255). All except *E. histolytica* are associated with the presence of large numbers of fecal leukocytes. Amebiasis can be diagnosed by finding erythrophagocytic trophozoites in the stool (see Chap. 173).

Other laboratory studies are nonspecific and may disclose a moderate neutrophilic leukocytosis, anemia due to blood loss with hemorrhagic diarrhea, prerenal azotemia, or a hyperchloremic acidosis if watery diarrhea has been pronounced. Laboratory findings in shigellosis complicated by the HUS are discussed above.

TREATMENT The mild to moderate dehydration in shigellosis is readily corrected with oral rehydration solutions (see Chap. 120). The role of antibiotic therapy is variable and dependent on the organism and severity of disease. Since *S. sonnei* infection is usually self-limited, culture results generally do not become available until the patient is better and there is little clinical need for further therapy. The use of antibiotics in more severe cases with bloody diarrhea or dysentery will reduce the duration of illness and can shorten the duration of the carriage state. Resistance to sulfonamides, streptomycin, chloramphenicol, and tetracyclines is almost universal, and many *Shigella* are now also resistant to ampicillin and trimethoprim-sulfamethoxazole. Knowledge of the pattern of resistance in a given population, which can change with time, is useful. In the United States, multiresistant strains are most likely acquired during travel abroad, and either ampicillin, 50 to 100 mg/kg per day in children or 2 g/d in adults in divided doses, or trimethoprim-sulfamethoxazole, 8/40 mg/kg per day in children or 2 regular-strength tablets twice a day in adults, given for 5 days, is generally recommended. Amoxicillin should *not* be substituted for ampicillin because it is not effective treatment for shigellosis. In developing countries, where resistance to both these drugs is commonplace, the drug of choice for the treatment of multiresistant *S. dysenteriae* type 1 infections has been nalidixic acid, 55 mg/kg per day for 5 days; however, resistance is increasing in prevalence. The 4-fluoroquinolones (e.g., ciprofloxacin) are highly effective for all strains (see Chap. 100) but are currently too costly for the third world and in the United States are not yet approved for use in children under 17 because of the concern for cartilage toxicity. Alternative drugs shown to be effective include oral pivamdinocillin (but not yet available in the United States) and intravenous ceftriaxone, 50 mg/kg per day for 5 days. In small clinical trials, cephalexin has had no effect in limiting symptoms; single doses of ceftriaxone may be effective, but more information is needed. No antibiotic treatment is recommended for the convalescent carriage state, since this is usually limited to only several weeks' duration. Patients with AIDS may develop chronic carriage of shigella and be subject to relapsing infection with bacteremia (see Chap. 279). This cycle may be interrupted by prolonged (several weeks) treatment with a quinolone.

The role of antimotility agents such as atropine sulfate and diphenoxylate (Lomotil) and loperamide (Imodium) in the early phases of shigellosis remains unclear. They may reduce the diarrhea without provoking more severe disease through delayed excretion of organisms. There is no indication for their use in the dysenteric phase of disease, however, and they are not recommended.

Treatment of complications of shigellosis often differs in developed and developing countries. For example, antibiotic-unresponsive toxic megacolon, with or without perforation, is often managed by colectomy in the United States. Surgery is less often employed in developing countries because of lack of availability or difficulties in ileostomy management. Hemolytic-uremic syndrome often requires dialysis. In developing countries this may be less commonly needed because azotemia is slow to develop and the risk of significant hyperkalemia is often diminished because of the preexisting deficiency in total-body potassium with malnutrition and wasting of lean body mass. The management of hyponatremia, usually caused by inappropriate secretion of antidiuretic hormone (vasopressin), is governed by its severity and the symptomatic state of the patient as outlined in Chap. 45. Infusion of glucose can reverse clinical manifestations caused by hypoglycemia, and responses can be monitored by finger-stick blood glucose tests if no biochemistry laboratory is available. Optimal nutritional management is needed to correct the deficiencies due to underlying malnutrition and the superimposed catabolic stress and protein-losing enteropathy of shigellosis. This should begin during the acute illness and may require months of nutritional support afterwards (see Chap. 76).

PREVENTION Direct contact transmission of shigellosis can be prevented by appropriate environmental and personal hygiene. Hand washing with soap and water, decontamination of water supplies, use of sanitary latrines or toilets, and protection of food preparation and its storage can all reduce the primary and secondary transmission of *Shigella* infection. In the highly endemic developing countries, infants are protected during the period of exclusive breast feeding, and this should be encouraged. Any measures that also reduce the burden of malnutrition will have a favorable effect on the population as well. Hospitalized patients should be put on stool precautions to ensure safe disposal of infected excreta and linens, and hospital personnel must wash their hands and medical instruments such as stethoscopes after each contact with an infected patient. Cohorting of asymptomatic infected children, use of antibiotics to reduce infectiousness, and scrupulous attention to hygiene are usually successful in hospital outbreaks. Children in day-care must be kept at home while clinically ill and ideally should have a negative stool culture before returning to the group. Food handlers who develop shigellosis also should be required to be culture-negative before being allowed to return to work. Antibiotic treatment is not indicated for the asymptomatic carriage state. No effective vaccine is available.

REFERENCES

BASKIN DH et al: *Shigella* becteremia in patients with the acquired immune deficiency syndrome. Am J Gastroenterol 82:338, 1987

BENNISH ML: Potentially lethal complications of shigellosis. Rev Infect Dis 13(suppl):S319, 1991

——— et al: Hypoglycemia during diarrhea in childhood: Prevalence, pathophysiology, and outcome. N Engl J Med 322:1357, 1990

CLEMENTS JD et al: Breast feeding as a determinant of severity in shigellosis. Am J Epidemiol 123:710, 1986

COHEN D et al: Prospective study of the association between serum antibodies to lipopolysaccharide O antigen and the attack rate of shigellosis. J Clin Microbiol 29:386, 1991

GRIFFIN PM et al: Emergence of highly trimethoprim-sulfamethoxazole–resistant *Shigella* in a native American population: An epidemiologic study. Am J Epidemiol 129:1042, 1989

HALE TL: Genetic basis of virulence in *Shigella* species. Microbiol Rev 55:206, 1991

HALPERN Z et al: Shigellosis in adults: Epidemiologic, clinical, and laboratory features. Medicine 68:210, 1989

HOFFMAN RE, SHILLAM PJ: The use of hygiene, cohorting, and antimicrobial therapy to control an outbreak of shigellosis. Am J Dis Child 144:219, 1990

LEE LA et al: Hyperendemic shigellosis in the United States: A review of surveillance data for 1967–1988. J Infect Dis 164:894, 1991

LEVINE OS, LEVINE MM: Houseflies *(Musca domestica)* as mechanical vectors of shigellosis. Rev Infect Dis 13:688, 1991

SALAM MA, BENNISH ML: Antimicrobial therapy for shigellosis. Rev Infect Dis 13(suppl):S332, 1991

SANSONETTI PJ et al: *Pathogenesis of Shigellosis.* Berlin, Springer-Verlag, 1992

SORVILLO FJ et al: Shigellosis associated with recreational water contact in Los Angeles County. Am J Trop Med Hyg 38:613, 1988

TAUXE RV et al: Antimicrobial resistance of *Shigella* isolates in the USA: The importance of international travelers. J Infect Dis 162:1107, 1990

VARSANO I et al: Comparative efficacy of ceftriaxone and ampicillin for treatment of severe shigellosis in children. J Pediatr 118:627, 1991

ZVULUNOV A et al: The prognosis of convulsions during childhood shigellosis. Eur J Pediatr 149:293, 1990

119 CAMPYLOBACTER INFECTIONS

MARTIN J. BLASER

DEFINITION *Campylobacteriosis* refers to the group of pyogenic infections caused by bacteria of the genus *Campylobacter*. Although acute diarrheal illnesses are most common, these organisms may cause infections in virtually all parts of the body, especially in compromised hosts, and there may be late nonsuppurative sequelae. The designation *Campylobacter* comes from the Greek for "curved rod" and refers to the organism's vibrio-like morphology.

ETIOLOGY Campylobacters are motile, non-spore-forming, curved gram-negative rods. Originally known as *Vibrio fetus*, these bacilli were reclassified as a new genus in 1973 after it was recognized that they were quite dissimilar from other vibrios. Since then, more than 15 different *Campylobacter* species have been identified. However, not all these species are pathogens of humans. The human pathogens can be divided into two major groups: those that primarily cause diarrheal disease and those that cause extraintestinal infection. The principal diarrheal pathogen is *C. jejuni*, which accounts for 80 to 90 percent of all recognized illness due to campylobacters. Other organisms that cause diarrheal disease include *C. coli*, *C. upsaliensis*, *C. lari*, and *C. fetus*. The major species causing extraintestinal illnesses is *C. fetus;* however, any of the diarrheal agents may cause systemic or localized infection as well. Neither aerobes nor strict anaerobes, these microaerophilic organisms are adapted for survival in the gastrointestinal mucous layer. This chapter will focus on *C. jejuni* and *C. fetus* as the major pathogens and prototypes for their groups.

EPIDEMIOLOGY Campylobacters are found within the gastrointestinal tract of many animals used for food production (including poultry, cattle, sheep, and swine) and of household pets (including birds, dogs, and cats). However, these microorganisms usually do not cause illness in their animal hosts. In most cases, campylobacters are transmitted to humans in raw or undercooked food products or through direct contact with infected animals. In the United States and other developed countries, ingestion of contaminated poultry that has not been sufficiently cooked is the most common means of acquiring infection (50 to 70 percent of cases). Other modes of transmission include ingestion of raw (unpasteurized) milk or untreated water, contact with infected household pets, travel to developing countries (campylobacters being among the causes of traveler's diarrhea), and occasionally, contact with an index case who is incontinent of stool.

Campylobacter infections are not rare. Several studies indicate that in the United States diarrheal disease due to campylobacters is more common than that due to *Salmonella* and *Shigella* combined. Infections occur throughout the year, but their incidence peaks during summer and early autumn. Persons of all ages are affected; however, attack rates for *C. jejuni* are highest among young children and young adults, while those for *C. fetus* are highest at the extremes of ages. Systemic infections due to *C. fetus* (and other *Campylobacter* species) are most common in compromised hosts. Persons at increased risk include those with AIDS, hypogammaglobulinemia, neoplasia, liver disease, diabetes mellitus, and generalized atherosclerosis and pregnant women. However, apparently healthy, nonpregnant persons occasionally develop transient *Campylobacter* bacteremia.

In developing countries, *C. jejuni* infections are hyperendemic, with the highest rates in very young children (<2 years old). Infection rates fall with age, as does the illness-to-infection ratio; these observations suggest that frequent exposure to *C. jejuni* leads to the acquisition of immunity.

PATHOLOGY AND PATHOGENESIS Many *C. jejuni* infections are subclinical, especially in partially immune hosts. Most illnesses occur within 2 to 4 days (range 1 to 7 days) of exposure to the organism in food or water. The sites of tissue injury include the jejunum, ileum, and colon. Biopsies show an acute nonspecific inflammatory reaction, with neutrophils, monocytes, and eosinophils in the lamina propria, as well as damage to the epithelium, including loss of mucus, glandular degeneration, and crypt abscesses. Biopsy findings may be consistent with Crohn's disease or ulcerative colitis, but these "idiopathic" chronic inflammatory diseases should not be diagnosed unless infectious colitis, *specifically including* that due to infection with *Campylobacter*, has been ruled out.

The high frequency of *C. jejuni* infections and their severity and recurrence among hypogammaglobulinemic patients suggest that antibodies are important in protective immunity. The pathogenesis of infection is uncertain. Motility and adherence of the strain to host tissues both appear to favor disease, but classic enterotoxins and cytotoxins (although described) do not appear to play a role in tissue injury or disease production. The documentation of a significant tissue response and occasionally of *C. jejuni* bacteremia suggests that tissue invasion may occur, but this point has not been resolved satisfactorily.

The pathogenesis of *C. fetus* infections is better defined. Virtually all clinical isolates of *C. fetus* possess a proteinaceous capsule-like structure (S-layer) that renders the organism resistant to complement-mediated killing and opsonization. As a result, *C. fetus* can be bacteremic beyond the intestinal tract and can seed systemic sites. The ability of the organism to switch S-layer proteins, a phenomenon that induces antigenic variability, may contribute to the chronicity and high rate of recurrence of these infections in compromised hosts.

CLINICAL MANIFESTATIONS OF *C. JEJUNI* AND *C. FETUS* INFECTIONS The clinical features of infections due to all of the *Campylobacter* species causing enteric disease appear identical. There is often a prodrome with fever, headache, myalgia, and/or malaise 12 to 48 h before the onset of diarrheal symptoms. The most common symptoms of the intestinal phase are diarrhea, abdominal pain, and fever. The degree of diarrhea varies from several loose stools to grossly bloody stools; most patients presenting for medical attention have 10 or more bowel movements on the worst day of illness. Abdominal pain usually consists of cramping and may be the most prominent symptom. Pain usually is generalized but may become localized; *C. jejuni* infection may cause pseudoappendicitis. Fever may be the only initial manifestation of *C. jejuni* infection, a situation mimicking the early stages of typhoid fever. Febrile young children may develop convulsions. *Campylobacter* enteritis generally is self-limited; however, symptoms persist for longer than 1 week in 10 to 20 percent of patients seeking medical attention, and relapses occur in 5 to 10 percent of untreated patients.

C. fetus may cause a diarrheal illness similar to that due to *C.*

jejuni, especially in normal hosts, or may cause either intermittent diarrhea or nonspecific abdominal pain without localizing signs. Sequelae are uncommon, and outcome is benign. *C. fetus* also may cause a prolonged relapsing systemic illness (with fever, chills, and myalgias) that has no obvious primary source; this manifestation is especially common in compromised hosts. Secondary seeding of an organ (including meninges, brain, bone, urinary tract, and soft tissue) complicates the course, which may be fulminant. *C. fetus* infections have a tropism for vascular sites; endocarditis, mycotic aneurysm, and septic thrombophlebitis all may occur. Infection during pregnancy often leads to fetal death.

COMPLICATIONS Bacteremia is uncommon, developing most often in immunocompromised hosts and at the extremes of age. Three patterns of extraintestinal infection have been noted: (1) Transient bacteremia in a normal host with enteritis. The course is benign, and no specific treatment is needed. (2) Sustained bacteremia or focal infection in a normal host. Bacteremia originates from enteritis, and patients respond well to antimicrobial therapy. (3) Sustained bacteremia or focal infection in a compromised host. Enteritis may not be present. Antimicrobial therapy, possibly prolonged, is necessary for suppression or cure of the infection.

Campylobacter infections in patients with AIDS or hypogammaglobulinemia may be severe, persistent, and extraintestinal; relapse after cessation of therapy is common. Hypogammaglobulinemic patients also may develop osteomyelitis and an erysipelas-like rash.

Local suppurative complications of infection include cholecystitis, pancreatitis, and cystitis, and distant complications include meningitis, endocarditis, arthritis, peritonitis, or septic abortion; all are rare. Hepatitis, interstitial nephritis, and the hemolytic-uremic syndrome occasionally complicate acute infection. Reactive arthritis and other rheumatologic complaints may develop several weeks after infection, especially in persons with the HLA-B27 phenotype. Guillain-Barré syndrome follows *Campylobacter* infection uncommonly (i.e., in 1 of every 1000 to 2000 cases). However, because of the high incidence of infection due to campylobacters, it is now estimated that *Campylobacter* infections may trigger 10 to 30 percent of all cases of Guillain-Barré syndrome.

LABORATORY FINDINGS In patients with *Campylobacter* enteritis, peripheral leukocyte counts reflect the severity of the inflammatory process. However, stools contain leukocytes or erythrocytes in nearly all patients presenting for medical attention in the United States. Fecal smears should be stained with Gram's or Wright's stain and examined in all suspected cases. Diagnosis of *Campylobacter* enteritis is established by visualization of organisms with characteristic vibrioid morphology on direct microscopic examination of stools with Gram's staining (or the use of phase-contrast or dark-field microscopy to identify the characteristic "darting" motility) or by isolation of the organism from fecal culture. Confirmation of the diagnosis of *Campylobacter* infection is based on identification of an isolate from cultures of stool, blood, or another site. Since all *Campylobacter* species are fastidious, they will not be isolated unless selective media or other selective techniques are used. Not all media are equally useful for isolation of the broad array of campylobacters; therefore, failure to isolate campylobacters from stool does not entirely rule out their presence. The presence of the organism almost always implies infection; there is a brief period of postconvalescent fecal carriage and no commensalism. In contrast, *C. sputorum* and related organisms found in the oral cavity are commensals without known pathogenic significance.

DIFFERENTIAL DIAGNOSIS The symptoms of *Campylobacter* enteritis are not unusual enough to distinguish this illness from that due to *Salmonella*, *Shigella*, or *Yersinia*, among other pathogens. The combination of fever and fecal leukocytes or erythrocytes is indicative of inflammatory diarrhea, and definitive diagnosis is based on culture. Similarly, extraintestinal *Campylobacter* illness is diagnosed by culture. Infection due to *Campylobacter* should be suspected in the setting of septic abortion and that due to *C. fetus* specifically in the setting of septic thrombophlebitis. It is important to reiterate that the presentation of *Campylobacter* enteritis may mimic that of ulcerative colitis or Crohn's disease, that *Campylobacter* enteritis is much more common than either of the latter (especially among young adults), and that biopsy may not distinguish among these entities. Thus a diagnosis of inflammatory bowel disease should not be made until *Campylobacter* infection has been ruled out, especially in persons with a history of foreign travel, significant animal contact, immunodeficiency, or practices incurring a high risk of transmission.

TREATMENT Fluid and electrolyte replacement is central to the treatment of diarrheal illnesses (see Chap. 87). Even among patients presenting for medical attention with *Campylobacter* enteritis, fewer than half will clearly benefit from specific antimicrobial therapy. Indications for such therapy include high fever, bloody diarrhea, severe diarrhea, persistence for more than 1 week, and worsening of symptoms. A 5- to 7-day course of erythromycin (250 mg PO four times daily, or 30 to 50 mg/kg per day in divided doses for children) is the regimen of choice. Although not studied in clinical trials, the in vitro susceptibility of *Campylobacter* species to macrolides, such as clarithromycin and azithromycin, suggest that they also would be useful therapeutic agents. An alternative regimen for adults is ciprofloxacin (500 mg PO twice daily) for 5 to 7 days. Other alternatives include tetracycline, norfloxacin, and furazolidone. Use of antimotility agents, which may prolong the duration of symptoms and have been associated with deaths, is not recommended.

For systemic infections, treatment with an aminoglycoside such as gentamicin, a third-generation cephalosporin such as cefotaxime, or chloramphenicol should be started empirically, but susceptibility testing should then be performed. Erythromycin and amoxicillin/clavulanate are alternative agents. For immunocompromised patients with systemic infections due to *C. fetus*, prolonged therapy is usually necessary.

PROGNOSIS Nearly all patients recover fully from *Campylobacter* enteritis, either spontaneously or after antimicrobial therapy. Volume depletion likely contributes to the few deaths that are reported. As stated above, occasional patients develop reactive arthritis or Guillain-Barré syndrome. Systemic infection with *C. fetus* is much more often fatal; this higher mortality reflects in part the population affected. Prognosis is dependent on the rapidity with which appropriate therapy is begun. Normal hosts usually survive *C. fetus* infections without sequelae.

REFERENCES

Blaser MJ et al: *Campylobacter* enteritis: Clinical and epidemiologic features. Ann Intern Med 91:179, 1979
——— et al: *Campylobacter* enteritis in the United States: A multicenter study. Ann Intern Med 98:360, 1983
Nachamkin I et al (eds): *Campylobacter jejuni: Current Strategy and Future Trends.* Washington, American Society for Microbiology, 1992, pp 1–300
Perlman DM et al: Persistent *Campylobacter jejuni* infections in patients infected with the human immunodeficiency virus. Ann Intern Med 108:540, 1988

120 CHOLERA AND OTHER VIBRIOSES

GERALD T. KEUSCH / ROBERT L. DERESIEWICZ

Members of the genus *Vibrio* cause a number of important infectious syndromes. Classic among them is that caused by *V. cholerae* group O1, cholera, a devastating diarrheal disease responsible for seven world pandemics and much suffering over the past two centuries. Epidemic cholera remains a major public health concern and is dealt with at length in this chapter. Recently, other vibrioses have been described, including syndromes of diarrhea, soft-tissue infection, or primary sepsis caused by additional named species within the genus *Vibrio*. Those, too, are considered below.

All members of the genus are actively motile, facultatively anaerobic, curved gram-negative rods with one or more polar flagella. With the exception of *V. cholerae* and *V. mimicus,* all require salt for growth ("halophilic vibrios"). In nature they most commonly reside in tidal rivers and bays under conditions of moderate salinity. They proliferate in the summer months when water temperatures exceed about 20°C. As might be expected, the illnesses they cause also increase in frequency during the warm months. Some isolates of certain species within the genus share important determinants of virulence, in particular the ability to produce a potent protein enterotoxin (O1 and non-O1 *V. cholerae, V. mimicus,* and *V. fluvialis*).

CHOLERA

DEFINITION Cholera is an acute diarrheal disease that can, in a matter of hours, result in profound, rapidly progressive dehydration and death. Accordingly, cholera gravis (the severe form of cholera) is a much feared disease, particularly in its epidemic presentation. Fortunately, prompt, aggressive fluid repletion and supportive care can obviate the high mortality that it has historically wrought. The term *cholera* has occasionally been applied to any severely dehydrating secretory diarrheal illness whether due to *V. cholerae* or not and, indeed, whether infectious in etiology or not (including, for example, diarrhea due to endocrine syndromes such as vasoactive intestinal peptide–secreting tumors).

ETIOLOGY AND EPIDEMIOLOGY The species *V. cholerae* comprises a host of organisms classified on the basis of their somatic O antigen. Those which agglutinate in O group 1 antiserum cause the majority of cases of clinical cholera. Some 70 other members of the species are recognized and are collectively known as non-O1 *V. cholerae*. While some of the latter also can cause diarrhea, only rarely do they cause cholera gravis.

V. cholerae O1 exists in two biotypes, *classical* and *El Tor,* that are distinguished on the basis of a number of characteristics, including phage susceptibility and hemolysin production. Each biotype is further subdivided into two serotypes, termed *Inaba* and *Ogawa.* Serotyping is a useful tool in field epidemiologic studies.

Cholera is native to the Ganges delta in the Indian subcontinent. Since 1817, seven world pandemics have occurred. Before 1991, the last to reach the United States was in 1911, when the sixth pandemic made brief entry into New York and Massachusetts. In the past decade, sporadic endemic infection due to consumption of contaminated shellfish has been recognized along the Gulf Coasts of Louisiana and Texas. As well, small outbreaks associated with contaminated drinking water have occurred aboard offshore oil rigs.

In January 1991, epidemic cholera struck in Latin America. Beginning in Peru, the disease was carried by fisherman to Ecuador and Colombia and then by travelers to virtually all of South and Central America, to Mexico, and to the United States. Nearly 400,000 cases were reported in the first year of the outbreak, greatly exceeding the number of cases reported to the World Health Organization (WHO) worldwide in any previous year of record keeping. The epidemic continues, although at a much lower incidence. While the overall mortality rate has been about 1 percent, it approached 20 to 30 percent in the communities first affected, where a lack of familiarity with the disease led initially to the employment of draconian and wholly ineffective therapeutic measures. Intensive education of health providers and of the community at large has enhanced awareness of the disease and its appropriate management and has greatly diminished mortality. Of note, the epidemic reached the United States via illegally transported boiled crab meat, affecting eight people at a family party in New Jersey. This underscores the need for vigilance among health professionals, even in locations remote from the epicenter of an outbreak.

As it did in Africa in the 1970s, the organism has proven capable of establishing itself in inland waters rather than in its classical niche of coastal salt waters and has already become endemic in many of the countries into which it was recently introduced.

In 1993, an outbreak of severe clinical cholera occurred in Bangladesh and in India, affecting all age groups. The organism turned out to be a non-O1 *V. cholerae* and was designated *O139 Bengal*. The initial characterization of O139 Bengal has demonstrated the same major virulence attributes as in O1 *V. cholera*, including the key virulence regulatory genes. The only apparent difference in epidemiologic behavior between O139 Bengal and O1 *V. cholerae* is that prior immunity to the latter seems not to be effective in protecting individuals against the former. Accordingly, the population at risk is behaving as a virgin population with respect to severe, lethal cholera, and the same devastating epidemiology and clinical outcome seen in prior global pandemics of O1 *V. cholerae*, including the epidemic in the Americas in 1991, is being repeated in Asia. The isolate is resistant to trimethoprim-sulfamethoxazole but, at least at the outset, is sensitive to tetracycline.

Ingestion of water soiled by infected human feces is the most common means of transmission, but consumption of contaminated food in the home, in restaurants, or from street vendors also can contribute to spread. There is no known animal reservoir. The infectious dose is relatively high but is markedly reduced in hypochlorhydric subjects, in those using antacids, and when gastric acidity is buffered by a meal. In endemic areas, cholera is predominantly a pediatric disease, but it affects adults and children equally when newly introduced into a population. In endemic areas the disease is more common in the summer and fall months. While not fully explained, this seasonality may be due to environmental conditions that affect the multiplication of vibrios or to seasonal alterations in human behavior that affect their contact with water. Asymptomatic infections are frequent and are more common with the El Tor than with the classical biotype. In endemic areas, children under 2 years of age are less likely to develop severe cholera than are older children, perhaps due to passive immunity acquired from breast milk. For unexplained reasons, susceptibility to cholera is significantly influenced by ABO blood group status; those with type O are at greatest risk, while those with group AB are at least risk.

PATHOGENESIS Once ingested, the organism must safely traverse the acidic gastric environment. If successful, it next colonizes the upper small bowel. Attachment is mediated principally by the toxin coregulated pilus (TCP), so named because its synthesis is regulated in parallel with that of cholera toxin (CT). Several other properties of the organism enhance its ability to colonize, including its motility, chemotaxis, and hemagglutinin/protease production. The last, formerly termed *cholera lectin*, is closely related to the *Pseudomonas aeruginosa* elastase. It is both an agglutinin and a zinc-dependent protease and is able to cleave mucin and fibronectin, as well as the A subunit of cholera toxin. It also may serve to detach organisms so that they can attack distal intestinal sites or be excreted.

CT, TCP, and several other putative virulence factors, including an accessory colonization factor and various hemagglutinins, are coordinately regulated by the *tox*R gene product. ToxR protein is a "master switch" that modulates the expression of virulence genes in response to signals that it senses in the environment, the most important of which, at least in vitro, are changes in osmolarity, pH, and the presence of certain free amino acids. Coordinate regulation presumably enables the organism to tailor its repertoire of proteins to suit its needs as it passes from microenvironment to microenvironment. Regulation of the toxR type has become a paradigm for similar systems that have been discovered in a wide range of pathogenic bacteria.

Once established, the organism produces CT, a protein toxin that is the principal cause of the watery diarrhea characteristic of cholera. CT consists of a monomeric enzymatic moiety (the A subunit) and a pentameric binding moiety (the B subunit). The B pentamer binds to G_{MI} ganglioside, a glycolipid receptor on the surface of jejunal epithelial cells, and so delivers the A subunit to its cytosolic target. The activated A subunit (A_1) irreversibly transfers ADP-ribose from nicotinamide adenine dinucleotide (NAD) to its specific target protein, the GTP-binding regulatory component of adenylate cyclase in intestinal epithelial cells. When ADP-ribosylated, this so-called G protein up-regulates the cyclase catalytic subunit, which results in the intracellular accumulation of high levels of cyclic AMP (cAMP). cAMP, in turn, inhibits the absorptive sodium transport system in villus cells and activates the excretory chloride transport system in crypt cells, leading to the accumulation of sodium chloride in the intestinal lumen. Since water moves passively to maintain osmolality, isotonic fluid accumulates in the lumen. When the volume of that fluid exceeds the capacity of the rest of the gut to resorb it, watery diarrhea results. Unless the wasted fluid and electrolytes are adequately replaced, shock (due to profound dehydration) and acidosis (due to loss of bicarbonate) follow.

The nature of the immune response to cholera is poorly understood. Protection seems to be mediated primarily by an antibacterial effect at the mucosal surface and secondarily by antitoxin antibodies of the secretory IgA class. Serum antibody, though a marker for prior exposure, is not protective.

CLINICAL MANIFESTATIONS After a 24- to 48-h incubation period, cholera begins with the sudden onset of painless watery diarrhea that may quickly become voluminous and is often soon followed by vomiting. In severe cases, stool volume can exceed 250 mL/kg in the first 24 h. If fluids and electrolytes are not replaced, hypovolemic shock and death ensue. Fever is usually absent. Muscle cramps due to electrolyte disturbances are common. The stool has a characteristic appearance: a nonbilious, gray, slightly cloudy fluid with flecks of mucus, no blood, and a somewhat sweet, inoffensive odor. It has been referred to by the sobriquet "rice water" stool because of its resemblance to the water in which rice has been washed. Clinical symptoms parallel volume contraction: At losses of 3 to 5 percent of normal body weight, thirst occurs; at 5 to 8 percent, postural hypotension, weakness, tachycardia, and decreased skin turgor; above 10 percent, oliguria, weak to absent pulses, sunken eyes and (in infants) sunken fontanelles, wrinkled ("washerwoman") skin, somnolence, and coma. Complications derive exclusively from the effects of volume and electrolyte depletion and include, for example, renal failure due to acute tubular necrosis. Thus, if the patient is adequately treated with fluid and salt, complications are averted and the process self-limited, resolving in a few days.

Laboratory data usually reveal an elevated hematocrit in nonanemic patients (due to hemoconcentration); mild neutrophilic leukocytosis; elevations of BUN and creatinine consistent with prerenal azotemia; normal sodium, potassium, and chloride levels; a markedly reduced bicarbonate level (<15 mmol/L); and an elevated anion gap (due to coexistent increases in serum lactate, protein, and phosphate). Arterial pH is usually low (about 7.2).

DIAGNOSIS The clinical suspicion of cholera can be confirmed by the identification of the organism in stool. In experienced hands, the organism can be detected directly by dark-field microscopy on a wet mount of fresh stool, and its serotype discerned by immobilization with Inaba- or Ogawa-specific antiserum. The best selective culture medium is thiosulfate–citrate–bile salts–sucrose (TCBS) agar, on which the organism grows as a flat yellow colony. If a delay in sample processing is expected, Carey-Blair transport medium and/or alkaline-peptone water-enrichment medium should be inoculated as well. In endemic areas there is little need for biochemical characterization, though it may be worthwhile in places where *V. cholerae* is an uncommon isolate. Standard microbiologic biochemical testing for Enterobacteriaceae will suffice for identification of *V. cholerae*. All vibrios are oxidase-positive. *V. cholerae* can be distinguished from the otherwise similar *V. mimicus* by its ability to ferment sucrose.

TREATMENT Cholera is simple to treat, needing only the rapid and adequate replacement of fluids, electrolytes, and base. The mortality rate is usually less than 1 percent. It has been proven conclusively that fluid may be given orally, thereby taking advantage of the hexose-Na$^+$ cotransport mechanism to move Na$^+$ across the gut mucosa together with an actively transported molecule such as glucose. Since Na$^+$ losses in the stool are high, a fluid containing 90 mmol/L Na$^+$ has been recommended by the WHO (Table 120-1). That amount of Na$^+$ is higher than needed to treat diarrhea due to most other causes. The solution is safe, even in infants, if alternated with sodium-free fluid such as breast milk or water. For the sake of simplicity, WHO advises routine use of this single solution for diarrheal disease rather than attempting to select from multiple formulations according to etiology. In the future, cereal-based oral rehydration solutions may be more widely recommended. For severely dehydrated patients, the intravenous route of fluid replacement, if available, is preferable for initial management. Because profound acidosis (pH < 7.2) is common in that group, Ringer's lactate is the best choice among commercial products (Table 120-2). It requires the use of additional potassium supplements, preferably given by mouth. The total fluid deficit (usually estimated at 10 percent of body weight in severely dehydrated patients) can be replaced safely within the first 4 h of therapy, half within the first hour. Thereafter, oral therapy usually can be initiated, with the goal of maintaining fluid intake equal to output. However, patients with continued large-volume diarrhea may require prolonged intravenous treatment to keep up with gastrointestinal fluid losses. Severe hypokalemia can be present but will respond to potassium given either intravenously or orally. In the absence of adequate staff to monitor the patient's progress, the oral route of rehydration and potassium repletion is safer than the intravenous route and is physiologically regulated by thirst and urine output.

Though not necessary to achieve cure, the use of an antibiotic to which the organism is susceptible will diminish the duration and volume of fluid loss and will hasten clearance of the organism from the stool. Single-dose tetracycline (2 g) or doxycycline (300 mg) is effective in adults but is not recommended for children under 8 years of age because of possible deposition in bone and developing teeth. Trimethoprim-sulfamethoxazole (5 mg/kg of trimethoprim and 25 mg/kg of sulfamethoxazole given bid for 3 days) is a suitable alternative for young children. Other antibiotics, including ampicillin and the new 4-fluoroquinolones, are also active. Emerging drug resistance is a concern.

CONTROL   In outbreaks, efforts should first be made to identify case contacts and to treat incubating carriers. Next, epidemiologic study should be undertaken to establish the modes of transmission in order to define the best strategy to interrupt them. Rehydration centers should be established and rehydration techniques taught, both of which are essential to reducing mortality.

PREVENTION   Provision of safe water, facilities for sanitary disposal of feces, improved nutrition, and attention to food preparation and storage in the household could significantly reduce the incidence of cholera. Much effort has been devoted to the development of a cholera vaccine over the past two decades, focusing particularly on the use of live oral vaccine strains. Traditional killed cholera vaccine given intramuscularly provides little protection to nonimmune subjects

TABLE 120-2   Electrolyte composition of cholera stool and of intravenous rehydration solution

	Concentration, mmol/L			
Substance	Na$^+$	K$^+$	Cl$^-$	Base
Stool				
Adult	135	15	90	30
Child	100	25	90	30
Ringer's lactate	130	4*	109	28

* Potassium supplements, preferably administered by mouth, are required to replete the usual potassium losses from stool.

and predictably causes adverse effects, including pain at the injection site, malaise, and fever. A new approach, the oral administration of killed whole bacterial cells either with or without cholera toxin B subunit (BS-WC vaccine or WC vaccine), has shown promise. In trials in Bangladesh, both vaccines conferred about 50 percent protection compared with placebo over a 3-year evaluation period. Protective efficacy of BS-WC was superior to that of WC during the initial 8 months of follow-up (69 versus 41 percent) but equivalent or inferior thereafter. Immunity was relatively sustained in persons vaccinated above the age of 5 years but only poorly so in younger vaccinees. Several laboratories are now bringing the powerful techniques of molecular biology to bear on this problem and offer the hope that an inexpensive, easily administered, and broadly efficacious vaccine will one day be available. Although one case per week of travel-associated cholera is presently being reported in the United States, it is estimated that using the existing intramuscular vaccine and assuming 1 case per 500,000 trips, a routine vaccination program for travelers from North America to endemic areas would cost over $28 million for each case of cholera prevented and would produce over 100 vaccine-associated adverse events. Vaccine is therefore not recommended for Americans traveling in cholera-endemic areas unless mandated by the country to be visited. Travelers should observe careful hygiene and eating and drinking habits that reduce the likelihood of their encountering the organism.

OTHER *VIBRIO* SPECIES

In recent years, the taxonomic, epidemiologic, pathophysiologic, and clinical features of the non-O1 vibrios have been increasingly well understood. Ten human pathogens are currently recognized within the genus *Vibrio*. Included are species associated primarily with gastrointestinal illness (*V. parahaemolyticus*, non-O1 *V. cholerae*, *V. mimicus*, *V. fluvialis*, *V. hollisae*, and *V. furnissii*) and species associated primarily with soft tissue infections (*V. vulnificus*, *V. alginolyticus*, and *V. damsela*). As well, *V. vulnificus* has emerged as a cause of primary sepsis in certain compromised hosts. Vibrios are abundant in coastal waters the world over and tend to concentrate in the tissues of filter-feeding mollusks. Under optimal conditions some can double in as little as 9 minutes. Consequently, seawater and raw or undercooked shellfish are important sources of human infection (Table 120-3). Vibrios grow best at temperatures between about 28 and 44°C but not at all below 4°C or above 60°C. Most can be cultured on blood or MacConkey agar, each of which contains enough salt to support the growth of the halophilic organisms (≥0.5 percent). As with *V. cholerae*, TCBS is the best selective medium. The species can be differentiated in the laboratory by standard biochemical tests. The most important members of the group are *V. parahaemolyticus*, a major cause of gastroenteritis in the Far East, and *V. vulnificus*, a notable cause of sepsis in certain immunosuppressed patients in the United States. These and other select species are considered below in greater detail.

SPECIES ASSOCIATED PRIMARILY WITH GASTROINTESTINAL ILLNESS   *V. parahaemolyticus*   First implicated as a cause of enteritis by Japanese workers in 1953, *V. parahaemolyticus* is now

TABLE 120-1   Composition of World Health Organization oral rehydration solution (WHO ORS)*,†

	Concentration, mmol/L				
	Na$^+$	K$^+$	Cl$^-$	Citrate‡	Glucose
WHO ORS	90	20	80	10	111

* Contains NaCl 3.5 g, Na$_3$C$_6$H$_5$O$_7$·2H$_2$O 2.9 g, KCl 1.5 g, and glucose 20 g per package, to be added to 1 L of drinking water.
† If prepackaged ORS is unavailable, a simple homemade alternative can be prepared by combining 5 g NaCl (about 1 level teaspoon) and either 50 g precooked rice cereal or 40 g sucrose in 1 L of drinking water. In that case, potassium must be supplied separately (e.g., orange juice or coconut water).
‡ 10 mmol of citrate per liter, which supplies 30 mmol of HCO$_3$ per liter.

TABLE 120-3   Features of select noncholera vibrioses

Organism	Vehicle or activity	Host at risk	Syndrome
V. parahaemolyticus	Shellfish, seawater	Normal	Gastroenteritis
	Seawater	Normal	Wound infection
Non-O1 V. cholerae	Shellfish, travel	Normal	Gastroenteritis
	Seawater	Normal	Wound infection, otitis media
V. vulnificus	Shellfish	Immunosuppressed*	Sepsis, secondary cellulitis
	Seawater	Normal	Wound infection, cellulitis
V. alginolyticus	Seawater	Normal	Wound infection, cellulitis, otitis
	Seawater	Burn, other immunosuppressed	Sepsis

* Especially liver disease or hemochromatosis.

recognized as an important intestinal pathogen in many parts of the world. In one study from Japan, 24 percent of reported cases of food poisoning were attributed to it, presumably owing to the widespread consumption of raw seafood there. In the United States it has been responsible for several well-documented common-source outbreaks of diarrhea, typically linked to ingestion of undercooked or improperly handled seafood or to other foods that have been contaminated by seawater. Most reports have come from the Atlantic Coast, the Gulf of Mexico, or Hawaii. The organism is ubiquitous in marine environments and is able to grow in saline concentrations up to about 8 to 10 percent. The ability to cause hemolysis on Wagatsuma agar (the so-called Kanagawa phenomenon) is closely linked to enteropathogenicity. In one study, 96.5 percent of isolates from patients with diarrhea were hemolytic versus only about 1 percent of isolates from seawater. Hemolysis is attributed to a 42-kDa heat-stable protein, the exact pathophysiologic role of which is uncertain. The mechanism by which V. parahaemolyticus causes diarrhea is uncertain.

V. parahaemolyticus has been associated with two distinct gastrointestinal presentations. Most common is a syndrome of watery diarrhea, usually accompanied by abdominal cramps, nausea, and vomiting, and by fever and chills in about one-quarter of cases. The incubation period ranges from 4 h to 4 days, and the symptomatic period persists for a median duration of 3 days. The vast majority of North American cases have been of this type. A less common syndrome is one of dysentery described in India and Bangladesh and characterized by severe abdominal cramps, nausea, vomiting, and bloody or mucoid stools. Most cases of either type are self-limited and require neither antimicrobials nor hospitalization. The occasional severe case should be treated with fluid repletion and antibiotics, as described above for cholera. Mortality is very rare. There are no reliable differential diagnostic features. V. parahaemolyticus should be considered in all cases of diarrhea that can be epidemiologically linked to seafood consumption or to the sea.

In addition to gastrointestinal disease, V. parahaemolyticus is a rare cause of extraintestinal infections, including wound infections, otitis, and, very rarely, sepsis.

Non-O1 V. cholerae   The non-O1 V. cholerae are a heterogeneous group of organisms that on routine testing are biochemically indistinguishable from V. cholerae O1 but that fail to agglutinate in O1 antiserum. They have been responsible for several well-described food-borne outbreaks of gastroenteritis, as well as sporadic cases of otitis media, wound infection, and bacteremia. About half the U.S. isolates are obtained from stool specimens. Like other vibrios, they are widely distributed in marine environments, but unlike most, they require only trace amounts of NaCl to survive (nonhalophilic). Recognized U.S. cases have invariably been associated either with the consumption of raw oysters or with recent travel, typically to Mexico. The clinical spectrum of diarrheal disease that they cause is broad and likely reflects the heterogeneous virulence attributes among members of the group. Occasional isolates make a protein enterotoxin very similar to cholera toxin. Others make cytotoxins, hemolysins, or invasins.

Gastroenteritis due to non-O1 V. cholerae typically has an incubation period of less than 2 days. Stools may be copious and watery and may leave the patient severely dehydrated, as with cholera, or they may be partly formed, of lesser volume, and bloody or mucoid. Abdominal cramps, nausea, vomiting, and fever are often present. In one series, 11 percent of patients were hospitalized; in another, 50 percent. The duration of illness ranges from about 2 to 7 days. As with cholera, patients with significant dehydration should be treated with oral or intravenous fluids. The role of antibiotics is uncertain.

Wound infections and otitis media each account for about 10 percent of non-O1 V. cholerae isolates. Bacteremias account for another 20 percent. Patients with extraintestinal infection often have a history of occupational or recreational exposure to seawater. Bacteremia is more likely in those with liver disease. Extraintestinal infections should be treated with antibiotics. There is a paucity of data by which to guide one's choice of a specific agent and schedule. Most strains are sensitive in vitro to tetracycline, chloramphenicol, and other agents.

SPECIES ASSOCIATED PRIMARILY WITH SOFT TISSUE INFECTIONS OR BACTEREMIA   V. vulnificus   Though it represents only a minority of the Vibrio species found in nature (4 percent of Atlantic coast isolates in one study), V. vulnificus is perhaps the most important cause of severe Vibrio infections in the United States (0.8 cases per 100,000 population in one study from Louisiana). Formerly grouped in the species V. parahaemolyticus, V. vulnificus was distinguished in the 1970s by its ability to ferment lactose and by recognition of the distinct clinical syndromes that it causes. Like most vibrios, it proliferates in the warm summer months. It requires saline for growth but prefers concentrations (range up to about 8 percent, optimal about 1 percent) lower than do V. parahaemolyticus and V. alginolyticus. Human infections typically occur in coastal states between the months of May and October, most often in men over age 40. It has been unequivocally linked to two distinct syndromes: primary sepsis, typically in patients with antecedent liver disease, and primary wound infections, usually in people without underlying disease. Some have suggested that it causes gastroenteritis, but the evidence for this is tenuous.

The organism is remarkably invasive in animal models. It is endowed with a number of virulence attributes, including an antiphagocytic capsule, serum resistance, a cytotoxin/hemolysin (it is Kanagawa-positive), collagenase, elastolytic protease, phospholipase, and siderophores. Its virulence, as measured by the 50 percent lethal dose (LD_{50}) in mice, is markedly enhanced under conditions of iron overload, a fact consonant with its propensity to infect patients with hemochromatosis.

Primary sepsis occurs most commonly in patients with cirrhosis or hemochromatosis but also has been observed in patients with hematopoietic disorders or chronic renal insufficiency, in those using immunosuppressive medications or alcohol, and rarely, in those without apparent underlying disease. Most have ingested raw oysters within 2 days of onset (median incubation period 16 h). The process begins precipitously with malaise, chills, fever (mean 39.8°C), and prostration. Hypotension develops in one-third of cases, often by the time of admission. Cutaneous manifestations, which develop in three-quarters of cases usually by 36 h after onset, typically are on the extremities, lower more often than upper. A common sequence is the evolution of erythematous patches followed by ecchymoses, vesicles, and bullae. (Indeed, the presence of sepsis and bullous skin lesions should suggest the diagnosis in the appropriate setting.) Necrosis and sloughing may occur. Laboratory study reveals leukopenia more often than leukocytosis, thrombocytopenia, and occasionally, elevated fibrin split products. The organism can be cultured from blood or cutaneous lesions. Mortality approaches 50 percent, usually due to uncontrolled sepsis. Accordingly, prompt treatment is critical and should include empirical antibiotics, aggressive debridement, and general supportive care. The organism is sensitive to a number of antimicrobials in vitro, including tetracycline, gentamicin, and third-generation cephalosporins. There are no compelling clinical data in humans to support the use of any particular one of these agents. Tetracycline is demonstrably superior in a murine model and is considered the drug of choice (0.5 to 1 g IV every 12 h), either alone or in combination with gentamicin. The duration of therapy is guided by the clinical response.

Wound infections occur in patients with or without underlying disease and invariably follow contact of seawater with either an existing or a fresh wound. The incubation period is brief (4 h to 4 days, mean 12 h). The disease begins with swelling, erythema, and often intense pain around the wound. A rapidly spreading cellulitis follows, with vesicular, bullous, or necrotic lesions developing in some. Metastatic events do not generally occur. Fever (median 38.9°C) and leukocytosis are present in most. The organism can be cultured from the skin lesions and occasionally from blood. Prompt antibiotic therapy and debridement are usually curative.

V. alginolyticus This species was first recognized as a human pathogen in 1973 and is now known to cause occasional wound, ear, and eye infections. It is the most salt-tolerant of the vibrios, able to grow in concentrations exceeding 10 percent. Most clinical isolates come from superinfected wounds presumably contaminated at the beach. Infection varies in severity but is generally not serious and responds well to antibiotics and drainage. A few reports describe otitis externa, otitis media, or conjunctivitis. Therapy with tetracycline is usually curative. The organism is a rare cause of bacteremia in immunocompromised hosts.

REFERENCES

BLAKE PA et al: Disease of humans (other than cholera) caused by vibrios. Annu Rev Microbiol 34:341, 1980

CARPENTER CCJ: The treatment of cholera: Clinical science at the bedside. J Infect Dis 166:2, 1992

CENTERS FOR DISEASE CONTROL: Update: Cholera—Western hemisphere, and recommendation for treatment of cholera. Morb Mort Week Rep 40:562, 1991

————: Cholera associated with international travel—1992. Morb Mort Week Rep 41:664, 1992

CLEMENS JD et al: ABO blood groups and cholera: New observations on specificity of risk and modification of vaccine efficacy. J Infect Dis 159:770, 1989

———— et al: Field trial of oral cholera vaccines in Bangladesh: Results from three-year follow-up. Lancet 335:270, 1990

GLASS RI et al: Epidemic cholera in the Americas. Science 256:1524, 1992

HIRSHHORN N, GREENOUGH WB: Progress in oral rehydration therapy. Sci Am 264:50, 1991

LEVINE MM, EDELMAN R: Future vaccines against enteric pathogens. Infect Dis Clin North Am 4:105, 1990

LOWRY PW et al: Cholera in Louisiana: Widening spectrum of seafood vehicles. Arch Intern Med 149:2079, 1989

MACPHERSON DW, TONKIN M: Cholera vaccination: A decision analysis. Can Med Assoc J 146:1947, 1992

MORRIS JG JR: Non-O1 *V. cholerae*: A look at the epidemiology of an occasional pathogen. Epidemiol Rev 12:179, 1990

MORRIS JG, BLACK RE: Cholera and other vibrioses in the United States. N Engl J Med 312:343, 1985

Prevention and treatment of cholera. Med Lett 33:107, 1991

SWERDLOW DL et al: Waterborne transmission of epidemic cholera in Trujillo, Peru: Lessons for a continent at risk. Lancet 340:28, 1992

TACKET CO et al: Cholera vaccines. Biotechnology 20:53, 1992

VANDEN BROUCKE JP et al: Who made John Snow a hero? Am J Epidemiol 133:967, 1991

121 BRUCELLOSIS

DONALD KAYE

DEFINITION Brucellosis is an infection caused by bacteria of the genus *Brucella*. Human infection results from occupational contact with an infected animal or from ingestion of infected milk, milk products, or tissues. The symptoms of brucellosis are often nonspecific and include fever, malaise, and weight loss, often without physical findings.

ETIOLOGY There are four species of *Brucella* that cause infection in humans. The most pathogenic is *B. melitensis*, followed by *B. suis*, *B. abortus*, and *B. canis*. While each of these tends to produce infection in a specific animal host (*B. melitensis* in sheep and goats, *B. suis* in swine, *B. abortus* in cattle, and *B. canis* in dogs), cross-species infection occurs (e.g., *B. abortus* in sheep) and other animals may become infected.

Brucella are small, nonmotile, nonencapsulated, gram-negative coccobacilli which do not form spores. *Brucella* grow best at 37°C under increased CO_2 tension and are separated from each other by biochemical and serologic techniques. Strains with decreased lipopolysaccharide in the outer membrane have reduced virulence.

EPIDEMIOLOGY Animals acquire brucellosis either sexually or by ingesting contaminated milk or other animal products. Humans develop disease following ingestion of contaminated animal food products, by contact of *Brucella* with abraded skin, through the conjunctivae, or by inhalation. Person-to-person transmission rarely, if ever, occurs.

While there are 500,000 new cases of brucellosis reported annually worldwide, it has become a rare disease in the United States, with fewer than 200 cases reported each year. However, it is estimated that only about 4 percent of cases are recognized and reported. *B. abortus* and *B. suis* cause most cases in the United States; *B. melitensis* and *B. canis* are rare. In the United States, brucellosis is mainly an occupational disease, with most cases occurring in working-age males who are abattoir workers, butchers, or farmers. Veterinarians may become infected by accidental inoculation of live attenuated *B. abortus* vaccine, which causes mild disease. In most instances of brucellosis acquired in the United States from ingestion of contaminated milk products, the foods came from other parts of the world (Mexico, Mediterranean countries, the Far East, and South America).

Worldwide, *B. melitensis* is the most frequent cause of brucellosis. There are tremendous differences in the yearly incidence of human brucellosis in different countries, mainly depending on the extent of animal brucellosis. The areas with the highest prevalence are the Mediterranean countries, Asia, and Central and South America.

PATHOGENESIS AND PATHOLOGY After invading the body, *Brucella* are phagocytized by polymorphonuclear leukocytes and macrophages. Some *Brucella* are killed, but others multiply within these cells and destroy them. *Brucella* are able to survive inside phagocytes by inhibiting degranulation of myeloperoxidase-containing granules and thus interfering with myeloperoxidase-dependent bactericidal mechanisms.

Organisms spread via lymphatics to regional lymph nodes and, if not contained, to the bloodstream. Bacteremia may result in foci in cells of the reticuloendothelial system in the liver, spleen, and bone marrow and in other organs such as the kidneys. *Brucella* inside phagocytic cells (as in the reticuloendothelial system and tissue macrophages) are protected against antibody and many antibiotics.

The reaction of tissues to *Brucella* is the formation of granulomas with epithelioid cells, giant cells, lymphocytes, and plasma cells. *B. abortus* usually causes mild disease with noncaseating granulomas in the liver and other reticuloendothelial organs. *B. suis* causes more severe disease with local suppurative complications and granulomas that may caseate. *B. melitensis* produces the most severe acute disease with symptoms that may be disabling. *B. canis* results in mild disease similar to that seen with *B. abortus*. Activated macrophages can kill *Brucella*, and this is the probable mechanism by which spontaneous cure and immunity occur. Granulomas in brucellosis eventually heal with fibrosis and often calcification.

Brucella localize to the placenta in pregnant ungulates due to the presence of erythritol, which enhances the growth of the bacteria. Abortion may ensue. However, erythritol is not found in significant concentrations in humans, and abortions do not occur any more frequently with this disease than with other bacteremias.

MANIFESTATIONS Brucellosis may be asymptomatic, with only serologic evidence of infection. Children are particularly prone to subclinical infection. The manifestations of symptomatic brucellosis may be divided into acute brucellosis, localized disease, and chronic brucellosis.

Acute brucellosis The incubation period of acute brucellosis usually varies between 7 and 21 days but may be months. The onset is often insidious, with a low-grade fever and no localizing complaints. Malaise, weakness, fatigue, headache, backache, myalgias, sweats, and chills are often prominent. Most patients are anorectic and lose weight. With *B. melitensis* infection, the onset may be acute with high fever.

Typically, there are a multitude of complaints but a paucity of physical findings. When physical findings occur, the major manifestations are splenomegaly (which occurs in 10 to 20 percent of patients), lymphadenopathy (15 percent of patients), and hepatomegaly (less than 10 percent).

Localized brucellosis Localized disease may occur at almost any anatomic location, but osteomyelitis, splenic abscess, genitourinary tract infection, pulmonary disease, and endocarditis are among the more common. Osteomyelitis usually occurs in the vertebrae, with the lumbosacral area the most frequent site. There is a disc space infection with involvement of both adjacent vertebrae. Bone scans are positive early, followed by roentgenographic evidence of osteoporosis, anterior vertebral plate erosion, and formation of "parrot-beaked" osteophytes. Arthritis, which is much less common than osteomyelitis, most often involves the knee. Splenic abscesses may occur and result in areas of calcification. Epididymoorchitis and less often clinically apparent prostatic or renal infection may be observed. Neurologic complications are uncommon and include meningoencephalitis, myelitis, radiculitis, and peripheral neuropathy. Pleural effusion and pneumonia are occasional manifestations.

Endocarditis is the most common cause of mortality among patients with brucellosis. It has been reported predominantly in males, most often involves the aortic valve, has an indolent onset, results in bulky and ulcerative vegetations, is accompanied by a high rate of congestive heart failure and arterial embolization, and has usually required both valve replacement and antibiotic therapy to achieve cure.

Chronic brucellosis Chronic brucellosis is defined as ill health for more than 1 year following onset of brucellosis. It has mixed manifestations and includes patients with relapsing illness, with or without localized infection, as well as those who have no objective signs of infection (e.g., no fever) and no evidence of active brucellosis (by serology or culture). While the former clearly have brucellosis, it is doubtful that the latter have active brucellosis. Their complaints, fatigue and weakness, are more likely functional.

An unusual complication that occurs in veterinarians removing placentas from infected animals consists of an erythematous macular, papular, or pustular rash on the hands and arms, which is presumed to be a hypersensitivity reaction to *Brucella* antigens.

DIAGNOSIS Brucellosis is a relatively rare disease, and there are many common illnesses that may mimic the most frequent presentation (i.e., fever without localizing symptoms or physical findings). Among them are infectious mononucleosis, toxoplasmosis, tuberculosis, hepatitis, systemic lupus erythematosus, typhoid fever, and many others. The clinical suspicion that the patient has brucellosis should be higher in farmers, abattoir workers, veterinarians, and others exposed to infected tissues or animal products. Most routine laboratory tests are not helpful. The white blood cell count is usually normal or low, and the erythrocyte sedimentation rate may be normal.

Cultures The definitive evidence of *Brucella* infection consists of isolating *Brucella* from the patient. However, culturing *Brucella* organisms may be dangerous to laboratory personnel. Therefore, specimens should be labeled as "suspected brucellosis" and should be processed only in laboratories that have biosafety level 3 facilities. Up to half the untreated patients studied early in the course of infection will have *Brucella* in the blood when a culture is grown in trypticase soy broth for 1 to 3 weeks in the presence of 5 to 10% CO_2. Optimally, Casteñeda's medium (a biphasic trypticase soy broth and agar medium) should be used and incubated for 4 weeks. Bone marrow cultures are often positive in acute brucellosis when blood cultures are not. They are also more likely to remain positive later in the course of the disease and in spite of administration of antimicrobial agents. As the illness progresses, bacteremia is less frequent, and organisms may then be isolated from infected lymph nodes or granulomas involving the spleen, liver, and bone. Altogether, only 15 to 20 percent of cases of brucellosis are confirmed by culture. In localized brucellosis, biopsy and isolation of *Brucella* may be necessary for diagnosis. In the majority of cases of brucellosis, the diagnosis is made serologically.

Serology The standard tube *Brucella* agglutination test (STA) has been used most in the diagnosis of brucellosis. It measures antibodies directed primarily at *Brucella* lipopolysaccharide antigens. A titer of $\geq 1:160$ is considered positive and indicates past or present exposure to *Brucella* organisms or antigens that cross-react with *Brucella* species (*Brucella* skin tests, cholera vaccination, and infection with *Vibrio cholerae*, *Francisella tularensis*, or *Yersinia enterocolitica*). A fourfold or greater rise in titer of antibody in serum specimens drawn 1 to 4 weeks apart is indicative of recent exposure to *Brucella* or *Brucella*-like antigens. Paired specimens should be tested on the same day in the same laboratory. Most patients develop a rise in titer, as measured by the STA, within 1 to 2 weeks of illness, and by 3 weeks virtually all patients will show seroconversion. If there is strong clinical suspicion of brucellosis, dilutions as high as 1:1280 should be made, because false-negative tests due to blocking antibodies have been reported with blocking antibody titers as high as 1:640. True STA titers below 1:160 are strong evidence against active brucellosis.

The methods for serologic diagnosis of brucellosis use *B. abortus* antigens, because antibodies to *B. melitensis* and *B. suis* cross-react with *B. abortus*. However, antibodies to *B. canis* will not react with *B. abortus* antigen, and specialized serologic studies are necessary to detect these antibodies.

IgM antibody titers rise early in brucellosis (usually in the first week of infection), peak at about 3 months, and then fall gradually. However, high titers may persist for years. IgG antibodies appear 2 to 3 weeks after onset of illness, peak in about 8 weeks, and persist as long as the infection is active. With cure, IgG antibody titers decrease rapidly and usually disappear within 1 year. The persistence of IgG antibody indicates continuing active infection. With relapse, both IgM and IgG titers increase. Use of 2-mercaptoethanol (2-ME) in the STA destroys the agglutinating activity of IgM antibodies and allows measurement of only the IgG-agglutinating antibody. In contrast to elevated IgM antibodies, a single titer of $\geq 1:160$ in the 2-ME STA is good evidence of either current or very recent infection.

The *Brucella* skin test is only a measure of past infection. Because it may cause a rise in antibody titers, confusing the interpretation of the STA, it should not be performed.

TREATMENT The combination of doxycycline 100 mg every 12 hours or tetracycline 30 mg/kg per day in four equally divided doses, orally, for 3 to 6 weeks plus streptomycin 15 mg/kg every 12 h intramuscularly for the first 2 weeks is considered the treatment of choice for brucellosis. The longer duration of a tetracycline is recommended for patients with localized brucellosis. Patients who relapse are usually cured with retreatment. Tetracyclines should not be used in pregnant women or children below the age of 8 because of the danger of staining developing teeth. Streptomycin may cause eighth-nerve toxicity, and the dose must be decreased in patients with renal insufficiency.

A variety of other regimens, including a tetracycline plus gentamicin or rifampin in lieu of streptomycin or trimethoprim-sulfamethoxazole alone, have been tried in an attempt to decrease relapses and toxicity, but none has been superior to the tetracycline-streptomycin combination. When a tetracycline plus streptomycin cannot be used, trimethoprim-sulfamethoxazole (480/2400 mg/d) for 4 weeks is a reasonable substitute, although relapses are common. Addition of rifampin (900 mg/d) to the basic tetracycline-streptomycin or trimethoprim-sulfamethoxazole regimen may improve results when response is poor or when meningitis or endocarditis is present. Despite in vitro activity against *Brucella*, ciprofloxacin has resulted in a high relapse rate and should not be used. Successful therapy of endocarditis has usually required valve replacement in addition to one of the above antimicrobial regimens. The role of the third-generation cephalosporins in brucellosis remains to be determined, despite their apparent in vitro activity against strains of *Brucella*.

Abscesses should be drained when indicated. Splenectomy has been performed in some patients with splenomegaly and multiple relapses and has apparently been successful in preventing further relapses. Headache, backache, and generalized aches and pains should be treated with analgesics.

PROGNOSIS Even before the advent of antimicrobial treatment, the mortality rate of brucellosis was less than 5 percent, and only 15 percent of patients had an illness exceeding 3 months in duration. With chemotherapy, the mortality rate is less than 2 percent, and long illnesses and complications are rare. When the morbidity exceeds 1 to 2 months, other causes, previously unsuspected underlying disease, or a complication of brucellosis should be considered.

PREVENTION The key to elimination of brucellosis in humans is the eradication of animal brucellosis. This can be accomplished by immunization of animals with a live attenuated *Brucella* vaccine, which produces immunity. No vaccine is available for human immunization in the United States. The risk of acquiring brucellosis can be decreased by use of pasteurized milk and pasteurized milk products, by guarding against exposure to tissue from infected animals, and by protecting potential portals of entry in high-risk individuals (veterinarians, meat inspectors, slaughterhouse workers) with protective bandages over cuts and the use of protective clothing, gloves, and goggles.

REFERENCES

CASTILLO JD et al: Comparative trial of doxycycline plus streptomycin versus doxycycline plus rifampin for the therapy of human brucellosis. Chemotherapy 35:146, 1989

CISNEROS JM et al: Multicenter prospective study of treatment of *Brucella melitensis* brucellosis with doxycycline for 6 weeks plus streptomycin for 2 weeks. Antimicrob Agents Chemother 34(5):881, 1990

GOTUZZO E et al: An evaluation of diagnostic methods for brucellosis—The value of bone marrow culture. J Infect Dis 153(1):122, 1986

JACOBS F et al: Brucella endocarditis: The role of combined medical and surgical treatment. Rev Infect Dis 12(5):740, 1990

LANG R et al: Failure of prolonged treatment with ciprofloxacin in acute infections due to *Brucella melitensis*. J Antimicrob Chemother 26:841, 1990

MIKOLICH, DJ, BOYCE, JM: Brucella species, in *Principles and Practice of Infectious Diseases*, 3d ed. GL Mandell et al (eds). New York, Churchill Livingstone, 1990

SHEHABI A et al: Diagnosis and treatment of 106 cases of human brucellosis. J Infect 20:5, 1990

SMITH LD, FICHT TA: Pathogenesis of brucella. Clin Rev Microbiol 17(3):209, 1990

STASZKIEWICZ J et al: Outbreak of *Brucella melitensis* among microbiology laboratory workers in a community hospital. J Clin Microbiol 29(2):287, 1991

YOUNG EJ: Serologic diagnosis of human brucellosis: Analysis of 214 cases by agglutination tests and review of the literature. Rev Infect Dis 13:359, 1991

122 TULAREMIA

DONALD KAYE

DEFINITION Tularemia (rabbit fever, deer fly fever) is an infection caused by *Francisella tularensis*. *F. tularensis* is found in many animals and is transmitted to human beings by direct contact or via an insect vector. The illness is characterized by an ulcerative lesion at the site of inoculation with regional lymphadenopathy, by pneumonia, or by fever without localizing findings.

ETIOLOGY *F. tularensis* is a small, nonmotile, pleomorphic, gram-negative, aerobic coccobacillus. It grows poorly in many media but will grow well in glucose-cysteine blood agar, thioglycolate broth, and other media supplemented with cysteine. *F. tularensis* is found only in the northern hemisphere. There are two types of *F. tularensis*. Type A is distributed solely in North America, is virulent for humans and rabbits, produces citrulline ureidase, and ferments glycerol. Type B is found in North America, Europe, and Asia, causes no or mild disease in humans and rabbits, does not produce citrulline ureidase, and does not ferment glycerol. *F. tularensis* cross-reacts serologically with *Brucella* species and *Yersinia pestis*.

EPIDEMIOLOGY *F. tularensis* has been found in many mammals, including rabbits, squirrels, muskrats, beavers, deer, cattle, and sheep; in birds; in amphibians; and in fish. Tularemia can result from skin contact with any of these species. Tularemia also has been caused by cat bite. Ticks and deer flies can transmit the bacterium. Ticks pass *F. tularensis* to their offspring via a transovarian route. The organism is found in tick feces but not in salivary glands. In the United States, the disease can be carried by *Dermacentor andersoni* (Rocky Mountain wood tick), *Dermacentor variabilis* (American dog tick), *Dermacentor occidentalis* (Pacific Coast dog tick), and *Amblyomma americanum* (Lone Star tick). *F. tularensis* also has been recovered from streams.

In the United States, most cases of tularemia result from skin contact with infected wild rabbits (especially cottontail rabbits) or tick feces. Infection occasionally results from ingestion or inhalation of infected material. Hunters and trappers are at greatest risk. Tularemia is most likely to occur in adult males, and person-to-person transmission rarely, if ever, occurs.

Tularemia has been reported from all parts of the United States, but mostly from Arkansas, Missouri, Texas, Oklahoma, and Tennessee. Fewer than 200 cases are reported annually in the United States. Arthropod-borne disease occurs mainly in the spring and summer, and rabbit-produced infection occurs mainly in the winter.

PATHOGENESIS AND PATHOLOGY In human infection, the most common portal of entry is through the skin or mucous membranes either directly through inapparent abrasions or via the bite of a tick or other arthropod. Inhalation or ingestion of *F. tularensis* also can result in infection. Fewer than 50 organisms will result in infection when injected into the skin or inhaled, whereas more than 10^8 are usually required to produce infection via the oral route.

Following inoculation into the skin, the bacteria multiply locally and after 2 to 5 days (occasionally 1 to 10 days) produce an erythematous, tender, or pruritic papule. The papule rapidly enlarges and forms an ulcer with a black base. The bacteria spread to regional lymph nodes, producing lymphadenopathy, and further spread with bacteremia may occur. With bacteremia, organisms are cleared from the blood by phagocytic cells of the reticuloendothelial system (mainly in the liver and spleen) and may survive intracellularly for long periods of time.

Affected organs (liver, spleen, lymph nodes) demonstrate areas of focal necrosis initially surrounded mainly by polymorphonuclear leukocytes. Subsequently, granulomas form with epithelioid cells and lymphocytes and sometimes multinucleated giant cells surrounding the areas of necrosis, which may resemble caseation necrosis.

Coalescence of granulomas can lead to formation of abscesses. Nodes may occasionally become fluctuant and even rupture. Healing occurs with fibrosis and calcification of the granulomas. While antibody to *F. tularensis* is formed, it probably plays a minor role in immunity and containment of infection. Cell-mediated immunity, which develops over a 2- to 4-week period, plays the major role. Macrophages, once activated, are capable of killing *F. tularensis*.

Contamination of the conjunctiva can result in infection of the eye with regional lymph node enlargement. Aerosolization and inhalation of *F. tularensis* can result in pneumonia. Pneumonia also can occur via the hematogenous route. There is an inflammatory reaction with foci of alveolar necrosis and initially polymorphonuclear leukocytic and later mononuclear cell infiltration with granuloma formation. Chest roentgenograms usually reveal bilateral patchy infiltrates rather than large areas of consolidation. Mediastinal or other regional lymphadenopathy may occur.

Pharyngitis with cervical lymphadenopathy or gastrointestinal tularemia with mesenteric lymphadenopathy may follow ingestion of large numbers of *F. tularensis*. Typhoidal tularemia, which is characterized by fever and no localizing signs, is uncommon; the portal of entry is unknown.

CLINICAL MANIFESTATIONS   Tularemia usually has an incubation period of 2 to 5 days, after which there is onset of one of a number of syndromes (listed below), all of which are usually associated with fever and chills and often with headache, myalgias, and malaise. Tender hepatosplenomegaly is common. About 20 percent of patients develop a generalized maculopapular rash which may occasionally become pustular, and some report erythema nodosum.

Ulceroglandular tularemia   Most patients with tularemia (75 to 85 percent) develop infection secondary to inoculation of the skin. In cases related to rabbits, the portal of entry is usually on the finger or hand. In tick-related cases, the site of inoculation is usually on the lower extremities, inguinal or axillary areas, scalp, abdomen, or chest.

At time of onset of illness the patient usually has an erythematous papule that may be tender or pruritic, or an ulcer is already present at the portal of entry of the organism. If there is a papule, it evolves over a period of several days to form a punched-out ulcer with sharply dermarcated edges and a yellow exudate. The ulcer gradually develops a black base. The patient has very tender, large regional lymphadenopathy (usually axillary or epitrochlear with tularemia from rabbits and inguinal or femoral lymphadenopathy with tick-borne disease). The nodes may become fluctuant and drain spontaneously. In 5 to 10 percent of patients, the skin lesion may be inapparent and the lymphadenopathy the only physical finding. This has been called "glandular tularemia."

Oculoglandular tularemia   In about 1 percent of patients, the conjunctiva serves as the portal of entry for the organism. Purulent conjunctivitis with regional lymphadenopathy (preauricular, submandibular, or cervical) is present. Corneal perforation may occur.

Oropharyngeal and gastrointestinal tularemia   Rarely, tularemia occurs after ingestion of *F. tularensis* (usually in undercooked meat), resulting in acute exudative or membranous pharyngitis associated with cervical lymphadenopathy or ulcerative intestinal lesions with associated mesenteric lymphadenopathy, diarrhea, abdominal pain, nausea, vomiting, and gastrointestinal bleeding.

Pulmonary tularemia   Tularemia pneumonia can present as an atypical pneumonia and must be considered in the differential diagnosis of atypical pneumonia. Involvement of the lung can result from inhalation of *F. tularensis* or as a part of the bacteremia caused by tularemia at another site. Inhalation pulmonary disease occurs most often in laboratory workers and is a serious infection with high mortality. Pulmonary involvement occurs in 10 to 15 percent of patients with ulceroglandular tularemia and in about half the patients with typhoidal tularemia. The patient has cough, which is usually nonproductive, and may have dyspnea or pleuritic chest pain. Most often the physical examination is normal. Roentgenograms of the chest usually reveal bilateral patchy infiltrates which have been described as "ovoid densities." Lobar pneumonia may occur, and pleural effusion(s) with a polymorphonuclear leukocytic (rarely mononuclear) exudate may be present.

Typhoidal tularemia   In about 10 percent of cases of tularemia, fever develops without apparent skin lesion or lymphadenopathy. In the absence of a history of possible contact with a vector of the disease, diagnosis is extremely difficult.

Other manifestations   Meningitis, pericarditis, peritonitis, endocarditis, and osteomyelitis have been reported. The meningitis causes a lymphocytic response in the spinal fluid. Bacteremia may be associated with acute rhabdomyolysis.

DIAGNOSIS   Differential diagnosis   In patients with fever and large, tender lymphadenopathy, the possibility of tularemia should be strongly considered, and an attempt should be made to determine if there was an appropriate animal or arthropod vector contact. The suspicion of tularemia should be especially high in hunters, trappers, game wardens, veterinarians, and laboratory workers. However, in up to 40 percent of patients with tularemia, no history of epidemiologic contact with an animal or arthropod vector can be elicited.

Ulceroglandular tularemia is often so characteristic that it does not present a problem in differential diagnosis, but on occasion it must be differentiated from other diseases. The skin lesion may resemble those seen in sporotrichosis, skin infection with coagulase-positive staphylococci or group A streptococci, syphilis, anthrax, rat-bite fever (caused by *Spirillum minus*), rickettsial infections (such as scrub typhus), and *Mycobacterium marinum* infection. However, the regional lymphadenopathy in these diseases is usually not as impressive as in tularemia.

The lymphadenopathy of tularemia must be differentiated from that of plague (see Chap. 123), lymphogranuloma venereum (see Chap. 140), and cat-scratch disease (see Chap. 95). However, in these infections there is usually no local lesion resembling the ulcer of tularemia.

Typhoidal tularemia may resemble typhoid fever, other *Salmonella* bacteremias, rickettsial infections (such as Rocky Mountain spotted fever), brucellosis, infectious mononucleosis, toxoplasmosis, miliary tuberculosis, sarcoid, or hematologic malignancies. Tularemia pneumonia may resemble pneumonias caused by other bacteria as well as viral or *Mycoplasma* pneumonia.

Laboratory diagnosis   Blood cultures are usually negative, and the diagnosis is most frequently made serologically by agglutination methods. A significant rise in titer (i.e., fourfold or greater) in paired serum specimens over a 2- to 3-week period is diagnostic. Agglutinating antibody appears after 1 to 2 weeks of illness. Fifty percent of patients have antibody in the second week, and the rest develop antibody later in the course. Titers peak at 4 to 8 weeks and may remain elevated for years. A single agglutinating titer of ≥1:160 in a patient who has been ill for at least 2 weeks is highly suggestive of tularemia but may only indicate old infection. Antibodies to *F. tularensis* may cross-react with *Brucella*, but the titers to *Brucella* are usually much lower than the titers to *F. tularensis*. In the future, enzyme-linked immunosorbent assay (ELISA) tests may offer an advantage because they tend to turn positive earlier than agglutinating antibody tests.

F. tularensis is rarely observed on Gram stains of skin lesions, sputum, or aspirates of nodes. However, the organisms can often be demonstrated by staining with a modified Dieterle stain or by fluorescent antibody staining techniques. Cultures of these materials or blood may be positive if processed on appropriate media, but there is a major risk of infection in laboratory personnel. Cultivation of *F. tularensis* should only be attempted in laboratories with adequate isolation techniques and experienced personnel.

Isolation of *F. tularensis* can be achieved by inoculation intraperitoneally into guinea pigs, which will die within 10 days, and by direct plating onto glucose-cysteine blood agar. Agents such as cycloheximide, polymyxin B, and penicillin are frequently added to media to suppress other organisms in specimens that may overgrow *F. tularensis*.

A delayed-type skin test (similar to the tuberculin test) with *F. tularensis* antigen or killed whole bacilli turns positive during the first week of illness, prior to the appearance of agglutinating antibody, and persists for years. However, the skin test antigen is not available commercially and can boost titers of agglutinating antibodies.

The white blood cell count is usually normal, and the erythrocyte sedimentation rate may be normal as well. Pyuria is common.

TREATMENT Streptomycin, in a dose of 7.5 to 10 mg/kg every 12 h intramuscularly, is considered the drug of choice. In severe infections, 15 mg/kg every 12 h may be used for the first 48 to 72 h. Therapy is continued for 7 to 10 days. Gentamicin, in a dose of 1.7 mg/kg, intramuscularly or intravenously, every 8 h, is also effective. Virtually all strains are susceptible to streptomycin and gentamicin. Temperature response occurs within 2 days, but skin lesions and lymph nodes may take 1 to 2 weeks to heal. When therapy is not initiated until several weeks of illness have elapsed, the temperature response may be delayed. Relapses are very uncommon with streptomycin therapy.

Tetracycline or chloramphenicol, 30 mg/kg per day in four divided doses for 14 days, also has been used to treat tularemia. While response to these agents is good, the relapse rate is unacceptably high, occurring in up to 20 percent of patients. The newer fluoroquinolones such as ciprofloxacin seem promising in preliminary reports.

If fluctuant nodes require aspiration or drainage, at least several days of antibiotic therapy should be given first to avoid exposure of medical personnel to aerosolization of infected material.

PREVENTION Prevention of tularemia is based on avoidance of exposure and vaccination of high-risk populations. Avoidance of skinning wild mammals, especially rabbits, and wearing gloves while handling rabbit carcasses will decrease the risk of transmission. Use of insect repellents and prompt removal of ticks will help prevent transmission by ticks in tick-infested areas.

A multiple-puncture intradermal vaccine made from live attenuated *F. tularensis* and available from the Centers for Disease Control is effective in decreasing the frequency and severity of disease but will not totally prevent tularemia. Protection is long-lasting. Veterinarians, hunters, trappers, game wardens, and others who are likely to come in contact with infected wild mammals are candidates for immunization. Laboratory workers who handle specimens containing *F. tularensis* should be immunized. Prophylactic treatment with streptomycin will prevent development of clinical disease in patients who are incubating *F. tularensis*.

PROGNOSIS If untreated, symptoms of tularemia usually last 1 to 4 weeks but may continue for months. The mortality of severe untreated infection (which includes all untreated tularemia pneumonia) can be as high as 30 percent. However, the overall mortality rate for untreated tularemia is less than 8 percent. Mortality is about 1 percent with appropriate therapy and is often associated with long delays in diagnosis and treatment. Following tularemia there is usually lifelong immunity.

REFERENCES

BOYCE JM: *Francisella tularensis* (Tularemia), in *Principles and Practice of Infectious Diseases*, 3d ed, GL Mandell et al (eds). New York, Churchill Livingstone, 1990

CRAVEN RB, BARNES AM: Plague and tularemia. Infect Dis Clin North Am 5(1):165, 1991

PENN RL, KINASEWITZ GT: Factors associated with a poor outcome in tularemia. Arch Intern Med 147:265, 1987

SYRJÄLÄ H et al: In vitro susceptibility of *Francisella tularensis* to fluoroquinolones and treatment of tularemia with norfloxacin and ciprofloxacin. Eur J Clin Microbiol Infect Dis 10:68, 1991

TAYLOR JP et al: Epidemiologic characteristics of human tularemia in the southwest-central states, 1981–1987. Am J Epidemiol 133(10):1032, 1991

TARNVIK A: Nature of protective immunity to *Francisella tularenis*. Rev Infect Dis 11(3):440, 1989

123 PLAGUE AND OTHER *YERSINIA* INFECTIONS

DARWIN L. PALMER

DEFINITION Plague is an acute infectious illness of humans, rodents, and their ectoparasites which is caused by the gram-negative bacillus *Yersinia pestis*. The disease persists because of its firm entrenchment in both wild and domestic rodent-flea ecosystems throughout the world. In the United States, wild rodent contact leads to sporadic human disease; the historically explosive Asian and European urban epidemics resulted from transmission of disease by rats. Human plague follows bites by rodent fleas; after several days, painful febrile lymphadenitis (the bubo) occurs. If untreated, it results in death in more than 50 percent of cases with sepsis and multiorgan involvement. Primary plague pneumonia is transmitted between humans by cough-generated aerosols, has a fulminant course, and is almost universally fatal if untreated.

EPIDEMIOLOGY Sylvatic plague involves more than 200 species of wild rodents and is found in the southwestern United States, Russia, India, Vietnam, and Africa. In the United States, field and burrowing rodents, especially ground squirrels, rock squirrels, wood rats, and prairie dogs, are potential carriers. Rodent disease is characterized by occurrence in the spring and summer, year-to-year variations in disease activity, chronicity in the populations involved, slow regional spread, and rare geographic regression. The epizootic disease results in cyclic rodent population die-offs, leaving both resistant survivors and infected fleas seeking another host. Disease also persists in natural foci because of latent infection during animal hibernation, by prolonged viability of *Y. pestis* in soil of rodent burrows, by survival of infected fleas (and possibly ticks), and by persistent infection in relatively resistant rodents. Rodent predators also may spread plague; felines, such as domestic cats, generally die when infected with *Y. pestis*, whereas canines (e.g., foxes, coyotes, dogs) and bears often recover and may serve as serologic sentinels of wild rodent disease. Human disease can be readily acquired from domestic pets when the pets become infected or catch and return plague-infected rodents or their fleas to rural homes. Hares and rabbits are occasional nonrodent sources of the disease in humans, especially during the winter hunting season.

Rodent fleas are critical to the natural plague cycle and are implicated in about 85 percent of human cases. After infection, fleas develop obstruction of the foregut, causing regurgitation of plague bacilli during the next blood meal. The rat flea, *Xenopsylla cheopis*, is an especially efficient plague vector both between rats and between rodents and humans. Transmission without fleas may occur by ingestion of infected carcasses by predators, possibly by contact with infected tissue through an open wound, or by inhalation of infected aerosols. Human body lice as well as ticks also are capable of interhuman or person-to-person transmission.

In the last four decades there has been a fluctuating incidence of sporadic human plague originating in the western United States, varying from 40 cases per year to none. An overall death rate of 16 percent is double that seen in large outbreaks and reflects delay in the diagnosis or incorrect therapy. Travel during the incubation period out of plague endemic areas and failure to elicit a history of animal exposure are common diagnostic problems. Sporadic human plague occurs most frequently in the spring and summer, especially in males, children, or youths under age 20, reflecting outdoor activities and risk of wild rodent contact. While urban rat-related human outbreaks are rare in the United States, they are still important sources of human disease in Asia and Africa. Spread from sylvatic rodents into urban rats was documented as recently as 1983 in Los Angeles. Primary plague pneumonia arises as a hematogenous disseminated pulmonary infection during bubonic/septicemic disease. It may thereafter result in person-to-person spread via infectious aerosols. In close quarters it is rapidly transmitted. A primary pneumonic plague outbreak in the United States last occurred in 1919, when 13 cases with 12 deaths (including two physicians and one nurse) developed before the disease was recognized and halted by case isolation. Cases of primary human pneumonic plague also have been acquired from domestic cats dying of plague pneumonia.

ETIOLOGY *Yersinia pestis* is a member of family Enterobacteriaceae. It is a pleomorphic, gram-negative, nonmotile, aerobic bacillus which grows optimally at 28°C. The organism is a facultative intracellular parasite, but it grows readily, although slowly, on routine media, and cultures should not be discarded before 72 h. Although weakly gram-negative, *Y. pestis* stains best with Giemsa's or Wayson's stains, with which it shows prominent bipolar "safety pin" microscopic morphology. Related virulence-associated plasmids are found in several *Yersinia* species which encode determinants for temperature requirements and calcium dependence. These plasmids appear to enable the organism to grow inside macrophages during the early incubation period. The same virulence plasmids encode for production of outer membrane proteins and V and W antigens which confer resistance to phagocytic intracellular killing. Other virulence factors include pesticin, fibrinolysin, coagulase, and lipopolysaccharide endotoxin. No separate serotypes are recognized, but biotypes *antigua*, *orientalis*, and *mediaevalis* have geographic distributions which presumably mark historic epidemic spread. The organism is relatively resistant to drying and may maintain its viability in cool, moist conditions, such as the soil of an animal burrow, for many months. Antibiotic resistance can be developed in the laboratory and has been noted in wild strains, but significant resistance to streptomycin and tetracycline has not been seen in clinical outbreaks.

PATHOGENESIS After *Y. pestis* is inoculated into the skin by a flea bite, bacteria migrate to local lymph nodes, where they are taken up but not killed by mononuclear cells. Intracellular multiplication results in development of capsular envelopes containing envelope antigen (fraction 1 protein); toxins are elaborated. An acute inflammatory response is provoked in the lymph node in the ensuing 2 to 6 days, resulting in the bubo. At this stage, the organisms are relatively resistant to phagocytosis by polymorphonuclear leukocytes because the bacteria are protected by increased elaboration of envelope antigen and the lack of specific opsonic antibody. Characteristically, hemorrhagic necrosis of lymph nodes with lysis of macrophages next occurs, from which large numbers of bacteria gain access to the bloodstream and other organs. Extensions along lymphatics involve superficial nodes at the site of inoculation, the spleen, and nodes in the abdomen, mediastinum, or perihilar areas. The lung is secondarily infected in 10 to 20 percent of patients, generally as a rapidly progressive, multilobar pneumonia, often with pleural exudate. The early acute inflammatory reaction is followed by lobar consolidation and hemorrhagic necrosis and, if death does not intervene, may progress to abscess formation. Fibrin thrombi may be extensive in the pulmonary vessels as well as in glomeruli and vessels of skin and other organs. Secondarily, the adult respiratory distress syndrome or a rise in pulmonary artery pressure may be seen. Pericarditis with a small amount of seropurulent exudate is frequent, and meningitis may occur late in partially or untreated bubonic plague. In 5 to 15 percent of patients, the skin, predominantly of the extremities, is involved with purpuric lesions due to thrombocytopenia and vasculitis. Late in the disease, buboes may become fluctuant and occasionally may become superinfected with other bacteria. Endotoxemia may result in both septic shock and disseminated intravascular coagulation.

MANIFESTATIONS Bubonic plague has an incubation period of 2 to 7 days from flea bite to onset of illness. Although many patients do not remember an insect contact, a small eschar may be found at the bite site. Patients present with a painful bubo and fever accompanied by headache, prostration, and abdominal distress. The bubo, a tender enlarged lymph node or nodes, ranges in size from 1 to 10 cm and is found in the groin in 70 percent of patients; alternatively, buboes may develop in axillary or cervical nodes or in several lymphatic

chains simultaneously. Buboes are extremely tender and not fixed to skin or underlying structures, and overlying skin is often erythematous. Fever and rigors are prominent and occasionally precede appearance of a bubo by 1 to 3 days. Gastrointestinal symptoms are present in more than half the patients, with abdominal pain often extending from the groin bubo and accompanied by anorexia, nausea, vomiting, and diarrhea, which may be bloody. Cutaneous petechiae and hemorrhages occur in 5 to 50 percent of patients and may be extensive late in the disease. Disseminated intravascular coagulation occurs in subclinical form in as many as 86 percent of patients, 5 to 10 percent of whom have clinical manifestations, including gangrene of the skin, fingers, toes, and penis. If untreated, bubonic disease may proceed without other organ system involvement to generalized sepsis, prostration, hypotension, and death within the next 2 to 10 days. Some patients have very prominent early signs of sepsis with high-density bacteremia and no demonstrable bubo. This represents a form of bubonic plague in which lymphatic involvement is limited to deep structures or where the buboes are so small as to be overlooked in the presence of overwhelming signs of infection. Septicemic disease may progress rapidly with chills, fever, rapid pulse, severe headache, nausea, vomiting, delirium, and death within 48 h. The case fatality rate may exceed one-third. In such fulminant sepsis, bacteremia is so prominent that buffy coat blood smear may readily show *Y. pestis* on Gram stain.

Other than the lymphatics, the lung is the organ most commonly involved, with development of secondary pneumonia in 10 to 20 percent of all patients. Cough, fever, and tachypnea appear on days 2 to 3 of illness, accompanied by minimal pulmonary infiltrates. Later, or less commonly, from the start, symptoms worsen rapidly, with marked dyspnea, bloody sputum, and evidence of respiratory failure. There may be multilobar involvement, with variable degrees of consolidation, the sputum may teem with *Y. pestis* and is highly contagious when disseminated by cough-generated aerosols. Primary plague pneumonia is a fulminant illness; time from the initial contact to death ranges from 2 to 6 days. The adult respiratory distress syndrome (ARDS), characterized by noncardiac pulmonary edema, anoxia, and respiratory failure, also occurs as a manifestation of plague sepsis and may be indistinguishable from plague pneumonia except for absence of bacteria in respiratory secretions. Both *Y. pestis* pneumonia and the ARDS form of illness have a mortality in excess of 75 percent, despite appropriate antimicrobial and supportive therapy. Less commonly, marked perihilar adenopathy may present alone or accompany pneumonia.

Plague meningitis, as a late complication that occurs in 6 percent of untreated patients, is characterized by nuchal rigidity, headache, confusion, and coma and is often preceded or accompanied by bacteremia. Most meningitis cases have been described in patients treated with antibiotics that do not readily cross the blood-brain barrier, such as tetracycline and streptomycin. Other contributory factors seem to be late or inadequate therapy. Meningitis due to plague is indistinguishable from that caused by other bacteria.

Rarely, patients with plague have a very mild illness manifested chiefly by low-grade fever and adenopathy. In this group are patients with tonsillar plague, who have positive throat cultures, serologic conversion, and minimal illness. Other, less common late complications include persistent hectic fever despite appropriate therapy, fluctuance and spontaneous drainage from buboes, and pulmonary cavitation with abscess formation.

LABORATORY FINDINGS With the exception of definitive microbiologic studies, laboratory tests are of little diagnostic help. A polymorphonuclear leukocytosis of 15 to 20 cells $\times 10^9$ per liter is common, and the white cells may show toxic changes. Rarely, a marked leukemoid reaction with more than 100×10^9 white cells per liter is seen. Modest elevations of serum aminotransferases are common, but otherwise, liver function studies are normal. Evidence of disseminated intravascular coagulation with low platelet counts, prolonged partial thromboplastin times, and positive fibrin degradation products in the serum is common. The electrocardiogram is usually normal but may show right axis deviation and peaked P waves indicative of acute cor pulmonale. The chest x-ray will show infiltrates, often with pleural effusion, in secondary or primary plague pneumonia or evidence of pulmonary edema in patients with ARDS. In meningitis, examination of cerebrospinal fluid demonstrates polymorphonuclear pleocytosis, low sugar, elevated protein, and gram-negative coccobacillary organisms, although culture may demonstrate *Y. pestis* more reliably.

Confirmation of the clinical suspicion of bubonic plague may be obtained by needle aspiration of a bubo with direct staining of the aspirated material. With either Wayson's or Giemsa's stain, the characteristic bipolar-staining, "safety pin" forms are seen. By fluorescent antibody staining, a presumptive diagnosis may be specifically confirmed in about 80 percent of cases. Cultures of aspirated material, as well as sputum, pleural fluid, and blood, will be positive in a high percentage of patients. Microscopic examination of buffy coat smear may show *Y. pestis* in septicemic cases. A serologic response with a fourfold or greater rise is detected in the second week of illness by complement fixation, hemagglutination, or indirect immunofluorescent antibody.

DIAGNOSIS Bubonic plague must be suspected in any febrile patient with painful adenopathy who has a history of wild animal exposure in a plague endemic area, but it may be confused with other illnesses. Presentation with fever and a painful groin bubo can mimic lymphogranuloma venereum or syphilis or, when more severe, an acute abdominal crisis such as incarcerated inguinal hernia, appendicitis, or a ruptured viscus. Abdominal pain and bloody diarrhea can be mistaken for shigellosis or other acute diarrheal processes. With an axillary or cervical bubo, acute streptococcal or staphylococcal lymphadenitis, tularemia, cat-scratch fever, lymphogranuloma venereum, or syphilis need to be considered. Bubonic/septicemic disease with an absent or small bubo suggests typhoid fever or bacteremia due to other causes. Primary or secondary pneumonic plague may mimic bacterial pneumonia from any cause.

When plague is suspected, diagnostic maneuvers must include aspiration of buboes with appropriate stains and cultures, as well as blood cultures and cultures from other sources. Cultures should not be discarded early because the organism grows slowly and may only appear in 48 to 72 h. A serologic rise by passive hemagglutination is evident by day 5 and peaks by day 14. Newer serologic methods such as enzyme-linked immunosorbent assay compare well in sensitivity with standard passive hemagglutination tests and are more rapid.

TREATMENT If plague is strongly suspected on clinical and/or epidemiologic grounds, therapy must be started immediately, prior to completion of diagnostic studies. Antibiotic and supportive treatment should reduce the 40 to 100 percent mortality of untreated bubonic or pneumonic plague to 5 to 10 percent. Effective antibiotics include streptomycin, tetracycline, and chloramphenicol. Streptomycin, the most effective therapy, should be given in a dosage of 7.5 to 15 mg/kg every 12 h intramuscularly for a total of 10 days. Streptomycin is in limited supply and is available only through state health departments. Tetracycline, for patients who cannot tolerate streptomycin, may be given orally or intravenously at 10 to 20 mg/kg every 6 h. Tetracycline may be started concurrently and streptomycin discontinued after 3 days without fever but should be continued for a total of 5 to 7 days after the fever has disappeared. In less severely ill patients, tetracycline alone at 5 to 10 mg/kg every 6 h may be given by mouth. Chloramphenicol in a dose of 12.5 to 25 mg/kg given intravenously every 6 h should be substituted for streptomycin or tetracycline in patients with meningitis (because of its better central nervous system penetration) or in hypotensive patients. In hypotensive patients, intravenous chloramphenicol or gentamicin are effective and rapidly distributed. Tetracycline or trimethoprim-sulfamethoxazole can be used for the prophylaxis of case contacts and should be given orally for 5 days. Local treatment of the bubo is not indicated unless fluctuance or spontaneous drainage occurs, when cultures should be obtained to detect staphylococci. Ventilatory support for patients with plague pneumonia or ARDS may be necessary and lifesaving.

PREVENTION AND CONTROL Individuals working in high-risk occupations in plague endemic areas or conducting laboratory work with *Y. pestis* should consider use of the formalin-killed whole-bacteria vaccine; however, the vaccine must be readministered every 6 months owing to rapidly waning immunity. Individuals briefly visiting a plague epidemic area should use insect repellant and garments to cover the arms and legs and may take tetracycline or trimethoprim-sulfamethoxazole prophylaxis. Following the presumptive diagnosis of pneumonic plague, patients should be placed in respiratory isolation; simple hand-washing precautions suffice for bubonic cases. Contacts of a patient with plague pneumonia should be given oral tetracycline prophylaxis, 250 mg four times daily by mouth, and should be advised to seek medical attention if respiratory symptoms or fever develop. Possibly due to such precautions, tramsmission of primary plague pneumonia has not occurred in the United States for many years.

The potential for spread of plague into urban rat populations from sylvatic rodent sources is an ever-present risk. Prevention depends on control of urban rat populations and their exclusion from dwellings, as well as surveillance of sylvatic rodents and of their local predators. Picnickers, hikers, and others traveling into plague endemic regions during the spring-summer seasons should be warned that plague is a potential danger. They should avoid touching carcasses or sick rodents and should restrain and treat pets with flea-repellent powders. No practical measures exist for eliminating plague from wild rodent sources. Reducing rodent harborage and use of insecticides around rural homes in endemic regions is important. Killing rodents around rural dwellings with rodenticides should be preceded by insect control to prevent displaced rodent fleas from seeking humans or domestic pets.

OTHER *YERSINIA* INFECTIONS (*Y. PSEUDOTUBERCULOSIS* AND *Y. ENTEROCOLITICA*)

ETIOLOGY *Y. enterocolitica* and *Y. pseudotuberculosis* are both non-lactose-fermenting, gram-negative, aerobic bacilli related to one another and to *Y. pestis* and are members of the Enterobacteriaceae. Other *Yersinia* species have been discovered but do not appear to be pathogenic for humans. Both organisms grow slowly on media used for the detection of other enteric bacteria, and their detection can be enhanced by cold enrichment incubation at 20 to 25°C. Strains can be distinguished from one another and from *Y. pestis* on the basis of serologic and biochemical reactions as well as by antibiotic sensitivities. As in *Y. pestis*, both organisms elaborate W and V virulence factors which confer dependency on calcium for growth at 37°C and enable the organisms to survive intracellularly. This requirement is transmitted by a 70-kilobase plasmid which is common to all invasive *Yersinia*. Invasive strains of *Y. enterocolitica* also carry a plasmid-mediated outer membrane protein which enhances both attachment and cell invasion. These strains evoke a keratoconjunctivitis of guinea pigs (Sereney test) and produce a suppurative infection of Peyer's patches and mesenteric lymph nodes. They invade further to cause systemic infection of lung, liver, and spleen, especially in the presence of excess iron, since they normally lack siderophores. Both organisms produce an endotoxin, and *Y. enterocolitica* elaborates a heat-stable enterotoxin which may be of significance in food-borne illness. A large number of serotypes of both organisms exist causing disease in many animal species, but most human infections are caused by a limited number of strains. Strain and disease differences exist between Europe and the United States; American strains appear more invasive but less likely to cause postinfectious sequelae.

MANIFESTATIONS Although recognized most commonly in northern Europe and North America, *Y. enterocolitica* causes enteric infection worldwide and accounts for approximately 1 to 3 percent of all cases of acute bacterial enteritis. The origin of the disease is often unclear, although the portal of entry is the oropharynx or gastrointestinal tract, and outbreaks traced to both food and water have been reported; person-to-person as well as animal-to-person transmission is common. Manifestations of the disease vary with age. In infants and young children, the predominant symptom is acute watery diarrhea lasting 3 to 14 days; 5 percent of children have blood in the stool. In older children and young adults, a syndrome of right lower quadrant pain accompanied by fever and moderate leukocytosis indistinguishable from acute appendicitis occurs. In adults, especially in women over age 40, erythema nodosum often follows enteritis by 1 to 2 weeks. Adults in Scandinavia may develop a monarticular arthritis of the knee, foot, or hand with or without preceding enteritis. Rarely, a severe, disabling suppurative arthritis is seen. Among patients with arthritis, 65 percent have histocompatibility group HLA-B27. A high prevalence of antibodies to *Y. enterocolitica* membrane antigens has been reported in individuals with Graves' disease. *Y. enterocolitica* also causes bacteremia, mostly in individuals with underlying illness such as diabetes mellitus, severe anemia, cirrhosis, or malignancy or in conditions of iron overload. Septicemic patients complain of headache, fever, and abdominal pain with or without diarrhea and frequently develop abscesses in multiple organs. Exudative pharyngitis with *Y. enterocolitica* was found in adult patients during the course of an outbreak of milk-borne yersiniosis.

Pseudotuberculosis is a rare illness acquired from humans or domestic and wild animals, presumably by fecal-oral contact. Most cases are sporadic and occur in the young, with males more commonly affected than females and with a peak in the winter months corresponding to the peak occurrence in animals. After ingestion, the organisms apparently penetrate the ileal mucosa, localize in the ileocecal lymph nodes, and produce an acute mesenteric adenitis which is generally accompanied by vomiting, abdominal pain, and diarrhea. Fever is usually high, and leukocytosis is common. At laparotomy, the appendix appears normal, but enlarged mesenteric lymph nodes and inflammation of the terminal ileum may be seen. Complications appear in adults less commonly than with *Y. enterocolitica* but include arthritis, erythema nodosum, and septicemia.

DIAGNOSIS   *Y. enterocolitica* is much more frequent as a human pathogen than *Y. pseudotuberculosis*. They cause similar signs and symptoms but may have different reservoirs; the first is characterized primarily by diarrhea and the second by mesenteric adenitis. Therefore, *Y. enterocolitica* causes disease similar to other bacterial diarrheas and must be distinguished from them by microbiologic means. Laboratory detection of the organism depends on special cultural techniques. The diagnosis is made best by isolation of the organism from stool in patients with enteritis or atypical cases of appendicitis, erythema nodosum, or reactive arthritis. Cultures of pharyngeal exudate, blood, peritoneal fluid, and other body fluids should be obtained where clinically indicated. Hemagglutination titers peak in 8 to 10 days and remain elevated for 18 months after infection. Cross-reactivity with some *Brucella*, *Salmonella*, and *Vibrio cholerae* antigens occurs. The diagnosis of *Y. pseudotuberculosis* is also made by culture of stool and mesenteric lymph nodes.

THERAPY AND PREVENTION   *Y. enterocolitica* organisms are susceptible in vitro to aminoglycosides, chloramphenicol, tetracycline, trimethoprim-sulfamethoxazole, and the third-generation cephalosporins but are generally resistant to the penicillins and first-generation cephalosporins. However, the value of antimicrobial therapy is unclear, because most cases of enteritis are self-limited. Patients with very severe illness or septicemia should be treated, because treatment may shorten both the duration of disease and the shedding of organisms. *Y. pseudotuberculosis* is usually sensitive to ampicillin, tetracycline, chloramphenicol, and cephalosporins. No controlled clinical trials demonstrate efficacy of treatment, although patients with septicemic disease should receive ampicillin or tetracycline because severe infection has a high mortality. Prevention depends on reducing contamination from animal reservoirs and hygienic measures such as careful food handling, availability of clean drinking water, and hand washing to prevent spread within families or other human contacts.

REFERENCES

Plague

CENTERS FOR DISEASE CONTROL: Human plague—United States, 1988. Morb Mort Week Rep 37:653, 1988

BECKER TB et al: Plague meningitis. A retrospective analysis of cases reported in the U.S., 1970–79. West J Med 147:554, 1987

BUTLER T: A clinical study of bubonic plague: Observations on the 1970 Vietnam epidemic with emphasis on coagulation studies, skin histology, and electrocardiograms. Am J Med 53:268, 1972

KAUFMAN AF et al: Public health implications of plague in domestic cats. Am J Vet Assoc 179:875, 1981

REED WP et al: Bubonic plague in the southwestern United States: A review of recent experience. Medicine 49:465, 1970

SIMPSON WJ et al: Recombinant capsular antigen (fraction 1) from *Yersinia pestis* induces a protective antibody response in *Balb/c* mice. Am J Trop Med Hyg b3:389, 1990

Other *Yersinia* infections

BUTLER T: *Yersinia* species (including plague), in *Principles and Practice of Infectious Diseases*, 3d ed, GL Mandell et al (eds). New York, Wiley, 1990, pp 1748–1756

MILLER VL, et al: Nucleotide sequence of the *Yersinia enterocolitica ail* gene and characterization of the Ail protein product. J Bacteriol 172:1062, 1990

COVER TL, ABER RC: *Yersinia enterocolitica.* N Engl J Med 321:16, 1989

TACKET CO et al: *Yersinia enterocolitica* pharyngitis. Ann Intern Med 99:40, 1983

TERTTI R et al: An outbreak of *Yersinia pseudotuberculosis* infection. J Infect Dis 149:245, 1984

124   BARTONELLOSIS AND BACILLARY ANGIOMATOSIS

LUCY STUART TOMPKINS

BARTONELLOSIS

DEFINITION   Bartonellosis consists of two clinical manifestations produced by infection with *Bartonella bacilliformis*, a member of the rickettsia group closely related to *Rochalimaea quintana* and *R. henselae*, the bacterial agent of bacillary angiomatosis. The disease occurs almost exclusively in the Andes Mountains of Peru, Ecuador, and Colombia. Initial infection in nonimmune persons produces Oroya fever, characterized by fever, profound anemia, and a high mortality rate; lesions called *verruga peruana* develop during the convalescent phase or during chronic infection. Daniel Carrion, a Peruvian medical student, inoculated himself with blood from a patient with verruga peruana and subsequently died from Oroya fever, thus proving that both diseases are caused by a single agent. As a result, bartonellosis is also known as *Carrion's disease*.

Carrion's disease is rarely seen outside South America because of the geographic localization of the arthropod vector. However, the disorder is similar in many ways to two disorders that do occur in the United States—cutaneous bacillary angiomatosis and the angiogenic response engendered by *Rochalimaea* species.

CLINICAL MANIFESTATIONS   Oroya fever occurs following the bite of the sandfly vector, *Phlebotomus*, an insect found in the river valleys of the Andes Mountains at altitudes from 600 to 2500 m. The disease has rarely been described in the United States. Onset of symptoms may be either insidious or abrupt after an incubation period of approximately 3 weeks. In the subacute presentation, low-grade fever, malaise, headache, and anorexia may be present. Sudden-onset disease characterized by high fever, chills, diaphoresis, headaches, and changes in mental status is followed by the sudden development of profound anemia due to a marked decrease in numbers of erythrocytes associated with macrocytic changes in poikilocytosis, Howell-Jolly bodies, nucleated erythrocytes, and immature myeloid cells. The leukocyte differential usually shifts to the left, although the total count may be normal. The erythrocyte count may fall to extremely low levels. Numerous microorganisms can be seen adhering to most erythrocytes in eosin/thiazine-stained peripheral blood smears.

During the acute phase, muscle and joint pain and headache may be severe; central nervous system changes also occur, including insomnia, delerium, and decreased level of consciousness. Thrombocytopenic purpura may develop. If the patient survives, a convalescent phase ensues characterized by the sudden disappearance of bacteria from blood smears, declining fever, and increase in erythrocyte count. While much of the mortality is due to profound anemia and toxicity, bacterial secondary infections, including salmonellosis and other enteric infections, malaria, and tuberculosis, often contribute substantially.

After convalescence from acute Oroya fever, verrugas may develop. The red or purple cutaneous lesions may be tiny and sessile or large, pedunculated, and nodular. They bear a marked resemblance to the lesions in bacillary angiomatosis. Both types of cutaneous lesion may resemble Kaposi's sarcoma.

PATHOLOGY During initial infection in the nonimmune host, *B. bacilliformis* cells adhere to erythrocytes and produce indentations in the cell membrane, with subsequent intracellular entry and persistent deformation of the cellular cytoskeleton. The parasitized erythrocytes are phagocytosed and destroyed. Although the life span of infected erythrocytes is markedly decreased, not all of this change can be attributed to the mechanical fragility induced by internalization, and decreased bone marrow erythropoiesis also contributes to the anemia. Bacteria can be cultured in vitro from the blood during acute infection. The hallmark of verruga peruana is the formation of new blood vessels (angiogenesis) at the sites of bacterial replication.

TREATMENT Oroya fever responds to a variety of antimicrobial agents, including chloramphenicol, tetracyclines, penicillin, and streptomycin. Chloramphenicol is most often used because of its efficacy against most *Salmonella* infections, which may occur intercurrently. Verruga peruana may respond similarly; failure of response or relapse is common.

BACILLARY ANGIOMATOSIS

DEFINITION Bacillary angiomatosis was initially described as an infectious complication of human immunodeficiency virus (HIV) diseases that causes cutaneous lesions resembling Kaposi's sarcoma. The infectious microorganism *Rochalimaea henselae* causes three clinical syndromes: chronic bacteremia, bacillary peliosis hepatis, and cutaneous or disseminated bacillary angiomatosis. Immunocompromised individuals, especially those with HIV infection or those with AIDS, are at particularly high risk of infection; rarely, patients are not obviously immunosuppressed. A recent study has shown that *Rochalimaea quintana*, the agent of trench fever, can also cause bacillary angiomatosis in HIV-positive patients. Several recently described studies have implicated *R. henselae* as a cause of typical cat scratch disease (CSD) in immunocompetent individuals.

CLINICAL MANIFESTATIONS The skin lesions of bacillary angiomatosis (also called *epithelioid angiomatosis*) are vascular nodules, papules, or tumors of variable size, ranging from tiny lesions resembling cherry angiomas or pyogenic granulomas to large, pedunculated, exophytic masses (Fig. 124-1). Characteristically, the lesions are red or purple, resembling Kaposi's sarcoma; they may be surrounded by an epithelial collarette, may be located anywhere on the skin, and also may involve mucous membranes. The overlying epidermis may be focally ulcerated, and underlying bone may be invaded and destroyed.

Dissemination of *R. henselae* infection occurs primarily in patients with cellular immune defects. The liver, spleen, bone marrow, and lymph nodes are primarily affected. In addition, HIV-infected patients may develop CNS abnormalities (including psychiatric disorders and brain lesions) responsive to antibiotic therapy. Skin lesions are usually not present in patients with disseminated infection. Involvement of

FIGURE 124-1 Characteristic skin lesion of bacillary angiomatosis in an HIV-positive young woman. This large, pedunculated tumor exhibits the typical angiomatous appearance. The patient was treated with oral erythromycin, with nearly complete resolution of the lesion; however, upon discontinuation of antibiotic therapy after a 4-week course, the lesion recurred.

the liver or spleen may produce bacillary peliosis hepatis. Clinical manifestations accompanying dissemination are often nonspecific and include persistent fever, abdominal pain, weight loss, and malaise. Patients with peliosis hepatis may have localized pain on palpation of the abdomen. Nodular lesions of variable size can be demonstrated by CT scan or MRI, with or without contrast agents.

Koehler and colleagues described three cases of bacillary angiomatosis caused by *R. quintana* in patients with HIV infection.

Infection also may present as prolonged fever and bacteremia in the absence of cutaneous lesions. Two patients reportedly developed chronic bacteremia following tick bites. Although symptoms generally abate after appropriate antibiotic therapy, relapse and recrudescence may occur. This clinical picture is quite similar to trench fever, a febrile illness initially described during World War I, which is caused by *R. quintana* transmitted by the human body louse.

Recent serologic studies demonstrated that most patients with typical CSD had antibodies which specifically reacted with *R. henselae*. Furthermore, *R. henselae* has been isolated from lymph nodes of patients with CSD. Therefore, the role of *Afipia felis*, the putative agent of CSD, is presently uncertain.

DIFFERENTIAL DIAGNOSIS The differential diagnosis of cutaneous lesions includes Kaposi's sarcoma, angiomas, and pyogenic granulomas. These can be distinguished by histopathologic examination of biopsied material. Cases of persistent fever following an insect bite must be differentiated from trench fever and other rickettsial infections by identification of bacteria from blood cultures and by negative results of appropriate serologic tests for rickettsial species.

MICROBIOLOGY The etiologic microorganisms can be demonstrated in tissue by Warthin-Starry silver stain and morphologically resemble *Apifia felis*, the agent of CSD. Clumps and clusters of small pleomorphic bacilli appear as purple deposits in tissue stained with hematoxylin and eosin. The nature of the bacilli was first recognized by Relman and colleagues, who used molecular techniques to analyze DNA extracted from tissue samples. The bacteria also have been isolated from blood and from other sites. Bacterial colonies develop after prolonged incubation; bacterial cells are gram-negative. Taxonomic studies have revealed that *R. henselae* is closely related to *R. quintana*, the agent of trench fever, and also to *B. bacilliformis*; it is less closely related to *A. felis* which was isolated from patients with CSD. Unlike other rickettsiae, *R. henselae* is not an obligate intracellular parasite and does not appear inside endothelial cells.

EPIDEMIOLOGY Most infections of bacillary angiomatosis occur in patients with HIV disease or other types of immunosuppression; thus an immune deficiency of T cells is implicated. Cutaneous

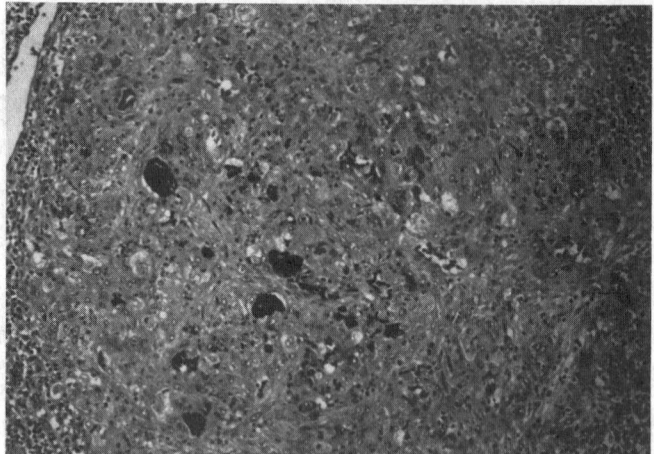

FIGURE 124-2 Histopathologic appearance of bacillary angiomatosis involving the skin. Characteristic features include nodules composed of epithelioid endothelial cells forming irregular, poorly formed vascular channels and large amounts of collagen. An neutrophilic inflammatory response is also present. Bacillary bacterial forms can be seen upon Warthin-Starry staining (hematoxylin and eosin; original magnification ×200).

infections occur primarily in urban areas of the United States in which HIV infection is most prevalent. However, tick-associated cases have been reported in Oklahoma. The prevalence of specific antibodies among healthy individuals is not established. Because of the tick-associated cases and the close taxonomic relationship of *R. henselae* to *R. quintana* and *Bartonella*, both of which are transmitted by insects, an insect vector has been postulated. Exposure to cats is a risk factor for bacillary angiomatosis and CSD.

PATHOGENESIS AND PATHOLOGY   Bacillary angiomatosis is characterized by a lobular proliferation of new blood vessels (angiogenesis) and a neutrophilic inflammatory response to myriad bacilli located within collagen-rich microscopic and macroscopic nodules (Fig. 124-2). The endothelial cells lining the vascular spaces have a typical epithelioid appearance, and the lesions may resemble Kaposi's sarcoma histopathologically, although the characteristic spindle cell of the latter disease is usually absent. Of note is the striking similarity between bacillary angiomatosis and verruga peruana. The bacterial and eucaryotic host factors that elicit the pathologic response are unknown. The pathologic response of immunocompetent patients with CSD consists of granulomas and microabscesses in lymph nodes draining the site of inoculation. Angiogenesis is not seen in CSD in otherwise healthy individuals.

TREATMENT   Cutaneous lesions have been treated with a wide variety of antimicrobial drugs, including macrolides and tetracyclines, and *R. henselae* is susceptible to most antibiotics in vitro. Erythromycin given orally over a 3-week course is usually efficacious; however, relapse may require prolonged therapy. Patients with peliosis hepatis should be treated with intravenous antibiotics, and those with disseminated disease or bacteremia should be treated with a prolonged course of oral antibiotics, such as macrolides, cephalosporins, or norfloxacin. Relapses may require prolonged treatment with antibiotics that reach an intracellular compartment, such as macrolides or floxacins. Cutaneous lesions may regress spontaneously, an event perhaps reflecting the status of the host's immunity.

REFERENCES

ARIAS-STELLA J et al: Histology, immunhistochemistry, and ultrastructure of the verruga in Carrion's disease. Am J Surg Pathol 10:595, 1986

BENSON LA et al: Entry of *Bartonella bacilliformis* into erythrocytes. Infect Immun 54:347, 1986

COCKERELL CJ, LEBOIT PE: Bacillary angiomatosis: A newly characterized, pseudoneoplastic, infectious, cutaneous vascular disorder. J Am Acad Dermatol 22:501, 1990

——— et al: Epithelioid angiomatosis: A distinct vascular disorder in patients with the acquired immunodeficiency syndrome of AIDS-related complex. Lancet 2:654, 1987

KEMPER CA et al: Visceral bacillary epithelioid angiomatosis: Possible manifestations of disseminated cat scratch disease in the immunocompromised host: A report of two cases. Am J Med 89:449, 1990

KOEHLER JE et al: Isolation of *Rochalimaea* species from cutaneous and osseous lesions of bacillary angiomatosis. New Engl J Med 327:1625, 1992

LEBOIT PE et al: Bacillary angiomatosis: The histopathology and differential diagnosis of pseudoneoplastic infection in patients with human immunodeficiency virus disease. Am J Surg Pathol 13:909, 1989

LUCEY D et al: Relapsing illness due to *Rochalimaea henselae* in immunocompetent hosts: Implication for therapy and new epidemiological associations. Clin Infect Dis 14:683, 1992

O'CONNOR SP et al: 16S rRNA sequences of *Bartonella bacilliformis* and cat scratch disease bacillus reveal phylogenetic relationships with the alpha-2 subgroup of the class *Proteobacteria*. J Clin Microbiol 29:2144, 1991

PERKOCHA LA et al: Clinical and pathological features of bacillary peliosis hepatis in association with human immunodeficiency virus infection. N Engl J Med 323:1581, 1990

REGNERY RL et al: Characterization of a novel *Rochalimaea* species, *R. henselae* sp. nov., isolated from blood of a febrile, human immunodeficiency virus-positive patient. J Clin Microbiol 30:265, 1992

——— et al: Serological response to "*Rochalimaea henselae*" antigen in suspected cat-scratch disease. Lancet 339:1443–45, 1992

RELMAN DA et al: The organism causing bacillary angiomatosis, peliosis hepatis, and fever and bacteremia in immunocompromised patients. N Engl J Med 324:1514, 1991

——— et al: The agent of bacillary angiomatosis: An approach to the identification of uncultured pathogens. N Engl J Med 323:1573, 1990

RICKETTS WE: Clinical manifestations of Carrion's disease. Arch Intern Med 84:751, 1949

SLATER LN et al: A newly recognized fastidious gram-negative pathogen as a cause of fever and bacteremia. N Engl J Med 323:1587, 1990

---

125   DONOVANOSIS (GRANULOMA INGUINALE)

KING K. HOLMES

DEFINITION   Donovanosis (granuloma inguinale) is a mildly contagious, chronic, indolent, progressive, autoinoculable, ulcerative disease involving the skin and lymphatics of the genital or perianal areas. The disease appears to be sexually transmitted and is associated with the presence in affected tissues of an intracellular microorganism, identified morphologically as the Donovan body.

ETIOLOGY   Donovanosis was described by McLeod in India in 1882, and in 1905 Donovan described the intracellular bodies which are thought to cause the disease. During the 1940s, encapsulated bacteria resembling Donovan bodies were recovered from pseudo-buboes of granuloma inguinale by inoculation of chick embryo yolk sacs or yolk-agar medium. These bacteria, which are known as *Calymmatobacterium granulomatis*, measure 1.5 by 0.7 μm. Such isolates are no longer available, *C. granulomatis* has not been cultivable in recent years, and the organism has not yet been characterized. Electron microscopic studies of Donovan bodies show their morphologic resemblance to gram-negative bacteria.

EPIDEMIOLOGY   Donovanosis is endemic in the tropics, particularly in Papua, New Guinea, southern India, and southern Africa. In the United States, the disease is rare. In reported cases, the sex ratio of males to females is nearly 10:1. The disease is uncommon in Caucasians. The frequency of donovanosis in sexual partners of chronically infected patients is highly variable, ranging from 1 to over 50 percent. Evidence for sexual transmission includes the age-specific incidence, which corresponds to that of other sexually transmitted diseases, the frequent concomitant presence of syphilis, the predilection for genital involvement in heterosexuals and for anorectal infection in homosexually active men, and the fact that outbreaks of clusters of cases of donovanosis have been traced to sexual exposure to a single-source contact. A significant association of HIV infection with donovanosis has been found among men in Durban, South Africa.

CLINICAL MANIFESTATIONS   The incubation period ranges from 8 days to 12 weeks, but most lesions appear within 30 days after sexual exposure.

Donovanosis begins as a papule that ulcerates and develops into a painless elevated zone of clean, beefy-red, friable granulation tissue. The edges are irregular and spread by continuity or by autoinoculation of approximated skin surfaces. Secondary anaerobic infection may produce pain and a foul-smelling exudate. Less common complications of the disease include deep ulcerations, chronic cicatricial lesions, phimosis, lymphedema, and exuberant epithelial proliferation which grossly resembles carcinoma. In men, the lesions are usually located on the glans, prepuce, or shaft of the penis or the perianal area, while infection of the labia is most common in women. Lesions in women often arise at the fourchette and progress anteriorly in a V shape along the vulva. Extragenital lesions may occur, involving the face, neck, mouth, and other sites. The chronicity of the disease is of diagnostic importance, since several months often elapse before patients seek treatment. Extension to the inguinal region by autoinoculation, by continuity, or via the lymphatics results in a diffuse intradermal and subcutaneous swelling or suppuration known as a *pseudobubo* because involvement of the underlying lymph nodes is minimal. Locally destructive lesions and secondary infection may produce severe morbidity or death. Fatal disseminated disease, involving the bones, joints, or liver, has been reported. Disseminated infection apparently occurs more frequently during pregnancy. The relationship of donovanosis to subsequent carcinoma of the genitalia is uncertain.

DIAGNOSIS   Early donovanosis may be mistaken for the primary chancre or condyloma latum of syphilis. Epithelial proliferation resembling carcinoma in the genital or perianal region in a young individual should always raise the suspicion of donovanosis if unnecessary destructive surgery is to be avoided. Chronic ulcerative or cicatricial changes may resemble lymphogranuloma venereum.

Amebiasis can produce penile lesions resembling donovanosis. In the United States, *Haemophilis ducreyi* frequently has been isolated from lesions resembling donovanosis, which have been termed *pseudo-granuloma inguinale–chancroid*. Histologic studies in donovanosis reveal marked acanthosis and pseudoepitheliomatous hyperplasia. The dermis contains an inflammatory infiltrate consisting mainly of plasma cells and histiocytes. Because Donovan bodies are seldom detectable in sections stained with hematoxylin and eosin, these changes may lead to an erroneous diagnosis of carcinoma and to unnecessary destructive surgery. Although silver impregnation techniques are useful for demonstration of Donovan bodies in sections, the diagnosis is best made by examination of impression smears prepared from specimens obtained by punch biopsy of granulation tissue from the periphery of a lesion; the deep portion of the specimen is removed, crushed between two slides which are air-dried and fixed in methanol, and stained with Wright-Giemsa stain. With this method, Donovan bodies appear as very rounded coccobacilli, 1 by 2 μm in size, which lie within cystic spaces in the cytoplasm of large mononuclear cells. The capsule stains as a dense acidophilic zone surrounding the bacterium, which resembles a closed safety pin because of bipolar condensation of chromatin. The pathognomonic mononuclear cell is 25 to 90 μm in diameter and has many cystic areas containing Donovan bodies. Donovan bodies also have been identified in histiocytes in cervical Papanicolaou smears.

Perianal donovanosis may resemble condylomata lata of secondary syphilis. Other venereal diseases, particularly syphilis, frequently coexist with donovanosis. Repeated negative dark-field examinations of lesions and negative serologic tests will exclude syphilis but should not be rigidly required while treatment is withheld from potentially noncompliant patients. In countries where donovanosis is endemic, the persistence of suspected condylomata lata after appropriate penicillin therapy for syphilis is highly suggestive of donovanosis.

TREATMENT   The antimicrobials currently effective in the treatment of donovanosis in various parts of the world include trimethoprim-sulfamethoxazole, tetracycline, erythromycin, newer quinolones, gentamicin, and chloramphenicol or the related drug thiamphenicol (not available in the United States). Streptomycin, once commonly used for this condition, is not widely used today. Ampicillin is not recommended for donovanosis. Unfortunately, no comparative trials have been conducted with the currently used antimicrobials, and in vitro susceptibility testing is not possible. The minimum duration of treatment is not well established, and it is common protocol to continue therapy until lesions have completely healed over. Thus treatment for large lesions is generally more prolonged. Healing of small lesions is usually apparent within 3 weeks, as the lesions become pale and flatter and peripheral reepithelialization begins. Lack of objective clinical response within 7 days should lead to reassessment of the diagnosis and therapy. Donovan bodies disappear from lesions within a few days after onset of therapy. Typical dosages of the commonly used drugs include tetracycline or erythromycin, 500 mg four times daily, or trimethoprim-sulfamethoxazole (trimethoprim 160 mg, sulfamethoxazole 800 mg) twice daily.

REFERENCES

FREINKEL AL et al: A serologic test for granuloma inguinale. Genitourin Med 68:269, 1992

KRAUS SJ et al: Pseudogranuloma inguinale caused by *Haemophilus ducreyi*. Arch Dermatol 118:494, 1982

KUBERSKI T: Granuloma inguinale (donovanosis). Sex Transm Dis 7:29, 1980

O'FARRELL N: Clinico-epidemiological study of donovanosis in Durban, South Africa. Genitourin Med 69:108

——— et al: A rapid stain for the diagnosis of granuloma inguinale. Genitourin Med 66:200, 1990

——— et al: HIV-1 infection among heterosexual attendees of a sexually transmitted disease clinic in Durban. S Afr Med J 80:17, 1991

RICHENS J: The diagnosis and treatment of donovanosis (granuloma inguinale). Genitourin Med 67:441, 1991

ROSEN T et al: Granuloma inguinale. J Am Acad Dermatol 11:433, 1984

SCHNEIDER J et al: Extragenital donovanosis: Three cases from Western Australia. Genitourin Med 62:196, 1966

section 7 Miscellaneous bacterial infections

126 NOCARDIOSIS

GREGORY A. FILICE

DEFINITION *Nocardia* species are aerobic actinomycetes associated with several characteristic syndromes. Pneumonia and disseminated disease, both thought to follow inhalation of fragmented bacterial mycelia, are most common. Three syndromes follow transcutaneous inoculation: cellulitis, a lymphocutaneous syndrome, and mycetoma. Keratitis occurs after inoculation into the eye, usually after corneal trauma.

MICROBIOLOGY *Nocardia* species are common inhabitants of soil, where they contribute to decay of organic matter. Only three species are well-documented human pathogens, *N. asteroides, N. brasiliensis,* and *N. otitidiscaviarum* (formerly *N. caviae*). *N. farcinica* and *N. nova* are species of uncertain or controversial pathogenic status that have been isolated from humans. *N. transvalensis* has been reported in association with disseminated infection in three patients with host defense defects and has been isolated from a few cases of mycetoma.

EPIDEMIOLOGY Nocardiosis occurs throughout the world, and approximately 1000 cases of infection are diagnosed annually in the United States, 85 percent of them pulmonary and/or systemic. The disease is more common in adults and in males. Epidemics are rare, and person-to-person spread has not been established.

The risk for pulmonary or disseminated disease is increased in people with deficient cell-mediated immunity, especially deficiency associated with lymphoma or transplantation. Nocardiosis has been reported in people with AIDS, although nocardiosis is not as common as some other opportunistic infections in this group (see Chap. 279). Nocardiosis also has been associated with pulmonary alveolar proteinosis, tuberculosis, and chronic granulomatous disease.

Nocardia species are among several aerobic actinomycetes associated with mycetoma (see below). Cases of mycetoma occur mainly in tropical and subtropical regions, especially Mexico, Central and South America, Africa, and India. The most important risk factor for mycetoma is frequent contact with soil or vegetable matter.

PATHOLOGY The characteristic histologic feature of pulmonary or systemic *Nocardia* infection is an abscess infiltrated extensively with neutrophils. Granulation tissue usually surrounds the lesions, but extensive fibrosis or encapsulation is uncommon. Nocardial mycetoma is characterized by suppurative inflammation with sinus tract formation. Mycetoma lesions and their drainage contain granules composed of dense masses of bacterial filaments.

CLINICAL MANIFESTATIONS Pulmonary disease Nocardial infection typically presents as a subacute pneumonia with symptoms developing over a few days to several weeks. Nocardiosis may occur in a more acute form in immunosuppressed patients. Cough is prominent and is often productive of small amounts of thick, purulent nonmalodorous sputum. Fever, anorexia, weight loss, and malaise are common. Dyspnea, pleuritic pain, and hemoptysis occur in some patients. Tracheitis and bronchitis are rare. Remissions and exacerbations over periods of several weeks are frequent.

Roentgenographic patterns of pulmonary nocardiosis are variable. Infiltrates or nodules of varying size and density are typical, occurring in any lobe. Cavitation is common, and empyema is present in one-third of cases.

Pulmonary nocardiosis may spread directly from the lungs to involve adjacent tissue, causing pericarditis, mediastinitis, and superior vena caval obstruction. Spread through the chest wall is rare.

Nocardia species are sometimes isolated from respiratory secretions of patients without apparent nocardial disease. Most of these patients have underlying pulmonary disease with abnormal chest roentgenograms. A positive sputum culture in the presence of symptoms and signs of pulmonary infection must be considered indicative of nocardial pneumonia. In the absence of clear evidence of pneumonia, the presence of nocardiae on Gram stain and the ability to isolate nocardiae in multiple cultures are factors suggesting an increased likelihood of nocardial disease. A positive sputum culture in an immunosuppressed patient usually reflects disease, not colonization.

Extrapulmonary dissemination In one-half of cases of pulmonary nocardiosis, disease appears in disseminated form outside the lungs. One-fifth of patients present only with disease outside the lungs, which is assumed to have spread hematogenously from an inapparent or healed pulmonary focus. The most commonly infected sites outside the lungs are brain, skin and supporting structures, kidneys, bone, and muscle, but dissemination to nearly every organ has occurred. Peritonitis and endocarditis have been reported. The typical manifestation of extrapulmonary dissemination is a subacute or chronic abscess. A minority of abscesses outside the lungs or central nervous system (CNS) form fistulas and discharge small amounts of pus.

The CNS is the most common location for disseminated disease. Usually there are one or more supratentorial brain abscesses, often multiloculated. The symptoms and signs are somewhat more indolent than those of other cases of bacterial brain abscess. Brain abscesses sometimes burrow into the ventricles or out into the subarachnoid space and result in meningitis. Occasional patients present with meningitis, but many of these are found to have brain abscesses by careful clinical evaluation or by imaging studies. The organism is not easily recovered from cerebrospinal fluid (CSF) even in cases with meningitis.

Transcutaneous inoculation Infection following transcutaneous inoculation usually occurs in patients with intact immune systems and takes one of three forms: cellulitis, lymphocutaneous syndrome, or mycetoma. In the United States, cellulitis is most common, followed by the lymphocutaneous syndrome, and finally by mycetoma.

Cellulitis usually begins 1 to 3 weeks after a recognized breach of the skin. Often, there has been obvious contamination of the wound with soil. A subacute cellulitis with pain, swelling, erythema, and warmth develops over a period of days to weeks. The lesions are usually firm and nonfluctuant. The process may progress to involve underlying muscle, tendon, bones, and joints. Dissemination is rare. In colder climates, most cases are associated with *N. asteroides;* in warmer climates, *N. brasiliensis* is more common.

In the lymphocutaneous form, there is typically a pyodermatous lesion at the site of inoculation with central ulceration and purulent or honey-colored drainage. Subcutaneous nodules may appear along lymphatics that drain the primary lesion. The lymphangitic form closely resembles lymphocutaneous sporotrichosis (see Chap. 169). Most cases of the lymphocutaneous syndrome are associated with *N. brasiliensis.*

Mycetoma usually begins with a nodular swelling, sometimes with a history of local trauma. Lesions typically occur on the feet or the hands but may involve the posterior part of the neck, the upper back, the head, and other locations. The nodule eventually forms one or more fistulas. The fistulas tend to come and go, with new ones forming as old ones disappear. The discharge is serous or purulent and may be bloody; it often contains 0.1- to 2-mm white granules which consist of masses of mycelia. The lesions spread slowly along fascial planes to involve adjacent areas of skin, subcutaneous tissue, and bone. Over a period of months to years, there may be extensive deformation of the affected part. Pain is minimal in lesions involving soft tissues but may be severe if lesions affect bones or joints. Systemic symptoms of fever and malaise are absent or minimal. Infection rarely disseminates from a mycetoma, and lesions on the hands and feet usually cause only local disability. Lesions on the head, neck, and trunk can invade locally to involve deep organs and result in severe disability or death.

Keratitis *Nocardia* species, usually *N. asteroides,* are uncommon causes of subacute keratitis. The infection usually follows eye trauma. Nocardial infection of lacrimal glands has been reported. Disease involving deeper eye structures is usually a manifestation of disseminated disease.

DIAGNOSIS The first step is examination of sputum or pus for crooked, branching, beaded, gram-positive filaments 1 μm in width and up to 50 μm in length. Most nocardiae are acid-fast in direct smears if a weak acid is used for decolorization, as with the modified Kinyoun, Ziehl-Neelsen, or Fite-Faraco methods. Nocardiae often take up silver stains. Nocardiae grow relatively slowly; colonies may take up to 2 weeks to appear and may not develop their characteristic appearance for up to 4 weeks. Growth is so different from more common pathogens that the laboratory should always be alerted when *Nocardia* is suspected so that the likelihood of recovering it is maximized. In difficult cases, paraffin baiting can be employed, since nocardiae are among the few aerobic microorganisms that can use paraffin as a carbon source.

When smears are negative, it is often necessary to pursue the diagnosis by more invasive procedures. For pulmonary cases, bronchoscopy, needle aspiration, and open lung biopsy are all effective. Transtracheal aspiration should be avoided because it frequently leads to nocardial cellulitis in tissues around the puncture wound.

All patients with nocardial pneumonia should be evaluated for disseminated disease with a careful history and physical examination. Suggestive symptoms or signs should be pursued with further diagnostic tests. Computed tomography or magnetic resonance imaging of the head with and without contrast material should be done if there are signs or symptoms suggesting brain involvement.

Biphasic culture bottles (liquid medium over agar) incubated aerobically for up to 30 days often yield nocardiae, but routine blood cultures are usually negative. If clinically indicated, specimens of CSF or urine should be concentrated and then cultured. In mycetoma cases, an effort should be made to find granules in the discharge. Suspect particles should be washed in saline, examined microscopically, and cultured.

Several presumptive diagnostic tests have been studied, including tests for antibodies and nocardial metabolites in serum or CSF. None is ready for clinical use at this time.

THERAPY Sulfonamides are the drugs of choice. Sulfadiazine or sulfisoxazole, 6 to 8 g/d in four divided doses, is commonly administered, but doses from 4 to 12 g/d have been given. In difficult cases, sulfonamide blood levels should be measured and dosages adjusted to keep serum levels between 100 and 150 μg/mL. The combination of sulfamethoxazole and trimethoprim has been associated with similar success with a modestly increased risk of hematologic toxicity. Trimethoprim, 5 to 20 mg/kg, and sulfamethoxazole, 25 to 100 mg/kg, should be given each day in two divided doses. Nocardiosis has been rare among transplant recipients receiving sulfamethoxazole and trimethoprim for prophylaxis against other infectious diseases,

which has suggested that the combination may prevent nocardiosis as well.

Minocycline is the best-established alternative orally administered drug and should be given in doses of 100 to 200 mg twice a day. There is little clinical evidence that other tetracyclines are reliably effective. Amoxicillin and clavulanic acid have been effective in some cases and would be a reasonable choice in patients who cannot be treated with sulfonamides or minocycline. Other orally administered antimicrobials have been used, but there is less experience with them. Chloramphenicol (1 g four times a day), cycloserine (250 mg three times a day), and ampicillin (1 g four times a day) have appeared effective in some cases, often used together with sulfonamides. Ampicillin and erythromycin (500 to 750 mg four times a day) may be effective when used together, but erythromycin alone is not usually effective.

Amikacin is the best-established parental drug, given in doses of 5 to 7.5 mg/kg every 12 h. Serum levels should be monitored with prolonged therapy, in the face of diminished renal function, or in the elderly. Limited experience with newer β-lactam antibiotics, including cefotaxime, ceftizoxime, and imipenem, suggests that they may be helpful alone or in combination with other antimicrobials.

Antimicrobial susceptibility testing of *Nocardia* species has not been developed to the point where clinical relevance is ensured, and ordinarily, choices of antimicrobials should be based on published clinical experience. In cases in which the usual antimicrobials fail or cannot be used, susceptibility testing may be used to guide the choice of alternative agents. Sulfonamides, most aminoglycosides, minocycline, fusidic acid, and some newly developed β-lactam antibiotics appear active against most strains. Sulbactam and clavulanic acid inactivate nocardial β-lactamases, but the potential clinical effectiveness of combinations including β-lactamase inhibitors is unknown.

In many cases, two or more antimicrobials have been used to treat nocardiosis, often in combinations including a sulfonamide or minocycline. Whether therapy with two or more agents is better than therapy with a single agent is not known, and therapy with multiple drugs increases the risk of toxicity.

Brain abscesses should be treated surgically if the diagnosis is unclear, if an abscess is large and accessible, or if an abscess fails to respond to chemotherapy. Aspiration, excision, and drainage are all effective. Small abscesses and abscesses in inaccessible or critical locations should be treated medically. In cases managed medically, results should be monitored with repeated imaging.

Antimicrobial therapy usually suffices for treatment of nocardial mycetoma. In deep or extensive cases, drainage or excision of heavily involved tissue may facilitate healing, but structure and function should be preserved whenever possible.

Immunosuppressive therapy should be continued if necessary for treatment of an underlying disease or to prevent rejection of a transplanted organ. In other cases, it seems prudent to reduce or eliminate immunosuppressive therapy.

Nocardial infections tend to relapse, and long courses of antimicrobial therapy are necessary. Nocardiosis is particularly tenacious and likely to relapse in people with chronic granulomatous disease. For nonimmunosuppressed patients, treatment of pulmonary or systemic nocardiosis outside the CNS should be continued for 6 to 12 months. Ordinarily, treatment of CNS nocardiosis should be continued for 1 year. If all apparent disease has been excised, the duration of therapy may be reduced to 6 months. For immunosuppressed patients, treatment of pulmonary or systemic nocardiosis should be continued for 1 year. If nocardial disease is unusually extensive, or if the response to therapy is slow, these recommendations should be exceeded.

Patients with cellulitis or the lymphocutaneous syndrome should be treated for 2 months if infection is limited to soft tissues and for 4 months if bone is involved. Unusually extensive cases or cases in immunosuppressed people should be treated longer, depending on degrees of involvement and of immunosuppression. Therapy of mycetoma should be continued for 6 to 12 months after clinical cure. Keratitis should be treated with oral and topical sulfonamides until the infection appears cured and then with oral sulfonamides alone for an additional 2 to 4 months.

The mortality for pulmonary or disseminated nocardiosis outside the CNS should be less than 5 percent. CNS disease increases the risk of death. Patients should be followed carefully for at least 6 months after therapy has ended. Any child with nocardiosis and no known cause of immunosuppression should have tests performed to determine the adequacy of the child's phagocytic respiratory burst.

REFERENCES

BERKEY P, BODEY GP: Nocardial infection in patients with neoplastic disease. Rev Infect Dis 11:407, 1989

BROSS JE, GORDON G: Nocardial meningitis: Case reports and review. Rev Infect Dis 13:160, 1991

JAVALY K et al: Nocardiosis in patients with human immunodeficiency virus infection: Report of 2 cases and review of the literature. Medicine 71:128, 1992

KIM J et al: Nocardial infection as a complication of AIDS: Report of six cases and review. Rev Infect Dis 13:624, 1991

PALMER DL et al: Diagnostic and therapeutic considerations in *Nocardia asteroides* infection. Medicine 53:391, 1974

PETERSON EA et al: Minocycline treatment of pulmonary nocardiosis. JAMA 250:930, 1983

SATTERWHITE TK, WALLACE RJ JR: Primary cutaneous nocardiosis. JAMA 242:333, 1979

TIGHT RR, BARTLETT MS: Actinomycetoma in the United States. Rev Infect Dis 3:1139, 1981

WALLACE RJ et al: Antimicrobial susceptility patterns of *Nocardia asteroides*. Antimicrob Agents Chemother 32:1776, 1988

127 ACTINOMYCOSIS

PHILLIP I. LERNER

Actinomycosis is caused by filamentous, gram-positive bacteria that are part of the normal oral flora. In this chronic, suppurative, fibrosing infection, external sinuses often discharge tiny colonies of organisms that are referred to as *sulfur granules* because of their resemblance to elemental pharmaceutical sulfur particles. After oral commensals have invaded the face, neck, lungs, and/or ileocecal region, infection spreads to contiguous structures, unrestricted by normal tissue plane barriers. The indolent course resembling that of fungal infection, tuberculosis, or malignancy can confound early diagnosis. In fact, the diagnosis can be stubbornly elusive, often being made only after months or even years. Between three and four times as many men as women develop actinomycosis. Prolonged antibiotic therapy coupled with removal of foreign bodies and drainage of suppurative sites is usually necessary for its eradication.

AGENTS OF ACTINOMYCOSIS Classic actinomycosis is caused most often by *Actinomyces israelii* (78 percent) but also can be attributed to other anaerobic and microaerophilic oral commensals, including *A. naeslundii*, *A. viscosus*, *A. odontolyticus*, *A. meyeri*, and *Propionibacterium* (formerly *Arachnia*) *propionica*. In the microbiology laboratory, all species of *Actinomyces* (except *A. viscosus*) and *Propionibacterium propionica* require extended anaerobic or microaerophilic (6% to 10% CO_2) incubation. The best attainable culture sensitivity is only 50 percent for samples of frank pus or tissue free of contamination from mucosal surfaces. Thus laboratory personnel must be alerted when actinomycosis is suspected. Pathologists must be diligent in sectioning and examining resected tissues for diagnostic granules. In early or acute infections, organisms may appear as separate gram-positive, branching filaments rather than the characteristic colonies or granules typical of advanced lesions. Fluorescein isothiocyanate species-specific conjugate antisera can identify all major *Actinomyces* species, *P. propionica*, and even mixed species in granules.

Actinomycotic lesions characteristically include "associates"—other members of the endogenous oral or gastrointestinal flora that cannot be separated from the actinomycetes in culture. These organisms usually are not considered in the selection of antibiotic therapy. *Actinobacillus actinomycetemcomitans*, *Haemophilus* species, fusobacteria, streptococci, micrococci, staphylococci, *Eikenella corrodens*, and oral *Bacteroides* species can be found in cervicofacial and thoracic actinomycosis, while coliforms and intestinal anaerobes are the associated microbes in abdominal actinomycosis. Although there is probably an essential synergy between the actinomycetes and these associates, this relationship is not understood.

PATHOGENESIS AND PATHOLOGY The species of *Actinomyces* and *Propionibacterium* that cause actinomycosis are endogenous oral saprophytes of low virulence that dwell in periodontal pockets, carious teeth, dental plaque, and tonsillar crypts; they also can be isolated from the lower gastrointestinal and female genital tracts. Thus the growth of actinomycetes in cultures from these sites is nondiagnostic. After trauma, surgery, or another infection that alters the host's mucosal barriers, these organisms advance to invade surrounding tissues. The process is usually chronic and fibrosing, and the frequent absence of clinical findings associated with bacterial infections (e.g., fever, leukocytosis, and anemia) raises suspicions of a fungal or mycobacterial infection or a malignancy. Lesions may be indurated masses or soft and loculated. Sinus tracts extending from these lesions to skin, mucous membranes, or internal organs permit further spread of the infection, particularly in the abdomen and pelvis. The actinomycetes are only rarely opportunists in immunocompromised states such as leukemia, solid tumor malignancies, renal failure, and AIDS.

Histologic examination generally reveals pus surrounded by acute or chronic fibrosing granulation tissue, although fibrosis may not be evident in pulmonary infections or any early process. In advanced lesions, classic yellow, brown, or dull white granules may form in pockets of suppuration or collect on gauze dressings over draining sinuses. These so-called sulfur granules occur only in vivo and are actually mineralized bacterial filaments encased in calcium phosphate as a result of alkaline phosphatase activity in inflamed host tissues. While other infectious agents, including fungi, *Nocardia*, *Streptomyces*, and *Staphylococcus*, can form similar aggregates, only the granules of actinomycosis feature surface "clubs" visible by light microscopy. Granules (diameter, 1 to 2 mm) from pus or surgical dressings can be stained and crushed between microscope slides. Upon staining with 1% methylene blue at low magnification, the distinctive cauliflower-like granules become visible; Gram staining at high magnification reveals the thin (diameter ≤ 1 μm), branching, gram-positive filaments of the organisms. These granules may be sparse; careful examination of multiple histologic sections of abscess wall, sinus tract, or tumor masses is often required for the diagnosis of actinomycosis.

CLINICAL SYNDROMES Cervicofacial actinomycosis Between 50 and 96 percent of cases of human actinomycosis affect the head and neck region. The clinician should suspect actinomycosis when a patient has acute, subacute, or chronic phlegmon of the skin or soft tissue or swelling of the head and neck, especially if a draining sinus develops. A dental portal is usually implicated; infection is often preceded by a tooth extraction, and evidence of poor dental hygiene, tooth decay or abscess, or periodontal disease is frequently found. Even a simple molar eruption or nonpenetrating jaw trauma can interrupt mucosal integrity enough to precipitate infection.

Clinically, there are two patterns of cervicofacial actinomycosis. In the more indolent form, a painless, fluctuant, bluish or purplish lesion enlarges slowly, often where the facial artery and vein cross the lower border of the mandible. In this slowly evolving form, patients eventually develop trismus and oral or cutaneous fistulas. The second form, which is more acute and painfully suppurative, can occur anywhere in the head and neck; it involves the submandibular area, the angle of the mandible, and the parotid region particularly often. Isolated infection, with or without fistulas, can appear in the scalp, orbit, lacrimal glands, middle ear, mastoid, paranasal sinuses, thyroid, or trachea, with no clue as to the original site of oral mucosal entry. Infection spreads without regard for fascial tissue planes or lymphatic channels. In this acute, rapidly progressive form, subcutaneous abscesses and trismus develop, and impressive edema of involved tissues is often documented. The incidence of spontaneous abscess rupture in acute cervicofacial disease has decreased in the antibiotic era. An acute abscess, inflammatory nodule, or infiltrating mass resembling a tumor may involve the pharyngeal and laryngeal structures. If the infection reaches the bone, periostitis is followed by lytic destruction with surrounding hyperdensity.

Thoracic and disseminated actinomycosis Actinomycosis can involve the lungs, pleura, and mediastinal structures. Infection at these sites follows aspiration, direct extension from the neck or esophagus, or retroperitoneal spread from the abdomen. Antecedent chronic lung disease predisposes to pulmonary actinomycosis. Diagnosis can be extremely difficult: symptoms such as fever or cough are often minimal or absent, and the common use of empirical antibiotic therapy may limit spread to the lungs, preventing the appearance of a classic granule-discharging sinus in the chest wall.

Pulmonary actinomycosis is usually a debilitating illness resembling tuberculosis or carcinoma. Chest radiography may show a fibrocavitary process with a loss of volume, an alveolar process, or a mass compressing or invading a bronchus. Actinomycosis and tuberculosis can coexist. Since *Actinomyces* species can proliferate in necrotic tumors, a positive sputum culture alone is not diagnostic.

Radiographic features suggestive of thoracic actinomycosis include (1) lung lesions eroding the chest wall, (2) periostitis or lysis of ribs, sternum, or shoulder girdle adjacent to a chronic lung process, (3) pulmonary infiltrate crossing an interlobar fissure, and (4) vertebral destruction with sparing of the disk space and erosion of both the body and the processes of the affected vertebra and adjacent ribs. Mediastinal infection can obstruct the superior vena cava or provoke a transesophageal or systemic-to-pulmonary venous fistula. Fewer than 2 percent of cases of actinomycosis include pleuropulmonary involvement, and massive empyema is rare.

Disseminated actinomycosis generally occurs in conjunction with thoracic disease and is quite unusual. Vasculitic lesions in the skin, subcutaneous tissue, or muscle can harbor both actinomycetes and associated microorganisms. Concomitant pulmonary disease may assume a miliary pattern. Rarely occurring primary actinomycosis of the extremity is preceded by trauma—e.g., a human bite or fist fight (punch actinomycosis)—in 60 percent of cases.

Abdominal and pelvic actinomycosis Most abdominal actinomycotic infections are preceded by surgery, e.g., laparotomy for acute appendicitis, perforated diverticulum or ulcer, cholecystitis, perforating trauma, or another abdominal catastrophe. Rarely, nonpenetrating trauma initiates the process. Infection usually begins in the gastrointestinal tract and spreads to the peritoneal cavity and abdominal wall or extends paracecally to the subphrenic space or pouch of Douglas. Sinus tracts are common; true bowel fistulas are not. The interval between inoculation and diagnosis can be months or even years. Actinomycotic lesions may be mistaken for Crohn's disease, malignancy, tuberculosis, amebiasis, or chronic appendicitis.

Gastric actinomycosis follows perforation of or surgery for gastric ulcer and can itself mimic peptic ulcer disease or carcinoma. Hepatic involvement, seen in 15 percent of cases, occurs via the portal vein, by direct extension from contiguous viscera, or (rarely) via the hepatic artery during disseminated infection; in turn, hepatic infection can extend to the abdominal wall or diaphragm, adjacent viscera, or retroperitoneum. Hepatic involvement may appear as single or multiple hepatic lesions or as a miliary process.

Pelvic actinomycosis may originate in an anal crypt and spread posterolaterally to the gluteal region or extend to the anorectal region from elsewhere in the pelvis, causing recurrent draining sinuses, anal fistulas, and rectal fissures. Endometrial infection is uncommon unless it is introduced directly during abortion, from an intrauterine device (IUD), or through infected pessaries or retained surgical sutures. IUD-associated actinomycosis ranges from vaginal discharge to pelvic inflammatory disease with tuboovarian abscess, ureteral obstruction, or a "frozen pelvis" mimicking malignancy. *Actinomyces*-like organisms seen in Papanicolaou smears from IUD users neither signal pathology nor mandate IUD removal. Five percent of healthy women without IUDs also harbor *Actinomyces*-like organisms in the genital tract.

Actinomycosis of the central nervous system The CNS is involved in 10 percent of all cases of actinomycosis. Infections spreading hematogenously from the mouth, lungs, abdomen, or pelvis numerically exceed those extending from a cervicofacial primary site. CNS disease usually presents as a single, multiloculated hemispheric abscess; multiple lesions occur in 15 percent of cases. A primary focus for CNS actinomycosis may not exist. Meningeal involvement may produce only chronic lymphocytic meningitis. Infection can reach the vertebral canal via the intervertebral foramina from a cervicofacial, thoracic, or abdominal focus and cause epidural abscess and cord compression.

THERAPY Actinomycosis should be suspected when a recurrent pattern of exacerbation and remission of infection develops during empirical antibiotic therapy. Since the 1960s, the treatment of choice has been a prolonged course of high-dose intravenous benzylpenicillin coupled with appropriate surgical drainage, bony curettage, foreign body removal, debridement, or radical sinus tract excision. Occasionally, a complete response of acute disease (particularly early cervicofacial infection) to therapy with intravenous penicillin alone eliminates the need for surgery or allows better definition of fascial planes and renders subsequent surgery less extensive. Penicillin G (10 to 20 million units per day for 2 to 6 weeks), followed by oral penicillin V (e.g., phenoxymethyl penicillin, 2 to 4 g/d, to the limits of the patient's tolerance for 3 to 6 additional months), is an accepted regimen for most deep-seated infections. The likelihood of relapse diminishes with at least 2 to 4 months of therapy in early or mild cases and with 6 to 12 months of antibiotic treatment in severe or chronic actinomycosis. Erythromycin and clindamycin also can be used. Tetracyclines are as effective as penicillin G for cervicofacial disease. Metronidazole, oral cephalosporins, oral antistaphylococcal penicillins, and quinolone antibiotics should not be used.

In vivo acquisition of resistance by *Actinomyces* species, particularly that to penicillin G, is not a problem. When the response to therapy is poor or a relapse occurs, an undrained abscess or resistant bacterial associate should be sought. In general, the susceptibility of associated organisms is not considered when antibiotics are prescribed, but some investigators prefer ampicillin or amoxicillin initially because associated bacteria are less susceptible to penicillin G. Metronidazole or clindamycin may be added to the regimen when *Bacteroides* species (e.g., *B. fragilis*, *B. thetaiotamicron*) are isolated.

REFERENCES

BERARDI RS: Abdominal actinomycosis. Surg Gynecol Obstet 149:257, 1979
BENNHOFF DF: Actinomycosis: Diagnostic and therapeutic considerations. Laryngoscope 94:1198, 1984
BURDEN P: Actinomycosis. J Infect 19:95, 1989
LERNER PI: The lumpy jaw: Cervicofacial actinomycosis. Infect Dis Clin North Am 2:203, 1988
PEABODY JW, SEABURY JH: Actinomycosis and nocardiosis. Am J Med 28:99, 1960
RICHTSMEIER WJ, JOHNS ME: Actinomycosis of the head and neck. CRC Crit Rev Clin Lab Sci 11:175, 1979
SCHAAL KP: The genera *Actinomyces*, *Arcanobacterium*, and *Rothia*, in *Prokaryotes 2*, A Balows et al (eds). New York, Springer-Verlag, 1992, chap 38
SMEGO RA JR: Actinomycosis of the central nervous system. Rev Infect Dis 9:855, 1987

128 INFECTIONS DUE TO MIXED ANAEROBIC ORGANISMS

DENNIS L. KASPER

DEFINITIONS *Anaerobic* bacteria are organisms that require reduced oxygen tension for growth, failing to grow on the surface of solid media in 10% CO_2 in air. *Microaerophilic* bacteria can grow in 10% CO_2 in air or under anaerobic or aerobic conditions. *Facultative* bacteria can grow in the presence or absence of air. This chapter describes infections caused by nonsporulating anaerobic bacteria. In general, anaerobes associated with human infections are relatively aerotolerant. They can survive for as long as 72 h in the presence of oxygen, although generally they will not multiply in this environment. Many fewer pathogenic anaerobic bacteria, which are also part of the normal flora, die after brief contact with oxygen, even in low concentrations.

The nonsporulating anaerobic bacteria exist as normal flora on the mucosal surfaces of humans and animals. The major reservoirs of these bacteria are the mouth, gastrointestinal tract, skin, and the female genital tract. Of the oral flora, anaerobes are the predominant commensal organisms, ranging in concentrations from 10^9 per milliliter in saliva to 10^{12} in gingival scrapings. In the oral cavity the relative concentration of anaerobic to aerobic bacteria ranges from 1:1 on the surface of a tooth to 1000:1 in the gingival crevice. Anaerobic bacteria are not found in appreciable numbers in the normal intestine until the distal ileum. In the colon, the proportion of anaerobes increases significantly, as does the overall bacterial count. For example, in the colon there are 10^{11} to 10^{12} organisms per gram of stool, with a ratio of anaerobes to aerobes of approximately 1000:1. In the female genital tract there are approximately 10^9 organisms per milliliter of secretions, with a ratio of anaerobes to aerobes of approximately 10:1. Hundreds of species of anaerobic bacteria have been identified as part of the normal flora of humans. Identification of as many as 500 different anaerobic species in fecal specimens reflects the diversity of the anaerobic flora. Despite the complex array of bacteria which exist in the normal flora, relatively few species are isolated commonly from human infection.

Anaerobic infections occur when the harmonious relationship between the host and bacteria is disrupted. Any site in the body is susceptible to infection with these indigenous organisms when a mucosal barrier or the skin is compromised by surgery, trauma, tumor, or ischemia or necrosis, which reduces local tissue redox potentials. Because the sites that are colonized by anaerobic bacteria contain many species of bacteria, disruption of anatomic barriers allows penetration of many organisms, resulting in mixed infections involving multiple species of anaerobes combined with facultative or microaerophilic organisms. Such mixed infections are seen in the head and neck (chronic sinusitis, chronic otitis media, Ludwig's angina, and periodontal abscesses). Brain abscesses and subdural empyema are the most frequent anaerobic infections of the central nervous system. Anaerobes are responsible for pleuropulmonary diseases such as aspiration pneumonia, necrotizing pneumonia, lung abscesses, and empyema. Anaerobes play an important role in various intraabdominal infections such as peritonitis and intraabdominal and liver abscesses (see Chap. 86). They are isolated frequently in female genital tract infections such as salpingitis, pelvic peritonitis, tuboovarian abscess, vulvovaginal abscesses, septic abortions, and endometritis (see Chaps. 88 and 89). Anaerobic bacteria also are frequently found in infections of the skin, soft tissue, and bones and in bacteremia.

ETIOLOGY The major anaerobic gram-positive cocci producing disease are *Peptostreptococcus* species. The major species involved in infections are *P. magnus*, *P. asaccharolyticus*, *P. anaerobius*, and *P. prevotii*. Clostridia are gram-positive rods which are isolated from wounds, abscesses, abdominal infections, and bacteremias; they are discussed in Chap. 108. The principal anaerobic gram-negative bacilli are the *Bacteroides* "family," which includes the *Bacteroides fragilis* group, fusobacteria, *Prevotella*, and *Porphyromonas*. The *B. fragilis* group contains the anaerobic pathogens most frequently isolated from clinical infections. Members of this group are part of the normal bowel flora. The group comprises several distinct species, including *B. fragilis*, *B. thetaiotaomicron*, *B. distasonis*, *B. vulgatus*, *B. uniformis*, and *B. ovatus*. Of this group, *B. fragilis* is the most important clinical isolate. However, in the normal fecal flora, the frequency with which *B. fragilis* is isolated is low compared with other *Bacteroides* species. A second major group of phenotypically similar organisms is part of the indigenous oral flora. These are primarily pigment-producing bacteria which were previously classified under the species *B. melaninogenicus*, now known as *Prevatella melaninogenica*. The terminology of this group has changed so that several distinct species are recognized, including *Porphyromonas gingivalis*, *Porphyromonas asaccharolyticus*, and *P. melaninogenica*. In female genital tract infections, *Prevotella bivius* and *Prevotella disiens* are the most frequent isolates, although *B. fragilis* is not uncommon. Fusobacteria are also isolated from clinical infections, including necrotizing pneumonia and abscesses.

Infections due to anaerobic bacteria most frequently are mixed infections with more than one organism. They may be due to one or several anaerobic species or a combination of anaerobic organisms and aerobic bacteria acting synergistically.

APPROACH TO THE PATIENT WITH ANAEROBIC BACTERIAL INFECTIONS There are several features to remember when approaching the patient with presumptive infection due to anaerobic bacteria. (1) Most of these organisms are harmless commensals, and very few cause disease. (2) In order for these organisms to cause infection, they must spread beyond the normal mucosal barriers. (3) Conditions favoring the propagation of these bacteria, particularly a lowered oxidation-reduction potential, are necessary. These include sites of trauma, tissue destruction, compromised vascular supply, or complication of preexisting infection that produces necrosis. (4) There is a complex array of infecting flora. For example, as many as 12 different types of organisms can be isolated from a suppurative site. (5) Anaerobic organisms tend to be found in abscess cavities or in necrotic tissue. The detection of an abscess in a patient which fails to yield organisms on routine culture is the clue that the abscess is likely to contain anaerobic bacteria. Often smears of this "sterile pus" are teeming with bacteria on Gram's stain. The malodorous nature of the pus should suggest anaerobic infections. Although some facultative organisms, such as *Staphylococcus aureus*, also are capable of causing abscesses, abscesses in organs or within deeper body tissues should call to mind anaerobic infection. (6) Treatment need not be directed at all the organisms in the infectious site. However, some species in particular require specific therapy. The best example of this principle is the need to treat the *B. fragilis* group. Many of these synergistic infections can be cured with antibiotics directed at some, but not all, of the organisms. Antibiotic therapy, combined with drainage, disrupts the interdependent relationship among the bacteria, and species which are resistant to the antibiotic do not survive without the coinfective organisms. (7) Manifestations of disseminated intravascular coagulation are unusual in patients with anaerobic infection.

EPIDEMIOLOGY Difficulties in obtaining appropriate cultures, contamination of cultures by aerobic bacteria or normal flora, and the lack of readily available reliable culture techniques have made accurate incidence or prevalence data on anaerobic infections unavailable. However, these infections are encountered frequently in hospitals with active surgical, trauma, and obstetric and gynecologic services. In some centers, anaerobic bacteria, particularly *B. fragilis*, account for approximately 8 to 10 percent of positive blood cultures.

PATHOGENESIS Anaerobic bacterial infections usually occur when an anatomic barrier becomes disrupted and the local flora enter a site which was previously sterile. The bacteria which are isolated from infected sites have survived changes in oxidation-reduction potential and exposure to host defenses. Because of the specific growth requirements of anaerobic organisms and their presence as commensals on mucosal surfaces, conditions must arise which allow these organisms to penetrate mucosal barriers and enter tissue with a lowered oxidation-reduction potential. Therefore, tissue ischemia, trauma, surgery, perforated viscus, shock, or aspiration provide environments conducive to the proliferation of anaerobes. Some highly fastidious anaerobes lack the enzyme superoxide dismutase (SOD) that in other organisms reduces toxic superoxide radicals, thereby lessening the potentially lethal effects of superoxide. In the case of a perforated viscus, hundreds of species of anaerobic bacteria are spilled into the peritoneal cavity, but many of these organisms are unable to survive because the highly vascularized tissue provides an adequate oxygen supply. The entry of oxygen into the environment results in selection of aerotolerant organisms.

The ability of an organism to adhere to host tissues is important to the establishment of infection. Some oral species adhere to crevicular epithelium in the oral cavity. *P. melaninogenica* actually attach to other microorganisms. *P. gingivalis* is a common isolate in periodontal disease. These organisms have been shown to have fimbriae which facilitate attachment. Some unencapsulated *Bacteroides* strains appear to be piliated, which may account for their ability to adhere.

The most extensively studied virulence factor of the nonsporulating anaerobes is the polysaccharide capsule of *B. fragilis*. These polysaccharides possess distinct biologic properties such as the ability to promote abscess formation in a rodent model of intraabdominal sepsis. Abscess induction is a T cell–dependent phenomenon requiring CD4+, CD8+ T cells. Immunization with the capsule confers protection against abscess induction following challenge with whole *B. fragilis* and is mediated by a non-major histocompatibility complex–restricted T cell circuit. Although some clinicians have viewed abscess formation as a protective host response to localize and contain infecting bacteria, abscess formation in patients with sepsis often results in severe and chronic illness that requires surgical drainage in combination with extensive antimicrobial therapy.

Anaerobic bacteria produce a number of exoenzymes which are capable of enhancing their virulence. These enzymes include a heparinase elaborated by *B. fragilis* which may contribute to intravascular clotting and lead to a requirement for increased doses of heparin in patients on heparin therapy. Collagenase, produced by *P. gingivalis*, may enhance tissue destruction. Both *B. fragilis* and *P. melaninogenica* possess lipopolysaccharides (endotoxins) which lack the biologic potency characteristic of endotoxins associated with aerobic gram-negative bacteria. The biologic inactivity of the endotoxin may account for the rarity of disseminated intravascular coagulation and purpura in *Bacteroides* bacteremia compared with facultative and aerobic gram-negative rod bacteremia.

CLINICAL MANIFESTATIONS Anaerobic infections of the mouth, head, and neck (See Chap. 84) Infections of the mouth can be divided into those infections which arise from the supragingival or subgingival dental plaque. Supragingival plaque formation begins with the adherence of gram-positive bacteria to the tooth surface. This form of plaque is influenced by salivary and dietary components, oral hygiene, and local host factors. Once established, the acquisition of pathogenic bacteria as well as an increase in the amount of plaque is responsible for the ultimate development of gingivitis. Early bacteriologic changes in the supragingival plaque initiate an inflammatory response in the gingiva, including edema, swelling, and increase in gingival fluid, and are responsible for the development of caries and endodontic (pulp) infections. Also, these changes contribute to the subsequent pathogenic alteration in the subgingival plaque which arises from poor or inadequate oral hygiene. Subgingival plaque is associated with periodontal disease and disseminated infection arising from the oral cavity. Bacteria that colonize the subgingival area are

primarily anaerobic. The black-pigmented gram-negative anaerobic bacilli, principally *P. gingivalis* and *P. melaninogenica*, are the most important. Infections in this area are frequently mixed and involve both anaerobic and aerobic bacteria. After establishment of local infection either in root canals or in the periodontal area, infection may extend into the mandible, causing osteomyelitis; to the maxillary sinuses; or to local tissues in the submandibular or submental spaces, depending on which teeth are involved. Periodontitis also may result in spreading infection that can involve adjacent bone or soft tissues.

GINGIVITIS Gingivitis may become a necrotizing infection (trench mouth, Vincent's stomatitis). The onset of disease is usually sudden and is associated with tender bleeding gums, foul breath, and a bad taste. The gingival mucosa, especially the papillae between the teeth, become ulcerated and may be covered by a gray exudate which is removable with gentle pressure. These patients may become systemically ill, developing fever, cervical lymphadenopathy, and leukocytosis. Occasionally, ulcerative gingivitis can spread to the buccal mucosa, the teeth, and the mandible or maxilla, resulting in widespread destruction of bone and soft tissue. This infection is termed *acute necrotizing ulcerative mucositis* (cancrum oris, noma). It destroys tissue rapidly, causing the teeth to fall out and large areas of bone, even the whole mandible, to be sloughed. A strong putrid odor frequently is present, although the lesions are not painful. The gangrenous lesions eventually heal, leaving large disfiguring defects. This infection is seen most commonly following a debilitating illness or in severely malnourished children in underdeveloped areas. It has been known to complicate leukemia or to develop in individuals with a genetic deficiency of catalase.

ACUTE NECROTIZING INFECTIONS OF THE PHARYNX These usually occur in association with ulcerative gingivitis. Symptoms include an extremely sore throat, foul breath, and a bad taste in the mouth, accompanied by a sensation of choking and fever. Examination of the pharynx demonstrates that the tonsillar pillars are swollen, red, and ulcerated and covered with a grayish membrane that peels easily. Lymphadenopathy and leukocytosis are common. The disease may last for only a few days or may persist for weeks if not treated. Lesions begin unilaterally but may spread to the other side of the pharynx or the larynx. Aspiration of the infected material by the patient can result in lung abscesses. Soft tissue infection of the oral-facial area may or may not be odontogenic in origin. *Ludwig's angina*, a periodontal infection usually arising from the third molar, may produce submandibular cellulitis that results in marked local swelling of tissues with pain, trismus, and superior and posterior displacement of the tongue. Submandibular swelling of the neck develops, which can impair swallowing and cause respiratory obstruction. In some cases tracheotomy may be life-saving.

FASCIAL INFECTIONS These arise from the spread of organisms originating in the upper airways to potential spaces formed by the fascial planes of the head and neck. Perimandibular space infection most commonly involves the submandibular, peritonsillar, and parapharyngeal spaces. Peritonsillar abscesses occur in association with pharyngitis. Complicated dental infections spread to the submandibular and buccal spaces. Both portals of entry can result in parapharyngeal space infections. Although there are few well-documented reports on the microbiology of these syndromes, anaerobes from the oral flora have been implicated in many cases. *Staphylococcus aureus* and *Streptococcus pyogenes* infections may arise from boils or impetigo, whereas anaerobes are associated with space infections arising from diseases of the mucous membranes or dental manipulations or occurring spontaneously.

SINUSITIS AND OTITIS The role of anaerobic bacteria in acute sinusitis may be underestimated because of improper collection of specimens. In chronic sinusitis, anaerobic bacteria were found in 52 percent of specimens collected during external frontoethmoidotomy or radical antrotomy. Anaerobic bacteria are much more easily implicated in chronic suppurative otitis media than in acute otitis media. Purulent exudate from chronically draining ears has been found to contain anaerobes, particularly *Bacteroides* species, in up to 50 percent of patients. In contrast to other infections of the head and neck, *B. fragilis* has been isolated from up to 28 percent of patients with chronic otitis media.

COMPLICATIONS OF ANAEROBIC HEAD AND NECK INFECTIONS Contiguous spread of these infections craniad may result in osteomyelitis of the skull or mandible or in intracranial infections such as brain abscesses and subdural empyema. Caudad spread can produce mediastinitis or pleuropulmonary infections. Hematogenous complications also may result from anaerobic infections of the head and neck. Bacteremia, which can occasionally be polymicrobial, can lead to endocarditis or other distant infections. When infections spread to produce suppurative thrombophlebitis of the internal jugular vein, a destructive syndrome with prolonged fever, bacteremia, septic emboli to both the lung and brain, and multiple metastatic foci of suppurative infection may develop. This syndrome has been reported with septicemia from species of *Fusobacterium* following exudative pharyngitis but is uncommon in this era of antimicrobial agents.

Central nervous system infections   Brain abscesses are frequently associated with anaerobic bacteria (see Chap. 374). If optimal bacteriologic techniques are employed, as many as 85 percent of brain abscesses yield anaerobic bacteria. The anaerobic bacteria found most often in these infections are anaerobic gram-positive cocci, followed in frequency by fusobacteria and *Bacteroides* species. Frequently, facultative or microaerophilic streptococci and coliforms are involved in brain abscesses as mixed infections.

Pleuropulmonary infections   Anaerobic pleuropulmonary infections result from the aspiration of oropharyngeal contents, which is often associated with an altered state of consciousness or absent gag reflex. There are four clinical syndromes associated with anaerobic pleuropulmonary infection produced by aspiration: simple aspiration pneumonia, necrotizing pneumonia, lung abscess, and empyema.

ASPIRATION PNEUMONITIS   Aspiration pneumonitis must be distinguished from two other types of aspiration pneumonitis, neither of which is bacterial. One aspiration syndrome results from aspiration of solids, usually food. Obstruction of major airways with resulting atelectasis is typical. Moderate nonspecific inflammation occurs. Therapy consists of removal of the foreign body.

A second aspiration syndrome is more easily confused with bacterial aspiration. This is the so-called Mendelson's syndrome, resulting from regurgitation of stomach contents and aspiration of chemical material, usually gastric juices. Pulmonary inflammation including destruction of alveolar lining with transudation of fluid into the alveolar space occurs with remarkable rapidity. Typically this syndrome develops within hours, often following anesthesia when the gag reflex is depressed. The patient becomes tachypneic, hypoxic, and febrile. The leukocyte count may rise, and the chest x-ray may evolve suddenly from normal to a complete whiteout bilaterally within 8 to 24 h. Minimal sputum production occurs. The pulmonary signs and symptoms can resolve quickly with symptomatic therapy or result in respiratory failure with subsequent development of bacterial superinfection over a period of days. Antibiotic therapy is not indicated unless bacterial infection supervenes. The signs of bacterial infection include sputum, persistent fever, leukocytosis, and clinical evidence of sepsis.

In contrast to these syndromes, bacterial aspiration pneumonia develops more slowly. It is seen in patients who are hospitalized and have a depressed gag reflex, elderly patients, or those with transient impaired consciousness in the wake of seizures or alcoholic blackouts. Patients who enter the hospital with this syndrome typically have been ill for several days and generally complain of low-grade fever, malaise, and sputum production. Usually the history reveals a predisposition for aspiration, such as alcohol overdose or residence in a nursing home. Sputum characteristically is not malodorous unless the process has been present for at least a week. Mixed bacterial flora with many polymorphonuclear leukocytes are present on Gram's stain; reliable cultures can be obtained only by avoiding contamination with normal oral flora, i.e., by transtracheal aspiration. In general, this procedure is not indicated in the evaluation of these patients.

Chest x-rays show consolidation in dependent pulmonary segments. These are the basilar segments of the lower lobes if the patient aspirated while upright or sitting, or the posterior segment of the upper lobe, usually on the right side, or the superior segment of the lower lobe if aspiration has occurred in the supine position. Organisms isolated reflect the pharyngeal flora; *P. melaninogenica*, *Fusobacterium* species, and anaerobic cocci are the most frequent isolates. The patient who aspirates in a hospital setting also may have mixed infection involving enteric gram-negative rods.

NECROTIZING PNEUMONITIS   This is a form of anaerobic pneumonitis characterized by numerous small abscesses which spread to involve several pulmonary segments. The process can be indolent or fulminating. This syndrome is less common than either aspiration pneumonia or lung abscess and includes features of both types of infection.

ANAEROBIC LUNG ABSCESSES   These result from subacute anaerobic pulmonary infection. The clinical syndrome typically involves a history of constitutional symptoms including malaise, weight loss, fever, chills, and foul-smelling sputum which may occur over a period of weeks (see Chap. 220). Patients who develop lung abscesses characteristically have dental infection and periodontitis, but there are reports of lung abscesses in patients who are edentulous. Abscess cavities may be single or multiple and generally occur in dependent pulmonary segments. Anaerobic abscesses must be distinguished from tuberculosis, neoplasia, and other causes of lung abscess, despite the fact that the clinical syndrome is usually typical. Oral anaerobes predominate, although *B. fragilis* is isolated in up to 10 percent of cases. *S. aureus* may be found as well. For many years penicillin was considered the gold standard of therapy for lung abscesses. Recent clinical trials have shown that clindamycin therapy results in a better clinical outcome than penicillin, presumably because of the enhanced spectrum of activity of clindamycin against oral anaerobes. Thus a combination of penicillin and metronidazole or other antibiotic combinations that treat both oral anaerobes and aerobes are likely to be as effective as clindamycin. Bronchoscopy is indicated only to rule out the presence of airway obstruction but should be delayed until the antimicrobial has begun to affect the disease process so that it does not spread the infection. Bronchoscopy has no role in enhancing drainage. Surgery is almost never indicated because of the danger of spilling the abscess contents into the lungs.

Empyema   Empyema is a manifestation of long-standing anaerobic pulmonary infection. The clinical presentation resembles other anaerobic pulmonary infections including the presence of foul-smelling sputum. Patients may complain of pleuritic chest pain and marked chest wall tenderness.

Empyema may be masked by overlying pneumonitis and should be considered especially in cases of persistent fever in a patient receiving antibiotic therapy. Diligent physical examination and the use of ultrasound to localize a loculated empyema are important diagnostic tools. The presence of a foul-smelling exudate obtained by thoracentesis is typical. Drainage is required. Defervescence, a return to a feeling of well-being, and resolution of the process may require several months.

Extension from a subdiaphragmatic infection also may result in an anaerobic empyema. Septic pulmonary emboli may originate from intraabdominal or female genital tract infections and can produce anaerobic pneumonia.

Intraabdominal infections (See Chap. 86)

Pelvic infections   The vagina of a healthy woman is one of the major reservoirs of anaerobic and aerobic bacteria. In the normal flora of the female genital tract, anaerobes outnumber aerobes by a ratio of approximately 10:1 and include anaerobic gram-positive cocci and *Bacteroides* species. Anaerobes are isolated from the majority of patients with infections of the genital tract, when infection is not caused by a sexually transmitted pathogen. The major anaerobic pathogens are *B. fragilis*, *P. bivius*, *P. disiens*, *P. melaninogenica*, anaerobic cocci, and clostridial species. Anaerobes frequently are encountered in tuboovarian abscess, septic abortion, pelvic abscess, endometritis, and postoperative wound infection, particularly following hysterectomy. Although these infections are frequently mixed, involving both anaerobes and coliforms, pure anaerobic infections without coliform or other facultative bacterial species occur more often in pelvic infections than in intraabdominal infections and are characterized by drainage of foul-smelling pus or blood from the uterus, generalized uterine or local pelvic tenderness, and continued fever and chills. Suppurative thrombophlebitis of the pelvic veins may complicate the infections and lead to repeated episodes of septic pulmonary emboli. Anaerobic bacteria have been the presumed cause of bacterial vaginosis, but some observers believe it is the anaerobic gram-negative coccobacillus belonging to the genus *Mobiluncus*. This hypothesis is not universally accepted, and others believe that an imbalance in the normal microbial flora of the female genital tract is key.

Skin and soft tissue infections   Injury to skin, bone, or soft tissue by trauma, ischemia, or surgery creates a suitable environment for anaerobic infections. These infections are most frequently found when the site is prone to contamination with feces or upper airway secretions. Examples include wounds associated with intestinal surgery, decubitus ulcers, and human bites. Anaerobic bacteria can be isolated in cases of crepitant cellulitis, synergistic cellulitis, or gangrene and necrotizing fasciitis. These organisms have been isolated from cutaneous abscesses, rectal abscesses, and axillary sweat gland infections (hydradenitis suppurativa). Anaerobes frequently have been cultured from foot ulcers in diabetic patients.

These soft tissue or skin infections are usually polymicrobial. A mean of 4.8 bacterial species can be isolated with a roughly 3:2 ratio of anaerobes to aerobes. The most frequently isolated organisms include *Bacteroides* species, anaerobic streptococci, enterococci, clostridial species, and *Proteus* species. The presence of anaerobes in these types of infections is associated with a higher frequency of fever, foul-smelling lesions, or a visible foot ulcer.

Anaerobic bacterial *synergistic gangrene* (Meleney's) is exquisitely painful, red, and swollen, followed by induration. Erythema surrounds a central zone of necrosis. A granulating ulcer which may heal forms at the original center as necrosis and erythema extend outward. Symptoms are limited to pain. Fever is not typical. These infections usually involve a combination of anaerobic cocci and *S. aureus*. Treatment includes surgical removal of necrotic tissue and antimicrobial therapy.

NECROTIZING FASCIITIS   This is a rapidly spreading destructive disease of the fascia, usually attributed to group A streptococci, but it can be caused by anaerobic bacteria including *Peptostreptococcus* and *Bacteroides* species. Similarly, myonecrosis can be associated with mixed anaerobic infection. Fournier's gangrene is an anaerobic cellulitis involving the scrotum, perineum, and anterior abdominal wall in which mixed anaerobic organisms spread along deep external fascial planes and cause extensive loss of skin.

Bone and joint infections   Although *actinomycosis* (see Chap. 127) accounts on a worldwide basis for the majority of anaerobic infections in bone, other organisms, including anaerobic or microaerophilic cocci, *Bacteroides* species, *Fusobacterium*, and *Clostridium* species, can be found. These infections frequently arise adjacent to soft tissue infections. Hematogenous seeding of bone is uncommon. Oral *Bacteroides* are seen in infections involving the maxilla and mandible, whereas *Clostridium* species have been reported as anaerobic pathogens in cases of osteomyelitis of the long bones, following fracture or trauma. Fusobacteria have been isolated in pure culture from osteomyelitis adjacent to the perinasal sinuses. Anaerobic and microaerophilic cocci have been reported as significant pathogens in infections involving the skull or mastoid.

In cases of anaerobic septic arthritis, the most common isolates are *Fusobacterium* species. Most of these patients have uncontrolled peritonsillar infections progressing to septic cervical venous thrombophlebitis and resulting in hematogenous dissemination which shows a predilection for the joints. Following the introduction of antibiotics, the isolation of *Fusobacterium* species from joints has been less

common. Unlike anaerobic osteomyelitis, most cases of pyoarthritis caused by anaerobes are not polymicrobial and may be acquired hematogenously. Anaerobes are important pathogens in infections involving prosthetic joints; in these infections, the causative organisms are part of the normal skin flora, such as anaerobic gram-positive cocci and *P. acnes*.

In patients with osteomyelitis (see Chap. 92), the most reliable source of culture is a bone biopsy obtained free from normal uninfected skin and subcutaneous tissue. If mixed flora is isolated from a bone biopsy, all isolates should be treated. When an anaerobic isolate is recognized as a major or sole pathogen involving a joint, the duration of treatment should be similar to that for arthritis caused by aerobic bacteria. Therapy includes management of underlying disease states, appropriate antimicrobial therapy, temporary joint immobilization, percutaneous drainage of effusions, and usually removal of infected prostheses or internal fixation devices. Surgical drainage and debridement such as sequestrectomy are essential for removal of necrotic tissue that would sustain anaerobic infections.

Bacteremia   Transient bacteremia is a well-known event that occurs in healthy people when the anatomic mucosal barriers are injured (e.g., dental extractions or dental scaling). These bacteremic episodes, which are often due to anaerobes, have no pathologic consequences. However, anaerobic bacteria are found in blood cultures from clinically ill patients when proper culture techniques are used. *B. fragilis* is the single most frequent anaerobic isolate. In recent years, the isolation rate for anaerobic bacteria from blood cultures has been decreasing. Studies from the 1970s and early 1980s reported that 10 to 15 percent of positive blood cultures grew anaerobes. More recently, similar surveys have yielded lower rates. The cause of this change is not defined but may relate to antibiotic prophylaxis before intestinal surgery, earlier recognition of localized infections, and the empirical use of broad-spectrum antibiotics for presumed infection.

The portal of bloodstream entry can frequently be deduced along with the likely underlying problem that led to seeding of the bloodstream by identification of the organism and understanding its place of normal residence. For example, mixed anaerobic bacteremia including *B. fragilis* usually implies colonic pathology with mucosal disruption from neoplasia, diverticulitis, or some other inflammatory lesion. The initial manifestations are determined by the portal of entry and reflect the localized condition. When bloodstream invasion occurs, patients can become extremely ill with rigors and hectic fevers ranging up to 40.6°C (105°F). The clinical picture may be quite similar to that seen in sepsis with aerobic gram-negative bacilli. Although other complications of anaerobic bacteremia such as septic thrombophlebitis and septic shock have been reported, the incidence of these complications in association with anaerobic bacteremia is low. Anaerobic bacteremia is potentially fatal and requires rapid diagnosis and appropriate therapy. Mortality appears to increase with the age of the patient (reported over 66 percent in patients over 60 years of age), polymicrobial bloodstream isolates, and failure to surgically remove a focus of infection.

ENDOCARDITIS (See Chap. 85)   Endocarditis due to anaerobes is uncommon. However, anaerobic streptococci, which are often classified incorrectly, are responsible for this disease more frequently than is appreciated. Gram-negative anaerobes are unusual causes of endocarditis.

DIAGNOSIS   Because of the time and difficulty involved in the isolation of anaerobic bacteria, diagnosis of these infections must frequently be made on presumptive evidence. Certain clinical settings such as avascular, necrotic tissues with lowered oxidation-reduction potential favor the diagnosis of an anaerobic infection. When infections occur in proximity to mucosal surfaces normally harboring anaerobic flora, such as the gastrointestinal tract, female genital tract, or oropharynx, anaerobes should be considered as potential etiologic agents. A foul odor often is present, since anaerobes produce certain organic acids as they proliferate in necrotic tissue. Although the presence of these odors is nearly pathognomonic for anaerobic infection, the absence of odor does not exclude these organisms as potential etiologic agents. Because anaerobes often coexist with other bacteria to form a mixed or synergistic infection, Gram-stained exudate frequently reveals numerous pleomorphic cocci and bacilli suggestive of anaerobes. Sometimes these organisms will have morphologic characteristics associated with specific species.

The presence of gas in tissues is highly suggestive, but not diagnostic, of anaerobes. Culture reports from obviously infected sites which yield no growth or only streptococci or a single aerobic species such as E. coli, when a Gram's stain reveals mixed flora, imply that the anaerobic microorganisms failed to grow because of inadequate transport and/or culture techniques. Failure of a patient to respond to antibiotics that are not active against anaerobes, e.g., aminoglycosides and, in some circumstances, penicillin, cephalosporins, or tetracyclines, suggests the possibility of anaerobic infection.

There are three critical steps to diagnose anaerobic infection: (1) proper specimen collection, (2) rapid transportation of these specimens to the microbiology laboratory, preferably in anaerobic transport media, and (3) proper handling of these specimens by the laboratory. Collection of specimens must be performed by meticulously sampling infected sites and avoiding contamination with normal flora. When there is a likely contamination of a specimen with normal flora, the specimen is unacceptable for processing by the bacteriology laboratory. Examples of unacceptable specimens for anaerobic culture include (1) sputum collected by expectoration or nasal tracheal suction, (2) bronchoscopy specimens, (3) direct collections through the vaginal vault, (4) collections of urine by voided specimen, and (5) feces. Specimens which can be cultured for anaerobes include blood, pleural fluid, transtracheal aspirates, pus obtained by direct aspiration from an abscess cavity, fluid obtained by culdocentesis, suprapubic bladder aspirates, cerebrospinal fluid, and lung puncture specimens.

Because even brief exposure to oxygen may kill some anaerobic organisms and result in failure to isolate them in the laboratory, abscess cavities which are aspirated with a syringe should have the air expelled and the needle capped with a sterile rubber stopper. Proper precautions should be utilized when handling contaminated needles. Specimens can be injected into transport bottles containing a reduced medium or brought immediately in syringes to the laboratory for direct culture on anaerobic media. In general, swabs should not be used. If a swab must be used, it should be placed in a reduced semisolid carrying medium before transport to the laboratory. Delays in transportation may lead to failure to isolate anaerobes due to exposure to oxygen or overgrowth of facultative organisms, which may eliminate or obscure the anaerobes that are present. All clinical specimens from suspected anaerobic infections should be Gram-stained and examined for organisms with characteristic morphology. It is not unusual for organisms to be observed on Gram's stain but not isolated in culture. If purulent materials are found to be sterile or organisms are seen on Gram's stain but do not grow in the culture, suspicion should be raised that anaerobes are involved.

TREATMENT Successful therapy of anaerobic infections involves a combination of appropriate antibiotics, surgical resection, and drainage. Perforations must be closed promptly, devitalized tissues removed, closed spaces drained, tissue compartments decompressed, and adequate blood supply established. Drainage of abscess cavities should be carried out as soon as fluctuation or localization occurs. While surgery was formerly required to establish drainage, with the advent of CT, MRI, and ultrasound, diagnostic radiologists now are able to perform percutaneous drainage of a number of abscess sites.

Patients with infections due to anaerobic bacteria require appropriate antibiotics. Antibiotic susceptibility testing of anaerobic bacteria has been difficult and controversial. The slow growth rate of many anaerobes, lack of standardized methodology, lack of clinically related standards for resistance, and generally good results with empirical therapy have resulted in susceptibility testing being recommended only for studying resistance patterns in regional centers or local hospitals, predicting efficacy of new antibiotics, and helping to manage selected patients. The selection of initial antibiotic therapy should be based on knowledge of the pathogens likely to be present in a specific clinical setting, in combination with the Gram-stain findings, which should suggest the likelihood of certain species of organisms. Because many anaerobic infections tend to be mixed with coliforms and other facultative organisms, it is advisable, in general, to use drugs active against both aerobic and anaerobic components. If anaerobes are suspected, the choice of empirical antibiotics can nearly always be made reliably, since patterns of antimicrobial susceptibility are usually predictable (see Chap. 100 and Table 128-1).

Organisms belonging to the B. fragilis group are resistant to penicillin. This clinically significant resistance mandates that anaerobic infections arising below the diaphragm be treated with specific therapy directed at B. fragilis (see Table 128-1). Recently, β-lactamase production has been reported in strains which are usually isolated from infections originating above the diaphragm. Forty to sixty percent of the clinical isolates classified at Prevotella and Porphyromonas, non–B. fragilis species of Bacteroides, and Fusobacterium species have been reported as producing β-lactamase. The clinical implications of this resistance has not been completely clarified, and most oral anaerobic infections and anaerobic pneumonia respond to penicillin therapy. However, clindamycin does appear to be superior to penicillin for the treatment of lung abscesses. Some infections due to oral organisms fail to respond to penicillin treatment, and in these cases the use of a drug which is effective against penicillin-resistant anaerobes is recommended (see Table 128-1). It is imperative that other appropriate antibiotics be used in conjunction with metronidazole in the treatment of mixed anaerobic and aerobic infections. Metronidazole is inactive against aerobic bacteria, Actinomyces, and Propionibacterium. The sensitivity of peptostreptococci to metronidazole is unpredictable. Therapy of intraabdominal sepsis (see Chap. 86) must include drugs active against the aerobic flora of the bowel. Combinations of antibiotics used in the treatment of mixed infections of oral origin must include antibiotics active against the aerobic flora of the mouth.

Infections arising from a colonic source are likely to contain B. fragilis. Many therapeutic failures have been noted in patients with documented B. fragilis infection who are treated with penicillin or first-generation cephalosporins. In intraabdominal sepsis, the use of antibiotics effective against anaerobes has clearly reduced the incidence of postoperative infection and serious infectious complications. The number of antimicrobial agents effective against B. fragilis has expanded, and there are currently several choices which are useful (see Table 128-1). In general, greater than 80 percent cure rates can be achieved in patients with B. fragilis infection when treated with appropriate antimicrobial therapy and drainage.

TABLE 128-1 Antimicrobial therapy for infections involving Bacteroides fragilis group, non–B. fragilis Bacteroides, and penicillin-resistant Prevotella, Porphyromonas, and Fusobacterium species, according to antimicrobial resistance

Group 1 (<1% resistance)	Group 2 (<15% resistance)	Group 3 (variable resistance)	Group 4 (resistant)
Metronidazole*	Clindamycin	Penicillin	Aminoglycosides
Ampicillin-sulbactam	Cefoxitin	Cephalosporins	Quinolones
or	High-dose	Tetracycline	Monobactams
Ticarcillin-clavulanic acid	antipseudomonal	Vancomycin	
Imipenem	penicillins	Erythromycin	
Chloramphenicol			

* Usually need to give in combination with aerobic bacterial coverage. For infections originating below the diaphragm, aerobic gram-negative coverage is essential. For infections from an oral source, aerobic gram-positive coverage is added. Metronidazole is also not active against Actinomyces or Propionibacterium and is unreliable against peptostreptococci.

Antibiotic recommendations for treatment of anaerobes is usually based on known resistance patterns in certain species and the likelihood of encountering a given species in the clinical setting at hand. Antibiotics active against the *B. fragilis* group, penicillin-resistant *Prevotella* and *Porphyromonas*, non–*B. fragilis* species of *Bacteroides*, and *Fusobacterium* species can be grouped into four categories based on their predicted activity against anaerobes (see Table 128-1).

Resistance of *B. fragilis* to metronidazole has been reported rarely. This well-tolerated drug achieves significant serum levels and also can be found in high levels within abscess cavities. It should be considered first-line therapy against *B. fragilis* infection. If a patient fails to respond to one of the group 1 or 2 drugs (Table 128-1), consideration should be given to alternative therapy and to determining the resistance patterns among *B. fragilis* group isolates. Although in vitro resistance to chloramphenicol has not been reported, this drug may not be as effective as other group 1 drugs. Among newer drugs, ampicillin-sulbactam, ticarcillin-clavulanic acid, and imipenem have been excellent in the treatment of *B. fragilis* infection. Penicillin remains the drug of choice for peptostreptococci.

Specific regimens must be tailored to the initial infecting site in clinical situations. In the treatment of intraabdominal sepsis, a group 1 drug must be included in the broad-spectrum coverage (see Chap. 86). If gram-positive bacteria are suspected, an appropriate penicillin should be added. Chloramphenicol can be used successfully in patients with anaerobic central nervous system infections at a dose of 30 to 60 mg/kg per day depending on the severity of illness. However, penicillin G and metronidazole also cross the blood-brain barrier and are bactericidal for many anaerobic organisms (see Chap. 374).

Nearly all the drugs mentioned have toxic side effects. These are described in detail in Chap. 100.

Anaerobic infections that have failed to respond to treatment or that relapse should be reassessed. Consideration should be given to additional surgical drainage or debridement. Superinfections with resistant gram-negative facultative or aerobic bacteria should be ruled out. Drug resistance also must be entertained; repeated cultures should yield the pathogenic organism.

Other supportive measures in the management of anaerobic infections include careful attention to fluid and electrolyte balance, since extensive local edema formation may lead to hypoalbuminemia; hemodynamic support for septic shock; immobilization of infected extremities; maintenance of adequate nutrition during chronic infections by parenteral hyperalimentation; relief of pain; and anticoagulation with heparin for thrombophlebitis. Hyperbaric oxygen therapy is advocated by some experts but is of no proven value.

REFERENCES

APPELBAUM PC et al: β-Lactamase production and susceptibilities to amoxicillin, amoxicillin-clavulanate, ticarcillin, ticarcillin-clavulanate, cefoxitin, imipenem, and metronidazole of 320 non–*Bacteroides fragilis Bacteroides* isolates and 129 fusobacteria from 28 U.S. Centers. Antimicrob Agents Chemother 34:1546, 1990

BARTLETT JG: Infections caused by anaerobic bacteria, in *Infectious Diseases*, SL Gorbach et al (eds). Philadelphia, Saunders, 1992

——, FINEGOLD SM: Anaerobic infections of the lung and pleural space. Am Rev Respir Dis 110:56, 1974

CRABB JH et al: T-cell regulation of *Bacteroides fragilis*–induced intraabdominal abscesses. Rev Infect Dis 12:S178, 1990

DORSHER CW et al: Anaerobic bacteremia: Decreasing rate over a 15-year period. Rev Infect Dis 13:633, 1991

FINEGOLD SM: Anaerobes: Problems and controversies in bacteriology, infections, and susceptibility testing. Rev Infect Dis 12:S223, 1990

——, GEORGE WL: *Anaerobic Infections in Humans*, San Diego, Academic, 1989

GIBBS RS: Microbiology of the female genital tract. Am J Obstet Gynecol 156:491, 1987

GORBACH SL: Anaerobic bacteria, in *Principles and Practices of Infectious Diseases*, 3d ed, GL Mandell et al (eds). New York, Wiley, 1990

HORN J et al: Role of anaerobic bacteria in permandibular space infections. Ann Otol Rhinol Laryngol Suppl 154:34, 1991

LEVIN S, GOODMAN LJ: Selected overview of nongynecologic surgical intraabdominal infections: Prophylaxis and therapy. Am J Med 79:146, 1985

MATHISEN GE et al: Brain abscess and cerebritis. Rev Infect Dis 6:5101, 1984

NAKATA MN, LEWIS RP: Anaerobic bacteria in bone and joint infections. Rev Infect Dis 6:5165, 1984

NEWMAN MG: Anaerobic oral and dental infections. Rev Infect Dis 6:5107, 1984

ONDERDONK AB et al: Animal model system for studying virulence of and host response to *Bacteroides fragilis*. Rev Infect Dis 12:S169, 1990

PANTOSTI A et al: Immunochemical characterization of two surface polysaccharides of *Bacteroides fragilis*. Infect Immun 59(5):1690, 1991

THORNSBERRY C: Antimicrobial susceptibility testing of anaerobic bacteria: Review and update on the role of the National Committee for Clinical Laboratory Standards. Rev Infect Dis 12:S218, 1990

TZIANABOS AO et al: Structural features of polysaccharides that induce intra-abdominal abscesses. Science 262:416, 1993

ZALEZNIK DF: Role of bacterial virulence factors in pathogenesis of anaerobic infections, in *Anaerobic Infections in Humans*, S. Finegold (ed). Orlando, Academic, 1989

——, KASPER DL: *Bacteroides* species, in *Principles and Practice of Infectious Diseases*, 3d ed, GL Mandell et al (eds). New York, Wiley, 1990

section 8 Mycobacterial diseases

129 ANTIMYCOBACTERIAL AGENTS

PAUL W. WRIGHT / RICHARD J. WALLACE

The physician is greatly challenged to provide optimal therapy for mycobacterial illnesses because of the advent of AIDS, the increase in both drug-susceptible and multidrug-resistant tuberculosis, and the plethora of new antibiotics with antimycobacterial potential. This chapter reviews the therapeutic agents used for treatment of tuberculosis, leprosy (Hansen's disease), and diseases caused by the pathogenic nontuberculous mycobacteria, including *M. avium-intracellulare* (MAI), *M. kansasii*, the rapidly growing mycobacteria, and *M. marinum*.

TUBERCULOSIS

Drugs used to treat tuberculosis have been classified into first-line and second-line agents. *First-line* antituberculous agents are the most effective and are considered essential for any short-course therapeutic regimen. The two drugs in this category are isoniazid and rifampin. First-line supplemental agents either can further shorten chemotherapy (e.g., pyrazinamide) or are considered highly effective, with infrequent toxicity (ethambutol and streptomycin). *Second-line* antituberculous drugs are clinically much less effective and have a much higher incidence of severe drug reactions. These drugs are used rarely in therapy and then only by individuals experienced in their use. They include *para*-aminosalicylic acid, ethionamide, cycloserine, kanamycin, amikacin, capreomycin, and thiacetazone.

FIRST-LINE ANTITUBERCULOUS DRUGS Isoniazid Perhaps the best antituberculous drug currently available, isoniazid should be included in all tuberculosis treatment regimens unless the organism is resistant. It is inexpensive, readily synthesized and available worldwide, very selective for mycobacteria, and well tolerated, with only 5 percent of patients exhibiting any adverse effects. In the United States it is usually given in combination form with rifampin.

MECHANISM OF ACTION Isoniazid is the hydrazide of isonicotinic acid, a small, water-soluble molecule that easily penetrates the cell. Its mechanism of action is inhibition of mycolic acid cell wall synthesis at unidentified sites. Isoniazid is bacteriostatic against resting bacilli and bactericidal against rapidly multiplying organisms, both extracellularly and intracellularly. Wild-type (untreated) strains of *M. tuberculosis* have minimal inhibitory concentrations (MICs) of <0.1 µg/mL, while *M. kansasii* usually has MICs in the range of 0.5 to 2.0 µg/mL. The MICs for other mycobacteria are much higher.

PHARMACOLOGY Both oral and intramuscular preparations are readily absorbed; a 300-mg oral dose produces peak serum levels that are usually within the 3 to 5 µg/mL range. Isoniazid diffuses well throughout the body and provides therapeutic concentrations in serum, cerebrospinal fluid (CSF), and infected tissue, including caseous granulomas. Isoniazid is metabolized in the liver via acetylation and hydrolysis, with the metabolites being excreted into the urine. The rate of acetylation is genetically controlled. The usual daily dosage for tuberculosis is 5 mg/kg for adults and 10 to 20 mg/kg for children, to a maximum daily dose of 300 mg for both groups. Even in moderate to severe renal failure, the adult dose rarely needs reduction below 200 mg/d.

ADVERSE EFFECTS (Table 129-1) The two most important adverse effects of isoniazid therapy are hepatotoxicity and peripheral neuropathy. Other adverse effects are either rare or less significant and include rash (2 percent), fever (1.2 percent), anemia, acne, arthritic symptoms, optic atrophy, seizures, and psychiatric symptoms. Isoniazid-associated hepatitis is idiosyncratic and increases in incidence with age. It occurs in 0.3 percent of those under 35 years of age, 1.2 percent of those under 49 years of age, and 2.3 percent of those over 50 years of age. An increased risk of isoniazid-related hepatitis is associated with daily alcohol consumption, concomitant rifampin administration, and slow acetylation of isoniazid (Table 129-2). Mortality from isoniazid-induced hepatitis has been reported to be 6 to 12 percent, but the real risk is certainly much lower, since this rate occurred in high-risk patients who continued taking the drug despite progressive symptoms of hepatitis and without monitoring of liver enzymes. Liver enzymes are routinely monitored in most current settings among all high-risk patients. No specific guidelines have been proposed, but a reasonable approach would be to determine serum AST or ALT at baseline, at 2 and 4 weeks, and monthly thereafter for up to 6 months. An ALT or AST level is mandatory, however, whenever a patient notices the onset of symptoms suggestive of isoniazid hepatitis (i.e., fever, anorexia, nausea, flulike syndrome, etc.), with immediate discontinuation of the drug until the relationship between the two is determined. Isoniazid also should be discontinued whenever an asymptomatic AST or ALT level exceeds 150 to 200 IU. When these guidelines are followed, death from isoniazid-associated hepatitis has occurred at a rate of only 14 per 100,000 treated patients. Twelve percent of patients taking isoniazid may experience transient elevations of AST. If the AST elevation persists, if AST is elevated more than three to five times normal, or if symptoms of hepatitis occur, drug withdrawal is required.

Peripheral neuritis associated with isoniazid occurs at a dose-dependent rate of 2 to 20 percent; this rate can be reduced to 0.2 percent with the prophylactic administration of 10 to 50 mg pyridoxine (vitamin B_6) daily.

RESISTANCE Isoniazid-resistant mutants of *M. tuberculosis* occur spontaneously at a rate of 1 in 10^5 to 10^6 organisms. The mechanism and molecular site of isoniazid resistance developed in the laboratory or in vivo are unknown. However, recent molecular genetic studies of some mycobacterial strains demonstrate an association of isoniazid resistance with reduced catalase and peroxidase activity. These studies demonstrated restored or increased bacterial sensitivities to isoniazid in an isoniazid-resistant strain of *M. smegmatis* and some strains of *Escherichia coli*, which were genetically engineered with a single *M. tuberculosis* gene encoding for both catalase and peroxidase. Conversely, they showed isoniazid resistance in two clinical isolates of *M. tuberculosis* from which this same gene was deleted. Primary drug resistance occurs in previously untreated patients at a rate of 7 percent in native U. S. populations but may approach 50 percent in immigrant populations from Southeast Asia. To prevent secondary drug resistance, isoniazid should be given in combination with one or more effective antituberculous drugs.

Rifampin Rifampin, a semisynthetic derivative of *Streptomyces mediterranei*, is the second most important antituberculous agent with efficacy against *M. tuberculosis* comparable with that of isoniazid. It is also active against a wide spectrum of other organisms, including some gram-positive and gram-negative bacteria, *Legionella* species, *M. kansasii*, *M. marinum*, and some strains of MAI.

PHARMACOLOGY Rifampin is a fat-soluble complex macrocyclic antibiotic that is absorbed readily either orally or intravenously. Serum levels of 10 to 20 µg/mL are achieved after a standard oral dose of 600 mg. Rifampin distributes well throughout most body tissues, including inflamed meninges. It turns body fluids (urine, saliva, sputum, tears) to a red-orange color, thereby providing a simple and inexpensive check on patient compliance. Rifampin is excreted primarily through the bile and enterohepatic circulation, while 30 to 40 percent is excreted via the kidneys. It is administered once daily, usually 600 mg for adults (10 mg/kg) and 10 to 20 mg/kg for children.

MECHANISM OF ACTION Rifampin has both intracellular and extracellular bactericidal activity. It blocks RNA synthesis by specifically binding and inhibiting DNA-dependent RNA polymerase. Susceptible strains of *M. tuberculosis* as well as *M. kansasii* and *M. marinum* are inhibited by 1 µg/mL or less.

ADVERSE EFFECTS (Table 129-1) Even though the drug is generally well tolerated, patients with chronic liver disease, especially alcoholism and old age, appear to be at higher risk for the most common adverse drug reaction, which is hepatotoxicity. Other adverse effects include a flulike syndrome (20 percent, primarily with intermittent therapy), nausea and vomiting (1.5 percent), rash (0.8 percent), hemolytic anemia (<1 percent), renal failure due to interstitial nephritis or acute tubular necrosis (<1 percent), and immunosuppression of questionable clinical importance. Rifampin induces hepatic microsomal enzyme production and thereby decreases the half-life of a number of drugs, including digoxin, warfarin, prednisone,

TABLE 129-1 Monitoring adverse effects of common antituberculosis drugs

Drug	Adverse effect	What to monitor/management
Isoniazid	Hepatitis	AST/limit alcohol consumption/ monitor for hepatitis symptoms
	Peripheral neuritis	Administer vitamin B_6
	Optic neuritis	Administer vitamin B_6
	Seizures	Administer vitamin B_6
Rifampin	Rash	Observation
	Liver dysfunction	AST/limit alcohol consumption/ monitor for hepatitis symptoms
	Flulike syndrome	Administer twice or more weekly
	Red-orange urine	Reassure patient
	Drug interaction	Consider monitoring drug levels, when possible, especially with contraceptives, anticoagulants, chloramphenicol, and digoxin.
Pyrazinamide	Hepatitis	AST/limit dosage to 15–30 mg/ kg per day
	Hyperuricemia	Monitor uric acid level only if symptomatic with gout or renal failure
Ethambutol	Optic neuritis	Use lower dose (15 g/kg per day) when possible; monitor visual acuity and color vision monthly; educate patient about this side effect.
Streptomycin	Ototoxicity	Limit dose and length of therapy as possible; BUN, serum creatinine, audiometry before and (as needed) during therapy; screen patients for tinnitus, nausea, and vertigo, and decreased hearing; Measure levels if possible.

propranolol, cyclosporine, methadone, oral contraceptives, and quinidine (Table 129-2).

RESISTANCE Rifampin resistance occurs as a result of spontaneous mutations that presumably affect either cell wall transport (low-level resistance) or the RNA polymerase (high-level resistance). Recent studies with rifampin resistant *M. leprae* showed 8 of 9 strains to have a mutation involving a serine residue in the rpoB gene, which encodes the beta subunit of RNA polymerase.

FIRST-LINE SUPPLEMENTAL DRUGS Pyrazinamide (PZA) A derivative of nicotinic acid, pyrazinamide is an important bactericidal drug used in short-course chemotherapy of tuberculosis.

PHARMACOLOGY Pyrazinamide is well absorbed after oral administration, with a plasma concentration of 45 μg/mL in 2 h and excellent distribution throughout the body. It is hydrolyzed in the liver into several metabolites, one of which, pyrazinoic acid, is considered the active form of the drug. Pyrazinoic acid is then hydroxylated to 5-hydroxypyrazinoic acid, which is subsequently excreted by renal glomerular filtration.

MECHANISM OF ACTION Pyrazinamide is similar to isoniazid in its narrow spectrum of antibacterial activity against essentially only *M. tuberculosis*. The drug is considered primarily effective against slowly metabolizing organisms located within the acid environment of the phagocyte or caseous granuloma, since it is active only at a pH below 6.0. The mechanism of action is unknown.

ADVERSE EFFECTS (Table 129-1) With the high dosages used in the past, hepatotoxicity was a major complication of pyrazinamide therapy. However, at the current recommended dosages of 15 to 30 mg/kg with a maximum of 2 g/d (may be given in one daily dose), the occurrence of hepatotoxicity is not increased over that observed with concomitant isoniazid and rifampin therapy. Hyperuricemia is a common adverse effect of pyrazinamide therapy that is probably reduced by concurrent rifampin therapy. Clinical gout is only rarely seen in patients receiving pyrazinamide; polyarthralgias are not uncommonly encountered but are not related to the hyperuricemia.

Ethambutol A derivative of ethylenediamine, ethambutol is a water-soluble compound that is active only against mycobacteria. Susceptible species include *M. tuberculosis*, *M. marinum*, *M. kansasii*, and MAI. Among first-line drugs, it is the least potent against *M. tuberculosis*. It is used most often with rifampin in the treatment of tuberculosis in patients who are unable to tolerate isoniazid or who are suspected or known to be infected with isoniazid-resistant organisms.

MECHANISM OF ACTION Ethambutol is bacteriostatic against rapidly growing mycobacteria. The mechanisms of action and resistance to ethambutol are unknown.

PHARMACOLOGY After oral administration, 75 to 80 percent of the drug is absorbed from the gastrointestinal route and produces peak serum levels of 2 to 4 μg/mL 2 to 4 h after the usual 15 mg/kg dose. Distribution throughout the body is adequate except in the CSF, where it achieves only low levels. Almost all the drug is excreted by the kidneys within 24 h of ingestion, either unchanged or as metabolites. The usual adult dosage of ethambutol is 15 mg/kg (may be given in one daily dose) in initial treatment regimens and 25 mg/kg in retreatment regimens (usually 800 to 1600 mg daily) or for the initial 6 to 8 weeks on the four-drug regimen for suspected drug-resistant tuberculosis. These dosages must be lowered in patients with renal insufficiency (creatinine clearance of <25 mL/min) to prevent drug accumulation and toxicity.

ADVERSE EFFECTS (Table 129-1) The drug is usually well tolerated, with optic neuritis (usually retrobulbar) being the most serious adverse effect. Axial or central neuritis, the only form of retrobulbar optic neuritis reported in patients taking daily doses of <30 mg/kg, involves the papillomacular bundle of fibers and results in reduced visual acuity, central scotoma, and loss of ability to see green. Symptoms of ocular toxicity typically occur several months after initiation of therapy, but rapid-onset optic neuritis has been reported. Optic neuritis is dependent on dose and duration of therapy and occurs in 5 percent of patients receiving 25 mg/kg but less than 1 percent of patients on a dose of 15 mg/kg. Patients should be tested monthly for visual acuity and red-green color discrimination. Optic neuritis with the associated visual loss is usually reversible, but recovery may take up to 6 months.

Other adverse effects with ethambutol are infrequent. Hyperuricemia occurs but is usually asymptomatic. The drug is not recommended for young children in whom visual complications would be difficult to monitor.

Streptomycin Streptomycin is an aminoglycoside which was isolated from *Streptomyces griseus*. It is available for intramuscular administration only. In the United States it is the least used first-line supplemental drug for tuberculosis because of its toxicity, the difficulty in obtaining serum levels, and the inconvenience of intramuscular administration. In developing countries, however, it is frequently used because of its low cost. Streptomycin is active against untreated strains of *M. tuberculosis*, *M. kansasii*, and *M. marinum* and some strains of MAI at readily achievable serum levels.

PHARMACOLOGY The drug achieves peak serum levels of 25 to 40 μg/mL after a 1.0-g dose. Streptomycin is bactericidal for rapidly dividing extracellular mycobacteria but is ineffective in the acid environment within the macrophage. It diffuses poorly into the meninges and achieves CSF levels in patients with meningitis that are only 20 percent of the serum drug level.

The usual adult dose is 0.5 to 1.0 g/d (10 to 15 mg/kg) or five times per week; the pediatric dose is 20 to 40 mg/kg per day, with a maximum of 1.0 g/d. Dosage must be lowered in most patients over 50 years of age and in any patient with renal impairment because streptomycin is almost exclusively eliminated by the kidneys.

MECHANISM OF ACTION Streptomycin inhibits protein synthesis by disruption of ribosomal function.

ADVERSE EFFECTS (Table 129-1) Adverse effects from streptomycin therapy occur in 10 to 20 percent of patients, with ototoxicity and renal toxicity being the most common and serious. Renal toxicity, usually manifested as nonoliguric renal failure, is less common with streptomycin than with other commonly used aminoglycosides such as gentamicin. Ototoxicity involves both hearing loss and vestibular dysfunction. The latter is more common and includes nausea, vertigo, and tinnitus. Patients receiving streptomycin must be monitored carefully for these adverse effects. Less serious effects include eosinophilia, rash, and drug fever.

TABLE 129-2 Major antituberculous drug interactions

Rifampin	Isoniazid	Pyrazinamide	Ethambutol	Streptomycin
Warfarin	Warfarin	Probenecid	Antacids	Methicillin
Glucocorticoids	Glucocorticoids			
Cyclosporine	Alcohol			
Digoxin	Antacids			
Quinidine	PAS			
Oral contraceptives	Oral contraceptives			
Oral hypoglycemic agents	Levodopa			
Ketoconazole	Ketoconazole			
Narcotics	Meperidine			
Halothane	Enflurane			
Barbiturates	Aspirin			
Diazepam	Benzodiazepines			
Beta blockers	Propranolol			
Analgesics				
Verapamil				
Clofibrate				
Progestins				
Disopyramide				
Mexiletine				
Theophylline				
Chloramphenicol				
Anticonvulsants				
Probenecid				
Dapsone				

RESISTANCE   Streptomycin resistance in mycobacteria is believed to be similar in mechanism to resistance in other bacteria. It develops rapidly with one-drug therapy, and random mutational resistance occurs in 1 in 10^5 organisms. Low-level resistance can result from alterations in cellular transport, while high-level resistance is secondary to alteration in the ribosomal binding protein. Isolates of *M. tuberculosis* resistant to streptomycin are not cross-resistant to capreomycin or amikacin.

SECOND-LINE ANTITUBERCULOUS DRUGS   Second-line antituberculous drugs are used either for drug-resistant tuberculosis or when first-line supplemental drugs are not available. The more important second-line drugs are discussed below.

***Para*-aminosalicylic acid (PAS)**   PAS is rarely indicated because of its low antituberculous activity and its high gastrointestinal toxicity (consisting of nausea, vomiting, diarrhea) and occasional hepatitis. Adult dosage is 10 to 12 g/d in several doses and requires the patient to swallow 20 to 24 large and unpleasant-tasting tablets. PAS is well absorbed from oral administration and is distributed throughout the body, but it has low concentrations in the CSF. The drug has a short half-life of 1 h, and 80 percent is excreted in the urine.

Ethionamide   Another derivative of isonicotinic acid (as are isoniazid and PZA), ethionamide exerts bactericidal activity against metabolizing *M. tuberculosis* and some nontuberculous mycobacteria. It is most useful in the therapy of multidrug-resistant tuberculosis. However, drug use is severely limited by its toxicity and frequent adverse effects that include intense gastrointestinal intolerance (anorexia, vomiting, and dysgeusia), serious neurologic reactions, reversible hepatitis (5 percent), hypersensitivity reactions, and hypothyroidism. It is well absorbed orally and widely distributed throughout the body, including the CSF. Ethionamide is excreted primarily through the kidneys, with 99 percent of the drug being excreted as a metabolite. Adult patients initially are given 250-mg tablets twice daily and then increased to 250 mg four times daily (15 mg/kg per day with 1 g/d maximum) as tolerated. Pyridoxine should be administered with ethionamide.

Cycloserine   Cycloserine, D-4-amino-3-isoxazolidinone, is produced by *Streptomyces orchidaceus* and has activity against a broad spectrum of bacteria as well as *M. tuberculosis*. It has excellent oral absorption and is widely distributed throughout body fluids, including the CSF. Serious adverse effects limit the use of this drug and include psychosis even resulting in suicide, seizures, peripheral neuropathy, headaches, somnolence, and allergic reactions. Because excretion is primarily renal, dosage must be adjusted in patients with reduced renal function. The usual adult dose is 250 mg three times per day (15 to 20 mg/kg). Plasma concentrations should be maintained below 30 μg/mL to reduce toxicity. However, the assay for determination of plasma levels is not performed in most hospital laboratories. Pyridoxine should be administered with this drug. Cycloserine should not be given to patients with epilepsy, active alcohol abuse, severe renal insufficiency, or a history of depression or psychosis.

Capreomycin   Capreomycin is a complex cyclic polypeptide antibiotic derived from *Streptomyces capreolus*. This drug is similar to streptomycin in dosing, mechanism of action, pharmacology, and toxicity. It is administered only by the intramuscular route in doses of 10 to 15 mg/kg per day or five times per week (maximum daily dose of 1 g), with peak blood levels of 20 to 40 μg/mL. Patients should be monitored closely for renal and eighth cranial nerve toxicity, which are of major concern with this drug. Dosage must be reduced in patients over 50 years of age and those with renal insufficiency. Cross-resistance with kanamycin and amikacin is common, but not with streptomycin. Capreomycin is the injectable drug of choice for tuberculosis in patients unable to tolerate streptomycin due to hypersensitivity or whose isolate is streptomycin-resistant.

Kanamycin and amikacin   These are well-known aminoglycosides that are bactericidal to extracellular organisms. Kanamycin is rarely used because of greater toxicity. Amikacin is active against *M. tuberculosis* and several of the nontuberculous species, including the rapidly growing mycobacteria, *M. scrofulaceum*, MAI, and *M. leprae*.

The usual dosage is 10 mg/kg intramuscularly or intravenously three to five times a week, with a maximum daily dose of 0.5 g.

Thiacetazone   This drug is not available in the United States but is widely used in combination with isoniazid to treat tuberculosis in the developing world because it is inexpensive and readily available. It is usually given in a dosage of 150 mg/d in combination with 300 mg isoniazid in a single tablet. Thiacetazone is structurally related to isoniazid but is bacteriostatic and more toxic.

Rifabutin   This is a recently approved derivative of rifamycin that is related to rifampin. It is bactericidal against *M. tuberculosis*, MAI, and other nontuberculous mycobacteria. Rifabutin appears to have efficacy in treating both tuberculosis and nontuberculous mycobacterial infections. Usual adult dosage will probably be 300 to 600 mg/d. The drug produces much lower serum levels than rifampin but has a much longer half-life and is much more active against isolates of MAI. Isolates of *M. tuberculosis* resistant to rifampin are usually cross-resistant to rifabutin.

Quinolones   Two newer fluorinated quinolones, ciprofloxacin and ofloxacin, show activity against many of the mycobacteria, especially *M. tuberculosis*, *M. marinum*, *M. kansasii*, and *M. fortuitum*. These two drugs are well absorbed orally, reach high serum levels, and distribute well to body tissues and fluid. Adverse effects, which are uncommon (0.5 to 3 percent), include gastrointestinal intolerance, skin rashes, or CNS problems such as headache, insomnia, and dizziness. The quinolones prevent DNA synthesis by inhibiting DNA gyrase. Resistance, from either a change in the permeability of the organism or a change in the DNA gyrase, develops rapidly with mycobacteria as with bacterial species.

LEPROSY (HANSEN'S DISEASE)

Therapy for leprosy remains difficult, especially in developing countries, because of the length of therapy required, the cost and availability of drugs, frequent adverse effects, acquired drug resistance, and the difficulty of susceptibility testing given the inability to grow the organism in vitro. While many drugs show activity against *M. leprae*, only dapsone, rifampin, and clofazimine are part of standard World Health Organization (WHO) therapy for paucibacillary and multibacillary leprosy.

DAPSONE (DDS)   Dapsone (4,4'-diaminodiphenylsulfone), a sulfone, inhibits bacterial folic acid synthesis. It is considered the drug of first choice in most cases of Hansen's disease because of its availability, low cost, low toxicity, and the susceptibility of untreated strains of *M. lepra* to very low concentrations of the drug.

Pharmacology   The drug is well absorbed orally and distributes well throughout the body. The usual adult daily dosage is 100 mg and 1.0 to 1.5 mg per kg for children. Peak plasma concentrations occur within 1 to 3 h, and the median half-life of elimination is 22 h. Dapsone is cleared by acetylation in the liver, with genetic variation similar to the acetylation of isoniazid. The drug is 70 percent bound to plasma protein. Usual daily doses produce serum concentrations of 10 to 15 μg/mL that far exceed the MIC for *M. leprae* of 0.01 to 0.001 μg/mL.

Adverse effects   Hemolysis and methemoglobinemia are common untoward reactions to dapsone. Patients should be screened for glucose-6-phosphate dehydrogenase deficiency to prevent drug-induced hemolysis. However, most patients tolerate dapsone therapy well with adequate clinical and laboratory supervision. Other adverse effects include gastrointestinal intolerance, headache, pruritus, agranulocytosis, fever, and rash. In lepromatous leprosy, erythema nodosum leprosum (ENL) may occur and may be difficult to distinguish from allergic reactions to the drug (dapsone syndrome).

RIFAMPIN   Rifampin, the second most useful drug in leprosy therapy, has the major limitation worldwide of cost. It is bactericidal against *M. leprae* and rapidly reduces the number of viable bacilli in patient tissue. It must be combined with other antileprosy drugs to prevent the development of resistance. For cost reasons the drug is given 600 mg once a month (supervised) outside the United States but is given daily in the United States.

CLOFAZIMINE A phenazine iminoquinone dye, clofazimine is weakly bactericidal against *M. leprae*. It is useful in treating dapsone-resistant leprosy and may lessen ENL. Clofazimine's mode of action is not well understood, but it may inhibit DNA binding. The drug is absorbed orally and distributed to the fatty tissues and the reticuloendothelial system. Its serum half-life is about 60 to 70 days, with only a small amount being excreted daily into the urine or bile. Bactericidal activity occurs very slowly and may be observed about 50 days after administration. Usual adult dosage is 50 to 100 mg/d, 100 mg three times a week, or 300 mg/d for treatment of ENL. Untoward effects include skin discoloration and, less commonly, gastrointestinal intolerance. Clofazimine also has in vitro activity against some of the nontuberculous mycobacterial species, including MAI, *M. kansasii*, *M. simiae*, and *M. abscessus*.

OTHER AGENTS A number of other drugs show significant activity against *M. leprae*, but clinical experience with these agents is lacking. Thalidomide may be useful in suppressing ENL but acts as a tranquilizer and is also extremely teratogenic; it is no longer available in the United States. Second-line drugs for the treatment of leprosy include ethionamide, prothionamide, and amithiozone (a thiosemicarbazone).

The newer macrolide antibiotics, particularly clarithromycin, and minocycline, a long-acting tetracycline, and a number of the fluoroquinolones have recently shown bactericidal activity against *M. leprae* in mice. Ofloxacin appears to be the most bactericidal agent among the newer quinolones. These new drugs show considerable promise for leprosy therapy because of their low toxicity and various modes of action that differ from the established drugs. Rifabutin has similar activity to rifampin, but its longer half-life may facilitate less frequent dosing.

NONTUBERCULOUS MYCOBACTERIA (NTM)

The nontuberculous mycobacteria are of low pathogenicity but cause pulmonary, skin, bone and joint, lymph node, and soft tissue infection and disseminated disease in immunocompromised hosts, including patients with AIDS. MAI and *M. kansasii* are the two most common causes of NTM pulmonary infection; up to 40 percent of AIDS patients develop disseminated disease with MAI.

MAI Therapy for MAI is controversial because of the lack of controlled clinical trials. First-line antituberculous drugs are much less active against MAI than against *M. tuberculosis*. Cycloserine and ethionamide show the best in vitro activity but are markedly limited by their toxicity. The American Thoracic Society recommends the following initial daily therapy for MAI lung disease (HIV-negative patients) for 18 to 24 months: isoniazid (300 mg), rifampin (600 mg), ethambutol (25 g/kg and 15 mg/kg from the third month on), with 0.5 to 1.0 g streptomycin. The streptomycin therapy should be 5 days per week for the first 6 to 12 weeks and then two to three times per week for a total of 3 to 6 months of therapy as tolerated. Because of the relatively poor in vivo and in vitro activity of isoniazid and its higher incidence of toxicity in the elderly population, replacement of isoniazid with one of the newer macrolides has been suggested by some experts but has not been studied by clinical trial. For disseminated disease in AIDS, commonly used drugs include one of the newer macrolides (clarithromycin or azithromycin) plus rifampin, ethambutol, and/or clofazimine. Alternative drugs include ciprofloxacin, amikacin, ethionamide, and cycloserine. Rifabutin at a dose of 300 mg/d was recently approved for prophylaxis of disseminated MAI in AIDS patients with CD4 counts of less than 100.

MYCOBACTERIUM KANSASII *M. kansasii* is usually sensitive to most antituberculous drugs, with the major exception of pyrazinamide. Current recommendations for therapy of pulmonary disease are 18 to 24 months of daily isoniazid (300 mg), rifampin (600 mg), and ethambutol (15 mg/kg).

RAPIDLY GROWING MYCOBACTERIA (RGM) *M. fortuitum*, *M. abscessus*, and *M. chelonae* account for more than 80 percent of clinical disease due to the RGM. They are resistant to antituberculous agents other than amikacin but are variably susceptible to several traditional antibiotics, including amikacin (80 to 100 percent), cefoxitin (80 percent of *M. abscessus* and *M. fortuitum*), doxycycline (50 percent of *M. fortuitum*), imipenem (100 percent of *M. fortuitum*, 70 percent of *M. chelonae* and *M. abscessus*), and the fluorinated quinolones (ciprofloxacin and ofloxacin, 100 percent of *M. fortuitum*), and sulfonamides (90 percent of *M. fortuitum*).

MYCOBACTERIUM MARINUM *M. marinum*, a photochromogen, is typically susceptible to minocycline, rifampin, ethambutol, clarithromycin, and trimethoprim/sulfamethoxazole.

CLARITHROMYCIN Clarithromycin, 6-O-methylerythromycin, is a new macrolide that is similar to erythromycin in mechanism of action. However, unlike erythromycin, it is well absorbed with or without meals and has little gastrointestinal intolerance at low doses. It distributes well into body tissues and fluids, but there are no data about its penetration into the CSF. The drug is metabolized in the liver, with approximately 30 percent excreted in the urine. Standard dosage for bacterial infections is 250 to 500 mg twice daily. Dosage should be reduced if the creatinine clearance is 30 mL/min or less. As with erythromycin, the drug binds with plasma proteins (65 to 70 percent) and can raise the levels of drugs such as theophylline and carbamazepine. Clarithromycin appears to be the best single drug for therapy of MAI infections, especially disseminated disease in AIDS patients. However, because the organism may acquire drug resistance, the drug should be combined with other antimycobacterial agents such as ethambutol and rifampin. The drug is also highly active against *M. marinum*, *M. kansasii*, *M. chelonae*, and most isolates of *M. fortuitum*. Standard antimycobacterial drug doses have been 500 mg twice daily, with doses of 1000 mg twice daily generally being used in disseminated MAI disease in AIDS patients. The more common adverse effects seen with high doses include nausea, vomiting, a bitter taste, and occasionally abnormal liver function tests. The drug is teratogenic in laboratory animals and is rated category C for pregnancy. Azithromycin, another new macrolide, appears to have similar activity in vitro, but less is known about its clinical activity against mycobacteria.

REFERENCES

EDWARDS E, KIRKPATRICK CH: The immunology of mycobacterial disease. Am Rev Respir Dis 134:1062, 1986

HASTINGS RC et al: Leprosy. Clin Microbiol Rev 1:330, 1988

HEIFETS LB et al: Clarithromycin minimal inhibitory and bactericidal concentrations against *Mycobacterium avium*. Am Rev Respir Dis 145:856, 1992

JACOBS RF, ABERNATHY RS: Management of tuberculosis in pregnancy and the newborn. Clin Perinatol 15:305, 1988.

LEIBOLD JE: The ocular toxicity of ethambutol and its relation to dose. Ann NY Acad Sci 135:904, 1966

MACKAY AD, COLE RB: The problems of tuberculosis in the elderly. Q J Med 53:497, 1984

O'BRIEN RJ: Present chemotherapy of tuberculosis. Semin Respir Infect 4:216, 1989

REYNOLDS JEF (ed): *Martindale The Extra Pharmacopoeia*, 29th ed. London, The Pharmaceutical Press, 1989

SCHILD HS et al: Rapid reversible ocular toxicity from ethambutol therapy. Am J Med 90:404, 1991

STAKRE JR et al: Medical Progress: Resurgence of tuberculosis in children. J Pediatr 120:839, 1992

UNDERLIED CB: Antimycobacterial agents: in vitro susceptibility testing, spectrums of activity, mechanism of action and resistance, and assays for activity in biological fluid, in *Antibiotics in Laboratory Medicine*, 3d ed, V Lorian (ed). Baltimore, Williams & Wilkins, 1991, pp 134–197

WALLACE RJ JR et al: Diagnosis and treatment of disease caused by nontuberculous mycobacteria. Am Rev Respir Dis 142:940, 1990

WAYNE LG, SRAMEK HA: Agents of newly recognized or infrequently encountered mycobacterial diseases. Clin Microbiol Rev 5:1, 1992

WOLINSKY E: Nontuberculous mycobacteria and associated diseases. Am Rev Respir Dis 119:107, 1979

YODER LJ: Leprosy. Curr Opin Infect Dis 4:302, 1991

ZHANG Y et al: The catalase-peroxidase gene and isoniazid resistance of *Mycobacterium tuberculosis*. Nature 358:591, 1992

130 TUBERCULOSIS

THOMAS M. DANIEL

DEFINITION　Tuberculosis is a chronic bacterial infection caused by *Mycobacterium tuberculosis* and characterized by the formation of granulomas in infected tissues and by cell-mediated hypersensitivity. The usual site of disease is the lungs, but other organs may be involved. In the absence of effective treatment for active disease, a chronic wasting course is usual, and death ultimately supervenes.

ETIOLOGY　*Mycobacterium tuberculosis*, the tubercle bacillus, is one of more than 30 well-characterized and many unclassified members of the genus *Mycobacterium*. Along with the closely related *M. bovis*, it causes tuberculosis. *M. leprae* is the etiologic agent of leprosy (see Chap. 131). *M. avium* and a number of other mycobacterial species produce less common human diseases (see Chap. 132). Most mycobacteria are not pathogenic for humans, and many are readily isolated from environmental sources.

Mycobacteria are distinguished by their surface lipids, which render them acid-fast so that they cannot be decolorized with acid alcohol after staining. Because of this lipid, heat or detergents are usually necessary to accomplish primary staining.

Important to understanding the pathogenesis of tuberculosis is recognition that *M. tuberculosis* contains many immunoreactive substances. Surface lipids of mycobacteria and water-soluble components of cell wall peptidoglycan are important adjuvants that may exert their effects through their primary actions on host macrophages. Mycobacteria contain an array of protein and polysaccharide antigens, some probably species-specific but others clearly sharing epitopes broadly throughout the genus. Cell-mediated hypersensitivity is characteristic of tuberculosis and is an important determinant of the disease's pathogenesis.

EPIDEMIOLOGY　Tuberculosis continues as an important cause of death. In 1991, a total of 26,283 cases of tuberculosis were reported in the United States, a case rate of 10.4 per 100,000 per year. The case rate had been falling at a rate of 5 to 6 percent per year, but since 1985 this trend has reversed, with the rate having increased by 15.8 percent in the ensuing 5 years. It is estimated that 10 million Americans have a positive tuberculin test but that fewer than 1 percent of American children are tuberculin reactors. Tuberculosis in North America tends to be a disease of the elderly, of the urban poor, of minority groups, and of patients with AIDS. At all ages, case rates among nonwhites tend to be twice those in whites. Hispanic, Haitian, and Southeast Asian immigrants may have case rates as high as those of the countries from which they come, and in these individuals the frequency of disease among younger persons reflects its occurrence in young individuals in those countries. The geographic distribution of tuberculosis in the United States reflects the distribution of the populations in which this disease is prevalent. New York, including New York City, has been particularly affected by the recent increase in tuberculosis in the United States, with a 30.4 percent increase from 1985 to 1990.

Because in the United States tuberculosis has become a disease of the elderly, it is frequently seen in nursing homes. Although transmission of infection can occur at any age, most disease in older persons represents a legacy of previous times. The elderly of today were children when transmission of tubercle bacilli occurred much more frequently. Of those who were infected, many developed disease in young adulthood. Some, especially males, did not and are only now developing reactivation disease in their late years. However, an increasing portion of elderly persons have never been infected and have acquired nosocomial new infections in nursing homes.

In much of the world, transmission of tuberculous infection is declining, but in many impoverished nations this is not true. In some countries, estimated new case rates are as high as 400 per 100,000 per year. As in North America and Europe, poverty and tuberculosis go hand in hand. In high-prevalence areas, tuberculosis is seen with equal prevalence in rural and urban settings and afflicts chiefly young adults. In countries where human immunodeficiency virus (HIV) infection is endemic, tuberculosis is commonly the single most important cause of morbidity and mortality in AIDS patients. A reasonable estimate of the magnitude of tuberculosis in the world is that one-third of the population of the world is infected with *M. tuberculosis*, that there are 30 million cases of active tuberculosis in the world, that 10 million new cases occur annually, and that 3 million people die of tuberculosis each year. Tuberculosis probably causes 6 percent of all deaths worldwide.

TRANSMISSION　*M. tuberculosis* is transmitted from person to person via the respiratory route. Although other routes of transmission are possible and have been documented on occasion, none is of major importance. Tubercle bacilli in respiratory secretions form nuclei for liquid droplets expelled during coughing, sneezing, and vocalizing. Droplets evaporate within a short distance from the mouth, and thereafter desiccated bacilli remain airborne for long periods. Infection of a susceptible host occurs when a few of these bacilli are inhaled. The number of bacilli excreted by most infected persons is not large; typically, household contact of many months is required for transmission. However, patients with laryngeal tuberculosis, endobronchial disease, recent transbronchial spread of tuberculosis, and extensive cavitary pulmonary disease are often highly contagious. Infectiousness correlates with the number of organisms in the expectorated sputum, extent of pulmonary disease, and frequency of cough. Mycobacteria are susceptible to ultraviolet irradiation, and outdoor transmission of infection rarely occurs in daylight. Adequate ventilation is the most important measure to reduce the infectiousness of the environment. Fomites are not important in the transmission of tuberculosis. Most patients become noninfectious within 2 weeks after the institution of appropriate chemotherapy because of a decrease in the number of organisms excreted and a decrease in cough.

Transmission of infection with *M. bovis* has long been associated with the consumption of contaminated cow's milk. This organism is no longer a major cause of human disease in most of the world.

PATHOGENESIS　The initial entry of tubercle bacilli into the lungs or another site in a previously uninfected individual elicits a nonspecific acute inflammatory response which is rarely noted and is usually accompanied by few or no symptoms. Bacilli are then ingested by macrophages and transported to the regional lymph nodes. If spread of the organism is not contained at the level of regional lymph nodes, then tubercle bacilli reach the bloodstream and widespread dissemination ensues. Most lesions of disseminated tuberculosis heal, as do most primary pulmonary lesions, although they remain potential foci of later reactivation. Dissemination may result in miliary or meningeal tuberculosis—illnesses with potential for major morbidity and mortality, especially in infants and young children.

During the 2 to 8 weeks after primary infection, while bacilli continue to multiply in their intracellular environment, cell-mediated hypersensitivity develops in the infected host. Immunologically competent lymphocytes enter areas of infection, where they elaborate chemotactic factors, interleukins, and lymphokines. In response, monocytes enter the area and undergo transformation into macrophages and subsequently into specialized histiocytic cells, which become organized into granulomas. Mycobacteria may persist within macrophages for many years despite increased lysozyme production within these cells, but their further multiplication and spread are usually confined. Healing then occurs, often with late calcification of the granulomas that sometimes leaves a residual lesion visible on chest radiograph. The combination of a calcified peripheral lung lesion and calcified hilar lymph node is known as a *Ghon complex*.

In the United States, 90 to 95 percent of immunocompetent individuals undergo complete healing of primary tuberculous lesions with no subsequent evidence of disease. In other populations, where infective inocula may be higher and where nutritional status and other host factors may be less propitious, failure of complete healing may occur in more than 5 to 10 percent of individuals. Famine and many intercurrent diseases adversely affect healing and threaten the stability of healed tuberculous lesions.

Tuberculosis—the clinical disease—develops in the minority who do not successfully contain their primary infections. In some individuals, tuberculosis develops within weeks after primary infection; in most, organisms lie dormant for many years before entering a phase of exponential multiplication leading to disease. Among many, age can be identified as a significant factor determining the course of tuberculosis. In infants, tuberculous infection frequently progresses rapidly to disease, and the risk of disseminated disease, including meningitis and miliary tuberculosis, is high. In children older than 1 or 2 years up to about the age of puberty, primary tuberculous lesions almost always heal; most of those destined to develop tuberculosis do so during adolescence or young adulthood. Individuals infected in adulthood are at greatest risk of developing tuberculosis within approximately 3 years following infection. Tuberculous disease is more common in young adult women, whereas it is more common in men later in life.

IMMUNOLOGY **Immunity** Humans display native immunity to tuberculosis, with substantial individual variation. Studies of twins have demonstrated that tuberculosis is more likely to occur in both members of monozygotic sibships than in dizygotic sibships or other family relationships. Attempts to link susceptibility to tuberculosis to HLA phenotype have produced conflicting data. Although susceptibility to tuberculosis has been associated with race, the evidence is largely anecdotal and is not convincing. As noted, age is an important determinant of native immunity to tuberculosis. Although specific data on nutrition and tuberculosis immunity are lacking, the association of tuberculosis with famine is clear.

Acquired immunity follows primary tuberculous infection. Disease due to exogenous reinfection is probably rare in North America and Europe; it may be more frequent in populations of high prevalence, where the risk of repeated exposure is great. It is useful to recall that *immunity*, in the classic sense of the word, refers to resistance to infection, whereas *hypersensitivity* describes a state of altered host reactivity. In this sense, immunity also may result from vaccination with bacillus Calmette-Guérin (BCG) or from infection with other species of mycobacteria.

In animal models, antigen-specific immunity is T lymphocyte–dependent and can be transferred adoptively with lymphocytes. It closely parallels cutaneous-type delayed hypersensitivity in its development.

Tuberculin hypersensitivity Tuberculin hypersensitivity is antigen-specific in nature and follows primary infection. It is chiefly or perhaps entirely directed against protein antigens. It is mediated by T lymphocytes through secretion of lymphokines, which act on effector monocytes.

Mycobacterial antigens have been subjected to extensive immunochemical study. It is clear that there is no single dominant antigen and that infected and artificially sensitized hosts develop hypersensitivity to an array of mycobacterial proteins. Tuberculin purified protein derivative (PPD), the antigen preparation most frequently employed clinically and epidemiologically to demonstrate tuberculin hypersensitivity, is a crude mixture of largely denatured antigens and is a poor representative of native antigens. Nevertheless, its use has yielded much information.

Antigen recognition by the sensitized host follows processing by macrophages and depends on expression by the macrophage—at its surface—of antigen-specific epitopes in association with Ia antigen, a gene product of the major histocompatibility locus. This complex is recognized by specific T lymphocytes. Macrophage synthesis and secretion of interleukin 1 are also necessary for T lymphocyte response to the presented antigen. Following antigen presentation, T lymphocyte clonal expansion occurs. Specific subsets of T lymphocytes develop that have antigen-specific immunoregulatory functions and that modulate the immune response (see Chap. 277).

Immunoreactive lymphocytes secrete mediators, and in response macrophages become activated and serve as the principal effector cells of tuberculin hypersensitivity. Peripheral blood monocytes from tuberculous patients have been shown to have several features characteristic of activated macrophages, including increased hexose monophosphate shunt activity, augmented surface adhesiveness, expression of characteristic membrane structures, and increased bactericidal activity. Animal studies have demonstrated that these features are T lymphocyte–dependent. Activated monocytes/macrophages are important immunoregulatory cells possessing suppressor functions.

In tuberculosis, aberrations of this carefully modulated state of hypersensitivity occur with some frequency and are recognizable in 15 percent of acutely ill patients. This has given rise to the suggestion that tuberculosis may present with an immunologic spectrum similar to that seen in leprosy but more subtly expressed. At one pole are patients with chronic cavitary disease, relatively chronic courses, and florid expression of tuberculin hypersensitivity. At the other pole are the rarely seen patients with cutaneous anergy, a few of whom have absence of granuloma formation and all other manifestations of cellular hypersensitivity, pancytopenia, widely disseminated disease, and a progressive downhill course. Although the delayed tuberculin skin reaction is the best-known manifestation of tuberculin hypersensitivity (see below), granuloma formation is probably its central and most important expression because it is important in containing the spread of infection.

Production of antibodies to protein and polysaccharide antigens of mycobacteria is readily demonstrated in tuberculosis. There is no evidence that these antibodies play a role in immunity, hypersensitivity, or pathogenesis.

CLINICAL MANIFESTATIONS **Primary tuberculosis** Primary tuberculous infection is usually asymptomatic. A nonspecific pneumonitis typically occurs in the lower or midlung zones. Hilar lymph node enlargement is usual and in children is sometimes sufficient to produce bronchial obstruction. In low-prevalence areas, primary infection may not occur until adulthood. It may progress directly to clinical disease that has the pathologic features of reactivation disease. In these persons, presentation as subapical pneumonia is common.

Reactivation tuberculosis Reactivation tuberculosis is a chronic wasting disease, and in pulmonary tuberculosis, constitutional manifestations are often more prominent than respiratory symptoms. Weight loss and low-grade fever are common. Many patients present with typical drenching night sweats over the upper half of the body several times a week.

Pulmonary tuberculosis Reactivation-type pulmonary tuberculosis has a predilection for the apical posterior segments of the upper lobes and the superior segments of the lower lobes of the lungs. The extent of disease varies from minimal infiltrates that produce no clinical illness and that are barely discernible on chest radiographs to massive involvement with extensive cavitation and debilitating constitutional and respiratory symptoms. In the absence of effective therapy, pulmonary tuberculosis pursues a chronic and progressive course. There are often long periods of stability and relative well-being, but in most patients these give way to episodes of disease progression with increasing involvement of lung parenchyma.

The onset of pulmonary tuberculosis is usually insidious, and illness may not be noted by the patient for some time. However, it is incorrect to view this onset as one of slow progression. In fact, pulmonary tuberculosis usually reaches its full extent within a few weeks. About one-third of patients will live long lives with chronic illness interspersed with periods of relative well-being. The overall death rate of untreated pulmonary tuberculosis approaches 60 percent, and the median course to death is about $2\frac{1}{2}$ years.

As pulmonary lesions progress, central necrosis occurs with development of caseation, so named because of the cheesy nature of necrotic material that only partly liquefies. Satellite lesions develop concomitantly. They can usually be recognized on chest x-ray films and are often helpful in distinguishing tuberculosis from pulmonary neoplasms. Necrotic material may empty into bronchi, with resulting cavitation of the nodular disease. Other parts of the lung may be seeded transbronchially, with the development of exudative lesions. In some patients, tuberculous pneumonia develops in a lobar or segmental pulmonary distribution. Occasionally, transbronchial spread following rupture of a tuberculous peribronchial lymph node into a bronchus leads to tuberculous pneumonia in the absence of other obvious disease. With the progression of pulmonary tuberculosis, the normal pulmonary architecture is lost. Fibrosis, volume loss, and upward contraction are typical. However, recently diseased areas may heal with relatively little destruction when effective chemotherapy is administered.

Pulmonary cavities may persist even though effective chemotherapy has resulted in apparent cure. In the absence of therapy, persistence of cavities is to be expected. Cavities may be a source of major hemoptysis, especially in the presence of continued active disease. Persistent terminal pulmonary arteries within cavities may be a source of profound bleeding (Rasmussen's aneurysm). Another cause of bleeding is an aspergilloma in a chronic tuberculous cavity, and bleeding in this instance may occur without persisting tuberculous disease. Rupture of a tuberculous cavity into the pleural space may lead to tuberculous empyema and bronchopleural fistula.

Chronic cough is the principal respiratory symptom. Sputum is usually scant and nonpurulent. Hemoptysis is frequent and is usually limited to blood streaking of the sputum. Massive, life-threatening hemoptysis is rare.

Findings on physical examination of the lung in patients with pulmonary tuberculosis are typically few and generally can be appreciated only in the presence of extensive disease. Rales that are accentuated or heard only posttussively are characteristic of apical disease. With extensive cavitation, amphoric breath sounds may be present. Dullness to percussion may sometimes be recognized in Krönig's isthmus and at the clavicles, reflecting extensive apical disease.

Extrapulmonary tuberculosis　PLEURISY WITH EFFUSION　Pleurisy with effusion results when the pleural space is seeded with *M. tuberculosis*. Following a peripheral primary infection, the pleural space may be contaminated by organisms that are transported lymphogenously to the pleura and then across the surface of the lung to the hilum. Pleural effusion occurs, sometimes massively, usually with substantial pleuritic pain. The onset of symptoms is often abrupt. The effusion is most frequently, but not invariably, unilateral. Classically, tuberculous pleurisy with effusion occurs in younger individuals in the absence of pulmonary tuberculosis. However, in the United States this disease presents in many individuals past the age of 35, and simultaneous pulmonary tuberculosis is present in about one-third of patients. The effusion is exudative in nature, and a protein concentration greater than 3.0 g/dL is the most characteristic feature of the pleural fluid. Lymphocytes usually, but not invariably, predominate among the pleural fluid cells. Mesothelial cells are rare. Needle biopsy of the parietal pleura may reveal granulomas, confirming the diagnosis of tuberculous pleurisy. The tuberculin skin test is negative in one-third of patients, either because the disease presents early before tuberculin reactivity develops or because this form of tuberculosis is particularly prone to aberrations of immunoregulation. Untreated, tuberculous pleurisy usually remits, but active pulmonary tuberculosis develops within 5 years in two-thirds of cases. Response to chemotherapy is good. Complete removal of pleural fluid is not necessary. There is rarely a need for surgical decortication.

Bronchopleural fistula and tuberculous empyema are catastrophic complications of untreated tuberculosis resulting from rupture of a pulmonary lesion into the pleural space. The diagnosis is usually not difficult, and acid-fast bacilli are usually readily demonstrated in the pleural exudate. Treatment consists of adequate surgical drainage and chemotherapy.

TUBERCULOUS PERICARDITIS AND PERITONITIS　The pericardium and peritoneum may be the sites of tuberculosis. Pericarditis sometimes occurs in association with pleurisy and may represent an extension of that process. More commonly, the pericardium is seeded by drainage from an infected lymph node. Exudative effusion occurs,

and patients present with fever and pericardial pain. A friction rub may be present. Cardiac tamponade occasionally occurs. Chronic constrictive pericarditis is a late sequel. The diagnosis of tuberculous pericarditis is often difficult and sometimes requires thoracotomy for pericardial biopsy.

Tuberculous peritonitis results from hematogenous seeding of the peritoneum or entry of bacilli from an abdominal lymphatic or genitourinary organ source. As with other serositis, an exudative effusion occurs. The onset is usually insidious, and the disease is often mistaken for hepatic cirrhosis in alcoholic patients. As with tuberculous pericarditis, the diagnosis is often difficult, and recovery of the organism from paracentesis fluid is possible only in a minority of cases. Surgical biopsy may be necessary for diagnosis.

LARYNGEAL AND ENDOBRONCHIAL TUBERCULOSIS　Tuberculosis of the larynx is usually seen in association with far-advanced pulmonary disease. Occasionally it occurs with only minimal pulmonary involvement. It results from seeding of the mucosal surface during expectoration. The disease progresses from a superficial laryngitis to ulceration and granuloma formation. The epiglottis and hypopharynx are occasionally involved. Hoarseness is the principal symptom of tuberculous laryngitis. In a similar fashion, the bronchial mucosa may be seeded, with resultant tuberculous bronchitis. Indeed, localized bronchitis in segmental bronchi leading to diseased portions of lung is common. Cough and minor hemoptysis are the chief clinical manifestations. Patients with tuberculous laryngitis and extensive bronchitis are usually highly infectious. These forms of disease respond rapidly to chemotherapy and have a favorable prognosis with treatment.

TUBERCULOUS ADENITIS　*Scrofula* is chronic tuberculous lymphadenitis of the cervical lymph nodes. Any of the cervical nodes may be involved, but the anterior triangle of the neck just below the mandible is the most frequent site of disease. Tuberculous nodes are usually rubbery and not tender. With progression, they become harder and matted. Chronic draining fistulas may develop, but these are rare, and the course of this form of tuberculosis is usually indolent. The diagnosis is commonly established by surgical biopsy. Lymph node biopsy specimens obtained for this purpose should always be submitted for culture as well as histologic examination, and chemotherapy should be instituted at or before the time of surgery to avoid postoperative fistulas in the surgical wound site. Lymph nodes other than those in the cervical regions are less commonly involved in tuberculosis and account for about 35 percent of tuberculous adenitis.

In children, *M. scrofulaceum* and *M. intracellulare* are frequently the cause of scrofula. The onset of this disease is usually before 5 years of age. As with tuberculosis, lymph nodes high in the neck are most frequently involved. A single enlarged node is commonly the presenting manifestation. Constitutional symptoms are absent, and the adenitis usually is not tender. Progression is common, with necrosis of the node and the development of fistulous sinus tracts. The organisms involved are usually not susceptible to drugs, and treatment, if necessary, is surgical excision. Spontaneous resolution is usual after puberty.

SKELETAL TUBERCULOSIS　Bone and joint disease is a not-infrequent manifestation of tuberculosis. Pott's disease, tuberculosis of the spine, usually involves the midthoracic spine. Tubercle bacilli reach the spine hematogenously or through lymphatic channels from the pleural space to paravertebral lymph nodes. Anterior erosion of vertebral bodies leads to collapse. The result is a sharply angulated kyphosis without scoliosis (gibbus deformity). Paraplegia may result. If there is no neurologic compromise, Pott's disease can be treated with chemotherapy. If the spine is unstable, surgical stabilization may be necessary. In the face of new paraparesis, immediate orthopedic consultation should be obtained. Paravertebral ''cold abcesses'' are a frequent concomitant of tuberculous spondylitis. They usually do not need to be drained, if adequate chemotherapy is given, unless they are very large. They may extend along fascial planes and point in the inguinal region or in other remote sites.

Tuberculosis of joints most frequently affects large weight-bearing joints such as the hips and knees. It responds well to immobilization and chemotherapy. Tuberculous synovitis may occur alone or in association with tuberculous arthritis.

GENITOURINARY TUBERCULOSIS Genitourinary tuberculosis may involve any part of either the male or female genitourinary system. Renal tuberculosis usually presents initially as microscopic pyuria and hematuria with a sterile routine urine culture. The diagnosis may be established by finding tubercle bacilli on culture of the urine. As the disease progresses, cavitation of the renal parenchyma occurs. In the past, nephrectomy was often performed for renal tuberculosis. However, with adequate chemotherapy, surgical removal of a kidney is almost never necessary. The ureters and bladder may be infected by tubular spread of the organism, and ureteral stricture may result.

Tuberculous salpingitis often results in female sterility. Genital tuberculosis in the male most commonly involves the prostate, seminal vesicles, and epididymis. Prostatic and epididymal tuberculosis is characterized by nontender nodular induration detectable by physical examination. The presentation of genital tuberculosis in both males and females is insidious, with chronic or subacute symptoms. The diagnosis is usually made by culture of acid-fast bacilli.

MENINGEAL TUBERCULOSIS The leptomeninges are relatively frequently seeded by organisms that disseminate during primary infection. In young children, tuberculous meningitis may develop at this time. This chronic infection is manifested not only by meningeal signs but also frequently by cranial nerve signs, reflecting a tendency for basilar distribution of the infection. High protein content, low glucose, and lymphocytosis are characteristic of the cerebrospinal fluid. Prior to the advent of effective chemotherapy, this disease was almost always fatal. Chemotherapy with isoniazid, rifampin, and ethambutol is effective. Intrathecal drug administration is not necessary. Late reactivation of meningeal tuberculous foci may produce disease in adults who have no evidence of pulmonary tuberculosis. Tuberculomas of the meninges or brain may become evident in adult life many years after primary infection, and seizures are often their major clinical manifestation.

OCULAR TUBERCULOSIS Tuberculosis may involve almost any part of the eye. Chorioretinitis and uveitis are the most common manifestations. The diagnosis of tuberculosis of the eye is extremely difficult to establish, and most diagnoses are presumptive. The manifestations cannot be distinguished clinically from sarcoidosis or systemic mycoses, but phlyctenular keratitis strongly suggests tuberculosis. Phlyctenular lesions are thought to represent manifestations of tuberculin hypersensitivity rather than bacterial infection. Choroid tubercles are often present in patients with miliary tuberculosis, and their recognition may be helpful in the diagnosis of miliary tuberculosis. Ocular tuberculosis responds well to standard chemotherapy.

GASTROINTESTINAL TUBERCULOSIS The stomach is extremely resistant to tuberculous infection, and a large number of virulent tubercle bacilli can be swallowed without establishing an infection. Rarely, usually concomitantly with extensive cavitary pulmonary disease and severe debility, swallowed organisms reach the terminal ileum and cecum and tuberculous ileitis develops. Chronic diarrhea and fistula development are the principal manifestations, and the disease is difficult to distinguish from Crohn's disease. Tuberculosis of the liver can occur as an isolated event, but it is usually a manifestation of miliary tuberculosis.

ADRENAL TUBERCULOSIS Hematogenous seeding of the adrenal gland is probably fairly common, but disease due to this infection is rare and usually seen only in association with long-standing and extensive pulmonary tuberculosis. The cortex is most frequently involved, and adrenal insufficiency may result. In contrast, carcinomatous involvement of the adrenal cortex, even though very extensive, rarely produces clinical adrenal insufficiency.

CUTANEOUS TUBERCULOSIS Tuberculous infection of the skin is rare in the absence of long-standing, untreated disease elsewhere. Lupus vulgaris is a granulomatous disease of the skin, and it responds well to treatment. Diagnosis is made by skin biopsy. Tuberculin

hypersensitivity manifestations are common. Erythema nodosum may be present, although it much more commonly results from other granulomatous diseases, including sarcoidosis and systemic mycoses. Tuberculids are poorly understood papular lesions of tuberculin hypersensitivity.

MILIARY TUBERCULOSIS Miliary tuberculosis results from widespread hematogenous dissemination. It often presents as a perplexing fever, sometimes with a double quotidian curve, often accompanied by anemia and splenomegaly. Miliary tuberculosis is apt to be more fulminating in children than in adults.

Classically, miliary tuberculosis develops following hematogenous dissemination at the time of primary infection, and patients present with no antecedent history of tuberculosis. Lesions develop synchronously throughout the body. Patients become ill before radiographic changes, which take 4 to 6 weeks to become recognizable, appear. The typical radiologic findings are soft, uniformly distributed, fine nodules throughout both lung fields. They often can be recognized first on a lateral chest film or an underpenetrated posteroanterior radiograph. The diagnosis is difficult, and expectorated sputum rarely contains organisms. Transbronchial biopsy and liver biopsy are usually, but not invariably, positive. Bone marrow biopsy is positive in approximately two-thirds of patients.

When hematogenous dissemination occurs in a previously diseased individual, a much more fulminant course results. Prostration is common. Diffuse but ragged nodular infiltrates develop within a few weeks, and the sputum is often positive. The diagnosis is rarely difficult.

The subacute form and the rare chronic form of miliary tuberculosis often present major problems in diagnosis. These types of disease are usually attributed to repeated seeding of the bloodstream from a tuberculous focus. A very rare form of disseminated tuberculosis occurs with widespread dissemination of disease, a massive number of bacteria in tissues, complete absence of granuloma formation, and pancytopenia. It is termed *disseminated nonreactive tuberculosis* and has a poor prognosis, even with chemotherapy.

Tuberculin anergy is common in miliary tuberculosis, and a negative skin test should not be a deterrent to considering this diagnosis. Anergy may or may not extend to other delayed hypersensitivity antigens. In vitro cultured leukocyte studies also demonstrate hyporesponsiveness, and experimental data suggest that this anergy is mediated by monocytes with suppressor function. With treatment and stabilization of patients with miliary tuberculosis, tuberculin hypersensitivity is restored.

Without treatment, the prognosis for miliary tuberculosis is grave. This disease responds well to chemotherapy, however, and can be treated with the same drug regimens employed for other forms of tuberculosis.

SILICOTUBERCULOSIS Tuberculosis occurs with increased frequency in patients with silicosis and possibly in patients with some other pneumoconioses. The diagnosis is often difficult because of confounding radiographic changes due to the underlying pneumoconiosis. Even with therapy, the prognosis is less favorable than in other patients. Patients with silicotuberculosis should be treated for longer than customary periods. Patients with silicosis who are tuberculin-positive should be considered for isoniazid prophylaxis even when they do not meet other criteria for this form of therapy. Isoniazid prophylaxis may be less effective in persons with silicosis.

TUBERCULOSIS IN AIDS Tuberculosis is a major opportunistic infection of HIV-infected persons. For individuals infected first with *M. tuberculosis* and then with HIV, the risk of developing tuberculosis is 5 to 10 percent per year. When these infections are acquired in the reverse order, the association is even more dramatic: Tuberculosis develops in as many as half of HIV-infected persons following primary infection with *M. tuberculosis*, usually within a few months. In the United States, 3 to 4 percent of tuberculosis patients are HIV-seropositive. In a survey in New York City, 42 percent of hospitalized males with tuberculosis were HIV-seropositive; intravenous drug users made up the majority of these patients. In Africa, tuberculosis is the single most important infectious complication of AIDS, and in Kampala, Uganda, 66 percent of hospitalized tuberculosis patients are HIV-seropositive. In the Ivory Coast, death has been attributed to tuberculosis in 40 percent of autopsied patients with AIDS. The potential epidemiologic impact of the HIV pandemic on the incidence of tuberculosis in areas of high tuberculosis prevalence can scarcely be overstated. New case rates for tuberculosis may be as high as 2000 per 100,000 population by the end of the twentieth century in some parts of sub-Saharan Africa.

Lymphocytes and monocytes, the primary defense cells mustered against tuberculous infection, are destroyed by HIV. What is remarkable, however, is that the failure of antituberculous immunity is manifest early, before severe depletion of CD4 T lymphocytes. Tuberculin skin test reactivity may be lost by HIV-infected individuals who are still healthy and free of clinical AIDS, yet as many as two-thirds of HIV-infected patients with tuberculosis have positive tuberculin skin tests. Although tuberculosis may develop at any time during the course of HIV infection in persons also infected with *M. tuberculosis*, it commonly precedes the first other AIDS-defining opportunistic infection by 1 to 3 months. CD4 T lymphocyte counts in HIV-seropositive tuberculosis patients are typically in the range of 150 to 200 cells per cubic millimeter, with considerable individual variation.

Nearly half of AIDS patients with tuberculosis have extrapulmonary forms of the disease, with tuberculous lymphadenitis, usually in the anterior neck, predominating. Among AIDS patients with pulmonary tuberculosis, nearly half have atypical roentgenographic findings, with diffuse fine infiltrates, pneumonic infiltrates, hilar adenopathy and perihilar infiltrates, and pleural effusions frequently seen. Some AIDS patients with sputum-positive tuberculosis have normal chest radiographs. Mycobacterial infections other than tuberculosis are frequently seen in patients with AIDS. In the United States, approximately half of AIDS patients develop disseminated disease due to *M. avium*, usually late in the course of AIDS (see Chap. 279). *M. avium* disease is virtually unknown among AIDS patients in sub-Saharan Africa.

DIAGNOSIS Bacteriology The diagnosis of tuberculosis is established when tubercle bacilli are identified in the sputum, urine, body fluids, or tissues of the patient. For the majority of patients who have pulmonary tuberculosis, the diagnosis can be established most readily by sputum examination. The staining characteristics of *M. tuberculosis* allow its ready identification in clinical specimens, although it is usually present in small numbers so that prolonged study of stained slides is necessary. A slender (less than 0.5 μm diameter), sometimes curved, often polychromatically beaded rod, it frequently presents in clinical specimens as pairs or clumps of a few organisms lying side by side. When stained with fluorescent auramine-rhodamine, tubercle bacilli can be seen under usual high-dry (100×) magnification. A more definitive stain consists of carbolfuchsin; this stain requires meticulous scanning with oil-immersion (1000×) microscopy. Sputum culture adds to the diagnostic yield and also permits the specific identification of acid-fast bacilli and the determination of drug susceptibility. Primary isolation from clinical specimens usually requires 4 to 8 weeks on classical media. Radiometric techniques using highly selective media allow cultivation in 1 or 2 weeks, but confirmation of the identity of an isolated organism may require additional time. Mycobacteria are aerobes. Modern culture techniques are excellent, and there is no longer reason to inoculate guinea pigs for primary isolation. Niacin production characterizes *M. tuberculosis* and helps to distinguish it from other species. Nucleic acid hybridization probes have been developed for the rapid identification of mycobacteria in cultures.

If expectorated sputum is not readily available for examination, expectoration may be induced or samples obtained by nasotracheal aspiration. Early-morning gastric aspiration provides excellent material for culture and for smear examination. Although nonpathogenic mycobacteria are occasionally found in gastric aspirates, their number is so small as to preclude their appearance in smears of gastric aspirates. Bronchoscopy has a high yield in the diagnosis of tuberculosis, but in the absence of other considerations, it should not be undertaken unless multiple attempts by simpler means have failed and the diagnosis remains obscure.

The diagnostic yield of sputum smear and culture is directly related to the extent of pulmonary disease. About one-third of patients in whom a positive sputum culture can be obtained will have acid-fast bacilli identified on an initial sputum smear. With repeated examinations on separate days, this figure rises to about two-thirds. There is rarely an indication for obtaining more than five sputum examinations. However, only about one-third of patients with minimal pulmonary tuberculosis will have a positive sputum smear, even after multiple examinations. If there is no lesion visible on the chest radiograph, then there is usually little reason to obtain sputum examinations for tubercle bacilli. Conversely, if a patient with extensive cavitary disease or an exudative pneumonic process has a negative sputum smear, diagnoses other than tuberculosis should be sought.

Newer methods of rapid diagnosis Serologic tests for the diagnosis of tuberculosis that are based on the recognition of serum IgG antibody to selected mycobacterial antigens and that use enzyme-linked immunosorbent (ELISA) techniques have been developed and appear to offer promise, with sensitivity similar to that of sputum microscopy. Serology may have its greatest application in children and in patients with extrapulmonary tuberculosis–i.e., in cases where sputum is not available. Gene amplification by the polymerase chain reaction (PCR) has been used with great sensitivity and specificity to identify mycobacterial DNA. If this technique can be applied successfully in routine clinical laboratories, it offers great promise for rapid diagnosis. In reference laboratories with sufficient instrumentation, high-performance chromatographic techniques are capable of rapidly identifying mycobacteria by their characteristic lipids.

Radiology The chest radiograph is an important tool for both diagnosis and evaluation of tuberculosis. Healed primary lesions may leave a small peripheral nodule that may calcify with the passing of years. The Ghon complex comprises a calcified peripheral nodule together with a calcified hilar lymph node. Similar lesions result from histoplasmosis and coccidioidomycosis, and it is not possible to distinguish radiologically between healed primary lesions of these diseases. Calcification of right paratracheal lymph nodes is seen more commonly in histoplasmosis.

Multinodular infiltration in the apical posterior segments of the upper lobes and superior segments of the lower lobes is the most typical lesion of pulmonary tuberculosis. Cavitation is frequently present and is usually accompanied by substantial amounts of infiltration in the same pulmonary segments. Laminagrams are often helpful in recognizing satellite nodular lesions, which are characteristic of tuberculosis and not usually seen in carcinoma. Lordotic views may be of help in evaluating disease obscured by the intersection of the third or fourth posterior rib, second anterior rib, and clavicle. They are of little use in evaluating disease located elsewhere. As tuberculosis becomes inactive or heals, fibrotic scarring becomes apparent on the chest radiograph. There is frequently volume loss in the involved upper lobes, and upward and medial retraction of hilar markings is common. Fibrotic lesions may develop calcifications. The activity of tuberculosis may be judged from serial films. It is never wise to judge tuberculosis to be inactive on the basis of a single chest radiograph.

Clinical pathology Other than bacteriologic examinations, clinical laboratory tests contribute relatively little to the diagnosis of tuberculosis. Peripheral blood monocytosis in the range of 8 to 12 percent is common. The erythrocyte sedimentation rate is usually elevated, and modest anemia may be present.

Tuberculin test The intracutaneous tuberculin skin test is a reliable means of recognizing prior mycobacterial infection. The preferred antigen is tuberculin purified protein derivative (PPD), and the intermediate-strength dose should be used. In North America this is 5 tuberculin units of material, which is standardized by bioassay (bioequivalent) against reference antigen designated PPD-S. In other parts of the world, PPD lot RT-23, prepared in Denmark and widely distributed by the World Health Organization, is available. A gravimetric unit has been assigned to this material, and 2 units of this PPD is equivalent to 5 units of PPD-S. Diluents for PPD should contain polysorbate 80, which decreases loss of potency due to adsorption onto glass and plastic surfaces. Multiple puncture devices offer much convenience but do so at the cost of decreased specificity. They can be recommended only as screening tests, and positive tests should be repeated using intracutaneous PPD.

The tuberculin test is usually applied on the forearm. Reactions should be read by measuring the transverse diameter of induration as detected by gentle palpation at 48 to 72 h. Patients with tuberculosis have normally distributed reaction sizes, with the mean and mode at 17 mm. Infected but healthy, nondiseased individuals have similarly distributed reactions. A reaction to PPD is presumptive evidence of current or prior mycobacterial infection.

Tuberculin hypersensitivity may result from contact with nonpathogenic environmental mycobacteria, and this nonspecific reactivity may confound the interpretation of tuberculin tests. Nonspecific tuberculin reactivity is rarely found in northern climates, and in such areas all reactivity to PPD can be considered to reflect infection with M. tuberculosis. In many warm and humid climatic zones, including all the coastal areas of the southeastern United States, nonspecific tuberculin reactivity is common. In such regions it is customary to consider reactions smaller than 10 mm as not significant and attribute them to cross reactivity with environmental mycobacterial antigens. However, considering smaller reactions as not significant always incurs the risk of missing some reactions which bespeak infection with M. tuberculosis. A reasonable and pragmatic approach to the interpretation of tuberculin skin test reactions is to consider any reaction positive in HIV-infected persons; any reaction of ≥5 mm positive in persons likely to be infected, especially household contacts of tuberculous patients; reactions of ≥10 mm positive in persons from population groups at elevated risk of tuberculosis; and reactions of ≥15 mm positive in persons from low-risk general populations, especially in geographic areas known to have a high prevalence of nonspecific tuberculin reactivity.

Repeated skin testing may boost reaction size, whether the primary reactivity was directed to M. tuberculosis or was nonspecific. Caution must be used in attributing a small increase in reactivity to new infection. It is well established, however, that repeated skin testing with PPD does not lead to positive reactions in uninfected persons. Positive reactions do not occur as a result of allergy to components of the diluent. Tuberculin reactivity wanes with advancing age, and the booster phenomenon may be useful in this situation. For example, if an older person fails to react to initial testing, repeat testing with intermediate-strength PPD may be done after 7 to 10 days. A reaction at this time should be accepted as significant.

PPD is also available in a second strength that contains 50 times the amount of PPD in intermediate-strength material. Except as a test for anergy, this product has little use. Because PPD at this strength so readily elicits nonspecific reactivity, a positive reaction to second-strength PPD is much more apt to give misinformation than to contribute to the correct diagnosis. A first-strength PPD is also available. It contains one-fifth the amount of PPD of intermediate PPD and is not useful clinically.

Anergy is the paradoxical absence of dermal tuberculin reactivity in infected persons. It occurs in association with a number of disease states and in immunosuppressed individuals. It also occurs in as many as 15 percent of tuberculous patients with newly active pulmonary disease. In these persons, tuberculin reactivity reappears with stabilization of the disease process. One-half of patients with miliary tuberculosis and one-third of patients with newly diagnosed tuberculous pleurisy have negative tuberculin tests. It has become common practice in many medical centers to use a battery of delayed hypersensitivity antigens as controls for tuberculin tests in demonstrating anergy. However, antigens standardized for this purpose are not available, and tuberculin anergy may be antigen-specific. False-negative tuberculin tests may result from technical errors, including subcutaneous injection, use of outdated PPD, and permitting PPD to remain in syringes before use. Such errors should not be mistaken for anergy.

TREATMENT The modern treatment of tuberculosis is based on the administration of effective drugs. In the presence of adequate chemotherapy, hospitalization, rest, and improved diet do not contribute to achieving cures. In order to prevent the emergence of drug-resistant mutants, which are present initially in very small numbers, at least two effective drugs are always required. Because of the long generation time of mycobacteria and their long periods of metabolic inactivity, prolonged courses of drug therapy are always necessary. Treatment regimens do not differ for pulmonary and extrapulmonary tuberculosis.

Table 130-1 presents dosage and toxicity information on drugs currently in use for the treatment of tuberculosis. Table 130-2 describes several effective treatment regimens. Daily therapy with regimens including isoniazid and rifampin for 9 to 12 months represents the most effective treatment available and is capable of achieving a favorable outcome in 99 percent of patients. Many experts add a third drug initially until the results of sensitivity tests become available; pyrazinamide is the optimal third drug, and ethambutol is also effective. In developing countries where drug costs are a limiting factor, the extremely low-cost combination of isoniazid and thioacetazone for 12 to 18 months provides a regimen that can achieve 80 to 90 percent cure rates.

An accepted hypothesis states that tubercle bacilli exist in tuberculous patients in three pools—a metabolically active extracellular pool and relatively metabolically inactive intracellular and necrotic caseum pools. Only rifampin is bactericidal for all these pools, and it may not be necessary to continue rifampin-containing regimens for as long as other regimens that rely on organisms entering the metabolically active pool to achieve sterilization. Isoniazid and streptomycin are both bactericidal against extracellular, metabolically active organisms. Against intracellular organisms, isoniazid and pyrazinamide are bactericidal and streptomycin is inactive. In clinical trials, pyrazinamide has been found to be particularly useful during the first 2 months of treatment. Ethambutol is only bacteriostatic.

TABLE 130-1 Drugs used in the treatment of tuberculosis

Drug	Usual daily adult dose	Major toxicity
Isoniazid	300 mg	Hepatitis, peripheral neuropathy, drug fever
Rifampin	600 mg	Hepatitis, influenza-like syndrome, thrombocytopenia (rare)
Streptomycin	0.75–1 g	Deafness, loss of vestibular function, loss of renal function
Pyrazinamide	1.5–2 g	Hepatitis, hyperuricemia
Ethambutol	15 mg/kg	Optic neuritis (extremely rare at this dose)
p-Aminosalicylic acid	12 g	Diarrhea, hepatitis, hypersensitivity reactions
Ethionamide	1 g	Hepatitis
Cycloserine	1 g	Depression, personality changes, psychosis, convulsions
Thioacetazone	150 mg	Exfoliative dermatitis, hepatitis
Kanamycin	1 g	Deafness, loss of renal function, loss of vestibular function (rare)
Capreomycin	1 g	Deafness, loss of vestibular function, loss of renal function
Viomycin	1 g	Deafness, loss of vestibular function, loss of renal function

TABLE 130-2 Effective drug regimens for the treatment of tuberculosis

Regimen (adult drug dose)	Comment
Isoniazid (300 mg) and rifampin (600 mg) daily for 9–12 months	An effective regimen for initial treatment of patients unless drug resistance is suspected.
Isoniazid (300 mg) and ethambutol (15 mg/kg) daily for 12–18 months	The least toxic effective regimen. Suitable for patients with minimal disease.
Isoniazid (300 mg) and thioacetazone (150 mg) daily for 12–18 months	The least expensive effective regimen. Streptomycin (0.75–1 g) may be added daily for the first 8 weeks to increase effectiveness, but this doubles both cost and toxicity.
Isoniazid (300 mg), rifampin (600 mg), pyrazinamide (2 g), with or without streptomycin (1 g) or ethambutol (15 mg/kg) daily for 2 months followed by one of the following: a Isoniazid (300 mg) and rifampin (600 g) daily for 4 months	Initial intensive phase for short-course regimens. Short-course regimens have only been demonstrated to be effective under conditions of close patient supervision.
b Isoniazid (300 mg), rifampin (600 mg), and streptomycin (1 g) twice weekly for 6 months	Suitable for fully supervised therapy.
c Isoniazid (300 mg) and thioacetazone (150 mg) daily for 6 months	Inexpensive.
Isoniazid (300 mg) and rifampin (600 mg) daily for 1 month followed by isoniazid (900 mg) and rifampin (600 mg) twice weekly for 8 months	Effectiveness demonstrated in ambulatory treatment programs in Arkansas. Has not been compared with other regimens in clinical trials.

The major problem in tuberculosis treatment programs is patient default. It is unusual for a tuberculosis clinic to achieve a default rate of less than 15 percent, and default rates of 40 to 60 percent are common. Unfortunately, these rates tend to be highest in those parts of the world where high tuberculosis prevalence is coupled with limited resources. Default leads not only to treatment failure but also to the emergence and transmission of drug-resistant organisms. Since most patient defaults occur within the first 6 months of the treatment program, short-course therapy has been employed to mitigate the consequences of default. This strategy will be successful only if the resources conserved by shortening treatment are used to maintain patient compliance. Completely supervised regimens are often successful for noncompliant patients, but their widespread use is costly. Twice-weekly drug administration is effective and facilitates patient supervision.

Short-course treatment programs are best considered as consisting of two phases. An initial 2-month intensive phase of daily therapy should include isoniazid, rifampin, and pyrazinamide and also may include either streptomycin or ethambutol. A consolidation phase of daily therapy with isoniazid and one other drug should be continued for an additional 4 months, and preferably 6 months. In the United States, a regimen of isoniazid 300 mg and rifampin 600 mg daily for 1 month, followed by isoniazid 900 mg and rifampin 600 mg twice weekly for 8 months, has been highly effective. Patients with AIDS should be treated in the same manner as immunocompetent individuals with tuberculosis. Response to therapy is favorable in these patients, although they have more frequent drug reactions, particularly skin rashes. The optimal duration of therapy for these patients is not known, although it is probably wise to avoid short regimens. AIDS patients should be followed for relapse after therapy for the rest of their lives.

Relapses after successful therapy should be less than 1 percent. Since these few relapses usually present with symptoms and are almost never found by routine x-rays, patients may be discharged from follow-up at the completion of therapy. Relapses are more frequent after short-course therapy, usually occurring within the first year, and follow-up for such patients for 1 or 2 years is justified.

Symptomatic improvement occurs within the first 2 to 3 weeks in most patients. Clearing of infiltrates on the chest radiograph may not occur within the first month but usually is rapidly recognized between the second and fourth months. Most patients reach a point of radiologic stability between 3 and 6 months. Therapy usually should be continued for 6 months after this point of stability is reached, even if this means prolonging the planned period of treatment. Sputum conversion occurs in most patients within the first 2 months. The fact that an individual patient responds more slowly than the norm should not necessarily be a cause for concern, provided the patient is taking effective drugs.

Since there are alternative effective drug regimens, toxicity becomes a factor in choice of therapy. Major individual drug toxicities are listed in Table 130-1; the toxicity of greatest concern is hepatitis. Toxicity sufficient to require change in regimen occurs in 3 to 5 percent of patients taking isoniazid and rifampin and in about 1.5 percent of patients taking isoniazid and ethambutol. The toxicity of isoniazid and thioacetazone appears to vary with the racial characteristics of the patient population. It reaches about 30 percent in Oriental groups but is only 2 to 5 percent in other populations. It approaches 25 percent in HIV-infected persons. Routine monitoring of serum enzymes or other blood tests reflecting liver disease is of little use and is not recommended. Normal values do not predict absence of toxicity, and serum enzymes in patients taking isoniazid may rise transiently to three times normal values without the subsequent development of hepatitis. A well-educated patient and an alert treatment supervisor are the principal safeguards against drug hepatitis. If medication is discontinued during the prodromal phase or promptly with the onset of jaundice, drug hepatitis can be expected to resolve without untoward incident. Isoniazid toxicity is probably due to toxic metabolites of acetyl isoniazid. Induction of cytochrome P-450 enzymes by alcohol or long-acting barbiturates predisposes to isoniazid hepatitis. Isoniazid also causes a peripheral neuropathy that is preventable and reversible by the administration of pyridoxine. Patients with such predisposing factors as old age, diabetes, alcoholism, and malnutrition should be given pyridoxine concomitantly with isoniazid; the usual dose is 50 mg/d.

Isoniazid is safe in pregnant patients. Data are less complete for other drugs but suggest that both ethambutol and rifampin are acceptable. Rifampin should always be used if the tuberculosis is disseminated or very extensive. Streptomycin should not be used in pregnancy because of the risk of fetal ototoxicity. Tuberculosis often pursues an unfavorable course during and just after pregnancy, and treatment of a pregnant woman should never be deferred. It is reasonable, however, to postpone isoniazid prophylaxis until just after delivery.

Patients with chronic renal failure also present special treatment problems, and these patients have tuberculosis case rates approximately 10 times those of the general population. Isoniazid is acetylated to an inactive form by the liver and then excreted by the kidney. Acetyl isoniazid is the precursor of hydrazines, which are probably hepatotoxic. Both isoniazid and acetyl isoniazid are not bound by plasma proteins and are dialyzable. In patients with renal failure, isoniazid should be reduced to 5 mg/kg body weight (300 mg in adults) two or three times weekly. Patients on dialysis should receive the drug following each dialysis. Ethambutol behaves like isoniazid, except that it is excreted by the kidney as the active drug. As with isoniazid, the usual daily dose should be given at longer intervals, and administration should follow dialysis. Optic nerve toxicity of ethambutol appears to be related not to intermittent high drug levels but to sustained high drug levels. Patients with renal failure who are receiving ethambutol should have their color vision and visual acuity monitored regularly. Rifampin is protein-bound, nondialyzable, and excreted in the bile by the liver. No change in dose or interval is necessary in the presence of renal failure. Caution should be exercised in using rifampin in patients with hepatic failure.

Faced with relapse in a previously treated patient, a major concern should be the possibility of drug resistance, and resistance studies of the organism should be obtained in a competent reference laboratory. In one-third of patients who relapse after adequate regular drug therapy, the relapse is caused by drug-resistant organisms. If, however, the patient took the drug sporadically or the previous regimen was inadequate, then the likelihood of drug resistance is about two chances in three. Therapy for presumed drug-resistant tuberculosis should be instituted with two drugs that the patient has not taken previously, provided that one of these two new drugs is isoniazid or rifampin. Otherwise, four drugs should be used, including as many new drugs as possible. When resistance studies become available, the regimen should be modified appropriately. It is beneficial to continue isoniazid even when laboratory studies indicate drug resistance. In general, all retreatment regimens should be closely supervised and directed by physicians with special experience with this problem.

Primary drug resistance should be suspected in patients who appear to have contracted their infection from patients with known drug resistance or with known noncompliance and in patients who come from areas where drug resistance is common. In the United States, this group includes immigrants from Haiti, Southeast Asia, and many areas of Latin America. Multidrug-resistant strains of tuberculosis have been seen with increasing frequency in the United States, especially in New York City, where 20 to 25 percent of newly diagnosed patients with tuberculosis currently have organisms resistant to both isoniazid and rifampin. While laboratory resistance studies are pending, drug therapy should be dictated by the prior treatment of the suspected index case. In immigrant populations, most of the drug resistance of concern is to isoniazid. In this circumstance, therapy should be initiated with isoniazid, rifampin, pyrazinamide, and ethambutol. One or two of these drugs may be discontinued when resistance studies become available. Treatment of suspected multidrug-resistant tuberculosis is difficult and should only be made on consultation with local experts or public health authorities. Some experts recommend that a fluoroquinolone be added to initial regimens, with final decisions on therapy made when drug resistance studies are completed. Other possibilities for a fifth drug include streptomycin, cycloserine, or ethionamide.

PREVENTION Chemoprophylaxis In one of the largest controlled clinical trials ever conducted, 1 year of isoniazid has been shown to be effective in reducing the incidence of tuberculosis in tuberculin-positive individuals presumed to have been infected with *M. tuberculosis*. The benefit of isoniazid prophylaxis · has been demonstrated so clearly that the question of its use now hinges primarily on the risk of drug toxicity, chiefly hepatitis.

In administering isoniazid prophylaxis, highest priority should be assigned to treating immunosuppressed and HIV-infected persons, household contacts of persons with active tuberculosis, and persons known to have become infected within the preceding year. The risks of developing tuberculosis in these three groups are, respectively, 5 to 10 percent per year, 0.5 percent per year, and 3 percent during the first year. Particular attention should be given to treating children in these categories. Prophylaxis of childhood household contacts with isoniazid should be started immediately. After 3 months of therapy, the child should be skin-tested with intermediate-strength PPD. If the skin test is negative at that time, isoniazid may be discontinued. If it is positive, 12 months of prophylaxis should be completed.

Younger individuals benefit most from isoniazid prophylaxis because the drug is most effective when the infection is recent and because older individuals often have already outlived a substantial part of their risk. The risk of hepatitis rises with age, reaching approximately 2 percent by the seventh decade. Cost-benefit analyses with large data bases have shown that there is a 1:1 ratio of cases of tuberculosis prevented and hepatitis caused at age 45 when individuals without added risks are considered. Based on this calculation, there is a general consensus that all persons younger than age 35 with a positive tuberculin reaction should receive isoniazid 300 mg/d for 1 year.

It is also possible to develop criteria for the prophylactic use of isoniazid in older persons with remote tuberculosis, either known historically or evident radiographically, who have never received adequate chemotherapy. The annual risk of tuberculosis in such persons is at least 0.5 percent. Isoniazid 300 mg/d should be given for 1 year to all persons in this category who have a life expectancy greater than 10 years. In compliant adults with fibrotic residuals of untreated tuberculosis visible on roentgenograms, 1 year of isoniazid prophylaxis reduced disease during the subsequent 5 years by 75 percent, and 6 months of isoniazid reduced disease by 65 percent. Others at high risk for the development of tuberculosis include tuberculin-positive individuals with AIDS or Hodgkin's disease (both of which alter T lymphocyte–mediated immunity), patients with silicosis (which affects macrophage function), and persons who are (1) receiving immunosuppressive agents or glucocorticoids chronically or (2) suffering from renal failure. As with therapy for active tuberculosis, monitoring serum enzymes is not useful in patients receiving isoniazid prophylaxis.

BCG vaccination Bacillus Calmette-Guérin (BCG) is an attenuated strain of *M. bovis* that has been given to more than 2 billion persons as a vaccine against tuberculosis. It is clearly safe, but its efficacy is in some dispute. In some controlled studies it offered little or no protection. However, even then, the disseminated forms of tuberculosis, which have such high mortalities among children, were virtually eliminated. While final judgment on the efficacy of BCG must be reserved, its continued use in high-prevalence areas appears justified.

BCG vaccination induces tuberculin hypersensitivity. However, the dermal reaction to PPD is usually not as large as that which follows natural infection, usually does not persist as long, and varies from strain to strain of vaccine. Individuals with large PPD reactions persisting for many years after vaccination should be viewed as infected and considered for isoniazid prophylaxis.

CONTROL PROGRAMS In most low-prevalence areas, such as North America, resources are relatively abundant and disease occurrence is mostly sporadic. Increasingly, tuberculosis is being seen in microepidemics, often centered in family groups or congregate housing facilities. Immigrant groups and residents and employees of nursing homes are at high risk. Homeless shelters and correctional institutions are frequent sites of transmission of infection. Central to any program is an efficient case-reporting and registry system. Contact investigation must be carried out effectively and is especially important when index cases occur in children. The major modality for decreasing the spread of infection is chemotherapy for all infectious patients. Chemoprophylaxis is necessary for contacts.

At the other end of the spectrum are high-prevalence areas with few or no resources for tuberculosis control. The single most effective measure in this setting is a network of ambulatory tuberculosis treatment centers that provide diagnosis by direct sputum smear and standardized drug therapy. Successful treatment must entail no cost to the patient. Tuberculosis diagnostic and treatment programs should be integrated into national health programs, under expert supervision. Treatment records should be maintained, but complex registries are of little value.

In high-prevalence areas, BCG vaccine should be offered to every individual under age 15 or 20 without prior tuberculin testing. Older individuals can be assumed to have been infected already. Before a mass BCG campaign is initiated, planning should begin for continuing vaccination of newborns or young schoolchildren. Community-wide isoniazid prophylaxis programs have not been successful.

REFERENCES

AMERICAN THORACIC SOCIETY: Treatment of tuberculosis and tuberculosis infection in adults and children. Am Rev Respir Dis 134:355, 1986
———: Mycobacterioses and the acquired immunodeficiency syndrome. Am Rev Respir Dis 136:492, 1987
———: Diagnostic standards and classification of tuberculosis. Am Rev Respir Dis 142:725, 1990

BRUDNEY K, DOBKIN J: Resurgent tuberculosis in New York City: Human immunodeficiency virus, homelessness, and the decline of tuberculosis control programs. Am Rev Respir Dis 144:745, 1991

COMSTOCK GW, EDWARDS PQ: The competing risks of tuberculosis and hepatitis for adult tuberculin reactors. Am Rev Respir Dis 111:573, 1975

———— et al: The tuberculin skin test. Am Rev Respir Dis 124:356, 1981

————: Epidemiology of tuberculosis. Am Rev Respir Dis 125(suppl):8, 1982

EDWARDS LB et al: An atlas of sensitivity to tuberculin, PPD-B, and histoplasmin in the United States. Am Rev Respir Dis 99(suppl):1, 1969

GLASSROTH J et al: Tuberculosis in the 1980s. N Engl J Med 302:1441, 1980

GROSSET J: Bacteriologic basis of short-course chemotherapy for tuberculosis. Clin Chest Med 1:231, 1980

GRZYBOWSKI S, ENARSON DA: The fate of cases of pulmonary tuberculosis under various treatment programmes. Bull Int Union Tuberc 53:70, 1978

MURRAY JF: The white plague: Down and out, or up and coming. Am Rev Respir Dis 140:1788, 1989

————: Cursed duet: HIV infection and tuberculosis. Respiration 57:210, 1990

SELWYN PA et al: A prospective study of the risk of tuberculosis among intravenous users with human immunodeficiency virus infection. N Engl J Med 320:545, 1989

SNIDER DE, JR: The tuberculin skin test. Am Rev Respir Dis 125(suppl):108, 1982

STEAD WW et al: Tuberculosis as an endemic and nosocomial infection among the elderly in nursing homes. N Engl J Med 312:1483, 1985

TENDAM HG et al: Present knowledge of immunization against tuberculosis. Bull WHO 54:255, 1976

131 LEPROSY (HANSEN'S DISEASE)

RICHARD A. MILLER

DEFINITION AND ETIOLOGY Leprosy (Hansen's disease) is a chronic granulomatous infection of humans which attacks superficial tissues, especially the skin and peripheral nerves. *Mycobacterium leprae* is the causal agent of leprosy. It is an acid-fast rod assigned to the family Mycobacteriaceae on the basis of morphologic, biochemical, antigenic, and genetic similarities to other mycobacteria. Although it has not been cultivated in artificial media or tissue culture, it can be propagated in armadillos and in the foot pads of mice. The bacillus multiplies exceedingly slowly, with an estimated optimal doubling time of 11 to 13 days during logarithmic growth in mouse foot pads. The mouse model has been used extensively for the study of antileprosy drugs, and the high bacterial yield from armadillos has been crucial for immunologic and genetic studies.

The cellular components of *M. leprae* which are responsible for its pathogenicity and ability to survive within the host are poorly understood. The best-characterized virulence factor is phenolic glycolipid I, a prominent surface lipid specific to *M. leprae*. Phenolic glycolipid I can bind to complement component C3, which in turn mediates phagocytosis of the bacterium by mononuclear phagocytes via CR1, CR3, and CR4 receptors on their cell surfaces. Once inside the phagocyte, phenolic glycolipid I helps to protect the bacterium from oxidative killing by chemically scavenging hydroxyl radicals and superoxide anions.

EPIDEMIOLOGY There are probably 10 to 20 million persons affected with leprosy in the world. The disease is more common in tropical countries, in many of which the prevalence rate is 1 to 2 percent of the population. A warm environment is not critical for transmission, and leprosy also occurs in certain regions with cooler climates, such as Korea and central Mexico. Distribution of infected individuals within countries is very nonhomogeneous, and districts in which 20 percent of the population is affected can be found. The distribution of cases across the spectrum of leprosy also varies between countries, with lepromatous disease predominating in some countries, such as Mexico, and tuberculoid disease in others, such as India. Ninety percent of the cases diagnosed in the United States in the past two decades have occurred in immigrants from leprosy-endemic countries. Indigenous transmission occurs primarily in Hawaii, the Pacific Island territories, and sporadically along the Gulf Coast. The incidence of leprosy in the United States has fallen from a peak of

360 cases in 1985, associated with the influx of immigrants from Southeast Asia, to 139 cases in 1991.

Leprosy can present at any age, although cases in infants less than 1 year of age are extremely rare. The age-specific incidence peaks during childhood in most developing countries; up to 20 percent of cases occur in children under 10. Since leprosy is most prevalent in poorer socioeconomic groups, this may simply reflect the age distribution of the high-risk population. The sex ratio of leprosy presenting during childhood is 1:1, but males predominate by a 2:1 ratio in adults.

It is humbling to realize how little is known concerning the modes of transmission and acquisition of leprosy, given that the communicable nature of the infection has been recognized for millennia and that the etiologic agent was identified over 100 years ago. Direct human-to-human transmission is believed responsible for most cases of leprosy, although a history of prior exposure can be elicited from fewer than half of all patients. Animal reservoirs exist among feral armadillos and possibly among nonhuman primates, but in only a few human cases has zoonotic transmission been implicated. Among close family contacts of untreated lepromatous patients, the risk of disease is increased approximately eightfold, and the attack rate can be as high as 10 percent. Development of clinical disease in contacts of tuberculoid patients is less common, although immunologic tests suggest that most of these contacts have been sensitized to *M. leprae*. The site of entry remains a matter of conjecture but is probably either the skin or the mucosa of the upper respiratory tract. The chief portal of exit is thought to be the nasal mucosa of untreated lepromatous patients.

The incubation period is frequently 3 to 5 years but has been reported to range from 6 months to several decades.

PATHOGENESIS The early events following the entry of *M. leprae* into the body have not been described in humans. The bacilli are surrounded by a dense, nearly inert lipid capsule, produce no exotoxins, and engender little inflammatory response. Immunologic and epidemiologic studies suggest that only a small fraction, possibly 10 to 20 percent, of those infected will develop signs of indeterminate leprosy and that only about 50 percent of those with indeterminate disease will progress to full-blown clinical leprosy.

The intensity of the specific cell-mediated immune response to *M. leprae* correlates with the clinical and histologic disease class. Individuals with polar tuberculoid disease have an intense cellular response to *M. leprae* and a low bacillary load, whereas patients with lepromatous leprosy have no detectable cellular immunity to the leprosy bacillus. There is evidence from family studies that specific HLA-associated genes may be linked to different classes of disease. HLA-DR2 is inherited preferentially by children with polar tuberculoid disease, whereas HLA-MT1 is associated with polar lepromatous disease. The effect of the HLA-associated genes is limited to influencing the type of leprosy; there is no association between HLA haplotypes and overall susceptibility to leprosy.

The defect in cell-mediated immunity in lepromatous patients is extremely specific. They do not suffer increased morbidity following infection by pathogens such as viruses, protozoa, or fungi for which cellular immunity is important, and they do not have an increased risk of neoplasia. Patients with lepromatous leprosy have been shown to have an increased number of circulating CD8+ ("suppressor") lymphocytes which can be specifically activated by *M. leprae* antigens, and the lymphocytes present in their cutaneous granulomas are almost exclusively CD8+. In contrast, CD4+4B4+ ("helper") cells predominate among the T cells in the cutaneous lesions of tuberculoid patients. In lepromatous leprosy, cells of the monocyte-macrophage family become engorged with *M. leprae* and are unable to kill or digest the organisms. However, when studied in vitro, monocytes from these patients respond normally to cytokines and display normal phagocytic and microbicidal activity. These results suggest that an underlying defect in regulation of T lymphocyte subpopulations is responsible for the immunologic tolerance characteristic of lepromatous leprosy.

Intense bacillemia is very common in lepromatous leprosy, and organisms can often be seen in stained smears of peripheral blood or buffy coats, but high fever and signs of systemic toxicity are absent. Even in the most advanced cases, destructive lesions are limited to the skin, peripheral nerves, anterior portions of the eyes, upper respiratory passages above the larynx, testes, and structures of the hands and feet. One feature common to these sites is that they are all usually several degrees cooler than 37°C. Two sites of preferential involvement are the ulnar nerves near the elbow and the peroneal nerves where they pass around the head of the fibula; above and below these areas, where these nerves take deeper courses, they are less severely involved. In patients with lepromatous leprosy, collections of bacilli are also found in the liver, spleen, and bone marrow, but no visceral organ system dysfunction has been associated with the presence of these bacilli.

CLINICAL AND HISTOPATHOLOGIC MANIFESTATIONS The variable immune response to infection with *M. leprae* results in a wide spectrum of histologic and clinical manifestations. There is a strong concordance between the clinical findings and the dermal histopathology, and they will be discussed together.

Early or indeterminate leprosy The first signs of leprosy are usually cutaneous. The lesions of indeterminate leprosy are very subtle and are most commonly diagnosed in examination of contacts of known leprosy patients. One or more hypopigmented or hyperpigmented macules or plaques may be seen. Often an anesthetic or paresthetic patch is the first symptom noted by the patient, but on careful examination, skin involvement can be found. Sensation is often preserved in these early lesions, particularly those on the face. The lesions may clear spontaneously in a year or two, but specific treatment is recommended.

Tuberculoid leprosy The initial lesion of tuberculoid leprosy, one of the "poles" of the clinical and immunologic spectrum, is often a hypopigmented macule which is sharply demarcated and hypesthetic. Later the lesions enlarge by peripheral spread, and the margins become elevated and circinate or gyrate (Fig. 131-1). The central area in turn becomes atrophic and depressed. Fully developed lesions are densely anesthetic and have lost the normal skin organs (sweat glands and hair follicles). The lesions are single or few in number. Nerve involvement occurs early, and the superficial nerves leading from the lesions may be enlarged. The larger peripheral nerves (especially the ulnar, peroneal, and greater auricular nerves) may be palpably and visibly enlarged, particularly those closest to the skin lesion. There may be severe neuritic pain. Neural involvement leads to muscle atrophy, especially of the small muscles of the hand. Contractures of the hand and foot are frequent. Trauma, especially from burns and splinters and from excessive pressure, leads to secondary infection of the hands and to plantar ulcers. Later, resorption and loss of phalanges may supervene. When the facial nerves are involved, there may be lagophthalmos, exposure keratitis, and corneal ulceration leading to blindness.

The histologic picture consists of noncaseating granulomas comprising lymphocytes, epithelioid cells, and perhaps giant cells; bacilli are frequently absent or difficult to demonstrate.

Lepromatous leprosy Lepromatous leprosy is the other polar form. The cutaneous involvement is extensive and roughly bilaterally symmetric across the midline of the host. Individual skin lesions are highly variable and can include macules, nodules, plaques, or papules. The borders of the lesions are ill defined, and the centers of raised lesions are indurated and convex (rather than concave, as in tuberculoid disease). There is diffuse infiltration of the dermis between discrete lesions, and apparently normal skin will usually contain bacilli demonstrable by staining. The sites of predilection are the face (cheeks, nose, brows), ears, wrists, elbows, buttocks, and knees. At times, involvement with infiltration and little or no nodulation may progress so subtly that the disease goes unnoticed. Loss of the lateral portions of the eyebrows is common. Much later the skin of the face and forehead becomes thickened and corrugated (leonine facies), and the earlobes become pendulous.

Nasal "stuffiness," epistaxis, and obstructed breathing are common early symptoms. Complete nasal obstruction, laryngitis, and hoarseness also occur. Septal perforation and nasal collapse lead to saddlenose. Invasion of the anterior portion of the eye can result in keratitis and iridocyclitis. Painless inguinal and axillary lymphadenopathy occurs. In adult males infiltration and scarring of the testes lead to sterility. Gynecomastia is common.

Involvement of the major nerve trunks is less prominent in the lepromatous form, but diffuse hypesthesia involving the peripheral portions of the extremities is common in advanced disease. Pathologically, the peripheral nerves are heavily infected but often better preserved than in the tuberculoid form.

Histologically, there is a diffuse granulomatous reaction with macrophages, large foam (Virchow or lepra) cells, and many intracellular bacilli, frequently in spheroidal masses (globi). Epithelioid cells and giant cells are not found.

Borderline leprosy The borderline portion of the spectrum lies between the tuberculoid and lepromatous poles and is usually subdivided into borderline tuberculoid, borderline (or dimorphous), and borderline lepromatous classes. Classification within the borderline region of the spectrum is less precise than at the poles. Lesions tend to increase in number and heterogeneity but decrease in individual size as the lepromatous pole is approached. The skin lesions of borderline tuberculoid leprosy generally resemble those of tuberculoid disease but are greater in number and have less well defined borders. Involvement of multiple peripheral nerve trunks is more common than in polar tuberculoid disease.

Increasing variability in the appearance of the skin lesions is characteristic of borderline leprosy. Papules and plaques may coexist with macular lesions. Anesthesia is less prominent than in tuberculoid disease. The earlobes may be slightly thickened, but the eyebrows and nasal regions are spared. Skin lesions become even more numerous in borderline lepromatous disease, but the distribution lacks the bilateral symmetry typical of polar lepromatous disease (Fig. 131-2).

The histopathology of the granulomas in borderline leprosy changes from an epithelioid cell predominance in borderline tuberculoid disease to a macrophage predominance as the lepromatous pole is approached. The presence and number of lymphocytes are variable

FIGURE 131-1 Tuberculoid leprosy. Large, solitary lesion with a raised, indurated border. The central clear area of the lesion is hypesthetic with thinning of the dermis and loss of dermal structures such as sweat glands and hair follicles.

FIGURE 131-2 Borderline lepromatous leprosy. Multiple macules, papules, and nodules with an asymmetric distribution. Individual lesions are small but may become confluent.

and correlate poorly with the disease class. Bacilli are present in large numbers in the skin granulomas of borderline and borderline lepromatous patients. For this reason, these groups, together with polar lepromatous leprosy, are referred to as *multibacillary leprosy*. Borderline tuberculoid, polar tuberculoid, and indeterminate classes are grouped together as *paucibacillary leprosy*.

The borderline disease states are unstable and may shift toward the lepromatous form in the untreated patient or toward the tuberculoid pole during treatment. Change of either polar type to the other is exceedingly rare.

In all forms of leprosy, peripheral nerve involvement is a constant feature. In any histologic section, involvement of nerves will tend to be more severe than involvement of other tissues. Much of the neural destruction appears to result from the granulomatous reaction of the host rather than from an innate neurotoxic property of the bacillus. Though uncommon, neural involvement can occur in the absence of cutaneous lesions (pure neural leprosy).

REACTIONAL STATES The general course of leprosy is indolent, but it may be interrupted by two types of reaction. Both forms of reactions can occur in untreated patients but more often emerge as complications of chemotherapy.

Erythema nodosum leprosum Erythema nodosum leprosum (ENL), or type 2 lepra reaction, occurs in lepromatous and borderline lepromatous patients, most frequently in the latter half of the initial year of treatment. Tender, inflamed subcutaneous nodules develop, usually in crops. Each nodule lasts a week or two, but new crops may appear. ENL may last only a week or two, or it may persist for long periods. Fever, lymphadenopathy, and arthralgias can accompany severe ENL. Histologically, ENL is characterized by polymorphonu-

clear infiltration and deposits of IgG and complement, resembling an Arthus reaction.

Reversal reaction Reversal reaction, or type 1 lepra reaction, can complicate all three borderline categories. Existing skin lesions develop erythema and swelling, and new lesions may appear. An early influx of lymphocytes into existing lesions is followed by edema and a shift toward tuberculoid histology. Cellular immunity increases. Reversal reactions can be differentiated from disease progression or relapse by mouse inoculations to test bacillary viability and by histologic studies. Downgrading reactions, which clinically mimic reversal reactions, are most common in untreated patients and in women during the third trimester of pregnancy. Skin biopsies reveal a shift toward lepromatous histology and reflect a decrease in cellular immunity.

COMPLICATIONS Leprosy is probably the most frequent cause of crippling of the hand in the world (Fig. 131-3). Trauma and secondary chronic infections can lead to loss of digits or distal extremities. Blindness is also common.

The *Lucio phenomenon*, characterized by arteritis, is limited to patients with diffuse, infiltrative, nonnodular lepromatous disease. Severe cases clinically resemble other forms of necrotizing vasculitis and are associated with a high mortality rate.

Secondary amyloidosis is a complication of severe lepromatous disease, especially in chronic ENL.

Leprosy and human immunodeficiency virus (HIV) infection Surprisingly, given the experience with other mycobacterial diseases and the intricate immune response to *M. leprae*, concurrent infection with HIV appears to have little effect on the clinical manifestations or natural history of leprosy. Anecdotal reports suggest that the relapse rate after completion of therapy for paucibacillary disease may be slightly increased in HIV-infected patients, and HIV-positive patients with early or subclinical leprosy may be more likely to develop overt disease. Concurrent leprosy also may accelerate the course of HIV disease.

DIAGNOSIS The demonstration of acid-fast bacilli in skin smears made by the scraped-incision method is strong evidence for leprosy, but in tuberculoid disease bacilli may not be demonstrable. Wherever possible, a skin biopsy specimen from the affected area should be sent to a pathologist knowledgeable in leprosy. The histologic involvement of peripheral nerves is pathognomonic, even in the absence of bacilli. Work is underway on the development of tests using genetic probes for the rapid identification and speciation of mycobacteria in clinical specimens.

FIGURE 131-3 Borderline tuberculoid leprosy. Bilateral claw hand deformities resulting from ulnar and median nerve damage. Note the severe loss of muscle tissue in the forearms secondary to neuropathic and disuse atrophy.

Hematologic and blood chemistry tests are of little help in establishing the diagnosis. Lepromatous patients frequently have mild anemia, an elevated erythrocyte sedimentation rate, and hyperglobulinemia. Between 10 and 20 percent of lepromatous patients have low-titer false-positive serologic tests for syphilis or autoantibodies directed against nuclear or cellular antigens.

Lepromin is a suspension of killed *M. leprae* prepared from heavily infected human or armadillo tissue. Intradermal injection elicits, somewhat variably, a tuberculin-like reaction at 48 h (Fernandez's reaction) and, more consistently, a papular reaction at 3 to 4 weeks (Mitsuda's reaction). The Mitsuda reaction is usually positive in tuberculoid patients and is always negative in lepromatous patients. However, because it is also positive in nearly all normal adults, even those residing in areas free of endemic leprosy, it has no diagnostic value. Lepromin is not commercially available.

A specific serodiagnostic test for leprosy has been developed. Based on the detection of antibody to phenolic glycolipid I, this assay has a sensitivity of over 95 percent in polar lepromatous disease and about 30 percent in tuberculoid disease. The level of antibody appears to correlate with the bacillary load, which explains the high false-negative rate in polar tuberculoid disease. Despite this limitation, the near 100 percent specificity of this assay makes it potentially useful for confirming the diagnosis of leprosy and as an epidemiologic tool for studying disease incubation and transmission.

The differential diagnosis includes lupus erythematosus, lupus vulgaris, sarcoidosis, yaws, dermal leishmaniasis, and a host of banal skin diseases. The skin lesions of leprosy, especially of turberculoid disease, are characterized by hypesthesia, and peripheral nerve involvement can always be demonstrated. Peripheral neuropathy from other causes and syringomyelia may be confused with leprosy, although skin involvement is not a feature of other diseases causing peripheral neuropathy. The combination of a chronic skin disease and peripheral nerve involvement should always lead to the consideration of leprosy.

TREATMENT The management of leprosy involves a broad, multidisciplinary approach, including consultative services such as orthopedic surgery, ophthalmology, and physical therapy in addition to antimicrobial chemotherapy.

Specific chemotherapy *Dapsone* (4,4'-diaminodiphenylsulfone, DDS, diphenylsulfone), a folate antagonist, is the mainstay of therapy. The daily dosage is 50 to 100 mg in adults. Dapsone is very inexpensive, safe in pregnancy, and has a long serum half-life of about 24 h, allowing once daily administration. Major side effects, which are relatively uncommon, include hemolysis, agranulocytosis, hepatitis, and potentially fatal exfoliative dermatitis. In lepromatous disease, enough bacilli are killed during the first 10 to 12 weeks of dapsone monotherapy to render mouse foot pad inoculations negative. However, in this form of the disease nonviable bacilli disappear slowly and may be found in the tissues for 5 to 10 years. Moreover, a few viable bacilli (persisters) may survive in the tissues for many years and cause a relapse if treatment is discontinued.

Years of dapsone monotherapy led to the emergence of dapsone-resistant strains of *M. leprae*. Secondary resistance occurs in 2 to 30 percent of lepromatous patients receiving dapsone monotherapy. It presents as a clinical and bacteriologic relapse after several years of apparently successful, regular therapy. Primary dapsone resistance in previously untreated patients has complicated empiric therapy in many parts of the world but remains uncommon (less than 3 percent) in the United States. To counteract this problem, the World Health Organization, in 1982, recommended the use of multiple-drug therapy for all leprosy patients.

Rifampin is the most rapidly mycobactericidal drug known for *M. leprae*. The viability of skin bacilli falls to undetectable levels within 5 days following a single 1500-mg dose of oral rifampin. The usual dosage is 600 mg/d. The high cost of rifampin has limited its use in the developing world and has led to regimens in which it is given at a dosage of 600 or 900 mg once per month. Many leprologists prefer to treat with daily or twice-weekly rifampin if cost is not a crucial issue. Rare cases of rifampin-resistant *M. leprae* have been reported. Rifampin has not been approved for the intermittent treatment of leprosy by the Food and Drug Administration.

Clofazimine is a compound derived from a phenazine dye. It is highly lipophilic and accumulates in the skin, the gastrointestinal tract, and macrophages and monocytes. It is usually given in a dosage of 50 to 200 mg/d and has an apparent half-life of over 70 days. Major toxicity is restricted to the skin and the intestinal tract. The reddish skin pigmentation, often accompanied by ichthyosis, is unacceptable to many light-skinned patients and can lead to poor compliance. The intestinal toxicity is also dose-related and is reflected in diarrhea and cramping abdominal pain. Clofazimine is not safe for use during pregnancy.

There are several older agents with limited activity against *M. leprae* which have been used in certain clinical situations, including ethionamide, prothionamide, thiambutosine, and amithiozone. All these drugs have significant toxicities, and none has been approved for this purpose by the Food and Drug Administration. An extremely important and exciting development in the last few years has been the identification of several new antimicrobials with impressive activity against *M. leprae*. The most promising agents are minocycline, ofloxacin, and clarithromycin. Fusidic acid, ampicillin/clavulanic acid, and brodimoprim also have shown activity against *M. leprae* in vitro or in mice. Clinical trials of many of these new drugs are now underway, but all should be considered investigational, and none has been approved for the treatment of leprosy by the Food and Drug Administration.

Therapy for multibacillary disease should consist of three drugs, usually dapsone, rifampin, and clofazimine. If the organism is known to be dapsone-sensitive, the combination of dapsone and rifampin may be adequate for borderline and borderline lepromatous cases, but the likelihood of secondary dapsone resistance makes the addition of a third drug advisable in lepromatous disease. Objective measures of response to therapy, including skin scrapings and biopsies, should be monitored and therapy continued at least until morphologically intact bacilli are consistently absent and the inflammatory cell infiltrate has resolved. The optimal duration of therapy is unknown, but a minimum of 2 years is recommended. Indefinite therapy may be required in some cases of lepromatous disease.

Therapeutic regimens containing two drugs, usually dapsone and rifampin, are adequate for paucibacillary leprosy. The World Health Organization recommends a 6-month course and reports an annual failure rate after completion of only 0.1 percent. Standard practice in the United States is to treat with dapsone and rifampin for the first 6 to 12 months (depending on the clinical response), followed by dapsone alone to complete a total of 24 months of therapy.

Evidence of clinical improvement should be visible by the second or third month of treatment. The clinical response to therapy may be confused by intercurrent reactional states, but the disease stops progressing and the skin lesions gradually improve. Recovery from neurologic impairment is limited.

Treatment of reactional states Mild ENL is managed with antipyretics and analgesics. Severe cases can be rapidly controlled with high dosages of prednisone (60 to 120 mg/d). Antimicrobial therapy should be continued, since glucocorticoid therapy promotes the viability of *M. leprae* in mice not given antileprosy drugs. Rifampin enhances the metabolism of glucocorticoids by the liver, necessitating administration of larger doses to achieve a given therapeutic effect. Thalidomide is the most effective drug for ENL. The usual initial dosage is 200 mg twice a day, which can be gradually tapered to a maintenance dosage of 50 to 100 mg/d for patients with chronic ENL. Thalidomide is absolutely contraindicated in women of childbearing age because of its teratogenicity but has proved relatively free of major side effects in other leprosy patients. This drug has not been approved by the Food and Drug Administration but is available through the Hansen's Disease Center, Carville, Louisiana, as an investigational agent. Clofazimine has anti-inflammatory properties as well as antimycobacterial activity and can be valuable in the treatment of chronic ENL, but it requires at least 3 to 4 weeks to reach effective levels, making it of little use in acute attacks. Other anti-inflammatory agents, including chloroquine, cyclosporine, and cytotoxic drugs, have been used in difficult cases; in general, these unusual situations should be managed in consultation with a leprosy specialist.

Reversal reactions are often acute and can lead to rapid and irreversible neurologic damage. Glucocorticoids are indicated for severe reversal reactions. Clofazimine is of some use in chronic situations, but it is generally necessary to continue glucocorticoids as well. Reversal reactions do not respond to thalidomide.

Other measures   Many of the deformities and disabilities of leprosy are preventable. Plantar ulcers, which are very common, may be prevented by rigid-soled footwear or walking plaster casts, and contractures of the hand may be prevented by physical therapy and application of casts. Reconstructive surgery is sometimes helpful. Nerve and tendon transplants and release of contractures can give patients more functional ability. Vocational retraining is often necessary for those with permanent disability. Plastic repair of facial deformities assists acceptance of patients in society. The psychological trauma which resulted from prolonged segregation is now minimized by home therapy in virtually all cases.

CONTROL   Case finding and chemotherapy form the present basis of control. Infectiousness can be quickly suppressed with chemotherapy, making early detection of cases important. In endemic countries, this means establishing local clinics or traveling teams. Family and other close contacts need to be examined regularly for leprosy. A benefit of the short (6- to 24-month) multidrug treatment regimens is that patients can be certified disease-free much sooner than was possible with dapsone monotherapy. This permits leprosy case workers to devote proportionately more effort to contact screening and case detection. In the United States, patients are eligible for treatment by the Public Health Service, and special clinics are located in several major cities. Risk of transmission is very low, even in untreated patients, and no unusual infection control precautions are required when patients are hospitalized. Chemoprophylaxis with lowered doses of dapsone may be effective, but contact screening by yearly physical examinations is preferred to empiric therapy in most situations. Vaccine trials with bacillus Calmette-Guérin in endemic areas have yielded conflicting results with, at most, modest efficacy. At least four new experimental vaccines are currently in field trials in India and South America.

REFERENCES

BLAKE LA et al: Environmental nonhuman sources of leprosy. Rev Infect Dis 9:562, 1987

BLOOM BR, GODAL T: Selective primary health care: Strategies for the control of disease in the developing world. V. Leprosy. Rev Infect Dis 5:765, 1983

BULLOCK WE: *Mycobacterium leprae* (leprosy), in *Principles and Practice of Infectious Diseases*, 3d ed, GL Mandell et al (eds). New York, Wiley, 1990, pp 1906–1914

EDITORIAL: Serological tests for leprosy. Lancet 1:533, 1986

GOODLESS DR et al: Reactional states in Hansen's disease: Practical aspects of emergency management. South Med J 84:237, 1991

HASTINGS RC (ed): *Leprosy*. New York, Churchill Livingstone, 1985

JACOBSON R: The face of leprosy in the United States today. Arch Dermatol 126:1627, 1990

MASTRO TD et al: Leprosy in the United States, 1971–1988. Am J Public Health 82:1127, 1992

MILLER RA: Leprosy and AIDS. Int J Lepr Other Mycobact Dis 59:639, 1991

SCHLESINGER LS et al: Phenolic glycolipid-1 of *Mycobacterium leprae* binds complement component C3 in serum and mediates phagocytosis by human monocytes. J Exp Med 174:1031, 1991

SHIELDS ED et al: Genetic epidemiology of the susceptibility to leprosy. J Clin Invest 79:1139, 1987

132   MYCOBACTERIUM AVIUM COMPLEX AND OTHER NONTUBERCULOUS MYCOBACTERIAL INFECTIONS

FERRIC C. FANG / STANLEY D. FREEDMAN

Mycobacteria other than the tubercle bacillus have been known to be agents of human disease since the 1950s. A classification of these organisms based on colonial morphology and growth characteristics was provided by Runyon. He classified mycobacteria as photochromogens (pigment production induced by light), scotochromogens (constitutive pigment production), nonchromogens (absent pigment production), or rapid growers. These bacteria are widely distributed in nature as saprophytes, primarily in soil and water. Animals can be infected and may serve as reservoirs for infection of humans. Person-to-person transmission occurs rarely, if at all. Skin tests with tuberculins from the various species have demonstrated the extent of infection in the United States and other countries, as well as notable geographic variability among species. These bacteria have been referred to as *atypical mycobacteria* or *anonymous mycobacteria*, reflecting the emphasis of earlier microbiologists on *Mycobacterium tuberculosis*. Currently preferred designations are *nontuberculous mycobacteria* (NTM), *mycobacteria other than tuberculosis* (MOTT), and *environmental mycobacteria*. The frequency with which they are found in the environment requires that repeated isolation from a diseased site or isolation from blood or bone marrow be achieved before nontuberculous mycobacteria can be definitively identified as the cause of disease. In some cases, pathologic evidence of a granulomatous inflammatory process also may be required before a disease process can be attributed unequivocally to a nontuberculous mycobacterium. With recent improvements in laboratory techniques, such as radiometric culture systems and nucleic acid probes, species designations are becoming increasingly familiar (Table 132-1). Although of lesser virulence than the tubercle bacillus, these organisms may be important pathogens in compromised individuals, particularly those with impaired cellular immunity or underlying lung disease. The recognition of serious disseminated nontuberculous mycobacterial infections in patients with AIDS has given new significance to the nontuberculous mycobacteria. Although infections with *M. asiaticum*, *M. flavescens*, *M. fortuitum*/*M. chelonae*, *M. gordonae*, *M. haemophilum*, *M. kansasii*, *M. malmoense*, *M. marinum*, *M. scrofulaceum*, *M. simiae*, *M. smegmatis*, *M. szulgai*, *M. ulcerans*, and *M. xenopi* have

TABLE 132-1   Human mycobacterial pathogens other than *M. tuberculosis* and *M. leprae*

Mycobacterium	Pigmentation*	Usual site of disease	Environmental source
M. avium complex	N	Disseminated, lungs, lymph nodes	Water, soil, ? Animals
M. fortuitum/ *M. chelonae*	N	Skin, lungs	Water, soil
M. haemophilum	N	Skin	Unknown
M. kansasii	P	Lungs	? Water, ? animals
M. marinum	P	Skin	Water, fish
M. scrofulaceum	S	Lymph nodes	Water, soil
M. szulgai	S†	Lungs	? Fish
M. ulcerans	N	Skin	Tropical grasses
M. xenopi	S	Lungs	Water, animals
M. asiaticum	P	Lungs	? Animals
M. malmoense	N	Lungs	Unknown
M. shimoidei	N	Lungs	Unknown
M. simiae	P (weak)	Lungs	Water, ? animals

* P = photochromogen, N = nonchromogen, S = scotochromogen
† Scotochromogen at 37°C, photochromogen at 25°C

been reported in association with AIDS, more than 95 percent of nontuberculous mycobacterial infections in AIDS are caused by *M. avium* complex (MAC).

MYCOBACTERIUM AVIUM COMPLEX Although a variety of technical methods can distinguish *M. avium* from *M. intracellulare*, species distinction by routine culture methods is difficult, and they are often considered as a complex (MAC); alternatively, this group of organisms may be referred to collectively as *Mycobacterium avium-intracellulare* (MAI). Commercially available specific nucleic acid probes now permit rapid and convenient differentiation of *M. avium* and *M. intracellulare*. These ubiquitous organisms are particularly prevalent in the southeastern United States and, overall, are the most commonly isolated mycobacteria. They can be isolated from soil, water (including tap water), house dust, food, and animals. MAC organisms are classified as nonchromogens, but some strains are lightly pigmented.

The lungs are the most important site of localized infection due to MAC. Aerosols are thought to be an important mode of acquisition of respiratory disease. Colonization and inapparent infection are common. When the lungs are involved, the clinical picture frequently resembles pulmonary tuberculosis. Alternatively, patients may present with lower zone nodular subpleural shadowing, bronchiectasis, or solitary nodules. Underlying pulmonary disease, collagen-vascular disease, a possible genetic predilection, and advanced age are risk factors. When a MAC organism is isolated from a patient with pulmonary disease, it is important to be certain of the pathogenic role of the organism in the disease process, because chemotherapy is often associated with morbidity.

Skin involvement and musculoskeletal infections including vertebral osteomyelitis that resembles Pott's disease have been described. MAC is the major mycobacterial cause of cervical lymphadenitis in American children and is especially common between 1 and 5 years of age. Genitourinary disease, meningitis, gastrointestinal ulcers, panniculitis, pericarditis, and otomastoiditis also have been reported. Disseminated MAC infection can occur in children and adults, mostly in association with severe underlying diseases.

MAC in AIDS There is a striking association between disseminated *Mycobacterium avium* complex infection and AIDS (see Chap. 279). MAC infection is diagnosed in 10 to 30 percent of AIDS patients antemortem and in 50 percent at autopsy. MAC infection occurs fairly uniformly among different AIDS risk groups; the most important risk factor appears to be a CD4 count less than 100 cells per microliter of blood. Massive involvement of the gastrointestinal tract has suggested the possibility of an oral route of infection from contaminated water, and experimental evidence supporting this hypothesis has been obtained in the beige mouse model. Nevertheless, the relationship between colonization and the development of disseminated infection remains uncertain at present, and respiratory colonization appears to precede disseminated illness in some cases. The organism burden is extremely high, with up to 10^6 bacteria per milliliter of blood and 10^{10} bacteria per gram of tissue. The cellular inflammatory response, granulomatous or otherwise, is minimal. It has been speculated that the fibrillar peptidoglycolipid sheath of MAC organisms both protects the microbe from host defenses and prevents activation of inflammatory mediators by shielding toxic sulfatides and cord factor in the organism's cell wall.

Fever, weight loss, and cytopenias are common. Involvement of the small intestine may produce watery diarrhea and malabsorption. The histopathology resembles that of Whipple's disease; acid-fast stains reveal that the macrophages filling the intestinal lamina propria are packed with mycobacteria. In other organs these macrophages may resemble lepra cells. Colonic involvement may produce severe abdominal pain. Hepatic infiltration is frequent and may result in marked elevation of the serum alkaline phosphatase. The findings of hepatosplenomegaly, thickening of the small bowel wall, and bulky lymphadenopathy on abdominal CT scan suggest MAC infection. Although endobronchial lesions with airway narrowing may occur and bacteria are frequently present in the respiratory secretions

of infected patients, pulmonary parenchymal disease is curiously uncommon.

The diagnosis of disseminated MAC infection is made by isolation of organisms from blood, bone marrow, or liver tissue. Radiometric blood culture systems can quickly confirm the diagnosis in the vast majority of patients with disseminated disease, and nucleic acid probes can facilitate rapid speciation. MAC organisms may be recovered from the blood in as few as 5 to 14 days. The compound NAP (*p*-nitro-α-acetylamino-β-hydroxypropiophenone) selectively inhibits species of the *M. tuberculosis* complex in culture, and its inclusion in radiometric cultures may aid in presumptive identification. Bone marrow biopsy, liver biopsy, or intestinal biopsy also may provide a diagnosis of disseminated MAC infection. Culture of MAC organisms from these tissues by routine methods usually takes 4 weeks. The presence of heavy acid-fast bacilli on touch preparations of tissue or stool smear is highly suggestive. It has been reported that buffy coat acid-fast smears are positive in approximately one-third of patients. MAC organisms also have been found in the lymph nodes, eye, thyroid, esophagus, mediastinum, pericardium, pancreas, adrenal, kidney, muscle, brain, joint, bone, and skin of infected patients. The usual survival is only 4 to 10 months once the diagnosis of disseminated MAC infection has been made in a patient with AIDS, but therapy reduces morbidity in some patients and may extend survival.

Both microbial and host factors appear to be critical to the development of disseminated MAC infection in AIDS. *M. avium* is isolated from 97 percent of AIDS patients with MAC infection, whereas *M. intracellulare* accounts for 40 percent of MAC infections in patients without AIDS. Furthermore, strains of *M. avium* from patients with AIDS are more likely to be from serovars 1, 4, and 8; produce pigment; contain plasmids; and have a particular RFLP (restriction fragment length polymorphism) pattern. MAC organisms have been demonstrated to inhibit phagosome-lysosome fusion and superoxide production by macrophages. Although no difference has been found in the ability of normal or AIDS-infected macrophages to phagocytose and kill MAC organisms, the characteristic pathologic finding of macrophages stuffed with acid-fast bacilli is consistent with the idea that impaired T cell function results in an inability of host macrophages to control MAC replication. MAC growth is suppressed in macrophages cocultivated with sensitized T cells or natural killer cells. Recent studies have indicated that MAC growth in macrophages also may be modulated by cytokines and serum factors that are deficient in some patients with AIDS.

Treatment of MAC infections Treatment of these infections is difficult and often unsatisfactory. The organisms are usually resistant to most conventional antimycobacterial agents. Multiple-drug therapy sometimes appears to be of benefit, possibly reflecting synergy between agents which are not individually very active. The value of in vitro susceptibility studies is controversial. Nonetheless, it seems prudent to select an antimicrobial regimen that includes drugs to which an isolate is susceptible. For pulmonary disease thought to warrant treatment, the American Thoracic Society has recommended isoniazid, rifampin, ethambutol, and the initial use of streptomycin. These recommendations were made on the basis of limited clinical studies but may require modification as experience with newer antimycobacterial agents accumulates. Surgical excision is the treatment of choice for lymphadenitis and is a reasonable alternative for a few other localized infections.

Because it has been difficult to demonstrate clinical benefit of antimicrobial therapy in many AIDS patients with disseminated MAC infection, treatment usually has been reserved for highly symptomatic patients. Agents which may be useful in this setting include ethambutol, rifampin, rifabutin (ansamycin), ciprofloxacin, clofazimine, streptomycin, amikacin, clarithromycin, azithromycin, and sparfloxacin. Ethionamide and cycloserine also have activity against some MAC isolates but are often poorly tolerated. The new macrolides clarithromycin and azithromycin appear to be particularly useful against MAC organisms and have shown encouraging results in early clinical trials. Among the attractive features of these agents is their ability to be concentrated within phagocytic cells. When used as monotherapy, the new macrolides give rise to resistance fairly rapidly. This is not surprising in view of the organism load in infected patients and underscores the importance of using multiple agents in the treatment of mycobacterial infections. The new fluoroquinolone sparfloxacin is also active against MAC in vitro, but clinical studies are pending. Clarithromycin, sparfloxacin, and, to a lesser extent, azithromycin slow intracellular MAC replication in macrophages in vitro; the addition of ethambutol or rifampin provides synergy. Other investigational agents such as rifapentine, WIN57273, thiacetazone, and liposomal amikacin are undergoing evaluation.

Therapy of symptomatic patients with disseminated MAC infection may improve the quality of their lives. Until studies define the optimal regimen, initial therapy with one of the newer macrolides plus two other agents, e.g., ethambutol and rifampin, should be considered. Rifabutin (ansamycin) is active against the majority of *M. avium* isolates and is being evaluated as a prophylactic agent in AIDS patients with less than 200 CD4 cells per microliter. Early results from these studies are promising. Use of combination therapy for prophylaxis is also under investigation.

Other MAC organisms   *M. avium* ssp. *paratuberculosis* is the etiologic agent of Johne's disease in ruminants. It is dependent on mycobactin, an iron-chelating factor, for in vitro growth. A mycobactin-dependent mycobacterium resembling *M. avium* ssp. *paratuberculosis* has been isolated from the terminal ileum of a small number of patients with Crohn's disease, but the significance of this finding remains highly controversial.

MYCOBACTERIUM FORTUITUM/CHELONAE AND OTHER RAPID GROWERS

The distinguishing feature of these acid-fast bacteria is their rapid growth. Initial growth may take as long as 1 to 5 weeks, but subsequent subcultures generally grow within 1 to 3 days. Their distinction from more slowly growing mycobacteria has been supported by rRNA sequence analysis. These gram-positive, nonpigmented organisms are readily cultured on most media and may be confused with diphtheroids. Unlike other mycobacteria, they may not stain with auramine-rhodamine used in fluorescence microscopy. Although geographically widespread, these organisms are isolated most frequently in the southern United States from Georgia to Texas.

M. fortuitum and *M. chelonae* account for more than 95 percent of the reported infections due to rapid growers. Rare infections have been reported with other rapid-growing mycobacteria such as *M. smegmatis*, *M. thermoresistibile*, *M. flavescens*, and *M. neoaurum*. *M. smegmatis* can be part of the normal urogenital flora and is sometimes responsible for misleading positive acid-fast smears of urine. *M. fortuitum* is frequently associated with posttraumatic and postoperative skin and soft tissue infection. Most pulmonary infections and disseminated disease have been attributed to *M. chelonae*. Three biovars of *M. fortuitum* and three subspecies of *M. chelonae* have been described, but subspeciation is not necessary for clinical purposes. Since they are widespread in nature and in hospital environments and are highly resistant to antibiotics, antiseptics, and disinfectants, rapid growers are important nosocomial pathogens. Contamination of equipment, solutions, or water in the hospital setting also may lead to "pseudoepidemics."

Most skin infections are associated with interruption of the integument and injury or alteration of the soft tissues. Surgery, accidental trauma, or injections are important risk factors. Cutaneous infection may result in pyogenic abscesses, chronic ulcers, or sporotrichoid lesions. Although a chronic granulomatous reaction with caseation may occur, the typical pathologic process is suppurative with formation of microabscesses, and diphtheroid-like organisms may be seen on Gram's stain. In contrast to patients with lung infection caused by other nontuberculous mycobacteria, most patients with *M. chelonae* or *M. fortuitum* pulmonary infections have no underlying lung disease. The majority of these patients are women over 50 years of age. Cavitation is less frequent than in other mycobacterial lung infections. Other reported clinical manifestations include bone and joint infection, otitis media, intravascular or

peritoneal catheter infection, shunt infection, lymphadenitis, ocular infection, intraoral or facial infection, pericarditis, mediastinitis, hepatitis, gastrointestinal infection, prostatitis, meningitis, and endocarditis involving porcine, prosthetic, or natural valves. Hematogenous dissemination is uncommon and affects primarily those with impaired host defenses. Infections have followed cardiothoracic surgery, augmentation mammaplasty, arthroplasty, ocular surgery, and dialysis.

Adequate debridement and drainage with removal of foreign bodies are indicated whenever possible. Many of these organisms are highly resistant to antimicrobial agents, but antimicrobial susceptibility testing is indicated because it may be a more reliable determinant of appropriate chemotherapy than it is in infections with other nontuberculous mycobacteria. *M. chelonae* tends to be more drug-resistant than *M. fortuitum* but is generally sensitive to cefoxitin and amikacin. Other drugs sometimes useful in the treatment of infections caused by rapidly growing mycobacteria include erythromycin, doxycycline, minocycline, ciprofloxacin, ofloxacin, ethionamide, tobramycin, imipenem, sulfonamides, and rifabutin. Relapses are not unusual, and prolonged therapy (12 to 16 weeks) is often recommended. Clarithromycin and other new macrolides are active in vitro, and preliminary anecdotal clinical reports are encouraging.

MYCOBACTERIUM HAEMOPHILUM

This organism is a very fastidious, slow-growing, nonpigmented mycobacterium which requires hemin (factor X) or ferric ammonium citrate for in vitro growth. Optimal growth occurs at 30°C in 10% CO_2. *M. haemophilum* has been associated principally with chronic nodular skin lesions of the extremities, most often in immunocompromised patients (AIDS, lymphoma, transplant patients). The skin lesions may ulcerate. Arthritis, tenosynovitis, osteomyelitis, and occasionally lymphadenitis also have been reported. Some isolates have been susceptible to rifampin, rifabutin, PAS (*para*-amino salicylate), ciprofloxacin, cycloserine, kanamycin, minocycline, doxycycline, and trimethoprim-sulfamethoxazole. Surgical debridement has been helpful in some instances.

MYCOBACTERIUM KANSASII

M. kansasii is nearly always photochromogenic, grows optimally at 37°C, and characteristically appears long and thick with prominent transverse banding on acid-fast smear. Infections are most common in the central United States, Japan, England, and Wales; most patients in the United States have originated in Louisiana, Texas, California, Illinois, or Florida. The reasons for these geographic variations are unknown but likely relate to subtle ecologic preferences of these organisms. *M. kansasii* has been isolated from tap and natural water sources, as well as from cattle and swine. Person-to-person spread is not recognized. The incidence of infection is highest in white adult males.

Pulmonary disease is the most frequent manifestation of infection with this organism, and the clinical picture closely resembles pulmonary tuberculosis, although signs and symptoms are milder. Pneumoconiosis and chronic obstructive pulmonary disease (COPD) are important predisposing conditions. Thin-walled cavities with minimal inflammatory reaction are typical roentgenographic findings. Pleural effusions are uncommon. Abnormalities usually progress slowly in the absence of therapy. As with other nontuberculous mycobacteria, isolation of *M. kansasii* does not necessarily indicate the presence of disease; 25 to 50 percent of positive sputum cultures are thought to represent colonization.

Skin and soft tissue involvement may mimic *M. marinum* infections. Tenosynovitis, osteomyelitis, lymphadenitis, pericarditis, and genitourinary tract infections have been reported. Disseminated disease is now recognized as an important manifestation of *M. kansasii* infections. Hematogenous spread is associated with hairy cell leukemia, malignancies, AIDS, and bone marrow and renal transplantation. Fever and signs and symptoms of multiple organ system involvement occur. Pancytopenia has been reported in disseminated infection.

Localized disease due to *M. kansasii* responds well to treatment. Rifampin appears to be the most effective drug and should be used in all initial regimens. Ethambutol and isoniazid are usually the other drugs administered. Typical strains demonstrate low-level resistance to isoniazid and streptomycin, but approximately 95 percent of patients respond to a 15- to 18-month course of isoniazid, rifampin, and ethambutol. The addition of ethambutol is important because the acquisition of rifampin resistance greatly complicates management. Other potentially active agents include sulfonamides, ciprofloxacin, ofloxacin, ethionamide, cycloserine, erythromycin, rifabutin, amikacin, and minocycline. Surgery is occasionally useful but seldom required.

MYCOBACTERIUM MARINUM This organism, previously known as *M. balnei*, is a photochromogen which inhabits fresh and salt water, grows best at 30°C, and causes disease in fish. Human infections are usually associated with some aquatic activity, such as working with fish tanks or swimming. *M. marinum* is relatively common along the Gulf Coast of the United States. The organism enters abraded skin and may form a nodule, which can spread along lymphatics in a pattern suggesting sporotrichosis, cause verrucous lesions, or, less commonly, ulcerate. The pathology consists of a granulomatous lesion which lacks caseation—the so-called swimming pool or fishtank granuloma. On acid-fast smear, *M. marinum* are relatively long organisms with frequent cross-barring, but primary smears reveal organisms in only a minority of patients. Infection is frequently associated with a positive tuberculin test reflecting shared antigens with *M. tuberculosis*. Because the differential diagnosis includes sporotrichosis as well as other mycobacterial infections, appropriate cultures at an incubation temperature of 28 to 32°C are critical. As with other mycobacteria associated with cutaneous disease (e.g., *M. haemophilum*, *M. ulcerans*), the inability of *M. marinum* to grow at 37°C explains its limitation to superficial tissues. Infections of tendon sheaths, bone, and synovium have been described in association with penetrating injuries. An unusual case involving the eye and a possible case of visceral involvement have been reported. Cutaneous ulcerations similar to those caused by *M. ulcerans*, as well as disseminated skin lesions, have been reported in immunocompromised patients. Minor lesions may resolve spontaneously. The organism is often sensitive in vitro to rifampin and ethambutol, and these drugs have been curative.

Tetracyclines, especially minocycline, and trimethoprim-sulfamethoxazole also have been used with favorable results. Prior steroid injections into infected sites are associated with an unfavorable prognosis. Surgical debridement is sometimes required.

MYCOBACTERIUM SCROFULACEUM This bacillus, which forms yellow-orange pigment even in the dark (scotochromogenic), is a cause of lymphadenitis in children. Environmental isolation has been reported from soil, water, raw milk, and oysters. *M. scrofulaceum* appears to be decreasing in incidence in the United States. Submandibular nodes are typically involved, in contrast to *M. tuberculosis*, which more frequently involves tonsillar, anterior cervical, or supraclavicular nodes, and associated systemic symptoms are rare. Definitive diagnosis requires culture, and definitive therapy requires total excision of the node and sinus tract, if present. There are a few reports of pulmonary disease, osseous and soft tissue infections, conjunctivitis, meningitis, and hepatitis. Dissemination usually is associated with serious underlying conditions. Surgery remains the mainstay of therapy. *M. scrofulaceum* is typically resistant to many drugs in vitro, and multiple-drug regimens have been used. Some isolates are sensitive to isoniazid, rifampin, streptomycin, cycloserine, sulfonamides, erythromycin, ethambutol, or ethionamide.

MYCOBACTERIUM SZULGAI At 37°C this organism is scotochromogenic and can be confused with more common tap water contaminants; at 25°C it is photochromogenic. It has been isolated from snails and tropical fish. *M. szulgai* is more than 99 percent homologous to *M. malmoense* at the RNA sequence level. *M. szulgai* was initially recognized as an uncommon pulmonary pathogen producing disease similar to *M. tuberculosis*. Bursitis, lymphadenitis, tenosynovitis, skin lesions, osteomyelitis, and disseminated disease also have been reported. Most isolates are sensitive to rifampin and

ethionamide. Isoniazid, ethambutol, streptomycin, erythromycin, tetracycline, trimethoprim-sulfamethoxazole, cefoxitin, and amikacin also may be active. As with other mycobacterial infections, combination therapy is advisable. Surgery may be required for definitive management.

MYCOBACTERIUM ULCERANS *M. ulcerans* is the etiologic agent of the Buruli or Bairnsdale ulcer. It is a nonchromogen which grows only at 30 to 33°C. Colonies may require 6 to 12 weeks to appear; isolation may be enhanced by inoculation of mouse footpads. A disease of the tropics, it is concentrated in Australia and Africa; foci in Malaysia, Papua (New Guinea), Guyana, and Mexico also have been recognized. The organism may be cultured from grass and is believed to be introduced into the skin via grass cuts. The first sign of infection with *M. ulcerans* is a small painless nodule developing into an extensive granulomatous ulceration, usually affecting the extensor surfaces of the extremities. Characteristically, the ulcer is deep with a necrotic base and undermined edges. Satellite lesions may develop. Tissue destruction may be mediated by a soluble bacterial toxin that appears to mute the host response. Patients do not exhibit constitutional symptoms. Wide surgical excision with skin grafting is curative; there are no clear data regarding chemotherapy. Dapsone and streptomycin with or without ethambutol may be used as adjunctive therapy. Isoniazid, trimethoprim-sulfamethoxazole, rifampin, oxytetracycline, minocycline, and clofazimine also may be active, but treatment failures have been reported despite in vitro drug susceptibility.

MYCOBACTERIUM XENOPI *M. xenopi* is a slow-growing scotochromogen. Although the mycobacterium was first isolated from a toad, birds may be an important reservoir in nature. Geographic foci with increased rates of isolation have been described in Ontario, southeast England, and Scandinavia. Although *M. xenopi* may grow in hot or cold water, it grows optimally at 42°C, and some strains will grow only at 42 to 45°C. Clusters of cases have occurred in association with contaminated hot water generators. *M. xenopi* infrequently causes tuberculosis-like pulmonary disease in humans, usually in association with underlying diseases. Cavitary disease is particularly common. Extrapulmonary disease is rare, but prosthetic joint, sinus tract, epididymis, osseous, and lymph node isolates have been described. Reports of disseminated disease are becoming more common, notably in patients with AIDS. Unlike a number of nontuberculous mycobacteria, it is sensitive to most of the antituberculous drugs in vitro, but some pulmonary infections have not responded well to antimicrobial therapy. Active agents include isoniazid, rifampin, ethambutol, streptomycin, ethionamide, cycloserine, and ciprofloxacin; some isolates are susceptible to vancomycin, cefuroxime, and erythromycin.

OTHER MYCOBACTERIA *M. asiaticum* is a photochromogen first isolated from monkeys. It is an uncommon cause of lung disease which resembles pulmonary tuberculosis but occurs predominantly in individuals with preexisting lung disease. The first reports of human disease due to *M. asiaticum* originated in Australia, and the organism is rarely isolated in the United States. Agents used in treatment have included isoniazid, rifampin, ethambutol, pyrazinamide, capreomycin, PAS, and streptomycin. Some isolates have been reported to be susceptible in vitro to cycloserine, kanamycin, and ciprofloxacin, although *M. asiaticum* appears to be somewhat less sensitive to fluoroquinolones than other nontuberculous mycobacteria.

M. malmoense is nonpigmented, microaerophilic, and slow growing. It grows poorly on conventional mycobacterial media; isolation can be facilitated by adjusting the pH to 6 to 6.5 and substituting 0.4% sodium pyruvate for glycerol. The organism can be confused microbiologically with nonpathogenic *M. terrae* or *M. gastri* species. Although a rare isolate in the United States, *M. malmoense* has been reported as a cause of chronic pulmonary disease in Scandinavia, Switzerland, Germany, Belgium, and the United Kingdom. Cases of lymphadenitis and dissemination in patients with AIDS or leukemia also have been described. Some isolates are susceptible to ethambutol, ethionamide, kanamycin, cycloserine, and erythromycin, but in vitro susceptibility has not correlated well with clinical outcome. Prolonged therapy of 18 months or more has been recommended, and some patients have required surgical excision of diseased areas.

M. shimoidei was first reported in Japan. It is nonpigmented and can be confused with the nonpathogenic species *M. terrae*. *M. shimoidei* has been associated with cavitary pulmonary disease, but very few infections have been reported. Most isolates have been sensitive to ciprofloxacin, but they may be resistant to isoniazid and rifampin.

Like *M. asiaticum*, *M. simiae* was originally isolated from monkeys. *M. simiae* is a weak photochromogen and can resemble MAC organisms in culture if pigment production is scant. Two-thirds of strains are niacin-positive, a feature that distinguishes them from most nontuberculous mycobacteria. Geographically localized clusters of *M. simiae* isolation have been reported from Israel and the southwestern United States. Some clusters have been associated with water sources. Most *M. simiae* isolates are not associated with disease, but pulmonary, osseous, renal, and peritoneal infections have been described. A few infections have been reported in patients with AIDS. The organism is highly resistant to antituberculous agents in vitro and is typically susceptible only to ethionamide and cycloserine.

Some other environmental mycobacterial species have been implicated in but not definitively proven to cause human disease. *M. gastri*, a nonpigmented organism found in soil and water, has been implicated in dialysis-associated peritonitis and pulmonary infections. *M. gordonae* is an extremely common environmental isolate found in ice, tap water, and surface water. It is scotochromogenic and of questionable or very low pathogenicity. A commercially available nucleic acid probe facilitates rapid identification. "Pseudoepidemics" due to contaminated laboratory reagents have been described. Possible associations with pulmonary, skeletal, peritoneal, genitourinary, prosthetic heart valve, cutaneous, shunt, ocular, and disseminated infections have been reported. Because it is ubiquitous in the environment and rarely causes disease, however, each purported infection with *M. gordonae* must be viewed with great caution and skepticism. *M. nonchromogenicum* is a nonpigmented mycobacterium that has been reported to be associated with pulmonary disease. The

M. terrae–M. triviale complex organisms are nonpigmented residents of soil and water which have occasionally been implicated in pulmonary, skeletal, intestinal, and disseminated infections. Finally, in 1988, an unidentified acid-fast bacillus was reported as the cause of fatal disseminated infection in an AIDS patient in Switzerland. The organism could not be cultivated on artificial media but multiplied in nude mice. Electron microscopic and chromatographic analyses suggested that the organism was a *Mycobacterium*. More recently, the organism has been cultivated successfully from other patients with AIDS, and has been designated *M. genavense*.

REFERENCES

CHIODINI RJ: Crohn's disease and the mycobacterioses: A review and comparison of two disease entities. Clin Microbiol Rev 2:90, 1989

COYLE MB et al: Laboratory aspects of '*Mycobacterium genavense*', a proposed species isolated from AIDS patients. J Clin Microbiol 30:3206, 1992

DAUTZENBERG G et al: Activity of clarithromycin against *Mycobacterium avium* infection in patients with the acquired immune deficiency syndrome: A controlled clinical trial. Am Rev Respir Dis 144:564, 1991

ELLNER JJ et al: *Mycobacterium avium* infection and AIDS. J Infect Dis 163:1326, 1991

HIRSCHEL B et al: Fatal infection with a novel, unidentified mycobacterium in a man with the acquired immunodeficiency syndrome. N Engl J Med 323:109, 1990

KRISTJANSSON M et al: *Mycobacterium haemophilum* infection in immunocompromised patients: Case report and review of the literature. Rev Infect Dis 13:906, 1991

NIGHTINGALE SD et al: Incidence of *Mycobacterium avium-intracellulare* complex bacteremia in human immunodeficiency virus–positive patients. J Infect Dis 165:1082, 1992

PITCHENIK AE, FERTEL D: Medical management of AIDS patients: Tuberculosis and nontuberculous mycobacterial disease. Med Clin North Am 76:121, 1992

SHIRATSUCHI H et al: Bidirectional effects of cytokines on the growth of *Mycobacterium avium* within human monocytes. J Immunol 146:3165, 1991

WALLACE RJ, SWENSON JM: Spectrum of disease due to rapidly growing mycobacteria. Rev Infect Dis 5:657, 1983

—— et al: Diagnosis and treatment of disease caused by nontuberculous mycobacteria. Am Rev Respir Dis 142:940, 1990

WAYNE LG, SRAMEK HA: Agents of newly recognized or infrequently encountered mycobacterial diseases. Clin Microbiol Rev 5:1, 1992

WOLINSKY E: Nontuberculous mycobacteria and associated diseases. Am Rev Respir Dis 119:107, 1979

WOODS GL, WASHINGTON JA: Mycobacteria other than *Mycobacterium tuberculosis*: Review of microbiologic and clinical aspects. Rev Infect Dis 9:275, 1987

section 9 Spirochetal diseases

133 SYPHILIS

SHEILA A. LUKEHART / KING K. HOLMES

DEFINITION Syphilis is a chronic systemic infection caused by *Treponema pallidum* subspecies *pallidum*, is usually sexually transmitted, and is characterized by episodes of active disease interrupted by periods of latency. Following an incubation period averaging 3 weeks, a primary lesion appears and is often associated with regional lymphadenopathy; a secondary bacteremic stage is associated with generalized mucocutaneous lesions and generalized lymphadenopathy, followed by a latent period of subclinical infection lasting many years. In about one-third of untreated cases, the tertiary stage is characterized by progressive destructive mucocutaneous, musculoskeletal or parenchymal lesions, aortitis, or symptomatic central nervous system disease.

ETIOLOGY The discovery of *Treponema pallidum* in syphilitic material was made by Schaudinn and Hoffman in 1905. *Treponema*

pallidum is one of the many spiral-shaped microorganisms which propel themselves by spinning around their longitudinal axis. The Spirochaetales include three genera which are pathogenic for humans and for a variety of other animals: the *Leptospira*, which cause human leptospirosis; the *Borrelia*, including *B. recurrentis* and *B. vincentii*, which cause relapsing fever and Vincent's angina, respectively, as well as *B. burgdorferi*, the causative agent of Lyme disease; and the *Treponema*, which are responsible for the diseases known as treponematoses. The *Treponema* include *T. pallidum* subspecies *pallidum* (hereafter called *T. pallidum*), which causes venereal syphilis; *T. pallidum* subspecies *pertenue*, which causes yaws; *T. pallidum* subspecies *endemicum*, which causes endemic syphilis or bejel; *T. carateum*, which causes pinta (see Chap. 134); and *T. paraluiscuniculi*, the cause of rabbit syphilis. Other *Treponema* species are found in the human mouth, genital mucosa, and gastrointestinal tract but have no proven pathogenic role. These can be confused with *T. pallidum* on dark-field examination. Recently, a new oral treponeme was described by Riviere and coworkers. This organism is very closely related to *T. pallidum* antigenically and is significantly associated with periodontitis and acute necrotizing ulcerative gingivitis. Its etiologic role in these gum diseases is unknown.

T. pallidum is a thin, delicate organism with 6 to 14 spirals and tapered ends measuring 6 to 15 μm in total length and 0.2 μm in width. The cytoplasm is surrounded by a trilaminar cytoplasmic membrane, which in turn is surrounded by a delicate peptidoglycan layer providing some structural rigidity. The outer membrane is rich in lipid and contains relatively few integral membrane proteins. Six endoflagella wind around the cell body in a space between the inner cell wall and the outer membrane and may be the contractile elements responsible for motility. None of the four pathogenic treponemes has yet been cultured in vitro in quantity, and no convincing morphologic, serologic, or metabolic differences between them have been discerned. They are distinguished primarily according to the clinical syndrome they produce. The only known natural host for *T. pallidum* is the human. Many mammals can be infected with *T. pallidum*, but only humans, higher apes, and a few laboratory animals regularly develop syphilitic lesions. Virulent strains of *T. pallidum* are maintained in rabbits.

EPIDEMIOLOGY   Nearly all cases of syphilis are acquired by sexual contact with infectious lesions (i.e., the chancre, mucous patch, skin rash, or condyloma latum). Less common modes of transmission include nonsexual personal contact and infection in utero or following blood transfusions.

The total number of cases of syphilis reported annually in the United States (Fig. 133-1) fell steadily from 575,593 in 1943 to a low of 64,621 in 1977, an 88 percent decrease, but then increased to 134,255 in 1990, with a 97 percent increase from 1986 through 1990. The number of new cases of infectious syphilis reached a peak in 1947 and then fell to approximately 6000 in 1956; since then, there has been a rather steady increase in infectious syphilis punctuated by three periods of rapid growth: 10,000 more new cases by 1960 compared with 1956; 13,000 more new cases by 1982 compared with 1979; and from 1986 through 1990, an increase of 22,340 new infectious cases within only 4 years. In 1990, there were 50,223 reported cases of primary and secondary syphilis and 55,132 cases of early latent syphilis; the number of undiagnosed cases is estimated to be much greater.

The populations at highest risk for acquiring syphilis have changed. Between 1977 and 1982, approximately half of all patients with early syphilis in the United States were homosexual or bisexual men. Largely because of changing sexual practices in this population due to the AIDS epidemic, the proportion of early syphilis cases involving homosexual and bisexual men has decreased. The current epidemic of syphilis is occurring predominantly in black heterosexual men and women (Fig. 133-2), largely in urban areas. In some cities, infectious syphilis is significantly correlated with exchange of sex for "crack"

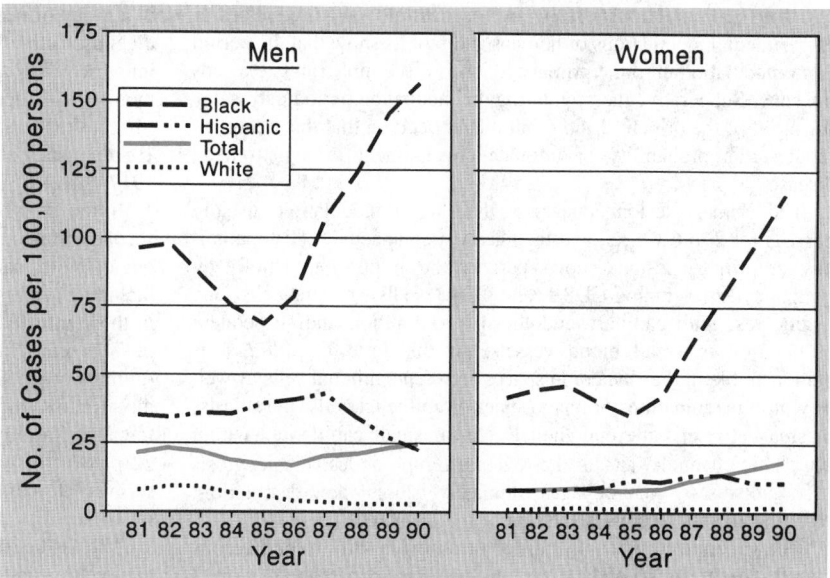

FIGURE 133-1   Number of cases of total syphilis and primary and secondary syphilis reported annually in the United States, 1940–1990. (*From Centers for Disease Control.*)

cocaine. The peak incidence of syphilis occurs in the age group 15 to 34. Although the reported incidence of syphilis is much higher in blacks and Hispanics than in whites and is higher in urban than in rural areas, these differences in part may reflect the fact that many members of urban minority groups are treated at public clinics, where case reporting is more complete. The case rates of early syphilis are highest in large urban population centers, including New York City, parts of Florida and Texas, Los Angeles, and the District of Columbia.

The incidence of congenital syphilis roughly parallels that of infectious syphilis in females. The number of reported cases of congenital syphilis in infants ≤1 year of age was lowest (107 cases)

FIGURE 133-2   Rate of primary and secondary syphilis in men and women in the United States, by ethnic origin, 1981–1990. (*From Centers for Disease Control.*)

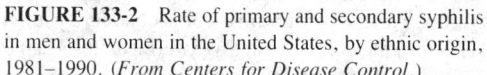

in 1978, when infectious syphilis was most prevalent in homosexual and bisexual men. The dramatic increase in primary and secondary syphilis in women from 1986 to 1990 has resulted in a proportional increase in the number of infants born with congenital syphilis, to 2899 infants in 1990. It is important to note, however, that the case definition for congenital syphilis was broadened in 1989 and now includes all live or stillborn infants delivered to women with untreated or inadequately treated syphilis at delivery.

Approximately one of two individuals named as sexual contacts of persons with infectious syphilis becomes infected. Many sexual contacts will have already developed manifestations of syphilis when they are first seen, and about 30 percent of apparently uninfected contacts who are examined within 30 days of exposure will actually be in the incubation stage and will themselves develop infectious syphilis if not treated. Because of this, the identification and "epidemiologic" treatment of all recently exposed sexual contacts has become an important aspect of syphilis control. For every sex partner notified of exposure to syphilis during 1991, the CDC estimates that approximately 0.2 developed new previously untreated syphilis and received treatment and that 0.5 were exposed but seronegative and received prophylactic treatment. Also important is the identification of infected persons by serologic testing of pregnant women, hospital admissions, military inductees, and persons undergoing examination in physicians' offices. More controversial are laws and regulations requiring routine premarital serologic testing for syphilis, where the yield is undoubtedly lower, though national data are not available.

NATURAL COURSE AND PATHOGENESIS OF UNTREATED SYPHILIS *T. pallidum* rapidly penetrates intact mucous membranes or abraded skin and within a few hours enters the lymphatics and blood to produce systemic infection and metastatic foci long before the appearance of a primary lesion. Blood from a patient with incubating or early syphilis is infectious. The generation time of *T. pallidum* during early active disease in vivo is estimated to be 30 to 33 h, and the incubation period of syphilis is inversely proportional to the number of organisms inoculated. The concentration of treponemes generally reaches at least 10^7 per gram of tissue before the appearance of a clinical lesion. In experimental infection in rabbits or humans, very low numbers of treponemes can initiate infection which leads to a discernible lesion only after several weeks, although histopathologic changes are evident earlier; intradermal injection of 10^6 organisms usually produces a lesion within 72 h. The number of organisms required for production of symptomatic infection in humans was determined by intradermal injection of three graded doses of *T. pallidum* simultaneously at separate inoculation sites into each of eight volunteers; based on these results, the 50 percent infectious dose (ID_{50}) was calculated to be 57 organisms. The median incubation period in humans of about 21 days suggests an average inoculum of 500 to 1000 infectious organisms for naturally acquired disease. Experimental inoculations of humans and rabbits show that the period from inoculation until the primary lesion is discernible rarely exceeds 6 weeks. Subcurative therapy during the incubation period may delay the onset of the primary lesion, but it is not certain that this treatment reduces the probability of ultimate development of symptomatic disease.

The primary lesion appears at the site of inoculation, usually persists for 2 to 6 weeks, and then heals spontaneously. Histopathology of primary lesions shows perivascular infiltration, chiefly by lymphocytes (including CD8+ and CD4+ cells), plasma cells, and histiocytes, with capillary endothelial proliferation and subsequent obliteration of small blood vessels. At this time *T. pallidum* is demonstrable in the chancre in spaces between epithelial cells as well as within invaginations or phagosomes of epithelial cells, fibroblasts, plasma cells, and the endothelial cells of small capillaries, within lymphatic channels, and in the regional lymph nodes. Phagocytosis of organisms by macrophages ultimately causes their destruction, resulting in spontaneous resolution of the chancre.

The generalized parenchymal, constitutional, and mucocutaneous manifestations of secondary syphilis usually appear about 6 to 8 weeks after healing of the chancre, although 15 percent of patients with secondary syphilis have persisting or healing chancres. In other patients, secondary lesions may appear several months after the chancre has healed, and some patients may enter the latent stage without ever developing secondary lesions. Secondary maculopapular skin lesions show histopathologic features of hyperkeratosis of the epidermis, capillary proliferation with endothelial swelling in the superficial corium, and dermal papillae with transmigration of polymorphonuclear leukocytes and, in the deeper corium, perivascular infiltration by monocytes, plasma cells, and lymphocytes. Treponemes are found in many tissues, including the aqueous humor of the eye and the cerebrospinal fluid. Invasion of the central nervous system by *T. pallidum* occurs during the first weeks or months of infection, and cerebrospinal fluid abnormalities are detected in as many as 40 percent of patients during the secondary stage. Clinical hepatitis and immune complex–induced membranous glomerulonephritis are relatively rare but recognized manifestations of secondary syphilis; abnormal liver function tests may be demonstrated in up to a quarter of patients with early syphilis. Generalized lymphadenopathy is present in 85 percent of patients with secondary syphilis and is characterized by marked follicular hyperplasia, with histiocytic infiltration and lymphocyte depletion of the paracortical areas, where treponemes are present in greatest numbers. The reason for the paradoxical appearance of secondary manifestations in the face of high antibody titers (including immobilizing antibody) to *T. pallidum* is unknown. The secondary lesions subside within 2 to 6 weeks, and the patient enters the latent stage, which is detectable only by serologic testing. In the preantibiotic era, up to 25 percent of untreated patients experienced one or more subsequent generalized or localized mucocutaneous relapses at some time during the first 2 to 4 years after infection. Since 50 percent of such infectious relapses occur during the first year, identification and examination of sexual contacts are most important for patients with syphilis of less than 1 year's duration. Recurrent generalized rash is now rare.

In the preantibiotic era, about one-third of patients with untreated latent syphilis developed clinically apparent tertiary disease; today specific treatment and coincidental therapy of early and latent syphilis have greatly reduced the apparent incidence of tertiary disease. In the past, the most common type of tertiary disease was the gumma, a usually benign granulomatous lesion. Today, gummas are very uncommon. The tertiary lesions are caused by obliterative small-vessel endarteritis, which usually involves the vasa vasorum of the ascending aorta and, less often, the central nervous system. Asymptomatic CNS involvement is demonstrable in up to 25 percent of patients with late latent syphilis. Factors which determine development and progression of tertiary disease are unknown.

The course of untreated syphilis has been studied retrospectively in a group of nearly 2000 patients with primary or secondary syphilis diagnosed clinically, before the dark-field and Wassermann tests came into use (the Oslo Study, 1891–1951); prospectively in 431 black men with seropositive latent syphilis of 3 or more years' duration (the Tuskegee Study, 1932–1972); and retrospectively in a review of 198 autopsies of patients with untreated syphilis (the Rosahn Study, 1917–1942).

In the Oslo Study, 24 percent of the patients developed relapsing secondary lesions within 4 years, and 28 percent eventually developed one or more manifestations of late syphilis. Cardiovascular syphilis, including aortitis, was detected in 10 percent, with no cases occurring in those infected before age 15; symptomatic neurosyphilis occurred in 7 percent, and 16 percent developed benign tertiary syphilis (gumma of the skin, mucous membranes, and skeleton). Syphilis was the primary cause of death in 15 percent of males and 8 percent of females. Cardiovascular syphilis was found in 35 percent of men and 22 percent of women who eventually came to autopsy. In general, serious late complications were nearly twice as common in men as in women.

The Tuskegee Study showed that the death rate of untreated black men with syphilis, 25 to 50 years of age, was 17 percent greater than in uninfected subjects and that 30 percent of all deaths were attributable to cardiovascular or CNS syphilis. The ethical issues raised by this study, begun in the preantibiotic era but continuing into the early 1970s, had a major influence on development of current guidelines for human medical experimentation. By far the most important factor in increased mortality was cardiovascular syphilis. Anatomic evidence of aortitis was found in 40 to 60 percent of autopsied subjects with syphilis (versus 15 percent of controls), while CNS syphilis was found in only 4 percent. Hypertension also was increased in the infected subjects. These studies each show that about one-third of patients with untreated syphilis develop clinical or pathologic evidence of tertiary syphilis, about one-fourth die as a direct result of tertiary syphilis, and additional excess mortality not directly attributable to tertiary syphilis is also seen.

MANIFESTATIONS Primary syphilis The typical primary chancre usually begins as a single painless papule which rapidly becomes eroded and usually, but not always, is indurated, with a characteristic cartilaginous consistency on palpation of the edge and base of the ulcer (Fig. 133-3). Histologic examination of the ulcer shows lymphocytic and histiocytic infiltrates with obliterative endarteritis and periarteritis of small vessels. *T. pallidum* is seen by electron microscopy to lie in interstitial perivascular spaces and within invaginations or phagosomes of macrophages, neutrophils, endothelial cells, and plasma cells.

The chancre is usually located on the penis in heterosexual men, whereas in homosexual men it is often found in the anal canal or rectum, within the mouth, or on the external genitalia. In women, common primary sites are the cervix and labia. Consequently, primary syphilis may go unrecognized in women and homosexual men.

Atypical primary lesions are common. The clinical appearance depends on the number of treponemes inoculated and on the immunologic status of the patient. A large inoculum produces a dark-field–positive ulcerative lesion in nonimmune volunteers but may produce a small dark-field–negative papule, an asymptomatic but seropositive latent infection, or no response at all in individuals with a history of syphilis. A small inoculum usually produces only a papular lesion, even in nonimmune humans. Therefore, syphilis should be considered even in the evaluation of trivial or atypical, dark-field–negative genital lesions. The most common genital lesions which must be differentiated from primary syphilis include traumatic superinfected lesions, genital herpes simplex virus infection (see Chap. 143), and chancroid (see Chap. 112). *Primary genital herpes* may produce inguinal adenopathy, but the nodes are tender and associated with multiple painful vesicles, which later ulcerate and which are often accompanied by systemic symptoms including fever; *recurrent genital herpes* typically begins with a cluster of painful vesicles, usually without associated adenopa-

thy. *Chancroid* produces painful, superficial exudative, nonindurated, more often multiple ulcers; adenopathy is either unilateral or bilateral, is tender, and may suppurate.

Regional lymphadenopathy usually accompanies the primary syphilitic lesion, appearing within 1 week of the onset of the lesion. The nodes are firm, nonsuppurative, and painless. Inguinal lymphadenopathy is bilateral and may occur with anal as well as with external genital chancres, since lymphatic drainage of the anus involves inguinal nodes. Rectal chancres result in perirectal lymphadenopathy, while chancres of the cervix and vagina result in iliac or perirectal adenopathy. The chancre generally heals within 4 to 6 weeks (range 2 to 12 weeks), but the lymphadenopathy may persist for months.

Secondary syphilis The manifestations of the secondary stage are protean but usually include localized or diffuse symmetric mucocutaneous lesions and generalized nontender lymphadenopathy. The healing primary chancre is still present in 15 percent of cases. The skin rash consists of macular, papular, papulosquamous, and occasionally pustular syphilides, often with one or more forms present simultaneously. The eruption may be very subtle, and approximately 25 percent of patients with a discernible rash of secondary syphilis may be unaware that they have dermatologic manifestations. Initial lesions are bilaterally symmetric, pale red or pink, nonpruritic, discrete, round macules, 5 to 10 mm in diameter, distributed on the trunk and proximal extremities (Fig. 133-4). After several days or weeks, red papular lesions 3 to 10 mm in diameter also appear. These may progress to necrotic lesions (resembling pustules) in association with increasing endarteritis and perivascular mononuclear infiltration. These lesions are distributed widely, frequently involve the palms and soles (Fig. 133-5), and may occur on the face and scalp. Tiny papular *follicular syphilides* involving hair follicles may result in patchy alopecia (alopecia areata) and loss of scalp hair, eyebrows, or beard in up to 5 percent of patients. Nonpatchy hair loss also occurs

FIGURE 133-4 Maculopapular rash of secondary syphilis. (*Reprinted, with permission, from Sexually Transmitted Diseases, Prof. Dr. E. Stolz, Rotterdam, ©Boehringer Ingelheim International, 1977.*)

FIGURE 133-3 Primary chancre on the penis. (*Reprinted, with permission, from Sexually Transmitted Diseases, Prof. Dr. E. Stolz, Rotterdam, ©Boehringer Ingelheim International, 1977.*)

FIGURE 133-5 Secondary rash on palms and soles. (*From Ronald Roddy; reprinted, with permission, from Gynecology and Obstetrics, JW Sciarra (ed), New York, Harper & Row, 1985.*)

FIGURE 133-6 Mucous patches on the tongue. (*From Ronald Roddy; reprinted, with permission, from Sexually Transmitted Diseases, 2d ed, KK Holmes et al (eds), New York, McGraw-Hill, 1990.*)

in secondary syphilis. Progressive endarteritis obliterans and ischemia result in superficial scaling of papules (*papulosquamous syphilides*) and eventually may lead to central necrosis (*pustular syphilides*). In warm, moist, intertriginous areas, including the perianal area, vulva, scrotum, inner thighs, axillae, and the skin under pendulous breasts, papules enlarge and become eroded to produce broad, moist, pink or gray-white, highly infectious lesions called *condylomata lata*, which are seen in 10 percent of patients with secondary syphilis. Superficial mucosal erosions, called *mucous patches*, occur in 10 to 15 percent of patients and may involve lips, oral mucosa, tongue (Fig. 133-6), palate, pharynx, vulva and vagina, glans penis, or inner prepuce. The typical mucous patch is a silver-gray erosion surrounded by a red periphery and is usually painless.

During relapses of secondary syphilis, condylomata lata are particularly common, and skin lesions tend to be asymmetrically distributed and more infiltrated, resembling skin lesions of late syphilis, perhaps reflecting increasing cellular immunity.

Constitutional symptoms which may accompany or precede secondary syphilis include sore throat (15 to 30 percent), fever (5 to 8 percent), weight loss (2 to 20 percent), malaise (25 percent), anorexia (2 to 10 percent), headache (10 percent), and meningismus (5 percent). *Acute meningitis* occurs in only 1 to 2 percent of patients, but increased cells and protein have been found in the cerebrospinal fluid in 30 percent or more. *T. pallidum* also has been recovered from CSF during primary and secondary syphilis in 30 percent of patients; this finding is often correlated with other CSF abnormalities but may be seen in patients with otherwise normal CSF.

Other less common complications of secondary syphilis include hepatitis, nephropathy, gastrointestinal involvement (hypertrophic gastritis, patchy proctitis, ulcerative colitis, or a rectosigmoid mass), arthritis and periostitis, and iridocyclitis. Ocular findings which suggest secondary syphilis include otherwise unexplained pupillary abnormalities, optic neuritis, and a retinitis pigmentosa syndrome, as well as the classic iritis (especially granulomatous iritis) or uveitis. The diagnosis of secondary syphilis is often considered only after failure to respond to steroid therapy. Anterior uveitis has been reported in 5 to 10 percent of patients with secondary syphilis, and *T. pallidum* has been demonstrated in the aqueous humor from these patients. *Syphilitic hepatitis* is distinguished by an unusually high serum alkaline phosphatase level and by a nonspecific histologic appearance which is unlike viral hepatitis and includes moderate inflammation with polymorphonuclear leukocytes and lymphocytes, some hepatocellular damage, and no cholestasis. The *renal involvement* is associated with proteinuria, with an acute nephrotic syndrome, or rarely with hemorrhagic glomerulonephritis and is characterized by subepithelial electron-dense deposits and glomerular immune complexes—findings

suggesting that this complication is a form of immune-complex glomerulonephritis.

Latent syphilis   A diagnosis of latent syphilis is established by the finding of a positive specific treponemal antibody test for syphilis together with a normal CSF examination and the absence of clinical manifestations of syphilis on physical examination and chest films. The diagnosis is often suspected on the basis of a history of primary or secondary lesions, history of exposure to syphilis, or delivery of an infant with congenital syphilis. A previous negative serologic test and a history of lesions or exposure may help establish the duration of latent infection. *Early latent* syphilis encompasses the first year after infection, while *late latent* syphilis beginning 1 year after infection in the untreated patient is associated with relative immunity to infectious relapse and with increasing resistance to reinfection. *T. pallidum* may still intermittently seed the bloodstream during this stage; pregnant women with latent syphilis may infect the fetus in utero; and transfusion syphilis has been transmitted from patients with latent syphilis of many years' duration. It was thought that untreated late latent syphilis had three possible outcomes: (1) it could persist throughout the life of the infected individual, (2) it could end in development of late syphilis, or (3) it could end with spontaneous cure of infection, with reversion of serologic tests to negative. It is now apparent, however, that the more sensitive treponemal antibody tests rarely, if ever, become negative. About 70 percent of untreated patients with latent syphilis never develop clinically evident late syphilis, but the occurrence of spontaneous cure is in doubt.

Late syphilis   The onset of slowly progressive inflammatory disease leading to the tertiary stage begins early during the pathogenesis of syphilis, although it may not be clinically apparent for years. Evidence of early syphilitic aortitis is present soon after the secondary lesions subside, and it is patients who develop CSF abnormalities during the early stages of syphilis who appear to be at highest risk of late neurologic complications.

ASYMPTOMATIC NEUROSYPHILIS   Central nervous system syphilis represents a continuum of early invasion, usually within the first weeks or months of infection, and asymptomatic involvement, which may or may not result in neurologic manifestations. Traditionally, the diagnosis of asymptomatic neurosyphilis has been made in patients who no longer have manifestations of primary or secondary syphilis, who lack neurologic symptoms and signs, and who have certain CSF abnormalities. Such abnormalities are found in up to one-quarter of patients with untreated late latent syphilis, and it is these patients who are known to be at risk for neurologic complications. However, evidence of CNS involvement can include isolation of *T. pallidum* from CSF even in the absence of other CSF abnormalities, and approximately 40 percent of patients with primary and secondary syphilis have had *T. pallidum* isolated from the CSF, abnormalities of the CSF consistent with asymptomatic neurosyphilis, or both. Although the therapeutic implications of these findings in early syphilis are uncertain, it seems appropriate to conclude that patients with early syphilis who have such findings do indeed have asymptomatic neurosyphilis. In patients with untreated asymptomatic neurosyphilis, the overall cumulative probability of progression to clinical neurosyphilis is about 20 percent in the first 10 years but increases with passing time and is highest in those who show the greatest degree of pleocytosis or protein elevation. Patients with untreated latent syphilis and normal CSF probably have no future risk of subsequently developing neurosyphilis.

SYMPTOMATIC NEUROSYPHILIS   Although mixed features are common, the major clinical categories of symptomatic neurosyphilis include meningeal, meningovascular, and parenchymatous syphilis. The last category includes general paresis and tabes dorsalis. The interval from infection to onset of symptoms is a few months to 20 years for meningeal syphilis (usually in the first year) and for meningovascular syphilis (average 7 years), 20 years for general paresis, and 25 to 30 years for tabes dorsalis. However, many patients with symptomatic neurosyphilis, particularly in the antibiotic era, do not present a classic picture but have mixed and subtle or incomplete syndromes. *Meningeal syphilis* may involve either the brain or spinal cord, and patients may present with headache, nausea, vomiting, neck stiffness, cranial nerve palsies, seizures, and changes in mental status. *Meningovascular syphilis* is associated with diffuse inflammation of the pia and arachnoid, together with evidence of focal or widespread arterial involvement of small, medium, or large vessels. The most common presentation is a stroke syndrome in a relatively young adult involving the middle cerebral artery; however, unlike the usual thrombotic or embolic stroke syndrome of sudden onset, meningovascular syphilis often presents after a subacute encephalitic prodrome with headaches, vertigo, insomnia, and psychological abnormalities followed by a gradually progressive vascular syndrome. The manifestations of *general paresis* reflect widespread parenchymal damage and include abnormalities corresponding to the mnemonic *paresis* [*p*ersonality, *a*ffect, *r*eflexes (hyperactive), *e*ye (e.g., Argyll Robertson pupils), *s*ensorium (illusions, delusions, hallucinations), *i*ntellect (decreased recent memory, orientation, calculations, judgment, insight), and *s*peech]. *Tabes dorsalis* presents symptoms and signs of demyelination of the posterior columns, dorsal roots, and dorsal root ganglia. Symptoms include ataxic wide-based gait and footslap, paresthesias, bladder disturbances, impotence, areflexia, and loss of position, deep pain, and temperature sensation. Trophic joint degeneration (Charcot's joints) and perforating ulceration of the feet can result from loss of pain sensation. The Argyll Robertson pupil, seen in both tabes dorsalis and paresis, is a small, irregular pupil which reacts to accommodation but not to light. *Optic atrophy* also occurs frequently in association with tabes.

CARDIOVASCULAR SYPHILIS   Cardiovascular manifestations are limited to the large vessels in which the blood supply is provided by vasa vasorum. Endarteritis obliterans of the vasa vasorum produces medial necrosis with destruction of elastic tissue, particularly in the ascending and transverse segments of the aortic arch, resulting in uncomplicated aortitis, aortic regurgitation, saccular aneurysm, or coronary ostial stenosis. The onset of symptoms occurs from 10 to 40 years after infection. Cardiovascular complications are more common and occur at an earlier age in men than in women and may be more common in blacks than in whites. In the preantibiotic era, the incidence of symptomatic cardiovascular complications in late untreated syphilis was approximately 10 percent, with aortic regurgitation being two to four times as common as aneurysm. However, syphilitic aortitis was demonstrated at autopsy in about one-half of black men with untreated syphilis.

Asymptomatic syphilitic aortitis may be suspected if linear calcification of the ascending aorta is demonstrated on chest x-ray films, since arteriosclerotic disease seldom produces this sign. Aortic dilatation and a tambour quality of the sound of aortic closure are unreliable signs of aortitis. Syphilitic aneurysms are usually saccular, occasionally fusiform, and do not lead to dissection. Approximately 1 in 10 aortic aneurysms of syphilitic origin may involve the abdominal aorta, but these aneurysms tend to occur above the renal arteries, whereas arteriosclerotic abdominal aneurysms usually are found below the renal arteries. With increasing age, the nervous system is also affected in up to 40 percent of patients with cardiovascular syphilis.

LATE LESIONS OF THE EYES   Iritis associated with pain, photophobia, and dimness of vision or chorioretinitis occurs not only during secondary syphilis but also as a relatively common manifestation of late syphilis. Adhesions of the iris to the anterior lens may produce a fixed pupil, not to be confused with Argyll Robertson pupil.

LATE BENIGN SYPHILIS (GUMMA)   Gummas may be multiple or diffuse but are usually solitary lesions which range from microscopic size to several centimeters in diameter and histologically consist of granulomatous inflammation with central necrosis surrounded by mononuclear, epithelioid, and fibroblastic cells, occasional giant cells, and perivasculitis. Although *T. pallidum* is rarely demonstrated microscopically, it has reportedly been recovered from the lesions. The most commonly involved sites are the skin and skeletal systems, mouth and upper respiratory tract, larynx, liver, and stomach, although any organ may be involved. Gummas of skin produce painless nodular, papulosquamous, or ulcerative lesions, which are indurated and form characteristic circles or arcs, with peripheral hyperpigmentation. The lesions are usually indolent and may heal spontaneously with scarring, but they also may be explosive in onset and are often destructive. These lesions may resemble many other chronic granulomatous conditions, including tuberculosis and sarcoidosis, leprosy, and deep fungal infections. Skeletal gummas involve long bones of the legs with greatest frequency, although any bone may be affected. Trauma may predispose to involvement of a specific site. Presenting symptoms usually include focal pain and tenderness. When sufficiently advanced to produce radiographic abnormalities, the findings may include periostitis or destructive or sclerosing osteitis. Gummas of the upper respiratory tract can lead to perforation of the nasal septum or palate. Gummatous hepatitis may produce epigastric pain and tenderness and low-grade fever and may be associated with splenomegaly and anemia.

The histopathology and extensive tissue necrosis associated with gummas suggest that delayed hypersensitivity to *T. pallidum* produces these lesions. Certain individuals appear to develop an exaggerated delayed-hypersensitivity response to *T. pallidum*, presumably mediated by sensitized T lymphocytes and macrophages. Since the histologic changes may be suggestive but are nonspecific, the diagnosis of late benign syphilis is confirmed by serologic testing and by therapeutic trial. Treatment with penicillin results in rapid healing of active gummatous lesions.

Congenital syphilis   Transmission of *T. pallidum* from a syphilitic woman to her fetus across the placenta may occur at any stage of pregnancy, but the lesions of congenital syphilis develop generally after the fourth month of gestation, when immunologic competence begins to develop. This timing suggests that the pathogenesis of congenital syphilis may depend on the immune response of the host rather than on a direct toxic effect of *T. pallidum*. The risk of infection of the fetus during untreated early maternal syphilis is estimated to be 75 to 95 percent, decreasing to about 35 percent for maternal syphilis of longer than 2 years' duration, with the risk of fetal infection apparently continuing throughout late latent maternal syphilis. Adequate treatment of the mother before the sixteenth week of pregnancy should prevent fetal damage. Untreated maternal infection may result in up to 40 percent fetal loss (stillbirth is more common than abortion, because of the late onset of fetal pathology), prematurity, neonatal death, or nonfatal congenital syphilis. Of mothers with untreated syphilis of less than 2 years' duration, 21 percent aborted or had a stillbirth, 13 percent had infants who died within 2 months, 43 percent had infants with syphilis alive at 2 months, and 23 percent had nonsyphilitic infants. Only fulminant cases of congenital syphilis are clinically apparent in live infants at birth, and these babies have a very poor prognosis. The most common clinical problem is the healthy-appearing baby born to a mother who has a positive serologic test. Routine serologic testing in early pregnancy is considered cost-effective in virtually all populations, even in areas of low prenatal prevalence of syphilis. In noncompliant individuals, rapid plasma reagin (RPR) screening should be performed when pregnancy is detected to ensure prompt treatment. Where the prevalence of syphilis is high, and in high-risk patients, syphilis serology should be repeated in the third trimester and at delivery.

The manifestations of congenital syphilis can be divided into (1) early manifestations, which appear within the first 2 years of life, often between 2 and 10 weeks of age, are infectious, and resemble severe secondary syphilis in the adult; (2) late manifestations, which appear after 2 years and are noninfectious; and (3) the residual stigmata of congenital syphilis. During 1990, 87 percent of reported cases of congenital syphilis were diagnosed during the first year of life.

The earliest sign of congenital syphilis is usually rhinitis (''snuffles''), soon followed by other mucocutaneous lesions. These may include bullae (syphilitic pemphigus), vesicles, superficial desquamation, petechiae, and later, papulosquamous lesions, mucous patches, and condylomata lata. The most common early manifestations are osteochondritis and osteitis, particularly involving the metaphyses of long bones, progressing in severity during the first 6 months of life and then spontaneously subsiding; and periostitis, which continues to progress after the first 6 months. Hepatosplenomegaly, lymphadenopathy, anemia, jaundice, thrombocytopenia, and leukocytosis are common. The anemia is usually hypoproliferative but may be hemolytic (paroxysmal cold hemoglobinuria due to Donath-Landsteiner antibody, an IgG antibody that binds to the P antigen of red cells at low temperatures). The nephrotic syndrome in early congenital syphilis, as in adult secondary syphilis, represents an immune-complex–induced glomerulonephritis. A compilation of clinical presentations of congenital syphilis in nine studies involving a total of 212 infants included abnormal bone x-rays (61 percent), hepatomegaly (51 percent), splenomegaly (49 percent), petechiae (41 percent), other skin rash (35 percent), anemia (34 percent), lymphadenopathy (32 percent), jaundice (30 percent), pseudoparalysis (28 percent), and snuffles (23 percent).

Neonatal congenital syphilis must be differentiated from other generalized congenital infections, including rubella, cytomegalovirus or herpes simplex virus infection, and toxoplasmosis, as well as from erythroblastosis fetalis. Neonatal death is usually due to pulmonary hemorrhage, secondary bacterial infection, or severe hepatitis. Pathologic findings include interstitial and perivascular inflammation, followed by variable fibroblastic proliferation, involving skin, bones, liver, kidneys, pancreas, spleen, lungs, and intestines, and by extramedullary hematopoiesis.

Late congenital syphilis is defined as congenital syphilis which remains untreated after 2 years of age. In perhaps 60 percent of cases, the infection remains subclinical, while the clinical spectrum in the remainder differs in certain respects from that of acquired late syphilis in the adult. For example, cardiovascular syphilis rarely develops in late congenital syphilis, whereas interstitial keratitis is much more common and occurs between ages 5 and 25. The onset is acute, with photophobia, pain, and circumcorneal injection, followed by superficial and deep vascularization of the cornea, which progresses despite antibiotic therapy and eventually becomes bilateral. The symptoms and signs may be suppressed with glucocorticoid therapy. Although treponemes have occasionally been demonstrated in aqueous humor in interstitial keratitis, the pathogenesis is obscure and is ascribed to ''hypersensitivity.'' Other manifestations associated with interstitial keratitis are eighth-nerve deafness and recurrent arthropathy. Bilateral knee effusions are known as *Clutton's joints*. Examination of CSF discloses asymptomatic neurosyphilis in about one-third of untreated patients without other late clinical manifestations, and clinical neurosyphilis occurs in a quarter of untreated individuals with

congenital syphilis over 6 years of age. The clinical manifestations of congenital neurosyphilis correspond to those seen in adult neurosyphilis. Gummatous periostitis occurs between ages 5 and 20 and, as in nonvenereal endemic childhood syphilis, tends to cause destructive lesions of the palate and nasal septum.

Characteristic stigmata include *Hutchinson's teeth*, the centrally notched, widely spaced, peg-shaped upper central incisors and ''mulberry'' molars, sixth-year molars which have multiple, poorly developed cusps, numbering more than the usual four. The abnormal facies of congenital syphilis, which includes frontal bossing, saddlenose, and poorly developed maxillae, also may be seen in congenital ectodermal dysplasia. Saber shins, or anterior tibial bowing, are rare but were probably more common in the past when syphilitic periostitis of the anterior tibia was accompanied by vitamin D deficiency. *Rhagades* are linear scars at the angles of the mouth and nose caused by secondary bacterial infection of the early facial eruption. Other stigmata include unexplained nerve deafness, old chorioretinitis, optic atrophy, and corneal opacities due to past interstitial keratitis.

LABORATORY EXAMINATIONS   Dark-field examination technique   Dark-field examination is essential in evaluating cutaneous lesions, such as the chancre of primary syphilis or condylomata lata of secondary syphilis. Although it is often difficult to demonstrate *T. pallidum* in dry maculopapular lesions in secondary syphilis by dark-field examination, the organism may be demonstrated by saline aspiration of lymph nodes during this stage. The surface of the suspected ulcerated lesion should be cleaned with saline and gauze and then gently abraded further with dry gauze without production of bleeding. The lesion is then squeezed to express a serous transudate, and a drop of the transudate is picked up on the surface of a glass slide. A drop of saline (without bacteriostatic additives) may be mixed with the transudate if necessary, and this preparation is then covered with a coverslip and examined immediately for *T. pallidum* with a dark-field or phase-contrast microscope by an experienced individual. The identification of a single characteristic motile organism by a trained observer is sufficient for diagnosis. Examination of oral lesions by this method is not recommended, and it is also difficult to differentiate *T. pallidum* from other spirochetes that may be present in anal ulcers. A single negative examination does not exclude syphilis, since at least 10^4 treponemes per microliter of transudate must be present to be seen, and prior use of topical antiseptic or cleansing by the patient may obfuscate the results. Cleansing or use of topical medication should therefore be avoided, and ideally, the dark-field examination should be repeated on three successive days before being considered negative.

Direct immunofluorescence   Most syphilis is diagnosed in private physicians' offices where dark-field microscopy is not available; alternative methods for the identification of *T. pallidum* in exudate are needed. The direct fluorescent antibody *T. pallidum* (DFA-TP) test, available at central laboratories, uses fluorescein-conjugated polyclonal antitreponemal antibody for detection of *T. pallidum* in fixed smears prepared from suspect lesions. Because of cross-reactive antibodies which also will stain commensal nonpathogenic spirochetes, the antiserum is extensively absorbed with cultured treponemes in an effort to produce a specific reagent.

A refinement of this technique using a monoclonal antibody which is specific only for the pathogenic treponemes has been developed but is not yet commercially available. It has been shown in clinical trials to be as sensitive and specific as dark-field microscopy for examination of suspicious lesions. A new monoclonal antibody–based ELISA test, which detects *T. pallidum* in swab specimens from primary and secondary lesions, is currently being evaluated.

Demonstration of T. pallidum in tissue   It is often necessary to demonstrate *T. pallidum* in tissue when clinical or histopathologic features suggest the diagnosis of syphilis. Although the organism can be found in tissue by appropriate silver stains, these results should be interpreted with caution, because artifacts resembling *T. pallidum* are often seen. Treponemes can be demonstrated more reliably in tissue by immunofluorescence or immunohistochemistry using specific monoclonal or polyclonal antibodies to *T. pallidum*.

Serologic tests for syphilis The profusion of serologic tests for syphilis causes much unnecessary confusion. Syphilitic infection produces two types of antibodies, the nonspecific *reaginic* antibody and specific antitreponemal antibody, which are measured by the nontreponemal and treponemal tests, respectively (Table 133-1). The treponemal tests, as well as the nontreponemal tests, are reactive in persons with any treponemal infection, including yaws, pinta, and endemic syphilis.

The nontreponemal antibodies produced in syphilis contain both IgG and IgM immunoglobulins directed against a lipoidal antigen that results from the interaction of *T. pallidum* with host tissues and possibly against a lipoidal antigen of *T. pallidum* itself. The term *reagin* is unfortunate, since the unrelated IgE antibody involved in certain allergic phenomena is also known as reagin. The most widely used nontreponemal or reagin antibody tests for syphilis are the RPR test, which can be automated (ART), and the Venereal Disease Research Laboratory (VDRL) slide test. Other, less frequently used nontreponemal tests include the unheated serum reagin (USR) and the reagin screen test (RST). In these tests, antibody is detected by the microscopic (VDRL, USR) or macroscopic (RPR, RST) flocculation of the antigen suspension (see Table 133-1).

The RPR is often more expensive than the VDRL test but is easier to perform and uses unheated serum; it is the test of choice for rapid serologic diagnosis in a clinic or office setting. The VDRL reagents are less expensive but must be prepared fresh daily. Although the development of the simpler macroscopic tests has resulted in the replacement of the VDRL by the RPR test for examination of serum in many laboratories, the VDRL test remains the standard for use with CSF.

RPR and VDRL tests are equally sensitive and may be used for initial screening or for quantitation of serum reagin antibody titer. The reagin titer reflects the activity of the disease. A fourfold or greater rise in titer may be seen during the evolution of primary syphilis; VDRL titers usually reach 1:32 or higher in secondary syphilis; a persistent fall in titer following treatment of early syphilis provides essential evidence of an adequate response to therapy. VDRL titers do not correspond directly to RPR titers, and sequential quantitative testing (as for response to therapy) must employ a single test.

There are two standard treponemal tests: the fluorescent treponemal antibody–absorption (FTA-ABS) test and the microhemagglutination assay for antibodies to *T. pallidum* (MHA-TP). Another hemagglutination test, the TPHA, is widely used in Europe but is not available in the United States.

For the FTA-ABS test, the patient's serum is first diluted with a substance containing nonpathogenic treponemal antigens (sorbent) to bind group-specific antibodies which may be produced against saprophytic oral and genital treponemes. The patient's absorbed serum is then placed on a slide which contains fixed *T. pallidum*. If specific antibody to *T. pallidum* is present in the patient's serum, it is bound to the dried treponemes and is then detected by the addition of fluorescein-labeled antihuman gamma globulin and subsequent examination of the slide by fluorescence microscopy. The *T. pallidum*

hemagglutination tests (MHA-TP and TPHA) also use a sorbent-like diluent for binding treponemal group antibodies. *T. pallidum*–specific antibody is detected by agglutination of *T. pallidum*–coated sheep or turkey erythrocytes. These hemagglutination tests are more commonly used than the FTA-ABS test. The *T. pallidum* immobilization (TPI) test, in which immobilization of live *T. pallidum* is produced by immune serum plus complement, is the most specific treponemal test but is more laborious and, in the United States, is available only in research laboratories. Both the hemagglutination and FTA-ABS tests are very specific and, when used for confirmation of positive reaginic antibody tests, have a very high positive predictive value for the diagnosis of syphilis. However, even these tests give false-positive rates as high as 1 to 2 percent when used for screening normal populations.

The relative sensitivities of the VDRL, FTA-ABS, and MHA-TP tests in the various stages of syphilis are shown in Table 133-2. The nontreponemal tests are nonreactive in nearly one-third of patients with primary or late syphilis. In early primary syphilis, the detection of antibody can be maximized either by performing an FTA-ABS test or simply by repeating a VDRL test after 1 to 2 weeks if the initial VDRL was negative. However, obtaining a reagin antibody test alone is not sufficient in evaluating late symptomatic syphilis; the more sensitive FTA-ABS test should be obtained routinely in suspected late syphilis. The hemagglutination tests are even less sensitive than the reagin tests in primary syphilis but are as sensitive as the FTA-ABS test in other stages. All treponemal and nontreponemal tests are reactive during secondary syphilis, and a nonreactive result virtually excludes syphilis in a patient with otherwise compatible mucocutaneous lesions. (Less than 1 percent of patients with secondary syphilis have a nonreactive or weakly reactive VDRL test with undiluted serum which becomes positive in higher dilutions—the *prozone* phenomenon.) While the nontreponemal tests will become negative or decline in titer following therapy for early syphilis, the treponemal tests will often remain reactive after therapy and are not helpful in determining the infection status in persons with past syphilis.

The presence of specific IgM antibody has been proposed as a marker for active syphilis, with the claim that IgM disappears following adequate therapy. The rate at which IgM declines after therapy is quite variable from patient to patient, and the use of this criterion for cure is not universally accepted. A new 19S IgM FTA-ABS test for syphilis has been approved for use by the Centers for Disease Control and is recommended for evaluation of infants with suspected congenital syphilis.

False-positive serologic tests for syphilis Because the antigen used in the nontreponemal tests is found in other tissues, the tests may be reactive in persons without treponemal infection, although rarely in titers exceeding 1:8. In a population which has been selected for screening because of clinical suspicion, history of exposure, or increased risk for sexually transmitted infections, <2 percent of reactive tests are falsely positive. False-positive reagin tests are classified as acute if they become negative within 6 months and may occur during a variety of acute infections, such as viral diseases, *Mycoplasma* pneumonia, and malaria, and following certain immuni-

---

TABLE 133-1 Common serologic tests for syphilis

Nontreponemal (reagin) tests
  Microscopic flocculation: Venereal Disease Research Laboratory (VDRL)
  Macroscopic flocculation: rapid plasma reagin (RPR)

Treponemal tests
  Immunofluorescence: fluorescent treponemal antibody-absorption (FTA-ABS)
  Hemagglutination: *T. pallidum* hemagglutination assay (MHA-TP, TPHA)

TABLE 133-2 Reactivity of serodiagnostic tests in untreated syphilis

Test	Stage of disease, % positive*			
	Primary	Secondary	Latent	Tertiary
VDRL	59–87	100	73–91	37–94
FTA-ABS	86–100	99–100	96–99	96–100
MHA-TP	64–87	96–100	96–100	94–100

* Percentage figures provided should not be interpreted as absolute values because there are small numbers in certain categories and test results vary from study to study.
SOURCE: Modified (with permission) from H Jaffe, D Musher, Management of the reactive syphilis serology, in *Sexually Transmitted Diseases*, KK Holmes et al (eds), 2d ed. New York, McGraw-Hill, 1990, p 935.

zations. Chronic reactions, which persist 6 months or longer, occur in intravenous drug addiction, in autoimmune diseases, and with aging. False-positive reagin tests occur in 25 percent of narcotic addicts and in 10 to 20 percent of patients with active systemic lupus erythematosus. The autoimmune nature of the false-positive reagin test is suggested by the occurrence of systemic lupus erythematosus or other connective tissue diseases in 15 to 45 percent of chronic false-positive reactors. Other antibodies which have been found with great frequency in sera from chronic false-positive reactors include antinuclear, antithyroid, and antimitochondrial antibodies as well as rheumatoid factor and cryoglobulins. The Donath-Landsteiner antibody responsible for paroxysmal cold hemoglobinuria is an autoimmune hemolysin which appears in syphilis. The prevalence of false-positive reagin tests increases with advancing age, and 10 percent of people over 70 years of age have false-positive reactions. Other diseases associated with hyperglobulinemia, such as leprosy, also may produce chronic false-positive reactions.

In the patient with a false-positive reagin test, syphilis is excluded by obtaining a nonreactive treponemal test. A typical *reactive* FTA-ABS test occurs infrequently in conditions other than syphilis. Although false-positive FTA-ABS tests have been reported in 15 percent of patients with active systemic lupus erythematosus, the fluorescent staining is often weak or has an atypical "beaded" appearance which is recognized by the technician. For practical purposes, most clinicians need to be familiar with the three uses of serologic tests for syphilis: (1) for testing large numbers of sera for screening or diagnostic purposes (e.g., RPR or VDRL), (2) for quantitative measurement of reaginic antibody titer in order to assess the clinical activity of syphilis or to follow the reagin titer in response to therapy (e.g., VDRL or RPR), and (3) for confirmation of the diagnosis of syphilis in a patient with a positive reagin antibody test or with a suspected clinical diagnosis of syphilis (e.g., FTA-ABS or MHA-TP).

Evaluation for asymptomatic neurosyphilis Asymptomatic involvement of the central nervous system is detected by examination of cerebrospinal fluid. CSF abnormalities are very infrequent in the primary stage, but pleocytosis or elevated protein can be demonstrated in CSF from up to 40 percent of patients with secondary or latent syphilis. *T. pallidum* has been recovered by rabbit inoculation from up to 40 percent of those with primary and secondary syphilis but rarely from those with latent syphilis. The demonstration of *T. pallidum* in CSF is often associated with other CSF abnormalities; however, organisms can be recovered from patients without pleocytosis or elevated protein. In the prepenicillin era, the risk of developing clinical neurosyphilis was roughly proportional to the intensity of CSF changes in early syphilis. CSF examination is essential in any seropositive patient with neurologic signs and symptoms and is recommended in all patients with untreated syphilis of unknown duration or of greater than 1 year's duration. The possibility that asymptomatic neurosyphilis is present in some patients with secondary and early latent disease is not addressed by these recommendations. Because standard penicillin G benzathine (benzathine benzylpenicillin) therapy for early syphilis fails to result in treponemicidal levels in the CSF, some experts advise lumbar puncture in secondary and early latent syphilis, with follow-up examinations for patients with abnormalities.

CSF is examined for pleocytosis, increased protein concentration, and VDRL reactivity. The CSF VDRL test is very specific if the fluid is not contaminated with blood. The CSF VDRL test is relatively insensitive, however, and may be nonreactive even in progressive symptomatic neurosyphilis. Highest sensitivities are seen in meningovascular syphilis and paresis; lower sensitivities are seen in asymptomatic neurosyphilis and tabes dorsalis. The unabsorbed FTA test on CSF is reactive far more often than the CSF VDRL test in all stages of syphilis, but FTA reactivity may reflect passive transfer of serum antibody into the CSF. Most specialists do not recommend performing an FTA test on CSF. Similarly, the finding of a reactive CSF FTA-ABS test without other CSF abnormalities in a patient with nonspecific

neurologic findings does not prove a diagnosis of neurosyphilis. Even in the absence of confirmatory CSF examination, a therapeutic trial of penicillin in doses adequate for neurosyphilis is warranted in any patient with a positive serum treponemal antibody test who also has neurologic findings consistent with neurosyphilis.

Attempts to identify a more sensitive and specific marker for neurosyphilis have included CSF oligoclonal banding and measurement of intrathecal production of antitreponemal IgM and IgG. CSF from 80 percent of patients with multiple sclerosis and approximately 40 percent of patients with other inflammatory CNS diseases (including neurosyphilis, bacterial meningitis, viral encephalitis, subacute sclerosing panencephalitis) has discrete oligoclonal immunoglobulin bands in the gamma globulin region following agarose gel electrophoresis. These antibodies are thought to be intrathecally produced and have specificity for the etiologic agent (e.g., *T. pallidum* in syphilis and measles virus in subacute sclerosing panencephalitis); however, an oligoclonal banding pattern per se is not specific for neurosyphilis in a seropositive patient.

Evaluation for syphilis in patients concurrently infected with human immunodeficiency virus (HIV) Because persons at highest risk for acquiring syphilis (inner-city populations and homosexually active men) are also at high risk for acquisition of HIV, these infections are frequently found in the same patient. There is evidence that syphilis and other genital ulcer diseases may be important risk factors for acquisition and transmission of HIV infection. Several studies propose that the manifestations of syphilis may be altered in patients with concurrent HIV infection, and multiple cases of neurologic relapse following standard therapy have been reported in HIV-infected patients. *T. pallidum* has been isolated from the CSF of patients following therapy for early syphilis with penicillin G benzathine. One case of VDRL and FTA-ABS seronegative secondary syphilis has been reported in a patient with AIDS; this patient finally seroconverted prior to therapy after weeks of secondary manifestations. In contrast, HIV-infected patients with unusually high VDRL or RPR titers also have been described. It should be emphasized that the nature and extent of the interaction between HIV infection and syphilis have not been well defined. The frequency of unusual clinical and laboratory manifestations of syphilis in patients coinfected with HIV is unknown, and such changes may be dependent on the stage of HIV infection and degree of immunosuppression. There is no clear evidence that the sensitivity of serologic tests for syphilis or the serologic response to therapy is different in the vast majority of HIV-infected patients, and interpretation of serologic results in these patients should be the same as for HIV-uninfected individuals.

The evaluation of all syphilis patients should include serologic testing for HIV, with the patient's consent. Conversely, persons with newly diagnosed HIV infection should be tested for syphilis. Examination of CSF for evidence of neurosyphilis is recommended by some authorities for all coinfected patients, regardless of the clinical stage of syphilis. If CSF abnormalities are found, or if CSF examination is not performed, therapy adequate for neurosyphilis should be administered regardless of the apparent stage of infection. Serologic testing following treatment is important for all patients with syphilis and particularly for those also infected with HIV.

TREATMENT OF ACQUIRED SYPHILIS Penicillin G is the drug of choice for all stages of syphilis. *T. pallidum* is killed by very low concentrations of penicillin G, although a long period of exposure to penicillin is required for treatment because of the unusually slow rate of multiplication of the organism. The efficacy of penicillin for syphilis remains undiminished after nearly 50 years of use. Other antibiotics which are effective in syphilis include the tetracyclines, erythromycin, and the cephalosporins. Aminoglycosides and spectinomycin inhibit *T. pallidum* only in very large doses, and the sulfonamides and the quinolones are inactive. The optimal dose and duration of therapy have not been established definitively for any antimicrobial for any stage of syphilis.

It is necessary to achieve serum levels of penicillin G of 0.03 μg/mL or more for at least 7 days to cure early syphilis. Recurrence rates for a given regimen increase as infection progresses from incubating syphilis to seronegative primary to seropositive primary to secondary to late syphilis. Therefore, it is probable, but unproved, that a longer duration of therapy is required to effect cure as the infection progresses. For these reasons, some authorities use more prolonged penicillin therapy than that recommended by the U.S. Public Health Service when treating secondary, latent, or late syphilis.

The treatment regimens recommended for syphilis are summarized in Table 133-3 and are described below.

Early syphilis Preventive (abortive, "epidemiologic") treatment is recommended for seronegative individuals without signs of syphilis who have been exposed to infectious syphilis within the previous 3 months. Before treatment is given, every effort should be made to establish a diagnosis by examination and serologic testing. *The regimens recommended for preventive treatment are the same as those recommended for early syphilis.*

For patients who have no known exposure to syphilis but who are undergoing treatment for other sexually transmitted diseases, most currently recommended STD regimens involving β-lactam or tetracycline antibiotics are probably also effective for very early incubating syphilis. It is likely that the regimen currently recommended for treating gonorrhea [ceftriaxone 250 mg intramuscularly followed by doxycycline or tetracycline orally for 1 week (see Chap. 110)] is effective against incubating syphilis.

Penicillin G benzathine is the most widely used form of treatment for early syphilis, including primary, secondary, and early latent syphilis, although it is more painful on injection than penicillin G procaine. A single dose of 2.4 million units cures over 95 percent of cases of primary syphilis. Because efficacy for secondary syphilis may be slightly lower, some physicians administer a second dose of 2.4 million units 1 week after the initial dose for secondary syphilis. There are reports of treatment failure following penicillin G benzathine in patients coinfected with HIV and early syphilis. Therapeutic recommendations should be guided by knowledge of CSF abnormalities in such patients. CSF examination in HIV-seropositive individuals with syphilis of any stage is recommended. Patients without HIV infection also may benefit from CSF examination. Some experts recommend treatment with regimens effective against neurosyphilis for all HIV-seropositive individuals with syphilis of any stage.

Late latent and late syphilis Lumbar puncture should be performed in the evaluation of latent syphilis of more than 1 year's duration, in suspected neurosyphilis, and also in late complications other than symptomatic neurosyphilis, since asymptomatic neurosyphilis may coexist with other late complications. In older asymptomatic individuals, the yield of lumbar puncture is relatively low. CSF examination is most clearly indicated in the following situations: neurologic signs or symptoms, treatment failure, serum reagin titer $\geq 1:32$; HIV antibody positivity, other evidence of active syphilis (e.g., aortitis, gumma, visual or hearing changes), or nonpenicillin therapy planned. Recommended treatment for late latent syphilis with normal CSF, for cardiovascular syphilis, and for late benign syphilis (gumma) is penicillin G benzathine, 2.4 million units intramuscularly once a week for 3 successive weeks (7.2 million units total). If CSF abnormalities are found, the patient should be treated for neurosyphilis.

No studies of penicillin G benzathine for cardiovascular syphilis have been reported, and the efficacy of penicillin therapy in any form for cardiovascular syphilis has not been proved. The response of cardiovascular syphilis to penicillin is seldom dramatic because aortic aneurysm and aortic regurgitation cannot be reversed by antibiotic treatment, although further progression of these lesions may be arrested. In contrast, the response of benign tertiary syphilis and of meningovascular syphilis to penicillin G is usually impressive. The response of parenchymal neurosyphilis has been variable. In a cooperative study of the treatment of 1086 general paretics with penicillin, the frequency of clinical improvement or termination of progression ranged from 38 percent of those with severe involvement to 81 percent of those with mild involvement. Tabes dorsalis or optic atrophy responds less often. In general, treatment of inactive neurosyphilis in which neurologic damage has already occurred may not produce any clinical change, and retreatment of such cases is not warranted. However, persistence of CSF pleocytosis or recurrence of pleocytosis following initial response to treatment indicates continuing active infection, which should respond to additional treatment. The 1989 Centers for Disease Control treatment guidelines for neurosyphilis are presented in Table 133-3. Because penicillin G benzathine given in doses of up to 7.2 million units to adults or 50,000 units per kilogram to infants does not produce detectable concentrations of penicillin G in CSF, this form of penicillin is unreliable for the treatment of neurosyphilis in the adult or infant, and asymptomatic neurosyphilis has been found to relapse in up to one-quarter of patients treated with 2.4 million units of penicillin G benzathine. Therefore, use of penicillin G benzathine alone for treatment of neurosyphilis is not recommended. On the other hand, administration of intravenous penicillin G in doses of 12 million units or more per day for 10 days or longer ensures treponemicidal concentrations of penicillin G in CSF and occasionally cures patients who failed to respond to other therapy. There are no data to support the use of antibiotics other than penicillin G for the treatment of

---

TABLE 133-3 Recommendations for therapy of syphilis*

Stage of syphilis	Patients without penicillin allergy	Patients with confirmed penicillin allergy
Primary, secondary, or early latent	Benzathine penicillin G, 2.4 million units single dose IM (1.2 million units in each buttock)	Tetracycline hydrochloride, 500 mg PO 4 times daily; or doxycycline, 100 mg PO twice daily, for two weeks
Late latent (or latent of uncertain duration), cardiovascular, or benign tertiary	Lumbar puncture CSF normal: Benzathine penicillin G, 2.4 million units IM weekly for 3 weeks CSF abnormal: Treat as neurosyphilis	Lumbar puncture CSF normal: Tetracycline hydrochloride, 500 mg PO 4 times daily; or doxycycline, 100 mg PO twice daily, for 4 weeks CSF abnormal: Treat as neurosyphilis
Neurosyphilis† (asymptomatic or symptomatic)	Aqueous penicillin G, 12–24 million units per day IV for 10–14 days *Or* Aqueous procaine penicillin G, 2.4 million units IM daily, plus oral probenecid, 500 mg 4 times each day, both for 10–14 days	Confirm penicillin allergy by skin-testing; if confirmed, desensitize and treat with penicillin
Syphilis in pregnancy	According to stage	Confirm penicillin allergy by skin-testing; if confirmed, desensitize and treat with penicillin

* See text for discussion of syphilis therapy in HIV-infected individuals.
† Some authorities recommend following these regimens with three doses of 2.4 million units of benzathine penicillin G, given IM one week apart. Benzathine penicillin G alone has given inferior results for treatment of neurosyphilis. Drugs other than penicillin are not recommended. Many patients who give a history of penicillin allergy prove negative when skin-tested for immediate hypersensitivity to penicillin and could be given aqueous crystalline penicillin G for CNS syphilis under close supervision in the hospital.
SOURCE: These recommendations are modified from Centers for Disease Control, 1989.

neurosyphilis; however, some of the third-generation cephalosporins may deserve further evaluation. In patients with penicillin allergy documented by skin testing, desensitization may be the best course (see Chap. 85).

Management of syphilis in pregnancy   Every pregnant woman should undergo a nontreponemal test at her first prenatal visit, and women who are at high risk for acquiring STDs should have a repeat test in the third trimester and at delivery. In the pregnant patient with presumed syphilis (evidenced by a reactive serology, with or without clinical manifestations) and with no history of treatment for syphilis, expeditious evaluation and initiation of treatment are essential. Therapy should be administered according to stage of the disease, as for nonpregnant patients. Patients should be warned of the risk of a Jarisch-Herxheimer reaction, which may be associated with mild premature contractions but rarely results in premature delivery.

Penicillin is the only recommended therapy for syphilis in pregnancy. If the patient has well-documented penicillin allergy, and this is confirmed by demonstration of an immediate wheal-and-flare response to skin testing with penicilloyl polylysine or penicillin G minor determinant mixture, desensitization and penicillin treatment should be carried out in a hospital using the 1989 STD guidelines issued by the Centers for Disease Control. After treatment, a quantitative reagin test should be repeated monthly throughout pregnancy, and if a fourfold rise in titer occurs, treatment should be repeated. Treated women who do not show a fourfold decrease in titer in a 3-month period also should be retreated.

Evaluation and management of congenital syphilis   Newborn infants of mothers with reactive VDRL or FTA-ABS tests may themselves have reactive tests, whether or not they have become infected, because of transplacental transfer of maternal IgG antibody. Rising or persistent titers indicate infection, and the infant should be treated. If the seropositive mother received inadequate penicillin treatment or treatment other than penicillin, if her treatment status is unknown, or if the infant may be difficult to follow, the infant should be treated at birth. It is unwise to require proof of diagnosis before treatment in such cases. The CSF should be examined as a baseline before treatment of such infants. Penicillin is the only recommended drug for syphilis in infants. The calculation of penicillin dosage for treatment of late congenital syphilis is the same as that used in the infant, until dosage based on weight reaches that used for adult neurosyphilis. Specific recommendations for treatment of infants can be found in the 1989 Centers for Disease Control treatment guidelines. Neonatal IgM antibody can be detected in cord or neonatal sera in the 19S IgM FTA-ABS test, in which IgM is enriched by column chromatography (to remove IgG) and detected by fluorescein-labeled antihuman IgM. This test avoids the specificity and sensitivity problems associated with earlier versions of the IgM FTA-ABS test. Alternatively, monthly quantitative reagin tests may be performed on asymptomatic infants born to women who were treated adequately with penicillin during pregnancy.

Jarisch-Herxheimer reaction   A dramatic, though usually mild, reaction consisting of fever (average temperature elevation 1.5°C), chills, myalgias, headache, tachycardia, increased respiratory rate, increased circulating neutrophil count (average total white blood cell count 12,500 per microliter), and vasodilatation with mild hypotension may occur following initiation of treatment for syphilis. This reaction occurs in approximately 50 percent of patients with primary syphilis, 90 percent with secondary syphilis, and 25 percent with early latent syphilis. The onset occurs within 2 h of treatment, the peak temperature occurs at about 7 h, and defervescence takes place within 12 to 24 h. The reaction is more delayed in neurosyphilis, with peak fever occurring after 12 to 14 h. In patients with secondary syphilis, an increase in erythema and edema of the mucocutaneous lesions occurs; occasionally, subclinical or early mucocutaneous lesions may first become apparent during the reaction. The pathogenesis of this reaction is undefined. Patients should be warned to expect such symptoms, which can be managed by bed rest and aspirin. Adjunctive steroid

therapy has not been shown to prevent the Jarisch-Herxheimer reaction in syphilis and is not recommended.

Follow-up evaluation of responses to therapy for all stages of syphilis   The response of early syphilis to treatment should be determined by following the quantitative VDRL or RPR titer 1, 3, 6, and 12 months after treatment. More frequent serologic examination (1, 2, 3, 6, 9, and 12 months) is recommended for patients concurrently infected with HIV. Because the FTA-ABS and hemagglutination tests remain positive in most patients treated for seropositive early syphilis, these tests are not useful in following the response to therapy. After successful treatment of seropositive first-episode primary or secondary syphilis, the VDRL titer progressively declines, becoming negative by 12 months in 40 to 75 percent of seropositive primary cases and 20 to 40 percent of secondary cases. Two years after treatment for first-episode primary syphilis, ≥60 percent of patients have a negative VDRL, although 25 to 58 percent of patients with secondary disease and a higher proportion of those treated for early latent syphilis maintain low reagin titers. Patients with a history of syphilis have less rapid declines in titer and are less likely to become VDRL- or RPR-negative. If the VDRL becomes negative or reaches a fixed low titer within 1 or 2 years, performing a lumbar puncture is unnecessary at that time, since the CSF examination is almost invariably normal and there is little risk of subsequent neurosyphilis. However, if a VDRL titer of 1:8 or more fails to fall at least fourfold within 12 months, if the VDRL titer rises fourfold, or if clinical symptoms persist or recur, retreatment is indicated. Every effort should be made to differentiate treatment failure from reinfection, and the CSF should be examined. Patients with suspected treatment failure, especially those with abnormal CSF, should be treated as described for neurosyphilis. If the patient remains seropositive but asymptomatic after such retreatment, no further therapy is necessary. Patients treated for late latent syphilis frequently have a low-titered VDRL test prior to therapy and may not demonstrate a fourfold drop following therapy with penicillin; about half of these patients remain seropositive in low titer for years following therapy. Retreatment is not warranted unless the titer rises or signs and symptoms of syphilis recur.

The activity of neurosyphilis correlates best with the degree of CSF pleocytosis. Changes in the CSF cell count and, to a lesser extent, in CSF protein concentration provide the most sensitive index of response to treatment. CSF examination should be performed every 3 to 6 months for 3 years after treatment of asymptomatic or symptomatic neurosyphilis. An elevated CSF cell count falls to 10 or fewer per microliter within 3 to 12 months in 95 percent of adequately treated cases and becomes normal in all cases within 2 to 4 years. Elevated levels of CSF protein fall more slowly, and the CSF reagin titer declines slowly over a period of several years.

Persistence of treponemal forms   The persistence of *T. pallidum* in the aqueous humor, CSF, lymph nodes, brain, inflamed temporal arteries, and other tissues following "adequate" penicillin treatment of latent or late syphilis has been suggested by dark-field microscopy, immunofluorescent antibody and silver staining techniques, and rabbit inoculation. Because the data on persisting treponemes are scanty, no modification of the treatment recommendations for latent or late syphilis seems warranted. Adherence to recommendations regarding CSF examination prior to selection of therapy should minimize the possibility of *T. pallidum* persistence.

IMMUNITY AND PREVENTION OF SYPHILIS   About 50 percent of the named contacts of patients with primary and secondary syphilis become infected, but the actual risk of infection from a single exposure is probably much lower. The rate of development of acquired resistance to *T. pallidum* following natural or experimental infection is quantitatively related to the amount of the antigenic stimulus, which depends on both the size of the infecting inoculum and the duration of infection prior to treatment. The role of serum antibody in conferring immunity to syphilis remains controversial. Reagin (VDRL) antibody is not protective. Passively administered antibody from rabbits recovering from experimental syphilis prevents or delays appearance of clinical manifestations of syphilis; it does not prevent infection. Cellular immunity is considered to be of major importance in the healing of early lesions and control of syphilis infection. The cellular infiltration of early lesions is predominantly composed of T lymphocytes and macrophages, and specifically sensitized T lymphocytes develop early in the course of infection in humans and experimentally infected rabbits. Clearance of organisms from early lesions is mediated by macrophages. Specific antibody enhances phagocytosis and is required for macrophage-mediated killing of *T. pallidum*.

Inability to cultivate pathogenic treponemes in vitro has hindered analysis, purification, and concentration of treponemal antigens. Attempts to induce immunity to syphilis by vaccination have shown limited promise, although several specific antigens have been identified and characterized. The outer membrane of *T. pallidum* contains few integral membrane proteins, and no surface-exposed antigens have been definitively identified. Many of the major antigens are lipoproteins, which are probably associated via their lipid tail with the inner membrane, projecting into the periplasmic space. Repeated injection of rabbits with gamma-irradiated motile strains has conferred immunity to a rechallenge. Until a practical and effective vaccine is developed, the prevention of syphilis will depend on use of condoms and antiseptic prophylactic agents and the detection and treatment of infectious cases.

REFERENCES

BAKER-ZANDER et al: Macrophage-mediated killing of opsonized *T. pallidum*. J Infect Dis 165:69, 1992

BERRY CD et al: Neurologic relapse after benzathine penicillin therapy for secondary syphilis in a patient with HIV infection. N Engl J Med 316:1587, 1987

CENTERS FOR DISEASE CONTROL: Guidelines for the prevention and control of congenital syphilis. Morb Mort Week Rep (Suppl) 37(S-1):1, 1988

———: Recommendations for diagnosing and treating syphilis in HIV-infected individuals. Morb Mort Week Rep 37:600, 1988

———: Regional and temporal trends in the surveillance of syphilis, United States 1986–1990. Morb Mort Week Rep 40 (SS-3):29, 1991

———: 1989 Sexually transmitted diseases treatment guidelines. Morb Mort Week Rep 38(Suppl 8):1, 1989

CHAPEL T: The signs and symptoms of secondary syphilis. Sex Trans Dis 7:161, 1980

GREENE BM et al: Failure of penicillin G benzathine in the treatment of neurosyphilis. Arch Intern Med 140:1117, 1980

HOOK EW III et al: Detection of *Treponema pallidum* in lesion exudate with a pathogen-specific monoclonal antibody. J Clin Microbiol 22:241, 1985

HOTSON JR: Modern neurosyphilis: A partially treated chronic meningitis. West J Med 135:191, 1981

KATZ DA et al: Neurosyphilis in acquired immunodeficiency syndrome. Arch Neurol 46:895, 1989

LUGER A et al: Diagnosis of neurosyphilis by examination of the cerebrospinal fluid. Br J Vener Dis 57:232, 1981

LUKEHART SA et al: Invasion of the central nervous system by *Treponema pallidum*: Implications for diagnosis and treatment. Ann Intern Med 109:855, 1988

McLEISH WM et al: The ocular manifestations of syphilis in the human immunodeficiency virus type I–infected host. Ophthalmology 97:196, 1990

MOHR JA et al: Neurosyphilis and penicillin in cerebrospinal fluid. JAMA 236:2208, 1976

MULLER F, MOSKOPHIDIS M: Estimation of the local production of antibodies to *Treponema pallidum* in the central nervous system of patients with neurosyphilis. Br J Vener Dis 59:80, 1983

MUSHER DM et al: Effect of human immunodeficiency virus infection on the course of syphilis and on the response to treatment. Ann Intern Med 113:872, 1990

RADOLF JD et al: Outer membrane ultrastructure explains the limited antigenicity of virulent *Treponema pallidum*. Proc Natl Acad Sci 86:2051, 1989

RIVIERE GR et al: Identification of spirochetes related to *Treponema pallidum* in necrotizing ulcerative gingivitis and chronic periodontitis. N Engl J Med 325:539, 1991

ROMANOWSKI B et al: Serologic response to treatment of infectious syphilis. Ann Intern Med 114:1005, 1991

SIMON RP: Neurosyphilis. Arch Neurol 42:606, 1985

WENDEL GD et al: Penicillin allergy and desensitization in serious infections during pregnancy. N Engl J Med 312:1229, 1985

134 ENDEMIC TREPONEMATOSES

PETER L. PERINE

GENERAL CONSIDERATIONS Nonvenereal treponematoses occur in remote, impoverished areas of the world. Yaws, pinta, and endemic syphilis are distinguished from venereal syphilis solely by clinical and epidemiologic features. Yaws, pinta, and endemic syphilis are caused by treponemes which have no demonstrated significant morphologic or genetic differences from *T. pallidum*. The etiologic agents of endemic syphilis and yaws are generally held to be identical with *T. pallidum* and have been designated as *T. pallidum* ssp. *endemicum* and ssp. *pertenue*, respectively. Pinta is caused by *T. carateum* and involves the skin alone; yaws affects skin and bones; and endemic syphilis involves the skin, bone, and mucous membranes. Each disease tends to progress by stages, but these are neither as distinct nor as predictable as in syphilis. Congenital infections and cardiovascular and central nervous system involvement occur rarely, if ever, in the nonvenereal treponematoses but are common in syphilis. It is unclear whether the clinical and epidemiologic differences among yaws, pinta, endemic syphilis, and venereal syphilis are solely determined by environmental and host factors or are attributable to undefined biologic differences among the causal treponemes. The relationship of the treponematoses is summarized in Table 134-1.

EPIDEMIOLOGY Treponemal antibodies are demonstrable in some proportion of nonhuman primates in regions of Africa where human yaws and endemic syphilis are common, and pathogenic treponemes have been found in skin lesions and lymph nodes of seropositive animals. These treponemes have produced yawslike lesions in susceptible monkeys and hamsters. There is no epidemiologic evidence to indicate that these treponemes play a significant role in the epidemiology of yaws in humans.

Yaws and endemic syphilis are diseases of young children. Yaws occurs throughout the world between the Tropics of Cancer and Capricorn in humid, warm environments. Transmission of yaws among children is favored by scanty clothing, poor hygiene, and frequent skin trauma. Spread occurs by direct contact with infected lesions and perhaps by passive transfer of treponemes by insects. Endemic syphilis occurs in arid subtropical or temperate climates in Africa, the eastern Mediterranean, the Arabian peninsula, and central Asia. It is not observed in the Western Hemisphere. Skin-to-skin transmission is less important than in yaws; instead, infection of mucous membranes results from direct mouth-to-mouth contact or from contaminated fomites, such as shared drinking or eating utensils. Venereal syphilis can spread by nonvenereal contact among children and cause household outbreaks in modern cities when crowding and poverty favor transmission of *T. pallidum*.

Although cutaneous pigmentary changes resembling late stages of pinta occur in yaws or endemic syphilis, pinta is a separate, more benign disease which occurs only in the Western Hemisphere. The onset is typically later than in yaws or endemic syphilis, usually when the person is between 10 and 20 years of age. Pinta is not very contagious, and its mode of transmission is not well defined.

The WHO/UNICEF-assisted mass campaign for eradication of endemic nonvenereal treponematosis from 1948 to 1969 was an unusually successful public health campaign. Over 160 million people were examined in 46 countries, and approximately 50 million cases, contacts, and latent infections were treated. The impact of this program was remarkable. The prevalence of active yaws lesions was reduced from over 20 percent to less than 1 percent in many rural areas. In Bosnia, formerly part of Yugoslavia, endemic syphilis was eradicated—the only example of eradication of an endemic treponematosis.

Relaxation of active surveillance activities after the mass campaigns has led to a resurgence of yaws, particularly in Africa. Yaws has not

TABLE 134-1 Etiology, epidemiology, and clinical manifestations of the treponematoses

	Venereal syphilis	Endemic syphilis	Yaws	Pinta
Organism	*T. pallidum* ssp. *pallidum*	*T. pallidum* ssp. *endemicum*	*T. pallidum* ssp. *pertenue*	*T. carateum*
Transmission	Sexual, transplacental*	Household contacts: mouth-to-mouth or via drinking, eating utensils	Skin-to-skin ? Insect vector	Skin-to-skin ? Insect vector
Usual age	Adult	Early childhood	Early childhood	Adolescent
Primary lesion	Cutaneous ulcer (chancre)	Rarely seen	Framboise (raspberry), or "mother yaw"	Nonulcerating papule with satellites
Secondary lesion	Mucocutaneous; occasional periostitis	Florid mucocutaneous lesions (mucous patch, split papule, condyloma latum); osteoperiostitis	Cutaneous papulosquamous lesions; osteoperiostitis	Pintides
Tertiary	Gumma, cardiovascular, and CNS lues	Destructive cutaneous osteoarticular gummas	Destructive cutaneous osteoarticular gummas	Dyschromic, achromic macules

* Since the nonvenereal treponematoses are usually acquired in childhood and treponemal bacteremia ceases with time, only in adult-onset venereal syphilis is there any likelihood of a mother giving birth to an infected child.

been eradicated in any large area. A large reservoir of yaws persists in West Africa which includes the Ivory Coast, Ghana, Togo, Benin, and the pygmies of Zaire and the Central African Republic. Yaws is also prevalent in Indonesia; Papua, New Guinea; and the Solomon Islands of the western Pacific. The Sahelian African nations of Mali, Niger, Burkina Faso, and Senegal have prevalence rates in some areas of 10 to 15 percent for endemic syphilis. These rates exceed those reported before the mass treatment campaigns. Seroactivity and late manifestations of endemic syphilis continue to occur among nomads in Saudi Arabia. The resurgence of yaws and endemic syphilis led to a new yaws campaign in Ghana in 1980, and other national campaigns are planned to control resurgent yaws and endemic syphilis in Africa.

Antitreponemal and reaginic seroreactivity has been detected in a small percentage of children without clinical disease born after the mass campaigns in some areas (e.g., Nigeria, New Guinea, and Bosnia). This may represent attenuated or asymptomatic infection or may simply reflect the decreased predictive value of serologic tests (probability that disease is present if the test is positive) when the prevalence of disease is sharply reduced.

In the Americas, foci of yaws persist in Haiti; Dominica, St. Lucia, and St. Vincent; Peru, Colombia, and Ecuador; a few areas of Brazil; and Guyana and Surinam. Pinta is confined to Central America and northern South America, where it appears to have regressed to remote Indian villages. Its prevalence today is probably less than 1 percent of that found 20 years ago.

BIOLOGIC RELATIONSHIPS Specific humoral antibodies to *T. pallidum* are produced in individuals with yaws, pinta, or endemic syphilis, but the time of appearance of antibodies after onset of infections is variable. The fluorescent treponemal antibody absorption (FTA-ABS) test, the *T. pallidum* hemagglutination test (TPHA), and the *T. pallidum* immobilization (TPI) test cannot differentiate among the treponematoses.

In addition to the clinical and epidemiologic differences among the treponematoses in humans, the range of susceptible animal hosts and some manifestations of experimental infection are also different. In particular, *T. carateum* has produced an infection in chimpanzees which resembles pinta, but attempts to infect other experimental animals have been unsuccessful. Individuals who have had yaws or pinta are considered relatively immune to syphilis, and persons with active pinta or syphilis cannot be superinfected with *T. pallidum* ssp. *pertenue* by experimental inoculation.

CLINICAL MANIFESTATIONS Yaws Also known as *pian*, *framboesia*, or *bubas*, yaws is a chronic infectious disease of childhood caused by *T. pallidum* ssp. *pertenue*. The disease is characterized by an initial skin lesion(s) followed by relapsing, nondestructive,

secondary lesions of skin and bone. In the late stages, destructive lesions of skin, bone, and joints occur.

The incubation period following experimental inoculation of susceptible human beings is 3 to 4 weeks. Disruption of the skin by insect bites, abrasions, or injuries promotes acquisition of natural infection from infected contacts, most likely by fingers contaminated directly or indirectly with material from early yaws lesions. The initial early lesion is a single papule which is usually located on a leg. The lesion enlarges and becomes papillomatous (Fig. 134-1). This lesion also is known as a *framboesioma* (raspberry), or "mother yaw." It becomes superficially eroded and covered by a thin yellow crust of serous exudate containing *T. pallidum* ssp. *pertenue*. Erythema and induration do not occur. The lesion is mildly pruritic, and regional lymphadenopathy occurs. The initial lesion usually heals in 6 months. As a result of treponemal bacteremia and autoinoculation, a generalized secondary eruption of similar lesions appears either before or after the initial lesion has healed and is most extensive on the exposed surfaces of the body. These early cutaneous lesions of yaws have a variety of forms, including desquamative macular and papular as well as papillomatous types. Painful papillomata on the soles of the feet result in a crablike gait referred to as "crab yaws." Early lesions are infectious and heal slowly; they may result in scarring, hyperpigmentation, or depigmentation, resembling the pigmentary changes seen in pinta. Histologic findings are mononuclear cell infiltration, acanthosis, hyperkeratosis, and the presence of many treponemes.

Other manifestations of early yaws include lymphadenopathy and nocturnal bone pain and polydactylitis due to periostitis. Fever and other constitutional symptoms are rare, however, unless lesions become secondarily infected. Infectious cutaneous relapses are characteristic during the first 5 years after infection. Late yaws lesions occur in about 10 percent of cases, starting 5 years or more after infection, and differ histologically from early lesions in showing endarteritis. Late lesions include gummas of the skin and long bones, particularly of the legs, hyperkeratoses of the soles and palms, osteitis, periostitis, juxtaarticular fibromatous nodes, and hydrarthrosis.

Late lesions of yaws are characteristically extensive and usually destructive. Destruction of the nose, maxilla, palate, and pharynx, termed *gangosa*, or *rhinopharyngitis mutilans*, occurs in late yaws, as well as in leprosy and leishmaniasis. Hypertrophic paranasal maxillary osteitis produces distinctive facies known as *goundou*.

The clinical features of yaws have become less reliable for diagnosis as the prevalence of yaws has decreased, necessitating the use of easily performed serologic tests, such as the rapid plasma reagin (RPR) card test. *T. pallidum* ssp. *pertenue* can be demonstrated by dark-field examination in early cutaneous lesions but should not be confused with other spirochetes found in tropical ulcers. The serum

FIGURE 134-1 Young man with squamous micro-papules of early yaws with papillomas in the left axilla and scapular area.

reagin antibody tests become positive after 1 month, and the FTA-ABS test is also positive.

Endemic syphilis Synonyms for endemic syphilis are Bejel, Siti, Dichuchwa, Njovera, and Skerljevo. It is a chronic nonvenereal treponemal infection of childhood characterized by early mucous membrane or mucocutaneous lesions, a latent period of indeterminate duration, and late complications including gummas of bone and skin. The causative organism, *T. pallidum* ssp. *endemicum*, is indistinguishable from *T. pallidum* ssp. *pallidum*. Endemic syphilis differs from congenital syphilis in that dental changes, interstitial keratitis, and neurosyphilis rarely, if ever, occur. Cardiovascular complications are considered rare in both endemic and congenital syphilis.

Primary cutaneous lesions are infrequent and, when present, are extragenital. The earliest manifestation of endemic syphilis is usually an intraoral mucous patch or mucocutaneous lesion resembling the split papules or condylomata of secondary syphilis. Periostitis is common. Regional lymphadenopathy occurs, but generalized lymphadenopathy is unusual. Treponemes are abundant in the moist early lesions and in aspirates from regional lymph nodes. After a variable latent period, late lesions may develop and are the most frequent clinical manifestations. These resemble the lesions of late benign syphilis and include osseous or cutaneous gummas. Destructive gummas, osteitis, and gangosa are more common than in late yaws. Gummas occur on the nipples of mothers who have themselves previously had endemic syphilis and who breastfeed infants with oral lesions. Both early and late forms of endemic syphilis thus may coexist in the same family. The tertiary lesions of endemic syphilis sometimes may be a consequence of repeated exposure of a previously sensitized host to reinfection.

Pinta Also known as *mal del pinto*, *carate*, *azul*, or *purupuru*, pinta is an infectious disease of the skin caused by *T. carateum*. This disease has three cutaneous stages characterized by marked changes in the skin color, does not involve osseous tissue or viscera, and causes no disability other than that associated with cosmetic disfigurement.

The initial lesion is a small papule which appears 7 to 30 days after exposure and is located most often on the extremities, face, neck, or buttocks. It increases in size slowly by peripheral extension and by coalescing with smaller satellite papules. Regional lymphadenopathy occurs. A secondary eruption not associated with generalized lymphadenopathy appears 1 month to 1 year after the appearance of the initial lesion. The secondary lesions are termed *pintides*, may be numerous, and evolve into a psoriatic or circinate configuration.

Pintides are initially red but become deeply pigmented, reaching a slate-blue color after a period of time which is related to exposure to sun. Pigmentation occurs most rapidly on the exposed parts of the body. These pigmented lesions are known as dyschromic macules and contain treponemes which are located principally in the epidermis in older lesions. Histologically, there is deposition of pigment in the dermis with decreased melanin pigment in the basal cell layer. Within 3 months to a year, most of the pintides show varying degrees of depigmentation, becoming brown and finally white and giving the skin a mottled appearance. The porcelain-white achromic lesions represent the "late" stage of the disease in which the epidermis is atrophic, and melanocytes and melanin are absent. *T. carateum* can be demonstrated in transudates from initial, early secondary, or dyschromic lesions. Reaginic and antitreponemal antibody tests are positive but may take four times longer to become positive in pinta than in venereal syphilis.

TREATMENT Treatment is similar for all the endemic treponematoses. Intramuscular injection of 2.4 million units of benzathine penicillin G in adults and half this dose in children results in rapid resolution of lesions and prevents recurrence. Procaine penicillin G in oil and 2% aluminum monostearate (PAM) has been used extensively. In persons who are allergic to penicillin, tetracycline hydrochloride in a dose similar to that used for infectious syphilis (see Chap. 133) is effective. In areas where less than 5 percent of the population has active disease, cases are managed on an individual basis, and all contacts of infected persons are treated with antibiotics.

PREVENTION Although the nonvenereal treponematoses are less amenable to eradication than smallpox, the resurgence of yaws has led some authorities to suggest that the application of *selective epidemiologic control* as used in smallpox eradication be applied to yaws control. This strategy would emphasize ongoing active surveillance, investigation of outbreaks, and treatment of active cases and their contacts rather than mass treatment. There is concern that the epidemiology and course of yaws and endemic syphilis will be adversely affected by the HIV pandemic in Africa and Asia. Cutaneous lesions may be prolonged, be more easily secondarily infected, and serve as a portal for nonvenereal transmission of HIV.

REFERENCES

BURKE JP et al (eds): International symposium on yaws and other endemic treponematoses. Rev Infect Dis 7:S217, 1985
ENGELKENS HJH et al: Endemic treponematosis. Int J Dermatol 30:77, 1991

GUTHE T: Clinical, serological and epidemiological features of framboesia tropica (yaws) and its control in rural communities. Acta Dermatol Venereol 49:343, 1969

NOORDHOEK GT, VAN EMBDEN JDA: Yaws, an endemic treponematosis reconsidered in the HIV era. Eur J Clin Microbiol Infect Dis 10:4, 1991

MEHEUS A, ANTAL GM: Endemic treponematoses: Not yet eradicated. World Health Stat Q 45:228, 1992

PERINE PL et al: Handbook of Endemic Treponematoses. Geneva, WHO, 1984

Treponematoses Research: Report of a WHO Scientific Group, WHO Technical Report Series 674, 1982

135   LEPTOSPIROSIS

JAY P. SANFORD

DEFINITION *Leptospirosis* is a term applied to disease caused by all leptospiras regardless of specific serotype. Correlation of clinical syndromes with infection by differing serotypes leads to the conclusion that a single serotype of *Leptospira* may be responsible for a variety of clinical features; conversely, a single syndrome, e.g., aseptic meningitis, may be caused by multiple serotypes. Hence there is a preference for the general term *leptospirosis* rather than the synonyms such as *Weil's disease* and *canicola fever*.

ETIOLOGY The genus *Leptospira* contains only one species, *L. interrogans*, which may be subdivided into two complexes, interrogans and biflexa. The interrogans complex includes the pathogenic strains, while the biflexa complex includes saprophytic strains. Within each complex the organisms show antigenic variations that are stable and allow them to be classed as serotypes (serovars). Serotypes with common antigens are arranged in serogroups (varieties). Despite contrary common usage, an example of the correct designation of *Leptospira* is as follows: Pomona serogroup of *L. interrogans* or *L. interrogans* var. pomona, not *L. pomona*. The interrogans complex now contains about 240 serotypes arranged in 23 serogroups (the number in parentheses refers to number of serotypes within the serogroup): Icterohemorrhagiae (18), Hebdomadis (30), Autumnalis (17), Canicola (12), Australis (12), Tarassovi (17), Pyrogenes (12), Bataviae (10), Javanica (8), Pomona (8), Ballum (3), Cynopteri (3), Celledoni (3), Grippotyphosa (5), Panama (2), Shermani (1), Ranarum (2), and Bufonis (1). At least 27 serotypes of *Leptospira* occur naturally in the United States.

EPIDEMIOLOGY Leptospirosis is thought to be the most widespread zoonosis in the world. Cases are regularly reported from all continents except Antarctica and are especially prevalent in the tropics. Although leptospirosis is not a common disease, it has been reported from all regions of the United States, including arid areas such as Arizona. Between 1987 and 1992, 43 to 93 cases were reported annually. Infection in humans is an incidental occurrence and is not essential to the maintenance of leptospirosis. The disease occurs in a wide range of domestic and wild animal hosts, including poikilothermic vertebrates. In many species, such as opossums, skunks, raccoons, and foxes, infectivity ratios in the range of 10 to 50 percent are not unusual. Interspecies spread of specific serotypes of leptospiras between animal hosts is frequent; e.g., Pomona, a serotype principally associated with livestock, has been demonstrated in dogs. Infection in animals may vary from inapparent illness to severe, fatal disease. Even asymptomatic animals may carry high numbers ($>10^{10}$ organisms per gram) in their kidneys. The carrier state, in which the host may shed leptospiras in its urine for months to years, may develop in many animals. Immunization of dogs may not prevent the carrier, or shedder, state.

Survival of pathogenic leptospiras in nature is governed by such factors as pH of the urine of the host, pH of soil or water into which they are shed, and ambient temperature. Leptospiras in most "urine spots" in soil retain infectivity for 6 to 48 h. Acid urine permits only limited survival; however, if the urine is neutral or alkaline and is shed into a similar moist environment which has low salinity, is not badly polluted with microorganisms or detergents, and has a temperature above 22°C, leptospiras may survive for several weeks. Human infections can occur either by direct contact with urine or tissue of an infected animal or indirectly through contaminated water, soil, or vegetation. The usual portals of entry in humans are abraded skin, particularly about the feet, and exposed conjunctival, nasal, and oral mucous membranes. Swallowing contaminated water during immersion has been associated with high attack rates. The previously held concept that organisms could penetrate intact skin has been questioned. While leptospiras have been isolated from ticks, these arthropods appear to be unimportant in transmission.

With the ubiquitous infection of animals, leptospirosis in human beings can occur in all age groups, at all seasons, and in both sexes. However, it is primarily a disease of teenage children and young adults (about one-half of patients are between the ages of 10 and 39), occurs predominantly in males (80 percent), and develops most frequently in hot weather (in the United States one-half of infections occur from July to October). The wide spectrum of animal hosts results in both urban and rural human disease. Leptospirosis has been considered an occupational disease; however, improved methods of rat control and better standards of hygiene have reduced the incidence among occupational groups such as coal miners and people who work in sewers. The epidemiologic pattern has changed; in the United States, the United Kingdom, Europe, and Israel, water-associated and cattle-associated leptospirosis is most common. Fewer than 20 percent of patients have had direct contact with animals; they are mostly farmers, trappers, or abattoir workers. In the majority of patients, exposure is incidental; two-thirds of cases occur in children, students, or housewives. Swimming or partial immersion in contaminated water, e.g., riding motorcycles through contaminated pools of water, has been implicated in one-fifth of patients and has accounted for most of the recognized common-source outbreaks. In Hawaii, one-fourth of cases have been associated with aquaculture industries; in the United Kingdom, fish; while in Italy, farm workers are at increased risk; leptospirosis remains common in the rice-growing areas of the Po River Valley (a serologic survey of railway workers in the area showed an antibody prevalence of 10 percent).

PATHOLOGY In patients who have died with hepatorenal involvement (Weil's syndrome), the significant gross changes include hemorrhages and bile staining of tissues. The hemorrhages, which vary from petechial to ecchymotic, are widespread and are most prominent in skeletal muscle, kidneys, adrenals, liver, stomach, spleen, and lungs.

In skeletal muscle, focal, necrotic, and necrobiotic changes typical of leptospirosis occur. Biopsies early in the illness demonstrate swelling and vacuolation. Leptospiral antigen has been demonstrated in these lesions by the fluorescent antibody technique. Healing ensues by the formation of new myofibrils with minimal fibrosis. The renal lesions in the acute phase involve predominantly the tubules and vary from simple dilatation of distal convoluted tubules to degeneration, necrosis, and basement membrane rupture. Interstitial edema and cellular infiltrates consisting of lymphocytes, neutrophilic leukocytes, histiocytes, and plasma cells are uniformly present. Glomerular lesions either are absent or consist of mesangial hyperplasia and focal foot process fusion, which are interpreted as representing nonspecific changes associated with acute inflammation and protein filtration. Microscopic alterations in the liver are not diagnostic and correlate poorly with the degree of functional impairment. The changes include cloudy swelling of parenchymal cells, disruption of liver cords, enlargement of Kupffer cells, and bile stasis in biliary canaliculi. The changes in the brain and meninges are also minimal and are not diagnostic. Microscopic evidence of myocarditis has been recorded. Pulmonary findings consist of a patchy, localized hemorrhagic pneumonitis. Special staining techniques utilizing silver impregnation methods have demonstrated organisms in the lumina of renal tubules but rarely in other organs.

PATHOGENESIS Leptospirosis is one of the recognized human spirochetal diseases; other diseases in this group include syphilis, pinta, yaws, bejel, relapsing fever (due to *Borrelia* species), Lyme disease, and rat-bite fever (due to *Spirillum minus*). Despite differences in epidemiology, there are many similarities among these entities. Spirochetemia develops soon after the entry of leptospiras through the skin or mucous membranes, with wide dessemination throughout tissue and body fluid. Coincident with an immune response (both humoral and cellular), spirochetemia either terminates or is greatly reduced; however, organisms may persist in immunologically isolated areas. With leptospirosis, persistence in the kidney and shedding of leptospiras in urine are integral to epidemiology. Later manifestations, e.g., aseptic meningitis and iridocyclitis, are thought to be immuno-pathologically mediated. Such occurrences are features in each of the spirochetal diseases.

The cell wall of *L. interrogans* contains lipopolysaccharide (endotoxin). With initiation of antimicrobial therapy in leptospirosis, a Jarisch-Herxheimer–like reaction (J-HR) similar to that seen with other spirochetal diseases may occur. It had been postulated that the J-HR was due to release of endotoxin; however, in the clinically most predictable and severe J-HR (that associated with louse-borne relapsing fever), limulus amebocyte lysate (LAL) assays for endotoxin were negative, and it was concluded that endotoxin, if present, had leaked into the circulation from intestinal gram-negative organisms.

Watt and associates studied 24 patients with proven leptospirosis who were treated with penicillin. While none had J-HR, 78 percent had endotoxemia, as measured by LAL assays. Patients with positive LAL specimens had significantly higher leukocyte counts and levels of serum creatinine and bilirubin than did patients with negative LAL assays. The authors postulated delayed hepatic clearance of endotoxin due to hepatic dysfunction. Recently, in patients with proven *Borrelia recurrentis* infection who experienced J-HR with penicillin treatment, the peak of the J-HR was strongly associated with high plasma levels of tumor necrosis factor (TNF). Peaks of interleukin 6 and interleukin 8 occurred just after that of TNF. Extrapolation of these data to leptospirosis suggests that cytokine release through rapid phagocytosis of *L. interrogans* in response to antibody or therapy may mediate many of the symptoms, especially in the secondary phase.

CLINICAL MANIFESTATIONS **General features** The incubation period following immersion or accidental laboratory exposure has shown extremes of 2 to 26 days, the usual range being 7 to 13 days and the average 10 days.

Leptospirosis is a typically biphasic illness. *During the lepto-spiremic, or first, phase*, leptospiras are present in the blood and cerebrospinal fluid (CSF). The onset is typically abrupt, and initial symptoms include headache, which is usually frontal, is less often retroorbital, but occasionally may be bitemporal or occipital. Severe muscle aching occurs in most patients, the muscles of the thighs and lumbar areas being most prominently involved, and often is accompanied by severe pain on palpation. Patients often complain of leg pain with walking. The myalgia may be accompanied by extreme cutaneous hyperesthesia (causalgia). Chills followed by a rapidly rising temperature are prominent. Following the abrupt onset, the leptospiremic phase typically lasts 4 to 9 days. Features during this interval include recurrent chills, high spiking temperatures [usually 38.9°C (102°F) or greater], headache, and continued severe myalgia. Involvement of one organ system may predominate, often leading to initial misdiagnosis. Such symptom complexes most commonly include hepatitis, nephritis, atypical pneumonia, influenza, or "viral" gastroenteritis. Anorexia, nausea, and vomiting are encountered in one-half or more of patients. Occasional patients have diarrhea. Pulmonary manifestations, usually either cough or chest pain, have varied in frequency of occurrence from less than 25 percent to 86 percent. Hemoptysis occurs uncommonly in the United States and Europe but is a common feature in Korea and China, being noted in 40 percent of patients. Examination during this phase reveals an acutely ill, febrile patient, with a relative bradycardia and normal blood pressure. Disturbances in sensorium may be encountered in up

to 25 percent of all patients and in one-half of patients with icteric disease. Transient cerebral ischemic attacks in children associated with leptospiral arteritis have been reported from China.

The most characteristic physical sign is conjunctival suffusion, which usually first appears on the third or fourth day. It may be lacking in some patients but more often is overlooked. It may be associated with photophobia, but serous or purulent secretion is unusual. Less common findings may include pharyngeal injection, cutaneous hemorrhages, and skin rashes that, even when they occur, are not prominent. The rashes may be macular, maculopapular, or urticarial and usually occur on the trunk. Uncommon findings are splenomegaly, hepatomegaly, lymphadenopathy, or jaundice. The first phase terminates after 4 to 9 days, usually with defervescence and improvement in symptoms. This coincides with the disappearance of leptospiras from the blood and CSF.

The second phase has been characterized as the "immune" phase and correlates with the appearance of circulating IgM antibodies; the concentration of C3 in serum remains normal. The clinical manifestations of this phase show greater variability than those during the first phase. After a relatively asymptomatic period of 1 to 3 days, the fever and earlier symptoms recur, and meningismus may develop. The fever rarely exceeds 38.9°C (102°F) and is usually of 1 to 3 days' duration. It is not uncommon for fever to be absent or quite transient. Even when symptoms or signs of meningeal irritation are absent, routine examination of CSF after the seventh day has revealed pleocytosis in 50 to 90 percent of patients. Less common features include iridocyclitis, optic neuritis, and other nervous system manifestations, including encephalitis, myelitis, and peripheral neuropathy. Leptospirosis during pregnancy may be associated with an increased risk of fetal loss.

Specific features WEIL'S SYNDROME *Weil's syndrome*, which may be due to serotypes other than Icterohemorrhagiae, is defined as severe leptospirosis with jaundice, usually accompanied by azotemia, hemorrhages, anemia, disturbances in consciousness, and continued fever. It occurs in 1 to 6 percent of patients with leptospirosis, although the figure may have been as high as 62 percent in a recent series from Portugal. There is uncertainty as to the pathogenesis of the syndrome, i.e., whether it represents direct toxic damage due to leptospiras or is the consequence of immune response to leptospiral antigens. The consensus favors toxic damage.

The onset and first stage are identical with the less severe forms of leptospirosis. The distinctive features of Weil's syndrome appear from the third to the sixth days but do not reach their peak until well into the second stage. As in milder forms of leptospirosis, there is a tendency for defervescence about the seventh day; however, with recurrence, fever is marked and may persist for several weeks. Either renal or hepatic manifestations may predominate. Hepatic disturbances include tenderness in the right upper quadrant and hepatic enlargement, both of which are common when jaundice is present. Serum aspartate aminotransferase (AST) values are rarely increased more than fivefold regardless of the degree of hyperbilirubinemia (in which conjugated bilirubin predominates). The predominant mechanism appears to be an intracellular block to bilirubin excretion.

Renal manifestations of Weil's syndrome consist primarily of proteinuria, pyuria, hematuria, and azotemia. Dysuria is rare. Serious renal damage usually occurs in the form of acute tubular necrosis associated with oliguria. The peak elevation of blood urea nitrogen usually is seen on the fifth to seventh day. Hemorrhagic manifestations are most prevalent in this group of patients and include epistaxis, hemoptysis, gastrointestinal bleeding, hemorrhage into the adrenal glands, hemorrhagic pneumonitis, and subarachnoid hemorrhage. These have been explained on the basis of diffuse vasculitis with capillary injury. In addition, in some patients hypoprothrombinemia, thrombocytopenia, and thrombotic thrombocytopenic purpura have been observed.

HEMORRHAGIC FEVER WITH RENAL SYNDROME Studies on the epidemiology of Hantavirus (Chap. 159) have shown that for the initial 24 to 72 h there is significant overlap in the clinical features of leptospirosis, hemorrhagic fever with renal syndrome (HFRS), and scrub typhus (H.W. Lee, personal communication). In Korea, where all three diseases are prevalent, 21 percent of the blood samples submitted for Hantavirus serology had antibody to *Leptospira* antigens and 6 percent to *Rickettsia tsutsugamushi*. Conversely, among 261 patients in Singapore clinically suspected of having leptospirosis, 3 percent had serologic evidence of Hantavirus infection. Hantavirus disease, which varies from mild (nephropathica epidemica) to severe (Balkan nephropathy), is common in Europe and Scandinavia. Because of the similarity in epidemiology and clinical presentation and the potential for dual infections, it has been recommended that blood be submitted for Hantavirus serology in all cases of suspected leptospirosis. Clinically, the term *lepthangamushi syndrome* has been used to describe this overlap syndrome.

ATYPICAL PNEUMONIA SYNDROME   Pulmonary symptoms and signs are common in patients with leptospirosis; even the adult respiratory distress syndrome (ARDS) has been reported. While this association is not fully appreciated in the United States, leptospirosis is recognized in other parts of the world as an important differential diagnostic consideration in the patient with fever, chills, headache, severe myalgia, and bilateral bronchopneumonia, with or without an associated "active" urine sediment. In Italy, respiratory or influenza-like symptoms were the only clinical signs of illness in 21 percent of more than 300 patients with confirmed leptospirosis. In a group of 37 Korean patients with pulmonary radiographic findings, 21 had small nodular densities, 10 had a diffuse ground glass pattern, and 6 had large confluent areas of consolidation. Abnormalities were bilateral and nonlobar in all. In surviving patients, resolution occurred within 15 days. Given appropriate epidemiologic circumstances, leptospirosis should be added to the differential diagnosis of "atypical" pneumonia.

ASEPTIC MENINGOENCEPHALITIS   A leptospiral etiology has been incriminated in 5 to 13 percent of sporadic cases of aseptic meningitis. Pleocytosis is not present before the immune phase but then develops rapidly. There are usually tens to hundreds of leukocytes, occasionally 1000, per microliter, among which neutrophils or mononuclear cells may predominate. CSF glucose concentration is almost always normal, but occasional instances of lowered glucose levels have been recorded. CSF protein may exceed 1 g/L (100 mg/dL) early in the course. Xanthochromic CSF has been observed in the presence of jaundice. Neurologic manifestations may include encephalitis and, in rare cases, hemiparesis. Each of the serotypes of *Leptospira* that is pathogenic for humans is probably capable of causing aseptic meningitis. The most prevalent serotypes have been Canicola, Icterohemorrhagiae, and Pomona.

MYOCARDITIS   Cardiac arrhythmias, including paroxysmal atrial fibrillation, atrial flutter, ventricular tachycardia, and premature ventricular contractions, have been described but are usually of little clinical significance. However, on rare occasions pericarditis and definite cardiac dilatation with acute left ventricular failure have been observed. Associated manifestations have included jaundice (occurring in 95 percent of cases described in a recent report), pulmonary infiltrates, arthritis, and skin rashes. The serotypes thus far incriminated have included Icterohemorrhagiae, Autumnalis, Pomona, and Grippotyphosa.

CHILDREN   Several clinical features that are not seen or are very rare in adults occur in children: hypertension, acalculous cholecystitis (five of nine children in one series), pancreatitis, abdominal causalgia, and peripheral desquamation of a rash that may be associated with gangrene and cardiopulmonary arrest. The features of desquamation, myocardial involvement, and hydrops of the gallbladder suggest Kawasaki syndrome [mucocutaneous lymph node syndrome (see Chap. 58)].

LABORATORY FEATURES   Leukocyte counts vary from leukopenic levels to mild elevations in the anicteric patients. In patients with jaundice, leukocytosis—with as many as 70,000 cells per microliter—may be present. However, regardless of the total leukocyte count, neutrophilia (greater than 70 percent neutrophils) is very frequently encountered during the first stage.

Hemolytic substances have been demonstrated in cultures of pathogenic leptospiras. In contrast to many hemolysins of bacterial origin which are not hemolytic in vivo, the leptospiral hemolysins appear to be active in vivo. In patients with jaundice, anemia may be severe and is most characteristically due to intravascular hemolysis. Other mechanisms of anemia include azotemia and blood loss secondary to hemorrhage. Anemia due to leptospirosis is unusual in anicteric patients.

Thrombocytopenia sufficient to be associated with bleeding (less than 30,000 platelets per microliter) may be encountered. Additional hematologic abnormalities include elevation of the erythrocyte sedimentation rate in over one-half of patients (usually less than 50 mm/h).

Urinalysis during the leptospiremic phase reveals mild proteinuria, casts, and an increase in cellular elements. In anicteric infections, these abnormalities rapidly disappear after the first week. Proteinuria and abnormalities in the urine sediment usually are not associated with elevations in blood urea nitrogen. Since the anicteric form of the disease often has gone undiagnosed, estimates of the frequency of azotemia and jaundice are probably high. Azotemia has been reported in approximately one-fourth of patients. In three-fourths of these patients, the blood urea nitrogen level is less than 36 mmol/L (100 mg/dL). Azotemia is usually associated with jaundice. The serum bilirubin levels may reach 1110 µmol/L (65 mg/dL); however, in two-thirds of patients the levels are less than 340 µmol/L (20 mg/dL). During the first phase, one-half of patients have increased serum creatine phosphokinase (CK) levels, with mean values of five times normal. Such increases are not seen in viral hepatitis, and a slight increase in transaminase with a definite increase in CK suggests leptospirosis rather than viral hepatitis.

DIAGNOSIS   Diagnosis is based on culture of the organism or serologic proof of its existence. The most common initial diagnostic impressions in patients with leptospirosis are meningitis, hepatitis, nephritis, fever of undetermined origin (FUO), influenza, Kawasaki syndrome, toxic shock syndrome, and Legionnaires' disease. Leptospiras may be isolated quite readily during the first phase from blood and CSF or during the second phase from the urine. Leptospiras may be excreted in the urine for up to 11 months after the onset of illness and may persist despite antimicrobial therapy. Whole blood should be inoculated immediately into tubes containing semisolid medium, such as Fletcher's or EMJH medium. If culture medium is not available, leptospiras reportedly will remain viable up to 11 days in blood to which anticoagulants, preferably sodium oxalate, have been added. Animal inoculation (preferably either suckling hamsters or guinea pigs) may be used and is of particular value if specimens are contaminated. Direct examination of blood or urine by dark-field methods has been employed; *however, this method so frequently results in failure or misdiagnosis that it should not be employed*. Serologic methods are applicable during the second phase; antibodies appear from the sixth to the twelfth days of illness. Two serologic methods are commonly used: a macroscopic or slide agglutination test, which is easy to perform but lacks specificity and sensitivity and hence is suitable for screening only, and the microscopic agglutination test, which is more complicated but also more specific. An IgM-specific dot-ELISA has been effective in diagnosing leptospirosis in an endemic area. Serologic criteria for diagnosis include a fourfold or greater rise in titer during the course of illness. Cross-agglutination reactions between various serotypes commonly occur so that the infection serotype often cannot be determined with certainty without isolation of leptospiras.

PROGNOSIS   The prognosis is dependent on both the virulence of the organism and the general condition of the patient. The mortality rate in reported cases in the United States has varied annually between 2.5 and 16.4 percent, averaging 7.1 percent. Age is the most significant host factor related to increased mortality. In a representative series, the mortality rate rose from 10 percent in men less than 50 years of age to 56 percent in those over 51 years of age. The virulence of the infecting leptospiras correlates best with the development of jaundice. In anicteric patients, death is extremely rare, but with the development of jaundice, the mortality rate in various series has ranged from 15 to 48 percent. Death is usually secondary to hemorrhage (especially gastrointestinal) or to renal failure. The long-term prognosis following the acute renal lesion of leptospirosis is good. Glomerular filtration rates have returned to normal, usually within 2 months; however, a few patients show residual tubular dysfunction such as a defect in concentrating capacity.

TREATMENT A variety of antimicrobial drugs, including penicillin, streptomycin, the tetracycline congeners, chloramphenicol, erythromycin, and ciprofloxacin, have been effective in vitro and in experimental leptospiral infections. Data concerning the efficacy of antibiotics in human beings have been conflicting. Within 4 to 6 h after initiation of penicillin G therapy, a Jarisch-Herxheimer type of reaction, which suggests antileptospiral activity, may occur. A controlled trial of intravenous penicillin (1.5 million units every 6 h for 7 days) clearly demonstrated shortening of duration of fever and creatinine elevation, shortening of hospitalization, and prevention of leptospiruria, even when treatment was started after the fifth day of illness. In contrast, a randomized trial of high-dose penicillin was not beneficial in jaundiced patients. Doxycycline (100 mg orally taken twice daily for 7 days), when started within 4 days of onset of symptoms, significantly shortened the duration of fever and most other symptoms and decreased the frequency of leptospiruria in patients with mild illness. Doxycycline (200 mg orally taken once per week) is also highly effective in preventing disease in an area of high prevalence. Azotemia and jaundice require meticulous attention to fluid and electrolyte therapy. Since the renal damage is reversible, patients with azotemia should be considered for peritoneal hemodialysis. Exchange transfusion may be beneficial in the management of patients with extreme hyperbilirubinemia.

REFERENCES

CICERONI L et al: Recent trends in human leptospirosis in Italy. Eur J Epidemiol 4:49, 1988

CORWIN A et al: Waterborne outbreak of leptospirosis among United States military personnel in Okinawa, Japan. Int J Epidemiol 19:743, 1990

EDWARDS CN et al:Leptospirosis in Barbados: A clinical study. West Indian Med J 39:27, 1990

FEIGIN RD, ANDERSON DC: Human leptospirosis. CRC Crit Rev Clin Lab Sci 5:413, 1975

GILKS CF et al: Failure of penicillin prophylaxis in laboratory acquired leptospirosis. Postgrad Med J 64:236, 1988

GRIFFIN GE: New insights into the pathophysiology of the Jarisch-Herxheimer reaction. J Antimicrob Chemother 29:613, 1992

HINDRICHSEN S et al: Hantavirus infection in Brazilian patients from Recife with suspected leptospirosis. Lancet 341:50, 1993

IM JG et al: Leptospirosis of the lung: Radiographic findings in 58 patients. AJR 152:955, 1989

JACKSON LA et al: Outbreak of leptospirosis associated with swimming. Pediatric Infect Dis J 12:48, 1993

JOHNSON WD JR et al: Serum creatine phosphokinase in leptospirosis. JAMA 233:981, 1975

KUDESIA G et al: Dual infection with Leptospira and Hantavirus. Lancet 1:1397, 1988

LECOUR H et al: Human leptospirosis—A review of 50 cases. Infection 17:8, 1989

MCCLAIN JB et al: Doxycycline therapy for leptospirosis. Ann Intern Med 100:696, 1984

PARK SK et al: Leptospirosis in Chonbuk Province of Korea in 1987: A study of 97 patients. Am J Trop Med Hyg 41:345, 1989

SCHMID GP: Epidemiology and clinical similarities of human spirochetal disease. Rev Infect Dis 11(suppl 6):S1460, 1989

TAKAFUJI ET et al: An efficacy trial of doxycycline chemoprophylaxis against leptospirosis. N Engl J Med 310:497, 1984

TURNER JS, WILLCOX PA: Respiratory failure in leptospirosis. Q J Med 72:841, 1989

WATT G: Leptospirosis. Curr Opin Infect Dis 5:659, 1992

——— et al: Placebo-controlled trial of intravenous penicillin for severe and late leptospirosis. Lancet 1:433, 1988

——— et al: Rapid diagnosis of leptospirosis: Prospective comparison of dot-ELISA and genus specific microscopic agglutination test at different stages of illness. J Infect Dis 157:840, 1988

——— et al: Central nervous system leptospirosis in the Philippines. Southeast Asian J Trop Med Public Health 20:265, 1989

——— et al: Limulus lysate positivity and Herxheimer-like reactions in leptospirosis: A placebo-controlled study. J Infect Dis 162:564, 1990

WINEARLS CG et al: Acute renal failure due to leptospirosis: Clinical features and outcome in six cases. Q J Med 53:487, 1984

WONG ML et al: Leptospirosis: A childhood disease. J Pediatr 90:532, 1977

136 RELAPSING FEVER

BAYU TEKLU / PETER L. PERINE

DEFINITION Relapsing fever is an acute spirochetal infection characterized by recurrent episodes of fever alternating with apyrexial intervals. The disease is caused by spirochetes of the genus *Borrelia* and has two epidemiologic varieties—louse-borne and tick-borne.

ETIOLOGY Borreliae are motile, spiral-shaped organisms 8 to 20 μm long and 0.2 to 0.45 μm thick. Their length may vary, but their thickness remains constant. They have an inner and an outer cell membrane with an interposed flagellum, which makes them unique morphologically. They are microaerophilic and grow and multiply easily in their vertebrate and invertebrate hosts. Several species can be cultured in embryonated eggs or Kelly's medium. After several passages in the laboratory, cultured strains may lose their infectivity. While *B. recurrentis* is the sole cause of louse-borne relapsing fever, there are over a dozen species of borreliae causing tick-borne relapsing fever.

EPIDEMIOLOGY The body louse is the only vector of louse-borne relapsing fever, and humans are the only known host, although other primates may be experimentally infected. The louse ingests blood from an infected person, and the spirochetes multiply in its tissues. Body lice travel from one another in conditions of crowding and poor hygiene and cause intense itching. Infection takes place when the louse is crushed intentionally or accidentally and its body fluids enter the bloodstream through the bite site, skin abrasions caused by scratching, or occasionally through mucous membranes. Accidental touching of the conjunctivae with contaminated fingernails is also known to produce infection.

Louse-borne relapsing fever is endemic in Central and East Africa and is thought to exist in Peru and China. In this century, epidemics destroyed large populations in Africa, Asia, and Europe during both world wars. Louse-borne relapsing fever is endemic in the highlands of Ethiopia and neighboring Sudan, where there is a steep increase in the incidence during the rainy season when the poor and louse-ridden huddle together in crowded shelters; an estimated 10,000 cases of louse-borne relapsing fever occur annually. Imported cases of louse-borne relapsing fever are seen occasionally in Europe and North America.

Tick-borne relapsing fever has a worldwide distribution, occurring in all the continents except Australasia. Soft-shelled argasid ticks belonging to the genus *Ornithodoros* are the vectors of the spirochetes, and small rodents act as their natural host. These ticks are nocturnal feeders and become infected by taking a blood meal from an infected rodent or human. The spirochetes multiply in the midgut and then enter the salivary glands and reproductive organs, where they remain alive and infective for years. Ticks of both sexes transmit the spirochetes, and female ticks infect their progeny transovarially. Humans become infected by a tick bite when the salivary and coxal secretions containing spirochetes are injected into the bloodstream. Urine and milk of infected rodents also contain live spirochetes, and contact of their infected urine with the mucous membranes of the mouth, nose, or conjunctivae also can cause infection.

B. duttoni is the most common species of borreliae causing tick-borne disease in Africa. In North America, the main species responsible are *B. hermsii*, *B. parkeri*, and *B. turicatae*, each species being named for the species of tick that transmits the spirochete. In North America, relapsing fever is prevalent in spring and summer in the western states, when people are out of doors and ticks and rodents are active. Most infections are acquired by staying overnight in log cabins infested with *Borrelia*-infected ticks. In Africa and Asia, borreliae are transmitted by domestic ticks living in the cracks of walls and mud floors. Once established, a reservoir of *Borrelia*-infected ticks can last for decades unless eradicated by insecticides.

PATHOGENESIS AND PATHOLOGY The spirochetes live and multiply with ease in the arthropods, which are devoid of an immune system. Spirochetes have survived throughout the years in their rodent reservoirs through *serologic mutation*. In this phenomenon, spirochetes constantly change their surface antigens to avoid destruction by the immune system. By the time spirochetemia peaks, antibodies have developed to clear the blood of opsonized parasites by phagocytosis. However, a few organisms with spontaneously derived mutant surface antigens escape phagocytosis, rapidly multiply, and produce another relapse in 5 to 10 days.

A large number of different *Borrelia* serotypes emerge spontaneously by multiphasic antigenitic variation during the course of untreated relapsing fever. Serotype specificity is determined by variable antigens in the outer membrane of *Borrelia* called *Vmp lipoproteins*. A variant spirochete carrying a new Vmp appears spontaneously at a frequency of 10^{-4} to 10^{-3} per cell generation and will flourish until the host responds with serotype-specific antibodies. There are at least 25 different serotypes of HSI strain of *B. hermsi* prevalent in the western United States.

Once spirochetes enter the bloodstream, they rapidly multiply and reach 10^5 to 10^8 per cubic milliliter of blood. Fever is the first clinical manifestation and begins 3 to 12 days after infection. The severity of illness and injury is proportional to the number of spirochetes in the blood. Most injury occurs intravascularly with extensive endothelial damage, extravasation of blood into the mucous membranes and skin, and disseminated intravascular coagulation. Spirochetes also invade the brain and kidneys and may appear in the cerebrospinal fluid and urine.

At autopsy, splenic microabscesses, serosal petechiae, intracranial hemorrhages, diffuse histiocytic myocarditis, and hepatitis with focal necrosis are common. Spirochetes cross the placenta and may cause abortion or relapsing fever in the neonate.

CLINICAL MANIFESTATIONS Louse-borne relapsing fever runs a more severe clinical course than tick-borne fever. After an incubation period of 3 to 18 days, those with louse-borne relapsing fever experience an abrupt onset of rigors with fever, usually remittent, headaches, arthralgia, and myalgias. Abdominal pain, nausea, vomiting, and mental confusion are common. Dry cough and signs of heart failure may develop. Epistaxis occurs in 10 to 40 percent of cases, jaundice in 15 to 45 percent, and skin petechiae or ecchymoses in up to 60 percent. Subconjunctival and retinal hemorrhages occur rarely, and hemoptysis and hematuria are infrequent. Meningismus is seen in 40 percent of cases.

The first attack lasts 3 to 6 days and ends by crisis characterized by rigors, with abruptly rising body temperature, blood pressure, pulse, and respiratory rate lasting 10 to 20 minutes. Peak core body temperature rapidly increases and may reach 44°C. This is followed by profuse sweating, falling temperature, and hypotension which may last several hours. The patient either recovers or dies during crisis from a combination of hyperpyrexia, severe hypotension, and intractable heart failure due to myocarditis. If recovery occurs, the patient may feel reasonably well for 5 to 10 days until less severe relapse occurs; additional relapses are rare. The decreased number of spirochetes during relapses is attributed to the increasingly effective host immune response. Although fewer in number, the spirochetes producing relapses are as virulent as those producing first attacks in a susceptible host.

In tick-borne relapsing fever, neurologic sequelae occur more frequently. Deafness and unilateral blindness secondary to panophthalmitis or iridocyclitis and other neurologic deficits are seen in subsequent relapses. Splenomegaly occurs in 41 percent, hepatomegaly in 18 percent. Jaundice or neurologic features are seen in 8 percent. Skin rash is seen in 28 percent and epistaxis in only 2 percent. Convulsions occur frequently in children. Up to 10 relapses have been documented; each tends to be less severe and symptomatic. In pregnant women, relapsing fever can cause abortion and stillbirth.

LABORATORY FINDINGS A mild anemia and thrombocytopenia are frequent findings. The white cell count is usually normal. Transient elevations of blood urea and creatinine are seen. Elevations in alanine aminotransferase, serum bilirubin, prothrombin time, and activated partial thromboplastin time are common. The majority of patients develop agglutinins to *Proteus* OXK and OX19. Proteinuria and microscopic hematuria may occur. A chest x-ray may show cardiomegaly and pulmonary edema. The ECG shows a prolongation of QTc interval and premature ventricular contractions.

Definitive diagnosis is made by demonstrating borreliae in peripheral blood films, thin or thick, stained with Wright's, Giemsa, or Leishman's stain. Motile borreliae also may be demonstrated in wet preparations with dark-field or phase-contrast microscopy. If spirochetemia is light, a peripheral blood smear may be negative, and repeated examinations are usually necessary, especially of samples collected during spikes of fever. If the smear is negative and there is a strong suspicion of the tick-borne disease, blood may be injected into mice and their blood examined subsequently for spirochetes. In patients with meningeal signs, the cerebrospinal fluid may show increased protein and mononuclear pleocytosis; in rare cases borreliae are seen by dark-field or phase-contrast microscopy.

DIFFERENTIAL DIAGNOSIS In both varieties of relapsing fever, the differential diagnosis includes malaria, typhoid fever, typhus, Lyme disease, rat-bite fever, leptospirosis, meningococcal disease, and hepatitis. In tick-borne relapsing fever, brucellosis, tularemia, juvenile rheumatoid arthritis, dengue fever, and Rocky Mountain spotted fever also should be considered.

TREATMENT Borreliae are highly susceptible to a variety of antimicrobials, including penicillins, tetracycline, chloramphenicol, and erythromycin, but are resistant to rifampicin and sulfonamides. Before administration of intravenous antibiotic, a good peripheral or preferably a central venous line should be secured. In louse-borne relapsing fever, the drug of choice is tetracycline, 500 mg, intravenously or orally, as a single dose, which clears the blood of spirochetes within a few hours. The same dose may be used for chloramphenicol or erythromycin with similar results. All antibiotics precipitate the Jarisch-Herxheimer reaction (J-HR). If intravenous tetracycline is used, patients with louse-borne relapsing fever invariably develop a severe J-HR within 1 h of drug administration. The initial "chill" phase, in which the patient abruptly becomes agitated with severe rigors, lasts about 1 h. During this phase, blood pressure, pulse, and respiratory rate rise sharply and the patient develops hyperpyrexia, usually over 40°C and lasting up to 1 h. Severe abdominal pain, vomiting, and diarrhea with urinary incontinence also may occur. Serial blood films show that spirochetes rapidly decrease in number, accompanied by leukopenia and thrombocytopenia. Hyperpyrexia should be treated promptly with tepid sponging or acetaminophen. A "flush" phase follows that is characterized by profound vasodilation, drenching sweats, and falling vital signs. Systolic blood pressure may reach 70 mmHg or less, and congestive heart failure or pulmonary edema may ensue. Failure can be managed by judicious use of saline infusions and digoxin, 0.5 mg intravenously. Hypotension and listlessness may last several hours and, rarely, contribute to multiple organ failure and death.

The crisis and Jarisch-Herxheimer reaction in louse-borne relapsing fever have recently been shown to be temporally associated with high circulating levels of the monokines tumor necrosis factor α, interleukin 6 (IL-6), and IL-8. It may be possible to block the reaction by pretreatment with human anti-TNF antibody.

Aspirin, acetaminophen, high-dose oral or intravenous corticosteroids, or intravenous naloxone administered during the reaction or before antibiotic administration do not prevent or ameliorate the J-HR. Meptazinol, an opioid antagonist with some agonist properties, in a dose of 300 to 500 mg intravenously, reduces the severity of the J-HR. Since relapses have occasionally been noted after ampicillin or penicillin treatment, this treatment should be followed by a single 500-mg oral dose of tetracycline, chloramphenicol, or erythromycin after the crisis has ended. If the peripheral smear is negative for *Borrelia* and there is a strong clinical suspicion of louse-borne relapsing fever, 500 mg tetracycline either intravenously or orally can be given as a therapeutic trial. Occurrence of the crisis confirms the diagnosis, while its absence virtually excludes the disease. Typhoid fever, typhus, malaria, Kala-azar, rickettsiosis, and tuberculosis may occur concomitantly.

The treatment of choice for tick-borne relapsing fever is tetracycline, 500 mg, orally every 6 h for 10 days, or in those not tolerating tetracycline, erythromycin in the same dose may be substituted. Doxycycline, 100 mg, twice daily for 10 days, is equally effective. J-HR occurs in one-third of cases of tick-borne relapsing fever following administration of antibiotics.

Improved personal hygiene and living conditions should eradicate louse-borne relapsing fever. Because patients with the disease are usually infected with lice, they should be bathed, their scalp hair shaved, and 1% lindane or lysol solution or DDT powder applied. Cohabitants should be deloused in a similar manner. If buildings and cracks in walls are sprayed with 2% benzene hydrochloride, and if campers avoid tick-infested areas, the incidence of tick-borne relapsing fever can be reduced. Camping in tents is safer than sleeping in rodent-infested log cabins. A novel means of eradicating ticks in rodent burrows is to scatter pyrethrin-impregnated cotton balls on the ground around dwellings known to harbor *Borrelia*-infected ticks; rodents collect these cotton balls and carry them back to their burrows as nesting material. The insecticide-impregnated cotton kills ticks living in the borrow.

PROGNOSIS The mortality from louse-borne relapsing fever in the preantibiotic era was 30 to 70 percent, but with antibiotic therapy, mortality in hospitals and at refugee camps ranges from 0 to 5 percent. Poor prognostic signs include coma, deep jaundice, hemorrhage, and evidence of myocarditis.

In tick-borne relapsing fever, mortality varies from 0 to 8 percent. Fatalities usually occur in young children and congenitally infected neonates.

REFERENCES

BARBOUR AG: Antigenic variation of a relapsing fever borrelia species. Annu Rev Microbiol 44:155, 1990

HORTON JM, BLASER MJ: The spectrum of relapsing fever in Rocky Mountains. Arch Intern Med 145:871, 1985

JUDGE DM et al: Louse-borne relapsing fever in man. Arch Pathol 97:136, 1974

NEGUSSIE Y et al: Detection of plasma tumor necrosis factor, interleukins 6 and 8 during the Jarisch-Herxheimer reaction of relapsing fever. J Exp Med 175:1207, 1992

TEKLU B et al: Meptazinol diminishes the Jarisch-Herxheimer reaction of relapsing fever. Lancet 1:835, 1983

137 LYME BORRELIOSIS

ALLEN C. STEERE

DEFINITION Lyme borreliosis, a tick-transmitted spirochetal illness, usually begins with a characteristic expanding skin lesion, erythema migrans (EM) (stage 1, localized infection). After several days to weeks, the spirochete may spread hematogenously to many different sites (stage 2, disseminated infection). Possible manifestations of disseminated infection include secondary annular skin lesions, meningitis, cranial or peripheral neuritis, carditis, or migratory musculoskeletal pain. Months to years later, usually following periods of latent infection, intermittent or chronic arthritis or chronic neurologic or skin abnormalities may develop (stage 3, persistent infection). Although there are regional variations, the basic stages of the illness are similar worldwide.

ETIOLOGY *Borrelia burgdorferi*, the causative agent of the disease, is a fastidious, microaerophilic bacterium that grows best at 33°C in a complex liquid medium called Barbour, Stoenner, Kelly (BSK) medium. Except in the case of erythema migrans skin lesions, culture of the spirochete from clinical specimens has been difficult. Three genomic subgroups of *B. burgdorferi* have recently been defined. To date, American isolates have been genomic subgroup 1, whereas European isolates have included all 3 subgroups. These differences probably account for the clinical variations in the disease in different geographic regions.

EPIDEMIOLOGY The distribution of Lyme disease correlates primarily with the geographic ranges of certain ixodid ticks–*Ixodes dammini*, *I. pacificus*, *I. ricinus*, and *I. persulcatus*. *I. dammini* is the principal vector in the northeastern United States (from Massachusetts to Maryland) and in the Midwest (Wisconsin and Minnesota). In surveys of *I. dammini* in these states, 20 percent or more of the ticks have been infected with *B. burgdorferi*, and most cases of Lyme disease in the United States have occurred in these areas. *I. pacificus* is the vector in the western United States. The disease may be acquired throughout Europe—from Great Britain to Scandinavia to Russia—where *I. ricinus* is the vector; in Asia, where *I. persulcatus* is the vector; and in Australia. The ticks have different animal hosts; for *I. dammini*, the white-footed mouse is the preferred host of the immature tick and the white-tailed deer of the mature tick.

Most new cases have onsets during the summer months. Cases have occurred in association with hiking, camping, and hunting trips or among people living in wooded or rural areas. Patients of any age and both sexes are affected. Cases have been reported in 47 states, and more than 1000 people now acquire the infection in the United States each summer.

PATHOGENESIS After injection into the skin, *B. burgdorferi* may migrate outward, producing EM, and may spread hematogenously to other organs. The spirochete has been cultured from blood, skin (EM), cerebrospinal fluid, and joint fluid and has been seen in most affected tissues. These findings and the response of all stages of the disease to antibiotic therapy suggest that the organism invades and persists in affected tissues throughout the illness.

Initially, the immune response seems to be suppressed. The mononuclear cells of patients respond minimally to *B. burgdorferi* antigens and less than normally to mitogens. After the first several weeks of infection, mononuclear cells generally have heightened responsiveness to *B. burgdorferi* antigens and to mitogens, and evidence of B cell hyperactivity—elevated total serum IgM levels, cryoprecipitates, and circulating immune complexes. The specific antibody response to the spirochete develops gradually over months to years and is directed at an increasing array of spirochetal polypeptides. Specific IgM antibody titers to *B. burgdorferi* peak between the third and sixth week after disease onset; specific IgG antibody titers rise slowly and are generally highest months or years later, when arthritis is present. By that time, antigen-reactive mononuclear cells and immune complexes are found in the joint fluid. Patients with chronic arthritis have an increased frequency of the class II major histocompatibility complex alleles HLA-DR4 and, secondarily, HLA-DR2. These alleles may determine a host immune response to *B. burgdorferi* that has autoreactive features.

CLINICAL MANIFESTATIONS Early infection: Stage 1 (localized infection) After an incubation period of 3 to 32 days, EM, which occurs at the site of the tick bite, usually begins as a red macule or papule that expands to form a large annular lesion, most often with a bright-red outer border and partial central clearing. Because of the small size of ixodid ticks, most patients do not remember the preceding tick bite. The center of the lesion sometimes becomes intensely erythematous and indurated, vesicular, or necrotic. In other instances, the expanding lesion remains an even, intense red; several red rings are found within the outside one; or the central area turns blue before it clears. Although the lesion can be located anywhere, the thigh, groin, and axilla are particularly common sites. The lesion is warm but not often painful. Skin biopsies show perivascular infiltrates or lymphocytes and histiocytes. Perhaps as many as 25 percent of patients lack this characteristic skin manifestation of the disorder.

Early infection: Stage 2 (disseminated infection) Within days after the onset of EM, the organism often spreads hematogenously to many different sites. Such patients frequently develop secondary annular skin lesions which are similar in appearance to the initial lesion. Skin involvement is often accompanied by severe headache, mild neck stiffness, fever, chills, migratory musculoskeletal pain, arthralgias, and profound malaise and fatigue. Less common manifestations include generalized lymphadenopathy or splenomegaly, hepatitis, sore throat, nonproductive cough, conjunctivitis, iritis, or testicular swelling. Except for fatigue and lethargy, which are often constant, the early signs and symptoms of Lyme disease are typically intermittent and changing. Even in untreated patients, the early symptoms usually improve or disappear within several weeks.

Symptoms suggestive of meningeal irritation may occur early in Lyme disease, when EM is present, but are usually not associated with a spinal fluid pleocytosis or objective neurologic deficit. After several weeks to months, about 15 percent of patients develop frank neurologic abnormalities, including meningitis, subtle encephalitic signs, cranial neuritis (including bilateral facial palsy), motor or sensory radiculoneuropathy, mononeuritis multiplex, chorea, or myelitis, alone or in various combinations. The usual pattern consists of fluctuating symptoms of meningitis accompanied by facial palsy and peripheral radiculoneuropathy. Cerebrospinal fluid shows a lymphocytic pleocytosis (about 100 cells per microliter), often with elevated protein, and normal or slightly low glucose. In Europe, the first neurologic sign is characteristically radicular pain, which is followed by the development of a cerebrospinal fluid pleocytosis (called Bannwarth's syndrome), but meningeal or encephalitic signs are frequently absent. These early neurologic abnormalities usually resolve completely within months, but chronic neurologic disease may occur later.

Within several weeks after the onset of illness, about 8 percent of patients develop cardiac involvement. The most common abnormality is fluctuating degrees of atrioventricular block (first-degree, Wenckebach, or complete heart block). Some patients have more diffuse cardiac involvement, including electrocardiographic changes of acute myopericarditis, left ventricular dysfunction on radionuclide scans, or, rarely, cardiomegaly or pancarditis. Cardiac involvement usually lasts only a few weeks but may recur. One case of chronic cardiomyopathy caused by *B. burgdorferi* has been reported.

During this stage, musculoskeletal pain is common. The typical pattern is migratory pain in joints, tendons, bursae, muscle, or bone, usually without joint swelling, lasting hours or days in one or two locations at a time.

Late infection: Stage 3 (persistent infection) Months after the onset of infection, about 60 percent of patients in the United States who have received no antibiotic treatment develop frank arthritis. The typical pattern is intermittent attacks of oligoarticular arthritis in large joints, especially knees, lasting weeks to months in a given joint. Small joints and periarticular sites also may be affected, primarily during early attacks. The number of patients who continue to have recurrent attacks decreases each year. However, in a small percentage of patients, involvement in large joints, usually one or both knees, becomes chronic and may lead to erosion of cartilage and bone. The involvement of joints seems to be a more frequent manifestation of the illness in the United States than in Europe.

Joint fluid white cell counts range from 500 to 110,000 cells per microliter (average, 25,000 cells per microliter), mostly polymorphonuclear leukocytes. Tests for rheumatoid factor or antinuclear antibodies are usually negative. Synovial biopsies show fibrin deposits, villous hypertrophy, vascular proliferation, microangiopathic lesions, and a heavy infiltration of lymphocytes and plasma cells.

Although less common, chronic neurologic or skin involvement (acrodermatitis chronica atrophicans) also may occur months to years after the onset of infection, sometimes following long periods of latent infection. This late skin manifestation of the disorder has been observed primarily in Europe. The most common form of chronic central nervous system involvement is a subtle encephalopathy affecting memory, mood, or sleep. These patients often have evidence of memory impairment on neuropsychological tests and abnormal CSF analyses. The encephalopathy is frequently accompanied by an axonal polyneuropathy manifested as either distal paresthesias or spinal or radicular pain. Electromyography generally shows extensive abnormalities of proximal and distal nerve segments. Leukoencephalitis, a rare manifestation of Lyme borreliosis, is a severe neurologic disorder that may include spastic parapareses, upper motor neuron bladder dysfunction, and lesions in the periventricular white matter. Acrodermatitis begins with red-violaceous lesions that become sclerotic or atrophic over a period of years. This chronic skin disorder has been observed primarily in elderly women.

DIAGNOSIS Lyme disease is diagnosed by recognition of a characteristic clinical picture with serologic confirmation. Although serologic testing may be negative during the first several weeks of infection, most patients have a positive antibody response to *B. burgdorferi*, determined by ELISA, after that time. Western blotting is often helpful in sorting out false-positive results in patients who have indeterminate responses by ELISA. However, patients with previous Lyme disease often remain seropositive, and a small percentage of patients have asymptomatic infection. If these patients develop another illness, the positive serologic test for Lyme disease may cause diagnostic confusion. In about 5 percent of patients who receive antibiotic therapy during the first several weeks of infection, the spirochete may still survive in protected niches and cause subtle joint or neurologic symptoms. In these patients, the humoral immune response may be aborted, but a cellular immune response to the spirochete can usually be demonstrated by proliferative assay.

TREATMENT The various manifestations of Lyme disease can usually be treated successfully with oral antibiotic therapy, except for objective neurologic abnormalities, which seem to require intravenous therapy. For early Lyme disease, doxycycline, 100 mg twice a day, or amoxicillin, 500 mg four times a day, is effective therapy, but doxycycline should not be given to children or pregnant women. Cefuroxime, 500 mg twice a day, seems to be an equally effective alternative in patients with penicillin allergy. Erythromycin, 250 mg four times a day, is less effective clinically but is another alternative in patients with allergies to the other medications. In children, amoxicillin is effective (50 mg/kg per day); in cases of penicillin allergy, erythromycin (30 mg/kg per day) can be given. For patients with infection localized to the skin, 10 days of therapy is generally sufficient. For patients with disseminated infection, a course of 20 to 30 days may be needed. Approximately 15 percent of patients experience a Jarisch-Herxheimer–like reaction during the first 24 h of therapy.

These oral antibiotic regimens, when given for 30 days, also may be effective for the treatment of Lyme arthritis. However, the response to therapy may be slow. A small percentage of patients with arthritis, particularly those with the HLA-DR4 allele and an immune response to the OspA or OspB proteins of the spirochete, do not respond to antimicrobial therapy. Synovectomy may be successful in these patients.

For objective neurologic abnormalities, with the possible exception of facial palsy alone, parenteral antibiotic therapy seems to be necessary. Intravenous ceftriaxone, 2 g/d for 2 to 4 weeks, is most commonly used for this purpose, but intravenous penicillin G, 20 million units/d in divided doses, also may be effective. In patients with high-degree atrioventricular block or a PR interval of greater than 0.3 s, intravenous ceftriaxone, 2 g/d, or intravenous penicillin, 10 to 20 million units/d for at least 10 days, and cardiac monitoring are recommended. In patients with complete heart block or congestive heart failure, glucocorticoids may be of benefit if the patient does not improve on antimicrobial therapy alone within 24 h.

In a small percentage of patients, infection with *B. burgdorferi* may trigger fibromyalgia, which is thought to be a variant of the chronic fatigue syndrome. It is important to distinguish this diffuse pain syndrome from active Lyme disease, since the pain syndrome does not respond to antibiotic therapy. The risk of infection with *B. burgdorferi* after a recognized tick bite is so low that prophylactic antimicrobial treatment is not routinely indicated. If the patient is quite anxious or if the tick is engorged, 10 days of amoxicillin or doxycycline therapy is likely to prevent the occurrence of Lyme disease.

PROGNOSIS The response to treatment is best early in the illness. Treatment of Lyme borreliosis later in the course of illness often results in months of convalescence. Eventually, complete recovery ensues in the majority of patients.

REFERENCES

BARANTON G et al: Delineation of *Borrelia burgdorferi* sensu stricto, *Borrellia garinii* sp. nov., and group VS461 associated with Lyme borreliosis. Int J Sys Bact 42:378, 1992

BARBOUR AG, HAYES SF: Biology of *Borrelia* species. Microbiol Rev 50:381, 1986

LOGIGIAN EL et al: Chronic neurologic manifestations of Lyme disease. N Engl J Med 323:1438, 1990

MASSAROTTI EM et al: The treatment of early Lyme disease. Am J Med 92:396, 1992

PACHNER AR, STEERE AC: The triad of neurologic manifestations of Lyme disease: Meningitis, cranial neuritis, and radiculoneuritis. Neurology 35:47, 1985

————: Lyme disease. N Engl J Med 321:586, 1989

———— et al: Lyme carditis: Cardiac abnormalities of Lyme disease. Ann Intern Med 93:8, 1980

———— et al: The early clinical manifestations of Lyme disease. Ann Intern Med 99:76, 1983

———— et al: The clinical evolution of Lyme arthritis. Ann Intern Med 107:725, 1987

section 10 *Rickettsia, Mycoplasma, and Chlamydia*

138 RICKETTSIAL DISEASES

THEODORE E. WOODWARD

The rickettsial diseases of humans consist of a variety of clinical entities caused by microorganisms of the family Rickettsiaceae. The rickettsias are obligate intracellular parasites about the size of bacteria and are usually seen microscopically as pleomorphic coccobacilli. Each of the rickettsias pathogenic for humans is capable of multiplying in one or more species of arthropod as well as in animals and humans. Indeed, the majority of the rickettsias are maintained in nature by a cycle which involves an insect vector and an animal reservoir, and infection of humans is unimportant in the cycle. Epidemic typhus presents a number of points of dissimilarity to most of the other rickettsioses. Until recently, the natural cycle of infection was thought to involve only humans and lice. The finding of a sylvatic reservoir in flying squirrels associated with a human illness which resembles classic typhus emphasizes that there are other mechanisms.

A compendium of information on the rickettsial diseases is given in Table 138-1.

Of all the afflictions of the human race, the rickettsial diseases, particularly epidemic typhus, rank among the foremost as a cause of suffering and death. The record of deaths from epidemic typhus in this century in the Balkan countries and in Poland and Russia reached astounding figures. Typhus ravaged Russia and eastern Poland from 1915 to 1922, infecting 30 million inhabitants and causing an estimated 3 million deaths. It is currently quite prevalent in Ethiopia.

The past two decades have seen the development of excellent methods for the prevention and treatment of rickettsioses. In fact, these measures have been so successful that the rickettsioses have become of minor importance in the United States and in many other countries. Although conquered, these infections have not been eliminated, and they could again become rampant if the will to control them, the present high standards of sanitation, and the necessary industrial capacities for production of effective insecticides and therapeutic agents should be compromised.

PATHOGENESIS Rickettsial diseases develop after infection through the skin or the respiratory tract. Agents of the typhus and spotted fever groups are introduced through the bite of the infected arthropod vector. Ticks and mites, which transmit the agents of spotted fever and scrub typhus, inoculate the rickettsias directly into the dermis during feeding. The louse and flea, which transmit epidemic and murine typhus, respectively, deposit infected feces on the skin; infection occurs when organisms are rubbed into the puncture wound made by the arthropod. The rickettsias of Q fever gain entry through the respiratory tract when infected dust is inhaled; the respiratory route is also occasionally implicated in epidemic typhus when infection results from inhalation of dried infected louse feces.

Although organisms probably multiply at the original site of entry in all instances, local lesions appear with regularity only in certain diseases, namely, the initial cutaneous lesions of scrub typhus, rickettsialpox, and boutonneuse fever and the pneumonitis which develops in about half the persons with Q fever.

Volunteers infected with either scrub typhus or Q fever develop rickettsemia late in the incubation period, often some hours before the onset of fever. Similar events probably occur in all the rickettsial diseases; circulating rickettsias can be detected during the early febrile period in practically all patients. Little is known about the pathogenesis of infection during the midportion of the incubation period. However, it is reasonable to assume that during this time, in patients with typhus or spotted fever, a transient low-grade rickettsemia results from release of organisms multiplying at the initial site of infection and that this seeds infection in the endothelial cells of the vascular tree. Vascular lesions developing at such sites account for the pathologic changes, including the rash.

Rickettsias apparently invade and proliferate in the endothelial cells of small blood vessels. Raoult separated endothelial cells from the blood of patients with Mediterranean spotted fever. By means of antiendothelial antibody, endothelial cells were bound to magnetized beads; the rickettsias were identified by the immunofluorescence technique. Endothelial cell destruction results from the proliferation of organisms and eventual disruption. Rickettsias may exert a cytotoxic effect on endothelial cells; in mice the rickettsial toxin causes a remarkable increase in capillary permeability, independent of

TABLE 138-1   Rickettsial diseases

Disease		Geographic distribution	Natural cycle		Principal means of transmission to humans	Serologic diagnosis	
Type	Agent		Arthropod	Mammal		Weil-Felix reaction	CF, MA, and IFA reactions*
SPOTTED FEVER GROUP							
Rocky Mountain spotted fever	R. rickettsii	Western hemisphere	Ticks	Wild rodents, dogs	Tick bite	Positive OX-19 OX-2	Positive Group- and type-specific
Boutonneuse fever	R. conorii	Africa, Europe, Middle East, India	Ticks	Rodents, dogs	Tick bite	Positive OX-19 OX-2	Positive Group- and type-specific
Queensland tick typhus	R. australis	Australia	Ticks	Marsupials, wild rodents	Tick bite	Positive OX-19 OX-2	Positive Group- and type-specific
North Asian tick-borne rickettsiosis	R. sibirica	Siberia, Mongolia	Ticks	Wild rodents	Tick bite	Positive OX-19 OX-2	Positive Group- and type-specific
Rickettsialpox	R. akari	United States, Russia, Africa	Blood-sucking mites	House mice, other rodents	Mite bite	Negative	Positive Group- and type-specific
TYPHUS GROUP							
Endemic (murine)	R. typhi	Worldwide	Fleas	Small rodents	Infected flea feces into broken skin	Positive OX-19	Positive Group- and type-specific
Epidemic	R. prowazekii	Worldwide	Body lice	Humans, flying squirrels	Infected louse feces into broken skin	Positive OX-19	
	R. canada	North America	Ticks			Positive OX-19	
Brill-Zinsser disease	R. prowazekii	Worldwide	Recurrence years after original attack of epidemic typhus			Usually negative	Positive
Scrub	R. tsutsugamushi	Asia, Australia, Pacific islands	Trombiculid mites	Wild rodents	Mite bite	Positive OX-K	Positive in about 50% of patients
OTHER RICKETTSIAL DISEASES							
Q fever	R. burnetii	Worldwide	Ticks	Small mammals, cattle, sheep, goats	Inhalation of dried infected material	Negative	Positive
Trench fever	R. quintana†	Europe, Africa, North America	Body lice	Humans	Infected louse feces into broken skin	Negative	None available

* CF = complement fixation; MA = microscopic agglutination; IFA = immunofluorescent antibody.
† Some authorities no longer place the agent in the genus *Rickettsia* because it can be cultured on artificial media.

proliferation. The anatomic location of multiple microscopic lesions and the numerous foci of rickettsial vascular changes with rickettsias present coincide well with the organs examined microscopically such as the kidney, lung, heart, and liver. These findings confirm Wolbach's original conclusion that "the lesions of the blood vessel are due to the presence of the parasite." Absence of inflammatory cell reactions in fulminant Rocky Mountain spotted fever tends to exclude several host-mediated immunopathogenetic mechanisms. The underlying cause of the toxic-febrile state which characterizes the rickettsial diseases remains unknown. Several rickettsial species contain type-specific toxins which are lethal for mice, and these may play a role in humans. Careful studies of *Rickettsia*-infected cells and macrophages maintained in tissue culture may help explain the mechanisms of the increased permeability which typifies Rocky Mountain spotted fever and severe typhus fever. Increased release of prostaglandins (PG_1 and PG_2) and leukotrienes (LTB_4) by damaged endothelial cells and macrophages has suggested a possible mechanism to explain capillary leakage. If confirmed, corrective strategies might be developed to diminish production of arachidonate metabolites.

PATHOLOGIC PHYSIOLOGY   Peripheral vascular collapse results in death in fulminating cases during the first week, with capillary dilatation and pooling of blood without increased capillary permeability or loss of fluid into extravascular spaces. Proliferative and thrombotic lesions develop in small vessels, resulting in necrosis and increased capillary permeability, with loss of water, electrolytes, proteins, and erythrocytes. These events in turn result in a decrease in blood volume, together with an increase in the extravascular space and clinical edema, particularly during the later stages of illness (stage III). Edema, anoxia of the myocardium, and histologic evidence of myocarditis are disclosed by electrocardiographic abnormalities, including serious arrhythmias. Liver function is impaired. The azotemia which develops in seriously ill patients late in illness appears to be prerenal. Clinical manifestations resulting from the peripheral vascular collapse are oliguria and anuria, azotemia, anemia, hypoproteinemia, hyponatremia, edema, and coma. In spotted fever and typhus patients with hemorrhagic skin lesions, consumptive coagulopathy is present. All these alterations are absent or minimal in patients with mild cases or in those who are given specific treatment early.

PATHOLOGY The basic changes in the spotted and typhus fever groups are vascular, with resultant widespread lesions in adjacent parenchymatous organs. They are most common in the skin, muscles, heart, lung, and brain. The most conspicuous and diverse are found in Rocky Mountain spotted fever, where swelling, proliferation, and degeneration of the endothelial cells occur, frequently with thrombus formation which partially or completely occludes the lumen. The muscle cells of the arterioles undergo swelling and fibrinoid changes. The adventitial tissues are infiltrated with mononuclear leukocytes, lymphocytes, and plasma cells. The vascular damage is scattered along arteries, veins, and capillaries, with normal architecture prevailing throughout most of the vascular bed. The changes in murine, epidemic, and scrub typhus fevers resemble those in Rocky Mountain spotted fever, but thrombosis is uncommon and involvement of the musculature is rare.

Interstitial myocarditis occurs in each of these diseases but is usually most extensive in Rocky Mountain spotted fever and scrub typhus. In the brain, glial nodules are found in all members of the group, but microinfarcts in the brain tissue or in the myocardium are most often observed in spotted fever. By immunofluorescence techniques, rickettsias can be identified in brain, lung, myocardium, and other tissues.

Rickettsial pneumonitis occurs, at least to some extent, in many patients with spotted or typhus fever and is characteristic in patients with Q fever. The process is patchy and consists microscopically of areas of congestion and edema. Within the consolidated areas the alveoli are filled with compact fibrinocellular exudate containing lymphocytes, plasma cells, large mononuclear cells, and erythrocytes but few, if any, polymorphonuclear leukocytes.

Rickettsias can occasionally be observed microscopically in sections of tissue such as brain, myocardium, and lung. Failure to demonstrate them is of no diagnostic significance. They are readily identifiable by the immunofluorescence technique, even after 50 years of fixation.

LABORATORY DIAGNOSIS Diagnostic procedures which depend on isolation of the etiologic agent from blood or other clinical material are expensive, time-consuming, and hazardous to laboratory personnel. Primary isolation of rickettsias by chick embryo inoculation or tissue culture usually fails because of the small number of organisms in the patient's blood. Rickettsias have been identified in stained cultured monocytes of infected monkeys and by direct or indirect immunofluorescence of infected animal tissues. Except in unusual circumstances, however, currently available serologic tests are adequate for laboratory confirmation of the clinical diagnosis in each of the rickettsial diseases. The demonstration of a rise in titer of specific

antibody during convalescence is of prime importance in establishing laboratory confirmation. Table 138-2 summarizes the serologic results usually encountered in persons who have rickettsial diseases in the United States. The Weil-Felix test employing *Proteus* strains OX-19 and OX-2 gives positive results in patients with spotted fever and murine typhus and negative results in those with rickettsialpox and Q fever. It is useful as a screening procedure but cannot be relied on to differentiate spotted fever from murine typhus. In patients with Brill-Zinsser disease, the *Proteus* OX-19 reaction is usually negative or low in titer.

Serologic tests employing group-specific rickettsial antigens provide data which clearly differentiate the most common infections, i.e., epidemic typhus, murine typhus, Rocky Mountain spotted fever, and Q fever. Type-specific rickettsial antigens generally make it possible to distinguish rickettsialpox from spotted fever and Brill-Zinsser disease from murine typhus.

The type of immunoglobulin in acute (IgM) and late or recurrent (IgG) illness is helpful in identifying recrudescent typhus (Brill-Zinsser disease). In general, the Weil-Felix and complement fixation tests are useful for routine diagnosis; microscopic agglutination, immunofluorescent antibody, and hemagglutination reactions are valuable for specific identification.

Specific antibiotic therapy has little effect on the time of appearance of antibodies or on their ultimate titer, provided treatment is instituted some days after onset of the illness. However, if the illness is cut short by early and vigorous treatment, antibody production may be delayed for a week or so, and the maximum titers attained may be below those illustrated in Table 138-2. Under these circumstances, a sample of blood taken 4 to 6 weeks after onset of illness also should be tested.

The immunofluorescent antibody test is very useful for detecting *Rickettsia* in the tissues of patients with the typhus group of rickettsioses, the spotted fevers, and Q fever. Identifiable rickettsias have been visualized in skin lesions of patients with Rocky Mountain spotted fever as early as the fourth day of illness and as late as the tenth day. Rickettsias may be visualized in human tissues several days after administration of chloramphenicol or tetracycline. The technique also visualizes rickettsias in ticks and in animal tissues, including those fixed with paraffin.

Normochromic anemia occurs in patients severely ill with rickettsial diseases. The white blood cell count in Rocky Mountain spotted fever, rickettsialpox, murine and epidemic typhus, Brill-Zinsser disease, Q fever, and other rickettsial diseases is usually within the normal range: 6000 to 10,000 cells per microliter. Leukopenia is occasionally observed, and in the presence of complications, such as

---

TABLE 138-2 Serologic diagnosis of rickettsial diseases in the United States

Group	Disease	Weil-Felix reaction				Complement fixation tests with type-specific antigen				
		Proteus	Illustrative titer		Cases with diagnostic titer	Rickettsial antigen	Illustrative titer			Cases with diagnostic titer
			10th day	20th day			10th day	20th day	30th day	
Spotted fever	Rocky Mountain spotted fever	OX-19	40	320	Most	*R. rickettsii*	20	160	80	Most
		OX-2	20	160						
	Rickettsialpox	OX-19	0	0	None	*R. akari*	0	64	128	Most
		OX-2	0	0						
Typhus	Murine typhus	OX-19	160	640	Most	*R. typhi*	0	160	160	Most
		OX-2	10	40						
	Epidemic typhus, squirrel related	OX-19	160	640	Most	*R. prowazekii*	0	160	160	Most
		OX-2	10	40						
	Brill-Zinsser disease	OX-19	160	20	Few	*R. prowazekii*	1280	640	320	Most
		OX-2	0	0						
	Q fever	OX-19	0	0	None	*R. burnetii*	10	80	160	Most
		OX-2	0	0						

superimposed infections and extensive vascular lesions, moderate leukocytosis occurs. The differential blood cell count is usually normal. Thrombocytopenia occurs in severely ill patients with spotted and scrub typhus fever and extensive vascular lesions; hypofibrinogenemia, prolonged prothrombin and partial thromboplastin times, and other clotting abnormalities occur.

TREATMENT   Patients seriously ill with one of the diseases of the typhus–spotted fever group may show circulatory collapse, coma, oliguria and anuria, azotemia, anemia, hypoproteinemia, hypochloremia and hyponatremia, and edema. These alterations are often absent in the mildly ill, and in them management is much less complicated. The therapeutic principles necessary for treatment of all rickettsioses are (1) specific chemotherapy and (2) supportive care. Attention to both is mandatory for the seriously ill patient first recognized late in the disease. During the first week in the moderately ill patient, supportive therapy may need to be less energetic, because specific chemotherapy usually suffices. The early mild case may be successfully treated at home; more severely ill patients should receive hospital care because manifestations can progress rapidly in fulminant cases.

Specific therapy   Specific therapy is most effective when initiated during the early stages of disease coincident with the appearance of the rash. When therapy is delayed until the rash has become hemorrhagic and widespread, the response is less dramatic. The antibiotics of choice are chloramphenicol and the tetracyclines, which are effective because of their rickettsiostatic properties. They are not rickettsiocidal. Ciprofloxacin therapy is effective in patients with Mediterranean spotted fever. Its value for other rickettsial diseases is unknown.

The following antibiotic regimen is considered optimal: for chloramphenicol, an initial dose of 50 mg/kg of body weight, and for tetracycline, 25 mg/kg. Subsequent daily doses are the same as the initial loading dose, with the requirement divided equally and given at 6- to 8-h intervals. Antibiotic treatment is continued until the patient has improved and has been afebrile approximately 24 h. The decision to stop specific therapy is based on careful assessment of the patient's status coupled with good clinical judgment. In patients too ill to take oral medication, an intravenous preparation of one of the antimicrobials should be employed.

Adrenal cortical hormones may be needed for their antitoxemic effects in patients first observed late in the course of severe illness. Large doses for brief periods of about 3 days, in combination with specific antibiotics, are recommended in critically ill patients.

In uncomplicated cases of spotted fever, there is symptomatic improvement within 24 h, and the temperature becomes normal in 60 to 72 h.

Supportive care   Frequent turning of the patient relieves pressure from prominent bony parts and also militates against the development of aspiration pneumonia. Proper mouth care, with frequent swabbing of the oral cavity, may avert the development of parotitis and gingivitis. Sucking of the juice of a lemon or the oral use of glycerin or mineral oil is helpful. Usually food is well tolerated by patients with rickettsial disease, and the daily diet should provide 1 to 2 g protein per kilogram of normal body weight; the diet may need to be supplemented with oral or parenteral hyperalimentation (see Chap. 76).

When indicated, red cell transfusions given slowly are helpful. The support of the hypotensive patient with rickettsial disease is similar to that of other patients with shock (see Chap. 83). Dialysis is indicated when there is clear-cut evidence of acute renal failure.

ROCKY MOUNTAIN SPOTTED FEVER   Definition   Rocky Mountain spotted fever is an acute febrile illness caused by *Rickettsia rickettsii*. It is transmitted to humans by ticks. The disease is characterized by sudden onset with headache and chills and by fever which persists for 2 to 3 weeks. A characteristic exanthem appears on the extremities and trunk about the fourth day of illness. Delirium, shock, and renal failure occur in severely ill patients.

Etiology and epidemiology   The causative microbe, *R. rickettsii*, is the prototype for the rickettsial group of agents. The minute organisms are purple when stained by Giemsa's method or red by Macchiavello's technique; most of them are gram-negative. These organisms often occur in pairs and possess a cell wall similar in structure and chemical composition to that of gram-negative bacteria; there are a cell membrane, cytoplasmic granules corresponding to ribosomes, and prokaryotic organization of nuclear material. The cell membrane is selectively permeable; the cell wall is the focus of important antigens and an endotoxin-like substance.

The rickettsias grow in the nucleus and the cytoplasm of infected cells of ticks, mammals, and embryonated eggs; the intranuclear situation of the organisms is shared by the other members of the spotted fever group but not by rickettsias of the typhus group. *Rickettsia rickettsii* is readily distinguishable from the agents of the typhus fevers by cross-immunity tests in guinea pigs and by complement fixation tests employing antigens prepared from infected yolk sac tissues. The differentiation of *R. rickettsii* from closely related members of the spotted fever group frequently requires elaborate procedures. Strains of the agent of Rocky Mountain spotted fever vary considerably in their virulence for humans and animals.

The first reports of spotted fever in Idaho and Montana during the final decade of the last century led to the name *Rocky Mountain spotted fever*. However, the disease has been reported from all states (except Maine, Alaska, and Hawaii), as well as from Canada, Mexico, Colombia, and Brazil. Although related diseases are found on other continents, this particular infection is limited to the Western Hemisphere. From 1981 to 1986, an average of 933 cases per year were reported in the United States, while more recently (1987–1990), the yearly average has decreased to 621 cases. Why this decrease has occurred is not known. The mortality rate was about 20 percent in the days before specific therapy but has decreased to about 7 percent. More than half the cases occur in the South Atlantic and South Central states, with the greatest number in North Carolina, Virginia, Georgia, Maryland, Tennessee, and Oklahoma.

An unusual outbreak of "urban" spotted fever occurred in New York City's Bronx borough during the summer of 1987. Eight percent of dog ticks were positive for *R. rickettsii*.

A number of species of ticks are found infected with *R. rickettsii* in nature, but only two are important in transmitting spotted fever to humans. These are *Dermacentor andersoni*, the wood tick, which is the principal vector in the West, and *D. variabilis*, the dog tick, which assumes this role in the East. *Amblyomma americanum*, the lone star tick, and *D. variabilis* are the common vectors in the west South Central states. Infected female ticks transmit the agent transovarially to at least some of their offspring. Ticks which become infected, either through the egg or at one of the stages during their development cycle by feeding on an infected mammal, harbor the rickettsias throughout their lifetime, which may be several years; thus the tick is a reservoir as well as a vector. Small wild mammals are suspected of playing an important role in spreading the rickettsias in nature by infecting ticks which feed on them during rickettsemia.

Disease in humans is generally acquired from the bite of an infected tick. Transmission is unlikely unless the tick remains attached for a number of hours. Infection also may be acquired through abrasions in the skin which become contaminated with infected tick feces or tissue juices, hence the hazard associated with crushing ticks between the fingers when removing them from persons or animals. The agent of Rocky Mountain spotted fever has been transmitted accidentally to humans by transfusion of blood taken from a donor just before onset of illness.

There are seasonal variations in the incidence of cases of spotted fever, as well as differences in age and sex distribution of cases. In each instance these differences are related to exposure to ticks. Most cases are seen during the period of maximal tick activity, i.e., April to September, and 60 percent of cases occur in individuals under 20 years of age. This age distribution is undoubtedly influenced by propinquity to the wood and dog ticks. The mortality rate increases with the age of the patient.

Rocky Mountain spotted fever has been acquired by laboratory workers via aerosol transmission, and special precautions are necessary when the agent is handled in the laboratory.

Clinical manifestations INCUBATION PERIOD AND PRODROMATA A history of tick bite is elicited in approximately 80 percent of patients. The incubation period varies between 3 and 12 days, with a mean of 7 days. A short incubation period usually indicates a more serious infection.

ONSET In nonvaccinated persons, the onset is usually abrupt, with severe headache, a sudden shaking rigor, prostration, generalized myalgia (especially in the back and leg muscles), nausea with occasional vomiting, and fever which reaches 39.4 to 40°C (103 to 104°F) within the first 2 days. Pain in the abdominal muscles may be severe, and arthralgia is not uncommon. Deep muscle palpation often elicits tenderness. Occasionally, the debut of illness in children and adults is mild, accompanied by lethargy, anorexia, headache, and low-grade fever. These symptoms are similar to those of many acute infectious diseases, and specific diagnosis is therefore difficult during the first few days. The course of illness is occasionally rapid, with death 6 or 7 days after onset.

PYREXIA Fever continues for approximately 15 to 20 days in untreated cases. The febrile course in children may be shorter. Hyperthermia of 40.5°C (105°F) or greater is of unfavorable prognostic significance, although fatalities may occur when the patient is hypothermic, with concurrent vasomotor collapse. Fever generally terminates by lysis over a period of several days but rarely does so by crisis. Recurrent fever is uncommon except in the presence of secondary pyrogenic complications.

The *headache* is generalized and excruciating and frequently most intense over the frontal area. It persists throughout the first and second weeks of illness in untreated cases. Occasionally, headache is mild. Malaise continues for the first week; irritability is notable, and the patient shuns distractions such as questioning and examination.

CUTANEOUS MANIFESTATIONS The rash which is present in practically all cases is the most characteristic and helpful diagnostic sign. It usually appears on the fourth febrile day; the range is 2 to 6 days. Faint-pink macules which fade on pressure have been noted on the first febrile day. The initial lesions are on the wrists, ankles, palms, soles, and forearms. The first lesions are macular, nonfixed, pink, irregularly defined, and measure 2 to 6 mm. A warm compress applied to the extremity accentuates the rash in the early stages. The exanthem is most prominent when the temperature is elevated. After 6 to 12 h, the rash extends centripetally to the axilla, buttocks, trunk, neck, and face. (This is in contrast to the eruption of typhus fever, which begins on the trunk and spreads centrifugally, rarely involving the face, palms, or soles.) The rash becomes maculopapular after 2 to 3 days (it may be felt by light palpation) and assumes a deeper red hue. By about the fourth day it is petechial and fails to fade on pressure. Not uncommonly, the hemorrhagic lesions coalesce to form large ecchymotic blemishes; these lesions tend to form over bony prominences and may ultimately slough to form indolent, slow-healing ulcers. Patients who have had the typical rash show brownish discolorations at the site for several weeks during convalescence. In milder cases, the rash does not become purpuric and may disappear within a few days. Antibiotic therapy may abort the early exanthem; the later fixed lesion fades less rapidly with specific therapy. Occasionally, a rash does not occur or is unnoticed, particularly in dark-skinned patients.

The application of tourniquets for several minutes or the occasional taking of the blood pressure may provoke additional petechiae (Rumpel-Leede phenomenon), further evidence of capillary abnormalities.

CARDIOVASCULAR AND RESPIRATORY FEATURES During the early stages, the pulse is full and regular and is accelerated in proportion to the height of the temperature, and the blood pressure is well sustained. During the peak of illness in seriously ill patients, the pulse is rapid and feeble, and hypotension of 90 mmHg or less is common. If circulatory failure is sustained, the resultant hypoxia and shock lead to agitation and delirium and contribute to the formation of ecchymoses and gangrene of fingers, toes, genitalia, buttocks, earlobes, and nose. Cyanosis of the peripheral parts of the body is common. A reduction of the total blood volume is found occasionally, late in the course of illness. The ECG shows low voltage, minor ST-segment deflections, and, occasionally, delay in atrioventricular conduction. These changes are transient and nonspecific. Severely ill patients have a puffy appearance of the face, hands, ankles, feet, and lower parts of the sacrum. Occasionally, a severe arrhythmia associated with myocarditis results in sudden death.

Respirations are either normal or slightly accelerated. Cough may be harassing and nonproductive, and localized pneumonitis may occur, but pulmonary consolidation is extremely rare. Pulmonary edema may develop after injudicious use of intravenous fluids.

HEPATIC AND RENAL MANIFESTATIONS In the majority of patients there is little alteration in renal or hepatic function. The liver may be enlarged, but jaundice is unusual. Oliguria and anuria commonly occur in seriously ill patients. Azotemia is common; when marked, it is a very unfavorable sign. Abnormalities in liver function include hypoproteinemia, with reduction in the albumin fraction.

NEUROLOGIC MANIFESTATIONS The principal neurologic manifestations are headache, restlessness, and varying degrees of insomnia. Stiffness of the back is common. The cerebrospinal fluid (CSF) is clear, with normal dynamics and normal chemical constituents. Occasionally, the CSF pressure is elevated; there may be a slight increase in mononuclear cells. Coma and muscular rigidity may occur. Athetoid movements, convulsive seizures, and hemiplegia are grave manifestations. Deafness during the active stages of the disease is not uncommon. As a rule, all neurologic signs abate without residua. Findings based on follow-up examinations and electroencephalograms may be interpreted as indicative of minor residual brain damage for a year or more following recovery of some patients from Rocky Mountain spotted fever.

OTHER PHYSICAL MANIFESTATIONS Patients become dehydrated, with extreme dryness of the lips, gums, tongue, and pharynx. The skin is hot and dry; the conjunctivae are frequently injected and the eyes suffused. Photophobia is common in the early stages of illness. Petechial hemorrhages may be noted in the conjunctivae or in the retina. The spleen is enlarged in approximately one-half the cases and is firm and nontender. Usually there is abdominal distention and some degree of intestinal ileus. Occasionally, the severity of abdominal discomfort associated with muscle spasm may suggest the diagnosis of acute appendicitis, cholecystitis, and localized peritonitis. An elevated leukocyte count suggests an inflammatory reaction. Vasculitis involving small vessels is probably responsible for the conflicting symptoms.

Course In patients with mild and moderately severe cases who are given no specific antibiotic therapy, the disease abates within 2 weeks, and convalescence is rapid. In fatal cases, death usually occurs during the latter part of the second week as a result of toxemia, vasomotor collapse and shock, or renal failure. In a few patients, the course is fulminant, with death occurring as early as the sixth day of illness.

In vaccinated individuals who contract the disease, the illness is mild, with a short febrile course and an atypical rash.

Prognosis If the serious manifestations of spotted fever are regarded as intrinsic parts of the disease, then complications are uncommon and consist mainly of secondary bacterial infections such as bronchopneumonia, otitis media, and parotitis. Thrombosis of major blood vessels may result in gangrene of a portion of an extremity. Hemiplegia and peripheral neuritis are rare sequelae.

The overall mortality rate for spotted fever was formerly about 20 percent. Death occurred in more than half of persons over 40 years of age, but the mortality rate was much lower in children and young adults. Since the introduction of the broad-spectrum antibiotics and the development of more precise knowledge regarding correction of the physiologic abnormalities which develop during the disease, fewer deaths occur. Some of the fatalities can be attributed to failure to consider spotted fever in the differential diagnosis and resultant delay in instituting appropriate treatment.

Differential diagnosis During the early stages of infection, before the rash has appeared, differentiation from other acute infections is difficult. A history of tick bite while living or traveling in wooded or bushy sites known to be in a highly endemic area is helpful. The rash of meningococcemia (see Chap. 109) resembles Rocky Mountain spotted fever in certain aspects, because it is macular, maculopapular, or petechial in the chronic form and petechial, confluent, or ecchymotic in the fulminant type. The meningococcal skin lesion is tender and develops with extreme rapidity in the fulminant form, whereas the rickettsial rash occurs on about the fourth day of disease and gradually becomes petechial. *Spotted fever is often confused with measles.* The exanthem of rubeola rapidly becomes confluent, while that of rubella *usually remains discrete.* In boutonneuse fever, Mediterranean spotted fever, and related diseases, there is often an eschar along with enlarged glands at the site of the tick attachment; the rash is typically red, is distinctly maculopapular, and may become hemorrhagic.

Murine typhus is a milder disease than Rocky Mountain spotted fever; the rash is less extensive, nonpurpuric, and nonconfluent, and renal and vascular complications are uncommon. Not infrequently, differentiation of these two rickettsial infections must await the results of specific serologic tests. Epidemic typhus fever is capable of causing all the pronounced clinical, physiologic, and anatomic alterations seen in patients with Rocky Mountain spotted fever, i.e., hypotension, peripheral vascular collapse, cyanosis, skin necrosis and gangrene of digits, renal failure and azotemia, and neurologic manifestations. However, the rash of classic typhus is noted initially in the axillary folds of the trunk and later extends peripherally, rarely involving the palms, soles, or face. The serologic patterns in these two diseases are distinctive when specific rickettsial antigens are employed. Moreover, louse-borne typhus is now recognized in the United States as a flying squirrel–related illness which occurs sporadically and as Brill-Zinsser disease (recrudescent typhus fever). Rickettsialpox, although caused by a member of the spotted fever group, is usually readily differentiated from Rocky Mountain spotted fever by the initial lesion, the relative mildness of the illness, and the early vesiculation of the maculopapular rash. The Weil-Felix reaction is positive in Rocky Mountain spotted fever and in murine and epidemic typhus but is negative in rickettsialpox. Agglutinins against *Proteus* OX-19 and OX-2 appear in the sera of patients with spotted fever, but only those against OX-19 are generally found in murine and epidemic typhus. In Lyme disease, the typical skin lesion, erythema chronicum migrans, consists of concentric annular rings with clear centers.

Complications *Pyogenic complications*, including otitis media and parotitis, are encountered in patients severely ill with Rocky Mountain spotted fever and other rickettsioses. These localized infections respond to therapy with appropriate antibiotics combined with surgical measures.

Pneumonitis may develop as a result of specific rickettsial action or as a bacterial superinfection. The sputum is scanty and should be examined to determine whether superimposed bacterial infection is present. Specific therapy is guided by the results of these laboratory studies. The pneumonitis generally responds to the antibiotic therapy the patient is receiving, but if staphylococcal pneumonia is suspected, a penicillinase-resistant penicillin or a cephalosporin should be added to the tetracycline or chloramphenicol.

Circulatory failure of peripheral or central origin is treated with careful administration of plasma expanders and fluids (see Chaps. 34 and 83). When the clinical signs reveal unmistakable evidence of cardiac failure, digitalis, diuretics, and other cardiac drugs should be employed as indicated (see Chap. 195).

Prevention Prevention is attained primarily by avoidance of tick-infested areas. When this is impractical, prophylactic measures include (1) spraying the ground with dieldrin or chlordane for area control of ticks (although there are environmental objections to the use of residual insecticides in area control of ticks, under special conditions such procedures may be warranted), (2) application of repellents such as diethyltoluamide or dimethylphthalate to clothing and exposed parts of the body or in very heavily infested areas the wearing of clothing which interferes with the attachment of ticks, i.e., boots and a one-piece outer garment, preferably impregnated with repellent, and (3) daily inspection of the entire body, including the hairy parts, to detect and remove attached ticks. In removing attached ticks, great care should be taken to avoid crushing the arthropod with resultant contamination of the bite wound. Gentle traction with tweezers applied close to the mouthparts may be necessary; the skin area should be disinfected with soap and water or other antiseptics. Similarly, precautions should be employed in removing engorged ticks from dogs and other animals, because infection through minor abrasions on the hands is possible. Improved vaccines containing inactivated *R. rickettsii* are under development and when available commercially should be used for those at great risk, namely, persons frequenting highly endemic areas and laboratory workers exposed to the agent. Because the broad-spectrum antibiotics are such excellent therapeutic agents in spotted fever, there has been less impetus for vaccination of persons who run only a minor risk of infection.

After a tick bite in a known endemic area, an exposed person should be observed for signs of fever, headache, prostration, and rash; therapy is very effective early in the infection.

MURINE (ENDEMIC) TYPHUS FEVER **Definition** Murine typhus fever is an acute febrile disease caused by *Rickettsia typhi (mooseri)* and transmitted to humans by fleas. The clinical illness is characterized by fever of 9 to 14 days, headache, a maculopapular rash appearing on the third to fifth day, and myalgia.

Etiology and epidemiology *R. typhi* resembles other rickettsias in morphologic properties, staining characteristics, and intracellular parasitism. Under the electron microscope, *R. typhi* is seen to contain dense masses of nuclear material in a less dense homogeneous protoplasmic substance, the whole of which is surrounded by a limiting membrane. It differs from *R. rickettsii* in that it always multiplies within the cytoplasm of cells, in contrast to the intranuclear and cytoplasmic positions of spotted fever rickettsias.

Invasion of the body by *R. typhi* provokes specific and nonspecific immunologic responses. With highly purified antigens, specific antibodies may be demonstrated readily by complement fixation, microscopic agglutination, and immunofluorescent antibody reactions. The positive Weil-Felix reaction that occurs in this disease is nonspecific because it is attributable to the presence of common carbohydrate antigens.

The common vector of *R. typhi* for rats and humans is the rat flea (*Xenopsylla cheopis*). In nature, the rat louse (*Polypax spinulosis*) may transmit the agent among rodents. Customarily, rat fleas become infected on ingestion of blood from diseased rats; the rickettsias multiply within the intestinal cells of the arthropod and are excreted in the feces. Infection in humans occurs after the flea bite and contamination of the broken skin by *Rickettsia*-laden feces. Dried flea feces also may infect via the conjunctivae or the upper part of the respiratory tract.

Rats and mice are naturally infected with murine typhus, and although the rodent disease is nonfatal, viable rickettsias persist in the brain for variable periods.

Murine typhus is one of the most benign and widespread of the rickettsioses in the United States. Prevalent in the southeastern and Gulf Coast states, it has been identified in most of the other states and in harbor centers throughout the world wherever rats and fleas abound. In the early 1940s, 2000 to 5000 cases of murine typhus were reported annually. This contrasts with between 50 and 69 cases reported in the United States yearly between 1986 and 1990. This sharp reduction was achieved by control of rats and their fleas in known areas of high prevalence. In urban areas the disease is more prevalent during the summer and fall and occurs predominantly among persons working in proximity to granaries or food depots. There has been an extension to certain rural areas when changing agricultural practices have provided rats with ready access to adequate food supplies. Endemic typhus has been reported in laboratory workers. This emphasizes the importance of taking special precautions when working with rickettsial organisms in the laboratory.

Clinical manifestations INCUBATION PERIOD AND PRODROMATA The incubation period ranges from 8 to 16 days, with a mean of 10 days. Common prodromata are headache, backache, arthralgia, and chilly sensations. Nausea, malaise, and transient temperature rises may precede the true onset of disease.

ONSET AND GENERAL SYMPTOMS A frank shaking chill and repeated rigors are present at the onset, associated with a severe frontal headache and fever. This triad of headache, chill, and pyrexia is usually followed within a few hours by nausea and vomiting. Prostration, malaise, and weakness are sufficient to enforce cessation of activity in adults, in contrast to children, whose illness is less severe. Occasionally, mild symptoms make it difficult to define the actual onset.

PYREXIA The usual febrile course in murine typhus lasts for about 12 days in adults; the temperature ranges from 38.8 to 40°C (102 to 104°F) but may reach 40.5 to 41.1°C (105 to 106°F) in children. The temperature may reach high levels abruptly after onset or ascend in a stepwise manner during the first few days. With the appearance of the rash, fever is usually sustained, with partial daily remissions which occasionally reach normal levels in the morning. Defervescence is generally by lysis over several days but sometimes occurs by crisis. Transient mild fever of 37.7°C (100°F) is not uncommon during early convalescence. A few patients experience only low-grade fever throughout, but this does not necessarily connote a mild illness.

CUTANEOUS MANIFESTATIONS The early lesions, which are sparse and discrete, are hidden in the axillae and inner surface of the arm. Most patients then develop with surprising suddenness a generalized, dull-red macular rash of the upper part of the abdomen, shoulders, chest, arms, and thighs. The individual lesions are discrete and pea-sized, with an ill-defined border, and fade on pressure during the first 24 h. They later become maculopapular, in contrast to the exanthem of epidemic typhus, which is persistently macular. The distribution over the trunk with sparse involvement of the extremities, palms, soles, and face differs from the peripheral distribution and facial involvement of Rocky Mountain spotted fever. The murine rash generally appears initially on the fifth febrile day, but rarely it is seen concurrently with the onset of fever or develops as late as the seventh day.

Eighty percent of patients develop a rash which persists for 4 to 8 days and fades before defervescence. The cutaneous manifestations vary greatly in intensity and duration and may be fleeting. They are readily overlooked in dark-skinned patients, in whom they should be sought by light palpation and indirect lighting.

CARDIOVASCULAR AND RESPIRATORY FEATURES An irritating, nonproductive cough is frequent and is occasionally associated with moderate hemoptysis. Early in the second week, rales may be detected in the basilar lung areas. These changes are generally a result of the primary rickettsial infection rather than bacterial superinfection. Pulmonary congestion occurs in extremely ill and elderly patients.

Accelerated pulse and hypotension occur, although less frequently than in patients with epidemic typhus or Rocky Mountain spotted fever. Rickettsial endocarditis is thought, by some, to be a rare complication of murine typhus.

NEUROLOGIC MANIFESTATIONS Headache is the most common neurologic manifestation of murine typhus and may dominate the clinical picture. It is frontal and continues into the second week of illness. Stupor and prostration may occur in the second week, and in severe cases there may be delirium, extreme agitation, or coma.

Coma in elderly patients after 2 weeks of illness presages death. Nuchal rigidity and general spasticity often suggest meningitis, although the CSF is normal except for slight increases in pressure and the presence of lymphocytes (5 to 30 per microliter). Transient partial deafness occurs occasionally, but rarely is there localized neuritis or hemiplegia. Neurologic sequelae are unusual. Children experience minimal neurologic changes.

OTHER PHYSICAL MANIFESTATIONS During the first 2 days of illness the patient may be nauseated and vomit, but vomiting later in the illness should arouse suspicion of a complication. Abdominal pain is bothersome; when associated with diarrhea or ileus, it responds to intravenous alimentation. Hepatomegaly and jaundice are unusual. There is splenomegaly in approximately 25 percent of patients.

Photophobia, retroocular pain, and suffusion of the conjunctivae are common but are less severe than in the other typhus and spotted fevers.

Renal function is usually unaltered except in elderly patients with prolonged hypotension. Under these circumstances, azotemia may develop to the degree observed in epidemic typhus. In severe murine typhus, as in the epidemic typhus, hyponatremia and hypoalbuminemia are encountered.

Course After defervescence, murine typhus patients recover rapidly. Fatalities occur between the ninth and twelfth days in elderly or debilitated patients, usually as a result of circulatory and renal failure or intercurrent bacterial infection.

Prognosis The mortality rate in murine typhus was low even before the introduction of specific therapy (<1 percent).

Differential diagnosis Because murine typhus and Rocky Mountain spotted fever occur in many of the same states, the problem of differential diagnosis often arises. Flea-borne murine typhus, which is predominantly an urban disease, is more likely to occur in late summer and autumn. In contrast, spotted fever is a rural and suburban disease in which exposure to ticks is important. Most cases occur in the spring and summer.

Treatment and prevention Both chloramphenicol and the tetracycline antibiotics have controlled the disease (see above). Prevention of murine typhus in humans is attained by reducing the natural reservoir and vector by applying measures for eliminating rodents and employing appropriate insecticides in rat-infested areas to control fleas. Spraying of rat burrows with DDT effectively reduces the population of the vector.

EPIDEMIC (LOUSE-BORNE) TYPHUS FEVER **Definition** Classic epidemic typhus is a severe, febrile disease caused by R. prowazekii and transmitted to humans by the body louse. Intense headache, continuous pyrexia of about 2 weeks, a macular skin eruption appearing on about the fifth febrile day, malaise, and vascular and neurologic disturbances represent the principal clinical features. Confirmation of the diagnosis is made by demonstration of Proteus OX-19 agglutinins and of specific complement-fixing antibodies in convalescence. The broad-spectrum antibiotics are specific therapeutic agents.

Etiology and epidemiology The causative microbe, R. prowazekii, is closely related to R. typhi, which causes murine typhus; indeed, the two have a number of common antigens.

Human beings generally are infected when Rickettsia-laden louse feces are rubbed into the broken skin; scratching the louse bite facilitates this process. Pediculus humanus corporis, which is peculiarly adapted to humans, is the only important vector of epidemic typhus. It dies of its infection and fails to transmit rickettsias to its offspring. R. prowazekii has been isolated from flying squirrels, and the organism probably infests their ectoparasites. Generally, however, the organism is maintained by a cycle involving human-louse-human. New epidemics apparently originate from patients with Brill-Zinsser disease (recurrent epidemic typhus). Flying squirrels can serve as a potential host to initiate an outbreak of epidemic typhus, provided an avid human vector, such as the body louse, is prevalent. Pathogenic rickettsias reside for long periods in patients with epidemic typhus as well as Rocky Mountain spotted fever and scrub typhus. Lice readily become infected when they feed on patients with recurrent typhus. Inhalation of dust containing dried louse feces may cause infection. An established nonhuman reservoir such as flying squirrels poses a serious threat.

If uncontrolled, epidemic typhus behaves as a cyclic disease in a susceptible population, extending over a 3-year period. During the first year there is a gradual seeding of cases throughout the group, during the second there is epidemic spread, and during the third the epidemic tapers off, because the majority of persons have become immune. Outbreaks of epidemic typhus last occurred in the United States in the nineteenth century, and its presence is now recognized in the form of Brill-Zinsser disease and flying squirrel–related typhus. Cases of epidemic typhus now occur in significant numbers in Ethiopia and probably in highland areas of other impoverished countries.

Clinical manifestations   Epidemic typhus resembles murine typhus but is more severe. After an incubation period of about 7 days, an abrupt onset of headache, chill, and rapidly mounting fever ushers in the illness. Headache, malaise, and prostration continue unabated until the rash appears on the fifth febrile day. It is initially macular in the axillary folds but ultimately invades the trunk and extremities as a pink, irregular macular lesion which becomes fixed, petechial, and confluent in the later stages.

Neurologic features range from headache and general spasticity to extreme agitation, stupor, and coma. Circulatory disturbances consisting of tachycardia, hypotension, and cyanosis are more profound than those observed in murine typhus and are almost as severe as in Rocky Mountain spotted fever. Ultimately, in untreated cases, azotemia often reaches high levels as a result of vascular and renal failure, and death occurs late in the second week of illness. Thrombosis of major blood vessels and cutaneous gangrene develop in a manner similar to that seen in the virulent form of Rocky Mountain spotted fever.

The complications and sequelae of epidemic typhus are more severe than those in murine typhus but not as severe as those in Rocky Mountain spotted fever. However, during certain outbreaks, epidemic typhus was fatal in 60 percent of those infected, and convalescence in survivors was prolonged. The use of chloramphenicol or tetracycline has almost eradicated mortality in this dread disease, provided therapy is instituted before irreversible organ system changes occur.

Differential diagnosis   Differentiation of epidemic typhus from the various rickettsioses and other diseases with which it may be confused was described earlier. The disease is not known to occur in epidemic form in the absence of louse infestation in the general population. Under the conditions in which typhus epidemics are likely to occur, other diseases which may cause confusion include malaria, relapsing fever, pneumonia, and tuberculosis. Classic typhus contracted by a previously vaccinated person is usually mild and may be clinically indistinguishable from murine typhus except by serologic methods.

Treatment and prevention   Both chloramphenicol and the tetracycline antibiotics have been found to be highly efficient therapeutic agents in epidemic typhus. Usually the patient becomes afebrile after 2 days of treatment. Under field conditions, 100 mg doxycycline in a single oral dose resulted in abatement of clinical manifestations and defervescence in epidemic typhus.

The most effective measures for controlling epidemic typhus are those which eliminate lice. DDT or lindane powder when dusted into clothing is suitable for this purpose. If resistant lice are found, malathion or carbaryl may prove effective.

A commercially available vaccine prepared from formalin-treated suspensions of infected yolk sac tissue is an effective immunizing agent.

BRILL-ZINSSER DISEASE (RECRUDESCENT TYPHUS)   Brill-Zinsser disease is a recrudescent episode of epidemic typhus fever that occurs years after the initial attack. *R. prowazekii* has been isolated from lice feeding on patients during the active stages of illness.

The clinical entity, not always mild, resembles epidemic typhus in the character of the rash, circulatory disturbances, and hepatic, renal, and nervous system changes. Recovery is the rule. The Weil-Felix reaction with the various *Proteus* antigens is usually negative or positive in very low titer. The specific complement fixation, microscopic agglutination, and immunofluorescent antibody reactions are valuable in establishing the diagnosis. In Brill-Zinsser disease the specific complement-fixing antibodies appear as early as the fourth day after the onset of illness; antibodies are IgG, and the peak response is attained by the eighth to tenth days. Specific antibody titers in the primary attack of epidemic typhus begin later, about the eighth to twelfth day, with maximum titers on about the sixteenth day after onset. Treatment is the same as for other rickettsial infections.

SCRUB TYPHUS   Definition   Scrub typhus is limited to eastern and southeastern Asia, India, northern Australia, and the adjacent islands. It is common in northern Thailand. It is caused by *R. tsutsugamushi* and is characterized by a primary lesion at the site of the bite of an infected mite, a fever of about 2 weeks' duration, a cutaneous rash which develops about the fifth day, and the appearance late in the second week of agglutinins against the OX-K strain of *Proteus* bacillus. Antibiotics similar to those used for other rickettsial infections are specific therapeutic agents.

Etiology   The agent of scrub typhus resembles other rickettsias in its physical properties but differs from them in antigenic structure, vector, and reservoir. The disease is transmitted by larvae of several species of mites, especially *Leptotrombidium* (*Trombicula*) *akamushi* and *L. deliense*. These tiny chiggers attach themselves to the skin and during the process of obtaining a meal of tissue juice may acquire infection from the host or transmit rickettsias to the vertebrate. The infection is maintained in nature by a cycle involving mites and small rodents and by transovarial transmission in mites; human infection represents an accident attributable to propinquity.

Clinical manifestations   About 10 to 12 days after infection, illness begins abruptly with chilliness, severe headache, fever, conjunctival injection, and moderate generalized lymphadenopathy, which is most prominent in the nodes draining the area of the primary lesion. The initial lesion at the beginning of fever is evidenced by an erythematous indurated area 1 cm in diameter, surmounted by a multiloculated vesicle; within a few days the vesicle ulcerates and becomes covered with a black crust.

Fever increases progressively during the first week, generally reaching 40 to 40.5°C (104 to 105°F), but the pulse remains relatively slow, 70 to 100 beats per minute. The red macular rash, which begins on the trunk about the fifth day and spreads to the extremities, sometimes becomes maculopapular but usually fades in a few days. The course of the disease and the complications resemble those of endemic and epidemic typhus; however, interstitial myocarditis is more prominent than in the other typhus fevers.

Prognosis   Before the introduction of chloramphenicol and tetracycline, the mortality rate varied from 1 to 60 percent, depending on the geographic area and the virulence of the local strains of *R. tsutsugamushi*, and convalescence was prolonged. With modern therapeutic methods, deaths are rare and convalescence is short.

Differential diagnosis   Scrub typhus must be differentiated from the other members of the typhus and spotted fever group of diseases as well as from measles, typhoid fever, and the meningococcal infections. The geographic localization of scrub typhus, the primary lesion, and the occurrence of OX-K agglutinins are especially useful in establishing the diagnosis.

Treatment and prevention   Chloramphenicol and the tetracycline antibiotics are extremely effective in scrub typhus. Scrub typhus is more amenable to drugs than are the other rickettsial infections, and patients with this disease regularly become afebrile and are decidedly improved within 24 to 36 h after beginning treatment, irrespective of the stage of disease. Antibiotic treatment may be discontinued after several afebrile days.

Relapse of clinical illness is unusual unless specific treatment is initiated early, such as before the fifth febrile day. Under these circumstances, recrudescence is prevented by giving the antibiotic for several days and resuming treatment about 5 days after cessation of the initial course of therapy.

Prevention of disease in the individual is accomplished by the application of miticidal chemicals (dibutyl phthalate, benzyl benzoate, diethyltoluamide, and others) to clothing and the skin. There is no satisfactory vaccine. Chemoprophylactic studies conducted in highly endemic infested areas of scrub typhus showed that single oral doses of chloramphenicol or tetracycline given every 5 days for a total of 35 days (seven doses with 5-day nontreatment intervals) prevent scrub typhus and result in active immunity. This procedure is recommended under special circumstances. A long-acting tetracycline (doxycycline) serves the same purpose.

TRENCH FEVER Trench fever is a rare febrile disease transmitted between humans by the body louse, *Pediculus humanus corporis*. It is characterized by a sudden onset with headache and severe pain in the muscles, bones, and joints. In most cases the fever and other symptoms assume a relapsing character. Fatalities are rare. The disease is also known as shin bone fever, Volhynia fever, His-Werner disease, and quintan fever. Because of its rarity in the United States, textbooks of rickettsiology should be consulted for a detailed description.

RICKETTSIALPOX **Definition** Rickettsialpox is a mild, nonfatal, self-limited, febrile illness caused by *R. akari*, which is transmitted from mice to humans by mites. It is characterized by an initial skin lesion at the mite bite, a week's febrile course, and a papulovesicular rash.

Etiology and epidemiology Rickettsialpox was first recognized in New York City in 1946, and about 180 cases were reported annually for several years thereafter. It has been diagnosed in several other areas of the United States, and outbreaks have been reported in European Russia. A possible new focus has been identified in Baltimore, Md. The vector is a small, colorless mite, *Allodermanyssus sanguineus* (Hirst), which infests small mice and rodents. House mice serve as the reservoir of infection.

R. akari is morphologically and biologically similar to other rickettsias and is antigenically related to, but distinct from, *R. rickettsii*, the cause of Rocky Mountain spotted fever.

Clinical manifestations The initial skin lesion appears about 7 to 10 days after the mite bite as a firm red papule 1 to 1.5 cm in diameter. In a few days, the center vesiculates, and the papule is surrounded by an area of erythema. The regional lymph glands are moderately enlarged. The primary lesion, which is not painful, becomes covered with a black scab; it heals slowly, and a small scar is visible on separation of the crust.

The febrile phase begins 3 to 7 days after the initial lesion, and an exanthem may accompany the fever or begin several days later. The onset of fever is sudden, with chilly sensations or frank chills, headache, sweats, myalgia, anorexia, and photophobia. The pyrexia ranges from 39.4 to 40°C (103 to 104°F) and continues for about a week, occasionally with morning remissions.

The exanthem is maculopapular-vesicular, is generalized in distribution, and may be abundant or scant. The lesions may involve the oral cavity but not the palms or soles. In a week, the vesicles dry and form scabs which eventually scale but leave no scar.

The constitutional symptoms are generally mild, and the course of illness is uncomplicated. No fatal cases have been reported.

The disease may be confused with chickenpox, which is different because it occurs usually in childhood and has no initial lesion and the papular cutaneous lesion is entirely transformed into a vesicle. Variola (smallpox) is accompanied by a more severe constitutional reaction, and the vesicles become pustules. The skin lesions of the other rickettsioses differ in their lack of vesiculation. The Weil-Felix

reaction is usually negative in this rickettsial disease, but specific complement fixation, microscopic agglutination, and immunofluorescence antibody reactions are useful diagnostic aids even though there is considerable antigenic crossing with Rocky Mountain spotted fever.

Treatment and prevention Chloramphenicol and the tetracycline antibiotics are all effective for treating patients with rickettsialpox. The temperature reaches normal levels in about 2 days, and recovery is rapid.

Control measures should be directed toward elimination of house mice and the vector mites responsible for transmitting the disease.

OTHER TICK-BORNE RICKETTSIAL DISEASES **Definition** Boutonneuse fever, North Asian tick-borne rickettsiosis, and Queensland tick typhus, three diseases occurring in the Eastern Hemisphere, are caused by rickettsias closely related to one another and to the agent of Rocky Mountain spotted fever. Each is transmitted by the bite of an ixodid tick. These mild to moderately severe illnesses are characterized by an initial lesion (called *tache noire* in boutonneuse fever), a fever of several days to 2 weeks, and a generalized maculopapular erythematous rash which appears on about the fifth day and usually involves the palms and soles. Specific complement-fixing antibodies appear in the patients' sera during convalescence, but agglutinins to *Proteus* OX-19 (Weil-Felix reaction) are frequently found only in low titer.

Etiology and epidemiology The etiologic agents of these three diseases are all members of the spotted fever group of rickettsias. Together with *R. rickettsii* and *R. akari* they possess common group antigens which are readily demonstrated by agglutination, complement fixation, microscopic agglutination, and immunofluorescent antibody reactions.

Boutonneuse fever (Mediterranean spotted fever), which may be regarded as the prototype of the three, is caused by *R. conorii*. Modern serologic methods employing specific rickettsial antigens have shown this *Rickettsia* to be the causative agent for a single widely disseminated disease known by various local names. Information on the distribution and etiology of the various tick-borne rickettsial diseases is contained in Table 138-1.

In general, the epidemiology of these tick-borne rickettsioses resembles that of spotted fever in the Western Hemisphere. Ixodid ticks and small wild animals maintain the rickettsias in nature; if humans intrude accidentally into the cycle, they become a dead end in the transmission chain. In certain areas, the cycle of boutonneuse fever involves domiciliary environments, with the brown dog tick, *Rhipicephalus sanguineus*, as the dominant vector.

Clinical manifestations These three tick-borne rickettsioses resemble one another closely. The clinical course is usually milder than that of spotted fever, with a shorter febrile period and fewer severe complications; fatalities are rare and generally limited to the aged and debilitated. Boutonneuse fever is not always mild; fulminant cases with death are reported. The initial lesion, which is present in most cases at the onset of fever, heals slowly; the regional lymph nodes are enlarged. The rash usually remains papular and only in severe cases becomes hemorrhagic.

The clinical picture (including the primary lesion), the geographic location, and epidemiologic considerations are helpful in establishing the diagnosis. The typhus fevers, meningococcal infections, leptospirosis, and measles must be considered in the differential diagnosis; the Weil-Felix and complement fixation tests are of value here.

Treatment and prevention Chloramphenicol and the tetracyclines are effective therapeutic agents, patients generally become afebrile after 2 to 3 days of treatment, and recovery is rapid. Ciprofloxacin is effective but is not regarded as the first choice.

The major effective methods of control are concerned with avoidance of tick bites; these include application of repellents and prompt removal of attached ticks. Effective vaccines are not available commercially.

Q FEVER **Definition** Q fever is an acute infectious disease caused by *Coxiella burnetii* and characterized by a sudden onset of fever, malaise, headache, weakness, anorexia, and interstitial pneumonitis. Rickettsemia occurs during the febrile period, and specific complement-fixing antibodies are present during convalescence. In contrast to the other rickettsioses, the disease is not associated with a cutaneous exanthem or agglutinins for the *Proteus* bacteria (Weil-Felix reaction).

Etiology and epidemiology *C. burnetii* possesses the general properties of other rickettsias but is somewhat more resistant to inactivation in unfavorable environments and more pleomorphic than the others. Its infectivity after drying under natural conditions is of importance in the spread of infection to humans. *C. burnetii* has a wide host range in nature, but guinea pigs and embryonated eggs are the common laboratory hosts employed for its propagation.

C. burnetii undergoes antigenic phase variation similar to the rough-smooth dissociation of bacteria. Phase I organisms are found in nature; they possess a cell wall–associated surface antigen that is probably related to virulence and is antiphagocytic. The phase II variant is a laboratory artifact that follows adaptation of phase I in chick embryos. Complement-fixing antibodies to phase I antigen reflect a recent acute infection; they appear in 7 to 10 days, peak at about 20 days, and slowly decline.

Human Q fever is contracted by inhalation of infected dusts, by handling infected materials, possibly by drinking milk contaminated with *C. burnetii*, and, in one instance, by blood transfusion. The disease in Australia is enzootic in animals, especially bandicoots, and is transmitted in nature by ticks. *Rickettsia*-laden tick feces may contaminate cattle hides, and inhalation of this material has caused infection in humans. In the United States, a number of species of ticks are naturally infected, among them *Dermacentor andersoni* and *Amblyomma americanum*, and in North Africa, transovarial transmission of the agent in indigenous ticks has been demonstrated. Sheep, goats, and cows have been found to be naturally infected in North America and in Europe, and *C. burnetii* has been recovered from the milk of such animals. Both milk and infected excretions from livestock probably account for certain outbreaks of human disease following inhalation by cows of infected dust from barns and pens. The airborne route of dried contaminated material is the most likely method of spread. A number of epidemics have occurred among laboratory workers engaged in studies on *C. burnetii*. The disease is not transmitted between humans.

Slaughterhouse workers are often exposed to infected aerosols; in 1985, five cases of hepatitis occurred at a meat packing plant that processed sheep in California. A serologic survey of approximately 100 employees, conducted to identify the extent of the outbreak, revealed a total of 31 persons with evidence of infection. The primary reservoirs of *C. burnetii* are cattle, sheep, goats, and ticks. Many wild and domestic animals are susceptible to infection. In Uruguay, there were 14 outbreaks of Q fever between 1975 and 1985, comprising 1358 clinically suspected cases, all of which occurred in workers at meat processing plants; 814 were serologically confirmed.

An "urban" outbreak of Q fever occurred in 12 poker players in Halifax, Nova Scotia. Presumably the disease was transmitted by a parturient cat.

Clinical manifestations After incubation for approximately 19 days (range 14 to 26 days), the disease begins with headache, chilly sensations, fever, malaise, myalgia, and anorexia. For several days, the temperature ranges from 38.3 to 40°C (101 to 104°F); the entire course rarely exceeds 2 weeks and usually ranges from 3 to 6 days. There may be wide fluctuations in the fever. Respiratory and gastrointestinal symptoms are not conspicuous in the early stages. Headache and fever predominate. A dry cough and chest pain occur after about 5 days, when rales are usually audible. Roentgenographic findings indistinguishable from those of primary atypical pneumonia are present usually by the third to fourth day of disease, first as patchy areas of consolidation involving a portion of one lobe, giving a homogeneous ground-glass appearance. Occasionally, a homogeneous localized infiltration may resemble a tumor mass. These manifestations persist beyond the febrile period and may appear in patients who are unaware of pulmonary involvement. Complications are rare, and coincident with defervescence the appetite begins to return. Convalescence progresses slowly for several weeks, during which time the principal disability is weakness. It is not uncommon for patients to lose 7 to 9 kg during the active stages of disease. The disease may be protracted in approximately 20 percent of cases, with fever persisting for longer than 4 weeks, particularly in elderly patients. Occasionally, relapse occurs, especially in patients treated with antibiotics during the first several days of disease.

Hepatitis, with the development of clinically detectable icterus, occurs in approximately one-third of patients with the protracted form. This form of Q fever is characterized by fever, malaise, absence of headache or respiratory signs, and hepatomegaly with right upper quadrant pain. Liver biopsy specimens show diffuse granulomatous changes with multinucleated giant cells and scattered infiltrations of polymorphonuclear leukocytes, lymphocytes, and macrophages. *C. burnetii* may be demonstrated in such specimens with the fluorescent antibody technique. Q fever must be included in the differential diagnosis of patients with hepatitis and those with hepatic granulomas such as tuberculosis, sarcoidosis, histoplasmosis, brucellosis, tularemia, syphilis, and others.

Endocarditis with *C. burnetii* has been identified by smear and isolation of the *Rickettsia* in vegetations on the heart valves obtained at operation or autopsy. The aortic valve is most commonly involved, often with large vegetations. It is important to suspect Q fever in cases of apparent subacute bacterial endocarditis with persistently negative blood cultures. Operative intervention with replacement of damaged valves is usually necessary for recovery because the available antibiotics are not rickettsicidal. In some instances, long-term antibiotic therapy has been successful.

A high complement-fixing antibody titer to phase I antigen is present in patients with endocarditis and granulomatous hepatitis.

Prognosis Few fatalities have been recorded, and except for the patient with protracted illness and hepatic involvement or endocarditis, the course of disease is generally uncomplicated and benign.

Treatment and control The tetracycline antibiotics and chloramphenicol are effective in the treatment of patients with Q fever. Most patients, when treated early in the course of disease, respond promptly and recover without relapses. The therapeutic procedures are comparable with those used in spotted fever.

Control of Q fever depends primarily on immunization of susceptible persons with specific vaccines. Vaccines made from phase I rickettsias are potent and afford considerable protection to slaughterhouse and dairy workers, herders, rendering-plant workers, wool sorters, tanners, laboratory workers, and others at risk. To avoid side reactions, it is important that the vaccine be given only to persons who are skin test negative. Measures should be taken to avoid exposure to infected aerosols; milk from infected domestic livestock must be pasteurized or boiled.

EHRLICHIOSIS Clinical manifestations range from the asymptomatic to an abrupt onset illness with fever, chills, headache, and malaise present in most cases. Some patients exhibit a maculopapular or petechial rash involving the trunk and extremities. Abdominal pain, vomiting, and diarrhea may occur. Important hematologic and hepatic abnormalities include leukopenia, thrombocytopenia, and elevated levels of transaminase and alkaline phosphatase. In severe cases, disseminated intravascular coagulation, renal and bone marrow failure, hepatitis and disorientation can develop.

The causative agents, *Ehrlichia*, are *Rickettsia*-like bacteria transmitted to humans by ticks. Often specific confirmation is made only by serologic procedures using the indirect fluorescent antibody test (IFA) to detect IgG antibodies against *Ehrlichia*. Patients with ehrlichiosis respond well to the tetracycline antibiotics and chloramphenicol, similar to the response in Rocky Mountain spotted fever. Hence the physician who cannot distinguish clearly between the two diseases should initiate treatment in order to ensure against late sequelae.

REFERENCES

BOZEMAN FM et al: Serologic evidence of *Rickettsia canada* infection in man. J Infect Dis 121:367, 1970

——— et al: Epidemic typhus rickettsiae isolated from flying squirrels. Nature 255:545, 1975

CENTERS FOR DISEASE CONTROL: Summary of notifiable diseases, United States, 1987. Morb Mort Week Rep 36:54, 1987

DERRICK EH: The epidemiology of Q fever: A review. Med J Aust 1:245, 1953

DUMLER JS et al: Rapid immunoperoxidase demonstration of *Rickettsia rickettsii* in fixed cutaneous specimens from patients with Rocky Mountain spotted fever. Am J Clin Pathol 93:410, 1990

FERGUSON IC et al: Clinical, virological and pathological findings in a fatal case of Q fever endocarditis. Br J Clin Pathol 15:235, 1962

GAMBRILL MR, WISSEMAN CL JR: Mechanisms of immunity in typhus infections. Infect Immun 8:519, 1973

HARRELL GT: Rickettsial involvement of the nervous system. Med Clin North Am 37:395, 1953

HATTWICK MAW et al: Rocky Mountain spotted fever: Epidemiology of an increasing problem. Ann Intern Med 84:732, 1976

KOSTER FT et al: Cellular immunity in Q fever: Specific lymphocyte unresponsiveness in Q fever endocarditis. J Infect Dis 152:1283, 1985

LANGLEY J et al: Poker player's pneumonia: An urban outbreak of Q fever following exposure to a parturient cat. N Engl J Med 319:354, 1988

MURRAY ES et al: Brill's disease: I. Clinical and laboratory diagnosis. JAMA 142:1059, 1950

———, Snyder JC: Brill's disease: II. Etiology. Am J Hyg 53:22, 1951

ORMSBEE RA et al: The influence of phase on the protective potency of Q fever vaccine. J Immunol 92:404, 1964

——— et al: Serologic diagnosis of epidemic typhus fever. Am J Epidemiol 105:261, 1977

PEDERSEN CE et al: Demonstration of *Rickettsia rickettsii* in Rhesus monkeys by immune fluorescence microscopy. J Clin Microbiol 2:121, 1975

PERINE PL et al: A clinico-epidemiological study of epidemic typhus in Africa. Clin Infect Dis 14:1149, 1992

PHILIP RN et al: A comparison of serologic methods for diagnosis of Rocky Mountain spotted fever. Am J Epidemiol 105:56, 1977

RAOULT D et al: Ciprofloxacin therapy for Mediterranean spotted fever. Antimicrob Agents Chemother 30:606, 1986

ROSE HM: The clinical manifestations and laboratory diagnosis of rickettsialpox. Ann Intern Med 31:871, 1949

SALGO MP et al: A focus of Rocky Mountain Spotted Fever within New York City. N Engl J Med 318:345, 1988

SMADEL JE: Influence of antibiotics on immunologic responses in scrub typhus. Am J Med 17:246, 1954

——— (ED): *Symposium on Q Fever*, Medical Science Publication 6. Washington, DC, Walter Reed Army Institute of Research, 1959

SOMENSHINE DE et al: Epizootiology of epidemic typhus (*Rickettsia prowazekii*) in flying squirrels. Am J Trop Med Hyg 27:339, 1978

SOMMA-MOREIRA RE et al: Analysis of Q fever in Uruguay. Rev Infect Dis 9:386, 1987

VINSON JW: Etiology of trench fever in Mexico, in *Industry and Tropical Health*, vol V. Boston, Harvard School of Public Health, 1964, p 109

WALKER DH, CAIN BG: A method for specific diagnosis of Rocky Mountain spotted fever on fixed, paraffin-embedded tissue by immunofluorescence. J Infect Dis 137:206, 1978

———, BRADFORD WD: Rocky Mountain spotted fever in childhood, in *Perspectives in Pediatric Pathology*, vol 6, HS Rosenberg, J Bernstein (eds). New York, Masson Publishing, 1981, pp 35–61

——— et al: Histopathology and immunohistologic demonstration of the distribution of *Rickettsia typhi* in fatal murine typhus. Am J Clin Pathol 91:720, 1989

WOODWARD TE: A historical account of the rickettsial diseases with a discussion of unsolved problems. J Infect Dis 127:583, 1973

———: Identification of *Rickettsia* in skin tissues. J Infect Dis 134:297, 1976

——— et al: The remarkable contributions of S. Burt Wolbach on rickettsial vasculitis updated. Trans Am Clin Climatol Assoc vol CIII, pp 78–94 1992

139 MYCOPLASMA INFECTIONS

WALLACE A. CLYDE, JR.

The mycoplasmas are a heterogeneous group of unusual bacteria belonging to microbial class Mollicutes ("soft skin"). They differ from classical bacteria by lacking rigid cell wall structures, being contained instead by trilaminar unit membranes. This property confers on mycoplasmas an inability to react with organic dyes, such as those in the Gram stain, and an absolute insensitivity to the penicillins, since there are no cell wall receptor sites for these antibiotics.

The mycoplasma genome is roughly one-sixth the size of that in *Escherichia coli*, making the mycoplasmas fastidious species requiring many precursor substances for growth in artificial media. With maximum dimensions of 0.15 to 0.5 μm, less than some of the larger viruses, mycoplasmas are the smallest organisms known that are capable of extracellular existence.

Mycoplasmas are ubiquitous in nature and cause a wide variety of diseases among animals, birds, plants, and insects. In humans the most important pathogen is *Mycoplasma pneumoniae*, a common cause of respiratory tract infections. *M. hominis* and *Ureaplasma urealyticum* also are implicated in disease involving mainly the genitourinary system. A newly described species having many pathogenic properties, *M. genitalium*, is of uncertain significance. In addition to these organisms, there are eight other distinct species that are components of the normal microflora on the oropharyngeal and genital mucosal surfaces.

MYCOPLASMA PNEUMONIAE

DEFINITION *M. pneumoniae* produces an influenza-like respiratory illness of gradual onset with headache, malaise, fever, and cough. When pneumonia is present, physical findings may be minimal despite extensive changes seen in chest x-rays. Synonyms include Eaton agent pneumonia, cold hemagglutinin–positive pneumonia, atypical or primary atypical pneumonia, and "walking" pneumonia. Asymptomatic infections also occur, especially in young children and partially immune adults.

ETIOLOGY *M. pneumoniae* was discovered by Eaton in 1941 and related to the syndrome of atypical pneumonia. It is a minute, motile filament, measuring approximately 0.1 by 2 μm, that has one differentiated pole where a specialized adhesin (P1) mediates attachment to respiratory epithelial cells. Production of peroxide and an inhibitor of host cell catalase are thought to be major mediators of parasitized cell injury. The organism may be isolated from respiratory secretions using complex artificial media, requiring usually 1 to 3 weeks or more for growth and identification procedures. New rapid diagnostic techniques, based on antigen detection or nucleic acid probes used directly on specimens, appear promising.

Invasive disease caused by *M. pneumoniae* has been reported—albeit only rarely—in severe or complicated cases. The usual clinical manifestations thus are mediated by surface parasitism of respiratory epithelial cells. Peribronchial accumulations of lymphoid and plasma cells develop, and intraluminal recruitment of macrophages and polymorphonuclear leukocytes takes place. In addition to sIgA, IgA, IgM, and IgG antibodies, a variety of autoantibodies develop in many patients. These include antibodies reactive with brain, heart, and muscle; erythrocyte I antigen; intermediate filaments; and mitotic spindles of dividing cells. Polyclonal B cell activation and suppression of delayed hypersensitivity also have been described. It is not clear that any of the various nonrespiratory complications of *M. pneumoniae* disease are due to these immunologic aberrations.

EPIDEMIOLOGY Communicability of *M. pneumoniae* infections is thought to be via large droplets of respiratory secretions; close indoor contact such as in household, institutional, or dormitory settings facilitates spread. The incubation period has been estimated at 2 to 3 weeks. Disease occurs most commonly in elementary school children, adolescents, and young adults. Infections can be found during any season of the year, although epidemic disease tends to occur during the fall and early winter months in temperate countries. Many studies have shown a periodicity of 3 to 5 years in the occurrence of major outbreaks. In Seattle, Washington, it was found that the average incidence of disease across all years and age groups was 2 per 1000 population per year. This occurrence doubled during epidemic years and was higher in the age groups between 5 and 40 years. In adolescent patients, 15 to 20 percent of all pneumonias could be attributed to *M. pneumoniae*. The organism has been implicated in up to 50 percent of pneumonia episodes in college students and in 20 to 30 percent of cases occurring in military recruits.

CLINICAL MANIFESTATIONS The most common clinical syndrome associated with *M. pneumoniae* infection is that of an acute or subacute tracheobronchitis. Symptoms appearing over several days' time include headache, malaise, feverishness, scratchy sore throat, and dry cough. The cough may be paroxysmal, often disturbing sleep, and gradually becomes productive of mucoid or mucopurulent sputum. Physical findings may be minimal, other than temperature elevation rarely exceeding 38.9°C (102°F). If pneumonia is present, isolated crackles or areas of wheezing may be heard, usually over one of the lower lobes. Areas of subsegmental atelectasis and small pleural effusions that may be seen on chest x-rays rarely are detectable by physical examination.

Most *M. pneumoniae* disease is mild and self-limited, running its course in 2 to 4 weeks without treatment. Appropriate antibiotics in controlled clinical trials have been shown to shorten significantly the duration of fever, hospitalization, and x-ray manifestations. Rarely, severe, life-threatening, or fatal episodes can occur.

A wide variety of respiratory and nonrespiratory tract complications may be encountered. Otitis media may be seen in children, while sinusitis is commonly present in adults. Occasional patients develop the syndrome of bullous myringitis. Nondescript maculopapular skin rashes are frequent in children, and *M. pneumoniae* infections have been associated with erythema multiforme and the Stevens-Johnson syndrome. Central nervous system complications of meningoencephalitis, cerebellar ataxia, and various radiculopathies have been described. Other rare complications include monarticular arthritis, myocarditis, pericarditis, coagulopathies, hemolytic anemia, and noncardiogenic pulmonary edema.

ROENTGENOGRAPHIC FINDINGS X-ray manifestations of *M. pneumoniae* pneumonia are protean and nonspecific. The most frequent pattern is one of bronchial thickening with areas of interstitial infiltration and subsegmental atelectasis involving one of the lower lobes. Another common finding is the occurrence of ''platelike'' atelectasis, often seen to best advantage on lateral views. Other changes include areas of small nodular densities, which can be confused with tuberculosis, and hilar adenopathy suggesting a variety of other entities. Lobular or lobar consolidation and massive pleural effusions are uncommon.

LABORATORY FINDINGS Total blood leukocyte and differential cell counts are usually normal, but the erythrocyte sedimentation rate is often elevated and C-reactive proteins may be demonstrated. There are no characteristic findings in urinalysis, liver or renal function tests, serum electrolytes, or electrocardiograms, although abnormalities may be seen with some of the disease complications. Specific diagnostic tests include recovery of *M. pneumoniae* from respiratory secretions or demonstration of fourfold titer changes between paired sera using a variety of methods, of which the complement fixation technique is the most widely available. However, these test results are not available promptly enough to assist therapeutic decision making. New rapid diagnostic tests of four types have been marketed. One depends on detection of *M. pneumoniae* rRNA by a nucleic acid hybridization technique. A second detects a major protein present in the organisms. The polymerase chain reaction has been applied—with promising results—to the diagnosis of *M. pneumoniae* infection and may prove useful clinically if costs and difficulties caused by in-laboratory contamination can be controlled. The fourth test detects *M. pneumoniae*–specific IgM antibody by agglutination. False-positive results may be obtained if antibody from a prior infection is detected; false-negative results may be obtained if the test is done too early in the course of infection or in an adult in whom prior infection has elicited a predominantly IgG response. The usefulness of these rapid tests will be determined as greater clinical experience with them accrues.

Another helpful test is cold hemagglutination serology, because of its rapidity and simplicity. These IgM class antibodies directed toward the I antigen of erythrocyte membranes develop during the first or second week of illness in up to 80 percent of patients with pneumonia (95 percent of those below age 20) and may be present in high or rising titers when patients first present. Single titers of ≥64 or fourfold or greater titer changes in sera collected ≥5 days apart are considered significant. False-positive cold hemagglutinin reactions may be seen in rubeola, infectious mononucleosis, adenovirus pneumonias, and several tropical diseases, and, more rarely, in collagen vascular disease. As in some of these entities, polyclonal B lymphocyte activation and T cell suppression occurring during *M. pneumoniae* infections may explain the appearance of various host tissue autoantibodies and of transient anergy in some patients.

DIFFERENTIAL DIAGNOSIS Because of its common occurrence, *M. pneumoniae* should be considered in all cases of pneumonia. Generally, patients with mycoplasma pneumonia have milder illnesses than are caused by classical bacteria, less dense pulmonary infiltrations on x-rays, and normal blood leukocyte values. Epidemiologic data are especially useful: age (5 to 40 years), season (fall months predominantly), year (3- to 5-year epidemic cycles), and contact history with other cases. Other infections requiring special consideration are influenza virus pneumonia or its secondary bacterial complications (during epidemic periods) (see Chap. 152), adenovirus pneumonias (see Chap. 150) (particularly in military recruits), and mild forms of community-acquired *Legionella pneumophila* (see Chap. 113) pneumonia. The agent *Chlamydia pneumoniae* (TWAR) may produce disease clinically indistinguishable from that due to *M. pneumoniae*. TWAR infection is estimated to occur half as frequently as mycoplasma pneumonia.

TREATMENT Erythromycin and tetracycline derivatives are effective in reducing the morbidity of *M. pneumoniae* disease. For adults, erythromycin (0.5 g every 6 h orally), tetracycline (250 mg every 6 h orally), or doxycycline (100 mg once daily orally) in 10- to 14-day courses is usually prescribed. In severely ill patients, intravenous erythromycin may be selected, but tetracycline is not recommended by this route. For children less than 8 to 10 years old, erythromycin (30 to 50 mg/kg per day orally for 14 days) is the primary choice; tetracycline and doxycycline are alternatives for older patients. Relapses occasionally occur upon cessation of therapy but respond to retreatment. In cases where *Legionella* infection cannot be excluded, erythromycin should be chosen for therapy. If *Chlamydia pneumoniae* pneumonia is a consideration, the use of tetracycline or doxycycline is recommended.

OTHER MYCOPLASMAL INFECTIONS

A growing body of literature documents evidence of other human mycoplasma infections, including a variety of genitourinary syndromes in both sexes and perinatal diseases. Mycoplasma infection should be considered in suppurative processes where classical bacterial cultures are negative; examples include urethritis, salpingitis, amnionitis, pyelonephritis, postpartum sepsis, and neonatal pneumonia or meningitis. Mycoplasmal abcesses or arthritis may occur in immunocompromised patients. Recent interest has focused on isolation of fastidious strains of *M. fermentans* from some patients with AIDS; the significance of this association is presently unknown. Sexually transmitted diseases associated with mycoplasmas are considered in Chaps. 88 and 89.

In these infections, the species most commonly encountered are *M. hominis* and *U. urealyticum*. Standard bacteriologic media may support growth of *M. hominis* as minute colonies, especially media for anaerobic bacteria that are incubated for several days. Selective media for *Ureaplasma* species are available that may permit their identification in 24 to 48 h. Cultural facilities for *Mycoplasma* species are available in some diagnostic microbiology laboratories, whereas serodiagnosis of infections other than those due to *M. pneumoniae* is not routine. Specimens may be transported on wet ice (within 24 h) or dry ice (greater than 24 h) to reference laboratories for assistance. For *M. hominis* infections, tetracycline and clindamycin are effective antibiotics; this species is insensitive to erythromycin. Erythromycin or tetracycline may be used for *Ureaplasma* infections. Resistance of both species to the recommended antibiotics occurs and is a problem requiring special laboratory guidance. It has been shown in vitro that *M. hominis* is sensitive to ciprofloxacin, but ureaplasmas have limited susceptibility to quinolones currently on the market. Since mycoplasmas do not synthesize folic acid, they are insensitive to trimethoprim-sulfamethoxazole.

REFERENCES

BROUGHTON RA: Infections due to *Mycoplasma pneumoniae* in childhood. Pediatr Infect Dis J 5:71, 1986

CASSELL GH (ed): Ureaplasmas of humans: With emphasis upon maternal and neonatal infections. Pediatr Infect Dis J 5:S221, 1986

CLYDE WA JR: Mycoplasmal infections, in *Diagnostic Procedures for Bacterial Infections*, 7th ed, BB Wentworth (ed). Washington, DC, American Public Health Association, 1987, pp 391–405

GRAYSTON JT et al: A new respiratory pathogen: *Chlamydia pneumoniae* strain TWAR. J Infect Dis 161:618, 1990

MÅRDH P-A et al (eds): International symposium on *Mycoplasma hominis*—a human pathogen. Sex Transm Dis 10(Suppl):225, 1983

MCCRACKEN GH JR: Current status of antibiotic treatment for *Mycoplasma pneumoniae* disease. Pediatr Infect Dis J 5:167, 1986

NAGAYAMA Y et al: Isolation of *Mycoplasma pneumoniae* from children with lower-respiratory-tract infections. J Infect Dis 157:911, 1988

140 CHLAMYDIAL INFECTIONS

WALTER E. STAMM / KING K. HOLMES

The genus *Chlamydia* contains three species: *C. psittaci, C. trachomatis,* and *C. pneumoniae* (formerly the TWAR agent). *C. psittaci* is widely distributed in nature, producing genital, conjunctival, intestinal, or respiratory infections in many mammalian and avian species. Genital infections with *C. psittaci* have been well characterized in several species and cause complications such as abortion and infertility. Although mammalian strains of *C. psittaci* are not known to infect humans, avian strains occasionally infect humans, causing pneumonia and the systemic illness known as psittacosis.

C. pneumoniae is a fastidious chlamydial species that appears to be a frequent cause of upper respiratory tract infection and pneumonia, primarily in children and young adults. No animal reservoir has been identified for *C. pneumoniae*, and it appears to be a human pathogen spread by close personal contact.

C. trachomatis is exclusively a human pathogen and was recognized as the cause of trachoma in the 1940s. Since then, *C. trachomatis* has been recognized as a major cause of sexually transmitted and perinatal infection.

Chlamydiae are obligate, intracellular parasites. They possess both DNA and RNA, have a cell wall and ribosomes similar to those of gram-negative bacteria, and are inhibited by antibiotics such as tetracycline. Chlamydiae are classified as bacteria belonging to their own order (Chlamydiales).

A unique feature of all chlamydiae is their complex reproductive cycle. Two forms of the microorganism—the extracellular elementary body and the intracellular reticulate body—participate in this cycle. The elementary body is adapted for extracellular survival and is the infective form transmitted from one person to another. Elementary bodies attach to susceptible target cells (usually columnar or transitional epithelial cells) and enter the cells within a phagosome. Within 8 h, the elementary bodies reorganize into reticulate bodies. These forms are adapted to intracellular survival and multiplication. They undergo binary fission, eventually producing numerous replicates contained within the membrane-bound ''inclusion body,'' which occupies much of the infected host cell. Chlamydial inclusions resist lysosomal fusion until late in the developmental cycle. After 24 h, the reticulate bodies condense and form elementary bodies still contained within the inclusion. The inclusion then ruptures, releasing elementary bodies from the cell to initiate infection of adjacent cells.

C. psittaci, C. pneumoniae, and *C. trachomatis* share a genus-specific or group lipopolysaccharide antigen. Antibody to this antigen is measured in the complement fixation (CF) serologic test available in most state health departments. With a microimmunofluorescence test, *C. trachomatis* strains can be further characterized serologically on the basis of antibody to their major outer-membrane protein (MOMP). Recent studies using monoclonal antibodies to MOMP and nucleotide sequencing of MOMP have delineated at least 20 serotypes of *C. trachomatis*. According to the serovar classification system of Wang and Grayston, strains associated with trachoma have generally been those of the A, B, Ba, and C serovars, while serovars D through K have been largely associated with sexually transmitted and perinatally acquired infections. Serovars L_1, L_2, and L_3 produce lymphogranuloma venereum (LGV) and hemorrhagic proctocolitis. The LGV strains demonstrate unique biologic behavior in that they are more invasive than the other serovars, produce disease in lymphatic tissue, grow readily in cell culture systems and macrophages, and are fatal when inoculated intracerebrally into mice and monkeys. Non-LGV strains of *C. trachomatis* characteristically produce superficial infections involving the columnar epithelium of the eye, genitalia, and respiratory tract.

C. trachomatis has been reported as an infrequent cause of subacute endocarditis, peritonitis, pleuritis, and possibly periappendicitis and may occasionally cause respiratory infections in older children and adults. Immunosuppressed patients with pneumonia have had, in some cases, either serologic or cultural evidence of *C. trachomatis* infection, but more data are necessary to define the role of *Chlamydia* in these patients.

SEXUALLY TRANSMITTED AND PERINATAL INFECTIONS DUE TO *C. TRACHOMATIS*

SPECTRUM OF *C. TRACHOMATIS* GENITAL INFECTIONS Genital infections caused by *C. trachomatis* represent the most common bacterial sexually transmitted disease (STD) in the United States. An estimated 3 to 4 million cases occur each year. In adults the clinical spectrum of sexually transmitted *C. trachomatis* infections parallels the spectrum of gonococcal infections (Table 140-1). Chlamydial and gonococcal infections have been associated with urethritis, proctitis, and conjunctivitis in both sexes; with epididymitis in men; and with mucopurulent cervicitis, acute salpingitis, bartholinitis, and the Fitz-Hugh–Curtis syndrome (perihepatitis) in women. Moreover, both types of infection can be associated with systemic complications, particularly arthritis. In general, however, chlamydial infections produce fewer symptoms and signs than corresponding gonococcal infections at the same site; in fact, the former are often totally asymptomatic. Increasing evidence suggests that many chlamydial infections of the genital tract, especially in women, persist for months without producing symptoms. Simultaneous infection with *C. trachomatis* occurs in up to 30 to 50 percent of women with cervical gonococcal infection and in up to 25 percent of heterosexual men with gonococcal urethritis.

EPIDEMIOLOGY Infections due to *C. trachomatis* have been made reportable in many states, and national incidence data show steadily rising numbers of reported infections, probably reflecting both increased testing and reporting. The annual occurrence of nongonococcal urethritis (NGU) has been measured by surveys of diagnoses made by physicians in private practice and has been used as a surrogate measure of trends in chlamydial infection. The incidence of NGU increased dramatically during the 1960s and 1970s, a period when chlamydiae caused 30 to 50 percent of such cases. Even as the incidence of gonococcal urethritis fell during the 1980s, the incidence of NGU stabilized in the United States, probably reflecting the relative

TABLE 140-1   Clinical parallels between sexually transmitted infections due to _Neisseria gonorrhoeae_ and _Chlamydia trachomatis_

Site of infection	Resulting clinical syndrome	
	N. gonorrhoeae	_C. trachomatis_
MEN		
Urethra	Urethritis	Nongonococcal or post-gonococcal urethritis
Epididymis	Epididymitis	Epididymitis
Rectum	Proctitis	Proctitis
Conjunctiva	Conjunctivitis	Conjunctivitis
Systemic	Disseminated gonococcal infection	Reiter's syndrome
WOMEN		
Urethra	Acute urethral syndrome	Acute urethral syndrome
Bartholin's gland	Bartholinitis	Bartholinitis
Cervix	Cervicitis	Cervicitis
Endometrium	Endometritis	Endometritis
Fallopian tube	Salpingitis	Salpingitis
Conjunctiva	Conjunctivitis	Conjunctivitis
Liver capsule	Perihepatitis	Perihepatitis
Systemic	Disseminated gonococcal infection	Reiter's syndrome

lack of implementation of programs to control chlamydial infections. More recently, implementation of chlamydial control programs in some regions has been associated with a decline in the proportion of NGU cases caused by chlamydiae; thus trends in NGU may be less reliable as a surrogate for trends in the incidence of chlamydial infection.

The age of peak incidence of genital _C. trachomatis_ infections is the late teens and early twenties, as in other sexually transmitted infections. The prevalence of chlamydial urethral infection in young men ranges from 3 to 5 percent of men seen in general medical settings, to over 10 percent of asymptomatic soldiers undergoing routine physical examination, to 15 to 20 percent of heterosexual men seen in STD clinics. Urethral chlamydial infection is less common among homosexual than among heterosexual men, but rectal infections occur in homosexual men who practice receptive anorectal intercourse without condoms. The ratio of chlamydial to gonococcal urethritis is highest for heterosexual men and for those with high socioeconomic status and is lowest for homosexual men and indigent populations.

The incidence of cervical infection in women has ranged from approximately 5 percent among asymptomatic college students or prenatal patients in the United States, to over 10 percent of women seen in family planning clinics, to over 20 percent of women seen in STD clinics. In the United States, the prevalence of _C. trachomatis_ in the cervix of pregnant women is 5 to 10 times higher than that of _Neisseria gonorrhoeae_. The prevalence of genital infection with either agent is highest in individuals who are single, nonwhite (primarily black or hispanic), and between ages 18 and 24. Oral contraceptive use also confers an increased risk of chlamydial infection. The proportion of infections that are asymptomatic appears to be higher for _C. trachomatis_ than for _N. gonorrhoeae,_ and symptomatic _C. trachomatis_ infections are clinically less severe. It is suspected that mild or asymptomatic chlamydial infections of the fallopian tubes may nonetheless cause ongoing tubal damage and infertility. Furthermore, because the total number of _C. trachomatis_ infections exceeds that of _N. gonorrhoeae_ infections in industrialized countries, the total morbidity caused by _C. trachomatis_ genital infections in these countries equals or exceeds that caused by _N. gonorrhoeae._ The prevalence of _C. trachomatis_ is higher than that of _N. gonorrhoeae_ in industrialized countries, in part because measures such as treatment

of sex partners and routine cultures for case detection in asymptomatic individuals have been applied much more effectively to the control of gonorrhea than to that of _C. trachomatis_ infection.

CLINICAL MANIFESTATIONS   Nongonococcal and postgonococcal urethritis   Nongonococcal urethritis is a diagnosis of exclusion that is applied to men with symptoms and/or signs of urethritis who do not have gonorrhea. Postgonococcal urethritis (PGU) refers to nongonococcal urethritis developing 2 to 3 weeks after treatment of gonococcal urethritis in men with single-dose regimens such as amoxicillin or cephalosporins that lack sufficient activity against chlamydia. Since treatment for gonorrhea now also includes 7 days of tetracycline or doxycycline for concomitant chlamydial infection, both the incidence of PGU and the causative role of chlamydiae in this syndrome have declined. _C. trachomatis_ causes 20 to 50 percent of the cases of NGU and PGU in heterosexual men but is less commonly isolated from homosexual men with these syndromes. The cause of most of the remaining cases is uncertain, although considerable evidence suggests that _Ureaplasma urealyticum_ causes many of these infections, while _Trichomonas vaginalis_ and herpes simplex virus cause some cases of NGU.

Nongonococcal urethritis is diagnosed by documentation of a leukocytic urethral exudate and by exclusion of gonorrhea by Gram's stain or culture. _C. trachomatis_ urethritis is generally less severe than gonococcal urethritis, although in an individual patient these two forms of urethritis cannot be reliably differentiated solely on clinical grounds. Symptoms include urethral discharge, dysuria (often whitish and mucoid rather than frankly purulent), and urethral itching. The examination may show meatal erythema and tenderness and a urethral exudate that is often demonstrable only by stripping of the urethra. At least one-third of males with _C. trachomatis_ urethral infection have no demonstrable signs or symptoms of urethritis. Asymptomatic chlamydial urethritis has been demonstrated in 5 to 10 percent of sexually active adolescent males screened in teen clinics. Such patients frequently have first-glass pyuria ($\geq$15 leukocytes per $400\times$ microscopic field in the sediment of first-voided urine), a positive leukocyte esterase test, or an increased number of leukocytes on Gram-stained smear prepared from a urogenital swab inserted 1 to 2 cm into the anterior urethra. For the enumeration of leukocytes, the smear is first scanned at low power to identify areas of the slide containing the highest concentration of leukocytes. These areas are then examined under oil-immersion ($1000\times$). An average of four or more leukocytes in at least three of five $1000\times$ (oil-immersion) fields is indicative of urethritis and correlates with recovery of _C. trachomatis_. To differentiate between true urethritis and functional symptoms among symptomatic patients or to make a presumptive diagnosis of _C. trachomatis_ infection in asymptomatic men (e.g., male patients in STD clinics, sex partners of women with nongonococcal salpingitis or mucopurulent cervicitis, fathers of children with inclusion conjunctivitis), the examination of an endourethral specimen for increased leukocytes is useful if specific diagnostic tests for chlamydiae are not available. Alternatively, noninvasive screening for urethritis can be accomplished by testing a first-void urine sample for pyuria either by microscopy or by the leukocyte esterase test.

Epididymitis   _C. trachomatis_ is the major cause of epididymitis in sexually active heterosexual men under 35 years of age, accounting for about 70 percent of cases. _N. gonorrhoeae_ causes most of the remaining cases, and some men have simultaneous infections with both pathogens. Asymptomatic urethritis as defined above is usually present in these patients. In homosexual men, sexually transmitted coliform infection acquired via rectal intercourse may cause epididymitis. Coliform bacteria and _Pseudomonas aeruginosa_ are the most common causes of epididymitis in men over 35, usually in association with preceding urologic instrumentation or surgery. These men typically present with unilateral scrotal pain, fever, and epididymal tenderness or swelling on examination. The illness may be mild enough to treat in the outpatient setting or severe enough to require hospitalization. Testicular torsion should be promptly excluded by radionuclide scan, Doppler flow study, or surgical exploration in a teenager or young adult who presents with acute unilateral testicular pain without urethritis. Testicular tumor or chronic infection (e.g., tuberculosis) should be excluded in the patient with unilateral intrascrotal pain and swelling who does not respond to appropriate antimicrobial therapy.

Reiter's syndrome   Reiter's syndrome consists of conjunctivitis, urethritis (or cervicitis in females), arthritis, and characteristic mucocutaneous lesions (see Chap. 289). *C. trachomatis* has been recovered from the urethra of up to 70 percent of men with untreated nondiarrheal Reiter's syndrome and associated urethritis. In the absence of overt urethritis, it is important to exclude subclinical urethritis in the men in whom this diagnosis is suspected.

The pathogenesis of Reiter's syndrome remains obscure. However, since more than 80 percent of affected patients have HLA-B27 and since other mucosal infections (*Salmonella, Shigella,* or *Campylobacter,* for example) produce an identical syndrome, chlamydial infection is thought to initiate an aberrant and hyperactive immune response that produces inflammation at the involved target organs in these genetically predisposed individuals. Evidence of exaggerated cell-mediated and humoral immune responses to chlamydial antigens in Reiter's syndrome supports this hypothesis. The presumptive demonstration of chlamydial elementary bodies and chlamydial DNA in the joint fluid and synovial tissue of patients with Reiter's syndrome suggests that chlamydiae may actually spread from genital to joint tissues in these patients.

Proctitis   *C. trachomatis* of either the genital immunotypes D through K or the LGV immunotype L_2 causes proctitis in homosexual men who practice receptive anorectal intercourse. The vast majority of cases are due to immunotypes D through K and present either as asymptomatic infection or as mild proctitis not unlike gonococcal proctitis. These infections may be seen in heterosexual women as well. Clinically, these patients present with mild rectal pain, mucous discharge, tenesmus, and occasionally bleeding. Nearly all have neutrophils in their rectal Gram's stain. Anoscopy in these non-LGV cases of chlamydial proctitis reveals mild, patchy mucosal friability and mucopurulent discharge, and the disease process is limited to the distal rectum. LGV strains produce a more severe ulcerative proctitis or proctocolitis that can be confused clinically with herpes simplex virus proctitis (severe rectal pain, bleeding, discharge, and tenesmus) and that histologically resembles Crohn's disease in that giant-cell formation and granulomas can be seen (see Chap. 255). In the United States, these cases occur almost exclusively in homosexual men.

Mucopurulent cervicitis   *C. trachomatis* has been isolated from the cervix of 20 percent or more of women with gonorrhea or a history of contact with men who have gonorrhea or NGU and from the cervix of 10 to 20 percent of women attending STD clinics who do not have a history of contact with a partner with urethritis. Women who have cervical ectopy or who use oral contraceptives appear to have an increased prevalence of cervical infection with *C. trachomatis.*

Although many women with *C. trachomatis* infection of the cervix have no symptoms or signs, a careful speculum examination will demonstrate evidence of mucopurulent cervicitis in 30 to 50 percent. As discussed more fully in Chap. 89, mucopurulent cervicitis is associated with yellow mucopurulent discharge from the endocervical columnar epithelium and with $\geq$20 neutrophils per 1000$\times$ microscopic field within strands of cervical mucus on a thinly smeared, Gram-stained preparation of endocervical exudate. Other characteristic findings include edema of the zone of cervical ectopy and a propensity of the mucosa to bleed on minor trauma, e.g., when specimens are collected with a swab. Pap smear shows increased numbers of neutrophils as well as a characteristic pattern of mononuclear inflammatory cells, including plasma cells, transformed lymphocytes, and histiocytes. Cervical biopsy shows predominantly a mononuclear infiltrate of the subepithelial stroma, often with a follicular cervicitis.

Pelvic inflammatory disease (PID)   *C. trachomatis* plays an important causative role in salpingitis. *C. trachomatis* infection has been demonstrated in laparoscopically verified salpingitis, the organism has been recovered from the fallopian tubes in the absence of other pathogens, and serologic evidence of recent *C. trachomatis* infection has been found in women with PID. In the United States *C. trachomatis* has been identified in the fallopian tubes or endometrium in up to 50 percent of women with PID, and its role as an important etiologic agent in this syndrome is well accepted.

Pelvic inflammatory disease occurs via ascending intraluminal spread of *C. trachomatis* from the lower genital tract. Mucopurulent cervicitis is thus followed by endometritis, endosalpingitis, and finally pelvic peritonitis. Evidence of mucopurulent cervicitis is usually present in women with laparoscopically verified salpingitis. Similarly, endometritis, demonstrated by endometrial biopsy showing plasma cell infiltration of the endometrial epithelium, is present in most women with laparoscopically verified chlamydial (or gonococcal) salpingitis. Chlamydial endometritis also can occur in the absence of clinical evidence of salpingitis: approximately 40 to 50 percent of women with mucopurulent cervicitis have plasma cell endometritis. Histologic evidence of endometritis has been correlated with an "endometritis syndrome," consisting of vaginal bleeding, lower abdominal pain, and uterine tenderness in the absence of adnexal tenderness, and with peripheral blood leukocytosis. It is not known what proportion of those with chlamydial endometritis without adnexal tenderness had salpingitis. However, chlamydial salpingitis may produce milder symptoms than does gonococcal salpingitis and may be associated with less marked adnexal tenderness. The presence of mild adnexal or uterine tenderness in sexually active women with cervicitis suggests PID.

Infertility associated with fallopian tube scarring has been strongly linked to antecedent *C. trachomatis* infection in serologic studies. Since many infertile women with tubal scarring and antichlamydial antibody have no history of PID, is appears that subclinical tubal infection ("silent salpingitis") may produce scarring. Ectopic pregnancy, which occurs in over 70,000 women in the United States annually, is also thought to be related to *Chlamydia*-induced tubal scarring in many cases.

Perihepatitis, or the Fitz-Hugh–Curtis syndrome, was originally described as a complication of gonococcal PID. However, cultural and/or serologic evidence of *C. trachomatis* infection is found in three-quarters of women with this syndrome. *C. trachomatis* has also been cultured from exudate on the hepatic capsule in laparoscopically verified cases. This syndrome should be suspected whenever a young, sexually active woman presents with an illness resembling cholecystitis (fever and right upper quadrant pain of subacute or acute onset). Symptoms and signs of salpingitis may be minimal. High titers of antichlamydial antibodies are generally present.

Urethral syndrome in women   In the absence of infection with uropathogens such as coliforms or *Staphylococcus saprophyticus, C. trachomatis* is the pathogen most commonly isolated from college women with dysuria, frequency, and pyuria (see Chap. 90). *Chlamydia* also can be isolated from the urethra of women without symptoms of urethritis, and up to 25 percent of female STD clinic patients with chlamydial urogenital infection have had positive *C. trachomatis* cultures from the urethra only.

C. trachomatis infection in pregnancy   *C. trachomatis* in pregnancy has been associated in some studies (but not in others) with premature delivery and with postpartum endometritis. Whether these complications are in part attributable to *C. trachomatis* is not clear.

PERINATAL INFECTIONS: INCLUSION CONJUNCTIVITIS AND PNEUMONIA Epidemiology   Studies in the United States have demonstrated that 5 to 25 percent of pregnant women have *C. trachomatis* infections of the cervix. In these studies, approximately one-half to two-thirds of the children who were exposed during birth acquired *C. trachomatis* infection. Roughly half of the infected infants (or 25 percent of the group exposed) developed clinical evidence of inclusion conjunctivitis. In addition to being found in eye infection, *C. trachomatis* has been isolated frequently and persistently from the nasopharynx, the rectum, and the vagina, occasionally for periods exceeding 1 year in the absence of treatment. Pneumonia occurs in about 10 percent of children infected perinatally, and otitis media may in some cases result from perinatally acquired chlamydial infection.

Inclusion conjunctivitis of the newborn (neonatal chlamydial conjunctivitis) Neonatal chlamydial conjunctivitis has an acute onset and often produces a profuse mucopurulent discharge. In the newborn, chlamydial conjunctivitis generally has a longer incubation period than gonococcal conjunctivitis (usually 5 to 14 days vs. 1 to 3 days); however, this guideline is not reliable for the diagnosis of individual cases, and in any event it is impossible to differentiate chlamydial conjunctivitis from other forms of neonatal bacterial conjunctivitis clinically. Instead, laboratory diagnosis is required. Besides *C. trachomatis* and *N. gonorrhoeae*, the other important infectious causes of conjunctivitis in newborns include *Haemophilus influenzae, Streptococcus pneumoniae*, and herpes simplex virus. Inclusions within epithelial cells often can be demonstrated in Giemsa-stained conjunctival smears, but these smears are less sensitive than cultures or antigen detection tests. Gram-stained smears may show gonococci or occasional small gram-negative coccobacilli in *Haemophilus* conjunctivitis, but smears should be accompanied by cultures for these agents. Very rarely a trachoma-like eye disease occurs in children who have chlamydial infection and live in areas that do not have endemic trachoma. If neonatal chlamydial conjunctivitis is not treated appropriately with oral antimicrobials, it may be followed by chlamydial pneumonia.

Infant pneumonia *C. trachomatis* causes a distinctive pneumonia syndrome in infants. Recent epidemiologic studies have linked chlamydial pulmonary infection in infants with increased occurrence of subacute lung disease (bronchitis, asthma, wheezing) in later childhood. For details, consult standard textbooks of pediatrics.

LYMPHOGRANULOMA VENEREUM Definition Lymphogranuloma venereum is a sexually transmitted infection caused by *C. trachomatis* strains of the L_1, L_2, and L_3 serovars. Most cases are caused by L_2 organisms. Acute LGV in heterosexual men is characterized by a transient primary genital lesion followed by multilocular suppurative regional lymphadenopathy. Women, homosexual men, and—in occasional instances—heterosexual men may develop hemorrhagic proctitis with regional lymphadenitis. Acute LGV is almost always associated with systemic symptoms such as fever and leukocytosis and is rarely associated with systemic complications such as meningoencephalitis. After a latent period of years, late complications include genital elephantiasis due to lymphatic involvement, strictures, and fistulas of the penis, urethra, and rectum.

EPIDEMIOLOGY LGV is usually sexually transmitted, but occasional transmission by nonsexual personal contact, fomites, or laboratory accidents has been documented. Laboratory work involving creation of aerosols of the causative organisms (e.g., sonication, homogenization) must be conducted with appropriate biologic containment.

The peak incidence of LGV corresponds to the age of greatest sexual activity, the second and third decades of life. The worldwide incidence of LGV is falling, but the disease is still endemic and a major cause of morbidity in Asia, Africa, South America, and parts of the Caribbean. In the Bahamas, an apparent outbreak of LGV has been described in association with a concurrent increase in heterosexual human immunodeficiency virus (HIV) infection. However, only 277 cases were reported in the United States in 1990.

The frequency of infection following exposure is believed to be much lower than that associated with gonorrhea and syphilis. Early manifestations are recognized far more often in men than in women, who usually present with late complications. In the United States, where the reported sex ratio is 3.4 males to 1 female, most cases have involved homosexually active men and travelers, seamen, and military personnel returning from abroad. The main reservoir of infection is presumed to be asymptomatically infected individuals, although such a reservoir has not been directly demonstrated.

Clinical manifestations In heterosexuals, a *primary genital lesion* develops from 3 days to 3 weeks after exposure. It is a small, painless vesicle or nonindurated ulcer or papule located on the penis

in men and on the labia, posterior vagina, or fourchette in women. The primary lesion is noticed by less than one-third of men with LGV and only rarely by women. It heals in a few days without scarring and, even when noticed, is usually not recognized as LGV except in retrospect. LGV strains of *C. trachomatis* have occasionally been recovered from genital ulcers, and also from the urethra of men and the endocervix of women who present with inguinal adenopathy; these areas may be the primary site of infection in some cases.

In women and homosexual men, *primary anal or rectal infection* develops following receptive anorectal intercourse. In women, rectal infection with LGV (or non-LGV) strains of *C. trachomatis* presumably can also arise either via contiguous spread of infected secretions along the perineum (as with rectal gonococcal infection in women) or perhaps by spread to the rectum via the pelvic lymphatics.

From the site of the primary urethral, genital, anal, or rectal infection, the organism spreads via the regional lymphatics. Penile, vulvar, and anal infection can lead to inguinal and femoral lymphadenitis. Rectal infection produces hypogastric and deep iliac lymphadenitis. Upper vaginal or cervical infection results in enlargement of the obturator and iliac nodes.

The most common presenting picture in heterosexual men is the *inguinal syndrome*, which is characterized by painful inguinal lymphadenopathy beginning 2 to 6 weeks after presumed exposure; rarely the onset occurs after a few months. The inguinal adenopathy is unilateral in two-thirds of cases, and palpable enlargement of the iliac and femoral nodes is often evident on the same side as the enlarged inguinal nodes. The nodes are initially discrete, but progressive periadenitis results in a matted mass of nodes that becomes fluctuant and suppurative. The overlying skin becomes fixed, inflamed, and thinned and finally develops multiple draining fistulas. Extensive enlargement of chains of inguinal nodes above and below the inguinal ligament (''the sign of the groove'') is common but not specific and is documented in only a minority of cases. Histologically, infected nodes initially show characteristic small stellate abscesses surrounded by histiocytes. These abscesses coalesce to form large, necrotic, suppurative foci. Spontaneous healing usually occurs after several months; inguinal scars or granulomatous masses of varying size persist for life. Massive pelvic lymphadenopathy in women or homosexual men may lead to exploratory laparotomy.

As cultures and serologic tests for *C. trachomatis* are being used more often, increasing numbers of cases of LGV proctitis are being recognized in homosexual men. Such patients present with anorectal pain and mucopurulent, bloody rectal discharge. Although patients may complain of diarrhea, the condition usually represents frequent, painful, unsuccessful attempts at defecation (tenesmus). Sigmoidoscopy reveals ulcerative proctitis or proctocolitis, with purulent exudate and mucosal bleeding. The histopathologic findings in the rectal mucosa include granulomas with giant cells, along with crypt abscesses and extensive inflammation. These clinical, sigmoidoscopic, and histopathologic findings may closely resemble Crohn's disease of the rectum.

Constitutional symptoms are common during the stage of regional lymphadenopathy and, in the presence of proctitis, may include fever, chills, headache, meningismus, anorexia, myalgias, and arthralgias. These findings in the presence of lymphadenopathy are sometimes mistaken for malignant lymphoma. Other systemic complications are infrequent but include arthritis with sterile effusion, aseptic meningitis, meningoencephalitis, conjunctivitis, hepatitis, and erythema nodosum. Chlamydiae have been recovered from the cerebrospinal fluid and in one case were isolated from the blood of a patient with severe constitutional symptoms, indicating the occurrence of disseminated infection. Laboratory-acquired infections suspected of being due to inhalation of aerosols have been associated with mediastinal lymphadenitis, pneumonitis, and pleural effusion.

Complications of untreated anorectal infection include perirectal abscess, fistula in ano, and rectovaginal, rectovesical, and ischiorectal fistulas. Secondary bacterial infection probably contributes to these complications. Rectal stricture is a late complication of anorectal infection and usually occurs 2 to 6 cm from the anal orifice, within reach on digital rectal examination. Proximal extension of the stricture for several centimeters may lead to a mistaken clinical and radiographic diagnosis of carcinoma.

A small percentage of cases of LGV in men present as chronic progressive infiltrative, ulcerative, or fistular lesions of the penis, urethra, or scrotum. Associated lymphatic obstruction may produce elephantiasis. When urethral stricture occurs it usually involves the posterior urethra and causes incontinence or difficulty with urination.

APPROACH TO THE DIAGNOSIS AND TREATMENT OF *C. TRACHOMATIS* GENITAL INFECTIONS

Four types of laboratory procedures are available to confirm *C. trachomatis* infection. These are direct microscopic examination of tissue scrapings for typical intracytoplasmic inclusions; isolation of the organism in cell cultures; detection of chlamydial antigens or nucleic acid by immunologic or hybridization methods; and detection of antibody in the serum or in local secretions.

Except in conjunctivitis, direct microscopic examination of Giemsa-stained cell scrapings for typical inclusions has an unacceptably low sensitivity, and false-positive interpretations by inexperienced observers are common. But even for conjunctivitis this approach has been replaced by direct fluorescent antibody staining of conjunctival smears to identify chlamydial elementary bodies (see below).

Cell culture techniques are available in most large medical centers for isolation of *C. trachomatis*. While LGV strains grow well in many cell lines, the other *C. trachomatis* strains are much more difficult to culture. Although culture remains the gold standard for diagnosis of chlamydial infection, it is expensive, technically demanding, and not available to most clinicians. Therefore, nonculture methods utilizing antigen detection or nucleic acid hybridization have been developed that can be used instead of cultures. In the immunofluorescent slide test, potentially infected genital or ocular secretions are smeared on a slide, fixed, and stained with fluorescein-conjugated monoclonal antibody specific for chlamydial antigens. The observation of fluorescing elementary bodies confirms the diagnosis. Compared with culture, this test is 80 to 90 percent sensitive, and it is quite specific when used for confirmation of urethral, cervical, or ocular infection in high-risk patients with suspected *C. trachomatis* infection. The apparently lower sensitivity of the test in low-risk populations, along with its relatively labor-intensive nature, limits its value as a screening tool.

Enzyme-linked immunosorbent assay (ELISA) techniques for chlamydial antigen detection provide another alternative to culture. The reported sensitivity and specificity of these tests for genital infections have been 70 to 95 percent and 94 to 99 percent, respectively, in high-risk populations. Sensitivities have generally been higher in cervical infection (80 to 90 percent) and lower in urethritis among males (70 to 85 percent). Like the direct fluorescence antibody slide test, ELISA is less accurate in low-prevalence populations. ELISAs are better suited than culture to screening because large numbers of specimens can be easily processed. Newer diagnostic tests in which the polymerase chain reaction (PCR) is used to amplify small amounts of chlamydial DNA in samples are now being investigated and may offer greater sensitivity than current nonculture diagnostic methods for some purposes (e.g., for diagnosis of asymptomatic urethral infection in men). However, as such tests become commercially available, they are expected to be expensive, and their role remains to be defined.

Serologic tests have limited usefulness in the diagnosis of chlamydial oculogenital infections. The CF test with the heat-stable genus-specific antigen has been used to diagnose LGV with some success, but it is insensitive in non-LGV *C. trachomatis* infections. The microimmunofluorescence (micro-IF) test with *C. trachomatis* antigens is more sensitive but is generally available only in research laboratories. The test measures antibodies by serovar specificity and by immunoglobulin class (IgM, IgG, IgA, secretory IgA) in both serum and local secretions. Serologic diagnosis using the micro-IF test may be useful in infant pneumonia (in which high-titer IgM antibody and/or fourfold titer rises can often be demonstrated), in chlamydial salpingitis (especially Fitz-Hugh–Curtis syndrome), and in LGV.

Table 140-2 summarizes the diagnostic tests of choice for patients with suspected chlamydial infection. With few exceptions, the most suitable method for diagnosis is demonstration of the agent in cell culture or by antigen detection methods. Selection of the most appropriate of these tests depends upon local availability and expertise. In patients in whom medico-legal considerations may apply (victims of sexual or child abuse), cultures should always be used. Since *C. trachomatis* is an intracellular pathogen, adequate specimens for chlamydial culture must include epithelial cells. Cultures of pus result in fewer isolations of the organism. In urethritis, a thin-shafted urogenital swab should be inserted at least 2 cm into the urethra to obtain an appropriate specimen. Although cultures of urine for chlamydiae are less sensitive than urethral cultures, recent studies suggest that an ELISA for chlamydial antigen or a PCR test on a first-void urine specimen from men may be a reasonably sensitive diagnostic alternative to the more invasive urethral swab-based tests. When a cervical sample is taken for culture, the external os should first be cleaned of debris and purulent material; a plastic-shafted swab should then be inserted into the cervix, rotated slowly several times, and withdrawn. When conjunctival specimens are sought, the epithelium should be swabbed to remove cells rather than simply purulent material. All specimens for chlamydial culture should be placed immediately into transport medium and then either refrigerated (if they will reach the laboratory within 12 to 18 h) or frozen at $-70°C$ (if longer storage is anticipated). A major advantage of antigen detection techniques is their less rigid transport requirements.

From a public health viewpoint, the most effective use of chlamydial diagnostic testing has not been established and will vary depending upon clincial population, local resources, and laboratory expertise. The Centers for Disease Control and Prevention have recommended empiric treatment (without diagnostic testing if resources are not available for testing) of selected high-risk groups. These include men with NGU or sexually transmitted epididymitis; women with mucopurulent cervicitis (MPC) or PID; asymptomatic sex partners of patients with these syndromes; women and heterosexual men with gonorrhea (because of the high proportion of these patients who also have *C. trachomatis* infection); and sexual contacts of men or women with gonorrhea. Diagnostic testing has several potential benefits in these patients, including confirmation of infection and support of the clinical diagnosis (especially in women with MPC and PID), enhancement of sex partner referral and compliance with drug therapy, determination of prognosis, and education of physicians regarding the correlation of signs and symptoms with culture results. As chlamydial diagnostic testing becomes more widely available, its use for specific diagnosis in such patients should be promoted. Where diagnostic testing must be rationed because of limited resources, the highest priority should be given to the screening of asymptomatic high-risk women who would not otherwise receive treatment for presumptive chlamydial infection, especially those seen in high-risk settings (i.e., STD clinics, abortion clinics) and those with a high-risk profile (e.g., sexually active and ≤21 years of age, new sex partner within past 2 months, or more than one current sex partner).

ANTIMICROBIAL SUSCEPTIBILITY In laboratory tests that evaluate the growth of chlamydiae in cell cultures, the tetracyclines, erythromycin, rifampin, certain fluoroquinolones (especially ofloxacin), and the new macrolide azithromycin are all highly active against these organisms. Sulfonamides and clindamycin are also active against *C. trachomatis,* but to a lesser degree. Penicillin and ampicillin suppress chlamydial multiplication but do not eradicate the organism in vitro. The cephalosporins also appear relatively ineffective against *C. trachomatis*. Streptomycin, gentamicin, neomycin, kanamycin, vancomycin, ristocetin, spectinomycin, and nystatin are not effective

TABLE 140-2 Diagnostic tests in *C. trachomatis* infection

Infection	Suggestive signs/symptoms	Presumptive diagnosis*	Confirmatory test of choice
MEN			
Nongonococcal urethritis, postgonococcal urethritis	Discharge, dysuria	Gram's stain with more than four neutrophils per oil-immersion field, no gonococci	Urethral culture or antigen detection test for *C. trachomatis*
Epididymitis	Unilateral intrascrotal swelling, pain, tenderness; fever; nongonococcal urethritis	Gram stain with more than four neutrophils per oil immersion field, no gonococci	Urethral culture or antigen detection test for *C. trachomatis*
WOMEN			
Cervicitis	Mucopurulent cervical discharge, bleeding and edema of the zone of cervical ectopy	Cervical Gram's stain with ≥20 neutrophils per oil-immersion field in cervical mucus	Cervical culture or antigen detection test for *C. trachomatis*
Salpingitis	Lower abdominal pain, cervical motion tenderness, adnexal tenderness or masses	*C. trachomatis* always potentially present in salpingitis	Cervical culture or antigen detection test for *C. trachomatis*
Urethritis	Dysuria and frequency without urgency or hematuria	Mucopurulent cervicitis, sterile pyuria, negative routine urine culture	Urethral and cervical cultures or antigen detection test for *C. trachomatis*
ADULTS OF EITHER SEX			
Proctitis	Rectal pain, discharge, tenesmus, bleeding; history of receptive anorectal intercourse	Negative gonococcal culture and Gram's stain; at least one neutrophil in rectal Gram's stain	Rectal culture or direct immunofluorescence test for *C. trachomatis*
Reiter's syndrome	Nongonococcal urethritis, arthritis, conjunctivitis, typical skin lesions	Gram's stain with more than four neutrophils per oil-immersion field, no gonococci indicates nongonococcal urethritis	Urethral culture or antigen detection test for *C. trachomatis*
LGV	Regional adenopathy, primary lesion, proctitis, systemic symptoms	None	Isolation of LGV strain from node or rectum, occasionally from urethra or cervix; LGV CF titer, ≥1:64; micro-IF titer, ≥1:512
NEONATES			
Conjunctivitis	Purulent conjunctival discharge 6 to 18 days postdelivery	Negative cultures and Gram stains for gonococci, *Haemophilus* sp., pneumococci, staphylococci	Conjunctival culture or antigen detection test for *C. trachomatis;* Giemsa-stained scraping of conjunctival material can provide more rapid diagnosis but is less sensitive
Infant pneumonia	Afebrile, staccato cough, diffuse rales, bilateral hyperinflation, interstitial infiltrates	None	Chlamydial culture of sputum, pharynx, eye, rectum; micro-IF antibody to *C. trachomatis*—fourfold change in IgG or IgM antibody

* A presumptive diagnosis of chlamydial infection is often made in the syndromes listed when gonococci are not found. A positive test for *Neisseria gonorrhoeae* does not exclude *C. trachomatis,* which often is also present in patients with gonorrhea.

at concentrations inhibitory for most bacteria and fungi. There does not appear to be much strain-to-strain variation in susceptibility to antibiotics, and clinically significant antimicrobial resistance in chlamydiae has not been described. Thus antimicrobial susceptibility testing is not needed in the routine management of patients with chlamydial infection.

TREATMENT Until the introduction of azithromycin, chlamydial infections could not be eradicated by single-dose or short-term antimicrobial regimens. In most situations in adults, 7 days of treatment with doxycycline or tetracycline should be given for uncomplicated genital infections, but 2 weeks of therapy is recommended for complicated chlamydial infections (e.g., PID, epididymitis) and for LGV. Failure after treatment of genital infections with a tetracycline usually indicates poor compliance or reinfection.

Therapy for *C. trachomatis* urethritis is more effective than therapy for other forms of NGU. *C. trachomatis* is eradicated from the urethra by treatment with tetracycline hydrochloride, 500 mg qid for 7 days, or doxycycline, 100 mg by mouth bid for 7 days. An effective alternative regimen is erythromycin, 500 mg qid for 7 days.

Eradiction of *C. trachomatis* from the cervix has been demonstrated with similar doses and durations of tetracycline, doxycycline, and erythromycin. Erythromycin base, 500 mg qid for 10 to 14 days, is the regimen of choice for pregnant women with *C. trachomatis* infection. Amoxicillin, 500 mg tid for 10 days, has also been used successfully in one study of pregnant women. Tetracycline hydrochloride, 500 mg qid, or doxycycline, 100 mg bid, for 14 days, produces clinical and microbiologic cure of epididymitis and PID associated with *C. trachomatis* infection, but in this situation tetracycline should always be used together with a drug that is highly effective against gonorrhea.

Two relatively new antimicrobial agents have recently been approved for treatment of uncomplicated chlamydial genital infections in men and women. Ofloxacin, 300 mg orally twice daily for 7 days, is as effective as doxycycline for treatment of chlamydial infection and appears to be safe and well tolerated. It cannot be used in pregnancy. Azithromycin, a macrolide, has been effective in uncomplicated chlamydial infection as a 1-g single dose. It causes fewer adverse gastrointestinal reactions than do older macrolides like erythromycin. Both ofloxacin and azithromycin offer alternatives for treatment that may be of value in selected patients allergic to or intolerant of tetracyclines and erythromycin, but they are considerably more expensive than these standard regimens. The single-dose regimen of azithromycin has great appeal for the treatment of patients with a history of poor compliance, particularly those seen in urgent-care settings (e.g., emergency rooms), where follow-up is not assured.

Treatment of sex partners The continued high prevalence of chlamydial infections in most parts of the United States is due primarily to the failure to diagnose—and therefore treat—patients with symptomatic or asymptomatic infection and their sex partners. Cases of NGU, epididymitis, Reiter's syndrome, and mucopurulent endocervicitis are sometimes not treated with antimicrobials, and sex partners are treated even less often. *C. trachomatis* urethral or cervical infection has been well documented in a high proportion of the sex partners of patients with NGU, epididymitis, Reiter's syndrome, salpingitis, or endocervicitis. If possible, confirmatory laboratory tests for *Chlamydia* should be undertaken in such patients, but even those without evidence of clinical disease who have recently been exposed to proven or possible chlamydial infection (for example, NGU) should be offered therapy.

In neonates with conjunctivitis or infants with pneumonia, erythromycin ethylsuccinate or estolate can be given orally in a dose of 50 mg/kg per day, preferably as 122.5 mg/kg qid, for 2 weeks. Careful attention must be given to compliance with therapy—a frequent problem. Relapses of eye infection are common following treatment with topical erythromycin or tetracycline opthalmic ointment and may also occur after oral erythromycin therapy. Thus follow-up cultures should be obtained after treatment. Both parents should be examined for *C. trachomatis* infection and, if diagnostic tests are not readily available, should be treated with a tetracycline.

PREVENTION Early diagnosis and treatment shorten the duration of infectiousness of the carrier and therefore constitute primary prevention of chlamydial infection. By the early 1990s, one of the 10 regions of the United States (region X, the Pacific Northwest) had formally undertaken a chlamydial control program utilizing widespread testing. Approximately 500,000 tests per year were undertaken in 150 family planning clinics throughout the region in women meeting criteria for high risk. Within 5 years, the prevalence of chlamydial infection had fallen from 10 percent to 5 percent. It is appalling that, as of 1992, no other U.S. region had attempted a similar control effort. Moreover, throughout the nation, many public STD clinics still were not offering chlamydial testing, which has been performed for as little as $5 per test in region X.

TRACHOMA AND ADULT INCLUSION CONJUNCTIVITIS

DEFINITION Trachoma is a chronic conjunctivitis associated with infection by *C. trachomatis* serovars A, B, Ba, and C. It has produced an estimated 20 million cases of blindness throughout the world and remains an important preventable cause of blindness. Inclusion conjunctivitis is an acute ocular infection caused by sexually transmitted *C. trachomatis* strains (usually serovars D through K) in adults exposed to infected genital secretions and in their newborn offspring.

EPIDEMIOLOGY Epidemiologically, two types of eye disease are caused by *C. trachomatis*. In trachoma-endemic areas where the classic eye disease is seen, transmission is from eye to eye via hands, flies, towels, and other fomites and usually involves serovar A, B, Ba, or C. In nonendemic areas, organisms of serovars D through K can be transmitted from the genital tract to the eye, usually causing only the inclusion conjunctivitis syndrome, occasionally with keratitis. Rarely the eye disease acquired in this way progresses with the development of pannus and scars similar to those seen in endemic trachoma. These cases may be referred to as paratrachoma to differentiate them epidemiologically from eye-to-eye-transmitted endemic trachoma.

The worldwide incidence and severity of trachoma have decreased dramatically during the past 35 years in areas with improving hygienic and economic conditions. Endemic trachoma is still the major cause of preventable blindness in north Africa, sub-Saharan Africa, the Middle East, and parts of Asia. Transmission of the endemic disease occurs primarily through close personal contact, particularly among young children in rural communities with limited water supplies. In endemic areas, trachoma is associated with repeated exposure and reinfection, but the infection can also be latent. In the United States a mild form of endemic trachoma still occurs in Mexican Americans as well as in immigrants from areas where trachoma is endemic. Acute relapse of old trachoma occasionally follows treatment with cortisone eye ointment or develops in very old persons who were exposed in their youth.

CLINICAL MANIFESTATIONS Both endemic trachoma and adult inclusion conjunctivitis present initially as a conjunctivitis characterized by small lymphoid follicles in the conjunctiva. In regions with hyperendemic classic blinding trachoma, the disease usually starts insidiously before the age of 2 years. Reinfection is common and probably contributes to the pathogenesis of trachoma. Studies using PCR techniques indicate that chlamydial DNA is often present in the ocular secretions of patients with trachoma, even in the absence of positive cultures. Thus persistent infection may be more common than was previously thought.

The cornea becomes involved with inflammatory leukocytic infiltrations and superficial vascularization (pannus formation). As the inflammation continues, conjunctival scarring eventually distorts the eyelids, causing them to turn inward so that the inturned lashes constantly abrade the eyeball (trichiasis and entropion); eventually the corneal epithelium is abraded and may ulcerate, with subsequent corneal scarring and blindness. Destruction of the conjunctival goblet cells, lacrimal ducts, and lacrimal gland may produce a ''dry-eye'' syndrome, with resultant corneal opacity due to drying (xerosis) or secondary bacterial corneal ulcers.

Communities with blinding trachoma often experience seasonal epidemics of conjunctivitis due to *Haemophilus influenzae* that contribute to the intensity of the inflammatory process. In such areas the active infectious process usually resolves spontaneously in affected persons between 10 and 15 years of age, but the conjunctival scars continue to shrink, producing trichiasis and entropion and subsequent corneal scarring in adults. In areas with milder and less prevalent disease, the process may be much slower, with active disease continuing into adulthood; blindness is rare in these cases.

Eye infection with genital *C. trachomatis* strains in sexually active young adults presents as the acute onset of unilateral follicular conjunctivitis and preauricular lymphadenopathy similar to that seen in acute adenovirus or herpesvirus conjunctivitis. If untreated, the disease may persist for 6 weeks to 2 years. It is frequently associated with corneal inflammation in the form of discrete opacities (''infiltrates''), punctate epithelial erosions, and minor degrees of superficial corneal vascularization. Very rarely conjunctival scarring and eyelid distortion occur, particularly in patients treated for many months with topical glucocorticoids. Recurrent eye infections develop most often in patients whose sexual consorts are not treated with antimicrobials.

DIAGNOSIS The clinical diagnosis of classic trachoma can be made if two of the following signs are present:

1 Lymphoid follicles on the upper tarsal conjunctiva
2 Typical conjunctival scarring
3 Vascular pannus
4 Limbal follicles or their sequelae, Herbert's pits

The clinical diagnosis of endemic trachoma should be confirmed by laboratory tests in children with more marked degrees of inflammation. Intracytoplasmic chlamydial inclusions are found in 10 to 60 percent of Giemsa-stained conjunctival smears in such populations, but isolation in cell cultures, newer antigen detection tests, or chlamydial PCR is more sensitive. Follicular conjunctivitis in adult Europeans or Americans living in trachomatous regions is rarely due to trachoma.

Sporadic cases of adult inclusion conjunctivitis must be differentiated from adenovirus and herpes simplex virus keratoconjunctivitis during the first 15 days after onset and from other forms of chronic follicular conjunctivitis later. Demonstration of chlamydial infection by Giemsa- or immunofluorescent-stained smears or by isolation in cell cultures constitutes definitive evidence of infection. Genital examination and tests for genital chlamydial infection are indicated. Serum antibody does not constitute evidence of chlamydial eye infection since many sexually active adults have acquired serum antibody from genital infection. A practical diagnostic procedure in cases with chronic follicular conjunctivitis is treatment for 6 days with an oral tetracycline or erythromycin; a marked response of symptoms within 3 to 4 days is highly suggestive of inclusion conjunctivitis, and treatment should be continued for at least 3 weeks.

DIFFERENTIAL DIAGNOSIS OF CONJUNCTIVITIS AND KERATOCONJUNCTIVITIS The eye and its adnexa may be infected during the course of many cutaneous and systemic viral diseases. Sometimes these ocular infections produce minor manifestations, such as the transient loss of accommodation in dengue and the milder forms of conjunctivitis in systemic adenovirus infections. Other virus infections, however, such as herpes simplex (see Chap. 143), herpes zoster (see Chap. 144), measles (see Chap. 155), and vaccinia (see Chap. 147), occasionally produce serious and permanent visual loss. In addition, congenital infections are an important cause of blindness, particularly rubella, which leads to cataracts and microphthalmus; cytomegalic inclusion disease with retinal involvement; and syphilis with interstitial keratitis or optic neuritis. Among the viral infections limited to the outer eye and manifested as a follicular conjunctivitis are epidemic keratoconjunctivitis, herpes simplex keratoconjunctivitis, Newcastle disease virus conjunctivitis, and acute hemorrhagic conjunctivitis.

TREATMENT Public health control programs for endemic trachoma have consisted of the mass application of tetracycline or erythromycin ointment to the eyes of all children in affected communities for 21 to 60 days or on an intermittent schedule. These programs also include surgical correction of inturned eyelids by a mobile surgical team that visits each locality. Oral erythromycin, but none of the oral tetracyclines, offers an alternative method of mass antibiotic treatment for trachoma of young children and pregnant women.

Adult inclusion conjunctivitis responds well to treatment with full doses of systemic tetracycline or erythromycin for 3 weeks. Treating all sexual consorts of the patient simultaneously is also necessary to prevent ocular reinfection and to avoid the genital diseases due to chlamydial infection. Topical antibiotic treatment is not required for patients treated with systemic antibiotics.

PREVENTION Efforts to develop a trachoma vaccine have not yet been successful. General hygienic measures associated with improved living standards are effective in the elimination of endemic trachoma. Adequate water supply for personal cleanliness may be a key factor. In some areas the reduction of flies in the household is important.

PSITTACOSIS

DEFINITION Psittacosis is primarily an infectious disease of birds that is caused by *Chlamydia psittaci*. Transmission of infection from birds to humans results in a febrile illness characterized by pneumonitis and systemic manifestations. Inapparent infections or mild influenza-like illnesses may also occur. The term *ornithosis* is sometimes applied to infections contracted from birds other than parrots or parakeets, but *psittacosis* is the preferred generic term for all forms of the disease.

EPIDEMIOLOGY Almost any avian species can harbor *C. psittaci*. Psittacine birds (parrots, parakeets, budgerigars) are most commonly infected, but human cases have been traced to contact with pigeons, ducks, turkeys, chickens, and many other birds. Psittacosis may be considered an occupational disease of pet-shop owners, poultry workers, pigeon fanciers, taxidermists, veterinarians, and zoo attendants. During the past 20 years, there has been an increase in incidence, with cases and outbreaks occurring primarily among employees of poultry processing plants. It is suspected that many cases are undiagnosed and not reported. The disease appears to be more common in England, where budgerigars are popular household pets and where restrictions on the importation of these birds have been eased.

The agent is present in nasal secretions, excreta, tissues, and feathers of infected birds. Although the disease can be fatal, infected birds frequently show only minor evidence of illness, such as ruffled feathers, lethargy, and anorexia. Asymptomatic avian carriers are common, and complete recovery may be followed by continued shedding of the organism for many months.

Psittacosis is almost always transmitted to humans by the respiratory route. On rare occasions the disease may be acquired from the bite of a pet bird. Prolonged contact is not essential for transmission of the disease; a few minutes spent in an environment previously occupied by an infected bird has resulted in human infection. The severity of the disease in humans bears no apparent relationship to closeness or duration of contact, although sick birds are more likely to transmit infection than healthy ones. A psittacosis-like agent has been transmitted among hospital personnel, with severe and sometimes fatal infections. There is evidence that these "human" strains are more virulent than avian organisms. There is no record of infection acquired by eating poultry products.

PATHOGENESIS The psittacosis agent gains entrance to the body through the upper part of the respiratory tract, spreads via the bloodstream, and eventually localizes in the pulmonary alveoli and in the reticuloendothelial cells of the spleen and liver. Invasion of the lung probably takes place by way of the bloodstream rather than by direct extension from the upper air passages. A lymphocytic inflammatory response occurs on both the interstitial and the respiratory surfaces of the alveoli as well as in the perivascular spaces. The alveolar walls and interstitial tissues of the lung are thickened, edematous, necrotic, and occasionally hemorrhagic. Histologically, the affected areas show alveolar spaces filled with fluid, erythrocytes, and lymphocytes. The picture is not pathognomonic of psittacosis unless macrophages containing characteristic cytoplasmic inclusion bodies (LCL bodies) can be identified. The respiratory epithelium of the bronchi and bronchioles usually remains intact.

CLINICAL MANIFESTATIONS The clinical manifestations and course of psittacosis are extremely variable. After an incubation period of 7 to 14 days or longer, the disease may start abruptly with shaking chills and fever ranging as high as 40.5°C (105°F), but the onset is often gradual with fever increasing over a 3- to 4-day period. Headache is almost always a prominent symptom; it is usually diffuse and excruciating and is often the patient's chief complaint.

Many patients present with a dry hacking cough that is usually nonproductive, but small amounts of mucoid or bloody sputum may be raised as the disease progresses. Cough may begin early in the course of the disease or as late as 5 days after the onset of fever. Chest pain, pleurisy with effusion, or a friction rub may all occur but are rare. Pericarditis and myocarditis have been reported. Most patients have a normal or slightly increased respiratory rate; marked dyspnea with cyanosis occurs only in severe psittacosis with extensive pulmonary involvement. In psittacosis, as in most nonbacterial pneumonias, the physical signs of pneumonitis tend to be less prominent than symptoms and x-ray findings would suggest. The initial examination may reveal fine sibilant rales, or clinical evidence of pneumonia may be completely lacking. Rales usually become audible and more numerous as the illness progresses. Signs of frank pulmonary consolidation are usually absent. Symptoms of upper respiratory tract infection are not prominent, although mild sore throat, pharyngitis, and cervical adenopathy are often present; on occasion the last may be the only manifestations of illness. Epistaxis is encountered early in the course of nearly one-fourth of cases. Photophobia is also a common complaint.

Patients often report generalized myalgia, and spasm and stiffness of the muscles of the back and neck may lead to an erroneous diagnosis of meningitis. Lethargy, mental depression, agitation, insomnia, and disorientation have been prominent features of the illness in some epidemics but not in others; delirium and stupor develop near the end of the first week in severe cases. Occasional patients are comatose when first seen, and the diagnosis of psittacosis may be elusive in these cases. Gastrointestinal problems such as abdominal pain, nausea, vomiting, or diarrhea are noted in some cases; constipation and abdominal distention sometimes occur as late complications. Icterus, the result of severe hepatic involvement, is a rare and ominous finding. A faint macular rash (Horder's spots) simulating the rose spots of typhoid fever has been described.

Patients without cough or other clinical evidence of respiratory involvement present with fever of unknown origin (see Chap. 16). The pulse rate is slow in relation to the fever. When splenomegaly is present in a patient with acute pneumonitis, psittacosis should be considered; the reported incidence of splenomegaly in this disease ranges from 10 to 70 percent. Nontender hepatic enlargement also occurs, but jaundice is rare. Thrombophlebitis is not unusual during convalescence; indeed, pulmonary infarction is sometimes a late complication and may be fatal.

In untreated cases of psittacosis, sustained or mildly remittent fever persists for 10 days to 3 weeks or occasionally for as long as 3 months. Over this period, the respiratory manifestations gradually abate. Psittacosis contracted from parrots or parakeets is more likely to be a severe, prolonged illness than infection acquired from pigeons or barnyard fowl. Relapses occur but are rare. Occasional patients develop endocarditis, and *C. psittaci* infection should be considered in cases of culture-negative endocarditis. Secondary bacterial infections are uncommon. Immunity to reinfection is probably permanent.

LABORATORY FINDINGS The chest x-ray in psittacosis mimics that in a great variety of pulmonary diseases. The pneumonic lesions are usually patchy in appearance but can be hazy, diffuse, homogeneous, lobar, atelectatic, wedge-shaped, nodular, or miliary. The white blood cell count is normal or moderately decreased in the acute phase of the disease but may rise in convalescence. The erythrocyte sedimentation rate is frequently not elevated. Transient proteinuria is common. The cerebrospinal fluid sometimes contains a few mononuclear cells but is otherwise normal. Despite hepatomegaly, the results of liver function tests are generally normal.

The diagnosis can be confirmed only by isolation of the causative microorganism or by serologic studies. The agent is present in the blood during the acute phase of the disease and in the bronchial secretions for weeks or sometimes years after infection, but it is difficult to isolate. Further, the organism is hazardous to work with in the laboratory, and most clinical laboratories do not offer culture for *C. psittaci*. Thus psittacosis is most readily diagnosed by the demonstration of a rising titer of CF antibody in the serum of a patient with a compatible clinical syndrome. Both an acute-phase and a convalescent-phase specimen should always be tested. *C. trachomatis*, *C. psittaci*, and *C. pneumoniae* all share a genus-specific "group" antigen, which is the basis of the CF test. Thus acute infections with *C. trachomatis* or *C. pneumoniae* can also produce titer rises in the CF test. However, these three species have different MOMPs that are the principal antigens in the micro-IF test. If there is doubt as to the interpretation of the CF test, the micro-IF test can therefore be used to differentiate among them. The prompt initiation of treatment with tetracycline has been shown to delay an antibody rise in convalescence for several weeks or months.

DIFFERENTIAL DIAGNOSIS A history of exposure to birds may be the only clinical basis for differentiating psittacosis from a variety of infectious and noninfectious febrile disorders. A partial list of pulmonary diseases that may be confused with psittacosis includes *Mycoplasma* pneumonia, *C. pneumoniae* pneumonia, legionellosis, viral pneumonia, Q fever, coccidioidomycosis, tuberculosis, enteroviral infection, carcinoma of the lung with bronchial obstruction, and common bacterial pneumonias. In the early stages, before pneumonitis appears, psittacosis may be mistaken for influenza, typhoid fever, miliary tuberculosis, and infectious mononucleosis.

TREATMENT The tetracyclines are consistently effective in the treatment of psittacosis. Defervescence and alleviation of symptoms usually take place within 24 to 48 h after the institution of therapy with 2 g daily in four divided doses. To avoid relapse, treatment should probably be continued for at least 7 to 14 days after defervescence. In severe cases, hospitalization and pulmonary intensive care may be indicated. Sulfonamides are not active against *C. psittaci*. Erythromycin can be used in patients allergic to or intolerant of tetracyclines.

C. PNEUMONIAE INFECTIONS

A third chlamydial species, *C. pneumoniae*, has been described. *C. pneumoniae* can be distinguished from the other two species on the basis of DNA hybridization and restriction endonuclease analyses. Although *C. pneumoniae* can be grown in a variety of cell cultures, it is considerably more difficult to culture than other chlamydiae, especially from clinical specimens. Fewer than 50 isolates have been obtained from patients worldwide. HL cells appear to be the most effective cell line for isolation of *C. pneumoniae*.

Knowledge of the epidemiology of *C. pneumoniae* infections has been derived primarily from serologic studies. Infections begin to occur in late childhood and adolescence and continue throughout adult life. Seroprevalence in the many adult populations that have been tested throughout the world exceeds 40 percent—a figure suggesting that *C. pneumoniae* infections are ubiquitous. Secondary episodes (reinfections) appear to occur in older adults throughout life. In Scandinavia, *C. pneumoniae* produces epidemics of pneumonia and respiratory illness followed by periods of infrequent infection. The incidence of infections outside of epidemics remains poorly defined. Transmission appears to be from person to person, probably primarily in schools and family units.

The clinical spectrum of *C. pneumoniae* infection includes acute pharyngitis, sinusitis, bronchitis, and pneumonitis, primarily in young adults. The clinical manifestations seen in primary infection appear to be more severe and prolonged than those seen in reinfection. The pneumonitis resembles *Mycoplasma pneumoniae* pneumonia in that leukocytosis is frequently absent and patients often have prominent antecedent upper respiratory tract symptoms, fever, nonproductive cough, mild to moderate degree of illness, minimal findings on chest auscultation, and small segmental infiltrates on chest x-ray. In elderly patients, pneumonia due to *C. pneumoniae* can be especially severe and may necessitate hospitalization and respiratory support.

Epidemiologic studies have demonstrated an association between serologic evidence of *C. pneumoniae* infection and coronary atherosclerotic disease. In addition, *C. pneumoniae* has been identified in atherosclerotic plaques by electron microscopy, DNA hybridization, and immunostaining. The clinical significance of these findings is not yet clear.

Diagnosis of *C. pneumoniae* infection is currently difficult because cell culture techniques are not available for routine clinical use and noncultural tests using antigen detection methods or DNA probes have not been developed. Acute- and convalescent-phase sera can be tested for chlamydial CF antibody to make a retrospective diagnosis. However, this test does not distinguish *C. pneumoniae* infection from infection due to *C. trachomatis* or *C. psittaci*. Although controlled treatment trials have not been conducted, *C. pneumoniae* is inhibited in vitro by erythromycin and tetracycline. Recommended therapy is 2 g/d of either agent for 10 to 14 days.

REFERENCES

Cates W Jr, Wasserheit JN: Genital chlamydial infections: Epidemiology and reproductive sequelae. Am J Obstet Gynecol 164:1771, 1991

Centers for Disease Control: *Chlamydia trachomatis* infections: Policy guidelines for prevention and control. MMWR 34:535, 1985

CHERNESKY M et al: Detection of *Chlamydia trachomatis* antigens in urine as an alternative to swabs and cultures. J Infect Dis 161:124, 1989

COULTS II et al: Clinical and radiographic features of psittacosis infection. Thorax 40:530, 1985

GRAYSTON JT: Infections caused by *Chlamydia pneumoniae*, strain TWAR. Clin Infect Dis 15:757, 1992

——— et al: A new *Chlamydia psittaci* strain, TWAR, isolated in acute respiratory tract infections. N Engl J Med 315:161, 1986

HANDSFIELD HH et al: Criteria for selective screening for *Chlamydia trachomatis* infection in women attending family planning clinics. JAMA 255:1730, 1986

HOLMES KK: Lower genital tract infections in women: Cystitis, urethritis, vulvovaginitis, and cervicitis, in *Sexually Transmitted Diseases*, 2d ed, KK Holmes et al (eds). New York, McGraw-Hill, 1990

JONES RB: Treatment of *Chlamydia trachomatis* infections of the urogenital tract, in *Chlamydial Infections*, WE Bowie et al (eds). London, Cambridge University Press, 1990, pp 509–519

MARTIN DH et al: A controlled trial of a single dose of azithromycin for the treatment of chlamydial urethritis and cervicitis. N Engl J Med 327: 921, 1992

RETTIG PJ: Perinatal infections with *Chlamydia trachomatis*. Clin Perinatol 15:321, 1988

SCHACHTER J et al: Experience with the routine use of erythromycin for chlamydial infections in pregnancy. N Engl J Med 314:276, 1986

SHAFER MA et al: Urinary leukocyte esterase test for asymptomatic chlamydia and gonococcal infections in males. JAMA 262:2562, 1989

STAMM WE: Diagnosis of *Chlamydia trachomatis* genitourinary infections. Ann Intern Med 108:710, 1988

———, HOLMES KK: *Chlamydia trachomatis* infections in adults, in *Sexually Transmitted Diseases*, 2d, ed KK Holmes et al (eds). New York, McGraw-Hill, 1990

——— et al: *Chlamydia trachomatis* urethral infections in men. Prevalence, risk factors, and clinical manifestations. Ann Intern Med 100:47, 1984

TOOMEY KE, BARNES RC: Treatment of *Chlamydia trachomatis* genital infections. Rev Infect Dis 12 (suppl 6):S645, 1990

section 11   Viral diseases

141   THE BIOLOGY OF VIRUSES

KENNETH L. TYLER / BERNARD N. FIELDS

STRUCTURE AND CLASSIFICATION OF VIRUSES   A typical virus particle (*virion*) contains a core of nucleic acid of either DNA or RNA. There is considerable variability in the structure and size of animal viruses and their associated nucleic acids (Table 141-1 and Fig. 141-1). The genomes of smallest molecular weight, such as those of the Parvoviridae, encode three or four proteins, whereas the larger genomes, such as those of the Poxviridae, encode more than 100 structural proteins and enzymes. The number of proteins encoded by a viral genome may be greater than predicted from the genome's molecular weight because of the presence of multiple open reading frames and/or overlapping regions of nucleic acid that can be transcribed into several distinct messenger RNAs. Extensive nucleotide sequence data are available for part or all of the genomes of many viruses.

The viral nucleic acid is surrounded by either a single or double protein shell (*capsid*). The viral nucleic acid plus the capsid are referred to as the *nucleocapsid*. The viral capsids are composed of smaller repetitive subunits (*capsomers*) arranged in symmetric constructions. The repeating subunits facilitate assembly of viral proteins into mature virions and reduce the amount of genomic information required to encode structural proteins. Capsids are formed by self-assembly of their structural subunits.

The two fundamental patterns of capsid structural symmetry are icosahedral and helical. Some of the largest viruses, such as the poxviruses, have more complex structural patterns. The retroviruses appear to have icosahedral capsid symmetry and helical core symmetry. Viruses with icosahedral capsid symmetry generally follow principles of physical organization that specify the total allowable number of structural subunits. The nucleic acid in icosahedral viruses is usually in a condensed form and is geometrically independent of the surrounding capsid structure.

Animal viruses with helical symmetry have RNA genomes. A general feature of animal viruses is the binding of protein subunits of the capsid in a regular, periodic fashion along the viral RNA. This close interaction between the capsid proteins and nucleic acid is in sharp contrast to the loose interactions in viruses with icosahedral symmetry and imposes different constraints for viral assembly.

Many viruses have an envelope surrounding the nucleocapsid. The viral envelope is composed of virus-specific proteins and of lipids and carbohydrates derived from host cell membranes. The host cell components are added as the virus buds through the host cell nuclear membrane, endoplasmic reticulum, Golgi apparatus, or cytoplasmic membrane. Different viruses utilize distinctive types of host cell membranes for budding. The factors that determine this specificity are incompletely understood. In some cases, virus-specific envelope proteins may include a matrix protein (*M protein*), which lines the inner side of the envelope and is in contact with the nucleocapsid. Virus-specific glycoproteins protrude from the outer surface of the envelope (e.g., as "spikes") and may in some cases contain hydrophobic domains, which span the lipid bilayer of the envelope, as well as internal domains, which may contact the M proteins.

Viral proteins, referred to as *structural* or *virion proteins*, can form the viral capsid, can be a major component of viral envelopes, or can be associated with the viral nucleic acid (*core proteins*). A number of viruses contain surface glycoproteins that agglutinate red blood cells (*hemagglutinins*) by binding to receptors on the red cell surface. Many viruses contain proteins with enzymatic activity. In many cases these enzymes are required for the synthesis of messenger RNA (mRNA) of the appropriate (+) polarity for translation into protein or for replication of the viral genome.

The earliest classifications of viruses were based solely on their ability to pass through filters with small pore sizes. Subsequent classifications stressed pathogenic properties, specific organ tropisms (e.g., enteroviruses), or epidemiologic characteristics (e.g., arboviruses). Current classifications of viruses are based on a combination of genetic, physicochemical, and biologic factors. These include the type and structure of the viral nucleic acid; the nature of virion ultrastructure, including size, type of capsid symmetry, capsid composition; and the presence or absence of an envelope; as well as the strategy used by the virus for genome replication. The reliance on morphologic criteria often means that electron-micrographic studies provide sufficient information to identify both the family and the genus to which a virus belongs. Subdivisions within major viral taxonomic groups may be based on immunologic, cytopathologic, pathogenetic, or epidemiologic features. The application of recombinant DNA techniques will require revision of these classifications based on degrees of genetic relatedness.

REPLICATION   *Replication* refers to the process by which viruses infect susceptible cells, reproduce their genomic material and proteins, and assemble and release infectious progeny. The diversity among viruses in terms of structure and type of genomic material is reflected by the large number of replicative strategies.

The first stage of viral infection of target cells begins with adsorption of the virus particles and ends when the infectious progeny

TABLE 141-1 Structure of viral nucleic acid

Family	Example	Type of nucleic acid	Genome size, kilobases or kilobase pairs	Envelope	Capsid symmetry
Picornaviridae	Poliovirus	ss(+)RNA	7.2–8.4	No	I
Caliciviridae	Norwalk virus	ss(+)RNA	8	No	I
Togaviridae	Rubella virus	ss(+)RNA	12	Yes	I
Flaviviridae	Yellow fever virus	ss(+)RNA	10	Yes	UNK
Coronaviridae	Coronaviruses	ss(+)RNA	16–21	Yes	H
Rhabdoviridae	Rabies virus	ss(−)RNA	13–16	Yes	H
Filoviridae	Marburg virus	ss(−)RNA	13	Yes	H
Paramyxoviridae	Measles virus	ss(−)RNA	16–20	Yes	H
Orthomyxoviridae	Influenza viruses	8 ss(−)RNA segments*	14	Yes	H
Bunyaviridae	California encephalitis virus	3 circular ss(−)RNA segments	13–21	Yes	H
Arenaviridae	Lymphocytic choriomeningitis virus	2 circular ss(−)RNA segments	10–14	Yes	H
Reoviridae	Rotaviruses	10–12 dsRNA† segments	16–27	No	I
Retroviridae	HIV-1	2 identical ss(+)RNA segments	3–9	Yes	I-capsid H-nucleocapsid (probable)
Hepadnaviridae	Hepatitis B virus	dsDNA with ss portions	3	Yes	UNK
Parvoviridae	Human parvovirus B-19	ss(+) or (−) DNA	5	No	I
Papovaviridae	JC virus	Circular dsDNA	5–8	No	I
Adenoviridae	Human adenoviruses	dsDNA	36–38	No	I
Herpesviridae	Herpes simplex virus	dsDNA	120–200	Yes	I
Poxviridae	Vaccinia virus	dsDNA with covalently closed ends	130–280	Yes	Complex

* Influenza C = 7 segments.
† Reovirus, orbivirus = 10 segments; rotavirus = 11 segments; Colorado tick fever virus = 12 segments.
NOTE: ds = double-stranded; ss = single-stranded; (+) message sense; (−) anti-message sense; I = icosahedral; H = helical; UNK = unknown.
SOURCE: FA Murphy, DW Kingsbury, in *Fields' Virology*, BN Fields, DM Knipe (eds), New York, Raven Press, 1990.

virus begins to form. This stage is often referred to as the *eclipse period* and may last from a few hours (picornaviruses) to more than 72 h (some herpesviruses). From the beginning of this period (adsorption) to the end (formation of infectious progeny virus), there is a dramatic drop in the amount of infectious virus that can be recovered from disrupted cells.

Adsorption appears to be a process that is initially reversible, resulting from random collisions between viruses and target cells. It has been estimated that only 1 in 10^3 to 10^4 such collisions leads to tighter binding (*attachment*). Attachment is facilitated by the appropriate ionic and pH conditions but is largely temperature-independent and does not require energy. Adsorption of virus to a target cell may involve specific binding of viral proteins to receptors on the cell surface. The virion structure mediating cell attachment has been identified for a number of viruses. For enveloped viruses, the viral attachment protein is typically one of the "spikes" inserted on the outer surface of the viral envelope such as the hemagglutinin (HA) of influenza viruses or the gp120 protein of human immunodeficiency virus (HIV). For some enveloped viruses, such as the herpesviruses and vaccinia virus, attachment may be mediated by several proteins acting together. In nonenveloped viruses, surface polypeptides, such as the fiber protein of adenovirus and the hemagglutinin (σ1) protein of reovirus, often function as attachment proteins.

The exact nature of the cellular receptors for animal viruses is known in only a few specific cases. Among the putative cell surface receptors for viruses are sialic acid residues (influenza virus), epidermal growth factor receptor (vaccinia virus), lymphocyte antigen CD4 (HIV), complement receptor CR2 (Epstein-Barr virus), intercellular adhesion molecule ICAM-1 (human rhinovirus 14), heparan sulfate (herpes simplex virus), and an immunoglobulin superfamily protein (poliovirus) (Table 141-2). Even when the specific receptor

is still unknown, it has been possible to identify "families" or classes of viral receptors using competition binding studies. Viruses of the same species but different serotypes may compete for the same receptor class (e.g., poliovirus serotypes 1, 2, 3) or for different receptor classes (e.g., human rhinovirus 2 and 14). Viruses from

TABLE 141-2 Putative viral receptors

Virus	Receptor
Cytomegalovirus	Beta-2-microglobulin/MHC
Echovirus 1	Integrin VLA-2
Ecotropic murine leukemia virus	y$^+$, membrane amino acid transporter
Encephalomyocarditis virus	Glycophorin A (RBCs)
Epstein-Barr virus	C3d receptor (CR2) (CD21)
Herpes simplex virus	Heparan sulfate proteoglycans
Human coronavirus 229E	Human aminopeptidase N
Human immunodeficiency virus	CD4 (T4 antigen)
Human rhinovirus 14	ICAM-1 (CD54)
Influenza virus	Glycophorin A (RBCs) Sialic acid
Lactate dehydrogenase elevating virus	Ia
Mouse hepatitis virus	CEA family glycoprotein
Poliovirus	Immunoglobulin superfamily protein
Rabies virus	Acetylcholine receptor
Reovirus type 3 (Dearing)	Glycophorin A (RBCs), sialic acid residues
Semliki Forest virus	HLA, H-2 antigens
Sendai virus	Sialic acid
Sindbis virus	Laminin receptor
SV40	Class I MHC
Vaccinia virus	Epidermal growth factor receptor
Vesicular stomatitis virus	Phospho- or glycolipids

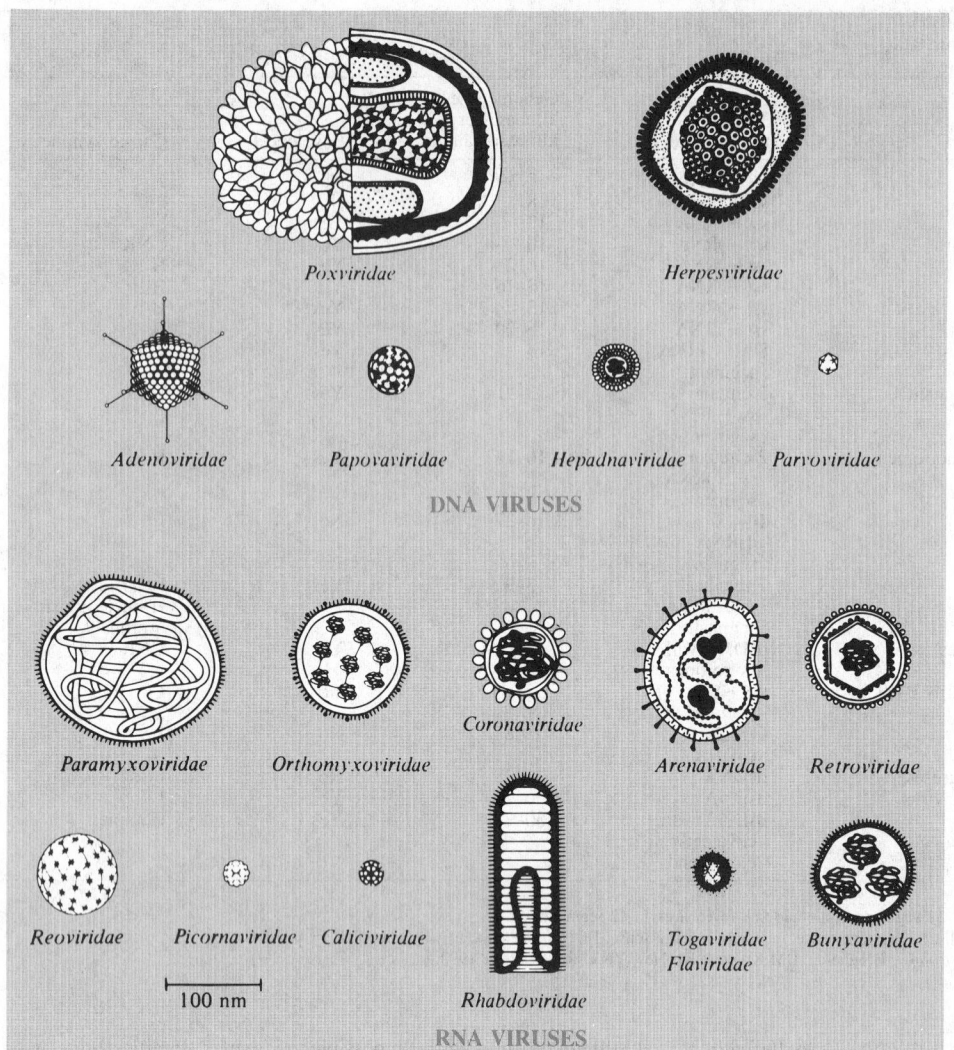

Poxviridae

Herpesviridae

Adenoviridae　　Papovaviridae　　Hepadnaviridae　　Parvoviridae

DNA VIRUSES

Paramyxoviridae　　Orthomyxoviridae　　Coronaviridae　　Arenaviridae　　Retroviridae

Reoviridae　　Picornaviridae　　Caliciviridae

Rhabdoviridae

Togaviridae
Flaviridae

Bunyaviridae

100 nm

RNA VIRUSES

FIGURE 141-1 Structure of DNA and RNA viruses. (*From White DO, Fenner FJ: Medical Virology, 3d ed. Orlando, Academic Press, 1986. Reprinted by permission.*)

different families (e.g., coxsackievirus B3 and adenovirus 2) also may compete for the same class of receptor. These types of binding studies suggest that there are generally 10^4 to 10^6 viral binding sites (receptors) per cell.

Once attachment has occurred, the entire virion or a substructure containing the viral genome and any virion polymerases required for its initial transcription must be translocated across the plasma membrane of the cell. The rate of penetration varies depending on the nature of the virus, the type of cells being infected, and environmental factors such as temperature. Some nonenveloped viruses such as poliovirus and reovirus undergo a process of receptor-mediated endocytosis (*viropexis*) and appear in the cytoplasm inside endocytic vesicles. Other nonenveloped viruses may be able to cross the plasma membrane directly and appear free in the cytoplasm without entering endocytic vesicles.

Enveloped viruses also utilize at least two strategies for penetration. The first is exemplified by Semliki Forest virus (SFV). SFV, a togavirus, binds to specific cell surface receptors, which then aggregate at distinct sites on the plasma membrane (*coated pits*) and are internalized by receptor-mediated endocytosis. They subsequently appear inside clathrin-coated vesicles within the cell cytoplasm. Fusion between the viral envelope and the endosomal membrane causes release of the viral nucleocapsid into the cytoplasm. A second mechanism for penetration of enveloped viruses occurs with paramyxoviruses (e.g., Sendai). The viral envelope fuses directly with the cell plasma membrane, and the viral nucleocapsid is discharged free into the cytoplasm.

Uncoating is the process of removing or disaggregating part or all of the viral protein capsid in preparation for transcription and translation of the viral genome. In many cases penetration and uncoating are part of a single process. Some picornaviruses, for example, seem to undergo an alteration in capsid structure and integrity and loss of an internal protein as they are translocated across the plasma membrane. The structural alterations associated with loss of the protein may facilitate entry of the viral RNA into the cytoplasm.

Nonenveloped viruses which enter endosomes, such as adenovirus, may induce fusion of lysosomes with the endosome and have their capsid removed by lysosomal enzymes. In the case of reoviruses, intraendosomal proteases sequentially remove the three outer capsid proteins to produce an "infectious subviral particle." Further proteolytic processing to a "core particle" leads to activation of the viral transcriptase. Uncoating of poxviruses, such as vaccinia virus, may require virus-induced uncoating proteins with trypsin-like activity.

A number of strategies have evolved for *transcription* of viral genomes into mRNA and *translation* of mRNA into protein. One approach is for viruses to contain mRNA that is translated into a large precursor polyprotein, which is then cleaved to produce the various virion proteins (e.g., in picornaviruses). In the case of both the picornaviruses and the togaviruses, a virally encoded RNA polymerase synthesizes a complementary RNA using the genomic RNA as template. In turn, the newly synthesized RNA serves as template for the synthesis of more genomic RNA.

Viruses which contain linear or segmented RNA produce unique mRNAs for each viral protein rather than a single large mRNA molecule. A transcriptase enzyme contained in the virion (the virion polymerase) is required to produce mRNAs from the genomic RNA. The presence of multiple mRNAs allows regulation of the amount of each protein synthesized. A single region of genomic RNA may have multiple reading frames, each of which is transcribed into unique mRNAs, which are in turn translated into distinct proteins. Genomic $(-)$ single-stranded (ss)RNA is replicated via a $(+)$ssRNA intermediate, which then serves as a template to synthesize more $(-)$ss genomic RNA.

Reoviruses contain an RNA-dependent RNA polymerase that transcribes $(+)$ssRNAs from the $(-)$ strand of each double-stranded (ds) RNA segment. These $(+)$ssRNAs are extruded from the viral core through channels in the core spike and serve as mRNAs for translation into viral proteins. The viral RNA polymerase also synthesizes $(+)$ssRNAs, which in turn serve as templates for the complementary $(-)$ strand during replication of the viral genome.

The retroviruses utilize a unique replicative strategy. Viral $(+)$ssRNA serves as a template for the virion RNA-dependent DNA polymerase (reverse transcriptase) and primer transfer RNAs (tRNAs). An ssDNA copy is produced which is initially hydrogen bonded to its complementary $(+)$ssRNA. A virally encoded ribonuclease digests the ssRNA, and a complementary DNA strand is synthesized. Then dsDNA is integrated into chromosomal DNA in the host cell nucleus. Transcription of this integrated viral DNA is under the control of the host cell transcriptases.

DNA viruses such as papovaviruses, adenoviruses, and herpesviruses use replicative strategies in which transcription of viral DNA into mRNA occurs in the nucleus of the host cell and depends on host cell enzymes. The viral mRNA encodes a DNA polymerase that replicates the viral DNA. Protein synthesis occurs in a series of sequential stages in which the first (early) proteins synthesized include regulatory proteins and proteins involved in DNA replication. Viral structural proteins are synthesized subsequently.

Poxviruses are the most complicated of the known animal viruses, and their replicative cycle is correspondingly complex. All the initial steps of transcription and translation appear to occur in the host cell cytoplasm; thus the virus must contain its own DNA-dependent RNA polymerase to initiate transcription. Replication, transcription, and later viral assembly all occur in virus-initiated "factories" within the host cell cytoplasm. Sequential groups of virus-specified proteins can be detected in infected cells. Early proteins include a number of enzymes (e.g., a DNA polymerase and a thymidine kinase), as well as some structural proteins. As infection proceeds, DNA replication begins, the synthesis of the early nonstructural proteins ceases, and the synthesis of late proteins begins. Many of the late proteins are structural proteins; other late proteins include enzymes and proteins that may play a role in viral assembly.

Once replication of the viral genome and synthesis of the viral proteins have been completed, intact virions must then be assembled and released from the host cells. Assembly of the nonenveloped viruses and the nucleocapsid of enveloped viruses often appears to proceed in a crystallization-like fashion which depends on the self-assembly of viral capsomers.

In most cases, nonenveloped virions accumulate within the infected cell and are released together when the cell lyses. The events leading to cell disruption include inhibition of the synthesis of host cell protein, lipid, and nucleic acids; disorganization of the host cell cytoskeleton; and alteration of host cell membrane structure. Membrane disruption may result in increased cell permeability and the release of proteolytic enzymes from lysosomes. The failure to replenish energy-rich substrate molecules inhibits the function of ion transport pumps and disturbs transport of essential nutrients and cellular waste products.

Enveloped viruses are typically released from infected cells by budding. This process may be lethal to the cell. In all cases, virus-specified proteins are inserted into host cell membranes in a fashion that restructures the membrane by displacing some of its normal protein components. Viral capsids may then bind to virus-specified matrix proteins which line the cytoplasmic side of these altered patches of membrane. In the case of the smallest enveloped viruses, the togaviruses, the capsids bind to the intracytoplasmic domains of viral proteins inserted in the host cell membrane rather than to matrix proteins.

Release of certain enveloped and nonenveloped viruses occurs preferentially from particular surfaces of certain types of polarized cells, such as epithelial cells. In the case of enveloped viruses, selective insertion of envelope glycoproteins into either the apical or the basolateral cell membrane precedes polarized release. Recent studies suggest that specific amino acid sequences within the viral envelope proteins may determine their insertion at a particular cell surface. The mechanisms responsible for polarized release of nonenveloped viruses remain to be determined. Polarized release may have important implications for pathogenesis. Release of virus at apical surfaces may facilitate local spread of infection, whereas release at the basolateral surface may facilitate systemic invasion.

PATHOGENESIS The signs and symptoms of disease are the result of the culmination of a series of interactions between the virus and the host. A virus must first be able to enter the host, then undergo a period of primary replication, followed by spread to its final target tissue. Once a virus reaches its target organs, it must then infect and successfully replicate in a susceptible population of host cells. The outcome of this last step may be a productive infection with or without cell injury, latent infection, or persistent infection. To transmit infectious virus to the next host, the virus must successfully avoid or overcome the host immune response and a wide variety of other host defense mechanisms. A great deal of viral replication can occur before any signs or symptoms of clinical illness are detectable. This "incubation period" can vary from a few days (e.g., influenza) to weeks (e.g., measles, varicella) to months (e.g., rabies, hepatitis) to years (e.g., slow viruses).

Most viral diseases result from exposure to exogenous virus. However, in some cases disease results from the reactivation of endogenous virus that has been latent within specific host cells. Examples of infections caused by reactivated endogenous viruses include shingles (herpes zoster), progressive multifocal leukoencephalopathy (JC or BK papovaviruses), recurrent labial and genital herpes (herpes simplex), and some types of cytomegalovirus (CMV) infections.

In the majority of cases, transmission of viral illnesses occurs between members of a susceptible host population (*horizontal spread*). *Vertical spread* of infection occurs when the fetus becomes infected in utero through virus carried in the germ cell line, virus infecting the placenta, or virus in the maternal birth canal. HIV, rubella virus, CMV, herpes simplex virus, varicella-zoster virus, and hepatitis B virus can all produce vertically transmitted congenital infections.

The age and genetic background of the host can have important implications for the outcome of viral infections. Newborns, for example, are particularly susceptible to severe, disseminated herpes simplex virus infections. In contrast, many of the exanthematous illnesses, poliovirus infection, and EBV infection are typically more severe in older individuals than in children. In mice, specific genes help determine susceptibility to certain viral infections. These genes may act through effects on the immune system, interferon production, or viral receptors. Inadequate host nutritional status may increase susceptibility to infections such as measles, perhaps by depressing cell-mediated immunity. The host also can influence viral infections in ways that are still poorly understood. Stress may trigger recurrent herpes labialis. Strenuous exercise may have an adverse effect on the course of polio.

Viral infection begins with *entry* into the host, which may occur via a number of routes. The stratum corneum of the skin provides both a physical and a biologic barrier against the entry of viruses. Some viruses overcome the skin barrier by being directly inoculated via insect or animal bites or mechanical devices such as needles. The arthropod-borne viruses are directly inoculated into the bloodstream when an infected tick or mosquito takes a blood meal. Rabies virus and herpesvirus simiae (monkey B virus) enter tissues after an animal bite. Iatrogenic inoculation allows entry of a large number of viruses. Hepatitis B virus, CMV, and HIV-1 may all be present in contaminated blood products used for transfusion. Parenteral vaccination using live attenuated virus represents another category of iatrogenic inoculation.

A large number of viruses enter the host by crossing mucosal barriers in the respiratory and gastrointestinal tracts. Respiratory infection can be transmitted by means of aerosol droplets, nasal secretions, or saliva. Entry via either the respiratory or the enteric route requires that the virus overcome a formidable series of host defenses. In the lung, immunologic defenses include secretory IgA, natural killer (NK) cells, and macrophages. Nonspecific glycoprotein viral inhibitors are present in tracheobronchial mucus. Ciliated respiratory epithelial cells continually move mucus away from the lower respiratory tract. The harsh acidic environment of the stomach inactivates acid-labile viruses such as rhinoviruses. Bile salts, present in the lumen of the small intestine, can destroy the lipid envelope of many viruses and may account for the fact that entry via the gastrointestinal route is limited largely to nonenveloped viruses. Proteolytic enzymes and secretory IgA contribute to host antiviral defenses in the gastrointestinal tract. Specific viral capsid proteins may allow some viruses to withstand proteolytic digestion in the gut.

For some enteric viruses, passage across the mucosal barrier of the gut is mediated by a specific population of cells overlying Peyer's patches known as *microfold (M) cells*. These cells, and perhaps their analogues in bronchial lymphoid tissue, facilitate transport of some viruses, including reoviruses and polioviruses, to the abluminal surface of the small intestine.

Venereal transmission with entry across the genitourinary or rectal mucosa appears to be important for herpes simplex virus type 2, CMV, hepatitis B virus, and HIV-1.

For some viruses, the processes of entry, primary replication, and tissue tropism all occur at the same anatomic site. Examples of this type of viral illness include the upper and lower respiratory infections caused by the rhinoviruses, orthomyxoviruses, and paramyxoviruses; the enteritis caused by rotaviruses; and the dermatologic lesions induced by human papillomavirus (warts) and paravaccinia virus (milker's nodules). In other cases, a virus enters at one site and must subsequently spread to a distant area, such as the central nervous system, to produce disease. Enteroviruses enter via the gastrointestinal tract but must spread to the CNS to produce meningitis, encephalitis, and poliomyelitis. Measles virus and varicella virus enter the body through the respiratory tract but then spread to produce skin disease (exanthem) and often generalized organ involvement.

Neural, hematogenous, and lymphatic pathways are all utilized by viruses to spread to target tissues. Rabies virus, herpes simplex virus, herpesvirus simiae (monkey B), varicella-zoster virus, reovirus type 3, and certain coronaviruses spread via nerves. Herpes simplex virus appears to enter nerves via receptors located primarily near synaptic endings rather than on the nerve cell body. Rabies virus accumulates at the motor end plate of the neuromuscular junction (NMJ), as do La Crosse bunyavirus and the togavirus Sindbis. Rabies virus can infect muscle and then spread via motor and sensory nerves to the spinal cord. The kinetics of neural spread for rabies virus, herpes simplex virus, reovirus, and poliovirus strongly suggest that these agents utilize intraneuronal mechanisms involved with fast axonal transport. Infection of Schwann cells may provide another "neural" pathway to the CNS. Axonal transport also provides a pathway for spread of viruses within the CNS and from it to the periphery.

The olfactory pathway represents a special category of neural spread. The rod processes of olfactory receptor cells lie exposed in the olfactory mucosa. These cells synapse directly with the mitral cells in the olfactory bulb within the CNS. Under experimental conditions, intranasal or aerosol inoculations of rabies virus, herpes simplex virus, poliovirus, and some togaviruses can lead to CNS infection via the olfactory route. This route may provide a pathway to the CNS in humans for rabies and possibly other viruses in circumstances where high-titer aerosols are present, such as in caves occupied by large numbers of rabid bats or in accidental laboratory-acquired infections. An olfactory route of spread might be one explanation for the localization of herpes simplex virus to the orbitofrontal and medial temporal cortex in cases of herpes simplex encephalitis.

Hematogenous spread is important for many viruses. A period of primary replication usually precedes the initial viremia and can be asymptomatic or result in prodromal symptoms. For enteric viruses, primary replication occurs in Peyer's patches and peritonsillar lymphatic tissue. Primary replication of respiratory viruses occurs in epithelial or alveolar cells and for many enteroviruses and togaviruses in skeletal muscle. In some cases virus travels from the site of initial multiplication via lymphatics to regional lymph nodes before entering the bloodstream. The initial (*primary*) viremia often disseminates virus to tissues such as the spleen and liver, where continued multiplication in parenchymal cells leads to an amplified secondary viremia. Growth in endothelial cells may help sustain the viremic phase in some togavirus infections. Sustained secondary amplification of the viremia is required if a virus is to overcome clearance by reticuloendothelial cells.

Blood-borne virus can travel free or in association with cellular elements. Hepatitis B virus, picornaviruses, and togaviruses all travel free within plasma; Colorado tick fever virus and Rift Valley fever virus are associated with red blood cells; EBV, CMV, rubella virus, and HIV are lymphocyte- or monocyte-associated.

In some cases, viruses use different pathways of spread at different stages in the infectious cycle. Varicella-zoster virus disseminates to the skin by the hematogenous route to produce chickenpox. The virus then spreads centripetally along nerves from the skin to the dorsal root ganglion, where it remains latent. Reactivation results in centrifugal spread of virus down sensory nerves to their skin dermatome and the production of shingles (zoster).

Once a virus has spread from its site of primary replication to a target organ, it must infect a population of susceptible cells. This requires the interaction between specific viral structures (*viral attachment proteins*) and viral receptors on cells. Virus-encoded tissue-specific enhancers may in part mediate viral injury to specific cell populations. Lytic infection also requires that all the subsequent steps in the viral replicative cycle be successfully completed.

HOST FACTORS   The antibody response   Most viruses make good antigens for stimulating the immune response because they contain a large number of foreign proteins, each of which may contain multiple antigenic sites. In addition, although the amount of viral antigenic material may initially be quite small, there is amplification in its quantity due to viral replication. Few of the antibodies play a significant role in protecting the host against infection, and in some cases they may themselves be implicated in disease pathogenesis.

The immunogenicity of viruses depends on the nature of the virus itself and on a variety of host factors. The route of viral infection also may play a role in immunity. In experimental influenza infections, intravenous inoculation is more immunogenic than intraperitoneal inoculation, which in turn exceeds the subcutaneous route.

Antibodies which destroy the infectivity of virus are referred to as *neutralizing antibodies (Nab)*. The binding of Nab to virus is generally a reversible reaction. Viral infectivity may be reduced because Nab inhibits attachment, penetration, or uncoating of virus; produces aggregation of virions; accelerates viral degradation in vesicles; or enhances viral opsonization and subsequent phagocytosis. In the case of poliovirus, Nab binding appears to induce a conformational rearrangement of the viral outer capsid which blocks viral uncoating but not attachment. It is important to recognize that some antibodies which fail to neutralize viral infectivity in vitro may still protect against viral infection in vivo and that, conversely, not all Nab is protective in vivo.

Complement   Viruses can trigger activation of both the alternate and classical pathways of complement in the absence of an antibody response. Activated complement components (e.g., C3b) may act as opsonins that enhance phagocytosis of viruses. Activation of the alternate complement pathway, in combination with antibody, may produce lysis of enveloped viruses or virus-infected cells. Although the complement system plays a role in the protection against viral infection in animals, human complement-deficiency states are not typically associated with an increase in the frequency or severity of viral illnesses.

Cell-mediated immunity Virus-infected cells can be lysed by lymphocytes and other cells through both antibody-dependent and antibody-independent pathways. NK cells are large granular lymphocytes that bind to infected target cells and then secrete cytotoxic molecules contained in azurophilic granular vesicles. NK activity is increased by interferons and possibly by some viral glycoproteins and does not require antibody. NK cytotoxicity provides one of the earliest host defenses against viral infection (peak activity at 2 to 3 days) and precedes the appearance of antibody (7 days), cytotoxic T lymphocytes (CTLs), and delayed-type hypersensitivity (DTH). Activated NK cells have been identified in human viral infections caused by CMV, EBV, measles virus, and mumps virus.

Antibody-dependent lysis of infected cells can occur via antibody-dependent cell-mediated cytotoxicity (ADCC). In ADCC reactions, virus-specific antibody bound to antigens on an infected cell interacts with Fc receptors for IgG on the surface of leukocytes, and this interaction results in the activation of these leukocytes and their subsequent killing of the target cell.

Lysis of infected cells mediated by CTLs is typically class I histocompatibility antigen–restricted, although examples of class II–restricted CTLs have been described. CTLs must be activated by antigen presented by macrophages or other antigen-presenting cells (APCs). The nature of the specific epitopes expressed on the surface of infected cells that CTLs recognize has been defined for some viruses, such as influenza. In contrast to the specificity of neutralizing antibodies, which typically recognize epitopes on intact viral surface proteins, CTLs recognize antigens presented as short peptides derived from both viral surface and internal proteins. The pathways by which these peptides are processed, appear on the surface of infected cells, and interact with major histocompatibility complex (MHC) antigens are subjects of active investigation.

Interferons Leukocytes produce more than a dozen alpha (''leukocyte'') interferons that share about 77 percent amino acid sequence homology. Beta (''fibroblast'') interferon is produced by fibroblasts and epithelial cells and has 30 percent homology to α-interferons. Both α- and β-interferons are acid-stable (pH = 2) and relatively heat resistant. ''Immune'' (γ-) interferon is produced by both sensitized and unsensitized lymphocytes, has different physicochemical properties and different inducers, and uses a different cellular receptor from α- and β-interferons. Genes encoding interferons are located on human chromosomes 9(α and β) and 12(γ).

Interferons can be induced by both active and inactivated viruses, by dsRNA, and by a number of other compounds. The amount of interferon produced may vary with different viruses. All the interferons have extremely high specific activity and are generally most active in cells of the species in which they are induced (''species-specific''), presumably because of variation in the nature of the interferon receptor. Interferon production appears to involve a derepression of cellular genes induced by the presence of viral nucleic acid in the host cell cytoplasm. This results in the rapid production of mRNAs for interferon and subsequent interferon synthesis.

Newly produced interferon is released into extracellular fluid and then binds to a specific receptor on adjacent cells. The gene encoding the glycoprotein receptor for α- and β-interferon is on human chromosome 21, and that for γ-interferon is on chromosome 6. Binding of interferon to its receptor results in a complex variety of subsequent events. A protein kinase is synthesized and phosphorylates a protein synthesis initiation factor (eIF$_2$), resulting in inhibition of initiation complex formation and hence of viral protein synthesis. An induced 2,5-oligoisoadenylate synthetase produces 2,5-oligoadenylates, which in turn activate a cellular ribonuclease (RNase L) that cleaves viral mRNAs. Inhibition of methyltransferase reactions decreases methylation of mRNAs and thereby interferes with viral protein synthesis. In addition to these actions, changes in target cell surface antigens result in enhanced expression of both class I and class II histocompatibility antigens. Interferons also increase the activity of NK cells, CTLs, and cells involved in ADCC reactions. The relative importance of each of these activities in creating the interferon-induced antiviral state is not established.

Virus-induced immunopathology Viruses can combine with virus-specific antibodies to produce circulating immune complexes which may be involved in immunopathogenesis. Virus stimulation of B lymphocytes may result in the production of polyclonal antibodies to antigens unrelated to the inciting virus. Viruses also can induce cross-reacting antibodies to normal host structures which contain antigenic regions similar to those of the virus (*molecular mimicry*). These types of autoantibodies also may lead to immune-complex formation. Immune complexes can become trapped in basement membranes at a variety of sites, including the skin, the kidney, the choroid plexus, and the walls of blood vessels. These immune complexes result in tissue injury by attracting and activating a variety of inflammatory mediators.

Autoantibodies produced by virus infection also may result in direct tissue injury. Autoantibodies to lymphocytes, platelets, smooth muscle, intermediate filaments, immunoglobulins, and myelin basic protein are usually transient and of low titer. These autoantibodies could result from a variety of mechanisms, including (1) incorporation of host antigens into viral structures or virus-induced alteration of host antigens, (2) virus-induced alterations in immunoregulatory systems, (3) cross reactivity between virus antigens and normal host cell structures (molecular mimicry), and (4) elicitation of anti-idiotypic antibodies which stimulate host cell receptors.

EPIDEMIOLOGY Viral epidemiology includes the study of the causes, distribution, frequency, modes of transmission, and spread of viral diseases. Accurate enumeration of the incidence and prevalence of viral diseases is an important aspect of epidemiology. *Incidence* can be defined as the number of *new* cases of a particular disease that appear during a defined period of time, and *prevalence* as the *total* number of cases. It is often useful to refer to incidence and prevalence *rates*, which are obtained by dividing incidence or prevalence numbers by the size of the total population at risk. Terms such as *epidemic* and *outbreak* are arbitrary and simply indicate that a greater than expected number of cases of a particular disease has occurred in a specific population, geographic location, or time period.

The appearance of an acute viral disease indicates that an infected host has come into contact with a susceptible individual under conditions that permit the transmission of a particular viral agent. The time interval between exposure to a virus and the development of signs and symptoms of disease is referred to as the *incubation period* and can vary from a few days (e.g., influenza) to years (slow virus diseases). Viral infection does not always lead to overt clinical disease. The percentage of those infected who develop overt disease ranges from 100 percent (e.g., rabies, measles) to 0 percent (BK, JC papovaviruses). In most cases, symptomatic disease is less common in children than in adults (e.g., EBV mononucleosis, paralytic poliomyelitis, hepatitis A virus).

Transmission of a virus from an infected host to a susceptible individual can take a variety of forms. Human-to-human transmission can occur from an acutely ill individual, from a chronic carrier, or from mother to fetus. The method of spread can involve respiratory aerosols, fecal-oral contamination, sexual contact, or direct inoculation via infected needles or blood products.

Respiratory aerosolization usually occurs via coughing or sneezing. A sneeze may generate up to 2 million aerosol particles and a cough up to 90,000. The fate of these particles depends on both ambient environmental conditions (e.g., humidity, wind currents) and particle size. Small particles remain airborne longer and can escape the filtering action of the nose, which traps particles larger than 6 μm in diameter. The number of viral particles aerosolized may vary for different strains of the same virus.

For most viruses it is unclear how many viral particles are required to initiate a respiratory infection. For influenza A virus, adenovirus, or coxsackievirus A21, as few as 10 particles may be sufficient. Aerosolization is not the only possible route of respiratory transmission. EBV is typically spread by saliva during kissing. A critical pathway of spread for rhinoviruses, which cause the common cold, is from hands to eyes, nose, or mouth—a cycle which can be interrupted by hand washing.

Gastrointestinal transmission occurs when virus shed in feces contaminates food or water and is then ingested by a susceptible individual (fecal-oral spread). Stool-tainted hands, resulting from poor personal hygiene, provide another vehicle of spread for enteric viruses. The high incidence of enteric virus infections in infant day-care centers and institutions for the mentally retarded reflects the difficulty of maintaining hygiene in these settings.

In many types of viral disease the vector is an insect or infected animal. In dengue fever there is a continuing cycle between humans and infected mosquitoes. Dengue virus multiplies in the gut of the *Aedes aegypti* mosquito, spreads to its salivary glands, and is injected into a human during the mosquito's blood meal. The infected person develops a high-titer viremia which is sufficient to transmit virus to an uninfected mosquito during biting. In other arbovirus infections the human being is a "dead-end host" because the degree of viremia in infected individuals is insufficient to transmit infection to a new group of insect vectors. Examples of this type of cycle are provided by togaviruses, such as eastern, western, and St. Louis encephalitis viruses. The normal animal reservoirs for arboviruses include small birds and mammals. The horse, like humans, is usually a dead-end host, although in Venezuelan equine encephalitis, horses may be a reservoir of virus.

Some arthropod-borne infections do not require a viremic vertebrate intermediate host. Virus can be passed in transovarian fashion to the progeny of an infected tick or mosquito or by venereal transmission between male and female mosquitoes. Transovarian transmission may allow survival of arthropod viruses through the winter months.

Zoonotic infections illustrate another mechanism of disease transmission. In the case of rabies, transmission results from the bite of an infected animal. Many human infections occur when humans are exposed to the excreta (feces, urine, saliva) of infected rodents. Examples include arenavirus infections and the hemorrhagic fevers with renal disease caused by the bunyaviruses.

DIAGNOSIS OF VIRAL DISEASES A reasonably accurate diagnosis of some viral illnesses, such as measles, can be made on clinical grounds alone. In other cases the best that can be done clinically is to identify a group of viruses that are likely pathogens for specific categories of illness. More definitive diagnosis is often necessary because of availability of antiviral agents with activity limited only to certain types of viruses. Definitive diagnosis requires isolation of the virus in animals or in tissue culture, identification of the virus or detection of virus-specified antigens or viral nucleic acids in tissues or body fluids, or documentation of specific serologic responses. The physician must ensure that the appropriate specimens are obtained for diagnostic studies during a suitable phase of the illness, that they are rapidly transported, and that adequate clinical information is provided to the diagnostic laboratories.

In the case of diarrheal or gastrointestinal illness where a viral etiology is suspected, a fresh *stool sample* is the specimen of choice for virus isolation. In diseases of the respiratory system, including pharyngitis, croup, bronchiolitis, and pneumonia, nasopharyngeal or tracheal *aspirates* provide the best specimens. Nasopharyngeal and throat *swabs* are less satisfactory. When a vesicular rash is present, a needle aspirate of vesicular fluid provides the optimal specimen. When the rash is petechial or maculopapular, both nasopharyngeal aspirates and a stool sample should be obtained. In patients with CNS diseases of suspected viral etiology, including meningitis, encephalitis, myelitis, and Guillain-Barré syndrome, a nasopharyngeal aspirate and stool and cerebrospinal fluid specimens should be obtained. A urine sample may be helpful when infection due to CMV, measles virus, mumps virus, or papovaviruses is suspected. Blood specimens may be useful for the detection of some arboviruses, herpesviruses, and lymphocytic choriomeningitis (LCM) virus. Saliva has been used for the detection of rabies and mumps viruses. A brain biopsy specimen is often required for the definitive diagnosis of herpes simplex encephalitis, progressive multifocal leukoencephalopathy, subacute sclerosing panencephalitis (SSPE), and progressive rubella panencephalitis.

Nasopharyngeal or rectal swab specimens should be placed in an appropriate transport medium. In general, this consists of a few milliliters of a neutral isotonic salt solution to which a small amount of protein or animal serum has been added. Antibiotics should be added to inhibit bacterial contaminants. Specimens can be placed in a thermos flask filled with crushed ice if any delay in transport is anticipated. Ideally, specimens should be inoculated into the appropriate culture systems on arrival in the virology laboratory. Storage up to 48 h can often be done safely at refrigerator temperature (4°C), and longer storage should be at −70°C. Many viruses quickly lose infectivity if repeatedly frozen and thawed.

Isolation of virus from clinical specimens is done in cell cultures, embryonated eggs, and animals such as suckling mice. Cell culture techniques involve the use of primary cultures of cells prepared from organs of freshly killed animals (e.g., monkey kidney cells), human diploid cell lines such as WI-38 embryo fibroblasts, and continuous (heterodiploid) cell lines such as HeLa, HEp-2, BHK-21, and Vero. Some viruses grow better on certain cell lines than others. Inoculation into the amniotic cavity or the allantoic cavity of embryonated chicken eggs is useful in the isolation of influenza virus. Intraperitoneal and intracerebral inoculation into neonatal mice may be necessary for isolation of coxsackievirus A and may help in the isolation of many arboviruses, rabies virus, arenaviruses, and orbiviruses. Adult mice or guinea pigs can be used to isolate LCM virus. Special isolation techniques using brain tissue explants are required to identify measles virus in cases of SSPE or rubella virus in cases of progressive rubella panencephalitis.

Once cell culture inoculation has been performed, the specimens are examined for distinctive patterns of cytopathic effect (CPE). Viruses such as HSV and many enteroviruses produce early CPE, whereas cultures may need to be followed for weeks and even subcultured to detect CPE due to CMV, rubella virus, and some adenoviruses. Cultured cells are examined for cell lysis and vacuolization. The presence of syncytia suggests HSV, respiratory syncytial virus (RSV), measles virus, or mumps virus. Cytomegaly is seen with HSV, varicella-zoster virus (VZV), and CMV. Detection of inclusion bodies is aided by the use of Giemsa or other stains. Immunocytochemical staining of cell cultures to detect viral antigens using fluorescein or enzyme-conjugated specific antiviral antibodies can aid in the detection and identification of many viruses. Some viruses produce minimal or no detectable CPE. Orthoviruses and paramyxoviruses (influenza, parainfluenza, measles, mumps) can be detected by the ability of infected cultures to adsorb certain red blood cells (*hemadsorption*). Infection with rubella virus can be detected by the ability of infected cultures to block the CPE produced by infection with a second challenge virus (*interference*).

Identification of virus particles or antigens in tissue specimens provides another important method of viral diagnosis. Skin scrapings from the base of vesicles can be stained with Wright or Giemsa stain according to the Tzanck method to help identify HSV or VZV. Similar techniques may help identify CMV-infected cells in urine sediment or measles virus–infected cells in scrapings from Koplik spots. In some cases, examination of appropriately prepared specimens by electron microscopy (EM) is of diagnostic value; high concentrations of virus must be present. A special technique which concentrates virus in specimens by adsorbing excess fluid and salts on an agarose surface may enable detection of as few as 10^4 particles per milliliter (pseudoreplica technique). EM easily distinguishes between vaccinia virus and VZV in vesicular fluid negatively stained with phosphotung-stic acid and may be extremely useful in identifying skin viruses such as human papilloma virus, orf virus, and molluscum contagiosum virus. The use of specific antisera to aggregate virus in prepared stool specimens facilitates EM detection of rotaviruses, hepatitis A virus, and the Norwalk agent. EM examination of brain biopsy specimens may allow identification of herpes simplex encephalitis, progressive multifocal leukoencephalopathy (PML), and SSPE.

Detection of virus-specific antigens is facilitated by immunofluo-rescence and immunocytochemical techniques. These procedures are particularly valuable in diagnosing rabies, herpes infection, PML, and SSPE from brain biopsy specimens; herpes keratitis from corneal scrapings; HSV, VZV, and vaccinia virus infections from vesicle scrapings; parainfluenza virus, influenza virus, and RSV infections from nasopharyngeal aspirates; hepatitis B virus infections from liver biopsy specimens; and Colorado tick fever virus infection from blood clots. Radioimmunoassays and immunoassays in which viral antibody coupled to a solid support (ELISA) is used to detect viral antigens have proved useful in the diagnosis of hepatitis A and B virus, rotavirus, and adenovirus infections.

The detection of a fourfold or greater increase in antibody titer to a specific viral agent in a patient's acute and convalescent (3 to 4 weeks later) sera can usually be considered diagnostic of acute infection. A single serum specimen is only occasionally useful in viral diagnosis. A high antibody titer against a rare agent in a typical clinical setting or a distinct pattern of antibody titers to viral antigens of specific types may provide presumptive evidence of acute infection. Blood for serology should be collected in anticoagulant- and preserva-tive-free glass tubes and allowed to clot. Serum should be separated out and stored frozen. A number of different types of antibodies, including neutralizing (N), complement-fixing (CF), and hemaggluti-nation-inhibiting (HI) antibodies, are routinely assayed. The time course of these antibody responses and their sensitivity and specificity differ greatly.

Restriction enzyme analysis of the genomes of DNA viruses (e.g., HSV, VZV, CMV) and oligonucleotide fingerprinting of ribonuclease T_1 cleaved genomes of RNA viruses (e.g., influenza virus, dengue enterovirus) are valuable in epidemiologic studies and in establishing the origin of certain types of viral isolates. In situ hybridization and the polymerase chain reaction technique may enable the detection of even single copies of virus genomes in tissue samples or cells from body fluids.

VACCINES FOR THE PREVENTION OF VIRAL ILLNESS Cur-rently available vaccines utilize inactivated virus, attenuated virus, or virus subunits to induce active immunization. Formalin-inactivated vaccines are available for rabies virus, influenza virus, and poliovirus. A highly purified subunit vaccine preparation containing the surface antigen of hepatitis B virus is also available. Strains used in the inactivated influenza whole-virus vaccine are specified yearly by the FDA. The vaccine is composed of formalin-inactivated natural isolates of influenza virus and laboratory-designed reassortant strains containing the hemagglutinin and neuraminidase genes of the influenza viruses that are currently circulating. As many as 60 to 80 percent of those immunized show a reduction in the frequency or severity of influenzal illness. Guillain-Barré syndrome occurred in 1 in 100,000 individuals vaccinated with the swine influenza vaccine in 1976 to 1977 but has not been associated with subsequent influenza vaccine preparations. Killed polio vaccine is widely used in Sweden, Finland, and the Netherlands; is used in combination with live vaccine in Denmark; but in the United States is reserved for immunization of immunodeficient individuals and their household contacts, immuniza-tion of pregnant women, and adult primary immunization in certain other instances.

Inactivated virus vaccines have advantages and disadvantages compared with live vaccines. The absence of live virus results in immunization without active infection. Since there is no live virus present, reversion to virulence does not occur, although improperly prepared vaccines can contain virulent virus or adventitious viral contaminants (e.g., SV40, avian leukosis virus). Effective local immunity does not develop, so vaccinated individuals may still transmit virus to the community. In rare cases (measles virus, RSV), inactivated vaccines have resulted in atypical immunologic re-sponses which potentiated rather than prevented subsequent natural infections.

The attenuated live virus vaccines in current use have been developed either from naturally occurring attenuated viruses (e.g., poliovirus type 2 strain 712) or from viruses after serial passage in tissue culture cells or embryonated eggs. These passage-selected viruses have mutations when compared with their wild-type parents. For example, the vaccine strain of poliovirus type 1 differs in 21 amino acids from the original parent virus. On some vaccine viruses, the largest number of mutations are located in genes coding for viral surface proteins such as VP1 (polio) or V3 (yellow fever). However, in the case of the type 1 polio vaccine strain, mutations responsible for attenuation appear to be distributed throughout the viral genome, including the 5'noncoding region. In other cases (e.g., mumps virus) a clear marker for the vaccine virus strain has not been identified.

Following immunization with the oral Sabin polio vaccine, the vaccinated person excretes virus which can infect other individuals in the community. In rare cases, the excreted virus appears to be more virulent than the vaccine strain and may account for some of the rare cases of paralytic polio in close contacts of vaccinees. Reversion to virulence by the vaccine strain of virus also may cause paralytic polio in vaccinees. Approximately 1 in 10 million vaccinated individuals develops paralytic polio, and there are 3 cases of paralytic polio per 10 million household and community contacts of recent vaccinees. These risks are small and are probably overestimates which include coincidental as well as causal associations. In rare settings, where exposure to polio occurs at a very young age, a combined program using both inactivated (killed) and attenuated vaccines may be of benefit (see also Chap. 154).

Live attenuated measles, mumps, and rubella vaccines can be administered together (MMR) without any loss in immunizing capacity (>90 percent). Of individuals who receive the measles vaccine alone (Schwarz strain), 10 to 30 percent have mild clinical reactions, and there are rare cases of encephalitis (<1 in 1 million). Widespread use of measles vaccine has been associated with a dramatic reduction in the incidence of SSPE. Children and nonimmune adults (except for pregnant women and immunocompromised individuals) should be vaccinated. The attenuated Jeryl Lynn B strain is used in the live mumps virus vaccine, which should be given to all children except those with immunodeficiency or a history of anaphylactic reactions to eggs. Adverse effects are rare and include allergic reactions as well as CNS complications. The most commonly used rubella vaccine strain (RA 27/3) was attenuated by multiple passages through the WI-38 line of cultured human diploid fibroblasts. The most notable complications are transient arthralgia and rare cases of arthritis. The vaccine is extremely effective, and all immunocompetent children should be immunized. It is essential to ensure that women of childbearing age are immune; nonpregnant women should be revacci-nated if there is any ambiguity concerning their immune status.

A live attenuated vaccine for yellow fever has been prepared using virus derived from passage through chicken embryos. Of those vaccinated intradermally, 95 percent develop an immune response. Serious adverse reactions occur in fewer than 1 in 1 million cases. The vaccine is currently indicated only for travelers going to yellow fever-endemic areas.

A novel approach to vaccination is illustrated by the adenovirus vaccine. In this case, the live vaccine virus strains (4, 7) are not attenuated, but the route of administration (via oral ingestion of an enteric coated tablet) results in an asymptomatic infection with subsequent immunity. Ingested virus does not reach the respiratory tract but produces an intestinal infection that stimulates an immune response against subsequent adenovirus-induced respiratory infections. This vaccine is extremely effective, and side effects are very rare. It is used primarily in military recruits to prevent outbreaks of acute respiratory disease.

Two vaccines utilize virus subunits rather than whole virus to induce immunity. The influenza subunit vaccine is composed of purified envelope glycoproteins. It appears to be less toxic than live whole virus vaccine but also less antigenic. The hepatitis B vaccine uses HBsAg protein derived from cloned viral DNA expressed in yeast. The vaccine appears to be extremely effective, with few associated adverse effects. It should be given to people at high risk of exposure to hepatitis B, including health care workers, hemodialysis patients, certain institutionalized individuals, intimate contacts of hepatitis B chronic carriers, and intravenous drug users.

With the eradication of smallpox, routine vaccination with live attenuated vaccinia virus is no longer necessary. Its use should be limited to researchers working with vaccinia or related viruses.

ANTIVIRAL THERAPY **Immune globulins** The role in antiviral therapy of immunoglobulins extracted from pooled lots of adult plasma is limited. Antibody titers to specific viruses in different pooled lots of gamma globulin vary over a tenfold range. Intramuscular administration of immune globulin at the time of exposure to hepatitis A virus can prevent infection or decrease the severity of subsequent illness. A similar beneficial effect has been reported for measles virus infection and possibly for hepatitis B virus infection.

Specific immune globulins are made from plasma with high antibody titer against specific viruses. When given within 72 h of exposure to VZV, varicella-zoster immune globulin can prevent or modify subsequent infection. Such therapy is of value in exposed immunocompromised individuals, pregnant women, and newborn infants of mothers who develop chickenpox or of nonimmune mothers exposed to chickenpox. Hepatitis B immune globulin is useful in preventing infection of individuals exposed to HBsAg-positive material (e.g., a needle stick) or of infants born to hepatitis B–infected mothers. Rabies immune globulin is an integral part of postexposure prophylaxis of rabies. Other immune globulins are available but are not widely used.

Antiviral chemotherapy See Chap. 142.

REFERENCES

Evans AS (ed): *Viral Infections of Humans: Epidemiology and Control*, 3d ed. New York, Plenum Press, 1989

Fields BN et al (eds): *Virology*, 2d ed. New York, Raven Press, 1990

Galasso GJ et al (eds): *Antiviral Agents and Viral Diseases of Man*, 3d ed. New York, Raven Press, 1990

Lennette EH et al (eds): *Laboratory Diagnosis of Infectious Diseases, Principles and Practice*, vol 2, *Viral, Rickettsial and Chlamydial Diseases*. New York, Springer-Verlag, 1988

Mandell GL et al (eds): *Principles and Practice of Infectious Diseases*, 3d ed. New York, Churchill Livingstone, 1990

Mims CA, White DO: *Viral Pathogenesis and Immunology*. Oxford, Blackwell, 1984

Notkins AL, Oldstone MBA (eds): *Concepts in Viral Pathogenesis*. New York, Springer-Verlag, 1984

———: *Concepts in Viral Pathogenesis II*. New York, Springer-Verlag, 1986

———: *Concepts in Viral Pathogenesis III*. New York, Springer-Verlag, 1989

142 ANTIVIRAL CHEMOTHERAPY

RAPHAEL DOLIN

The use of antiviral compounds for chemotherapy and chemoprophylaxis of viral diseases is a relatively new development in the field of infectious diseases, particularly when compared with the more than 45 years of experience with antibacterial antibiotics. The principles which underlie the use of antiviral compounds have been modeled after those successfully employed in the treatment of bacterial

infections, as outlined in Chap. 100. However, application of these principles to antiviral chemotherapy and chemoprophylaxis presents a number of unique problems.

First, antiviral compounds must possess a high degree of selectivity because of the biologic properties of viruses. Bacteria can replicate extracellularly and have evolved metabolic and structural features which differ considerably from those of mammalian cells. However, viruses must replicate intracellularly and often employ host cell enzymes, macromolecules, and organelles for the synthesis of virus particles. Therefore, safe and effective antiviral compounds must be able to discriminate with a high degree of efficiency between cellular and virus-specific functions. Inhibitors of virus replication which lack this selectivity are likely to be too toxic for clinical use.

Second, because of the nature of virus replication, evaluation of the in vitro sensitivity of virus isolates to antiviral compounds must be carried out in a complex culture system consisting of living cells (e.g., tissue culture). The results from such assay systems vary widely according to the type of tissue culture cells which are employed and the conditions of assay. Furthermore, the precise relationship between the in vitro sensitivity of an isolate and the outcome of antiviral therapy is not well worked out for many viral infections.

Third, information regarding the pharmacokinetics of antiviral compounds, particularly in diverse clinical settings, is limited, particularly when compared with that available for antibacterial antibiotics. For compounds such as acyclovir, considerable detailed pharmacokinetic data are available, while for others such as amantadine, relatively little information exists. Assays to determine concentrations of antivirals, particularly of active moieties within cells, are not widely available. There are few guidelines with which to adjust dosage levels to maximize antiviral activity and to minimize toxicity. Therefore, clinical use of antiviral compounds must be accompanied by particular vigilance for unanticipated side effects or toxicities.

Fourth, it is clear that highly complex host defense systems play critical roles in the course of viral infections. The presence or absence of preexisting immunity and the ability to mount humoral and/or cell-mediated immune responses are especially important determinants in the outcome of viral infections. For example, profound "immunosuppression" may result in infections in which prolonged viral replication is present, and inhibition of such replication by antiviral compounds may be particularly useful. On the other hand, if host defenses are severely depressed, as in bone marrow transplants, antiviral therapy may be relatively ineffective. The state of host defenses and their interactions with antiviral compounds need to be considered when antivirals are utilized or evaluated.

Finally, as with antibacterial antibiotics, the optimal use of antiviral compounds requires that a specific and timely diagnosis be made. For some viral infections, such as herpes zoster, the clinical manifestations are so characteristic that a diagnosis can be made on clinical grounds alone. For other viral infections, such as influenza A, epidemiologic information (i.e., community-wide outbreaks) can be utilized to make a presumptive diagnosis with a high degree of accuracy. However, for most other viral infections, including herpes simplex encephalitis, cytomegalovirus infections, and acute viral gastroenteritis, diagnosis on clinical grounds alone cannot be accomplished with certainty. For such infections, rapid, noninvasive viral diagnostic techniques are sorely needed, and considerable effort is being expended to develop such tests.

Despite the preceding complexities, the efficacy of several antiviral compounds has been clearly established in rigorously conducted and controlled studies. The compounds which are currently licensed or likely to be licensed in the immediate future for clinical use are discussed below and summarized in Table 142-1.

AMANTADINE AND RIMANTADINE Amantadine (1-adamantanamine hydrochloride) and the closely related compound rimantadine (α-methyl-1-adamantanemethylamine hydrochloride) are primary symmetric amines with antiviral activity limited to influenza A viruses. They inhibit influenza A virus replication by interfering with uncoating of virus after infection of the cell has occurred through interaction with the influenza A M2 matrix protein. A substitution of a single amino acid in the M2 protein can result in a virus which is resistant to amantadine and rimantadine.

Amantadine and rimantadine have been demonstrated to be effective in the prophylaxis of influenza A in large-scale studies in young adults and in less extensive studies in children and elderly subjects. In such studies, efficacy rates of 55 to 80 percent in prevention of influenza-like illness were noted, and even higher rates were reported when virus-specific attack rates were calculated. Amantadine and rimantadine also have been demonstrated to be effective in the treatment of influenza A infection in studies carried out predominantly in young adults and, to a lesser extent, in children. Administration of these compounds within 24 to 72 h after the onset of illness has resulted in a reduction of duration of signs and symptoms by approximately 50 percent when compared with a placebo-treated group. The effect on signs and symptoms of illness has been demonstrated to be superior to that of commonly used antipyretic-analgesics. Only anecdotal reports are available concerning the efficacy of amantadine or rimantadine in the prevention or treatment of complications of influenza (e.g., pneumonia).

Amantadine and rimantadine are available only in oral formulations and are ordinarily administered in a dose of 200 mg/d for adults, given once or twice daily. Despite their structural similarities, the pharmacokinetics of the two compounds are different. Amantadine is not metabolized and is excreted almost entirely by the kidney, with a half-life of 12 to 17 h and peak plasma concentrations of 0.4 μg/mL. Rimantadine is extensively metabolized to hydroxylated derivatives and has a half-life of 30 h. Only 30 percent of an orally administered dose is recovered in the urine. The peak plasma levels of rimantadine are approximately one-half those of amantadine, but rimantadine is concentrated in respiratory secretions to a greater extent than amantadine. For prophylaxis, the compounds must be administered daily for the period at risk (i.e., the peak duration of the outbreak). For therapy, amantadine or rimantadine is generally administered for 5 to 7 days.

Although these compounds are generally well tolerated, 5 to 10 percent of amantadine recipients experience mild central nervous system side effects, consisting primarily of dizziness, anxiety, insomnia, and difficulty in concentrating. These side effects are rapidly reversible upon cessation of the drug. In a dose of 200 mg/d, rimantadine is better tolerated than amantadine, and in a large-scale study in young adults, side effects were no more frequent in rimantadine recipients than in placebo recipients. Seizures and worsening of congestive heart failure also have been reported in patients treated with amantadine, although a causal relationship has not been established. Because amantadine is excreted primarily by the kidney, dosage should be reduced in patients with renal failure and in the elderly, for whom a dose of 100 mg/d is recommended.

Resistance to amantadine and rimantadine can be induced readily in vitro. The emergence and probable transmission of virus resistance to these drugs also have been noted in vivo after treatment of children or adults with rimantadine or amantadine. Amantadine is licensed for the prophylaxis and therapy of influenza A in the United States, while rimantadine remains experimental.

RIBAVIRIN Ribavirin is a synthetic nucleoside analogue that inhibits a wide range of RNA and DNA viruses. The mechanism of action of ribavirin is not completely defined and may be different for different groups of viruses. Ribavirin-5'-monophosphate blocks the conversion of inosine-5'-monophosphate to xanthosine-5'-monophosphate and interferes with the synthesis of guanine nucleotides and both RNA and DNA synthesis. Ribavirin-5'-monophosphate also inhibits capping of virus-specific messenger RNA in certain viral systems. In studies demonstrating the effectiveness of ribavirin, the compound has been administered as a small-particle aerosol. It has been utilized to treat respiratory syncytial virus (RSV) infection in infants and, to a lesser extent, parainfluenza infections in children and influenza A and B infection in young adults. In RSV infection in infants, ribavirin administered by continuous aerosol for 3 to 6

days resulted in more rapid resolution of illness, lower respiratory tract signs, and less arterial oxygen desaturation when compared with placebo-treated groups. It also has had beneficial clinical effect in infants with RSV who required mechanical ventilation. Aerosolized ribavirin has been administered to adults with severe RSV infections, but the benefit, if any, is unclear. Orally administered ribavirin has not been effective in the treatment of influenza A infections. Intravenous or oral ribavirin has reduced mortality in patients with Lassa fever, particularly when given within the first 6 days of illness.

Large doses of ribavirin administered orally (800 to 1000 mg/d) have been associated with reversible hematopoietic toxicity, but this has not been observed with aerosolized ribavirin, apparently because little drug is absorbed systemically. Aerosolized administration of ribavirin is generally well tolerated but can be associated with occasional bronchospasm, rash, or conjunctival irritation. Aerosolized ribavirin has been licensed for treatment of RSV infection in infants. Because of the need for aerosolized administration, the drug can only be given for this indication under close supervision. Health care workers exposed to the drug have experienced minor toxicity, including eye and respiratory tract irritation.

ACYCLOVIR Acyclovir, 9-[(2-hydroxyethoxy)methyl]guanine, is a highly potent and selective inhibitor of replication of certain herpesviruses, including herpes simplex 1 (HSV-1), herpes simplex 2 (HSV-2), varicella-zoster virus (VZV), and Epstein-Barr virus (EBV). It is relatively ineffective in human cytomegalovirus (CMV) infections.

The high degree of selectivity of acyclovir is related to its mechanism of action, which requires that the compound first be phosphorylated to acyclovir monophosphate. This phosphorylation occurs efficiently in herpesvirus-infected cells by means of a virus-coded thymidine kinase. In uninfected mammalian cells, little phosphorylation of acyclovir occurs, and therefore, the drug is concentrated in herpesvirus-infected cells. Acyclovir monophosphate is subsequently converted by host cell kinases to a triphosphate which is a potent inhibitor of virus-induced DNA polymerase but has relatively little effect on host cell DNA polymerase. Acyclovir triphosphate also can be incorporated into viral DNA, with early chain termination.

Acyclovir is available in intravenous, oral, and topically administered forms. Intravenous acyclovir has been demonstrated to be markedly effective in the therapy of mucocutaneous HSV infections in immunocompromised hosts, reducing time to healing, duration of pain, and virus shedding. When administered prophylactically during periods of intense immunosuppression such as chemotherapy for leukemia or transplantation, but before lesions are present, intravenous acyclovir also has reduced the frequency of HSV-associated disease. After prophylaxis was discontinued, recurrent HSV lesions developed. Intravenous acyclovir also has been demonstrated to be effective in the treatment of HSV encephalitis, and two comparative trials have indicated that acyclovir is more effective than vidarabine for treatment of the latter infection (see below). Varicella-zoster virus (VZV) is generally less sensitive to acyclovir than is HSV, so higher doses of acyclovir must be used to treat VZV infections. In immunocompromised patients with herpes zoster, intravenous acyclovir reduced the frequency of cutaneous dissemination and visceral complications and was more effective than vidarabine in one comparative trial. Acyclovir administered orally at doses of 800 mg five times a day had a modest beneficial effect on localized herpes zoster lesions in both immunocompromised and immunocompetent patients and is being further evaluated in large-scale collaborative trials. Orally administered acyclovir (600 mg five times a day) reduced complications of herpes zoster ophthalmicus in a placebo-controlled trial.

In normal children with chickenpox, acyclovir administered at 20 mg/kg four times a day up to a maximum of 800 mg four times a day within 24 h of the onset of rash resulted in a modest overall clinical benefit. Intravenous acyclovir also has been reported to be effective in the therapy of immunocompromised children with chickenpox.

The most widespread use of acyclovir is in the therapy of

TABLE 142-1   Antiviral chemotherapy and chemoprophylaxis

Infection	Antiviral drug	Administration	Dosage	Comment
Influenza A (prophylaxis)	Amantadine	Oral	Adults: 200 mg/d for period at risk Children ≤9 yrs: 4.4–8.8 mg/kg per day not to exceed 150 mg/d	Needs to be administered for the duration of the outbreak. Dosage should be reduced in renal failure and in the elderly. Can be administered along with vaccine.
Influenza A (therapy)	Amantadine	Oral	As above for 5–7 days	Both amantadine and rimantadine are effective in uncomplicated influenza. Neither drug has been demonstrated to be effective in complicated influenza (e.g., pneumonia).
Respiratory syncytial virus	Ribavirin	Aerosol	Administered continuously by small-particle aerosol from a reservoir containing 20 mg/mL for 3–6 days	Utilized for treatment of infants and young children hospitalized with RSV pneumonia and bronchiolitis.
Herpes simplex encephalitis	Acyclovir or vidarabine	IV IV	10 mg/kg q 8 h for 10 days 15 mg/kg per day as a continous infusion for 12 h for 10 days	Acyclovir is the drug of choice for this infection on the basis of comparative trials vs. vidarabine. Optimal results are obtained when therapy is initiated early in illness.
Neonatal herpes simplex	Vidarabine or acyclovir	IV IV	30 mg/kg per day given as a continuous infusion over 12 h per day for 14–21 days 10 mg/kg q 8 h for 14–21 days	Vidarabine and acyclovir are equivalent in clinical efficacy. Serious morbidity is frequent despite therapy.
Genital herpes simplex: primary infection	Acyclovir	IV Oral Topical	5 mg/kg q 8 h for 5–10 days 200 mg 5 times per day for 10 days 5% ointment; 4–6 applications per day for 7–10 days	IV route is preferred if infection is of sufficient severity to warrant hospitalization, or if neurologic complications are present. Preferred route of administration for patients who do not warrant hospitalization. Adequate hydration should be maintained. Largely supplanted by oral therapy. May be of use in pregnant women in order to avoid systemic therapy. Systemic symptoms and untreated areas are not affected.
Genital herpes simplex: recurrent infections (therapy)	Acyclovir	Oral	200 mg 5 times per day for 5 days	Clinical effect is modest and is enhanced if therapy is initiated early. No effect on subsequent recurrence rates.
Genital herpes simplex: recurrent infections (suppression)	Acyclovir	Oral	400 mg 2 times per day for 12 months or longer	Suppressive therapy is recommended only for patients with frequent recurrences, at least 6 to 10 per year. Occasional "breakthrough" may occur, and asymptomatic shedding of virus occurs. Need for suppressive therapy should be reevaluated after 1 year.
Mucocutaneous herpes simplex in immunocompromised patients (treatment)	Acyclovir or vidarabine	IV Oral Topical IV	250 mg/m² q 8 h for 7 days 400 mg PO 5 times per day for 10 days 5% ointment; 4–6 applications per day for 7 days or until healed 10 mg/kg per day for 7 days given as a 12-h infusion	Choice of intravenous or oral route will depend on severity of infection and whether patient can take oral medication. Oral or IV administration has supplanted topical therapy except for small, easily accessible lesions. Efficacy has been demonstrated in HSV-1 infections and in patients who were older than 40. Appears to be less useful than acyclovir in this setting.
Herpes zoster ophthalmicus	Acyclovir	Oral	600 mg PO 5 times a day for 10 days	Reduces ocular complications including ocular keratitis and uveitis.
Cytomegalovirus retinitis in immunosuppressed patients	Ganciclovir or foscarnet	IV IV	5 mg/kg twice a day for 14–21 days, then 5 mg/kg per day as maintenance 60 mg/kg q 8 h for 14–21 days, then 90–120 mg/kg per day as maintenance	Both ganciclovir and foscarnet are licensed for treatment of CMV retinitis in immunosuppressed patients, including those with AIDS. Effectiveness in colitis, pneumonia, or "wasting" syndromes associated with CMV is uncertain. Foscarnet is not myelosuppressive and is active against acyclovir- and ganciclovir-resistant strains of herpesviruses.
HIV infection	Zidovudine or didanosine or	Oral Oral	200 mg PO q 8 h 125–200 mg (tablets) PO twice per day.	Licensed for treatment of patients with HIV infection and CD4 counts less than 500 per microliter. Lower doses (500–600 mg/d) are equally effective and less toxic than higher doses. ddI is licensed for patients with HIV infection who are intolerant of or failing on ZDV. Studies comparing ddI and ZDV are underway.

TABLE 142-1   Antiviral chemotherapy and chemoprophylaxis *(continued)*

Infection	Antiviral drug	Administration	Dosage	Comment
	zalcitabine	Oral	0.75 mg PO q 8 h	Licensed for use in combination with ZDV in patients with advanced infection who are failing on ZDV alone.
Mucocutaneous herpes simplex in immunocompromised patients (prevention of recurrences during periods of intense immunosuppression)	Acyclovir	Oral	200 mg 4 times per day	Acyclovir is administered during periods when intense immunosuppression is expected, e.g., antitumor chemotherapy, after transplantation. After therapy is discontinued, lesions recur.
		IV	5 mg/kg q 12 h	
Herpes simplex keratitis	Trifluorothymidine	Topical	One drop of 0.1% ophthalmic solution every 2 h while awake (maximum 9 drops per day)	Therapy should be undertaken in consultation with an ophthalmologist.
	or			
	vidarabine	Topical	0.5-in ribbon of 3% ophthalmic ointment 5 times per day	As above
Varicella in normal hosts	Acyclovir	Oral	20 mg/kg (up to a maximum of 800 mg), 4 times per day for 5 days.	Modest clinical benefit when administered within 24 h of onset of rash.
Varicella in immunocompromised patients	Acyclovir	IV	500 mg/m² every 8 h for 7 days	Studies comparing IV acyclovir with vidarabine in the treatment of varicella have not been performed. Limited placebo-controlled studies suggest the effects of both drugs on varicella are similar.
	or	IV		
	vidarabine		10 mg/kg per day in a 12-h infusion for 5 days	
Herpes zoster in immunocompromised patients	Acyclovir	IV	500 mg/m² q 8 h for 7 days	Efficacy of acyclovir and vidarabine are established for localized zoster, particularly when treated early, and acyclovir appears to be more effective. Studies of the effectiveness of the two drugs in treatment of disseminated zoster are underway. Oral acyclovir (4 g/d) is under study in herpes zoster in immunosuppressed patients.
	or	IV		
	vidarabine		10 mg/kg per day in a 12-h infusion for 5 days.	
Herpes zoster in immunocompetent hosts	Acyclovir	Oral	800 mg 5 times per day for 7–10 days	Acyclovir accelerated resolution of skin lesions and provided some acute symptomatic relief.
Condyloma acuminatum	Interferon α2b	Intralesional	1 million units per wart (maximum of 5) 3 times per week for 3 weeks	Intralesional treatment results in frequent clearance of warts, but lesions often recur. Parenteral administration may be useful if lesions are numerous.
	or			
	interferon αn3	Intralesional	250,000 units per wart (maximum of 10) 2 times per week for up to 8 weeks.	
Chronic hepatitis, non-A, non-B/C	Interferon α2b	SC or IM	3 million units 3 times/week for 24 weeks	Normalization of serum ALT values occur in 40 percent, but half will relapse when treatment is stopped. Optimal duration and regimens of treatment are under study.
Chronic hepatitis B	Interferon α2b	SC or IM	5 million units per day for 16 weeks	Loss of HBeAg and HBV DNA occurs in 40 to 50 percent of patients. Histopathologic improvement is also seen.

genital HSV infections. Both intravenous and oral formulations have shortened the duration of symptoms, reduced virus shedding, and accelerated healing when employed for the treatment of primary genital HSV infections. Oral acyclovir also had a modest effect in the therapy of recurrent genital HSV infections. However, treatment of either primary or recurrent disease did not reduce the frequency of subsequent recurrences, indicating that acyclovir was ineffective in elimination of latent infection. Chronically administered oral acyclovir for periods ranging from 1 to 6 years has been shown to reduce the frequency of recurrences markedly while on therapy, although once the drug was discontinued, lesions recurred. In AIDS patients, chronic or intermittent administration of acyclovir has been associated with the development of HSV and VZV strains resistant to the action of the drug and with clinical failures. The most common mechanism of resistance is a deficiency of the virus-induced thymidine kinase. Patients with HSV or VZV infections resistant to acyclovir have frequently responded to foscarnet.

With the availability of the oral and intravenous forms, there are few indications for topical acyclovir, although treatment with this formulation has shown modest beneficial effects in the therapy of primary genital HSV infections and of mucocutaneous HSV infections in immunocompromised hosts.

Overall, acyclovir is remarkably well tolerated and generally free of toxicity. The most frequently encountered toxicity has been occasional renal dysfunction, particularly after rapid intravenous administration or when patients have been inadequately hydrated. Central nervous system changes, including lethargy and tremors, occasionally have been reported, primarily in immunosuppressed patients. However, whether these changes are related to acyclovir, to concurrent administration of other therapy, or to underlying infection remains unclear. Acyclovir is excreted primarily unmetabolized by the kidney, by both glomerular filtration and tubular secretion. Approximately 15 percent of a dose of acyclovir is metabolized to 9-[(carboxymethoxy)methyl]guanine or other minor metabolites. Reduction in dosage is indicated in patients with creatinine clearance less than 50 mL/min per 1.73 m². The half-life of acyclovir is approximately 3 h in normal adults, and the peak plasma concentration after a 1-h infusion employing a 5 mg/kg dose is 9.8 μg/mL. Approximately 22 percent of acyclovir administered orally is absorbed, and peak plasma concentrations of 0.3 to 0.9 μg/mL are attained after administration of a 200-mg dose. Acyclovir penetrates relatively well into the cerebrospinal fluid, with CSF concentrations approaching one-half of those found in plasma.

GANCICLOVIR An analogue of acyclovir, ganciclovir, 9-[(1,3-dihydroxy-2-propoxy)methyl]guanine, has activity against all herpesviruses but markedly increased activity against CMV. Ganciclovir triphosphate inhibits CMV DNA polymerases and can be incorporated into CMV DNA with eventual termination of elongation of viral DNA. CMV, unlike HSV, does not code for its own thymidine kinase, but ganciclovir is phosphorylated by a virus-coded protein kinase and/or cellular kinases. Ganciclovir triphosphate is present in tenfold greater concentrations in CMV-infected cells than in uninfected cells. Ganciclovir has been utilized extensively in the treatment of CMV infection in AIDS and otherwise immunosuppressed patients and has been licensed for the treatment of CMV retinitis in immunocompromised patients. It also has been used to treat other CMV-associated syndromes, such as CMV colitis, "wasting" syndrome, and pneumonitis, but its efficacy for these infections remains to be established.

Ganciclovir is available only for intravenous administration. It has a plasma half-life of 2.9 ± 1.3 h and is excreted primarily by the kidney, unmetabolized. The most commonly employed dosage for initial therapy is 5 mg/kg twice a day for 14 to 21 days, followed by a maintenance dose of 5 mg/kg per day or 5 times per week, possibly for as long as the immunosuppression persists. Administration of ganciclovir has been associated with profound bone marrow suppression, particularly neutropenia, which represents a major limitation of its use in many patients. Bone marrow toxicity is potentiated when other bone marrow suppressants such as zidovudine are used concomitantly. CMV isolates resistant to ganciclovir have been reported in AIDS patients receiving the drug.

FOSCARNET Foscarnet (phosphonoformic acid) is a pyrophosphate-containing compound which is a potent inhibitor of herpesviruses, including CMV. It inhibits viral DNA polymerases at the pyrophosphate binding site at concentrations which have relatively little effect on cellular polymerases. Because foscarnet does not require phosphorylation to exert its antiviral activity, it is active against herpesviruses that are resistant to acyclovir because of deficiencies in thymidine kinase and against ganciclovir-resistant strains of CMV. Foscarnet also inhibits the reverse transcriptase of HIV and is active against HIV in vivo.

Foscarnet is poorly soluble and must be administered intravenously in a dilute solution infused over 1 to 2 h. The plasma half-life of foscarnet is 3 to 5 h and increases with decreasing renal function, since the drug is primarily eliminated by the kidneys. It has been estimated that 10 to 28 percent of a dose may be deposited in bone, where it can persist for months. The most common initial dosage of foscarnet is 60 mg/kg every 8 h for 14 to 21 days, followed by a maintenance dose of 90 to 120 mg/kg given once a day.

Foscarnet is licensed for the treatment of CMV retinitis in patients with AIDS. In a comparative clinical trial, it appeared to have efficacy similar to that of ganciclovir against CMV retinitis but was associated with a longer survival, which is as yet unexplained. It also has been used to treat acyclovir-resistant HSV and VZV infections and ganciclovir-resistant CMV infections.

The major toxicity of foscarnet is renal impairment, and renal function should be monitored closely, particularly during the initial phase of therapy. Since foscarnet binds divalent metal ions, hypocalcemia, hypomagnesemia, hypokalemia, and hypo- or hyperphosphatemia can occur. Although hematologic abnormalities also have been observed, foscarnet is not generally myelosuppressive and may

be administered concomitantly with myelosuppressive medications such as zidovudine.

ZIDOVUDINE Zidovudine (ZDV), also known as azidothymidine (AZT), inhibits the replication of HIV through a competitive inhibition of HIV reverse transcriptase by AZT triphosphate, and through chain termination of viral DNA synthesis as well. ZDV is administered orally and has a plasma half-life of approximately 1 h. Ninety percent of a dose is recovered as ZDV or its metabolite in urine. A large-scale placebo-controlled trial carried out in 1987 in patients with AIDS or with advanced AIDS-related complex (ARC) demonstrated that administration of ZDV was associated with prolonged survival and with a decreased frequency and severity of opportunistic infections. Subsequently, placebo-controlled trials in patients with less advanced HIV disease, including patients with early symptomatic disease (CD4 counts of 200 to 800 per microliter and oral thrush, hairy leukoplakia, or intermittent diarrhea) and asymptomatic patients with CD4 counts of less than or equal to 500 per microliter demonstrated lower rates of progression of HIV disease in ZDV recipients. Studies in asymptomatic patients with CD4 counts greater than 500 per microliter are currently underway.

ZDV is currently licensed for treatment of patients with HIV infection who have 500 or fewer CD4 lymphocytes per microliter in peripheral blood. In patients with advanced disease, the beneficial clinical effects of ZDV appear, for unclear reasons, to wane after 12 to 18 months of therapy. HIV isolates obtained from patients with advanced disease who have received ZDV for more than 6 months show high rates of resistance to ZDV in vitro, which may play a role in clinical failures of ZDV. The development of resistance appears to be less frequent in asymptomatic patients or in patients with less advanced disease. ZDV resistance is associated with specific amino acid substitutions in the HIV reverse transcriptase.

The most frequently employed dosage of ZDV is 200 mg by mouth every 8 h, and comparative dosage studies indicate that total daily doses of 500 to 600 mg are as effective and less toxic than higher doses which had been previously recommended. The major toxicities of ZDV are hematopoietic, particularly anemia and granulocytopenia, which occur more frequently in patients with more advanced HIV disease. Nausea, headache, and malaise are also encountered frequently, and a ZDV-related myopathy also can occur.

DIDANOSINE Didanosine (or ddI) is a nucleoside analogue with antiviral activity against HIV-1 and HIV-2. It is an inhibitor of the HIV reverse transcriptase and also can act as a chain terminator for viral DNA elongation. ddI is phosphorylated and converted to ddATP, which is the active antiviral moiety. ddI is active in vitro against most HIV isolates which are resistant to ZDV.

ddI is given orally and is highly acid labile, so it must be administered with buffers against stomach acidity. These buffers are incorporated into the powder or tablet preparations. ddI in tablets is 20 to 25 percent more bioavailable than in powder. The plasma half-life of ddI is 1.5 h, and approximately 50 percent of a dose is cleared by renal mechanisms. The intracellular half-life of ddATP is considerably longer (8 to 24 h) and provides the rationale for the recommended dosing schedule of every 12 h.

ddI has been carefully studied in phase I trials and has received extensive use in a large-scale "expanded access" program under which more than 22,000 patients with HIV infection have received the drug. On the basis of a favorable effect on circulating CD4 counts and serum p24 concentrations in the phase I studies and of an interim analysis of an ongoing phase II study, ddI has been licensed for patients who are intolerant of ZDV therapy or who are failing clinically or immunologically on ZDV treatment. Controlled studies comparing ddI and ZDV are nearing completion and should provide important information regarding the clinical efficacy and appropriate use of this drug.

The major toxicities encountered in the use of ddI have been pancreatitis and peripheral neuropathy. Overall rates of pancreatitis in recipients of ddI have been estimated to be 5 to 9 percent, and cases occur more frequently in patients with advanced HIV disease.

Most cases are mild to moderate in severity, but fatal cases have occurred, though rarely. Painful peripheral neuropathy, primarily involving the lower extremities, also may develop and is generally reversible if recognized early and if drug administration is stopped. Medications or other factors which can cause pancreatitis or peripheral neuropathy should be avoided in patients who are taking ddI. ddI has not been associated with consistent hematopoietic toxicity, and in fact, hemoglobin, white blood cell, and platelet counts frequently improve on ddI therapy. Thus ddI may be particularly useful in the setting where hematopoietic suppression is present or anticipated, either from drugs or from underlying diseases.

ZALCITABINE AND OTHER ANTIRETROVIRAL DRUGS Zalcitabine (or ddC) is a nucleoside analogue which is a potent inhibitor of HIV. The triphosphate of ddC (ddCTP) inhibits HIV reverse transcriptase activity and also acts as a chain terminator. ddC is administered orally, has a plasma half-life of 1.2 h, and is excreted primarily by the kidney. A recently concluded study comparing ddC with ZDV in patients who had received less than 3 months of ZDV showed that ddC was less effective than ZDV in prevention of opportunistic infections and neoplasms. The major toxicities of ddC are a dose-related peripheral neuropathy and aphthous stomatitis. Hematologic toxicities, as manifested by anemia and neutropenia, were not major problems. Recently, phase I studies of combinations of ZDV and ddC have demonstrated a favorable effect on CD4 counts and p24 concentrations, and large-scale clinical trials of this combination are underway. ddC has recently been licensed for use in combination with ZDV to treat patients with advanced HIV infection who are failing clinically or immunologically on ZDV alone.

A variety of other antiretroviral drugs are at various stages of preclinical and early (phase I) clinical development. These include reverse transcriptase inhibitors of the nucleoside analogue class such as d4T and nonnucleoside inhibitors such as TIBO or BI-RG-587. Compounds that interfere with HIV binding or with replication at other sites such as inhibitors of viral protease, inhibitors of protein glycosylation (N-butyl-deoxynojirimycin), and inhibitors of HIV tat protein are also under development.

VIDARABINE Vidarabine (9-β-D-arabinofuranosyladenine) is a purine nucleoside analogue with activity against HSV-1, HSV-2, VZV, and EBV. Vidarabine inhibits viral DNA synthesis through its 5'-triphosphorylated metabolite, although the precise molecular mechanisms of action are not completely understood. In the therapy of herpes zoster in immunosuppressed patients, vidarabine, administered in a dose of 10 mg/kg per day for 5 days, resulted in reduction of rates of cutaneous and visceral dissemination and of postherpetic neuralgia but was less effective overall than acyclovir in a comparative trial. Beneficial effects also have been observed in the treatment of varicella in immunosuppressed patients. Vidarabine administered in a higher dose (15 mg/kg per day for 10 days) was demonstrated to be effective in the therapy of herpes simplex encephalitis in a placebo-controlled study, but comparative studies indicate that acyclovir (30 mg/kg per day) is the drug of choice for this infection. Vidarabine appears to be equal in efficacy to acyclovir in the treatment of neonatal herpes simplex infection. The ophthalmic ointment of vidarabine (3%) is effective in the treatment of HSV keratitis.

For systemic administration, vidarabine is available only as an intravenous preparation with poor solubility and is administered as a constant 12-h infusion, so a substantial fluid load can result which may be a significant problem in central nervous system infections. Vidarabine at doses of 10 to 15 mg/kg per day is generally well tolerated, but at somewhat higher doses (20 mg/kg per day) the drug has been associated with hematopoietic side effects, including anemia, leukopenia, and thrombocytopenia. Neurotoxicity also has been reported, particularly with high dosages and in patients with hepatic or renal insufficiency.

TOPICAL ANTIVIRALS IUdR (5'-iodo-2'-deoxyuridine) is an inhibitor of DNA virus replication, including herpesviruses and poxviruses. It was formerly used systemically to treat herpesvirus infections, including HSV encephalitis, but because of associated toxicity and lack of demonstrated efficacy, its systemic use has largely been abandoned. Topical IUdR has been effective in the treatment of HSV keratitis, particularly in superficial epithelial infections, but has been largely supplanted by topically applied trifluorothymidine or vidarabine.

Trifluorothymidine (TFT) is an analogue of deoxythymidine, which is also effective against herpesvirus infections. Because of bone marrow suppression, its use is restricted to topical application in the eye, where it appears to be somewhat more effective and better tolerated than IUdR and at least as effective as vidarabine. TFT also has been effective in some patients who had not responded clinically to topical IUdR or vidarabine.

INTERFERONS From its earliest descriptions, considerable interest has existed in the application of interferon to the prophylaxis and/or therapy of viral infections. Interferons are cytokines with broad antiviral activities, as well as immunomodulating and antiproliferative properties. Early studies with human leukocyte interferon demonstrated an effect in the prophylaxis of experimentally induced rhinovirus infections in humans and in the treatment of varicella-zoster infections in immunosuppressed patients. DNA recombinant technology has made available highly purified α-, β-, and γ-interferons, which have been evaluated in a variety of viral infections. Results of such trials have confirmed the effectiveness of intranasally administered interferon in the prophylaxis of rhinovirus infections, although its use has been associated with nasal mucosal irritation. Recent studies also have demonstrated a beneficial effect of parenterally administered interferons on genital warts, primarily in reduction of size of lesions, and this mode of therapy may be useful in individuals who have numerous warts which cannot easily be treated by individual intralesional injection. However, lesions frequently recur after intralesional or parenteral interferon therapy is discontinued.

Interferons also have received extensive study in the therapy of chronic hepatitis B infection. Interferon α2b administered to patients with stable chronic hepatitis B infection resulted in loss of markers of HBV replication, such as HBeAg and HBV DNA, in 40 to 50 percent of patients who received daily doses of 5 million units for 16 weeks; 10 to 20 percent of patients also became HBsAg negative. More than 80 percent of patients who lose HBeAg and HBV DNA markers will have return of serum aminotransferases to normal levels, and both short- and long-term improvement in liver histopathology has been described. Predictors of a favorable response to therapy include low pretherapy HBV DNA levels, high pretherapy serum ALT levels, short duration of chronic hepatitis B infection, and active liver histopathology. Adverse effects of the preceding dose of interferon are common and include fever, chills, myalgia, and fatigue. Approximately 25 percent of patients receiving a daily dose of 5 million units will require dose reduction, but fewer than 5 percent will require discontinuation of therapy.

Several interferon preparations, including α2a, α2b, and αL (lymphoblastoid) have been studied as therapy for chronic non-A, non-B/C infections. A variety of dose regimens have been employed, of which the most common is 1 or 3 million units three times per week for 6 months. A complete response, defined as a return to normal serum ALT values at the end of treatment, has been observed in approximately 40 percent of patients. Liver biopsies also showed decrease of lobular and periportal inflammation. However, relapse occurred in half or more of the patients when therapy was discontinued. Relapses have generally responded quickly to retreatment. Additional clinical studies to develop more effective regimens of therapy and to define prognostic variables in this patient population are currently underway.

Interferon is licensed in the United States for the treatment of chronic hepatitis B (α2b), chronic hepatitis non-A, non-B/C infection (α2b), condyloma acuminatum (α2b, αn3), hairy-cell leukemia (α2a, α2b) and Kaposi's sarcoma (α2a, α2b). Interferon-γ (γ1b) is licensed for the treatment of patients with chronic granulomatous disease.

REFERENCES

DAVIS GL et al: Treatment of chronic hepatitis with recombinant interferon alfa: A multicenter randomized, controlled trial. N Engl J Med 32:1501, 1989

DOLIN R et al: A controlled trial of amantadine and rimantadine in the prophylaxis of influenza A infection. N Engl J Med 307:580, 1982

FAULDS D, HEEL RC: Ganciclovir: A review of its antiviral activity, pharmacokinetic properties, and therapeutic efficacy in cytomegalovirus infections. Drugs 39:597, 1990

FISCHL M et al: The efficacy of azidothymidine (AZT) in the treatment of patients with AIDS and AIDS-related complex; a double blind placebo-controlled trial. N Engl J Med 317:185, 1987

HALL CB et al: Aerosolized ribavirin treatment of infants with respiratory syncytial viral infection: A randomized double blind study. N Engl J Med 308:1443, 1983

MERTZ GJ et al: Double blind placebo-controlled trial of oral acyclovir in first episode genital herpes simplex infection. JAMA 252:147, 1984

PALESTINE AG et al: A randomized, controlled trial in the treatment of cytomegalovirus retinitis in patients with AIDS. Ann Intern Med 115:669, 1991

PERILLO RP et al: A randomized, controlled trial of interferon alfa-2b alone and after prednisone withdrawal, in the treatment of chronic hepatitis B infection. N Engl J Med 323:295, 1990

REICHMAN·RL et al: Treatment of condyloma acuminatum with three different interferons administered intralesionally: A double-blind, placebo-controlled trial. Ann Intern Med 108:675, 1988

VOLBERDING P et al: Zidovudine in asymptomatic human immunodeficiency virus infection: A controlled trial in persons with fewer than 500 CD4-positive cells per cubic millimeter. N Engl J Med 322:941, 1990

WHITLEY RJ et al and the NIAID Collaborative Antiviral Study Group: Herpes simplex encephalitis: Adenine arabinoside versus acyclovir therapies. N Engl J Med 314:144, 1986

YARCHOAN R et al: Long term toxicity/activity profile of 2'3'-dideoxyinosine in AIDS and AIDS related complex. Lancet 336:526, 1990

section 12   DNA viruses

143   HERPES SIMPLEX VIRUSES

LAWRENCE COREY

DEFINITION Herpes simplex viruses (HSV-1, HSV-2; *Herpesvirus hominis*) produce a variety of infections involving mucocutaneous surfaces, the central nervous system, and occasionally visceral organs. The advent of effective antiviral chemotherapy for HSV infections has made prompt recognition of these syndromes of clinical importance.

ETIOLOGY The genome of herpes simplex virus is a linear, double-stranded DNA molecule (about 100×10^6 in molecular weight) that encodes for more than 60 gene products. The genomic structures of the two HSV subtypes are similar, and the overall sequence homology between HSV-1 and HSV-2 is about 50 percent. The homologous sequences are distributed over the entire genome map, and most of the polypeptides specified by one viral type are antigenically related to polypeptides of the other viral type. Many type-specific regions unique to HSV-1 and HSV-2 proteins do exist, however, and many of these regions appear to be important in host immunity. Restriction endonuclease analysis of viral DNA can be utilized to distinguish between the two subtypes and among strains of the two subtypes. The variability of nucleotide sequences from clinical strains of HSV-1 and HSV-2 is such that HSV isolates obtained from two individuals can be differentiated by restriction enzyme patterns unless the isolates are from epidemiologically related sources, such as sexual partners, mother-infant pairs, or common-source outbreaks.

The viral genome is packaged within a regular icosahedral protein shell (capsid) composed of 162 capsomers. The outer covering of the virus is a lipid-containing membrane (envelope) derived from modified cell membrane and acquired as the DNA-containing capsid buds through the inner nuclear membrane of the host cell. Between the capsid and lipid bilayer of the envelope is the tegument, composed of a number of viral proteins whose properties and functions are largely unknown. Viral replication has both nuclear and cytoplasmic phases. The initial steps of replication include attachment, fusion between the viral envelope and a cell membrane to liberate the nucleocapsid into the cytoplasm of the cell, and disassembly of the nucleocapsid to release the viral DNA. Replication of HSV is highly regulated. Following fusion of the virion envelope with the host cell membrane, two proteins are released from the HSV virion. HSV shuts off host protein synthesis, and α TIF, a γ gene product, "turns on" transcription of the α genes (immediate early). The presence of the α-gene products is required for synthesis of the subsequent polypeptide group, the β polypeptides, many of which are regulatory proteins and enzymes required for DNA replication. Most current antiviral drugs interrupt β proteins such as the viral DNA polymerase enzyme. The third (γ) class of HSV genes requires viral DNA replication for expression and constitutes most of the structural proteins specified by the virus.

Following replication of the viral genome and synthesis of structural proteins, nucleocapsids are assembled in the nucleus of the cell. Envelopment occurs as the nucleocapsids bud through the inner nuclear membrane into the perinuclear space. In some cells, viral replication within the nucleus forms two types of inclusion bodies: type A basophilic Feulgen-positive bodies that contain viral DNA and an eosinophilic inclusion body that is devoid of viral nucleic acid or protein and represents a "scar" of viral infection. Virions are then transported via the endoplasmic reticulum and the Golgi apparatus to the cell surface.

HSV infection of some neuronal cells does not result in cell death. Instead, viral genomes are maintained by the cell in a repressed state compatible with survival and normal activities of the cell, a process called *latency*. Subsequently, activation of the viral genome may occur, resulting in viral replication and, in some cases, the redevelopment of herpetic lesions, a process termed *reactivation*. Whereas infectious virus rarely can be recovered from sensory or autonomic nervous system ganglia dissected from cadavers, maintenance and growth of the neural cells in tissue culture result in production of infectious virions, a process called *explanation*, and subsequent permissive infection of susceptible cells, a process called *cocultivation*. Virus replication was first detected in neurons during reactivation in vitro, suggesting that the neuron harbors the latent virus in vivo. Subsequently, viral DNA has been found in neural tissue at times when infectious virus cannot be isolated. HSV DNA extracted from latently infected neural tissue differs from HSV DNA in cells with actively replicating virus. In latently infected cells, only partial transcription of viral proteins occurs. Two RNA transcripts which overlap the immediate early (α) gene product, called ICP-o, are found in abundance in the nuclei of latently infected neurons. The coding of these RNA transcripts in an "antisense" direction suggests that they may be a factor in inhibiting the subsequent transcription of β and γ proteins. Deletion mutants of this region have been made. While these viruses can become latent, the efficiency of their subsequent reactivation is reduced; thus the "antisense" transcripts may play a role in maintaining rather than in establishing latency. Understanding molecular mechanisms of latency may lead to new therapies to prevent reactivation of HSV.

PATHOGENESIS Exposure to virus at mucosal surfaces or abraded skin permits entry of virus and initiation of replication in cells of the epidermis and dermis. Whether or not clinically apparent lesions develop, sufficient viral replication to permit infection of either sensory or autonomic nerve endings may occur. Whether latency always results from peripheral mucosal infection is unclear. Virus—or, more likely, nucleocapsid—is then thought to be transported intraaxonally to the nerve cell bodies in ganglia. In humans, the time from inoculation of virus in peripheral tissue to spread to the ganglia is unknown. During the initial phase of infection, viral replication occurs in ganglia and contiguous neural tissue. Virus then spreads to other mucosal skin surfaces through centrifugal migration of infectious virions via peripheral sensory nerves. This spread of virus to the skin from peripheral sensory nerves helps explain the large surface area, the high frequency of new lesions distant from the initial crop of vesicles which are characteristic in patients with primary genital or oral-labial HSV infection, and the recovery of virus from neural tissue distant from neurons innervating the inoculation site. Contiguous spread of locally inoculated virus also may occur and allow further mucosal extension of disease.

Following resolution of primary disease, infectious virus can no longer be recovered in the ganglia. The mechanisms by which various stimuli cause reactivation of HSV infection are unknown. Ultraviolet light, immunosuppression, and trauma to the skin or ganglia are associated with reactivation.

Analysis of the HSV DNA from sequentially isolated strains of HSV or from multiple infected ganglia in any one individual has revealed identical restriction endonuclease patterns in most persons. Occasionally, and more frequently in immunocompromised persons, multiple strains of the same viral subtype can be detected in the same person. This finding suggests that exogenous infection with different strains of the same subtype is possible.

IMMUNITY Host responses to infection influence the acquisition of disease, severity of infection, resistance to development of latency, maintenance of latency, and frequency of HSV recurrences. Both antibody-mediated and cell-mediated reactions are clinically important. Immunocompromised patients with defects in cell-mediated immunity experience more severe and extensive HSV infections than those with deficits in humoral immunity such as agammaglobulinemia. Experimental ablation of lymphocytes indicates that T cells play a major role in preventing lethal disseminated disease, although antibodies help reduce virus titers in neural tissue. Some aspects of the pathogenesis of disease also may be related to the host immune response, e.g., stromal opacities associated with recurrent herpetic keratitis. The surface viral glycoproteins have been shown to be antigens recognized by antibodies mediating neutralization and immune-mediated cytolysis (antibody-dependent cell-mediated cytotoxicity, ADCC). Monoclonal antibodies specific for each of the known viral glycoproteins have, in experimental infections, conferred protection against subsequent neurologic disease or ganglionic latency. Multiple cell populations, including natural killer (NK) cells, macrophages, a variety of T lymphocyte populations, and lymphokines generated by these cells, play a role in host defenses to HSV infections. In animals, passive transfer of primed lymphocytes confers protection from subsequent challenge. Maximum protection usually requires the activation of multiple T cell subpopulations, including cytotoxic T cells and T cells responsible for delayed hypersensitivity. The latter cells may confer protection by the antigen-stimulated release of lymphokines (e.g., interferons), which may have a direct antiviral effect or activate other nonspecific effector cells.

EPIDEMIOLOGY Seroepidemiologic studies have shown that HSV infections are found worldwide. Because much of the humoral immune response to HSV is to type-common antigenic determinants, it is difficult to detect HSV-2 antibodies in persons with prior HSV-1 infection and HSV-1 antibodies in those with prior HSV-2 infections. Serologic assays which utilize whole-virus antigen preparations, such as complement fixation, neutralization, indirect immunofluorescence assay (IFA), passive hemagglutination (PHA), radioimmunoassay (RIA), and enzyme-linked immunosorbent assay (ELISA), do not reliably distinguish between the two viral subtypes. Recently, serologic assays which identify antibodies to type-specific surface proteins of the two viruses have been developed. These assays can reliably distinguish the human antibody response between HSV-1 and HSV-2. These assays are based on demonstrating antibodies to type-specific epitopes of the virus; the most commonly utilized are those which measure antibodies to glycoprotein G of HSV-1 (gG1) and HSV-2 (gG2). At present, these assays are available only in a limited number of laboratories.

Infection with HSV-1 is acquired more frequently and earlier than infection with HSV-2. Over 90 percent of adults have antibodies to HSV-1 by the fifth decade. In lower socioeconomic populations, most persons will acquire HSV-1 infection before the third decade.

Antibodies to HSV-2 are not routinely detected until puberty. Antibody prevalence rates correlate with past sexual activity and vary greatly among different population groups. In most routine obstetrical and family planning clinics, 20 to 30 percent of women possess HSV-2 antibodies, although only 10 percent report a history of genital lesions. As many as 50 percent of heterosexual adults attending STD clinics possess HSV-2 antibodies. In university clinics, HSV antibody prevalence may be as low as 3 to 8 percent. Antibody prevalence rates average about 5 percent higher in women than in men. The large reservoir of unidentified carriers of HSV-2 and the frequent asymptomatic reactivation of virus from the genital tract have fostered the continued spread of genital herpes throughout the world. HSV-2 infection has been shown to be a risk factor for the acquisition and transmission of infection with human immunodeficiency virus type 1 (HIV-1).

HSV infections occur throughout the year. The incubation period ranges from 1 to 26 days (median 6 to 8 days). Contact with active ulcerative lesions or asymptomatically excreting patients can result in transmission. Asymptomatic salivary excretion of HSV-1 has been reported in 2 to 9 percent of adults and 5 to 8 percent of children. HSV-2 has been isolated from the genital tract of 0.3 to 6 percent of males and 1.5 to 13 percent of females attending STD clinics. The titer of HSV in cultures from lesions is 100 to 1000 times higher than from salivary or genital tract secretions in asymptomatically excreting persons. The efficiency of transmission is greater during symptomatic than asymptomatic periods of viral excretion.

CLINICAL SPECTRUM HSV has been isolated from nearly all visceral or mucocutaneous sites. The clinical manifestations and course of HSV depend on the anatomic site of the infection, the age and immune status of the host, and the antigenic type of the virus. First episodes of HSV disease, especially primary infections (i.e., first infections with either HSV-1 or HSV-2 in which the host lacks HSV antibodies in acute-phase sera), are frequently accompanied by systemic signs and symptoms, involve both mucosal and extramucosal sites, and have a longer duration of symptoms, a longer time during which virus is isolated from lesions, and a higher rate of complications than recurrent episodes of disease. Both viral subtypes can cause genital and oral-facial infections, and these infections are clinically indistinguishable. However, the frequency of future reactivations of infection is influenced by the anatomic site and virus type. Genital HSV-2 infection is twice as likely to reactivate and will recur 8 to 10 times more frequently than genital HSV-1 infection. Conversely, oral-labial HSV-1 infections will recur more frequently than oral-labial HSV-2 infections.

Oral-facial HSV infections Gingivostomatitis and pharyngitis are the most frequent clinical manifestations of first-episode HSV-1 infection, while recurrent herpes labialis is the most frequent clinical manifestation of reactivation HSV infection. HSV pharyngitis and gingivostomatitis usually result from primary infection and are most commonly seen in children and young adults. Clinical symptoms and signs include fever, malaise, myalgias, inability to eat, irritability, and cervical adenopathy, which may last from 3 to 14 days. Lesions may involve the hard and soft palate, gingiva, tongue, lip, and facial area. HSV-1 or HSV-2 infection of the pharynx usually results in exudative or ulcerative lesions of the posterior pharynx and/or tonsillar pillars. Concomitant lesions of the tongue, buccal mucosa, or gingiva may occur later in the course in one-third of cases. Fever lasting from 2 to 7 days and cervical adenopathy are common. The clinical differentiation of HSV pharyngitis from bacterial pharyngitis, *Mycoplasma pneumoniae* infections, and noninfectious causes of pharyngeal ulcerations such as Stevens-Johnson syndrome may be difficult. No substantial evidence suggests that reactivation oral-labial HSV infection is associated with symptomatic recurrent pharyngitis.

Reactivation of HSV from the trigeminal ganglia may be associated with asymptomatic excretion in the saliva, development of intraoral mucosal ulcerations, or herpetic ulcerations on the vermilion border of the lip or external facial skin. About 50 to 70 percent of seropositive patients undergoing trigeminal nerve root decompression and 10 to 15 percent of those undergoing dental extraction will develop oral-labial HSV infection a median of 3 days after these procedures.

In immunosuppressed patients infection may extend into mucosal and deep cutaneous layers. Friability, necrosis, bleeding, severe pain, and inability to eat or drink may result. HSV mucositis is clinically similar to mucosal lesions due to cytotoxic drug therapy, trauma, or fungal or bacterial infections. Persistent ulcerative HSV infections are among the most common infections in patients with AIDS. Concomitant HSV and *Candida* infections also occur commonly. Systemic acyclovir therapy speeds the rate of healing and relieves the pain of mucosal HSV infections in immunosuppressed patients. Patients with atopic eczema also may develop severe oral-facial HSV infections (eczema herpeticum) which may rapidly involve extensive areas of skin and occasionally disseminate to visceral organs. Prompt resolution of extensive eczema herpeticum has been achieved with the administration of intravenous acyclovir. Erythema multiforme (EM) also may be associated with HSV infections, and some evidence suggests that HSV infection is the precipitating event in about 75 percent of cases of cutaneous EM. HSV antigen has been demonstrated both in circulatory immune complexes and in skin lesion biopsy of these patients. Patients with severe HSV-associated EM are candidates for chronic suppressive oral acyclovir therapy.

Genital HSV infections   First-episode primary genital herpes is characterized by fever, headache, malaise, and myalgias. Pain, itching, dysuria, vaginal and urethral discharge, and tender inguinal lymphadenopathy are the predominant local symptoms. Characteristically, widely spaced bilateral lesions of the external genitalia are seen. Lesions may be present in varying stages, including vesicles, pustules, or painful erythematous ulcers. Involvement of the cervix and urethra is seen in over 80 percent of women with first-episode infections. First episodes of genital herpes in patients who have had prior HSV-1 infection are associated with less frequent systemic symptoms and faster healing than primary genital herpes. The clinical courses of acute first-episode genital herpes among patients with HSV-1 and HSV-2 infections are similar. However, the recurrence rates of genital disease differ. About 90 percent of patients with first-episode HSV-2 infection will have a recurrence within 12 months (median number of recurrences, four) compared with 55 percent of those with primary HSV-1 infections (median number of recurrences, less than one). Recurrence rates of genital HSV-2 infections vary greatly between individuals and over time within the same individual. HSV has been isolated from the urethra and urine of men and women without concomitant external genital lesions. A clear mucoid discharge and dysuria are characteristics of symptomatic HSV urethritis. HSV has been isolated from the urethra of 5 percent of women with the dysuria-frequency syndrome. Occasionally, genital tract disease manifested by HSV endometritis and salpingitis in women and HSV prostatitis in men may occur.

Both HSV-1 and HSV-2 can cause symptomatic or asymptomatic rectal and perianal infections. Symptoms of HSV proctitis include anorectal pain, anorectal discharge, tenesmus, and constipation. Sigmoidoscopy reveals ulcerative lesions of the distal 10 cm of the rectal mucosa. Rectal biopsies show mucosal ulceration, necrosis, polymorphonuclear and lymphocytic infiltration of the lamina propria, and occasionally multinucleated intranuclear inclusion–bearing cells. Perianal herpetic lesions are also seen in immunosuppressed patients receiving cytotoxic therapy. Either HSV-1 or HSV-2 can cause perianal herpes. The HSV-1 strains isolated from perianal lesions are often identical to those found in the oropharynx. This finding suggests that the mode of spread is autoinoculation of the perianal area from HSV-infected saliva and/or finger lesions. Replication of HSV-2 from sacral nerve root ganglia may lead to extensive perianal herpetic lesions and/or HSV proctitis among patients with HIV infection or those undergoing transplantation. Chronic acyclovir therapy is often used to suppress such recurrences.

Herpetic whitlow   Herpetic whitlow, HSV infection of the finger, may occur as a complication of primary oral or genital herpes by inoculation of virus via a break in the epidermal surface or by direct introduction of virus into the hand through occupational or other exposure. Clinical signs and symptoms include the abrupt onset of edema, erythema, and localized tenderness of the infected finger. Vesicular or pustular lesions of the fingertip indistinguishable from pyogenic bacterial infection are seen. Fever, lymphadenitis, and epitrochlear and axillary lymphadenopathy are common. The infection may recur. Prompt diagnosis to avoid unnecessary and potentially exacerbating surgical therapy and/or transmission is essential.

Herpes gladiatorum   HSV may infect almost any area of skin. Mucocutaneous HSV infections of the thorax, ears, face, and hands have been described among wrestlers. Transmission of these infections is facilitated by trauma to the skin sustained during wrestling. Prompt diagnosis and therapy are required to contain spread of this infection.

Herpetic eye infections   HSV infection of the eye is the most frequent cause of corneal blindness in the United States. HSV keratitis presents with acute onset of pain, blurring of vision, chemosis, conjunctivitis, and characteristic dendritic lesions of the cornea. Use of topical corticosteroids may exacerbate symptoms and lead to involvement of deep structures of the eye. Debridement, topical antiviral treatment, and/or interferon therapy hastens healing. However, recurrences are common, and immunopathologic injury of the deeper structures of the eye may occur. Chorioretinitis, usually as a manifestation of disseminated HSV infection, may occur in neonates or in patients with HIV infection. Acute necrotizing retinitis due to HSV is an uncommon but severe manifestation of HSV infection.

Central and peripheral nervous system infections with HSV-1 and HSV-2   HSV encephalitis is the most common identified cause of acute, sporadic viral encephalitis in the United States, comprising 10 to 20 percent of all cases. The estimated incidence is about 2.3 cases per million persons per year. Cases are distributed throughout the year, and the age distribution appears biphasic, with peaks at 5 to 30 and >50 years of age. HSV-1 accounts for more than 95 percent of cases. The pathogenesis of HSV encephalitis varies. In children and young adults, primary HSV infection may result in encephalitis; presumably, exogenously acquired virus enters the CNS by neurotropic spread from the periphery via the olfactory bulb. However, most adults with HSV encephalitis have clinical or serologic evidence of mucocutaneous HSV-1 infection prior to the onset of the CNS symptoms. In about 25 percent of the cases examined, the HSV-1 strains from the oropharynx and brain tissue of the same patient differ; thus some cases may result from reinfection with another strain of HSV-1 that reaches the CNS. Two theories have been proposed to explain the development of actively replicating HSV in localized areas of the CNS in persons from whom the ganglionic and CNS isolates are similar. Reactivation of latent trigeminal or autonomic nerve root HSV-1 infection may be associated with extension of virus into the CNS via nerves innervating the middle cranial fossa. HSV DNA has been demonstrated by DNA hybridization in human autopsy brain tissue. Reactivation of long-standing latent CNS infection may be another potential mechanism for the development of HSV encephalitis.

The clinical hallmark of HSV encephalitis has been the acute onset of fever and focal neurologic, especially temporal lobe, symptoms. Differentiation of HSV encephalitis from other viral encephalitides, as well as from other focal infections and noninfectious processes, is difficult. An increase in CSF and serum antibodies to HSV does occur with most cases of HSV encephalitis. However, these increased antibody titers rarely are present prior to 10 days into the illness and, while useful retrospectively, are usually not helpful in establishing the clinical diagnosis early in the course of disease. Demonstration of HSV antigen or DNA in brain biopsy has a high sensitivity and a low complication rate and also provides the best opportunity to diagnose and establish alternative, potentially treatable causes of encephalitis. The most sensitive early noninvasive method for diagnosing HSV encephalitis is the demonstration of HSV DNA in CSF by polymerase chain reaction (PCR). Antiviral chemotherapy reduces the mortality of HSV encephalitis, and intravenous acyclovir is more effective than vidarabine. Even with therapy, however, neurologic sequelae are frequent, especially in those over 35 years of age. Most authorities recommend initiating intravenous acyclovir treatment in patients with presumed HSV encephalitis until the diagnosis is confirmed or an alternative diagnosis is made.

HSV has been isolated from the cerebrospinal fluid (CSF) of 0.5 to 3 percent of patients presenting to the hospital with aseptic meningitis. HSV meningitis is usually seen in association with primary genital HSV infection. HSV meningitis is an acute, self-limited disease manifested by headache, fever, and mild photophobia and lasting from 2 to 7 days. A lymphocytic pleocytosis in the CSF is characteristic. Neurologic sequelae are rare. Recurrent bouts of aseptic meningitis related to reactivation of HSV have been reported.

Autonomic nervous system dysfunction, especially of the sacral region, has been reported in association with both HSV and varicella-zoster infections. Numbness, tingling of the buttock or perineal areas, urinary retention, constipation, CSF pleocytosis, and impotence in males may occur. Symptoms appear to resolve slowly over a period of days to weeks. Occasionally, hypesthesia and/or weakness of the lower extremities may persist for many months. Rarely, transverse myelitis manifested by a rapidly progressive symmetric paralysis of the lower extremities or a Guillain-Barré syndrome may occur after HSV infection. Similarly, peripheral nervous system involvement [idiopathic facial paralysis (Bell's palsy)] or cranial polyneuritis also may be related to reactivation of HSV-1 infection. Transitory hypesthesia of the area of skin innervated by the trigeminal nerve and vestibular system dysfunction as measured by electronystagmography are the predominant signs of disease. Studies to determine if antiviral chemotherapy may abort or alleviate the frequency and severity of these signs are unavailable.

Visceral infections HSV infection of visceral organs usually results from viremia, and multiple organ involvement is common. Occasionally, however, the clinical manifestations of HSV infection may involve only the esophagus, lung, or liver. HSV esophagitis may result from direct extension of oral-pharyngeal HSV infection into the esophagus or may occur de novo by reactivation of HSV and spread of virus to the esophageal mucosa via the vagus nerve. The predominant symptoms of HSV esophagitis are odynophagia, dysphagia, substernal pain, and weight loss. There are multiple oval ulcerations on an erythematous base with or without a patchy white pseudomembrane. The distal esophagus is most commonly involved. With extensive disease, diffuse friability may spread to the entire esophagus. Neither endoscopic nor barium examination can differentiate HSV esophagitis from *Candida* esophagitis or from esophageal ulcerations due to thermal injury, radiation, and corrosives. Endoscopically obtained secretions for cytologic examination and culture provide the most useful material for diagnosis. Systemic antiviral chemotherapy usually reduces symptoms and heals esophageal ulcerations.

HSV pneumonitis is uncommon except in severely immunosuppressed patients and may result from extension of herpetic tracheobronchitis into lung parenchyma. Focal necrotizing pneumonitis usually results. Hematogenous dissemination of virus from oral or genital mucocutaneous disease also may occur and produce a bilateral interstitial pneumonitis. Concomitant bacterial, fungal, and parasitic

pathogens are common in HSV pneumonitis. Since the mortality of HSV pneumonia in immunosuppressed patients is high (>80 percent), these patients should be candidates for antiviral chemotherapy. HSV also has been isolated from the lower respiratory tract of persons with acute respiratory distress syndrome (ARDS). However, the relationship between isolation of HSV and the pathogenesis of the respiratory distress syndrome is unclear.

HSV is an uncommon cause of hepatitis in immunocompetent patients. HSV infection of the liver is associated with fever, abrupt elevations of bilirubin and the serum transaminases, and leukopenia (white blood cells <4000 per microliter). Disseminated intravascular coagulation also may be present.

Other isolated but reported complications of HSV include monarticular arthritis, adrenal necrosis, idiopathic thrombocytopenia, and glomerulonephritis. Disseminated HSV infection in the immunocompetent patient is rare. In immunocompromised, burn, or malnourished patients, dissemination of HSV to other visceral organs such as adrenal glands, pancreas, small and large intestine, and bone marrow may occur occasionally. Rarely, primary HSV infection in pregnancy may disseminate and may be associated with mortality in both mother and fetus. This uncommon event is usually associated with acquisition of primary infection in the third trimester.

Neonatal HSV infection Neonates (<6 weeks of age) have the highest frequency of visceral and/or CNS infection of any HSV-infected patient population. Untreated, over 70 percent of neonatal herpes cases will disseminate or develop into CNS infection. Without therapy, the overall mortality of neonatal herpes is 65 percent, and less than 10 percent of neonates with CNS infection experience normal development. While skin lesions are the most commonly recognized features of disease, many infants do not develop lesions until well into the course of disease. Seventy percent of neonatal HSV cases are caused by HSV-2 infection, almost all of which result from contact via infected genital secretions at the time of delivery. However, congenitally infected infants have been reported, usually from mothers who acquired primary HSV infection during pregnancy. Neonatal HSV-1 infections may be acquired from genital HSV-1 infection in the mother, through postnatal contact with immediate family members with symptomatic or asymptomatic oral-labial HSV-1 infection, or from nosocomial transmission within the hospital. Antiviral chemotherapy has reduced the mortality of neonatal herpes to 25 percent. However, the morbidity, especially in infants with HSV-2 CNS involvement, is still very high.

DIAGNOSIS Both clinical and laboratory criteria are useful for establishing the diagnosis of HSV infections. Clinical diagnosis can be made accurately where characteristic multiple vesicular lesions on an erythematous base are present. Scrapings of the base of the lesions and subsequent staining with Wright, Giemsa (Tzanck preparation), or Papanicolaou's stain will demonstrate characteristic giant cells or intranuclear inclusions of a herpesvirus infection. These cytologic techniques are often useful as a quick office procedure to confirm the diagnosis. Limitations of this method are that it does not differentiate between HSV and varicella-zoster infections and is only about 60 percent as sensitive as viral isolation. The laboratory confirmation of HSV infection is best performed by isolation of virus in tissue culture or demonstration of HSV antigens in scrapings from lesions. HSV causes a discernible cytopathic effect in a variety of cell culture systems, and most specimens can be identified within 48 to 96 h after inoculation. Spin-amplified culture with subsequent staining for HSV antigen has shortened the time needed to identify HSV to less than 24 h. The sensitivity of viral isolation varies with the stage of lesions (higher in vesicular than in ulcerative lesions), whether the patient has a first or recurrent episode of the disease (higher in first episodes), and whether the sample is from an immunosuppressed or immunocompetent patient (more antigen in immunosuppressed). IFA, ELISA, and some DNA hybridization procedures have approached the sensitivity of viral isolation for detecting HSV from genital or oral-labial lesions but appear only about 50 percent as sensitive as viral isolation for the detection of asymptomatic HSV in cervical or salivary secretions. HSV PCR techniques may be more sensitive than viral isolation. Laboratory confirmation allows for subtyping the virus, which may be useful epidemiologically as well as in helping to predict the frequency of reactivation after first-episode oral-labial or genital HSV infection. Restriction endonuclease analysis of viral DNA can be used to differentiate between HSV-1 and HSV-2 as well as to differentiate between strains within the same subtypes; the latter information may be very useful in identifying common-source outbreaks of HSV.

Acute and convalescent serum can be useful in documenting seroconversion during primary HSV-1 or HSV-2 infection. However, only 5 percent of patients with recurrent mucocutaneous HSV infections show a fourfold or greater rise in anti-HSV antibodies between acute and convalescent sera. Serologic assays, especially type-specific assays, should be utilized to identify asymptomatic carriers of HSV-1 or HSV-2 infection, and such carriers should be counseled about the risk of transmission.

THERAPY   Many aspects of mucocutaneous and visceral HSV infections are amenable to antiviral chemotherapy. For mucocutaneous infections, acyclovir has been the mainstay of therapy. Several antivirals are available for topical use in HSV eye infections: idoxuridine, trifluorothymidine, and topical vidarabine. For HSV encephalitis, intravenous acyclovir is the treatment of choice. For neonatal HSV infections, high-dose intravenous vidarabine and acyclovir are effective.

Acyclovir has been shown to be effective in shortening the duration of symptoms and lesions of mucocutaneous HSV infections in immunocompromised patients and first-episode genital herpes in immunocompetent patients (Table 143-1). Intravenous and oral acyclovir also will prevent reactivation of HSV in seropositive immunocompromised patients during induction chemotherapy for acute leukemia or in the period immediately following bone marrow transplantation.

Oral acyclovir also has been shown to speed the healing and resolution of symptoms in first and recurrent episodes of genital HSV-1 and HSV-2 infections. The benefit of treating acute episodes of recurrent genital disease with oral acyclovir is modest, and thus routine use for recurrent episodes of disease, especially for mild episodes, is not recommended. Chronic daily suppressive therapy reduces the frequency of reactivation disease among patients with frequent genital herpes. Chronic suppressive oral acyclovir does not eliminate sacral ganglionic latency, and reactivation of genital herpes occurs after discontinuation of therapy. Oral acyclovir is of benefit in primary gingivostomatitis but has limited benefit in the treatment of recurrent oral-labial lesions; lesions are not aborted and total healing time is not reduced. If started early, the duration of the ulcerative stage of the lip lesion may be reduced.

Both intravenous vidarabine 15 mg/kg per day over 12 h and intravenous acyclovir 30 mg/kg per day given as 10 mg/kg infusion over 1 h at 8-hourly intervals have been shown to be effective in reducing the mortality of HSV encephalitis. Primary determinants of outcome include young age and early therapy. Comparative trials of the two drugs for the treatment of HSV encephalitis have indicated a lower mortality rate and fewer neurologic sequelae with intravenous acyclovir. The major side effect associated with intravenous acyclovir is transient renal insufficiency, usually due to crystallization of the compound in the renal parenchyma. This can be avoided if the medication is given slowly over 1 h and the patient is well-hydrated. Because CSF levels of acyclovir average only 30 to 50 percent of plasma levels, the dosage of acyclovir used for treatment of CNS infection (30 mg/kg per day) is double that used for treatment of mucocutaneous or visceral disease (15 mg/kg per day). Vidarabine at doses of 15 mg/kg per day tends to produce more hematopoietic and hepatic toxicity than acyclovir, but this is usually not a limiting problem in treating severe neonatal or CNS infections.

Acyclovir-resistant strains are being identified with increasing frequency, especially in HIV-infected persons. Almost all clinically significant acyclovir resistance has been seen in immunocompromised

---

TABLE 143-1   Antiviral chemotherapy of HSV infection

Mucocutaneous HSV infections

A Immunosuppressed patients

1 Acute symptomatic first or recurrent episodes: IV acyclovir (5 mg/kg every 8 h) or oral acyclovir (400 mg PO 4 times per day for 7 to 10 days) relieves pain and speeds healing. With localized external lesions 5% topical acyclovir ointment applied 4 to 6 times daily may be beneficial.

2 Suppression of reactivation disease: IV (5 mg/kg every 8 h) or oral acyclovir (400 mg PO 3 to 5 times per day) will prevent recurrences during high-risk periods, e.g., the immediate posttransplantation period.

B 1 Genital herpes

a First episodes: Oral acyclovir (200 mg PO 5 times per day for 10 to 14 days) is the treatment of choice. IV acyclovir (5 mg/kg every 8 h for 5 days) is given for severe disease or neurologic complications such as aseptic meningitis. Topical 5% ointment or cream applied 4 to 6 times daily for 7 to 10 days may be beneficial in patients without cervical, urethral, or pharyngeal involvement.

b Symptomatic recurrent genital herpes: Oral acyclovir (200 mg PO 5 times per day for 5 days) has modest benefit in shortening lesion duration and viral excretion time. Routine use for all episodes is not recommended.

c Suppression of recurrent genital herpes: Daily oral acyclovir (200-mg capsules 2 or 3 times daily, 400 mg PO 2 times daily, or 800 mg PO once daily) will prevent reactivation of symptomatic recurrences.

d Suppression of reactivation of oral-labial HSV: Oral acyclovir (400 mg PO 2 times per day), if started before exposure and continued for the duration of exposure (usually 5 to 10 days), will prevent reactivation of recurrent oral-labial HSV associated with severe sun exposure.

2 Oral-labial HSV infections

a First episode: Oral acyclovir 200 mg is given 4 or 5 times per day.
Recurrent episodes: Topical acyclovir ointment is of no clinical benefit. Oral acyclovir has minimal benefit.

3 Herpetic whitlow: Oral acyclovir 200 mg is given 5 times daily for 7 to 10 days.

4 HSV proctitis: Oral acyclovir (400 mg PO 5 times per day) is useful in shortening course of infection. In immunosuppressed patients or in patients with severe infection, IV acyclovir 5 mg/kg every 8 h may be useful.

C Herpetic eye infections: In acute keratitis, topical trifluorothymidine, vidarabine, idoxuridine, acyclovir, and interferon are all beneficial. Debridement may be required; topical steroids may worsen disease.

CNS HSV infections

A HSV encephalitis: Intravenous acyclovir 10 mg/kg every 8 h (30 mg/kg per day) for 10 days or vidarabine (15 mg/kg per day) decreases mortality; acyclovir is the preferred agent.

B HSV aseptic meningitis: No studies of systemic antiviral chemotherapy exist. If therapy is to be given IV, acyclovir at 15 to 30 mg/kg per day should be utilized.

C Autonomic radiculopathy: No studies are available.

Neonatal HSV infections: Intravenous vidarabine (30 mg/kg per day) or acyclovir (30 mg/kg per day) is given. Neonates appear to tolerate this high dose of vidarabine.

Visceral HSV infections

A HSV esophagitis: Systemic acyclovir (15 mg/kg per day) should be considered. In some patients with milder forms of immunosuppression, 800 mg 3 times daily will relieve symptoms.

B HSV pneumonitis: No controlled studies exist. Systemic acyclovir (15 mg/kg per day) should be considered.

Disseminated HSV infections: No controlled studies exist. Intravenous acyclovir or vidarabine should be attempted. Because of reduced side effects, acyclovir is preferred. No definite evidence indicates that therapy will decrease mortality.

Erythema multiforme associated with HSV: Anecdotal observations suggest that oral acyclovir capsules 2 to 3 times daily will suppress EM.

Infections due to acyclovir-resistant viruses: Foscarnet 40 mg/kg IV every 8 h should be given until lesions heal. The optimal duration of therapy and the usefulness of its continuation to suppress lesions are unclear. Some patients may benefit from cutaneous application of trifluorothymidine.

---

patients who have received multiple intermittent courses of therapy. The frequent reactivation of virus and high virus titers in the lesions of immunocompromised patients in combination with the use of the medication selects out these resistant variants. Most acyclovir-resistant strains of HSV have an altered substrate specificity for phosphorylating acyclovir. Thus intracellular levels of acyclovir triphosphate are low. In some patients, higher doses of acyclovir will be associated with clearing of lesions. In others, clinical disease will progress despite high-dose therapy. Isolation of HSV from persisting lesions despite adequate dosages and blood levels of acyclovir should raise the suspicion of acyclovir resistance. Therapy with the antiviral drug foscarnet is useful (see Chap. 142). Because of its toxicity and cost, this drug is usually reserved for patients with extensive mucocutaneous infections.

PREVENTION The large reservoir of persons with asymptomatic HSV-1 and HSV-2 infections indicates that control of HSV disease through suppressive antiviral chemotherapy and/or educational programs will be limited. Control of HSV infection will require prevention of infection, a goal most likely achievable by vaccination. Effective HSV vaccines are not currently available. Heterologous vaccines such as smallpox, bacillus Calmette-Guérin, and influenza, which have been used as therapies for genital HSV infection, have been ineffective.

Barrier forms of contraception, especially condoms, decrease transmission of disease, especially during periods of asymptomatic viral excretion. When lesions are present, the disease may be transmitted despite the use of a condom, and patients should be instructed to avoid sexual activity during these intervals.

REFERENCES

ASHLEY R et al: Inability of enzyme immunoassays to accurately discriminate between infections with herpes simplex virus types 1 and 2. Ann Intern Med 115:520, 1991

BROWN ZA et al: Neonatal herpes simplex virus infection in relation to asymptomatic maternal infection at the time of labor. N Engl J Med 324:1247, 1991

COREY L, SPEAR P: Infections with herpes simplex viruses. N Engl J Med 314:686, 1986

ERLICH KS et al: Acyclovir-resistant herpes simplex virus infections in patients with the acquired immunodeficiency syndrome. N Engl J Med 320:293, 1989

HOOK EW et al: Herpes simplex virus infection as a risk factor for human immunodeficiency virus infection in heterosexuals. J Infect Dis 165:251, 1992

MERTZ GJ et al: Risk factors for the sexual transmission of genital herpes. Ann Intern Med 116:197, 1992

SAFRIN S et al: A controlled trial comparing foscarnet with vidarabine for acyclovir-resistant mucocutaneous herpes simplex in the acquired immunodeficiency syndrome. N Engl J Med 325:551, 1991

STONE KM, WHITTINGTON WL: Treatment of genital herpes. Rev Infect Dis 12:S610, 1990

WHITLEY R, GNANN JW: Acyclovir: A decade of experience. N Engl J Med (in press)

144 VARICELLA-ZOSTER VIRUS INFECTIONS

RICHARD J. WHITLEY

DEFINITION Varicella-zoster virus (VZV) causes two distinct clinical entities: varicella, or chickenpox, and herpes zoster, or shingles. Chickenpox, a ubiquitous and extremely contagious infection, is usually a benign illness of childhood characterized by an exanthematous, vesicular rash. With reactivation of latent VZV, more common after the sixth decade of life, the disease presents as a dermatomal, vesicular rash which is usually associated with severe pain.

ETIOLOGY A clinical association between varicella and herpes zoster has been recognized for nearly 100 years. Early in the twentieth century, similarities in the histopathologic findings of skin lesions resulting from varicella and herpes zoster were demonstrated. Viral isolates from patients with chickenpox and herpes zoster produced similar alterations in tissue culture, specifically the appearance of eosinophilic intranuclear inclusions and multinucleated giant cells, suggesting that the viruses were biologically similar. Restriction endonuclease analyses of viral DNA from a patient with chickenpox who subsequently developed herpes zoster verified the molecular identity of the two viruses responsible for these differing clinical

presentations. Varicella-zoster virus is a member of the herpesvirus family, sharing such similar structural characteristics as a lipid envelope surrounding a nucleocapsid with icosahedral symmetry, a total size of approximately 150 to 200 nm, and centrally located double-stranded DNA with a molecular weight of approximately 80 million. Only enveloped virions are infectious.

PATHOGENESIS AND PATHOLOGY   Primary infection Transmission is most likely by the respiratory route, followed by localized replication at an undefined site, presumably the nasopharynx, and leading to seeding of the reticuloendothelial system with, ultimately, viremia. The occurrence of viremia in patients with chickenpox is supported by the diffuse and scattered nature of the skin lesions and can be verified in selected cases by the recovery of virus from the blood. Vesicles involve the corium and dermis, with degenerative changes characterized by ballooning, multinucleated giant cells, and eosinophilic intranuclear inclusions. Infection may involve localized blood vessels of the skin, resulting in necrosis and epidermal hemorrhage. With disease evolution, vesicular fluid becomes cloudy with the recruitment of polymorphonuclear leukocytes, degenerated cells, and fibrin. Ultimately, the vesicles rupture and release their fluid contents, which include infectious virus, or are gradually reabsorbed.

Recurrent infection The mechanism of reactivation of VZV that results in herpes zoster is unknown. It is presumed that virus infects the dorsal root ganglia during chickenpox, where it remains latent until reactivated. Histopathologic examination of the representative dorsal root ganglia during active herpes zoster demonstrates hemorrhage, edema, and lymphocytic infiltration.

Active VZV replication can occur in other organs, such as the lung or brain, during either chickenpox or herpes zoster but is uncommon in the immune-competent host. Lung involvement is characterized by interstitial pneumonitis, multinucleated giant cell formation, intranuclear inclusions, and pulmonary hemorrhage. Central nervous system (CNS) infection leads to histopathologic evidence of perivascular cuffing similar to that encountered with measles and other viral encephalitides. Focal hemorrhagic necrosis of the brain, characteristic of herpes simplex virus encephalitis, is uncommon with VZV infection.

EPIDEMIOLOGY AND CLINICAL PRESENTATION   Chickenpox Humans are the only known reservoir for VZV. Chickenpox is highly contagious, with an attack rate of at least 90 percent among susceptible or seronegative individuals. Both sexes and individuals of all races are infected equally. The virus is endemic in the population at large; however, it becomes epidemic among susceptible individuals during seasonal periods, namely, late winter and early spring in the temperate zone. Children between the ages of 5 and 9 are most commonly affected and account for 50 percent of all cases. Most other cases occur between the ages of 1 to 4 and 10 to 14. Over the age of 15, approximately 10 percent of the population of the United States is susceptible to infection.

The incubation period of chickenpox ranges between 10 and 21 days but is usually between 14 and 17 days. Secondary attack rates in susceptible siblings within a household are between 70 and 90 percent. Patients are infectious approximately 48 h prior to the onset of the vesicular rash, during the period of vesicle formation (generally 4 to 5 days), and until all vesicles are crusted.

Clinically, chickenpox presents as a rash, low-grade fever, and malaise, although a few patients will develop a prodrome 1 to 2 days prior to the onset of the exanthem. In the immune-competent, this is usually a benign illness that is associated with lassitude and fever from 37.8 to 39.4°C (100 to 103°F) of 3 to 5 days' duration. The skin lesions, the hallmark of the infection, consist of maculopapules, vesicles, and scabs in varying stages of evolution. The evolution of lesions from maculopapules to vesicles occurs over a matter of hours to days. The lesions appear on the trunk and face and rapidly involve other areas of the body. Most are small and have an erythematous base with a diameter of 5 to 10 mm. Successive crops appear over a 2- to 4-day period. Lesions also can be found on the mucosa of the pharynx or the vagina. Their severity varies from individual to individual. Some individuals have very few lesions, while others can have as many as 2000. Younger children tend to have fewer vesicles than older individuals. Immunocompromised individuals, both children and adults, particularly those with leukemia, have more numerous lesions, often with a hemorrhagic base, and the lesions take longer to heal. These individuals also are at greater risk for visceral complications, which occur in 30 to 50 percent of cases and which are fatal in 15 percent.

The most common infectious complication of varicella is secondary bacterial superinfection of the skin, which is usually caused by *Streptococcus pyogenes* or *Staphylococcus aureus*. This may result from excoriation of skin lesions following scratching. Gram stain of skin lesions should help clarify the etiology of unusually erythematous and pustulated lesions.

The most common extracutaneous site of involvement in children is the central nervous system. The syndrome consists of acute cerebellar ataxia and meningeal irritation which generally appears approximately 21 days after the onset of the rash and rarely occurs in the preeruptive phase. The cerebrospinal fluid contains lymphocytes and elevated levels of protein. This is a benign complication of VZV infection in children and does not generally require hospitalization. Aseptic meningitis, encephalitis, transverse myelitis, Guillain-Barré syndrome, and Reye's syndrome also can occur. Encephalitis is reported in 0.1 to 0.2 percent of children with chickenpox. No specific therapy, other than supportive care, is available for patients with CNS involvement caused by VZV.

Varicella pneumonia is the most serious complication following chickenpox, occurring more commonly in adults (up to 20 percent) than in children. It usually appears 3 to 5 days into the course of illness and is associated with tachypnea, cough, dyspnea, and fever. Cyanosis, pleuritic chest pain, and hemoptysis are frequent. Roentgenographic evidence of disease consists of nodular infiltrates and an interstitial pneumonitis. Resolution of pneumonitis parallels improvement of skin rash; however, patients may have persistent fever and compromised pulmonary function for weeks.

Other complications of chickenpox include myocarditis, corneal lesions, nephritis, arthritis, bleeding diatheses, acute glomerulonephritis, and hepatitis. Hepatic involvement, distinct from Reye's syndrome, is common in chickenpox and is usually characterized by an elevation of liver enzymes, particularly aspartate aminotransferase (AST) and alanine aminotransferase (ALT). Hepatic involvement is usually asymptomatic.

Perinatal varicella is associated with a high mortality rate when maternal disease develops within 5 days before delivery and 48 h post partum. Because the newborn does not receive protective transplacental antibodies and has an immature immune system, illness may be exaggerated. The mortality rate has been reported as high as 30 percent in this group. Congenital varicella with clinical manifestations at birth is extremely uncommon.

Herpes zoster   Herpes zoster, a sporadic disease, is the consequence of reactivation of latent virus from the dorsal root ganglia. It occurs at all ages but mainly among the elderly. Most patients have no history of exposure to other individuals with VZV infection. The highest incidence is between 5 and 10 cases per 1000 persons for individuals in the sixth through the eighth decades of life. It has been suggested that approximately 2 percent of herpes zoster patients will develop a second episode of infection.

Herpes zoster, or "shingles," is characterized by a unilateral vesicular eruption within a dermatome, often associated with severe pain. The dermatomes from T3 to L3 are most frequently involved. If the ophthalmic branch of the trigeminal nerve is involved, zoster ophthalmicus results. The factors responsible for reactivation of virus are not known. In children, reactivation is usually benign, whereas in adults, acute neuritis and postherpetic neuralgia can be particularly debilitating. The onset of disease is heralded by pain within the dermatome that may precede lesions by 48 to 72 h, followed by an erythematous maculopapular rash which evolves rapidly to vesicular

lesions. In the normal host, these lesions may remain few in number and continue to form only for a period of 3 to 5 days. The total duration of disease is generally between 7 and 10 days; however, it may take as long as 2 to 4 weeks before the skin returns to normal. In a few patients, characteristic localization of pain to a dermatome with serologic evidence of herpes zoster has been reported in the absence of skin lesions. When branches of the trigeminal nerve are involved, lesions may appear on the face, in the mouth, in the eye, or on the tongue. Lesions appear on the ear canal and tongue when the sensory branch of the facial nerve is involved (Ramsay Hunt syndrome).

The most debilitating complication of herpes zoster, in both the normal and the immunocompromised host, is pain associated with acute neuritis and postherpetic neuralgia. Postherpetic neuralgia is uncommon in young individuals; however, at least 50 percent of patients over age 50 with zoster will report pain in the involved dermatome months after resolution of cutaneous disease. Changes in sensation within the dermatome, resulting in either hypo- or hyperesthesia, are common.

Central nervous system involvement following localized herpes zoster may occur. Many patients without signs of meningeal irritation will have cerebrospinal fluid pleocytosis and moderately elevated levels of CSF protein. Symptomatic meningoencephalitis is characterized by headache, fever, photophobia, meningitis, and vomiting. A rare manifestation of CNS involvement is granulomatous angiitis with contralateral hemiplegia, which can be diagnosed by cerebral arteriography. Other neurologic manifestations include transverse myelitis with or without motor paralysis.

As with chickenpox, herpes zoster in the immunocompromised host is more severe than in the normal individual. Lesion formation continues for over a week, and total scabbing does not develop in the majority of patients until 3 weeks into the course of illness. Patients with Hodgkin's disease and non-Hodgkin's lymphoma are at greatest risk for progressive herpes zoster because cutaneous dissemination develops in about 40 percent of these patients. Among patients with cutaneous dissemination, there is a 5 to 10 percent increased risk of pneumonitis, meningoencephalitis, hepatitis, and other serious complications. However, even in immunocompromised patients, disseminated zoster is rarely fatal.

Patients who have had a bone marrow transplant are at particular risk of VZV infection. Thirty percent of cases of posttransplant VZV infections occur within 1 year (50 percent of these within 9 months), and 45 percent of such patients have cutaneous or visceral dissemination. The mortality rate is 10 percent, and postherpetic neuralgia, scarring, and bacterial superinfection are more frequent in VZV infections occurring within 9 months of a transplant. Among infected patients, concomitant graft-versus-host disease increases the chance for dissemination and/or a fatal outcome.

TABLE 144-1   Recommendations for VZIG utilization

Exposure
- *A* Both exposure to person with chickenpox or zoster as:
  - *1* Continuous household contact
  - *2* Playmate for >1 h indoors
  - *3* Hospital contact (same room or prolonged face-to-face)
  - *4* Newborn exposure whereby mother had onset of chickenpox <5 days before delivery to 48 h post partum
- *B* And time elapsed ≤96 h (preferably sooner)

Candidates (provided significant exposure) include
- *A* Immunocompromised susceptible children
- *B* Normal susceptible adolescents (>15 years) and adults, especially pregnant women
- *C* Newborn infants of mothers with onset of chickenpox 5 days before or 2 days after delivery
- *D* Hospitalized premature infants
  - *1* ≥28 weeks' gestation when mother has no history of chickenpox
  - *2* <28 weeks' gestation and/or birth weight of ≤1000 g regardless of maternal history

SOURCE: Adapted from *1991 Redbook*, American Academy of Pediatrics.

DIFFERENTIAL DIAGNOSIS The diagnosis of chickenpox is not difficult. The characteristic rash of chickenpox and the epidemiologic history of recent exposure should lead to prompt diagnosis. Other viral infections which can mimic chickenpox include disseminated herpes simplex virus infection in patients with atopic dermatitis and the disseminated vesiculopapular lesions sometimes associated with coxsackievirus, echovirus, or atypical measles infections. These rashes are more commonly morbilliform with a hemorrhagic component rather than vesicular or vesiculopustular. Rickettsialpox can be confused with chickenpox; however, it can be easily distinguished by finding the "herald spot" at the site of the mite bite and a more pronounced headache. Serologic testing is useful in differentiating rickettsialpox from varicella.

Unilateral vesicular lesions in a dermatomal pattern should lead rapidly to the diagnosis of herpes zoster. Both herpes simplex virus and coxsackievirus infections can be a cause of dermatomal vesicular lesions. In such situations, a Tzanck smear with supportive diagnostic virology will be helpful in ensuring the proper diagnosis. In the prodromal stage of herpes zoster, the diagnosis can be exceedingly difficult and may only be achieved once lesions have appeared or by retrospective serologic assessment.

LABORATORY FINDINGS Unequivocal confirmation of the diagnosis is possible only through the isolation of virus in susceptible tissue culture cell lines or by the demonstration of seroconversion or a fourfold or greater antibody rise in convalescent versus acute specimens. A rapid impression can be obtained by a Tzanck smear, performed by scraping the base of the lesions in an attempt to demonstrate multinucleated giant cells. Direct immunofluorescent staining of cells from the skin base or detection of viral antigens by other assays (immunoperoxidase) also can be utilized, although such tests are not commercially available. The most frequently employed serologic tools for assessing host response are immunofluorescent detection of antibodies to VZV membrane antigens, the fluorescent antibody to membrane antigen (FAMA) test, immune adherence hemagglutination, and enzyme-linked immunosorbent assay (ELISA). The FAMA and ELISA tests appear to be the most sensitive.

PROPHYLAXIS In the normal host, prophylaxis and treatment of chickenpox are of relatively little value because the disease is usually benign. However, the immunocompromised individual is at significant risk for developing progressive varicella; modalities of prevention include passive immunization or experimental administration of a live attenuated vaccine. Immune prophylaxis can be accomplished by the administration of specific zoster immune globulin (ZIG) derived from patients with herpes zoster, varicella-zoster immune globulin (VZIG), or the intravenous formulation of zoster immune plasma (ZIP). Both ZIG and VZIG should be given within 96 h, but preferably within 72 h, of exposure in order to be effective. It is likely that ZIP can be given somewhat later. Indications for the administration of ZIG or VZIG are summarized in Table 144-1. VZIG should be administered to immunodeficient patients under age 15 who have a negative or unknown history of chickenpox, who have not been vaccinated against VZV, and who have had a contact in a household, with a playmate for more than 1 h indoors, or in a shared hospital room. It also should be administered to the newborn whose mother had an onset of chickenpox within less than 5 days before delivery and 48 h post partum. VZIG should be administered to normal susceptible adolescents (≥15 years of age) and adults, especially pregnant women; however, serologic evaluation of immune status is advised. Finally, AZIG is recommended for hospitalized premature infants of ≥28 weeks' gestation whose mother has no history of chickenpox and those of <28 weeks' gestation regardless of maternal history when exposure is significant.

Clinical trials in Japan and the United States have demonstrated the efficacy of live attenuated vaccine (OKA) both in normal individuals and in immunocompromised hosts. This live attenuated VZV vaccine may be licensed in the United States in the near future.

TREATMENT Medical management of chickenpox in the normal host is directed toward preventing avoidable complications. Obvi-

ously, good hygiene should include daily bathing and soaks. Secondary bacterial infection of the skin can be avoided by meticulous skin care, particularly with close cropping of fingernails. Pruritus can be decreased with topical dressings or the administration of antipruritic drugs. Tepid water baths and wet compresses are better than drying lotions for the relief of itching. Domeboro soaks for the management of herpes zoster can be both soothing and cleansing. Administration of aspirin should be avoided in children with chickenpox because of the recent association between aspirin derivatives and the development of Reye's syndrome. In addition, acyclovir therapy (800 mg PO five times daily for 5 to 7 days) is recommended for adolescents and adults with chickenpox of ≤24 h duration. Acyclovir therapy for children <12 years of age may be of benefit if initiated early in the disease (<24 h) at a dose of 20 mg/kg every 6 h.

Patients with varicella pneumonia may require removal of bronchial secretions and ventilatory support. Zoster ophthalmicus should be referred promptly and immediately to an ophthalmologist. Therapy consists of administration of analgesics for severe pain and the use of atropine. The administration of acyclovir in the management of zoster ophthalmicus will accelerate healing. Patients with herpes zoster may benefit from acyclovir therapy, as evidenced by accelerated cutaneous healing. The dose is 800 mg PO five times daily for 7 to 10 days.

Both chickenpox and herpes zoster in the immunocompromised host should be treated with intravenous vidarabine or, preferably, acyclovir. Acyclovir is used preferentially over vidarabine because of decreased toxicity, especially in immunocompromised patients. Intravenous acyclovir leads to the decreased occurrence of visceral complications but has no effect on healing of skin lesions or pain. The dose is 10 to 12.5 mg/kg every 8 h for 7 days. These treatment recommendations apply to immunocompromised patients with disseminated herpes zoster as well. Oral acyclovir therapy is not recommended for treatment of VZV infections in immune-compromised patients. Concomitant with the administration of intravenous acyclovir to the immunosuppressed host, it is desirable to attempt to wean patients from immunosuppressive treatment.

Management of acute neuritis and/or postherpetic neuralgia can be particularly difficult. In addition to the judicious use of analgesics, ranging from nonnarcotic to narcotic derivatives, drugs such as amitriptyline hydrochloride and fluphenazine hydrochloride have been reported to be beneficial for pain relief. Glucocorticoids have been reported in some studies to be useful when administered early in the course for prevention of postherpetic neuralgia. This approach remains controversial.

REFERENCES

BRUNELL PA et al: Prevention of varicella by zoster immune globulin. N Engl J Med 280:1191, 1969

BALFOUR HH JR et al: Acyclovir treatment of varicella in otherwise healthy adolescents. J Pediatr 120:627–633, 1992

DUNKLE LM et al: A controlled trial of acyclovir for chickenpox in normal children. N Engl J Med 325:1539, 1991

ESSMAN V et al: Prednisone does not prevent postherpetic neuralgia. Lancet 2:126, 1987

GERSHON AA et al: Live attenuated varicella vaccine. JAMA 252:355, 1984

HOPE-SIMPSON RE: The nature of herpes zoster: A long-term study and a new hypothesis. Proc R Soc Med 58:9, 1965

LOCKSLEY RM et al: Infection with varicella-zoster virus after marrow transplantation. J Infect Dis 152:1172, 1985

PROBER CG et al: Acyclovir therapy of chickenpox in immunosuppressed children—a collaborative study. J Pediatr 101:622, 1982

SHEPP D et al: Treatment of varicella-zoster virus in severely immunocompromised patients: A randomized comparison of acyclovir and vidarabine. N Engl J Med 314:208, 1987

WEIBEL RE et al: Live attenuated varicella versus vaccine: Efficacy trail in healthy children. N Engl J Med 310:1409, 1984

WELLER TH: Varicella and herpes zoster: Changing concepts of the natural history, control, and importance of a not-so-benign virus. N Engl J Med 309:1362, 1983

WHITLEY RJ et al: Early vidarabine therapy to control the complications of herpes zoster in immunosuppressed patients. N Engl J Med 307:971, 1982

———— et al: Vidarabine therapy of varicella in immunosuppressed patients. J Pediatr 1:125, 1982

———— et al: Varicella-zoster virus infections, in *Antiviral Agents and Viral Diseases of Man*, vol 2, GJ Galasso et al (eds). New York, Raven, 1984, pp 517–542

———— et al: Disseminated herpes zoster in the immunocompromised host: A comparative trial of acyclovir and vidarabine. J Infect Dis 165:450, 1992

ZAIA JA et al: Evaluation of varicella-zoster immune globulin: Protection of immunosuppressed children after household exposure to varicella. J Infect Dis 147:737, 1983

145   EPSTEIN-BARR VIRUS INFECTIONS, INCLUDING INFECTIOUS MONONUCLEOSIS

ROBERT T. SCHOOLEY

DEFINITION Epstein-Barr virus (EBV) is a B lymphotropic human herpesvirus which is worldwide in distribution. Primary infection with EBV during childhood is usually subclinical. Between 25 and 70 percent of adolescents and adults who undergo a primary EBV infection develop the clinical syndrome of infectious mononucleosis. Infectious mononucleosis is defined by the clinical triad of fever, lymphadenopathy, and pharyngitis combined with the transient appearance of heterophil antibodies and an atypical lymphocytosis. EBV is also associated with nasopharyngeal carcinoma and certain B cell lymphomas.

EPIDEMIOLOGY OF EBV INFECTIONS EBV is a ubiquitous agent that has been found in all population groups surveyed to date. The virus was initially described by Epstein, Achong, and Barr, who noted, by electron microscopy, the presence of particles similar in morphology to herpes simplex virus in continuous cell lines which had arisen from tumor tissue obtained from patients with Burkitt's lymphoma. Following an observation by the Henles of antibodies to EBV in a patient with infectious mononucleosis, large-scale serologic surveys confirmed EBV as the etiologic agent for infectious mononucleosis.

EBV is transmitted primarily in saliva or, less commonly, by blood transfusion. Primary infection tends to occur at an earlier age among lower socioeconomic groups and in developing countries. In industrialized countries, approximately 50 percent of individuals have experienced a primary EBV infection by adolescence. These early infections are usually mild and nonspecific or clinically inapparent. A second wave of seroconversions to EBV occurs with the onset of the social activity associated with adolescence and young adulthood. Primary EBV infection among this age group accounts for most cases of infectious mononucleosis. The peak incidence of infectious mononucleosis occurs between 14 and 16 years of age for girls and between 16 and 18 years of age for boys. By adulthood, most individuals are EBV-seropositive.

EBV is shed from the oropharynx for up to 18 months following primary infection; thereafter it is shed intermittently by all EBV-seropositive individuals in the absence of a clinical illness. EBV can be isolated from the oropharyngeal washings of 15 to 25 percent of healthy EBV-seropositive individuals. Immunosuppressed individuals shed the virus more frequently. EBV can be isolated from 25 to 50 percent of the oropharyngeal washings obtained from renal allograft recipients and from virtually all patients with AIDS. Asymptomatic shedding of EBV by healthy individuals accounts for most of the spread to uninfected members of the population despite the fact that it is not highly contagious. Transmission is largely dependent on salivary contact (e.g., kissing). It is not likely to be transmitted by aerosol or fomites. Thus isolation restrictions on patients with mononucleosis or individuals likely to be shedding EBV are not appropriate.

ETIOLOGY AND PATHOGENESIS OF INFECTIOUS MONONU-CLEOSIS By electron microscopy, EBV appears as an icosahedral nucleocapsid surrounded by a complex envelope and is indistinguish-able from other members of the human herpesvirus group. The double-stranded EBV DNA has a molecular weight of approximately 101×10^6 and encodes for at least 30 polypeptides. Two types of EBV (types A and B) have been recognized on the basis of divergence of several of the Epstein-Barr nuclear antigens (see below). Type B virus is less efficient at transforming B lymphocytes and was initially thought to be prevalent primarily in central Africa and New Guinea. Type A virus is found in a greater number of individuals worldwide and is the type most frequently isolated from throat washings obtained from healthy members of the western community. Recent work suggests that type B virus is found more widely geographically than was previously appreciated and is found more frequently in immunocompromised individuals, especially those with HIV-1 infection. In such individuals, dual infection with both types of EBV has been demonstrated. There is currently no evidence that type differences account for the wide range of clinical conditions associated with EBV infection.

When EBV is transmitted by saliva, the initial site of replication is the oropharynx. EBV grows productively in B lymphocytes and oropharyngeal epithelial cells of patients with infectious mononucleosis; both cell types have specific surface receptors for EBV. During the acute phase of the illness, EBV antigens can be demonstrated within the nuclei of up to 20 percent of circulating B lymphocytes. After the infection subsides, the virus can be isolated from a small number of B lymphocytes of EBV-seropositive individuals and also resides within nasopharyngeal epithelial cells.

Virus-host interactions EBV infection has both direct and indirect effects on the cellular and humoral immune responses. Within 18 to 24 h after entry of EBV into B lymphocytes by means of the C3d receptor (also known as CD21), Epstein-Barr nuclear antigens (EBNA) are detectable within the nucleus of the infected cell. The six antigens which comprise EBNA (EBNA 1, 2, 3a, 3b, 3c, and leader protein) are responsible for conferring the transformed phenotype on EBV-infected B lymphocytes. Immortalized B lymphocytes can be propagated continuously in vitro and are polyclonally stimulated by EBV to produce immunoglobulin. Antibodies reactive with sheep red blood cells (heterophil) and antibodies with several other specificities are manifestations of polyclonal immunoglobulin production and may mediate several of the complications of infectious mononucleosis. A minority of EBV-infected B lymphocytes enter the lytic cycle (production of mature progeny virus and death of the host cell) and produce EBV antigens that are detected during virus replication. These are divided into the early antigen (EA) complex and viral capsid antigens (VCA). The EA complex consists of two groups of antigens: (1) diffuse (EA-D), which are detectable in both the cytoplasm and the nucleus of cells in the lytic cycle, and (2) restricted (EA-R), which are demonstrable only in the cytoplasm. These antigens serve as markers of infection at the cellular level; the pattern of the antibody response to these antigens is useful diagnostically in the identification of EBV-associated disease states (Table 145-1). After the appearance of VCA, the host cell dies and virions are released, which can infect and transform additional B lymphocytes.

An effective immune response to EBV involves humoral and cellular components. Neutralizing antibodies which inactivate cell-free virus and antibodies to VCA and EBNA appear during primary infection in all patients; antibodies to EA-D appear in most patients. The cellular immune response is largely responsible for controlling B cell proliferation and polyclonal immunoglobulin production triggered by EBV and is composed primarily of T lymphocytes having functional and surface phenotypic characteristics of activated, suppressor-cytotoxic T lymphocytes (CD8+, Ia+). These EBV-specific cytotoxic T lymphocytes appear to be directed primarily at several epitopes within the EBNA complex. As the illness progresses, memory T lymphocytes capable of limiting proliferation of autologous EBV-infected B lymphocytes are demonstrable. These memory T lymphocytes persist for life. However, latent EBV remains in a small

TABLE 145-1 EBV-specific antibodies

Antibody specificity	Time of appearance in IM	Persistence	Percent of IM patients with antibody	Comments
VCA:				
IgM	At clinical presentation	1–2 months	100	Best indicator of primary infection; not present with reactivation
IgG	At clinical presentation	Lifelong	100	Standard "EBV titer" reported by most commercial and state labs; major utility is as a marker for prior or current infection in epidemiologic studies
EA:				
EA-D	Peaks 3–4 weeks after onset	3–6 months	70	Presence correlates with more severe disease in patients with IM; present in nasopharyngeal carcinoma; IgA anti-EA-D antibodies useful for prediction of NPC in high-risk populations
EA-R	Several weeks after onset	Months to years		Present in high titer in African Burkitt's lymphoma; may be useful as an indicator of reactivation of EBV in immunosuppressed patients
EBNA	3–6 weeks after onset	Lifelong	100	Late appearance of anti-EBNA antibodies in IM makes seroconversion a useful marker for primary infection if IgM anti-VCA antibody studies are not available

NOTE: IM = infectious mononucleosis; VCA = viral capsid antigen; EA = early antigens; EA-D = diffuse early antigens; EA-R = restricted early antigens; EBNA = Epstein-Barr nuclear antigens; NPC = nasopharyngeal carcinoma.

proportion of B lymphocytes and also in epithelial cells in the oropharynx.

During the primary immune response to EBV, global cellular immune hyporesponsiveness is readily demonstrable. This resolves after resolution of the illness, but reactivation of EBV is facilitated by conditions which interfere with the cellular immune response (immunosuppressive drugs, especially cyclosporin A, and disorders associated with cellular immunodeficiency, such as HIV-1 infection). EBV and cytomegalovirus (CMV) reactivation in immunosuppressed patients is frequently associated with a return of the immunoregulatory abnormalities characteristic of the primary immune response to these viruses. In the case of CMV particularly, this hyporesponsiveness may contribute to many of the superinfections which frequently accompany CMV infections in immunocompromised hosts. The cellular hyporesponsiveness associated with EBV reactivation is generally less intense and less prolonged than that associated with CMV but also may contribute to morbidity in immunocompromised individuals.

CLINICAL MANIFESTATIONS Symptoms and signs After an incubation period of 4 to 8 weeks, prodromal symptoms of malaise, anorexia, and chills frequently precede the onset of pharyngitis, fever, and lymphadenopathy by several days. Severe pharyngitis is the symptom which most frequently prompts patients to seek medical attention. Occasionally, patients will note only fever or lymphadenopathy or will present with one of the complications of infectious mononucleosis. Most patients also complain of headache and malaise. Abdominal pain is infrequent in the absence of splenic rupture.

Physical examination Fever is present in 90 percent of patients and may reach 39 to 40°C. Periorbital edema may be seen. The pharyngitis is usually diffuse; an exudate is observed in one-third of patients. Palatal petechiae also may be observed. Posterior and/or anterior cervical adenopathy is noted in 90 percent of patients with infectious mononucleosis. Individual nodes are rarely painful but may be moderately tender to palpation. Hepatomegaly is infrequent, although mild hepatic tenderness is present in up to half the patients. Approximately half of all patients have splenomegaly, which is usually maximal in the second or third week of illness. In 5 percent of patients, a macular, petechial, scarlatiniform, urticarial, or erythema multiforme–like rash may appear. Administration of ampicillin results in a pruritic, maculopapular eruption in 90 to 100 percent of patients.

Clinical course Infectious mononucleosis is a self-limited illness in the vast majority of cases. The pharyngitis is maximal for 5 to 7 days and then resolves over the subsequent 7 to 10 days. Fever usually persists for 7 to 14 days but occasionally may continue somewhat longer. The course of the lymphadenopathy is variable but rarely exceeds 3 weeks. The most persistent symptom is malaise. Most patients are well enough to return to work or school within 3 to 4 weeks, but occasional patients remain exhausted, have difficulty concentrating, and are unable to return to full activities for months. This subgroup is often found among those who present with a less acute onset without severe pharyngitis and high fever.

Occasional patients have been reported in whom recurrent pharyngitis and fever are accompanied by persistent or resurgent heterophil antibodies. A group of patients has been described with nonspecific symptoms which may include malaise, fatigue, pharyngitis, fever, lymphadenopathy, and difficulty with higher cognitive function. These patients are usually heterophil-negative. The demonstration that some of these patients have anti-VCA and anti-EA-R titers which are higher and anti-EBNA titers which are lower than median titers for the general population has led to the speculation that this symptom complex may be a manifestation of ongoing replication of EBV. However, since healthy members of the general population may have antibodies to EA-R antigens, there is no reason to apply the diagnosis of chronic active EBV infection to patients with these nonspecific symptoms simply on the basis of the presence of anti-EA-R antibodies. Several studies have demonstrated the lack of utility of EBV-specific antibodies in the evaluation of patients with chronic fatigue and malaise. A blinded, placebo-controlled crossover study demonstrated no benefit from acyclovir therapy in this patient population. The group of patients formerly given the diagnosis of chronic active EBV infection has been included in a larger diagnostic category termed the *chronic fatigue syndrome* (see Chap. 388) to reflect the uncertain pathogenesis of this illness. Occasional patients have been reported in whom mortality or severe morbidity (pneumonitis, fever, pancytopenia) is associated with evidence of ongoing EBV replication. Such patients are extremely rare, and specific antiviral therapy may be useful in their management.

Complications Complications of infectious mononucleosis occur infrequently but may be so dramatic as to be the predominant manifestation of the illness (Table 145-2). Hematologic complications

TABLE 145-2　Complications of infectious mononucleosis

Hematologic complications:
　Autoimmune hemolytic anemia
　Thrombocytopenia
　Granulocytopenia
Splenic rupture
Neurologic complications:
　Encephalitis
　Cranial nerve palsies, especially Bell's palsy
　Meningoencephalitis
　Guillain-Barré syndrome
　Seizures
　Mononeuritis multiplex
　Transverse myelitis
　Psychosis
Hepatic complications:
　Hepatitis
Cardiac complications:
　Pericarditis
　Myocarditis
Pulmonary complications:
　Airway obstruction
　Interstitial pneumonitis

include autoimmune hemolytic anemia, which may be mediated by IgM antibodies with anti-i specificity. Hemolytic anemia usually subsides over a 1- to 2-month period. Mild thrombocytopenia occurs in up to 50 percent of cases; profound thrombocytopenia is a rare but well-recognized complication and is frequently antibody-mediated. Mild granulocytopenia is frequently observed in uncomplicated infectious mononucleosis, and severe granulocytopenia associated with infection or death has been reported. Antibodies which react with granulocytes have been detected in up to 80 percent of patients and may contribute to the profound granulocytopenia which is occasionally observed. Both the thrombocytopenia and the granulocytopenia are usually self-limited and resolve over 3 to 6 weeks. Glucocorticoids have been advocated for treatment of both hemolytic anemia and thrombocytopenia associated with infectious mononucleosis, but efficacy has not been proved in controlled studies. Splenic rupture is an infrequent complication of infectious mononucleosis, often accompanied by the insidious or abrupt onset of abdominal pain, and is usually observed during the second or third week of illness. Surgery, usually splenectomy or splenorrhaphy, is the only effective management.

Neurologic complications of infectious mononucleosis may be the presenting or sole manifestation of the illness. Heterophil antibodies may be absent, and atypical lymphocytes may not be present at the onset of the neurologic event. The most frequent neurologic complications are cranial nerve palsies and encephalitis which may present initially with cerebellar findings. The onset of the encephalitis is usually abrupt. Cerebrospinal fluid findings are not diagnostic, and localization by noninvasive neurodiagnostic studies may suggest herpes simplex encephalitis. Eighty-five percent of patients with EBV-associated neurologic findings recover spontaneously.

Hepatitis is a common component of infectious mononucleosis. Almost 90 percent of patients have mild elevation of hepatic transaminases. Although more serious hepatic sequelae have been reported, severe or permanent hepatic dysfunction is exceedingly rare.

Cardiac abnormalities are uncommon but may include pericarditis, myocarditis, coronary artery spasm, and electrocardiographic abnormalities.

Airway obstruction from pharyngeal or paratracheal adenopathy can occur. This may require surgical intervention but is usually quite sensitive to glucocorticoid therapy. Pulmonary parenchymal abnormalities such as interstitial infiltrates are noted infrequently in adults but appear to be more common among children.

Infectious mononucleosis is rarely fatal. Neurologic complications, airway obstruction, and splenic rupture are the most frequent causes of death in previously healthy individuals with primary EBV infection. Sporadic or X-linked cases of overwhelming EBV infection accompanied by lymphoproliferation and hepatic dysfunction have been reported.

The X-linked condition known as *X-linked lymphoproliferative (XLP)* or *Duncan's syndrome* (see Chap. 278) results in the death of 40 percent of affected males during primary EBV infection. In addition to overwhelming lymphoproliferation, XLP patients may manifest severe immunologic or hematologic sequelae such as agammaglobulinemia, aplastic anemia, or lymphocytic lymphoma. The pathophysiology of the XLP syndrome has not yet been completely elucidated, but an X-linked defect in the immune response to EBV may result in failure to control EBV replication or in disordered immunoregulation which leads to the other immunologic sequelae observed in this syndrome.

LABORATORY MANIFESTATIONS Heterophil antibodies Antibodies to sheep erythrocytes which can be removed by prior absorption with beef red blood cells, but not with guinea pig kidney, are termed *heterophil antibodies*. Heterophil antibodies are demonstrated in 50 percent of children and 90 to 95 percent of adolescents and adults with mononucleosis. Although the classic tube heterophil titer is still performed in many laboratories, the "monospot" test using a commerical kit is sensitive, specific, easily performed, and more routinely employed. The frequency of heterophil positivity associated with infectious mononucleosis depends on the test used, the age of the patient population, and the time during the illness at which the test is performed. Monospot tests may be slightly more sensitive than heterophil titers. Ten to fifteen percent of patients with mononucleosis may be heterophil-negative if tested only during the first week of the illness. If the clinical suspicion of mononucleosis is high enough, retesting for heterophil antibodies during the second or third week of illness is warranted. Heterophil antibodies decline in titer after the acute illness has resolved but may be detectable for up to 9 months after the onset of the illness.

Atypical lymphocytosis A relative and absolute lymphocytosis is present in about 75 percent of cases of infectious mononucleosis. The lymphocytosis usually peaks in the second or third week of illness and is characterized by cells with atypical morphology. These atypical lymphocytes, which are primarily activated T lymphocytes, are larger than mature lymphocytes and often contain eccentrically placed lobulated nuclei with nucleoli and vacuolated cytoplasm with rolled up edges. Mild neutropenia and thrombocytopenia are frequent. Other laboratory abnormalities include a mild polyclonal increase in immunoglobulins of the IgM, IgG, and IgA classes and mild elevations of hepatocellular enzymes.

EBV-specific antibody response Antibodies to several EBV-specific antigens arise during primary EBV infection (see Table 145-1). Proper utilization of EBV-specific antibody studies may facilitate the diagnosis of primary EBV infection in clinically atypical or heterophil-negative cases. IgM antibodies to the VCA are diagnostic of a primary EBV infection. IgG anti-VCA antibodies are present at clinical presentation in almost all patients and remain detectable for life. IgG anti-VCA antibodies are useful mainly as a test for susceptibility to EBV and are not useful for the diagnosis of primary infection. Approximately 70 percent of patients with infectious mononucleosis make antibodies to EA-D. Anti-EA-D antibodies usually peak 3 to 4 weeks after the onset of illness and usually disappear after recovery. Antibodies to EBNA appear 6 to 8 weeks into the illness and persist for life. The presence of IgM anti-VCA antibodies and seroconversion to EBNA are diagnostic of a primary EBV infection. Patients with defects in cellular immunity may fail to make antibodies to EBNA.

DIAGNOSIS The diagnosis of infectious mononucleosis is not difficult in the vast majority of cases. The constellation of fever, pharyngitis, and lymphadenopathy coupled with an atypical lymphocytosis and heterophil antibodies is virtually always due to primary EBV infection and requires no further laboratory studies. Certain patients with EBV-induced mononucleosis, particularly preadolescents or those with neurologic complications, may be heterophil-negative or may lack an atypical lymphocytosis. Primary EBV infection can be diagnosed with certainty in these patients with the proper use of EBV-specific serologic studies (see above). Culturing EBV from oropharyngeal washings or peripheral blood mononuclear cells is laborious, and because of the ubiquity of the virus among EBV-seropositive individuals, it is not diagnostic of primary EBV infection.

Primary CMV infection is the illness most frequently confused with EBV-induced infectious mononucleosis. About two-thirds of adults with heterophil-negative mononucleosis have CMV-induced mononucleosis. Patients with CMV mononucleosis are, on average, slightly older than those with EBV-induced infectious mononucleosis and usually have an illness characterized predominantly by fever and malaise. Pharyngitis and lymphadenopathy are less common than with infectious mononucleosis. CMV-induced mononucleosis is usually more insidious in onset and slower to resolve than EBV-induced mononucleosis. The diagnosis can be made by the isolation of CMV from the peripheral blood and the demonstration of seroconversion or a fourfold or greater rise in antibody titer to CMV. Although CMV is also shed in saliva and urine by patients with CMV mononucleosis, demonstration of the agent in the blood is a more specific, but less sensitive, indicator of CMV-induced morbidity.

Severe pharyngitis also may be caused by another virus (e.g., herpes simplex) or by group A beta-hemolytic streptococci. Since group A beta-hemolytic streptococci can be isolated from the throat of up to 30 percent of patients with infectious mononucleosis, isolation of this organism does not rule out the diagnosis of infectious mononucleosis. Atypical lymphocytes also may be observed in a number of other conditions, including rubella, hepatitis, toxoplasmosis, mumps, and drug reactions. These conditions rarely pose major differential diagnostic problems when careful attention is paid to the other clinical and laboratory features of these illnesses.

TREATMENT Infectious mononucleosis usually requires only supportive management. Patients should be advised to obtain adequate rest; there is no evidence that forced bed rest hastens recovery. Fever and pharyngitis are usually ameliorated by acetaminophen. Because of the infrequent complication of splenic rupture, patients should be advised to avoid contact sports for 6 to 8 weeks after the onset of illness. The timing of return to school or work is determined solely by symptoms. Patients with mild illness may not require any major changes in routine. Occasional patients with protracted illness may not return to a full school or work schedule for several months. Recovery from mononucleosis is often gradual, and the malaise may wax and wane for some time.

Although glucocorticoids may hasten defervescence and the resolution of pharyngitis, they are indicated only for certain specific complications of mononucleosis; airway obstruction usually responds dramatically to parenteral glucocorticoids. Glucocorticoids also may hasten the recovery of patients with severe hemolytic anemia or thrombocytopenia. There is no evidence that glucocorticoids are beneficial for the neurologic complications of the illness. Occasional selected patients with protracted illness may benefit from a short course of prednisone, but glucocorticoids should be avoided in the majority of patients with infectious mononucleosis.

Acyclovir, α-interferon, and 9-[2-hydroxy-1-(hydroxymethyl)ethoxy]methyl guanine (ganciclovir) are active inhibitors of EBV replication in vitro. α-Interferon has antiviral activity and can decrease shedding of EBV by renal allograft recipients treated with antithymocyte globulin. Administration of intravenous or high-dose oral acyclovir halts oropharyngeal shedding of EBV in patients with acute infectious mononucleosis; however, clinical benefits are minimal or inapparent.

EBV-ASSOCIATED MALIGNANCY Since the initial description of EBV in patients with African Burkitt's lymphoma, the virus has been detected in association with several other malignancies. EBV DNA sequences have been detected in tumor tissue from more than 90 percent of patients with African Burkitt's lymphomas. American Burkitt's lymphoma, which often affects older children and more often presents as an intraabdominal tumor, is EBV-associated in only 15 percent of cases. Anaplastic nasopharyngeal carcinoma, a common

neoplasm in southeast China, is highly associated with EBV; virtually all adequately studied patients with this malignancy have evidence of EBV in tumor tissue.

There is increasing evidence that implicates EBV in the pathogenesis of certain cases of lymphocytic lymphoma in the immunoincompetent host (see Chap. 311). B cell lymphoma is greatly overrepresented among malignancies developing in immunosuppressed individuals such as organ allograft recipients, patients with ataxia telangiectasia, and patients with AIDS. Immunologically privileged areas such as the central nervous system also appear to be particularly susceptible to EBV-associated B cell lymphomas. Cardiac allograft recipients treated with cyclosporin A appear to be particularly susceptible to B cell lymphoma. EBV sequences are detectable in up to half the B cell malignancies encountered in immunosuppressed individuals. The pathogenesis of B cell lymphoma is complex. In some cases, EBV-driven B cell transformation may be an early event; in others, transformation may be driven primarily by cytokines such as interleukin 6. The process, which may be polyclonal initially, becomes oligoclonal or monoclonal with a second-step chromosomal translocation made more likely by the increased number of proliferating B lymphocytes. The biologic behavior of these tumors does not always correlate with clonality as defined by conventional techniques. Patients have been described who have succumbed to lymphoproliferative processes which appear to be polyclonal by surface immunoglobulin studies. More sensitive techniques of defining clonality, such as that utilizing immunoglobulin gene rearrangement, may reveal that a larger proportion of the polyclonal lymphomas are in fact oligo- or monoclonal. The response of these B cell lymphomas to conventional chemotherapy is often disappointing. On occasion, these lymphoproliferative syndromes are reversible if the immunosuppression is decreased. There are case reports of apparent responses to acyclovir therapy; in most cases, however, such tumors do not respond to acyclovir, and conventional combination chemotherapy is required. Studies of larger numbers of these patients for the presence of EBV sequences and for the progression from a polyclonal to an oligoclonal or monoclonal disorder will shed more light on the role of EBV in oncogenesis in both immunoincompetent and immunologically normal hosts.

REFERENCES

GROSE C et al: Primary Epstein-Barr virus infections in acute neurologic diseases. N Engl J Med 292:392, 1975

HENLE W et al: Epstein-Barr virus specific diagnostic tests in infectious mononucleosis. Hum Pathol 5:551, 1974

HOLMES GP et al: Chronic fatigue syndrome: A working case definition. Ann Intern Med 108:387, 1989

MEEKER TC et al: Evidence for molecular subtypes of HIV-associated lymphoma: Division into peripheral monoclonal, polyclonal, and central nervous system lymphoma. AIDS 5:669, 1991

MILLER G et al: Selective lack of antibody to a component of EB nuclear antigen in patients with chronic active Epstein-Barr virus infection. J Infect Dis 156:26, 1987

MURRAY RJ et al: Human cytotoxic T-cell responses against Epstein-Barr virus nuclear antigens demonstrated by using recombinant vaccinia vectors. Proc Natl Acad Sci USA 87:2906, 1990

SCHOOLEY RT et al: Chronic Epstein-Barr virus infection associated with fever and interstitial pneumonitis. Ann Intern Med 104:636, 1986

SCULLEY TB et al: Coinfection with A-type and B-type Epstein-Barr virus in human immunodeficiency virus–positive subjects. J Infect Dis 162:643, 1990

SIXBY JW et al: Epstein-Barr virus replication in oropharyngeal epithelial cells. N Engl J Med 310:1225, 1984

STRAUS SE et al: Treatment of the chronic fatigue syndrome with acyclovir: Lack of efficacy in a placebo-controlled trial. N Engl J Med 319:1692–1698, 1988

146   CYTOMEGALOVIRUS INFECTION

MARTIN S. HIRSCH

DEFINITION   Cytomegalovirus (CMV), which was initially isolated from patients with congenital cytomegalic inclusion disease, is now recognized as an important pathogen in all age groups. In addition to inducing severe birth defects, CMV causes a wide spectrum of disorders in older children and adults, ranging from an asymptomatic, subclinical infection to a mononucleosis syndrome in healthy individuals to disseminated disease in the immunocompromised. Human CMV is one of several related species-specific viruses that cause similar diseases in various animals. All are associated with the production of characteristic enlarged cells, hence the name *cytomegalovirus.*

ETIOLOGY   CMV is a member of the beta herpesvirus group and contains double-stranded DNA, a protein capsid, and a lipoprotein envelope. Like other members of the herpesvirus group, CMV demonstrates icosahedral symmetry, replicates in the cell nucleus, and can cause either a lytic and productive or a latent infection. CMV can be distinguished from other herpesviruses by certain biologic properties such as host range and the type of cytopathology induced. Virus replication is associated with the production of large intranuclear inclusions and smaller cytoplasmic inclusions. The virus appears to replicate in a variety of cell types in vivo; in tissue culture it grows preferentially in fibroblasts. It is unclear whether CMV is oncogenic in vivo. However, the virus can rarely transform fibroblasts, and genomic transforming fragments have been identified.

EPIDEMIOLOGY   CMV has a worldwide distribution. Approximately 1 percent of newborns in the United States are infected with CMV, and the percentage is higher in many less-developed countries. Communal living and poor personal hygiene facilitate early spread. Perinatal and early childhood infections are common. Virus may be present in milk, saliva, feces, and urine. Transmission of CMV has been identified among young children in day-care centers and has been traced from infected toddler to pregnant mother to developing fetus. When an infected child introduces CMV into a household, 50 percent of susceptible family members seroconvert within 6 months.

The virus is not readily spread by casual contact but requires repeated or prolonged intimate exposure for transmission. In late adolescence and young adulthood, CMV is often transmitted sexually, and asymptomatic viral carriage in semen or cervical secretions is common. The rate of detectable CMV antibody titers approaches 100 percent in female prostitutes and in sexually active homosexual men. Sexually active adults may harbor several strains of CMV simultaneously. Transfusion of whole blood or certain blood products containing viable leukocytes also may transmit CMV with a frequency of 0.14 to 10 percent per unit transfused.

Once infected, an individual probably carries the virus for life. Most commonly these infections remain latent. However, with compromise of T lymphocyte–mediated immunity, as occurs following organ transplantation or in association with lymphoid neoplasms and certain acquired immunodeficiencies (in particular, that caused by infection with the human immunodeficiency virus, or HIV; see Chap. 279), CMV reactivation syndromes develop frequently. Most primary CMV infections in organ transplant recipients result from transmission of the virus in the graft itself. In CMV-seropositive transplant recipients, infection results from reactivation of latent virus or, less commonly, from reinfection by a new strain of CMV.

PATHOGENESIS   Congenital CMV infection can follow either primary or reactivation infection of the mother. However, clinical disease in the fetus or newborn is almost exclusively related to primary maternal infections (Table 146-1). Factors determining the severity of congenital infection are unknown; a deficient capacity to produce precipitating antibodies and to mount T cell responses to CMV is associated with more severe disease.

Primary infection in late childhood or adulthood is often associated with a vigorous T lymphocyte response that may contribute to the development of a mononucleosis syndrome similar to that observed following Epstein-Barr virus infection (see Chap. 145). The hallmarks of such infections are the appearance of atypical lymphocytes in the peripheral blood; these cells are predominantly activated T lymphocytes of cytotoxic-suppressor phenotype. Polyclonal activation of B cells by the virus contributes to the development of rheumatoid factors and other autoantibodies during CMV mononucleosis.

Once acquired during symptomatic or asymptomatic primary infection, CMV persists indefinitely in tissues of the host. The sites of persistent or latent infection are unclear but probably include multiple cell types and various organs. Transmission following blood transfusion or organ transplantation is due to silent infections in these tissues. Autopsy studies suggest that salivary glands and bowel also may be areas of latent infection.

If T cell responses of the host become compromised by disease or by iatrogenic immunosuppression, latent virus can be reactivated to cause a variety of syndromes. Chronic antigenic stimulation (as occurs following tissue transplantation) in the presence of immunosuppression appears to be an ideal setting for CMV activation and CMV-induced disease. Certain particularly potent suppressants of T cell immunity, such as antithymocyte globulin, are associated with a high rate of clinical CMV syndromes, which may follow either primary or reactivation infection. CMV may itself contribute to further T lymphocyte hyporesponsiveness, which often precedes superinfection with other opportunistic pathogens, such as *Pneumocystis carinii.* CMV and pneumocystis are frequently found together in immunosuppressed patients with severe interstitial pneumonia. CMV may function as a cofactor to activate latent HIV infection.

PATHOLOGY   Cytomegalic cells in vivo are presumed to be infected epithelial cells. They are two to four times larger than

---

TABLE 146-1   CMV in the immunocompromised host

Population	Risk factors	Principal syndromes	Treatment	Prevention
Fetus	Primary maternal infection/ early pregnancy	Cytomegalic inclusion disease	None	Avoidance of exposure
Organ transplant recipient	Seropositive donor, seronegative recipient; intensive immunosuppression, particularly with antilymphocyte globulins, cyclosporine	Febrile leukopenia; pneumonia; gastrointestinal disease	Ganciclovir	Donor-matching; CMV immunoglobulin; ganciclovir or high-dose acyclovir
Bone marrow transplant recipient	Graft-vs-host disease; older age; seropositive recipient; viremia	Pneumonia; gastrointestinal disease	Ganciclovir plus CMV immunoglobulin	Ganciclovir or high-dose acyclovir
Person with AIDS	<100 CD4 cells/mm³; CMV seropositivity	Retinitis; gastrointestinal disease	Foscarnet or ganciclovir	Trials under way

surrounding cells and often contain an 8- to 10-μm intranuclear inclusion that is eccentrically placed and surrounded by a clear halo resulting in an "owl's eye" appearance. Smaller granular cytoplasmic inclusions also may be demonstrated occasionally. Cytomegalic cells are found in a wide variety of organs, including salivary glands, lung, liver, kidney, intestines, pancreas, adrenal glands, and the central nervous system.

The cellular inflammatory response to infection consists of plasma cells, lymphocytes, and monocyte-macrophages. Granulomatous reactions are occasionally observed, particularly in the liver. Immunopathologic reactions may contribute to CMV disease. Immune complexes have been described in infected infants, sometimes associated with CMV-related glomerulopathies. Immune-complex glomerulopathy has been observed in some CMV-infected patients following renal transplantation.

CLINICAL MANIFESTATIONS **Congenital CMV infection** Fetal infections range from inapparent to severe and disseminated. Cytomegalic inclusion disease develops in approximately 5 percent of infected fetuses and is seen almost exclusively in infants born to mothers who develop primary infections during pregnancy. Petechiae, hepatosplenomegaly, and jaundice are the most common presenting features (60 to 80 percent). Microcephaly with or without cerebral calcifications, intrauterine growth retardation, and prematurity are noted in 30 to 50 percent of patients. Inguinal hernias and chorioretinitis occur less commonly. Laboratory abnormalities, in decreasing order of frequency, include an increase in serum IgM to >0.20 g/L (>20 mg/dL), atypical lymphocytosis, elevated liver transaminases, thrombocytopenia, hyperbilirubinemia, and an increase in cerebrospinal fluid protein to >0.20 g/L (>20 mg/dL). Prognosis among severely infected infants is poor, with mortality rates of 20 to 30 percent; few patients escape intellectual or hearing difficulties in later years. Differential diagnoses of cytomegalic inclusion disease in infants include syphilis, rubella, toxoplasmosis, herpes simplex or enterovirus infection, and bacterial sepsis.

Most congenital CMV infections are clinically inapparent at birth. Between 5 and 25 percent of asymptomatically infected infants develop significant psychomotor, hearing, ocular, or dental abnormalities over the next several years.

Perinatal CMV infection The newborn may acquire CMV at the time of delivery by passage through an infected birth canal or by postnatal contact with maternal milk or other secretions. Approximately 40 to 60 percent of infants who are breast-fed for over 1 month by seropositive mothers will become infected. Iatrogenic transmission also can result from neonatal blood transfusion. Screening of blood products prior to transfusion into low-birth-weight seronegative infants or seronegative pregnant women will decrease the risk of infection. The great majority of infants infected at or after delivery will remain asymptomatic. However, protracted interstitial pneumonitis has been associated with perinatally acquired CMV infection, particularly in premature infants, occasionally associated with *Chlamydia trachomatis*, *P. carinii*, or *Ureaplasma urealyticum* infections. Poor weight gain, adenopathy, rash, hepatitis, anemia, and atypical lymphocytosis also may be present, and CMV excretion often persists for months to years.

CMV mononucleosis The most common clinical manifestation of CMV infection in normal hosts beyond the neonatal period is a heterophil-antibody-negative mononucleosis syndrome. This may occur spontaneously or following the transfusion of leukocyte-containing blood products. Although the syndrome occurs at all ages, sexually active young adults are most often involved. Incubation periods range from 20 to 60 days, and the illness generally lasts 2 to 6 weeks. Prolonged high fevers, sometimes accompanied by chills, profound fatigue, and malaise, characterize this disorder. Myalgias, headache, and splenomegaly are frequent, but in CMV mononucleosis (as opposed to infectious mononucleosis caused by Epstein-Barr virus), exudative pharyngitis and cervical lymphadenopathy are rare. Occasional patients will develop rubelliform rashes, often after exposure to ampicillin. Less commonly observed are interstitial or segmental pneumonia, myocarditis, pleuritis, arthritis, or encephalitis. Rarely, Guillain-Barré syndrome may complicate CMV mononucleosis. The characteristic laboratory abnormality is a peripheral blood relative lymphocytosis with greater than 10 percent atypical lymphocytes. Total leukocyte counts may be low, normal, or markedly elevated. Although significant jaundice is uncommon, moderately elevated serum transaminase and alkaline phosphatase levels are often present. Heterophil antibodies are absent; however, transient immunologic abnormalities are common. These may include the presence of cryoglobulins, rheumatoid factors, cold agglutinins, and antinuclear antibodies. Rarely, hemolytic anemia, thrombocytopenia, and granulocytopenia complicate recovery.

Most patients recover without sequelae, although postviral asthenia may persist for months. CMV excretion in urine, genital secretions, or saliva often continues for months to years. Rare patients have recurrent episodes of fever and malaise, sometimes associated with autonomic nervous system dysfunction, e.g., attacks of sweating or flushing.

CMV infection in the immunocompromised host (See also Table 146-1) CMV appears to be the most frequent and important viral pathogen complicating organ transplantation. In renal, cardiac, lung, and liver transplant recipients, CMV induces a variety of syndromes, including fever and leukopenia, hepatitis, pneumonitis, esophagitis, gastritis, colitis, and retinitis. The maximal period of risk is between 1 and 4 months after transplantation, although retinitis may be a later complication. The risk of disease appears greater following primary infection. In addition, molecular studies indicate that seropositive transplant recipients are susceptible to reinfection with donor-derived, genotypically variant CMV, which often results in disease. Reactivation infection, although frequent, is less likely to be important clinically. Clinical disease is related to various factors (see Table 146-1), such as the degree of immunosuppression; patients receiving certain immunosuppressive agents, such as antithymocyte globulin, appear more likely to have severe infections than those receiving other agents, such as cyclosporin A. The transplanted organ is particularly vulnerable as a target for CMV infection; i.e., CMV hepatitis follows liver transplantation, and CMV pneumonitis more commonly follows lung transplantation.

CMV pneumonia occurs in nearly 15 to 20 percent of bone marrow transplant recipients, with a case-fatality rate of 84 to 88 percent. The risk is greatest between 5 and 13 weeks after transplantation, and several risk factors have been identified. These include type of immunosuppression, acute graft-versus-host disease, older age, viremia, and seropositivity before transplantation.

CMV has become recognized as an important pathogen in patients with AIDS (see Chap. 279). CMV infection is nearly ubiquitous in patients with AIDS and often causes retinitis or disseminated disease, contributing to death. CMV-induced immunosuppression probably also contributes to the T lymphocyte deficiency initiated by the etiologic retrovirus.

CMV syndromes in the immunocompromised host often begin with prolonged fever, malaise, anorexia, fatigue, night sweats, and arthralgias or myalgias. Liver function abnormalities, leukopenia, thrombocytopenia, and atypical lymphocytosis may be observed during these episodes. The development of tachypnea, hypoxia, and unproductive cough signals respiratory involvement. Radiologic examination of the lung often demonstrates bilateral interstitial or reticulonodular infiltrates, beginning in the periphery of the lower lobes and spreading centrally and superiorly; localized segmental, nodular, or alveolar patterns are less commonly observed. Diagnosis requires lung biopsy or bronchoalveolar lavage, since neither peripheral virus excretion nor high antibody titers provide sufficient information to prove etiology. The differential diagnoses include *P. carinii*; other viral, bacterial, or fungal pathogens; pulmonary hemorrhage; and injury secondary to radiation or cytotoxic drugs.

Gastrointestinal CMV involvement may be localized or extensive and occurs almost exclusively in compromised hosts. Ulcers of the esophagus, stomach, small intestine, or colon may result in bleeding or perforation. CMV infection may lead to exacerbations of underlying ulcerative colitis. Hepatitis occurs frequently, particularly following liver transplantation, and CMV-associated acalculous cholecystitis has been described.

CMV rarely causes meningoencephalitis in otherwise healthy individuals. Although CMV antigens and inclusions are observed occasionally in brains of patients dying from AIDS encephalopathy, the relative roles and interactions of CMV and HIV in this disorder are unclear. In immunocompromised patients, CMV can cause a subacute progressive polyradiculopathy, which is often reversible if recognized and treated promptly.

CMV retinitis is an important cause of blindness in immunocompromised patients, particularly patients with AIDS. Early lesions consist of small, opaque, white areas of granular retinal necrosis that spread in a centrifugal manner and are later accompanied by hemorrhages, vessel sheathing, and retinal edema (see Fig. A8-14). CMV must be distinguished from other causes of retinopathy, including toxoplasmosis, candidiasis, and herpes simplex virus infection.

Fatal CMV infections are often associated with persistent viremia and multiple organ system involvement. Progressive pulmonary infiltrates, pancytopenia, hyperamylasemia, and hypotension are characteristic, often with a terminal bacterial, fungal, or protozoan superinfection. Extensive adrenal necrosis with CMV inclusions is often present at autopsy, as is CMV involvement of many other organs.

DIAGNOSIS The diagnosis of CMV infection usually cannot be made reliably on clinical grounds alone. Virus isolation from appropriate clinical specimens, together with demonstration of a fourfold or greater antibody rise or persistently elevated antibody titers, is the preferred diagnostic approach. Virus excretion or viremia is readily detected by culture of appropriate specimens on human fibroblast monolayers. If virus titers are high, as is frequently the case in congenital disseminated infection or in patients with AIDS, characteristic cytopathic effects may be detected within a few days. However, in some situations, e.g., CMV mononucleosis, virus titers are low, and cytopathic effects may take several weeks to appear. Many laboratories expedite diagnosis by using an overnight tissue culture method (shell vial assay) involving centrifugation and an immunocytochemical detection technique employing monoclonal antibodies to an immediate early CMV antigen. Virus isolation from urine or saliva by itself does not prove acute infection, since excretion from these sites may continue for months to years following illness. Detection of CMV viremia is a better predictor of acute infection. Detection of CMV immediate-early antigens or DNA in peripheral blood leukocytes may hasten the diagnosis of CMV disease in certain populations, e.g., organ transplant recipients. Positivity in such assays may antedate culture positivity by several days.

A variety of serologic assays (complement fixation, immunofluorescence, indirect hemagglutination, ELISA) are available to detect antibody rises to CMV antigens. Antibody rises may not be detectable for up to 4 weeks after primary infection, and titers often remain high for years after infection. For this reason, single-sample antibody determinations are of no value in assessing the acuteness of infection. Detection of CMV-specific IgM is sometimes useful in the diagnosis of recent or active infection; circulating rheumatoid factors may result in occasional false-positive IgM tests.

PREVENTION AND TREATMENT Several prophylactic measures are useful to prevent CMV infection in patients at high risk. The use of blood from seronegative donors or blood that was frozen, thawed, and deglycerolized greatly decreases transfusion-associated transmission of CMV. Similarly, matching of organ or bone marrow transplants by CMV serology, using only organs from seronegative donors for seronegative recipients, reduces primary infections following transplantation.

CMV immune globulin has been reported to reduce CMV-associated syndromes and fungal or parasitic superinfections in seronegative renal transplant recipients. Similar studies in bone marrow transplant recipients have produced conflicting results. Prophylactic acyclovir has been demonstrated to reduce CMV infection and disease in seronegative renal transplant recipients; acyclovir is not effective in treatment of active CMV disease, however.

Ganciclovir (dihydroxypropoxymethyl guanine, DHPG) is a guanosine derivative with considerably more activity against CMV than its congener, acyclovir. After intracellular conversion, ganciclovir triphosphate is a selective inhibitor of CMV DNA polymerase. Several clinical studies have indicated response rates of 70 to 90 percent among patients with AIDS given ganciclovir for the treatment of CMV retinitis or colitis. In bone marrow transplant recipients with CMV pneumonia, ganciclovir is less effective when given alone, but a favorable clinical response occurs 50 to 70 percent of the time when it is combined with CMV immune globulin. Prophylactic or suppressive ganciclovir may be useful in high-risk bone marrow or organ transplant recipients e.g., those who are CMV-seropositive pretransplant or who are CMV culture-positive posttransplant. In many patients with AIDS and CMV disease, clinical and virologic relapses occur if treatment with ganciclovir is discontinued. Therefore, prolonged maintenance regimens are recommended. Resistance to ganciclovir is common in patients treated for more than 3 months. Usual induction courses for CMV retinitis are 5 mg/kg IV twice daily for 14 to 21 days followed by 5 mg/kg daily for 5 to 7 days per week. Peripheral blood neutropenia, the major toxic effect of ganciclovir, often can be ameliorated by the concomitant use of granulocyte colony-stimulating factor or granulocyte-macrophage colony-stimulating factor.

Foscarnet (sodium phosphonoformate) also acts against CMV infection by inhibiting the viral DNA polymerase. Because this agent does not require phosphorylation to be active, it is also effective against ganciclovir-resistant CMV isolates. A comparative trial of foscarnet and ganciclovir in 234 patients with AIDS and CMV retinitis demonstrated equivalent activity against retinitis but longer survival (12.6 versus 8.5 months) in the foscarnet group. Although the reasons for the survival differences are unclear, the antiretroviral activity of foscarnet and the greater use of zidovudine in foscarnet recipients are strong possibilities. Foscarnet exhibits considerable toxicity, including renal dysfunction, hypomagnesemia, hypokalemia, hypocalcemia, seizures, fever, and rash, each occurring in more than 5 percent of recipients. Moreover, foscarnet administration requires the use of an infusion pump and close clinical monitoring. The recommended regimen of foscarnet for CMV retinitis is induction with 60 mg/kg IV every 8 h for 14 to 21 days, followed by daily maintenance infusions of 90 to 120 mg/kg.

REFERENCES

BALFOUR HH et al: A randomized, placebo-controlled trial of oral acyclovir for the prevention of cytomegalovirus disease in recipients of renal allografts. N Engl J Med 320:1381, 1989

BOWDEN RA et al: Cytomegalovirus (CMV)-specific intravenous immunoglobulin for the prevention of primary CMV infection and disease after marrow transplant. J Infect Dis 164:483, 1991

BUHLES WC et al: Ganciclovir treatment of life- or sight-threatening cytomegalovirus infection: Experience in 314 immunocompromised patients. Rev Infect Dis 10:S495, 1988

CHOU S: Newer methods for diagnosis of cytomegalovirus infection. Rev Infect Dis 12:5727, 1990

DREW WL: Cytomegalovirus infection in patients with AIDS. J Infect Dis 158:449, 1988
———— et al: Prevalence of resistance in patients receiving ganciclovir for serious cytomegalovirus infection. J Infect Dis 163:716, 1991

EMMANUEL D et al: Cytomegalovirus pneumonia after bone marrow transplantation successfully treated with the combination of ganciclovir and high-dose intravenous immunoglobulin. Ann Intern Med 109:777, 1988

GERNA G et al: Monitoring of human cytomegalovirus infections and ganciclovir treatment in heart transplant recipients by determination of viremia, antigens and DNA emia. J Infect Dis 164:488, 1991

GRUNDY JE et al: Symptomatic cytomegalovirus infection in seropositive kidney recipients: Reinfection with donor virus rather than reactivation of recipient virus. Lancet 2:132, 1988

HIRSCH MS: Cytomegalovirus and its role in the pathogenesis of acquired immunodeficiency syndrome. Transplant Proc 23:S118, 1991
————: The treatment of cytomegalovirus in AIDS: More than meets the eye. N Engl J Med 326:264, 1992

Ho M: *Cytomegalovirus: Biology and Infection*. New York, Plenum Press, 1982

Horwitz CA et al: Clinical and laboratory evaluation of cytomegalovirus-induced mononucleeosis in previously healthy patients. Medicine 65:124, 1986.

Jacobson MA, Mills J: Serious cytomegalovirus disease in the acquired immunodeficiency syndrome (AIDS). Ann Intern Med 108:585, 1988

Merigan TC et al: A controlled trial of ganciclovir to prevent cytomegalovirus disease after heart transplantation. N Engl J Med 326:1182, 1992

Meyers JD et al: Cytomegalovirus excretion as a predictor of cytomegalovirus disease after marrow transplantation: Importance of cytomegalovirus viremia. J Infect Dis 162:373, 1990

Miller, RG et al: Ganciclovir in the treatment of progressive AIDS-related polyradiculopathy. Neurology 40:569, 1990

Onorato IM et al: Epidemiology of cytomegaloviral infections: Recommendations for prevention and control. Rev Infect Dis 7:479, 1985

Pass RF et al: Young children as a probable source of maternal and congenital cytomegalovirus infection. N Engl J Med 316:1366, 1987

Preiksaitis JK et al: The risk of cytomegalovirus infection in seronegative transfusion recipients not receiving exogenous immunosuppression. J Infect Dis 157:523, 1988

Reed EC et al: Treatment of cytomegalovirus pneumonia with ganciclovir and intravenous cytomegalovirus immunoglobulin in patients with bone marrow transplants. Ann Intern Med 109:783, 1988

Schmidt GM et al: A randomized controlled trail of prophylactic ganciclovir for cytomegalovirus pulmonary infection in recipients of allogeneic bone marrow transplants. N Engl J Med 324:1005, 1991

Schooley RE: Cytomegalovirus in the setting of the infection with human immunodeficiency virus. Rev Infect Dis 12:5811, 1990

Smyth RL et al: Cytomegalovirus infection in heart-lung transplant recipients: Risk factors, clinical associations, and response to treatment. J Infect Dis 164:1045, 1991

Snydman DR et al: Use of cytomegalovirus immune globulin to prevent cytomegalovirus disease in renal transplant recipients. N Engl J Med 317:1049, 1987

Studies of Ocular Complication of AIDS Research Group, AIDS Clinical Trials Group: Mortality in patients with the acquired immunodeficiency syndrome treated with either foscarnet or ganciclovir for cytomegalovirus retinitis. N Engl J Med 326:213, 1992

van den Berg AP et al: Antigenemia in the diagnosis and monitoring of active cytomegalovirus infection after liver transplantation. J Infect Dis 164:265, 1991

147 SMALLPOX, VACCINIA, AND OTHER POXVIRUSES

HARVEY M. FRIEDMAN

Poxviruses that infect humans share the common feature of producing cutaneous vesicular eruptions. They are brick-shaped, double-stranded DNA viruses and are the largest of the animal viruses. Human pathogens include variola, vaccinia, monkeypox, cowpox, milker's node virus, and molluscum contagiosum. These viruses can be distinguished from one another by antigenic differences, clinical manifestations of infection, and pox morphology when inoculated onto chick embryo chorioallantoic membranes. Global eradication of smallpox and the concomitant reduction in smallpox vaccination programs have changed the epidemiology of variola and vaccinia and have modified their importance in modern medicine.

SMALLPOX

DEFINITION Smallpox (variola major) is a highly contagious disease characterized by fever, a vesicular and pustular eruption, and a high mortality rate. A milder form (variola minor) may be caused by the same virus.

The global eradication of smallpox was officially announced in 1979, marking one of the greatest achievements of modern medicine. Smallpox has not reappeared for over a decade. If this pattern persists, a disease that once accounted for 10 percent of all deaths will become an illness mainly of historical interest.

ETIOLOGY Variola virus, the causative agent of smallpox, is an orthopoxvirus within the Poxviridae family. Variola is a large (200 to 400 nm) DNA virus differing from other DNA viruses in that it lacks icosahedral symmetry. When viewed by electron microscopy, it has a complex structure and appears brick-shaped. It has an outer membrane, two lateral bodies, and a dumbbell-shaped core that contains a single molecule of double-stranded DNA.

PATHOGENESIS AND PATHOLOGY The oropharynx of infected patients serves as the main source for virus spread. Contacts become infected by inhaling virus which enters the respiratory tract and multiplies locally, probably within macrophages. Virus is carried within macrophages into the circulation and to regional lymph nodes. Multiplication occurs within lymphoid organs, and a secondary viremia develops. Virus localizes within small dermal blood vessels, leading to endothelial swelling and infection of epidermal cells. Intraepidermal vesicles form in skin and mucous membranes. When stained with hematoxylin and eosin, the cytoplasm of infected cells contains faintly basophilic or acidophilic inclusions (Guarnieri bodies). Extension of infection into the corium and sebaceous glands produces pockmarks, or scars, which, upon healing, are characteristic of smallpox infection.

Virus infection stimulates cytotoxic T cell responses, neutralizing antibodies, and the production of interferons. These responses restrict viral replication and induce prolonged immunity if the patient recovers. The infection is likely to be most severe in impaired hosts, particularly those with T cell deficits. Milder forms of the infection have been observed in immunized patients, although it remains unclear why variola minor may be produced by the same virus in the unimmunized.

EPIDEMIOLOGY Smallpox was described in Asia during the first century A.D., in Europe and Africa around 700 A.D., and in Central, South, and North America during the sixteenth and seventeenth centuries. Endemic variola major was eradicated from the United States in 1926, and variola minor during the 1940s. Eradication was slower in Asia, Africa, and parts of the Americas. The last naturally occurring smallpox infection occurred in Somalia, Africa, in October 1977. The last known case developed 1 year later in Birmingham, England, in September 1978, and was the result of a laboratory accident. The ability to eradicate this disease by an effective worldwide vaccination program appears to be centrally related to the facts that human beings were the only known reservoir for the variola virus; that no asymptomatic carrier state existed, facilitating surveillance; and that early diagnosis and prevention of disease or modification of the course by rapid vaccination of contacts were possible.

In temperate climates, endemic smallpox occurred in winter and spring. It was mainly a disease of children and young adults. Spread in unvaccinated family contacts was approximately 58 percent, compared with 4 percent in vaccinees. Patients were usually severely ill and confined to bed, which restricted transmission to immediate family contacts. Index cases rarely infected more than five patients, most commonly those sharing living quarters. Transmission intervals were 2 to 3 weeks apart, and new cases would appear in a community or region over many months.

CLINICAL FEATURES Smallpox was endemic in every country of the world and existed as two forms, variola major, which was a serious illness with a mortality rate of >20 percent in the unvaccinated, and variola minor, which was a milder infection with a mortality of <1 percent. Both were caused by the same virus. On an individual case basis, it may be difficult to distinguish variola minor from a mild case of variola major. The severity of an entire outbreak is generally required to differentiate the two. The evolution of rash in variola minor is more rapid, similar to accelerated smallpox.

Variola major has been classified into five clinical categories:

1 *Ordinary type:* This comprised >70 percent of cases. It is characterized by raised pustular skin lesions which can be divided into three categories: (a) *confluent* rash present on face and forearms, (b) *semiconfluent* rash present on face with discrete rash elsewhere, and (c) *discrete* rash on all involved areas with normal skin between pustules. In unvaccinated patients, mortality was 62 percent for confluent infection, 37 percent for semiconfluent, and 9 percent for discrete infection.

2 *Modified type:* This form of smallpox is similar to ordinary disease, except that the course is accelerated and pustular lesions are

smaller. Modified smallpox was common in vaccinated patients who developed lesions, in health care workers exposed by accidental inoculation, and in those intentionally infected by variolation, a procedure once widely used as a method of vaccination.

3 Variola sine eruptione: Patients have fever but no rash. This was seen in vaccinated patients or those previously infected. Laboratory testing is required for confirmation of the diagnosis.

4 Flat type: Pustules remain flat and are usually confluent or semiconfluent in distribution. This form of infection occurred mainly in children and was often fatal.

5 Hemorrhagic type: Skin lesions and mucous membranes become hemorrhagic. Pregnant women were predisposed to this form of smallpox, which was rare but severe. Profound prostration, heart failure, diffuse bleeding, and bone marrow suppression resulted, and most infections were fatal within 3 to 4 days, earning the name "sledgehammer smallpox."

In a typical case of ordinary type smallpox, the incubation period is 7 to 19 days, with a mean of 12. A preeruptive phase lasting 2 to 4 days is characterized by sudden onset of fever, severe headache, backache, and malaise. Vomiting occurs in 50 percent and diarrhea in 10 percent of patients. The rash first appears as minute red spots on the tongue and palate and as small macules (herald spots) on the face. Spread is centrifugal, involving the face, proximal extremities, trunk, and then distal extremities. Intraoral rash evolves from papules to vesicles, which break down and release large amounts of virus. The enanthem is an important source of virus spread. On the skin, macules evolve to papules by day 2, vesicles by days 4 to 5, and pustules by day 7 of rash. Fever may recur during the pustular phase. Lesions, which range from few to thousands, have a shotty, hard feel to them. Crusts develop by day 14 and heal leaving depigmented areas.

LABORATORY FINDINGS Virus isolation Virus can be isolated from skin lesions (until scabs form), oropharynx, conjunctiva, and urine. Viremia precedes the rash and clears in most patients when the rash appears. Virus particles can be seen by negative-staining electron microscopy performed on fluid obtained from skin lesions. This form of diagnosis was used to identify cases during the intensified eradication programs carried out in the 1960s and 1970s.

Serology Antibodies appear by days 6 to 8 of infection. Antibody titer rises can be detected by testing paired serum samples drawn 2 to 3 weeks apart. Methods used to measure antibodies include hemagglutination inhibition, complement fixation, neutralization, and gel precipitation.

Hematology Granulocytopenia, thrombocytopenia, and lymphocytosis are common during the prodromal and early rash phase. Leukocytosis occurs with pustulation of the vesicles. A profile consistent with disseminated intravascular coagulation is seen in patients with hemorrhagic smallpox.

DIFFERENTIAL DIAGNOSIS Distinguishing varicella from smallpox was particularly difficult during epidemics of variola minor or when mild smallpox infection developed in vaccinated patients. Dense rash on the trunk and appearance of lesions in crops are features of varicella not seen in smallpox. Human monkeypox, seen in western and central Africa, is difficult to distinguish from smallpox. Monkeypox is associated with more lymphadenopathy than smallpox. In the past, virus isolation was required to differentiate the two. On occasion, virus isolation also was required to distinguish disseminated vaccinia infection from smallpox.

COMPLICATIONS AND SEQUELAE Complications include secondary bacterial infections of the skin, keratitis and corneal ulcerations, viral arthritis and osteomyelitis, bacterial pneumonia, orchitis, and encephalitis. Sequelae include blindness from corneal scarring, limb deformities, and pockmarks, which appear hypopigmented in dark-skinned individuals and hyperpigmented in light-skinned patients.

TREATMENT AND OUTCOME In the past, mortality was highest in infants and the elderly. Infection in pregnant women led to abortion rates of >60 percent. Vaccination during the first week of incubation modified the course of disease by protecting many and reducing the severity of infection in others. This constituted an important method for control of smallpox. Immunotherapy with vaccinia immune globulin given during the incubation period of infection modified disease; however, supplies were too limited for this form of therapy to be widely applicable. Several different thiosemicarbazones, a class of antiviral compounds, were tried for treatment, but no benefit was detected in controlled human trials. One thiosemicarbazone, metisazone, was found to be useful as preventive therapy following exposure. Vaccinia immune globulin also was effective in postexposure prophylaxis without the side effects of metisazone. The mainstay of treatment was good nursing care, which was often provided by family members at home or in hospitals.

CONTROL Attempts at control of smallpox began once it was noted that accidental exposure to smallpox by scratch on the skin resulted in less severe infection. This led to the practice of variolation, which began in China and India in the tenth century. Variolation involved intentional administration of pustular fluids or scabs to uninfected persons. In 1796, Edward Jenner showed that inoculation with cowpox virus protected against smallpox and carried less risk of illness than variolation. Subsequently, vaccination was modified to use of vaccinia virus for smallpox control. The origins of vaccinia virus are uncertain, but many strains existed which were apparently derived from either variola or cowpox virus. Successful vaccination provided high levels of protection for 5 years and some protection for 20 years. Periodic revaccination was necessary for optimal protection. Postexposure vaccination lowered the incidence and reduced the severity of infection when administered within 1 week after exposure.

In 1959, the World Health Assembly adopted a program aimed at global eradication of smallpox. The development of stable freeze-dried vaccine meant that vaccination programs could reach less developed tropical countries. Efforts were intensified by 1967 and were built on the principles of surveillance and containment involving case detection, quarantine of infected patients, and vaccination of contacts and others living in the immediate area. Surveillance and contact vaccination were extremely important for the eventual success of the program. This approach was successful because smallpox has a long incubation period that allows vaccination to modify the course of the illness. The lack of a reservoir for variola, other than humans, the ease of clinical diagnosis; and the fact that variola does not establish latent or persistent infection were important contributors to the success of the eradication program.

VACCINIA

DEFINITION AND ETIOLOGY Vaccinia is a localized skin infection caused by inoculation of vaccinia virus. In immunosuppressed patients it may occasionally disseminate and produce severe disease. Vaccinia virus is thought to be derived from either variola, cowpox, or perhaps a hybrid of the two. "Vaccination" with vaccinia induces immunity to variola and was the method used to control or prevent smallpox. Endemic smallpox was eradicated from the United States in 1949, which led to the eventual discontinuation of routine childhood immunization by 1972. Evidence of immunization against smallpox is no longer required for international travel.

COMPLICATIONS OF VACCINATION Vaccine is applied to the skin, which is punctured several times by a sterile needle to penetrate the epidermis. Primary vaccination results in formation of a papule in 4 to 5 days that becomes a vesicle 2 to 3 days later. Mild fever and localized lymphadenopathy are often present at this stage. Within 2 weeks, a scab forms that leaves a scar when healing is complete. The response during revaccination is accelerated and generally is not associated with fever or lymphadenopathy.

Vaccinia virus never underwent controlled trials to establish safety and efficacy before licensing. Nevertheless, the vaccine was highly effective, despite considerable adverse effects. *Complications* included: (1) *Progressive vaccinia* (vaccinia gangrenosum) developed in patients who were agammaglobulinemic, T cell deficient, or receiving immunosuppressive therapy. Destruction of local areas of skin, subcutaneous tissue, and other underlying structures occurred, with metastatic lesions appearing at other cutaneous sites and in viscera and bone. This complication developed in approximately 1 patient per million during primary or revaccination and was usually fatal over a period of several months. (2) *Eczema vaccinatum* involved wide cutaneous spread of vaccinia virus in vaccinees and their contacts who had eczema or other chronic skin diseases. It developed in 1 per 100,000 primary vaccinations or 1 per million revaccinations and was sometimes fatal; bacterial superinfection often complicated eczema vaccinatum. (3) *Generalized vaccinia*, characterized by satellite lesions around the inoculation site or more widely disseminated pox, occasionally occurred in immunocompetent individuals and developed in 3 per 100,000 primary vaccinations or 1 per million revaccinations. This complication had a good prognosis. (4) *Accidental inoculation*, especially of eyelids, perineum, and vulva, occurred in 3 per 100,000 to 1 million vaccinees. The consequences were generally not serious. (5) *Postvaccinial encephalitis* was a serious complication which occurred in 3 per million patients after primary vaccination. It usually developed 6 to 15 days after vaccination and had a violent onset. Features included convulsions, hemiplegia, and aphasia. Spinal fluid analysis was normal except for increased pressure. Recovery was often incomplete, and neurologic sequelae ensued.

Contraindications to vaccination include B or T cell immune disorders, neoplasms of the reticuloendothelial system, concomitant use of immunosuppressive drugs, eczema, pregnancy, and disorders of the central nervous system. When complications developed due to uncontrolled or progressive vaccinia infection, some were treated effectively with vaccinia immune globulin. This treatment is not effective for postvaccinial encephalitis. A role for antivirals, such as thiosemicarbazones, has not been definitely established.

Interest has reemerged in vaccinia as a vehicle for vaccination. Genes from herpes simplex virus, hepatitis B virus, human immunodeficiency virus, and malaria have been introduced into the vaccinia genome. Proteins encoded by these genes are expressed during vaccinia infection, which indicates that this virus potentially could serve as a vector for multiple vaccines. Should this approach prove successful, then the same precautions should be followed as in vaccination to prevent smallpox.

OTHER POXVIRUSES

HUMAN MONKEYPOX   The monkeypox virus is a member of the *Orthopoxvirus* genus. Human monkeypox is a rare zoonosis that occurs in tropical rain forests of west and central Africa. This disease was first recognized in the 1960s during smallpox eradication efforts. Identification resulted from attempts to confirm suspected cases of smallpox by laboratory methods. Infection does not spread from person to person, which accounts for the low number of cases, less than 100, identified so far. The clinical features of infection are similar to smallpox, except that cervical and inguinal lymphadenopathy are more prominent in human monkeypox. The diagnosis can be established by the characteristic pox morphology when virus is inoculated onto chorioallantoic membrane cultures.

COWPOX   Cowpox virus is another member of the genus *Orthopoxvirus*. Infection develops by hand contact with infected ulcers on the teats of cows. The virus is also found in wild rodents, which may serve as a reservoir for some human infections. After exposure, one or more skin lesions develop, most often on the hands. The evolution of a lesion is similar to that seen during primary smallpox vaccination: a vesicle progresses to a pustule that later scabs. The rash does not become generalized. It is often associated with lymphangitis and localized lymphadenopathy. The disease may be confused with milker's nodule (see below). Laboratory confirmation can be estab-

lished by the characteristic pox that develop when virus is isolated on chorioallantoic membranes.

MILKER'S NODE VIRUS   This infection is caused by a parapoxvirus and is sometimes referred to as pseudocowpox or paravaccinia. It is acquired by contact with infected cows. Lesions appear as red nodules that progress to firm purple papules. The lack of vesicles or pustules distinguishes it from cowpox. Lesions are relatively painless and generally resolve in 4 to 6 weeks.

ORF   This is a disease of sheep that is sometimes referred to as contagious pustular dermatitis. It is caused by a parapoxvirus. Human infection is acquired by contact with sheep infected around the mouth, nose, or eyes. Human infection usually occurs at abrasion sites on the hands. Single or multiple painful large vesicles develop and are often associated with lymphadenopathy. Resolution occurs within several weeks.

MOLLUSCUM CONTAGIOSUM   This infection occurs only in humans and is caused by an unclassified poxvirus that cannot be cultured in vitro. Lesions occur anywhere on the body, except on the palms and soles, and appear as pearly, flesh-colored, raised, umbilicated nodules 2 to 5 mm in diameter. Lesions develop in crops, are painless, and resolve over a period of weeks to several years. Spread is probably by direct contact, which accounts for the commonly observed genital distribution of lesions in sexually active adults. An increased incidence of molluscum contagiosum is seen in patients infected with the human immunodeficiency virus. No specific therapy is available, although lesions can be removed by curettage.

REFERENCES

BAXBY D: The origins of vaccinia virus. J Infect Dis 136:453, 1977
BREMAN JG, ARITA I: The confirmation and maintenance of smallpox eradication. N Engl J Med 303:1263, 1980
FENNER F: Poxviruses, in *Virology*, 2d ed, BN Fields et al (eds). New York, Raven, 1990, pp 2113–2133
——— et al: *Smallpox and Its Eradication*. Geneva, World Health Organization, 1988
MOSS B: Poxviridae and their replication, in *Virology*, 2d ed, BN Fields et al (eds). New York, Raven, 1990, pp 2079–2111
———: Vaccinia virus: A tool for research and vaccine development. Science 252:1662, 1991

148   PARVOVIRUS

NEIL R. BLACKLOW

DEFINITION   The parvovirus group includes several species-specific viruses of animals. One parvovirus, designated B19, is known to be a human pathogen. B19 is a small (diameter 20 to 25 nm), icosahedral, nonenveloped, single-stranded DNA virus with an outer capsid formed by two structural proteins. Individual virus particles contain DNA strands of positive or negative polarity. The virus is stable and retains infectivity after incubation at 60°C for 16 h. It has failed to grow in conventional cell culture lines and animal model systems but does replicate in vitro in erythroid progenitor cells derived from human bone marrow, umbilical cord, peripheral blood, or fetal liver sources.

During the 1980s, it was discovered that B19 causes a variety of disorders ranging from erythema infectiosum and acute arthropathy in otherwise healthy hosts to transient aplastic crisis and chronic anemia in compromised patients to fetal infection manifested by death or hydrops fetalis. Many of the severe manifestations of B19 viremia relate to the propensity of the virus to infect and lyse erythroid precursor cells in the bone marrow. The name B19 is derived from the code number of the human serum in which the virus was discovered.

PATHOGENESIS Two studies of adult volunteers have provided a basis for understanding the pathogenesis of B19 infection, which has two phases. The first phase is characterized by viremia that develops approximately 6 days after intranasal inoculation of B19 into susceptible individuals who lack serum antibodies to the virus. The viremia lasts about 1 week; its clearance is correlated with the development of IgM antibodies to B19 that remain detectable for up to a few months. IgG antibodies develop several days later and persist indefinitely. Nonspecific systemic symptoms lasting 2 or 3 days occur early during the viremic phase; these symptoms include headache, malaise, myalgia, fever, chills, and pruritus and are accompanied by reticulocytopenia and excretion of the virus from the respiratory tract. Several days after the onset of symptoms, a clinically insignificant decline in hemoglobin concentration is noted; the decreased level is maintained for 7 to 10 days, during which time examination of bone marrow samples reveals a marked depletion of erythroid precursor cells. Transient mild lymphopenia, neutropenia, and a drop in platelet count also may be documented. A second phase of illness begins around 17 or 18 days after virus inoculation (after the clearance of viremia, the cessation of viral shedding in throat secretions, and the resolution of reticulocytopenia). This illness mimics erythema infectiosum in adults, with 2 to 3 days of fine maculopapular rash accompanied by arthralgias and arthritis that last another 1 or 2 days. This phase occurs in the presence of rising serum titers of antibody to B19.

The studies just described indicate that B19 disease in the otherwise *healthy host*, manifested by self-limited erythema infectiosum and/or arthropathy, is almost certainly an immune-complex disorder. This concept is supported by the induction of erythema infectiosum through the infusion of immunoglobulins into chronically viremic patients. In contrast, B19 disease in the *compromised host* (chronic hemolytic disease or immunodeficiency syndromes) is often serious, resulting from the destruction by B19 of erythroid precursor cells. Normal hosts can tolerate 7 to 10 days of shutoff of erythropoiesis; however, patients with hemolytic disease who require increased production of erythrocytes do not tolerate erythroid cell destruction and thus usually develop severe transient aplastic crisis. Patients who are immunodeficient may fail to clear B19 viremia, the results being persistent infection of red blood cells and chronic severe anemia. The fetus requires increased production of red blood cells and possesses an immature immune system; both these factors could explain B19-induced hydrops fetalis.

EPIDEMIOLOGY Although B19 infections occur year round, they appear most commonly as outbreaks of erythema infectiosum in schools during winter and spring months. Between 20 and 60 percent of children in outbreaks are symptomatic, and 10 percent have asymptomatic infection. Seroepidemiologic studies indicate that approximately half of adults possess serum antibodies to B19, with antibody prevalence (reflecting prior exposure and probable immunity to the virus) rising rapidly between the ages of 5 and 18. B19 can be detected in throat swabbings, respiratory tract secretions, and serum, and its detection at these sites probably correlates with infectiousness. Thus patients with transient aplastic crisis are highly infectious. Their infectivity has been well documented as the source of one well-defined nosocomial outbreak of erythema infectiosum among nurses. In contrast, individuals with erythema infectiosum are much less infectious. The usual route of viral transmission under natural conditions is unknown but may be respiratory or through direct contact. B19 can be transmitted during therapy with clotting factor concentrate, even after exposure to steam or dry heat.

CLINICAL MANIFESTATIONS Erythema infectiosum Erythema infectiosum is the most common manifestation of B19 infection and occurs predominantly in children. This entity is also called *fifth disease* because it was classified in the late nineteenth century as the fifth in a series of six exanthems of childhood. Normally a mild illness, erythema infectiosum typically presents as a facial rash with a "slapped-cheek" appearance that is sometimes preceded by low-grade fever. The rash may develop quickly on the arms and legs and

usually has a lacy, reticular, erythematous appearance. The trunk, palms, and soles are less commonly involved. Occasionally, the rash appears with maculopapular, morbilliform, vesicular, purpuric, or pruritic characteristics. The typical rash resolves in about a week but can recur intermittently for several weeks, particularly after stress, exercise, exposure to sunlight, bathing, or change in environmental temperature. Arthralgia and arthritis are uncommon among children but are frequent among adults, in whom the rash is often absent or nonspecific, with a lack of the characteristic facial erythema.

Arthropathy B19 infection in adults most commonly presents as acute arthralgias and arthritis, sometimes accompanied by rash. The arthritis is characteristically symmetric and peripheral, involving the wrists, hands, and knees most frequently. It normally resolves in about 3 weeks and is nondestructive. However, a small percentage of patients have arthritis persisting for months or even (in rare cases) for years. It is not known whether these individuals have persistent infection or an abnormal immune response to the virus. Several case reports have suggested a link—as yet unproven—between B19 and vascular purpura and vasculitis, idiopathic thrombocytopenic purpura, virus-associated hemophagocytic syndrome with pancytopenia, Lyme-like arthritis, recurrent paresthesias, rheumatoid arthritis, fibromyalgia, periarteritis nodosa, and systemic lupus erythematosus.

Transient aplastic crisis B19 infection is the cause in most instances of transient aplastic crisis developing suddenly in patients with chronic hemolytic disease. Nearly all hemolytic conditions can be affected by B19 infection, including sickle cell disease, erythrocyte enzyme deficiencies, hereditary spherocytosis, thalassemias, paroxysmal nocturnal hemoglobinuria, and autoimmune hemolysis. B19-induced aplastic crisis also can occur in the setting of acute blood loss. Patients present with weakness, lethargy, pallor, and severe anemia, a syndrome often preceded by a few days of nonspecific symptoms. These patients have intense reticulocytopenia lasting 7 to 10 days, and their bone marrow contains no erythroid precursor cells despite a normal myeloid series. Transient aplastic crisis can produce life-threatening anemia and may require urgent transfusion therapy. Unlike patients with erythema infectiosum or arthropathy, those with transient aplastic crisis are viremic and can readily transmit B19 virus infection to other people.

Chronic anemia in immunodeficient patients Immunodeficient patients may be unable to eliminate B19 infection, probably because they cannot produce adequate levels of virus-specific IgG antibodies. The result is persistent infection with destruction of erythroid precursor cells in the bone marrow and chronic transfusion-dependent anemia. This condition has been described in patients with immunodeficiency related to infection with human immunodeficiency virus, congenital immunodeficiencies, and acute lymphocytic leukemia during maintenance chemotherapy, as well as in recipients of bone marrow transplants. B19-induced chronic anemia also may be the presenting finding of an otherwise unrecognized immunodeficiency. Chronic anemia may fluctuate in intensity over time and may be cured or controlled by immunoglobulin therapy. Both the spectrum of immunodeficiencies associated with B19-induced chronic anemia and the frequency of the association remain to be determined.

Fetal infection Maternal B19 infections usually do not adversely affect the fetus; more often than not, in fact, the fetus remains uninfected. It is estimated that fewer than 10 percent of maternal B19 infections lead to fetal death; when fetal death does occur, it is usually attributable to the development of nonimmune hydrops fetalis, wherein the fetus succumbs to severe anemia and congestive heart failure. B19 virus can be detected in fetal tissues, with predominant infection of erythroblasts. Some hydropic fetuses survive B19 infection and appear normal at delivery. There is no evidence that B19 infection produces congenital abnormalities. A pregnant woman is not likely to become infected with B19 after exposure to a child with erythema infectiosum because the infectious stage of this disease is probably over by the time the classic rash develops.

DIAGNOSIS Diagnosis most commonly relies on measurements of B19 virus–specific IgM and IgG antibodies. The virus, its DNA, or its antigens are also detected in the serum or infected tissues of some patients. Acute infection can be proven by B19-compatible symptoms and the presence of IgM antibodies or virus itself, whereas past infection is documented by IgG antibodies. Individuals with erythema infectiosum and acute arthropathy usually have IgM antibodies without detectable virus in serum. Those with transient aplastic crisis may have IgM antibodies but typically possess high titers of virus and its DNA in serum. Immunodeficient patients with anemia often lack readily detectable antibodies but have viral particles and DNA in serum. Fetal infection may be recognized by hydrops fetalis and the presence of B19 DNA in amniotic fluid or fetal blood. Until recently, serologic tests required the use of B19 virus itself (collected from the blood of infected patients); this requirement restricted the use of these assays to a few laboratories, such as those at the Centers for Disease Control and Prevention. The expression of genetically engineered B19 capsids in infected cell cultures should lead to an ample supply of reagents and the ready availability of immunoassay kits for IgM antibodies.

TREATMENT AND PREVENTION Erythema infectiosum usually requires no treatment; the same is true for many cases of arthropathy. More severe cases of arthritis, particularly those involving chronic symptoms, can be treated with nonsteroidal anti-inflammatory agents. Transient aplastic crisis is usually treated with erythrocyte transfusions. In immunodeficient anemic patients, B19 infection should be treated with commercial intravenous immunoglobulin, which is known to contain IgG antibodies to B19. This therapy controls and may cure B19 infection. Prophylaxis of B19 infection should be considered for patients with chronic hemolysis or immunodeficiency and for pregnant women. The risk of infection for these persons may be reduced by hand washing before eating or after contact with respiratory or other secretions when B19 is known to be present in a community. Patients with transient aplastic crisis or chronic B19 infection (but not those with erythema infectiosum or arthropathy) pose a serious risk for nosocomial transmission of infection. They should be hospitalized in a private room with contact and respiratory isolation precautions. It is not known whether pre- or postexposure administration of immunoglobulin prevents infection. No vaccine for B19 is available; however, a baculovirus-infected insect cell line that expresses noninfectious B19 capsid proteins could serve as a prototype vaccine candidate.

REFERENCES

ANAND A et al: Human parvovirus infection in pregnancy and hydrops fetalis. N Engl J Med 316:183, 1987

ANDERSON LJ: Human parvoviruses. J Infect Dis 161:603, 1990

ANDERSON MJ et al: Experimental parvoviral infection in humans. J Infect Dis 152:257, 1985

BELL LM et al: Human parvovirus B19 infection among hospital staff members after contact with infected patients. N Engl J Med 321:485, 1989

BLACKLOW NR: Adeno-associated viruses of man, in *Parvoviruses and Human Disease*, JR Pattison (ed). Boca Raton, CRC Press, 1988, pp 165–174

CENTERS FOR DISEASE CONTROL: Risks associated with human parvovirus B19 infection. Morb Mort Week Rep 38:81, 1989

FRICKHOFEN N et al: Persistent B19 parvovirus infection in patients infected with human immunodeficiency virus type 1 (HIV-1): A treatable cause of anemia in AIDS. Ann Intern Med 113:926, 1990

HARRIS JW: Parvovirus B19 for the hematologist. Am J Hematol 39:119, 1992

KAJIGAYA S et al: Self-assembled B19 parvovirus capsids, produced in a baculovirus system, are antigenically and immunologically similar to native virions. Proc Natl Acad Sci USA 88:4646, 1991

KURTZMAN G et al: Pure red-cell aplasia of 10 years' duration due to persistent parvovirus B19 infection and its cure with immunoglobulin therapy. N Engl J Med 321:519, 1989

NAIDES SJ et al: Rheumatologic manifestations of human parvovirus B19 infection in adults: Initial two-year clinical experience. Arthritis Rheum 33:1297, 1990

PLUMMER FA et al: An erythema infectiosum-like illness caused by human parvovirus infection. N Engl J Med 313:74, 1985

POTTER CG et al: Variation of erythroid and myeloid precursors in the marrow and peripheral blood of volunteer subjects infected with human parvovirus (B19). J Clin Invest 79:1486, 1987

TOROK TJ et al: Prenatal diagnosis of intrauterine infection with parvovirus B19 by the polymerase chain reaction technique. Clin Infect Dis 14:149, 1992

149 HUMAN PAPILLOMAVIRUS INFECTIONS

RICHARD C. REICHMAN

DEFINITION Human papillomaviruses (HPV) selectively infect the epithelium of skin or mucous membranes. These infections may be asymptomatic, produce warts, or be associated with a variety of both benign and malignant neoplasias.

ETIOLOGY HPV, members of the A genus of the family Papovaviridae, are nonenveloped viruses, 50 to 55 nm in diameter, with icosahedral capsids composed of 72 capsomers. They contain a double-stranded, circular DNA genome of about 7900 base pairs. Papillomaviruses (PV) are species-specific, and HPV have not been propagated in tissue culture or in standard experimental animals. Although virus particles of HPV types 1 and 11 can be produced in human tissues implanted beneath the renal capsule of athymic mice, significant quantities of other HPV types are difficult to obtain. At least partly because of these problems, HPV have been only incompletely characterized. Structural viral proteins make up 88 percent of the mass of PV virions. A major capsid protein with a molecular weight of 56,000 and a minor capsid protein which migrates at 76,000 have been identified by sodium dodecyl sulfate–polyacrylamide gel electrophoresis. Viral DNA is complexed with cellular histones. Type-specific antigenic determinants appear to be located on the virion surface. Antisera produced by immunization of experimental animals with disrupted PV virions are broadly cross-reactive.

The genomic organization of all PV is similar. Types and subtypes are defined by degree of DNA hybridization under stringent conditions. DNA of a distinct PV type cross-hybridizes less than 50 percent with DNAs of other classified viruses. More than 60 types of HPV are recognized. Individual types are associated with specific clinical manifestations (Table 149-1).

EPIDEMIOLOGY There are few good studies of the incidence or prevalence of human warts in well-defined populations. Common warts are found in as many as 25 percent of some groups and are most prevalent among young children. Plantar warts are also widely prevalent and occur most commonly among adolescents and young adults. The incidence of venereal warts (condylomata acuminata) has risen dramatically in the last 15 to 20 years, and condyloma acuminatum is one of the most common sexually transmitted diseases

TABLE 149-1 Correlation of human papillomavirus (HPV) type with disease

Disease	Associated HPV type(s)*
Deep plantar warts	1, 2, 4
Common warts	1, 2, 4, 26, 27, 29, 41, 57
Common warts of meat handlers	7
Flat warts	3, 10, 27, 28, 41, 49
Intermediate warts	10, 26, 28
Epidermodysplasia verruciformis	5, 8, 9, 12, 14, 15, 17, 19–25, 36, 46, 47, 50
Condylomata acuminata	6, 11, 30, 42–45, 51, 54
Intraepithelial neoplasias, unspecified	30, 33–35, 39, 40, 42–45, 51–53, 56–59, 66
Bowen's disease	16, 31, 34
Bowenoid papulosis	16, 34, 39, 42, 55
High-grade dysplasias	16, 18
Low-grade dysplasias	6, 11, 31, 42, 45, 51
Cervical carcinoma	16, 18, 31, 33, 35, 39, 45, 51, 52, 56, 58
Laryngeal papillomas	6, 11, 30
Focal epithelial hyperplasia of Heck	13, 32
Conjunctival papillomas	6, 11
Others	36–38, 41, 46, 48, 60

*Types 61 to 65 have been identified but have not yet been described in the literature.

in the United States. HPV infection of the uterine cervix produces the most commonly detected squamous cell abnormalities on Papanicolaou smears.

DNA hybridization analyses of specimens from patients have provided important insights into the epidemiology and clinical spectrum of genital tract HPV infection. DNA of HPV can be detected in a significant proportion of cytologically normal cervical specimens obtained from sexually active women. This finding suggests that many HPV infections are latent. Seroepidemiologic studies of HPV infections have been hampered severely by lack of appropriate antigens. However, recent studies using intact HPV type 11 particles in an ELISA have demonstrated specific antibodies in sera of patients with condyloma acuminatum or recurrent respiratory papillomatosis.

CLINICAL MANIFESTATIONS   Until the mid-1970s, it was generally believed that there was only one type of HPV and that clinical and pathologic differences among warts were a function of the nature of the squamous epithelium at the site of infection. With the discovery of multiple HPV types, it has become clear that the specific HPV is an important determinant of the nature of the lesion. Thus clinical manifestations of HPV infection depend on location of lesions and virus type. Common warts (verrucae vulgaris) usually occur on the hands and are flesh-colored to brown, exophytic, hyperkeratotic papules. Plantar warts (verrucae plantaris) may be quite painful and can be differentiated from callus by paring the surface to reveal thrombosed capillaries. Flat warts (verrucae plana) are most common among children and occur on the face, neck, chest, and flexor surfaces of forearms and legs.

Anogenital warts (condylomata acuminata, or venereal warts) occur on skin and mucosal surfaces of external genitalia and perianal areas. The differential diagnosis of anogenital warts includes condylomata lata of secondary syphilis, molluscum contagiosum, pearly penile papules, fibroepitheliomas, and a variety of benign and malignant mucocutaneous neoplasms. Anogenital warts are sexually transmitted and have an incubation period of 1 to 6 months. In men, condylomata are found most frequently at the frenum or coronal sulcus, but they may affect any part of the penis. They occur commonly at the urethral meatus and may extend proximally. Perianal warts are common among homosexual men but appear in heterosexual men as well. In women, warts appear first at the posterior introitus and adjacent labia. They then spread to other parts of the vulva and commonly involve the perineum and anus. Condylomata frequently involve the vagina and cervix. These lesions may be present in the absence of external warts. Respiratory papillomatosis is uncommon, occurs predominantly in preschool children, and may result from acquisition of virus at the time of delivery through an infected birth canal. These lesions are typically multiple and may produce life-threatening airway obstruction. Disease in adults may be acquired by orogenital sexual contact.

Immunosuppressed patients, particularly those undergoing organ transplantation, often develop pityriasis versicolor–like lesions from which DNA of several HPV types has been extracted. Occasionally, such lesions appear to undergo malignant transformation. Patients infected with human immunodeficiency virus (HIV) have more severe clinical manifestations of HPV infection and appear to be at higher risk of developing cervical and anal malignancies.

Epidermodysplasia verruciformis is a rare, autosomal recessive disease characterized by the inability to control HPV infection. The patients involved often are infected with unusual HPV types and frequently develop cutaneous squamous cell malignancies, particularly in sun-exposed areas. Lesions resemble flat warts or macules similar to those of pityriasis versicolor.

Complications of warts include itching and occasionally bleeding. Rarely, warts may become secondarily infected with bacteria or fungi. Large masses of warts may produce mechanical problems such as obstruction of the birth canal.

Epidemiologic, cytopathologic, virologic, and histologic data have established a strong association of HPV infection with dysplasia and carcinoma of the uterine cervix. HPV nucleic acids have been detected in cervical scrapings and biopsy specimens from patients with these diseases. In addition, squamous carcinomas and dysplasias of the penis, anus, vagina, and vulva have been associated with HPV infection. HPV types 16 and 18 are the most frequently detected types in dysplasias and carcinomas of the genital tract, whereas HPV types 6 and 11 are most commonly associated with condyloma acuminatum.

PATHOGENESIS   HPV infection is transmitted by close personal contact and is facilitated by minor trauma at the site of inoculation. It may result from direct contact with another individual or, less commonly, from autoinoculation or contact with fomites. All types of squamous epithelium may be infected by HPV, and gross and histologic appearances of individual lesions vary with site of infection and virus type. Exophytic warts are characterized by papillomatosis, hyperkeratosis, and parakeratosis. Acanthosis, an increase in cellularity, occurs in the prickle cell layer in association with viral DNA synthesis. Late gene expression, manifested by the appearance of structural proteins and assembled virions, is evident within nuclei of cells in the granular layer, where koilocytosis develops. Koilocytes are large round cells with pyknotic nuclei and large areas of perinuclear vacuolization surrounded by a ring of dense amphophilic cytoplasm. Histologically normal epithelium may contain HPV DNA. The presence of residual DNA after treatment may produce recurrent disease.

Host defense responses to HPV infection are poorly understood. Most immunologic studies are difficult to interpret because of a lack of standardized antigen preparations and assay techniques. The relative importance of type-specific and genus-specific responses in resolution of and protection from disease has not been adequately evaluated. Virus-specific IgM and IgG antibodies have been demonstrated in patients with and without clinical evidence of active infection. Cell-mediated immune responses to HPV antigens also have been measured, and patients with defects in cell-mediated immunity appear to be more susceptible than normal individuals to HPV infections. Such patients occasionally develop extensive HPV disease.

DIAGNOSIS   Most warts that are visible to the naked eye can be diagnosed correctly by history and physical examination alone. Colposcopy is invaluable in assessing vaginal and cervical lesions and is helpful in the diagnosis of oral and cutaneous HPV disease as well. Papanicolaou smears prepared from cervical scrapings often show cytologic evidence of HPV infection. Persistent or atypical lesions should be biopsied and examined by routine histologic methods. In addition, genus-specific capsid antigens can be identified in tissue sections by immunohistochemical techniques, and virus type can be determined by nucleic acid hybridization.

TREATMENT   Therapy should be initiated with the knowledge that no treatment of proven safety and efficacy is currently available and that many HPV lesions resolve spontaneously. Frequently used therapies include cryosurgery, application of caustic agents, electrodesiccation, surgical excision, and ablation with laser. Topical antimetabolites such as 5-fluorouracil also have been used. Failure as well as recurrence have been well-documented following all these methods of treatment. The high frequency of recurrence may be explained by the presence of HPV DNA in normal-appearing tissue adjacent to lesions and in previously involved areas during periods of remission. Cryosurgery is the initial treatment of choice for condyloma acuminatum. Topically applied podophyllum preparations also have been used, and recently, a well-characterized preparation of the active ingredient, podophyllotoxin, has become available in the United States. Different interferon preparations have been employed with modest success in the treatment of respiratory papillomatosis and condyloma acuminatum. Two α-interferon preparations are currently licensed in the United States for intralesional therapy of anogenital warts.

At the present time, no effective methods of prevention are available for HPV infections other than avoiding contact with infectious lesions. Barrier methods of contraception may be helpful in preventing transmission of condyloma acuminatum and other HPV-associated diseases of the genital tract.

REFERENCES

BONNEZ W et al: Antibody response to human papillomavirus (HPV) type 11 in children with juvenile-onset recurrent respiratory papillomatosis (RRP). Virology 188:384, 1992

DE VILLIERS E-M: Heterogeneity of the human papillomavirus group. J Virol 63:4898, 1989

———— et al: Human papillomavirus infections in women with and without abnormal cervical cytology. Lancet 2:703, 1987

KOUTSKY LA, WOLNER-HANSSEN P: Genital human papillomavirus infections: Current knowledge and future prospects. Obstet Gynecol Clin North Am 16:541, 1989

REICHMAN RC et al: Treatment of condyloma acuminatum with three different alpha interferon preparations administered parenterally: A double-blind, placebo-controlled trial. J Infect Dis 162:1270, 1990

———, BONNEZ W: Papillomaviruses, in Principles and Practice of Infectious Diseases, GL Mandell et al (eds). New York, Wiley, 1990

ROSE RC et al: Expression of the full-length products of the HPV-6b and HPV-11 L2 open reading frames by recombinant baculovirus, and antigenic comparisons with HPV-11 whole virus particles. J Gen Virol 71:2725, 1990

SHAH KV, HOWLEY PM: Papillomaviruses, in Virology, BN Fields (ed). New York, Raven Press, 1990

STOLER MH et al: Infectious cycle of human papillomavirus type 11 in human foreskin xenografts in nude mice. J Virol 64:3310, 1990

section 13 DNA and RNA respiratory viruses

150 COMMON VIRAL RESPIRATORY INFECTIONS

RAPHAEL DOLIN

GENERAL CONSIDERATIONS Acute viral respiratory illnesses are among the most common of human diseases, accounting for one-half or more of all acute illnesses. The incidence of acute respiratory disease in the United States is from 3 to 5.6 cases per person per year. The highest rates occur in children under 1 (6.1 to 8.3 cases per year), and the rates remain high until age 6, when a progressive decrease is noted. Adults have 3 to 4 cases per person per year. Morbidity from acute respiratory illnesses accounts for 30 to 50 percent of time lost from work by adults and from 60 to 80 percent of time lost from school by children.

It has been estimated that two-thirds to three-fourths of cases of acute respiratory illnesses are caused by viruses. More than 200 antigenically distinct viruses from 8 different genera have been reported to cause acute respiratory illness, and it is likely that additional agents will be described in the future. The vast majority of these viral infections involve the upper respiratory tract, but lower respiratory tract disease also can occur, particularly in younger age groups and in certain epidemiologic settings.

The illnesses caused by respiratory viruses traditionally have been divided into multiple distinct syndromes, such as the "common cold," pharyngitis, croup (laryngotracheobronchitis), tracheitis, bronchiolitis, bronchitis, and pneumonia. These general categories of illnesses have a certain epidemiologic and clinical utility; e.g., croup occurs exclusively in very young children and has a characteristic clinical course. Some types of respiratory illnesses are more likely to be associated with certain viruses, e.g., the "common cold" with rhinoviruses, while others occupy characteristic epidemiologic niches, such as adenoviruses in military recruits. The syndromes most commonly associated with infection with the major respiratory virus groups are summarized in Table 150-1. Despite these associations, it is clear that most respiratory viruses have the potential to cause more than one type of respiratory illness, and frequently features of several types of illness may be present in the same patient. Moreover, the clinical illnesses induced by these viruses are rarely sufficiently distinctive to enable an etiologic diagnosis to be made on clinical grounds alone, although the epidemiologic setting increases the likelihood that one group of viruses rather than another may be involved. In general, laboratory methods must be relied on to establish a specific viral diagnosis.

This chapter will review viral infections caused by five of the major groups of respiratory viruses: rhinoviruses, coronaviruses, respiratory syncytial viruses, parainfluenza viruses, and adenoviruses. Influenza viruses, which are a major cause of mortality as well as morbidity, are reviewed in Chap. 152. Herpesviruses, which occasionally cause pharyngitis and which also cause lower respiratory

TABLE 150-1 Illnesses associated with respiratory viruses

Frequency of respiratory syndromes associated with virus groups

Virus	Most frequent	Occasional	Infrequent
Rhinoviruses	Common cold	Exacerbation of chronic bronchitis and asthma	Pneumonia (children)
Coronaviruses	Common cold	Exacerbation of chronic bronchitis and asthma	Pneumonia and bronchiolitis
Respiratory syncytial virus	Pneumonia and bronchiolitis in young children	Common cold in adults	Pneumonia in elderly
Parainfluenza viruses	Croup and lower respiratory tract disease in young children	Pharyngitis and common cold	Tracheobronchitis in adults
Adenoviruses	Common cold and pharyngitis in children	Outbreaks of ARD in military recruits*	Pneumonia in children and immunosuppressed patients
Influenza A viruses	"Influenza-like illness"†	Pneumonia and excess mortality in "high-risk" patients	Pneumonia in healthy individuals
Influenza B viruses	"Influenza-like illness"†	Rhinitis and pharyngitis alone	Pneumonia
Enteroviruses	Acute undifferentiated febrile illnesses‡	Rhinitis and pharyngitis	Pneumonia
Herpes simplex viruses	Gingivostomatitis (children) Pharyngotonsillitis (adults)	Tracheitis and pneumonia in immunocompromised patients	Disseminated infection in immunocompromised patients

* Serotypes 4 and 7.
† Fever, cough, myalgia, malaise.
‡ May or may not have a respiratory component.

tract disease in immunosuppressed patients, are reviewed in Chap. 143. Enteroviruses, which account for occasional respiratory illnesses during the summer months, are reviewed in Chap. 154.

RHINOVIRUS INFECTIONS

ETIOLOGY   Rhinoviruses are members of the Picornaviridae family, which are small (15 to 30 nm), nonenveloped viruses which contain a single-stranded RNA genome. In contrast to other members of the picornavirus family, such as enteroviruses, rhinoviruses are acid-labile and are almost completely inactivated at pH 3 or lower. Rhinoviruses grow preferentially at 33 to 34°C, which is the temperature of nasal passages in humans, rather than the higher temperature (37°C) of the lower respiratory tract. One hundred distinct serotypes and one subtype of rhinoviruses are recognized.

EPIDEMIOLOGY   Rhinoviruses are a major cause of the common cold and have been isolated from 15 to 40 percent of adults with common cold–like illnesses. Overall infection rates with rhinoviruses are higher among infants and young children and decrease with increasing age. Rhinovirus infections occur throughout the year, but seasonal peaks occur in early fall and spring in temperate climates. Rhinovirus infections are most often introduced into families by preschool or grade school children below 6 years of age. Between 25 and 70 percent of initial illnesses in family settings are followed by secondary cases, with the highest attack rates occurring in the youngest siblings at home. Attack rates also increase with increasing size of families.

The spread of rhinoviruses appears to be by direct contact with infected secretions, usually respiratory droplets. In some volunteer studies, transmission was most efficient by hand-to-hand contact, with subsequent self-inoculation of the conjunctival or nasal mucosa. In other studies, aerosol transmission appeared to be more important. Virus also can be recovered from plastic surfaces inoculated 1 to 3 h previously, suggesting that environmental surfaces also may contribute to transmission. In studies conducted in married couples in which serum antibody was not present in either partner, transmission was associated with prolonged contact (122 h or more) during a 7-day period. Transmission was infrequent unless virus was recoverable from the donor's hands and nasal mucosa, at least 1000 TCID$_{50}$ of virus was present in nasal washes of the donor, and the donor was at least moderately symptomatic with the "cold." Despite anecdotal observations, exposure to cold temperatures, fatigue, or sleep deprivation has not been associated with increased rates of rhinovirus-induced illness in volunteers.

Infection with rhinoviruses is worldwide in distribution, and by the time they reach adulthood, nearly all individuals have neutralizing antibodies to multiple serotypes, although the prevalence of antibody to any one serotype varies widely. Multiple serotypes circulate simultaneously, and generally no single serotype or group of serotypes has emerged as being more prevalent than others.

PATHOGENESIS   Rhinoviruses infect cells via attachment to specific cellular receptors; the major group of such receptors has been recently recognized to be intercellular adhesion molecule 1(ICAM-1). Relatively limited information is available on the histopathology and pathogenesis of acute rhinovirus infections in humans. Biopsies performed in experimentally induced and in naturally occurring illness indicate that the nasal mucosa is edematous, often hyperemic, and, during acute illness, is covered by a mucoid discharge. There is a mild infiltrate with inflammatory cells, including neutrophils, lymphocytes, plasma cells, and eosinophils. Mucus-secreting glands in the submucosa appear hyperactive; the nasal turbinates are engorged, which may lead to obstruction of nearby openings of sinus cavities.

The incubation period for rhinovirus illness is short, generally ranging from 1 to 2 days. Virus shedding coincides with the onset of illness or may begin shortly before symptoms develop. The mechanisms of immunity to rhinovirus are not well worked out. In some studies, the presence of homotypic antibody significantly reduced the rates of subsequent infection and illness, but conflicting data exist as to the relative importance of serum and local antibody in protection from rhinovirus infection.

CLINICAL MANIFESTATIONS   The most common clinical manifestations of rhinovirus infections are those of the common cold. Initially, illness begins with rhinorrhea and sneezing, accompanied by nasal congestion. Sore throat is frequently present and in some cases may be the initial complaint. Systemic signs and symptoms, such as malaise and headache, are mild or absent, and fever is unusual. Illness generally lasts for 4 to 9 days and resolves spontaneously without sequelae. In children, bronchitis, bronchiolitis, and bronchopneumonia have been reported, although it appears that rhinoviruses are not major causes of lower respiratory tract disease in children. Rhinoviruses also may cause exacerbations of asthma and chronic pulmonary disease in adults. The vast majority of rhinovirus infections resolve without sequelae, but complications related to obstruction of the eustachian tubes or sinus ostia, including otitis media or acute sinusitis, can occur.

DIAGNOSIS   Although rhinoviruses are the most frequently recognized cause of the common cold, similar illnesses may be caused by a variety of other viruses, and the etiologic diagnosis cannot be made on clinical grounds alone. The diagnosis of rhinovirus infection is made by isolation of virus from nasal washes or nasal secretions in tissue culture. In practice, this procedure is rarely carried out because of the benign, self-limited nature of the illness. Because of the large number of serotypes of rhinovirus, diagnosis of rhinovirus infections by serum antibody tests is currently not practical. Common laboratory tests such as white cell count and sedimentation rate are not helpful in the diagnosis of rhinovirus infection.

TREATMENT AND PREVENTION   Rhinovirus infections are generally mild and self-limited, so treatment is not necessary. Some patients may benefit from the use of analgesics and nasal decongestants, and reduction of activity is prudent if significant discomfort or fatigability is present. Antibacterial antibiotics should only be used if bacterial complications such as otitis media or sinusitis develop. Specific antiviral therapy is not available. Application of interferon sprays intranasally has been effective in the prophylaxis of rhinovirus infections but is also associated with local irritation of nasal mucosa. Prevention of rhinovirus infection by antibodies directed against rhinovirus receptors or by the use of the soluble purified receptors themselves is under study. Experimental vaccines to certain rhinovirus serotypes have been prepared, but their utility is questionable because of the existence of the large number of serotypes and the uncertainty regarding the mechanisms of immunity. Thorough hand washing or barrier protection against autoinoculation may help to reduce transmission of infection.

CORONAVIRUS INFECTIONS

ETIOLOGY   Coronaviruses are pleomorphic, single-stranded RNA viruses, 80 to 160 nm in diameter, with clublike projections emanating from the virus envelope, resulting in an appearance which resembles that of the solar "corona," from which their name is derived. Three distinct coronavirus serotypes, designated B814, 229E, and OC43, have been isolated from humans. Coronaviruses are fastidious and are difficult to culture in vitro. Some strains will grow only in human tracheal organ cultures rather than in tissue culture.

EPIDEMIOLOGY   Only limited seroepidemiologic studies have been carried out in coronavirus infections. Seroprevalence studies of two of the serotypes, 229E and OC43, have yielded variable rates of serum antibodies, ranging from 12 to more than 80 percent in various populations. Overall, coronaviruses account for 10 to 20 percent of common colds. Coronavirus infections appear to be particularly prevalent in late fall, winter, and early spring, at a time when rhinovirus infections are less common. Depending on the serotype, a cyclical pattern for outbreaks of coronavirus infection has been suggested, which ranges from every 2 years for OC43 to every 2 to 4 years with 229E.

CLINICAL FEATURES The clinical features of illness caused by coronaviruses are similar to those caused by rhinoviruses. In volunteer studies, the mean incubation period of illness induced by coronaviruses (3 days) is somewhat longer than that caused by rhinoviruses, and the duration of illness is somewhat shorter, with a mean of 6 to 7 days. In some studies, the amount of nasal discharge was somewhat greater in colds induced by coronaviruses than in those induced by rhinoviruses. Coronaviruses also have been recovered from infants with pneumonia and from military recruits with lower respiratory tract disease and also have been associated with worsening of chronic bronchitis. However, the overall significance of coronaviruses in lower respiratory tract disease in humans is unclear.

TREATMENT AND PREVENTION The approach to the treatment of common colds caused by coronaviruses is similar to that discussed above for rhinovirus-induced illnesses. Because of the uncertainty regarding the number and relative importance of coronavirus serotypes and the mechanisms of immunity, vaccines against coronaviruses have not been developed.

RESPIRATORY SYNCYTIAL VIRUS INFECTIONS

ETIOLOGY Respiratory syncytial virus (RSV) is a member of the Paramyxoviridae family and comprises the genus *Pneumovirus*. RSV is an enveloped virus, approximately 150 to 300 nm in size, so named because virus replication leads to fusion of neighboring cells into large multinucleated syncytia. The single-stranded RNA genome codes for 10 virus-specific proteins. Viral RNA is contained in a helical nucleocapsid surrounded by a lipid envelope bearing two glycoproteins, one of which is the G protein by which the virus attaches to cells, and the other is the F, or fusion, protein which facilitates entry of virus into the cell by fusing host and viral membranes. Respiratory syncytial viruses have been considered to be of a single antigenic type, but it has been found that two distinct subtypes (A and B) exist. The epidemiologic and clinical significance of subtype differences are being investigated.

EPIDEMIOLOGY RSV is the major respiratory pathogen of young children and is the major cause of lower respiratory disease in infants. Infection with RSV is seen throughout the world in annual epidemics which occur in either late fall, winter, or spring and can last up to 5 months. The virus is rarely encountered during the summer. The highest rates of illness occur in infants between 1 and 6 months of age, with peak rates occurring between 2 and 3 months of age. The attack rates among susceptibles are extraordinarily high, approaching 100 percent in settings such as day-care centers where large numbers of susceptible infants are present. RSV accounts for 20 to 25 percent of hospital admissions for pneumonia of young infants and children and up to 75 percent of cases of bronchiolitis in this age group. It has been estimated that more than half of infants who are at risk will become infected during an RSV epidemic.

In older children and adults, reinfection with RSV is frequent, but disease is milder than in infancy. A "common cold–like syndrome" is the illness most commonly associated with RSV infection in adults. Severe lower respiratory tract disease with pneumonitis can occur in elderly, often institutionalized, adults or those with immunocompromising disorders or treatment. RSV infection is more severe and prolonged in immunocompromised children. RSV is also an important nosocomial pathogen and can infect pediatric patients and up to 25 to 50 percent of the staff on pediatric wards during an RSV outbreak. The spread of virus among families is also efficient, and up to 40 percent of siblings may become infected when RSV is introduced into the family setting.

RSV is transmitted primarily by close contact with contaminated fingers or fomites and by self-inoculation of the conjunctiva or anterior nares. Virus also may be spread by coarse aerosols produced by coughing or sneezing but is inefficiently spread by fine-particle aerosols. The incubation period of illness is approximately 4 to 6 days, and virus shedding may last for 2 weeks or longer in children and for shorter periods of time in adults.

PATHOGENESIS Little is known about the histopathology of minor RSV infection. In severe bronchiolitis or pneumonia, there is necrosis of the bronchiolar epithelium and a peribronchiolar infiltrate of lymphocytes and mononuclear cells. Interalveolar thickening and filling of alveolar spaces with fluid also can occur. The characteristics of the immune response to RSV are not well elucidated. Because reinfection occurs frequently and is often associated with illness, the immunity that develops after single episodes of infection is not complete or long-lasting. However, the cumulative effect of multiple reinfections ameliorates subsequent disease and provides some temporary measure of protection against infection. Studies of experimentally induced disease in normal volunteers indicate that the presence of nasal IgA neutralizing antibody correlates more closely with protection than does the presence of serum antibody. Studies in infants, however, suggest that maternally acquired antibody provides some protection from lower respiratory tract disease, although severe illness also may occur in infants who have moderate levels of maternally derived serum antibody.

CLINICAL MANIFESTATIONS RSV infection leads to a wide spectrum of respiratory illnesses. In infants, 25 to 40 percent of infections result in lower respiratory tract involvement, including pneumonia, bronchiolitis, and tracheobronchitis. In infants, illness begins most frequently with rhinorrhea, low-grade fever, and mild systemic symptoms, often accompanied by cough and wheezing. Most patients gradually recover in 1 to 2 weeks. In more severe illness, tachypnea and dyspnea develop, and eventually frank hypoxia, cyanosis, and apnea can ensue. Physical examination may reveal diffuse wheezing, rhonchi, and rales. Chest x-ray shows hyperexpansion, peribronchial thickening, and variable infiltrates ranging from diffuse interstitial infiltrates to segmental or lobar consolidation. Illness may be particularly severe in children with congenital cardiac disease, bronchopulmonary dysplasia, or immunosuppression. One study documented a 37 percent mortality rate for infants with RSV pneumonia and congenital cardiac disease.

In adults, the most common symptoms of RSV infection are those of the common cold, with rhinorrhea, sore throat, and cough. Illness may occasionally be associated with moderate systemic symptoms such as malaise, headache, and fever. RSV also has been reported to cause febrile lower respiratory tract disease in adults, including severe pneumonia in the elderly.

LABORATORY FINDINGS AND DIAGNOSIS The diagnosis of RSV infection can be suspected on the basis of the epidemiologic setting, i.e., severe illness in infants during an outbreak of RSV in the community. Infections in older children and adults cannot be differentiated with certainty from those caused by other respiratory viruses. The specific diagnosis is established by isolation of RSV from respiratory secretions, including sputum, throat swabs, or nasopharyngeal washes. Virus is detected in tissue culture and identified specifically by immunologic reactions employing immunofluorescence, enzyme-linked immunosorbent assay (ELISA), or other techniques. Immunofluorescence microscopy of nasal scrapings or washings provides a rapid diagnostic method that is in use in many diagnostic virology laboratories. Serologic tests which depend on fourfold or greater rises in complement fixing or neutralizing antibody titers are useful for diagnosis in older children and adults but are less sensitive in children under 4 months of age. Compared with complement fixation or neutralization tests, ELISA detects serum antibody with more sensitivity. As with other serologic tests, diagnosis requires comparison of acute and convalescent serum specimens and is therefore not useful during the acute illness.

TREATMENT AND PREVENTION Treatment of upper respiratory tract RSV infection consists primarily of symptomatic therapy similar to that for other upper respiratory tract viral infections. For lower respiratory tract infections, treatment consists of respiratory therapy, including hydration, suctioning of secretions, and administration of humidified oxygen and antibronchospastic agents as needed. If severe hypoxia is present, intubation and ventilatory assistance may be required. Studies of infants with RSV infection who were given aerosolized ribavirin, a nucleoside analogue which is active in vitro against RSV, have demonstrated a beneficial effect on the resolution of lower respiratory tract illness, including improvement of blood gases. Similar studies have not been performed in adults with RSV pneumonitis, and the benefit of ribavirin in these patients is unknown.

Considerable interest exists in the development of an effective vaccine against RSV. Inactivated whole-virus vaccines have either been ineffective or, in one study, potentiated the disease in infants. Other approaches to vaccine development include immunization with purified F and G surface glycoproteins of RSV or generation of stable, live attenuated virus vaccines. In the settings where high rates of transmission occur, such as pediatric wards, barrier methods of protection of hands and conjunctivae may be useful in reducing the spread of virus.

PARAINFLUENZA VIRUS INFECTIONS

ETIOLOGY   Parainfluenza viruses are members of the Paramyxoviridae family and comprise the genus *Paramyxovirus*. Parainfluenza viruses are 150 to 250 nm in diameter, enveloped, and contain a single-stranded RNA genome. The envelope is studded with two glycoproteins, one of which possesses both hemagglutinin and neuraminidase activity, while the other glycoprotein contains the fusion activity. The viral RNA genome is enclosed in a helical nucleocapsid and codes for eight or nine virus-specific proteins. There are four distinct serotypes of parainfluenza viruses, all of which share certain common antigens with other members of the Paramyxoviridae family, including mumps and Newcastle disease virus.

EPIDEMIOLOGY   Parainfluenza viruses are distributed throughout the world, although type 4 has been reported less widely, probably because it is more difficult to grow in tissue culture. Infection occurs in early childhood so that by 8 years of age most children show antibodies to serotypes 1, 2, and 3. Parainfluenza types 1 and 2 cause epidemics during the fall, primarily in odd-numbered years. Type 3 infection has been detected during all seasons of the year, but epidemics of type 3 virus have occurred annually in the spring.

The contribution of parainfluenza infections to respiratory disease is variable according to both the location and year. In studies carried out in the United States, parainfluenza virus infections accounted for 4.3 to 22 percent of respiratory illnesses in children. In adults, parainfluenza infections are generally mild and account for less than 5 percent of respiratory illnesses. The major importance of parainfluenza viruses is as a cause of respiratory illness in young children, where they are second only to RSV as causes of lower respiratory tract illness. Parainfluenza type 1 is the most frequent cause of croup (laryngotracheobronchitis) in children, while serotype 2 causes similar, although generally less severe, disease. Parainfluenza type 3 is an important cause of bronchiolitis and pneumonia in infants, while illnesses associated with parainfluenza type 4 have been generally mild. Parainfluenza type 3, but not types 1 and 2, frequently causes illness during the first month of life, while passively acquired maternal antibody is still present. Parainfluenza viruses are spread through infected respiratory secretions, primarily by person-to-person contact and/or by large droplets. In experimental studies, the incubation period has varied from 3 to 6 days but may be somewhat shorter in naturally occurring disease in children.

PATHOGENESIS   Immunity to parainfluenza viruses is incompletely understood, but there is suggestive evidence that immunity to infections with serotypes 1 and 2 is mediated by local IgA antibodies in the respiratory tract. Passively acquired serum-neutralizing antibodies also confer some protection against infection with parainfluenza types 1, 2, and, to a lesser degree, 3.

CLINICAL MANIFESTATIONS   Parainfluenza virus infections occur most frequently in children, in whom initial infection with serotypes 1, 2, or 3 is associated with an acute febrile illness in 50 to 80 percent of cases. Children may present with coryza, sore throat, hoarseness, and cough, which may or may not be croupy. In severe croup, fever persists, with worsening coryza and sore throat. A brassy or barking cough may be noted and may progress to frank stridor. In most children, recovery will occur over the next 1 to 2 days, although progressive airway obstruction and hypoxia may ensue occasionally. If bronchiolitis or pneumonia develops, progressive cough accompanied by wheezing, tachypnea, and intercostal retractions may be present. In this setting, a moderate increase in sputum production can be seen. Physical examination shows nasopharyngeal discharge and oropharyngeal injection, along with rhonchi, wheezes, or coarse breath sounds. Chest x-rays can show air trapping and, occasionally, interstitial infiltrates.

In older children and adults, parainfluenza infections tend to be milder, presenting most frequently as the common cold or hoarseness, with or without cough. Lower respiratory tract involvement in older children and adults is uncommon, but tracheobronchitis in adults has been reported. More severe and prolonged parainfluenza infection has been reported in children with severe immunosuppression.

LABORATORY FINDINGS AND DIAGNOSIS   As with other respiratory viral diseases, the clinical syndromes caused by parainfluenza viruses are not sufficiently distinctive to permit a diagnosis to be made on clinical grounds alone, with the possible exception of croup in young children. A specific diagnosis is established by detection of virus in respiratory tract secretions, throat swabs, or nasopharyngeal washings. Virus is detected by growth in tissue culture, either by hemagglutination or by cytopathic effect, or by immunofluorescence of viral antigens in exfoliated cells from the respiratory tract. Serologic diagnosis can be made by fourfold or greater rises in acute and convalescent serum specimens as detected by hemagglutination inhibition or complement fixation or neutralization tests. However, frequent heterotypic responses occur among the parainfluenza serotypes, so identification of the serotype which causes the illness often cannot be made by serologic techniques alone.

Acute epiglottitis caused by *Haemophilus influenzae* type B (bacterial croup) must be differentiated from viral croup. Influenza A virus also is a common cause of croup during epidemic periods.

TREATMENT AND PREVENTION   For upper respiratory tract illness, symptomatic therapy can be employed as discussed for other viral respiratory tract illnesses. If complications such as sinusitis, otitis, or superimposed bacterial bronchitis develop, appropriate antibiotics should be administered. Mild cases of croup should be treated with bed rest and moist air as generated by vaporizers. More severe cases require hospitalization and close observation for the development of respiratory distress. If acute respiratory distress develops, humidified oxygen and intermittent racemic epinephrine are usually administered. High-dose systemic glucocorticoids also may be of benefit. There is no specific antiviral therapy available, although ribavirin has activity against parainfluenza viruses in vitro and is being evaluated clinically. Effective vaccines against parainfluenza viruses have not been developed.

ADENOVIRUS INFECTIONS

ETIOLOGY   Adenoviruses are complex DNA viruses which are 70 to 80 nm in diameter. Human adenoviruses belong to the genus *Mastadenovirus*, of which 47 serotypes are recognized. Adenoviruses have a characteristic morphology consisting of an icosahedral shell composed of 20 equilateral triangular faces and 12 vertices. The protein coat ("capsid") consists of hexon subunits with group-specific and type-specific antigenic determinants and penton subunits at each vertex primarily containing group-specific antigens. From each penton, a fiber with a knob at the end projects, which contains type-specific and some group-specific antigens. Adenoviruses have been divided into six or seven subgroups based on the homology of DNA genomes. The adenovirus genome is a linear double-stranded DNA which codes for structural and nonstructural polypeptides. The replicative cycle of adenovirus may result either in lytic infection of cells or in the establishment of a latent infection (primarily involving lymphoid cells). Some adenovirus types can induce oncogenic transformation, and tumor formation has been observed in rodents, but despite intensive investigation, adenoviruses have not been associated with tumors in humans.

EPIDEMIOLOGY Adenovirus infections occur most frequently in infants and children. Infections occur throughout the year but are most commonly noted from fall to spring. Large-scale surveys have shown that adenoviruses account for 3 to 5 percent of acute respiratory infections in children. Infections are less frequent in adults and account for less than 2 percent of respiratory illness in civilians. Nearly 100 percent of adults have serum antibody against multiple serotypes, indicating that infection is common in childhood. Types 1, 2, 3, and 5 are the most frequent isolates obtained from children. Certain adenovirus serotypes, particularly 4 and 7, but also 3, 14, and 21, are associated with outbreaks of acute respiratory disease (ARD) in military recruits which occur in winter and spring. Transmission of adenovirus infection can occur by inhalation of aerosolized virus, by inoculation of virus in conjunctival sacs, and probably by the fecal-oral route as well. Type-specific antibody generally develops after infection and is associated with protection against infection with the same serotype.

CLINICAL MANIFESTATIONS In children, adenoviruses cause a variety of clinical syndromes. The most common is an acute upper respiratory tract infection, with prominent rhinitis. On occasion, lower respiratory tract disease, including bronchiolitis and pneumonia, also can be seen. Adenoviruses, particularly types 3 and 7, cause pharyngoconjunctival fever, a characteristic acute febrile illness of children which occurs in outbreaks, most often in summer camps. The syndrome is marked by bilateral conjunctivitis in which the bulbar and palpebral conjunctiva have a granular appearance. Low-grade fever is frequently present, along with rhinitis, sore throat, and cervical adenopathy. The illness generally lasts for 1 to 2 weeks and resolves spontaneously. Febrile pharyngitis without conjunctivitis also has been associated with adenovirus infection. Adenoviruses also have been isolated from cases of whooping cough with or without *Bordetella pertussis*; the significance of adenovirus in that disease is unknown.

In adults, the most frequently reported illness has been ARD in military recruits caused by adenovirus types 4 and 7. This illness is marked by a prominent sore throat and the gradual onset of fever, often reaching 39°C on the second or third day of illness. Cough is almost always present, and coryza and regional lymphadenopathy are also frequently seen. Physical examination may show pharyngeal edema, injection, and tonsillar enlargement with little or no exudate. If pneumonia is present, auscultation of the chest and x-ray may indicate areas of patchy infiltration.

Adenoviruses also have been associated with a number of nonrespiratory tract diseases, including acute diarrheal illness in young children caused by adenovirus types 40 and 41 and hemorrhagic cystitis caused by adenoviruses 11 and 21. Epidemic keratoconjunctivitis, caused most frequently by adenovirus types 8, 19, and 37, has been associated with contaminated common sources such as ophthalmic solutions and roller towels. Adenoviruses also have been associated with disseminated disease and pneumonia in immunosuppressed patients, including patients with acquired immunodeficiency syndrome (AIDS).

LABORATORY FINDINGS AND DIAGNOSIS Adenovirus infection should be suspected in the epidemiologic setting of ARD and in certain of the clinical syndromes such as pharyngoconjunctival fever or epidemic keratoconjunctivitis in which outbreaks of characteristic illnesses occur. In the majority of cases, however, illnesses caused by adenovirus infection cannot be differentiated from those caused by a number of other viral respiratory agents and *Mycoplasma pneumoniae*. A definitive diagnosis of adenovirus infection is established by culture or detection of virus from sites such as the conjunctiva and oropharynx or from sputum, urine, or stool. Virus may be detected in tissue culture by cytopathic changes and specifically identified by immunofluorescence or other immunologic techniques. Adenovirus types 40 and 41, which have been associated with diarrheal disease in children, require special tissue culture cells for isolation, and these serotypes are most commonly detected by direct ELISA of stool. Serum antibody rises can be demonstrated by complement fixation or neutralization, ELISA, or radioimmunoassays. Hemagglutination inhibition tests also may be done for those adenoviruses which hemagglutinate red cells.

TREATMENT AND PREVENTION Only symptomatic and supportive therapy is available for adenovirus infections, and no clinically useful antiviral compounds have emerged. Live vaccines have been developed against adenovirus types 4 and 7 and are widely utilized to control this illness in military recruits. These vaccines consist of live, unattenuated virus which is administered in enteric coated capsules. Infection of the gastrointestinal tract with types 4 and 7 does not cause disease but stimulates local and systemic antibodies which protect against subsequent ARD with those serotypes. Vaccines prepared from purified subunits of adenovirus are currently under investigation.

REFERENCES

Rhinoviruses

GREVE JM et al: The major human rhinovirus receptor is ICAM-1. Cell 56:809, 1989
GWALTNEY JM: Rhinoviruses, in *Principles and Practice of Infectious Diseases*, 3d ed, GF Mandell et al (eds). New York, Churchill Livingstone, 1990, pp 1399–1404
ROSSMAN MG et al: Structure of a human common cold virus and functional relationships to other picornaviruses. Nature 317:145, 1985
TYRRELL DAJ: Common colds. Intervirology 25:177, 1986

Coronaviruses

BRADBURNE AF et al: Effects of a "new" human respiratory virus in volunteers. Br Med J 3:767, 1967
LARSON HE et al: Isolation of rhinoviruses and coronaviruses from 38 colds in adults. J Med Virol 5:221, 1980
MCINTOSH K: Coronaviruses, in *Virology*, 2d ed, BN Fields (ed). New York, Raven, 1989, pp 857–864

Respiratory syncytial virus

ENGLUND JA et al: Respiratory syncytial virus infection in immunocompromised adults. Ann Intern Med 109:203, 1988
GLEZEN WP et al: Risk of primary infection and reinfection with respiratory syncytial virus. Am J Dis Child 140:543, 1986
HALL CB et al: Aerosolized ribavirin treatment of infants with respiratory syncytial viral infection. A randomized double blind study. N Engl J Med 308:1443, 1983
HENDERSON FW et al: Respiratory syncytial virus infections, reinfections and immunity. N Engl J Med 300:530, 1979
MUFSON MA et al: Respiratory syncytial virus epidemics: Variable dominance of subgroups A and B strains among children, 1981–1986. J Infect Dis 1:143, 1988
SMITH DW et al: A controlled trial of aerosolized ribavarin in infants receiving mechanical ventilation for severe respiratory syncytial virus infection. N Engl J Med 325:24, 1991

Parainfluenza viruses

DENNY FW et al: Croup: An 11 year study in a pediatric practice. Pediatrics 71:871, 1983
HEILMAN CA: Respiratory syncytial and parainfluenza viruses. J Infect Dis 161:402, 1990
WRIGHT PF: Parainfluenzaviruses, in *Textbook of Human Virology*, 2d ed, RB Belshe (ed). St. Louis, Mosby, 1991, pp 342–350

Adenoviruses

BAUM SG: Adenoviruses, in *Principles and Practice of Infectious Diseases*, 3d ed, G Mandell et al (eds). New York, Churchill Livingstone, 1990, pp 1185–1190
FOX JP et al: The Seattle virus watch. VII. Observations of adenovirus infections. Am J Epidemiol 105:362, 1977
WIGAND R et al: Adenoviridae: Second report. Intervirology 18:169, 1982
ZAHRADNIK JM et al: Adenovirus infection in the immunosuppressed patient. Am J Med 68:725, 1980

section 14   RNA viruses

151   THE HUMAN RETROVIRUSES

ROBERT C. GALLO / ANTHONY S. FAUCI

Retroviruses were first described at the beginning of the century as filterable agents that caused transmissible tumors in chickens; the first recognized mammalian retroviruses were isolated from mice with leukemia in the 1950s. However, despite extensive investigation, the first human retrovirus, HTLV-I, was not isolated until 1978. Isolation became possible only after the discovery of RNA-to-DNA transcription by viruses and through the use of reverse transcriptase (RT) as a sensitive "footprint" for these viruses. In addition, the obligate requirement of a T cell growth factor, interleukin 2 (IL-2) (see Chap. 277), for growth of T cells in culture helped make isolation possible. There are now four well-characterized pathogenic human retroviruses belonging to two distinct groups: the human T cell leukemia retroviruses, HTLV-I and HTLV-II, and the human immunodeficiency viruses, HIV-1 and HIV-2.

Although retroviruses are sometimes categorized as oncogenic viruses, lentiviruses, and spumaviruses, they also may be grouped by the disease they cause, their electron-microscopic appearance, and their biologic effects. In contrast to the infectious retroviruses, some, called *endogenous retroviruses,* are transmitted in the germ line. Although there is limited homology of the genomes of animal retroviruses to some sequences in the human genome, there are no known human endogenous viruses. The spumaviruses are known for their ability to produce a characteristic foamy cytopathic effect in tissue culture, but their existence and biologic role in human beings are still debatable. The lentiviruses, first recognized in ungulates, until recently were associated only with nonmalignant disease, particularly neurologic disorders (visna virus), immune-complex disease (equine infectious anemia virus), encephalitis and arthritis (caprine arthritis encephalitis virus), and immunodeficiencies (feline immunodeficiency virus, simian immunodeficiency virus, HIV). These viruses are "slow-acting" only by comparison with viruses that cause acute infections, such as influenza virus, but not by comparison with other retroviruses. Retroviruses associated with malignant disease include HTLV-I and HTLV-II, some of the closely related simian viruses (STLV-I), feline leukemia virus (FeLV), bovine leukemia virus (BLV), gibbon ape leukemia virus (GaLV), and many avian and murine viruses. These viruses also may induce nonmalignant disease. For example, FeLV, which can cause T cell leukemia, more frequently causes immunodeficiency in cats, mimicking human AIDS. It appears that a change in the envelope of the virus is correlated with a change in the kind of disease induced by the virus.

When retroviruses cause malignant disease, they do so by one of several molecular mechanisms; in each case, however, the mechanism is direct in that the DNA proviral sequences are integrated in clonal fashion in each cell of the tumor. Recent evidence indicates that retroviruses sometimes greatly facilitate the development of certain neoplasms by indirect mechanisms wherein the virus-infected cell is not transformed but influences tumor development in some uninfected cell. HIV-1–associated B cell lymphomas and Kaposi's sarcoma are examples.

GENERAL BIOLOGY OF RETROVIRUSES   Retroviruses are enveloped viruses, usually about 100 nm in diameter, that form by budding from cell membranes (Fig. 151-1). An electron-dense central core surrounds two identical copies of the single-stranded viral RNA genome; thus retroviruses are diploid—a structure unusual among viruses (see Chap. 141). However, it is the DNA polymerase, known as *reverse transcriptase,* that is the distinguishing feature of a retrovirus. Complexed to an RNA in the viral core, this enzyme catalyzes the transcription of the RNA genome into a double-stranded DNA form that migrates from the cytoplasm to the nucleus and integrates into the host cell DNA. In this form, known as the *provirus,* the viral genes remain integrated for the lifetime of the cell. They are duplicated with the cell DNA during the S phase of the cell cycle. Therefore, once established, infection of an organism is generally lifelong. When the provirus is expressed, viral RNA and proteins are

FIGURE 151-1   Electron micrographs of the characterized human retroviruses. The viruses are shown as they replicate by budding from a cell membrane *(upper panels)* and as mature infectious extracellular virions *(lower panels).*

HTLV-I   HTLV-II

HIV-1   HIV-2

found in the cell cytoplasm and assembled at the cell membrane, where budding and release of infectious virions complete the replication cycle (Fig. 151-2).

The molecular mechanisms by which retroviruses alter the life cycle of infected cells are strikingly diverse and often depend on the organization of the viral genome. All retroviruses contain three essential genes for virus replication: *gag, pol,* and *env* (Fig. 151-3). *Gag* codes for a polyprotein precursor that is cleaved by a viral protease into three or four structural proteins; *pol* codes for RT and the viral protease and integrase; *env* codes for the transmembrane and outer glycoprotein of the virus. The properties of the envelope have a major influence on the kind of cell the virus can infect (though they are not the sole determinant of infectivity), and production of antibodies to the envelope is one of the essential features sought in a vaccine. At either end of the provirus, the long terminal repeats (LTRs) are covalently joined to the cellular DNA; they contain regulatory elements that influence the expression of the viral genes and sometimes nearby cellular genes. The LTRs share features in common with movable genetic elements such as retrotransposons.

Examples of retroviruses that contain only these three genes are FeLV, murine leukemia virus (MuLV), GaLV, and avian leukosis virus (ALV). These are the chronic leukemia viruses. They are all replication competent, take a long time to cause disease, and are relatively common in nature. There is some evidence that they cause leukemia by integration into a specific region of a chromosome so that the associated LTRs act to promote continual expression of a nearby cellular gene involved in growth (a proto-oncogene) (see Chap. 63). The best-studied examples of this *cis* mechanism is in chickens, where the LTRs of avian leukosis virus promote expression of the cellular proto-oncogene *myc,* believed to be the first step in the induction of B cell leukemia by this virus. Since integration by retroviruses is random, a high rate of replication increases the chance of integration into regions sufficiently near the cellular oncogene to effect its expression. There are no known human viruses of this type.

When a retrovirus acquires a host cell gene that rapidly transforms cells and induces acute malignancies, the virus is often called an *acute leukemia* or *sarcoma virus,* and the acquired gene (i.e., host proto-oncogene) is called a *viral onc gene.* This type of change almost always leads to an incomplete viral genome that forms defective viral particles. The virus then needs the addition of a helper virus and in vitro manipulation by the virologist for its propagation. Viruses with *onc* genes are thought to be rare in nature and are of interest in animals chiefly as tools for investigating mechanisms of neoplastic transformation rather than as causes of naturally occurring cancer. An example relates to FeLV. In addition to the mechanism of specific integration near a proto-oncogene and subsequent activation of this gene, the relatively frequent acquisition of cell-derived oncogenes may enable FeLV to cause malignancies. Every cell infected by these viruses can be transformed (giving rise to polyclonal tumors) because the product of the viral *onc* gene directly transforms the cells. Therefore, a common site of integration or a second genetic event to trigger transformation is not needed. The development of the malignancy is usually rapid and sometimes occurs within months of infection. Human viruses of this type have not been found.

FEATURES OF HUMAN RETROVIRUSES The known human and some related animal retroviruses can be regarded as unique categories of retroviruses. Human T lymphotropic (or leukemia) viruses (HTLV-I and HTLV-II) transform cells in culture, while human immunodeficiency viruses (HIV-1 and -2) are cytopathic in culture. While the two groups have little sequence homology and major differences, they also have some striking similarities.

Shown in Fig. 151-4 is the structure of an HIV-1 virion, or virus particle, with the location of the virion proteins as indicated. The envelope proteins can be seen as a rod and sphere protruding from the viral lipid bilayer. Just inside the lipid shell is the matrix protein. The major capsid protein, p24, makes up the outer surface of the core, which contains the viral genome and the proteins necessary for replication and integration of the viral genome, such as RT.

In addition to the usual viral structural genes, all the human retroviruses contain extra genes that provide regulatory signals essential to the replication and biologic activities of the virus. Such genes were found first in HTLV-I and HTLV-II and more recently in HIV-2 and HIV-1, the well-known causes of AIDS.

One of these genes, called *tax*-1 in HTLV-I and *tat*-1 in HIV-1, codes for proteins that activate the expression of viral and some cellular genes. Another gene, *rex* in HTLV-I and *rev* in HIV-1, codes

FIGURE 151-2 Life cycle of a retrovirus (as represented by HIV-1). Intact virions are endocytosed via a specific cellular receptor. The uncoated viral single-stranded RNA is then transcribed into double-stranded DNA, enters the cell nucleus, and integrates into the host genome. The DNA provirus in some conditions is unexpressed. In other cases it is transcribed, giving rise to viral RNA encoding viral proteins and genome-length viral RNA molecules, which then reassemble with viral proteins to make complete virions. These progeny are released by budding from the cell membrane. All known infectious retroviruses follow these steps. The specific molecules described pertain only to HIV-1 (the CD4 receptor with Vif, Tat, and Rev viral proteins).

FIGURE 151-3 Genomic structure of human retroviruses. Viral proteins may be translated in each of three reading frames. RNA is transcribed from viral DNA and processed by viral and cellular enzymes, giving rise to both genomic viral RNA and mRNA. Arrows indicate double-spliced mRNA. LTR, long terminal repeat; *gag,* core proteins; *pol,* polymerase (RT); *env,* envelope. Viral genes shown in color code for regulatory proteins.

for proteins that favor the expression of unspliced or single-spliced viral mRNA; in their absence only small, double-spliced or multiply spliced mRNAs are made. The *rev/rex* proteins are localized in the nucleus and appear to increase transport of the larger mRNAs, which encode structural proteins, to the cytoplasm. Conversely, they diminish the availability of the mRNA for *rev* or *rex* and for the other regulatory proteins. For each virus these proteins are structurally distinct but have similar functions.

HIV-1 follows many of the same regulatory strategies as HTLV-I, but its genome is even more complex. By deletion analysis the function of several other genes has been evaluated.

The *nef* gene product appears to be a negative regulator of viral production under some conditions, while under other conditions it appears to have no effect or a positive effect. *Nef* appears to be required

FIGURE 151-4 Structure of an HIV-1 virion, shown schematically. The gp120 and gp41 are the two envelope proteins; p17 is present in the matrix, just inside the lipid bilayer; and p24, the major core structural protein, encapsulates the viral RNA, RT (p66), and integrase (p32).

SU (gp120)
TM (gp41)
CA (p24)
RNA
MA (p17)
RT (p66)
IN (p32)
NC (p7)
PR (p12)

for the maintenance of a high load of simian immunodeficiency virus (SIV), an HIV-related virus of monkeys, in vivo and for the production of disease by this virus. The *vif* gene affects the ability of virus particles to infect target cells but does not affect viral expression or transmission by cell-to-cell contact. The *vpu* gene has been reported to modestly enhance the exit of virus from the cell in vitro and to destabilize the complex formed in the endoplasmic reticulum between newly synthesized envelope-protein precursor and intracellular CD4, the cell surface receptor for incoming virus (see below). This destabilization appears to facilitate envelope precursor processing, which may be how *vpu* enhances transmission by virions. The *vpr* gene has been reported to stimulate the promoter region of the virus and is the only one of these extra gene products to be contained in virions. In reality, the functions of these genes are poorly understood and their in vivo relevance is unclear.

All four known human retroviruses preferentially infect the CD4 + T lymphocyte (T4 cell), and the diseases they cause involve this cell, often resulting in profound biologic consequences. Ironically, the cellular receptor for HIV is the CD4 molecule itself (see Fig. 151-2). (See Chap. 277 for discussion of the function of CD4.) The remarkably high affinity of gp120 envelope protein for this molecule probably determines the host range of the virus, the nature of target cell populations, the mode of virus transmission, and the ability of the virus to be efficiently transmitted and contributes to the cytopathic effect both through the formation of syncytia and through effects on virus production. A region of the transmembrane protein gp41 facilitates entry of the virus into the cell by fusing with the target cell membrane. The cellular receptor(s) for the HTLVs is not known, but its gene is on chromosome 17. HTLV-I usually can be transmitted only by cell-to-cell contact, probably because its envelope does not function efficiently, while the HIVs can be transmitted both in this manner and as extracellular virus. The limited mode of transmission of HTLV-I suffices because the virus is able to immortalize its host cell, the replication of which is sufficient to propagate the HTLV-I genome. In contrast, HIV-1 sometimes kills its host cell and needs to be able to infect new cells efficiently.

The monocyte-macrophage is also a major target for HIV-1. As for lymphocytes, entry requires attachment to CD4 molecules expressed on the cell surface and may be enhanced by Fc receptor–

mediated endocytosis, although this point has been disputed. Infected monocytes are believed to play a major role in the disease by acting as reservoirs for the virus, as vehicles for its spread, and as inappropriate producers of growth factors and other cytokines. Related cells are infected in the brain, lymph node, skin, lung, and gastrointestinal tract. HIV infection induces certain cytokines. Cytokine production by infected monocytes and T cells may play a direct role in the induction of malignancy, neurologic disease, and perhaps other clinical manifestations such as enteritis, arthritis, and lymphoid interstitial pneumonitis. Moreover, many cytokines are able to induce virus production from latently infected cells (see Chap. 279).

DISEASES ASSOCIATED WITH HTLV-I INFECTION HTLV-I rapidly induces transformation of human T cells in vitro; it has neither an *onc* gene nor a single integration site, yet it results in monoclonal malignancies. The majority of HTLV-I-induced leukemias or lymphomas involve the CD4+ cell. Infection of CD4+ cells by HTLV-I or HTLV-II leads to the transformation of some of the infected cells, and the properties of such transformed cells are similar. The infected cells often exhibit extensive "cerebriform" lobulation of the nuclei and form giant multinucleated cells in culture. They constitutively express increased numbers of receptors for IL-2 (IL-2R), which can be found on circulating CD4+ cells. Increased receptor expression may be due to the *tax* gene product, which can up-regulate the receptor, transform T cells when transfected, and induce tumors in transgenic animals. The maintenance of malignancy is not believed to require additional viral gene products since the HTLV-I genes are not highly expressed in the leukemic cells in vivo by the time the leukemia is clinically evident. The reason that only some individuals develop malignancy is not known. Since cells other than T4 lymphocytes can be infected, the reason for the frequency of transformation of the CD4+ cell is unclear. The relatively high incidence of adult T cell leukemia/lymphoma (ATLL) (lifetime risk of 1 to 3 percent) independent of geographic location suggests that a specific environmental cofactor is not necessary to produce disease. In contrast, lymphoma associated with Epstein-Barr virus (EBV) develops at a much lower rate and only in certain areas such as the "Burkitt lymphoma belt" in Africa, where specific environmental cofactors are present.

Leukemias/lymphomas caused by HTLV-I are characterized by an aggressive course, frequent hypercalcemia (associated with tumor necrosis factor β and parathyroid hormone induction by the Tax protein), opportunistic infection, and in over one-half of cases, leukemic skin infiltrates. HTLV-I also may be involved in T4 cell leukemias/lymphomas that exhibit a more chronic course (15 to 20 percent of cases) involving progression from polyclonal T cell proliferation to an expansion of a particular clone to frank clinical malignancy. The latter malignancies, in contrast to adult T cell leukemia (ATL), may be indistinguishable pathologically or clinically from chronic T cell lymphocytic leukemia (CLL), diffuse histiocytic lymphoma, large and mixed cell lymphomas, and mycosis fungoides or Sézary leukemias (see Chaps. 310 and 311). Typical ATL cases recognized worldwide are almost always HTLV-I–positive. In the United States, only a small percentage of T cell malignancies are HTLV-I–positive. In contrast, in endemic areas, almost all T4 cell malignancies are virus-positive.

In areas of the world where HTLV-I is endemic, some B cell lymphoid malignancies and certain other cancers are associated with HTLV-I infection more frequently than would be expected from the prevalence of the virus in the general population. In contrast to virus-positive T cell leukemias, where the viral genes are integrated into the DNA of the leukemic cell, these B cell tumors have no HTLV-I in their DNA. Instead, the virus is present in the normal T cells of these patients, and the role of the virus must be indirect, as in HIV-1 and B cell lymphomas and Kaposi's sarcoma. Several of these B cell neoplasms have been shown to make specific antibody to HTLV-I; thus years of stimulation of some B cell populations by HTLV-I proteins may be involved in their malignant transformation.

The etiologic association of HTLV-I with ATL was firmly established by the epidemiology and serology in endemic areas and by the presence of proviral DNA integrated in the host chromosomes in a monoclonal manner in the tumor. The integration of proviral DNA indicated that the first transformed cell contained the provirus rather than the tumor being infected later in an opportunistic manner. The ability of HTLV-I to immortalize target T cells in vitro is also consistent with its role in vivo as a transforming virus. Considerable data in animals show that exogenous type C retroviruses are usually leukemogenic. This finding predicted that HTLVs also would be leukemogenic in human beings.

An interesting aspect of HTLV-I is the association of this virus with a demyelinating disorder, tropical spastic paraparesis (TSP) (see Chap. 375). This syndrome also has been referred to as *HTLV-I–associated myelopathy* (HAM). It is a chronic progressive encephalomyelopathy with symmetric upper motor neuron disease, prominent lower extremity weakness, and hyperreflexia, with sphincter and sensory abnormalities that may resemble a spinal cord variant of multiple sclerosis. Central nervous system lesions are seen on magnetic resonance imaging (MRI) scans. The pathogenesis is not certain, but the high antibody responses to HTLV-I, the presence of spontaneously proliferating ("activated") CD8+ cytotoxic T lymphocytes directed against HTLV-I Env, Tax, and Rex proteins in peripheral blood, and the improvement with glucocorticoids suggest an autoimmune disease mechanism. A few individuals have both ATL and neurologic disease. While the lifetime risk of developing ATL appears to be between 1 and 3 percent in HTLV-I–infected individuals, the attack rate of TSP in some areas such as Colombia may be higher. Several other diseases may be associated with HTLV-I infection in endemic areas, including infectious dermatitis, polymyositis, Bell's palsy, Guillain-Barré syndrome, and rheumatoid arthritis.

HTLV-II, which is 55 percent identical to HTLV-I at the nucleotide sequence level, was first isolated from a cell line derived from a patient with hairy cell leukemia. In contrast to HTLV-I, HTLV-II has been associated only with several cases of T cell variants of hairy cell leukemia and an increase in bacterial infections. The difference from HTLV-I is surprising, since HTLV-II appears to have the same biologic properties in vitro as HTLV-I. This difference suggests that host factors are more successful in preventing pathogenesis by HTLV-II than by HTLV-I.

There are two major considerations in the treatment of HTLV-I infection. First, the time from infection to disease may be 20 years or more. Second, when ATL develops, the virus is often transcriptionally silent in the peripheral blood leukemic cells. Treatment for asymptomatic seropositive individuals at present is limited to periodic evaluation for neurologic and hematologic disease, screening of family members at risk, and avoidance of infection transmitted by breast feeding, sexual activity, and transfusion. Thus far, no regimen of chemotherapy has been demonstrated to increase survival in ATL, though there are case reports of remission obtained with zidovudine (AZT) combined with interferon-α. Several experimental approaches are currently being evaluated in clinical trials, including targeting of the IL-2 receptor on leukemic cells with toxin-coupled antibody. Since virus is generally not replicating, antiviral chemotherapy seems unlikely to be effective. Thus the success in a few cases of ATL with AZT and interferon-α is puzzling. Several reports have indicated that high-dose glucocorticoids benefit TSP patients, but well-controlled trials have not been done.

ORIGIN AND EPIDEMIOLOGY OF HTLV-I AND HTLV-II Originally discovered in two black patients with T cell malignancies in the United States, HTLV-I was, within a year, associated with clusters of a newly described T cell malignancy (ATL) in some southwestern islands of Japan and in Caribbean-born blacks. It may have been brought to both areas from Africa centuries ago by merchants and slave traders. HTLV-I occurs worldwide but tends to be highly restricted or clustered geographically. Recent studies show evidence of ancient infections of some South Pacific tribal bush populations, but the HTLV-I of these regions appears to be of a unique subtype that differs significantly from cosmopolitan HTLV-I found in cities all over the world, which is highly conserved (Fig. 151-5). In endemic areas the fraction of infected individuals ranges from 5 to 25 percent. Transmission is by sexual contact, by blood or blood products, and by breast feeding (and perhaps by infection of the developing fetus in utero). Because of increased travel, changes in sexual habits, intravenous drug abuse (blood-contaminated needles), and wide use of blood and blood products, the prevalence of HTLV in nonendemic areas may be increasing.

Until recently, it has been difficult to distinguish HTLV-II from HTLV-I in seropositive individuals. With the advent of polymerase chain reaction (PCR) amplification technology, it has become relatively simple to amplify the viral DNA sequences in peripheral blood and to distinguish whether the amplified DNA is derived from HTLV-I or HTLV-II. Data obtained with this technique have shown that much of the HTLV-I seropositivity in drug addict populations is due to HTLV-II. HTLV-II seems to be the major infecting type among seropositive new world indians, including those from Alaska, New Mexico, and Central America and nonacculturated tribes from South America. HTLV-II thus appears to be primarily a new world virus and, in light of its wide prevalence, has likely been so for a long time. It is apparently far less pathogenic than HTLV-I, a characteristic suggesting that it is well adapted to its hosts.

It was through analyses of PCR-amplified DNA from HTLV-I–infected people that variants of HTLV-I that were much more divergent than previously reported strains were discovered in parts of the South Pacific, such as Papua New Guinea. The discovery of these viruses raises the possibility that in some areas viruses equally related to HTLV-I and HTLV-II may exist—or even that a continuous genetic spectrum of these viruses exists.

DISEASES ASSOCIATED WITH HIV INFECTION (See also Chap. 279) Just as the discovery of the tuberculosis bacillus or the spirochete of syphilis unified diverse disease manifestations, the

FIGURE 151-5 Phylogenetic tree of HTLV-I and HTLV-II. This dendrogram was constructed on the basis of the DNA sequence of the HTLV-I and HTLV-II envelope encompassing the carboxy terminus of gp46 and almost all of gp21. The cosmopolitan HTLV-I group includes most of the HTLV-I strains from the Americas, West Africa, Europe, and Japan, with an average nucleotide divergence among themselves of approximately 2 percent. HTLV-I from the equatorial region of Zaire constitutes a quasi-species, since a discrete divergence is found among the genotypes present in the same host. The members of this group of viruses diverge from the cosmopolitan HTLV-I by 3 percent. HTLV-I variants from Melanesia and Australia are another quasi-species whose members differ among themselves by approximately 4 percent and diverge from the two other HTLV-I groups by 8 percent. HTLV-II strains can be divided genetically in two subgroups and diverge from all HTLV-I strains by approximately 30 percent.

spectrum of disease associated with AIDS has been interpreted in the context of the biology and epidemiology of HIV-1 infection. HIV-2, the most recently described human retrovirus, has about 40 percent genetic identity with HIV-1. It is even more closely related to some members of a group of viruses causing immune deficiency in simians (SIV). HIV-2 has been isolated from patients with immunodeficiency and has been detected serologically in western Africa in populations (different from those with HIV-1 infection) in whom AIDS is not endemic. It appears to be a relatively uncommon and inefficient cause of AIDS and is not spreading with the rapidity of HIV-1.

HIV-1–infected patients have an increased incidence of certain B cell lymphomas, Hodgkin's disease, certain carcinomas, and Kaposi's sarcoma (KS) (see Chap. 279). The reason for the increase in these malignancies is not completely understood, but it is not necessarily associated with the degree of immune impairment, especially in the case of KS. HIV-1 is not the direct cause of any of these tumors because viral sequences are not found in the DNA from the majority of tumor cells. For the B cell lymphomas, the mechanism may be similar to the indirect role described above for HTLV-I.

Infection with HIV-1 induces a variety of cytokines, and various protein factors have been shown to augment the growth of cells in cultures of tissue from KS lesions. HIV-1 also may play a more direct role. Viral Tat protein has been shown to be secreted by HIV-1–infected cells and taken up in an active form by other cells. Tat appears to act as a growth promoter for KS-derived cells and could play a similar role in vivo. Additional support for this concept is the appearance of KS-like lesions in transgenic male mice expressing the Tat protein. Thus the role of HIV-1 in KS may be dual: it may augment the production of a number of cytokine growth factors [e.g., tumor necrosis factor (TNF), IL-1, IL-6, oncostatin, platelet-derived growth factor (PDGF), and basic fibroblast growth factor (bFGF)] that facilitate growth of KS spindle cells and angiogenesis, and it may exert effects similar to those of the HIV-1 protein Tat.

MOLECULAR HETEROGENEITY OF HIV Analysis at the molecular level of various HIV isolates reveals variation of nucleotide sequences of certain parts of the genome, especially in the envelope gene. In different isolates the amino acid sequence of the envelope proteins ranges from very closely related (1 to 2 percent variation) to variation by 25 to 30 percent. These changes tend to cluster in hypervariable regions. One such region, called V3, is a target for neutralizing antibodies and contains recognition sites for T cell responses. Variability in this region is almost certainly due to selective pressure from the host immune system.

A single individual (and perhaps intimate contacts) is usually infected with a "swarm" of closely related viruses that may constitute a single "strain." Shown in Fig. 151-6 is a dendrogram, or genetic tree, graphically representing the relative genetic differences among strains of HIV-1. The group encompassing the LW strains and the HXB2, HXB3, BH8, and BH10 strains include virus isolates from a single individual. The BAL-1, JRFL, SC, MN, NY5CG, and RF strains, which are isolates from different individuals in the United States, are more distant on the tree. The African isolates are yet more distant, reflecting increased variability. SIV$_{cpz}$, and HIV-1–related virus from a chimpanzee, is least related to the other HIV-1 strains. Even a very small difference, called *microheterogeneity*, may exert a profound influence on the biology of the virus. Variation within an individual appears to increase with time, perhaps as a result of selective pressure exerted by the host immune response. Transmission from one individual to another also appears to select subpopulations from the virus swarm in the transmitter. Both prolonged duration of infection and multiple rounds of person-to-person transmission contribute to the diversity seen in HIV-1. The greater interstrain variability in Africa than in Europe or the United States suggests an earlier origin from a limited focus of infection in Africa. Variation does not occur to any great extent during prolonged tissue culture of a single molecularly cloned virus; thus these changes may occur during transcription of the viral RNA genome to the DNA form and/or during the recombinational process when the DNA provirus

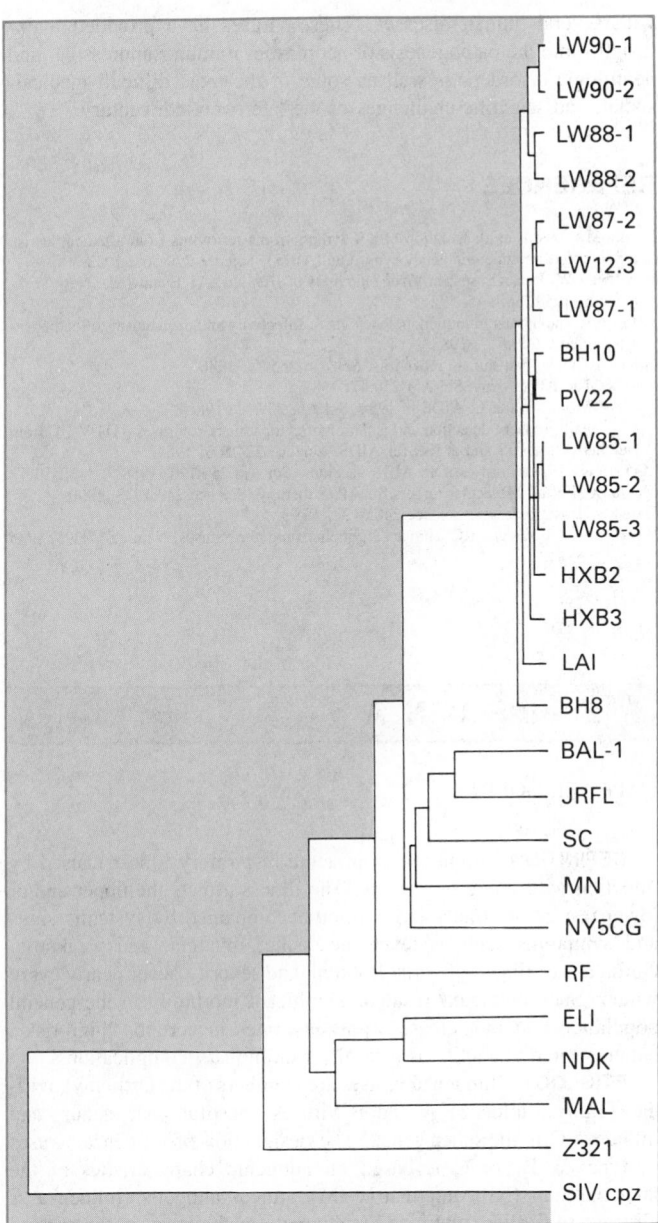

FIGURE 151-6 Dendrogram showing the relative genetic distances of HIV-1 isolates. The LW isolates and BH8, BH10, HXB2, HXB3, PV22, and LAI are variants within the same strain. BAL-1, JRFL, SC, MN, NY5CG, and RF are U.S. strains, and ELI, NDK, MAL, and Z321 are African strains. SIV$_{cpz}$ is an HIV-1–related isolate from a chimpanzee and is the most distant from the HIV-1 isolates.

least costly and most effective way of preventing infectious disease, especially those caused by viruses, but there are special problems with HIV: (1) Because of the integration of viral genes, a limited number of viral particles may be sufficient to establish infection, and therefore, the demands on a vaccine may be very stringent. (2) CD4 + T cells are the principal cells that induce protection against a virus, and these are the cells destroyed by the virus. (3) Envelope heterogeneity, as mentioned above, allows the escape from neutralizing antibodies; several conserved areas of the envelope gene are being studied as subunit vaccines. (4) The nature of a protective immune response is not yet clear. Most infected individuals develop progressive disease despite the presence of neutralizing antibodies and cytotoxic T cells. The expectation is that immunization prior to infection may prevent disease. Some encouragement comes from the finding that for most infections of a single individual only one strain of the virus has been found. This fact suggests that an individual is infected only once despite repeated exposure. (5) Animal models for vaccine development against HIV are limited, but the development of animal systems with SIV, which can produce AIDS in macaques, is likely to be very helpful. Protection against infection by low doses of the strain of killed virus used for vaccination has been achieved with SIV in monkeys. Chimpanzees similarly have been protected from HIV-1 by a regimen of inoculations with native viral envelope proteins and peptides representing the V3 loop. The protection of chimps by passive immunization with neutralizing antibodies suggests that such antibodies are effective if they are already present at the time of infection. Indeed, in most of the successful animal vaccine studies to date, the protected animal was challenged only at the time of the peak immune response following vaccination and only with a single virus strain. The difficulty of maintaining a high-level immune response and the variability of the virus remain major obstacles.

Another issue that needs to be taken into account in vaccine design is the extent to which mucosal transmission takes place, particularly during sexual activity. One piece of evidence that this issue may prove important is the high rate of heterosexual transmission in Africa and Thailand. Heterosexual contact is less likely to produce trauma leading to exposure of the blood than is homosexual contact; heterosexual transmission is thus more likely to be purely mucosal. The argument that heterosexual contact may be less risky is weakened by the higher rate of venereal diseases associated with genital lesions in these areas than in the United States and Europe. Transmission of SIV by swabbing of virus onto the vaginal mucosa of monkeys also has been demonstrated. This transmission, however, required a high dose of virus. The preceding information suggests that mucosal transmission may occur but that it is inefficient. If this should be a common route, vaccines will have to be designed so that they elicit mucosal immunity.

Antiviral therapy is based on a detailed understanding of the viral replication cycle, and almost every definable step offers the possibility of interfering with replication of virus (see Chap. 279). Approaches are available, beginning with HIV binding to the cell. Recombinant CD4 is being tested that acts as a "molecular decoy" for the virus by competing with cellular receptors for binding viral gp120 envelope proteins. This approach has been effective in vitro but has not been of any clinical benefit. Two likely reasons are the very short half-life of recombinant CD4 in the circulation and the greater resistance of field strains of HIV-1 than of laboratory strains to inhibition by CD4. The most successful agents to date affect the next stage, formation of the DNA provirus, by inhibiting RT. These agents include zidovudine and other nucleoside analogues such as dideoxyinosine (ddI) and dideoxycytidine (ddC). The next targets are the synthesis, maturation, and transport from nucleus to cytoplasm of viral RNA from proviral DNA, for which inhibitors of *tat* and *rev* function are being studied. Viral mRNA must be translated, and on an experimental basis this step can be inhibited specifically with antisense DNA. Lastly, viral proteins must assemble to form new virus, and this step depends on a specific viral protease. This protein has been crystallized, and inhibitors have been shown to be effective in vitro.

integrates into the host cell DNA. RT tends to be error-prone because, unlike cellular DNA polymerases, it lacks a proofreading mechanism. The RT of HIV may be particularly error-prone. Variation of other genes is generally far less frequent than that of the envelope. It is possible that strain variation may account for a difference in the clinical course of an HIV-infected person; experimental studies have revealed significant biologic variations among strains, including target cell tropism and response to neutralizing antibody. A variant that can avoid elimination by antibodies or cytotoxic CD8 + T cells could lead more easily to progressive disease. For example, selection pressure on cultured viruses in the presence of human neutralizing antisera has resulted in viruses with one amino acid change that is no longer neutralized by the selecting sera.

PREVENTION AND TREATMENT OF RETROVIRUS INFECTION

There are three major approaches to the control of human retroviral disease: vaccination, antiviral therapy, and education and public health measures (see Chap. 279). Vaccines have proved to be the

Because infection with HIV probably always means integration of the viral genes into the DNA of the infected cells, it is likely that lifelong treatment will be required. To minimize toxicity and reduce the chance for viral resistance, it may be necessary to use a combination of compounds with different mechanisms of action. Another approach would be to kill infected cells; success would depend on elimination of all infected cells. However, this may not be possible with human retroviruses because most infected cells do not express viral proteins and are therefore not distinguishable from uninfected cells. Moreover, infected macrophages appear to act as reservoirs for the virus and may release additional virions from intracellular vacuolar membranes when killed.

A different approach to treating people who are already infected involves the genetic alteration of uninfected target cells so that they are no longer susceptible to infection or of infected cells so that they are incapable of producing virus. For example, CD4+ peripheral blood cells altered ex vivo could be placed back into the patient, comprising an HIV-1–resistant population whose presence might slow the decline in the immune system. A more attractive possibility would be to do the same thing with pluripotent hematopoietic stem cells in the bone marrow so that the immune system might be able to reconstitute itself. To date, however, only stem cells from mice have been sufficiently well studied to permit their unambiguous isolation from mouse marrow.

There are a number of genes whose products have been shown to interfere with the production of HIV-1 in vitro and could thereby protect target cells. One such gene produces an RNA transcript containing multiple tandem copies of a region on viral RNA, called the *tat activation region* (TAR), that must bind with the HIV-1 Tat protein for efficient RNA expression. In vitro, the multiple TAR outcompetes viral RNA for Tat and strongly inhibits virus production. Another gene makes a defective copy of one of the viral structural core proteins. Even a few copies of this protein inserted into an otherwise-normal virus core prevent the formation of infectious virus. There are also mutants of *rev* and *tat* that not only are nonfunctional but actually interfere with normal *rev* and *tat* function and inhibit virus expression. These are called *trans*-dominant negative mutants. All these genes have been shown to be effective in vitro.

OTHER DISEASES ASSOCIATED WITH HUMAN RETROVIRAL INFECTION The possibility that several well-described human diseases are associated with retroviral infection should be considered carefully. While the potential of many candidate viruses to cause disease has not been realized, the number of retroviruses with diverse mechanisms of disease found in other species suggests a wide range of possibilities. A report of RT activity in non-A, non-B hepatitis has not been substantiated, and a new flavivirus has been discovered as the probable cause. T activity has been detected in patients with Kawasaki disease, but neither a virus nor viral sequences have been found, and there has been no confirmation of the original reports. Mammary tumors in mice have been transmitted via breast milk infected with mammary tumor virus. Despite sporadic reports of electron-micrographic evidence of virus in human tumors, no human equivalent has been isolated and characterized. Retroviruses are known to produce neurologic disease in some species (e.g., visna in sheep and murine leukemia in some mice); HIV-1 infects the central nervous system; and HTLV-I is associated with a demyelinating disease. A retroviral etiology of multiple sclerosis has been considered. Sequences related to HTLV-I have been reported in the peripheral blood of patients with multiple sclerosis by in situ hybridization or polymerase chain reaction. Differentiation of these sequences from those endogenous to cells and recovery of intact virus are needed to confirm the significance of these associations. An HTLV-II–related retrovirus has been reported to be linked to the chronic fatigue syndrome by nucleic acid and serologic studies. This link has not been confirmed, and no virus has been isolated.

The discovery of the HTLV-I occurred at a time when many thought that there would be no human retroviruses. In the ensuing decade, four human retroviruses have been discovered and associated with several human diseases. These viruses have provided major insights into the pathogenesis of neoplastic, immunosuppressive, and neurologic disorders as well as some of the most difficult medical, social, and scientific challenges of the late twentieth century.

REFERENCES

BAARE-SINOUSSI F et al: Isolation of a T lymphotropic retrovirus from a patient at risk for acquired immune deficiency syndrome (AIDS). Science 220:868, 1983

BLATTNER W: Retroviruses, in *Viral Infections of Humans*, AS Evans (ed). New York, Plenum, 1989, pp. 545–592

FAUCI AS: The human immunodeficiency virus: Infectivity and mechanisms of pathogenesis. Science 239:617, 1988

GALLO RC: The first human retrovirus. Sci Am 255:88, 1986

———: The AIDS virus. Sci Am 256:47, 1987

———, MONTAGNIER L: AIDS in 1988. Sci Am 259:41, 1988

——— et al: Frequent detection and isolation of cytopathic retroviruses (HTLV-III) from patients with AIDS and at risk for AIDS. Science 224:500, 1984

MATTHEWS TJ, BOLOGNESI DP: AIDS vaccines. Sci Am 259:120, 1988

MITSUYA H et al: Molecular targets for AIDS therapy. Science 249:1533, 1990

VARMUS H: Retroviruses. Science 240:1427, 1988

WONG-STAAL F, GALLO RC: Human T-lymphotropic retroviruses. Nature 317:395, 1985

152 INFLUENZA

RAPHAEL DOLIN

DEFINITION Influenza is an acute respiratory illness caused by infection with influenza viruses. The illness affects the upper and/or lower respiratory tracts and is often accompanied by systemic signs and symptoms such as fever, headache, myalgia, and weakness. Outbreaks of illness of variable extent and severity occur nearly every winter. Such outbreaks result in significant morbidity in the general population and in increased mortality rates in certain "high-risk" patients, predominantly as a result of pulmonary complications.

ETIOLOGY Influenza viruses are members of the Orthomyxoviridae family. Influenza A and B viruses constitute one genus, and influenza C is the other genus. The designation of influenza viruses as type A, B, or C is based on antigenic characteristics of the nucleoprotein (NP) and matrix (M) protein antigens. Influenza A viruses are further subdivided (subtyped) on the basis of the surface hemagglutinin (H) and neuraminidase (N) antigens (see below). Individual strains are also designated according to the site of origin, isolate number, year of isolation, and subtype (e.g., influenza A/Victoria/3/79 H3N2). Influenza B and C viruses are similarly designated, but H and N antigens from these viruses do not receive subtype designations, since intratypic variations in H and N antigens of influenza B and C viruses are less extensive.

Most of the information regarding the molecular biology of influenza viruses has been generated from studies of influenza A viruses, and less is known about the replicative cycle of influenza B and C viruses. Morphologically, influenza viruses A, B, and C are similar. The virions are irregularly shaped spherical particles, 80 to 120 nm in diameter, that contain a lipid envelope from whose surface the hemagglutinin and neuraminidase glycoproteins project. The hemagglutinin serves as the site by which virus binds to cell receptors, while the neuraminidase degrades the receptor and probably plays a role in release of virus from infected cells after replication has taken place. Antibodies directed against the H antigen are the major determinants of immunity against influenza virus, while antineuraminidase antibodies limit viral spread and contribute to reduction of the infection. The inner surface of the lipid envelope contains the matrix proteins (M1 and M2), whose functions are incompletely understood but which may be involved in virus assembly and stabilization of the lipid envelope. The virion also contains the nucleoprotein (NP) with which the genome of the virus is associated, as well as three polymerase (P) proteins which are essential for transcription and synthesis of viral RNA. Two nonstructural (NS) proteins of unknown function are also present in infected cells.

The genome of influenza A virus consists of eight single-stranded segments of viral RNA, which code for the structural and nonstructural proteins. Because the genome is segmented, the opportunity for reassortment of genes during infection is high, and reassortment has been noted to occur frequently during infection of cells with more than one influenza A virus.

EPIDEMIOLOGY Influenza outbreaks occur virtually every year, although the extent and severity of such outbreaks vary widely. Localized outbreaks occur at variable intervals, usually every 1 to 3 years. Global epidemics or pandemics have occurred approximately every 10 to 15 years since the 1918–1919 pandemic (Table 152-1).

The most extensive and severe outbreaks are caused by influenza A viruses. In part, this is a result of the remarkable propensity of the hemagglutinin and neuraminidase antigens of influenza A virus to undergo periodic antigenic variation. Major antigenic variations are referred to as *antigenic shifts*, which most likely occur from reassortment of genome segments between viral strains. Antigenic shifts may be associated with pandemics and are restricted to influenza A viruses. Minor variations are called *antigenic drifts* and likely arise from point mutations. These antigenic changes may involve the hemagglutinin alone or both the hemagglutinin and the neuraminidase. In human infections, three major antigenic subtypes of hemagglutinins (H1, H2, and H3) and two neuraminidases (N1, N2) have been recognized. The hemagglutinins formerly designated as H0 and Hsw1 are now classified as variants of H1. An example of an antigenic shift which involved both the hemagglutinin and neuraminidase occurred in 1957, when the predominant influenza A virus subtype shifted from H1N1 to H2N2, and resulted in a severe pandemic, with an estimated 70,000 *excess deaths*, i.e., deaths in excess of the number expected without an influenza epidemic, in the United States alone. In 1968, an antigenic shift occurred which involved only the hemagglutinin (H2N2 to H3N2), and the subsequent pandemic was less severe than that seen in 1957. In 1977, an A/H1N1 virus emerged which caused a pandemic that primarily affected younger individuals, i.e., those born after 1957. As can be seen in Table 152-1, H1N1 viruses circulated from 1918 to 1956, so individuals born prior to 1957 would be expected to possess some degree of immunity to H1N1 viruses. During most outbreaks of influenza A, a single subtype has circulated at a time. However, since 1977, both A/H1N1 and A/H3N2 viruses have circulated simultaneously, resulting in outbreaks of varying severity. In some outbreaks influenza B viruses also circulated simultaneously with influenza A viruses.

The origin of pandemic strains is unknown. Because of the marked differences between the primary structures of the hemagglutinins of different subtypes of influenza A viruses (H1, H2, or H3), it is believed unlikely that antigenic shifts result from spontaneous mutations in the hemagglutinin gene. Because the segmented genome of influenza viruses may result in high rates of reassortment, it has been suggested that pandemic strains may emerge by reassortment of genes between human and animal influenza viruses. Influenza B viruses do not have an animal reservoir and do not undergo antigenic shifts, although antigenic drifting occurs.

Although pandemics provide the most dramatic evidence of the impact of influenza, illnesses that occur between pandemics account for an even greater total in mortality and morbidity, albeit over a longer period of time. Since 1957, interpandemic illness has been associated with 10,000 or more excess deaths on 20 occasions in the United States, resulting in an accumulated mortality of more than 500,000 over that period of time. Influenza A viruses that circulate between pandemics demonstrate antigenic drifts in the hemagglutinin antigen. These antigenic drifts apparently result from point mutations which involve the RNA segment that codes for the hemagglutinin. Amino acid analysis of "drifted" hemagglutinins indicates that changes in a single amino acid have little effect on the antigenic properties of the hemagglutinin. Epidemiologically significant strains, i.e., those which have potential for causing widespread outbreaks, have changes in amino acids in at least two of the four major antigenic sites in the HA molecule. Since two-point mutations are unlikely to occur simultaneously, it is believed that antigenic drifts result from point mutations which occur sequentially during the spread of virus from person to person. Antigenic drifts have occurred nearly annually since 1977 for A/H1N1 viruses and since 1968 for A/H3N2 viruses.

Influenza A epidemics begin abruptly, reach a peak over a 2- to 3-week period, generally last for 2 to 3 months, and often subside almost as rapidly as they began. The first indication of influenza activity in a community is an increase in the number of children with febrile respiratory illnesses who present for medical attention. This is followed by increases in influenza-like illnesses among adults and eventually by an increase in hospital admissions for patients with pneumonia, worsening of congestive heart failure, and exacerbations of chronic pulmonary disease. Rises in industrial and school absenteeism also occur at this time. An increase in the number of deaths caused by pneumonia and influenza is generally a late observation in an outbreak. Attack rates have been highly variable from outbreak to outbreak but most commonly are in the range of 10 to 20 percent of the general population. During the pandemic of 1957, it was estimated that the attack rate of clinical influenza exceeded 50 percent in urban populations and that an additional 25 percent or more may have been subclinically infected with influenza A virus. Among institutionalized populations and in semiclosed settings where a large number of susceptible individuals are present, even higher attack rates have been reported.

Epidemics of influenza occur almost exclusively during the winter months in the Northern and Southern Hemispheres. It is highly unusual to detect influenza A virus at times other than those in which an outbreak occurs, although rarely serologic rises have been noted at other times of the year. Where or how influenza A virus persists between outbreaks is unknown. A possible explanation is that influenza A viruses are maintained in the human population on a worldwide basis by person-to-person transmission and that large population clusters might be able to support a low level of interepidemic transmission. Alternatively, human strains may persist in animal reservoirs, but convincing evidence to support either explanation is not available. In the modern era, rapid modes of transportation may contribute to the transmission of viruses from widespread geographic locales.

The factors which result in the inception and termination of outbreaks of influenza are also incompletely understood. A major determinant of the extent and severity of an outbreak is the level of immunity present in the population at risk. When an antigenically novel influenza virus emerges to which little or no antibody is present in a community, extensive outbreaks may occur. When the absence of antibody is worldwide, epidemic disease may spread around the globe, resulting in a pandemic. Such pandemic waves can occur for

TABLE 152-1 Emergence of antigenic subtypes of influenza A associated with pandemic or epidemic disease

Year	Subtype of influenza A	Extent of outbreak
1889–90	H2N8*	Severe pandemic
1900–03	H3N8*	?Moderate epidemic
1918–19	H1N1† (formerly HswN1)	Severe pandemic
1933–35	H1N1† (formerly H0N1)	Mild epidemic
1946–47	H1N1	Mild epidemic
1957–58	H2N2	Severe pandemic
1968–69	H3N2	Moderate pandemic
1977–78‡	H1N1	Mild pandemic

* As determined by retrospective serologic survey of individuals alive during those years ("seroarcheology").
† Hemagglutinins formerly designated as Hsw and H0 are now classified as variants of H1.
‡ From this time until the present (1991–92), new antigenic subtypes of influenza A have not emerged. Rather, viruses of H1N1 or H3N2 subtypes have circulated either in alternating years or concurrently.

several years, until immunity in the population reaches a high level. In the years following pandemic influenza, antigenic drifts among influenza viruses result in outbreaks of variable severity in populations that have high levels of immunity to the pandemic strain which circulated earlier. This situation persists until another antigenically novel pandemic strain emerges. On the other hand, outbreaks also may terminate despite the persistence of a large pool of susceptible individuals in the population. Occasionally, the emergence of a significantly different antigenic variant will result only in a localized outbreak. The "swine influenza outbreak" of 1976 in the United States, caused by an A/H1N1 virus antigenically similar to the virus which circulated in 1918–1919 (see Table 152-1), may be an example of this, although this outbreak may simply represent the introduction of a swine influenza virus into a crowded human population without spread beyond that setting. It also has been suggested that certain viruses, such as recently circulating A/H1N1 strains, may be intrinsically less virulent and cause less severe disease, even in immunologically virgin subjects, suggesting that other undefined factors besides the level of preexisting immunity play a role in the epidemiology of influenza.

Influenza B causes outbreaks which are generally less extensive and are associated with less severe disease than those caused by influenza A virus. The hemagglutinin and neuraminidase of influenza B virus undergo less frequent and less extensive variation than is seen in influenza A viruses, which may account, in part, for the observation of less extensive disease. Influenza B outbreaks are seen most frequently in schools and military camps, although occasional outbreaks in institutions in which elderly individuals reside also have been noted. The most serious complication of influenza B virus infection is Reye's syndrome (see below). Influenza C has been infrequently associated with human disease, although the prevalence of serum antibody to influenza C virus is widespread, which indicates that asymptomatic infection may be common.

The morbidity and mortality of influenza outbreaks continue to be substantial. Mortality occurs primarily in individuals with underlying diseases who have been characterized as being at "high risk" for complications of influenza. Excess hospitalizations for adults with "high risk" medical conditions have reached rates of 800 per 100,000 during recent outbreaks of influenza. These high-risk conditions are primarily chronic cardiac and pulmonary diseases, as well as increased age. Increased mortality rates also have been observed among individuals with chronic metabolic, renal, and certain immunosuppressive diseases, although to a lesser extent than among those with chronic cardiopulmonary diseases. In addition to the excess mortality, the morbidity of influenza in the general population is also extensive. For each of three outbreaks in the United States that were studied during the 1960s, it has been estimated that direct and indirect economic costs ranged from 1.5 to 3.5 billion dollars and that today such costs would be much greater.

PATHOGENESIS   The initial event in influenza is infection of the respiratory epithelium with influenza virus, which is acquired from respiratory secretions of acutely infected individuals. In all likelihood, this occurs via aerosols generated by coughs and sneezes, although hand-to-hand, other personal contact, and even fomite transmission may occur. Experimental evidence suggests that infection by small-particle aerosol (less than 10 μm in diameter) is more efficient than that produced by larger droplets. Initially, viral infection involves the ciliated columnar epithelial cells, but it also may involve other respiratory tract cells, including alveolar cells, mucous gland cells, and macrophages. In infected cells, virus replication takes place within 4 to 6 h, after which infectious virus is released to infect adjacent or nearby cells. This results in spread of infection from a few foci to a large number of respiratory cells over several hours. In experimentally induced infection, the incubation period of illness has ranged from 18 to 72 h, depending on the size of the virus inoculum. Histopathologically, degenerative changes can be seen in infected ciliated cells, including granulation, vacuolization, swelling, and

pyknotic nuclei. The cells eventually become necrotic and desquamate, and in some areas, previously columnar epithelium is replaced by flattened and metaplastic epithelial cells. The severity of illness is correlated with the quantity of virus shed in secretions, suggesting that the degree of viral replication itself may be an important mechanism in the pathogenesis of illness. Despite the frequent presence of systemic signs and symptoms such as fever, headache, and myalgias, influenza virus has only rarely been detected in extrapulmonary sites, including the bloodstream, and the pathogenesis of systemic symptoms in influenza remains unknown.

The host response to influenza infections involves a complex interplay of humoral antibody, local antibody, cell-mediated immune responses, interferon, and other host defenses. Serum antibody responses may be measured by a variety of techniques and can be detected by the second week after primary infection with influenza virus. Such antibodies may be measured by hemagglutination inhibition (HAI), complement fixation (CF), neutralization, enzyme-linked immunosorbent assays (ELISA), and antineuraminidase antibody assays. Antibodies directed against the hemagglutinin appear to be the most important mediators of immunity, and in several studies, HAI titers of 40 or greater have been associated with protection from infection. Secretory antibodies produced in the respiratory tract are predominantly of the IgA class and also play a major role in protection against infection. Secretory antibody neutralization titers of 4 or higher also have been associated with protection. A variety of cell-mediated immune responses, both antigen-specific and non-antigen-specific, can be detected early after infection, depending on prior immunity of the host. These responses include T cell proliferative, T cell cytotoxic, and natural killer cell activity. Interferons have been detected in respiratory secretions shortly after shedding of virus has begun, and rises in interferon titers coincide with decreases in virus shedding.

The host defense factors responsible for cessation of virus shedding and resolution of illness have not been defined specifically. Virus shedding generally stops within 2 to 5 days after symptoms first appear, at a time when serum and local antibody responses are often not detectable by conventional techniques, although antibody rises may be detected earlier by use of highly sensitive techniques, particularly in individuals with previous immunity to the virus. It has been suggested that interferon, cell-mediated immune responses, or nonspecific inflammatory responses may be important in the resolution of illness.

MANIFESTATIONS   Influenza has been most frequently described as an illness characterized by the abrupt onset of systemic symptoms such as headache, feverishness, chilliness, myalgia, or malaise, accompanied by respiratory tract signs, particularly cough and sore throat. In many cases, the onset is so abrupt that patients can recall the precise time of the onset of illness. A typical case of naturally occurring influenza is depicted in Fig. 152-1. However, a wide spectrum of clinical presentations may occur. These can range from mild, afebrile respiratory illnesses similar to the common cold, with either gradual or abrupt onset, to illnesses in which severe prostration with relatively few respiratory signs and symptoms may be present. In the majority of cases which come to a physician's attention, fever is present, and temperatures can range from 38°C to as high as 41°C. The temperature rises rapidly within the first 24 h of illness and is generally followed by a gradual defervescence over a 2- to 3-day period, although, on occasion, fever may last for as long as a week. Patients complain of a feverish feeling and chilliness, but true rigors are rare. Headache, either generalized or frontal, is often a particularly troublesome complaint. Myalgias may involve any part of the body but are most common in the legs and lumbosacral area. Arthralgias also may be present.

Respiratory complaints often become more prominent as systemic symptoms subside. Many patients complain of a sore throat or persistent cough, which may last for a week or more and which is often accompanied by substernal discomfort. Ocular signs and

FIGURE 152-1 Clinical characteristics of a naturally occurring case of influenza A in an otherwise healthy 28-year-old male. (*From R Dolin, Am Fam Phys 14:74, 1976.*)

symptoms include pain on motion of the eyes, photophobia, and burning of the eyes.

Physical findings are usually minimal in cases of uncomplicated influenza. Early in the illness, the patient appears flushed, and the skin is hot and dry, although diaphoresis and mottled extremities, particularly in older patients, may occur. Examination of the pharynx may be surprisingly unremarkable despite a severe sore throat, but injection of the mucous membranes and postnasal discharge can be present. Mild cervical lymphadenopathy may be noted, particularly in younger individuals. Chest examination is largely negative in uncomplicated influenza, although rhonchi, wheezes, and scattered rales have been reported with variable frequency in different outbreaks. Frank dyspnea, hyperpnea, cyanosis, diffuse rales, and signs of consolidation are evidence of pulmonary complications. Patients with apparently uncomplicated influenza have been reported to have a variety of mild ventilatory defects and increased alveolar-capillary diffusion gradients, indicating that subclinical pulmonary involvement may be more frequent than is appreciated.

In uncomplicated influenza, the acute illness generally resolves over a 2- to 5-day period, and most patients have largely recovered in 1 week. In a significant minority, however, symptoms of weakness or lassitude (''postinfluenzal asthenia'') may persist for several weeks, particularly in the elderly, and may prove troublesome for those who wish to return to full activity promptly. The pathogenetic basis for this ''asthenia'' is unknown, although pulmonary function abnormalities may persist for several weeks after uncomplicated influenza.

COMPLICATIONS OF INFLUENZA The most common complication of influenza is pneumonia, which may occur either as ''primary'' influenza viral pneumonia, secondary bacterial pneumonia, or mixed viral and bacterial pneumonia. Primary influenza viral pneumonia is the least common but most severe of the pneumonic complications. It presents as acute influenza which does not resolve but instead relentlessly progresses with persistent fever, dyspnea, and eventual cyanosis. Sputum production is generally scanty but can contain blood, and few physical signs may be present early in the illness. In more advanced cases, diffuse rales may be noted, and chest x-ray findings consistent with diffuse interstitial infiltrates and/or acute respiratory distress syndrome may be present. In such cases, arterial blood gases show marked hypoxia. Viral cultures, particularly if taken early in illness, show high titers of virus in respiratory secretions and in the lung parenchyma. Histopathology of fatal cases of primary viral pneumonia shows a marked inflammatory reaction in the alveolar septa, with edema and infiltration with lymphocytes, macrophages, occasional plasma cells, and variable numbers of neutrophils. Fibrin thrombi in alveolar capillaries, along with necrosis and hemorrhage, also have been noted. Eosinophilic hyaline membranes also can be found lining alveoli and alveolar ducts.

Primary influenza viral pneumonia has a predilection for individuals with cardiac disease, particularly those with mitral stenosis, but also has been reported in otherwise healthy young adults, as well as in older individuals with chronic pulmonary disorders. In some epidemics of influenza (notably 1918 and 1957), pregnancy increased the risk of the development of primary influenza pneumonia.

Secondary bacterial pneumonia is a complication in which bacterial infection develops following a case of acute influenza. With this illness, patients experience a period of improvement for 2 to 3 days after acute influenza, followed by a reappearance of fever, along with clinical signs and symptoms of bacterial pneumonia. These include cough, production of purulent sputum, and physical and x-ray signs of consolidation. The most common bacterial pathogens in this setting are *Streptococcus pneumoniae*, *Staphylococcus aureus*, and *Haemophilus influenzae*, organisms that can colonize the nasopharynx and that cause infection in the wake of changes in bronchopulmonary defenses. The etiology can often be determined by Gram's stain and culture of an appropriately obtained sputum specimen. Secondary bacterial pneumonia occurs most frequently in high-risk individuals with chronic pulmonary and cardiac disease and in elderly individuals. Patients with secondary bacterial pneumonias will often respond to antibiotic therapy when it is instituted promptly.

Perhaps the most common of the pneumonic complications that occur during outbreaks of influenza are mixed viral and bacterial pneumonias. The clinical course of this complication contains features of both primary and secondary pneumonias. Patients may have a gradual progression of their acute illness or may show a transient improvement followed by a clinical worsening, with eventual manifestation of the clinical features of a bacterial pneumonia. Sputum cultures may contain both influenza A virus and one of the bacterial pathogens described above. Patchy infiltrates or areas of consolidation may be noted by physical examination and chest x-ray. Patients with mixed viral and bacterial pneumonias generally have less widespread involvement of the lung than those with primary viral pneumonia, and their bacterial infections may respond to appropriate antibiotics. Mixed viral and bacterial pneumonias occur primarily in patients with chronic cardiovascular and pulmonary diseases.

In addition to the pulmonary complications of influenza, a number of extrapulmonary complications may occur. *Reye's syndrome* is a serious complication of influenza B and to a lesser extent of influenza A virus infection, as well as of varicella-zoster virus infection. It occurs in children most commonly between the ages of 2 and 16 and follows several days after a generally unremarkable viral illness. Reye's syndrome is marked by the onset of nausea and vomiting for 1 to 2 days, after which central nervous system symptoms appear. These are most frequently changes in mental status, ranging from lethargy to coma, and can include delirium and seizures. Hepatomegaly is noted, along with a marked elevation of AST, ALT, and LDH levels. Bilirubin values are only moderately elevated, so the children are not jaundiced, but blood ammonia levels are elevated in virtually all patients. Hypoglycemia can occur, especially after varicella-zoster virus infection or after viral gastrointestinal illnesses. Children are usually afebrile, and while lumbar puncture generally shows an elevated pressure, the cerebrospinal fluid is quite unremarkable, indicating that an encephalopathy rather than a meningoencephalitis is present. The mortality of the syndrome is related to the state of consciousness on admission and has decreased from more than 40 percent, when the syndrome was originally described, to approximately 10 percent, reflecting earlier recognition and improved management of cerebral edema and hypoglycemia. Histopathology demonstrates little in the way of inflammatory changes in either the liver or the central nervous system. Liver biopsy shows diffuse fatty infiltration of hepatocytes and swelling and pleomorphism in mitochondria. Cerebral edema and anoxic changes in neurons are the only pathologic changes detected in the central nervous system. The pathogenesis of Reye's syndrome is unknown, but the virus is almost never found in the affected liver and brain. An epidemiologic association with aspirin therapy for the antecedent viral infection has been noted, and the incidence of Reye's syndrome has decreased markedly with widespread warnings regarding the use of aspirin in children with acute viral respiratory infections.

Myositis, rhabdomyolysis, and myoglobinuria also have been reported as occasional complications of influenza infection. Although myalgias are exceedingly common in influenza, true myositis is rare. Patients with acute myositis have exquisite tenderness of the affected muscles, most commonly in the legs, and may not be able to tolerate even the slightest pressure, such as the touch of bed sheets. In the most severe cases, there is frank swelling and bogginess of muscles. Markedly elevated serum creatine phosphokinase and aldolase levels are present, and an occasional patient has developed renal failure from myoglobinuria. The pathogenesis of influenza-associated myositis is also unclear, although the presence of influenza virus in affected muscles has been reported.

Myocarditis and pericarditis in association with influenza virus infection was reported during the 1918–1919 pandemic, based largely on histopathologic findings, and has been documented infrequently since that time. Electrocardiographic changes during acute influenza are commonly noted in patients who have cardiac disease, but these have been most often ascribed to exacerbations of the underlying cardiac disease rather than to direct involvement of the myocardium with influenza virus.

Central nervous system disease also has been reported during influenza, including encephalitis, transverse myelitis, and Guillain-Barré syndrome. The etiologic relationship of influenza virus to such CNS illnesses remains unestablished. "Toxic shock" syndrome caused by S. aureus infection following acute influenza infection has been reported recently (see Chap. 102).

In addition to complications involving the specific organ systems described above, every influenza outbreak includes a number of elderly and other high-risk individuals who develop influenza and who subsequently experience a gradual deterioration of underlying cardiovascular, pulmonary, or renal function, occasionally leading to irreversible changes and death. These fatalities contribute to the overall toll of excess mortality associated with influenza A outbreaks.

LABORATORY FINDINGS Laboratory diagnosis is accomplished during the acute illness by isolation of virus from throat swabs, nasopharyngeal washes, or sputum. Virus is usually detected in tissue culture or less commonly in the amniotic cavity of chick embryos within 48 to 72 h after inoculation. Viral antigens may be detected somewhat earlier by use of immunodiagnostic techniques in tissue culture or directly in exfoliated nasopharyngeal cells obtained by washings, although this technique is less sensitive than isolation of virus in tissue culture. The type of influenza virus (A or B) may be identified by either immunofluorescence or hemagglutination inhibition techniques, and the hemagglutinin subtype of influenza A virus (H1, H2, or H3) may be identified by hemagglutination inhibition using subtype-specific antisera. Serologic methods for diagnosis require comparison of antibody titers in sera obtained during the acute illness with those obtained 10 to 14 days after the onset of illness and are useful primarily in retrospect. Fourfold or greater titer rises as detected by hemagglutination inhibition or complement fixation or significant rises in antibody levels as measured by ELISA techniques are diagnostic of acute infection. Complement fixation tests are generally less sensitive than other serologic techniques, but since they

detect type-specific antigens, they may be particularly useful when subtype-specific reagents are not available.

Other laboratory tests are generally not helpful in making a specific diagnosis of influenza virus infection. Leukocyte counts are variable, being frequently low early in illness and normal or slightly elevated later. Severe leukopenia has been described in overwhelming viral or bacterial infection, while leukocytosis with counts of greater than 15,000 cells per microliter should raise the suspicion that secondary bacterial infection is present.

DIFFERENTIAL DIAGNOSIS On clinical grounds alone, an individual case of influenza may be difficult to differentiate from an acute respiratory illness caused by a variety of respiratory viruses or by *Mycoplasma pneumoniae*. Severe streptococcal pharyngitis or early bacterial pneumonia may mimic acute influenza, although bacterial pneumonias generally do not run a self-limited course. The presence of purulent sputum in which a bacterial pathogen can be detected by Gram's stain is an important diagnostic feature in bacterial pneumonia. The fact that influenza occurs in characteristic outbreaks during the winter months may be helpful in making a clinical diagnosis. When local health authorities indicate that influenza is present in the community, the etiology of an acute febrile respiratory illness can be attributed to influenza with a high degree of certainty, particularly if the typical features of abrupt onset and systemic symptoms are present.

TREATMENT In uncomplicated cases of influenza, symptomatic therapy for headache, myalgia, and fever may be considered, employing either acetaminophen or salicylates, but salicylates should be avoided in children below 18 years of age because of the possible association of salicylates with Reye's syndrome. Since cough is ordinarily self-limited, treatment with cough suppressants generally is not indicated, although codeine-containing compounds may be employed if the cough is particularly troublesome. Patients should be advised to rest and maintain hydration during acute illness and should return to full activity only gradually after the illness has resolved, particularly if illness has been severe.

The only specific antiviral therapy available for influenza is amantadine. Amantadine is active only against influenza A viruses and has been licensed for the prophylaxis and therapy of influenza A virus infections in the United States. If begun within 48 h of the onset of illness, amantadine reduces the duration of systemic and respiratory symptoms of influenza by approximately 50 percent, and in one study, it was superior to aspirin. From 5 to 10 percent of individuals who receive amantadine will experience mild central nervous system side effects, primarily jitteriness, anxiety, insomnia, or difficulty in concentrating. These side effects disappear promptly upon cessation of the drug. The dose of amantadine for adults is 200 mg/d for 3 to 5 days or up to 48 h after illness has resolved. Because amantadine is excreted almost entirely by the kidneys, the dose should be reduced in individuals with renal insufficiency. Rimantadine, an experimental drug which is a closely related analogue of amantadine, appears to be equally efficacious and is associated with less frequent central nervous system side effects than is amantadine. Ribavirin, a nucleoside analogue with activity against a variety of viral agents, has been reported to be effective against both influenza A and B virus infections when administered as an aerosol, although it is relatively ineffective when administered orally.

Studies demonstrating the therapeutic efficacy of antiviral compounds in influenza have been carried out almost exclusively in uncomplicated disease in young adults, and it is not known whether such compounds are effective in the treatment of complications such as influenza pneumonia. Therapy for primary influenza pneumonia is directed at maintaining oxygenation and is most appropriately managed in an intensive care unit, with aggressive respiratory and hemodynamic support as needed. Bypass membrane oxygenators have been employed in this setting with variable results. When an acute respiratory distress syndrome develops, fluids must be administered cautiously, with close monitoring of blood gases and hemodynamic function.

Antibacterial drugs should be reserved for the therapy of bacterial complications of acute influenza such as secondary bacterial pneumonia. The choice of antibiotics should be guided by Gram's stain and culture of appropriate specimens of respiratory secretions, such as sputum or transtracheal aspirates. If the etiology of a bacterial pneumonia is unclear from examination of respiratory secretions, empiric antibiotics should be selected which are effective against the most common bacterial pathogens in this setting, namely, *S. pneumoniae*, *S. aureus*, and *H. influenzae* (see Chaps. 101, 102, and 119).

PROPHYLAXIS The major public health measure for prevention of influenza has been the use of inactivated influenza vaccines. These vaccines are derived from influenza A and B viruses which circulated during the previous influenza season. If the vaccine and currently circulating viruses are closely related, such vaccines would be expected to provide 50 to 80 percent protection against influenza. Currently available vaccines have been highly purified and are associated with few reactions. Up to 5 percent of individuals will experience low-grade fever and mild systemic symptoms 8 to 24 h after vaccination, and up to one-third may have mild redness or tenderness at the vaccination site. Since the vaccine is produced in eggs, individuals with true hypersensitivity to egg products either should be desensitized or should not receive vaccine. Although the 1976 swine influenza vaccine appears to have been associated with an increased frequency of Guillain-Barré syndrome, influenza vaccines administered since 1976 have not been associated with Guillain-Barré syndrome. Live attenuated ("cold-adapted") influenza A vaccines also have been developed and appear to be promising in ongoing studies in adults and children. Such vaccines are administered intranasally and stimulate local antibody production more efficiently than conventional inactivated vaccines.

The U.S. Public Health Service recommends influenza vaccination for any individual older than 6 months of age who is at an increased risk for complications of influenza. These include individuals with chronic cardiovascular or pulmonary disorders (including asthma) and residents of nursing homes and other chronic care facilities. Other populations for whom the vaccine is recommended include otherwise healthy individuals over 65 years of age and individuals who have required regular medical attention for diabetes mellitus, renal disease, hemoglobinopathies, or immunosuppression. Individuals who provide care for high-risk patients or who come into frequent contact with such patients, including household members, also should receive vaccine to reduce the likelihood of transmission of infection. Since commercially available vaccines are inactivated ("killed"), they may be administered safely to immunocompromised patients. Influenza vaccination is not associated with exacerbations of chronic nervous system diseases such as multiple sclerosis. Vaccination should be administered early in the autumn before influenza outbreaks occur and should be administered on an annual basis to maintain immunity against the most current influenza virus strains.

Amantadine and rimantadine also have been demonstrated to be effective in the prophylaxis of influenza A. Studies have demonstrated 70 to 100 percent effectiveness of these drugs in preventing illness associated with influenza A virus infection. The major use for prophylaxis with amantadine or rimantadine is likely to be for high-risk individuals who have not received influenza vaccine or when the vaccines previously administered are relatively ineffective because of antigenic changes in the circulating virus. If vaccination is performed during an outbreak, amantadine can be administered simultaneously with inactivated vaccine, since it will not interfere with an immune response to the vaccine. There is also evidence that the protective effects of amantadine and vaccine may be additive. Amantadine also has been employed to control nosocomial outbreaks of influenza A. For prophylaxis, amantadine or rimantadine should be instituted promptly when influenza A activity is detected and must be administered daily for the duration of the outbreak. The dosage most frequently employed has been 200 mg/d for adults, but the dose of amantadine should be reduced in patients with renal insufficiency and in the elderly. Viruses resistant to both amantadine and rimantadine can emerge quickly after therapy with these drugs.

REFERENCES

CENTERS FOR DISEASE CONTROL: Prevention and control of influenza. Morb Mort Week Rep 40:1, 1991

DOLIN R et al: A controlled trial of amantadine and rimantadine in the prophylaxis of influenza A infection. N Engl J Med 307:580, 1982

DOUGLAS RG JR (ed): Prevention, management, and control of influenza: A mandate for the 1980s. Am J Med 82 (suppl 6A), 1987

GLEZEN WP: Serious morbidity and mortality associated with influenza epidemics. Epidemiol Rev 4:25, 1982

MURPHY BR, WEBSTER RG: Orthomyxoviruses, in *Virology*, 2d ed, BN Fields (ed). New York, Raven Press, 1990, pp 1091-1152

YINNON AM, DOLIN R: Using antivirals to fight influenza in 1991–1992. J Respir Dis 12:1146, 1991

153 VIRAL GASTROENTERITIS

HARRY B. GREENBERG

In less developed countries, acute infectious diarrheal disease is a leading cause of morbidity in all age groups and of mortality in infants and young children. In developed countries, acute diarrheal illness remains an important cause of morbidity among both children and adults. Two distinct groups of viruses—the rotaviruses and the enteric caliciviruses such as Norwalk virus—as well as a variety of bacterial pathogens (see Chap. 87) have emerged as important etiologic agents of gastroenteritis. The rotaviruses are primarily pathogens of young children. The Norwalk and related enteric caliciviruses affect predominantly older children and adults.

ROTAVIRUS Classification and characterization Rotaviruses are members of the Reoviridae family. The rotavirus virion consists of a 70-nm double-shelled icosahedral capsid which surrounds a genome composed of 11 segments of double-stranded RNA. The virus has two surface proteins which are both involved with viral neutralization. Because rotaviruses have a segmented genome, they are capable of undergoing gene reassortment at very high frequency. The role of gene reassortment in generating rotavirus antigenic diversity is not known. In humans, rotavirus infection is characterized by replication that is localized almost exclusively in the small intestinal epithelial cells.

Epidemiology Rotavirus infection occurs worldwide. By the age of 3, virtually every individual has been infected by rotaviruses at least once. In areas with a temperate climate, rotavirus infection is seasonal, occurring in the cooler winter months. In the United States, the annual seasonal rotavirus epidemic tends to spread from West to East, starting in California and ending in New England. In tropical areas, rotavirus infection tends to occur throughout the year, with some increase in incidence during the cooler rainy season. Rotaviruses are the single most important cause of severe dehydrating diarrhea in infants and young children under age 3 in both developed and less developed countries and account for between 30 and 50 percent of all cases of diarrhea requiring hospitalization or intensive rehydration therapy. Although rotavirus infections are primarily confined to infants and small children, they are frequently associated with diarrhea in adults, particularly family members of affected infants, geriatric patients, and immunocompromised hosts. They account for up to 10 percent of traveler's diarrhea (see Chap. 87). Rotaviruses also may be responsible for some cases of acute and chronic diarrhea in patients with AIDS. Subclinical infections or mild gastrointestinal illnesses which do not require hospitalization account for the majority of rotavirus infections. Subclinical infections also have been documented in neonates; these infections were shown to protect against severe rotavirus gastroenteritis for up to 3 years. At least eight distinct serotypes of human rotavirus have been described, but only four types are commonly encountered. The relationship of the frequency of infection with these serotypes to host immune status is unclear. A large variety of other mammals and avian species can be infected by rotavirus, but it does not appear that these animal rotavirus strains cause disease in humans under most conditions. Rotaviruses are shed in very large numbers (up to 10^{10} particles per gram of feces) in the stool; it is presumed that transmission occurs via fecal-oral spread.

Pathophysiology   Rotavirus infects and kills the mature villous tip cells of the small intestine. The mature epithelial cells are replaced by immature absorptive cells that cannot absorb carbohydrates or other nutrients efficiently. Rotavirus infection leads to an osmotic diarrhea due to nutrient malabsorption. Changes in intracellular cyclic adenosine monophosphate or guanosine monophosphate are not involved in the etiology of rotavirus diarrhea.

Manifestations   These range from subclinical infections to mild diarrhea to severe, occasionally fatal illness. Most information concerning the signs and symptoms of rotavirus infection has been derived from studies of hospitalized young children. The onset of illness is usually abrupt. Vomiting, followed by diarrhea, occurs in over 80 percent of affected children. About one-third of hospitalized children will have a temperature greater than 39°C (102.2°F). Gastrointestinal symptoms usually last between 2 and 6 days. Mucus is commonly found in the stool, but white and red blood cells are present in less than 15 percent of cases. Rotavirus infection frequently occurs in conjunction with respiratory tract symptoms, but there is little evidence to indicate that rotavirus replicates in the respiratory tract. Rotavirus infection has been observed in association with a wide variety of other clinical syndromes, including sudden infant death syndrome, Reye's syndrome, encephalitis, aseptic meningitis, pneumonia, exanthem subitum, Kawasaki's syndrome, necrotizing enterocolitis, intussusception, Schönlein-Henoch purpura, hemolytic uremic syndrome, disseminated intravascular coagulation, and Crohn's disease. The etiologic relationship between these clinical syndromes and rotavirus infection is probably coincidental rather than causal. Rotavirus infection may be especially severe, and even fatal, in immunocompromised children.

Clinical immunity   Relative immunity to rotavirus illness is acquired following infection early in childhood. Immunity is not complete, and adults with low levels of antibody can be symptomatically infected. Local immunity appears to be a critical determinant in protection, and cellular immune mechanisms appear to be involved as well.

Diagnosis   Because rotavirus is shed in large amounts in the stool, detection is relatively easy. A variety of specific commercial immunoassays are available to detect rotavirus antigen in fecal specimens. DNA probe diagnosis also appears to be sensitive and specific. There are no pathognomonic signs or symptoms of rotavirus infection, but rotavirus infection is more frequently associated with severe dehydration than are infections caused by other enteric bacterial or viral pathogens.

Treatment and prevention   Despite the fact that rotavirus diarrhea is caused by intestinal epithelial cell lysis and death, it can be adequately treated by standard oral rehydration therapy. Only rarely is intravenous rehydration required. Since rotavirus infections have persisted in developed countries with advanced sanitation facilities and widely available clean water, it is unlikely that the viral infection will be preventable by hygienic measures alone. Progress with a number of candidate live attenuated vaccines suggests that prevention through vaccination may be feasible in the future.

NORWALK AND RELATED ENTERIC CALICIVIRUSES   Classification and characterization   A variety of round 27- to 32-nm particles, some with clearly defined ultrastructure, have been identified in the stools of individuals with acute nonbacterial gastroenteritis. These agents have not been definitely classified because they are shed in the stool in small amounts for only a few days, and they have not been adapted to cell culture or to animal models. The Norwalk virus represents the most extensively studied and best characterized member of this group of agents, which also includes such serologically distinct viruses as the Hawaii agent, the Snow Mountain agent, the W-Ditchling agent, and a number of agents described as calicivirus-like.

The Norwalk virus and the Snow Mountain virus appear to have a protein structure similar to that of typical caliciviruses. Recently, the genome of Norwalk virus has been cloned and partially sequenced. It is a plus-stranded RNA molecule of approximately 7.5 kilobases.

Epidemiology   Norwalk infection occurs year round and is common. From 58 to 70 percent of adults in both developed and less developed countries have antibodies to this virus. Antibody acquisition occurs at a considerably younger age in children in less developed countries than in those in developed areas, consistent with the presumption that Norwalk virus is spread by the fecal-oral route. In developed countries, the virus is responsible for approximately one-third of all epidemics of nonbacterial gastroenteritis. Norwalk virus has been incriminated in a variety of food-borne epidemics, and transmission vehicles have included oysters, green salad, and chocolate icing. The virus is a common cause of waterborne epidemics of gastroenteritis and has been shown to be the etiologic agent in nursing home, cruise ship, and institutional (summer camps and schools) outbreaks. Norwalk virus is also responsible for a small proportion of cases of traveler's diarrhea.

In less developed countries, the role of Norwalk virus infection in the etiology of diarrhea has not been thoroughly investigated. Preliminary studies indicate that Norwalk virus can cause mild diarrhea in young children, but it does not appear to cause severe illness in infants in either developed or less developed countries. The other serologically distinct calicivirus-like gastroenteritis agents must be studied in more detail before their epidemiology can be distinguished from that of Norwalk virus. It appears, however, that some human caliciviruses, especially those with well-defined ultrastructure, are primarily pathogens of young children rather than adults.

Pathophysiology   Following infection with Norwalk or Hawaii virus, the proximal small intestinal architecture is altered, with villus shortening, crypt hyperplasia, and lamina propria infiltration by polymorphonuclear and mononuclear cells. Changes are not observed in the stomach or colon. The cells in which viral replication occurs have not been identified. The histologic alterations are accompanied by mild steatorrhea, carbohydrate malabsorption, and decreased levels of some brush border enzymes. Changes in adenylate cyclase activity have not been observed.

Manifestations   Norwalk illness has an incubation period of between 18 and 72 h. Disease is characterized by the abrupt onset of nausea and abdominal cramps followed by vomiting and/or diarrhea. Vomiting occurs more frequently in children than adults. Low-grade fever [above 37.5°C (99.5°F)] is seen in about half of affected individuals. Headache, myalgias, and abdominal pain are common. The white blood cell count is normal; rarely, there is leukocytosis with a relative lymphopenia. Red and white cells are not found in the stool. The illness is usually mild and self-limited, lasting 24 to 48 h.

Clinical immunity   For most people, long-term (2 years or greater) resistance to Norwalk reinfection does not occur. In volunteers challenged with Norwalk agent, there is a paradoxical relationship between the level of antibody to Norwalk virus and susceptibility to illness. Low levels of Norwalk antibody in the serum and intestine are associated with clinical resistance to illness. It appears, therefore, that immune mechanisms are not the primary determinants of protection from Norwalk virus.

Diagnosis, treatment, and prevention   Radioimmunoassays and an enzyme-linked immunosorbent assay (ELISA) have been developed for Norwalk virus and several other 27- to 30-nm gastroenteritis agents. These tests are not yet available commercially. Recently, detection assays based on nucleic acid probing and the polymerase chain reaction also have been developed. Norwalk illness is acute and self-limited; treatment is not usually required. In the rare case of severe vomiting or diarrhea, oral or intravenous rehydration is indicated. Because long-term immunity to Norwalk illness does not usually follow natural infection, it seems unlikely that a vaccine will be developed.

MISCELLANEOUS ENTERIC VIRAL PATHOGENS   Enteric adenoviruses are a minor (10 percent) cause of diarrheal illness in infants and children. These viruses differ from other adenovirus strains in a variety of ways, including neutralization serotype, restriction endonuclease digestion pattern, and ability to grow in tissue culture. The role of enteric adenovirus illness in adults or in persons in less developed countries is not known.

Several strains of antigenically distinct rotaviruses, presently called "atypical rotaviruses" or group B and C rotaviruses, have been identified as the cause of occasional episodes of diarrhea in humans and animals.

Preliminary epidemiologic studies have indicated that astroviruses are a relatively frequent cause of mild to moderate diarrhea in young children in developed and less developed countries, accounting for about half as much illness as group A rotaviruses. Astroviruses are 27 to 32 nm in diameter, have a characteristic icosahedral ultrastructure, and contain a plus-stranded RNA genome with a size of approximately 7.8 kilobases. The recent availability of sensitive and specific diagnostic assays should facilitate more complete assessment of the importance of these agents.

Coronaviruses are frequent causes of diarrheal disease in a variety of animals. Several investigators, using electron microscopy, have identified putative coronavirus-like particles in the stools of patients with diarrhea. In most cases, however, these particles do not have the typical morphologic features of coronaviruses and may represent bacterial breakdown products or cellular fragments.

REFERENCES

BLACK RE et al: A two-year study of bacterial, viral and parasitic agents associated with diarrhea in rural Bangladesh. J Infect Dis 142:660, 1980

BLACKLOW NR, GREENBERG HB: Viral gastroenteritis. N Engl J Med 325:252, 1991

HO M et al: Rotavirus as a cause of diarrheal morbidity and mortality in the United States. J Infect Dis 158:1112, 1988

JIANG X et al: Norwalk virus genome cloning and characterization. Science 250:1580, 1990

KAPIKIAN AZ, CHANOCK RM: Rotaviruses, in *Virology*, vol 2, 2d ed, BN Fields, DM Knipe, RM Chanock, MS Hirsch, JL Melnick, TP Monath (eds). New York, Raven, 1990, p 1353

LEBARON CW et al: Annual rotavirus epidemic patterns in North America. JAMA 264:983, 1990

MATSUI SM et al: The isolation and characterization of a Norwalk virus-specific cDNA. J Clin Invest 87:1456, 1991

154 ENTEROVIRUSES AND REOVIRUSES

C. GEORGE RAY

GENERAL CONSIDERATIONS

Enteroviruses consist of a major subgroup of picornaviruses that include the polioviruses, coxsackieviruses, echoviruses, and more recently discovered agents that are simply designated enteroviruses. The number of serotypes that infect humans is nearly 70, and more are likely to be found in the future. Their name is derived from their ability to infect intestinal tract epithelial and lymphoid tissues and to be shed into the feces.

Enteroviruses can cause paralytic disease, encephalitis and acute aseptic meningitis syndromes, pleurodynia, exanthems, pericarditis, myocarditis, nonspecific febrile illness, and occasional fulminant disease in the newborn. The spectrum of disease may be even broader. Some infections can lead to permanent damage, and others may trigger chronic, active disease processes.

Since these viruses have many features in common, they will first be considered as a group. Some of the special features of important serotypes will be discussed in detail later in this chapter.

CHARACTERISTICS OF ENTEROVIRUSES As a group, the picornaviruses are extremely small (22 to 30 nm in diameter), single-stranded RNA viruses with icosahedral symmetry. In contrast to the rhinoviruses, the enterovirus subgroup is resistant to ether, acid pH (3.0), and bile. Another feature is cationic stability; in the presence of magnesium chloride, the viruses become more resistant to thermal inactivation. They can survive for prolonged periods in sewage and even in chlorinated water if sufficient organic debris is present. Although some of the enterovirus serotypes share antigens, there are no significant serologic relationships between the major classes listed in Table 154-1; however, a single, highly conserved epitope may be shared by virtually all serotypes. Genetic variation within specific strains occurs, and mutants which exhibit antigenic drift and altered tropism for specific cell types have been recognized. Definitive identification of isolates usually requires neutralization tests.

Most of these agents can be isolated in primate (human or simian) cell cultures; however, some strains, such as several coxsackievirus group A serotypes, are grown with difficulty in vitro, and inoculation of newborn mice may be necessary for detection. This latter procedure was one basis for the original classification of group A and B coxsackieviruses. After the mice have been inoculated, at 24 h of age or less, and observed for 2 to 12 days, group A viruses primarily have a widespread, inflammatory, necrotic effect on skeletal muscle, leading to flaccid paralysis and usually death; similar inoculation of group B viruses causes encephalitis, resulting in spasticity and occasionally convulsions. Other organs are variably affected, and histopathologic examination is sometimes helpful in distinguishing the two. Echoviruses and polioviruses rarely have an adverse effect on mice, unless special adaptation procedures are employed. The higher-numbered enteroviruses (types 68 to 71), which have overlapping growth and host characteristics, have been classified separately.

Humans are the major natural host for the polioviruses, coxsackieviruses, and echoviruses. There are enteroviruses of other animals with limited host ranges that do not appear to extend to humans. Conversely, viruses thought to be identical or related to human enteroviruses have been isolated from dogs and cats. Whether these agents cause disease in the animals is debatable, and there is no evidence of spread from animals to humans.

EPIDEMIOLOGY The enteroviruses have a worldwide distribution, and asymptomatic infection is common. The proportion of infected individuals who will develop illness varies from 2 to 100 percent depending on the serotype or strain involved, prior immune status, and age of the patient. Secondary infections in households are common and range as high as 40 to 70 percent depending on factors such as family size, crowding, and sanitary conditions.

There is a seasonal predilection; epidemics are usually observed during the summer and fall. In subtropical and tropical climates, the duration of greatest transmission sometimes extends into the winter. Certain serotypes emerge as dominant strains during some years; they then may wane, only to reappear in epidemics years later.

Direct or indirect fecal-oral transmission is considered the most common mode of spread. After infection, the virus persists in the oropharynx for 1 to 4 weeks, and it can be shed in the feces for 1 to 18 weeks. Sewage-contaminated water, contaminated foods, or insect

TABLE 154-1 Enteroviruses that infect humans

Class	Number of serotypes
Poliovirus	3
Coxsackievirus	
Group A	23*
Group B	6
Echovirus	31
Enterovirus	Types 68–71†

* Includes several subtypes; coxsackievirus A23 is the same as echovirus 9.
† The classification of the more recently described enteroviruses is based on overlapping biologic characteristics. These are identified numerically.

vectors (flies, cockroaches) may occasionally be the source of infection. More commonly, however, spread is directly from person to person. Approximately two-thirds of all isolates are from children 9 years of age or younger.

Incubation periods vary, but relatively short intervals (2 to 10 days) are the rule. Illness is often seen concurrently in more than one family member, and the clinical features may vary within the household.

PATHOGENESIS AND PATHOLOGY After primary replication in the epithelial cells and lymphoid tissues in the upper respiratory and gastrointestinal tracts, viremic spread to other sites can occur. Potential target organs vary according to the virus strain and its tropism but may include the central nervous system, heart, vascular endothelium, liver, pancreas, gonads, lungs, skeletal muscles, synovial tissues, skin, and mucous membranes. Histopathologic findings include cell necrosis and mononuclear cell inflammatory infiltrates; in the central nervous system, the inflammatory cells are localized most prominently in perivascular sites. The initial tissue damage is thought to result from the lytic cycle of virus replication. Viremia is usually undetectable when symptoms appear, and termination of virus replication commences with the appearance of circulating interferon, neutralizing antibody, and mononuclear cell infiltrations of infected tissue. The early antibody response is mainly immunoglobulin M–specific and usually wanes 6 to 12 weeks after onset to be replaced by IgG-specific antibodies.

Although initial acute tissue damage may be caused by the lytic effects of the virus on the cell, many of the secondary sequelae appear to be immunologically mediated. Enterovirus-caused poliomyelitis, disseminated disease of the newborn, aseptic meningitis, encephalitis, exanthems, and acute respiratory illnesses, thought to represent primary lytic infections, can usually be identified through routine methods of virus isolation and determination of specific antibody titer changes. On the other hand, syndromes such as myopericarditis, nephritis, and myositis have been associated with enteroviruses primarily by serologic evidence and the use of cDNA probes to detect viral RNA in tissues. Viral isolation is the exception. The pathogenesis of these illnesses involves cell-mediated immunologic responses to tissue injury by the virus or to viral or virus-induced antigens that persist in the affected tissues.

Infection by a specific serotype in an immunologically normal host is followed by a humoral antibody response, which can often be detected by neutralization methods for many years thereafter. There is relative immunity to reinfection by the same serotype; however, reinfection has been reported, usually resulting in subclinical infection or mild illness. Although there is some antigenic sharing between serotypes in some of the enterovirus classes (e.g., group B coxsackieviruses), there is no evidence of significant heterotypic immunity to infection by different serotypes.

LABORATORY DIAGNOSIS In acute enteroviral infections, the diagnosis is most readily established by virus isolation from throat swabs, stool or rectal swabs, body fluids, and occasionally tissues. Except in young infants, viremia is usually not detected. When there is central nervous system involvement, cerebrospinal fluid (CSF) cultures taken during the acute phase of the disease may be positive in 10 to 85 percent of cases (except in poliovirus infections, in which virus recovery from this site is rare) depending on the stage of illness and the serotype involved. Direct isolation of virus from affected tissues or body fluids in enclosed spaces (e.g., pleural, pericardial, or CSF) usually confirms the diagnosis. Isolation of an enterovirus from the throat is suggestive of an etiologic association because the virus is usually detectable at this site for only 2 days to 2 weeks after infection; isolation of virus from fecal specimens only must be interpreted more cautiously because asymptomatic shedding from the bowel may persist for as long as 4 months.

The diagnosis may be further supported by a fourfold or greater neutralizing antibody titer increase in paired acute and convalescent serum samples. This method is expensive and cumbersome, requiring careful selection of serotypes for use as antigens. Serodiagnosis is generally reserved for critical situations in which the etiology is questionable, such as isolation of a virus only from a peripheral source such as the feces or, in illnesses such as myopericarditis, in which the yield on routine culture is low and the number of serotypes that might be expected to be involved is limited. Quantitative interpretations of antibody titers on single serum samples are rarely helpful because of the high prevalence and wide range of titers to different serotypes that can be found in healthy individuals. In acute poliovirus infections, complement-fixing antibody titer determinations on acute and convalescent sera can aid in diagnosis.

Recently, it has been shown that common enteroviral RNA sequences can be revealed by the polymerase chain reaction, enhancing and often speeding detection in tissue and CSF. However, routine diagnostic testing for enterovirus infections by this method is not currently available.

White blood cell counts and the erythrocyte sedimentation rates are usually only mildly elevated. If there is necrosis (e.g., liver, lung), a neutrophilic reaction may be noted. Hyperbilirubinemia and elevated transaminase and alkaline phosphatase levels may be seen in patients with hepatitis. Albuminuria often occurs transiently, but hematuria is rare.

PROPHYLAXIS AND TREATMENT Vaccines, which are available only for the prevention of poliovirus infections, will be discussed in detail below. Although proper disposal of feces and careful personal hygiene are recommended, the usual quarantine or isolation measures are relatively ineffective in controlling the spread of enteroviruses in the family or community.

None of the currently available antiviral agents or immune serum globulins has been effective in treatment or prophylaxis of enterovirus infections. The only exception may be the intravenous or intraventricular use of high-titered immunoglobulin in the treatment of chronic enteroviral encephalitis in antibody-deficient patients. Otherwise, treatment is entirely symptomatic and supportive. Glucocorticoids are contraindicated.

POLIOVIRUS INFECTIONS

The most important enteroviruses are the three poliovirus serotypes (types 1, 2, and 3). They first emerged as important causes of disease in developed temperate-zone countries during the latter part of the nineteenth century and continue to be a serious public health problem in some developing countries. In 1988, the World Health Organization committed itself to the global elimination of poliomyelitis by the year 2000. Thus far, eradication efforts have been particularly successful in the Western Hemisphere, where reported cases of wild-type poliovirus infections dropped to a low of 9 in 1991 and none during the first 9 months of 1992; most recently, these have all been localized in areas of Colombia and Peru.

The particular tropism of polioviruses for the central nervous system, which they usually reach by passage across the blood-CNS barrier, is perhaps favored by reflex dilatation of capillaries supplying the affected motor centers of the anterior horn of the brainstem or spinal cord. An alternate pathway may be via entry into motor neurons at peripheral neuromuscular junctions. Motor neurons are particularly vulnerable to infection and variable degrees of destruction. The histopathologic findings in the brainstem and spinal cord include necrosis of neuronal cells and perivascular "cuffing" by infiltration with mononuclear cells, primarily lymphocytes.

CLINICAL MANIFESTATIONS Most infections (perhaps 90 percent) are either subclinical or extremely mild. When disease does result, the incubation period can be from 4 to 35 days but is usually between 7 and 14 days. The disease falls into three classes: The first, *abortive poliomyelitis*, is a nonspecific febrile illness of 2- to 3-day duration with no signs of CNS localization. A second group of patients will additionally develop *aseptic meningitis*. Recovery is rapid and complete, usually within a few days. The third class, *paralytic poliomyelitis*, is the major possible outcome of infection and is often preceded by a period of fever and "minor illness." Classically, after several days, symptoms disappear. In 5 to 10 days fever recurs, and signs of meningeal irritation and asymmetric flaccid paralysis ensue. Cramping muscle pain and spasm as well as coarse twitching in affected parts follows. The maximum extent of involvement is apparent within a few days after first paralysis. In children under 5 years, paralysis of one leg is most common. In patients 5 to 15 years of age, weakness of one arm or paraplegia is frequent, while in adults, quadriplegia is more likely to occur. Urinary bladder and respiratory muscle dysfunction are also frequent in adults. Encephalitis is rare.

Tendon reflexes are diminished or absent. Sensation is intact, in contrast to the usually symmetric paralysis and mild sensory disturbance of the Guillain-Barré syndrome. Paralysis due to heavy metal poisoning also may be difficult to distinguish clinically from poliomyelitis.

Among paralytic cases, 6 to 25 percent may be bulbar. Myocarditis, hypertension, pulmonary edema, shock, nosocomial gram-negative or staphylococcal pneumonias, urinary tract infections, and emotional problems are among the complications of severe paralytic disease. Treatment is supportive. About 2 to 5 percent of children and 15 to 30 percent of adults with paralyzing infection die. As temporarily damaged neurons regain their function, recovery begins and may continue for as long as 6 months. Paralysis persisting beyond that time is permanent and may be associated with complaints of severe pain in the affected areas that sometimes recurs years after the illness.

Some patients develop progressive muscle weakness, usually beginning 20 to 30 years later. This is called *postpoliomyelitis neuromuscular atrophy*, or the *postpolio syndrome*. Symptoms vary from mild to moderate deterioration of function, with fatigue, muscle pain, fasciculations, and weakness that may stabilize or progress to muscle atrophy. The limbs are often affected; in addition, clinical or subclinical involvement of the bulbar and respiratory musculature can sometimes lead to severe dysphagia, choking episodes, aspiration, or sleep apnea. The pathogenesis is usually considered to involve a dysfunction of surviving motor neurons with slow disintegration of axon terminals, leading to late denervation of muscle. There is also evidence suggesting that reactivation of latent or persistent poliovirus in the central nervous system may occur in some patients.

PREVENTION Two types of poliovirus vaccines are currently licensed in the United States: inactivated polio vaccine and live, oral, attenuated virus vaccine. Each contains the three serotypes of poliomyelitis virus.

Inactivated polio vaccine (IPV) has been used extensively in some countries, notably Sweden, Finland, and the Netherlands, and its efficacy has been excellent. The current product is considered safe, with no significant deleterious side effects. In 1988, a more potent IPV, which is produced in human diploid cells, was licensed. This enhanced-potency IPV has been shown to produce 99 to 100 percent seropositivity for all three poliovirus types after two doses in infants. Primary vaccination with three subcutaneous doses (two doses 4 to 8 weeks apart and the third 6 to 12 months later) is recommended for unimmunized children and adults. A booster dose at the time of school entry is recommended for children. The duration of protection is at least 5 years and may be considerably longer.

Oral polio vaccine (OPV) is composed of live, attenuated viruses. The vaccine is given as a primary series of three doses (the first two doses usually 6 to 8 weeks apart and the third 8 to 12 months later) and produces antibodies to all three serotypes in more than 95 percent of recipients. As with IPV, recall boosters are recommended to maintain adequate antibody levels. Like wild poliovirus, OPV viruses infect and replicate in the oropharynx and intestinal tract and may be shed into the feces for 6 weeks or longer.

One disadvantage of OPV is the remote risk of vaccine-associated paralytic disease in some recipients, such as immunocompromised persons; susceptible adults are at a higher risk than children. The incidence of vaccine-associated paralytic poliomyelitis is estimated to be approximately 1 per 2.6 million doses distributed and 1 per 520,000 after the first dose. Of the 138 cases of paralytic poliomyelitis

reported in the United States from 1973 through 1984, 105 were vaccine-associated (35 in healthy recipients, 50 in close contacts, 14 with immune-deficiency conditions, and 6 with no history of vaccination or contact).

The major advantages of OPV include ease of administration and secondary immunization of nonimmune contacts through shedding of vaccine virus into the intestinal tract, resulting in more widespread immunity in the population. It is also theorized that during outbreaks, transient vaccine virus colonization results in the induction of mucosal immunity (primarily through secretory IgA), which may interfere with subsequent acquisition and spread of wild poliovirus.

The choice between IPV and OPV for routine primary immunization is widely debated; however, it is clear that both are highly effective vaccines and that immunization with one or the other is important in the prevention of disease. Ideally, immunization should commence in infancy. A susceptible adult at risk of exposure to infection because of occupation or travel to an endemic area should receive complete immunization, preferably with IPV. Persons with immunodeficiency or altered immune status should not be exposed to OPV, either directly or by household contact, because of the increased risk of vaccine-associated paralysis. Other situations where IPV· immunization is specifically indicated include persons with compromised immunity who are unimmunized or partially immunized, human immunodeficiency virus–infected patients, whether or not symptomatic, household contacts of either of the above groups, and partially immunized or unimmunized adults (or other close contacts) in households of children to be given OPV, but only if timely immunization of the child can be ensured.

Although there are no currently recognized areas of wild poliovirus prevalence in the United States, importation of these strains can occur from endemic areas in developing nations. Once introduced into a community, the virus can spread rapidly among susceptible individuals. For this reason, continuing immunization programs are of utmost importance in preventing spread of this disease.

COXSACKIEVIRUSES AND ECHOVIRUSES

The coxsackieviruses and echoviruses are widespread throughout the world. The basic features of their epidemiology and pathogenesis are the same as those of the polioviruses. Unlike polioviruses, they have a tendency to affect the meninges and occasionally the cerebrum, and only rarely do they affect anterior horn cells.

The consequences of infection with these agents are highly variable and related only in part to virus subgroup and serotype. Up to 60 percent of infections are subclinical. The main interest in these agents stems from their ability to cause more serious illness, which becomes most evident during epidemics.

Inapparent infection is common, but it varies with the infecting strain and the host involved. The manifestations of illness range from mild to lethal and from acute to chronic. Table 154-2 lists the major syndromes and serotypes commonly associated with each. Considerable overlap occurs, however, and it is not surprising to find different enteroviral serotypes associated with any specific syndrome. The group B coxsackieviruses generally have the greatest latitude with regard to tissue tropism.

ASEPTIC MENINGITIS (See Chap. 375) In terms of relative frequency, aseptic meningitis is the most important illness associated with enterovirus infections. This syndrome can be mild and self-limiting; however, it is occasionally accompanied by encephalitis, which can lead to permanent sequelae, particularly in infants. Overall, enteroviruses cause the majority of all nonbacterial CNS infections now observed in the United States.

There may be a mild prodromal malaise, but major illness usually begins with fever, headache, and stiff neck. Kernig's and Brudzinski's signs may be present. Localizing sensory or motor deficits are unusual. Confusion and delirium are common. These acute findings may persist for 4 to 7 days. Cerebrospinal pleocytosis is usually less than 500

TABLE 154-2 Clinical syndromes reported to be commonly associated with enterovirus serotypes

Syndrome	Coxsackievirus Group A	Coxsackievirus Group B	Echovirus and enterovirus (E)
Aseptic meningitis, encephalitis	2,4,7,9,10	1,2,3,4,5	4,6,9,11,16,30; E70,E71
Muscle weakness and paralysis (poliomyelitis-like disease)	7,9	2,3,4,5	2,4,6,9,11,30;E71
Cerebellar ataxia	2,4,9	3,4	4,6,9
Generalized disease (infants)	——	1,2,3,4,5	3,6,9,11,14,17,19
Exanthems and enanthems	4,5,6,9,10,16	2,3,4,5	2,4,5,6,9,11,16,18, 25;E71
Pericarditis, myocarditis	4,16	2,3,4,5	1,6,8,9,19
Epidemic myalgia (pleurodynia), orchitis	9	1,2,3,4,5	1,6,9
Respiratory symptoms	9,16,21,24	1,3,4,5	4,9,11,20,25
Conjunctivitis	24	1,5	7;E70

cells per microliter. Early, there may be as many as 90 percent polymorphonuclear leukocytes, but within 48 h the cellular response usually becomes predominantly or totally mononuclear. Persistence of polymorphonuclear leukocytes in the CSF suggests pyogenic meningitis or intracerebral, subdural, or epidural abscess. Gram's stain and appropriate CSF cultures must be done to exclude bacterial meningitis, tuberculosis, or mycotic meningitis. Protein concentration in the CSF is moderately elevated, but glucose is usually normal. Early in the illness enteroviruses may be isolated from CSF, even in the absence of significant pleocytosis. It usually takes several weeks before the CSF reverts to normal. An occasional patient may develop a transient syndrome of inappropriate secretion of antidiuretic hormone. In hypo- or agammaglobulinemic syndromes echoviruses have persisted in CSF for months to years, producing a progressive encephalitis or polymyositis.

For attempts at virus isolation, throat, stool, and CSF specimens should be collected as early in the course as possible. Acute and convalescent sera also can be studied for rises in type-specific neutralizing antibodies in patients in whom viral isolation results are negative or equivocal.

It is often not possible to distinguish clinically between aseptic meningitis due to various enteroviruses, arboviruses, Epstein-Barr virus, human immunodeficiency virus type 1, or mumps. Localizing findings, hemiplegia, oculogyric crises, coma, and bloody CSF favor the diagnosis of type 1 herpes simplex virus encephalitis (see Chap. 143). Although enterovirus aseptic meningitis most often is self-limited and recovery in persons afflicted after the first year of life is usually complete within 1 to 2 weeks, about 10 percent of patients have more serious involvement of the central nervous system. Minor muscle weakness with reflex changes may persist for weeks to months, but over 90 percent of patients recover completely within a year. Occasionally, choreiform movements, ataxia, nystagmus, transverse myelitis, Guillain-Barré syndrome, poliomyelitis-like symptoms, coma, bulbar involvement, and death occur.

OTHER ENTEROVIRAL ILLNESSES *Generalized disease of the newborn* is a highly lethal expression of enteroviral infection in which the infant may be overwhelmed by simultaneous virus infection of the heart, liver, adrenals, brain, and other organs.

Acute myocarditis and/or pericarditis can be caused by a variety of viral agents; however, it is estimated that as many as 50 percent of cases are associated with infection by coxsackievirus B. Such infections are usually self-limited, but they can lead to a fatal outcome (arrhythmia or heart failure) or cause chronic heart disease (see Chaps. 205 and 206).

The exanthems may or may not be associated with CNS inflammation. The rashes can resemble rubella, roseola infantum, or adenovirus

exanthems. They are usually macular or maculopapular, with sparing of the palmar and plantar surfaces. This latter feature contrasts with the frequently prominent distal extremity involvement seen with otherwise similar-appearing eruptions caused by some drugs, Kawasaki disease, syphilis, rickettsial infections, staphylococcal and streptococcal toxins, and rat-bite fevers. Vesicular or hemangioma-like lesions also have been associated with enterovirus infections. Hand-foot-and-mouth disease usually affects children and is characterized by a vesicular eruption over the extremities and the anterior oral cavity. Coxsackievirus A16 is the specific agent most frequently implicated, but others, such as enterovirus 71, can cause a similar illness.

Herpangina is an enanthematous (mucous membrane) disease characterized by the acute onset of fever and sore throat. Characteristic small vesicles or white papules (lymphonodules) surrounded by a red halo are seen over the posterior half of the palate, pharynx, and tonsillar areas. This mild, self-limiting (1 to 2 weeks) illness usually has been associated with infection by several different group A coxsackievirus serotypes.

Epidemic myalgia (pleurodynia, or Bornholm disease) is characterized by fever and sudden onset of intense upper abdominal or lower thoracic pain, often accompanied by a frontal headache. The pain may be aggravated by movement, such as breathing or coughing, and usually persists for 3 to 14 days. Group B coxsackieviruses are most frequently implicated.

A variety of other illnesses also may result from infections by this subgroup. Epidemic acute hemorrhagic keratoconjunctivitis associated with enterovirus 70 has been reported in Asia and the United States, and outbreaks of disease resembling paralytic poliomyelitis caused by enterovirus 71 infection have occurred in Bulgaria, Australia, and the United States. Sporadic cases of poliomyelitis-like disease also have been reported with other enterovirus infections, notably coxsackievirus A7 and several echovirus serotypes. There is some evidence that certain enteroviruses may participate in the pathogenesis of at least some cases of insulin-dependent diabetes mellitus, acute arthritis, polymyositis, hemolytic-uremic syndrome, and idiopathic acute nephritis.

REOVIRUS INFECTIONS

The reoviruses (respiratory enteric orphans) are naked virions that contain double-stranded RNA. They have been found in humans, simians, cattle, rodents, and a variety of other hosts. Three serotypes are known to infect humans; however, their role and relative importance in causing disease remain uncertain. Sporadic cases of febrile upper respiratory infections, exanthems, pneumonia, hepatitis, encephalitis, and gastroenteritis have all been reported to be associated with these viruses. Reovirus type 3 has been implicated as a possible cause of biliary atresia and neonatal hepatitis, but this relationship remains uncertain. Asymptomatic shedding of reoviruses often makes it difficult to prove association with disease. Reoviruses can be isolated in cell cultures, particularly primary monkey kidney or human kidney monolayers.

REFERENCES

BARAK Y, SCHWARTZ JF: Acute transverse myelitis associated with echo type 5 infection. Am J Dis Child 142:128, 1988

BOWLES NE et al: Detection of coxsackie-B-virus-specific RNA sequences in myocardial biopsy samples from patients with myocarditis and dilated cardiomyopathy. Lancet 1:1120, 1986

——— et al: Dermatomyositis, polymyositis, and coxsackie-B-virus infection. Lancet 1:1004, 1987

BROWN WR et al: Lack of correlation between infection with reovirus 3 and extrahepatic biliary atresia or neonatal hepatitis. J Pediatr 113:670, 1988

HAYWARD JC et al: Outbreak of poliomyelitis-like paralysis associated with enterovirus 71. Pediatr Infect Dis J 8:611, 1989

JOSSELSON J et al: Acute rhabdomyolysis associated with an echovirus infection. Arch Intern Med 140:1671, 1980

KAPLAN MH et al: Group B coxsackievirus infections in infants younger than three months of age: A serious childhood illness. Rev Infect Dis 5:1019, 1983

MCKINNEY RE JR et al: Chronic enteroviral meningoencephalitis in agammaglobulinemia patients. Rev Infect Dis 9:334, 1987

ONORATO IM et al: Mucosal immunity induced by enhanced-potency inactivated and oral polio vaccines. J Infect Dis 163:1, 1991

QUERFURTH H, SWANSON PD: Vaccine-associated paralytic poliomyelitis: Regional case series and review. Arch Neurol 47:541, 1990

REN R, RACANIELLO VR: Poliovirus spreads from muscle to the central nervous system by neural pathways. J Infect Dis 166:747, 1992

ROTBART HA: Diagnosis of enteroviral meningitis with the polymerase chain reaction. J Pediatr 117:85, 1990

SHARIEF MK et al: Intrathecal immune response in patients with the post-polio syndrome. N Engl J Med 325:749, 1991

SHARPE AH, FIELDS BN: Pathogenesis of viral infections: Basic concepts derived from the reovirus model. N Engl J Med 312:486, 1985

SONIES BC, DALAKOS MD: Dysphagia in patients with the post-polio syndrome. N Engl J Med 324:1162, 1991

WRIGHT PF et al: Strategies for the global eradication of poliomyelitis by the year 2000. N Engl J Med 325:1774, 1991

155 MEASLES (RUBEOLA)

C. GEORGE RAY

DEFINITION Measles, or rubeola, is an acute febrile eruption which has been one of the most common diseases of civilization. Despite the development of an effective vaccine, it remains a worldwide health problem.

ETIOLOGY The measles virion is composed of a central core of ribonucleic acid with a helically arranged protein coat surrounded by a lipoprotein envelope with small, spikelike structures. The virion is 120 to 200 nm in diameter and is classified as a morbillivirus in the paramyxovirus family. There are at least six virion structural proteins, three of which are in the envelope. These latter include the matrix (M) protein that is important in virus assembly and two glycoprotein projections (peplomers); the hemagglutinin (H) mediates attachment to host cells, and the other (F) mediates cell fusion and viral entry into cells.

EPIDEMIOLOGY Measles occurs naturally only in human beings, although infection with the virus can be demonstrated in laboratory colonies of monkeys exposed to infected individuals. Before active immunization was available, epidemics of measles occurred in 2- to 3-year cycles, usually during the spring months, and about 95 percent of urban dwellers developed the disease before the age of 15. The virus is transmitted by transfer of nasopharyngeal secretions, either directly or in airborne droplets, to the respiratory mucous membranes or conjunctivae of susceptible individuals. Persons infected with the virus may transmit the disease during a period which extends from 5 days after exposure until 5 days after skin lesions have appeared. The virus is highly contagious, with secondary attack rates among susceptible household contacts usually exceeding 90 percent; asymptomatic primary infections are rare. In the United States, the number of reported measles cases reached an all-time low of 1492 in 1983. However, this has since increased substantially, particularly in 1990, when nearly 28,000 cases occurred. This rise has been associated with outbreaks among unvaccinated infants and preschool children; other outbreaks have involved groups of high school and college students, where the immunization rates were often 95 percent or greater. Recent data also indicate shifts in age-specific attack rates away from the previous high frequency among children in the 5- to 14-year age group. In 1990, 22 percent of cases occurred in adults 20 years of age or older, and nearly half were in unvaccinated preschool children, mostly minorities.

PATHOGENESIS AND PATHOLOGY Once access has been gained to the respiratory tract epithelium, virus replication com-

mences. This process damages or destroys susceptible cells and promotes cell fusion with formation of syncytia, disruption of the cellular cytoskeleton, chromosomal disorganization, and appearance of nuclear and cytoplasmic inclusion bodies. Initial replication is followed by viremic (and probably lymphatic) dissemination to other sites, including lymphoid tissues, bone marrow, liver and other viscera, eyes, and skin. Viremia is detectable during the prodromal phase, and viruria persists for as long as 4 days after onset of the rash. Virus replication in thymic Hassall's corpuscles, capillary endothelium, and hepatic endothelium also occurs. During viremia, measles can infect T and B lymphocytes, macrophages, and polymorphonuclear leukocytes. These latter events do not cause significant cytolysis but can impair critical general defense functions such as immunoglobulin synthesis and generation of oxygen radicals by polymorphonuclear leukocytes and macrophages. In the early stages of infection, natural killer cells and cytotoxic T cells play a role in limiting virus replication. These, and cytokines produced as a result of immune activation, also play a role in mediating the inflammatory responses observed in the early acute phase. At rash onset, specific antibody becomes detectable, and effector lymphocytes are found in areas of viral replication in the skin and mucosal lesions. This event usually heralds the onset of viral clearance and clinical recovery, as well as the development of anergy; there is depressed hypersensitivity to skin test antigens such as tuberculin and reduced in vitro lymphoproliferation and cytokine production in response to mitogenic stimuli. Anergy can persist for several weeks and is also seen in recipients of live, attenuated measles virus vaccine.

The mucous membrane lesions (Koplik's spots) consist of vesicle formation and epithelial necrosis. Histology of the Koplik's spots reveals cytoplasmic and intranuclear inclusions, giant cells, and intercellular edema. Large multinucleated epithelial giant cells that show inclusion bodies within the nucleus and cytoplasm can be found during the prodrome and acute stages of illness in the buccal mucosa, pharynx, tracheobronchial mucosa, and occasionally the urine. In addition, reticuloendothelial giant cells (Warthin-Finkeldey cells) are found in hyperplastic lymphoid tissues, including lymph nodes, tonsils, spleen, and thymus. The epithelium of the respiratory passages can become necrotic and slough off, leading to secondary bacterial infection; interstitial pneumonia with giant cell infiltration may be observed. Changes in the brain of patients with encephalomyelitis resemble those seen in other postviral encephalitides and consist of focal hemorrhage, congestion, and perivenous demyelination. Levels of soluble CD8 are elevated in the cerebrospinal fluid during the acute phase of postmeasles encephalomyelitis, but virus cannot be detected. The pathogenesis is probably related to infiltration of CD8+ cytotoxic T cells in the brain, which react with target cells—either myelin-forming cells or virus-infected cells.

MANIFESTATIONS The time from exposure to the development of the first symptoms of measles infection is usually 8 to 12 days and from exposure to the appearance of rash about 2 weeks. The initial manifestations of the disease are malaise, irritability, temperature as high as 40.6°C (105°F), conjunctivitis with excessive lacrimation, edema of the eyelids and photophobia, moderately severe hacking cough, and nasal discharge. The prodromal period usually lasts 3 to 4 days, with a range of 1 to 8 days before the onset of a rash. Koplik's spots—small, red, irregular lesions with blue-white centers—appear 1 or 2 days before the onset of the rash on the mucous membranes of the mouth and occasionally on the conjunctivae or intestinal mucosa. The findings of the prodromal illness subside or disappear within 1 or 2 days after the appearance of skin lesions, although the cough may persist throughout the course of the disease.

The red maculopapular rash of measles breaks out first on the forehead, spreads downward over the face, neck, and trunk, and appears on the feet on the third day. The density of lesions is greatest on the forehead, face, and shoulders, where coalescence of individual spots usually occurs. The lesions in each area persist for about 3 days and disappear in the same order in which they appeared, resulting in total duration of rash of about 6 days. As the maculopapules fade, a brown discoloration of the skin may be noticed, and finely granular desquamation may occur. In adults the duration of fever may be longer, the rash more prominent, and the incidence of complications higher.

The course of measles can be altered by the administration of gamma globulin soon after exposure. The incubation period may be prolonged for as long as 20 days. The prodromal period of the modified disease may be shorter; the fever, respiratory symptoms, and conjunctivitis milder; the rash less marked; and Koplik's spots may not be present.

COMPLICATIONS Measles, usually a benign self-limited disease, may be complicated by a number of illnesses. Viral involvement of the respiratory tract may lead to croup, bronchitis, bronchiolitis, or rarely to *interstitial giant cell pneumonia*. The last is seen most often in children suffering from severe systemic disease such as leukemia, congenital or acquired immunodeficiency, or severe malnutrition and is characterized by severe respiratory symptoms, pulmonary infiltration, and multinucleated giant cells in the pulmonary parenchyma. Pneumonitis may occur in the absence of the typical measles exanthem. *Conjunctivitis*, which is seen regularly in the course of uncomplicated measles, may occasionally progress to corneal ulceration, keratitis, and blindness. *Myocarditis*, characterized by transient changes in the electrocardiogram, occurs in about 20 percent of patients with measles, but clinical evidence of cardiac dysfunction is rare. Viral involvement of the mesenteric lymph nodes and appendix may result in abdominal pain and signs of peritoneal inflammation so severe that surgical exploration is considered. The situation is especially confusing if evidence of appendiceal involvement becomes manifest during the preeruptive phase of the disease. *Hepatitis*, usually without clinical signs, also frequently occurs. It is usually detected by the presence of a transient elevation of AST or ALT values during the acute phase of illness. Transient *acute glomerulonephritis* also has been observed during the acute phase of illness. In adults, mild to moderate hypocalcemia and musculoskeletal symptoms with elevated CPK levels have each been reported to occur in one-third or more of cases. Measles infection of pregnant women can be particularly severe and also results in death of the fetus in about 20 percent of the cases; however, a teratogenic effect such as that observed in rubella has not been demonstrated.

Superimposed bacterial pneumonia caused by streptococci, pneumococci, staphylococci, or *Haemophilus influenzae* is considerably more common than giant cell pneumonia and occasionally may progress to empyema or lung abscess. Bacterial otitis media is a frequent sequel of measles infection in children. In tropical areas, stomatitis, probably of bacterial origin, progressing to cancrum oris may be encountered during the course of the disease.

Clinically apparent *encephalomyelitis* occurs in 1 of 1000 patients with measles. It usually begins 4 to 7 days after the appearance of the eruption but may precede the rash by 10 days or follow it by 24 days. It is characterized by high fever, headache, drowsiness, and coma and in some patients by focal brain or spinal cord involvement. Death occurs in about 10 percent of affected individuals, and persistent signs of central nervous system damage, including mental changes, epilepsy, and paralysis, are encountered. Electroencephalographic abnormalities without other signs of CNS dysfunction have been detected in 50 percent of patients with otherwise uncomplicated measles. A progressive, fatal encephalitis has been described in children with lymphatic malignancies treated with immunosuppressive drugs, with onset 1 to 6 months after an episode of measles. Other, more unusual neurologic complications include transverse myelitis and ascending myelitis. An extremely rare condition, *subacute sclerosing panencephalitis* (see Chap. 375), is probably a late complication of measles. *Thrombocytopenia* may occur 3 to 15 days after the onset of symptoms and results in purpura as well as bleeding from mouth, intestine, and genitourinary tract. Measles is also associated with exacerbation of existing tuberculosis and an increased incidence of new tuberculous infections.

LABORATORY FINDINGS Leukopenia is frequent in the prodromal phase of measles, and the appearance of leukocytosis suggests bacterial superinfection or another complication. Extreme lymphopenia (fewer than 2000 lymphocytes per microliter) is considered to be a poor prognostic sign. During the prodrome and in the early eruptive phase, multinucleated giant cells can be identified in stained preparations of sputum, nasal secretions, or urine, and the measles virus can be isolated by inoculation of the same materials onto appropriate cell cultures. Measles antigen can often be detected quickly by fluorescent antibody staining of infected respiratory or urinary epithelial cells. Complement fixation, enzyme immunoassay, immunofluorescent, and hemagglutination inhibition tests are available for serologic confirmation of measles. Spinal fluid protein of patients with encephalomyelitis ranges from 48 to 240 mg/dL, and lymphocyte counts are usually in a range of 5 to 99 cells per microliter, although counts as high as 1000 cells per microliter have been reported. Bacterial infection can be identified by appropriate cultures.

DIFFERENTIAL DIAGNOSIS With its prodrome, Koplik's spots, and characteristic rash, measles is infrequently confused with other diseases. Rubella is a milder disease of shorter duration with mild or no respiratory complaints. Infectious mononucleosis and toxoplasmosis can be identified by the presence of atypical lymphocytes and by serologic tests. Secondary syphilis may show skin lesions similar to the measles rash. Other infections which can sometimes mimic measles include those caused by adenoviruses, enteroviruses, *Mycoplasma pneumoniae*, *Staphylococcus aureus* (toxic shock syndrome), and *Streptococcus pyogenes* (scarlet fever). Drug reactions, particularly those associated with ampicillin and phenytoin, and Kawasaki syndrome also can produce a morbilliform rash.

ATYPICAL MEASLES During the period 1963–1967, a formalin-inactivated ("killed") measles vaccine was given to an estimated 600,000 to 900,000 recipients in the United States. Distribution of this vaccine was discontinued after 1967, but use continued in Canada through 1970. Between 1965 and 1968, there were multiple reports of a severe, atypical illness in children exposed to wild virus who had received killed measles vaccine 2 to 4 years earlier. Subsequently, a similar, although somewhat more variable, syndrome has been described among young adults who were immunized with killed measles vaccine 20 or more years previously. There are also reports of atypical measles among a few individuals who had received live measles vaccine.

The pathogenesis of atypical measles is thought to be related to formalin inactivation of F glycoprotein with preservation of H antigenicity. The resultant lack of antibodies to F may allow cell-to-cell spread of virus by fusion, and the antigens produced could generate immune complexes, cytotoxic cell-mediated responses, or both.

In atypical measles, the incubation period is similar to that of typical measles, but the prodromal period often develops abruptly. High fever, headaches, myalgias, abdominal pain, and a nonproductive cough usually last for 1 to 3 days, followed by an eruption which can be urticarial, maculopapular, hemorrhagic, and/or vesicular. In contrast to natural measles, the rash begins on the hands and feet and progresses toward the head. It is especially prominent on the legs and in the body creases. Koplik's spots are rarely seen. Pneumonia, often associated with extremity edema, frequently occurs. The pneumonia is lobar or segmental; hilar lymphadenopathy and pleural effusion are common. Ill-defined nodular shadows may persist at the periphery of the lung for as long as 2 years. Symptoms often last for 2 weeks or longer. The severity of illness, abruptness of onset, and unique clinical findings that are variably observed have sometimes suggested diagnoses such as Rocky Mountain spotted fever, varicella pneumonia, scarlet fever, or meningococcemia; in the prodromal phase, acute appendicitis and bacterial pneumonia have been considered.

The diagnosis of atypical measles is based on clinical, epidemiologic, and serologic grounds. Unlike typical measles, virus-isolation attempts are generally unsuccessful. Antibodies rapidly increase from undetectable or low levels to very high titers that usually exceed those observed in convalescence from typical measles.

PROPHYLAXIS Active immunity can be induced by the use of live, attenuated measles virus, which does not spread to contacts of vaccinated individuals. The vaccine of choice, even in adults, is measles-mumps-rubella (MMR). Vaccination induces immunity in more than 95 percent of individuals inoculated at 15 months of age or older; this immunity extends for more than 20 years and is probably lifelong. The vaccine also usually provides protection if given within 3 days after exposure. Routine immunization in infancy is begun at 15 months of age; a second dose is recommended at ages 11 to 12 years. Most persons born before 1957 can be considered immune and usually do not need to be vaccinated; however, a small portion of such persons are in fact susceptible and should be considered for immunization unless there is documented proof of immunity, particularly if they are involved in a high-risk outbreak setting. Entrants into colleges and universities and health care workers who do not have clear proof of immunity (physician-diagnosed measles or laboratory evidence of immunity) should be required to provide documentation of two doses of measles vaccine commencing on or after their first birthday; if there has been no previous measles immunization, then the second dose should follow the first by no less than 1 month.

Persons who received killed measles vaccine in the past should be considered unprotected and, in fact, at high risk of severe atypical measles if exposed to wild virus. At least one dose of live vaccine should be given to them as well as to anyone who received vaccine of unknown type in 1963–1967. Measles reimmunization is also recommended for persons who received killed vaccine followed in 3 months by live vaccine, were immunized before their first birthday, or received further attenuated (Schwartz or Moraten strains) or unknown vaccine with immunoglobulin. Asymptomatic (and probably also symptomatic) HIV-infected persons also should be immunized if they are susceptible.

Live measles vaccine should not be given to pregnant women, to patients with untreated tuberculosis, to patients with leukemia or lymphoma, or to those whose immune responsiveness is depressed. However, persons with leukemia who are in remission and have not received chemotherapy for at least 3 months and HIV-infected persons can be vaccinated. All children infected with HIV should be immunized on schedule; the degree of protection is uncertain. Hypersensitivity reactions to the vaccine even among egg-sensitive individuals have been rare; however, extreme caution should be observed in persons with a history of anaphylactic reactions following egg ingestion or receipt of neomycin. Except in unusual circumstances, vaccination should not be given in the first 13 months of life. If epidemiologic circumstances suggest a risk to infants less than 15 months of age, monovalent vaccine or MMR may be given as early as 6 months of age, followed by a dose of MMR vaccine at 15 months of age.

Approximately 5 to 15 percent of nonimmune vaccinees will develop temperatures of 103°F (39.4°C) or higher, usually beginning 5 to 12 days after vaccination and lasting 1 to 2 days; rarely, fever can continue for up to 5 days. The prevalence of vaccine-induced rash is approximately 5 percent. Encephalitis after measles vaccination is extremely rare; it has not been possible to discern its risk from the background prevalence of encephalitis of unknown cause. Prior recipients of killed measles vaccine have a risk of up to 50 percent for reactions to live vaccine. Most such reactions are mild, consisting of local swelling, erythema, and low-grade fever for 1 to 2 days. Rarely, more severe reactions such as lymphadenopathy, prolonged fever, and extensive local Arthus-like reactions are seen. However, recipients of killed measles vaccine are likely to have significantly more serious illness when exposed to natural measles than that which may occur with live vaccine. There is no evidence suggesting an increased risk of adverse effects from measles or MMR vaccines among persons who are already immune.

Measles can be modified or prevented by the intramuscular administration of gamma globulin, 0.25 mL/kg (not to exceed 15 mL), within 6 days of exposure. This approach is not recommended for outbreak control but is useful in situations where measles vaccine is contraindicated (e.g., susceptible pregnant women, persons receiving cancer chemotherapy) or where vaccine-induced immunity cannot be ensured (e.g., HIV-infected patients). If measles immunoglobulins are administered, in either gamma globulin or other blood products, vaccination should be deferred for at least 3 months.

TREATMENT No therapy is indicated for uncomplicated measles. Gamma globulin, although effective in prophylaxis, is of no value once symptoms are evident. In areas where nutritional deficiencies and severe measles are common, vitamin A supplementation (400,000 IU orally) on two successive days as soon as measles is diagnosed may reduce the risk of delayed mortality and blindness. Patients should be monitored for the development of bacterial superinfections, which require appropriate antibiotics on the basis of clinical and bacteriologic findings. Aerosolized ribavirin also has been used for treatment of severe measles pneumonia; however, reports of efficacy have thus far been anecdotal.

REFERENCES

ATMAR RL et al: Complications of measles during pregnancy. Clin Infect Dis 14:217, 1992

BLOCH AB et al: Measles outbreak in a pediatric practice: Airborne transmission in an office setting. Pediatrics 75:676, 1985

CENTERS FOR DISEASE CONTROL: Update on adult immunization: Recommendations of the Immunization Practices Advisory Committee (ACIP). Morb Mort Week Rep 40(no. RR-12):19, 1991

CHERRY JD et al: Atypical measles in children previously immunized with attenuated measles virus vaccines. Pediatrics 50:712, 1972

DERMSTADT GL, HALSEY NA: Measles in mother-infant pairs. Pediatr Infect Dis J 11:492, 1992

FULGINITI VA, HELFER RE: Atypical measles in adolescent siblings 16 years after killed measles virus vaccine. JAMA 244:804, 1980

GAVISH D et al: Hepatitis and jaundice associated with measles in young adults. Arch Intern Med 143, 1983

GILADI M et al: Measles in adults: A prospective study of 291 consecutive cases. Br Med J 295:1314, 1987

GRIFFIN DE et al: Immune activation in measles. N Engl J Med 320:1667, 1989

GUSTAFSON TL et al: Measles outbreak in a fully immunized secondary-school population. N Engl J Med 317:771, 1987

HUSSEY GD, KLEIN M: A randomized, controlled trial of vitamin A in children with severe measles. N Engl J Med 323:160, 1990

LAVI S et al: Administration of measles, mumps, and rubella virus vaccine (live) to egg-allergic children. JAMA 263:269, 1990

MARKOWITZ LE et al: Persistence of measles antibody after revaccination. J Infect Dis 166:205, 1992

MINNICH LL et al: Use of immunofluorescence to identify measles virus infections. J Clin Microbiol 29:1148, 1991

MOUALLEM M et al: Measles epidemic in young adults. Arch Intern Med 147:1111, 1987

NATIONAL VACCINE ADVISORY COMMITTEE: The measles epidemic: The problems, barriers, and recommendations. JAMA 266:1547, 1991

RIVERA ME et al: Nosocomial measles infection in a pediatric hospital during a community-wide epidemic. J Pediatr 119:183, 1991

156 RUBELLA ("GERMAN MEASLES") AND OTHER VIRAL EXANTHEMS

C. GEORGE RAY

RUBELLA

DEFINITION Rubella ("German measles," "3-day measles") is usually a benign febrile exanthem, but when it occurs in pregnant women, it may lead to serious chronic fetal infection and malformations.

ETIOLOGY   In the late 1930s and 1940s rubella was transmitted experimentally to humans and monkeys, and in 1962 a viral agent was recovered in cell cultures inoculated with nasopharyngeal secretions of infected persons. The rubella virion, 60 to 70 nm in diameter, is a somewhat spheroidal RNA virus which has been classified in the togavirus family.

PATHOGENESIS AND PATHOLOGY   Rubella can be induced in susceptible persons by the instillation of virus into the nasopharynx, and natural infection is probably induced in the same way. Initial replication of the virus in the respiratory tract is followed by spread via the bloodstream. Viremia has been detected for as long as 8 days before and up to 2 days after appearance of the rash, and shedding of virus from the oropharynx persists for up to 8 days after the onset of symptoms.

Congenital rubella results from transplacental transmission of virus to the fetus from an infected mother and may be associated with growth retardation, infiltration of liver and spleen by hematopoietic tissue, interstitial pneumonia, a decreased number of megakaryocytes in the bone marrow, and various structural malformations of the cardiovascular and central nervous systems. The virus can persist in the fetus during intrauterine life and may be excreted for 6 to 31 months after birth.

EPIDEMIOLOGY   Rubella is not as contagious as measles, and immunity to the disease is not so widespread. Estimates of susceptibility to rubella among young adults now range from 6 to 11 percent. The number of reported rubella cases in the United States steadily declined from more than 56,000 in 1969, when routine vaccination began, to a low of 225 in 1988. Of the more than 900 cases reported in 1990, approximately 57 percent occurred in persons ≥15 years of age. In addition, at least 20 cases of congenital rubella syndrome were diagnosed among infants born in 1990. Limited outbreaks continue to occur in colleges and work environments (e.g., hospitals), further reflecting an epidemiologic shift away from young children.

MANIFESTATIONS   The time from exposure to the appearance of the rash of rubella is 14 to 21 days, usually about 18 days. In adults there may be a prodromal illness preceding the exanthem by 1 to 7 days. The prodrome consists of malaise, headache, fever, mild conjunctivitis, and lymphadenopathy. In children the rash may be the first manifestation of disease. It is apparent from serologic studies that 25 to 50 percent of infections are subclinical or result in only lymph node enlargement without skin lesions; however, rash without lymphadenopathy is uncommon. Respiratory symptoms are mild or absent. Small, red lesions (Forschheimer spots) occasionally appear on the soft palate but are not pathognomonic of the disease.

The rash begins on the forehead and face and spreads downward to the trunk and extremities. The small maculopapular lesions, of lighter hue than those of measles, are usually discrete but can coalesce to form a diffuse erythema suggestive of scarlet fever. The rash may last from 1 to 5 days but is most commonly present for 3 days. Enlarged, tender lymph nodes appear before the rash, are most impressive during the early eruptive phase, and often persist several days after the rash has disappeared. Splenomegaly or generalized lymphadenopathy may occur, but the postauricular and suboccipital nodes are most strikingly involved. Arthralgias and slight joint swellings sometimes accompany rubella, especially in young women. The pain and swelling, involving wrists, fingers, and knees, are most marked during the period of rash and may persist for 1 to 14 days after other manifestations of rubella have disappeared. Recurring joint symptoms for a year or more also have been reported. Purpura with or without thrombocytopenia may occur and can be associated with hemorrhage. Encephalomyelitis following rubella resembles other postinfectious encephalitides but is much less common than encephalitis following measles. Testicular pain is also occasionally reported in young adults.

Congenital rubella   The syndrome of congenital rubella has conventionally been thought to consist of heart malformations—patent ductus arteriosus, interventricular septal defect, or pulmonic stenosis; eye lesions—corneal clouding, cataracts, chorioretinitis, and micro-

phthalmia; microcephaly; mental retardation; and deafness. In the American epidemic of 1964, thrombocytopenic purpura, hepatosplenomegaly, intrauterine growth retardation, interstitial pneumonia, myocarditis or myocardial necrosis, and metaphyseal bone lesions were encountered frequently in association with the previously recognized manifestations, leading to the term *expanded rubella syndrome*. Some infants also have been found to have significant humoral and/or cellular immunodeficiency, which generally resolves as chronic viral excretion diminishes and eventually ceases. Any combination of lesions may be seen in an individual infant, and the severity is highly variable.

Later complications include an apparent higher risk of development of diabetes mellitus. There are reports of patients with congenital rubella who develop a progressive, subacute panencephalitis, with onset in the second decade of life. It is characterized by intellectual deterioration, ataxia, seizures, and spasticity. T cell abnormalities, including slightly decreased T4/T8 ratios and other minor subset defects, sometimes persist into adulthood.

Congenital rubella is usually the result of maternal infection during the first trimester of pregnancy, although well-documented cases have resulted from infection several days before conception; deafness may occur as a result of infection in the fourth month. The greatest risk to the fetus is when maternal infection develops 3 to 6 weeks after conception. Asymptomatic maternal rubella can result in severe fetal disease. It is therefore desirable to ascertain the immune status of every woman either before conception or as early in the pregnancy as possible by history of previous immunization or by serologic testing. If rubella antibodies are present before or within 10 days after exposure, the patient is considered immune, and the risk of fetal damage is virtually nil. If antibodies are not detectable and exposure has occurred, acute and convalescent antibody titers should be determined simultaneously on sera obtained 2 to 4 weeks apart, with the exact interval depending on the time after exposure when the acute sample was drawn.

DIAGNOSIS   Rubella is frequently confused with other diseases associated with maculopapular exanthems, with infectious mononucleosis (see Chap. 145), as well as with drug eruptions and scarlet fever. *A certain diagnosis of rubella can be made only by virus isolation and identification or by changes in antibody titers.* Rubella antibodies may be detectable by the second day of rash and increase in titer over the next 10 to 21 days. A variety of serologic tests are available for diagnosis or determination of immune status. The presence of IgM-specific antibodies suggests recent rubella infection (within 2 months); however, they have been known to persist as long as 1 year in some cases. There are no other laboratory findings helpful in the diagnosis of rubella, although lymphocytosis with atypical lymphocytes often occurs.

Patients with the congenital rubella syndrome may lose antibodies at age 3 or 4 years. Therefore, a negative serologic test in a child over 3 years of age does not exclude the possibility of congenital rubella. Congenital rubella should be differentiated from congenital syphilis by appropriate serologic tests (see Chap. 133), toxoplasmosis (see Chap. 177), and cytomegalic inclusion virus disease (see Chap. 146). IgM-specific antibodies are often found early in the first year of life in infants with congenital rubella, but virus isolation is the most reliable way to confirm the diagnosis.

PREVENTION   In adults and children, rubella is usually a mild disease with infrequent complications. However, the severity of congenital infection has prompted efforts to prevent the disease. Administration of gamma globulin to exposed persons can abort the clinical disease, but seroconversion and transmission of the disease from mother to fetus may occur despite the administration of large amounts of gamma globulin soon after exposure.

Active immunization with live, attenuated rubella vaccines has been practiced in this country since 1969, especially among young children. The aim has been to decrease the frequency of the infection in the population and to decrease the chance that susceptible pregnant women will be exposed. Vaccination is strongly recommended for adolescents and adults, particularly females, unless there is proof of immunity (i.e., positive results in serologic tests or documentation of rubella vaccination on or after the first birthday). The only exceptions are persons in whom vaccination is specifically contraindicated, as noted below. Persons working in hospitals or clinics who might contract rubella from infected patients or who, if infected, might transmit the infection to pregnant patients should be required to have proof of immunity.

The attenuated virus can be detected in the respiratory secretions of vaccinees for as long as 4 weeks after immunization, but transmission to other susceptible individuals has never been documented during more than 20 years of experience. The vaccine induces detectable antibodies that persist at least 16 years and probably for a lifetime in about 95 percent of recipients. After heavy exposure in closed populations, vaccinated individuals sometimes develop subclinical infections (diagnosed by antibody rises and virus isolation). However, the failure to demonstrate viremia in immunized persons suggests that previously vaccinated pregnant women will not infect their fetuses even if they acquire subclinical rubella.

Side effects of fever, rash, lymphadenopathy, polyneuropathy, or arthralgias occur very seldom in vaccinated children; joint pain and swelling or paresthesias are seen in less than 2 percent of women with vaccines prepared in human embryonic fibroblast cell cultures (RA 27/3 vaccine). The joint symptoms usually begin 1 to 3 weeks after vaccination and may be confused with other forms of arthritis. *Rubella vaccine must never be given to pregnant women or to those who may become pregnant within 3 months of immunization.* Although no infant with the congenital rubella syndrome has been reported to have been born to a woman inadvertently vaccinated during pregnancy, the theoretical risk of vaccine virus–induced fetal damage remains. Vaccine is contraindicated in patients who have immune-deficiency diseases or who are taking immunosuppressive drugs. One exception is HIV infection. Rubella vaccination should be provided to asymptomatic HIV-infected children and adults. Furthermore, the presence of HIV-related symptoms is not a contraindication with regard to rubella vaccination (or, more commonly, mumps-measles-rubella vaccination) of children, and vaccination also should be considered for symptomatic adults. If immunoglobulin (Ig) is being used, the vaccine should be given at least 14 days before Ig administration or deferred until a minimum of 6 weeks (preferably 3 months) afterward. Postpartum rubella immunization is not contraindicated when whole-blood or human anti-Rho(D)Ig has recently been used, but follow-up testing 6 to 8 weeks later is advised to ensure that seroconversion has occurred.

OTHER VIRAL EXANTHEMS

In addition to the diseases such as measles, rubella, and chickenpox that historically have been associated with prominent skin lesions, there are other virus infections in which skin manifestations may occur. Table 156-1 lists the most commonly recognized causes of maculopapular eruptions. Some of them, particularly the enteroviruses, also can occasionally cause papulovesicular or petechial rashes; others are capable of provoking erythema multiforme–like eruptions. One helpful aspect of the physical examination is the observation that virus-caused maculopapular (not vesicular) exanthems usually *relatively* spare the palms and soles. This is in contrast to eruptions associated with drug reactions, bacteria, *Mycoplasma*, and *Rickettsia*, in which a prominent palmar or plantar eruption is often noted.

EXANTHEM SUBITUM (ROSEOLA INFANTUM) Exanthem subitum is a benign disease of infants 6 months to 4 years of age that is characterized by a high fever and rash. Several different agents, such as enteroviruses and adenoviruses, may produce a similar illness; however, human herpesvirus type 6 (HHV-6) has been implicated as the major cause. The first manifestations of disease, after an estimated incubation period of 5 to 15 days, are the abrupt onset of irritability and fever, which last for 3 to 5 days; the temperature can be as high

TABLE 156-1 Causes of maculopapular eruptions

Viral	Other
Measles	*Mycoplasma pneumoniae*
Rubella	Syphilis
Exanthem subitum: human herpesvirus type 6	Typhoid fever
	Bacterial toxins:
Erythema infectiosum: human parvovirus B19	streptococci and staphylococci
	Rat-bite fever
Enteroviruses	*Rickettsia*
Epstein-Barr virus	Live-virus vaccines
Adenoviruses	Drug eruptions
Reoviruses	Mucocutaneous lymph node
Arboviruses	syndrome

as 40.6°C (105°F). There may be mild pharyngitis and slight lymph node enlargement; convulsions sometimes occur during the height of the fever. On the fourth to fifth day of illness, there is a sudden drop in temperature to normal or below normal; several hours before or after defervescence, the rash suddenly appears. It is characterized by faint 2- to 3-mm macules or maculopapules over the neck and trunk and may extend to the thighs and buttocks; it lasts for a few hours to 1 to 2 days. Leukopenia is frequently noted later in the febrile period. The disease is benign and very rarely associated with complications. In the early, preeruptive phase, the disease may be difficult to differentiate from an acute bacteremia, particularly one associated with *Streptococcus pneumoniae*. Although a leukocytosis with an increase in band forms is often seen in bacteremias presenting in this fashion, blood cultures are necessary to make the diagnosis.

Recent laboratory and clinical studies indicate that HHV-6 infection is widespread; by 3 to 5 years of age, up to 95 percent of children have serologic evidence of infection. Seroprevalence rates decline to ≤55 percent after the fourth decade of life. The virus has been found in saliva from more than 90 percent of healthy adults studied; this reservoir is very likely a major source of transmission. In immunocompetent older children and adults, HHV-6 infection has been associated with mononucleosis-like symptoms, afebrile lymphadenopathy, and acute hepatitis. The virus also has been implicated in interstitial pneumonitis in bone marrow transplant recipients. Further investigations are necessary to clearly define the pathogenesis of HHV-6–related illnesses. At present, the infection is most commonly diagnosed by serologic testing; molecular and immunologic probe methods are also being employed increasingly.

ENTEROVIRAL EXANTHEMS Many individual enteroviruses have been associated with rash. Most commonly implicated have been echovirus serotypes 1–7, 9, 11, 12, 14, 16, 18–20, 25, and 30 and coxsackievirus serotypes A4–A6, A9, A10, A16, B2, B3, and B5. Except in hand-foot-and-mouth disease, usually associated with coxsackievirus A16 or enterovirus 71 infection (see Chap. 154), there is no set of clinical or epidemiologic features that aids in differentiating the specific enteroviral agent involved in a specific case. All are capable of producing maculopapular rashes which vary in intensity and duration and also can occasionally produce petechial or papulovesicular exanthems and enanthems. In community and household outbreaks, younger children and infants are usually more likely to have exanthems, while other features of enteroviral infection, such as fever, myalgia, and aseptic meningitis, are more prominent among older children and young adults. Two enterovirus serotypes that have been particularly associated with outbreaks of febrile exanthems are echoviruses 9 and 16.

ERYTHEMA INFECTIOSUM (FIFTH DISEASE) See Chap. 148.

REFERENCES

ASANO Y et al: Viremia and neutralizing antibody response in infants with exanthem subitum. J Pediatr 114:535, 1989

CARRIGAN DR et al: Interstitial pneumonitis associated with human herpesvirus-6 infection after marrow transplantation. Lancet 338:147, 1991

CENTERS FOR DISEASE CONTROL: Update on adult immunization: Recommendations of the Immunization Practices Advisory Committee (ACIP). Morb Mort Week Rep 40:1, 1991

ENDERS G et al: Outcome of confirmed periconceptional rubella. Lancet 1:1445, 1988

HERRMANN KL: Available rubella serologic tests. Rev Infect Dis 7:S108, 1985

LEE SH et al: Resurgence of congenital rubella syndrome in the 1990s. JAMA 267:2616, 1992

LEVY JA et al: Frequent isolation of HHV-6 from saliva and high seroprevalence of the virus in the population. Lancet 335:1047, 1990

MCINTOSH EDG, MENSER MA: A fifty-year follow-up of congenital rubella. Lancet 340:414, 1992

NAIDES SJ et al: Human parvovirus B19-induced vesiculopustular skin eruption. Am J Med 84:968, 1988

STEEPER TA et al: The spectrum of clinical and laboratory findings resulting from human herpesvirus-6 (HHV-6) in patients with mononucleosis-like illnesses not resulting from Epstein-Barr virus or cytomegalovirus. Am J Clin Pathol 93:776, 1990

TOWNSEND JJ et al: Progressive rubella panencephalitis: Late onset after congenital rubella. N Engl J Med 292:990, 1975

157   MUMPS

C. GEORGE RAY

DEFINITION   Mumps is an acute communicable disease of viral origin characterized by painful enlargement of the salivary glands and sometimes by involvement of the gonads, meninges, pancreas, and other organs.

ETIOLOGY   The causative agent of mumps is a paramyxovirus of intermediate size (120 to 200 nm in diameter). It has a tight helical inner core (single-stranded RNA) enclosed in an outer envelope of lipid and glycoproteins. Only one antigenic type is known.

EPIDEMIOLOGY   Human beings are the only natural host for mumps. The disease is worldwide in distribution and is endemic in urban communities. Epidemics are relatively infrequent and are usually confined to closely associated groups who live in orphanages, army camps, or schools. The disease is most frequent in the spring, particularly during April and May. Although mumps is generally considered less "contagious" than measles and chickenpox, this difference may be more apparent than real because many mumps infections (at least 25 percent) tend to be inapparent clinically. In some surveys, 80 to 90 percent of an adult population had serologic evidence of previous mumps. Approximately 5000 mumps cases were reported annually in the United States in 1988, 1989, and 1990. There has been an apparent upward shift in the age groups affected. In 1989, 38 percent of patients were ≥15 years of age; in 1977, the figure was only 12 percent.

Infections are rare before the age of 2 years. The virus is transmitted in infected salivary secretions, although its isolation from urine suggests that it also may spread via this route. The saliva is infectious for approximately 6 days prior to the onset of parotitis, and virus has been recovered from this site for as long as 2 weeks after onset of parotid swelling. Viruria also persists for 2 to 3 weeks in some patients. Despite this prolonged secretion of virus, the period of greatest infectivity is from a day or two before onset of parotitis to 5 days after the appearance of glandular enlargement. Patients are usually no longer contagious 9 days after onset of parotid swelling.

One attack of clinical or subclinical mumps confers lasting immunity, and second attacks are most unusual. Unilateral parotitis affords protection just as effectively as does bilateral disease.

PATHOGENESIS   The virus enters via the respiratory route; during the incubation period of 12 to 25 days, it presumably replicates in the upper respiratory tract and cervical lymph nodes, from which it is disseminated via the bloodstream to target tissues such as the parotid glands and meninges. After initial replication in these sites, a secondary viremia may occur, resulting in variable involvement of organs such as the gonads, pancreas, thyroid, breasts, liver, heart,

and kidneys. The salivary adenitis is thought by many to be secondary to initial viremia, but direct spread from the respiratory tract has not been ruled out as an alternative mechanism. Viruria is common; nearly all infections are associated with discernible impairment of renal function.

Immunity is correlated with the presence of neutralizing antibody. Cellular immune mechanisms are thought to contribute both to the pathogenesis of the acute disease and to recovery. Like other systemic viral infections, mumps can cause a transient suppression of delayed-type hypersensitivity to previously recognized antigens, such as tuberculin protein.

MANIFESTATIONS   Salivary adenitis   The onset of parotitis is usually sudden, although it may be preceded by a prodromal period of malaise, anorexia, chilly sensations, feverishness, sore throat, and tenderness at the angle of the jaw. In many cases, however, parotid swelling is the first indication of illness. The glands enlarge progressively over a period of 1 to 3 days, and the swelling resolves within a week after maximal enlargement. The swollen gland extends from the ear to the lower portion of the mandibular ramus and to the inferior portion of the zygomatic arch, often displacing the ear upward and outward. The skin over the gland is usually not warm or erythematous, in contrast to the findings in bacterial parotitis. There may be reddening and pouting of the orifice of Stensen's duct. Usually, pain and tenderness are marked, although at times they are absent. The edema of mumps has been described as "gelatinous," and when the involved gland is tweaked, it rolls like jelly. Swelling may involve only the submaxillary and sublingual glands and may extend over the anterior part of the chest, producing *presternal edema*. Involvement of submaxillary glands alone can cause difficulty in distinguishing mumps from acute cervical adenitis. Swelling of the glottis occurs rarely but may require tracheostomy. Parotitis is bilateral in two-thirds of cases and remains confined to one side in the remainder. The second gland tends to swell as the first is subsiding, usually 4 to 5 days after onset. In general, parotitis is accompanied by a temperature of 37.8 to 39.4°C (100 to 103°F), malaise, headache, and anorexia, but systemic symptoms may be virtually absent, particularly in children. In most patients, the chief complaints are difficulty in eating, swallowing, and talking.

Epididymoorchitis   Mumps is complicated by orchitis in 20 to 30 percent of postpubertal males. Testicular involvement usually appears 7 to 10 days after onset of parotitis, although it may precede it or appear simultaneously. Occasionally, orchitis occurs in the absence of parotitis. Gonadal involvement is bilateral in 3 to 17 percent of patients with epididymoorchitis. Orchitis is heralded by recrudescence of malaise and appearance of chilly sensations, headache, nausea, and vomiting. Shaking chills and high fevers, with temperatures between 39.4 and 41.1°C (103 and 106°F), are frequent. The testicle becomes greatly swollen and acutely painful. The epididymis is often palpable as a swollen tender cord. Occasionally there may be epididymitis without orchitis. Swelling, pain, and tenderness persist for 3 to 7 days and gradually subside; lysis of fever usually parallels abatement of swelling. The temperature occasionally falls by crisis. Mumps orchitis is followed by progressive atrophy of the testicle in one-half of cases. Even after bilateral orchitis, sterility is unusual, provided no significant atrophy has taken place. However, if bilateral testicular atrophy occurs after mumps, sterility or subnormal sperm counts are quite common. Plasma testosterone levels are depressed during acute orchitis but return to normal with recovery. *Pulmonary infarction* has been noted to follow mumps orchitis. This may be the result of thrombosis of the veins in the prostatic and pelvic plexuses in association with the testicular inflammation. Priapism is a rare but painful complication of mumps orchitis.

Pancreatitis   Pancreatic involvement is a potentially serious manifestation of mumps, which may rarely be complicated by shock or pseudocyst formation. It should be suspected in patients with abdominal pain and tenderness together with clinical or epidemiologic evidence of mumps. It is difficult to document, since hyperamylasemia, the hallmark of pancreatitis, is also often present in parotitis.

Many times the symptoms resemble those of gastroenteritis. Although diabetes or pancreatic insufficiency rarely follows mumps pancreatitis, several children have developed "brittle" diabetes a few weeks after mumps.

Central nervous system involvement Approximately 60 percent of patients with clinical mumps have an increased number of cells, usually lymphocytes, in the cerebrospinal fluid (CSF), while 10 percent have symptoms of meningitis: stiff neck, headache, and drowsiness. In typical cases, the onset of overt central nervous system signs and symptoms occurs 3 to 10 days after the onset of parotitis; however, CNS mumps may develop prior to the parotitis or 2 to 3 weeks later. In approximately 30 to 40 percent of laboratory-proven cases, there is *no* associated salivary gland involvement at any time in the course of illness. The CSF protein is moderately elevated, and CSF glucose tends to be normal, although in as many as 10 percent of patients low CSF glucose concentrations, in the range of 1.1 to 2.8 mmol/L (20 to 50 mg/dL), may be seen. True encephalitis is unusual, although it is responsible for most of the CNS sequelae, including behavioral disturbances, headaches, seizures, deafness (usually unilateral), and visual disturbances. Mumps also should be recognized as capable of presenting a picture of mild paralytic poliomyelitis; definition of the cause depends on isolation of virus or serologic confirmation of mumps in the absence of changing antibody titers to poliomyelitis viruses. Rarely, mumps may produce a transverse myelitis, cerebellar ataxia, or the Guillain-Barré syndrome. Mumps meningitis, without clinical encephalitis, is generally benign.

Other manifestations Mumps virus tends to involve glandular tissues; inflammation of the lacrimal glands, thymus, thyroid, breasts, and ovaries occurs occasionally. *Oophoritis* may be recognized by persistence of pain in the lower part of the abdomen and fever. It does not result in sterility. Mumps virus has been implicated in the causation of subacute thyroiditis; occasionally the virus can be isolated from the thyroid gland. Myxedema following mumps thyroiditis has been reported. Ocular manifestations of mumps include dacryoadenitis, optic neuritis, keratitis, iritis, conjunctivitis, and episcleritis. Although these conditions may transiently interfere with vision, complete resolution is the rule. Mumps *myocarditis* is evidenced primarily by transient abnormalities in the electrocardiogram. It does not usually produce symptomatic disease or impair cardiac function, but rare deaths have been reported. Similarly, *hepatic* involvement may be manifested by mild abnormalities in liver function, but icterus and other clinical signs of hepatic damage are extremely rare. *Thrombocytopenic purpura* as a complication of mumps has been described, and an occasional patient has a leukemoid reaction involving predominantly lymphocytes. Tracheobronchitis and interstitial pneumonia also have been associated with mumps infection, particularly among young children.

Other rare but interesting manifestations of mumps include *polyarthritis* which is often migratory. Monarticular arthritis is most common in males between the ages of 20 and 30. Joint symptoms begin 1 to 2 weeks after subsidence of parotitis; usually the large joints are involved, especially the hip or knee. The illness lasts 1 to 12 weeks, and complete recovery is the rule. The pathogenesis of mumps-associated arthritis is unclear. The usual delayed onset after parotitis and the failure to isolate the virus from synovial fluid suggest an immunologically mediated mechanism.

Acute hemorrhagic glomerulonephritis in the absence of streptococcosis has been reported after mumps. The relationship of these two diseases is not clear.

Late complications With the exception of the rare CNS complications and occasional sterility following bilateral testicular involvement, mumps leaves no sequelae. However, persistent mumps infection may be a cause of inclusion-body myositis, a chronic inflammatory myopathy that occurs primarily in the sixth decade. There is no firm evidence that offspring with congenital defects are more common among mothers who have mumps during pregnancy. Mumps illness during the first trimester of pregnancy has been associated with an increased risk of spontaneous abortion, however.

LABORATORY FINDINGS In uncomplicated parotitis, the blood leukocyte count is normal, although there may be mild leukopenia with relative lymphocytosis. Patients with mumps orchitis, however, may have a marked leukocytosis with a shift to the left. In meningoencephalitis, the white blood cell count is usually within normal limits. The erythrocyte sedimentation rate is usually normal but may rise with testicular or pancreatic involvement. The serum amylase level is elevated both in pancreatitis and in salivary adenitis. It also may be elevated in some patients in whom the sole evidence of mumps is meningoencephalitis, and such elevation probably reflects subclinical involvement of the salivary glands. In contrast to the amylase level, the serum lipase level is elevated only in pancreatitis, in which hyperglycemia and glucosuria also may occur. The CSF contains up to 2000 cells per microliter, almost all mononuclear, although occasionally polymorphonuclear cells will predominate in the early stages. The pleocytosis in mumps meningitis tends to be greater than in aseptic meningitides caused by the enteroviruses. There is no relationship between the cell count and the severity of CNS involvement. Transient hematuria and mild reversible abnormalities in renal function, including inability to concentrate the urine maximally and to clear creatinine, occur in association with the viruria of mumps.

DIAGNOSIS The definitive diagnosis of mumps depends on isolation of the virus from blood, throat swabs, secretions from Stensen's duct, CSF, or urine. In addition, immunofluorescence can be utilized for rapid detection of the viral antigen directly in oropharyngeal cells. Serologic determination of acute infection or susceptibility can be done by a variety of methods. The best test is the enzyme-linked immunosorbent assay (ELISA). Immunofluorescent assays also can be used for identification of IgM- and IgG-specific antibody responses. The complement fixation test can be employed to quantitate antibody responses to the S and V antigenic components for the diagnosis of acute or recent mumps infection. Antibodies to the S antigen develop rather rapidly, often reaching a peak within 1 week after the onset of symptoms, and usually disappear in 6 to 12 months. Complement-fixing antibodies to the V antigen reach a peak titer within 2 to 3 weeks after onset, remain elevated for at least 6 weeks, and then persist at lower levels for years afterward. Paired sera obtained 2 to 3 weeks apart are recommended. A fourfold increase in titer by any standard assay confirms recent infection. When an acute serum is not obtained until later in the course of illness, either an elevation of antibodies to the S antigen to a titer that exceeds the V antibody titer or the presence of IgM-specific antibody suggests recent infection. The *skin test* consists of intradermal injection of killed mumps virus; previous exposure will result in a delayed reaction of the tuberculin type and an anamnestic antibody titer rise to mumps. The skin test is unreliable for determining the mumps immune status of an individual; if this information is needed, ELISA or neutralization assays should be used.

The diagnosis of mumps during an epidemic is usually obvious. Sporadic cases, however, must be distinguished from other causes of parotid enlargement. Parotitis may be caused by other viruses, notably parainfluenza, influenza, and coxsackieviruses. *Bacterial parotitis* usually occurs in debilitated patients with severe underlying diseases. The parotid glands are swollen, warm, and tender, and pus can be expressed from the orifices of Stensen's ducts. Marked polymorphonuclear leukocytosis is present. *Staphylococcus aureus* is the usual causative organism. Dehydration followed by inspissation of secretions in the salivary ducts is an important predisposing factor. *Calculus* in a salivary duct is usually detectable by palpation or by injection of radiopaque media into Stensen's duct. *Drug reactions* may produce tender swelling of the parotid and other salivary glands. "Iodine mumps" is the most common type; it may follow such procedures as intravenous urography. The antihypertensive agent guanethidine also may cause parotid enlargement and tenderness. A careful history usually serves to clarify the cause of these reactions. *Cervical adenitis* caused by streptococci, "bullneck" diphtheria, infectious mononucleosis, cat-scratch disease, sublingual cellulitis (Ludwig's angina), or cellulitis of the external auditory canal is usually easy to distinguish from mumps by careful examination. Parotid tumors and chronic infections such as actinomycosis tend to follow a more indolent course, with slowly progressive swelling. The common "mixed tumor" of the parotid is well-circumscribed, nontender, and very firm (almost cartilaginous) on palpation. Parotid swelling and fever, often accompanied by lacrimal adenitis and uveitis (Mikulicz's syndrome), may occur in tuberculosis, leukemia, Hodgkin's disease, and lupus erythematosus. The onset may be sudden, but the process is usually painless and of long duration. Uveoparotid fever of similar type may be the first manifestation of sarcoidosis; in this disease, parotid swelling is frequently accompanied by single or multiple palsies of cranial nerves, particularly the facial nerve, and is referred to as *Heerfordt's syndrome*. Presternal edema also may be a manifestation of malignant lymphoma involving retrosternal lymph nodes. Bilateral painless parotid swelling unassociated with fever is found in patients with Laennec's cirrhosis, chronic alcoholism, malnutrition, diabetes mellitus, pregnancy and lactation, and hypertriglyceridemia.

Sjögren's syndrome (see Chap. 288) is a chronic inflammation of the parotid and other salivary glands which is often associated with atrophy of the lacrimal glands and occurs most commonly in women past the menopause. With cessation of lacrimal and salivary function, there may be striking dryness of the conjunctiva and the cornea (keratoconjunctivitis sicca) and of the mouth (xerostomia). These patients also may have a variety of systemic manifestations, including rheumatoid arthritis, splenomegaly, leukopenia, and hemolytic anemia. The chronicity of the process and its occurrence in elderly women make confusion with mumps unlikely. Finally, benign hypertrophy of both masseter muscles, presumably due to habitual clenching and grinding of teeth, may be confused with painless parotid swelling.

The causes of aseptic meningitis are discussed in Chap. 375.

Orchitis occurring in the absence of parotitis is likely to remain undiagnosed. Serologic testing may later confirm the diagnosis of mumps. Orchitis may occur in association with acute bacterial prostatitis and seminal vesiculitis. It is a rare complication of gonorrhea. Occasionally, testicular inflammation accompanies pleurodynia, leptospirosis, melioidosis, tuberculosis, relapsing fever, chickenpox, brucellosis, and lymphocytic choriomeningitis. *Chlamydia trachomatis* also should be considered in the differential diagnosis of epididymitis, particularly among young adults.

TREATMENT   There is no specific treatment for infections with the mumps virus. Patients with parotitis should receive mouth care, analgesics, and a bland diet. Bed rest is advisable only as long as the patient is febrile; contrary to popular belief, physical activity has no influence on the development of orchitis or other complications. Patients with epididymoorchitis may be acutely ill and in great pain. Many forms of treatment, including surgical decompression of the testicle, infiltration of the spermatic cord with local anesthetics, and administration of estrogens, convalescent serum, and broad-spectrum antibiotics, have not been regularly effective. Despite failure to document their effectiveness in controlled studies, glucocorticoids have been of apparent benefit in diminishing fever and testicular pain and swelling. A large daily dose corresponding to 60 mg of prednisone is given initially; then the dose is tapered over 7 to 10 days. Glucocorticoids have not exerted an adverse effect on concomitant pancreatitis or meningitis, although they have not benefited patients with meningeal involvement, and their withdrawal usually has been accompanied by a recrudescence of symptoms. They have not prevented the appearance of parotid involvement on the contralateral side. Mumps arthritis is usually responsive to ibuprofen but not to salicylates. Mumps thyroiditis may subside spontaneously, but excellent relief has been obtained with glucocorticoids.

PREVENTION   A live, attenuated mumps virus vaccine (Jeryl Lynn strain) has been highly effective in producing significant rises in mumps antibody in individuals who are seronegative prior to vaccination and has afforded 75 to 95 percent protection to individuals subsequently exposed to mumps. The vaccine also has boosted antibody levels in vaccinated individuals who are seropositive. The vaccine produces an inapparent, noncommunicable infection. Parotitis

or fever after vaccination has been reported only rarely, and CNS dysfunction has not been proved to be a complication in the United States. The vaccine has conferred excellent protection for at least 17 years and has not interfered with vaccines against measles, rubella, and poliomyelitis or with smallpox vaccine given simultaneously.

Live mumps vaccine can be administered at any time after 1 year of age, and vaccination should be considered particularly for children approaching puberty, adolescents, and adults born after 1956 who have not had clinical mumps or live mumps vaccine in the past. Individuals living in groups or in institutions should be vaccinated, particularly because it has been shown that physical isolation of mumps patients does not effectively prevent transmission of the infection. Vaccination is also recommended for asymptomatic HIV-infected persons and may be considered for those who are symptomatic. Killed mumps vaccine was available from 1950 until 1978; persons who received this vaccine might benefit from revaccination with a live-virus product. There is no evidence for an increased risk of adverse reactions to live mumps vaccine among persons who are already immune to mumps.

Vaccination is contraindicated in babies under the age of 1 year because of the interfering effect of maternal antibody; in individuals with a history of hypersensitivity to vaccine components; in patients with febrile illnesses, leukemia, lymphoma, or generalized malignancies; in those receiving glucocorticoids, alkylating drugs, antimetabolites, or irradiation; and in pregnant women.

It is not known whether the vaccine will prevent infection when administered after exposure, but no contraindication to its use in this situation exists. Neither mumps immune globulin nor ordinary gamma globulin has been shown to be effective in postexposure prophylaxis, and neither is recommended.

REFERENCES

BEARD CM et al: The incidence and outcome of mumps orchitis in Rochester, Minnesota, 1935 to 1974. Mayo Clin Proc 52:3, 1977

CENTERS FOR DISEASE CONTROL: Update on adult immunization: Recommendations of the Immunization Practices Advisory Committee (ACIP). Morb Mort Week Rep 40:22, 1991

CHAUDARY S, JASKI BE: Fulminant mumps myocarditis. Ann Intern Med 110:569, 1989

CHOU SM: Inclusion body myositis: A chronic persistent mumps myositis? Hum Pathol 17:765, 1986

COHEN AA et al: Mumps-associated acute cerebellar ataxia. Am J Dis Child 146:930, 1992

GORDON SC, LAUTER CB: Mumps arthritis: Unusual presentation as adult Still's disease. Ann Intern Med 97:45, 1982

HAREL L et al: Mumps arthritis in children. Pediatr Infect Dis J 9:928, 1990

HERSH BS et al: Mumps outbreak in a highly vaccinated population. J Pediatr 119:187, 1991

LEVITT LP et al: Central nervous system mumps: A review of 64 cases. Neurology 20:829, 1970

MCDONALD JC et al: Clinical and epidemiologic features of mumps meningoencephalitis and possible vaccine-related disease. Pediatr Infect Dis J 8:751, 1989

158   RABIES, RHABDOVIRUSES, AND MARBURG-LIKE AGENTS

LAWRENCE COREY

RABIES

DEFINITION   Rabies is an acute viral disease of the central nervous system that affects all mammals and that is transmitted by infected secretions, usually saliva. Most exposures to rabies are through the bite of an infected animal, but on occasion a virus aerosol or the ingestion or transplantation of infected tissues may initiate the disease process.

ETIOLOGY The rabies virus is a bullet-shaped, enveloped, single-stranded ribonucleic acid virus of 75- to 80-nm diameter belonging to the rhabdovirus group. The envelope glycoproteins are arranged in knoblike structures which cover the surface of the virion. The viral glycoproteins bind to acetylcholine receptors, contribute to the neurovirulence of rabies virus, elicit neutralizing and hemagglutination-inhibiting antibodies, and stimulate T cell immunity. The nucleocapsid antigen induces a complement-fixing antibody. Neutralizing antibodies to the surface glycoproteins appear to be protective. Antirabies antibodies used in diagnostic immunofluorescence assays are generally directed against the nucleocapsid antigens. Isolates of rabies virus from different animal species and locales differ in their antigenic and biologic properties. These variations may account for differences in virulence between isolates. Interferon is induced by rabies virus, particularly in those tissues with high virus concentrations, and may play some role in retarding progressive infection.

EPIDEMIOLOGY Rabies exists in two epidemiologic forms: *urban*, propagated chiefly by unimmunized domestic dogs and/or cats, and *sylvatic*, propagated by skunks, foxes, raccoons, mongooses, wolves, and bats. Infection in domestic animals usually represents a "spillover" from sylvatic reservoirs of infection, and human beings can be infected by either. Hence human infection tends to occur in locales where rabies is enzootic or epizootic, where there is a large population of unimmunized domestic animals, and where human contact with the outdoors is common. While only about 1000 rabies deaths are reported to the World Health Organization (WHO) each year, the worldwide incidence of rabies is approximated at over 30,000 cases per year. Southeast Asia, the Philippines, Africa, the Indian subcontinent, and tropical South America are areas where the disease is especially common. In some endemic areas 1 to 2 percent of autopsied patients show evidence of rabies. Increased spread of terrestrial rabies and increased travel to countries where urban rabies is present have made recognition of clinical rabies and its prevention of increasing importance. In the United States, human rabies is exceedingly rare, and most cases now originate from animal bite exposures in countries where canine rabies is endemic.

In most areas of the world, the dog is the important vector of rabies virus for humans. However, the wolf (eastern Europe, arctic regions), the mongoose (South Africa, the Caribbean), the fox (western Europe), and the vampire bat (Latin America) also may be prominent vectors of the disease. In the United States, cat rabies is now reported more frequently than dog rabies; thus the vaccination of domestic cats is extremely important. Rodents and lagomorphs are rarely infected with rabies. In the United States, rabies in wildlife accounts for about 85 percent of the reported animal rabies, with dogs and cats comprising only about 2 and 3 percent, respectively. However, most cases of postexposure prophylaxis are associated with dog or cat bites.

Several cases of human-to-human transmission of rabies through corneal transplantation also have been documented.

PATHOGENESIS The first event is the introduction of live virus through the epidermis or onto a mucous membrane. Initial viral replication appears to occur within striated muscle cells at the site of inoculation. The peripheral nervous system is exposed at the neuromuscular and/or neurotendinal spindles. The virus then spreads centripetally up the nerve to the central nervous system, probably via peripheral nerve axoplasm. Experimentally, viremia has been shown to occur but is not thought to play a role in naturally acquired disease. Once the virus reaches the central nervous system, it replicates almost exclusively within the gray matter and then passes centrifugally along autonomic nerves to reach other tissue—the salivary glands, adrenal medulla, kidney, lung, liver, skeletal muscle, skin, and heart. Passage into the salivary glands facilitates further transmission of the disease via infected saliva. The incubation period of rabies is exceedingly variable, ranging from 10 days to over 1 year (mean 1 to 2 months). The time period appears to depend on the amount of virus introduced, the amount of tissue involved, host defense mechanisms, and the actual distance that the virus has to travel from the site of inoculation

to the central nervous system. Cases of human rabies with an extended incubation period (2 to 7 years) have been reported, but they are rare. Host immune responses and viral strains also may influence disease expression. Cell-mediated immune responses were noted in patients with rabies encephalitis but were absent in patients with paralytic rabies.

The neuropathology of rabies resembles other viral diseases of the central nervous system: hyperemia, varying degrees of chromatolysis, nuclear pyknosis, and neuronophagia of the nerve cells; infiltration by lymphocytes and plasma cells of the Virchow-Robin space; microglial infiltration; and parenchymal areas of nerve cell destruction. In experimental animal models, adenohypophyseal infection with rabies virus, with reduction in growth hormone and vasopressin release, is common. The pathognomonic lesion of rabies is the Negri body. This eosinophilic mass, approximately 10 nm in size, is made up of a finely fibrillar matrix and rabies virus particles. Negri bodies are distributed throughout the brain, particularly in Ammon's horn, the cerebral cortex, the brainstem, the hypothalamus, the Purkinje cells of the cerebellum, and the dorsal spinal ganglia. Negri bodies are not demonstrated in at least 20 percent of cases of rabies, and their absence from brain material does not rule out the diagnosis.

MANIFESTATIONS The clinical manifestations of rabies can be divided into four stages: (1) a nonspecific prodrome, (2) an acute encephalitis similar to other viral encephalitides, (3) a profound dysfunction of brainstem centers that produces the classic features of rabies encephalitis, and (4) rarely, recovery.

The prodromal period usually persists for 1 to 4 days and is marked by fever, headache, malaise, myalgias, increased fatigability, anorexia, nausea and vomiting, sore throat, and a nonproductive cough. The prodromal symptom suggestive of rabies is the complaint of paresthesias and/or fasciculations at or about the site of inoculation of virus and may be related to the multiplication of virus in the dorsal root ganglion of the sensory nerve supplying the area of the bite. This symptom is present in 50 to 80 percent of patients.

The encephalitic phase is usually ushered in by periods of excessive motor activity, excitation, and agitation. Quickly, confusion, hallucinations, combativeness, bizarre aberrations of thought, muscle spasms, meningismus, opisthotonic posturing, seizures, and focal paralysis appear. Characteristically, the periods of mental aberration are interspersed with completely lucid periods, but as the disease progresses, the lucid periods get shorter until the patient lapses into coma. Hyperesthesia, with excessive sensitivity to bright light, loud noise, touch, and even gentle breezes, is very common. On physical examination, the temperature may be found to be as high as 40.6°C (105°F). Abnormalities of the autonomic nervous system include dilated irregular pupils, increased lacrimation, salivation, perspiration, and postural hypotension. Evidence of upper motor neuron paralysis with weakness, increased deep tendon reflexes, and extensor plantar responses is the rule. Paralysis of the vocal cords is common.

The manifestations of brainstem dysfunction begin shortly after the onset of the encephalitic phase. Cranial nerve involvement causes diplopia, facial palsies, optic neuritis, and the characteristic difficulty with deglutition. The combination of excessive salivation and difficulty in swallowing produces the traditional picture of "foaming at the mouth." Hydrophobia, the painful, violent, involuntary contraction of the diaphragm, accessory respiratory, pharyngeal, and laryngeal muscles initiated by swallowing liquids, is seen in about 50 percent of cases. Involvement of the amygdaloid nucleus may result in priapism and spontaneous ejaculation. The patient lapses into coma, and involvement of the respiratory center produces an apneic death. The prominence of early brainstem dysfunction distinguishes rabies from other viral encephalitides and accounts for the rapid downhill course. The median survival after the onset of symptoms is 4 days, with a maximum of 20, unless artificial supporting measures are instituted.

If intensive respiratory support is used, a number of late complications may appear and include inappropriate secretion of antidiuretic hormone, diabetes insipidus, cardiac arrythmias, vascular instability, adult respiratory distress syndrome, gastrointestinal bleeding, thrombocytopenia, and paralytic ileus. Recovery is very rare and, when it occurs, gradual.

Occasionally, rabies may present as an ascending paralysis resembling the Landry-Guillain-Barré syndrome (dumb rabies, *rage tranquille*). This clinical pattern occurs most frequently in those who are bitten by vampire bats or who have received postexposure rabies prophylaxis.

The difficulty of suspecting rabies when it is associated with ascending paralysis is illustrated by the documentation of person-to-person transmission of the virus by tissue transplantation. Corneal transplants from two donors who died of presumed Landry-Guillain-Barré syndrome produced clinical rabies and death in the recipients. Retrospective pathologic examinations of the brains of both recipients demonstrated Negri bodies, and rabies virus was subsequently isolated from each donor's frozen eye.

LABORATORY FINDINGS   Early in the disease the hemoglobin and routine blood chemistries are normal, but abnormalities occur as hypothalamic dysfunction, gastrointestinal bleeding, and other complications ensue. The peripheral white blood cell count is usually slightly elevated (12,000 to 17,000 cells per microliter) but may be normal or as high as 30,000 cells per microliter.

As in any viral infection, the specific diagnosis of rabies depends on (1) the isolation of virus from infected secretions [saliva, rarely cerebrospinal fluid (CSF), or tissue (brain)], (2) the serologic demonstration of acute infection, or (3) the demonstration of viral antigen in infected tissue, e.g., corneal impression smears, skin biopsies, or brain. Samples of brain obtained either on postmortem examination or at brain biopsy should be subjected to (1) mouse inoculation studies for virus isolation, (2) fluorescent antibody (FA) staining for viral antigen, and (3) histologic and/or electron-microscopic examination for Negri bodies. While the mouse inoculation studies for virus isolation and direct FA staining for viral antigen are quite reliable and sensitive, "autosterilization" may occur and these tests may be negative if the patient's life has been prolonged and high levels of neutralizing antibody are present in serum and CSF. The use of FA staining of skin biopsies, corneal impression smears, and saliva for evidence of rabies antigen has been helpful in diagnosing rabies during life. Confirmation of these findings either serologically or by demonstration of virus in brain should be sought.

If the patient has not received antirabies immunization, a fourfold rise in neutralizing antibody to rabies virus in serial serum samples is diagnostic. If the patient has received rabies vaccination, a clue to the diagnosis may be obtained from the absolute titers of serum-neutralizing antibody and the presence of neutralizing antibody to rabies in CSF. Postexposure rabies prophylaxis rarely produces CSF-neutralizing antibody to rabies. If present, it is usually in low titer, e.g., less than 1:64, whereas CSF titers in human rabies may vary from 1:200 to 1:160,000.

DIFFERENTIAL DIAGNOSIS   There is little to distinguish rabies from other viral encephalitides, and the most helpful point in diagnosis is the history of exposure. Other problems to be considered include hysterical reactions to animal bites (pseudohydrophobia), Landry-Guillain-Barré syndrome, poliomyelitis, and allergic encephalomyelitis to rabies vaccine. The latter occurs most commonly after use of nerve tissue–derived vaccine and usually begins 1 to 4 weeks after vaccination.

PREVENTION AND TREATMENT   Each year more than 1 million Americans are bitten by animals. In each instance, a decision must be made whether to initiate postexposure rabies prophylaxis. When deciding whether to institute rabies prophylaxis, the following considerations apply: (1) whether the individual came into physical contact with saliva or another substance likely to contain rabies virus, (2) whether rabies is known or suspected in the species and area associated with the exposure (e.g., all persons within the continental United States bitten by a bat that then escapes should receive postexposure prophylaxis), (3) the circumstances surrounding the exposure, and (4)

the treatment alternative and complications. A guide for postexposure rabies prophylaxis is illustrated in Fig. 158-1.

If rabies is known to be present or suspected to be present in the animal species involved in a human exposure, the animal should be captured, if possible. Wild animals or any ill, unvaccinated, or stray domestic animal involved in a rabies exposure, particularly any animal involved in an unprovoked bite, exhibiting abnormal behavior, or suspected of being rabid, should be humanely killed, and the head should be sent immediately to an appropriate laboratory for rabies FA examination. If examination of the brain by the FA technique is negative for rabies, it can be assumed that the saliva contains no virus, and the exposed person need not be treated. Persons exposed to escaped wild animals capable of carrying rabies (bats, skunks, coyotes, foxes, raccoons, etc.) in an area where rabies is known or suspected to be present should receive both passive and active immunization against rabies.

If a healthy dog or cat bites a person, the animal should be captured, confined, and observed for 10 days. If any illness or abnormal behavior develops in the animal during the observation period, it should be killed for FA examination. Experimental and epidemiologic evidence suggests that animals that remain healthy for 10 days after a bite will not have transmitted rabies virus at the time of the bite.

Postexposure prophylaxis   Once a decision regarding the necessity to initiate postexposure rabies prophylaxis has been made, the general principle of postexposure therapy is to minimize the amount of virus at the site of inoculation with local treatment of the wound and to establish an early and long-lasting neutralizing antibody titer to rabies virus. In most instances, postexposure therapy includes administration of globulin and vaccines. The following is a therapeutic regimen:

1 *Local wound therapy*. This is an important part of rabies prevention. The wound should be scrubbed with soap and then flushed with water. Both mechanical and chemical cleansing are important. Quaternary ammonium compounds such as 1 to 4% benzalkonium chloride or 1% cetrimonium bromide are useful because they inactivate the rabies virus. However, 0.1% benzalkonium solutions

FIGURE 158-1   Postexposure rabies prophylaxis algorithm.

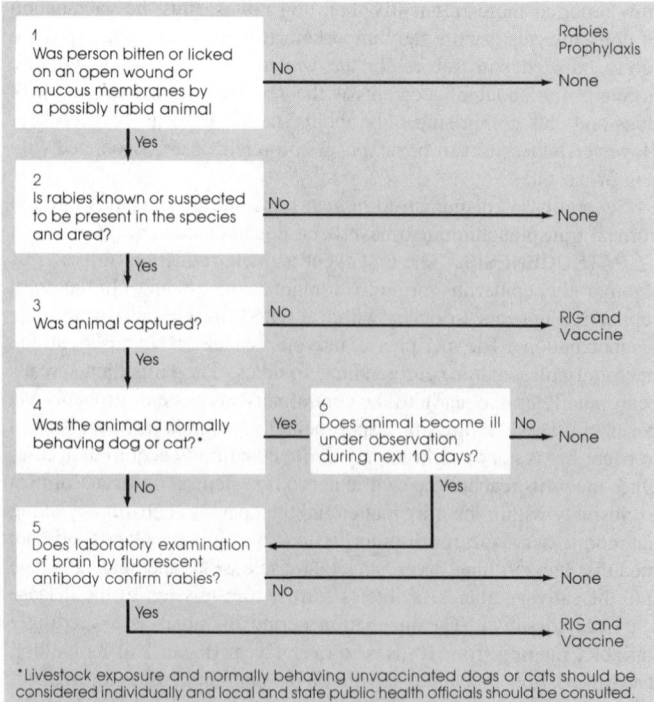

*Livestock exposure and normally behaving unvaccinated dogs or cats should be considered individually and local and state public health officials should be consulted.

are less effective than 20% soap solutions. Usually tetanus toxoid and antibiotics should be administered.

2 *Passive immunization with antirabies antiserum* of either equine or human origin. Human rabies immune globulin (HRIG) is preferred because equine antiserum may cause serum sickness. Fifty percent of the total dose of 20 units per kilogram for HRIG and 40 units per kilogram for the equine antiserum is given by local infiltration of the wound, and the rest is administered intramuscularly into the gluteal region.

3 *Active immunization with antirabies vaccine.* Human diploid cell vaccine (HDCV) is the recommended rabies vaccine. In the United States, two products are licensed. One vaccine contains the Pitman-Moure strain of virus (Pasteur-Meriux; Imovax) that is grown on human diploid cell cultures and inactivated with β-propiolactone. The other vaccine, rabies vaccine absorbed (RVA), is distributed by the Biologics Products Program, Michigan Department of Public Health, and is prepared from the Kissling strain of virus adapted to fetal rhesus lung diploid cells. Both vaccines are considered equally efficacious and safe. Severe reactions to HDCV are uncommon. Immediate hypersensitivity responses such as urticaria have been reported in approximately 1 in 650 recipients. Systemic reactions such as fever, headache, and nausea are generally mild and are reported in 1 to 4 percent of recipients. Local reactions such as swelling, erythema, and induration at the injection site occur in 15 to 20 percent of vaccinees.

Five 1-mL doses of HDCV are given intramuscularly, preferably in the deltoid or anterolateral thigh area, as soon as possible after exposure. The first dose (day 0) also should be accompanied by antirabies serum (HRIG) in the gluteal area. Five doses should be administered within 28 days on the following schedule: days 0, 3, 7, 14, and 28. The WHO also recommends a 21- and 90-day course.

The combination of HRIG and HDCV produces high titers of neutralizing antibodies in almost all recipients. Only rarely has this regimen proved unsuccessful in preventing the subsequent development of rabies. The administration of vaccine alone appears to be associated with a higher failure rate than HRIG and HDCV, especially in severe bite exposures. The combination of HRIG plus 0.1-mL intradermal doses at eight sites on day 0, four sites on day 7, and one site on days 28 and 91 produces good antibody responses, although the clinical experience with this regimen is less than with intramuscular administration.

Preexposure prophylaxis Individuals with a high risk of contact with rabies virus—veterinarians, cave explorers, laboratory workers, and animal handlers—should have preexposure prophylaxis with rabies vaccine. HDCV is the preferred vaccine for preexposure prophylaxis; three IM or three 0.1-mL intradermal injections on days 0, 7, and 28 should be administered. RVA should not be used intradermally. A neutralizing antibody titer should be checked after vaccination. Concomitant chloroquine administration interferes with the antibody response to vaccine. Depending on risk, serologic testing should be done at 2- to 6-year intervals. When neutralizing titers fall below 1:5, booster doses should be given. Booster doses may be administered either as a single 1-mL intramuscular or 0.1-mL intradermal injection. Postexposure prophylaxis in individuals previously given preexposure therapy consists of HDCV alone (two IM doses of HDCV on days 0 and 3 are usually adequate).

Booster doses of HDCV are associated with fever, headache, muscle aches, and joint pains in about 20 percent of recipients. Up to 6 percent of persons receiving IM booster doses of HDCV have developed an immune-complex–like reaction characterized by urticaria, arthritis, nausea, vomiting, and, occasionally, angioedema. These reactions have been self-limited and appear to be associated with the presence of β-propriolactone-altered human serum albumin in the vaccine and the development of IgE antibodies to this antigen. Persons who work in high-risk areas should undergo periodic measurement of antibodies, and booster doses are recommended for those with low antibody titers. Those at very low risk may elect not to receive routine booster doses but only to receive active immunization with any substantive exposure.

MOKOLA VIRUS

Mokola virus was first isolated from wild shrews captured in Nigeria and subsequently was shown to be related morphologically and serologically to rabies virus. However, neither of the two reported cases of human disease (both in children) demonstrated classic clinical features of rabies. One patient had a nonfatal illness characterized by fever, pharyngitis, and convulsions. Mokola virus was recovered from her cerebrospinal fluid (CSF). The second patient initially had fever, cough, and vomiting, followed in several days by drowsiness, confusion, and generalized flaccid weakness. Her CSF was normal. She progressed to deep coma and died within 10 days of onset. Mokola virus was isolated from her brain, and histopathologic sections revealed finely granular cytoplasmic inclusions that were distinguishable from Negri bodies in many neurons.

VESICULAR STOMATITIS VIRUS

Vesicular stomatitis is a viral illness of animals that occasionally affects humans. It presents as an acute, self-limited, influenza-like disease. The disease in animals is found in the United States and South America and affects chiefly domestic cattle, horses, swine, wild deer, raccoons, skunks, and bobcats.

In animals, vesicular stomatitis is characterized by the development of vesicles on the oral mucosa, particularly the tongue, udders, and heels. The mode of spread is probably by direct contact; however, epidemics tend to occur in warm weather, and isolation of the virus from *Phlebotomus* sandflies in Panama and *Aedes* species in New Mexico suggests these as possible vectors. Two distinct serotypes, New Jersey and Indiana, have been recognized, and most of the outbreaks in North America have been attributed to the New Jersey strain. The disease is most common in laboratory workers, and in one report, three-fourths of laboratory personnel handling experimentally infected animals or manipulating the virus developed neutralizing antibodies. The disease is transmissible, however, under natural conditions among workers having direct contact with infected animals, especially cattle. The incubation period ranges from 1 to 6 days. This is followed by the sudden onset of fever up to 40°C (104°F), chills, profuse sweating, myalgias, malaise, headache, and pain on ocular movement. One-third to one-half of patients have sore throat and cervical and/or submandibular adenopathy. Small raised vesicular lesions may appear on the buccal mucosa. Conjunctivitis and coryza are present in about 20 percent of cases. Occasionally, small subcorneal, intraepithelial vesicles may appear on the fingers, usually associated with direct inoculation of the virus. Symptoms generally last 3 to 4 days, but occasionally a diphasic course may occur. Inapparent infection is common, and among laboratory workers with serologic evidence of infection, only about one-half reported clinical symptoms. In some areas of Panama, 17 to 35 percent of the population have neutralizing antibodies against vesicular stomatitis virus.

The differential diagnosis includes hand-foot-and-mouth disease, herpangina, primary herpetic pharyngitis and other mucocutaneous syndromes, and influenza. Viral isolation from patients is not common; however, a rise in complement fixation and/or neutralizing antibodies to vesicular stomatitis virus between acute and convalescent sera will help to confirm the diagnosis. Treatment is nonspecific.

MARBURG VIRUS DISEASE

DEFINITION Marburg virus causes an acute systemic febrile illness characterized by the abrupt onset of headache, myalgias, pharyngitis, rash, and hemorrhagic manifestations. It was recognized first in 1967 when it caused simultaneous outbreaks in the Federal Republic of Germany and Yugoslavia among laboratory workers exposed to imported African green monkeys (*Cercopithecus aethiops*). Outbreaks have been reported from Kenya. The clinical manifestations are similar to those of other hemorrhagic fevers of the arenavirus class or flavivirus group (Argentinian and Bolivian hemorrhagic fever; Chap. 160). The high case-fatality rate and demonstrated ability for nosocomial spread have made recognition of this rare agent an important worldwide public health concern.

ETIOLOGY The Marburg virus has been isolated in guinea pig and various cell culture systems such as vervet monkey kidney. The virus particle contains lipid and RNA, and under the electron microscope the virus appears as an 80- to 100-nm elongated filamentous particle with occasional "blister-like excrescences." Marburg and Ebola viruses have been included in a new family of viruses called Filoviridae. These viruses are biosafety level 4 pathogens, and maximum biologic containment facilities are recommended.

EPIDEMIOLOGY The initial outbreak affected 31 patients in Marburg and Frankfurt, Germany, and Belgrade, Yugoslavia, and was epidemiologically linked to monkeys imported from the same source in Uganda. Virus was isolated from the blood and tissue of these monkeys. Of the 25 primary infections, there were seven deaths and six secondary cases, most of which appeared related to accidental needle sticks or abrasions. The wife of one patient developed Marburg virus disease. Marburg virus was demonstrated in semen of the original patient, despite the presence of circulating antibody, and this secondary case is believed to have been acquired through sexual intercourse. Recently, Marburg and Ebola viruses have been isolated from cynomolgus monkeys imported into the United States; these isolates are morphologically similar but genetically distinct from the viruses isolated in Europe in 1967. Human disease has not yet been associated with these latter strains.

PATHOLOGY Marburg virus appears "pantropic" and produces lesions in almost all organs, including lymphoid tissue, liver, spleen, pancreas, adrenals, thyroid, kidney, testes, skin, and brain. In lymphoid tissue, focal necrosis with degeneration is apparent. In the liver, eosinophilic cytoplasmic bodies resembling the Councilman bodies of yellow fever have been noted. The lungs may show interstitial pneumonitis, as well as vascular lesions in small arterioles, indicative of endarteritis. Neuropathologic changes consist of multiple small hemorrhagic infarcts with glial proliferation.

CLINICAL MANIFESTATIONS After an incubation period of 3 to 9 days, patients develop frontal and temporal headache, malaise, myalgias (especially in the lumbar area), nausea, and vomiting. Fever of 39.4 to 40°C (103 to 104°F) is characteristic, and about half the patients have conjunctivitis. Between 1 and 3 days after onset, watery diarrhea (often severe), lethargy, and a change in mentation are noted. An enanthem of the palate and tonsils and cervical lymphadenopathy also may be noted during the first week of illness. The most reliable clinical feature is the appearance of nonpruritic maculopapular rash, which begins on the fifth to seventh day on the face and neck and spreads centrifugally to involve the extremities. A fine desquamation of the affected skin, especially the palms and soles, appears 4 to 5 days later. Hemorrhagic manifestations, including gastrointestinal, renal, vaginal, and/or conjunctival hemorrhages, generally develop between days 5 and 7 of disease.

During the first week, the temperature continues in the vicinity of 40°C (104°F), falling by lysis during the second week, to increase again between the twelfth and fourteenth days. Other clinical signs apparent in the second week of disease include splenomegaly, hepatomegaly, facial edema, and scrotal or labial reddening. Complications include orchitis, which may lead to testicular atrophy; myocarditis with irregular pulse and electrocardiographic abnormalities; and pancreatitis. The overall case-fatality rate has been about 25 percent, with death usually occurring during the eighth to sixteenth days of illness. Recovery is often protracted over a 3- to 4-week period, and during this period, loss of hair, intermittent abdominal pain, poor appetite, and prolonged psychotic disturbances have been noted. Late sequelae, including transverse myelitis and uveitis, have been reported. Marburg virus has been isolated from the anterior eye chamber and semen nearly 3 months after onset of disease.

LABORATORY FINDINGS Abnormalities in granulocyte function are found, and leukopenia is detected as early as the first day, with leukocyte counts as low as 1000 cells per microliter and a neutrophilia by the fourth day. Subsequently, atypical lymphocytes, as well as neutrophils exhibiting the characteristic of the Pelger-Huët anomaly, may appear. Thrombocytopenia appears early and is most marked, often less than 10,000 cells per microliter, between the sixth and twelfth days. In fatal cases, evidence of disseminated intravascular coagulation can be demonstrated. Hypoproteinemia, proteinuria, and azotemia may occur. Elevations in aspartate aminotransferase (SGOT) and alanine aminotransferase (SGPT) are usual. Lumbar puncture may be normal or reveal a minimal pleocytosis. The erythrocyte sedimentation rate is usually low.

DIAGNOSIS The characteristic clinical course and epidemiologic features are the basis of the diagnosis. Specific diagnosis requires isolation of the virus or serologic evidence of infection in paired serum samples. Viremia coincides with the febrile state of disease, and virus has been isolated from tissue as well as urine, semen, and throat and rectal swabs. Attempts to isolate virus must be carried out only in *specialized high-security laboratories*. All patients should be kept in strict isolation, and all specimens should be handled and shipped according to World Health Organization guidelines.

TREATMENT Patients have received a multiplicity of drugs without apparent influence on the course of the illness. Convalescent serum was administered to four patients, whose subsequent disease followed a mild course. However, similarly benign outcomes were observed in patients who did not receive serum.

EBOLA VIRUS

Between July and November 1976, simultaneous outbreaks of an acute febrile hemorrhagic disease occurred in southern Sudan and northern Zaire. "Secondary and tertiary" spread of infection, particularly among hospital staff, was noted. In the Sudan over 300 cases with 151 deaths and in Zaire 237 cases with 211 fatalities were reported. The virus isolated from these patients was morphologically similar to but antigenically distinct from the Marburg agent. The name *Ebola virus*, after the river in Zaire located near the epidemic, has been proposed. Biologic and antigenic differences between strains of Ebola viruses isolated in Zaire and the Sudan may account for the differences in mortality between the two outbreaks. Sporadic cases of disease also appear to occur, and a serosurvey revealed a prevalence rate of 7 percent for antibodies to Ebola virus in endemic areas. As with other hemorrhagic fevers, neutrophil leukocytosis, hypofibrinogenemia, thrombocytopenia, and microangiopathic hemolytic anemia are features of the illness.

Ebola virus has been propagated in tissue culture (Vero cells) and in suckling mice and guinea pigs. The source of the outbreak in both the Sudan and Zaire is unknown; however, as with other viral hemorrhagic fevers, peridomestic rodents are suspected as being a reservoir of the infection, and serologic evidence of Ebola virus infection was detected in a domestic guinea pig trapped in Zaire. More recently, the isolation of Ebola virus from Asian macaques has suggested that these animals are the natural reservoir of infection. Once established, nosocomial as well as community-acquired cases occur, especially among persons who have close and prolonged contact with infected individuals. Parenteral exposure to the virus through disinfected rather than sterilized needles may have played a role in transmission. Barrier nursing and strict isolation precautions with use of protective clothing appeared to decrease the number of nosocomial cases.

CLINICAL MANIFESTATIONS Clinically, the disease is similar to Marburg virus disease. The incubation period ranges from 4 to 6 days. Patients usually present on the fifth day of illness with a history of abrupt onset of headache, malaise, myalgias, high fever, diarrhea, abdominal pain, dehydration, and lethargy. Pleuritic chest pain, a dry hacking cough, and a pronounced pharyngitis also have been noted. A maculopapular eruption develops between days 5 and 7 of illness. On black skins the rash is often faint and not recognized until desquamation occurs. Hematemesis, melena, and bleeding from the nose, gums, and vagina are common. Abortion and massive metrorrhagia are frequent complications among pregnant women. Death usually occurs in the second week of illness and is preceded by severe blood loss and shock.

TREATMENT Patients should be isolated until virologic studies indicate they are free of virus, usually 21 days from onset of illness. The frequent detection of malaria parasites in blood films of patients with Ebola virus infection in the Sudan indicated that parasitemia does not rule out concomitant viral illness. Treatment with plasma containing Ebola virus–specific antibodies has resulted in diminished levels of viremia; however, further tests are required to establish the effectiveness of this form of therapy. Requests for viral isolation as well as convalescent plasma should be addressed to WHO Regional Centers in Atlanta or Geneva.

REFERENCES

Rabies

BAER GM: Research towards rabies prevention: Overview. Rev Infect Dis 10(suppl 4):S576, 1988

———, FISHBEIN DB: Rabies post exposure prophylaxis. N Engl J Med 316:1270, 1987

BERNARD KW et al: Preexposure immunization with intradermal human diploid cell rabies vaccine. JAMA 257:1059, 1987

HOUFF SA et al: Human-to-human transmission of rabies virus by a corneal transplant. N Engl J Med 300:603, 1979

NICHOLSON KG: Rabies. Lancet 335:1201, 1990

PAPPAIVANOU M et al: Antibody response to preexposure diploid-cell rabies vaccine given concurrently with chloroquine. N Engl J Med 314:280, 1986

Recommendations of the Public Health Service, Immunization Practices Advisory Committee (ACIP): Rabies prevention. United States, 1991. Morb Mort Week Rep 40(RR-3):1, 1991

SMITH JS et al: Unexplained rabies in three immigrants to the United States. N Engl J Med 324:205, 1991

WARRELL DA, WARRELL MJ: Human rabies and its prevention: An overview. Rev Infect Dis 10 (Suppl 4):S726, 1988

Mokola virus

FAMILUSI JB: Fatal human infection with Mokola virus. Am J Trop Med Hyg 21:959, 1972

Marburg virus

Filovirus infections among persons with occupational exposure to nonhuman primates. Morb Mort Week Rep 39:266, 1990

SIMPSON DH: Marburg and Ebola virus infections: A guide for their diagnosis, management and control. Geneva, WHO Offset Publication 36, 1977

SMITH DH et al: Marburg-virus disease in Kenya. Lancet 1:816, 1982

Ebola virus

JAHRLING PB: Preliminary report: Isolation of Ebola virus from monkeys imported to USA. Lancet 335:502, 1990

McCORMICK JB et al: Biologic differences between strains of Ebola virus from Zaire and Sudan. J Infect Dis 147:264, 1983

STANSFIELD SK: Antibody to Ebola virus in guinea pigs: Tandala, Zaire. J Infect Dis 146:483, 1982

159 ARBOVIRUS INFECTIONS

JAY P. SANFORD

DEFINITION AND CLASSIFICATION The definition of an arthropod-borne virus (arbovirus) was published in 1967 by the World Health Organization:

Arboviruses are viruses which are maintained in nature principally, or to an important extent, through biological transmission between susceptible vertebrate hosts by hematophagous arthropods; they multiply and produce viremia in the vertebrates, multiply in the tissues of arthropods, and are passed on to new vertebrates by the bites of arthropods after a period of extrinsic incubation.

From this definition it can be appreciated that the term *arbovirus* is used in the ecologic sense. Transmission by vectors is not correlated with virus architecture. Current approaches to taxonomy are based on viral morphology, structure, and function. As a result, for taxonomic purposes, the term *arbovirus* has been eliminated. The purpose of this chapter is to define viral illness transmitted to humans by biting insects. Because the number of agents is large, mention will be made of those which have been best documented, have demonstrated unusual features, or seem to be of greatest potential public health importance.

The more than 530 antigenically distinct "arboviruses" are now grouped into six families (Table 159-1). The majority of agents contain single-stranded RNA, although some, such as the Reoviridae, contain double-stranded RNA. Sixty arboviruses have been isolated in the United States and Canada, of which 16 are associated with human disease.

"Arboviruses" are of importance in both temperate and tropical zones. Representative viruses have been isolated in almost every geographic area outside the polar regions.

"Arbovirus" infection of vertebrates is usually asymptomatic. The viremia stimulates an immune response which sharply limits the duration of the viremia. In "arbovirus" infections other than urban yellow fever, phlebotomus fever, chikungunya, o'nyong-nyong, mayaro, oropouche, and dengue, infection of humans represents an incidental occurrence which is tangential to the basic maintenance cycle of the virus. Hence the isolation of virus from arthropod vectors or the detection of infection in the natural vertebrate host may provide a means for early detection and enable control of epizootic infection before significant spread to humans occurs.

Most human "arbovirus" infections are asymptomatic. When disease is produced, the spectrum of clinical illness is varied both in predominant features and in severity. Most commonly, disease is self-limited with symptoms of fever, headache, malaise, and myalgia. Associated rash and lymphadenopathy may be features. "Arboviruses" which may cause three major clinical syndromes—arthralgia-arthritis, encephalitis–aseptic meningitis, or hemorrhagic disease—are tabulated in Table 159-2.

INFECTIONS PRESENTING CHIEFLY WITH FEVER, MALAISE, HEADACHE, AND MYALGIA

VENEZUELAN EQUINE ENCEPHALITIS Venezuelan equine encephalitis (VEE) was first noted in equines in Colombia in 1935.

Etiology Like other alphaviruses, the causative agent of VEE is a 40- to 45-nm, single-stranded RNA virus. Based on serologic tests and oligonucleotide fingerprints, a complex of Venezuelan encephalitis viruses has been established: VE subtypes IA to IE, II (Everglades), III (Mucambo), and IV (Pixuna). IA was the original epidemic strain which occurred in Venezuela, and IB, which was recognized in Ecuador in 1963, spread through Central America into Mexico and was responsible for the epidemic in Mexico in 1971 which spread into southern Texas, with the occurrence of at least 76 laboratory-

TABLE 159-1 Virus taxonomy and arboviruses-arenaviruses*

Family	Genus	Virus "English vernacular name"[†]	Family	Genus	Virus "English vernacular name"[†]

Reoviridae	Orbivirus	Colorado tick fever[‡]
		Orungo
		Kemerovo
		  Lipovnik
		  Tribec
			Rhabdoviridae	Vesiculovirus	Vesicular stomatitis Indiana[‡]
					Vesicular stomatitis New Jersey[‡]
					Chandipura
					Piry
					Isfahan

Togaviridae	Alphavirus (group A)	*Associated with encephalitis*
		Eastern equine encephalitis[‡]
		Venezuelan encephalitis[‡]
		Western equine encephalitis[‡]
		Associated with acute arthropathy
		Sindbis
		  Okelbo (Pogosta and Karelian fevers)
		  Babanki
		Semliki Forest complex
		  Chikungunya[‡]
		  O'nyong-nyong
		  Igbo Ora
		  Ross River[‡]
		  Barmah Forest
		  Mayaro
				Lyssavirus	Rabies[‡]
					Mokola
					Duvenhage

			Filoviridae		Marburg[‡] Ebola[‡] Reston strain

Flavivirdae	Flavivirus (group B)	*Associated with encephalitis*
		St. Louis encephalitis[‡]
		Japanese encephalitis[‡]
		Murray Valley encephalitis[‡]
		Tick-borne encephalitis complex[‡]
		  Russian spring-summer encephalitis
		  Central European encephalitis
		  Negishi
		  Powassan[‡]
		  Louping-ill
		  Rocio
		Associated with fever-arthralgia-rash
		Dengue fever[‡]
		West Nile fever[‡]
		Ten other agents—of less public health importance
		Associated with hemorrhagic fever
		Yellow fever[‡]
		Dengue fever[‡]
		  Omsk hemorrhagic fever
		Kyasanur Forest disease
			Bunyaviridae	Bunyavirus (16 serogroups)	Twenty-four agents may cause fever, fever-rash. None cause death. None in United States.
					California serogroup
					  LaCrosse[‡]
					  Snowshoe hare
					  Jamestown Canyon
					  California encephalitis
					  Tahyna

				Phlebovirus	Thirty-seven phleboviruses isolated from human beings; none cause death except Rift Valley fever virus. Sandfly fever–Naples[‡] Sandfly fever–Sicilian[‡] Toscana Rift Valley fever[‡]
				Nairovirus	Crimean-Congo hemorrhagic fever[‡]
				Hantavirus	Hantaan[‡] Puumala[‡] Seoul[‡] Porogia[‡]
			Arenaviridae	Arenavirus	Lymphocytic choriomeningitis[‡] Lassa[‡] Machupo[‡] Junin[‡] Guanarito[‡]

* Only agents which have been shown to naturally infect humans are tabulated.
[†] Virus species have not yet been designated formally. The International Committee on

Taxonomy of Viruses lists species under the term "English vernacular name."
[‡] Viruses found in the United States and/or of major public health importance.

---

confirmed human cases. In early 1973, almost 4000 cases occurred in Peru.

Epidemiology VEE has been primarily a disease of equines and other mammals, although occasionally the agent has infected humans. Evidence of human infection (virus isolation or specific neutralizing antibodies) has been found in Colombia, Ecuador, Panama, Surinam, Guyana, French Guiana, Mexico, Brazil, Curaçao, Trinidad, Argentina, Peru, Florida, and Texas. Each subtype of VE virus is unique to its enzootic vector and does not replicate well in other vectors. Most common is an enzootic cycle between *Culex* mosquitoes and forest rodents. Enzootic VEE infects people who enter the rain forest or swamps, rubber tappers, forestry workers, and military personnel on jungle maneuvers. During an epizootic, many species of mosquitoes can transmit virus, especially *Aedes*, *Mansonia*, and *Psorophora*. The virus has a wide host range in wild mammals, with at least 20 genera, including capuchin monkeys, rats, mice, opossum, jackrabbit, fox, and bats, being naturally infected. Domestic animals other than equines which have been shown to be infected include cattle and pigs in Mexico and goats and sheep in Venezuela. VEE appears to multiply well in mammals with high titers of virus in the blood; e.g., infected horses may have titers of up to $10^{7.5}$ mouse intraperitoneal lethal doses per milliliter of blood. Although 29 species of wild birds have been shown to be naturally infected with VEE (20 percent of which

are colonial nestling herons and related species), whether the VEE-viremia levels in birds are high enough to infect vector mosquitoes is not known. During the initial 3 days of illness, viremia has been detected in approximately two-thirds of patients. The levels of viremia are sufficiently high that humans could serve as a reservoir. VEE virus also has been isolated by pharyngeal swab in a few patients, suggesting the potential for person-to-person transmission. The available observations make it reasonable to consider that the natural vector is a mosquito, with the primary reservoir being either wild or domestic terrestrial mammals. However, natural infection can probably take place without an arthropod vector. Laboratory infections have occurred and are probably due to inhalation of aerosols.

Clinical manifestations In humans, infection with VEE virus usually results in a mild acute febrile illness without neurologic complications. No age is spared, and there is no sex preponderance. The incubation period is 2 to 5 days, followed by the abrupt onset of headache, fever often associated with rigors, malaise, and myalgia. Other common symptoms may include nausea, vomiting, diarrhea, and sore throat. Uncommon features include photophobia, seizures, mental confusion, coma, tremors, and diplopia. Lymphadenopathy occurs in one-third of patients. On laboratory examination initial leukocyte counts are normal with 80 percent neutrophils. By the third day leukopenia occurs in two-thirds of patients. The cerebrospinal

TABLE 159-2 Major clinical syndromes,* associated arboviruses-arenaviruses, and major geographic distribution

Virus	Geographic distribution	Virus	Geographic distribution
FEVER, MALAISE, MYALGIA		**ENCEPHALITIS/ASEPTIC MENINGITIS** (*continued*)	
Phlebotomus (Sandfly) fever	Mediterranean, Middle East, northwest India, Central and South America, East Africa, southern China	Japanese encephalitis	Japan, Korea, China, India, Philippines, Southeast Asia, Thailand, Former Soviet Union
Colorado tick fever	Rocky Mountain region of United States and Canada	Murray Valley encephalitis	Australia, New Guinea
		Rocio	Brazil
Venezuelan equine encephalitis	South and Central America, Florida and Texas	Omsk hemorrhagic fever	Former Soviet Union
		Kyasanur Forest disease complex	India
Rift Valley fever	Eastern and South Africa, Egypt	Negishi	Japan
		Powassan	New York, eastern Canada
FEVER, MALAISE, LYMPHADENOPATHY, AND RASH		Louping ill	United Kingdom, Ireland
		Russian spring-summer encephalitis	Western Siberia
Dengue	Tropical Asia, Oceania, Africa, Australia, Americas	Central European encephalitis	Eastern Europe, Scandinavia, France, Switzerland
West Nile fever	Africa, Middle East, former Soviet Union, France, India, Indonesia	California group (except Tahyna)	North America
		Tahyna	Europe
FEVER, ACUTE ARTHOPATHY		Rift Valley fever	Eastern and South Africa, Senegal, Mauritania
Chikungunya	Africa, Southeast Asia	Lymphocytic choriomeningitis	United States, Germany, Hungary, Argentina
O'nyong-nyong	Eastern Africa (? central Africa)		
Ross River	Australia, Papua, New Guinea, Fiji, Somoa, Cook Islands	**HEMORRHAGIC FEVER**	
Barmah Forest	Eastern Australia	Yellow fever	South America, Africa
Mayaro	South and Central America	Dengue	Caribbean, Southeast Asia, China
Sindbis	Africa, former Soviet Union, Finland, Sweden, South and Central America	Chikungunya	Southeast Asia
		Kyasanur Forest disease	India
Igbo Ora	Central Africa, Nigeria, Ivory Coast	Omsk hemorrhagic fever	Former Soviet Union
		Crimean-Congo hemorrhagic fever	Africa, eastern Europe, Middle East, Asia
ENCEPHALITIS/ASEPTIC MENINGITIS		Hantaan	Korea, Japan, eastern China, Manchuria, former Soviet Union, central Europe
Kemerovo	Central Europe, former Soviet Union	Seoul	Korea, Japan
Eastern equine encephalitis	Atlantic, Gulf coasts, United States, upper New York, Caribbean, western Michigan	Puumala	Scandinavia, central Europe
		Porogia	Balkan area of Europe
Venezuelan equine encephalitis	Northern South America, Central America, Mexico, Florida	Marburg	Uganda, Kenya, Zimbabwe (consider sub-Saharan Africa)
Western equine encephalitis	United States, Canada, Central and South America	Ebola	Zaire, Sudan (under sub-Saharan Africa)
		Lassa fever	West Africa
St. Louis encephalitis	United States, Caribbean	Machupo	Bolivia
		Junin	Argentina
		Guanarito	Venezuela

* Most agents are more often associated with undifferentiated febrile illness than with the specific syndromes. See text for exceptions.

fluid (CSF) may reveal pleocytosis with modest increases in protein and normal glucose concentration. Virus may be isolated both from blood and from CSF. The symptoms usually last 3 to 5 days in mild cases and up to 8 days in more severe cases. A biphasic course of illness may be encountered, with recrudescence of symptoms on the sixth to the ninth day. In an epidemic in Venezuela in 1962, almost 16,000 cases of acute disease were evaluated; 38 percent were classified as encephalitis, but only 3 to 4 percent had severe neurologic abnormalities: convulsions, nystagmus, drowsiness, delirium, or meningitis. The mortality rate was estimated to be less than 0.5 percent, and nearly all deaths occurred in young children.

PHLEBOTOMUS FEVER Phlebotomus (sandfly, pappataci, or 3-day) fever is an acute, relatively mild, self-limited infection caused by at least seven immunologically distinct phleboviruses (Naples, Sicilian, Punta Toro, Alenquer, Toscana, Chagres, and Candiru). Humans, the only known host, probably serve as a dead-end host. The virus is likely maintained by transovarial transmission in sandflies, with vertebrate hosts having little role in the transmission cycle.

Prevalence The disease occurs throughout the Mediterranean basin, the Balkans, the Near and Middle East, the eastern part of Africa, the former Soviet republics of central Asia, Pakistan, parts of India, Panama, Brazil, and possibly certain parts of southern China. In the Middle East and central Asia, native populations acquire the disease at an early age and develop and maintain high levels of immunity. Cases in Panama and Brazil are sporadic, occurring mainly in persons entering the forest. The apparent absence of phlebotomus

fever in indigenous adult populations residing in areas where sandflies are abundant may present a deceptive picture of the actual risk to susceptible persons.

Epidemiology In the Middle East and central Asia, the disease occurs during the hot, dry season (summer or autumn months) and is transmitted to human beings by the bite of infected sandflies (*Phlebotomus* spp.), which are small (2- to 3-mm) urban flies, highly anthropophilic, that can penetrate ordinary house screens. Only the female bites and usually does so during the night. In persons who are not sensitive, there is neither pain nor local irritation after the bite; hence only about 1 percent of patients will remember having been bitten. In contrast, most of the human-biting sandflies (*Lutzomyia* spp.) of tropical America are sylvan in their habits, infrequently entering houses to bite people. In humans, the incubation period averages 3 to 5 days. Viremia is present for at least 24 h before the onset of fever but is not detectable for more than 2 days after the onset of illness. Following recovery, the patient has lifelong immunity to the infecting virus but not to heterologous serotypes. Hence an individual can have illnesses several times.

Clinical manifestations The onset of symptoms is abrupt in over 90 percent of patients, with the temperature rapidly rising to its highest point, which may vary from 37.8 to 40.1°C (100 to 105°F). Headache is nearly always present and often is accompanied by pain on moving the eyes and retroorbital pain. Myalgia is common and may be localized to the chest, resembling pleurodynia, or to the abdomen. Other symptoms may include vomiting, photophobia, giddiness, neck stiffness, alteration or loss of taste, and arthralgia. Conjunctival injection is present in approximately one-third of patients. Small vesicles may be seen on the palate, and macular or urticarial rashes occur. The spleen is rarely palpable, and lymphadenopathy is absent. The pulse rate may be elevated in proportion to the temperature on the first day; thereafter, bradycardia is often present. The fever persists 3 days in most patients, with gradual defervescence. Giddiness, weakness, and feelings of depression are frequently encountered during convalescence. Second attacks 2 to 12 weeks after the first occur in 15 percent of cases.

In common with other "arbovirus" infections, phlebotomus fever may be associated with *aseptic meningitis*. In one series, 12 percent of patients had symptoms and signs sufficient to warrant a lumbar puncture. Findings in these patients included pleocytosis, with an average cell count of 90 per microliter and a predominance of either polymorphonuclear or mononuclear leukocytes. CSF protein concentration ranged from 0.2 to 1.3 g/L (20 to 130 mg/dL). In another series, mild papilledema was observed in a few patients with severe illness.

Laboratory findings The changes in leukocyte count constitute the only positive laboratory findings. Total leukocyte counts of less than 5000 cells per microliter are observed in 90 percent of patients if daily counts are done during the febrile period and convalescence. The leukopenia may not appear until the last day of fever or even after defervescence. The differential leukocyte count will reveal an absolute decrease in lymphocytes on the first day, accompanied by an increase in nonsegmented neutrophils. During the second or third day, the number of lymphocytes begins to return to normal and may constitute 40 to 65 percent of the total count. Concurrently, there is a reversal in proportion of segmented and band neutrophils. The differential count usually returns to normal within 5 to 8 days after defervescence. Erythrocyte values and urinalyses are usually normal.

Diagnosis In the absence of a readily available serologic test, the diagnosis must be made on clinical and epidemiologic grounds.

Treatment The disease is self-limited, and no specific therapy is available. Symptomatic care, including bed rest, adequate fluid intake, and analgesia with aspirin, is recommended. Convalescence may require a week or longer.

Prognosis No fatalities have been recorded among tens of thousands of cases.

COLORADO TICK FEVER Colorado tick fever is one of the two tick-transmitted viral diseases of humans recognized in the United States and Canada, Powassan virus being the other. Though "mountain fever" had been described ever since the advent of immigrants to the Rocky Mountain region, it must be differentiated from mild Rocky Mountain spotted fever. Once the clinical picture of disease had been established, it was renamed Colorado tick fever. A second serotype of the Colorado tick fever serogroup (Eyach virus) was isolated from *Ixodes ricinus* ticks near the village of Eyach in Germany and in France. This agent has not been clearly associated with human disease.

Etiology Colorado tick fever virus is grouped as an "arbovirus" because it replicates in ticks. It is a double-stranded RNA virus belonging to the orbivirus genus of the Reoviridae family (see Table 159-1).

Prevalence The disease has been contracted in mountain forest areas at 4000 to 10,000 ft in the Rocky Mountain region of the United States and Canada. The possibility exists that Colorado tick fever may occur over a wider geographic area. Mild and clinically inapparent forms of the disease occur. Up to 15 percent of perennial campers have neutralizing antibodies. The number of cases of Colorado tick fever reported in Colorado is 20 times greater than that of Rocky Mountain spotted fever. In fact, almost one-half of the patients diagnosed as having Rocky Mountain spotted fever in Utah were subsequently shown to have Colorado tick fever.

Epidemiology Colorado tick fever is transmitted to humans by the adult hard-shelled wood tick, *Dermacentor andersoni*. The virus has been found in 10 to 25 percent of this species of ticks collected in endemic areas. Transovarial transmission of the virus in the tick has been established. Illness occurs from late March through

September, mostly in May and June. Virus can be recovered from blood for 2 weeks in most patients, for at least 1 month in nearly one-half, and from CSF during the acute illness. The virus persists within erythrocytes of convalescent patients for as long as 120 days and can be readily isolated from washed erythrocytes 100 days following infection. Transfusion-associated Colorado tick fever has been reported.

Clinical manifestations The incubation period is usually 3 to 6 days, and in 90 percent a history of tick contact within 10 days of onset of illness can be obtained. Failure to obtain such a history militates against the diagnosis. Persons affected usually are those whose occupational or recreational activities bring them in contact with ticks. The disease may occur at any age, although 40 percent in one series were 20 to 29 years of age. The clinical picture is characterized by the sudden onset of severe aching of the muscles of the back and legs, chilliness without true rigors, a rapid increase in temperature, which usually reaches 38.9 to 40°C (102 to 104°F), headache with pain on ocular movement, retroorbital pain, and photophobia. Abdominal pain and vomiting occur in one-fourth of patients; diarrhea is rare. The physical findings are not specific. Tachycardia in proportion to the temperature, flushed facies, and variable conjunctival injection may be present. Occasionally, the spleen is palpable. Rash occurs in 5 to 12 percent of patients, but on occasion, a petechial rash involving primarily the arms and legs or a maculopapular rash over the entire body may occur. Rarely, punched-out ulcers may form at the site of tick bite. The fever with the associated symptoms lasts about 2 days and then abruptly lyses to normal or subnormal, leaving the patient very weak. After an afebrile period of about 2 days, the fever recurs, may be higher than in the first phase, and may last as long as 3 days. One-half of patients show this saddleback pattern of temperature. Rarely there may be three febrile phases. Convalescence of more than 3 weeks is reported in 70 percent of patients over age 30, while symptoms last less than 1 week in 60 percent of patients under 20. Prolonged convalescence has no relationship to persistent viremia.

Evidence of central nervous system involvement has been recorded in a few patients (3 to 7 percent). The findings are those of either an aseptic meningitis with stiffness of the neck or encephalitis with clouding of the sensorium, delirium, and coma. Hemorrhagic fever with epistaxis, gastrointestinal bleeding, and purpura have been observed in children. Rarer complications include epididymoorchitis and patchy pneumonitis.

Laboratory findings The most important laboratory feature is moderate to marked leukopenia, although in one-third of confirmed cases leukocyte counts remain about 4500 cells per microliter. On the first day of illness, the total leukocyte count may be at normal levels, but usually by the fifth or sixth day there has been a decrease to 2000 to 3000 cells per microliter. Characteristically, there is a proportionate decrease in lymphocytes and granulocytes. Toxic changes in neutrophils are often conspicuous, and "virocyte" types of lymphocytes are frequently observed. Bone marrow examination reveals "maturation arrest" in the granulocytic series. Erythrocyte values remain normal. The blood picture returns to normal within a week after the fever subsides. Mild elevations in serum aspartate aminotransferase and creatine phosphokinase are reported.

Diagnosis The diagnosis of Colorado tick fever is suspected on the basis of the epidemiologic history and clinical findings. Because of the infrequency of rash, patients who develop fever and rash after tick bites should be suspected of having Rocky Mountain spotted fever. The usual methods for confirming Colorado tick fever are mouse inoculation and fluorescent antibody (FA) staining of patients' erythrocytes; a combination of the two is best. Special handling of blood is not necessary for the FA test, which remains positive for several weeks after clinical illness.

Prognosis Three deaths have been reported, all with hemorrhagic signs.

RIFT VALLEY FEVER Rift Valley fever is an acute disease principally of livestock, sheep, goats, cattle, and camels which is widespread throughout eastern and South Africa. It was first described in humans during an extensive epizootic of hepatitis in sheep in the Rift Valley in Kenya. During an epizootic in South Africa in 1950–1951, an estimated 20,000 humans became infected. Fatal human disease, four cases of hemorrhagic illness and hepatitis, was first reported during an epizootic in South Africa in 1975. In 1977 Rift Valley fever jumped the Sahara to Egypt with a major outbreak. Cases occurred in subsequent years until 1980; an estimated 200,000 cases with 598 reported deaths occurred in 1977.

Virus has been found in several species of mosquitoes: *Culex pipiens*, *Eretmapodites chrysogaster*, *Aedes caballus*, *Aedes circumluteolus*, and *Culex theileri*. *Culex pipiens* has been suggested as the vector in Egypt. While antibodies to Rift Valley fever have been found in wild field rats in Uganda, the reservoir is unknown. It has been suggested that the virus may be maintained by transovarial transmission in floodwater *Aedes*. Although humans presumably can be infected by arthropods, many infections occur as a result of handling infected animal tissues. In addition, laboratory-acquired infections have been common, suggesting a respiratory route of transmission.

The incubation period is usually 3 to 6 days. The onset is abrupt, with malaise, chilly sensation or rigors, headache, retroorbital pain, and generalized aching and backache. The temperature rises rapidly to 38.3 to 40°C (101 to 104°F). Later complaints include anorexia, loss of taste, epigastric pain, and photophobia. Findings on examination are usually unremarkable except for flushing of the face and conjunctival injection. The temperature curve is often saddleback in type, with an initial elevation lasting 2 to 3 days, followed by a remission and second febrile period. Convalescence is typically rapid. Prior to the outbreak in Egypt, Rift Valley fever was a benign illness with almost no fatalities. In Egypt, approximately 1 percent of patients developed severe complications, such as encephalitis, retinopathy, or hemorrhagic manifestations. Encephalitis appeared as the acute infection waned and was severe with serious residua in some survivors. Generalized hemorrhages and icterus appeared as the disease evolved. Deaths from massive hepatic necrosis occurred 7 to 10 days after onset of illness. The fatality rate in severely ill patients may exceed 50 percent. Visual loss, including light perception, occurred 2 to 7 days after the onset of fever. Macular edema, hemorrhage, vasculitis, retinitis, and vascular occlusion were noted. One-half of patients had some permanent loss of visual acuity. A characteristic finding is an initial normal total leukocyte count followed by leukopenia with a decrease in neutrophils associated with an increase in band forms. The diagnosis is made by isolating the virus from the blood by inoculation of mice. Three-fourths of patients are viremic (up to 10^8 mouse intraperitoneal lethal doses per milliliter blood) when first seen. Neutralizing antibodies have been demonstrated as early as 4 days after onset. There is no specific treatment. A killed vaccine which had been stockpiled in the United States is being utilized.

HANTAVIRUS DISEASE—UNITED STATES Acute hantavirus infection was recognized in at least 30 people in 1993 in the New Mexico-Arizona-Colorado region. Patients presented with fever, myalgia, headache, and cough followed by rapid development of respiratory failure and noncardiogenic pulmonary edema. Approximately two-thirds of the cases were fatal. Examination of trapped rodents indicated that *Peromyscus maniculatis* (deer mouse) was the most likely vector through exposure to its excreta. Diagnosis can be confirmed by serologic (IgM) response, polymerase chain reaction, or immunohistochemical stains of infected tissues.

INFECTIONS PRESENTING CHIEFLY WITH FEVER, MALAISE, LYMPHADENOPATHY, AND RASH

DENGUE FEVER Dengue is endemic over large areas of the tropics and subtropics, Asia, Oceania, Africa, Australia, and the Americas. Outbreaks of dengue have occurred in the Caribbean,

including Puerto Rico and the U.S. Virgin Islands, since 1969. Indigenous infection occurred in the United States for the first time in 35 years in 1980. Eleven cases have been recognized in residents of the Rio Grande Valley of Texas. In the summer of 1981, almost 350,000 cases of dengue with 158 deaths occurred in Cuba. *Aedes aegypti*, the vector, has reappeared along the U.S. Gulf Coast; hence the threat of dengue along the Gulf Coast is real. Dengue is emerging as an important disease of travelers, with 102 cases reported in U.S. residents in 1990.

Etiology There are four serotypes of dengue viruses, all of which are flaviviruses. In the Caribbean, type 1 was associated with the 1977–1978 outbreak, type 2 in 1968–1969, type 3 in 1963–1964, and type 4 was documented in the Western Hemisphere for the first time in 1981.

Epidemiology Dengue infections in nature involve primarily humans and *Aedes* mosquitoes. Dengue transmission involving monkeys and forest *Aedes* spp. has been documented in Malaysia and West Africa. *Aedes aegypti* is the most important worldwide vector species. This species, as well as the less common vector species, is peridomestic, biting humans readily or even preferentially and breeding in small collections of water such as cisterns and backyard litter. Surveys in Texas have revealed containers with water in which *A. aegypti* were breeding in up to 25 percent of premises. They fly during the day. Humans appear to be uniformly susceptible, and susceptibility is not influenced by age, sex, or race. During outbreaks, attack rates may be very high; in Puerto Rico and the U.S. Virgin Islands, the overall rate of clinical illness was 20 percent, with infection rates as determined by serologic survey as high as 79 per 100.

Clinical manifestations Dengue viruses frequently produce inapparent infections in humans. When symptoms develop, three broad clinical patterns may be encountered: classic dengue, hemorrhagic fever (see below), and a mild atypical form. Classic dengue (breakbone fever) occurs primarily in nonimmune individuals, specifically nonindigenous adults and children. The usual incubation period is 5 to 8 days. Prodromal symptoms such as mild conjunctivitis or coryza may occur, followed in hours by the abrupt onset of a severe splitting headache, retroorbital pain, backache, especially in the lumbar area, and leg and joint pains. The headache is aggravated by movement. At least three-fourths of patients have ocular soreness, with pain on moving the eyes. A few have mild photophobia. Though true rigors are common during the course, they are usually not present at the onset. Additional symptoms include insomnia, anorexia with loss of taste or bitter taste, and weakness. Mild transient rhinopharyngitis occurs in as many as one-quarter of the individuals. Cough is almost never seen. Some patients present with epistaxis, gingival bleeding, hematuria, or melena. In a study of 26 patients with upper gastrointestinal bleeding, 13 percent had gastric or duodenal ulcers and hemorrhagic gastritis on endoscopy. Examination reveals scleral injection (90 percent), tenderness upon pressure on the ocular globe, and nontender posterior cervical, epitrochlear, and inguinal lymphadenopathy. Over one-half of patients have an enanthem characterized initially by pinpoint-sized vesicles over the posterior half of the soft palate. The tongue is often coated. Skin rashes, varying from diffuse flushing to scarlatiniform and morbilliform, are frequently present over the thorax and inner aspects of the arms. These are transient and fade, only to be followed by a more definite maculopapular rash which appears on the trunk on the third to the fifth day and spreads peripherally. The rash may be pruritic and generally terminates with desquamation. Extreme bradycardia is not observed. Within 2 to 3 days after the onset, the temperature may decrease to nearly normal and other symptoms disappear. The remission typically lasts 2 days and is followed by return of fever and the other symptoms, although they are generally less severe than during the initial phase. This saddleback diphasic febrile course is considered characteristic but often is not encountered. The febrile illness usually lasts 5 to 6 days and terminates abruptly. Complaints of fatigue for several weeks after infection are common.

In addition to this "classic" syndrome, an atypically mild illness may occur. Symptoms include fever, anorexia, headache, and myalgia. On examination, evanescent rashes may be seen, but lymphadenopathy is usually absent. The course is usually less than 72 h in duration.

At the onset both in classic and in mild dengue, the leukocyte counts may be low or normal; however, by the third to the fifth day, leukopenia, usually with counts of less than 5000 leukocytes per microliter, and neutropenia are the rule. Occasionally albuminuria of moderate degree occurs.

Diagnosis Inoculation of blood obtained within the first 3 to 5 days onto mosquito tissue cell cultures or inoculation into mosquitoes is used for primary viral isolation. Diagnosis can be made by serologic tests employing paired serums for hemagglutination inhibition tests and complement fixation tests. IgM antibodies are produced in primary dengue infections. Specific serologic diagnosis is complicated by cross-reactions with other flavivirus antibodies such as those following immunization with yellow fever vaccine.

Treatment Treatment is entirely symptomatic.

Prognosis In the absence of the dengue hemorrhagic fever or dengue shock syndrome, mortality is nil.

Prevention An attenuated vaccine for dengue type 2 is undergoing experimental evaluation. Control depends on mosquito abatement.

WEST NILE FEVER West Nile virus is distributed throughout Africa, the Middle East, parts of Europe (Camargue, France), the former Soviet Union, India, and Indonesia. It produces a clinical picture closely resembling dengue. Outbreaks of disease involving several hundred patients occurred in Israel in 1950 to 1952. In one outbreak, over 60 percent of the population developed overt disease.

Epidemiology The disease is highly endemic in Egypt but goes largely unrecognized. Presumably most of the adult population is immune, and the infection in childhood is an undifferentiated mild febrile illness, whereas in Israel it mainly affects adults. The infection occurs in the summer both in Israel and in Egypt. The transmission cycle in the Middle East is bird-mosquito-bird, with *Culex univittatus* and *Culex pipiens molestus* being the principal vectors. *Culex tritaeniorhynchus* is an important vector in Asia. Although humans and a variety of other vertebrates are infected by the virus, their involvement is tangential.

Clinical manifestations The incubation period is 1 to 6 days. Most of the patients in Israel have been young adults, with neither sex predominating. The onset is usually abrupt and without prodromal symptoms. The temperature quickly rises to 38.3 to 40°C (101 to 104°F), with chills occurring in one-third of patients. Symptoms include drowsiness, severe frontal headache, ocular pain, and pain in the abdomen and back. A small number of patients have anorexia, nausea, and dryness of the throat. Cough is uncommon. There are flushing of the face, conjunctival injection, and coating of the tongue. The prominent finding is general enlargement of lymph nodes, which are of moderate size but are not hard and are only slightly tender. Occipital, axillary, and inguinal nodes are usually involved. The spleen and liver are slightly enlarged in a small proportion of patients. In one-half of patients a rash may appear from the second to the fifth day of illness and may persist for several hours or until defervescence. The rash occurs predominantly over the trunk and consists of pale roseolar maculopapular lesions. The illness is self-limited and lasts 3 to 5 days in 80 percent of patients.

In a few patients, transitory meningeal involvement may be encountered. CSF examinations may reveal a pleocytosis and some increase in protein concentration.

Leukopenia occurs in the majority of patients, and total leukocyte counts are lower than 4000 cells per microliter in one-third. Differential counts vary from a moderate shift to the left to a slight lymphocytosis.

Convalescence is often prolonged, lasting 1 to 2 weeks, with prominent symptoms of fatigue. Enlargement of lymph nodes subsides over several months. Only rarely have complications, sequelae, or fatalities been seen in natural infections, although in one outbreak in a group of elderly patients a high proportion of patients developed meningoencephalitis, and four fatalities ensued.

Accurate diagnosis rests on virus isolation, which can be accomplished because viremia persists for as long as 6 days, or the demonstration of a rising specific antibody titer.

The treatment is symptomatic.

INFECTIONS PRESENTING CHIEFLY WITH FEVER, ACUTE ARTHROPATHY, AND RASH

CHIKUNGUNYA This term is a local tribal word meaning "that which bends up" which was used to describe an epidemic of acute arthropathy in Tanzania in 1952–1953 shown to be caused by a togovirus of the alphavirus genus (Table 159-1). It is likely that chikungunya (CHIK) virus caused epidemics in Southeast Asia, India, Africa, and possibly the southern United States in the 1800s and early 1900s. Today, CHIK is responsible for extensive *A. aegyti*–transmitted disease in cities in Africa and Asia. With the increase in *A. aegypti* and introduction of *A. albopictus* in the United States, the possibility of CHIK exists today.

Clinical manifestations The incubation period is usually 2 to 3 days (range 1 to 12 days) followed by the abrupt onset of fever (often to 40°C), rigors, and acute joint pain. The arthalgias are polyarticular and predominantly affect the smaller joints of the hands, wrists, ankles, and feet. Swelling (periarticular) is common, but joint effusions are not. Generalized myalgia is frequent. The acute phase typically lasts 2 to 3 days, with the fever remitting. A maculopapular rash involving the trunk and limbs is typical, usually appearing with defervescence. The rash lasts 1 to 5 days. Constitutional symptoms and signs are common but do not dominate the clinical picture. Conjunctival suffusion is common. Two-thirds of patients will have joint symptoms for several weeks. About 5 percent, usually older patients, have persistent joint pain for 3 to 5 years. In Asia, the clinical syndrome differs, being seen predominantly in children who present with fever, headache, pharyngitis, vomiting, abdominal pain, constipation, or diarrhea, and cough. A maculopapular rash and conjunctival injection are common, but arthritis and arthralgia are not seen. In Bangkok, about 10 percent of patients with the dengue–hemorrhagic fever syndrome have CHIK infection.

O'NYONG-NYONG FEVER O'nyong-nyong fever was first noted as an epidemic illness characterized by joint pains, rash, and lymphadenopathy in the northern province of Uganda in 1959. The agent is an alphavirus which shows close antigenic relationships with chikungunya viruses. The original outbreak was associated with an explosive epidemic which spread to Tanzania and other areas in east Africa. By 1961, 2 million cases were recorded. In some areas, 78 percent of the population had either clinical disease or inapparent infection. Local outbreaks extended over the entire year. All age groups were affected. The most likely vectors are *Anopheles funestus* and *Anopheles gambiae*. The clinical features are similar to those of chikungunya virus infection. The disease disappeared in 1962. While the virus was isolated from *A. funestus* in Kenya in 1978, no further outbreaks have been recognized.

SINDBIS VIRUS Sindbis virus, once thought rarely to present as clinical disease, has been recognized in Africa (Uganda, Zimbabwe, central Africa, and South Africa), Australia, Malaysia, and Europe (former Soviet Union, Finland, and Sweden). In the former Soviet Union it is known as Karelian fever, in Sweden as Okelbo disease, and in Finland as Pogosta disease. Clinically, fever is low-grade and accompanied by malaise, myalgia, and arthralgia involving joints and tendons. The most striking feature is a maculopapular rash appearing on the trunk and extremities but usually sparing the face. Unlike the rash of chikungunya or o'nyong-nyong, the rash often becomes vesicular, especially on the feet and hands. Joint disease is usually multiple—ankles, knees, and wrists. Periarticular involvement is common. Persistent or recurrent joint pains lasted for 2 years in one-third of patients in a Swedish series. Permanent joint deformity is not described.

ROSS RIVER VIRUS Epidemics of polyarthritis associated with rashes have been observed in Australia since 1928. Outbreaks occur almost entirely in the period December to June. Ross River virus infection was limited to Australia, New Guinea, and the Solomon Islands until 1979, when a major outbreak occurred in Fiji which spread to the Samoan, Cook, and some Melanesian Islands. In the Fiji outbreak in 1979, infection rates were equal at all ages and in both sexes, but clinical attack rates were 4 percent in patients under 20 years and 42 percent in adults, and the clinical attack rate of males to females was 1:1.7. The onset is usually sudden and the initial symptom usually joint pain. Initially, fever may be absent or minimal [highest 38°C (100.4°F)]. In about one-half of patients, arthritis, involving mainly the small joints, wrists, and ankles and sometimes associated with swelling, and paresthesias precede a rash by 1 to 15 days. In the other half, the rash precedes the arthralgia. The rash, which lasts 2 to 10 days, is usually maculopapular, appears on the cheeks and forehead, occasionally spreads to the trunk, or may be restricted to the limbs. The rash may be pruritic. Vesicles occur rarely. Tender lymphadenopathy occurs in one-fifth of the patients. Joint symptoms persist for 3 weeks to 3 months. The virus has been isolated from *Culex annulirostris* and *Aedes vigilax*. Animals may serve as reservoir hosts in Australia. In the Pacific, person-mosquito-person transmission seems likely.

BARMAH FOREST VIRUS Barmah Forest virus is an alphavirus in Australia (Queensland, New South Wales, Victoria) which recently has been recognized as a cause of fever (two-thirds of patients), chills (one-third), arthritis/arthralgia (three-quarters), rash (one-half, occasionally vesicular), myalgia (two-thirds), and respiratory symptoms (one-fifth). Desquamation has been noted as the rash resolves. The virus has been isolated from the same vector mosquitoes as Ross River virus. There is serologic evidence of extensive infection in Queensland (0.23 percent of the population per year). It is likely that Barmah Forest virus has been misdiagnosed as Ross River virus as one of the causes of epidemic polyarthritis.

MAYARO VIRUS Three epidemics have been described, two in Brazil in the Amazon region and one in Bolivia. In the outbreak in Belterra, Brazil, the attack rate was high (20 percent), with a high proportion of individuals having symptomatic disease. The symptoms and signs were similar in occurrence and frequency to those noted with other alphavirus infections.

INFECTIONS WITH CNS INVOLVEMENT

Four "arboviruses" are presently recognized as numerically important causes of central nervous system disease in the United States: St. Louis encephalitis virus (SLE), eastern equine encephalitis virus (EEE), western equine encephalitis virus (WEE), and the California serogroup (CE) viruses. The spectrum of infection caused by these agents includes inapparent infection, fever with headache, aseptic meningitis, and encephalitis. Some 1500 to 2000 cases of encephalitis are reported in the United States each year. In the absence of epidemics, 5 to 10 percent of these (75 to 200 cases) are confirmed as "arboviral" in cause. In nonepidemic years, California serogroup viruses (predominantly LaCrosse virus) represent two-thirds to three-fourths of the cases.

Etiology Despite the diversity of specific viral causes (see Table 159-2), in individual patients the clinical manifestations of aseptic meningitis and encephalitis are very similar and preclude an etiologic diagnosis without ancillary information regarding epidemiologic and serologic features (Table 159-3). The clinical features of aseptic meningitis due to "arboviruses" are indistinguishable from those due to the more prevalent enteroviruses. Since transmission to humans in the United States and Canada involves arthropods, specifically mosquitoes, except for Powassan and Colorado tick fever, indigenously acquired disease occurs at times when mosquitoes are prevalent, such as late spring through early fall.

Clinical manifestations The clinical features of "arbovirus" encephalitis differ among age groups. In infants under 1 year of age, the only consistently noted symptoms are sudden onset of fever, which is often accompanied by convulsions. Convulsions may be generalized or focal. Typically, fever ranges between 38.9 and 40°C (102 and 104°F). Other physical findings may include bulging of the fontanelle, rigidity of the extremities, and abnormal reflexes.

In children between 5 and 14 years of age, subjective symptoms are more easily elicited. Headache, fever, and drowsiness of 2 to 3 days' duration before medical attention is sought are common. The symptoms may then subside or become more intense and may be associated with nausea, vomiting, muscular pain, photophobia, and, less frequently, convulsions (less than 10 percent except in California encephalitis). The child is found to be acutely ill, febrile, and lethargic. Nuchal rigidity and intention tremors are often present, and on occasion muscular weakness can be demonstrated.

In adults, the initial symptoms commonly include the fairly abrupt onset of fever, nausea with vomiting, and severe headache. The headache is most often frontal but may be occipital or diffuse. Mental aberrations, represented by confusion and disorientation, usually appear within the subsequent 24 h. Other symptoms may include diffuse myalgia and photophobia. The abnormalities found on physical examination predominantly relate to the neurologic examination, although conjunctival suffusion is frequently seen and skin rashes may occur. Disturbances in mentation are among the most outstanding clinical features. These range from coma through severe disorientation to subtle abnormalities detected only by cerebral function tests such as the subtraction of serial 7s. A small proportion of patients show only lethargy, lying quietly, apparently asleep unless stimulated.

TABLE 159-3 Features of arboviral encephalitides common in the United States

	Geographic predominance in the United States	Urban/rural	Age, years	Sex	Unique clinical features	Mortality, %	Residua
California encephalitis	Midwest	Rural	5–10	M	Seizures	2	Seizures (one-fourth who had them in acute phase), behavioral problems (15%)
Eastern equine encephalitis	Eastern seaboard	Both	<5 >55	=	CSF may have >1000 WBC/μL	50	Children <10 years have emotional lability, retardation, convulsions
St. Louis encephalitis	Eastern and midwest	Both	>35	=	Dysuria	2–12	Ataxia, speech difficulties (5%)
Western equine encephalitis	Entire	Both	<1 >55	=	None	3	Children <3 months have behavioral problems, convulsions

Tremor is common and is observed more frequently in individuals over 40 years of age. The tremors vary in location and may be continuous or intention in type. Cranial nerve abnormalities resulting in oculomotor muscle paresis and nystagmus, facial weakness, and difficulty in deglutition may occur and are usually present within the initial several days. Objective sensory changes are unusual. Hemiparesis or monoparesis may occur. Reflex abnormalities are also common; these include exaggerated palmomental reflexes and suck and snout reflexes. Superficial abdominal and cremasteric reflexes are usually absent. Changes in the tendon reflexes are variable and inconstant. The plantar response may be extensor and fluctuates almost hourly. Dysdiadochokinesia often exists.

The duration of the fever and neurologic symptoms and signs varies from several days to a month but usually ranges from 4 to 14 days. Clinical improvement generally follows the subsidence of the fever within several days unless irreversible anatomic changes have occurred.

Laboratory findings Erythrocytes are usually normal. Total leukocyte counts often reveal both a slight to moderate leukocytosis (occasionally greater than 20,000 leukocytes per microliter) and neutrophilia. Examination of the CSF usually reveals several hundred cells per microliter, but on occasion cloudy CSF with cells in excess of 1000 per microliter may be seen. Within the first several days of illness, polymorphonuclear neutrophils may predominate. The initial CSF protein is usually only slightly elevated but on occasion may exceed 1.0 g/L (100 mg/dL). The level of CSF sugar is normal; a significant decrease should raise serious consideration of an alternative diagnosis. As the illness progresses, mononuclear cells in the CSF tend to increase so that they predominate and the protein concentration may increase. Other laboratory studies have been reported only sporadically, but abnormalities may include hyponatremia, often due to the inappropriate secretion of antidiuretic hormone, and elevations in serum creatine phosphokinase.

Diagnosis Specific diagnosis requires the isolation of the virus or detection of antibodies with a rising titer between the acute phase of disease and convalescence. Antibodies can be detected by hemagglutination inhibition, complement fixation, or virus neutralization techniques.

Treatment Treatment is entirely supportive and requires meticulous attention in the comatose patient.

LACROSSE ENCEPHALITIS A previously undescribed virus was isolated in 1943 from mosquitoes in Kern County, California. Since 1963, a large number of agents now designated as the California group of viruses have been isolated (see Table 159-1). LaCrosse, Snowshoe hare, Jamestown Canyon, California encephalitis, and Trivittatus viruses cause human encephalitis in North America. Tahyna and Inkoo viruses are associated with febrile and, rarely, encephalitic disease in Europe. Since 1966 in midwestern United States, LaCrosse virus (California) encephalitis has been incriminated in 5 to 6 percent of cases of acute central nervous system disease, ranking above all agents except the enteroviruses.

Epidemiology LaCrosse virus infection occurs in the North Central states, in New York, in wooded areas of eastern Texas and Louisiana, and along the Eastern Seaboard. The virus is maintained by transovarial transmission in woodland mosquitoes, *Aedes triseratus*, which breed in tree holes in hardwood forests and have adapted to discarded tires. The virus is present in seminal fluid of male mosquitoes and is transmitted to the female. The virus overwinters in eggs of *A. triseratus*. Chipmunks and gray squirrels serve as amplifier hosts. LaCrosse virus (California) encephalitis occurs during the summer months (June to October), most often involving boys (60 percent) 5 to 10 years of age (60 percent) who live in rural areas.

Clinical manifestations Two clinical patterns of LaCrosse virus disease have been defined. One is a mild form with a 2- to 3-day prodrome of fever, headache, malaise, and gastrointestinal symptoms. About the third day the temperature increases to 40°C (104°F), and the patient becomes lethargic and develops meningeal signs. These findings abate gradually over a 7- to 8-day period without overt

sequelae. The second pattern, a severe form which occurs in at least one-half of patients, begins abruptly with fever, headache, and vomiting, followed shortly by lethargy and disorientation. During the first 2 to 4 days, the course is rapidly progressive, with the occurrence of seizures (50 to 60 percent), focal neurologic signs (20 percent), pathologic reflexes (10 percent), and coma (10 percent). Focal neurologic signs may include asymmetric flaccid paralysis. Uncommon findings have included arthralgia and rash. Clinical laboratory features include peripheral leukocyte counts ranging from 7000 to 30,000 cells per microliter (median 16,000 cells per microliter) with neutrophilia. CSF examination reveals 10 to 500 cells per microliter, usually with a predominance of mononuclear cells, protein concentrations of less than 1.0 g/L (100 mg/dL), and normal sugar concentrations. Electroencephalograms (EEGs) are abnormal in at least 80 percent of patients, revealing slow delta-wave activity. In one-half of patients the abnormality is asymmetric, suggesting focal destructive lesions. Brain scans using ^{99m}Tc-pertechnetate and computed tomography (CT) also may be abnormal, and temporal lobe localization has been observed. Beginning about the fourth day and proceeding over the next 3 to 7 days, there is progressive improvement, with almost all patients becoming afebrile, seizure-free, and ready for discharge from the hospital within 2 weeks after onset.

Diagnosis Serum and CSF should be tested for LaCrosse virus IgM antibodies. Serum capture IgM enzyme-linked immunosorbent assay (ELISA) tests detected 83 percent of cases on admission in LaCrosse encephalitis. Early specific diagnosis eliminates the need for brain biopsy to exclude herpes encephalitis, which is suggested by the temporal lobe localization.

Treatment Initial seizure activity is frequently prolonged and difficult to control. The most effective anticonvulsant medication has been parenteral diazepam. Patients with the severe form of disease should be discharged on anticonvulsants such as phenobarbital for 6 to 12 months.

Prognosis The case-fatality ratio is low (2 percent or less); however, one-third of patients may have abnormal neurologic findings at the time of discharge. During the early convalescent period, emotional lability and irritability are common. In one series, recurrent seizures occurred in one-quarter of the patients who had seizures during the acute phase. In this same series, EEGs were abnormal in one-third of patients evaluated 1 to 8 years after their acute illness. In another series, 15 percent had sequelae, predominantly personality or behavioral problems.

OTHER CALIFORNIA GROUP ENCEPHALITIDES Jamestown Canyon encephalitis is uncommon but, in contrast to LaCrosse encephalitis, usually occurs in adults. Snowshoe hare virus has been isolated from mosquitoes throughout Canada and from Alaska. Encephalitis has been reported from the eastern provinces. In the Midwest, antibodies to Trivittatus virus are common, but only one case of human illness has been reported. Clinical features of Tahyna virus disease, which has been seen in children in Europe, include fever, pharyngitis, pneumonitis, gastrointestinal symptoms, and aseptic meningitis. Neither mortality nor sequelae are reported.

EASTERN EQUINE ENCEPHALITIS Eastern equine encephalitis (EEE), an alphavirus, was first isolated in 1933 from the brain tissue of horses during an outbreak of equine illness in New Jersey. The first recognized human outbreak occurred in Massachusetts in 1938.

Epidemiology The virus is distributed along the East Coast of the Americas from northeastern United States to Argentina. Foci have been found in the Syracuse region of New York, Ontario, Canada, western Michigan, and South Dakota. Viral isolations also have been reported in the Philippines, Thailand, Czechoslovakia, Poland, and the former Soviet Union, but the question of type specificity has not been resolved. In the northeastern United States, epidemics occur in the late summer and early fall. Epizootics in horses precede the occurrence of human cases by 1 to 2 weeks. The disease affects mainly infants, children, and adults over 55 years of age. There is no sex preponderance. Inapparent infection occurs in all age groups, suggesting that the decreased likelihood of developing overt infection in the 15- to

54-year age group is not the result of decreased exposure. The ratio of inapparent infection to overt encephalitis approximates 25:1.

The transmission of EEE involves *Culiseta melanura* mosquitoes and swamp-dwelling birds, e.g., red-winged blackbirds, sparrows, pheasants. Transmission by pecking has been shown in domestic pheasant flocks. *C. melanura* rarely feed on horses or humans, and other mosquitoes, especially *Aedes sollicitans*, a salt-marsh mosquito which is an avid human feeder, have been postulated as the epidemic vector. In June 1991, EEE virus was isolated from *A. albopictus* in Florida. *A. albopictus* has the potential for becoming an important epidemic vector. The epidemiology of overwintering and maintenance between outbreaks remains unknown. Equine animals and human beings are "dead ends" in the transmission cycle, and infection in them is accidental.

Clinical manifestations   Though human infections have been thought usually to result in serious, if not fatal, central nervous system involvement, the detection of inapparent infection as well as relatively mild disease establishes the occurrence of milder forms. In many patients, the CSF is cloudy and contains in excess of 1000 cells per microliter.

Diagnosis   ELISA tests for the detection of specific IgM antibodies in CSF or serum permit early diagnosis, although absence of IgM does not exclude infection. Confirmation can be obtained by a fourfold or more rise or fall in complement fixation (CF), hemagglutination inhibition, or virus neutralization tests.

Prognosis   The mortality rate in clinical infection exceeds 50 percent. In the most severe cases, death occurs between the third and fifth days. Children under 10 years of age have a greater likelihood of surviving the acute illness, but they also have a greater likelihood of developing severe disabling residuals: mental retardation, convulsions, emotional lability, blindness, deafness, speech disorders, and hemiplegia.

ST. LOUIS ENCEPHALITIS   St. Louis encephalitis (SLE) was first recognized as an entity during a major outbreak in St. Louis, Missouri, in 1933. Subsequently, sporadic, unpredictable outbreaks have occurred in the Ohio-Mississippi Valley, eastern Texas, Florida, Kansas, Colorado, and California. The attack rate in Greenville, Mississippi, in 1975 was the highest which has been encountered, 10 per 10,000 population.

Epidemiology   In the United States, epidemics of SLE fall into two epidemiologic patterns. One pattern is found in the West, where mixed outbreaks of western equine encephalitis and SLE have occurred primarily in irrigated rural areas. The vector has been *Culex tarsalis*. The second pattern occurred in the original St. Louis outbreak and the numerous subsequent epidemics in the Midwest, Texas, New Jersey, and Florida. These outbreaks have been more urban in location and are characterized by occurrence of encephalitis in older persons. In such urban-suburban epidemics, the epidemic vectors have been mosquitoes of the *Culex pipiens-quinquefasciatus* complex with the exception of the Florida epidemic, in which *Culex nigripalpus* was incriminated. The presence of SLE virus outside the United States has been proved by isolations in Trinidad, Panama, Jamaica, Brazil, and Argentina. However, except for Jamaica, SLE has not been reported outside the United States. The basic transmission cycle is that of wild bird–mosquito–wild bird. The virus survives the winter in female mosquitoes which ingest a blood meal from a viremic bird before overwintering. The disease in humans usually appears in midsummer to early fall. In urban epidemics, there is no sex predominance, while among sporadic cases in the West, men predominate 2:1 due to greater occupational exposure. The human represents an accidental host and plays no role in the basic transmission cycle. Serologic studies following most urban epidemics indicate that infection rates are similar in all age groups and that the increasing age-specific attack rate for clinical encephalitis which is typical of urban St. Louis encephalitis is probably due to age differences in host susceptibility to overt disease rather than to a higher rate of infection.

Clinical manifestations   Infection with SLE virus most commonly results in an inapparent infection. Of the patients with confirmed disease, approximately three-fourths have clinical encephalitis; the remainder present with aseptic meningitis, febrile headaches, or nonspecific illness. Virtually all patients over 40 years have encephalitic manifestations. Urinary frequency and dysuria have been symptoms in approximately 20 percent of patients despite sterile routine aerobic urine cultures. SLE virus antigen has been demonstrated in urine; viruria may account for the occurrence of urinary tract symptoms.

Diagnosis   The occurrence of either encephalitis or aseptic meningitis as manifested by febrile illness with CSF pleocytosis in the months of June through September in an adult, especially over 35 years of age, should raise the suspicion of St. Louis encephalitis. Because approximately 40 percent of patients with SLE have antibodies detectable by hemagglutination inhibition at the onset of illness, acute serum for serologic studies should be submitted promptly to a competent laboratory. ELISA tests for the detection of specific IgM antibodies in CSF or serum provide a means of early specific diagnosis.

Prognosis   The case-fatality ratio in the original St. Louis epidemic was 20 percent. In most subsequent outbreaks the mortality rate has varied from 2 to 12 percent. Subjective complaints, including nervousness, headaches, and easy fatigability and excitability, appear to be the most common residuals. Late organic defects such as speech defects, difficulty in walking, and disturbances in vision were demonstrated in approximately 5 percent of patients 3 years following infection.

WESTERN EQUINE ENCEPHALITIS   Western equine encephalitis (WEE) virus is an alphavirus that was isolated in 1930 in California from horses with encephalitis. In 1938 it was recovered from a fatal human infection.

Epidemiology   WEE virus has been isolated in the United States, Canada, Brazil, Guyana, and Argentina. Human disease has been diagnosed in the United States, Canada, and Brazil. In the United States, the virus is found in virtually all geographic areas. The central valley of California represents an important endemic area. The disease occurs mainly in early and midsummer. Wild birds, which develop viremia of sufficiently high titer to be able to infect mosquitoes that feed on them, are the basic reservoir. *Culex tarsalis* is the principal vector in the western United States. In areas east of the Appalachian Mountains, the virus has been repeatedly isolated from *Culiseta melanura;* however, the importance of this species has been questioned, since it is not primarily a human-biting mosquito. The overwintering mechanism is not known. The ratio of inapparent infection to disease, as evidenced by serologic survey studies, varies from 1:1 in infants to 58:1 in children to 1150:1 in adults. Approximately one-fourth of patients are less than 1 year of age. The highest attack rates occur in persons 55 years or older.

Prognosis   The case-fatality rate approximates 3 percent in laboratory-confirmed cases. The incidence and severity of sequelae are related to age. Sequelae among very young infants are frequent (appearing in 61 percent of a group of patients less than 3 months old) and severe; they consist of upper motor neuron impairment, involving the pyramidal tracts, extrapyramidal structures, and cerebellum, and result in behavioral problems and convulsions. Both the incidence and severity of sequelae diminish rapidly after 1 year of age. Adults may complain of nervousness, irritability, easy fatigability, and tremulousness for 6 months or longer after the acute illness. Probably not more than 5 percent of adults have sequelae which are sufficiently severe to be of practical significance. Postencephalitic seizures are rare.

JAPANESE ENCEPHALITIS   The name *Japanese B encephalitis* was employed during an epidemic which occurred in 1924 to distinguish it from von Economo's disease, which was designated as type A encephalitis. The designation as Japanese B no longer seems useful, and the term *Japanese encephalitis* (JE) is used.

Epidemiology   JE virus infection is known to occur in eastern Siberia, China, Korea, Japan, all of Southeast Asia, Guam, Nepal, and India. Since the late 1960s, JE has virtually disappeared in Japan

(<20 cases annually) and is declining in China (still >10,000 cases annually). JE remains a major problem in northern Thailand (attack rates of 10 to 20 per 100,000 annually). In temperate climates, the disease shows a late-summer–early-fall seasonal incidence. In tropical climates, epidemics occur mainly in the summer monsoon months. The mosquito *Culex tritaeniorhynchus* is the major vector species. It is a rural mosquito which breeds in rice fields and preferentially bites large domestic animals, such as pigs, but also feeds on birds and humans. The human is an accidental host in the transmission cycle. In endemic areas, children ages 3 to 15 are primarily affected. Epidemics in nonendemic areas have affected all age groups, but young children and older adults predominate. The ratio of inapparent infection, as evidenced by a serologic survey study of Australian troops in Vietnam, was 210:1.

Clinical manifestations The incubation period is 5 to 15 days. As with SLE, illness may present as encephalitis, aseptic meningitis, or febrile headache. The occurrence of severe rigors at the onset has been noted in almost 90 percent of patients. On admission, most patients are alert, but deterioration of mental status occurs in about three-fourths of patients within 3 to 4 days. Localized paresis is found more often than with other "arboviral" encephalitides, e.g., in 31 percent of cases, with predominantly upper extremity involvement; however, it resolves rapidly with defervescence. Convulsions are frequent in children but occur in less than 10 percent of adults. Severe hyperthermia may occur and require treatment. A peripheral leukocytosis with 50 to 90 percent neutrophils is common. Weight loss has been very striking. The failure of the temperature to lyse, appearance of diaphoresis, tachypnea, and the accumulation of bronchial secretions are grave prognostic signs.

Prognosis The immediate mortality rate has varied from 7 to 50 percent and is highest in young children and persons over 65. The occurrence of sequelae varies inversely with the case-fatality rate; in those series with high case-fatality rates (33 percent), sequelae occurred in 3 to 14 percent. In another series with a case-fatality rate of 7.4 percent, the rate of adverse sequelae was 32 percent. Individuals who had neurologic abnormalities during the acute phase but survived have no more than an 80 percent chance for complete recovery. Sequelae consist of seizures, persistent paralysis, ataxia, mental retardation, and behavioral disorders.

Prevention Cases have been reported among U.S. citizens traveling to endemic areas (Southeast Asia, China). In 1983, the Centers for Disease Control obtained an investigational new drug exemption from the Food and Drug Administration to evaluate the BIKEN JE vaccine. The vaccine is inactivated and prepared in mouse brain. Protective efficacy has been 80 percent or more, with adverse effects occurring in fewer than 1 percent of vaccinees. Millions of doses have been administered. In non-Asian adults, a three-dose immunization schedule probably affords the best protection. JE vaccine is still not licensed and available in the United States, but it is available in Canada and many European countries. Vaccine should be considered for travelers during summer monsoon months whose activities will include travel into rural farming areas or sleeping in unscreened quarters.

OTHER "ARBOVIRUSES" WITH CENTRAL NERVOUS SYSTEM INVOLVEMENT A large number of additional "arboviruses" have been associated with encephalitis or aseptic meningitis. Some of these agents are listed in Table 159-2. Though the epidemiologic picture of each of these agents is unique, the general features are sufficiently similar to require laboratory support for their differentiation.

DISEASES PRESENTING CHIEFLY WITH HEMORRHAGIC MANIFESTATIONS

For 300 years, yellow fever was the only epidemic viral disease known to be accompanied by grave hemorrhagic manifestations. Since the 1930s, diverse viral etiologies of the hemorrhagic fever syndrome have been recognized (see Table 159-2). Additional agents include members of several families and genera: flavivirus, Filoviri-

dae, phlebovirus, Nairovirus, Hantavirus, and arenavirus (see Chap. 160). Despite diverse causes, there are many similar clinical manifestations. The onset is usually sudden, with headache, backache, generalized myalgia, conjunctivitis, and prostration. From approximately the third day, the initial stage is followed by hypotension, and hemorrhagic manifestations may occur; these are characterized by bleeding gums, epistaxis, hemoptysis, hematemesis, melena, petechiae, ecchymoses, and hemorrhages into most visceral organs. Mild leukopenia develops early, but with the appearance of hemorrhagic manifestations, leukocytosis may occur. The pathophysiology of the cardinal signs is attributable to hematopoietic and capillary damage, with variable localization of lesions. On the basis of limited confirmatory observations, variable degrees of disseminated intravascular coagulation may be in part responsible for the pathophysiology of the hemorrhagic fever syndromes. Death usually occurs in the second week of disease, at which time a high titer of antibody has developed and the patient may have become afebrile. Death is usually associated with coma, which is due not to encephalitis but to an encephalopathy. The pathologic changes may be similar despite diverse viral causes, with midzonal hepatic necrosis and acidophilic cytoplasmic inclusions similar to the Councilman bodies of yellow fever.

YELLOW FEVER Yellow fever is an acute infectious disease of short duration and extremely variable severity; it is caused by a flavivirus and is followed by lifelong immunity. The classic triad of symptoms—jaundice, hemorrhages, and intense albuminuria—is present only in severe infections, which make up only a small proportion of the total.

Prevalence For more than 200 years, after the first identifiable outbreak occurred in Yucatan in 1648, yellow fever was one of the great plagues of the world. As late as 1905, New Orleans and other southern United States ports experienced at least 5000 cases and 1000 deaths. Because of the existence of the sylvatic form of the disease, protective measures must be maintained against human disease. During the past 20 years, outbreaks and extensive epidemics have occurred in South America (Bolivia, Brazil, Colombia, Ecuador, Peru, Venezuela) and Africa (Burkino Faso, Gambia, Ghana, Nigeria, Senegal). In southern Ethiopia from 1962 to 1964 there were over 100,000 cases with some 30,000 deaths. In Gambia the attack rate was 2.6 to 4.4 percent, with a case-fatality rate of 19 percent. Yellow fever has never occurred in Asia.

Epidemiology Human infection results from two different cycles of virus transmission, urban and sylvatic. The urban cycle is human-mosquito-human, i.e., *Aedes aegypti*–transmitted yellow fever. After a 2-week extrinsic incubation period, mosquitoes can transmit infection. Sylvan yellow fever differs under various ecologic circumstances. In the rain forests of South and Central America, species of treetop *Haemagogus* or *Sabethes* mosquitoes maintain transmission in wild primates. Once infected, the mosquito vector remains infectious for life; hence it may serve as a reservoir as well as a vector. When humans come into proximity with the forest-canopy mosquitoes, sporadic cases or focal outbreaks may occur. With sylvan yellow fever, males predominate. Focal outbreaks may be quite extensive; in Brazil in 1973 at least 21,000 persons out of 1.5 million (1.4 percent) were infected. In east Africa, the mosquito-primate cycle is maintained by the forest-canopy mosquito *A. africanus*, which seldom feeds on humans. The peridomestic mosquito *A. simpsoni* feeds on primates entering the village gardens and can then in turn transmit the virus to humans. Once yellow fever is reintroduced into urban areas, the *A. aegypti*–borne urban cycle can be reinitiated, with the potential for epidemic disease. In the Americas, *A. aegypti* outbreaks have not occurred for 30 years, while in Africa, both sylvan and urban epidemics have occurred.

Clinical manifestations The incubation period is usually 3 to 6 days. In accidental laboratory- or hospital-acquired infections, longer incubation periods (10 to 13 days) have been reported. In mild yellow fever the only symptoms may be the abrupt onset of fever and headache. Additional symptoms may include nausea, epistaxis, relative bradycardia known as *Faget's sign* [e.g., with a temperature of 38.9°C (102°F) the pulse may be only 48 to 52 beats per minute], and slight albuminuria. The mild illness lasts only 1 to 3 days and resembles influenza except that coryzal symptoms are lacking.

Moderately severe and malignant attacks of yellow fever are characterized by three distinct clinical periods: the period of infection, the period of remission, and the period of intoxication. Prodromal symptoms are usually absent. The onset is characteristically sudden, with headache, dizziness, and temperature elevations to 40°C (104°F) without a relative bradycardia. Young children may have febrile convulsions. The headache is followed quickly by pains in the neck, back, and legs. Often there is nausea with vomiting and retching. Examination reveals a flushed face and injection of the conjunctivae. The congestion of the eyes persists until the third day. The tongue characteristically shows bright-red margins and tip and a white furred center. Faget's sign appears by the second day. Epistaxis and gingival bleeding are common. On the third day of illness the fever may fall by crisis and the patient enters remission, or in the malignant form, copious hemorrhages, anuria, or delirium may occur. The stage of remission lasts from several hours to several days. In the third stage, the "classic" symptoms develop; the fever returns, but the pulse remains slow. Jaundice becomes detectable about the third day; however, jaundice often is not prominent even in fatal illnesses. Increased epistaxis, melena, and uterine hemorrhages are common, but gross hematuria is rare. Of the classic signs, "black vomit" is more characteristic than is jaundice. Hematemesis usually does not occur before the fourth day and is often associated with a fatal outcome. Albuminuria, which rarely develops before the third day, occurs in 90 percent of patients and may be quite marked (3 to 20 g albumin per liter). Despite this massive albuminuria, edema or ascites has not been reported. In malignant infections, coma frequently occurs 2 to 3 days before death. Shortly before death, which usually occurs between the fourth and the sixth days, the patient becomes delirious and wildly agitated. Though the duration of fever in the third stage is usually 5 to 7 days, the period of intoxication is the most variable of the stages and may last up to 2 weeks. Yellow fever is relatively free from complications, suppurative parotitis being the most striking of those which do occur. Clinical relapses are not characteristic of yellow fever.

Laboratory findings Early in the disease, progressive leukopenia may occur. By the fifth day, total leukocyte counts of 1500 to 2500 cells per microliter often are found, the decrease being due mostly to a decrease in neutrophils. Total leukocyte counts return to normal by the tenth day, and in fatal cases there may be a marked terminal leukocytosis. Hemoglobin values remain normal except terminally, when hemoconcentration or bleeding may occur. Platelet counts are normal or decreased. Prolongation of clotting, prothrombin, and partial thromboplastin times is marked in patients with jaundice. Increases in total and conjugated bilirubin occur. In icteric patients, marked elevations of serum glutamic oxaloacetic transaminase occur. Hypoglycemia has been seen in patients with severe hepatic damage. Electrocardiograms may show T-wave changes. The CSF is normal.

Diagnosis Inoculation onto mosquito cell cultures and intrathoracically into mosquitoes are methods of choice for virus isolation from blood. Isolation is most likely from specimens obtained during the first 3 days of illness. Serologic methods include plaque reduction neutralization tests on paired sera and detection of yellow fever IgM antibodies and antigen usually by ELISA methods. The ELISA method enables confirmation in the field within 3 h.

Treatment The management has been symptomatic and supportive and should be based on assessment and correction of the circulatory abnormalities. Close attention to fluids and electrolytes is essential. As with all the hemorrhagic fevers, aspirin is contraindicated. Ribavirin has in vitro antiviral activity against yellow fever virus, but trials in experimentally infected monkeys showed no therapeutic effect.

Prognosis The overall fatality rate in yellow fever is between 5 and 10 percent of clinical cases; it may be even less, since many infections are mild or inapparent.

Prevention Effective control measures are available. Immunization with the 17 Da vaccine has been effective in the prevention of outbreaks. With the occurrence of sylvatic outbreaks, work in the area of epizootic activity should be discontinued, and intensive mosquito abatement measures should be instituted. These measures may provide the time necessary for a mass immunization program.

DENGUE HEMORRHAGIC FEVER All four dengue virus serotypes can cause dengue hemorrhagic fever (DHF) and dengue shock syndrome (DSS). Infection with dengue 1, 3, or 4 followed within a few years by dengue 2 may be especially important in the pathogenesis. There is consensus that DHF is an immunologically mediated disease. Enhanced growth of dengue 2 virus occurs in peripheral blood mononuclear phagocytes obtained from dengue immune donors or in cells from normal donors in the presence of subneutralizing concentrations of dengue or cross-reacting heterotypic flavivirus antibodies. Infectious virus-antibody complexes attach and enter mononuclear phagocytes by way of Fc receptors. Increased replication of virus in macrophages may result in clinical "sepsis" due to excessive production of tumor necrosis factor, interleukins, and platelet-activating factor.

Prevalence The reasons for the apparent sudden "appearance" of the syndrome in the past 40 years are completely obscure. However, during the 1922 epidemic of dengue fever in Louisiana, hemorrhagic manifestations, including epistaxis, bleeding gums, melena, menorrhagia, and even "black vomit," were observed. DHF is now a leading cause of morbidity and mortality in tropical Asia. Over 500,000 cases of DHF have been officially reported, with major epidemics in the People's Republic of China, Vietnam, Indonesia, Thailand, and Cuba. In the Cuban outbreak in 1981, almost 350,000 persons developed dengue, approximately 10,000 had hemorrhagic manifestations, and 158 died (1.6 percent mortality). DHF in Asia is a disease of childhood, with one peak observed in children under 1 year and a second in children ages 3 to 5. The disease in infants is associated with primary infection in the presence of maternal antibody. Studies in Thailand have estimated the frequency of DSS as 11 cases per 1000 secondary dengue infections. DSS occurs more frequently in girls than in boys. Dengue hemorrhagic fever occurs almost exclusively in indigenous populations; it has been observed only rarely in whites of European descent, despite the frequent occurrence of classic dengue in this group.

Clinical manifestations Illness begins abruptly, with a minor stage characterized by fever, cough, pharyngitis, headache, anorexia, nausea, vomiting, and abdominal pain which is often severe. This continues for 2 to 4 days. In contrast to classic dengue, myalgia, arthralgia, and bone pain are unusual. Physical signs include fever varying from 38.3 to 40.6°C (101 to 105°F), injection of the tonsils and pharynx, and palpable lymph nodes and liver. The initial state is followed by abrupt deterioration, with the rapid onset of lassitude and weakness (Table 159-4). On examination, the child is found to be restless and to have cold clammy extremities with a warm trunk and a pallid face with circumoral cyanosis. Petechiae, most frequently

TABLE 159-4 World Health Organization's clinical classification of dengue hemorrhagic fever

	Grade	Clinical features	Laboratory findings
DHF* {	I	Fever, constitutional symptoms, positive tourniquet test	Hemoconcentration Thrombocytopenia
	II	Grade I plus spontaneous bleeding (e.g., skin, gums, gastrointestinal tract)	Hemoconcentration Thrombocytopenia
DSS* {	III	Grade II plus circulatory failure, agitation	Hemoconcentration Thrombocytopenia
	IV	Grade II plus profound shock (blood pressure = 0)	Hemoconcentration Thrombocytopenia

* DHF, dengue hemorrhagic fever; DSS, dengue shock syndrome.

located on the forehead and distal extremities, are seen in half the cases. Occasionally there may be a macular or maculopapular rash. The extremities are frequently cyanotic. Hypotension, with narrowing of the pulse pressure, and tachycardia occur. Pathologic reflexes may be present. Most fatalities occur in the fourth or fifth day of illness; melena, hematemesis, coma, or unresponsive shock are poor prognostic signs. Cyanosis, dyspnea, and convulsions are terminal manifestations. Following this critical period, survivors show steady and rapid improvement.

Laboratory findings In one study, hemoconcentration was found in one-fifth of the children. The majority had leukocyte counts between 5000 and 10,000 cells per microliter, with one-third showing a leukocytosis. Only 10 percent of children had a true leukopenia. The most characteristic findings were thrombocytopenia, rarely with blood platelets under 75,000 cells per microliter, positive tourniquet test, and prolonged bleeding time. Prothrombin time and partial thromboplastin times were usually near normal values. Depression of clotting factors V, VII, IX, and X may be present. Bone marrow examination may reveal maturation arrest of megakaryocytes. In Manila or Bangkok, hematuria has been infrequent even with other serious bleeding manifestations; however, in Tahiti, gross hematuria was common. CSF examinations are usually normal. Other abnormal laboratory findings may include hyponatremia, acidosis, elevated blood urea nitrogen levels, elevation in serum glutamic oxalacetic transaminase levels, mild hyperbilirubinemia, and hypoproteinemia. Electrocardiograms may reveal diffuse myocardial abnormalities. Two-thirds of patients have radiologic evidence of bronchopneumonia, with many showing pleural effusions. Ultrasonography is useful in detecting pleural effusions, ascites, and thickening of the gallbladder wall.

Diagnosis The World Health Organization (WHO) has established criteria for the diagnosis of DHF: fever—acute onset, high, continuous, and lasting for 2 to 7 days; hemorrhagic manifestations, including at least a positive tourniquet test and any of the following: petechiae, purpura, ecchymoses, epistaxis, bleeding gums, hematemesis, or melena; enlargement of the liver; thrombocytopenia, ≤100,000 cells per microliter; hemoconcentration, hematocrit increased by ≥20 percent. Criteria for DSS are a rapid, weak pulse with narrowing of the pulse pressure (≤20 mmHg) or hypotension with cold, clammy skin and restlessness. The WHO classification includes a grading of severity (see Table 159-4). Minor hemorrhagic manifestations may be seen during the course of classic dengue fever without meeting WHO criteria for DHF. These cases should be termed *dengue fever with hemorrhage*, not DHF.

Treatment The mainstay is correction of circulatory collapse while avoiding fluid overload. Administration of 5% glucose in 0.5 N saline at a rate of 40 mL/kg restored blood pressure within 1 to 2 h in one-half of patients. When stable, the rate of administration of intravenous fluids was slowed to 10 mL/kg per hour. If improvement did not occur, plasma or a plasma expander (20 mL/kg) was administered. Transfusion of whole blood is not recommended. Oxygen should be administered. Glucocorticoids have been used, but doses of 25 mg/kg have not resulted in significant improvement. Since the evidence for severe disseminated intravascular coagulation is questionable, use of heparin is not clear-cut, although in a group of Filipino children with type 3 dengue virus, administration of heparin (1 mg sodium heparin per kilogram) was associated with a dramatic rise in number of platelets and level of plasma fibrinogen. Antibiotics are not indicated; sympathomimetic amines and salicylates are contraindicated. Recovery from vascular collapse usually occurs within 24 to 48 h, at which time diuretics and digitalis may be necessary. An uncontrolled trial of interferon was conducted during the 1981 epidemic in Cuba with some indication of efficacy.

Prognosis Mortality has varied from 1 to 23 percent. Deaths have been most common in infants under 1 year of age.

Prevention At present, vector control is the only method available to prevent hemorrhagic fever.

TICK-BORNE HEMORRHAGIC FEVERS **Crimean-Congo hemorrhagic fever** At the close of World War II, a new disease entity was recognized in the Crimea region of the former Soviet Union. Retrospective studies demonstrated that an almost identical syndrome had been recognized in the south central Asian republics of the former Soviet Union for many years. Soviet workers repeatedly isolated virus strains during 1967 to 1969.

The virus of Crimean hemorrhagic fever (CHF) is antigenically identical with Congo virus, which was isolated from patients, cattle, and ticks in Kenya, Uganda, Zaire, and Nigeria. Crimean-Congo hemorrhagic fever (CCHF) virus is now known in South Africa, throughout most of subsaharan Africa, eastern Europe, the Middle East, and Asia as far as the Xinjiang Province of China. CCHF occurs where *Hyalomma* ticks are found.

The cases occur between April and September. The sex distribution of CCHF is equal, and 80 percent of the cases occur in the 20- to 60-year age group, with the majority occurring in dairy and agricultural workers. The major arthropod vectors for transmission to humans are ticks which belong to the genus *Hyalomma*. Cattle and wild hares appear to be important reservoirs, and rooks and other birds have been implicated. Once a case of human CCHF occurs, person-to-person transmission is possible. Nosocomial outbreaks have occurred in the former Soviet Union, Pakistan, India, and Iraq. Transmission is presumed to occur through direct contact with infected blood. There are no data to suggest airborne transmission.

After an incubation period of 3 to 6 days, the onset is abrupt, with temperatures to 40°C (104°F), dizziness, headache, and diffuse myalgia. The course of fever is occasionally biphasic, with an average duration of 8 days. Findings include flushing of the face, conjunctival injection, vomiting, and, on occasion, epigastric pain. Hepatomegaly occurs in half the patients. Splenomegaly has been reported in 2 to 25 percent of patients. Respiratory symptoms or signs are unusual. Hemorrhagic manifestations generally begin on the fourth day, with petechiae on the oral mucosa and skin, epistaxis, gingival bleeding, hematemesis, and melena. Neurologic abnormalities, seen in 10 to 25 percent of patients, include nuchal rigidity, excitation, and coma. Laboratory findings show leukopenia, with the number of white blood cells falling as low as 1000 cells per microliter, and thrombocytopenia, which is often severe. Proteinuria and microscopic hematuria are common, but azotemia and oliguria are not. Convalescence may be prolonged. Death is usually attributed to shock or intercurrent infection. Sequelae include transient alopecia and mono- or polyneuritis.

The major approach to therapy has been supportive. Convalescent immune serum has shown promise if administered during the first 3 days of illness. Patients should be isolated, with contact restricted to hospital staff and immediate family. Masks and gowns should be worn, and blood and body fluids should be handled as infectious. The reported mortality rate has varied between 9 and 50 percent.

Omsk hemorrhagic fever Omsk hemorrhagic fever (OHF) is an acute febrile disease which occurs in the Omsk and Novosibirsk oblasts in the former Soviet Union and is caused by a flavivirus. OHF is transmitted to humans either by the bite of infected ticks, *Ixodes apronophorus*, or by the handling of infected muskrats. Epidemics occurred from 1945 to 1948, but recently the disease has been less prevalent.

Following an incubation interval of 3 to 8 days, illness begins abruptly with fever, headache, and hemorrhagic manifestations, which include epistaxis and gastrointestinal and uterine bleeding. OHF has a low case-fatality rate (0.5 to 3.0 percent).

Kyasanur Forest disease Kyasanur Forest disease was shown to be due to a flavivirus. Kyasanur Forest disease occurs following occupational exposure to *Haemaphysalis spinigera* ticks in the tropical forests of western Mysore in southern India. Laboratory-associated infections have been common.

The major symptoms include abrupt onset of fever, headache, fatigue, myalgia (especially of the lumbar area and calf muscles), and retroorbital pain. Cough and abdominal pain occur in half the patients. On examination, findings include relative bradycardia, conjunctival injection, and generalized lymphadenopathy. Fine and coarse rales are frequently heard. The fever usually lasts from 6 to 11 days. After an afebrile period of 9 to 21 days, approximately half the patients may develop a second phase, which lasts from 2 to 12 days. This is manifested by recurrence of fever, severe headache, neck stiffness, mental disturbance, coarse tremors, giddiness, and abnormalities in reflexes, as well as by recurrence of many of the initial symptoms. No sequelae have been observed, but convalescence is often prolonged.

Only limited laboratory studies have been reported. During the initial phase, leukopenia is a constant feature. During the second phase, there is a mild leukocytosis. Lumbar puncture during the second phase has shown a pattern of aseptic meningitis. Diagnosis is based upon virus isolation from blood. Serologic tests of paired sera also can be performed. The management is supportive. The mortality rate is approximately 5 percent.

HEMORRHAGIC FEVER WITH RENAL SYNDROME

Synonyms for this disease (HFRS) include *Korean hemorrhagic fever*, *Far Eastern hemorrhagic fever*, endemic or *epidemic nephroso-nephritis*, *Manchurian epidemic hemorrhagic fever*, *Songo fever*, and *Churilov's disease*. A similar but milder disease in Scandinavia has been called *nephropathia epidemica* or *epidemic nephritis* (EN).

ETIOLOGY In 1976, the antigen of HFRS was demonstrated in the lungs of the rodent *Apodemus agrarius coreae*. Diagnostic increases in immunofluorescent antibodies were demonstrated in 113 of 116 cases of severe HFRS. The agent designated *Hantaan virus* is a single-stranded RNA virus belonging to the family Bunyaviridae, genus Hantavirus (see Table 159-1). The genus consists of at least five species: Hantaan virus (Korean hemorrhagic fever), Seoul virus, Puumala virus (nephropathia epidemica), Porogia virus (Balkan HFRS), and Prospect Hill virus (isolated from meadow voles in Maryland and associated with human infection, not disease).

PREVALENCE In Korea between April 1951 and January 1953, 2070 cases of epidemic hemorrhagic fever were reported among United Nations personnel. In a recent analysis of sera collected in 1951–1954 from 245 clinically diagnosed patients, 94 percent had specific IgM antibody against Hantaan virus. The disease usually occurs as an isolated event; hence overall attack rates have relatively less meaning. With this reservation, attack rates in two United States Army divisions stationed in Korea varied between 1.9 and 2.9 cases per 1000 persons per epidemic season. Approximately 800 cases per year have continued to occur; however, most cases are now seen in Korean civilians and military, with less than 10 cases per year in U.S. military personnel. During the past 15 years, the disease has increased in prevalence in Korea, urban Japan, and China. In the People's Republic of China, over 100,000 cases of HFRS are reported annually; the incidence is increasing. Hundreds of cases of EN have occurred annually in Finland and other Scandinavian countries since the 1930s. In 1953 a severe form of HFRS was recognized in the Balkan countries, and in 1982, in Greece and France. Antibody studies indicate worldwide distribution. Antibodies in human sera have been found in Argentina, Brazil, Colombia, Europe, Canada, the United States (including Hawaii and Alaska), Southeast Asia, Egypt, and central Africa.

EPIDEMIOLOGY In Korea, the majority of cases occur in May to June and in October to November. These peaks coincide with rodent population density. Hantaan virus is present in rodent urine, feces, and saliva in high titer. Transmission from rodent to rodent is primarily respiratory, with transmission to people through inhalation of virus-containing dried excreta. There is no evidence for person-to-person transmission. The urban reservoir appears to be the house rat. Laboratory-acquired cases have occurred in the former Soviet Union,

Korea, Japan, and Europe, with rats implicated in Korea, Japan, and the United Kingdom.

CLINICAL MANIFESTATIONS There are two forms of disease, a mild illness characteristically diagnosed in Scandinavia as epidemic nephritis (EN) and the more severe HFRS seen especially in the Far East and central Europe.

EN is characterized by sudden onset of high fever, backache, headache, and abdominal pain. On the third or fourth day, hemorrhagic manifestations may occur, and conjunctival hemorrhages, palatine petechiae, and a petechial rash appear on the trunk. About one patient in five is "toxic" and mentally obtunded. Oliguria and azotemia develop. Urinalysis reveals proteinuria, hematuria, and leukocyturia. After about 3 days the rash subsides, the patient develops polyuria, and recovers in several weeks.

Hemorrhagic fever with renal syndrome (HFRS) The incubation period in HFRS is usually 10 to 25 days, with possible extremes of 7 and 36 days. Visitors who contract the disease in an endemic area may not develop illness until after their return home.

The clinical course of HFRS may be divided into phases on the basis of the underlying physiologic aberrations: febrile, hypotensive, oliguric, diuretic, and convalescent. There is considerable variation among patients in the severity of the illness. In one study, two-thirds of the 264 cases studied were classified as mild, while 14 percent were termed severe.

FEBRILE (INVASIVE) PHASE From 10 to 20 percent of patients describe vague prodromal symptoms resembling mild upper respiratory infections. The onset is then usually abrupt, often initiated by a chill and accompanied by fever, headache, backache, abdominal pain, and generalized myalgia. Anorexia and thirst are almost universal, while nausea and vomiting are common, although not constant, symptoms. The headache is most commonly frontal or retroorbital. Eye symptoms, especially mild photophobia and pain on movement of the eyes, are characteristic. Diarrhea is not a feature. Fever is present in almost all patients; the temperature ranges from 37.8 to 41.1°C (100 to 106°F), reaches a peak on the third or fourth day after onset, and falls by lysis on the fourth to seventh day. There is a relative bradycardia. Initially the blood pressure is normal. One of the most typical early findings is a diffuse reddening of the skin, most marked over the face and V area of the neck, that may resemble a severe sunburn. The erythema blanches on pressure. Dermographism can be demonstrated in over 90 percent of patients at the same time as the flush. Slight edema of the upper eyelids causes a bleary-eyed appearance. Bulbar and palpebral conjunctivae show injection. Conjunctival petechiae may develop by the third or fifth day of illness. Subconjunctival hemorrhages may be striking. Intense pharyngeal reddening without significant sore throat is typical. The first location for petechiae is usually the palate, where they occur in half the patients. Within 12 to 24 h, petechiae appear at pressure areas such as the axillary folds, lateral chest wall, belt line, hips, and thighs. Retinal hemorrhages occur rarely. Cervical, axillary, and inguinal nodes are moderately enlarged but nontender. Abdominal and costovertebral tenderness is almost a constant finding. Splenomegaly is unusual. The degree of flush, fever, and conjunctival injection and the number of petechiae correlate quite well with the overall severity of illness.

Laboratory studies during this phase are often not striking. Initial hemoglobin and hematocrit values are usually normal. Prior to the fourth day, leukocyte counts range from 3600 to 6000 cells per microliter but are associated with neutrophilia. Early in the course urine specific gravity may be high. Albuminuria, which is an almost universal finding, appears, often abruptly, between the second and fifth days of illness. The urinary sediment reveals microscopic hematuria and hyaline, granular, red blood cell casts, and/or white blood cell casts. Erythrocyte sedimentation rates are normal during the first week. Capillary fragility tests are usually positive at the time of admission and become most abnormal by the ninth day. Electrocardiographic abnormalities may be seen in 15 to 30 percent of patients; these include sinus bradycardia and low or inverted T waves. Lumbar punctures may reveal gross blood in the spinal fluid.

HYPOTENSIVE PHASE   On about the fifth day of illness, during the last 24 to 48 h of the febrile phase, hypotension or shock may occur. In mild cases, only a transient fall in blood pressure occurs; among moderately and severely ill patients, shock may persist for 1 to 3 days. In 828 patients, 16.5 percent had clinical shock, and another 14 percent had hypotension without shock. Headache often diminishes, but thirst persists. In the beginning of the hypotensive phase, most patients have warm, dry skin and extremities. As the systolic blood pressure decreases and pulse pressure narrows, the skin becomes cool and moist. Tachycardia replaces the relative bradycardia.

At this stage an increase in hematocrit with no change in total serum protein level is found. This is thought to reflect a loss of plasma through damaged capillaries. On about the fifth day, all patients develop marked proteinuria. The previously normal urine specific gravity begins to fall and in 2 to 3 days is usually around 1.010. Blood urea nitrogen concentrations begin to increase. Other laboratory findings include leukocytosis with white blood cell counts of 10,000 to 56,000 per microliter with neutrophilia and toxic granulation. The number of platelets often decreases to less than 70,000 per microliter.

OLIGURIC PHASE (HEMORRHAGIC OR TOXIC PHASE)   About the eighth day of illness, blood pressure returns to the normal range and in some instances increases to hypertensive levels. While oliguria may have appeared during the shock phase, it now becomes a prominent feature. Oliguria develops even though hypotension was not recognized. Symptomatically, patients continue to feel weak and thirsty and have more severe backache. Protracted vomiting and hiccups may ensue.

Blood urea nitrogen levels increase rapidly and are associated with hyperkalemia, hyperphosphatemia, and hypocalcemia. Metabolic acidosis is rarely severe. Although platelets begin to return to normal, hemorrhagic manifestations become more prominent and include petechiae, hematemesis (analogous to "black vomit" in yellow fever), melena, hemoptysis, gross hematuria, and hemorrhages into the central nervous system. The enlarged lymph nodes may now become tender.

With the onset of diuresis on about the seventh to the eleventh day, symptoms of fluid and electrolyte abnormalities and central nervous system or pulmonary complications may appear. Central nervous system symptoms include disorientation, extreme restlessness, lethargy, paranoid delusions, and hallucinations. Grand mal seizures, pulmonary edema, and pulmonary infection occur in some patients.

DIURETIC PHASE   With the onset of diuresis, progressive improvement is the rule. Most patients begin to eat and regain their strength. In fatal cases, the diuretic phase is associated with a daily urine output of less than 4 L and often less than 2 L, in contrast to larger volumes in surviving patients.

CONVALESCENT PHASE   The convalescent phase lasts 3 to 6 weeks. Weight is regained slowly. Complaints include muscular weakness, intention tremor, and lack of stamina. Hyposthenuria and polyuria are present; however, within 2 months most patients are able to concentrate their urine to a specific gravity of 1.023 or greater after a 12-h period of water deprivation.

DIAGNOSIS   Diagnosis is based on demonstration of specific IgM antibodies by ELISA or a fourfold change in immune adherence hemagglutination titers in paired sera. Studies on the epidemiology of Hantavirus have shown that during the initial 24 to 72 h (febrile phase) there is significant overlap in the clinical features of leptospirosis, HFRS, and scrub typhus. In Korea, where all three diseases are prevalent, of blood samples submitted for Hantavirus serology, 21 percent had antibody to leptospira antigens and 6 percent to *Rickettsia tsutsugamushi*. Because of the similarity in epidemiology and clinical presentation and the potential for dual infections, it has been recommended that blood be submitted for Hantavirus serology in all cases of suspected leptospirosis (see Chap. 135).

TREATMENT   Clinical management primarily revolves around meticulous supportive care. Trials with a variety of agents, including antibiotics, glucocorticoids, antihistamines, convalescent serum, and interferon-α, were without significant beneficial effect during the Korean epidemics. In a controlled U.S./Chinese clinical trial in the People's Republic of China, ribavirin was shown to have efficacy.

PROGNOSIS   The experience in the former Soviet Union indicates a mortality rate of 3 to 32 percent; in China, the case-fatality ratio was 7 to 15 percent. Between April 1951 and December 1976, the overall case-fatality ratio in Korea was 6.6 percent.

Residua are uncommon. Of 783 surviving patients cared for at the Hemorrhagic Fever Center in Korea between April and December 1952, only 16 were unable to return to duty within a period of 4 months. Fifteen of these individuals still had hyposthenuria. Follow-up studies on patients 3 to 5 years later showed that they had many more subsequent hospital admissions for urologic problems than did a control group and that the relative frequency correlated with the severity of the acute episode of HFRS.

REFERENCES

"Arboviruses": Definition, classification, and general review

FIELDS BN et al (eds): *Virology*, 2d ed. New York, Raven, 1990
HALSTEAD SB: Dengue fever, viral hemorrhagic fever, and rabies. Curr Opin Infect Dis. 5:332, 1992
MONATH TP (ed): *The Arboviruses: Epidemiology and Ecology*, vols 2 to 4. Boca Raton, CRC Press, 1988, 1989
TSAI TF: Arboviral infections in the United States. Infect Dis Clin North Am 5:73, 1991

Infections characterized by fever, malaise, headaches, and myalgia

BOWEN GS et al: Clinical aspects of human Venezuelan equine encephalitis in Texas, 1971. Bull Pan Am Health Org 10:46, 1976
BRICENO ROSSIE AL: Rural epidemic encephalitis in Venezuela caused by a group A arbovirus (VEE). Prog Med Virol 9:176, 1967
DIETZ WH JR et al: Ten clinical cases of human infection with Venezuelan equine encephalomyelitis virus, subtype I–D. Am J Trop Med Hyg 28:329, 1979
FLEMING J et al: Sandfly fever. Review of 664 cases. Lancet 1:443, 1947
GOODPASTURE HC et al: Colorado tick fever: Clinical, epidemiologic and laboratory aspects of 228 cases in Colorado in 1973–1974. Ann Intern Med 88:303, 1978
HUGHES LE et al: Persistence of Colorado tick fever virus in red blood cells. Am J Trop Med Hyg 23:530, 1974
LAUGHLIN LW et al: Epidemic Rift Valley fever in Egypt: Observations of the spectrum of human illness. Trans R Soc Trop Med Hyg 73:630, 1979
LENNETTE EH, KOPROWSKI H: Human infection with Venezuelan equine encephalomyelitis virus. JAMA 123:1088, 1943
SCHERER WF et al: Ecologic studies of Venezuelan encephalitis virus in Southeastern Mexico: VII. Infection of man. Am J Trop Med 21:79, 1972
SIAM AL et al: Rift Valley fever ocular manifestations: Observations during 1977 epidemic in Egypt. Br J Ophthalmol 64:366, 1980

Infections presenting chiefly with fever, malaise, lymphadenopathy, and rash

ALVAREZ MD, RAMÍREZ-RONDA CH: Dengue and hepatic failure. Am J Med 79:670, 1985
CENTERS FOR DISEASE CONTROL: Dengue epidemic, Peru 1990. Morb Mort Week Rep 40:145, 1991
MICKS DW, MOON WB: *Aedes aegypti* in a Texas coastal county as an index of dengue fever receptivity and control. Am J Trop Med Hyg 29:1382, 1980
TSAI CJ et al: Upper gastrointestinal bleeding in Dengue fever. Am J Gastroenterol 86:33, 1991

Infections presenting chiefly with fever, acute arthropathy, and rash

AASKOV JG et al: An epidemic of Ross River virus infection in Fiji, 1979. Am J Trop Med Hyg 30:1053, 1981
CLARK JA et al: Annually recurrent epidemic polyarthritis and Ross River virus activity in a coastal area of New South Wales. I. Occurrence of the disease. Am J Trop Med Hyg 22:543, 1973
DELLER JJ JR, RUSSELL PK: Chikungunya disease. Am J Trop Med 17:107, 1968
PHILLIPS DA et al: Clinical and subclinical Barmah Forest virus infection in Queensland. Med J Aust 152:463, 1990
PINHEIRO FP et al: An outbreak of Mayaro virus disease in Belterra, Brazil: I. Clinical and virological findings. Am J Trop Med Hyg 30:674, 1981
ROBINSON MC: An epidemic of virus disease in Southern Province, Tanganyika territory in 1952–53: I. Clinical features. Trans R Soc Trop Med Hyg 49:28, 1955

SHORE H: O'nyong-nyong fever: An epidemic virus disease in East Africa: III. Some clinical and epidemiological observations in the Northern Province of Uganda. Trans R Soc Trop Med Hyg 55:361, 1961

Infections presenting chiefly with central nervous system involvement

BALFOUR HH JR et al: California arbovirus (LaCrosse) infections. Pediatrics 52:680, 1973

BURKE DS, LEAKE CJ: Japanese encephalitis, in *Arboviruses: Epidemiology and Ecology*, vol 3, TP Monath (ed). Boca Raton, CRC Press, 1998, p 63

CENTERS FOR DISEASE CONTROL: Eastern equine encephalitis virus associated with *Aedes albopictus*, Florida, 1991. Morb Mort Week Rep 41:115, 1992

DICKERSON RB et al: Diagnosis and immediate prognosis of Japanese B encephalitis. Observations based on more than 200 patients with detailed analysis of 65 serologically confirmed cases. Am J Med 12:277, 1952

FINLEY KH et al: Western equine and St. Louis encephalitis. Preliminary report of a clinical follow-up study in California. Neurology 5:223, 1955

GRABOW JD et al: The electroencephalogram and clinical sequelae of California arbovirus encephalitis. Neurology 19:394, 1969

HILTY MD et al: California encephalitis in children. Am J Dis Child 124:530, 1972

KETEL WB, OGNIBENE AJ: Japanese B encephalitis in Vietnam. Am J Med Sci 261:271, 1971

LUBY JP et al: The epidemiology of St. Louis encephalitis (SLE): A review. Ann Rev Med 20:329, 1969

————: Antigenemia in St. Louis encephalitis. Am J Trop Med Hyg 29:265, 1980

POLAND JD et al: Evaluation of potency and safety of inactivated Japanese encephalitis vaccine in U.S. inhabitants. J Infect Dis 161:878, 1990

SCHNEIDER RJ et al: Clinical sequelae after Japanese encephalitis: One year follow-up study in Thailand. Southeast Asian J Trop Med Public Health 5:560, 1974

Diseases presenting primarily with hemorrhagic manifestations

BRUNO P et al: Hemorrhagic fever with renal syndrome imported to Hawaii from West Germany. Am J Med 89:232, 1990

BURNEY MI et al: Nosocomial outbreak of viral hemorrhagic fever caused by Crimean hemorrhagic fever—Congo virus in Pakistan, January 1976. Am J Trop Med Hyg 29:941, 1980

CENTERS FOR DISEASE CONTROL: Viral hemorrhagic fever. Initial management of suspected and confirmed cases. Ann Intern Med 101:73, 1984

————: Korean hemorrhagic fever. JAMA 259:1622, 1988

DENNIS LH et al: The original hemorrhagic fever: Yellow fever. Blood 30:858, 1967

GARTNER L: Hantaan virus infection (Korean hemorrhagic fever) as a cause of acute renal failure. Dtsch Med Wochenschr 113:937, 1988

HALSTEAD SB, O'ROURKE EF: Dengue viruses and mononuclear phagocytes: I. Infection enhancement by non-neutralizing antibody. J Exp Med 146:201, 1977

————: The pathogenesis of dengue: Molecular epidemiology in infectious disease. Am J Epidemiol 114:632, 1981

KLIKS SC et al: Antibody-dependant enhancement of dengue virus growth in human monocytes as a risk factor for dengue hemorrhagic fever. Am J Trop Med Hyg 40:444, 1989

KUDESIA G et al: Dual infection with leptospira and Hantavirus. Lancet 1:1397, 1988

LEDUC JW et al: A retrospective analysis of sera collected by the Hemorrhagic Fever Commission during the Korean Conflict. J Infect Dis 162:182, 1990

LEE HW et al: Isolation of the etiologic agent of Korean hemorrhagic fever. J Infect Dis 137:298, 1978

MONATH TP et al: Yellow fever in the Gambia, 1978–1979: Epidemiologic aspects with observations on the occurrence of Orongo virus infections. Am J Trop Med Hyg 29:912, 1980

NELSON ER: Hemorrhagic fever in children in Thailand: Report of 69 cases. J Pediatr 56:101, 1960

PILASKI J et al: Haemorrhagic fever with renal syndrome in Germany. Lancet 337:111, 1991

PINHEIRO FP et al: An epidemic of yellow fever in Central Brazil 1972–1973: I. Epidemiological studies. Am J Trop Med Hyg 27:125, 1978

WORLD HEALTH ORGANIZATION: *Dengue hemorrhagic fever: Diagnosis, treatment and control*. Geneva, 1986

————: Hemorrhagic fever with renal syndrome: Memorandum from a WHO meeting. Bull WHO 61:269, 1983

160   ARENAVIRUS INFECTIONS

JAY P. SANFORD

DEFINITION AND CLASSIFICATION   The term *arenavirus* is the designation for a group of RNA viruses which have unique morphology. The virions are pleomorphic, with diameters between 50 and 300 nm, and contain an electron-dense membrane with projections and 2 to 10 inclusion-like dense particles (resembling ribosomes) that give the virion an appearance of having been sprinkled with sand (Latin *arenaceus*, "sandy"). Fifteen distinct arenaviruses have been described (Table 160-1). All except Tacaribe are parasites of rodents, and most are unique to tropical America. A special property of arenaviruses that cause disease in humans is the capacity of congenitally or newborn acquired infections to persist in their reservoir hosts with no ill effects and in the absence of an immune response.

LYMPHOCYTIC CHORIOMENINGITIS   The first-recognized arenavirus was lymphocytic choriomeningitis (LCM) virus. It was recognized early that LCM was carried by apparently healthy laboratory mice. Clinically, LCM has been considered primarily in the context of aseptic meningitis; however, it is associated with at least two clinical syndromes in humans: central nervous system (CNS) and influenza-like illness which may be associated with rash, arthritis, or orchitis. LCM virus has provided a valuable model for the study of chronic, persistent, and generally symptomless viral infections in laboratory animals.

Prevalence   In the United States, human infection with LCM virus is rare; however, seroepidemiologic studies on specimens obtained in 1935 to 1940 from persons with no history of CNS disease

TABLE 160-1   Classification of arenaviruses

Virus	Clinical disease	Reservoir	Known geographic range
OLD WORLD SPECIES			
Lymphocytic choriomeningitis	Aseptic meningitis, meningoencephalitis, influenzal syndrome, orchitis, arthritis	Mice, hamsters	Worldwide except Australia
Lassa	Lassa fever	*Mastomys natalensis*	Nigeria, Liberia, Sierra Leone, Republic of Guinea, Central African Republic
Ippy		*Arvicanthis* spp.	Central African Republic
Mobala		*Praomys jacksoni*	Central African Republic
Mopeia		*Mastomys natalensis*	Mozambique
NEW WORLD SPECIES: TACARIBE COMPLEX			
Tacaribe		Bats	Trinidad
Junin	Argentinian hemorrhagic fever	*Calomys musculinus*	Argentina
Machupo	Bolivian hemorrhagic fever	*Calomys callosus*	Northeast Bolivia
Guanarito	Venezuelan hemorrhagic fever	*Sigmodon hispidus* (cotton rat) *Oryzomys* spp. (rice rat)	Northwest Venezuela
Amapari			Brazil
Latino			Bolivia
Parana			Paraguay
Pichinde			Colombia
Tamiami			Florida
Flexal		*Orzomys* spp.	Brazil

from all parts of the United States revealed neutralizing antibodies in 10 to 28 percent. In recent years, the prevalence of infection seems to have decreased markedly.

Epidemiology   The virus of LCM is worldwide in distribution. Foci of LCM virus have been defined in Germany, Hungary, and elsewhere in Europe. Scandinavia appears to be LCM virus–free, as are most of the Americas except Argentina. Although infection can be induced in a variety of animals, mice are the major natural reservoir as well as the primary host in which latent, asymptomatic infection occurs. The latency of infection in the mouse depends on immunologic tolerance. Animals infected in utero or shortly after birth excrete LCM virus for life without overt disease. Human infections are secondary to contact with an infected rodent. The mode of transmission is thought to be via airborne spread or contact with excrement from infected animals. In the past, most cases have arisen in persons living in rodent-infested houses, but lately outbreaks of LCM virus disease in humans have been reported from Germany and the United States in which the source of infection was traced to laboratory animals and household pets, specifically hamsters, which, like mice, can shed LCM virus in urine and stool. LCM occurs throughout the year but has been more frequent in the colder months. Person-to-person transmission has not been demonstrated.

Pathogenesis   In natural infection, the portal of entry of the LCM virus is probably the respiratory tract. Virus multiplication occurs initially in the respiratory epithelium, and an influenza-like illness develops. Dissemination of virus to extrapulmonary sites, presumably to reticuloendothelial cells with multiplication, and viremia occur. LCM virus crosses the blood-brain barrier. In mice, the resulting meningitis is attributed to a cell-mediated immune reaction. Support for this hypothesis derives from observations that disease but not infection can be prevented in experimental animals by neonatal thymectomy, irradiation, or immunodepressant drugs such as cyclophosphamide. Similar pathogenetic mechanisms may operate in humans, although isolation of LCM virus from the cerebrospinal fluid (CSF) of patients with aseptic meningitis is quite common.

Clinical manifestations   The exact incubation period is not known. Following experimental inoculation of LCM virus into volunteers, fever occurred in $1\frac{1}{2}$ to 3 days, while an influenza-like constellation of symptoms developed 5 to 10 days after exposure. An influenza-like illness is the most common clinical pattern. In some patients the illness may be biphasic, with subsequent aseptic meningitis or encephalomyelitis. Fever, usually from 38.3 to 40°C (101 to 104°F), associated with rigors, is uniformly noted. Other symptoms which are encountered in over one-half of patients include malaise, weakness, myalgia (especially lumbar aching), retroorbital headache, photophobia, anorexia, nausea, and light-headedness. Symptoms which occur in one-fourth to one-half of patients include sore throat, vomiting, and dysesthesias. Later, arthralgias, especially in the hands, occur. Less common complaints (up to one-quarter of patients) include aching pain in the chest, associated with pneumonitis; increased hair loss progressing to generalized alopecia, 2 or 3 weeks after the onset of illness; testicular pain or frank orchitis, usually unilateral, 1 to 3 weeks after onset; and parotid pain, which may lead to a misdiagnosis of mumps. Physical findings in the first week of illness are few. Patients often have a relative bradycardia. Pharyngeal injection without exudate is common (60 percent). Mild nontender cervical or axillary lymphadenopathy may occur. The initial phase lasts from 5 days to 3 weeks, followed by improvement. After a remission of 1 to 2 days, many patients relapse with recurrent fever and more prominent headache. Physical signs may include skin rashes, swelling of metacarpophalangeal and proximal interphalangeal joints, meningeal signs, orchitis, parotitis, and alopecia. Convalescence generally is of 1 to 4 weeks' duration, characterized by easy fatigability, an excessive need for sleep, dysesthesias, and occasional dizziness. Patients with aseptic meningitis almost always recover without sequelae. With encephalitis, 25 to 30 percent of patients have neurologic residua.

Laboratory findings   Leukopenia and thrombocytopenia are almost uniform during the first week of illness. Although leukocyte counts usually vary between 2000 and 3000 cells per microliter, counts as low as 600 cells per microliter have been recorded. Differential counts generally show slight relative lymphocytosis. Platelet counts are usually between 50,000 and 100,000 per microliter. Anemia is not encountered. The erythrocyte sedimentation rate often is normal. Mild elevations of serum aspartate aminotransferase and lactic dehydrogenase (LDH) may occur. Chest radiographs may suggest basilar pneumonias. In patients with meningeal signs, examination of the CSF usually reveals several hundred cells per microliter, although cell counts in excess of 1000 per microliter are reported in half the patients in some series. Lymphocytes predominate (greater than 80 percent) even early. The initial CSF protein is usually slightly elevated, but on occasion levels may exceed 1.5 g/L (150 mg/dL). Although a normal CSF glucose level is considered the hallmark of viral meningitides, low CSF glucose has been observed in up to 27 percent of patients with LCM.

Diagnosis   The diagnosis of LCM can be established with certainty by recovery of the virus from blood or spinal fluid; however, this procedure requires a biosafety level 3 facility. The simplest method is a direct immunofluorescent assay (IFA) of infected cells fixed on a microscopic slide. ELISA or radioimmunoassay also may be used. IgG antibodies appear by 7 to 10 days. Neutralizing antibodies appear after 6 to 8 weeks, increase in titer slowly, and remain high for years. The clinical manifestations of LCM cannot be differentiated from those produced by numerous other viruses.

Treatment   There is no specific treatment.

ARGENTINIAN AND BOLIVIAN HEMORRHAGIC FEVERS   The first cases of a new American hemorrhagic disease were seen near the Argentinian town of Junin near Buenos Aires in 1953. A virus was isolated from patients' blood and from local rodents and their mites. In 1959, cases of a disease thought to resemble severe epidemic typhus were noted among rural workers in northeastern Bolivia. The similarity between these syndromes was recognized. In 1963, the causal virus was isolated from patients and rodents and named the *Machupo virus*. Machupo virus is serologically related to but distinct from Junin virus.

Prevalence   Junin virus infections, Argentinian hemorrhagic fever (AHF), have occurred in epidemic form since 1958, with between 100 and 3500 cases reported annually. Since initial recognition, AHF has spread more widely. In contrast, Bolivian hemorrhagic fever (BHF) has not spread to other geographic areas, and virtually no cases have been reported in the past 10 years.

Epidemiology   AHF occurs in sharply endemic seasonal form (February to August), mostly among male rural workers, especially those exposed to fields at the time of the maize harvest. Virus is transmitted in the urine of rodents with chronic infection and viruria. Humans acquire the virus through contact with items or foodstuffs which have been contaminated with infected rodent urine. The main reservoir is two species of rodents, *Calomys laucha* and *C. musculinus*.

BHF is similarly transmitted by the urine of *C. callosus* (a mouselike rodent) chronically infected with Machupo virus. Direct person-to-person transmission is possible and may have occurred in the outbreak in Cochabamba. Disease has not occurred in medical personnel attending infected patients.

Clinical features   AHF presents manifestations of renal, cardiovascular, and hematologic involvement. Inapparent infections are rare. The incubation period is estimated to be 7 to 16 days, followed by a gradual onset of chills, fever, headache, malaise, myalgia, anorexia, nausea, and vomiting. The temperature reaches 38.9 to 40°C (102 to 104°F), facial flushing may be prominent, and there is a painless enanthem of the pharynx. Lymphadenopathy and splenomegaly are not present. From 3 to 5 days after the onset, the signs and symptoms worsen, with the appearance of dehydration, relative bradycardia, hypotension to 50 to 100 mmHg, and oliguria. In the more severe cases, hemorrhagic manifestations, including bleeding from the gums, hematemesis, hematuria, and melena, occur. At this phase, one-half of patients will have neurologic symptoms: cranial nerve weakness, oculogyric crises, and tremor of the tongue and extremities. Some patients develop psychic manifestations, with agitation, delirium, or stupor. Progressive shock, hypothermia, gallop rhythm, or gastrointestinal bleeding may occur from the seventh to tenth days. In fatal cases, pulmonary edema usually is the cause of death. During convalescence, temporary alopecia has been noted. Erythrocyte counts are normal or elevated. The total leukocyte counts drop to less than 1000 cells per microliter, and platelet counts of less than 100,000 per microliter are invariable. Disseminated intravascular coagulation does not seem to be the mechanism responsible for the hemorrhagic manifestations. Intense proteinuria is common, and microscopic hematuria also occurs. Blood urea nitrogen levels rise rapidly.

The clinical picture of BHF is similar to that of AHF, although epistaxis and hematemesis at the onset are more common in BHF.

Diagnosis IgG antibodies, which appear within 7 to 10 days, are detected by IFA.

Treatment Treatment consists of supportive measures, including peritoneal dialysis or hemodialysis-filtration to correct both the azotemia and the pulmonary edema. In AHF, a double-blind trial with immune plasma reduced mortality from 16 to 1 percent. However, 10 percent of treated patients developed neurologic symptoms 4 to 6 weeks after treatment. The neurologic syndrome included fever, headache, ataxia, and intention tremors but lasted less than 1 week. Preliminary studies suggest that ribavirin may be effective in both experimental BHF and AHF. Treatment protects against the acute hemorrhagic phase but does not prevent the late neurologic disease. Since Junin virus is seldom isolated from the CNS in fatal human AHF, evaluation of ribavirin in humans with AHF seems justified.

Prognosis The mortality rate among patients with AHF is usually 3 to 15 percent, while that in BHF is 5 to 30 percent.

Prevention In Bolivia, rodent control measures directed primarily against *C. callosus* populations in the houses has resulted in a prompt and dramatic cessation of human cases. In Argentina, the wide dispersal of infected hosts renders rodent control measures futile.

VENEZUELAN HEMORRHAGIC FEVER An outbreak of severe hemorrhagic illness occurred in Guanarito, Venezuela, in September 1989.

Epidemiology Although preliminary transmission through contact with infected rodents or their excretions is likely, a newly identified agent, Guanarito virus, a new member of the Tacaribe complex of Arenaviridae, was isolated from the cotton rat, and antibodies were identified in the rice rat. Infection rate was low in family contacts (10 percent had antibodies), and illness was not recognized in hospital personnel who cared for over 100 patients with the disease. Transmission seems to occur in and around houses, as with BHF and Lassa fever.

Clinical features Patients range in age from 6 to 54 years, with sexes equally affected. Duration of illness at the time of admission to hospital was 3 to 12 days. The most common presenting symptoms included fever (93 percent), headache (60 percent), diarrhea (46 percent), cough (40 percent), and hemorrhagic manifestations (86 percent): epistaxis, bleeding gums, menorrhagia, and melena. Clinical signs included pharyngitis (some with tonsillar exudate), marked conjunctival injection, facial edema, cervical lymphadenopathy, scattered pulmonary rales, and petechiae. Among 104 presumed cases there were 26 deaths, while 9 (60 percent) of 15 patients with confirmed cases died. Among the 6 survivors, one had temporary alopecia and one a mild hearing loss. Convalescence was lengthy, lasting several months.

Laboratory features Hemoglobin and hematocrit values were normal. Leukopenia (1100 to 3900 cells per microliter) was noted in two-thirds of patients. Platelet counts were less than 100,000 per microliter in one-half; serum creatinine levels were elevated in one-third.

Diagnosis The virus was isolated from serum and spleen by tissue culture on vero cells. In surviving patients, antibodies were measured by IFA tests.

Treatment While treatment is still undefined, an approach similar to that for AHF seems appropriate.

LASSA FEVER A virus disease which is both highly contagious and virulent occurred in a missionary nurse in Lassa, a town in northeast Nigeria, in 1969.

Epidemiology Since the initial outbreak at Lassa in 1969, during which one of the patients was transferred to New York City, there have been other outbreaks near Jos in northern Nigeria in 1970 (32 suspected cases with 10 deaths), in Zorzor, Liberia, in 1972 (11 cases with 4 deaths), and in the eastern province of Sierra Leone with 63 suspected cases admitted to two hospitals between 1970 and 1972. Lassa fever occurs as an endemic disease in eastern Sierra Leone. Population surveys showed more than one-half of older adults had antibodies. Other countries in west Africa having clinical or serologic evidence of Lassa fever include Senegal, Gambia, Guinea, Ghana, Burkina Faso (formerly Upper Volta), Mali, and Ivory Coast. Lassa-related viruses (Mopeia, Mobala) have been isolated from rodents in Mozambique, Zimbabwe, and the Central African Republic; however, they have not been associated with human illness. In Jos and Zorzor, outbreaks apparently resulted from person-to-person nosocomial spread from the index case to hospital workers or other patients. In Sierra Leone, the great majority of cases were acquired outside the hospital, although hospital workers were at risk. *Mastomys natalensis*, a multimammate rat widespread in Africa, is the animal reservoir, and primary human cases result from contamination of foodstuffs with rodent urine. Human-to-human transmission may occur through contact with urine, feces, vomitus, or saliva through droplets, and particularly through wounds contaminated with blood. Intrafamilial outbreaks have occurred around several cases. There are a number of cases which have been acquired through accidental autoinoculation with needles while starting intravenous fluids. At least one laboratory-acquired infection has occurred. In Sierra Leone 6 percent of the population surveyed had complement fixing antibody against Lassa virus, while only 0.2 percent had recognized disease, suggesting mild disease or inapparent infection. In Liberia 10 percent of hospital personnel had antibodies. In west Africa the incidence is estimated to be greater than 250,000 cases per year.

Clinical features The incubation period is usually 7 to 18 days. Patients have ranged from 5 months to 46 years of age; approximately two-thirds are women. Three of eight women in one series were 22 to 28 weeks pregnant during their illness. The apparent predilection for women may relate to exposure to contaminated food or work in hospitals rather than to differences in susceptibility. The onset of illness was described by most patients as insidious. The most frequent initial symptoms were fever (100 percent), chilliness and true rigors, headache (50 percent), malaise (100 percent), and myalgia (50 percent). Most patients did not seek medical attention for 4 to 9 days after onset. Symptoms of a systemic viral illness then developed with anorexia, nausea, vomiting, myalgia, and pain in the chest, epigastrium, and lumbar area. Headache was usually present. Two-thirds of patients developed a dry nonproductive cough. Early examination revealed fever and flushing of the face and V area of the neck. Pharyngitis developed in 70 percent and became progressively more severe during the first week; patients expectorated saliva because swallowing was so painful. Examination often revealed raised patches of whitish exudate occurring on the palatine arches, which occasionally coalesced into a pseudomembrane. Oral ulcerations have been noted in up to one-half of cases. Generalized nontender lymphadenopathy occurred in one-half of patients. During the second week, severe lower abdominal pain and intractable vomiting were common, and facial and neck swelling with conjunctival edema and infection frequently developed. Occasionally patients had tinnitus, epistaxis, bleeding from the gums and venipuncture sites, maculopapular rashes, and dizziness. During the acute stage, systolic blood pressures of less than 90 mmHg, with pulse pressures less than 20 mmHg, occurred in 60 to 80 percent of patients. Initially, relative bradycardia was common. During the second week, the patients who recovered defervesced, while the patients who died often developed signs of shock, clouding of the sensorium, rales, signs of pleural effusion, agitation, and, on occasion, grand mal seizures. The duration of illness in surviving patients ranged from 7 to 31 days (average 15 days), while that in fatal cases was 7 to 26 days (average 12 days). The mortality rates in Jos and Zorzor were 52 and 36 percent, respectively, while in Sierra Leone the rate was 8 percent. During convalescence, occasional flurries of rapid involuntary eye movement (oculogyric crises) occurred. Late sequelae included deafness (29 percent) and alopecia.

Laboratory features The hematologic findings include relatively normal hematocrit values and early leukopenia (less than 4000 cells per microliter in 36 percent) with a relative neutrophilia and immature forms of leukocytes. In two cases in which it was recorded, the erythrocyte sedimentation rate was normal. Urinalyses revealed proteinuria, which was often massive. Chest radiographs may suggest basilar pneumonitis and pleural effusions. Electrocardiographic abnormalities compatible with diffuse myocardial disease have been encountered. Levels of serum enzymes, SGOT, creatinine phosphokinase (CPK), and LDH have been elevated. An SGOT of > 150 IU/L is associated with a case-fatality rate of 50 percent. A viremia of $> 1 \times 10^{3.0}$ TCID$_{50}$ per milliliter is associated with increased mortality. Both factors together carry a risk of death of 80 percent. Lassa virus may be recovered from CSF.

Diagnosis Diagnosis can be made by demonstrating a fourfold rise in antibody titer to Lassa virus between acute-phase and convalescent-phase serum specimens with the IFA technique or with Lassa IgM antibodies. The diagnosis is unlikely if IgM antibodies are absent by the fourteenth day of illness.

Treatment The management has been supportive. Infusion of immune plasma from convalescent patients resulted in a dramatic effect in three of four patients. Because of the self-limited nature of the disease, these results cannot be assessed easily. In a study of the antiviral agent ribavirin, 19 of 20 patients treated intravenously within 6 days of onset with a 2.0-g loading dose, followed by 1.0 g every 6 h for 4 days, then 0.5 g every 8 h for another 6 days, survived, whereas 11 of 18 who received no therapy and 10 of 16 who received convalescent plasma died. In view of the hospital association and the presence of virus in pharyngeal secretions and urine, respiratory and enteric isolation and blood precautions are required. With reasonable isolation practices, nosocomial spread need not be as feared as previously.

OTHER HEMORRHAGIC FEVERS Ebola hemorrhagic fever and Marburg virus disease are caused by members of the family Filoviridae and are discussed in Chap. 158 and summarized in Table 159-1.

REFERENCES

BAUM SG et al: Epidemic non-meningitic lymphocytic-choriomeningitis virus infection. N Engl J Med 274:934, 1966

CASALS J: Arenaviruses. Yale J Biol Med 48:115, 1975

CENTERS FOR DISEASE CONTROL: Viral hemorrhagic fever. Initial management of suspected and confirmed cases. Ann Intern Med 101:73, 1984

CUMMINS D et al: Acute sensorineural deafness in Lassa fever. JAMA 264:2093, 1990

FIELDS BN et al (eds): Virology, 2d ed. New York, Raven, 1990

FRAME JD et al: Lassa fever, a new virus disease of man from West Africa: I. Clinical description and pathological findings. Am J Trop Med Hyg 19:670, 1970

JOHNSON KM et al: Hemorrhagic fever of Southeast Asia and South America. A comparative approach. Prog Med Virol 9:105, 1967

McCORMICK JB et al: Lassa fever: Effective therapy with ribavirin. N Engl J Med 314:20, 1986

McKEE KT JR et al: Ribavirin prophylaxis and therapy for experimental Argentine hemorrhagic fever. Antimicrob Agents Chemother 32:1304, 1988

MacKENZIE RB et al: Epidemic hemorrhagic fever in Bolivia: 1. A preliminary report of the epidemiologic and clinical findings in a new epidemic area in South America. Am J Trop Med Hyg 13:620, 1964

MERTENS PE et al: Clinical presentation of Lassa fever cases during the hospital epidemic at Zorzor, Liberia, March–April 1972. Am J Trop Med Hyg 22:780, 1973

MONATH TP et al: Lassa fever in the Eastern Province of Sierra Leone, 1970–1972: II. Clinical observations and virological studies on selected hospital cases. Am J Trop Med Hyg 23:1140, 1974

SALAS R et al: Venezuelan hemorrhagic fever. Lancet 338:1033, 1991

VANZEE BE et al: Lymphocytic choriomeningitis in University hospital personnel. Clinical features. Am J Med 58:803, 1975

section 15 Fungal infections

161 DIAGNOSIS AND THERAPY OF FUNGAL INFECTIONS

JOHN E. BENNETT

DIAGNOSIS

Many fungi can be identified as to genus or even species by microscopic examination of smears or biopsies. Calcofluor white stain with fluorescent microscopy is a sensitive technique for smear of sputum, bronchoalveolar lavage, or pus. India ink smear remains the choice for detecting cryptococci in cerebrospinal fluid (CSF). Smears of vaginal or oral lesions for *Candida* pseudohyphae can be done by wet mount or Gram's stain. For histopathology slides, Gomori methenamine silver and a neutral counterstain are preferred.

Methodology has a marked effect on rapidity and sensitivity of blood cultures for fungi, except that *Candida* species are relatively easy to grow. For most other fungi, concentrating blood by lysis centrifugation and culturing on solid medium constitute the optimal technique. Commercially available nucleic acid hybridization techniques can speed the identification of slow-growing molds, such as *Histoplasma capsulatum*. Serology has limited value, but testing serum or CSF for cryptococcal antigen or antibody to *Coccidioides immitis* can be diagnostic. Skin testing with fungal antigens is not useful in detecting active infection.

ANTIFUNGAL THERAPY

TOPICAL AGENTS Imidazoles and triazoles These synthetic compounds act by inhibiting ergosterol synthesis in the fungal cell wall and when given topically may cause direct damage to the cytoplasmic membrane. Drug resistance rarely arises in the previously sensitive strains. Imidazoles available for cutaneous application include clotrimazole, econazole, ketoconazole, sulconazole, oxiconazole, and miconazole. Vaginal formulations include four imidazoles—miconazole, clotrimazole, tioconazole, and butoconazole—and one triazole—terconazole. Miconazole lotion and vaginal preparations of both miconazole and clotrimazole are available without prescription. As yet, no substantial difference in efficacy or local intolerance among the topical azoles has appeared. All are effective in treatment of cutaneous candidiasis, tinea versicolor, and mild to moderately severe ringworm of the glabrous skin. Vaginal formulations are effective in vulvovaginal candidiasis. Clotrimazole is poorly absorbed from the gastrointestinal tract, but the oral troche is useful as a topical treatment for oral and esophageal candidiasis.

Polyene macrolide antibiotics These broad-spectrum antifungal agents combine with sterol in the fungal cytoplasmic membrane, increasing membrane permeability. Topically, they are not active against ringworm but are effective against candidiasis of the skin and mucous membranes. Nystatin suspension is effective in oral thrush, and vaginal troches are effective in vulvovaginal candidiasis. Both nystatin and amphotericin B are available in topical preparations for cutaneous candidiasis. Natamycin ophthalmic suspension is marketed in some countries (but not in the United States) for mycotic keratitis and conjunctivitis.

Other topical antifungals Ciclopirox olamine, haloprogin, and naftifine have the same clinical spectrum among the cutaneous mycoses as the imidazoles. Tolnaftate and undecylenic acid are effective against ringworm but not candidiasis. Keratolytic agents, such as salicylic acid, are helpful as accessory drugs for some hyperkeratotic skin lesions.

SYSTEMIC ANTIFUNGALS Griseofulvin Griseofulvin is a useful drug in treating certain kinds of ringworm; however, it is ineffective in treating candidiasis. The microcrystalline and ultramicrocrystalline preparations differ in dose but not in efficacy. Absorption of both is enhanced when ingested with fat-containing foods. Griseofulvin interacts with phenobarbital and coumarin-type anticoagulants.

Imidazoles and triazoles KETOCONAZOLE Absorption of ketoconazole is variable among individuals, is not affected by food, and is poor in patients with AIDS and those taking cimetidine or other H-2 blocking agents. Simultaneous administration of antacids also can impair absorption. Metabolism is chiefly hepatic, but substantial liver disease has minimal effect on plasma ketoconazole concentrations. Ketoconazole plasma levels are decreased in patients taking rifampin and also in some taking isoniazid. Ketoconazole administration can elevate cyclosporine blood levels, can increase the likelihood of terfenadine or astemizole cardiotoxicity, and, occasionally, can enhance the anticoagulant effect of warfarin. The drug is contraindicated during pregnancy and, because it appears in breast milk, during breast-feeding. Neither renal disease nor hemodialysis affects the metabolism of ketoconazole. The most common toxicities of ketoconazole are dose-related nausea, anorexia, and occasionally, vomiting. Hepatotoxicity is idiosyncratic and usually mild but rarely can be serious and fatal. Several dose-related, temporary endocrine effects have been observed: decreased adrenal cortical reserve; gynecomastia; decreased serum testosterone, libido, and potency in males; and menstrual irregularity in females. Pruritus or rash also may occur. Ketoconazole is effective in blastomycosis, histoplasmosis, paracoccidioidomycosis, chronic mucocutaneous candidiasis, esophageal candidiasis, and some forms of disseminated coccidioidomycosis and pseudallescheriasis. The usual adult dose is 400 mg, taken once daily. Partial improvement may be seen in cutaneous sporotrichosis and chromoblastomycosis. Although vulvovaginal candidiasis, ringworm, and tinea versicolor are responsive to the drug, the toxicity of oral ketoconazole makes topical imidazoles or other drugs preferable for these indications.

ITRACONAZOLE This triazole analogue of ketoconazole is superior to the parent compound in safety and efficacy. Hormonal suppression and hepatotoxicity are less with itraconazole than with ketoconazole. Clinical indications for itraconazole include all those for ketoconazole but also selected patients with sporotrichosis, cryptococcosis, and aspergillosis. The drug is marketed as 100-mg capsules. No parenteral formulation is available. The usual dose is 200 mg, once or twice a day by mouth. Itraconazole is metabolized in the liver, with the hydroxy metabolite retaining antifungal activity. Concurrent therapy with rifampin, carbamazepine, and H-2 receptor antagonists or phenytoin decreases itraconazole blood levels. Cardiotoxicity due to terfenadine or astemizole and cyclosporine nephrotoxicity may occur during concomitant itraconazole therapy.

FLUCONAZOLE This triazole can be administered as oral tablets or intravenous infusion. With a half-life of about 31 h, fluconazole can be given once a day. Bioavailability by the oral route is excellent and unimpaired by lack of gastric acid or presence of food. Fluconazole therapy can elevate blood levels of phenytoin, cyclosporine, warfarin, and sulfonylureas. Approximately 80 percent of the drug is excreted unchanged in the urine. Patients with creatinine clearance of 21 to 50 and 11 to 20 mL/min should have their fluconazole dose reduced by 50 and 75 percent, respectively. Penetration of drug into the CSF and other body fluids is very good. Aside from nausea and allergic reactions, toxicity has been unusual. Fluconazole is useful in certain forms of candidiasis, cryptococcosis, and coccidioidomycosis.

Amphotericin B A colloidal preparation of this drug is available for intravenous or intrathecal administration. The drug cannot be given intramuscularly and is not absorbed orally. Sodium or potassium salts must not be added to the infusion solutions because the colloidal drug will precipitate out of solution. In-line filters with 0.22-μm pore diameter may trap some of the colloid. Catabolism is extremely slow and is not influenced by renal failure, hepatic failure, or hemodialysis. Penetration into CSF and vitreous humor is poor; however, concentrations in pleural, peritoneal, and articular exudates are adequate for many mycoses. Histoplasmosis, blastomycosis, paracoccidioidomycosis, candidiasis, and cryptococcosis are the most responsive mycoses. Coccidioidomycosis, extraarticular sporotrichosis, aspergillosis, and mucormycosis are less responsive; chromoblastomycosis, mycetoma, and pseudallescheriasis show little, if any, response. The usual course is 8 to 10 weeks of 0.4 to 0.6 mg/kg daily. Infusions are generally given in 5% dextrose over 2 to 4 h. Severe febrile reactions to initial doses generally prompt use of an initial test dose with 1 mg, followed by escalating doses based on the gravity of the patient's infection and tolerance of the drug. Virtually all patients show toxic reactions that are related to the dose and duration of therapy. These side effects include azotemia, anemia, hypokalemia, nausea, anorexia, weight loss, phlebitis, and occasionally, hypomagnesemia. Intrathecal amphotericin B is indicated in coccidioidal meningitis and refractory cryptococcal meningitis, although this therapy is associated with considerable toxicity. Doses of 0.1 to 0.5 mg are given three times per week initially, then with decreasing frequency. Several new intravenous formulations of amphotericin B with reduced nephrotoxicity are in clinical trial, but their efficacy is as yet unknown.

Flucytosine Flucytosine (5-fluorocytosine) is a synthetic oral drug useful in cryptococcosis, candidiasis, and chromoblastomycosis. Within the fungal cell, flucytosine is converted to the antimetabolite 5-fluorouracil. Drug resistance appears rather rapidly when flucytosine is used alone. For this reason, the drug is generally used in combination with amphotericin B, permitting a lower dose of the latter. The usual regimen is amphotericin B 0.3 mg/kg daily and flucytosine 37.5 mg/kg every 6 h. Flucytosine is well absorbed from the gastrointestinal tract, even in the presence of food. The drug penetrates well into the CSF and is excreted unchanged in the urine. Hemodialysis results in significant drug removal. Even modest reductions in renal function may elevate flucytosine blood levels into the toxic range, ≥ 100 to 125 μg/mL. Elevated levels are associated with a significant incidence of neutropenia and thrombocytopenia. Elevated flucytosine blood levels also seem to predispose to colitis, the other major toxicity of this drug. Hepatotoxicity is idiosyncratic and uncommon. An allergic rash also may occur.

REFERENCES

General

KWON-CHUNG KJ, BENNETT JE: *Medical Mycology*. Philadelphia, Lea & Febiger, 1992

Therapy

Bennett JE: Antifungal agents, in *Goodman and Gilman's The Pharmacological Basis of Therapeutics*, AG Gilman et al (eds). New York, Pergamon, 1990, pp 1165–1181

Goodman JL et al: A controlled trial of fluconazole to prevent fungal infections in patients undergoing bone marrow transplantation. N Engl J Med 326:845, 1992

Lazar JD, Hilligoss DM: The clinical pharmacology of fluconazole. Semin Oncol 17:14, 1990

Tucker RM et al: Adverse events associated with itraconazole in 189 patients on chronic therapy. J Antimicrob Chemother 26:561, 1991

Wingard JR et al: Increase in *Candida krusei* infection among patients with bone marrow transplantation and neutropenia treated prophylactically with fluconazole. N Engl J Med 325:1274, 1991

162   HISTOPLASMOSIS

JOHN E. BENNETT

ETIOLOGY *Histoplasma capsulatum* is a dimorphic fungus that grows as a mold in nature or on Sabouraud's agar at room temperature. Hyphae bear both large and small spores, which are used for identification. *H. capsulatum* grows as a small budding yeast in host tissue and on enriched agar, such as blood cysteine glucose, at 37°C. Despite the name, the fungus is unencapsulated. Coculture of isolates with the opposite mating type can produce the perfect state called *Ajellomyces capsulatus*.

PATHOGENESIS AND PATHOLOGY Infection with *H. capsulatum* has been encountered in many areas of the world but is much more frequent in certain areas. Within the United States, infection is most common in the southeastern, midatlantic, and central states. Endemic areas are probably determined by the availability of proper conditions in nature for growth of the fungus. *H. capsulatum* prefers moist surface soil, particularly when it is enriched by droppings of certain birds and bats. The fungus has not only been isolated repeatedly from such sites, but many case clusters have occurred 5 to 18 days after groups were exposed to such dust, e.g., by raking, cleaning dirt-floored chicken coops, bulldozing, or cave exploring. Judging by skin test reactivity in many endemic areas, 80 percent or more of residents over age 16 have been exposed.

Microconidia, or small spores, of *H. capsulatum* are small enough to reach the alveoli on inhalation and are transformed to budding forms. With time, an intense granulomatous reaction occurs. Caseation necrosis or calcification may mimic tuberculosis. The primary infection in children usually heals completely but may leave spotty calcification in the hilar nodes or lung. Transient dissemination may leave calcified granulomas in the spleen. In adults, a rounded mass of scar tissue, with or without central calcification, may remain in the lung. This has been called a *histoplasmoma*. Previous exposure is thought to confer some protection against reinfection, but infection in persons with prior positive skin tests clearly has occurred.

In a small proportion of patients, histoplasmosis becomes a progressive, potentially fatal infection. The disease occurs either as chronic fibrocavitary pneumonia or, less commonly, as disseminated infection. Patients with either form lack a history of acute primary pulmonary histoplasmosis. Chronic pulmonary infection favors otherwise healthy males over the age of 40. A history of cigarette use can be elicited from nearly all patients with chronic progressive pulmonary histoplasmosis. An acute, rapidly fatal course is most likely to be encountered in young children and immunosuppressed patients, including those with AIDS. A more chronic but equally lethal disseminated infection is more common in previously healthy adults.

CLINICAL MANIFESTATIONS The vast majority of infections are either asymptomatic or mild, and the diagnosis is elusive. Cough, fever, malaise, and chest x-ray findings of hilar adenopathy with or without one or more areas of pneumonitis occur. Erythema nodosum and erythema multiforme have been reported in a few outbreaks.

Hilar adenopathy may cause temporary compression of the right middle lobe bronchus in children and young adults. Subacute pericarditis may occur, probably by extension from contiguous lymph nodes. Rarely, hilar nodes undergo a caseous, granulomatous reaction with perinodal fibrosis. Mediastinal structures become encased by progressive fibrosis, and over many years, compression of the pulmonary veins, superior vena cava, pulmonary arteries, and esophagus may occur. Late in mediastinal disease only rare nonviable histoplasma can be found in caseous residua of lymph nodes.

Patients with *chronic pulmonary histoplasmosis* have a gradual onset over weeks or months of increasing productive cough, weight loss, and sometimes night sweats. Chest x-ray reveals uni- or bilateral fibronodular apical infiltrates. Approximately one-third of cases will stabilize or improve spontaneously early in the course. The remainder show insidious progression. Retraction and cavitation of the upper lobes occur with spread to the apex of the lower lobes and other areas of the lung. Emphysema and bullae formation further compromise pulmonary function. Death from cor pulmonale, bacterial pneumonia, or histoplasmosis occurs after months or years.

Acute disseminated histoplasmosis may be mistaken for miliary tuberculosis (see Chap. 130). Common findings include fever, emaciation, hepatosplenomegaly, lymphadenopathy, jaundice, anemia, leukopenia, and thrombocytopenia. All these features may occur in chronic dissemination as well, but the disease tends to be more localized. Indurated ulcers of the mouth, tongue, nose, or larynx occur in about a fourth of patients. Other focal findings include granulomatous hepatitis, Addison's disease, gastrointestinal ulceration, endocarditis, and chronic meningitis. Chest x-ray abnormalities occur in half the cases and show discrete nodules or a miliary pattern.

The presumed *ocular histoplasmosis* syndrome is a distinct clinical form of uveitis. Although a positive histoplasmin skin test is a requisite for diagnosis, none of these patients has had active histoplasmosis.

Infection with *H. capsulatum var. duboisii* is rare outside of Africa. The yeast form is larger in tissue than *H. capsulatum*. Clinical manifestations resemble blastomycosis more than histoplasmosis because skin and bone lesions are very common.

DIAGNOSIS Histoplasmosis may be suspected by serologic tests and clinical manifestations, but definitive diagnosis requires demonstration of the organism by culture or histology. Serologic tests are performed on serum or cerebrospinal fluid (CSF) using either a culture filtrate called *histoplasmin* or whole yeast form cells. The results are interchangeable. Complement fixation is quantifiable and is the best test. An agar gel diffusion test with histoplasmin is useful but not quantifiable. An H band on agar gel testing is more diagnostic of active histoplasmosis than an M band. Frequent false-negative and false-positive results limit all current serologic tests. Serologic conversion is helpful but occurs rarely except in acute pulmonary histoplasmosis. High complement fixation titers, such as 1:32 or greater, are suggestive of the diagnosis, but no titer is diagnostic. Cross-reactions with serologic tests for blastomycosis are common. A 5-mm or more diameter area of induration 24 to 48 h after skin testing with histoplasmin has been very helpful in identifying prior exposure to *Histoplasma*, but false-negative and false-positive results are so frequent that skin testing has little value in the study of ill patients. Further, a positive skin test can cause seroconversion.

Culture of *H. capsulatum* from sputum is difficult but is the procedure of choice in chronic pulmonary histoplasmosis. Digestion by proteolytic enzymes and centrifugation of sputum are helpful.

In patients with chronic pulmonary histoplasmosis, organisms may be infrequent in lung biopsies and lead to a mistaken diagnosis of lymphomatoid granulomatosis or Wegener's granulomatosis. Examination of several sections stained with methenamine silver may be necessary.

Acute disseminated histoplasmosis is difficult to diagnose in AIDS patients because fever, weight loss, leukopenia, and thrombocytopenia may occur with either infection. These patients also may have a diffuse pulmonary infiltrate resembling *Pneumocystis carinii* pneumonia. Patients may no longer be living in the endemic area, so the diagnosis may not be considered. Culture of blood by the lysis centrifugation technique, culture of bone marrow aspirate or bronchoalveolar lavage fluid, and Giemsa-stained smears of these specimens are important in detecting histoplasmosis. Radioimmunoassay for *Histoplasma* antigen in urine and serum has been helpful in diagnosis and in following results of therapy, but the test is not commercially available. Histologic examination of mucosal, skin, liver, or lymph node biopsy specimens can expedite diagnosis.

TREATMENT Acute pulmonary histoplasmosis requires no therapy. Patients with mediastinal fibrosis may benefit by surgery, but the ultimate prognosis is poor. All patients with disseminated or chronic fibronodular pulmonary histoplasmosis should receive chemotherapy. The indications for using ketoconazole or itraconazole, as well as the treatment regimen, are the same as those given in Chap. 164 for blastomycosis. Amphotericin B is given as 0.4 to 0.5 mg/kg per day or double that on alternate days and is continued for at least 10 weeks. AIDS patients with disseminated histoplasmosis respond poorly to ketoconazole and should be treated with amphotericin B. After an initial intensive course, these patients are given amphotericin B, 1 mg/kg once a week, or itraconazole, 200 mg once daily, to prevent relapse. In chronic pulmonary histoplasmosis, chest x-ray abnormalities improve somewhat, but pulmonary function improves very little. Successful therapy prevents progression. Addisonian crisis is a preventable cause of death in disseminated histoplasmosis.

REFERENCES

McKinsey DS et al: Long-term amphotericin B therapy for disseminated histoplasmosis in patients with the acquired immunodeficiency syndrome (AIDS). Ann Intern Med 111:655, 1989

Wheat JL et al: Disseminated histoplasmosis in the acquired immune deficiency syndrome: Clinical findings, diagnosis and treatment, and review of the literature. Medicine 69:361, 1990

163 COCCIDIOIDOMYCOSIS AND PARACOCCIDIOIDOMYCOSIS

JOHN E. BENNETT

COCCIDIOIDOMYCOSIS

ETIOLOGY *Coccidioides immitis* has two forms, growing as a white fluffy mold on most culture media but as a nonbudding spherical form, a spherule, in host tissue or under specialized conditions. Reproduction in the host tissue is by formation of small endospores within mature spherules. After rupture of the spherule, the released endospores enlarge, become spherules, and repeat the cycle. The fungus is identified by its appearance and by formation of thick-walled, barrel-shaped spores, called *arthrospores*, in the hyphae of the mold form.

PATHOGENESIS AND PATHOLOGY *C. immitis* is a soil saprophyte in certain arid regions of the United States, Mexico, Central America, and South America. Within the United States, most cases are acquired in California, Arizona, western Texas, and New Mexico. A few cases are acquired in bordering areas and by exposure to fomites from endemic areas, such as in cotton bales.

Infection in humans and animals results from inhalation of windborne arthrospores arising from soil sites. This primary pulmonary infection is symptomatic in only 40 percent of individuals, with symptoms ranging from a mild, influenza-like illness to severe pneumonia. Mild, self-limited infections may come to medical attention because of case clusters or hypersensitivity reactions:

erythema nodosum, erythema multiforme, toxic erythema, arthralgia, arthritis, conjunctivitis, or episcleritis. Case clusters occur 10 to 14 days after a group of susceptible individuals is exposed to dust in an endemic area through such activities as unearthing Indian relics, rock hunting, military maneuvers, or construction. Wind storms can carry spores to adjacent nonendemic areas and cause case clusters. The usual course of primary pulmonary infection is complete healing, although an area of pneumonitis on x-ray may heal by forming a coinlike lesion, or *coccidioidoma*. Less commonly, a single thin-walled cavity remains as a chronic sequela in the area of consolidation. The consolidation may persist as a chronic pneumonia or progress to fibronodular, cavitary disease.

Pleural effusion may be the only manifestation of primary infection. Self-healing of this form is common.

An uncommon but dreaded complication of coccidioidomycosis is dissemination beyond the lung and hilar lymph nodes. Dissemination is more frequent in blacks, Filipinos, Native Americans, Mexican-Americans, and pregnant or immunosuppressed patients, including those with AIDS.

C. immitis incites a chronic granulomatous reaction in host tissue, often with caseation necrosis. Lung and hilar node lesions may show calcification. Both IgM and IgG antibodies against *C. immitis* are induced by infection, but neither appears protective. The amount of specific IgG antibody is a rough measure of the antigenic mass, i.e., of the amount of infection, and a high titer is a poor prognostic sign. Appearance of delayed hypersensitivity to antigens of *C. immitis* is most common in those clinical forms of disease with a good prognosis, such as self-limited primary pulmonary disease. Negative skin tests to *Coccidioides* antigens occur in roughly half the patients with disseminated disease and portend a poor prognosis.

CLINICAL MANIFESTATIONS Symptomatic primary pulmonary infection is manifested by fever, cough, chest pain, malaise, and sometimes hypersensitivity reactions. Chest x-ray may show an infiltrate, hilar adenopathy, or pleural effusion. Peripheral blood may show a mild eosinophilia. Spontaneous improvement begins after several days to 2 weeks of illness and usually culminates in complete recovery.

The symptoms of a chronic thin-walled cavity include cough or hemoptysis in half the cases; the other patients are asymptomatic. Chronic progressive pulmonary coccidioidomycosis produces cough, sputum, variable degrees of fever, and weight loss. The first indications of dissemination usually appear during the primary infection. Reactivation with dissemination in later years occurs occasionally, especially if Hodgkin's disease, non-Hodgkin's lymphoma, renal transplantation, AIDS, or other immunosuppression has supervened. Dissemination should be suspected when fever, malaise, hilar or paratracheal lymphadenopathy, elevated sedimentation rate, and high complement fixation titers show abnormal persistence in patients with primary pulmonary coccidioidomycosis. With time, lesions appear in the bone, skin, subcutaneous tissue, meninges, joints, and other sites. Without therapy, dissemination may progress rapidly to death or wax and wane for years.

DIAGNOSIS When coccidioidomycosis is suspected, sputum, urine, and pus should be examined for *C. immitis* by wet smear and culture. *The laboratory request should indicate clearly that coccidioidomycosis is suspected because the mold form must be handled with extreme care to prevent infection of laboratory personnel.* On biopsy, smaller spherules must be distinguished from nonbudding forms of *Blastomyces* and *Cryptococcus*, but appearance of the mature spherule is diagnostic.

Serologic tests are very helpful in coccidioidomycosis. Latex agglutination and agar gel diffusion tests are useful in screening sera for antibody to *Coccidioides*. The complement fixation test is used on cerebrospinal fluid (CSF) and to confirm and quantitate serum antibody detected by screening tests. The number of cases with a positive complement fixation test will depend on the severity of disease and on the laboratory performing the test. Positive tests are least common in patients with solitary pulmonary cavities or primary pulmonary infection, while sera from patients with multiorgan disseminated disease are nearly all positive. Seroconversion is helpful in primary pulmonary coccidioidomycosis but may not occur for up to 8 weeks after onset. A positive complement fixation test in unconcentrated CSF is diagnostic of meningitis. Rarely, a parameningeal focus will cause a positive CSF serology.

Conversion of the skin test from negative to positive (≥ 5 mm induration at 24 or 48 h) with either coccidioidin or spherulin, the two commercially available antigens, may occur between the third and twenty-first days of symptoms in primary pulmonary coccidioidomycosis. Skin testing also can be helpful in epidemiologic studies, such as investigation of case clusters or definition of endemic areas. The utility of skin testing as a diagnostic tool is limited by the presence of persistent positive tests resulting from remote exposures to *Coccidioides* and by the frequency of negative skin tests in many patients with either thin-walled cavities or disseminated coccidioidomycosis.

TREATMENT   Primary pulmonary coccidioidomycosis usually resolves spontaneously. Some physicians give a few weeks of intravenous amphotericin B when patients show an unusually severe or protracted primary infection, hoping to abort disseminated or chronic pulmonary disease. There is no solid evidence to support this practice, but the stronger the suspicion of dissemination becomes in any given patient, the more logical this approach appears. Once evidence for dissemination becomes incontrovertible, amphotericin B may be palliative rather than curative.

Patients with severe or rapidly progressing disseminated coccidioidomycosis are begun on intravenous amphotericin B, 0.5 to 0.7 mg/ kg daily. Patients who have improved after amphotericin B or who have more indolent disseminated infection are given ketoconazole, 400 to 800 mg/d, or itraconazole, 200 to 400 mg/d. These oral agents are useful for long-term suppression of infection and should be continued for years. Patients with coccidioidal meningitis are usually begun on fluconazole 400 mg daily but may require intrathecal amphotericin B. Hydrocephalus is a frequent complication of uncontrolled meningitis. Surgical debridement of bone lesions or drainage of abscesses can be helpful. Prognosis for ultimate cure of disseminated coccidioidomycosis is guarded.

Resection of chronic progressive pulmonary lesions is a helpful adjunct to chemotherapy when infection is confined to the lung and to one lobe. A single thin-walled cavity tends to close spontaneously and ordinarily is not resected. Such a cavity responds poorly to chemotherapy.

PARACOCCIDIOIDOMYCOSIS

ETIOLOGY   Formerly called *South American blastomycosis,* this is the mycosis caused by *Paracoccidioides brasiliensis.* A dimorphic fungus, *P. brasiliensis* grows as a budding yeast in tissue but may be grown as either yeast or mold on a culture medium. Identification is by gross and microscopic appearance. A superficial resemblance to *Blastomyces dermatitidis* may cause misdiagnosis.

PATHOGENESIS AND PATHOLOGY   Infection is thought to be acquired by inhalation of spores from environmental sources, but the reservoir in nature remains obscure. Pulmonary infection produces few symptoms initially. Hematogenous spread to the mucous membranes of the mouth and nose, the lymph nodes, and other sites brings the patient to medical attention. Fatal cases show spread to the adrenal, the gastrointestinal tract, and many other viscera.

CLINICAL MANIFESTATIONS   Common symptoms include indurated ulcers of the mouth, oropharynx, larynx, and nose; enlarged and draining lymph nodes; lesions of the skin and genitalia; and productive cough, weight loss, dyspnea, and sometimes fever. Acquisition of infection is restricted to South America, Central America, and Mexico, but the extreme indolence of this infection may lead to recognition many years after the patient has left the endemic area. Chest x-ray most often shows a bilateral patchy pneumonia.

DIAGNOSIS   Cultures of sputum, pus, and mucosal lesions are often diagnostic. The diagnosis can be made by smear or histologic section, though confirmation by culture is preferable. Serologic tests are useful in suggesting the diagnosis and monitoring therapy.

TREATMENT   Milder cases may be cured by one year's treatment with oral ketoconazole, 200 to 400 mg daily. Itraconazole appears to give comparable results. More advanced cases are given intravenous amphotericin B, followed by ketoconazole.

REFERENCES

AMPEL NM et al: Coccidioidomycosis: Clinical update. Rev Infect Dis 11:897, 1989

BAKOS I et al: Disseminated paracoccidioidomycosis with skin lesions in a patient with acquired immunodeficiency syndrome. Am Acad Dermatol 20:854, 1989

GALGIANI JN et al: Ketoconazole therapy of progressive coccidioidomycosis. Comparison of 400 and 800 mg doses and observations at higher doses. Am J Med 84:603, 1988

GRAYBILL JR et al: Itraconazole treatment of coccidioidomycosis. Am J Med 89:282, 1990

RESTREPO A et al: Itraconazole in the treatment of paracoccidioidomycosis: A primary report. Rev Infect Dis 9(suppl 1):51, 1987

SUGAR AM et al: Paracoccidioidomycosis in the immunosuppressed host: Report of a case and review of the literature. Am Rev Respir Dis 129:340, 1984

TUCKER RM et al: Treatment of coccidioidal meningitis with fluconazole. Rev Infect Dis 12:S380, 1990

164   BLASTOMYCOSIS

JOHN E. BENNETT

ETIOLOGY   *Blastomyces dermatitidis* is a dimorphic fungus that grows at room temperature as a white or tan mold but grows within the host or at 37°C as budding, round yeastlike cells. The fungus is identified by its appearance, its dimorphism, and the appearance of small spores borne on hyphae of the mold form. When isolates of the two opposite mating types are grown closely together on specialized culture media, sporulating structures appear which characterize the perfect form, *Ajellomyces dermatitidis.*

PATHOGENESIS AND PATHOLOGY   The infection is restricted by geography and age. Blastomycosis is uncommon in any locality, but the majority of cases occur in the southeast, central, and midatlantic areas of the United States, with occasional cases in other localities in the United States and Canada. Cases also have been encountered in Africa, Mexico, Central America, and, rarely, South America. Most patients are between 20 and 69 years old. The male/ female ratio is about 10:1. There is no occupational predisposition.

Infection appears to be acquired by inhalation of the fungus from soil, decomposed vegetation, or rotting wood. Several case clusters have occurred during recreational activities in wooded areas along waterways. Infection is not transmissible from person to person. The initial pulmonary infection may heal spontaneously or become chronic. Spread to other portions of the lung, cavitation, or endobronchial lesions may appear in chronic cases. Whether or not the lung lesion resolves spontaneously, infection commonly spreads hematogenously to skin, subcutaneous tissue, bone, prostate, epididymis, or mucosa of the nose, mouth, or larynx. Less commonly, infection spreads to the brain, meninges, liver, lymph nodes, or spleen. Dissemination may not be evident for weeks or years after the appearance of the lung lesion. Progressive infection is only rarely attributable to an underlying disease or immunosuppressive treatment. The inflammatory response includes lymphocytes, giant cells, and neutrophils. Pseudoepitheliomatous hyperplasia may be striking and lead to a mistaken diagnosis of squamous cell carcinoma.

CLINICAL MANIFESTATIONS   A small number of patients have an acute, self-limited pneumonia. Fever, productive cough, myalgia, and malaise usually have resolved within a month. Pulmonary infiltrates have cleared slowly as *B. dermatitidis* disappeared from the sputum.

The vast majority of patients with blastomycosis have an indolent onset and a chronically progressive course. Fever, cough, weight loss, lassitude, skin lesions, and chest ache are common symptoms. Skin lesions favor exposed areas and enlarge over many weeks from a pimple to a well-circumscribed, verrucous, crusted, or ulcerated lesion. Pain and regional lymphadenopathy are minimal. Large chronic lesions may show central healing with scarring and contracture. Mucous membrane lesions resemble squamous cell carcinoma. Chest x-ray is abnormal in two-thirds of cases, with one or more pneumonic or nodular infiltrates. Calcification, hilar adenopathy, and large pleural effusions are rare. Osteolytic lesions may occur in nearly any bone and present as cold abscess or a draining sinus. Extension to a contiguous joint may cause indolent swelling, pain, and restricted motion. Prostatic and epididymal lesions resemble tuberculosis clinically.

DIAGNOSIS The diagnosis is made by demonstrating the fungus in culture of sputum, pus, or urine. In experienced hands, diagnosis by appearance of the organism in wet smear or histopathologic section is adequate. The fungus may be visible in a sputum cytology smear but is easily overlooked.

TREATMENT A few patients have been observed with transitory lung lesions, but no guidelines are known to distinguish these patients from those whose disease will progress locally or disseminate. Therefore, every patient should receive treatment. Intravenous amphotericin B is the drug of choice for patients with rapidly progressive infections, severe illness, or meningitis. Skin and noncavitary lung lesions should be treated for about 8 to 10 weeks. The recommended total dose for an adult is about 2.0 g. Cavitary lung disease or infection beyond the lung and skin should be treated for about 10 to 12 weeks with 2.5 g or more. Ketoconazole is an effective drug in patients with indolent nonmeningeal blastomycosis of mild to moderate severity and who take the drug reliably. The initial adult dose is 400 mg once daily, raised after a month to 600 or 800 mg daily if improvement is suboptimal. Itraconazole, 200 mg PO once or twice daily, is an effective alternative agent. Therapy is continued for 6 to 12 months. The mortality rate in appropriately treated cases is 15 percent or less.

REFERENCES

BRADSHER RW: Blastomycosis: Fungal infections of the lung. Update 1989. Semin Respir Infect 5:105, 1990

KLEIN BS et al: Serological tests for blastomycosis: Assessments during a large point-source outbreak in Wisconsin. J Infect Dis 155:262, 1989

165 CRYPTOCOCCOSIS

JOHN E. BENNETT

ETIOLOGY Cryptococcosis is an infection caused by the yeastlike fungus *Cryptococcus neoformans*. *C. neoformans* reproduces by budding and forms round, yeastlike cells 4 to 6 μm in diameter. Within the host and on certain culture media, a large polysaccharide capsule surrounds each yeast cell. The fungus grows well as smooth, creamy white colonies on Sabouraud's or other simple media at 20 to 37°C. Certain culture media for ringworm contain cycloheximide, which inhibits *C. neoformans*. Identification is based on gross and microscopic appearance, biochemical tests, and growth at 37°C. The fungus has four capsular serotypes, designated A, B, C, and D. There

are also two mating types. Coculture of opposite mating types creates a transient diploid state called *Filobasidiella neoformans* for serotypes A or D and *Filobasidiella bacillispora* for serotypes B or C.

Weathered pigeon droppings commonly contain serotype A or D *Cryptococcus neoformans*. Serotypes B or C have been rarely found in nature, with the exception of flowering *Eucalyptus camaldulensis* trees in Australia. Transmission of infection to man from a specific natural site or from another patient has never been clearly documented, except for transplantation of an infected kidney, cornea, or other organ. Currently, more than half the cases in the United States are in AIDS patients. Cryptococcosis is a grave complication of late HIV infection at a time when the CD4 count is below 200 per cubic microliter. Among the cryptococcosis patients who are not infected with HIV, more than half are immunosuppressed. Corticosteroid therapy, but not neutropenia or immunoglobulin deficiency, predisposes to cryptococcosis. The male-to-female ratio in the non-AIDS patients is 2:1. Infection before puberty is uncommon.

PATHOGENESIS AND PATHOLOGY Infection is thought to be acquired by inhalation of fungus into the lungs. Pulmonary infection has a tendency toward spontaneous resolution and is frequently asymptomatic. Silent hematogenous spread to the brain leads to clusters of cryptococci in the perivascular areas of cortical gray matter, basal ganglia, and, to a lesser extent, other areas of the central nervous system. Inflammatory response around these foci is usually scant. In the more chronic cases, a dense basilar arachnoiditis occurs. Lung lesions show an intense granulomatous inflammation. Cryptococci are best seen in tissue by staining with methenamine silver or periodic acid Schiff. A strongly positive mucicarmine stain of the organism in tissue is diagnostic, but staining varies from intense to absent.

CLINICAL MANIFESTATIONS The majority of patients have *meningoencephalitis* at the time of diagnosis. This form of the infection is invariably fatal without appropriate therapy, and death occurs anywhere from 2 weeks to several years from onset of symptoms. Early manifestations include headache, nausea, staggering gait, dementia, irritability, confusion, and blurred vision. Both fever and nuchal rigidity are often mild or absent. Papilledema is present in one-third of patients at the time of diagnosis. Cranial nerve palsies, typically asymmetric, occur in about one-fourth of the patients. Other lateralizing signs are rare. With progression of the infection, deepening coma and signs of brainstem compression appear. Autopsy often reveals cerebral edema in the more acute cases or hydrocephalus in more chronic cases.

Pulmonary cryptococcosis causes chest pain in about 40 percent of patients and cough in 20 percent. Chest x-ray shows one or more dense infiltrates, which are often well circumscribed. Cavitation, pleural effusions, and hilar adenopathy are infrequent. Calcification is not present, and fibrotic stranding is rarely noticeable.

Skin lesions are present in 10 percent of patients with cryptococcosis, and the vast majority of patients with skin lesions have disseminated infection. One or a few asymptomatic tiny papular lesions appear, slowly enlarge, and tend to show central softening leading to ulceration. Osteolytic bone lesions occur in 4 percent of patients and usually present as a cold abscess. Rare manifestations of cryptococcosis include prostatitis, endophthalmitis, hepatitis, pericarditis, endocarditis, and renal abscess.

DIAGNOSIS Fever and headache in a patient with AIDS or with risk factors for HIV infection should suggest the possibility of cryptococcosis, toxoplasmosis, or central nervous system lymphoma. Presence of a focal lesion on magnetic resonance imaging (MRI) is unusual in cryptococcosis. In patients without AIDS, meningitis due to *C. neoformans* resembles that due to *M. tuberculosis*, *Histoplasma capsulatum*, *Coccidioides immitis*, or metastatic cancer. Lumbar puncture is the single most useful test. An india ink smear of centrifuged spinal fluid sediment reveals encapsulated yeast in more than half the cases, although artifacts can cause confusion. In patients without AIDS, cerebrospinal fluid glucose is reduced in half the cases, protein is usually increased, and a lymphocytic pleocytosis is usually present. CSF abnormalities are less pronounced in patients with AIDS, though india ink smear is more often positive.

Approximately 90 percent of patients with cryptococcal meningoencephalitis, including all those with a positive CSF smear, will have capsular antigen detectable in CSF or serum by latex agglutination. False-positive tests occur occasionally, making culture the definitive diagnostic test. *C. neoformans* is often present in urine from patients with meningoencephalitis. Fungemia occurs in 10 to 30 percent of patients and is particularly common in AIDS patients.

Pulmonary cryptococcosis mimics malignancy by x-ray and symptoms. Sputum culture is positive in only 10 percent, and serum antigen tests are positive in only a third. Occasionally, *C. neoformans* appears in one or multiple sputum specimens as an endobronchial saprophyte. Biopsy is usually required for diagnosis of pulmonary cryptococcosis. Cutaneous cryptococcosis may be mistaken for a comedo, basal cell carcinoma, or sarcoidosis. In AIDS patients, skin lesions may be numerous and mistaken for molluscum contagiosum. Biopsy reveals a myriad of cryptococci. Osseous cryptococcosis resembles tuberculosis.

TREATMENT Patients with AIDS and cryptococcosis are treated initially with intravenous amphotericin B with or without flucytosine and then changed to fluconazole. During active infection, fluconazole, 400 mg, is given once daily. After infection is controlled, fluconazole, 200 mg daily, is continued indefinitely. Itraconazole is being evaluated for maintenance therapy as an alternative to fluconazole.

In patients without AIDS cryptococcosis may be treated with amphotericin B alone or in combination with flucytosine. Amphotericin B is given as 0.5 to 0.6 mg/kg per day when used alone or as 0.3 mg/kg per day in combination therapy. With either regimen, double-dose therapy on alternate days may be employed. Flucytosine is given initially as 37.5 mg/kg every 6 h to patients with normal renal function. Although nomograms are available for adjusting flucytosine dosage in the presence of reduced renal function, frequent measurement of serum levels and maintenance between 50 and 100 μg/mL offer the best chance of preventing toxicity.

Duration of therapy is based on the results of lumbar punctures. These are best done weekly until culture conversion is clearly documented. Six weeks of therapy may be adequate for patients with at least four weekly cultures of 2 to 4 mL CSF, whose india ink smear has become negative, and whose CSF glucose is normal. Approximately 50 to 70 percent of non-AIDS patients are cured.

Hydrocephalus may be an early or late complication of cryptococcosis. Blindness, dementia, and personality change are other sequelae.

Patients with extraneural cryptococcosis most often require intravenous amphotericin B, with or without flucytosine. Observation or excision of lesions may suffice for some patients who are previously normal, who have a single focus in lung, skin, or bone, and who have no cryptococci in the cerebrospinal fluid, urine, or blood.

REFERENCES

CHUCK SL, SANDE MA: Infections with *Cryptococcus neoformans* in the acquired immunodeficiency syndrome. N Engl J Med 321:794, 1989

POWDERLY WG et al: A controlled trial of fluconazole or amphotericin B to prevent relapse of cryptococcal meningitis in patients with the acquired immunodeficiency syndrome. N Engl J Med 326:793, 1992

SAAG MS et al: Comparison of amphotericin B with fluconazole in the treatment of acute AIDS-associated cryptococcal meningitis. N Engl J Med 326:83, 1992

SUGAR AM et al: Overview: Treatment of cryptococcal meningitis. Rev Infect Dis 12:S338, 1990

166 CANDIDIASIS

JOHN E. BENNETT

ETIOLOGY *Candida albicans* is the most common cause of candidiasis, but *C. tropicalis*, *C. parapsilosis*, *C. guilliermondii*, *C. glabrata*, *C. krusei*, and a few other species can cause deep candidiasis and may even be fatal. *C. parapsilosis* is particularly notable for its ability to cause endocarditis. *C. tropicalis* accounts for about one-third of the cases of deep candidiasis in neutropenic patients. All *Candida* species pathogenic for humans are also encountered as commensals of humans, particularly in the mouth, stool, and vagina. These species grow rapidly at 25 to 37°C on simple media as oval, budding cells. In specialized culture media, hyphae or elongated branching structures called *pseudohyphae* are formed. *C. glabrata*, formerly called *Torulopsis glabrata*, differs from other members of the genus in that no true hyphae or pseudohyphae are formed in vitro or in infected tissue. *C. albicans* can be identified presumptively by its ability to form germ tubes in serum or by the formation of thick-walled large spores, called *chlamydospores*. Final identification of all species requires biochemical tests.

PATHOGENESIS AND PATHOLOGY Either local or systemic factors may lead to tissue invasion by *Candida*. Chronic maceration predisposes to cutaneous candidiasis, as in diaper rash, intertrigo in obese patients, or paronychia in bartenders or cannery workers. Age is important because neonatal colonization often leads to oral candidiasis (thrush). Women in the third trimester of pregnancy are prone to vulvovaginal thrush. Patients with diabetes mellitus or hematologic malignancy or those receiving broad-spectrum antibiotics or high doses of adrenal corticosteroids are especially susceptible to candidiasis. Oral thrush is common any time in the course of HIV infection. As the number of CD4 cells declines, *Candida* esophagitis is also common. Breaks in the integrity of the skin or mucous membranes may provide access to deeper tissues. Examples include perforation of the gastrointestinal tract by trauma, surgery, and peptic ulceration; indwelling catheters for intravenous alimentation, peritoneal dialysis, and urinary tract drainage; severe burns; and intravenous drug abuse. In many hospitals, candidemia is the sixth most common cause of sepsis due to intravenous catheters.

Candida species, except *C. glabrata*, appear in tissue as both yeast and pseudohyphae. In any single lesion, only one form may be present. With *C. glabrata*, only yeast cells are present. Visceral lesions are characterized by necrosis and a neutrophilic inflammatory response. Neutrophils kill *Candida* yeast cells and damage segments of pseudohyphae in vitro, and visceral candidiasis complicates neutropenia, suggesting a major role for the neutrophil in host defense against this fungus. Visceral lesions show a preference for kidney, brain, spleen, heart, eye, and liver.

CLINICAL MANIFESTATIONS *Oral thrush* presents as discrete and confluent adherent white plaques on the oral and pharyngeal mucosa, particularly in the mouth and tongue. These lesions are usually painless, but fissuring at the corners of the mouth can be painful. *Cutaneous candidiasis* presents as red, macerated intertriginous areas, paronychia, balanitis, or pruritus ani. Candidiasis of the perineal and scrotal skin may be accompanied by discrete pustular lesions on the inner aspects of the thighs. *Chronic mucocutaneous candidiasis* or *Candida granuloma* typically presents as circumscribed hyperkeratotic skin lesions, crumbling dystrophic nails, partial alopecia in areas of scalp lesions, and both oral and vaginal thrush. Systemic infection is very rare, but disfigurement of the face and hands can be severe. Other findings may include chronic epidermophytosis, dental dysplasia, and hypofunction of the parathyroid, adrenal, or thyroid glands. A variety of defects in T cell function have been described in these patients. Vulvovaginal thrush causes pruritus, discharge, and sometimes pain on intercourse or urination. Speculum examination reveals an inflamed mucosa and a thin exudate, often with white curds.

From one to multiple small shallow ulcerations due to *Candida* may appear in the esophagus or gastrointestinal tract. Esophageal lesions favor the distal third and may cause dysphagia or substernal pain. Other such lesions tend to be asymptomatic but assume importance in the leukemic patient as a portal for disseminated candidiasis. Within the urinary tract, the most common lesions are either hematogenous renal abscesses, which can cause azotemia, or bladder thrush. Bladder invasion usually follows catheterization or instrumentation of a patient with diabetes mellitus or who is receiving broad-spectrum antibiotics. This lesion generally is asymptomatic and benign. Rarely, retrograde invasion of the renal pelvis leads to renal papillary necrosis.

Hematogenous dissemination of Candida presents with fever and toxicity but with few localizing findings. One or more retinal abscesses may appear and extend slowly into the vitreous humor. The patient may note orbital pain, blurred vision, scotoma, or opacities floating across the visual field. Pulmonary candidiasis is almost always hematogenous and is visible on chest x-ray only when the abscesses are numerous enough to cause a diffuse, vaguely nodular infiltrate. Candidiasis of the endocardium or around intracardiac prostheses resembles bacterial infection of these sites. Chronic *Candida* meningitis or arthritis may occur, from either disseminated disease or insertion of a prosthesis in the case of arthritis or ventriculoperitoneal shunt infection. Rare focal manifestations of disseminated disease include osteomyelitis, pustular skin lesions, myositis, and brain abscess.

DIAGNOSIS Demonstration of pseudohyphae on wet smear with confirmation by culture is the procedure of choice for diagnosing superficial candidiasis. Scrapings for the smear may be obtained from skin, nails, and oral and vaginal mucosa. Culture alone is not diagnostic; however, recovery of *Candida* species from multiple superficial sites in immunosuppressed patients may portend visceral invasion.

Deeper lesions of *Candida* may be diagnosed by histologic section of biopsy specimens or by culture of cerebrospinal fluid, blood, joint fluid, or surgical specimens. Blood cultures are very useful in *Candida* endocarditis and intravenous catheter–induced sepsis but are positive less often in other forms of disseminated disease. Serologic tests for antibody or antigen are not useful.

TREATMENT Cutaneous candidiasis of macerated areas responds to measures which reduce moisture and chafing plus a topically applied antifungal agent in a nonocclusive base. Nystatin powder or a cream with ciclopirox or an azole is useful. Clotrimazole, miconazole, econazole, ketoconazole, sulconazole, and oxiconazole are available as creams or lotions. *Candida* vulvovaginitis responds better to an azole than to nystatin suppositories. There is little difference in efficacy among miconazole, clotrimazole, tioconazole, butoconazole, and terconazole vaginal formulations. Systemic treatment of *Candida* vulvovaginitis with ketoconazole or fluconazole is more convenient that topical treatment, but the potential for adverse effects is higher. Clotrimazole troches, used five times a day, are more effective in oral and esophageal candidiasis than nystatin suspension. Ketoconazole, 200 to 400 mg daily, is also useful in *Candida* esophagitis, but many of the patients absorb the drug poorly because they are receiving H-2 receptor antagonists or have AIDS. In AIDS patients, fluconazole, 100 to 200 mg daily, is the most effective azole for oral and esophageal candidiasis.

When esophageal symptoms are pronounced, a 5- to 10-day course of intravenous amphotericin B, 0.3 mg/kg per day, may be beneficial. Bladder thrush responds to bladder irrigations with amphotericin B, 50 μg/mL for 5 days. If no bladder catheter is present, oral fluconazole can be used to control candiduria. In all forms of superficial candidiasis, relapse after successful treatment is common unless the underlying factor can be eliminated.

Intravenous amphotericin B is the drug of choice in disseminated candidiasis. The drug is usually given as 0.4 to 0.5 mg/kg every day or as a double dose on alternate days for several weeks. In patients with no contraindication to the use of flucytosine, administration of that drug in dosage of 100 to 150 mg/kg per day plus amphotericin B, 0.3 mg/kg per day, is an effective alternative. Ketoconazole in an adult dose of 200 mg daily is probably the drug of choice for chronic mucocutaneous candidiasis.

Candida isolated from a properly obtained blood culture should be considered significant; true false-positives are rare. All patients with *Candida* cultured from peripheral blood should receive intravenous amphotericin B to treat acute infection and prevent late sequelae. In patients without neutropenia, endocarditis, or other deep focus, treatment for 2 weeks is often adequate. Funduscopic examination through a dilated pupil is invaluable in detecting endophthalmitis before permanent loss of vision has occurred. Removal of an infected intravenous catheter is usually required to effect cure. If a catheter has caused suppurative phlebitis of a peripheral vein, excision of the infected portion of the vein is usually required.

In one study of bone marrow transplant recipients, daily prophylaxis with fluconazole, 400 mg, appeared to decrease the number of cases of deep candidiasis. Fluconazole also can be used to complete treatment of chronic disseminated (''hepatosplenic'') candidiasis if amphotericin B is given until the patient is no longer neutropenic. A comparison of fluconazole with intravenous amphotericin B in the nonneutropenic patient with catheter-acquired candidemia is currently underway. *C. krusei* appears to be resistant to fluconazole.

REFERENCES

AHONEN P et al: Clinical variation of autoimmune polyendocrinopathy-candidiasis-ectodermal dystrophy in a series of 68 patients. N Engl J Med 322:1829, 1991

ANAISSIE E et al: Fluconazole therapy for chronic disseminated candidiasis in patients with leukemia and prior amphotericin B therapy. Am J Med 91:142, 1991

DUPONT B, DROUHET E: Fluconazole in the management of oropharyngeal candidosis in a predominantly HIV antibody-positive group of patients. J Med Vet Mycol 26:67, 1988

MEUNIER F: Candidiasis. Eur J Clin Microbiol Infect Dis 8:438, 1989

ODD FC: *Candida and Candidosis*. Philadelphia, Saunders, 1988

THALER M et al: Hepatic candidiasis in cancer patients: The evolving picture of the syndrome. Ann Intern Med 198:88, 1988

167 ASPERGILLOSIS

JOHN E. BENNETT

ETIOLOGY *Aspergillus fumigatus* is the most common pathogen, but *A. flavus*, *A. niger*, and several other species can cause disease. *Aspergillus* is a mold with septate hyphae about 2 to 4 μm in diameter. The fungus is identified by its gross and microscopic appearance in culture.

PATHOGENESIS AND PATHOLOGY All the common species of *Aspergillus* which cause disease in humans are ubiquitous in the environment, growing on dead leaves, stored grain, compost piles, hay, and other decaying vegetation. Inhalation of *Aspergillus* spores must be extremely common, but disease is rare. Invasion of lung tissue is almost entirely confined to immunosuppressed patients. Roughly 90 percent will have two of these three conditions: fewer than 500 granulocytes per microliter of peripheral blood, supraphysiologic doses of adrenal corticosteroids, and a history of cytotoxic drugs such as azathioprine. Invasive aspergillosis is an occasional complication of HIV infection, usually concurrent with neutropenia and CD4 cell depletion. Infection is characterized by hyphal invasion of blood vessels, thrombosis, necrosis, and hemorrhagic infarction. Chronic granulomatous disease of childhood also predisposes to invasive pulmonary aspergillosis, but here the inflammatory response is granulomatous and blood vessel invasion is rare.

Massive inhalation of *Aspergillus* spores by normal persons can lead to an acute, diffuse, self-limited pneumonitis. Epithelioid granulomas with giant cells and central pyogenic areas containing hyphae are seen. Spontaneous recovery taking several weeks is the usual course.

Aspergillus can colonize the damaged bronchial tree, pulmonary cysts, or cavities of patients with underlying lung disease. Balls of hyphae within cysts or cavities may reach several centimeters in diameter and be visible on chest x-ray. Tissue invasion does not occur. The term *allergic bronchial aspergillosis* denotes the condition of patients with preexisting asthma who have eosinophilia, IgE antibody to *Aspergillus*, and fleeting pulmonary infiltrates from bronchial plugging (see Chap. 218).

CLINICAL MANIFESTATIONS *Endobronchial pulmonary aspergillosis* presents as chronic productive cough and often hemoptysis in a patient with prior chronic lung disease, such as tuberculosis, sarcoidosis, bronchiectasis, or histoplasmosis. *Aspergilloma* refers to a ball of hyphae within a lung cyst or cavity, usually in the upper lobe. *Aspergillus* may be spread from its endocavitary or endobronchial site to the pleura during the course of bacterial lung abscess or surgery.

Invasive aspergillosis in the immunosuppressed host presents as an acute pneumonia and has a tendency to cavitation. Infection progresses by hematogenous spread as well as extension to surrounding lung and other contiguous structures. Occasionally, the portal of infection in the immunosuppressed host is the paranasal sinus, gastrointestinal tract, skin, or palate.

Aspergillus sinusitis in nonimmunosuppressed patients may take two forms. A ball of hyphae may form in a chronically obstructed paranasal sinus, without tissue invasion. Much less commonly, a chronic, fibrosing granulomatous inflammation with *Aspergillus* hyphae within tissue may begin in the sinus and spread slowly to the orbit and brain.

Growth of *Aspergillus* on cerumen and detritus within the external auditory canal is termed *otomycosis*. Trauma to the cornea may cause *Aspergillus* keratitis. Endophthalmitis follows introduction of *Aspergillus* into the globe by trauma or surgery. *Aspergillus* may infect intracardiac or intravascular prostheses.

DIAGNOSIS Repeated isolation of *Aspergillus* from sputum or demonstration of hyphae in sputum or bronchial brushing specimens suggests endobronchial colonization or infection. Even a single isolation of *Aspergillus* from the sputum of a neutropenic patient with pneumonia, particularly a child or nonsmoker, suggests the diagnosis of invasive aspergillosis. Fungus ball of the lung is usually detectable by chest x-ray. Antibody of the IgG class to *Aspergillus* antigens is demonstrable in the serum of many colonized patients and of virtually all patients with fungus ball.

Biopsy is usually required to diagnose invasive aspergillosis of the lung, paranasal sinus, or sites of dissemination. Blood cultures are rarely positive, even in patients with infected cardiac prosthetic valves. *Aspergillus* hyphae can be identified presumptively by histology, but culture is required for confirmation and determination of species.

TREATMENT Patients with severe hemoptysis due to fungus ball of the lung may benefit by lobectomy. Poor pulmonary function in residual lung and dense pleural adhesions around the lesion can complicate the resection. Systemic chemotherapy is of no value in endobronchial or endocavitary aspergillosis.

Intravenous amphotericin B has resulted in arrest or cure of invasive aspergillosis when immunosuppression is not severe. Combined flucytosine–amphotericin B may be useful in nonneutropenic patients with invasive aspergillosis. Itraconazole, 200 mg bid, is useful in some of the less immunosuppressed patients with indolent or slowly progressive invasive aspergillosis.

REFERENCES

DENNING DW, STEVENS DA: Antifungal and surgical treatment of invasive aspergillosis: Review of 2121 published cases. Rev Infect Dis 12:1147, 1990
——— et al: Treatment of invasive aspergillosis with itraconazole. Am J Med 86:791, 1989
SHIRAKUSA T et al: Surgical treatment of pulmonary aspergilloma and *Aspergillus* empyema. Ann Thorac Surg 48:779, 1989
TALBOT GH et al: Invasive *Aspergillus* rhinosinusitis in patients with acute leukemia. Rev Infect Dis 13:219, 1991

168   MUCORMYCOSIS

JOHN E. BENNETT

ETIOLOGY Species of *Rhizopus*, *Rhizomucor*, and *Cunninghamella* are most common, but species of *Apophysomyces*, *Saksenaea*, *Mucor*, and *Absidia* occasionally cause mucormycosis. These molds have broad, rarely septate hyphae of uneven diameter, ranging from 6 to 50 µm. The fungus is inexplicably difficult to grow from infected tissue. When it occurs, growth is rapid and profuse on most media at room temperature. Identification is based on gross and microscopic appearance of the mold.

Zygomycosis is a term that includes mucormycosis and entomophthoramycosis. The latter is a tropical infection of the subcutaneous tissue or paranasal sinuses caused by species of *Basidiobolus* or *Conidiobolus*.

PATHOGENESIS AND PATHOLOGY *Rhizopus* and *Rhizomucor* species are ubiquitous, appearing on decaying vegetation, dung, and foods of high sugar content. Infection is uncommon and is largely confined to patients with serious preexisting diseases. Mucormycosis originating in the paranasal sinuses and nose occurs predominantly in patients with poorly controlled diabetes mellitus. Patients with organ transplantation, hematologic malignancy, or who are receiving long-term deferoxamine therapy are predisposed to mucormycosis of either sinus or lung. Gastrointestinal mucormycosis occurs in a variety of conditions, including uremia, severe malnutrition, and diarrheal diseases. Infection is acquired from nature, with no person-to-person spread. In all forms of mucormycosis, vascular invasion by hyphae is prominent. Ischemic or hemorrhagic necrosis is the predominant histologic finding.

CLINICAL MANIFESTATIONS Mucormycosis originating in the nose and paranasal sinuses produces a characteristic clinical picture. Low-grade fever, dull sinus pain, and sometimes nasal congestion or a thin, bloody nasal discharge are followed in a few days by double vision, increasing fever, and obtundation. Examination reveals a unilateral generalized reduction of ocular motion, chemosis, and proptosis. The nasal turbinates on the involved side may be dusky red or necrotic. A sharply delineated area of necrosis, strictly respecting the midline, may appear in the hard palate. The skin of the cheek may become inflamed. Fungal invasion of the globe or ophthalmic artery leads to blindness. Opacification of one or more sinuses is found on CT scan or by magnetic resonance imaging. Carotid arteriogram may show invasion or obstruction of the carotid siphon. Coma is due to direct invasion of the frontal lobe. Early symptoms mimic bacterial sinusitis. Clouding of the sensorium may be attributed to diabetic acidosis. Cavernous sinus thrombosis may be considered when orbital invasion occurs. Without treatment, death may occur in a few days to a few weeks.

Pulmonary mucormycosis is a progressive severe pneumonia, accompanied by high fever and toxicity. The necrotic center of large infiltrates may cavitate. Hematogenous spread to other areas of the lung, as well as to brain and other organs, is common. Survival beyond 2 weeks is unusual. Gastrointestinal invasion presents as one or more ulcers which tend to perforate. Hematogenous dissemination can originate from the gastrointestinal tract, lung, or paranasal sinuses. Sometimes no portal of entry can be found.

DIAGNOSIS Lesions of the lung and craniofacial structures are best diagnosed by biopsy and histologic section. Cultural confirmation should be attempted. Wet smear of crushed tissue can provide rapid diagnosis. Cultures of blood and cerebrospinal fluid are negative. Smear and culture of sputum may be positive during cavitation of a lung lesion.

TREATMENT Regulation of diabetes mellitus and decreasing the dose of immunosuppressive drugs aid in the treatment. Extensive debridement of craniofacial lesions appears to be very important. Orbital exenteration may be required. Intravenous amphotericin B is clearly of value in craniofacial mucormycosis and should be employed in the other forms of mucormycosis as well. Maximum tolerated doses are given until progression is halted. The drug is continued for a total of 10 to 12 weeks. Appropriate management results in cure of about half the craniofacial infections. Survival of patients with pulmonary, gastrointestinal, or disseminated mucormycosis is rare.

REFERENCES

GALETTA SL et al: Rhinocerebral mucormycosis: management and survival after carotid occlusion. Ann Neurol 28:103, 1990

INGRAM CW et al: Disseminated zygomycosis: Report of four cases and review. Rev Infect Dis 11:741, 1989

VLASVELD TL, VAN ASBECK BS: Treatment with deferoxamine: A real risk factor for mucormycosis? Nephron 571:487, 1991

169 MISCELLANEOUS MYCOSES

JOHN E. BENNETT

CHROMOBLASTOMYCOSIS This chronic subcutaneous mycosis is rarely seen in the United States but presents as a verrucoid, ulcerated, or crusted skin lesion. Disease originates when thorns or bits of vegetation introduce the fungus into the subcutaneous tissue. Infection spreads over ensuing months and years to contiguous tissue, causing very few symptoms. Appearance of the thick-walled dark-colored rounded forms (''copper pennies'') in tissue is diagnostic. No satisfactory treatment is available.

DERMATOPHYTOSIS **Definition** Dermatophytosis, also known as ringworm or tinea, is a chronic fungal infection of the skin, hair, or nails.

Etiology Species of *Trichophyton*, *Microsporum*, and *Epidermophyton* are called *dermatophytes*. They grow in and remain confined to the keratinous structures of the body. Other mycoses can show fungal invasion of keratinous structures, such as candidiasis, pityriasis versicolor, and tinea nigra, but are traditionally not termed *dermatophytoses*.

Pathology and pathogenesis Dermatophyte species are called *anthropophilic*, *zoophilic*, or *geophilic* depending on whether their usual reservoir within nature appears to be humans, animals, or soil. Infectivity of all these sources is low, and group outbreaks are largely confined to an occasional case clustering of scalp infections in children. Acquisition of a dermatophytosis appears to be favored by minor trauma, maceration, and poor hygiene of the skin. Infection does not seem to confer solid immunity. Repeated infection with the same species is common, particularly with anthropophilic species. Infrequency of scalp infection in adults has been attributed to local factors rather than immunity.

Invasion of the stratum corneum by dermatophytes may cause little inflammation, or, particularly with zoophilic fungi, inflammation can be intense. Shedding of the stratum corneum is increased by inflammation. To the extent that fungal growth cannot keep up with shedding, inflammation may help terminate infection. Conversely, infection is probably favored when shedding is reduced by glucocorticoids and cytotoxic drugs. Antifungal drugs interfere with the ability of fungal growth to keep up with shedding.

Clinical manifestations The disease varies with the site of infection and fungal species. Foot infection (athlete's foot, tinea pedis) may present as fissuring of the toe webs, scaling of the plantar surfaces, or vesicles around the toe webs and soles. Interdigital lesions may be pruritic or, when bacterial superinfection occurs, may be painful. Hand infection is less common but resembles foot infection. Scalp dermatophytosis (tinea capitis) is characterized by areas of alopecia and scaling. In so-called endothrix infection, the hair shaft breaks off at the skin surface, leaving the hairs visible as black dots in the scalp. With some forms of scalp infection, an intense boggy suppuration occurs, called a *kerion*. Dermatophytosis of the glabrous skin (tinea corporis) presents as circumscribed lesions with a wide variety of appearances. Scales, vesicles, or pustules may appear. Inflammation may be minimal or intense. Central healing of less inflamed lesions may be seen. The serpiginous border of inflammation is the source of the name *ringworm*. Dermatophytosis of the bearded area (tinea barbae) appears as a pustular folliculitis. Onychomycosis (tinea unguium) presents as white discolored nails or thickened, chalky, crumbling nails. Peeling and fissuring of the paronychia or keratotic debris under the nail edge also may be seen.

Diagnosis Discolored hairs, scales, and keratotic debris under infected nails should be collected for KOH smear and culture. In the scraping of skin lesions, a drop of water on the skin site may keep the removed scales from flying off and aid in their collection. Culture is important in distinguishing dermatophytes from *Candida* and fungal saprophytes growing in keratinaceous debris.

Treatment Noninflammatory lesions of the trunk, groin, hands, and feet usually respond to twice-daily applications of clotrimazole, miconazole, ketoconazole, econazole, or ciclopirox olamine cream. Hyperkeratotic lesions of the palms and soles respond slowly to these agents and may benefit from Whitfield's ointment initially to thin the keratin. Ointment should not be used between the toes or in the groin or gluteal crease because maceration permits bacterial infection.

Ringworm that is moderately severe, that is unresponsive to topical therapy, or that involves the scalp, nails, or bearded area should be treated systemically. The drug of choice is griseofulvin. Either 500 mg of the microcrystalline form or 375 mg of the ultramicrocrystalline form is given once daily or divided into two doses, given with meals. Double this amount has been recommended for refractory infections. Treatment must be continued until all infected keratin is gone. Cutting of infected hair, epilating nails, and cleansing interdigital webs can expedite cure. Secondary bacterial infection of the foot may require soaks or antibacterial agents. Relapse of dermatophyte foot infections may be decreased by measures to keep the feet clean and dry. Griseofulvin-resistant cases may respond to oral ketoconazole, 200 to 400 mg daily.

FUSARIOSIS Fusarium species can cause localized or hematogenously disseminated infection. Almost all patients with the latter have had hematopoietic malignancy and neutropenia. Abrupt onset of fever, sometimes with myalgia, is followed by distinctive skin lesions in two-thirds of cases. The lesions resemble ecthyma gangrenosum, tend to be multiple, progressively expand in size, and favor the extremities. A portal of infection is not usually apparent. Blood cultures have been positive in 59 percent of cases. Amphotericin B is probably the drug of choice, but recovery depends on diminution of neutropenia.

MALASSEZIA INFECTION (PITYRIASIS) *Malassezia furfur* is part of the normal human skin flora but can cause tinea (pityriasis) versicolor or catheter-acquired sepsis. Tinea versicolor appears as asymptomatic well-delineated hyperpigmented or hypopigmented macules, centered on the upper trunk and upper arms. Confluence of lesions may cover large areas, making the border difficult to find. A fine branny scale or folliculitis is sometimes visible. Skin scrapings examined microscopically by KOH mount show characteristic round and elongated cells. On inspection with Wood's light, lesions either do not fluoresce or appear yellow-green. Erythrasma resembles tinea versicolor but has gram-positive bacilli on smear and fluoresces coral red. Azole creams are effective treatment for small areas of tinea versicolor, but application of selenium sulfide shampoo (Selsun) for 10 min daily, followed by showering to remove the shampoo, is more practical for large areas. Oral ketoconazole is also effective. Catheter-acquired sepsis occurs in patients receiving intravenous lipid, particularly neonates, requires special culture conditions for growth, and is cured by catheter removal.

MYCETOMA　Etiology *Actinomycetoma* refers to infection by actinomycetes of the genera *Nocardia*, *Nocardiopsis*, *Streptomyces*, and *Actinomadura*. *Eumycetoma* is caused by true fungi of many different genera. The most common agent varies with the locality.

Pathogenesis and pathology　The pathogens live in the soil and enter the skin through minor trauma. The most common site of infection is the foot. Infection runs a relentless course over many years, with destruction of contiguous bone and fascia. Grains are found in purulent foci, surrounded by fibrosis and a mononuclear cell inflammatory response.

Clinical manifestations　*Mycetoma* is a chronic suppurative infection originating in subcutaneous tissue and characterized by the presence of grains, which are tightly clumped colonies of the causative agent. The infected site shows painless swelling, woody induration, and sinus tracts which discharge pus intermittently. Systemic symptoms and spread to distant sites in the body are not seen.

Diagnosis　The clinical picture is characteristic, but confusion with chronic osteomyelitis or botryomycosis may occur. The diagnosis requires demonstration of grains in pus from the draining sinus or in biopsy sections. Many histologic sections may need to be examined to locate a grain.

Treatment　Actinomycetoma may respond to prolonged combination chemotherapy, such as streptomycin and either dapsone or trimethoprim-sulfamethoxazole. Eumycetoma rarely has responded to chemotherapy. As a possible exception, some cases infected with *Madurella mycetomatis* have appeared to respond to ketoconazole.

PHAEOHYPHOMYCOSIS　This is the name given to infections caused by fungi with dark-walled hyphae, excluding those infections which can be given conventional names such as chromoblastomycosis. Although an extraordinary variety of fungi and clinical syndromes are encompassed by this definition, the majority of patients have brain abscess, subcutaneous abscess, or allergic fungal sinusitis. Most of the brain abscesses are due to *Cladosporium trichoides* and occur in previously normal persons. Subcutaneous abscesses are usually single, arise at the site of minor trauma, and occur in both immunosuppressed and previously normal persons.

Allergic fungal sinusitis occurs in patients with allergic rhinitis and presents as an expanding mucoid mass in one or more paranasal sinuses. The tenacious mucus contains eosinophils, Charcot-Leyden crystals, and occasional hyphae. Surgical excision of phaeohyphomycotic lesions is important; response to antifungal therapy is often unsatisfactory.

PSEUDALLESCHERIASIS　Etiology　Also called *Petriellidium boydii*, *Pseudallescheria boydii* is a mold frequently found in soil. When the fungus is isolated in the imperfect state, it is called *Scedosporium apiospermum*.

Pathogenesis and pathology　Wind-borne spores of *P. boydii*, arising in soil, are the presumed source of infection. The fungus grows as a mold within tissue, causing necrosis and abscess formation.

Clinical manifestations　*P. boydii* resembles *Aspergillus* in its ability to colonize the endobronchial tree, to form fungus balls in the lung or paranasal sinuses, and to invade the cornea or globe following trauma or surgery and by its propensity to invade the immunosuppressed host. Hyphae of *P. boydii* in tissue may be difficult to distinguish from *Aspergillus*. Infection with *P. boydii* is much less common than with *Aspergillus*. *P. boydii* is the single most common

cause in the United States of mycetoma. Intravascular hyphae, a hallmark of invasive aspergillosis, also can be found in pseudallescheriasis. Occasional normal patients have developed necrotizing pneumonia or abscesses in brain or other organs due to *P. boydii*.

Diagnosis　Demonstration of hyphae in tissue and culture confirmation are required for diagnosis.

Treatment　Intravenous miconazole, itraconazole, or ketoconazole is recommended, but therapeutic response to all drugs has been poor.

SPOROTRICHOSIS　Etiology　*Sporothrix schenckii* lives as a saprophyte on plants in many areas of the world. In nature and on culture at room temperature the fungus grows as a mold, but within host tissue or at 37°C on enriched media it grows as a budding yeast. Identification is by appearance of the fungus in mold and yeast forms.

Pathogenesis and pathology　Infection results when minor trauma inoculates the fungus into subcutaneous tissue. Nursery workers, florists, and gardeners acquire the illness from roses, sphagnum moss, and other plants. Infection may be limited to the site of inoculation (plaque sporotrichosis) or extend along proximal lymphatic channels (lymphangitic sporotrichosis). Spread beyond an extremity, the usual site of infection, is rare, and hematogenous dissemination from the skin remains unproven. The portal for osteoarticular, pulmonary, and other extracutaneous forms of sporotrichosis is unknown but is likely the lung.

Untreated sporotrichosis shows little evidence of self-healing and is capable of extreme chronicity. The inflammatory response contains both clusters of neutrophils and a marked granulomatous response with epithelioid cells and giant cells.

Clinical manifestations　Lymphangitic sporotrichosis, by far the most common manifestation, forms a nearly painless red papule at the site of inoculation. Over the next several weeks, similar nodules form along proximal lymphatic channels. Nodules intermittently discharge small amounts of pus. Ulceration may occur. The proximal extension of these lesions, often with skip areas, is quite distinctive but may be mimicked by lesions of *Nocardia brasiliensis*, *Mycobacterium marinum*, or, on rare occasions, by *Leishmania brasiliensis* or *M. kansasii*.

Plaque sporotrichosis is a nontender red maculopapular granuloma confined to the site of inoculation. Osteoarticular sporotrichosis presents as mono- or polyarticular arthritis of indolent onset and progression over months or years involving the elbows, knees, wrists, ankles, and, rarely, smaller joints of the extremities. Periarticular bone develops areas of demineralization on x-ray, and draining sinuses may appear over joints and bursae. Hematogenous spread to the skin may be observed during polyarticular disease, but none of the skin lesions shows lymphangitic spread. Immunosuppression, including advanced HIV infection, predisposes to hematogenous spread. Pulmonary sporotrichosis usually presents as a single chronic cavitary upper-lobe lung lesion.

Diagnosis　Culture of pus, joint fluid, sputum, or skin biopsy specimen is the preferred method of diagnosis. Appearance of *S. schenckii* in tissue is quite variable. In skin lesions, the organisms are hard to find.

Treatment　Cutaneous sporotrichosis can be cured with oral administration of a saturated solution of potassium iodide given in increasing divided daily doses up to 4.5 to 9 mL/d for adults, as tolerated. Gastrointestinal disturbance or acneiform rash over the cape area and face is common, but therapy should be continued for 1 month after resolution of all lesions. Patients with serious allergic reactions to iodides may respond to local heat, particularly when plaque sporotrichosis is the only form of disease. Itraconazole, an experimental drug, may be of value. Extracutaneous sporotrichosis rarely responds to iodides, but cures have been obtained in over half such patients with prolonged courses of intravenous amphotericin B. Itraconazole is effective in lymphocutaneous sporotrichosis and in some cases of extracutaneous sporotrichosis.

TRICHOSPORONOSIS　*Trichosporon beigelii* causes asymptomatic small white concretions on hair shafts, a condition called *white* *piedra*, but can cause hematogenously disseminated infection in neutropenic patients, mostly leukemics. Multiple erythematous or purpuric papules accompany the fungemia. The lesions can evolve into large, tense hemorrhagic bullae. Blood cultures are usually positive. Prosthetic valve endocarditis due to *T. beigelii* is also well described. Intravenous amphotericin B is the drug of choice.

REFERENCES

Chromoblastomycosis

TUFFANELLI L, MILBURN PB: Treatment of chromoblastomycosis. J Am Acad Dermatol 23:728, 1990

Dermatophytosis

WRIGHT DC et al: Generalized chronic dermatophytosis in patients with human immunodeficiency virus type I infection and CD4 depletion. Arch Dermatol 127:265, 1991

Fusariosis

ANAISSIE E et al: New spectrum of fungal infections in patients with cancer. Rev Infect Dis 11:369, 1989
GAMIS AS et al: Disseminated infection with *Fusarium* in recipients of bone marrow transplants. Rev Infect Dis 13:1077, 1991

Malassezia infection (pityriasis)

DANKER WM et al: *Malassezia* fungemia in neonates and adults: Complication of hyperalimentation. Rev Infect Dis 9:743, 1987

JACINTO-JAMORA S et al: *Pityrosporum* folliculitis in the Philippines: Diagnosis, prevalence and management. J Am Acad Dermatol 24:693, 1991

Mycetoma

GUMAA SA et al: Mycetoma of the head and neck. Am J Trop Med Hyg 35:594, 1986
TIGHT RR, BARTLETT MS: Actinomycetoma in the United States. Rev Infect Dis 3:1139, 1981

Phaeohyphomycosis

WASHBURN RG et al: Chronic fungal sinusitis in apparently normal hosts. Medicine 67:231, 1988

Pseudallescheriasis

BERENGUER J et al: Central nervous system infection caused by *Pseudallescheria boydii*: Case report and review. Rev Infect Dis 11:890, 1989
GALGIANI JN et al: *Pseudallescheria boydii* infections treated with ketoconazole. Chest 86:219, 1984
TRAVIS LB et al: Clinical significance of *Pseudallescheria boydii*: A review of 10 years' experience. Mayo Clin Proc 60:531, 1985

Sporotrichosis

BULLPITT P, WEEDON D: Sporotrichosis: A review of 39 cases. Pathology 10:249, 1978
ENGLAND DM, HOCHHOLZER L: Primary pulmonary sporotrichosis. Am J Surg Pathol 9:193, 1985
FRIEDMAN SJ, DOYLE JA: Extracutaneous sporotrichosis. Int J Dermatol 22:171, 1983
PLUSS JL, OPAL SM: Pulmonary sporotrichosis: Review of treatment and outcome. Medicine 65:143, 1986
SHAW JC et al: Sporotrichosis in the acquired immunodeficiency syndrome. J Am Acad Dermatol 21:1145, 1989

Trichosporonosis

WALSH TJ et al: Trichosporonosis in patients with neoplastic disease. Medicine 65:268, 1986

section 16   Protozoal and helminthic infections: General considerations

170   MOLECULAR BIOLOGY AND IMMUNOLOGY OF PARASITIC INFECTIONS

JOHN R. DAVID / LEO X. LIU

Protozoan and helminthic parasites have caused incalculable human suffering and death through the ages, and their global impact on human health remains enormous today. Every year several hundred million people contract malaria, the most serious human protozoal disease, and close to a million children die of falciparum malaria in Africa alone. Another protozoan, *Trypanosoma cruzi*, is a major cause of heart disease in South America. Protozoal parasites such as *Toxoplasma* and *Cryptosporidium* have emerged as important opportunistic pathogens in patients with AIDS and other immunocompromised conditions. Schistosomiasis, a helminthic fluke disease transmitted via snails, affects 200 to 300 million persons worldwide. Filarial nematode parasites infect a similar number of people, and one of these, *Onchocerca volvulus*, is the second most common infectious cause of blindness in the world. Over one *billion* people harbor intestinal nematode parasites, including *Ascaris*, hookworm, and *Trichuris*.

Many traditional control measures have failed to curb the magnitude of parasitic infections. Nowhere is this more evident and serious than in the case of malaria. In the middle of this century there was widespread optimism that malaria could be eradicated by spraying homes with DDT against mosquitoes and by treating infected people with chloroquine. However, the development of widespread insecticide resistance in mosquitoes and chloroquine resistance in *Plasmodium falciparum* has contributed to an alarming resurgence of malaria in the last two decades. For example, in Sri Lanka, the annual number of reported malaria cases in the 1960s rose from 18 to over half a million! Furthermore, modernization efforts in many developing countries have paradoxically increased the spread of certain parasitic infections. Dams constructed in Egypt and Ghana to provide industrial energy have vastly expanded the amount of lake coastline available for the transmission of schistosomiasis to local residents by infected snails. Irrigation schemes in Asia for rice cultivation have multiplied the number of breeding sites for mosquitoes that carry malaria. Clearing of the Amazon rainforest has greatly increased human contact with indigenous sandflies that transmit leishmaniasis.

PARASITE BIOLOGY   The term *parasite* derives from the Greek παρασιτοσ, meaning literally "one who eats at the table of another." In a broad sense, all infectious microorganisms can be considered parasites, since they depend on the host organism for essential nutrients and impart some degree of harm. Nevertheless, by convention, *parasitic infections* refer to those caused by protozoa and helminths. What distinguish these eukaryotic parasites are complex life cycles and long-lived chronic infections of the human host. A typical parasite life cycle comprises sequential developmental stages which can include parasitic life-styles in more than one host and in some instances a period of free-living existence. Nonhuman hosts involved in the rather bewildering variety of parasite life cycles include insects, mollusks, and mammals. Transmission by these biologic vectors or infected intermediate hosts is a crucial feature of

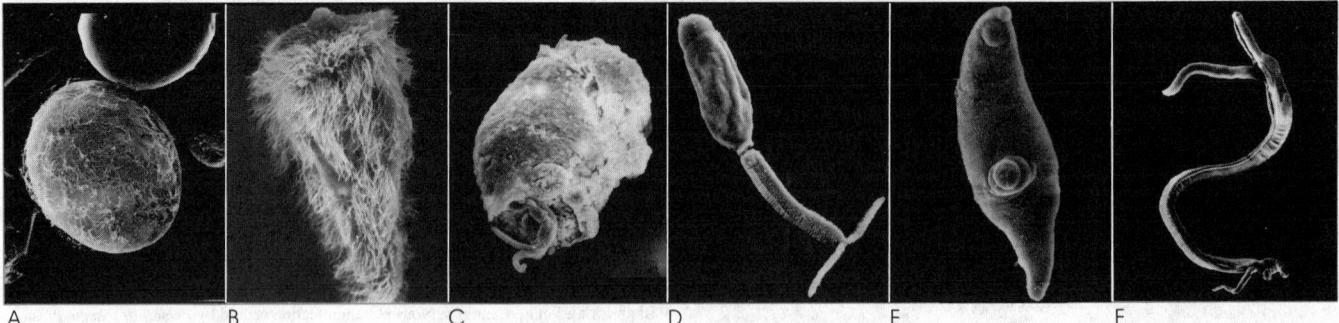

A   Egg in human tissues and stool

B   Miracidium in water

C   Sporocyst in snail

D   Cercaria in water and human skin

E   Schistosomulum in human tissues and blood

F   Adult worms in mesenteric veins

FIGURE 170-1 Morphologic transformations of schistosome parasites in the course of their life cycle. (*Scanning electron micrographs of Schistosome* *japonicum and S. mekongi courtesy of Prasert Sobhon, Ph.D., Mahidol University, Thailand.*)

many parasitic infections. The functional adaptations required of a parasite to negotiate completely different environments results in parasite stages which are morphologically and biochemically distinct from one another. Each transition from one parasite stage to another should be envisioned as an all-encompassing transformation no less radical than the metamorphosis of a caterpillar to a butterfly (Fig. 170-1). Compared with viruses and bacteria, parasites are antigenically complex. Each developmental stage is antigenically different, which has direct implications for the nature of immune responses in parasitic infections.

GENERAL FEATURES OF PARASITIC INFECTIONS   There are important differences between protozoal and helminthic parasites. Protozoal parasites are unicellular and replicate directly within the human host by asexual division. Helminthic parasites, on the other hand, are relatively large, multicellular worms which (with rare exceptions) cannot directly multiply in humans. Protozoans, being of small size, can be intracellular or extracellular parasites, whereas helminths are almost exclusively extracellular parasites of tissue, blood, or the gastrointestinal tract. Like viruses and bacteria, protozoal parasites replicate directly within the host, without having to pass through the outside environment or through intermediate hosts. In malaria, for example, infective sporozoites multiply as merozoites in the liver, and merozoites subsequently infect host erythrocytes with repeating amplification cycles of parasite replication and reinvasion. Thus even a single infectious mosquito bite can ultimately result in severe morbidity or death from malaria. In contrast, helminth parasites typically reproduce sexually in the host to generate eggs or larvae which must be passed out (via the feces, urine, or a biting insect vector) in order to continue development. Further parasite development in the environment or an intermediate host is then required to reach a stage infective for humans. Thus many helminthic infections, unlike malaria, require repeated exposures to infectious larvae or eggs in order for a heavy burden of parasites to develop. This usually entails prolonged residence in an area of ongoing transmission. Even in an endemic area, most individuals are only lightly infected and often asymptomatic, whereas helminthic *disease* develops mainly in those individuals who bear heavy worm burdens.

Chronicity is a predominant characteristic of infections with protozoa and helminths and is related to the remarkable ability of parasites to counteract or evade host immune responses. Immediate mortality is unusual in parasitic infections except for severe malaria, visceral leishmaniasis and trypanosomiasis. Some parasites (such as *Toxoplasma* and *Trichinella*) become latent after the initial phase of invasion. Pathologic changes and clinical disease take years to develop in many parasitic infections, such as Chagas' disease and most helminthic infections.

Whereas in many instances, immunity to viruses and bacteria can

be complete and lifelong after only a single exposure to the pathogen, such sterilizing immunity is rare among protozoa and nonexistent for helminth parasites. For many protozoal and helminthic infections, protection from serious infection is rarely, if ever, complete, becomes maximal only after repeated infection, and declines in the absence of further exposure. For certain parasites such as the intestinal nematodes, naturally acquired immunity does not appear to develop at all. Finally, detrimental host immune responses can lead to immunopathologic tissue damage that typifies some parasitic diseases such as schistosomiasis and lymphatic filariasis.

The scientific understanding of parasitic protozoa and helminths has lagged behind that of viruses and bacteria in part because their complex structures and life cycles make parasites more difficult to study in the laboratory. Furthermore, most serious parasitic infections are largely confined to the developing countries of Africa, Asia, and South America. The last two decades, however, have witnessed a resurgence of scientific interest in medically important parasites, leading to impressive progress in understanding their biology. The development of DNA cloning techniques and monoclonal antibodies, as well as in vitro culture methods for certain protozoa such as malaria, has made it possible to study parasites at a molecular level. The enormous public health impact of parasitic infections and the failure of classic control programs have stimulated a search for better ways to treat and control these diseases using modern immunologic and molecular biology methods.

MOLECULAR MECHANISMS OF PARASITE INVASION

Parasites can enter the human body by only a few infective routes, including oral ingestion, skin penetration, and bites of insect vectors. Virtually any host organ or tissue can become parasitized, however, and most parasites are highly specific in the selection of host sites in which they become established. Parasitic protozoa and helminths have evolved a variety of exquisite adaptations to recognize, invade, and survive in specific host cells and tissues (Table 170-1). For intracellular protozoa such as *Plasmodium* and *Leishmania* spp., attachment to a specific host cell is followed by membrane invagination or endocytosis that allows the parasite to enter that cell. Attachment to host cell membranes is also vital to extracellular protozoal parasites such as *Entamoeba histolytica,* which uses an adherence protein (a galactose-inhibitable lectin) that binds to colonic mucins. Other extracellular parasites have developed specialized structures, such as the adhesive ventral disk of *Giardia* trophozoites, to affix themselves to host tissues.

TABLE 170-1 Some molecular mechanisms of parasite invasion and establishment

Parasite	Cell or tissue target	Proposed mediators	
		Host cell organelle or molecule	Parasite-derived factors
INTRACELLULAR PARASITES			
Leishmania promastigote	Macrophage	Complement receptors CR1 and CR3	LPG (lipophosphoglycan, gp63)
		Mannose-fucose receptor advance glycosylation end-product receptor	
Plasmodium sporozoite	Liver hepatocyte	Basolateral membrane	CSP (circumsporozoite protein)
P. vivax merozoite	Reticulocytes only		PvRBP 1 and 2 (reticulocyte-binding proteins)
	Duffy (+) erythrocytes only	Duffy group antigen	PvDAP-1 (Duffy adhesion protein)
P. falciparum merozoite	All erythrocytes	Glycophorins	SABP (sialic acid–binding protein)
			MSP-I (merozoite surface protein-I)
P. falciparum–infected RBCs	Endothelium	ICAM-1, CD36, thrombospondin	PfEMP-1, PfHRP-2
Trypanosoma cruzi	Macrophage	Vacuolar membrane	TC-TOX, a C9-like pore-forming protein
	Fibroblast	Surface adhesion	Penetrin, a heparin-binding protein
	Many cell types	Membrane surface glycoproteins	*trans*-Sialidase
	Many cell types	Fibronectin	GP85, a fibronectin receptor
Trichinella spiralis	Skeletal muscle	Induction of muscle cell dedifferentiation	Unknown
EXTRACELLULAR PARASITES			
Entamoeba histolytica	Colonic mucosa	Surface mucinous glycoproteins	Galactose-inhibitable lectin
Giardia lamblia	Gut epithelium	Surface glycans	Trypsin-activated lectin
Schistosoma cercariae	Skin		Elastase
Hookworms	Skin penetration, anticoagulant		Metalloproteinase

MOLECULAR PARASITE-HOST INTERACTIONS IN MALARIA

Malarial parasites furnish elegant examples of host cell recognition, attachment, and invasion by successive parasite stages. Malaria is transmitted by the bite of an infected anopheline mosquito. Malarial sporozoites injected into the bloodstream from the mosquito salivary gland soon invade the liver, where each parasite divides asexually to produce many merozoites. These burst out of the hepatocytes into the bloodstream and invade erythrocytes. The parasite further divides within the erythrocyte to generate more merozoites, which eventually rupture the cell and invade other erythrocytes in repeating cycles that are responsible for much of the clinical disease. Some merozoites develop into gametocytes that are taken up by another mosquito when it bites an infected person, leading to the development of sporozoites which are infective for humans.

The surface membrane of the malarial sporozoite is covered by a stage-specific protein called the *circumsporozoite protein* (CSP), which has been intensively investigated in the quest for a malaria vaccine (see below). In addition to an immunogenic central domain, CSP also contains a carboxyl-terminal region (termed *region II*) whose amino acid sequence is similar to a known cell adhesion domain of the bridging protein thrombospondin. Recent studies have shown that CSP binds exclusively to hepatocytes and not to other cells or organs and in particular attaches to the basolateral segment of the hepatocyte membrane which is exposed to the bloodstream. Synthetic region II peptides can block not only the binding of recombinant CSP to hepatocytes but also the penetration of live sporozoites into liver cells, indicating that this adhesive motif of the parasite molecule is critical for recognition and invasion of the target host cell.

Bloodstream infection begins when *Plasmodium* merozoites invade red blood cells. In addition to adhering to the erythrocyte surface, the merozoite must orient itself so that its apical end (containing key organelles for invasion) faces the host cell membrane. After the parasite and erythrocyte membranes form a tight junction, the erythrocyte membrane invaginates to form a parasitophorous vacuole that engulfs the merozoite. Different malarial species prefer different types of erythrocytes; for example, *P. vivax* primarily invades the reticulocyte (immature) subpopulation, whereas *P. falciparum* invades all types of red blood cells. How do these species recognize different types of erythrocytes? In the case of *P. falciparum*, the merozoites

appear to exploit sialic acid residues of glycophorins (which are integral membrane proteins of *all* erythrocytes) as cell-surface receptors. Two *P. falciparum* proteins have been discovered to date that bind erythrocyte sialic acid. *P. vivax* merozoites, on the other hand, require Duffy blood group glycoproteins for erythrocyte attachment and entry. Indeed, the resistance of most black Africans to *P. vivax* malaria can be explained by the absence of Duffy group antigens on their erythrocytes. Research into this phenomenon has uncovered merozoite apical complex proteins which mediate specific binding to Duffy glycoproteins, as well as others which bind only to reticulocytes.

Malaria has exerted a more profound influence on human genetics than any other infectious disease, as is evident from the variety of genetic polymorphisms (such as the thalassemias and hemoglobin S) that confer protection against fatal falciparum malaria in heterozygous individuals. Recently, specific HLA haplotypes also have been shown to confer protection against severe falciparum malaria; these are the first known examples of immune-response genes that protect against a fatal infectious agent. One reason *P. falciparum* is so dangerous is that parasitized erythrocytes are sequestered in deep vascular beds of the brain, giving rise to cerebral malaria. This sequestration is caused by the adherence of parasite-derived proteins on the surface of infected erythrocytes to endothelial cells. Intercellular adhesion molecule-1 (ICAM-1, which also binds leukocytes and human rhinoviruses) has been identified as an endothelial cytoadhesion receptor for *P. falciparum*–infected erythrocytes. Other endothelial molecules which bind parasitized red blood cells include CD36, an integral membrane glycoprotein, and thrombospondin, a protein thought to bridge cells together by linking membrane-associated proteins.

INVASION STRATEGIES OF OTHER INTRACELLULAR PARASITES

Many other remarkable tactics are used by parasites to invade host cells. *Leishmania* parasites occupy what is seemingly the most inhospitable site for any infectious organism, namely, the phagolysosome of macrophages. To reach this unusual niche, infective *Leishmania* promastigotes actually activate serum complement and become opsonized with C3b, which promotes their uptake into macrophages. How do these parasites manage to avoid being killed by the activated complement pathway? *Leishmania* promastigotes are covered by a complex polysaccharide called *lipophosphoglycan* (LPG), which is the major C3 acceptor on the parasite surface. In virulent promastigotes, an elongated form of LPG (created by the addition of repeated oligosaccharide subunits) prevents the insertion of the terminal C5–C9 membrane attack complex into the parasite membrane. Both LPG and a surface protease called *gp63* mediate the in vitro uptake of promastigotes via complement receptors on the macrophage surface. Once inside the phagolysosome, the parasite appears to survive by inactivating lysosomal enzymes and toxic oxidative metabolites. Here again, LPG plays an important role by inhibiting the macrophage oxidative burst and by scavenging oxygen radicals.

T. cruzi, the cause of Chagas' disease, can invade many different types of host cells. The invasive trypomastigote stage possesses a surface enzyme, required for host cell entry, which has the unique ability to transfer sialic acid residues from host glycoproteins to the parasite's own surface. Shortly after entering the host cell inside a parasitophorous vacuole, the parasite disrupts the vacuolar membrane to reach the cytoplasm, where it multiplies. This escape may be effected by another *T. cruzi* protein that forms a pore in the vacuolar membrane and is structurally similar to C9, the terminal pore-forming complement component.

The ancient disease known as *trichinosis* is caused by *Trichinella spiralis* larvae ingested by humans when they eat infected meat. These multicellular worms have the extraordinary ability to invade a skeletal muscle cell and completely transform the host cell morphology and gene expression, with an increase in cell size and nuclei numbers coupled with the loss of contractile proteins. *Trichinella* appears to have evolved mechanisms to take over the transcriptional machinery of myocytes, causing the muscle cell to redifferentiate into a nurse cell which sustains the larva.

INVASION OF HOST TISSUES BY HELMINTH PARASITES Helminth parasites elaborate a complex variety of enzymes and other substances which allow them to penetrate host tissues. Invasive larvae of nematodes and trematodes, such as hookworm larvae or schistosome cercariae, secrete proteolytic enzymes which help to penetrate the skin. Once inside the host, helminth parasites use a variety of mechanisms to remain fixed in their preferred anatomic locale. *Trichuris* whipworms, for example, thread themselves into the superficial colonic epithelium, whereas *Ancylostoma* hookworms use buccal teeth to fasten onto small bowel mucosa. Worms which live in a vascular or gut lumen presumably "swim" by active motility to resist being swept downstream. These include adult filariae in the lymphatic channels and *Ascaris* roundworms in the gut. Still other parasites, such as *Trichinella* larvae and *Onchocerca* adult worms, envelop themselves with a specialized structure which protects them from immune attack. The molecular basis of locating an appropriate host, tissue tropism, and tissue invasion by helminth parasites remains largely unexplored, however. In vitro culture systems like those taken for granted in the study of viruses and bacteria have not yet been realized for parasitic helminths, which can be experimentally propagated only through host animals and invertebrate vectors. Once parasitic helminths do invade the host, they unveil a sophisticated array of mechanisms to evade host immune responses, and some of these have been elucidated as described below.

PARASITE BIOCHEMISTRY

DRUG RESISTANCE The development of drug resistance in parasites, as for pathogenic viruses and bacteria, has become a serious issue. The situation is most grave for the treatment and prophylaxis of malaria. Chloroquine resistance in *P. falciparum*, the most malignant form of human malaria, is so widespread that it is no longer the exception but the rule. Resistance to chloroquine appears to be due to enhanced efflux of the drug out of the malarial cell. *Leishmania* spp. can become resistant to antimetabolite drugs by a process of gene amplification, in which they overproduce the target parasite enzymes to overcome inhibition by the drugs. Other known mechanisms by which parasites become resistant include reduced drug

uptake, increased drug inactivation, and alteration and loss of receptor sites and target molecules for a drug. Drug resistance has already developed to relatively new antiparasitic agents such as mefloquine for malaria, praziquantel for schistosomiasis, and ivermectin for nematode infections. Unfortunately, the actual site and mechanism of action of these and many other useful drugs are still unknown, which hinders the understanding of drug resistance and attempts to overcome it by chemical modifications to the parent compound.

DRUG DESIGN A better understanding of parasite biochemistry also may suggest new targets for antiparasite chemotherapy. Because many parasites by their nature depend on host metabolism, some of their own biochemical pathways have degenerated. For example, parasitic protozoa and helminths are unable to synthesize their own purines and must depend on intricate purine salvage pathways. In other cases, parasites may have evolved unique enzymes which are employed exclusively in essential parasitic behaviors. It may be possible to rationally exploit such differences between parasite and host biochemistry and metabolism to develop new drugs which act selectively against a parasite without incurring host toxicity. Unfortunately, there are limited commercial incentives to develop drugs that are most needed in poor tropical countries. For example, only a few new drugs are undergoing clinical testing for malaria (a disease that causes 1 to 3 million deaths yearly), and none of these is being developed by U.S. pharmaceutical companies. In contrast, almost 100 drugs are currently in testing for AIDS, a disease of rich countries as well as poor.

DIAGNOSTIC TESTS Contemporary molecular and immunologic techniques provide a new generation of sensitive tools suitable for clinical diagnosis and epidemiologic studies. Immunodiagnostic assays can be designed to detect either parasite antigens or host antiparasite antibodies. The enzyme-linked immunosorbent assay (ELISA), for example, is useful for detecting tissue parasites, such as *Toxoplasma* and cysticerci, that cannot be isolated readily from body fluids of patients. Serologic cross-reactions are common in parasitic infections, a fact which limits the usefulness of immunoassays in endemic areas where people are commonly exposed to many kinds of parasites. This problem can be overcome by the use of monoclonal antibodies to parasite antigens which are species-specific. Extremely sensitive detection of parasite DNA is possible with DNA hybridization techniques and the polymerase chain reaction. For example, using specific DNA probes, it is possible not only to detect *Leishmania* in skin biopsies but also to determine the particular species involved. Other clinical applications of parasite DNA detection include the diagnosis of low-grade malaria or screening of donor blood in areas where *T. cruzi* is endemic. Such methods are also useful in epidemiologic field surveys of infected humans or vectors as part of mass control programs.

IMMUNE EVASION BY PARASITES

Parasites have evolved a variety of ingenious ways to evade immune responses of the host. Some of these are listed in Table 170-2. For intracellular pathogens such as those discussed above, invasion and immune evasion are often two sides of the same coin, for seclusion within a host cell can provide a privileged site inaccessible to immunologic surveillance. Other protozoa besides *Leishmania* manage to avoid lysis by complement. The virulent trypomastigotes of *T. cruzi*, for example, release an inhibitor of C3 convertase activity, thereby limiting complement activation on the parasite surface. *Toxoplasma* parasites, after being engulfed by a macrophage, block fusion of the phagosome with lysosomes and prevent the acidification of the phagosome. A number of parasites induce suppressor mechanisms which dampen or eliminate an effective host immune response. Other parasites can destroy mediators of inflammation involved in an effective immune response. For example, *Taenia* cestodes destroy complement components, and amebae produce factors that neutralize macrophage chemotaxis. Nematodes possess metabolically active

TABLE 170-2 Some mechanisms of parasite immune evasion

Parasite	Mechanism
Trypanosoma brucei, Giardia, Plasmodium merozoites	Antigenic variation
Plasmodium, Leishmania, T. cruzi	Escape into host cells
Toxoplasma gondii	Prevention of lysosome-phago-some fusion
Leishmania, Toxoplasma, T. brucei, T. cruzi	Inhibition of complement
Leishmania amastigotes	Prevention of lysosomal toxic action
Schistosomes	Acquisition of host molecules
Schistosomes	Antigenic mimicry
Schistosomes, Trichinella	Shedding of surface antigens
Schistosomes, filariae	Immune suppression
Schistosomes, Fasciola, T. cruzi	Cleavage of bound immunoglobulins
Schistosomes, parasitic nematodes	Surface and secreted antioxidant enzymes
Many tissue nematodes	Shedding of mucinous surface coat
Taenia, amebae	Inactivation of inflammatory mediators

cuticles which can absorb extrinsic molecules and secrete abundant quantities of parasite enzymes which may be important in evading innate and antibody-mediated host defenses. Many nematode parasites are also covered by an outermost surface glycocalyx which is rapidly turned over and can be sloughed off in the event of antibody-mediated leukocyte attachment.

ANTIGENIC VARIATION IN AFRICAN TRYPANOSOMES The protozoa that cause African sleeping sickness display a particularly fascinating and formidable mechanism of immune evasion. *T. brucei* possesses a thick surface coat made up of $>10^7$ molecules of a single antigenic glycoprotein. When laboratory animals are experimentally injected with cloned trypanosomes, all bearing the same surface antigen, successive waves of parasites appear in the blood similar to those seen when a human is bitten by an infected tsetse fly. Each wave consists mainly of organisms expressing a single variant surface glycoprotein (VSG) antigen that is different from VSGs expressed in previous peaks in the same infection. Each peak of parasitemia induces soluble antibody directed at the major VSG. However, the parasites escape immune destruction by periodically switching from one surface VSG to another VSG. A single trypanosome clone can sequentially produce hundreds of different VSGs! VSGs are linked to the parasite membrane by a glycosylphosphotidyl inositol (GPI) anchor, which allows rapid turnover of the exposed protein by the cleavage action of a specific phospholipase. Indeed, GPI anchoring of membrane surface proteins was first discovered in these parasite antigens. Molecular studies have shown that each VSG is encoded by a distinct gene and that only one VSG gene is usually expressed at a time from the hundreds available in the trypanosome genome. A VSG gene can be expressed following several different types of novel gene rearrangements. For example, a particular VSG gene to be expressed can be copied and transposed to a telomeric site on another chromosome which is used for expression. Only the duplicate gene, referred to as an *expression-linked copy*, is then expressed. If each VSG gene is visualized as a tape cassette in a library, then a selected VSG gene cassette is duplicated, and the duplicate cassette is removed from the library and inserted into a genetic tape deck to be played. Basic research on trypanosomes has led to the discovery of other unique molecular mechanisms that have expanded existing concepts of eukaryotic gene expression, including *trans* splicing and RNA editing. In the phenomenon of *trans* splicing, mRNAs from two noncontiguous segments of nuclear DNA, an invariant miniature exon and the protein-coding exon, are spliced together to produce a chimeric mRNA. RNA editing, which occurs in mitochondrial (kinetoplast) transcripts, entails the addition or deletion of uridine bases to mRNA, which results in the modification of noncoding primary transcripts (specified in the DNA) to mature mRNA molecules which do code

for proteins. Whether these novel molecular processes contribute to parasitism or could provide specific targets for antiparasite drug development is as yet unknown.

IMMUNE EVASION BY SCHISTOSOMES In schistosomiasis, the adult worms can live for decades in the human vasculature despite direct exposure to effector elements of the immune system, such as B and T lymphocytes and myelocytes. Schistosomes provide the most intensively studied examples of immune evasion among helminth parasites. Their battery of evasion strategies includes molecular mimicry, antigenic disguise, suppression of immune responses, and blocking antibodies. Following invasion, schistosomes can disguise themselves by acquiring host antigens that are incorporated into the outer lipid bilayer of the parasite tegument. These include blood group antigens, MHC glycoproteins, fibronectin, immunoglobulins, a C1q receptor, antiproteases, and a molecule resembling human decay accelerating factor. Schistosomes also produce a surface protein that mimics host alpha$_2$-macroglobulin. Their tegumental membrane is periodically turned over, and areas containing bound immunoglobulin can be shed. Schistosomes also produce immunomodulatory molecules such as β-endorphin as well as proteases that cleave immunoglobulins and interfere with complement action. Finally, ongoing antigenic stimulation by schistosome molecules can result in the preferential generation of IgM and irrelevant IgG antibodies (blocking antibodies) that may down-regulate effective humoral or cytotoxic cellular responses against the parasite.

IMMUNOLOGIC RESPONSES TO PARASITIC INFECTIONS

A variety of humoral and cell-mediated immune mechanisms have been found to be effective against parasites in vitro. However, the nature of protective immunity in vivo against most parasites is highly elusive. Protozoal and helminthic parasites present a complex panoply of antigens to the host. Different stages of the same parasite usually occupy different sites in the body, and each stage displays a distinct repertoire of antigens so that the parasite in effect presents a moving target to the host immune system. Furthermore, as discussed above, parasites have evolved numerous ways of escaping host defenses. In a typical chronic parasitic infection, the host mounts a series of immunologic responses which are unable to eliminate the parasite and in some cases lead to immunopathologic damage to host tissues. Few if any of these diverse host immune responses may prevent reinfection or limit the expression of clinical disease. For many parasitic infections, the evidence for acquired immunity rests on empirical epidemiologic observations. For example, population studies suggest that age-related resistance develops in schistosomiasis because adults have less intense infections and are less likely to become reinfected than children following curative chemotherapy. The dissection of protective immune responses, i.e., those which parasites *cannot* evade, is the central challenge of parasite immunology.

IMMUNE EFFECTOR MECHANISMS AGAINST PARASITES These include antibodies, antibody-dependent cell-mediated cytotoxicity, activated macrophages, CD8+ cytotoxic T cells, and possibly natural killer cells. Antibodies can be effective against intracellular protozoa by blocking receptors involved in host cell entry. For example, antibodies against some of the malarial merozoite proteins mentioned above can block erythrocyte invasion, and antibodies against gp63 can prevent *Leishmania* from infecting macrophages in vitro. Antibodies are also an integral component of the classical complement pathway, in which lytic killing of target cells follows opsonization by antibody. African trypanosomes can be lysed in vitro by serum complement in the presence of antibodies against VSG, but complement-mediated killing is probably not significant in actual human infection with trypanosomes and most other parasites.

In the laboratory, purified eosinophils will kill schistosomules of *S. mansoni* if the schistosomules have been coated previously with specific antiparasite IgG antibodies, a phenomenon known as *antibody-dependent cell-mediated cytotoxicity* (ADCC). This mechanism entails the attachment of eosinophils to the Fc portion of the IgG via an Fc receptor, followed by the release of toxic eosinophil granule proteins which kill the schistosome larvae. If antibodies contact the parasite surface, macrophages and even platelets can be shown in vitro to attach to these antibodies through their Fc receptors and kill parasites. Interferon-γ (IFN-γ) and other cytokines such as migration inhibitory factor (MIF) and tumor necrosis factor α (TNFα) can activate effector cells to enhance antibody-dependent parasite killing.

IMMUNOREGULATION BY T CELLS AND CYTOKINES Some of the most exciting new developments in immunology research concern T lymphocytes and their secreted cytokines, which have been shown to strongly influence both protective immunity and immunopathology in parasitic infections. CD4 + helper T cells can be classified into two major subsets, T_{H1} and T_{H2}, based on differential profiles of cytokine secretion, according to evidence derived from murine models and recently extended to cultured human T cells. T_{H1} cells produce IFN-γ and interleukin 2 (IL-2) and are responsible for cell-mediated immune reactions such as delayed-type hypersensitivity. IFN-γ provides a key signal that activates macrophages to kill intracellular organisms by reactive oxygen intermediates and nitric oxide. Animals injected with antibodies to IFN-γ or transgenic mice with disrupted genes for IFN-γ or the IFN-γ receptor are highly susceptible to *Leishmania,* mycobacteria, and other intracellular pathogens. T_{H2} cells, on the other hand, release IL-4, IL-5, and other cytokines which result in eosinophilia, elevated serum IgE, and mastocytosis, which are seen in both allergic reactions and helminthic infections.

Experimental infections with *L. major,* a cause of cutaneous leishmaniasis, have provided the strongest evidence of genetically controlled T cell–mediated resistance to a parasitic infection. Cutaneous infection of most inbred mouse strains with *L. major* provides a T_{H1} response with abundant local generation of IFN-γ, which in turn results in a limited skin lesion that heals spontaneously and confers resistance to reinfection. Certain other inbred mouse strains instead mount a T_{H2}-type response upon infection, with very little production of IFN-γ, and here the infection progresses to a disseminated and ultimately fatal form of leishmaniasis. CD8 + T cells, which produce high levels of IFN-γ and can kill infected host cells, also appear to play an important role in protecting against certain intracellular protozoa. In experimental models CD8 + T cells have recently been shown to confer resistance against *T. cruzi, T. gondii,* and the preerythryocytic liver stages of malaria. Whereas T_{H1} cells play a protective role against *Leishmania* and shistosomes, T_{H2} cells protect against certain nematodes.

EOSINOPHILS, IgE, AND IMMUNITY IN HELMINTHIC INFECTIONS The immunologic hallmarks of chronic infection with parasitic helminths include eosinophilia, elevated IgE levels, and in certain cases mastocytosis. These responses appear to be induced mainly by T_{H2} cytokines: IL-5 stimulates eosinophilopoiesis, IL-4 induces immunoglobulin isotype switching to IgE, and IL-4 and other cytokines stimulate mastocytosis. Eosinophils have been thought to play a protective function in helminthic infections because of their potency in killing schistosomes and other helminths via ADCC. Helminthic parasites also can be killed in vitro by IgE-mediated activation of macrophages and other cytotoxic cells. It is unclear, however, whether eosinophils and IgE protect against helminthic infections in vivo. Field studies of schistosomiasis in Africa showed that adults, who had high levels of antiparasite IgE, were far less likely to become reinfected following chemotherapy than children, who had low levels of antischistosome IgE, despite comparable exposure to infection through cercariae-infested waters. Rats made specifically IgE-deficient by repeated injections of antiepsilon chain antibodies show a markedly impaired resistance to *Trichinella* infection. However, the depletion in rodents of IgE by injection of monoclonal antibodies to IL-4 does not influence resistance to *S. mansoni* and other helminthic infections. Similarly, administration of monoclonal antibodies to IL-5 drastically reduces blood and tissue eosinophils in rodents but does not alter their worm burden or resistance to reinfection with schistosomes or *Trichinella.*

In animals that have established chronic infections with adult schistosome worms, new invading cercariae are destroyed while the adult worms remain unaffected—an unusual form of immunity called *concomitant immunity.* Of note, T_{H1}-type responses, characterized by high IFN-γ and IL-2 levels, predominate early in schistosome infection and are also associated with protective immunity induced by vaccination with irradiated cercariae. On the other hand, a T_{H2} pattern of response (with high levels of IL-4 but low levels of IFN-γ) characterizes the granulomatous reaction to schistosome eggs in the liver and may thus contribute to the immunopathology of hepatosplenic schistosomiasis. These disparate immunologic features of the same disease may be somewhat reconciled by considering that different parasite stages, localized to different organs, may stimulate different T cell–mediated immune responses that can result in organ-specific sequelae ranging from true protection to tolerance to immunopathology.

IMMUNOPATHOLOGY Schistosomiasis can be considered an immunologic disease, i.e., host immune responses to the parasite are largely responsible for disease manifestations. Cercarial dermatitis is believed to be due to a hypersensitivity reaction to cercarial proteins. Acute schistosomiasis or Katayama fever is a serum sickness–like syndrome characterized by fever, hepatosplenomegaly, and urticaria. The intense eosinophilia, complement activation, and immune-complex formation in this syndrome are due to immediate hypersensitivity reactions to egg antigens once adult worms begin to lay eggs. Local and systemic allergic reactions are encountered in the course of many other tissue helminthic infections, including hydatid cyst rupture, tropical pulmonary eosinophilia (occult filariasis), pulmonary ascariasis, acute trichinosis, and the larva migrans syndromes. Compelling evidence indicates that the lesions of chronic hepatosplenic schistosomiasis are due to T cell–mediated granulomatous reactions to schistosomal egg antigens. Indeed, tumor necrosis factor alpha (TNFα), a T cell–derived cytokine, has recently been found to trigger the granulomatous response to schistosome eggs in severe combined immunodeficient mice (which lack functional B and T cells). Interestingly, egg output by adult female worms increases dramatically both in vitro and vivo upon administration of TNFα, suggesting that schistosomes exploit the cytokine network for their own reproduction. Chronic delayed-type hypersensitivity responses are also the basis of lymphatic destruction leading to elephantiasis in filarial infection. Host responses may be further modified by anti-idiotypic antibodies or anti-idiotypic T cells, which arise when the antigen binding site (idiotype) of the original antiparasite antibody induces antibodies or T cells whose antigen combining site recognizes the idiotype.

VACCINES AGAINST PARASITIC DISEASES?

The reawakening of scientific interest in parasite biology has stimulated immunologic approaches to the control of parasitic infections. The preceding discussion makes it clear that the development of antiparasite vaccines will not be an easy task, and in fact, no vaccine against any human parasitic disease has yet been successfully produced. Because the nature of protective immunity in parasitic infections is poorly understood, approaches to vaccine development have been essentially empirical. Such approaches must consider the entire repertoire of stage-specific parasite antigens and host immune responses to those antigens. Development of a vaccine against filariasis, for example, must take into account the fact that the disease largely results from deleterious host immune responses rather than toxic effects of the parasite itself. The use of killed or attenuated organisms, as for many viral and bacterial vaccines, is not practicable for human parasites because they cannot be produced in the industrial quantities necessary for mass immunization. Subunit vaccines based on parasite protein or carbohydrate antigens are therefore desirable and could be produced with use of recombinant DNA or peptide synthesis technologies. Some of these scientific issues are illustrated in the ongoing saga of vaccine development for malaria.

MALARIA VACCINE Intensive work is under way on vaccines for *P. falciparum*, the most malignant malaria parasite. Following initial infection, humoral immune responses are minimal until the merozoite stage. These asexual blood stages are antigenically diverse and can undergo antigenic variation with each successive erythrocytic cycle. It is unclear whether any of the antibodies generated to merozoite antigens are protective or correlate with less severe disease. The best evidence for the existence of immunity in humans is in areas that are highly endemic for malaria. Here, repeatedly infected individuals develop a more chronic, benign infection with low parasitemia and often no symptoms, in contrast to severe parasitemia and attendant complications that occur in young children or immigrants and travelers to the area.

Sporozoite vaccine The cardinal impetus for the development of a sporozoite vaccine was the demonstration that humans and experimental animals can be protected against sporozoite infection by prior vaccination with irradiated sporozoites. This "vaccination" was accomplished by allowing irradiated infected mosquitoes (containing irradiated sporozoites incapable of dividing) to bite volunteers. Laboratory studies showed that antibodies from protected individuals neutralized sporozoites by binding specifically to the CSP. Furthermore, monoclonal antibodies to CSP could passively transfer protection against malaria in naive mice and monkeys. Molecular cloning of the CSP gene revealed the target epitopes of protective antibodies to be a central domain consisting of 23 repeats of the amino acid sequence NANP or NVDP. However, trials of recombinant or synthetic sporozoite vaccines in humans have been disappointing because the vaccines elicited poor antibody responses, and parasitemia was prevented in only a few individuals who had high titers of antibody. Efforts are underway to enhance immunogenicity by using new adjuvants and by combining the CSP repeat sequence with potent T cell epitopes found elsewhere in the molecule.

Accumulating experimental evidence indicates that cell-mediated immune responses are important in protection against malaria. For example, IFN-γ and CD8+ cytotoxic T cells inhibit the early liver stages of malarial parasites. Furthermore, an oral vaccine consisting of an attenuated strain of *Salmonella typhimurium* transfected with the CSP gene induced cellular and not humoral responses in mice and yet protected them from challenge with live sporozoites. Incorporating T cell immunogens into a genetically engineered peptide vaccine also would allow natural boosting of immunity in endemic areas by infective mosquito bites. However, individual T cell epitopes may be limited by the MHC-restricted responsiveness to peptide epitopes in human populations. Finally, an antisporozoite vaccine would have to be virtually 100 percent effective to prevent disease, since a person can still develop malaria even if only a few sporozoites manage to escape immune destruction.

Blood-stage vaccine Other potential targets for a malaria vaccine are the asexual blood stages that are responsible for the clinical symptoms and pathology. Unlike a sporozoite vaccine, a vaccine directed against blood stages would still be beneficial if parasitemia were only partially reduced. A large number of merozoite and infected erythrocyte antigens have been identified and cloned. Monoclonal antibodies to some of these blood-stage antigens confer passive protection in rodent malaria, and antigens purified with use of these antibodies can induce protective immunity. Some success has been achieved in protecting primates with blood-stage vaccines by the use of recombinant or synthesized antigens combined with complete Freund's adjuvant.

In an unconventional approach pioneered in Colombia, a blood-stage vaccine was chemically synthesized by polymerization of three different merozoite antigens together with the NANP repeat peptide of CSP. This polymeric vaccine, known as SPf66, substantially reduced the risk of falciparum malaria in immunized volunteers in a recent large Colombian field trial and will undergo further trials in

Africa and Southeast Asia. Of note, there was no correlation between antibody levels and protection, and continual natural boosting by mosquito bites in the malarious region was necessary to establish strong immunity, thus strongly suggesting a key role for cell-mediated immune mechanisms. This exciting new development represents one of the most encouraging results to date of prototype malaria vaccines.

Gametocyte vaccine Gametocytes, the sexual stages of malaria, do not cause clinical symptoms but are responsible for malaria transmission via mosquitoes in the population at large. Antibodies to gametocytes would be taken up in the mosquito blood meal and block further sexual development within the mosquito. Several monoclonal antibodies to isolated gametocyte antigens do prevent the fertilization of gametocytes in the mosquito. Transmission-blocking vaccines will not protect the individual but could substantially reduce the incidence and prevalence of malaria in certain endemic areas.

Antidisease vaccine Host cytokines that are generated in response to specific malarial antigens can contribute to the clinical manifestations of malaria. In particular, TNFα, produced by activated macrophages, has been found to potentiate many of the complications of malaria such as anemia and cytoadherence. Thus an "antidisease" vaccine directed against TNF-inducing antigens, as opposed to an "antiparasite" vaccine, might be effective in preventing such pathologic consequences. Indeed, animals immunized with a *P. falciparum* antigen responsible for TNF production survive high levels of parasitemia that kill unvaccinated animals. Alternatively, a vaccine that could block the cytoadherence of *P. falciparum*–infected erythrocytes to endothelium might prevent cerebral malaria, which is often lethal.

Conclusion An effective malaria vaccine will probably have to comprise a cocktail of antigens from several stages of the parasite life cycle, together with epitopes that stimulate T cells and possibly immunomodulators that stimulate protective cytokines. A highly successful recombinant vaccine has recently been developed against a veterinary parasite, the cestode *Taenia ovis* in sheep. In this case, a fusion protein consisting of a recombinant defined cestode antigen linked to a schistosome glutathione-*S*-transferase proved to be highly protective against challenge infection. This achievement demonstrates the feasibility of employing modern immunologic and molecular approaches in the development of antiparasite vaccines. Such vaccines could prove a highly cost-effective means of protecting the great masses of humanity who are exposed to serious parasitic infections.

REFERENCES

Ash C, Gallagher RB (eds): *Immunoparasitology Today.* Cambridge, Elsevier Trends Journals, 1991

David JR: Host-parasite interface: immune invasion, in *Tropical and Geographic Medicine,* 2d ed, KS Warren, AAF Mahmoud (eds). New York, McGraw-Hill, 1990, p 117

Englund PT, Sher A (eds): *The Biology of Parasitism.* New York, Liss, 1988

Mahmoud AAF: Parasitic protozoa and helminths: Biological and immunological challenges. Science 246:1015, 1989

Maizels RM et al: Immunological modulation and evasion by helminth parasites in human populations. Nature 365:797, 1993

Mendis KN: Malaria vaccine research: a game of chess, in *Malaria: Waiting for the Vaccine,* GAT Targett (ed). New York, Wiley, 1992, p 183

Sher A, Coffman RL: Regulation of immunity to parasites by T cells and T cell–derived cytokines. Annu Rev Immunol 10:385, 1992

Wang CC (ed): *Molecular and Immunological Aspects of Parasitism.* Washington, American Association for the Advancement of Science, 1991

Warren KS (ed): *Immunology and Molecular Biology of Parasitic Infections,* 3d ed. Oxford, Blackwell, 1993

Wyler DJ (ed): *Modern Parasite Biology: Cellular, Immunological, and Molecular Aspects.* New York, Freeman, 1990

171 LABORATORY DIAGNOSIS OF PARASITIC INFECTIONS

CHARLES E. DAVIS

The cornerstone for the diagnosis of parasitic infections is a careful history of the patient's illness. Epidemiologic aspects of the illness are especially important because the risks of acquiring many parasites are closely related to occupation, recreation, or travel to areas of high endemicity. Without a basic knowledge of the epidemiology and life cycles of the major parasites, it is difficult to approach the diagnosis of parasitic infections systematically. Accordingly, the medical classification of important human parasites in this chapter emphasizes their geographic distribution, their transmission, and the anatomic location and stages of the life cycle that occur in people. The text and tables are intended to serve as a guide to the correct diagnostic procedures for the major parasitic infections and to direct the reader to subsequent chapters which contain more comprehensive information about each infection. Tables 171-1 to 171-3 summarize the geographic distributions, anatomic locations, and the laboratory methods employed for the diagnosis of parasitic infections.

In addition to selecting the correct diagnostic procedures, physicians also must counsel their patients to ensure that specimens are collected properly and arrive at the laboratory promptly. For example, the diagnosis of Bancroftian filariasis is unlikely to be confirmed by laboratory personnel unless blood is drawn near midnight when the nocturnal microfilariae are active. The motile, erythrophagocytic trophozoites of *Entamoeba histolytica* are fragile and will not be detected in fecal specimens that arrive at the laboratory several hours after collection. Laboratory personnel and surgical pathologists should be notified in advance when a parasitic infection is suspected. Continuing interaction with the laboratory staff and the surgical pathologists helps to ensure that parasites in body fluids or biopsy specimens are examined carefully by the most capable individuals.

INTESTINAL PARASITES Most helminths and protozoa exit the body in the fecal stream. The patient or attendant should be instructed

TABLE 171-1 Flatworm infections

| Parasite | Geographic distribution | Life-cycle hosts | | Parasite stage | Diagnosis | | |
		Intermediate (transmission)	Definitive		Body fluid or tissue	Serologic test	Other
TAPEWORMS (CESTODES)							
Intestinal tapeworms							
Taenia saginata (beef tapeworm)	Worldwide	Beef	Humans	Ova, segments	Feces	—	Motile segments
Hymenolepis nana (dwarf tapeworm)	Worldwide	Grain beetle	Humans, mouse*	Ova	Feces	—	—
Diphyllobothrium latum (fish tapeworm)	Worldwide	Copepods–fish‡	Humans, other mammals	Ova, segments	Feces	—	Megaloblastic anemia in 1%
Taenia solium† (pork tapeworm)	Worldwide	Swine	Humans	Ova, segments	Feces	WB	Esp. Mexico, C. and S. America, Africa
Somatic tapeworms							
Echinococcus granulosus (hydatid disease)	Sheep raising and hunting areas	Sheep, camels, humans, others	Dogs	Hydatid	Lung, liver	WB	Chest x-ray, CT, MRI
Echinococcus multilocularis (hydatid disease)	Subarctic	Rodents, humans	Fox, dog, cat	Hydatid	Liver	—	May resemble cholangiocellular Ca
Taenia solium† (pork tapeworm)	Worldwide	Swine, humans	Humans	Cysticercus	Muscles, CNS	WB	CT, MRI, x-ray
FLUKES (TREMATODES)							
Intestinal flukes							
Fasciolopsis buski	China, India	Snail–water chestnut	Humans	Ova	Feces	—	—
Heterophyes heterophyes	Far East, India	Snail–fish	Humans	Ova	Feces	—	—
Metagonimus yokogawai	Focal in Europe and N. Africa	Snail–fish	Humans	Ova	Feces	—	—
Liver flukes							
Clonorchis sinensis	China, S.E. Asia	Snail–fish	Humans	Ova	Feces, bile	—	Recurrent bacterial cholangitis
Fasciola hepatica	Sheep raising areas	Snail–watercress	Humans, sheep	Ova	Feces, bile	—	Cirrhosis, portal hypertension
Lung flukes							
Paragonimus spp.	Orient, Africa, S. America	Snail–crabs/crayfish	Humans, other mammals	Adults, ova	Lung, sputum, CNS	WB	Chest x-ray, CT, MRI
Blood flukes							
Schistosoma mansoni	Africa, C. and S. America, W. Indies	Snail	Humans	Ova, adults	Feces	EIA	Rectal snips, liver biopsy
Schistosoma haematobium	Africa	Snail	Humans	Ova, adults	Urine	EIA	Liver, urine, or bladder biopsy
Schistosoma japonicum	Far East	Snail	Humans	Ova, adults	Feces	EIA	Liver biopsy

NOTE: WB = Western blot; CF = complement fixation; EIA = enzyme immunoassay; serologic tests listed in Tables 171-1, 171-2, and 171-3 are available from the Centers for Disease Control and Prevention (CDC), Atlanta, Ga.
* Larvae also can mature in intestinal villi of humans and mice.
† *Taenia solium* can cause either intestinal infections or cysticercosis. Ova are identical to *T. saginata;* scolices and segments differ.
‡ When there are two intermediate hosts, the first is separated from the second by a hyphen. Definitive hosts are infected by the second intermediate host.

TABLE 171-2 Roundworm infections

Parasite	Geographic distribution	Life-cycle hosts		Diagnosis			
		Intermediate (transmission)	Definitive	Parasite stage	Body fluid or tissue	Serologic tests	Other
INTESTINAL ROUNDWORMS							
Enterobius vermicularis (pinworm)	Temperate and tropical zones	Fecal-oral	Humans	Ova	Perianal skin	—	"Scotch tape" test
Trichuris trichiura (whipworm)	Temperate and tropical zones	Soil, fecal-oral	Humans	Ova	Feces	—	Rectal prolapse
Ascaris lumbricoides (roundworm of man)	Temperate and tropical zones	Soil, fecal-oral	Humans	Ova	Feces		Sx of pulmonary migration
Ancylostoma duodenale (old world hookworm)	EuroAsia, Africa, Pacific	Soil→skin	Humans	Ova/larvae	Feces	—	Sx of pulmonary migration, anemia
Necator americanus (new world hookworm)	U.S., Africa, worldwide	Soil→skin	Humans	Ova/larvae	Feces	—	Sx of pulmonary migration, anemia
Strongyloides stercoralis (strongylodiasis)	Moist tropics and subtropics	Soil→skin	Humans	Larvae	Feces, sputum, duodenal fluid	EIA	Dissemination in immunodeficiency
TISSUE ROUNDWORMS							
Trichinella spiralis (trichinosis)	Worldwide	Swine/humans	Swine/humans	Larvae	Muscle	BF	Muscle biopsy
Wuchereria bancrofti (filariasis)	Coastal in tropics and subtropics	Mosquito	Humans	Microfilariae	Blood, lymph nodes	—	Nocturnal periodicity*
Brugia malayi (filariasis)	Asia, Indian subcontinent	Mosquito	Humans	Microfilariae	Blood	—	Nocturnal
Loa loa (African eye worm)	West and Central Africa	Mango fly (chrysops)	Humans	Microfilariae	Blood	—	May be visible in eye, diurnal
Onchocerca volvulus (river blindness)	Africa, Mexico, C. and S. America	Black flies	Humans	Adults/larvae	Skin/eye	—	Examine nodules or skin snips
Dracunculus medinensis (guinea worm)	Orient, Africa, W. Indies, Brazil	Cyclops	Humans	Adults/larvae	Skin	—	May be visible in lesion
LARVA MIGRANS SYNDROMES							
Ancylostoma braziliensis (creeping eruption)	Tropical and temperate zones	Soil→skin	Dog/cat, humans	Larvae	Skin	—	Dog and cat hookworm
Toxocara canis and *cati* (visceral larva migrans)	Tropical and temperate zones	Soil, fecal-oral	Dog/cat, humans	Larvae	Viscera, CNS, eye	EIA	Also caused by roundworms of other spp.

NOTE: BF = bentonite flocculation
* Blood should be drawn at midnight, except for infection acquired in the South Pacific.

to collect feces in a clean cardboard container and to record the time of collection on the container. Contamination with water, which could contain free-living protozoa, or urine should be avoided. Fecal samples should be collected before ingestion of barium or other contrast agents for radiologic procedures and before treatment with antidiarrheal agents and antacids because these substances change the consistency of the feces and interfere with microscopic detection of parasites. Cyclic shedding of most parasites in the feces requires examination of a minimum of three samples collected on alternate days. When delays in transport to the laboratory are unavoidable or specimens must be shipped by mail, fecal samples should be kept in polyvinyl alcohol to preserve protozoal trophozoites. Refrigeration also will preserve trophozoites for a few hours and protozoal cysts and helminth ova for several days.

Analysis of fecal samples consists of both a macroscopic and a microscopic examination. Watery or loose stools are more likely to contain protozoal trophozoites, but protozoal cysts and all stages of helminths may be found in formed feces. If adult worms or tapeworm segments are observed in the physician's office or on the wards, they should be transported promptly to the laboratory or washed and preserved in fixative for later examination. The only tapeworm with

motile segments is *Taenia saginata*, the beef tapeworm, which patients will sometimes bring to the physician. Motility is an important distinction, because the ova of *T. saginata* and *T. solium*, the cause of cysticercosis, are indistinguishable.

Microscopic examination of the feces (See also Table 171-4) Microscopic examination of feces is not complete until direct wet mounts, concentration techniques, and permanent stains have been examined. The physician should insist that the laboratory conduct each of these procedures before accepting the final report as negative for ova and parasites. Some intestinal parasites are more readily detected in anatomic locations other than feces. For example, the string test or its commercial substitutes to sample duodenal contents is sometimes necessary to detect *Giardia lamblia* and *Cryptosporidium*. The "Scotch tape" technique to detect pinworm ova on the perianal skin will sometimes reveal ova of *T. saginata* deposited perianally when the motile segments disintegrate (see Table 171-4).

Two routine solutions are used to make wet mounts for the identification of the various life stages of helminths and protozoa: physiologic saline for trophozoites, cysts, ova, and larvae and dilute iodine solution for staining protozoal cysts and ova. Iodine solution

TABLE 171-3 Protozoal infections

Parasite	Geographic distribution	Life-cycle hosts		Diagnosis			
		Intermediate (transmission)	Definitive	Parasite stage	Body fluid or tissue	Serologic tests	Other
INTESTINAL PROTOZOANS							
Entamoeba histolytica (amebiasis)	Worldwide, esp. tropics	Fecal-oral	Humans	Troph, cyst	Feces, liver	ID,* IHA	Ultrasound, CT liver
Giardia lamblia (giardiasis)	Worldwide	Fecal-oral	Humans	Troph, cyst	Feces	AG detection	String test
Isospora belli	Worldwide	Fecal-oral	Humans	Oocysts	Feces	—	Acid-fast
Cryptosporidium	Worldwide	Fecal-oral	Humans and animals	Oocysts	Feces	AG detection	Acid-fast, biopsy
Enterocytozoon bieneusi (microsporidiosis)	Worldwide?	?	Animals, humans	Spores	Feces	—	Modified trichrome, biopsy
FREE-LIVING AMEBAS							
Naegleria	Worldwide	Warm water	Humans	Troph, cyst	CNS, nares	—	Biopsy, nasal swab
Acanthamoeba	Worldwide	Soil, water	Humans	Troph, cyst	CNS, skin, cornea	—	Biopsy, scrapings
BLOOD AND TISSUE PROTOZOANS							
Plasmodium spp. (malaria)	Subtropics and tropics	Mosquito	Humans	Asexual	Blood	Little use	—
Babesia microti (babesiosis)	U.S., esp. New England	Tick	Rodents, humans	Asexual	Blood	IIF	Animal spp. in asplenia
Trypanosoma rhodesiense (Afr. sleeping sickness)	Subsaharan E. Africa	Tsetse fly	Humans, herbivores	Tryp	Blood, CSF	Card agglut, IIF†	Also chancre, lymph nodes
Trypanosoma gambiense (Afr. sleeping sickness)	Subsaharan W. Africa	Tsetse fly	Humans, swine	Tryp	Blood, CSF	Card agglut, IIF†	Also chancre, lymph nodes
Trypanosoma cruzi (Chagas disease)	Mexico→S. America	Reduviid bugs (triatomes)	Humans, dogs and wild animals	Amastigotes, Tryp	Multiple organs/blood	CF, IIF	Reactivation in immunosuppressed
Leishmania tropica, etc.	Widespread in tropics and subtropics	Sand flies (phlebotomus)	Humans, dogs, rodents	Amastigotes	Skin	EIA‡	Biopsy, scraping, culture
Leishmania braziliensis (mucocutaneous)	Mexico→S. America	Sand flies (lutzomyia)	Humans, dogs, rodents	Amastigotes	Skin mucous membranes	EIA‡	Biopsy, scraping, culture
Leishmania donovani (kala-azar)	Widespread in tropics and subtropics	Sand flies (phlebotomus)	Humans, dogs, wild animals	Amastigotes	RE system	EIA‡	Biopsy, culture
Toxoplasma gondii (toxoplasmosis)	Worldwide	Humans, other mammals	Cats	Cyst, troph	CNS, eye, muscles, other	EIA, IIF	Reactivation in immunosuppressed
Pneumocystis carinii	Worldwide	?	Humans	Cyst, troph	Lung, Other	—	Induced sputum, biopsy

* ID = immunodiffusion by commerical kit (not available at the CDC); IHA = indirect hemagglutination; AG = antigen; CF = complement fixation; Troph = trophozoite; Tryp = trypomastigote form; IIF = indirect immunofluorescence

† Card agglutination provided to endemic countries by the World Health Organization; IIF available intermittently—contact the WHO or CDC.

‡ Limited specificity.

must never be used to examine specimens for trophozoites because it kills the parasites and destroys their characteristic motility.

The two most common concentration procedures for detecting small numbers of cysts and ova are formalin-ether sedimentation and zinc sulfate flotation. The formalin-ether technique is preferable because all parasites sediment, but not all float. Permanently stained slides for trophozoites should be prepared before concentration. Additional stained slides for cysts and ova may be made from the concentrate.

In many instances, especially in differentiation of *E. histolytica* from other amebae, identification from wet mounts or concentrates must be considered tentative. Permanently stained smears allow study of the cellular detail necessary for definitive identification. The iron-hematoxylin stain is excellent for critical work, but the trichrome stain, which can be completed in 1 h, is a satisfactory alternative that also stains parasites in specimens preserved in PVA fixative.

BLOOD AND TISSUE PARASITES   Protozoa and helminths invading the tissues present a more difficult problem in the choice of

diagnostic techniques. For example, physicians must understand that aspiration of an amebic liver abscess rarely reveals *E. histolytica* because the trophozoites are located primarily in the abscess wall. They must remember to order an examination of the sputum for ova of *Paragonimus westermani* in the Southeast Asian immigrant with a cystic lung lesion (Table 171-5) and know that the urine sediment offers the best opportunity to detect *Schistosoma haematobium* in the Ethiopian youngster or American traveler who returns from Africa with hematuria (Table 171-6). Tables 171-1, 171-2, and 171-3, which offer a quick guide to the geographic distribution and anatomic locations of the major tissue parasites, should help the physician to select the appropriate body fluid or biopsy site for microscopic examination. Tables 171-5 through 171-8 provide additional information about identification of parasites in samples from specific anatomic locations. The laboratory procedures for detection of parasites from other body fluids are similar to those used in the examination of feces. The physician should insist on wet mounts, concentration techniques, and permanent stains of all body fluids. The trichrome or iron-

TABLE 171-4 Laboratory diagnosis of parasites found in feces*

Parasites and fecal stages	Alternative diagnostic procedures
TAPEWORMS (CESTODES)	
Taenia saginata ova and segments	Perianal "Scotch tape" test for ova
Hymenolepis nana ova	None
Diphyllobothrium ova and segments	None
Taenia solium ova and segments	Brain bx for neurocysticercosis; serology
FLUKES (TREMATODES)	
Fasciolopsis buski ova	None
Heterophyes heterophyes ova	None
Metagonimus yokogawai ova	None
Clonorchis sinensis ova	Examine bile for ova and adults in cholangitis
Fasciola hepatica ova	Examine bile for ova and adults in cholangitis
Paragonimus spp. ova	Sputum, lung bx, or brain bx for ova; serology
Schistosoma ova	Rectal snips (esp. *S. mansoni*), urine (*S. haematobium*), liver bx, and serology for all
ROUNDWORMS	
Enterobius vermicularis ova and adults	Perianal "Scotch tape" test for ova and adults
Trichuris trichiura ova	None
Ascaris lumbricoides ova and adults	Examine sputum for larvae in lung disease
Hookworm ova and occasional larvae	Examine sputum for larvae in lung disease
Strongyloides larvae	Duodenal asp. or jejunal bx‡; sputum or lung bx for filariform larvae in disseminated disease; serology
Capillaria phillipinensis ova†	None
PROTOZOANS	
Entamoeba histolytica trophs and cysts	Liver bx for trophs; serology
Giardia lamblia trophs and cysts	Duodenal aspirate or jejunal bx‡
Isospora belli oocysts	Duodenal aspirate or jejunal bx‡
Cryptosporidium oocysts	Duodenal aspirate or jejunal bx‡
Enterocytozoon bieneusi spores	Duodenal aspirate or jejunal bx‡

* Stains and concentration techniques are discussed in the text.
† Can be confused with *Trichuris trichiura*.
‡ Commercial string test or Crosby capsule are satisfactory; *Isospora* and *Cryptosporidium* are acid-fast.

TABLE 171-5 Laboratory diagnosis of parasitic infections of the lungs

	Parasite stage(s)	Stains
SPUTUM*/BRONCHOALVEOLAR LAVAGE		
Pneumocystis carinii	Trophs and cysts	Methenamine silver, toluidine blue, indirect immunofluorescence test
Ascaris lumbricoides	Third-stage larvae	Wet mount, trichrome, iron-hematoxylin, Giemsa
Hookworms	Filariform larvae	Same as *Ascaris*
Strongyloides	Filariform larvae	Same as *Ascaris*
Paragonimus spp.	Ova	Same as *Ascaris*
Entamoeba histolytica	Trophozoites	Same as *Ascaris*
Echinococcus	Scolices	Wet mount, acid-fast
Toxocara species	Larvae	Same as *Ascaris*
LUNG BIOPSY (OPEN OR TRANSBRONCHIAL)		
Pneumocystis carinii	Trophs and cysts	H&E‡ and as above
Paragonimus spp.	Adults and ova	H&E, iron-hematoxylin
Entamoeba histolytica	Trophozoites	Same as *Paragonimus*
Echinococcus	Hydatid, scolices	H&E‡, iron-hematoxylin, acid-fast
Schistosoma spp.	Ova	H&E, iron-hematoxylin
Brugia and *Wuchereria*†	Microfilariae	H&E, Giemsa
Toxocara spp.	Larvae	Same as *Paragonimus*

* Induced sputum for *Pneumocystis*. There are no data for the efficacy of induced sputum or BAL in the diagnosis of the other parasites. Transbronchial brush may be included in BAL.
† In lymphatic filariasis and tropical pulmonary eosinophilia.
‡ Hematoxylin and eosin for typical histopathology and for detection of all parasites except *Pneumocystis*.

TABLE 171-6 Identification of parasites in blood and other body fluids

	Enrichment/stain	Culture technique
BLOOD		
Plasmodium spp.	Thick and thin smears/ Giemsa or Wright's	Not useful for diagnosis
Leishmania spp.	Buffy coat/Giemsa	Media available from CDC
African trypanosomes*	Buffy coat, anion column/wet mount, and Giemsa	Mouse or rat inoculation*
Trypanosoma cruzi†	As for African species	As above and xenodiagnosis
Toxoplasma gondii	Buffy coat/Giemsa	Fibroblast cell lines
Microfilariae‡	Nuclepore filtration/ wet mount, and Giemsa	None
URINE§		
Schistosoma haematobium	Centrifugation/wet mount	None
Microfilariae (in chyluria)	As for blood	None
SPINAL FLUID		
African trypanosomes	Centrifugation, anion column/wet mount, and Giemsa	As for blood
Naegleria fowleri	Centrifugation/wet mount, and Giemsa or trichrome	Nonnutrient agar overlaid with *E. coli*

* *T. rhodesiense* and *T. gambiense*. Inject mice intraperitoneally with 0.2 mL whole heparinized blood (0.5 mL for rats). After 5 days, tail blood should be checked daily for trypanosomes as described above.
† Detectable in blood by conventional techniques only during acute disease. Xenodiagnosis is successful in about 50 percent of patients with chronic Chagas' disease.
‡ Day (1000–1400) and night (2200–0200) blood should be drawn to maximize the chance of detecting *Wuchereria* (nocturnal except for Pacific strains), *Brugia* (nocturnal), and *Loa Loa* (diurnal).
§ *Trichomonas vaginalis* is often detectable in urine, but examination of vaginal secretions is probably the preferable technique.

hematoxylin stains are satisfactory for all tissue helminths in body fluids other than blood, but microfilarial worms and the blood protozoa are more easily visualized when stained with Giemsa or Wright's stain.

The most common parasites detected in Giemsa-stained blood smears are the plasmodia, microfilariae, and African trypanosomes (see Table 171-6). Most patients with Chagas' disease present in the chronic phase when *T. cruzi* is no longer microscopically detectable in blood smears. Wet mounts are sometimes more sensitive than stained smears for the detection of microfilariae and the African trypanosomes because these active parasites cause noticeable movement of the erythrocytes in the microscopic field. Nuclepore filtration of blood facilitates detection of microfilariae. The intracellular amastigote forms of *Leishmania* spp. and *T. cruzi* can sometimes be visualized in stained smears of peripheral blood, but aspirates of the bone marrow, liver, and spleen are the best sources for microscopic detection and culture of *Leishmania* in kala-azar and *T. cruzi* in chronic Chagas' disease.

The diagnosis of malaria and the critical differentiation among the *Plasmodium* spp. is made by microscopic examination of stained thick and thin blood films (see Table 171-7). Most malariologists

TABLE 171-7   Differential diagnosis of *Plasmodium* species in blood smears

	Falciparum	*Vivax*	*Malariae*	*Ovale*
FEATURE OF RBC				
Size	All sizes	Large (young)	Small (old)	Large (young)
Shape	Round; may be crenated	Round or oval	Round	Round or pear-shaped, fimbriated
Stippling	Maurer's clefts: large, red (up to 20)	Schuffner's dots: numerous, small red dots	None	Schuffner's dots
FEATURE OF PARASITE				
Ring trophozoite	Thread-like, multiple infections, double chromatin dots, accole forms*	Thicker	Compact	Compact
Mature trophozoites	Absent	Ameboid, may fill cell	More regular, smaller, band forms†	Less ameboid and smaller than vivax
Schizonts	Absent	12 to 24 merozoites	8 to 12 merozoites often rosetted around pigment	8 to 12 merozoites
Gametocytes	Banana-shaped, central chromatin (female) or diffuse (male)	Round, fills cell, pigment often central	Round, large, coarse pigment	Smaller and oval, but similar to vivax
DIAGNOSTIC KEYS				
	Gametocyte, multiple rings, double chromatin dots, accole forms, heavy infections	Schizont, large RBCs, ameboid forms	Schizont, small RBCs, band forms	Schizont and large RBCs, pear-shaped, fimbriated RBCs

* At periphery of RBC; may be flattened into rod shape.
† Stretch across RBC, but not banana-shaped.

prefer Giemsa stain because of its overall high quality, suitability for staining both thick and thin smears, and stability in tropical climates. Wright's stain can produce high-quality thin smears and is widely used in the Americas, but it deteriorates rapidly in the tropics because its methanol base is highly hygroscopic. Specimens of capillary or venous blood should be obtained every 4 to 12 h until a diagnosis is established. The thin smear is made on clean slides exactly like a blood film for a white blood cell differential. The thick film is made by placing one drop of blood on the slide and stirring it in a circular motion to a diameter of about 2 cm. The erythrocytes in the thick film are lysed with water, but the thin film is fixed in methanol to preserve erythrocyte morphology.

Although most tissue parasites stain with the traditional hematoxylin and eosin stain, surgical biopsy specimens also should be stained with appropriate special stains. The surgical pathologist who is accustomed to staining induced sputum and transbronchial biopsies with silver stains for *Pneumocystis carinii* may have to be reminded to examine wet mounts and iron-hematoxylin stains of pulmonary

specimens for helminth ova and *E. histolytica* (see Table 171-5). The clinician also should be able to advise the surgeon and pathologist about optimal techniques for identification of parasites from specimens obtained by certain specialized minor procedures (see Table 171-8). For example, the excision of skin snips for the diagnosis of onchocerciasis, rectal snips for the diagnosis of schistosomiasis, and punch biopsies of skin lesions for the identification and culture of cutaneous and mucocutaneous species of *Leishmania* are simple procedures, but the diagnosis can be missed if the specimens are improperly obtained or processed.

NONSPECIFIC TESTS   Eosinophilia is a common accompaniment of infections with most of the tissue helminths and may reach high absolute numbers in trichinosis and the migratory phases of filariasis (Table 171-9). Intestinal helminths provoke eosinophilia only during pulmonary migration of the larval stages. Eosinophilia is not a manifestation of protozoal infections, with the possible exceptions of *Isospora* and *Dientamoeba fragilis*.

Like the hypochromic, microcytic anemia of heavy hookworm

TABLE 171-8   Minor procedures for diagnosis of parasitic infections

Procedure	Parasite(s) and stage
Skin snips: Lift skin with a needle and excise about 1 mg to a depth of 0.5 mm from several sites. Weigh each, place in 0.5 mL saline for 4 h, and examine wet mounts and Giemsa stains of the saline either directly or after filtration. Count microfilariae.*	*Onchocerca volvulus* and *Mansonella streptocerca* microfilariae
Biopsies of subcutaneous nodules: Giemsa stains of routine histopathologic sections and impression smears.	*Loa loa* adults and *Onchocerca volvulus* adults and microfilariae
Muscle biopsies: Excise about 1.0 g of deltoid or gastrocnemius m. and squash between two glass slides for direct microscopic examination.	*Trichinella spiralis* larvae (*Taenia solium* cysticerci may be detected)
Rectal snips: From four areas of mucosa take 2-mg snips, tease onto a glass slide, and flatten with a second slide before direct exam at 10X. May be fixed in alcohol or stained.	*Schistosoma* ova of all species, but esp. *S. mansoni*
Aspirate of chancre or lymph node†: Aspirate center with 18-gauge needle, place a drop on a slide, and examine for motile forms. Insufficient material may be Giemsa stained.	*Trypanosoma gambiense* and *Trypanosoma rhodesiense* trypomastigotes
Corneal scrapings: Obtain sample from opthalmologist for immediate Giemsa stain and culture on nutrient agar overlaid with *E. coli*.	*Acanthamoeba* species trophozoites or cysts
Swabs, aspirates, or punch biopsies of skin lesions: Obtain specimen from margin of lesion for Giemsa stain of impression smears and section and culture on special media from CDC.	Cutaneous and mucocutaneous species of *Leishmania*

* Counts of >100 per milligram are associated with significant risk of complications.
† Lymph node aspiration is contraindicated in some infections and should be used judiciously.

TABLE 171-9 Parasites frequently associated with eosinophilia*

Parasite	Comment
TAPEWORMS (CESTODES)	
Echinococcus granulosus	When hydatid cyst leaks
Taenia solium	During muscle encystation and in CSF with neurocysticercosis
FLUKES (TREMATODES)	
Paragonimus spp.	Uniformly high in acute stage
Fasciola hepatica	May be high in acute stage
Clonorchis sinensis	Variable
Schistosoma mansoni	50% of infected travelers
Schistosoma haematobium	25% of infected travelers
Schistosoma japonicum	Up to 6000 per microliter in acute infection
ROUNDWORMS	
Ascaris lumbricoides	During larval migration
Hookworm species	During larval migration
Strongyloides stercoralis	Profound during migration and early years of infection
Trichinella spiralis	Up to 7000 per microliter
Wuchereria bancrofti	From normal to 2500 per cubic microliter†
Brugia spp.	Similar to *Wuchereria*†
Loa loa	Varies but can reach 5000 to 8000 per microliter
Onchocerca volvulus	May exceed 5000 per microliter
Toxocara spp.	>3000 per microliter
Ancylostoma braziliensis	With extensive cutaneous eruption
Gnathostoma spinigerum	In VLM and eosinophilic meningitis
Angiostrongylus cantonensis	In eosinophilic meningitis
Angiostrongylus costaricensis	During larval migration in mesenteric vessels
POSSIBLE PROTOZOAL CAUSES	
Isospora belli	A few reports of profound eosinophilia
Dientamoeba fragilis	Possible pathogenicity and eosinophilia

* Virtually every helminth has been associated with eosinophilia. This table includes both common and uncommon parasites that frequently elicit eosinophilia during infection.
† Also in tropical pulmonary eosinophilia, where eosinophilia, fleeting infiltrates, and asthma may be the only manifestations of filariasis.

TABLE 171-10 Serologic tests for parasitic infections

Infections with	Antibody tests	Antigen tests
TAPEWORMS		
Echinococcosis	WB, IHA	
Cysticercosis	WB	
FLUKES		
Paragonimiasis	WB	
Schistosomiasis	EIA, WB	
ROUNDWORMS		
Strongyloidiasis	EIA	
Trichinellosis	BF	
Toxocariasis	EIA	
PROTOZOANS		
Amebiasis	IHA	
Giardiasis		EIA, IIF
Cryptosporidiosis		IIF
Malaria (all species)*	IIF	
Babesiosis (*B. microti*)	IIF	
Chagas' disease	IIF, CF	
Leishmaniasis	IIF, CF	
Toxoplasmosis	IIF, EIA-IgM	
Pneumocystosis		IIF

NOTE: BF = bentonite flocculation; CF = complement fixation; EIA = enzyme immunoassay; WB = western blot; IHA = indirect hemagglutination; IIF = indirect immunofluorescence. All antibody tests listed are available from the CDC. Antigen and parasite detection kits are available commercially.
* Of use primarily for screening blood donors.

infections, other nonspecific laboratory abnormalities may suggest parasitic infection in patients with appropriate geographic and/or environmental exposures. Biochemical evidence of cirrhosis or an abnormal urine sediment in an African immigrant certainly raises the possibility of schistosomiasis. Megaloblastic anemia can be the presenting manifestation of the fish tapeworm (*Diphyllobothrium latum*), and anemia and thrombocytopenia in a febrile traveler or immigrant are among the hallmarks of malaria. Computed tomography and magnetic resonance imaging also contribute to the diagnosis of infections with many tissue parasites and have become invaluable adjuncts to the diagnosis of neurocysticercosis and cerebral toxoplasmosis.

ANTIBODY AND ANTIGEN DETECTION As shown in Table 171-10, there are useful antibody assays for many of the important tissue parasites. The filarial worms are a notable exception. Although filariae provoke a strong immune response and many antibody assays have been used, none has proved sensitive and specific enough for universal adoption. The detection of antibody to plasmodia is primarily an epidemiologic tool of limited use for the diagnosis of malaria in individual patients. The limited geographic distribution of many of the tropical parasites increases the usefulness of antibody detection as a means of establishing diagnoses in travelers from industrialized countries. On the other hand, a large proportion of the world has been exposed to *T. gondii*, and the presence of IgG antibody does not establish the presence of active disease. One or more of the antibody assays listed in the tables are available at the Centers for Disease Control and Prevention (CDC) in Atlanta, Georgia. The

results of most serologic tests not listed in the tables nor offered by the CDC should be interpreted with caution.

Many fewer antibody assays are available for the diagnosis of intestinal parasites. Although most stimulate coproantibodies and humoral antibodies, problems of cross-reactivity between parasites, lack of efficient cultivation techniques, and the ability to establish diagnoses without invasive procedures have discouraged intensive investigation. *E. histolytica* is the major exception. The availability of sensitive specific serologic tests is an invaluable aid in the diagnosis of amebiasis. Commercial kits for the detection of antigen by ELISA and whole organisms by fluorescent antibody are now available for the diagnosis of giardiasis and cryptosporidiosis.

MOLECULAR TECHNIQUES DNA hybridization with probes that are repeated many times in the genome of a specific parasite and amplification of a specific DNA fragment by the polymerase chain reaction (PCR) are promising techniques for the diagnosis of infections with parasites and other infectious agents. DNA probes for hybridization to *P. falciparum*, *T. cruzi*, the African trypanosomes, and lymphatic filariae are already being used for detection of these agents in infected insect vectors and are being applied investigationally in animal models and human trials. Although none is available for routine use in patients at this time, DNA probes and PCR should become important additions to our future diagnostic armamentarium.

REFERENCES

DESPOMMIER DD, KARAPELEU JW: *Parasite Life Cycles.* New York, Springer-Verlag, 1987

FLECK SL, MOODY AH: *Diagnostic Techniques in Medical Parasitology.* London, Wright, 1988

GUTIERREZ V, LITTLE MD (eds): *Clinics in Laboratory Medicine: Diagnosis of Important Parasitic Diseases,* vol 11. Philadelphia, Saunders, 1991

TOMECKI KJ (ed): *Dermatologic Clinics: Systemic Mycoses and Parasitic Diseases,* vol 7. Philadelphia, Saunders, 1989

WEBER R et al: Improved light-microscopical detection of microsporidia spores in stool and duodenal aspirates. N Engl J Med 326:161, 1992

WELLER PF: Eosinophilia in travelers, in *The Medical Clinics of North America: Travel Medicine,* vol 76, MS Wolfe (guest ed). Philadelphia, Saunders, 1992

WILSON M, SCHANTZ P: Nonmorphologic diagnosis of parasitic infections, in *Manual of Clinical Microbiology,* 5th ed, A Balows (ed). Washington, American Society of Microbiology, 1991

172   THERAPY FOR PARASITIC INFECTIONS

LEO X. LIU / PETER F. WELLER

Chemotherapy for parasitic diseases is beset with potential problems. Knowledge of the fundamental biology and metabolism of eukaryotic parasites is still rudimentary. Many essential antiparasitic drugs, such as chloroquine or diethylcarbamazine, have been used for decades without our having a full understanding of their mechanisms of action. For a disease such as falciparum malaria, which causes tremendous suffering and death worldwide, the emergence of drug resistance poses an urgent problem. Because most parasitic infections primarily affect populations in poor developing countries, commercial incentives to develop and market antiparasitic drugs are limited. Nevertheless, the introduction in recent years of several new agents such as mefloquine, praziquantel, and ivermectin has improved the therapy for several parasitic infections. Table 172-1 summarizes drug therapy for the more common parasitic diseases. Information regarding indications, adverse effects, and contraindications of selected drugs follows below. Drugs considered investigational by the Food and Drug Administration (FDA) for a given parasitic indication are marked with an asterisk (*). Other drugs, marked with a dagger (†), may not be generally available in the United States but may be obtained through the Centers for Disease Control and Prevention Drug Service, Atlanta, GA 30333 (telephone 404-639-3670). Antiparasitic drug treatment for children and pregnant women or in certain unusual circumstances is detailed in the references.

Albendazole* This new benzimidazole derivative is active against a variety of helminthic parasites but is currently available only from the manufacturer (Smith-Kline Beecham). Albendazole is the drug of choice for the medical treatment of hydatid cysts and is also useful as an adjunct to surgical therapy. It is effective for cysticercosis, is also promising for many intestinal and tissue nematode infections, and is less toxic than the older benzimidazoles. Adverse reactions to albendazole include occasional diarrhea and abdominal pain, and its use during pregnancy is contraindicated.

Benznidazole* This nitroimidazole derivative, not presently available in the United States, can ameliorate the course of acute

TABLE 172-1   Treatment of parasitic infections

Infection	Treatment of choice	Alternative regimen
Amebiasis *(Entamoeba histolytica)*		
Asymptomatic	Diloxanide furoate 500 mg tid for 10 days	Iodoquinolol 650 mg tid for 20 days; **or** paromomycin 25–30 mg/kg/d in 3 doses for 7 days
Mild to moderate disease	Metronidazole 750 mg tid for 10 days followed by iodoquinolol 650 mg tid for 20 days	Paromomycin as above **or** tinidazole 2 g/d; either followed by iodoquinolol as above
Severe intestinal disease	Metronidazole as above **or** tinidazole 600 mg bid for 5 days followed by iodoquinolol as above	Dehydroemetine 1–1.5 mg/kg/d (max 90 mg/d) IM up to 5 days; **or** paromomycin as above; either followed by iodoquinolol as above
Hepatic abscess	Metronidazole as above **or** tinidazole 800 mg tid for 5 days followed by iodoquinolol as above	Dehydroemetine as above, followed by chloroquine phosphate 600 mg base (1 g)/d for 2 days, then 300 mg base (500 mg)/d for 2–3 weeks plus iodoquinolol as above
Amebic meningoencephalitis *(Naegleria)*	Amphotericin B 1 mg/kg/d IV for uncertain duration	
Angiostrongyliasis *(Angiostrongylus cantonensis)*	Supportive therapy and glucocorticoids as needed	
(Angiostrongylus costaricensis)	Thiabendazole 75 mg/kg/d in 3 doses for 3 days (max 3 g/d)	
Anisakiasis *(Anisakis)*	Surgical or endoscopic removal	
Ascariasis *(Ascaris lumbricoides)*	Mebendazole 100 mg bid for 3 days; **or** piperazine 75 mg/kg (max 3.5 g) for 2 days	Pyrantel pamoate 11 mg/kg (max 1 g); **or** albendazole 400 mg once
Babesiosis *(Babesia)*	Clindamycin 1.2 g bid IV; **or** 600 mg tid PO for 7 days, plus quinine 650 mg tid PO for 7 days	
Balantidiasis *(Balantidium coli)*	Tetracycline 500 mg qid for 10 days	Metronidazole 750 mg tid for 5 days
Capillariasis *(Capillaria philippinensis)*	Mebendazole 200 mg bid for 20 days	Albendazole 200 mg bid for 10 days; **or** thiabendazole 25 mg/kg/d in 2 doses for 30 days
Cryptosporidiosis *(Cryptosporidium)*	No effective specific therapy; self-limited in normal hosts	
Cutaneous larva migrans (creeping eruption)	Thiabendazole 10% suspension topically qid; **or** 25 mg/kg for 2–5 days	Cryotherapy
Cysticercosis *(Cysticercus cellulosae)*	Praziquantel 50 mg/kg/d in 3 doses for 15 days; **or** albendazole 15 mg/kg/d in 3 doses for 8 days, repeated as necessary, with concurrent glucocorticoids for CNS disease	Surgery
Dracunculiasis *(Dracunculus medinensis)*	Metronidazole 250 mg tid for 10 days plus worm removal	Thiabendazole 50–75 mg/kg/d in 2 doses for 3 days plus worm removal

TABLE 172-1   Treatment of parasitic infections (*continued*)

Infection	Treatment of choice	Alternative regimen
Echinococcosis		
Echinococcus granulosus (hydatid cyst)	Surgical excision plus preoperative albendazole	Albendazole 400 mg bid for 28 days, repeated as necessary
Echinococcus multilocularis	Surgical excision	
Enterobiasis		
(*Enterobius vermicularis,* pinworm)	Pyrantel pamoate 11 mg/kg once (max 1 g) **or** mebendazole 100 mg once **or** albendazole 400 mg once; each repeated after 2 weeks	
Filariasis		
Lymphatic filariasis (*Wuchereria bancrofti, Brugia malayi*)	Diethylcarbamazine Day 1: 50 mg PO Day 2: 50 mg tid Day 3: 100 mg tid Days 4–21: 6 mg/kg/d in 3 doses	
Loaisis (*Loa loa*)	Diethylcarbamazine Day 1: 50 mg PO Day 2: 50 mg tid Day 3: 100 mg tid Days 4–21:9 mg/kg/d in 3 doses	
Mansonella ozzardi	Ivermectin 25–200 μg/kg single dose	
Mansonella perstans	Mebendazole 100 mg bid for 30 days	Ivermectin 25–200 μg/kg single dose
Mansonella streptocerca	Diethylcarbamazine as for lymphatic filariasis	
Tropical pulmonary eosinophilia	Diethylcarbamazine 6 mg/kg/d in 3 doses for 21 days	
Onchocerciasis *Onchocerca volvulus*	Ivermectin 150 μg/kg once, repeated every 6–12 months	
Fluke infections		
Liver flukes (*Clonorchis sinensis; Opisthorchis viverrini*)	Praziquantel 75 mg/kg/d in 3 doses for 1 day	
Sheep liver fluke (*Fasciola hepatica*)	Bithionol 30–50 mg/kg on alternate days for 10–15 doses	
Intestinal flukes (*Fasciolopsis buski, Heterophyes heterophyes, Metagonimus yokogawai*)	Praziquantel 75 mg/kg/d in 3 doses for 1 day	
Lung fluke (*Paragonimus westermani*)	Praziquantel 75 mg/kg/d in 3 doses for 2 days	Bithionol 30–50 mg/kg on alternate days for 10–15 doses
Giardiasis (*Giardia lamblia*)	Metronidazole 250 mg tid for 5 days; **or** quinacrine HCl 100 mg tid for 5 days	Tinidazole 2 g once; **or** paromomycin 25–30 mg/kg/d in 3 doses for 7 days; **or** furazolidone 100 mg qid for 7–10 days
Gnathostomiasis (*Gnathostoma spinigerum*)	Surgical removal; **or** mebendazole 200 mg q3h for 6 days	
Hookworm (*Ancylostoma duodenale, Necator americanus*)	Mebendazole 100 mg bid for 3 days; **or** pyrantel pamoate 11 mg/kg (max 1 g) for 3 days	Albendazole 400 mg once
Isosporiasis (*Isospora belli*)	Trimethoprim-sulfamethoxazole (160/800 mg) qid for 10 days, then bid for 3 weeks	Pyrimethamine 50–75 mg once daily for 3 weeks
Leishmaniasis —cutaneous, mucocutaneous, or visceral (*L. braziliensis, L. mexicana, L. tropica, L. major, L. donovani*)	Stibogluconate sodium 20 mg/kg/d (max 800 mg/d) IV or IM for 28 days; **or** meglumine antimoniate 20 mg/kg/d for 20–28 days; may be repeated or continued until response	Amphotericin B 0.25—1 mg/kg slow infusion daily or every 2 days for up to 8 weeks; **or** pentamidine isethionate 2–4 mg/kg/d IM up to 15 doses
Malaria treatment (*Plasmodium falciparum, P. ovale, P. vivax, P. malariae*)		
All except chloroquine-resistant *P. falciparum*		
Oral	Chloroquine phosphate 600 mg base (1 g) then 300 mg base (500 mg) at 6, 24, and 48 h	
Parenteral	Quinidine gluconate 10 mg/kg loading dose (max 600 mg) over 1 h followed by continuous infusion of 0.02 mg/kg/min for 3 d maximum	Chloroquine HCl 200 mg base (250 mg) IM q6h if oral therapy cannot be started
Followed by (for *P. vivax* & *P. ovale* only)	Primaquine phosphate 15 mg base (26.3 mg)/d for 14 days or 45 mg base (79 mg)/wk for 8 weeks	
Chloroquine-resistant *P. falciparum*		
Oral	Quinine sulfate 650 mg tid for 3 days plus pyrimethamine-sulfadoxine 3 tablets at once on last day of quinine; **or** plus tetracycline 250 mg qid for 7 days; **or** plus clindamycin 900 mg tid for 3 days	Mefloquine 1250 mg once; **or** halofantrine 500 mg q6h for 3 doses
Parenteral	Quinidine gluconate as above	
Malaria prophylaxis		
Chloroquine-sensitive areas	Chloroquine phosphate 300 mg base (500 mg salt) orally, once/wk beginning 1 wk before and continuing for 4 weeks after last exposure	

(*continued*)

TABLE 172-1   Treatment of parasitic infections (*continued*)

Infection	Treatment of choice	Alternative regimen
Chloroquine-resistant areas	Mefloquine 250 mg oral once/week continuing for 4 weeks after last exposure; **or** doxycycline 100 mg daily during exposure and for 4 weeks afterwards; **or** chloroquine phosphate as above plus pyrimethamine-sulfadoxine for presumptive treatment **or** plus proguanil 200 mg daily for sub-Saharan Africa during exposure and for 4 weeks afterward	
***Pneumocystis* pneumonia** (*Pneumocystis carinii*)	Trimethoprim-sulfamethoxazole (20/100 mg/kg/d) oral or IV in 4 doses for 14–21 days; **or** pentamidine isethionate 4 mg/kg/d IV for 14–21 days plus prednisone for severe pneumonia	Trimethoprim 5 mg/kg PO q6h for 21 days plus dapsone 100 mg PO once daily for 21 days; **or** primaquine 15 mg base PO once daily for 21 days plus clindamycin 300–450 mg PO q6h for 21 days; **or** trimetrexate 45 mg/m² IV once daily for 21 days plus folinic acid 20 mg/m² PO or IV q6h for 21 days
Schistosomiasis *S. mansoni*	Praziquantel 40 mg/kg/d in 2 doses for 1 day	Oxamniquine 15 mg/kg once; 30 mg/kg once for East Africa; 30 mg/kg once daily for 2 days for Egypt and South Africa
S. haematobium	Praziquantel 40 mg/kg/d in 2 doses for 1 day	
S. japonicum, S. mekongi	Praziquantel 60 mg/kg/d in 3 doses for 1 day	
Strongyloidiasis (*Strongyloides stercoralis*)	Thiabendazole 50 mg/kg/d in 2 doses (max 3 g/d) for 2 days; for disseminated disease continue for 7d, or longer if immunocompromised	Ivermectin 200 μg/kg/d for 1–2 days; **or** Albendazole 400 mg once daily for 3 days
Tapeworm intestinal infections *Diphyllobothrium latum*—fish; *Taenia saginata*—beef; *T. solium*—pork; *Dipylidium caninum*—dog *Hymenolepis nana* (dwarf tapeworm)	Praziquantel 10–20 mg/kg once; or niclosamide single dose of 4 tablets (2 g), chewed thoroughly Praziquantel 25 mg/kg once; or niclosamide, single dose of 4 tablets (2 g) chewed thoroughly then 2 tablets daily for 6 days	
Toxoplasmosis (*Toxoplasma gondii*)	Pyrimethamine 75 mg/d plus sulfadiazine 2–4 g/d	Clindamycin 450 g/d tid plus pyrimethamine 75 mg/d
Trichinosis (*Trichinella spiralis*)	Glucocorticoids for severe symptoms plus mebendazole 200–400 mg tid for 3 days, then 400–500 mg tid for 10 days	
Trichomoniasis (*Trichomonas vaginalis*)	Metronidazole 2 g once or 250 mg tid PO for 7 days; **or** tinidazole 2 g once	
Trichostrongyliasis (*Trichostrongylus*)	Pyrantel pamoate 11 mg/kg once (max 1 g)	Mebendazole 100 mg bid for four days; **or** albendazole 400 mg once
Trichuriasis (whipworm) (*Trichuris trichiura*)	Mebendazole 100 mg bid for 3 days; **or** albendazole 400 mg once	
Trypanosomiasis *T. cruzi* (Chagas' disease)	Nifurtimox 8–10 mg/kg/d PO in 4 doses for 120 days	Benznidazole 5–7 mg/kg/d for 30–120 days
T. brucei gambiense, T.b. rhodesiense (sleeping sickness) Hemolymphatic stage	Suramin 100–200 mg test dose IV, then 1 g IV on days 1, 3, 7, 14, 21; **or** eflornithine 100 mg/kg qid for 14 days, then 300 mg/kg/d PO for 3–4 weeks	Pentamidine isethionate 4 mg/kg/d for 10 days
Late stage with CNS involvement	Melarsoprol 2–3.6 mg/kg/d IV for 3 doses; after 1 week 3.6 mg/kg/d IV for 3 doses; repeat after 10–21 days; **or** eflornithine 100 mg/kg qid for 14 days, then 300 mg/kg/d PO for 3–4 weeks	Tryparsamide 30 mg/kg (max 2 g) IV q5d to total of 12 injections; may repeat after 1 month, plus suramin 10 mg/kg IV q5d to total of 12 injections; may be repeated after 1 month
Visceral larva migrans (toxocariasis)	Supportive therapy and glucocorticoids	Diethylcarbamazine 2 mg/kg tid for 7–10 days; **or** mebendazole 100–200 mg bid for 5 doses; **or** thiabendazole 50 mg/kg/d in 2 doses for 5 days (max 3 g/d)

Chagas' disease. Frequent side effects include rashes, nausea, and peripheral neuritis.

Bithionol†   This drug is used for the treatment of fascioliasis and paragonimiasis. Adverse cutaneous and gastrointestinal effects are common.

Chloroquine   This mainstay oral antimalarial drug is a 4-amino-

quinolone that rapidly kills schizonts and gametocytes of *Plasmodium vivax, P. ovale, P. malariae,* and susceptible strains of *P. falciparum.* Unfortunately, in many areas *P. falciparum* is resistant to chloroquine, and in Oceania resistance has emerged in *P. vivax.* Chloroquine is still effective in the treatment and prophylaxis of malaria in areas where resistance is not yet established. Chloroquine phosphate is available as generic and commercial tablets in the United States; chloroquine sulfate is also available outside the United States. Hydroxychloroquine sulfate, more familiarly used as an antiarthritic agent, also has been used effectively. Chloroquine is safe in children and pregnant women. Side effects may include abdominal discomfort, headache, and dizziness.

Dehydroemetine† This is an ipecac alkaloid used as an alternative treatment for invasive amebiasis. Dehydroemetine is highly irritating and should only be administered by intramuscular injection. Pain, cellulitis, or abscess formation at the injection site is frequent. Cardiac arrhythmias, chest pain, and hypotension are common and limit the use of this drug to a monitored setting. Dehydroemetine is contraindicated in pregnancy.

Diethylcarbamazine† This piperazine derivative remains the drug of choice for lymphatic filariasis despite adverse reactions and a cumbersome dosage schedule. The mechanism of action of diethylcarbamazine is unclear, but it is microfilaricidal in vivo. Side effects are generally proportional to the microfilarial burden and include fever, headache, dizziness, and transient exacerbation of lymphangitis. In onchocerciasis, the drug elicits prominent pruritus and ocular and constitutional symptoms (Mazzotti reaction) and has been supplanted by ivermectin. Diethylcarbamazine is effective for treatment and prophylaxis of *Loa loa* infection and has been used for visceral larva migrans. The drug is not commercially available in the United States; limited amounts may be obtained from the manufacturer (Lederle).

Diloxanide furoate† This amebicidal agent is poorly absorbed and is active only against luminal amebas. Its mode of action is unknown. Mild side effects include flatulence and gastrointestinal discomfort.

Eflornithine Commonly known as difluoromethylornithine or DFMO, this drug is effective in both hemolymphatic and central nervous system stages of *Trypanosoma brucei gambiense* infections (African trypanosomiasis). Eflornithine is available in the United States only from the manufacturer (Merrell Dow). It acts by irreversible inhibition of the trypanosomal ornithine decarboxylase, although *Trypanosoma brucei rhodesiense* is relatively insensitive. Side effects of diarrhea, anemia, and leukopenia are frequent but reversible.

Furazolidone This nitrofuran derivative is used as an alternative drug for giardiasis. Unlike other drugs for giardiasis, it is not bitter and is available in a liquid form useful for young children. Nausea, vomiting, and allergic reactions occur. The drug is a monoamine oxidase (MAO) inhibitor and also produces a disulfiram-like reaction when taken with alcohol.

Halofantrine This new oral antimalarial drug, recently available in the United States, has been used to treat malaria due to chloroquine-resistant *P. falciparum*. Adverse effects include abdominal pain, diarrhea, and pruritus. It should not be used in pregnancy.

Iodoquinol This halogenated oxyquinolone is used for noninvasive amebiasis and *Dientamoeba fragilis* infection and as an alternative for *Balantidium coli* infection. Adverse effects are uncommon, but optic neuritis has been observed with prolonged use of excessively high doses.

Ivermectin† This semisynthetic derivative of avermectin is now the drug of choice for *Onchocerca volvulus* infections. A single oral dose of ivermectin is active against microfilariae but has no effect on the adult worms. Its mechanism of action has not been conclusively identified. Ivermectin also is active against a range of intestinal nematodes and is under investigation for the treatment of lymphatic filariasis. The drug is safe and well-tolerated in children and adults, but its safety in pregnancy has not been specifically addressed.

Mebendazole This benzimidazole derivative is effective against a spectrum of intestinal and tissue nematodes, including *Ascaris*, hookworm, *Enterobius*, and *Trichuris*, and is an investigational drug for *Capillaria*. Benzimidazoles may act by binding β-tubulin to disrupt microtubule formation and glucose uptake. Side effects include mild abdominal pain and diarrhea. Benzimidazoles can be teratogenic in experimental animals and so are avoided during pregnancy.

Mefloquine This new antimalarial agent is active against the blood stages of all malarial species and the schizonts of *P. falciparum*. A 4-aminoquinolone derivative, mefloquine is the currently preferred agent for the prophylaxis and oral treatment of chloroquine-resistant malaria. Adverse effects are generally dose-related and include nausea and dizziness and, more rarely, vomiting, diarrhea, psychosis, and seizures. Because it has been associated with sinus bradycardia, mefloquine is contraindicated in persons taking beta-adrenoreceptor and calcium-channel blocking agents and should not be given concurrently with quinine or quinidine. Mefloquine resistance of *P. falciparum* occurs in parts of Southeast Asia and Africa and will present a growing problem. Since its safety in pregnancy has not been established, mefloquine should be avoided during pregnancy.

Melarsoprol† This organic arsenical compound is used only to treat late-stage African trypanosomiasis involving the central nervous system. Only after intravenous administration does enough drug enter the cerebrospinal fluid to kill the trypanosomes. Severe adverse effects are common, including myocarditis, encephalopathy, and Herxheimer reactions.

Metrifonate This organophosphate compound is active against *Schistosoma haematobium*. Adverse effects include abdominal pain, nausea, vomiting, diarrhea, headache, and vertigo. It should not be used during pregnancy.

Metronidazole This 5-nitroimidazole has potent activity against anaerobic bacteria and several protozoa, including *Entamoeba histolytica*, *Giardia lamblia*, *Trichomonas vaginalis*, and *Balantidium coli*. Metronidazole is the drug of choice for giardiasis (although not FDA approved for this indication) and the initial treatment of invasive amebiasis. It is generally well tolerated, but mild abdominal pain, headache, nausea, and a persistent metallic taste are common. The drug is teratogenic in animals and should be avoided in early pregnancy. Because it produces a disulfiram-like reaction, abstinence from alcohol is advisable.

Niclosamide Niclosamide is safe and highly effective against intestinal tapeworms when given as a single oral dose and chewed thoroughly before it is washed down with water. Intestinal reactions are minimal, and there are no contraindications to its use. Since it is not absorbed from the gastrointestinal tract, niclosamide is not active against larval cestodes.

Nifurtimox† This is a synthetic nitrofuran compound active in acute *Trypanosoma cruzi* infection. Response rates are variable, and the drug has little effect in chronic Chagas' disease. Adverse reactions, including nausea, vomiting, insomnia, headache, vertigo, tremor, paresthesias, and convulsions, are common and dose-dependent.

Oxamniquine This tetrahydroquinolone derivative is used as an alternative agent for *Schistosoma mansoni* infection. Higher doses are needed in Egypt and South Africa, and resistant strains also have been encountered. Oxamniquine is well tolerated, with occasional side effects of headache, dizziness, drowsiness, and gastrointestinal disturbances. It should not be used in pregnancy.

Paromomycin This oral, poorly absorbed aminoglycoside is used as an alternative treatment for noninvasive amebiasis. Though not approved for the purpose, paromomycin also has been used in lieu of metronidazole to treat amebiasis and giardiasis in pregnant women.

Pentamidine isethionate This is a stable aromatic diamine compound active against *Pneumocystis carinii* and several protozoal pathogens, including *Leishmania* spp. and *T. brucei gambiense*. Its mechanism of action remains uncertain. Adverse reactions to parenteral pentamidine are common, including reversible nephrotoxicity, acute hypotension, pancreatitis, hypoglycemia, cardiac arrhythmias, blood dyscrasias, and sterile abscesses at the injection site. Aerosolized pentamidine used for the prophylaxis of *Pneumocystis* pneumonia in susceptible patients is associated with local adverse effects, including sore throat, oral paresthesias, metallic taste, cough, and bronchospasm.

Piperazine This inexpensive drug, widely used in developing countries for the treatment of ascariasis and enterobiasis, is an anticholinergic agent that acts by paralyzing the worms, allowing them to be flushed out by peristalsis. Intestinal disturbances, hypersensitivity reactions, and dizziness are occasional adverse reactions. Piperazine and pyrantel pamoate have antagonistic modes of action and should not be administered together.

Praziquantel   This novel agent is the drug of choice for most trematode (fluke) and many cestode infections. Its mechanism of action is unknown, but in schistosomes it causes paralysis and tegumental disruption, which may then permit a synergistic host immune response. Praziquantel is highly active against all human schistosome parasites, intestinal tapeworms, cysticercosis, and other flukes exclusive of *Fasciola hepatica*. Side effects include headache, dizziness, drowsiness, and abdominal discomfort. Higher doses and adjunctive anti-inflammatory corticosteroids are recommended for neurocysticercosis.

Primaquine   This 8-aminoquinolone derivative is the only standard drug active against the intrahepatic hypnozoite forms of malarial species and is used for the radical cure of *P. vivax* and *P. ovale* malaria following schizonticidal therapy. It is also an effective gametocidal agent. A potent oxidant, primaquine causes acute hemolysis in the presence of glucose-6-phosphate dehydrogenase deficiency, and at-risk patients should be screened before such therapy is instituted. Primaquine is contraindicated during pregnancy.

Proguanil*   This pyrimidine derivative is active against the preerythrocytic intrahepatic forms of *P. falciparum* and possibly *P. vivax*. Its use is largely limited to malaria prophylaxis, in combination with chloroquine, in parts of Africa where chloroquine-resistant *P. falciparum* is not yet widely prevalent. However, foci of proguanil resistance also exist in many regions, and clinical failures with proguanil are common. Proguanil is not licensed in the United States but is sold in Europe and Africa.

Pyrantel   This well-tolerated pyrimidine derivative acts against intestinal nematodes by inducing neuromuscular paralysis in the worms, allowing them to be expelled. A single dose is usually curative for ascariasis, enterobiasis, and trichostrongyliasis, but several doses are recommended for hookworm infection. It is safe for use in pregnancy.

Pyrimethamine-sulfonamides   Pyrimethamine combined with sulfadiazine is used in the treatment of toxoplasmosis. The high doses required for the latter often result in significant folate deficiency, necessitating folinic acid replacement. Abdominal symptoms and rashes are also common. Pyrimethamine combined with sulfadoxine is active against most strains of *P. falciparum*, although drug resistance is becoming more widespread. Pyrimethamine-sulfadoxine, as an adjunct to quinine, is still useful in the oral treatment of chloroquine-resistant *P. falciparum* malaria, but it is no longer recommended for malarial prophylaxis because of occasional severe and fatal skin hypersensitivity reactions and hepatitis.

Quinacrine   This acridine dye used to treat giardiasis is well absorbed and may impart a yellow color to the urine and, rarely, to the skin or sclerae. Adverse effects include headache, dizziness, vomiting, diarrhea, and, less commonly, psychotic episodes. Distribution of this drug has ceased within the United States.

Quinine and quinidine   These cinchona alkaloids have reemerged as first-line drugs for treatment of falciparum malaria because of widespread chloroquine resistance. Quinine plus a second orally active drug (to reduce the likelihood of recurrence) is recommended

for oral therapy for *P. falciparum* malaria. For severe infections requiring intravenous therapy, only quinidine gluconate (which is at least as effective as parenteral quinine) is available in the United States. Cardiac monitoring during quinidine infusion is mandatory, and oral quinine should be substituted as soon as the patient is able to take it. Both quinine and quinidine can cause hypoglycemia. Symptoms of cinchonism, including tinnitus, headache, visual disturbances, nausea, and abdominal pain, often develop with treatment but are rarely grounds for discontinuing the drug. Oral quinine also is used with clindamycin to treat babesiosis.

Spiramycin   This is an alternative to antifolates in the treatment of toxoplasmosis, particularly for pregnant women, in whom it is safe. This agent is available from the FDA.

Stibogluconate sodium† (sodium antimony gluconate)   This pentavalent antimonial parenteral solution is the drug of choice for all forms of leishmaniasis. Its mechanism of action is unknown. Adverse effects include muscle pain, joint stiffness, nausea, vomiting, and, less commonly, rash and cardiac or hepatic toxicity. Meglumine antimoniate, another pentavalent antimonial drug, is used in many French- and Spanish-speaking countries.

Suramin†   This complex derivative of urea is the drug of choice for treating early African trypanosomiasis and is the only available drug active against adult *Onchocerca volvulus* worms. It must be given intravenously and is excreted very slowly. Adverse effects are common and can be severe, including vomiting, pruritus, urticaria, paresthesias, photophobia, peripheral neuropathy, anaphylaxis, and renal damage.

Tetracycline, doxycycline   Tetracycline is effective against *Balantidium coli* and *Dientamoeba fragilis* and also is used as an adjunct to quinine in treating chloroquine-resistant falciparum malaria. Doxycycline, a once-daily form, may be used for chemoprophylaxis of chloroquine-resistant falciparum malaria. Tooth staining in children and photosensitivity are potential hazards.

Thiabendazole   This older benzimidazole derivative is active against a variety of nematode parasites, but frequent and severe side effects limit its primary systemic use to treatment of strongyloidiasis. These adverse reactions include dizziness, nausea, vomiting, drowsiness, pruritus, headache, neuropsychiatric disturbances, hepatitis, and hypersensitivity reactions, including Stevens-Johnson syndrome. A topical suspension of thiabendazole is used for cutaneous larva migrans.

Tinidazole*   This nitroimidazole is available only outside the United States for the treatment of amebiasis, giardiasis, and vaginal trichomoniasis. Tinidazole appears to be more effective and better tolerated than metronidazole.

Trimethoprim-sulfamethoxazole   This antifolate combination is active in *P. carinii* pneumonia and *Isospora belli* infection in immunocompromised patients. Adverse effects are predominantly due to the sulfamethoxazole and include skin, liver, and bone marrow toxicity.

REFERENCES

Drugs for parasitic infections. Med Lett Drugs Ther 34:17, 1992

ROSENBLATT JE: Antiparasitic agents. Mayo Clin Proc 67:276, 1992

WORLD HEALTH ORGANIZATION: *Model Prescribing Information: Drugs Used in Parasitic Diseases*. Geneva: WHO, 1990

section 17   Protozoal infections

173   AMEBIASIS AND INFECTION WITH FREE-LIVING AMEBAS

SHARON L. REED

AMEBIASIS

DEFINITION   Amebiasis is an infection with the intestinal protozoan *Entamoeba histolytica*. About 90 percent of infections are asymptomatic, and the remaining 10 percent display a spectrum of clinical syndromes ranging from dysentery to abscesses of the liver or other organs.

LIFE CYCLE AND TRANSMISSION   *E. histolytica* is acquired by ingestion of viable cysts from fecally contaminated water, food, or hands. Food-borne exposure is most prevalent, particularly when handlers are shedding cysts or food is grown in fecally contaminated soil, fertilizer, or water. Less common sources include waterborne transmission, oral and anal sexual practices, and, rarely, direct rectal inoculation through colonic irrigation devices. Motile trophozoites are released from cysts in the small intestine, where they remain as harmless commensals in the large bowel of most patients. After encystation, infectious cysts are shed in the stool and can survive for several weeks in a moist environment. In some patients, the trophozoites invade either the bowel mucosa, causing symptomatic colitis, or the bloodstream, causing distant abscesses of the liver, lungs, or brain. The trophozoites may not encyst in patients with active dysentery, and motile, hematophagous trophozoites are frequently present in fresh stools. Trophozoites are rapidly killed by exposure to air or stomach acid, however, and therefore cannot cause infection.

EPIDEMIOLOGY   About 10 percent of the world's population is infected with *E. histolytica*; amebiasis is the third cause of death from parasitic disease after schistosomiasis and malaria. Areas of highest incidence include most developing countries in the tropics due to inadequate sanitation and crowding, particularly in Mexico, Central and South America, India, tropical Asia, and Africa. The main groups at risk in developed countries are travelers, recent immigrants, homosexual men, and inmates of institutions.

All *E. histolytica* trophozoites and cysts are morphologically identical, but the wide spectrum of clinical disease is determined by the virulence of the infecting strain. Isolates of *E. histolytica* from patients with invasive amebiasis have unique isoenzymes, surface antigens, DNA markers, and virulence properties (including the production of extracellular proteinases and resistance to complement-mediated lysis).

Most asymptomatic carriers, including homosexual men and AIDS patients, harbor nonpathogenic strains and have self-limited infections. These findings suggest that nonpathogenic strains of *E. histolytica* are incapable of causing invasive disease, since *Cryptosporidium* and *Isospora belli*, which also cause only self-limited illnesses in immunocompetent people, cause devastating diarrhea in AIDS patients. Some asymptomatic individuals are infected with strains that are pathogenic, as shown by isoenzyme patterns. In one study, 10 percent of asymptomatic patients who were colonized with pathogenic strains went on to develop amebic colitis, while the rest remained asymptomatic and cleared the infection within 1 year. Host factors play a role as well, since some patients infected with pathogenic strains do not develop invasive amebiasis.

FIGURE 173-1   Cyst of *E. histolytica* showing three of the four nuclei (trichrome stain).

PATHOGENESIS AND PATHOLOGY   Both cysts (Fig. 173-1) and trophozoites (Fig. 173-2) are found in the intestinal lumen, but only trophozoites invade tissue. The trophozoite is 20 to 60 μm in diameter and contains vacuoles and a nucleus with a characteristic central karyosome. In animals, depletion of intestinal mucus, diffuse inflammation, and disruption of the epithelial barrier occur before trophozoites actually come into contact with the colonic mucosa. Trophozoites attach to the interglandular epithelium by surface lectins. The earliest intestinal lesions are microulcerations of the mucosa of the cecum, sigmoid colon, or rectum that release erythrocytes, inflammatory cells, and epithelial cells. Proctoscopy reveals small ulcers with heaped up margins and normal intervening mucosa. Submucosal extension of ulcerations under viable-appearing surface mucosa causes the classic "flask-shaped" ulcer containing trophozoites at the margins of dead and viable tissues. Although neutrophilic

FIGURE 173-2   Trophozoite of *E. histolytica* demonstrating a single nucleus with a central, dotlike karyosome (trichrome stain).

infiltrates may accompany the early lesions in animals, human intestinal infection is marked by a paucity of inflammatory cells, probably in part because of the killing of neutrophils by trophozoites. Treated ulcers characteristically heal with little or no scarring. Occasionally, however, full-thickness necrosis and perforation occur.

Rarely, intestinal infection results in the formation of a mass lesion or ameboma in the bowel lumen. The overlying mucosa is usually thin and ulcerated, while other layers of the wall are thickened, edematous, and hemorrhagic, resulting in exuberant formation of granulation tissue with little fibrous tissue response.

A number of virulence factors have been linked to the ability of amebas to invade through the interglandular epithelium. One is an extracellular proteinase that degrades collagen, elastin, and components of the extracellular matrix. Other enzymes may disrupt glycoprotein bonds between mucosal epithelial cells in the gut. Amebas can lyse neutrophils, monocytes, lymphocytes, and colonic and hepatic cell lines. The cytolytic effect of amebas appears to require direct contact with target cells and may be linked to the release of phospholipase A and pore-forming peptides.

Liver abscesses are always preceded by intestinal colonization that may be asymptomatic. Blood vessels may be compromised early by lysis of the wall and thrombus formation. Trophozoites invade veins to reach the liver through the portal venous system. Pathogenic isolates are resistant to complement-mediated lysis, a property critical to survival in the bloodstream. In contrast, nonpathogenic strains are rapidly lysed by complement and are thus restricted to the bowel lumen. Inoculation of amebas into the portal system of hamsters results in an acute cellular infiltrate consisting predominantly of neutrophils. Later, the neutrophils are lysed by contact with amebas, and the release of neutrophil toxins may contribute to necrosis of hepatocytes. The liver parenchyma is replaced by necrotic material that is surrounded by a thin rim of congested liver tissue. The necrotic contents of a liver abscess are classically described as "anchovy paste," although the fluid is variable in color and is composed of bacteriologically sterile granular debris with few or no cells. Amebas, if seen, tend to be found only near the capsule of the abscess.

Clinical infection does not induce immunity to recurrent colonization with E. histolytica, but repeated episodes of colitis or liver abscess are unusual. Antibody is not protective; titers correlate with the length of illness rather than with the severity of disease. Studies of animals suggest that cell-mediated immunity may be important for protection, although patients with AIDS do not appear to be predisposed to more severe disease.

CLINICAL SYNDROMES   Intestinal amebiasis   The most common type of amebic infection is that of asymptomatic cyst passage. Even in highly endemic areas, most patients harbor nonpathogenic strains.

Symptomatic amebic colitis develops 2 to 6 weeks after the ingestion of infectious cysts. Lower abdominal pain and mild diarrhea develop gradually and are followed by malaise, weight loss, and diffuse lower abdominal or back pain. Cecal involvement may mimic acute appendicitis. Patients with full-blown dysentery may have 10 to 12 stools per day. The stools contain little fecal material and consist mainly of blood and mucus. In contrast to those with bacterial diarrhea, fewer than 40 percent of patients with amebic dysentery are febrile. Virtually all patients have heme-positive stools.

More fulminant intestinal infection, with severe abdominal pain, high fevers, and profuse diarrhea, is rare and occurs predominantly in children. Patients may develop toxic megacolon, which is severe bowel dilatation with intramural air. Patients receiving glucocorticoids are at risk for more severe amebiasis. Uncommonly, patients develop a chronic form of amebic colitis, which can be confused with inflammatory bowel disease. The positive association between severe complications of amebiasis and steroid therapy emphasizes that amebiasis must be excluded in any patient in whom inflammatory bowel disease is suspected. Amebomas are inflammatory mass lesions that develop due to chronic intestinal forms of amebiasis. An occasional patient presents only with an asymptomatic or tender abdominal mass caused by an ameboma, which is easily confused with cancer on barium studies. A positive serologic test or biopsy can prevent unnecessary surgery in this setting. The syndrome of postamebic colitis, persistent diarrhea following documented cure of amebic colitis, is controversial; no evidence of recurrent amebic infection can be found, and retreatment usually has no effect.

Amebic liver abscess   Extraintestinal infection by E. histolytica most often involves the liver. Of travelers who develop an amebic liver abscess after leaving an endemic area, 95 percent do so within 5 months. Young patients with an amebic liver abscess are more likely to present acutely with prominent symptoms of less than 10 days' duration. The majority of patients are febrile and have right upper quadrant pain, which may be dull or pleuritic in nature and radiate to the shoulder. Point tenderness over the liver and right pleural effusion are common. Jaundice is rare. Although the initial site of infection is the colon, fewer than one-third of patients with an amebic abscess have active diarrhea. Older patients from endemic areas are more likely to have a subacute course lasting 6 months, with weight loss and hepatomegaly. About one-third of patients with chronic presentations are febrile. Thus the clinical diagnosis of an amebic liver abscess may be difficult to establish because the symptoms and signs are often nonspecific. Since 10 to 15 percent of patients present only with fever, amebic liver abscess must be considered in the differential diagnosis of fever of unknown origin.

Complications of amebic liver abscess   Pleuropulmonary involvement, which occurs in 20 to 30 percent of patients, is the most frequent complication of amebic liver abscess. Manifestations include sterile effusions, contiguous spread from the liver, and rupture into the pleural space. Sterile effusions and contiguous spread usually resolve with medical therapy, but frank rupture into the pleural space requires drainage. An hepatobronchial fistula may cause cough productive of large amounts of necrotic material that may contain amebas. This dramatic complication carries a good prognosis. Abscesses that rupture into the peritoneum may present as an indolent leak or an acute abdomen and require both percutaneous catheter drainage and medical therapy. Rupture into the pericardium, usually from abscesses of the left lobe of the liver, carries the gravest prognosis, can occur during medical therapy, and requires surgical drainage.

Other extraintestinal sites   Involvement of the genitourinary tract may occur by direct extension from the colon or hematogenous spread. Painful genital ulcers, characterized by a punched-out appearance and profuse discharge, may develop secondary to extension from either the intestine or the liver. Both these conditions respond well to medical therapy. Cerebral involvement occurs in fewer than 0.1 percent of patients in large clinical series. Symptoms and prognosis depend on the size and location of the lesion.

DIAGNOSTIC TESTS   Laboratory diagnosis   Stool examinations, serology, and noninvasive imaging of the liver are the most important tests to establish the diagnosis. Fecal findings suggestive of amebic colitis include a positive test for heme, a paucity of neutrophils, and the presence of Charcot-Leyden crystal protein (double pyramid-shaped crystals normally found in the cytoplasm of eosinophils). The cornerstone of the diagnosis of amebic colitis, however, is the demonstration of the hematophagous trophozoites or the cysts of E. histolytica (Figs. 173-1 and 173-2). Because trophozoites are rapidly killed by water, drying, or barium, it is important to examine at least three fresh stool specimens. Examination of a combination of wet mounts, iodine-stained concentrates, and trichrome stains of fresh stool and concentrates confirms the diagnosis in 75 to 95 percent of cases. Cultures of amebas are more sensitive but are not routinely available. If stool examinations are negative, sigmoidoscopy with biopsy of the edge of ulcers may increase the yield but is risky during fulminant colitis because of the risk of perforation. Trophozoites in the biopsy of a colonic mass confirm the diagnosis of ameboma, but trophozoites are rare in liver aspirates. Accurate diagnosis requires experience, since trophozoites may be confused with neutrophils and the cysts must be differentiated

A   B

FIGURE 173-3 *A*. Cyst of *E. hartmanni* showing the smaller size with a single nucleus and eccentric karyosome. *B*. Cyst of *E. coli* showing five of the seven nuclei. *(A and B from FM Spencer, LS Monroe, Color Atlas of Intestinal Parasites, Springfield, Ill, Charles C Thomas, 1982.)*

morphologically from *E. hartmanni* and *E. coli* (Fig. 173-3 *A* and *B*) and from *Endolimax nana*, which do not cause clinical disease and do not warrant therapy. Unfortunately, the cysts of pathogenic and nonpathogenic *E. histolytica* cannot be distinguished microscopically.

Serology is helpful in the diagnosis of invasive amebiasis. Kits for the performance of counterimmunodiffusion, agar gel diffusion, and ELISA assays are commercially available, and the results of these tests are positive in more than 90 percent of patients with colitis, amebomas, or liver abscess. Positive results suggest active disease because serologies usually revert to negative within 6 to 12 months. Even in highly endemic areas such as South Africa, fewer than 10 percent of asymptomatic people have a positive amebic serology. The interpretation of the indirect hemagglutination (IHA) test is more difficult because titers may remain positive for as long as 10 years. Up to 10 percent of patients with acute amebic liver abscess may have a negative serology; in suspected cases, testing should be repeated in a week. In contrast to carriers of nonpathogenic strains, most asymptomatic carriers of pathogenic strains develop antibodies. Thus serologic tests are helpful in assessing the risk of invasive amebiasis in an asymptomatic patient. Serologies also should be assessed in patients with ulcerative colitis before the institution of steroid therapy to prevent the development of severe colitis or toxic megacolon during unsuspected amebiasis.

Routine hematology and chemistry tests are usually not very helpful in the diagnosis of invasive amebiasis. About three-fourths of patients with an amebic liver abscess have leukocytosis (>10,000 cells per cubic millimeter); this condition is particularly likely if symptoms are acute or complications have developed. Invasive amebiasis does not elicit eosinophilia. Anemia, if present, is usually multifactorial. Even with large liver abscesses, liver enzymes are normal or minimally elevated. The alkaline phosphatase level is most often elevated and may remain so for months. Transaminase elevations suggest acute disease or a complication.

Radiographic studies Radiographic barium studies are potentially dangerous in acute amebic colitis. Amebomas are usually identified first by a barium enema, but biopsy is necessary for differentiation from carcinoma.

Newer radiographic techniques have improved the detection of amebic liver abscesses. Liver scans, ultrasonography, computed tomography, and magnetic resonance imaging are all useful for detection of the round or oval hypoechoic cyst. More than 80 percent of patients who have had symptoms for more than 10 days have a single abscess of the right lobe of the liver. Approximately 50 percent of patients who have had symptoms for less than 10 days have multiple abscesses. Findings associated with complications include large abscesses (>10 cm) in the superior part of the right lobe, which

may rupture into the pleural space; multiple lesions, which must be differentiated from pyogenic abscesses; and lesions of the left lobe, which may rupture into the pericardium. Because abscesses resolve slowly and may increase in size in patients who are responding clinically to therapy, frequent follow-up ultrasonography may prove confusing. Complete resolution of a liver abscess within 6 months can be anticipated in two-thirds of patients, but 10 percent may have persistent abnormalities for a year.

DIFFERENTIAL DIAGNOSIS The differential diagnosis of intestinal amebiasis includes bacterial diarrheas caused by *Campylobacter*, enteroinvasive *Escherichia coli*, and *Shigella*, *Salmonella*, and *Vibrio* species. Although the typical patient with amebic colitis has less prominent fever and heme-positive stools with few neutrophils, bacterial cultures, microscopic examination of stools, and amebic serology are essential for correct diagnosis. Amebiasis must be ruled out in any patient thought to have inflammatory bowel disease.

Because of the variety of presenting signs and symptoms, amebic liver abscess can easily be confused with pulmonary or gallbladder disease or with any febrile illness with few localizing signs, e.g., malaria or typhoid fever. The diagnosis should be considered in high-risk groups with a history of recent travel outside the United States and in inmates of institutions. Once radiographic studies have identified an abscess in the liver, the most important differential is between amebic and pyogenic abscess. The patient with pyogenic abscess typically is older and has a history of underlying bowel disease or recent surgery. Amebic serology is helpful, but aspiration of the abscess, with Gram stains and cultures of the material, may be required to differentiate the two diseases.

TREATMENT Intestinal disease Drugs to treat amebiasis can be classified according to their primary site of action. Luminal amebicides are poorly absorbed and reach high concentrations within the bowel, but their activity is limited to cysts and trophozoites close to the mucosa. Three luminal drugs are available in the United States: iodoquinol, paromomycin, and diloxanide furoate (Table 173-1). Indications for the use of luminal agents include eradication of cysts in patients with colitis or a liver abscess and treatment of asymptomatic carriers. Until probes are available for differentiating nonpathogenic from pathogenic cysts, it is prudent to treat asymptomatic individuals who pass cysts.

Tissue amebicides reach high concentrations in the blood and tissue after oral or parenteral administration. The development of nitroimidazole compounds, especially metronidazole, was a major advance in the treatment of invasive amebiasis. Patients with amebic colitis should be treated with metronidazole, 750 mg, three times daily, IV or orally, for 10 days. Side effects include nausea, vomiting,

TABLE 173-1 Drug therapy for amebiasis

	Dosage
ASYMPTOMATIC CARRIER (LUMINAL AGENTS)	
Iodoquinol (650-mg tablets)	650 mg tid for 20 days
Diloxanide furoate* (500-mg tablets)	500 mg tid for 10 days
Paromomycin (250-mg tablets)	500 mg tid for 10 days
ACUTE COLITIS	
Metronidazole (250- or 500-mg tablets)	750 mg PO or IV tid for 5–10 days
plus	
Luminal agent as above	
AMEBIC LIVER ABSCESS	
Metronidazole	750 mg PO or IV tid for 5–10 days
Tinidazole†	2 g PO
Ornidazole†	2 g PO
plus	
Luminal agent as above	

* Available only through the CDC at telephone number (404) 639-3356.
† Not available in the United States.

abdominal discomfort, and a disulfiram-like effect. Other imidazole compounds such as tinidazole and ornidazole are as effective but are not available in the United States. All patients should receive a full course of therapy with a luminal agent, since metronidazole does not eradicate cysts. Resistance to metronidazole has not been identified. Relapses probably represent reinfection or failure to eradicate amebas from the bowel because of inadequate dosage or duration of therapy.

Amebic liver abscess Metronidazole is the drug of choice for amebic liver abscess. The usefulness of nitroimidazoles in single-dose or abbreviated regimens is important in endemic areas with limited access to hospitalization. With early diagnosis and therapy, mortality from uncomplicated amebic liver abscess is less than 1 percent. Second-line therapeutic agents such as emetine and chloroquine should be avoided if possible because of the potential cardiovascular and gastrointestinal side effects of the former and the higher relapse rates with the latter. There is no evidence that combined therapy with two drugs is more effective than the single-drug regimen. Studies of South Africans with liver abscesses demonstrated that 72 percent of patients without intestinal symptoms were colonized asymptomatically with pathogenic strains; thus all treatment regimens should include a luminal agent to eradicate cysts and prevent further transmission. Amebic liver abscess recurs rarely.

Aspiration of liver abscesses More than 90 percent of patients respond dramatically to metronidazole therapy with decreases in both pain and fever within 72 h. Indications for aspiration of liver abscesses are (1) the need to rule out a pyogenic abscess, particularly in patients with multiple lesions, (2) the failure to respond clinically in 3 to 5 days, (3) the threat of imminent rupture, and (4) the prevention of rupture of left lobe abscesses into the pericardium. There is no evidence that aspiration, even of large abscesses (up to 10 cm), leads to more rapid healing. Percutaneous drainage may be successful even if the liver abscess has already ruptured. Surgery should be reserved for instances of bowel perforation and rupture into the pericardium.

PREVENTION Amebic infection is spread by ingestion of food or water contaminated with cysts. Since an asymptomatic carrier may excrete up to 15 million cysts a day, prevention of infection requires adequate sanitation and eradication of cyst carriage. In high-risk areas, infection can be minimized by avoiding unpeeled fruits and vegetables and using bottled water. Because cysts are resistant to readily attainable levels of chlorine, disinfection by iodination (tetraglycine hydroperiodide) is recommended. There is no effective prophylaxis.

INFECTION WITH FREE-LIVING AMEBAS

EPIDEMIOLOGY Free-living amebas of the genera *Acanthamoeba* and *Naegleria* are distributed throughout the world and have been isolated from a wide variety of fresh and brackish water, including that from lakes, taps, hot springs, swimming pools, and heating and air-conditioning units, and even from the nasal passages of healthy children. Encystation may protect the protozoa from desiccation and food deprivation. The persistence of *Legionella pneumophila* in water supplies may be attributable in part to chronic infection of free-living amebas, particularly *Naegleria*.

***NAEGLERIA* INFECTIONS** More than 100 cases of primary amebic meningoencephalitis from *Naegleria fowleri* have been reported. Infection follows the aspiration of water contaminated with trophozoites or cysts or the inhalation of dust leading to invasion of the olfactory neuroepithelium. After an incubation period of 2 to 15 days, severe headache, high fever, nausea, vomiting, and meningismus occur. Photophobia and palsies of the third, fourth, and sixth cranial nerves are common. Rapid progression to seizures and coma may follow, and most patients die within a week. Infection is most common in otherwise healthy children or young adults, who often report recent swimming in lakes or heated swimming pools, particularly in July and August.

Diagnosis depends on the detection of motile trophozoites in wet mounts of fresh spinal fluid. Other laboratory findings resemble those of fulminant bacterial meningitis, with elevated intracranial pressure, high white blood cell counts (up to 20,000 cells per cubic millimeter), elevated spinal fluid protein concentration, and low glucose levels. The diagnosis should be considered in any patient who has purulent meningitis without evidence of bacteria by Gram stain, antigen detection, and culture. The prognosis is uniformly poor. Only four survivors, treated with high-dose amphotericin B and rifampin, have been reported. Antibodies to *Naegleria* spp. have been detected in normal adults, and serology is not useful in the acute diagnosis.

***ACANTHAMOEBA* INFECTIONS Granulomatous amebic encephalitis** Infection with *Acanthamoeba* species follows a more indolent course and occurs typically in chronically ill or debilitated patients. Risk factors include lymphoproliferative disorders, chemotherapy, glucocorticoid therapy, lupus erythematosus, and AIDS. Infection usually reaches the central nervous system hematogenously from a primary focus in the skin or lungs. The onset is insidious and often mimics a space-occupying lesion. Altered mental status, headache, and stiff neck may be accompanied by focal findings such as cranial nerve palsies, ataxia, and hemiparesis. Cutaneous ulcers or hard nodules containing amebas were detected in 9 of the 30 patients reported in the United States.

Examination of the cerebrospinal fluid for trophozoites may be helpful, but lumbar puncture may be contraindicated because of increased intracerebral pressure. Computed tomography frequently reveals cortical and subcortical lesions of decreased density consistent with embolic infarcts. Demonstration of the trophozoites and cysts of *Acanthamoeba* in biopsies establishes the diagnosis. Fluorescein-labeled antiserum is available from the Centers for Disease Control to be used in detecting protozoa in biopsy specimens. At least nine cases of granulomatous amebic encephalitis have been reported in patients with AIDS, who may have an accelerated course because of their difficulty in forming granulomas. Although studies in animals suggest that rifampin may be useful, the infection is almost uniformly fatal. A similar syndrome may be caused by a leptomyxid ameba.

Keratitis The incidence of keratitis caused by *Acanthamoeba* has increased in the past 15 years; more than 250 infections have been reported to the Centers for Disease Control. The first recognized infections were associated with trauma to the eye and exposure to contaminated water. At present, most infections are linked to extended-wear contact lenses. Risk factors include the use of homemade saline, wearing lenses while swimming, and inadequate disinfection. Since contact lenses presumably cause microscopic trauma, the early corneal findings may be nonspecific. The first symptoms usually include tearing and the painful sensation of a foreign body. Once infection is established, progression is rapid, and the characteristic clinical sign is an annular, paracentral corneal ring representing a corneal abscess. Deeper corneal invasion and loss of vision may follow.

The differential diagnosis includes bacterial, mycobacterial, and herpetic infection. The irregular, polygonal cysts of *Acanthamoeba* may be identified in corneal scrapings or biopsy material, and trophozoites can be grown on special media. Cysts are resistant to available drugs, and the results of medical therapy are disappointing. Some reports have suggested partial responses to the combination of propamidine isethionate eyedrops and topical steroids. Severe infections usually require keratoplasty.

REFERENCES

Amebiasis

ALLASON-JONES E et al: *Entamoeba histolytica* as a commensal intestinal parasite in homosexual men. N Engl J Med 315:353, 1986

IRUSEN EM et al: Asymptomatic intestinal colonization by pathogenic *Entamoeba histolytica* in amebic liver abscess: Prevalence, response to therapy, and pathogenic potential. Clin Infect Dis 14:889, 1992

KATZENSTEIN D et al: New concepts of amebic liver abscess derived from hepatic imaging, serodiagnosis, and hepatic enzymes in 67 consecutive cases in San Diego. Medicine 61:237, 1982

RAVDIN JL (ed): *Amebiasis: Human Infection by Entamoeba histolytica.* New York, Wiley, 1988

REED SL: Amebiasis: an update. Clin Infect Dis 14:385, 1992

———— et al: *Entamoeba histolytica* infection and AIDS. Am J Med 90:269, 1991

SARGEAUNT PG: The reliability of *Entamoeba histolytica* zymodemes in clinical diagnosis. Parasitol Today 3:40, 1987

THOMPSON JE et al: Amebic liver abscess: A therapeutic approach. Rev Infect Dis 7:171, 1985

Acanthamoeba and *Naegleria*

MA P et al: *Naegleria* and *Acanthamoeba* infections: Review. Rev Infect Dis 12:490, 1990

STEHR-GREEN JK et al: *Acanthamoeba* keratitis in soft contact lens wearers: A case-control study. JAMA 258:57, 1987

VISVESVARA GS, STEHR-GREEN JK: Epidemiology of free-living ameba infections. J Protozool 37:25S, 1990

WILEY CA et al: Acanthamoeba meningoencephalitis in a patient with AIDS. J Infect Dis 155:130, 1987

174 MALARIA AND BABESIOSIS

NICHOLAS J. WHITE / JOEL G. BREMAN

MALARIA

Malaria is a protozoan disease transmitted by the bite of *Anopheles* mosquitoes. It is the most important of the parasitic diseases of humans, affecting 103 endemic countries with a population of over 2.5 billion people and causing between 1 and 3 million deaths each year. Malaria has now been eradicated from North America, Europe, and Russia; however, despite enormous control efforts, there has been a resurgence of the disease in many parts of the tropics. In addition, drug resistance poses increasing problems in most malarious areas. Malaria remains today, as it has for centuries, a major burden on tropical communities and a danger to travelers.

ETIOLOGY Four species of the genus *Plasmodium* infect humans. These are *P. vivax, P. ovale, P. malariae,* and *P. falciparum* (Table 174-1). Almost all deaths from malaria are caused by *P. falciparum.* Human infection begins when a female anopheline mosquito inoculates sporozoites from its salivary glands during a blood meal (Fig. 174-1). These small motile forms are carried rapidly via the bloodstream to the liver, where they target hepatic parenchymal cells, invade, and begin a period of asexual reproduction. By this amplification process (known as *intrahepatic* or *pre-erythrocytic merogony*), a single sporozoite eventually produces several thousand daughter merozoites. The swollen liver cell eventually bursts, discharging merozoites into the bloodstream—an event that initiates the symptomatic stage of the infection. In *P. vivax* and *P. ovale* infections, a proportion of the intrahepatic forms do not divide immediately but remain dormant for months before reproduction begins. These

"sleeping" forms, or hypnozoites, are the cause of the relapses that characterize infection with these two species.

After entering the bloodstream, merozoites rapidly invade erythrocytes. Attachment is mediated by a specific erythrocyte surface receptor. In *P. vivax* this receptor is related to the Duffy blood group antigen Fy^a or Fy^b. Most West Africans (or people with origins in that region) carry the Duffy-negative Fy phenotype and are therefore resistant to *P. vivax* malaria. The glycophorins, a family of membrane sialoglycoproteins, are the red cell attachment sites for the merozoites of *P. falciparum.* During the early stage of development, the small "ring forms" of the four parasite species appear similar under light microscopy. As the trophozoites enlarge, species-specific characteristics become evident, pigment becomes visible, and the parasite assumes an irregular or ameboid shape. By the end of the 48-h cycle (72 h for *P. malariae*), the parasite has grown to occupy most of the red cell. Multiple nuclear fission (merogony) then takes place, and the red cell ruptures to release 6 to 32 daughter merozoites, each of which is capable of invading a new red cell and repeating the cycle. After a period of asexual reproduction, a proportion of the parasites develop into morphologically distinct sexual forms (gametocytes) that are long-lived and are not associated with illness.

After ingestion of a blood meal by a biting female anopheline mosquito, male and female gametocytes fuse in the insect's midgut to form a zygote. This stage matures to form an ookinete, which penetrates and encysts in the mosquito's gut wall. The resulting oocyst expands by asexual division until it bursts to liberate myriad motile sporozoites, which migrate to the mosquito's salivary gland to await inoculation into humans at the next feeding.

The disease in humans is attributable to the direct effects of red cell invasion and destruction and the host's reaction to this process.

EPIDEMIOLOGY Malaria occurs throughout most of the tropical regions of the world. *P. falciparum* predominates in sub-Saharan Africa, New Guinea, and Haiti. While *P. vivax* is more common in Central America and the Indian subcontinent, an increase in *P. falciparum* infections has occurred in India over the past decade. The prevalence of these two species is approximately equal in South America, eastern Asia, and Oceania. *P. malariae* is found in most areas (particularly in West and Central Africa) but is less common. *P. ovale* infection is relatively unusual outside Africa.

The epidemiology of malaria may vary even within small geographic areas. Major epidemiologic determinants are the immunologic and genetic makeup of the population, the species of parasite and mosquito in the community at risk, the level of rainfall, the temperature, the distribution of mosquito breeding sites, the use of antimalarial drugs, and the application of other control measures that could decrease transmission.

Endemicity has been defined in terms of prevalence of parasitemia and a palpable spleen in children less than 9 years of age, although these figures can vary with the season and with the presence of other endemic diseases causing splenomegaly. An area is considered to be hypoendemic if fewer than 10 percent of children have parasitemia

TABLE 174-1 Characteristics of *Plasmodium* species infecting humans

Characteristic	*P. falciparum*	*P. vivax*	*P. ovale*	*P. malariae*
Duration of intrahepatic phase (days)	5–7	7–8	9	14–16
Duration of erythrocytic cycle (hours)	48	48	50	72
Red cell preference	Younger cells, but can invade cells of all ages	Reticulocytes	Reticulocytes	Older cells
Morphology	Usually only ring forms; parasitemia level may exceed 2 percent, with multiple infections of a single erythrocyte; banana-shaped gametocytes	Irregularly shaped, large rings and trophozoites; enlarged erythrocytes; Schüffner's dots	Infected erythrocytes enlarged and oval; Schüffner's dots	Band or rectangular forms of trophozoites common
Pigment color	Black	Yellow-brown	Dark brown	Brown-black
Relapses	No	Yes	Yes	No

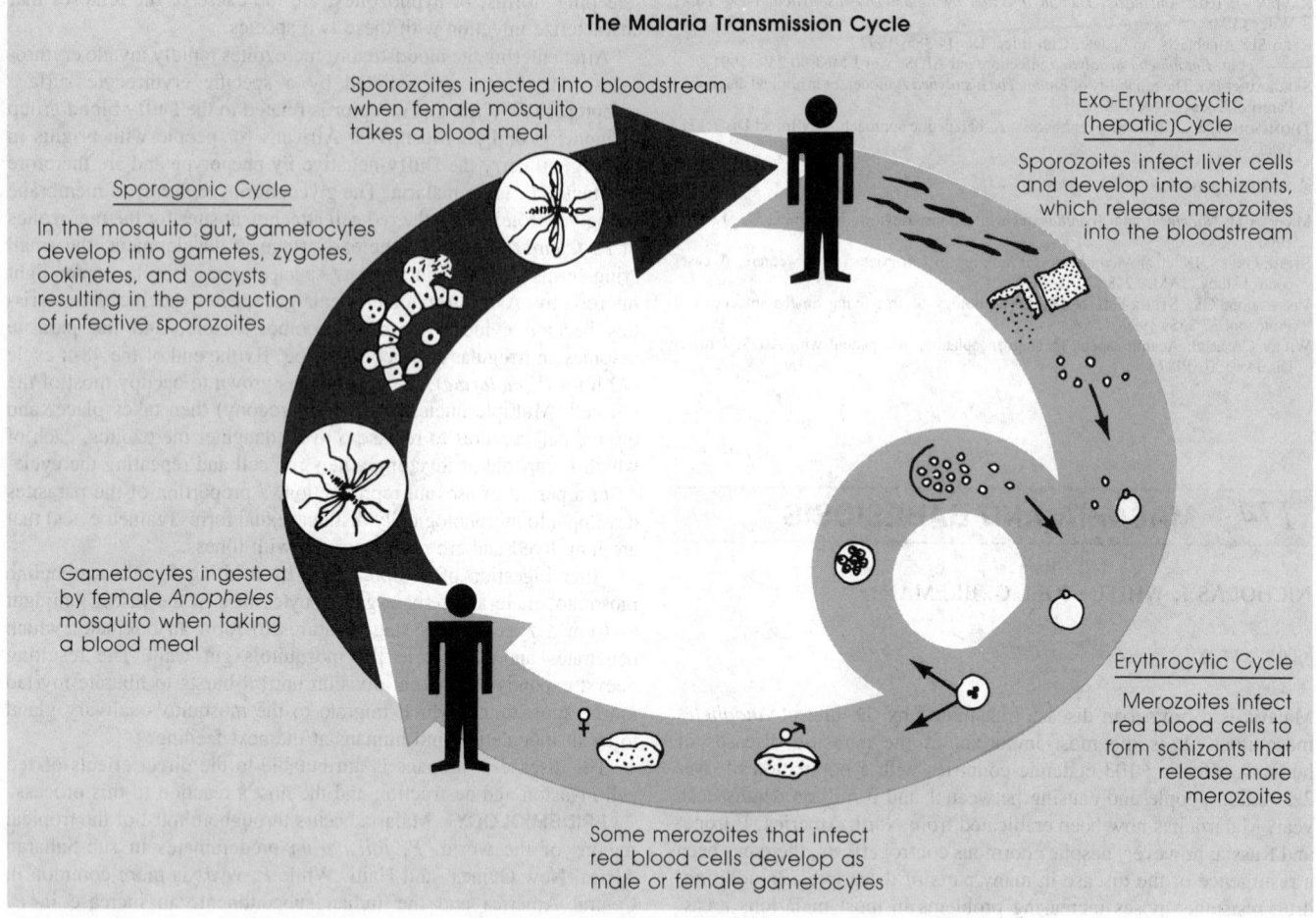

FIGURE 174-1 The malaria transmission cycle. (From Breman and Steketee.)

and a palpable spleen, mesoendemic if the figures are 11 to 50 percent, hyperendemic if they are 51 to 75 percent, and holoendemic if they are greater than 75 percent. In holo- and hyperendemic areas (e.g., much of tropical Africa and coastal New Guinea), where *P. falciparum* transmission is intense, persons are infected repeatedly throughout their lives. Malaria causes illness and death during childhood. The development of immunity is perilous, but by adulthood malaria infections are largely asymptomatic. This situation is termed *stable malaria*. In areas in which transmission is low, erratic, or focal, the chance that one infected person will transmit malaria to another is relatively small, full immunity is not acquired, and symptomatic disease may occur at any age. This situation is termed *unstable malaria*. Even in areas with stable malaria, seasonal variations in disease coincide with increased breeding of mosquitoes during the rainy season. Malaria can behave like an epidemic disease in some areas (such as northern India, Sri Lanka, Madagascar, and northwestern Brazil) when refugees or workers migrate from a nonmalarious region to areas of high transmission or when malaria control measures (mainly household spraying with insecticides) are stopped abruptly. Epidemics of falciparum malaria can produce considerable mortality at all ages.

The principal determinants of malaria transmission are the sporozoite rates, (proportion of potential vectors with sporozoites in the salivary glands), biting habits, longevity, and density of the mosquito vectors. In general, the rate of malaria transmission is directly proportional to (1) the density of the vector, (2) the square of the number of human bites per day per mosquito, and (3) the tenth power of the probability of a mosquito surviving for 1 day. Because the extrinsic cycle from gametocyte ingestion to subsequent sporozoite inoculation takes a minimum of 7 days (with the exact interval depending on ambient temperature), mosquito longevity is particularly important.

Therefore, the most effective mosquito vectors are long-lived, occur in high densities, and bite humans frequently (e.g., *Anopheles gambiae* in West Africa). The entomologic inoculation rate, which is used as a measure of the intensity of malaria transmission, is the number of sporozoite-positive mosquito bites per person per unit time.

ERYTHROCYTE CHANGES   After invasion, the growing parasite progressively consumes and degrades intracellular proteins, principally hemoglobin, and alters the red cell membrane by changing its transport properties, exposing cryptic surface antigens, and inserting new parasite-derived proteins. The red cell becomes more spherical and less deformable. In *P. falciparum* infections, membrane protuberances appear on the erythrocyte surface in the second 24 h of the asexual cycle. These "knobs" overlie accretions of electron-dense, histidine-rich parasite proteins. They extrude a strain-specific, adhesive-variant protein of high molecular weight that mediates red cell attachment to receptors on venular and capillary endothelium, causing a phenomenon called *cytoadherence*. *P. falciparum*–infected red cells also adhere to uninfected red cells to form rosettes. This event occurs at the same stage of parasite development as cytoadherence and has been linked to cerebral malaria. Cytoadherence and rosetting are central to the pathogenesis of falciparum malaria. These processes result in the formation of red cell aggregates and the intravascular sequestration of red cells that contain mature forms of the parasite in vital organs (particularly the brain and heart). Aggregated and sequestered red cells interfere with microcirculatory flow and metabolism and allow parasite development away from the principal host defense, splenic processing and filtration. As a consequence, only the younger ring forms of the asexual parasites are seen in the peripheral blood in falciparum malaria, and the peripheral parasitemia (which can reach high levels) is an underestimate of the true number of parasites within the body. With *P. vivax, P. malariae,* and *P. ovale,* sequestration does not take place, all stages of parasite development may be seen on peripheral blood smears, and levels of parasitemia seldom exceed 1 to 2 percent. These species show a marked predilection for either old red cells *(P. malariae)* or reticulocytes *(P. vivax)* (see Table 174-1).

HOST RESPONSE The initial response to infection in a nonimmune person is the activation of nonspecific host defense mechanisms. Immunologic and filtrative functions of the spleen are augmented, with accelerated removal of both parasitized and uninfected erythrocytes. The parasitized cells that escape splenic removal are destroyed when the schizont (meront) ruptures. The material released induces the activation of macrophages and the release of mononuclear cell–derived cytokines (including tumor necrosis factor) and, in succession, interleukins 1, 6, and 8, which cause fever and other pathologic effects. High serum concentrations of tumor necrosis factor are associated with a poor prognosis in severe malaria, although whether or not tumor necrosis factor is directly lethal in malaria remains to be determined. Temperatures of 40°C or higher are schizontocidal, leading to the synchronization of the parasite cycle and to production of the regular fever spikes and rigors that were once used to characterize the different malarias (quotidian, daily fever spike; tertian, every 2 days; quartan, every 3 days). These regular fever patterns are seldom seen in patients who receive prompt, effective antimalarial treatment.

The distribution of sickle cell disease, thalassemia, and glucose-6-phosphate dehydrogenase (G6PD) deficiency in the world closely resembles that of malaria before the introduction of control measures. This correlation implies that these genetic disorders may confer protection against death from malaria. This has been confirmed in the case of sickle cell trait, but the mechanism of protection has not been elucidated, except in Melanesian ovalocytosis, in which the rigid erythrocytes resist merozoite invasion and the intraerythrocytic electrolyte milieu is hostile to the parasite.

The specific immune response to malaria limits the level of parasitemia and, with repeated exposure to a sufficient number of strains, eventually confers protection from disease but not from infection. This state of premunition is specific for both the species and the strain of the infecting malaria parasite. Both humoral and cellular immune systems participate, but the mechanisms are incompletely understood. Immune individuals have a polyclonal increase in serum IgM, IgG, and IgA, although much of this antibody is unrelated to protection. Antibodies and cellular immune responses to parasite antigens expressed both on the merozoite surface (leading to agglutination) and on the erythrocyte surface (leading to parasite killing and erythrophagocytosis) presumably act in concert to limit in vivo parasite replication. Passive transfer IgG from immune mothers reduces the level of parasitemia in children. Passive transfer of maternal antibody also contributes to the relative protection of the infant from severe malaria during the first months of life.

Factors that retard the development of cellular immunity include the absence of major histocompatibility antigens on the surface of infected red cells, which precludes direct α and β T cell recognition; malaria antigen–specific immune unresponsiveness coupled with nonspecific parasite-induced mitogenic activity that produces an "immunologic smokescreen"; and the diversity of malarial strains and their ability to express antigens on the erythrocyte surface that change during the course of infection. Hence no individual is ever immune to all strains. Parasites may persist in the blood for months—or, in the case of *P. malariae,* for years—if untreated. Because of the complex immune response in malaria, the diversity of the parasites' evasive mechanisms, and the lack of a good means of in vitro assessment of clinical immunity, no effective vaccine is available yet.

GENERAL CLINICAL FEATURES The first symptoms are nonspecific and similar to those of a minor viral illness, with malaise, headache, fatigue, abdominal discomfort, and muscle aches, followed by fever and chills. In some cases, a prominence of headache, chest pain, nausea, vomiting, abdominal pain, arthralgia, myalgia, or diarrhea may suggest other illnesses. The classic malarial paroxysms in which fever spikes, chills, and rigors (tremors induced by chills) occur at regular intervals are rare. True rigors are more common with *P. vivax* and *P. ovale* than with *P. falciparum.* More often, the fever is irregular at first; in nonimmune adults or children, nausea, vomiting, and orthostatic hypotension are common. Most patients with uncomplicated acute infections have few abnormal physical findings other than mild anemia and in some cases a palpable spleen.

SEVERE FALCIPARUM MALARIA (See Table 174-2) **Cerebral malaria** Coma is a characteristic and ominous feature of severe falciparum malaria and, despite treatment, is associated with a mortality of approximately 20 percent in adults and 15 percent in children. Lesser degrees of obtundation, delirium, or abnormal behavior also should be addressed with urgency because deterioration can be rapid. The onset of coma may be gradual or sudden following a convulsion. Cerebral malaria is a diffuse symmetric encephalopathy; focal neurologic signs are unusual. Although there may be passive resistance to head flexion, signs of meningeal irritation are absent. The eyes may be divergent, and a pout reflex is common, but other primitive reflexes are usually absent. The corneal reflexes are preserved except in deep coma. Muscle tone may be increased or decreased. The tendon reflexes are variable, and the plantar reflexes may be flexor or extensor; abdominal and cremasteric reflexes are absent. Flexor or extensor posturing may occur. Approximately 15 percent of patients have retinal hemorrhages. Anemia and jaundice are common. Convulsions, which are usually generalized, are common in children with cerebral malaria and in about half of adults. Seizures are associated with high temperatures (≥40°C). Approximately 10 percent of children who survive cerebral malaria, particularly those

---

TABLE 174-2 Manifestations of severe malaria

MAJOR SIGNS

Unarousable coma/ cerebral malaria	Failure to localize or respond appropriately to noxious stimuli; coma should persist for >30 min after generalized convulsion
Severe normochromic, normocytic anemia	Hematocrit <15 percent or hemoglobin <5 g/dL with parasitemia level >10,000 per microliter
Renal failure	Urine output <400 mL/24 h in adults or 12 mL/kg per 24 h in children; no improvement with rehydration; serum creatinine >265 μmol/L (>3.0 mg/dL)
Pulmonary edema/ adult respiratory distress syndrome	
Hypoglycemia	Glucose <2.2 mmol/L (<40 mg/dL)
Hypotension/shock	Systolic blood pressure <50 mmHg in children 1–5 years or <80 mmHg in adults; core skin temperature difference >10°C.
Bleeding/disseminated intravascular coagulation	Significant bleeding and hemorrhage from the gums, nose, gastrointestinal tract, and/or evidence of disseminated intravascular coagulation.
Convulsions	More than two generalized seizures in 24 h
Acidemia/acidosis	Arterial pH <7.25 or plasma bicarbonate <15 mmol/L, venous lactate >6 mmol/L
Hemoglobinuria	Macroscopic black, brown, or red urine; not associated with effects of oxidant drugs and red blood cell enzyme defects (such as G6PD deficiency)

OTHER SIGNS

Impaired consciousness/ arousable	
Extreme weakness	
Hyperparasitemia	Parasitemia >5 percent in nonimmune patients
Jaundice	Serum bilirubin level >50 mmol/L (>3.0 mg/dL)
Hyperpyrexia	Rectal temperature >40°C.

with hypoglycemia, severe anemia, repeated seizures, and deep coma, have persistent neurologic deficits. Residual deficits are unusual in adults (< 3 percent).

Hypoglycemia Hypoglycemia is associated with a poor prognosis. Children and pregnant women are at special risk. Hypoglycemia results from failure of hepatic gluconeogenesis and increased consumption of glucose by the host and the parasites. Plasma concentrations of the principal gluconeogenic substrates, lactate and alanine, are increased. To compound the situation, quinine and quinidine, the drugs of choice for the treatment of severe chloroquine-resistant malaria, are powerful stimulants to pancreatic insulin secretion; pregnant women who receive quinine are especially prone to hypoglycemia. Clinical diagnosis of severe hypoglycemia is difficult because the adrenergic signs (sweating, gooseflesh, tachycardia) may be absent and neurologic impairment attributable to hypoglycemia cannot be distinguished from that of malaria itself.

Lactic acidosis Anaerobic glycolysis occurs in tissues where sequestered parasitized erythrocytes interfere with microcirculatory flow. This phenomenon, together with hypotension and a failure of hepatic lactate clearance, causes lactic acidosis. Hyperventilation is usually followed by circulatory failure refractory to volume expansion and to inotropic drugs. The prognosis of lactic acidosis is poor.

Noncardiogenic pulmonary edema Adult respiratory distress syndrome (ARDS) may develop in adults with severe falciparum malaria, even after several days of antimalarial therapy and clearance of parasites. The pathogenesis is unclear, but the mortality rate of established ARDS is over 80 percent.

Renal impairment Renal impairment is common among adults with severe falciparum malaria but rare among children. Renal failure is associated with high mortality. The pathogenesis is unclear but may be related to sequestration of parasitized erythrocytes and reduction of renal microcirculatory flow. Clinically and pathologically, malaria-induced renal failure resembles acute tubular necrosis; if the anuric patient survives the acute phase and effective dialysis is undertaken, the flow of urine usually recommences in about 4 days, and the serum creatinine level returns to normal in 2 to 3 weeks (see Chap. 236).

Hematologic abnormalities Anemia is caused by accelerated destruction and removal of red cells by the spleen and by suppression of the bone marrow with ineffective erythropoiesis. Anemia can develop rapidly, and transfusion is often required. Anemia is a particular problem in children. In some patients with *P. falciparum*, massive hemolysis causes hemoglobinemia, black urine, and renal failure (blackwater fever). Coagulation defects occur in falciparum malaria. Bleeding is significant in fewer than 5 percent of patients with cerebral malaria and is usually associated with disseminated intravascular coagulation. Hematemesis, presumably from stress ulceration or acute gastric erosions, also may occur.

Other complications People with malaria are predisposed to bacterial superinfection. Aspiration pneumonia following convulsions is an important cause of death in cerebral malaria. Pneumonia and catheter-induced urinary tract infections are common in unconscious patients. In Africa, falciparum malaria has been associated with *Salmonella* septicemia.

MALARIA IN PREGNANCY *P. falciparum* infection of the placenta of pregnant women is associated with low birth weight, particularly in the primigravida. In areas with stable and intense transmission, pregnant women generally remain asymptomatic despite sequestration of parasitized erythrocytes in the placental microcirculation. In areas that have unstable transmission (hypo- or mesoendemic), pregnant women are prone to severe infections and are particularly vulnerable to the development of high levels of parasitemia, anemia, hypoglycemia, and acute pulmonary edema. Fetal distress, premature labor, spontaneous abortion, and stillbirth are common. Congenital malaria occurs in fewer than 5 percent of newborns whose mothers are infected and is related directly to the parasite density in the placenta.

MALARIA IN CHILDREN Most of the 1 to 3 million who die each year from falciparum malaria are children, mainly in Africa. Convulsions, coma, hypoglycemia, metabolic acidosis, and severe anemia are relatively common among children with severe malaria, whereas severe jaundice, acute renal failure, and acute pulmonary edema are unusual. In general, children tolerate antimalarial drugs well and respond rapidly to treatment.

TRANSFUSION MALARIA Malaria can be transmitted by blood transfusion or by needle sharing between infected intravenous drug users. *P. malariae* and *P. falciparum* are the most common etiologic agents in such cases. The incubation period is often short because there is no pre-erythrocytic development. Clinical features and management are similar to those of naturally acquired infections, although falciparum malaria tends to be especially severe in drug addicts. Radical chemotherapy with primaquine in infections due to *P. vivax* or *P. ovale* is unnecessary because intrahepatic merogony does not take place in transfusion-induced malaria.

TROPICAL SPLENOMEGALY (HYPERREACTIVE MALARIOUS SPLENOMEGALY) Some residents of endemic areas exhibit an abnormal immunolological response to repeated malarial infections that results in massive splenomegaly, hepatomegaly, marked elevations in serum levels of IgM and malaria antibody, hepatic sinusoidal lymphocytosis, and—in Africa—10 percent develop peripheral (B cell) lymphocytosis. This immune response is associated with the production of cytotoxic IgM antisuppressor lymphocyte (CD8 +) antibodies, which leads to uninhibited B cell production of IgM and the formation of cryoglobulins (IgM aggregates and immune complexes). This process then stimulates reticuloendothelial hyperplasia and clearance activity and eventually produces splenomegaly. Patients with hyperactive malarial splenomegaly have an abdominal mass or experience a dragging sensation in the abdomen with occasional sharp abdominal pains that suggests perisplenitis. Patients are usually anemic and exhibit some degree of pancytopenia. In most cases, malaria parasites cannot be found in peripheral blood smears. Patients with hyperreactive malarious splenomegaly are particularly vulnerable to infections, and have an increased mortality. Hyperreactive malarious splenomegaly usually responds to antimalarial prophylaxis. In patients who are refractory to therapy, clonal lymphoproliferation may occur, resulting in a malignant lymphoproliferative disorder.

QUARTAN MALARIAL NEPHROPATHY Chronic or repeated infections with *P. malariae* may cause soluble immune-complex injury to the renal glomeruli, resulting in the nephrotic syndrome. Other factors contribute because only a small proportion of infected persons develops renal disease. The histologic appearance of the glomeruli is of focal or segmental glomerulonephritis with splitting of the capillary basement membrane. Dense subendothelial deposits are seen on electron microscopy, and immunofluorescence reveals deposits of complement and immunoglobulins; in children, *P. malariae* antigens are often seen. Patients who have a coarse granular pattern of basement-membrane immunofluorescent deposits (predominantly IgG3) and selective proteinuria have a better prognosis than those with a fine, granular, predominantly IgG2 pattern and nonselective proteinuria. Quartan nephropathy usually does not respond to treatment with either antimalarial agents or glucocorticoids and cytotoxic drugs.

DIAGNOSIS The diagnosis of malaria rests on the demonstration of asexual form of the parasite in peripheral blood smears stained preferably with Giemsa (see Chap. 171). Other Romanowsky stains (Wright's, Field's or Leishman's) are less reliable. Both thin and thick blood smears should be made with great care on clean slides. The thin smear should be air dried rapidly, fixed in anhydrous methanol, and stained. The red cells in the tail of the film should be examined under oil immersion microscopy. The level of parasitemia is expressed as the number of parasitized erythrocytes per 1000 red blood cells, and this figure is then converted to the number per microliter of blood.

The thick smear should be dried thoroughly and stained (also with Giemsa) without alcohol fixation. Since many layers of erythrocytes overlie one another and are lysed during the staining procedure, the thick film concentrates the parasites up to 40 times that of the thin smear, thereby increasing the sensitivity of diagnosis. Both parasites and white blood cells are counted, and the number of parasites per unit volume is calculated from the total leukocyte count. A minimum of 200 white cells should be counted. Interpretation of thick films requires experience because artifacts are common. Phagocytosed malaria pigment may be visible inside peripheral blood monocytes or polymorphonuclear leukocytes and may provide a clue to recent infection if malaria parasites are not seen. Occasionally, parasites and pigment are evident in bone marrow aspirates or smears obtained from fluid expressed after intradermal puncture, but not on peripheral blood smears. Staining of the parasites with the fluorescent dye acridine orange allows a more rapid diagnosis when levels of parasitemia are low. Compared with microscopy, this technique is less accurate for species identification and for quantitation of parasitemia. The relation between the level of parasitemia and the prognosis is complex; in general, patients with parasitemia levels in excess of 10^5 per microliter (~2 percent) are more likely to die. However, nonimmune patients may die with relatively low parasite densities, and partially immune persons may tolerate relatively high levels with minor symptoms. At any level of parasitemia, a predominance of more mature parasites (i.e., >20 percent of parasites with visible pigment) or circulating *P. falciparum* schizonts (meronts) carries a poor prognosis.

LABORATORY FINDINGS Normochromic, normocytic anemia is the rule. The leukocyte count is low to normal, although it may be elevated in severe infections. The erythrocyte sedimentation rate, plasma viscosity, and C-reactive protein level are high. The platelet count is usually moderately reduced (to about 100,000 per microliter). In severe infections, the prothrombin and partial thromboplastin times may be prolonged, and thrombocytopenia may be severe. Levels of antithrombin III are reduced even in mild infection. In uncomplicated malaria, plasma concentrations of electrolytes, blood urea nitrogen, and creatinine are usually normal. In severe falciparum malaria, metabolic acidosis may be present with low plasma concentrations of glucose, sodium, bicarbonate, calcium, phosphate, and albumin and elevated plasma levels of lactate, blood urea nitrogen, creatinine, urate, muscle and liver enzymes, and conjugated and unconjugated bilirubin. Hypergammaglobulinemia is usual in immune and semi-immune patients. In adults with cerebral malaria, the mean opening pressure at lumbar puncture is normal or mildly elevated. Approximately 20 percent of adult patients have elevated CSF pressure (>200 mm of CSF); in contrast, approximately 80 percent of children have raised CSF pressure (>100 mm H_2O; the normal range is lower than in adults). The CSF protein level is usually normal or slightly elevated (<100 mg/dL). In cerebral malaria, the white blood cell count often varies between 9000 and 11,000 per microliter but can be higher than 20,000 per microliter; the differential count is usually normal. The CSF glucose level in cerebral malaria is about two-thirds of the blood glucose level, which, in about 10 percent of patients, is low. Low glucose [<2.2 mmol/L(40mg/dL] and high lactate [>6mmol/L(54 mg/dL)] concentrations in blood or CSF indicate a poor prognosis.

PREVENTION In most of the rural tropics, eradication of malaria is not feasible because of the paucity of resources and the incomplete understanding of the biologic and epidemiologic features of the infection and the disease. Over the past decade, there has been an increased focus on the reduction of malaria mortality by effective management of patients rather than by prevention, particularly in tropical Africa, where most malaria cases occur. Where practical, the disease is contained by judicious use of insecticides to kill the mosquito vector and of chemoprophylaxis in high-risk groups (e.g., pregnant women, nonimmune travelers, military personnel, and workers on priority economic projects). Treating bed nets with permethrin, a residual synthetic pyretroid, reduces the incidence of malaria and reduces overall mortality in West Africa. Despite massive investment aimed at the development of a malaria vaccine, and despite major advances in understanding the biology and immunology of malaria, a safe, effective, and long-lasting vaccine is unlikely to be available in the near future.

PERSONAL PROTECTION AGAINST MALARIA Measures to reduce the frequency of mosquito bites can be effective. These include avoiding exposure at peak mosquito feeding times (usually from dusk to dawn), wearing clothing that covers the skin, and using insect repellents. Sleeping in areas that are distant from breeding sites and in rooms that are air-conditioned and screened against mosquitoes is also advised. Use of bed nets, especially those impregnated with insecticide, is advised for persons in endemic areas, as is the use of insecticide spray for flying insects in sleeping quarters.

CHEMOPROPHYLAXIS (See also Table 174-3) Recommendations for prophylaxis rely on knowledge of the drug sensitivity of local parasites and the likelihood of acquiring infection. Chemoprophylaxis is never entirely effective, and malaria should always be considered in the differential diagnosis of fever in patients who have traveled to endemic areas, even if they have taken prophylactic antimalarial drugs.

With chloroquine-resistant *P. falciparum* present throughout most of the malarious world (Fig. 174-2), mefloquine (250 mg weekly for adults) is the drug of choice for prophylaxis for nonimmune individuals traveling to such areas. Mefloquine is effective and well tolerated, although nausea, dizziness, and abdominal pain may occur. Rarely (1:10,000), prophylaxis with mefloquine is associated with an acute reversible neuropsychiatric reaction manifested by confusion, psychosis, convulsions, or encephalopathy. Large-scale assessments of the side effects experienced by Swiss travelers who took mefloquine indicated that these effects are similar to those of chloroquine. The safety of mefloquine prophylaxis in pregnancy has not been established. Daily administration of doxycycline (100 mg maximum) is an effective alternative. Doxycycline is generally well tolerated but may cause *Candida* infections, diarrhea, and photosensitivity. Doxycycline cannot be used during pregnancy or given to children less than 8 years of age. Women who are pregnant or intending to become so should avoid travel to areas with chloroquine-resistant *P. falciparum* because there is no completely safe and effective antimalarial prophylaxis in pregnancy.

Because of the increasing spread and intensity of chloroquine resistance in Africa and other areas of the world, the Centers for Disease Control and Prevention (CDC, which recommend weekly mefloquine for all travelers to such areas except for pregnant women) maintain an updated 24-h malaria information audiotape that can be accessed by touch-tone telephone (404-332-4555) and an interactive international travel information service that responds by fax (404-332-4565).

Chloroquine (5 mg of base per kilogram per week, 300 mg maximum) is the drug of choice for the prevention of infection with drug-sensitive *P. falciparum* (in the few areas where such sensitivity still exists; see Fig. 174-2) and with other species. Chloroquine is generally well tolerated, although some patients cannot take the drug because of dysphoria, headache, or (in black patients) pruritus. Chloroquine is considered relatively safe in pregnancy. In adults, cumulative prophylactic doses of more than 100 g are associated with retinopathy; this complication is rare and occurs more often with treatment for rheumatoid arthritis than with prophylaxis of malaria. Skeletal and cardiac myopathy may occur but are also more likely with the high doses of 4-aminoquinoline drugs (e.g., hydroxychloroquine) used in the treatment of rheumatoid arthritis. Neuropsychiatric reactions and skin rashes are unusual. Another 4-aminoquinoline drug, amodiaquine, can cause agranulocytosis and is not recommended. The recent reports of chloroquine-resistant strains of *P. vivax* from Papua New Guinea and Indonesia indicate that no drug is 100 percent effective against malaria.

TABLE 174-3 Recommended regimens for malaria prophylaxis

Drugs	Adult dosage	Pediatric dosage
AREAS WITH CHLOROQUINE-RESISTANT *P. falciparum*		
Mefloquine*	250 mg (250 mg base, 1 tablet), once weekly for 1 week before exposure, during exposure, and for 4 weeks after exposure	15–19 kg: ¼ tab per week 20–30 kg: ½ tab per week 31–45 kg: ¾ tab per week >45 kg: 1 tab per week
Alternatives (1) Doxycycline†	100 mg daily for 1–2 days before exposure, during exposure, and for 4 weeks after exposure	>7 years: 2 mg/kg daily up to adult dose
or (2) Chloroquine	300 mg of base once weekly for 1 week before exposure, during exposure, and for 4 weeks after exposure	5 mg of base per kilogram once weekly up to 300 mg of base
plus (a) Proguanil‡	200 mg daily for 1–2 days before exposure, during exposure, and for 4 weeks after exposure	<2 years: 50 mg/d 2–6 years: 100 mg/d 7–9 years: 150 mg/d >9 years: 200 mg/d
Carry (b) Pyrimethamine-sulfadoxine	Carry single dose of 3 tablets (25 mg pyrimethamine and 500 mg sulfadoxine per tab) for self-treatment of febrile illness when medical treatment is not immediately available	<1 year: ¼ tab 1–3 years: ½ tab 4–8 years: 1 tab 9–14 years 2 tabs >14 years: 3 tabs
AREAS WITH CHLOROQUINE-SENSITIVE *P. falciparum*		
Chloroquine	300 mg of base once weekly for 1 week before exposure, during exposure and for 4 weeks after exposure	5 mg of base per kilogram once weekly up to 300 mg of base

* Mefloquine should not be used by children who weigh <15 kg, by pregnant women, or by patients with a history of psychiatric or seizure disorders (see Table 174-4). Caution should be used in administering mefloquine to persons with underlying cardiac conduction abnormalities who are taking beta blockers, or to persons requiring critical motor skills, such as pilots.
† Doxycycline should not be given to pregnant women or children <8 years of age.
‡ Proguanil is not available in the United States but may be obtained in the United Kingdom and some disease-endemic countries.

FIGURE 174-2 Distribution of malaria and chloroquine-resistant *Plasmodium falciparum*, 1993.

⊞ Chloroquine-resistant *P. falciparum*

● Chloroquine-sensitive malaria

In the past, the dihydrofolate reductase inhibitors pyrimethamine and proguanil (chloroguanide) were used for malaria prophylaxis, but resistant strains of both *P. falciparum* and *P. vivax* limit their efficacy. Whereas the quinoline antimalarials, such as chloroquine, act only on the erythrocyte stage of parasite development, the dihydrofolate reductase inhibitors also inhibit pre-erythrocytic growth in the liver (causal prophylaxis) and development in the mosquito (sporontocidal activity). The prophylactic use of the combination of pyrimethamine and sulfadoxine is not recommended because of severe toxicity, including exfoliative dermatitis and other skin rashes, agranulocytosis, hepatitis, and pulmonary eosinophilia. An alternative for persons who cannot take mefloquine or doxycycline is chloroquine weekly and proguanil (3 mg/kg daily, 200 mg maximum), but this regimen appears to be failing increasingly, particularly in East Africa. The combination of pyrimethamine with dapsone (0.2/1.5 mg/kg weekly, 25/200 mg maximum) is also used in areas with chloroquine-resistant *P. falciparum*. The combination is generally well tolerated, although resistance is increasing and dapsone may cause methemoglobinemia, allergic reactions, and (with higher doses) agranulocytosis.

Travelers should start taking antimalarial drugs at least 1 week (1 to 2 days for doxycycline) before arrival in an endemic area to allow time for the detection of untoward reactions and for the attainment of therapeutic blood levels; prophylaxis should continue for 4 weeks after departure from this area. Individuals who were born in malarious countries but live away from these areas for many years lose their immunity. These persons, particularly children, are at risk when they return to their homeland; thus they should receive chemoprophylaxis and take other preventive measures against malaria.

TREATMENT Patients in or from malarious areas who develop fever should have thick and thin blood smears made promptly to confirm the diagnosis and identify the species of infecting parasite. In endemic areas, uncomplicated infections may be treated on an outpatient basis. Patients with severe malaria or those unable to take oral drugs should receive parenteral antimalarial treatment. If there is any doubt about drug resistance, then quinine or quinidine should be given. Several drugs are available for oral treatment, and the choice of drug depends on the likely sensitivity of the infecting parasites. Despite recent reports of chloroquine-resistant *P. vivax* from Oceania and Indonesia, chloroquine is still the treatment of choice for *P. vivax*, *P. malariae*, and *P. ovale*. Recommended regimens are detailed in Table 174-4, and the characteristics of various agents are given in Table 174-5.

Uncomplicated malaria Infections due to *P. vivax*, *P. malariae*, *P. ovale*, or known sensitive strains of *P. falciparum* (Table 174-4) should be treated with oral chloroquine (25 mg of base per kilogram) given over 48 h. Where there is resistance to chloroquine, either quinine plus tetracycline or quinine plus pyrimethamine-sulfadoxine should be used; tetracycline should not be given to pregnant women or children less than 8 years of age. Oral quinine is extremely bitter and regularly produces the symptom complex of cinchonism which comprises tinnitus, high-tone deafness, nausea, vomiting, and dysphoria. Therefore, a 7-day course of quinine given with a 7-day course of tetracycline or a single dose of pyrimethamine-sulfadoxine. Chloroquine-resistant strains are sensitive to a single dose of pyrimethamine-sulfadoxine in some areas (e.g., Africa). All the quinoline antimalarials (chloroquine, mefloquine, and quinine) may exacerbate the orthostatic hypotension of malaria, and all are tolerated better by children than by adults. Symptomatic treatment with tepid sponging and acetaminophen lowers fever and reduces the propensity to vomit the oral antimalarial drugs. While mefloquine is effective against multidrug-resistant strains of *P. falciparum*, therapeutic doses (25 mg/kg) cause neuropsychiatric reactions in about 0.01–0.1 percent of patients. In addition, significant resistance of *P. falciparum* to mefloquine has been reported in Thailand, Burma, and Cambodia. Halofantrine, which is also effective against multidrug-resistant strains of *P. falciparum*, is used in some parts of Europe, Africa, and Asia but is not available in the United States. Although the drug is generally

well tolerated, it has variable bioavailability, and the optimal regimen remains to be determined. The principal adverse effects of halofantrine are diarrhea and a quinidine-like effect on the myocardium (prolonged electrocardiographic QT_c interval).

The Chinese compound artemisinin (quinghaosu) and its derivatives artemether and artesunate are being used increasingly in Asia. These drugs are effective against multidrug-resistant infections with *P. falciparum* and are rapid acting and appear to be safe. They are not available in the United States.

Pregnant women, young children, patients unable to tolerate oral therapy, and nonimmune persons (e.g., travelers) with malaria should be hospitalized. If the identity of the malaria species is doubtful, treatment should be given for chloroquine-resistant falciparum malaria. Since one negative smear does not rule out malaria, repeat thick blood films should be taken at least every 6 to 12 h at least 2 days to exclude the diagnosis. Following treatment, nonimmune persons with malaria should have daily parasite counts until thick films are negative. If the level of parasitemia does not fall below 25 percent of the admission value in 48 h, or if parasitemia has not cleared by 7 days, drug resistance is likely, and treatment should be changed.

Primaquine (0.3 mg of base per kilogram, 15 mg maximum) should be given daily for 14 days in *P. vivax* or *P. ovale* infection after G6PD deficiency is excluded. If the patient has a mild variant of G6PD deficiency, then primaquine can be given in a dose of 0.6 mg of base per kilogram (45 mg maximum) once weekly for 6 weeks.

Severe malaria Severe falciparum malaria (see Table 174-4) is a medical emergency that requires intensive nursing care and careful management. Patients should be weighed; if comatose, their blood glucose should be checked, and they should be positioned on their side and given a single intramuscular dose of phenobarbital (5 to 7 mg/kg) to prevent convulsions. Frequent evaluation is essential. Ancillary drugs such as high-dose glucocorticoids, mannitol, urea, heparin, and dextran are of no value.

The choice of drug dosage and route of administration depend on the prevailing sensitivity of *P. falciparum* to antimalarial drugs, the condition of the patient, and the place where treatment is given. The cinchona alkaloids (quinidine or quinine) are the mainstays of treatment because of their activity against chloroquine-resistant strains of *P. falciparum*. Quinidine gluconate is as effective as quinine and is more readily available outside tropical areas. In the United States, quinidine has replaced quinine for the parenteral treatment of severe malaria. Because quinidine is more cardiotoxic than quinine, its administration must be closely monitored if dysrhythmia or hypotension is to be avoided. A blood level in excess of 22 μmol/L (7 mg/L), an electrocardiographic QT interval of >0.55 s, or a QRS prolongation of >50 percent or QT_c >25 percent of baseline is an indication for slowing infusion rates. If arrhythmia or saline-unresponsive hypotension develops, quinidine should be discontinued. The dosage for quinidine is provided in Table 174-4.

Cardiovascular monitoring is not required routinely during quinine treatment. An initial loading dose (Table 174-4) should be given so that therapeutic concentrations are reached as soon as possible, but such a dose is not necessary if adequate treatment is started before admission to the hospital. The clearance and volume of distribution of these alkaloids are reduced in severe malaria, but plasma protein binding is increased and blood concentrations after a given dose are raised in proportion to disease severity. If the patient remains seriously ill or in acute renal failure for 3 days, the maintenance doses should be reduced by one-third to one-half to prevent accumulation of the drugs to toxic levels. (The initial doses should not be reduced.) If chloroquine is given, dose reduction is unnecessary even in renal failure.

In unconscious patients, the blood glucose value should be measured every 4 to 6 h; if the blood glucose value falls below 2.2 mmol/L (40 mg/dL), the patient should receive intravenous dextrose (0.3 g/kg). All patients given intravenous quinine or quinidine should receive a continuous infusion of 5% to 10% dextrose. The parasite

TABLE 174-4   Recommended regimens for the treatment of uncomplicated and severe malaria

Chloroquine-resistant *P. falciparum*	Chloroquine-sensitive *P. falciparum*, *P. vivax*, *P. malariae*, and *P. ovale*

UNCOMPLICATED, CAN BE TREATED ANYWHERE

Quinine sulfate, 650 mg (salt) tid orally for 7 days; pediatric dosage, 10 mg (salt)/kg tid for 7 days *plus either* Tetracycline, 250 mg qid orally for 7 days; pediatric dosage, 5 mg/kg qid for 7 days[a] *or* Pyrimethamine/sulfadoxine, 3 tablets (25 mg pyrimethamine and 500 mg sulfadoxine per tab) in single dose; pediatric dose 6–11 months, ¼ tab; 1–3 years, ½ tab; 4–8 years, 1 tab; 9–14 years, 2 tabs; >14 years, 3 tabs *Alternative treatments:* Mefloquine, 15–25 mg of base per kilogram, single dose (maximum 1500 mg)[c] Halofantrine, 8 mg of base per kilogram every h for 3 doses (maximum 500 mg per dose); dosage repeated after 7 days for nonimmune persons[d]	Chloroquine, 10 mg of base per kilogram (maximum 600 mg), followed by 5 mg of base per kilogram (maximum 300 mg) at 6, 24, and 48 h (or 10 mg of base per kilogram daily for 3 days) *plus* Primaquine phosphate, 0.3 mg of base per kilogram (maximum 15 mg) daily for 14 days for *P. vivax* or *P. ovale* infections[b]

SEVERE, AT HOSPITALS (WITH NURSING FACILITIES)

Quinidine gluconate, 10 mg of base per kilogram infused IV as loading dose over 1–2 h, followed by 0.02 mg/kg per min, keeping quinidine blood levels at 3–7 mg/L until parasitemia is <1 percent and patient can take drugs orally[e]; complete with quinine sulfate tablets for 3–7 days and tetracycline or pyrimethamine-sulfadoxine as indicated above *or* Quinine, 7 mg of salt per kilogram infused IV at a constant rate over 30 min as a loading dose, followed immediately by 10 mg of salt per kilogram over 4 h; after a 4-h interval, infusions of 10 mg of salt per kilogram over 8 h or until patient can complete 3–7 days of treatment orally with quinine sulfate tablets; tetracycline or pyrimethamine-sulfadoxine also should be given as indicated above *Alternative treatment* Artemether and related compounds, 3.2 mg/kg IM, followed by 1.6 mg/kg IM every 12–24 h until patient awakes[f,g] *plus* Exchange transfusion for very high parasitemia (>10 percent) and altered mental status	Chloroquine, 10 mg of base per kilogram (maximum 600 mg) infused IV at a constant rate over 8 h, followed by 15 mg of base per kilogram (maximum 900 mg) infused over 24 h[e] *plus* Exchange transfusion as for chloroquine-resistant malaria

SEVERE, AT RURAL CLINICS (NO NURSING FACILITIES)[h]

Quinine, 20 mg of salt per kilogram IM, followed by 10 mg of salt per kilogram every 8 h given by deep IM injection Quinine concentration should be 60–100 mg of salt per milliliter, and first dose should be split, with one-half the dose given deep IM in each thigh. Evacuate patient as soon as possible (when stable). When patient can take drugs orally, complete 3–7 days with quinine sulfate and tetracycline or pyrimethamine-sulfadoxine as indicated above	Chloroquine, 3.5 mg of base per kilogram (maximum 200 mg) every 6 h or 2.5 mg of base per kilogram every 4 h (maximum 150 mg) by either SC or IM injection; when patient can take medicines orally, complete treatment with chloroquine as above; total doses, 25 mg/kg of base (maximum 1500 mg)

[a]Tetracycline should not be given to pregnant women or to children <8 years of age.
[b]Patients who require primaquine should be screened for G6PD deficiency before treatment; patients with mild variants of G6PD deficiency can receive primaquine phosphate 0.75 mg of base per kilogram (maximum 45 mg) once weekly for 6 weeks. Primaquine should not be given during pregnancy.
[c]Treatment with mefloquine is associated with very infrequent neuropsychiatric side effects; this drug should not be used by children who weigh <15 kg, by pregnant women, by persons with underlying cardiac conduction abnormalities or are taking beta blockers, or by patients with a history of psychiatric or seizure disorders. Caution should be used in administering mefloquine to persons requiring critical motor skills, such as pilots.
[d]Halofantrine should not be given to persons with underlying cardiac conduction abnormalities or a long ECG QT interval.
[e]Infusion should be stopped temporarily if the electrocardiograph QRS interval is prolonged by >50 percent of the baseline or the QT_c instead is prolonged by >25 percent of the baseline; oral treatment should be substituted for parenteral treatment when the patient can swallow satisfactorily.
[f]This drug has not been approved by the Food and Drug Administration at the time of this publication.
[g]Artemether is only available in some countries in Asia, Africa, and South America.
[h]Nasogastric administration of oral antimalarials should be attempted if parenteral treatment is not possible, pending transfer to a hospital.

count and hematocrit should be measured every 12 h. If the hematocrit falls below 15 to 20 percent, then whole blood (preferably fresh) or packed cells should be transfused slowly, with careful attention to circulatory status; judicious use of diuretics may be required to prevent fluid overload. Renal function should be assessed daily. Management of fluid balance is difficult in severe malaria because there is a thin dividing line between overhydration, which can lead to pulmonary edema, and underhydration, which can contribute to renal impairment. If necessary, pulmonary arterial wedge pressure should be measured and maintained in the low to normal range. As soon as the patient can take fluids, oral antimalarials should be substituted.

COMPLICATIONS   Acute renal failure   If blood urea nitrogen or creatinine levels rise despite adequate rehydration, fluid administration should be restricted to prevent volume overload. The indications for

dialysis are the same as those in other forms of hypercatabolic acute renal failure (see Chap. 236). Although peritoneal dialysis is adequate, hemodialysis is preferable when available and where secondary bacterial infections are common. Some patients pass small volumes of urine sufficient to allow control of fluid balance and may be managed conservatively if other indications for dialysis do not arise. Renal function usually improves within days but may not recover fully for weeks.

Acute pulmonary edema   Patients should be positioned in bed at a 45° angle and given oxygen and intravenous diuretics. Their pulmonary arterial wedge pressure may be normal, indicating increased pulmonary capillary permeability. Positive-pressure ventilation should be started if these immediate measures fail (see Chap. 231).

TABLE 174-5 Characteristics of antimalarial drugs

Drug	Pharmacokinetic properties	Antimalarial activity	Minor toxicity	Major toxicity
Quinidine and quinine	Absorption: *Oral*: good. *Intramuscular*: good. Cl* and V_d† decreased, but plasma protein binding increased (90%) in malaria. $t_{1/2}$: 16 h in malaria, 11 h in healthy persons.	Acts mainly on mature trophozoite blood stage. Gametocytocidal against *P. vivax, P. ovale,* and *P. malariae*; no action on liver stages.	Bitter tasting. *Common*: "Cinchonism," tinnitus, high-tone hearing loss, nausea, vomiting, dysphoria, postural hypotension. prolonged electrocardiographic QT_c interval. *Rare*: Diarrhea, visual disturbance, rashes.	*Common*: Hypoglycemia. *Rare*: Hypotension, blindness, deafness, cardiac arrhythmias, thrombocytopenia, hemolysis, cholestatic hepatitis, neuromuscular paralysis. Quinidine more cardiotoxic.
Chloroquine	Absorption: *Oral*: good. *Intramuscular* and *subcutaneous*: very rapid. Complex pharmacokinetics. Enormous Cl and V_d (unaffected by malaria). Distribution processes determine blood concentration profile in malaria. $t_{1/2}$: 1–2 months.	Acts on ring-stage parasites. As for quinine	Bitter tasting. Well-tolerated. *Common*: Nausea, dysphoria, pruritus in dark-skinned patients, postural hypotension. *Rare*: Accommodation difficulties, rash.	*Acute*: Hypotensive shock (parenteral), cardiac arrhythmias, neuropsychiatric reactions. *Chronic*: Rare retinopathy (cumulative dose >100 g), skeletal and cardiac myopathy.
Mefloquine	Absorption: *Oral*: good. No parenteral preparation. $t_{1/2}$: 20 days.	As for quinine.	*Common*: Nausea, giddiness, dysphoria, postural hypotension.	Neuropsychiatric reactions infrequent; convulsions, encephalopathy.
Halofantrine‡	Absorption: variable, increased by fats. $t_{1/2}$: 1–3 days. Active desbutyl metabolite. $t_{1/2}$ 3–7 days.	As for quinine but more rapid.	Diarrhea, prolonged electrocardiographic QT_c interval.	Cardiac arrhythmias
Artemisinin and derivatives (artemether, artesunate)‡	Absorption: good. Rapid biotransformation to active metabolite dihydroartemisinin, which is eliminated rapidly.	Broader stage specificity and more rapid than other drugs; no action on liver stages.	Drug-induced pyrexia.	Neurotoxicity documented in animals.
Pyrimethamine	Absorption: *Oral*: good. *Intramuscular*: variable. $t_{1/2}$: 4 days.	For blood stages acts mainly on mature forms.	Well-tolerated.	Megaloblastic anemia, pancytopenia, pulmonary infiltration.
Proguanil (chloroguanide)	Absorption: *Oral*: good. biotransformed to active metabolite, cycloguanil. $t_{1/2}$: 16 h.	Causal prophylactic; not used for treatment.	Well-tolerated. *Rare*: Mouth ulcers, hair loss.	Megaloblastic anemia in renal failure.
Primaquine	Absorption: *Oral*: complete. Active compound not known. $t_{1/2}$:7 h.	Radical cure eradicates exoerythrocytic forms of *P. vivax* and *P. ovale*. Gametocytocidal against *P. falciparum*.	Nausea, vomiting, diarrhea, abdominal pain, hemolysis, methemoglobinemia.	Massive hemolysis in subjects with severe G6PD deficiency.

*Cl = systemic clearance.
†V_d = total apparent volume of distribution.
‡Not been approved by the U.S. Food and Drug Administration at the time of this publication.

Hypoglycemia An initial slow injection of 50% dextrose (0.5 g/kg) should be followed by an infusion of 10% dextrose (0.10 g/kg per hour). The blood glucose value should be monitored regularly thereafter, since recurrent hypoglycemia is common, particularly in patients who are receiving quinine or quinidine. In severely ill patients, hypoglycemia commonly occurs with lactic acidosis and may prove fatal.

Other complications Patients who develop spontaneous bleeding should be given fresh blood and intravenous vitamin K. Convulsions should be treated with intravenous (or rectal) diazepam. Aspiration pneumonia should be suspected in any unconscious patient with convulsions, particularly if he or she has persistent hyperventilation (see Chap. 100). Hypoglycemia or gram-negative septicemia should be suspected in any patient whose condition deteriorates for no obvious reason during antimalarial treatment. Exchange transfusion should be considered for patients with a parasitemia level of greater than 10 percent and deteriorating neurologic status.

Physicians who have questions about the management of patients with malaria can call the Malaria Branch, CDC, 404-488-4046 (nights and weekends, 404-639-2888).

BABESIOSIS

Babesiosis is a protozoan disease of animals that is transmitted by ticks; humans are infected incidentally and develop initially a nonspecific febrile illness. *Babesia* organisms enter red blood cells and resemble malaria parasites morphologically, thus posing a diagnostic problem.

ETIOLOGY AND NATURAL CYCLE Of the more than 70 species of *Babesia, B. microti* and *B. divergens* cause most human infections. Ixodid (or hard-bodied) ticks, in particular *Ixodes dammini* and *I. ricinus,* are vectors. Ticks ingest *Babesia* while feeding, and the parasites multiply within the gut wall of the vector. The organisms then spread to the salivary glands; their inoculation into a vertebrate host by a tick larva, nymph, or adult completes the transmission cycle. Asexual reproduction of *Babesia* within red blood cells produces two to four parasites. Transovarial transmission occurs in *I. ricinus* infected with *B. bovis,* a parasite of cattle that is slightly larger than *B. divergens* and is usually located on the margin of the red blood cell.

EPIDEMIOLOGY While *Babesia* infections in wild and domestic animals are distributed globally, almost all *B. microti* infections in the United States occur along the northeastern coast, including Nantucket Island and Martha's Vineyard in Massachusetts, Long Island and Shelter Island in New York, and the nearby mainland, including Connecticut. Cases also have been reported from California and Wisconsin. The deer tick, *I. dammini,* is the vector associated with *B. microti.*

Transfusions also have been the source of babesiosis. In several such cases, parasites were not detected in the donors, but serologic testing of the donor's blood for *Babesia* gave a positive result.

B. divergens infections have occurred sporadically in previously splenectomized patients in several countries of Europe. *I. ricinus* is probably the vector in these cases, as it is for transmission of this organism among cattle. The infected persons had been splenectomized and thus were predisposed to illness.

I. dammini feeds on rodents during its larval and nymphal stages and on deer as an adult; nymphs are abundant during the spring and summer and feed on humans readily. In some endemic areas, the seroprevalence in the human population may be greater than 2 percent, which indicates that asymptomatic infection is more frequent than is generally thought.

CLINICAL PRESENTATION　　The incubation period for *B. microti* is about 1 to 4 weeks. Splenectomized individuals and the elderly have the most severe illness. The clinical presentation varies widely; symptoms and signs include gradual onset of irregular fever, chills, sweating, muscle pain, and fatigue. Mild hepatosplenomegaly and mild hemolytic anemia may occur. The level of parasitemia may exceed 10 percent. The illness may continue for weeks or months.

Patients infected with *B. divergens* have a more severe illness, with rapid onset of chills, fever, nausea, vomiting, and hemolytic anemia progressing to jaundice, hemoglobinemia, and renal failure. *B. divergens* infections are often fatal.

DIAGNOSIS　　Whether or not they have a history of exposure to ticks or tick bites, febrile persons living in endemic areas should have Giemsa-stained thick and thin blood films made and examined for small intraerythrocytic parasites. *B. microti* appears as a small ring form similar to *P. falciparum.* Unlike infection with *Plasmodium,* that with *Babesia* does not cause the production of pigment in red blood cells, nor are schizonts or gametocytes formed. *B. microti,* dividing within red blood cells, can form four daughter parasites attached by strands of cytoplasm; these "tetrad" forms are seen infrequently in human blood films but are a distinguishing feature. An immunofluorescence antibody test is useful for the diagnosis of infection with *B. microti* but does not replace the blood smear. The serum antibody titer rises 2 to 4 weeks after the onset of illness and then wanes over 6 to 12 months; cross-reactions can occur with other species of *Babesia* and with *Plasmodium.* About half of patients infected with *B. microti* have antibody to *Borrelia burgdorferi,* the agent of Lyme disease (Chap. 137). Mixed infections occur, since both organisms are transmitted by *I. dammini.* Intraperitoneal inoculation of blood from patients with babesiosis into hamsters or gerbils has resulted in detectable parasitemia within 2 to 4 weeks.

TREATMENT　　*B. microti* infections in patients with intact spleens are generally self-limiting without treatment. The combination of quinine sulfate (650 mg of salt PO tid) and clindamycin (600 mg PO tid or 1.2 g parenterally bid) for 7 to 10 days is effective in some cases but may not eliminate parasites. Symptoms may persist for months with or without treatment, although there are no permanent sequelae. More severe infections with high levels of *B. microti* parasitemia in asplenic patients have been successfully treated with exchange transfusions in addition to quinine and clindamycin.

Massive exchange transfusion, intravenous clindamycin, and oral chloroquine have been used successfully for the treatment of infection caused by *B. divergens,* a species that has been most refractory to therapy. Pentamidine (not approved by the Food and Drug Administration for this use) may be an alternative agent, since it is effective against several species of *Babesia* in animals.

REFERENCES

BREMAN JG, STEKETEE RW: Malaria, in *Maxcy-Rosenau-Last Public Health and Preventive Medicine,* 13th ed, JM Last, RB Wallace (eds). Norwalk, Conn, Appleton and Lange, 1992, pp 240–253

BRUCE CHWATT LJ: *Essential Malariology,* 2d ed. New York, Wiley, 1985

CENTERS FOR DISEASE CONTROL: Information for International Travelers. Washington, Public Health Service, U.S. Department of Health and Human Services, Publication No. 93-8280, 1993

GARNHAM PCC: Malaria parasites of man: Life cycles and morphology (excluding ultrastructure) in malaria, in *Principles and Practice of Malariology,* WH Wernsdorfer, I McGregor (eds). Edinburgh, Churchill Livingstone, 1988, pp. 61–96

HEALY G, RISTIC M: Human babesiosis, in *Babesiosis of Domestic Animals and Man,* M Ristic (ed). Boca Raton, Fla, CRC Press, 1988, pp 209–225

HOWARD RJ, GILLADOGGA AD: Molecular studies related to the pathogenesis of cerebral malaria. Blood 74:2603, 1989

KITCHEN SF: Symptomatology: General considerations and falciparum malaria, in *Malariology,* Vol 2. MF Boyd (ed). Philadelphia, Saunders, 1949, pp 966–1016

MILLER KD et al: Treatment of severe malaria in the United States with a continuous infusion of quinidine gluconate and exchange transfusion. N Engl J Med 321:65, 1989

MOLINEAUX L, GRAMICCIA G: *The Garki Project: Research on the Epidemiology and Control of Malaria in the Sudan Savannah of West Africa.* Geneva, World Health Organization, 1980

OAKS SC JR et al (eds): *Malaria: Obstacles and Opportunities,* CS Carpenter, CS Oaks (eds). Washington, National Academy Press, 1991

ROSNER F et al: Babesiosis in splenectomized adults: Review of 22 reported cases. Am J Trop Med Hyg 76:696, 1984

SPITZ S: Pathology of acute falciparum malaria. Military Med 99:555, 1946

STEFFEN R et al: Mefloquine compared with other malaria chemoprophylactic regimens in tourists visiting East Africa. Lancet 341:1299, 1993

WARRELL DA et al: Dexamethasone proves deleterious in cerebral malaria: A double-blind trial in 100 comatose patients. N Engl J Med 306:313, 1982

WHITE NJ: Drug treatment and prevention of malaria. Eur J Clin Pharmacol 34:1, 1988

———, HO M: The pathophysiology of malaria. Adv Parasitol 31:84, 1992

WORLD HEALTH ORGANIZATION, DIVISION OF CONTROL OF TROPICAL DISEASES: Severe and complicated malaria. Trans R Soc Trop Med Hyg 84(suppl 2): 1, 1990

175　LEISHMANIASIS

RICHARD M. LOCKSLEY

DEFINITION　　*Leishmaniasis* denotes disease caused by any of a number of species of protozoa in the genus *Leishmania.* There are four major clinical syndromes—visceral leishmaniasis (kala azar), cutaneous leishmaniasis of the old and new worlds, mucocutaneous leishmaniasis (espundia), and diffuse cutaneous leishmaniasis. Most commonly, these parasites are transmitted from animal reservoirs to human hosts by the bite of phlebotomine sandflies.

ETIOLOGY　　Different *Leishmania* species appear identical and are generally distinguished by clinical and geographic characteristics. Modern speciation by isoenzyme patterns, monoclonal antibodies, DNA hybridization, DNA restriction endonuclease fragment analysis, and chromosomal karyotyping is continuing to delineate new species, particularly in the new world, and to demonstrate the capacity of different species to cause similar clinical syndromes.

In the sandfly and in culture media, *Leishmania* exist as motile, spindle-shaped promastigotes (1.5 to 4 μm by 14 to 20 μm) with a single anterior flagellum. On inoculation into a mammalian host, the organisms enter mononuclear phagocytes, lose their flagella, and multiply as small (2 by 5 μm), oval, obligate intracellular amastigotes (Leishman-Donovan bodies).

EPIDEMIOLOGY　　Leishmaniasis is a zoonotic infection which involves the rodents, canines, and various forest mammals of every inhabited continent except Australia. The disease is spread when female sandflies of the genus *Phlebotomus* (old world) or *Lutzomyia* (new world) ingest amastigotes while taking a blood meal from an infected mammal. These transform into promastigotes within the insect's gut, migrate to the salivary glands, and are deposited on the skin of the new host when the insect next engorges. Phlebotomines breed in warm, humid microclimates and are typically found in rodent burrows, termite hills, and rotting vegetation. Humans may acquire the disease when they encroach on this sylvatic cycle. Establishment of infection in the domestic dog provides an important urban reservoir of leishmaniasis. Animal reservoirs have not been identified in the central East African and Indian forms of kala azar. It is estimated that worldwide over 12 million people are infected.

PATHOGENESIS Promastigotes are deposited on the skin into a small pool of blood drawn by the probing sandfly. Products from the fly salivary gland promote vasodilation and infectivity, in part via peptides that deactivate host macrophages. Complement is activated by the classical and/or alternative pathways, depending on the species, and is deposited onto the major outer membrane molecules of the promastigote—a 63-kDa molecular weight glycoprotein protease (gp63) and lipophosphoglycan (LPG). LPG and gp63 either directly or through bound C3b or C3bi target the organisms to macrophages via the complement receptors CR3 and CR1. The promastigotes transform into amastigotes within phagolysosomes and replicate by binary fission. They eventually rupture the cell and invade adjacent macrophages.

The course of the subsequent disease is determined by the host's cellular immunity as well as the species of the parasite. In cutaneous leishmaniasis, there is a marked lymphocytic infiltration associated with a reduction in the number of parasites, the development of a delayed skin test (leishmanin or Montenegro) reaction, and frequently, spontaneous cure. In mucocutaneous disease, the complete or partial resolution of the primary lesion may be followed by metastatic mucocutaneous lesions at a later date. In diffuse cutaneous leishmaniasis there is no infiltration by lymphocytes or reduction in the number of parasites, the leishmanin reaction remains negative, and the skin lesions become chronic, progressive, and disseminated. The patients have a selective anergy to *Leishmania* antigens. In visceral leishmaniasis, the parasites spread to macrophages throughout the body, perhaps due to the greater resistance of *L. donovani* to the spontaneous cidal activity present in normal serum.

Cure of visceral leishmaniasis has been correlated with the capacity of sensitized T lymphocytes from the patient to release macrophage-activating cytokines, particularly interferon-γ (IFN-γ). Macrophage activation results in induction of nitric oxide synthase and the production of nitric oxide, which is toxic for the intracellular amastigotes. Cure is thought to confer immunity to the infecting strain. Failure to cure has been related not only to the absence of production of IFN-γ but also to the release of macrophage-deactivating cytokines, such as interleukins 4 and 10 and transforming growth factor beta, in response to *Leishmania* antigens. Antibodies reach high levels in disseminated disease but are not protective against the intracellular organisms. In mucosal leishmaniasis, IFN-γ is produced, but concurrent production of deactivating cytokines leads to the inability to completely clear the parasite and to continuous inflammation, thus contributing to severe tissue destruction.

DIAGNOSIS Diagnosis of leishmaniasis requires demonstrating the organism by smear or culture of aspirates or tissue. Although Novy-MacNeal-Nicolle (NNN) medium traditionally has been used to culture *Leishmania*, several commercially available liquid media offer improved storage capability and enhanced recovery of organisms. Cultures are maintained at 22 to 28°C for 21 days and examined microscopically for the presence of the motile promastigotes. Inoculation of hamsters with infected clinical material results in infections after a period of weeks.

Species-specific diagnosis of human cutaneous new world isolates has been achieved by use of monoclonal antibodies or by hybridization of tissue touch blots with radiolabeled kinetoplast DNA probes.

Antibodies are detectable in all forms of leishmaniasis but are most useful in visceral leishmaniasis where cutaneous lesions are not present. The direct agglutination test detects IgM antibody and is a sensitive indicator of acute disease. The test is group-specific, but the titer is generally greatest to the homologous strain. A positive test

($> 1:32$) varies from 97 percent in visceral leishmaniasis to 81 percent in new world cutaneous leishmaniasis. Direct agglutination antibodies decline and may disappear with cure. ELISAs also have been developed that are highly sensitive and specific in visceral leishmaniasis.

The Montenegro skin test using promastigote antigens is negative in visceral leishmaniasis. It is generally nonstandardized and is used only for epidemiologic purposes.

VISCERAL LEISHMANIASIS (KALA AZAR) *Leishmania donovani* causes kala azar, a disease that may be endemic, epidemic, or sporadic. *African kala azar* is found in the eastern half of Africa from the Sahara in the north to the equator in the south. Sporadic cases have been reported from West Africa. It is a disease of older children and young adults (10 to 25 years); males are involved more commonly than females. It is endemic in dogs and several wild carnivores in many areas and is more resistant to therapy with antimony compounds than the forms of kala azar found in the rest of the world.

Mediterranean, or infantile, kala azar is seen primarily in the Mediterranean area, China, and Latin America. It is a disease of children under the age of 4, but adults, particularly travelers to endemic areas, are not spared. Dogs, jackals, and foxes serve as reservoirs. Rats have been identified as a potential reservoir in Italy. The strains responsible for the Mediterranean and American disease are sometimes referred to as *L. infantum* and *L. chagasi*, respectively.

Indian kala azar has an age and sex distribution similar to African kala azar. Humans are the only known reservoir, and transmission is carried out by anthropophilic sandflies.

Manifestations The incubation period is generally about 3 months (3 weeks to 18 months). A primary cutaneous lesion (leishmanioma) is not uncommon in Africa. The onset of disease may be insidious or abrupt; the latter occurs more frequently in individuals from nonendemic areas. Failure to thrive is common among infected infants and children. Fever, typically nocturnal and occasionally double-quotidian, is almost universal and is accompanied by tachycardia without signs of toxemia. Diarrhea and cough are frequent. Nontender splenomegaly becomes dramatic by the third month. The liver enlarges less conspicuously. Cirrhosis and portal hypertension occur in about 10 percent of patients. Lymphadenopathy accompanies some cases of African kala azar. Asymptomatic and prolonged, subclinical forms of infection are common in endemic areas; malnutrition is a risk factor for the progression to full-blown disease. Fulminant kala azar has been described in patients with AIDS.

Pancytopenia is characteristic. Anemia is multifactorial: autoimmune hemolysis, splenomegaly, and gastrointestinal blood loss all contribute. The latter is exacerbated by thrombocytopenia. Agranulocytosis, cancrum oris, and superinfections complicate untreated cases. Extensive leishmanial infiltration of the gastrointestinal tract may lead to malabsorption. Hypoalbuminemia and polyclonal hypergammaglobulinemia (IgG and IgM) are constant features. Circulating immune complexes are frequently present. Immune-complex glomerulonephritis and interstitial nephritis have been described. Edema, cachexia, and hyperpigmentation (*kala azar* means "black fever") are late manifestations. Without treatment, death occurs within 3 to 20 months in 90 to 95 percent of adults and 75 to 85 percent of children, usually from superinfections or gastrointestinal hemorrhage.

After successful treatment, 3 to 10 percent of cases develop post–kala azar dermal leishmaniasis (PKDL), characterized by a spectrum of lesions ranging from depigmented macules to wartlike nodules over the face and extensor surfaces of the limbs. PKDL appears shortly after symptoms subside in African cases and typically disappears after several weeks. In the Indian disease, PKDL appears after a latent period of 1 to 2 years and may last for years, creating a persistent human reservoir. A clinical variant of *L. chagasi* causing papular cutaneous lesions without visceral involvement occurs in Honduras.

Diagnosis Bone marrow aspirate and biopsy are positive in over 85 percent of cases. In Brazil and Africa, splenic aspiration (95 percent) has proved quite safe and has been used serially to assess the response to therapy. In general, however, aspiration of the spleen or liver (75 percent) is not recommended because of the risk of hemorrhage. Aspirates or biopsy of enlarged lymph nodes will show parasites in 60 percent of cases. Suspicious skin lesions should be biopsied as well. The direct agglutination test is positive early in the disease. The leishmanin skin test becomes positive 6 to 8 weeks after recovery. Other causes of fever in the tropics, including malaria, brucellosis, tuberculosis, typhoid, and hepatic abscess, can be distinguished by appropriate testing. PKDL must be differentiated from leprosy, syphilis, and yaws.

Treatment Transfusions and treatment of complicating superinfections must supplement specific therapy. Pentavalent antimonials are highly effective against *Leishmania* and are relatively nontoxic. Sodium antimony gluconate (Pentostam; 100 mg Sb^{5+} per milliliter) is given intravenously or intramuscularly in a single daily dose of 20 mg/kg for 28 days. Meglumine antimoniate (Glucantime; 85 mg Sb^{5+} per milliliter) also can be used. Therapy should be repeated using 20 mg/kg for 40 to 60 days in patients with relapses or incomplete responses. Periodic electrocardiographic monitoring is recommended during prolonged therapy. The addition of oral allopurinol (20 to 30 mg/kg per day in three divided doses) has been effective. Incomplete therapy of the initial illness remains the major risk factor for relapse with drug-resistant organisms. Such cases must be treated with intravenous amphotericin B (0.5 to 1 mg/kg on alternate days) or pentamidine (3 to 4 mg/kg three times per week for 5 to 25 weeks, depending on the response). Adjunctive splenectomy has been successful in some cases of drug-resistant kala azar. Mortality remains 15 to 25 percent in advanced cases, although the cure rate is over 90 percent when therapy is given early. Follow-up at 3 and 12 months is recommended to detect relapses. PKDL should be treated in the same fashion as the initial illness. Recombinant human interferon-γ has shown promise as adjunctive therapy with pentavalent antimony in previous treatment failures or in seriously ill patients with kala azar.

Prevention Preventive measures include early treatment of human cases, elimination of diseased dogs, and the use of DDT against sandflies. Application of insect repellents and the use of permethrin-coated fine netting are important for travelers. There are no useful prophylactic agents.

CUTANEOUS AND MUCOCUTANEOUS LEISHMANIASIS This form of leishmaniasis is caused by a number of species in both the old world and the new world. Disease is characterized by the development of single or multiple localized lesions on exposed areas of skin that typically ulcerate. Although spontaneous healing is the rule for old world cutaneous leishmaniasis, this is less common in new world disease.

Old world cutaneous leishmaniasis *L. tropica* causes anthroponotic (urban, chronic, dry) cutaneous leishmaniasis, an endemic disease of children and young adults in areas bordering the Mediterranean, the Middle East, The Republic of Georgia, and India. The principal reservoirs are humans, although domestic dogs are synanthropic hosts. The incubation period ranges from 2 to 24 months. Usually the lesion begins as a single, red pruritic papule on the face (oriental sore). The central area ulcerates and slowly enlarges centrifugally, reaching a size of approximately 2 cm. Lymphadenopathy is unusual. Healing occurs over 1 to 2 years and leaves a small depigmented scar. The disease can be complicated by the development of leishmaniasis recidiva, a condition marked by persistent facial lesions containing a scant number of parasites and by an exaggerated delayed hypersensitivity response to parasite antigens. Rarely, the organism may spread to the viscera and present as fever of unknown origin (viscerotropic leishmaniasis) or as typical kala azar.

L. major causes zoonotic (rural, acute, moist) cutaneous leishmaniasis, which is endemic across the desert areas of the Middle East to Afghanistan and in Africa. The reservoir is maintained in burrowing rodents. The incubation period ranges from 2 to 6 weeks. The initial lesions are often multiple and located on the lower extremities. Regional lymphadenopathy and satellite lesions are common. Healing

with scarring occurs within 3 to 6 months. *L. major* has been implicated in cases of mucocutaneous leishmaniasis in Saudi Arabia.

L. aethiopica, maintained in rock hyraxes of the Ethiopian and Kenyan highlands, causes cutaneous leishmaniasis which may pursue a relatively prolonged course and can be complicated by the development of diffuse cutaneous leishmaniasis (see below).

DIAGNOSIS Lesions should first be cleansed with alcohol to reduce bacterial contamination, which hinders recovery of the organisms. Aspirates should be obtained from the outer edge of the ulcer. If the aspirated smears are negative, full-thickness skin biopsies from the ulcer margin should be taken for touch smears, histology, and culture. The direct agglutination test and the leishmanin skin test become positive within 4 to 6 weeks.

TREATMENT Specific therapy should be withheld in endemic areas until ulceration takes place, thereby conferring immunity. Exceptions include disfiguring or disabling lesions and lesions persisting for longer than 6 months. Imidazoles have some efficacy, and ketoconazole (600 mg/d orally for 4 weeks) has been recommended prior to use of antimonials when possible. Treatment with antimonials is as described for kala azar, although shorter courses (20 days) are effective. Higher doses of antimony may be required for *L. aethiopica* infections (20 mg/kg twice a day for 30 days). Ulcers should be covered to prevent infection of vectors and other canine and human hosts.

New world cutaneous and mucocutaneous leishmaniasis Leishmanias causing new world cutaneous disease are divided into numerous subspecies within the *L. mexicana* and *L. braziliensis* groups (Table 175-1). Spontaneous healing occurs more commonly in disease due to *L. mexicana*. The natural reservoirs for these organisms include a wide variety of mammals inhabiting the forests of South and Central America. Disease is most prevalent in the Amazon basin but occurs throughout the Americas as far north as south-central Texas.

L. mexicana causes chiclero's ulcer, or bay sore. Chicle gatherers who work in forests during the rainy season when sandflies are abundant develop isolated cutaneous lesions on the hand or head. These show little tendency to ulcerate and generally heal spontaneously within 6 months. Ear lesions, however, may persist and cause extensive destruction of the pinna.

L. venezuelensis causes indolent nodular lesions. *L. amazonensis* causes persistent lesions that may be multiple and seldom heal spontaneously. *L. amazonensis* also may cause diffuse cutaneous leishmaniasis (see below), visceral leishmaniasis, and mucocutaneous leishmaniasis.

L. peruviana causes uta, a disease consisting of single or multiple ulcers typically on the face. Spontaneous healing within 3 months to a year is the rule. The reservoir is the domestic dog. The disease occurs on the western slopes of the Peruvian Andes at altitudes above 600 m (2000 ft). Species of *L. mexicana* and new world *L. major*-like organisms also have been implicated in uta.

Mucocutaneous leishmaniasis, or espundia, is caused primarily by *L. braziliensis*, which typically produces one or several lesions on the lower extremities that undergo extensive ulceration; complete healing may or may not occur spontaneously. After months to years, metastatic lesions appear in the nasopharynx in 2 to 5 percent of patients. Less frequently, lesions occur in the perineum. Multiple, large antecedent skin lesions and insufficient antimony therapy for the primary infection are risk factors. Nasal obstruction and epistaxis are frequent presenting symptoms. Extensive destruction of soft tissue structures ensues, with painful mutilating erosions (espundia). Fever, anemia, and weight loss are common. Death is caused by bacterial infection, inanition, aspiration, and respiratory obstruction.

L. panamensis causes nonhealing ulcerative lesions, and *L. guyanensis* causes nodular lesions that persist and metastasize along lymphatics (pian bois). These strains can cause mucocutaneous leishmaniasis.

DIAGNOSIS Speciation of the infecting organism should be attempted for prognostic and epidemiologic purposes. Regional interna-

TABLE 175-1 New world *Leishmania* Species

Species	Geographic distribution	Reservoir	Clinical syndrome*
L. chagasi	Mexico, Honduras, Guatemala, Surinam, El Salvador, Colombia, Venezuela, Ecuador, Brazil, Bolivia, Paraguay, Argentina, Martinique, Guadeloupe	Canines	VL, CL, PKDL
L. mexicana complex			
L. mexicana	Mexico, Guatemala, Belize, Costa Rica, Panama, Colombia, Ecuador, Texas (U.S.A.)	Forest rodents	CL, DCL
L. amazonensis	Brazil, Costa Rica, Panama, Colombia, French Guyana, Ecuador, Peru, Bolivia, Venezuela	Rodents, marsupials	CL, VL, PKDL, MCL, DCL
L. venezuelensis	Venezuela	?	CL
L. braziliensis complex			
L. braziliensis	Brazil, Guatemala, Honduras, Belize, Colombia, Venezuela, Peru, Bolivia, Paraguay, Ecuador	Forest rodents	CL, MCL
L. guyanensis	Colombia, Brazil, Surinam, French Guyana, Guyana, Ecuador	Sloths, anteaters	CL, MCL
L. panamensis	Panama, Honduras, Colombia, Ecuador	Sloths	CL, MCL
L. peruviana	Peru	Canines	CL
L. lainsoni	Brazil	?	CL
L. naiffi	Brazil	?	CL
L. colombiensis	Colombia, Panama, Venezuela	Sloths	CL
L. major–like isolates	Venezuela, Ecuador	?Canines	CL, DCL

* VL = visceral leishmaniasis; CL = cutaneous leishmaniasis; PKDL = post–kala azar dermal leishmaniasis; MCL = mucocutaneous leishmaniasis; DCL = diffuse cutaneous leishmaniasis.

tional reference laboratories for speciation have been identified by the World Health Organization (Geneva). Skin biopsies are the preferred means of obtaining tissue for stains and culture. Parasites may be scant, particularly in mucocutaneous lesions. The direct agglutination test and the leishmanin skin test become positive within 4 to 6 weeks. Syphilis, yaws, blastomycosis, paracoccidioidomycosis, sporotrichosis, leprosy, and carcinoma must be considered in the differential diagnosis.

TREATMENT In general, cutaneous lesions should be treated with systemic antimonials for 20 days in order to decrease the subsequent risk of mucocutaneous disease. Local heat (40 to 41°C) may accelerate healing. Oral ketoconazole (600 mg/d for 28 days) has been efficacious in cutaneous lesions caused by *L. mexicana*.

Espundia should be treated with antimonials (20 mg/kg per day) for 28 days, although long-term cure may be difficult, particularly among patients with severe disease. Failures should be treated with amphotericin. Reconstructive facial prostheses should not be used until the disease has been in remission for at least 1 year without therapy. A rising antibody titer may predict relapse and indicate that further therapy is required.

Diffuse cutaneous leishmaniasis Diffuse cutaneous leishmaniasis is found in Venezuela, Peru, Brazil, Mexico, and the Dominican Republic in the new world and in Ethiopia in the old world. Patients display a specific deficiency of cell-mediated immunity to leishmanial antigens. Organisms from the *L. mexicana* complex have been implicated in the Americas, and *L. aethiopica* in Africa. Disease is characterized by massive dissemination of skin lesions without visceral involvement. The clinical picture often bears a striking resemblance to lepromatous leprosy. The diagnosis is not difficult, because the lesions contain large numbers of organisms. In contrast to all other types of cutaneous leishmaniasis, the leishmanin skin test remains negative. The disease is progressive and very refractory to treatment. High doses of antimony (20 mg/kg twice a day for 30 days) and multiple courses of amphotericin or pentamidine are often required to produce remission, but cures are rare. Immunotherapy with a combination of BCG and *Leishmania* antigens and administration of recombinant IFN-γ have been promising.

REFERENCES

BADARO R et al: Treatment of visceral leishmaniasis with pentavalent antimony and interferon-gamma. N Engl J Med 322:16, 1990

BARRAL A et al: Leishmaniasis in Bahia, Brazil: Evidence that *Leishmania amazonensis* produces a wide spectrum of clinical disease. Am J Trop Med Hyg 44:536, 1991

CARVALHO EM et al: Immunologic markers of clinical evolution in children recently infected with *Leishmania donovani chagasi*. J Infect Dis 165:535, 1992

FRANKE ED et al: Efficacy and toxicity of sodium stibogluconate for mucosal leishmaniasis. Ann Intern Med 113:934, 1990

GRIMALDI G JR et al: A review of the geographic distribution and epidemiology of leishmaniasis in the new world. Am J Trop Med Hyg 41:687, 1989

HERWALDT BL et al: The natural history of cutaneous leishmaniasis in Guatemala. J Infect Dis 165:518, 1992

HERWALDT BL, BERMAN JD: Recommendations for treating leishmaniasis with sodium stibogluconate (Pentostam) and review of pertinent clinic studies. Am J Trop Med Hyg 46:296, 1992

MELBY PC et al: Cutaneous leishmaniasis: Review of 59 cases seen at the National Institutes of Health. Clin Infect Dis 15:924, 1992

NAVIN TR et al: Placebo-controlled clinical trial of sodium stibogluconate (Pentostam) versus ketoconazole for treating cutaneous leishmaniasis in Guatemala. J Infect Dis 165:528, 1992

176 TRYPANOSOMIASIS

LOUIS V. KIRCHHOFF

CHAGAS' DISEASE

DEFINITION Chagas' disease, or American trypanosomiasis, is a zoonosis caused by the protozoan parasite *Trypanosoma cruzi*. Acute Chagas' disease is generally a mild, febrile illness that results from initial infection with the organism. Following spontaneous resolution of the acute illness, most infected individuals remain for life in the indeterminate phase of chronic Chagas' disease, which is characterized by subpatent parasitemia, high levels of anti-*T. cruzi* antibodies, and an absence of symptoms. In a minority of chronically infected individuals, cardiac and gastrointestinal lesions develop that can result in serious morbidity and even death.

LIFE CYCLE AND TRANSMISSION *T. cruzi* is transmitted among its mammalian hosts by hematophagous triatomine insects, or reduviid bugs. The insects become infected by sucking blood from animals or humans who have circulating parasites. Ingested organisms multiply in the gut of the reduviids, and infective forms are discharged with the feces at the time of subsequent blood meals. Transmission to a second vertebrate host occurs when breaks in the skin, mucous membranes, or conjunctivae are contaminated with bug feces that contain infective parasites. *T. cruzi* also can be transmitted by transfusion of blood donated by infected persons, and congenital infections occur as well.

PATHOLOGY　An indurated inflammatory lesion called a *chagoma* often appears at the site of the parasite's entry. Local histologic changes include intracellular parasites in leukocytes and cells of subcutaneous tissues, interstitial edema, lymphocytic infiltration, and reactive hyperplasia of adjacent lymph nodes. After dissemination through the lymphatics and the bloodstream, muscles, including the myocardium, may be heavily parasitized. The characteristic pseudocysts seen in sections of infected tissues are intracellular aggregates of multiplying parasites.

The pathogenesis of chronic Chagas' disease is poorly understood. The heart is the organ most commonly affected, and changes include biventricular enlargement, thinning of the ventricular walls, apical aneurysms, and mural thrombi. Widespread lymphocytic infiltration, diffuse interstitial fibrosis, and atrophy of myocardial cells are often present, but parasites are rarely demonstrated in myocardial tissue. Conduction system involvement most frequently affects the right branch and the left anterior branch of the bundle of His. In chronic Chagas' disease of the gastrointestinal tract (megadisease), the esophagus and colon may be enormously dilated and hypertrophied. On microscopic examination, focal inflammatory lesions with lymphocytic infiltration are seen, and the number of neurons in the myenteric plexus is reduced.

EPIDEMIOLOGY　*T. cruzi* is found only in the Americas. Wild and domestic mammals harboring *T. cruzi* and infected reduviids are found in spotty distributions from the southern United States to southern Argentina. Humans become involved in the cycle of transmission when infected vectors take up residence in the primitive wood, adobe, and stone houses common in much of Latin America. Thus human *T. cruzi* infection is primarily a health problem among the poor in rural areas of Central and South America. Most new *T. cruzi* infections in rural settings occur in children, but the incidence is unknown because most go undiagnosed. Thousands of individuals also become infected every year through blood transfusions in urban areas. Currently, it is estimated that 16 million people, more than a third of whom live in Brazil, are chronically infected with *T. cruzi*. Chronic Chagas' disease is a major cause of morbidity and mortality in many Latin American countries, including Mexico, since many chronically infected individuals eventually develop symptomatic cardiac lesions or gastrointestinal disease.

Acute Chagas' disease is rare in the United States. Four cases of autochthonous transmission have been described, and recently, three instances of transmission by blood transfusion have occurred. In addition, between 1971 and 1992, seven laboratory-acquired infections and nine imported cases of acute Chagas' disease have been reported to the Centers for Disease Control and Prevention. In contrast, the prevalence of chronic *T. cruzi* infections in the United States has increased considerably in recent years. Since the mid-1970s enormous numbers of Central Americans have emigrated to the United States, and in one study done in Washington, D.C., 5 percent of Salvadoran and Nicaraguan immigrants were found to have chronic *T. cruzi* infections. Conservative estimates place the total number of infected immigrants now living here at more than 50,000. The presence of these carriers of *T. cruzi* poses a significant risk of transmission by blood transfusion, as evidenced by the occurrence of the three transfusion-associated cases.

CLINICAL COURSE　The first signs of acute Chagas' disease occur at least 1 week after invasion by the parasites. When the organisms have entered through a break in the skin, an indurated area of erythema and swelling, the *chagoma*, may appear, accompanied by local lymphadenopathy. Romaña's sign, the classic finding in acute Chagas' disease, consists of unilateral painless edema of the palpebrae and periocular tissues that can result when the conjunctiva

is the portal of entry. These initial local signs are followed by malaise, fever, anorexia, and edema of the face and lower extremities. Generalized lymphadenopathy and mild hepatosplenomegaly may appear. Severe myocarditis develops rarely, and most deaths in acute Chagas' disease are due to heart failure. Neurologic signs are not common, but meningoencephalitis has been reported. The acute symptoms resolve spontaneously in virtually all patients, who then enter the asymptomatic or indeterminate phase of chronic *T. cruzi* infection.

Symptomatic chronic Chagas' disease becomes apparent years or even decades after the initial infection. The heart is commonly involved, and symptoms are caused by rhythm disturbances, cardiomyopathy, and thromboembolism. Right bundle branch block is the most common electrocardiographic abnormality, but other types of atrioventricular block, premature ventricular contractions, and tachy- and bradyarrhythmias are seen frequently. Cardiomyopathy often results in right-sided or biventricular heart failure. Embolization of mural thrombi to the brain or other areas may occur. Patients with megaesophagus suffer from dysphagia, odynophagia, chest pain, and regurgitation. Aspiration can occur, especially during sleep, and repeated episodes of aspiration pneumonitis are common. Weight loss, cachexia, and pulmonary infection can result in death. Patients with megacolon are plagued by abdominal pain and chronic constipation, and advanced megacolon can cause obstruction, perforation, septicemia, and death.

DIAGNOSIS　The diagnosis of Chagas' disease requires the detection of parasites. Microscopic examination of fresh anticoagulated blood or of the buffy coat is the simplest way to see the motile organisms. Parasites also can be seen in Giemsa-stained thin and thick blood smears. When repeated attempts to visualize the organisms are unsuccessful, mouse inoculation and culture of blood in specialized media should be performed. As a last resort, xenodiagnosis should be attempted. In this technique, uninfected reduviid bugs are allowed to feed on the patient's blood. Approximately 30 days after the blood meal, the intestinal contents of the bugs are examined for parasites. When done properly, this method is positive in virtually all patients with acute Chagas' disease and in approximately half of those with chronic infections. Since early treatment of acute Chagas' disease is extremely important, however, the decision to initiate anti-*T. cruzi* therapy in a patient with negative wet preparations and smears must be made on clinical and epidemiologic grounds before the results of these indirect methods become available. Serologic testing is of limited usefulness in diagnosing acute Chagas' disease.

The diagnosis of chronic Chagas' disease is made by detecting antibodies that bind to *T. cruzi* antigens. Demonstration of the parasite is not of primary importance. Several highly sensitive serologic tests for the detection of anti-*T. cruzi* antibodies are used widely in Latin America, including complement fixation and immunofluorescence assays and enzyme-linked immunosorbent assay (ELISA). However, a persistent problem with these conventional assays is the occurrence of false-positive reactions, typically with sera from patients with diseases such as leishmaniasis. For this reason, it is generally recommended that positivity in one assay be confirmed in two other tests and that well-characterized positive and negative comparison sera be included in each run. A highly sensitive and specific method for detecting anti-*T. cruzi* antibodies that employs immunoprecipitation of radiolabeled *T. cruzi* antigens has been described. This assay effectively deals with the problem of false-positive reactions and is available in the author's laboratory, but it has not been adapted for mass screening. Serodiagnostic assays that employ recombinant *T. cruzi* proteins as target antigens are being developed, as are tests based on polymerase chain reaction amplification of *T. cruzi* DNA sequences, but they are not yet available for general use.

TREATMENT　Therapy for Chagas' disease is unsatisfactory. Nifurtimox is the only drug active against *T. cruzi* that is available in the United States. In acute Chagas' disease, nifurtimox markedly reduces the duration of symptoms and parasitemia and decreases mortality. Nevertheless, its ability to eradicate parasites is limited, since patients treated with nifurtimox during the acute phase may have positive xenodiagnoses after full courses of the drug. Nifurtimox treatment should be initiated as early as possible in acute Chagas' disease. Moreover, when laboratory accidents occur in which it appears likely that *T. cruzi* infection could become established, nifurtimox therapy should be initiated without waiting for clinical or parasitologic indications of infection.

The usefulness of nifurtimox in individuals with indeterminate phase or symptomatic chronic Chagas' disease has not been established. There is no evidence that patients in the indeterminate phase are less likely to develop symptomatic disease after treatment with nifurtimox, and likewise, it has not been shown to have any effect on symptomatic chronic disease. Moreover, posttreatment xenodiagnoses are also positive in a large proportion of chronically infected patients given this drug. Hence there is no indication for treating individuals with chronic *T. cruzi* infections with nifurtimox.

Common adverse effects of nifurtimox include abdominal pain, anorexia, nausea, vomiting, and weight loss. Neurologic symptoms may include restlessness, disorientation, insomnia, twitching, paresthesia, polyneuritis, and seizures. These symptoms usually disappear when the dosage is reduced or treatment is discontinued. The recommended dosage for adults is 8 to 10 mg/kg body weight per day. The dosage for adolescents is 12.5 to 15 mg/kg per day, and for children 1 to 10 years of age, 15 to 20 mg/kg per day. The drug should be given orally in four divided doses each day, and therapy should be continued for 90 to 120 days. Nifurtimox is available from the Drug Service of the CDC, Atlanta, Georgia (telephone no. 404-639-3670).

Benznidazole is a second agent used to treat Chagas' disease. Its efficacy is similar to that of nifurtimox, and adverse effects include peripheral neuropathy, rash, and granulocytopenia. The recommended oral dosage is 5 mg/kg per day for 60 days. Benznidazole is used widely in Latin America, but it is not available in the United States.

Limited studies in experimental systems and in humans have suggested that allopurinol may be useful for treating chronic Chagas' disease. Currently, its efficacy is being evaluated in trials in humans. In addition, studies in mice have shown that recombinant interferon-γ decreases the duration and severity of acute *T. cruzi* infection, but its usefulness in persons with acute Chagas' disease has not been evaluated systematically.

PREVENTION Since drug therapy is unsatisfactory and vaccines are not available, the control of *T. cruzi* transmission in endemic countries must depend on reduction of domiciliary vector populations by spraying of insecticides and improvement in housing. Also, in endemic areas, expansion and improvement of programs for screening donated blood for the presence of *T. cruzi* are necessary to reduce transmission by transfusion. Tourists traveling in endemic areas should avoid sleeping in dilapidated houses outside urban areas. Mosquito nets and insect repellent will provide additional protection.

In the United States, blood donations should not be accepted from immigrants from regions in which Chagas' disease is endemic, unless serologic assays indicate that the donor is not infected with *T. cruzi*. Moreover, all immigrants from endemic regions should be screened for serologic evidence of infection with the parasite. Identification of infected individuals in this group is important not only to prevent transmission by blood transfusion but also to enable physicians who care for these patients to undertake appropriate diagnostic monitoring and supportive therapy when indicated. Laboratory personnel should wear gloves and eye protection when working with *T. cruzi* and infected vectors. Patients with end-stage chagasic cardiopathies should not undergo cardiac transplantation because the immunosuppression required after surgery often leads to reactivation of *T. cruzi* infection with serious consequences and even death.

SLEEPING SICKNESS

DEFINITION Sleeping sickness, or African trypanosomiasis, is caused by flagellated protozoan parasites belonging to the *Trypano-* *soma brucei* complex that are transmitted to humans by tsetse flies. In untreated patients, the trypanosomes first cause a febrile illness that is followed months or years later by progressive neurologic impairment and death.

THE PARASITES AND THEIR TRANSMISSION The East African (*rhodesiense*) and the West African (*gambiense*) forms of sleeping sickness are caused, respectively, by two trypanosome subspecies, *T. brucei rhodesiense* and *T. brucei gambiense*. These subspecies are indistinguishable morphologically but cause illnesses that are epidemiologically and clinically distinct. The parasites are transmitted by blood-sucking tsetse flies of the genus *Glossina*. The insects acquire the infection when they ingest blood from infected mammalian hosts. After many cycles of multiplication in the midgut of the vector, the parasites migrate to the salivary glands, and transmission takes place when they are inoculated during a subsequent blood meal. The injected trypanosomes multiply in the blood and other extracellular spaces and evade immune destruction in mammalian hosts for long periods by undergoing antigenic variation, a process by which the antigenic structure of their surface coat of glycoproteins changes periodically.

PATHOGENESIS AND PATHOLOGY A self-limited inflammatory lesion (trypanosomal chancre) may appear a week or so after the bite of an infected tsetse fly. A systemic febrile illness then evolves as the parasites are disseminated through the lymphatics and bloodstream. Systemic African trypanosomiasis without central nervous system (CNS) involvement is generally referred to as *stage I disease*. In this stage, there is widespread lymphadenopathy and splenomegaly, reflecting marked lymphocytic and histiocytic proliferation and invasion of morular cells, which are plasmacytes that may be involved in the production of IgM. An endarteritis with perivascular infiltration of both parasites and lymphocytes may develop in lymph nodes and spleen. Myocarditis develops frequently in patients with stage I disease, especially with *T. b. rhodesiense* infections.

Hematologic manifestations that accompany stage I trypanosomiasis include a moderate leukocytosis, thrombocytopenia, and anemia. High levels of immunoglobulins, consisting primarily of polyclonal IgM, are a constant feature, and heterophile antibodies, anti-DNA antibodies, and rheumatoid factor are often detected. High levels of antigen-antibody complexes may play a role in the tissue damage and increased vascular permeability that facilitate dissemination of the parasites.

Stage II trypanosomiasis involves invasion of the CNS. The presence of trypanosomes in perivascular areas is accompanied by intense infiltration of mononuclear cells. Cerebrospinal fluid (CSF) abnormalities include increased pressure, elevated total protein concentration, and pleocytosis. Trypanosomes also are frequently present in the CSF.

EPIDEMIOLOGY The trypanosomes that cause sleeping sickness are found only in Africa. Approximately 20,000 new cases are reported each year, but this number is surely an underestimate. Humans are the only reservoir of *T. b. gambiense*, and infections occur in widely distributed foci in tropical rain forests of Central and West Africa. Gambiense trypanosomiasis is primarily a problem in rural populations, and tourists rarely become infected. Trypanotolerant antelope species in savanna and woodland areas of Central and East Africa are the principal reservoir of *T. b. rhodesiense*. Cattle also can become infected but generally succumb to the parasite. Humans acquire *T. b. rhodesiense* infection only incidentally, since for the most part risk results from contact with tsetse flies that feed on wild animals. Thus the disease is an occupational hazard for persons who work in areas where infected game and vectors are present. In addition, occasional cases of *T. b. rhodesiense* infection occur among visitors to game parks in East Africa. During the past two decades, 16 cases of imported African trypanosomiasis have been reported to the CDC, most of which were caused by *T. b. rhodesiense*.

CLINICAL COURSE A painful trypanosomal chancre appears in some patients at the site where parasites were inoculated. Hematogenous and lymphatic dissemination (stage I disease) is marked by the onset of fever, and typically, bouts of high temperatures lasting several days are separated by afebrile periods. Lymphadenopathy is prominent in *T. b. gambiense* trypanosomiasis. The nodes are discrete, movable, rubbery, and nontender. Cervical nodes are often visible, and enlargement of the nodes of the posterior cervical triangle, or Winterbottom's sign, is a classic finding in individuals infected with *T. b. gambiense*. Pruritus is frequent, and a circinate rash is often present. Inconstant findings include malaise, headache, arthralgias, weight loss, edema, hepatosplenomegaly, and tachycardia.

CNS invasion (stage II disease) is characterized by the insidious development of protean neurologic manifestations, accompanied by progressive abnormalities in the CSF. A picture of progressive indifference and daytime somnolence (sleeping sickness) develops, sometimes alternating with restlessness and insomnia at night. A listless gaze accompanies a loss of spontaneity, and speech may become halting and indistinct. Extrapyramidal signs may include choreiform movements, tremors, and fasciculations. Ataxia is frequent, and the patient may appear to have Parkinson's disease with a shuffling gait, hypertonia, and tremors. In the final phase, progressive neurologic impairment ends in coma and death.

The most striking difference between the West African and East African trypanosomiases is that the latter illness tends to follow a more acute course. Typically, in tourists, systemic signs of infection such as fever, malaise, and headache may appear before the end of the trip or shortly after their return home. Persistent tachycardia unrelated to fever is common early in the course of *T. b. rhodesiense* trypanosomiasis, and death may result from arrhythmias and congestive heart failure before CNS disease develops. In general, untreated East African trypanosomiasis leads to death in a matter of weeks to months, often without a clear distinction between the hemolymphatic and CNS stages.

DIAGNOSIS A definitive diagnosis of African trypanosomiasis requires detection of the parasite. If a chancre is present, fluid should be expressed and examined directly by light microscopy for the highly motile trypanosomes. The fluid also should be fixed and stained with Giemsa. Material obtained by needle aspiration of lymph nodes early in the course of the illness should be examined similarly. Examination of wet preparations and Giemsa-stained thin and thick films of serial blood samples is also useful. If parasites are not found by these methods, the buffy coat from 10 to 15 mL anticoagulated blood or the pellet obtained by centrifugation of the eluate from 25 to 50 mL blood passed through a DEAE-cellulose column should be examined. Trypanosomes also may be seen in material aspirated from the bone marrow, and the aspirate can be inoculated into liquid culture medium, as can blood, buffy coat, lymph node aspirates, and CSF. Finally, *T. b. rhodesiense* infection can be detected by inoculation of these specimens into mice or rats, resulting in patent parasitemias in a week or two. This is a highly sensitive method for the detection of *T. b. rhodesiense*, but unfortunately, due to host specificity, *T. b. gambiense* cannot be detected by this technique.

Examination of the CSF is mandatory in all patients suspected of having African trypanosomiasis. An increase in the CSF cell count is the first abnormality to be detected, and increased opening pressure, as well as total protein and IgM levels, develops later. Trypanosomes may be seen in the sediment of centrifuged CSF. Any CSF abnormality in a patient in whom trypanosomes have been found in specimens from other sites must be viewed as pathognomonic for CNS involvement, and thus specific treatment for CNS disease must be given.

A number of serologic assays are available to aid in the diagnosis of African trypanosomiasis, but their variable sensitivity and specificity mandate that treatment decisions be based on demonstration of the parasite. These tests are of value for epidemiologic surveys.

TREATMENT The drugs traditionally used for treatment of African trypanosomiasis are suramin, pentamidine, and organic arsenicals. A recent addition to this list is eflornithine (difluoromethylornithine), which was approved by the U.S. Food and Drug Administration (FDA) in November 1990 for treatment of West African trypanosomiasis. In the United States these drugs can be obtained

from the CDC. Therapy for African trypanosomiasis must be individualized on the basis of the infecting organism (*T. b. gambiense* or *T. b. rhodesiense*), the presence or absence of CNS disease, adverse reactions, and occasionally, drug resistance. The choices of drugs for treatment of African trypanosomiasis are summarized as follows.

Stage I (normal CSF) West African trypanosomiasis (*T. b. gambiense*) should be treated with either suramin or eflornithine. Pentamidine can be used as an alternative drug. Stage II West African trypanosomiasis (abnormal CSF) should be treated with eflornithine.

Stage I East African trypanosomiasis (*T. b. rhodesiense*) should be treated with suramin, and pentamidine can be used as an alternative drug. Since suramin and pentamidine do not penetrate the CNS well and eflornithine has variable efficacy against *T. b. rhodesiense*, stage II East African trypanosomiasis should be treated with melarsoprol, and patients who cannot tolerate the latter drug should be treated with tryparsamide plus suramin.

Suramin is highly effective against stage I disease, but it can cause serious adverse effects and must be administered under the close supervision of a physician. A 100- to 200-mg intravenous test dose should be administered to detect hypersensitivity. The dosage for adults is 1 g intravenously on days 1, 3, 7, 14, and 21. The regimen for children is 20 mg/kg body weight (maximum dose is 1 g) intravenously on days 1, 3, 7, 14, and 21. The drug is given by slow intravenous infusion of a freshly prepared 10% aqueous solution. Approximately 1 patient in 20,000 has an immediate, severe, and potentially fatal reaction to the drug consisting of nausea, vomiting, shock, and seizures. Less severe reactions include fever, photophobia, pruritus, arthralgias, and skin eruptions. Renal damage is the most common important adverse effect of suramin. Transient proteinuria often appears during treatment. Urinalysis should be done before each dose, and the drug should be discontinued if proteinuria increases or casts and red cells appear in the sediment. Suramin should not be used in patients with renal insufficiency.

Eflornithine is highly effective for treatment of both stages of West African trypanosomiasis. In the trials on which the FDA based its approval, it cured more than 90 percent of 600 stage II patients. The recommended treatment schedule is 400 mg/kg per day intravenously in four divided doses for 2 weeks. This should be followed by oral treatment with 300 mg/kg per day for 3 to 4 weeks. Adverse effects include diarrhea, anemia, thrombocytopenia, seizures, and hearing loss. The efficacy of eflornithine in *T. b. rhodesiense* infection has not been determined. The high dosage and long duration of therapy are disadvantages that may make widespread use of eflornithine difficult.

Pentamidine isethionate is the alternative drug for patients with stage I African trypanosomiasis, but it should be kept in mind that some *T. b. rhodesiense* infections are unresponsive to this drug. The dose for both adults and children is 4 mg/kg per day intramuscularly or intravenously for 10 days. Frequent, immediate adverse reactions include nausea, vomiting, tachycardia, and hypotension. These reactions are usually transient and do not warrant cessation of therapy. Other adverse reactions include nephrotoxicity, abnormal liver function tests, neutropenia, rashes, hypoglycemia, and sterile abscesses.

The arsenical melarsoprol is the drug of choice for therapy of East African trypanosomiasis with CNS involvement. Melarsoprol will cure both stages of the disease, and thus it is also indicated for treatment of stage I patients in whom suramin and/or pentamidine have failed or are not tolerated. However, melarsoprol should never be the first choice for therapy of stage I disease because of its relatively high toxicity. In adults the drug should be given in three courses of 3 days each. The dosage is 2 to 3.6 mg/kg per day intravenously in three divided doses for 3 days, followed 1 week later by 3.6 mg/kg per day, also in three divided doses and for 3 days. The latter course is then repeated 10 to 21 days later. In debilitated patients, 2 to 4 days of suramin treatment are administered before starting melarsoprol, and an 18-mg initial dose of the latter drug, followed by progressive increases to the standard dose, has been recommended. For children, a total of 18 to 25 mg/kg should be given over 1 month. A starting dose of 0.36 mg/kg intravenously should be increased gradually to a maximum of 3.6 mg/kg at 1- to 5-day intervals for a total of 9 to 10 doses.

Melarsoprol is highly toxic and should be administered with great care. The incidence of reactive encephalopathy has been reported to be as high as 18 percent in some series. Clinical manifestations of reactive encephalopathy include high fever, headache, tremor, impaired speech, seizures, and even coma and death. Melarsoprol should be discontinued at the first sign of encephalopathy but may be restarted cautiously with small doses a few days after the signs have resolved. Extravasation of the drug results in intense local reactions, and vomiting, abdominal pain, nephrotoxicity, and myocardial damage can occur.

The treatment for patients with stage II East African disease who cannot tolerate melarsoprol is problematic. The combination of the arsenical tryparsamide and suramin is one possible approach, but its efficacy is limited because suramin does not penetrate the CNS and tryparsamide is much less effective against *T. b. rhodesiense* than it is against *T. b. gambiense*. The dose of tryparsamide is 30 mg/kg body weight (maximum 2 g) in a single intravenous dose every 5 days for a total of 12 doses, and that for suramin is 10 mg/kg every 5 days, also for a total of 12 injections. Tryparsamide can cause encephalopathy, fever, vomiting, abdominal pain, rash, tinnitus, and a variety of ocular symptoms. Alternatively, eflornithine can be administered as outlined above to patients who cannot tolerate melarsoprol, but as noted, its effectiveness against *T. b. rhodesiense* is variable.

PREVENTION The trypanosomiases constitute complex public health and epizootic problems in Africa. Considerable progress has been made in some areas through control programs that focus on eradication of vectors and drug treatment of infected humans, but there is no consensus on the best approach to solving the overall problem. Individuals can reduce the risk of acquiring trypanosomiasis by avoiding areas known to harbor infected insects, by wearing protective clothing, and by using insect repellent. Chemoprophylaxis is not recommended, and no vaccine is available to prevent transmission of the parasites.

REFERENCES

Chagas' disease

BRENER Z: Biology of *Trypanosoma cruzi*. Annu Rev Microbiol 27:347, 1973
HAGAR JM, RAHIMTOOLA SH: Chagas' heart disease in the United States. N Engl J Med 325:763, 1991
KIRCHHOFF LV: Is *Trypanosoma cruzi* a new threat to our blood supply? Ann Intern Med 111:773, 1989
————: American trypanosomiasis (Chagas disease): A persistent problem in Latin America now affects the United States. N Engl J Med (in press)
———— et al: American trypanosomiasis (Chagas' disease) in Central American immigrants. Am J Med 82:915, 1987
———— et al: Increased specificity of serodiagnosis of Chagas' disease by detection of antibody to the 72- and 90-kilodalton glycoproteins of *Trypanosoma cruzi*. J Infect Dis 155:561, 1987
MARR JJ et al: Chemotherapy for Chagas' disease: A perspective on current therapy and considerations for future research. Rev Infect Dis 8:884, 1986
SALAZAR SCHETTINO PM et al: Chagas disease in Mexico. Parasitol Today 4:348, 1988
SCHIFFLER RJ et al: Indigenous Chagas' disease (American trypanosomiasis) in California. JAMA 251:2983, 1984
SCHMUNIS GA: *Trypanosoma cruzi*, the etiologic agent of Chagas' disease: Status in the blood supply in endemic and nonendemic countries. Transfusion 31:547, 1991

Sleeping sickness

BRYAN RT et al: African trypanosomiasis in American travelers: A 20 year review, in *International Travel Medicine*, R Steffen (ed). Berlin, Springer-Verlag, 1990
DONELSON JE et al: Molecular biology of trypanosome antigenic variation. Microbiol Rev 49:107, 1985
DOUA F et al: Treatment of human late-stage gambiense trypanosomiasis with alpha-difluoromethylornithine (eflornithine): Efficacy and tolerance in 14 cases in Cote D'Ivoire. Am J Trop Med Hyg 37:525, 1987
JORDAN AM: *Trypanosomiasis Control and African Rural Development*. London, Longmans, 1986
POLTERA AA: Pathology of human African trypanosomiasis with reference to experimental African trypanosomiasis and infections of the central nervous system. Br Med Bull 41:169, 1985
VICKERMAN K: Developmental cycles and biology of pathogenic trypanosomes. Br Med Bull 41:105, 1985

---

177 TOXOPLASMA INFECTION AND TOXOPLASMOSIS

LLOYD H. KASPER

DEFINITION Toxoplasmosis is the disease caused by infection with the obligate intracellular parasite *Toxoplasma gondii*. *Toxoplasma* infection refers to the presence of the parasite in the infected person. Acute *Toxoplasma* infection acquired after birth is usually asymptomatic. This condition should be distinguished from chronic *Toxoplasma* infection, which describes the persistence of tissue cysts containing parasites in clinically asymptomatic individuals. Both acute and chronic toxoplasmosis are conditions in which the parasite is responsible for the development of clinical signs and symptoms (i.e., encephalitis, myocarditis, pneumonitis). Acute toxoplasmosis in the immunocompetent host usually is self-limited, is of short duration, and results in chronic toxoplasmosis. This condition is generally asymptomatic but can result in the recrudescence of clinical signs and symptoms if the immune response is compromised. Congenital toxoplasmosis is an infection of newborns resulting from the transplacental passage of parasites from an infected mother to the fetus. These infants usually are asymptomatic at birth but later manifest a wide range of signs and symptoms, including chorioretinitis, strabismus, epilepsy, and psychomotor retardation.

ETIOLOGY *T. gondii*, is an intracellular coccidian that infects both birds and mammals. There are two distinct aspects of the life cycle of *T. gondii*: a nonfeline and a feline cycle. The nonfeline, asexual tachyzoite form of this parasite occurs within intermediate hosts such as humans, mice, sheep, and swine. *T. gondii* are able to grow in all mammalian cells except red blood cells, which they enter but do not divide in. During acute infection, parasites can be found in many organs of the body. Once the parasite attaches to and actively penetrates the host cell, it forms a parasitophorous vacuole and begins to divide by endodyogeny, a process akin to binary fission. Division time is usually 6 to 8 h for the more virulent strains. When the number of parasites within the infected cell approaches the critical mass (usually 64 to 128 in culture), the cell ruptures, releasing tachyzoites that infect adjoining cells. In this manner, an infected organ soon shows evidence of a cytopathic process. Most of the tachyzoites are eliminated by means of humoral and cell-mediated immune responses of the host. Tissue cysts containing many bradyzoites develop 7 to 10 days after the systemic tachyzoite infection. These tissue cysts occur in a variety of host organs but principally within the central nervous system (CNS) and muscle, where they may exist for the lifetime of the host. When cysts are ingested (e.g., humans eat undercooked meat products), the cyst membrane undergoes rapid digestion in the presence of acidic pH gastric secretions. In nonfeline hosts, the ingested bradyzoites enter the small intestinal epithelium and transform into rapidly dividing tachyzoites. This acute, systemic tachyzoite infection is followed by the formation of tissue cysts that contain slowly replicating bradyzoites. The development of this chronic stage completes the nonfeline cycle. Active infection in the immunocompromised host is most likely due to the spontaneous release of encysted parasites that undergo rapid transformation into tachyzoites within the CNS.

The principal life cycle of the parasite is in the cat (the definitive host) and its prey. The sexual life cycle of the parasite is defined by the formation of oocysts within the feline host. This enteroepithelial cycle begins with the ingestion of the bradyzoite tissue cysts and culminates after several intermediate stages in the production of micro- and macrogametes. The microgamete is flagellated, which allows the parasite to seek a macrogamete. Gamete fusion produces a zygote, which envelopes itself in a rigid wall and is secreted in the feces as an unsporulated oocyst. After 2 to 3 days of exposure to air at ambient temperature, the noninfectious oocyst sporulates to produce eight sporozoite progeny. The sporulated oocyst can be ingested by an intermediate host such as a pregnant woman emptying a cat's litter box, a pig rummaging in the barnyard, or perhaps a mouse. Once freed from the oocysts by digestion, the released sporozoites infect the intestinal epithelium of the nonfeline host, producing rapidly growing asexual tachyzoites and ultimately bradyzoites.

EPIDEMIOLOGY Because of its ability to infect virtually any nucleated host cell, T. gondii is able to infect a wide range of mammals and birds. The seroprevalence is dependent on locale and age of the population. Generally, hot, arid climatic conditions are associated with a low prevalence of infection. In the United States and most European countries, the prevalence of seroconversion increases with age and exposure. For example, in the United States, 5 to 30 percent of individuals 10 to 19 years old and 10 to 67 percent of those over the age of 50 years show serologic evidence of prior exposure. The increase in seroprevalence is approximately 1 percent per year. In Central America, France, Turkey, and Brazil, the seroprevalence is much higher, approaching 90 percent by the time adults reach age 40.

ORAL TRANSMISSION The principal source of transmission in human *Toxoplasma* infection remains uncertain. Transmission in acquired infection is primarily oral and can occur by ingestion of either sporulated oocysts from contaminated soil or bradyzoites from undercooked meat. During acute feline infection, a cat may excrete as many as 100 million parasites per day. About 1 percent of the cat population sheds oocysts in their feces. These very stable sporozoite-containing oocysts are highly infectious and may remain viable for many years in the soil. Humans infected during a well-documented outbreak of oocyst-transmitted infection develop stage-specific antibodies to the oocyst/sporozoite.

Children and adults also can acquire infection from tissue cysts containing bradyzoites. The ingestion of a single cyst is all that is required for human infection. Underprepared meat or insufficient freezing is an important source of infection in the developed world. In the United States, 10 to 20 percent of lamb and 25 to 35 percent of pork meat products show evidence of cysts that contain bradyzoites. The incidence in beef is much lower and may be as low as 1 percent. Direct ingestion of bradyzoite cysts in these various meat products will lead to acute infection. The recent identification of stage-specific bradyzoite antigens may allow for better determination of the source for oral transmission.

In addition to oral transmission, there is a low incidence of direct transmission of the parasite by blood or organ products during transplantation. Viable parasites can be cultured from refrigerated, anticoagulated blood and may be a source of infection in individuals receiving blood transfusions. T. gondii infection also has been reported to occur in kidney and heart transplant recipients who were uninfected before transplantation.

TRANSPLACENTAL TRANSMISSION T. gondii can be transmitted to the fetus if the mother acquires primary infection during pregnancy. About one-third of all women infected during pregnancy will transmit the parasite to the fetus. Of the various factors that may determine fetal outcome, gestational age at the time of infection is most critical. There are few data to support a role for recrudescent maternal infection as the source of congenital disease. Thus women who are seropositive before pregnancy usually are protected against acute infection and do not give birth to congenitally infected neonates.

The following general guidelines can be used to evaluate congenital infection. There is essentially no risk if the mother is infected 6 months or more before conception. If infection occurs less than 6 months before conception, the likelihood of transplacental infection increases as the interval between infection and conception decreases. Most women infected during pregnancy give birth to normal, uninfected babies. About one-third of women infected during pregnancy will transmit the infection to their offspring. If infection occurs during the first trimester, the incidence of transplacental infection is lowest (about 15 percent), but the disease in the neonate is the most severe. If infection occurs during the third trimester, the incidence of transplacental infection is greatest (65 percent), but the infant is usually asymptomatic at birth. Recent evidence, however, suggests that those infants which are infected and normal at birth may have a higher incidence of learning disabilities and chronic neurologic sequelae than uninfected children. Only a small number of women (20 percent) infected with T. gondii show clinical signs of infection. Often the diagnosis is first appreciated when routine postconception serologic tests show evidence of specific antibody.

PATHOGENESIS Upon the ingestion by the host of either tissue cysts containing bradyzoites or oocysts containing sporozoites, the parasites are released from the cyst by a digestive process. Bradyzoites are resistant to the effect of pepsin and quickly invade and multiply within the gastrointestinal tract of the host. Within the enterocytes, the parasites undergo morphologic transformation, giving rise to invasive tachyzoites. In mice, these tachyzoites are able to induce host secretory immunity, as evidenced by increased levels of parasite-specific IgA. These asexual parasites soon rupture the invaded host cell and then are disseminated to a variety of organs, particularly lymphatic tissue, skeletal muscle, myocardium, retina, placenta, and most frequently, the CNS. In these organs, the parasite infects host cells, replicates by endodyogeny, ruptures the cells, and goes on to invade the adjoining cells. In this fashion, cell death and focal necrosis surrounded by an acute inflammatory response become the hallmarks of infection. In the normal immune host, both the humoral and cellular immune responses are important in controlling infection. Tachyzoites are sequestered by a variety of immune mechanisms, including induction of parasiticidal antibody, activation of macrophages, production of interferon-γ (IFN-γ), and stimulation of cytotoxic T cells (CTLs) of the CD8+ phenotype. These antigen-specific CTLs are capable of killing both extracellular parasites and target cells infected with parasites. Once the tachyzoites are cleared from the acutely infected host, tissue cysts containing bradyzoites begin to appear, usually within the CNS and retina. A number of immune factors, including altered antibody levels within the CNS, IFN-γ, and CD4+ and CD8+ T cells, have been implicated in modulating the persistence of infection within the normal host. In the immunocompromised or fetal host, the immune factors necessary to control the spread of tachyzoite infection are lacking. This altered immune state gives rise to a progression of focal destruction that results in organ failure (i.e., necrotizing encephalitis, pneumonia, and myocarditis).

Persistence of infection in the normal host by cysts containing bradyzoites is common. This lifelong infection usually remains subclinical. Although bradyzoites are in a slow metabolic phase, degeneration and rupture of cysts do occur within the CNS. This degenerative process, with the development of new bradyzoite-containing cysts, is the most likely source of persistent antibody titers in the normal host. Degeneration of these cysts is the most probable source of recrudescent infection in immunocompromised individuals.

PATHOLOGY Cell death and focal necrosis by replicating tachyzoites induce an intense mononuclear inflammatory response in any tissue or cell type infected. Tachyzoites rarely can be visualized by routine histopathologic staining of these inflammatory lesions. However, immunofluorescence staining with parasite antigen–specific antibodies can be positive for the organism or reveal evidence of antigenemia. In contrast to this inflammatory process caused by tachyzoites, the bradyzoite-containing cysts exhibit evidence of inflammation only at the early stages of development, perhaps in response to the presence of tachyzoite antigens. Once the cyst reaches maturity, the inflammatory process can no longer be detected, and the cysts remain immunologically quiescent within the brain matrix until they rupture.

Lymph nodes During acute infection, lymph node biopsy will demonstrate characteristic findings, including follicular hyperplasia and irregular clusters of tissue macrophages with eosinophilic cytoplasm. Granulomas rarely are seen in these specimens. Although tachyzoites are not usually observed, their presence can be assessed either by subinoculation of infected tissue into mice, with resultant disease, or by the polymerase chain reaction (PCR). PCR amplification of DNA fragments representing either the p30 (SAG-1) or p22 (SAG-2) antigens has been shown to be an effective and sensitive assay for establishing infection of lymph node tissue by tachyzoites.

Ocular In the eye, infiltrates of monocytes, lymphocytes, and plasma cells may produce uni- or multifocal lesions. Granulomatous lesions and retinochoroiditis can be observed in the posterior chamber following acute necrotizing retinitis. Other ocular complications of infection include iridocyclitis, cataracts, and glaucoma.

Central nervous system During CNS involvement, both focal and diffuse meningoencephalitis can be observed, with evidence of necrosis and microglial nodules. Necrotizing encephalitis in the patient without AIDS is characterized by small, diffuse lesions with perivascular cuffing in contiguous areas. In the AIDS population, polymorphonuclear leukocytes may be present in addition to monocytes, lymphocytes, and plasma cells. Cysts containing bradyzoites frequently are found contiguous with the necrotic tissue border. In the mouse model, parasite DNA has been detected by PCR amplification in association with reactivation of CNS toxoplasmosis.

Pulmonary Among patients with AIDS who die of toxoplasmosis, 40 to 70 percent have involvement of the heart and lung. Interstitial pneumonitis can occur in the neonate and the immunocompromised patient. Thickened and edematous alveolar septa infiltrated with mononuclear and plasma cells are observed. This inflammation may extend to the endothelial walls. Tachyzoites and bradyzoite-containing cysts have been observed within the alveolar membrane. A superimposed bronchopneumonia can be caused by other microbial agents.

Heart Cysts and aggregates of parasites in cardiac muscle tissue can be seen in patients with AIDS who die of toxoplasmosis. Focal necrosis surrounded by inflammatory cells is associated with hyaline necrosis and disrupted myocardial cells. Pericarditis is an infrequent but reported condition associated with toxoplasmosis in some patients.

Pathologic changes during disseminated infection are similar to those described for the lymph nodes, eye, and CNS. In patients with AIDS, involvement of the skeletal muscle, pancreas, stomach, and kidneys consists of necrosis, invasion by inflammatory cells, and the rare observation of tachyzoites by routine staining. Large necrotic lesions may cause direct tissue destruction. In addition, secondary effects from acute infection of these various organs, including pancreatitis, myositis, and glomerulonephritis, have been reported.

HOST IMMUNE RESPONSE Acute *Toxoplasma* infection evokes a cascade of protective immune responses in the normal host. *Toxoplasma* enter the host at the gut mucosal level and evoke the production of IgA antibody. This isotype, which constitutes more than 80 percent of all antibody in the mucosa, has now been shown to be a potentially important modulator of protection and indicator of infection. Titers of serum IgA antibody directed at p30 (SAG-1) have been shown to be useful human serum markers of congenital and acute toxoplasmosis. Milk whey IgA from acutely infected mothers shows a high titer of antibody to *T. gondii* and is able to block infection of enterocyte cells in vitro. The predominant parasite antigen recognized by the whey IgA is p30. In mice, IgA intestinal secretions directed at the parasite are abundant and associated with the induction of mucosal T cells.

If the parasite is able to evade the host mucosal response, both humoral and cellular immunity is evoked. *T. gondii* rapidly induces detectable levels of both IgM and IgG antibodies in serum. Monoclonal gammopathy of the IgG class can occur in congenital infected infants. IgM levels may be increased in the newborn with congenital infection. The polyclonal IgG antibodies evoked by infection are parasiticidal in vitro in the presence of serum complement and are the basis for the Sabin-Feldman dye test. However, cell-mediated immunity is the major protective response evoked by the parasite during host infection. Macrophages are activated following phagocytosis of antibody-opsonized parasites. This activation can lead to death of the parasite by either an oxygen-dependent or an oxygen-independent process. In addition, T cells are activated by a variety of parasite antigens. These antigens can be either membrane-associated or cytoplasmic. The CD4+ and CD8+ T cell responses are antigen-specific and further stimulate the production of a variety of important lymphokines that expand the T cell and natural killer cell repertoire. Studies in mice indicate that INF-γ is an important factor in eliciting host immune protection against *Toxoplasma* infection. Antibody to this molecule converts an avirulent infection into a lethal one. T cells exhibiting both T_{H1} (IFN-γ) and T_{H2} (interleukin 4) have been identified during murine infection. The role of CD8+ cells appears critical to host immunity in experimental toxoplasmosis. In humans, prolonged alteration in T cell subpopulations is associated with *T. gondii* infection. Both asymptomatic patients and those with active infection may show a depression in the ratio of helper to suppressor lymphocytes. This shift may be correlated with disease syndrome but is not necessarily correlated with disease outcome. Several human T cell clones of both CD4+ and CD8+ phenotype have recently been isolated and characterized. Some of the human CD8+ T cell clones have been shown to be cytolytic against parasite-infected target cells. These T cell clones produce a wide range of cytokines, including INF-γ, interleukin 2 (IL-2), and tumor necrosis factor (TNF). In mice IL-12, a modulator of NK cells, appears to be important during acute infection by upregulating the production of IFN-γ.

In patients with AIDS, both the humoral and cellular responses to *T. gondii* are altered. Although infection in the patient with AIDS is believed to be recrudescent, determination of antibody titers is not helpful in establishing reactivation. Because of the severe depletion in CD4+ T cells, quite frequently there is no observed increase in antibody titer during exacerbation of infection. In regard to cytokines, T cells from AIDS patients with reactivation of toxoplasmosis fail to secrete both INF-γ and IL-2. This alteration in the production of these critical immune cytokines contributes to the persistence of infection. *Toxoplasma* infection frequently occurs late in the course of AIDS, when the loss of T cell–dependent protective mechanisms, particularly CD8+ T cells, becomes most pronounced.

CLINICAL MANIFESTATIONS In the person whose immune system is intact, acute toxoplasmosis is usually asymptomatic and self-limited. This condition can go unrecognized in 80 to 90 percent of adults and children with acquired infection. The asymptomatic nature of this infection makes diagnosis difficult in mothers infected during pregnancy. The wide range of clinical manifestations observed in congenitally infected children includes severe neurologic complications such as hydrocephalus, microcephaly, mental retardation, and retinochoroiditis. If prenatal infection is severe, multiorgan failure and subsequent intrauterine fetal death can occur. In children and adults, chronic infection can persist throughout life, with little consequence to the immunocompetent host.

Toxoplasmosis in the immunocompetent person The most common manifestation of acute toxoplasmosis is cervical lymphadenopathy. The nodes may be single or multiple, are usually nontender, are discrete, and vary in firmness. Lymphadenopathy also may be found in suboccipital, supraclavicular, inguinal, and mediastinal areas. Generalized lymphadenopathy occurs in 20 to 30 percent of symptomatic patients. Between 20 and 40 percent of patients with lymphadenopathy have headache, malaise, fatigue, and fever (usually <40°C). A smaller number of symptomatic individuals have myalgia, sore throat, abdominal pain, maculopapular rash, meningoencephalitis, and confusion. Rare complications associated with infection in the normal immune host include pneumonia, myocarditis, encephalopathy, pericarditis, and polymyositis. Symptoms associated with acute infection usually resolve within several weeks, although the lymphadenopathy may persist for some months. In a recent epidemic, toxoplasmosis was diagnosed correctly in only 3 of the 25 patients who consulted physicians. If toxoplasmosis is considered in the differential diagnosis, routine laboratory and serologic screening should be performed before node biopsy.

Routine laboratory studies are usually unremarkable, except for minimal lymphocytosis, elevated sedimentation rate, and nominal increase in liver transaminases. Evaluation of cerebrospinal fluid (CSF) in the patient with evidence of encephalopathy or meningoencephalitis shows an elevation of intracranial pressure, mononuclear pleocytosis (10 to 50 cells per milliliter), a slight increase in protein concentration, and occasionally an increase in the gamma globulin level. PCR amplification of the *Toxoplasma* DNA target sequence in the CSF may be beneficial. The CSF in chronically infected individuals is normal.

Ocular infection　Infection with *T. gondii* is estimated to cause 35 percent of all cases of chorioretinitis in the United States and Europe. Although most ocular involvement is believed to be due to congenital infection, there is a very low incidence following acquired infection. Individuals with AIDS also can develop debilitating chorioretinitis. A variety of ocular manifestations can be observed, including blurred vision, scotoma, photophobia, and eye pain. Macular involvement occurs with loss of central vision, and nystagmus is secondary to poor fixation. Involvement of the extraocular muscles may lead to disorders of convergence and to strabismus. Ophthalmologic examination should be undertaken in newborns with suspected congenital infection. As the inflammation resolves, vision improves, but episodic flare-ups of chorioretinitis, which progressively destroy retinal tissue and lead to glaucoma, are common.

The ophthalmologic examination will reveal lesions of yellow-white, cotton-like patches with indistinct margins of hyperemia. As the lesions age, white plaques with distinct borders and black spots within the retinal pigment become more apparent. Lesions usually are located near the posterior pole of the retina; they may be single but are more commonly multiple. Congenital lesions may be unilateral or bilateral and will show evidence of massive chorioretinal degeneration with extensive fibrosis. Surrounding these areas of involvement will be normal retina and vasculature. In patients with AIDS, retinal lesions are often large with diffuse necrosis of the retina and reveal both free tachyzoites and cysts containing bradyzoites.

Infection of the immunocompromised person　Patients with AIDS and those receiving immunosuppressive therapy for lymphoproliferative disorders are the most at risk for developing acute toxoplasmosis. This predilection may be due either to reactivation of latent infection or to acquisition of parasites from exogenous sources such as blood or transplanted organs. In individuals with AIDS, more than 95 percent of cases of *Toxoplasma* encephalitis are believed to be due to recrudescent infection. In most of these cases, encephalitis develops when the CD4+ cell count falls below 100 cells per cubic millimeter. In the immunocompromised individual, the disease may be rapidly fatal if untreated. Thus accurate diagnosis and initiation of appropriate therapy are necessary to prevent fulminant infection.

Toxoplasmosis is the major opportunistic infection of the CNS in persons with AIDS. Between 20,000 and 40,000 patients with AIDS will have developed *Toxoplasma* encephalitis by 1993. Although geographic origin may be related to frequency of infection, it has no correlation with the severity of disease in the immunocompromised host. Individuals with AIDS who are seropositive for *T. gondii* are at a very high risk for developing encephalitis. In the United States, about one-third of the 15 to 40 percent of adult patients with AIDS who are latently infected with the parasite will develop *Toxoplasma* encephalitis.

The signs and symptoms of acute toxoplasmosis in the immunocompromised patient are principally within the CNS. Over 50 percent of patients with clinical manifestations have intracerebral involvement. Clinical findings at the time of presentation can range from nonfocal to focal dysfunction. These findings include encephalopathy, meningoencephalitis, and mass lesions. Patients may present with altered mental status (75 percent), fever (10 to 72 percent), seizures (33 percent), headaches (56 percent), and focal neurologic findings (60 percent), including motor deficits, cranial nerve palsies, movement disorders, dysmetria, visual-field loss, and aphasia. Patients who present with evidence of diffuse cortical dysfunction develop evidence of focal neurologic disease as the infection progresses. This altered condition is due not only to the necrotizing encephalitis caused by direct invasion of the parasite but also to secondary effects, including vasculitis, edema, and hemorrhage. Onset of infection can range from an insidious onset over several weeks to an acute confusional state with fulminant focal deficits, including hemiparesis, hemiplegia, visual-field defects, localized headache, and focal seizures.

Although lesions within the CNS can occur anywhere, the areas most involved appear to be the brainstem, basal ganglia, pituitary gland, and corticomedullary junction. Brainstem involvement will give rise to a variety of neurologic dysfunctions, including cranial nerve palsy, dysmetria, and ataxia. With basal ganglia infection, patients may develop hydrocephalus, choreiform movements, and choreoathetosis. Because *Toxoplasma* usually causes encephalitis, meningeal involvement is unusual, and thus CSF findings may be unremarkable or perhaps show a modest increase in cell count and protein—but not in glucose—concentration.

Cerebral toxoplasmosis needs to be differentiated from other opportunistic infections or tumors within the CNS of those afflicted with AIDS. This would include herpes simplex encephalitis, cryptococcal meningitis, progressive multifocal leukoencephalopathy, and primary CNS lymphoma. Involvement of the pituitary gland can give rise to panhypopituitarism and hyponatremia from inappropriate secretion of vasopressin (antidiuretic hormone). AIDS-dementia complex may present as cognitive impairment, attention loss, and altered memory. Brain biopsy in those patients who have been treated for *Toxoplasma* encephalitis but who continue to exhibit neurologic dysfunction often fails to identify organisms.

Autopsies of patients infected with *Toxoplasma* have demonstrated multiple organ involvement with or without CNS disease. The organs infected include the lungs, gastrointestinal tract, pancreas, skin, eyes, heart, and liver. *Toxoplasma* pneumonia can occur and can be confused with *Pneumocystis carinii* infection. Respiratory involvement usually will present as dyspnea, fever, and a nonproductive cough, which may rapidly progress to acute respiratory failure with hemoptysis, metabolic acidosis, hypotension, and occasionally disseminated intravascular coagulation. Histopathologic studies will demonstrate necrosis and a mixed cellular infiltrate. The presence of organisms is a helpful diagnostic indicator, but organisms can also be found in healthy tissue. Most commonly, myocardial infection is asymptomatic. However, infection of the heart can be associated with cardiac tamponade or biventricular failure. As discussed previously, ocular involvement can occur without concomitant encephalitis. This infection should be distinguished from chorioretinitis caused by cytomegalovirus, which is usually more hemorrhagic in character. Toxoplasmic retinochoroiditis may be a prodrome to the development of encephalitis.

A presumptive clinical diagnosis of toxoplasmic encephalitis in patients with AIDS is based on clinical presentation, history of exposure as evidenced by positive serology, and radiologic evaluation. When these criteria are used, the predictive value is as high as 80 percent. More than 97 percent of patients with AIDS and toxoplasmosis have IgG antibody to the parasite in their sera. IgM serum antibody is usually not demonstrable. Intrathecal antibody to *T. gondii* may be present. Neuroradiologic evaluation should include a double-dose contrast computed tomographic (CT) scan of the head. By this test, single and frequently multiple contrast-enhancing lesions (<2 cm) may be identified. Magnetic resonance imaging (MRI) usually will demonstrate multiple lesions and will provide a more sensitive evaluation of efficacy of therapy. Patients with primary CNS lymphoma are four times more likely than patients with *Toxoplasma* encephalitis to have solitary lesions on an MRI scan. A therapeutic trial of anti-*Toxoplasma* medications frequently is used to assess the diagnosis. Recent studies have shown that treatment of presumptive *Toxoplasma* encephalitis with pyrimethamine-clindamycin results in a quantifiable clinical improvement in more than 50 percent of patients by day 3. By day 7, over 90 percent of patients successfully treated show evidence of improvement. In contrast, if patients fail to respond or have lymphoma, clinical signs and symptoms worsen by day 7. Thus patients in this category require brain biopsy with or without a change in therapy. This procedure can now be performed by a stereotactic CT-guided method that can reduce potential complications. Brain biopsy for the presence of *T. gondii* identifies organisms in 50 to 75 percent of cases. More recent studies indicate that PCR amplification of target genes significantly increases the sensitivity for detection of parasites.

DIAGNOSIS **Tissue and body fluid** The diagnosis of acute toxoplasmosis can be made by isolation of the parasite from either blood or other body fluids after subinoculation of the body fluid into the peritoneal cavity of mice. Mice should be tested for organisms in the peritoneal fluid 6 to 10 days postinfection. If no parasites are found in the mouse's peritoneal fluid, its anti-*Toxoplasma* serum titer can be evaluated 4 to 6 weeks following inoculation. Isolation of *T. gondii* from the patient's body fluids reflects acute infection, whereas isolation from biopsy tissue is an indication only of the presence of tissue cysts and should not be misinterpreted as acute toxoplasmosis. Persistent parasitemia in patients with latent, asymptomatic infection is rare. Histologic examination of lymph nodes may suggest the characteristic changes described above. Demonstration of tachyzoites in lymph nodes will establish the diagnosis of acute toxoplasmosis. As with subinoculation into mice, demonstration of cysts containing bradyzoites in histologic specimens confirms only prior infection with *T. gondii* but is nondiagnostic for acute infection.

Serology The preceding procedures have great diagnostic value but are limited because of the difficulty either in growing parasites in vivo or in identifying tachyzoites by histochemical methods. Serologic diagnosis has become the routine method. A wide range of serologic tests that can be used to measure antibody to *T. gondii* are available commercially. The reader is referred to the excellent review by Remington and McLeod discussing the various serologic tests currently available.

Diagnosis of acute infection with *T. gondii* can be established by determining the simultaneous presence of IgG and IgM antibody to *Toxoplasma* in the patient. The presence of circulating IgA favors the diagnosis of an acute infection. The Sabin-Feldman dye test, indirect fluorescent antibody test (IFA), and enzyme linked immunoassay (ELISA) all satisfactorily measure the presence of circulating IgG antibody to *Toxoplasma*. Positive IgG titers ($>$1:10) can be detected as early as 2 to 3 weeks after infection. These titers usually peak at 6 to 8 weeks and slowly decline to a new baseline, which remains elevated for life. It is necessary to obtain a serum IgM titer in concert with the IgG titer to better establish the time of infection. The methods currently available for this determination are the double-sandwich ELISA-IgM and the IgM-immunosorbent assay (IgM-ISAGA). Both these assays are specific, sensitive, and avoid false-positive results associated with rheumatoid factor and antinuclear antibody. The double-sandwich IgA-ELISA is more sensitive than the IgM-ELISA for detecting congenital infection in the fetus and newborn.

The immunocompetent adult or child For the patient who presents with lymphadenopathy only, a positive IgM titer is an indication of acute infection and for therapy if that is clinically warranted (see "Treatment," below). The serum titer should be determined again in 3 weeks. An elevation in the IgG titer without an increase in the IgM titer suggests that infection is present, but that it is not acute. If there is a borderline increase in either IgG or IgM, the titers should be assessed again in 3 to 4 weeks.

Ocular toxoplasmosis Because of the congenital nature of this infection, the serum titer may not correlate with presence of active lesions in the fundus. In general, if there is a positive IgG titer (on undiluted serum if necessary) and typical lesions, the diagnosis is established. If lesions are atypical and the titer is in the low-positive range, the diagnosis is presumptive.

Immunocompromised host As discussed above, in patients with AIDS, the presence of IgG and radiologic findings consistent with toxoplasmosis determine a presumptive diagnosis. Evaluation of rising IgG titers or attempts at identifying whether IgM is present are unreliable. Serologic evidence of infection is present in virtually all patients before they develop *Toxoplasma* encephalitis. It is therefore important to determine antibody status in all HIV-infected patients. Antibody titers may range from negative to 1:1024 in patients with AIDS and *Toxoplasma* encephalitis. Fewer than 3 percent of patients have no demonstrable antibody to *Toxoplasma* at the time of diagnosis. Determination of intrathecal antibody titer may be useful in identifying prior infection. PCR amplification of genetic material of the parasite found within the CSF may prove beneficial in the future.

Patients with toxoplasmic encephalitis will have focal or multifocal abnormalities demonstrable on CT or MRI scan. These findings are not pathognomonic of *Toxoplasma* infection since 40 percent of CNS lymphomas are multifocal and 50 percent are ring-enhancing. Lesions on CT scan are multiple and located in both hemispheres, with the basal ganglia and corticomedullary junction most commonly involved. A CT scan may underestimate the degree of inflammation during early disease. Double-dose contrast enhancement may increase the sensitivity of diagnosis. For both MRI and CT scans, the rate of false-negative results is approximately 10 percent. The finding of a single lesion on an MRI scan increases the suspicion of primary lymphoma and strengthens the argument for performing a brain biopsy. An MRI should be performed if the CT scan shows only a single lesion. CT and MRI scans are important for the assessment of response to therapy. As with other conditions, the radiologic response may lag behind the clinical response. Resolution of lesions may take from 3 weeks to 6 months. Some patients may show clinical improvement in the presence of worsening radiographic findings.

A presumptive diagnosis of *Toxoplasma* encephalitis should initiate prompt therapy. Patients should be monitored for neurologic deterioration during the first 7 days. After this time, successful therapy should result in stabilization or improvement in clinical status. After 3 weeks, repeat radiologic studies should identify improvement. If glucocorticoids have been administered, radiologic studies should be repeated at the time of discontinuation to determine if exacerbation of disease has occurred. If the patient's clinical conditions becomes worse, performance of a biopsy must be a strong consideration.

Congenital infection Serologic diagnosis of acute toxoplasmosis in the neonate is based either on persistence of IgG antibody or on a positive IgM titer (after the first week to exclude the possibility of placental leak). The determination of IgG titer should be repeated every 6 to 12 weeks to establish the pattern of response. An increase in IgM titer that extends beyond the first week is indicative of acute infection (the half-life of maternal IgM is 3 to 5 days).

TREATMENT Immunologically competent adults and older children who have only lymphadenopathy do not require specific therapy unless they have persistent and severe symptoms. Because of the high virulence of *Toxoplasma* strains used in the laboratory, it is advisable to treat patients with laboratory acquired infections. Patients with ocular toxoplasmosis should be treated for 1 month with sulfadiazine and pyramethamine. A large percentage of patients with chorioretinitis have shown clinical improvement. The alternative therapeutic agents for patients with ocular involvement include a combination of clindamycin and pyrimethamine.

Patients with AIDS should be treated for acute toxoplasmosis. Current therapeutic protocols are directed at folate metabolism, protein synthesis, or nucleic acid synthesis of the parasite. Pyrimethamine and trimethoprim are directed at the enzyme dihydrofolate reductase. The gene encoding this molecule has been cloned recently and expressed in vitro, making rational development of other folate inhibitors feasible. Inhibitors of protein synthesis, including clindamycin, chlortetracycline, and azithromycin, have been shown to affect growth of the parasite. Inhibitors of purine synthesis, such as arprinocid, may prove to be important. The antimicrobial agent hydroxynaphthoquinone (BW566C80), which blocks pyrimidine salvage, has demonstrated potent toxoplasmacidal activity against both the tachyzoite and cyst.

In the immunocompromised patient, toxoplasmosis is rapidly fatal if untreated. The mainstay of treatment for *Toxoplasma* encephalitis is combination therapy. Pyrimethamine and sulfadiazine administered together block folic acid metabolism and successfully reduce the parasite burden. Folinic acid (leucovorin) is given as an adjunct to prevent the bone marrow toxicity associated with pyrimethamine. Both pyrimethamine and sulfadiazine cross the blood-brain barrier. A major consequence of dual therapy is the high incidence of associated toxicity (40 percent). Rash may occur during the first 3 weeks in up to 20 percent of patients but does not preclude the use of this combination. Other complications include hematologic effects, crystalluria, hematuria, radiolucent renal stones, and nephrotoxicity. During therapy, serum levels of these drugs may be erratic, but such fluctuations have not been correlated with these potential complications. The current medication regimen includes pyrimethamine, a 200-mg loading dose followed by 50 to 75 mg/d, plus sulfadiazine, 4 to 6 g/d in four divided doses. In addition, the administration of calcium folinate, 10 to 15 mg/d for 6 weeks, is required. These agents are active only against the tachyzoite stage of the parasite. Thus, after these patients complete the initial course (4 to 6 weeks or until the radiologic improvement), they must receive lifelong suppressive therapy with pyramethamine (25 to 50 mg) and sulfadiazine (2 to 4 g). If sulfadiazine cannot be tolerated, a combination of pyrimethamine (75 mg/d) plus clindamycin (450 mg tid) can be used. It is possible that pyrimethamine (50 to 75 mg/d) is sufficient for chronic suppressive therapy. Congenitally infected neonates are treated with oral pyrimethamine (0.5 to 1 mg/kg) and sulfadiazine (100 mg/kg). In addition, therapy with spiramycin (100 mg/kg) plus prednisone (1 mg/kg) has been shown to be efficacious for congenital infection.

Alternative therapies have been established because of the toxicity associated with the long-term antimicrobial therapy necessary for many individuals infected with *T. gondii*. Although effective in animal models, trimethoprim-sulfamethoxazole has not yet been fully established as beneficial for humans. Dapsone (diamino-diphenyl sulfone) is a potent sulfone effective against murine toxoplasmosis. As with pyrimethamine, dapsone has no effect on the tissue cyst. Dapsone, because of its longer serum half-life and decreased toxicity, may be an effective alternative to sulfadiazine. Spiramycin has been used in Europe to treat pregnant women. Presumably, this medication is able to reduce transplacental transmission, although supporting evidence is not yet conclusive. Spiramycin has been ineffective as primary prophylaxis in patients with AIDS. Clindamycin is effective in treating murine toxoplasmosis. It is well absorbed from the gastrointestinal tract, and peak serum levels occur 1 to 2 h after administration. Recent data suggest that the combination of oral pyrimethamine (25 to 75 mg/d) plus intravenous clindamycin (1200 to 4800 mg/d) is effective in treating patients with AIDS who have *Toxoplasma* encephalitis. It is not clear if this treatment regimen is superior to that of pyrimethamine and sulfadiazine. Toxic effects from clindamycin include nausea, vomiting, neutropenia, rash, and pseudomembranous colitis. Macrolides in addition to spiramycin that have been evaluated in the murine system include roxithromycin, clarithromycin, and azithromycin. A combination of pyrimethamine and clarithromycin appears to be effective in a small number of patients evaluated to date. There is no evidence suggesting that the macrolides are beneficial by themselves. The agent hydroxynaphthoquinone (BW566C80) may be effective against the cysts containing bradyzoites and has sustained prolonged remission of the disease in an experimental model. Glucocorticoids can be used to treat intracerebral edema, but their benefit is not yet established. It is difficult to assess the benefit of glucocorticoids when they are administered in conjunction with anti-*Toxoplasma* medication. Anticonvulsants are sometimes necessary for treatment of seizures, but attention should be given to the potential interaction between sulfadiazine and phenytoin. There is currently no indication for primary prophylactic treatment in those who are seropositive for *T. gondii* and are at risk of developing *Toxoplasma* encephalitis.

PREVENTION Primary infection with *Toxoplasma* can be reduced by not eating undercooked meat and by avoiding oocyst-contaminated material (i.e., the cat's litter box). Meat should be heated to 60°C or frozen to kill cysts. Hands should be washed thoroughly after work in the garden, and all fruits and vegetables should be washed. Blood intended for transfusion into seronegative immunocompromised individuals should be screened for antibody to *T. gondii*. Although such serologic screening is not routinely performed, seronegative women should be screened for evidence of infection several times during pregnancy if they are exposed to environmental conditions that put them at risk for infection with *T. gondii*.

REFERENCES

BROOKS RG et al: Role of serology in the diagnosis of toxoplasmic lymphadenopathy. Rev Infect Dis 9:1055, 1987

BURG JL et al: Direct and sensitive detection of a pathogenic protozoan, *Toxoplasma gondii*, by polymerase chain reaction. J Clin Microbiol 27:1787, 1989

DAFFOS F et al: Prenatal management of 746 pregnancies at risk for congenital toxoplasmosis. N Engl J Med 318:271, 1988

DECOSTER A et al: IgA antibodies against P30 as markers of congenital and acute toxoplasmosis. Lancet 2:1104, 1988

GROVER CM et al: Rapid prenatal diagnosis of congenital *Toxoplasma* infection by using polymerase chain reaction and amniotic fluid. J Clin Microbiol 10:2297, 1990

KASPER LH et al: Antigen-specific (p30) mouse CD8+ T cells are cytotoxic against *Toxoplasma gondii*–infected peritoneal macrophages. J Immunol 148:1493, 1992

KHAN IA et al: Induction of antigen-specific human cytotoxic T cells by *Toxoplasma gondii*. J Clin Invest 85:1879, 1990

LUFT BJ, REMINGTON JS: Toxoplasmic encephalitis in AIDS. Clin Infect Dis 15:211, 1992

McCABE RE, REMINGTON JS: Toxoplasmosis: The time has come. N Engl J Med 318:313, 1988

MACK DG, McLEOD R: Human *Toxoplasma gondii*–specific secretory immunoglobulin A reduces *T. gondii* infection of enterocytes in vitro. J Clin Invest 90:2585, 1992

Prophylaxis for toxoplasma encephalitis. Infect Dis Alert 11:164, 1992

REMINGTON JS, McLEOD R: Toxoplasmosis, in *Infectious Diseases in Medicine and Surgery*, J Bartlett, S Gorbach, N Blacklow (eds). Philadelphia, Saunders, 1992

178 PNEUMOCYSTIS CARINII PNEUMONIA

PETER D. WALZER

DEFINITION *Pneumocystis carinii* is an opportunistic pathogen whose natural habitat is the lung. The organism is an important cause of pneumonia in the compromised host.

The taxonomy of *P. carinii* has long been controversial; however, recent studies favor placement in the fungal kingdom. Analysis of gene sequences of ribosomal RNA, mitochondrial proteins, and major enzymes (thymidylate synthase, dihydrofolate reductase) has demonstrated that *P. carinii* is more closely related to fungi than to protozoa. Biochemical studies have suggested that the cell wall of *P. carinii* contains glucans; drugs which inhibit 1,3-β-glucan synthesis in fungi are highly active against *P. carinii* in animal models.

ETIOLOGY Knowledge of the basic biology of *P. carinii* has been severely hampered by the lack of a reliable in vitro cultivation system. Major developmental stages of the organism include the small (1- to 4-μm) pleomorphic trophozoite or trophic form; the 5- to 8-μm cyst, which has a thick cell wall and contains up to eight intracystic bodies; and the precyst, an intermediate stage. The life cycle of *P. carinii* probably involves asexual replication by the trophic form and sexual reproduction by the cyst which ends in release of the intracystic bodies; an intracellular stage has not been identified. Ultrastructurally, *P. carinii* has a primitive organelle system, but little is known about its metabolism.

P. carinii has two major groups of antigens: a 110- to 120-kDa surface glycoprotein (gp120), which appears to mediate adherence to host cells, and a moiety of 35 to 45 kDa in human-derived and of 45 to 55 kDa in rat-derived organisms, respectively, which is the antigen most commonly recognized by the host.

EPIDEMIOLOGY   *P. carinii* has a worldwide distribution among humans and has been found in a variety of animals. Organisms for these hosts are morphologically identical, but species or strain differences exist. Data about the fungal nature of *P. carinii* raise intriguing questions about new developmental stages and environmental sources of the organism. Serologic surveys indicate that most normal children have been exposed to the organism by 3 to 4 years of age. Animal model experiments have demonstrated that *P. carinii* is transmitted by the airborne route. Human-to-human transmission has been suggested by the occurrence of outbreaks of pneumocystosis among institutionalized debilitated infants and in hospitals caring for immunosuppressed patients. On the basis of animal studies, the incubation period is thought to be 4 to 8 weeks.

PATHOGENESIS AND PATHOLOGY   *P. carinii* pneumonia occurs in the following hosts: premature, malnourished infants; children with primary immunodeficiency diseases; patients receiving immunosuppressive therapy (particularly corticosteroids) for cancer, organ transplantation, and other disorders; and people with AIDS. Pneumocystosis is a leading opportunistic infection and cause of death in AIDS patients in the United States and other industrialized countries, but it is less common in AIDS patients in tropical and developing countries. The reasons for this difference are unclear but may relate to the occurrence of more virulent infections (e.g., tuberculosis) in populations from the developing world.

The major host factor which predisposes to *P. carinii* pneumonia is impaired cellular immunity. The incidence of pneumocystosis among HIV patients can be correlated with the number of circulating CD4 cells. However, there is increasing evidence that antibodies also play a role in host defenses against this organism. It is generally thought that *P. carinii* pneumonia develops by reactivation of latent infection with immunosuppressive drugs or progressive breakdown of the immune system in AIDS. An alternative view is that the host is periodically exposed to new sources of *P. carinii*. Resolution of this argument awaits the development of better markers of the organism.

Within the lung, *P. carinii* attaches firmly to the alveolar type I pneumocyte. In vitro studies suggest several possible mechanisms of adherence to host cells, including the binding of gp120 to fibronectin or to mannose receptors. Animal models have shown that *P. carinii* organisms propagate slowly, gradually filling the alveoli; this phenomenon is accompanied by a series of complex changes in the microenvironment, such as increased alveolar-capillary permeability and alterations in surfactant constituents, which culminate in damage to the type I cell.

On hematoxylin and eosin–stained lung sections, the alveoli are filled with the typical foamy, vacuolated exudate. With severe disease there may be interstitial edema, fibrosis, and hyaline membrane formation. The host inflammatory changes usually consist of hypertrophy of alveolar type II cells, a typical reparative response, and a mild mononuclear cell interstitial infiltrate. Malnourished infants display an intense plasma cell infiltrate which gave the disease its early name of "interstitial plasma cell pneumonia."

CLINICAL FEATURES   Patients with *P. carinii* pneumonia complain of dyspnea, fever, and nonproductive cough. Symptoms in non-AIDS patients often begin after the glucocorticoid dose has been tapered and typically last 1 to 2 weeks. AIDS patients are usually ill for several weeks or longer and have more subtle manifestations. However, the clinical picture in individual patients is quite variable, and thus a high index of suspicion and careful history are key features to early detection.

Physical findings include tachypnea, tachycardia, and cyanosis, but lung auscultation reveals few abnormalities. The white blood count is variable and usually governed by the patient's underlying disease. Arterial blood gases demonstrate hypoxia, increased alveolar-arterial oxygen gradient ($Pa_{O_2} - Pa_{O_2}$), and respiratory alkalosis.

There also may be changes in pulmonary function tests (diffusing capacity) and increased uptake with nuclear imaging techniques (gallium scan). Elevated serum lactate dehydrogenase (LDH) has been reported, probably reflecting lung parenchymal damage, but is not specific for *P. carinii*. In general, the laboratory abnormalities are less severe in AIDS patients.

The classic findings on chest radiograph consist of bilateral diffuse infiltrates beginning in the perihilar regions, but a variety of atypical manifestations (nodular densities, cavitary lesions) also have been reported. Patients who receive aerosol pentamidine have an increased frequency of upper lobe infiltrates and pneumothorax. Early in the course of pneumocystosis, the chest radiograph may be normal.

DIAGNOSIS   Since the clinical picture of *P. carinii* can be produced by many different infectious and noninfectious agents, diagnosis must be made by specific identification of the organism. Definitive diagnosis is made by histopathologic staining. Traditional stains have included reagents (methenamine silver, toluidine blue, cresyl echt violet) which selectively stain the wall of *P. carinii* cysts and reagents (Wright-Giemsa) which stain the nuclei of all developmental stages. Immunofluorescence and immunoperoxidase staining, which are somewhat more sensitive, have gained in popularity as monoclonal antibodies to *P. carinii* became commercially available. Other reagents include nonspecific fluorochrome stains (calofluor white) and the Papanicolaou stain. Selection of these staining techniques is largely a matter of personal preference; frequently, more than one reagent is used to make the diagnosis. Molecular probes and the polymerase chain reaction offer promise in *P. carinii* diagnosis, but little progress has been made with culture or antigen and antibody detection techniques.

Successful diagnosis of pneumocystosis requires an aggressive approach to obtain proper specimens. In general, the yield from different diagnostic procedures is higher in AIDS patients than in non-AIDS patients; this probably reflects the higher organism burden in people with AIDS. In recent years, induced sputum has gained popularity as a simple, noninvasive technique; this procedure requires trained and dedicated personnel, and success in using it has varied at different institutions. Fiberoptic bronchoscopy with bronchoalveolar lavage (BAL), which is more sensitive and invasive than induced sputum, is the mainstay of *P. carinii* diagnosis. This procedure provides information about the organism burden, host inflammatory response, and the presence of other opportunistic infections. Transbronchial biopsy and open lung biopsy, which are the most invasive procedures, are reserved for situations when a diagnosis cannot be made by lavage.

COURSE AND PROGNOSIS   Although *P. carinii* usually remains confined to the lungs, cases of disseminated infection have occurred in AIDS and non-AIDS patients. Estimates of the frequency of extrapulmonary pneumocystosis have ranged from <1 to 3 percent in different series. One risk factor in HIV patients appears to be the administration of aerosol pentamidine. The most common sites of involvement have been lymph nodes, liver, spleen, and bone marrow. Disseminated *P. carinii* infection can occur without clinical evidence of pneumonia.

In the typical case of untreated *P. carinii* pneumonia, there is progressive respiratory embarrassment leading to death. Therapy is most effective when instituted early in the course of the disease, before there is extensive alveolar damage. The most widely used prognostic indicators have been the arterial oxygen pressure and alveolar-arterial oxygen gradient. Other factors which may influence survival include the organism burden, percentage of neutrophils in BAL fluid, chest radiograph abnormalities, serum LDH and albumin levels, and the expertise of the hospital in caring for AIDS patients. Concurrent pulmonary infections also complicate management, but the presence of cytomegalovirus does not affect the outcome of pneumocystosis.

TREATMENT   The two major drugs used in the treatment of *P. carinii* pneumonia have been trimethoprim-sulfamethoxazole (TMP-SMX) and pentamidine isethionate. These agents are equally contain four nuclei. Trophozoites are readily recognized as pear-shaped, dorsally convex, flattened parasites with two nuclei and four pairs of flagella. The diagnosis is sometimes difficult to establish. Direct examination of fresh or properly preserved stools as well as concentration methods should be used. Because cyst excretion is variable and may be undetectable at times, repeated stool examinations, sampling of duodenal fluid, and small intestinal biopsy may be required to detect the parasite. Tests to detect parasite antigen in stool, now commercially available, are as sensitive and specific as good microscopic examinations and easier to perform but are relatively expensive. All of these methods may uncommonly yield false-negative results.

Treatment   Metronidazole (250 mg tid for 5 days) and quinacrine (100 mg bid for 5 days) treatments are equally effective, but furazolidone (100 mg qid for 7 to 10 days) is somewhat less effective. Cure rates are usually greater than 80 percent. Those who fail initial treatment can be retreated with another drug or a longer course of the same drug. Almost all patients respond to therapy and are cured, although some with chronic giardiasis experience delayed resolution of symptoms even after eradication of *Giardia*. Those who remain infected after repeated treatments should be evaluated for the possibility of reinfection from family members, close personal contacts, and environmental sources, as well as for the presence of hypogammaglobulinemia. In cases refractory to multiple treatment courses, combined therapy with metronidazole (750 mg tid for 21 days) and quinacrine (100 mg bid for 21 days) has been successful. Tinidazole, not available in the United States, is considered more effective than metronidazole or quinacrine. Frequently, children attending day care centers infect the entire family, and in this situation, treatment of all infected family members, including asymptomatic carriers, may be required to prevent reinfection. Paromomycin, an oral aminoglycoside that is not well absorbed, can be used in symptomatic pregnant women, although sufficient experience is not available to judge how frequently this agent either eradicates infection or ameliorates symptoms.

Prevention   Although *Giardia* is extremely infectious, disease can be prevented by eating and drinking noncontaminated food and water. Cooking food adequately or boiling or filtering potentially contaminated water prevents infection. Transmission between heterosexual adults is not common when hygienic practices are employed.

CRYPTOSPORIDIOSIS   The coccidian parasite *Cryptosporidium* has become recognized in the last decade to cause human diarrheal disease in normal hosts and especially those with AIDS or other forms of immunodeficiency.

Life cycle and epidemiology   Infections are acquired by consumption of oocysts, which excyst to liberate sporozoites, which in turn enter and infect intestinal epithelial cells. Further development occurs by both asexual and sexual cycles, which produce forms capable of infecting other epithelial cells and of generating oocysts that are passed in the feces. *Cryptosporidium* spp. infect a number of animals and can spread from infected animals to humans. Oocysts are infectious when passed in feces, so person-to-person transmission occurs within day-care centers and among household contacts and medical providers. As with giardiasis, waterborne transmission accounts for infections in travelers and for common-source epidemics. Oocysts are quite hardy and resist killing by routine chlorination.

Pathophysiology   Although intestinal epithelial cells harbor the parasite in an intracellular vacuole, the means by which secretory diarrhea is elicited remain uncertain. No characteristic pathologic changes are found on biopsies. The distribution of infection can be spotty within the principal site of infection, the small bowel. In some patients, cryptosporidia are found in the pharynx, stomach, and large bowel and have been recovered from the respiratory tract, although the pathogenicity of the infection for human respiratory epithelium has not been determined. Involvement of the biliary tract can cause papillary stenosis, sclerosing cholangitis, or cholecystitis.

Clinical manifestations   Asymptomatic infections can occur in both normal and immunocompromised hosts. In normal hosts, symp-

toms develop after an incubation period of about a week and consist principally of watery, nonbloody diarrhea at times with abdominal pain, nausea, anorexia, fever, or weight loss. In these hosts, the illness usually subsides after 1 to 2 weeks, whereas in immunocompromised hosts, especially those with AIDS, diarrhea can be chronic, persistent, and remarkably profuse, leading to clinically significant fluid and electrolyte depletion. Stool volumes may range from 1 to 25 L/d. Weight loss, wasting, and abdominal pain may be severe. Biliary tract involvement can manifest as midepigastric or right upper quadrant pain.

Diagnosis   Evaluation usually starts with fecal examination for the small oocysts 4 to 5 μm in diameter. While these are smaller than the fecal stages of most other parasites, experienced microscopists can recognize them. Detection is enhanced by evaluation of stools obtained on multiple days and by several staining techniques, including modified acid-fast stains. If low numbers of oocysts are being excreted, Sheather's cover-slip flotation method concentrates oocysts for examination. Cryptosporidia also can be identified by light and electron microscopy at the apical surfaces of intestinal epithelium from biopsies of small bowel and less frequently large bowel. Serologic tests are available but have as yet undefined value in diagnosing either acute infections or infections in immunocompromised patients.

Treatment and prevention   To date, no effective chemotherapeutic agents have been identified. Treatment therefore consists of supportive care with fluid and electrolyte replacement and antidiarrheal agents. Biliary tract obstruction may require papillotomy or T-tube placement. Prevention requires minimizing exposure to infectious oocysts in human or animal feces.

TRICHOMONIASIS

Although different species of trichomonads can be found in the mouth in association with periodontitis and occasionally in the gastrointestinal tract, *Trichomonas vaginalis*, one of the most prevalent protozoal parasites in the United States, is a pathogen of the genitourinary tract and a major cause of symptomatic vaginitis.

Life cycle and epidemiology   *T. vaginalis* is a pear-shaped, actively motile organism, about 10 by 7 μm in size, that replicates by binary fission and inhabits the lower genital tract in females and the urethra and prostate in males. In the United States, it accounts for about 3 million infections per year in women. While the organism can survive for a few hours in moist environments and could be acquired by direct contact, person-to-person venereal transmission accounts for virtually all cases of trichomoniasis. Its prevalence is greatest among those with multiple sexual partners and those with other sexually transmitted diseases.

Clinical manifestations   Most men are asymptomatic, although a few will experience urethritis and rarely epididymitis or prostatitis. In contrast, following an incubation period of 5 to 28 days, infection develops in women that is usually symptomatic and manifest by an often yellow-colored malodorous vaginal discharge, vulvular erythema and itching, dysuria or urinary frequency (in 30 to 50 percent), and dyspareunia. These manifestations, however, do not clearly distinguish trichomoniasis from other causes of infectious vaginitis.

Diagnosis   Detection of motile trichomonads by microscopy of wet mounts of vaginal or prostatic secretions has been the conventional means of diagnosis, and although such microscopy has the advantage of providing an immediate diagnosis, the sensitivity of detecting *T. vaginalis* is only about 50 to 60 percent in routine evaluations of vaginal secretions. Culture of the parasite is the most sensitive means of detection but is not readily available and takes 3 to 7 days. Direct immunofluorescent antibody staining is more sensitive (70 to 90 percent) than wet mount examinations. *T. vaginalis* can be recovered from the urethra of both males and females and is detectable in males following prostatic massage.

Treatment and prevention   Metronidazole is the mainstay of treatment and may be given as either a single 2-g dose or 250 mg tid for 7 days. It is important that all sexual partners be treated concurrently to prevent reinfection, especially from asymptomatic males. Metronidazole should be avoided in the first trimester of pregnancy and if possible later in pregnancy. Alternative therapies during pregnancy are not readily available, although use of 100-mg clotrimazole vaginal suppositories nightly for 2 weeks may cure some infections during pregnancy. Although reinfection often accounts for apparent treatment failures, strains of *T. vaginalis* exhibiting high-level resistance to metronidazole have been encountered. Successful treatment of these resistant infections has been achieved with metronidazole given in higher oral doses, in parenteral doses, or in concurrent oral and vaginal doses.

OTHER INTESTINAL PROTOZOA **Balantidiasis** *Balantidium coli* is a large ciliated protozoal parasite which can produce a spectrum of large intestinal disease analogous to amebiasis. The parasite is widely distributed in the world. Since the parasite infects pigs, human cases are more common where pigs are raised; in Muslim countries, rodents may be important carriers. Transmission of infective cysts can occur by person-to-person contact and by waterborne transmission, but many cases are recognized as being due to ingestion of cysts derived from porcine feces, as may occur in association with slaughtering, with use of pig feces for fertilizer, or when pig feces contaminate water supplies.

Ingested cysts liberate trophozoites which reside and replicate in the large bowel. Many patients remain asymptomatic, but some will have persisting intermittent diarrhea and a few may develop more fulminant dysentery. In those with symptoms, the pathology in the bowel both grossly and microscopically is similar to that with amebiasis, with varying degrees of mucosal invasion, focal necrosis, and ulceration. Balantidiasis, unlike amebiasis, does not spread hematogenously to other organs. The diagnosis is made by detecting usually the trophozoite stage in stool or sampled colonic tissue. Tetracycline (500 mg qid for 10 days) is effective therapy.

***Blastocystis hominis* infection** *Blastocystis hominis,* long considered a nonpathogenic yeast, is believed by some to be a protozoan capable of causing intestinal disease, although its taxonomy and inherent pathogenicity remain areas of uncertainty. Some patients found to be passing *B. hominis* in their stools will be asymptomatic, whereas others will have diarrhea and associated intestinal symptoms. Among those with symptoms, diligent evaluation can detect other potential bacterial, viral, or protozoan causes of diarrhea in some but not all patients. Because of the uncertainty of whether *B. hominis* is pathogenic, and because therapy of *Blastocystis* is neither specific nor uniformly effective, patients with prominent intestinal symptoms should be fully evaluated for other infectious etiologies for diarrhea. If diarrheal symptoms associated with *Blastocystis* are prominent, either metronidazole (750 mg tid for 10 days) or iodoquinol (650 mg tid for 20 days) can be used.

***Dientamoeba fragilis* infection** *Dientamoeba fragilis* is unique among intestinal protozoa in that it has a trophozoite, but not a cyst, stage. The means by which trophozoites survive to transmit infection are not known, but heightened prevalence of *D. fragilis* in those with pinworm infection raises the possibility that eggs or larvae of *Enterobius* may facilitate transmission of *D. fragilis*. When symptoms are present with *D. fragilis*, they are generally mild and include intermittent diarrhea, abdominal pain, and anorexia. Diagnosis is made by finding trophozoites in stool, but the lability of these forms accounts for the greater yield found when fecal samples are preserved immediately after collection. Fecal excretion rates vary so that examination of several samples obtained on alternate days increases detection. Treatment can be with iodoquinol (650 mg tid for 20 days), paromomycin (25 to 30 mg/kg per day in three doses for 7 days), or tetracycline (500 mg qid for 10 days).

Isosporiasis The coccidian parasite *Isospora belli* causes human intestinal disease. Infections are acquired by consumption of oocysts, after which the parasite invades intestinal epithelium cells and undergoes both sexual and asexual cycles of development. Oocysts excreted in stool are not immediately infectious but must undergo

further maturation. Although *I. belli* infects many animals, little is yet known about the epidemiology or prevalence of this parasite in humans. It appears to be more common in tropical and subtropical countries. Acute infections can begin abruptly with fever, abdominal pain, and watery nonbloody diarrhea and may last for weeks or months. In patients with AIDS or other immunocompromise, infections are often not self-limited but rather may resemble cryptosporidiosis with chronic, profuse watery diarrhea. Eosinophilia, not found with other enteric protozoan infections, may be present. The diagnosis is usually made by detecting in stool the large (~25 μm diameter) oocysts, which stain with modified acid-fast stains. Oocyst excretion may be low and intermittent, and if repeated stool examinations are unrevealing, sampling of duodenal contents by aspiration or a string test (Enterotest) or a small bowel biopsy often with electron microscopic examination may be necessary.

In contrast to cryptosporidiosis, isosporiasis responds to chemotherapy. Trimethoprim-sulfamethoxazole (160/800 mg qid for 10 days and then bid for 3 weeks) has been effective; for those intolerant of sulfonamides, pyrimethamine (50 to 75 mg/d) can be used. Relapses occur in those with AIDS and necessitate maintenance therapy with trimethoprim-sulfamethoxazole (160/800 mg 3 times a week) or combined sulfadoxine (500 mg) and pyrimethamine (25 mg) once weekly.

Microsporidiosis Microsporidia are obligate intracellular spore-forming protozoa known to infect many animals. Only recently have four genera of microsporidia, *Encephalitozoon*, *Pleistophora*, *Nosema*, and *Enterocytozoon*, been recognized as causes of human disease, especially in those immunocompromised with AIDS. The different microsporidia are distinguished on the basis of size, nuclear morphology, mode of division, and whether intracellular proliferating forms are sequestered within membrane-bound vacuoles or are in direct contact with the cytoplasm. Little is known about how humans become infected and whether microsporidia cause self-limited disease in normal hosts. In patients with AIDS, intestinal infections with *Enterocytozoon bieneusi* are increasingly recognized in association with chronic diarrhea. Patients with AIDS also have developed keratoconjunctivitis with a coarse punctate epithelial keratopathy due to *Encephalitozoon* spp., whereas stromal keratitis due to *Nosema* spp. has been identified in a few HIV-seronegative patients. Peritonitis and hepatitis due to *Encephalitozoon* microsporidia have occurred in patients with AIDS, and an HIV-seronegative immunocompromised patient developed myositis with a *Pleistophora* species.

Microsporidia are small gram-positive organisms with mature spores measuring 0.5 to 2 μm by 1 to 4 μm. Diagnosis of microsporidial infections within tissue often has required electron microscopy, although on light microscopy intracellular spores can be visualized with hematoxylin-eosin, Giemsa, or tissue Gram's stains. For diagnosing intestinal microsporidiosis, recently developed chromotrope-based staining enables spores to be detected in smears of feces or duodenal aspirates. Specific therapy for microsporidial infections has not been established.

Sarcosporidiosis Various *Sarcocystis* spp. of coccidian parasites are widely distributed causative agents of infections in numerous animals. These parasites have an obligatory cycle of development involving two hosts. Sexual reproduction occurs in the intestine and leads to passage of sporocysts in feces. Asexual multiplication leads to development of muscle cysts. Humans, apparently infrequently, can develop intestinal infections by ingesting muscle-stage cysts present in undercooked pork or beef. While the full spectrum of the intestinal disease is not defined, a diarrheal illness can ensue, and sporocysts are found in the stool. Alternatively, ingestion of fecally derived sporocysts can lead to development of muscle cysts found in human striated or cardiac muscle. Some patients have experienced muscle pain and swelling, but the frequency and nature of symptoms elicited by muscle involvement are not clear, and these cysts, measuring 100 to 325 μm in size, also have been found incidentally in muscle specimens. Muscle-stage infections do not lead to further spread within the infected human. Specific therapy for either intestinal or muscle-stage *Sarcocystis* infections in humans is not available.

REFERENCES

Giardiasis

ADAM RD: The biology of *Giardia* spp. Microbiol Rev 55:706, 1991

ERLANDSEN SL, MEYER EA (eds): *Giardia* and Giardiasis: Biology, Pathogenesis, and Epidemology, New York, Plenum, 1984

Cryptosporidiosis

WOLFSON JS et al: Cryptosporidiosis in immunocompetent patients. N Engl J Med 312:1278, 1985

FAYER R, UNGAR BLP: *Cryptosporidium* spp. and cryptosporidiosis. Microbiol Rev 50:458, 1986

Trichomoniasis

LOSSICK JG, KENT HL: Trichomoniasis: Trends in diagnosis and management. Am J Obstet Gynecol 165:1217, 1991

WØLNER-HANSSEN P et al: Clinical manifestations of vaginal trichomoniasis. JAMA 261:571, 1989

Other intestinal protozoa

WEBER R et al: Improved light-microscopical detection of microsporidia spores in stool and duodenal aspirates. N Engl J Med 326:161, 1992

section 18   Helminthic infections

180   TRICHINOSIS AND TISSUE NEMATODES

LEO X. LIU / PETER F. WELLER

Nematodes are elongated symmetric roundworms that constitute one of the largest phyla in the animal kingdom. Most nematode species are free-living, but some have evolved into parasites of plants and animals, including humans. Parasitic nematodes of medical significance may be broadly classified into intestinal and tissue nematodes, but such a classification system is imperfect. This chapter covers trichinosis, visceral and ocular larva migrans, cutaneous larva migrans, cerebral angiostrongyliasis, and gnathostomiasis. All are zoonotic infections caused by incidental exposures to infectious parasites; clinical symptoms are largely due to invasive larval stages that (with the exception of *Trichinella*) do not reach maturity in humans.

TRICHINOSIS   Trichinosis develops after the ingestion of infected pork or other meat of carnivores containing cysts of *Trichinella spiralis*. While most infections are mild and asymptomatic, heavy infections can cause severe enteritis, periorbital edema, myositis, and (in rare cases) death.

Life cycle and epidemiology   *T. spiralis* is found worldwide in a great variety of carnivorous and omnivorous animals. After the consumption of trichinous meat, encysted larvae are liberated by digestive acid and pepsin. The larvae invade the small bowel mucosa and mature rapidly into adult worms. After about 1 week, female worms release newborn larvae that migrate via the circulation to striated muscle cells. The larvae then encyst by inducing a radical transformation of the muscle cell architecture. Although host immune responses may help to expel the adult worms, they have little effect on the encysted larvae.

Most human trichinosis is caused by the ingestion of infected pork products and thus can occur in almost any location where domestic or wild swine meat is eaten. Human trichinosis also may be acquired from the meat of other animals, including dog meat in parts of Asia and Africa, horse meat in Italy and France, and bear and walrus meat in northern regions. Although cattle (being herbivores) are not natural hosts of *Trichinella*, beef has been implicated in outbreaks when contaminated or adulterated with trichinous pork. Laws that prohibit the feeding of uncooked garbage to pigs have greatly reduced the transmission of the disease in the United States. About 50 to 100 cases of trichinosis are reported annually in the United States, but most mild cases probably remain undiagnosed. Recent American outbreaks have been attributable to undercooked ethnic pork dishes, homemade and commercial sausage, wild boar meat, and walrus meat.

Pathogenesis and clinical features   Clinical symptoms of trichinosis arise from the successive phases of parasite enteric invasion, larval migration, and muscle encystment. Most light infections (<10 larvae per gram of muscle) are asymptomatic, whereas heavy infections (which can involve >50 larvae per gram of muscle) can be life-threatening. Parasites invading the gut in the first week after infection occasionally provoke diarrhea in heavy infections. Abdominal pain, constipation, nausea, or vomiting also may be prominent. Prolonged and fulminant diarrhea has been noted with arctic trichinosis, probably reflecting a response to repeated infection.

Symptoms due to larval migration and muscle invasion begin to appear in the second week after infection. The migrating *Trichinella* larvae provoke a marked local and systemic hypersensitivity reaction with fever and hypereosinophilia. Periorbital and facial edema is common, as are hemorrhages in the subconjunctivae, retina, and nail beds ("splinter" hemorrhages). A maculopapular rash, headache, cough, dyspnea, or dysphagia is sometimes present. Myocarditis with tachyarrhythmias or heart failure—and, less commonly, encephalitis or pneumonitis—may develop and account for most fatalities in trichinosis.

Upon onset of larval encystment in muscle about 2 to 3 weeks after infection, symptoms of myositis with myalgias, muscle edema, and weakness develop, usually overlapping with the inflammatory reactions to migrating larvae. The most commonly involved muscle groups include the extraocular muscles, jaw, neck, biceps, lower back, and diaphragm. Peaking about 3 weeks after infection, symptoms subside only gradually during a prolonged convalescence.

Laboratory findings and diagnosis   Blood eosinophila develops in more than 90 percent of patients with symptomatic trichinosis and may peak at a level of greater than 50 percent between 2 and 4 weeks after infection. Serum levels of IgE and muscle enzymes, including creatine phosphokinase, lactate dehydrogenase, and aspartate aminotransferase, are elevated in most symptomatic patients. Patients should be thoroughly questioned regarding their consumption of pork and wild animal meat and whether other individuals became ill after eating a common meat. A presumptive clinical diagnosis can be based on fevers, eosinophilia, periorbital edema, and myalgias after a suspect meal. A rise in titers of parasite-specific antibody (assayed in the bentonite flocculation test), which is usually delayed until after the third week of infection, confirms the diagnosis. Alternatively, a definitive diagnosis requires surgical biopsy of at least 1 g of involved muscle, with the highest yields near tendinous insertions. The fresh muscle tissue should be compressed between glass slides and examined microscopically because routine histopathologic sectioning alone may miss larvae.

Treatment Current anthelmintic drugs are ineffective against *Trichinella* larvae in muscle. Fortunately, most lightly infected patients recover uneventfully with bed rest, antipyretics, and analgesics. Glucocorticoids like prednisone (1 mg/kg daily for 5 days) are beneficial for severe myositis and myocarditis. Mebendazole, like thiabendazole, appears to be active against enteric stages of the parasite, but its efficacy against encysted larvae has not been conclusively demonstrated.

Prevention Larvae may be killed by cooking pork until it is no longer pink or by freezing at −15°C for 3 weeks. However, arctic strains (*T. spiralis* var. *nativa*) in walrus or bear meat are more resistant and may remain viable despite freezing.

VISCERAL AND OCULAR LARVA MIGRANS Visceral larva migrans is a syndrome caused by nematodes that are normally parasitic for other host species. In humans, the nematode larvae do not typically develop into adult worms but instead migrate through host tissues and elicit eosinophilic inflammation. The most common form of visceral larva migrans is toxocariasis due to larvae of the canine ascarid *Toxocara canis* and less commonly the feline ascarid *T. cati*. Rare cases with eosinophilic meningoencephalitis have been caused by the raccoon ascarid *Baylisascaris procyonis*.

Life cycle and epidemiology The canine roundworm *T. canis* is distributed among dogs worldwide. Ingestion of infective eggs by dogs is followed by liberation of *Toxocara* larvae. Some larvae pass through tissues and return to the intestinal tract to develop into adult worms, which produce eggs released in the feces. The progress of other larvae is arrested. These organisms become dormant in canine tissues; they resume migration in pregnant bitches and infect puppies prenatally (via transplacental transmission) and after birth (via suckling). As a result, most puppies and lactating bitches shed *T. canis* eggs in their stools. Humans acquire toxocariasis mainly by eating soil contaminated by puppy feces containing infective eggs. Visceral larva migrans is most common among children with the habit of eating dirt, but most toxocaral infections are subclinical. Reported rates of *Toxocara* seropositivity range from 2 percent in an unselected American population to greater than 20 percent among kindergarten children in the United States and England.

Pathogenesis and clinical features Clinical disease most commonly afflicts preschool children. After humans ingest *Toxocara* eggs, the larvae hatch and penetrate the intestinal mucosa to be carried by the circulation to a wide variety of organs and tissues. The larvae invade the liver, lungs, central nervous system, and other sites, releasing toxic products and provoking intense local eosinophilic granulomatous responses. The degree of clinical illness depends on larval number and tissue distribution, reinfection, and host immune responses. Most light infections are asymptomatic and may be manifest only by blood eosinophilia. Characteristic symptoms of visceral larva migrans include fever, malaise, anorexia and weight loss, cough, wheezing, and rashes. Hepatosplenomegaly is common. These features are often accompanied by extraordinary peripheral eosinophilia that may approach 90 percent. Uncommonly, seizures or behavioral disorders may occur. The rare deaths in this disease are due to severe neurologic, pneumonic, or myocardial involvement.

Diagnosis and treatment In addition to prominent eosinophilia, leukocytosis and hypergammaglobulinemia are usually evident. Transient pulmonary infiltrates on chest x-ray are found in about half of patients with symptoms of pneumonitis. The clinical diagnosis can be confirmed by ELISA for toxocaral antibodies. Stool examination, while important in the evaluation of unexplained eosinophilia, is worthless for toxocariasis, since the larvae do not develop into egg-producing adults in humans. The vast majority of infections are self-limited and resolve without specific therapy. In patients with severe myocardial, central nervous system, or pulmonary involvement, glucocorticoids may be employed to reduce inflammatory complications. Available anthelmintic drugs, including diethylcarbamazine and thiabendazole, have not been conclusively shown to alter the course of larva migrans. Control measures include prohibiting dog excreta in public parks and playgrounds, deworming dogs, and preventing pica in children.

The ocular form of the larva migrans syndrome occurs when *Toxocara* larvae invade the eye. An eosinophilic granulomatous mass, most commonly in the posterior pole of the retina, develops around the entrapped larva. The retinal lesion can mimic retinoblastoma in appearance, and mistaken diagnosis of the latter condition can lead to unnecessary enucleation. The spectrum of eye involvement also includes endophthalmitis, uveitis, and chorioretinitis. Unilateral visual disturbances, strabismus, and eye pain are the most common presenting symptoms. In contrast to visceral larva migrans, ocular toxocariasis usually develops in older children or young adults with no history of pica; these patients seldom have eosinophilia or visceral manifestations. Treatment is unsatisfactory, and the role of glucocorticoids or anthelmintic drugs in management is controversial.

CUTANEOUS LARVA MIGRANS Cutaneous larva migrans ("creeping eruption") is a serpiginous skin eruption caused by burrowing larvae of animal hookworms, usually the dog and cat hookworm *Ancylostoma braziliense*. The larvae hatch from eggs passed in dog and cat feces and mature in the soil. Humans become infected after skin contact with soil in areas frequented by dogs and cats, such as underneath house porches or scrub vegetation. Cutaneous larva migrans is more prevalent among children and in warm, humid climates, including the southeastern United States.

After larvae penetrate the skin, erythematous lesions form along the tortuous tracts of larvae migrating through the dermal-epidermal junction, advancing several centimeters in a day. These intensely pruritic lesions may occur anywhere on the body and can be numerous if the patient has lain on the ground. Vesicles and bullae may form later. The animal hookworm larvae do not mature in humans and left untreated will die out after several weeks, with resolution of skin lesions. The diagnosis is made readily on clinical grounds, and a skin biopsy only rarely yields diagnostic parasite material. Symptoms can be alleviated by thiabendazole administered orally (25 mg/kg bid) or topically (10% aqueous or petroleum jelly suspension) for 2 to 5 days.

***ANGIOSTRONGYLUS CANTONENSIS* INFECTION** *Angiostrongylus cantonensis,* the rat lungworm, is the most common cause of human eosinophilic meningitis.

Life cycle and epidemiology This infection occurs principally in Southeast Asia and the Pacific Basin. *A. cantonensis* larvae produced by adult worms in the rat lung migrate to the gastrointestinal tract and are expelled with the feces. They develop into infective larvae within land snails and slugs. Humans acquire the infection by ingesting raw infected mollusks, vegetables contaminated by mollusk slime, or crabs, freshwater shrimp, and certain marine fish that have themselves eaten infected mollusks. The larvae then migrate to the brain.

Pathogenesis and clinical features The parasites eventually die in the central nervous system, but not before initiating pathologic consequences which in heavy infections can result in permanent neurologic sequelae or death. Migrating larvae cause proteolytic damage and marked local eosinophilic inflammation and hemorrhage, with subsequent necrosis and granuloma formation around dying worms. Clinical symptoms develop between 2 and 35 days after ingestion of larvae. Patients usually present with an insidious or abrupt excruciating frontal, occipital, or bitemporal headache. Neck stiffness, nausea and vomiting, and paresthesias are also common. Fever is usually absent. Cranial and extraocular nerve palsies, seizures, paralysis, and lethargy are uncommon.

Laboratory findings and treatment Examination of the cerebrospinal fluid is mandatory in suspected cases and usually reveals an elevated opening pressure, a white blood cell count of 150 to 2000 cells per microliter, and an eosinophilic pleocytosis of >20 percent. The protein concentration is usually elevated and the glucose level normal. The motile larvae of *A. cantonensis* are only rarely seen in the cerebrospinal fluid. Peripheral blood eosinophilia may be mild.

Angiostrongylus eggs. In nonsurgical cases, the diagnosis rests solely on clinical grounds because larvae and eggs cannot be detected in the stool. Medical therapy for abdominal angiostrongyliasis is unsatisfactory. Careful observation and surgical resection for severe symptoms are the mainstays of treatment.

REFERENCES

Ash LR, Orihel TC: *Atlas of Human Parasitology,* 3d ed. Chicago, ASCP Press, 1990

Cooper ES, Bundy DAP: Trichuris is not trivial. Parasitol Today 4:301, 1988

Cross JH: Intestinal capillariasis. Clin Microbiol Rev 5:120, 1992

Genta RM et al: Strongyloidiasis in US veterans of the Vietnam and other wars. JAMA 258:49, 1987

Khuroo MS et al: Hepatobiliary and pancreatic ascariasis in India. Lancet 335:1503, 1990

Leighton PM, MacSween HM: *Strongyloides stercoralis:* The cause of an urticarial-like eruption of 65 years' duration. Arch Intern Med 150:1747, 1990

Longworth DL, Weller PF: Hyperinfection syndrome with strongyloidiasis, in *Current Clinical Topics in Infectious Diseases,* vol 7, JS Remington, MN Swartz (eds). New York, McGraw-Hill, 1986, p 1

Ochoa B: Surgical complications of ascariasis. World J Surg 15:222, 1991

Schad GA, Warren KS (eds): *Hookworm Disease: Current Status and New Directions.* London, Taylor and Francis, 1990

Schantz PM: The dangers of eating raw fish (editorial). N Engl J Med 320:1143, 1989

182   FILARIASIS AND RELATED INFECTIONS (LOIASIS, ONCHOCERCIASIS, AND DRACUNCULIASIS)

THOMAS B. NUTMAN / PETER F. WELLER

Filarial worms are nematodes that dwell in the subcutaneous tissues and the lymphatics. Eight filarial species infect humans (Table 182-1); of these, four—*Wuchereria bancrofti, Brugia malayi, Onchocerca volvulus,* and *Loa loa*—are responsible for most serious filarial infections. Filarial parasites, which infect an estimated 140 million persons worldwide, are transmitted by specific species of mosquitoes or other arthropods and have a complex life cycle that includes infective larval stages that are carried by insects and adult worms that reside in either lymphatic or subcutaneous tissues of humans. The offspring of adults are microfilariae, which, depending on their species, are 200 to 250 μm long and 5 to 7 μm wide, may or may not be enveloped in a loose sheath, and either circulate in the blood or migrate through the skin (see Table 182-1). To complete the life cycle, microfilariae are ingested by the arthropod vector and develop over 1 to 2 weeks into new infective larvae. Adult worms live many years, whereas microfilariae survive from 3 to 36 months.

Usually, infection is only established with repeated and prolonged exposures to infective larvae. Since the clinical manifestations of filarial diseases develop relatively slowly, these infections should be considered chronic diseases with possible long-term debilitating effects. In terms of the nature, severity, and timing of clinical manifestations, patients with filariasis who are native to endemic areas and have lifelong exposures may differ significantly from those who are travelers or who have recently moved to these same areas. Characteristically, the disease is more acute and intense in newly exposed individuals than in natives of endemic areas.

LYMPHATIC FILARIASIS

Lymphatic filariasis is caused by *W. bancrofti, B. malayi,* or *B. timori.* The threadlike adult parasites reside in either lymphatic channels or lymph nodes, where they may remain viable for more than two decades.

EPIDEMIOLOGY   *W. bancrofti,* the most widely distributed human filarial parasite, affects an estimated 80 million people and is found throughout the tropics and subtropics, including Asia and the Pacific Islands, Africa, areas of South America, and the Caribbean basin. Humans are the only definitive host for the parasite. Nocturnally periodic forms of microfilariae are scarce in peripheral blood by day and increase at night, whereas with subperiodic forms microfilariae are present in peripheral blood at all times and reach maximal levels in the afternoon. Generally, the subperiodic form is found only in the Pacific Islands; elsewhere, *W. bancrofti* is nocturnally periodic. Natural vectors are *Culex fatigans* mosquitoes in urban settings and anopheline or aedean mosquitoes in rural areas.

Brugian filariasis due to *B. malayi* occurs primarily in China, India, Indonesia, Korea, Japan, Malaysia, and the Philippines. *B. malayi* also has two forms distinguished by the periodicity of microfilaremia. The more common nocturnal form is transmitted in areas of coastal rice fields, while the subperiodic form is found in forests. *B. malayi* naturally infects cats as well as human hosts. *B. timori* exists only on two islands in Indonesia.

TABLE 182-1   Characteristics of the filariae

Organism	Periodicity	Distribution	Vector	Location of adult	Microfilarial location	Sheath
Wuchereria bancrofti	Nocturnal	Cosmopolitan Mainly India China, Indonesia	*Culex* (mosquitoes) *Anopheles* (mosquitoes) *Aedes* (mosquitoes)	Lymphatic	Blood	+
	Subperiodic	Eastern Pacific	*Aedes* (mosquitoes)	Lymphatic	Blood	+
Brugia malayi	Nocturnal	Southeast Asia, Indonesia, India	*Mansonia, Anopheles* (mosquitoes)	Lymphatic	Blood	+
	Subperiodic	Indonesia, Southeast Asia	*Coquilletidia* (mosquitoes) Mansonia (mosquitoes)	Lymphatic	Blood	+
Brugia timori	Nocturnal	Indonesia	*Anopheles* (mosquitoes)	Lymphatic	Blood	+
Loa loa	Diurnal	West and Central Africa	*Chrysops* (deerflies)	Subcutaneous	Blood	+
Mansonella ozzardi	None	South and Central America Carribean	*Culicoides* (midges) *Simulium* (blackflies)	Undetermined	Blood	−
Mansonella perstans	None	South and Central America, Africa	*Culicoides* (midges)	Body cavities, mesentery, perirenal	Blood	−
Mansonella streptocerca	None	West and Central Africa	*Culicoides* (midges)	Subcutaneous	Skin	−
Onchocerca volvulus	None	South and Central America, Africa	*Simulium* (blackflies)	Subcutaneous	Skin, eye	−

PATHOLOGY The principal pathologic changes result from inflammatory damage to the lymphatics caused by adult worm and not by microfilariae. Adult worms live in afferent lymphatics or sinuses of lymph nodes and cause lymphatic dilatation and thickening of the vessel walls. Plasma cells, eosinophils, and macrophages infiltrate in and around the infected vessels and, with endothelial and connective tissue proliferation, lead to tortuosity of the lymphatics and damaged or incompetent lymph valves. Lymphedema and chronic stasis changes with hard or brawny edema develop in the overlying skin. These consequences of filariasis are not due to simple lymphatic obstruction by resident adult worms but rather to the immune response of the host to the parasite. These immune responses are believed to cause the granulomatous and proliferative processes that precede lymphatic obstruction. It is thought that as long as the worm remains viable, the vessel remains patent and that death of the worm leads to an enhanced granulomatous reaction and fibrosis. Lymphatic obstruction results, and despite collateralization of the lymphatics, lymphatic function is compromised.

CLINICAL FEATURES The common manifestations of lymphatic filariasis are asymptomatic microfilaremia, filarial fevers, and lymphatic obstruction. Asymptomatic microfilaremia is found in the majority of infected individuals who are clinically well. Filarial fevers are acute episodes in which high fever is often accompanied by shaking chills, lymphatic inflammation (lymphangitis and lymphadenitis), and transient local edema. Episodes can recur as frequently as 10 times per year and usually abate spontaneously after 7 to 10 days. The lymphangitis characteristically develops in a retrograde or descending fashion, extending peripherally from the draining node where the parasite presumably resides. Regional lymph nodes are often enlarged, and the entire lymphatic channel can become indurated and inflamed. Concomitant local thrombophlebitis can develop. In brugian filariasis, a local abscess may form over a lymphatic tract and rupture. Lymphadenitis and lymphangitis occur in both upper and lower extremities with bancroftian and brugian filariasis, but genital lymphatic involvement develops almost exclusively with *W. bancrofti* infection. Genital involvement can be manifested by funiculitis, epididymitis, and scrotal pain and tenderness.

If lymphatic damage progresses into lymphatic obstruction, the permanent changes associated with elephantiasis may follow. Brawny edema follows early pitting edema. With thickening of subcutaneous tissues, hyperkeratosis, fissuring of the skin, and hyperplastic changes develop. Bacterial superinfection of the poorly vascularized tissues is common. In bancroftian filariasis, scrotal lymphedema or hydrocele formation can occur. If the retroperitoneal lymphatics become obstructed, increased pressure leads to the rupture of renal lymphatics and the development of chyluria, which is usually intermittent and most prominent in the morning.

The clinical manifestations of filarial infections in travelers or transmigrants who have recently entered an endemic region are distinctive. Given a sufficient number of bites by infected vectors, usually over a 3- to 6-month period, recently exposed patients can develop acute lymphatic or scrotal inflammation with or without urticaria and localized angioedema. Lymphadenitis of epitrochlear, axillary, femoral, or inguinal lymph nodes is often followed by retrogradely evolving lymphangitis. Acute attacks are short-lived and, in contrast to filarial fevers in patients native to endemic areas, are usually not accompanied by fever. With prolonged exposures to infected mosquitoes, these attacks, if untreated, become more severe and lead to permanent lymphatic inflammation and obstruction.

DIAGNOSIS The definitive diagnosis can be made only by detection of the parasites and hence can be problematic. Adult worms localized in lymphatic vessels or nodes are largely inaccessible, and biopsies usually are not revealing and therefore not indicated. Microfilariae can be found in blood, in hydrocele fluid, or (occasionally) in other body fluids. Such fluids can be examined microscopically—either directly or with greater sensitivity after concentration of the parasites by filtration of fluids through a polycarbonate cylindrical pore filter (pore size 3 μm) or by centrifugation of fluid fixed in 2% formalin (Knott's concentration technique). Many infected individuals do not have microfilaremia, and definitive diagnosis in such patients can be difficult; in some instances, the diagnosis must be made on clinical grounds. In acute episodes, lymphatic filariasis must be distinguished from thrombophlebitis, infection, and trauma. Retrogradely evolving lymphangitis is a characteristic feature that helps distinguish filarial lymphangitis from typically ascending bacterial lymphangitis. Chronic filarial lymphedema must be distinguished from the lymphedema of malignancy, postoperative scarring, trauma, chronic edematous states, and congenital lymphatic-system abnormalities. Eosinophilia and elevations of serum IgE and antifilarial antibody concentrations support the diagnosis of lymphatic filariasis. There is, however, extensive cross-reactivity between filarial antigens and antigens of other helminths, including the common intestinal roundworms; thus interpretations of serologic findings can be difficult. In addition, residents of endemic areas can become sensitized to filarial antigens through exposure to infected mosquitoes without having patent filarial infections. Thus most serologic and skin tests are of less diagnostic value in individuals native to endemic areas than in travelers or short-term visitors.

TREATMENT Treatment for lymphatic filariasis is currently limited to diethylcarbamazine (DEC) given at 6 mg/kg per day in either single or divided doses for 2 to 3 weeks. This regimen clears microfilariae from the blood and has a limited but definite effect on adult parasites. If at least some adult parasites survive, as is often the case, microfilaremia along with clinical symptoms can recur within months after therapy. There is some evidence that several courses of DEC or chronic administration of low-dose DEC may effect a cure. Ivermectin, a drug active in onchocerciasis, has been used in trials of therapy for lymphatic filariasis; in a single dose (not approved by the FDA), it appears to be as effective as DEC at clearing microfilariae. Side effects of DEC (or ivermectin) treatment include fever, chills, arthralgia, headaches, nausea, and vomiting. Both the development and the severity of these reactions, which may reflect an acute reaction to antigens released by dying parasites, are related directly to the number of microfilariae circulating in the blood. To avoid these side effects, one can either initiate treatment with a small dose of DEC and increase to a full dose over a few days or premedicate the patient with glucocorticoids.

Treatment of chronic lymphatic obstruction is difficult but may be helpful. Elevation of the infected limb, use of elastic stockings, and local foot care eliminate some of the associated symptoms. Surgical decompression with a nodovenous shunt may provide relief for severely affected limbs. Hydroceles can be drained or managed surgically. The management of filarial chyluria is unsatisfactory; neither surgical intervention nor sclerosis of infected lymphatics is effective.

PREVENTION Avoidance of mosquito bites usually is not feasible for residents of endemic areas, but visitors should use insect repellent and mosquito nets. DEC can kill developing filarial larvae and is useful as a prophylactic agent, although the optimal regimen for prophylaxis has not been ascertained. Mass treatment with DEC may reduce community levels of microfilariae so as to interrupt vector-borne transmission among humans.

TROPICAL PULMONARY EOSINOPHILIA

Tropical pulmonary eosinophilia (TPE) is a distinct syndrome that develops in some individuals infected with lymphatic filarial species. This syndrome affects males and females at a ratio of 4:1, often during the third decade of life. The majority of cases have been reported from India, Pakistan, Sri Lanka, Brazil, and Southeast Asia.

CLINICAL FEATURES The main features include a history of residence in filarial endemic regions, paroxysmal cough and wheezing that are usually nocturnal (and probably related to the nocturnal periodicity of microfilariae), weight loss, low-grade fever, adenopathy, and pronounced blood eosinophilia (>3000 per microliter). Chest x-rays may be normal but generally show increased bronchovascular markings; diffuse miliary lesions or mottled opacities may be present in the middle and lower lung fields. Tests of pulmonary function show restrictive abnormalities in half and obstructive defects in most. Total serum IgE levels (10,000 to 100,000 ng/mL) and antifilarial antibody titers are characteristically elevated.

PATHOLOGY In TPE there is rapid immune-mediated clearance of microfilariae from the bloodstream into the lungs, and the clinical symptoms result from allergic and inflammatory reactions elicited by the cleared parasites. In some subjects, microfilarial trapping in other reticuloendothelial organs can cause hepatomegaly, splenomegaly, or lymphadenopathy. A prominent, eosinophil-enriched, intraalveolar infiltrate is often present. In the absence of successful treatment, interstitial fibrosis can lead to progressive pulmonary damage.

DIFFERENTIAL DIAGNOSIS TPE must be distinguished from asthma, Löffler's syndrome, allergic bronchopulmonary aspergillosis, allergic granulomatosis with angiitis (Churg-Strauss syndrome), the systemic vasculitides (most notably periarteritis nodosa and Wegener's granulomatosis), chronic eosinophilic pneumonia, and the idiopathic hypereosinophilic syndrome. In addition to a geographic history of filarial exposure, useful features for distinguishing TPE include wheezing that is solely nocturnal, very high levels of antifilarial antibodies, and a rapid initial response to treatment with DEC.

TREATMENT DEC is used at a dosage of 4 to 6 mg/kg of body weight per day for 14 days. Symptoms usually resolve within 3 to 7 days after initiating therapy. Relapse, which occurs in approximately 12 to 25 percent of individuals (sometimes after an interval of years), requires retreatment.

ONCHOCERCIASIS

Onchocerciasis ("river blindness") is caused by the filarial nematode *Onchocerca volvulus*, which infects an estimated 13 million individuals, primarily in equatorial Africa and Latin America. Onchocerciasis is the second leading cause of infectious blindness worldwide.

ETIOLOGY AND EPIDEMIOLOGY Infection in humans begins with the deposition of infective larvae onto the skin by the bite of an infected blackfly. Infected larvae develop into adults that are typically found in subcutaneous nodules. About 7 months to 3 years after infection, the gravid female releases microfilariae that migrate out of the nodule and throughout the tissues, concentrating in the dermis. Infection is transmitted to other persons when a female fly ingests microfilariae from the host's skin and these microfilariae then develop into infective larvae. Adult *O. volvulus* females and males are about 40 to 60 cm and 3 to 6 cm in length, respectively. The life span of adults can be up to 18 years, with an average of approximately 9 years. Because the blackfly vector breeds along free-flowing rivers and streams (particularly in rapids) and generally restricts its flight to within several kilometers from these breeding sites, both biting and disease transmission are most intense at these locations. The majority of individuals infected with *O. volvulus* are in the equatorial region of Africa extending from the Atlantic coast to the Red Sea. About 70,000 persons are infected in Guatemala and Mexico, with smaller foci in Venezuela, Colombia, Brazil, Ecuador, Yemen, and Saudi Arabia.

PATHOLOGY Onchocerciasis affects primarily the skin, eyes, and lymph nodes. In contrast to lymphatic filariasis, the damage in onchocerciasis is elicited by microfilariae and not by adults. In the skin, there are mild but chronic inflammatory changes that can eventuate in loss of elastic fibers, atrophy, and fibrosis. The subcutaneous nodules, or onchocercomata, consist primarily of fibrous tissues surrounding the adult worm, often with a peripheral ring of inflammatory cells. In the eye, neovascularization and corneal scarring lead to corneal opacities and blindness. Inflammation in the anterior and posterior chambers frequently can result in anterior uveitis, chorioretinitis, and optic atrophy. Although punctate opacities are due to an inflammatory reaction surrounding dead or dying microfilariae, the pathogenesis of most manifestations of onchocerciasis is still unclear.

CLINICAL FEATURES Skin Pruritus, the most frequent manifestation of onchocercal dermatitis, can be incapacitating even when skin microfilariae are rare. Long-term infection results in exaggerated and premature wrinkling of the skin, loss of elastic fibers, and epidermal atrophy that can lead to loose, redundant skin and hypo- or hyperpigmentation. A localized eczematoid dermatitis can cause hyperkeratosis, scaling, and pigmentary changes. Such lesions are often seen in the lower extremities but can be distributed more extensively.

Onchocercomata These subcutaneous nodules, which can be palpable or visible, contain the adult worm. In Africa they are common over the coccyx and sacrum, the trochanter of the femur, the lateral anterior crest, and other bony prominences. In Latin America, the subcutaneous nodules tend to be found preferentially in the upper part of the body, particularly the head, neck, and shoulders. Nodules vary in size and characteristically are firm and not tender. It has been estimated that for every palpable nodule there are four deeper, nonpalpable ones.

Ocular tissue Visual impairment is the most serious complication of onchocerciasis and usually affects only those persons with moderate or heavy infections. Lesions may be present in all parts of the eye. The most common early finding is conjunctivitis with photophobia. In the cornea, punctate keratitis—acute inflammatory reactions surrounding dying microfilariae manifested as "snowflake" opacities—is frequent in younger age groups and resolves without apparent complications. Sclerosing keratitis occurs in approximately 5 percent of persons infected with savannah strains and 1 percent of those infected with forest strains and is the leading cause of onchocercal blindness in Africa. Anterior uveitis and iridocyclitis develop in about 5 percent of infected persons in Africa. In Latin America, complications of the anterior uveal tract (pupillary deformity) may cause secondary glaucoma. Characteristic chorioretinal lesions develop as a result of atrophy and hyperpigmentation of the retinal pigment epithelium and the choriopapillaris. Constriction of the visual field and frank optic atrophy may occur.

Lymph nodes Mild to moderate lymphadenopathy is frequent, particularly in the inguinal and femoral areas, where enlargement of nodes may be gravitationally dependent ("hanging groin") and may predispose to inguinal and femoral hernias.

Systemic manifestations Some heavily infected individuals develop cachexia with loss of adipose tissue and muscle mass. In adults who become blind, there is a three- to fourfold increase in the mortality rate.

DIAGNOSIS Definitive diagnosis depends on the detection of an adult worm in an excised nodule or, more commonly, microfilariae in a skin snip. Skin snips are most readily obtained with a corneal-scleral punch, which collects a blood-free skin biopsy sample extending just below the epidermis. The biopsy tissue is incubated in tissue culture medium or in saline on a glass slide or flat-bottomed microtiter plate. After incubation for 2 to 4 h (or occasionally overnight in light infections), microfilariae emergent from the skin can be seen under a microscope.

TREATMENT The major goals of therapy are to prevent irreversible lesions and alleviate symptoms. Surgical excision is recommended when nodules are located on the head because of the proximity of microfilaria-producing adult worms to the eye, but chemotherapy is the mainstay of management. Ivermectin, a semisynthetic macrocyclic lactone active against microfilariae, is the first-line agent for the treatment of onchocerciasis. It is given orally in a single dose of 150 μg/kg, either yearly or semiannually. After treatment, most individuals have few or no reactions. Pruritus, cutaneous edema, and/or maculopapular rash occurs in approximately 1 to 10 percent of treated individuals. Contraindications to treatment include pregnancy, breast feeding, central nervous system disorders that may increase the penetration of ivermectin into the CNS (e.g., meningitis), and an age of less than 5 years. Although ivermectin treatment results in a marked drop in microfilarial density, its effect may last only 6 months. Suramin, a potent but potentially toxic macrofilaricidal agent, is recommended only if total cure is necessary. First, ivermectin is given to reduce the microfilarial load; then suramin is administered intravenously after a test dose. Weekly doses are started at 200 mg and increased by 200-mg increments until a total dose of 60 to 70 mg/kg is reached. Because of the drug's nephrotoxicity, renal function must be monitored closely. After suramin therapy, an additional course of ivermectin is customarily given to eliminate any remaining microfilariae.

PREVENTION Vector control has been beneficial in highly endemic areas with breeding sites that are vulnerable to insecticide spraying, but most endemic areas for onchocerciasis are not suited for this type of control. While persons working in fly-infested areas can minimize the number of bites they sustain by wearing protective garments, this approach is not feasible for the large majority of individuals in endemic foci. No drug has been shown to prevent infection with *O. volvulus*.

LOIASIS

ETIOLOGY AND EPIDEMIOLOGY Loiasis (the African eye worm) is caused by *Loa loa*, which is present in the rain forests of West and Central Africa. Adult parasites (females, 50 to 70 mm long and 0.5 mm wide; males, 25 to 35 mm long and 0.25 mm wide) live in subcutaneous tissues; microfilariae circulate in the blood with a diurnal periodicity that peaks between 12:00 noon and 2:00 P.M.

CLINICAL FEATURES Manifestations in natives of endemic areas may differ from those in temporary residents or visitors. Among the indigenous population, loiasis is often an asymptomatic infection with microfilaremia. Infection may be recognized only after subconjunctival migration of an adult worm (the so-called eye worm) or manifested as episodic Calabar swellings, evanescent localized areas of angioedema and erythema on the extremities and less frequently elsewhere. Nephropathy, encephalopathy, and cardiomyopathy are rare. In nonresidents, allergic symptoms predominate. The episodes of Calabar swelling tend to be more frequent and debilitating; microfilaremia is rare, and eosinophilia and increased levels of antifilarial antibodies are characteristic.

PATHOLOGY The pathogenesis of the manifestations is poorly understood. Calabar swellings are thought to result from a hypersensitivity reaction to the adult worm.

DIAGNOSIS Definitive diagnosis requires detection of microfilariae in the peripheral blood or isolation of the adult worm from the eye or from a subcutaneous biopsy at a site of swelling developing after treatment. In practice, the diagnosis must often be based on a characteristic history and clinical presentation, blood eosinophilia, and elevated levels of antifilarial antibodies, particularly in travelers to the endemic region, who are usually a microfilaremic. Other clinical findings in the latter individuals include hypergammaglobulinemia, elevated levels of serum IgE, and elevated leukocyte and eosinophil counts.

TREATMENT AND PREVENTION DEC (8 to 10 mg/kg per day for 21 days) is effective against both the adult and the microfilarial forms of *L. loa*, but multiple courses are frequently necessary before disease resolves completely. In cases of heavy microfilaremia, allergic or other inflammatory reactions can occur during treatment, including CNS involvement with coma and encephalitis. Heavy infections are treated initially with low doses of DEC (0.5 mg/kg per day) and glucocorticoids (40 to 60 mg prednisone per day). If there are no adverse effects from the antifilarial treatment, prednisone can be rapidly tapered and the dose of DEC gradually increased to 4 to 8 mg/kg per day.

STREPTOCERCIASIS

Mansonella streptocerca, found mainly in the tropical forest belt of Africa from Ghana to Zaire, is transmitted by biting midges. The major clinical manifestations involve the skin and include pruritus, papular rashes, and pigmentation changes. Many infected individuals have inguinal adenopathy, although the majority are asymptomatic. The diagnosis is made by detection of the characteristic microfilariae in skin snips. DEC (6 mg/kg per day in divided doses for 14 to 21 days) is effective in killing both microfilariae and adults. As in onchocerciasis, urticaria, arthralgias, myalgias, headaches, and abdominal discomfort may accompany treatment.

MANSONELLA PERSTANS INFECTION

Mansonella perstans, distributed across the center of Africa and in northeastern South America, is transmitted by midges. Adult worms reside in serous cavities—pericardial, pleural, and peritoneal—as well as in the mesentery and the perirenal and retroperitoneal tissues. Microfilariae circulate in the blood without periodicity. The clinical and pathologic features are poorly defined. Most patients appear to be asymptomatic, but manifestations may include transient angioedema and pruritus of the arms, face, or other parts of the body (analogous to Calabar swellings of loiasis), fever, headache, arthralgias, and right upper quadrant pain. Occasionally, pericarditis and hepatitis occur. The diagnosis is based on the demonstration of microfilariae in blood or serosal effusions. Perstans filariasis is often associated with peripheral blood eosinophilia and antifilarial antibody elevations. Although DEC (8 to 10 mg/kg per day for 21 days) is the standard therapy, there is little evidence that it is efficacious. If cure is obtained, symptoms and eosinophilia disappear; multiple courses of therapy are usually required. Mebendazole (100 mg twice daily for 30 days) also has been reported to be effective.

MANSONELLA OZZARDI INFECTION

The distribution of *Mansonella ozzardi* is restricted to Central and South America and certain Caribbean islands. Adult worms are rarely recovered from humans. Microfilariae circulate in the blood without periodicity. Although many consider this organism to be nonpathogenic, headache, articular pain, fever, pulmonary symptoms, adenopathy, hepatomegaly, pruritus, and eosinophilia have been ascribed to *M. ozzardi* infection. Diagnosis is made by the detection of microfilariae in peripheral blood. No drug is proven to be effective; ivermectin was effective in a single case report.

DRACUNCULIASIS (GUINEA WORM INFECTION)

ETIOLOGY AND EPIDEMIOLOGY Dracunculiasis, caused by *Dracunculus medinensis*, affects approximately 5 million people in the Middle East, Africa, India, and Pakistan. Humans acquire this infection when they ingest water containing infective larvae derived from the *Cyclops*, a crustacean that is the intermediate host. Larvae penetrate the stomach or intestinal wall, mate, and mature. The adult male probably dies; the female *Dracunculus* develops over a year and migrates to subcutaneous tissues, usually in the lower extremity. As the thin female *Dracunculus*, ranging in length from 300 cm to 1 m, approaches the skin, a blister forms that, over days, breaks down and forms an ulcer. When the blister opens, large numbers of motile, rhabditiform larvae can be released into stagnant water; ingestion by the *Cyclops* completes the life cycle.

CLINICAL FEATURES Few or no clinical manifestations are evident until just before the blister forms, when there is the onset of fever and generalized allergic symptoms, including periorbital edema, wheezing, and urticaria. The emergence of the worm is associated with local pain and swelling. When the blister ruptures (usually as a result of immersion in water), the adult releases larva-rich fluid, and this release is associated with a relief of symptoms. The shallow ulcer surrounding the emerging adult worm heals over weeks to months.

Such ulcers, however, can become secondarily infected, the result being cellulitis, local inflammation, abscess formation, or (uncommonly) tetanus. Occasionally, the adult worm does not emerge but becomes encapsulated and calcified.

DIAGNOSIS   The diagnosis is based on the findings developing with the emergence of the adult worm.

TREATMENT AND PREVENTION   Gradual extraction of the worm by winding of a few centimeters on a stick each day remains the common and effective practice. Worms may be excised surgically. Thiabendazole (25 mg/kg twice daily for 3 days) or metronidazole (250 mg three times daily for 10 days) may relieve symptoms but have no proven activity against the worm. Prevention, which remains the only real control measure, depends on the provision of safe drinking water.

ZOONOTIC FILARIAL INFECTIONS

Dirofilariae that affect primarily dogs, cats, and raccoons and *Brugia* parasites that affect small mammals occasionally infect humans incidentally. Because humans are an abnormal host, the parasites never fully develop. Pulmonary dirofilarial infection caused by the canine heartworm *Dirofilaria immitis* generally presents in humans as a solitary pulmonary nodule. Chest pain, hemoptysis, or cough is uncommon. Infections with *D. repens* (from dogs) or *D. tenuis* (from raccoons) can cause local subcutaneous nodules in humans. Zoonotic *Brugia* infection can produce isolated lymph node enlargement. Eosinophilia and antifilarial antibodies are not commonly elevated. Excisional biopsy is both diagnostic and curative; these infections usually do not respond to chemotherapy.

REFERENCES

EBERHARD ML, LAMMIE PJ: Laboratory diagnosis of filariasis. Clin Lab Med 11:977, 1991

Lymphatic filariasis

Filariasis. Ciba Found Symp 127:1, 1985
WHO EXPERT COMMITTEE ON LYMPHATIC FILARIASIS: Fifth report. Technical Report Series No. 821, Geneva, WHO 1993

Tropical pulmonary eosinophilia

OTTESEN EA, NUTMAN TB: Tropical pulmonary eosinophilia. Annu Rev Med 43:417, 1992

Onchocerciasis

WHO EXPERT COMMITTEE ON ONCHOCERCIASIS: Third report. Technical Report Series No. 752, Geneva, WHO, 1987

Loiasis

KLION AD et al: Loiasis in endemic and non-endemic populations: Immunologically mediated differences in clinical presentation. J Infect Dis 163:1318, 1991

Other filarial infections

ADOLPH PE et al: Diagnosis and treatment of *Acanthocheilonema perstans* filariasis. Am J Trop Med Hyg 11:76, 1962
MARINKELLE CJ, GERMAN E: Mansonelliasis in the Comisaria del Vaupes of Colombia. Trop Georgr Med 22:101, 1970
MEYERS WM et al: Human streptocerciasis: A clinicopathologic study of 40 Africans (Zairians) including identification of the adult filaria. Am J Trop Med Hyg 21:528, 1972

Dracunculiasis

RANQUE P, HOPKINS D: Current status of the global campaign to eradicate dracunculiasis (guinea worm disease) Ann Parasitol Hum Comp 66(suppl 1):37, 1991

Zoonotic filarial infections

RO JY et al: Pulmonary dirofilariasis: The great imitator of primary or metastatic lung tumor. A clinicopathologic analysis of seven cases and a review of the literature. Hum Pathol 20:69, 1989

183   SCHISTOSOMIASIS AND OTHER TREMATODE INFECTIONS

THEODORE E. NASH

The trematodes (flukes) that commonly infect humans live in the intestines, biliary tract, lungs, and venules of intestines or genitourinary tract. With the exception of the intestinal schistosomes, which cause a unique type of liver fibrosis, disease is limited primarily to the organs where the parasites reside. The pathophysiology of disease differs among the trematodes. Schistosomiasis is the best understood, and some of the factors important in disease development in this infection appear to apply to infections caused by many of the other trematodes. In endemic areas, large proportions of the population are infected but asymptomatic; the disease is mostly limited to heavily infected persons. Distinct acute and chronic syndromes are recognizable, as are predictable pathologic changes over time. Eosinophilia and fever are common findings in acute disease. Because many of these parasites follow complicated migration routes and/or are poorly adapted to suvival in a human host, infections in ectopic locations are an important cause of morbidity.

Infections in humans are limited to digenetic trematodes, i.e., those which undergo sexual reproduction and produce eggs in mammalian definitive hosts and asexual reproduction in snails. After eggs reach water, they either hatch immediately or undergo maturation before releasing a free-swimming *miracidium* which seeks out the appropriate intermediate snail host or is ingested by the snail. After a number of cycles of multiplication in the snail, free-swimming *cercariae* are released and, depending on the species, can (1) infect the definitive host, (2) seek out a second intermediate host such as fish or crustacea, or (3) encyst on vegetation. The encysted cercaria, or *metacercaria*, is a dormant, relatively resistant form which infects the host following ingestion. With the exception of schistosomes, most trematodes are flat, leaf-shaped parasites that vary in length from 1 mm to 7 cm. They possess two grasping organs called *suckers* and lack a body cavity. The gut usually lacks an anus, and digested food is regurgitated through the oral opening. The surfaces of trematodes are covered by a syncytium of cells or tegument through which nutrients are absorbed. Schistosomes differ from the other trematodes infecting humans in a number of important ways. Most trematodes are hermaphroditic, but the sexes are separate in the schistosomes, and completion of the sexual cycle requires the presence of male and female worms. The adult schistosomes reside in the bloodstream, whereas the other trematodes dwell in the liver, lung, or intestines. In schistosomiasis, humans become infected by free-swimming cercariae that invade the skin; in contrast, in the other trematode infections, humans become infected after ingestion. The eggs of hermaphroditic trematodes possess a characteristic operculum, or caplike structure. The morphology of schistosome ova differs from that of other trematode ova, as described below.

A large number of trematodes can infect humans. With the exception of some species of schistosomes, most trematodes have domestic or wild animals as definitive hosts, and humans are accidentally infected. In highly endemic situations or under particularly advantageous circumstances, humans are able to maintain the life cycle in the absence of the usual definitive host. Some infections are rare or occur in populations in limited geographic areas, while others affect large numbers of persons over extensive areas or produce recognizable syndromes.

A pertinent history is important to determine the diagnosis. Persons from endemic areas; travelers who are exposed to fresh water or ingest undercooked fish, crustacea, or potentially contaminated vegetation; or others who ingest locally obtained but potentially contaminated vegetation such as watercress or undercooked, pickled, or smoked fish can be infected. Eosinophilia is common in acute invasive trematode infections. The definitive diagnosis is established by demonstrating eggs in stool or sputum or by biopsy of the affected tissue. Serologic tests are available for schistosomiasis, fascioliasis, and paragonimiasis; a positive test is indicative of infection. Serologic tests for other trematode infections may be available in endemic areas or research laboratories.

SCHISTOSOMIASIS

Three major schistosome species, *Schistosoma mansoni*, *Schistosoma haematobium*, and *Schistosoma japonicum*, and a number of less prevalent species of the genus *Schistosoma* infect humans. Both *S. mansoni* and *S. japonicum* adults reside in the venules of the intestine, and the major disease manifestations of these parasites are hepatic. *S. mansoni* is found in parts of South America (Brazil, Venezuela, and Surinam), some Caribbean islands, Africa, and the Middle East, while infections with *S. japonicum* occur in the Far East, mostly in China and the Philippines. *S. haematobium* adults are found mostly in the venules of the urinary tract and cause lesions primarily of the ureters and bladder. Infections with this species occur in Africa and the Middle East. Of lesser importance are *S. mekongi*, a parasite related to *S. japonicum* which is found along the Mekong River in Indochina, and *S. intercalatum*, found in certain areas of central West Africa. Worldwide, as many as 200 million persons may be infected, and infection of entire communities is common. However, most infected persons experience few, if any, signs and symptoms, and only a small minority develop significant disease.

LIFE CYCLE The schistosome species infecting humans all share the same basic life cycle but are unique in ways which account for some of the different clinical and pathologic findings. Important differences include the length of time before egg laying begins (prepatent period), location of the adult worms, number of eggs produced by each pair of worms, response by the host to the ova, and eventual fate of retained eggs. The morphology of the parasites and the types of intermediate host snail are also distinct. Humans become infected after contact with water containing the infective stage of the parasite, called a *cercaria*, which is a microscopic form of the schistosome possessing a forked tail used for swimming and a head which is the anlage of the worm. Cercariae penetrate the unbroken skin, with the help of secreted enzymes, and in the skin transform into *schistosomules*, or developing schistosomes. After 2 to 3 days, the schistosomules migrate to the lungs and then to the portal vein, probably by an intravascular route. In the portal vein the maturing male and female schistosomes pair and migrate to the venules of the mesentery, bladder, or ureters, depending on the species of schistosome, and begin to deposit eggs. The time spent in migration and maturation differs. *S. mansoni* and *S. japonicum* begin depositing eggs around 4 to 5 weeks after infection, while egg deposition begins after 2 to 3 months for *S. haematobium*. Adult worms are about 1 to 2 cm in length and migrate in the blood vessels without eliciting a local inflammatory reaction. Adult worms do not multiply in humans, and immunosuppressive therapy does not result in increased numbers of worms. Once released, eggs are either retained in the tissues at the site of deposition or swept back, mostly to the liver, by way of the venous portal system in the case of the intestinal schistosomes. Eggs are deposited mainly in the bladder and ureters by *S. haematobium*. A portion of the mature schistosome ova are extruded into the lumen of the intestines, bladder, or ureters and, after contact with water, hatch, releasing a miracidium. This free-swimming ciliated stage seeks out the proper intermediate snail vector and burrows into the soft tissues of the snail. After 1 to 2 months, depending on the species, the miracidium develops into a primary and then secondary sporocyst which, after further development, begins releasing cercariae into the surrounding water. Thousands of cercariae can be released daily from each infected snail. Therefore, one miracidium produces many cercariae, and this amplifies the number of infective parasites and the risk of infection. Cercariae are most infectious immediately after shedding and are not viable 48 h

after release, so storing water for 48 h before contact prevents exposure and infection. Unlike most other trematodes, the sexes are separate in schistosomes, but this is only evident in the adult stage. Ova are laid only when males and females infect the same individual.

PATHOPHYSIOLOGY A number of factors govern the disease manifestations. These include the duration and intensity of infection, location of egg deposition, host genetics, concurrent infections, and other still undefined factors.

In individuals from endemic areas, initial infection goes unnoticed. There are a number of possible reasons for this, including age at initial exposure, manner of exposure, and transfer of antigens, antibodies, and anti-idiotypes from the mother. In visitors to endemic areas, initial infection with schistosomes commonly results in an acute febrile illness (Katayama fever or acute schistosomiasis) which is most likely a manifestation of the immune response to the developing schistosomes and eggs. There is a vigorous hypersensitivity response which becomes modulated. These individuals have elevated levels of eosinophils and immune complexes and react markedly to schistosome antigens, as measured by lymphocyte blastogenesis. Despite ongoing infection, symptoms subside, as do blastogenic responses to schistosome antigens but not to unrelated antigens such as purified protein derivative of tuberculin (PPD). The exudative acute granulomatous response to schistosome eggs is also modulated.

A major factor in determining the development of disease in humans is the worm burden of the host, which determines the number of eggs produced. The inflammatory and fibrotic response to these eggs is responsible for most of the morbidity and mortality associated with schistosomiasis. Factors which limit parasite survival will limit the development of disease. Immunity exists in experimental animals, but in human schistosome infections it has not been clearly established that protective immunity develops; however, immunity is thought to develop because reinfection rates in previously treated humans are reduced in older populations despite similar amounts of water contact. In the first few days after infection, the schistosomule is relatively susceptible to immune attack. A number of systems employing antibody and/or eosinophils, neutrophils, macrophages, and complement have been used to kill schistosomules in vitro. However, as the schistosomules mature, they become refractory to these immune responses. In addition, schistosomes coat their tegument with host proteins and evade recognition by the host. A number of antibodies which block effective killing also may result in enhanced parasite survival. Schistosomule and adult antigens have been defined with the hope of developing vaccines; the administration of murine monoclonal antibodies to some of these antigens has reduced worm burdens in challenge infections by about 50 percent, and immunization of rodents with a number of defined antigens produced similar levels of protection. Successful vaccination with anti-idiotypes also has been reported.

All schistosome eggs elicit a granulomatous response which is best understood in *S. mansoni* infections. The host becomes sensitized to the egg proteins by a T cell–mediated mechanism which induces a larger granuloma. However, with continued infection the granuloma decreases in size due to the recruitment of suppressor T cells, while antibody has no effect on granuloma size. The regulation of granulomas due to *S. japonicum* eggs differs from that of granulomas from *S. mansoni* eggs. Immune modulation is mediated by serum factors, including anti-idiotype networks, at least in the chronic stage of infection. Both eggs and granulomas release factors which induce fibroblast proliferation in vitro. The early cellular response induced by granulomas is followed by fibrosis in vivo; however, liver fibrosis in humans probably involves more than simple fusion of fibrotic granulomas. After years of continued infection, some heavily infected individuals develop end-stage fibrotic lesions, mainly portal fibrosis (Symmers' fibrosis), sometimes resulting in esophageal varices and splenomegaly in *S. mansoni*, *S. japonicum*, and *S. mekongi* infections and fibrosis of the ureters and bladder in *S. haematobium* infections. After the development of portal fibrosis, eggs are shunted to the lungs via portal-systemic collateral veins, resulting in cor pulmonale in infected patients. Serologic tests are available and may be particularly useful in lightly infected individuals or those with suspected ectopic lesions. In acute disease, the presence of eggs may not be detected until 2 to 3 months after exposure. Praziquantel is the treatment of choice at 25 mg/kg tid, for 2 days. Bithionol is also effective but more toxic.

LIVER-DWELLING TREMATODES, *FASCIOLA HEPATICA*   Humans are accidently infected with this parasite of sheep, cattle, and other ruminants. Acute manifestations are a combination of systemic symptoms and signs and manifestations directly referable to invasion of the liver. Chronic disease has many features indistinguishable from that caused by the other liver flukes.

Life cycle   Ruminants become infected after ingestion of metacercariae encysted on aquatic vegetation. Watercress is commonly implicated in human infections. Metacercariae excyst in the duodenum, pass through the intestine into the peritoneum, invade the liver through Glisson's capsule, and eventually reside in the biliary ducts. In humans, the flukes require at least 3 to 4 months to mature, but eggs may not be detected in stool. Adults are relatively large, measuring 30 by 13 mm. Infections occur worldwide in areas where sheep and cattle are raised, including Europe, Australia, and other developed countries. Endogenously acquired infections are rare in the continental United States but occur in Puerto Rico.

Pathophysiology   The severity of infection depends on the intensity and duration of infection and responses of the host. Early manifestations are due to migration of the flukes through the tissues. Punctuate hemorrhages, tracts, and nodules are seen on the surface of the liver and are points of entry, migration routes, and areas of encapsulated eosinophilic abscesses, respectively. Granulomatous reactions also occur around eggs themselves. In chronic infections, worms reside in the biliary system, and the anatomic changes caused by the worms generally resemble those of the other liver flukes. However, intermittent obstruction of the biliary passages by worms appears more common in fascioliasis and leads to periods of jaundice.

Clinical findings   Fever, hepatomegaly and/or abdominal pain, and eosinophilia are the hallmark of acute fascioliasis, which usually begins within 2 to 3 months following ingestion. Nausea, diarrhea, cough, and urticaria are also frequent. Elevation of liver function tests is inconstant, anemia is usually present, and the erythrocyte sedimentation rate is commonly elevated. Untreated, the disease lasts from months to years, but the manifestations change and with time more closely resemble those of other liver flukes, including intermittent obstruction, gallbladder and biliary duct thickening, cholecystitis, lithiasis, and the development of strictures. Ectopic localizations of flukes is also relatively common and leads to findings related to the invaded tissue. In contrast to the other liver flukes, there is no apparent association with cholangiocarcinoma. Because exposure is sometimes long-standing, acute and chronic manifestations may occur at the same time. Computed tomographic scans show multiple, hypodense, irregular lesions in the liver; ultrasonography fails to detect these lesions but is helpful in detecting resulting biliary duct pathology.

Diagnosis and treatment   The presence of fever, eosinophilia, and hepatomegaly or liver pain in the proper clinical setting should suggest the diagnosis. Definitive diagnosis is established by detecting ova in the feces and/or by serologic tests. Ova may not be detected in the feces because disease manifestation occurs before patency, because of the inability of ova to pass into the biliary system, or because of ectopic location or low level of ova excretion. Therefore, stool concentration methods should be employed. The ova are immature in the feces, measure 130 to 150 μm by 90 μm, and are indistinguishable from those of *Fasciolopsis buski*. Although effective in other trematode infections, praziquantel does not appear to be very effective in *F. hepatica* infection, and bithionol at 30 to 50 mg/kg on alternate days for 10 to 15 doses is the treatment of choice. Infections also have been treated successfully with the experimental drugs triclabendazole and albendazole.

INTESTINE-DWELLING   TREMATODES   *Fasciolopsis   buski*   One of the largest parasites that infect humans, *F. buski* measures 20

to 70 mm by 8 to 20 mm by 0.5 to 3 mm and resides in the small intestine and occasionally in the colon or pylorus. It is confined to the Far East. The adults attach to the intestinal epithelium, causing ulcerations and localized inflammation. Light infections are generally asymptomatic, but persons heavily infected complain of diarrhea, fever, and abdominal pain and may develop ascites, anasarca, and intestinal obstruction. The pathophysiology has not been well studied. The diagnosis is established by detecting ova (indistinguishable from those of *F. hepatica*) in the feces. The treatment of choice is praziquantel, 25 mg/kg tid for 1 day.

Heterophyes heterophyes **and** *Metagonimus yokogawai*   Both are tiny (about 1 mm) intestine-dwelling parasites whose major clinical manifestation is diarrhea. Humans acquire infection after the ingestion of undercooked freshwater fish. *H. heterophyes* and *M. yokogawai* are found in the Far East, but the former is also common in the Nile Delta and present in other areas of the Middle East. The worms attach to and at times burrow into the intestinal mucosa, eliciting inflammatory responses. Ova of *H. heterophyes* have been found in the heart and other organs and have reportedly caused clinically significant myocarditis. The diagnosis is established by detecting ova in the feces; the ova of both species are identical and resemble those of *C. sinensis* and related parasites. Praziquantel is the drug of choice, at 25 mg/kg tid for 1 day.

Nanophyetus salmincola   This tiny small-intestine–dwelling trematode has recently infected humans in the Pacific Northwest. It was previously known to infect humans in eastern Siberia. Infections occur after ingestion of undercooked, smoked, or raw fish, usually salmon or trout. Symptoms vary from asymptomatic carriage to watery diarrhea, abdominal pain, bloating, and other gastrointestinal complaints. Eosinophilia is found in a majority but is not universal. Unembryonated ova (64 to 97 μm by 34 to 55 μm) appear in the feces after 1 week but are excreted in low numbers so that concentration techniques are needed. The treatment of choice is praziquantel, 20 mg/kg tid for 1 day.

REFERENCES

Schistosomes

CHEEVER AW, ANDRADE ZA: Pathological lesions associated with *Schistosoma mansoni* infection in man. Trans R Soc Trop Med Hyg 61:626, 1968

FORSYTH DM: A longitudinal study of endemic urinary schistosomiasis in a small East African community. Bull WHO 40:771, 1969

HAGAN P: Reinfection, exposure and immunity in human schistosomiasis. Parasitol Today 8:12, 1992

HIAT RA et al: Factors in the pathogenesis of acute schistosomiasis mansoni. J Infect Dis 139:659, 1979

HOMEIDA M et al: Morbidity associated with *Schistosoma mansoni* infection as determined by ultrasound: A study in Gezira, Sudan. Am J Trop Med Hyg 39:196, 1988

———: Diagnosis of pathologically confirmed Symmers' periportal fibrosis by ultrasonography: A prospective blinded study. Am J Trop Med Hyg 39:86, 1988

HOMEIDA MA et al: Association of the therapeutic activity of praziquantel with the reversal of Symmers' fibrosis induced by *Schistosoma mansoni*. Am J Trop Med Hyg 45:360, 1991

JORDAN P, WEBBE G (eds): *Schistosomiasis, Epidemiology, Treatment and Control*. London, Heinemann Medical, 1982

LEHMAN JS et al: Urinary schistosomiasis in Egypt: Clinical, radiological, bacteriological, and parasitological correlations. Trans R Soc Trop Med Hyg 67:384, 1973

NASH TE et al: Schistosome infections in humans: Perspective and recent findings. Ann Intern Med 97:740, 1982

ROLLINSON O, SIMPSON AJG (eds): *The Biology of Schistosomes. From Genes to Latrines*. New York, Academic, 1987

SAAD AMA et al: Oesophageal varices in region of the Sudan endemic for *Schistosoma mansoni*. Br J Surg 78:1252, 1991

Other trematodes

BEAVER PC et al: *Clinical Parasitology*, 9th ed. Philadelphia, Lea & Febiger, 1984

ELKINS DB et al: A high frequency of hepatobiliary disease and suspected cholangiocarcinoma associated with heavy *Opisthorchis viverrini* infection in a small community in northeast Thailand. Trains R Soc Trop Med Hyg 84:715, 1990

FACEY MB et al: Fascioliasis in man: An outbreak in Hampshire. Br Med J ii:619, 1960

FRITSCHE TR et al: Praziquantel for treatment of human *Nanophyetus salmincola* (*Troglotrema salmincola*) infection. J Infect Dis 160:896, 1989

GUTIERREZ Y: *Diagnostic Pathology of Parasitic Infections with Clinical Correlations*. Philadelphia, Lea & Febiger, 1990

Hou P-C: The pathology of *Clonorchis sinensis* infestation of the liver. J Pathol Bacteriol 70:53, 1955

Koenigstein RP: Observations on the epidemiology of infections with *Clonorchis sinensis*. Trans R Soc Trop Med Hyg 42:503, 1949

Sadun EH, Buck AA: Paragonimiasis in South Korea—Immunodiagnostic, epidemiologic, clinical, roentgenologic and therapeutic studies. Am J Trop Med Hyg 9:562, 1960

———, Maiphoom C: Studies in the epidemiology of the human intestinal fluke, *Fasciolopsis buski* (Lankester) in Central Thailand. Am J Trop Med Hyg 2:1084, 1953

Singh TS et al: Pulmonary paragonimiasis: Clinical features, diagnosis and treatment of 39 cases in Manipur. Trans R Soc Trop Med Hyg 80:967, 1986

Sithithaworn P et al: Quantitative post-mortem study of *Opisthorchis viverrini* in man in northeast Thailand. Trans R Soc Trop Med Hyg 85:765, 1991

Takeyama N et al: Computed tomography findings of hepatic lesions in human fascioliasis: Report of two cases. Am J Gastroenterol 81:1078, 1986

Yokogawa M: Epidemiology and control of paragonimiasis, in *Parasitic Diseases*, EM Sasa (ed). Tokyo, International Medical Foundation of Japan, 1974, pp 137–149

184 CESTODES

THOMAS B. NUTMAN / PETER F. WELLER

Cestodes, or tapeworms, are segmented worms. The adults reside in the gastrointestinal tract, but the larvae can be found in almost any organ. Human tapeworm infections can be divided into two major clinical groups. In one group, humans are the definitive hosts, and the adult tapeworms live in the gastrointestinal tract (*Taenia saginata*, *Diphyllobothrium*, *Hymenolepis*, and *Dipylidium caninum*). In the other, humans are intermediate hosts, and larval-stage parasites are present in the tissues. Diseases in this category include echinococcosis, sparganosis, and coenurosis. For *Taenia solium*, the human may be either the definitive or the intermediate host.

The ribbon-shaped tapeworm attaches to the intestinal mucosa by means of sucking cups or grooves located on the head (scolex). Behind the scolex is a short, narrow neck from which proglottids (or segments) form. As each proglottid matures, it is displaced further back from the neck by new, less mature segments. The progressively elongated chain of attached proglottids, called the *strobila*, constitutes the bulk of the tapeworm and may contain over 1000 proglottids and be several meters in length. As each proglottid becomes gravid, eggs are released. Since eggs of different *Taenia* spp. are morphologically identical, differences in the morphology of the scolex or proglottids provide the only basis for diagnostic identification of the tapeworm species. Most human tapeworms require at least one intermediate host for complete larval development. After ingestion by an intermediate host, an egg develops into a larval oncosphere capable of penetrating the intestinal mucosa. The oncosphere migrates to tissues and develops into an encysted form known as a *cysticercus* (single scolex), a *coenerus* (multiple scolices), or a *hydatid* (cyst with daughter cysts each containing several scolices). Ingestion by the definitive host of tissues containing a cyst enables a scolex to develop into a tapeworm.

TAENIASIS SAGINATA The beef tapeworm, *Taenia saginata*, occurs in all countries where raw or undercooked beef is eaten and is more prevalent in sub-Saharan African and Middle Eastern countries.

Etiology and pathogenesis Humans are the only definitive host for the adult stage of *T. saginata*. This 3- to 10-meter-long tapeworm inhabits the upper jejunum and has a scolex with four prominent suckers and 1000 to 2000 proglottids. Each gravid segment has 15 to 30 uterine branches (in contrast to 8 to 12 with *T. solium*). The eggs are indistinguishable from those of *T. solium*, each measuring 30 to 40 μm, with a thick, brown striated shell containing a fully developed embryo. Eggs deposited on vegetation can live for months to years until they are ingested by cattle or other herbivores. The embryo released after ingestion invades the intestinal wall and is carried to striated muscle predominantly in the hindlimbs, diaphragm,

and tongue, where it transforms into a cysticercus. When ingested in raw or undercooked beef, this form can infect humans. After the cysticercus is ingested, it takes about 2 months for an adult worm to develop.

Clinical manifestations Patients become aware of the infection most commonly by noting passage of proglottids in their feces, and they may experience a discomforting perianal sensation when proglottids are discharged. Although usually minimal or mild, abdominal pain or discomfort, nausea, change in appetite, weakness, and weight loss can occur with *T. saginata* infection.

Diagnosis The diagnosis is made by detecting eggs or proglottids in the stool as soon as about 3 months after infection. Eggs also may be present on the perianal area, so if proglottids or eggs are not found in the stool, the perianal region should be examined with use of a cellophane-tape swab, as is done for pinworm infection. Separation of this infection from *T. solium* requires examination of mature proglottids or the scolex. Serologic tests are not helpful diagnostically. Eosinophilia and elevations of serum IgE may be present.

Treatment and prevention Either niclosamide (a single dose of four 0.5-g tablets chewed thoroughly) or a single dose of praziquantel (10 to 20 mg/kg) is highly effective therapy. The major means of preventing beef tapeworm infection involves the adequate cooking of beef; temperatures as low as 56°C for 5 min will destroy cysticerci. Refrigeration or salting for long periods or freezing at −10°C for 9 days also kills cysticerci in beef. General preventive measures include beef inspection and proper disposal of human feces.

TAENIASIS SOLIUM AND CYSTICERCOSIS The pork tapeworm, *Taenia solium*, can cause two distinct forms of infection, depending on whether humans are infected with adult tapeworms in the intestine or with larval forms in the tissues (cysticercosis). Humans are the only definitive hosts for *T. solium*, and pigs are the usual intermediate hosts, although dogs, cats, and sheep may harbor the larval forms. *T. solium* exists worldwide but is most prevalent in Mexico, Africa, Southeast Asia, eastern Europe, and South America. Cysticercosis occurs in industrialized nations largely as a result of the immigration of infected persons from endemic areas.

Etiology and pathogenesis The adult tapeworm generally resides in the upper jejunum, and its globular scolex attaches by both sucking disks and two rows of hooklets. Often only one adult worm is present but may live for up to 25 years. The tapeworm, usually about 3 m in length, may have as many as 1000 proglottids, each of which produces up to 50,000 eggs. Groups of 3 to 5 proglottids generally are released and excreted into the feces, and the eggs in these proglottids are infective for both humans and animals. The eggs survive in the environment for several months. After ingestion by the intermediate host, eggs embryonate, penetrate the intestinal wall, and are carried to many tissues, with a predilection for striated muscle of the neck, tongue, and trunk. Within 60 to 90 days, the encysted larval stage develops. These cysticerci can survive for long periods. Infections of humans that lead to intestinal tapeworms occur by ingestion of undercooked pork containing cysticerci. Infections that cause human cysticercosis occur after the ingestion of *T. solium* eggs, usually from fecally contaminated food. Autoinfection may occur if an individual with an egg-producing tapeworm unhygienically ingests eggs derived from his or her own feces or potentially if eggs reflux from the intestine into the stomach.

Clinical manifestations Intestinal infections with *T. solium* may be asymptomatic. Complaints of epigastric discomfort, nausea, sensation of hunger, weight loss, and diarrhea are infrequent. Fecal passage of proglottids may be noted by patients.

In cysticercosis, the clinical manifestations are entirely different. Since cysticerci can be found anywhere in the body (most commonly in the brain and the skeletal muscle), the location and size of cysticerci determine the clinical presentation. The manifestations of cysticercosis reflect two distinct processes, the local inflammatory response induced by the parasite and the local effect of the space-occupying lesions. Neurologic manifestations are the most common presentation. When inflammation surrounds lesions, seizures and focal neurologic deficits are frequent, and communicating and noncommunicating hydrocephalus and meningitis also can be seen. Generalized, focal, or Jacksonian seizures occur in most. Signs of increased intracranial pressure, including headache, nausea, vomiting, changes in vision, dizziness, ataxia, and confusion, often are present. In patients with hydrocephalus, papilledema and alteration in mental status may occur. An unusual form of cyticercosis is the racemose form, which consists of grapelike clusters of proliferating larval membranes. Characteristically, this form occurs at the base of the brain or in the subarachnoid space and causes chronic meningitis and arachnoiditis. Communicating or noncommunicating hydrocephalus frequently develops. The clinical presentation of neurocysticercosis, therefore, depends on the number, form, and location of cysticerci, the extent of cyst-associated inflammatory responses, and the duration of disease.

Diagnosis The diagnosis of intestinal *T. solium* infection is made by finding eggs or proglottids, as described for *T. saginata*. For cysticercosis, definitive diagnosis requires examination of the cysticercus within an involved tissue, but a diagnosis often can be based on the clinical presentation and results of compatible radiographic, especially computed tomographic (CT) and magnetic resonance imaging (MRI), studies and serologic tests.

For soft-tissue involvement, plain films may reveal multiple calcified "puffed-rice" lesions. For cerebral cysticercosis, CT studies demonstrate parenchymal lesions of varying number and size that are either cystic or solid and may exhibit contrast enhancement. On CT studies, some or many of the lesions may be calcified, so multiple punctate calcifications are common findings in neurocysticercosis. Ventricular dilatation may be demonstrable, but the CT finding of multiple calcified or noncalcified cystic lesions is strongly suggestive of cerebral cysticercosis. MRI detects cystic structures on T_1- and T_2-weighted images and high-intensity rims around cysts, particularly on T_2-weighted images. Because CT is more sensitive in identifying calcified lesions and MRI is better at identifying small cystic lesions, both techniques are useful in evaluating neurocysticercosis.

Most patients with cerebral cysticercosis show a cerebrospinal fluid (CSF) pleocytosis with a mononuclear cell predominance. In CSF, glucose is often decreased, and protein is elevated. Serologic tests of CSF and sera are helpful in establishing the diagnosis. A variety of serologic assays have been used, but many were complicated by cross-reactivity with other tapeworm, filarial and echinococcal infections. However, an immunoblotting technique has improved specificity to 98 percent, with sensitivities reaching 91 percent. Even with this technique, however, patients with single intracranial neurocysticercotic lesions may be seronegative.

Treatment and prevention Intestinal *T. solium* infection is treated with niclosamide or praziquantel, as specified for *T. saginata* infection. With the latter drug, however, there is the possible risk of evoking an inflammatory response in the central nervous system if concomitant cryptic cysticercosis is present. Preventive measures regarding pork are similar to those for beef and *T. saginata* above.

The therapy for cysticercosis can involve chemotherapy, surgery, and supportive medical treatment. Asymptomatic patients with calcified soft tissue or neural lesions generally require no treatment. For symptomatic patients with neurocysticercosis, both praziquantel (50 mg/kg per day in three doses for 15 days) and albendazole (15 mg/kg per day in three doses for 8 days) are effective. Because both agents provoke inflammatory responses around dying cysticerci, patients receiving either drug should be hospitalized and given high doses of glucocorticoids during treatment. Efficacy of therapy can be monitored by radiographic imaging, with a decrease in the size of active lesions expected within 3 to 6 months. For ocular and spinal lesions, drug-induced inflammation may cause irreversible damage; thus these lesions, as well as those within the ventricles, are best managed by surgical resection. Ventricular obstruction may require a ventriculostomy or ventriculoperitoneal shunting. Not all neurologic deficits resolve after therapy, and some patients may require continued anticonvulsive therapy. Prevention of cysticercosis involves minimizing the opportunities for ingestion of fecally derived eggs by

means of good personal hygiene, improvements in fecal disposal, and treatment and prevention of human intestinal infections.

ECHINOCOCCOSIS Echinococcosis is an infection of humans caused by the larval stage of *Echinococcus granulosus, E. multilocularis,* or *E. vogeli. E. granulosus,* which produces unilocular cystic lesions, is prevalent in areas where livestock is raised in association with dogs. It is found in Australia, Argentina, Chile, Africa, eastern Europe, the Middle East, New Zealand, and the Mediterranean, particularly Lebanon and Greece. *E. multilocularis,* which causes multilocular, alveolar lesions which are locally invasive, is found in subarctic or arctic regions, including Canada, the United States, and northern Europe and Asia. *E. vogeli* causes polycystic hydatid disease and is found only in Central and South America. As with other cestode infections, echinococcal species have both intermediate and definitive hosts. The definitive hosts are dogs that pass eggs in their feces. When the intermediate hosts—sheep, cattle, humans, goats, camels, and horses for *E. granulosus* and mice or other rodents for *E. multilocularis*—ingest the eggs, cysts develop within these hosts. When a dog ingests beef or lamb containing cysts, the life cycle is completed.

Etiology The small, 5-mm-long adult *E. granulosus* worm, which is resident with a 5- to 20-month lifespan in the jejunum of dogs, has only three proglottids—one immature, one mature, and one gravid. The gravid segment splits to release eggs morphologically indistinguishable from *Taenia* eggs and extremely hardy. After humans ingest the eggs, embryos escape from the eggs, penetrate the intestinal mucosa, enter the portal circulation, and are carried to various organs, most commonly the liver and lungs. Larvae develop into fluid-filled unilocular hydatid cysts which consist of an external membrane and an inner germinal layer. Daughter cysts develop from the inner aspect of the germinal layer, as do germinating cystic structures called *brood capsules*. New larvae, called *scolices,* develop in large numbers within the brood capsule. The cysts expand slowly over a period of years. The life cycle of *E. multilocularis* is similar except that small rodents serve as intermediate hosts. The cyst, however, is quite different, in that the larval form remains in the proliferative phase, the hydatid cyst is always multilocular, and vesicles progressively invade the host tissue by peripheral extension of processes from the germinal layer.

Clinical manifestations Slowly enlarging echinococcal cysts generally remain asymptomatic until their expanding size or their space-occupying effect in an involved organ elicits symptoms. Liver and lung are the most common sites. Since 5 to 20 years often elapses before cysts enlarge sufficiently to cause symptoms, the cysts may be discovered as an incidental finding on a routine x-ray or ultrasound study. Patients with hepatic echinococcosis who are symptomatic most often present with abdominal pain or a palpable mass in the right upper quadrant. Compression of a bile duct or leakage of cyst fluid into the biliary tree may mimic recurrent cholelithiasis, and biliary obstruction can result in jaundice. Rupture or episodic leakage from an hydatid cyst may produce fever, pruritus, urticaria, eosinophilia, or fatal anaphylaxis. Pulmonary hydatid cysts may rupture into the bronchial tree or peritoneal cavity and produce cough, chest pain, or hemoptysis. Rupture of hydatid cysts, by spreading the multitude of infectious scolices, leads to multifocal dissemination of new cyst-forming elements and can occur spontaneously or at surgery, especially when a cyst is not recognized to be of echinococcal etiology. Cysts may involve any organ, and other presentations are due to those in bone (invasion of the medullary cavity with slow bone erosion producing pathologic fractures), the central nervous system (space-occupying lesions), and the heart (conduction defects, pericarditis).

The cysts of *E. multilocularis* characteristically present as a slowly growing hepatic tumor with progressive destruction of the liver and extension into vital structures. Patients commonly complain of upper quadrant and epigastric pain, and obstructive jaundice may be present. A minority of patients will have metastatic lesions to the lung and brain.

Diagnosis Radiographic and related imaging studies are important in detecting and evaluating echinococcal cysts. Plain films will define pulmonary cysts, usually as rounded, irregular masses of uniform density, but may miss other cysts in other organs unless there is cyst wall calcification, as occurs in the liver. CT scans and ultrasound reveal well-defined cysts with thick or thin walls. If older cysts contain a layer of hydatid sand that is rich in accumulated scolices, these imaging methods may detect this fluid layer of different density, but the most pathognomonic finding, if demonstrable, is the visualization of daughter cysts within the larger cyst. This finding, as well as eggshell, or mural, calcification, indicates *E. granulosus* infection and helps to distinguish the cyst from carcinomas, bacterial or amebic liver abscesses, or hemangiomas. With alveolar hydatid cysts, CT reveals indistinct solid masses with central necrosis and plaquelike calcifications.

Specific diagnosis could be made by examination of aspirated fluids for the presence of scoliceal hooklets, but diagnostic aspiration is not conventionally recommended because of the risks from fluid leakage either by disseminating infection or provoking anaphylactic reactions. However, CT-guided aspiration of hydatid cysts for diagnosis has been utilized successfully in some centers in conjunction with installation of ethanol after aspiration. Pretreatment with albendazole (1-month course) is believed to minimize possible biopsy complications. Serodiagnostic assays can be useful, although a negative test does not exclude the diagnosis of echinococcosis. While cysts in the liver are more likely to elicit positive antibody responses than those in the lungs, up to 50 percent of infected individuals may have negative serology. Detection of antibody to a specific echinococcal antigen (antigen 5 or arc 5) has the highest degree of specificity, although false-positive findings may be present in cysticercosis.

Treatment Therapy for echinococcosis is based on considerations of the size, location, and manifestations of cysts and the overall health of the patient. Surgery, when feasible, is the principal definitive method of treatment by excising *E. granulosus* cysts or resecting tissue containing *E. multilocularis* cysts. Risks at surgery from leakage of fluid include anaphylaxis and dissemination of infectious scolices. The latter has been minimized by instilling scolicidal solutions such as hypertonic saline or ethanol. These may cause hypernatremia, ethanol intoxication, or possibly sclerosing cholangitis. Albendazole, which has antiechinococcal activity, can be administered adjunctively in the perioperative period and may be useful for medical treatment of echinococcosis. While albendazole has shown efficacy, the exact role of chemotherapy, potentially combined with percutaneous drainage, remains to be defined. As medical therapy, albendazole, given at 400 mg twice a day for 28 days and repeated from 1 to 8 times, separated by drug-free intervals of 2 to 3 weeks, is most efficacious for those with hepatic and/or pulmonary cysts.

Prevention In endemic areas, echinococcosis can be prevented by praziquantel treatment of infected dogs and by denying dogs access to butchering sites or offal of infected animals. Limitation of the number of stray dogs is helpful in reducing the prevalence of human infection.

HYMENOLEPIASIS NANA *Hymenolepis nana*, the dwarf tapeworm, is the most common of all the cestode infections. *H. nana* is endemic in both temperate and tropical regions of the world. Infection is spread by fecal/oral contamination and is common in institutionalized children.

Etiology and pathogenesis *H. nana* is the only cestode of humans that does not require an intermediate host. Both the larval and adult phases occur in the human. The adult, the smallest tapeworm parasitizing humans, is about 2 cm long and dwells in the proximal ileum. Proglottids, which are quite small and rarely seen in the stool, release spherical eggs 30 to 44 μm in diameter that each contain an oncosphere with six hooklets. The eggs are immediately infective and are unable to survive in the external environment for more than 10 days. *H. nana* also can be acquired by the ingestion of insects (especially larval meal worms and larval fleas) infected with the

parasite. When the egg is ingested by a new host, the oncosphere is freed and penetrates the intestinal villi, becoming a cysticercoid larva. Larvae migrate back into the intestinal lumen, attach to the mucosa, and mature over 10 to 12 days into adult worms. Eggs also may hatch before passing into the stool, causing internal autoinfection with increasing numbers of intestinal worms. Although the lifespan of adult *H. nana* is only about 4 to 10 weeks, the autoinfection cycle perpetuates the infection.

Clinical manifestations *H. nana* infection, even with many intestinal worms, is usually asymptomatic. When infection is intense, anorexia, abdominal pain, and diarrhea occur.

Diagnosis, treatment, and prevention Infection is diagnosed by finding eggs in the stool. Praziquantel (25 mg/kg once) is the treatment of choice, since it acts against both the adult worms and the cysticercoids in the intestinal villi. The alternative, niclosamide (2 g on day 1 and 1 g/d for 6 more days), must be given over a week, since it is ineffective against the cysticercoid stage. The dosage for children must be adjusted for body weight. Good personal hygiene and improved sanitation can eradicate the disease. Epidemics have been controlled by the use of mass chemotherapy coupled with improved hygiene.

HYMENOLEPIASIS DIMINUTA *Hymenolepis diminuta*, a cestode of rodents, occasionally infects small children, who become infected with the adult worm after ingesting uncooked cereal foods contaminated by fleas and other insects in which larval development occurs. Infection is usually asymptomatic and is diagnosed by finding the eggs in the stool. Niclosamide or praziquantel results in cure in most individuals.

DIPHYLLOBOTHRIASIS *Diphyllobothrium latum* and other *Diphyllobothrium* spp. can be found in the lakes, rivers, and deltas of the Northern Hemisphere, Central Africa, and Chile.

Etiology and pathogenesis The adult worm, the longest tapeworm, reaches lengths up to 25 m. It attaches to the ileal and occasionally to the jejunal mucosa by its suckers, which are located on its elongated scolex. The adult worm has 3000 to 4000 proglottids, which release approximately 1 million eggs daily into the feces. If an egg reaches water, it hatches and releases a free-swimming embryo that can be eaten by small freshwater crustaceans (*Cyclops* or *Diaptomus* spp.). After this infected crustacean containing a developed procercoid is swallowed by a fish, the larva migrate into the fish's flesh and grows into a plerocercoid, or sparganum larva. Humans acquire the infection by ingesting infected raw fish. Within 3 to 5 weeks, the tapeworm matures in the human intestine into an adult.

Clinical manifestations The majority of *D. latum* infections are asymptomatic, although manifestations may include transient abdominal discomfort, diarrhea, vomiting, weakness, and weight loss. Occasionally, infection can cause acute abdominal pain and intestinal obstruction; in rare cases cholangitis or cholecystitis may be caused by migrating proglottids. Because the tapeworm absorbs large quantities of vitamin B_{12} and interferes with ileal B_{12} absorption, vitamin B_{12} deficiency can develop. Up to 2 percent of infected patients, especially the elderly, have a megaloblastic anemia resembling pernicious anemia and may exhibit neurologic sequelae of B_{12} deficiency.

Diagnosis The diagnosis is made readily by detecting in the stool the characteristic eggs, which possess a single shell with an operculum at one end and a knob on the other. Mild to moderate eosinophilia may be present.

Treatment and prevention Praziquantel (10 to 20 mg/kg once) and niclosamide (a single 2-g dose) are highly effective. Parenteral vitamin B_{12} should be given if B_{12} deficiency is manifest. Infection can be prevented by heating fish to 54°C for 5 min or by freezing it at −18°C for 24 h. Placing fish in brine with a high salt concentration for long periods kills the eggs.

DIPYLIDIASIS *Dipylidium caninum*, a common tapeworm of dogs and cats, may accidentally infect humans. Dogs, cats, and occasionally humans become infected by ingesting fleas harboring cysticercoids. Children are more likely to become infected than adults.

Most infections are asymptomatic, but abdominal pain, diarrhea, anal pruritus, urticaria, and eosinophilia can occur. Diagnosis is made by detecting proglottids in the stool. Therapy is with praziquantel or niclosamide as for *D. latum* infection. Prevention requires antihelminthic treatment and flea control for pet dogs or cats.

SPARGANOSIS   Humans can be infected by sparganum, or plerocercoid larva, of another diphyllobothrid tapeworm of the genus *Spirometra.* Infection can be acquired by drinking water containing infected *Cyclops,* by ingesting infected snakes, birds, or other mammals, or by the application of infected flesh as poultices. The worm will migrate slowly in tissues, and infection commonly presents as a subcutaneous swelling. Periorbital tissues can be involved, and ocular sparganosis may destroy the eye. Surgical excision is used to treat localized sparganosis.

COENUROSIS   This rare infection of humans by the larval (or coenurus) stage of the dog tapeworm *Taenia multiceps* results in a space-occupying cystic lesion. As in cysticercosis, involvement of the central nervous system and subcutaneous tissue is most common. Both definitive diagnosis and treatment require surgical excision of the lesion. Chemotherapeutic agents are not effective.

REFERENCES

HORTON RJ: Chemotherapy of *Echinococcus* infection in man with albendazole. Aust NZ J Surg 59:665, 1989

RICHARDS F JR, SCHANTZ PM: Laboratory diagnosis of cysticercosis. Clin Lab Med 11:1011, 1991

SCHAEFER JW, KHAN MY: Echinococcosis (hydatid disease): Lessons from experience with 59 patients. Rev Infect Dis 13:243, 1991

SCHANTZ PM, OKELO GBA: Echinococcosis (hydatidosis), in *Tropical and Geographical Medicine,* 2d ed, KS Warren, AAF Mahmoud (eds). New York, McGraw-Hill, 1990, p 505

SCHARF D: Neurocysticercosis: Two hundred thirty eight cases from a California hospital. Arch Neurol 46:77, 1989

TEITELBAUM GP et al: MR imaging of neurocysticercosis. AJR 153:857, 1989

section 19   Ectoparasites

185   ECTOPARASITE INFESTATIONS

JAMES H. MAGUIRE / ANDREW SPIELMAN

Ectoparasites are arthropods or helminths that *infest* the skin of other animals from which they derive sustenance. They may penetrate beneath the surface of the host or attach superficially by their mouthparts. These organisms damage their hosts by direct injury, by eliciting a hypersensitivity reaction, or by inoculating toxins or pathogens. The main medically important ectoparasites are arachnids (including mites and ticks), insects (including lice, fleas, and flies), pentastomes (tongue worms), and leeches.

SCABIES

The human itch mite, *Sarcoptes scabiei,* which infests some 300 million persons each year, is one of the most common causes of itching dermatoses throughout the world. Gravid female mites measuring 0.3 to 0.4 mm in length burrow for a month superficially beneath the stratum corneum, where they deposit two to three eggs a day. Larvae that hatch from these eggs mature in a series of molts in about 2 weeks and then emerge to the surface of the skin, where they mate and subsequently reinvade the skin of the same or another host. Transfer of newly fertilized female mites from person to person occurs by intimate personal contact and is facilitated by crowding, uncleanliness, and sexual promiscuity. Medical practitioners are at particular risk of infestation. Transmission via sharing of contaminated bedding or clothing occurs only infrequently because these mites cannot survive much more than a day without host contact. In the United States, scabies may account for 2 to 5 percent of visits to dermatologists, particularly involving children, immigrants from developing countries, and close household contacts. Outbreaks occur in nursing homes, mental institutions, and hospitals.

The itching and rash associated with scabies derive from a sensitization reaction directed against the excreta that the mite deposits in its burrow. For this reason, an initial infestation remains asymptomatic for 4 to 6 weeks, and a reinfestation produces a hypersensitivity reaction without delay. Scratching generally destroys the burrowing mite, but symptoms remain even in its absence. Burrows become surrounded by infiltrates of eosinophils, lymphocytes, and histiocytes, and a generalized hypersensitivity rash later develops in remote sites. By destroying these pathogens, immunity and associated scratching limit most infestations to less than 15 mites per person. Hyperinfestation with thousands or millions or mites, a condition known as *crusted* (or *Norwegian*) *scabies,* may result from glucocorticoid use, immunodeficiency disease including AIDS, and neurologic and psychiatric illnesses that interfere with itching and scratching.

Patients with scabies complain of intense itching that worsens at night and after a hot shower. Typical burrows may be difficult to find because they are few in number and may be obscured by excoriations. Burrows appear as dark wavy lines in the epidermis measuring 3 to 15 mm and ending in a small pearly bleb which contains the female mite. In the majority of patients they occur on the volar wrists, between the fingers, on the elbows, and on the penis. Small papules and vesicles, often accompanied by eczematous plaques, pustules, or nodules, are symmetrically distributed in these sites and in skin folds under the breasts and around the navel, axillae, belt line, buttocks, upper thighs, and scrotum. Except in infants, the face, scalp, neck, palms, and soles are spared. Burrows and other typical lesions may be sparse in persons who wash frequently, and topical corticosteroids and bacterial superinfection may alter the appearance of the rash. Superinfection with nephritogenic strains of streptococci has led to acute glomerulonephritis. Crusted scabies resembles psoriasis because of the widespread erythema, thick keratotic crusts, scaling, and dystrophic nails. Characteristic burrows are not seen, and patients usually do not itch, although they are highly contagious and have been responsible for outbreaks of classic scabies in hospitals.

Diagnosis of scabies should be considered in patients with pruritus and symmetric polymorphic skin lesions in characteristic locations, particularly if there is a history of household contact. Burrows should be sought and unroofed with a sterile needle or scalpel blade, and the scrapings should be examined microscopically for the mite, its eggs, or its fecal pellets. A drop of mineral oil facilitates removal of the sample. Biopsies or scrapings of papulovesicular lesions also may be diagnostic. In the absence of identifiable mites or mite products, the diagnosis is based on the clinical presentation and history. Other sexually transmitted diseases should be excluded in adults with scabies.

The 5% permethrin cream that is the treatment of choice for

scabies is less toxic than the commonly used 1% lindane preparations and is effective against lindane-tolerant infestations. Both scabicides are applied from the neck down after bathing and are removed 8 h later by means of soap and water. Lindane is absorbed through the skin, and its overuse has led to seizures and aplastic anemia. It should not be applied to pregnant women or infants. Alternatives include topical crotamiton cream, benzyl benzoate, and sulfur ointments.

Although effectively treated scabies infestations become noninfectious within a day, itching and rash due to hypersensitivity frequently persist for weeks or months. Unnecessary retreatment of such patients may provoke a contact dermatitis. Antihistamines, salicylates, and calamine lotion relieve itching during treatment, and topical glucocorticoids are useful for the pruritus that lingers after effective treatment. An oral antibiotic may be necessary for bacterial superinfections that fail to resolve with antiscabietic therapy. To prevent reinfestations, bedding and clothing should be washed in hot water, and close contacts, even if asymptomatic, should be treated simultaneously.

SARCOPTIC MANGE (ANIMAL SCABIES)

Persons who have close contact with dogs and to a lesser extent cats and horses may become transiently infested by zoonotic scabies. Such mites are unable to propagate on the human host or to produce their elongate burrows, and the characteristic pruritic papulovesicular rash is self-limited.

CHIGGERS AND OTHER MITE INFESTATIONS

Chiggers are the larvae of trombiculid (harvest) mites that normally feed on mice in grassy or brush-covered sites in the tropics and subtropics. They quest for hosts on low vegetation and attach themselves to passing animals or to people. The larva then pierces the skin of its host and deposits a tubelike structure in the dermis through which it imbibes lymph and tissue juices. This highly antigenic "stylosotome" serves as the focus of an exceptionally pruritic papule that may be 2 cm in diameter and that develops within hours of attachment in persons previously sensitized to mite antigen. Scratching invariably destroys the body of a mite attached to a person. These lesions generally vesiculate and develop a hemorrhagic base. Itching and burning last for weeks. The rash is most common on the ankles or near tight-fitting clothes that obstruct the mites' movements.

Certain mesostigmatid mites that infest the nests of mice or birds feed on human beings when their normal hosts have been displaced. Intense episodes of itching dermatitis, for example, may follow removal of trash from a human residence or departure of pigeons that have been nesting on a window air-conditioner. Other mites that infest grain, straw, cheese, or other animal products occasionally produce similar episodes. Diagnosis of mite-induced dermatitides (including chiggers) leans heavily on a history of exposure to the source of the mite, since the tiny mite may escape notice or may already have fallen off or been scratched off the lesions. Antihistamines or topical steroids effectively reduce mite-induced pruritus.

Chiggers are the agents of scrub typhus in tropical and subtropical parts of Asia, and mouse mites are the agents of rickettsialpox in the cities of the northeastern United States. Repellants are useful for preventing chigger bite and sanitary measures for rickettsialpox.

TICK INFESTATIONS AND TICK PARALYSIS

Hard ticks (Ixodidae), including dog ticks and deer ticks, have become increasingly abundant since the mid-1900s, and their bites have come to be associated with diverse debilitating diseases. Because soft ticks (Argasidae) rarely attack human hosts in the United States, the following discussion deals with hard ticks. Ticks attach and feed painlessly; blood is their only food. Their secretions, however,

produce local reactions, a febrile illness, or paralysis. Local reactions to tick bites vary from small pruritic papules to chronic nodules, or "tick granulomas," reaching several centimeters in diameter. Tick-induced fever, associated with headache, nausea, and malaise, usually resolves within 24 to 36 h after the tick is removed. Tick paralysis is an ascending flaccid paralysis believed to be caused by a toxin in tick saliva that causes neuromuscular block and decreased nerve conduction. This rare complication has occurred following bites of the dog and wood ticks (*Dermacentor variabilis* and *D. andersoni*) in the United States and various other kinds of ticks elsewhere in North America and the world. Weakness begins in the lower extremities 5 to 6 days after the tick has been attached and ascends symmetrically over several days to result in complete paralysis of the extremities and cranial nerves. Deep tendon reflexes are diminished or absent, but sensory examination and findings on lumbar puncture are typically normal. Removal of the tick results in improvement within an hour and usually complete recovery after several days. Failure to remove the tick may lead to death from aspiration or respiratory paralysis. Diagnosis depends on finding the tick, which often is hidden beneath hair. Ticks should be removed by firm traction with a forceps placed near their point of attachment. Rupture of their bodies may permit the escape of fluids containing pathogenic viruses, rickettsiae, borelliae, or the agent of tularemia. An antiserum to saliva of *Ixodes holocyclus*, the usual cause of tick paralysis in Australia, effectively reverses paralysis caused by these ticks.

PEDICULOSIS (LICE INFESTATIONS)

All three species of human lice feed at least once a day on human blood. *Pediculus humanus* var. *capitis* infests the head, *P. humanus* var. *corporis* the clothing, and *Pthirus pubis* mainly the hair of the pubis. Females firmly cement their eggs to hair or clothing. The saliva of lice produces an intensely irritating maculopapular or urticarial rash in sensitized persons.

Head lice are transmitted directly from person to person and occasionally by shared headgear and grooming implements. Prevalence is greatest in school-aged girls who wear long hair; black children are less frequently infested than other children. Excoriations of pruritic lesions on the scalp, neck, and shoulders lead to oozing, crusting, matting of hair, bacterial infections, and regional lymphadenopathy.

Body lice remain in clothing except when feeding and are unable to survive more than a few hours away from the human host. It follows, therefore, that *P. humanus* var. *corporis* mainly infests disaster victims or indigent persons who do not change their clothes. Transmission by direct contact or sharing of clothing and beds is enhanced under crowded conditions. Body lice leave febrile persons or corpses as they become cold, thus facilitating transmission of typhus, louse-borne relapsing fever, and trench fever (see Chap. 138). Pruritic lesions are particularly common around the neckline. Chronic infestations result in postinflammatory hyperpigmentation and thickening of skin known as *vagabond disease*.

The cosmopolitan crab or pubic louse is transmitted mainly by sexual contact but can infest eyelashes, axillary hair, and hair in other sites as well as pubic hair. Intensely pruritic lesions and 2- to 3-mm blue macules (maculae ceruleae) develop at the site of bites. Blepharitis commonly accompanies infestations of the eyelashes.

A suspected diagnosis of pediculosis is confirmed by the finding of nits or adult lice on hairs or in clothing. The preferred treatment is topical permethrin (1%) or 0.5% malathion, which kills both eggs and lice. Alternative agents such as the more toxic 1% lindane and pyrethrins with piperonyl butoxide are not ovicidal and require a second application 1 week later to kill hatching nymphs. Lindane-resistant head lice have been reported. After louse infestations have been treated with insecticide, the hair should be combed with a fine-toothed nit comb to remove nits. Combs and brushes should be disinfected in hot water at 65°C for 5 min or soaked in insecticide for 1 h. Body lice can be eliminated by bathing and topical pediculicides applied from head to foot. Clothes and bedding are deloused by heat sterilization in a dryer at 65°C for 30 min or by fumigation. Pubic lice are treated with topical pediculicides except on the eyelashes, where a coating of petrolatum should be applied for 3 to 4 days.

FLEA INFESTATIONS AND TUNGIASIS

Fleas are wingless insects 2 to 4 mm long that feed on the blood of human beings and other warm-bodied animals. Common human-biting fleas include the dog and cat fleas (*Ctenocephalides* spp.) and the rat flea (*Xenopsylla cheopis*), which inhabit the nests and resting sites of their hosts. Larval fleas feed on pellets of dried host blood that the adult fleas eject from their rectums while feeding. The high-jumping adults attack human beings or other available warm-bodied animals when the usual host abandons or is driven from its nest. The human flea (*Pulex irritans*) infests human bedding and furniture but mainly in relatively humid buildings that lack central heating. Sensitized persons develop erythematous, pruritic papules, urticaria, and occasionally vesicles and bacterial superinfection at the site of the bite. Treatment consists of antihistamines and antipruritics.

Fleas transmit plague, murine typhus, and rat and dog tapeworms. Infestations by fleas are eliminated by frequent cleaning of the nesting sites and bedding of the host or judicious dusting or spraying of insecticides such as pyrethrin, DDT, or malathion.

Human infestations with *Tunga penetrans*, the chigoe flea, sand flea, or jigger, occur in tropical regions of Africa and the Americas. Adults live in sandy soil and burrow under the skin between toes, under nails, or on the soles of bare feet. The fleas engorge on blood and grow from pinpoint to pea size over a 2-week period. The lesions resemble a white pustule with a central black depression and may be pruritic or painful. Occasional complications include tetanus, bacterial infections, and autoamputation of toes. Tungiasis is treated by removal of the intact flea with a sterile needle or scalpel.

MYIASIS

Myiasis refers to infestations by maggots, mainly due to the larvae of metallic-colored screw-worm flies or botflies. Maggots invade living or necrotic tissue or body cavities and produce different clinical syndromes depending on the species of fly.

FURUNCULAR MYIASIS   In forested parts of Central and South America, larvae of *Dermatobia hominis*, the human botfly, produce boil-like subcutaneous nodules 2 to 3 cm in diameter. The adult female captures a mosquito or other bloodsucking insect and deposits her eggs beneath its abdomen. When the carrier insect attacks a human or bovine host several days later, the warmth and moisture of the host's surface stimulate the larvae to hatch and penetrate the skin. After 6 to 12 weeks, the larvae mature and drop to the ground, where they pupate. The African tumbu fly, *Cordylobia anthropophaga*, produces similar lesions. Dozens of eggs are deposited on sand or drying laundry that is contaminated with urine or sweat. Larvae hatch on contact with the body, penetrate the skin, and produce boils from which they emerge 8 or 9 days later. Diagnosis of furuncular myiasis is suggested by discomforting lesions with a central breathing pore that emits bubbles when submerged in water. Tumbu fly larvae can be removed by manual expression after the air pore is coated with petrolatum to suffocate the larvae and induce them to emerge. *Dermatobium* larvae often require surgical excision.

CREEPING DERMAL MYIASIS   Maggots of the horse botfly, *Gasterophilus intestinalis*, do not mature after penetrating human skin but migrate for weeks in the epidermis. The resulting pruritic and serpiginous eruption resembles cutaneous larva migrans caused by *Ancylostoma braziliense*. Horseback riders become infested when

eggs deposited on the flank of the horse hatch against their bare legs. The black spines of the larvae can be identified after mineral oil is smeared over the lesion. Larva are removed with a needle. The larvae of the cattle botfly (*Hypoderma* spp.) invade more deeply and produce boil-like swellings.

WOUND AND BODY CAVITY MYIASIS   Certain flies are attracted to blood and pus, and their newly hatched larvae enter wounds or diseased skin. Some larvae remain superficial and confined to necrotic tissue and were used in the past to debride purulent wounds. Other species, including the screw-worms, *Chrysomyia bezziana* in Asia and Africa and *Cochliomyia hominivorax*, and the flesh fly, *Wohlfahrtia vigil*, in the Americas, invade more deeply into viable tissue and produce large, suppurating lesions. Larvae that infest wounds also may infest body cavities such as the mouth, nose, ears, sinuses, anus, vagina, and lower urinary tract, particularly in unconscious or otherwise debilitated patients. The consequences range from harmless colonization to destruction of the nose, meningitis, and deafness. Treatment involves removal of maggots and debridement of tissue.

OTHER FORMS OF MYIASIS   The maggots responsible for furuncular and wound myiasis also may cause ophthalmomyiasis. Sequelae include nodules in the eyelid, retinal detachment, and destruction of the globe. In addition, the adult sheep botfly, *Oestrus ovis*, may oviposit larvae into the eyes of persons tending sheep and goats and produce a conjunctival infestation and acute conjunctivitis. True intestinal myiasis occurs when fly eggs or larvae of the drone fly, *Eristalis tenax*, are ingested with contaminated food and mature in the gut and cause an enteritis. Most instances in which maggots are found in human feces are the result of larviposition by flesh flies on recently passed stools.

PENTASTOMIASIS

Pentastomids, or tongue worms, are parasites with characteristics of both helminths and arthropods and are classified in a separate phylum. The wormlike adults inhabit the respiratory passages of reptiles and carnivorous mammals. Human infestation with *Linguatula serrata* is common in the Middle East and occurs in the Sudan following ingestion of encysted larval stages in raw liver or lymph nodes of sheep and goats, the intermediate hosts. The larvae migrate to the nasopharynx and produce an acute self-limiting syndrome known as halzoun (Marrara in the Sudan), which is characterized by pain and itching of the throat and ears, coughing, hoarseness, dysphagia, and dyspnea. Severe edema may cause obstruction and necessitate tracheostomy, and ocular invasion has been described. Diagnostic larvae measuring 5 to 10 mm in length are found in the copious nasal discharge or vomitus. Human beings become infected with *Armillifer armillatus* by ingestion of eggs in contaminated food or drink or after handling the definitive host, the African python. Larvae encyst in various organs and rarely cause symptoms unless they compress vital structures or perforate an organ during migration. Cysts occasionally require surgical removal as they enlarge while molting, but they are usually encountered as an incidental finding at autopsy. There are reports of the cutaneous larva migrans syndrome due to other pentastomes (*Reighardia* and *Sebekia* spp.) in Southeast Asia and Central America.

LEECH INFESTATIONS

Medically important leeches are annelid worms that attach to their hosts with chitinous cutting jaws and draw blood with muscular suckers. The medicinal leech, *Hirudo medicinalis*, is still occasionally used to reduce venous congestion in surgical flaps or replanted body parts. This practice has been complicated by wound infections, myonecrosis, and sepsis due to *Aeromonas hydrophila*, which colonizes the gullets of commercially available leeches.

Ubiquitous aquatic leeches that parasitize fish, frogs, and turtles readily attach to the skin of human beings and avidly suck blood. More notorious are the land leeches (*Haemadipsa*) that live in moist vegetation of tropical rain forests. Attachment is usually painless. Hidrudinin, a powerful anticoagulant secreted by the leech, causes continued bleeding after the leech has fallen off. Healing of the wound is slow, and bacterial infections are not uncommon. Several species of aquatic leeches in Africa, Asia, and southern Europe can enter through the mouth, nose, and genitourinary tract and attach to mucosal surfaces as deep as in the esophagus and trachea. Bleeding may be intense. Externally attached leeches are removed by steady gentle traction. Removal is hastened by application of alcohol, salt, vinegar, or a flame to the leech. Internal attachments may be relieved by saline gargles or removal by forceps.

REFERENCES

CHODOSH J, CLARRIDGE J: Ophthalmomyiasis: A review with special reference to *Cochliomyia hominivorax*. Clin Infect Dis 14:444, 1992

DONABEDIAN H, KHAZAN U: Norwegian scabies in a patient with AIDS. Clin Infect Dis 14:162, 1992

DRABICK JJ: Pentastomiasis. Rev Infect Dis 9:1087, 1987

HARWOOD RF, JAMES MT: *Entomology in Human and Animal Health*. New York, Macmillan, 1979.

LINEAWEAVER WC: *Aeromonas hydrophila* infections following clinical use of medicinal leeches: A review of published cases. Blood Coag Fibrinol 2:201, 1991

MEINKING TL, TAPLIN D: Advances in pediculosis, scabies, and other mite infestations. Adv Dermatol 5:131, 1990

SANUSI ID et al: Tungiasis: Report of one case and review of the 14 reported cases in the United States. J Am Acad Dermatol 20:941, 1989

SCHULTZ MW et al: Comparative study of 5% permethrin cream and 1% lindane lotion for the treatment of scabies. Arch Dermatol 126:167, 1990

STRICKLAND GT (ed): *Hunter's Tropical Medicine*, 7th ed. Philadelphia, Saunders, 1991

section 1   Disorders of the heart

186   APPROACH TO THE PATIENT WITH HEART DISEASE

EUGENE BRAUNWALD

The symptoms caused by heart disease result most commonly from myocardial ischemia, from disturbance of the contraction and/or relaxation of the myocardium, from obstruction to blood flow, or from an abnormal cardiac rhythm or rate. Ischemia is manifest most frequently as chest discomfort, while reduction of the pumping ability of the heart commonly leads to weakness and fatigability or, when severe, produces cyanosis, hypotension, syncope, and elevated intravascular pressure behind a failing ventricle; the latter results in abnormal fluid accumulation, which in turn leads to dyspnea, orthopnea, and systemic or pulmonary edema. Obstruction to blood flow, as in valvular stenosis, can cause symptoms resembling those resulting from congestive heart failure, despite normal or near-normal myocardial function. Cardiac arrhythmias often develop suddenly, and the resulting signs and symptoms—palpitation, dyspnea, angina, hypotension, and syncope—generally occur abruptly and may disappear as rapidly as they develop.

A cardinal principle useful in the evaluation of the patient with suspected heart disease is that myocardial or coronary function which may be adequate at rest may be inadequate during exertion. Thus a history of chest discomfort and/or dyspnea which appears only during activity is characteristic of heart disease, while the opposite pattern, i.e., the appearance of these symptoms at rest and their remission during exertion, is rarely observed in patients with organic heart disease.

Patients with cardiocirculatory disease also may be asymptomatic, both at rest and during exertion, but may present an abnormal physical finding, such as a heart murmur, elevated systemic arterial pressure, or an abnormality of the electrocardiogram or of the cardiac silhouette on the chest roentgenogram. Patients may exhibit asymptomatic ischemia on an exercise stress test or an ambulatory electrocardiogram.

Diseases of the heart and circulation are so common and the laity is so well acquainted with the major symptoms resulting from these disorders that patients, and occasionally physicians, erroneously attribute many noncardiac complaints to organic cardiovascular disease. The combination of the widespread fear of heart disease with the deep-seated emotional connotations concerning this organ's function results in the frequent development of symptoms which mimic those of organic disease in persons with normal cardiovascular systems. Sometimes it is difficult to interpret correctly the symptoms of patients with recognized organic cardiovascular disturbances. Such patients, in addition to having symptoms resulting from their disease, also may develop functional complaints referable to the cardiovascular system. The unraveling of symptoms and signs due to organic heart disease from those which are not directly related is an important and challenging task in these patients.

Dyspnea, one of the cardinal manifestations of diminished cardiac reserve, is not limited to disease of the heart but is also characteristic of conditions as diverse as pulmonary disease, marked obesity, and anxiety (Chap. 31). Similarly, chest discomfort may result from a variety of causes other than myocardial ischemia (Chap. 12). Whether heart disease is responsible for these symptoms can frequently be determined by carrying out a careful clinical examination. Noninvasive testing using electrocardiography at rest and during exercise (Chap. 189), echocardiography, roentgenography, and myocardial imaging (Chap. 190) usually provides important additional information to permit the correct interpretation of symptoms; more specialized invasive examinations (catheterization and angiography) are occasionally necessary.

DIAGNOSIS   In every branch of medicine the development of a rational plan of management and the assessment of prognosis are based on a correct diagnostic appraisal. In patients with disorders of the cardiocirculatory system, particular care must be taken to establish not only a correct but also a *complete* diagnosis. As outlined by the New York Heart Association, the elements of a complete cardiac diagnosis include consideration of

1 *The underlying etiology.* Is the disease congenital, infectious, hypertensive, or ischemic in origin?
2 *The anatomic abnormalities.* Which chambers are involved? Which valves are affected? Is there pericardial involvement? Has there been a myocardial infarction?
3 *The physiologic disturbances.* Is an arrhythmia present? Is there evidence of congestive heart failure or of myocardial ischemia?
4 *The extent of functional disability.* How strenuous is the physical activity required to elicit symptoms? The latter should be evaluated in the light of the intensity of therapy.

Two simple examples may serve to illustrate the importance of establishing a complete diagnosis: (1) The identification of myocardial ischemia as the cause of exertional chest discomfort is of great clinical importance. However, the recognition of ischemia is insufficient to develop either a therapeutic strategy or prognosis until the underlying disease process responsible for the myocardial ischemia, e.g., coronary atherosclerosis or aortic stenosis, is identified and a judgment made as to whether other factors which cause an imbalance between myocardial oxygen supply and demand, such as severe anemia, thyrotoxicosis, or supraventricular tachycardia play a contributory role. (2) Determining that heart disease is congenital provides an important starting point, but the decision about whether surgical treatment is advisable depends on the specific anatomic defect present and often on the nature of the physiologic disturbance and the functional impairment as well.

The establishment of a correct and complete cardiac diagnosis often requires the use of six different methods of examination: (1)

history, (2) physical examination (Chap. 188), (3) electrocardiogram (Chap. 189), (4) chest roentgenogram (Chap. 190), (5) noninvasive graphic examinations (echocardiogram, radionuclide and other noninvasive imaging techniques) (Chaps. 190 and 191), and occasionally (6) specialized invasive examinations, i.e., cardiac catheterization, angiocardiography, and coronary arteriography (Chap. 192). In order to be most effective, the results obtained from each of these six modalities should be analyzed independently of one another as well as with the information derived from the other methods clearly in mind. Only in this way can one avoid overlooking a subtle, though important, finding. For example, an electrocardiogram should be obtained in every patient suspected of having heart disease. It may provide the critical clue in establishing the correct diagnosis, e.g., the finding of a moderate atrioventricular conduction disturbance in a patient with unexplained syncope, even when all other methods of examination reveal no abnormal findings. On the other hand, when combined intelligently with the results of other methods of examination, the electrocardiogram may provide essential confirmatory data. Thus the knowledge that a patient has an apical diastolic rumbling murmur may direct particular attention to the P waves, and the recognition of left atrial enlargement electrocardiographically supports the suggestion that the murmur is caused by mitral stenosis. Under these circumstances, the additional finding on the electrocardiogram of right ventricular hypertrophy suggests that pulmonary hypertension is present and that the mitral stenosis is severe.

Family history In obtaining the history of a patient with known or suspected cardiovascular disease, particular attention should be directed to the family history. Familial clustering is common in many forms of heart disease. Genetic transmission may occur, as in hypertrophic cardiomyopathy (Chap. 205), the Marfan syndrome (Chap. 351), and sudden death associated with a prolonged QT syndrome (Chap. 198). In patients with essential hypertension or coronary atherosclerosis, the genetic component may be less obvious but is also of considerable importance. Familial clustering of cardiovascular diseases may occur not only on a genetic basis but also may be related to familial dietary or behavior patterns, such as excessive ingestion of salt or calories or cigarette smoking.

Assessment of functional impairment When an attempt is made to ascertain the severity of functional impairment in a patient with heart disease, it is helpful to ascertain the level of activity and the rate at which it is performed before symptoms develop. Thus breathlessness which occurs after running up two long flights of stairs denotes far less functional impairment than similar symptoms occurring after taking a few steps on the level. Also, the degree of customary physical activity at work and during recreation should be considered. The development of two-flight dyspnea in a marathon runner may be far more significant than the development of one-flight dyspnea in a previously sedentary person. Similarly, the history must include a detailed consideration of the patient's therapeutic regimen. For example, the persistence or development of edema, breathlessness, and other manifestations of heart failure in a patient whose diet is rigidly restricted in sodium content and who is receiving optimal doses of diuretics must be interpreted quite differently from the development of similar manifestations of heart failure in the absence of these measures. In an effort to ascertain the rate of progression of symptoms, and thereby of the severity of the underlying illness, it may be useful to ascertain what, if any, specific tasks the patient could carry out 1 year earlier which he or she cannot carry out now.

Electrocardiogram Although the electrocardiogram is an invaluable aspect of every cardiovascular examination, with the exception of the identification of arrhythmias and of many instances of acute myocardial infarction, it rarely permits establishment of a specific diagnosis. In the absence of other abnormal findings, electrocardiographic changes must not be overinterpreted. The range of normal electrocardiographic findings is wide, and the tracing can be affected significantly by many noncardiac factors, such as age, body habitus, and serum electrolyte concentrations.

Natural history The natural history of cardiovascular disease must be appreciated. Cardiovascular disorders often present acutely, as in a previously asymptomatic patient with extensive coronary atherosclerosis who develops an acute myocardial infarction or the previously asymptomatic patient with hypertrophic cardiomyopathy whose first clinical manifestation is syncope or even sudden death. However, in both instances, the alert physician may recognize the patient at risk of these complications long before they occur and can often take measures to prevent their occurrence. For example, the patient with acute myocardial infarction may well have had risk factors for atherosclerosis for many years. Had these been recognized, their elimination or reduction might have delayed or even prevented the infarction. Similarly, the patient with hypertrophic cardiomyopathy may have had the familial form of this disorder, and a careful family history might have led to an echocardiographic examination and the recognition of the condition long before the acute manifestations.

PITFALLS IN CARDIOVASCULAR MEDICINE Increasing subspecialization in internal medicine and the perfection of advanced diagnostic techniques in cardiology can lead to several undesirable consequences, which can be summarized as follows:

1 Failure by the *noncardiologist* to recognize cardiac manifestations of systemic illnesses. Examples of the latter are (*a*) the Down syndrome (associated with endocardial cushion defect); (*b*) gonadal dysgenesis, i.e., the Turner syndrome (associated with a variety of congenital cardiovascular defects, particularly coarctation of the aorta); (*c*) bony abnormalities of the upper extremities (associated with atrial septal defect in the Holt-Oram syndrome); (*d*) muscular dystrophies (associated with cardiomyopathy); (*e*) hemochromatosis and glycogen storage disease (associated with myocardial infiltration and restrictive cardiomyopathy); (*f*) congenital deafness (associated with prolonged QT interval and serious cardiac arrhythmias); (*g*) Raynaud's disease (associated with primary pulmonary hypertension and coronary vasospasm); (*h*) connective tissue disorders, i.e., the Marfan syndrome, Ehlers-Danlos and Hurler syndromes, and related disorders of mucopolysaccharide metabolism (aortic dilatation, prolapsed mitral valve, a variety of arterial abnormalities); (*i*) chronic hemolytic anemia (cardiac dilatation); (*j*) Refsum's disease (myocardial failure and conduction defects); (*k*) acromegaly (hypertension, accelerated coronary atherosclerosis, conduction defects, cardiomyopathy); (*l*) hyperthyroidism (heart failure, atrial fibrillation); (*m*) hypothyroidism (pericardial effusion, coronary artery disease); (*n*) rheumatoid arthritis (pericarditis, aortic valve disease); (*o*) Whipple's disease (pericarditis and endocarditis); (*p*) scleroderma (cor pulmonale, myocardial fibrosis, pericarditis); (*q*) systemic lupus erythematosus (valvulitis, myocarditis, pericarditis); (*r*) polymyositis (pericarditis, myocarditis); (*s*) sarcoidosis (arrhythmias, cardiomyopathy); (*t*) Fabry's disease (myocardial ischemia, heart failure); and (*u*) exfoliative dermatitis (high-output heart failure). In patients with these and other systemic disorders a detailed clinical and noninvasive examination of the cardiovascular system should be carried out to identify cardiovascular involvement.
2 Failure by the cardiologist to recognize an underlying systemic illness, such as those listed above, among patients with a cardiac disorder. Patients known or suspected of having heart disease require a detailed general assessment and a search for the frequent *noncardiac* manifestations of systemic disorders with cardiovascular manifestations. For example, infective endocarditis should be considered in patients with known congenital or valvular heart disease with fever, anemia, or albuminuria. A cardiovascular abnormality may provide the clue critical to the recognition of some systemic disorders. For instance, in an elderly person, unexplained atrial fibrillation may provide the first clue to the diagnosis of thyrotoxicosis.
3 Overreliance on and overutilization of laboratory tests, particularly invasive techniques for the examination of the cardiovascular system. Catheterization of the right and left sides of the heart,

selective angiography, and coronary arteriography (Chap. 192) provide precise diagnostic information under many circumstances. For example, they aid in establishing a specific anatomic diagnosis and in determining the physiologic consequences of the abnormalities in patients with chest pain of uncertain cause in whom ischemic heart disease is suspected, and in determining the functional significance of valvular abnormalities in patients with rheumatic heart disease being considered for surgical treatment. Although a great deal of attention has been lavished on these specialized examinations, it should be recognized that they serve to *supplement*, not *supplant*, a careful examination carried out by clinical and noninvasive examination. There is an unfortunate tendency to carry out procedures such as coronary arteriography in patients with chest pain suspected of having ischemic heart disease instead of taking a detailed and thoughtful history; although coronary arteriography may establish whether the coronary arteries are obstructed, the results often do not provide a definite answer to the question of whether a patient's complaint of chest pain is clearly attributable to coronary arteriosclerosis. Coronary arteriography is also often carried out unnecessarily in patients with symptoms and signs of mild myocardial ischemia and normal left ventricular function who are not likely to be candidates for coronary bypass surgery. Similarly, catheterization of the left side of the heart is all too frequently employed to determine whether operative treatment of valvular disease is indicated, even before the patient has had a trial of medical therapy.

Despite the enormous value of these invasive tests it must not be overlooked that they entail some small risk to the patient, involve discomfort and substantial cost, and place a strain on existing medical facilities. Therefore, *they should be carried out not as part of a "fishing expedition" or as evidence to the patient and the family that "everything is being done," but only if, after detailed clinical examination and assessment by noninvasive tests, the results of the invasive examination can be expected to modify or aid in the patient's management.*

MANAGEMENT After a complete diagnosis has been established, a number of therapeutic options are usually available. Several examples may be used to demonstrate some of the principles of modern cardiovascular therapeutics:

1 In the absence of evidence for the existence of heart disease, a clear, definitive statement to that effect should be made and the patient should *not* be asked to return at intervals for repeated examinations. If there is no evidence for disease, such attention may lead to the patient developing inappropriate anxiety and fixation on the heart.

2 If there is no evidence of cardiovascular disease but the patient has one or more risk factors for the development of ischemic heart disease (Chap. 208), a plan for their reduction should be developed and the patient should be retested at intervals to assess that he or she is complying and that these risk factors are in fact being reduced.

3 Asymptomatic or mildly symptomatic patients with established valvular heart disease should be evaluated periodically, every 6 to 12 months, by clinical and noninvasive examinations (Chap. 190). Early signs of deterioration of ventricular function can be detected in this manner and in appropriate patients may signify the need for cardiac catheterization and surgical treatment before the development of disabling symptoms, irreversible myocardial damage, and an excessive risk of surgical treatment (Chap. 201).

4 It is critical to establish clear criteria for deciding on the form of treatment (medical, angioplasty, or surgical revascularization) in patients with ischemic heart disease (Chap. 203). Surgical treatment represents a major therapeutic advance in the treatment of this most common form of heart disease, but operation has probably been employed too widely in the United States; the mere presence of angina pectoris and/or the demonstration of critical coronary arterial

narrowing at angiography should not reflexly evoke a decision to treat the patient surgically. Instead, this form of treatment should be limited to those patients with ischemic heart disease in whom it has been demonstrated that surgical treatment is superior to medical treatment.

REFERENCES

BRAUNWALD E (ED): *Heart Disease*, 4th ed. Philadelphia, Saunders, 1992

CHRISTIE LG, CONTI CR: Systematic approach to the evaluation of angina-like chest pain. Am Heart J 102:897, 1981

GOLDMAN L et al: Pitfalls in the serial assessment of cardiac functional status. How a reduction in "ordinary" activity may reduce the apparent degree of cardiac compromise and give a misleading impression of improvement. J Chronic Dis. 35:763, 1982

NEW YORK HEART ASSOCIATION, CRITERIA COMMITTEE: *Nomenclature and Criteria for Diagnosis of Diseases of the Heart and Great Vessels*, 8th ed. Boston, Little, Brown, 1981

PERLOFF K (ED): *Physical Examination of the Heart and Circulation*, 2d ed. Philadelphia, Saunders, 1990.

SAPIRA JD: The history, in *The Art and Science of Bedside Diagnosis*. Baltimore, Urban Schwartzenberg, 1990, pp 9–45

SCHMITT BP et al: The diagnostic usefulness of the history of the patient with dyspnea. J Gen Intern Med 1:386, 1986

SUTTON GC: Symptoms of heart disease, in *Diseases of the Heart*, DG Julian (ed). London, Balliere Tindall, 1989, pp 89–99

187 CELLULAR AND MOLECULAR BIOLOGY OF CARDIOVASCULAR DISEASE

EUGENE BRAUNWALD

Because the principal function of the heart is to serve as a pump, clinical cardiology, since the era of William Harvey, has been deeply rooted in physiology and hemodynamics. The development of electrocardiography at the beginning of this century and the recognition of clinical disturbances of cardiac rhythm led to increasing interest in electrophysiology. Since both the mechanical and the electrical properties of the heart can be altered profoundly by drugs, pharmacology also has provided strong scientific underpinnings to clinical cardiology.

A fuller understanding of cardiac function and dysfunction will ultimately require studies at the cellular, molecular, and genetic levels. However, such investigations have been retarded by the absence of any cell line of adult, fully differentiated myocytes that can be readily grown in vitro, manipulated, and studied. Perhaps for this reason, cellular biology and molecular genetics have been slower to have an impact on cardiovascular disease than on some other branches of medicine, such as hematology, oncology, endocrinology, and infectious diseases. However, application of these techniques to cardiovascular science has now gained momentum, and these efforts are beginning to influence the care of patients with cardiovascular disease. Several examples of this influence are considered in this chapter and include advances in understanding the process of myocardial hypertrophy, the constituents of the bloodstream such as apolipoproteins, and noncardiac cells, including vascular smooth-muscle cells, endothelial cells, and platelets. Discussed elsewhere (Chap. 316) are advances in thrombolytic therapy which also have resulted from studies at the cellular and molecular levels.

HYPERTROPHY

MYOCARDIAL HYPERTROPHY One of the most remarkable and important capacities of the heart is to adapt both acutely and chronically to changes in hemodynamic load. *Acute* adaptations are mediated by the two mechanisms discussed in Chap. 194: (1) an alteration in the number of cross-bridges that cycle between the actin and myosin myofilaments, which in turn is dependent on the length of the myocardial sarcomeres (this adaptation expresses, at the molecular level, Starling's law of the heart), and (2) changes in contractility mediated by the adrenergic neurotransmitter norepinephrine via adrenergic receptors. The degree of activation of these receptors ultimately regulates the concentration of calcium ions near the contractile proteins and, thereby, myocardial contractility. In contrast, with *chronic* hemodynamic overload, as in hypertension, valvular heart disease, and many forms of congenital heart disease, *myocardial hypertrophy* is the major adaptive response. As the ventricle hypertrophies, new sarcomeres are added to each myocyte, protein synthesis is augmented, and sometimes protein degradation declines. The fraction of total cardiac protein composed of myofibrillar proteins increases in hypertrophy and subsequently declines as heart failure supervenes. Exactly how mechanical load is converted into growth, a process that might be termed *mechanogrowth coupling*, is not fully understood. When myocytes are stretched in vitro, an increase in mRNA and protein synthesis takes place. Thus myocytes appear to be able to *sense* external load and to undergo hypertrophy, perhaps involving a release of growth factors.

The imposition of a pressure load on the ventricle is accompanied by an increase in the expression of messenger RNA (mRNA) that codes for various contractile proteins, and these increased levels of mRNA are responsible for the increase in myocardial protein synthesis. Proteins often occur in families of closely related isoforms, the expression of which is regulated in a tissue-specific and developmentally specific manner. In experimental animals, the hypertrophic response to pressure overload involves the reappearance in the adult heart of contractile protein isoforms characteristic of the fetus such as the V_3 form of beta-myosin heavy chain ("slow myosin"), which has a low ATPase activity and promotes a slower, more sustained contraction requiring less energy than the V_1 form ("fast myosin"). The fetal isoforms of alpha actin and tropomyosin and the mRNA of atrial natriuretic peptide (ANP) are also reexpressed when left ventricular hypertrophy is induced. This reexpression of fetal protein genes appears to represent a general adaptive response to hemodynamic overload in experimental animals.

The mechanisms of hypertrophy depend on the inciting stimulus. In contrast to the cardiac hypertrophy resulting from hemodynamic overload, the hypertrophy of hyperthyroidism is *not* accompanied by the induction of fetal forms of contractile protein genes or of the ANP gene. Thyroid hormone acts directly via nuclear receptors to regulate myosin heavy chain gene expression at the transcriptional level, causing an accumulation of alpha-myosin heavy chain mRNA, and inhibits the expression of beta-myosin heavy chain mRNA, thereby increasing the level of myosin isoenzyme V_1 and bringing about a more rapid contraction. Hypothyroid hearts have higher levels of beta-myosin heavy chain mRNA and the V_3 myosin isoform and lower levels of the mRNA encoding Ca^{2+} ATPase and Ca^{2+} release channels of sarcoplasmic reticulum.

Some of the changes in gene expression in ventricular hypertrophy may involve proto-oncogenes, which are normal cellular homologues of transforming genes carried by oncogenic retroviruses (Chap. 63). Three major classes of proto-oncogenes are induced rapidly by pressure overload: (1) proto-oncogenes such as c-*cis* that encode peptide growth factors, such as the beta chain of platelet-derived growth factor (PDGF), (2) proto-oncogenes such as c-*myc* and c-*fos*, which code for nuclear proteins that regulate transcription of a variety of genes which influence cell growth, and (3) proto-oncogenes such as c-*ras*, which code for cytoplasmic proteins that bind to guanine nucleotides and regulate other intracellular signaling systems. The reinduction of genes normally expressed in fetal life, such as the fetal isoforms of myosin and ANP (in the ventricle), is a later event.

Stimuli that increase intracellular cyclic AMP (cAMP) and intracellular Ca^{2+} (such as beta-adrenergic agonists) or those which enhance the turnover of inositol phospholipids (such as angiotensin II and alpha-adrenergic agonists) have direct trophic effect on cardiac myocytes when studied in vitro. Norepinephrine and angiotensin II augment expression of proto-oncogenes, stimulate protein synthesis, and induce the synthesis of fetal isoforms of actin and myosin. This action of the alpha-adrenergic agonists and angiotensin II occurs though G protein–coupled receptors and the subsequent activation of phospholipases and the protein kinase cascade (see below).

In addition to the growth of myocytes, the interstitium also participates in pressure-overload hypertrophy, which is associated with hyperplasia of fibroblasts and the deposition of excess and altered types of extracellular collagen. The relief of hemodynamic overload, either surgically or pharmacologically, usually results in partial regression of myocyte hypertrophy but not necessarily in regression of interstitial proliferation.

There are many potential applications to cardiology of the growing understanding of the mechanisms involved in myocyte hypertrophy. For example, overexpression of the c-*myc* proto-oncogene in the heart of transgenic mice results in cardiac enlargement due to myocyte hyperplasia. Treatment of animals with angiotensin-converting enzyme (ACE) inhibitors has been shown to cause regression of cardiac hypertrophy and interstitial fibrosis induced by hemodynamic overload. Investigation of these phenomena also might reveal the mechanism by which compensatory hypertrophy sometimes leads to myocardial failure and could suggest measures to prevent this complication. Ultimately, this knowledge also could lead to the development of a method for stimulating myocardial hypertrophy or even myocyte hyperplasia after cell death has occurred consequent to myocardial infarction or viral myocarditis.

VASCULAR WALL   The renin-angiotensin system in the vascular wall may be involved in the development of hypertrophy of vascular smooth muscle. Angiotensinogen mRNA in blood vessel walls may be elevated in chronic hypertension. The addition of angiotensin II to cultures of vascular smooth-muscle cells causes the rapid activation of the c-*fos* proto-oncogene, which may mediate angiotensin II–induced hypertrophy in smooth-muscle cells in vivo. Indeed, angiotensin II induces hypertrophy of arterial smooth-muscle cells in vitro, in association with rapid induction in c-*fos*, c-*myc*, and c-*jun* mRNA levels followed by marked increases in the expression of the α chain of PDGF. This hypertrophy of vascular smooth muscle can be blocked by ACE inhibitors. The gene for the PDGF receptor has been cloned; the PDGF receptor mediates the mitogenic effects of this substance on vascular smooth-muscle (and other) cells. The PDGF receptor has a structure similar to a family of growth factor receptors that have tyrosine kinase activity. The PDGF receptor interacts with the c-*ras* proto-oncogene product and activates phospholipase C.

Many growth factors for vascular smooth muscle, such as angiotensin II, vasopressin, PDGF, and epidermal growth factor, are also vasoconstrictors. These considerations may be of significance in selecting or designing antihypertensive drugs. Indeed, ACE inhibitors are more potent in causing regression of left ventricular hypertrophy than are direct-acting vasodilators such as hydralazine.

INHERITED DISORDERS OF THE CARDIOVASCULAR SYSTEM

A number of disorders of the cardiovascular system are inherited as single-gene disorders, but many more are multigene disorders. Efforts are underway to identify the genes responsible for hypertrophy using the technique of genetic linkage (or cosegregation) analysis (see Chap. 61). This technique is used to map the loci of genes that are tightly linked to a specific phenotype by making use of restriction fragment length polymorphisms (RFLPs) which are due to DNA sequence differences between individuals.

HYPERTROPHIC CARDIOMYOPATHY (See Chap. 205) This condition is familial in slightly more than half of all patients; it is transmitted as an autosomal dominant trait with almost complete

FIGURE 187-1   A diagram of the beta cardiac (myosin heavy chain) gene and the location of ten different missense mutations that cause (familial hypertrophic cardiomyopathy). The gene is divided into 40 exons (*small boxes*), and the locations of the exons that encode the head and rod regions of the myosin heavy chain polypeptide are indicated. Sequences that encode the initiation of gene transcription (ATG), ATPase activity (ATP), actin binding (actin I and actin II), myosin light chain binding (MLC), and hinge function (Hinge) are indicated. Mutations result in amino acid substitutions (designated by triple-letter code) and usually result in a change in charge (indicated). The ban above exon 40 represents a deletion. (*Modified from CE Seidman et al, in E Braunwald (ed), Heart Disease: Clinical Update 4, 4th ed, Philadelphia, Saunders, 1992; modified from H Watkins et al, N Engl J Med 326:1108, 1992.*)

penetrance. Linkage analysis for markers of variations in DNA sequence in affected family members has identified mutations in band 1 of chromosome 14 in about half of all patients with familial hypertrophic cardiomyopathy (FHC). One of the principal genes that encodes adult ventricular myosin heavy chain (MHC), the cardiac MHC gene, is also located in band 1 of chromosome 14, and it appears that mutations in this gene are associated with those cases of FHC linked to this chromosome (Fig. 187-1). Eight missense mutations involving a change of a single nucleotide base pair that alters an amino acid in the beta cardiac MHC have been described. When found in one family member, the same mutation occurs in all affected family members, and identical mutations have been observed in different family members. FHC is genetically heterogeneous; approximately one-half of the cases of FHC are *not* linked to mutations of the beta cardiac MHC gene on chromosome 14, and the absence of a mutation in this gene does not exclude the diagnosis of FHC. There is a wide range of phenotypic expressions of FHC, and genetic typing using circulating lymphocytes has identified mutations of the beta cardiac MHC gene associated with more serious clinical outcomes, including early death.

FHC with clinical features indistinguishable from those with mutations in the beta cardiac MHC gene also has been mapped to chromosome 1. Three genes encoding contractile proteins on the short arm of chromosome 1 (isoforms of actin, tropomyosin, and troponin) are possible genes for this FHC locus.

Genetic typing of FHC should make possible prenatal diagnosis, the identification of asymptomatic persons with FHC, prognostic stratification, genetic counseling, and ultimately, the early initiation of treatment.

DUCHENNE'S MUSCULAR DYSTROPHY (See also Chap. 385) This X-linked recessive skeletal muscle disorder is sometimes associated with cardiomyopathy and heart failure, as well as with atrioventricular and interventricular conduction disorders and a variety of arrhythmias and sudden death. The gene responsible for this disorder has been mapped to the X chromosome; it is large, spans more than 2.5×10^6 base pairs, and encodes a large (427 kDa) protein termed *dystrophin*. Mutations of this gene may cause dystrophin to be absent from the transverse tubules of skeletal and cardiac muscle of patients

with Duchenne's muscular dystrophy. Its absence in the myocardium is directly or indirectly responsible for the cardiomyopathy that frequently occurs in this condition.

MYOTONIC MUSCULAR DYSTROPHY (See also Chap. 385) This autosomal dominant defect is frequently associated with replacement of the cardiac conduction system with fatty and fibrous tissue resulting in cardiac conduction disturbances and sudden death and occasionally in a cardiomyopathy. The responsible gene has been mapped to chromosome 19. The abnormal protein responsible for myotonic dystrophy has not yet been isolated, but its identification should provide new insights into the mechanism of conduction disturbances in the Purkinje tissue.

LONG QT SYNDROME (See also Chap. 198)   This autosomal dominant disorder predisposes to ventricular tachycardia and fibrillation, episodes of syncope, and sudden death. In one large family the syndrome has been linked to the Harvey *ras*-1 gene located on chromosome 11. This gene is involved in the regulation of cardiac potassium channels and may thereby be responsible for delayed repolarization, the hallmark of this syndrome.

MARFAN SYNDROME (See also Chap. 351)   This condition exhibits simple Mendelian autosomal dominant inheritance with variable expression; approximately 15 percent of patients represent de novo mutations. This disorder of connective tissue is associated with numerous life-threatening cardiovascular manifestations, including aortic dissection, aortic aneurysm, myxomatous degeneration, and regurgitation of the aortic and mitral valves.

The connective tissue of patients with the Marfan syndrome has reduced content of microfibrils, of which a large (350 kDa) connective tissue glycoprotein *fibrillin* is an important constituent. The gene for fibrillin has been mapped to chromosome 15 and is tightly linked to the Marfan syndrome. There appears to be genetic heterogeneity of fibrillins, which may be responsible for the phenotypic variations in the Marfan syndrome. Mutation of a second gene for fibrillin, on chromosome 5, is responsible for a condition resembling the Marfan syndrome.

The identification of the genetic defects in the Marfan syndrome should allow genetic diagnosis and the commencement of therapy prior to the development of clinical manifestations.

ADRENERGIC AND MUSCARINIC RECEPTORS AND G PROTEINS (See also Chaps. 68 and 69 and Fig. 187-2)

Cardiac automaticity, excitability, and contractility are controlled by transmembrane signals, which involve four components: (1) cell surface receptors which are coupled to (2) guanine nucleotide regulatory (G) proteins, which in turn activate (3) effectors, such as ion channels or intracellular enzymes, which generate (4) the second messengers cAMP and inositol trisphosphate. Plasma membrane receptors bind ligands, including drugs and neurotransmitters, and mediate their interaction with cells (see Chap. 69). There are important functional and topographic analogies and amino acid sequence homologues between beta-adrenergic receptors, muscarinic (cholinergic) receptors, and rhodopsin, the light receptor in the rods of the retina. These receptors are all glycoproteins with seven membrane-spanning domains (Fig. 187-3). The receptors exist in multiple forms (isoforms), each with either a specific location or function. For example, the beta-adrenergic receptor exists in three forms with localization of the beta$_1$ receptor in the heart, beta$_2$ receptors in the airways, and beta$_3$ receptors in adipocytes. The genes coding for all three isoforms of beta-adrenergic receptors and the five muscarinic receptors have been cloned.

Beta-adrenergic and alpha$_1$-adrenergic receptors are coupled to different classes of G proteins. The binding of agonists such as norepinephrine released by adrenergic neurons or of infused dobutamine to the beta-adrenergic receptor—G protein complex results in a conformational change of the G stimulatory protein (G$_s$). This change in turn activates effectors such as adenylate cyclase that increase cAMP, a stimulant of myocardial contractility. G proteins couple alpha$_1$-adrenergic receptors to the activation of phospholipase C, which in turn breaks down a cell membrane phospholipid (PIP$_2$) into inositol trisphosphate (IP$_3$) and diacylglycerol. IP$_3$ in turn liberates calcium ions from intracellular stores and thereby stimulates cardiac contractility. Diacylglycerol activates a Ca^{2+}-sensitive protein kinase

C which appears to regulate myocyte ion channels, myocardial hypertrophy, and gene expression. Stimulation of muscarinic and adenosine receptors [through the inhibitory G protein (G$_i$)] inhibits adenylate cyclase and reduces the formation of cAMP.

Prolonged binding of beta-adrenergic agonists to beta receptors results in the phosphorylation of portions of the carboxy-terminal intracellular domain of the receptor, which in turn interacts with a cellular protein, *arrestin;* this protein interferes with beta receptor–G protein association and hence desensitizes the receptor. More prolonged agonist exposure results in receptor degradation or down-regulation. This process occurs in chronic heart failure (Chap. 194) consequent to the chronic exposure of the failing heart to excessive concentrations of the adrenergic agonist norepinephrine. The reduced beta-adrenergic responsiveness seen in chronic heart failure is also associated with increased levels of G$_i$, which may play a role in the pathogenesis of heart failure.

An understanding of the molecular structure of cardiac receptors and of the genes which encode them is likely to lead to more rational design of drugs that can modify cardiac function by acting on these receptors.

CALCIUM CHANNELS   Calcium ions play a unique role in a variety of cellular functions, in particular contraction of cardiac and vascular smooth muscle (Chap. 194). Calcium enters cardiac cells through voltage-sensitive calcium channels (see Fig. 187-2) that are controlled by transmembrane electrical potentials and open during depolarization of the sarcolemma. Interaction of the Ca^{2+} channel with the catalytic subunit of cAMP-dependent protein kinase results in activation of the calcium channels, increasing the probability of their opening and thereby increasing influx of calcium into myocytes and enhancing the force of cardiac contraction. This explains, in part, the positive inotropic actions of the beta-adrenergic agonists and of the phosphodiesterase inhibitors, both of which enhance levels of cAMP.

The (L-type) cardiac calcium channels appear to be large aqueous

---

FIGURE 187-2   Ion transport through the sarcolemma of a myocyte. The Na$^+$ channel of the heart muscle cell opens briefly at the start of an action potential, permitting an influx of Na$^+$. The Na$^+$ channel can be blocked by tetrodotoxin (TTX) or by type I antiarrhythmic agents (see Chap. 198). Depolarization of the sarcolemma leads to Ca^{2+} influx through the Ca^{2+} channel, which is sensitive to the change in potential. The Ca^{2+} channel can be blocked by the calcium entry blockers. D, diltiazem; V, verapamil; DHP, dihydropyridines. Repolarization of the membrane results principally from the opening of K$^+$ channels and the efflux of K$^+$. Ca^{2+} is removed from the cell by the Na$^+$/Ca^{2+} exchanger and by a Ca^{2+}-ATPase (an energy-requiring process). The Na$^+$ pump (Na$^+$,K$^+$-ATPase) removes Na$^+$ which has flowed into the cell and returns K$^+$ to the cell by an energy-requiring process; it may be blocked by digitalis (DIG).

Two types of receptors modulate ionic pathways. Beta-adrenergic receptors (which are one kind of type 2 receptor) stimulate the production of the second messenger cyclic AMP which by causing phosphorylation (P) allows the Ca^{2+} channel to open. Muscarinic cholinergic receptors (one kind of type 1 receptor) inhibit cyclic AMP production and also activate phospholipase C, the enzyme producing the second messenger inositol trisphosphate (IP$_3$), which in smooth-muscle cells mobilizes intracellular calcium.

Abbreviations: DIG, digitalis glycoside (Na$^+$,K$^+$-ATPase inhibitor); R$_1$ and R$_2$, binding proteins for the respective receptor types; AC, adenylate cyclase; Ni (AC-inhibiting) and Ns (AC-stimulating) nucleotide binding G proteins (G$_i$ and G$_s$, respectively); PhC, phospholipase C; PIP$_2$, phosphotidylinositol diphosphate, a membrane phospholipid. *(Reproduced with permission from U Ruegg, Sandorama 2:5, 1987.)*

FIGURE 187-3 Structure of the human beta₂-adrenergic receptor as it may be organized within the membrane. Open circles represent amino acids that are identical to those of hamster beta₂-adrenergic receptor. *(Reproduced with permission from Dohlman et al, Biochemistry 26:2664, 1987.)*

pores through which the calcium ions move, probably in single file. Their primary structure has been elucidated by cDNA cloning. These channels are quite selective for calcium ions under physiologic conditions and are composed of several subunits, the largest of which has a molecular weight of 243 kDa and binds calcium channel antagonists. Prolongation of the action potential occurs often in hypertrophied myocytes and may be responsible for arrhythmias in patients with heart failure. This prolongation may be due to delays in the inactivation of the L-type calcium channels. Three physically associated but distinct sites in the channels bind the three classes of calcium antagonists—nifedipine, verapamil, and diltiazem (Chap. 203). The cDNAs (DNAs complementary to their mRNA) encoding the calcium channels have been cloned, and their predicted sequences have been determined. This new understanding of the structure and function of calcium channels should make possible the design of drugs to influence the function of these channels with greater specificity, thereby increasing the ability to control function of the myocardium and of vascular smooth muscle.

SARCOLEMMAL ATPase One of the most important membrane proteins is the Na⁺,K⁺-ATPase (see Fig. 187-2) which plays a critical role in establishing sodium and potassium gradients across cell membranes. This enzyme catalyzes the reaction that extrudes sodium and transports potassium into the cell against concentration gradients. This process requires the hydrolysis of ATP and is critical to the function of cardiac (and other excitable) tissue by controlling membrane potentials. Phosphorylation and ATP binding sites are on the cytoplasmic component of the enzyme, and the cardiac glycoside binding site is located on the extracellular component. Knowledge of the primary structure of the enzyme may allow the design of inhibitors perhaps more potent and/or more selective than the cardiac glycosides.

APOLIPOPROTEINS AND ATHEROGENESIS

Abnormalities in the number or function of the low-density lipoprotein (LDL) receptors are responsible for some forms of atherosclerosis (Chaps. 208 and 344). Abnormalities of the *apolipoproteins,* many

of which are genetic, may play more frequent roles in atherogenesis. At least 10 apolipoproteins are embedded in the surface of the spherical lipoprotein particles that carry the lipids in the bloodstream and are encoded by genes localized to chromosomes 1, 2, 6, 11, and 19 (the LDL receptor gene is also on chromosome 19). Amino acid sequences suggest that several of these apolipoproteins are derived from a common ancestral gene. The major functions of apolipoproteins are to serve as (1) ligands that interact with cellular receptors for the lipoprotein particles, (2) cofactors of enzymes involved in lipid metabolism, and (3) structural components of the lipoproteins.

High-density lipoproteins (HDL) take up excess cholesterol from cells, and the risk of the development of ischemic heart disease is related inversely to the concentration of circulating HDL (Chaps. 208 and 344). Apolipoproteins (apo) AI, CIII, and AIV are three HDL apolipoproteins encoded by genes clustered on chromosome 11. Several disorders are associated with mutations of these apolipoproteins, leading to a defect in the synthesis or function of HDL and the development of premature atherosclerosis. For example, apo AI serves as a cofactor for the enzyme lecithin cholesterol acyl transferase (LCAT) which catalyzes the reaction that converts cholesterol taken up by the HDL particle into the form in which it is transported, i.e., cholesteryl ester. Some variants of apo AI are defective for this cofactor activity, thereby preventing the normal function of HDL and causing premature atherosclerosis.

Apo E is one of the principal constituents of very low density lipoproteins (VLDL) and of chylomicron remnants, the latter particles having potential atherogenic activity. Three alleles of the apo E gene, located on chromosome 19, have been described. Subjects who are homozygous for the E^2 allele, which encodes apo E², have decreased clearance of VLDL and chylomicron remnants from the circulation, presumably because apo E² fails to bind normally to lipoprotein receptors. In addition, persons with an E^2 allele have reduced lipolytic conversion of VLDL to LDL with lower plasma concentrations of the latter. Since apo E³ and apo E⁴ normally activate lipoprotein lipase, normolipidemic persons with the apo E phenotype E²/E² or E²/E³ have higher VLDL and lower LDL levels than persons with E³/E³ phenotype. The E^4 allele enhances conversion of VLDL to LDL, leading to decreased VLDL and increased LDL levels in phenotypes E³/E⁴ and E⁴/E⁴. Epidemiologic studies have found that apo E⁴ rather than apo E² is associated with coronary heart disease. The E^2 allele plays a permissive role in the development of type 3 hyperlipoproteinemia, a condition associated with the development of xanthomas and premature atherosclerosis (Chap. 208).

Elevation of the plasma concentration of Lp(a) (referred to as "lipoprotein little a") appears to be another risk factor for the development of premature atherosclerosis. Its protein components consist of apo B100 linked to apo(a). It shares similarities with LDL as a B100 cholesterol-rich lipoprotein. Six inherited apo(a) isoproteins and a series of alleles at a single gene locus control the apo(a) phenotypes and appear to determine the Lp(a) concentration. An interesting clue to the mechanism by which Lp(a) accelerates atherosclerosis has emerged. Through cDNA cloning and the deduced protein structure, it has been shown that apo(a) is a deformed relative of plasminogen, the precursor of the proteolytic enzyme plasmin, which dissolves fibrin clots (Chap. 316). Apo(a) contains multiple copies of kringle 4 (a portion of the plasminogen molecule in the shape of the Danish pastry known as *kringle*) followed by kringle 5 and the protease domain. This strong resemblance between a lipoprotein and plasminogen may provide a link between lipids, the clotting system, and atherogenesis. Microthrombi containing fibrin on the vessel wall become incorporated into atherosclerotic plaques. Kringle 4 of plasminogen normally binds to fibrin during fibrinolysis. Apo(a), with many copies of this kringle, also could bind to fibrin in microthrombi in the vessel wall. Following endothelial damage, Lp(a) may insinuate itself into the arterial wall, inhibiting the cleavage of fibrin in microthrombi by competing with plasminogen for access to fibrin.

Discussed above are just three of many possible examples showing how the genes encoding apolipoproteins can play a critical role in determining the risk for the development of atherosclerosis. Eventually, it may prove to be cost-effective to attempt to identify genetic defects of apolipoproteins (as well as of the LDL receptor) in childhood and to use a preventive approach on these subjects.

ENDOTHELIUM

For many years the endothelium, the monolayer of cells in direct contact with blood, was considered to be a relatively inert, smooth boundary between the blood and the vascular wall (Fig. 187-4). In fact, endothelial cells are quite active metabolically and normally produce a number of substances that affect the vascular lumen as well as platelets.

The first and best known of the endothelial vasodilators is prostacyclin (PGI_2) (see Chap. 70), which also inhibits the aggregation of platelets. The action of PGI_2 involves the activation of adenylyl cyclase and formation of cAMP. When stimulated by a large number of substances, including ATP and ADP, acetylcholine, thrombin, neurotransmitters, and serotonin, the normal endothelium also releases a labile, highly diffusible vasodilator termed *endothelium-derived relaxing factor* (EDRF), which appears to be nitric oxide (NO) or a relatively more stable adduct thereof. Normal endothelium also releases EDRF when stimulated by the shear stress of flowing blood, thereby controlling the lumen of arteries and arterioles in relation to the blood flow through the vessel. EDRF stimulates soluble guanylyl cyclase, which catalyzes the formation of cyclic GMP (cGMP) and, in turn, relaxes vascular smooth muscle. EDRF also inhibits adhesion

FIGURE 187-4 Current concepts of endothelium-derived factors and their modulation of vascular smooth-muscle contraction: Endothelium-derived relaxing factor (EDRF), a potent vasodilator of the underlying smooth muscle, increases cyclic GMP (cGMP) levels through activation of soluble guanylate cyclase. Prostacyclin (PGI_2) is another vasodilator released from the endothelium but whose effects depend on elevation of cyclic AMP (cAMP) through activation of adenylate cyclase. EDRF and PGI_2 may act synergistically in relaxing vascular smooth muscle and inhibiting platelet aggregation. The endothelial cells also secrete a hyperpolarizing factor (EDHF), the exact nature of which is unknown and which also has a vasodilator action. There are at least two endothelium-derived contracting factors; one is indomethacin-insensitive ($EDCF_1$) and may be endothelin, while the other is indomethacin-sensitive ($EDCF_2$) and may be superoxide anion. ACh, acetylcholine; 5-HT, 5-hydroxytryptamine (serotonin); ADP, adenosine diphosphate; AA, arachidonic acid; +, synergism or facilitation; −, inhibition; ?, exact nature unknown; M, muscarinic receptor; S, serotoninergic receptor; P, purinergic receptor; T, thrombin receptor; V, vasopressinergic receptor. *(Reproduced with permission from P Vanhoutte and Shimokawa, Circulation 80:1, 1989.)*

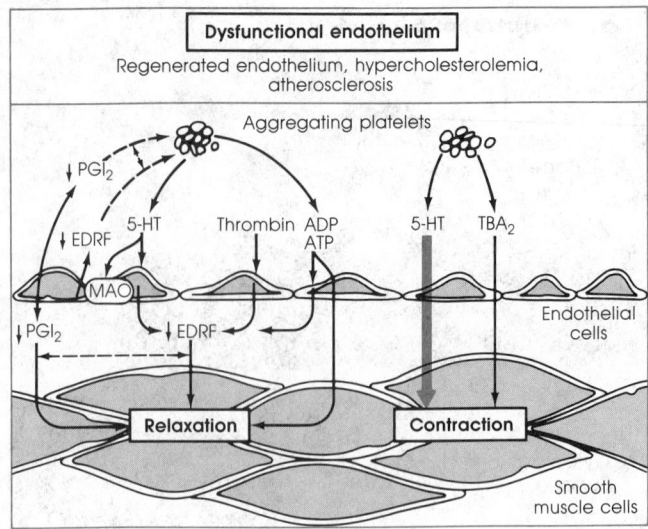

FIGURE 187-5 Responses of dysfunctional endothelium. The endothelium is dysfunctional when it is in a regenerated state, in the presence of hypercholesterolemia, hypertension, or atherosclerosis, releasing less endothelium-derived relaxing factor (EDRF), whereas the ability of the smooth muscle to contract is unaltered. As a result, in endothelial dysfunction smooth-muscle contraction predominates. In atherosclerosis, the production of both EDRF and prostacyclin (PGI_2) are reduced, and their synergistic actions against aggregating platelets may not occur, enhancing platelet aggregation. This may lead to thrombus formation, enhanced vascular contraction, and atherogenesis. 5-HT, 5-hydroxytryptamine (serotonin); ADP, adenosine diphosphate; ATP, adenosine triphosphate; TBA2, thromboxane A_2; MAO, monomine oxidase; ms, inhibition; +, synergism. *(Reproduced with permission from Vanhoutte and Shimokawa, Circulation 80:1, 1989.)*

and aggregation of platelets, an action apparently also mediated by cGMP. EDRF and prostacyclin interact synergistically to dilate blood vessels and inhibit platelet aggregation.

When the endothelium is destroyed or damaged (Fig. 187-5), as in atherosclerotic plaques, EDRF production may be impaired, thereby permitting coronary vasoconstriction in the vicinity of such plaques. Moreover, subtle damage to the endothelium, as in hypertension, some forms of hyperlipidemia, reperfusion after ischemia, and regenerating endothelium after mechanical trauma, leads to defective release of EDRF. On the other hand, the eicosapentaenoic and docosahexaenoic acids in fish oils stimulate the production of EDRF, perhaps explaining the putative antiatherogenic properties of these substances. A third endothelial product with antiplatelet properties is the ectoADPase located on the luminal surface. This enzyme degrades ADP, thereby limiting its access to and activation of platelets.

Endothelium also synthesizes *thrombomodulin*, a glycoprotein with a molecular weight of 105 kDa which is localized to the luminal side of the vascular endothelium and which serves as an endothelial receptor for thrombin. When bound to thrombomodulin, thrombin loses its hemostatic activity (conversion of fibrinogen to fibrin, stimulation of platelets), the rate at which it is inactivated by antithrombin is accelerated, and its activation of protein C, a naturally occurring anticoagulant and profibrinolytic substance, is enhanced.

Endothelium releases at least two vasoconstrictors. One is a product of cyclooxygenase activity that appears to be responsible for hypoxia-induced vascular contraction, while the other is an extremely potent 21-amino-acid peptide called *endothelin*. The expression of the gene for endothelin appears to be inhibited by the shear stress of flowing blood, a mechanism that acts in concert with the release of EDRF by the same stimulus to enhance vessel diameter as flow increases. In hypertension, EDRF release is impaired, whereas the release of endothelin may be augmented, presumably aggravating this condition. Like PDGF, endothelin is both a vasoconstrictor and a smooth-muscle mitogen.

In early atherosclerosis, endothelial injury or dysfunction leads to attenuated vasodilator responses and to enhanced platelet deposition on the arterial wall. If unopposed by EDRF and prostacyclin, serotonin and thromboxane A_2 released from the deposited platelets cause arterial constriction and spasm in the coronary arterial system. The adhesion and aggregation of platelets and the enhancement of the atherosclerotic process are also promoted by the release of these platelet products.

ANGIOGENESIS

Endothelial cells also secrete a group of growth factors that are mitogenic for endothelium and can induce formation of new blood vessels (angiogenesis). Angiogenic stimuli cause the elongation and proliferation of endothelial cells and the generation of new vessels. A group of angiogenic mitogens, which are heparin-binding peptides related to endothelial cell growth factors, has been identified. The amino acid sequences of several of these growth factors have been deduced by cloning and analysis of their genes.

Angiogenesis is of considerable pathogenic significance. Folkman has postulated that the growth of tumors depends on an adequate blood supply, which in turn is dependent on the growth of new vessels into the tumors; the latter is stimulated by angiogenesis factor(s) secreted by the tumor. Inhibition of angiogenesis can cause tumor regression in animal models. Abnormal angiogenesis may be involved in diverse disease states, including diabetic retinopathy, neovascular glaucoma, rheumatoid arthritis, and psoriasis.

The development of new vessels in the heart, i.e., of the coronary collateral circulation, is of critical importance in protecting the myocardium from the consequences of coronary obstruction. The extent of the collateral circulation varies enormously among patients with similar degrees of coronary arterial narrowing, and this difference may be related in part to differences in the production of angiogenic factors. It has been speculated that the introduction of purified angiogenic factors directly into ischemic myocardium might enhance the development of collaterals, accelerate the healing of the necrotic tissue, and prevent infarct expansion and cardiac dilatation. Angiogenesis also may be deleterious. Coronary atheroma are highly vascularized by a fragile capillary network, and rupture of these newly formed capillaries when they are exposed to high intravascular pressures may lead to hemorrhage into atherosclerotic plaques and coronary occlusion.

CONCLUSIONS

The applications of cellular and molecular biology to studies of the myocardium, vascular wall, platelets, and lipoproteins have already increased greatly our understanding of the fundamental abnormalities in cardiovascular disease. In the future these approaches are likely to improve the diagnosis of patients with genetic disorders causing cardiac disease, help to identify individuals at risk of developing these disorders, thereby leading to the institution of preventive measures, and provide new agents for the treatment and prevention of cardiovascular diseases.

REFERENCES

BOHELER KR, SCHWARTZ K: Gene expression in cardiac hypertrophy. Trends Cardiovasc Med 2:176, 1992

BRAUNWALD E: On future directions for cardiology: The Paul Dudley White lecture. Circulation 77:13, 1988

CHIEN KR: Molecular advances in cardiovascular biology. Science 260:916, 1993

COHEN SA, BARCHI RL: Cardiac sodium channel structure and function. Trends Cardiovasc Med 2:133, 1992

DIETZ HC et al: Marfan syndrome caused by a recurrent de novo missense mutation in the fibrillin gene. Nature 352:337, 1991

FOLKMAN J, WEISZ PB: Control of angiogenesis, in Biocatalysis and Biometrics, JD Burrington, DS Clark (eds). Washington, American Chemical Society, ACS Symposium Series 392, 1989, pp 19–32

GENEST J JR: Genetic lipid disorders in cardiovascular disease. Trends Cardiovasc Med 2:140, 1992

KEATING M et al: Linkage of a cardiac arrhythmia, the long QT syndrome, and the Harvey ras-1 gene. Science 252:704, 1991

KLUG D et al: Role of mechanical and hormonal factors in cardiac remodeling and the biologic limits of myocardial adaptation. Am J Cardiol 71:46A, 1993

NADAL-GINARD B, MAHDAVI V: General principles of cardiovascular cellular and molecular biology, in Heart Disease, 4th ed, E Braunwald (ed). Philadelphia, Saunders, 1992

NEER EJ, CLAPHAM DE: Signal transduction through G proteins in the cardiac myocyte. Trends Cardiovasc Med 2:6, 1992

PETTERSSON K et al: Endothelial integrity and injury in atherogenesis. Transplant Proc 25:2054, 1993

ROBERTS R (ed): Molecular Basis of Cardiology. Boston, Blackwell Scientific, 1992

SOLOMON SD et al: Left ventricular hypertrophy and morphology in familial hypertrophic cardiomyopathy associated with mutations of the β-myosin heavy chain gene. J Am Coll Cardiol (in press)

THOMPSON WG: Apoproteins, lipoprotein subfractions, and the risk of coronary artery disease. South Med J 86:194, 1993

188 PHYSICAL EXAMINATION OF THE CARDIOVASCULAR SYSTEM

ROBERT A. O'ROURKE / EUGENE BRAUNWALD

A careful physical examination is a relatively low cost method for an accurate assessment of the cardiovascular system and often provides important information for the appropriate selection of additional tests. First, the general physical appearance should be evaluated. The patient may appear tired because of a chronic low cardiac output; the respiratory rate may be rapid, indicating pulmonary venous congestion. Central cyanosis, often associated with clubbing of the fingers and toes, indicates right-to-left cardiac or extracardiac shunting or inadequate oxygenation of blood by the lungs. Cyanosis in the distal extremities, cool skin, and increased sweating result from vasoconstriction in patients with severe heart failure (Chap. 32). Noncardiovascular details can be equally important. For example, the diagnosis of infective endocarditis is highly likely in patients with petechiae, Osler's nodes, and Janeway lesions (Chap. 85).

The blood pressure should be taken in both arms and with the patient supine and upright; the heart rate should be timed for 1 min. Orthostatic hypotension and tachycardia may indicate a reduced blood volume, while resting tachycardia may be a clue to the presence of severe heart failure.

Careful examination of the optic fundi is essential (Chap. 209), and the retinal vessels may show evidence of systemic hypertension, arteriosclerosis, or embolism. The latter may result from atherosclerosis in larger arteries (e.g., carotid) or may represent a complication of valvular heart disease (e.g., endocarditis).

Palpation of the peripheral arterial pulses in the upper and lower extremities is necessary to define the adequacy of systemic blood flow and to detect the presence of occlusive arterial lesions. It is also important to examine both legs for evidence of edema, varicose veins, or thrombophlebitis (Chap. 211). The cardiovascular examination includes careful evaluation of both the carotid arterial and the jugular venous pulses, as well as deliberate precordial palpation and attentive cardiac auscultation. An understanding of the events of the cardiac cycle is vital to performing an accurate cardiovascular examination.

ARTERIAL PRESSURE PULSE The normal central aortic pulse wave is characterized by a fairly rapid rise to a somewhat rounded peak (Fig. 188-1). The anacrotic shoulder, present on the ascending limb, occurs at the time of peak rate of aortic flow just before maximum pressure is reached. The less steep descending limb is interrupted by a sharp downward deflection, synchronous with aortic valve closure, called the *incisura*. As the pulse wave is transmitted peripherally, the initial upstroke becomes steeper, the anacrotic shoulder becomes less apparent, and the incisura is replaced by the smoother dicrotic notch. Accordingly, palpation of a peripheral

FIGURE 188-1 *A.* Schematic representation of electrocardiogram, aortic pressure pulse (AOP), phonocardiogram recorded at the apex, and apexcardiogram (ACG). On the phonocardiogram, S_1, S_2, S_3, and S_4 represent the first through fourth heart sounds; OS represents the opening snap of the mitral valve, which occurs coincident with the O point of the apexcardiogram. S_3 occurs coincident with the termination of the rapid-filling wave (RFW) of the ACG, while S_4 occurs coincident with the a wave of the ACG. *B.* Simultaneous recording of electrocardiogram, indirect carotid pulse (CP), phonocardiogram along the left sternal border (LSB), and indirect jugular venous pulse (JVP). ES, ejection sound; SC, systolic click.

arterial pulse (e.g., radial) frequently gives less information than examination of a more central pulse (e.g., carotid) regarding alterations in left ventricular ejection or aortic valve function. However, certain findings such as the hyperkinetic pulse of aortic regurgitation or pulsus alternans are more readily evident in peripheral than in central arteries (Fig. 188-2). The carotid pulse usually is best examined with the sternocleidomastoid muscle relaxed and with the head rotated slightly toward the examiner. In palpating the brachial arterial pulse, the examiner can support the subject's relaxed elbow with the right arm while compressing the brachial pulse with the thumb. The usual technique for palpating the pulse is to compress the artery with the thumb or forefinger until the maximum pulse is sensed. Varying degrees of pressure should then be applied while concentrating on the separate phases of the pulse wave. This method, known as *trisection*, is useful for assessing the sharpness of the upstroke, systolic peak, and diastolic slope of the arterial pulse. In most normal persons a dicrotic wave is not palpable.

A small weak pulse, *pulsus parvus*, is frequently present in conditions with a diminished left ventricular stroke volume, a narrow pulse pressure, and increased peripheral vascular resistance (Fig. 188-2). A *hypokinetic* pulse may be due to hypovolemia, to left ventricular failure secondary to myocardial disease or myocardial infarction, to restrictive pericardial disease, or to mitral valve stenosis. In aortic valve stenosis the delayed systolic peak, *pulsus tardus*, is the result of mechanical obstruction to left ventricular ejection and is often

accompanied by the transmission of a coarse systolic thrill. In contrast, a large bounding, or *hyperkinetic*, pulse is usually associated with an increased left ventricular stroke volume, a wide pulse pressure, and a decrease in peripheral vascular resistance. This occurs characteristically in patients with abnormally elevated stroke volumes, as in complete heart block, hyperkinetic circulation due to anxiety, anemia, exercise, or fever, or in patients with an abnormally rapid runoff of blood from the arterial system (patent ductus arteriosus, peripheral arteriovenous fistula). Patients with mitral regurgitation or a ventricular septal defect also may have a bounding pulse, since vigorous left ventricular ejection produces a rapid upstroke in the arterial pulse even though the duration of systole and the forward stroke volume may be diminished. In aortic regurgitation, the rapidly rising, bounding arterial pulse results from increased left ventricular stroke volume and the associated increased rate of ventricular ejection.

The *bisferiens pulse*, which consists of two systolic peaks, is characteristic of aortic regurgitation (with or without accompanying stenosis) and of hypertrophic cardiomyopathy (Chap. 205). In the latter the pulse wave upstroke rises rapidly and forcefully, producing the first systolic peak ("percussion wave"). A brief decline in pressure follows because of the sudden decrease in the rate of left ventricular ejection during midsystole, when severe obstruction often develops. This pressure trough is followed by a smaller and more slowly rising positive pulse wave ("tidal wave") produced by continued ventricular ejection and by reflected waves from the periphery. The *dicrotic pulse* has two palpable waves, one in systole and one in diastole. It occurs most frequently in patients with a very low stroke volume, particularly in those with dilated (congestive) cardiomyopathy.

Pulsus alternans refers to a pattern in which there is regular alteration of the pressure pulse amplitude, despite a regular rhythm (Fig. 188-2). It is due to alternating left ventricular contractile force, usually denotes severe impairment of left ventricular function, and commonly occurs in patients who also have a loud third heart sound. Pulsus alternans also may occur during or following paroxysmal tachycardia or for several beats following a premature beat in patients without heart disease. In *pulsus bigeminus* there is also regular alteration of pressure pulse amplitude, but it is caused by a premature ventricular contraction that follows each regular beat. *Pulsus paradoxus* is an accentuation of the decrease in systolic arterial pressure accompanying the reduced amplitude of the arterial pulse which normally occurs during inspiration. In patients with pericardial tamponade (Chap. 206), airway obstruction, or superior vena cava obstruction, the decrease in systolic arterial pressure frequently exceeds the normal of 10 mmHg (1.33 kPa) and the peripheral pulse may disappear completely during inspiration.

Simultaneous palpation of the radial and femoral arterial pulses, which normally are virtually coincident, is important to rule out aortic coarctation, in which the latter is weaker and delayed (Chap. 199).

JUGULAR VENOUS PULSE (JVP)   The two main objectives of the bedside examination of the neck veins are inspection of their waveform and estimation of the central venous pressure (CVP). In

FIGURE 188-2 Schematic representation of arterial pulse waveforms that occur with alterations in cardiac hemodynamics which may result from normal physiologic responses or may be due to cardiac disease. S, systole; D, diastole. (*Modified from RA O'Rourke, in JW Hurst et al, eds. The Heart, 7th ed, New York, McGraw-Hill, 1990, with permission.*)

most patients, the right internal jugular vein is superior for both purposes. Usually, the maximum pulsation of the internal jugular vein is observed when the trunk is inclined by less than 30°. In patients with elevated venous pressure it may be necessary to elevate the trunk further, sometimes to as much as 90°. When the neck muscles are relaxed, shining a beam of light tangentially across the skin overlying the vein exposes the pulsations of the internal jugular vein. Simultaneous palpation of the left carotid artery aids the examiner in deciding which pulsations are venous and in relating the venous pulsations to their timing in the cardiac cycle.

The normal JVP reflects phasic pressure changes in the right atrium and consists of two or sometimes three positive waves and two negative troughs (Fig. 188-1). The positive presystolic a wave is produced by venous distention due to right atrial contraction and is the dominant wave in the JVP, particularly during inspiration. Large a waves indicate that the right atrium is contracting against an increased resistance (Fig. 188-3), such as occurs with tricuspid stenosis or more commonly with increased resistance to right ventricular filling (pulmonary hypertension or pulmonic stenosis). Large a waves also occur during arrhythmias whenever the right atrium contracts while the tricuspid valve is closed by right ventricular systole. Such "cannon" a waves may occur regularly (as during junctional rhythm) or irregularly (as in atrioventricular dissociation with ventricular tachycardia or complete heart block). The a wave is absent in patients with atrial fibrillation, and there is an increased temporal delay between the a wave and the carotid arterial pulse in patients with first-degree atrioventricular block.

The c wave, often but not invariably observed in the JVP, is a positive wave produced by the bulging of the tricuspid valve into the right atrium during right ventricular isovolumetric systole and by the impact of the carotid artery adjacent to the jugular vein. The x descent is due to a combination of atrial relaxation and the downward displacement of the tricuspid valve during ventricular systole. In patients with constrictive pericarditis (Fig. 188-3), there is often increased prominence of the x descent wave during systole, but this wave is reduced with right ventricular dilatation and often is reversed in tricuspid regurgitation. The positive, late systolic v wave results from the increasing volume of blood in the venae cavae and right atrium during ventricular systole when the tricuspid valve is closed. With tricuspid regurgitation the v wave is more prominent, and when tricuspid regurgitation becomes severe, the combination of a prominent v wave and obliteration of the x descent results in a single large positive systolic wave. After the peak of the v wave is reached, the right atrial pressure falls because of the decreased bulging of the tricuspid valve into the right atrium as right ventricular pressure declines and the tricuspid valve opens (Fig. 188-3).

This negative descending limb, referred to as the y descent of the JVP, is produced mainly by the tricuspid valve opening and the subsequent rapid inflow of blood into the right ventricle. A rapid, deep y descent in early diastole occurs with severe tricuspid regurgitation. A venous pulse characterized by a sharp y descent, a deep y trough, and a rapid ascent to the baseline is seen in patients with constrictive pericarditis or with severe failure of the right side of the heart and a high venous pressure. A slow y descent in the JVP suggests an obstruction to right ventricular filling, as occurs with tricuspid stenosis or right atrial myxoma.

For accurate estimation of the central venous pressure, the right internal jugular vein is best utilized, with the sternal angle as the reference point, since in the average patient the center of the right atrium lies approximately 5 cm below the sternal angle, regardless of body position. The patient is examined at the optimal degree of trunk elevation for visualization of venous pulsations. The vertical distance between the top of the oscillating venous column and the level of the sternal angle is determined and generally found to be less than 3 cm (3 cm + 5 cm = 8 cm blood). The most common cause of an elevated venous pressure is an elevated right ventricular diastolic pressure. In patients suspected of having right ventricular failure who have a normal CVP at rest, the abdominojugular reflux test may be helpful. The palm of the hand is placed over the abdomen, and firm pressure is applied for 10 s or more. Normally, the jugular venous pressure is not significantly altered, but with impaired function of the right side of the heart the upper level of venous pulsation usually increases. A positive abdominojugular test is best defined as an increase in JVP during 10 s of firm midabdominal compression followed by a rapid drop in pressure of 4 cm blood on release of the compression. The most common cause of a positive test is right-sided heart failure secondary to elevated left heart filling pressures. Also, abdominal compression may elicit the typical JVP of tricuspid regurgitation when the resting pulse wave is normal. Kussmaul's sign, an increase rather than the normal decrease in the CVP during inspiration, is most commonly caused by severe right-sided heart failure; it is a frequent finding in patients with constrictive pericarditis or right ventricular infarction.

PRECORDIAL PALPATION The location, amplitude, duration, and direction of the cardiac impulse usually can be best appreciated with the fingertips. The normal left ventricular apex impulse is located at or medial to the left midclavicular line in the fourth or fifth intercostal space and is a tapping, early systolic outward thrust localized to a point not more than 3 cm in diameter. It is due primarily to recoil of the heart as blood is ejected and should be evaluated with the patient supine and in the left lateral decubitus position. Left ventricular hypertrophy results in an exaggerated amplitude, duration, and often size of the normal left ventricular thrust. The impulse may be displaced laterally and downward into the sixth or seventh interspace, particularly in patients with a left ventricular volume load such as occurs in aortic regurgitation and in those with a dilated cardiomyopathy.

Additional abnormal features of the left ventricular apex include marked presystolic distention of the left ventricle, often accompanying a fourth heart sound in patients with an excessive left ventricular pressure load or myocardial ischemia/infarction, and a prominent early diastolic rapid-filling wave, often accompanying a third heart sound in patients with left ventricular failure or mitral valve regurgitation (Fig. 188-1). A double systolic apical impulse is frequently palpable in patients with hypertrophic cardiomyopathy.

Right ventricular hypertrophy results in a sustained systolic lift at the lower left parasternal area which starts in early systole and is synchronous with the left ventricular apical impulse. In patients with chronic obstructive pulmonary disease, a right ventricular impulse often may be detected by sliding the fingers up under the rib cage just beneath the sternum. The enlarged right ventricle strikes the ends of the fingertips as an inferiorly directed movement.

Abnormal precordial pulsations occur during systole in patients with left ventricular dyssynergy due to ischemic heart disease or to diffuse myocardial disease from some other cause. These pulsations often occur in patients with a recent transmural myocardial infarction

FIGURE 188-3 Abnormal jugular venous pulse waveforms commonly present in patients with cardiac disease and/or arrhythmias. See text. (*Modified from RA O'Rourke, in JW Hurst et al, eds. The Heart, 7th ed, New York, McGraw-Hill, 1990, with permission.*)

A. Tricuspid Stenosis   B. Constrictive Pericarditis   C. Tricuspid Regurgitation

D. Complete AV Block   E. Atrial Fibrillation

and may be present in some patients only during episodes of anginal pain. They are most commonly felt in the left midprecordium one or two interspaces above and/or 1 to 2 cm medial to the left ventricular apex. When a systolic bulge occurs in the region of the apex, it is difficult to distinguish from the impulse of left ventricular hypertrophy.

A left parasternal lift is present frequently in patients with severe mitral regurgitation. This pulsation occurs distinctly later than the left ventricular apical impulse, is synchronous with the *v* wave in the left atrial pressure curve, and is due to anterior displacement of the right ventricle by an enlarged, expanding left atrium. A similar impulse occurs to the right of the sternum in some patients with severe tricuspid regurgitation and a giant right atrium. Pulsation of the right sternoclavicular joint may indicate a right-sided aortic arch or aneurysmal dilatation of the ascending aorta. Pulmonary artery pulsation is often visible and palpable in the second left intercostal space and may be normal in children or thin young adults. However, this pulsation usually denotes pulmonary hypertension, increased pulmonary blood flow, or poststenotic pulmonary artery dilatation. Abnormally forceful valve closure can be palpated as a tap, and it occurs most commonly in the second left intercostal space in patients with pulmonary hypertension, in the second right intercostal space in patients with systemic hypertension, and at the cardiac apex in patients with mitral stenosis.

Thrills are palpable, low-frequency vibrations associated with heart murmurs. The systolic murmur of mitral regurgitation may be palpated at the cardiac apex. When the palm of the hand is placed over the precordium, the thrill of aortic stenosis crosses the palm of the hand toward the right side of the neck, while the thrill of pulmonic stenosis radiates more often to the left side of the neck. The thrill due to a ventricular septal defect is usually located in the third and fourth intercostal spaces near the left sternal border.

Percussion should be performed in each patient to identify normal or abnormal position of the heart, stomach, and liver. However, in patients with a normal cardiac situs, percussion adds little to careful inspection and palpation in the recognition of cardiac enlargement.

CARDIAC AUSCULTATION

To obtain maximal information from cardiac auscultation, the observer should keep in mind several principles: (1) It should be carried out in a quiet room to avoid the distractions caused by the noises of normal activity. (2) In order to hear a faint heart sound or murmur, attention must be focused on that phase of the cardiac cycle during which the auscultatory event may be expected to occur. (3) The accurate timing of a heart sound or murmur necessarily involves determining its relation to other observable events in the cardiac cycle—the carotid arterial pulse, the apical impulse, or the JVP. (4) To define the significance of a cardiac sound or murmur, it is often necessary to observe alterations in its timing or intensity during various physiologic and/or pharmacologic interventions (Table 188-1).

HEART SOUNDS   The major components of heart sounds are vibrations associated with the abrupt acceleration or deceleration of blood within the cardiovascular system, but there is continuing controversy regarding the relative significance of the vibrations of valves, muscles, vessels, and supporting structures in the production of the heart sounds. Studies using simultaneous echocardiographic-phonocardiographic recordings indicate that the first and second heart sounds are produced primarily by the closure of the AV and semilunar valves and the events that accompany these closures. The intensity of the *first heart sound* (S_1) is influenced by (1) the position of the mitral leaflets at the onset of ventricular systole, (2) the rate of rise of the left ventricular pressure pulse, (3) the presence or absence of structural disease of the mitral valve, and (4) the amount of tissue, air, or fluid between the heart and the stethoscope. S_1 is louder if diastole is shortened because of tachycardia, if atrioventricular flow is increased because of high cardiac output or prolonged because of

---

TABLE 188-1   Effects of physiologic and pharmacologic interventions on the intensity of heart murmurs and sounds*

RESPIRATION

Systolic murmurs due to TR or pulmonic blood flow through a normal or stenotic valve and diastolic murmurs of TS or PR generally increase with inspiration as do right-sided S_3 and S_4. Left-sided murmurs and sounds usually are louder during expiration.

VALSALVA MANEUVER

Most murmurs decrease in length and intensity. Two exceptions are the systolic murmur of HCM, which usually becomes much louder, and that of MVP, which becomes longer and often louder. Following release of the Valsalva, right-sided murmurs tend to return to control intensity earlier than left-sided murmurs.

POST VPB OR AF

Murmurs originating at normal or stenotic semilunar valves increase in the cardiac cycle following a VPB or in the cycle after a long cycle length in AF. By contrast, systolic murmurs due to AV valve regurgitation do not change, diminish (papillary muscle dysfunction), or become shorter (MVP).

POSITIONAL CHANGES

With *standing* most murmurs diminish, two exceptions being the murmur of HCM, which becomes louder, and that of MVP, which lengthens and often is intensified. With *squatting* most murmurs become louder but those of HCM and MVP usually soften and may disappear.

EXERCISE

Murmurs due to blood flow across normal or obstructed valves (e.g., PS, MS) become louder with both isotonic and submaximal isometric (handgrip) exercise. Murmurs of MR, VSD, and AR also increase with handgrip exercise. However, the murmur of HCM often decreases with near maximum handgrip exercise. Left-sided S_4 and S_3 are often accentuated by exercise, particularly when due to ischemic heart disease.

PHARMACOLOGIC INTERVENTIONS

During the initial relative hypotension following amyl nitrite inhalation, murmurs of MR, VSD, and AR decrease while murmurs of aortic stenosis or sclerosis increase. During the later tachycardia phase, murmurs of MS and right-sided lesions also increase. The response in MVP often is biphasic (softer then louder than control). The arterial constrictor phenylephrine tends to produce the opposite effects.

TRANSIENT ARTERIAL OCCLUSION

Transient external compression of both arms by bilateral cuff inflation to 20 mmHg > peak systolic pressure augments the murmurs of MR, VSD, and AR but not murmurs due to other causes.

* TR, tricuspid regurgitation; TS, tricuspid stenosis; PR, pulmonic regurgitation; HCM, hypertrophic cardiomyopathy; MVP, mitral valve prolapse; PS, pulmonic stenosis; MS, mitral stenosis; MR, mitral regurgitation; VSD, ventricular septal defect; AR, aortic regurgitation; VPB, ventricular premature beat; and AF, atrial fibrillation.

---

mitral stenosis, or if atrial precedes ventricular contraction by an unusually short interval, reflected in a short PR interval. The loud S_1 in mitral stenosis usually signifies that the valve is pliable and that it remains open at the onset of isovolumetric contraction because of the elevated left atrial pressure. A reduction in the intensity of S_1 may be due to poor conduction of sound through the chest wall, a slow rise of the left ventricular pressure pulse, a long PR interval, or imperfect closure due to reduced valve substance, as in mitral regurgitation. S_1 is also soft when the anterior mitral leaflet is immobile because of rigidity and calcification even in the presence of predominant mitral stenosis.

Splitting of the two high-pitched components of S_1 by 10 to 30 ms is a normal phenomenon (Fig. 188-1). The first component of S_1 normally is attributed to mitral valve closure and the second to tricuspid valve closure. A widened split of S_1 is most often due to complete right bundle branch block and the resulting delay in onset of the right ventricular pressure pulse. Reversed splitting of the S_1 with the mitral component following the tricuspid component may be present in patients with severe mitral stenosis, left atrial myxoma, and complete left bundle branch block.

Splitting of S_2 into audibly distinct aortic (A_2) and pulmonic (P_2) components occurs normally during inspiration when augmented inflow into the right ventricle increases its stroke volume and ejection period and delays closure of the pulmonic valve. P_2 is coincident with the incisura of the pulmonary artery pressure curve, which is separated from the right ventricular pressure tracing by an interval termed the "hangout time." The absolute value of this interval reflects the resistance to pulmonary blood flow and the impedance characteristics of the pulmonary vascular bed. This interval is prolonged and physiologic splitting of S_2 is accentuated in conditions associated with right ventricular volume overload and a distensible pulmonary vascular bed. However, in patients with an increase in pulmonary vascular resistance, the hangout time is markedly reduced and narrow splitting of S_2 is present. Splitting that persists with expiration, heard best at the pulmonic area or left sternal border, is usually abnormal when the patient is in the upright position. Such splitting may be due to a number of causes: delayed activation of the right ventricle (right bundle branch block); left ventricular ectopic beats; a left ventricular pacemaker; prolongation of right ventricular contraction with an increased right ventricular pressure load (pulmonary embolism or pulmonic stenosis); or delayed pulmonic valve closure because of right ventricular volume overload associated with right ventricular failure or diminished impedance of the pulmonary vascular bed and a prolonged hangout time (atrial septal defect).

In pulmonary hypertension, P_2 is increased in intensity, and splitting of the second heart sound may be diminished, normal, or accentuated depending on the cause of the pulmonary hypertension, the pulmonary vascular resistance, and the presence or absence of right ventricular decompensation. Early aortic valve closure, occurring with mitral regurgitation or a ventricular septal defect, also may produce splitting that persists during expiration. It also may occur with constrictive pericarditis. In patients with atrial septal defect the proportion of right atrial filling contributed by the left atrium and the venae cavae varies reciprocally during the respiratory cycle so that right atrial inflow remains relatively constant. Therefore, the volume and duration of right ventricular ejection are not significantly increased by inspiration, and there is little inspiratory exaggeration of the splitting of S_2. This phenomenon, termed *fixed splitting* of the second heart sound, is of considerable diagnostic value.

A delay in aortic valve closure causing P_2 to precede A_2 results in so-called reversed (paradoxic) splitting of S_2. Splitting is then maximal in expiration and decreases during inspiration with the normal delay of pulmonic valve closure. The most common causes of reversed splitting of S_2 are left bundle branch block and delayed excitation of the left ventricle from a right ventricular ectopic beat. Mechanical prolongation of left ventricular systole, resulting in reversed splitting of S_2, also may be caused by severe aortic outflow obstruction, a large aorta-to-pulmonary artery shunt, systolic hypertension, and ischemic heart disease or cardiomyopathy with left ventricular failure. P_2 is normally softer than A_2 in the second left intercostal space; when P_2 is greater than A_2 in this area, it suggests pulmonary hypertension, except in patients with atrial septal defect.

The *third heart sound* (S_3) is a low-pitched sound produced in the ventricle 0.14 to 0.16 s after A_2, at the termination of rapid filling. This sound is frequent in normal children and in patients with high cardiac output. However, in patients over 40 years of age, an S_3 usually indicates impairment of ventricular function, AV valve regurgitation, or other conditions which increase the rate or volume of ventricular filling. The left-sided S_3 is best heard with the bell piece of the stethoscope at the left ventricular apex during expiration and with the patient in the left lateral position. The right-sided S_3 is best heard at the left sternal border or just beneath the xiphoid and is increased with inspiration. Often it is accompanied by the systolic murmur of functional tricuspid regurgitation. Third heart sounds often disappear with treatment of heart failure.

An earlier (0.10 to 0.12 s after A_2), higher-pitched third heart sound (pericardial knock) often occurs in patients with constrictive pericarditis; its presence is dependent on the restrictive effect of the adherent pericardium, which halts diastolic filling abruptly.

The *opening snap* (OS) is a brief, high-pitched, early diastolic sound which is usually due to stenosis of an AV valve, more commonly the mitral valve. It is usually heard best at the lower left sternal border and radiates well to the base of the heart. The A_2-OS interval is inversely related to the height of the mean left atrial pressure and ranges from 0.04 to 0.12 s. In the second intercostal space an OS is often confused with P_2. However, careful auscultation at the upper left sternal border will reveal both components of S_2, followed by the OS. The OS of tricuspid stenosis occurs later in diastole than the mitral OS. Since most patients with tricuspid stenosis also have severe mitral valve disease, the tricuspid OS is often overshadowed by the diastolic rumble and OS originating in the stenotic mitral valve. An OS also may occur when there is increased flow across an AV valve, such as exists with left-to-right intracardiac shunts and mitral or tricuspid regurgitation.

The *fourth heart sound* (S_4) is a low-pitched, presystolic sound produced in the ventricle during ventricular filling; it is associated with an effective atrial contraction and is heard best with the bell piece of the stethoscope. The sound is absent in patients with atrial fibrillation. The S_4 occurs when diminished ventricular compliance increases the resistance to ventricular filling, and it is present frequently in patients with systemic hypertension, aortic stenosis, hypertrophic cardiomyopathy, ischemic heart disease, and acute mitral regurgitation. Most patients with an acute myocardial infarction and sinus rhythm have an audible S_4. The fourth heart sound is frequently accompanied by visible and palpable presystolic distention of the left ventricle. It is maximal in intensity at the left ventricular apex with the patient in the left lateral position and is accentuated by mild isotonic or isometric exercise in the supine position. The right-sided S_4 is present in patients with right ventricular hypertrophy secondary to either pulmonic stenosis or pulmonary hypertension and frequently accompanies a prominent presystolic a wave in the JVP.

An S_4 frequently accompanies delayed AV conduction even in the absence of clinically detectable heart disease. The incidence of an audible S_4 increases with increasing age. Whether an audible S_4 in adults without other evidence of cardiac disease is abnormal remains controversial.

The *ejection sound* is a sharp, high-pitched event occurring in early systole closely following the first heart sound. Ejection sounds occur in the presence of semilunar valve stenosis, when there are opening snaps of the aortic or pulmonic valves, and in conditions associated with dilation of the aorta or pulmonary artery. The aortic ejection sound is usually heard best at the left ventricular apex and the second right interspace; the pulmonary ejection sound is of maximal intensity at the upper left sternal border. The latter, unlike most other right-sided acoustical events, is heard better during expiration.

Nonejection or midsystolic clicks, occurring with or without a late systolic murmur, often denote prolapse of one or both leaflets of the mitral valve. They also may be caused by tricuspid valve prolapse. They probably result from functionally unequal length of the chordae tendineae of either or both AV valves and are heard best along the lower left sternal border and at the left ventricular apex. Systolic clicks may be single or multiple, and they may occur at any time in systole but usually later than the systolic ejection sound. Frequently the midsystolic click is misinterpreted as S_2, and the actual second heart sound is called an OS or S_3.

HEART MURMURS Cardiac murmurs result from vibrations set up in the bloodstream and the surrounding heart and great vessels as a result of turbulent blood flow, the formation of eddies, and cavitation (bubble formation as a result of sudden decrease in pressure).

The intensity (loudness) of murmurs may be graded from I to VI. A grade I murmur is so faint that it can be heard only with special effort, a grade IV murmur is commonly accompanied by a thrill, and a grade VI murmur is audible with the stethoscope removed from but are usually only systolic. Continuous murmurs may also be due to disturbances of flow pattern in constricted systemic (e.g., renal) or pulmonary arteries when marked pressure differences between the two sides of the narrow segment persist; a continuous murmur in the back may be present in *coarctation of the aorta; pulmonary embolism* may cause continuous murmurs in partially occluded vessels.

In nonconstricted arteries, continuous murmurs may be due to rapid flow through a tortuous bed. Such murmurs typically occur within the bronchial arterial collateral circulation in cyanotic patients with severe pulmonary outflow obstruction. The "mammary souffle," an innocent murmur heard over the breasts during late pregnancy and early postpartum, may be systolic or continuous. The innocent cervical venous hum is a continuous murmur usually audible over the medial aspect of the right supraclavicular fossa with the patient upright. The hum is usually louder during diastole and can be instantaneously abolished by digital compression of the ipsilateral internal jugular vein. Transmission of a loud venous hum to the area below the clavicles may result in a mistaken diagnosis of patent ductus arteriosus.

The *pericardial friction rub,* which may have presystolic, systolic, and early diastolic scratchy components, may be confused with a murmur or extracardiac sound when heard only in systole. It is best appreciated with the patient upright and leaning forward and may be accentuated during inspiration.

REFERENCES

ABRAMS J: *Essentials of Cardiac Physical Diagnosis.* Philadelphia, Lea & Febiger, 1987

BRAUNWALD E: Physical examination, in *Heart Disease,* 4th ed, E Braunwald (ed). Philadelphia, Saunders, 1992, p. 13

CRAWFORD MH: *Examination of the Heart,* part 2: *Inspection and Palpation of Venous and Arterial Pulses.* Chicago, American Heart Association, 1990

EILEN SD, CRAWFORD MH, O'ROURKE RA: Accuracy of precordial palpation for detecting increased left ventricular volume. Ann Intern Med 99:628, 1983

EWY GA: The abdominojugular test: Technique and hemodynamic correlates. Ann Intern Med 109:456, 1988

GREWE K et al: Differentiation of cardiac murmurs by auscultation. Curr Probl Cardiol 13(10):699, 1988

LEMBO NJ ET AL: Bedside diagnosis of systolic murmurs. N Engl J Med 318:1572, 1988

PERLOFF JK (ED): *Physical Examination of the Heart and Circulation,* 2d ed. Philadelphia, Saunders, 1990

———: Heart sounds and murmurs: Physiological mechanisms, in *Heart Disease,* 4th ed, E Braunwald (ed). Philadelphia, Saunders, 1992, p 43

SHAVER JA et al: Normal and abnormal heart sounds in cardiac diagnosis, Part I: Systolic sounds. Curr Probl Cardiol 10(3):1, 1985

189 ELECTROCARDIOGRAPHY

ARY L. GOLDBERGER

The electrocardiogram (ECG or EKG) is a graphic recording of electric potentials generated by the heart. The signals are detected by means of metal electrodes attached to the extremities and chest wall and are then amplified by a sensitive voltmeter such as the electrocardiograph. ECG *leads* actually record the instantaneous *differences* in potential between these electrodes.

The clinical utility of the ECG derives from its immediate availability as a noninvasive, inexpensive, and highly versatile test. In addition to the detection of arrhythmias, conduction disturbances, and myocardial ischemia, electrocardiography may reveal other findings related to life-threatening metabolic disturbances (e.g., hyperkalemia) or increased susceptibility to sudden cardiac death (e.g., QT prolongation syndromes). The advent of coronary thrombolysis in the early therapy of acute myocardial infarction (Chap. 189) has refocused particular attention on the sensitivity and specificity of ECG signs of myocardial ischemia.

ELECTROPHYSIOLOGY (See also Chaps. 197 and 198) Depolarization of the heart is the initiating event for cardiac contraction. The electric currents which spread through the heart are produced by three components: cardiac pacemaker cells, specialized conduction tissue, and the heart muscle itself. The ECG, however, records only the depolarization (stimulation) and repolarization (recovery) potentials generated by the atrial and ventricular myocardium. Under resting conditions, myocardial cells are *polarized*; i.e., they carry an electric charge on their surface due to transmembrane ion concentration differences. The charge measured across atrial and ventricular cell membranes is about 90 mV, with the inside negative relative to the outside. When these cells are stimulated above a critical threshold potential, they rapidly depolarize and transiently reverse their membrane polarity. This depolarization process spreads in a wavelike manner through the atria and ventricles. The return of myocardial fibers to their original resting state occurs during repolarization.

The depolarization stimulus for the normal heartbeat originates in the *sinoatrial* (SA) or *sinus node,* a collection of *pacemaker* cells which fire spontaneously; i.e., they exhibit *automaticity* (Fig. 189-1). The first phase of cardiac electrical activation is spread of the depolarization wave through the right and left atria, followed by atrial contraction. Next, the impulse stimulates pacemaker and specialized conduction tissues in the atrioventricular (AV) nodal and His-bundle areas; together, these two regions constitute the AV junction. The bundle of His bifurcates into two main branches, the right and the left bundles, that rapidly transmit depolarization wavefronts to the right and left ventricular myocardium by way of Purkinje fibers. The main left bundle bifurcates into two primary subdivisions, a left anterior fascicle and a left posterior fascicle. The depolarization wavefronts then spread through the ventricular wall, from endocardium to epicardium, triggering ventricular contraction.

Since the cardiac depolarization and repolarization waves have direction and magnitude, they can be represented by vectors. *Vectorcardiograms* that measure and display these instantaneous potentials are no longer used much in clinical practice. However, the general principles of vector analysis remain fundamental to understanding the genesis of normal and pathologic ECG waveforms. Vector analysis illustrates a central concept of electrocardiography—namely, that the ECG records the complex spatial and temporal summation of electrical potentials from multiple myocardial fibers conducted to the surface of the body. This principle accounts for inherent limitations in both ECG *sensitivity* (activity from certain cardiac regions may be canceled out or not of sufficient magnitude to be recorded) and *specificity* (the

FIGURE 189-1 Schematic of the cardiac conduction system.

FIGURE 189-2 Basic ECG waveforms and intervals. Not shown is the R-R interval, the time between consecutive QRS complexes.

FIGURE 189-3 The QRS-T cycle corresponds to different phases of the ventricular action potential.

same vectorial sum can result from either a selective gain or loss of forces in opposite directions).

ECG WAVEFORMS AND INTERVALS The ECG waveforms are labeled alphabetically beginning with the P wave, which represents atrial depolarization (Fig. 189-2). The QRS complex represents ventricular depolarization, and the ST-T-U complex (ST segment, T wave, and U wave) represents ventricular repolarization. The J point is the junction between the end of the QRS complex and the beginning of the ST segment. Atrial repolarization is usually of too low an amplitude to be detected, but it may become apparent in such conditions as acute pericarditis or atrial infarction.

The QRS-T waveforms of the surface (extracellular) ECG correspond in a general way with the different phases of simultaneously obtained ventricular *action potentials*, the intracellular recordings from single myocardial fibers (Fig. 189-3) (see also Chap. 197). The rapid upstroke (phase 0) of the action potential corresponds to the onset of QRS. The plateau (phase 2) corresponds to the isoelectric ST segment and active repolarization (phase 3) to the inscription of the T wave. Factors that decrease the slope of phase 0 by impairing the influx of Na^+ (e.g., drugs such as quinidine or procainamide, or hyperkalemia) tend to increase QRS duration. Conditions that prolong

phase 2 (amiodarone, hypocalcemia) increase the QT interval. In contrast, shortening of ventricular repolarization (phase 2), by digitalis or hypercalcemia, abbreviates the ST segment.

The electrocardiogram is ordinarily recorded on special graph paper which is divided into 1-mm^2 gridlike boxes (Fig. 189-4). Since the ECG paper speed is generally 25 mm/s, the smallest (1 mm) horizontal divisions correspond to 0.04 s (40 ms), with heavier lines at intervals of 0.20 s (200 ms). Vertically, the ECG graph measures the amplitude of a given wave or deflection (1 mV = 10 mm with standard calibration; the voltage criteria for hypertrophy mentioned below are given in millimeters). There are four major ECG intervals: R-R, PR, QRS, and QT (Fig. 189-2). The heart rate (beats per minute) can be readily computed from the interbeat (R-R) interval by dividing the number of large (0.20 s) time units between consecutive R waves into 300 or the number of small (0.04 s) units into 1500. The PR interval (normally 120 to 200 ms) measures the time (normally 120 to 200 ms) between atrial and ventricular depolarization, which

FIGURE 189-4 The ECG graph paper records the time (interval) between cardiac electrical events along the horizontal axis and their amplitude (voltage) along the vertical axis.

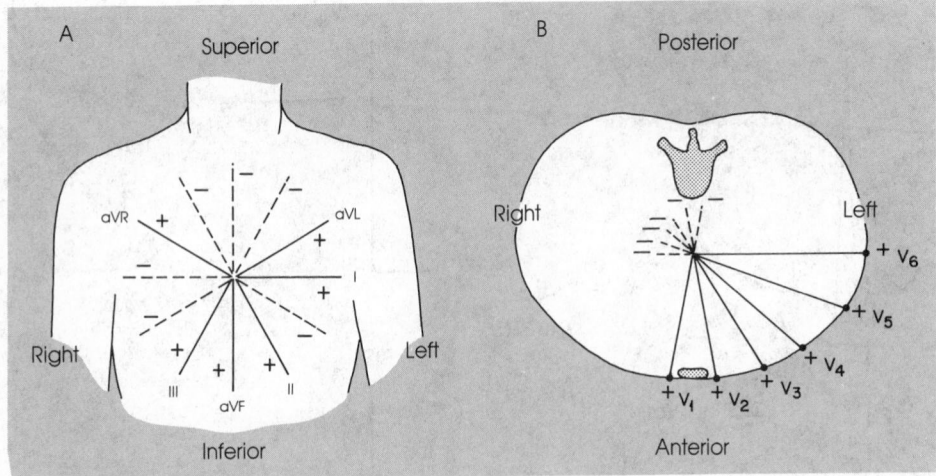

FIGURE 189-5   The six frontal plane (*A*) and six horizontal plane (*B*) leads provide a three-dimensional representation of cardiac electrical activity.

includes the physiologic delay imposed by stimulation of cells in the AV junction area. The QRS interval (normally 100 ms or less) reflects the duration of ventricular depolarization. The QT interval includes both ventricular depolarization and repolarization times and varies inversely with the heart rate. A rate-related ("corrected") QT interval, or QT_c, can be calculated as $QT/\sqrt{R\text{-}R}$ and normally is ≤ 0.44 s.

The QRS complex is subdivided into specific deflections or waves. If the initial QRS deflection in a given lead is negative, it is termed a *Q wave*; the first positive deflection is termed an *R wave*. A negative deflection after an R wave is an *S wave*. Subsequent positive or negative waves are labeled *R'* and *S'*, respectively. Lowercase letters (qrs) are used for relatively small amplitude waves. An entirely negative QRS complex is termed a *QS wave*.

ECG LEADS   The 12 conventional ECG leads record the difference in potential between electrodes placed on the surface of the body. These leads are divided into two groups; six extremity (limb) leads and six chest (precordial) leads. The extremity leads record potentials transmitted onto the *frontal plane* (Fig. 189-5*A*), and the chest leads record potentials transmitted onto the *horizontal plane* (Fig. 189-5*B*). The six extremity leads are further subdivided into three *bipolar* leads (I, II, and III) and three *unipolar* leads (aVR, aVL, and aVF). Each bipolar lead measures the difference in potential between electrodes at two extremities: lead I = left arm − right arm voltages, lead II = left leg − right arm, and lead III = left leg − left arm. The unipolar leads measure the voltage (V) at one locus relative to an electrode (called the *central terminal* or *indifferent electrode*) that has approximately zero potential. Thus aVR = right arm, aVL = left arm, and aVF = left leg (foot). The lower case *a* indicates that these unipolar potentials are electrically augmented by 50 percent. The right leg electrode functions as a ground. The spatial orientation and polarity of the six frontal plane leads is represented on the hexaxial diagram (Fig. 189-6).

The six chest leads (Fig. 189-7) are unipolar recordings obtained by electrodes in the following positions: lead V_1, fourth intercostal space, just to the right of the sternum; lead V_2, fourth intercostal space, just to the left of the sternum; lead V_3, midway between V_2 and V_4; lead V_4, midclavicular line, fifth intercostal space; lead V_5, anterior axillary line, same level as V_4; and lead V_6, midaxillary line, same level as V_4 and V_5.

Together, the frontal and horizontal plane electrodes provide a three-dimensional representation of cardiac electrical activity. Each lead can be likened to a different camera angle "looking" at the same events—atrial and ventricular depolarization and repolarization—from different spatial orientations. The conventional 12-lead ECG

can be supplemented with additional leads under special circumstances. For example, right precordial leads V_3R, V_4R, etc. are useful in detecting evidence of acute right ventricular ischemia. Esophageal leads may reveal atrial activity not detectable on the surface ECG. Bedside telemetry units and ambulatory ECG (Holter) recordings usually employ only one or two modified leads, respectively. Intracardiac electrocardiography and electrophysiologic testing are discussed in Chaps. 197 and 198.

The ECG leads are configured so that a positive (upright) deflection will be recorded in a lead if a wave of depolarization spreads toward the positive pole of that lead and a negative deflection if the wave spreads toward the negative pole. If the mean orientation of the

FIGURE 189-6   The frontal plane (extremity or limb) leads are represented on a hexaxial diagram. Each ECG lead has a specific spatial orientation and polarity. The positive pole of each lead axis (*solid line*) and negative pole (*hatched line*) are designated by their angular position relative to the positive pole of lead I ($0°$). The mean electrical axis of the QRS complex is measured with respect to this display.

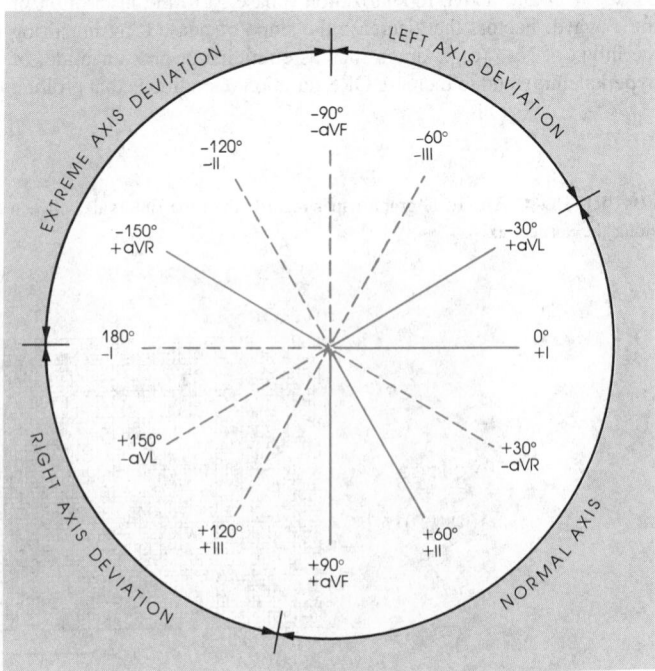

depolarization vector is at right angles to a given lead axis, a small biphasic (equally positive and negative) deflection will be recorded.

GENESIS OF THE NORMAL ECG

P WAVE The normal atrial depolarization vector is oriented downward and toward the subject's left, reflecting the spread of depolarization from the sinus node to the right and then the left atrial myocardium. Since this vector points toward the positive pole of lead II and toward the negative pole of lead aVR, the normal P wave will be positive in lead II and negative in lead aVR. By contrast, activation of the atria from an ectopic pacemaker in the lower part of either atrium or in the AV junction region may produce retrograde P waves (negative in lead II, positive in lead aVR).

QRS COMPLEX Normal ventricular depolarization proceeds as a rapid, continuous spread of activation wavefronts. This complex process can be divided into two major, sequential phases, and each phase can be represented by a mean vector (Fig. 189-8). The first phase is depolarization of the interventricular septum from the left to the right (vector 1). The second results from the simultaneous depolarization of the main mass of the right and left ventricles and is normally dominated by the more massive left ventricle so that vector 2 points leftward and posteriorly. Therefore, a right precordial lead (V_1) will record this biphasic depolarization process with a small positive deflection (septal r wave) followed by a larger negative deflection (S wave). A left precordial lead, e.g., V_6, will record the

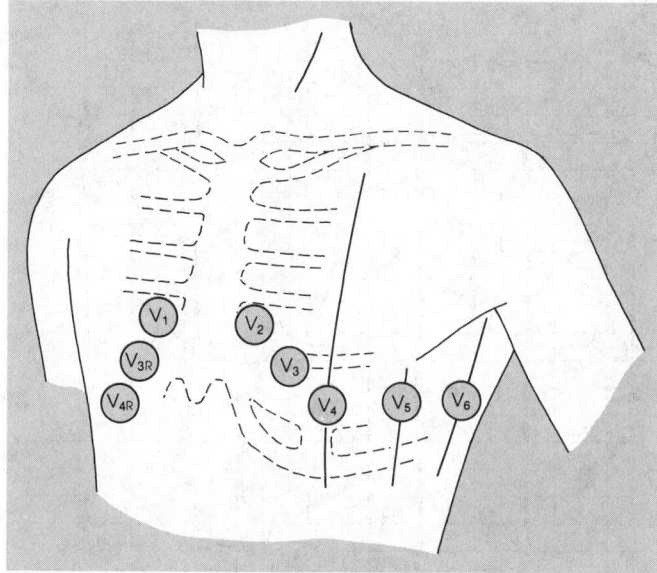

FIGURE 189-7 The horizontal plane (chest or precordial) leads are obtained with electrodes in the designated locations.

FIGURE 189-8 Ventricular depolarization can be divided into two major phases, each represented by a vector. *A.* The first phase (*arrow 1*) denotes depolarization of the ventricular septum, beginning on the left side and spreading to the right. This process is represented by a small "septal" r wave in lead V_1 and a small septal q wave in lead V_6. *B.* Simultaneous depolarization of the left and right ventricles (LV and RV) constitutes the second phase. Vector 2 is oriented to the left and posteriorly, reflecting the electrical predominance of the LV. *C.* Vectors (*arrows*) representing these two phases are shown in reference to the horizontal plane leads. *(After Goldberger and Goldberger.)*

FIGURE 189-9 Normal electrocardiogram from a healthy subject. Sinus rhythm is present with a heart rate of 75 beats per minute. PR interval is 0.16 s; QRS interval (duration) is 0.08 s; QT interval is 0.36 s; the mean QRS axis is about $+70°$. The precordial leads show normal R-wave progression with the transition zone (R wave = S wave) in lead V_3.

same sequence with a small negative deflection (septal q wave) followed by a relatively tall positive deflection (R wave). Intermediate leads show a relative increase in R-wave amplitude (normal R-wave progression) and a decrease in S-wave amplitude progressing across the chest from the right to left. The precordial lead where the R and S waves are of approximately equal amplitude is referred to as the *transition zone* (usually V_3 or V_4) (Fig. 189-9).

The QRS pattern in the extremity leads may vary considerably from one normal subject to another depending on the *electrical axis* of the QRS, which describes the mean orientation of the QRS vector with reference to the six frontal plane leads. Normally, the QRS axis ranges from -30 to $+100°$ (Fig. 189-7). An axis more negative than $-30°$ is referred to as *left axis deviation*, while an axis more positive than $+100°$ is referred to as *right axis deviation*. Left axis deviation may occur as a normal variant but is more commonly associated with left ventricular hypertrophy, a block in the anterior fascicle of the left bundle system (left anterior fascicular block or hemiblock), or inferior myocardial infarction. Right axis deviation also may occur as a normal variant (particularly in children and young adults), as a spurious finding due to reversal of the left and right arm electrodes, or in conditions such as right ventricular overload (acute or chronic), infarction of the lateral wall of the left ventricle, dextrocardia, left pneumothorax, or left posterior fascicular block.

T WAVE AND U WAVE   Normally, the mean T-wave vector is oriented roughly concordant with the mean QRS vector. Since depolarization and repolarization are electrically opposite processes, this normal QRS–T-wave vector concordance indicates that repolarization must normally proceed in the reverse direction from depolarization (i.e., from epicardium to endocardium or from cardiac apex to base). The normal U wave is a small rounded deflection (≤ 1 mm) following the T wave, usually having the same polarity as the T wave. An abnormal increase in U-wave amplitude is most commonly due to drugs (e.g., quinidine, procainamide, disopyramide) or hypokalemia. Very prominent U waves are a marker of increased susceptibility to

FIGURE 189-10   Right atrial (RA) overload may cause tall, peaked P waves in the limb or precordial leads. Left atrial (LA) abnormality may cause broad, often notched P waves in the limb leads and a biphasic P wave in lead V_1 with a prominent negative component representing delayed depolarization of the LA. *(After Park MK, Guntheroth WG, How to Read Pediatric ECGs, 2d ed, St. Louis, Mosby–Year Book, 1987.)*

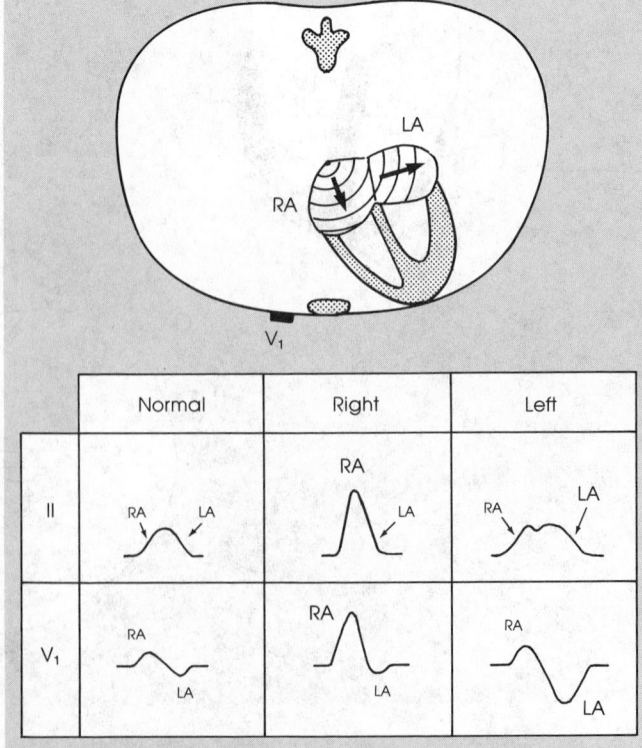

the *torsades de pointes* type of ventricular tachycardia (Chap. 198). Inversion of the U wave in the precordial leads is abnormal and may be a subtle sign of ischemia.

MAJOR ECG ABNORMALITIES

CARDIAC ENLARGEMENT AND HYPERTROPHY Right atrial overload (acute or chronic) may lead to an increase in P-wave amplitude (≥ 2.5 mm) (Fig. 189-10). Left atrial overload typically produces a biphasic P wave in V_1 with a broad negative component or a broad (≥ 120 ms), often notched P wave in one or more limb leads (Fig, 189-10). This pattern also may occur with left atrial conduction delays in the absence of actual atrial enlargement, leading to the more general designation of *left atrial abnormality*.

Right ventricular hypertrophy due to a pressure load (e.g., pulmonic valve stenosis or pulmonary artery hypertension) is characterized by a relatively tall R wave in lead V_1 (R $\geq$ S wave) usually with right axis deviation (Fig. 189-11); alternatively, there may be a qR pattern in V_1 or V_3R. ST depression and T-wave inversion in the right to midprecordial leads are also often present. This so-called ventricular strain pattern is attributed to repolarization abnormalities in hypertrophied muscle. Right ventricular hypertrophy due to ostium secundum type atrial septal defects, with the accompanying right ventricular volume overload, is commonly associated with an incomplete or complete right bundle branch block pattern with a rightward QRS axis.

Acute cor pulmonale due to pulmonary embolism, for example, may be associated with a normal ECG or a variety of abnormalities.

Sinus tachycardia is the most common arrhythmia, although other tachyarrhythmias such as atrial fibrillation or flutter may occur. The QRS axis may shift to the right, sometimes in concert with the so-called $S_1Q_3T_3$ pattern (prominence of the S wave in lead I, Q wave in lead III, with T-wave inversions in lead III). Acute right ventricular dilatation also may be associated with poor R-wave progression and T-wave inversions in V_1 to V_4 (right ventricular strain) simulating acute anterior infarction. A right ventricular conduction disturbance may appear.

Chronic cor pulmonale due to obstructive lung disease usually does not produce the classic ECG patterns of right ventricular hypertrophy noted above. Instead of tall right precordial R waves, chronic lung disease more typically is associated with small R waves in right to midprecordial leads (poor R-wave progression) due in part to downward displacement of the diaphragm and the heart. Low-voltage complexes are commonly present due to hyperaeration of the lungs.

A number of different voltage criteria for *left ventricular hypertrophy* (Fig. 189-11) have been proposed based on the presence of tall left precordial R waves and deep right precordial S waves (e.g., SV_1 + RV_5 or $RV_6 \geq 35$ mm; or RV_5 or $V_6 \geq 25$ mm). Repolarization abnormalities (ST depression with T-wave inversions) also may appear (left ventricular strain pattern) in leads with prominent R waves. However, prominent precordial voltages may occur as a normal variant, especially in athletic or thin-chested individuals. Left ventricular hypertrophy may increase limb lead voltage (e.g., RaVL ≥ 11 to 13 mm, RaVF ≥ 20 mm; R_I + $S_{III} \geq 25$ mm) with or without increased precordial voltage. The presence of left atrial abnormality increases the likelihood of underlying left ventricular hypertrophy in

FIGURE 189-11 Left ventricular hypertrophy (LVH) increases the amplitude of electrical forces directed to the left and posteriorly. In addition, repolarization abnormalities may cause ST-segment depression and T-wave inversion in leads with a prominent R wave strain pattern. Right ventricular hypertrophy (RVH) may shift the QRS vector to the right, usually associated with an R, RS, or qR complex in lead V_1. T-wave inversions may be present in right precordial leads (''strain'' pattern).

QRS in Hypertrophy

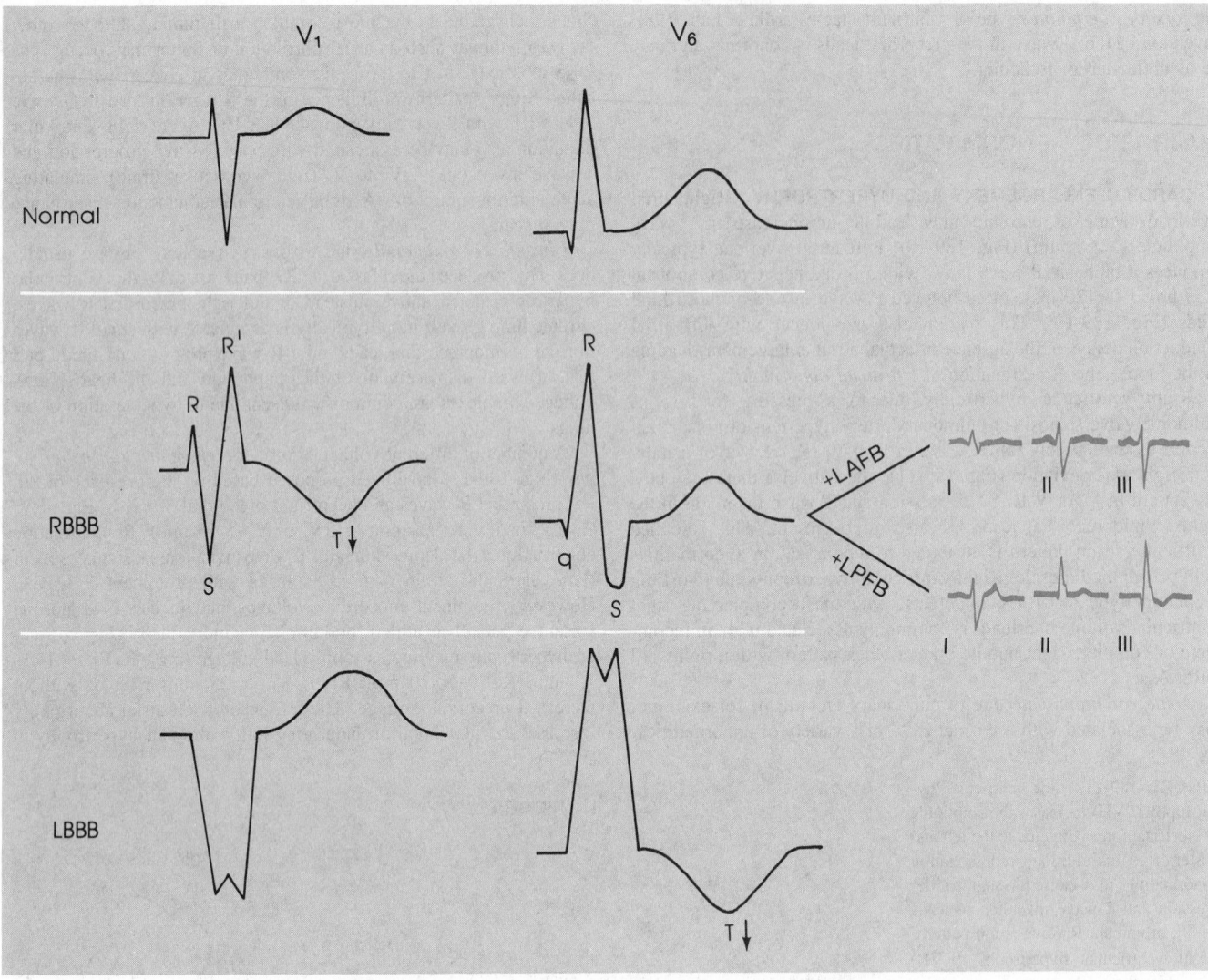

FIGURE 189-12 Comparison of typical QRS-T patterns in right bundle branch block (RBBB) and left bundle branch block (LBBB) compared to normal in leads V_1 and V_6. Note the secondary T-wave inversions (*arrows*) in leads with an rSR' complex with RBBB and in leads with a wide R wave with LBBB. RBBB with left axis deviation due to left anterior fascicular block (LAFB) and right axis deviation due to left posterior fascicular block (LPFB) are examples of bifascicular block.

cases with borderline voltage criteria. Left ventricular hypertrophy often progresses to incomplete or complete left bundle branch block. The sensitivity of conventional voltage criteria for left ventricular hypertrophy is decreased in the obese and in women. ECG evidence for left ventricular hypertrophy is a major noninvasive marker of increased risk of cardiovascular morbidity and mortality, including sudden cardiac death. However, because of false-positive and false-negative diagnoses, the ECG is of limited utility in diagnosing atrial or ventricular enlargement. More definitive information is provided by echocardiography (Chap. 190).

BUNDLE BRANCH BLOCKS Intrinsic impairment of conduction in either the right or left bundle system (intraventricular conduction disturbances) leads to prolongation of the QRS interval. With complete bundle branch blocks the QRS interval is ≥ 120 ms in duration; with incomplete blocks the QRS interval is between 100 and 120 ms. The QRS vector is usually oriented in the direction of the myocardial region where depolarization is delayed (Fig. 189-12). Thus with right bundle branch block the terminal QRS vector is oriented anteriorly and to the right (rSR' in V_1 and qRS in V_6, typically). Left bundle branch block alters both early and later phases of ventricular depolarization. The major QRS vector is directed to the left and posteriorly. In addition, the normal early left-to-right pattern of septal activation is disrupted such that septal depolarization proceeds from right to left as well. As a result, left bundle branch block generates wide, predominantly negative (QS) complexes in lead V_1 and entirely positive (R) complexes in lead V_6. A pattern identical to that of left bundle branch block, preceded by a sharp spike, is seen in most cases of electronic right ventricular pacing because of the relative delay in left ventricular activation.

Bundle branch block may occur in a variety of conditions. Right bundle branch block is seen more commonly in subjects without structural heart disease than left bundle branch block. Right bundle branch block also occurs with congenital (e.g., atrial septal defect) and acquired (e.g., valvular, ischemic) heart disease. Left bundle branch block is often a marker of one of four underlying conditions: ischemic heart disease, long-standing hypertension, severe aortic valve disease, or cardiomyopathy. Bundle branch blocks may be chronic or intermittent. Bundle branch block may be rate-related; e.g. it often occurs when the heart rate exceeds some critical value.

Bundle branch blocks and depolarization abnormalities secondary to artificial pacemakers not only affect ventricular depolarization (QRS) but are also characteristically associated with *secondary repolarization* (ST-T) abnormalities. With bundle branch blocks, the T wave is typically opposite in polarity to the last deflection of the QRS (Fig. 189-12). This discordance of the QRS–T-wave vectors is caused by the altered sequence of repolarization that occurs secondary

- Short PR
- Wide QRS
- Delta Wave (arrow)

FIGURE 189-13 Wolff-Parkinson-White pattern, due to ventricular preexcitation, causes a characteristic ECG triad.

TABLE 189-1 Differential diagnosis of a wide QRS complex
Intrinsic intraventricular delay (IVCD)*
A Left bundle branch block and variants
B Right bundle branch block and variants
C Other nonspecific IVCD patterns
Extrinsic IVCD
A Hyperkalemia
B Drug-induced: type I antiarrhythmias and related agents (tricyclics, phenothiazines)
Ventricular beat (premature, escape, paced)
Ventricular preexcitation Wolff-Parkinson-White (WPW) pattern and variants

* Bundle branch block patterns may occur transiently. Note also that a spuriously wide QRS will occur if the ECG is unintentionally recorded at fast paper speeds (50 or 100 mm/s).

to altered depolarization. In contrast, *primary repolarization* abnormalities are independent of QRS changes and are related instead to actual alterations in the electrical properties of the myocardial fibers themselves (e.g., resting membrane potential or action potential duration), not just to changes in the sequence of repolarization. Ischemia, electrolyte imbalance, and drugs such as digitalis all cause such primary ST–T-wave changes. Primary and secondary T-wave changes may coexist. For example, T-wave inversions in the right precordial leads with left bundle branch block or in the left precordial leads with right bundle branch block may be important markers of underlying ischemia or other abnormalities.

Partial blocks (''hemiblocks'') in the left bundle system (left anterior or posterior fascicular blocks) generally do not prolong QRS duration substantially but instead are associated with shifts in the frontal plane QRS axis (leftward or rightward, respectively). More complex combinations of fascicular and bundle branch blocks may occur involving the left and right bundle system. Examples of *bifascicular block* include right bundle branch block and left posterior fascicular block, right bundle branch block with left anterior fascicular block, and complete left bundle branch block. Chronic bifascicular block in an asymptomatic individual is associated with a relatively low risk of progression to high-degree AV heart block. In contrast, new bifascicular block with acute anterior myocardial infarction carries a much greater risk of complete heart block. Alternation of right and left bundle branch block is a sign of *trifascicular disease*. However, the presence of a prolonged PR interval and bifascicular block does not necessarily indicate trifascicular involvement, since this combination may arise with AV node disease and bifascicular block. Intraventricular conduction delays also can be caused by extrinsic (toxic) factors that slow ventricular conduction, particularly hyperkalemia or drugs (type 1 antiarrhythmic agents, tricyclic antidepressants, phenothiazines).

Prolongation of QRS duration does not necessarily indicate a conduction delay but may be due to *preexcitation* of the ventricles via a bypass tract, as in the Wolff-Parkinson-White (WPW) syndrome (Fig. 189-13) and related variants. The diagnostic triad of WPW consists of a wide QRS complex associated with a relatively short PR interval and slurring of the initial part of the QRS (delta wave), the latter due to aberrant activation of ventricular myocardium. The presence of a bypass tract predisposes to reentrant supraventricular tachyarrhythmias (Chap. 198). The differential diagnosis of a wide QRS complex is summarized in Table 189-1.

MYOCARDIAL ISCHEMIA AND INFARCTION The ECG is a cornerstone in the diagnosis of acute and chronic ischemic heart disease. The findings depend on several key factors: the nature of the process [reversible (i.e., ischemia) versus irreversible (i.e., infarction)], the duration (acute versus chronic), extent (transmural versus subendocardial), and localization (anterior versus inferoposterior), as well as the presence of other underlying abnormalities (ventricular hypertrophy, conduction defects).

Ischemia exerts complex time-dependent effects on the electrical properties of myocardial cells. Severe, acute ischemia lowers the resting membrane potential and shortens the duration of the action potential. Such changes cause a voltage gradient between normal and ischemic zones. As a consequence, current flows between these regions. These so-called currents of injury are represented on the surface ECG by deviation of the ST segment (Fig. 189-14). When the acute ischemia is *transmural*, the ST vector is usually shifted in the direction of the outer (epicardial) layers, producing ST elevations and sometimes, in the earliest stages of ischemia, tall, positive so-called hyperacute T waves over the ischemic zone. With ischemia confined primarily to the *subendocardium*, the ST vector typically shifts toward the subendocardium and ventricular cavity so that overlying (e.g., anterior precordial) leads show ST-segment depression (with ST elevation in lead aVR). Multiple factors affect the amplitude of acute ischemic ST deviations. Profound ST elevation or depression in multiple leads usually indicates very severe ischemia. Complete resolution of ST elevation promptly following thrombolytic therapy is a relatively specific, though not sensitive, marker of successful reperfusion.

The ECG leads are more helpful in localizing regions of Q wave than non-Q wave ischemia. For example, acute anterior wall ischemia leading to Q wave infarction is reflected by ST elevations or increased T-wave positivity (Fig. 189-15) in one or more of the precordial leads (V_1 to V_6) and leads I and aVL. Anteroseptal ischemia produces these changes in leads V_1 to V_3, apical or lateral ischemia in leads V_4 to V_6. Inferior wall ischemia produces changes in leads II, III, and aVF. Posterior wall ischemia may be indirectly recognized by *reciprocal* ST depressions in leads V_1 to V_3. Prominent reciprocal ST depressions in these leads also occur with certain inferior wall infarcts, particularly those with posterior or lateral wall extension. Right ventricular ischemia usually produces ST elevations in right-sided chest leads

FIGURE 189-14 Acute ischemia causes a current of injury. With predominant subendocardial ischemia, the resultant ST vector will be directed toward the inner layer of the affected ventricle and the ventricular cavity. Overlying leads therefore will record ST depression. With ischemia involving the outer ventricular layer (transmural or epicardial injury), the ST vector will be directed outward. Overlying leads will record ST elevation.

FIGURE 189-15 Hyperacute phase of anteroseptal myocardial infarction (MI). Note the tall positive T waves (V_2 to V_3) along with ST-segment elevations and Q waves (V_1 to V_3).

repolarization (ST-T) abnormalities. Necrosis of sufficient myocardial tissue may lead to decreased R-wave amplitude or frank abnormal Q waves in the anterior or inferior leads (Fig. 189-17). Previously, abnormal Q waves were considered to be markers of transmural myocardial infarction, while subendocardial infarcts were thought not to produce Q waves. However, careful ECG-pathologic correlative studies have indicated that transmural infarcts may occur without Q waves and that subendocardial (nontransmural) infarcts may sometimes be associated with Q waves. Therefore, infarcts are more appropriately classified as "Q-wave" or "non-Q-wave". The major acute ECG changes in syndromes of ischemic heart disease are schematically summarized in Fig. 189-18. Loss of depolarization forces due to posterior or lateral infarction may cause reciprocal increases in R-wave amplitude in leads V_1 and V_2 without diagnostic Q waves in any of the conventional leads. Atrial infarction may be associated with PR-segment deviations due to an atrial current of injury, changes in P-wave morphology, or atrial arrhythmias. In the weeks and months following infarction, these ECG changes may persist or begin to resolve. Complete normalization of the ECG following Q-wave infarction is uncommon but may occur, particularly with smaller infarcts. In contrast, persistent ST-segment elevations several weeks or more after a Q-wave infarct usually correlate with a severe underlying wall motion disorder (akinetic or dyskinetic zone), although not necessarily a frank ventricular aneurysm.

ECG changes due to ischemia may occur spontaneously or may be provoked by various exercise protocols (stress electrocardiography) (Chap. 203). In patients with severe ischemic heart disease, exercise testing is most likely to elicit signs of subendocardial ischemia (horizontal or downsloping ST depression in multiple leads). ST-segment elevation during exercise is most often observed after a Q-wave infarct. This repolarization change does not necessarily indicate active ischemia but correlates strongly with the presence of an underlying ventricular wall motion abnormality. However, in patients *without* prior infarction, transient ST-segment elevation with exercise is a reliable sign of transmural ischemia.

The ECG has important limitations in both sensitivity and specificity in the diagnosis of ischemic heart disease. Although a single normal ECG does not exclude ischemia or even acute infarction, a normal ECG *throughout* the course of an acute infarct is distinctly uncommon. Prolonged chest pain without diagnostic ECG changes, therefore, should always prompt a careful search for other noncoronary causes of chest pain (see Chap. 12). Furthermore, the diagnostic changes of acute or evolving ischemia are often masked by the presence of left bundle branch block, electronic ventricular pacemaker patterns, and WPW preexcitation. On the other hand, clinicians may overdiagnose ischemia or infarction based on the presence of ST-segment elevations or depressions, T-wave inversions, tall positive T waves, or Q waves *not* related to ischemic heart disease (pseudoinfarct patterns). For example, ST-segment elevations simulating ischemia may occur with acute pericarditis (Fig. 189-19) or myocarditis or as a normal variant ("early repolarization" pattern). Similarly, tall positive T waves do not invariably represent hyperacute ischemic changes but also may be due to normal variants, hyperkalemia, cerebrovascular injury, and left ventricular volume overload due to mitral or aortic regurgitation, among other causes. ST-segment elevations and tall, positive T waves are common findings in leads

(Fig. 189-7). When ischemic ST elevations occur as the earliest sign of acute infarction, they are typically followed within a period ranging from hours to days by evolving T-wave inversions and often by Q waves occurring in the same lead distribution. (T-wave inversions due to evolving or chronic ischemia correlate with prolongation of repolarization and are often associated with QT lengthening.) Reversible transmural ischemia, e.g., due to coronary vasospasm (Prinzmetal's variant angina), may cause transient ST-segment elevations without development of Q waves. Depending on the severity and duration of such ischemia, the ST elevations may either resolve completely within minutes or be followed by T-wave inversions that persist for hours or even days. Patients with ischemic chest pain who present with deep T-wave inversions in multiple precordial leads (e.g., V_1 to V_4) with or without cardiac enzyme elevations typically have severe obstruction in the left anterior descending coronary artery system (Fig. 189-16). In contrast, patients whose baseline ECG already shows abnormal T-wave inversions may develop T-wave normalization (pseudonormalization) during episodes of acute transmural ischemia.

With infarction, depolarization (QRS) changes often accompany

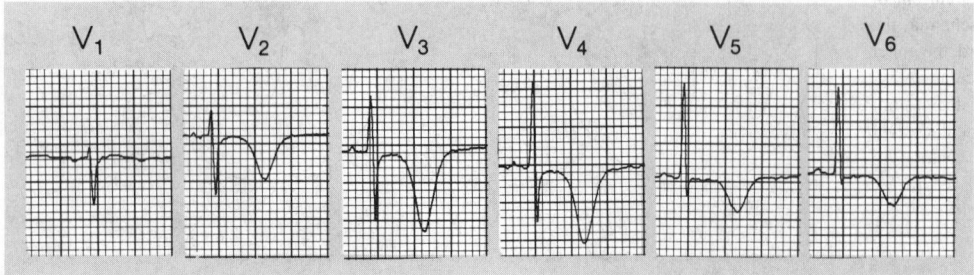

FIGURE 189-16 Severe anterior wall ischemia (with or without infarction) may cause prominent T-wave inversions in the precordial leads. This pattern is usually associated with a high-grade stenosis of the left anterior descending coronary artery.

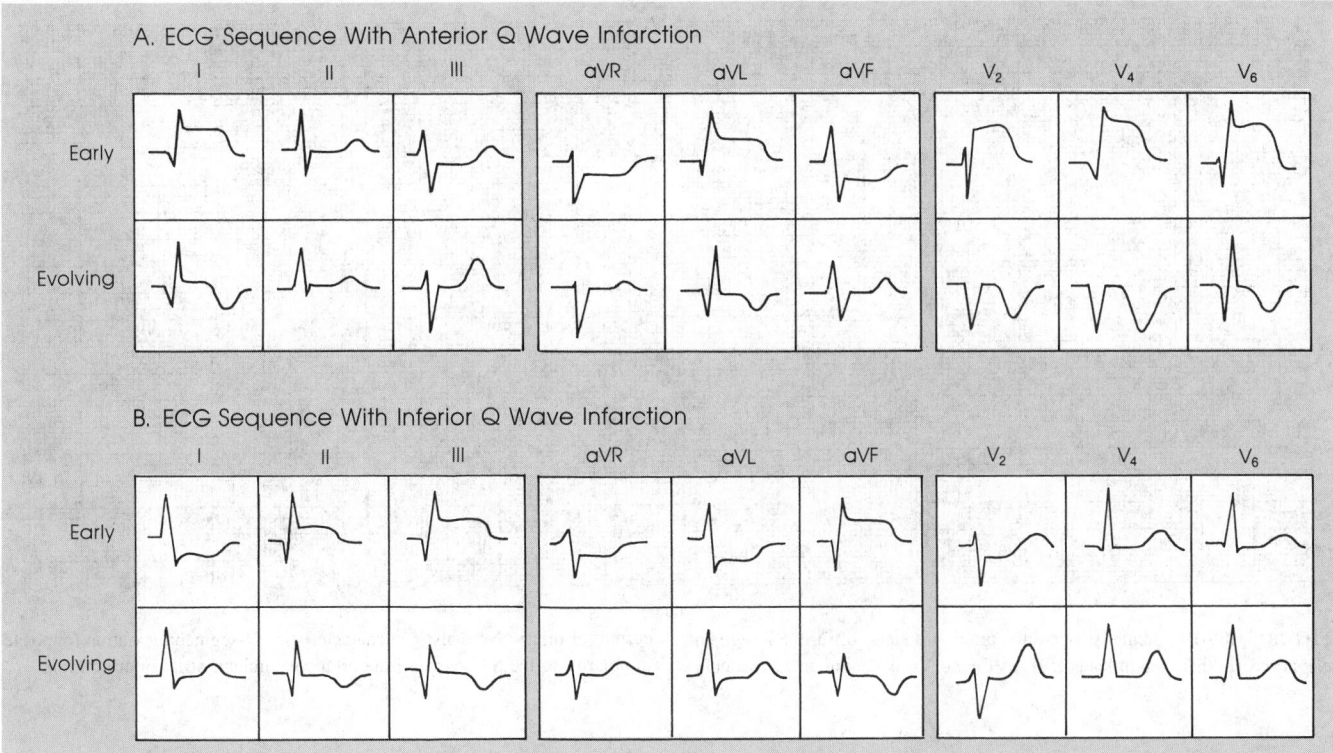

A. ECG Sequence With Anterior Q Wave Infarction

B. ECG Sequence With Inferior Q Wave Infarction

FIGURE 189-17 Sequence of depolarization and repolarization changes with (A) acute anterior and (B) acute inferior wall Q-wave infarctions. With anterior infarcts, ST elevation in leads I, aVL, and the precordial leads may be accompanied by reciprocal ST depressions in leads II, III, and aVF. Conversely, acute inferior (or posterior) infarcts may be associated with reciprocal ST depressions in leads V_1 to V_3. (After Goldberger and Goldberger.)

V_1 and V_2 in left bundle branch or left ventricular hypertrophy in the absence of ischemia. The differential diagnosis of Q waves (Table 189-2) includes physiologic or positional variants, ventricular hypertrophy, acute or chronic noncoronary myocardial injury, hypertrophic cardiomyopathy, and ventricular conduction disorders. Digitalis, ventricular hypertrophy, hypokalemia, and a variety of other factors may cause ST-segment depression mimicking subendocardial ischemia. Prominent T-wave inversion may occur with ventricular hypertrophy, cardiomyopathy, myocarditis, and cerebrovascular injury (particularly intracranial bleeds; Fig. 189-20), among many other conditions.

METABOLIC FACTORS AND DRUG EFFECTS A variety of metabolic and pharmacologic agents alter the ECG and in particular cause changes in repolarization (ST-T-U) and sometimes QRS prolongation (Table 189-1). Certain life-threatening electrolyte disturbances may be diagnosed initially and monitored from the ECG. *Hyperkalemia* produces a sequence of changes usually beginning with narrowing and peaking (tenting) of the T waves. Further elevation of extracellular K^+ leads to AV conduction disturbances, diminution in P-wave amplitude, and widening of the QRS interval. Severe hyperkalemia eventually causes cardiac arrest with a slow sinusoidal type of mechanism ("sinewave" pattern) followed by asystole. *Hypokalemia* (Fig. 189-20) prolongs ventricular repolarization, often with prominent U waves. Prolongation of the QT interval (Fig. 189-20) is also seen with drugs that increase the duration of the ventricular action potential: type 1A antiarrhythmic agents and related drugs (e.g., quinidine, disopyramide, procainamide, tricyclic antidepressants, phenothiazines) and type III agents (amiodarone, sotalol). Marked QT prolongation, sometimes with deep, wide T-wave inversions, may occur with intracranial bleeds, particularly subarachnoid hemorrhage ("CVA T-wave" pattern) (Fig. 189-20). Systemic *hypothermia* (Fig. 189-20) also prolongs repolarization, usually with a distinctive convex elevation of the J point (Osborn wave). *Hypocalcemia* typically prolongs the QT interval (ST portion),

FIGURE 189-18 Variability of ECG patterns with myocardial ischemia. The ECG also may be normal or nonspecifically abnormal. Furthermore, these categorizations are not mutually exclusive. For example, a non-Q-wave infarct may evolve into a Q-wave infarct, ST elevations may be followed by a non-Q-wave infarct, or ST depressions and T-wave inversions may be followed by a Q wave infarct. (After Goldberger.)

FIGURE 189-19 Acute pericarditis often produces diffuse ST-segment elevations (in this case in leads I, II, aVF, and V₂ to V₆) due to a ventricular current of injury. Note also the characteristic PR-segment deviation (opposite in polarity to the ST segment) due to a concomitant atrial injury current.

FIGURE 189-20 A variety of metabolic derangements, drug effects, and other factors may prolong ventricular repolarization with QT prolongation or prominent U waves. Repolarization prolongation, particularly due to hypokalemia or pharmacologic agents, indicates increased susceptibility to torsades de pointes type ventricular tachycardia. Hypothermia is associated with a distinctive convex "hump" at the J point (Osborn wave, *arrow*). Note QRS and QT prolongation along with sinus tachycardia in tricyclic antidepressant overdose.

TABLE 189-2 Differential diagnosis of Q waves (with selected examples)

Physiologic or positional factors
A Normal variant "septal" q waves
B Normal variant Q waves in V_1 to V_2, aVL, III, and aVF
C Left pneumothorax or dextrocardia: loss of lateral R-wave progression
Myocardial injury or infiltration
A Acute processes: myocardial ischemia or infarction, myocarditis, hyperkalemia
B Chronic processes: myocardial infarction, idiopathic cardiomyopathy, myocarditis, amyloid, tumor, sarcoid, scleroderma, Chagas' disease, echinococcus cyst
Ventricular hypertrophy/enlargement
A Left ventricular (poor R-wave progression*)
B Right ventricular (reversed R-wave progression[†] or poor R-wave progression, particularly with chronic obstructive lung disease)
C Hypertrophic cardiomyopathy (may simulate anterior, inferior, posterior or lateral infarcts)
Conduction abnormalities
A Left bundle branch block (poor R-wave progression*)
B Wolff-Parkinson-White patterns

---

* Small or absent R waves in the right to midprecordial leads.
[†] Progressive decrease in R-wave amplitude from V_1 to the mid- or lateral precordial leads.
SOURCE: *After Goldberger.*

FIGURE 189-21 Prolongation of the Q-T interval (ST-segment portion) typical of hypocalcemia. Hypercalcemia may cause abbreviation of the ST segment and shortening of the QT interval.

while *hypercalcemia* shortens it (Fig. 189-21). Digitalis glycosides also shorten the QT interval, often with a characteristic "scooping" of the ST–T-wave complex (*digitalis effect*).

ELECTRICAL ALTERNANS Electrical alternans, i.e., a beat-to-beat alternation in one or more components of the ECG signal, is a common type of nonlinear cardiovascular response to a variety of perturbations. For example, total electrical alternans (P-QRS-T) with sinus tachycardia is a relatively specific sign of pericardial effusion, often with cardiac tamponade (Fig. 189-22). The mechanism relates to a periodic swinging motion of the heart in the effusion at a frequency exactly one-half the heart rate. Alternation of the QRS complex (and sometimes R-R intervals) has been reported with rapid paroxysmal supraventricular tachycardias, usually involving a concealed bypass tract (Chap. 198). ST-segment alternans is a specific sign of severe transmural myocardial ischemia and may precede ventricular fibrillation. U-wave alternans may occur with idiopathic or acquired QT prolongation syndromes prior to the onset of *torsades de pointes* tachycardia (Chap. 198).

Many other factors are associated with ECG changes, particularly alterations in ventricular repolarization. T-wave flattening, minimal T-wave inversions or slight ST-segment depression ("nonspecific ST–T-wave changes") may occur with a variety of electrolyte and acid-base disturbances, a variety of infectious processes, central nervous system disorders, endocrine abnormalities, many drugs, ischemia, hypoxia, and virtually any type of cardiopulmonary abnormality. While subtle ST–T-wave changes may be markers of ischemia, transient nonspecific repolarization changes also may occur following a meal or with postural (orthostatic) change, hyperventilation, or exercise in healthy individuals.

CLINICAL INTERPRETATION OF THE ECG Accurate analysis of ECGs require thoroughness and care. Interpretation should always be done in the context of the patient's age, gender, and clinical status. For example, T-wave inversions in leads V_1 to V_3, are more likely to represent a normal variant in a healthy, young adult woman ("persistent juvenile T-wave pattern") than similar findings in an elderly male with chest discomfort. Similarly, the likelihood that ST-segment depression during exercise testing represents ischemia must be considered in light of the prior probability of coronary artery disease (Chap. 10).

Many mistakes in ECG interpretation are errors of omission. Therefore, a systematic approach is desirable. The following 14 points should be analyzed carefully in every ECG: (1) standardization (calibration) and technical features (including lead placement and artifact), (2) heart rate, (3) rhythm, (4) PR interval, (5) QRS interval, (6) QT interval, (7) P waves, (8) QRS voltages, (9) mean QRS electrical axis, (10) precordial R-wave progression, (11) abnormal Q waves, (12) ST segments, (13) T waves, and (14) U waves.

Only after analyzing all these points should the interpretation be formulated. Where appropriate, important clinical correlates or inferences should be mentioned. For example, prolonged ventricular repolarization with prominent U waves should suggest hypokalemia or drug toxicity (e.g., due to quinidine or procainamide) (see Fig. 189-20). The combination of left atrial abnormality (enlargement) and signs of right ventricular hypertrophy suggests mitral stenosis. Low voltage with sinus tachycardia raises consideration of pericardial tamponade or chronic obstructive lung disease. Sinus tachycardia with QRS and QT (U) prolongation suggests tricyclic antidepressant overdose (Fig. 189-20). Comparison with previous ECGs is essential. The diagnosis and management of specific cardiac arrhythmias and conduction disturbances are discussed in Chaps. 197 and 198.

FIGURE 189-22 Beat-to-beat alternation in QRS axis/amplitude with sinus tachycardia is a highly specific, though not particularly sensitive, sign of pericardial effusion with cardiac tamponade.

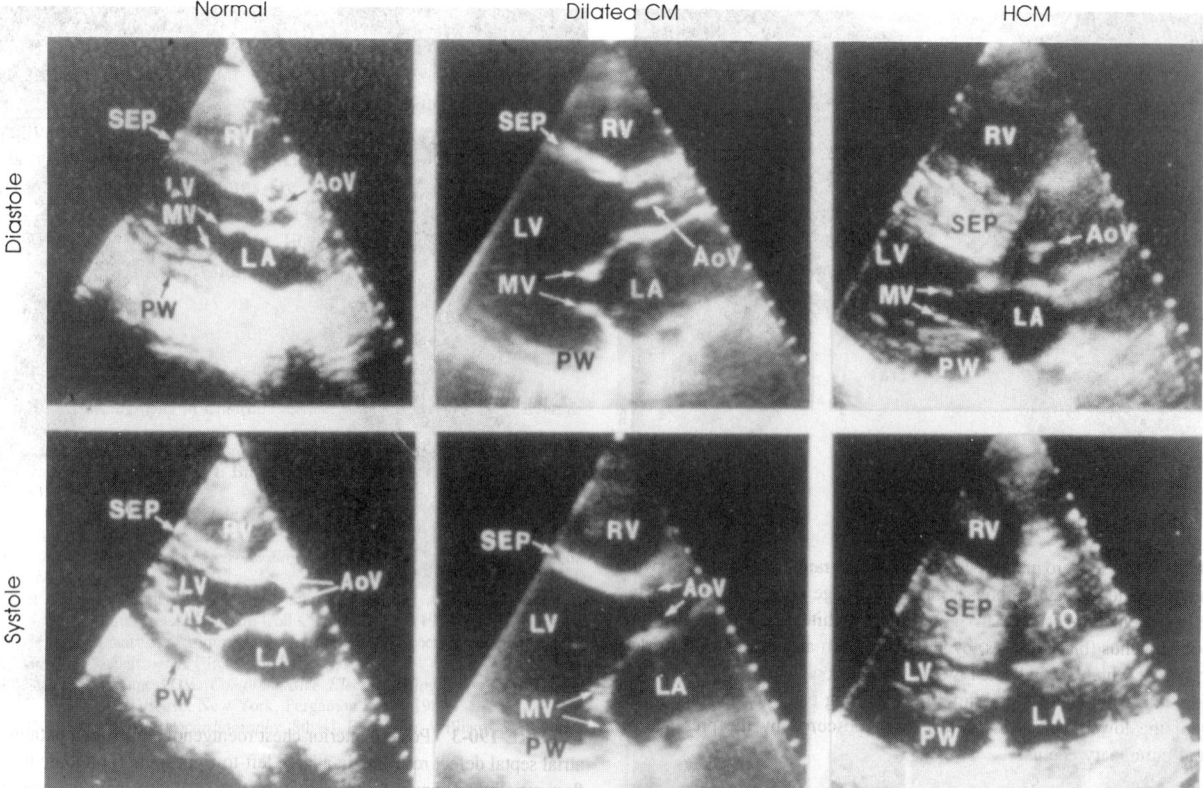

FIGURE 190-5 Long-axis parasternal views of the left ventricle in diastole and systole in a normal individual and in patients with dilated cardiomyopathy (CM) and hypertrophic cardiomyopathy (HCM). Normal diastolic wall thicknesses and normal systolic wall thickening and excursion are illustrated in the left panels. In the patient with dilated CM, left ventricular (LV) and left atrial (LA) diameters are increased, and there is markedly reduced systolic thickening and excursion of the septum (SEP) and posterior wall (PW). In the patient with HCM, the SEP is abnormally thick and highly echogenic. The LV cavity is small in diastole and almost disappears during systolic contraction. RV = right ventricle; MV = mitral valve; AoV = aortic valve.

with high-frequency transducers. Transesophageal echocardiography, therefore, may facilitate cardiac evaluation of patients with suboptimal transthoracic scans, such as ventilated patients or those with obesity or emphysema. Compared with transthoracic echocardiography, transesophageal echocardiography is more sensitive for detection of prosthetic valve dysfunction, atrial thrombus and other masses, atrial septal defects (especially of the sinus venosus type), aortic dissection, and complications of infective endocarditis (Fig. 190-6). It is used intraoperatively to monitor myocardial function and to assess the results of valvular repair and correction of congenital heart defects.

Doppler echocardiography (Fig. 190-7) detects blood flow velocity and turbulence. When sound encounters moving red blood cells, the frequency of its reflected signal is altered. The magnitude of the change *(Doppler shift)* indicates the velocity V of blood flow with respect to the sound beam:

$$V = \frac{C \times (\text{Doppler shift})}{(2 \times \text{emitted frequency}) \cos \theta}$$

where C is the speed of sound in tissue, and θ is the angle between the Doppler beam and the mean axis of blood flow. An upward shift (increased frequency of the reflected sound) indicates blood motion toward the transducer and a downward shift, motion away.

There are several types of Doppler studies, all of which can be performed using a single probe. Pulsed Doppler echocardiography,

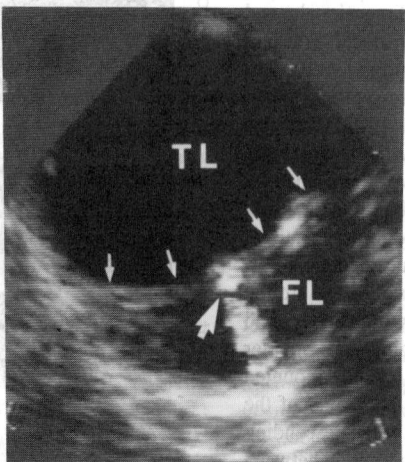

FIGURE 190-6 Transesophageal echocardiograms.

A. An image in systole from a patient with a Medtronic Hall mitral valve prosthesis who presented with a cerebral embolus. Thrombi (TH) are seen to arise from the annular insertion points of the prosthesis. The small white arrow indicates part of the prosthesis. LA = left atrium; LV = left ventricle; AO = aortic root.

B. Transverse view of the descending thoracic aorta in a patient presenting with aortic dissection. Color flow imaging (white) demonstrates flow from the true lumen (TL) into the false lumen (FL). The site of an initimal tear is indicated by the larger white arrow. The small white arrows indicate the intimal flap.

FIGURE 190-7 Continuous-wave Doppler studies, performed with the probe positioned at the apex, from one patient (*A, B*) with aortic stenosis (AS), aortic insufficiency (AI), and mitral regurgitation (MR) and from another patient (*C, D*) with mital stenosis (MS), severe MR, and AI. Flow away from the transducer, in the AS and MR jets, is depicted below the center (zero flow) line, while flow toward the transducer, in the AI and MS jets, is depicted above the center line. Flow velocity (*V*) in meters per second is given on the right side of each panel. As expected from knowledge of points of crossover between aortic, left ventricular, and left atrial pressures, the AS signal is shorter in duration than the MR signal and has a lower velocity. The AI signal is of longer duration than the MS signal. Instantaneous pressure gradients (*P*) across the valves can be calculated using the equation, $P = 4V^2$. Peak *V* of 5.1 m/s in the AS jet indicates a peak left ventricular to aortic *P* of 104 mmHg, while the peak *V* of 6.8 m/s in the MR jet indicates a left ventricular to left atrial systolic *P* of 185 mmHg. Peak aortic to left ventricular diastolic *P* in the AI jet is 81 mmHg, and peak left atrial to left ventricular *P* in the MS jet is 40 mmHg. Mean gradient, calculated using an off-line computer system, in the MS jet was markedly elevated at 26 mmHg.

which uses a single crystal to assess flow velocity and turbulence within operator-selected areas of interest in the heart and great vessels, permits excellent spatial localization of flow disturbances resulting from valvular stenosis and regurgitation and from shunts. Quantitation of high-flow velocity requires a continuous-wave transducer with two separate, adjacent crystals, one that continuously transmits sound and one that continuously receives reflected sound. Since continuous-wave transducers cannot spatially localize flow disturbances, optimal assessment of flow within the heart and vessels generally requires both pulsed- and continuous-wave technology. Combined two-dimensional echocardiography and pulsed Doppler techniques permit calculation of flow volumes across cardiac valves and, therefore, of cardiac output, pulmonic-to-systemic flow ratios, and regurgitant fractions. Pressure gradients (*P*) across restrictive orifices such as cardiac valves can be calculated using the modified Bernoulli equation, $P = 4V^2$, where *P* is the pressure gradient in mmHg and *V* the velocity in m/s.

Doppler color flow imaging is a complicated, combined imaging and Doppler technique in which blood flow direction, relative velocity, and turbulence are depicted by various colors superimposed on a two-dimensional image of the heart. It should be recognized, however, that color Doppler is extremely sensitive for regurgitation. Small signs of mitral, tricuspid, and pulmonic insufficiency are imaged in the majority of even normal individuals.

VALVULAR HEART DISEASE Imaging echocardiography can detect abnormalities of valve thickness and movement responsible for stenosis and regurgitation. In addition, the heart's response to pressure

or volume overload can be assessed in terms of chamber dilatation, hypertrophy, and wall movement. Doppler techniques permit evaluation of regurgitation and stenosis (see also Chap. 201.)

Mitral stenosis The echocardiographic appearance of a restricted valve opening, due to leaflet thickening and commissural fusion, and of shortened, thickened chordae is virtually diagnostic of rheumatic deformity (Fig. 190-4, *left*). Planimetry of the mitral area in the diastolic short-axis view and evaluation of the rate of falloff of the estimated transmitral diastolic pressure gradient by Doppler permit quite reliable estimation of valve area. Using the Doppler technique, mitral valve area (MVA) in square centimeters can be estimated with the equation MVA = 220 divided by duration of time (in milliseconds) necessary for the peak diastolic pressure gradient to decrease by 50 percent. Other causes of inflow obstruction, such as atrial myxoma (Fig. 190-4, *right*) or thrombus, massive annular calcification, supravalvular ring, cor triatriatum, and parachute mitral valve also may be detected.

Mitral regurgitation Systolic mitral competence depends on normal function of the mitral leaflets and their supporting structures, including the annulus, chordae tendineae, papillary muscles, and surrounding myocardium. Two-dimensional transthoracic or transesophageal techniques are useful for recognizing the etiology of mitral regurgitation, which includes rheumatic disease, prolapse, flail leaflets resulting from chordal or papillary muscle rupture, annular calcification, atrioventricular canal defects, myxomas, endocarditis, hypertrophic cardiomyopathy, and ventricular dysfunction. Doppler mapping provides a gross estimate of the severity of regurgitation.

Aortic stenosis Subvalvular, valvular, and supravalvular obstruction can generally be detected by two-dimensional echocardiography. Systolic leaflet doming and an unusual number or size of cusps (two in a bicuspid valve) suggest congenital valve disease. Acquired fibrosis and calcification cause valve thickening. Doppler detection of high-flow velocity across the valve, corresponding to a high transvalvular gradient, indicates the presence of stenosis. Lesser flow velocities do not, however, exclude stenosis because both reduced stroke volume and inability to position the Doppler beam parallel to flow may appreciably decrease measured velocities. If velocity can be reliably measured, aortic valve area (AVA) can be quantitated.

Aortic regurgitation Dilatation of the aortic root and aortic dissection can be distinguished from valve leaflet abnormalities causing regurgitation, including congenital disease, sclerosis, endocarditis, prolapse, and flail cusps. The presence and spatial extent of regurgitation is evaluated by Doppler study.

Tricuspid and pulmonary valve disease Two-dimensional echocardiography allows visualization of right-sided valves and can detect changes in structure and movement due to rheumatic deformity, Ebstein's malformation, prolapse, flail cusps, endocarditis, congenital dysplasia, and thickening due to carcinoid, amyloid, Loeffler's endocarditis, or endocardial fibrosis. Systolic doming of the pulmonic valve is characteristic of pulmonic stenosis. Stenosis and regurgitation are assessed by Doppler techniques. The flow velocity in a tricuspid regurgitant jet can be used to estimate right ventricular and pulmonary arterial systolic pressures.

Prosthetic valves (Fig. 190-6) Mechanical prostheses are difficult to evaluate, because their intrinsically high echogenicity often interferes with recognition of valve motion, vegetations, thrombi, and regurgitation. Abnormalities of bioprostheses, including fibrosis, calcification, vegetations, tears, and regurgitation, are more easily recognized. Transesophageal echocardiography should be considered strongly in patients with suspected prosthetic mitral valve dysfunction when transthoracic evaluation is nonrevealing. Angiography and hemodynamic study may be necessary for full evaluation.

Endocarditis Valvular vegetations, characterized by masses of shaggy-appearing echoes, are evident in most patients with native valve endocarditis (Chap. 85). They are less commonly identified in prosthetic valve endocarditis. Transesophageal techniques are more sensitive and, additionally, can readily detect perivalvular abscesses.

Left ventricle   A combination of M-mode and two-dimensional echocardiography is widely used to measure left ventricular size, wall thickness, and function. The rate of wall thinning in diastole may permit assessment of diastolic function, and the percentage of shortening of the minor axis, normally greater than 28 percent, and the mean velocity of circumferential fiber shortening are useful measurements of systolic performance. These indexes of systolic performance are influenced, however, by preload and afterload as well as by myocardial contractility. Analyses of end-systolic pressure-dimension relations, which are independent of preload and incorporate afterload, provide better information regarding contractile function. Estimates of global ventricular performance, based on icepick M-mode views, are useful, however, only when ventricular shape is normal and systolic movement relatively symmetric in extent and timing. Two-dimensional echocardiography, which images the ventricle in a number of different planes, improves assessment of volumes and function, particularly in patients with asymmetric contraction resulting from ischemic heart disease, in whom localized regional wall motion can be present. The left ventricular apex can be visualized only by two-dimensional techniques. Complications of infarction, including wall movement abnormalities, true and false aneurysms, myocardial rupture (septal, papillary muscle, or free wall), thrombi, and mitral regurgitation, may be detected. In patients being evaluated for ischemic heart disease, two-dimensional images can be recorded during exercise or pacing stress or during pharmacologic challenge with vasodilators (adenosine or dipyridamole) or with the beta agonist dobutamine. The development of one or more wall movement abnormalities, not present at rest, provides a highly sensitive and specific means of recognizing ischemia.

Echocardiography permits recognition of *cardiomyopathy* (Chap. 205), and classification into dilated, hypertrophic, and restrictive-obliterative types (Fig. 190-5). In dilated cardiomyopathy, both ventricles are generally enlarged and poorly contracting, and wall thicknesses are normal or only slightly increased. In contrast, appreciable ventricular hypertrophy (usually involving the septum asymmetrically), small ventricular size, enhanced systolic performance, and impaired diastolic relaxation characterize hypertrophic cardiomyopathy. Systolic anterior movement of the mitral valve to abut the septum, partial midsystolic aortic valve closure, and increased left ventricular outflow tract velocity correlate with dynamic obstruction. Increased wall thickness, biatrial enlargement, mitral and tricuspid regurgitation, and slowed diastolic filling characterize infiltrative disorders. In patients presenting with heart failure, echocardiographic recognition of whether ventricular dysfunction is predominantly systolic or diastolic has important prognostic and therapeutic implications.

Pericardial effusion   Echocardiography can detect effusions as small as 15 mL. Diastolic compression of heart chambers, usually the right atrium and ventricle, and exaggerated respiratory variation in transvalvular flow velocities may suggest tamponade.

Cardiac masses   Most masses involving the heart and pericardium are easily recognized. They include myxomas (Fig. 190-4), other primary and secondary tumors, and thrombi. The left atrium and its appendage are best studied by transesophageal echocardiography.

Congenital heart disease   Since valvular abnormalities and relationships of atria, valves, ventricles, and great vessels can easily be recognized by two-dimensional echocardiography, this technique has revolutionized the diagnosis of congenital heart disease. Contrast and Doppler echocardiography, especially color flow mapping, facilitate detection of shunts and of valvular stenosis and regurgitation.

RADIONUCLIDE IMAGING OF THE HEART

There are five major clinical indications for radionuclide study of the heart: (1) assessment of systolic and diastolic ventricular function using radionuclide ventriculography, (2) identification and quantification of intracardiac shunts using radioangiocardiography, (3) assessment of myocardial perfusion using ionic tracers, principally thallium 201, (4) detection of acute myocardial necrosis with infarct-avid radionuclides, and (5) assessment of myocardial metabolism by means of positron emission tomography (see Chap. 191).

VENTRICULAR PERFORMANCE   Radionuclide ventriculography (RVG) uses a radioactive intravascular indicator, usually technetium 99m attached to red blood cells, to delineate heart chambers and great vessels (Fig. 190-8). RVGs may be performed using two different methods. In the *first-pass* technique, radiotracer is injected intravenously, and a scintillation camera tracks its transit through the right heart, lungs, and left heart. In the *equilibrium*, or *gated*, method, counts are recorded in at least two views from several hundred cardiac cycles following uniform distribution of radiotracer throughout the blood pool. The scintigraphic information in each cycle is divided into multiple frames (often 30 or more), using the ECG as a timing reference. Counts from corresponding frames of each cycle are then summed by computer to provide images of the spatial distribution and density of counts over time. Gated scans are frequently obtained after first-pass scans, since no additional injection of radionuclide is required. Because detected counts, after background subtraction, are proportional to blood volume, these studies permit accurate estimation of chamber volumes, rates of ventricular ejection and filling, left-to-right ventricular stroke volume ratios, and ventricular ejection fractions. Using a time-activity curve generated from a region of interest over the left ventricle, left ventricular ejection fraction (LVEF), a widely used index of left ventricular function (Chap. 194), can be calculated as LVEF = EDC − ESC/EDC, where EDC is end-diastolic counts and ESC is end-systolic counts. Repeated scans can be obtained up to 20 h after injection, permitting assessment of the effects of interventions, such as exercise and drugs, on ventricular performance.

RVG may be used to detect patients with chronic ischemic heart disease. Since resting function may be normal, exercise is often used to provoke ischemia. Scans are obtained at rest and at peak exercise.

FIGURE 190-8   End-diastolic and end-systolic gated blood pool images from a normal individual (with estimated left and right ventricular ejection fractions of 69 and 45 percent, respectively) and from a patient with idiopathic dilated cardiomyopathy and marked, global reduction of left ventricular systolic function (left ventricular ejection fraction of 23 percent). In the patient with cardiomyopathy, there is very little change in left ventricular cavity size or count density from diastole to systole. The right ventricle, however, shows normal function, with an ejection fraction of 57 percent. RV = right ventricle; LV = left ventricle.

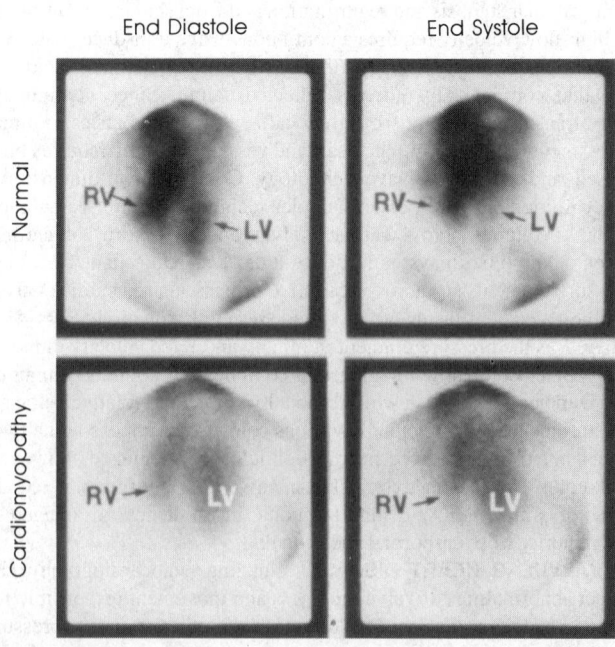

Failure to increase left ventricular ejection fraction by at least 5 units (e.g., from 40 to 45 percent) and development of one or more regional wall movement abnormalities have a sensitivity and specificity of approximately 90 and 60 percent, respectively, for detection of significant ischemic heart disease. The test is most helpful in patients with an intermediate pretest probability of disease. Low resting ejection fractions after acute infarction have been correlated with increased short- and long-term morbidity and mortality. Mitral regurgitation, septal rupture, and aneurysms resulting from infarction also may be detected. RVG can assess systolic and diastolic function in patients with cardiomyopathy (Fig. 190-8) or volume overload. A reduced resting ejection fraction correlates with a poor prognosis in patients with mitral or aortic regurgitation, even after valve replacement. The added value of exercise RVG in detecting reduced myocardial reserve due to volume overload remains controversial. Thrombi and other tumors may be recognized, but RVG is less sensitive than echocardiography.

SHUNT SCINTIGRAPHY   Assessment of left-to-right shunts utilizes a modification of the first-pass RVG in which the "region of interest" is focused over an area of lung. Following rapid injection of radiotracer into a large vein, usually the external jugular, the pulmonary time-activity curve is recorded by a gamma camera–computer system. Normally, counts increase sharply as the bolus reaches the lung underlying the detector. Following peak activity, there is a smooth descent and a later, smaller increase in counts representing normal recirculation of the radiotracer following systemic circulation. Left-to-right shunts cause premature interruption of the descent due to early reappearance of radioactivity within the lung. Computer analysis of the areas under the curve permits reliable determination of the ratio of pulmonic-to-systemic blood flow. Right-to-left shunts also may be recognized and quantified.

MYOCARDIAL PERFUSION IMAGING   The potassium analogue thallium 201, cyclotron-produced with a half-life of 72 h, is the most commonly used agent to assess myocardial perfusion. Its active uptake by normal myocardial cells is proportional to regional blood flow. Areas of myocardial necrosis, fibrosis, and ischemia show reduced thallium accumulation ("cold spots") on images obtained soon after injection. Following its initial accumulation within cells, however, thallium 201 continues to exchange with the systemic pool. After several hours, equilibration occurs; viable myocardial cells having intact membrane function contain nearly equal concentrations.

Thallium 201 scintigraphy is used most commonly to detect exercise-induced ischemia (Fig. 190-9). Thallium is injected intravenously at peak exercise, and images are obtained 5 to 10 minutes later in several projections using either planar imaging or single photon emission computed tomography (SPECT). The images may be analyzed qualitatively or quantitatively using computer algorithms. Normal scans show relatively homogeneous distribution of activity, while those of patients with infarction or ischemia typically demonstrate one or more "cold spots." Because of continued exchange of thallium between viable cells and the systemic pool, however, most initial defects due to ischemia "fill in" on repeat imaging several hours later. Some, however, require up to 24 h for redistribution or are best identified following reinjection of thallium 4 h after exercise, but areas of infarction demonstrate persistent reduction of uptake.

Compared with routine exercise electrocardiography, exercise thallium scintigraphy increases the sensitivity for detection of coronary disease from approximately 60 to 80 percent and increases specificity slightly from about 80 to 90 percent. It is most useful in patients with atypical chest pain in whom the exercise ECG is nondiagnostic or uninterpretable due to baseline ST abnormalities, left bundle branch block, ventricular hypertrophy, or drug and electrolyte effects; in patients who fail to achieve 85 percent of predicted maximal heart rate; and in patients with a high likelihood of a false-positive exercise ECG study. Thallium scanning improves localization of ischemia and provides prognostic information, since the presence and number of redistributing defects correlate with the incidence of future cardiac events. Thallium scintigraphy also has been used to detect ischemia

FIGURE 190-9   Serial thallium 201 scintigrams obtained in the 45° LAO projection in a patient undergoing exercise testing for evaluation of chest pain. The immediate postexercise image (*left*) demonstrates decreased perfusion of the septum. The 1- and 2-h delayed images (*middle and right*) demonstrate "filling in" of the defect, reflecting redistribution. The computer-derived time-activity curves (*bottom*) confirm the significant reduction in initial counts in the septum, relative to the posterolateral wall, and demonstrate near equalization of activity by 2 h. S = septum; PL = posterolateral wall. [*From PC Come (ed), Diagnostic Cardiology. Reprinted with permission of George A. Beller, M.D., and J.B. Lippincott Company*, 1985]

during spontaneous pain, pacing, and adenosine- and dipyridamole-induced coronary vasodilation. Dipyridamole thallium imaging appears to be as sensitive and specific as exercise thallium scintigraphy for detection of ischemic heart disease. It should be considered for patients unable to exercise, including those with peripheral vascular disease who have an increased risk of cardiac morbidity and mortality with vascular surgery.

Thallium scanning does not distinguish new from old infarcts and is less accurate than serum enzyme analysis in detecting acute necrosis. It does, however, offer prognostic information. Patients with smaller defects have better survival rates. On submaximal exercise thallium tests following infarction, the presence of multiple fixed or redistributing defects and/or increased lung uptake of thallium (probably representing transudation into the lung during periods of high pulmonary capillary pressure) identifies patients at higher risk for postinfarction morbidity and mortality.

The new perfusion imaging agents technetium 99m Sesta-MIBI and technetium 99m teboroxime offer some advantages over thallium 201. They are generator-produced, permitting continuous on-site availability. Image resolution is enhanced by both the ideal energy of technetium 99m for standard gamma camera imaging and its shorter half-life, which permits use of higher doses of radioactivity. Given the high count rates achieved, first-pass imaging for assessment of ejection fraction can be performed in addition to perfusion imaging. Redistribution of Sesta-MIBI is minimal, allowing scanning to be performed for up to 6 h after injection. Patients suspected of having acute infarction can therefore be injected at the bedside and stabilized or even treated with a thrombolytic agent prior to imaging. The image, of course, reflects the distribution of coronary blood flow at the time of injection, not at the time of imaging. However, separate injections are required to differentiate perfusion abnormalities due to ischemia from those due to infarction. Teboroxime has rapid washout from the myocardium, permitting dual-injection rest and exercise studies to be completed within 1 h. Alternatively, taking advantage of the different energy spectra of thallium 201 and technetium 99m, thallium can be injected at rest and Sesta-MIBI during exercise for dual postexercise imaging.

IMAGING OF NECROTIC MYOCARDIUM   Pyrophosphate scintigraphy   Pyrophosphate labeled with technetium 99m binds to calcium and organic macromolecules in irreversibly damaged myocardial cells, producing an image with increased uptake (''hot spot''). Scans are most likely to be positive when injections are performed 48 to 72 h after suspected infarction, when the elevated creatine kinase activity often has returned to normal. The major clinical indication is the detection of acute infarction in those rare patients in whom traditional diagnostic methods cannot be interpreted or have provided equivocal results or in patients who present too late to show an enzyme elevation. Sensitivity and specificity for transmural infarcts are both about 90 percent. Uptake is often fainter and more poorly localized in subendocardial infarcts, and myocardial damage from causes other than coronary disease may result in a positive scan.

Antimyosin imaging   Radiolabeled fragments of antibodies specific for cardiac myosin localize in areas of acute myocardial necrosis. Planar imaging or single photon emission computed tomography (SPECT) is performed 48 h after intravenous injection, following disappearance of the radionuclide from the blood pool. This technique can detect, localize, and quantitate acute myocardial infarction and also appears promising for detection of acute myocarditis and for prediction of cardiac transplant rejection.

POSITRON EMISSION TOMOGRAPHY   See Chap. 191.

REFERENCES

BANSAL RC et al: Biplane transesophageal echocardiography: Technique, image orientation, and preliminary experience in 131 patients. J Am Soc Echocardiogr 3:348, 1990

FREEMAN MR et al: Role of resting thallium 201 perfusion in predicting coronary anatomy, left ventricular wall motion, and hospital outcome in unstable angina pectoris. Am Heart J 117:306, 1989

MARCUS ML et al (eds): *Cardiac Imaging: A Companion to Braunwald's Heart Disease.* Philadelphia, Saunders, 1991

PACE L et al: Evaluation of myocardial perfusion and function by technetium-99m methoxy isobutyl isonitrile before and after percutaneous transluminal coronary angioplasty. Preliminary results. Clin Nucl Med 18:286, 1993

ROSE EL, et al: Prognostic value of noninvasive cardiac tests in the assessment of patients with peripheral vascular disease. Am J Cardiol 71:40, 1993

SCHECHTER D et al: Left ventricular thrombus identification. A scintigraphic and echocardiographic correlation. Clin Nucl Med 18:353, 1993

SEWARD JB et al: Biplanar transesophageal echocardiography: Anatomic correlations, image orientation, and clinical applications. Mayo Clin Proc 65:1193, 1990

191   NEW CARDIAC IMAGING TECHNIQUES

CHARLES B. HIGGINS

The strategy for applying cardiac imaging techniques to the diagnosis of cardiovascular disease is currently in transition. Echocardiography and cardiac scintigraphy (Chap. 190) have been used with increasing frequency during the past decade. Initially, these techniques were used for preliminary diagnosis, but definitive therapy was generally based upon cardiac catheterization and angiography. Echocardiographic findings now have been accepted as sufficiently reliable and definitive for preoperative evaluation of most cardiac lesions. The emergence of the new noninvasive tomographic techniques, which include cine computed tomography (cine-CT), magnetic resonance imaging (MRI), and positron emission tomography (PET), should further encourage the trend away from catheterization as a requisite for definitive therapy. The strength of cine-CT and MRI lies in their being comprehensive cardiac imaging techniques for evaluation of both cardiac anatomy and function. Because of the good contrast and spatial resolution and the capacity to image the entire heart in a tomographic fashion, quantitation of dimensions and function is achieved by cine-CT and MRI to a degree even exceeding that possible with cardiac angiography. Each technique can be applied in a manner that produces a three-dimensional data set from which precise and reproducible volumetric and functional measurements can be done. Myocardial metabolism can now be assessed with PET and magnetic resonance spectroscopy (MRS). Because these new techniques are still in the stage of development and evaluation, they are not available at many hospitals at the current time. The most readily available of the new techniques is MRI, but many of these instruments are still not fully adapted for cardiac diagnosis.

ULTRAFAST COMPUTED TOMOGRAPHY (CINE-CT)

The unique design of the cine-CT scanner accomplishes the x-ray exposure for a complete tomogram in 50 ms. This short exposure time offsets the degrading effects of cardiac motion. Moreover, tomograms at the same level can be obtained sequentially after a delay of only 8 ms and initiated by, as well as related precisely to, the time in the cardiac cycle. The multiple sequential images can all be obtained within a single cardiac cycle and thus provide a true real-time image; these images are laced together in a closed-loop cinematic format, termed a *cine-CT display*.

The tomograms are approximately 10 mm in thickness, so that 12 to 14 adjacent tomograms are required to encompass the average adult heart. Eight tomographic levels can be acquired during a single imaging sequence. The maximum number of images is 80 per sequence. When tomographic images encompassing the entire heart are required, cine-CT becomes a three-dimensional imaging technique. Consequently, highly accurate and reproducible measurements of ventricular volume are possible. Such precision is possible because chamber volumes can be measured directly by planimetry of the blood pool on each tomogram encompassing the various cardiac chambers, rather than estimating volumes through assumed geometric models derived from measurements in one or two planes. Cine-CT and MRI are the only techniques that can quantify right ventricular as well as left ventricular mass.

Several other types of fast CT scanners have been introduced in the past few years. These scanners are called *spiral* CT scanners; this name derives from the continuous clockwise rotation of the scanner gantry. Standard scanners rotate in one direction during the transmission and detection of x-rays and then rotate back to the initial position before another scan is acquired. The standard scanner acquires a tomogram at a single anatomic level in 2 to 4 s and the time between scans is 2.5 s, whereas the spiral (helical) CT scanner obtains a tomogram in 1 s with virtually no interscan delay. Although the spiral CT scanner lacks the temporal resolution for the evaluation of cardiac function, the images of the heart and great vessels are adequate for the assessment of cardiovascular morphology. The spiral CT scanners are more readily available than the cine-CT scanners, and in a few years will be present in most large hospitals.

The blood pool is distinguished from the myocardium after the intravenous injection of iodinated contrast medium. Because the latter and ionizing radiation are used, cine-CT is not a true noninvasive cardiac imaging technique, like echocardiography and MRI. Cine-CT is effective for the diagnosis of many congenital and acquired cardiac abnormalities, but its role is limited because of the high diagnostic yield achieved by other totally noninvasive techniques.

INDICATIONS   The principal indications for the use of cine-CT in the diagnosis of heart disease are given in Table 191-1. In ischemic heart disease, cine-CT demonstrates regional wall thinning and absence of systolic wall thickening at the site of prior myocardial infarction. It is most effective for demonstrating complications of infarction such as mural thrombi and true and false aneurysms of the left ventricle. A mural thrombus produces a filling defect projecting into the left ventricular blood pool; it is usually attached to the wall thinned by prior infarction. An aneurysm produces a regional evagination of the left ventricular wall in diastole and paradoxical motion during systole.

TABLE 191-1 Principal indications for the new imaging modalities for cardiovascular diagnosis

FAST COMPUTED TOMOGRAPHY

Thoracic aortic diseases
  Dissection
  Aneurysm
Pulmonary arterial disease
  Pulmonary embolism
  Pulmonary arterial aneurysm
  Intrinsic and extrinsic tumors
Pericardial disease
  Constrictive diseases
  Pericardial cysts, tumors
Paracardiac and intracardiac masses
  Primary tumors
  Secondary tumors
  Intracardiac thrombus
Coronary artery bypass graft patency
Complications of myocardial infarctions
  Left ventricular aneurysms
  Left ventricular thrombus
Identification of coronary arterial calcification as an indicator of atherosclerotic disease
Analysis of ventricular function
  Global and regional left ventricular function (volume and wall thickness)
  Global right ventricular function (volume and wall thickness)
  Distribution of ventricular hypertrophy (assessment of hypertrophic cardiomyopathy)
  Ventricular function during interventions (exercise, drug interventions)
  Regional myocardial perfusion (under evaluation)

MAGNETIC RESONANCE IMAGING

Thoracic aortic diseases
  Dissection
  Aneurysm
  Thrombus
  Aortitis
  Aortic hemorrhage
Pericardial diseases
  Constrictive disease
  Effusion, hemorrhagic vs. nonhemorrhagic
  Pericardial cyst, tumor
Paracardiac and intracardiac masses
  Primary tumors (myxoma, etc.)
  Secondary tumors (lung, mediastinal, metastatic)
  Intracardiac thrombus
Hypertrophic cardiomyopathy
  Variant forms (distribution of hypertrophy)
Complications of myocardial infarction
  Left ventricular aneurysm and pseudoaneurysm
  Left ventricular thrombus
Regional myocardial perfusion using fast cine-MRI and MR constant media (under evaluation)
Congenital heart disease
  Thoracic aortic anomalies
    Arch anomalies
    Coarctation
  Pulmonary arterial anomalies
    Pulmonary atresia (presence and size of central pulmonary arteries)
    Unilateral absence (atresia)
    Peripheral pulmonary stenoses
  Complex lesions
    Univentricular atrioventricular connections
    Volume of ventricles
    Presence and size of ventricular septum
    Status of extracardiac operative procedures: Fontan, Rastelli, Jatene, etc.
Analysis of ventricular function
  Ventricular volumes and mass
  Regional left ventricular function
  Detection and quantities of valvular regurgitation
Obstructive arterial disease
  Intracranial and extracranial carotid arteries
  Renal arterial stenosis (under evaluation)
  Aortoiliac and lower limb arteries
  Coronary arteries (under evaluation)

POSITRON EMISSION TOMOGRAPHY

Ischemic heart disease
  Recognition of viable myocardium
  Regional myocardial perfusion

Cine-CT has a diagnostic accuracy of greater than 90 percent in the determination of patency of coronary arterial bypass grafts (Fig. 191-1). After intravenous injection of contrast medium, scans are exposed sequentially; the bypass grafts are opacified simultaneously with the ascending aorta. The technique is not usually capable of identifying stenosis of the graft or adequacy of blood flow through the graft, but there is hope that flow abnormalities might be detectable by analysis of contrast-dilution curves or contrast transit times in the grafts.

Computed tomography is considerably more sensitive and specific than x-ray fluoroscopy in both the identification and precise localization of vascular calcification. Consequently, cine-CT has been used to detect coronary arterial calcification (Fig. 191-2) as a screening test to identify patients at increased risk for obstructive coronary arterial disease (CAD). Cine-CT can quantify the density and the extent of coronary calcification. A three-dimensional map of the extent of coronary arterial calcification can be produced. Studies using fluoroscopy and cine-CT have shown that coronary arterial calcification increases with age. However, a recent report has indicated that the total calcium score, a product of density and volume of calcium, on cine-CT is substantially higher in patients with significant CAD when compared with those without CAD at each decade of age extending from 30 to 70 years. At each decade of age nearly all patients with significant CAD, demonstrated by angiography, had calcification detected by cine-CT. Calcification, though to a lesser extent, was also detected in patients without hemodynamically significant CAD. The absence of coronary arterial calcification indicates that the risk of significant CAD is very low. These early results have now led to the proposal that cine-CT might be used as a screening test to identify patients at increased risk for the presence of significant CAD and future coronary events.

Cine-CT can be used in the evaluation of hypertrophic and congestive cardiomyopathies by quantitating ventricular volumes and myocardial mass. Because of the wide field of view and three-

FIGURE 191-1 Cine-CT images at the level of the proximal ascending aorta acquired on sequential heart beats during passage of contrast medium throughout the central cardiovascular structures. The bypass grafts to the right (arrow) and left anterior descending (arrow) coronary arteries opacify simultaneously with the ascending aorta (A). Images from upper left to lower right display sequential opacification from pulmonary artery to the aorta.

FIGURE 191-2 Cine-CT scans at four adjacent levels at the base of the heart. No contrast medium was used, and tomograms are 3 mm in thickness. Heavy calcification (circled) is identified at multiple sites in the left anterior descending (a,b,c,d) and circumflex coronary arteries (e,f).

dimensional scope of this technique, it can depict the distribution of ventricular hypertrophy. This is particularly useful for depiction of the various forms of hypertrophic cardiomyopathy and for quantifying the increase in myocardial mass.

The role of cine-CT in valvular heart disease is limited when compared to echo Doppler and color flow mapping and cine-MRI. Although both cine-MRI and echo Doppler can demonstrate the regurgitant flow, estimate its volume, and estimate the gradient across valvular stenoses, cine-CT can evaluate only indirectly the severity of regurgitation (see below).

For the evaluation of pericardial disease, standard CT or cine-CT can be used to visualize and measure the thickness of the pericardium. The diagnosis of constrictive pericarditis is supported by demonstrating pericardial thickness exceeding 4 mm and, sometimes, calcification (Fig. 191-3). Other indirect signs of this disease shown by CT are: (1) dilated atria and inferior vena cava; (2) small ventricular chambers; and (3) a sigmoid-shaped ventricular septum. Pericardial thickening is also observed for a variable period of time after cardiac surgery and in patients experiencing the postpericardiotomy syndrome (Dressler's syndrome). CT can also be used to demonstrate pericardial effusions and pericardial masses. Standard CT has been used to evaluate intracardiac and paracardiac masses and to define possible cardiac involvement by mediastinal and lung tumors. The capability is considerably enhanced by cine-CT, although MRI seems to be superior to both standard and cine-CT for the evaluation of intra- and paracardiac masses.

The role of CT for the evaluation of congenital heart disease is very limited when considered in relation to the availability and success of echocardiography and MRI. Encouraging results have been shown for cine-CT, but the results add little to echocardiography in the display of intracardiac anatomy and seem to be inferior to MRI for defining congenital abnormalities of the thoracic aorta and pulmonary artery.

Standard CT as well as cine-CT are effective for the diagnosis of diseases of the aorta (Chap. 210). The accuracy of CT for the diagnosis of aortic dissection exceeds 90 percent and in some series

is nearly 100 percent. The definitive diagnosis of aortic dissection is based upon the demonstration of displacement of the inner portion of the aortic wall into the lumen (intimal flap) and/or differential enhancement of the true and false aortic channels.

FIGURE 191-3 CT image shows calcification (arrow) and thickening of the pericardium in a patient with constrictive pericarditis.

EVALUATION OF CARDIAC FUNCTION WITH CINE-CT The exposure time of 50 ms attained by cine-CT is adequate for quantitating many aspects of cardiac function. The three-dimensional nature of the technique permits precise measurement of chamber volume. Right and left ventricular volumes can be assessed with equal accuracy. A disparity in the stroke volumes of the two ventricles is caused by shunts and valvular regurgitation, which can be measured by cine-CT. Cine-CT can also be used for monitoring the effect of interventions on the right and left ventricles. Cine-CT performed at peak effort during supine bicycle exercise has been used to identify the *abnormal* response in patients with suspected coronary arterial stenoses. Most patients with severe lung disease and pulmonary arterial hypertension also display an abnormal response to exercise. Cine-CT has also been proposed as a method for measuring regional myocardial perfusion at rest and following interventions that increase myocardial blood flow, such as exercise and vasodilators. Perfusion is estimated by monitoring density values of the myocardium over time on CT scans exposed sequentially during peak opacification and wash-out of contrast medium from the myocardium.

MAGNETIC RESONANCE IMAGING

This noninvasive technique uses no ionizing radiation or contrast medium for cardiovascular imaging. MR images are based upon the radiofrequency (RF) signal emitted by hydrogen nuclei of tissues after they have been perturbed by RF pulses in the presence of a strong magnetic field. The RF signal emitted has certain characteristics called *relaxation times*, consisting of T1 relaxation time (longitudinal magnetization) and T2 relaxation time (transverse magnetization). These properties are variable among tissues and are the predominant factors responsible for contrast among tissues. The signal intensity of one tissue compared to another (contrast) can be manipulated by varying the elapsed time between application of RF pulses (repetition time) and the time between an RF pulse and sampling the emitted signal (echo delay time).

The techniques used in MR imaging of the heart depend upon the primary goal of the procedure. When the evaluation of anatomic abnormalities is paramount, the use of ECG-gated spin echo technique provides static images with high signal-to-noise ratio. When the primary goal is to assess cardiac contractile function, cine gradient echo imaging (cine-GRE) is used. The cardiac cycle can be divided into more than 60 time frames with this latter technique, although the framing rate used is usually no greater than 30. By lacing these together in a cinematic format, tomograms of the beating heart (cine-MRI) are obtained.

The blood pool has a unique signal on both spin echo and gradient echo images. The blood pool on the ECG-gated spin echo images is generally a signal void, which provides high contrast between blood and the myocardial wall (Fig. 191-4). On the other hand, the blood pool produces a very bright signal when the gradient echo technique is used (Fig. 191-5). This also causes high contrast between the blood pool and the myocardial wall.

Blood flow velocity can be measured using a technique called flow velocity mapping because of the existence of a linear relationship between the motion of protons in blood and the magnitude of the shift in phase of the signal of moving protons relative to stationary ones. When this sequence is applied as part of the cine-GRE technique, a series of images is acquired at evenly spaced intervals (usually 15 to 20 time segments) throughout the cardiac cycle. This sequence, called *velocity-encoded cine-MRI*, can be used to produce velocity vs. time curves and volume flow vs. time curves as the product of velocity and cross-sectional areas of the flow region. Integration of the flow values measured on cross-sectional images of the proximal aorta and pulmonary artery provides a direct measurement of stroke volume of the right and left ventricles and the disparity between the two stroke volumes in left-to-right shunts. Because the technique distinguishes between antegrade and retrograde flow, it can be used

to quantify pathologic flow, such as valvular regurgitation. The technique has many practical similarities to Doppler echocardiography and, like Doppler, can be applied for estimating the gradient across valvular stenoses using the modified Bernoulli equation. The peak velocity (V) beyond the valvular stenosis is measured from the flow channel distal to the valve and used in the formula: peak gradient $= 4V^2$.

EVALUATION OF PATHOANATOMY MRI has been shown to be effective and useful in the diagnosis of a wide variety of cardiovascular abnormalities (Table 191-1). Patients with congenital heart disease are evaluated initially with the use of two-dimensional echocardiography, and in many congenital lesions MR is a secondary diagnostic technique in which the anatomy is displayed with the precision of angiography. In anomalies of the aortic arch and

FIGURE 191-4 *A.* ECG gated spin echo MRI in the cardiac short axis plane. Arrows = papillary muscles; L = left ventricle; RO = right ventricular outflow tract. *(From Higgins CB et al with permission) B.* Transaxial spin echo MR image demonstrates a mass in the left atrium (arrow). The wide area of attachment of the mass to the left atrial wall suggests a sarcoma rather than a benign myxoma. A = aorta; LA = left atrium; RA = right atrium; RV = right ventricle.

A

B

FIGURE 191-5 Series of cine gradient echo images at end-diastole for sequential anatomic levels extending from base (upper left) to apex (lower right) of the left ventricle. These tomograms provide a three-dimensional data set for measuring right and left ventricular volumes and masses.

coarctation, MR can be considered the procedure of choice. Also MRI is often the most useful study for the demonstration of pulmonary arterial abnormalities; for evaluating the status of the pulmonary arteries after systemic-pulmonary shunts have been surgically produced; for the evaluation of a single ventricle; and in the evaluation of pulmonary venous abnormalities.

The major use of MRI in ischemic heart disease has been to demonstrate complications of acute myocardial infarction, such as true and false aneurysms of the left ventricle and intraventricular thrombi (Fig. 191-6). However, in the future, MRI may assume a broader role in ischemic heart disease by demonstrating: (1) residual viable myocardium in a region involved by a previous infarct; (2) patency (or lack thereof) of coronary artery bypass grafts; and (3) regional perfusion using MR contrast media.

MRI has been used to define the extent and distribution of abnormal muscle in patients with hypertrophic cardiomyopathy. It provides accurate and reproducible measurement of myocardial mass, which can be used in monitoring response to therapy. It provides direct imaging of the pericardium, so that a diagnosis of abnormal pericardial thickness can be made. MRI is the procedure of choice for establishing the diagnosis of constrictive pericarditis.

MRI has been found to be effective for demonstrating intracardiac thrombi and tumors (Figs. 191-4B and 191-6). The utility of the technique has been shown in the demonstration of primary and metastatic cardiac tumors and tumors within the mediastinum invading or compressing central cardiovascular structures. The most frequent

indication for the use of MRI in evaluating an intracardiac mass is when echocardiography raises a question regarding abnormal echogenicity within the cardiac chambers.

Thoracic aortic diseases are evaluated best with MR. In patients with aortic dissection, MRI displays the intimal flap and the extent of the dissection within the aorta (Fig. 191-7). It can also identify a thrombus in the false channel and involvement of the arch and visceral arterial branches. In the search for the source of arterial embolism, MRI can be applied to identify a thrombus in the left atrium, left ventricle, or aorta.

EVALUATION OF CARDIAC FUNCTION Functional evaluation of the cardiovascular system is now practical using cine-MRI. By achieving a temporal resolution of 30 images per cardiac cycle, cine-MRI successfully captures end diastole and end systole, such that end-diastolic and end-systolic volumes, stroke volume, and ejection

FIGURE 191-6 ECG-gated spin echo MR images acquired in transverse plane demonstrate complications of myocardial infarctions. True aneurysm and mural thrombus (T) *(top)*. False aneurysm (A) *(bottom)*. The ostium is nearly as wide as the fundus of the true aneurysm, while the ostium is smaller than the fundus for the false aneurysm.

A

B

Faster gradient echo techniques have been developed in recent years so that it is now possible to obtain 15 or more images evenly spaced throughout a cardiac cycle during a single breath-hold period. Another new technique called *echoplanar imaging* acquires an image in 30 to 50 ms, so that images at multiple phases of the cardiac cycle can be obtained during a single heart beat, which constitutes real-time imaging of the heart. These innovations should extend the capability of MRI for the evaluation of cardiac function.

QUANTITATION OF VALVULAR LESIONS   The blood pool usually has a homogeneous high signal intensity throughout most of the cardiac cycle on cine-MR. Stenosis of or regurgitation through either the atrioventricular or semilunar valves is associated with a high-velocity jet that causes a signal void within the otherwise high-signal-intensity chamber (Fig. 191-8). This void can be used to identify the presence of valvular regurgitation. In aortic regurgitation, the signal void is in continuity with the closed aortic valve, whereas in mitral regurgitation it is in continuity with the closed mitral valve. Quantitation of the severity of valvular regurgitation can be accomplished by measuring the right and left ventricular stroke volumes and using these measurements to calculate regurgitant fraction or regurgitant volume. The volume of the signal void caused by regurgitation can also be measured on the images and used to estimate the severity of regurgitation. The velocity-encoded cine-MRI technique can be used to measure the volume of valvular regurgitation and to estimate the peak gradient across valvular stenosis (see below).

Velocity-encoded cine-MRI has been applied for the quantification of blood flow in the heart and great vessels in a variety of diseases. It has been used to measure the retrograde flow in the ascending aorta in diastole in order to directly quantify the regurgitant volume in aortic regurgitation. It has also been shown to provide an accurate measurement of the stoke volume of the right and left ventricles by quantifying systolic flow in the main pulmonary artery and aorta, respectively. The volume of regurgitant lesions is calculated as the difference in stroke volume of the two ventricles. Valvular and arterial stenoses can be estimated from the modified Bernoulli equation by measuring the peak flow velocity across the stenosis. This technique can be used to measure flow separately in the right and left pulmonary arteries; such measurements may be useful in the assessment of pulmonary blood flow in treated and untreated patients with congenital heart disease.

FIGURE 191-7   ECG-referenced gradient echo image in transaxial plane at the level of the aortic arch demonstrates an intimal flap (arrows) in the ascending and descending aorta. *(From Higgins CB et al, with permission)*

fraction can be calculated accurately. The temporal resolution of cine-MRI does not capture a single cardiac cycle, but rather separates an "average" cycle, acquired over 256 cardiac cycles, into many component images. A good correlation has been found between left ventricular volumes calculated from cine-MRI and those measured by angiography. Measurement of left ventricular mass using MRI has shown a close correlation with postmortem measurements in animals and estimates from angiography in human beings. Accurate measurement of left ventricular mass is important, as changes in mass may be the most effective way to monitor the response to therapy in diseases causing left ventricular hypertrophy. MRI has also been shown to provide measurement of right ventricular mass. Functional evaluation in ischemic heart disease by MRI is achieved by monitoring wall thickening during the cardiac cycle. The site of previous myocardial infarction can be recognized by the absence or diminution of wall thickening during systole.

FIGURE 191-8   Coronal cine-MR images in a patient with aortic regurgitation (*A*) and another with aortic stenosis (*B*). Regurgitation causes a signal void in the left ventricle during diastole. Aortic stenosis causes a signal void (arrow) starting at the valve level (arrow) and extending into the ascending aorta in systole. A = aorta; LV = left ventricle; P = pulmonary artery; RA = right atrium.

A

B

MR SPECTROSCOPY

MR spectroscopy is used for the evaluation of myocardial metabolism. It may eventually be used to assess the early response of the myocardium to various therapeutic and pharmacologic interventions, establish myocardial viability, assess beneficial or detrimental effects of reperfusion on the ischemically injured myocardium, and investigate the link between myocardial function and metabolism.

MR spectroscopy operates upon the same principle as MRI in that the nuclei of some atoms (those with an odd number of nuclear particles) resonate when radiofrequency energy is applied at a frequency specific for a particular atom. After this energy is applied, the nuclei resonate at a characteristic frequency so that the presence of a particular atom within a chemical compound or tissue can be identified by MR. In distinction to imaging, which is usually only sensitive to the presence of a certain atom within a compound, MR spectroscopy can provide a map of the various sites where an atom exists within a compound. MR spectroscopy depicts the very slight difference in resonant frequencies of the same nuclei when they exist in different compounds. This slight variation in resonant frequencies is called *chemical shift*, and the graphic display of the various frequencies is the MR spectrum of the nuclei. An example of this is the MR spectrum of phosphorus 31 (^{31}P), where the multiple spectral peak represent ^{31}P in the compounds inorganic phosphate, creatine phosphate, adenosine triphosphate, etc. (Fig. 191-9). The MR spectra are displayed in a convention whereby the position of the peak in the spectrum (horizontal axis) indicates the specific compounds, e.g., creatine phosphate, and the height of the peak (vertical axis) indicates the relative concentration of the compound.

The nuclei for which MR spectroscopy seems to be the most useful for diagnostic purposes are hydrogen 1, carbon 13, and phosphorus 31. Hydrogen 1 (proton) spectroscopy has been used to detect lactate in ischemic tissue and lipid accumulation in ischemically injured tissue. Metabolism of energy substrates in the myocardium has been approached using carbon 13; the technique has the potential for monitoring the utilization of fat and glucose by the myocardium and the manner in which ischemia influences their utilization. At this time most attention has been devoted to phosphorus 31 MR spectroscopy as a method for studying high-energy phosphate stores in various myocardial disease states and alterations of high-energy phosphate stores in response to therapeutic interventions.

FIGURE 191-9 Phosphorus 31 magnetic resonance spectrum from a normal subject. The important spectral peaks are inorganic phosphate, not seen; creatine phosphate (PCr); and the three for ATP, labeled α, β, and γ. The 2,3-diphosphoglycerate (DPG) peak indicates that the signal is partially derived from intracavitary blood as well as from myocardium. PD = phosphodiester.

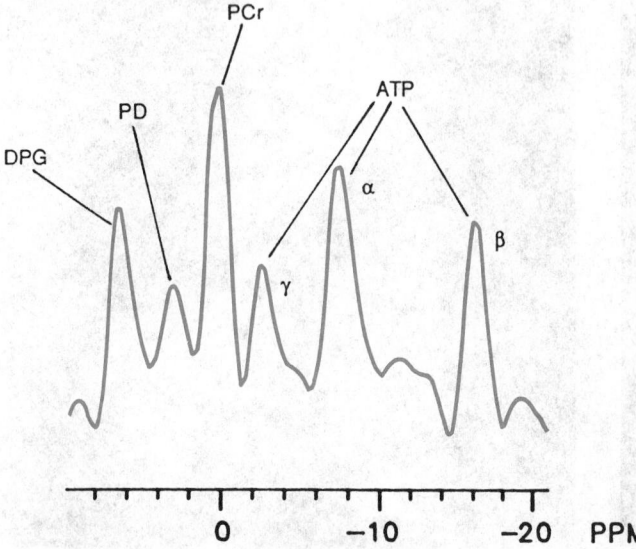

In experimental preparations, phosphorus 31 spectroscopy has been used to evaluate the influence of potentially toxic agents, such as adriamycin and ethanol, on the myocardium. Calcium channel antagonists have been found to enchance recovery of both function and high-energy phosphate stores of the ischemically injured myocardium. Phosphorus 31 MR spectroscopy may be used also in experimental preparations to determine whether ischemic myocardium which is reperfused is reversibly or irreversibly damaged. Abnormal ^{31}P spectra have been observed in patients with myocardial disease. However, the sensitivity, specificity, and, indeed, the clinical utility of ^{31}P MR spectroscopy has yet to be established.

POSITRON EMISSION TOMOGRAPHY

PET is a technique in which tomographic images are produced in relation to the concentration and position of positron emitters within the heart or any other organ. The positron is a positively charged electron produced during positron decay of a nucleus. After the positron interacts with a neighboring electron, a pair of photons are emitted in opposite directions. Because the photons simultaneously travel at equal speeds along paths at 180° to one another, photon detectors arrayed in a circle around the body can compute the precise site of origin of the pair. A substantial number of positron emitters are available for evaluating blood flow and various aspects of metabolic activity of the myocardium. Blood flow can be measured with ammonia labeled with nitrogen 13 (^{13}N), rubidium 82 (^{82}Rb), or oxygen 15 (^{15}O). Glucose utilization, fat utilization and metabolism, and myocardial oxygen consumption can be assessed by fluorine 18 (^{18}F)-labeled deoxyglucose (DG), carbon 11 (^{11}C)-labeled palmitate, and ^{11}C-labeled acetate, respectively.

PET can evaluate regional myocardial blood flow and metabolism. The transverse tomograms provide distinct spatial separation between various regions of the left ventricle, so that the uptake of metabolic markers can be assigned to the various myocardial regions. This technique may provide the capability of distinguishing between reversibly and irreversibly injured ischemic myocardium and predicting its response to reperfusion. By monitoring changes in metabolic patterns or substrate uptake, it may also prove capable of monitoring early response to therapy.

ASSESSMENT OF REGIONAL MYOCARDIAL BLOOD FLOW

Because the various regions of the left ventricle are separated from one another on the transverse tomographic images, PET scans using perfusion markers can be used to detect and localize coronary artery disease. Nitrogen 13 ammonia ([^{13}N]H$_3$), rubidium 82, and oxygen 15 have been used to assess regional myocardial blood flow at rest and in a hyperemic state induced by strong vasodilators such as dipyridamole and adenosine. This technique has shown regional reduction of the positron emitter in the presence of stenoses that reduce luminal diameter by more than 40 to 50 percent.

Myocardial metabolism   An unique feature of PET is the capability to measure regional myocardial substrate uptake and metabolic kinetics in a noninvasive and nonperturbing fashion. Specifically, it has been used to (1) measure regional myocardial uptake of exogenous glucose and free fatty acid; (2) quantitate free fatty acid metabolism in the myocardium in various physiologic states; (3) define the preferential myocardial energy source (fatty acid vs. glucose) in various physiologic states; and (4) evaluate myocardial chemical receptor sites.

PET employing [^{13}N]H$_3$ and [^{18}F]DG has been used to evaluate simultaneously regional myocardial perfusion and glucose uptake, respectively, in an effort to distinguish regions with a perfusion defect but containing viable myocardium from irreversibly infarcted myocardium. Using the combination of [^{13}N]H$_3$ (blood flow marker) and [^{18}F]DG (glucose uptake), several patterns of segmental myocardial metabolic abnormalities have been described in patients with various forms of ischemic heart disease. One is a "blood flow-metabolism match," in which a defect in the regional myocardial

[¹³]NH₃   [¹⁸]FDG   [¹³]NH₃   [¹⁸]FDG

FIGURE 191-10   Positron emission tomograms in two subjects: matched defects (*left*) and mismatched defects (*right*). Images show distribution for [¹³N]ammonium and [¹⁸F]deoxyglucose. The matched defects (arrowheads) in the anterior regions indicate a scar from a transmural infarct. The mismatched

defects show reduced perfusion (arrow) but persistent glucose uptake (arrow) consistent with viable (salvageable) myocardium. (*Images provided courtesy of Heinrich Schelbert, MD.*)

distribution of both isotopes is present. This pattern is usually caused by myocardial scar or nonviable myocardium (Fig. 191-10A). A second pattern is a "blood flow–metabolism mismatch," in which there is a segmental defect in [¹³N]H without a deficit in [¹⁸F]DG (Fig. 191-10B). This indicates reduced perfusion to a myocardial region but continued uptake of glucose. Both patterns have been observed in patients with wall motion abnormalities in the left ventricular region displaying the perfusion defects. This mismatch pattern is considered to be associated with ischemic but viable myocardium as surgical revascularization of patients with this pattern causes improved wall motion in a majority of such segments. Moreover, a substantial percentage of patients showing the mismatch pattern after acute myocardial infarction have demonstrated some recovery of regional function. On the other hand, the match pattern has been associated with no recovery of function after revascularization of akinetic segments.

PET using the positron emitter [¹¹C]palmitic acid has identified the consequences of myocardial ischemia and infarction on myocardial free fatty acid metabolism. These studies revealed that exogenous ¹¹C-labeled palmitic acid can enter two metabolic pools within the myocardium: a rapidly metabolized pool in which the fatty acid is immediately oxidized to CO_2 or a storage pool of triglycerides. During myocardial ischemia, myocardial uptake of [¹¹C]palmitic acid and its distribution into the two pools are altered. The free fatty acid pathway most vulnerable to ischemia is β oxidation, and consequently the amount of [¹¹C]palmitic acid entering this pathway is decreased initially.

Prediction of successful salvage of myocardium after thrombolysis has been achieved by PET imaging of [¹¹C]palmitic acid uptake in the jeopardized myocardium. Successful thrombolysis is associated with resumption of uptake of [¹¹C]palmitic acid in the jeopardized region. The principal indications for PET at the current time are to detect ischemic myocardium and to demonstrate potentially salvageable (viable) myocardium in the presence of acute or chronic myocardial ischemia.

REFERENCES

Cine-CT

AGATSON AS et al: Quantification of coronary arterial calcium using ultrafast computed tomography. J Am Coll Cardiol 1:827, 1990

MARCUS ML, WEISS RM: Evaluation of cardiac structure and function with ultrafast computed tomography, in *Cardiac Imaging*, ML Marcus et al (eds). Philadelphia, Saunders, 1991, p 669

STANFORD W et al: Sensitivity and specificity of assessing coronary bypass graft patency with ultrafast computed tomography. Results of a multicenter study. J Am Coll Cardiol 12:1, 1988

MR imaging

BARAKOS JA et al: Magnetic resonance imaging of cardiac and paracardiac masses. Pictorial essay. Am J Roentgenol 153:47, 1989

HIGGINS CB: MR of the heart: Anatomy, physiology and metabolism. Am J Roentgenol 151:239, 1988

———: Evaluation of valvular heart disease using cine GRE magnetic resonance imaging. Circulation (suppl) 84(3):I-194, 1991

——— et al: Magnetic resonance imaging in hypertrophic cardiomyopathy. Am J Cardiol 55:1121, 1985

——— et al: *Congenital Heart Disease. Echocardiography and Magnetic Resonance Imaging*. New York, Raven Press, 1990

——— et al (eds): *Magnetic Resonance Imaging of the Body*, 2d ed. New York, Raven Press, 1991

MacMILLAN RM: Cardiac magnetic resonance imaging. Cardiovasc Clin 23:125, 1993

SOMMERHOFF BA et al: Aortic dissection: Sensitivity and specificity of MR imaging. Radiology 3:651, 1988

UNDERWOOD R, FIRMIN D: *Magnetic Resonance of the Cardiovascular System*, Oxford, Blackwell Scientific, 1991

MR spectroscopy

MEYERHOFF DJ et al: Magnetic resonance spectroscopy, in *Magnetic Resonance Imaging of the Body*, 2d ed, CB Higgins et al (eds). New York, Raven Press, 1991

WEISS RG et al: Regional myocardial metabolism of high energy phosphates during isometric exercise in patients with coronary artery disease. N Engl J Med 323:1593, 1990

Positron Emission Tomography

ISADA L et al: Physiologic evaluation of coronary flow: The role of positron emission tomography. Cleve Clin J Med 60:19, 1993

SCHELBERT HR, BUXTON D: Insights into coronary artery disease gained from metabolic imaging. Circulation 78:496, 1988

SCHELBERT HR et al: Principles of positron emission tomography, in *Cardiac Imaging*, ML Marcus et al (eds). Philadelphia, Saunders, 1991, p 1140

192   DIAGNOSTIC CARDIAC CATHETERIZATION AND ANGIOGRAPHY

WILLIAM GROSSMAN / DONALD S. BAIM

Cardiac catheterization and angiography remain the gold standard for the assessment of both anatomy and physiology of the heart and vasculature. Initially developed in the animal laboratory, cardiac catheterization was first applied to humans in 1929 by Werner Forssmann, who at age 25 performed a right heart catheterization on himself. Forssmann's primary goal was to develop a therapeutic technique for the direct delivery of drugs into the heart. The potential

TABLE 192-1 Relative contraindications to cardiac catheterization and angiography

1 Uncontrolled ventricular irritability: increased risk of ventricular tachycardia and fibrillation during catheterization if ventricular irritability is uncontrolled
2 Uncorrected hypokalemia or digitalis toxicity
3 Uncorrected hypertension: predisposes to myocardial ischemia and/or heart failure during angiography
4 Intercurrent febrile illness
5 Decompensated heart failure: especially acute pulmonary edema, unless catheterization can be done with patient sitting up
6 Anticoagulated state: prothrombin time >18 s
7 Severe allergy to radiographic contrast agent
8 Severe renal insufficiency and/or anuria: unless dialysis is planned to remove fluid and radiographic contrast load

of Forssmann's technique as a diagnostic tool was appreciated by others, especially André Cournand and Dickinson Richards in New York, who shared the Nobel Prize with Forssmann in 1956 for the development of cardiac catheterization. Today, cardiac catheterization and angiography are performed as a combined procedure for diagnostic purposes, therapeutic intervention, or both. This chapter deals with cardiac catheterization as a diagnostic tool.

INDICATIONS AND CONTRAINDICATIONS Cardiac catheterization is recommended when there is a need to confirm the presence of a clinically suspected condition, define its anatomic and physiologic severity, and determine whether important associated conditions are present. This need most commonly arises when a patient is experiencing significant or increasing symptoms of cardiac dysfunction or when objective measures suggest that rapid deterioration, myocardial infarction, or other adverse events are imminent.

While there is debate as to whether cardiac catheterization is necessary in all patients being considered for cardiac surgery, cardiac catheterization and coronary arteriography remain the only techniques currently capable of defining coronary anatomy with sufficient precision to provide the data for decisions regarding coronary surgery or balloon angioplasty. In patients with other forms of heart disease (e.g., dilated cardiomyopathy, valvular heart disease), cardiac catheterization can provide hemodynamic characterization essential to the design of an appropriate medical regimen as well as assessment of prognosis. In some instances, however, decisions regarding cardiac surgery can be made without cardiac catheterization and angiography. Examples of such instances include children with simple congenital heart disease (e.g., patent ductus arteriosus, atrial septal defect), for whom a definitive diagnosis can be established by clinical examination and noninvasive studies.

Relative contraindications to cardiac catheterization are listed in Table 192-1.

TABLE 192-2 Patient characteristics associated with increased mortality from cardiac catheterization

1 *Age:* Infants (<1 month old) and the elderly (>80 years old) are at increased risk of death during cardiac catheterization. Elderly women appear to be at higher risk than elderly men.
2 *Functional class:* Mortality in class IV patients is more than 10 times greater than in class I–II patients.
3 *Severity of coronary obstruction:* Mortality for patients with left main disease is more than 10 times greater than in patients with one- or two-vessel disease.
4 *Valvular heart disease:* Especially when severe and combined with coronary disease is associated with a higher risk of death at cardiac catheterization than coronary artery disease alone.
5 *Left ventricular dysfunction:* Mortality in patients with left ventricular ejection < 30 percent is more than 10 times greater than in patients with ejection fraction ≥ 50 percent.
6 *Severe noncardiac disease:* Patients with renal insufficiency, insulin-requiring diabetes, advanced cerebrovascular and/or peripheral vascular disease, and severe pulmonary insufficiency have an increased incidence of death and other major complications from cardiac catheterization.

A history of *allergic reaction* to radiographic contrast agents, which may range from urticaria to frank anaphylactic reaction, is an important relative contraindication to cardiac catheterization, which requires appropriate pretreatment. Generally, pretreatment with glucocorticoids (prednisone 20 to 40 mg every 6 h), conventional antihistamines (e.g., diphenhydramine 25 mg every 6 h), and H-2 antagonists (cimetidine 300 mg every 6 h), starting 18 to 24 h prior to the procedure, is adequate. Alternatively, one of the newer nonionic contrast agents may be used with less risk of a severe allergic reaction. Despite these precautions, occasional individuals will still develop anaphylactic reactions during radiographic contrast angiography, and intravenous epinephrine must be at hand in such instances.

COMPLICATIONS OF CARDIAC CATHETERIZATION Since cardiac catheterization is an invasive technique, it is not surprising that potential complications include death, myocardial infarction, stroke, perforation of the heart or great vessels, and local vascular problems. Table 192-2 lists those characteristics associated with increased risk of death from cardiac catheterization.

TECHNIQUES

Cardiac catheterization is performed with the patient in the fasting state and awake, although sedated. Typical sedatives include diazepam (Valium 5 to 10 mg orally) and diphenhydramine (Benadryl 25 to 50 mg orally). Prophylactic antibiotics are not necessary. If patients have been anticoagulated chronically with warfarin, this agent must be discontinued for at least 48 h prior to the procedure, and the prothrombin time must be less than 18 s if the study is to be done safely. The technique of cardiac catheterization involves either direct exposure of artery and vein (usually the brachial artery and vein in the antecubital fossa) or catheterization by percutaneous approach (usually via the femoral artery and vein). Either technique can be used for right and/or left heart catheterization with coronary arteriography, but many procedures (e.g., intraaortic balloon pumping, mitral valve valvuloplasty, coronary atherectomy) require the femoral approach. For a procedure where either approach would be possible, the brachial approach has advantages in the patient with perpipheral vascular disease involving the abdominal aorta and iliac or femoral arteries and suspected thrombosis of the femoral or iliac vein or inferior vena cava. Advantages of the percutaneous femoral approach are that arteriotomy and arterial repair are not required; the procedure can be performed repeatedly in the same patient at intervals; infection and thrombophlebitis at the catheterization site are quite rare, and no scar is left.

RIGHT HEART CATHETERIZATION This is most commonly performed under fluoroscopic guidance utilizing a balloon flotation catheter which is advanced from a suitable vein (femoral, brachial, subclavian, or internal jugular) into the superior vena cava, where blood is sampled for oximetry. The catheter is then positioned in the right atrium, where pressure is measured. The balloon is inflated with air or carbon dioxide and advanced into the right ventricle, pulmonary artery, and pulmonary artery wedge positions. Pressures are recorded in each position, and the balloon is then deflated so that pulmonary artery pressure is monitored and blood sampled from the catheter tip. With a thermistor-tipped balloon catheter, cardiac output can be measured utilizing cold saline injection and a small computer (thermodilution technique). Comparison of oxygen saturations in the venae cavae, chambers of the right heart, and pulmonary artery blood permits assessment of the presence of a left-to-right shunt at the atrial, ventricular, or pulmonary artery level which will be manifested as an increase (''step-up'') in oxygen saturation of blood as it traverses these vessels and chambers. As discussed below, measurements of the pulmonary artery and aortic oxygen content and oxygen consumption allow calculation of the cardiac output by the Fick principle as an alternative to use of thermodilution.

The experienced operator will be alert to abnormalities in the course of the catheter during its passage through the right heart chambers, potentially providing information concerning the presence of congenital heart disease. For example, the catheter may pass directly from the right to the left atrium through an atrial septal defect, may enter an anomalous pulmonary vein draining into the right atrium, or may pass from the pulmonary artery directly into the aorta through a patent ductus arteriosus.

LEFT HEART CATHETERIZATION When left heart catheterization is done from the *brachial approach*, surgical cut-down is performed in the right (or left) antecubital fossa, with exposure of the brachial artery. An arteriotomy is made, and an appropriate catheter (e.g., Sones catheter) is advanced under fluoroscopic guidance to the central aorta, where pressure is measured and recorded. Next, the catheter is advanced in retrograde fashion across the aortic valve into the left ventricle, where pressure is measured. If a right heart catheter is in place, this is an appropriate time for simultaneous measurement and recording of left heart, right heart, and peripheral arterial pressures together with determination of cardiac output by either thermodilution or Fick principle. These measures allow assessment of possible pressure gradients across the mitral and aortic valves, and catheter pullback on the right side permits assessment of possible gradients across pulmonic and tricuspid valves. Simultaneous measurement of pressures and cardiac output provides the data for calculation of systemic and pulmonary vascular resistances.

The *percutaneous femoral approach* to left heart catheterization involves puncture of the right (or left) femoral artery with a Seldinger needle, passage of a J-tipped guidewire retrograde to the abdominal aorta under fluoroscopic guidance, and placement of an intraarterial sheath with a side arm port for flushing. An appropriate catheter (e.g., pigtail catheter) is then advanced over a guidewire to the descending aorta, at which time the guidewire is removed and the catheter aspirated and flushed vigorously. Under pressure monitoring and fluoroscopic guidance, the catheter is advanced to the ascending aorta, where pressure is recorded simultaneously with peripheral arterial pressure. Subsequent steps in the procedure are identical to those listed for the brachial approach.

An additional method of left heart catheterization is the *transseptal approach*. This approach, which is not commonly employed today except for special diagnostic problems or for purposes of therapeutic intervention (especially mitral valvuloplasty), involves a controlled puncture of the interatrial septum with a long stainless steel needle and advancement of a Teflon catheter or sheath over the needle into the left atrium. Rarely, direct catheterization of the left heart through the chest wall is necessary, by *left ventricular puncture* using a needle inserted into the cardiac apex.

CARDIAC ANGIOGRAPHY

Cardiac angiography involves injection of radiopaque contrast agent into a specific cardiac chamber or vessel using either hand injection or power injection through an automated syringe. Contrast agents utilized today are either nonionic or ionic; the nonionic contrast agents (and the ionic dimer ioxaglate) have less myocardial depressant effect but are substantially more expensive than traditional high-osmolar ionic agents. During injection, these low-osmolar contrast agents usually produce less vasodilatation and less sensation of marked warmth throughout the distribution of the injection than earlier high-osmolar agents.

CORONARY ANGIOGRAPHY This common procedure involves selective injection of radiographic contrast agent into the coronary arteries. Placement of the catheter tips into the right and left coronary arteries is carried out under fluoroscopic guidance, and contrast agent is injected by hand during recording of the radiographic image. Each coronary artery is usually viewed in several projections to permit assessment of severity of stenosis and to minimize overlap of adjacent vessels. In addition to the detection of coronary artery stenoses, coronary angiography is useful for the detection of congenital abnormalities of the coronary circulation, coronary arteriovenous fistulas, and patency of coronary artery bypass grafts. Examples of normal and abnormal coronary anatomy are seen in Figs. 192-1 to 192-3.

FIGURE 192-1 Representation of coronary anatomy relative to the interventricular and atrioventricular valve planes. Coronary branches are indicated as L Main (left main), LAD (left anterior descending), D (diagonal), S (septal), CX (circumflex), OM (obtuse marginal), RCA (right coronary artery), CB (conus branch), SN (sinus node), AcM (acute marginal), PD (posterior descending, PL (posterolateral left ventricular). RAO, right anterior oblique, LAO, left anterior oblique. (*From DS Baim, W Grossman, in W Grossman, DS Baim (eds), 1991, with permission.*)

CORONARY ANGIOGRAPHIC ANATOMY: REPRESENTATION IN STANDARD PRO

FIGURE 192-2   Coronary angiogram showing a right coronary artery (RCA) with a severe (95 percent) stenosis at its midpoint (*arrow*).

LEFT VENTRICULOGRAPHY   Injection of radiographic contrast material directly into the left ventricular cavity is an important part of routine left heart catheterization and yields important diagnostic information. Usually, a power injector is utilized to inject 30 to 45 mL of radiographic contrast material into the left ventricular chamber at an injection rate appropriate for the particular catheter being used. Angiographic assessment of the left ventricular silhouette at end-diastole and end-systole permits calculation of left ventricular chamber volumes and ejection fraction, as well as assessment of regional wall motion abnormalities. The normal left ventricle ejects 50 to 80 percent of its end-diastolic volume with each beat; i.e., its *ejection fraction* is 0.50 to 0.80. In adults, normal values for left ventricular volumes are end-diastolic volume, 72 ± 15 mL/m^2 (mean $\pm$ standard deviation), and end-systolic volume, 20 ± 8 mL/m^2. Regional abnormalities of wall motion are illustrated in Fig. 192-4 and include diminished inward motion of a myocardial segment (*hypokinesis*), no inward movement of a myocardial segment (*akinesis*), and paradoxical systolic expansion of a regional myocardial segment (*dyskinesis*).

FIGURE 192-3   Coronary angiogram of a left coronary artery (LCA) with a tight stenosis in the proximal left anterior descending (LAD) artery (*black arrow*) immediately prior to the origin of a large septal branch. The circumflex artery (CX) has two moderately severe stenoses (*white arrows*).

FIGURE 192-4   Diagrammatic representation of end-diastolic (*solid line*) and end-systolic (*dashed line*) silhouettes of left ventricular cineangiograms in various forms of localized wall motion disorder in patients with coronary heart disease. Normal wall motion is symmetric; a patient with *hypokinesis* exhibits reduced contraction, seen here over the anterior and apical surfaces; a patient with *akinesis* exhibits absent wall motion, seen here over the anteroapical surface; the patient with *dyskinesis* exhibits paradoxic bulging of a small portion of the anterior wall with systole.

Left ventriculography is usually performed in the right anterior oblique projection, which allows assessment of the mitral and aortic valves. Mitral regurgitation is easily visualized as the appearance of radiographic contrast material in the left atrium during left ventricular systole. Its severity can be estimated qualitatively using a grading system of 1+ (mild, radiographic contrast material clears with each beat and never opacifies the entire left atrium) to 4+ (severe, opacification of the entire left atrium occurs within one beat and contrast material can be seen refluxing into the pulmonary veins). *Regurgitant fraction* can be calculated by determining the total left ventricular stroke volume (left ventricular end-diastolic volume minus end-systolic volume), subtracting the forward stroke volume (determined by Fick or indicator-dilution technique), and dividing by the total stroke volume. The etiology of mitral regurgitation, such as myxomatous degeneration of the mitral leaflets and chordal rupture, may sometimes be identified from the left ventricular cineangiogram. Mitral and aortic stenosis can be *detected* by assessment of the speed and completeness with which the mitral and aortic leaflets open. Also important is an assessment of the thickness of the mitral and aortic leaflets and the presence and extent of calcification. These findings, however, are usually not useful in estimating the *severity* of physiologic stenosis.

Left ventriculography performed in the left anterior oblique projection permits detection of abnormal communications such as ventricular septal defect (Chap. 199). In the most common form of hypertrophic cardiomyopathy (Chap. 205) (idiopathic hypertrophic subaortic stenosis, IHSS), left ventriculography in this projection shows anterior motion of the anterior leaflet of the mitral valve during systole and bulging of the interventricular septum into the left ventricular cavity, especially in the subaortic region. Mural thrombi within the left ventricular chamber may be well visualized during left ventriculography. They occur most commonly in the left ventricular apex.

AORTOGRAPHY   Rapid injection of radiographic contrast material into the ascending aorta allows detection of abnormalities involving the aorta and aortic valve. It permits detection and qualitative

TABLE 192-3 Normal values for hemodynamic parameters

1 Pressures (mmHg)	
A Systemic arterial	
(*1*) Peak systolic/end-diastolic	100–140/60–90
(*2*) Mean	70–105
B Left ventricle	
(*1*) Peak systolic/end-diastolic	100–140/3–12
C Left atrium (or pulmonary capillary wedge)	
(*1*) Mean	2–10
(*2*) *a* wave	3–15
(*3*) *v* wave	3–15
D Pulmonary artery	
(*1*) Peak systolic/end-diastolic	15–30/4–12
(*2*) Mean	9–18
E Right ventricle	
(*1*) Peak systolic/end-diastolic	15–30/2–8
F Right atrium	
(*1*) Mean	2–8
(*2*) *a* wave	2–10
(*3*) *v* wave	2–10
2 Resistances [(dyn•s)/cm^5]	
(*1*) Systemic vascular resistance	700–1600
(*2*) Pulmonary vascular resistance	20–130
3 Cardiac index [(L/min)/m^2]	2.6–4.2
4 Oxygen consumption index [(L/min)/m^2]	110–150
5 Arteriovenous oxygen difference (mL/L)	30–50

assessment of the severity of aortic regurgitation utilizing a 1+ to 4+ scale, as for mitral regurgitation. Abnormal communications between the aorta and right side of the heart, such as patent ductus arteriosus or ruptured aneurysm of a sinus of Valsalva, may be visualized. Aortography can permit identification of aortic aneurysm and of aortic dissection (Chap. 210) and may visualize an intimal flap within the aortic lumen.

PRESSURE MEASUREMENTS

Pressures within the cardiac chambers and great vessels are recorded routinely during cardiac catheterization and provide important information concerning function of ventricular myocardium and cardiac valves. Normal values for pressures measured during cardiac catheterization are summarized in Table 192-3.

Simultaneous measurement of pressures in the left ventricle, aorta, and left atrium (or pulmonary capillary wedge position) permits assessment of mitral and aortic valve function. As seen in Fig. 192-5, left ventricular and aortic pressures are essentially equal during systole, while left atrial (pulmonary capillary wedge) and left ventricular pressures are equal during diastole in the normal heart. A pressure gradient between the left ventricle and aorta during systole may be due to obstruction at the level of the aortic valve (e.g., *calcific aortic stenosis*) or at the subaortic level (e.g., *hypertrophic obstructive cardiomyopathy*). A gradient between the left atrium (pulmonary capillary wedge) and left ventricle in diastole generally indicates *mitral stenosis*, although it also may be seen in rare conditions such as cor triatriatum and left atrial myxoma. An example of a large diastolic pressure gradient in a patient with mitral stenosis is seen in Fig. 192-6. As seen in Fig. 192-7, a prominent *v* wave in the pulmonary capillary wedge pressure will often increase substantially during modest exercise in a patient with significant mitral regurgitation. Severe *aortic regurgitation* produces a widening of the aortic pulse pressure, with equilibration of aortic and left ventricular pressures in diastole (Fig. 192-8). Right-sided pressures exhibit

FIGURE 192-5 Left ventricular (LV), radial artery, and pulmonary capillary wedge (PCW) pressures in a patient with normal cardiovascular function. Note the absence of a pressure gradient between the LV and radial artery in systole and between the LV and PCW in diastole.

FIGURE 192-6 Pulmonary capillary wedge (PCW) and left ventricular (LV) pressure tracings in a 40-year-old woman with mitral stenosis. This patient also had systemic hypertension and significant elevation of her LV diastolic pressure. *(From BA Carabello, W Grossman, in W Grossman, DS Baim (eds), 1991, with permission.)*

FIGURE 192-7 Hemodynamic findings at rest and during exercise in a patient with mitral regurgitation. Left ventricular (LV), pulmonary capillary wedge (PCW), and radial artery pressure tracings are shown before (*left*) and during (*right*) the sixth minute of supine bicycle exercise. PCW mean pressure and *v* wave increase substantially with exercise. (*From BH Lorell, W Grossman, in W Grossman, DS Baim (eds), 1991, with permission.*)

characteristic deformity in the presence of valvular heart disease affecting the tricuspid or pulmonic valves. In patients with severe *tricuspid regurgitation*, right atrial pressure resembles closely in appearance the right ventricular pressure. Mean right atrial pressure and right ventricular end-diastolic pressure are both elevated in tricuspid regurgitation. In *tricuspid stenosis* there is a pressure gradient between right atrium and ventricle during diastole.

Characteristic deformities of right and left ventricular diastolic pressures occur in patients with *cardiac tamponade* or *pericardial constriction*. In both conditions there is equalization of left and right ventricular diastolic pressures. However, in constrictive pericarditis, nearly all ventricular filling occurs shortly after mitral and tricuspid valve opening; following this period of rapid filling, ventricular volumes cannot increase further due to the limit of the constricting pericardium. This abnormality produces an abrupt early ventricular diastolic pressure rise with a mid and late ventricular pressure plateau, giving the so-called square root sign (Fig. 192-9). In contrast, in tamponade there is equalization of diastolic pressures with a gradual increase throughout diastole.

Congestive heart failure due to myocardial contractile dysfunction is associated with characteristic alterations in the ventricular pressure waveforms seen at cardiac catheterization. Both isovolumic pressure rise and pressure decline are not as steep as in the normal heart. The reduced slopes of pressure rise and decline are associated with an abbreviated ejection period, giving the left ventricular pressure tracing a triangular appearance (Fig. 192-10). Also, the pressure decline does not continue to zero, so the minimal left ventricular diastolic pressure may be elevated. This hemodynamic finding correlates with an increased ventricular end-systolic volume, which is a sign of depressed contractile function of the left ventricular myocardium.

MEASUREMENT OF FLOW

Systemic and pulmonary blood flows may be measured by either the Fick or indicator-dilution methods. In the normal heart, these flows are equal and are termed *cardiac output*. Specialized techniques have made it possible to measure coronary artery blood flow (catheter- or guidewire-tip-mounted Doppler flowmeter), coronary sinus blood flow (thermodilution technique), and renal, cerebral, and femoral blood flows as well.

Cardiac output is most commonly measured by the thermodilution technique, but the standard method, against which this technique and others are calibrated, remains the direct Fick oxygen method. In the direct Fick method, O_2 consumption is measured simultaneously with determination of arteriovenous oxygen difference across the lungs. Fick's principle states that

$$Q \text{ (L/min)} = \frac{O_2 \text{ consumption (mL/min)}}{\text{arteriovenous oxygen difference (mL/L)}}$$

In order to compare individuals of different body weights and sizes, O_2 consumption and cardiac output (Q) are commonly divided by body surface area. Normal values for O_2 consumption and cardiac output are given in Table 192-3. Cardiac output is calculated by dividing O_2 consumption by the arteriovenous O_2 difference across the lungs (estimated pulmonary venous–pulmonary arterial O_2 content); this actually provides a measure of *pulmonary blood flow* (Q_p). In patients with left-to-right shunts at the atrial, ventricular, or pulmonary artery levels, pulmonary blood flow exceeds systemic blood flow. In such cases, systemic blood flow (Q_s) is calculated by dividing O_2 consumption by the systemic arteriovenous O_2 difference. The latter is calculated as systemic arterial blood O_2 content minus mixed venous blood O_2 content using blood from the chamber immediately proximal to the level of the shunt. The Fick method is most dependable when the cardiac output is low and the arteriovenous oxygen difference is large.

For indicator-dilution measurement of cardiac output using the thermodilution technique, a thermistor is mounted on the tip of a

FIGURE 192-8 Severe aortic regurgitation. There is equilibration between the left ventricular (LV) and aortic or femoral artery (FA) pressures in diastole. Also, LV diastolic pressure exceeds pulmonary capillary wedge (PCW) pressure early in diastole, indicating premature closure of the mitral valve (a characteristic feature of severe aortic regurgitation). (*From W Grossman, in W Grossman, DS Baim (eds), 1991, with permission.*)

FIGURE 192-9   Left ventricular (LV), right ventricular (RV), and pulmonary capillary wedge (PCW) pressure tracings in a patient with severe constrictive pericarditis. Note the diastolic dip and plateau ("square root sign") pattern

for left and right ventricular diastolic pressures (*left*). The wedge pressure (*right*) shows early systolic and early diastolic dips.

balloon-flotation catheter, and the catheter is advanced so that the balloon tip and thermistor are located in the pulmonary artery. Cold dextrose solution or saline is injected via a proximal port on the catheter into the vena cava or right atrium, and the change in temperature monitored at the thermistor is integrated mathematically. This integral is inversely proportional to the volume flow rate past the thermistor, and if the temperatures of the injectate and pulmonary artery blood are measured, cardiac output (actually pulmonary blood flow) can be calculated. In contrast to the Fick method, the indicator-dilution method is least reliable when the cardiac output is low.

FIGURE 192-10   Left ventricular (LV) and aortic (Ao) pressures in a patient with advanced dilated cardiomyopathy. Marked slowing of the rates of left ventricular pressure rise and fall (impairment of contractility and relaxation) give the LV pressure pulse a triangular appearance. Also, the minimal value for left ventricular diastolic pressure is markedly elevated, suggesting an increased end-systolic volume and a reduced LV ejection fraction. *(From W Grossman, in W Grossman, DS Baim (eds), 1991, with permission.)*

Valve areas and resistances   Using simultaneous measures of pressure and flow, the resistance to blood flow across cardiac valves as well as the pulmonary and systemic arteriolar beds may be estimated. Valve areas are calculated using the Gorlin formula:

$$A = \frac{\text{flow}}{K \sqrt{\Delta P}}$$

where A = valve orifice area (cm^2), *flow* is the blood flow (mL/s) across the stenotic valve, ΔP is the mean pressure gradient (mmHg) during the period of blood flow, and K is a constant (44.3 for the aortic valve and 37.7 for the mitral valve).

The resistance to blood flow through the systemic vascular bed is

$$SVR = 80(MAP - RA)/SBF$$

where SVR is systemic vascular resistance [(dyn·s)/cm^5], MAP and RA are mean aortic and right atrial pressures (mmHg), 80 is a constant for converting to metric units, and SBF is systemic blood flow (L/min).

Resistance to blood flow through the pulmonary vascular bed is

$$PVR = 80(PA - PCW \text{ or } LA)/PBF$$

where PVR is pulmonary vascular resistance [(dyn·s)/cm^5]; PA, PCW, and LA are pulmonary artery, pulmonary capillary wedge, and left atrial mean pressures (mmHg); and PBF is pulmonary blood flow (L/min). Normal values for pulmonary and systemic vascular resistances are given in Table 192-3.

REFERENCES

GODLEWSKI KJ et al: Interpretation of cardiac pathophysiology from pressure waveform analysis: Acute aortic insufficiency. Cathet Cardiovasc Diagn 28:244, 1993

GROSSMAN W: Cardiac catheterization, in *Heart Disease*, 4th ed, E Braunwald (ed). Philadelphia, Saunders, 1992, p 180

———, BAIM DS (eds): *Cardiac Catheterization, Angiography, and Intervention*, 4th ed. Philadelphia, Lea & Febiger, 1991

JOHNSON LW, KRONE R: Cardiac catheterization 1991: A report of the Registry of the Society for Cardiac Angiography and Interventions (SCA&I). Cathet Cardiovasc Diagn 28:219, 1993

KERN MJ et al: Interpretation of cardiac pathophysiology from pressure waveform analysis: Simultaneous left and right ventricular pressure measurements. Cathet Cardiovasc Diagn 28:51, 1993

FIGURE 193-4 Eccentric, ulcerated lesion in the mid-left anterior descending coronary artery (*top*), being treated by directional atherectomy (*middle*), with a large and smooth luminal result (*bottom*).

FIGURE 193-5 Hemodynamic results of mitral valvuloplasty in a 38-year-old woman with mitral stenosis. The transmitral [left atrium (LA)–to–left ventricle (LV)] gradient, cardiac output, and calculated mitral valve area are shown before (*left panel*) and after (*right panel*) balloon dilatation.

75 to 15 mmHg. Balloon pulmonary valvuloplasty now stands as the preferred therapy for this lesion.

MITRAL VALVULOPLASTY The predominant application of balloon mitral valvuloplasty is in patients with rheumatic mitral stenosis, in whom stenosis results primarily from commissural fusion with associated leaflet thickening. Such patients previously would have undergone open or closed surgical commissurotomy but are now treated almost exclusively by balloon valvuloplasty. Other patients (with left atrial thrombus, mitral regurgitation, subvalvular disease, or leaflet thickening or rigidity) have less satisfactory results with either surgical commissurotomy or balloon valvuloplasty and are better treated by surgical valve replacement.

The usual approach to balloon mitral valvuloplasty is via transseptal puncture (right atrium to left atrium), followed by passage of a guidewire across the stenotic valve and into the left ventricle. One or more balloon catheters with a dilating area equivalent to a single 23- to 30-mm diameter balloon are advanced over this guidewire and inflated within the stenotic valve. Successful dilatation separates fused commissures and enhances leaflet compliance, thus increasing the effective diastolic valve area from 0.9 to 2.0 cm² or more (Fig. 193-5). Although this is still restricted compared with the 3.5- to 5-cm² area of a normal mitral valve, this increase in valve area provides excellent symptomatic relief and is equivalent to or approaches the increase in orifice size resulting from surgical mitral commissurotomy or prosthetic mitral valve replacement.

The main complications of balloon mitral valvuloplasty relate to the potential for cardiac perforation during transseptal puncture (approximately 2 percent of patients) and the chance of systemic embolization (approximately 1 percent of patients) despite preprocedure echocardiographic exclusion of patients with left atrial thrombus.

AORTIC VALVULOPLASTY Balloon aortic valvuloplasty may be performed in children with congenital aortic stenosis and in adults with rheumatic or acquired calcific aortic stenosis. Some patients with rheumatic aortic stenosis have leaflet fusion, but the problem in acquired calcific aortic stenosis is due more to rigidity of the valve leaflets themselves. In this latter group of patients, balloon valvuloplasty fractures leaflet calcium (providing new hinge points along which the valve leaflets can open) and temporarily expands the aortic annulus.

The most prevalent approach to balloon aortic valvuloplasty consists of femoral arterial puncture with retrograde passage of a guidewire and balloon (inflated diameter 18 to 23 mm) across the valve. Overdilatation of the valve annulus may cause leaflet avulsion and is generally avoided. Balloon aortic valvuloplasty typically increases the effective systolic valve area from 0.6 to 1.0 cm². The resultant valve area is still small compared with the area of a normal aortic valve (3 to 4 cm²) or with the effective area of an inflated 20-mm balloon (3.1 cm²), but it does relieve symptoms at rest or during mild to moderate exertion in most patients with critical aortic stenosis. Unfortunately, the relatively small effective orifice achieved and the high incidence of valvular restenosis (up to 50 percent within 1 year after dilatation) make balloon aortic valvuloplasty a temporary palliation most applicable to elderly patients who are poor risks for valve replacement or as a "bridge" to valve replacement.

TREATMENT OF CONGENITAL MALFORMATIONS

Pediatric interventional cardiologists have developed a number of innovative techniques to correct or palliate congenital cardiac lesions. Some techniques are those described above—i.e., balloon dilatation of stenotic pulmonary arteries, surgical shunts, or balloon valvuloplasty—but others are unique to the pediatric population.

ATRIAL SEPTOSTOMY In certain patients with cyanotic congenital heart disease, such as some with transposition of the great vessels, it is desirable to produce or enlarge an atrial septal defect in order to facilitate passage of oxygenated blood into the right side of the heart. This can be achieved by passage of a balloon catheter from right to left atrium across a patent foramen ovale, followed by forceful withdrawal of the inflated balloon. Alternatively, a catheter with a concealed blade can be passed across the septum. The blade can then be deployed in the left atrium to incise the septum as the catheter is withdrawn. The resulting septal incision can be widened by conventional balloon septostomy.

CLOSURE OF UNDESIRED SHUNTS OR COLLATERAL VESSELS A variety of appliances have been developed to close undesired intracardiac shunts, including defects in the atrial or ventricular septum and patent ductus arteriosus. These devices resemble a double (back-to-back) umbrella, which can be folded into a cylinder for containment in a catheter. Under fluoroscopic guidance, the delivery catheter can be positioned across the target defect so that the umbrella can be deployed to block undesired flow.

Smaller vascular shunts can be closed using special coils. These coils can be placed within a catheter and delivered to the undesired vessel. Once in place, the coil interferes with blood flow and promotes local thrombotic occlusion of the target vessel.

REFERENCES

BAIM DS: Interventional catheterization techniques: Percutaneous transluminal angioplasty, valvuloplasty and related procedures, in *Heart Disease*, 4th ed, E Braunwald (ed). Philadelphia, Saunders, 1992, p 1365

CARROZZA JP et al: Angiographic and clinical outcome of intracoronary stenting: Immediate and long-term results from a large single-center experience. J Am Coll Cardiol 20:328, 1992

DE FEYTER PJ et al: Balloon angioplasty for the treatment of lesions in saphenous vein bypass grafts. J Am Coll Cardiol 21:1539, 1993

FISHMAN R et al: Long-term results of coronary atherectomy—predictors of restenosis. J Am Coll Cardiol 20:1101, 1992

HANDENSCHILD CC: Pathobiology of restenosis after angioplasty. Am J Med 94:40S, 1993

JOHNSON MC et al: Repair of coarctation of the aorta in infancy. Comparison of surgical and balloon angioplasty. Am Heart J 125:464, 1993

KUNTZ RE et al: Predictors of event-free survival after balloon aortic valvuloplasty. N Engl J Med 325:17, 1991

LOCK JE et al: Transcatheter umbrella closure of congenital heart defects. Circulation 75:593, 1987

O'LAUGHLIN MP et al: Transcatheter closure of residual atrial septal defect following cardiac transplantation. Cathet Cardiovasc Diagn 28:162, 1993

194 NORMAL AND ABNORMAL MYOCARDIAL FUNCTION

EUGENE BRAUNWALD

CELLULAR BASIS OF CARDIAC CONTRACTION

The *myocardium* is composed of individual striated muscle cells (fibers), normally 10 to 15 μm in diameter and 30 to 60 μm in length (Fig. 194-1A). Each fiber contains multiple cross-banded strands (myofibrils) that run the length of the fiber and are, in turn, composed of serially repeating structures, the sarcomeres. The cytoplasm between the myofibrils contains other cell constituents, such as the single centrally located nucleus, numerous mitochondria, and intracellular membrane system, the sarcoplasmic reticulum.

The *sarcomere*, the structural and functional unit of contraction, is delimited by two adjacent dark lines, the Z lines (Fig. 194-1). The distance between Z lines varies with the degree of contraction or stretch of the muscle and ranges between 1.6 and 2.2 μm. Within the confines of the sarcomere are alternating light and dark bands, giving the myocardial fibers their striated appearance under the light microscope. At the center of the sarcomere is a dark band of constant width (1.5 μm), the A band, which is flanked by two lighter bands,

the I bands, which are of variable width. The sarcomere of heart muscle, like that of skeletal muscle, is made up of two sets of interdigitating myofilaments. Thicker filaments, composed principally of the protein myosin, traverse and are limited to the A band. They are about 10 nm (100 Å) in diameter, with tapered ends, and measure 1.5 to 1.6 μm in length. Thinner filaments, composed primarily of actin, course from the Z line through the I band into the A band. They are approximately 5 nm (50 Å) in diameter and 1.0 μm in length. Thus there is overlapping of thick and thin filaments only within the A band, while the I band contains only thin filaments (Fig. 194-1). On electron-microscopic examination, bridges may be seen to extend between the thick and thin filaments within the A band.

THE CONTRACTILE PROCESS The "sliding" model for muscle rests on the fundamental observation that the thick and thin filaments are constant in overall length during both contraction and relaxation. With activation, repeated interactions take place at the bridges between the actin and myosin filaments, and the actin filaments are propelled further into the A band. In the process, the A band remains constant in width, whereas the I band becomes more narrow and the Z lines move toward one another.

The myosin molecule is a complex, asymmetric fibrous protein with a molecular weight of about 500,000; it has a rod-like portion that is about 150 nm (1500 Å) in length with a globular portion at its end. This globular portion of the myosin is the site of adenosine triphosphatase (ATPase) activity and also forms the bridges between the myosin and actin. In forming the thick myofilament, which is composed of 300 longitudinally stacked myosin molecules, the rod-like segments of the myosin molecules are laid down in an orderly, polarized manner, leaving the globular portions projecting outward so that they can interact with actin to generate force and shortening (Fig. 194-2A). Actin has a molecular weight of 47,000. The thin filament is composed of a double helix of two chains of actin molecules wound about each other, intimately associated with two regulatory proteins, tropomyosin and troponin (Fig. 194-2B); the latter can be separated into three components, troponins C, I, and T (Fig. 194-2C). In contrast to myosin, actin has no intrinsic enzymatic activity, but it has the ability to combine reversibly with myosin in the presence of ATP and Mg^{2+}, which activates the myosin ATPase. In relaxed muscle this interaction is inhibited by tropomyosin.

During activation Ca^{2+} becomes attached to troponin C, which results in a conformational change in the regulatory protein tropomyosin, which in turn exposes the actin cross-bridge interaction sites. This results in sliding of the actin along the myosin filaments, ultimately causing muscle shortening and/or the development of tension. The splitting of ATP then dissociates the myosin cross-bridge from the actin. In the presence of ATP linkages between actin and myosin filaments are made and broken cyclically as long as sufficient Ca^{2+} is present; these linkages are broken when Ca^{2+} concentration falls below a critical level, and the troponin-tropomyosin complex once more prevents interactions between the myosin cross-bridges and the actin filaments. Ionic calcium is a principal mediator of the inotropic state of the heart; most positive inotropic drugs, including the digitalis glycosides and catecholamines, act by increasing the concentrations of Ca^{2+} in the vicinity of the myofilaments.

The *sarcoplasmic reticulum* (Fig. 194-1B) is a complex network of anastomosing intracellular channels that invests the myofibrils. It is less profuse in cardiac than in skeletal muscle. Its longitudinally disposed membrane-lined tubules are closely applied to the surfaces of individual sarcomeres but have no direct continuity with the outside of the cell. However, closely related to the sarcoplasmic reticulum, both structurally and functionally, are the transverse tubules or T system, formed by tubelike invaginations of the sarcolemma that extend into the myocardial fiber along the Z lines, i.e., the ends of the sarcomeres.

CARDIAC ACTIVATION At rest, the cardiac cell is polarized; i.e., the interior has a negative charge relative to the outside of the cell, with a transmembrane potential of −80 to −100 mV (Chap. 197). The sarcolemma, which in the resting state is largely imperme-

FIGURE 194-1 Microscopic structure of heart muscle. *A.* Myocardium as seen under the light microscope. Branching of fibers is evident. Each fiber, or cell, contains a centrally located nucleus. *B.* Myocardial cell, reconstructed from electron micrographs. Each cell is composed of multiple parallel fibrils. Each fibril is composed of serially connected sarcomeres (N, nucleus). *C.* Sarcomere from a myofibril, with diagrammatic representation of myofilaments. Thick filaments (1.5 μm long, composed of myosin) form the A band, and thin filaments (1 μm long, composed primarily of actin) extend from the Z line through the I band into the A band. The overlapping of thick and thin filaments is seen only in the A band. *D.* Cross sections of the sarcomere indicate the specific lattice arrangements of the myofilaments. In the center of the sarcomere only the thick, or myosin, filaments arranged in a hexagonal array are seen. In the distal portions of the A band, both thick and thin, or actin, filaments are found, with each thick filament surrounded by six thin filaments. In the I band only thin filaments are present. *(From Braunwald E, ed, Heart Disease, 4th ed, 1992, p 353.)*

able to Na$^+$, has a Na$^+$- and K$^+$-stimulating pump requiring ATP that extrudes Na$^+$ from the cell; the pump plays a critical role in establishing this resting potential. Thus on the inside of the cell [K$^+$] is relatively high and [Na$^+$] is far lower, while in the extracellular milieu [Na$^+$] is high and [K$^+$] is low. At the same time, in the resting state, the extracellular [Ca^{2+}] greatly exceeds the free intracellular [Ca^{2+}].

During the plateau of the action potential (phase 2) there is a slow inward current which reflects primarily a movement of Ca^{2+} into the cell (Fig. 194-3), although the absolute quantity of Ca^{2+} that crosses

the surface membrane is relatively small and itself appears to be incapable of bringing about full activation of the contractile apparatus. The depolarizing current not only extends across the surface of the cell but penetrates deeply into the cell by way of the ramifying T system; this current triggers the release of much larger quantities of Ca^{2+} from the sarcoplasmic reticulum, a process termed "regenerative release" of Ca^{2+}. This rise in intracellular Ca^{2+} is the key step in initiating contraction.

The Ca^{2+} released from the sarcoplasmic reticulum then diffuses toward the sarcomere, and as already described, combines with

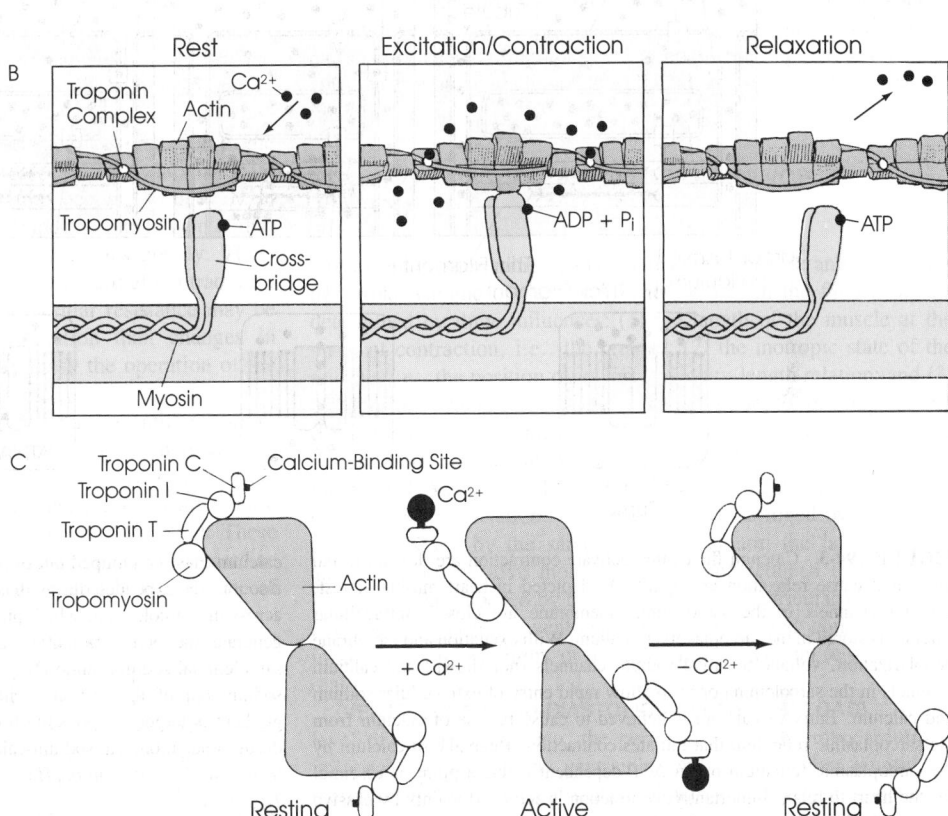

FIGURE 194-2 Contractile protein interactions and the role of calcium as activator messenger are shown schematically: *A*. Contractile proteins (myosin and actin) and regulatory proteins (troponin complex and tropomyosin) are shown in relative positions on myofilaments. *B*. Contraction takes place when the heads of myosin molecules, which form cross-bridges of thick filament, bind to actin, followed by shift in orientation of cross-bridge that pulls thin filament toward center of sarcomere. Activation requires calcium binding to troponin complex, reversing inhibition of interaction between myosin and actin. In the cycle of chemical reactions underlying contraction, hydrolysis of ATP produces the cross-bridge motion. Relaxation occurs when calcium becomes dissociated from troponin. *C*. Molecular rearrangements at the level of the thin filament involve regulatory proteins (tropomyosin and troponins C, I, T) in an allosteric effect. Calcium binding to troponin C loosens bond linking troponin I to actin; resulting dissociation of troponin T from actin backbone of thin filament displaces tropomyosin, exposing active sites for interaction with myosin. [*Reproduced by permission, from AM Katz, VE Smith, Hosp Prac, 19(1):69, 1984. Illustration by Bunji Tagawa.*]

troponin C. By repressing this inhibitor of contraction Ca^{2+} activates the myofilaments to produce contraction. During repolarization the sarcoplasmic reticulum reaccumulates Ca^{2+} against a concentration gradient. This is an energy-requiring process which lowers the concentration of Ca^{2+} in the vicinity of the myofibrils to a level that inhibits the actin-myosin interaction responsible for contraction and in this manner leads to relaxation. Thus, the cell membrane, transverse tubules, and sarcoplasmic reticulum, with their ability to transmit an action potential, to release and then reaccumulate Ca^{2+}, appear to play a fundamental role in the rhythmic contraction and relaxation of heart muscle.

The ATP formed from substrate oxidation is the principal source of energy for almost all of the mechanical work of contraction performed by the myocardial cell. The high-energy phosphate stores in ATP are in equilibrium with those in the form of creatine phosphate. The activity of myosin ATPase determines the rate of forming and breaking of the actin-myosin cross-bridges and ultimately the velocity of muscle contraction.

THE ROLE OF MUSCLE LENGTH In all striated muscle, including cardiac muscle, the force of contraction depends on initial muscle length. The sarcomere length associated with the most forceful contraction is approximately 2.2 μm. At this length the two sets of myofilaments of the sarcomere are situated to provide the greatest area for their interaction. In support of the sliding-filament hypothesis,

force development diminishes in direct proportion to the decrease in the overlap between thick and thin filaments and the resultant reduction in the number of reactive sites. The length of the sarcomere also appears to regulate the extent of activation of the contractile system, i.e., its sensitivity to Ca^{2+}, which is also greatest at approximately 2.2 μm. When sarcomere length is increased to 3.65 μm, the thin filaments are entirely withdrawn from the A band, and no tension can be developed. Similarly, when the sarcomeres are shorter than 2.0 μm, the thin filaments bypass one another, doubly overlapping each other and so reducing both the sensitivity of the contractile sites to Ca^{2+} and the capacity for force development.

The relation between the initial length of the muscle fibers and the developed force is of prime importance for the function of heart muscle. This forms the basis of the Frank-Starling relation (Starling's law of the heart), which states that, within limits, the force of ventricular contraction is a function of the end-diastolic length of the cardiac muscle, which in turn is closely related to the ventricular end-diastolic volume. In heart muscle, operating along the ascending limb of the length-active tension curve sarcomere length is directly proportional to muscle length. As muscle length decreases to the point at which sarcomere length approaches 1.5 μm and at which developed tension approaches zero, the I bands at first narrow, then disappear while the A band remains constant in length. At this latter point, the Z lines abut the edges of the A bands. Thus the sarcomere cardiac filling, and the resultant reduction in ventricular diastolic volume lowers stroke volume and ventricular work.

4 *Venous tone.* The venous system is not a simple system of passive conduits between the systemic capillary bed and the right atrium. Instead, the smooth muscle in the walls of the venules and veins responds to a variety of neural and humoral stimuli. Venoconstriction occurs during muscular exercise, deep respiration, fright, or marked hypotension, tending to diminish extrathoracic and to augment intrathoracic and intraventricular blood volumes and ventricular performance.

5 *The pumping action of skeletal muscle.* During muscular exercise the contracting skeletal muscles squeeze blood out of the venous bed and, with the aid of the venous valves, displace it centrally, thereby increasing intrathoracic blood volume, ventricular end-diastolic volume, and ventricular work.

Atrial contraction   Vigorous, appropriately timed atrial contraction augments ventricular filling and end-diastolic volume. The atrial contribution to ventricular filling is of particular importance in patients with concentric ventricular hypertrophy, in whom the loss of atrial systole (as in atrial fibrillation) tends to reduce ventricular end-diastolic pressure and volume, ultimately lowering myocardial performance. The atrial contribution to ventricular filling may be reduced by atrioventricular dissociation, prolongation or abbreviation of the P-R interval, and depression of the inotropic state of the atrium.

INOTROPIC STATE (MYOCARDIAL CONTRACTILITY)   A number of factors determine the level of ventricular performance at any given ventricular end-diastolic volume, i.e., the position of the ventricular function curve. These influences may be considered to operate by modifying myocardial force-velocity-length relations. In the final analysis, most of these influences act by altering the concentration of Ca^{2+} in the vicinity of the myofilaments.

Adrenergic nerve activity (See also Chap. 68)   The quantity of norepinephrine released by adrenergic nerve endings in the heart is, under ordinary circumstances, dependent on the adrenergic nerve impulse traffic, and alterations in the frequency of nerve impulses modify the quantity of norepinephrine released and acting on the beta-adrenergic receptors in the myocardium. This mechanism is the most important one which acutely modifies the position of the force-velocity and ventricular function curves under physiologic conditions.

Circulating catecholamines (See also Chap. 68)   The adrenal medulla and other sympathetic ganglia outside the heart, when stimulated by adrenergic nerve impulses, release catecholamines, which, when they reach the heart, augment the inotropic state and the frequency of contraction.

The force-frequency relation   The position of the myocardial force-velocity curve also is influenced by the rate and rhythm of cardiac contraction; e.g., ventricular extrasystoles result in post-extrasystolic potentiation, presumably by increasing the Ca^{2+} which enters the cardiac cell.

Exogenously administered inotropic agents   The cardiac glycosides, isoproterenol, dopamine, dobutamine, and other sympatho-mimetic agents, calcium, caffeine, theophylline, and their derivatives, all improve the myocardial force-velocity relation and therefore may be used therapeutically to augment ventricular performance at any given ventricular end-diastolic volume.

Physiologic depressants   Included among these are severe myocardial hypoxia, hypercapnia, ischemia, and acidosis. Acting either singly or in combination, these influences exert a depressant effect on the myocardial force-velocity curve and depress left ventricular work at any given ventricular end-diastolic volume.

Pharmacologic depressants   These include quinidine, procainamide, disopyramide, high doses of certain calcium antagonists, barbiturates, alcohol, and other local and general anesthetics, as well as many other drugs.

Loss of ventricular substance   When a sufficiently large portion of ventricular myocardium becomes nonfunctional or necrotic, as occurs transiently during ischemia (Chap. 203) and permanently in

myocardial infarction (Chap. 202), total ventricular performance at any given level of end-diastolic volume may become depressed.

Intrinsic myocardial depression   Although the fundamental mechanisms responsible for depression of myocardial contractility in most cases of chronic congestive heart failure remain to be elucidated, it is now apparent that in this condition the inotropic state of each unit of myocardium is depressed and that the level of ventricular performance at any ventricular end-diastolic volume is thereby lowered.

VENTRICULAR AFTERLOAD   The stroke volume is ultimately a function of the extent of ventricular fiber shortening. In the intact heart, as in isolated cardiac muscle, the velocity and extent of shortening of ventricular muscle fibers at any given level of diastolic fiber length and myocardial inotropic state are inversely related to the load which opposes shortening, i.e., the afterload. The afterload on the intact heart may be defined as the tension or stress developed in the wall of the ventricle during ejection. Therefore, the afterload on the ventricular muscle fibers also is dependent on the level of aortic pressure as well as on the volume and thickness of the ventricular cavity, since Laplace's law indicates that the tension of the myocardial fiber is a function of the product of the intracavitary ventricular pressure and ventricular radius divided by the wall thickness. Thus, at the same level of aortic pressure, the afterload faced by a dilated left ventricle is higher than that encountered by a ventricle of normal size. Conversely, at the same aortic pressure and ventricular diastolic volume the afterload of a thick-walled ventricle is lower than of a thin-walled chamber. The aortic pressure, in turn, is influenced largely by the peripheral vascular resistance, the physical characteristics of the arterial tree, and the volume of blood it contains at the onset of ejection. At any given ventricular end-diastolic volume and level of the inotropic state, the left ventricular stroke volume is related inversely to the afterload.

The critical role played by the ventricular afterload in cardiovascular regulation is shown in Fig. 194-4. As already noted, increases in both preload and contractility increase myocardial fiber shortening, while increases in afterload reduce it. The extent of myocardial fiber shortening and left ventricular size are the determinants of stroke volume. Arterial pressure, in turn, is related to the product of cardiac output and systemic vascular resistance, while afterload is a function of left ventricular volume, wall thickness, and arterial pressure. An increase in arterial pressure induced by vasoconstriction, for example, augments afterload, which opposes myocardial fiber shortening, reducing stroke volume, and cardiac output; this in turn tends to restore arterial pressure to its previous level.

When left ventricular function becomes impaired and the chamber dilates, i.e., when there is little or no preload reserve, left ventricular afterload becomes increasingly important in determining cardiac performance. Increases in afterload may result from the influence on the arterial bed of neural, humoral, or structural changes which can occur in response to a fall in cardiac output. This increased afterload may reduce cardiac output further while myocardial oxygen requirements are increased. Treatment with vasodilators (Chap. 195) has the opposite effect. In this way, alterations in the peripheral vascular bed probably play an important role in the hemodynamic and metabolic events which usually are attributed to progressive impairment of the myocardium.

All of the influences acting on cardiac performance enumerated above interact in a complex fashion to maintain cardiac output at a level appropriate to the requirements of the metabolizing tissues, and in a normal person interference with one of these mechanisms may not influence the cardiac output. For example, a moderate reduction of blood volume *or* the loss of the atrial contribution to ventricular contraction can ordinarily be sustained without a reduction in the resting cardiac output. Other factors, such as an increase in the frequency of adrenergic nerve impulses to the heart and an increase in heart rate, will, in a normal individual, augment contractility and sustain cardiac output. Mechanisms are also available that prevent elevation of the cardiac output when there is no physiologic demand

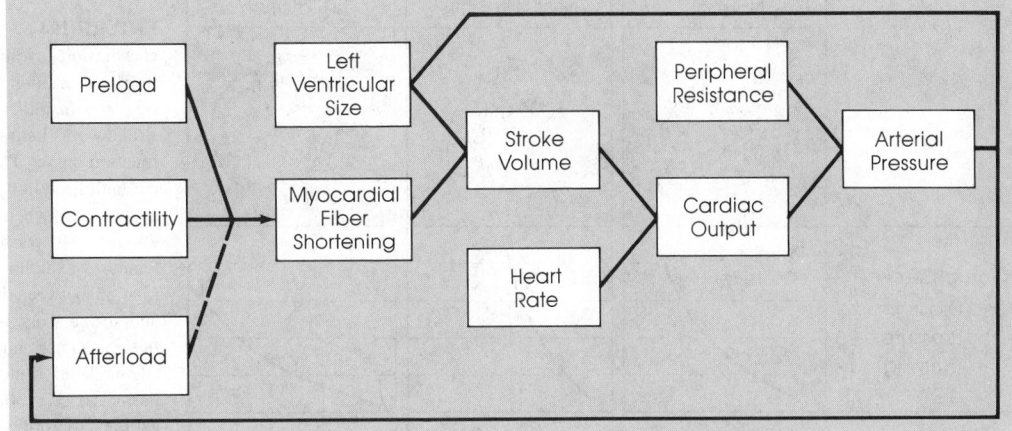

FIGURE 194-4 Scheme of interactions among various components that regulate cardiac activity. Solid lines indicate an augmenting effect; broken line represents an inhibiting effect. *(From Braunwald E: Regulation of the Circulation. N Engl J Med 290:1124–1129, 1420–1425, 1974.)*

for augmented flow. For example, augmentation of myocardial contractility by means of cardiac glycosides does not increase the cardiac output in normal humans. Thus, in analyzing the effect of an intervention on cardiac output, it is important to recognize that it is the preload, which in turn is related to the volume of blood available for filling the heart, rather than the inotropic state of the myocardium or the afterload which limits cardiac output in the normal individual. An improvement of myocardial contractility by a drug such as digitalis or the reduction of afterload with nitroprusside would not be expected to elevate the output in a normal subject. On the other hand, in the presence of congestive heart failure, the cardiac output usually is limited by the depressed contractile state of the myocardium, and a

FIGURE 194-5 Diagram showing the interrelations among influences on ventricular end-diastolic volume (EDV) through stretching of the myocardium and the contractile state of the myocardium. Levels of ventricular EDV associated with filling pressures that result in dyspnea and pulmonary edema are shown on the abscissa. Levels of ventricular performance required when the subject is at rest, while walking, and during maximal activity are designated on the ordinate. The broken lines are the descending limbs of the ventricular-performance curves, which are rarely seen during life but which show the level of ventricular performance if end-diastolic volume could be elevated to very high levels. For further explanation see text. *(From Braunwald E, ed, Heart Disease, 4th ed, 1992, p 413).*

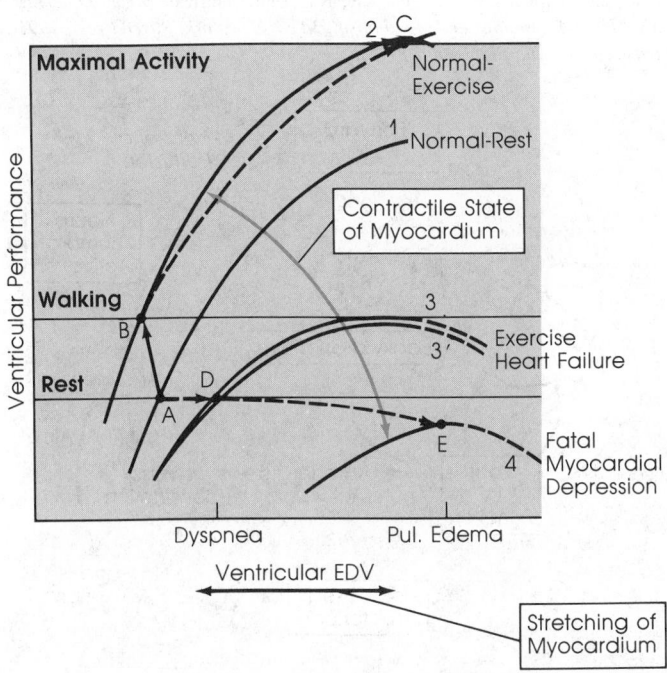

positive inotropic drug and/or reduction of afterload raises cardiac output (Chap. 195).

EXERCISE The hemodynamic changes which normally occur during exercise in the upright position are complex (Fig. 194-5). The hyperventilation, the pumping action of the exercising muscles, and the venoconstriction which occur all tend to augment venous return and hence ventricular filling and preload. Simultaneously, the increase in the adrenergic nerve impulses to the myocardium, the increased concentration of circulating catecholamines, and the tachycardia which occur during exercise all combine to augment the contractile state of the myocardium (Fig. 194-5, curves 1 and 2) and lead to an elevation of stroke work and stroke volume, with no change or even a decrease of end-diastolic pressure and volume (Fig. 194-5, points A and B). Vasodilation occurs in the exercising muscles, thus tending to counteract the marked increase in arterial pressure which would otherwise occur as cardiac output rises. This ultimately allows the achievement of a greatly elevated cardiac output during exercise, at an arterial pressure only moderately higher than in the resting state.

THE FAILING HEART

Though heart failure may be readily described as a clinical syndrome, characterized by well-known symptoms and physical signs, a precise physiologic or biochemical definition is far more difficult. However, from the clinical point of view, heart failure may be considered to be the condition in which *an abnormality of cardiac function is responsible for the inability of the heart to pump blood at a rate commensurate with the requirements of the metabolizing tissues and/or can do so only from an abnormally elevated ventricular diastolic volume.* Abnormalities during systole and/or diastole may be present in heart failure (Fig. 194-6). In so-called *systolic heart failure,* i.e., classic heart failure, an impaired inotropic state causes weakened systolic contraction, which leads, ultimately, to a reduction in stroke volume, inadequate ventricular emptying, cardiac dilatation, and often elevation of ventricular diastolic pressure. Idiopathic dilated cardiomyopathy (Chap. 205) is the prototype of systolic heart failure.

In *diastolic heart failure* (p. 1000) the principal abnormality involves impaired relaxation of the ventricle and leads to an elevation of ventricular diastolic pressure at any given diastolic volume. Failure of relaxation can be functional, i.e., as during transient ischemia, or it can be caused by a stiffened, thickened ventricle. Typical conditions in which diastolic failure occurs are restrictive cardiomyopathy secondary to infiltrative conditions, such as amyloidosis or hemochromatosis, as well as hypertrophic cardiomyopathy (Chap. 205). In many patients with cardiac hypertrophy and dilatation, systolic and diastolic failure coexist; the ventricle both empties and fills abnormally. There may be cardiac dilatation, but the ventricle's pressure-volume relation is shifted, raising the ventricular diastolic pressure at any given volume.

| Normal | Hypertrophy | Dilatation |

FIGURE 194-6 Relationship between left ventricular end-diastolic volume and (1) end-diastolic pressure (top), describing the *compliance* of the left ventricle, i.e., its *diastolic* properties; and (2) left ventricular stroke work (bottom), describing the ventricle's *systolic* function curve. The normal left ventricle (left) reaches an end-diastolic pressure of 30 mmHg (pulmonary edema level) when its end-diastolic volume is elevated to 200 mL. The concentrically hypertrophied left ventricle (center), exhibits normal systolic function since the relation between left ventricular end-diastolic volume and stroke work is unchanged, but there is "diastolic failure" in that end-diastolic pressure reaches pulmonary edema level (i.e., 30 mmHg) at a lower level than normal (i.e., 130 mL). The dilated ventricle (right) exhibits "systolic failure" in that the maximal stroke work and the stroke volume at any level of end-diastolic volume are depressed. The left ventricle displays increased diastolic compliance, i.e., distensibility, with a higher than normal end-diastolic volume (280 mL) required to reach the pulmonary edema level. *(Reprinted with permission from Gorlin R, Prim Cardiol 6:84, 1980.)*

Though a defect in myocardial contraction is characteristic of systolic heart failure, this defect may result from a primary abnormality in the heart muscle, as in cardiomyopathy, or it may be secondary to a chronic excessive work load as in hypertension and valvular heart disease. In ischemic heart disease systolic heart failure results from a loss in the quantity of normally contracting cells.

It is important to distinguish heart failure from (1) states of circulatory insufficiency in which myocardial function is not primarily impaired, such as cardiac tamponade or hemorrhagic shock; (2) conditions in which there is circulatory congestion because of abnormal salt and water retention but in which there is no serious disturbance of the heart's function, and (3) conditions in which a normal myocardium is suddenly presented with a load which exceeds its capacity, e.g., accelerated hypertension or rupture of a valve cusp secondary to infective endocarditis.

Adaptive mechanisms A series of mechanisms aid the heart faced with an increased hemodynamic burden, such as pressure or volume overload, or which has lost myocardial substance. These adaptive mechanisms include: (1) the Frank-Starling mechanism operating through an increase in preload (p. 991); (2) the development of myocardial hypertrophy, which restores elevated ventricular wall stress to normal; (3) redistribution of a subnormal cardiac output away from the skin, skeletal muscle, and kidneys with maintenance of blood flow to vital organs such as the brain and the heart itself; and (4) neurohumoral adjustments, which tend to maintain arterial pressure and are discussed on p. 997 and in Chap. 68.

The intrinsic contractile state of myocardium removed from failing animal hearts has been shown to be depressed soon after the imposition of a pressure overload. The laying down of more myofibrils often restores contractility to normal, but when the overload is maintained for prolonged periods, intrinsic myocardial contractility again declines. This state is often characterized by a relative reduction in the ratio of mitochondria to myofibrils.

In papillary muscles removed from the left ventricles of patients with heart failure the maximum degree of active tension which they can develop is reduced. Electron-microscopic analysis of failing cat papillary muscles fixed at the apexes of the length–active tension curves revealed sarcomere lengths averaging 2.2 μm. Thus, the abnormalities of contractility do *not* appear to be produced by an alteration in the overlap of filaments within the sarcomere.

The failing ventricle may still eject a normal or nearly normal stroke volume despite considerable depression of function, when its end-diastolic volume increases, i.e., through the operation of the Frank-Starling mechanism. As outlined above, an increase in the initial volume of the ventricle is associated with stretching of the sarcomere, a process that augments the number of sites at which the actin and myosin filaments can interact and/or which increases their sensitivity to Ca^{2+}. Furthermore, the development of ventricular hypertrophy may be considered to provide additional contractile units and thereby constitutes an important compensatory mechanism when the myocardium's intrinsic inotropic state is depressed.

CARDIAC METABOLISM IN HEART FAILURE There is no unifying theory providing a biochemical basis for heart failure. The common forms of low-output heart failure, secondary to coronary atherosclerosis, hypertension, cardiomyopathy, and certain valvular

FIGURE 194-7 Features of forward and backward failure. Note association of forward failure with hypotension and neurohumoral activation with consequent afterload increase. Note also the association of backward failure with pulmonary congestion. Backward failure is associated with abnormalities of left atrial emptying or LV relaxation. α, alpha adrenergic; β, beta adrenergic; aldo, aldosterone; LV, left ventricle; RV, right ventricle. *(From Opie LH: The Heart: Physiology and Metabolism, 2d ed, New York, Raven Press, 1991, p 411. Used with permission.)*

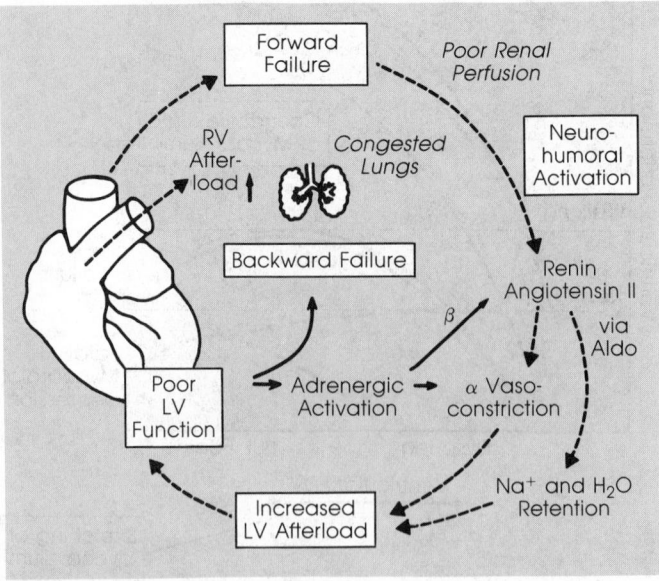

and congenital lesions, are characterized by an absolute or a relative reduction in the external work delivered by the heart, although myocardial oxygen consumption remains normal. Therefore, the external efficiency, i.e., the ratio of external work performed to energy consumed, is often depressed. When heart failure occurs in the absence of myocardial ischemia, there appears to be no abnormality of ATP generation or ATP use. When heart failure occurs in the presence of acute or chronic ischemia it can be attributed to reduced myocardial energy supplies.

Although some controversy concerning myocardial metabolism in heart failure persists, it now appears that severe impairment of myocardial performance may occur *without* disturbances of mitochondrial function or reduction of high-energy phosphate stores, although abnormalities in these processes have been shown to occur in some forms of experimental (and perhaps of clinical) heart failure.

Substantial evidence supports the view that in many forms of heart failure there is an *abnormality of excitation-contraction coupling,* which reduces the delivery of Ca^{2+} to the contractile sites, thereby impairing cardiac performance. However, the molecular basis of this abnormality, indeed the subcellular structures involved, i.e., the sarcolemma, T tubules, and/or sarcoplasmic reticulum, have yet to be defined. One attractive hypothesis involves reduced uptake of Ca^{2+} by the sarcoplasmic reticulum. This can impair myocardial relaxation and contribute to the development of diastolic heart failure. In addition, a reduction of Ca^{2+} in the sarcoplasmic reticulum can also lower Ca^{2+} released to the myofilaments during activation, thereby causing systolic heart failure.

NEUROHUMORAL ADJUSTMENTS   A reduction in cardiac performance evokes a series of neurohumoral adjustments which may be considered to be "two-edged swords" (Fig. 194-7). Although they are useful because they maintain arterial perfusion pressure in the face of a reduction of cardiac output, they increase the hemodynamic burden and oxygen requirements of the failing ventricle.

The renin-angiotensin-aldosterone system   When cardiac output declines, the renin-angiotensin-aldosterone system (Chap. 335) is activated. Concentrations of circulating angiotensin II and aldosterone are both increased, the former contributing to excess vasoconstriction and the latter to the retention of salt and water. Patients with chronic heart failure are usually improved by blocking this system with angiotensin-converting enzyme inhibitors and by aldosterone antagonists (Chap. 195).

The adrenergic nervous system   In patients with heart failure the levels of circulating norepinephrine may be markedly elevated, indicating that the activity of adrenergic neurons is augmented; the prognosis varies inversely with the concentration. This increased activity of the adrenergic neurons supports ventricular contractility in congestive heart failure. Heart failure is intensified when large doses of beta-adrenergic blocking agents are administered to such patients.

The density of adrenergic receptors and concentration of cardiac norepinephrine (NE) are both reduced in chronic, severe heart failure.

FIGURE 194-8 Schematic representation of influences on intramyocardial Ca^{2+} concentration and excitation-contraction coupling. The action potential is associated with intracellular entry of Na^+ and the extrusion of K^+ (not shown) and the entry of Ca^{2+} (shown). The Na^+-Ca^{2+} exchanger depends on concentration gradients and does not require ATP. Not shown is the energy-dependent sarcolemmal Ca^{2+} pump which extrudes Ca^{2+} from the cell. Isoproterenol and norepinephrine, the latter shown intraneuronally, stimulate the beta-adrenergic receptor in the outer sarcolemma. The beta receptor is coupled to G (guanine nucleotide–binding regulatory) proteins (GR), which in turn activate the catalytic adenylate cyclase (AC). The latter catalyzes the production of cyclic AMP from ATP. AC can be stimulated directly by the administration of forskolin, which bypasses both the beta receptor and the G proteins. Cyclic AMP activates protein kinase, which in turn enhances the phosphorylation of the Ca^{2+} channel, increasing transarcolemmal Ca^{2+} influx. Activated protein kinase also phosphorylates phospholamban, which in its phosphorylated form enhances the uptake of Ca^{2+} by the sarcoplasmic tubular network. Phosphodiesterase catalyzes the breakdown of cyclic AMP to AMP while milrinone, caffeine, and isobutylmethylxanthine inhibit phosphodiesterase, thereby augmenting cyclic AMP concentration. Digoxin inhibits the Na^+, K^+-ATPase in the sarcolemma, inhibiting Na^+ efflux from and K^+ influx into the cell. As a consequence the intracellular Na^+ concentration falls and Na^+-Ca^{2+} exchange is reduced, thereby raising intracellular Ca^{2+}. P represents phosphorylation. *(From Feldman AMD et al, by permission of the American Heart Association, Inc.)*

These changes are accompanied by a reduction in the activity of adenylate cyclase, which may lower the intracellular concentration of cyclic AMP. The latter in turn reduces the activation of protein kinase, the phosphorylation of Ca^{2+} channels, transarcolemmal Ca^{2+} entry, as well as the phosphorylation of phospholamban, a protein in the sarcoplasmic reticulum, thereby depressing the reuptake of Ca^{2+} by the latter (Fig. 194-8). Changes in the G (guanine regulatory) proteins, which couple the beta receptor to the catalytic adenylate cyclase (which is responsible for the production of cyclic AMP), may also occur in heart failure, with increased activity of the inhibitory subunit and/or reduced activity of the stimulatory subunit of the G proteins. The reduction of cardiac NE stores and the down-regulation of myocardial beta receptors in heart failure may be responsible for loss of the much-needed adrenergic support in the failing heart. On the other hand, the increased adrenergic stimulation and rise in circulating catecholamines may exert undesirable side effects by elevating vascular resistance and thereby presenting the heart with an afterload which is higher than optimal. It may also enhance the likelihood of ventricular arrhythmias. The survival of patients with congestive heart failure varies inversely with the concentration of circulating NE.

In the final analysis, in heart failure, the fundamental abnormality resides in depressions of the myocardial force-velocity relationship and of the length–active tension curve, reflecting reductions in the contractile state of the myocardium (Fig. 194-5, curves 1 to 3). In many instances, cardiac output and external ventricular performance at rest are within normal limits but are maintained at these levels only by an increased end-diastolic fiber length and an elevated ventricular end-diastolic volume, i.e., through the operation of the Frank-Starling mechanism (Fig. 194-5, points A to D). The elevation of left ventricular preload is associated with similar changes in the pulmonary capillary pressure, contributing to the dyspnea experienced by patients with heart failure. The normal improvement of contractility due to augmented adrenergic activity during exercise is attenuated or even prevented by NE depletion which occurs in severe heart failure (Fig. 194-5, curves 3 and 3'). The factors which tend to augment ventricular filling during exercise in the normal subject push the failing myocardium along its flattened length–active tension curve, and although the left ventricle may perform somewhat better, this occurs only as a consequence of an inordinate elevation of ventricular end-diastolic volume and pressure and, therefore, of the pulmonary capillary pressure. The elevation of the latter intensifies dyspnea and therefore plays an important role in limiting the intensity of exercise which the patient can perform. Left ventricular failure becomes fatal when the myocardial length–active tension curve is depressed (Fig. 194-5, curve 4) to the point at which cardiac performance fails to satisfy the requirements of the peripheral tissues even at rest, and/or the left ventricular end-diastolic and pulmonary capillary pressures are elevated to levels which result in pulmonary edema (Fig. 194-5, point E).

REFERENCES

BRAUNWALD E et al (eds): *Congestive Heart Failure: Current Research and Clinical Applications.* New York, Grune & Stratton, 1982

——— et al (eds): Contraction of the normal heart, in *Heart Disease,* 4th ed, E Braunwald (ed). Philadelphia, Saunders, 1992, pp 370–382

BRISTOW MR et al: Myocardial α and β-adrenergic receptors in heart failure: Is cardiac-derived norepinephrine the regulatory signal? Eur Heart J 9(Suppl H):35, 1988

COHN JN et al: Plasma norepinephrine as a guide to prognosis in patients with chronic congestive heart failure. N Engl J Med 311:819, 1984

EDES I et al: Sarcoplasmic reticulum function in normal heart and in cardiac disease. Heart Failure 6:221, 1991

GIBBONS WR, ZYGMUNT AC: Excitation-contraction coupling in the heart, in *The Heart and Cardiovascular System,* 2d ed, HA Fozzard et al (eds). New York, Raven, 1991, pp 1249–1352

GUTH BD et al: Time course and mechanisms of contractile dysfunction during acute myocardial ischemia. Circulation 87:IV35–42, 1993

HOLT W et al: Mechanism for depressed cardiac function in left ventricular volume overload. Am Heart J 121:531, 1991

KATZ AM: Cardiomyopathy of overload: A major determinant of prognosis in congestive heart failure. N Engl J Med 322:100, 1990

———: Heart failure, in *Physiology of the Heart,* 2d ed. New York, Raven, 1992, pp 638–668

OM A, HESS ML: Inotropic therapy of the failing myocardium. Clin Cardiol 16:5, 1993

SMITH V-E, ZILE MR: Relaxation and diastolic properties of the heart, in *The Heart and Cardiovascular System,* 2d ed, HA Fozzard et al (eds). New York, Raven, 1991, pp 1353–1368

195　HEART FAILURE

EUGENE BRAUNWALD

While a number of definitions of heart failure are commonly employed, here we consider heart failure to be the pathophysiologic state in which an abnormality of *cardiac* function is responsible for the failure of the heart to pump blood at a rate commensurate with the requirements of the metabolizing tissues *and/or* its ability to do so requires an abnormally elevated filling pressure. Heart failure is frequently, but not always, caused by a defect in myocardial contraction, and then the term *myocardial failure* is appropriate. The latter may result from a primary abnormality in heart muscle, as occurs in the cardiomyopathies (Chap. 205). Myocardial failure also may result from extramyocardial abnormalities, such as coronary atherosclerosis which leads to myocardial ischemia and infarction, as well as from abnormalities of the heart valves in which the heart muscle is damaged by the long-standing excessive hemodynamic burden imposed by the valvular abnormality, and/or by the rheumatic process (Chap. 200). In patients with chronic constrictive pericarditis, myocardial damage resulting from infiltration of the heart muscle by pericardial inflammation and calcification is common (Chap. 206).

In other patients with heart failure, however, a similar clinical syndrome is present, but without any detectable abnormality of *myocardial* function. In some of these patients the normal heart is suddenly presented with a load that exceeds its capacity, such as an acute hypertensive crisis, rupture of an aortic valve cusp, or massive pulmonary embolism. Heart failure, in the presence of normal myocardial function, also occurs in chronic conditions in which there is impairment of filling of the ventricles due to tricuspid and/or mitral stenosis, constrictive pericarditis without myocardial involvement, endocardial fibrosis, and some forms of hypertrophic cardiomyopathy.

Heart failure should be distinguished from (1) conditions in which there is circulatory congestion consequent to abnormal salt and water retention but in which there is no disturbance of cardiac function per se (the latter syndrome, termed the *congested state,* may result from the abnormal salt and water retention of renal failure or from excess parenteral administration of fluids and electrolytes) and (2) noncardiac causes of inadequate cardiac output, including shock due to hypovolemia and redistribution of blood volume (Chap. 34).

The ventricles respond to a chronically increased hemodynamic burden with the development of hypertrophy. With volume overload when the ventricle is called on to deliver an elevated cardiac output for prolonged periods, as in valvular regurgitation, it develops *eccentric* hypertrophy, i.e., cavity dilatation, with an increase in muscle mass so that the ratio between wall thickness and ventricular cavity size remains relatively constant. With chronic pressure overload, as in valvular aortic stenosis or untreated hypertension, it develops *concentric* hypertrophy, in which the ratio between wall thickness and ventricular cavity size increases. In both conditions, a stable hyperfunctioning state may exist for many years, but myocardial function may ultimately deteriorate, leading to heart failure.

CAUSES OF HEART FAILURE

In evaluating patients with heart failure, it is important to identify not only the *underlying cause* of the heart disease but also the *precipitating cause* of heart failure. The cardiac abnormality produced by a congenital or acquired lesion such as valvular aortic stenosis may exist for many years and produce no clinical disability. Frequently, however, clinical manifestations of heart failure appear for the first time in the course of some acute disturbance which places an additional load on a myocardium that chronically is excessively burdened. The heart may be compensated but have no additional reserve, and a precipitating cause results in further deterioration of cardiac function. Identification of such precipitating causes is of critical importance because their prompt alleviation may be lifesaving. However, in the absence of underlying heart disease, these acute disturbances do not usually, by themselves, lead to heart failure.

PRECIPITATING CAUSES

1 *Pulmonary embolism.* Physically inactive patients with low cardiac output are at increased risk of developing thrombi in the veins of the lower extremities or the pelvis. Pulmonary emboli may result in further elevation of pulmonary arterial pressure, which in turn may produce or intensify ventricular failure. In the presence of pulmonary vascular congestion, such emboli also may cause pulmonary infarction (Chap. 226).

2 *Infection.* Patients with pulmonary vascular congestion are also more susceptible to pulmonary infections; any infection may precipitate heart failure. The resulting fever, tachycardia, and hypoxemia and the increased metabolic demands may place a further burden on the overloaded, but compensated myocardium of a patient with chronic heart disease.

3 *Anemia.* The oxygen needs of the metabolizing tissues can be met only by an increase in the cardiac output in the presence of anemia (Chap. 56); though such an increase in cardiac output can be sustained by a normal heart, a diseased, overloaded, but otherwise compensated heart may be unable to augment sufficiently the volume of blood which it delivers to the periphery. In this manner, the combination of anemia and previously compensated heart disease can lead to inadequate oxygen delivery to the periphery and precipitate heart failure.

4 *Thyrotoxicosis and pregnancy.* As in anemia and fever, in thyrotoxicosis and pregnancy, adequate tissue perfusion requires an increased cardiac output. The development or intensification of heart failure may actually be one of the first clinical manifestations of hyperthyroidism in a patient with underlying heart disease which was previously compensated (Chap. 334). Similarly, heart failure not infrequently occurs for the first time during pregnancy in women with rheumatic valvular disease, in whom cardiac compensation may return following delivery.

5 *Arrhythmias.* In patients with compensated heart disease, arrhythmias are among the most frequent precipitating causes of heart failure. They exert a deleterious effect for a variety of reasons: (*a*) Tachyarrhythmias reduce the time period available for ventricular filling. In patients with ischemic heart disease, tachyarrhythmias also may cause ischemic myocardial dysfunction. (*b*) The dissociation between atrial and ventricular contractions characteristic of many arrhythmias results in the loss of the atrial booster pump mechanism, thereby raising atrial pressures. (*c*) In any arrhythmia associated with abnormal intraventricular conduction, myocardial performance may become further impaired because of the loss of normal synchronicity of ventricular contraction. (*d*) Marked bradycardia associated with complete atrioventricular block or other severe bradyarrhythmias will reduce cardiac output unless stroke volume rises reciprocally; this compensatory response cannot occur with serious myocardial dysfunction even in the absence of heart failure.

6 *Rheumatic and other forms of myocarditis.* Acute rheumatic fever and a variety of other inflammatory or infectious processes affecting the myocardium may impair myocardial function in patients with or without preexisting heart disease (Chaps. 200 and 205).

7 *Infective endocarditis.* The additional valvular damage, anemia, fever, and myocarditis which often occur as a consequence of

infective endocarditis may, singly or in concert, precipitate heart failure (Chap. 85).

8 *Physical, dietary, fluid, environmental, and emotional excesses.* The augmentation of sodium intake, the inappropriate discontinuation of medications to treat heart failure, blood transfusions, physical overexertion, excessive environmental heat or humidity, and emotional crises all may precipitate heart failure in patients with heart disease who were previously compensated.

9 *Systemic hypertension.* Rapid elevation of arterial pressure, as may occur in some instances of hypertension of renal origin or upon discontinuation of antihypertensive medication, may result in cardiac decompensation (Chap. 209).

10 *Myocardial infarction.* In patients with chronic but compensated ischemic heart disease, a fresh infarct, sometimes otherwise silent clinically, may further impair ventricular function and precipitate heart failure (Chap. 202).

A systematic search for these precipitating causes should be made in every patient with the new development or recent intensification of heart failure, particularly if it is refractory to the usual methods of therapy. If properly recognized, the precipitating cause of heart failure usually can be treated more effectively than the underlying cause. Therefore, the prognosis in patients with heart failure in whom a precipitating cause can be identified, treated, and eliminated is more favorable than in patients in whom the underlying disease process has advanced to the point of producing heart failure.

FORMS OF HEART FAILURE

Heart failure may be described as *high-output* or *low-output*, *acute* or *chronic*, *right-sided* or *left-sided*, *forward* or *backward*, and *systolic* or *diastolic*. These descriptors are often useful in a clinical setting, particularly early in the patient's course, but late in the course of chronic heart failure the differences between them often become blurred.

HIGH-OUTPUT VERSUS LOW-OUTPUT HEART FAILURE It is useful to classify patients with heart failure into those with a low cardiac output, i.e., *low-output heart failure*, and those with an elevated cardiac output, i.e., *high-output heart failure*. The former occurs secondary to ischemic heart disease, hypertension, dilated cardiomyopathy, valvular and pericardial disease, but the latter is seen in patients with heart failure and hyperthyroidism, anemia, pregnancy, arteriovenous fistulas, beriberi, and Paget's disease. In clinical practice, however, low-output and high-output heart failure cannot always be readily distinguished. The normal range of cardiac output is wide [2.5 to 3.8 (L/min)/m^2], and in many patients with so-called low-output heart failure the cardiac output may actually be just within the normal range at rest (although it is lower than it had been previously), but it fails to rise normally during exertion. On the other hand, in patients with so-called high-output heart failure the output may not exceed the upper limits of normal (although it would have been elevated had it been measured before heart failure supervened), but rather it may be close to the upper limit of normal. Regardless of the *absolute* level of the cardiac output, however, cardiac failure may be said to be present when the characteristic clinical manifestations described below are accompanied by a depression of the curve relating ventricular end-diastolic volume to cardiac performance (see Fig. 194-5, p. 995).

An integral physiologic component of *systolic* heart failure (p. 995) is the finding that the heart does not deliver the quantity of oxygen required by the metabolizing tissues. In the absence of peripheral shunting of blood, such inadequate delivery of oxygen to the metabolizing tissues is reflected in an abnormal widening of the normal arterial–mixed venous oxygen difference (35 to 50 mL/L in the basal state). In mild cases, such an abnormality may not be present at rest but becomes evident only during exertion or other hypermetabolic states. In patients with high cardiac output states, such as those associated with arteriovenous fistula, beriberi, thyrotoxicosis, deliver oxygen to the exercising muscle. Anorexia and nausea associated with abdominal pain and fullness are frequent complaints which may be related to the congested liver and portal venous system.

Cerebral symptoms   In severe heart failure, particularly in elderly patients with accompanying cerebral arteriosclerosis, reduced cerebral perfusion, and arterial hypoxemia, there may be alterations in the mental state characterized by confusion, difficulty in concentration, impairment of memory, headache, insomnia, and anxiety. *Nocturia* is common in heart failure and may contribute to insomnia.

PHYSICAL FINDINGS (See Chap. 188)   In moderate heart failure, the patient appears to be in no distress at rest except that he or she may be uncomfortable when lying flat for more than a few minutes. In more severe heart failure, the pulse pressure may be diminished, reflecting a reduction in stroke volume, and occasionally, the diastolic arterial pressure is elevated as a consequence of generalized vasoconstriction. In acute heart failure, hypotension may be prominent. There may be cyanosis of the lips and nail beds and sinus tachycardia, and the patient may insist on sitting upright. *Systemic venous pressure* is often abnormally elevated in heart failure and may be recognized by observing the extent of distention of the jugular veins. In the early stages of heart failure, the venous pressure may be normal at rest but may become abnormally elevated during and immediately after exertion as well as with sustained pressure on the abdomen (positive abdominojugular reflux).

Third and fourth heart sounds are often audible but are not specific for heart failure, and *pulsus alternans*, i.e., a regular rhythm in which there is alternation of strong and weak cardiac contractions and therefore alternation in the strength of the peripheral pulses, may be present. Pulsus alternans may be detected by sphygmomanometry and in more severe instances by palpation; it frequently follows an extrasystole and is observed most commonly in patients with cardiomyopathy or hypertensive or ischemic heart disease. It is a sign of severe heart failure and is caused by a reduction in the number of contractile units during weak contractions and/or by alternation in the ventricular end-diastolic volume.

Pulmonary rales   Moist, inspiratory, crepitant rales and dullness to percussion over the lung bases are common in patients with heart failure and elevated pulmonary venous and capillary pressures. In patients with pulmonary edema, rales may be heard widely over both lung fields; they are frequently coarse and sibilant and may be accompanied by expiratory wheezing. Rales may, however, be caused by many conditions other than left ventricular failure. Some patients with long-standing heart failure have no rales because of increased lymphatic drainage of alveolar fluid.

Cardiac edema   Cardiac edema is usually dependent, occurring in the legs symmetrically, particularly in the pretibial region and ankles in ambulatory patients, in whom it is most prominent in the evening, and in the sacral region of individuals at bed rest. Pitting edema of the arms and face occurs rarely and then only late in the course of heart failure.

Hydrothorax and ascites   Pleural effusion in congestive heart failure results from the elevation of pleural capillary pressure and transudation of fluid into the pleural cavities. Since the pleural veins drain into *both* the systemic and pulmonary veins, hydrothorax occurs most commonly with marked elevation of pressure in both venous systems but also may be seen with marked elevation of pressure in either venous bed. It is more frequent in the right pleural cavity than in the left. *Ascites* also occurs as a consequence of transudation and results from increased pressure in the hepatic veins and the veins draining the peritoneum (Chap. 43). Marked ascites occurs most frequently in patients with tricuspid valve disease and constrictive pericarditis.

Congestive hepatomegaly   An enlarged, tender, pulsating liver also accompanies systemic venous hypertension and is observed not only in the same conditions in which ascites occurs but also in milder forms of heart failure from any cause. With prolonged, severe hepatomegaly, as in patients with tricuspid valve disease or chronic constrictive pericarditis, enlargement of the spleen, i.e., congestive splenomegaly, also may occur.

Jaundice   This is a late finding in congestive heart failure and is associated with elevations of both the direct- and indirect-reacting bilirubin; it results from impairment of hepatic function secondary to hepatic congestion and the hepatocellular hypoxia associated with central lobular atrophy. Serum transaminase concentrations are frequently elevated. If hepatic congestion occurs acutely, the jaundice may be severe and the enzymes strikingly elevated.

Cardiac cachexia   With severe chronic heart failure there may be serious weight loss and cachexia because of (1) elevation of circulating concentrations of tumor necrosis factor, (2) elevation of the metabolic rate, which results in part from the extra work performed by the respiratory muscles, the increased oxygen needs of the hypertrophied heart, and/or the discomfort associated with severe heart failure, (3) anorexia, nausea, and vomiting due to central causes, to digitalis intoxication, or to congestive hepatomegaly and abdominal fullness, (4) impairment of intestinal absorption due to congestion of the intestinal veins, and (5) rarely, in patients with particularly severe failure of the right side of the heart, a protein-losing enteropathy.

Other manifestations   With reduction of blood flow, the extremities may be cold, pale, and diaphoretic. Urine flow is depressed, and the urine contains albumin and has a high specific gravity and a low concentration of sodium. In addition, prerenal azotemia may be present. In patients with long-standing severe heart failure, impotence and depression are common.

ROENTGENOGRAPHIC FINDINGS   In addition to the enlargement of the particular chambers characteristic of the lesion responsible for heart failure, distention of pulmonary veins and redistribution to the apices is common in patients with heart failure and elevated pulmonary vascular pressures (Chap. 190). Also, pleural effusions may be evident and associated with interlobar effusions.

DIFFERENTIAL DIAGNOSIS   The diagnosis of congestive heart failure may be established by observing some combination of the clinical manifestations of heart failure described above, together with the findings characteristic of one of the etiologic forms of heart disease. Since chronic heart failure is often associated with cardiac enlargement, the diagnosis should be questioned, but is by no means excluded, when all chambers are normal in size. Two-dimensional echocardiography is particularly useful in assessing the dimensions of each cardiac chamber. Heart failure may be difficult to distinguish from pulmonary disease, and the differential diagnosis is discussed in Chap. 31. Pulmonary embolism also presents many of the manifestations of heart failure, but hemoptysis, pleuritic chest pain, a right ventricular lift, and the characteristic mismatch between ventilation and perfusion on lung scan should point to this diagnosis (see Chap. 226).

Ankle edema may be due to varicose veins, cyclic edema, or gravitational effects (Chap. 33), but in these patients there is no jugular venous hypertension at rest or with pressure over the abdomen. Edema secondary to renal disease can usually be recognized by appropriate renal function tests and urinalysis and is rarely associated with elevation of venous pressure. Enlargement of the liver and ascites occur in patients with hepatic cirrhosis and also may be distinguished from heart failure by normal jugular venous pressure and absence of a positive abdominojugular reflux.

TREATMENT OF HEART FAILURE

The treatment of heart failure may be divided logically into three components: (1) removal of the precipitating cause, (2) correction of the underlying cause, and (3) control of the congestive heart failure state. The first two are discussed in other chapters together with each specific disease entity or complication. An example is the treatment of pneumococcal pneumonia and acute heart failure (removal of the precipitating cause) followed by mitral valvotomy (correction of the underlying cause) in a patient with mitral stenosis. In many instances, surgical treatment will correct or at least alleviate the underlying cause. The third component of the treatment of heart failure, i.e., control of the congestive heart failure state, may, in turn, be divided into three categories: (1) reduction of cardiac work load, including both the preload and the afterload, (2) control of excessive retention of salt and water, and (3) enhancement of myocardial contractility. The vigor with which each of these measures is pursued in any individual patient should depend on the severity of heart failure. Following effective treatment, recurrence of the clinical manifestations of heart failure can often be prevented by continuing those measures which were originally effective.

While a simple rule for the treatment of all patients with heart failure cannot be formulated because of the varied etiologies, hemodynamic features, clinical manifestations, and severity of heart failure, insofar as the treatment of chronic congestive failure is concerned, simple measures such as moderate restriction of activity and sodium intake should be tried first. If these are insufficient, therapy with a combination of a diuretic; a vasodilator, preferably an angiotensin-converting enzyme inhibitor; and usually a digitalis glycoside is then begun. The next step is more rigorous restriction of salt intake and higher doses of loop diuretics, sometimes accompanied by other diuretics. If heart failure persists, hospitalization with rigid salt restriction, bed rest, intravenous vasodilators, and positive inotropic agents comes next. In some patients, the order in which these measures are applied may be altered.

REDUCTION OF CARDIAC WORK LOAD   This consists of reducing physical activity, instituting emotional rest, and reducing afterload. Modest restriction of physical activity in mild cases and rest in bed or in a chair in severe failure remain cornerstones in the treatment of heart failure. Meals should be small in quantity but perhaps more frequent, and every effort should be made to diminish the patient's anxiety; sometimes drugs such as diazepam (2–5 mg tid) for several days are useful. Physical and emotional rest tends to lower arterial pressure and reduce the load on the myocardium by diminishing the requirements for cardiac output. These influences act in concert to diminish the need for redistribution of the cardiac output, and in many patients, particularly those with mild heart failure, simple bed rest and mild sedation often result in an effective diuresis.

Rest at home or in the hospital should be maintained for 1 to 2 weeks in patients with overt congestive failure and should be continued for several days after the patient's condition has stabilized. The hazards of phlebothrombosis and pulmonary embolism which occur with bed rest may be reduced with anticoagulants, leg exercises, and elastic stockings. *Absolute* bed rest rarely is required or advisable and the patient should be encouraged to sit in a chair and be given toilet privileges unless heart failure is extreme. Heavy sedation should be avoided, but small doses of tranquilizers may be helpful in calming the emotionally disturbed patient during the first few days of therapy and in permitting much-needed sleep. In patients with chronic, moderately severe heart failure, additional periods of bed rest on weekends will frequently allow continuation of gainful employment. Following recovery from heart failure, the patient's activities must be carefully assessed, and often, professional, community, and/or family responsibilities must be curtailed. Intermittent rest during the day (e.g., a scheduled 1-h nap or rest following lunch) and the avoidance of strenuous exertion are often helpful once compensation has been restored. Weight reduction by restriction of caloric intake in obese patients with heart failure also diminishes cardiac work load and is an essential component of the therapeutic program. Vasodilator therapy (p. 1004) may be considered a form of reduction of the cardiac work load. This form of therapy has been shown not only to ameliorate heart failure but also to retard its development in patients with left ventricular dysfunction.

CONTROL OF EXCESSIVE FLUID   Many of the clinical manifestations of heart failure result from hypervolemia and expansion of the interstitial fluid volume. By the time fluid retention due to heart failure becomes clinically evident, most commonly as edema, considerable expansion of the extracellular space has already occurred, and heart failure usually is already advanced. Exertional dypsnea and orthopnea may be caused by displacement of fluid from the systemic to the pulmonary vascular bed. Treatment aimed at reducing extracellular fluid volume is dependent primarily on lowering total-body sodium stores, while fluid restriction is of less importance. A negative sodium balance can be achieved by reducing the dietary intake and increasing the urinary excretion of this ion with the aid of diuretics. In severe heart failure, mechanical removal of extracellular fluid by means of thoracentesis, paracentesis, and rarely hemodialysis or peritoneal dialysis also may be employed.

Diet   In patients with mild heart failure, considerable improvement in symptoms may result simply from reducing the sodium intake, particularly if accompanied by periods of physical rest. In patients with more severe heart failure, the sodium intake must be controlled more rigidly, and other measures, such as diuretics, vasodilators, and glycosides, are used. Even following recovery from a bout of heart failure, if the underlying cause has not been corrected, at least moderate sodium restriction should be maintained. The normal diet contains approximately 6 to 10 g sodium chloride; this intake can be reduced by half simply by excluding salt-rich foods and salt which is added at the table. Reduction of the ordinary dietary intake to approximately one-fourth of normal may be achieved if, in addition, all salt is omitted from cooking. In patients with severe heart failure, in whom the daily sodium chloride intake should be reduced to between 500 and 1000 mg, milk, cheese, bread, cereals, canned vegetables and soups, some salted cuts of meat, and some fresh vegetables, including spinach, celery, and beets, must be eliminated. A variety of fresh fruit, green vegetables, specially processed breads and milk, and salt substitutes are permissible, but it is difficult to keep such diets palatable over the long term. Water intake may be ad libitum in all but the most severe forms of congestive heart failure. Late in the course of heart failure, dilutional hyponatremia may develop in patients who are unable to excrete a water load, sometimes because of excessive secretion of antidiuretic hormone. In such cases, water intake as well as sodium intake must be restricted.

Attention also must be directed to the caloric content of the diet. Calories should be restricted in obese patients with heart failure. On the other hand, in patients with severe heart failure and cardiac cachexia, an attempt must be made to maintain nutritional intake and to avoid caloric and vitamin deficiencies; nutritional supplements may be in order.

Diuretics   A variety of diuretic agents is available, and in patients with mild heart failure, almost all are effective. However, in the more severe forms of heart failure, the selection of diuretics is more difficult, and any existing abnormalities in serum electrolytes must be taken into account. Overtreatment must be avoided, since the resultant hypovolemia may reduce cardiac output, interfere with renal function, and produce profound weakness and lethargy.

THIAZIDE DIURETICS   These agents are used widely in clinical practice because of their effectiveness when administered orally. In patients with chronic heart failure of mild or moderate severity, the continued administration of a thiazide diuretic abolishes or diminishes the need for rigid dietary sodium restriction, although salty foods and table salt still should be avoided. Thiazides are well absorbed following oral administration; chlorothiazide and hydrochlorothiazide reach their peak action in 4 h, and diuresis persists for approximately 12 h. Thiazide diuretics reduce the reabsorption of sodium and chloride in the first half of the distal convoluted tubule and a portion of the cortical ascending limb of the loop of Henle, and water follows the unreabsorbed salt. Thiazides fail to increase free water clearance, and in some instances reduce it, supporting the hypothesis that these drugs inhibit selective reabsorption of sodium chloride in the distal cortical diluting segment, at a site where the urine is normally diluted (Chap. 235). This may result in the excretion of a hypertonic urine and may contribute to dilutional hyponatremia. As a consequence of increased delivery of sodium to the distal nephron, sodium-potassium ion exchange is enhanced, and kaliuresis results. In contrast to the loop diuretics which enhance calcium excretion, the thiazides have the opposite effect. These drugs are effective and useful in the treatment of heart failure as long as the glomerular filtration rate exceeds approximately 50 percent of normal.

Chlorothiazide is administered in doses of up to 500 mg every 6 h. Many derivatives of this compound are available but differ principally in dosage and duration of action and therefore offer few, if any, significant advantages over the parent compound, except for chlorthalidone, which may be administered once daily. Potassium depletion and metabolic alkalosis (the latter due to increased H^+ secretion as a substitute for the depleted intracellular stores of potassium and increased proximal tubular reabsorption of filtered HCO_3^- when there is relative depletion of the extracellular fluid volume) are the chief adverse metabolic effects following prolonged administration of the thiazides, of metolazone, and of the loop diuretics. Hypokalemia may enhance seriously the dangers of digitalis intoxication, induce fatigue and lethargy, and may be prevented by the oral supplementation of potassium chloride. However, the solution is not palatable and may be hazardous in patients with renal failure. Therefore, to prevent potassium depletion in patients receiving thiazide diuretics, intermittent dosage schedules, e.g., omitting the diuretic every third day, and the addition of a potassium-retaining diuretic, such as a spironolactone or triamterene, may be preferable. Other side effects of thiazides include reduction of the excretion of uric acid, which may lead to hyperuricemia, and a hyperglycemic effect, which rarely may precipitate hyperosmolar coma in the poorly regulated diabetic. Skin rashes, thrombocytopenia, and granulocytopenia also have been reported.

METOLAZONE   This quinethazone derivative has a site of action and potency similar to those of the thiazides but has been reported to be effective in the presence of moderate renal failure. The usual dose is 5 to 10 mg/d.

FUROSEMIDE, BUMETANIDE, AND ETHACRYNIC ACID   These ''loop'' diuretics are similar physiologically but differ chemically. These extremely powerful diuretics reversibly inhibit the reabsorption of sodium, potassium, and chloride in the thick ascending limb of Henle's loop, apparently by blocking a cotransport system in the luminal membrane. They may induce renal cortical vasodilatation and can produce rates of urine formation which may be as high as one-fourth of the glomerular filtration rate. While other diuretics lose their effectiveness as blood volume is restored to normal levels, the loop diuretics remain effective despite the elimination of excessive extracellular fluid volume. The major side effects of these agents are due to this marked diuretic potency, which on rare occasions may result in contraction of the plasma volume, circulatory collapse, reductions in the renal blood flow and glomerular filtration rate, and the development of prerenal azotemia. Metabolic alkalosis is produced by a large increase in the urinary excretion of chloride, hydrogen, and potassium ions. Hypokalemia (see discussion of thiazides, above) and hyponatremia may occur, and hyperuricemia and hyperglycemia are observed occasionally, as with thiazide diuretics. The reabsorption of free water is decreased.

All three drugs are readily absorbed orally and are excreted in the bile and urine. They are usually effective by mouth and intravenously. Weakness, nausea, and dizziness may complicate the administration of all loop diuretics; ethacrynic acid has been associated with transient or even permanent deafness as well as with skin rash and granulocytopenia.

These extremely effective diuretics are useful in all forms of heart failure, particularly in otherwise refractory heart failure and pulmonary edema. They have been shown to be effective in patients with hypoalbuminemia, hyponatremia, hypochloremia, hypokalemia, and reductions in the glomerular filtration rate and to produce a diuresis in patients in whom thiazide diuretics and aldosterone antagonists, alone and in combination, are ineffective.

In patients with refractory heart failure, the action of furosemide, bumetanide, and ethacrynic acid may be potentiated by intravenous administration and the addition of all other diuretics, i.e., thiazides, carbonic anhydrase inhibitors, osmotic diuretics, and the potassium-sparing diuretics—spironolactone, triamterene, and amiloride. These latter agents act on the cortical collecting ducts, are relatively weak, and therefore are rarely indicated as sole agents. However, their potassium-sparing properties make them particularly useful in conjunction with the more potent kaliuretic agents, the loop diuretics and thiazides. The potassium-sparing agents fall into two classes, as noted below.

ALDOSTERONE ANTAGONISTS   The 17-spironolactones resemble aldosterone structurally and act on the distal half of the convoluted tubule and the cortical portion of the collecting duct by competitive inhibition of aldosterone, thereby blocking the exchange between sodium and both potassium and hydrogen in the distal tubules and collecting ducts. These agents produce a sodium diuresis, and in contrast to the thiazides, ethacrynic acid, and furosemide, they result in potassium retention. Although secondary hyperaldosteronism exists in some patients with congestive heart failure, the spironolactones are effective even in patients in whom the serum aldosterone concentration is within normal limits. Aldactone A may be administered in doses of 25 to 100 mg three to four times daily by mouth. The maximal effect of this regimen is not observed for approximately 4 days. Spironolactones are most effective when administered in combination with thiazide and/or loop diuretics. The opposing action of these drugs on urine and serum potassium makes possible a sodium diuresis without either hyper- or hypokalemia when spironolactone and one of these other agents are administered in combination. Also, since spironolactone, triamterene, and amiloride act on the distal tubule, they are particularly effective when used in combination with one of these other diuretics which acts more proximally.

Spironolactone, triamterene, and amiloride should not be administered alone to patients with hyperkalemia, renal failure, or hyponatremia. Reported complications include nausea, epigastric distress, mental confusion, drowsiness, gynecomastia, and erythematous eruptions.

TRIAMTERENE AND AMILORIDE   These two drugs exert renal effects similar to those of the spironolactones; i.e., they block sodium reabsorption and secondarily inhibit potassium secretion in the distal tubules. However, their fundamental mechanism of action differs from that of the spironolactones, since they are active in adrenalectomized animals and their action does not depend on the presence of aldosterone. The effective dose of triamterene is 100 mg once or twice daily, and that of amiloride is 5 mg daily. Side effects include nausea, vomiting, diarrhea, headache, granulocytopenia, eosinophilia, and skin rash. Both triamterene and the chemically unrelated diuretic amiloride resemble Aldactone A in that their diuretic potency is not great, but they are effective in preventing the hypokalemia characteristic of the administration of thiazides, furosemide, and ethacrynic acid. A number of diuretic preparations contain a combination of a thiazide and either triamterene or amiloride in a single capsule. They may be useful in patients who develop hypokalemia with a thiazide but should not be used in patients with impaired renal function and/or hyperkalemia.

CHOICE OF DIURETICS   Orally administered thiazides and metolazone are the agents of choice in the treatment of chronic cardiac edema of mild to moderate degree in patients without hyperglycemia, hyperuricemia, or hypokalemia. Spironolactones, triamterene, and amiloride are not potent diuretics when used alone, but they potentiate other diuretics, particularly the thiazide and loop diuretics. However, in patients with heart failure and severe secondary hyperaldosteronism, spironolactone may be quite effective. Ethacrynic acid, bumetanide, and furosemide, given alone or with spironolactone or triamterene, are the agents of choice in patients with severe heart failure refractory to other diuretics. In very severe heart failure, the combination of a thiazide, a loop diuretic, and a potassium-sparing diuretic is required.

VASODILATOR THERAPY   In many patients with heart failure, left ventricular afterload is increased as a consequence of the several neural and humoral influences which act to constrict the peripheral vascular bed. These include the previously mentioned increased activity of the adrenergic nervous system, elevation of circulating catecholamines, and activation of the renin-angiotensin system, and perhaps increased circulating antidiuretic hormone. In addition to the vasoconstriction, the ventricular end-diastolic volume rises in heart failure. As a consequence of the operation of Laplace's law, which relates myocardial wall tension to the product of intraventricular pressure and radius (both of which may become elevated in heart failure), the aortic impedance, i.e., the force which opposes left ventricular ejection, or the ventricular afterload, rises. Vasoconstriction is generally considered to be a useful compensatory mechanism that allows blood flow to vital organs to persist in the presence of hypovolemia and many forms of shock associated with reduction of the total cardiac output (Chap. 34). However, in the presence of severely impaired cardiac function, the increase in afterload may reduce cardiac output further.

As shown in Fig. 194-4, afterload is a major determinant of cardiac function. When cardiac function is normal, a moderate elevation in afterload does not reduce stroke volume significantly, because the resultant increase in left ventricular end-diastolic volume, i.e., preload, can be tolerated easily. However, when myocardial function is impaired, such an increase in preload evoked by an elevation of afterload may raise ventricular end-diastolic and pulmonary capillary pressures to levels that may produce severe pulmonary congestion or even pulmonary edema. In many patients with heart failure, the ventricle is already operating at the peak, flat portion of its Frank-Starling curve (Fig. 194-5), and any additional increase in aortic impedance (afterload) will reduce stroke volume (p. 994). Conversely, a modest reduction of afterload will not have a significant effect on stroke volume in normal subjects, but in patients with heart failure it will tend to restore hemodynamics to normal by elevating the stroke volume of the failing ventricle and may reduce the elevated ventricular filling pressure.

The pharmacologic reduction of impedance to left ventricular ejection with vasodilator drugs represents an important adjunct in the management of heart failure. This approach may be particularly helpful but is by no means limited to patients with acute heart failure due to myocardial infarction (Chap. 202), valvular regurgitation (Chap. 201), elevated systemic vascular resistance and/or arterial pressure, and marked cardiac dilatation. The reduction of afterload by means of a variety of vasodilators reduces left ventricular end-diastolic pressure, volume, and oxygen consumption while raising stroke volume and cardiac output and causing only modest reduction in aortic pressure. Vasodilators should, of course, not be used in patients with hypotension.

In patients with both acute and chronic heart failure secondary to ischemic heart disease, cardiomyopathy, or valvular regurgitation who are treated with vasodilators, cardiac output increases, the pulmonary wedge pressure falls, the signs and symptoms of heart failure are relieved, and a new steady state is achieved in which cardiac output is higher and afterload lower with no or only mild reduction of arterial pressure (Fig. 195-1). Furthermore, the reduction of an elevated left end-diastolic pressure may improve subendocardial perfusion.

Vasodilator therapy is useful in the treatment of all forms of heart failure, ranging from the mild-chronic to the severe-acute forms.

The several available vasodilators vary in their hemodynamic effects, locus and duration of action, and mode of administration. Some vasodilators, such as hydralazine, minoxidil, and the alpha-adrenergic blocking agents, such as prazosin, act predominantly on the arterial bed and primarily increase stroke volume; others, such as nitroglycerin and isosorbide dinitrate, act almost entirely on the venous side of the circulation. The latter agents cause pooling of blood in the venous bed and act primarily to reduce ventricular filling pressures. Angiotensin-converting enzyme inhibitors, prazosin, and sodium nitroprusside are "balanced vasodilators" i.e., they act on both the arterial and venous beds. Some agents, such as sodium nitroprusside, must be administered by continuous intravenous infusion; nitroglycerin requires administration in ointment patch or intravenous forms when a prolonged effect is desired; and isosorbide

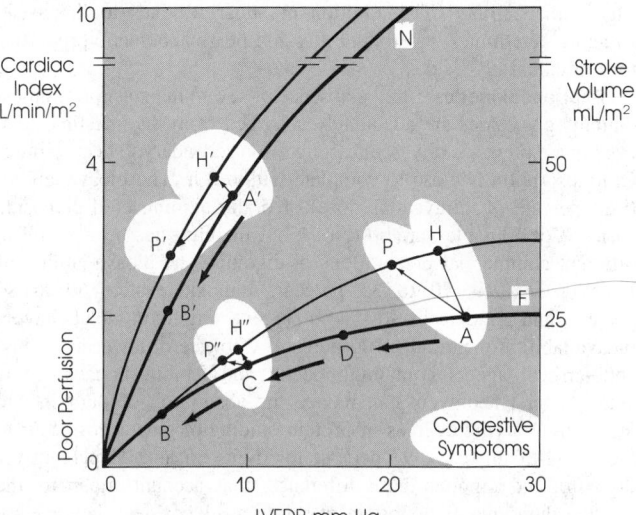

FIGURE 195-1 Effects of various vasodilators on the relationship between left ventricular end-diastolic pressure (LVEDP) and cardiac index or stroke volume in normal (N) and failing (F) hearts. H represents hydralazine or any other pure arterial dilator. It produces only a minimal increase in cardiac index in the normal subject (A' → H') or in the patient with heart failure with normal LVEDP (C → H''). In contrast, it elevates output in the patient with heart failure and elevated LVEDP (A → H). P represents a balanced vasodilator, such as sodium nitroprusside or an ACE inhibitor. It reduces filling pressure in all patients, elevates cardiac output in patients with heart failure and elevated LVEDP (A → P), lowers cardiac output in normal subjects (A' → P'), and has little effect on cardiac output in heart failure patients with normal filling pressures (C → P''). *(Reprinted with permission from TW Smith et al.)*

dinitrate is most effective when it is administered by the sublingual route.

The ideal vasodilator for the treatment of *acute* heart failure should have a rapid onset and brief duration of action when administered by intravenous infusion; sodium nitroprusside qualifies as such a drug, but its use requires careful monitoring of the arterial pressure and electrocardiogram and, if possible, of the pulmonary artery wedge pressure in an intensive care unit. For the treatment of chronic congestive heart failure, the agent should be effective on oral administration, and its action should persist for at least 6 h. Angiotensin-converting enzyme (ACE) inhibitors satisfy these requirements and have, quite properly, become the most useful and widely used vasodilators. It is advisable to commence therapy with very low doses, particularly in patients receiving diuretics, in order to avoid hypotension and gradually increase the dose.

Vasodilators are potent and effective in acutely improving the deranged hemodynamics of heart failure, and there is evidence in favor of a beneficial chronic effect as well. Studies with ACE inhibitors have demonstrated a favorable long-term reduction of symptoms and enhancement of exercise tolerance. Importantly, these drugs and, to a lesser extent, the combination of hydralazine and isosorbide dinitrate prolong survival of patients with heart failure. The administration of ACE inhibitors has been shown to prevent or retard the development of heart failure in patients with left ventricular dysfunction but without heart failure and to reduce long-term mortality when it is begun in such patients shortly after acute myocardial infarction.

ENHANCEMENT OF MYOCARDIAL CONTRACTILITY—DIGITALIS

The improvement of myocardial contractility by means of cardiac glycosides is an important component in the control of heart failure. The basic molecular structure of digitalis glycosides is a steroid nucleus to which an unsaturated lactone ring is attached at C-17. These two elements together are called *aglycone* or *genin*, and it is this portion of the molecule which is responsible for the cardiotonic activity. The addition of sugar residues to this basic structure determines water solubility and pharmacokinetic properties for individual glycosides.

Pharmacokinetics   In the absence of severe malabsorption, most digitalis glycosides are adequately absorbed from the intestinal tract even in the presence of vascular congestion secondary to heart failure. Oral absorption is close to complete within 2 h. The bioavailability (i.e., percent of intravenous dose) of orally administered glycoside varies. Considerable variability of bioavailability has been found in different commercial preparations of digoxin. The bioavailability of Lanoxin elixir is 70 to 85 percent, Lanoxin tablets 60 to 80 percent, and Lanoxicaps 90 to 100 percent. Digitoxin tablets have a bioavailability of virtually 100 percent. Cholesterol-lowering resins, antidiarrheal agents containing pectin and kaolin, nonabsorbable antacids, and neomycin can reduce the absorption of digoxin and digitoxin. Varying degrees of protein-binding of glycosides occur in the bloodstream (e.g., 97 percent for digitoxin and 25 percent for digoxin), and although these differences may account in part for the varying durations of the effect of different glycosides, they are not related to the speed of action of these drugs. The plasma contains only approximately 1 percent of the body stores of digoxin; therefore, digoxin is not effectively removed from the body by dialysis, exchange transfusions, or during cardiopulmonary bypass, presumably because of tissue binding. The major fraction of the glycosides is directly bound by various tissues, including the heart, in which the concentration is approximately 30 times that in the plasma for digoxin and 7 times for digitoxin; the latter is less polar and more lipid-soluble than digoxin.

Digoxin, which has a half-life of 1.6 days, is filtered in the glomeruli and secreted by the renal tubules; 85 percent is excreted in the urine, most in unchanged form; only 10 to 15 percent of digoxin is eliminated in the stool through biliary excretion in the presence of normal renal function. The ratio of digoxin clearance to endogenous creatinine clearance is 0.8, and the percentage of the body's total stores of digoxin lost per day can be calculated as $(14 \pm 0.2) \times$ creatinine clearance in milliliters per minute. In patients with normal renal function, a plateau concentration in the blood and tissue is reached after 5 days of daily maintenance treatment without a loading dose (see Fig. 66-2). Therefore, significant reductions of the glomerular filtration rate reduce the elimination of digoxin (but not of digitoxin) and, therefore, may prolong digoxin's effect, allowing it to accumulate to toxic levels if it is administered in patients with impaired renal function. The administration of most diuretics does not alter the excretion of digoxin significantly, but spironolactone can inhibit tubular secretion of digoxin, resulting in significant accumulation of the drug. *Digitoxin*, with a half-life of approximately 5 days, is metabolized chiefly in the liver; only 15 percent is excreted in the urine unchanged and an equal fraction in the stool. Drugs such as phenobarbital and phenylbutazone that increase the activity of hepatic microsomal enzymes accelerate the metabolism of digitoxin. To reach a steady state, digitoxin requires maintenance doses for 3 to 4 weeks. *Ouabain* is very rapidly acting, exhibiting an onset of action in 5 to 10 min and a peak effect within 60 min following intravenous injection. It is poorly and irregularly absorbed from the gastrointestinal tract, is excreted by the kidneys, has a half-life of 21 h, and is useful in emergencies.

Mechanism of action   The cardiac actions of all digitalis glycosides are alike. The clinical effects result from augmenting myocardial contractility and from prolonging the refractory period of the atrioventricular node.

The most important effect of digitalis on cardiac muscle is to shift its force-velocity relation upward (Chap. 194). This positive inotropic effect is exhibited in normal, nonfailing hypertrophied, and failing hearts. In the absence of heart failure, however, when cardiac output is not limited by cardiac contractility, the drug does not elevate the output.

Excitation-contraction coupling is the membrane and intracellular process most likely involved in producing the positive inotropic effect

of digitalis glycosides. These drugs inhibit transmembrane sodium and potassium movement by inhibition of the monovalent cation transport enzyme–coupled Na^+,K^+-ATPase. The latter, localized to the sarcolemma, appears to be the receptor for cardioactive glycosides, whose action results in an increase in intracellular sodium content; this, in turn, increases intracellular calcium concentration through a Na^+-Ca^{2+} exchange carrier mechanism. The increased myocardial uptake of calcium augments calcium released to the myofilaments during excitation (p. 989) and, therefore, invokes a positive inotropic response. There is a correlation between the degree of Na^+,K^+-ATPase inhibition and the inotropic potency of the glycoside.

Cardiac glycosides also produce alterations in the electrical properties of both the contractile cells and the specialized automatic cells. While low concentrations of glycosides produce little effect on the action potential, high concentrations result in a reduction in the resting potential (phase 4, see Fig. 197-2) and an augmented rate of diastolic depolarization. The reduction in the resting potential brings the cell closer to the threshold for depolarization. These two effects lead to increased automaticity and ectopic impulse activity. With the lowering of the resting potential, the rate of rise of the action potential is reduced, resulting in a slowing of conduction velocity, which is conducive to the development of reentry. Thus the known electrophysiologic effects of digitalis glycosides are capable of explaining the development of both reentry and ectopic foci and the resultant arrhythmias associated with digitalis intoxication.

The glycosides also prolong the effective *refractory period* of the atrioventricular node, largely as a result of an enhanced vagal effect. Digitalis also shortens the refractory period of the atrial and ventricular muscle. Small action potentials are propagated in a decremental fashion in the atrioventricular junction. Most do not reach the ventricles but leave some of the atrioventricular junctional cells in a refractory state. This helps to explain the slowing of ventricular rate produced by digitalis in supraventricular tachycardias. In atrial fibrillation, the slowing of ventricular rate is explained by prolongation of the effective refractory period of the atrioventricular node and increased concealed conduction. These actions reduce the frequency at which impulses penetrate the atrioventricular junction owing to both vagal and possibly direct effects of glycosides on junctional tissue.

Digitalis exerts a clinically significant negative chronotropic action, usually only in the setting of ventricular failure. In heart failure, slowing of the sinus rate following the administration of digitalis results also from withdrawal of sympathetic activity secondary to general improvement in circulatory status due to the positive inotropic effect of the glycoside. In the nonfailing heart, the slowing effect is negligible, and digitalis should not be used for the treatment of sinus tachycardia unless heart failure is present. The apparent suppression of pacemaker activity which may take place following large doses of digitalis is probably due not to arrest of the pacemaker but rather to a sinoatrial block related to a depression of conduction of impulses out of the sinus node.

In addition, the digitalis glycosides also exert an action on the peripheral vasculature, causing venous and arterial constriction in normal individuals and reflex dilatation resulting from withdrawal of sympathetic constrictor activity in patients with congestive heart failure.

Use in heart failure   By stimulating myocardial contractility moderately, digitalis improves ventricular emptying; i.e., it increases cardiac output, augments the ejection fraction, promotes diuresis, and reduces the elevated diastolic pressure and volume and end-systolic volume of the failing ventricle with consequent reduction of symptoms resulting from pulmonary vascular congestion and elevated systemic venous pressure. It is most beneficial in patients in whom ventricular contractility is impaired secondary to chronic ischemic heart disease or when hypertensive, valvular, or congenital heart disease imposes an excessive volume or pressure load. It is particularly helpful in the treatment of heart failure accompanied by atrial flutter and fibrillation and a rapid ventricular rate. It is of relatively little value in most forms of cardiomyopathy, myocarditis, beriberi with heart failure, mitral stenosis, thyrotoxicosis (all with sinus rhythm), cor pulmonale when the lung disease is not being treated concurrently (Chap. 204), and chronic constrictive pericarditis (Chap. 206). Nonetheless, when used in proper doses, it is not contraindicated in these disorders and is frequently used because it may exert a beneficial effect, albeit not a striking one.

Digitalis intoxication Although digitalis is one of the cornerstones of the treatment for heart failure, it is a two-edged sword, because intoxication due to digitalis excess is a serious and potentially fatal complication. The therapeutic-to-toxic ratios are similar for all cardiac glycosides. In most patients with heart failure, the lethal dose of most glycosides is probably 5 to 10 times the minimal effective dose and only about twice the dose which leads to minor toxic manifestations. In addition, advanced age, acute myocardial infarction or ischemia, hypoxemia, magnesium depletion, renal insufficiency, hypercalcemia, electrical cardioversion, and hypothyroidism all may reduce the tolerance of the patient to the digitalis glycosides or provoke latent digitalis intoxication. The most common precipitating cause of digitalis intoxication, however, is depletion of potassium stores, which often occurs as a result of diuretic therapy and secondary hyperaldosteronism. Since it is not necessary for a patient to receive a maximally tolerated dose of digitalis to derive a beneficial effect, even small doses provide some therapeutic action; this point should be considered if these drugs are to be used in patients prone to toxicity, particularly the elderly.

Anorexia, nausea, and vomiting, which are among the earliest signs of digitalis intoxication, are caused by direct stimulation of centers in the medulla and are not of gastrointestinal origin. The most frequent disturbance of cardiac rhythm caused by digitalis is premature ventricular beats, which may take the form of bigeminy because of increased myocardial irritability or facilitation of reentry. Atrioventricular block of varying degrees of severity may occur. Nonparoxysmal atrial tachycardia with variable atrioventricular block is quite characteristic of digitalis intoxication. Sinus arrhythmia, sinoatrial block, sinus arrest, and atrioventricular junctional and multifocal ventricular tachycardia also may occur. These arrhythmias are due to action of the glycoside both on cardiac tissues and on the central nervous system. Chronic digitalis intoxication may be insidious in onset and characterized by exacerbations of heart failure, weight loss, cachexia, neuralgias, gynecomastia, yellow vision, and delirium. Digitalis-toxic cardiac arrhythmias precede extracardiac (gastrointestinal or central nervous system) toxicity in about one-half of cases.

The administration of quinidine to patients receiving digoxin raises the serum concentration of the latter by reducing both the renal and nonrenal elimination of digoxin and by reducing its volume of distribution and thereby increasing the propensity to digitalis intoxication. The calcium channel antagonist verapamil and the antiarrhythmic agent amiodarone also appear to raise serum digoxin levels. Therefore, serum digoxin concentrations and electrocardiograms should be followed carefully when these drugs are administered to digitalized patients. The radioimmunoassays for digoxin and digitoxin make possible the correlation of serum glycoside levels with the presence of toxicity. In patients receiving standard maintenance doses of digoxin and digitoxin and in whom no sign of intoxication is present, serum concentrations approximate 1 to 1.5 and 20 to 25 ng/mL, respectively. When signs of intoxication are present, serum levels of more than 2 and 30 ng/mL, respectively, of these glycosides are often found. Since many factors other than the serum concentration determine digitalis intoxication, and since there is considerable overlap in serum glycoside concentrations in patients with and without toxicity, these levels cannot be used as a sole guide to digitalis dosage. However, when taken together with findings on the clinical examination and electrocardiogram, they add useful information to the clinical evaluations of digitalis intoxication. In addition, they will indicate whether a patient for whom the history of digitalis intake is in doubt has, in fact, been receiving the drug.

Treatment of digitalis intoxication When tachyarrhythmias result from digitalis intoxication, withdrawal of the drug and treatment

with potassium, phenytoin, a beta-adrenoceptor blocker, or lidocaine are indicated. Potassium should be administered cautiously and by the oral route whenever possible if hypokalemia is present, but *small* doses also may be helpful when serum potassium levels are normal; *potassium must not be employed in the presence of atrioventricular block or hyperkalemia.* A beta-adrenoceptor should not be used to treat digitalis toxicity in the presence of severe heart failure or atrioventricular block but may be useful otherwise; lidocaine is effective in the treatment of digitalis-induced ventricular tachyarrhythmias in the absence of preceding atrioventricular block. A cardiac pacemaker may be required in digitalis-induced atrioventricular block. Electrical conversion may not only be ineffective in treating digitalis-caused tachyarrhythmias but also may induce more serious arrhythmias. However, it may be lifesaving in digitalis-induced ventricular fibrillation. Quinidine and procainamide are of limited value in the treatment of digitalis intoxication. Fab fragments of purified, intact digitalis antibodies are a potentially lifesaving approach to the treatment of severe intoxication.

SYMPATHOMIMETIC AMINES (See also Chap. 68) Five sympathomimetic amines which act largely on beta-adrenergic receptors—norepinephrine, epinephrine, isoproterenol (isoprenaline), dopamine, and dobutamine—improve myocardial contractility in various forms of heart failure. The latter two agents appear to be most effective in the management of heart failure; they must be administered by constant intravenous infusion and are useful in patients with intractable heart failure, particularly those with a reversible component, such as exists in patients who have undergone cardiac surgery, and in some instances of myocardial infarction and shock or pulmonary edema. While they improve the hemodynamics in these conditions, it is not clear that they improve survival. Their administration should be accompanied by careful and continuous monitoring of the electrocardiogram, arterial pressure, and, if possible, pulmonary artery wedge pressure.

Dopamine (p. 420), the naturally occurring immediate precursor of norepinephrine, has a combination of actions which makes it particularly useful in the treatment of a variety of hypotensive states and congestive heart failure. At very low doses, i.e., 1 to 2 (μg/kg)/min, it dilates renal and mesenteric blood vessels through stimulation of specific dopaminergic receptors, thereby augmenting renal and mesenteric blood flow and sodium excretion. In the range of 2 to 10 (μg/kg)/min, dopamine stimulates myocardial beta receptors but induces relatively little tachycardia, while at higher doses it also stimulates alpha-adrenergic receptors and elevates arterial pressure.

Dobutamine is a synthetic catecholamine which acts on beta$_1$, beta$_2$, and alpha receptors. It exerts a potent inotropic action, has only a modest cardioaccelerating effect, and lowers peripheral vascular resistance, but since it simultaneously raises cardiac output, it has little effect on systemic arterial pressure. Dobutamine, given in continuous infusions of 2.5 to 10 (μg/kg)/min, is useful in the treatment of acute heart failure without hypotension. Like the other sympathomimetic amines, it may be particularly valuable in the management of patients requiring relatively short-term inotropic support—up to 1 week—in conditions which are reversible, such as the cardiac depression which sometimes follows open-heart surgery, or in patients with acute heart failure who are being prepared for operation. Adverse effects include sinus tachycardia, tachyarrhythmias, and hypertension.

A major problem with all sympathomimetics is the loss of responsiveness, apparently due to "downregulation" of adrenergic receptors, which becomes evident within 8 h of continuous administration. This problem may be managed by intermittent therapy.

Amrinone This bipyridine, a noncatecholamine, nonglycoside exerts both positive inotropic and vasodilator actions by inhibiting a specific phosphodiesterase. It is suitable for intravenous use only, and by simultaneously stimulating cardiac contractility and dilating the systemic vascular bed it reverses the major hemodynamic abnormalities associated with heart failure.

REFRACTORY HEART FAILURE   When the response to ordinary treatment is inadequate, heart failure is considered to be refractory. Before assuming that this condition simply reflects advanced, perhaps preterminal, myocardial depression, careful consideration must be given to several possibilities: (1) an underlying and overlooked cause of the heart disease that may be amenable to specific surgical or medical therapy, such as silent aortic or mitral stenosis, constrictive pericarditis, infective endocarditis, hypertension, or thyrotoxicosis, (2) one or a combination of the precipitating causes of heart failure, such as pulmonary or urinary tract infection, recurrent pulmonary emboli, arterial hypoxemia, anemia, or arrhythmia, and (3) complications of overly vigorous therapy, such as digitalis intoxication, hypovolemia, or electrolyte imbalance.

Recognition and proper treatment of the aforementioned complications are likely to make the patient responsive to therapy again. Perhaps the most common complication results from overzealous treatment with diuretics. When administered too rapidly, these drugs can produce sudden hypovolemia before edema fluid can be mobilized to replace the loss of blood volume, the result being a shocklike state with evidence of systemic hypoperfusion in the presence of edema. The chronically excessively diuresed patient may have exchanged the hazards of pulmonary edema and the inconvenience of systemic edema for a persistently depressed cardiac output with its associated weakness, lethargy, prerenal azotemia, and sometimes cardiac cachexia. Temporarily easing up on salt restriction and diuretic administration may overcome this difficulty, but as heart failure worsens, this course of action may lead to increased pulmonary congestion, which is equally unacceptable.

Hyponatremia is a late manifestation of refractory heart failure. It, too, may be a complication of overaggressive diuresis leading to reduced glomerular filtration rate and decreased delivery of NaCl to the diluting sites in the distal tubule. Hyponatremia also may result from nonosmotic stimuli for the continued secretion of antidiuretic hormone. Therapy involves improvement of the cardiovascular status, if possible (sometimes requiring the administration of a sympathomimetic amine such as dopamine or dobutamine), as well as temporary cessation of diuretic therapy and restriction of oral water intake. Hypertonic saline is very rarely indicated because total-body sodium is usually elevated, not depressed, in heart failure.

The combination of an intravenously administered vasodilator, such as sodium nitroprusside, along with a potent sympathomimetic amine, such as dopamine or dobutamine, often results in an additive effect, raising cardiac output and lowering filling pressure. Intravenous amrinone, sometimes accompanied by the administration of a converting enzyme inhibitor, also may be useful in patients with refractory heart failure.

Cardiac transplantation   When patients with heart failure become unresponsive to a combination of all the aforementioned therapeutic measures, are in New York Heart Association class IV, and are deemed unlikely to survive 1 year, they should be considered for cardiac transplantation (see Chap. 196).

TREATMENT OF ACUTE PULMONARY EDEMA   Pulmonary edema secondary to left ventricular failure or mitral stenosis is described in Chap. 31. It is life-threatening and must be considered a medical emergency. As is the case for the more chronic forms of heart failure, in the treatment of pulmonary edema, attention must be directed to identifying and removing any precipitating causes of decompensation, such as an arrhythmia or infection. However, because of the acute nature of the problem, a number of additional nonspecific measures are necessary. If it does not delay treatment unduly, recording pulmonary vascular pressures through a Swan-Ganz catheter and intraarterial pressure directly is advisable. The first six measures listed below are ordinarily applied simultaneously or nearly so.

1 Morphine is administered intravenously repetitively, as needed, in doses from 2 to 5 mg. This drug reduces anxiety, reduces adrenergic vasoconstrictor stimuli to the arteriolar and venous beds, and thereby helps to break a vicious cycle. Naloxone should be available in case respiratory depression occurs.

2 Because the alveolar fluid interferes with oxygen diffusion, resulting in arterial hypoxemia, 100% oxygen should be administered, preferably under positive pressure. The latter increases intraalveolar pressure and therefore reduces transudation of fluid from the alveolar capillaries and impedes venous return to the thorax, reducing pulmonary capillary pressure.

3 The patient should be maintained in the sitting position, with the legs dangling along the side of the bed, if possible, which also tends to reduce venous return.

4 Intravenous loop diuretics, such as furosemide or ethacrynic acid (40 to 100 mg), or bumetanide (1 mg) will, by rapidly establishing a diuresis, reduce circulating blood volume and thereby hasten the relief of pulmonary edema. In addition, when given intravenously, furosemide also exerts a venodilator action, reduces venous return, and reduces pulmonary edema even before the diuresis commences.

5 Afterload reduction is achieved with intravenous sodium nitroprusside at 20 to 30 μg/min in patients whose systolic arterial pressures exceed 100 mmHg.

6 If digitalis has not been administered previously, three-fourths of a full dose of a rapidly acting glycoside, such as ouabain, digoxin, or lanatoside C, should be administered intravenously.

7 Sometimes, aminophylline (theophylline ethylenediamine), 240 to 480 mg intravenously, is effective in diminishing bronchoconstriction, increasing renal blood flow and sodium excretion, and augmenting myocardial contractility.

8 If the above-mentioned measures are not sufficient, rotating tourniquets should be applied to the extremities.

After these emergency therapeutic measures have been instituted and the precipitating factors treated, the diagnosis of the underlying cardiac disorder responsible for the pulmonary edema must be established if it is not already known. After stabilization of the patient's condition, a long-range strategy for prevention of future episodes of pulmonary edema must be established, and this may require surgical treatment.

PROGNOSIS

The prognosis in heart failure depends primarily on the nature of the underlying heart disease and on the presence or absence of a precipitating factor which can be treated. When one of the latter can be identified and removed, the outlook for immediate survival is far better than if heart failure occurs without any obvious precipitating cause. In the latter situation, survival usually ranges between 6 months and 4 years depending on the severity of the heart failure. Also, the long-term prognosis for heart failure is most favorable when the underlying forms of heart disease can be treated. The prognosis also can be estimated by observing the response to treatment. When clinical improvement occurs with only modest dietary sodium restriction and small doses of diuretics or digitalis, then the outlook is far better than if, in addition to these measures, intensive diuretic therapy and vasodilators are necessary. Other factors which have been shown to be associated with a poor prognosis in heart failure include short (<3 min) exercise time, reduced (<133 mEq/L) serum sodium concentration, reduced (<3 mEq/L) serum potassium concentration, elevated circulating atrial natriuretic peptide and norepinephrine concentrations, as well as frequent ventricular extrasystoles on Holter monitoring. A large fraction of patients with congestive heart failure die suddenly, presumably of ventricular fibrillation. Unfortunately, there is no evidence that this complication can be prevented by the administration of antiarrhythmic agents.

REFERENCES

Bonow RO, Udelson JE: Left ventricular diastolic dysfunction as a cause of congestive heart failure: mechanisms and management. Ann Intern Med 117: 502, 1992

Braunwald E: ACE inhibitors: A cornerstone of the treatment of heart failure. N Engl J Med 325:351, 1991

———, Grossman W: Clinical aspects of heart failure, in *Heart Disease*, 4th ed, E Braunwald (ed). Philadelphia, Saunders, 1992, pp 444–463

Cody RJ: Optimising ACE inhibitor therapy of congestive heart failure. Clin Pharmacokinet 24:59, 1993

Cohn JN et al: A comparison of enalapril with hydralazine-isosorbide dinitrate in the treatment of chronic congestive heart failure. N Engl J Med 325:303, 1991

Francis GS et al: Comparison of neuroendocrine activation in patients with left ventricular dysfunction with and without congestive heart failure: A substudy of the Studies of Left Ventricular Dysfunction (SOLVD). Circulation 82:1724, 1990

——— et al: Neurohumoral activation in preclinical heart failure. Remodeling and the potential for intervention. Circulation 87 (suppl 5):IV90, 1993

Gilman A (ed): Cardiovascular drugs, in *Goodman and Gilman's The Pharmacological Basis of Therapeutics*, 8th ed. New York, Macmillan, 1990, pp 749–896

Groden DL: Vasodilator therapy for congestive heart failure. Lessons from mortality trials. Arch Intern Med 153:445, 1993

Iskandrian AS et al: Predicting left ventricular function: Bedside examination. Prim Cardiol (Suppl) 10:3A, 1984

Kannel WB: Epidemiologic aspects of heart failure, in *Heart Failure: Current Concepts and Management*, Cardiology Clinics Series 7/1, Weber KT (ed). Philadelphia, Saunders, 1989

Packer P: The neurohormonal hypothesis: A theory to explain the mechanism of disease progression in heart failure. J Am Coll Cardiol 20:248, 1992

Smith TW et al: Management of heart failure, in *Heart Disease*, 4th ed, E Braunwald (ed). Philadelphia, Saunders, 1992, p. 464

SOLVD Investigators: Effect of enalapril on survival in patients with reduced left ventricular ejection fractions and congestive heart failure. N Engl J Med 325:293, 1991

Swedberg K: Reduction in mortality by pharmacological therapy in congestive ehart failure. Circulation 87 (suppl 5):IV126, 1993

Wilcox CS: Diuretics, in *The Kidney*, 4th ed., BM Brenner, FC Rector Jr (eds). Philadelphia, Saunders, 1991, pp 2123–2148

196 CARDIAC TRANSPLANTATION

JOHN S. SCHROEDER

Orthotopic allograft cadaver cardiac transplantation as a treatment for end-stage cardiac disease achieved its twenty-fifth anniversary on December 7, 1992. On that day in 1967 Dr. Christiaan Barnard accomplished the first successful cardiac transplant in man, quickly followed by Drs. Norman Shumway and Richard Lower at Stanford University. After an initial early wave of enthusiasm, the problems of immunosuppression slowed application of the procedure until the introduction of cyclosporine in 1980. A subsequent worldwide expansion of cardiac transplantation has resulted in approximately 2500 cardiac transplants per year, with further increases limited only by the donor supply. Current 1- and 5-year survival rates of 95 and 70 percent indicate that cardiac transplantation is the therapy of choice in patients with end-stage heart disease who are unlikely to survive the next 6 to 12 months. This chapter reviews the procedure, indications, short- and long-term immunosuppressive therapy, and complications.

Since the introduction of cyclosporine in 1980 and the development of "low-dose" triple immunosuppressive regimens using azathioprine and prednisone, 1-year survival is reported at 80 to 90 percent and 5-year survival at 60 to 70 percent. The longest survivor has now lived 22 years after transplantation. Therefore, these survival statistics must be compared with those for other medical or surgical therapies in considering alternative therapies for end-stage heart disease.

INDICATIONS AND SELECTION OF CANDIDATES The limited donor supply and relatively high cost of cardiac transplantation have restricted it to patients most likely to survive and resume a functional life after transplantation. It is estimated that only 2000 potential donors in the United States, for a pool of at least 20,000 candidates based on current guidelines, become available yearly. Attempts to increase donor awareness in both physicians and the public are being made. Optimal candidates for this procedure are those who would be expected to return to a functional life if their hearts were replaced. This requires a mentally vigorous, medically compliant person who has not suffered extensive other end-stage organ damage from cardiac failure or does not have other systemic disease such as severe diabetes mellitus, collagen vascular disease, or HIV positivity. Long-standing pulmonary hypertension or recurrent pulmonary emboli and infarction may result in irreversible pulmonary hypertension leading to intraoperative death. Several heart transplant centers have initiated cardiac transplantation for newborns with left ventricular hypoplasia, but long-term survival experience is still very limited.

Timing of the recommendation to undergo cardiac transplantation can be difficult and requires assessment of the patient's current disability, stability of course, and likelihood of surviving the next 6 to 12 months. Generally, left ventricular ejection fractions under 15 to 20 percent and presence of serious ventricular arrhythmias indicate a 1-year survival rate of 50 percent or less. The increasing acceptance of cardiac transplantation as a treatment modality for heart failure without a corresponding increase in donor availability has led to prolonged waiting times of as much as 2 years or more. This longer waiting time has led to more rigorous medical care of the patient awaiting transplant with meticulous monitoring of electrolytes, fluid status, and overall well-being. Recurrent hospitalizations may be required. Patients may become dopamine/dobutamine-dependent to maintain adequate cardiac output. This dependency moves the patient to the highest ("status I") priority for a donor heart.

In addition to these pharmacologic bridges to transplantation, mechanical bridges are occasionally used where pharmacologic therapy is no longer effective. Three approaches are currently used. The first is intraaortic balloon pumping, which can increase cardiac output by 15 to 20 percent. The second is a left ventricular assist device (LVAD), which empties blood via a tube placed in the apex of the left ventricle and pumps it with an electrically driven "bellows-type" mechanism into the abdominal aorta. This approach is highly effective and has been used for up to 60 days with successful subsequent transplantation. Limitations include right ventricular failure and/or high pulmonary vascular resistance, since the LVAD does not "unload" the right ventricle. Blood clotting in the device remains a problem, in addition to the obvious problems of infection. Finally, total mechanical heart replacement is also applied in some transplant centers. This complete replacement circumvents the problem of right ventricular failure but is limited by the greater complexity of the device, which can lead to clotting and systemic emboli. Patients who underwent mechanical assistance *and* received a donor heart have 1-year survival statistics similar to those who went directly to transplantation. Tissue cross-matching between donor and recipient has generally not been done because of difficulty in obtaining good matches and lack of correlation between match and outcome. Size, ABO matching, negative lymphocyte cross-match, and avoidance of a transplantation from a cytomegalovirus (CMV)–positive donor to a CMV-negative recipient are more important.

OPERATIVE PROCEDURE The operative technique for orthotopic transplantation developed in animals in the early 1960s by Shumway and Lower remains little changed. In this technique, the surgeon removes the diseased heart but leaves the posterior wall of the right atrium in place and the superior and inferior venae cavae intact. The posterior wall of the left atrium is also left in situ with pulmonary veins intact. The donor heart is then removed in toto with the posterior wall of the right and left atria incised, which allows suturing of left atrial donor rim to recipient rim and right atrial donor rim to recipient rim, with anastomosis of the aorta and pulmonary artery.

IMMUNOSUPPRESSION AND REJECTION Controlling rejection while avoiding the adverse side effects of immunosuppressive agents is pivotal to successful transplantation. Rejection is characterized by perivascular infiltration of killer T lymphocytes, which migrate into the myocardium and cause cellular necrosis if not checked. Since early rejection can be silent, it is important to detect it before necrosis occurs. Immunologic monitoring of activated T lymphocytes in peripheral blood offers clues to the timing of a rejection process but has not been sufficiently reliable to dictate antirejection therapy. Therefore, repeated percutaneous transvenous right ventricular endomyocardial biopsies via the right internal jugular vein are required for histologic determination of the state of immunosuppression and rejection.

Billingham and associates have graded the stages of rejection as cannot rule out rejection, mild early rejection, moderate rejection, and severe rejection. Serial biopsies are taken every 1 to 2 weeks early after transplantation, with gradually widening intervals depending on the patient's course and rejection history. Prolongation of isovolumic relaxation time measured by echocardiography also may provide early clues to rejection.

Immunosuppressive therapy regimens vary but usually include triple therapy with cyclosporine, azathioprine, and prednisone. Prophylactic courses of monoclonal antibody OKT3 or antithymocyte globulin also may be given early after transplantation. Careful monitoring of the adverse side effects of these agents is extremely important because they include nephrotoxicity, bone marrow suppression, and opportunistic infections.

EARLY COURSE AND COMPLICATIONS   It is rare for a cardiac transplant patient to have a completely uncomplicated postoperative course. In the immediate postoperative period, right-sided heart failure due to pulmonary vascular disease is most life-threatening. During the 2 to 3 weeks after transplantation, the patient is hospitalized with meticulous monitoring for evidence of rejection and infections, repeated percutaneous transvenous endomyocardial biopsies, and adjustment of immunosuppressive drugs. During the ensuing 4 to 6 weeks, infectious complications, including bacterial, viral, and protozoan infections, are common. A successful transplant program requires a highly aggressive and sophisticated approach to diagnosis and therapy of infections in the immunocompromised host. Depending on the degree of cardiac cachexia preoperatively, the patient is usually functional at 1 week and discharged from the hospital at 2 to 3 weeks if no major complication occurs.

The average first-year cost ranges from $100,000 to $150,000, depending on the need for repeated hospitalization and cardiac biopsies, and is occasionally much higher. Yearly costs for immunosuppressive agents range from $5000 to $10,000, in addition to the expense of medical surveillance for rejection or complications.

PHYSIOLOGY AND FUNCTION   Since the allografted heart remains denervated, cardiac function differs from that of the innervated heart during both rest and exercise. The electrocardiogram in Fig. 196-1 shows two P waves. The P wave of the recipient's heart reflects the residual sinus node and posterior walls of the remaining native atria but is dissociated from the QRS, since the depolarization impulse does not cross the suture line. Although it does not control donor heart rate, the recipient's sinus node remains innervated and under the influence of the autonomic nervous system. The donor sinus node controls the rate of the transplanted heart. The donor heart's P wave has a regular PR interval, reflecting conduction to the ventricles. Since the controlling sinus node is denervated, it maintains a heart rate of 100 to 110 beats per minute, and rate increase depends on alterations in chronotropic agents perfusing the sinus node. Partial reinnervation may occur in some patients late after transplantation. This is manifested primarily by the occurrence of angina-like symptoms in patients who have developed accelerated graft atherosclerosis (see below).

Ventricular function in response to isometric and isotonic exercise has been studied extensively. The early response to exercise is more dependent on the Frank-Starling mechanism and change in ventricular volume and filling pressure. As exercise proceeds and catecholamines are released with their positive inotropic effects, cardiac output begins to rise. The cardiac transplant recipient can achieve approximately

FIGURE 196-1 Electrocardiogram in a patient with a transplanted heart. The arrows denote the P wave generated by the recipient's atrium. The P wave just preceding the QRS complex is generated by the donor heart.

70 percent of the maximal cardiac output expected for his or her age, easily sufficient for the stresses of everyday life.

LATE COURSE AND COMPLICATIONS   Although the rejection process partially subsides, lifelong administration of immunosuppressive drugs, albeit at lower doses, is still required and remains a hazard. Infectious complications and unsuspected rejection continue to occur, requiring ongoing surveillance and monitoring. Cardiac biopsies are performed at 3-month intervals to assess the response to rejection treatment. Figure 196-2 shows the causes of death by time posttransplantation from the Registry of the International Society for Heart and Lung Transplantation: Eighth Official Report, 1991. Acute rejection or infection predominates in the first year after transplantation. Subsequently, chronic rejection (i.e., accelerated coronary vascular disease) becomes the most important cause of death. In addition to the well-known hazards of long-term glucocorticoid usage, the immunosuppressed patient is at increased risk for neoplasia. Angina is rare, and patients may present with sudden death or silent myocardial infarction. This diffuse accelerated vascular process affects both distal and proximal coronary vessels so that standard approaches, such as angioplasty or coronary artery bypass grafting, are not generally useful.

Accelerated coronary vascular disease appears to be one of the major factors limiting longer-term survival. The process is a fibrointimal hyperplasia which can go undetected by coronary arteriography at first and then cause diffuse atherosclerotic changes. Risk factors for its development may include number of rejection episodes and elevated lipids. An unusual form of lymphoma can occur frequently in extranodal locations, which is linked to prior Epstein-Barr viral infection. This lymphoma may be polyclonal or monoclonal, is associated with excessive immunosuppression, and

FIGURE 196-2 Relationship between cause of death and survival interval in heart recipients. (*From Kreitt and Kaye.*)

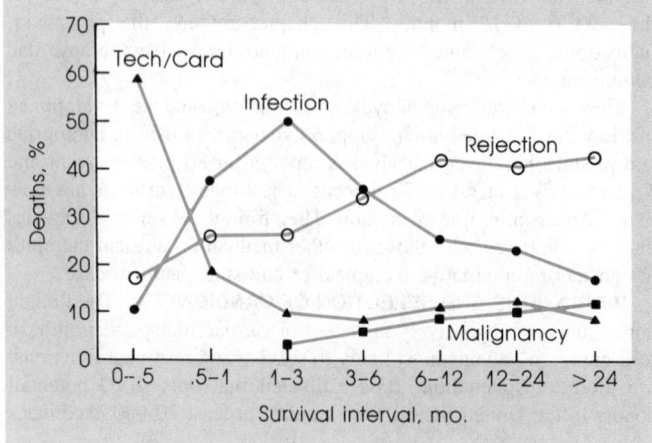

may respond to simply lowering doses of cyclosporine and administration of acyclovir rather than requiring more aggressive chemo- or radiotherapy. Many cases regress fully and do not recur. Retransplantation has been employed for some patients with severe graft atherosclerosis but it is limited by the scarcity of donors and poorer survival expectations after the second transplant. Dilitazem has been reported to reduce the severity and occurrence of this accelerated vascular process when started at the time of transplantation. CMV infections also have been associated with higher frequency of this disease. Uncontrolled trials with anticoagulation, aspirin, and improved immunosuppression with cyclosporine have done little to lower this frequency; 40 to 50 percent of patients show arteriographic evidence of coronary vascular disease 5 years after transplantation.

HEART-LUNG TRANSPLANTATION

Patients with congenital heart disease with Eisenmenger's complex (Chap. 199) or primary pulmonary hypertension (Chap. 225) are now considered for heart-lung transplantation. The surgical technique is similar to that for heart transplantation, except that the pulmonary venous attachments to the left atrium are left intact, and a tracheal anastomosis is required. The postoperative period is more complex, since the lungs may be rejected separately from the heart, requiring repeated endobronchoscopic biopsies when rejection is suspected. The immunosuppressive regimen is similar to that for heart transplants. Long-term survival has in the past been limited by obliterative bronchiolitis due to chronic unrecognized rejection; survival rates have been approximately 60 percent at 1 year and 50 percent at 2 years but appear to be improving. Heart-lung transplants also have been applied to primary pulmonary hypertension, but more recent experience with single-lung transplants for these patients has been satisfactory, thus utilizing scarce donors more effectively. Single-lung transplants are also being applied increasingly for patients with advanced emphysema. Double-lung transplants for patients with cystic fibrosis also have become the operation of choice for this group (see also Chap. 232).

REFERENCES

CAREY NR: Diagnostic criteria of chronic rejetion in transplanted hearts. Transplant Proc 25:2026, 1993

COPELAND JG et al: Orthotopic total artificial heart bridge to transplantation: Preliminary results. J Heart Transplant 8:124, 1989

GAO S-Z et al: Progressive coronary luminal narrowing after cardiac transplantation. Circulation 82(suppl IV):IV-269, 1990

GRATTAN MT et al: Cytomegalovirus infection is associated with cardiac allograft rejection and atherosclerosis. JAMA 261:3561, 1989

KRIETT JM, KAYE MP: The Registry of the International Society for Heart and Lung Transplantation: Eighth Official Report, 1991. J Heart Lung Transplant 10:491, 1991

LEVENSON JL, OLSBRISCH ME: Psychiatric aspects of heart transplantation. Psychosomatics 34:114, 1993

REEDY JE et al: Bridge to heart transplantation: Importance of patient selection. J Heart Transplant 9:475, 1990

SCHROEDER JS, HUNT SA: Cardiac transplantation: Update 1987. JAMA 258:3142, 1987

—— et al: A preliminary study of diltiazem in the prevention of coronary artery disease in heart-transplant recipients. N Engl J Med 328:30, 1993

STEVENSON LW et al: Poor survival of patients with idiopathic cardiomyopathy considered too well for transplantation. Am J Med 83:871, 1987

TANIO JW, EISEN HJ: Medical aspects of cardiac transplantation. Hosp Pract 28:61, 1993

197 **THE BRADYARRHYTHMIAS: DISORDERS OF SINUS NODE FUNCTION AND AV CONDUCTION DISTURBANCES**

MARK E. JOSEPHSON / FRANCIS E. MARCHLINSKI / ALFRED E. BUXTON

ANATOMY OF THE CONDUCTING SYSTEM   Under normal conditions, the pacemaker function of the heart resides in the sinoatrial (SA) node, which lies at the junction of the right atrium and superior vena cava. The SA node is approximately $1\frac{1}{2}$ cm long and 2 to 3 mm wide and is supplied by the sinus node artery, which arises from either the right coronary artery (60 percent of cases) or the left circumflex coronary artery (40 percent). Once the impulse exits the sinus node and perinodal tissue, it traverses the atrium until it reaches the atrioventricular (AV) node. The blood supply of the AV node is derived from the posterior descending coronary artery (90 percent of cases), which lies at the base of the interatrial septum just above the tricuspid annulus and anterior to the coronary sinus. The electrophysiologic properties of the AV node result in slow conduction, which is responsible for the normal delay in AV conduction, i.e., the PR interval.

The bundle of His emerges from the AV node, enters the fibrous skeleton of the heart, and courses anteriorly across the membranous interventricular septum. It has a dual blood supply from the AV nodal artery and a branch of the anterior descending coronary artery. The branching (distal) portion of the bundle of His gives rise to a broad sheet of fibers that course over the left side of the interventricular septum to form the left bundle branch and a narrow cable-like structure on the right side that forms the right bundle branch. The arborization of both the right and left bundle branches gives rise to the distal His-Purkinje system, which ultimately extends throughout the endocardium of the right and left ventricles.

The sinus node, atrium, and AV node are significantly influenced by autonomic tone. Vagal influences depress automaticity of the sinus node, depress conduction, and prolong refractoriness in the tissue surrounding the sinus node; inhomogeneously decrease atrial refractoriness and slow atrial conduction; and prolong AV nodal conduction and refractoriness. Sympathetic influences exert the opposite effect.

ELECTROPHYSIOLOGIC PRINCIPLES

In the resting state, the interior of most cardiac cells, with the exception of the sinus and AV nodes, is approximately -80 to -90 mV, negative with respect to a reference extracellular electrode. The resting membrane potential is determined primarily by the concentration gradient of potassium across the cell membrane. Activation of cardiac cells results from movement of ions across the cell membrane, causing a transient depolarization known as the *action potential*. The ionic species responsible for the action potential varies among the cardiac tissues, and the configuration of the action potential is therefore unique to each tissue (Fig. 197-1).

The action potential of the His-Purkinje system and ventricular myocardium has five phases (Fig. 197-2). The rapid depolarizing current (phase 0) is mainly determined by an influx of sodium into myocardial cells followed by a secondary (slower) influx of calcium which produces a slow inward current. The repolarization phases of the action potential (phases 1 to 3) are primarily related to outward flux of potassium. The resting membrane potential is phase 4.

The bradyarrhythmias result from abnormalities either of impulse formation, i.e., automaticity, or of conduction. *Automaticity*, which is normally observed in the sinus node, the specialized fibers of the His-Purkinje system, and some specialized atrial fibers, is the property

FIGURE 197-1 Action potential configurations in different regions of the mammalian heart. (*From AM Katz, Physiology of the Heart, New York, Raven, 1977.*)

of a cardiac cell which causes it to depolarize spontaneously during phase 4 of the action potential, leading to the generation of an impulse. To exhibit automaticity, the resting membrane potential must decrease spontaneously until threshold potential is reached and an all-or-none regenerative response occurs. The ionic components producing spontaneous diastolic depolarization appear to involve the inward current of either sodium or calcium. The velocity of *conduction*, i.e., impulse propagation through cardiac tissues, depends on

FIGURE 197-2 Schematic representation of the action potential in normal ventricle depicting the direction, strength, and period of flow of the ionic currents underlying the action potential. The arrow's direction and size indicate whether current is inward- or outward-directed and the approximate current strength of the ion identified at the arrow's base. The horizontal position of the arrow corresponds to the same moment in the time course of action potential (see text). The five phases of the action potential are indicated by the numerals placed along the waveform. (*From Ten Eick et al, Progress in Cardiovascular Diseases 24(2):157, 1981; used with permission.*)

the magnitude of inward current, which is directly related to the rate of rise and amplitude of phase 0 of the action potential. The more positive the threshold potential and the slower the rate of depolarization toward threshold, the slower is the rate of rise of phase 0 of the action potential and the slower is the conduction velocity. Disease states or drugs may result in lower rates of rise of phase 0 at any given membrane potential. Passive membrane properties (e.g., intracellular resistance and intercellular coupling) also can affect impulse propagation. Propagation is more rapid parallel to fiber orientation than transverse to it, a property termed *anisotropic conduction*.

Refractoriness is a property of cardiac cells which defines the period of recovery that cells require after being discharged before they can be reexcited by a stimulus. The *absolute refractory period* is defined by that portion of the action potential during which no stimulus, regardless of its strength, can evoke another response. The *effective refractory period* is that part of the action potential during which a stimulus can evoke only a local, nonpropagated response. The *relative refractory period* extends from the end of the effective refractory period to the time that the tissue is fully recovered. During this time, a stimulus of greater than threshold strength is required to evoke a response which is propagated more slowly than normal. In the normal His-Purkinje system or ventricular myocytes, excitability is recovered following completion of the action potential, and evoked responses have characteristics similar to the spontaneous normal response. In the AV node, recovery of excitability occurs well after completion of the action potential.

INTRACARDIAC RECORDINGS OF THE SPECIALIZED CONDUCTING SYSTEM Electrode catheters allow the recording of activation of portions of the specialized conducting system, including the bundle of His. To obtain a recording from the bundle of His, the electrode catheter is positioned across the tricuspid valve (Fig. 197-3). The interval from local atrial depolarization in the His bundle recording to the onset of depolarization of the His bundle deflection is called the *AH interval* (normal = 60 to 125 ms) and represents an indirect method of assessing AV nodal conduction time. The interval from the beginning of the His bundle deflection to the earliest onset of ventricular activation, as measured from any of multiple-surface electrocardiogram (ECG) leads or the intracardiac ventricular electrogram, is called the *HV interval* (normal = 35 to 55 ms) and represents conduction time through the His-Purkinje system. Electrode catheters can be positioned in the area of the sinus node to record high right atrial activity. Left atrial activity may be recorded directly via a catheter placed across a patent foramen ovale or indirectly using a catheter inserted into the coronary sinus. The atrial activation sequence may be "mapped", and sites of intra- and interatrial conduction abnormalities may be ascertained.

SINUS NODE DYSFUNCTION

The sinus node is normally the dominant cardiac pacemaker because its intrinsic discharge rate is the highest of all potential cardiac pacemakers. Its responsiveness to alterations in autonomic nervous system tone is responsible for the normal acceleration of heart rate during exercise and the slowing that occurs during rest and sleep. Increases in sinus rate normally result from an increase in sympathetic tone acting via beta-adrenergic receptors and/or a decrease in parasympathetic tone acting via muscarinic receptors. Slowing of the heart rate is normally due to opposite alterations. In adults, the normal sinus rate under basal conditions is 60 to 100 beats per minute. Sinus bradycardia is said to exist when the sinus rate is less than 60 beats per minute, and sinus tachycardia when it exceeds 100 beats per minute. However, there is wide variation among individuals, and rates less than 60 beats per minute do not necessarily indicate pathologic states. For example, trained athletes often exhibit resting rates under 50 beats per minute due to increases in vagal tone. Normal elderly individuals also may show marked sinus bradycardia at rest.

ETIOLOGY Sinus node dysfunction most often is found in the elderly as an isolated phenomenon. Although interruption of the blood

FIGURE 197-3 Normal intracardiac recording. Surface ECG leads I, II, and V₁ are displayed with intracardiac ECGs from the high right atrium (HRA), left atrium from the coronary sinus (CS), and AV junction to obtain a His bundle electrogram (HBE). T = time lines. A = atrial activation; H = His bundle activation; V = ventricular activation. Atrial activation begins in the high right atrium and spreads inferiorly to the low atrial septum, as recorded in the HBE, and the left atrium, as recorded in the CS. The AH and HV intervals represent AV nodal and His-Purkinje conduction times, respectively. Vertical lines = 0.10 s. (*From ME Josephson, SF Seides, Clinical Cardiac Electrophysiology: Techniques and Interpretations. Philadelphia, Lea & Febiger, 1979.*)

supply to the sinus node may produce dysfunction, the correlation between obstruction of the sinus node artery and clinical evidence of sinus node dysfunction is poor. Specific disease states associated with sinus node dysfunction include senile amyloidosis and other conditions associated with infiltration of the atrial myocardium. Sinus bradycardia is associated with hypothyroidism, advanced liver disease, hypothermia, typhoid fever, and brucellosis; it occurs during episodes of hypervagotonia (vasovagal syncope), severe hypoxia, hypercapnia, acidemia, and acute hypertension. However, in most cases of sinus node dysfunction a specific cause cannot be identified.

MANIFESTATIONS Although marked (≤50 beats per minute) sinus bradycardia may cause fatigue and other symptoms due to

inadequate cardiac output, more commonly sinus node dysfunction is manifest as paroxysmal dizziness, presyncope, or syncope. These symptoms usually result from abrupt, prolonged sinus pauses caused by failure of sinus impulse formation (sinus arrest) or block of conduction of sinus impulses to the surrounding atrial tissue (sinus exit block). In either case, the ECG manifestation is a prolonged period (>3 s) of atrial asystole. In some patients, sinus node dysfunction is accompanied by abnormalities in AV conduction. In addition to the absence of atrial activity, lower pacemakers fail to emerge during the sinus pauses, resulting in periods of ventricular asystole and syncope. Occasionally, sinus node dysfunction is manifested initially by the failure of the sinus rate to accelerate in response to conditions such as exercise or fever that normally cause increases in the sinus rate. In some patients, sinus node dysfunction may become manifest only in the presence of certain cardioactive drugs: cardiac glycosides, beta-adrenergic blocking drugs, verapamil, quinidine, and other antiarrhythmic agents. These agents, which do not cause sinus node dysfunction in normal people, may unmask evidence of sinus node dysfunction in susceptible individuals.

The *sick sinus syndrome* refers to a combination of symptoms (dizziness, confusion, fatigue, syncope, and congestive heart failure) caused by sinus node dysfunction and manifested by marked sinus bradycardia, sinoatrial block, or sinus arrest. Because these symptoms are nonspecific, and because ECG manifestations of sinus node dysfunction are not infrequently intermittent, it may be difficult to prove that such symptoms are actually caused by sinus node dysfunction.

Atrial tachyarrhythmias such as atrial fibrillation, atrial flutter, or atrial tachycardia may be accompanied by sinus node dysfunction. The *bradycardia-tachycardia syndrome* refers to paroxysmal atrial arrhythmia which upon termination is followed by prolonged sinus pauses (Fig. 197-4) or in which there are alternating periods of tachyarrhythmia and bradyarrhythmia. Syncope or presyncope may result from failure of the sinus node to recover function following suppression of automaticity by atrial tachyarrhythmia.

DIAGNOSIS *First-degree sinoatrial exit block* denotes a prolonged conduction time from the sinus node to the surrounding atrial tissue. It cannot be recognized on a standard (surface) ECG but requires invasive intracardiac recordings (see below). *Second-degree sinoatrial exit block* denotes the intermittent failure of conduction of sinus impulses to the surrounding atrial tissue; it is manifested as the intermittent absence of P waves (Fig. 197-5). *Third-degree*, or *complete, sinoatrial block* is characterized by a lack of atrial activity or by the presence of an ectopic subsidiary atrial pacemaker. On the standard ECG it cannot be distinguished from sinus arrest, but direct intracardiac recordings of sinus node activity permit this distinction. The *bradycardia-tachycardia syndrome* is manifested on the standard ECG as tachyarrhythmias (see Fig. 197-4). Most often these are atrial flutter or fibrillation, although any tachycardia with retrograde conduction to the atria may cause overdrive suppression of the sinus node resulting in clinical appearance of this syndrome.

The most important step in the diagnosis is to correlate symptoms with ECG evidence of sinus node dysfunction. While ambulatory ECG (Holter) monitoring remains a mainstay in evaluating sinus node function, most episodes of syncope are paroxysmal and unpredictable. Single and even multiple 24-h Holter monitor recordings may fail to include a symptomatic episode. Therefore, noting the response to carotid sinus pressure and pharmacologic autonomic "denervation"

FIGURE 197-4 Tachycardia-bradycardia syndrome. Rhythm strip of ECG lead II showing spontaneous cessation of supraventricular tachycardia followed by a 5.6-s pause prior to resumption of sinus activity. The patient was

asymptomatic during supraventricular tachycardia, but the sinus pause caused severe light-headedness.

FIGURE 197-5 Second-degree sinoatrial exit block. Surface ECG denoting abrupt absence of P wave during sinus rhythm. Prior to the pause, the sinus rate is regular. The interval of the pause is exactly twice the basal sinus cycle length. The arrow marks the appropriate location for the absent P wave.

of the heart is frequently helpful. Carotid sinus pressure is particularly useful in patients in whom paroxysmal dizziness or syncope is compatible with the hypersensitive carotid sinus syndrome (see Chap. 17). In such patients, the response can be dramatic, and sinus pauses in excess of 5 s may occur. Normally, a sinus pause of ≤3 s results from 5 s of unilateral carotid sinus massage. However, in elderly patients, pauses >3 s are common and do not necessarily signify a diagnostic response. In all individuals it is important to correlate symptoms with such ECG phenomena. If atropine can prevent the effects of carotid sinus pressure, autonomic dysfunction, not primary (intrinsic) sinus node dysfunction, is responsible. The other noninvasive test of sinus node function involves the use of pharmacologic agents to manipulate the autonomic nervous system and assess the balance of parasympathetic and sympathetic activity on the sinus node. Physiologic or pharmacologic maneuvers which are vagomimetic (Valsalva maneuver or phenylephrine-induced hypertension), vagolytic (atropine), sympathomimetic (isoproterenol or hypotension by nitroprusside), or sympatholytic (beta-adrenergic blocking agents) can be utilized, singly and in combination. These studies are designed to test the response of the sinus node to autonomic stimulation and inhibition and thereby characterize the status of autonomic regulation of the sinus node. Abnormalities of the autonomic control of sinus function are particularly common in patients in whom the only presenting arrhythmia is sinus bradycardia.

Intrinsic heart rate This is a manifestation of the primary activity of the sinus node, and its determination requires chemical autonomic blockade of the heart. Complete autonomic blockade is achieved with 0.2 mg/kg propranolol intravenously, followed after 10 min by 0.04 mg/kg atropine sulfate intravenously. Normal values of intrinsic heart rate (in beats per minute) are calculated by the formula $118.1 - (0.57 \times$ age). The use of autonomic blockade can separate patients with asymptomatic sinus bradycardia into a group with primary sinus node dysfunction (slow intrinsic heart rate) and a group with autonomic imbalance (normal intrinsic heart rate). Autonomic blockade is particularly useful when combined with invasive assessment of sinus node function (see below). Autonomic blockade may depress conduction in patients with intrinsic disease of the conduction system and should be carried out only in a setting where arrhythmias can be monitored and rapidly treated.

Sinus node recovery time Sinus node recovery time is evaluated by assessing the response of the sinus node to rapid atrial pacing (Fig. 197-6). When atrial pacing is discontinued, a pause, the *sinus node recovery time*, occurs prior to resumption of spontaneous sinus

FIGURE 197-6 Example of sinus node recovery time in a patient with symptomatic sinus node dysfunction. Cessation of atrial pacing at 150 beats per minute (cycle length 400 ms) results in a prolonged sinus pause (2.8 s). Surface ECG leads V_1 and V_6 are shown in addition to intracardiac recordings at the high right atrium (A), which demonstrates atrial pacing rate.

rhythm. When the sinus recovery time is prolonged, the results of this test mimic the prolonged sinus pauses seen following termination of atrial tachyarrhythmias in the bradycardia-tachycardia syndrome (see Fig. 197-4). The corrected sinus node recovery time (sinus recovery time − sinus cycle length) normally is less than 550 ms, and the uncorrected sinus node recovery time is less than 150 percent of the spontaneous cycle length. In patients with symptomatic sinus node dysfunction, prolongation of the sinus node recovery time is often observed. Patients with abnormally slow intrinsic heart rates usually have abnormal sinus node recovery times, while those with normal intrinsic heart rates have normal recovery times.

Sinoatrial conduction time Determination of the conduction time from the sinus node to the atrium allows for the differentiation of abnormalities of sinoatrial conduction from abnormalities of sinus impulse formation. The conduction time equals one-half the difference between the pause following termination of brief periods of pacing and the sinus cycle length. Alternatively, the sinus node electrogram can be recorded directly by a catheter electrode placed near the sinoatrial node.

EVALUATION The electrophysiologic investigation of sinus node dysfunction should be undertaken in patients who have had symptoms compatible with sinus node dysfunction and in whom no documentation of the arrhythmia responsible for these symptoms has been obtained by prolonged Holter monitoring. Asymptomatic patients with sinus bradycardia need *not* be tested, since no therapy is indicated. Similarly, symptomatic patients with ECG documentation of asystole, sinoatrial block or arrest, or the bradycardia-tachycardia syndrome do not require electrophysiologic tests for diagnosis. However, in symptomatic patients without documentation of an arrhythmia, electrophysiologic assessment of sinus node function can yield information that may be used to guide appropriate therapy. If a pacemaker is indicated, the side of pacemaker implantation for maximum hemodynamic effects can be guided by the results of electrophysiologic investigation. However, the results of tests of sinus node function must be interpreted with caution. Sinus node dysfunction coexists frequently with other disorders such as AV conduction disturbances which may cause symptoms such as syncope. Electrophysiologic evaluation of patients with symptoms such as undiagnosed syncope must not stop with the demonstration of abnormalities of sinus node dysfunction or carotid sinus hypersensitivity. Instead, complete evaluation, including His bundle recordings and programmed atrial and ventricular stimulation (see Chap. 198), is necessary to search for additional electrophysiologic abnormalities which could be responsible for symptoms.

TREATMENT Permanent pacemakers (see p. 1017) are the mainstay of therapy for patients with symptomatic sinus node dysfunction. Patients with intermittent paroxysms of bradycardia or sinus arrest and with the cardioinhibitory form of the hypersensitive carotid sinus syndrome are usually adequately treated by demand ventricular pacemakers. These devices are reliable, relatively inexpensive, and suffice to prevent episodic symptoms due to abrupt bradycardia. Patients with symptomatic chronic sinus bradycardia or frequent prolonged episodes of sinus node dysfunction do better with dual-chamber pacemakers that preserve the normal AV activation sequence. Although theoretically an atrial demand pacemaker should be adequate for patients with sinus node dysfunction, the frequent accompaniment of dysfunction in other portions of the cardiac conduction system usually mandates placement of a pacemaker capable of ventricular pacing. Recent studies suggest that AV sequential pacing also may be useful in preventing atrial fibrillation, an important component of the bradycardia-tachycardia syndrome.

AV CONDUCTION DISTURBANCES

The specialized cardiac conducting system normally ensures synchronous conduction of each sinus impulse from the atria to the ventricles. Abnormalities of conduction of the sinus impulse to the ventricles may portend the development of heart block, which can ultimately lead to syncope or cardiac arrest. In order to evaluate the clinical significance of conduction abnormalities, the physician must assess (1) the site of conduction disturbance, (2) the risk of progression to complete block, and (3) the probability that a subsidiary escape rhythm arising distal to the site of block will be electrophysiologically and hemodynamically stable. This latter point is perhaps the most important, since the rate and stability of the escape pacemaker determine what symptoms result from heart block. The escape pacemaker following AV nodal block is usually in the His bundle, which generally has a stable rate of 40 to 60 beats per minute and is associated with a QRS complex of normal duration (in the absence of a preexisting intraventricular conduction defect). This contrasts with escape rhythms arising in the distal His-Purkinje system, which have lower intrinsic rates (25 to 45 beats per minute), manifest wide QRS complexes with prolonged duration, and are unstable. Although prolonged QRS complexes are invariable when the distal His-Purkinje pacemakers form the escape mechanism, wide QRS complexes also can coexist with AV nodal block and a His bundle rhythm. Therefore, QRS morphology alone may not be adequate to identify the site of block.

ETIOLOGY The AV node is supplied by the parasympathetic and sympathetic nervous systems and is sensitive to variations in autonomic tone. Chronic slowing of AV nodal conduction may be seen in highly trained athletes who have hypervagotonia at rest. A variety of diseases also can influence AV nodal conduction. These include acute processes such as myocardial infarction (particularly inferior), coronary spasm (usually of the right coronary artery), digitalis intoxication, excesses of beta and/or calcium blockers, acute infections such as viral myocarditis, acute rheumatic fever, infectious mononucleosis, and miscellaneous disorders such as Lyme disease, sarcoidosis, amyloidosis, and neoplasms, particularly cardiac mesotheliomas. AV nodal block also may be congenital.

Two degenerative diseases are commonly responsible for damage to the specialized conducting system and produce AV block usually associated with bundle branch block (see Chap. 189). In *Lev's disease*, there is calcification and sclerosis of the fibrous cardiac skeleton, which frequently involves the aortic and mitral valves, the central fibrous body, and the summit of the ventricular septum. *Lenegre's disease* appears to be a primary sclerodegenerative disease within the conducting system itself with no involvement of the myocardium or the fibrous skeleton of the heart. These two diseases are probably the most common causes of isolated chronic heart block in adults. Hypertension and aortic and/or mitral stenosis are specific disorders that either accelerate the degeneration of the conducting system or have a direct effect by calcification and fibrosis involving the conducting system.

First-degree AV block, more properly termed *prolonged AV conduction*, is characterized by a PR interval >0.20 s. Since the PR interval is determined by atrial, AV nodal, and His-Purkinje activation, delay in any one or more of these structures can contribute to a prolonged PR interval. In the presence of a QRS complex of normal duration, a PR interval >0.24 s almost invariably is due to a delay within the AV node. If the QRS is prolonged, delays may be present at any of the levels mentioned above. Delay within the His-Purkinje system is always accompanied by a prolonged QRS duration in addition to a prolonged PR interval. However, as indicated below, it is only with intracardiac recordings that the exact site of delay can be determined.

Second-degree heart block (intermittent AV block) is present when some atrial impulses fail to conduct to the ventricles. Mobitz type I second-degree AV block (AV Wenckebach block) is characterized by progressive PR interval prolongation prior to block of an atrial impulse (Fig. 197-7A). The pause that follows is less than fully compensatory (i.e., is less than two normal sinus intervals), and the PR interval of the first conducted impulse is shorter than the last conducted atrial impulse prior to the blocked P wave. This type of block is almost always localized to the AV node and associated with a normal QRS

FIGURE 197-7 *A.* Mobitz type I second-degree AV block. Intracardiac recordings demonstrate that the PR prolongation (320, 615 ms) is localized to the AV node (AH 240, 535 ms, respectively). HBE = His bundle electrogram; A = atrium; H = His; V = ventricle. Time lines (T) = 100 ms (*From ME Josephson, SF Seides, Clinical Cardiac Electrophysiology: Techniques and Interpretations. Philadelphia, Lea & Febiger, 1979.*) *B.* Mobitz type II second-degree AV block. Intracardiac recordings document block below the His bundle.

duration. It is seen most often as a transient abnormality with inferior wall infarction or with drug intoxication, particularly digitalis, beta blockers, and occasionally calcium channel antagonists. This type of block also can be observed in normal individuals with heightened vagal tone. Although Mobitz type I block can progress to complete heart block, this is uncommon. Even when it does, however, the heart block is usually well tolerated because the escape pacemaker usually arises in the proximal His bundle and provides a stable rhythm. As a result, the presence of Mobitz type I second-degree AV block usually does not mandate aggressive therapy. Therapeutic decisions depend on the ventricular response and the symptoms of the patient. If the ventricular rate is adequate and the patient is asymptomatic, observation is sufficient.

In Mobitz type II second-degree AV block, conduction fails suddenly and unexpectedly without a preceding change in PR intervals (Fig. 197-7B). It is usually due to disease of the His-Purkinje system and is most often associated with a prolonged QRS duration. It is important to recognize this type of block because it has a high incidence of progression to complete heart block with an unstable, slow, lower escape pacemaker. Therefore, pacemaker implantation is necessary in this condition. Mobitz type II block may occur in the setting of anteroseptal infarction or in the primary or secondary sclerodegenerative or calcific disorders of the fibrous skeleton of the heart. In so-called high-degree AV block there are periods of two or more consecutively blocked P waves. Regardless of the site of origin of the escape rhythm, if it is slow and the patient is symptomatic, a cardiac pacemaker is mandatory.

Third-degree AV block is present when no atrial impulse propagates to the ventricles. If the QRS complex of the escape rhythm is of normal duration, occurs at a rate of 40 to 55 beats per minute, and increases with atropine or exercise, AV nodal block is probable. Congenital complete AV block is usually localized to the AV node (Fig. 197-8). If the block is within the His bundle, the escape

FIGURE 197-8 Third-degree AV block. Complete heart block with a slow, wide complex escape rhythm is present. Block in this instance is usually intra-His.

pacemaker usually is less responsive to these perturbations. If the escape rhythm of the QRS is wide and associated with rates ≤40 beats per minute, block is usually localized in, or distal to, the His bundle and mandates a pacemaker, since the escape rhythm in this setting is unreliable. Some patients with infra-His bundle block are capable of retrograde conduction. In such patients, a "pacemaker syndrome" (see below) may develop if a simple ventricular pacemaker is used. Dual-chambered pacemakers eliminate this potential problem.

AV DISSOCIATION   AV dissociation exists whenever the atria and ventricles are under the control of two separate pacemakers and, while present in complete AV block, can occur in the absence of a primary conduction disturbance. AV dissociation unrelated to heart block may occur under two circumstances: First, it may develop with an AV junctional rhythm in response to severe sinus bradycardia. When the sinus rate and the escape rate are similar and the P waves occur just before, in, or following the QRS complex, *isorhythmic AV dissociation* is said to be present. Treatment usually consists of removal of the offending cause of sinus bradycardia (i.e., discontinuation of digitalis, beta blockers, or calcium antagonists), accelerating the sinus node by vagolytic agents, or insertion of a pacemaker if the escape rhythm is slow and results in symptoms. Second, AV dissociation can be caused by an enhanced lower (junctional or ventricular) pacemaker which competes with normal sinus rhythm and frequently exceeds it. This has been called *interference AV dissociation* because the rapid lower pacemaker results in bombardment of the AV node in a retrograde fashion, rendering it refractory to the normal sinus impulses. Thus failure of antegrade conduction is a physiologic response in this circumstance. Interference dissociation commonly occurs during ventricular tachycardia, accelerated junctional or ventricular rhythms seen with digitalis intoxication, myocardial ischemia and/or infarction, or local irritation following cardiac surgery. The accelerated rhythm should be treated with either antiarrhythmic drugs (see Chap. 198), removal of an offending drug, or correction of the metabolic abnormality or ischemia.

INTRACARDIAC ELECTROCARDIOGRAPHIC RECORDINGS IN DIAGNOSIS AND MANAGEMENT   The main therapeutic decision in patients with AV conduction disturbance is whether or not a permanent pacemaker is required, and a number of circumstances exist in which His bundle electrocardiography can be a useful diagnostic tool upon which to base this decision. It is unquestionable that patients with *symptomatic* second- or third-degree AV block should be paced, and therefore, these patients do not require electrophysiologic study. However, intracardiac ECG recordings can be useful in at least the following three groups of patients:

1 Patients with syncope and bundle branch or bifascicular block without documentation of AV block. In such patients, the demonstration of marked infra-His bundle conduction disturbances, i.e., a prolonged HV interval (>100 ms), may usually be taken as an indication of the need for the insertion of the permanent pacemaker. With intervals ranging from 60 to 100 ms, the indications for pacing are equivocal. Block below the His bundle developing during atrial pacing at rates of less than 150 beats per minute and the development of an infra-His bundle block or HV prolongation >100 ms following 1 g procainamide intravenously also signify that the patient is at high risk for the development of subsequent AV block and that a pacemaker is indicated. Complete electrophysiologic evaluation, including atrial and ventricular programmed stimulation, is indicated to help identify other possible cardiac etiologies for the syncope. Since the incidence of significant advanced AV block is low in *asymptomatic* patients who have bifascicular block, electrophysiologic evaluation or permanent

pacemakers are not cost-effective. In this group, observation appears most reasonable.

2 Patients with 2:1 atrioventricular conduction. Intracardiac recordings are necessary to ascertain the site of the conduction disturbance because the typical ECG features of Mobitz type I or Mobitz type II block cannot be discerned during a 2:1 pattern of AV conduction on the surface ECG. Intracardiac recordings may demonstrate that AV nodal block, intra-His bundle block, infra-His bundle block, or combinations of block may be responsible. A surface electrocardiogram finding that suggests an infra-His bundle lesion is the presence of alternating bundle branch block associated with changing PR intervals. Intracardiac recordings in such patients confirm that the block is almost always in the His-Purkinje system. The finding of infra-His bundle block in patients with asymptomatic second-degree AV block mandates pacemaker therapy because of the high likelihood of their developing symptomatic high-grade AV block and syncope.

3 Asymptomatic patients with third-degree AV block. In such patients, electrophysiologic studies may be useful in assessing the stability of the junctional pacemaker. Pacing is indicated when the His bundle escape pacemaker is shown to be unstable by an inadequate response to exercise, atropine, or isoproterenol or by a prolonged junctional recovery time following ventricular pacing.

MANAGEMENT OF BRADYARRHYTHMIAS

PHARMACOLOGIC THERAPY   Pharmacologic therapy is usually reserved for acute situations. Atropine (0.05 to 2.0 mg intravenously) and isoproterenol (1 to 4 μg/min intravenously) are useful in increasing heart rate and decreasing symptoms in patients with sinus bradycardia or AV block localized to the AV node. They have an insignificant effect on lower pacemakers. In patients with neurovascular syncope, beta blockers and disopyramide have been suggested as methods to depress left ventricular function and decrease mechanoreceptor-related reflexes. Mineralocorticords, ephedrine, and theophylline also have been reported to be of benefit to occasional patients. Unfortunately, no controlled study has shown that any of these pharmacologic modalities works in a predictable fashion in all patients. Further work on delineating different mechanisms in different patient groups may allow us to apply pharmacologic agents more appropriately. Recently, theophylline has been suggested in patients with vasovagal syncope. Long-term therapy of bradyarrhythmias is best accomplished by pacemakers.

PACEMAKERS   External energy sources can be used to stimulate the heart when disorders in impulse formation and/or transmission lead to symptomatic bradyarrhythmias. Pacer stimuli can be applied to the atria and/or ventricles. Indications for pacemaker insertion are listed in Table 197-1.

Temporary pacing   This is usually instituted to provide immediate stabilization prior to permanent pacemaker placement or to provide pacemaker support when a bradycardia is precipitated by what is presumed to be a transient event such as ischemia or drug toxicity. Temporary pacing is usually achieved by the transvenous insertion of an electrode catheter with the catheter positioned in the right ventricular apex and attached to an external generator. This procedure is associated with a small risk of cardiac perforation, infection at the insertion site, and thromboembolism; the risk of the latter two complications increases markedly if the pacing wire is left in place for more than 48 h. The development of an entirely external transthoracic cardiac pacing system may preclude the need for transvenous pacing in selected patients. However, occasional failure

TABLE 197-1   Indications for permanent pacing*

ACQUIRED AV BLOCK IN ADULTS

Class I

A Complete heart block, permanent or intermittent, at any anatomic level, associated with any anatomic level, associated with any one of the following complications:
  1 Symptomatic bradycardia. In the presence of complete heart block, symptoms must be presumed to be due to the heart block unless proved to be otherwise.
  2 Congestive heart failure.
  3 Ectopic rhythms and other medical conditions that require drugs that suppress the automaticity of escape pacemakers and result in symptomatic bradycardia.
  4 Documented periods of asystole ≥ 3.0 s or any escape rate < 40 beats per minute in symptom-free patients.
  5 Confusional states that clear with temporary pacing.
  6 Post-AV junction ablation, myotonic dystrophy.
B Second-degree AV block, permanent or intermittent, regardless of the type or the site of block, with symptomatic bradycardia.
C Atrial fibrillation, atrial flutter, or rare cases of supraventricular tachycardia with complete heart block or advanced AV block, bradycardia, and any of the conditions described under *IA*. The bradycardia must be related to digitalis or drugs known to impair AV conduction.

Class II

A Asymptomatic complete heart block, permanent or intermittent, at any anatomic site, with ventricular rates of 40 beats per minute or faster.
B Asymptomatic type II second-degree AV block, permanent or intermittent.
C Asymptomatic type I second-degree AV block at intra-His or intra-His levels.

Class III

A First-degree AV block.
B Asymptomatic type I second-degree AV block at the supra-His (AV node) level.

AFTER MYOCARDIAL INFARCTION

Class I

A Persistent advanced second-degree AV block or complete heart block after acute myocardial infarction with block in the His-Purkinje system (bilateral bundle branch block).
B Patients with transient advanced AV block and associated bundle branch block.

Class II

A Patients with persistent advanced block at the AV node.

Class III

A Transient AV conduction disturbances in the absence of intraventricular conduction defects.
B Transient AV block in the presence of isolated left anterior hemiblock.
C Acquired left anterior hemiblock in the absence of AV block.
D Patients with persistent first degree AV block in the presence of bundle branch block not demonstrated previously.

BIFASCICULAR AND TRIFASCICULAR BLOCK

Class I

A Bifascicular block with intermittent complete heart block associated with symptomatic bradycardia.
B Bifascicular or trifascicular block with intermittent type II second-degree AV block without symptoms attributable to the heart block.

Class II

A Bifascicular or trifascicular block with syncope that is not proved to be due to complete heart block, but other possible causes for syncope are not identifiable.
B Markedly prolonged HV (>100 ms).
C Pacing-induced infra-His block.

Class III

A Fascicular block without AV block or symptoms.
B Fascicular block with first-degree AV block without symptoms.

SINUS NODE DYSFUNCTION

Class I

A Sinus node dysfunction with documented symptomatic bradycardia. In some patients this will occur as a consequence of long-term (essential) drug therapy of a type and dose for which there are no acceptable alternatives.

Class II

A Sinus node dysfunction, occurring spontaneously or as a result of necessary drug therapy, with heart rates < 40 beats per minute when a clear association between significant symptoms consistent with bradycardia and the actual presence of bradycardia has not been documented.

SINUS NODE DYSFUNCTION (continued)

Class III

A Sinus node dysfunction in asymptomatic patients, including those in whom substantial sinus bradycardia (heart rate < 40 beats per minute) is a consequence of long-term drug treatment.
B Sinus node dysfunction in patients in whom symptoms suggestive of bradycardia are clearly documented not to be associated with a slow heart rate.

HYPERSENSITIVE CAROTID SINUS AND NEUROVASCULAR SYNDROMES

Class I

A Recurrent syncope associated with clear, spontaneous events provoked by carotid sinus stimulation; minimal carotid sinus pressure induces asystole of >3 s duration in the absence of any medication that depresses the sinus node or AV conduction.

Class II

A Recurrent syncope without clear, provocative events and with a hypersensitive cardioinhibitory response.
B Syncope with associated bradycardia reproduced by a head-up tilt with or without isoproterenol or other forms of provocative maneuvers and in which a temporary pacemaker and a second provocative test can establish the likely benefits of a permanent pacemaker.

Class III

A A hyperactive cardioinhibitory response to carotid sinus stimulation in the absence of symptoms.
B Vague symptoms, such as dizziness, light-headedness, or both, with a hyperactive cardioinhibitory response to carotid sinus stimulation.
C Recurrent syncope, light-headedness, or dizziness in the absence of a cardioinhibitory response.

SOURCE: Dreifus LS et al.

* Class I: agreement that permanent pacemaker should be implanted. Class II: divergence of opinion regarding need for implantation. Class III: agreement that pacemaker is unnecessary.

---

of ventricular capture and significant discomfort related to the large current required for effective transthoracic ventricular stimulation preclude the uniform use of this approach.

Permanent pacing   This mode of pacing is instituted for persistent or intermittent symptomatic bradycardia not related to a self-limiting precipitating factor or for documented infranodal second- or third-degree AV block. Permanent pacing leads are usually inserted transvenously through the subclavian or cephalic vein with the leads positioned in the right atrial appendage for atrial pacing and the right ventricular apex for ventricular pacing. The leads are then attached to the pulse generator, which is inserted into a subcutaneous pocket below the clavicle. Epicardial lead placement is used when (1) transvenous access cannot be obtained, (2) the chest is already open, i.e., in the course of a cardiac operation, and (3) adequate endocardial lead placement cannot be achieved. Most pacemaker generators are powered by lithium batteries. The life expectancy of the generator is related to (1) current output required for capture, (2) requirement for incessant or intermittent pacing, and (3) number of cardiac chambers paced. Life expectancy of the simple ventricular demand pacemaker can exceed 10 years.

Pacing code   A code consisting of three to five letters has been developed for describing pacemaker type and function (Table 197-2). The first letter indicates the chamber(s) paced and is designated *V* for ventricular pacing, *A* for atrial pacing, or *D* for dual-chamber (both atrial and ventricular) pacing. The second letter indicates the chamber in which electrical activity is sensed and is also indicated by *A*, *V*, or *D*. An additional designation, *O*, has been used when pacemaker discharge is not dependent on a sensed electrical activity. The third letter refers to the response to a sensed electric signal. The letter *O* represents no response to an underlying electric signal, usually related to the absence of associated sensing function; *I* represents inhibition of pacing function; *T* represents triggering of pacing function; and *D* indicates a dual response, i.e., spontaneous atrial and ventricular activity inhibiting atrial and ventricular pacing and

TABLE 197-2   The NASPE/BPEG generic pacemaker code

Position category	I Chamber(s) paced	II Chamber(s) sensed	III Response to sensing	IV Programmability, rate modulation	V Antitachyarrhythmia function(s)
	O = None A = Atrium V = Ventricle D = Dual (A + V)	O = None A = Atrium V = Ventricle D = Dual (A + V)	O = None T = Triggered I = Inhibited D = Dual (T + I)	O = None P = Simple programmable M = Multiprogrammable C = Communicating R = Rate modulation	O = None P = pacing (antitachyarrhythmia) S = Shock D = Dual (P + S)
Manufacturer's designation	S = single (A or V)	S = (A or V)			

SOURCE: Zipes DP

atrial activity triggering a ventricular response. Additional fourth and fifth letters of the pacing code have been recommended to indicate whether the pacemaker is programmable and has rate modulation (fourth) and whether special antitachycardia functions are available (i.e., antitachycardia pacing, *T*, and delivery of high- or low-energy shocks). In the fourth category, *M* represents multiprogrammability and *R* represents rate response ("physiologic") pacing. It follows from the described code that the standard VVIR (ventricular demand pacemaker) paces the ventricle, senses the ventricle, is inhibited by sensed spontaneous ventricular activity, and has rate modulation, while the DDDR pulse generator is capable of sensing and pacing both the atria and ventricles and has a dual response to the sensed atrial and ventricular activity as described above (Fig. 197-9). Both pacemakers have rate modulation (*R*). "Physiologic" pacemakers use sensors (e.g., muscular activity, respiratory rate, temperature, O$_2$ saturation, QT interval, etc.) as methods to allow the pacemaker to increase the heart rate in response to physiologic demands, i.e., exercise. These pacemakers are essential when chronotropic incompetence is present and an increase in heart rate is required to enhance physiologic performance. Studies have shown that such "physiologic" pacemakers improve exercise tolerance and relieve symptoms to a greater degree than fixed-rate pacemakers.

FIGURE 197-9 Normally functioning DDD pacemaker. All three panels show a lead II rhythm strip at 50 mm/s. The programmed lower rate is approximately 55 beats per minute. (*Top*) AV sequential pacing with a paced AV interval of 160 ms is shown for the first two complexes. A VPC occurs and is sensed, resetting the cycle. (*Middle*) The first beat is AV paced, but spontaneous sinus P waves and APC trigger a ventricular paced complex with a sensed P to QRS of 120 ms. (*Bottom*) After the first AV paced complex, a paced atrial complex conducts to the ventricle with a PR of 120 ms, inhibiting the ventricular pacemaker.

Selection of the appropriate pacemaker and pacing mode depends on the clinical condition and the type of bradyarrhythmia being treated. The two most common pacing mode selections are DDD and VVI. DDD provides AV sequential pacing, which is ideally suited for the relatively young and active patient who has intact sinus node function or intermittent dysfunction and high-grade persistent or intermittent AV block. The DDD mode will allow for physiologic atrial sensed and ventricular paced rates and improve exercise tolerance. AV synchrony and dual-chamber pacing also may be desirable in patients with borderline hemodynamic reserve who are dependent on atrial contribution to cardiac output and in those patients who develop the pacemaker syndrome (see below) in response to ventricular demand pacing. Rate-responsive DDD (i.e., DDDR) pacing is indicated when chronotropic incompetence is present in a patient who requires AV synchrony. The DDD pacing mode is contraindicated in chronic atrial fibrillation or flutter, because rapid and irregular ventricular pacing will occur to the upper rate limit. In some cases this will produce a more rapid ventricular rate than the patient's own rate in the absence of a pacemaker. DDD pacemakers must either automatically switch or be reprogrammed to the VVI mode. Almost all such pacemakers are now combined with some form of rate responsiveness so that when the device functions in the VVI mode, it also will respond to physiologic demands (VVIR). Chronotropic insufficiency is a contraindication, since a DDD pacemaker will act as a "fixed-rate" pacemaker at the upper rate cutoff. In these situations, a rate-adaptive or "physiologic" pacemaker is indicated (VVIR or DDDR). In patients with impaired sinus node function or chronic atrial fibrillation, a sensor-driven, rate-adaptive pacemaker must be implanted. As mentioned earlier, these pacemakers automatically adjust ventricular pacing rates to a sensed indicator of exertion. The DDD pacing mode also may be contraindicated in patients with intermittent or persistent ventriculoatrial (VA) conduction, who may develop pacemaker-mediated tachycardia (see below).

Programmability of pacemakers   This allows for modification of pacing function after implantation and for adaptation to changes in clinical needs. Pacemaker programming is accomplished by activation of the programming head positioned over the implanted pulse generator after making the desired changes in programmable parameters (see Table 197-2). A radio frequency system is routinely used to communicate the program to the pacemaker. A high degree of sophistication is required to recognize the presence and causes of pacemaker malfunction and their treatment.

Complications   Adverse effects of permanent pacing are usually associated with failure or malfunction of the pacing system. These problems are usually secondary to over- or undersensing, output failure, and/or lead fracture or displacement. Two other problems may occur. The *pacemaker syndrome* consists of fatigue, dizziness, syncope, and distressing pulsations in the neck and chest and can be associated with adverse hemodynamic effects. The pathophysiologic contributors to the pacemaker syndrome include (1) loss of atrial contribution to ventricular systole, (2) vasodepressor reflex initiated by cannon *a* waves which are caused by atrial contractions against a closed tricuspid valve and observed in the jugular venous pulse (Chap.

188), and (3) systemic and pulmonary venous regurgitation due to atrial contraction against a closed AV valve. The symptoms associated with the pacemaker syndrome can be prevented by maintaining AV synchrony by dual-chamber pacing or, in the case of a ventricular demand pacemaker, by programming a hysteresis escape rate 15 to 20 beats per minute below that of the paced rate. As a result of this programming, sinus activity and thus atrial contraction will be less likely to occur at the same time as ventricular pacing and ventricular contraction. The second major problem peculiar to dual-chamber pacemakers is the development of *pacemaker-mediated tachycardia*. In this instance, retrograde depolarization of the atria, resulting from a premature ventricular depolarization or a paced ventricular complex, is sensed and leads to subsequent triggering of ventricular pacing. This, in turn, can result in repetition of the phenomenon of ventriculoatrial conduction with the development of an endless-loop, pacemaker-mediated tachycardia. It may be corrected by reprogramming the atrial refractory period.

REFERENCES

BAROLD SS, ZIPES DP: Cardiac pacemakers and antiarrhythmia devices, in *Heart Disease: A Textbook of Cardiovascular Medicine*, 4th ed, E Braunwald (ed). Philadelphia, Saunders, 1992, p 726

BAROLD SS et al: Electrocardiography of contemporary DDD pacemakers. Basic concepts: Upper rate response, retrograde ventriculoatrial conduction and differential diagnosis of pacemaker tachycardias, in *Electrical Therapy for Cardiac Arrhythmias: Pacing, Antitachycardia Devices, Catheter Ablation*, S Saksena, N Goldschlager (eds). Philadelphia, Saunders, 1990, p 225

BERNSTEIN AD et al: The NASPE/BPEG generic pacemaker code for antibradyarrhythmias and adaptive-rate pacing and antitachyarrhythmia devices. PACE 10:794, 1987

DREIFUS LS et al: Guidelines for implantation of cardiac pacemakers and antiarrhythmic devices: A report of the American College of Cardiology/American Heart Association Task Force on Assessment of Diagnostic and Therapeutic Cardiovascular Procedures (Committee on Pacemaker Implantation). J Am Coll Cardiol 18:1, 1991

ELLENBOGEN KA et al: New insights into pacemaker syndrome gained from hemodynamic, humoral and vascular responses during ventriculo-atrial pacing. Am J Cardiol 65(1):53, 1990

HUANG SK et al: Carotid sinus hypersensitivity in patients with unexplained syncope: Clinical, electrophysiologic and long-term follow-up observations. Am Heart J 116:989, 1988

JOSEPHSON ME: *Clinical Electrophysiology*, 2d ed. Philadelphia, Lea and Febiger, 1992, chaps 4, 5, 6, 13

MENDES LA, DAVIDOFF R: Cardiogenic seizure with bradyarrhythmia: Documentation of the mechanism during asystole. Am Heart J 125:1786, 1993

SRA JS et al: Comparison of cardiac pacing with drug therapy in the treatment of neurocardiogenic (vasovagal) syncope with bradycardia or asytole,. N Engl J Med 328:1085, 1993

WALLER BF et al: Anatomy, histology and pathology of the cardiac conduction system: Part II. Clin Cardiol 16:347, 1993

198 THE TACHYARRHYTHMIAS

MARK E. JOSEPHSON / ALFRED E. BUXTON / FRANCIS E. MARCHLINSKI

MECHANISMS OF TACHYARRHYTHMIAS

Tachyarrhythmias may be divided into disorders of impulse propagation and disorders of impulse formation. Disorders of impulse propagation (reentry) are generally considered to be the most common mechanism of sustained paroxysmal tachyarrhythmia. The requirements for initiating reentry include (1) electrophysiologic inhomogeneity (i.e., differences in conduction and/or refractoriness) in two or more regions of the heart connected with each other to form a potentially closed loop, (2) unidirectional block in one pathway, (3) slow conduction over an alternative pathway, allowing time for the initially blocked pathway to recover excitability, and (4) reexcitation of the initially blocked pathway to complete a loop of activation (Fig. 198-1). Repetitive circulation of the impulse over this loop can

FIGURE 198-1 Schema of reentry. Y branching of the Purkinje system to ventricular muscle is shown in panels *A* through *C*. The right limb (*hatched area*) of the Purkinje system has a longer refractory period than the left. *A*. During a slow stimulated rate (S_1), conduction proceeds normally over both Purkinje fibers, resulting in collision in the ventricular muscle. *B*. An early premature stimulus (S_2) results in block in the Purkinje fiber on the right and slow conduction down the left. The impulse conducts through the ventricle and attempts to reenter the initial site of block but fails because this site has not fully recovered excitability. *C*. An earlier stimulus (S_3) again results in block on the left. The resulting slower propagation down the left fiber provides enough time for the initial site of block to recur and allows the impulse to conduct through it to produce a reentrant circuit.

produce a sustained tachyarrhythmia. While anatomic obstacles may underlie reentry and provide an inexcitable center around which the impulse can circulate, they are not essential. Reentrant arrhythmias can be reproducibly initiated and terminated by premature complexes and rapid stimulation. The response of these arrhythmias to stimulation can help distinguish them from arrhythmias caused by triggered activity.

Disorders of impulse formation can be subdivided into tachyarrhythmias caused by enhanced automaticity and those caused by triggered activity. In addition to the sinus node, automatic pacemaker activity can be observed in specialized atrial fibers, fibers of the atrioventricular (AV) junction, and Purkinje fibers (see Chap. 197). Myocardial cells do not normally possess pacemaker activity. Enhancement of normal automaticity in latent pacemaker fibers or the development of abnormal automaticity due to partial depolarization of the resting membrane occurs as a consequence of a variety of pathophysiologic states, which include (1) increased endogenous or exogenous catecholamines, (2) electrolyte disturbances (e.g., hyperkalemia), (3) hypoxia or ischemia, (4) mechanical effects (e.g., stretch), and (5) drugs (e.g., digitalis). Tachycardia caused by automaticity cannot be started or stopped by pacing.

Triggered activities are events that do not occur spontaneously but require a change in cardiac frequency as a trigger. Triggered activity may be caused by early afterdepolarizations, which occur during phases 2 and 3 of the action potential, or delayed afterdepolarizations, which occur following completion of phase 3 of the action potential (Fig. 198-2). Triggered activity has been observed in atrial, ventricular, and His-Purkinje tissue under conditions such as increased local catecholamine concentration, hyperkalemia, hypercalcemia, and digitalis intoxication (delayed afterdepolarizations) or during bradycardia, hypokalemia, or other situations prolonging action potential duration (early afterdepolarizations). All these conditions produce an accumulation of intracellular calcium, which causes depolarizations during phase 2 or 3 of the action potential or following the action potential, termed *afterdepolarizations* (see Fig. 198-2). With increasing amplitude of the afterdepolarizations, threshold can be reached and repetitive activity produced. The exact role of triggered activity in spontaneous clinical arrhythmias is unknown, but tachyarrhythmias associated with digitalis intoxication, accelerated idioventricular rhythm in acute infarction, and exercise-induced ventricular tachycardia (VT) may be caused by triggered activity due to delayed afterdepolarizations. Torsades de pointes (polymorphic VT associated with long QT intervals) may be caused by triggered activity due to early afterdepolarizations.

The use of electrophysiologic studies, i.e., intracardiac recordings and programmed stimulation, has greatly expanded the understanding

FIGURE 198-2 Early and late afterdepolarizations.

of the mechanisms of tachyarrhythmias. In addition to helping diagnose arrhythmias, these techniques may be of value in determining the most appropriate types of therapy because they allow the physician to observe the hemodynamic and symptomatic consequences of the arrhythmia in the presence or absence of therapy. EP studies of tachycardias require the positioning of multiple electrode catheters at critical areas within the heart. These electrodes must be capable of both stimulating and recording from multiple sites in the atria and/or ventricles.

PREMATURE COMPLEXES

ATRIAL PREMATURE COMPLEXES (APCs) APCs can be found on 24-h Holter monitoring in over 60 percent of normal adults. APCs are usually asymptomatic and benign, although at times they may be associated with palpitations. In susceptible patients, they can initiate paroxysmal supraventricular tachycardias. APCs may originate from

any location in either atrium, and they are recognized on the ECG as early P waves with a morphology which differs from the sinus P wave (Fig. 198-3A). While APCs usually conduct to the ventricles when they occur late in the cardiac cycle, early APCs may reach the AV conduction system while it is still in its relative refractory period, resulting in a conduction delay manifested by prolonged PR interval following the premature P wave (Fig. 198-3A). Very early APCs may even block in the AV node if this structure is encountered during its effective refractory period. APCs, whether conducted or not, are usually followed by a pause before a return to sinus activity. Most commonly, an APC enters and resets the sinus node, so the sum of the pre- and postextrasystolic PP intervals is less than the sum of two sinus PP intervals (Fig. 198-3A). In this case, the pause is said to be less than fully compensatory. The QRS complex following most APCs is normal, although early APCs may be followed by aberrantly conducted QRS complexes due to the premature complex falling within the relative refractory period of the His-Purkinje system.

Since most APCs are asymptomatic, treatment is not required. When they cause palpitations or trigger paroxysmal supraventricular tachycardias (see below), treatment may be useful. Factors that precipitate APCs, such as alcohol, tobacco, or adrenergic stimulants, should be identified and eliminated, and in their absence, mild sedation or the use of a beta blocker may be tried. If this fails, quinidine or other type I agents may be used.

AV JUNCTIONAL COMPLEXES The site of origin of these complexes is thought to be in the bundle of His, since the normal AV node in vivo possesses no automaticity (p. 1012). AV junctional complexes are less common than either atrial or ventricular premature complexes and are more often associated with cardiac disease or digitalis intoxication. Junctional premature impulses can conduct both antegradely to the ventricles and retrogradely to the atrium and, on rare occasions, may fail to conduct in either direction. Premature AV junctional complexes can be recognized by normal-appearing QRS complexes that are not preceded by a P wave. Retrograde P waves (inverted in leads II, III, and aVF) may be observed after the QRS complex.

While often asymptomatic, junctional premature complexes may be associated with palpitations and cause cannon *a* waves which may result in distressing pulsations in the neck. When symptomatic, they should be treated like APCs.

FIGURE 198-3 *A*. ECG lead II. Sinus rhythm with two atrial premature complexes (*arrows*). Note the difference in P-wave configuration between sinus and the premature atrial complexes. In addition, note that the PR interval of the premature complexes is prolonged, due to slowed conduction of the premature impulse through the AV conduction system. *B*. ECG lead V_1. Atrial tachycardia with varying degrees of AV block, typical of digitalis toxicity. *C*. ECG lead II. Atrial flutter. Note the characteristic sawtooth baseline seen in the inferior ECG leads during atrial flutter. Variable degrees of AV conduction block are present. *D*. ECG lead II. Atrial fibrillation. Note the irregular wavy baseline without discrete atrial activity. The ventricular response is irregularly irregular. *E*. ECG leads I, aVR, and V_1. Atrial fibrillation in a patient with Wolff-Parkinson-White syndrome. Note the extremely rapid, grossly irregular ventricular rate with wide, bizarre QRS complexes.

VENTRICULAR PREMATURE COMPLEXES (VPCs) These are among the most common arrhythmias and occur in patients with and without heart disease. Of adult males ≥60 percent will exhibit VPCs during a 24-h Holter monitoring. In patients without heart disease, VPCs have not been shown to be associated with any increased incidence in mortality or morbidity. VPCs may occur in up to 80 percent of patients with previous myocardial infarction, and in this setting, if frequent (>10 per hour) and/or complex (occurring in couplets), they have been associated with increased mortality. However, cardiac mortality in such patients usually occurs in association with significantly impaired ventricular function. While frequent and complex ventricular ectopy is an independent risk factor, it is not as strong a risk factor as is impaired ventricular function. Moreover, even though ventricular tachycardia and/or fibrillation may be the basis for the sudden death in these patients, this does not a priori establish a cause-and-effect relation between spontaneous ectopy and life-threatening ventricular tachycardia or fibrillation. Very early cycle (R or T) VPCs have been stated by some to increase the risk of sudden death. Although this has been observed during acute ischemia and in the setting of QT prolongation, frequently, ventricular tachycardia or fibrillation is precipitated by VPCs which occur after the T wave of the prior beat.

VPCs are recognized by wide (usually >0.14 s), bizarre QRS complexes that are not preceded by P waves (Fig. 198-4A). Often they bear a relatively fixed relationship to the preceding sinus complex and are thus considered fixed coupled VPCs. When fixed coupling is not present and the interval between VPCs has a common denominator, *ventricular parasystole* is said to be present (Fig. 198-5). Under these circumstances, the VPCs are a manifestation of abnormal automaticity of a protected ventricular focus; because it is not penetrated by sinus impulses, it is not reset by them, and the interectopic intervals remain relatively fixed (≤120 ms variation of mean RR cycle length).

VPCs may occur singly; in patterns of bigeminy, in which every sinus beat is followed by a VPC; in trigeminy, in which two sinus beats are followed by a VPC; in quadrigeminy, etc. Two successive VPCs are termed *pairs* or *couplets*, while three or more consecutive VPCs are termed *ventricular tachycardia* when the rate exceeds 100 beats per minute. VPCs may have similar morphologies (monomorphic, or uniform) or different morphologies (polymorphic, or multiformed) (Fig. 198-4C).

Most commonly, VPCs are not conducted retrogradely to the atrium to reset the sinoatrial node. Thus they produce a fully compensatory pause; i.e., the interval between conducted sinus beats which bracket the VPC equals two basic RR intervals. Ventricular impulses also may manifest retrograde conduction to the atrium and cause inverted P waves in leads II, III, and aVF. The pause that results may therefore be less than compensatory. In many instances, the QRS complex will not be associated with retrograde ventriculoatrial (VA) conduction but may block in the AV node. This renders the AV node refractory to the subsequent sinus beat and causes slowed conduction (i.e., prolonged PR interval) or block of the next sinus P wave. This prolonged PR interval is said to be a manifestation of concealed retrograde conduction of the ventricular impulse into the AV node. A VPC that does not produce any manifestation of retrograde concealed conduction and fails to influence the oncoming sinus impulse is termed an *interpolated VPC*.

VPCs can cause palpitations or neck pulsations secondary to either the occurrence of cannon a waves or the increased force of contraction due to postextrasystolic potentiation of ventricular contractility. Patients with frequent VPCs or bigeminy may rarely develop syncope because the VPCs do not result in an adequate stroke volume and the cardiac output is reduced by the "halving" of the heart rate.

Management In the absence of cardiac disease, isolated asymptomatic VPCs, regardless of configuration and frequency, need no treatment. When arrhythmias are symptomatic, the symptoms should first be addressed by either allaying the patient's anxiety or, if this is not successful, reducing the frequency of the VPCs with antiarrhythmic agents. Beta-adrenergic blockers may be successful in managing

FIGURE 198-4 *A.* Single ventricular ectopy. During sinus rhythm, two premature ventricular complexes (*arrows*) occur. Note that the QRS configuration is bizarre, different from that during sinus rhythm. The premature ventricular complexes are not preceded by P waves. The QRS width of the premature complexes is approximately 160 ms. The pause surrounding the premature complexes is fully compensatory, the sinus beat after the premature complex occurring on time. *B.* A 5-beat run of nonsustained ventricular tachycardia having a uniform morphology (*dots*). Although intraventricular conduction during sinus rhythm is slightly prolonged, during the run of ventricular tachycardia the QRS duration is further prolonged. Note that 2:1 VA conduction is present during ventricular tachycardia. Retrograde P waves are denoted by the arrows. *C.* Simultaneous recordings of ECG leads I, aVF, and V₁. A 4-beat run of polymorphic nonsustained ventricular tachycardia is demonstrated. No two consecutive QRS complexes are the same. Polymorphic VT is not associated with a prolonged QT interval in this case.

VPCs that occur primarily in the daytime or under stressful situations and in specific settings such as mitral valve prolapse and thyrotoxicosis. Quinidine or quinidine-like agents may be tried should this be unsuccessful. In patients with cardiac disease, frequent VPCs are often associated with an increased risk of sudden and nonsudden cardiac death, and many physicians have attempted to eliminate or reduce the frequency of these VPCs in an attempt to reduce this risk. However, the cause-and-effect relationship of the VPCs to fatal events has never been established. The ability of pharmacologic antiarrhythmic therapy guided by continuous ECG monitoring to reduce the risk of sudden death in patients with frequent (≥6 per minute) VPCs was tested by the Cardiac Arrhythmia Suppression Trial (CAST). This study compared mortality in patients whose ectopy was suppressed by one of three agents (encainide, flecainide, or moricizine) and then randomized to treat with either the "effective" drug or placebo. After a mean follow-up of 2 years, the study was discontinued because both the sudden death and overall mortality rate was significantly increased in patients receiving antiarrhythmic agents. This study has shown that in patients having the characteristics of the study population, abolition of ventricular ectopy by pharmacologic

FIGURE 198-5 Ventricular parasystole. At varying sinus cycle lengths during exercise, interectopic intervals remain constant at 1620 to 1640 ms. However, the coupling intervals between sinus and ectopic complexes vary between 510 and 310 ms.

therapy cannot be used as a marker to define reduction of the risk of sudden death after myocardial infarction. Ongoing studies are examining the ability of more advanced techniques, such as electrophysiologic testing, to reduce the rate of sudden death in higher-risk patients, i.e., those with left ventricular ejection fractions of ≤40 and nonsustained VT (≥3 consecutive VPCs).

Antiarrhythmic agents also can produce the lethal arrhythmias which they are given to prevent (proarrhythmic effects). Thus therapy directed toward VPCs in the setting of chronic cardiac disease may result in an inappropriate and costly use of agents without proven efficacy and with potential side effects in many patients. The high incidence of side effects and the frequent exacerbation of arrhythmias caused by all antiarrhythmic drugs make it mandatory to monitor patients being treated with such agents.

In acute myocardial infarction, the greatest incidence of primary ventricular fibrillation occurs within the first 24 h (Chap. 202). Temporary prophylactic antiarrhythmic therapy with lidocaine has therefore been recommended for all patients with acute infarction, regardless of the presence or degree of spontaneous ectopy. However, recently, recognition of the toxicity of lidocaine has led to a reevaluation of this practice. Most physicians now recommend prophylactic lidocaine administration only to young patients with complicated infarctions, where a favorable risk-benefit ratio may be obtained. Other studies have shown that intravenous beta blockers also may reduce the incidence of primary ventricular fibrillation.

TACHYCARDIAS

Tachycardias refer to arrhythmias with three or more complexes at rates exceeding 100 beats per minute; they occur more often in structurally diseased than in normal hearts. Those paroxysmal tachycardias that are initiated by APCs or VPCs are considered to be due to reentry, except some of the digitalis-induced tachyarrhythmias, which are probably due to triggered activity (see below).

If the patient is hemodynamically stable, an attempt should be made to determine the mechanism and origin of the tachycardia, since this will usually lead to an appropriate therapeutic decision. Information to be obtained from the ECG includes (1) the presence, frequency, morphology, and regularity of P waves and QRS complexes, (2) the relationship between atrial and ventricular activity, (3) a comparison of the QRS morphology during sinus rhythm and during the tachycardia, and (4) the response to carotid sinus massage or other vagal maneuvers. It is useful first to compare the ECG during the tachycardia with one recorded during sinus rhythm, and it is often

desirable to record long rhythm strips using surface leads with the largest P waves, usually leads II or V_1. One also can utilize the electrodes situated at the end of a flexible pacing catheter inserted into the esophagus behind the left atrium to record atrial activity.

Carotid sinus pressure should only be applied while the patient is electrocardiographically monitored with resuscitative equipment available to manage the rare episode of asystole and/or ventricular fibrillation associated with this procedure. Carotid sinus massage should not be performed in patients with carotid arterial bruits. The patient should be positioned flat with the neck extended. Massage of one carotid bulb at a time should be performed by applying firm pressure just underneath the angle of the jaw for up to 5 s. Alternative vagomimetic maneuvers include the Valsalva maneuver, immersion of the face in cold water, and administration of 5 to 10 mg edrophonium.

Observation of the jugular venous pulse can provide clues to the presence of atrial activity and its relationship to ventricular ectopy. Intermittent cannon *a* waves suggest AV dissociation, while persistent cannon *a* waves suggest 1:1 VA conduction. Flutter waves may be seen or no atrial activity may be apparent, as in the presence of atrial flutter and fibrillation, respectively. The arterial pulse also may manifest AV dissociation or atrial fibrillation by demonstrating variations in amplitude. A first heart sound of variable intensity during a regular rhythm also suggests AV dissociation or atrial fibrillation.

SINUS TACHYCARDIA In the adult, sinus tachycardia is said to be present when the heart rate exceeds 100 beats per minute; sinus tachycardia rarely exceeds 200 beats per minute and is not a primary arrhythmia; instead, it represents a physiologic response to a variety of stresses, such as fever, volume depletion, anxiety, exercise, thyrotoxicosis, hypoxemia, hypotension, or congestive heart failure. Sinus tachycardia has a gradual onset and offset. The ECG demonstrates P waves with sinus contour preceding each QRS complex. Carotid sinus pressure usually produces modest slowing with a gradual return to the previous rate upon cessation. This contrasts with the response of paroxysmal supraventricular tachycardias, which may slow slightly and terminate abruptly.

Sinus tachycardia should not be treated as a primary arrhythmia, since it is almost always a physiologic response to a demand placed on the heart. As such, the therapy should be directed to the primary disorder. This may involve institution of digitalis and/or diuretics for heart failure and oxygen for hypoxemia, treatment of thyrotoxicosis, volume repletion, aspirin for fever, or tranquilizers for emotional upset.

ATRIAL FIBRILLATION (AF) This common arrhythmia may occur in paroxysmal and persistent forms. It may be seen in normal subjects, particularly during emotional stress or following surgery, exercise, or acute alcoholic intoxication. It also may occur in patients with heart or lung disease who develop acute hypoxia, hypercapnia, or metabolic or hemodynamic derangements. Persistent AF usually occurs in patients with cardiovascular disease, most commonly rheumatic heart disease, nonrheumatic mitral valve disease, hypertensive cardiovascular disease, chronic lung disease, atrial septal defect, and a variety of miscellaneous cardiac abnormalities. AF may be the presenting finding in thyrotoxicosis. So-called lone AF, which occurs in patients without underlying heart disease, is considered to represent the tachycardia phase of the tachycardia-bradycardia syndrome (p. 1013).

The morbidity associated with AF is related to (1) excessive ventricular rate, which in turn may lead to hypotension, pulmonary congestion, or angina pectoris in susceptible individuals, (2) the pause following cessation of AF, which can cause syncope, (3) systemic embolization, which occurs most commonly in patients with rheumatic heart disease, (4) loss of the contribution of atrial contraction to cardiac output, which may cause fatigue, and (5) anxiety secondary to palpitations. In patients with severe cardiac dysfunction, particularly those with hypertrophied, noncompliant ventricles, the combination of the loss of the atrial contribution to ventricular filling and the abbreviated filling period due to the rapid ventricular rate in AF can produce marked hemodynamic embarrassment, resulting in hypotension, syncope, or heart failure. In patients with mitral stenosis, in whom ventricular filling time is critical, development of AF with a rapid ventricular rate may precipitate pulmonary edema (see Chap. 201).

AF is characterized by disorganized atrial activity without discrete P waves on the surface ECG (Fig. 198-3D). Atrial activation is manifested by an undulating baseline or by more sharply inscribed atrial deflections of varying amplitude and frequency ranging from 350 to 600 beats per minute. The ventricular response is irregularly irregular. This results from the large number of atrial impulses which penetrate the AV node, making it partially refractory to subsequent impulses. This effect of nonconducted atrial impulses to influence the response to subsequent atrial impulses is termed *concealed conduction*. As a result, the ventricular response is relatively slow, considering the actual atrial rate. AF may convert to atrial flutter, especially in response to antiarrhythmic drugs like quinidine or flecainide. If AF converts to atrial flutter, which has a slower atrial rate, the effect of concealed conduction may be diminished, and a paradoxic increase in the ventricular response may occur. The main factor determining the rate of the ventricular response is the functional refractory period of the AV node or the most rapid paced rate at which 1:1 conduction through the AV node can be observed.

If, in the presence of AF, the ventricular rhythm becomes regular and slow (e.g., 30 to 60 beats per minute), complete heart block is suggested, and if the ventricular rhythm is regular and rapid (e.g., ≥100 beats per minute), a tachycardia arising in the AV junction or ventricle should be suspected. Digitalis intoxication is a common cause of both phenomena.

Patients with AF exhibit a loss of *a* waves in the jugular venous pulse and variable pulse pressures in the carotid arterial pulse. The first heart sound usually varies in intensity. On echocardiography, the left atrium is frequently enlarged, and in patients in whom the left atrial diameter exceeds 4.5 cm, it may not be possible to convert AF to sinus rhythm or to maintain the latter despite therapy.

Management In acute AF, a precipitating factor such as fever, pneumonia, alcoholic intoxication, thyrotoxicosis, pulmonary emboli, congestive heart failure, or pericarditis should be sought. When such a factor is present, therapy should be directed toward the primary abnormality. If the patient's clinical status is severely compromised, electrical cardioversion is the treatment of choice. In the absence of severe cardiovascular compromise, slowing of ventricular rate becomes the initial therapeutic goal. This may be accomplished with digitalis, calcium channel antagonists, or beta-adrenergic blockers, all of which prolong the refractory period of the AV node and slow conduction within it. Intravenous verapamil usually gives the most rapid response. However, in cases where catecholamine levels or sympathetic nervous system tone is likely to be elevated, beta blockers may be favored. Conversion to sinus rhythm may then be attempted, using quinidine-like (type IA) drugs or flecainide or other type IC drugs (Table 198-1). It is important to increase AV node refractoriness prior to administering such drugs because their vagolytic effect and their ability to convert AF to atrial flutter may reduce the concealed conduction and lead to an excessively rapid ventricular response. Beta-adrenergic blockers are especially useful in this regard. If medical therapy fails to convert AF, electrical cardioversion is useful; it generally requires 100 to 200 W·s of energy. Anticoagulation should be started at least 2 weeks prior to and continued for 2 weeks following any attempt at cardioversion, either pharmacologic or electrical, in patients with long-standing AF. Anticoagulation appears to decrease the incidence of systemic embolization associated with cardioversion. It is less likely for chronic AF to convert to or remain in sinus rhythm in the presence of long-standing rheumatic heart disease and/or when the atria are markedly enlarged. It is also unlikely for patients with lone AF to be converted to and maintained in sinus rhythm.

The goal of therapy in patients in whom AF cannot be converted to sinus rhythm is control of the ventricular response. This can usually

---

TABLE 198-1 Classification of antiarrhythmic drugs

Type I Drugs that reduce maximal velocity of phase of depolarization (V_{max}) due to block of inward Na^+ current in tissue with fast response action potentials

    A ↓ V_{max} at all heart rates and ↑ action potential duration, e.g., quinidine, procainamide, disopyramide

    B Little effect at slow rates on V_{max} in normal tissue; ↓ V_{max} in partially depolarized cells with fast response action potentials
       Effects increased at faster rates
       No change or ↓ in action potential duration, e.g., lidocaine, phenytoin, tocainide, mexiletine

    C ↓ V_{max} at normal rates in normal tissue
       Minimal effect on action potential duration, e.g., flecainide, propafenone, moricizine

Type II Antisympathetic agents, e.g., propranolol and other beta-adrenergic blockers: ↓ SA nodal automaticity, ↑ AV nodal refractoriness, and ↓ AV nodal conduction velocity

Type III Agents that prolong action potential duration in tissue with fast-response action potentials, e.g., bretylium, amiodarone, sotalol

Type IV Calcium (slow) channel blocking agents: ↓ conduction velocity and ↑ refractoriness in tissue with slow-response action potentials, e.g., verapamil, diltiazem

Drugs that cannot be classified by this schema:
    Digitalis
    Adenosine

---

be accomplished by digitalis, beta blockers, or calcium channel blockers singly or in combination. In occasional patients, the ventricular response cannot be controlled by pharmacologic therapy alone. In such patients, the creation of complete heart block by radiofrequency catheter ablation of the AV junction followed by permanent pacemaker implantation is appropriate. Surgical or direct-current catheter ablation of the AV junction is rarely required to achieve AV block.

If sinus rhythm is restored electrically or pharmacologically, quinidine or related agents as well as the type IC agents (e.g., flecainide) or amiodarone may be used to prevent recurrence. In patients in whom cardioversion is unsuccessful or in whom AF is likely to recur, it is probably wisest to allow the patient to remain in AF and to control the ventricular response with calcium antagonists, beta-adrenergic blockers, or digitalis glycosides. Since such patients are always at risk of systemic embolization, chronic anticoagulation must be considered. Several studies have now demonstrated conclusively that the incidence of embolization in patients with AF not associated with valvular heart disease is reduced by chronic anticoagulation with warfarin-like agents. Aspirin also may be effective for this purpose, but the data supporting its use are less extensive.

ATRIAL FLUTTER This arrhythmia occurs most often in patients with organic heart disease. Flutter may be paroxysmal, in which case there is usually a precipitating factor, such as pericarditis or acute respiratory failure, or it may be persistent. Atrial flutter (as well as AF) is very common during the first week following open heart surgery. Atrial flutter is usually less long-lived than is AF, although on occasion it may persist for months to years. Most commonly, if it lasts for more than a week, atrial flutter will convert to AF. Systemic embolization is less common in atrial flutter than in AF.

Atrial flutter is characterized by an atrial rate between 250 and 350 beats per minute. Typically, the ventricular rate is half the atrial rate, i.e., approximately 150 beats per minute. If the atrial rate is slowed to <220 beats per minute by antiarrhythmic agents such as quinidine, which also possess vagolytic properties, the ventricular rate may rise suddenly because of the development of 1:1 AV conduction. Classically, flutter waves are seen as regular sawtooth-like atrial activity, most prominent in the inferior leads (Fig. 198-3C). When the ventricular response is regular and not a simple fraction of the atrial rate, complete AV block is present, which may be a manifestation of digitalis toxicity. Activation mapping suggests that atrial flutter is a form of atrial reentry localized to the low right atrium.

Management The most effective treatment of atrial flutter is direct-current cardioversion, which can be accomplished at low energy

(10 to 50 W·s) under mild sedation. In patients who develop atrial flutter following open-heart surgery or recurrent flutter in the setting of acute myocardial infarction, particularly when they are being treated with digitalis, atrial pacing (using temporary pacing wires implanted at the time of operation or a pacing lead inserted into the atrium pervenously) at rates of 115 to 130 percent of the atrial flutter rate can usually convert the atrial flutter to sinus rhythm. Atrial pacing also may result in the conversion of atrial flutter to AF, which allows for easier control of the ventricular response. If immediate conversion of atrial flutter is not mandated by the patient's clinical status, the ventricular response should first be slowed by blocking the AV node with a beta blocker, calcium antagonist, or digitalis; the last drug occasionally converts atrial flutter into AF. Once AV nodal conduction is slowed with any of these drugs, an attempt to convert flutter to sinus rhythm using quinidine or quinidine-like agents should be made. Increasing doses of the drug selected are administered until the rhythm converts or side effects occur.

Quinidine, quinidine-like drugs, flecainide, propafenone, and amiodarone (Table 198-2) may be useful in preventing recurrences of both atrial flutter and atrial fibrillation.

PAROXYSMAL SUPRAVENTRICULAR TACHYCARDIAS (PSVT)
In most cases, functional differences in conduction and refractoriness in the AV node or the presence of an AV bypass tract provide the substrate for the development of PSVT (previously termed *paroxysmal atrial tachycardia*). Electrophysiologic studies have demonstrated that reentry is the mechanism responsible for the vast majority of cases of PSVT (Fig. 198-6). Reentry has been localized to the sinus node, atrium, AV node, or a macroreentrant circuit involving conduction in the antegrade direction through the AV node and retrograde through an AV bypass tract. Such a bypass tract also may conduct antegradely, in which case the Wolff-Parkinson-White (WPW) syndrome is said to be present. More frequently, however, the bypass tract manifests only retrograde conduction, and therefore it is termed a *concealed bypass tract* (Fig. 198-6B). In these cases, the QRS complex during sinus rhythm is normal. In the absence of the WPW syndrome, reentry through the AV node or through a concealed bypass tract makes up more than 90 percent of all PSVTs.

AV NODAL REENTRANT TACHYCARDIA
There is no age or disease predisposition for the development of AV nodal reentrant tachycardia, the most common cause of supraventricular tachycardia. It is, however, more commonly observed in women. It usually presents as a narrow QRS complex with regular rates ranging from 120 to 250 beats per minute. APCs that initiate the arrhythmia are almost always associated with a prolonged PR interval. Retrograde P waves may be absent, buried in the QRS complex, or appear as distortions at the terminal parts of the QRS complex (Fig. 198-6A).

AV nodal reentrant PSVT (Fig. 198-7) can be reproducibly initiated and terminated by appropriately timed atrial premature extrastimuli. The onset of the tachycardia is almost always associated with prolongation of the PR interval due to marked AV nodal conduction delay (prolonged AH interval) following the APC that is critical for the genesis of the arrhythmia. The sudden prolongation of the AH interval is consistent with the concept of dual AV nodal pathways: (1) a beta (fast) pathway, which exhibits rapid conduction and a long refractory period, and (2) an alpha (slow) pathway, which has a short refractory period but conducts slowly. During sinus rhythm, only conduction over the fast pathway is manifest, resulting in a normal PR interval. The normal sinus impulse, which simultaneously conducts down the slow pathway, reaches the His bundle after it has been depolarized and is therefore refractory. Atrial extrastimuli at a

critical coupling interval are blocked in the beta pathway because of its longer refractory period and are conducted slowly through the alpha pathway. If conduction down the alpha pathway is slow enough to allow the previously refractory beta pathway time to recover excitability, a single atrial echo or sustained tachycardia ensues. A critical balance between conduction velocity and refractoriness within the node is required to sustain AV nodal reentry. Retrograde atrial and antegrade ventricular activation occur simultaneously, explaining why P waves may not be apparent on the surface ECG.

Clinical features   AV nodal reentry may produce palpitations, syncope, and heart failure depending on the rate and duration of the arrhythmia and the presence and severity of any underlying heart disease. Hypotension and syncope may occur because of the sudden loss of the atrial contribution to ventricular filling; this also can lead to a marked increase in atrial pressure, acute pulmonary edema, and a reduction in ventricular filling. Simultaneous atrial and ventricular contraction produces cannon *a* waves with each heartbeat.

Treatment   In patients without hypotension, vagal maneuvers, particularly carotid sinus massage, can terminate the arrhythmia in 80 percent of cases. If hypotension is present, raising the blood pressure by the cautious use of intravenous phenylephrine in 0.1-mg increments may terminate the arrhythmia alone or in combination with carotid sinus pressure. If these maneuvers are unsuccessful, verapamil (2.5 to 10 mg intravenously) or adenosine (6 to 12 mg intravenously) is the agent of choice. We prefer to use adenosine because of its extremely short half-life, lessening the consequences of any side effects. Propranolol (0.05 to 0.2 mg/kg intravenously) or other beta blockers also may be used to slow or terminate the tachycardia but are agents of second choice. Digitalis glycosides have a slower onset of action and should not be used for acute therapy. When these drugs fail to terminate the tachycardia, or when the tachycardia is recurrent, atrial or ventricular pacing via a temporary pacemaker inserted pervenously may be used to terminate the arrhythmia. However, if severe ischemia and/or hypotension is caused by the tachycardia, dc cardioversion should be considered.

AV nodal reentry can usually be prevented by the use of drugs that act primarily on the antegrade slow pathway (such as digitalis, beta blockers, or calcium channel antagonists) or on the fast pathway (such as quinidine-like agents and newer drugs such as flecainide, propafenone, and amiodarone). We favor as initial therapy digitalis, beta blockers, or calcium channel antagonists because the risk-benefit ratio associated with treatment with these agents is more favorable than that of IA or IC agents. Drugs most likely to avert recurrences prevent induction of the arrhythmias by programmed stimulation. This technique utilizes temporary pacemaker catheters connected to a physiologic stimulator capable of variable rate pacing and stimulation with one or more precisely timed premature impulses. In symptomatic patients who require chronic therapy, radiofrequency catheter modification of AV nodal function has recently acquired first-line treatment status. This technique can cure AV nodal reeentry in >90 percent of cases and has been proven to be safe, although a 1 to 5 percent risk of AV block requiring a permanent pacemaker exists.

AV REENTRANT TACHYCARDIA
PSVT due to AV reentry incorporates a concealed AV bypass tract (i.e., one that conducts only retrogradely) as part of the tachycardia circuit. Thus the impulse passes antegradely from the atria through the AV node and His-Purkinje system to the ventricles and then retrogradely through the (concealed) bypass tract back to the atrium. Patients with this disorder manifest the same type of PSVT as do patients with the WPW syndrome (see below), but the bypass tract cannot conduct in an

FIGURE 198-6 Examples of reentrant PSVT. *A.* AV nodal reentry. No P waves are visible. *B.* AV reentry using a concealed bypass tract. Inverted retrograde P waves are superimposed on the T wave. *C.* Intraatrial reentry. P waves precede the QRS complex.

FIGURE 198-7 Mechanism of AV nodal reentry: The atrium, AV node (AVN), and His bundle are shown schematically. The AV node is longitudinally dissociated into two pathways, with different functional properties. The alpha pathway conducts relatively slowly while the beta pathway conducts rapidly (see text). In each panel of this diagram, heavy lines denote excitation in the AV node which is manifest on the surface electrocardiogram, while light lines denote conduction which is concealed and not apparent on the surface electrocardiogram. *A.* During sinus rhythm (NSR) the impulse from the atrium conducts down both pathways. However, only conduction over the fast (beta) pathway is manifest on the surface ECG, producing a normal PR interval of 0.16 s. *B.* An atrial premature depolarization (APD) blocks in the beta pathway. The impulse conducts over the alpha pathway to the His bundle and ventricles, producing a PR interval of 0.24 s. Because the impulse is premature, conduction over the alpha pathway occurs more slowly than it would during sinus rhythm. *C.* A more premature atrial impulse blocks in the beta pathway, conducting with increased delay in the alpha pathway, producing a PR interval of 0.28 s. The impulse conducts retrogradely up the beta pathway producing a single atrial echo. Sustained reentry is prevented by subsequent block in the alpha pathway. *D.* A still more premature atrial impulse blocks initially in the beta pathway, conducting over the alpha pathway with increasing delay producing a PR interval of 0.36 s. Retrograde conduction occurs over the beta pathway and reentry occurs, producing a sustained tachycardia (SVT). (*After Josephson.*)

antegrade direction during sinus rhythm or other atrial tachyarrhythmias.

AV reentrant tachycardia can be initiated and terminated by either APCs or VPCs. Alternation of the QRS complexes and/or T wave occurs in approximately one-third of such tachycardias. Since atrial activation must follow ventricular activation during AV reentry, the P wave usually occurs after the QRS complex (see Fig. 198-6*B*).

Atrial activation mapping is of major value in evaluating the origin of these tachycardias. Most concealed bypass tracts are left-sided. Thus, during supraventricular tachycardia or during ventricular pacing, the earliest activation sequence is recorded in the left atrium, usually via a catheter in the coronary sinus (Fig. 198-8). This eccentric atrial activation is quite distinct from the normal retrograde activation sequence in which the earliest activation of the atria is in the area of the AV junction. The ability of a ventricular stimulus to conduct to the atrium at a time when the bundle of His is refractory and the termination of the tachycardia by a ventricular stimulus that does not reach the atrium are diagnostic of retrograde conduction over a concealed bypass tract.

Treatment is similar to that for AV nodal reentry tachycardia. Although pharmacologic agents may be used, at this time, patients who require chronic therapy should be considered candidates for radiofrequency catheter ablation of the bypass tract. This requires detailed electrophysiologic study to exclude other arrhythmias which may be responsible for patients' symptoms and to determine the location of the bypass tract(s). The efficacy of this procedure exceeds 90 percent, with minimal risks. In the remaining small number of patients failing catheter ablation, surgical ablation should be considered.

SINUS NODE REENTRY AND OTHER ATRIAL TACHYCARDIAS
Reentry in the region of the sinus node or within the atria is invariably initiated by APCs. These arrhythmias are less common than AV nodal or AV reentry and are more often associated with underlying cardiac disease. During sinus node reentry, the P-wave morphology is identical to that occurring in sinus rhythm, but the PR interval is prolonged. This is in contrast to sinus tachycardia, in which the PR interval tends to shorten. With intraatrial reentry, the P-wave configuration differs from that during sinus rhythm, and the PR interval is prolonged (see Fig. 198-6*C*).

Treatment Sinus node and atrial reentrant arrhythmias are managed like other reentrant PSVTs except that catheter ablation is less successful because multiple foci may be present.

NONREENTRANT ATRIAL TACHYCARDIAS
These may be a manifestation of digitalis intoxication or may be associated with severe pulmonary or cardiac disease, with hypokalemia, or with the administration of theophylline or adrenergic drugs. The last frequently present as multifocal atrial tachycardias (MAT) (Fig. 198-9). By definition, MAT requires three or more consecutive P waves of different morphologies at rates greater than 100 beats per minute. MAT usually has an irregular ventricular rate because of varying AV conduction. There is a high incidence of atrial fibrillation (50 to 70 percent) in patients with MAT. Treatment should be directed at the underlying disorder. The digitalis-induced arrhythmias may be caused by triggered activity and/or enhanced automaticity. In such atrial

TABLE 198-2 Drugs used to treat cardiac tachyarrhythmias

Drug	Sinus node	Atrium and ventricle	AV node	His-Purkinje system	AV bypass tracts
ELECTROPHYSIOLOGIC EFFECTS					
Digoxin and other cardiac glycosides	NC; pts with sinus node disease may develop sinus exit block or arrest	Controversial	↑ ERP, ↓ conduction velocity, due to drug action and vagomimetic effects	NC	NC or ↓ ERP
Adenosine	↓ automaticity	Atrium: ↓ ERP Ventricle: no effect	↓ conduction velocity		
Quinidine (type IA)	NC; may suppress sinus node if node disease exists	↑ ERP; ↓ conduction velocity	↓ or NC in ERP; NC in conduction velocity	↓ automaticity; ↓ conduction velocity; ↑ ERP	↑ ERP may abolish all conduction
Procainamide (type IA)	NC	↑ ERP; ↓ conduction velocity	↓ or NC in ERP; ↓ or NC in conduction velocity	↓ automaticity; ↓ conduction velocity; ↑ ERP	↑ ERP may abolish conduction
Disopyramide (type IIA)	NC	↑ ERP; ↓ conduction velocity	↓ or NC in ERP; NC in conduction velocity	↓ automaticity; ↑ ERP; ↓ conduction velocity	↑ ERP may abolish conduction
Lidocaine (type IB)	NC	NC in ERP	NC or ↓ in ERP	NC or ↓ ERP	NC, ↓, or ↑ in ERP
Phenytoin (type IB)	NC	NC in ERP	NC or ↓ in ERP; NC or ↑ in conduction velocity	↓ in ERP; ↓ automaticity	
Tocainide (type IB)	NC	NC	NC	NC; ↓ automaticity	↑ ERP
Mexiletine (type IB)	NC; pts with sinus node disease may develop sinus arrest	NC	Variable and inconsistent effects on conduction and refractoriness	↑ ERP; NC or ↓ conduction velocity	
Flecainide (type IC)	NC; pts with sinus node disease may develop exit block or arrest	↓ conduction velocity; ↑ ERP	↓ conduction velocity; ↑ ERP	↓ conduction velocity	↓ conduction velocity; ↑ ERP; may abolish all conduction
Propafenone (type IC) (also beta blocker)	No significant effect	↓ conduction velocity; ↑ ERP	↓ in conduction velocity; ↑ ERP	↓ conduction velocity; ↑ ERP	↑ ERP
Moricizine (type 1C)	No significant effect	Atrium: NC in ERP; ↓ conduction velocity Ventricle: slight increase in ERP; ↓ conduction velocity	↓ conduction velocity	↓ conduction velocity	
Propranolol (type II)	↓ sinus rate; ↑ sinus node recovery time	NC	↑ ERP; ↓ conduction velocity	NC	NC
Bretylium (type III)	Initial increase in sinus rate, followed by decrease	↑ ERP	NC	NC	
Amiodarone (type III)	↓ sinus rate	↑ ERP	↑ ERP; ↓ conduction velocity	↑ ERP; ↓ conduction velocity	↑ ERP
Sotalol (type III) (also beta blocker)	↓ sinus rate	↑ ERP	↑ ERP; ↓ conduction velocity	↑ ERP	↑ ERP

ABBREVIATIONS: NC = no change; ↑ = increase; ↓ = decrease.

TABLE 198-2 Drugs used to treat cardiac tachyarrhythmias *(continued)*

Indications	Side effects and toxicity

CLINICAL EFFECTS

Slowing of ventricular rate during AF, flutter, and other atrial tachycardias in the absence of preexcitation; slowing, termination and/or prevention of SVT due to AV nodal reentry and AV reentry utilizing bypass tracts; may terminate or prevent intraatrial reentrant tachycardias; ineffective in prevention of automatic atrial tachycardias	Atrial tachycardia, VT, AV nodal block, accelerated junctional rhythms, atrial and ventricular premature depolarizations, VT, VF, anorexia, nausea, vomiting, acceleration of ventricular rate during AF/flutter in the presence of preexcitation causing VF
Acute termination of regular reentrant SVT involving the AV node	Transient atrial standstill following termination of SVT; transient hypotension
Atrial and ventricular extrasystoles; atrial and ventricular tachyarrhythmias; all types of SVT; control of ventricular rate in pts with preexcitation and AF and flutter	Anorexia, nausea, vomiting, diarrhea, cinchonism, tinnitus, confusion, hearing and visual changes; thrombocytopenia, hemolytic anemia, rash, drug interactions, elevation of digoxin levels; phenytoin and phenobarbital will decrease quinidine levels; QT prolongation associated with polymorphic VT (torsades de pointes); conversion of nonsustained to sustained acceleration of ventricular response to atrial flutter and fibrillation
Same as quinidine	Anorexia, nausea, confusion, hallucinations, agranulocytosis, and lupus erythematosus–like syndrome; QT prolongation associated with polymorphic VT (torsades de pointes); marked elevations in the primary metabolic rate (NAPA); may be more likely to cause polymorphic VT; conversion of nonsustained to sustained VT; acceleration of ventricular response to atrial flutter and fibrillation
Same as quinidine	Anticholinergic actions, including dry mouth, blurred vision, urinary retention, hesitancy, constipation, narrow-angle glaucoma, congestive heart failure, especially in patient with abnormal ventricular function and QT prolongation associated with polymorphic VT (torsades de pointes)
Same as quinidine	Dizziness, paresthesias, confusion, delirium, seizures, coma; may depress sinus node in pts with underlying sinus node disease; may suppress escape foci in pts with complete heart block; congestive heart failure or liver disease increases risk of side effects
VT and VF, especially during acute ischemia and myocardial infarction	Gingival hypertrophy, rash, blood dyscrasias, nystagmus, ataxia, stupor, coma, lupus erythematosus syndrome, lymph node hyperplasia, peripheral neuropathy, hypocalcemia, hyperglycemia, phlebitis, and hypotension during IV administration
Tachyarrhythmias induced by digitalis; occasionally effective for ventricular tachyarrhythmias not induced by digitalis, alone or in combination with other antiarrhythmic agents; polymorphic VT associated with increased QT	Ataxia, tremor, paresthesias, light-headedness, nausea, rash, lupus erythematosus syndrome, pulmonary fibrosis, bone marrow suppression; may exacerbate heart failure in pts with ventricular dysfunction
VT, VF, frequent VPCs	Nausea, vomiting, ataxia, tremor, gait disturbances, rash
Refractory atrial and ventricular tachyarrhythmias; SVT due to AV node reentry and AV bypass tracts	Refractory polymorphic VT without increased QT if dose is increased too rapidly or in pts with abnormal conduction system; sinus arrest in pts with normal sinus node function; nausea, dizziness, blurred vision; may precipitate heart failure in pts with ventricular dysfunction
Refractory atrial and ventricular tachyarrhythmias; SVT due to AV node reentry and AV bypass tracts	May exacerbate arrhythmias (increase frequency, convert nonsustained to sustained tachycardias); negative inotropic actions may worsen CHF; beta-blocking activity may worsen asthma, AV block, visual blurring, dizziness, paresthesias, taste disturbances
Atrial tachyarrhythmias including AF, SVT (not approved by the FDA for therapy of these arrhythmias), ventricular tachycardias	Increase in VPCs, new VT, sudden death (very rare), sinus pause, sinus arrest; prolongation of P-R and QRS intervals, nausea, headache, dizziness
Slowing of ventricular rate during AF, atrial flutter, and other atrial tachycardias in the absence of preexcitation; SVT due to AV nodal reentry, reentry utilizing bypass tracts; arrhythmias induced by exercise; arrhythmias occurring in the presence of hyperthyroidism; polymorphic VT associated with congenital long QT syndrome.	Sinus bradycardia, AV node block, congestive heart failure, bronchospasm, masking symptoms of hypoglycemia
Atrial and ventricular tachyarrhythmias (not FDA approved for atrial arrhythmias)	May exacerbate ventricular tachycardia; dizziness, nausea
Refractory VT and VF, especially due to acute ischemia	Initially, transient hypertension; subsequent hypotension increased in upright position; the hypotensive effect can be prevented by tricyclic drugs; nausea, vomiting
Refractory atrial and ventricular tachyarrhythmias; refractory SVT due to AV nodal reentry and AV reentry utilizing bypass tracts; not approved by FDA for atrial arrhythmias; atrial and ventricular extrasystoles and tachyrhythmias (not yet approved by the FDA)	Marked sinus bradycardia, complete heart block; IV administration may cause hypotension; increased QT associated with polymorphic VT; increased T_4, hypo- and hyperthyroidism; peripheral neuropathy; proximal myopathy, pulmonary fibrosis; increased liver enzymes; hepatitis; blue-gray skin discoloration; corneal microdeposits; elevation of digoxin levels; potential of oral coagulants; exacerbation of CHF, polymorphic VT associated with QT prolongation

FIGURE 198-8 Intracardiac recordings during supraventricular tachycardia using a left-sided AV bypass tract. Intracardiac recordings during sinus rhythm (NSR) and in supraventricular tachycardia (SVT) are shown. ECG leads I, aVF, and V_1 are displayed with electrograms from the high right atrium (HRA), coronary sinus (CS), His bundle (HBE), and right ventricle (RV). During NSR, the QRS complex and the AH and HV intervals are normal. During SVT the retrograde atrial activation sequence is abnormal. The earliest site of atrial activation is in the CS, which is followed by activation in the HBE and HRA. This activation sequence is diagnostic of a left-sided AV bypass tract conduction retrogradely from ventricle to atrium *[From ME Josephson, in Update IV, Harrison's Principles of Internal Medicine, KJ Isselbacher et al (eds), New York, McGraw-Hill, 1983; used with permission.]*

tachycardias with AV block secondary to digitalis intoxication (see Fig. 198-3*B*), the atrial rate rarely exceeds 180 beats per minute, and typically 2:1 block is present. Atrial arrhythmias precipitated by digitalis usually can be treated by withdrawal of the drug.

Automatic atrial tachycardias not caused by digitalis are difficult to terminate, and in such cases the main goal of therapy should be to control the ventricular response, either by drugs which affect the AV node, such as digitalis, beta blockers, or calcium channel antagonists, or by ablation techniques. Catheter ablation and surgery have been employed to eradicate the arrhythmia's focus or create heart block for rate control.

PREEXCITATION (WPW) SYNDROME The most frequently encountered type of ventricular preexcitation is that associated with AV bypass tracts. These connections are composed of strands of atrial-like muscle which may occur almost anywhere around the AV rings. The term *Wolff-Parkinson-White (WPW) syndrome* is applied to patients with both preexcitation on the ECG and paroxysmal tachycardias. AV bypass tracts can be associated with certain congenital abnormalities, the most important of which is Ebstein's anomaly.

AV bypass tracts that conduct in an antegrade direction produce a typical ECG pattern of a short PR interval (<0.12 s), a slurred upstroke of the QRS complex (delta wave), and a wide QRS complex. This pattern results from a fusion of activation of the ventricles over both the bypass tract and the AV nodal His-Purkinje system (Fig. 198-10). The relative contribution of activation over each system determines the amount of preexcitation.

During PSVT in WPW, the impulse is usually conducted antegradely over the normal AV system and retrogradely through the bypass tract. The characteristics are identical to those described on p. 1024. Rarely (approximately 5 percent), tachycardias occurring in patients with WPW will exhibit a reverse pattern with antegrade conduction through the bypass tract and retrograde conduction through the normal AV system. This produces a tachycardia with a wide QRS complex in which the ventricles are totally activated by the bypass

tract. Atrial flutter and AF also occur commonly in patients with WPW syndrome. Since the bypass tract does not have the same decremental conducting properties as the AV node, the ventricular responses during atrial flutter or fibrillation may be unusually rapid (see Fig. 198-3*E*) and may cause ventricular fibrillation.

The goals of electrophysiologic evaluation in patients suspected of having the WPW syndrome are (1) to confirm the diagnosis, (2) to localize the bypass tract and determine how many bypass tracts are present, (3) to demonstrate the role of the bypass tract in the genesis of the arrhythmias, (4) to determine the potential for the development of possibly life-threatening rates during atrial flutter or fibrillation, and (5) to evaluate therapeutic options.

Management Pharmacologic therapy is aimed at altering the electrophysiologic properties (i.e., refractoriness or conduction velocity) of one or more components of the reentrant circuit. This is most often accomplished by agents such as beta blockers or calcium channel blockers that slow conduction and increase refractoriness of the AV node or by agents such as quinidine or flecainide that slow conduction and increase refractoriness primarily in the bypass tract. Some drugs may affect multiple sites (Fig. 198-11).

Acute management of episodes of PSVT in patients with WPW syndrome is similar to that of PSVT in patients with concealed bypass tracts.

In patients with the WPW syndrome and AF, dc cardioversion should be carried out if there is a life-threatening, rapid ventricular response. Alternatively, lidocaine (3 to 5 mg/kg) or procainamide (15 mg/kg) administered intravenously over 15 to 20 min will usually slow the ventricular response. Caution should be employed when using digitalis or intravenous verapamil in patients with the WPW syndrome and AF, since these drugs can shorten the refractory period of the accessory pathway and can increase the ventricular rate, thereby placing the patient at increased risk for ventricular fibrillation. Chronic oral therapy with verapamil is not associated with this risk. In addition to these drugs, beta-blocking agents are of no utility in controlling

FIGURE 198-9 Multifocal atrial tachycardia. A lead I rhythm strip demonstrates a multifocal atrial tachycardia defined by ≥3 consecutive P waves of variable morphology and rate >100 beats per minute (*arrows*).

FIGURE 198-10 ECG in WPW syndrome. There is a short PR interval (0.11 s), a wide QRS complex (0.12 s), and slurring on the upstroke of the QRS produced by early ventricular activation over the bypass tract (delta wave, d in lead I). The negative delta waves in V_1 are diagnostic of a right-sided bypass tract. Note the Q wave (negative delta wave) in lead III, mimicking myocardial infarction.

the ventricular response during AF when conduction proceeds over the bypass tract. Although atrial or ventricular pacing can almost always terminate PSVT in patients with the WPW syndrome, they can induce AF. As such, chronic pacemaker therapy is to be discouraged.

Successful surgical ablation of bypass tracts is possible in more than 90 percent of cases and offers a permanent cure of SVT and most AFs associated with SVT. However, with the advent of radiofrequency catheter ablation, the need for surgery has been virtually eliminated. Catheter ablation of bypass tracts is possible in more than 90 percent of patients and is the treatment of choice in patients with symptomatic arrhythmias. It is safer, more cost-effective, and just as successful as surgery. Nevertheless, surgical ablation may be required in the occasional patient in whom catheter ablation fails.

NONPAROXYSMAL JUNCTIONAL TACHYCARDIA This rhythm usually results from conditions that produce enhanced automaticity or triggered activity in the AV junction and is most commonly due to digitalis intoxication, inferior wall myocardial infarction,

FIGURE 198-11 Site of action of antiarrhythmic agents in the WPW syndrome. The atrium, ventricle, antegrade conduction through the AV node (↓), retrograde conduction through the AV node (↑), and the bypass tract are shown. Drugs on the left affect antegrade AV nodal conduction. Type IA drugs on the upper right affect retrograde conduction over the node and antegrade conduction over the bypass tract. Drugs on the lower right affect conduction in both directions in the AV node and the bypass tract.

myocarditis, endogenous or exogenous catecholamine excess, acute rheumatic fever, or aftereffects of valve surgery.

The onset of nonparoxysmal junctional tachycardia is usually gradual, with a "warm-up" period prior to stabilization of the rate, which can range from 70 to 150 beats per minute, faster rates usually being associated with digitalis intoxication. Nonparoxysmal junctional tachycardia is recognized by a QRS complex identical to that of sinus rhythm. The rate can be influenced by autonomic tone and can be increased by catecholamines, vagolytic agents, or exercise and slowed somewhat by carotid sinus pressure. When this rhythm is due to digitalis intoxication, it usually is associated with AV block and/or dissociation. Soon after cardiac surgery, retrograde conduction is more likely to be present because of the heightened sympathetic state.

Management This is directed toward elimination of the underlying etiologic factors. Since digitalis is the most common cause of this rhythm, discontinuation of this drug is indicated. If the rhythm is associated with other serious manifestations of digitalis intoxication, such as ventricular or atrial irritability, active intervention with lidocaine or a beta blocker may be useful, and in some instances, use of digitalis antibodies (Fab fragments) should be considered. Cardioversion of this rhythm should not be attempted, particularly in the setting of digitalis intoxication. When AV conduction is intact, atrial pacing can capture and override the junctional focus and provide the AV synchrony necessary to maximize cardiac output. Nonparoxysmal junctional tachycardia usually is not a chronic, recurrent problem, and attention to the acute precipitating events can often resolve the tachycardia.

VENTRICULAR TACHYCARDIA (VT) *Sustained VT* is defined as *ventricular tachycardia* that persists for more than 30 s or requires termination because of hemodynamic collapse. VT generally accompanies some form of structural heart disease, most commonly chronic ischemic heart disease associated with a prior myocardial infarction. Sustained VT also may be associated with nonischemic cardiomyopathies, metabolic disorders, drug toxicity, or prolonged QT syndrome, and it occurs occasionally in the absence of heart disease or other predisposing factors. Nonsustained VT (three beats per 30 s) is also associated with cardiac disease but occurs in its absence more often than the sustained arrhythmia. While nonsustained VT usually does not produce symptoms, sustained VT is almost always symptomatic and is often associated with marked hemodynamic embarrassment and/or the development of myocardial ischemia. A fixed anatomic substrate, not acute ischemia, is responsible for most recurrent episodes of sustained uniform VT. Acute ischemia appears to have little role in the genesis of sustained uniform VT associated with chronic infarction but may play a role in the degeneration of stable VT into ventricular fibrillation (VF) or initiation of polymorphic VT. Most episodes of VF begin with VT.

The ECG diagnosis of VT is suggested by a wide-complex QRS tachycardia at a rate exceeding 100 beats per minute. The QRS configuration during any episode of VT may be uniform (monomorphic) (Figs. 198-4*B* and 198-12), or it may vary from beat to beat (polymorphic) (Fig. 198-4*C*). *Bidirectional tachycardia* refers to VT that shows an alternation in QRS amplitude and axis. Typically this appears as a QRS with a right bundle branch block pattern with alternating superior and inferior axes. While the rhythm is usually quite regular, slight irregularity may exist. Atrial activity may be dissociated from ventricular activity (Fig. 198-13), or the atria may be depolarized retrogradely. The onset of the tachycardia is generally abrupt, but in nonparoxysmal tachycardias it can be gradual. Paroxysmal VT is usually initiated by a VPC.

It is important to distinguish supraventricular tachycardia with aberration of intraventricular conduction from VT because the clinical implications and management of these two arrhythmias are totally different (Fig. 198-14). The most important clinical predictor of VT is the presence of structural heart disease. In a majority of cases, the diagnosis can and should be made by close examination of the 12-lead ECG. Pharmacologic maneuvers, such as administration of intravenous verapamil or adenosine, can be hazardous and should be

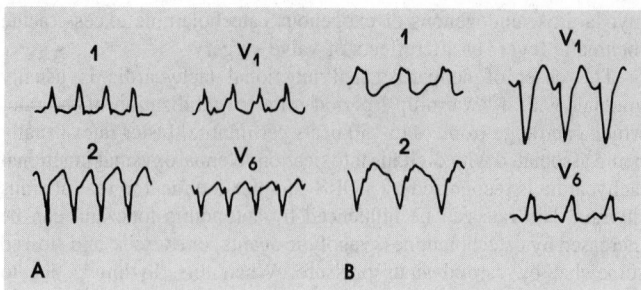

FIGURE 198-12 *A.* Sustained ventricular tachycardia having a uniform morphology. The QRS configuration in V_1 is a right bundle branch block type of configuration. Marked leftward frontal plane axis is present, denoted by the QS complex in lead II. The R/S ratio in lead V_6 is less than 1. The QRS width is greater than 140 ms. Note that 2:1 VA conduction is present with retrograde P waves present after every other QRS complex (best seen in leads I and V_1). *B.* Sustained ventricular tachycardia with a uniform, left bundle branch block type morphology (lead V_1). The QRS width is greater than 160 ms, and there are a Q wave in lead V_6 and a broad initial R wave in V_1, all favoring ventricular tachycardia rather than supraventricular tachycardia with aberrant conduction.

avoided. It is always useful to have a 12-lead ECG recorded during sinus rhythm for comparison with that during tachycardia. When the tracing obtained during sinus rhythm demonstrates a bundle branch block pattern with the same morphologic features as those during the tachycardia, the diagnosis of supraventricular tachycardia is favored. An infarction pattern on the sinus rhythm tracing suggests the potential presence of the anatomic substrate necessary for VT. Characteristics of the 12-lead ECG during the tachycardia that suggest a ventricular origin for the arrhythmia are (1) a QRS complex >0.14 s in the absence of antiarrhythmic therapy, (2) AV dissociation (with or without fusion or captured beats) or variable retrograde conduction, (3) a superior QRS axis in the presence of a right bundle branch block pattern, (4) concordance of the QRS pattern in all precordial leads (i.e., all positive or all negative deflections), and (5) other QRS patterns with prolonged duration that are inconsistent with typical right or left bundle branch block patterns. A wide, complex, bizarre tachycardia that is very irregular suggests AF with conduction over an AV bypass tract (see Fig. 198-3E). Similarly, a QRS complex in excess of 0.20 s is uncommon during VT in the absence of drug therapy and is more common with preexcitation. Intravenous verapamil will stop most recalcitrant supraventricular tachycardias involving the AV junction, but it is rarely effective for ventricular tachycardia. Because of this property, verapamil has been utilized to attempt to differentiate supraventricular tachycardia with aberrant conduction from ventricular tachycardia. However, this is extremely hazardous, since intravenous verapamil frequently precipitates cardiac arrest in patients with ventricular tachycardias.

FIGURE 198-13 Ventricular tachycardia with AV dissociation. P waves which are totally dissociated from the underlying ventricular rhythm are noted in lead III by arrows. AV dissociation is highly suggestive of ventricular tachycardia. In V_1 fusion complexes are present and denoted by arrows, confirming AV dissociation.

FIGURE 198-14 Intracardiac recordings distinguishing supraventricular tachycardia from ventricular tachycardia. ECG leads I, aVF, and V_1 are shown with a His bundle electrogram (HBE) and time line (TL). Wide QRS complex tachycardia with a right bundle branch block morphology are shown on the left and right panels. On the left, supraventricular tachycardia is diagnosed by the presence of His deflection (H) preceding each QRS complex, with normal HV interval. On the right, during ventricular tachycardia no His bundle deflections can be seen (*arrow*) and AV dissociation is observed (note single atrial deflection, A). *(From JA Kastor et al, N Engl J Med 304:1004, 1981; reprinted by permission.)*

The diagnosis of VT can be confirmed by analyzing the relationship between the electrogram recording from the His bundle and ventricular activity. In most cases of VT, the His deflection is not easily seen, but when visible, the interval from the His deflection to the onset of ventricular activation (HV interval) is less than that recorded during sinus rhythm, or negative due to retrograde activation over the His-Purkinje system, or is dissociated from ventricular activation (see Fig. 198-14). During SVT with aberrant conduction, the HV interval is greater than or equal to that recorded during sinus rhythm. In patients with a wide QRS complex tachycardia, the diagnosis of VT is confirmed when atrial pacing at rates equal to or greater than that of the tachycardia produces normalization of the QRS complex with a normal HV interval. Regardless of QRS morphology [left or right bundle branch block patterns (see Fig. 198-12)], VT due to ischemic heart disease arises from the *left* ventricle, in most instances near the subendocardium.

It has been possible to replicate sustained uniform VT in more than 95 percent of patients with this arrhythmia using programmed stimulation. In most patients the tachycardia is initiated with ventricular premature stimuli. A sustained monomorphic VT with a morphology identical to that of the spontaneous arrhythmia is the rule. The clinical significance of polymorphic VT initiated by programmed stimulation is not clear. It has been shown that when more aggressive stimulation is performed (i.e., the use of three or four extrastimuli), polymorphic VT and even VF can be induced in some normal subjects and in patients who have never had a clinical arrhythmia.

Sustained uniform VT can be terminated by programmed stimulation or rapid pacing in at least 75 percent of patients; the remainder require cardioversion. The ability to initiate and terminate a sustained, uniform VT reproducibly permits assessment of pharmacologic and electrical therapy of these arrhythmias. Serial testing of antiarrhythmic agents over a period of several days can be accomplished and predicts the likelihood of success of the agents or devices tested.

The reproducible termination of VT by programmed stimulation permits evaluation of the effectiveness of antitachycardia pacemakers for long-term therapy of paroxysmal episodes of arrhythmia. Unfortunately, rapid pacing, the most effective form of therapy, can accelerate the tachycardia and/or produce ventricular fibrillation. Therefore, antitachycardia pacing is a viable form of therapy only when the pacing device includes backup defibrillation capabilities.

Clinical features   Symptoms resulting from VT depend on the ventricular rate, duration of the tachycardia, and presence and extent of underlying cardiac disease. When the tachycardia is rapid and associated with severe myocardial dysfunction and cerebrovascular disease, hypotension and syncope are common. However, the presence of hemodynamic stability does not preclude a diagnosis of VT. The loss of the atrial contribution to ventricular filling and an abnormal sequence of ventricular activation are important factors producing a decreased cardiac output during VT.

The *prognosis* of VT depends on the underlying disease state. If sustained VT develops within the first 6 weeks following acute myocardial infarction, the prognosis is poor, with a 75 percent mortality rate at 1 year. Patients with nonsustained VT following myocardial infarction have a threefold greater risk of death than a comparable group of patients without this arrhythmia. However, a cause-and-effect relationship between the nonsustained tachycardia and subsequent sudden death has not been established. Patients without heart disease who have uniform VT have a good prognosis and have an extremely low risk of sudden death.

Management The risk-benefit ratio of treating each specific type of VT should be considered before beginning therapy. This is important because antiarrhythmic agents can produce or exacerbate the very arrhythmias which they are given to prevent. In general, patients with VT but without organic heart disease have a benign course; such patients with asymptomatic, nonsustained VT need not be treated because their prognosis will not be affected. An exception is the patient with congenital long QT syndrome. Such patients have recurrent polymorphic VT and a high mortality from sudden death if untreated. Patients with sustained VT in the absence of heart disease usually require therapy because the arrhythmia causes symptoms. These tachycardias may respond to beta blockers, verapamil, or quinidine-like agents. In patients with VT and organic heart disease, if marked hemodynamic embarrassment is present or if there is evidence of ischemia, congestive heart failure, or central nervous system hypoperfusion, the rhythm should be promptly terminated by dc cardioversion (see below). If the patient with organic heart disease tolerates the VT well, pharmacologic therapy may be tried. Procainamide is probably the most effective agent for acute therapy. It may or may not terminate the tachycardia but almost always slows the rate. In stable patients in whom these drugs do not terminate the arrhythmia, a pacing catheter can be inserted pervenously into the right ventricular apex, and the tachycardia can be terminated by overdrive pacing.

Programmed stimulation is probably the most efficacious way to select the appropriate antiarrhythmic agent to prevent recurrent, sustained VT. After demonstrating that the tachycardia can be initiated reproducibly in the absence of antiarrhythmic agents, drugs can be studied serially, and the drug that prevents initiation of the tachycardia can be selected; long-term successful prevention of the arrhythmia can than be expected in 90 percent of patients. Drug levels demonstrated to be successful in the laboratory need to be maintained chronically. Unfortunately, prevention of inducible VT is expected in only 50 percent of cases.

Antitachycardia pacing has been used as a means to terminate drug-resistant tachycardia. This usually requires that the tachycardia be stable and slow and that the patient be aware of it. Automatic antitachycardia pacing devices are not used alone because pacing during VT may accelerate tachycardia, converting a stable arrhythmia into an unstable one and resulting in severe hemodynamic compromise. However, devices combining antitachycardia pacing with an implantable cardioverter defibrillator (ICD) (see below) afford a "backup" means of terminating unstable arrhythmias. Radiofrequency pacemakers, which are best activated by a physician, have been used in occasional patients.

The advent of endocardial catheter and intraoperative mapping led to the development of surgical techniques for the management of VT. Activation mapping permits localization of the site of origin of the arrhythmia. In centers in which expertise in mapping is available, operation has been successfully employed to cure tachycardias in the majority of patients in whom it has been undertaken. Even though most patients with VT and ischemic heart disease have markedly impaired left ventricular function and multivessel coronary artery disease, the operative mortality rate has ranged between 8 and 15 percent. Following operation, more than 90 percent of survivors are controlled either off (two-thirds of patients) or on (one-third) antiarrhythmic agents that were previously ineffective in controlling these rhythms.

Specific types of VT TORSADES DE POINTES *Torsades de pointes* ("twisting of the points") (Fig. 198-15) refers to VT characterized by polymorphic QRS complexes that change in amplitude and cycle length, giving the appearance of oscillations around the baseline. This rhythm is, by definition, associated with QT prolongation. The latter may result from electrolyte disturbances (particularly hypokalemia and hypomagnesemia), use of a variety of antiarrhythmic drugs (especially quinidine), phenothiazines and tricyclic antidepressants, liquid protein diets, intracranial events, and bradyarrhythmias, particularly third-degree AV block. It also may occur as an isolated idiopathic congenital or acquired anomaly.

The electrocardiographic hallmark is polymorphic VT preceded by marked QT prolongation, often in excess of 0.60 s. These patients often have multiple episodes of nonsustained polymorphic VT associated with recurrent syncope, but they also may develop VF and sudden cardiac death.

Therapy should be directed at removing the precipitating factors, i.e., correcting metabolic abnormalities and removing drugs which have induced the prolonged QT interval. In the setting of drug-induced torsades de pointes, atrial or ventricular overdrive pacing and the administration of magnesium also have been useful in terminating and preventing the arrhythmia. For patients with the congenital prolonged QT interval syndrome, beta-adrenergic blocking agents have been the mainstay of therapy; agents which shorten the QT interval also may be useful (e.g., phenytoin). Cervicothoracic sympathectomy has been proposed as a form of therapy for congenital prolonged QT syndrome, but it is not often effective as the sole therapy.

Polymorphic tachycardias associated with normal QT intervals in patients with ischemic heart disease that are initiated by "R-on-T" VPCs are probably caused by reentry, and their treatment is totally different. This is not true torsades de pointes. In such cases, quinidine-like agents may be the most effective form of therapy and should be administered in full antiarrhythmic doses. However, these arrhythmias also may result from acute, severe ischemia and will only respond to abolition of the ischemia, usually by revascularization.

ACCELERATED IDIOVENTRICULAR RHYTHM This arrhythmia, also termed slow VT, with a rate which ranges from 60 to 120 beats per minute, usually occurs in acute myocardial infarction, often during reperfusion. It also may be seen following cardiac operations, in patients with cardiomyopathy, rheumatic fever, or digitalis intoxication, as well as in patients with no evidence of heart disease. The rhythm is usually transient and rarely causes significant hemodynamic compromise or symptoms.

Treatment is rarely necessary and should usually be considered only if symptoms arise due to impaired hemodynamics, most commonly due to AV dissociation. In most cases, atropine can accelerate the sinus rate to overdrive the ventricular rhythm.

FIGURE 198-15 Torsades de pointes. During sinus rhythm (lead II) a markedly prolonged QT interval was present. Lead V_1 shows polymorphic VT.

FIGURE 198-16 Ventricular fibrillation. In a patient with coronary disease ventricular fibrillation is initiated by a VPC that produces a rapid polymorphic ventricular tachycardia which rapidly degenerates to ventricular fibrillation (note the undulating baseline with indistinguishable systole and diastole).

VENTRICULAR FLUTTER AND VENTRICULAR FIBRILLATION

(VF) (See Fig. 198-16; see also Chap. 35) These arrhythmias occur most often in patients with ischemic heart disease. They also occur following administration of antiarrhythmic drugs, particularly those which induce prolonged QT intervals and torsades de pointes (see above), in patients with severe hypoxia or ischemia, and in those with WPW who develop AF with an extremely rapid ventricular response (see p. 1028). Electrical accidents frequently cause cardiac arrest due to the development of VF. The onset of these arrhythmias is rapidly followed by loss of consciousness and, if untreated, death. Episodes of cardiac arrest recorded during Holter monitoring reveal that approximately three-fourths of the sudden deaths are due to VT or VF.

In patients with VF, the onset almost always begins with a short run of rapid VT, which is initiated by a relatively late coupled VPC. In patients with acute myocardial infarction or ischemia, however, VF is usually precipitated by a single early ventricular complex beat falling on the T wave (the vulnerable period), which produces a rapid VT which degenerates into VF (see Fig. 198-16).

The clinical setting in which VF occurs is important. Most patients who have primary VF within the first 48 h of the onset of acute infarction have a good long-term prognosis, with a very low rate of recurrence or sudden cardiac death. Their short-term mortality may, however, be slightly increased. In contrast, patients who experience VF unassociated with the development of acute myocardial infarction have a recurrence rate of 20 to 30 percent in the year following the event (see Chap. 35).

Ventricular flutter usually appears as a sine wave with a rate between 150 and 300 beats per minute. These oscillations make it impossible to assign a specific morphology to the arrhythmia and in some cases to distinguish it from rapid VT. VF is recognized by grossly irregular undulations of varying amplitudes, contours, and rates (see Fig. 198-16). Electrophysiologic studies have demonstrated that regardless of the apparent gross irregularity on the surface ECG, VF usually starts out with a rapid repetitive sequence of VT which ultimately breaks down into multiple wavelets of reentry.

Electrophysiologic studies have been useful in patients who have been resuscitated from cardiac arrest. Programmed stimulation has demonstrated that in approximately 70 percent of such patients one can reproducibly initiate a sustained VT. Treatment is discussed in Chap. 35.

PHARMACOLOGIC ANTIARRHYTHMIC THERAPY

Prior to initiation of pharmacologic antiarrhythmic therapy, potential aggravating factors such as transient metabolic abnormalities, congestive heart failure, or acute ischemia must be corrected; in some cases this may suffice to control arrhythmias. In addition, the potential role of drugs as a cause or exacerbating factor in the development of the arrhythmia must be considered. Despite their name, it must be recognized that we do not have a good understanding of the effects of antiarrhythmic agents on the spontaneous onset of tachyarrhythmias. In some cases, they may facilitate the onset.

Antiarrhythmic drugs are used in three principal situations: (1) to terminate an acute arrhythmia, (2) to prevent recurrence of an arrhythmia, and (3) to prevent a life-threatening arrhythmia for which the patient is perceived to be at risk but which has never occurred. (The acute pharmacologic therapy of tachyarrythmias is summarized in Table 198-3.)

Most currently available antiarrhythmic agents have a relatively low toxic/therapeutic ratio; all can exert proarrhythmic effects, and

TABLE 198-3 Acute pharmacologic therapy of tachyarrhythmias

Arrhythmia	Drug	Dose
Atrial tachyarrhythmias (including AF and atrial flutter) in patients without preexcitation	Initially verapamil or beta-blocking agent to control ventricular response, then procainamide or quinidine	Verapamil: IV, 2.5–10 mg bolus (may precede by IV calcium gluconate or chloride to prevent hypotension)
		Propranolol: IV, 1-mg increments until desired effect achieved or side effects
		Metoprolol: IV, 5–10 mg
		Esmolol: IV, loading dose of 500 µg/kg/min for 1 min, followed by maintenance infusion of 50 µg/kg/min for 4 min; if effect is inadequate, repeat load followed by maintenance of 100 µg/kg/min, up to maximum maintenance of 200 µg/kg/min
		Procainamide: IV, up to 15 mg/kg at 25–50 mg/min until arrhythmia terminates; monitor BP q 5 min
		Quinidine sulfate: PO, 200–400 mg
Atrial tachyarrhythmias (including AF and atrial flutter) in patients with preexcitation	Procainamide	IV up to 15 mg/kg at 25–50 mg/min; monitor BP q 5 min
SVT with regular rate and narrow QRS complex	Adenosine	IV, 6-mg bolus initially; if no effect within 60 s, give 12 mg; onset of action immediate
	Verapamil	IV, 5–10 mg over 2–3 min; onset of action within 12 min; peak effect in 10–15 min
Sustained monomorphic VT	Procainamide	IV, infusion at 25–50 mg/min up to 15 mg/kg; monitor BP q 5 min
	Lidocaine	IV, bolus of 1 mg/kg followed by a second bolus of 0.5 mg/kg 5 min later; at time of initial bolus, begin maintenance infusion of 1–4 mg/min

therefore they may exacerbate underlying arrhythmias. Serum levels can be determined for most currently available antiarrhythmic agents. Standards for therapeutic and toxic levels can serve only as a rough guide for selecting the appropriate dose in any individual patient. In the final analysis, the therapeutic level in a given patient is that concentration which achieves the desired antiarrhythmic effect, and the toxic level for each patient is that concentration at which undesirable side effects occur. Since many adverse effects are directly related to drug concentrations, the lowest serum level which achieves an effective antiarrhythmic response should be chosen.

In order to determine the therapeutic level for a patient, one must have a standard to judge drug efficacy. For a patient with an incessant arrhythmia, antiarrhythmic drugs may be administered empirically until the arrhythmia is suppressed. If a reproducible precipitating factor such as exercise can be identified, serial drug testing during such a provocative maneuver may be performed. Unfortunately, most arrhythmias are sporadic and occur unpredictably without identifiable precipitating factors. In these cases, if one waits to observe spontaneous recurrences on each antiarrhythmic drug, assessment of drug efficacy may require months. This type of assessment of efficacy may be adequate for arrhythmias which are not life-threatening. However, this mode of assessment is inadequate for arrhythmias that compromise hemodynamic stability, result in syncope, or cause cardiac arrest. In such cases, two methods for determination of arrhythmic drug efficacy have been utilized. The first, which consists of continuous ECG monitoring in the control state and then in the presence of antiarrhythmic drugs, has been used in order to determine the effect that each drug has on spontaneous atrial or ventricular ectopy. This method presupposes that the mechanism responsible for sustained arrhythmias is the same as that causing isolated premature depolarizations (which may or may not be true) and that therefore eradication of isolated ectopy will correlate with prevention of sustained arrhythmias. This method has a number of limitations. First, patients frequently show marked degrees of spontaneous variation in frequency of ectopy, which may mimic antiarrhythmic drug effects. Second, 25 to 30 percent of patients with sustained ventricular arrhythmias such as VT or VF demonstrate only rare spontaneous ectopy. Finally, many patients demonstrate a dissociation between the effects of antiarrhythmic agents on spontaneous ectopy and the effects of the same agent on sustained arrhythmias.

An alternative method to assess drug efficacy is programmed stimulation. Numerous studies have demonstrated that most clinically occurring supraventricular and ventricular tachyarrhythmias may be reproducibly initiated and terminated safely using this technique. Studies are performed initially in a baseline state in the absence of antiarrhythmic drugs (Fig. 198-17). If the patient's clinical arrhythmia can be reproducibly initiated, then the ability of individual antiarrhythmic drugs to prevent reinduction of the arrhythmia can be assessed either after the drug is administered intravenously or after several days of oral loading in order to achieve a steady state serum concentration. Use of this method assumes that (1) the induced and spontaneous arrhythmias are identical and (2) prevention of induction of arrhythmias will correlate with prevention of recurrent spontaneous tachycardias on the same drug regimen. This technique has been validated in patients with a variety of reentrant PSVTs, VT, and VF. The technique is safe when carefully performed, the potential complications being those of any intravascular catheterization. Appropriate interpretation of the results of programmed stimulation is critically dependent on correlating the patient's spontaneous arrhythmias with those induced in the laboratory, with regard to rate and morphology, in order to be certain that the arrhythmia induced in the laboratory represents the same arrhythmia that occurred spontaneously and caused symptoms.

Classification of antiarrhythmic drugs   A number of classifications of antiarrhythmic drugs have been proposed, the most frequently used of which is a modification of one proposed by Vaughan-Williams (see Table 198-1). This classification is based in part on the ability of antiarrhythmic drugs to modify the cardiac cellular (1) excitatory

FIGURE 198-17   Selections of an effective antiarrhythmic drug for ventricular tachycardia by programmed stimulation. From top to bottom, the effects of programmed stimulation during the control state and following administration of several antiarrhythmic agents. During the control state two ventricular extrastimuli initiate the ventricular tachycardia at a rate of 230 per minute. Lidocaine, phenytoin, and disopyramide at the plasma levels shown failed to prevent induction of the tachycardia. Both procainamide and quinidine at the plasma levels shown prevented initiation of sustained tachycardia. Chronic oral quinidine therapy effectively prevented recurrences of the arrhythmia. *(From JA Kastor et al, N Engl J Med 304:1004, 1981; reprinted by permission.)*

currents (Na$^+$ or Ca^{2+}), (2) action potential duration, and (3) automaticity (phase 4 depolarization). These effects of the drugs on isolated cardiac cells are thought to account for some of the antiarrhythmic properties of the drugs. Thus depression of excitatory currents by type I and type IV antiarrhythmics results in slowing of conduction velocity and may interrupt arrhythmias by blocking conduction in areas of marginal excitability, where conduction velocity is already slow. Type III antiarrhythmics allegedly exert their action by increasing refractoriness through prolongation of the action potential duration. However, this classification has a number of limitations. The electrophysiologic effects of these drugs in vivo may differ from their effects on isolated cells. Also, the effects of heart rate and fiber

TABLE 198-4   Dose, serum half-life ($t_{\frac{1}{2}}$) following oral administration, and route of metabolism of drugs used in treatment of arrhythmias

Drug	Mode of administration	$t_{\frac{1}{2}}$ (oral), h	Route of metabolism
Digoxin	IV, 0.25–1.5 mg Oral, 0.75–1.5 mg loading dose over 12–24 h Maintenance, 0.23–0.50 mg/d	36	Renal
Propranolol	IV, 0.5–1 mg/min to total dose of 0.15–0.2 mg/kg Oral, 10–200 mg q 6 h	3–6	Hepatic
Verapamil	IV, 2.5–10 mg over 1–2 min to total of 0.15 mg/kg Oral, 80–120 mg q 6–8 h	3–8	Hepatic
Quinidine	IV, 20 mg/min to total of 10–15 mg/kg Oral, 200–400 mg q 6 h	5–9	Hepatic: 80% Renal: 20%
Procainamide	IV, 40–50 mg/min to total of 10–20 mg/kg Oral, 500–1000 mg q 4 h	3–5	Hepatic: 50% Renal: 50%
Disopyramide	Oral, 100–300 mg q 6–8 h	8–9	Renal: 50% Hepatic: 50%
Lidocaine	IV, 20–50 mg/min to total of 5-mg/kg loading dose followed by 1–4 mg/kg	1–2	Hepatic: 100%
Phenytoin	IV, 20 mg/min total dose to 1000 mg Oral, 1000-mg loading over 24 h Maintenance, 100–400 mg/d	18–36	Hepatic
Tocainide	Oral, 400–600 mg q 8–12 h	10–17	Hepatic-renal
Bretylium	IV, 1–2 (mg/kg)/min to total of 5–10 mg/kg Maintenance, 0.5–2 mg/min	8–14	Renal
Amiodarone	IV, 5–10 mg/kg Oral, load 800–1400 mg/d for 1–2 weeks Maintenance, 100–600 mg/d	Unknown	Unknown
Moricizine	Oral, 200–400 mg q 8 h	2–6	Hepatic
Propafenone	Oral, 450–900 mg q 8 h	5–8	Hepatic
Sotalol			
Adenosine	IV bolus, 6–12 mg	< 10 s	
Mexiletine	Oral, 100–300 mg q 6–8 h	9–12	Hepatic: 100%
Flecainide	Oral, begin at 50–100 mg bid; increase by no more than 50 mg not more often than every 4 days to a maximum of 400 mg daily	7–23	Hepatic: 75% Renal: 25%

geometry are not considered. Not all drugs (e.g., adenosine) fit into the classifications. Finally, some drugs (e.g., amiodarone) exhibit properties consistent with multiple classes. The uses and actions of currently available antiarrhythmic drugs are summarized in Tables 198-2 and 198-4.

ELECTRICAL THERAPY OF TACHYARRHYTHMIAS

PACEMAKERS   Cardiac pacing can be used to terminate and in selected cases prevent recurrent supraventricular and ventricular arrhythmias. Because many tachyarrhythmias appear to be due to a reentrant mechanism with the impulse traveling in a circuit, a properly timed paced impulse can penetrate and prematurely depolarize part of the circuit, rendering it refractory to the next circulating wavefront and thereby interrupting the circus movement. Pacing therapy for arrhythmias is generally reserved for patients whose arrhythmias are refractory to drug therapy and who remain hemodynamically stable during the tachycardia. All forms of pacing therapy require repeated demonstration of their effectiveness and reliability in terminating the arrhythmias during electrophysiologic testing prior to implantation of the pacing device.

The type of pacing device and modality selected for arrhythmia termination depends on (1) the rate of the tachycardia (rates >160 beats per minute are rarely terminated by a single premature stimulus), (2) the type of the arrhythmia (atrial flutter and VT are rarely terminated by single extrastimuli), and (3) concomitant drug therapy. Underdrive pacing, i.e., pacing at a rate slower than the tachycardia, can be used when a single premature stimulus has been demonstrated to reproducibly terminate a tachycardia. It is rarely used today because

pacemakers are available which can deliver timed stimuli or an increasing number of stimuli.

Because many tachycardias cannot be terminated by single premature stimuli, pacemakers have been developed which allow for multiple extrastimuli (burst pacing) to be introduced. In reentrant tachycardias involving an accessory AV connection, sequential, near-simultaneous activation of the heart from both the atria and the ventricle using a dual-chamber pacemaker will increase the likelihood of bidirectional block and termination of the tachycardia. However, the use of antitachycardia pacing for supraventricular arrhythmias has been rendered almost obsolete by the advent of radiofrequency catheter ablation.

Cardiac pacing also has been used to prevent ventricular tachyarrhythmias. Polymorphic VT associated with a long QT interval and bradycardia (torsades de pointes, p. 1021) is most likely to respond. Pacing the atrium and/or ventricle at rates between 90 and 120 beats per minute appears to increase the homogeneity of electrical recovery and markedly reduces the propensity for a recurrence of arrhythmias.

Pacemakers may be self-contained or energized by an external radiofrequency source. The self-contained pacemaker may function automatically [i.e., it incorporates an arrhythmia recognition program (circuit)], or it may be activated by an external magnet. The major advantage of a fully automatic system is that there is no need for the patient to recognize the arrhythmia in order for termination to occur. The advantages of the externally activated system include (1) the decreased risk of unnecessary treatment because of faulty sensing and (2) the opportunity to initiate monitoring at the time of attempted termination of arrhythmia. This type of monitoring is frequently helpful if pacing techniques are employed to terminate VT, given the risk of acceleration of the arrhythmia by pacing.

The limitations of pacing therapy are primarily related to (1) the changes in the characteristics of the arrhythmia over time such that programmed pacing parameters no longer terminate the tachycardia, (2) the risk of acceleration of the tachycardia with the development of AF when stimulating the atrium and the development of rapid VT and VF when stimulating the ventricles, and (3) inappropriate recognition of supraventricular tachyarrhythmias as ventricular tachycardias, leading to delivery of therapy unnecessarily, which can initiate VT or VF. Future pacing generators which also can deliver a larger amount of energy and perform cardioversion and defibrillation of accelerated arrhythmias have been approved by the U.S. Food and Drug Administration and will increase the applicability of pacing therapy for the treatment of arrhythmias (see below).

CARDIOVERSION AND DEFIBRILLATION Electrical cardioversion and defibrillation remain the most reliable methods for terminating arrhythmias. By depolarizing all or at least a large portion of excitable myocardium in a near homogeneous fashion, the electrical shock can interrupt reentrant arrhythmias. External cardioversion is routinely performed by placing two paddles 12 cm in diameter in firm contact with the chest wall, with one paddle usually located to the right of the sternum at the level of the second rib and the other in the left midclavicular line in the fifth intercostal space. If the patient is conscious, a short-acting barbiturate to act as an anesthetic or an amnesic drug such as diazepam should be administered to prevent patient discomfort. A person skilled in maintaining an airway should be present.

Energy is delivered synchronously with the QRS complex for all arrhythmias except ventricular flutter and VF, since asynchronous shocks can produce VF. The amount of energy used will vary with the type of tachycardia being treated. With the exception of AF, supraventricular tachycardias can frequently be terminated with energy levels in the range of 25 to 50 W·s, while AF usually requires ≥100 W·s for termination. For terminating VT, energy levels ≥100 W·s should probably be employed. While energies as low as 25 W·s may be used successfully, they also have a higher incidence of producing VF. At least 200 W·s of energy should be used for initial attempts at terminating VF. If the initial shock fails, all repeated attempts at defibrillation should be with the maximum energy that the defibrillator is capable of delivering (320 to 400 W·s).

Indications for cardioversion depend on the clinical setting and the patient's general condition. Any tachycardia (except sinus tachycardia) that produces hypotension, myocardial ischemia, or heart failure warrants consideration of prompt termination using external cardioversion. Arrhythmias that fail to terminate with pharmacologic therapy also may be terminated by electrical cardioversion. Transient bradycardias and supraventricular and ventricular irritability following cardioversion are common and usually do not warrant antiarrhythmic intervention.

IMPLANTED CARDIOVERSION/DEFIBRILLATION Implantable cardioverter/defibrillator devices have been developed that will promptly recognize and terminate life-threatening ventricular arrhythmias. These devices can deliver <1 to 40 W·s, the amount of which can be programmed. Newer devices have antitachycardia pacing capabilities such that VT can be sensed and terminated without resorting to a painful shock. In such devices, high-energy shocks are reserved for hypotensive VT, acceleration of VT, or failure to terminate VT after a programmed duration (see Fig. 198-18). Clinical trials testing the function of these devices in patients with drug-refractory ventricular arrhythmias have demonstrated survival from sudden death at 1 year ranging between 92 and 100 percent. At the time of writing, use of the FDA-approved devices should be reserved for patients with VT which is not hemodynamically tolerated or for patients with VF whose arrhythmias are refractory to drug therapy. The most frequent problem with the device has been its inappropriate discharge in the absence of sustained ventricular arrhythmias. Additional potential problems include an increase in defibrillation threshold and decrease in tachycardia rates below the rate cut-off of the device in response to many antiarrhythmic drugs. Permanently implanted

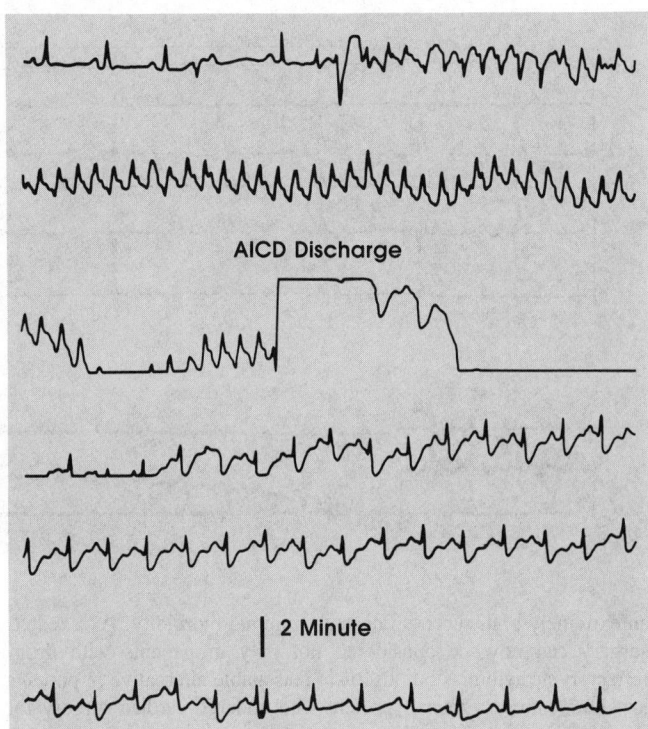

FIGURE 198-18 Normally functioning implantable defibrillators. A continuous Holter monitoring tracing is shown. On the top strip, a rapid polymorphic tachycardia is initiated which beats more uniformly. The automatic implantable cardioverter-defibrillator (AICD) senses the rhythm and delivers a shock which restores sinus rhythm.

ventricular pacemakers may interfere with the device's ability to sense VF. Many of these problems will be circumvented by advanced devices which are currently under investigation. These newer devices have the capability to take a "second look" prior to shock delivery and thus may abort delivery for self-terminating arrhythmias. In addition, the range of candidates suitable for implantation will be expanded because the newer devices have the capability of shock therapy for patients whose arrhythmias do not cause loss of consciousness. More advanced systems are being developed which can be implanted transvenously, thus avoiding the need to perform thoracotomy.

CATHETER ABLATION FOR ARRHYTHMIAS Catheter ablation techniques are now the procedures of choice for symptomatic patients with (1) concealed or manifest (WPW) bypass tracts, (2) AV nodal reentrant SVT, and (3) poorly controlled ventricular responses to atrial tachyarrhythmias, most commonly atrial fibrillation. Successful ablation of bypass tracts and modifications of the AV node by radiofrequency energy are extremely successful and cost-effective and are the procedure of choice for patients with recurrent episodes (see Figs. 198-19 and 198-20). The creation of AV block with implantation of a pacemaker is the method of choice in managing patients with atrial fibrillation and poorly controlled ventricular response.

SURGICAL TREATMENT OF ARRHYTHMIAS

Programmed stimulation and endocardial activation mapping have provided a better understanding of the mechanisms and sites of origin of many supraventricular and ventricular tachyarrhythmias so that in selected patients surgical treatment may be considered.

WOLFF-PARKINSON-WHITE SYNDROME Until the development of catheter ablation, surgery was the preferred form of therapy in patients with recurrent arrhythmias. However, advances made in the localization and surgical ablation of bypass tracts now allow for

FIGURE 198-19   Radiofrequency ablation in Wolff-Parkinson-White syndrome. Leads I, II, III, V_1, V_2, and V_6 are shown. Preexcitation using a left lateral bypass tract is present in the final four complexes. Following the third complex, radiofrequency energy is applied. By the second beat, preexcitation is lost as the bypass tract is destroyed.

FIGURE 198-20   Ablation of AV nodal reentrant tachycardia. Leads II and V_1, along with a right append-age electrode (RAA), are shown. AV nodal reentry is present at the time radiofrequency energy is delivered between the coronary sinus and tricuspid valve. The tachycardia slows and is terminated by block in the slow pathway. (*After Calkins et al.*)

an extremely high success rate with minimal morbidity. As a result, surgery can now be considered not only in patients with drug-refractory arrhythmias but also as a reasonable alternative in patients in whom a bypass tract is present who undergo cardiac surgery for other reasons.

SUPRAVENTRICULAR TACHYCARDIA AND OTHER ATRIAL AR-RHYTHMIAS   Although atrial flutter, AF, and PSVT are usually not life-threatening, they may be refractory to pharmacologic or pacing interventions. In such cases, surgery may be considered as a method of removing the abnormal focus, interrupting the reentry circuits, and curing the tachycardia or controlling the ventricular response by creating AV block. However, radiofrequency catheter ablation is now the therapy of choice for these arrhythmias. In atrial flutter and AF, the pathophysiologic substrate cannot be identified; thus the only option is to destroy the AV node–His bundle region by cryosurgery or transvenous catheter electroablation. Surgery, cryoablation, or electrode catheter ablation requires concomitant implantation of a permanent pacemaker. Focal atrial tachycardias have been treated surgically by discrete resection or ablation by cryothermal injury. Mapping the tachycardia is mandatory if a primary direct approach on the arrhythmia is to be performed. Surgery is for patients with arrhythmias refractory to other treatments and only when the tachycardia has been localized.

VENTRICULAR TACHYCARDIA   The demonstration that VT due to ischemic heart disease can often be reliably induced by programmed stimulation and that the arrhythmia is localized to a small region of endocardium in the area of prior infarction has permitted the development of specific surgical techniques for the cure of the arrhythmia.

Preoperatively, all morphologically distinct tachycardias that occur spontaneously are induced by programmed stimulation, and their respective sites of origin are determined by catheter activation mapping. Catheter mapping may be supplemented by intraoperative mapping, involving similar techniques. These studies have shown that tachycardias arise in the scar tissue near the endocardium.

Subendocardial resection and endocardial encircling ventriculo-tomy or cryoablation, the surgical techniques that have been applied to the management of ventricular tachycardia, are aimed at removing or isolating the pathophysiologic substrate of the arrhythmia, as identified by mapping. The major criterion for surgical success is the ability to localize the site from which the arrhythmias arise.

BAROLD SS, ZIPES DP: Cardiac pacemakers and antiarrhythmic devices, in *Heart Disease: A Textbook of Cardiovascular Medicine*, 4th ed, E Braunwald (ed). Philadelphia, Saunders, 1992, pp 726–755

BRUGADA J et al: The complexity of mechanisms in ventricular tachycardia. PACE Pacing Clin Electrophysiol 16:680, 1993

CALKINS H et al: Diagnosis and cure of the Wolff-Parkinson-White syndrome or paroxsymal supraventricular tachycardias during a single electrophysiologic test. N Engl J Med 324:1612, 1991

COX JL: Surgical management of cardiac arrhythmias, in *Cardiac Pacing and Electrophysi-ology*. N El-Sherif, P Samet (eds). Philadelphia, Saunders, 1991, p 436

DREIFUS LS: Guidelines for implantation of cardiac pacemakers and antiarrhythmic devices: A report of the American College of Cardiology/American Heart Association Task Force on Assessment of Diagnostic and Therapeutic Cardiovascular Procedures (Committee on Pacemaker Implantation). J Am Coll Cardiol 18:1, 1991

ECHT DS et al: Mortality and morbidity in patients receiving encainide, flecainide, or placebo: The Cardiac Arrhythmia Suppression Trial (CAST). N Engl J Med 324:781, 1991

GUARDIAN MULTICENTER INVESTIGATORS GROUP: Long term multicenter experience with a second-generation implantable pacemaker-defibrillator in patients with malignant ventricular tachyarrhythmias. J Am Coll Cardiol 19:490, 1992

GUIRAUDON GM et al: Surgery for atrial flutter, atrial fibrillation, and atrial tachycardia, in *Cardiac Electrophysiology: From Cell to Bedside*, DP Zipes, J Jalife (eds). Philadelphia, Saunders, 1990, p 915

JACKMAN WM et al: Catheter ablation of accessory atrioventricular pathways (Wolff-Parkinson-White syndrome) by radiofrequency current. N Engl J Med 324: 1605, 1991

JOSEPHSON ME: *Clinical Cardiac Electrophysiology*, 2d ed. Philadelphia, Lea & Febiger, 1993

KIM YH et al: Nonpharmacologic therapies in patients with ventricular tachyarrhythmias. Catheter ablation and ventricular tachycardia surgery. Cardiol Clin 11:85, 1993

KUTALEK SP, DREIFUS LS: Implantable cardioverter-defibrillators. Adv Intern Med 38:421, 1993

PRITCHETT ELC: Management of atrial fibrillation. N Engl J Med 326:1264, 1991

RODEN DM: Treatment of cardiovascular diseases: Arrhythmias, in *Clinical Pharmacol-ogy: Basic Principles in Therapeutics*, KL Melmon et al (eds). New York, McGraw-Hill, 1992, pp 151–185

SCHEINMAN MM et al: Current role of catheter ablation procedures in patients with cardiac arrhythmias: A report for health professionals from the Subcommittee on Electrocardiography and Electrophysiology, American Heart Association. Circulation 83:2146, 1991

WYSE DG: Pharmacologic therapy in patients with ventricular tachyarrhythmias. Cardiol Clin 11:65, 1993

ZIPES DP: Specific arrhythmias: Diagnosis and treatment, in *Heart Disease: A Textbook of Cardiovascular Medicine*, 4th ed, E Braunwald (ed). Philadelphia, Saunders, 1992, pp 667–725

———: Genesis of cardiac arrhythmias: Electrophysiological considerations, in *Heart Disease: A Textbook of Cardiovascular Medicine*, 4th ed, E Braunwald (ed). Philadelphia, Saunders, 1992, pp 588–627

———: Management of cardiac arrhythmias: Pharmacological, electrical, and surgical techniques, in *Heart Disease: A Textbook of Cardiovascular Medicine*, 4th ed, E Braunwald (ed). Philadelphia, Saunders, 1992, pp 628–667

REFERENCES

ALMENDRAL J et al: The importance of antitachycardia pacing for patients presenting with ventricular tachycardia. PACE Pacing Clin Electrophysiol 16:535, 1993

199 CONGENITAL HEART DISEASE IN THE ADULT

WILLIAM F. FRIEDMAN / JOHN S. CHILD

Congenital heart disease complicates approximately 1 percent of all live births. Substantial numbers of affected infants reach adulthood because of successful medical and/or surgical management, or because the alteration caused in cardiovascular physiology is well tolerated.

GENERAL CONSIDERATIONS

ETIOLOGY AND PREVENTION Congenital cardiovascular malformations are generally the result of aberrant embryonic development of a normal structure, or failure of such a structure to progress beyond an early stage of embryonic or fetal development. Malformations are due to complex multifactorial genetic and environmental causes. Recognized chromosomal aberrations and mutations of single genes account for less than 10 percent of all cardiac malformations (Table 199-1).

The presence of a cardiac malformation as one component of the multiple system involvement in Down's, Turner's, and the trisomy 13-15(D_1) and 17-18 (E) syndromes may be anticipated in occasional pregnancies by detection of abnormal chromosomes in fetal cells obtained from amniotic fluid or chorionic villus biopsy. Identification in such cells of the enzyme disorders characteristic of Hurler's syndrome, homocystinuria, or type II glycogen storage disease may also allow one to predict cardiac disease.

The feasibility of preventive programs will depend upon what is learned in the future about the cause of the majority of cardiovascular anomalies for which no cause is known. An effective rubella vaccine is available, and immunization of children with this vaccine may lessen maternal rubella and its cardiac consequences. Strict testing in animals of new drugs that can be teratogenic when taken early in pregnancy may reduce the chances of another thalidomide tragedy. In this regard, no medications should be taken during pregnancy without prior consultation with a physician. Physicians should be aware of known teratogens, as well as of drugs for which inadequate information exists as to teratogenic potential. Appropriate use of radiologic equipment and techniques for reducing gonadal and fetal radiation exposure should always be employed to reduce the hazards of birth defects.

PATHOPHYSIOLOGY The anatomic and physiologic changes in the heart and circulation due to any specific congenital cardiocirculatory lesion are not static, but rather progress from prenatal life to adulthood. Thus, malformations which are benign, or escape detection in childhood, may become clinically significant in the adult. For example, the functionally normal, congenitally bicuspid aortic valve may thicken and calcify with time, resulting in significant aortic stenosis; or the well-tolerated left-to-right shunt of an atrial septal defect may not result in cardiac decompensation, with or without pulmonary hypertension, until the fourth or fifth decade.

There are issues of particular concern to the *adult* with congenital heart disease that we will discuss separately in this chapter, including pulmonary hypertension and Eisenmenger syndrome of pulmonary vascular obstruction, the hematologic consequences of cyanotic heart disease, the special considerations of pregnancy in the woman with congenital heart disease, and problems involving employability and insurability.

Pulmonary hypertension This is a common accompaniment of many congenital cardiac lesions, and the status of the pulmonary vascular bed is often the principal determinant of the clinical manifestations, the course, and the feasibility of surgical repair. Increases in pulmonary arterial pressure result from elevation of pulmonary blood flow and/or resistance, the latter due sometimes to an increase in vascular tone but usually the result of obstructive, obliterative structural changes within the pulmonary vascular bed. Because pulmonary vascular obstructive disease can be the determining factor in assessing the advisability of operation, it is important to quantify and compare pulmonary to systemic flows and resistances in patients with severe pulmonary hypertension. The causes of pulmonary vascular obstructive disease are unknown, although increased pulmonary blood flow, increased pulmonary arterial blood pressure, elevated pulmonary venous pressure, polycythemia, systemic hypoxemia, acidosis, and the bronchial circulation have been implicated. The designation *Eisenmenger syndrome* is applied to patients with a large communication between the two circulations at the aortopulmonary, ventricular, or atrial levels and bidirectional or predominantly right-to-left shunts because of high-resistance and obstructive pulmonary hypertension. No specific treatment has proved beneficial for obstructive pulmonary vascular disease, although single lung transplantation and intracardiac defect repair, or total heart-lung transplantation show promise (see Chaps. 196 and 232).

Erythrocytosis The chronic hypoxemia in cyanotic congenital heart disease results in *erythrocytosis* due to increased erythropoietin production (see Chap. 32). The commonly used term *polycythemia* is a misnomer because white cell counts are normal and platelet counts are normal to decreased. Cyanotic patients with erythrocytosis may have compensated or decompensated hematocrits. Compensated erythrocytosis with iron-replete equilibrium hematocrits rarely results in symptoms of hyperviscosity at hematocrits less than 65 percent and occasionally with hematocrits of 70 percent or more. Therapeutic phlebotomy is rarely required in compensated erythrocytosis. In contrast, patients with decompensated erythrocytosis fail to establish equilibrium with unstable, rising hematocrits and recurrent hyperviscosity symptoms. Therapeutic phlebotomy, a two-edged sword, allows temporary relief of symptoms but begets instability of the hematocrit and compounds the problem by iron depletion. Iron-deficiency symptoms are usually indistinguishable from those of hyperviscosity; progressive symptoms after recurrent phlebotomy are usually due to iron depletion with hypochromic microcytosis. Iron depletion results in a larger number of smaller (microcytic) hypochromic red cells that are less capable of carrying oxygen and less deformable in the microcirculation. Because these microcytes are less deformable in the microcirculation and there are more of them relative to the plasma volume, the viscosity is greater than for an equivalent hematocrit with fewer, larger, iron-replete, deformable cells. As such, iron-depleted erythrocytosis results in increasing symptoms due to decreased oxygen delivery to the tissues.

Hemostasis is abnormal in cyanotic congenital heart disease, due in part to the increased blood volume and engorged capillaries, abnormalities in platelet function and sensitivity to aspirin or nonsteroidal anti-inflammatory agents, and abnormalities of the extrinsic and intrinsic coagulation system. Oral contraceptives are contraindicated for cyanotic women because of the enhanced risk of vascular thrombosis.

The risk of stroke is greatest in children less than 4 years old with cyanotic heart disease and iron deficiency, often with dehydration as an aggravating cause. In contrast, adults with cyanotic congenital heart disease do not appear to be at increased risk for stroke, unless there are excessive, injudicious phlebotomies or inappropriate use of aspirin or anticoagulants.

Symptoms of hyperviscosity can be produced in any cyanotic patient with erythrocytosis if dehydration causes a reduction of plasma volume. Phlebotomy, when required for symptoms of hyperviscosity not due to dehydration or iron deficiency, is a simple outpatient removal of 500 mL of blood over 45 min with isovolumetric replacement with isotonic saline (5% dextrose if congestive heart failure exists). Acute phlebotomy without volume replacement is contraindicated. Iron repletion in decompensated iron-depleted erythrocytosis ameliorates iron-deficiency symptoms but must be done gradually to avoid a sudden excessive rise in hematocrit and resultant hyperviscosity.

TABLE 199-1 Syndromes with associated cardiovascular involvement

Syndrome	Major cardiovascular manifestations	Major noncardiac abnormalities
HERITABLE AND POSSIBLY HERITABLE		
Ellis–van Creveld	Single atrium or atrial septal defect	Chondrodystrophic dwarfism, nail dysplasia, polydactyly
TAR (thrombocytopenia-absent radius)	Atrial septal defect, tetralogy of Fallot	Radial aplasia or hypoplasia, thrombocytopenia
Holt-Oram	Atrial septal defect (other defects common)	Skeletal upper limb defect, hypoplasia of clavicles
Kartagener	Dextrocardia	Situs inversus, sinusitis, bronchiectasis
Laurence-Moon-Biedl	Variable defects	Retinal pigmentation, obesity, polydactyly
Noonan	Pulmonary valve dysplasia, cardiomyopathy (usually hypertrophic)	Webbed neck, pectus excavatum, cryptorchidism
Tuberous sclerosis	Rhabdomyoma, cardiomyopathy	Phakomatosis, bone lesions, hamartomatous skin lesions
Multiple lentigines (leopard) syndrome	Pulmonic stenosis	Basal cell nevi, broad facies, rib anomalies
Rubenstein-Taybi	Patent ductus arteriosus (others)	Broad thumbs and toes, hypoplastic maxilla, slanted palpebral fissures
Familial deafness	Arrhythmias, sudden death	Sensorineural deafness
Osler-Rendu-Weber	Arteriovenous fistulas (lung, liver, mucous membranes)	Multiple telangiectasia
Apert	Ventricular septal defect	Craniosynostosis, midfacial hypoplasia, syndactyly
Incontinentia pigmenti	Patent ductus arteriosus	Irregular pigmented skin lesions, patchy alopecia, hypodontia
Alagille (arteriohepatic dysplasia)	Peripheral pulmonic stenosis, pulmonic stenosis	Biliary hypoplasia, vertebral anomalies, prominent forehead, deep-set eyes
DiGeorge	Interrupted aortic arch, tetralogy of Fallot, truncus arteriosus	Thymic hypoplasia or aplasia, parathyroid aplasia or hypoplasia, ear anomalies
Friedreich's ataxia	Cardiomyopathy and conduction defects	Ataxia, speech defect, degeneration of spinal cord dorsal columns
Muscular dystrophy	Cardiomyopathy	Pseudohypertrophy of calf muscles, weakness of trunk and proximal limb muscles
Cystic fibrosis	Cor pulmonale	Pancreatic insufficiency, malabsorption, chronic lung disease
Sickle cell anemia	Cardiomyopathy, mitral regurgitation	Hemoglobin SS
Conradi-Hünermann	Ventricular septal defect, patent ductus arteriosus	Asymmetric limb shortness, early punctate mineralization, large skin pores
Cockayne	Accelerated atherosclerosis	Cachectic dwarfism, retinal pigment abnormalities, photosensitivity dermatitis
Progeria	Accelerated atherosclerosis	Premature aging, alopecia, atrophy of subcutaneous fat, skeletal hypoplasia
CONNECTIVE TISSUE DISORDERS		
Cutis laxa	Peripheral pulmonic stenosis	Generalized disruption of elastic fibers, diminished skin resilience, hernias
Ehlers-Danlos	Arterial dilatation and rupture, mitral regurgitation	Hyperextensible joints, hyperelastic and friable skin
Marfan	Aortic dilatation, aortic and mitral incompetence	Gracile habitus, arachnodactyly with hyperextensibility, lens subluxation
Osteogenesis imperfecta	Aortic incompetence	Fragile bones, blue sclera
Pseudoxanthoma elasticum	Peripheral and coronary arterial disease	Degeneration of elastic fibers in skin, retinal angioid streaks
INBORN ERRORS OF METABOLISM		
Pompe's disease	Glycogen storage disease of heart	Acid maltase deficiency, muscular weakness
Homocystinuria	Aortic and pulmonary arterial dilatation, intravascular thrombosis	Cystathionine synthetase deficiency, lens subluxation, osteoporosis
Mucopolysaccharidosis: Hurler, Hunter	Multivalvular and coronary and great artery disease, cardiomyopathy	Hurler: Deficiency of α-L-iduronidase, corneal clouding, coarse features, growth and mental retardation Hunter: Deficiency of L-iduranosulfate sulfatase, coarse facies, clear cornea, growth and mental retardation
Morquio, Scheie, Maroteaux-Lamy	Aortic incompetence	Morquio: Deficiency of N-acetylhexosamine sulfate sulfatase, cloudy cornea, normal intelligence, severe bony changes involving vertebrae and epiphyses Scheie: Deficiency of α-L-iduronidase, cloudy cornea, normal intelligence, peculiar facies Maroteaux-Lamy: Deficiency of arylsulfatase B, cloudy cornea, osseous changes, normal intelligence
CHROMOSOMAL ABNORMALITIES		
Trisomy 21 (Down's syndrome)	Endocardial cushion defect, atrial or ventricular septal defect, tetralogy of Fallot	Hypotonia, hyperextensible joints, mongoloid facies, mental retardation
Trisomy 13 (D)	Ventricular septal defect, patent ductus arteriosus, double-outlet right ventricle	Single midline intracerebral ventricle with midfacial defects, polydactyly, nail changes, mental retardation

TABLE 199-1 Syndromes with associated cardiovascular involvement (*continued*)

Syndrome	Major cardiovascular manifestations	Major noncardiac abnormalities
CHROMOSOMAL ABNORMALITIES (*continued*)		
Trisomy 18 (E)	Congenital polyvalvular dysplasia, ventricular septal defect, patent ductus arteriosus	Clenched hand, short sternum, low-arch dermal-ridge pattern on fingertips, mental retardation
Cri-du-chat (short-arm deletion-5)	Ventricular septal defect	Cat cry, microcephaly, antimongoloid slant of palpebral fissures, mental retardation
XO (Turner)	Coarctation of aorta, bicuspid aortic valve	Short female, broad chest, lymphedema, webbed neck
XXXY and XXXXX	Patent ductus arteriosus	XXXY: hypogenitalism, mental retardation, radial-ulnar synostosis XXXXX: small hands, incurving of fifth fingers, mental retardation
SPORADIC DISORDERS		
VATER association	Ventricular septal defect	Vertebral anomalies, anal atresia, tracheo-esophageal fistula, radial and renal anomalies
CHARGE association	Tetralogy of Fallot (other defects common)	Colobomas, choanal atresia, mental and growth deficiency, genital and ear anomalies
Williams	Supravalvular aortic stenosis, peripheral pulmonic stenosis	Mental deficiency, "elfin" facies, loquacious personality, hoarse voice
Cornelia de Lange	Ventricular septal defect	Micromelia, synophrys, mental and growth deficiency
Shprintzen (velocardiofacial)	Ventricular septal defect, tetralogy of Fallot, right aortic arch	Cleft palate, prominent nose, slender hands, learning disability
TERATOGENIC DISORDERS		
Rubella	Patent ductus arteriosus, pulmonic valvular and/or arterial stenosis, atrial septal defect	Cataracts, deafness, microcephaly
Alcohol-induced	Ventricular septal defect (other defects)	Microcephaly, growth and mental deficiency, short palpebral fissures, smooth philtrum, thin upper lip
Phenytoin-induced	Pulmonic stenosis, aortic stenosis, coarctation, patent ductus arteriosus	Hypertelorism, growth and mental deficiency, short phalanges, bowed upper lip
Thalidomide-induced	Variable	Phocomelia
Lithium-induced	Ebstein's anomaly, tricuspid atresia	None

PREGNANCY The presence of congenital heart disease or its consequences may pose special problems for the pregnant woman. Thus, pregnant women with pulmonary vascular obstruction, whether pre- or postoperative, are at risk of dying during delivery or in the immediate postpartum period. The cause of the increased mortality rate is poorly understood. A particularly high mortality rate has been reported for those undergoing a cesarean section, although such surgery should cause less cardiovascular stress than that of labor and vaginal delivery. Irrespective of approach to delivery, some simple guidelines include both continuous administration of oxygen and avoidance of inhalant anesthetic agents. Arterial blood gases and, if possible, pulmonary arterial and systemic blood pressure should be monitored serially throughout delivery and the early postpartum period. Some physicians advise early abortion in women with marked pulmonary vascular obstruction because of the risks of pregnancy, and all such women should receive counseling on birth control. Intrauterine devices should be avoided because of the risks of bleeding and infection; oral contraceptive agents are contraindicated because they are associated with a tendency to develop pulmonary vascular or cerebrovascular thrombosis. Use of a barrier method of birth control is preferable. Prevention of pregnancy is safer than any form of management during pregnancy, labor, delivery, and the postpartum period.

In women with regurgitant or obstructive left-side valvular lesions, the increased volume and/or pressure load on the left atrium or left ventricle imposed by the augmentation in blood volume during pregnancy may result in pulmonary edema, requiring vigorous cardiac decongestive measures (Chap. 31). With medical control of the pulmonary edema, a normal vaginal delivery with careful local and epidural anesthesia is preferable to nonvaginal delivery.

A unique problem exists in women whose congenital heart disease has been corrected with the use of a prosthetic cardiac valve and/or conduit. Such women are at risk for thromboembolism and/or obstruction of their conduits or valves, and are thus, usually, on anticoagulants. Early in pregnancy, coumarin derivatives cause an increase in abortion and stillbirth and in craniofacial, neurologic, and other birth defects. Moreover, the transplacental passage of oral anticoagulants places the fetus at risk of intracranial hemorrhage during delivery. Accordingly, coumarin derivatives should be avoided early (before 10 weeks) and late (after 32 weeks) in pregnancy, and subcutaneous or intravenous heparin should be substituted, although heparin, to a lesser degree, also has been associated with adverse fetal outcome.

INFECTIVE ENDOCARDITIS (See also Chap. 85) Routine antimicrobial prophylaxis is recommended for all patients with congenital heart disease and for the majority of patients after operative repair of the lesion, but it should be recognized that antibiotic prophylaxis is not uniformly effective. Nonetheless, it is recommended for all dental procedures, gastrointestinal and genitourinary surgery, and diagnostic procedures such as proctosigmoidoscopy and cystoscopy. The clinical and bacteriologic profile of infective endocarditis in patients with congenital heart disease has changed with the advent of intracardiac surgery and of prosthetic devices. Two major predisposing causes of infective endocarditis are a susceptible cardiovascular substrate and a source of bacteremia. Prophylaxis includes both chemotherapeutic (antimicrobial) and nonchemotherapeutic (hygienic) measures. Meticulous dental and skin care is required.

EXERCISE Advice on athletics and exercise is governed by the nature of the exercise and by the type and severity of the congenital cardiovascular lesion. Patients with lesions characterized by left ventricular outflow tract obstruction, if more than mild to moderate, or pulmonary vascular disease risk syncope or even sudden death. In Fallot's tetralogy, isotonic exercise–induced decrease in systemic vascular resistance relative to the right ventricular outflow obstruction in the membranous portion of the septum. The functional disturbance is dependent primarily on its size and on the status of the pulmonary vascular bed, rather than on the location of the defect. Only small or moderate-size defects are usually seen initially in adulthood as the vast majority of patients with isolated large defects come to medical and, often, surgical attention very early in life.

A wide spectrum exists in the natural history of ventricular septal defect, ranging from spontaneous closure to congestive cardiac failure and death in early infancy. Within this spectrum is the possible development of pulmonary vascular obstruction, right ventricular outflow tract obstruction, aortic regurgitation, and infective endocarditis. Spontaneous closure is more common in patients born with a small ventricular septal defect and occurs in early childhood in most patients.

Patients with large ventricular septal defects and pulmonary hypertension are those at greatest risk for developing pulmonary vascular obstruction. Thus, large defects should be corrected surgically early in life when pulmonary vascular disease is still reversible or not yet developed. In patients with severe pulmonary vascular obstruction (Eisenmenger syndrome), symptoms in adult life consist of exertional dyspnea, chest pain, syncope, and hemoptysis. The right-to-left shunt leads to cyanosis, clubbing, and erythrocytosis. In all patients, the degree to which pulmonary vascular resistance is elevated before operation is a critical factor determining prognosis. If the pulmonary vascular resistance is one-third or less of the systemic value, progression of pulmonary vascular disease after operation is unusual. However, if a moderate to severe increase in pulmonary vascular resistance exists preoperatively, either no change or a progression of pulmonary vascular disease is common post-operatively.

Right ventricular outflow tract obstruction develops in approximately 5 to 10 percent of patients who present in infancy with a moderate to large left-to-right shunt. With time, as subvalvular right ventricular outflow tract obstruction progresses, the findings in these patients begin to resemble more closely those of the cyanotic tetralogy of Fallot.

In approximately 5 percent of patients, incompetence of the aortic valve results from insufficient cusp tissue or prolapse of the cusp through the interventricular defect; the aortic regurgitation then complicates and usually dominates the clinical course.

Two-dimensional *echocardiography* with conventional or color Doppler examination can usually define the number and location of defects in the ventricular septum and detect associated anomalies. Hemodynamic and angiographic study may be employed to assess the status of the pulmonary vascular bed and clarify details of the altered anatomy.

Management Surgery is not recommended for patients with normal pulmonary arterial pressures with small shunts (pulmonary-to-systemic flow ratios of less than 1.5 to 2.0:1.0). Operative correction is indicated when there is a moderate to large left-to-right shunt with a pulmonary-to-systemic flow ratio that exceeds 1.5:1.0 or 2.0:1.0, in the absence of prohibitively high levels of pulmonary vascular resistance.

PATENT DUCTUS ARTERIOSUS The ductus arteriosus is a vessel leading from the bifurcation of the pulmonary artery to the aorta just distal to the left subclavian artery. The vascular channel is open normally in the fetus but closes immediately after birth. The flow across the ductus is determined by the pressure and resistance relationships between the systemic and pulmonary circulations and by the cross-sectional area and length of the ductus. In most adults with this anomaly, pulmonary pressures are normal and a gradient and shunt from aorta to pulmonary artery persist throughout the cardiac cycle, resulting in a characteristic thrill and a continuous ''machinery'' murmur with a late systolic accentuation at the upper left sternal edge. In adults who were born with a large left-to-right shunt through the ductus arteriosus, pulmonary vascular obstruction (Eisenmenger syndrome) with pulmonary hypertension, right-to-left shunting, and cyanosis have usually developed. Severe pulmonary

vascular disease results in reversal of flow through the ductus, unoxygenated blood is shunted to the descending aorta, and the toes, but not the fingers, become cyanotic and clubbed, a finding termed *differential cyanosis*. The leading causes of death in adults with patent ductus are cardiac failure and infective endocarditis; occasionally severe pulmonary vascular obstruction may cause aneurysmal dilatation, calcification, and rupture of the ductus. In the absence of severe pulmonary vascular disease and predominant left-to-right shunting of blood, the patent ductus should be surgically ligated or divided. Operation should be deferred for several months in patients treated successfully for infective endocarditis, because the ductus may remain somewhat edematous and friable.

AORTIC ROOT TO RIGHT HEART SHUNTS The three most common causes of aortic root to right heart shunts are congenital aneurysm of an aortic sinus of Valsalva with fistula, coronary arteriovenous fistula, and anomalous origin of the left coronary artery from the pulmonary trunk. *Aneurysm of an aortic sinus of Valsalva* consists of a separation or lack of fusion between the media of the aorta and the annulus fibrosis of the aortic valve. Rupture usually occurs in the third or fourth decade of life; most often the aorticocardiac fistula is between the right coronary cusp and the right ventricle, but occasionally, when the noncoronary cusp is involved, the fistula drains into the right atrium. Abrupt rupture causes chest pain, bounding pulses, a continuous murmur accentuated in diastole, and volume overload of the heart. Diagnosis is confirmed by two-dimensional and Doppler echocardiographic studies; cardiac catheterization quantifies the left-to-right shunt, and thoracic aortography visualizes the fistula. Medical management is directed at cardiac failure, arrhythmias, or endocarditis. At operation, the aneurysm is closed and amputated, and the aortic wall is reunited with the heart, either by direct suture or with a prosthesis.

Coronary arteriovenous fistula, an unusual anomaly, consists of a communication between a coronary artery and another cardiac chamber, usually the coronary sinus or right atrium or ventricle. The shunt is usually of small magnitude, and myocardial blood flow is not usually compromised. Potential complications include infective endocarditis, thrombus formation with occlusion or distal embolization, rupture of an aneurysmal fistula, and rarely, pulmonary hypertension and congestive failure. A loud, superficial, continuous murmur at the lower or midsternal border usually prompts a further evaluation of asymptomatic patients. Doppler echocardiography demonstrates the site of drainage; if the site of origin is proximal, it may be detectable by two-dimensional echocardiography. Retrograde thoracic aortography or coronary arteriography permits identification of the size and anatomic features of the fistulous tract, which may be closed by suture obliteration.

The third anomaly causing a shunt from the aortic root to the right heart is *anomalous origin of the left coronary artery from the pulmonary artery*. As the elevated pulmonary vascular resistance declines immediately after birth, perfusion of the left coronary artery from the pulmonary artery ceases, and the direction of flow in the anomalous vessel reverses. Total myocardial perfusion must pass through the right coronary artery and may be sufficient if adequate collateral channels develop between the two coronary circulations. Myocardial infarction and fibrosis commonly lead to death within the first year, though up to 20 percent of patients survive to adolescence and beyond without surgical correction. In older children or adults, mitral regurgitation may result from dysfunction of ischemic or infarcted papillary muscles. The diagnosis of anomalous origin of the coronary artery is supported by the electrocardiographic findings of an anterolateral myocardial infarction. Aortic root or coronary angiography demonstrates the retrograde drainage of the coronary vessel into the pulmonary artery and the presence of a single right coronary artery arising from the aorta. Operative management of adults consists of coronary artery bypass with an internal mammary artery graft or saphenous vein–coronary artery graft. The outcome and prognosis are determined largely by the degree of preoperative myocardial damage.

ACYANOTIC CONGENITAL HEART DISEASE WITHOUT A SHUNT

CONGENITAL AORTIC STENOSIS Malformations that cause obstruction to left ventricular outflow include congenital valvular aortic stenosis, discrete subaortic stenosis, supervalvular aortic stenosis, and hypertrophic obstructive cardiomyopathy (Chap. 205).

Valvular aortic stenosis Valvular aortic stenosis occurs three to four times more often in males than in females. The congenital bicuspid aortic valve, which is not necessarily stenotic, is one of the most common congenital malformations of the heart, although it may go undetected in early life. Because bicuspid valves may become stenotic with time or be the site of infective endocarditis, the lesion may be difficult to distinguish in adults from acquired rheumatic or degenerative calcific aortic stenosis.

The dynamics of blood flow associated with a congenitally deformed, rigid aortic valve commonly lead to thickening of the cusps and, in later life, to calcification. Hemodynamically significant obstruction causes concentric hypertrophy of the left ventricular wall and dilatation of the ascending aorta.

The hemodynamic abnormalities are discussed in Chap. 201. A peak systolic pressure gradient exceeding 70 mmHg, in association with abnormal cardiac output, or an effective aortic orifice less than 0.6 cm² per square meter of body surface, is considered to represent critical obstruction to left ventricular outflow. In adults, the resting cardiac output is generally normal but often fails to rise normally during muscular exercise.

Many patients with congenital aortic stenosis are asymptomatic. Usually, a murmur is detected on a routine examination. Moderately severe obstruction should be suspected if there is a history of fatigability and exertional dyspnea. With severe obstruction, the inability of the left ventricle to increase its output and maintain cerebral flow during exercise may result in exertional syncope, and the disparity between the oxygen supply and myocardial oxygen requirements may cause angina. The symptomatic patient with valvular aortic stenosis generally has critical stenosis, although a lack of symptoms does not preclude the presence of moderately severe obstruction. Sudden death occurs in patients with critical stenosis, and ventricular arrhythmias, perhaps initiated by acute myocardial ischemia, may be responsible.

Hemodynamically significant obstruction is associated with a sustained left ventricular apical impulse and a precordial systolic thrill over the base of the heart with transmission to the jugular notch and along the carotid arteries. Presystolic apical expansion is often palpable. A systolic aortic ejection sound, signifying opening of the aortic valve, is typically heard best at the cardiac apex when the valve is mobile, particularly with mild to moderate stenosis. A fourth heart sound is generally associated with severe obstruction. The systolic murmur starts after the completion of left ventricular isometric contraction, is crescendo-decrescendo or diamond-shaped, loud, harsh, and best heard at the base of the heart. The murmur, like the thrill, radiates to the jugular notch and carotid vessels and to the apex. An early diastolic blowing murmur of aortic regurgitation may be present, but unless the valve has been eroded by infective endocarditis the regurgitation is usually not hemodynamically significant; rarely, in patients with a congenital bicuspid valve, severe aortic regurgitation may be the dominant hemodynamic lesion.

Electrocardiographic evidence of left ventricular hypertrophy tends to reflect the severity of obstruction, although a normal or near-normal electrocardiogram does not exclude severe aortic stenosis. The left ventricular "strain pattern" generally indicates that severe aortic stenosis is present. Two-dimensional echocardiography demonstrates the aortic valve morphology; Doppler echocardiography is the most accurate means of noninvasively estimating the magnitude of obstruction and valvular regurgitation if present. Cardiac catheterization and coronary angiography are indicated particularly if coronary artery disease is suspected.

TREATMENT The medical management of congenital valvular aortic stenosis includes prophylaxis against infective endocarditis and, in patients with diminished cardiac reserve, the administration of digitalis and diuretics and sodium restriction while awaiting operation. If severe aortic stenosis is present, strenuous physical activity should be avoided even when the patient is asymptomatic, and participation in competitive sports should probably be restricted in patients with milder degrees of obstruction. Aortic valve replacement is indicated in asymptomatic adults with severe obstruction or in patients who are symptomatic with an aortic valve area less than 1.0 cm². If surgery is contraindicated because of a complicating medical problem such as malignancy or renal or hepatic failure, balloon valvuloplasty may provide short-term improvement.

Subaortic stenosis The most common form of subaortic stenosis is the *idiopathic hypertrophic* variety, also termed *hypertrophic cardiomyopathy*, which is present at birth in about one-third of the patients and is discussed in Chap. 205. Both clinically and physiologically, the *discrete* form of subaortic stenosis resembles valvular aortic stenosis. The lesion usually consists of a membranous diaphragm or fibrous ring encircling the left ventricular outflow tract just beneath the base of the aortic valve. Echocardiography demonstrates the subaortic obstruction; Doppler studies show turbulence proximal to the aortic valve and also detect and quantify the pressure gradient and severity of aortic regurgitation. Treatment consists of excision of the membrane or fibrous ridge.

Supravalvular aortic stenosis This anomaly consists of a localized or diffuse narrowing of the ascending aorta originating just above the level of the coronary arteries at the superior margin of the sinuses of Valsalva. In contrast to other forms of aortic stenosis, the coronary arteries are subjected to the elevated pressures that exist within the left ventricle and are often dilated and tortuous.

COARCTATION OF THE AORTA Narrowing or constriction of the lumen of the aorta may occur anywhere along its length but is most common distal to the origin of the left subclavian artery near the insertion of the ligamentum arteriosum. Coarctation occurs in about 7 percent of patients with congenital heart disease and is twice as common in males as in females, although the lesion occurs frequently in patients with gonadal dysgenesis. Clinical manifestations depend on the site and extent of obstruction and the presence of associated cardiac anomalies, most commonly a bicuspid aortic valve. Aneurysmal arterial dilatation of the circle of Willis produces a high risk of sudden rupture and death.

Most children and young adults with isolated, discrete coarctation are asymptomatic. Headache, epistaxis, cold extremities, and claudication with exercise may occur, and attention is usually directed to the cardiovascular system when a heart murmur or hypertension in the upper extremities and absence, marked diminution, or delayed pulsations in the femoral arteries are detected on physical examination. Enlarged and pulsatile collateral vessels may be palpated in the intercostal spaces anteriorly, in the axillae, or posteriorly in the interscapular area. The upper extremities and thorax may be more developed than the lower extremities. A midsystolic murmur over the anterior part of the chest, back, and spinous processes may become continuous if the lumen is narrowed sufficiently to result in a high-velocity jet across the lesion throughout the cardiac cycle. Additional systolic and continuous murmurs over the lateral thoracic wall may reflect increased flow through dilated and tortuous collateral vessels. The electrocardiogram reveals left ventricular hypertrophy of varying degree. Roentgenograms may show a dilated left subclavian artery high on the left mediastinal border and a dilated ascending aorta. Indentation of the aorta at the site of coarctation and pre- and poststenotic dilatation (the "3" sign) along the left paramediastinal shadow are almost pathognomonic. Notching of the ribs, an important radiographic sign, is due to erosion by dilated collateral vessels. Two-dimensional echocardiography from para- or suprasternal windows identifies the site and length of coarctation, while Doppler studies record and quantify the pressure gradient. Transesophageal echocardiography and magnetic resonance imaging or digital angiography allow visualization of the length and severity of the obstruction and the associated collateral arteries. In adults, cardiac catheterization is indicated primarily to evaluate the coronary arteries.

The chief hazards result from severe hypertension and include the development of cerebral aneurysms and hemorrhage, rupture of the aorta, left ventricular failure, and infective endocarditis.

Management   This is usually surgical; resection and end-to-end anastomosis or subclavian flap angioplasty are employed commonly, although it may be necessary to use a tubular graft, patch, or bypass conduit if the narrowed segment is long. Systemic hypertension postoperatively, in the absence of residual coarctation, appears to be related to the duration of preoperative hypertension. Postsurgical recoarctation may be successfully treated with percutaneous balloon dilatation.

PULMONARY STENOSIS WITH INTACT VENTRICULAR SEPTUM
Obstruction to right ventricular outflow may be localized to the supravalvular, valvular, or subvalvular levels or occur at a combination of these sites. Multiple sites of narrowing of the peripheral pulmonary arteries are a feature of *rubella embryopathy* and may occur with both the familial and sporadic forms of supravalvular aortic stenosis. Valvular pulmonic stenosis is the most common form of isolated right ventricular obstruction.

The severity of the obstructing lesion, rather than the site of narrowing, is the most important determinant of the clinical course. In the presence of a normal cardiac output, a peak systolic transvalvular pressure gradient between 50 and 80 mmHg is considered to be moderate stenosis; levels below and above that range are classified as mild and severe, respectively. Patients with mild pulmonic stenosis are generally asymptomatic and demonstrate little or no progression in the severity of obstruction with age. In patients with more significant stenosis, the severity may increase with time. Symptoms vary with the degree of obstruction. Fatigue, dyspnea, right ventricular failure, and syncope may limit the activity of older patients, in whom moderate or severe obstruction may prevent an augmentation of cardiac output with exercise. In patients with severe obstruction, the systolic pressure in the right ventricle may exceed that in the left ventricle, since the ventricular septum is intact. Right ventricular ejection is prolonged with moderate or severe stenosis, and the sound of pulmonary valve closure is delayed and soft. Right ventricular hypertrophy reduces the compliance of that chamber, and a forceful right atrial contraction is necessary to augment right ventricular filling. A fourth heart sound, prominent *a* waves in the jugular venous pulse, and, occasionally, presystolic pulsations of the liver reflect vigorous atrial contraction. The clinical diagnosis is supported by a right parasternal lift and harsh systolic ejection murmur and thrill at the upper left sternal border, typically preceded by a systolic ejection sound, if the obstruction is valvular. The holosystolic decrescendo murmur of tricuspid regurgitation may accompany severe pulmonic stenosis, especially in the presence of congestive heart failure. Cyanosis usually reflects venoarterial shunting through a patent foramen ovale or atrial septal defect. In patients with supravalvular or peripheral pulmonary arterial stenosis, the murmur is systolic or continuous and is best heard over the area of narrowing, with radiation to the peripheral lung fields.

The *electrocardiogram* may be helpful in assessing the degree of right ventricular obstruction. In mild cases, the electrocardiogram is often normal, whereas moderate and severe stenoses are associated with right axis deviation and right ventricular hypertrophy. A ventricular strain pattern, as well as high-amplitude P waves in leads II and V_1, indicating right atrial enlargement, is associated with severe stenosis. The chest roentgenogram with mild or moderate pulmonic stenosis often shows a heart of normal size and normal vascularity of the lungs. In the presence of valvular stenosis, poststenotic dilatation of the main and left pulmonary arteries may be evident. With severe obstruction and resultant right ventricular failure, right atrial and ventricular enlargement are generally evident. The pulmonary vascularity may be reduced with severe stenosis, right ventricular failure, and/or a venoarterial shunt at the atrial level. Two-dimensional *echocardiography* visualizes pulmonary valve morphology; the out-

flow tract pressure gradient can be estimated by Doppler ultrasonography.

Management   The cardiac catheter technique of balloon valvuloplasty (Chap. 192) is usually effective. Direct surgical relief of moderate and severe obstruction may be accomplished at a low risk. Multiple stenoses of the peripheral pulmonary arteries are usually inoperable, but narrowing of a single branch or at the bifurcation of the main pulmonary trunk may be corrected.

CYANOTIC CONGENITAL HEART DISEASE WITH INCREASED PULMONARY BLOOD FLOW

COMPLETE TRANSPOSITION OF THE GREAT ARTERIES   In this condition the aorta arises from the right ventricle to the right of and anterior to the pulmonary artery, which emerges from the left ventricle. This results in two separate and parallel circulations, and some communication between the two circulations must exist after birth to sustain life. Most patients have an interatrial communication, two-thirds have a patent ductus arteriosus, and about one-third have an associated ventricular septal defect. Transposition is more common in males and accounts for approximately 10 percent of cyanotic heart disease.

The course is determined by the degree of tissue hypoxia, the ability of each ventricle to sustain an increased work load in the presence of reduced coronary arterial oxygenation, the nature of the associated cardiovascular anomalies, and the status of the pulmonary vascular bed. Severe morphologic alterations develop in the pulmonary vascular bed by 1 to 2 years of age in most patients who also have an associated large ventricular septal defect or large patent ductus arteriosus in the absence of obstruction to left ventricular outflow.

Surgical treatment   The creation or enlargement of an interatrial communication is the simplest procedure for providing increased intracardiac mixing of systemic and pulmonary venous blood; it may be achieved surgically or, preferably, by rupturing the valve of the foramen ovale with a balloon catheter during cardiac catheterization (Rashkind procedure). Systemic–pulmonary artery anastomosis may be indicated in the patient with severe obstruction to left ventricular outflow and diminished pulmonary blood flow. Intracardiac repair may be accomplished by rearranging the venous returns so that the systemic venous blood is directed to the mitral valve and thence to the left ventricle and pulmonary artery, while the pulmonary venous blood is diverted through the tricuspid valve and right ventricle to the aorta (Mustard or Senning operation). Many surgeons now prefer to correct this malformation in infancy by transposing both coronary arteries to the posterior artery and transecting, contraposing, and anastomosing the aorta and pulmonary arteries (Jatene or arterial switch operation). For those patients with a ventricular septal defect in whom it is necessary to bypass a severely obstructed left ventricular outflow tract, corrective operation employs an intracardiac ventricular baffle and extracardiac prosthetic conduit to replace the pulmonary artery (Rastelli procedure). Patients with a large ventricular septal defect require closure of the ventricular septal defect and the atrial switch operation early in infancy. There are now many adults who underwent venous switch repair early in life who are experiencing the long-term complications of that operation, including arrhythmias, baffle leaks, or obstruction and reduced performance of the systemic right ventricle.

TOTAL ANOMALOUS PULMONARY VENOUS CONNECTION   In this malformation all the pulmonary veins connect either to the right atrium directly or to the systemic veins or their tributaries. Because all venous blood returns to the right atrium, an interatrial communication is an integral part of this malformation. Most unoperated patients surviving to adult life have pulmonary vascular obstructive disease, a reduction in pulmonary blood flow, and cyanosis.

SINGLE VENTRICLE   This designation applies to a family of complex lesions with both atrioventricular valves or a common atrioventricular valve opening to a single ventricular chamber. In most patients, the single ventricle morphologically resembles a left ventricular chamber that is separated from an infundibular outlet chamber by a bulboventricular septum; in these cases the anomaly is often referred to as double-inlet left ventricle. Associated anomalies are common and include abnormal great artery positional relationships, pulmonic valvular or subvalvular stenosis, and subaortic stenosis.

Depending upon the associated anomalies, the clinical presentation of single ventricle mimics other conditions in which cyanosis and decreased (or increased) pulmonary blood flow coexist, e.g., tetralogy of Fallot in the former instance and complete transposition of the great arteries in the latter. Survival to adulthood depends upon a relatively normal pulmonary blood flow and good ventricular function. Correction of the defect usually consists of creation of a right atrial–pulmonary conduit (the Fontan procedure); some patients are candidates for a septation operation in which the single ventricle is partitioned with a prosthetic patch.

CYANOTIC CONGENITAL HEART DISEASE WITH DECREASED PULMONARY BLOOD FLOW

TRICUSPID ATRESIA Atresia of the tricuspid valve, an interatrial communication, and, frequently, hypoplasia of the right ventricle and pulmonary artery exist in this malformation. Because of the small or nearly absent right ventricle, this anomaly is basically a "univentricular" heart with a single inlet (mitral) to the left ventricle. The clinical picture is usually dominated by severe cyanosis due to obligatory admixture of systemic and pulmonary venous blood in the left ventricle. The electrocardiogram characteristically shows right atrial enlargement, left axis deviation, and left ventricular hypertrophy.

Atrial septostomy and palliative operations to increase pulmonary blood flow, often by anastomosis of a systemic artery or vein to a pulmonary artery, may allow survival to the second or third decade. A Fontan atriopulmonary connection may then allow functional correction in those patients with normal or low pulmonary arterial resistance pressure and good left ventricular function.

EBSTEIN'S ANOMALY This malformation is characterized by a downward displacement of the tricuspid valve into the right ventricle, due to anomalous attachment of the tricuspid leaflets. Tricuspid valve tissue is dysplastic; a variable portion of the septal and inferior cusps adhere to the right ventricular wall some distance away from the atrioventricular junction. The abnormally situated tricuspid orifice produces a portion of the right ventricle lying between the atrioventricular ring and the origin of the valve, which is continuous with the right atrial chamber. This proximal segment is "atrialized," and the distal ventricular chamber is small. The degree of impairment of right ventricular function depends primarily on the extent to which the right ventricular inflow portion is atrialized and on the magnitude of tricuspid valve regurgitation. Most patients survive at least to the third decade. Although the clinical manifestations are variable, some patients come to initial attention because of progressive cyanosis from right-to-left atrial shunting, or symptoms due to tricuspid regurgitation and right ventricular dysfunction, or paroxysmal atrial tachyarrhythmias with or without bypass tracts (type B Wolff-Parkinson-White syndrome is common). Diagnostic findings by two-dimensional echocardiography include the abnormal positional relation between the tricuspid and mitral valves with apical displacement of the septal tricuspid leaflet. Tricuspid regurgitation is detected and quantified by Doppler examination. Surgical approaches have included prosthetic replacement of the tricuspid valve when the leaflets are tethered, or, in patients with an elongated mobile anterior leaflet, creation of a competent, unicuspid valve by insertion of the elongated anterior leaflet into the original tricuspid annulus and plication of the atrialized right ventricle. Transection of bypass tracts may be necessary to abolish atrial tachyarrhythmias.

TETRALOGY OF FALLOT This malformation accounts for about 10 percent of all forms of congenital heart disease and is the most common cause of cyanotic forms. The four components of the tetralogy of Fallot are ventricular septal defect, obstruction to right ventricular outflow, aortic override (straddle) of the ventricular septal defect, and right ventricular hypertrophy. The basic anomaly results from an anterior and superior deviation of the infundibular ventricular septum away from its usual location in the heart between the limbs of the trabecular septum. This displacement causes subpulmonary obstruction, aortic "override," and a large, nonrestrictive, malalignment-type ventricular septal defect.

The severity of right ventricular outflow obstruction determines the clinical presentation. The severity of hypoplasia of the right ventricular outflow tract varies from mild to complete (pulmonary atresia). Pulmonary valve stenosis and supravalvular and peripheral pulmonary arterial obstruction may coexist; rarely there is unilateral absence of a pulmonary artery (usually the left). A right-sided aortic arch and descending aorta occur in about 25 percent of patients with tetralogy. The coronary arteries may have variations that are surgically important. The anterior descending artery sometimes originates from the right coronary artery, which may also give rise to a left branch coursing anterior to the infundibulum; a single left coronary artery may give rise to a branch that crosses the outflow tract of the right ventricle.

The relationship between the resistance to blood flow from the ventricles into the aorta and into the pulmonary vessels plays a major role in determining the hemodynamic and clinical picture. Thus, the severity of obstruction to right ventricular outflow is of fundamental significance. In many infants and children the obstruction is mild but progressive. When the obstruction is severe, the pulmonary blood flow is reduced markedly, and a large volume of desaturated systemic venous blood is shunted from right to left across the ventricular septal defect. Severe cyanosis and erythrocytosis occur, and symptoms and sequelae of systemic hypoxemia are prominent.

The *electrocardiogram* ordinarily shows right ventricular and, less often, right atrial hypertrophy. Radiologic examination characteristically reveals a normal-sized, boot-shaped heart (*coeur en sabot*) with prominence of the right ventricle and a concavity in the region of the pulmonary conus. The pulmonary vascular markings are typically diminished, and the aortic arch and knob may be on the right side. Two-dimensional echocardiography from the parasternal or subcostal windows demonstrates the malalignment of the ventricular septal defect and the subpulmonary stenosis. The presence or absence of stenoses at the origins of the main branch pulmonary arteries can also be assessed. Selective angiocardiography with right ventricular injection provides architectural details of the right ventricular outflow tract, pulmonary valve and annulus, and caliber of the main branches of the pulmonary artery; coronary arteriography identifies the anatomy and course of the coronary arteries.

Management Factors that may complicate the treatment of patients with tetralogy of Fallot include infective endocarditis, paradoxic embolism, excessive erythrocytosis, coagulation defects, and cerebral infarction or abscess. Corrective operation is advisable at some point for almost all patients with this anomaly. Successful correction avoids progressive infundibular obstruction, delayed growth, and complications due to hypoxemia and excessive erythrocytosis. The size of the pulmonary arteries rather than the age or size of the infant or child is the most important determinant in establishing candidacy for primary repair. Pronounced hypoplasia of the pulmonary arteries is a relative contraindication for an early corrective surgical procedure. When this problem is present, a palliative operation, such as creation of a systemic arterial–pulmonary arterial shunt, is carried out and is usually followed by complete correction, which can be carried out at a lower risk later in childhood.

OTHER FORMS OF CONGENITAL HEART DISEASES

CONGENITALLY CORRECTED TRANSPOSITION The two fundamental anatomic abnormalities in this malformation are transposition of the ascending aorta and pulmonary trunk and inversion of the ventricles. This arrangement results in desaturated systemic venous blood passing from the right atrium through the mitral valve to the left ventricle and into the pulmonary trunk, whereas arterialized pulmonary venous blood flows from the left atrium through the tricuspid valve to the right ventricle and into the aorta. Thus, the circulation is corrected functionally. The clinical presentation, course, and prognosis of patients with congenitally corrected transposition vary depending on the nature and severity of any complicating intracardiac anomalies. Ebstein-type anomalies of the left-side tricuspid atrioventricular valve, ventricular septal defect, obstruction to outflow from the venous ventricle, and congenital heart block are often associated with corrected transposition. The diagnosis of the malformation and associated lesions can often be established by two-dimensional echocardiography and Doppler examination.

MALPOSITIONS OF THE HEART Positional anomalies refer to conditions in which the cardiac apex is in the right side of the chest (dextrocardia), or at the midline (mesocardia), or in which there is a normal location of the heart in the left side of the chest but abnormal position of the viscera (isolated levocardia). Knowledge of the position of the abdominal organs and of the branching pattern of the main stem bronchi is important in categorizing these malpositions. When dextrocardia occurs *without* situs inversus, when the *visceral situs is indeterminate*, or if *isolated levocardia* is present, associated, often complex, multiple cardiac anomalies are usually present. In contrast, mirror-image dextrocardia is usually observed with complete situs inversus, which occurs most frequently in individuals whose hearts are otherwise normal.

SURGICALLY MODIFIED CONGENITAL HEART DISEASE

Because of the enormous strides in cardiovascular surgical techniques that have occurred in the past 15 years, a large number of long-term survivors of corrective operations in infancy and childhood have reached adulthood. These patients are often challenging because of the diversity of anatomic, hemodynamic, and electrophysiologic residua and sequelae of cardiac operations.

The proper care of the survivor of operation for congenital heart disease requires that the clinician understand the details of the malformation prior to operation, pay meticulous attention to the details of the operative procedure, and recognize the postoperative residua (conditions left totally or partially uncorrected), sequelae (conditions caused by surgery), and the complications that may have resulted from the operation. With the exception of ligation and division of an uncomplicated patent ductus arteriosus, almost every other surgical repair of an anomaly leaves behind or causes some abnormality of the heart and circulation that may range from trivial to serious. Intraoperative transesophageal echocardiography assists in detecting unsuspected lesions, in monitoring the repair, and in verifying a satisfactory result or directing further repair. Thus, even with results that are considered clinically to be good to excellent, continued long-term postoperative follow-up is advisable.

Table 199-3 lists the categories of common late postoperative problems. Several of these residua, sequelae, and complications deserve special mention. Thus, cardiac operations importantly involving the atria, such as closure of atrial septal defect, repair of total or partial anomalous pulmonary venous return, or venous switch corrections of complete transposition of the great arteries (the Mustard or Senning operations), may be followed years later by sinus node or atrioventricular node dysfunction or by atrial arrhythmias. Intraventricular surgery may also result in electrophysiologic consequences, including complete heart block necessitating pacemaker insertion to avoid sudden death. In addition, valvular problems may arise late after initial cardiac operation. An example is the progressive stenosis of an initially nonobstructive bicuspid aortic valve in the patient who underwent aortic coarctation repair. Such aortic valves may also be

TABLE 199-3 Potential late postoperative problems

Residual shunts
Residual ventricular outflow obstruction
Residual valvular anomalies
Systemic arterial hypertension
Pulmonary vascular obstruction
Arrhythmias and conduction defects
Myocardial dysfunction
Prosthetic valve malfunction
Prosthetic conduit obstruction
Infective endocarditis

the site of infective endocarditis. After repair of the ostium primum atrial septal defect, the cleft mitral valve may become progressively incompetent. Low-pressure pulmonary regurgitation is common and well tolerated in most patients with repaired tetralogy of Fallot. However, in such patients with significant residual peripheral pulmonary arterial stenoses, severe pulmonary valvular regurgitation may result in right ventricular failure and tricuspid regurgitation. Tricuspid regurgitation may also be progressive in the postoperative patient with tetralogy of Fallot if right ventricular outflow tract obstruction was not relieved adequately at initial surgery. In many patients, inadequate relief of an obstructive lesion, or a residual regurgitant lesion, or a residual shunt will cause or hasten the onset of clinical signs and symptoms of myocardial dysfunction. In many patients, particularly those who were cyanotic for many years before operation, a preexisting compromise in ventricular performance is due to the original underlying malformation. A final category of postoperative problems involves the use of prosthetic valves, patches, or conduits in the operative repair. The special risks in such patients include infective endocarditis, thrombus formation, and premature degeneration and calcification of the prosthetic materials. There are many patients in whom extracardiac conduits are required to correct the circulation functionally and often to carry blood to the lungs from the right atrium or right ventricle. These conduits may develop intraluminal obstruction and, if they include a prosthetic valve, it may show progressive calcification and thickening.

REFERENCES

CHILD JS: Echo-Doppler and color-flow imaging in congenital heart disease. Cardiol Clin 8:289, 1990

CROWLEY JJ et al: Telltale signs of congential heart disease. Radiol Clin North Am 31:573, 1993

FRIEDMAN WF: Congenital heart disease in infancy and childhood, in *Heart Disease*, 4th ed, E Braunwald (ed). Philadelphia, Saunders, 1992, p 887

NORA JJ: Causes of congenital heart diseases: Old and new modes, mechanisms and models. Am Heart J 125:1409, 1993

PERLOFF JK: *The Clinical Recognition of Congenital Heart Disease*, 3d ed. Philadelphia, Saunders, 1987

———, CHILD JS: *Congenital Heart Disease in Adults*. Philadelphia, Saunders, 1991

——— et al: 22nd Bethesda Conference: Congenital heart disease after childhood; an expanding patient population. J Am Coll Cardiol 18:311, 1991

WEIDMAN WH: Second natural history study of congenital heart defects. Circulation 87:II, 1993

WEINTRAUB R et al: Transesophageal echocardiography in infants and children with congenital heart disease. Circulation 86:711, 1992

200 RHEUMATIC FEVER

GENE H. STOLLERMAN

DEFINITION Rheumatic fever is an inflammatory disease which occurs as a delayed sequel to pharyngeal infection with group A streptococci. It involves principally the heart, joints, central nervous system, skin, and subcutaneous tissues. The usual manifestations in the acute form are migratory polyarthritis, fever, and carditis.

Sydenham's chorea, subcutaneous nodules, and erythema marginatum may occur as other typical manifestations. No single symptom, sign, or laboratory test is pathognomonic of rheumatic fever, although several combinations of them are diagnostic. Although the name *acute rheumatic fever* emphasizes involvement of the joints, rheumatic fever owes its importance to the involvement of the heart, which can be fatal during the acute stage or lead to rheumatic heart disease, a chronic condition due to scarring and deformity of the heart valves.

ETIOLOGY AND PATHOGENESIS The etiologic relationship of group A streptococci to rheumatic fever can be summarized briefly as follows: (1) Numerous clinical and epidemiologic studies have shown a close association of group A streptococcal infections and rheumatic fever. (2) Antecedent streptococcal infection can almost always be demonstrated immunologically in the acute stage of rheumatic fever by increased titers of antibodies to streptococcal antigens. Moreover, in long-term prospective follow-up studies, rheumatic fever recurs only as a result of intercurrent streptococcal infections. (3) Both primary and secondary attacks of the disease can be prevented by prompt treatment or prevention of streptococcal infections with antimicrobial therapy. (4) The site of infection is critical. The pharyngeal route of infection is necessary to initiate the rheumatic process. Streptococcal skin or soft tissue infections do not do so. (5) Not all strains of group A streptococci cause the disease. The so-called skin strains that cause streptococcal pyoderma do not cause rheumatic fever, even when infecting the throat. The strains that have been clearly associated with rheumatic fever outbreaks have distinct virulence properties when freshly isolated from the pharynx. They are very rich in the extractable serotypic surface M protein and contain large hyaluronic acid capsules that are responsible for the formation of mucoid colonies on blood agar plates. Such strains usually belong to certain serotypes, notably M types 3, 5, 18, 19, 24, and others. All strains within these serotypes, however, are not always in this phase of virulence and are not always rheumatogenic. The M protein of rheumatogenic strains forms an unusually large, extended molecule consisting of repeating peptide subunits not found in other strains of group A streptococci so far studied.

The mechanism by which the group A streptococcus initiates the disease process remains unknown. A relatively small percentage of persons who suffer from streptococcal sore throats subsequently develop rheumatic fever. The organism is not demonstrable in the lesions when rheumatic fever appears after a characteristic latent period of 1 to 5 weeks after the acute pharyngeal streptococcal infection. No one product of the streptococcus has been incriminated as a cause of the lesions, either as a direct tissue toxin or as an antigen inducing hypersensitivity. Several streptococcal antigens have demonstrated cross-reactivity with cardiac and other tissues. Notably, epitopes within the non-type-specific peptides of the M protein of rheumatogenic strains cross-react immunologically with myosin, keratin, and other coiled proteins found in cardiac tissues. Although the hyaluronic acid of group A streptococcal capsules and that of human host tissues are chemically identical, autoantibodies to this substance are demonstrable. Such findings suggest that a ''molecular mimicry'' type of autoimmunity may relate to the pathogenesis of rheumatic fever, perhaps induced by the strong immunologic adjuvant properties of some parts of the M protein molecule that have superantigen-like activity, i.e., the capability of activating lymphocyte receptors directly. Such properties may invoke autoimmune responses in susceptible hosts and also may explain the finding that all streptococcal antibodies so far studied tend to be higher in patients with acute rheumatic fever than in those who do not develop the disease following a bout of streptococcal pharyngitis.

INCIDENCE AND EPIDEMIOLOGY Although rheumatic fever may occur at any age, it is extremely rare in infancy; it appears most commonly between the ages of 5 and 15 years, when streptococcal infection is most frequent and intense. Similarly, the geographic distribution, incidence, and severity of rheumatic fever are, in general, a reflection of the frequency and severity of streptococcal pharyngitis. The attack rate of rheumatic fever following exudative streptococcal

pharyngitis in epidemics averages approximately 3 percent. When streptococcal pharyngitis is sporadic and mild or due to strains of lesser or no rheumatic potential, the attack rate of rheumatic fever may be very much lower. Strains of group A streptococci that cause epidemics of streptococcal pharyngitis are most likely to be rheumatogenic. Following such infections, the attack rate of rheumatic fever is directly correlated with the magnitude of the streptococcal immune response. Analysis of reported epidemics of acute rheumatic fever caused by a variety of serotypes shows some, such as type 5, to be overrepresented and others to be conspicuously absent. In some populations, such as in Trinidad, strains responsible for rheumatic fever and acute glomerulonephritis are serotypically distinct.

Environmental, bacterial, and host factors which appear to play a role in the development of rheumatic fever are important primarily because they are related to the incidence and severity of preceding streptococcal infection. Such factors as latitude, altitude, dampness, economic factors, and age all affect the incidence of rheumatic fever because they are related to the incidence of streptococcal infection in general. Crowding is, however, the major environmental factor relating to the occurrence of this disease because, regardless of other variables, it promotes interpersonal spread of the most virulent group A streptococcal strains. Such crowding as occurs in military barracks, closed institutions, large families in small quarters, and those massed in the densely populated core of major urban centers is most likely to be associated with an increase in incidence of rheumatic fever.

The attack rate of rheumatic fever following streptococcal infections by rheumatogenic strains in patients who have had previous attacks of rheumatic fever is increased to as high as 5 to 50 percent and is also related to the virulence of the reactivating infection. Furthermore, the frequency of rheumatic recurrences following streptococcal infection is consistently greater in those with rheumatic heart disease than in those who escaped cardiac injury during prior attacks. The tendency to suffer recurrences of rheumatic fever following streptococcal infections declines with the passage of years since the preceding attack. It appears, therefore, that certain host variables, as well as qualitative and quantitative differences in the nature of the antecedent streptococcal infection, also influence the development of rheumatic fever. To what extent such variables are genetic or acquired has not been settled. It is common to obtain a family history of rheumatic fever as well as to encounter multiple cases among siblings of a single family. However, the concordance of rheumatic fever in identical twins is approximately 20 percent, suggesting only a limited penetrance of genetic predisposition to rheumatic fever. Although investigations of the distribution of haplotypes in rheumatic hosts have been limited in scope and number, there have been so far no class I and somewhat limited class II HLA-DR associations occurring along racial lines, particularly in those who have developed rheumatic carditis. Recently, B lymphocyte allotypic antigens have been found to be strikingly overrepresented in patients with rheumatic heart disease. Their nature and relation to pathogenesis, however, are not yet known.

The mortality of acute rheumatic fever has been declining steadily for the past 30 years. It is still, however, a major cause of death and disability in children and adolescents in socioeconomically depressed areas of the world. The incidence of rheumatic fever has been decreasing dramatically in countries where housing and economic conditions have been improving steadily. The rate of decrease in rheumatic fever may have been accelerated by the wide use of antimicrobial therapy. The decrease also may be due to a change in the prevalence of rheumatogenic streptococcal strains, which seemed to have disappeared in affluent societies, whereas the prevalence of streptococcal pharyngitis in school children remains the same. In recent years, however, local outbreaks of rheumatic fever have occurred in the United States in two military populations, one at the San Diego Naval Base, California, and the other at Fort Leonard Wood, Missouri. Outbreaks also have occurred among school children in Utah, Ohio, and Pennsylvania. Middle-class communities with relatively high standards of living and medical care have been affected.

Further investigations of the streptococcal strains causing pharyngitis in these communities have resulted in the recovery of "mucoid" strains of group A streptococci belonging to serotype M types 3 and 18. These strains were once prevalent in well-studied epidemics of rheumatic fever in the 1940s and 1950s, particularly in military populations. They have rarely been seen since then. The explanation for the reappearance of these strains in middle-class communities and in widely separated military bases is unclear and has caused a resurgence of interest in proper diagnosis and treatment of streptococcal sore throat. Rheumatic fever remains, however, a worldwide disease having its greatest incidence wherever poor economic conditions, overcrowding, and substandard housing are most common and where such conditions promote the transmission of rheumatogenic streptococci.

PATHOLOGY   The lesions of rheumatic fever are disseminated widely throughout the body, with special predilection for connective tissues. Focal inflammatory lesions occur particularly around small blood vessels.

Cardiovascular lesions   The heart is the site of the most characteristic and consequential involvement, and all its layers—endocardium, myocardium, and pericardium—may be involved. This generalized involvement gives rise to the term *rheumatic pancarditis*. The most characteristic and specific pattern of rheumatic inflammation is found in the *myocardial Aschoff body*, a submiliary granuloma. This lesion, when present in its classic form, is generally considered to be pathognomonic of rheumatic fever. In many areas the inflammatory lesion is accompanied by swelling and fragmentation of the collagen fibers and alteration in the staining properties of the ground substances of the connective tissues. This change is described as *fibrinoid degeneration of collagen*, but its chemical basis has not been established. Aschoff bodies with less exudative and more productive changes may persist for many years as the lingering traces of chronic rheumatic inflammation in patients with rheumatic heart disease, long after rheumatic fever has become clinically quiescent. The persistence of such lesions is most common in patients who develop severe mitral stenosis. Eventually, the Aschoff body is converted into a spindle-shaped or triangular scar lying between the muscle bundles and surrounding blood vessels.

Rheumatic endocarditis produces the verrucous valvulitis of acute rheumatic fever which leads to the most serious permanent cardiac damage. It may heal with fibrous thickening and adhesion of the valve commissures and chordae tendineae, leading to variable degrees of valvular regurgitation and stenosis. Deformity resulting in functional impairment of the heart occurs most commonly in the mitral and aortic valves, less frequently in the tricuspid valve, and almost never in the pulmonic valves. *Rheumatic pericarditis* (see Chap. 206) produces a serofibrinous effusion, with the deposit of shaggy elements of fibrin on the surface of the heart. The pericardium may become calcified, but pericardial constriction does not occur.

Extracardiac lesions   Involvement of the *joints* is characterized by exudative rather than proliferative changes, and healing of these structures occurs without significant scarring or deformity. *Subcutaneous nodules*, seen during the acute phase of the disease, are composed of granulomas with localized areas of "fibrinoid" swelling of subcutaneous collagen bundles and perivascular collections of large cells with pale nuclei and prominent nucleoli. Synovitis is usually mild and nonspecific. *Pulmonary* and *pleural* lesions are less definite and less characteristic. Fibrinous pleurisy and rheumatic pneumonitis may occur with exudative and proliferative lesions but without definite Aschoff bodies. Patients with active *chorea* rarely die. The pathologic findings which have been reported in the central nervous system are not consistent, and no characteristic lesion has been reported to explain this clinical manifestation. During active chorea, the spinal fluid remains normal, being free of cells, with no increase in total protein and no change in the relative concentration of various proteins.

CLINICAL FEATURES   The major clinical manifestations by which rheumatic fever can be recognized are polyarthritis, carditis, chorea, erythema marginatum, and subcutaneous nodules.

TABLE 200-1   Jones criteria, 1992 update

Major manifestations	Minor manifestations	Supporting evidence of antecedent group A streptococcal infection
Carditis	Clinical findings	Positive throat culture or rapid streptococcal antigen test
Polyarthritis	Arthralgia	
Chorea	Fever	
Erythema marginatum	Laboratory findings	Elevated or rising streptococcal antibody titer
Subcutaneous nodules	Elevated acute phase reactants	
	Erythrocyte sedimentation rate	
	C-reactive protein	
	Prolonged PR interval	

If supported by evidence of preceding group A streptococcal infection, the presence of two major manifestations or of one major and two minor manifestations indicates a high probability of acute rheumatic fever.

SOURCE: American Heart Association, 1992.

Arthritis   The classic attack of rheumatic fever appears as an acute migratory polyarthritis accompanied by signs and symptoms of an acute febrile illness. The large joints of the extremities are most frequently affected, but no joint is impervious to the inflammatory process; one may find arthritis of the hands and feet but only rarely of the spine or of the sternoclavicular or temporomandibular joints. Joint effusions occur but are not persistent. As pain and swelling subside in one joint, others tend to become involved. Although such "migratory" involvement is characteristic, it is not invariable, and several large joints may be inflamed at one time. To be acceptable as a criterion for the diagnosis of rheumatic fever, the polyarthritis should involve two or more joints, should be associated with at least two minor manifestations such as fever and elevation of sedimentation rate, and should be associated with high titer of antistreptolysin O or some other streptococcal antibody (Table 200-1). There is nothing distinctive about the arthritis of rheumatic fever, and other causes of migratory polyarthritis that may be associated only coincidentally with high streptococcal antibody levels must, of course, be excluded.

Acute rheumatic carditis   Acute rheumatic carditis first becomes manifest by the appearance of the heart murmurs of either mitral or aortic regurgitation, the former most frequently. Signs and symptoms of pericarditis and of congestive heart failure may supervene in more severe cases. Death may result from heart failure during the acute stage of the disease, or permanent valvular damage may be sustained which results ultimately in serious disability. Carditis may vary from a fulminating, fatal course to a low-grade, inapparent inflammation. *It is well to bear in mind that the vast majority of patients with carditis do not have symptoms referable to the heart.* The latter occur only in more severe cases when heart failure or pericardial effusions produce characteristic symptoms. For this reason, unless extracardiac manifestations, such as polyarthritis and chorea, are present, patients whose rheumatic fever is manifested only by carditis are frequently not diagnosed and in later life may be discovered to have rheumatic heart disease without a definite history of rheumatic fever.

When carditis is manifest, there is usually tachycardia disproportionate to the degree of fever, gallop rhythms are often heard, and the heart sounds may become fetal in character due to the loss of the muscular quality of the first heart sound. Occasionally, arrhythmias and/or a pericardial friction rub may be present. Prolongation of the conduction time may lead to dropped beats with varying degrees of heart block. Prolongation of the PR interval and other changes in the electrocardiogram are very common, but these findings, in the absence of clinical manifestations of carditis, have a benign prognosis. Therefore, changes in the electrocardiogram alone, unassociated with significant murmurs or cardiac enlargement, do not by themselves constitute an acceptable criterion for the diagnosis of rheumatic carditis. Pericarditis may cause precordial pain, and a friction rub may be audible.

A definite clinical diagnosis of carditis can be made if one or more of the following can be demonstrated: (1) the appearance of, or change in the character of, organic heart murmurs, (2) definite increase in heart size demonstrated by radiogram or fluoroscopy, (3) pericardial friction rub or effusion best demonstrated by echocardiography, or (4) signs of congestive heart failure. Rheumatic carditis is almost always associated with a significant murmur. The most common murmurs of acute rheumatic carditis are those due to mitral and aortic regurgitation caused by valvular inflammation. The former is usually a high-pitched holosystolic blowing murmur which must be carefully distinguished from the functional low-pitched, musical, apical flow murmur commonly heard with increased cardiac output in children and other thin-chested individuals. When more severe, mitral inflammation and left ventricular dilatation may produce, in addition to a blowing systolic murmur, a very low pitched, vibratory middiastolic murmur which often follows an accentuated third heart sound—the so-called Carey Coombs murmur. Aortic regurgitation murmurs are often associated with those of mitral origin, and in acute rheumatic fever, occasionally cooing or screeching ("seagull") murmurs are heard that reflect the turbulence formed around swollen and distorted valves during the acute inflammatory phase of carditis.

Subcutaneous nodules   These are usually small, pea-sized, painless swellings over bony prominences and therefore frequently go unnoticed by the patient. The skin moves freely over them. Characteristic locations are the extensor tendons of the hands and feet, the elbows, margins of the patellae, the scalp, over the scapulae, and over the spinous processes of the vertebrae.

Chorea (Sydenham's chorea, chorea minor, Saint Vitus' dance) This is a disorder of the central nervous system characterized by sudden, aimless, irregular movements, often accompanied by muscle weakness and emotional instability. Chorea is a delayed manifestation of rheumatic fever, and other manifestations may or may not still be present at the time it appears. Polyarthritis, when part of the same attack, almost always subsides before chorea appears. Carditis is often discovered for the first time when the presenting feature of rheumatic fever is chorea. Chorea usually appears after a long latent period (up to several months) from the antecedent streptococcal infection and at a time when all other manifestations of rheumatic fever have abated. When no previous rheumatic manifestations are noted, such cases are called *pure chorea.*

The clinical onset of chorea is often gradual. Patients may be unusually nervous and fidgety and may have difficulty in writing, drawing, and handiwork. They may stumble or fall, drop things, and grimace. As symptoms become more severe, spasmodic movements extend to all parts of the body, and muscular weakness may become so marked that patients cannot walk, talk, or sit up. Often the weakness is severe enough to simulate paralysis. The irregular, jerky, spasmodic movements may become so violent that cribs and beds must be padded to prevent injury. Symptoms are exaggerated by excitement, effort, or fatigue but subside during sleep. Emotional instability is almost invariable in patients with chorea. All degrees of speech disturbance are seen. Central nervous system stimulants exacerbate and sedatives suppress choreiform activity.

Erythema marginatum   This evanescent pink rash is characteristic of rheumatic fever. The erythematous areas often have clear centers and round or serpiginous margins. They vary greatly in size and occur mainly on the trunk and proximal part of the extremities, never on the face. The erythema is transient, migratory, and may be brought out by the application of heat; it is nonpruritic, not indurated, and blanches on pressure.

Minor clinical criteria   These include fever, arthralgia, abdominal pain, tachycardia, and epistaxis, clinical features which occur frequently in rheumatic fever but are also common to many other diseases and are therefore of minor diagnostic value.

LABORATORY FINDINGS   There is no specific laboratory test to indicate the presence of rheumatic fever. The appraisal of rheumatic activity by laboratory findings is, however, of value, since various tests may indicate *continued* rheumatic inflammation when clinical features are not apparent.

Streptococcal antibody tests to disclose preceding streptococcal infection   Streptococcal antibody titers differentiate preceding streptococcal from other acute respiratory infections and are increased following asymptomatic as well as symptomatic streptococcal infections. These antibody levels are increased in the early stages of acute rheumatic fever. They may be declining or low if the interval between the acute streptococcal infection and the detection of rheumatic fever has been longer than 2 months, a situation which occurs most often in patients whose presenting rheumatic manifestation is chorea. However, patients whose only major manifestation is rheumatic carditis also may have low antibody titers when first seen. Their rheumatic attack may have been in progress several months before becoming symptomatic and recognized. Except in these two instances, *one should be reluctant to make the diagnosis of acute rheumatic fever in the absence of serologic evidence of a recent streptococcal infection.* The antistreptolysin O (ASO) test is the most widely used and best-standardized streptococcal antibody test. In general, single titers of at least 250 Todd units in adults and at least 333 units in children over 5 years of age are considered to be increased. Depending on the general prevalence of streptococcal infections, a varying percentage of the normal population may show titers of this magnitude.

About 20 percent of patients in the early stages of acute rheumatic fever, and most patients who present with chorea, have a low or borderline ASO titer. In these instances, it is advisable to obtain a different streptococcal antibody test such as anti-DNase B or antihyaluronidase (AH). The antistreptozyme (ASTZ) test is a hemagglutination reaction to a concentrate of extracellular streptococcal antigens absorbed to red blood cells. It is a very sensitive indicator of recent streptococcal infection; virtually all patients with acute rheumatic fever have titers greater than 200 units per milliliter. A rise in titer of two dilution tubes or more can be demonstrated for at least one of the specific streptococcal antibodies in almost all recurrent as well as primary attacks of rheumatic fever. Increased streptococcal antibodies, however, do not reflect rheumatic activity per se, and their rate of decline is independent of the course of the rheumatic attack. Because it almost always occurs within the first 4 to 5 weeks of the antecedent streptococcal pharyngitis, polyarthritis is the clinical manifestation most promptly recognized and therefore most reliably associated with rising streptococcal antibody titers. The absence of increased or increasing streptococcal antibody titers in patients with acute polyarthritis therefore makes rheumatic fever a very unlikely cause.

Isolation of group A streptococci   Some patients continue to harbor group A streptococci at the onset of acute rheumatic fever, but these organisms are usually present in small numbers and may be difficult to isolate by a single throat culture. The administration of penicillin or other antibiotics also may result in failure to isolate the infecting organism. In addition, a significant number of *normal* individuals, particularly children, may harbor group A streptococci in the upper respiratory tract. For these reasons, throat cultures are less satisfactory than antibody tests as supporting evidence of recent streptococcal infection.

Acute phase reactants   These tests offer objective but nonspecific confirmation of the presence of an inflammatory process. The *erythrocyte sedimentation rate* (ESR) and the test for *C-reactive protein* (CRP) in serum are used most commonly. Unless the patient has received glucocorticoids or salicylates, these reactions are almost always abnormal in patients presenting with polyarthritis or acute carditis, whereas they are often normal in patients with "pure" chorea. Other laboratory findings which reflect inflammation include reactions such as leukocytosis and increases in serum complement, mucoproteins, and alpha$_2$ and gamma globulins. Prolongation of the PR interval of the electrocardiogram, although neither specific for rheumatic fever nor diagnostic of serious cardiac involvement, is frequent in acute rheumatic fever (about 25 percent of all cases), and other nonspecific electrocardiographic changes are also common. Anemia, due to the suppression of erythropoiesis characteristic of chronic inflammatory diseases, is another feature of rheumatic activity.

COURSE AND PROGNOSIS The course of rheumatic fever varies greatly and is impossible to predict at the onset of the disease. In general, however, approximately 75 percent of acute rheumatic attacks subside within 6 weeks, 90 percent within 12 weeks, and less than 5 percent persist more than 6 months. These last usually consist of severe, intractable forms of rheumatic carditis or stubborn, prolonged attacks of Sydenham's chorea, both of which may persist for as long as several years. Once acute rheumatic fever has subsided and more than 2 months has elapsed after withdrawal of treatment with salicylates or glucocorticoids, rheumatic fever does not recur in the absence of new streptococcal infections. Recurrences are most common within the first 5 years of the initial attack and tend to decline with increasing duration of freedom from rheumatic activity. The frequency of recurrences is dependent on the frequency and severity of streptococcal infection with strains of rheumatogenic potential, the presence or absence of rheumatic heart disease following an attack, and the duration of the interval since the last attack.

Approximately 70 percent of patients who develop carditis do so within the first week of the disease, 85 percent within the first 12 weeks of the disease, and almost all within 6 months from the onset of the acute attack. Thereafter, if significant murmurs have not appeared, the prognosis for a patient in whom recurrences are prevented is excellent.

Chronic rheumatic carditis and the course of rheumatic heart disease The remarkable variability in the course of rheumatic carditis and rheumatic valvular disease stems from several factors: (1) the variability in the duration and severity of the rheumatic inflammation, (2) the amount of scarring of the valves and myocardium following the abatement of the acute inflammation, (3) the location and severity of the hemodynamic lesion due to valvular insufficiency or stenosis, (4) the frequency of recurrent bouts of carditis, and (5) the progression of valvular calcification and sclerosis, which occurs as a secondary phenomenon in a deformed or injured valve without recurrent or persistent rheumatic inflammation (as seen in congenital valvular disease or following healed acute bacterial endocarditis). These factors, and possibly others not yet appreciated, produce striking variations in the clinical syndromes of rheumatic heart disease.

Chronic rheumatic myocarditis In this syndrome, the presenting picture is one of chronic heart failure in a patient with a markedly dilated heart and with physical, roentgenographic, and electrocardiographic findings of mitral and/or aortic and sometimes tricuspid regurgitation. The differentiation of this syndrome from other forms of chronic myocarditis may be very difficult, if not impossible, when the associated extracardiac features of rheumatic fever (chorea, polyarthritis, and so forth) are not present (Chap. 205). Although rheumatic fever does not produce *isolated* myocarditis and is almost invariably a pancarditis, the pericardial inflammation may not be clearly evident, and the mitral valvulitis may not be distinguishable from mitral regurgitation due to dilation of the mitral ring. In such cases, one must search diligently for an evanescent friction rub, evidence of pericardial effusion, appearance of a soft aortic regurgitation murmur, and extracardiac clues such as fever responding promptly to salicylates, arthralgias, transient subcutaneous nodules, evanescent erythema marginatum, and subtle signs of chorea.

The course of chronic rheumatic carditis may be intractable and end fatally after months or even several years. Often, however, the patient improves rather suddenly and even recovers cardiac reserve dramatically in association with the disappearance of systemic manifestations of the inflammatory process. The heart may remain large, may decrease somewhat in size, or in occasional instances may return to normal size with varying degrees of residual valvular deformity. Such a course signals the termination of the "toxic" phase of the rheumatic process, and thereafter the course of rheumatic heart disease depends on the variables in healing cited above.

DIFFERENTIAL DIAGNOSIS Early cases of rheumatic fever may be confused with other diseases which begin with acute polyarthritis. It is wise to exclude *bacteremia* by blood cultures, particularly because such infections may be masked by penicillin given for presumed acute rheumatic fever. Polyarthritis due to *infective endocarditis* in a patient with preexisting rheumatic heart disease may be mistaken for a recurrence of acute rheumatic fever. If streptococcal antibodies are not increased, polyarthritis should be attributed to some cause other than rheumatic fever. Gonococcal polyarthritis may be distinguished from rheumatic fever by the dramatic response of the former to a therapeutic trial of penicillin. In rheumatoid arthritis, joint involvement will persist and characteristic joint deformities may appear. The latter are not seen in rheumatic fever. The rheumatoid factor so characteristic of rheumatoid arthritis is not present in rheumatic fever. Antibodies against nuclear components and against IgG are absent in rheumatic fever. Rheumatic pericarditis and myocarditis, associated with cardiac enlargement and heart failure, are both almost invariably associated with valvular lesions which produce significant murmurs.

Overdiagnosis of rheumatic fever is a danger. Unless ill-defined febrile syndromes are clearly associated with a major manifestation of rheumatic fever, the diagnosis of rheumatic fever should not be made. A common error is the premature, vigorous administration of glucocorticoids or salicylates before the signs and symptoms of rheumatic fever are unmistakable. In the absence of a curative agent, one should not suppress the signs and symptoms of rheumatic fever until they are clearly expressed.

Particularly confusing in the differential diagnosis of rheumatic fever is the drug sensitivity with fever and polyarthritis which may occur after administration of penicillin for a previous pharyngitis. Urticaria or angioedema, if present, helps identify penicillin sensitivity in such cases. The abdominal pain of rheumatic fever may be mistaken for appendicitis, and the crisis of sickle cell anemia also may be associated with joint pain, enlargement of the heart, and cardiac murmurs. The rapidity with which the arthritis symptoms of rheumatic fever are controlled with salicylates is characteristic of this disease. Dramatic response to salicylates does not in itself, however, establish a diagnosis of rheumatic fever.

In order to help clarify the diagnosis of acute rheumatic fever, the American Heart Association has accepted and modified criteria usually referred to as the *Jones criteria* (see Table 200-1). They are not to be used as a substitute for good medical judgment but are recommended as a guide for careful study of questionable cases. The finding of two major criteria or of one major and two minor criteria indicates a high probability of the presence of rheumatic fever if supported by evidence of a preceding streptococcal infection. The absence of the latter should always make the diagnosis questionable, except in the situation in which rheumatic fever is first discovered after a long latent period from the antecedent infection (Sydenham's chorea or low-grade carditis). Because the prognosis may differ according to the major manifestations, for recording purposes the diagnosis of rheumatic fever should be followed by a list of the major manifestations present, e.g., rheumatic fever manifested by polyarthritis and carditis (Table 200-2). An indication of the severity of carditis in terms of presence or absence of congestive heart failure and cardiomegaly is also advisable.

TABLE 200-2   Ninety-nine cases of acute rheumatic fever indicated by three major manifestations of Jones Criteria

Major manifestations*	Percent
Carditis	14
Polyarthritis	14
Chorea	4
Carditis and polyarthritis	44
Carditis and chorea	14
Carditis, chorea, and polyarthritis	6
Polyarthritis and chorea	4
Total	**100**

* Categories are mutually exclusive.
SOURCE: Acute rheumatic fever—Utah. Morb Mort Week Rep 36:109, 1988

TREATMENT There is no specific cure for rheumatic fever, and no known measures change the course of the attack. Good supportive therapy, however, can reduce the mortality and morbidity of the disease.

Antibiotic therapy After rheumatic fever is first diagnosed, a course of penicillin should be given to eliminate group A streptococci. This course is advisable even if bacteriologic examination yields throat cultures negative for streptococci, since the organisms may be present in areas inaccessible to swabs. It is preferable to administer penicillin parenterally. An effective course is a single injection of 1.2 million units of benzathine penicillin intramuscularly or 600,000 units of procaine penicillin intramuscularly daily for 10 days. Attempts to reduce ultimate heart damage by administering larger doses of penicillin early in the acute rheumatic attack have not been successful. After completion of the therapeutic course of penicillin, continuous protection from reinfection with streptococci should be provided by instituting one of the prophylactic regimens described below.

Suppressive therapy For patients without carditis, treatment with glucocorticoids is unnecessary. Acute arthritis can be relieved with codeine or salicylate, the latter being preferable to reduce fever and joint inflammation. When salicylate is used in the therapy of rheumatic fever, the dosage should be increased until the drug produces either a clinical effect or systemic toxicity characterized by tinnitus, headache, or hyperpnea. A starting dose of 100 to 125 mg/kg per day in children and 6 to 8 g in adults given in four or five divided doses is recommended. Of the various salicylate preparations, ordinary aspirin is cheapest and most effective.

Many physicians prefer glucocorticoids to salicylates for the treatment of carditis, despite the lack of a demonstrated advantage of these adrenal hormones in controlled clinical trials. Glucocorticoids are more potent anti-inflammatory agents but are more likely to be followed by posttherapeutic "rebounds," and they have the additional disadvantage of more frequent side effects, particularly acne, hirsutism, and cushingoid changes in facies and habitus. For this reason it is preferable to begin treatment of patients who have carditis with salicylates; if these drugs fail to reduce fever and to ameliorate heart failure, therapy with glucocorticoids may be initiated promptly. Prednisone is administered in doses of 60 to 120 mg or higher when necessary in four divided doses daily. After the inflammation has been brought under control by either salicylates or glucocorticoids, treatment should be continued until the sedimentation rate approaches near-normal values and should be maintained for several weeks thereafter. To prevent poststeroid rebounds, an "overlap" course of salicylate therapy may be added when steroids are tapered off over a 2-week period. A useful method for tapering steroids is outlined in Chap. 335. Salicylates may then be continued for an additional 2 to 3 weeks. Rebounds of rheumatic activity are usually of short duration and, when mild, are best managed without resuming anti-inflammatory treatment because a second or even a third rebound may occur when suppressive therapy is discontinued. About 5 percent of rheumatic attacks persist for 6 months or longer, either in the form of spontaneous acute recrudescences or as posttherapeutic rebounds. These "chronic" attacks are most likely to occur in patients with cardiac damage and with previous rheumatic episodes. Weekly tests for C-reactive protein in blood and for erythrocyte sedimentation rate are useful in following the healing process, particularly while treatment with glucocorticoids or salicylates is gradually withdrawn.

Treatment of chorea The signs and symptoms of chorea usually do not respond well to treatment with antirheumatic agents. Because the patient with chorea is frequently emotionally unstable, and because the manifestations of chorea may be exaggerated by emotional trauma, complete mental and physical rest is essential. Patients with chorea should be kept in a quiet room and cared for by sympathetic attendants. Glucocorticoids or salicylates have little or no effect on chorea. Sedatives and tranquilizers, particularly diazepam and chlorpromazine, are useful. Chorea, no matter how severe, disappears during sleep, which should therefore be ensured by adequate sedation. Padded sideboards for the bed may be necessary to avoid injury to the patient. In the absence of other evidence of acute rheumatic disease, it is advisable to allow gradual resumption of physical activity when improvement is apparent rather than waiting for all choreiform movements to disappear, which may require many months.

Because of the great variability in the course of chorea, evaluating the effectiveness of various therapeutic measures is difficult. It is well to remember that chorea is a self-limited disease which is usually not followed by significant neurologic sequelae and that good results are almost invariably obtained by patient, attentive nursing care and conservative medical management.

PREVENTION OF RECURRENCE The resurgence of localized outbreaks of rheumatic fever in the United States in recent years has been blamed, in part, on less than faithful adherence to conventional recommendations for rigorous penicillin regimens known to be highly effective in the prevention of both primary and secondary rheumatic attacks. It is recommended, therefore, that these regimens continue to be employed. The most efficient regimen for continuous prophylaxis against group A streptococci is a monthly intramuscular injection of 1.2 million units of benzathine penicillin G. The disadvantages and discomfort of this regimen have to be weighed against the individual patient's susceptibility to recurrences. Those with rheumatic heart disease, recent rheumatic fever, and exposure to an environment in which the incidence of streptococcal infection is frequent deserve the most effective protection. As a second choice, prophylaxis may be administered orally with either 1 g sulfadiazine daily in a single dose or 200,000 units of penicillin given twice daily on an empty stomach. The duration of continuous prophylaxis cannot be fixed arbitrarily. Certainly, those under the age of 18 years should receive a continuous prophylactic regimen. A minimum period of 5 years is recommended for patients who develop rheumatic fever without carditis over the age of 18 years. The decision to continue prophylaxis beyond this period should take into account a number of variables. Patients with rheumatic heart disease are more susceptible to reactivation of rheumatic fever if they contract a streptococcal infection. Moreover, patients who have had carditis in a previous attack are much more likely to suffer carditis again in a subsequent attack. Climate, age, occupation, household situation, cardiac status, and length of time since the previous attack are all significant variables which influence the risk of recurrence. The decline in recurrence rates with increasing age is due to (1) decreased rate of rheumatogenic streptococcal infection and (2) decrease in the rate of rheumatic reactivation following streptococcal infection in older rheumatic subjects. Despite this decreased rate, however, the risk of rheumatic recurrence in adults remains relatively high when the streptococcal disease encountered is severe or epidemic and particularly when rheumatic fever, and thus rheumatogenic streptococci, are known to be extant in the population to which a rheumatic subject is exposed.

PREVENTION OF INITIAL RHEUMATIC ATTACKS Early and adequate treatment of pharyngeal infection due to group A streptococci will prevent initial attacks of rheumatic fever. If clinical streptococcal disease were properly detected by throat cultures and adequately treated, the spread of infection in a given population would be prevented, the epidemiology of streptococcal disease would be modified markedly, and the incidence of rheumatic fever in the community would be diminished. In communities where group A streptococcal disease has been diagnosed early and treated well and where socioeconomic standards are high, the group A organisms cultured frequently from school children's throats may be of relatively low virulence and may either not cause rheumatic fever at all or do so less frequently than more virulent strains prevalent in many epidemics. The appearance of rheumatic fever in a community, however, signals the presence of rheumatogenic streptococci whose spread must be interrupted by use of effective penicillin regimens. In a closed population, such as a military base or an institution, an outbreak of rheumatic fever is best treated by mass penicillin prophylaxis, i.e., treatment of all exposed individuals, whether or not symptomatic.

Streptococcal pharyngitis is adequately treated by a single intramuscular injection of 600,000 units of benzathine penicillin in children less than 10 years of age or 1.2 million units in older children and adults. Any alternative plan of parenteral therapy or combined parenteral and oral therapy should provide for treatment over a period of 10 days. If oral penicillin is employed, at least 800,000 units per day in four divided doses must be given for no less than 10 days to achieve results comparable with a single injection of benzathine penicillin. Erythromycin in daily doses of 1 g for 10 days may be substituted in penicillin-sensitive individuals. Tetracycline is not recommended because some strains of group A streptococci have acquired resistance to it. All group A streptococci have so far remained extremely sensitive to penicillin. When erythromycin has been used extensively in place of penicillin as the drug of choice to treat pharyngitis, erythromycin-resistant group A streptococci have emerged with high frequency. Penicillin therefore remains the treatment of choice for streptococcal sore throat.

REFERENCES

American Heart Association Committee on Rheumatic Fever, Endocarditis and Kawasaki Disease of the Council on Cardiovascular Disease: Prevention of rheumatic fever. Circulation 78:1082, 1988

Bisno AL: Group A streptococcal infections and acute rheumatic fever. N Engl J Med 35(11):783, 1991

Burge DJ, DeHoratius RJ: Acute rheumatic fever. Cardiovasc Clin 23:3, 1993

Feldman T: Rheumatic mitral stenosis. On the rise again. Postgrad Med 93:93, 99, 1993

Guidelines for the diagnosis of rheumatic fever—Jones criteria, 1992 update. JAMA 268(15):2069, 1992

Kaplan EL et al: Group A streptococcal serotypes isolated from patients and sibling contacts during the resurgence of rheumatic fever in the United States in the mid-1980s. J Infect Dis 159:101, 1989

Stollerman GH: Rheumatogenic group A streptococci and the return of rheumatic fever. Adv Intern Med 35:1, 1990

201   VALVULAR HEART DISEASE

EUGENE BRAUNWALD

The role of physical examination in the evaluation of patients with valvular disease is also considered in Chap. 188; of electrocardiography in Chap. 189; of roentgenography, echocardiography, and other noninvasive techniques in Chap. 190; of cardiac catheterization and angiography in Chap. 192; and of balloon valvuloplasty in Chap. 193.

MITRAL STENOSIS

ETIOLOGY AND PATHOLOGY   Two-thirds of all patients with mitral stenosis (MS) are females. MS is generally rheumatic in origin; rarely, it is congenital. Pure or predominant MS occurs in approximately 40 percent of all patients with rheumatic heart disease. The valve leaflets are diffusely thickened by fibrous tissue and/or calcific deposits. The mitral commissures fuse, the chordae tendineae fuse and shorten, the valvular cusps become rigid, and these changes, in turn, lead to narrowing at the apex of the funnel-shaped valve. While the initial insult to the mitral valve is rheumatic, the later changes may be a nonspecific process resulting from trauma to the valve caused by altered flow patterns due to the initial deformity. Calcification of the stenotic mitral valve immobilizes the leaflets and narrows the orifice further. Thrombus formation and arterial embolization may arise from the calcific valve itself.

PATHOPHYSIOLOGY   In normal adults the mitral valve orifice is 4 to 6 cm². In the presence of significant obstruction, i.e., when the orifice is less than approximately 2 cm², blood can flow from the left atrium to the left ventricle only if propelled by an abnormally elevated left atrioventricular pressure gradient (Fig. 192-6), the hemodynamic hallmark of MS. When the mitral valve opening is reduced to 1 cm², a left atrial pressure of approximately 25 mmHg is required to maintain a normal cardiac output. The elevated left atrial pressure, in turn, raises pulmonary venous and capillary pressures, reducing pulmonary compliance and causing exertional dyspnea. The first bouts of dyspnea are usually precipitated by clinical events which increase the rate of blood flow across the mitral orifice, which results in further elevation of the left atrial pressure (see below). In order to assess the severity of obstruction, it is essential to measure both the transvalvular pressure gradient and the flow rate (Chap. 192). The latter is dependent not only on the cardiac output but on the heart rate as well. An increase in heart rate shortens diastole proportionately more than systole and diminishes the time available for flow across the mitral valve. Therefore, at any given level of cardiac output, tachycardia augments the transvalvular gradient and elevates further the left atrial pressure.

The left ventricular diastolic pressure is normal in isolated MS; coexisting aortic valve disease, systemic hypertension, mitral regurgitation, ischemic heart disease and perhaps the residua of damage produced by rheumatic myocarditis are sometimes responsible for elevations which reflect impaired left ventricular function and/or reduced left ventricular compliance. Left ventricular dysfunction, as reflected in reduced ejection fraction and circumferential fiber shortening rate, occurs in about one-fourth of patients with severe MS. This may be a consequence of chronic reduction of preload and extension of the scarring from the valve into the adjacent myocardium. In pure MS and sinus rhythm, the mean left atrial and pulmonary artery wedge pressures are usually elevated, and the pressure pulse shows a prominent atrial contraction (*a* wave) and a gradual pressure decline after mitral valve opening (*y* descent). In patients with mild to moderate MS without elevation of the pulmonary vascular resistance, the pulmonary arterial pressure may be near the upper limits of normal at rest and may rise with exercise. In severe MS and whenever the pulmonary vascular resistance is significantly increased, the pulmonary arterial pressure is elevated even when the patient is at rest, and in extreme cases it may exceed the systemic arterial pressure. Further elevations of left atrial, pulmonary capillary, and pulmonary arterial pressures occur during exercise. When the pulmonary arterial systolic pressure exceeds approximately 50 mmHg in patients with MS, or for that matter with any lesion affecting the left side of the heart, the increased right ventricular afterload impedes the emptying of this chamber, and right ventricular end-diastolic pressure and volume usually rise as a compensatory mechanism.

Cardiac output   This varies considerably; the hemodynamic response to a given degree of mitral obstruction may range from a normal cardiac output at rest and a high left atrioventricular pressure gradient to a reduced cardiac output and low transvalvular pressure gradient at the opposite end of the hemodynamic spectrum. In a minority of patients with moderately severe MS, the cardiac output is normal at rest and rises normally during exertion; under these circumstances, the high atrioventricular pressure gradient elevates the left atrial and pulmonary capillary pressures markedly, and this elevation is responsible for symptoms of severe pulmonary congestion. In the majority of patients with moderate MS, however, the cardiac output is normal or almost so at rest but rises subnormally during exertion. In patients with severe MS, particularly those in whom the pulmonary vascular resistance is strikingly elevated, the cardiac output is subnormal at rest and may fail to rise or may even decline during activity. The depressed cardiac output in patients with MS is related primarily to the obstruction of the mitral orifice but also may be due to the impairment of the function of either ventricle.

Pulmonary hypertension   The clinical and hemodynamic features of MS are influenced importantly by the level of the pulmonary artery pressure. Pulmonary hypertension results from (1) the passive backward transmission of the elevated left atrial pressure, (2) pulmonary arteriolar constriction, which presumably is triggered by left atrial and pulmonary venous hypertension (reactive pulmonary hypertension), and (3) organic obliterative changes in the pulmonary vascular bed. The elevation of pulmonary vascular resistance may be considered to be a complication of long-standing and severe MS; in time, the resultant severe pulmonary hypertension results in tricuspid and pulmonary incompetence as well as right-sided heart failure. However, the changes in the pulmonary vascular bed also may be considered to exert a protective effect; the elevated precapillary resistance reduces the likelihood of symptoms of pulmonary congestion by reducing the surge of blood into the pulmonary capillary bed during activity which then dams up behind the stenotic mitral valve. However, this protection occurs at the expense of a decreased cardiac output.

SYMPTOMS AND COMPLICATIONS In temperate climates the latent period between the initial attack of rheumatic carditis (in the increasingly rare circumstances in which a history of one can be elicited) and the development of symptoms due to MS is generally on the order of two decades; most patients begin to experience disability in the fourth decade. Studies carried out prior to the development of mitral valvuloplasty revealed that once a patient with MS becomes seriously symptomatic, continuous progression of the disease to death usually occurs in 2 to 5 years. In economically deprived areas, particularly on the Indian subcontinent, in Central America, and the Middle East, MS tends to progress more rapidly and frequently causes serious symptoms before the age of 20 years. On the other hand, slowly progressive MS in the elderly is being recognized with increasing frequency in the United States and western Europe.

When valvular obstruction is mild, many of the physical signs of MS may be present in the absence of any symptoms. However, even in those patients whose mitral orifices are large enough to accommodate a normal blood flow with only mild elevations of left atrial pressure, extreme exertion, excitement, fever, severe anemia, paroxysmal tachycardia, sexual intercourse, pregnancy, and thyrotoxicosis all may precipitate elevations of pulmonary capillary pressure and lead to dyspnea and cough. As stenosis progresses, lesser stresses precipitate dyspnea, and the patient becomes limited in his or her daily activities. Redistribution of blood from the dependent portions of the body to the lungs, which occurs when the recumbent position is assumed, leads to orthopnea and paroxysmal nocturnal dyspnea. *Pulmonary edema* develops when there is a sudden surge in flow across a markedly narrowed mitral orifice (Chap. 31). When moderately severe MS has existed for several years, *atrial arrhythmias*—premature contractions, paroxysmal tachycardia, flutter, and fibrillation—occur with increasing frequency. The rapid ventricular rate associated with untreated or inadequately treated atrial fibrillation is frequently responsible for acute exacerbations of dyspnea. The development of permanent atrial fibrillation often marks a turning point in the patient's course and is generally associated with acceleration of the rate at which symptoms progress.

Hemoptysis (Chap. 30) results from rupture of pulmonary-bronchial venous connections secondary to pulmonary venous hypertension. It occurs most frequently in patients who have elevated left atrial pressures *without* markedly elevated pulmonary vascular resistances and is almost never fatal. True hemoptysis must be distinguished from the bloody sputum that occurs with pulmonary edema, pulmonary infarction, and bronchitis, three conditions that occur with increased frequency in the presence of MS.

As the condition progresses and the pulmonary vascular resistance rises or when tricuspid stenosis or regurgitation develops, symptoms secondary to pulmonary congestion sometimes diminish, and the episodes of acute pulmonary edema and hemoptysis become reduced in frequency and severity. Elevation of pulmonary vascular resistance further increases right ventricular systolic pressure, leading to right ventricular failure, fatigue, abdominal discomfort due to hepatic congestion, and edema.

Recurrent pulmonary emboli, sometimes with infarction (Chap. 226), are an important cause of morbidity and mortality late in the course of MS, occurring most frequently in patients with right ventricular failure. *Pulmonary infections*, i.e., bronchitis, bronchopneumonia, and lobar pneumonia, commonly complicate untreated MS. *Infective endocarditis* (Chap. 85) is rare in *pure* MS but is not uncommon in patients with combined stenosis and regurgitation. *Chest pain* occurs in about 10 percent of patients with severe MS; it may be due to pulmonary hypertension or myocardial ischemia secondary to coronary atherosclerosis; often the cause cannot be discovered.

Pulmonary and pulmonary vascular changes In addition to the aforementioned changes in the pulmonary vascular bed, fibrous thickening of the walls of the alveoli and pulmonary capillaries occurs commonly in MS. The vital capacity, total lung capacity, maximal breathing capacity, and oxygen uptake per unit of ventilation are reduced (Chap. 214), and in patients with severe MS, the latter fails to rise normally during exertion. The reduction of pulmonary compliance that occurs generally correlates directly with the severity of the dyspnea and with the heightened pulmonary capillary pressure, and these changes are intensified during exercise. In some patients, airway resistance is abnormally increased. These alterations in pulmonary mechanics contribute to an increase in the work of breathing and play an important role in the genesis of dyspnea. The changes in the lungs are due, in part, to increased transudation of fluid from the pulmonary capillaries into the interstitial and alveolar spaces as a consequence of the elevated pulmonary capillary pressure. The distribution of blood flow and ventilation may be uneven; as in other conditions in which left atrial pressure is elevated, pulmonary blood flow in the erect position is displaced from the basal to the apical segments of the lung (Chap. 214). The diffusing capacity may be reduced, particularly during exertion, as a result of structural changes in the diffusing surface and reduction of the pulmonary capillary blood volume. The thickening of the alveolar and capillary walls impedes the transudation of fluid into the alveoli and the development of pulmonary edema at times when the pulmonary capillary pressure exceeds the plasma oncotic pressure. The increased capacity of the pulmonary lymphatic system to drain excess fluid also retards the development of pulmonary edema.

Thrombi and emboli *Thrombi* may form in the left atria, particularly in the enlarged atrial appendages of patients with MS. If they *embolize*, they do so most commonly to the brain, kidneys, spleen, and extremities. Embolization occurs much more frequently in patients with atrial fibrillation or unstable rhythms, in older patients, and in those with a reduced cardiac output, and it is seen in patients with relatively mild, as well as in those with severe, obstruction. Thus systemic embolization may be the presenting complaint in otherwise asymptomatic patients with mild MS. At operation, thrombi are *not* found more frequently in the left atria of patients with a past history of embolization than in those without this complication, indicating that it is usually the freshly formed clots that dislodge. Patients who have had one or more systemic emboli have an increased predilection for further embolic episodes compared with patients with stenosis of comparable severity without previous embolization. Rarely, a large pedunculated thrombus or a free-floating clot may suddenly obstruct the stenotic mitral orifice. Such "ball valve" thrombi produce syncope, angina, and changing auscultatory signs with alterations in position, findings that resemble those produced by a left atrial myxoma (Chap. 207).

PHYSICAL FINDINGS (See also Chap. 188) **Inspection** Peripheral and facial *cyanosis* may occur in patients with extremely severe MS. In advanced cases there is a malar flush and the facies appear pinched and blue. The jugular venous pulse reveals prominent *a* waves due to vigorous right atrial systole in patients with sinus rhythm who have severe pulmonary hypertension or associated tricuspid stenosis. When atrial fibrillation is present, the jugular pulse reveals only a single expansion during systole (*c-v* wave). The systemic arterial pressure is usually normal or slightly low.

Palpation A right ventricular tap along the left sternal border signifies an enlarged right ventricle. The first heart sound may be palpable in patients with pliable valve leaflets. In patients with pulmonary hypertension, the impact of pulmonary valve closure can usually be felt in the second and third left intercostal spaces just left of the sternum; the left ventricle is not palpable in severe, pure MS. A diastolic thrill is frequently present at the cardiac apex, particularly if the patient is turned into the left lateral recumbent position.

Auscultation The first heart sound (S_1) is generally accentuated and snapping, and since the mitral valve does not close until the left ventricular pressure reaches the level of the elevated left atrial pressure, this sound is often slightly delayed on phonocardiography, causing a prolonged Q-S_1 interval, particularly in patients with severe stenosis. In patients with pulmonary hypertension, the pulmonary component of the second heart sound (P_2) is often accentuated, and the two components of the second heart sound are closely split. A pulmonary systolic ejection click may be heard in patients with severe pulmonary hypertension and marked dilatation of the pulmonary artery. The opening snap (OS) of the mitral valve is most readily audible in expiration at, or just medial to, the cardiac apex but also may be easily heard along the left sternal edge or at the base of the heart. This sound generally follows the sound of aortic valve closure (A_2) by 0.05 to 0.12 s; that is, it follows P_2. Since the OS occurs when the left ventricular pressure falls below the left atrial pressure, the time interval between A_2 closure and OS varies inversely with the severity of the MS. It tends to be short (0.05 to 0.07 s) in patients with severe obstruction, and long (0.10 to 0.12 s) in patients with mild MS. The intensities of the OS and S_1 correlate with the mobility of the anterior mitral leaflet.

The OS usually ushers in a low-pitched, rumbling, diastolic murmur, heard best at the apex with the patient in the left lateral recumbent position. It is accentuated by exercise carried out just before auscultation and reduced during the strain of a Valsalva maneuver. In general, the duration of this murmur correlates with the severity of the stenosis. In patients with sinus rhythm, the murmur often reappears or becomes reaccentuated during atrial systole, as atrial contraction reelevates the rate of blood flow across the narrowed orifice. Soft (grade I or II/VI) systolic murmurs are commonly heard at the apex or along the left sternal border in patients with pure MS and do not necessarily signify the presence of mitral regurgitation. Hepatomegaly, ankle edema, ascites, and pleural effusion, particularly in the right pleural cavity, may occur in patients with MS and right ventricular failure.

Associated lesions With severe pulmonary hypertension, a pansystolic murmur produced by functional tricuspid regurgitation may be audible along the left sternal border. Characteristically, this murmur is accentuated by inspiration, diminishes during forced expiration or during performance of the Valsalva maneuver, diminishes or disappears as pulmonary artery pressure declines, and should not be confused with the apical pansystolic murmur of mitral regurgitation, since management of the two valvular lesions is quite different.

The recognition of associated mitral regurgitation is of considerable clinical importance in patients with MS. A presystolic murmur and an accentuated first heart sound speak against the presence of serious associated mitral regurgitation, but when the first heart sound and/or the opening snap are soft or absent in a patient with mitral valve disease who also has an apical systolic murmur, it is likely that significant mitral regurgitation and/or serious calcification of the deformed mitral valve leaflets are present. A third heart sound at the apex often signifies that the mitral regurgitation is serious; this sound is generally duller, lower pitched, and follows the opening snap. Occasionally, in patients with pure MS, physical signs may falsely suggest mitral regurgitation. Thus, in the presence of severe pulmonary hypertension and right ventricular failure, a third heart sound may originate from the right ventricle. The enlarged right ventricle may rotate the heart in a clockwise direction and form the cardiac apex, giving the examiner the erroneous impression of left ventricular

enlargement. Under these circumstances, the rumbling diastolic murmur and the other auscultatory features of MS become less prominent or may even disappear and be replaced by the systolic murmur of functional tricuspid regurgitation which is mistaken for mitral regurgitation. When cardiac output is markedly reduced in a patient with MS, the typical auscultatory findings, including the diastolic rumbling murmur, may not be detectable (silent MS), but they may reappear as compensation is restored. Associated tricuspid stenosis also tends to obscure many of the physical signs of MS.

The Graham Steell murmur of pulmonary regurgitation, a high-pitched, diastolic, decrescendo blowing murmur along the left sternal border, results from dilatation of the pulmonary valve ring and occurs in patients with mitral valve disease and severe pulmonary hypertension. This murmur may be indistinguishable from the more common murmur produced by aortic regurgitation except that it is rarely audible at the second right intercostal space and may disappear following successful surgical treatment of the MS.

Electrocardiogram In MS and sinus rhythm, the P wave usually suggests left atrial enlargement (Chap. 189). It may become tall and peaked in lead II and upright in lead V_1 when severe pulmonary hypertension or tricuspid stenosis complicates MS and right atrial enlargement occurs. The QRS complex may be normal, even in patients with critical MS. However, with severe pulmonary hypertension, right axis deviation and right ventricular hypertrophy are usually found. When left ventricular hypertrophy is present in patients with MS, it generally indicates that an additional lesion which places a significant burden on the left ventricle, such as mitral regurgitation, aortic valve disease, or hypertension, is present.

Echocardiogram (See also Chap. 190) The echocardiogram is the most sensitive and specific noninvasive method for diagnosing MS. Two-dimensional color Doppler flow echocardiographic imaging and Doppler echocardiography (see Figs. 190-4 and 190-7) provide critical information, including an estimate of the transvalvular gradient and of mitral orifice size, the presence and severity of accompanying mitral regurgitation, the extent of restriction of valve leaflets, their thickness, and the degree of distortion of the subvalvular apparatus. In addition, echocardiography provides an assessment of the size of the cardiac chambers, an estimation of the pulmonary artery pressure, and an indication of the presence and severity of associated tricuspid and pulmonic regurgitation.

Roentgenogram (Chap. 190) The earliest changes are straightening of the left border of the cardiac silhouette, prominence of the main pulmonary arteries, dilatation of the upper lobe pulmonary veins, and backward displacement of the esophagus by an enlarged left atrium. In patients with mild or moderate MS, the heart is not grossly enlarged. In severe MS, however, all chambers and vessels upstream to the narrowed valve are prominent, including the two atria, the pulmonary arteries and veins, right ventricle, and superior vena cava. Kerley B lines are fine, dense, opaque, horizontal lines which are most prominent in the lower and midlung fields and which result from distention of interlobular septa and lymphatics with edema when the resting mean left atrial pressure exceeds approximately 20 mmHg. As the pulmonary arterial pressure rises, the smaller pulmonary arteries become attenuated, at first in the lower, then in the middle, and finally in the upper lung fields. In patients who have had multiple hemoptyses, hemosiderin-containing macrophages fill the air spaces, and if they become confluent, they result in a fine, diffuse nodulation most prominent in the lower lung fields.

DIFFERENTIAL DIAGNOSIS Significant mitral regurgitation may be associated with a prominent diastolic murmur at the apex, but this murmur commences slightly later than in patients with MS, and there is often clear-cut evidence of left ventricular enlargement on physical examination, roentgenography, and electrocardiography. In addition, an apical pansystolic murmur of at least grade III/VI intensity as well as a third heart sound should arouse the suspicion of significant associated regurgitation. Similarly, the apical middiastolic murmur associated with aortic regurgitation (Austin Flint murmur) may be mistaken for MS. However, in a patient with aortic regurgitation, the absence of an opening snap or of presystolic accentuation if sinus rhythm is present points to the *absence* of MS. Tricuspid stenosis, a valvular lesion that occurs very rarely in the absence of MS, may mask many of the clinical features of MS. Echocardiography is particularly useful in detecting MS in patients who have or are suspected of having other valve lesions and in defining the severity of the various lesions.

Exertional dyspnea and recurrent pulmonary infections may be falsely ascribed to pulmonary emphysema in patients with both *chronic lung disease* and MS. Careful auscultation, however, will generally reveal the characteristic opening snap and rumbling diastolic murmur. Similarly, the hemoptysis that occurs in many otherwise asymptomatic patients with MS may be improperly attributed to bronchiectasis or tuberculosis; the latter condition is uncommon in patients with significant mitral obstruction.

Primary pulmonary hypertension (Chap. 225) results in a number of the clinical and laboratory features observed in MS. It occurs most frequently in young women; however, the OS and diastolic rumbling murmur are absent, there is no left atrial enlargement, and the pulmonary artery wedge and left atrial pressures are normal, as is the size of the left atrium on echocardiography. *Atrial septal defect* (Chap. 199) also may be mistaken for MS; in both conditions there is often clinical, electrocardiographic, and roentgenographic evidence of right ventricular enlargement and accentuation of the pulmonary vascularity. The widely split S_2 of atrial septal defect may be confused with the mitral OS, and the diastolic flow murmur across the tricuspid valve may be mistaken for the mitral diastolic murmur. However, the absence of left atrial enlargement and of Kerley B lines and the demonstration of fixed splitting of S_2 favor atrial septal defect over MS. *Cor triatriatum* is an unusual congenital malformation that consists of a fibrous ring within the left atrium. It results in elevation of the pulmonary venous, capillary, and arterial pressures. This lesion can be recognized most readily by means of left atrial angiography.

Left atrial myxoma (Chap. 207) may obstruct left atrial emptying, causing dyspnea, a diastolic murmur, and hemodynamic changes resembling those of MS. However, patients with left atrial myxoma often demonstrate findings suggestive of a systemic disease, with weight loss, fever, anemia, systemic emboli, and elevated erythrocyte sedimentation rate and serum IgG concentration. Usually an OS is not audible, there is no clinical evidence of associated aortic valve disease, and the auscultatory findings frequently change with body position. The diagnosis can be established by demonstrating a characteristic echo-producing mass in the left atrium by two-dimensional echocardiography.

CARDIAC CATHETERIZATION AND ANGIOCARDIOGRAPHY Catheterization of the left side of the heart (Chap. 192) is extremely helpful in deciding whether valvulotomy is necessary in patients in whom it is difficult to estimate the severity of obstruction by clinical means and noninvasive tests. When combined with aortography and left ventricular angiocardiography, this procedure serves as the ultimate method for detecting and estimating associated mitral regurgitation and coexisting lesions such as aortic stenosis and regurgitation as well as left ventricular dysfunction. These "invasive" methods are also helpful in the detection of accompanying conditions, such as coronary artery disease, that impair left ventricular function and would thereby contraindicate or reduce the effectiveness of mitral valvulotomy. Catheterization is not usually necessary to aid in the decision regarding surgery in relatively young (<45 years for males, <50 for females) patients with typical findings of severe obstruction on clinical examination and echocardiography. In older patients, coronary angiography is usually advisable preoperatively, in order to detect patients with critical coronary obstructions which should be bypassed at the time of operation. Catheterization and left ventricular angiography are also indicated in most patients who have undergone previous mitral valve operations and who have redeveloped serious symptoms; in such patients, clinical assessment may be particularly difficult, and the hemodynamic studies allow determination of the severity of the lesion, intelligent planning of the operative procedure when it is indicated, and a more accurate estimate of the risk.

MANAGEMENT In the asymptomatic adolescent with mitral valve disease, penicillin prophylaxis of beta-hemolytic streptococcal infections (Chap. 200) and prophylaxis for infective endocarditis (Chap. 85) are important. In symptomatic patients, some improvement usually occurs with restriction of sodium intake and maintenance doses of oral diuretics. Digitalis glycosides do not alter the hemodynamics and usually do not benefit patients with pure stenosis and sinus rhythm, but they are necessary for slowing the ventricular rate of patients with atrial fibrillation and for reducing the manifestations of right-sided heart failure in the advanced stages of the disease. Small doses of beta blockers (e.g., atenolol 25 to 50 mg/d) may be added when cardiac glycosides fail to control ventricular rate in patients with atrial fibrillation or flutter. Particular attention should be directed toward detecting and treating any accompanying anemia and infections. Hemoptysis is treated by measures designed to diminish pulmonary venous pressure, including bed rest, the sitting position, salt restriction, and diuresis. Anticoagulants should be administered for at least 1 year in patients with MS who have suffered systemic and/or pulmonary embolization and continuously in those with atrial fibrillation.

If atrial fibrillation is of relatively recent origin in a patient whose MS is not severe enough to warrant surgical treatment, reversion to sinus rhythm pharmacologically or by means of electrical countershock is indicated. Usually this should be undertaken following 3 weeks of anticoagulant treatment. Conversion to sinus rhythm is rarely helpful in patients with severe MS, particularly those in whom the left atrium is especially enlarged or in whom atrial fibrillation has been present for more than 1 year, since reversion to atrial fibrillation is common.

Mitral valvulotomy Unless there is a specific contraindication, mitral valvulotomy is indicated in the symptomatic patient with pure MS whose effective orifice is less than approximately 1.3 cm² (or 0.8 cm²/m² of body surface area). Operation usually not only results in striking symptomatic and hemodynamic improvement but also prolongs survival. In uncomplicated cases, the surgical mortality rate should be 0 to 3 percent. However, there is no evidence that surgical treatment improves the prognosis of patients with slight or no functional impairment. Therefore, unless recurrent systemic embolization has occurred, valvulotomy is *not* recommended for patients who are entirely asymptomatic, regardless of hemodynamic findings. When there is little symptomatic improvement following valvulotomy, it is likely that the procedure was ineffective, that it induced mitral regurgitation, or that associated valvular or myocardial disease was present. The recurrence of symptoms several years after what appeared to be a satisfactory initial result is usually due to an inadequate valvulotomy, but progression of other valvular lesions, restenosis of the mitral valve, or some combination of these conditions also may be responsible. More than half of all patients undergoing mitral valvulotomy require reoperation by 10 years. In the *pregnant patient* with MS, operative treatment should be carried out if pulmonary congestion occurs despite intensive medical treatment.

An "open" operation using cardiopulmonary bypass is usually preferable to closed commissurotomy for patients with pure MS who have not been operated on previously. In addition to opening the valve commissures, it is important to loosen any subvalvular fusion of papillary muscles and chordae tendineae and to remove large deposits of calcium, thereby improving valvular function, and to remove atrial thrombi. In patients with significant associated mitral regurgitation, those in whom the valve has been severely distorted by previous operative manipulation, or those in whom the surgeon does not find it possible to improve valve function significantly, the valve may have to be replaced with a prosthesis. Since the operative mortality of replacement of the mitral valve is still approximately 5 percent, and since there are long-term complications of valve replacement, patients in whom preoperative evaluation suggests the possibility that replacement may be required should be operated on only if they have *critical* mitral stenosis, i.e., an orifice <1.0 cm², and are in the New York Heart Association class III, i.e., symptomatic with ordinary activity, despite optimal medical therapy.

Percutaneous balloon valvuloplasty, described on p. 987, is an alternative to surgical mitral valvuloplasty in patients with pure or predominant rheumatic mitral stenosis. Young patients without extensive valvular calcification or thickening or subvalvular deformity are the best candidates for this procedure; in them the results approach those of closed surgical commissurotomy with similar low mortality. It is particularly useful in pregnant women but also may be used in older patients with severe valvular deformity with serious extracardiac disease who are poor operative candidates.

VALVE REPLACEMENT The results of replacement of any valve are dependent primarily on (1) the patient's myocardial function at the time of operation, (2) the technical abilities of the operative team and the quality of the postoperative care, and (3) the durability, hemodynamic characteristics, and thrombogenicity of the prosthesis. Increased operative mortality is associated with the degree of preoperative functional disability and pulmonary hypertension. Late complications of replacement of any valve, which fortunately are declining in incidence, include paravalvular leakage, thromboemboli, bleeding due to anticoagulants, mechanical dysfunction of the prosthesis, and infective endocarditis.

The considerations regarding the choice between a bioprosthetic (tissue) and artificial mechanical valve are similar in the mitral and aortic positions and in the treatment of stenotic, regurgitant, or mixed lesions. All patients who have undergone replacement of any valve with a mechanical prosthesis must be maintained permanently on anticoagulants. The primary advantage of bioprostheses over mechanical prostheses is the reduction of thromboembolic complications, and except for patients with chronic atrial fibrillation, few such instances have been associated with their use. The major disadvantage of bioprosthetic valves is their mechanical deterioration. This results in the need to replace the prosthesis in 30 percent of patients by 10 years and 50 percent by 15 years. Bioprostheses are ordinarily not used in younger patients (<35 years) because of accelerated deterioration but are particularly useful in the elderly (>70 years), in whom there is more concern about chronic anticoagulation than about long-term (>15 years) valve durability. These valves are also indicated in women who expect to become pregnant, as well as others in whom anticoagulation may be contraindicated. In patients without such contraindications, particularly those under 65 years, a mechanical prosthesis may be preferable. Many surgeons now select the St. Jude prosthesis, a double-disk tilting prosthesis, for replacement of both aortic and mitral valves because of somewhat more favorable hemodynamic characteristics and a suggestion of lower thrombogenicity.

The overall 10-year survival of operative survivors following mitral valve replacement is approximately 60 percent. Long-term prognosis is worse in older patients and those with marked disability and striking depression of the cardiac index preoperatively.

MITRAL REGURGITATION

ETIOLOGY Chronic rheumatic heart disease is the cause of severe mitral regurgitation (MR) in about one-third of cases. In contrast to MS, rheumatic MR occurs more frequently in males. The rheumatic process produces rigidity, deformity, and retraction of the valve cusps and commissural fusion, as well as shortening, contraction, and fusion of the chordae tendineae. MR also may occur as a congenital anomaly (Chap. 199), most commonly as (1) a defect of the endocardial cushions or in association with (2) corrected transposition, (3) endocardial fibroelastosis, and (4) the "parachute" mitral valve deformity. MR may occur with fibrosis of a papillary muscle in patients with healed myocardial infarction as well as in patients with infarction involving the base of a papillary muscle. Transient regurgitation also may occur during periods of ischemia involving a papillary muscle or the adjacent myocardium and may accompany bouts of angina pectoris. MR may occur with marked left

ventricular enlargement of any cause in which dilatation of the mitral annulus and lateral displacement of the papillary muscles interfere with coaptation of the valve leaflets. In hypertrophic cardiomyopathy, the anterior leaflet of the mitral valve is displaced anteriorly during systole, leading to regurgitation (Chap. 205). Massive calcification of the mitral annulus of unknown cause, presumably degenerative, which occurs most commonly in elderly women, also can be responsible for significant MR. Systemic lupus erythematosus, rheumatoid arthritis, and ankylosing spondylitis are less common causes. *Acute* MR may occur secondary to infective endocarditis involving the valve or chordae tendineae, in acute myocardial infarction with rupture of a papillary muscle or one of its heads, as a consequence of trauma, or following apparently spontaneous chordal rupture.

Abnormal elongation of chordae tendineae and/or redundant posterior cusps of the mitral valve with prolapse of the cusps into the left atrium, the so-called floppy valve, leading to the syndrome of midsystolic click and midsystolic murmur, also referred to as the *prolapsing mitral valve leaflet syndrome* (see below), is another important cause of MR.

Regardless of cause, severe MR is often progressive, since enlargement of the left atrium places tension on the posterior mitral leaflet, pulling it away from the mitral orifice and thereby aggravating the valvular dysfunction. Similarly, the dilatation of the left ventricle increases the regurgitation, which in turn enlarges further the left atrium and ventricle, causing chordal rupture and resulting in a vicious cycle; hence the aphorism, "mitral regurgitation begets mitral regurgitation."

PATHOPHYSIOLOGY Since the regurgitant mitral orifice is in parallel with the aortic orifice, the resistance to left ventricular emptying is reduced in patients with MR. As a consequence, the left ventricle is decompressed into the left atrium during ejection, and with the reduction in left ventricular size there is a rapid decline in left ventricular tension, i.e., a progressive reduction in left ventricular afterload, allowing a greater proportion of the contractile activity of the left ventricle to be expended in shortening. The initial compensation to MR consists of more complete systolic emptying of the left ventricle. However, left ventricular volume increases progressively as the severity of the regurgitation increases and the function of the left ventricle deteriorates. This is often accompanied by a depressed forward cardiac output. The regurgitant volume varies directly with the left ventricular systolic pressure and the size of the regurgitant orifice; the latter, in turn, is influenced profoundly by the degree of left ventricular dilatation.

The atrial contraction wave in the left atrial pressure pulse (*a* wave) is not as prominent as it is in MS, but the *v* wave is usually taller, since it is inscribed during ventricular systole, when the left atrium fills from the pulmonary veins as well as from the left ventricle. During early diastole, as the distended left atrium suddenly empties, there is a particularly rapid *y* descent as long as there is no associated MS (Fig. 192-7, p. 984). Left ventricular end-diastolic pressure may be slightly elevated. However, in chronic MR, there is often an increase in left ventricular compliance, so ventricular volume may be increased with little elevation in end-diastolic pressure. The effective (forward) cardiac output usually declines in seriously symptomatic patients. Although a left atrioventricular pressure gradient persisting throughout diastole signifies the presence of significant associated MS, a brief, early diastolic gradient may occur in patients with pure regurgitation as a result of the torrential flow of blood across a normal-sized mitral orifice.

The prompt appearance of contrast material in the left atrium following its injection into the left ventricle signifies the presence of MR. The regurgitant volume can be measured by determining the difference between the total left ventricular stroke volume estimated angiocardiographically and the effective forward stroke volume determined by the Fick method (Chap. 192). The results of such studies suggest that in patients with severe regurgitation the regurgitant volume may be of the same magnitude as the effective forward stroke volume or may even exceed it. Qualitative, but clinically useful, estimates of the severity of regurgitation may be made by Doppler echocardiography, color Doppler flow echocardiographic imaging, and observation on cineangiograms of the degree of left atrial opacification following the injection of contrast material into the left ventricle.

The compliance, i.e., the pressure-volume relationship, of the left atrium and pulmonary venous bed affects the clinical picture. Patients with *normal or reduced compliance* usually have *acute* MR, little enlargement of the left atrium, but marked elevation of the left atrial pressure, particularly of the *v* wave. Pulmonary edema is common. After several months, the pulmonary vascular resistance may become markedly elevated, presumably as a consequence of the left atrial hypertension, and right-sided heart failure also may occur; sinus rhythm is usually present.

Patients with a *marked increase in left atrial compliance* are the opposite end of the spectrum, having severe long-standing severe MR, marked enlargement of the left atrium, and normal or only slightly elevated left atrial pressure, pulmonary artery pressure, and pulmonary vascular resistance. These patients usually complain of severe fatigue and exhaustion secondary to a low cardiac output, while symptoms resulting from pulmonary congestion are less prominent; atrial fibrillation is almost invariably present.

By far the most common group are patients whose clinical and hemodynamic features are between those in the other two groups with variable degrees of enlargement of the left atrium and with significant elevation of the left atrial pressure. Symptoms are secondary to both reduced cardiac output and pulmonary congestion.

SYMPTOMS Fatigue, exertional dyspnea, and orthopnea are the most prominent complaints in patients with chronic, severe MR. Since fluctuations of the mean pulmonary capillary pressure are less marked, symptoms resulting from pulmonary congestion tend to be less episodic in nature than in patients with chronic severe MR. Hemoptysis and systemic embolism also occur less frequently in MR than in MS. Right-sided heart failure, with painful hepatic congestion, ankle edema, distended neck veins, ascites, and tricuspid regurgitation, may be observed in patients with MR who have associated pulmonary vascular disease and marked pulmonary hypertension. In patients with *acute*, severe MR, left ventricular failure with acute pulmonary edema and/or cardiovascular collapse is common.

PHYSICAL FINDINGS The arterial pressure is usually normal, and in severe MR the arterial pulse is often characterized by a sharp upstroke. The jugular venous pulse shows abnormally prominent *a* waves in patients with sinus rhythm and marked pulmonary hypertension and prominent *v* waves in those with accompanying severe tricuspid regurgitation.

Palpation A systolic thrill is often palpable at the cardiac apex, the left ventricle is hyperdynamic with a brisk systolic impulse and a palpable rapid-filling wave, and the apex beat is often displaced laterally. When the left atrium is markedly enlarged, it may extend anteriorly, and its expansion may be palpable along the sternal border late during ventricular systole, resembling a right ventricular lift. The combination of retraction of the left ventricle and expansion of the left atrium during systole may produce a characteristic rocking motion of the chest with each cardiac cycle. A right ventricular tap and the shock of pulmonary valve closure may be palpable in patients with marked pulmonary hypertension.

Auscultation The first heart sound is generally absent, soft, or buried in the systolic murmur; an accentuated mitral closure sound is useful in excluding severe regurgitation. A pulmonary ejection sound is often audible in patients with associated pulmonary hypertension. In patients with severe MR, the aortic valve may close prematurely, resulting in wide splitting of the second heart sound. An OS indicates associated MS but does not exclude predominant regurgitation. A low-pitched third heart sound (S_3) occurring 0.12 to 0.17 s after the aortic valve closure sound, i.e. at the completion of the rapid-filling phase of the left ventricle, is believed to be caused by the sudden tensing of the papillary muscles, chordae tendineae, and valve leaflets and is an important auscultatory feature of severe MR. The absence

of an S_3 indicates that if MR exists, it may not be severe. The S_3 may be followed, often after a brief interval, by a short, rumbling, diastolic murmur, even in the absence of MS. A fourth heart sound is often audible in patients with acute, severe MR of recent onset who are in sinus rhythm. A presystolic murmur is not ordinarily heard in patients with pure MR and sinus rhythm but is present when there is significant associated MS.

A systolic murmur of at least grade III/VI intensity, is the most characteristic auscultatory finding in severe MR. It is usually holosystolic (Chap. 188), but it may be decrescendo in patients with acute, severe MR when the tall *v* wave in the left atrial pressure pulse reduces the late systolic left ventricular–atrial pressure gradient. In MR due to papillary muscle dysfunction or mitral valve prolapse, the systolic murmur commences in midsystole (see below). Although the systolic murmur is usually most prominent at the apex and radiates into the axilla, in a minority of patients, particularly those with ruptured chordae tendineae or primary involvement of the posterior mitral leaflet, the regurgitant jet strikes the left atrial wall adjacent to the aortic root, and the systolic murmur is transmitted to the base of the heart and therefore may be confused with the murmur of aortic stenosis. In patients with ruptured chordae tendineae the systolic murmur may have a cooing or "sea gull" quality; in patients with a flail leaflet the murmur may have a musical quality. The systolic murmur of MR is intensified by isometric strain but is reduced by the strain of the Valsalva maneuver.

Electrocardiogram In patients with sinus rhythm there is evidence of left atrial enlargement, but right atrial enlargement also may be present when pulmonary hypertension is severe. Chronic, severe MR with left atrial enlargement is generally associated with atrial fibrillation. In many patients there is no clear-cut electrocardiographic evidence of enlargement of either ventricle. In others the signs of left ventricular hypertrophy are often present, although in patients with pulmonary hypertension, combined ventricular hypertrophy may be noted.

Echocardiogram Doppler echocardiography and color Doppler flow echocardiography imaging are the most accurate noninvasive techniques for the detection and estimation of MR (see Fig. 190-7). The left atrium is usually enlarged and/or exhibits increased pulsations; the left ventricle may be hyperdynamic. With ruptured chordae tendineae or a flail leaflet coarse, erratic motion of the involved leaflets may be noted. Findings which help to determine the etiology of MR can often be identified. These include vegetations associated with infective endocarditis, incomplete coaptation of the anterior and posterior mitral leaflets, and annular calcification, as well as left ventricular dilatation, aneurysm, or dyskinesis. The echocardiogram in patients with mitral valve prolapse is described below.

Roentgenogram The left atrium and left ventricle are the dominant chambers; in chronic cases, the former may be massively enlarged and forms the right border of the cardiac silhouette. Pulmonary venous congestion, interstitial edema, and Kerley B lines are sometimes noted. Marked calcification of the mitral leaflets occurs commonly in patients with long-standing combined MR and MS. Calcification of the mitral annulus may be visualized. Contrast left ventriculography is useful in the quantification of MR.

TREATMENT **Medical** The nonsurgical management of MR is directed toward restricting those physical activities that regularly produce dyspnea and excessive fatigue, reducing sodium intake, and enhancing sodium excretion with the appropriate use of diuretics (Chap. 195). Vasodilators and digitalis glycosides increase the forward output of the failing left ventricle. Intravenous nitroprusside (Chap. 195) or nitroglycerin to reduce afterload and thereby the volume of regurgitant flow are useful in stabilizing patients with acute and/or severe MR. Angiotensin-converting enzyme inhibitors are given in chronic MR. The same considerations as in patients with MS apply to the reversion of atrial fibrillation to sinus rhythm. In the late stages of heart failure anticoagulants and leg binders are used to diminish the likelihood of venous thrombi and pulmonary emboli.

Surgical In the selection of patients for surgical treatment, the chronic, often slowly progressive nature of the disease must be balanced against the immediate risks and long-term uncertainties attendant on valve reconstruction or replacement. Patients with MR who are asymptomatic or who are limited only during strenuous exertion are not considered to be candidates for surgical treatment, since their condition may remain stable for many years. On the other hand, unless there are contraindications, surgical treatment should be offered to patients with severe MR whose limitations do not allow them to work full time or to perform normal household activities despite optimal medical management. Even in patients with mild symptoms, surgical treatment is indicated when left ventricular dysfunction is progressive. In patients with chronic heart failure, the risks of surgery rise sharply, the recovery of impaired left ventricular function is incomplete, and the long-term survival is reduced. However, conservative management has little to offer these patients, so operative treatment may be indicated even at an advanced stage of the disease, and occasionally, the clinical and hemodynamic improvement following surgical treatment in patients with advanced disease is dramatic. Though most patients who survive operation appear to be greatly improved, some degree of myocardial dysfunction may persist.

When surgical treatment is contemplated, right- and left-sided heart catheterization and left ventricular angiocardiography are generally indicated. These studies are helpful in confirming the presence of severe regurgitation and aid in the identification of patients with primary myocardial disease and relatively mild, functional MR, who usually do not benefit from operation. Hemodynamic studies are also helpful in detecting and assessing the severity of any associated valve lesions, which may have to be dealt with at the time of operation or which may limit the patient's ultimate improvement if they are left untreated. Coronary angiography identifies patients who require concomitant coronary revascularization.

Surgical treatment of MR, especially that caused by valves that are markedly deformed, with shrunken, calcified leaflets secondary to rheumatic fever, requires replacement of the valve with a prosthesis, although in an increasing fraction of patients, particularly those with severe annular dilatation, flail leaflets, mitral valve prolapse, ruptured chordae, or infective endocarditis, reconstruction of the mitral valve apparatus (mitral valvuloplasty) and/or mitral annuloplasty may be successful. Valve reconstruction should be carried out whenever feasible since the operative risk is about half (2 to 4 percent) of that associated with valve replacement. Also, reconstruction spares the patient the long-term adverse consequences of valve replacement (i.e., thromboembolic and hemorrhagic complications in the case of mechanical prostheses and late valve failure necessitating repeat valve replacement in the case of bioprostheses). In addition, by preserving the integrity of the papillary muscles and subvalvular apparatus, mitral valvuloplasty maintains left ventricular function.

MITRAL VALVE PROLAPSE

Mitral valve prolapse (MVP), also variously termed the *systolic click-murmur syndrome, Barlow's syndrome, floppy-valve syndrome,* and *billowing mitral leaflet syndrome,* is a common, but highly variable, clinical syndrome resulting from diverse pathogenic mechanisms of the mitral valve apparatus. Among these are excessive or redundant mitral leaflet tissue, which is commonly involved with myxomatous degeneration and greatly increased concentration of acid mucopolysaccharide. It is a frequent finding in patients who have the typical features of the Marfan syndrome or cystic medial necrosis (Chap. 210), although in most patients with MVP myxomatous degeneration is confined to the mitral valve leaflets without other clinical or pathologic manifestations of disease; the posterior leaflet is usually more affected than the anterior, and the mitral valve annulus is often greatly dilated. In many patients, elongated redundant chordae tendineae cause or contribute to the regurgitation.

In the majority of patients with MVP, the cause is unknown, but in some it appears to be a genetically determined collagen tissue disorder. A reduction in the production of type III collagen has been incriminated and electron microscopy has revealed fragmentation of collagen fibrils. MVP may be associated with thoracic skeletal deformities similar to but not as severe as those in the Marfan syndrome, including a high arched palate and alterations of the chest and thoracic spine. MVP also may occur as a sequel of acute rheumatic fever, in chronic rheumatic heart disease and following mitral valvulotomy, in ischemic heart disease, and in cardiomyopathies, as well as in 20 percent of patients with ostium secundum atrial septal defect.

MVP may lead to excessive stress on the papillary muscles, which in turn leads to dysfunction and ischemia of the papillary muscles and subjacent ventricular myocardium; rupture of chordae tendineae and progressive annular dilatation and calcification also contribute to valvular regurgitation, which then places more stress on the diseased mitral valve apparatus, thereby creating a vicious cycle. The electrocardiographic changes (see below) and ventricular arrhythmias appear to result from regional ventricular dysfunction related to increased stress placed on the papillary muscles.

MVP is more common in females and has been noted in a wide age range but most commonly between the ages of 14 and 30 years. There is an increased familial incidence in some patients suggesting an autosomal dominant form of inheritance. In many patients the echocardiographic abnormality is not accompanied by any other clinical manifestation of cardiac disease, and the significance of this finding is uncertain.

MVP encompasses a broad spectrum of severities, ranging from patients with only a systolic click and murmur and mild prolapse of the posterior leaflet of the mitral valve to those with severe MR due to chordal rupture and massive prolapse of both leaflets. In many patients, this condition progresses over years or decades.

Most patients are asymptomatic and remain so for their entire lives. Although severe MR is a relatively uncommon complication of MVP, the latter has become the most common cause of isolated *severe* MR. Arrythmias, most commonly ventricular premature contractions and paroxysmal supraventricular and ventricular tachycardia, have been reported and may cause palpitations, light-headedness, and syncope. Sudden death is a very rare complication. Many patients have chest pain which is difficult to evaluate. It is often substernal, prolonged, poorly related to exertion, and rarely resembles typical angina pectoris. Transient cerebral ischemic attacks secondary to emboli from the mitral valve with endothelial disruption have been reported. Infective endocarditis may occur in patients with MR associated with MVP.

PHYSICAL EXAMINATION   Auscultation   The most important finding is the mid- or late (nonejection) systolic click, which occurs 0.14 s or more after the first heart sound and is thought to be generated by the sudden tensing of slack, elongated chordae tendineae or by the prolapsing mitral leaflet when it reaches its maximum excursion. Systolic clicks may be multiple and may be followed by a high-pitched late systolic crescendo-decrescendo murmur, occasionally "whooping" or "honking," which is heard best at the apex. The click and murmur occur earlier with standing, the Valsalva maneuver, or inhalation of amyl nitrate, interventions which decrease left ventricular volume, exaggerating the propensity of mitral leaflet prolapse. Conversely, squatting and isometric exercise, which increase left ventricular end-diastolic volume, diminish the propensity for the mitral valve leaflets to prolapse, and the click-murmur complex is delayed and may even disappear. Some patients have a midsystolic click without the murmur; others have the murmur without a click.

LABORATORY EXAMINATION   The *electrocardiogram* most commonly is normal but may show biphasic or inverted T waves in leads II, III, and aVF and occasionally supraventricular or ventricular premature contractions. Two-dimensional echocardiography is particularly useful in identifying the abnormal position and prolapse of the mitral valve leaflets; a useful echocardiographic definition of MVP is systolic displacement (in the parasternal view) of the mitral valve leaflets into the left atrium with coaptation superior to the plane of the mitral annulus. Thickening of the mitral valve leaflets identifies a subgroup of patients at higher risk of infective endocarditis and the development of severe MR. Doppler studies are helpful in revealing and evaluating accompanying MR. *Angiocardiography* generally shows prolapse of the posterior and sometimes of both mitral valve leaflets and, rarely, severe MR. Some patients have bulging of the posteroinferior wall of the left ventricle into the left ventricular cavity during systole and/or hypokinesis of the anterolateral left ventricular wall. Others display prolapse of other valves, particularly the tricuspid, in addition to the mitral.

TREATMENT The management of patients with MVP consists of reassurance of the asymptomatic patient without severe MR or arrhythmias, the prevention of infective endocarditis with antibiotic prophylaxis in patients with a systolic murmur and/or the typical echocardiographic features, and the relief of the atypical chest pain; beta blockers have been found to be helpful in this regard, although their use is empirical. Antiarrhythmic agents may be administered if frequent ventricular premature contractions or tachyarrhythmias have caused symptoms. If the patient is symptomatic from severe MR, mitral valve repair (or rarely, replacement) is indicated. Antiplatelet aggregation agents such as aspirin should be given to patients with transient ischemic attacks, and if these are not effective, anticoagulants should be employed.

AORTIC STENOSIS

Aortic stenosis (AS) occurs in about one-fourth of all patients with chronic valvular heart disease; approximately 80 percent of adult patients with symptomatic valvular AS are male.

ETIOLOGY AS may be congenital in origin, it may be secondary to rheumatic inflammation of the aortic valve, or it may be due to degenerative calcification of the aortic cusps of unknown cause. The *congenitally affected valve* may already be stenotic at birth (see Chap. 199) and may become progressively more fibrotic, calcified, and stenotic. In others the valve may be congenitally deformed, usually bicuspid, without serious narrowing of the aortic orifice during childhood; its abnormal architecture makes its leaflets susceptible to otherwise ordinary hemodynamic stresses, which ultimately lead to valvular thickening, calcification, increased rigidity, and narrowing of the aortic orifice.

Rheumatic endocarditis of the aortic leaflets produces commissural fusion, resulting sometimes in a bicuspid valve. This, in turn, makes the leaflets more susceptible to trauma and ultimately leads to calcification and further narrowing. By the time the obstruction to left ventricular outflow causes serious clinical disability, the valve is usually a rigid calcified mass, and careful examination may make it difficult or even impossible to determine whether the underlying process was rheumatic or congenital. Rheumatic AS is almost always associated with rheumatic involvement of the mitral valve. A rheumatic etiology is favored by a history of active rheumatic fever and by associated severe aortic regurgitation.

Idiopathic calcific AS occurs most often in the elderly and may be associated with fibrosis and fusion of the valve cusps; the pathologic process is considered to be a degenerative one—a "wear-and-tear" phenomenon. It may produce many of the characteristic systolic murmurs of AS. However, the valvular obstruction is usually relatively mild and of little, if any, hemodynamic significance; it may, on occasion, produce critical obstruction.

OTHER FORMS OF OBSTRUCTION TO LEFT VENTRICULAR OUTFLOW Besides valvular AS, three other lesions may be responsible for obstruction to left ventricular outflow.

1 Hypertrophic cardiomyopathy. This condition is characterized by marked hypertrophy of the left ventricle, involving in particular the interventricular septum of the left ventricular outflow tract, and may cause subaortic obstruction, as described in Chap. 205.

2 Discrete congenital subvalvular AS. This congenital anomaly is produced by either a membranous diaphragm or a fibrous ridge just below the aortic valve (Chap. 199).

3 Supravalvular AS. This uncommon congenital anomaly is produced by narrowing of the ascending aorta or by a fibrous diaphragm with a small opening just above the aortic valve (Chap. 199).

PATHOPHYSIOLOGY The primary hemodynamic abnormality is obstruction to left ventricular outflow which causes a systolic pressure gradient between the left ventricle and aorta. When severe obstruction is suddenly produced experimentally, the left ventricle responds by dilatation and reduction of stroke volume. However, in patients the obstruction may be present at birth and/or increases gradually over the course of many years, and left ventricular output is maintained by the presence of left ventricular hypertrophy. This serves as a useful compensatory mechanism because it reduces toward normal the systolic stress developed by each segment of myocardium. A large transaortic valvular pressure gradient may exist for many years without a reduction of cardiac output, left ventricular dilatation, or the development of symptoms.

A peak systolic pressure gradient exceeding 50 mmHg in the face of a normal cardiac output or an effective aortic orifice less than approximately $0.5 \text{ cm}^2/\text{m}^2$ of body surface area, i.e., less than approximately one-third of the normal orifice, is generally considered to represent critical obstruction to left ventricular outflow. The left ventricular pressure pulse exhibits a rounded summit as the contraction of this chamber becomes progressively more isometric. The elevated left ventricular end-diastolic pressure observed in many patients with severe AS does not necessarily signify the presence of left ventricular dilatation or failure but may reflect diminished compliance of the hypertrophied left ventricular wall.

A large *a* wave in the left atrial pressure pulse is usually present in severe AS. Loss of an appropriately timed, vigorous atrial contraction, as occurs in atrial fibrillation or atrioventricular dissociation, may result in a rapid aggravation of symptoms.

Although the cardiac output at rest is within normal limits in the majority of patients with severe AS, it may fail to rise normally during exercise. Late in the course the cardiac output and left ventricular–aortic pressure gradient decline, and the mean left atrial, pulmonary artery wedge, pulmonary arterial, and right ventricular pressures rise.

The hypertrophied left ventricular muscle mass elevates myocardial oxygen requirements. In addition, even in the absence of obstructive coronary artery disease, there may be interference with coronary blood flow, because the pressure compressing the coronary arteries exceeds the coronary perfusion pressure. Metabolic evidence of myocardial ischemia can be demonstrated in patients with AS both in the presence and in the absence of coronary arterial narrowing.

A significant fraction of patients with rheumatic AS has associated mitral valve disease. AS intensifies the severity of mitral regurgitation by increasing the pressure driving blood from the left ventricle to the left atrium.

SYMPTOMS AS is rarely of hemodynamic or clinical importance until the valve orifice has narrowed to approximately one-third of normal, i.e., to 1 cm² in adults. Even critical AS may exist for many years without producing any symptoms because of the ability of the hypertrophied left ventricle to generate the elevated intraventricular pressures.

Most patients with pure or predominant AS have gradually increasing obstruction for years but do not become symptomatic until the fifth to seventh decades. Exertional dyspnea, angina pectoris, and syncope are the three cardinal symptoms. Often there is a history of insidious progression of fatigue and dyspnea associated with gradual curtailment of activities. *Dyspnea* results primarily from elevation of the pulmonary capillary pressure; the latter is caused by elevations of left atrial and left ventricular end-diastolic pressures secondary to reduced compliance and/or left ventricular dilatation. *Angina pectoris* usually develops somewhat later and reflects an imbalance between the augmented myocardial oxygen requirements and reduced oxygen availability; the former results from the increased myocardial mass and intraventricular pressure, while the latter may result from accompanying coronary artery disease, which is not uncommon in patients with AS, as well as from compression of the coronary vessels by the hypertrophied myocardium. Therefore, angina may occur in severe AS even without obstructive epicardial coronary artery disease. *Exertional syncope* may result from a decline in arterial pressure caused by vasodilatation in the exercising muscles and inadequate vasoconstriction in nonexercising muscles in the face of a fixed cardiac output or from a sudden fall in cardiac output produced by an arrhythmia.

Since the cardiac output at rest is usually well maintained until late in the course, marked fatigability, weakness, peripheral cyanosis, and other clinical manifestations of a low cardiac output are usually not prominent until this stage is reached. Orthopnea, paroxysmal nocturnal dyspnea, and pulmonary edema, i.e., symptoms of left ventricular failure, also occur only in the advanced stages of the disease. Severe pulmonary hypertension leading to right ventricular failure and systemic venous hypertension, hepatomegaly, atrial fibrillation, and tricuspid regurgitation are usually preterminal findings.

When AS and MS coexist, the latter lesion masks many of the clinical findings of the former. The reduction of cardiac output induced by MS lowers the pressure gradient across the aortic valve, diminishes the frequency of anginal episodes, and retards the development of severe left ventricular hypertrophy. On the other hand, symptoms considered more characteristic of MS, such as pulmonary congestion and hemoptysis, may be present. Physical, electrocardiographic, radiologic, and echocardiographic examinations in patients with combined AS and MS generally reveal more evidence of left ventricular enlargement than in patients with pure MS, and left heart catheterization is helpful in defining the relative importance of each valvular abnormality.

PHYSICAL FINDINGS   The systemic arterial pressure is usually within normal limits. In the late stages, however, when stroke volume declines, the systolic pressure may fall and the pulse pressure narrow. Systemic hypertension is unusual in patients with marked AS, and a basal systolic arterial pressure exceeding 200 mmHg practically excludes severe narrowing of this valve. The peripheral arterial pulse, as palpated in the carotid or brachial arteries, rises slowly to a delayed sustained peak. Indirect recordings of the carotid pulse exhibit a gradually ascending limb, often with a prominent anacrotic notch or shoulder on the upstroke, as well as a delayed peak, with coarse systolic vibrations. The left ventricular ejection period is prolonged, the preejection period is abbreviated, and the ratio of these two, i.e., the preejection period/systolic ejection period, is characteristically reduced. Late in the course of the disease, in the presence of heart failure, the ratio may return to normal. A palpable double systolic arterial pulse, the so-called bisferiens pulse, excludes pure or predominant AS and signifies dominant or pure aortic regurgitation or obstructive hypertrophic cardiomyopathy (Chap. 205). In the late stages of valvular AS, when the pulse pressure is reduced, the pulse amplitude may be so small that the anacrotic nature of the pulse and the delay in its upstroke may become difficult to appreciate. In many patients the *a* wave in the jugular venous pulse is accentuated. This results from the diminished distensibility of the right ventricular cavity caused by the bulging, hypertrophied interventricular septum and/or the presence of pulmonary hypertension.

Palpation   The apex beat is usually active and displaced laterally, reflecting the presence of left ventricular hypertrophy. A double apical impulse may be appreciated, particularly with the patient in the left lateral recumbent position; the first outward expansion occurs during atrial systole and reflects the important contribution made by atrial contraction to ventricular filling, while the second occurs during ventricular systole and usually is forceful and sustained during ejection. The right ventricle is palpable only when pulmonary hypertension develops in the late stages. A systolic thrill is generally present at the base of the heart, in the jugular notch, and along the carotid arteries, but occasionally it is palpable only during expiration and with the patient leaning forward. In patients who do not have marked pulmonary emphysema, a thick chest wall, thoracic deformity, or heart failure, the absence of a systolic thrill suggests that the aortic stenosis is relatively mild.

Auscultation   The rhythm is generally regular until very late in the course; at other times, atrial fibrillation should suggest the possibility of associated mitral valve disease. An early systolic ejection sound, actually the OS of the aortic valve, is frequently audible in children and adolescents with congenital *noncalcific* valvular AS. This sound usually disappears when the valve becomes calcified and rigid. The sound of aortic valve closure also can be identified most frequently in patients with AS who have pliable valves, and calcification diminishes the intensity of this sound as well. As AS increases in severity, left ventricular systole may become prolonged so that the aortic valve closure sound no longer precedes the pulmonic valve closure sound, and the two components may become synchronous, or aortic valve closure may even follow pulmonic valve closure, causing paradoxic splitting of the second heart sound (Chap. 188). The latter finding usually signifies severe obstruction to left ventricular outflow. Frequently, a fourth heart sound is audible at the apex in many patients with severe AS and reflects the presence of left ventricular hypertrophy and an elevated left ventricular end-diastolic pressure; a third heart sound generally occurs when the left ventricle dilates and fails.

The murmur of AS is characteristically an ejection systolic murmur which commences shortly after the first heart sound, increases in intensity to reach a peak toward the middle of ejection, and ends just before aortic valve closure (Chap. 188). It is usually low-pitched, rough, and rasping in character, loudest at the base of the heart, most commonly in the second right intercostal space. It is transmitted to the jugular notch and upward along the carotid arteries. Occasionally, it is transmitted downward and to the apex and may be confused with the systolic murmur of MR; however, the latter is usually holosystolic. In almost all patients with severe obstruction, the murmur is at least grade III/VI. In patients with mild degrees of obstruction or in those with severe stenosis with heart failure in whom the stroke volume and therefore the transvalvular flow rate are reduced, the murmur may be relatively soft and brief.

Electrocardiogram   This reveals left ventricular hypertrophy in the majority of patients with severe AS (Chap. 189). In advanced cases, ST-segment depression and T-wave inversion (left ventricular "strain") in standard leads I and aVL and in the left precordial leads are evident. However, there is no close correlation between the electrocardiogram and the hemodynamic severity of obstruction, and the absence of electrocardiographic signs of left ventricular hypertrophy does not exclude severe obstruction. The presence of left atrial enlargement should suggest the possibility of associated mitral valve disease.

Echocardiogram   The key findings are left ventricular hypertrophy and in patients with valvular calcification, multiple, bright, thick, echoes from within the aortic root. Eccentricity of the aortic valve cusps is characteristic of congenitally bicuspid valves. Left ventricular dilatation and reduced systolic shortening reflect impairment of left ventricular function. The transaortic valvular gradient can be estimated by Doppler echocardiography. Echocardiography is particularly useful for identifying valvular abnormalities such as MS and aortic regurgitation which sometimes accompany AS (Fig. 190–7), and for differentiating valvular from obstructive hypertrophic cardiomyopathy.

Roentgenogram   The chest roentgenogram may show no or little overall cardiac enlargement for many years, since the development of concentric left ventricular hypertrophy is the initial response to obstruction to left ventricular outflow. Hypertrophy without dilatation may produce some rounding of the cardiac apex in the frontal projection and slight backward displacement in the lateral view; critical AS is often associated with poststenotic dilatation of the ascending aorta. Aortic calcification is usually readily apparent on fluoroscopic examination with an image intensifier or by echocardiography; *the absence of valvular calcification in an adult suggests that severe valvular AS is not present.* In later stages of the disease as the left ventricle dilates, there is increasing evidence of left ventricular enlargement, roentgenographic signs of pulmonary congestion, as well as enlargement of the left atrium, pulmonary artery, and right side of the heart.

Catheterization and angiocardiography Catheterization of the left side of the heart and coronary arteriography should generally be carried out in patients suspected of having severe AS, particularly before a final decision concerning operative treatment is made. The goals are to (1) determine the severity of the aortic obstruction, often previously estimated by Doppler echocardiography, (2) assess the status of left ventricular function, and (3) determine the location of the left ventricular outflow obstruction. These investigations are especially indicated in the following:

1 Young, asymptomatic patients with noncalcific congenital AS (Chap. 199), in order to define the severity of obstruction to left ventricular outflow, since operation or balloon valvuloplasty may be indicated in them if severe AS is present, even in the absence of symptoms.
2 Patients in whom it is suspected that the obstruction to left ventricular outflow may not be at the aortic valve but rather in the sub- or supravalvular regions.
3 Patients with clinical signs of AS and symptoms of myocardial ischemia, in whom associated coronary artery disease is suspected. An effort should be made to determine whether aortic stenosis or coronary atherosclerosis is primarily responsible for the symptoms, and coronary arteriography should be carried out in addition to catheterization of the left side of the heart.
4 Patients with multivalvular disease, in whom the role played by each valvular deformity should be defined before operative treatment is planned.

Angiographic studies, while not mandatory, are helpful in defining the size of the left ventricular cavity, the thickness of the left ventricle, the site of obstruction, the degree of deformity and mobility of the aortic valve cusps, the diameter of the ascending aorta, and the presence and degree of accompanying mitral and aortic regurgitation and of obstructive coronary disease.

NATURAL HISTORY Death in patients with severe AS occurs most commonly in the seventh and eighth decades. Based on data obtained at postmortem examination in patients *not treated surgically*, the average time to death after the onset of various symptoms was as follows: angina pectoris, 3 years; syncope, 3 years; dyspnea, 2 years; and congestive heart failure, 1.5 to 2 years. Moreover, in more than 80 percent of patients who died with AS, symptoms had existed for less than 4 years. Congestive heart failure was considered to be the cause of death in one-half to two-thirds of patients. Among adults dying with valvular AS, sudden death, which presumably results from an arrhythmia, occurred in 10 to 20 percent and at an average age of 60 years.

TREATMENT All patients with moderate or severe AS require careful periodic follow-up. In patients with *severe* AS, strenuous physical activity should be avoided even in the asymptomatic stage. Digitalis glycosides, sodium restriction, and the cautious administration of diuretics are indicated in the treatment of congestive heart failure, but care must be taken to avoid volume depletion. While nitroglycerin is helpful in relieving angina pectoris, vasodilator therapy for heart failure is usually of little value. The most critical decision in the management of AS concerns the advisability of surgical treatment. The indications and results of operation, as well as the techniques, differ considerably, depending on the patient's age and the nature of the valvular deformity.

In children and adolescents with noncalcific congenital AS, considerable hemodynamic improvement can be anticipated from simple commissural incision under direct vision. This operation is recommended not only for symptomatic patients but also for asymptomatic children and adolescents with hemodynamic evidence of critical obstruction to left ventricular outflow, with a peak systolic pressure gradient exceeding 50 mmHg when the cardiac output is normal, or a calculated effective orifice less than 0.5 cm^2/m^2 of body surface area.

In the majority of adults with calcific AS and critical obstruction, replacement of the valve is necessary. In most instances, it is prudent to postpone operation in patients with severe calcific AS who are asymptomatic, since their future course is difficult to predict and they may continue to do well for many years. However, they should be followed carefully by clinical examination for the development of symptoms and by serial echocardiograms (Chap. 190) for evidence of deteriorating left ventricular function; operation is generally indicated in patients with severe AS and left ventricular dysfunction, even if they are asymptomatic. In patients without heart failure, the operative risk is approximately 5 percent. It is likely that as the results of surgical replacement of the aortic valve continue to improve, many asymptomatic patients with severe AS will become candidates for operation before their left ventricular function deteriorates. At present, replacement of the aortic valve should be undertaken in patients with hemodynamic evidence of severe obstruction and symptoms, even when these are relatively mild, or in those with progressive left ventricular dysfunction regardless of the presence or absence of symptoms. In such patients, the operative risk is relatively low (<5 percent) in experienced centers.

When angina pectoris, syncope, or left ventricular decompensation develops in adults with severe valvular AS, the outlook, despite medical treatment, is very poor and can be improved significantly by replacement of the aortic valve with an artificial valve. The operative risk in this group of patients, although relatively high (approximately 10 percent), is still considerably lower than the risk involved by nonoperative treatment; moreover, the symptomatic improvement in some survivors of operation has been remarkable.

Operation should, if possible, be carried out before frank left ventricular failure develops; at this late stage, the operative risk is high (15 to 20 percent), and evidence of myocardial disease may persist even when the operation is technically successful. Furthermore, long-term postoperative survival also correlates inversely with preoperative left ventricular dysfunction. Nonetheless, in view of the very poor prognosis of such patients when they are treated medically, there is usually little choice but to advise immediate surgical treatment. In patients in whom severe AS and coronary artery disease coexist, relief of the AS and revascularization of the myocardium by means of aortocoronary bypass grafting may result in striking clinical and hemodynamic improvement. Since many patients with calcific AS are elderly, particular attention must be directed to the adequacy of hepatic, renal, and pulmonary function before valve replacement is recommended. The mortality rate depends to a substantial extent on the patient's preoperative clinical and hemodynamic state. The 10-year survival rate of patients with aortic valve replacement is approximately 67 percent. Approximately 15 percent of bioprosthetic valves evidence primary valve failure in 10 years, requiring re-replacement, and an approximately equal percentage of patients with mechanical prostheses develop significant hemorrhagic complications as a consequence of treatment with anticoagulants. Fortunately, there is evidence that regression of left ventricular hypertrophy may occur following relief of obstruction.

Percutaneous balloon aortic valvuloplasty, described in Chap. 193, is an alternative to surgery in children and young adults with congenital aortic stenosis. It is not commonly employed in elderly patients with severe calcific aortic stenosis because of a high restenosis rate. Nonetheless, this procedure may be useful in patients who are too ill or frail to undergo surgery, in patients with life-threatening aortic stenosis and advanced extracardiac disease, and as a "bridge to surgery" in patients with severe left ventricular dysfunction.

AORTIC REGURGITATION

ETIOLOGY Approximately three-fourths of patients with pure or predominant aortic regurgitation (AR) are males; females predominate among patients with AR who have associated mitral valve disease. In approximately two-thirds of patients with AR the disease is rheumatic in origin, resulting in thickening, deformation, and shortening of the individual aortic valve cusps, changes which prevent their proper opening during systole and closure during diastole. A rheumatic origin is less common in patients with isolated AR. Acute AR also may result from infective endocarditis, which may attack a valve previously affected by rheumatic disease, a congenitally deformed valve, or rarely a normal aortic valve, and perforate or erode one or more of the leaflets. Patients with discrete membranous subaortic stenosis often develop thickening of the aortic valve leaflets, which in turn leads to mild or moderate degrees of AR and makes these valves particularly susceptible to endocarditis. AR also may occur in patients with congenital bicuspid aortic valves. Prolapse of an aortic cusp, resulting in progressive chronic AR, occurs in approximately 15 percent of patients with ventricular septal defect (Chap. 199). Congenital fenestrations of the aortic valve occasionally produce mild AR. Although traumatic rupture of the aortic valve is an uncommon cause of acute AR, it does represent the most frequent serious lesion observed in patients surviving nonpenetrating cardiac injuries. In patients with AR due to primary valvular disease, dilatation of the aortic annulus may occur secondarily and intensify the regurgitation.

AR, both acute and chronic, also may be due entirely to marked aortic dilatation, i.e., aortic root disease, without primary involvement of the valve leaflets; widening of the aortic annulus and separation of the aortic leaflets are responsible for the AR. Syphilis and ankylosing rheumatoid spondylitis may be associated with cellular infiltration and scarring of the media of the thoracic aorta, leading to aortic dilatation, aneurysm formation, and severe regurgitation. In syphilis of the aorta (Chap. 210), the involvement of the intima may narrow the coronary ostia, which in turn may be responsible for myocardial ischemia. Cystic medial necrosis of the ascending aorta, which may or may not be associated with other manifestations of the Marfan syndrome, idiopathic dilatation of the aorta, osteogenesis imperfecta, and severe hypertension all may widen the aortic annulus and lead to progressive AR. Occasionally, AR is caused by retrograde dissection of the aorta involving the aortic annulus.

The coexistence of hemodynamically significant AS with AR usually excludes all the rarer forms of AR because it occurs almost exclusively in patients whose AR is on a rheumatic or congenital basis.

PATHOPHYSIOLOGY The total stroke volume expelled by the left ventricle (i.e., the sum of the effective forward stroke volume and the volume of blood which regurgitates back into the left ventricle) is increased in AR. In patients with wide-open (*free*) AR, the volume of regurgitant flow may equal the effective forward stroke volume. In contrast to MR, in which a fraction of the left ventricular stroke volume is delivered into the low-pressure left atrium, in AR the entire left ventricular stroke volume must be ejected into a high-pressure zone, the aorta. However, the low aortic diastolic pressure (low afterload) facilitates early ventricular emptying. An increase in the left ventricular end-diastolic volume (increased preload) constitutes the major hemodynamic compensation for AR. The dilatation of the left ventricle allows this chamber to expel a larger stroke volume without requiring any increase in the relative shortening of each myofibril. Therefore, severe AR may occur with a normal effective forward stroke volume and a normal ejection fraction [total (forward plus regurgitant) stroke volume/end-diastolic volume], together with an elevated left ventricular end-diastolic pressure and volume. However, through the operation of Laplace's law (which indicates that myocardial wall tension is the product of intracavitary pressure and left ventricular radius), left ventricular dilatation increases the left ventricular systolic tension required to develop any given level of systolic pressure. As left ventricular function deteriorates, the end-

diastolic volume and the ejection fraction and forward stroke volume decline. Deterioration of left ventricular function often precedes the development of symptoms. Considerable thickening of the left ventricular wall also occurs with chronic AR, and at autopsy the hearts of these patients may be among the largest encountered, sometimes exceeding 1000 g in weight.

The reverse pressure gradient from aorta to left ventricle, which is responsible for the aortic regurgitant flow, falls progressively during diastole, accounting for the decrescendo nature of the diastolic murmur. Equilibration between aortic and left ventricular pressures may occur toward the end of diastole in patients with severe AR, particularly when the heart rate is slow, and the left ventricular end-diastolic pressure may be elevated, occasionally to extremely high levels (>40 mmHg). Rarely, the left ventricular pressure exceeds the left atrial pressure toward the end of diastole, and this reversed pressure gradient closes the mitral valve prematurely or causes diastolic mitral regurgitation.

In patients with free AR, the effective forward cardiac output usually is normal or only slightly reduced at rest, but often it fails to rise normally during exertion. Early signs of left ventricular dysfunction include reductions in the fraction of systolic shortening and in the ejection fraction, determined by echocardiography or radionuclide or contrast angiography. In advanced stages there may be considerable elevation of the left atrial, pulmonary artery wedge, pulmonary arterial, and right ventricular pressures and lowering of the forward cardiac output at rest.

Myocardial ischemia may occur in patients with AR because myocardial oxygen requirements are elevated by both left ventricular dilatation and elevated left ventricular systolic tension. However, the major portion of coronary blood flow occurs during diastole, when arterial pressure is subnormal, thereby reducing coronary perfusion pressure. The combination of increased oxygen demand and reduced supply may cause myocardial ischemia.

HISTORY A family history may frequently be elicited from patients with AR associated with the Marfan syndrome. Patients with AR of obscure cause should be questioned about a positive serologic test for syphilis and about prior chest trauma; a history compatible with infective endocarditis may sometimes be elicited from patients with rheumatic or congenital involvement of the aortic valve, and the infection often precipitates or seriously aggravates preexisting symptoms. Ankylosing spondylitis is usually self-evident.

Patients with severe AR may remain asymptomatic for as long as 10 to 15 years.

In chronic, severe AR, uncomfortable awareness of the heartbeat, especially on lying down, may be an early complaint. Sinus tachycardia during exertion or with emotion or premature ventricular contractions may produce particularly uncomfortable palpitations, as well as head pounding. These complaints may persist for many years before the development of exertional dyspnea, usually the first symptom of diminished cardiac reserve. This is followed by orthopnea, paroxysmal nocturnal dyspnea, and excessive diaphoresis. Chest pain occurs frequently, even in younger patients, and it is not necessary to invoke the presence of coronary artery disease to explain this symptom in patients with AR. It may be due to myocardial ischemia, or it may originate from excessive cardiac pounding on the chest wall. Anginal pain may develop at rest as well as during exertion. Nocturnal angina may be a particularly troublesome symptom, and it may be accompanied by marked diaphoresis. The anginal episodes can be prolonged and often do not respond satisfactorily to sublingual nitroglycerin. Late in the course of the disease, evidence of systemic fluid accumulation, including congestive hepatomegaly, ankle edema, and ascites, may develop. Patients with severe AR tolerate high fevers, infections, or cardiac arrhythmias poorly and may die in pulmonary edema as a result of one of these complications.

In patients with acute, severe AR, as may occur in trauma or infective endocarditis, the left ventricle rapidly exhausts its ability to dilate, and left ventricular diastolic pressure rises rapidly with associated elevations of left atrial and pulmonary capillary pressures.

PHYSICAL FINDINGS Even prior to the examination of the heart of the patient with free AR, the jarring of the entire body and the bobbing motion of the head with each systole can be appreciated, and the abrupt distention and collapse of the larger arteries are easily visible. The examination should be directed toward the detection of conditions predisposing to AR, such as the Marfan syndrome, rheumatoid spondylitis, syphilis, essential hypertension, and ventricular septal defect.

Arterial pulse A rapidly rising "water-hammer" pulse, which collapses suddenly as arterial pressure falls rapidly during late systole and diastole (Corrigan's pulse), and capillary pulsations, an alternate flushing and paling of the skin at the root of the nail while pressure is applied to the tip of the nail (Quincke's pulse), are characteristic of free AR. A booming, "pistol-shot" sound can be heard over the femoral arteries (Traube's sign), and a to-and-fro murmur (Duroziez's sign) is audible if the femoral artery is lightly compressed with a stethoscope.

The arterial pulse pressure is widened, with an elevation of the systolic pressure, sometimes to as high as 300 mmHg, and a depression of the diastolic pressure. The measurement of arterial diastolic pressure with a sphygmomanometer may be complicated by the fact that systolic sounds are frequently heard with the cuff completely deflated. However, the level of cuff pressure at the time of muffling of the Korotkoff sounds generally corresponds fairly closely to the true intraarterial diastolic pressure. The severity of AR does not always correlate directly with the arterial pulse pressure, and severe regurgitation may exist in patients with arterial pressures in the range of 140/60. As the disease progresses and the left ventricular end-diastolic pressure rises markedly, the arterial diastolic pressure may actually rise also, since the aortic diastolic pressure cannot fall below the left ventricular end-diastolic pressure.

Palpation The apex beat is heaving and displaced laterally and inferiorly. The systolic expansion and diastolic retraction of the apex are prominent and contrast sharply with the sustained systolic thrust characteristic of severe AS. A diastolic thrill is often palpable along the left sternal border, and a prominent systolic thrill may be palpable in the jugular notch and transmitted upward along the carotid arteries. This thrill and the accompanying systolic murmur are due to the markedly increased blood flow across the aortic orifice and do not necessarily signify the coexistence of AS. In many patients with pure AR or with combined AS and AR, palpation or recording of the carotid arterial pulse reveals it to be bisferiens, i.e., with two systolic waves separated by a trough.

Auscultation In patients with severe AR, the aortic valve closure sound is usually diminished or absent. A third heart sound is common, and occasionally, a fourth heart sound also may be heard. A loud systolic ejection sound is frequently audible; presumably it results from the sudden dilatation of the aorta by a greatly increased stroke volume. The murmur of AR is typically a high-pitched, blowing, decrescendo diastolic murmur which is usually heard best in the third left intercostal space. In patients with mild regurgitation, this murmur is brief, but as the severity increases, the murmur generally becomes louder and longer, and in patients with free AR it is usually holodiastolic. When the murmur is soft, it can be heard best with the diaphragm of the stethoscope and with the patient sitting up, leaning forward, and with the breath held in forced expiration. As it increases in intensity, it tends to radiate widely, particularly along the lower sternal edge. In patients in whom the AR is caused by primary valvular disease, the diastolic murmur is usually louder along the left than the right sternal border. However, when the decrescendo diastolic murmur is heard best along the right sternal border, it suggests that the AR is caused by aneurysmal dilatation of the aortic root. "Cooing" or musical diastolic murmurs suggest eversion of an aortic cusp vibrating in the regurgitant stream. Unless it is trivial in magnitude, the AR is usually accompanied by peripheral signs such as a widened pulse pressure or a collapsing pulse. On the other hand, with the Graham Steell murmur of pulmonary regurgitation, there usually is clinical evidence of severe pulmonary hypertension, in-cluding a loud and palpable pulmonary component of the second heart sound.

A midsystolic ejection murmur is frequently audible in AR. It is generally heard best at the base of the heart and is transmitted to the jugular notch and along the carotid vessels. This murmur may be quite loud without signifying organic obstruction; it is often higher pitched, shorter, and less rasping in quality than the ejection systolic murmur heard in patients with predominant AS. A third murmur which is frequently heard in patients with AR is the Austin Flint murmur, a soft, low-pitched, rumbling middiastolic or presystolic bruit. It is probably produced by the displacement of the anterior leaflet of the mitral valve by the aortic regurgitant stream but does not appear to be associated with hemodynamically significant mitral obstruction. Both the Austin Flint murmur and the rumbling diastolic murmur of MS are loudest at the apex, but the murmur of MS is usually accompanied by a loud first heart sound and immediately follows the opening snap of the mitral valve, while the Austin Flint murmur is often shorter in duration than the murmur of MS, and in patients with sinus rhythm the latter exhibits presystolic accentuation. The auscultatory features of AR are intensified by isometric exercise such as strenuous handgrip, which augments systemic resistance, and reduced by inhalation of amyl nitrite. A blowing holosystolic murmur at the apex, which is transmitted to the axilla, also may be heard in patients with AR who have marked left ventricular dilatation and functional mitral regurgitation.

In *acute*, severe AR, the elevation of left ventricular end-diastolic pressure may lead to early closure of the mitral valve, an associated middiastolic sound, a soft or absent S_1, a pulse pressure that is not particularly wide, and a soft, short diastolic murmur.

Electrocardiogram In patients with mild AR, there may be no electrocardiographic abnormalities, but with severe, chronic AR, the electrocardiographic signs of left ventricular hypertrophy become manifest (Chap. 189). In addition, these patients frequently exhibit ST-segment depressions and T-wave inversions in leads I, aVL, V_5, and V_6 ("left ventricular strain"). Left axis deviation and/or QRS prolongation denote diffuse myocardial disease, generally associated with patchy fibrosis, and usually signify a poor prognosis.

Echocardiogram This reveals increased systolic excursion of the posterior left ventricular wall; the extent and velocity of wall motion are normal or even supernormal, until myocardial contractility declines. A rapid, high-frequency fluttering of the anterior mitral leaflet produced by the impact of the aortic regurgitant jet is a characteristic finding. The echocardiogram is also useful in determining the cause of AR, by detecting dilatation of the aortic annulus. Thickening of the aortic valve and failure of coaptation of the leaflets also may be noted. Color Doppler flow echocardiographic imaging is very sensitive in the detection of AR, and Doppler echocardiography is helpful in assessing its severity (Fig. 190-7). Serial two-dimensional echocardiography is valuable in evaluating left ventricular performance and in detecting progressive myocardial dysfunction.

Roentgenogram In severe chronic AR the apex is displaced downward and to the left in the frontal projection, and frequently the cardiac shadow extends below the left diaphragm. Left ventricular enlargement also may be apparent in the left anterior oblique and lateral projections, in which the left ventricle is displaced posteriorly and encroaches on the spine. In patients in whom primary valvular disease is responsible for the AR, the ascending aorta and aortic knob may be moderately dilated. When AR is caused by primary disease of the aortic wall, aneurysmal dilatation of the aorta may be noted, and the aorta may fill the retrosternal space in the lateral view.

Cardiac catheterization and angiography These tests should be carried out to aid in the decision regarding surgical treatment. In addition to providing an accurate measurement of the magnitude of regurgitation and the status of left ventricular function, the condition of the coronary arterial bed may be evaluated.

TREATMENT Although operation constitutes the principal treatment of aortic regurgitation, and should be carried out before the development of heart failure, the latter usually does respond initially to treatment with digitalis glycosides, salt restriction, diuretics, and vasodilators, especially angiotensin-converting enzyme inhibitors. Digitalis also may be indicated in patients with severe regurgitation and dilated left ventricles without symptoms of frank left ventricular failure. Cardiac arrhythmias and infections are poorly tolerated in patients with free AR and must be treated promptly and vigorously. Although nitroglycerin and long-acting nitrates are not as helpful in relieving anginal pain as in patients with ischemic heart disease, they are worth a trial. Patients with syphilitic aortitis should receive a full course of penicillin therapy (Chap. 133).

In deciding on the advisability and proper timing of surgical treatment, two points should be kept in mind: (1) patients with chronic AR usually do not become symptomatic until *after* the development of myocardial dysfunction, and (2) surgical treatment often does not restore normal left ventricular function. Therefore, in patients with severe AR, careful clinical follow-up and noninvasive testing with echocardiography at approximately 6-month intervals are necessary if operation is to be undertaken at the optimal time, i.e., after the onset of left ventricular dysfunction but prior to the development of severe symptoms. Operation can be deferred as long as the patient remains asymptomatic *and* retains normal left ventricular function.

Replacement of the aortic valve with a suitable mechanical or tissue prosthesis is generally necessary in patients with rheumatic AR and in many patients with other forms of regurgitation. Rarely, when a leaflet has been perforated during an episode of infective endocarditis or torn from its attachments to the aortic annulus, surgical repair may be possible. When AR is due to aneurysmal dilatation of the annulus and ascending aorta rather than to primary valvular involvement, it may be possible to reduce the regurgitation by narrowing the annulus or by excising a portion of the aortic root without replacing the valve. More frequently, however, regurgitation can be eliminated only by replacing the aortic valve, excising the aneurysm responsible for the regurgitation, and replacing the latter with a graft. This formidable procedure entails a higher risk than aortic valve replacement alone.

As in patients with other valvular abnormalities, both the operative risk of aortic valve replacement and late mortality are largely dependent on the stage of the disease and on myocardial function at the time of operation; patients with marked cardiac enlargement and prolonged left ventricular dysfunction experience an operative mortality of approximately 10 percent and a late mortality of approximately 5 percent per year despite a technically satisfactory operation. Nonetheless, because of the poor prognosis with medical management, even patients with left ventricular failure should be considered for operation.

ACUTE AORTIC REGURGITATION   Infective endocarditis, aortic dissection, and trauma are the most common causes of severe, acute AR. Since the left ventricle has not had time to dilate, stroke volume declines and ventricular diastolic pressure rises markedly; the arterial pulse pressure is often not markedly widened, and the physical signs characteristic of severe chronic AR may be absent. Premature closure of the mitral valve is common and can be recognized by echocardiography. The first heart sound is soft or absent; the aortic diastolic murmur is characteristically brief. Patients present with pulmonary congestion and edema, as well as hypotension secondary to a low cardiac output. Acute, severe regurgitation requires prompt surgical treatment, which may be lifesaving.

TRICUSPID STENOSIS

Tricuspid stenosis (TS), a relatively uncommon valvular lesion in North America and western Europe, is more common on the Indian subcontinent. It is generally rheumatic in origin and is more common in women than in men. It does not usually occur as an isolated lesion or in patients with pure MR but is usually observed in association with MS. Hemodynamically significant TS occurs in 5 to 10 percent of patients with severe MS; rheumatic TS is commonly associated with some degree of regurgitation.

PATHOPHYSIOLOGY   A diastolic pressure gradient between the right atrium and ventricle can be recorded with a double-lumen cardiac catheter. It is augmented when the transvalvular blood flow increases during inspiration and is reduced during expiration. A *mean* diastolic pressure gradient exceeding 4 mmHg is usually sufficient to elevate the mean right atrial pressure to levels which result in systemic venous congestion and, unless sodium intake has been restricted and diuretics administered, it is associated with ascites and edema. In patients with sinus rhythm, the right atrial *a* wave may be extremely tall and may even approach the level of the right ventricular systolic pressure. The resting cardiac output is usually quite low and fails to rise during exercise. The low cardiac output is responsible for the normal or only slightly elevated left atrial, pulmonary arterial, and right ventricular systolic pressures despite the presence of MS.

SYMPTOMS   Since the development of MS generally precedes that of TS, many patients initially have symptoms of pulmonary congestion. Amelioration of the latter should raise the possibility that TS may be developing. Characteristically, patients complain of relatively little dyspnea for the degree of hepatomegaly, ascites, and edema which they present. Fatigue secondary to a low cardiac output and discomfort due to refractory edema, ascites, and marked hepatomegaly are common in patients with TS and/or regurgitation. In some patients, TS may be suspected for the first time when symptoms of right ventricular failure persist after an adequate mitral valvulotomy.

PHYSICAL FINDINGS   Since TS usually occurs in the presence of other obvious valvular disease, the diagnosis may be missed unless it is specifically considered and searched for. Severe TS is associated with marked hepatic congestion, often resulting in cirrhosis, jaundice, serious malnutrition, anasarca, and ascites. Congestive hepatomegaly and, in cases of severe tricuspid valve disease, splenomegaly are present. The jugular veins are distended, and in patients with sinus rhythm there may be giant *a* waves. The *v* waves are less conspicuous, and since tricuspid obstruction impedes right atrial emptying during diastole, there is a slow *y* descent. In patients with sinus rhythm there may be prominent presystolic pulsations of the enlarged liver as well.

The right ventricle and the shock of pulmonic valve closure are usually not palpable. Indeed, a giant *a* wave in the jugular venous pulse without palpatory evidence of pulmonary hypertension or right ventricular enlargement should suggest the possibility of TS. On auscultation, the pulmonic closure sound is not accentuated, and occasionally, an OS of the tricuspid valve may be heard approximately 0.06 s after pulmonic valve closure. The diastolic murmur of TS has many of the qualities of the diastolic murmur of MS, and since TS almost always occurs in the presence of MS, the less common valvular lesion may be missed. However, the tricuspid murmur is generally heard best along the left lower sternal margin and over the xiphoid process and is most prominent during presystole in patients with sinus rhythm. The diastolic murmur is reduced in amplitude as the stethoscope is inched laterally, only to intensify or reappear as the mitral murmur at the apex. The murmur is augmented during inspiration, and it is reduced during expiration and particularly during the Valsalva maneuver, when tricuspid blood flow is reduced. This finding (Carvallo's sign) is often most easily elicited when the patient is in the erect position.

Noninvasive examinations   The features of right atrial enlargement (Chap. 189) include tall, peaked P waves in lead II, as well as prominent, upright P waves in lead V_1. The *absence* of electrocardiographic evidence of right ventricular hypertrophy in a patient with right-sided heart failure who is believed to have MS should suggest associated tricuspid valve disease. The chest roentgenograms in patients with combined TS and MS show particular prominence of the right atrium and superior vena cava without much enlargement of the pulmonary artery and with less evidence of pulmonary vascular congestion than occurs in patients with isolated MS. On echocardiographic examination, the tricuspid valve is usually thickened; the transvalvular gradient can be estimated by Doppler echocardiography.

TREATMENT Patients with TS generally exhibit marked systemic venous congestion; intensive salt restriction and diuretic therapy are required during the preoperative period. Such a preparatory period may diminish hepatic congestion and thereby improve hepatic function sufficiently so that the risks of operation are diminished. Surgical treatment of the tricuspid valve is not ordinarily indicated at the time of mitral valve surgery in patients with *mild* TS. On the other hand, definitive surgical relief of the TS should be carried out, preferably at the time of mitral valvulotomy, in patients with moderate or severe TS who have mean diastolic pressure gradients exceeding 4 to 5 mmHg and tricuspid orifices less than 1.5 to 2.0 cm². TS is almost always accompanied by significant tricuspid regurgitation. Open-heart operations utilizing cardiopulmonary bypass may permit substantial improvement of tricuspid valve function. If this cannot be accomplished, the tricuspid valve may have to be replaced with a prosthesis, preferably a tissue valve.

TRICUSPID REGURGITATION

Most commonly, tricuspid regurgitation (TR) is functional and secondary to marked dilatation of the right ventricle and the tricuspid annulus. Functional TR may complicate right ventricular enlargement of any cause, including inferior wall infarcts that involve the right ventricle, and it is commonly seen in the late stages of heart failure due to rheumatic or congenital heart disease with severe pulmonary hypertension, as well as in ischemic heart disease, cardiomyopathy, and cor pulmonale. It is in part reversible if pulmonary hypertension is relieved. Rheumatic fever may produce organic TR, often associated with TS. Less commonly, regurgitation results from congenitally deformed tricuspid valves, and it occurs with defects of the atrioventricular canal, as well as with Ebstein's malformation of the tricuspid valve (Chap. 199). Infarction of right ventricular papillary muscles, tricuspid valve prolapse, carcinoid heart disease, endomyocardial fibrosis, infective endocarditis, and trauma all may produce TR.

As is the case for TS, the clinical features of TR result primarily from systemic venous congestion and reduction of cardiac output. With the onset of TR in patients with pulmonary hypertension, symptoms of pulmonary congestion diminish, but the clinical manifestations of right-sided heart failure become intensified. The neck veins are distended with prominent *v* waves, and marked hepatomegaly, ascites, pleural effusions, edema, systolic pulsations of the liver, and positive hepatojugular reflux are common. A prominent right ventricular pulsation along the left parasternal region and a blowing holosystolic murmur along the lower left sternal margin which may be intensified during inspiration and reduced during expiration or the Valsalva maneuver are characteristic findings; atrial fibrillation is usually present.

The electrocardiogram usually shows changes characteristic of the lesion responsible for the enlargement of the right ventricle which leads to TR and therefore is helpful in elucidating its cause. In the rare instances of isolated TR, the electrocardiogram often shows incomplete right bundle branch block. Roentgenographic examination usually reveals enlargement of both the right atrium and ventricle. Echocardiography may be helpful by demonstrating right ventricular dilatation and prolapsing or flail tricuspid leaflets; the diagnosis of tricuspid regurgitation can be made by color flow echocardiography and the severity estimated by Doppler examination. The latter is also useful in estimating pulmonary artery pressure.

In patients with severe TR, the cardiac output is usually markedly reduced, and the right atrial pressure pulse may exhibit no *x* descent during early systole but a prominent *c-v* wave with a rapid *y* descent. The mean right atrial and the right ventricular end-diastolic pressures are often elevated.

Isolated TR, without pulmonary hypertension, such as that occurring as a consequence of infective endocarditis or trauma, is usually well tolerated and does not require operation. Indeed, even total excision of an infected tricuspid valve is often well tolerated if the pulmonary artery pressure is normal. Treatment of the underlying cause of heart failure usually reduces the severity of functional TR. In patients with mitral valve disease and TR due to pulmonary hypertension and massive right ventricular enlargement, effective surgical correction of the mitral valvular abnormality results in lowering of the pulmonary vascular pressures and gradual reduction or disappearance of the TR without direct treatment of the tricuspid valve. However, recovery may be much more rapid in patients with severe secondary TR if, at the time of mitral valve replacement, tricuspid annuloplasty (often with the insertion of a plastic ring) or, in the rare instance of severe organic tricuspid valve disease, tricuspid valve replacement is performed. Surgical treatment of the TR also should be carried out in patients with severe regurgitation secondary to deformity of the tricuspid valve due to rheumatic fever, particularly those *without* severe pulmonary hypertension.

PULMONIC VALVE DISEASE

The pulmonic valve is affected by rheumatic fever far less frequently than are the other valves, and it is uncommonly the seat of infective endocarditis. The most common acquired abnormality affecting the pulmonic valve is regurgitation secondary to dilatation of the pulmonic valve ring as a consequence of severe pulmonary hypertension. This produces the Graham Steell murmur, a high-pitched, decrescendo, diastolic blowing murmur along the left sternal border, which is difficult to differentiate from the far more common murmur produced by aortic regurgitation. It is usually of little hemodynamic significance; indeed, surgical removal or destruction of the pulmonic valve by infective endocarditis does not produce heart failure unless serious pulmonary hypertension is also present. The *carcinoid syndrome* may cause pulmonic stenosis and/or regurgitation.

Congenital pulmonic stenosis is discussed in Chap. 199.

REFERENCES

BLOOMFIELD P et al: Twelve year comparison of a Bjork-Shiley mechanical heart valve with porcine bioprostheses. N Engl J Med 324:573, 1991

BOUDOULAS H, WOOLEY CF (eds): *The Mitral Valve Prolapse Syndrome*. Futura, Mount Kisco, NY 1988

BRAUNWALD E: Valvular heart disease, in *Heart Disease*, 4th ed, E Braunwald (ed). Philadelphia, Saunders, 1992, p 1007

FELDMAN T: Rheumatic mitral stenosis. On the rise again. Postgrad Med 93:93, 99, 1993

GRAY RJ, HELFANT RH: Timing of surgery for valvular heart disease. Casrdiovasc Clin 23:209, 1993

GRUNKEMEIER GL et al: Prosthetic heart valve performance: Long-term follow-up. Curr Probl Cardiol 17:331, 1992

HESS OM et al: Diastolic dysfunciotn in aortic stenosis. Circualtion 87(Suppl 5):IV73, 1993

JAMIESON WR: Modern cardiac valve devices—bioprostheses and mechanical prostheses: State of the art. J Card Surg 8:89, 1993

KIRKLIN JW, BARRATT-BOYES BG: Part III. Acquired valvular heart disease, in *Cardiac Surgery*, 2d ed, JW Kirklin, BG Barratt-Boyes (eds). New York, Wiley, 1993, p 425

KLUES HG, HANRATH P: Echocardiography in valvular heart disease. Curr Opin Cardiol 7:209, 1992

NAIR CK et al: Ten-year results with the St. Jude Medical Prosthesis. Am J Cardiol 65(3):217, 1990

PAN M et al: Factors determining late success after mitral balloon valvulotomy. Am J Cardiol 71:1181, 1993

RAVKILDE JL, HANSEN PS: Late results following closed mitral valvotomy in isolated mitral valve stenosis: Analysis of 35 years of follow-up in 240 patients using Cox regression. Thorac Cardiovasc Surg 39:133, 1991

REED D et al: Prediction of outcome after mitral valve replacement in patients with symptomatic chronic mitral regurgitation. Circ 84:23, 1991

RODRIGUEZ A et al: Factors influencing the outcome of balloon aortic valvuloplasty in the elderly. Am Heart J 120:373, 1990

SLATER J et al: Comparison of cardiac catheterization and Doppler echocardiography in the decision to operate in aortic and mitral valve disease. J Am Coll Cardiol 17:1026, 1991

STRONG MD 3d, BROCKMAN SK: Mitral valve reconstruction. Cardiovasc Clin 23:255, 1993

202 ACUTE MYOCARDIAL INFARCTION

RICHARD C. PASTERNAK / EUGENE BRAUNWALD

Myocardial infarction is one of the most common diagnoses occurring in hospitalized patients in western countries. In the United States, approximately 1.5 million myocardial infarctions occur each year. Mortality with acute infarction is approximately 30 percent, with more than half of the deaths occurring before the stricken individual reaches the hospital. Although survival following hospitalization has improved over the last two decades, an additional 5 to 10 percent of survivors die in the first year following myocardial infarction and the number of myocardial infarctions each year in the United States has remained largely unchanged since the early 1970s. Risk of excess mortality and recurrent nonfatal myocardial infarction persists in patients who recover.

Myocardial infarction generally occurs with the abrupt decrease in coronary blood flow that follows a thrombotic occlusion of a coronary artery previously narrowed by atherosclerosis. Progression of the atherosclerotic lesion to the point where thrombus formation occurs is a complex process related to vascular injury. This injury is produced or facilitated by factors such as cigarette smoking, hypertension, and lipid accumulation. In the majority of cases, infarction occurs when an atherosclerotic plaque fissures, ruptures, or ulcerates, and, with conditions favoring thrombogenesis (factors which may be local or systemic), a mural thrombus forms leading to coronary artery occlusion. In rare cases, infarction may be due to coronary artery occlusion secondary to coronary emboli, congenital abnormalities, coronary spasm, and a wide variety of systemic—particularly inflammatory—diseases. Ultimately, the amount of myocardial damage caused by coronary occlusion depends upon the territory supplied by the affected vessel, whether or not the vessel becomes totally occluded, native factors which can produce early spontaneous lysis of the occlusive thrombus, the quantity of blood supplied by collateral vessels to the affected tissue, and the demand for oxygen of the myocardium whose blood supply has been suddenly limited.

Patients at increased risk of developing acute myocardial infarction include those with unstable angina, multiple coronary risk factors (Chap. 208) and Prinzmetal's variant angina (Chap. 203). Less common etiologic factors include hypercoagulability, coronary emboli, collagen vascular disease, and cocaine abuse.

CLINICAL PRESENTATION

Although in roughly one-half of cases no precipitating factor appears to be present prior to myocardial infarction, triggers such as physical exercise, emotional stress, and medical or surgical illnesses can often be identified. The onset of myocardial infarction may be at any time of the day or night, but a higher frequency of onset occurs in the morning within a few hours of awakening. *Pain* is the most common presenting complaint in patients with myocardial infarction. In some instances, the discomfort may be severe enough to be described as the worst pain the patient has ever experienced (Chap. 12). The pain of myocardial infarction is deep and visceral; adjectives commonly used to describe it are *heavy, squeezing,* and *crushing.* It is similar in character to the discomfort of angina pectoris but is usually more severe and lasts longer. Typically the pain involves the central portion of the chest and/or epigastrium, and in about 30 percent of cases it radiates to the arms. Less common sites of radiation include the abdomen, back, lower jaw, and neck. The location of the pain beneath the xiphoid and patients' denial that they may be suffering a heart attack are chiefly responsible for the mistaken diagnosis of indigestion. The pain of myocardial infarction may radiate as high as the occipital area but not below the umbilicus. The pain is often accompanied by weakness, sweating, nausea, vomiting, giddiness, and anxiety. The discomfort usually commences with the patient at rest. When the pain begins during a period of exertion, in contrast to angina pectoris, it does not usually subside with cessation of activity. Approximately one-half of patients with myocardial infarction exhibit the prodrome of unstable angina (Chap. 203).

Although pain is the most common presenting complaint, it is by no means always present; a minimum of 15 to 20 percent of myocardial infarcts are *painless.* The incidence of painless infarcts is greater in women and patients with diabetes mellitus, and it increases with age. In the elderly, myocardial infarction may present as sudden-onset breathlessness, which may progress to pulmonary edema. Other less common presentations, with or without pain, include sudden loss of consciousness, a confusional state, a sensation of profound weakness, the appearance of an arrhythmia, evidence of peripheral embolism, or merely an unexplained drop in arterial pressure. The pain of myocardial infarction can be similar to pain from acute pericarditis (Chap. 206), pulmonary embolism (Chap. 226), acute aortic dissection (Chap. 210), or costochondritis. These conditions should be considered in the differential diagnosis.

PHYSICAL FINDINGS Most patients are anxious and restless, attempting to relieve the pain by moving about in bed, squirming, and stretching. Pallor is common and is often associated with perspiration and coolness of the extremities. The combination of substernal chest pain persistent for more than 30 min and diaphoresis strongly suggests acute myocardial infarction. Although many patients have a normal pulse rate and blood pressure, within the first hour of infarction about one-fourth of patients with anterior infarction have manifestations of sympathetic nervous system hyperactivity (tachycardia and/or hypertension), and up to one-half with inferior infarction show evidence of parasympathetic hyperactivity (bradycardia and/or hypotension).

The precordium is usually quiet, and the apical impulse may be difficult to palpate. In about one-fourth of patients with anterior wall infarction, an abnormal systolic pulsation caused by dyskinetic bulging of infarcted myocardium develops in the periapical area within the first days of the illness and then may resolve. Other physical signs of ventricular dysfunction that may be present include, in decreasing incidence, fourth (S_4) and third (S_3) heart sounds, decreased intensity of heart sounds, and, rarely, paradoxical splitting of the second heart sound (Chap. 188). A transient apical systolic murmur, presumably due to mitral regurgitation secondary to papillary muscle dysfunction during acute infarction, may be midsystolic or late systolic in timing. A pericardial friction rub is heard in many patients with transmural myocardial infarction at some time in their course if they are examined frequently. Jugular venous distention occurs commonly in patients with right ventricular infarction. The carotid pulse is often decreased in volume, reflecting reduced stroke volume. Temperature elevations up to 38°C may be observed during the first week following acute myocardial infarction; however, a temperature exceeding 38°C should prompt a search for other causes. The arterial pressure is variable; in most patients with transmural infarction systolic pressure declines approximately 10 to 15 mmHg from the preinfarction state.

LABORATORY FINDINGS

The laboratory tests of value in confirming the diagnosis of myocardial infarction may be divided into four groups: (1) nonspecific indexes of tissue necrosis and inflammation, (2) the electrocardiogram, (3) serum enzyme changes, and (4) cardiac imaging.

The *nonspecific reaction* to myocardial injury is associated with polymorphonuclear leukocytosis, which appears within a few hours after the onset of pain, persists for 3 to 7 days, and often reaches levels of 12,000 to 15,000 leukocytes per microliter. The erythrocyte sedimentation rate rises more slowly than the white blood cell count, peaking during the first week, and sometimes remaining elevated for 1 or 2 weeks.

The *electrocardiographic manifestations* of acute myocardial infarction are described in Chap. 189. Although electrocardiographic-pathologic correlations are not excellent, transmural infarction is often present if the electrocardiogram demonstrates Q waves or loss of R waves; nontransmural infarction may be present if the electrocardiogram shows only transient ST-segment and sustained T-wave changes. However, the latter changes are variable and nonspecific and should not form the sole basis for the diagnosis of infarction. Therefore, a more rational nomenclature for designating electrocardiographic infarction is now commonly in use, with the terms *Q-wave* or *non-Q-wave infarction* in place of the terms *transmural* or *nontransmural infarction*, respectively. In the past, the Q-wave/non-Q-wave dichotomy was held to be particularly useful for prognostic and management reasons; however, today this is widely recognized as an oversimplified distinction, useful primarily for descriptive purposes.

SERUM ENZYMES Enzymes are released in large quantities into the blood from necrotic heart muscle following myocardial infarction. The rate of liberation of specific enzymes differs following infarction, and the temporal pattern of enzyme release is of diagnostic importance. Creatine phosphokinase (CK) rises within 8 to 24 h and generally returns to normal by 48 to 72 h, except in the case of large infarctions, when CK clearance is delayed. Lactic dehydrogenase (LDH) rises later (24 to 48 h) and remains elevated for as long as 7 to 14 days. The serum aminotransferase enzymes AST and ALT (previously designated SGOT and SGPT) were utilized in the diagnosis of myocardial infarction for many years but have fallen out of favor because it has been recognized that their time course of elevation is intermediate between CK and LDH, thus offering little advantage, and because of lack of tissue specificity. The MB isoenzyme of CK has the advantage over CK and LDH in that it is not present in significant concentrations in extracardiac tissue and therefore is more specific. CK-MB isoenzymes are particularly useful when skeletal muscle and/or brain damage are suspected since both of these tissues contain large quantities of the CK enzyme but none of the MB isoenzyme. The myocardial specificity of the MB isoenzyme determination depends on the technique used for measurement. Radioimmunoassay techniques are most specific, but the more commonly employed gel electrophoresis technique is significantly less specific and therefore prone to more frequent false positives. Tissues differ with respect to the five specific LDH isoenzyme patterns. The isoenzyme which predominates in the heart is referred to as LDH_1, which rises before total LDH in patients with myocardial infarction and may rise when there is no change in total LDH. Therefore, increased LDH_1 is a more sensitive indicator of myocardial infarction than total LDH; sensitivity exceeds 95 percent. However, LDH isoenzymes need to be measured only when the initial CK or CK-MB elevation might have been missed (after 48 h), for they are not more sensitive than CK-MB and therefore only increase cost without increasing diagnostic accuracy.

A two- to threefold elevation of total CK (not CK-MB) may follow an intramuscular injection. This may lead to the erroneous diagnosis of myocardial infarction in a patient who has been given an intramuscular injection of a narcotic for chest pain of noncardiac origin. Other potential sources of total CK elevation worthy of note are (1) muscular diseases including muscular dystrophy, myopathies, and polymyositis, (2) electrical cardioversion, (3) cardiac catheterization, (4) hypothyroidism, (5) stroke, (6) surgery, and (7) skeletal muscle damage secondary to trauma, convulsions, and prolonged immobilization. Cardiac surgery, myocarditis, and electrical cardioversion often result in elevation of serum levels of MB isoenzyme.

While it has long been recognized that the *total* quantity of enzyme released correlates with the size of the infarct, the *peak* enzyme concentration is only weakly correlated with infarct size. Thus while the *area* under the CK-MB time curve is related to infarct size, the *absolute* value of the peak CK-MB and its time to peak are related to the kinetics of CK-MB washout from myocardium. The opening of a coronary artery occlusion (either spontaneously, or by mechanical or pharmacologic means) in the early hours of myocardial infarction will cause early and higher peaking (at about 8 to 12 h following

reperfusion) of both the CK and CK-MB time curves. Without reperfusion, the CK peak occurs at about 24 h.

Characteristic rises occur in serum enzyme concentration in more than 95 percent of patients with clinically proven myocardial infarction. CK and LDH levels generally do not rise in unstable angina. Many patients with suspected infarction have baseline enzyme levels that are normal and increase threefold in a pattern consistent with infarction, although the absolute level of enzyme in the blood never exceeds the upper limits of normal. These have been termed "microinfarctions," and such patients have a prognosis intermediate between that of unstable angina and that of proven myocardial infarction. Isoenzyme studies are particularly helpful in this situation.

CARDIAC IMAGING Several radionuclide imaging techniques are of value in the diagnosis or assessment of the patient with acute myocardial infarction (Chap. 190). Acute infarct scintigraphy ("hot-spot" imaging) is carried out with an infarct-avid imaging agent such as [^{99m}Tc]stannous pyrophosphate. Scans are usually positive 2 to 5 days after infarction, particularly in patients with transmural infarcts; although they aid in *localizing* infarcts and provide a measure of infarct size (Chap. 190), these scans are less sensitive than CK determination for making the *diagnosis* of myocardial infarction. Myocardial perfusion imaging with thallium 201 or technetium 99m Sesta-Mibi, which are distributed in proportion to myocardial blood flow and concentrated by viable myocardium, reveals a defect ("cold spot") in most patients during the first few hours after development of a transmural infarct (p. 971). However, since it is not possible to distinguish acute infarcts from chronic scars, perfusion scanning, although extremely *sensitive*, is not *specific* for the diagnosis of *acute* myocardial infarction. Through sequential [^{99m}Tc]Sesta-Mibi imaging (e.g., before and after thrombolysis) the area of myocardium at risk may be estimated; likewise, sequential scanning may permit assessment of the area of successful reperfusion and comparison of infarct size (late) with the area at risk (early). Radionuclide ventriculography, carried out with ^{99m}Tc-labeled red blood cells (p. 970), frequently demonstrates wall motion disorders and reduction in ventricular ejection fraction in patients with acute myocardial infarction. While of value in assessing the hemodynamic consequences of infarction, and in aiding in the diagnosis of right ventricular infarction when the right ventricular ejection fraction is depressed, this technique is also quite nonspecific, since many cardiac abnormalities other than myocardial infarction alter the radionuclide ventriculogram.

Two-dimensional echocardiography (Chap. 190) can also be of value in patients with acute myocardial infarction. Abnormalities of wall motion are almost universally present. Even with nontransmural myocardial infarction nearly two-thirds of patients have echocardiographically detectable wall motion abnormalities. Although acute infarction cannot be distinguished from old myocardial scar or from acute severe ischemia by an echocardiogram, the ease and safety of the procedure make its use appealing as a screening tool. In the emergency room setting, the early use of echocardiography can aid in management decisions such as whether or not thrombolytic agents should be administered (see later). Echocardiographic estimation of left ventricular function is relatively accurate and can be useful prognostically. Echocardiography may be particularly useful in the diagnosis of right ventricular infarction, ventricular aneurysm, pericardial effusion, and left ventricular thrombus. Additionally, Doppler echocardiography is useful in the detection of a ventricular septal defect and mitral regurgitation, complications of acute myocardial infarction.

Cardiac imaging employing newer technologies such as ultrafast computed tomography and magnetic resonance imaging (Chap. 191) is likely to be useful for many of the above-noted purposes in the future.

MANAGEMENT

The prognosis in acute myocardial infarction is largely related to the occurrence of two general classes of complications: (1) electrical (arrhythmias) and (2) mechanical ("pump failure"). Ventricular fibrillation is the most common form of arrhythmic death in acute myocardial infarction. The vast majority of deaths due to ventricular fibrillation occur within the first 24 h of the onset of symptoms, and of these deaths, over half occur in the first hour. Most out-of-hospital deaths from myocardial infarction are due to ventricular fibrillation. It may occur without warning symptoms or arrhythmias. Over the last 30 years, with careful monitoring and prompt attention to arrhythmias, the in-hospital mortality for acute myocardial infarction has been reduced from about 30 to between 10 and 15 percent, and death from in-hospital ventricular arrhythmia is now unusual.

Pump failure is now the primary cause of in-hospital death from acute myocardial infarction. The extent of ischemic necrosis correlates well with the degree of pump failure and with mortality, both early, i.e., within 10 days of infarction, and later as well. A classification dependent on the status of cardiac pump function, estimated clinically, originally proposed by Killip divides patients into four groups as follows: class I, no signs of pulmonary or venous congestion; class II, moderate heart failure as evidence by rales at the lung bases, S_3 gallop, tachypnea, or signs of failure of the right side of the heart including venous and hepatic congestion; class III, severe heart failure, pulmonary edema; and class IV, shock with systolic pressure less than 90 mmHg and evidence of peripheral vasoconstriction, peripheral cyanosis, mental confusion, and oliguria. The expected hospital mortality rate of patients in these clinical classes when this classification was established was as follows: class I, 0 to 5 percent; class II, 10 to 20 percent; class III, 35 to 45 percent; and class IV, 85 to 95 percent. With recent advances in management, mortality has fallen, perhaps by as much as one-third to one-half, in each class.

Given the information summarized above, the principal objectives of management of the patient with myocardial infarction are to prevent death from arrhythmia and to minimize the mass of infarcted tissue.

Arrhythmias can usually be managed successfully if trained personnel and appropriate equipment are available when this complication develops. Since mortality from arrhythmia is greatest during the first few hours after infarction, it is obvious that the effectiveness of treatment relates directly to the speed with which patients come under medical observation. The biggest delay usually is not in transportation to the hospital but rather between the onset of pain and the patient's decision to call for help. This delay can best be reduced by education of the public concerning the significance of chest pain and the importance of seeking early medical attention. Increasingly, monitoring and treatment are carried out by trained personnel in the ambulance, shortening even further the time between the onset of the infarction and appropriate care.

CORONARY CARE UNITS   These have resulted in improved care of patients with myocardial infarction, reduction in mortality rates, and major increases in knowledge about myocardial infarction. These units are routinely equipped with a system which permits continuous monitoring of the cardiac rhythm of *each* patient and hemodynamic monitoring in *selected* patients. Defibrillators, respirators, noninvasive transthoracic pacemakers, and facilities for introducing pacing catheters and flow-directed balloon-tipped catheters should be available. Equally important is the organization of a highly trained team of nurses who can recognize arrhythmias, adjust the dosage of antiarrhythmic, vasoactive, and anticoagulant drugs, and perform cardiac resuscitation, including electroshock, when necessary.

Patients should be admitted to these units early in their illness when they may expect to derive maximum benefit from the care provided. In the past, all patients with suspected myocardial infarction were admitted to the coronary care unit. Currently, however, several factors have led to a change in this rule. The availability of electrocardiographic monitoring and trained personnel in "intermediate care units" has allowed admission of lower-risk patients (e.g., those not hemodynamically compromised or without active arrhythmias) to such units. For economic reasons, and to utilize limited facilities optimally, many institutions have developed guidelines to aid in triaging patients with suspected myocardial infarction. While most

such patients in the United States are admitted to the hospital, in other countries, such as the United Kingdom, the patients at lowest risk may be cared for at home. Once admitted to the hospital the fraction of patients actually admitted to the coronary care unit may depend on a balance between the clinical status of the patient and bed availability. In some units beds are utilized primarily for patients with a complicated course, particularly those who require hemodynamic monitoring.

REPERFUSION   Thrombolysis   One of the most important developments in the care of patients with acute myocardial infarction derives from the recognition that early reperfusion of ischemic myocardium can potentially salvage tissue before it becomes irreversibly injured. Since most infarctions are caused by a relatively sudden thrombotic occlusion overlying an atherosclerotic plaque in a major epicardial coronary vessel, recent attention has been appropriately directed at techniques to pharmacologically or mechanically recanalize the "culprit" vessel. The thrombolytic agents streptokinase, anisoylated plasminogen streptokinase activator complex (APSAC), and tissue plasminogen activator (tPA) have been approved by the Federal Drug Administration for intravenous use in the setting of acute myocardial infarction. These agents, as well as other investigational ones, have been extensively studied in many clinical trials from which emerge important conclusions about the management of patients with acute myocardial infarction. Thrombolytic therapy can reduce in-hospital mortality for myocardial infarction by up to 50 percent when administered within the first hour of the onset of symptoms, with much of this benefit maintained for one or more years. Appropriately employed thrombolytic therapy appears to reduce infarct size and limit left ventricular dysfunction as well. Since salvage of myocardium can only occur before the myocardium is irreversibly injured, timing of thrombolytic therapy is of extreme importance in achieving maximum benefit. While an upper time limit depends on specific factors in individual patients, it is clear that "every minute counts" and that patients treated within 1 to 3 h of the onset of symptoms stand to benefit most. Although the reduction of mortality is more modest, institution of therapy remains of benefit in many patients seen 3 to 6 h after the onset of infarction, and some benefit appears possible up to 12 h, especially if chest discomfort is ongoing and ST segments remain elevated in electrocardiographic leads that do not yet demonstrate new Q waves. In addition to the possibility of early treatment, clinical factors that favor proceeding with thrombolytic therapy include: anterior wall injury, hemodynamically complicated infarction, and widespread ECG evidence of myocardial jeopardy.

tPA is more effective than streptokinase or APSAC at restoring coronary artery flow, and has a small edge in improving survival as well. The current recommended total dose of tPA is 100 mg, beginning with a 5 to 10 mg bolus followed by 60 mg intravenously over the first hour, followed by 20 mg each in the second and third hours. "Front-loaded" regimens utilizing a larger initial bolus, and weight-adjusted doses to minimize complications in smaller individuals, are being tested but thus far a consensus about an alternative to the FDA approved dose of tPA has not been reached. Streptokinase is administered as 1.5 million units intravenously over 1 h. APSAC has the benefit of being administered as a single dose of 30 mg over 2 to 5 min, making it an ideal agent when given out of the hospital. Anticoagulant and platelet regimens appear to aid in establishing and maintaining vessel patency, and aspirin has been shown to lower mortality when given with thrombolytic therapy. Recent studies suggest that 160 to 325 mg of aspirin and 5000 units of I.V. heparin should be given with the institution of thrombolytic therapy. This should be followed by 325 mg of aspirin daily and a continuous infusion of heparin for 2 to 5 days.

Clear contraindications to the use of thrombolytic agents include a history of cerebrovascular accident, a recent (within 2 weeks) invasive or surgical procedure (or prolonged cardiopulmonary resuscitation), marked hypertension (systolic arterial pressure greater than 180 mmHg and/or diastolic pressure greater than 100 mmHg) at any time during the acute presentation, and active peptic ulcer disease.

Other clinical reasons for an increased risk of bleeding should be sought and the potential benefit of such therapy weighed against expected risk before the decision to administer a thrombolytic agent is made. While advanced age is associated with an increase in hemorrhagic complications, the benefit of thrombolytic therapy in the elderly appears to merit its use in most cases, particularly if no other contraindications are present and the amount of myocardium in jeopardy appears to be substantial. Following thrombolytic therapy cardiac catheterization and coronary angiography should be carried out if there is evidence of coronary artery reocclusion (reelevation of ST segments and/or recurrent chest pain) or if recurrent ischemia develops (such as recurrent angina in the early hospital course or a positive exercise stress test prior to discharge). Under these circumstances, and if the coronary anatomy is suitable, coronary angioplasty should be performed. Coronary artery bypass surgery should be reserved for a small minority of patients whose coronary anatomy is unsuitable for angioplasty but in whom revascularization appears to be advisable because of extensive jeopardized myocardium or recurrent ischemia.

Repeat administration of a thrombolytic agent is an alternative to early mechanical revascularization. Although there is little to suggest how this might be best undertaken, one reasonable strategy is to give a half dose of tPA (50 mg over 4 h) if reocclusion occurs 12 to 24 h after the agent is initially given and a repeat full dose (100 mg over 3 h) if such an event occurs more than 24 h later. Both APSAC and streptokinase are antigenic; once one has been used, repeat administration with either agent should be avoided.

Allergic reactions to streptokinase or APSAC occur in approximately 2 percent of cases. While a minor degree of hypotension occurs in 4 to 10 percent of patients given these agents, marked hypotension occurs, though rarely, in association with severe allergic reactions. In such cases, in addition to specific treatment of the allergic response and stopping the infusion of the thrombolytic agent initially used, consideration should be given to the rapid additional use of tPA. Hemorrhage is the most frequent and potentially the most serious complication. Since bleeding episodes which require transfusion are more common when patients require invasive procedures, unnecessary venous or arterial intervention should be avoided in patients receiving thrombolytic agents. Hemorrhagic stroke is the most serious complication and occurs in approximately 0.4 percent of cases. This rate increases with advancing age, with patients greater than 70 years of age experiencing roughly twice the rate of intracranial hemorrhage as those less than 65 years of age. Large-scale intervention trials have suggested that the rate of intracranial hemorrhage with APSAC or tPA is slightly higher than that seen with streptokinase.

Primary percutaneous transluminal coronary angioplasty Primary PTCA without preceding thrombolysis is also effective in restoring perfusion in acute myocardial infarction. It has the advantages of being applicable to patients with contraindications to thrombolytic therapy; it appears to be more effective than thrombolysis in opening occluded coronary arteries and may be associated with a somewhat better clinical outcome. Subgroups of patients in which direct PTCA may provide a special benefit over thrombolytic therapy include patients with cardiogenic shock and others at high risk because of advanced age (>70 years) or hemodynamic compromise (systolic arterial pressure <100 mmHg). However, this technique is expensive in terms of personnel and facilities, and its applicability is seriously limited by logistic considerations.

The quantity of myocardium that becomes necrotic secondary to a coronary artery occlusion is determined by factors other than just the site of occlusion. One such important factor is the status of collateral blood supply to ischemic tissue. Myocardium well supplied by collaterals clearly has the capacity to survive hours longer than poorly collateralized areas following coronary occlusion. Infarct size is affected by a number of therapeutic agents currently in use. The balance between myocardial oxygen supply and demand in areas rendered ischemic determines the ultimate fate of these areas of jeopardized myocardium. While no routine therapeutic approach to

reduce infarct size in all patients is currently recommended, the realization that infarct size may be increased by interventions which adversely alter the supply-demand balance has prompted the reevaluation of previously accepted therapeutic maneuvers in the management of patients with acute infarction. Cardioactive sympathomimetic amines must be used sparingly and only for clear-cut indications. The early administration of nitrates and beta blockers, with or without thrombolytic therapy, appears to be of benefit.

ROUTINE TREATMENT OF THE PATIENT WITH MYOCARDIAL INFARCTION

ANALGESIA Since myocardial infarction usually presents with severe pain, one of the important initial therapeutic objectives is the relief of pain. Morphine is an extremely effective analgesic for the pain associated with myocardial infarction. However, it may reduce sympathetically mediated arteriolar and venous constriction. The resultant venous pooling may produce a reduction in cardiac output and arterial pressure. This must be recognized but does not necessarily contraindicate its use. Hypotension associated with venous pooling usually responds promptly to elevation of the legs, but in some patients volume expansion with intravenous saline is required. The patient may experience diaphoresis and nausea, but these events usually pass and are replaced by a feeling of well-being associated with the relief of pain. Morphine also has a vagotonic effect and may cause bradycardia or advanced degrees of heart block, particularly in patients with posteroinferior infarction. These side effects of morphine usually respond to atropine (0.5 mg intravenously). Morphine is routinely administered by repetitive (every 5 min) intravenous injection of small doses of drug (2 to 4 mg) rather than by administration of a larger quantity by the subcutaneous route, by which absorption may be unpredictable. Meperidine hydrochloride or hydromorphone hydrochloride may be effectively employed in place of morphine.

Prior to administering morphine, sublingual nitroglycerin can be given safely to most patients with myocardial infarction. As long as hypotension does not occur, up to three 0.4-mg doses should be administered at about 5-min intervals. In addition to diminishing or abolishing chest discomfort, this form of therapy, once considered contraindicated in the setting of acute myocardial infarction, may be capable of both decreasing myocardial oxygen demand (by lowering preload) and increasing myocardial oxygen supply (by dilating infarct-related coronary vessels or collateral vessels). However, therapy with nitrates should be avoided in patients who present with a low systolic arterial pressure (<100 mmHg). The potential for an idiosyncratic reaction to nitrates, consisting of sudden marked hypotension and bradycardia, should be recognized. This problem, occurring more frequently in patients with inferior wall infarction, can usually be promptly reversed by the rapid administration of intravenous atropine. In patients whose initially favorable response to sublingual nitroglycerin is followed by the return of chest pain, particularly if accompanied by other evidence of ongoing ischemia such as further ST-segment or T-wave shifts, the use of intravenous nitroglycerin should be considered.

Intravenous beta blockers are also useful in the control of the pain of acute myocardial infarction. These drugs have been shown to control pain effectively in some patients, presumably by diminishing ischemia consequent to lowering myocardial oxygen demand. More importantly, there is some evidence that intravenous beta blockers reduce in-hospital mortality, particularly in high-risk patients. Dosing similar to that used to treat the hyperdynamic state may be utilized.

Glucocorticoids and nonsteroidal anti-inflammatory agents, with the exception of aspirin, should be avoided in the setting of acute myocardial infarction. They can impair infarct healing and increase the risk of myocardial rupture, and may produce a larger infarct scar. Additionally, they can increase coronary vascular resistance, thereby potentially reducing flow to ischemic myocardium.

OXYGEN The routine use of oxygen is supported by the observation that the arterial P_{O_2} is reduced in many patients with myocardial infarction and that oxygen inhalation reduces the area of ischemic injury in experimental animals. Oxygen should be administered by face mask or nasal prongs for the first day or two after infarction.

ACTIVITY Factors which increase the work of the heart during the initial hours of infarction may increase the size of the infarct. Circumstances in which heart size, cardiac output, or myocardial contractility are increased should be avoided. It has been demonstrated that 6 to 8 weeks are required for complete healing, i.e., replacement of the infarcted myocardium by scar tissue. The purpose of a graded increase in physical activity is to provide the most favorable possible circumstances for this healing.

Most patients with myocardial infarction should be admitted to a coronary care unit or suitable monitoring facility and remain there, under constant observation by trained personnel utilizing continuous electrocardiographic monitoring, until clinical stability has been demonstrated (usually 1 to 3 days). A catheter should be introduced into a peripheral vein, firmly fixed so that it is not easily dislodged, and be kept open either by the slow infusion of isotonic glucose solution or by a closed heparin lock. In the absence of heart failure or other complications during the first 1 to 3 days, the patient should be in bed most of the day, with one or two periods of 15 to 30 min in a bedside chair. The patient should be bathed but may eat unassisted. Bedside commode privileges are given to all hemodynamically stable patients with a stable rhythm from the first day. The bed should be equipped with a footboard, against which the patient should push both feet regularly to prevent venous stasis and thromboembolism and to maintain muscle tone in the legs.

By the third or fourth day the patient with an uncomplicated course should be spending at least 30 to 60 min in a chair twice a day. At this time the patient's blood pressure should be measured when standing in order to be aware of postural hypotension, which may be a problem when ambulation is begun. Standing and gradual ambulation are usually begun between the second and fourth days post infarction in patients with uncomplicated myocardial infarction. Ambulation is progressively increased, eventually including walks about the hospital floor. In many hospitals a cardiac rehabilitation program with progressive exercise is initiated in the hospital and continued after discharge. Ideally, such programs should include an educational component which provides patients with information about their disease and its risk factors. The total duration of hospitalization in uncomplicated cases (Killip class I, see p. 1068) is usually 6 to 11 days. Patients in Killip class II or higher may require 2 or more weeks of hospitalization depending upon the rapidity with which heart failure resolves and the home situation to which the patient is returning. Many physicians perform heart rate–limited exercise tolerance tests just prior to discharge in the majority of patients with myocardial infarction. In some centers, symptom-limited (maximal) exercise tests are performed, as preliminary evidence suggests that this approach poses no increase in risk and it may be more sensitive for the detection of ischemia. Testing identifies high-risk patients as those who develop angina, S-T segment change, hypotension, or serious ventricular ectopic activity during or immediately following exercise. Such patients require special attention including measures such as beta-adrenoceptor blocking agents, long-acting nitrates, and/or calcium antagonists for evidence of ischemia. Selected patients may require further evaluation for possible antiarrhythmic therapy (p. 1072).

If ischemia occurs at rest, or if ischemia and/or hypotension occur during limited exercise, coronary arteriography should be carried out, except in the very elderly or in those for whom contraindications to invasive procedures exist. If a large quantity of viable myocardium, perfused by critically narrowed vessel(s), is found at angiography, then revascularization (either by angioplasty or by operation) may be required. Exercise tests also aid in formulating an individualized exercise prescription, which can be much more vigorous in patients who tolerate exercise without any of the above-mentioned adverse signs. Additionally, predischarge stress testing may provide an important psychological benefit related to building the patient's confidence through the demonstration of reasonable exercise tolerance.

Furthermore, particularly when no arrhythmias or signs of ischemia are identified, the patient benefits by the physician's reassurance that objective evidence suggests no immediate jeopardy.

The remainder of the convalescent phase of myocardial infarction may be accomplished at home. From 2 to 6 weeks, the patient should be encouraged to increase activity by walking about the house and outdoors in good weather. Patients should still spend 8 to 10 h in bed each night. Additional rest periods in the morning and afternoon may be advisable for selected patients. Normal sexual activity may be resumed during this period.

From 6 to 8 weeks onward, the physician must regulate the patient's activity on the basis of his or her exercise tolerance. It is during this period of increasing activity that the patient may become aware of profound fatigue. Postural hypotension may still be a problem. Most patients will be able to return to work after 12 weeks, and many patients much earlier. If not performed earlier, a maximal exercise test is frequently performed after 6 to 8 weeks or prior to returning to work. A trend toward earlier ambulation, hospital discharge, and resumption of full activity for patients recuperating from acute myocardial infarction has developed in recent years.

DIET During the first 4 or 5 days, a low-calorie diet divided into multiple small feedings is preferred. Cardiac output increases following ingestion of food, and therefore the quantity of individual feedings should be kept low. If heart failure is present, sodium intake should be restricted. Since constipation is common, it is reasonable to give average or even increased amounts of bulk in the diet. In addition, the ingestion of potassium-rich foods should be encouraged in patients receiving diuretics. During the second week, increasing amounts of food may be introduced into the diet. At this time, the importance of restriction of calories, cholesterol, and saturated fat may be explained to the patient, and he or she can be started on an appropriate diet. Willingness to accept dietary restriction and to discontinue cigarette smoking is usually never greater than it is during this early period of convalescence.

BOWELS Bed rest of 3 to 5 days and the effect of the narcotics utilized for the relief of pain often lead to constipation. A bedside commode, rather than a bed pan, a diet rich in bulk, and the routine use of a stool softener such as dioctyl sodium sulfosuccinate, 200 mg daily, are recommended. If the patient remains constipated despite these measures, a laxative can be safely used. It is safe to perform a gentle rectal examination on patients with acute myocardial infarction.

SEDATION Most patients require sedation during hospitalization in order to withstand the period of enforced inactivity with tranquility. Diazepam, 5 mg, oxazepam, 15 to 30 mg, or lorazepam, 0.5 to 2 mg, given three or four times daily, is usually effective. An additional dose of any of the above medications may be given at night to ensure adequate sleep. Attention to this problem is especially important during the first few days in the coronary care unit, where the atmosphere of 24-h vigilance may interfere with the patient's sleep. However, sedation is no substitute for reassuring, quiet surroundings.

ANTICOAGULANTS AND ANTIPLATELET AGENTS The use of anticoagulant therapy to retard the process of coronary occlusion during the initial phases of the illness is of accepted importance as a result of the recognition that thrombosis plays an important role in the pathogenesis of acute myocardial infarction. Data from trials employing aspirin and/or thrombolytic agents have led to increased consensus about the appropriate treatment regimens. At the time of thrombolytic therapy, unless contraindications exist, most patients with possible or probable myocardial infarction should be started on aspirin, 160 or 325 mg daily. This should be started immediately, e.g., by chewing an aspirin in the Emergency Room as thrombolytic therapy is begun. In the patient who is to receive a thrombolytic agent, conventional therapy in the United States includes a 5000-unit bolus of intravenous heparin, followed by a constant intravenous infusion beginning at 1000 units per hour adjusted to keep the partial thromboplastin time (PTT) at 1.5 to 2 times normal. Patients with acute myocardial infarction not undergoing thrombolytic therapy should also generally receive aspirin. This strategy has been shown to prevent some patients who present with unstable angina from progressing to myocardial infarction, and data suggest that in-hospital mortality is lowered even among patients who do develop myocardial infarction if they are given aspirin early in their course. Additionally, in order to prevent venous thrombosis in patients *not* treated with thrombolytic therapy, either intravenous heparin or small subcutaneous doses of heparin (5000 units every 8 to 12 h) should be employed as well.

Controversy persists about the use of oral anticoagulants once the patient is out of the intensive care area. Warfarin should be used for patients with congestive heart failure which persists for more than 3 to 4 days or for those with large anterior infarctions in whom the risk of developing a left ventricular thrombus is greater. The incidence of arterial embolism from a clot originating in the ventricle at the site of an infarction is small but definite. Two-dimensional echocardiography allows for the early detection of left ventricular thrombi in about one-third of patients with anterior wall infarction but rarely in patients with inferior or posterior infarction. Arterial embolism often presents as a major complication, such as hemiparesis when the cerebral circulation is involved, or hypertension if the renal circulation is compromised. The low incidence of these complications, contrasted with their severity, renders it impractical to establish firm guidelines for the use of anticoagulant drugs as prophylaxis against arterial embolism in acute myocardial infarction. The likelihood of arterial embolism appears to increase with the extent of infarction and the resultant inflammation and endocardial stasis due to akinesis. Therefore the indication for anticoagulation as prophylaxis against arterial embolism increases with the extent of infarction. When a thrombus has been clearly demonstrated by echocardiographic or other techniques, systemic anticoagulation should be undertaken (in the absence of contraindications), for the incidence of embolic complications appears to be markedly lowered by such therapy. The appropriate duration of therapy is unknown, but probably should be carried out for 3 to 6 months.

Evidence suggests that warfarin lowers late mortality and the incidence of reinfarction after an acute myocardial infarction. Since studies comparing aspirin and warfarin therapy separately or in combination have not yet been completed, the final choice of agents must be based on physician preferences, experience, and patient characteristics.

BETA-ADRENOCEPTOR BLOCKERS The chronic routine use of oral beta-adrenoceptor blockers for at least 2 years following acute myocardial infarction is supported by well-conducted placebo-controlled trials which have convincingly demonstrated reductions in total mortality, sudden death, and in some instances, reinfarction rate. While beta blockers are of benefit, even when started as late as 28 days following the acute event, additional benefit probably accrues to those patients who are started earlier, including patients receiving thrombolytic therapy. For patients presenting with the clear picture of a hyperdynamic state, in the absence of contraindications such as congestive heart failure, hypotension, bradycardia, atrioventricular block, or a history of asthma, an intravenous dose of a beta blocker such as metoprolol may be given (5 mg every 5 to 10 min for a total dose of 15 mg, stopping between doses if any complications arise). This is usually followed by an oral dose regimen of metoprolol (50 to 100 mg bid). Later in the hospital course, a long-acting beta blocker, such as atenolol (50 to 100 mg qd) can be prescribed. Beta blocker therapy is probably indicated for most patients after myocardial infarction, except those for whom its use is specifically contraindicated (patients with heart failure, heart block, orthostatic hypotension, or severely compromised left ventricular function, but without symptoms of heart failure or a history of asthma) and perhaps those whose excellent long-term prognosis (defined as mortality less than 1 percent per year) markedly diminishes any potential benefit (patients with normal ventricular function, no complex ventricular ectopy, no angina, and a negative maximal exercise stress test).

OTHER AGENTS On the basis of the recently completed SAVE trial, the administration of *angiotensin-converting enzyme (ACE)*

inhibitors can now be recommended for improvement in mortality as well as for prevention of heart failure and recurrent myocardial infarction in patients with ejection fractions of 40 percent or less. In such cases, captopril (target dose 50 mg tid) should be started once hemodynamic stability has been demonstrated. In pharmacologically equivalent doses, other ACE inhibitors are likely to be of benefit as well, but these agents have not yet been tested. However, the early (within 24 h) use of intravenous enalaprilat has been shown to be of no benefit, and should be avoided as excessive hypotension may be produced.

Magnesium appears to have favorable effects on cardiac arrhythmias, coronary blood flow, platelet aggregation, as well as myocardial metabolism. One relatively large trial and meta-analyses of many smaller trials strongly suggest that the early use of intravenous magnesium (8 mmol $MgSO_4$ over 15 min, followed by 65 mmol over the next 24 h) significantly reduces serious arrhythmias and total mortality after myocardial infarction. Such therapy is inexpensive, causes few side effects, and is easy to administer.

As noted earlier, *nitrates* (intravenous or oral) may be useful in the relief of pain associated with acute myocardial infarction. Favorable effects on the ischemic process and ventricular remodeling (see below) has led many physicians to routinely use intravenous nitroglycerin (5 to 10 μg/min initial dose and up to 200 μg/min as long as hemodynamic stability is maintained) for the first 24 to 48 h after the onset of infarction.

Results of multiple trials of different *calcium antagonists* have failed to convincingly establish a role for these agents in the treatment of most patients with myocardial infarction. Unlike the more consistent data which exists for other drugs (e.g., beta blockers, aspirin, thrombolytic therapy, and magnesium) the routine use of calcium antagonists cannot be recommended. They should be reserved for patients who develop recurrent myocardial ischemia.

COMPLICATIONS OF MYOCARDIAL INFARCTION AND THEIR TREATMENT

ARRHYTHMIAS (See also Chaps. 197 and 198) The prompt management of arrhythmias constitutes a most significant advance in the treatment of myocardial infarction.

Ventricular premature systoles Infrequent, sporadic ventricular premature depolarizations occur in almost all patients with infarction and do not require therapy. Whereas in the past, frequent, multifocal, or early diastolic ventricular extrasystoles (so-called warning arrhythmias) were routinely treated, pharmacologic therapy is now reserved for patients with sustained or symptomatic ventricular arrhythmias. Prophylactic antiarrhythmic therapy (either intravenous lidocaine early or oral agents later), in the absence of clinically important ventricular tachyarrhythmias, is contraindicated as such therapy may actually increase late mortality. Beta-adrenoceptor blocking agents are effective in abolishing ventricular ectopic activity in infarction patients and in the prevention of ventricular fibrillation. They should be used routinely in patients without contraindications. In addition, hypokalemia is a risk factor for ventricular fibrillation in patients with acute myocardial infarction, and the serum potassium concentration should be adjusted to approximately 4.5 mmol/L.

Ventricular tachycardia and ventricular fibrillation Within the first 24 h of myocardial infarction ventricular tachycardia and fibrillation can occur without prior warning arrhythmias. The occurrence of such primary arrhythmias can be reduced by prophylactic administration of intravenous lidocaine. However, use in this manner has never been shown to reduce overall mortality with acute myocardial infarction. In fact, in addition to noncardiac complications that may occur with lidocaine use, lidocaine may predispose to bradycardia and asystole. This may explain the trend toward increased mortality with lidocaine in meta-analyses of its prophylactic use. Furthermore, over the past 20 years the incidence of primary ventricular fibrillation appears to have fallen dramatically, perhaps by as much as a factor of 10. For these reasons, and with earlier treatment of active ischemia, more frequent use of beta-blocking agents, and the nearly universal success of electrical cardioversion or defibrillation, routine *prophylactic* antiarrhythmic drug therapy is no longer recommended. It should be reserved for patients who cannot reach a hospital or those treated in hospitals that lack the constant presence in the coronary care unit of a physician or nurse trained in the recognition and treatment of ventricular fibrillation. Sustained ventricular tachycardia is treated first with lidocaine, and if it cannot be terminated by one or two 50- to 100-mg doses, electroconversion should be employed (Chap. 198). Electroshock is used immediately in patients with ventricular fibrillation, or when ventricular tachycardia causes hemodynamic deterioration. If fibrillation has persisted for more than a few seconds, the first shock may be unsuccessful, and in this situation it is advisable to administer closed-chest massage and mouth-to-mouth respiration before attempting electroconversion again. Improvement of oxygenation and perfusion increase the likelihood of successful defibrillation. Bretylium is useful in the treatment of both refractory ventricular fibrillation and ventricular tachycardia. For ventricular fibrillation, bretylium is given as a 5-mg/kg bolus and defibrillation is again attempted. If the latter fails, a second bolus of 10 mg/kg is given to facilitate electroconversion of ventricular fibrillation. Ventricular tachycardia can be treated with bretylium 5 to 10 mg/kg injected slowly over 10 min. In either situation, the initial dose of bretylium may be followed by a continuous infusion of 2 mg/min if the arrhythmia is recurrent. Severe postural hypotension occurs after intravenous bretylium administration; therefore, patients should always be supine when and immediately after the drug is given, and intravenous fluids should be available for rapid administration if needed. Ventricular arrhythmias, including the unusual form of ventricular tachycardia known as *torsades de pointes* (Chap. 198) may occur in infarct patients as a consequence of other concurrent problems (such as hypoxia, hypokalemia, or other electrolyte disturbances) or due to the toxic effects of agents already being administered to the patient (such as digoxin or quinidine). A search for such secondary causes should always be undertaken.

Long-term survival is good (generally better than 90 percent at 1 year) in patients with *primary* ventricular fibrillation, i.e., ventricular fibrillation resulting as a primary response to acute ischemia and not associated with predisposing factors such as congestive heart failure, shock, bundle branch block, or ventricular aneurysm. This prognosis is in sharp contrast to that for patients who develop ventricular fibrillation *secondary* to severe pump failure. In patients who develop ventricular tachycardia or ventricular fibrillation late in their hospital course, the mortality in 1 year may be as high as 85 percent. Such patients may warrant electrophysiologic study (Chap. 198).

Accelerated idioventricular rhythm   Accelerated idioventricular rhythm (AIVR, "slow ventricular tachycardia"), a ventricular rhythm with a rate of 60 to 100 beats per minute, occurs in 25 percent of patients with myocardial infarction. It is especially frequent in inferoposterior infarction, where it is usually associated with sinus bradycardia. It often occurs transiently during thrombolytic therapy at the time of reperfusion. The rate of AIVR is usually similar to that of the sinus rhythm which precedes and follows it, and this similarity of rate and the relatively minor hemodynamic effects make this rhythm difficult to detect other than by electrocardiographic monitoring. For the most part, this rhythm is benign and does not presage the development of classic ventricular tachycardia. Most AIVR does not require treatment if the patient is monitored carefully since degeneration into a more serious arrhythmia is rare, and if it occurs, the AIVR can generally be readily treated with a drug which decreases the ventricular escape rate, such as mexiletine, and/or one that increases the sinus rate (atropine).

Supraventricular arrhythmias   Sinus tachycardia is the most common arrhythmia of this type. If it occurs secondary to other causes (such as anemia, fever, heart failure, or a metabolic derangement), the primary problem should be treated first. However, if sinus tachycardia appears to be due to sympathetic overstimulation, such

as is seen as part of a hyperdynamic state, then treatment with a relatively short acting beta blocker such as propranolol should be considered. Other common arrhythmias in this group are junctional rhythm and tachycardia, atrial tachycardia, atrial flutter, and atrial fibrillation. These rhythm disturbances are often secondary to left ventricular failure. The administration of digoxin is usually the treatment of choice for supraventricular arrhythmias if heart failure is present. If heart failure is absent, verapamil is an ideal alternative, as this agent may also help control ischemia. If the abnormal rhythm persists for more than 2 h with a ventricular rate in excess of 120 beats per minute, or at any time when tachycardia induces heart failure, shock, or ischemia (as manifested by recurrent pain or ECG changes), electroshock should be utilized.

Junctional arrhythmias are of diverse etiology, are not indicative of any specific abnormality, and from a therapeutic viewpoint must be considered on an individual basis. Digitalis excess must be ruled out as a cause of junctional tachycardia. In some patients with severely compromised left ventricular function, the loss of appropriately timed atrial systole results in a marked decrease in cardiac output. Right atrial or coronary sinus pacing is indicated in such instances.

Sinus bradycardia   Treatment of sinus bradycardia is indicated if hemodynamic compromise results from the slow heart rate. Elevation of the legs and/or the foot of the bed is frequently helpful in the treatment of sinus bradycardia. Atropine is the most useful drug for increasing heart rate and should be given intravenously in doses of 0.5 mg initially. If the rate remains below 60 beats per minute, additional doses of 0.2 mg, up to a total of 2.0 mg, may be given in divided doses. Persistent bradycardia (<40 beats per minute) despite atropine may be treated with electrical pacing. Isoproterenol should be avoided.

Atrioventricular and intraventricular conduction disturbances (See also Chap. 197)   The in-hospital mortality rate of patients with complete AV block in association with anterior infarction is markedly higher (60 to 75 percent) than that of patients who develop AV block with inferior infarction (25 to 40 percent), and the risk of subsequent death in those who survive to leave the hospital is also increased in the former group. This difference is related to the fact that heart block in inferior infarction is usually caused by AV nodal ischemia. The AV node is a small discrete structure, and thus a small amount of ischemia or necrosis can result in AV nodal dysfunction. In anterior wall infarction, heart block is usually related to ischemic malfunction of all three fascicles of the conduction system and thus commonly results only from extensive myocardial necrosis.

Electrical pacing provides an effective means of increasing the heart rate of patients with bradycardia due to AV block, but it is not possible to be sure that such acceleration is always beneficial. For example, in patients with anterior wall infarction and complete heart block, the large size of the infarct is the major factor determining the outcome, and correction of the conduction deficit may not improve the poor prognosis in this group. It should, however, be carried out if it improves hemodynamics. But pacing does appear to be beneficial in patients with inferoposterior infarction who have complete heart block associated with heart failure, hypotension, marked bradycardia, or significant ventricular ectopic activity. A subgroup of these patients, those with right ventricular infarction, often respond poorly to ventricular pacing because of the loss of the atrial "kick." In such patients, dual chamber, atrioventricular sequential pacing may be required.

In the past, prophylactic placement of a pacing catheter has been advocated for patients with conduction disturbances known to be precursors of complete heart block. However, the availability of reliable noninvasive (external) temporary pacing devices makes it possible to pace conscious patients without insertion of a transvenous pacemaker lead. Therefore, routine, prophylactic insertion of a pacing catheter is no longer necessary in most situations. Permanent pacing has been advocated for patients who develop combined persistent bifascicular and transient third-degree heart block during the acute phase of myocardial infarction. Retrospective studies in such patients suggest that the incidence of sudden death is decreased in those in whom permanent pacing was instituted.

HEART FAILURE Some degree of transient impairment of left ventricular function occurs in over half of patients with myocardial infarction. The most common clinical signs are pulmonary rales and S_3 and S_4 gallop rhythms. Pulmonary congestion is also frequently seen on the chest roentgenogram. Elevation of left ventricular filling pressure and pulmonary artery pressure are the characteristic hemodynamic findings, but it should be appreciated that these findings may result from a reduction of diastolic ventricular compliance (diastolic failure) and/or a reduction of stroke volume with secondary cardiac dilatation (systolic failure) (Chap. 194). The management of heart failure in association with myocardial infarction is similar to that of acute heart failure secondary to other forms of heart disease, with a few exceptions (Chap. 195). The major difference concerns the use of cardiac glycosides. The benefit following the administration of digitalis in acute myocardial infarction is unimpressive. This is not surprising since the function of the noninfarcted tissue may be normal and digitalis would not be expected to improve the systolic or diastolic dysfunction of infarcted or ischemic tissue. On the other hand, diuretic agents are extremely effective since they diminish pulmonary congestion in the presence of systolic and/or diastolic heart failure. A fall in left ventricular filling pressure and an improvement in orthopnea and dyspnea follow the intravenous administration of furosemide. This drug should be used with caution, however, as it can result in a massive diuresis with associated decrease in plasma volume, cardiac output, systemic blood pressure, and hence coronary perfusion. Nitrates in various forms may be used to decrease preload and congestive symptoms. Oral isosorbide dinitrate, topical nitroglycerin ointment, or intravenous nitroglycerin, all have the advantage over a diuretic of lowering preload through venodilatation without decreasing the total plasma volume. Additionally, nitrates may improve ventricular compliance if concurrent ischemia is present, since ischemia causes an elevation of left ventricular filling pressure. The patient with pulmonary edema is treated in the manner described in Chap. 195, but vasodilators must be used with caution to prevent serious hypotension.

Ventricular remodeling Soon after myocardial infarction, the left ventricle begins to dilate. Acutely, this occurs as the result of expansion of the infarct. Later, lengthening of the noninfarcted segments occurs as well. Overall chamber enlargement is related to the size of the infarction, with greater degrees of dilatation causing more marked hemodynamic impairment, more frequent heart failure, and a poorer prognosis as well. Progressive dilatation and its clinical consequences may be attenuated by afterload-reducing therapy such as vasodilatation induced by an ACE inhibitor. Thus, in patients with a depressed ejection fraction (less than 40 percent), regardless of whether or not heart failure is present, consideration should be given to captopril therapy (beginning with 6.25 mg tid and advancing to 25 to 50 mg tid as tolerated). Equivalent doses of other ACE inhibitors are probably of benefit as well.

Hemodynamic monitoring Hemodynamic evidence of abnormal left ventricular function becomes apparent when contraction is seriously impaired in 20 to 25 percent of the left ventricle. Infarction of 40 percent or more of the left ventricle usually results in the syndrome of cardiogenic shock (see below). Positioning of a balloon flotation catheter in the pulmonary artery permits monitoring of left ventricular filling pressure, a technique which is useful in patients who exhibit clinical evidence of hemodynamic abnormalities or instability. However, in view of the complications that can occur, insertion of a pulmonary artery catheter should be limited to those patients with hemodynamic instability. Cardiac output can also be determined with a pulmonary artery catheter. With the addition of intraarterial pressure monitoring, systemic vascular resistance can be calculated as a guide to adjusting vasopressor and vasodilator therapy. Some patients with acute myocardial infarction have markedly elevated left ventricular filling pressures (>22 mmHg) and normal cardiac indexes [>2.6 and <3.6 (L/min)/m²], while others have relatively low filling pressures

(<15 mmHg) and reduced cardiac indexes. The former usually benefit from diuresis, while the latter respond to volume expansion by means of intravenous administration of colloid-containing solutions.

Cardiogenic shock—power failure In recent years efforts to reduce infarct size and prompt treatment of ongoing ischemia and other complications of myocardial infarction appear to have reduced the incidence of cardiogenic shock.

It is useful to consider cardiogenic shock as a form of severe left ventricular failure. This syndrome is characterized by marked hypotension with systolic arterial pressure <80 mmHg and a marked reduction of cardiac index [<1.8 (L/min)m²] in the face of elevated left ventricular filling (pulmonary capillary wedge) pressure >18 mmHg. Hypotension alone is not a basis for the diagnosis of cardiogenic shock, because many patients who make an uneventful recovery will have serious hypotension (systolic pressure <80 mmHg) for several hours. Such patients often have low left ventricular filling pressures, and their hypotension usually resolves with the administration of intravenous fluids. In contrast to hypovolemic hypotension (see below) cardiogenic shock is generally associated with a mortality rate of >70 percent; however, recent efforts to restore coronary blood flow early in the course of infarction (with coronary angioplasty or surgical revascularization), suggests that this high mortality rate can be lowered by as much as one-half.

Cardiogenic shock may develop during the first hours of the infarct and be present at the time of initial hospitalization. Alternatively, it may appear after hospitalization—most commonly during the first day but sometimes as late as the sixth day. Risk factors for the in-hospital development of shock include advanced age, depressed left ventricular ejection fraction on admission, large infarct, history of diabetes mellitus, and previous myocardial infarction. Patients with several of these risk factors may be considered for cardiac catheterization and mechanical reperfusion (angioplasty or surgery) *before* the development of shock.

Pathophysiology of pump failure Marked reduction in the quantity of contracting myocardium is the cause of cardiogenic shock in myocardial infarction. The initial insult results in a decrease in arterial pressure and hence in coronary blood flow because of its dependence on aortic perfusion pressure (Fig. 202-1). The reduction in coronary perfusion pressure and myocardial blood flow further impairs myocardial function and may increase the size of the myocardial infarction. Arrhythmias and metabolic acidosis also contribute to this deterioration because they are the result of inadequate perfusion. It is this positive feedback loop which accounts for the high mortality rate associated with the shock syndrome.

A simple schematic diagram depicting the relationship between left ventricular work and filling pressure is seen in Fig. 202-2. The upper curve represents the familiar Frank-Starling relationship in the normal heart; the lower curve shows the relation which might be expected in the patient with shock secondary to myocardial infarction. It is obvious that, at all levels of end-diastolic pressure, the left ventricular work of the patient with myocardial infarction is depressed. At point C, the end-diastolic pressure is elevated, but at point B, it may be normal despite the fact that myocardial work is well below that expected of the normal heart at this diastolic pressure, as indicated by point A.

Treatment of pump failure The physiology and ominous prognosis associated with this condition dictate that all patients with shock should, if possible, have continuous monitoring of arterial pressure and of left ventricular filling pressure (as reflected in the pulmonary capillary wedge pressure measured with a pulmonary artery balloon catheter) as well as frequent determinations of cardiac output. When pulmonary edema coexists, endotracheal intubation may be necessary to ensure oxygenation. The relief of pain is important, as some vasodepressor reflex activity may be a response to severe pain. However, narcotics should be used cautiously in view of their propensity to lower arterial pressure.

The primary objective of treatment is to avoid the sequence depicted in Fig. 202-1, by attempting to maintain coronary perfusion

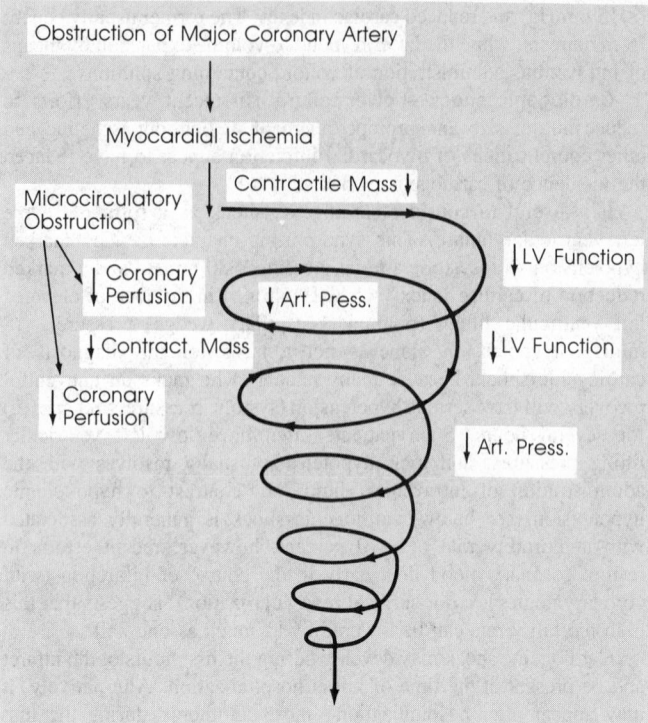

FIGURE 202-1 The sequence of events in the vicious cycle in which coronary artery obstruction leads to cardiogenic shock and progressive circulatory deterioration.

by raising the arterial blood pressure with vasopressors (see below), intraaortic balloon counterpulsation, and manipulation of blood volume to a level that ensures an optimum left ventricular filling pressure (approximately 20 mmHg). The latter may require either infusion of crystalloid or diuresis.

In patients seen within the first 4 to 8 h of the onset of infarction, reperfusion by thrombolytic therapy and/or PTCA (p. 1069) may improve left ventricular function dramatically, thereby interrupting the cycle of hemodynamic deterioration.

Hypovolemia This is an easily corrected condition which may contribute to the hypotension and vascular collapse associated with myocardial infarction in some patients. Hypovolemia may be secondary to previous diuretic use, to reduced fluid intake during the early

FIGURE 202-2 Schematic representation of the Frank-Starling relationship as applied to patients with the shock syndrome in myocardial infarction.

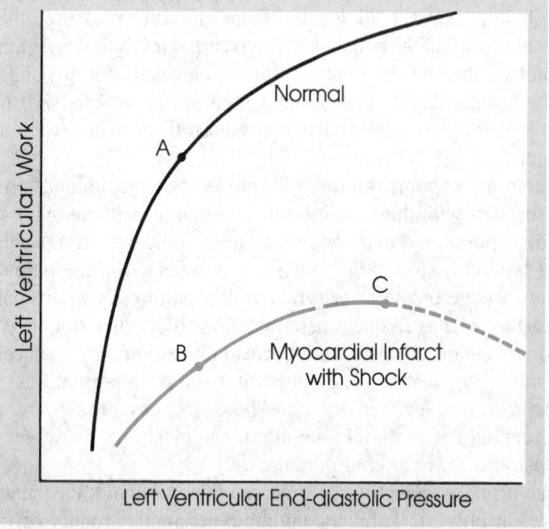

stages of the illness, and/or to vomiting associated with pain or medications. Consequently, hypovolemia should be identified and corrected in patients with acute myocardial infarction and hypotension before embarking upon more vigorous forms of therapy. The optimal left ventricular filling or pulmonary artery wedge pressure may vary considerably among different patients. Each patient's ideal level (generally at approximately 20 mmHg) is reached by cautious fluid administration during careful monitoring of oxygenation and cardiac output. When the cardiac output plateaus (Fig. 202-2, point C), further increases in left ventricular filling pressure will only increase congestive symptoms and decrease systemic oxygenation without raising arterial pressure. Central venous pressure reflects right rather than left ventricular filling pressure and is an inadequate guide for adjustment of blood volume, since left ventricular function is almost always affected much more adversely than right ventricular function in acute myocardial infarction.

Vasopressors A variety of intravenous drugs may be used to augment arterial pressure and cardiac output in patients with cardiogenic shock. Unfortunately, all have important disadvantages or problems associated with their use, and none have been shown to change the outcome in patients with established shock. *Isoproterenol* is a sympathomimetic amine which is now rarely used in the treatment of shock due to myocardial infarction. Although this agent increases contractility, it also produces peripheral vasodilatation and increases heart rate. The resultant increase in myocardial oxygen consumption and reduction of coronary perfusion pressure may extend the area of ischemic injury. *Norepinephrine* (p. 420) is a potent alpha-adrenergic agent with powerful vasoconstrictive properties which also possesses beta-adrenergic activity and therefore enhances contractility. Because the increase in afterload and contractility associated with its use causes a marked increase in myocardial oxygen consumption, it should be reserved for desperate situations or for patients with cardiogenic shock and lowered systemic vascular resistance. It should be started at 2 to 4 μg/min. If pressure cannot be maintained with a dosage of 15 μg/min, it is unlikely that a further increase will be beneficial.

Dopamine (Chap. 68) is useful in many patients with power failure. At low doses [2 to 10 (μg/kg)/min] the drug has positive chronotropic and inotropic effects as a consequence of beta receptor stimulation. At higher doses, a vasoconstrictive effect results from alpha receptor stimulation. At lower doses dopamine [≤2 (μg/kg)/min] also has the unique effect of dilating the renal and splanchnic vascular beds and apparently has little effect on myocardial oxygen consumption. Intravenous dopamine is started at an infusion rate of 2 to 5 (μg/kg)/min with increments in dosage every 2 to 5 min up to a maximum of 20 to 50 (μg/kg)/min. Systolic arterial blood pressure should be maintained at approximately 90 mmHg. *Dobutamine* is a synthetic sympathomimetic amine with positive inotropic action and minimal positive chronotropic or peripheral vasoconstrictive activity in the usual dosage range of 2.5 to 10 (μg/kg)/min. It should not be employed when a vasoconstrictor effect is required. However, in patients with less profound degrees of hypotension, dobutamine may be an extremely useful agent, particularly if positive chronotropy is to be avoided.

Amrinone is a positive inotropic agent without catecholamine structure or activity. It resembles dobutamine in its pharmacologic activity, although it has a more potent vasodilating action. Initially a loading dose of 0.75 mg/kg is given over 2 to 3 min. If effective, this is followed by an infusion of 5 to 10 (μg/kg)/min, followed if necessary 30 min later by an additional bolus of 0.75 mg/kg. If necessary, the dose may then be increased up to 15 (μg/kg)/min for short periods.

Cardiac glycosides (Chap. 195) Controlled studies have failed to demonstrate significant beneficial effects of cardiac glycoside therapy in the early phases (0 to 48 h) of acute myocardial infarction. Hemodynamic improvement has been documented at later times, but this effect, too, is marginal. Since cardiac glycosides cannot improve the function of necrotic myocardium and since pump failure is thought to be related to the total mass of infarcted tissue, digitalis therapy does not usually result in improvement in patients with acute myocardial infarction and sinus rhythm.

Aortic counterpulsation In cardiogenic shock mechanical assistance with an intraaortic balloon pumping system capable of augmenting both diastolic pressure and cardiac output can provide circulatory support. A sausage-shaped balloon at the end of a catheter is introduced percutaneously into the aorta via the femoral artery, and the balloon is automatically inflated during early diastole, thereby enhancing both coronary blood flow and peripheral perfusion. The balloon collapses in early systole, thereby reducing the afterload against which left ventricular ejection takes place. Improvement in hemodynamic status has been observed with balloon pumping in a large number of patients, but, in the absence of early revascularization, long-term survival following this mode of therapy in patients with cardiogenic shock is still disappointing. The balloon counterpulsation system may best be reserved for patients whose condition merits mechanical (surgery or angioplasty) intervention (e.g., patients with continuing ischemia, ventricular septal rupture, or mitral regurgitation) and in whom a successful result is likely to result in the reversal of cardiogenic shock. Intraaortic balloon pumping is contraindicated if aortic regurgitation is present or if aortic dissection is possible or suspected.

There is reason to believe that results of therapy of the shock syndrome secondary to myocardial infarction, while improving gradually as a result of meticulous attention to the details of therapy outlined above, will continue to be disappointing overall because a large fraction of patients with the syndrome have large areas of infarcted myocardium with severe, diffuse coronary atherosclerosis. Emerging evidence suggests that dramatic results can be achieved with emergency revascularization surgery, or, more commonly, coronary angioplasty. However, only a minority of patients developing cardiogenic shock have prompt access to these expensive technologies, and it is hoped that the widespread and early application of thrombolytic therapy will reduce the amount of myocardium which becomes necrotic and thereby reduce the incidence of this syndrome.

Other complications MITRAL REGURGITATION The reported incidence of apical systolic murmurs of mitral regurgitation during the first few days after the onset of a myocardial infarction varies widely (10 to 50 percent of patients) depending on the population studied and the acumen of the observers. In the first hours of infarction, mitral regurgitation can be demonstrated angiographically in approximately 15 percent of patients but is audible in only about one-tenth of those with positive angiograms. Whether audible or angiographically demonstrated, mitral regurgitation is of hemodynamic importance in only a minority of these patients.

The most common cause of mitral regurgitation following myocardial infarction is dysfunction of the papillary muscles of the left ventricle due to ischemia or infarction. Mitral regurgitation may also be the result of alteration in the size or shape of the ventricle due to impaired contractility or to aneurysm formation. Either papillary muscle may rupture, the posterior one twice as frequently as the anterior. Left ventricular function may deteriorate dramatically with superimposition of mitral regurgitation. The differential diagnosis includes perforation of the ventricular septum (see below), and the differentiation from mitral regurgitation is conveniently made at the bedside by color flow Doppler echocardiography. Surgical repair or replacement of the mitral valve may be followed by dramatic improvement in patients in whom acute heart failure results primarily from severe mitral regurgitation due to papillary muscle rupture or dysfunction and in whom myocardial function is relatively well preserved.

If aortic systolic pressure is lowered in patients with mitral regurgitation, a greater fraction of the left ventricular output will be ejected antegrade, thus lessening the regurgitant fraction. To this end, both intraaortic balloon counterpulsation, which lowers the aortic systolic pressure mechanically, and the infusion of sodium nitroprusside or nitroglycerin, which reduce systemic vascular resistance, have

been used with success for the interim management of patients with severe mitral regurgitation in the setting of acute myocardial infarction. Ideally, definitive operative treatment should be postponed for 4 to 6 weeks after the infarct. However, if the patient's hemodynamic and/or clinical condition does not improve or stabilize, surgical treatment should be undertaken, even in the acute stage.

Cardiac rupture Myocardial rupture is a dramatic complication of myocardial infarction most likely to occur during the first week after the onset of symptoms; its frequency increases with the age of the patient. First infarction, a history of hypertension, no history of angina pectoris, and relatively large Q-wave infarcts are associated with a higher incidence of cardiac rupture. The clinical presentation may often be that of a sudden disappearance of the pulse, blood pressure, and consciousness while the electrocardiogram continues to show sinus rhythm (*apparent* electromechanical dissociation). The myocardium continues to contract, but forward flow is not maintained as blood escapes into the pericardium. Cardiac tamponade (Chap. 206) ensues, and closed-chest massage is ineffective. This condition is almost universally fatal.

Septal perforation The pathogenesis of perforation of the ventricular septum is similar to that of external rupture of the myocardium, but the therapeutic potential is greater. Patients with ventricular septal rupture present with severe heart failure in association with the sudden appearance of a pansystolic murmur, often accompanied by a parasternal thrill. It is often impossible to differentiate this condition from rupture of a papillary muscle with resultant mitral regurgitation, and a tall *v* wave in the pulmonary capillary wedge pressure in both conditions further complicates the differentiation. The diagnosis can be established by the demonstration of a left-to-right shunt (i.e., an oxygen step-up at the level of the right ventricle) by limited cardiac catheterization performed at the bedside using a flow-directed balloon catheter. Color flow Doppler echocardiography can be extremely useful for making this diagnosis at the bedside. Rupture of the ventricular septum is amenable to immediate surgical treatment, albeit at a significant risk, but this form of therapy is ordinarily indicated on an urgent basis in patients whose condition cannot be stabilized rapidly. A prolonged period of hemodynamic compromise may produce end-organ damage and other complications that can be avoided by early intervention including nitroprusside infusion and intraaortic balloon counterpulsation.

The physiology of acute mitral regurgitation and acute ventricular septal perforation are similar in that the level of aortic systolic pressure determines in part the regurgitant volume, the principal difference being the chamber into which the regurgitant fraction is ejected. In septal perforation, a fraction of left ventricular output is ejected into the right ventricle. In a manner analogous to mitral regurgitation, lowering of aortic systolic pressure by mechanical (intraaortic balloon counterpulsation) and/or pharmacologic (nitroglycerin or nitroprusside) means can decrease the hemodynamic compromise caused by perforation.

Ventricular aneurysm The term *ventricular aneurysm* is usually used to describe *dyskinesis* or local expansile paradoxical wall motion. Normally functioning myocardial fibers must shorten more if stroke volume and cardiac output are to be maintained in patients with ventricular aneurysm, and if they are unable to do so, overall ventricular function is impaired. Aneurysms are composed of scar tissue and neither predispose to nor are associated with cardiac rupture.

The complications of left ventricular aneurysm do not usually occur for weeks to months following myocardial infarction; they include congestive heart failure, arterial embolism, and ventricular arrhythmias. Apical aneurysms are the most common and the most easily detected by clinical examination. The physical finding of greatest value is a double, diffuse, or displaced apical impulse. The electrocardiographic finding of ST-segment elevation at rest is present in precordial leads in 25 percent of patients with either apical or anterior aneurysms. Ventricular aneurysms are readily detectable by two-dimensional echocardiography, which may also reveal a mural thrombus within an aneurysm. Rarely, myocardial rupture may be contained by a local area of pericardium, along with organizing thrombus and hematoma. Over time this *pseudoaneurysm* enlarges, maintaining communication with the left ventricular cavity via a narrow neck. Because spontaneous rupture of a pseudoaneurysm often occurs, if recognized, it should be surgically repaired.

Right ventricular infarction   Approximately one-third of patients with inferoposterior infarction demonstrate at least a minor degree of right ventricular necrosis. An occasional patient with inferoposterior left ventricular infarction also has extensive right ventricular myocardial infarction, and rarely patients present with infarction limited to the right ventricle. These patients often present with signs of severe right ventricular failure (jugular venous distention, Kussmaul's sign, hepatomegaly) with or without hypotension. ST-segment elevations of the right-sided precordial electrocardiographic leads, particularly lead V_4R, are present in the majority of patients with right ventricular infarction. Radionuclide ventriculography and two-dimensional echocardiography are also sensitive in the detection of right ventricular dysfunction associated with acute myocardial infarction. Catheterization of the right side of the heart often reveals a distinctive hemodynamic pattern resembling cardiac tamponade or constrictive pericarditis (Chap. 206). Volume expansion is often successful in treating low cardiac output and hypotension associated with extensive right ventricular infarction.

Postinfarction ischemia and extension   Recurrent angina develops in approximately 25 percent of patients hospitalized for acute myocardial infarction. This percentage is even higher in patients undergoing successful thrombolysis. Since recurrent or persistent ischemia often heralds extension of the original infarct and is associated with a doubling of risk following acute myocardial infarction, patients with these symptoms should be considered for prompt coronary arteriography and mechanical revascularization.

Thromboembolism   Clinically apparent thromboembolism complicates acute myocardial infarction in approximately 10 percent of cases, but embolic lesions are found in 45 percent of patients in necropsy series, suggesting that thromboembolism is often clinically silent. Thromboembolism is considered to be at least an important contributing cause of death in 25 percent of infarct patients who die following admission to the hospital. Arterial emboli originate from left ventricular mural thrombi, while most pulmonary emboli arise in the leg veins. Thromboembolism most commonly occurs in association with large infarcts in the presence of heart failure. Thromboembolism occurs extremely commonly in patients with echocardiographic evidence of a left ventricular thrombus, but only rarely if a thrombus is not present on the echocardiogram. Although well-controlled trials do not exist, the incidence of embolization appears to be decreased by anticoagulation.

Pericarditis (See also Chap. 206)   Pericardial friction rubs and/or pericardial pain are frequently encountered in patients with acute transmural myocardial infarction. This complication can usually be managed with aspirin (650 mg qid). It is important to diagnose the chest pain of pericarditis accurately, since failure to appreciate it may lead to the erroneous diagnosis of recurrent ischemic pain and/or infarct extension with resultant inappropriate use of anticoagulants, nitrates, beta blockers, or coronary arteriography. The possibility exists that anticoagulants can cause tamponade in the presence of acute pericarditis, thus their use is contraindicated in patients with pericarditis, as manifested by either pain or persistent rub, unless there is a compelling indication.

Post-myocardial infarction syndrome—Dressler's syndrome (See also Chap. 206)   This syndrome, characterized by fever and pleuropericardial chest pain, is thought to be due to an autoimmune pericarditis, pleuritis, and/or pneumonitis. It may begin from a few days to 6 weeks after myocardial infarction. The occurrence of Dressler's syndrome may be etiologically related to the early use of anticoagulants and appears to have decreased markedly in the last decade as long-term anticoagulants are used less frequently in acute myocardial infarction. The syndrome usually responds promptly to

therapy with salicylates. On occasion, glucocorticoids may be required to relieve discomfort of an unusual, refractory nature. Effusions associated with Dressler's syndrome may become hemorrhagic if anticoagulants are administered.

POSTINFARCTION RISK STRATIFICATION AND MANAGEMENT

The goal of preventing reinfarction and death following recovery from myocardial infarction has led to strategies to evaluate risk following infarction. Early after infarction this generally involves use of non-invasive testing. As noted earlier, in stable patients submaximal exercise stress testing should be carried out prior to hospital discharge to detect residual ischemia and ventricular ectopy, and to provide the patient with a guideline for exercise in the early recovery period. Alternatively, or in addition, a maximal (symptom-limited) exercise stress test may be carried out 4 to 6 weeks following infarction. Evaluation of left ventricular function at rest and during exercise is usually warranted as well. Recognition of a depressed left ventricular ejection fraction by echocardiography or radionuclide ventriculography helps the physician with the selection of pharmacologic measures to improve long-term outcome (e.g., beta-blockers and/or ACE inhibitors) (pp. 424 and 1128, respectively). Patients with angina induced at relatively low workloads, those who have a large reversible defect on perfusion imaging or a depressed ejection fraction and demonstrable ischemia, and those in whom exercise provokes symptomatic ventricular arrhythmias should be considered at high risk for recurrent myocardial infarction or death from arrhythmia, and cardiac catheterization with coronary angiography and/or invasive electrophysiologic evaluation is advised, as discussed above.

Many clinical factors have been identified which are associated with an increase in cardiovascular risk following initial recovery from a myocardial infarction. Some of the most important factors, as already noted, include: ongoing symptoms of ischemia, depressed left ventricular ejection fraction (less than 40 percent), rales above the bases on physical examination or congestion on chest radiograph, and symptomatic ventricular arrhythmias. Other features associated with increased risk include history of previous myocardial infarction, age over 70 years, history of diabetes, prolonged sinus tachycardia, hypotension, the occurrence of ST-segment changes at rest without angina ("silent ischemia"), an abnormal signal-averaged electrocardiogram, nonpatency of the infarct-related coronary artery (if angiography is undertaken), and persistent advanced heart block or new intraventricular conduction abnormality on the electrocardiogram. Therapy must be individualized depending on the relative importance of the risk(s) present and the degree of benefit to be achieved by specific therapy including revascularization or the use of pharmacologic agents.

A variety of secondary preventive measures are at least partially responsible for the improved long-term mortality and morbidity following myocardial infarction. The benefits and use of beta blockers, antiplatelet agents and anticoagulants, and ACE inhibitors are discussed above. The relative limitations of calcium antagonists and antiarrhythmic agents have also been noted. Finally, risk factors for atherosclerosis (Table 208-4, p. 1110) should be discussed with the patient, and when possible, favorably modified. In particular, efforts should be made to ensure the cessation of smoking and the control of hypertension and hyperlipidemia. Additionally, regular physical exercise and reduction of emotional stress should be encouraged. Much of the above can be accomplished by referring the patient to a comprehensive cardiac rehabilitation program.

REFERENCES

ACC/AHA: Guidelines for the early management of patients with acute myocardial infarction: A report of the ACC/AHA task force on assessment of diagnostic and therapeutic cardiovascular procedures. Circulation 82:664, 1990

AMERICAN HEART ASSOCIATION: *1992 Heart and Stroke Facts.* Dallas, American Heart Association National Center, 1991, p. 1

ANTMAN EM, BERLIN JA: Declining incidence of ventricular fibrillation in myocardial infarction. Implications for the prophylactic use of lidocaine. Circulation 86:764, 1992

BATES ER: Expanding indications for thrombolytic therapy in acute myocardial infarction. Can J Cardiol 9:152, 1993

BENGTSON JR et al: Prognosis in cardiogenic shock after acute myocardial infarction in the interventional era. J Am Coll Cardiol 20:1482, 1992

EISENBERG MS et al: Thrombolytic therapy. Ann Emerg Med 22:417, 1993

ELDAR M et al: Primary ventricular tachycardia in acute myocardial infarction: Clinical characteristics and mortality. Ann Intern Med 117:31, 1992

FUSTER V et al: The pathogenesis of coronary artery disease and the acute coronary syndromes. N Engl J Med 326:242, 310, 1992

GIBBONS RJ: Technetium 99m sestamibi in the assessment of acute myocardial infarction. Semin Nucl Med 21:213, 1991

GOLDBERG RJ et al: Prognosis of acute myocardial infarction complicated by complete heart block (the Worcester Heart Attack Study). Am J Cardiol 69:1135, 1992

GOMES JA et al: Post-myocardial infarction stratification and the signal-averaged electrocardiogram. Prog Cardiovasc Dis 35:263, 1993

GOTTLIEB S et al: Interrelation of left ventricular ejection fraction, pulmonary congestion and outcome in acute myocardial infarction. Am J Cardiol 69:977, 1992

HORNER SM: Efficacy of intravenous magnesium in acute myocardial infarction in reducing arrhythmias and mortality. Meta-analysis of magnesium in acute myocardial infarction. Circulation 86:774, 1992

JUGDUTT BI: Role of nitrates after acute myocardial infarction. Am J Cardiol 70:82B, 1992

KRONE RJ: The role of risk stratification in the early management of a myocardial infarction. Ann Intern Med 116:223, 1992

LANGE RA, HILLIS LD: Immediate angioplasty for acute myocardial infarction. N Engl J Med 328:726, 1993

LEE L et al: Multicenter Registry of Angioplasty Therapy of Cardiogenic Shock: Initial and Long-term Survival. J Am Coll Cardiol 17:599, 1991

LEE TH, GOLDMAN L: Serum enzyme assays in the diagnosis of acute myocardial infarction. Ann Intern Med 105:221, 1986

LEHMANN KG et al: Mitral regurgitation in early myocardial infarction. Ann Intern Med 117:10, 1992

MAGGIONI AP et al: The risk of stroke in patients with acute myocardial infarction after thrombolytic and antithrombotic treatment. N Engl J Med 327:1, 1992

MUELLER HS et al: Predictors of early morbidity and mortality after thrombolytic therapy of acute myocardial infarction. Analyses of patient subgroups in the Thrombolysis in Myocardial Infarction (TIMI) trial, Phase II. Circulation 85:1254, 1992

MULTICENTER POSTINFARCTION RESEARCH GROUP: Low level exercise testing after myocardial infarction: Usefulness in enhancing clinical risk stratification. Circulation 71:80, 1985

PASTERNAK RC et al: Acute myocardial infarction, in *Heart Disease,* 4th ed, E Braunwald (ed). Philadelphia, Saunders, 1992, p. 1200

PFEFFER MA et al: Effect of captopril on mortality and morbidity in patients with left ventricular dysfunction after myocardial infarction. Results of the Survival and Ventricular Enlargement Trial. N Engl J Med 327:669, 1992

REEDER GS, GERSH BJ: Modern management of acute myocardial infarction. Curr Probl Cardiol 18:81, 1993

SIEGEL D et al: Risk factor modification after myocardial infarction. Ann Intern Med 109:213, 1988

TCHENG JE et al: Outcome of patients sustaining acute ischemic mitral regurgitation during myocardial infarction. Ann Intern Med 117:18, 1992

TENAGLIA AN, STACK RS: Angioplasty for acute coronary syndromes. Annu Rev Med 44:465, 1993

THIRD INTERNATIONAL STUDY OF INFARCT SURVIVAL COLLABORATIVE GROUP: ISIS-3: A randomized comparison of streptokinase vs tissue plasminogen activator vs anistreplase and of aspirin plus heparin vs aspirin alone among 41,299 cases of suspected acute myocardial infarction. Lancet 339:754, 1992

TIMI STUDY GROUP: Comparison of invasive and conservative strategies after treatment with intravenous tissue plasminogen activator in acute myocardial infarction. Results of the Thrombolysis in Myocardial Infarction (TIMI) Phase II Trial. N Engl J Med 320:618, 1989

TOFLER GH et al: Modifiers of timing and possible triggers of acute myocardial infarction in the Thrombolysis in Myocardial Infarction Phase II (TIMI II) study group. J Am Coll Cardiol 20:1049, 1992

203 ISCHEMIC HEART DISEASE

ANDREW P. SELWYN / EUGENE BRAUNWALD

Ischemia refers to a lack of oxygen due to inadequate perfusion. Ischemic heart disease is a condition of diverse etiologies, all having in common an imbalance between oxygen supply and demand.

ETIOLOGY AND PATHOPHYSIOLOGY

The most common cause of myocardial ischemia is atherosclerotic disease of epicardial coronary arteries. By reducing the lumen of these vessels, atherosclerosis causes an absolute decrease in myocardial perfusion in the basal state or limits appropriate increases in perfusion when the demand for flow is augmented. Coronary blood flow can also be limited by arterial thrombi, spasm, and rarely coronary emboli as well as by ostial narrowing due to luetic aortitis. Congenital abnormalities, such as anomalous origin of the left anterior descending coronary artery from the pulmonary artery, may cause myocardial ischemia and infarction in infancy, but this cause is very rare in adults. Myocardial ischemia can also occur if myocardial oxygen demands are abnormally increased, as in severe ventricular hypertrophy due to hypertension or aortic stenosis. The latter can present with angina that is indistinguishable from that caused by coronary atherosclerosis. A reduction in the oxygen-carrying capacity of the blood, as in extremely severe anemia or in the presence of carboxyhemoglobin, is a rare cause of myocardial ischemia. Not infrequently, two or more causes of ischemia will coexist, such as an increase in oxygen demand due to left ventricular hypertrophy and a reduction in oxygen supply secondary to coronary atherosclerosis.

The normal coronary circulation is dominated and controlled by the myocardial requirements for oxygen. This need is met by the heart's ability to vary coronary vascular resistance (and therefore blood flow) considerably while the myocardium extracts a high and relatively fixed percentage of oxygen (Chap. 12). Normally, intramyocardial resistance arterioles demonstrate an immense capacity for dilation. With exercise and emotional stress, the changing oxygen needs affect coronary vascular resistance and in this manner regulate the supply of blood and oxygen (metabolic regulation). These same vessels adapt to physiologic alterations in blood pressure in order to maintain coronary blood flow at levels appropriate to myocardial needs (autoregulation). Although the large epicardial coronary arteries are capable of constriction and relaxation, in healthy persons they serve as conduits and are referred to as *conductance vessels,* while the intramyocardial arterioles normally exhibit striking changes in tone and are therefore referred to as *resistance vessels.* Abnormal constriction or failure of normal dilation of the coronary resistance vessels also can cause ischemia. When it causes angina this condition is sometimes referred to as *microvascular angina.*

CORONARY ATHEROSCLEROSIS (See also Chap. 208) Epicardial coronary arteries are a major site of atherosclerotic disease. The major risk factors for atherosclerosis (high plasma LDL, low plasma HDL, cigarette smoking, diabetes mellitus, and hypertension) are thought to disturb the normal functions of the vascular endothelium. Dysfunction of vascular endothelium and an abnormal interaction with blood monocytes and platelets lead to subintimal collections of abnormal fat, cells, and debris (i.e., atherosclerotic plaques), which develop at irregular rates in different segments of the epicardial coronary tree and lead eventually to segmental reductions in cross-sectional area. The relationship between pulsatile flow and luminal stenosis is complex, but experiments have shown that when a stenosis reduces the cross-sectional area by approximately 75 percent, a full range of increases in flow to meet increased myocardial demand is not possible. When the luminal area is reduced by more than approximately 80 percent, blood flow at rest may be reduced, and further minor decreases in the stenotic orifice can reduce coronary flow dramatically and cause myocardial ischemia.

Segmental atherosclerotic narrowing of epicardial coronary arteries is caused most commonly by the formation of a plaque, which is subject to fissuring, hemorrhage, and thrombosis. Any of these events can temporarily worsen the obstruction, reduce coronary blood flow, and cause clinical manifestations of myocardial ischemia, as described below. The location of the obstruction will influence the quantity of myocardium rendered ischemic and thus determine the severity of the clinical manifestations. Severe coronary narrowing and myocardial ischemia are frequently accompanied by the development of collateral vessels, especially when the narrowing develops gradually. When well developed, such vessels can provide sufficient blood flow to sustain the viability of the myocardium at rest but not during conditions of increased demand.

Once severe stenosis of a proximal epicardial artery has reduced the cross-sectional area by more than approximately 70 percent, the distal resistance vessels (when they function normally) dilate to reduce vascular resistance and maintain coronary blood flow. A pressure gradient develops across the proximal stenosis, and poststenotic pressure falls. When the resistance vessels are maximally dilated, myocardial blood flow becomes dependent on the pressure in the coronary artery distal to the obstruction. In these circumstances alterations in myocardial oxygenation can be caused by changes in myocardial oxygen demand and changes in the caliber of the stenosed coronary artery due to physiologic vasomotion, pathologic spasm, or small platelet plugs. All these transient events can upset the critical balance between oxygen supply and demand and thus precipitate myocardial ischemia.

EFFECTS OF ISCHEMIA The inadequate oxygenation induced by coronary atherosclerosis may cause transient disturbances of the mechanical, biochemical, and electrical functions of the myocardium. The abrupt development of ischemia usually affects a segment of left ventricular myocardium with almost instantaneous failure of normal muscle contraction and relaxation. The relatively poor perfusion of the subendocardium causes more intense ischemia of this portion of the wall. Ischemia of large segments of the ventricle will cause transient left ventricular failure, and if the papillary muscles are involved, mitral regurgitation can complicate this event. When ischemic events are transient, they may be associated with angina pectoris; if prolonged, they can lead to myocardial necrosis and scarring with or without the clinical picture of acute myocardial infarction (see Chap. 202). Coronary atherosclerosis is a focal process that usually causes nonuniform ischemia. As a result, regional disturbances of ventricular contractility cause segmental bulging or dyskinesia and can greatly reduce the efficiency of myocardial pump function.

Underlying these mechanical disturbances are a wide range of abnormalities in cell metabolism, function, and structure. When oxygenated, the normal myocardium metabolizes fatty acids and glucose to carbon dioxide and water. With severe oxygen deprivation, fatty acids cannot be oxidized, and glucose is broken down to lactate; intracellular pH is reduced as are the myocardial stores of high-energy phosphates, adenosine triphosphate (ATP), and creatine phosphate. Impaired cell membrane function leads to potassium leakage and the uptake of sodium by myocytes. The severity and duration of the imbalance between myocardial oxygen supply and demand will determine whether the damage is reversible or whether it is permanent, with subsequent myocardial necrosis.

Ischemia also causes characteristic electrocardiographic changes such as repolarization abnormalities, as evidenced by inversion of the T wave and later by displacement of the ST segment (Chap. 189). Transient ST-segment depression often reflects subendocardial ischemia, while transient ST-segment elevation is thought to be caused by more severe transmural ischemia. Another important consequence of myocardial ischemia is electrical instability, since this may lead to ventricular tachycardia or ventricular fibrillation (Chap. 198). Most patients who die suddenly from ischemic heart disease do so as a result of ischemia-induced malignant ventricular tachyarrhythmias (Chap. 35).

CLINICAL MANIFESTATIONS

ASYMPTOMATIC VERSUS SYMPTOMATIC CORONARY ARTERY DISEASE Postmortem studies on accident victims and military casualties in western countries have shown that coronary atherosclerosis often begins to develop prior to age 20 and is widespread even among adults who were asymptomatic during life. Before the menopause women develop less coronary atherosclerosis and have a much lower incidence of the clinical manifestations of coronary artery disease (angina pectoris, myocardial infarction, and coronary death). This protection is lost progressively after the menopause. When all age groups are considered, ischemic heart disease is the most common cause of death not only in men but also in women (Chap. 5). Exercise stress tests in asymptomatic persons may show evidence of silent myocardial ischemia, i.e., exercise-induced electrocardiographic changes not accompanied by angina; coronary angiographic studies of such persons frequently reveal obstructive coronary artery disease. Postmortem examination of patients with obstructive coronary artery disease who had no history of any clinical manifestations of myocardial ischemia often shows macroscopic scars of myocardial infarction in regions supplied by diseased coronary arteries. According to population studies, approximately 25 percent of patients who survive acute myocardial infarction may not reach medical attention, and these patients carry the same adverse prognosis as those who present with the classic clinical syndrome (Chap. 202). Sudden death may be unheralded and is a common presenting manifestation of ischemic heart disease (Chap. 35). Patients can also present with cardiomegaly and heart failure secondary to ischemic damage of the left ventricular myocardium that caused no symptoms prior to the development of heart failure; this condition is referred to as *ischemic cardiomyopathy*. In contrast to the asymptomatic phase of ischemic heart disease, the symptomatic phase is characterized by chest discomfort due to either angina pectoris or acute myocardial infarction (Chap. 202). Having entered the symptomatic phase, the patient may exhibit a stable or progressive course, revert to the asymptomatic stage, or suddenly die.

CHRONIC STABLE ANGINA PECTORIS This episodic clinical syndrome is due to transient myocardial ischemia. Various diseases that cause myocardial ischemia as well as the numerous forms of discomfort with which it may be confused are discussed in Chap. 12. Males constitute approximately 70 percent of all patients with angina pectoris and an even greater fraction of those younger than 50 years of age. The typical patient with angina is a 50- to 60-year-old man or 65- to 75-year-old woman who seeks medical help for troublesome or frightening chest discomfort, usually described as heaviness, pressure, squeezing, smothering, or choking and only rarely as frank pain. When the patient is asked to localize the sensation, he or she will typically press on the sternum, sometimes with a clenched fist, to indicate a squeezing, central, substernal discomfort. This symptom is usually crescendo-decrescendo in nature and lasts 1 to 5 min. Angina can radiate to the left shoulder and to both arms, and especially to the ulnar surfaces of the forearm and hand. It can also arise in or radiate to the back, neck, jaw, teeth, and epigastrium.

Although episodes of angina are typically caused by exertion (e.g., exercise, hurrying, or sexual activity) or emotion (e.g., stress, anger, fright, or frustration) and are relieved by rest, they may also occur at rest (see "Unstable Angina Pectoris," below) and at night while the patient is recumbent (angina decubitus). The patient may be awakened at night distressed by typical chest discomfort and dyspnea. The pathophysiology of nocturnal angina is analogous to that of paroxysmal nocturnal dyspnea (Chap. 195), i.e., the expansion of the intrathoracic blood volume that occurs with recumbency causes an increase in cardiac size and myocardial oxygen demand that lead to ischemia and transient left ventricular failure.

The threshold for the development of angina pectoris varies from person to person and may vary by time of day and emotional state. A patient may report symptoms upon minor exertion in the morning (a short walk or shaving) yet by midday may be capable of much greater effort without symptoms. Angina may be precipitated by unfamiliar tasks, a heavy meal, or exposure to cold.

Sharp, fleeting chest pain or prolonged, dull aches localized to the left submammary area are rarely due to myocardial ischemia. However, angina pectoris may be atypical in location and may not be strictly related to provoking factors. In addition, this symptom may exacerbate and remit over days, weeks, or months, and its occurrence can be seasonal.

Systematic questioning of the patient with suspected ischemic heart disease is important to uncover a positive family history of ischemic heart disease, diabetes, hyperlipidemia, hypertension, cigarette smoking, and other risk factors for coronary atherosclerosis.

In *variant (Prinzmetal's) angina,* the chest discomfort characteristically occurs at rest or awakens the patient from sleep. It may be accompanied by palpitations or severe shortness of breath, explosive in onset, severe, and frightening. It may also be brought on by effort, although the workload at which it is precipitated usually varies considerably. Variant angina is caused by focal spasm of proximal epicardial coronary arteries; in approximately three-fourths of the patients atherosclerotic coronary artery obstruction is present, in which case the vasospasm occurs near the stenotic lesion.

Physical examination   The physical examination is often normal. The patient's general appearance may reveal signs of risk factors associated with coronary atherosclerosis such as xanthelasma, xanthomas (Chap. 208), or diabetic skin lesions. There may also be signs of anemia, thyroid disease, and nicotine stains on the fingertips from cigarette smoking. Palpation can reveal thickened or absent peripheral arteries, signs of cardiac enlargement, and abnormal contraction of the cardiac impulse (left ventricular akinesia or dyskinesia). Examination of the fundi may reveal increased light reflexes and arteriovenous nicking as evidence of hypertension (an important risk factor for ischemic heart disease), while auscultation can uncover arterial bruits, a third and/or fourth heart sound, and, if acute ischemia or previous infarction has impaired papillary muscle function, a late apical systolic murmur due to mitral regurgitation. These auscultatory signs are best appreciated with the patient in the left decubitus position. Aortic stenosis, aortic regurgitation (Chap. 201), and hypertrophic cardiomyopathy (Chap. 205) must be excluded, since these disorders may cause angina even in the absence of coronary artery disease. Examination during an anginal attack is useful, since ischemia can cause transient left ventricular failure with the appearance of a third and/or fourth heart sound, a dyskinetic cardiac apex, mitral regurgitation, and even pulmonary edema.

Laboratory examination   Although the diagnosis of ischemic heart disease can be made with confidence from a typical history, a number of simple laboratory tests can be helpful. The urine should be examined for evidence of diabetes mellitus and renal disease, since both these conditions may accelerate atherosclerosis. Similarly, examination of the blood should include measurements of lipids (cholesterol—total, low density, and high density), glucose, creatinine, hematocrit, and, if indicated based on the physical examination, thyroid function. A chest x-ray is important, since it may show the consequences of ischemic heart disease, i.e., cardiac enlargement, ventricular aneurysm, or signs of heart failure. Calcification of the coronary arteries can sometimes be identified on chest fluoroscopy. These signs can support the diagnosis of coronary artery disease and are important in assessing the degree of cardiac damage and the effects of treatment for heart failure.

Electrocardiogram   A normal ECG does not exclude the diagnosis of ischemic heart disease; however, certain characteristic abnormalities in tracings obtained at rest can confirm it. A 12-lead ECG recorded at rest is normal in about half the patients with typical angina pectoris, but there may be signs of an old myocardial infarction (Chap. 189). Serial tracings are particulary useful to look for past or evolving myocardial infarction. Although repolarization abnormalities, i.e., T-wave and ST-segment changes and intraventricular conduction disturbances at rest, are suggestive of ischemic heart disease, they are nonspecific, since they can also occur in pericardial, myocardial, and valvular heart disease or with anxiety, changes in posture, drugs, or esophageal disease. Typical ST-segment and T-wave changes that accompany episodes of angina pectoris and disappear thereafter are more specific. The most characteristic changes include displacement of the ST segment that is similar in every way to that induced during a stress test (see below). The ST segment is usually depressed during angina but may be elevated—sometimes strikingly so—as in the early stages of myocardial infarction and in Prinzmetal's angina.

Stress testing   The most widely used test in the diagnosis of ischemic heart disease involves recording the 12-lead ECG before, during, and after exercise on a treadmill or using a bicycle ergometer.

The test consists of a standardized incremental increase in external workload while the patient's ECG, symptoms, and arm blood pressure are continuously monitored. Performance is usually symptom-limited and the test is discontinued upon evidence of chest discomfort, severe shortness of breath, dizziness, fatigue, ST-segment depression of greater than 0.2 mV (2 mm), a fall in systolic blood pressure exceeding 15 mmHg, or the development of a ventricular tachyarrhythmia. This test seeks to discover any limitation in exercise performance and establish the relationship between chest discomfort and the typical electrocardiographic signs of myocardial ischemia. The ischemic ST-segment response is generally defined as flat depression of the ST segment of more than 0.1 mV below the baseline (i.e., the PR segment) and lasting longer than 0.08 s. This type of depression is designated "square wave" or "plateau" and is flat or downsloping. Upsloping or junctional ST-segment changes are not considered characteristic of ischemia and do not constitute a positive test. Although T-wave abnormalities, conduction disturbances, and ventricular arrhythmias that develop during exercise should be noted, they are also not diagnostic. Negative exercise tests in which the target heart rate (85 percent of maximal heart rate for age and sex) is not achieved are considered to be nondiagnostic.

Based on the above criteria, the rate of false-positive diagnoses, using the coronary arteriogram as the gold standard, is approximately 15 percent, and a similar percentage of patients with severe, multivessel coronary artery disease will not have a positive test (false-negative). According to Bayes' theorem, the probability that ischemic heart disease exists in the patient or population under study (pretest probability) must be considered in light of the diagnostic features of the test in order to interpret a positive or negative test result (Fig. 10-2, p. 46). For example, a positive result on exercise indicates that the likelihood of coronary artery disease is 98 percent in males above the age of 50 years with typical angina pectoris, but progressively lower in those with atypical chest pain, nonanginal chest pain, and asymptomatic persons. The incidence of false-positive tests is increased in asymptomatic men under the age of 40 years or premenopausal women without risk factors for premature atherosclerosis, in patients taking cardioactive drugs such as digitalis and quinidine, or in those with intraventricular conduction disturbances, resting abnormalities of the ST segment and the T wave, myocardial hypertrophy, or abnormal serum potassium levels. Obstructive disease limited to the circumflex coronary artery may result in a false-negative stress test since the posterior portion of the heart which this vessel supplies is not well represented on the surface 12-lead ECG.

The physician should be present throughout the exercise test, and it is important to measure total duration of exercise, the time to the onset of ischemic ST-segment change and chest discomfort, the external work performed, and the internal cardiac work performed; the last is represented by the heart rate–blood pressure product. The depth of the ST-segment depression and the time needed for recovery of these electrocardiographic changes are also important. Because the risks of exercise testing are small but real—estimated at one fatality and two nonfatal complications per 10,000 tests—equipment for resuscitation should be available. Modified (heart rate-limited rather than symptom-limited) exercise tests can be performed safely in patients as early as 7 days after myocardial infarction.

The normal response to exercise includes a progressive increase in heart rate and blood pressure. Failure of the blood pressure to increase or an actual decrease in blood pressure with signs of ischemia during the test is an important adverse prognostic sign, since it may reflect ischemia-induced global left ventricular dysfunction. The presence of pain or severe ST-segment depression at a low workload and ST-segment depression that persists for more than 5 min after the termination of exercise will increase the specificity of the test and suggests severe ischemic heart disease.

The exercise test can be enhanced by the intravenous administration of a radioisotope such as thallium 201 or Sesta-Mibi to assess regional myocardial perfusion by means of a gamma camera (p. 971). Technetium 99m can be used to label the blood pool for gated radioisotope angiography. This technique (Fig. 190-8, p. 970) can provide a measure of ventricular volume, ejection fraction, and regional ventricular wall motion at rest and during exercise, and can identify transient global and regional left ventricular dysfunction due to myocardial ischemia at rest or during ischemia. A reduction in ejection fraction during exercise with the appearance of regional wall motion abnormalities is an important sign and suggests the presence of severe ischemia and/or multivessel coronary disease.

An important fraction of patients who need noninvasive stress testing to identify myocardial ischemia and increased risk of coronary events cannot exercise because of peripheral vascular or musculoskeletal disease. In these circumstances intravenous dipyridamole or adenosine can be used in place of exercise. The electrocardiogram with a radionuclide such as thallium 201 is used to detect myocardial ischemia. Ambulatory monitoring of the electrocardiogram can assess myocardial ischemia as episodes of ST-segment depression. These new techniques are sensitive and capable of identifying patients with ischemia who are at increased risk of coronary events. Technetium 99-labeled Sesta-Mibi is a new radionuclide that has advantages over thallium 201.

The severity of ischemia in all of the tests described above has been shown to correlate with risk for future adverse coronary events (myocardial infarction and death).

Two-dimensional echocardiography records cross-sectional images of the left ventricle and can identify regional wall motion abnormalities due to myocardial infarction or persistent ischemia (Chap. 190). In this way, the test can also be used as an aid in the diagnosis of ischemic heart disease.

Coronary arteriography (Chap. 192) This invasive diagnostic method outlines the coronary anatomy and can be used to detect important evidence of coronary atherosclerosis or to exclude this condition. By this means, one can assess the severity of obstructive lesions and when combined with left ventricular angiocardiography can evaluate both global and regional function of the left ventricle. Coronary arteriography is indicated in (1) patients with chronic stable or unstable angina pectoris who are severely symptomatic despite medical therapy and who are being considered for revascularization, i.e., percutaneous transluminal coronary angioplasty or coronary artery bypass graft surgery; (2) patients with troublesome symptoms that present diagnostic difficulties in whom there is need to confirm or rule out the diagnosis of coronary artery disease; and (3) patients suspected of having left main stem or three-vessel coronary artery disease based on signs of severe ischemia on noninvasive testing, regardless of the presence or severity of symptoms.

Examples of other possible clinical situations include:

1 Patients with chest discomfort suggestive of angina pectoris but a negative exercise test who require a definitive diagnosis for guiding medical management, alleviating psychological stress, career or family planning, or insurance purposes.
2 Patients who have been admitted repeatedly to the hospital for suspected acute myocardial infarction but in whom this diagnosis has not been established and in whom the presence or absence of coronary artery disease should be determined.
3 Patients with careers that involve the safety of others (e.g., airline pilots) who have questionable symptoms, suspicious or positive noninvasive tests, and in whom there are reasonable doubts about the state of the coronary arteries.
4 Patients with aortic stenosis or hypertrophic cardiomyopathy and angina in whom the pain could be due to coronary artery disease.
5 Male patients aged 45 and females aged 55 years of age or older who will undergo valve replacement and who may or may not have clinical evidence of myocardial ischemia.
6 Patients who are at high risk after myocardial infarction because of the recurrence of angina, heart failure, frequent ventricular premature contractions, or signs of ischemia in the stress test.
7 Patients with angina pectoris, regardless of severity, in whom noninvasive testing reveals signs of severe ischemia, i.e., early

and/or marked (>2 mm) ST-segment depression, large or multiple perfusion defects and/or increased lung uptake on thallium 201 scintigrams following exercise, global left ventricular dysfunction precipitated by exercise, and/or exercise-induced hypotension.

PROGNOSIS

The principal prognostic indicators in patients with ischemic heart disease are the functional state of the left ventricle, the location and severity of coronary artery narrowing, and the severity or activity of myocardial ischemia. Angina pectoris of recent onset, unstable angina, angina which is unresponsive or poorly responsive to medical therapy or is accompanied by symptoms of congestive heart failure all indicate an increased risk for adverse coronary events. The same is true for the physical signs of heart failure, episodes of pulmonary edema, or roentgenographic evidence of cardiac enlargement. An abnormal resting ECG or positive evidence of myocardial ischemia during a stress test also indicate increased risk. Most importantly, the following signs during noninvasive testing indicate a high risk for coronary events: a strongly positive exercise test showing onset of myocardial ischemia at low workloads, large or multiple perfusion defects or increased lung uptake during stress thallium scanning, a decrease in left ventricular ejection fraction during exercise on radionuclide ventriculography, and hypotension with ischemia during stress testing.

On cardiac catheterization, elevations in left ventricular end-diastolic pressure and ventricular volume and a reduced ejection fraction are the most important signs of left ventricular dysfunction and are associated with a poor prognosis. Patients with chest discomfort but normal left ventricular function and normal coronary arteries have an excellent prognosis. In patients with normal left ventricular function and mild angina but with critical stenoses (≥70 percent luminal diameter) of one, two, or three epicardial coronary arteries, the 5-year mortality rates are approximately 2, 8, and 11 percent, respectively. Obstructive lesions of the proximal left anterior descending coronary artery are associated with a greater risk than are lesions of the right or left circumflex coronary artery, since the former vessel usually perfuses a greater quantity of myocardium. Critical stenosis of the left main coronary artery is associated with a mortality of about 15 percent per year.

With any degree of obstructive coronary artery disease, mortality is greatly increased when left ventricular function is impaired; conversely, at any level of left ventricular function, the prognosis is influenced importantly by the extent of myocardium perfused by the critically obstructed vessels. It is useful to consider that coronary atherosclerosis demonstrates its harmful potential by causing transient myocardial ischemia and by leading to myocardial infarction, which characteristically destroys myocardium, thereby reducing cardiac reserve at an unpredictable rate (or causing sudden death). The larger the amount of myocardial necrosis, the less the heart is able to withstand additional damage and the poorer the prognosis. In this light, the various indices of ischemic damage, such as the ECG showing evidence of an old infarction and symptoms or signs of heart failure or cardiac enlargement, should be taken as indications of myocardial damage.

The segmental atherosclerotic plaques in epicardial arteries go through phases of cellular activity, degeneration, endothelial instability, abnormal vasomotion, platelet aggregation, and fissuring or hemorrhage. These factors can temporarily worsen the stenosis and cause abnormal reactivity of the vessel wall thus exacerbating the manifestations of ischemia. The development of unstable angina and/or severe ischemia during stress testing reflects rapid progression.

MANAGEMENT

Each patient must be evaluated individually with respect to life patterns, risk factors, control of symptoms, and prevention of damage to left ventricular myocardium. The degree of the patient's disability and the specific physical and emotional stresses that precipitate pain must all be carefully recorded in order to set the proper goals for treatment. The management plan should consist of (1) explanation and reassurance, (2) reduction of risk factors in an attempt to slow the progression of coronary atherosclerosis, (3) treatment of coexisting conditions capable of aggravating angina, (4) sensible adaptations of activities to minimize anginal attacks, (5) a program of drug therapy, and (6) definition of end points that will indicate the need to consider mechanical revascularization.

EXPLANATION AND REASSURANCE Patients with ischemic heart disease need to understand their condition as best they can and to realize that a long and useful life is possible even though they suffer from angina pectoris or have experienced and recovered from an acute myocardial infarction. Offering case histories of persons in public life who have lived with coronary disease can be of great value when encouraging patients to resume or maintain activity and return to their occupation. A planned program of rehabilitation can encourage patients to lose weight, improve exercise tolerance, and control risk factors with more confidence.

REDUCTION OF RISK FACTORS (SECONDARY PREVENTION) (See also Chap. 208) The discontinuance of cigarette smoking is vital. The risk of coronary events is low when the total plasma cholesterol is less than 200 mg/100 mL, intermediate when it is 200 to 240 mg/100 mL, and abnormally increased when the plasma cholesterol is over 240 mg/100 mL. Clinical trials in selected patients seem to indicate that effective modification of risk factors (e.g., plasma lipid levels) can slow the growth of coronary atherosclerosis and decrease the morbidity and mortality due to coronary artery disease. Ideal weight should be attained and maintained. Aggravating factors (e.g., endocrine disorders, hypertension, and drugs such as glucocorticoids) should be treated and eliminated when possible (see Chaps. 208 and 344). After appropriate diet and exercise, drug therapy should be used in patients in an attempt to reduce the total plasma cholesterol (ideal value <200 mg/100 mL), reduce the plasma LDL fraction (ideal value <130 mg/100 mL) and increase the plasma HDL fraction (ideal value >45 mg/mL). The total cholesterol and LDL fraction are effectively reduced by bile acid binding resins (e.g., cholestyramine) and the HMG CoA reductase inhibitors of cholesterol synthesis (e.g., lovastatin) while the HDL is effectively increased by drugs such as niacin and gemfibrozil (see Chap. 344). Diabetes mellitus and hypertension, when present, should be treated. Unless angina is provoked by strenuous activity, the patient should be encouraged to engage in steady, dynamic exercise such as walking; isometric exercise may be hazardous. By maintaining good physical condition, the patient will be able to perform physical work more efficiently and at a lower pulse rate, thus reducing the frequency of angina pectoris. Patients in good physical condition may also have a better chance of surviving a myocardial infarction. The administration of estrogen to postmenopausal women appears to provide significant protection with a reduction in coronary events. Nevertheless, there is a modest increase in the occurrence of some malignancies and therefore therapy should be individualized.

ELIMINATION OF COEXISTING ILLNESS A number of illnesses that are not primarily cardiac in nature may either increase oxygen demand or decrease oxygen supply to the myocardium and may precipitate or exacerbate angina. In the former category, hypertension and hyperthyroidism may be treated successfully in order to reduce the frequency of anginal attacks. Decreased myocardial oxygen supply may be due to reduced oxygenation of the blood (e.g., in intrinsic pulmonary disease or, when carboxyhemoglobin is present, due to cigarette or cigar smoking) or decreased oxygen-carrying capacity (e.g., in anemia). Correction of these abnormalities, if present, may reduce or even eliminate anginal symptoms.

ADAPTATION OF ACTIVITIES Therapy of angina due to episodes of myocardial ischemia consists of eliminating the discrepancy between the demand of the heart muscle for oxygen and the ability of the coronary circulation to meet this demand. Most patients will

understand this fundamental concept and utilize it in the rational programming of activity. Many tasks that ordinarily evoke angina may be accomplished without symptoms simply by reducing the speed at which they are performed. Patients must appreciate the diurnal variation in their tolerance of certain activities and should reduce their energy requirements in the morning and immediately after meals. Sometimes it is helpful to alter the eating pattern, taking small and more frequent meals.

It may be necessary to recommend a change in employment or residence to avoid physical stress; however, with the exception of manual laborers, most patients with ischemic heart disease can usually continue to function merely by allowing more time to complete each task. In some patients, anger and frustration may be the most important factors precipitating myocardial ischemia. If these cannot be avoided, training in stress management may be useful. A treadmill exercise test to determine the approximate heart rate at which ischemic electrocardiographic changes or symptoms develop may be helpful in the development of a specific exercise program. Ambulatory electrocardiography during daily activities may also be helpful in this regard.

DRUG THERAPY The commonly used drugs for angina pectoris are summarized in Table 203-1.

Nitrates This valuable class of drugs in the management of angina pectoris acts by causing systemic venodilation, thereby reducing myocardial wall tension and oxygen requirements, as well as by dilating the epicardial coronary vessels and increasing blood flow in collateral vessels. The absorption of these agents (hence action) is most rapid and complete through the mucous membranes. For this reason, nitroglycerin is administered sublingually in tablets of 0.4 or 0.6 mg. Patients with angina should be instructed to take the

TABLE 203-1 Commonly used drugs for angina pectoris

Drug	Usual Dose	Side Effects	Contraindications
NITRATES			
Sublingual NTG	0.3–0.6 mg	Flushing, headache	Intolerance of side effects
Isosorbide dinitrate SR	40 mg	Flushing, headache, tolerance after 24 h	As above, worsening ischemia on withdrawal
Transdermal NTG	5–100 mg	Flushing, headache, tolerance after 24 h	As above, worsening ischemia on withdrawal
BETA ADRENOCEPTOR BLOCKING DRUGS			
Propranolol	20–80 mg qid	Depression, constipation, impotence, bronchospasm, heart failure, bradycardia	Asthma, AV conduction block, heart failure
Metoprolol	25–200 mg bid	As above	As above
Atenolol	50–150 mg once daily	As above	As above
CALCIUM CHANNEL BLOCKING DRUGS			
Nifedipine XL	30–90 mg once daily	Hypotension, flushing, edema, worsening angina	Hypotension, intolerance of side effects
Diltiazem SR	60–120 mg bid	Constipation, AV conduction block, worsening heart failure	AV conduction block, impaired LV function, bradycardia
Verapamil SR	180–240 mg once daily	Constipation, AV conduction block, worsening heart failure	AV conduction delay, impaired LV function, bradycardia

Abbreviations: SR = slow release, NTG = nitroglycerin, XL = slow release preparation.

medication both to relieve an attack and also in anticipation of stress (exercise or emotional) that is likely to induce an attack. The value of this prophylactic use of the drug cannot be overemphasized.

Headache and a pulsating feeling in the head are the most common side effects of nitroglycerin and fortunately only rarely become disturbing at the doses usually required to relieve or prevent angina. Nitroglycerin deteriorates with exposure to air, moisture, and sunlight, so that if the drug neither relieves discomfort or headache nor produces a slight sensation of burning at the sublingual site of absorption, the preparation may be inactive and a fresh supply should be obtained. If relief is not achieved after the first dose of nitroglycerin, a second or third dose may be given at 5-min intervals. If discomfort continues despite treatment, the patient should consult a physician or report promptly to a hospital emergency room for evaluation of possible unstable angina or acute myocardial infarction (Chap. 202).

Asking the patient with recently diagnosed angina pectoris to record the occurrence of pain relative to activity and other precipitating factors as well as nitroglycerin consumption is often helpful to the physician attempting to tailor a management program. Such a diary may also be valuable for detecting changes in the frequency or severity of discomfort that may signify the development of unstable angina pectoris and/or herald an impending myocardial infarction.

None of the long-acting nitrates is as effective as sublingual nitroglycerin for the acute relief of angina. These preparations can be swallowed, chewed, or administered as a patch or paste by the transdermal route. They can provide effective plasma levels for up to 24 h, but the therapeutic response is highly variable. Different preparations and/or administration during the daytime should be tried only to relieve discomfort in the individual patient while avoiding side effects such as headache and dizziness. Individual dose titration is important in order to prevent side effects. Useful preparations include isosorbide dinitrate (10 to 40 mg PO tid), nitroglycerin ointment (0.5 to 2.0 inches qid), or sustained-release transdermal patches (5 to 25 mg/d). Long-acting nitrates are relatively safe and can be used together with intermittent sublingual nitroglycerin to relieve discomfort and prevent attacks of angina. The nitrates likely bind to guanylate cyclase in vascular smooth muscle cells, oxidize sulfhydryl groups, and are converted to S-nitrosothiols. This leads to an increase in cyclic guanosine monophosphate which causes cell relaxation of vascular smooth muscle. Tolerance with loss of efficacy develop with 12 to 24 h of continuous exposure to all of the long-acting nitrates due to depletion of sulfhydryl groups and to counterregulatory alterations in intravascular fluid balance with fluid retention. In order to minimize the effects of tolerance, the minimum effective dose should be used and a minimum of 8 h each day kept free of the drug so as to restore any useful response(s).

Beta-adrenoceptor blockade (See also Chap. 68) Beta-adrenoceptor blockers represent an important component of the pharmacologic treatment of angina pectoris. These drugs reduce myocardial oxygen demand by inhibiting the increases in heart rate and myocardial contractility caused by adrenergic activity. Beta blockage reduces these variables most strikingly during exercise while causing only small reductions in heart rate, cardiac output, and arterial pressure at rest. Propranolol is usually administered in an initial dose of 20 to 40 mg four times a day and is increased as tolerated to 320 mg per day in divided doses. Long-acting beta-blocking drugs (atenolol, 50 to 100 mg/d, and nadolol, 40 to 80 mg/d) offer the advantage of once-a-day dosage (Table 68-1, p. 430). The therapeutic aims include relief of angina and ischemia. These drugs can also reduce mortality and reinfarction when given to patients after myocardial infarction. They can produce fatigue, impotence, cold extremities, intermittent claudication, and bradycardia and can worsen disturbed cardiac conduction, left ventricular failure, and bronchial asthma or intensify the hypoglycemia produced by oral hypoglycemic agents and insulin. Reducing the dose or even discontinuation of the drug may be necessary if these side effects develop and persist.

Calcium antagonists Nifedipine (10 to 40 mg qid), verapamil (80 to 120 mg tid), and diltiazem (30 to 90 mg qid) and other calcium antagonists are all coronary vasodilators that produce variable and dose-dependent reductions in myocardial oxygen demand, contractility, and arterial pressure. These combined pharmacologic effects are advantageous and make these agents quite effective in the treatment of angina pectoris. Verapamil and diltiazem may produce symptomatic disturbances in cardiac conduction and bradyarrhythmias, exert negative inotropic actions, and are more likely to worsen left ventricular failure, particularly when used in combination with beta blockers in patients with underlying left ventricular dysfunction. Although useful effects are usually achieved when calcium antagonists are combined with beta blockers and nitrates, careful individual titration of dose is essential with these potent combinations. Variant (Prinzmetal's) angina responds particularly well to calcium antagonists, supplemented when necessary by nitrates. The calcium antagonists are now formulated as long-acting preparations including nifedipine (30 to 90 mg once daily), diltiazem (60 to 120 mg twice daily), and verapamil (180 to 240 mg once daily). Verapamil should not be combined with beta-adrenoreceptor blocking drugs because of the combined effects on heart rate and contractility. Diltiazem can be combined with beta blockers with caution and only in patients with normal ventricular function and no conduction disturbances. Nifedipine and the beta blockers have complementary actions on coronary blood supply and myocardial oxygen demands. While the former decreases blood pressure and dilates coronary arteries the latter slows heart rate and decreases contractility.

Treatment of angina and heart failure Patients with angina pectoris may also have evidence of elevated left ventricular diastolic pressures and volumes due to transient ischemia. This transient left ventricular failure with angina can be controlled by the judicious use of nitrates, calcium antagonists, and even beta blockers. For patients with established congestive heart failure the increased left ventricular wall tension raises myocardial oxygen demand. Treatment of congestive heart failure with digitalis, angiotensin-converting enzyme inhibitors, and diuretics (Chap. 195) can help to decrease heart size, wall tension, and myocardial oxygen demands, which will help to control angina and ischemia. Nocturnal angina can often be relieved by these agents; however, there is no benefit—and possibly aggravation of angina—when these drugs are used in patients with a normal heart size and no evidence of heart failure. Nitrates are particularly useful and can improve the disturbed hemodynamics of congestive heart failure and relieve angina by preventing or reversing myocardial ischemia. The combination of congestive heart failure and angina in patients with coronary artery disease usually indicates a poor prognosis and warrants serious consideration of cardiac catheterization and mechanical revascularization, if possible.

Aspirin Aspirin is an irreversible inhibitor of platelet cyclooxygenase activity and thereby interferes with platelet activation. Chronic administration of 100 to 325 mg orally per day has been shown to reduce coronary events in asymptomatic adult men, patients with asymptomatic ischemia after myocardial infarction, patients with chronic stable angina, and patients who have survived unstable angina and myocardial infarction. Administration of this drug should be considered in all patients with coronary artery disease in the absence of side effects such as gastrointestinal bleeding, allergy, or dyspepsia.

MECHANICAL REVASCULARIZATION

It is important to appreciate that although the basic management of patients with a lifelong condition such as ischemic heart disease is medical, the years of medical management may be punctuated by mechanical revascularization procedures, as described below. These interventions should not replace the continuing need to ease symptoms and modify risk factors.

PERCUTANEOUS TRANSLUMINAL CORONARY ANGIOPLASTY

PTCA is a widely used method to achieve revascularization of the myocardium in patients with symptomatic ischemic heart disease and suitable stenoses of epicardial coronary arteries. Whereas patients with stenosis of the left main coronary artery and those with three-vessel coronary artery disease who require revascularization are best treated with coronary artery bypass surgery, PTCA is widely employed in patients with symptoms and evidence of ischemia due to stenoses of one or two vessels, and even selected patients with three-vessel disease, and may offer many advantages over surgery.

After a flexible guidewire is advanced into a coronary artery and across the stenosis to be dilated, a miniature balloon catheter is advanced over the guidewire and into the stenosis followed by repeated inflations until the stenosis is decreased or relieved. The development of a range of steerable guidewires, low-profile balloon catheters, and balloon catheters that also allow coronary flow during inflation have all helped to decrease complications, reach more distal lesions, and dilate more complex stenoses. (See also Chap. 193.)

Indications and patient selection The most common clinical indication for PTCA is angina pectoris, stable or unstable, which should be accompanied by evidence of ischemia in an exercise test. This symptom should be sufficiently severe to warrant the consideration of bypass graft surgery. PTCA is more effective than medical therapy for the relief of angina in patients with single-vessel coronary artery disease. The value of this procedure in improving outcome has not been established, and therefore it is not generally indicted in asymptomatic or mildly symptomatic patients. PTCA can also be used to dilate stenoses in native coronary arteries and in bypass grafts in patients who have recurrent angina following coronary artery surgery. This is an important indication when the technical difficulties and the increased mortality that accompanies reoperation are considered. Angioplasty has also been carried out in patients with recent total occlusion (within 3 months) of a coronary artery and severe angina; in this group the primary success rate is decreased to approximately 50 percent.

Risks When coronary stenoses are discrete and symmetrical, two and three vessels can be dilated in sequence. However, cautious case selection is essential in order to avoid a prohibitive risk of complications. Female gender, advanced age, the left anterior descending artery, stenoses with thrombus, left ventricular dysfunction, stenosis of an artery perfusing a large segment of myocardium without collaterals, long eccentric or irregular stenoses, and calcified plaques all increase the likelihood of complications. The major complications are usually due to dissection or thrombosis with vessel occlusion, uncontrolled ischemia, and ventricular failure. In experienced hands, the overall mortality rate should be less than 1 percent, the need for emergency coronary surgery less than 3 percent, and myocardial infarction in less than 3 percent of cases. Minor complications occur in 5 to 10 percent of patients and include occlusion of a branch of a coronary artery and complications of arterial catheterization.

Efficacy Primary success, i.e., adequate dilation with relief of angina, is achieved in 85 to 90 percent of cases. Recurrent stenosis of the dilated vessels occurs in 20 to 40 percent of cases within 6 months of the procedure, and angina will recur within 6 to 12 months in 25 percent of cases. This recurrence of symptoms and restenosis is more common in patients with diabetes mellitus, unstable angina, incomplete dilation of the stenosis, dilation of the left anterior descending coronary artery, and stenoses containing thrombi. Dilation of arteries which are totally occluded and of stenotic or occluded vein grafts also exhibit a high incidence of restenosis. It is usual clinical practice to administer aspirin and a calcium channel antagonist for months after the procedure. Although aspirin may help prevent acute coronary thrombosis during and immediately following PTCA, there are no controlled clinical trials that have demonstrated that these medications or any other can clearly reduce the incidence of restenosis.

If patients do not develop restenosis or angina within the first year after angioplasty, the prognosis for maintaining improvement over the subsequent 4 years is excellent. If restenosis occurs, PTCA can be repeated with the same success and risk, but the likelihood of restenosis increases with the third or subsequent attempt.

Between 30 and 50 percent of patients with symptomatic coronary artery disease who require revascularization can be treated by PTCA

and need not undergo coronary artery bypass surgery. Successful angioplasty is less invasive and expensive than coronary artery surgery, usually requires only two days in the hospital, and permits considerable savings in the cost of care. Successful PTCA also allows earlier return to work and the resumption of an active life.

CORONARY ARTERY BYPASS GRAFTING In this procedure, a section of a vein (usually the saphenous) is used to form a connection between the aorta and the coronary artery distal to the obstructive lesion. Alternatively, anastomosis of one or both of the internal mammary arteries to the coronary artery distal to the obstructive lesion may be employed.

Although some indications for coronary artery bypass surgery are controversial, certain areas of agreement exist:

1 The operation is relatively safe, with mortality rates less than 1 percent when the procedure is performed by an experienced surgical team in patients without serious comorbid disease and normal left ventricular function.

2 Intraoperative and postoperative mortality increases with the degree of ventricular dysfunction, comorbidities, and surgical inexperience. The effectiveness and risk of coronary artery bypass grafting vary widely depending on case selection and the skill and experience of the surgical team, so that the latter must be taken into account when a patient is being considered as a candidate for this procedure.

3 Occlusion of *vein grafts* is observed in 10 to 20 percent during the first postoperative year, and the incidence is approximately 2 percent per year during 5- to 7-year follow-up and 5 percent per year thereafter. Long-term patency rates are considerably higher for internal mammary artery implantations; in patients with left anterior descending coronary artery obstruction, survival is better when coronary bypass involves the internal mammary artery rather than a saphenous vein.

4 Angina is abolished or greatly reduced in approximately 85 percent of patients following complete revascularization. Although this is usually associated with graft patency and restoration of blood flow, the pain may also have been alleviated as a result of infarction of the ischemic segment or a placebo effect.

5 Coronary artery bypass grafting does not appear to reduce the incidence of myocardial infarction in patients with chronic ischemic heart disease; perioperative myocardial infarction occurs in 5 to 10 percent of cases, but in most instances these infarcts are small.

6 Mortality is reduced by operation in patients with stenosis of the left main coronary artery as well as in patients with three-vessel coronary artery disease and impaired left ventricular function. However, there is no evidence that coronary artery bypass surgery improves survival in patients with one- or two-vessel disease who have chronic stable angina and normal left ventricular function or in patients with one-vessel disease and impaired left ventricular function. Evidence is conflicting concerning the effects of operation on survival in patients with impaired left ventricular function and obstructive disease of two coronary arteries, one of which is the proximal left anterior descending artery.

Indications for coronary artery bypass grafting are usually based on the severity of symptoms, coronary anatomy, and ventricular function. The ideal candidate is male, less than 70 years of age, has no other complicating disease, has troublesome or disabling symptoms that are not adequately controlled by medical therapy, wishes to lead a more active life, and has severe stenoses of several epicardial coronary arteries with objective evidence of myocardial ischemia as a cause of the chest discomfort. Great symptomatic benefit can be anticipated in such patients. When the patient also has a disturbance of left ventricular function, coronary artery bypass grafting may, in addition, prolong life.

UNSTABLE ANGINA PECTORIS

The following three patient groups may be said to have unstable angina pectoris: (1) patients with new onset (<2 months) angina that is severe and/or frequent (≥3 episodes per day); (2) patients with accelerating angina, i.e., those with chronic stable angina who develop angina that is distinctly more frequent, severe, prolonged, or precipitated by less exertion than previously; (3) those with angina at rest. Unstable angina may be primary, i.e., occur in the absence of an extracardiac condition that has intensified myocardial ischemia, or it may be precipitated by a condition extrinsic to the coronary vascular bed that has intensified myocardial ischemia, such as anemia, fever, infection, tachyarrhythmias, emotional stress, or hypoxemia. Unstable angina may also develop shortly after myocardial infarction. Unstable angina, particularly when it is characterized by rest pain or occurs in the postinfarction state, carries an adverse prognosis, with significant risk of acute myocardial infarction or the development of intractable chronic stable angina.

When unstable angina is accompanied by objective electrocardiographic evidence of transient myocardial ischemia (ST-segment changes and/or T-wave inversions during episodes of chest pain), it is almost always associated with critical stenoses in one or more major epicardial coronary arteries. The atherosclerotic lesions may have a complicated morphology, with evidence of superimposed thrombosis in approximately 25 to 60 percent of cases. Segmental spasm in the vicinity of atherosclerotic plaques may also play a role in the development of unstable angina.

MANAGEMENT The patient should be admitted promptly to the hospital for observation, further diagnosis, and treatment. It is important to identify and treat concomitant conditions that can intensify ischemia, such as uncontrolled tachycardia, hypertension and diabetes mellitus, cardiomegaly, heart failure, arrhythmias, thyrotoxicosis, and any acute febrile illness. Acute myocardial infarction should be ruled out by means of serial ECGs and measurements of plasma cardiac enzyme activity.

Continuous electrocardiographic monitoring should be carried out and the patients should receive reassurance and sedation. Thrombus formation frequently complicates this condition. Therefore, intravenous heparin should be given for 3 to 5 days to maintain the partial thromboplastin time at 2 to 2.5 times control, together with or followed by oral aspirin at a dose of 325 mg/d. Beta-adrenoceptor blocking drugs and calcium antagonists should be administered, but with caution and an awareness of the possible side effects discussed above. Dosages must be titrated to avoid bradycardia, heart failure, and hypotension. Nitroglycerin should be given by the sublingual route as needed for symptoms. In addition, intravenous nitroglycerin is quite effective, although it requires continuous monitoring of arterial pressure. It is begun at a dosage of 10 μg/min and is raised in 5-μg/min increments to a level at which chest pain is abolished but systolic arterial pressure is maintained or reduced only slightly and other side effects are avoided.

The majority of patients improve with such treatment. However, the clinical outcome is highly variable. If angina and/or electrocardiographic evidence of ischemia do not diminish within 24 to 48 h of the comprehensive treatment described above in patients with no obvious contraindications for revascularization, then cardiac catheterization and coronary arteriography should be performed. If the anatomy is suitable, PTCA can be performed with surgical standby. PTCA in this condition, particularly in the presence of thrombus, is attended by increased risk of acute closure and ischemia. If angioplasty cannot be done, coronary artery bypass grafting should be considered to relieve symptoms and myocardial ischemia and as a means of preventing myocardial damage. If the patient's symptoms and signs are controlled on medical therapy, a diagnostic exercise ECG should be obtained near the time of hospital discharge. If there is evidence of severe myocardial ischemia, serious consideration should be given to catheterization and revascularization. It should be recognized that severe coronary artery disease is often present in patients with unstable angina who respond to medical therapy. Many patients in whom the unstable state is controlled are left with severe chronic stable angina and ultimately require mechanical revascularization.

ASYMPTOMATIC (SILENT) ISCHEMIA

Obstructive coronary artery disease, acute myocardial infarction, and transient myocardial ischemia are frequently asymptomatic. During continuous ambulatory electrocardiographic monitoring, the majority of ambulatory patients with typical chronic stable angina are found to have objective evidence of myocardial ischemia (ST-segment depression) during episodes of chest discomfort while they are active outside the hospital, but many of these patients also appear to have more frequent episodes of asymptomatic ischemia. In addition, there is a large (but as yet unknown) number of totally asymptomatic people with severe coronary atherosclerosis who exhibit ST-segment changes during activity. Evidence of frequent episodes of ischemia (symptomatic and asymptomatic) during daily life appears to indicate an increased likelihood of adverse coronary events such as death and myocardial infarction. The widespread use of exercise electrocardiography during routine examinations has also defined some of these heretofore unrecognized patients with asymptomatic coronary artery disease. Longitudinal studies have demonstrated an increased incidence of coronary events (sudden death, myocardial infarction, and angina) in asymptomatic patients with positive exercise tests. In addition, patients with asymptomatic ischemia after suffering a myocardial infarction are at far greater risk for a second coronary event. Patients who seek evaluation and who have asymptomatic ischemia should be subjected to a detailed noninvasive examination, utilizing stress electrocardiography and radionuclide scintigraphy.

MANAGEMENT The management of patients with asymptomatic ischemia must be individualized. Thus, the physician should consider the following: (1) the degree of positivity of the exercise test, particularly the stage of exercise at which electrocardiographic signs of ischemia appear, the magnitude and number of the perfusion defect(s) on thallium scintigraphy, and the change in left ventricular ejection fraction which occurs during ischemia and/or during exercise on radionuclide ventriculography; (2) the electrocardiographic leads showing a positive response, with changes in the anterior precordial leads indicating a less favorable prognosis than changes in the inferior leads; and (3) the patient's age, occupation, and general medical condition. Most would agree that an asymptomatic 45-year-old commercial airline pilot with 4-mm ST-segment depression in leads V_1 to V_4 during mild exercise should undergo coronary arteriography, whereas the asymptomatic, sedentary 75-year-old retiree with 1-mm ST-segment depression in leads II and III during maximal activity need not. However, there is no consensus about the appropriate procedure in the large majority of patients for whom the situation is less extreme. Patients with evidence of severe ischemia on noninvasive testing (as outlined earlier) should undergo coronary arteriography. Asymptomatic patients with silent ischemia, three-vessel coronary artery disease, and impaired left ventricular function may be considered appropriate candidates for coronary artery bypass surgery.

The chronic administration of aspirin to patients with asymptomatic ischemia after myocardial infarction has been shown to reduce adverse coronary events. While the incidence of asymptomatic ischemia can be reduced by treatment with beta blockers, calcium channel antagonists, and long-acting nitrates, it is not clear whether this is necessary or desirable in patients who have not suffered a myocardial infarction. However, there is evidence that beta-adrenoceptor blockade begun 7 to 35 days after acute myocardial infarction improves survival (Chap. 202).

REFERENCES

BELLER GA et al: Sensitivity, specificity and prognostic significance of noninvasive testing for occult or known coronary disease. Prog Cardiovasc Dis 24:241, 1987

BRAUNWALD E: Unstable angina—A classification. Circulation 80:410, 1989

———, SOBEL BE et al: Coronary blood flow and myocardial ischemia, in *Heart Disease*, 4th ed, E Braunwald (ed). Philadelphia, Saunders, 1992, pp 1161–1199

DEEDWANIA PC: Asymptomatic ischemia during predischarge Holter monitoring predicts poor prognosis in the postinfarction period. Am J Cardiol 71:859, 1993

——, CARBAJAL EV: Silent ischemia during daily life is an independent predictor of mortality in stable angina. Circulation 81:748, 1990

FAXON D: Percutaneous coronary angioplasty in stable and unstable angina. Cardiol Clin 9:99, 1991

FUSTER V et al: Mechanisms of disease: Pathophysiology of coronary artery disease and the acute coronary syndromes. N Engl J Med 326:24, 1992

GOTTO AM, FARMER JA: Risk factors for coronary artery disease, in *Heart Disease,* 4th ed, E. Braunwald (ed). Philadelphia, Saunders, 1992, pp 1125-1160

HAUDENSCHILD CC: Pathobiology of restenosis after angioplasty. Am J Med 94:40S, 1993

LEUNG WH: Coronary and circulatory support strategies for percutaneous transluminal coronary angioplasty in high-risk patients. Am Heart J 125:1727, 1993

NOBUYOSHI M et al: Restenosis after percutaneous transluminal coronary angioplasty: Pathologic observations in 20 patients 17:433, 1991

NYMAN I et al: Prevention of serious cardiac event by low-dose aspirin in patients with silent myocardial ischemia. Lancet 340:497, 1992

PARISI AF et al: A comparison of angioplasty with medical therapy in the treatment of single-vessel coronary artery disease. N Engl J Med 326:10, 1992

RIDKER PM et al: Low-dose aspirin therapy for chronic stable angina. Ann Intern Med 114:835, 1991

ROCCO MB et al: Prognostic importance of myocardial ischemia detected by ambulatory monitoring in patients with stable coronary artery disease. Circulation 78:877, 1988

RUTHERFORD JD et al: Chronic ischemic heart disease, in *Heart Disease,* 4th ed, E Braunwald (ed). Philadelphia, Saunders, 1992, pp 1292–1364

RYAN TJ et al: Guidelines for percutaneous transluminal coronary angioplasty. A report of the American College of Cardiology/American Heart Association Task Force on assessment of diagnostic and therapeutic cardiovascular procedures (Subcommittee on Percutaneous Transluminal Coronary Angioplasty). Circulation 78:486, 1988

SELWYN AP et al: Pathophysiology of ischemia in patients with coronary artery disease. Progr Cardiovasc Dis 35:1, 1992

Special Report: ACC/AHA guidelines and indications for coronary artery bypass graft surgery. A report of the American College of Cardiology/American Heart Association Task Force on Assessment of Diagnostic and Therapeutic Cardiovascular Procedures (Subcommittee on Coronary Artery Bypass Graft Surgery). Circulation 83:1125, 1991

STAMPFER MJ: Post menopausal estrogen therapy an cardiovascular disease. Ten year follow-up from the Nurses' Health Study. N Engl J Med 325:756, 1991

THEROUX P et al: Aspirin, heparin or both to treat acute unstable angina. N Engl J Med 319:1105, 1988

WILLERSON JT et al: Unstable angina pectoris and the progression to acute myocardial infarction: Role of platelets and platelet-derived mediators. Texas Heart Inst J 18:243, 1991

204   COR PULMONALE

JOHN BUTLER* / EUGENE BRAUNWALD

DEFINITIONS *Cor pulmonale* is enlargement of the right ventricle secondary to diseases of the lung, thorax, or pulmonary circulation. It is sometimes accompanied by right ventricular failure. In right ventricular failure there is an elevation of transmural right ventricular end-diastolic pressure which cannot be accounted for by an increase in right ventricular output. *Chronic* dysfunction of the right ventricular myocardium is rarely a cause of right heart failure but may occur when cor pulmonale and ischemic heart disease coexist. Approximately 20 percent of hospital admissions for heart failure are caused by right ventricular failure associated with cor pulmonale. More than half of the patients with chronic obstructive lung diseases have cor pulmonale, and this condition constitutes between 5 and 10 percent of all adult heart diseases in the United States. It constitutes a higher percentage of all forms of heart disease in countries such as the United Kingdom, where the incidence of obstructive lung disease is higher.

NORMAL FUNCTION OF THE PULMONARY CIRCULATION

The pulmonary circulation is interposed between the right and left ventricles for the purpose of gas exchange, the filtering out of particles, and the chemical "conditioning" of the blood, such as the conversion of angiotensin I to angiotensin II. Normally, flow through the pulmonary vascular bed depends not only on the pumping action of the right ventricle but also on respiratory movements and the

* Deceased

contraction of the left ventricle. Respiratory motion facilitates pulmonary blood flow by aspirating blood into the thorax on inhalation; the blood is then propelled forward by the positive pressure of exhalation acting on a one-way valved system.

The stroke volume of the right ventricle, as of the left, is regulated by its preload, contractility, and afterload (Chap. 194). Since the right ventricle is a compliant reservoir, acute changes in venous return (e.g., an increase with inhalation and decline with exhalation) are accommodated with little change in transmural right ventricular pressure. However, the ability of the right ventricle to increase its systolic pressure is limited. Normally, the right ventricular afterload, which is closely related to the pulmonary artery pressure, is low. The pulmonary artery pressure normally rises slightly when blood is displaced into the chest at the start of exercise, on assuming recumbency, or with cold, anxiety, or pain. A driving pressure of only about 5 cmH$_2$O between the pulmonary artery (15 cmH$_2$O) and the left atrium (10 cmH$_2$O) normally propels the entire cardiac output of approximately 5 L/min at rest through the lungs, and only a modest increase in pressure is necessary to drive a flow of up to 25 L/min through the pulmonary capillary bed during exercise.

The resistance of the pulmonary circulation (R), i.e., the pulmonary vascular resistance (p. 985), is calculated as the intravascular driving pressure (DP), i.e., pulmonary artery pressure minus pulmonary venous or left atrial pressure, divided by the pulmonary blood flow rate ($\dot{Q}$). The caliber of a distensible vessel depends on its transmural pressure. R increases when vessels collapse, narrow, or lengthen, or when the viscosity of the blood increases.

$$R = \frac{Kl\mu}{r^4}$$

where K = constant
l = length
r = radius
μ = viscosity

There is no single value of R which describes the pulmonary vascular bed, because the relationship between driving pressure and flow is not linear; calculated R decreases with increasing pulmonary blood flow because pulmonary vessels are distended and collapsed vessels are recruited (Fig. 204-1).

PATHOPHYSIOLOGY The severity of right ventricular enlargement in cor pulmonale is a function of the magnitude of the increase in afterload. When the pulmonary vascular resistance is increased and relatively fixed, as in pulmonary vascular or parenchymal lung disease, an elevation in cardiac output as occurs with physical exertion can elevate pulmonary artery pressure markedly. Right ventricular afterload is chronically augmented when lung volume is enlarged, as in chronic obstructive lung disease, due to the lengthening of the pulmonary vessels and the compression of the alveolar capillaries. Right ventricular afterload can also increase when lung volume is reduced following extensive pulmonary resection, as well as in restrictive lung diseases in which pulmonary vessels are compressed and distorted. Right ventricular afterload rises with hypoxic pulmonary vasoconstriction, which is an important cause of pulmonary hypertension. Hypoxic vasoconstriction in regions of the lung affected by disease distributes blood flow to normally ventilated regions. The elevation in pulmonary artery pressure becomes a significant stress on the right ventricle when the lung disease is diffuse or when the entire lung becomes hypoxic due to hypoventilation. Hypoxic vasoconstriction results from alveolar, rather than intravascular, hypoxia and is made worse by hypercarbia, probably because of the associated acidosis. When the hematocrit becomes markedly elevated with chronic hypoxemia, the increase in blood viscosity can intensify the pulmonary hypertension.

The elevation of right ventricular afterload responsible for cor pulmonale is caused principally by pulmonary vascular or parenchymal disease. The principal syndromes and their pathophysiologic mechanisms are summarized in Table 204-1.

FIGURE 204-1 Relationship between flow and driving pressure (''vascular resistance'') in the pulmonary circulation. Note that it does not pass through zero at the origin since an opening pressure must be overcome before flow starts. Thus the calculated vascular resistance (reciprocal of relationship of flow to pressure, dashed lines) falls (1 → 2) as flow increases. *(Modified from Graham et al: Dopamine, dobutamine and phentolamine effects on pulmonary vascular mechanics. J Appl Physiol 54:1277, 1983.)*

PULMONARY VASCULAR DISEASES

In these conditions the right ventricular afterload is elevated as a consequence of the restriction to pulmonary blood flow. In cor pulmonale secondary to pulmonary vascular disease pulmonary hypertension is usually more severe than in pulmonary parenchymal disease. Chronic cor pulmonale secondary to pulmonary vascular disease may result from repeated pulmonary emboli, pulmonary vasculitis, pulmonary vasoconstriction secondary to high altitude, as well as pulmonary venoocclusive disease. Disorders of pulmonary ventilation causing hypoxemia (Chap. 229) may also cause pulmonary hypertension and cor pulmonale. When the cause of elevated pulmonary vascular resistance is unknown the condition is referred to as *primary pulmonary hypertension* (Chap. 225).

COR PULMONALE DUE TO PULMONARY EMBOLI This condition is associated with two distinct syndromes.

Acute cor pulmonale It has been estimated that in the United States about 50,000 people die each year from embolic pulmonary vascular disease (Chap. 226). Probably half die within the first hour from acute right heart failure due to massive or multiple emboli. A large embolic burden causes a sudden, low-output state resulting from the right ventricle's inability to generate the pressure necessary to drive blood through the acutely compromised pulmonary vascular bed. Depression of cardiac output can also occur with a moderate-sized embolism if the pulmonary circulation has been critically compromised by previous pulmonary vascular or parenchymal disease. The right ventricle begins to fail when systolic pressure suddenly exceeds approximately 40 to 45 mmHg. Acute right ventricular failure secondary to pulmonary embolism is suggested by the history of the sudden onset of severe dyspnea and cardiovascular collapse in a patient with, or predisposed to, venous thrombosis. The low cardiac output causes pallor, sweating, hypotension, and a rapid pulse of small amplitude. The neck veins are distended and often exhibit the prominent *v* waves of tricuspid regurgitation. The liver may be pulsatile, distended, and tender. A systolic murmur of tricuspid regurgitation at the left sternal border may be accompanied by a

TABLE 204-1 Cor pulmonale

Mechanisms	Responses	Characteristics
PULMONARY VASCULAR DISEASES		
Emboli, large or multiple	Fall in output due to acute obstruction	Acute cor pulmonale Right ventricular distention Shock
Emboli, small; vasculitis; widespread lung damage (ARDS)	Pulmonary hypertension due to widespread hypoxia and microvascular obstruction High output	Subacute cor pulmonale Right ventricular distention Breathlessness and fever
Emboli, medium and recurrent; primary pulmonary hypertension; diet or drug vasopathy	Pulmonary hypertension due to vascular obstruction Low or normal output	Chronic cor pulmonale Right heart hypertrophy Breathlessness
RESPIRATORY DISEASES		
Obstructive		
A Chronic bronchitis and emphysema; chronic asthma	Pulmonary hypertension due to hypoxia, vascular stretching and loss Heart beat impeded externally by lung hyperinflation Normal or high output	Chronic cor pulmonale ''Blue bloater'' Underventilation
Restrictive		
A Intrinsic: interstitial fibrosis, lung resection	Hypertension due to hypoxia, vascular distortion and loss Normal or low output	Chronic cor pulmonale Breathlessness Overventilation
B Extrinsic: obesity, myxedema, muscle weakness, kyphoscoliosis, upper airway obstruction, diminished respiratory drive, high altitude	Hypertension due to alveolar hypoxia Normal or high output	Chronic cor pulmonale Peripheral edema Underventilation

presystolic (S_4) gallop sound. Arterial blood gases frequently show hypoxemia due to ventilation/perfusion mismatching and a low Pa_{CO_2} due to hyperventilation. If the cardiac output remains adequate to sustain the patient during the critical first two or three hours, the natural lytic response usually results in fragmentation of the clot so that the patient survives. Although it has been shown that treatment with thrombolytic agents lyses clots more rapidly than does heparin (Chap. 226), this therapy is probably indicated only when blood flow is critically reduced and not improving.

Chronic cor pulmonale secondary to pulmonary vascular disease In contrast to acute, massive thromboembolism, when the elevation in pulmonary vascular resistance and the development of right ventricular hypertrophy are gradual, higher pulmonary vascular pressures, sometimes even exceeding systemic arterial levels, may be generated. Chronic cor pulmonale can be caused by recurrent, medium-sized emboli that fail to lyse, but organize and recanalize. Particles from intravenous drug abuse, parasites, or tumor tissue which embolizes into the pulmonary vascular bed also may cause persistent pulmonary hypertension. Chronic cor pulmonale also can be caused by *primary pulmonary hypertension* (Chap. 225) or any chronic widespread vasculitis, such as occurs in association with the collagen vascular disorders, and that affects the pulmonary vascular bed, particularly the CREST syndrome (Chap. 286).

Symptoms and signs Breathlessness is a characteristic feature of pulmonary hypertension due to pulmonary vascular disease. It may be distressing during even mild exertion, and it is *not* relieved by sitting upright. An unproductive cough is another frequent complaint. Anterior chest pain, due to acute dilation of the root of the pulmonary artery or right ventricular ischemia, can occur. The elevation in systemic venous pressure can cause hepatomegaly and ankle edema.

Patients with pulmonary hypertension and cor pulmonale often have tachypnea that is evident both on mild exertion and at rest, and may even persist during sleep. Occasionally there is cyanosis due to arterial hypoxemia and low cardiac output. A right ventricular heave may be palpable along the left sternal border or in the epigastrium and a high-pitched pulmonary ejection click may be audible to the left of the upper sternum. The second (pulmonary) component of the second heart sound is intensified and may be palpable; fixed splitting of the second heart sound may be present and a right ventricular protodiastolic gallop (S_3) which increases during inspiration may be present. A systolic murmur of tricuspid regurgitation, which is augmented by inspiration (p. 952) is often audible; occasionally, a diastolic murmur of pulmonary regurgitation also is heard. Prominent *a* and *v* waves in the jugular venous pulse are evident. The onset of right ventricular failure is reflected by an increase of venous pressure, the development of larger *v* waves associated with worse tricuspid regurgitation, a hepatojugular reflux, and a gallop rhythm with both third and fourth heart sounds. These physical findings of right ventricular failure may be evanescent and can disappear rapidly when pulmonary artery pressure is suddenly reduced by relief of hypoxemia.

Hypocarbia due to alveolar hyperventilation is an important feature of chronic pulmonary hypertension secondary to pulmonary vascular disease. Usually there are no abnormalities on spirometry, but the ratio of dead space to tidal volume may be high, particularly when large-vessel obstruction is present. The diffusing capacity of the lung is reduced when a capillary vasculitis and/or loss of capillary blood volume is associated with pulmonary vascular disease. Typically, exercise causes a marked fall in Pa_{O_2}. The assessment of exercise capacity may be a useful way of following changes in the severity of pulmonary vascular disease in patients with chronic cor pulmonale because exercise ability is limited by cardiac output and the latter, in turn, by the severity of the pulmonary vascular obstruction.

On *radiologic examination* the pulmonary trunk and hilar vessels are enlarged. Widening of the hilum may be judged from the ratio of the distance between the start of the first divisions of the right and left main pulmonary arteries divided by the transverse diameter of the thorax; a ratio >0.36 suggests pulmonary hypertension. Another radiologic indicator of pulmonary hypertension is widening of the descending right pulmonary artery shadow, from a normal value of <16 mm to >20 mm. Ventilation and perfusion lung scans and systemic venography showing deep vein thrombosis are helpful in confirming the diagnosis of embolic pulmonary vascular disease. In the presence of severe pulmonary hypertension, the ECG shows P pulmonale, right axis deviation, and right ventricular hypertrophy.

Echocardiography allows measurement of the thickness of the right ventricular wall and, although volume changes cannot be measured, this technique can show enlargement of the right ventricular cavity in relation to that of the left. The interventricular septum may be displaced leftward. Right ventricular systolic pressure can be estimated from measurement of the peak tricuspid regurgitant flow and pulmonic regurgitant flow with Doppler echocardiography (Chap. 190).

Magnetic resonance imaging (Chap. 191) is useful for measuring right ventricular mass, wall thickness, cavity volume and ejection fraction.

Failure of the right ventricular ejection fraction (measured by radionuclide ventriculography) to increase on exercise appears to be a good indicator of pulmonary hypertension and/or intrinsic right ventricular dysfunction. Myocardial perfusion scintigraphy with thallium 201 or Sesta-Mibi is also useful for diagnosing cor pulmonale (Chap. 190), since the hypertrophied right ventricle is visualized by these radionuclides. (Normally the right ventricle is not imaged because of the much greater uptake by the left ventricle.)

Cardiac catheterization is necessary for the precise measurement of pulmonary vascular pressures, the determination of pulmonary vascular resistance, and its response to oxygen and vasodilators. Catheterization is sometimes indicated in patients with cor pulmonale to exclude congenital and left heart diseases, and it allows pulmonary angiography to be carried out to confirm the nature of the pulmonary vascular obstruction. Measurements of pulmonary vascular pressures and flow should also be made during exercise to look for abnormal pressure increments or poor responses of cardiac output.

Lung biopsy can be useful in demonstrating vasculitis in some types of pulmonary vascular disease such as the collagen vascular diseases, rheumatoid arthritis, and Wegener's granulomatosis.

PARENCHYMAL PULMONARY DISEASES

Cor pulmonale may be caused by both obstructive and restrictive lung diseases, more frequently the former. In these conditions there are usually only modest elevations of pulmonary artery pressure. The development of cor pulmonale confers a poor prognosis on patients with respiratory disease; in patients with cor pulmonale and right ventricular failure, the 3-year survival is approximately 40 percent. Respiratory diseases causing cor pulmonale are usually associated with distortions of the lung which affect the position of the heart, so that cardiac physical signs are altered.

CHRONIC OBSTRUCTIVE LUNG DISEASE (COLD) (See Chap. 223) This is the most common cause of chronic cor pulmonale. The enlargement of the right ventricle is attributed to the mild-to-moderate pulmonary hypertension which is common in severe obstructive bronchitis and emphysema. Pulmonary artery systolic pressure is typically in the range of 40 to 50 mmHg, far below the systemic levels which appear to be tolerated in patients with congenital heart disease and in those with primary pulmonary hypertension. Patients with cor pulmonale due to COLD usually have an advanced form of the disease with FEV_1 <1.0 L (Chap. 214) and Pa_{O_2} ≤60 mmHg. Right ventricular failure secondary to COLD often occurs when there is "acute-on-chronic" respiratory failure with intensification of hypoxemia.

Pulmonary hypertension in COLD is due to the generalized pulmonary vasoconstriction caused by the alveolar hypoxia, acidemia, and hypercarbia; by the mechanical effects of the high lung volume on the pulmonary vessels; by the loss of small vessels in the vascular bed in regions of emphysema; and sometimes by the increased blood viscosity caused by the associated polycythemia. Of these causes hypoxia is undoubtedly the most important. Pulmonary artery pressure rises further on exercise and often falls acutely on inspiration of 100% O_2. Cardiac output tends to be high in the absence of heart failure if hypoxia and hypercarbia are present. Because of the importance of hypoxic pulmonary vasoconstriction in causing pulmonary hypertension, the hypoventilating "blue bloater" with alveolar hypoxia and hypercarbia more frequently suffers from cor pulmonale than does the emphysematous "pink puffer," without alveolar hypoxia (p. 1201). Ischemic left-heart disease is a frequent accompaniment of patients with cor pulmonale secondary to COLD since they usually have a history of heavy cigarette smoking. The elevation of pulmonary artery pressure may be secondary, in part, to the increase in left atrial pressure resulting from left-heart dysfunction. Almost half of all patients who die with cor pulmonale due to COLD also have left ventricular hypertrophy on postmortem examination.

Right ventricular failure often complicates cor pulmonale when patients with COLD develop ventilatory failure with hypoxia and hypercarbia. When there is a worsening of the airflow due to increasing airway obstruction the resulting hypoxia and hypercarbia may increase cardiac output by their vasodilator effect on the systemic arteriolar bed. Hypoxic pulmonary vasoconstriction is intensified and both supraventricular and ventricular arrhythmias may occur. The liver becomes palpable and tender because it is engorged and displaced downward by the low diaphragm; a hepatojugular reflux may be present.

An exacerbation of airway obstruction elevates intrathoracic pressure, which impedes venous return, raises jugular venous pressure, and may cause peripheral edema, even in the absence of heart failure. This elevation of venous pressure secondary to airway obstruction is *not* associated with an increase in the transmural right ventricular pressure, the hallmark of right ventricular failure. The venous hypertension due to airflow obstruction declines, sometimes very rapidly, with relief of the obstruction.

Pathology In COLD right ventricular hypertrophy increases progressively. The main pulmonary arteries are enlarged and the muscular pulmonary arteries show prominent longitudinal muscle, fibrosis, and elastic changes that continue into the arterioles, where the media also becomes muscularized. The small vessels and capillaries are distorted or disappear in regions of lung hyperinflation.

Symptoms and signs A history of a productive cough and dyspnea, perhaps with wheezing, is frequently elicited. Breathlessness limits the patient's ability in the minor stresses of daily living. Frequently there is a history of emergency hospital admissions because of respiratory infection, sometimes necessitating mechanical ventilation. In breathing oxygen, there may be increasing somnolence or other symptoms of hypercarbia such as recurring headaches, confusion, and even vomiting which, when combined with blurred optic discs (also due to cerebral vasodilation), constitutes the "pseudo tumor cerebri" syndrome. Hypoxia due to hypoventilation is usually worse at night, particularly when severe snoring leads to obstructive apnea (Chap. 217).

Physical findings Often there is nicotine staining of the fingers, a tell-tale sign reflecting many years of heavy cigarette smoking. The skin may be warm and the arterial pulse bounding in the high cardiac output state induced by hypoxia and hypercarbia. The distention of the chest due to the airflow obstruction and the rhonchi and wheezes secondary to chronic bronchitis usually make cardiac auscultation difficult. A right-sided protodiastolic gallop sound (S_3) and a systolic murmur of tricuspid regurgitant may be audible. Signs of right-heart failure are, as discussed above, difficult to separate from those due to severe airflow obstruction. However, a sudden worsening of peripheral edema and rise of systemic venous pressure when atrial fibrillation occurs or when pulmonary infection supervenes is usually considered to be evidence of heart failure. This may be confirmed by the presence of a positive hepatojugular reflux. The distinction is important since patients can survive for years with the high systemic venous pressure and edema secondary to airflow obstruction but usually have a poor prognosis after right-heart failure develops.

Laboratory examinations *Pulmonary function studies* show marked airflow obstruction with hypoxemia and hypercarbia. Exercise is limited by ventilatory rather than cardiac dysfunction until right ventricular failure develops. The *chest roentgenogram* reveals hyperinflation, which makes the degree of right-heart enlargement difficult to assess. The central pulmonary arteries are large but the vessels are narrowed and disappear at the periphery, particularly in regions of the lungs which are markedly emphysematous. The ECG is relatively insensitive in demonstrating right-heart enlargement because the enlarged lungs are poor electrical conductors and the inspiratory position of the chest is associated with a vertically positioned heart. Arrhythmias, particularly atrial fibrillation and multifocal atrial tachycardia, are common.

Echocardiographic imaging is often difficult because of the air in the distended lungs but may reveal an increased cross section of the right ventricular cavity and abnormal thickening of the right ventricular wall. Myocardial perfusion scintigraphy shows an abnormally high ratio of right-to-left ventricular uptake.

Right heart catheterization can be carried out at the bedside with a balloon-tipped, flow-directed, multilumen catheter fitted with thermocouples for measuring cardiac output by thermodilution (Chap. 192). The pulmonary artery wedge pressure is usually normal in patients at rest who have uncomplicated cor pulmonale. Cardiac catheterization may be useful in assessing left ventricular function as well as the severity of the pulmonary hypertension and its response

to respiring oxygen. Pressure measurements during exercise study may be helpful, particularly in excluding left-heart dysfunction.

Treatment First, medical management of the acute and/or chronic lung disease must be optimal (Chaps. 223 and 230). Alveolar hypoxia should be corrected by improving alveolar ventilation through relieving the airflow obstruction and by judiciously increasing the inspired O_2 concentration. Long-term O_2 therapy is helpful in patients with severe COLD and reduces pulmonary artery pressure and pulmonary vascular resistance. When the lung disease improves and pulmonary vasoconstriction secondary to the alveolar hypoxia and hypercarbia are corrected, tachypnea and the signs attributed to right-heart failure are relieved. Bronchodilators and antibiotics lessen the airflow obstruction and diuretics relieve the edema. Loop diuretics must be used with care since they may cause a metabolic alkalosis and thereby blunt the respiratory drive. Digitalis should be used in the presence of overt right ventricular failure, and phlebotomy should be considered when the hematocrit exceeds 55 percent.

RESTRICTIVE LUNG DISEASES Cor pulmonale in restrictive lung disease is associated with two different clinical syndromes: (1) hyperventilation in patients with a variety of restrictive diseases intrinsic to the lungs (Chap. 224), and (2) hypoventilation in patients with extrinsic diseases, such as obesity, myxedema, musculoskeletal disorder, or neuromuscular dysfunction. Pulmonary hypertension is due to a combination of the hypoxemia and to the increased pulmonary vascular resistance resulting from compression of the pulmonary vessels. Again, oxygen is the main treatment, but specific therapy may be available for some of the underlying lung diseases.

REFERENCES

BEHAR JV et al: Performance of new criteria for right ventricular hypertrophy and myocardial infarction in patients with pulmonary hypertension due to cor pulmonale and mitral stenosis. J Electrocardiog 24:231, 1991

CARTER R et al: Altered exercise gas exchange and cardiac function in patients with mild chronic obstructive pulmonary disease. Chest 103:745, 1993

FERGUSON GT, CHERNIACK RM: Management of chronic obstructive pulmonary disease. N Engl J Med 328:1017, 1993

FISHMAN AP: Pulmonary hypertension and cor pulmonale, in *Pulmonary Diseases and Disorders*, 2d ed., AP Fishman (ed). New York, McGraw Hill, 1988, pp 999–1048

KLINGER JR, HILL NS: Right ventricular dysfunction in chronic obstructive pulmonary disease: Evaluation and management. Chest 99:715–23, 1991

McFADDEN ER, BRAUNWALD E: Cor pulmonale and pulmonary thromboembolism, in *Heart Disease*, 4th ed, E Braunwald (ed). Philadelphia, Saunders, 1992, pp 1581–1601

OLIVER RM et al: Right ventricular function at rest and during exercise in chronic obstructive pulmonary disease. 103:74, 1993

PATTYNAMA PMT et al: Early diagnosis of cor pulmonale with MR imaging of the right ventricle. Radiology 182:375, 1992

TRAMARIN R et al: Doppler echocardiographic evaluation of pulmonary artery pressure in chronic obstructive pulmonary disease. A European multicentre study. Eur Heart J 12:103, 1991

WEITZENBLUM E et al: Benefit from long-term O_2 therapy in chronic obstructive pulmonary disease patients. Respiration 59(suppl I):14–117, 1992

205 THE CARDIOMYOPATHIES AND MYOCARDITIDES

JOSHUA WYNNE / EUGENE BRAUNWALD

CARDIOMYOPATHIES

The cardiomyopathies are diseases that involve the myocardium primarily and are not the result of hypertension or congenital, valvular, coronary, arterial, or pericardial abnormalities.* When the

---

* Diffuse myocardial fibrosis secondary to multiple myocardial scars produced by extensive coronary arterial narrowing and occlusion can impair left ventricular function and is frequently referred to as *ischemic cardiomyopathy*. According to the definition given above, however, the term *cardiomyopathy* should be restricted to a condition *primarily* involving heart muscle. In ischemic "cardiomyopathy" the *primary* involvement is in the coronary vessels.

TABLE 205-1 Etiologic classification of cardiomyopathies

PRIMARY MYOCARDIAL INVOLVEMENT

A Idiopathic (D,R,H)
B Familial (D,H)
C Eosinophilic endomyocardial disease (R)
D Endomyocardial fibrosis (R)

SECONDARY MYOCARDIAL INVOLVEMENT

A Infective (D)
  1 Viral myocarditis
  2 Bacterial myocarditis
  3 Fungal myocarditis
  4 Protozoal myocarditis
  5 Metazoal myocarditis
  6 Spirochetal
  7 Rickettsial
B Metabolic (D)
C Familial storage disease (D,R)
  1 Glycogen storage disease
  2 Mucopolysaccharidoses
D Deficiency (D)
  1 Electrolytes
  2 Nutritional
E Connective tissue disorders (D)
  1 Systemic lupus erythematosus
  2 Polyarteritis nodosa
  3 Rheumatoid arthritis
  4 Progressive systemic sclerosis
  5 Dermatomyositis
F Infiltrations and granulomas (R,D)
  1 Amyloidosis
  2 Sarcoidosis
  3 Malignancy
  4 Hemochromatosis
G Neuromuscular (D)
  1 Muscular dystrophy
  2 Myotonic dystrophy
  3 Friedreich's ataxia (H,D)
  4 Refsum's disease
H Sensitivity and toxic reactions (D)
  1 Alcohol
  2 Radiation
  3 Drugs
I Peripartum heart disease (D)
J Endocardial fibroelastosis (R)

NOTE: The principal clinical manifestation(s) of each etiologic grouping is denoted by D (dilated), R (restrictive), or H (hypertrophic) cardiomyopathy.
SOURCE: Adapted from the WHO/ISFC task force report on the definition and classification of cardiomyopathies, 1980.

cardiomyopathies are classified on an etiologic basis, two fundamental forms are recognized: (1) a primary type, consisting of heart muscle disease of unknown cause, and (2) a secondary type, consisting of myocardial disease of known cause or associated with a disease involving other organ systems (Table 205-1). In many cases it is not possible to arrive at a specific etiologic diagnosis, and thus it is often more desirable to classify the cardiomyopathies on the basis of differences in their pathophysiology and clinical presentation (Tables 205-2 and 205-3).

DILATED (CONGESTIVE) CARDIOMYOPATHY In this condition, left and/or right ventricular systolic pump function is impaired, leading to cardiac enlargement and often producing symptoms of congestive heart failure. Mural thrombi are often present, particularly

TABLE 205-2 Clinical classification of cardiomyopathies

1 Dilated (congestive): Left and/or right ventricular enlargement, impaired systolic function, congestive heart failure, arrhythmias, emboli

2 Restrictive: Endomyocardial scarring or myocardial infiltration resulting in restriction to left and/or right ventricular filling

3 Hypertrophic: Disproportionate left ventricular hypertrophy, typically involving septum more than free wall, with or without an intraventricular systolic pressure gradient; usually of a nondilated left ventricular cavity

in the left ventricular apex. Histologic examination reveals extensive areas of interstitial and perivascular fibrosis, with minimal necrosis and cellular infiltration. Although no cause is apparent in many cases, dilated cardiomyopathy probably is the end result of myocardial damage produced by a variety of toxic, metabolic, or infectious agents. There is increasing evidence to suggest that in some patients dilated cardiomyopathy may be the late sequel of acute viral myocarditis, possibly mediated through an immunologic mechanism. Although most commonly a disease of middle-aged men, it may occur in any patient population. A reversible form of dilated cardiomyopathy may be found with alcohol, pregnancy, selenium deficiency, hypophosphatemia, hypocalcemia, and chronic uncontrolled tachycardia. A minority of patients (but probably more than usually suspected) have familial forms of the disease. *Right ventricular dysplasia* is a unique cardiomyopathy marked by progressive replacement of the right ventricular wall with adipose tissue. Often associated with ventricular arrhythmias, the clinical course is variable but sudden death is a constant threat.

Clinical manifestations Symptoms of left- and right-sided congestive failure, manifested by dyspnea on exertion, fatigue, orthopnea, paroxysmal nocturnal dyspnea, peripheral edema, and palpitations, develop gradually in most patients. Some patients have left ventricular dilatation for months or even years before becoming symptomatic. Although vague chest pain may be present, typical angina pectoris is unusual and suggests the presence of concomitant coronary artery disease.

Physical examination Variable degrees of cardiac enlargement and findings of congestive heart failure are noted. In patients with advanced disease, the pulse pressure is narrow, and the jugular venous pressure is elevated. Third and fourth heart sounds are common, and mitral or tricuspid regurgitation may occur. Diastolic murmurs, valvular calcification, and severe hypertension reduce the likelihood of cardiomyopathy.

Laboratory examinations The chest roentgenogram demonstrates left ventricular enlargement, although generalized cardiomegaly often is seen, sometimes due to a concomitant pericardial effusion. The lung fields may demonstrate evidence of pulmonary venous hypertension and interstitial or alveolar edema. The electrocardiogram often shows sinus tachycardia or atrial fibrillation, ventricular arrhythmias, left atrial enlargement, diffuse nonspecific ST-T wave abnormalities, and sometimes intraventricular conduction defects. Echocardiography (see Fig. 190-4) and radionuclide ventriculography (see Fig. 190-8) show left ventricular enlargement, with normal or minimally thickened or thinned walls, and systolic dysfunction (reduced ejection fraction); a pericardial effusion is often noted. Radioisotopic imaging with gallium 67 may identify patients with dilated cardiomyopathy and concomitant myocarditis.

Hemodynamic studies reveal a cardiac output that does not increase normally with exercise. The left ventricular end-diastolic, left atrial, and pulmonary capillary wedge pressures usually are elevated; when failure of the right side of the heart supervenes, the right ventricular end-diastolic, right atrial, and central venous pressures are also elevated. Angiography reveals a dilated, diffusely hypokinetic left ventricle, often with some degree of mitral regurgitation; the coronary arteries are normal, thereby excluding so-called ischemic cardiomyopathy. Transvenous endomyocardial biopsy (Chap. 192) may be helpful in excluding certain conditions such as myocardial infiltration by amyloid; in some patients there is biopsy evidence of myocardial round cell inflammation, suggesting previous viral myocarditis.

Treatment Most patients pursue an inexorably downhill course, and the majority, particularly those over 55 years of age, die within 2 years of the onset of symptoms, but spontaneous improvement or stabilization occurs in a minority. Death is due to either congestive heart failure or ventricular tachy- or bradyarrhythmia; sudden death is a constant threat. Systemic embolization is common, and all patients without contraindications should receive anticoagulants. Strenuous exertion should be interdicted. Treatment of heart failure in dilated cardiomyopathy is directed primarily toward improvement in symp-

TABLE 205-3 Laboratory evaluation of the cardiomyopathies

	Dilated (congestive)	Restrictive	Hypertrophic
Chest roentgenogram	Moderate to marked cardiac enlargement Pulmonary venous hypertension	Mild cardiac enlargement	Mild to moderate cardiac enlargement
Electrocardiogram	ST-segment and T-wave abnormalities	Low voltage, conduction defects	ST-segment and T-wave abnormalities Left ventricular hypertrophy Abnormal Q waves
Echocardiogram	Left ventricular dilatation and dysfunction	Increased left ventricular wall thickness Normal or mildly reduced systolic function	Asymmetric septal hypertrophy (ASH) Systolic anterior motion (SAM) of the mitral valve
Radionuclide studies	Left ventricular dilatation and dysfunction (RVG)	Normal or mildly reduced systolic function (RVG)	Vigorous systolic function (RVG) Asymmetric septal hypertrophy (RVG or ^{201}Tl)
Cardiac catheterization	Left ventricular dilatation and dysfunction Elevated left- and often right-sided filling pressures Diminished cardiac output	Normal or mildly reduced systolic function Elevated left- and right-sided filling pressures	Vigorous systolic function Dynamic left ventricular outflow obstruction Elevated left- and right-sided filling pressures

NOTE: RVG = radionuclide ventriculogram; ^{201}Tl = thallium 201.

toms; an improvement in survival is achieved with angiotensin-converting enzyme inhibitor therapy. Standard therapy of heart failure with salt restriction, diuretics, digitalis, and vasodilators may produce symptomatic improvement. Some patients with dilated cardiomyopathy who have evidence of myocardial inflammation have been treated with immunosuppressive therapy with variable but usually only transient benefit. Others have been treated cautiously with gradually increasing doses of beta-adrenergic blockers with apparent clinical benefit. Antiarrhythmic agents are best avoided for fear of proarrhythmic and other side effects, unless they are needed to treat symptomatic or serious arrhythmias. Alternative therapies, such as surgical interruption of the arrhythmic circuit or implantation of an automatic internal defibrillator, have gained favor. In patients with advanced disease who are refractory to medical therapy and who have no contraindications to the procedure, cardiac transplantation should be considered (Chap. 196).

Alcoholic cardiomyopathy Individuals who consume large quantities of alcohol over many years may develop a clinical picture identical to idiopathic dilated cardiomyopathy; indeed, alcoholic cardiomyopathy is the major form of secondary dilated cardiomyopathy in the western world. Ceasing alcohol consumption before severe heart failure has developed may halt the progression or even reverse the course of this disease, unlike the idiopathic variety, which is marked by progressive deterioration. Alcoholics with advanced heart failure have a poor prognosis, particularly if they continue to drink; less than one-quarter survive 3 years. The key to the treatment of alcoholic cardiomyopathy is total and permanent abstinence. Although thiamine deficiency may be present in some of these patients, alcoholic cardiomyopathy is associated with a low cardiac output and systemic vasoconstriction. In contrast, beriberi heart disease (Chaps. 77 and 207) is characterized by elevated cardiac output and diminished peripheral vascular resistance, so thiamine deficiency per se does not appear to cause alcoholic cardiomyopathy. The toxic effect of alcohol on striated muscle often extends beyond the heart to cause myopathy in skeletal muscles. A second presentation of alcoholic cardiotoxicity may be found in individuals without overt heart failure and consists of recurrent supraventricular or ventricular tachyarrhythmias. Termed the "holiday heart syndrome," it typically appears after a drinking binge; atrial fibrillation is seen most frequently, followed by atrial flutter and ventricular premature depolarizations. Other patients develop left ventricular hypertrophy, perhaps related to concomitant systemic hypertension; they may present with symptoms of pulmonary congestion due to abnormal diastolic stiffness (diminished compliance) of the left ventricle.

Peripartum cardiomyopathy Cardiac dilatation and congestive heart failure of unexplained cause may develop during the last month of pregnancy or within the first few months after delivery. The cause of this disorder is unknown but in some patients endomyocardial biopsy has shown evidence of a myocarditis. Necropsy shows cardiac enlargement, often with mural thrombi, along with histologic evidence of myocardial degeneration and fibrosis. The patient who develops peripartum cardiomyopathy typically is multiparous, black, and over the age of 30. While some patients are malnourished, there is no conclusive evidence that dietary deficiencies are etiologically involved. The symptoms, signs, and treatment are similar to those in patients with idiopathic dilated cardiomyopathy; pulmonary and systemic emboli are particularly common. The mortality rate is quite variable but may be as high as 25 to 50 percent. The prognosis in these patients appears to be closely related to whether the heart size returns to normal after the first episode of congestive heart failure. If it does, subsequent pregnancies may sometimes be well tolerated; if the heart remains enlarged, however, further pregnancies frequently produce increasing myocardial damage, ultimately leading to refractory congestive heart failure and death. Those who recover should be encouraged to avoid further pregnancies, particularly if cardiomegaly persists. Some patients with evidence of myocarditis on biopsy appear to respond to immunosuppressive therapy (although there is a high frequency of spontaneous clinical improvement in this condition).

Neuromuscular disease (See also Chap. 385) Cardiac involvement is common in many of the muscular dystrophies. In *Duchenne's progressive muscular dystrophy*, myocardial involvement is most frequently indicated by a distinctive and unique electrocardiographic pattern consisting of tall R waves in right precordial leads with an R/S ratio greater than 1.0, often associated with deep Q waves in the limb and lateral precordial leads, and is not found in other forms of muscular dystrophy. These electrocardiographic abnormalities appear to result from selective transmural necrosis of the posterobasal left ventricle and associated papillary muscle. A variety of supraventricular and ventricular arrhythmias is frequently found. Rapidly progressive congestive heart failure may develop despite extended periods of apparent circulatory stability during which the only detectable abnormalities are in the electrocardiogram. *Myotonic dystrophy* is characterized by a variety of electrocardiographic abnormalities, especially disorders of impulse formation and particularly conduction, but other overt clinical evidence of heart disease is uncommon. Because of the abnormalities of impulse generation and conduction, syncope and sudden death are major hazards; in appropriate patients, insertion of a permanent pacemaker may be efficacious. In *limb-girdle* and *fascioscapulohumeral dystrophy*, cardiac involvement is uncommon and seldom severe. Involvement of the heart is very common in *Friedreich's ataxia* (manifested by abnormal electrocardiographic or echocardiographic findings), with as many as half the patients developing cardiac symptoms. The electrocardiogram most commonly demonstrates ST-segment and T-wave abnormalities. The echocardiogram may demonstrate left ventricular hypertrophy, with either symmetric or asymmetric hypertrophy of the left ventricular septum compared with the free wall. Although morphologically similar to some cases of hypertrophic cardiomyopathy, cellular disarray is lacking.

Drugs A variety of pharmacologic agents may damage the myocardium acutely, producing a pattern of inflammation (myocarditis), or they may lead to chronic damage of the type seen with idiopathic dilated cardiomyopathy. Certain drugs produce only electrocardiographic abnormalities, while others may precipitate fulminant congestive heart failure and death. The anthracycline derivatives, particularly *doxorubicin* (Adriamycin), are powerful antineoplastic agents which, when given in high doses (more than 550 mg/m^2 for doxorubicin), may produce fatal heart failure. The incidence of heart failure is related not only to the dose of the drug but also to the presence or absence of several risk factors (cardiac irradiation, age greater than 70 years, underlying heart disease, hypertension, treatment with cyclophosphamide); at any dose patients with these risk factors have an eight- to tenfold greater frequency of developing heart failure than do patients lacking them. Radionuclide ventriculography (Chap. 190) may document preclinical deterioration of left ventricular function and allow appropriate dose adjustments; by so monitoring left ventricular function, it is often possible to continue doxorubicin even in patients at high risk for developing heart failure. Recent efforts to modify the dose schedule by giving the drug more slowly have further reduced the risk of cardiotoxicity.

Some patients with congestive heart failure, even those with severe depression of left ventricular function, have demonstrated recovery of cardiac function with aggressive management with digitalis, diuretics, and vasodilators. In others, late asymptomatic contractile dysfunction is common, even in those without initial cardiotoxicity. Children may demonstrate reduced myocardial hypertrophy and mass over time, presumably due to doxorubicin's inhibition of myocardial cell growth. High-dose *cyclophosphamide* may produce congestive heart failure acutely or within 2 weeks of administration; a characteristic histopathologic feature is myocardial edema and hemorrhagic necrosis. Rarely, patients treated with *5-fluorouracil* will develop chest pain and electrocardiographic changes of myocardial ischemia or infarction. Electrocardiographic changes and arrhythmias may result from treatment with tricyclic antidepressants, the phenothiazines, emetine, lithium, and various aerosol propellants. *Cocaine abuse* is associated with a variety of life-threatening cardiac complications, including sudden death, myocarditis, dilated cardiomyopathy, and acute myocardial infarction (resulting from coronary spasm and/or thrombosis with or without underlying coronary artery stenosis). Thrombolytic therapy has been effective in lysing coronary thrombi in patients with acute myocardial infarction. Nitrates and calcium antagonists have been used as well to treat a variety of cocaine-induced cardiotoxicities.

RESTRICTIVE CARDIOMYOPATHY The hallmark of the restrictive cardiomyopathies is abnormal diastolic function; the ventricular walls are excessively rigid and impede ventricular filling. Myocardial fibrosis, hypertrophy, or infiltration due to a variety of causes is usually responsible. The infiltrative diseases, which represent important causes for secondary restrictive cardiomyopathy, also may show some impairment of systolic function. Myocardial involvement with *amyloid* is a common cause of secondary restrictive cardiomyopathy, although restriction is also seen in hemochromatosis, glycogen deposition, endomyocardial fibrosis, fibroelastosis, the eosinophilias, neoplastic infiltration, and myocardial fibrosis of diverse causes. In many of these conditions, particularly those with substantial concomitant endocardial involvement, partial obliteration of the

ventricular cavity by fibrous tissue and thrombus contributes to the abnormally increased resistance to ventricular filling. As a result of persistently elevated venous pressure, these patients commonly have dependent edema, ascites, and an enlarged, tender liver. The jugular venous pressure is elevated and does not fall normally, or it may rise with inspiration (Kussmaul's sign). The heart sounds may be distant, and third and fourth heart sounds are common. In contrast to constrictive pericarditis, which these diseases resemble, the apex impulse is usually easily palpable, and mitral regurgitation is more common. The electrocardiogram shows low-voltage, nonspecific ST-T-wave changes and various arrhythmias. Pericardial calcification on x-ray, which would suggest constrictive pericarditis, is absent. Echocardiography typically reveals symmetrically thickened left ventricular walls and normal or slightly reduced systolic function. Doppler recordings demonstrate accentuated early diastolic filling. Cardiac catheterization shows a decreased cardiac output, elevation of the right and left ventricular end-diastolic pressures, and a dip-and-plateau configuration of the diastolic portion of the ventricular pressure pulse resembling that seen in constrictive pericarditis.

Differentiation from constrictive pericarditis, at the bedside and even after cardiac catheterization, may be difficult or impossible (Chaps. 192 and 206.) This distinction is of importance because the latter condition is potentially curable by operation. Helpful in the differentiation of these two diseases are right ventricular transvenous endomyocardial biopsy (by revealing interstitial infiltration or fibrosis in restrictive cardiomyopathy) and computed tomography or magnetic resonance imaging (by demonstrating a thickened pericardium in constrictive pericarditis).

Endomyocardial fibrosis This is a progressive disease of unknown cause that occurs most commonly in children and young adults residing in tropical and subtropical Africa, particularly Uganda and Nigeria. The disease is characterized by fibrous endocardial lesions of the inflow portion of the right or left ventricle (or both) and often involves the atrioventricular valves, producing valvular regurgitation. The apex of the ventricles may be obliterated by a mass of thrombus and fibrous tissue. In many ways this disease resembles eosinophilic endomyocardial disease, although they occur in quite different geographic areas and age groups. Endomyocardial fibrosis is a frequent cause of heart failure in Africa, accounting for up to one-quarter of deaths due to heart disease.

The clinical picture depends on which ventricle and atrioventricular valve show predominant involvement; left-sided involvement results in symptoms of pulmonary congestion, while predominant right-sided disease presents features of a restrictive cardiomyopathy. Medical treatment is often disappointing, and surgical excision of the fibrotic endocardium and replacement of the involved atrioventricular valve have led to substantial symptomatic improvement in a small number of patients.

Eosinophilic endomyocardial disease Also called *Loeffler's endocarditis* and *fibroplastic endocarditis*, this disease appears to be a subcategory of the hypereosinophilic syndrome in which the heart is predominantly involved, with cardiac damage the apparent result of the toxic effects of eosinophilic proteins. Typically, the endocardium of either or both ventricles thickens markedly, with involvement of the underlying myocardium. Large mural thrombi may develop in either ventricle, thereby compromising the size of the ventricular cavity and serving as a source of pulmonary and systemic emboli. Hepatosplenomegaly and localized eosinophilic infiltration of other organs are usually present. Routine management with digitalis, diuretics, afterload-reducing agents, and anticoagulation as indicated, in conjunction with glucocorticoids and cytotoxic drugs (hydroxyurea in particular), appears to have improved survival substantially.

Differential diagnosis Involvement of the heart is the most frequent cause of death in *primary amyloidosis* (Chap. 281), while clinically significant cardiac involvement is uncommon in the secondary form. Focal deposits of amyloid in elderly patients (*senile cardiac amyloidosis*) are common and usually clinically insignificant. In a minority of patients the clinical cardiac findings are identical to those of primary amyloidosis, the principal difference being the structural composition of the amyloid protein. Aspiration of abdominal fat or biopsy of the rectal mucosa, gingiva, liver, kidney, or myocardium permits the diagnosis to be made before death in over three-quarters of cases. The heart is firm, rubbery, and noncompliant, and four clinical presentations (alone or in combination) are seen: (1) diastolic dysfunction (restrictive cardiomyopathy), (2) systolic dysfunction, (3) arrhythmias, and (4) orthostatic hypotension. The two-dimensional echocardiogram may be helpful in making the diagnosis of amyloidosis and may show a thickened myocardial wall with a distinctive "speckled" appearance. *Hemochromatosis* (Chap. 345) should be suspected if cardiomyopathy occurs in the setting of diabetes mellitus, hepatic cirrhosis, and increased skin pigmentation. Phlebotomy may be of some benefit if employed early in the course of the disease. Continuous subcutaneous administration of deferoxamine may reduce body iron stores and result in clinical improvement. Myocardial *sarcoidosis* (Chap. 292) is generally associated with other manifestations of systemic disease and may have restrictive as well as congestive features, since cardiac infiltration by sarcoid granulomas results not only in increased stiffness of the myocardium but also in diminished systolic contractile function. A variety of arrhythmias, including atrioventricular block, have been noted.

HYPERTROPHIC CARDIOMYOPATHY   This disease is characterized by left ventricular hypertrophy, typically of a nondilated chamber, without obvious antecedent cause. The hypertrophy is thus not secondary to a cardiovascular or systemic disease, such as hypertension or aortic stenosis, that places a hemodynamic burden on the left ventricle. Two commonly found features of the disease have attracted the greatest attention: (1) heterogeneous left ventricular (LV) hypertrophy, often with asymmetric septal hypertrophy (ASH), wherein the upper portion of the interventricular septum is preferentially hypertrophied compared with the posterobasal left ventricular free wall, and (2) a dynamic left ventricular outflow tract pressure gradient, related to a narrowing of the subaortic area as a consequence of the midsystolic apposition of the anterior mitral valve leaflet against the hypertrophied septum, i.e., systolic anterior motion of the mitral valve (SAM). Initial studies of this disease emphasized the dynamic "obstructive" features, and it has been termed *idiopathic hypertrophic subaortic stenosis* (IHSS), *hypertrophic obstructive cardiomyopathy* (HOCM), and *muscular subaortic stenosis*. It has become clear, however, that only about one-quarter of patients with hypertrophic cardiomyopathy demonstrate an outflow tract gradient. The ubiquitous pathophysiologic abnormality is not systolic but rather *diastolic* dysfunction, characterized by increased stiffness of the hypertrophied muscle that results primarily from an abnormality in calcium handling with attendant intracellular calcium overload. This results in elevated diastolic filling pressures and is present despite a hyperdynamic left ventricle.

The pattern of hypertrophy is distinctive in hypertrophic cardiomyopathy and differs from that seen in secondary hypertrophy (as in hypertension). Most patients have striking regional variations in the extent of hypertrophy in different portions of the left ventricle, and the majority demonstrate a ventricular septum whose thickness is disproportionately increased when compared with the free wall. Other patients may demonstrate disproportionate involvement of the apex or left ventricular free wall; 10 percent or more of patients have concentric involvement of the ventricle. All, however, show a bizarre and disorganized arrangement of cardiac muscle cells in the septum, whether or not a gradient is present, along with a variable degree of myocardial fibrosis and abnormalities of the small intramural coronary arteries.

About half of all cases of hypertrophic cardiomyopathy are familially linked, and many are associated with one of several mutations of the beta cardiac myosin heavy chain gene on chromosome 14, with certain mutations associated with more malignant prognoses. The remainder of familial cases presumably are due to mutations of a different gene or genes. Echocardiographic studies have confirmed that about one-third of the first-degree relatives (i.e.,

parents, siblings, and children) of patients with familial hypertrophic cardiomyopathy have evidence of the disease, although in many of these patients the extent of hypertrophy is mild, no outflow tract pressure gradient is present, and symptoms are not prominent. Since the hypertrophic characteristics may not be apparent in childhood and only first appear in adolescence, a single normal echocardiogram in a child does not entirely exclude the presence of the disease. Genetic analysis of peripheral lymphocytes can identify the disease in subjects who demonstrate none of the gross morphologic features of the disease.

In contrast to the obstruction produced by a fixed narrowed orifice, such as valvular aortic stenosis, the pressure gradient in hypertrophic cardiomyopathy, when present, is dynamic and may change between examinations and even from beat to beat. Obstruction appears to result from further narrowing of an already small left ventricular outflow tract by systolic anterior motion of the mitral valve against the hypertrophied septum. While SAM may be found in a variety of other conditions besides hypertrophic cardiomyopathy, it is *always* found when obstruction is present in hypertrophic cardiomyopathy. Three basic mechanisms are involved in the production of the dynamic pressure gradient: (1) increased left ventricular contractility, which reduces ventricular systolic volume and increases the ejection velocity of the blood moving through the outflow tract, thus drawing the anterior mitral valve leaflet against the septum as a result of reduced distending pressure, (2) decreased ventricular volume (preload), which reduces further the size of the outflow tract, and (3) decreased aortic impedance and pressure (afterload), which increases the velocity of flow through the subaortic area and also reduces ventricular systolic volume. Interventions that increase myocardial contractility, such as exercise, isoproterenol, and digitalis glycosides, and those that reduce ventricular volume, such as the Valsalva maneuver, sudden standing, nitroglycerin, amyl nitrite, or tachycardia, all may cause an increase in the gradient and the murmur. Conversely, elevation of arterial pressure by phenylephrine, squatting, sustained handgrip, augmentation of venous return by passive leg raising, and expansion of the blood volume all increase ventricular volume and ameliorate the gradient and murmur.

Clinical features   Many patients with hypertrophic cardiomyopathy are asymptomatic and may be relatives of patients with known disease. Unfortunately, the first clinical manifestation of the disease may be sudden death, frequently occurring in children and young adults, often during or after physical exertion. In symptomatic patients, the most common complaint is dyspnea, largely due to increased stiffness of the left ventricular walls, which impairs ventricular filling and leads to elevated left ventricular diastolic and left atrial pressures. Other symptoms include angina pectoris, fatigue, syncope, and near-syncope ("graying-out spells"). Symptoms are not related to the presence or severity of an outflow gradient. Most patients with gradients demonstrate a double or triple apical impulse, a rapidly rising carotid arterial pulse, and a fourth heart sound. The hallmark of obstructive hypertrophic cardiomyopathy is a systolic murmur, which is typically harsh, diamond-shaped, and usually begins well after the first heart sound, since ejection is unimpeded early in systole. The murmur is best heard at the lower left sternal border as well as at the apex, where it is often more holosystolic and blowing in quality, no doubt due to the mitral regurgitation that usually accompanies obstructive hypertrophic cardiomyopathy.

Laboratory evaluation   The *electrocardiogram* commonly shows left ventricular hypertrophy and widespread, deep, broad Q waves that suggest an old myocardial infarction. Many patients demonstrate arrhythmias, both atrial (supraventricular tachycardia or atrial fibrillation) and ventricular (ventricular tachycardia), during ambulatory (Holter) monitoring. *Chest roentgenography* may be normal, although a mild to moderate increase in the cardiac silhouette is common. The mainstay of the diagnosis of hypertrophic cardiomyopathy is the *echocardiogram*, which demonstrates left ventricular hypertrophy, often with the septum 1.3 or more times the thickness of the high posterior left ventricular free wall. The septum may demonstrate an unusual ground glass appearance, probably related to its abnormal cellular architecture and myocardial fibrosis. Systolic anterior motion of the mitral valve is found in patients with pressure gradients. The left ventricular cavity typically is small in hypertrophic cardiomyopathy, with vigorous posterior wall motion but reduced septal excursion. A rare form of hypertrophic cardiomyopathy, characterized by apical hypertrophy, is often associated with giant negative T waves on the electrocardiogram and a "spade-shaped" left ventricular cavity on angiography, and usually has a benign clinical course. *Radionuclide scintigraphy* with thallium 201 frequently reveals evidence of myocardial perfusion defects even in asymptomatic patients.

The two typical *hemodynamic* features are an elevated left ventricular diastolic pressure due to diminished left ventricular compliance and, when obstruction is present, a systolic pressure gradient between the body of the left ventricle and the subaortic region. When a gradient is not present, it often can be induced by provocative maneuvers such as infusion of isoproterenol, inhalation of amyl nitrite, or the Valsalva maneuver.

Treatment Beta-adrenergic blockers often are used and may ameliorate to some degree the symptoms of angina pectoris and syncope in one-third to one-half of patients. Resting intraventricular pressure gradients usually are unchanged, although these drugs may limit the increase in the gradient that occurs during exercise. It is not known whether beta-adrenergic blockers offer any protection against sudden death, which presumably is arrhythmic in origin. It is not established whether any antiarrhythmic agent is efficacious in this setting. However, amiodarone appears to be effective in reducing the frequency of supraventricular as well as life-threatening ventricular arrhythmias. Verapamil and diltiazem may reduce the stiffness of the ventricle, reduce the elevated diastolic pressures, increase exercise tolerance, and, in some instances, reduce the severity of outflow tract gradients, although adverse side effects occur in about one-quarter of patients. Disopyramide has been used in some patients to reduce left ventricular contractility and the outflow gradient. Dual-chamber permanent pacing recently has gained favor because it improves symptoms and reduces the outflow gradient in patients with severe symptoms, presumably by altering the pattern of ventricular contraction. Surgical myotomy/myectomy of the hypertrophied septum may result in lasting symptomatic improvement in about three-quarters of operated patients, but the mortality of approximately 5 percent limits the operation to severely symptomatic patients with large pressure gradients who are unresponsive to medical management. Digitalis, diuretics, nitrates, and beta-adrenergic agonists are best avoided if possible, particularly in patients with known left ventricular outflow tract pressure gradients.

Prognosis The natural history of hypertrophic cardiomyopathy is variable, although many patients demonstrate an improvement or stabilization of symptoms with time. Atrial fibrillation is common late in the course of the disease; its onset may lead to an increase in symptoms, presumably due to loss of the atrial contribution to filling of the thickened ventricle. Infective endocarditis occurs in less than 10 percent of patients, and endocarditis prophylaxis is indicated, particularly in patients with resting obstruction and mitral regurgitation. Progression of hypertrophic cardiomyopathy to left ventricular dilatation and dysfunction without an outflow gradient has been reported but is unusual; in about 5 to 10 percent of patients, however, some degree of left ventricular systolic impairment, wall thinning, and chamber enlargement occurs over time. The major cause of mortality in hypertrophic cardiomyopathy is sudden death, which may occur in asymptomatic patients or interrupt an otherwise stable course in symptomatic ones. Predictors of sudden death include age less than 30 years, ventricular tachycardia on ambulatory monitoring, marked ventricular hypertrophy, syncope, and a family history of sudden death. There is no correlation between the risk of sudden death and the severity of symptoms or the presence or severity of an outflow tract pressure gradient. Since sudden death often occurs during or just after physical exertion, strenuous exercise should be avoided in all patients, regardless of symptoms. Hemodynamic factors

appear to play a role. It is likely that most deaths, particularly those that are sudden, are due to ventricular arrhythmias.

MYOCARDITIDES

Myocarditis is said to be present when the heart is involved in an inflammatory process. Most commonly the result of an infectious process, myocarditis also may be present in hypersensitivity states such as acute rheumatic fever (Chap. 200) or may be caused by radiation, chemicals, physical agents, and drugs. In an unknown number of cases, acute myocarditis progresses to chronic dilated cardiomyopathy. While almost every infectious agent is capable of producing myocarditis, clinically significant acute myocarditis in the United States is caused most commonly by viruses, especially coxsackievirus B. In most cases the clinical manifestations are nonspecific (fatigue, dyspnea), and the presence of myocarditis is inferred only by the finding of transient electrocardiographic ST-T-wave abnormalities, but arrhythmias, heart failure, and death may occur in fulminant cases, particularly in infants and pregnant women. In some patients myocarditis simulates acute myocardial infarction, with chest pain, electrocardiographic changes, and elevated serum levels of myocardial enzymes.

Physical examination may be normal in patients who have only electrocardiographic abnormalities, although more severe cases may show a muffled first heart sound, along with a third heart sound and a murmur of mitral regurgitation. A pericardial friction rub may be audible in patients with associated pericarditis.

Experimental studies suggest that exercise may be deleterious in patients with myocarditis, and strenuous activity should be proscribed until the electrocardiogram has returned to normal. Patients who develop congestive heart failure respond to the usual measures (digitalis, diuretics, salt restriction), but they appear to be unusually sensitive to digitalis. Arrhythmias are common and are occasionally difficult to manage. Deaths attributed to heart failure, tachyarrhythmias, and heart block have been reported, and it seems prudent to monitor the electrocardiogram of patients with arrhythmias, especially during the acute illness.

Though viral myocarditis is most often self-limited and without sequelae, severe involvement may recur, and it is likely that acute viral myocarditis occasionally progresses to a chronic form. Patients with viral myocarditis often give a history of a preceding upper respiratory febrile illness, and viral nasopharyngitis or tonsillitis may be evident clinically. The isolation of virus from the stool, pharyngeal washings, or other body fluids and changes in specific antibody titers are helpful clinically. Some instances of apparent *idiopathic* dilated cardiomyopathy (p. 1089) appear to arise from mild or subclinical episodes of myocarditis. While glucocorticoids may exacerbate heart damage in animals with acute viral myocarditis, a small number of patients with congestive heart failure and inflammatory myocarditis appear to have responded to immunosuppression. Serial right ventricular endomyocardial biopsies have shown regression of inflammatory infiltrates in some patients so treated. However, such therapy remains experimental at present.

Bacterial myocarditis Bacterial involvement of the heart is uncommon, but when it does occur, it is usually as a complication of bacterial endocarditis (typically due to *Staphylococcus aureus* and enterococci). Myocardial abscess formation may involve the valve rings and interventricular septum. *Diphtheritic myocarditis* develops in over one-quarter of the patients with diphtheria, is one of the most serious complications, and is the most common cause of death due to diphtheria (Chap. 104). Cardiac damage is due to the liberation of a toxin that inhibits protein synthesis and leads to a dilated, flabby, hypocontractile heart; the conducting system is frequently involved as well. Cardiomegaly and severe congestive heart failure typically appear after the first week of illness. Prompt therapy with antitoxin is crucial; antibiotic therapy is also indicated but is of less urgency.

Chagas' disease Chagas' disease, caused by the protozoan *Trypanosoma cruzi* and transmitted by an insect vector (Chap. 176), produces an extensive myocarditis that typically becomes evident years after the initial infection. It is one of the most common causes of heart disease encountered in Central and South America; in rural areas up to 20 percent of the population may be affected. An increasing number of cases are found in the United States as patients migrate from endemic areas. Although only a minority of infected individuals have an acute illness, upwards of one-third develop chronic myocardial damage. Electrocardiographic evidence of cardiac involvement may appear in adolescence, although symptoms often do not appear until adulthood. The chronic form is characterized by dilatation of several cardiac chambers, fibrosis and thinning of the ventricular wall, aneurysm formation in the areas of thinning (especially at the apex), and mural thrombi. Chronic progressive heart failure is the rule and is associated with reduced survival. The electrocardiogram typically shows right bundle branch block and left anterior hemiblock, which may progress to complete atrioventricular block. The echocardiogram may reveal a unique pattern of hypokinesis of the posterior left ventricular wall and relatively preserved septal motion. Ventricular arrhythmias are common and are seen especially during and after exertion; oral amiodarone appears to be particularly effective in treating ventricular tachyarrhythmias. The cause of death is either intractable congestive heart failure or an arrhythmia. Therapy is directed toward amelioration of the congestive heart failure and arrhythmias; progressive conduction system disease and heart block may require implantation of a pacemaker. Medical therapy is often unsatisfactory or unavailable, however, and a more promising tactic has been the institution of public health measures, particularly the use of insecticides to eliminate the vector.

Toxoplasmic myocarditis (See also Chap. 177)   This uncommon form of protozoal myocardial involvement occurs most frequently in immunosuppressed adults; congenital toxoplasmal infections are much more common, but myocarditis is not a prominent feature. Myocardial involvement may lead to cardiac dilatation, pericarditis, and pericardial effusion. Heart failure, arrhythmias, and conduction abnormalities may be seen. Because of the difficulty in diagnosing this condition, it may be a more common problem than is usually appreciated. Treatment is with pyrimethamine and sulfonamides, but the response to treatment is variable.

Giant cell myocarditis   This rare myocarditis of unknown cause is characterized by the presence of multinucleated giant cells in the myocardium. It usually causes rapidly fatal congestive heart failure and arrhythmia in young to middle-aged adults. At necropsy, the distinctive features include cardiac enlargement, ventricular thrombi, grossly visible serpiginous areas of myocardial necrosis in both ventricles, and microscopic evidence of giant cells within an extensive inflammatory infiltrate. The cause of giant cell myocarditis remains obscure, although it occurs in association with thymoma, systemic lupus erythematosus, and thyrotoxicosis. No therapy has been shown to be efficacious.

Lyme carditis (See also Chap. 137)   Lyme disease is caused by a tick-borne spirochete and is most common in the Northeast, upper Midwest and Pacific Coastal regions of the United States during the summer months. About 10 percent of patients develop symptomatic cardiac involvement, with conduction abnormalities the most common manifestations. Concomitant myopericarditis is not uncommon, and mild asymptomatic left ventricular dysfunction may occur. Intravenous ceftriaxone or penicillin is used in all but the mildest forms of Lyme carditis, in which case oral amoxicillin or doxycycline is employed. A temporary pacemaker may be needed for symptomatic heart block; the utility of glucocorticoids in reversing heart block is uncertain, but they are usually employed.

Human immunodeficiency virus myocarditis   Many HIV-infected patients have subclinical cardiac involvement, including pericardial effusion, right-sided chamber enlargement, and neoplastic involvement. The most common finding is left ventricular dysfunction, often due to myocarditis, that in some cases appears to be due to infiltration of the myocardium by the virus itself. The clinical manifestations of cardiac involvement may be incorrectly attributed to concurrent noncardiac problems such as pneumonia. This is unfortunate, since the dilated cardiomyopathy of HIV infection may respond at least transiently to standard therapy with digitalis, diuretics, and vasodilators.

REFERENCES

Cohn LH et al: Long-term follow-up of patients undergoing myotomy/myectomy for obstructive hypertrophic cardiomyopathy. Am J Cardiol 70:657, 1992

Fananapazir L et al: Impact of dual-chamber permanent pacing in patients with obstructive hypertrophic cardiomyopathy with symptoms refractory to verapamil and β-adrenergic blocker therapy. Circulation 85:2149, 1992

Friman G, Fohlman J: The epidemiology of viral heart disease. Scand J Infect Dis Suppl 88:7, 1993

Gilbert EM et al: Beta-adrenergic receptor regulation and left ventricular function in idiopathic dilated cardiomyopathy. Am J Cardiol 71:23C, 1993

Gwathmey JK et al: Diastolic dysfunction in hypertrophic cardiomyopathy. J Clin Invest 87:1023, 1991

Hagar JM, Rahimtoola SH: Chagas' heart disease in the United States. N Engl J Med 325:763, 1991

Jacob AJ et al: Effects of abstinence on alcoholic heart muscle disease. Am J Cardiol 68:805, 1991

Kloner RA et al: The effects of acute and chronic cocaine use on the heart. Circulation 85:407, 1992

Larsen L et al: Sudden death in idiopathic dilated cardiomyopathy: Role of ventricular arrhythmias. PACE Pacing Clin Electrophysiol 16:1051, 1993

Manolio TA et al: Prevalence and etiology of idiopathic dilated cardiomyopathy (summary of a National Heart, Lung, and Blood Institute workshop). Am J Cardiol 69:1458, 1992

Midei MG et al: Peripartum myocarditis and cardiomyopathy. Circulation 81:922, 1990

Narula J et al: Recognition of acute myocarditis masquerading as acute myocardial infarction. N Engl J Med 328:100, 1993

Watkins H et al: Characteristics and prognostic implications of myosin missense mutations in familial hypertrophic cardiomyopathy. N Engl J Med 326:1108, 1992

Wynne J, Braunwald E: The cardiomyopathies and myocarditides: Toxic, chemical and physical damage to the heart, in *Heart Disease*, 4th ed, E Braunwald (ed). Philadelphia, Saunders, 1992, pp 1394–1450

206   PERICARDIAL DISEASE

EUGENE BRAUNWALD

NORMAL FUNCTIONS OF THE PERICARDIUM   The visceral pericardium is a serous membrane which is separated by a small amount (15 to 50 mL) of fluid, an ultrafiltrate of plasma, from a fibrous sac, the parietal pericardium. The pericardium prevents sudden dilatation of the cardiac chambers during exercise and hypervolemia, and as the result of the development of a negative intrapericardial pressure during ejection, it facilitates atrial filling during ventricular systole. The pericardium also restricts the anatomic position of the heart, minimizes friction between the heart and surrounding structures, prevents displacement of the heart and kinking of the great vessels, and probably retards the spread of infections from the lungs and pleural cavities to the heart. Notwithstanding the foregoing, total absence of the pericardium does not produce obvious clinical disease. In partial left pericardial defects the main pulmonary artery and left atrium may bulge through the defect; very rarely, herniation and subsequent strangulation of the left atrium may cause sudden death.

ACUTE PERICARDITIS

It is useful to classify the types of pericarditis both clinically and etiologically (Table 206-1), since this disorder is by far the most common pathologic process involving the pericardium. Pain, a pericardial friction rub, electrocardiographic changes, and pericardial effusion with cardiac tamponade and paradoxic pulse are cardinal

TABLE 206-1 Classification of pericarditis

I Clinical classification
  A Acute pericarditis (<6 weeks)
    1 Fibrinous
    2 Effusive (or bloody)
  B Subacute pericarditis (6 weeks to 6 months)
    1 Constrictive
    2 Effusive-constrictive
  C Chronic pericarditis (>6 months)
    1 Constrictive
    2 Effusive
    3 Adhesive (nonconstrictive)
II Etiologic classification
  A Infectious pericarditis
    1 Viral
    2 Pyogenic
    3 Tuberculous
    4 Mycotic
    5 Other infections (syphilitic, parasitic)
  B Noninfectious pericarditis
    1 Acute myocardial infarction
    2 Uremia
    3 Neoplasia
      a Primary tumors (benign or malignant)
      b Tumors metastatic to pericardium
    4 Myxedema
    5 Cholesterol
    6 Chylopericardium
    7 Trauma
      a Penetrating chest wall
      b Nonpenetrating
    8 Aortic aneurysm (with leakage into pericardial sac)
    9 Postirradiation
    10 Associated with atrial septal defect
    11 Associated with severe chronic anemia
    12 Infectious mononucleosis
    13 Familial Mediterranean fever
    14 Familial pericarditis
      a Mulibrey nanism*
    15 Sarcoidosis
    16 Acute idiopathic
  C Pericarditis presumably related to hypersensitivity or autoimmunity
    1 Rheumatic fever
    2 Collagen vascular disease
      a Systemic lupus erythematosus
      b Rheumatoid arthritis
      c Scleroderma
    3 Drug-induced
      a Procainamide
      b Hydralazine
      c Other
    4 Postcardiac injury
      a Postmyocardial infarction (Dressler's syndrome)
      b Postpericardiotomy

* An autosomal recessive syndrome, characterized by growth failure, muscle hypotonia, hepatomegaly, ocular changes, enlarged cerebral ventricles, mental retardation, and chronic constrictive pericarditis.

manifestations of many forms of acute pericarditis and will be considered prior to a discussion of the most common forms of the disorder.

Chest pain is an important but not invariable symptom in various forms of acute pericarditis (Chap. 12); it is usually present in the acute infectious types and in many of the forms presumed to be related to hypersensitivity or autoimmunity. Pain is often absent in a slowly developing tuberculous, postirradiation, neoplastic, or uremic pericarditis. The pain of pericarditis is often severe. It is characteristically retrosternal and left precordial, referred to the back and the trapezius ridge. Often the pain is pleuritic consequent to accompanying pleural inflammation, i.e., sharp and aggravated by inspiration, coughing, and changes in body position, but sometimes it is a steady, constrictive pain which radiates into either arm or both arms and resembles that of myocardial ischemia; therefore, confusion with myocardial infarction is common. Characteristically, however, the pericardial pain may be relieved by sitting up and leaning forward. The differentiation of acute myocardial infarction from acute pericarditis becomes even more perplexing when, with acute pericarditis, the serum transaminase and creatine kinase levels rise, presumably

because of concomitant involvement of the epicardium. However, these enzyme elevations, if they occur, are quite modest, given the extensive electrocardiographic ST-segment elevation in pericarditis.

The *pericardial friction rub* is the most important physical sign; it may have up to three components per cardiac cycle and is high-pitched, scratching, and grating, as described in Chap. 188; it can sometimes be elicited only when firm pressure with the diaphragm of the stethoscope is applied to the chest wall at the left lower sternal border. It is heard most frequently during expiration with the patient in the sitting position, but an independent pleural friction rub may be audible during inspiration with the patient leaning forward or in the left lateral decubitus position. The rub is often inconstant and transitory, and a loud to-and-fro leathery sound may disappear within a few hours, possibly to reappear the following day.

Moderate elevations of the MB fraction of creatine phosphokinase may occur and reflect accompanying epimyocarditis.

The *electrocardiogram* in acute pericarditis without massive effusion usually displays changes secondary to acute subepicardial inflammation (see Fig. 189-19, p. 964). There is widespread elevation of the ST segments, involving two or three standard limb leads and V_2 to V_6, with reciprocal depressions only in aVR and sometimes V_1 and without significant changes in QRS complexes, except for some reduction in voltage in patients with large pericardial effusions. After several days, the ST segments return to normal, and only then do the T waves become inverted. In contrast, in acute myocardial infarction, reciprocal depression of ST segments is usually more prominent; QRS changes occur, particularly the development of Q waves, as well as notching and loss of the amplitude of R waves; and T-wave inversions usually occur within hours *before* the ST segments have become isoelectric. Sequential electrocardiograms are useful in distinguishing acute pericarditis from acute myocardial infarction. In the latter, elevated ST segments return to normal within hours. Early repolarization is a normal variant and also may cause widespread ST-segment elevation, most prominent in left precordial leads. However, in this condition the T waves are usually tall and the ST/T ratio is under 0.25, but it exceeds this number in acute pericarditis. Depression of the PQ segment (below the TP segment) also is common and reflects atrial involvement. With large pericardial effusions, the QRS voltage is reduced; atrial premature beats and atrial fibrillation are sometimes noted.

PERICARDIAL EFFUSION Usually associated with pain and/or the above-mentioned electrocardiographic changes characteristic of pericarditis and an enlargement of the cardiac silhouette, pericardial effusion is especially important clinically when it develops within a relatively short time, since it may lead to cardiac tamponade. Differentiation from cardiac enlargement may be difficult, but heart sounds tend to become faint; the friction rub may disappear or remain clearly audible, and the apex impulse may vanish, but sometimes it remains palpable albeit medial to the left border of cardiac dullness. The base of the left lung may be compressed by pericardial fluid, producing Ewart's sign, a patch of dullness beneath the angle of the left scapula. The chest roentgenogram may show a "water bottle" configuration of the cardiac silhouette, but it also may be normal or almost so. Lucent pericardial fat lines may be seen deep within the cardiopericardial silhouette. Fluoroscopic examination may show the ventricular pulsations to be diminished.

Diagnosis of pericardial effusion Echocardiography (Chap. 190) is the most effective diagnostic laboratory technique available, since it is sensitive, specific, simple, innocuous, noninvasive, and may be performed at the bedside. The presence of pericardial fluid is recorded by two-dimensional transthoracic echocardiography as a relatively echo-free space between the posterior pericardium and left ventricular epicardium in patients with small effusions and a space between the anterior right ventricle and the parietal pericardium just beneath the anterior chest wall with larger effusions (Fig. 206-1). In patients with large effusions the heart may swing freely within the pericardial sac; when severe, the extent of this motion alternates and may be associated with electrical alternans. Echocardiography

FIGURE 206-1 Two-dimensional (*upper panel*) and short-axis (*lower panel*) parasternal scans in systole in a patient with a large pericardial effusion surrounding the entire heart. Fluid is seen to extend behind the left atrium (*white arrowhead*) and anterior to the descending thoracic aorta (DA). AoV = aortic valve; LA = left atrium; LV = left ventricle; PE = pericardial effusion; RV = right ventricle. (*Modified from PC Come (ed), Diagnostic Cardiology: Noninvasive imaging techniques, Philadelphia, Lippincott, 1985.*)

also allows localization and estimation of the quantity of pericardial fluid. When pericardial effusion causes tamponade, during inspiration right ventricular diameter increases while left ventricular diameter and mitral valve opening decrease. Often the right ventricular cavity is reduced and there is late diastolic inward motion (collapse) of the right ventricular free wall and of the right atrium. Doppler ultrasound shows exaggerated tricuspid and pulmonic flow with reciprocal changes in mitral flow during inspiration. The diagnosis of pericardial fluid or thickening may be confirmed by computed tomography or magnetic resonance imaging (Chap 190); these techniques may be superior to echocardiography in detecting loculated pericardial effusions. At cardiac catheterization the catheter is introduced into the right atrium and rotated so that its tip makes contact with the lateral right atrial wall. In the presence of an effusion or pericardial thickening, the tip of the catheter is separated from the radiolucent lungs by an opaque band. When contrast medium is injected rapidly into the right atrium, the angiocardiogram also shows the lateral wall to be separated from the edge of the cardiac silhouette.

When it is deemed desirable to remove pericardial fluid for diagnostic and/or therapeutic purposes, a needle attached to a properly grounded electrocardiographic lead is inserted into the pericardial space, usually through a subxiphoid approach, and, if possible, using echocardiographic control. Intrapericardial pressure should be measured before fluid is withdrawn. Pericardial effusion nearly always has the physical characteristics of an exudate. Bloody fluid is commonly due to tuberculosis or tumor, but it also may be found in the effusion of rheumatic fever, in post-cardiac injury and post-myocardial infarction, especially following the administration of anticoagulants, and in uremic pericarditis.

CARDIAC TAMPONADE The accumulation of fluid in the pericardium in an amount sufficient to cause serious obstruction to the inflow of blood to the ventricles results in cardiac tamponade, a grave complication which may be fatal if it is not treated promptly. The three most common causes of tamponade are neoplastic disease, idiopathic pericarditis, and uremia, but it also results from bleeding into the pericardial space following cardiac operations, trauma (including cardiac perforation during diagnostic procedures), tuberculosis, and hemopericardium; the latter may result when a patient with any form of acute pericarditis is treated with anticoagulants. The three principal features of tamponade are elevation of intracardiac pressures, limitation of ventricular filling in diastole, and reduction of cardiac output. The amount of fluid necessary to produce this critical state may be as small as 200 mL when the fluid develops rapidly or over 2000 mL in slowly developing effusions when the pericardium has had the opportunity to stretch and adapt to the increasing volume of fluid. The volume of fluid required to produce tamponade also varies directly with the thickness of the ventricular myocardium and inversely with the thickness of the parietal pericardium.

Table 206-2 lists the features that distinguish cardiac tamponade from constrictive pericarditis. The classic findings of falling arterial pressure, rising venous pressure, and a small, quiet heart with faint heart sounds usually are seen only with severe, acute tamponade, as occurs with cardiac trauma or rupture. Tamponade may also develop more slowly, and the clinical manifestations resemble those of heart failure, including dyspnea, orthopnea, hepatic engorgement, and jugular venous hypertension. A high index of suspicion for cardiac tamponade is required, since, in many instances, no obvious cause for pericardial disease is apparent, and tamponade should be considered in any patient with hypotension and elevation of jugular venous pressure with a prominent x descent; in contrast to constrictive pericarditis, often the y descent is diminutive or absent. A positive Kussmaul sign (see below) is rare in cardiac tamponade, as is a pericardial knock. Their presence suggests that an organizing process and epicardial constriction are present in addition to effusion. A widening of the area of flatness to percussion across the anterior aspect of the chest wall, a paradoxical pulse (see below), relatively clear lung fields, diminished pulsations of the cardiac silhouette on fluoroscopy, enlargement of the cardiac silhouette (especially in subacute or chronic tamponade), reduction in amplitude of the QRS complexes, and *electrical alternans* of the P, QRS, and T waves should raise the suspicion of cardiac tamponade.

Since immediate treatment of tamponade may be lifesaving, prompt measures to establish the diagnosis, i.e., echocardiography sometimes followed by cardiac catheterization, should be undertaken. The latter reveals elevation of the right atrial pressure with prominence of the x but not of the y descent (Table 206-2). When measured, the pericardial pressure is also elevated and equal to the right atrial pressure. There is "equalization" of pressures, i.e., the pulmonary artery wedge is equal, or close, to right atrial, right ventricular, and pulmonary artery diastolic pressures. The "square root" sign in the ventricular pressure pulses and the prominent y descent in atrial and jugular venous pressure are characteristic of constrictive pericarditis (see below) and are usually absent in tamponade. In an emergency, pericardiocentesis may be carried out without cardiac catheterization but preferably after confirmation of the clinical diagnosis by echocardiography.

TABLE 206-2 Features that distinguish constrictive pericarditis from similar clinical disorders

Characteristic	Tamponade	Constrictive pericarditis	Restrictive cardiomyopathy	RVMI*
Clinical				
Pulsus paradoxus	Common	Usually absent	Rare	Rare
Jugular veins				
Prominent y descent	Absent	Usually present	Rare	Rare
Prominent x descent	Present	Usually absent	Present	Rare
Kussmaul's sign	Absent	Present	Absent	Absent
Third heart sound	Absent	Absent	Rare	May be present
Pericardial knock	Absent	Often present	Absent	Absent
Electrocardiogram				
Low ECG voltage	May be present	May be present	May be present	Absent
Electrical alternans	May be present	Absent	Absent	Absent
Echocardiography				
Thickened pericardium	Absent	Present	Absent	Absent
Pericardial calcification	Absent	Often present	Absent	Absent
Pericardial effusion	Present	Absent	Absent	Absent
RV size	Usually small	Usually normal	Usually normal	Enlarged
Myocardial thickness	Normal	Normal	Usually increased	Normal
Right atrial collapse and RVDC	Present	Absent	Absent	Absent
Increased early filling mitral flow velocity	Absent	Present	Present	May be present
Exaggerated respiratory variation in flow velocity	Present	Present	Absent	Absent
Computed tomography, Magnetic resonance imaging				
Thickened/calcific pericardium	Absent	Present	Absent	Absent
Cardiac catheterization				
Equalization of diastolic procedures	Usually present	Usually present	Usually absent	Absent or present
Cardiac biopsy helpful?	No	No	Somewhat	No

* RV = right ventricle, RVMI = right ventricular myocardial infarction, RVDC = right ventricular diastolic collapse, ECG = electrocardiograph
SOURCE: From GM Brockington et al, Cardiol Clin 8:645, 1990.

Paradoxical pulse This important clue to the presence of cardiac tamponade consists of *a greater than normal (10 mmHg) inspiratory decline in systolic arterial pressure.* When severe, it may be detected by palpating weakness or disappearance of the arterial pulse during inspiration, but usually sphygmomanometric measurement of systolic pressure during slow respiration is required (Fig. 206-2).

Since both ventricles share a tight incompressible covering, i.e., the pericardial sac, in cardiac tamponade the inspiratory enlargement of the right ventricle compresses and reduces left ventricular volume substantially; leftward bulging of the interventricular septum further reduces the left ventricular cavity as the right ventricle enlarges during inspiration. Thus in cardiac tamponade the normal inspiratory augmentation of right ventricular volume causes an exaggerated reciprocal reduction in left ventricular volume. Also, respiratory distress increases the fluctuations in intrathoracic pressure, which exaggerates the mechanism just described. Right ventricular infarction (Chap. 202) may resemble cardiac tamponade with hypotension, elevated jugular venous pressure, an absent y descent in the jugular venous pulse, and occasionally pulsus paradoxus. The differentiation between these two conditions is shown in Table 206-2.

Paradoxical pulse, a hallmark of cardiac tamponade, occurs in only approximately one-third of patients with *constrictive pericarditis.* It is important to bear in mind that paradoxical pulse is not pathognomonic of pericardial disease because it may be observed in various forms of restrictive cardiomyopathies (Chap. 205) and in some cases of hypovolemic shock, chronic obstructive airways disease, and severe bronchial asthma.

Low-pressure tamponade refers to mild tamponade in which the intrapericardial pressure is increased from its slightly subatmospheric levels to +5 to +10 mmHg; in some instances hypovolemia coexists. As a consequence, the central venous pressure is normal or only slightly elevated while arterial pressure is unaffected. The patients are asymptomatic or complain of mild weakness and dyspnea. The

diagnosis is aided by echocardiography, and both hemodynamic and clinical manifestations improve following pericardiocentesis.

TREATMENT Patients with acute pericarditis should be placed at bed rest until pain and fever have disappeared. Anticoagulants should be avoided. The patient should be observed frequently for the development of an effusion; if a moderate or large effusion is already present, the patient should be hospitalized and signs of tamponade must be watched for carefully. In the presence of an effusion, arterial and venous pressures and heart rate should be monitored continuously or followed carefully and serial echocardiograms obtained. If manifestations of tamponade appear, pericardiocentesis must be carried out at once, since relief of the intrapericardial pressure may be lifesaving. A small catheter advanced over the needle inserted into the pericardial cavity may be left in place to allow draining of the pericardial space if fluid reaccumulates. When a *diagnostic* pericardiocentesis of a large effusion is carried out, an attempt should be made to remove as much fluid as possible.

VIRAL OR IDIOPATHIC FORM OF ACUTE PERICARDITIS This disorder is an important clinical entity because of its frequency and because it may be confused with other, more serious illnesses. In some cases, an A or B coxsackievirus or the virus of influenza, echovirus type 8, mumps, herpes simplex, chickenpox, or adenovirus has been isolated from pericardial fluid and/or appropriate elevations in viral antibody titers have been noted; in many instances, acute pericarditis has occurred in association with illnesses of known viral origin and, presumably, was caused by the same agent. Commonly, there is an antecedent infection of the respiratory tract, but in many patients such an association is not evident and viral isolation and serologic studies are negative. Most frequently, a viral causation cannot be established, nor can it be excluded; the term *acute idiopathic pericarditis* is then appropriate.

Regardless of the specific causative factor, the clinical manifestations are similar. Acute pericarditis occurs at all ages but is more

FIGURE 206-2 Simultaneous recording of electrocardiogram (ECG), blood flow velocity in the superior vena cava (SVC), brachial arterial pressure (BA), and the pneumogram (Pneumo) in a patient with cardiac compression and paradoxical pulse. A downward deflection of the pneumogram denotes inspiration, when SVC blood velocity rises and arterial pressure falls (paradoxical pulse). Arterial pressure is maintained during prolonged expiratory pause.

frequent in young adults; it is often associated with pleural effusions and pneumonitis. The appearance of fever and precordial pain at about the same time, often 10 to 12 days after a presumed viral illness, constitutes an important feature in the differentiation of acute pericarditis from myocardial infarction, in which pain precedes fever. The constitutional symptoms are usually mild to moderate, but occasionally the initial symptoms are stormy, the temperature rising to 40°C. The disease ordinarily runs its course in a few days to 4 weeks, but one or more recurrences occur in about one-fourth of patients. Although accumulation of some pericardial fluid is common, tamponade is unusual, and constrictive pericarditis develops rarely. A pericardial friction rub is often audible. The ST-segment alterations in the electrocardiogram are usually transitory, but the abnormal T waves may persist for several years or indefinitely and be a source of confusion in persons without a clear history of pericarditis. Pleuritis and pneumonitis frequently accompany pericarditis. The erythrocyte sedimentation rate is elevated. Granulocytosis followed by lymphocytosis is common.

Management There is no specific therapy, but bed rest and anti-inflammatory treatment with aspirin, if necessary up to 900 mg qid, may be given. If this is ineffective, one of the nonsteroidal anti-inflammatory agents, such as indomethacin (25 to 75 mg qid) or a glucocorticoid (e.g., prednisone, 20 to 80 mg daily) effectively suppresses the clinical manifestations of the acute illness and may be useful in patients in whom the purulent and tuberculous forms of pericarditis have been excluded. After the patient has been asymptomatic and afebrile for about 1 week, the dose of the anti-inflammatory agent is gradually tapered. Occasionally, tamponade progression to chronic constrictive pericarditis occurs. When recurrences are multiple, frequent, disabling, and continue beyond 2 years, pericardiectomy may be effective in terminating the illness.

POST-CARDIAC INJURY SYNDROME An acute form of pericarditis may appear under a variety of circumstances which have one common feature: previous injury to the myocardium, with blood in the pericardial cavity. The syndrome has been observed when the injury has been induced in the course of a cardiac operation (postpericardiotomy syndrome). It also may follow myocardial infarction (Dressler's syndrome) (Chap. 202) or develop after trauma of the heart (Chap. 207), e.g., a stab wound, contusions after a nonpenetrating blow to the chest, or perforation of the heart with a catheter.

The principal symptom is the pain of acute pericarditis, which usually develops 1 to 4 weeks following the cardiac injury but sometimes appears only after a lapse of months. Recurrences are common and may occur up to 2 years or more after the injury. Fever to 40°C, pericarditis, pleuritis, and pneumonitis are the outstanding features, the bout of illness usually subsiding in 1 or 2 weeks. The pericarditis, which appears to be the most constant lesion, may be of

the fibrinous variety, or it may be a pericardial effusion, which is often serosanguineous, rarely causes tamponade, and is accompanied by arthralgias. Leukocytosis, an increased sedimentation rate, and electrocardiographic changes typical of acute pericarditis also may occur.

The mechanisms responsible for this syndrome have not been identified, but there is a likelihood that they are the result of a hypersensitivity reaction in which the antigen originates from injured myocardial tissue and/or pericardium; the suggested designation of post-cardiac injury syndrome for this group of disorders implies that they may have a common pathogenetic mechanism. Circulating autoantibodies to myocardium occur frequently, but their precise role in this syndrome has not been defined. Viral infection also may play an etiologic role, since antiviral antibodies are often elevated in patients who develop this syndrome following cardiac surgery.

The clinical picture of the post-cardiac injury syndrome mimics acute viral or acute idiopathic pericarditis. Moreover, it is possible that the recurrences that occur so frequently in the latter condition are not always caused by an exacerbation of the original (presumably viral) infection but that the original injury may have initiated the sequence of events that culminates in the post-cardiac injury syndrome.

Often no treatment is necessary aside from aspirin and analgesics. The management of pericardial effusion and tamponade has already been discussed. When the illness is followed by a series of disabling recurrences, therapy with a nonsteroidal anti-inflammatory agent or a glucocorticoid is usually effective.

DIFFERENTIAL DIAGNOSIS Since there is no specific test for *acute idiopathic pericarditis* the diagnosis is one of exclusion. Consequently, all other disorders that may be associated with acute fibrinous pericarditis must be considered. When associated with *acute myocardial infarction*, acute fibrinous pericarditis may be confused with acute viral or idiopathic pericarditis; this complication of infarction, described in Chap. 202 is characterized by the occurrence of fever, pain, and a friction rub in the first 4 days following the development of the infarct (to be distinguished from the pericarditis in Dressler's syndrome, which is a form of post-cardiac injury pericarditis and which occurs a week or two following myocardial infarction). Electrocardiographic abnormalities (such as the appearance of Q waves, brief ST-segment elevations with reciprocal changes, and earlier T-wave changes in myocardial infarction), the extent of the elevations of myocardial enzymes, and the total clinical picture are helpful in relating pericarditis to acute myocardial infarction. A common diagnostic error is assuming that acute viral or idiopathic pericarditis represents acute myocardial infarction and vice versa.

Acute pericarditis occurring as a component of the post-cardiac injury syndrome is most likely to be confused with acute idiopathic pericarditis. Pericarditis secondary to post-cardiac injury is differentiated from acute idiopathic pericarditis chiefly by timing. If it occurs within a few weeks of a myocardial infarction or a chest blow, it may be justified to conclude that the two are probably related. If the infarct has been silent or the chest blow forgotten, the relationship to the pericarditis may not be recognized.

It is important to distinguish *pericarditis due to collagen disease* from acute idiopathic pericarditis. Most important in the differential diagnosis is the pericarditis due to systemic lupus erythematosus (Chap. 284); often pain is present, sometimes the pericarditis appears as an asymptomatic effusion, and rarely, tamponade develops. Very rarely, when pericarditis occurs in the absence of other evidence of any underlying disorder, differentiation from acute viral and idiopathic pericarditis or tuberculous pericarditis may be made on discovery of lupus erythematosus (LE) cells, a rise in antinuclear antibodies, or by the specific methods for diagnosing tuberculosis (see below). Acute pericarditis may complicate the viral, pyogenic, mycobacterial, and fungal infections that occur in AIDS. Acute pericarditis is an occasional complication of *rheumatoid arthritis, scleroderma,* and *polyarteritis nodosa,* but again, other evidence of these diseases is usually obvious. Asymptomatic pericardial effusion is also frequent in these disorders. It is important to question every patient with acute pericarditis about the ingestion of procainamide, hydralazine, isoniazid, cromolyn, and minoxidil, since these drugs can cause this syndrome.

The pericarditis of *acute rheumatic fever* is generally associated with evidence of severe pancarditis and with cardiac murmurs (Chap. 200). *Pyogenic (purulent) pericarditis* is usually secondary to cardiothoracic operations, immunosuppressive therapy, rupture of the esophagus into the pericardial sac, or rupture of a ring abscess in a patient with infective endocarditis and with septicemia complicating aseptic pericarditis. It is now uncommonly due to pneumococcal pneumonia and pleuritis, previously the most common cause. *Tuberculous pericarditis* (see Chap. 130) may present as an acute pericarditis, associated with fever, weight loss, and other clinical manifestations of active systemic tuberculosis; the diagnosis may be aided by a positive tuberculin test and evidence of pulmonary or mediastinal tuberculosis. Tubercle bacilli can be cultured from the pericardial space only infrequently, and a biopsy of the pericardium with bacteriologic and histologic examination may be required. Alternatively, tuberculous pericarditis may present as a chronic asymptomatic effusion, as subacute effusive-constrictive pericarditis (see below), or as frank chronic constrictive pericarditis (see below).

Uremic pericarditis (Chap. 237) occurs in up to one-third of patients with chronic uremia and is seen most frequently in patients undergoing chronic hemodialysis. It may be fibrinous or associated with a bloody effusion. A friction rub is common, but pain is usually absent. Treatment with an anti-inflammatory agent and intensification of hemodialysis is usually adequate. Occasionally, tamponade occurs and pericardiocentesis is required. When uremic pericarditis is recurrent, persistent or very troubling pericardiectomy may be necessary. Pericarditis due to *neoplastic diseases* results from extension or invasion of primary or metastatic tumors (most commonly carcinoma of the lung and breast, malignant melanoma, lymphoma, and leukemia) to the pericardium; pain, atrial arrhythmias, and tamponade are complications which occur occasionally. *Mediastinal irradiation* for neoplasm may cause pericarditis after eradication of the tumor. Unusual causes of acute pericarditis include syphilis, fungal infection (histoplasmosis, blastomycosis, aspergillosis, and candidiasis), and parasitic infestation (amebiasis, toxoplasmosis, echinococcosis, trichinosis).

CHRONIC PERICARDIAL EFFUSIONS Chronic pericardial effusions are not infrequently encountered in patients without an antecedent history of acute pericarditis. They may cause few symptoms per se, and they may be suspected by finding an enlarged cardiac silhouette on chest roentgenogram which may be obtained in the course of the workup of a patient with symptoms related to the underlying illness.

Tuberculosis This is a common cause of chronic pericardial effusion, although less so in the United States than in other parts of the world (Chap. 130). The symptoms are often those of a chronic,

systemic illness in an individual with pericardial effusion. It is important to bear this condition in mind when a middle-aged or elderly person with fever has apparent enlargement of the cardiac silhouette of undetermined origin, with or without elevation of venous pressure. Weight loss, fever, and fatigability are sometimes observed. Inasmuch as treatment is quite effective, overlooking a tuberculous pericardial effusion may cause serious consequences. Consequently, no method of examination should be omitted to exclude this diagnosis in such patients. Included are chest roentgenograms for pulmonary tuberculosis and a search for tuberculosis in other organs; tuberculin skin tests, repeated after several weeks; and cultures and smears of gastric washings and of pleural and pericardial fluid. Finally, if the etiology of chronic pericardial effusion is still obscure, a pericardial biopsy, preferably by a limited thoracotomy, should be performed. If definitive evidence is then still lacking but the specimen shows caseation necrosis, antituberculous chemotherapy for at least 24 months is justified (Chap. 130). Pericardiectomy should be carried out in order to prevent the development of constriction if the biopsy specimen shows a thickened pericardium.

Other causes of chronic pericardial effusion *Myxedema* may be responsible for a pericardial effusion that is sometimes massive but rarely, if ever, causes cardiac tamponade. The other manifestations of myxedema should clarify the diagnosis, but unfortunately, even when they are present, the diagnosis is frequently overlooked. It is important, therefore, to carry out appropriate tests for thyroid function (Chap. 334) in patients with an enlarged cardiac outline of undetermined origin. The cardiac silhouette is markedly enlarged and an echocardiogram is necessary to distinguish cardiomegaly from pericardial effusion. *Cholesterol pericardial disease* produces large pericardial effusions with a high cholesterol content, which may induce an inflammatory response and constrictive pericarditis.

Neoplasms, systemic lupus erythematosus, rheumatoid arthritis, mycotic infections, radiation therapy, pyogenic infections, severe chronic anemia, and chylopericardium also may cause chronic pericardial effusion and should be considered and specifically looked for in such patients.

Aspiration and analysis of the pericardial fluid are often helpful in diagnosis. In infections the organism can often be identified by smear or culture. Grossly sanguineous pericardial fluid results most commonly from a neoplasm, tuberculosis, uremia, or slow leakage from an aortic aneurysm.

CHRONIC CONSTRICTIVE PERICARDITIS

This disorder results when the healing of an acute fibrinous or serofibrinous pericarditis or a chronic pericardial effusion is followed by obliteration of the pericardial cavity with the formation of granulation tissue. This gradually contracts and forms a firm scar, encasing the heart and interfering with filling of the ventricles. In some reports, a high percentage of all cases has been of tuberculous origin. In other series, particularly those reported in the United States in the last two decades, tuberculosis has been an infrequent cause. Chronic constrictive pericarditis also may follow purulent infection, trauma, cardiac operation of any type, mediastinal irradiation, histoplasmosis, neoplastic disease, and acute viral or idiopathic pericarditis, rheumatoid arthritis, lupus erythematosus, and chronic renal failure with uremia treated by chronic dialysis. In many patients the cause of the pericardial disease is undetermined, and in them an asymptomatic or forgotten bout of viral pericarditis, acute or idiopathic, may have been the inciting event. Routine radiographic examination may reveal calcification of the pericardium in a person who is free of all symptoms referable to the heart (calcific, not constrictive, pericarditis). The heart also may be constricted and compressed by malignant tumors or organized blood clot in the pericardial cavity.

The basic physiologic abnormality in symptomatic patients with chronic constrictive pericarditis, as in those with cardiac tamponade, is the inability of the ventricles to fill adequately during diastole because of the limitations imposed by the rigid, thickened pericardium or the tense pericardial fluid. However, in constrictive pericarditis ventricular filling is unimpeded during early diastole but is reduced abruptly when the elastic limit of the pericardium is reached, while in cardiac tamponade ventricular filling is impeded throughout diastole. In chronic constrictive pericarditis stroke volume is reduced, and the end-diastolic pressures in both ventricles and the mean pressures in the atria, pulmonic veins, and systemic veins are all elevated to about the same levels. Despite these hemodynamic changes, myocardial function may actually be normal or only slightly impaired; instead, the ventricles may be considered to be underloaded.

In constrictive pericarditis the central venous and right and left atrial pressure pulses display an M-shaped contour, with prominent x and y descents; the y descent (absent or diminished in cardiac tamponade) is the most prominent deflection and is interrupted by a rapid rise in pressure during early diastole, when ventricular filling is impeded by the constricting pericardium. These characteristic changes are transmitted to the jugular veins, where they may be recognized by inspection or recorded. In constrictive pericarditis, both ventricular pressure pulses exhibit characteristic "square root" signs during diastole. These hemodynamic changes, although characteristic, are not pathognomonic of constrictive pericarditis but also may be observed in cardiomyopathies characterized by restriction of ventricular filling, as discussed in Chap. 205.

CLINICAL FINDINGS (See Table 206-2) Weakness, fatigue, weight loss, and anorexia are common. The patient often appears to be chronically ill with decreased skeletal muscle mass and a protuberant abdomen. Contrary to a widely held impression, dyspnea, though absent or slight at rest, is often present on exertion, and orthopnea is common in chronic constrictive pericarditis, although it is not severe. However, attacks of acute left ventricular failure (acute pulmonary edema) practically never occur. The cervical veins are distended and may remain so even after intensive diuretic treatment, and venous pressure may fail to decline during inspiration (Kussmaul's sign). In about one-third of the cases a paradoxical pulse may be observed. Congestive hepatomegaly is pronounced and may impair hepatic function; ascites is common and is usually more prominent than dependent edema. In about half of patients the heart is normal in size; if it is enlarged, the enlargement is rarely extreme. The apical pulse is reduced in intensity, retracts in systole, and moves outward in diastole. The heart sounds may be distant; an early third heart sound, i.e., a pericardial knock, occurring 0.06 to 0.12 s after aortic valve closure which coincides with a sudden deceleration in ventricular filling, is often conspicuous; and murmurs are usually absent. The apex beat is poorly defined, and cardiac pulsations under fluoroscopic examination are diminished. Because of the high sustained venous pressure, congestive splenomegaly may make the spleen palpable. In the absence of infective endocarditis or tricuspid valve disease, splenomegaly in a patient with congestive heart failure should arouse suspicion of constrictive pericarditis. Protein-losing gastroenteropathy due to impaired lymphatic drainage from the small intestine, and the nephrotic syndrome, or marked proteinuria or hypoalbuminemia, may complicate chronic constrictive pericarditis.

The electrocardiogram frequently displays low voltage of the QRS complex and diffuse flattening or inversion of the T waves. P mitrale may be present in patients with sinus rhythm; atrial fibrillation is present in about one-third of patients. The echocardiogram usually, but not invariably, shows pericardial thickening and reduced amplitude of left ventricular wall motion, prominent early diastolic filling, and normal left ventricular size.

Systemic and/or pulmonary venous congestion is initially the result of impaired filling of the ventricles caused by the restrictive action of the inelastic pericardium. However, the fibrotic process may extend into the myocardium and cause myocardial scarring, and venous congestion may then be due to the combined effects of the myocardial and pericardial lesions. The interference with filling reduces the work of the heart, and perhaps this leads to myocardial atrophy. The latter

probably accounts for the delayed beneficial effects of operative treatment observed in some patients with advanced disease.

Inasmuch as the usual physical signs of cardiac disease (murmurs, cardiac enlargement) may be inconspicuous or absent in chronic constrictive pericarditis, hepatic enlargement and dysfunction associated with intractable ascites may lead to a mistaken diagnosis of cirrhosis of the liver. This error can be avoided if the neck veins are inspected carefully in all patients with ascites and hepatomegaly. *Given a clinical picture resembling hepatic cirrhosis, but with the added feature of distended neck veins, careful search for calcification of the pericardium by chest roentgenography, fluoroscopy, and echocardiography should be carried out and may disclose this curable or remediable form of heart disease.* Calcification occurs in only about one-half of these patients, usually in those with long-standing pericardial constriction. Most patients with chronic constrictive pericarditis show pericardial thickening on echocardiographic examination. However, echocardiography cannot definitively exclude the diagnosis. Magnetic resonance imaging and computed tomography are more accurate than echocardiography in establishing or excluding the presence of a thickened pericardium (Chap. 191). Pericardial thickening and even pericardial calcification, however, are not synonymous with constrictive pericarditis since they may occur without seriously impairing ventricular filling.

DIFFERENTIAL DIAGNOSIS Like cor pulmonale (Chap. 204), chronic constrictive pericarditis may be associated with severe systemic venous hypertension but with little or no pulmonary congestion; the heart usually is not enlarged, and a striking inspiratory fall in arterial pressure may be present. However, in cor pulmonale, advanced parenchymal pulmonary disease is usually obvious and venous pressure *falls* during inspiration; i.e., Kussmaul's sign is negative. *Tricuspid stenosis* (p. 1064) also may simulate chronic constrictive pericarditis; congestive hepatomegaly, splenomegaly, ascites, and venous distention may be equally prominent, and the manifestations of left-sided heart failure may be inconspicuous. However, in tricuspid stenosis, the characteristic murmur, the almost universal coexistence of mitral stenosis, the absence of a paradoxic pulse, and the absence, in the jugular venous pulse, of the steep, deep y descent followed by a rapid ascent (manifested by the diastolic shock on palpation and its audible equivalent, the pericardial knock) facilitate the clinical differentiation.

Because constrictive pericarditis can be corrected surgically it is important, though often difficult, to distinguish chronic constrictive pericarditis from various forms of heart disease which are characterized by a similar physiologic abnormality, i.e., restriction of ventricular filling. These restrictive cardiomyopathies, which may resemble pericarditis clinically, are described in Chap. 205 and include endomyocardial fibrosis and infiltrative cardiomyopathies such as amyloidosis, hemochromatosis, sarcoidosis, scleroderma, and idiopathic myocardial hypertrophy. In the last the marked thickening of the ventricular wall is responsible for the diminished compliance (Table 206-2).

The features favoring the diagnosis of one of the above forms of cardiomyopathy are a well-defined apex beat, enlargement of the heart, and pronounced orthopnea with attacks of acute left ventricular failure, left ventricular hypertrophy, gallop sounds (in place of a pericardial knock), bundle branch block, and in some cases significant Q waves in the electrocardiogram. The echocardiogram shows ventricular thickening. At catheterization, patients with chronic constrictive pericarditis usually have left atrial or pulmonary arterial wedge pressure equaling right atrial pressure, the latter often exceeding 15 mmHg despite intensive medical treatment for heart failure. The pulmonary artery systolic pressure is often less than 50 mmHg, and the right ventricular end-diastolic pressure often reaches one-third of the systolic pressure; the cardiac output is slightly depressed. In patients with cardiomyopathy, the left atrial usually exceeds the right atrial pressure by more than 5 mmHg, the mean right atrial pressure is often below 15 mmHg following intensive treatment with diuretics, the pulmonary artery systolic pressure often exceeds 50 mmHg, and the right ventricular end-diastolic pressure is usually less than one-third of the systolic pressure, while the cardiac output is markedly depressed. The volumes of both ventricles, as determined by angiography or echocardiography, are characteristically reduced or normal in constrictive pericarditis, and the ejection fractions are normal or almost so. The left ventricular end-diastolic volume also may be normal in some cardiomyopathies, but it is frequently elevated in others in which the ejection fraction is markedly reduced; the latter finding militates strongly against the diagnosis of constrictive pericarditis. The echocardiogram in chronic constrictive pericarditis characteristically shows pericardial thickening, i.e., a distinct echo posterior to the left ventricular wall, and paradoxical septal motion. The left ventricular wall moves sharply outward in early diastole and then remains flat. The definitive diagnosis of restrictive cardiomyopathy, when it is due to an infiltrative disease such as amyloidosis, can often be established by endomyocardial biopsy. CT scanning and MRI are very useful in distinguishing between restrictive cardiomyopathy and chronic constrictive pericarditis (Chap. 191).

When a patient has progressive, disabling, and unresponsive congestive failure, and if he or she displays any of the phenomena of constrictive heart disease, the most careful and detailed clinical and laboratory studies must be carried out in order to detect or exclude constrictive pericarditis, which is potentially a curable condition. Cardiac catheterization, selective angiocardiography, coronary arteriography, endomyocardial biopsy, and MRI may be required. However, in the very rare instance when even these examinations do not yield a definitive diagnosis, surgical exploration of the pericardium is the only decisive method of determining whether constrictive pericarditis is responsible for the clinical manifestations of heart failure.

Occult constrictive disease Patients with this condition may have unexplained fatigue, dyspnea, and chest pain. No overt manifestations of pericardial disease are present, but following the rapid intravenous infusion of 1 L saline solution, diastolic equilibration of intracardiac atrial and ventricular pressures found in overt constrictive pericarditis occur. Although symptomatic improvement may follow pericardiectomy, this procedure should not be carried out in asymptomatic persons.

TREATMENT Pericardial resection is the only definitive treatment of constrictive pericarditis, but dietary sodium restriction and diuretics are useful during preoperative preparation. Digitalis may be beneficial in the prevention of heart failure when resection of the thickened pericardium permits an increased inflow into the ventricles and hence places an enhanced burden on an atrophic myocardium. The benefits derived from cardiac decortication are often striking, and the improvement, though slight at first, usually is progressive over a period of many months. The risk of this operation depends on the extent of penetration of the myocardium by the calcific process, by the severity of myocardial atrophy, by the extent of secondary impairment of hepatic and/or renal function, and by the patient's general condition. Operative mortality is in the range of 7 to 15 percent; the patients with the most severe and/or advanced disease are at highest risk. Therefore, surgical treatment should be carried out relatively early in the course.

Many cases of constrictive pericarditis are of tuberculous origin. Antituberculous therapy during the phase of effusion may prevent the development of constriction, and such therapy should be carried out before and after operation, if a tuberculous origin is suspected or cannot be excluded in a patient with chronic constrictive pericarditis (Chap. 130).

SUBACUTE EFFUSIVE-CONSTRICTIVE PERICARDITIS This form of pericardial disease is characterized by the combination of a tense effusion in the pericardial space and constriction of the heart by thickened pericardium. It shares a number of features both with pericardial effusion producing cardiac compression and with pericardial constriction. It may be caused by tuberculosis, multiple attacks of acute idiopathic pericarditis, radiation, traumatic pericarditis, uremia, and scleroderma. The heart is generally enlarged, and

there are a paradoxical pulse and a prominent x descent (without a prominent y descent) in the atrial pressure pulse. Following pericardiocentesis, the physiologic findings may change from those of cardiac tamponade to those of pericardial constriction, with a "square root" sign in the ventricular pressure pulse and a prominent y descent in the atrial and jugular venous pressure pulses. Furthermore, the intrapericardial pressure and the central venous pressure may decline, but not to normal. In many patients the condition progresses to the chronic constrictive form of the disease. Wide excision of both the visceral and parietal pericardium is usually effective.

OTHER DISORDERS OF THE PERICARDIUM

Pericardial cysts appear as rounded or lobulated deformities of the cardiac silhouette, most commonly at the right cardiophrenic angle. They do not cause symptoms, and their major clinical significance lies in the possibility of confusion with a tumor, ventricular aneurysm, or massive cardiomegaly. *Tumors* involving the pericardium are most commonly secondary to malignant neoplasms originating in or invading the mediastinum, including carcinoma of the bronchus and breast, lymphoma, and melanoma. The most common *primary* malignant tumor is the mesothelioma. The usual clinical picture of malignant pericardial tumor is an insidiously developing, often bloody, pericardial effusion. Surgical exploration is required to establish a definitive diagnosis and to carry out definitive or, more commonly, palliative treatment.

REFERENCES

ARSENIAN MA: Cardiovascular sequelae of therapeutic thoracic radiation. Prog Cardiovasc Dis 33:299, 1991

DACSO CC: Pericarditis in AIDS. Cardiol Clin 8:697, 1990

FOWLER NO: Cardiac tamponade. A clinical or an echocardiographic diagnosis? 87:1738, 1993

———: Tuberculous pericarditis. JAMA 266:99, 1991

GOLD RG: Post-viral pericarditis. Eur Heart J 9:(G):175, 1988

HANCOCK EW: Subacute effusive-constrictive pericarditis. Circulation 43:183, 1971

KHAN AH: The postcardiac injury syndromes. Clin Cardiol 15:67, 1992

LORELL B, BRAUNWALD E: Pericardial disease, in *Heart Disease*, 4th ed, E Braunwald (ed). Philadelphia, Saunders, 1992, pp 1465–1516

MCCAUHGAN BC et al: Early and late results of pericardiectomy for constrictive pericarditis. J Thorac Cardiovasc Surg 89:340, 1985

VAITKUS PT, KUSSMAUL WG: Constrictive versus restrictive cardiomyopathy: A reappraisal and update of diagnostic criteria. Am Heart J 122:1431, 1991

ZISKIND AA et al: Percutaneous balloon pericardiotomy for the treatment of cardiac tamponade and large pericardial effusions; description of technique and report of the first 50 cases. J Am Coll Cardiol 21:1, 1993

207 CARDIAC TUMORS, CARDIAC MANIFESTATIONS OF SYSTEMIC DISEASES, AND TRAUMATIC CARDIAC INJURY

WILSON S. COLUCCI / EUGENE BRAUNWALD

TUMORS OF THE HEART

PRIMARY TUMORS Primary tumors of the heart are rare and are often classified as "benign" histologically (Table 207-1). However, since all cardiac tumors have the potential for causing life-threatening complications, and many are now curable by surgery, it is important that this diagnosis be made whenever possible. Approximately three-quarters are *histologically* benign, and the remainder are malignant, in almost all cases sarcomas.

TABLE 207-1 Relative incidence of primary tumors of the heart

Type	Percent
BENIGN	
Myxoma	30.5
Lipoma	10.5
Papillary fibroelastoma	9.9
Rhabdomyoma	8.5
Fibroma	4.0
Hemangioma	3.5
Teratoma	3.3
Mesothelioma of the AV node	2.8
Other benign tumors	2.1
Total	75.1
MALIGNANT	
Sarcomas	18.6
Lymphoma	1.6
Other malignant tumors	4.7
Total	24.9

source: Modified from HA McAllister, JJ Fenoglio, in *Atlas of Tumor Pathology*, Washington, Armed Forces Institute of Pathology, 1978, fasc 15, 2d series.

TABLE 207-2 Comparison of clinical features of sporadic myxoma and syndrome myxoma

Feature	Sporadic	Syndrome
Age (y) (range)	56 (39–82)	25 (10–56)
Female/male ratio	2·7:1	1·8:1
Patients (no.)	70	44
Cardiac myxomas (no.)	72	103
Distributions of myxomas (%):		
Atrial/ventricular	100/0	87/13
Single/multiple	99/1	50/50
Biatrial	0	23
Recurrent	0	18
Freckling (%)	0	68
Noncardiac tumors (%)	0	57
Endocrine neoplasm (%)	0	30
Familial (%)	0	14

source: HJ Vidaillet et al: "Syndrome myxoma:" A subset of patients with cardiac myxoma associated with pigmented skin lesions and peripheral and endocrine neoplasms. Br Heart J 57:247, 1987

Clinical presentation Cardiac tumors may present with a wide array of cardiac and noncardiac manifestations. There may be signs and symptoms of all the more common forms of heart disease, including chest pain, syncope, heart failure, murmurs, arrhythmias, conduction disturbances, and pericardial effusion or tamponade. The specific signs and symptoms produced are most closely related to the location of the tumor.

Myxoma Myxomas are the most common type of primary cardiac tumor for all age groups, accounting for one-third to one-half of all cases at postmortem, and for approximately three-quarters of the tumors that are treated surgically. They occur at all ages and show no sex preference. Although the large majority of myxomas are sporadic, some are familial with autosomal dominant transmission or are part of a syndrome that involves a complex of abnormalities including lentigines or pigmented nevi, primary nodular adrenal cortical disease with or without Cushing's syndrome, myxomatous mammary fibroadenomas, testicular tumors, and/or pituitary adenomas with gigantism or acromegaly. Certain constellations of findings have been referred to as the *NAME syndrome* (nevi, atrial myxoma, myxoid neurofibroma, and ephelides) or the *LAMB syndrome* (lentigines, atrial myxoma, and blue nevi). Approximately 7 percent of cardiac myxomas are familial or part of the *syndrome myxoma* with complex abnormalities described above.

Most authorities consider the myxoma a true neoplasm, while others have suggested that it is formed by organization of an intracardiac thrombus attached to the endocardium. The large majority of sporadic myxomas are solitary and located in the atria, particularly the left, where they arise from the interatrial septum in the vicinity of the fossa ovalis. Sporadic myxomas may also occur in the ventricles or may be found in multiple locations. In contrast to sporadic myxomas, familial or syndrome myxoma tumors tend to occur in younger individuals, are more often multiple in location, and are more likely to have postoperative recurrences, probably reflecting their multicentric nature (Table 207-2). Most are pedunculated on a fibrovascular stalk and average 4 to 8 cm in diameter. The most common clinical presentation resembles that of mitral valve disease, either stenosis as a result of tumor prolapse into the mitral orifice during diastole or regurgitation as a consequence of injury to the valve by tumor-induced trauma. Ventricular myxomas may cause outflow obstruction and may therefore mimic subaortic or subpulmonic stenosis. Characteristically, the symptoms and signs of atrial myxomas are highly dependent on position, intermittent, and sudden in onset as a result of changes in tumor position with gravity. On auscultation,

a characteristic low-pitched sound, termed a "tumor plop," is audible during early or middiastole and is thought to result from the tumor abruptly stopping as it strikes the ventricular wall. Myxomas may also present with peripheral or pulmonary emboli, or any of several noncardiac signs and symptoms including fever, weight loss, cachexia, malaise, arthralgia, rash, clubbing, Raynaud's phenomenon, hypergammaglobulinemia, anemia, polycythemia, leukocytosis, elevated erythrocyte sedimentation rate, thrombocytopenia, or thrombocytosis. Not surprisingly, myxomas are frequently misdiagnosed as endocarditis, collagen vascular disease, or noncardiac tumor.

Both M-mode and two-dimensional echocardiography (Fig. 190-4), are useful in the diagnosis of cardiac myxoma, the latter having the advantage of allowing determination of the site of tumor attachment and tumor size, important considerations in the planning of surgical excision. Computed tomography and particularly magnetic resonance imaging may provide important information regarding the size, shape, and surface characteristics of the tumor. Because myxomas may be familial, echocardiographic screening of first-degree relatives is appropriate, particularly if the patient is young and has multiple tumors or other evidence of syndrome myxoma. While cardiac catheterization and angiography are often performed prior to surgery, catheterization of the chamber from which the tumor originates is attended by the risk of dislodgment of tumor emboli. In many centers catheterization is no longer considered mandatory when adequate noninvasive information is available and other cardiac diseases (e.g., coronary artery disease) are not considered likely.

Surgical excision utilizing cardiopulmonary bypass is indicated and is generally curative. Occasional reports of tumor recurrence are most likely due to inadequate excision of multiple tumor sites not evident at the time of presentation.

Other benign tumors Cardiac *lipomas*, although relatively common, are usually incidental findings at postmortem examination and seldom result in symptoms. However, they may grow as large as 15 cm and present with symptoms due to mechanical interference with cardiac function, arrhythmias, or conduction disturbances, or as an abnormality of the cardiac silhouette on chest x-ray. *Papillary fibroelastomas*, similarly, are relatively common findings on cardiac valves or the adjacent endothelium at postmortem but seldom result in clinical symptoms. Occasionally, these growths may cause mechanical interference with valvular function. *Rhabdomyomas* and *fibromas*, the most frequent tumors in infants and children, most commonly occur in the ventricles, and therefore produce signs and symptoms by mechanical obstruction which may mimic valvular stenosis, congestive heart failure, restrictive or hypertrophic cardiomyopathy, and pericardial constriction. Rhabdomyomas are probably hamartomatous growths, are multiple in about 90 percent of cases, and may be associated with tuberous sclerosis, adenoma sebaceum, and benign kidney tumors in approximately 30 percent of patients. Calcification of a cardiac tumor strongly suggests that it is a fibroma, although myxomas and sarcomas may also be calcified. *Hemangiomas* and *mesotheliomas* are generally small tumors, most often intramyocardial in location, and may cause atrioventricular conduction disturbances and even sudden death as a result of their propensity for location in the region of the AV node.

Sarcomas Cardiac sarcomas may be of several histologic types, but in general are characterized by a rapidly downhill course leading to the patient's death in weeks to months from the time of presentation as a result of hemodynamic compromise, local invasion, or distant metastases. Sarcomas commonly involve the right side of the heart, and because of their rapid growth, invasion of the pericardial space and obstruction of the cardiac chambers or venae cavae are common. Sarcomas also can occur on the left side of the heart and they may be mistaken for myxomas. At the time of presentation these tumors have often spread too extensively for surgical excision. While there are scattered reports of palliation with surgery, radiotherapy, and/or chemotherapy, the overall experience with cardiac sarcomas is poor. The one exception to this appears to be cardiac lymphosarcomas, which may respond to a combination of chemo- and radiotherapy.

TUMORS METASTATIC TO THE HEART Tumors metastatic to the heart are several times more common than primary tumors, and as the life expectancy of patients with various forms of malignant neoplasms is extended by more effective therapy, it is likely that the frequency of cardiac metastases will also increase. Although cardiac metastases occur in 1 to 20 percent of all tumor types, the incidence is especially high in malignant melanoma, and to a somewhat lesser extent in leukemia and lymphoma. In absolute numbers, cardiac metastases are most common in carcinoma of the breast and lung, reflecting the high incidence of these cancers. Cardiac metastases almost always occur in the setting of widespread primary disease, and most often there is either primary or metastatic disease elsewhere in the thoracic cavity. Nevertheless, occasionally a cardiac metastasis may be the initial presentation of a tumor elsewhere in the body.

Cardiac metastases reach the heart via the bloodstream, lymphatics, or direct invasion and generally are small, firm nodules; diffuse infiltrations may also occur, especially with sarcomas or hematologic neoplasms. The pericardium is most often involved, followed by myocardial involvement of any chamber, and, rarely, by involvement of the endocardium or cardiac valves.

Cardiac metastases result in clinical manifestations only about 10 percent of the time, and rarely are they the cause of death. In most patients they are *not* the cause of the presenting clinical features but occur in the setting of a previously recognized malignant neoplasm. While cardiac metastases may present a large number of nonspecific signs and symptoms, the most common are dyspnea, signs of acute pericarditis, cardiac tamponade, a rapid increase in the cardiac silhouette on chest x-ray, the new onset of an ectopic tachyarrhythmia, AV block, and congestive heart failure. As with primary cardiac tumors, the clinical presentation is more closely related to the location and size of the tumor than to its histologic type. Many of these signs and symptoms may also occur with myocarditis, pericarditis, or cardiomyopathy resulting from radiotherapy or chemotherapy.

The electrocardiographic findings are entirely nonspecific and may include ST-T-wave changes, decreased QRS voltage, arrhythmias, and conduction disturbances. On chest roentgenography the cardiac silhouette is most often normal but may reveal a pericardial effusion or bizarre contour. Echocardiography is useful for the diagnosis of pericardial effusion and the visualization of larger metastases. Computed tomography, magnetic resonance imaging, and radionuclide imaging with gallium or thallium may provide useful anatomic information. Angiography may delineate discrete lesions, and pericardiocentesis can allow a specific cytologic diagnosis. Since most patients with cardiac metastases have widespread disease, therapy generally consists of pericardiocentesis when there is hemodynamic compromise and treatment directed at the primary tumor. The removal of a malignant effusion by pericardiocentesis, with or without concomitant instillation of a sclerosing agent (e.g., tetracycline), or placement of a pericardial window for drainage to the pleural space may palliate symptoms and delay or prevent reaccumulation of the effusion.

CARDIAC EFFECTS OF CANCER THERAPY See Chap. 205.

CARDIOVASCULAR MANIFESTATIONS OF SYSTEMIC DISEASES

DIABETES MELLITUS (See Chap. 337) In patients with insulin-dependent diabetes mellitus there is an increased incidence of large-vessel atherosclerosis and myocardial infarction, and diabetics are more likely to have an abnormal or absent pain response to myocardial ischemia, probably as a result of generalized autonomic nervous system dysfunction. Diabetic patients may also have myocardial dysfunction characteristic of a restrictive cardiomyopathy in the absence of large-vessel coronary artery disease, with abnormal relaxation of the myocardium, and evidenced clinically by elevated left ventricular filling pressures. Histologically, these patients have increased amounts of collagen, glycoprotein, triglycerides, and cholesterol in the myocardial interstitium, and in some cases intimal thickening, hyaline deposition, and inflammatory changes have been observed in small intramural arteries. Diabetic subjects have an increased risk of developing clinical heart failure, even after correction for the presence of coronary artery disease, hypertension, and obesity, and it is likely that diabetic cardiomyopathy contributes to excessive cardiovascular morbidity and mortality of these patients. There is some evidence that insulin therapy results in an amelioration of the myocardial dysfunction.

MALNUTRITION AND THIAMINE DEFICIENCY (BERIBERI) Malnutrition (See Chap. 72) In patients whose intake of protein, calories, or both is severely deficient, the heart may become thin, pale, and flabby with myofibrillar atrophy and interstitial edema. The systolic pressure and cardiac output are low and the pulse pressure narrow. Generalized edema is common and is due to a combination of factors, including reduced serum oncotic pressure and myocardial dysfunction. Such profound states of malnutrition, termed *marasmus* in the case of caloric deficiency or *kwashiorkor* in the case of relative protein deficiency, are most common in underdeveloped countries. However, significant nutritional heart disease may also occur in developed nations, particularly in patients with chronic diseases such as AIDS, in the semistarvation that can occur in anorexia nervosa, or in patients with severe cardiac failure in whom gastrointestinal hypoperfusion and venous congestion may cause anorexia and malabsorption. Open-heart surgery poses an increased risk in such patients, who may benefit from preoperative intensive hyperalimentation. Deficient nutrients and minerals should be replaced gradually since rapid expansion of the intravascular space may stress the weakened heart and result in overt congestive heart failure.

Thiamine deficiency (See Chap. 77) In many cases, malnutrition is accompanied by thiamine deficiency, although this hypovitaminosis may also occur in the presence of an adequate protein and caloric intake, particularly in the Far East, where polished rice deficient in thiamine may be a major dietary component. The widespread use of thiamine-enriched flour in western nations confines this disease primarily to alcoholics and food faddists. Clinically, there is usually evidence of generalized malnutrition, peripheral neuropathy, glossitis, and anemia. The characteristic cardiovascular syndrome is that of high-output heart failure with tachycardia, increased cardiac output, and often elevated filling pressures in the left and right sides of the heart. It appears that the major cause of the high-output state is vasomotor depression, the precise mechanism of which is not understood, but which leads to a reduced systemic vascular resistance. The cardiac examination reveals a wide pulse pressure, tachycardia, a third heart sound, and, frequently, a systolic murmur at the apex. The electrocardiogram may show decreased voltage, a prolonged QT interval, and T-wave abnormalities; the chest x-ray generally shows a large heart with signs of congestive heart failure. The response to thiamine is often dramatic, with an increase in systemic vascular resistance, decrease in cardiac output, clearing of pulmonary congestion, and a reduction in heart size often occurring in 12 to 48 h. Although the response to digitalis and diuretics may be poor prior to thiamine therapy, these agents may be important *after* thiamine is given, since the left ventricle may not be capable of dealing with the increased workload presented by the return of vascular tone.

OBESITY (See Chap. 73)   Although not defined as a disease per se, severe obesity, particularly when it occurs in an upper-body distribution, is associated with an increase in cardiovascular morbidity and mortality, due in part to hypertension, glucose intolerance, and atherosclerotic coronary artery disease, all of which are more prevalent in obese patients. In addition, these patients have a distinct abnormality of the cardiovascular system characterized by increases in total and central blood volumes, cardiac output, and left ventricular filling pressure. It appears that cardiac output is elevated in order to help supply the metabolic needs of the excessive adipose tissue. Left ventricular filling pressure is often at the upper limits of normal and rises excessively with exercise. As a result of chronic volume and pressure overload, eccentric cardiac hypertrophy with cardiac dilation and abnormal ventricular function may develop. Pathologically, there is left and, in some cases, right ventricular hypertrophy and generalized cardiac enlargement, which is not due simply to fatty infiltration of the myocardium. Clinically, these patients may develop pulmonary congestion, peripheral edema, and exercise intolerance, findings which may be difficult to recognize in massively obese patients. Weight reduction is the most effective therapy and results in reduction in blood volume and in return of cardiac output toward normal. However, rapid weight reduction may cause cardiac arrhythmias and sudden death due to electrolyte imbalance and may result in cardiac atrophy similar to that seen in malnutrition. Digitalis, sodium restriction, and diuretics may also be useful. This form of heart disease should be distinguished from the Pickwickian syndrome (Chap. 229), which may share several of the cardiovascular features but, in addition, frequently has components of central apnea, hypoxemia, pulmonary hypertension, and cor pulmonale.

THYROID DISEASE (See Chap. 334)   Thyroid hormone exerts a major influence on the cardiovascular system by a number of direct and indirect mechanisms, and not surprisingly, cardiovascular effects are prominent in both hypo- and hyperthyroidism. Thyroid hormone causes increases in total-body metabolism and oxygen consumption that indirectly place an increased workload on the heart. In addition, although the exact mechanism has not been defined, thyroid hormone exerts direct inotropic, chronotropic, and dromotropic effects that are similar to those seen with adrenergic stimulation (e.g., tachycardia, increased cardiac output). It has been shown that thyroid hormone increases the synthesis of myosin and of Na^+,K^+-ATPase, as well as the density of myocardial beta-adrenergic receptors.

Hyperthyroidism   Excess thyroid hormone results in increases in heart rate, cardiac output, stroke volume, pulse pressure, and measures of left ventricular contractility. Patients may present with palpitations, systolic hypertension, fatigue, or, in patients with underlying heart disease, angina or heart failure. Sinus tachycardia is found in about 40 percent of patients, and atrial fibrillation in about 15 percent. Other findings include a hyperactive precordium, an increase in the intensity of the first heart sound and the pulmonic component of the second heart sound, and a third heart sound. An increased incidence of mitral valve prolapse has been associated with hyperthyroidism, and in some cases there may be a midsystolic murmur heard best at the left sternal border with or without a systolic ejection click. A systolic scratchy sound, the *Means-Lerman scratch*, may occasionally be heard at the left second intercostal space during expiration and is thought to result from the rubbing of the hyperdynamic pericardium against the pleura. Elderly patients with hyperthyroidism may present with only the cardiovascular manifestations of thyrotoxicosis, such as atrial fibrillation, which may be resistant to therapy until the hyperthyroidism is controlled. Angina pectoris and congestive heart failure are unusual unless there is coexistent underlying heart disease, and in many cases will resolve with therapy of the hyperthyroidism.

Hypothyroidism   There is a reduction in cardiac output, stroke volume, heart rate, blood pressure, and pulse pressure. In about one-third of patients there is a pericardial effusion which only rarely results in tamponade. Increased capillary permeability results in pleural and pericardial effusions, but only rarely results in tamponade. Other clinical signs include cardiomegaly, bradycardia, weak arterial pulses, and distant heart sounds. As a result of earlier detection and treatment of hypothyroidism, these overt signs are commonly absent, and the major findings may be exertional dyspnea and easy fatigability. Although the signs and symptoms of myxedema may suggest the diagnosis of congestive heart failure, in the absence of other cardiac disease, myocardial failure is uncommon. Biochemical abnormalities, including elevations of creatine kinase, serum glutamic oxaloacetic transaminase, and lactic dehydrogenase, may lead to a mistaken diagnosis of myocardial infarction. The electrocardiogram generally shows sinus bradycardia and low voltage and may show prolongation of the QT interval, decreased P-wave voltage, prolonged AV conduction time, intraventricular conduction disturbances, and nonspecific ST-T-wave abnormalities. Chest x-ray may show cardiomegaly, often with a "water bottle" configuration, pleural effusions, and, in some cases, evidence of congestive heart failure. Pathologically, the heart is pale, dilated, and flabby, often with myofibrillar swelling, loss of striations, and interstitial fibrosis.

Patients with hypothyroidism frequently have elevations of cholesterol and triglycerides and severe atherosclerotic coronary artery disease. Prior to treatment with thyroid hormone, patients with hypothyroidism frequently do not have angina pectoris, presumably because of the low metabolic demands made by their condition. However, such patients, especially when elderly, are prone to angina and myocardial infarction during replacement of thyroid hormone, and this should always be done with extreme care, starting with very low doses which are increased gradually.

MALIGNANT CARCINOID (See Chap. 276)   These tumors elaborate a variety of vasoactive amines (e.g., serotonin), kinins, indoles, and other substances which are believed to be responsible for the diarrhea, flushing, and labile blood pressure seen in these patients. The cardiac lesions due to gastrointestinal carcinoids are almost exclusively in the right side of the heart and occur only when there are hepatic metastases, suggesting that the substance responsible for the cardiac lesions is inactivated by passage through the liver and lungs. Similar lesions occur in the left side of the heart when there is a right-to-left shunt or the tumor is located in the lungs. Fibrous plaques are found on the endothelium of the cardiac chambers, valves, and great vessels. These plaques, which result in distortion of the cardiac valves, consist of smooth muscle cells embedded in a stroma of acid mucopolysaccharide and collagen, and presumably result from healing of endothelial injury. The clinical syndrome is most often that of tricuspid regurgitation, pulmonic stenosis, or both. In some cases a high-output state may occur, presumably as a result of a decrease in systemic vascular resistance due to a vasoactive substance released by the tumor. Progression of the cardiac lesions does not appear to be affected by treatment with serotonin antagonists, and in some severely symptomatic patients valve replacement is indicated. Coronary artery spasm, presumably due to a circulating vasoactive substance, may occur in patients with carcinoid syndrome.

PHEOCHROMOCYTOMA (See Chap. 336)   In addition to causing hypertension, which may be labile or sustained, the high circulating levels of catecholamines may also cause direct myocardial injury. Focal myocardial necrosis and inflammatory cell infiltration are seen in about 50 percent of patients who die with pheochromocytoma and may contribute to clinically significant left ventricular failure and pulmonary edema. Left ventricular function and congestive heart failure may resolve after removal of the tumor. In addition, hypertension results in left ventricular hypertrophy.

RHEUMATOID ARTHRITIS AND THE COLLAGEN VASCULAR DISEASES   Rheumatoid arthritis (See Chap. 285)   There may be inflammation of any or all parts of the heart in patients with rheumatoid arthritis. *Pericarditis* is the most common cause of clinically apparent disease and may be found in 30 to 50 percent of all patients with rheumatoid arthritis, particularly those with subcutaneous nodules, if carefully searched for by echocardiography or at postmortem examination. However, only a small fraction of these patients will have clinical evidence of pericarditis, which usually follows a benign course, but occasionally may progress to cardiac tamponade or constrictive pericarditis. The pericardial fluid is generally an exudate, with decreased concentrations of complement and glucose and elevated cholesterol. Treatment is directed at the underlying rheumatoid arthritis and may include glucocorticoids. Pericardiectomy is usually required in cases of tamponade or persistent effusion. *Coronary arteritis* with intimal inflammation and edema is present in about 20 percent of cases but only rarely results in angina pectoris or myocardial infarction. The cardiac valves, most often the mitral and aortic, may be involved by inflammation and granuloma formation which in some cases may cause clinically significant regurgitation due to valve deformity. Myocarditis rarely results in cardiac dysfunction.

Seronegative arthropathies The seronegative arthropathies (Chaps. 289 and 298), ankylosing spondylitis, Reiter's syndrome, psoriatic arthritis, and the arthritides associated with ulcerative colitis and regional enteritis may be accompanied by a pancarditis and proximal aortitis; the latter may result in aortic regurgitation and may extend into the anterior mitral valve ring and/or AV node. Both aortic regurgitation and AV block are more common in patients with peripheral joint involvement and long-standing disease; treatment with aortic valve replacement and permanent pacemaker placement may be required. Up to one-fifth of patients with peripheral joint involvement and disease for more than 30 years have significant aortic regurgitation. Occasionally, aortic regurgitation precedes the onset of arthritis, and, therefore, the diagnosis of a seronegative arthritis should be considered in young males with isolated aortic regurgitation.

Systemic lupus erythematosus (SLE) (See Chap. 284) Pericarditis is common, occurring in about two-thirds of patients, and generally pursues a benign course, although rarely tamponade or constriction may result. The characteristic *endocardial lesions* of SLE, described by Libman and Sacks, consist of wartlike lesions most often located at the angles of the AV valves or on the ventricular surface of the mitral valve. Hemodynamically important valvular regurgitation is rare. Patients with SLE and elevated levels of antibody to cardiolipin appear to have a particularly high incidence of valvular disease, which is also more severe than in patients without these antibodies. Myocarditis generally parallels the activity of the disease, and although common histologically, seldom results in clinical heart failure unless associated with hypertension. Although arteritis of large coronary arteries may rarely result in myocardial ischemia, there is also an increased frequency of coronary atherosclerosis which may be related to hypertension or glucocorticoid therapy.

TRAUMATIC HEART DISEASE

Cardiac damage may be due to both penetrating and nonpenetrating injuries. The most frequent cause of a *nonpenetrating injury* is impact of the chest against the steering wheel of an automobile. Serious injury of the heart may ensue even though no external sign of thoracic trauma is evident. Although the commonest injury is myocardial contusion, any structure of the heart may be affected by the trauma. If the valvular apparatus is ruptured, a loud heart murmur produced by valvular regurgitation may appear, followed by the development of rapidly progressive heart failure. The most serious consequence of nonpenetrating injury is rupture, either of the atria or of the ventricles, which is generally fatal. Hemopericardium may also follow tearing of a pericardial vessel or coronary artery.

Myocardial contusion may cause arrhythmias, bundle branch block, or electrocardiographic abnormalities resembling those of infarction, and so it is important to bear trauma in mind as a cause

of otherwise unexplained electrocardiographic changes. Similarly, myocardial contusion may produce positive radionuclide scans and regional impairment of ventricular function, as occurs in myocardial infarction (Chap. 190). Pericardial effusion may occur weeks or even months after the accident. In these cases, the pericardial effusion is a manifestation of the postcardiac injury syndrome, which resembles the postpericardiotomy syndrome (Chap. 206).

Acute myocardial failure resulting from rupture of a valve usually requires operative correction. Myocardial infarction due to trauma is treated similarly to that due to ischemic heart disease (Chap. 202). Pericardial hemorrhage often leads to constriction which must be treated by decortication.

Penetrating injuries of the heart, produced by bullets or stab wounds, usually result in immediate or very rapid death because of hemopericardium or massive hemorrhage. However, sometimes the patient survives the acute incident and presents with a cardiac murmur and congestive heart failure. A left-to-right shunt due to traumatic ventricular septal defect, aortopulmonary artery fistula, or coronary arteriovenous fistula may be suspected and confirmed by cardiac catheterization and angiocardiography. Operation is indicated if hemodynamically significant abnormalities are present or if a foreign body, e.g., a bullet, is lodged in the heart. Immediate thoracotomy should be carried out if there is cardiac tamponade and/or shock, whether the trauma was penetrating or nonpenetrating. Pericardiocentesis may be helpful in patients with tamponade, but usually only as a holding maneuver. Patients who suffer penetrating injuries of the heart should be carefully examined several weeks after the event to rule out a ventricular septal defect or mitral regurgitation that may have gone undetected at the time of emergency surgery.

Rupture of the aorta is a common consequence of chest trauma. Indeed, rupture of the aorta at the isthmus or just above the aortic valve is the most common vascular deceleration injury. The clinical presentation is similar to that in aortic dissection (Chap. 210). The arterial pressure and pulse amplitude may be increased in the upper extremities and decreased in the lower extremities, and on chest roentgenogram there may be widening of the mediastinum. Occasionally, the rupture is limited by the aortic adventitia and results in a silent false aneurysm that may be discovered months or years after the injury. When great vessel rupture is due to a penetrating injury, there is usually a hemothorax and, less often, a hemopericardium. Hematoma formation may compress major vessels, and arteriovenous fistulae may be formed, sometimes resulting in high-output congestive heart failure.

REFERENCES

Actis Dato GM et al: Long-term follow-up of cardiac myxomas (7–31 years). J Cardiovasc Surg 34:141, 1993

Castells E et al: Cardiac myxomas: Surgical treatment, long-term results and recurrence. J Cardiovasc Surg 34:49, 1993

Cohn PF, Braunwald E: Traumatic heart disease, in *Heart Disease*, 4th ed, E Braunwald (ed). Philadelphia, Saunders, 1992, p 1517

Colucci WS, Braunwald E: Primary tumors of the heart, in *Heart Disease*, 4th ed, E Braunwald (ed). Philadelphia, Saunders, 1992 p 1451

Galve E et al: Prevalence, morphologic types, and evolution of cardiac valvular disease in systemic lupus erythematosus. N Engl J Med 319:817, 1988

Hara KS et al: Rheumatoid pericarditis: Clinical features and survival. Medicine (Baltimore) 69:81, 1990

Imperato-McGinley J et al: Reversibility of catecholamine-induced dilated cardiomyopathy in a child with a pheochromocytoma. N Engl J Med 316:793, 1987

Klein I: Thyroid hormone and the cardiovascular system. Am J Med 88:631, 1990

Lundin L: Carcinoid heart disease. A cardiologist's viewpoint. Acta Oncol 30:499, 1991

Nihoyannopoulos P et al: Cardiac abnormalities in systemic lupus erythematosus. Association with raised anticardiolipin antibodies. Circulation 82:369, 1990

O'Neill TW, Bresnihan B: The heart in ankylosing spondylitis. Ann Rheum Dis 51:705, 1992

Stollerman GH: Rheumatic fever and other rheumatic diseases of the heart, in *Heart Disease*, 4th ed, E Braunwald (ed). Philadelphia, Saunders, 1992, p 1721

Tazelaar HD et al: Pathology of surgically excised primary cardiac tumors. Mayo Clin Proc 67:957, 1992

Uusitupa MI et al: Diabetic heart muscle disease. Ann Med 22:377, 1990

Vidaillet HR Jr: Cardiac tumors associated with hereditary syndromes. Am J Cardiol 61:1355, 1988 section 2   **Disorders of the vascular system**

208   ATHEROSCLEROSIS AND OTHER FORMS OF ARTERIOSCLEROSIS

EDWIN L. BIERMAN

Arteriosclerosis, a generic term for thickening and hardening of the arterial wall, is responsible for the majority of deaths in the United States and most westernized societies. One type of arteriosclerosis is *atherosclerosis*, the disorder of the larger arteries that underlies most *coronary artery disease*, *aortic aneurysm*, and *arterial disease of the lower extremities* and also plays a major role in *cerebrovascular disease*. Atherosclerosis is by far the leading cause of death in the United States, both above and below age 65 and in both sexes (Table 208-1).

Other types of arteriosclerosis include focal calcific arteriosclerosis (*Mönckeberg's sclerosis*) and *arteriolosclerosis*. The major arterial diseases other than arteriosclerosis include *congenital structural defects*, *inflammatory* or *granulomatous* diseases (e.g., syphilitic aortitis), and disorders affecting mainly the smaller vessels, such as *hypersensitivity* or autoimmune diseases.

THE NORMAL ARTERY

STRUCTURE   The normal artery wall consists of three layers: the intima, the media, and the adventitia.

Intima   A single continuous layer of *endothelial cells* lines the lumen of all arteries. The intima is delimited on its outer aspect by a perforated tube of elastic tissue, the *internal elastic lamina*. This tube of elastic tissue is particularly prominent in the large elastic arteries and the medium-caliber muscular arteries, and it disappears in capillaries. The endothelial cells are attached to one another by a series of junctional complexes and are also attached, apparently somewhat tenuously, to an underlying meshwork of loose connective tissue, the *basal lamina*. These lining endothelial cells normally form a barrier that controls the entry of substances from the blood into the artery wall. Such substances usually enter the cells by specific transport systems. In addition, endothelial cells secrete a variety of substances that affect blood coagulation and the contraction and relaxation of the subjacent vascular smooth muscle (see below). Normally, no other cell type is present in the intima of most arteries.

Media   The media consists of only one cell type, the *smooth-muscle cell*, arranged in either a single layer (as in small muscular arteries) or multiple lamellae (as in elastic arteries). These cells are surrounded by small amounts of collagen and elastic fibers, which they elaborate, and usually take the pattern of diagonal concentric spirals through the vessel wall. They are closely apposed to one another and may be attached by junctional complexes. The smooth-muscle cell appears to be the major connective tissue–forming cell of the artery wall, producing collagen, elastic fibers, and proteoglycans. In this sense it is analogous to the fibroblast in skin, the osteoblast in bone, and the chondroblast in cartilage. The media is bounded on the luminal side by the *internal elastic lamina* and on the abluminal side by a less continuous sheet of elastic tissue, the *external elastic lamina*. In *elastic arteries*, such as the aorta and the

major pulmonary arteries, elastic lamellae are prominent. Such arteries expand and increase their elastic tension with the pulse of systole. In diastole, the elastic fibers recoil, helping to propel the blood distally and progressively damping the pulsatile character of flow toward more terminal vessels. In *muscular arteries*, in which smooth-muscle cells predominate, peripheral flow is regulated, particularly in arterioles, by contraction (vasoconstriction) and relaxation (vasodilatation). Located about midway through the media of most arteries is a "nutritional watershed." The outer portion is nourished from the small blood vessels (vasa vasorum) in the adventitia; the inner layers receive their nutrients from the lumen.

Adventitia   The outermost layer of the artery is the adventitia, which is delimited on the luminal aspect by the external elastic lamina. This external coat consists of a loose interwoven admixture of collagen bundles, elastic fibers, smooth-muscle cells, and fibroblasts. This layer also contains the vasa vasorum and nerves.

METABOLISM AND FUNCTION   The artery wall is a metabolically active organ that must meet a steady demand for energy to maintain smooth-muscle tension and endothelial cell function and to repair and replenish tissue constituents. The mechanical forces on the arterial wall are complex, and considerable tensile stresses are imposed on it, mainly by hydraulic force. Shear or frictional stresses are especially prominent near the entrance regions of branches. The form and manner in which these forces are dissipated depend on flow, the amount of elastic tension developed, and the tethering or external support provided by surrounding structures. Arteries are also permeable pipes, which constantly exchange fluid and solutes with the blood they carry.

Maintenance of the endothelial cell lining is critical. Endothelial cell turnover occurs at a slow rate but may be accelerated in focal areas by changing patterns of flow along the vessel wall. When intact, these cells selectively control the passage of circulating substances by active transport (endocytosis and exocytosis) through their cytoplasm, and they elaborate connective tissue components to form their own substratum. In addition, intact endothelial cells function to prevent clotting partly by elaboration of a particular prostaglandin (prostacyclin or PGI$_2$) that inhibits platelet function, thereby enhancing unimpeded flow of blood. When the lining is damaged, platelets adhere to it, in part as the result of production of a different class of prostaglandins, the thromboxanes, and form a clot; endothelial cells

---

TABLE 208-1   Deaths by cause in the United States, 1989

| | No. of deaths, thousands | | | |
| | Below age 65 | | Age 65 and above | |
Causes of death	Male	Female	Male	Female
All causes	394	217	721	717
All cardiovascular diseases	107	48	345	432
Ischemic heart disease	62	21	197	221
Cerebrovascular disease	10	9	47	78
All infectious disease	5	3	1	2
All cancer	85	77	177	158
Accidents	56	19	14	14

SOURCE: National Center of Health Statistics, *Vital Statistics Report, Final Mortality Statistics, 1989.*

function in the clotting process by elaboration of key substances, including factor VIII.

The metabolism of arteries reflects the biochemistry of smooth-muscle cells. Arterial smooth-muscle cells form abundant collagen, elastic fibers, soluble and insoluble elastin, and glucosaminoglycans (mainly dermatan sulfate). Multiple anabolic and catabolic pathways are present. These cells metabolize glucose by both anaerobic and aerobic glycolysis. A variety of catabolic enzymes are present, including fibrinolysins, mixed-function oxidases, and lysosomal hydrolases. Because of the prominence of lipids in atherosclerotic lesions, much attention has been directed to lipid metabolism in arteries. Arterial wall cells can synthesize fatty acids, cholesterol, phospholipids, and triglycerides from endogenous substrates to satisfy their structural needs (membrane replenishment), but smooth-muscle cells appear preferentially to utilize lipids from plasma lipoproteins transported into the wall. Circulating lipoproteins traverse endothelial cells in pinocytotic vesicles. Smooth-muscle cells possess specific high-affinity surface receptors for certain apoproteins on the surface of lipid-rich lipoproteins, thus facilitating the entry of lipoproteins into the cell by adsorptive endocytosis. As has been shown for cultured skin fibroblasts, in arterial smooth-muscle cells these vesicles fuse with lysosomes, resulting in catabolism of lipoprotein components (Chap. 344). Free cholesterol entering the cell in this manner inhibits endogenous cholesterol synthesis, facilitates its own esterification, and partially limits further entry of cholesterol by regulating the number of lipoprotein receptors. However, lipoprotein cholesterol can gain entry into arterial smooth-muscle cells by unregulated receptor-independent pathways, potentially causing cholesterol ester accumulation. Because of the importance of regulation of arterial smooth-muscle cell proliferation, interest also has focused on the elaboration of growth factors and growth inhibitors by arterial wall cells. Both endothelial cells and smooth-muscle cells are capable of elaborating a variety of growth regulatory molecules, functions that may be altered in disease. Further, endothelial cells can regulate vascular tone by elaboration of molecules that produce vasoconstriction or vasodilation (e.g., nitric oxide) and can elaborate cytokines and adhesion molecules that influence interactions with circulating blood cells.

Thus many complex and interrelated metabolic processes are present in arterial wall cells. Although some of these may play a role in the production of arteriosclerosis, no one biochemical reaction or cellular function can be singled out as culpable. Physiologic factors, such as transfer processes across the endothelial lining, the flux of oxygen and substrates from both the luminal and adventitial sides of the wall, and the reverse flow of catabolic products, need to be considered as well. The ability of the arterial wall to maintain the integrity of its endothelium, prevent platelet aggregation, prevent adherence of blood mononuclear cells, prevent cholesterol accumulation, prevent intimal smooth-muscle cell proliferation, and ensure the nutrition of its middle portion may be the critical determinants of the arteriosclerotic process.

CHANGES WITH AGING The major change that occurs with normal aging in the arterial wall in humans is a slow, apparently continuous, symmetric increase in the thickness of the intima. This intimal thickening results from a gradual accumulation of smooth-muscle cells surrounded by additional connective tissue. In the nondiseased artery wall, lipid content, mainly cholesterol ester and phospholipid (particularly sphingomyelin), also progressively increases with age. While most of the phospholipid in the normal artery wall appears to be derived from in situ synthesis, the cholesterol ester that accumulates with aging appears to be derived from plasma, since it contains principally linoleic acid, the major plasma cholesterol ester fatty acid. Furthermore, low-density lipoproteins are immunologically detectable in the intima of normal arteries in direct relation to their concentration in plasma. It has been estimated that between the second and sixth decade, the normal intima accumulates approximately 25 μmol (10 mg) cholesterol per gram of tissue. Thus, as the normal artery ages, smooth-muscle cells and connective tissue accumulate

diffusely in the intima, leading to progressive thickening, coupled with progressive accumulation of sphingomyelin and cholesterol linoleate. This diffuse age-related intima thickening is to be distinguished from focal discrete raised fibrous plaques, a characteristic feature of atherosclerosis.

Functionally, these changes with aging result in gradually increasing rigidity of vessels. The larger arteries may become dilated, elongated, and tortuous, and aneurysms may form in areas of an encroaching degenerating arteriosclerotic plaque. Such "wear-and-tear" changes are frequently proportional to the vessel diameter and correlated with branching, curvature, and anatomic points of attachment. The amount of external support also determines the ability of vessels, weakened by loss of elasticity, to withstand hydrostatic pressure. The unsupported cerebral arteries may be particularly vulnerable in this regard. Although senescence is accompanied by the intimal thickening that is a feature of localized atheromatosis, the changes of aging and arteriosclerosis appear to be separate and distinct processes.

NONATHEROMATOUS FORMS OF ARTERIOSCLEROSIS

Atherosclerosis involves primarily the intimal layer and occurs most commonly in the abdominal aorta and its large renal and lower extremity branches, the coronary arteries, and the cerebral vasculature. It may accompany or accelerate the other major forms of arteriosclerosis, *focal calcification* and *arteriolosclerosis* (Table 208-2).

FOCAL CALCIFICATION Not to be confused with atherosclerosis is focal calcification of the media, particularly in the medium-sized muscular arteries. This type of arteriosclerosis is called *Mönckeberg's sclerosis* and is common in the lower extremities, upper extremities, and the arterial supply of the genital tract in both sexes. This disorder is rare in individuals below age 50 and affects both sexes indiscriminately. The process involves degeneration of smooth-muscle cells followed by calcium deposition. The vessels become hard and tortuous so that palpable vessels such as the radial artery can be felt as rigid tubes. Its characteristic radiologic appearance consists of regular concentric calcifications in cross section and a "railroad track" in longitudinal section, commonly seen in vessels in the pelvis, legs, and feet. The medial changes alone do not narrow the lumen, have little effect on the circulation, and have relatively little clinical significance. However, in the lower extremities, medial arterial calcification is often associated with atherosclerosis, leading to arterial occlusion. These changes are common in the elderly and in patients

---

TABLE 208-2   Disorders associated with early arteriosclerosis

ATHEROSCLEROSIS

Diabetes mellitus
Hypertension
Familial hypercholesterolemia
Familial combined hyperlipidemia
Familial dysbetalipoproteinemia
Familial hypoalphalipoproteinemia
Hypothyroidism
Cholesterol ester storage disease
Systemic lupus erythematosus
Homocysteinemia

NONATHEROMATOUS ARTERIOSCLEROSIS

Diabetes mellitus
Chronic renal insufficiency
Chronic vitamin D intoxication
Pseudoxanthoma elasticum
Idiopathic arterial calcification in infancy
Aortic valvular calcification in the elderly
Werner's syndrome

on long-term glucocorticoid therapy, but in individuals with diabetes mellitus, focal calcification may be accelerated and severe. It is much more common in diabetics with neuropathy, and sympathetic denervation of medial smooth muscle has been implicated in its cause.

Focal calcification also can produce the arteriosclerotic aortic valve in the elderly. Progressive calcium deposition occurs on the aortic surface of normal trileaflet aortic valves with age, resulting in a spectrum of clinical findings ranging from an innocent systolic murmur to severe calcific aortic stenosis (Chap. 201).

ARTERIOLOSCLEROSIS This disorder involves hyaline and degenerative changes affecting both the intima and media of smooth arteries and arterioles, particularly in the spleen, pancreas, adrenal, and kidney. In the kidney, but not necessarily elsewhere, arteriosclerosis is almost invariably associated with hypertension. Lesser degrees of sustained hypertension characteristically cause *hyalinization* of renal arterioles; more severe or malignant hypertension produces a typical *fibrous and elastic hyperplasia*, and even necrosis, of the media and intima.

ATHEROSCLEROSIS

LESIONS   Morbid anatomy Atherosclerosis is a patchy nodular type of arteriosclerosis. The lesions are commonly classified as *early lesions* (*initial lesions* and *fatty streaks*), *intermediate lesions*, *fibrous plaques*, and *complicated lesions*.

Initial (fatty streak) and *intermediate lesions* are focal, small, and nonobstructive. Initial lesions may be detectable only chemically or microscopically, consist of lipid deposition in intimal macrophages (macrophage foam cells), and represent the first changes that have been found to evolve into lesions associated with clinical disease. Often found in children, they are located in atherosclerosis-susceptible regions of the arterial tree.

Fatty streaks are visible to the naked eye on the endothelial surface of the aorta and coronary arteries. They are still small and nonobstructive and contain a larger accumulation of lipid-filled smooth-muscle cells and macrophages (foam cells) and fibrous tissue in focal areas of the intima. They are stained distinctly by fat-soluble dyes but may be visible without staining as yellowish or whitish patches, streaks, or dots on the intimal surface. The lipid is mainly cholesterol oleate and is mainly intracellular.

Fatty streaks are visible in the aorta and coronary arteries of very young children and increase in the aorta at puberty. Whether or not these lesions progress to advanced lesions at particular sites depends largely on hemodynamic forces and the plasma levels of atherogenic lipoproteins. Those lesions that are prone to progression develop extracellular lipid and debris in the proteoglycan matrix so that lipid pools form among the layers of intimal smooth-muscle cells. At this stage, a single lipid core is not evident, cell death is not apparent, and cholesterol crystals are rarely found. These lesions are considered to be intermediate or preatheromatous, on the way to developing the lipid core characterizing the advanced lesion (atheroma or fibrous plaque).

Fibrous plaques are palpably elevated areas of intimal thickening and represent the most characteristic lesion of advancing atherosclerosis. These atheromatous lesions first appear in the abdominal aorta, coronary arteries, and carotid arteries in the third decade and increase progressively with age. They appear in men before women, in the aorta before the coronary arteries, and much later in the vertebral and intracranial cerebral arteries. Reasons for the difference in susceptibility of various segments of the arterial tree and the nonuniform distribution of lesions are not known. Typically, the fibrous plaque is firm, elevated, and dome-shaped, with an opaque glistening surface that bulges into the lumen. It consists of a central core of extracellular lipid (with cholesterol crystals) and necrotic cell debris ("gruel") covered by a fibromuscular layer or cap containing large numbers of smooth-muscle cells, macrophages, and collagen. Thus the plaque is much thicker than is normal intima. Although the lipid,

like that of fatty streaks, is mainly cholesterol ester, the principal esterified fatty acid is linoleic rather than oleic, reflecting its largely extracellular distribution. Thus plaque cholesterol ester composition differs from fatty streaks but resembles plasma lipoproteins.

The *complicated lesion* is a calcified fibrous plaque containing various degrees of necrosis, thrombosis, and ulceration. These are the lesions frequently associated with symptoms. With increasing necrosis and accumulation of gruel, the arterial wall progressively weakens, and rupture of the intima can occur, causing aneurysm and hemorrhage. Arterial emboli can form when fragments of plaque dislodge into the lumen. Stenosis and impaired organ function result from gradual occlusion as plaques thicken and thrombi form.

Localization Although the term *generalized atherosclerosis* is commonly used clinically, lesions are actually irregularly distributed; different vessels are involved at different ages and to varying degrees. The abdominal aorta is involved earliest and most severely by atherosclerotic lesions, and it is the bellwether of lesions elsewhere. The aorta is usually most heavily involved at or near the orifices of its branches (particularly at the level of the coronary and intercostal arteries), in the aortic arch, and frequently at its bifurcation into the iliac arteries. There is more atherosclerosis in the lower than in the upper limbs. In the legs, the incidence decreases peripherally as the musculoelastic vessels give way to large muscular arteries and these become smaller vessels, such as the plantar or digital arteries. Plaques and thromboses are particularly common in the *femoral* artery, in Hunter's canal, and in the *popliteal* artery just above the knee joint. The *anterior* and *posterior tibial* arteries are often occluded together, but in different sites—the posterior where it rounds the internal malleolus and the anterior where it is superficial and becomes the dorsalis pedis artery. The peroneal artery, which is well embedded in muscle, often escapes when other major vessels are occluded, and it may be the main blood supply to the extremity (*peroneal leg*). Atherosclerosis in abdominal branches, except for the renal and mesenteric arteries, causes less difficulty than in coronary and cerebral vessels.

In the *coronary arteries*, raised lesions are most prominent in the main stems, the highest incidence being a short distance beyond the ostia. Atherosclerosis is nearly always found in the epicardial (extramural) portions of the vessels, while the intramural coronary arteries are spared. Coronary atherosclerosis is often diffuse. The degree to which the lumen is narrowed varies, but once the process is present, all the intima of the extramural portions of the vessel is usually involved. A single tiny plaque occluding an otherwise normal coronary artery is rare. Selective involvement of the coronary arteries may relate to the unique hemodynamic forces, unlike those of other major arteries, resulting from greater flow in diastole than systole. The implications of these flow patterns for atherogenesis are as yet unknown. Typical atheromatous fibrous plaques also develop in saphenous vein aortocoronary bypass grafts.

In the cervical and cerebral arteries the distribution of atherosclerosis is patchy, as it may be in other arteries. It first appears in the base of the brain in the carotid, basilar, and vertebral arteries. The proximal portion of the internal carotid artery in the neck is a site of special predilection. There is a concentration of lesions near bifurcations. Atherosclerosis in the *pulmonary artery* bears no relation to the severity of the disease in the aorta or other systemic arteries. There is some involvement in about half of adults over 50 years of age who have no reason to have pulmonary hypertension. Pulmonary hypertension per se, however, is associated with medial hypertrophy, intimal thickening, and great acceleration of atheroma formation.

THEORIES OF ATHEROGENESIS A generally accepted theory for the pathogenesis of atherosclerosis consistent with a variety of experimental evidence is the *reaction to injury* hypothesis. According to this idea, the endothelial cells lining the intima are exposed to repeated or continuing insults to their integrity. The injury to the endothelium may be subtle or gross, resulting in a loss of the ability of the cells to function normally and act as a permeability barrier. In the extreme, the cells may desquamate. Examples of types of "injury" to the endothelium include metabolic injury, as in chronic hypercholesterolemia or homocysteinemia, mechanical stress associated with hypertension, and immunologic injury, as may be seen after cardiac or renal transplantation. Dysfunctional endothelial cells at susceptible sites in the arterial tree would lead to exposure of the subendothelial tissue to increased concentrations of plasma constituents. This may trigger a sequence of events including monocyte and platelet adherence, migration of monocytes into the intima to become macrophages, platelet aggregation and formation of microthrombi, and release of platelet and macrophage secretory products, including growth factors and cytokines (such as platelet-derived growth factor, interleukin 1, colony stimulating factors), in conjunction with plasma constituents, including lipoproteins and hormones such as insulin. This could stimulate the proliferation of intimal smooth-muscle cells at these sites of injury. These proliferating smooth-muscle cells would deposit a connective tissue matrix and accumulate lipid, a process that would be particularly enhanced with hyperlipidemia. Monocyte-derived macrophages also can accumulate lipids, some of which are in the form of lipid-protein complexes characteristic of oxidized lipoproteins. These cells are also capable of modifying lipoproteins in situ, favoring their uptake by scavenger receptors. Endothelial cells and macrophages can elaborate a chemoattractant protein that sustains accumulation of monocyte-derived macrophages.

Adherence of monocytes to altered endothelial cells and their migration into the arterial wall to become resident macrophages may be the earliest cellular abnormality in atherogenesis. Thus repeated or chronic injury could lead to a slowly progressing lesion involving a gradual increase in intimal smooth-muscle cells, macrophages, connective tissue, and lipid. Areas where the shearing stress on endothelial cells is increased, such as branch points or bifurcation of vessels, would be at greatest risk. As the lesions progress and the intima becomes thicker, blood flow over the sites will be altered and will potentially place the lining endothelial cells at even greater risk for further injury, leading to an inexorable cycle of events culminating in the complicated lesion. However, a single or a few injurious episodes may lead to a proliferative response that could regress, in contrast to continued or chronic injury. This hypothesis of reaction to injury thus is consistent with the known intimal thickening observed during normal aging, would explain how many of the etiologic factors implicated in atherogenesis might enhance lesion formation, might explain how inhibitors of platelet aggregation could interfere with lesion formation, and could elucidate how treatment targeted at risk-factor reduction can interrupt progression or even produce regression of atheromatous lesions.

Other theories of atherogenesis are not mutually exclusive. The *monoclonal hypothesis* suggests, on the basis of single isoenzyme types found in lesions, that the intimal proliferative lesions result from the multiplication of single, individual smooth-muscle cells, as do benign tumors. In this manner, mitogenic, and possibly mutagenic, factors that might stimulate smooth-muscle cell proliferation would act on single cells. Focal *clonal senescence* may explain how intrinsic aging processes contribute to atherosclerosis. According to this hypothesis, the intimal smooth-muscle cells that proliferate to form an atheroma are normally under feedback control by mitosis inhibitors formed by the smooth-muscle cells in the contiguous media, and this feedback control system tends to fail with age as these controlling cells die and are not adequately replaced. This is consistent with the observation that cultured human arterial medial smooth-muscle cells, like fibroblasts, show a decline in their ability to replicate as a function of donor age.

The *lysosomal theory* suggests that altered lysosomal function might contribute to atherogenesis. Since lysosomal enzymes can accomplish the generalized degradation of cellular components required for continuing renewal, this system has been implicated in cellular aging and the accumulation of lipofuscin or "age pigment." It has been suggested that increased deposition of cholesterol esters in arterial smooth-muscle cells may be related in part to a relative deficiency in the activity of lysosomal cholesterol ester hydrolase. Consonant with this idea, some patients with the rare cholesterol ester storage disease caused by a defect in lysosomal cholesterol ester hydrolase may have accelerated atherosclerosis. However, lipid droplets in foam cells are often cytoplasmic rather than lysosomal, and this theory is not now widely held.

RECOGNITION OF ATHEROSCLEROSIS Angiographic visualization of deformity in the lumen of a vessel remains the best presumptive test of silent atherosclerosis. Coronary angiography now permits visualization and assessment of arteries as small as 0.5 mm in diameter. Several sophisticated noninvasive techniques have been developed for demonstrating its presence. Doppler probes for measuring velocity and amount of blood flow have been used noninvasively and adapted to determine vessel outlines. Ultrasonic techniques are not yet clinically useful for detection of plaques in the coronary arteries.

Functional tests based on pathophysiologic or metabolic effects of a narrowed arterial lumen often give indirect clues. Assessment of electrocardiographic changes induced after standardized exercise is a relatively simple noninvasive aid to the diagnosis of coronary atherosclerosis with significant narrowing. Similarly, myocardial perfusion defects demonstrable with imaging techniques using radionuclides are usually attributable to atherosclerosis (Chap. 191). Digital plethysmography with exercise often unmasks significant atherosclerotic involvement of lower extremity arteries.

Radiographic demonstration of calcification in the location of arteries does not always indicate the presence of atherosclerosis. Although calcified coronary vessels usually indicate atherosclerosis, complete luminal obstruction may occur in the absence of any calcification. Calcification or beading of peripheral arteries is not correlated directly with atherosclerosis but more likely reflects medial sclerosis. Abnormalities in retinal arterioles evident on funduscopic examination are not well correlated with atherosclerosis in arteries. Thus, despite the availability of a variety of tests, detection of atherosclerosis usually awaits one of the clinical events attending a critical decrease of blood flow in an involved vessel. As yet there is no blood test for atherosclerosis. Knowledge of the prevalence and incidence of arteriosclerosis and most of the inferences concerning its causes are derived from tabulations of the appearance of its sequelae.

Ischemic heart disease (IHD), synonymous with *coronary heart disease* or *arteriosclerotic heart disease* (Chap. 203), is the most reliable indicator of atherosclerosis available today. Practically all patients with myocardial infarction, as defined by electrocardiographic and enzymatic changes, have coronary atherosclerosis. Rare exceptions are due to congenital anomalies of the coronary vessels, emboli, or ostial occlusion due to the other types of cardiac or vascular disease. Nontraumatic *sudden death* (Chap. 35) makes up a sizable portion of all deaths eventually certified as due to IHD. At autopsy, evidence of fresh myocardial infarction or of *coronary thrombosis* is usually absent. While ventricular fibrillation may have been due to sudden closure of a partially compromised vessel by a small thrombus or embolus or to *spasm*, none of these need have preceded a fatal arrhythmia. The majority of victims of sudden death have had a previous diagnosis of IHD; the number who had diabetes or hypertension is also significant. In epidemiologic studies of IHD, *angina pectoris* and electrocardiographic changes attributable to ischemia without infarction are considered "softer end points" and are treated separately.

Cerebrovascular disease (stroke) is a less reliable criterion for the presence of atherosclerosis. It includes *cerebral thrombosis* and *cerebral hemorrhage* (Chap. 368). Cerebral thrombosis, including infarction or softening without evidence of embolus, is usually due to atherosclerosis. On the other hand, cerebral hemorrhage is most often the result of congenital aneurysms or of vascular defects peculiar to hypertension and diabetes. Dissections of the aorta (Chap. 210), *peripheral vascular disease* (Chap. 211), thrombosis of other major vessels, and ischemic renal disease (Chap. 243) likewise are not used to determine the prevalence of atherosclerosis in a population or as an index of atherosclerosis elsewhere. Therefore, from an epidemiologic standpoint, consideration of atherosclerosis focuses on IHD.

INCIDENCE AND PREVALENCE According to the National Health Examination Survey, about 5 million Americans have IHD. It is the leading cause of death in males after age 35 and in all persons after age 45. Premature deaths from IHD, arbitrarily defined as those appearing before age 65, occur preponderantly in men, and a third of all deaths from IHD in males occur before age 65. In fact, nearly all the excess premature mortality in American males is due to IHD. Between the ages of 35 and 55, the death rate is five times higher in white men than in white women in the United States. The exceptions are women with hypertension, diabetes, hyperlipidemia, or premature (usually iatrogenic) menopause, who are at increased risk and often share the risk of the male. For both sexes, there is more than a fivefold increase in the average annual incidence of myocardial infarction between ages 40 and 60. A higher mortality rate in younger nonwhite women is probably due mainly to a greater incidence of hypertension in blacks. There is less difference between men and women in the prevalence of angina pectoris than in that of myocardial infarction; after age 65, more women than men have angina without a history of infarction.

Changing death rates In the United States death rates from IHD rose appreciably between 1940 and 1960. Mortality peaked in 1963 and started to decline, with the rate of decline accelerating in recent years for all ages, for both sexes, and for whites and nonwhites. This recent decline in mortality from coronary atherosclerosis (Table 208-3) is the first recorded in American history and is almost unique among industrialized countries. In other parts of the world, including Russia and many countries in eastern Europe, IHD death rates are still climbing. By contrast, in the United States, the IHD death rate declined by 57 percent between 1968 and 1990. The trend cannot be attributed to a single cause, but there has been a concurrent change in living habits, including reduced cigarette smoking among middle-aged men, decreased consumption of animal fats and cholesterol, better control of hypertension, and improved treatment of IHD.

International comparisons In most industrialized countries, IHD is the major single cause of premature cardiovascular deaths. There are, however, marked differences in premature death rates among them. The seven having the highest rates in men between 35 and 74 years of age are Finland, Scotland, Northern Ireland, Australia, New Zealand, England, and the United States. Much lower age-adjusted death rates from IHD are found in Latin America and Japan. The rates in Japan are about one-sixth those in the United States. Subsamples obtained in many countries convey the strong impression that upper socioeconomic classes that have adopted the culture of western industrialized countries have far more IHD than do lower socioeconomic classes. Among the most obvious cultural differences between these groups are total calories, fat content of the diet, and amount of physical work. Extensive epidemiologic studies have not revealed the reasons for differences between cultures that are superficially similar. Migrants to the United States tend to have a higher risk of death from premature IHD than do age-matched relatives who remain at home. Although there are many instances in which

TABLE 208-4 Risk factors for atherosclerosis

Male gender
Family history of premature IHD (before age 55 in a parent or sibling)
Hyperlipidemia
Cigarette smoking (currently smoking more than 10 cigarettes per day)
Hypertension
Low HDL cholesterol [below 0.9 mmol/L (35 mg/dL)]
Diabetes mellitus
Hyperinsulinemia
Abdominal obesity
High lipoprotein (a)
Personal history of cerebrovascular disease or occlusive peripheral vascular disease

different ethnic groups in the same locality have widely differing prevalences of IHD, the available data suggest that cultural factors are more important than genetic determination of IHD. Nevertheless, genetic heterogeneity undoubtedly underlies many of the striking differences in susceptibility seen among individuals sharing the same ethnic and cultural setting.

ETIOLOGIC FACTORS A number of conditions and habits present more frequently in individuals who develop atherosclerosis than in the general population; these factors have been termed *risk factors*. The majority of people below age 65 afflicted with atherosclerosis have one or more identifiable risk factors other than aging (Table 208-4). The risk-factor concept implies that a person with at least one risk factor is more likely to develop a clinical atherosclerotic event and is likely to do so earlier than a person with no risk factors. The presence of multiple risk factors further accelerates atherosclerosis. They vary in terms of importance in the population of the United States. Hypercholesterolemia, hypertension, and cigarette smoking may be the most potent factors involved in causation of atherosclerosis. Risk factors also vary in terms of their potential reversibility with current techniques of preventive management.

Thus age, gender, and genetic factors are currently considered to be irreversible risk factors, whereas continually emerging evidence suggests that elimination of cigarette smoking and treatment of hypertension reverses the high risk for atherosclerosis attributable to those factors. A major multicenter trial has shown that reduction of hypercholesterolemia reduces the risk of IHD. Life insurance policyholder data suggest that reduction of obesity reduces total mortality, presumably by diminishing the sequelae of atherosclerosis. Other potentially reversible factors are currently under study.

These factors are not mutually exclusive, since they clearly interact. For example, obesity, particularly of the abdominal type (assessed by the waist/hip circumference ratio), appears to be causally associated with hypertension, hyperglycemia, hypercholesterolemia, hypertriglyceridemia, and low high-density lipoprotein (HDL) cholesterol levels. Genetic factors may play a role by exerting direct effects on arterial wall cell structure and metabolism, or they may act indirectly via such factors as hypertension, hyperlipidemia, diabetes, and obesity. Aging appears to be one of the more complex factors associated with the development of atherosclerosis, since many of the risk factors in themselves are related to aging, e.g., elevated blood pressure, hyperglycemia, and hyperlipidemia. Thus, in addition to the possible involvement of intrinsic aging in atherogenesis (perhaps through effects on arterial wall metabolism), a variety of associated metabolic factors are also age-dependent.

Hyperlipidemia Both *hypercholesterolemia* and *hypertriglyceridemia* appear to be important risk factors for atherosclerosis. While there is no absolute quantitative definition of hyperlipidemia, statistical definitions, based on the upper 5 or 10 percent of the distribution of plasma lipid levels within a population, are often used. Such definitions are likely to detect affected individuals from families with one of the familial hyperlipidemias or having hyperlipidemia associated with other diseases or drugs; they also are useful for prediction of emergence of premature atherosclerosis and institution of preventive measures. However, these upper limits of "normality" are too high

TABLE 208-3 Age-adjusted death rates by cause in the United States, 1968, 1979, and 1990

	Rate per 100,000 population		
Cause of death	1968	1979	1990
All deaths	744	577	520
All cardiovascular diseases	362	254	190
Ischemic heart disease	242	150	103
Cerebrovascular disease	71	42	28
Cancer	129	131	135

SOURCE: The National Center for Health Statistics, *Monthly Vital Statistics Report, Advance Report of Final Mortality Statistics, 1990.*

for defining those cholesterol and triglyceride levels that are correlated with increasing risk of IHD in whole populations. Thus correlations between the cholesterol concentrations in young men in North America and the incidence of premature IHD indicate that an increasing risk can be detected when the cholesterol level is higher than 5.20 mmol/L (200 mg/dL), a value close to the median for men from 40 to 49 years of age in this population. Extrapolation of similar data from other populations suggests that the cholesterol level at birth averages 1.5 mmol/L (60 mg/dL). Within a month the average has risen to about 3 mmol/L (120 mg/dL) and by the first year to 4.5 mmol/L (175 mg/dL). A second rise begins in the third decade and continues to about age 50 in men and somewhat later in women.

A similar age-related increase in plasma triglyceride level is also observed. The increases in cholesterol are associated mainly with a rise in *low-density lipoprotein* (LDL) concentrations; the increases in triglyceride are associated with a rise in *very low density lipoproteins* (VLDL) and *remnants* of their catabolism (mainly intermediate-density lipoprotein, IDL). Adiposity may play a key role in this age-associated rise in triglyceride and cholesterol levels, since the increases in triglyceride, cholesterol, and body weight with age in whole populations occur concurrently. In primitive people who remain thin throughout adulthood, plasma lipids do not increase with age. Metabolic mechanisms have been postulated whereby abdominal obesity, which is associated with insulin resistance of peripheral tissues and compensatory hyperinsulinemia, promotes enhanced production of triglyceride- and cholesterol-rich lipoproteins by the liver and consequent hyperlipidemia, hypertension, and hyperglycemia (the insulin-resistance syndrome). Current concepts of plasma lipoprotein transport suggest that accumulation of cholesterol in the circulation may in part be secondary to excessive production of triglyceride-rich lipoproteins. Particle size of LDL (small, dense LDL or LDL subclass phenotype pattern B) has been implicated as a risk factor for IHD. LDL pattern B may be inherited as a dominant genetic trait and is also associated with high triglyceride and low HDL cholesterol levels, central obesity, and other features of the insulin-resistance syndrome. While closely associated with IHD in cross-sectional studies, LDL pattern B may not be an *independent* indicator of risk.

HYPERCHOLESTEROLEMIA   This is associated unequivocally with increased incidence of premature IHD; however, its importance varies in relation to age. In the Framingham Study, cholesterol levels in men below age 40 were closely related to the future development of IHD; this relation was less pronounced in older individuals. In the Multiple Risk Factor Intervention Trial (MRFIT), men with cholesterol levels above about 6 mmol/L (240 mg/dL) had more than a threefold increase in risk of IHD death compared with men with cholesterol levels below about 5 mmol/L (200 mg/dL). There is a continuous exponential gradient of risk as the cholesterol level ascends. These data are supported by comparisons of the prevalence of IHD and cholesterol (or LDL) in many other populations. The relationship of triglycerides and VLDL to IHD is confounded by a rise in cholesterol as VLDL increases. Nevertheless, in several, but not all, population studies, increased triglycerides (or VLDL) are independently correlated with premature IHD.

HYPERTRIGLYCERIDEMIA   This may be associated with premature atherosclerosis in some specific disorders; this association may not be apparent in studies of whole populations. Patients with high VLDL levels who come from families with familial combined hyperlipidemia appear to be at the same increased risk as those affected members of these families with elevated LDL levels. In contrast, patients with comparably elevated VLDL levels who come from families with pure monogenic familial hypertriglyceridemia do not appear to have an increased risk. In addition, high VLDL levels may increase the risk for premature atherosclerosis when associated with other risk factors for coronary artery disease, such as in diabetics and in patients on chronic hemodialysis who smoke and are hypertensive. Individuals in whom remnant lipoproteins accumulate, with resulting elevations in both cholesterol and triglycerides (Chap. 344), also seem to be at risk for early development of atherosclerosis.

Some of these relationships were clarified in a comprehensive study in Seattle of the role of the genetics of hyperlipidemia in clinical atherosclerosis in which 500 consecutive survivors of myocardial infarction were tested. Hyperlipidemia was present in about one-third of the group. Approximately one-half of the males and two-thirds of the females below age 50 had either hypertriglyceridemia, hypercholesterolemia, or both. On the other hand, in individuals over age 70, the prevalence of atherosclerotic coronary disease was very high, yet virtually no males (and only about one-fourth of the females) had hyperlipidemia. Thus in both sexes there appeared to be a progressive decline with age in the association of hyperlipidemia with myocardial infarction. More than half the hyperlipidemic atherosclerotic survivors appeared to have simple monogenic familial disorders inherited as an autosomal dominant trait (*familial combined hyperlipidemia* was the most common and *familial hypercholesterolemia* was the least common). These simply inherited hyperlipidemias were more frequent in myocardial infarction survivors below age 60 than in those who were older. In contrast, nonmonogenic forms of hyperlipidemia occurred with equal frequency above and below age 60. Thus it appears that genes associated with the simply inherited hyperlipidemias accelerate atherosclerosis. While all studies indicate that hyperlipidemia is a very meaningful risk factor below age 50 and that it operates independently of, and in addition to, hypertension, diabetes, obesity, and other factors, blood lipid levels continue to predict IHD in men and women over age 65.

SCREENING   When the screening of individuals for hyperlipidemia occurs after a myocardial infarction, it is several decades too late, although interruption of further progression of atherosclerosis now appears possible. Screening at birth or in childhood for genetic hyperlipidemia is not practical or useful except in the instance of familial hypercholesterolemia, which may affect about 1 in 1000 children. This is detectable by LDL elevations in cord blood when one already knows that a parent is affected. Other genetic or nongenetic primary hyperlipidemia often is not apparent until the third decade. *Today, screening measurement of blood cholesterol levels (nonfasting) by physicians is recommended for all adult patients. It is especially important in all young persons who have a family history of premature IHD.*

Hyperlipidemia is best confirmed by measurement of the concentration of total cholesterol and triglycerides and of HDL cholesterol in serum or plasma in a sample obtained after an overnight fast. The measurements should be made by a reliable laboratory that follows a program of standardization. Routine use of lipoprotein electrophoresis provides little additional information, is nonspecific, and is not recommended for screening or for management.

MANAGEMENT OF HYPERLIPIDEMIAS   In adults less than 65 years of age, a cholesterol concentration (C) greater than 6 mmol/L (240 mg/dL) or a triglyceride concentration (TG) greater than 2.8 mmol/L (250 mg/dL) clearly indicates hyperlipidemia sufficient to require some attention by the physician to the items listed in Table 208-5. Less severe degrees of hypercholesterolemia nevertheless can impart some degree of risk for IHD. The National Cholesterol Education Program (NCEP) has suggested that total cholesterol (C) > 6.2 mmol/L (240 mg/dL) is "high risk" and should prompt careful evaluation (see Table 208-5), estimation of LDL cholesterol, and some approach to cholesterol lowering. Cholesterol between 5.2 and 6.1 mmol/dL (200 and 239 mg/dL) is borderline high. The presence of two or more risk factors (independent of C or TG levels) listed in Table 208-4 or preexisting IHD puts these patients in the high-risk category. For treatment decisions, and when TG < 4.5 mmol/L (400 mg/dL), LDL cholesterol (LDL-C) levels can be estimated as total C − HDL-C − TG/5. Patients considered at high risk for IHD should be treated aggressively to lower blood cholesterol out of the high-risk range (Table 208-6). If C < 5.2 mmol/L (200 mg/dL), the tests need not be repeated for several years in an adult who maintains body weight and does not otherwise change in health or life-style. If causes of *secondary hyperlipidemia* or offending drugs are absent, attention to the origin of *primary hyperlipidemia* turns mainly to diet and

TABLE 208-5 **Factors to consider in patients with hyperlipidemia**

Disorders to which hyperlipidemia is secondary
  Uncontrolled diabetes mellitus (insulin deficiency)
  Hypothyroidism
  Uremia
  Nephrotic syndrome (hypoproteinemia)
  Obstructive liver disease
  Dysproteinemia (multiple myeloma, lupus erythematosus)
Drugs producing or aggravating hyperlipidemia
  Oral contraceptives
  Glucocorticoids
  Antihypertensives (thiazides and beta blockers)
Dietary factors
  Caloric intake (recent weight gain)
  Content of saturated fats and cholesterol
  Alcohol intake
Genetic disorders (primary hyperlipidemias)
  Family history of hyperlipidemia or xanthomas
  History of pancreatitis or recurrent abdominal pain

genetic causes. Severe hyperlipidemia [C > 7.8 mmol/L (300 mg/dL) or TG > 5.6 mmol/L (500 mg/dL)] usually reflects a genetic disorder; when xanthomas are present, it practically always does. Diagnosis always includes examination of first-degree relatives and proceeds according to information contained in Chap. 344.

Reduction of hypercholesterolemia results in a decrease in progression of atherosclerosis in humans and other primates. Several controlled trials of different diets which have been accompanied by a fall in mean cholesterol levels in small test populations have shown a favorable effect on incidence of the overall complications of IHD. The drug clofibrate given to a normal population reduced the incidence of nonfatal myocardial infarctions and was associated with a reduction of cholesterol levels; however, total mortality was not lowered. In the Lipid Research Clinics trial, the drug cholestyramine given to hypercholesterolemic asymptomatic men reduced morbidity and mortality from myocardial infarction in direct relation to the degree of cholesterol lowering; again, however, total mortality was not reduced. Lipid lowering by means of bile acid–binding resins (with niacin and diet therapy) also decreases progression and even induces regression of coronary lesions, as demonstrated by angiography in patients who have had coronary artery bypass graft surgery. Another fibric acid drug, gemfibrozil, has been shown to reduce mortality from IHD (but not total mortality) in association with lowered TG and C and raised HDL-C. Thus the weight of evidence strongly favors conservative measures to reduce cholesterol levels in patients through middle age and aggressive measures in patients who are frankly hypercholesterolemic, have clinical evidence of IHD, or are at high risk for progression of IHD.

Diet   The first step in treatment of primary hyperlipidemia is attention to diet. All patients with mild to moderate hyperlipidemia

TABLE 208-6 **Guidelines for treatment of high blood cholesterol in adults**

	Cholesterol, mmol/L (mg/dL)			
	Desirable	Borderline-high	High	Decision
Total C	<5.2 (200)	5.2–6.1 (200–239)*	>6.2 (240)	Estimate LDL-C if total C borderline or high
LDL-C	<3.4 (130)	3.4–4.1 (130–159)*	>4.1 (160)	Diet treatment if LDL-C borderline or high
			>4.9 (190) or >4.1 (160)* or >3.4 (130)†	Drug treatment if LDL-C exceeds cut points after diet

* Becomes high risk if more than two risk factors (see Table 208-4) are present.
† High risk if definite IHD is present
SOURCE: National Cholesterol Education Program.

should first be brought to normal weight if they exceed it and then be maintained on a diet emphasizing decreases in intake of saturated fat and cholesterol. If hypertriglyceridemia is present, alcohol intake should be limited or eliminated. A single dietary approach to all forms of hyperlipidemia, including reduced intake of calories, cholesterol (to less than 300 mg/d), and saturated fat (to less than 10 percent of total calories), is appropriate for most patients. The degree of dietary modification would be proportional to the degree and nature of the hyperlipidemia. In practice, such a modification translates into limitation of animal fats and substitution of vegetable oils, fish, and carbohydrates. Increased physical activity is often a useful adjunct to dietary management. The maximum effect of such a regimen will be observed within 3 months after body weight has stabilized.

Drug therapy   This often needs to be added for the management of the familial hyperlipidemias (Chap. 344) and for patients with a positive family history of atherosclerosis. Drug therapy is recommended by the NCEP for any adult patient whose LDL cholesterol level remains greater than 4.9 mmol/L (190 mg/dL) or greater than 4.1 mmol/L (160 mg/dL) in the presence of two or more risk factors (see Table 208-4) after an adequate trial of at least 3 months of diet therapy alone. A more aggressive approach is recommended for patients with clinically manifest IHD, with a suggested LDL cholesterol level of 3.4 mmol/L (130 mg/dL) or greater for initiation of drug therapy. A decision to start drug therapy should be made only after careful evaluation, since it usually commits patients to lifelong treatment. Continued follow-up and monitoring are essential. Drugs that act primarily by lowering LDL cholesterol (bile acid–binding resins, nicotinic acid, HMG-CoA reductase inhibitors; Table 208-7) are the drugs of choice for high-risk patients.

The resins act by enhancing sterol excretion and indirectly increasing LDL receptor–mediated catabolism of circulating LDL. They are minimally absorbed and have no systemic toxicity. Since there have been successful trials demonstrating safety and efficacy in primary prevention of IHD, they can be considered for use in children with familial hypercholesterolemia and for primary prevention in young adults. Nicotinic acid usage also has been associated with a reduction in recurrent IHD and total mortality in a secondary prevention trial and with regression of IHD in several angiographic studies. It uniquely lowers LDL and VLDL levels while raising HDL cholesterol (see below). It is the least expensive drug; side effects can be minimized by careful attention to very gradual increases in dosage. By blocking the rate-limiting step in cholesterol synthesis, the HMG-CoA reductase inhibitors (vastatins) enhance LDL receptor–mediated catabolism of LDL and are very effective in lowering LDL cholesterol levels. Side effects are minimal, and these drugs have been associated with regression of IHD in angiographic trials. Long-term efficacy and safety are being studied. Estrogen replacement therapy is effective in postmenopausal women with hypercholesterolemia and may be the first-choice agent in that patient group. Other LDL-lowering drugs (see Table 208-7) have had limited utility thus far. Aside from nicotinic acid, drugs that lower LDL cholesterol may increase VLDL, and conversely, drugs that lower VLDL may increase LDL in some patients. Thus LDL-lowering drugs alone are contraindicated in hypertriglyceridemia.

If TG remains greater than 3.4 mmol/L (300 mg/dL) after diet, a fibric acid derivative or nicotinic acid may be tried (see Table 208-7). Fibrates appear to decrease VLDL synthesis and enhance lipoprotein lipase–mediated catabolism of VLDL, thereby lowering TG and reciprocally raising HDL cholesterol levels. These drugs increase lithogenicity of bile and can produce myopathy. In a group of patients with high VLDL cholesterol, high LDL cholesterol, and low HDL cholesterol levels, gemfibrozil was effective in the primary prevention of IHD.

Two types of drugs may be used simultaneously if both C and TG are high. In patients with familial hypercholesterolemia (Chap. 344), combined therapy with a resin and nicotinic acid has achieved dramatic normalization of LDL cholesterol levels. Further studies are needed to define the long-term efficiency of various lipid-lowering agents in

TABLE 208-7 Drugs available for treatment of the hyperlipidemias

Class of drug	Drugs available	Major lipoprotein decreased	Mechanism	Usual daily dose	Common side effects	Reduces IHD risk
Fibric acid derivates	Clofibrate, gemfibrozil	VLDL	Decreases VLDL synthesis; enhances LPL action*	2 g 1–2 g	Gallstones, myopathy	Yes
Nicotinic acid	Nicotinic acid	VLDL, LDL	Decreases VLDL synthesis	2–6 g	Gastrointestinal symptoms, flushing, hyperglycemia, hepatic dysfunction	Yes
Bile acid–binding resins	Cholestyramine, cholestipol	LDL	Promotes sterol excretion; increases LDL receptor–mediated removal	4–24 g 5–20 g	Gastrointestinal symptoms, high VLDL	Yes
HMG-CoA reductase inhibitors	Lovastatin, simvastatin, pravastatin	LDL	Blocks cholesterol synthesis; increases LDL receptor–mediated removal	10–40 mg 5–20 mg 10–40 mg	Gastrointestinal symptoms, myopathy	Yes
Probucol	Probucol	LDL	Unknown	1 g	Diarrhea, low HDL	Unknown
Estrogens	Premarin, estradiol	LDL	Unknown	0.625 mg 2 mg	High VLDL, endometrial cancer	Yes

* LPL = lipoprotein lipase.

the prevention or reversal of atherosclerosis and its sequelae. The long-term effects of any of these drugs used before puberty are unknown, and their use during pregnancy is not advocated. There is a paucity of data to justify their use in the elderly, although studies are underway. In a revision of the NCEP, it was suggested that elderly individuals should not be excluded from treatment solely on the basis of age, since they are responsive to cholesterol-lowering regimens. As the first approach to this group, attention to multiple risk factors and hygienic measures (diet and physical activity) appears appropriate.

OTHER RISK FACTORS High-density lipoproteins (HDL) The level of HDL, a complex family of particles that carry about 20 percent of the total plasma cholesterol, is inversely associated with the development of premature atherosclerosis and therefore can be considered an "antirisk factor." HDL levels can be assessed simply by measurement of cholesterol in the supernatant fluid after the other lipoproteins in plasma have been precipitated. Thus individuals whose HDL cholesterol is elevated may be less likely to develop IHD; conversely, low HDL cholesterol is associated with increased risk of IHD. In the Framingham Study, low HDL cholesterol was a more potent lipid risk factor than was high total cholesterol or LDL. At least five diverse population studies have confirmed a close correlation between IHD and low HDL, independent of other factors.

Consistent with differences in risk between the sexes, HDL cholesterol averages about 25 percent higher in women than in men. Estrogens tend to raise and androgens tend to lower HDL levels. In women, low HDL, particularly when associated with diabetes and obesity, markedly raises the risk of IHD. Octogenarians tend to have high HDL, which may be partly familial. Of interest for preventive measures, cigarette smoking decreases and regular strenuous exercise increases HDL cholesterol. Regular exercise increases HDL even in individuals after myocardial infarction. A small daily intake of alcohol has been associated with both reduced risk of IHD and high HDL levels. Mechanisms for these effects remain unknown.

The utility of HDL cholesterol measurements as a single determinant of risk in individuals is limited because the analytical error in many laboratories exceeds the differences in HDL levels associated with risk. HDL measurements are most helpful for estimation of LDL cholesterol. Because of the close inverse relationship between plasma triglycerides (or VLDL) and HDL, HDL in most hypertriglyceridemic persons, with or without hypercholesterolemia, will be predictably low. Low HDL cholesterol is one of the factors that can place patients in a high-risk category for IHD (see Table 208-6).

Hypertension (See Chap. 209) High blood pressure is an important risk factor for atherosclerosis, mainly IHD and cerebrovascular disease. The risk increases progressively with increasing blood pressure; in the Framingham Study, IHD incidence in middle-aged men with blood pressures exceeding 160/95 was more than five times that in normotensive men (blood pressure 140/90 or less). Hypertensive men and women are both affected, with the diastolic pressure perhaps being more important. In industrialized populations, blood pressure appears to increase inexorably with age; however, the nature of this age relation varies among populations, since there are remote primitive populations that age without any changes in blood pressure levels. The age-associated blood pressure increase might be related to physical activity or dietary factors, particularly sodium and total caloric content. Hypertension appears to increase atherosclerosis throughout the age span.

Conversely, the risk for atherosclerosis appears diminished by therapeutic reduction of blood pressure. Recent intervention studies have shown convincingly that reduction of diastolic levels that had been greater than 105 mmHg significantly reduces the incidence of strokes, IHD, and congestive heart failure in men. Even when patients with diastolic pressures between 90 and 105 mmHg are similarly maintained on adequate treatment, the incidence of some of these complications may be reduced. A recent trial of treatment of isolated systolic hypertension in otherwise healthy elderly subjects showed that reduction of blood pressure substantially reduced both IHD and stroke. Special urgency for relief of hypertension obtains when hyperlipidemia, diabetes, or other risk factors are present.

Cigarette smoking Not only is cigarette smoking one of the more potent risk factors for atherosclerosis, it is also one of the factors that when reduced or eliminated clearly decreases the risk of developing atherosclerosis. Ample statistical evidence supports a mean increase of about 70 percent in the death rate and a three- to fivefold increase in risk of IHD in men who smoke one pack of cigarettes per day compared with nonsmokers. In general, the increase in death rate is proportional to the amount smoked and decreases with age. Excess morbidity from myocardial infarction is also present in women smokers, but the relationship is somewhat less firm than in men. However, there is an impressive accentuation of IHD mortality in women over age 35 taking oral contraceptives who in addition smoke cigarettes. In some atherosclerosis-prone populations, such as patients maintained on long-term hemodialysis, cigarette smoking interacts with other risk factors, resulting in a marked enhancement of atherosclerosis mortality. Such interaction is also likely for diabetic and hypertensive populations.

The association of smoking and increased IHD remains unexplained. Pipe and cigar smokers have a lesser increase in risk of IHD, presumably because less smoke is inhaled. Smokers dying of causes other than IHD have been found at autopsy to have more coronary atherosclerosis than nonsmokers. The major influence of smoking is on the incidence of sudden death, however. Those who stop smoking show a prompt decline in risk and may reach the risk level of nonsmokers as early as after 1 year of abstention.

Hyperglycemia and diabetes mellitus (See Chap. 337) Studies in a variety of populations have shown an association of hyperglycemia with clinically evident atherosclerotic disease, suggesting a role of hyperglycemia in atherogenesis. In known diabetics, both insulin-dependent (IDD) and non-insulin-dependent (NIDD) types, there is at least a twofold increase in incidence of myocardial infarction compared with nondiabetics. This risk is markedly increased in younger diabetics; recent data indicate that about one-third of patients with IDD die of IHD by age 55. Diabetic women are even more prone to IHD than are diabetic men. There is an increased tendency toward cerebral thrombosis and infarction but not toward cerebral hemorrhage in diabetes. Gangrene of the lower extremities has been variously estimated to be from 8 to 150 times as frequent in diabetics as in nondiabetics and is most often found in diabetics who smoke. Diabetes mellitus is associated with an increase in atherosclerosis observed at autopsy in a variety of populations worldwide, whether the prevalence of atherosclerosis in a particular population is high or low. Mortality from IHD in diabetes is increased even in populations in which the incidence of IHD is low, such as those in Asia. Data from MRFIT show that while IHD mortality increases as a function of the number and intensity of the major risk factors in diabetics, just as it does in nondiabetics, for every risk-factor level, diabetics have three- to fivefold higher IHD mortality rates.

The risk for atherosclerotic disease, however, does not appear to be grossly related to the degree of hyperglycemia among diabetics. Results in the University Group Diabetes Program Study have suggested that reduction of blood glucose by insulin does not appear to influence mortality from established atherosclerosis during a 5-year period. Thus hyperglycemia and atherosclerosis are associated, since there is an increased prevalence of large-vessel disease in known diabetics and, conversely, an increased prevalence of hyperglycemia in association with atherosclerotic disease. These associations remain unexplained and reversibility undocumented. Clinical and experimental studies also support a role for the insulin-resistance syndrome and high circulating insulin levels in IHD. The capillary microangiopathy, pathognomonic of diabetes mellitus and causing important dysfunction of the kidneys and retina, has unknown clinical significance in relation to atherosclerotic disease in larger arteries.

Obesity In general, morbidity and mortality from IHD are higher in direct relation to the degree of overweight beyond about 30 percent. Furthermore, from data obtained in the Framingham Study, it appears that obesity may accelerate atherosclerosis, since its effect is more apparent before age 50. Nevertheless, some of the major epidemiologic studies of coronary heart disease have not demonstrated an independent relationship between this condition and anything less than very severe obesity. A close relation between type of obesity (i.e., abdominal) and IHD has been identified. Furthermore, abdominal obesity is a disorder closely associated with several other potent risk factors, i.e., hypertriglyceridemia, hypercholesterolemia, hyperglycemia, and hypertension. This cluster defines the insulin-resistance syndrome. The relationship between obesity and atherosclerosis is thus multifaceted; since in practice obesity does not occur "independently," it is of considerable importance as a risk factor, particularly abdominal obesity.

Physical inactivity Study of the relationship of the prevalence of IHD to daily (occupational) physical activity is made difficult because so many variables are involved. Among prospective studies, the Framingham data do indicate that the less sedentary an individual is, the less susceptible that individual is to sudden death. Physical work may be the major determinant of greatly differing incidences of IHD in southern black and white males in the United States and in populations that move from rural areas to urbanized environments. How physical activity may operate to decrease death from IHD, or possibly to decrease atherogenesis, is not known. Beyond the amelioration of hyperlipidemia by increasing caloric expenditure, no mechanism has been demonstrated. The meaning of the physical activity–induced increase in HDL, the antirisk factor for IHD, remains mysterious. Physical training has been shown to improve exercise performance in patients with IHD and angina pectoris. Regular physical activity is supported as a desirable element in a program of preventive health maintenance.

Stress and personality There is a valid clinical impression that psychic or emotional stress and anxiety are associated with precipitation of overt IHD and sudden death. Debate continues as to whether there may be distinct personality types prone to or relatively immune to premature IHD (the so-called personality types A and B) and whether the presumably more deleterious type is amenable to correction beyond elimination of cigarette smoking and adverse dietary patterns and avoidance of stressful life situations. Many social and demographic analyses have so far failed to reach any agreement about the etiologic relationships of occupation and similar situational factors and the incidence of IHD.

Genetic factors Premature atherosclerosis often appears to be familial. In many instances this can be attributed to the inheritance of risk factors such as hypertension, diabetes mellitus, and hyperlipidemia. Occasionally, families with excessive premature vascular disease can be found in which none of the known risk factors appears to be operating. Genetic determinants of protective factors, such as HDL, and of nonlipid risk factors, such as apolipoprotein B and lipoprotein (a), need to be understood; undoubtedly other important determinants remain to be discovered. Nevertheless, family history is one of the more important factors to be weighed in assessment of risk, thereby helping the physician to avoid missing treatable risk factors and in institution of appropriate preventive measures.

ROLE OF DIET IN RISK FOR ATHEROSCLEROSIS The relationship of diet to IHD remains an area of intense interest and persistent controversy. In epidemiologic studies, no population habitually subsisting on a diet low in saturated fat and cholesterol has an appreciable amount of IHD. These populations also tend to have lower plasma lipid concentrations. There is a general upward shift of average cholesterol and triglyceride levels in highly developed countries, which is an effect of change in total culture and life-style as well as in diet. Dietary changes in migrant populations who move from more primitive to more industrialized societies commonly include increased intake of total calories, animal fats, cholesterol, and salt, leading to a diet-accentuated emergence of risk factors such as obesity, hyperlipidemia, diabetes, and hypertension. There is no question that the plasma cholesterol (and LDL) level is sensitive to the amount of saturated fat and cholesterol in the diet. The "average" adult male in the United States eats about 140 g fat per day and about 0.1 mmol (400 mg) cholesterol. The mixture of fats ingested usually contains about three times as much saturated fatty acids (mainly palmitic and stearic) as polyunsaturated fatty acids (mainly linoleic and linolenic). If a healthy young adult switches from this diet to one containing the same amount of total fat in which the ratio of polyunsaturates to saturates is closer to unity and the cholesterol content is less than 0.07 mmol (300 mg) per day, the cholesterol concentration will usually drop by 10 to 15 percent within 2 weeks and remain depressed on continuation of the diet.

The average cholesterol level in most populations is most closely related to the amount of animal fats (meat, eggs, and milk products, major sources of long-chain saturated fatty acids and cholesterol) in the diet. Increased animal fat consumption also tends to be correlated with a greater proportion of dietary fats being saturated and with lesser intake of complex carbohydrates and vegetable fibers; these are dietary changes that may lead to a rise in plasma cholesterol levels. The average triglyceride level is more sensitive to total caloric balance and to alcohol intake. It is important to note that physical activity, emotional stress, smoking, and intake of coffee or tea have only weak or indirect influences on total cholesterol and triglyceride concentrations.

In experimental animals, added dietary cholesterol and fat are essential for the production of atherosclerosis. Typical American diets fed to nonhuman primates produce aortic and coronary atherosclerosis which is reversible when a cholesterol-free diet is fed. Controlled metabolic studies in humans show a direct relation between dietary and plasma cholesterol below intakes of about 0.15 mmol (600 mg) per day; no relation is observed at higher intakes when plasma cholesterol is already high. There appear to be marked genetic variations in the ability of dietary cholesterol to influence plasma cholesterol level among individuals and among populations. The relation between dietary polyunsaturated/saturated fat ratio (P/S) and both cholesterol and triglyceride levels also has been amply established. The unique triglyceride-lowering effects of the particular long-chain polyunsaturated fatty acids in large ocean fish are currently under study.

A definitive prospective study of the effect of diet on IHD in the general population has never been undertaken. Nevertheless, reports of newer studies of alterations of diet in high-risk populations provide strong evidence of a reversible relation among diet, plasma lipids, and IHD. On this basis, numerous authoritative nutrition councils have recommended prudent dietary modifications for the general population of western countries to be instituted early in life and to include a caloric intake adjusted to achieve and maintain ideal body weight, a reduction in total fat calories to 30 to 35 percent of total calories achieved by a substantial reduction in dietary saturated fat to less than 10 percent of total calories, and a reduction in cholesterol intake to less than 300 mg/d. Although a causal relationship in humans between sodium intake and hypertension has not been firmly established, avoidance of excessive dietary sodium also has been recommended.

RISK FACTORS AND MECHANISMS OF ATHEROGENESIS

Adiposity produces insulin resistance in peripheral tissues (mainly muscle and adipose), which leads to compensatory hyperinsulinemia. The liver is not resistant to some effects of insulin, and enhanced production of triglyceride-rich lipoproteins results, leading to elevated plasma triglyceride and cholesterol levels. Thus it has been demonstrated that body weight is related not only to triglyceride levels but also to cholesterol levels. Concomitantly, obesity is associated with increased total-body cholesterol synthesis. Obesity, particularly the abdominal type, produces higher circulating levels of insulin, both in the basal state and after stimulation with glucose or other secretagogues. Since obesity is related to atherosclerosis—both directly and via hypertension, hypertriglyceridemia, hypercholesterolemia, and hyperglycemia—it is not surprising that many studies show a relationship between serum insulin levels, particularly after oral glucose intake, and atherosclerotic disease of the coronary and peripheral arteries. A few studies, however, suggest that this association between insulin and atherosclerosis occurs independently of obesity. It has been postulated that insulin may directly affect arterial wall metabolism, leading to increased endogenous lipid synthesis and thus predisposing to atherosclerosis. Insulin has been shown to stimulate proliferation of arterial smooth-muscle cells, enhance binding of LDL and VLDL, and decrease binding of HDL to cells; it therefore may be one of the plasma factors involved in atheroma formation.

Hypertension may enhance atherogenesis by directly producing injury via mechanical stress on endothelial cells at specific high-pressure sites in the arterial tree. The sequence of events in the chronic injury hypothesis of atherogenesis would follow. In addition, hypertension alters endothelial permeability and markedly increases lysosomal enzyme activity. Experimental hypertension also increases the thickness of the intimal smooth-muscle layer in the arterial wall and increases connective tissue elements. It is still not known if continued high pressure within the artery produces changes in the ability of smooth-muscle cells or stem cells to proliferate.

Diabetes could provide a unique contribution to atherogenesis. Although the fundamental genetic abnormality in either type of human diabetes mellitus remains unknown, it has been suggested that genetic diabetes in humans imparts a primary cellular abnormality intrinsic to all cells, resulting in a decreased life span of individual cells, which in turn results in increased cell turnover in tissues. If arterial endothelial and smooth-muscle cells are intrinsically defective in

diabetes, accelerated atherogenesis can be readily postulated on the basis of any one of the current theories of pathogenesis. Platelet dysfunction in diabetes also may play a role.

The role of glucose in atheroma formation, if any, is poorly understood. Hyperglycemia is known to affect aortic wall metabolism. Sorbitol, a product of the insulin-independent aldose reductase pathway of glucose metabolism (the polyol pathway), accumulates in the arterial wall in the presence of high glucose concentrations, resulting in osmotic effects, including increased cell water content and decreased oxygenation. Increased glucose also appears to stimulate proliferation of cultured arterial smooth-muscle cells. Glycosylation of apolipoproteins and other key proteins intrinsic to the arterial wall producing advanced glycosylated end products also may be involved. When deposited in the artery, these products may influence arterial wall cell function. For example, glycosylated collagen avidly binds and traps LDL. Glycosylated LDL can be formed which may be more susceptible to oxidation and more readily deliver cholesterol to arterial wall cells than native LDL.

The development of atherosclerosis accelerates in approximate quantitative relation to the degree of *hyperlipidemia*. A long-established theory suggests that the higher the circulating levels of lipoprotein, the more likely they are to gain entrance to the arterial wall. By an acceleration of the usual transendothelial transport, large concentrations of lipoproteins within the arterial wall could overwhelm the ability of smooth-muscle cells and monocyte-derived macrophages to metabolize them. Lipoproteins have been immunologically identified in atheroma, and in humans there is a close relationship between plasma cholesterol and arterial lipoprotein cholesterol concentration. High-density lipoproteins may be protective in relation to their ability to promote cholesterol efflux from artery wall cells. Chemically modified or oxidized lipoproteins, possibly produced in hyperlipidemic disorders, could gain access to the scavenger arterial wall macrophages, leading to formation of foam cells. It is possible that the lipid that accumulates in the arterial wall with increasing age results from infiltration of plasma lipoproteins which bind to matrix components. However, atheromatous lesions are associated with a more marked increase in arterial wall lipids, which may result in part from injury to the endothelium produced by chronic hyperlipidemia, as demonstrated in cholesterol-fed monkeys.

The effect of *chronic smoke inhalation* from cigarettes could result in repetitive toxic injury to endothelial cells, thereby accelerating atherogenesis. Hypoxia stimulates proliferation of cultured human arterial smooth-muscle cells; thus, since cigarette smoking is associated with high levels of carboxyhemoglobin and low oxygen delivery to tissues, another mechanism for atherogenesis is suggested. Hypoxia could produce diminished lysosomal enzyme degradative ability, as evidenced by impaired degradation of LDL by smooth-muscle cells, causing LDL-derived cholesterol to accumulate in the cells. Consistent with this suggestion is the fact that aortic lesions that resemble atheroma have been produced in experimental animals by systemic hypoxia, and lipid accumulation in the arterial wall of cholesterol-fed rabbits and monkeys appear to be increased by hypoxia.

RISK FACTOR REVERSAL AND REGRESSION OF ATHEROSCLEROSIS

By removal or reversal of a single risk factor or group of risk factors, the emergence of clinical consequences of atherosclerosis can be lessened, and the regression or interruption of progression of atherosclerosis, determined by direct or indirect examination of lesions, can be accomplished in humans. Recent studies of the size of coronary or peripheral artery atheromatous lesions by sequential arteriograms taken before and after a period of treatment aimed at risk-factor reversal strongly suggest that interruption of lesion progression and even regression of lesions are possible. Treatments that have been successful include lipid-lowering by single drugs, multiple drugs, diet alone, combinations of diet and drug therapy, and ileal bypass surgery. Advanced atherosclerotic lesions appear to respond more favorably when serum LDL cholesterol levels are reduced to the low levels that prevail in populations consuming a low-fat diet. There is also encouraging evidence in animals, most notably in primates, that relatively complicated plaques induced by hyperlipidemia will regress and that further progression of atherosclerosis will cease when hyperlipidemia is removed.

Risk factor reversal is feasible in asymptomatic individuals and should be encouraged. Through mass-media educational efforts, whole communities can be influenced to reduce smoking, change diet, and lower blood pressure levels. Adult males in the United States have lowered cigarette consumption, although increases among teenage girls are disappointing. There has been a trend toward lower cholesterol and saturated fat consumption in the United States, coupled with increasing attention to weight reduction and the use of exercise programs. Concomitantly, and perhaps causally, there has been the noted decline in IHD mortality. Therefore, efforts to prevent atherogenesis, to interrupt progression, and perhaps to promote regression of existing lesions by risk factor reduction seem warranted.

PREVENTION   Although premature IHD is overall the most costly and common of the untimely complications of atherosclerosis, preoccupation with IHD should not obscure the fact that angina pectoris and myocardial infarction are expressions of late-stage atherosclerotic lesions. Factors precipitating these clinical events may be independent of those leading to initiation of plaque formation or its progression to a complicated lesion. Steps taken to prevent recurrence of myocardial infarction or fatal arrhythmia, termed *secondary prevention*, will not necessarily be the same as those taken to delay or prevent formation of atherosclerosis (*primary prevention*). Since atherosclerotic plaques have been detected in the coronary arteries of American males as early as the second decade in autopsy studies of Korean and Vietnam war deaths, primary prevention of atherosclerosis must begin early in life, long before there is any suspicion of IHD.

Thus *prevention of atherosclerosis, rather than treatment, is the goal.* Although an effective program has not been established with certainty, enough is known to act as a guide both in identification of those with a higher risk and in development of conservative measures that probably will reduce that risk. Thus prevention currently is equated with risk-factor reduction.

The decline of American death rates from premature IHD coincides with two trends in health practices. One is the increasing recognition of the importance of detecting and attempting to correct some of the risk factors correlated with atherosclerosis. The other is a greater awareness of the dietary sources of cholesterol and saturated fats and a tendency of the public to restrict their intake somewhat. Whether these trends are causally related to the decline in death rate is not known. While a rigorous approach to changes in life-style for the general population may be debatable, it is desirable to continue finding and helping those most susceptible to early atherosclerosis. The physician's role in risk-factor reduction involves treatment of hypertension and hyperlipidemia and advice regarding diet, body weight, smoking, and exercise. Drug treatment of hyperlipidemia should be limited to those individuals at high risk who do not respond adequately to dietary management. Since pooled data from trials are encouraging, the long-term use of antiplatelet drugs to reduce the incidence of reinfarction or death in individuals with IHD has been advocated.

TREATMENT   There is no agent proven to have any value in "treatment" of atherosclerosis unless it clearly reduces severe hyperlipidemia or obvious hypertension. In fact, there is no treatment of atherosclerosis, only of its complications. While end-stage treatment technology has reduced morbidity, prevention remains the long-term goal of both research and medical practice.

REFERENCES

Austin MA: Plasma triglyceride and coronary heart disease. Arteriosclerosis Thrombosis. 11:2, 1991

Aviram M: Modified forms of low density lipoprotein and atherosclerosis. Atherosclerosis 98:1, 1993

Bierman EL: Atherogenesis in diabetes. Arteriosclerosis Thrombosis. 12:647, 1992

————: Aging and atherosclerosis, in *Principles of Geriatric Medicine and Gerontology*, 3d ed, WR Hazzard et al (eds). New York, McGraw-Hill, 1993

Brown G et al: Regression of coronary artery disease as a result of intensive lipid-lowering therapy in men with high levels of apolipoprotein B. N Engl J Med 323:1289, 1990

Clarke R et al: Hyperhomocysteinemia: An independent risk factor for vascular disease. N Engl J Med 324:1149, 1991

Everhart JE et al: Medial arterial calcification and its association with mortality and complications of diabetes. Diabetologia 31:16, 1988

Leone A: Cardiovascular damage from smoking: A fact or a belief? Int J Cardiol 38:113, 1993

National Cholesterol Education Program: Report of the National Cholesterol Education Program Expert Panel on Detection, Evaluation and Treatment of High Blood Cholesterol in Adults. JAMA 269:3015, 1993

Poothullil JM: Obesity, hyperlipidemia and non-insulin-dependent diabetes: A unified theory. Neurosci Biobehav Rev 17:85, 1993

Rifkind RB (ed): *Drug Treatment of Hyperlipidemia*. New York, Dekker, 1991

Ross R: The pathogenesis of atherosclerosis: A perspective for the 1990's. Nature 362:801, 1993

Sharrett AR: Invasive versus noninvasive studies of risk factors and atherosclerosis. Circulation 87:II48, 1993

Stampfer MJ et al: Postmenopausal estrogen therapy and cardiovascular disease. N Engl J Med 326:756, 1991

Stary HC et al: A definition of the intima of human arteries and of its atherosclerosis-prone regions. Circulation 85:391, 1992

Vos J et al: Retardation and arrest of progression or regression of coronary artery disease: A review. Prog Cardiovasc Dis 35:435, 1993

Wallace RB, Anderson RA: Blood lipids, lipid-related measures, and the risk of atherosclerotic cardiovascular disease. Epidemiol Rev 9:95, 1987

Yla Herttuala S: Biochemistry of the arterial wall in developing atherosclerosis. Ann NY Acad Sci 623:40, 1991

209   HYPERTENSIVE VASCULAR DISEASE

GORDON H. WILLIAMS

An elevated arterial pressure is probably the most important public health problem in developed countries. It is common, asymptomatic, readily detectable, usually easily treatable, and often leads to lethal complications if left untreated. As a result of extensive educational programs in the late 1960s and 1970s by both private and governmental agencies, the number of undiagnosed and/or untreated patients has been significantly reduced to a level of less than 20 percent. This factor may be the most important one responsible for the decline in cardiovascular mortality which has taken place during the past 20 years (Chap. 208). Although our understanding of the pathophysiology of an elevated arterial pressure has increased, in 90 to 95 percent of cases the etiology (and thus potentially the prevention or cure) is still largely unknown. As a consequence, in most cases the hypertension is treated nonspecifically, resulting in a large number of minor side effects and a relatively high (~50 percent) non-compliance rate.

DEFINITION   Since there is no dividing line between normal and high blood pressure, arbitrary levels have been established to define those who have an increased risk of developing a morbid cardiovascular event and/or will clearly benefit from medical therapy. These definitions should consider not only the level of diastolic pressure but also systolic pressure, age, sex, and race. For example, patients with a diastolic pressure greater than 90 mmHg will have a significant reduction in morbidity and mortality with adequate therapy. These, then, are patients who have hypertension and who should be considered for treatment.

The level of *systolic* pressure is also important in assessing arterial pressure's influence on cardiovascular morbidity. Males with normal diastolic pressures (<82 mmHg) but elevated systolic pressures (>158 mmHg) have a $2\frac{1}{2}$-fold increase in their cardiovascular mortality rates when compared with individuals with similar diastolic pressures but whose systolic pressures are normal (<130 mmHg). Reduction in mortality and morbidity with treatment, specifically in the elderly, has been documented in these patients. This beneficial effect is mainly secondary to a reduction in strokes and occurs in women as well. Other significant factors which modify blood pressure's influence on the frequency of morbid cardiovascular events are age, race, and sex, with young black males being most adversely affected by hypertension.

When hypertension is suspected, blood pressure should be measured at least twice during two separate examinations after the initial screening. In adults, a *diastolic* pressure below 85 mmHg is considered to be normal; between 85 and 89 is high normal; 90 to 104 is mild hypertension; 105 to 114 moderate hypertension; 115 or greater is severe hypertension. When the diastolic pressure is below 90 mmHg, a *systolic* pressure below 140 mmHg indicates normal blood pressure; between 140 and 159 is borderline isolated systolic hypertension; 160 or higher is isolated systolic hypertension. Increasing use of 12- or 24-h blood pressure monitoring may provide additional useful information in patients who are difficult to classify. However, normal values for this procedure and their utility in relationship to therapeutic outcomes are not currently available.

Arterial pressure fluctuates in most persons, whether they are normotensive or hypertensive. Those who are classified as having *labile* hypertension are patients who sometimes, but not always, have arterial pressures within the hypertensive range. These patients are often considered to have borderline hypertension.

Sustained hypertension can become accelerated or enter a malignant phase, although this is unusual in treated patients. Though a patient with *malignant hypertension* often has a blood pressure above 200/140, it is papilledema, usually accompanied by retinal hemorrhages and exudates, and not the absolute pressure level, that defines this condition. *Accelerated hypertension* signifies a significant recent increase over previous hypertensive levels associated with evidence of vascular damage on funduscopic examination but without papilledema.

PREVALENCE The prevalence of hypertension depends on both the racial composition of the population studied and the criteria used to define the condition. In a white suburban population like that in the Framingham Study, nearly one-fifth have blood pressures greater than 160/95, while almost one-half have pressures greater than 140/90. An even higher prevalence has been documented in the nonwhite population.

The prevalence of various forms of secondary hypertension depends on the nature of the population studied and how extensive the evaluation is. There are no available data to define the frequency of secondary hypertension in the general population, although in middle-aged males it has been reported to be 6 percent. On the other hand, in referral centers where patients undergo an extensive evaluation, it has been reported to be as high as 35 percent. The various forms of hypertension are outlined in Table 209-1, and their relative frequencies are given in Table 209-2.

ESSENTIAL HYPERTENSION

Patients with arterial hypertension and no definable cause are said to have *primary*, *essential*, or *idiopathic hypertension*. Undoubtedly, the primary difficulty in uncovering the mechanism(s) responsible for the hypertension in these patients is attributable to the variety of systems that are involved in the regulation of arterial pressure—peripheral and/or central adrenergic, renal, hormonal, and vascular—and to the complexity of the relationships of these systems to one another. Several abnormalities have been described in patients with essential hypertension, often with a claim that one or more of these are primarily responsible for the hypertension. While it is still uncertain whether these individual abnormalities are primary or secondary, varying expressions of a single disease process or reflective of separate disease entities, the accumulating data increasingly support the latter hypothesis. Therefore, just as pneumonia is caused by a variety of infectious agents, even though the clinical picture observed may be similar, so essential hypertension likely has a number of distinct causes. Thus the distinction between primary and secondary hypertension has become blurred, and the approach to both the diagnosis and therapy of hypertensive patients has been modified. For

---

TABLE 209-1   Classification of arterial hypertension

SYSTOLIC HYPERTENSION WITH WIDE PULSE PRESSURE

A Decreased compliance of aorta (arteriosclerosis)
B Increased stroke volume
  1 Aortic regurgitation
  2 Thyrotoxicosis
  3 Hyperkinetic heart syndrome
  4 Fever
  5 Arteriovenous fistula
  6 Patent ductus arteriosus

SYSTOLIC AND DIASTOLIC HYPERTENSION (INCREASED PERIPHERAL VASCULAR RESISTANCE)

A Renal
  1 Chronic pyelonephritis
  2 Acute and chronic glomerulonephritis
  3 Polycystic renal disease
  4 Renovascular stenosis or renal infarction
  5 Most other severe renal disease (arteriolar nephrosclerosis, diabetic nephropathy, etc.)
  6 Renin-producing tumors
B Endocrine
  1 Oral contraceptives
  2 Adrenocortical hyperfunction
    a Cushing's disease and syndrome
    b Primary hyperaldosteronism
    c Congenital or hereditary adrenogenital syndromes (17α-hydroxylase and 11β-hydroxylase defects)
  3 Pheochromocytoma
  4 Myxedema
  5 Acromegaly
C Neurogenic
  1 Psychogenic
  2 "Diencephalic syndrome"
  3 Familial dysautonomia (Riley-Day)
  4 Polyneuritis (acute porphyria, lead poisoning)
  5 Increased intracranial pressure (acute)
  6 Spinal cord section (acute)
D Miscellaneous
  1 Coarctation of aorta
  2 Increased intravascular volume (excessive transfusion, polycythemia vera)
  3 Polyarteritis nodosa
  4 Hypercalcemia
  5 Medications, e.g., glucocorticoids, cyclosporine
E Unknown etiology
  1 Essential hypertension (>90% of all cases of hypertension)
  2 Toxemia of pregnancy
  3 Acute intermittent porphyria

---

example, as a group of patients with essential hypertension is separated into a distinct subset (e.g., low-renin essential hypertension), such patients have not been reclassified as having a form of secondary hypertension but rather remain in the essential hypertensive group. In this chapter, those individuals with a specific structural organ defect responsible for hypertension are defined as having a *secondary* form of hypertension. In contrast, individuals who may have general-

---

TABLE 209-2   Prevalence of various forms of hypertension in the general population and in specialized referral clinics*

Diagnosis	General population, %	Specialty clinic, %
Essential hypertension	92–94	65–85
Renal hypertension:		
Parenchymal	2–3	4–5
Renovascular	1–2	4–16
Endocrine hypertension:		
Primary aldosteronism	0.3	0.5–12
Cushing's syndrome	<0.1	0.2
Pheochromocytoma	<0.1	0.2
Oral contraceptive–induced	2–4	1–2
Miscellaneous	0.2	1

* Estimates based on a number of reports in the literature.

ized or functional abnormalities causing their hypertension, even if discrete, are defined as having *essential* hypertension.

HEREDITY Genetic factors have long been assumed to be important in the genesis of hypertension. Data supporting this view can be found in animal studies as well as in population studies in humans. One approach has been to assess the correlation of blood pressure within families (familial aggregation). From these studies, the minimum size of the genetic factor can be expressed by a correlation coefficient of approximately 0.2. However, the variation in the size of the genetic factor in different studies reemphasizes the likely heterogeneous nature of the essential hypertensive population. Additionally, most studies support the concept that the inheritance is probably multifactorial or that a number of different genetic defects each have as one of their phenotypic expressions an elevated blood pressure. Finally, monogenic defects have now been reported which have as one of their consequences an increased arterial pressure, e.g., glucocorticoid-remediable aldosteronism (see below and Chap. 335).

ENVIRONMENT A number of environmental factors have been specifically implicated in the development of hypertension, including salt intake, obesity, occupation, alcohol intake, family size, and crowding. These factors have all been assumed to be important in the increase in blood pressure with age in more affluent societies, in contrast to the decline in blood pressure with age in more primitive cultures.

SALT SENSITIVITY The environmental factor which has received the greatest attention is salt intake. Even this factor illustrates the heterogeneous nature of the essential hypertensive population in that the blood pressure in only approximately 60 percent of hypertensives is particularly responsive to the level of sodium intake. The cause of this special sensitivity to salt varies, with primary aldosteronism, bilateral renal artery stenosis, renal parenchymal disease, or low-renin essential hypertension accounting for about half the patients. In the remainder, the pathophysiology is still uncertain, but recent postulated contributing factors include chloride, calcium, a generalized cellular membrane defect, insulin resistance, and "nonmodulation" (see below).

Role of renin Renin is an enzyme secreted by the juxtaglomerular cell of the kidney and linked with aldosterone in a negative feedback loop (see Chap. 335). While a variety of factors can modify this secretion, the primary determinant is the volume status of the individual, particularly as related to changes in dietary sodium intake. The end product of the action of renin on its substrate is the generation of the peptide angiotensin II. The response of target tissues to this peptide is uniquely determined by the prior dietary electrolyte intake. For example, sodium intake normally modulates adrenal and renal vascular responses to angiotensin II. With sodium restriction, adrenal responses are enhanced and the renal vascular responses reduced. Sodium loading has the opposite effect. The range of plasma renin activities observed in hypertensive subjects is more broad than in normotensive individuals. Thus some hypertensive patients have been defined as having low-renin and others as having high-renin essential hypertension.

LOW-RENIN ESSENTIAL HYPERTENSION Approximately 20 percent of patients who by all other criteria have essential hypertension have suppressed plasma renin activity. This occurs more frequently in black than in white patients. Though these patients are not hypokalemic, they have been reported to have expanded extracellular fluid volumes, and it is tempting to implicate sodium retention and renin suppression due to excessive production of an unidentified mineralocorticoid. Involvement of the adrenal cortex is suggested by the observation that large doses of spironolactone, the mineralocorticoid antagonist, and the inhibition of steroidogenesis by aminoglutethimide can result in sodium loss and lowering of blood pressure in these patients. A search for other mineralocorticoids has not proven fruitful. Some studies have suggested that the adrenal cortex of many of these patients has an increased sensitivity to angiotensin II as the underlying mechanism. Not only does this hypothesis potentially explain their low plasma renin activity, it also suggests the cause of their

hypertension. On a normal or high-sodium diet, they will not suppress aldosterone production normally, thus leading to a mild degree of hyperaldosteronism with its resultant increased sodium retention, volume expansion, and increase in blood pressure. Since this altered sensitivity has been reported even in patients with normal-renin hypertension, it is likely that patients with low-renin hypertension are not a distinct subset but rather form part of a continuum of patients with essential hypertension.

NONMODULATING ESSENTIAL HYPERTENSION In another subset of the hypertensive population, an adrenal defect the opposite of that observed in low-renin patients is present; i.e., the adrenal response to sodium restriction is reduced. In these individuals, sodium intake does not modulate either adrenal or renal vascular responses to angiotensin II. This subset of hypertensives has been termed *nonmodulators* because of the absence of the sodium-mediated modulation of target tissue responses to angiotensin II. These individuals comprise 25 to 30 percent of the hypertensive population, have normal or high plasma renin activity levels, and have a salt-sensitive form of hypertension because of a defect in the kidney's ability to excrete sodium appropriately. Furthermore, the abnormality appears to be genetically determined and can be corrected by the administration of a converting-enzyme inhibitor.

HIGH-RENIN ESSENTIAL HYPERTENSION Approximately 15 percent of patients with essential hypertension have plasma renin activity levels elevated above the normal range. It has been suggested that plasma renin plays an important role in the pathogenesis of the elevated arterial pressure in these patients. However, most studies have documented that saralasin (a competitive antagonist for angiotensin II) significantly reduces blood pressure in less than half these patients. This has led some investigators to postulate that the elevated renin levels and blood pressure may both be secondary to an increased activity of the adrenergic system. It has been proposed that in patients with angiotensin-dependent high-renin hypertension whose arterial pressures are lowered by saralasin, the mechanism responsible for the increased renin and, therefore, the hypertension is the nonmodulating defect.

Sodium ion vs. chloride or calcium Most studies assessing the role of salt in the hypertensive process have assumed that it is the sodium ion which is important. However, some investigators have suggested that the chloride ion may be equally important. This suggestion is based on the observation that feeding chloride-free sodium salts to salt-sensitive hypertensive animals fails to increase arterial pressure. Calcium also has been implicated in the pathogenesis of some forms of essential hypertension. A low calcium intake has been associated with an increase in blood pressure in epidemiologic studies; an increase in leukocyte cytosolic calcium levels has been reported in some hypertensives; and finally, calcium entry blockers are effective antihypertensive agents. Several studies have reported a potential link between the salt-sensitive forms of hypertension and calcium. It has been postulated that with salt loading and a defect in the kidney's ability to excrete it, a secondary increase in circulating natriuretic factors may occur. One of these, the so-called digitalis-like natriuretic factor, inhibits ouabain-sensitive sodium-potassium ATPase and thereby leads to intracellular calcium accumulation and a hyperreactive vascular smooth muscle.

Cell membrane defect Another postulated explanation for salt-sensitive hypertension is a generalized cell membrane defect. This hypothesis derives most of its data from studies on circulating blood elements, particularly red blood cells, in which abnormalities in the transport of sodium across the cell membrane have been documented. Since both increases and decreases in the activity of different transport systems have been reported, it is likely that some abnormalities are primary and some secondary processes. It has been assumed that this abnormality reflects an undefined alteration in the cellular membrane and that this defect occurs in many, perhaps all, cells of the body, particularly the vascular smooth muscle. Because of this defect, there is then an abnormal accumulation of calcium within vascular smooth muscle, resulting in a heightened vascular responsivity to vasoconstrictor agents. This defect has been proposed to be present in 35 to 50 percent of the essential hypertensive population based on studies using red cells. Other studies suggest that the abnormality in the red cell sodium transport is not a fixed abnormality but can be modified by environmental factors.

Each of these hypotheses has as a common final pathway an increase in cytosolic calcium resulting in increased vascular reactivity. However, as described above, several mechanisms might produce the increase in calcium accumulation.

INSULIN RESISTANCE Insulin resistance and/or hyperinsulinemia have been suggested as being responsible for the increased arterial pressure in some patients with hypertension. While it is clear that a substantial fraction of the hypertensive population has insulin resistance and hyperinsulinemia, it is less certain that this is more than an association. Insulin resistance is common in patients with type II diabetes mellitus or obesity. Both obesity and diabetes mellitus occur more frequently in hypertensive than normotensive subjects. However, several studies have documented that hyperinsulinemia and insulin resistance are present even in lean hypertensive patients free of diabetes mellitus, suggesting that this relationship is more than coincidence.

Hyperinsulinemia can increase arterial pressure by one or more of four mechanisms. An underlying assumption in each is that some, but not all, insulin target tissues are resistant to its effects. Specifically, tissues involved in glucose homeostasis are resistant (thereby producing the hyperinsulinemia), while tissues involved in the hypertensive process are not. First, hyperinsulinemia produces renal sodium retention (at least acutely) and increases sympathetic activity. Either or both of these could lead to an increase in arterial pressure. Another mechanism is vascular smooth-muscle hypertrophy secondary to insulin's mitogenic action. Finally, insulin also modifies ion transport across the cell membrane, thereby potentially increasing the cytosolic calcium levels of insulin-sensitive vascular or renal tissues. Via this mechanism, arterial pressure would be increased for reasons similar to those described above for the membrane-defect hypothesis. It is important to point out, however, that insulin's role in controlling arterial pressure is only vaguely understood, and therefore, its potential as a pathogenic factor in hypertension remains unclear.

FACTORS MODIFYING THE COURSE OF ESSENTIAL HYPERTENSION Age, race, sex, smoking, alcohol intake, serum cholesterol, glucose intolerance, and weight may all alter the prognosis of this disease. The younger the patient when hypertension is first noted, the greater is the reduction in life expectancy if the hypertension is left untreated. In the United States, urban blacks have about twice the prevalence rate for hypertension as whites and more than four times the hypertension-induced morbidity rate. At all ages and in both white and nonwhite populations, females with hypertension fare better than males, and the prevalence of hypertension in premenopausal females is substantially less than in age-matched males or postmenopausal females. Yet females with hypertension run the same relative risk of a morbid cardiovascular event compared with their normotensive counterparts as males do. Accelerated atherosclerosis is an invariable companion of hypertension. Thus it is not surprising that independent risk factors associated with the development of atherosclerosis, e.g., an elevated serum cholesterol, glucose intolerance, and/or cigarette smoking, significantly enhance the effect of hypertension on mortality rates regardless of age, sex, or race (Chap. 208). There also is no question that a positive correlation exists between obesity and arterial pressure. A gain in weight is associated with an increased frequency of hypertension in subjects with normal pressures, and weight loss in obese subjects with hypertension lowers their arterial pressure and, if they are being treated, the intensity of therapy required to maintain them normotensive. Whether these changes are mediated by changes in insulin resistance is unknown. However, there are no convincing data that obesity adversely affects the hypertension-associated mortality rate.

NATURAL HISTORY Because essential hypertension is a heterogeneous disorder, variables in addition to the level of arterial pressure

---

TABLE 209-3 Factors indicating an adverse prognosis in hypertension

Black race
Youth
Male
Persistent diastolic pressure >115 mmHg
Smoking
Diabetes mellitus
Hypercholesterolemia
Obesity
Excess alcohol intake
Evidence of end organ damage
  A Cardiac
    1 Cardiac enlargement
    2 ECG changes of ischemic or left ventricular strain
    3 Myocardial infarction
    4 Congestive heart failure
  B Eyes
    1 Retinal exudates and hemorrhages
    2 Papilledema
  C Renal: impaired renal function
  D Nervous system: cerebrovascular accident

---

modify its course. Thus the probability of developing a morbid cardiovascular event with a given arterial pressure may vary by as much as twentyfold depending on whether associated risk factors are present (Table 209-3). Although exceptions have been reported, most untreated adults with hypertension will develop further increases in their arterial pressure with time. Furthermore, both from actuarial data and from experience in the era prior to effective therapy, it has been documented that untreated hypertension is associated with a shortening of life by 10 to 20 years, usually related to an acceleration of the atherosclerotic process, with the rate of acceleration in part related to the severity of the hypertension. Even individuals with relatively mild disease, i.e., without evidence of end organ damage, left untreated for 7 to 10 years have a high risk of developing significant complications. Nearly 30 percent will exhibit atherosclerotic complications, and more than 50 percent will have end organ damage related to the hypertension itself, e.g., cardiomegaly, congestive heart failure, retinopathy, a cerebrovascular accident, and/or renal insufficiency. Thus, even in its mild forms, hypertension is a progressive and lethal disease if left untreated.

SECONDARY HYPERTENSION

As noted earlier, in only a small minority of patients with an elevated arterial pressure can a specific cause be identified. Yet these patients should not be ignored for at least two reasons: (1) with correction of the cause, their hypertension may be cured, and (2) the secondary forms may provide insight into the etiology of essential hypertension. Nearly all the secondary forms are related to an alteration in hormone secretion and/or renal function and are discussed in detail in other chapters.

RENAL HYPERTENSION (See also Chap. 243) Hypertension produced by renal disease is the result of either (1) a derangement in the renal handling of sodium and fluids leading to volume expansion or (2) an alteration in renal secretion of vasoactive materials resulting in a systemic or local change in arteriolar tone. The main subdivisions of renal hypertension are renovascular hypertension, including preeclampsia and eclampsia, and renal parenchymal hypertension. A simple explanation for *renal vascular hypertension* is that decreased perfusion of renal tissue due to stenosis of a main or branch renal artery activates the renin-angiotensin system, described in Chap. 335. Circulating angiotensin II elevates arterial pressure by direct vasoconstriction, by stimulation of aldosterone secretion with resultant sodium retention, and/or by stimulating the adrenergic nervous system. In actual practice, only about one-half of patients with renovascular hypertension have absolute elevations in renin activity in peripheral plasma, although when renin measurements are referenced against an index of sodium balance, a much higher fraction have inappropriately high values.

Activation of the renin-angiotensin system also has been offered as an explanation for the hypertension in both acute and chronic *renal parenchymal disease*. In this formulation, the only difference between renovascular and renal parenchymal hypertension is that the decreased perfusion of renal tissue in the latter case results from inflammatory and fibrotic changes involving multiple small intrarenal vessels. There are enough differences between the two conditions, however, to suggest that other mechanisms are active in renal parenchymal disease: (1) peripheral plasma renin activity is elevated far less frequently in renal parenchymal than in renovascular hypertension; (2) cardiac output is said to be normal in the renal parenchymal type (unless uremia and anemia are present) but slightly elevated in renovascular hypertension; (3) circulatory responses to tilting and to the Valsalva maneuver are exaggerated in the latter condition; and (4) blood volume tends to be high in patients with severe renal parenchymal disease and low in patients with severe renovascular hypertension. Alternative explanations for the hypertension in renal parenchymal disease include the possibilities that the damaged kidneys (1) produce an unidentified vasopressor substance other than renin, (2) fail to produce a necessary humoral vasodilator substance (perhaps prostaglandin or bradykinin), (3) fail to inactivate circulating vasopressor substances, and/or (4) are ineffective in disposing of sodium, and the retained sodium is responsible for the hypertension, as outlined earlier. Though all these explanations, including participation of the renin-angiotensin system, probably have some validity in individual patients, the hypothesis involving sodium retention is particularly attractive. It is supported by the observation that those patients with chronic pyelonephritis or polycystic renal disease who are salt wasters do not develop hypertension and by the observation that removal of salt and water by dialysis or diuretics is effective in controlling arterial pressure in the majority of patients with renal parenchymal disease.

A rare form of renal hypertension results from the excess secretion of renin by juxtaglomerular cell tumors or nephroblastomas. The initial presentation is similar to that of hyperaldosteronism with hypertension, hypokalemia, and overproduction of aldosterone. However, in contrast to primary aldosteronism, peripheral renin activity is *elevated instead of subnormal*. This disease can be distinguished from other forms of secondary aldosteronism by the presence of normal renal function and with unilateral increases in renal vein renin concentration without a renal artery lesion.

ENDOCRINE HYPERTENSION   Adrenal hypertension   Hypertension is a feature of a variety of adrenal cortical abnormalities. In *primary aldosteronism* (Chap. 335) there is a clear relationship between the aldosterone-induced sodium retention and the hypertension. Normal individuals given aldosterone develop hypertension only if they also ingest sodium. Since aldosterone causes sodium retention by stimulating renal tubular exchange of sodium for potassium, hypokalemia is a prominent feature in most patients with primary aldosteronism, and therefore, the measurement of serum potassium provides a simple screening test. The effect of sodium retention and volume expansion in chronically suppressing plasma renin activity is critically important for the definitive diagnosis. In most clinical situations, plasma renin activity and plasma or urinary aldosterone levels parallel each other, but in patients with primary aldosteronism, aldosterone levels are high and relatively fixed because of autonomous aldosterone secretion, while plasma renin activity levels are suppressed and respond sluggishly to sodium depletion. Primary aldosteronism may be secondary either to a tumor or to bilateral adrenal hyperplasia. It is important to distinguish between these two conditions preoperatively, since usually the hypertension in the latter is not modified by operation.

The sodium-retaining effect of large amounts of glucocorticoids also offers an explanation for the hypertension in severe cases of Cushing's syndrome (Chap. 335). Moreover, increased production of mineralocorticoids also has been documented in some patients with Cushing's syndrome. However, the hypertension in many cases of Cushing's syndrome does not seem volume-dependent, leading investigators to speculate that it may be secondary to glucocorticoid-induced production of renin substrate (angiotensin-mediated hypertension) or the increased cortisol levels saturating the 11-hydroxysteroid dehydrogenase enzyme system in the kidney. In the forms of the adrenogenital syndrome due to C-11 or C-17 hydroxylase deficiency (Chap. 335), deoxycorticosterone accounts for the sodium retention and the resultant hypertension, which is accompanied by suppression of plasma renin activity.

In patients with pheochromocytoma (Chap. 336), increased secretion of epinephrine and norepinephrine by a tumor most often located in the adrenal medulla causes excessive stimulation of adrenergic receptors, which results in peripheral vasoconstriction and cardiac stimulation. This diagnosis is confirmed by demonstrating increased urinary excretion of epinephrine and norepinephrine or their metabolites.

Acromegaly (See also Chap. 331)   Hypertension, coronary atherosclerosis, and cardiac hypertrophy are frequent complications of this condition.

Hypercalcemia (See also Chap. 356)   The hypertension which occurs in up to one-third of patients with hyperparathyroidism ordinarily can be attributed to renal parenchymal damage due to nephrolithiasis and nephrocalcinosis. However, increased calcium levels also can have a direct vasoconstrictive effect. In some cases, the hypertension disappears when the hypercalcemia is corrected. Thus, paradoxically, the increased serum calcium level in hyperparathyroidism raises blood pressure, while epidemiologic studies suggest that a high calcium intake lowers blood pressure. To further confuse the issue, calcium entry blocking agents are effective antihypertensive agents. Additional studies are needed to resolve these seemingly conflicting observations.

Oral contraceptives   The most common cause of endocrine hypertension is that resulting from the use of estrogen-containing oral contraceptives. Indeed, this may be the most common form of secondary hypertension. The mechanism producing the hypertension is likely to be secondary to activation of the renin-angiotensin-aldosterone system. Thus both volume (aldosterone) and vasoconstrictor (angiotensin II) factors are important. The estrogen component of oral contraceptive agents stimulates the hepatic synthesis of the renin substrate angiotensinogen, which in turn favors the increased production of angiotensin II and secondary aldosteronism. Women taking oral contraceptives have increased plasma concentrations of angiotensin II and aldosterone with some increase in arterial pressure. However, only about 5 percent actually have an increase in arterial pressure greater than 140/90, and in about half of these the hypertension will remit within 6 months of stopping the drug.

Why some women taking oral contraceptives develop hypertension and others do not is unclear but may be related to (1) increased vascular sensitivity to angiotensin II, (2) the presence of mild renal disease, (3) familial factors (over one-half have a positive family history for hypertension), (4) age (hypertension is significantly more prevalent in women over age 35), and/or (5) obesity. Indeed some investigators have suggested that the oral contraceptives are simply unmasking women with essential hypertension.

COARCTATION OF THE AORTA (See also Chap. 199)   The hypertension associated with coarctation may be caused by the constriction itself or perhaps by the changes in the renal circulation which result in an unusual form of renal arterial hypertension. The diagnosis of coarctation is usually evident from physical examination and routine x-ray findings.

EFFECTS OF HYPERTENSION

Patients with hypertension die prematurely; the most common cause of death is heart disease, with stroke and renal failure also frequent, particularly in those with significant retinopathy.

EFFECTS ON HEART   Cardiac compensation for the excessive work load imposed by increased systemic pressure is at first sustained by concentric left ventricular hypertrophy, characterized by an increase in wall thickness. Ultimately, the function of this chamber deteriorates, the cavity dilates, and the symptoms and signs of heart failure appear (Chap. 195). Angina pectoris also may occur because of the combination of accelerated coronary arterial disease and increased myocardial oxygen requirements as a consequence of the increased myocardial mass (Chap. 203). On physical examination, the heart is enlarged and has a prominent left ventricular impulse. The sound of aortic closure is accentuated, and there may be a faint murmur of aortic regurgitation. Presystolic (atrial, fourth) heart sounds appear frequently in hypertensive heart disease, and a protodiastolic (ventricular, third) heart sound or summation gallop rhythm may be present. Electrocardiographic changes of left ventricular hypertrophy (Chap. 189) may occur, but the electrocardiogram substantially underestimates the frequency of cardiac hypertrophy compared with that observed with the echocardiogram. Evidence of ischemia or infarction may be observed late in the disease. The majority of deaths due to hypertension result from myocardial infarction or congestive heart failure.

NEUROLOGIC EFFECTS   The neurologic effects of long-standing hypertension may be divided into retinal and central nervous system changes. Because the retina is the only tissue in which the arteries and arterioles can be examined directly, repeated ophthalmoscopic examination provides the opportunity to observe the progress of the vascular effects of hypertension (Table 209-4). The Keith-Wagener-Barker classification of the *retinal changes* in hypertension has provided a simple and excellent means for serial evaluation of hypertensive patients. Increasing severity of hypertension is associated with focal spasm and progressive general narrowing of the arterioles, as well as the appearance of hemorrhages, exudates, and papilledema. These retinal lesions often produce scotomata, blurred vision, and even blindness, especially in the presence of papilledema or hemorrhages of the macular area. Hypertensive lesions may develop acutely and, if therapy results in significant reduction of blood pressure, may show rapid resolution. Rarely, these lesions resolve without therapy. In contrast, retinal arteriolosclerosis results from endothelial and muscular proliferation, and it accurately reflects similar changes in other organs. Sclerotic changes do not develop as rapidly as hypertensive lesions, nor do they regress appreciably with therapy. As a consequence of increased wall thickness and rigidity, sclerotic arterioles distort and compress the veins as they cross within their common fibrous sheath, and the reflected light streak from the arterioles is changed by the increased opacity of the vessel wall.

Central nervous system dysfunction also occurs frequently in patients with hypertension. Occipital headaches, most often in the morning, are among the most prominent early symptoms of hypertension. Dizziness, light-headedness, vertigo, tinnitus, and dimmed vision or syncope also may be observed, but the more serious manifestations are due to vascular occlusion, hemorrhage, or encephalopathy (Chap. 368). The pathogeneses of the former two disorders are quite different. *Cerebral infarction* is secondary to the increased atherosclerosis observed in hypertensive patients, while *cerebral hemorrhage* is the result of both the elevated arterial pressure and the development of cerebral vascular microaneurysms (Charcot-Bouchard aneurysms). Only age and arterial pressure are known to influence the development of the microaneurysms. Thus it is not surprising that the association of arterial pressure with cerebral hemorrhage is much better than with either cerebral or myocardial infarction.

Hypertensive encephalopathy consists of the following symptom complex: severe hypertension, disordered consciousness, increased intracranial pressure, retinopathy with papilledema, and seizures. The pathogenesis is uncertain but probably not related to arteriolar spasm or cerebral edema. Focal neurologic signs are infrequent and, if present, suggest that infarction, hemorrhage, or transient ischemic attacks are more likely diagnoses. Although some investigators have suggested that prompt lowering of arterial pressure in these patients may adversely affect cerebral blood flow, most studies indicate that this is not the case.

RENAL EFFECTS (See also Chap. 243)   Arteriosclerotic lesions of the afferent and efferent arterioles and the glomerular capillary tufts are the most common renal vascular lesions in hypertension and result in decreased glomerular filtration rate and tubular dysfunction. Proteinuria and microscopic hematuria occur because of glomerular lesions, and approximately 10 percent of the deaths secondary to hypertension result from renal failure. Blood loss in hypertension occurs not only from renal lesions; epistaxis, hemoptysis, and metrorrhagia also occur frequently in these patients.

APPROACH TO THE PATIENT WITH HYPERTENSION

In evaluating patients with hypertension, the initial history, physical examination, and laboratory tests should be directed at (1) uncovering correctable secondary forms of hypertension (see Table 209-1), (2) establishing a pretreatment baseline, (3) assessing factors which may influence the type of therapy or which may be adversely modified by therapy, (4) determining if target organ damage is present, and (5) determining whether other risk factors for the development of arteriosclerotic cardiovascular disease are present (see Chap. 208).

TABLE 209-4   Classification of hypertensive and arteriolosclerotic retinopathy

| Degree | Hypertension | | | | | Arteriolosclerosis | |
| | Arterioles | | | | | | |
	General narrowing AV ratio*	Focal spasm†	Hemorrhages	Exudates	Papilledema	Arteriolar light reflex	AV crossing defects‡
Normal	3:4	1:1	0	0	0	Fine yellow line, red blood column	none
Grade I	1:2	1:1	0	0	0	Broadened yellow line, red blood column	Mild depression of vein
Grade II	1:3	2:3	0	0	0	Broad yellow line, "copper wire," blood column not visible	Depression or humping of vein
Grade III	1:4	1:3	+	+	0	Broad white line, "silver wire," blood column not visible	Right-angle deviation, tapering, and disappearance of vein under arteriole; distal dilatation of vein
Grade IV	Fine, fibrous cords	Obliteration of distal flow	+	+	+	Fibrous cords, blood column not visible	Same as grade III

* This is the ratio of arteriolar to venous diameters.
† This is the ratio of diameters of region of spasm to proximal arteriole.
‡ Arteriolar length and tortuosity increase with severity.

Ideally, this evaluation also would determine the underlying mechanism(s) in essential hypertension, particularly if such information leads to a more specific therapeutic program. Unfortunately, at the present time this aspect of the evaluation is limited either by lack of knowledge of the underlying mechanisms, uncertainty as to the specificity of therapy for a distinct subset even if the underlying mechanisms are known, or the prohibitive expense in defining a subset of hypertensive patients even if specific therapy were available. However, with the accumulation of additional information, a sixth component in the evaluation of patients with hypertension may become increasingly more important.

SYMPTOMS AND SIGNS The majority of patients with hypertension have no specific symptoms referable to their blood pressure elevation and will be identified only in the course of a physical examination. When symptoms do bring the patient to the physician, they fall into three categories. They are related to (1) the elevated pressure itself, (2) the hypertensive vascular disease, and (3) the underlying disease in the case of secondary hypertension. Though popularly considered a symptom of elevated arterial pressure, headache is characteristic only of severe hypertension; most commonly it is localized to the occipital region, is present when the patient awakens in the morning, and subsides spontaneously after several hours. Other possibly related complaints include dizziness, palpitations, easy fatigability, and impotence. Complaints referable to vascular disease include epistaxis, hematuria, blurring of vision owing to retinal changes, episodes of weakness or dizziness due to transient cerebral ischemia, angina pectoris, and dyspnea due to cardiac failure. Pain due to dissection of the aorta or to a leaking aneurysm is an occasional presenting symptom.

Examples of symptoms related to the underlying disease in secondary hypertension are polyuria, polydipsia, and muscle weakness secondary to hypokalemia in patients with primary aldosteronism or weight gain and emotional lability in patients with Cushing's syndrome. The patient with a pheochromocytoma may present with episodic headaches, palpitations, diaphoresis, and postural dizziness.

CLINICAL EVALUATION History A strong family history of hypertension, along with the reported finding of intermittent pressure elevation in the past, favors the diagnosis of essential hypertension. Secondary hypertension often develops before the age of 35 or after 55. The history of use of adrenal steroids or estrogens is of obvious significance. A history of repeated urinary tract infections suggests chronic pyelonephritis, although this condition may occur in the absence of symptoms; nocturia and polydipsia suggest renal or endocrine disease, while trauma to either flank or an episode of acute flank pain may be a clue to the presence of renal injury. A history of weight gain is compatible with Cushing's syndrome, and weight loss with pheochromocytoma. A number of aspects of the history aid in determining whether vascular disease has progressed to dangerous stages. These include angina pectoris and symptoms of cerebrovascular insufficiency, of congestive heart failure, and/or of peripheral vascular insufficiency. Other risk factors that should be elicited include cigarette smoking, diabetes mellitus, lipid disorders, and a family history of early deaths due to cardiovascular disease. Finally, aspects of the patient's lifestyle which could contribute to the hypertension or affect its treatment should be assessed, including diet, physical activity, family status, work, and educational level.

Physical examination The physical examination starts with the patient's general appearance. For instance, are the round face and trunkal obesity of Cushing's syndrome present? Is muscular development in the upper extremities out of proportion to that in the lower extremities, suggesting coarctation of the aorta? The next step is to compare the blood pressures and pulses in both upper extremities and in the supine and standing positions (for at least 2 min). A rise in diastolic pressure when the patient goes from the supine to the standing position is most compatible with essential hypertension; a fall, in the absence of antihypertensive medications, suggests secondary forms of hypertension. The patient's height and weight should be recorded. Detailed examination of the ocular fundi is mandatory,

since funduscopic findings provide one of the best indications of the duration of hypertension and of prognosis. A useful guide is the Keith-Wagener-Barker classification of funduscopic changes (Table 209-4; see also Atlas 8); the specific changes in each fundus should be recorded and a grade assigned. Palpation and auscultation of the carotid arteries for evidence of stenosis or occlusion are important; narrowing of a carotid artery may be a manifestation of hypertensive vascular disease, and it also may be a clue to the presence of a renal arterial lesion, since these two lesions may occur together. In examination of the heart and lungs, one should search for evidence of left ventricular hypertrophy and cardiac decompensation. Is there a left ventricular lift? Are third and fourth heart sounds present? Are there pulmonary rales? A third heart sound and pulmonary rales are unusual in uncomplicated hypertension. Their presence suggests ventricular dysfunction. Chest examination also includes a search for extracardiac murmurs and palpable collateral vessels that may result from coarctation of the aorta.

The most important part of the abdominal examination is auscultation for bruits originating in stenotic renal arteries. Bruits due to renal arterial narrowing nearly always have a diastolic component or may be continuous and are best heard just to the right or left of the midline above the umbilicus or in the flanks; they are present in many patients with renal artery stenosis due to fibrous dysplasia and in 40 to 50 percent of those with functionally significant stenosis due to arteriosclerosis. The abdomen also should be palpated for abdominal aneurysm and for the enlarged kidneys of polycystic renal disease. The femoral pulses must be carefully felt, and if they are decreased and/or delayed in comparison with the radial pulse, the blood pressure in the lower extremities must be measured. Even if the femoral pulse is normal to palpation, arterial pressure in the lower extremities should be recorded at least once in patients in whom hypertension is discovered before the age of 30 years. Finally, examination of the extremities for edema and a search for evidence of a previous cerebrovascular accident and/or other intracranial pathology should be performed.

Laboratory investigation Controversy exists as to what laboratory studies should be performed in patients presenting with hypertension. In general, the disagreement resides in how extensively to evaluate the patient for secondary forms of hypertension or subsets of essential hypertension. In the following discussion, laboratory studies are divided into those which should be performed in all patients with sustained hypertension (basic studies) and those which should be added if (1) from the initial evaluation a secondary form of hypertension is suggested and/or (2) arterial pressure is not controlled after initial therapy (secondary studies).

BASIC STUDIES Renal status is evaluated by assessing the presence of protein, blood, and glucose in the urine and measuring serum creatinine and/or blood urea nitrogen (BUN). Microscopic examination of the urine is also helpful. A serum potassium level is needed both as a screen for mineralocorticoid-induced hypertension and as a baseline prior to initiating diuretic therapy.

Other blood chemistries also may be useful, particularly since they often can be ordered as a battery of automated tests at minimal cost to the patient. For example, a blood glucose determination is helpful both because diabetes mellitus may be associated with accelerated arteriosclerosis, renal vascular disease, and diabetic nephropathy in patients with hypertension and because primary aldosteronism, Cushing's syndrome, and pheochromocytoma all may be associated with hyperglycemia. Furthermore, since antihypertensive therapy with diuretics, for example, can raise the blood glucose level, it is important to establish a baseline. The possibility of hypercalcemia also may be investigated. Serum uric acid determination is useful because of the increased incidence of hyperuricemia in patients with renal and essential hypertension and because, as with blood glucose, the level subsequently may be raised by treatment with diuretics. Serum cholesterol, HDL cholesterol, and triglycerides may be measured to identify other factors which predispose to the development of arteriosclerosis. An electrocardiogram should be obtained in all cases as an assessment of cardiac status, particularly if left ventricular hypertrophy is present, and as a baseline. The echocardiogram is more sensitive than either the electrocardiogram or physical examination in determining if cardiac hypertrophy is present. Thus, in some circumstances, this may be a useful addition in the *baseline* evaluation of a hypertensive patient, particularly since left ventricular hypertrophy is an independent cardiovascular risk factor and its presence suggests the need for vigorous antihypertensive therapy. Furthermore, while substantial increases in arterial pressure usually correlate with the presence or absence of left ventricular hypertrophy, mild increases may not. Thus one cannot use the level of blood pressure per se as a surrogate marker for the presence or absence of left ventricular hypertrophy. On the other hand, because of the cost of an echocardiogram and the uncertainty as to whether the resultant information would modify therapy, it is unclear that routine *follow-up* echocardiograms during therapy are justified. The chest roentgenogram also may be helpful by providing the opportunity to identify aortic dilatation or elongation and the rib notching that occurs in coarctation of the aorta.

SECONDARY STUDIES (Table 209-5)   Certain clues from the history, physical examination, and basic laboratory studies may suggest an unusual cause for the hypertension and dictate the need for special studies. For example, the abrupt onset of severe hypertension and/or the onset of hypertension of any severity under the age of 25 or after the age of 50 years should lead to laboratory tests to exclude renovascular hypertension and pheochromocytoma. A history of headaches, palpitations, anxiety attacks, unusual sweating, hyperglycemia, and weight loss also should lead to tests to exclude pheochromocytoma. The presence of an abdominal bruit should lead to workup for renovascular hypertension, and the finding of bilateral upper abdominal masses on physical examination, consistent with polycystic renal disease, should lead to the performance of an intravenous pyelogram. An elevated creatinine or blood urea nitrogen level, associated with proteinuria and hematuria, should initiate a detailed workup for renal insufficiency (Chap. 235). Special studies for secondary hypertension are also indicated if there is therapeutic failure with the initial drug program. The specific diagnostic measures depend on the most likely causes of secondary hypertension.

Pheochromocytoma   (See also Chap. 336)   The easiest and best screening procedure for pheochromocytoma is the measurement of catecholamines or their metabolites in a 24-h urine collected during the time the patient is hypertensive. Measurement of plasma catecholamine levels also may be useful. These tests may be indicated even in patients who do not have episodic hypertension, since over half the patients with pheochromocytoma have fixed hypertension.

TABLE 209-5 Laboratory tests and special studies for evaluation of hypertension

BASIC STUDIES

A Always included
  1 Urine for protein, blood, and glucose
  2 Hematocrit
  3 Serum potassium
  4 Serum creatinine and/or blood urea nitrogen
  5 Electrocardiogram
B Usually included, depending on cost and other factors
  1 Microscopic urinalysis
  2 White blood cell count
  3 Plasma/blood glucose, cholesterol, HDL cholesterol, and triglycerides
  4 Serum calcium, phosphate, and uric acid
  5 Chest x-ray

SPECIAL STUDIES TO SCREEN FOR SECONDARY HYPERTENSION

A Renovascular: digital subtraction angiogram or rapid sequence IVP
B Pheochromocytoma: 24-h urine for creatinine, metanephrines, and catecholamines or plasma catecholamines
C Cushing's syndrome: overnight dexamethasone suppression test or 24-h urine cortisol

---

Provocative tests are seldom, if ever, indicated, although occasionally a suppressive test may be useful.

Cushing's syndrome   (See also Chap. 335)   A 24-h urine test for cortisol or the administration of 1 mg dexamethasone at bedtime, followed by measurement of plasma cortisol at 7 to 10 A.M., is the best test for the presence of this condition. A urine cortisol level less than 2750 nmol (100 μg) or suppression of the plasma cortisol level to below 140 nmol/L (5 μg/dL) effectively rules out Cushing's syndrome.

Renovascular hypertension   (See also Chap. 243)   The standard screening test for renal vascular hypertension has been the rapid-sequence intravenous pyelogram (IVP). Features suggestive of renal ischemia include (1) unilateral delayed appearance and excretion of contrast material, (2) a difference in kidney size greater than 1.5 cm, (3) irregular contour of the renal silhouette, suggesting partial infarction or atrophy, (4) indentations on the ureter or renal pelvis, possibly due to dilated ureteral arteries (collateral notching), and (5) hyperconcentration of contrast medium in the collecting system of the smaller kidney. When these criteria are used, the false-positive rate is 11 percent and the false-negative rate 12 percent. The digital subtraction angiogram has been received with considerable enthusiasm as a more precise screening test for renal vascular disease. Its ultimate place as a screening test is unclear, however, because of its relatively high cost and the need for an arterial rather than a venous injection. The isotope renogram and saralasin infusion test, both enthusiastically endorsed in the past as screening procedures, are now used infrequently because of either lower sensitivity and specificity or limited availability. However, the captopril-induced renogram may be more useful. This test takes advantage of the dependency of the renal vasculature on angiotensin II. Thus, when individuals with renal artery stenosis are given a converting enzyme inhibitor (captopril) which reduces angiotensin II levels on the stenotic side, there will be renal blood flow pattern demonstrating a reduced uptake and delayed excretion as assessed by the isotope renogram.

The definitive test of surgically correctable renal disease is the combination of a renal angiogram and renal vein renin determinations. The renal arteriogram both establishes the presence of a renal arterial lesion and aids in determining whether the lesion is due to atherosclerosis or to one of the fibrous or fibromuscular dysplasias. It does not, however, prove that the lesion is responsible for the hypertension, nor does it permit prediction of the chances of surgical cure; it must be noted that (1) renal artery stenosis is a frequent finding by angiography and at postmortem in normotensive individuals, and (2) essential hypertension is a common condition and may occur in combination with renal arterial stenosis which actually may not be responsible for the hypertension. Bilateral renal vein catheterization for measurement of plasma renin activity is therefore used to assess the functional significance of any lesion noted on arteriography. When one kidney is ischemic and the other is normal, all the renin released comes from the involved kidney. In the most straightforward situation, the ischemic kidney has a significantly higher venous plasma renin activity than the normal kidney by a factor of 1.5 or more. Moreover, the renal venous blood draining the uninvolved kidney exhibits levels similar to those in the inferior vena cava below the entrance of the renal veins. Significant benefit from operative correction may be anticipated in at least 80 percent of patients with the findings described above if care is taken to prepare the patient properly prior to renal vein blood sampling, i.e., discontinuing renin-suppressing drugs, such as beta blockers, for at least 10 days, placing the patient on a low-sodium intake for 4 days, and/or giving a converting enzyme inhibitor for 24 h. When obstructing lesions in the *branches* of the renal arteries are demonstrated by arteriography, an attempt to obtain blood samples from the main *branches* of the renal vein should be made in an effort to identify a localized intrarenal arterial lesion responsible for the hypertension.

Primary aldosteronism   (See also Chap. 335)   These patients almost always exhibit hypokalemia. Diuretic therapy often complicates the picture when the hypokalemia is first observed and needs to be assessed. Given hypokalemia, the relation between plasma renin activity and the aldosterone level becomes the key to the diagnosis of primary aldosteronism. The aldosterone concentration or excretion is high and plasma renin activity is low in primary aldosteronism, and these levels are relatively unaffected by changes in sodium balance. A critical part of the evaluation after primary aldosteronism has been established is to determine whether unilateral or bilateral disease is present, since surgical removal of the lesion usually reduces arterial pressure only in those with unilateral disease.

Plasma renin activity measurements   Some studies have suggested that most hypertensive patients should have a plasma renin level measured and related to a 24-h urine sodium excretion rate to assess whether high, low, or normal levels are present. It has been proposed that this information may be important for both therapeutic and prognostic reasons. However, as noted earlier, it is unclear, on the basis of presently available data and treatment programs, that these random measurements are really useful except in patients with findings suggestive of renal vascular disease or mineralocorticoid excess in whom lateralizing renal vein renin levels or suppressed peripheral renin levels may be of diagnostic and/or therapeutic significance.

TREATMENT

Virtually every patient with a diastolic arterial pressure which persistently exceeds 90 mmHg, or any patient over 65 years of age with a systolic arterial pressure over 160 mmHg, is a candidate for diagnostic studies and for subsequent treatment. Furthermore, at any given level of blood pressure elevation, the ultimate risk of developing hypertensive vascular complications is greater in men than in women and in younger than in older persons. It may be argued, then, that it is hard to justify producing the uncomfortable side effects of therapy in, for example, an asymptomatic woman over 70 years of age with a diastolic pressure of 90 mmHg. On the other hand, it is easy to justify side effects in a man of 30 with a diastolic pressure exceeding 110 mmHg because such a person may be expected to receive the greatest benefit from therapy. Fortunately, the choice of treatment is such that a satisfactory program to control arterial pressure with minimal side effects can be developed for most patients, particularly as more studies assessing the impact of specific therapeutic agents on the patient's quality of life are reported. A reasonable guideline would be that all patients with diastolic pressure repeatedly above 90 mmHg should be treated unless specific contraindications exist. Patients with isolated *systolic* hypertension (levels greater than 160 mmHg) also should be treated if they are over age 65. It is uncertain that individuals under age 65 who have isolated systolic hypertension will benefit from therapy until the results of a well-controlled, perspective study are completed. Patients with labile hypertension or isolated systolic hypertension who are not treated should have regular follow-up examinations at 6-month intervals because of the frequent development of progressive and/or sustained hypertension.

The identification of an operable form of secondary hypertension does not automatically mean that surgical treatment is indicated. The decision depends on the age and general health of the patient, the natural history of the lesion, and the response of the arterial pressure to drug therapy. In patients with renovascular hypertension, the feasibility of renal angioplasty, surgical repair versus nephrectomy, and the degree of overall renal functional impairment must be considered. Age and general health are important in patients with renovascular hypertension due to arteriosclerosis, because there is no evidence that repair of the stenosis increases life expectancy in the elderly patient with other evidence of vascular disease. Knowledge of the natural history of the disease is especially important when approaching the decision in the young patient with renal artery stenosis due to fibrous dysplasia. If the arteriographic appearance suggests that the stenosis is due to intimal or subadventitial fibroplasia, the lesion may be expected to progress, and operation or angioplasty is required. Medial fibroplasia, on the other hand, often remains stable,

and operation or angioplasty may not be necessary if pressure can be controlled by drug therapy. The decision regarding operation also should be considered carefully in patients with primary aldosteronism when bilateral adrenal venography does not demonstrate a tumor, because such patients may prove to have multinodular hyperplasia. This means that bilateral adrenalectomy would be required to eliminate the aldosterone excess, and even then, hypertension usually persists. If hypokalemia can be controlled by spironolactone or other drug therapy and arterial pressure lowered with antihypertensive agents, then it is reasonable to withhold operative treatment.

GENERAL MEASURES   Nondrug therapeutic intervention is probably indicated in all patients with sustained hypertension and probably most with labile hypertension. The general measures employed include (1) relief of stress, (2) diet, (3) regular aerobic exercise, (4) weight reduction (if needed), and (5) control of other risk factors contributing to the development of arteriosclerosis. Relief of emotional and environmental stress is one of the reasons for the improvement in hypertension that occurs when a patient is hospitalized. Though it is usually impossible to extricate the hypertensive patient from all internal and external stresses, he or she should be advised to avoid any unnecessary tensions. In rare instances, it may be appropriate to recommend a change of job or of life-style. It has been suggested that relaxation techniques also may lower arterial pressure. However, it is uncertain that these techniques alone have much long-term effect.

Dietary management has three aspects:

1 Because of the documented efficacy of sodium restriction and volume contraction in lowering blood pressure, patients previously were instructed to curtail sodium intake drastically. Some investigators have suggested this is no longer necessary. They base their conclusion on two observations: (a) In many patients the blood pressure is not sensitive to the level of sodium intake, and (b) diuretics provide another method of decreasing body sodium stores in those individuals whose blood pressure may be sodium-sensitive. However, a number of reports have documented that while mild sodium restriction has little, if any, direct action on blood pressure, it significantly potentiates the efficacy of nearly all antihypertensive agents, and thus, by allowing blood pressure control with lower doses of drugs, side effects are reduced. In addition, it is quite clear that in some hypertensive patients, as noted above, the level of sodium intake does influence the blood pressure. Thus, since there is no apparent risk to mild sodium restriction, the most practical approach now is to advise mild dietary sodium restriction (up to 5 g NaCl per day), which can be achieved by eliminating all additions of salt to food which is prepared normally. Some studies also have reported lowering of arterial pressure by *increasing* potassium and/or calcium intake. While the advisability of this form of dietary alteration is still controversial, since a moderately high calcium intake (1.5 g elemental calcium daily) probably also reduces the extent of age-related osteoporosis, it is probably a useful adjunct.

2 Caloric restriction should be urged for the patient who is overweight. Some obese patients will show a significant reduction in pressure simply as a consequence of weight loss.

3 A restriction in intake of cholesterol and saturated fats is recommended, since such a diet may diminish the incidence of arteriosclerotic complications. Reducing or eliminating alcohol intake is also beneficial. Regular exercise is indicated within the limits of the patient's cardiovascular status. Not only is exercise helpful in controlling weight, but also there is evidence that physical conditioning itself may lower arterial pressure. Isotonic exercises (jogging, swimming) are better than isometric exercises (weight lifting) since, if anything, the latter raises arterial pressure. The dietary management outlined above is aimed at the control of other risk factors. Probably the most significant additional step that could be taken in this area would be to convince the smoker to give up cigarettes.

DRUG THERAPY (Table 209-6)   To make rational use of antihypertensive drugs, the sites and mechanisms of their action must be understood. In general, there are five classes of drugs: diuretics, antiadrenergic agents, vasodilators, calcium entry blockers, and angiotensin-converting enzyme (ACE) inhibitors.

Diuretics (See also Chap. 195)   The thiazides are the most frequently used and most extensively investigated members of this group, and their early effect certainly is related to sodium diuresis and volume depletion. A reduction in peripheral vascular resistance also has been reported by some workers to be important in the long term. Traditionally, thiazide diuretics have formed the cornerstone of most therapeutic programs designed to lower arterial pressure and are usually effective within 3 to 4 days. Furthermore, they have been shown to reduce mortality and morbidity in long-term trials. However, in recent years, increasing resistance to their routine use has occurred primarily because of their adverse metabolic effects, which include hypokalemia due to renal potassium loss, hyperuricemia due to uric acid retention, carbohydrate intolerance, and hyperlipidemia. The more potent loop-acting diuretics furosemide and bumetanide also have been shown to be antihypertensive but have been used less extensively for this purpose primarily because of their shorter duration of action. Spironolactone causes renal sodium loss by blocking the effect of mineralocorticoids, and therefore, it may be more effective in patients whose mineralocorticoids are present in excess, e.g., primary or secondary aldosteronism. Although they do not compete directly with aldosterone, triamterene and amiloride act at the same site as spironolactone to impede sodium reabsorption and are effective in the same situations as spironolactone, except triamterene has little intrinsic antihypertensive effect. Their major disadvantage is that they can produce hyperkalemia, particularly in patients with impaired renal function. Any of these three potassium-sparing diuretics also can be given along with thiazide diuretics to minimize renal potassium loss.

Antiadrenergic agents (See also Chap. 68)   These drugs act at one or more sites either centrally on the vasomotor center, in peripheral neurons modifying catecholamine release, or by blocking adrenergic receptor sites on target tissue. Drugs that appear to have predominant *central actions* are *clonidine, methyldopa, guanabenz,* and *guanfacine*. These drugs and their metabolites are predominantly alpha-receptor agonists. Stimulation of alpha$_2$ receptors in the vasomotor centers of the brain *reduces* sympathetic outflow, thereby reducing arterial pressure. Usually a fall in cardiac output and heart rate also occurs, more commonly with clonidine and guanabenz, but the baroreceptor reflex is intact. Thus postural symptoms are absent. However, rebound hypertension may occur rarely when these drugs, particularly clonidine and guanabenz, are stopped. This is probably secondary to the increase in norepinephrine release which had been inhibited by these agents secondary to their agonist effect on presynaptic alpha receptors.

Another class of antiadrenergic agents is the *ganglionic blocking* drugs, which have little effect when the patient is supine but prevent reflex vasoconstriction in the upright position. Ganglionic blocking agents interfere with parasympathetic as well as sympathetic function, and this results in such side effects as impairment of visual accommodation, paralytic ileus, retention of urine, and failure of erection and ejaculation. Because of these problems, ganglionic blocking agents are now usually reserved for the rapid lowering of arterial pressure by parenteral administration of the short-acting agent *trimethaphan* in patients with severe hypertension.

Various drugs act at *postganglionic adrenergic nerve endings*. The *rauwolfia alkaloids* such as reserpine are the oldest members of the group; their long-term effect results from their ability to inhibit the storage of norepinephrine within the vesicles in adrenergic nerve endings, thus leading to depletion of catecholamine stores. The frequent side effects, including depression, nasal congestion, diarrhea, impairment of sexual function, and increased gastric secretion, have limited the use of these drugs. Reserpine is contraindicated in patients with current or past depression. *Guanethidine* and its shorter-acting analogue guanadrel block the release of norepinephrine from adrener-gic nerve endings. They usually reduce cardiac output and lower systolic more than diastolic blood pressure. They also produce a greater postural effect than the other drugs that act at the nerve endings, and orthostatic hypotension is a frequent side effect, particularly if other factors promoting vasodilation are present, e.g., heat, exercise, alcohol ingestion. However, centrally mediated side effects (sedation, depression) are infrequently observed because these drugs are poorly soluble in lipids and therefore do not readily enter the central nervous system.

The last group of drugs affecting the adrenergic system are those which block the *peripheral adrenergic receptors*, alpha, beta, or both (see also Chap. 68). *Phentolamine* and *phenoxybenzamine* block the action of norepinephrine at *alpha*-adrenergic receptor sites. While the preceding two compounds block both presynaptic (alpha$_2$) and postsynaptic (alpha$_1$) alpha receptors, the former action accounts for the tolerance which develops, while *prazosin* is more effective because it selectively blocks only *postsynaptic alpha* receptors, i.e., alpha$_1$ receptors. Thus presynaptic alpha activity remains, suppressing norepinephrine release, and tolerance occurs only infrequently. Accordingly, prazosin produces less tachycardia but more postural hypotension than direct-acting vasodilators, e.g., hydralazine, and rarely can produce substantial hypotension following the first dose.

A number of effective *beta-adrenergic receptor blocking agents* are available which block sympathetic effects on the heart and should be most effective in reducing cardiac output and in lowering arterial pressure when there is increased cardiac sympathetic nerve activity. In addition, they block the adrenergic nerve–mediated release of renin from the renal juxtaglomerular cells, and this action may be an important component of their blood pressure–lowering action. Beta-adrenergic blockers are particularly useful when employed in conjunction with vascular smooth-muscle relaxants, which tend to evoke a reflex increase in heart rate, and with diuretics, the administration of which often results in an elevation of circulating renin activity. In practice, beta blockers appear to be effective even when there is no evidence of increased sympathetic tone, with about one-half or more of all hypertensive patients showing a fall in pressure. Furthermore, like diuretics, they have been shown to reduce morbidity and mortality in long-term clinical trials. However, these agents can precipitate congestive heart failure and asthma in susceptible individuals and must be used with caution in diabetics receiving hypoglycemic therapy because they inhibit the usual sympathetic responses to hypoglycemia. Cardioselective beta-blocking agents (so-called beta$_1$ blockers) have been developed (metoprolol, atenolol) which may be superior to nonselective beta blockers such as propranolol and timolol in patients with bronchospasm. Nadolol, a nonselective beta blocker, unlike other drugs of this class, is excreted unchanged in the urine and has a half-life of 14 to 20 h. Therefore, only one dose a day is required. Atenolol also usually only needs to be given once a day. Pindolol and acebutolol are nonselective beta blockers with partial agonist activity and, therefore, produce less bradycardia. Labetalol exerts both alpha- and beta-adrenergic blocking actions. Thus it lowers arterial pressure by the same complex actions as do beta blockers but also directly by reducing systemic vascular resistance. Usually it has a more rapid onset of action but produces more postural symptoms and chronic sexual dysfunction than the other beta blockers.

Vasodilators   *Hydralazine* is the most versatile of the drugs that cause direct relaxation of vascular smooth muscle; it is effective both orally and parenterally, acting mainly on arterial resistance rather than on venous capacitance vessels, as evidenced by lack of postural changes. Unfortunately, the effect of hydralazine on peripheral resistance is partly negated by reflex increases in sympathetic discharge that raise heart rate and cardiac output. This limits the usefulness of hydralazine, especially in patients with severe coronary artery disease. However, the efficacy of hydralazine can be increased if it is given in conjunction with beta blockers or drugs such as methyldopa or clonidine, all of which block reflex sympathetic stimulation of the heart. A serious side effect of doses of hydralazine exceeding 300 mg/d has been the production of a lupus erythematosus–like syndrome.

TABLE 209-6 Drugs used in treatment of hypertension—listed according to site of action

Site of action	Drug	Dosage	Indications	Contraindications	Frequent or peculiar side effects
DIURETICS					
Renal tubule	Thiazides: e.g., hydrochlorothiazide	Depends on specific drug Oral: 12.5–25 mg daily or twice daily	Mild hypertension, as adjunct in treatment of moderate to severe hypertension	Diabetes mellitus, hyperuricemia, primary aldosteronism	Potassium depletion, hyperglycemia, hyperuricemia, hypercholesterolemia, dermatitis, purpura, depression, hypercalcemia
	Loop acting: e.g., furosemide	Oral: 20–80 mg 2 or 3 times a day	Mild hypertension, as adjunct in severe or malignant hypertension particularly with renal failure	Hyperuricemia, primary aldosteronism	Potassium depletion, hyperuricemia, hyperglycemia, hypocalcemia, blood dyscrasias, rash, nausea, vomiting, diarrhea
	Potassium-sparing: Spironolactone	Oral: 25 mg 2 to 4 times daily	Hypertension due to hypermineralocorticoidism, adjunct to thiazide therapy	Renal failure	Hyperkalemia, diarrhea, gynecomastia, menstrual irregularities
	Triamterene	Oral: 50–100 mg 1 or 2 times daily			Hyperkalemia, nausea, vomiting, leg cramps, nephrolithiasis, GI disturbances
	Amiloride	Oral: 5–10 mg daily			
ANTIADRENERGIC AGENTS					
Central	Clonidine	Oral: 0.05–0.6 mg twice daily	Mild to moderate hypertension, renal disease with hypertension		Postural hypotension, drowsiness, dry mouth, rebound hypertension after abrupt withdrawal, insomnia
	Guanabenz	Oral: 4–16 mg twice daily			
	Guanfacine	Oral: 1–3 mg daily			
	Methyldopa (also acts by blocking sympathetic nerves)	Oral: 250–1000 mg twice daily IV: 250–1000 mg every 4–6 h (tolerance may develop)	Mild to moderate hypertension (oral), malignant hypertension (IV)	Pheochromocytoma, active hepatic disease (IV), during MAO inhibitor administration	Postural hypotension, sedation, fatigue, diarrhea, impaired ejaculation, fever, gynecomastia, lactation, positive Coombs' tests (occasionally associated with hemolysis), chronic hepatitis, acute ulcerative colitis, lupus-like syndrome
Autonomic ganglia	Trimethaphan	IV: 1–6 mg/min	Severe or malignant hypertension	Severe coronary artery disease, cerebrovascular insufficiency, diabetes mellitus (on hypoglycemic therapy), glaucoma, prostatism	Postural hypotension, visual symptoms, dry mouth, constipation, urinary retention, impotence
Nerve endings	Rauwolfia alkaloids: Reserpine	Oral: 0.05–0.25 mg daily	Mild to moderate hypertension in young patient	Pheochromocytoma, peptic ulcer, depression, during MAO inhibitor administration	Depression, nightmares, nasal congestion, dyspepsia, diarrhea, impotence
	Guanethidine	Oral: 10–150 mg daily	Moderate to severe hypertension	Pheochromocytoma, severe coronary artery disease, cerebrovascular insufficiency, during MAO inhibitor administration	Postural hypotension, bradycardia, dry mouth, diarrhea, impaired ejaculation, fluid retention, asthma
	Guanadrel	Oral 5–50 mg twice daily			
Alpha receptors	Phentolamine	IV: 1–5 mg bolus	Suspected or proved pheochromocytoma	Severe coronary artery disease	Tachycardia weakness, dizziness, flushing
	Phenoxybenzamine	Oral: 10–50 mg once or twice daily (tolerance may develop)	Proven pheochromocytoma		Postural hypotension, tachycardia, miosis, nasal congestion, dry mouth
	Prazosin	Oral: 1–10 mg twice daily	Mild to moderate hypertension	Use with caution in the elderly	Sudden syncope, headache, sedation dizziness, tachycardia anticholinergic effect, fluid retention
	Terazosin	Oral: 1–20 mg daily			
Beta receptors	Propranolol	Oral: 10–120 mg 2 to 4 times daily	Mild to moderate hypertension (especially with evidence for hyperdynamic circulation), adjunct to hydralazine therapy	Congestive heart failure, asthma, diabetes mellitus (on hypoglycemic therapy), during MAO inhibitor administration, COPD, sick sinus syndrome, 2d or 3d degree heart block	Dizziness, depression, bronchospasm, nausea, vomiting, diarrhea, constipation, heart failure, fatigue, Raynaud's phenomenon, hallucinations, hypertriglyceridemia, hypercholesterolemia, psoriasis; sudden withdrawal may precipitate angina or myocardial injury in patients with heart disease
	Metoprolol	Oral: 25–150 mg twice daily			
	Nadolol	Oral: 20–120 mg daily			
	Atenolol	Oral 25–100 mg daily			
	Timolol	Oral: 5–15 mg twice daily			

Site of action	Drug	Dosage	Indications	Contraindications	Frequent or peculiar side effects
ANTIADRENERGIC AGENTS (continued)					
	Betaxolol	Oral: 10–20 mg daily			
	Carteolol	Oral: 2.5–10 mg daily			
	Pindolol	Oral: 5–30 mg twice daily			Less resting bradycardia than other beta blockers
	Acebutolol	Oral: 200–600 mg twice daily			
alpha/beta receptor	Labetalol	Oral: 100–600 mg twice daily IV: 2 mg/min			Similar to beta blockers with more postural effects
VASODILATORS					
Vascular smooth muscle	Hydralazine	Oral: 10–75 mg 4 times daily IV or IM: 10–50 mg every 6 h (tolerance may develop)	As adjunct in treatment of moderate to severe hypertension (oral), malignant hypertension (IV or IM), renal disease with hypertension	Lupus erythematosus, severe coronary artery disease	Headache, tachycardia, angina pectoris, anorexia, nausea, vomiting, diarrhea, lupus-like syndrome, rash, fluid retention
	Minoxidil	Oral 2.5–40 mg twice daily	Severe hypertension	Severe coronary artery disease	Tachycardia, aggravates angina, marked fluid retention, hair growth on face and body, coarsening of facial features, possible pericardial effusions
	Diazoxide	IV: 1–3 mg/kg up to 150 mg rapidly	Severe or malignant hypertension	Diabetes mellitus, hyperuricemia, congestive heart failure	Hyperglycemia, hyperuricemia, sodium retention
	Nitroprusside	IV: 0.5–8 (μg/kg)/min	Malignant hypertension		Apprehension, weakness, diaphoresis, nausea, vomiting, muscle twitching, cyanide toxicity
ANGIOTENSIN-CONVERTING ENZYME INHIBITORS					
Converting enzyme	Captopril	Oral: 12.5–75 mg twice daily	Mild to severe hypertension, renal artery stenosis	Renal failure (reduction of dose), bilateral renal artery stenosis, pregnancy	Leukopenia, pancytopenia, hypotension, cough, angioedema, urticarial rash, fever, loss of taste, acute renal failure in bilateral renal artery stenosis, hyperkalemia
	Benazepril	Oral: 10–40 mg daily			Same as captopril, but little evidence for leukopenia, but perhaps increased frequency of cough and angioedema. All can be given once daily, but side effects are reduced if one-half dose is given twice daily. Fosinopril is excreted more in bile than others.
	Enalapril	Oral: 2.5–40 mg daily			
	Enalaprilat	IV: 0.625–1.25 mg over 5 minutes every 6–8 h			
	Fosinopril	Oral: 10–40 mg daily			
	Lisinopril	Oral: 5–40 mg daily			
	Quinapril	Oral: 10–80 mg daily			
	Ramipril	Oral: 2.5–20 mg daily			
CALCIUM CHANNEL ANTAGONISTS					
Vascular smooth muscle	Nifedipine	Oral: 10–30 mg 4 times daily or as XL form 30–90 mg daily	Mild to moderate hypertension	Heart failure, 2d or 3d degree heart block	Tachycardia, flushing, gastrointestinal disturbances, hyperkalemia, edema, headache
	Amlodipine	Oral: 2.5–10 mg daily			
	Felodipine XL	Oral: 5–10 mg daily			
	Isradipine	Oral: 2.5–10 mg daily			
	Nicardipine	Oral: 20–40 mg 3 times daily			
	Diltiazem	Oral: 30–90 mg 4 times daily or as CD form 180–300 mg daily			Same as nifidepine, except no tachycardia, but can cause heart block, constipation, and liver dysfunction
	Verapamil	Oral: 30–120 mg 4 times daily or as SR form 120–480 mg daily			

TABLE 209-7 Therapeutic agents used to treat malignant hypertension

Drug	Route	Starting dose	Onset	Peak	Duration	Oral preparation available
			\<Time course of action\>			
IMMEDIATE ONSET						
Nitroprusside	Continuous IV	0.25 (μg/kg)/min	\<1 min	1–2 min	2–5 min	No
Trimethaphan	Continuous IV	0.5 mg/min	\<1 min	1–2 min	2–5 min	No
Nitroglycerin	Continuous IV	5 μg/min	1–5 min	2–6 min	3–10 min	No
Diazoxide	IV bolus	50 mg q 5–10 min up to 600 mg	1–5 min	2–4 min	4–12 h	No
DELAYED ONSET						
Enalaprilat	IV	1.25 mg q 6 h	10–15 min	3–4 h	6–24 h	Yes
Hydralazine	IV, IM	5–10 mg q 20 min × 3	10–20 min	20–40 min	4–12 h	Yes
Labetalol	IV	20–80 mg q 10 min up to 300 mg	5 min	20–30 min	3–6 h	Yes
Nifedipine	SL	10–20 mg	5–15 min	30–60 min	3–6 h	Yes

Minoxidil is even more potent but unfortunately produces significant hypertrichosis and fluid retention and, therefore, is mainly limited to patients with severe hypertension and renal insufficiency.

Diazoxide, a thiazide derivative, is restricted in its application to acute situations. It is not a diuretic; in fact, it causes sodium retention. However, like other thiazides, it reduces carbohydrate tolerance. It must be given rapidly intravenously to guarantee effect. It begins to act immediately to lower blood pressure, and its effects may last for several hours. *Nitroprusside* given intravenously also acts as a direct vasodilator, with onset and offset of actions that are almost immediate. *Nitroglycerin* is a third direct-acting vasodilator useful as an intravenous agent. These latter three drugs are useful only for the treatment of hypertensive emergencies (Table 209-7).

ACE inhibitors Drugs from several of the categories discussed above have been shown to possess an additional action resulting in inhibition of renin secretion. These include clonidine, reserpine, methyldopa, and beta blockers. A second group of drugs in this class compress those which inhibit the enzyme converting angiotensin I into angiotensin II. These agents are useful because they not only inhibit the generation of a potent vasoconstrictor (angiotensin II) but also may retard the degradation of a potent vasodilator (bradykinin), alter prostaglandin production (most notably with captopril), and can modify the activity of the adrenergic nervous system. They are especially useful in renal or renovascular hypertension, as well as in accelerated and malignant hypertension. However, in patients with bilateral renal artery stenosis, rapid deterioration of renal function may occur. They are also as effective in mild, uncomplicated hypertension as beta blockers and thiazides—probably with fewer side effects, particularly those which adversely affect the patient's quality of life.

These drugs should be used with caution when the renin system is activated, e.g., with severe heart failure, prior diuretic therapy, or substantial salt restriction, in order to avoid profound hypotension. Usually diuretics are stopped 2 to 3 days before starting an ACE inhibitor and are added back later if needed.

Calcium channel antagonists These drugs modify the entry of calcium into cells by blocking the slow or voltage-dependent calcium channels, resulting in vasodilatation and, in the case of nifedipine and nicardipine, usually reflex tachycardia. Diltiazem and verapamil both can slow atrioventricular conduction—a feature not observed with nifedipine. While calcium channel antagonists are also useful in angina pectoris (see Chap. 203), because of their negative inotropic actions, they should be used with caution in hypertensive patients with heart failure.

APPROACH TO DRUG THERAPY (Fig. 209-1) The aim of drug therapy is to use the agents just described, alone or in combination, to return arterial pressure to normal levels with minimal side effects. Ideally, one would choose a therapeutic program which specifically corrects the underlying defect resulting in the elevated blood pressure,

e.g., spironolactone for patients with primary aldosteronism. As our knowledge of the mechanisms underlying the hypertension in individual patients increases, more specific drug programs will become available. This presumably will result in normalization of blood pressure with fewer side effects. In the absence of this information,

FIGURE 209-1 Schematic approach to the treatment of the patient with hypertension in whom a specific form of therapy is unavailable or unknown and volume expansion is not present.

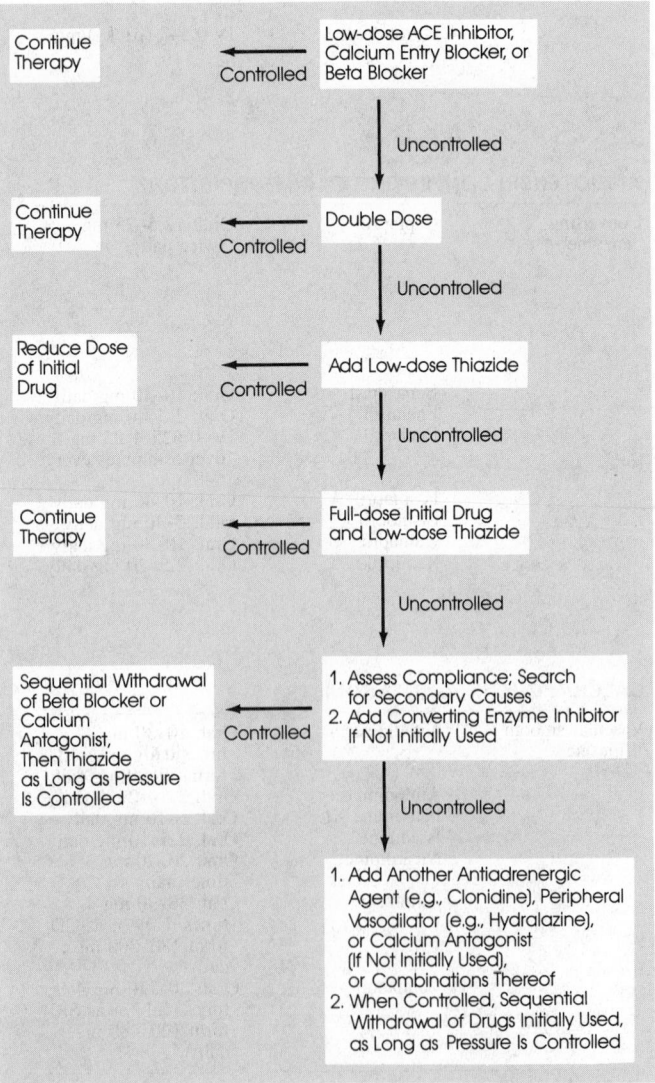

an empirical approach is used, which takes into consideration efficacy, safety, impact on the quality of life, compliance, ease of administration, and cost. When used in combination, drugs are chosen for their different sites of action. However, except for those patients with severe hypertension (average diastolic blood pressure >130 mmHg), in whom intensive therapy with several agents simultaneously usually is required, most patients should be treated *initially* with a single agent. Since many effective antihypertensive agents are available, a number of useful therapeutic regimens have been developed, with the ideal program still unclear. Initial therapy with a diuretic or beta blocker has been the usual first approach, particularly since they are the only agents proven to reduce mortality. However, this does not mean that other effective antihypertensives would fail to have the same beneficial effect if used in similar trials. Thus ACE inhibitors and calcium channel antagonists are also effective as first-line therapy, replacing the old stepped-care approach. The physician is therefore required to choose from four classes of agents for initial therapy with little evidence that one is more effective than another. Some have suggested that an ACE inhibitor or calcium channel blocker be used first, because of their reduced side effects, with a slight preference for ACE inhibitors because of their longer duration of action, potentially fewer adverse effects, and increased compliance rates. I agree with this suggestion. The reason for choosing one drug over the others is empirical, although, in general, older individuals and blacks may be particularly responsive to diuretics, while younger individuals and whites respond well to beta blockers, ACE inhibitors, and calcium channel antagonists.

The schema outlined in Fig. 209-1 takes into account the presently available data on effectiveness, adverse reactions, compliance, impact on quality of life, and economic impact (including cost, usage of health care resources, quality and quantity of work performance) in deciding when to use a given agent. This approach is applicable to all patients in whom an indication for a specific form of therapy is lacking. Because of its lower cost, low-dose thiazide therapy, e.g., 25 mg hydrochlorothiazide (or its equivalent) daily, often has been the first choice. However, three major concerns with widespread thiazide usage have arisen: relatively poor compliance rates (approximately 80 percent) probably reflecting an adverse effect on the patient's quality of life, adverse metabolic effects (hypokalemia, hypomagnesemia, hyperglycemia, and hypercholesterolemia), and potentially an increased frequency of cardiac arrhythmias including sudden death, probably secondary to the electrolyte disturbances. These concerns, coupled with the eight- to tenfold increase in cost associated with the frequent need for potassium supplementation or a potassium-sparing diuretic, have caused some to suggest that thiazides should play a more restricted role in initial antihypertensive therapy, limited to those individuals who are volume-expanded. Thus ACE inhibitors, beta blockers, and calcium channel antagonists are probably the preferred first-line therapy for hypertension, with beta blockers being particularly useful in patients with a hyperactive hemodynamic state, e.g., hypertension with an elevated heart rate.

Under any circumstance, the agent should be started at a low dose, e.g., 25 mg atenolol, 25 mg captopril, 5 mg enalapril, or 120 mg diltiazem (or their equivalents) in divided doses as needed (Table 209-6). If arterial pressure is lowered to less than 140/90 with any of these agents, no further therapy is indicated (see Fig. 209-1). If it is not after 1 to 3 months, the next step is to double the dose of the primary agent. If still not controlled, then 25 mg hydrochlorothiazide (or its equivalent) per day should be added. Thiazides potentiate the action of ACE inhibitors and probably of beta blockers and at least are additive to the antihypertensive effect of calcium channel antagonists. Combining diuretics with ACE inhibitors is particularly appealing because the adverse metabolic effects of the thiazide, in part, will be ameliorated by the ACE inhibitor. This is not true for beta blockers or calcium antagonists. Indeed, beta blockers and thiazides may actually potentiate each other's adverse effects insofar as electrolytes (hypokalemia) and metabolic actions (hypercholesterolemia) are concerned.

If therapy with two drugs does not achieve blood pressure control, the primary agent should be increased to full dose, e.g., 100 mg captopril or atenolol, 20 mg enalapril, or 360 mg diltiazem. While larger doses than these can be used, it is probably advisable to switch to another medication rather than increase the dose further. Occasionally, increasing the thiazide to the equivalent of 50 mg hydrochlorothiazide daily may bring about control of the hypertension; however, thiazide doses higher than this are seldom, if ever, warranted because they almost invariably produce significant side effects. If the blood pressure is still not controlled, then a detailed search for a secondary cause of hypertension, as outlined above, is indicated. If none is found, then a dietary assessment often will reveal a high sodium intake. With reduction in salt intake to 5 g/d or less, blood pressure often is controlled. If the blood pressure is still not controlled, then the primary agent should be switched, maintaining the thiazide. Caution should be used if an ACE inhibitor was not the original agent, since administration of such an agent to a patient who already is taking a diuretic may lead to profound hypotension. If none of the changes produce better control of arterial pressure, then the combination of a calcium channel antagonist and an ACE inhibitor or triple therapy usually with a diuretic, ACE inhibitor, and hydralazine may be effective.

If the blood pressure is controlled, then there should be stepwise reduction in the dose and/or withdrawal of some of the agents in order to determine the minimal therapeutic program that will maintain the blood pressure at 140/90 mmHg or less.

Fewer than 5 percent of patients will still be hypertensive at this point. In them, one first should consider the reasons for therapeutic failure, as shown in Table 209-8. If none can be identified, then one of the other agents such as a vasodilator listed in Table 209-6 (e.g., hydralazine) or an antiadrenergic agent (e.g., prazosin or clonidine) should be added. If blood pressure is controlled, previous drugs are sequentially withdrawn in order to determine the minimal therapeutic program that maintains a normal blood pressure.

While the recommendations outlined above are satisfactory for a large majority of patients, it is important to use a flexible approach, because individual patients may respond differently to individual drugs and drug combinations. For those patients requiring multiple drugs, once the appropriate combination has been found, the use of a single formulation with the appropriate combination of drugs may simplify the regimen and thereby increase compliance. Every effort should be made to reduce the number of times each day the patients must interrupt their schedules for the medication. Pharmacologic treatment of essential hypertension is usually lifelong, and since most patients are asymptomatic, compliance with a complex regimen may be a serious problem, particularly if the therapeutic regimen has a negative impact on the quality of the patient's life. Finally, what level of arterial pressure should be accepted as adequate control remains uncertain. It is clear that reducing diastolic blood pressure to below 90 mmHg is appropriate and beneficial in reducing morbidity and/or mortality. However, whether a reduction below 85 mmHg is warranted, particularly in elderly patients, remains controversial.

TABLE 209-8 Reasons for poor therapeutic response in patients with hypertension

Inadequate patient compliance
Volume expansion
  Excessive sodium intake
  Secondary to nondiuretic antihypertensive agent
Excessive weight gain
Inadequate doses
Drug antagonism
  Cold remedies
  Sympathomimetics
  Oral contraceptives (estrogens)
  Adrenal steroids
Secondary forms of hypertension

Special considerations Five groups of patients with hypertension require special consideration because of associated conditions.

RENAL DISEASE Reduction of arterial pressure in hypertensive patients with impaired renal function is often accompanied initially by an increase in serum creatinine. This change does not represent further structural renal damage and should not deter continuation of therapy, since achievement of blood pressure control may eventually reduce the value toward normal. However, if serum creatinine increases in patients treated with a converting enzyme inhibitor, care needs to be exercised because these patients may have bilateral renal artery disease. Their renal function will continue to deteriorate as long as the converting enzyme inhibitor is given. Thus converting enzyme inhibitors should be used cautiously in patients with impaired renal function, and renal function should be assessed frequently (every 4 to 5 days) for the first 3 weeks. While converting enzyme inhibitors are contraindicated in patients with bilateral renal artery stenosis, these are the drugs of choice in patients with unilateral renal artery stenosis and a normally functioning contralateral kidney and perhaps in patients with chronic renal failure.

CORONARY ARTERY DISEASE In these patients who also may be taking cardiac glycosides, thiazides should be used judiciously, and a reduction in serum potassium levels should be looked for and, if found, should be corrected rapidly. Beta blockers should be withdrawn carefully, if at all, in these patients. Finally, calcium channel antagonists and converting enzyme inhibitors may be useful in these patients because they minimize a number of potential adverse reactions accompanying other therapeutic agents, particularly nonspecific vasodilators.

DIABETES MELLITUS The diabetic patient with hypertension is particularly challenging because many of the agents used to lower blood pressure can affect glucose metabolism adversely. Converting enzyme inhibitors may be particularly useful in these individuals. They have no known adverse effects on glucose or lipid metabolism and may actually minimize the development of diabetic nephropathy by reducing renal vascular resistance and renal perfusion pressure— the primary factor underlying renal deterioration in these patients.

PREGNANCY The patient who is pregnant and hypertensive or who develops hypertension during pregnancy (pregnancy-induced hypertension, preeclampsia, eclampsia) is particularly difficult to treat. Because it is uncertain that autoregulation of uterine blood flow occurs, lowering blood pressure in the pregnant hypertensive may result in reduce placental and fetal perfusion. Thus a conservative approach to lowering blood pressure is usually indicated. In the second and third trimesters, antihypertensives often are not indicated unless the diastolic pressure exceeds 95 mmHg. In general, severe salt restriction and/or diuretics are not given because of the associated increase in fetal wastage. Beta blockers need to be used cautiously for similar reasons. Methyldopa and hydralazine, and to a lesser extent calcium channel antagonists, are the most frequent antihypertensives used because they have no known adverse effects on the fetus. Little is known about the safety of other antihypertensives in pregnancy except that nitroprusside and converting enzyme inhibitors may cause adverse effects on the fetus and are contraindicated.

ELDERLY PATIENTS The hypertensive patient who is over age 65, and particularly those over age 75, offers substantial challenges to the physician. Several recent studies have documented that in healthy elderly patients, whether male or female, there is a substantial reduction in strokes and stroke-related deaths in those treated with relatively modest doses of antihypertensive agents. This is true whether the patient has systolic and diastolic hypertension or isolated systolic hypertension. What is not clear from these studies is how broadly the results can be extrapolated, since they were performed in healthy elderly patients, while many such patients have other diseases. Thus, in the elderly hypertensive patient, individualization of therapy still seems warranted.

Probably fewer than one-third of hypertensive patients in the United States are being treated effectively. Only a small number of these failures are related to drug unresponsiveness. The majority are related to (1) failure to detect hypertension, (2) failure to institute effective treatment of the asymptomatic hypertensive subject, and (3) failure of the asymptomatic hypertensive subject to adhere to therapy. In order to improve this deficiency, patients must be educated to continue treatment once an effective regimen has been identified. Side effects and inconveniences of treatment must be minimized or counteracted in order to obtain the patient's continued cooperation.

MALIGNANT HYPERTENSION

In addition to marked blood pressure elevation in association with papilledema and retinal hemorrhages and exudates, the full-blown picture of malignant hypertension may include manifestations of hypertensive encephalopathy, such as severe headache, vomiting, visual disturbances (including transient blindness), transient paralyses, convulsions, stupor, and coma. These have been attributed to spasm of cerebral vessels and to cerebral edema. In some patients who have died, multiple small thrombi have been found in the cerebral vessels. Cardiac decompensation and rapidly declining renal function are other critical features of malignant hypertension. Oliguria may, in fact be the presenting feature. The vascular lesion characteristic of malignant hypertension is fibrinoid necrosis of the walls of small arteries and arterioles, and this can be reversed by effective antihypertensive therapy.

The pathogenesis of malignant hypertension is unknown. However, at least two independent processes, dilatation of cerebral arteries and generalized arteriolar fibrinoid necrosis, contribute to the associated signs and symptoms. The cerebral arteries dilate because the normal autoregulation of cerebral blood flow decompensates secondary to the markedly elevated arterial pressure. As a result, cerebral blood flow is excessive, producing the encephalopathy associated with malignant hypertension. Many patients also show evidence of a microangiopathic hemolytic anemia; this secondary phenomenon could contribute to the deterioration of renal function. Most patients also have elevated levels of peripheral plasma renin activity and increased aldosterone production, and these may be involved in causing vascular damage.

About 1 percent of hypertensive patients develop the malignant phase, which occurs in the course of both essential and secondary hypertension. Rarely it is the first recognized manifestation of the blood pressure problem, and it is unusual for it to occur in patients under treatment. The average age at diagnosis is 40, and men are more often affected than women. Prior to the availability of effective therapy, life expectancy after diagnosis of malignant hypertension was less than 2 years, with most deaths being due to renal failure, cerebral hemorrhage, or congestive heart failure. With the advent of effective antihypertensive therapy, at least half the patients survive for more than 5 years.

Malignant hypertension is a medical emergency that requires immediate therapy. However, it needs to be distinguished from severe hypertension, since overly aggressive therapy in malignant hypertension could result in a potentially hazardous reduction in myocardial and cerebral perfusion. The initial aim of therapy should be to reduce diastolic pressure by one-third, but not below 95 mmHg. The drugs available for treatment of malignant hypertension can be divided into two groups on the basis of time of onset of action (see Table 209-7). Those in the first group act within a few minutes but are not satisfactory for long-term management. If the patient is having convulsions, and if arterial pressure must be reduced rapidly, then one from the immediate-acting group should be used. The first three agents in this group require continuous infusion and close monitoring. *Nitroprusside* is given by continuous intravenous infusion at a dose of 0.25 to 8.0 (μg/kg)/min. It is probably the agent of choice in this condition since it dilates both arterioles and veins. It has the advantage over the ganglionic blockers of not being associated with the development of tachyphylaxis and can be utilized for days with few side effects. The dosage must be controlled with an infusion pump. *Trimethaphan*, a ganglionic blocker, is given at a rate of 0.5 to 5 mg/min. It also dilates arterioles and veins. The patient should be in the sitting position, and the pressure should be monitored closely, preferably in an intensive care unit. Monitoring may be more complex than with nitroprusside, but trimethaphan may be better therapy in acute aortic dissection. *Nitroglycerin* affects veins more than arterioles and is given by continuous infusion at a rate of 5 to 100 μg/min. It is particularly useful in treating hypertension following coronary bypass surgery. *Diazoxide* is the easiest to administer, for no individual titration of dosage is required. It primarily affects arteriolar and not venous tone. A dose of 50 to 150 mg is given rapidly intravenously, and the antihypertensive effect is noted in 1 to 5 min. The same dose can be repeated in 5 to 10 min, if necessary, or when the pressure begins to rise, usually after several hours. The total dose should not exceed 600 mg/d. In an occasional patient, pressure may drop below normal levels after diazoxide administration. It should not be used in patients in whom aortic dissection or myocardial infarction is suspected. Because it can increase the force of myocardial contraction, often a beta blocker is given concomitantly. *Enalaprilat*, an intravenous form of the ACE inhibitor *enalapril*, also has proven effective in preliminary studies. Finally, intravenous *labetalol* may be particularly useful in patients with a myocardial infarct or angina because it prevents an increase in heart rate. However, it may be ineffective in patients previously treated with beta blockers and is contraindicated in patients with heart failure, asthma, bradycardia, or heart block. It also may serve as an alternative therapy in patients with eclampsia who are unresponsive to hydralazine.

Patients given any of these agents also should receive other medications effective for long-term control. Those in the second group in Table 209-7 require 30 min or more to obtain full effect but have the advantage of being satisfactory for subsequent oral administration and for long-term management of the patient's hypertension. If such a delay in attainment of full effect is acceptable, intravenous *hydralazine* is effective in many patients within 10 min; an effective protocol involves giving 10-mg doses intravenously every 10 to 15 min until the desired effect has been obtained or until a total of 50 mg has been administered. The total required for response may then be repeated intramuscularly or intravenously every 6 h. Hydralazine should be used with caution in patients with significant coronary artery disease and should be avoided in patients evidencing myocardial ischemia or aortic dissection. It is effective in preeclampsia. Sublingual *nifedipine* has been reported to be useful in some cases, although it may produce tachycardia, and success has not been uniform.

Furosemide is an important adjunct to the therapy just discussed. Given either orally or intravenously, it serves to maintain sodium diuresis in the face of a falling arterial pressure and thus will speed recovery from encephalopathy and congestive heart failure as well as maintain sensitivity to the primary antihypertensive drug. Digitalis (Chap. 195) also may be indicated if there is evidence of cardiac decompensation.

In patients with malignant hypertension in whom the existence of pheochromocytoma is suspected, urine should be collected for measurement of the products of catecholamine metabolism, and drugs which might release additional catecholamines, such as methyldopa, reserpine, and guanethidine, must be avoided. The parenteral drug of choice in these patients is phentolamine, administered with care to avoid a precipitous reduction in arterial pressure.

There is hope even for patients who fail to respond sufficiently to any of the forms of therapy and who show progressive deterioration in renal function. In some, a period of peritoneal dialysis or hemodialysis to deplete extracellular fluid has resulted in better blood pressure control and eventual improvement in renal function. In other patients with refractory hypertension and renal failure who do not respond to volume depletion or hypotensive therapy, including minoxidil, particularly those with marked elevation of plasma renin activity, bilateral nephrectomy has resulted in amelioration of hypertension; subsequently, these patients have been maintained on chronic dialysis or have received renal homografts. However, bilateral nephrectomy should be avoided where possible because (1) the loss of renal erythropoietin will contribute to the associated anemia, (2) vitamin D metabolism may be adversely affected, and (3) all residual renal function will be lost.

REFERENCES

CALHOUN DA et al: Treatment of hypertensive crisis. N Engl J Med 323:1177, 1990

DAHLOF B et al: Morbidity and mortality in the Swedish Trial in Old Patients with Hypertension (STOP-Hypertension). Lancet 338:1281, 1991

DANNENBERG AL et al: Incidence of hypertension in the Framingham study. Am J Publ Health 78:676, 1988

FARNETT L et al: The J-curve phenomenon and the treatment of hypertension: Is there a point beyond which pressure reduction is dangerous? JAMA 265:489, 1991

GIFFORD RW et al: Office evaluation of hypertension: A statement for health professionals by a writing group of the Council for High Blood Pressure Research, American Heart Association. Circulation 79:283, 1989

GOTTDIENER JS et al: Left ventricular hypertrophy in men with normal blood pressure: Relation to exaggerated blood pressure response to exercise. Ann Intern Med 112(3):161, 1990

JOINT NATIONAL COMMITTEE ON DETECTION, EVALUATION AND TREATMENT OF HIGH BLOOD PRESSURE: The fifth report. Arch Intern Med 153:154, 1993

KEANE WF et al: Angiotensin-converting enzyme inhibitors and progressive renal insufficiency: Current experience and future directions. Ann Intern Med 111:503, 1989

KURTZ TW, SPENCE MA: Genetics of essential hypertension. Am J Med 94:77, 1993

LAVIE CJ et al: Regression of increased left ventricular mass by antihypertensives. Drugs 42:945, 1991

LIFTON RP, JEUNEMAITRE X: Finding genes that cause human hypertension. J Hypertens 11:231, 1993

LITTENBERG B et al: Screening for hypertension. Ann Intern Med 112(3):192, 1990

NALLY JV et al: Diagnostic criteria of renovascular hypertension with captopril renography: A consensus statement. Am J Hypertens 4:749S, 1991

OBERMAN A et al: Pharmacologic and nutritional treatment of mild hypertension: Changes in cardiovascular risk status. Ann Intern Med 112(2):89, 1990

PARATI G, MANCIA G: Calcium antagonists in the treatment of arterial hypertension. Am Heart J 125:642, 1993

SALVETTI A: Newer ACE inhibitors: A look at the future. Drugs 40:800, 1990

SHEP COOPERATIVE RESEARCH GROUP: Prevention of stroke by antihypertensive drug treatment in older persons with isolated systolic hypertension: Final results of the Systolic Hypertension in the Elderly Program (SHEP) JAMA 265:3255, 1991

STAMLER J et al: Blood pressure, systolic and diastolic, and cardiovascular risks. US population data. Arch Intern Med 153:598, 1993

SUBCOMMITTEE OF NON-PHARMACOLOGIC THERAPY OF THE JOINT NATIONAL COMMITTEE ON DETECTION, EVALUATION AND TREATMENT OF HIGH BLOOD PRESSURE: Non-pharmacological approaches to the control of high blood pressure: Final report. Hypertension 8:444, 1986

WEIDMANN P et al: Pathogenesis and treatment of hypertension associated with diabetes mellitus. Am Heart J 125:1498, 1993

WEINBERGER MH Racial differences in renal sodium excretion: Relationship to hypertension. Am J Kidney Dis 21:41, 1993

WILLIAMS GH: Quality of life and its impact on hypertensive patients. Am J Med 82:98, 1987

————: Converting enzyme inhibitors in the treatment of hypertension. N Engl J Med 319:1517, 1989

————, HOLLENBERG NK: Pathophysiology of essential hypertension, in *Cardiology*, vol 2, WW Parmley, J Chatterjee (eds). Philadelphia, Lippincott, 1990, chap 22

210   DISEASES OF THE AORTA

VICTOR J. DZAU / MARK A. CREAGER

The aorta is the conduit through which the blood ejected from the left ventricle is delivered to the systemic arterial bed. In adults, its diameter is approximately 3 cm at the origin, 2.5 cm in the descending portion in the thorax, and 1.8 to 2 cm in the abdomen. The aortic wall consists of a thin intima composed of endothelium, subendothelial connective tissue, and an internal elastic lamina; a thick tunica media composed of smooth-muscle cells and extracellular matrix; and an adventitia composed primarily of connective tissue and enclosing the vasa vasorum and nervi vascularis. In addition to its conduit function, the viscoelastic and compliant properties of the aorta also subserve a buffering function. The aorta is distended during systole to enable a

TABLE 210-1   Diseases of the aorta: Classification and etiology

Aortic aneurysm
   Atherosclerosis
   Cystic medial necrosis
   Syphilitic infection
   Mycotic infection
   Rheumatic aortitis
   Trauma
Aortic dissection
   Cystic medial necrosis
   Systemic hypertension
   Atherosclerosis
Aortic occlusion
   Atherosclerosis
   Thromboembolism
Aortitis
   Syphilitic aortitis
   Rheumatic aortitis
   Takayasu's arteritis and aortic arch syndromes
   Giant cell arteritis

portion of the stroke volume to be stored, and it recoils during diastole so that blood continues to flow to the periphery during diastole. Because of its continuous exposure to high pulsatile pressure and shear stress, the aorta is particularly prone to injury and disease resulting from mechanical trauma (Table 210-1). The aorta is also more prone to rupture than any other vessel, especially with the development of aneurysmal dilatation, since its wall tension, as governed by Laplace's law (i.e., proportional to the product of pressure and radius), is intrinsically high.

AORTIC ANEURYSM

An *aneurysm* is defined as a pathologic dilatation of a segment of a blood vessel. A *true* aneurysm involves all three layers of the vessel wall and is distinguished from a *pseudoaneurysm*, in which the intimal and medial layers are disrupted and the dilatation is lined by adventitia only and sometimes by perivascular clot. Aneurysms also may be classified according to their gross appearance. A *fusiform* aneurysm affects the entire circumference of a segment of the vessel, resulting in a diffusely dilated lesion. In contrast, a *saccular* aneurysm involves only a portion of the circumference, resulting in an outpouching of the vessel wall.

The most common pathologic condition associated with aortic aneurysm is atherosclerosis. It is controversial whether atherosclerosis itself actually causes aortic aneurysm or develops as a secondary event in the dilated aorta. Causality is inferred by studies that have shown that many patients with aortic aneurysms have coexisting risk factors and atherosclerosis in other blood vessels. Familial clusterings of abdominal aortic aneurysms occur in 20 percent of patients, suggesting a hereditary basis of the disease. Indeed, a mutation of the gene encoding type III procollagen has been implicated. Additional causes of aortic aneurysm include cystic medial necrosis, syphilis or other bacterial infections, rheumatic aortitis, and trauma. Congenital aortic aneurysms may be primary or associated with other anomalies, such as a bicuspid aortic valve or aortic coarctation.

Aortic aneurysms are also classified according to location, i.e., abdominal versus thoracic. Those in the abdominal aorta are almost always associated with atherosclerosis. Aneurysms of the ascending thoracic aorta may be related to cystic medial necrosis, atherosclerosis, syphilis, bacterial infections, or rheumatoid arthritis. Aneurysms of the descending thoracic aorta are usually contiguous with infradiaphragmatic aneurysms and, as with the latter, are associated with atherosclerosis.

Aortic aneurysms usually do not produce symptoms. However, as they expand, they may become painful. Compression or erosion of adjacent tissue by aneurysms also may cause symptoms. The formation

of mural thrombi within the aneurysm may predispose to peripheral embolization. Occasionally, an aneurysm may leak, leading to extravasation of blood into the vessel wall and the periadventitial area and causing acute pain and local tenderness. This is usually a harbinger of rupture and represents a medical emergency. More often, acute rupture occurs without any prior warning, and this complication is always life-threatening.

ATHEROSCLEROTIC ANEURYSMS   Seventy-five percent of atherosclerotic aneurysms are located in the distal abdominal aorta below the renal arteries. An abdominal aneurysm commonly produces no symptoms and is usually detected on routine examination as a palpable, pulsatile, and nontender mass, or it is an incidental finding during an abdominal x-ray or ultrasound performed for other reasons. Some patients may complain of strong pulsations in the abdomen, others of lower back pain. Rarely, there is leakage of the aneurysm with severe pain and tenderness. Acute pain and hypotension occur with rupture of the aneurysm, requiring emergency operation.

Abdominal radiography may demonstrate the calcified outline of the aneurysm. However, about 25 percent of aneurysms are not calcified and cannot be visualized by plain x-ray. A more accurate method of detection is ultrasound, which can delineate the transverse and longitudinal dimensions of the aneurysm; mural thrombus may be detected. Ultrasound is useful for serial documentation of aneurysm size. Both computed tomography (CT) with contrast and magnetic resonance imaging (MRI) have been introduced for the detection and follow-up of aortic aneurysm. These relatively expensive but noninvasive techniques provide higher resolution than ultrasound and have replaced the latter in some centers. Abdominal aortography remains the gold standard in evaluating patients with aneurysm for surgery, but this procedure carries a small risk of complications, such as bleeding, allergic reactions, and atheroembolism. This technique is useful in documenting the extent of the aneurysm, especially its upper and lower limits, and the extent of associated atherosclerotic vascular disease. However, since the presence of mural clots may reduce the laminal size, aortography may underestimate the diameter of an aneurysm.

Prognosis is related to both the size of the aneurysm and the severity of coexistent coronary artery and cerebral vascular diseases. The mortality of patients with abdominal aneurysms exceeding 6 cm in diameter who do not undergo surgical treatment is approximately 50 percent in 1 year, while in those with lesions between 4 and 6 cm, it is 25 percent. The risk of rupture increases with the size of the aneurysm. Most of the others succumb to coronary heart disease and stroke.

Operative excision with replacement with a graft is indicated for patients with abdominal aneurysms greater than 6 cm in diameter, as well as in symptomatic patients and in those with rapidly expanding aneurysms irrespective of the absolute diameter. Except for patients with exceptionally high operative risk, operation is also usually recommended in patients with aneurysm diameters of 5 to 6 cm. Serial noninvasive follow-up of smaller (<5 cm) aneurysms is an alternative to immediate surgery. In surgical candidates, careful preoperative cardiac and general medical evaluations (followed by appropriate therapy of complicating conditions) are essential. Preexisting coronary artery disease, congestive heart failure, pulmonary disease, diabetes and advanced age add to the risk of surgery. If clinically indicated, preoperative evaluation should identify high-risk coronary artery disease using an exercise stress test or dipyridamole thallium scanning. Noninvasive tests, such as stress echocardiography or ambulatory electrocardiographic monitoring for silent ischemia, are favored in some institutions. Perioperative management should include the placement of a Swan-Ganz catheter and arterial line to monitor and optimize left ventricular filling pressure, cardiac output, and arterial pressure, especially during clamping and declamping of aorta, as well as during the immediate postoperative period. With careful preoperative cardiac evaluation and postoperative care, which includes Swan-Ganz catheterization, operative mortality approximates

1 to 2 percent. Following acute rupture, the mortality of emergency operation is generally greater than 50 percent.

CYSTIC MEDIAL NECROSIS This is due to the degeneration of collagen and elastic fibers in the media of the aorta, which are replaced by multiple clefts of mucoid material. Cystic medial necrosis characteristically affects the proximal aorta, results in circumferential weakness and dilatation, and leads to the development of fusiform aneurysms involving the ascending aorta and the sinuses of Valsalva. This condition is particularly prevalent in patients with the Marfan syndrome and Ehlers-Danlos syndrome type IV (Chap. 351) but is also seen in pregnancy and hypertension and sometimes as an isolated condition in patients without any other apparent disease. The clinical manifestations include expanding aneurysms, rupture, and aortic regurgitation. Operative repair is indicated in patients in whom the diameter of the aortic root exceeds 6 cm to prevent dissection or rupture. Control of arterial pressure is an important part of the long-term management of this condition.

MYCOTIC ANEURYSM This rare condition develops as the result of staphylococcal, streptococcal, or salmonella infections of the aorta, usually at an atherosclerotic plaque. Blood cultures are usually positive and reveal the nature of the infecting agent. The aneurysms are usually saccular. Treatment requires parenteral antibiotics and surgical excision.

TRAUMA Aortic rupture may develop following penetrating injury or blunt trauma. Deceleration injury may tear the aortic isthmus at the site of insertion of the ligamentum arteriosum. Other causes of arotic aneurysm, such as syphilitic infection and rheumatic vasculitides, are discussed below under "Aortitis."

AORTIC DISSECTION

Aortic dissection is caused by a circumferential or transverse tear of the intima, usually along the right lateral wall of the ascending aorta where the hydraulic shear stress is high. It has been speculated that the initiating event is a medial hemorrhage that dissects into and disrupts the intima. Another common site is the descending thoracic aorta just below the ligamentum arteriosum. The pulsate aortic flow then dissects along the elastic lamellar plates of the aorta and creates a false lumen. The dissection usually propagates distally down the descending aorta and into its major branches, but it also may propagate proximally. In some cases, a secondary distal intimal disruption occurs, resulting in the reentry of blood from the false to the true lumen.

DeBakey and coworkers classified aortic dissections as type I, in which an intimal tear occurs in the ascending aorta but which involves the descending aorta as well, type II, in which the dissection is limited to the ascending aorta, and type III, in which the intimal tear is located in the descending area with distal propagation of the dissection (Fig. 210-1). Another classification (Stanford) is that of type A, in which the dissection involves the ascending aorta (proximal dissection), and type B, in which it is limited to the descending aorta (distal dissection). From a management standpoint, classification into type A or B is more practical and useful, since DeBakey types I and II are managed in a similar manner.

The factors that predispose to aortic dissection include systemic hypertension, a coexisting condition in 70 percent of patients, and cystic medial necrosis. Aortic dissection is the major cause of morbidity and mortality in patients with the Marfan syndrome (Chap. 351). The incidence is also increased in patients with congenital aortic valve anomalies (e.g., bicuspid valve), in those with coarctation of the aorta, and in otherwise normal women during the third trimester of pregnancy.

CLINICAL MANIFESTATIONS The presentations of aortic dissection are the consequences of intimal tear, dissecting hematoma, occlusion of involved arteries, and compression of adjacent tissues. Acute aortic dissection presents with the sudden onset of pain (Chap.

FIGURE 210-1 Classification of aortic dissections. Stanford classification: Top panels illustrate type A dissections that involve the ascending aorta independent of site of tear and distal extension; type B dissections (bottom panels) involve transverse and/or descending aorta without involvement of the ascending aorta. DeBakey classification: Type I dissection involves ascending to descending aorta (top left); type II dissection is limited to ascending or transverse aorta, without descending aorta (top center + top right); type III dissection involves descending aorta only (bottom left). (*From DC Miller, in RM Doroghazi, EE Slater (eds). Aortic Dissection. New York, McGraw-Hill, 1983, with permission.*)

12), which is often described as very severe and tearing and associated with diaphoresis. The pain may be localized to the front or back of the chest, often the interscapular region, and typically migrates with propagation of the dissection. Other symptoms include syncope, dyspnea, and weakness. Physical findings may include hypertension or hypotension, loss of pulses, aortic regurgitation, pulmonary edema, and neurologic findings due to carotid artery obstruction (hemiplegia, hemianesthesia) or spinal cord ischemia (paraplegia). Bowel ischemia, hematuria, and myocardial ischemia have all been observed. These clinical manifestations reflect complications resulting from the dissection occluding the major arteries. Furthermore, clinical manifestations may result from the compression of adjacent structures (e.g., superior cervical ganglia, superior vena cava, bronchus, esophagus) by the expanding dissection aneurysm and include Horner's syndrome, superior vena caval syndrome, hoarseness, dysphagia, and airway compromise. Hemopericardium and cardiac tamponade may complicate a type A lesion with retrograde dissection. Acute aortic regurgitation is an important and common (over 50 percent) complication of proximal dissection. This is the outcome of either a circumferential tear that widens the aortic root or a disruption of the annulus by dissecting hematoma that tears a leaflet(s) or displaces it below the line of closure. Signs of aortic regurgitation include bounding pulses, a wide pulse pressure, a diastolic murmur often radiating to the right sternal border, and evidence of congestive heart failure. The clinical manifestation depends on the severity of the regurgitation.

In dissections involving the ascending aorta, the chest x-ray often reveals a widened superior mediastinum. A pleural effusion (usually left-sided) also may be present. In dissections of the descending thoracic aorta, a widened mediastinum also may be observed on chest x-ray. In addition, the descending aorta may appear to be wider than the ascending portion. An electrocardiogram which shows no evidence of ischemia is helpful in distinguishing aortic dissection from myocardial infarction. Rarely, the dissection involves the right or left coronary ostium and causes acute myocardial infarction. The diagnosis of aortic dissection can be established by aortography or by the use of noninvasive techniques such as two-dimensional echocardiography, CT scan, or MRI (Chap. 191). Two-dimensional transthoracic echocardiography can be performed simply and rapidly and may diagnose 70 to 90 percent of proximal aortic dissections. It is less useful for detecting dissection of the arch and descending thoracic aorta. Transesophageal echocardiography requires greater skill and patient cooperation but is very accurate in identifying dissections of the ascending and descending thoracic aorta, but not the arch, achieving 98 percent sensitivity and specificity. CT scan and MRI are each highly accurate in identifying the intimal flap and the extent of the dissection. MRI also can detect blood flow, which may be useful in characterizing antegrade versus retrograde dissection. However, these procedures are time-consuming, costly, and are usually performed in a non-intensive-care setting. Presently, the gold standard is still aortography, which should be performed as soon as the diagnosis is seriously considered. It is important to identify the entry point, the intimal flap, and the false and true lumina and to establish the extent of dissection into the major arteries. Coronary angiography may be performed concomitantly in high-risk patients in the evaluation and preparation for surgery.

MANAGEMENT Medical therapy should be initiated as soon as the diagnosis is considered. The patient should be admitted to an intensive care unit for monitoring hemodynamics and urine output. Unless hypotension is present, therapy should be aimed at reducing cardiac contractility and systemic arterial pressure, and thereby shear stress. For acute dissection, unless contraindicated, beta-adrenergic blockers should be administered via the parenteral route, using either intravenous propranolol, metoprolol, or the short-acting esmolol to achieve a heart rate of approximately 60 beats per minute. This should be accompanied by sodium nitroprusside infusion to lower systolic blood pressure to 120 mmHg or less. Recently, labetalol (p. 1127), a drug with both beta- and alpha-adrenergic blocking properties, also has been used as a parenteral agent in the acute therapy of dissection. Trimethaphan, a ganglionic blocker, may be used if nitroprusside or labetalol cannot be employed. Experience with calcium antagonists is limited. Direct vasodilators, such as diazoxide and hydralazine, are contraindicated because these agents can increase hydraulic shear and may propagate dissection.

For ascending aortic dissection (type A), surgical correction, which includes reconstruction of the aortic wall, is the preferred treatment. Emergency operation carries a high operative mortality. Thus, if possible, surgery should be deferred for several days, allowing time for stabilization of the patient's clinical status. However, if pain continues and evidence of further dissection develops despite medical therapy, emergency surgery is indicated. The overall in-hospital mortality rate after surgical treatment of patients with aortic dissection is reported to be 15 to 20 percent. The major causes of perioperative mortality and morbidity include myocardial infarction, paraplegia, renal failure, tamponade, hemorrhage, and sepsis. For uncomplicated and stable distal dissection (type B), medical therapy is the preferred treatment unless there is clinical evidence of propagation, compromise of major branches of the aorta, impending rupture, or continued pain. The in-hospital mortality rate of medically treated patients with type B dissection is 15 to 20 percent. Long-term therapy for patients with aortic dissection (with or without surgery) consists of the control of hypertension and reduction of cardiac contractility with the use of beta blockers plus other antihypertensive agents such as angiotensin-converting enzyme inhibitor or calcium antagonist. The long-term prognosis for patients with treated dissections (with the exception of those with the Marfan syndrome) is generally good; the 10-year survival rate is approximately 60 percent.

AORTIC OCCLUSION

CHRONIC ARTERIOSCLEROTIC OCCLUSIVE DISEASE

Chronic occlusive disease usually involves the distal abdominal aorta below the renal arteries. Frequently the disease extends to the common iliac arteries, but it may spare the external iliac arteries. Because of the slowly progressive nature of the atherosclerotic process, the natural history of aortic occlusion is usually chronic and insidious. Claudication characteristically involves the lower back, buttocks, and thighs and may be associated with impotence in males (Leriche syndrome). The severity of the symptoms depends on the adequacy of collaterals. With sufficient collateral blood flow, a complete occlusion of the abdominal aorta may occur without the development of ischemic symptoms. The physical findings include absence of femoral and other distal pulses bilaterally and the detection of an audible bruit over the abdomen (usually at or below the umbilicus) and the common femoral arteries. Atrophic skin, loss of hair, and coolness of the lower extremities are usually observed. In advanced ischemia, rubor on dependency and pallor on elevation can be seen.

The diagnosis is usually established by the physical examination and noninvasive testing, including leg pressure measurements, Doppler velocity analysis, and pulse volume recordings. The anatomy may be defined by abdominal aortography prior to revascularization. Operative treatment is indicated in patients with debilitating symptoms and/or with the development of leg ischemia.

ACUTE OCCLUSION Acute occlusion in the distal abdominal aorta represents a medical emergency because it threatens the viability of the lower extremities. It usually results from an occlusive embolus that almost always originates from the heart. Rarely, acute occlusion may occur as the result of in situ thrombosis in a preexisting severely narrowed segment of the aorta or plaque rupture and hemorrhage into such an area.

The clinical picture is one of acute ischemia of the lower extremities. Severe rest pain, coolness, and pallor of the lower extremities and the absence of distal pulses bilaterally are the usual manifestations. Diagnosis should be established rapidly by aortography. Emergency thrombectomy or revascularization is indicated.

AORTITIS

Aortitis frequently affects the ascending aorta and may result in aneurysmal dilatation and aortic regurgitation; it occasionally obstructs branch vessels of the aorta.

SYPHILITIC AORTITIS This late manifestation of luetic infection (Chap. 133) usually affects the proximal ascending aorta, particularly the aortic root, resulting in aortic dilatation and aneurysm formation. Syphilitic aortitis may occasionally involve the aortic arch or the descending aorta. The aneurysms may be saccular or fusiform and are usually asymptomatic, but compression of and erosion into adjacent structures may result in symptoms; rupture also may occur.

The initial lesion is an obliterative endarteritis of the vasa vasorum, especially in the adventitia. This is an inflammatory response to the invasion of the adventitia by the spirochetes. Destruction of the aortic media occurs as the spirochetes spread into this layer, usually via the lymphatics accompanying the vasa vasorum. Destruction of collagen and elastic tissues leads to dilation of the aorta, scar formation, and calcification. These changes account for the characteristic radiographic appearance of a calcified ascending aortic aneurysm.

The disease typically presents as an incidental radiographic finding 15 to 30 years after initial infection. Symptoms may result from aortic regurgitation, narrowing of coronary ostia due to syphilitic aortitis, compression of adjacent structures (e.g., esophagus), or rupture. Diagnosis is established by a positive serologic test, i.e., VDRL or fluorescent treponemal antibody (see Chap. 133). Treatment includes penicillin and surgical excision and repair.

RHEUMATIC AORTITIS Rheumatoid arthritis (Chap. 285), ankylosing spondylitis (Chap. 289), psoriatic arthritis (Chap. 298), Reiter's syndrome (Chap. 289), Behçet's syndrome (Chap. 290), relapsing polychondritis, and inflammatory bowel disorders may all be associated with aortitis involving the ascending aorta. The inflammatory lesions usually involve the ascending aorta and may extend to the sinuses of Valsalva, the mitral valve leaflets, and adjacent myocardium. The clinical manifestations are aneurysm, aortic regurgitation, and involvement of the cardiac conduction system.

TAKAYASU'S ARTERITIS AND OTHER AORTIC ARCH SYNDROMES Inflammatory diseases of the aortic arch resulting in obstruction of the aorta and its major arteries characterize this major group of diseases. Takayasu's arteritis is also termed *pulseless disease* because of the frequent occlusion of the large arteries originating from the aorta. It also may involve the descending thoracic and abdominal aorta and occlude large branches such as the renal arteries. The pathology is a panarteritis with marked intimal hyperplasia, medial and adventitial thickening, and, in chronic form, fibrotic occlusion. The disease is most prevalent in young females of Asian descent. During the acute stage, fever, malaise, weight loss, and other systemic symptoms may be evident. An elevation of the erythrocyte sedimentation rate is common. The chronic stages of the disease present with symptoms related to large artery occlusion, such as upper extremity claudication, cerebral ischemia, and syncope. The chronic disease is intermittently active. Since the process is progressive and there is no definitive therapy, the prognosis is usually poor. Glucocorticoids and immunosuppressive agents have been reported to be effective in some patients during the acute phase. Occasionally, anticoagulation prevents thrombosis and complete occlusion of a large artery. Surgical bypass of a critically stenotic artery may be necessary.

GIANT CELL ARTERITIS (See Chap. 291) Primarily large and medium-sized arteries are affected. The pathology is that of focal granulomatous lesions involving the entire arterial wall. It may be associated with polymyalgia rheumatica (Chap. 23). Obstruction of medium-sized arteries (e.g., temporal and ophthalmic arteries) and of major branches of the aorta and the development of aortitis and aortic regurgitation are some of the complications of the disease. High-dose glucocorticoid therapy may be effective when given early.

REFERENCES

CIGARROA JE et al: Diagnostic imaging in the evaluation of suspected aortic dissection: Old standards and new directions. N Engl J Med 328:35, 1993

CREAGER MA et al: Aneurysmal disease of the aorta and its branches, in *Vascular Medicine*, J Loscalzo et al (eds). Boston, Little, Brown, 1992, pp 903–930

DeSANCTIS RW et al: Medical progress: Aortic dissection. N Engl J Med 317:1060, 1987

EAGLE KA, DeSANCTIS RW: Diseases of the aorta, in *Heart Disease*, 4th ed, E Braunwald (ed). Philadelphia, Saunders, 1992, pp 1528–1558

——— et al: Combining clinical and thallium data optimizes preoperative assessment of cardiac risk before major vascular surgery. Ann Intern Med 110:859, 1989

ERNST CB: Abdominal aortic aneurysm. N Engl J Med 328:1167, 1993

GUILMET D et al: Aortic dissection: Anatomic types and surgical approaches. J Cardiovasc Surg 34:23, 1993

HUNDER GG et al: Pathogenesis of giant cell arteritis. Arthritis Rheum 36:757, 1993

KULVANIEMI H et al: Genetic causes of aortic aneurysms: Unlearning at least part of what the textbooks say. J Clin Invest 88:1441, 1991

NEVITT MP et al: Prognosis of abdominal aortic aneurysys: A population based study. N Engl J Med 321:1009, 1989

NIENABER CA et al: The diagnosis of thoracic aortic dissection by noninvasive imaging procedures. N Engl J Med 328:1, 1993

REED D et al: Are aortic aneurysms caused by atherosclerosis? Circulation 85:205, 1992

211 VASCULAR DISEASES OF THE EXTREMITIES

MARK A. CREAGER / VICTOR J. DZAU

ARTERIAL DISORDERS

ATHEROSCLEROSIS OF THE EXTREMITIES Atherosclerosis (arteriosclerosis obliterans) is the leading cause of occlusive arterial disease of the extremities in patients over 40 years old; the highest incidence occurs in the sixth and seventh decades of life. As in patients with atherosclerosis of the coronary and cerebral vasculature, there is an increased prevalence of peripheral atherosclerotic occlusive disease in individuals with hypertension, hypercholesterolemia, and diabetes mellitus and in cigarette smokers. Atherosclerosis of the extremities is seen most frequently in elderly males.

Pathology (See Chap. 208) Segmental lesions causing stenosis or occlusion are usually localized in large and medium-sized vessels. The pathology of the lesions includes atherosclerotic plaques with calcium deposition, thinning of the media, patchy destruction of muscle and elastic fibers, fragmentation of the internal elastic lamina, and thrombi composed of platelets and fibrin. The primary sites of involvement are the abdominal aorta and iliac arteries in 30 percent of symptomatic patients, the femoral and popliteal arteries in 80 to 90 percent of patients, and the more distal vessels (including the tibial and peroneal arteries) in 40 to 50 percent of patients. Atherosclerotic lesions occur preferentially at arterial branch points, sites of increased turbulence, altered shear stress, and intimal injury. Involvement of the distal vasculature is most common in elderly individuals and patients with diabetes mellitus.

Clinical evaluation The most common *symptom* is intermittent claudication, which is defined as a pain, ache, cramp, numbness, or sense of fatigue in the muscles; it occurs during exercise but is relieved with rest. The site of claudication is distal to the location of the occlusive lesion. For example, buttock, hip, and thigh discomfort occurs in patients with aortoiliac disease (Leriche syndrome), whereas calf claudication develops in patients with femoral-popliteal disease. Symptoms are far more common in the lower than in the upper extremities because of the higher incidence of obstructive lesions. In patients with severe arterial occlusive disease, rest pain may develop. Patients will complain of pain or a feeling of cold or numbness in the foot and toes. Frequently these symptoms occur at night when the legs are in a "neutral" position and improve when the legs are in a dependent position. With severe ischemia, rest pain may be present.

Important *physical findings* of chronic arterial insufficiency include decreased or absent pulses distal to the obstruction, the presence of bruits over the narrowed artery, and muscle atrophy. With more severe disease, hair loss, thickened nails, smooth and shiny skin, reduced skin temperature, and pallor or cyanosis are frequent physical signs. In addition, ulcers or gangrene may occur. Elevation of the legs and repeated flexing of the calf muscles produce pallor of the soles of the feet, whereas rubor, secondary to reactive hyperemia, may develop when the legs are dependent. The duration of time for rubor to develop or for the veins in the foot to fill when the patient's legs are transferred from an elevated to a dependent position is related to the severity of the ischemia and presence of collateral vessels. Patients with severe ischemia may develop peripheral edema, because frequently they keep their legs in a dependent position. Ischemic neuritis can result in numbness and hyporeflexia.

Noninvasive testing The history and physical examination are usually sufficient to establish the diagnosis of peripheral arterial occlusive disease. Objective assessment of the severity of disease is obtained by noninvasive techniques. These include digital pulse volume recordings, Doppler flow velocity waveform analysis, duplex ultrasonography (which combines B-mode imaging and pulse-wave

Doppler examination), segmental pressure measurements, stress testing (usually using a treadmill), and tests of reactive hyperemia. In the presence of significant arterial occlusive disease, the volume displacement in the leg is decreased with each pulse, and the Doppler velocity contour becomes progressively flatter. Duplex ultrasonography is often useful in detecting stenotic lesions in native arteries and bypass grafts.

Arterial pressure can be recorded noninvasively along the legs by serial placement of sphygmomanometric cuffs and use of a Doppler device to auscultate or record blood flow. Normally, blood pressures in the legs and arms are similar. Indeed, ankle pressures may be slightly higher than arm pressures due to pulse-wave reflection. In the presence of hemodynamically significant stenoses, the arterial pressure in the leg is decreased. Thus, if one were to obtain a ratio of the ankle and brachial artery pressures, it would be >1.0 in normal individuals and <1.0 in patients with occlusive disease. A ratio of <0.5 is consistent with severe ischemia.

Treadmill testing allows the physician to assess functional limitations objectively. Decline of the ankle-brachial systolic pressure ratio immediately after exercise may provide further support for the diagnosis of arterial occlusive disease in patients with equivocal symptoms and findings on examination. Exercise testing also allows simultaneous evaluation for the presence of coronary artery disease.

Angiography should not be used for routine diagnostic testing but is performed prior to potential revascularization. It is useful for defining the anatomy to assist operative planning and is also indicated if nonsurgical interventions are being considered, such as percutaneous transluminal angioplasty or thrombolysis.

Prognosis The natural history of patients with peripheral arterial occlusive disease is influenced primarily by the extent of coexistent coronary artery and cerebral vascular disease. Studies utilizing coronary angiography have estimated that approximately one-half of patients with symptomatic peripheral arterial occlusive disease also have significant coronary artery disease. Life-table analysis has indicated that patients with claudication have a 70 percent 5-year and a 50 percent 10-year survival rate. The majority of deaths are either sudden or secondary to myocardial infarction. The likelihood of symptomatic progression of peripheral arterial occlusive disease appears less than the chance of succumbing to coronary artery disease. Approximately 70 percent of nondiabetic patients who present with mild to moderate claudication remain symptomatically stable. Improvement may occur in 10 to 15 percent of these patients; deterioration is likely to occur in the remainder, with approximately 5 percent of the group ultimately undergoing amputation. Prognosis is worse in those patients who continue to smoke cigarettes or have diabetes mellitus.

Management Therapeutic options include supportive measures, pharmacologic treatment, nonoperative interventions, and surgery. Supportive measures include meticulous care of the feet. The feet should be kept clean, and excessive drying should be prevented with the use of moisturizing creams. Well-fitting and protective shoes are advised to reduce trauma. Sandals and shoes made of synthetic materials that do not "breathe" should be avoided. Elastic support hose should be avoided, since these reduce blood flow to the skin. In patients with ischemia at rest, shock blocks under the head of the bed together with a canopy over the feet may improve perfusion pressure and ameliorate some of the rest pain.

Treatment of associated factors that contribute to the development of atherosclerosis should be initiated. The importance of discontinuing cigarette smoking cannot be overemphasized. The physician must assume a major role in this life-style modification. It is important to control blood pressure in hypertensive patients but to avoid hypotensive levels. Treatment of hypercholesterolemia is advocated, although reduction in cholesterol levels has not been shown unequivocally to reverse peripheral atherosclerotic lesions. However, it has been shown to prevent or to slow progression of the disease. Patients with claudication also should be encouraged to exercise regularly and to progressively increasing levels. Supervised exercise training

programs may improve muscle efficiency and prolong walking distance. Patients also should be advised to walk for 30 to 45 minutes daily, stopping at the onset of claudication and resting until the symptoms resolve before resuming ambulation. Other forms of exercise, such as bicycle riding and swimming, provide overall cardiovascular and psychological benefit and often are tolerated better than walking.

PHARMACOLOGIC MANAGEMENT This form of treatment of patients with peripheral arterial occlusive disease has not been as successful as the medical treatment of coronary artery disease (Chap. 203). In particular, vasodilators, as a class, have not proven to be beneficial. During exercise, peripheral vasodilation occurs normally distal to sites of significant arterial stenoses. As a result, perfusion pressure falls, often to levels less than that generated in the interstitial tissue by the exercising muscle. Unless vasodilators are able to improve collateral blood flow, it is unlikely that they would improve perfusion pressure and thereby increase blood supply to the exercising muscle. Drugs such as alpha-adrenergic blocking agents, calcium channel antagonists, papaverine, and other vasodilators have not been shown to be effective in patients with occlusive arterial disease. Pentoxifylline, a substituted xanthine derivative, has been reported to decrease blood viscosity and to increase red cell flexibility, thereby increasing blood flow to the microcirculation and enhancing tissue oxygenation. Several placebo-controlled studies have reported that pentoxifylline increased duration of exercise in patients with claudication, but its efficacy has not been confirmed in all clinical trials. Long-term parenteral administration of vasodilator prostaglandins may decrease pain and facilitate healing of ulcers in patients with severe limb ischemia.

Platelet inhibitors, particularly aspirin, have been reported to decrease progression of atherosclerosis in patients with peripheral arterial occlusive disease. Aspirin also reduces the risk of adverse cardiovascular events in patients with peripheral atherosclerosis. However, no study with aspirin has demonstrated any improvement in exercise capacity. Ticlopidine, a drug that inhibits platelet aggregation via its effect on ADP-dependent activation of glycoprotein IIb/IIIa, also reduces cardiovascular morbidity and mortality in patients with claudication. The anticoagulants heparin and warfarin have not been shown to be effective in patients with chronic arterial occlusive disease but may be useful in acute arterial obstruction secondary to thrombosis or systemic embolism. Similarly, thrombolytic intervention using drugs such as streptokinase, urokinase, or recombinant tissue plasminogen activator may have a role in the treatment of acute thrombotic arterial occlusion but is not effective in patients with chronic arterial occlusion secondary to atherosclerosis.

REVASCULARIZATION Such procedures, including nonoperative as well as operative interventions, are usually reserved for patients with progressive, severe, or disabling symptoms and ischemia at rest, as well as for those individuals who must be symptom-free because of their occupation. Angiography should be performed principally in those patients who are being considered for a revascularization procedure. Nonoperative interventions include percutaneous transluminal angioplasty (PTA), laser angioplasty, atherectomy, and stent placement. PTA of the iliac artery is associated with a higher success rate than PTA of the femoral and popliteal arteries. Approximately 90 to 95 percent of iliac PTAs are initially successful, and the 3-year patency rate is in excess of 75 percent. The initial success rate for femoral-popliteal PTA is approximately 80 percent, with a 60 percent 3-year patency rate. Patency rates are influenced by the severity of pretreatment stenoses; the prognosis of total occlusive lesions is worse than that of nonocclusive stenotic lesions. Laser angioplasty usually is used in conjunction with PTA and results in similar patency rates. The efficacy of percutaneous atherectomy and stent placement is being addressed in clinical trials.

Several operative procedures are available for treating patients with aortoiliac and femoral-popliteal artery disease. The preferred operative procedure depends on the location and extent of the obstruction(s) and general medical condition of the patient. Operative procedures for aortoiliac disease include aortobifemoral bypass, axillofemoral bypass, femoral-femoral bypass, and aortoiliac endarterectomy. The most commonly utilized procedure is the aortobifemoral bypass, using knitted Dacron grafts. Immediate graft patency approaches 99 percent, and 5- and 10-year graft patency in survivors is in excess of 90 and 80 percent, respectively. Operative complications include myocardial infarction and stroke, infection of the graft, peripheral embolization, and sexual dysfunction from interruption of autonomic nerves in the pelvis. Operative mortality ranges from 1 to 3 percent, mostly due to ischemic heart disease.

Operative therapy for femoral-popliteal artery disease includes in situ and reverse autogenous saphenous vein bypass grafts, polytetrafluoroethylene (PTFE) or other synthetic grafts, and thromboendarterectomy. Operative mortality ranges from 1 to 3 percent. Long-term patency rate is dependent on the type of graft utilized, the location of the distal anastomosis, and the patency of runoff vessels beyond the anastomosis. Patency rates of femoral-popliteal saphenous vein bypass grafts at 1 year approach 90 percent and at 5 years 70 to 80 percent. Five-year patency rates of infrapopliteal saphenous vein bypass grafts are 60 to 70 percent. In contrast, 5-year patency rates of infrapopliteal PTFE grafts are less than 30 percent. Lumbar sympathectomy alone or as an adjunct to aortofemoral reconstruction has fallen into disfavor. While this procedure may increase blood flow to the skin, it does not increase blood flow to muscle. There is no good clinical evidence that lumbar sympathectomy increases graft patency or improves limb survival.

Preoperative cardiac risk assessment may identify individuals most likely to experience an adverse cardiac event during the perioperative period. Patients with angina, prior myocardial infarction, ventricular ectopy, or heart failure are among those with increased risk. Noninvasive tests such as treadmill testing, if feasible, dipyridamole thallium or Sesta-MIBI scintigraphy, and ambulatory ischemia monitoring enable further stratification of patient risk. Patients with abnormal tests require close supervision and adjunctive management with antianginal medications. It is not known whether coronary angiography and coronary arterial revascularization reduce overall perioperative mortality in high-risk patients undergoing peripheral vascular surgery, but these procedures should be considered in patients suspected of having left main or three-vessel coronary artery disease.

FIBROMUSCULAR DYSPLASIA This is a hyperplastic disorder affecting medium-sized and small arteries. It occurs predominantly in females and usually involves renal and carotid arteries but can affect extremity vessels such as the iliac and subclavian arteries. The histologic classification includes intimal, medial, and periadventitial dysplasia. Medial dysplasia is the most common type and is characterized by hyperplasia of the media with or without fibrosis of the elastic membrane. It is identified angiographically by a "string of beads" appearance caused by thickened fibromuscular ridges contiguous with thin, less involved portions of the arterial wall. When limb vessels are involved, clinical manifestations are similar to those for atherosclerosis, including claudication and rest pain. PTA and surgical reconstruction have been beneficial in patients with debilitating symptoms or threatened limbs.

THROMBOANGIITIS OBLITERANS Thromboangiitis obliterans (Buerger's disease) is an inflammatory occlusive vascular disorder involving small and medium-sized arteries and veins in the distal upper and lower extremities. Cerebral, visceral, and coronary vessels also may be affected. This disorder develops most frequently in men under age 40. The prevalence is higher in Asians and individuals whose lineage originates in eastern Europe. While the cause of thromboangiitis obliterans is not known, there is a definite relationship to cigarette smoking and an increased incidence of HLA-B5 and -A9 antigens in patients with this disorder.

In the initial stages of thromboangiitis obliterans, polymorphonuclear leukocytes infiltrate the walls of the small and medium-sized arteries and veins. The internal elastic lamina is preserved, and thrombus may develop in the vascular lumen. As the disease progresses, mononuclear cells, fibroblasts, and giant cells replace the

neutrophils. Later stages are characterized by perivascular fibrosis and recanalization.

The clinical features of thromboangiitis obliterans often include a triad of claudication of the affected extremity, Raynaud's phenomenon (see below), and migratory superficial vein thrombophlebitis. Claudication is usually confined to the lower calves and feet or forearms and hands because this disorder primarily affects distal vessels. In the presence of severe digital ischemia, trophic nail changes, ulcerations, and gangrene may develop at the tips of the fingers. The physical examination shows normal brachial and popliteal pulses but reduced or absent radial, ulnar, and/or tibial pulses. Arteriography is helpful in making the diagnosis. Smooth, tapering segmental lesions in the distal vessels are characteristic, as are collateral vessels at sites of vascular occlusion. Proximal atherosclerotic disease is usually absent. The diagnosis can be confirmed by excisional biopsy and pathologic examination of an involved vessel.

There is no specific treatment except abstention from tobacco. The prognosis is worse in individuals who continue to smoke, but results are discouraging even in those who do stop smoking. Arterial bypass of the larger vessels may be used in selected instances, as well as local debridement, depending on symptoms and severity of ischemia. Antibiotics may be useful; anticoagulants and glucocorticoids are not helpful. If these measures fail, amputation may be required.

VASCULITIS Other vasculitides may affect the arteries supplying the upper and lower extremities. Takayasu's arteritis and giant cell (temporal) arteritis are discussed in Chap. 291.

ACUTE ARTERIAL OCCLUSION This results in the sudden cessation of blood flow to an extremity. The severity of ischemia and the viability of the extremity are dependent on the location and extent of the occlusion and the presence and subsequent development of collateral blood vessels. There are two principal causes of acute arterial occlusion: embolism and thrombus in situ.

The most common sources of arterial emboli are the heart, aorta, and large arteries. Cardiac disorders that cause thromboembolism include atrial fibrillation, both chronic and paroxysmal, and acute myocardial infarction, ventricular aneurysm, cardiomyopathy, infectious and marantic endocarditis, prosthetic heart valves, and atrial myxoma. Emboli to the distal vessels also may originate from proximal sites of atherosclerosis and aneurysms of the aorta and large vessels. Less frequently, an arterial occlusion may result paradoxically from a venous thrombus that has entered the systemic circulation via a patent foramen ovale or other septal defect. Arterial emboli tend to lodge at the bifurcation of vessels because the caliber of the vessel decreases at these sites; in the lower extremities, emboli lodge most frequently in the femoral artery, followed by the iliac artery, aorta, and popliteal and tibioperoneal arteries.

Acute arterial thrombosis in situ occurs most frequently in atherosclerotic vessels at the site of a stenosis or aneurysm and in arterial bypass grafts. Trauma to an artery also may result in the formation of an acute arterial thrombus. Arterial occlusion may complicate arterial punctures and placement of catheters. Less frequent causes include the thoracic outlet compression syndrome, causing subclavian artery occlusion, and entrapment of the popliteal artery by abnormal placement of the medial head of the gastrocnemius muscle. Polycythemia and hypercoagulable disorders (Chaps. 309 and 316) are also associated with acute arterial thrombosis.

Clinical features The symptoms of the acute arterial occlusion depend on the location, duration, and severity of the obstruction. Often, severe pain, paresthesias, numbness, and coldness develop in the involved extremity within 1 h. Paralysis may occur with severe and persistent ischemia. Physical findings include loss of pulses distal to the occlusion, cyanosis or pallor, mottling, decreased skin temperature, muscle stiffening, loss of sensation, weakness, and/or absent deep tendon reflexes. If acute arterial occlusion occurs in the presence of an adequate collateral circulation, as is often the case in acute graft occlusion, the symptoms and findings may be less impressive. In this situation, the patient complains about an abrupt decrease in the distance walked before claudication occurs or of modest pain and paresthesias. Pallor and coolness are evident, but sensory and motor functions are generally preserved. The diagnosis of acute arterial occlusion is usually apparent from the clinical presentation. Arteriography is useful for confirming the diagnosis and demonstrating the location and extent of occlusion.

Management Once the diagnosis is made, the patient should be anticoagulated with intravenous heparin to prevent propagation of the clot. In cases of severe ischemia of recent onset and particularly when limb viability is jeopardized, immediate intervention to ensure reperfusion is indicated. Surgical thromboembolectomy or arterial bypass procedures are used to restore blood flow to the ischemic extremity promptly, particularly when a large proximal vessel is occluded.

Intraarterial thrombolytic therapy is effective when acute arterial occlusion is caused by a thrombus in an atherosclerotic vessel or arterial bypass graft. Thrombolytic therapy also may be indicated when the patient's overall condition contraindicates surgical intervention or when smaller distal vessels are occluded, thus preventing surgical access. Intraarterial streptokinase is administered as a bolus injection of 25,000 to 250,000 IU followed by a continuous infusion of 5000 to 15,000 IU/h. One approach for administering intraarterial urokinase is to give a bolus of 60,000 to 120,000 IU followed by 240,000 IU/h for 2 h, 120,000 IU/h for 2 h, and then 60,000 IU/h. Clinical trials are now in progress to assess the efficacy of intraarterial recombinant tissue plasminogen activator (tPA). Meticulous observation for hemorrhagic complications is required during intraarterial thrombolytic therapy.

If the limb is not in jeopardy, a more conservative approach that includes observation and administration of anticoagulants may be taken. Anticoagulation prevents recurrent embolism and reduces the likelihood of thrombus propagation. It can be initiated with intravenous heparin and followed by oral warfarin. Recommended dosages are the same as those used in deep vein thrombosis (see later). Emboli resulting from infectious endocarditis, prosthetic heart valves, or atrial myxoma often require surgical intervention to remove the cause.

ATHEROEMBOLISM Atheroembolism constitutes a subset of acute arterial occlusion. In this condition, multiple small deposits of fibrin, platelet, and cholesterol debris embolize from proximal atherosclerotic lesions or aneurysmal sites. Atheroembolism may occur after intraarterial procedures. Since the emboli tend to lodge in the small vessels of the muscle and skin and may not occlude the large vessels, distal pulses usually remain palpable. Patients complain of acute pain and tenderness at the site of embolization. Digital vascular occlusion may result in ischemia and the "blue toe" syndrome; digital necrosis and gangrene may develop. Localized areas of tenderness, pallor, and livedo reticularis (see below) occur at sites of emboli. Skin or muscle biopsy may demonstrate cholesterol crystals.

Ischemia resulting from atheroemboli is notoriously difficult to treat. Usually neither surgical revascularization procedures nor thrombolytic therapy is helpful because of the multiplicity, composition, and distal location of the emboli. Some evidence suggests that platelet inhibitors prevent atheroembolism. Surgical intervention to remove or bypass the atherosclerotic vessel or aneurysm that causes the recurrent atheroemboli may be necessary.

THORACIC OUTLET COMPRESSION SYNDROME This refers to a symptom complex resulting from compression of the neurovascular bundle at the thoracic outlet (artery, vein, or nerves) as it courses through the neck and shoulder. Cervical ribs, abnormalities of the scalenus anticus muscle, the proximity of the clavicle to the first rib, or abnormal insertion of the pectoralis minor muscle may compress the subclavian artery and brachial plexus as these structures pass from the thorax to the arm. Patients may develop shoulder and arm pain, weakness, paresthesias, claudication, Raynaud's phenomenon, and even ischemic tissue loss and gangrene. Examination is often normal unless provocative maneuvers are performed. Occasionally, distal pulses are decreased or absent and digital cyanosis and ischemia may be evident. Tenderness may be present in the supraclavicular fossa.

Abducting the affected arm 90° and externally rotating the shoulder may precipitate symptoms. Several additional maneuvers are used to confirm the diagnosis of vascular compression and suggest the location of the abnormality. These include the scalene (extension of the neck and rotation of the head to the side of the symptoms), costoclavicular (posterior rotation of shoulders), and hyperabduction (raising the arm 180°) maneuvers which may cause subclavian bruits and loss of pulses in the arm. A chest x-ray will indicate the presence of cervical ribs. The electromyogram will be abnormal if the brachial plexus is involved.

Most patients can be managed conservatively. They should be advised to avoid those positions that cause symptoms. Many patients benefit from shoulder girdle exercises. Surgical procedures such as removal of the first rib or resection of the scalenus anticus muscle are necessary occasionally for relief of symptoms or treatment of ischemia.

ARTERIOVENOUS FISTULAS These abnormal communications between an artery and a vein, bypassing the capillary bed, may be congenital or acquired. Congenital arteriovenous fistulas are the result of persistent embryonic vessels that fail to differentiate into arteries and veins; these may be associated with birth marks, are located in almost every organ of the body, and frequently occur in the extremities. Acquired arteriovenous fistulas are either created to provide vascular access for hemodialysis or occur as a result of a penetrating injury such as a gunshot or knife wound or as complications of arterial catheterization or surgical dissection. An infrequent cause of arteriovenous fistula is rupture of an arterial aneurysm into a vein.

The clinical features depend on the location and size of the fistula. Frequently, a pulsatile mass is palpable, and a thrill and bruit lasting throughout systole and diastole are present over the fistula. With long-standing fistulas, clinical manifestations of chronic venous insufficiency, including peripheral edema, large tortuous varicose veins, and stasis pigmentation, become apparent because of the high venous pressure. Evidence of ischemia may occur in the distal portion of the extremity. Skin temperature is higher over the arteriovenous fistula. Large arteriovenous fistulas may result in an increased cardiac output with consequent cardiomegaly and high-output heart failure (Chap. 195).

Diagnosis This is often evident from the physical examination. Compression of a large arteriovenous fistula may cause reflex slowing of the heart rate (Nicoladoni-Branham sign). Arteriography can confirm the diagnosis and is useful in demonstrating the site and size of the arteriovenous fistula.

Management This may involve surgery, radiotherapy, or embolization. Congenital arteriovenous fistulas are often difficult to treat because the communications may be numerous and extensive and new ones frequently develop after ligation of the most obvious ones. Many of these lesions are best treated conservatively using elastic support hose to reduce the consequences of venous hypertension. Occasionally, embolization with autologous material, such as fat or muscle, or with hemostatic agents, such as gelatin sponges or silicon spheres, is used to obliterate the fistula. Acquired arteriovenous fistulas are usually amenable to surgical treatment that involves division or excision of the fistula. Occasionally this requires autogenous or synthetic grafting to reestablish continuity of the artery and vein.

RAYNAUD'S PHENOMENON Raynaud's phenomenon is characterized by episodic digital ischemia, manifested clinically by the sequential development of digital blanching, cyanosis, and rubor of the fingers or toes following cold exposure and subsequent rewarming. Emotional stress also may precipitate Raynaud's phenomenon. The color changes are usually well demarcated and are confined to the fingers or toes. Typically, one or more digits will appear white when the patient is exposed to a cold environment or touches a cold object. The blanching, or pallor, represents the ischemic phase of the phenomenon and is secondary to vasospasm of digital arteries. During the ischemic phase, capillaries and venules dilate, and cyanosis results from the deoxygenated blood that is present in these vessels. Sensation of cold, numbness, or paresthesias of the digits often accompany the phases of pallor cyanosis.

With rewarming, the digital vasospasm resolves, and blood flow into the dilated arterioles and capillaries increases dramatically. This "reactive hyperemia" imparts a bright red color to the digits. In addition to rubor and warmth, patients often experience a throbbing, painful sensation during the hyperemic phase. Although the triphasic color response is typical of Raynaud's phenomenon, some patients may develop only pallor and cyanosis; others may experience only cyanosis.

Pathophysiology Raynaud originally proposed that cold-induced episodic digital ischemia was secondary to exaggerated reflex sympathetic vasoconstriction. This theory is supported by the fact that adrenergic blocking drugs as well as sympathectomy decrease the frequency and severity of Raynaud's phenomenon in some patients. An alternative hypothesis is that there is enhanced digital vascular responsiveness to cold or to normal sympathetic stimuli. It is also possible that normal reflex sympathetic vasoconstriction is superimposed on local digital vascular disease or that there is enhanced adrenergic neuroeffector activity.

Raynaud's phenomenon is broadly separated into two categories: the idiopathic variety termed *Raynaud's disease* and the secondary variety, which is associated with other disease states or known causes of vasospasm (Table 211-1).

Raynaud's disease This appellation is applied when the secondary causes of Raynaud's phenomenon have been excluded. Over 50 percent of patients with Raynaud's phenomenon have Raynaud's disease. Women are affected about five times more often than men, and the age of presentation is usually between 20 and 40 years. The fingers are involved more frequently than the toes. Initial episodes may involve only one or two fingertips, but subsequent attacks may involve the entire finger and may include all the fingers. The toes are affected in 40 percent of patients. Although vasospasm of the toes usually occurs in patients with symptoms in the fingers, it may happen alone. Rarely, the earlobes and the tip of the nose are involved. Raynaud's phenomenon occurs frequently in patients who also have migraine headaches or variant angina. These associations suggest that there may be a common predisposing cause for the vasospasm.

The physical examination is often entirely normal; the radial, ulnar, and pedal pulses are normal. The fingers and toes may be cool between attacks and may perspire excessively. Thickening and tightening of the digital subcutaneous tissue, i.e., sclerodactyly, develop in 10 percent of patients. Angiography of the digits for diagnostic purposes is not indicated.

Patients with Raynaud's disease, in general, appear to have the milder forms of Raynaud's phenomenon. Less than 1 percent of these patients lose a part of a digit. After the diagnosis is made, the disease spontaneously improves in approximately 15 percent of patients and progresses in about 30 percent.

Secondary causes of Raynaud's phenomenon Raynaud's phenomenon occurs in 80 to 90 percent of patients with systemic sclerosis

---

TABLE 211-1 Classification of Raynaud's phenomenon

Primary or idiopathic Raynaud's phenomenon: Raynaud's disease
Secondary Raynaud's phenomenon
  Collagen vascular diseases: scleroderma, systemic lupus erythematosus, rheumatoid arthritis, dermatomyositis, polymyositis
  Arterial occlusive diseases: atherosclerosis of the extremities, thromboangiitis obliterans, acute arterial occlusion, thoracic outlet syndrome
  Pulmonary hypertension
  Neurologic disorders: invertebral disk disease, syringomyelia, spinal cord tumors, stroke, poliomyelitis, carpal tunnel syndrome
  Blood dyscrasias: cold agglutinins, cryoglobulinemia, cryofibrinogenemia, myeloproliferative disorders, Waldenström's macroglobulinemia
  Trauma: vibration injury, hammer hand syndrome, electric shock, cold injury, typing, piano playing
  Drugs: ergot derivatives, methysergide, beta-adrenergic receptor blockers, bleomycin, vinblastin, cisplatin

---

(scleroderma) and is the presenting symptom in 30 percent (Chap. 286). It may be the only symptom of scleroderma for many years. Abnormalities of the digital vessels may contribute to the development of Raynaud's phenomenon in this disorder. Ischemic fingertip ulcers may develop and progress to gangrene and autoamputation. About 20 percent of patients with systemic lupus erythematosus (SLE) have Raynaud's phenomenon (Chap. 284). Occasionally, persistent digital ischemia develops and may result in ulcers or gangrene. In most severe cases, the small vessels are occluded by a proliferative endarteritis. Raynaud's phenomenon occurs in about 30 percent of patients with dermatomyositis or polymyositis (Chap. 384). It frequently develops in patients with rheumatoid arthritis and may be related to the intimal proliferation that occurs in the digital arteries.

Atherosclerosis of the extremities is a frequent cause of Raynaud's phenomenon in men over age 50. Thromboangiitis obliterans is an uncommon cause of Raynaud's phenomenon but should be considered in young men, particularly in those who are cigarette smokers. The development of cold-induced pallor in these disorders may be confined to one or two digits of the involved extremity. Occasionally, Raynaud's phenomenon may occur following acute occlusion of large and medium-sized arteries by a thrombus or embolus. Embolization of atheroembolic debris may cause digital ischemia. The latter often involves one or two digits and should not be confused with Raynaud's phenomenon. In patients with the thoracic outlet syndrome, Raynaud's phenomenon may result from diminished intravascular pressure, stimulation of sympathetic fibers in the brachial plexus, or a combination of both. Raynaud's phenomenon occurs in patients with primary pulmonary hypertension (Chap. 225); this is more than coincidental and may reflect a neurohumoral abnormality that affects both the pulmonary and digital circulations.

A variety of blood dyscrasias may be associated with Raynaud's phenomenon. Cold-induced precipitation of plasma proteins, hyperviscosity, and aggregation of red cells and platelets may occur in patients with cold agglutinins, cryoglobulinemia, or cryofibrinogenemia. Hyperviscosity syndromes that accompany myeloproliferative disorders and Waldenström's macroglobulinemia also should be considered in the initial evaluation of patients with Raynaud's phenomenon.

Raynaud's phenomenon occurs often in patients whose vocations require the use of vibrating hand tools such as chain saws or jackhammers. The frequency of Raynaud's phenomenon also seems to be increased in pianists and typists. Electric shock injury to the hands and frostbite may lead to the later development of Raynaud's phenomenon.

Several drugs have been causally implicated in Raynaud's phenomenon. These include ergot preparations, methysergide, beta-adrenergic receptor antagonists, and the chemotherapeutic agents bleomycin, vinblastine, and cisplatin.

Management Most patients with Raynaud's phenomenon experience only mild and infrequent episodes. These patients need reassurance and should be instructed to dress warmly and avoid unnecessary cold exposure. In addition to gloves and mittens, patients should protect the trunk, head, and feet with warm clothing in order to prevent cold-induced reflex vasoconstriction. Tobacco use is contraindicated.

Drug treatment should be reserved for the severe cases. The calcium channel antagonists, especially nifedipine (10 to 30 mg tid) and diltiazem (30 to 90 mg tid), decrease the frequency and severity of Raynaud's phenomenon. Long-acting preparations of these drugs also may be effective. Adrenergic blocking agents, such as reserpine (0.25 to 0.5 mg qd), have been shown to increase nutritional blood flow to the fingers. Some, but not all, patients achieve satisfactory results with long-term reserpine therapy. Moreover, systemic use of this drug is limited by side effects of hypotension, nasal stuffiness, lethargy, and depression. The postsynaptic alpha$_1$-adrenergic antagonist prazosin (1 to 5 mg tid) has been used with favorable responses. Doxazosin and terazosin also may be effective. Other sympatholytic agents such as methyldopa, guanethidine, and phenoxybenzamine may be useful in some patients. Parenteral treatment with vasodilator prostaglandins is under investigation, but its potential utility is applicable more to severe digital ischemia than to episodic Raynaud's phenomenon. Surgical sympathectomy is helpful in some patients who are unresponsive to medical therapy, but benefit is often transient.

ACROCYANOSIS In this condition, there is arterial vasoconstriction and secondary dilatation of the capillaries and venules with resulting persistent cyanosis of the hands and, less frequently, the feet. Cyanosis may be intensified by exposure to a cold environment. Women are affected much more frequently than men, and the age of onset is usually less than 30 years. Generally patients are asymptomatic but seek medical attention because of the discoloration. Examination reveals normal pulses, peripheral cyanosis, and moist palms. Trophic skin changes and ulcerations do *not* occur. The disorder can be distinguished from Raynaud's phenomenon because it is persistent and not episodic, the discoloration extends proximally from the digits, and blanching does not occur. Ischemia secondary to arterial occlusive disease usually can be excluded by the presence of normal pulses. Central cyanosis and decreased arterial oxygen saturation are not present. Patients should be reassured and advised to dress warmly and avoid cold exposure. Pharmacologic intervention is not indicated.

LIVEDO RETICULARIS In this condition, localized areas of the extremities develop a mottled or netlike appearance of reddish to blue discoloration. The mottled appearance may be more prominent following cold exposure. The idiopathic form of this disorder occurs equally in men and women, and the most common age of onset is in the third decade. Patients with the idiopathic form usually are asymptomatic and seek attention for cosmetic reasons. Livedo reticularis also occurs following atheroembolism (see above). Rarely, skin ulcerations develop. Patients should be reassured and advised to avoid cold environments. No drug treatment is indicated.

PERNIO (CHILBLAINS) This is a vasculitic disorder associated with exposure to cold; acute forms have been described. Raised erythematous lesions develop on the lower part of the legs and feet in cold weather. These are associated with pruritus and a burning sensation, and they may blister and ulcerate. Pathologic examination demonstrates angiitis characterized by intimal proliferation and perivascular infiltration of mononuclear and polymorphonuclear leukocytes. Giant cells may be present in the subcutaneous tissue. Patients should avoid exposure to cold, and ulcers should be kept clean and protected with sterile dressings. Sympatholytic drugs may be effective in some patients.

ERYTHROMELALGIA (ERYTHERMALGIA) This disorder is characterized by burning pain and erythema of the extremities. The feet are involved more frequently than the hands, and males are affected more frequently than females. Erythromelalgia may occur at any age but is most common in middle age. It may be primary or secondary to disorders such as polycythemia vera and hypertension. Patients complain of burning in the extremities, precipitated by exposure to a warm environment and aggravated by the dependent position. The symptoms are relieved by exposing the affected area to cool air or water or by elevation. Erythromelalgia can be distinguished from ischemia secondary to arterial occlusive disorders and peripheral neuropathy because the peripheral pulses are present and the neurologic examination is normal. There is no specific treatment; aspirin may produce relief. Treatment of associated disorders in secondary erythromelalgia may be helpful.

FROSTBITE In this condition, tissue damage results from severe environmental cold exposure or from direct contact with a very cold object. Tissue injury results from both freezing and vasoconstriction. Frostbite usually affects the distal aspects of the extremities or exposed parts of the face, such as the ears, nose, chin, and cheeks. Superficial frostbite involves the skin and subcutaneous tissue. Patients experience pain or paresthesia, and the skin appears white and waxy. After rewarming, there is cyanosis and erythema, wheal and flare formation, edema, and superficial blisters. Deep frostbite involves muscle, nerves, and deeper blood vessels. It may result in edema of the hand or foot, vesicles and bullae, tissue necrosis, and gangrene.

Initial treatment is rewarming, performed in an environment where reexposure to freezing conditions will not occur. Rewarming is accomplished by immersion of the affected part in a water bath at temperatures of 40 to 44°C (104 to 111°F). Massage, application of ice water, and extreme heat are contraindicated. The injured area should be cleansed with soap or antiseptic and sterile dressings applied. Analgesics are often required during rewarming. Antibiotics are used if there is evidence of infection. The efficacy of sympathetic blocking drugs is not established. Following recovery, the affected extremity may exhibit increased sensitivity to cold.

VENOUS DISORDERS

Veins in the extremities can be broadly classified as either superficial or deep. In the lower extremity, the superficial venous system includes the greater and lesser saphenous veins and their tributaries. The deep veins of the leg accompany the major arteries. Perforating veins connect the superficial and the deep systems at multiple locations. Bicuspid valves are present throughout the venous system to direct the flow of venous blood centrally.

VENOUS THROMBOSIS The presence of thrombus within a superficial or deep vein and the accompanying inflammatory response in the vessel wall is termed *venous thrombosis* or *thrombophlebitis*. Initially, the thrombus is composed principally of platelets and fibrin. Red cells become interspersed with fibrin, and the thrombus tends to propagate in the direction of blood flow. The inflammatory response in the vessel wall may be minimal or characterized by granulocyte infiltration, loss of endothelium, and edema.

The factors that predispose to venous thrombosis were initially described by Virchow in 1856 and include stasis, vascular damage, and hypercoagulability. Accordingly, a variety of clinical situations are associated with increased risk of venous thrombosis (Table 211-2). Venous thrombosis may occur in more than 50 percent of patients having orthopedic surgical procedures, particularly those involving the hip or knee, and in 10 to 40 percent of patients who undergo abdominal or thoracic operations. The prevalence of venous thrombosis is particularly high in patients with cancer of the pancreas, lungs, genitourinary tract, stomach, and breast. Approximately 10 to 20 percent of patients with idiopathic deep vein thrombosis have or develop clinically overt cancer; there is no consensus on whether these individuals should be subjected to intensive diagnostic workup to search for occult malignancy. Risk of thrombosis is increased following trauma, such as fractures of the spine, pelvis, femur, and tibia. Immobilization, regardless of the underlying disease, is a major predisposing cause of venous thrombosis. This may account for the relatively high incidence in patients with acute myocardial infarction or congestive heart failure. The incidence of venous thrombosis is increased during pregnancy, particularly in the third trimester and in

---

TABLE 211-2 Conditions associated with an increased risk for development of venous thrombosis

Surgery
  Orthopedic, thoracic, abdominal, and genitourinary procedures
Neoplasms
  Pancreas, lung, ovary, testes, urinary tract, breast, stomach
Trauma
  Fractures of spine, pelvis, femur, tibia
Immobilization
  Acute myocardial infarction, congestive heart failure, stroke, postoperative convalescence
Pregnancy
Estrogen use (for replacement or contraception)
Hypercoagulable states
  Deficiencies of antithrombin III, protein C, or protein S; anticardiolipin antibodies; myeloproliferative diseases; dysfibrinogenemia; disseminated intravascular coagulation
Venulitis
  Thromboangiitis obliterans, Behçet's disease, homocysteinuria
Previous deep vein thrombosis

the first month postpartum, and in individuals who use estrogens. A variety of clinical disorders that produce systemic hypercoagulability, including antithrombin II, protein C, and protein S deficiencies, systemic lupus erythematosus, myeloproliferative diseases, dysfibrinogenemia, and disseminated intravascular coagulation, may cause venous thrombosis. Venulitis occurring in thromboangiitis obliterans, Behçet's disease, and homocysteinuria also may cause venous thrombosis.

DEEP VENOUS THROMBOSIS The most important consequences of this disorder are pulmonary embolism (Chap. 226) and the syndrome of chronic venous insufficiency. Deep thrombosis of the iliac, femoral, or popliteal veins is suggested by unilateral leg swelling, warmth, and erythema. Tenderness may be present along the course of the involved veins, and a cord may be palpable. There may be increased tissue turgor, distention of superficial veins, and the appearance of prominent venous collaterals. In some patients, deoxygenated hemoglobin in stagnant veins imparts a cyanotic hue to the limb, a condition called *phlegmasia cerulea dolens*. In markedly edematous legs, the interstitial tissue pressure may exceed the capillary perfusion pressure, causing pallor, a condition designated *phlegmasia alba dolens*.

The diagnosis of deep venous thrombosis of the calf is often difficult to make at the bedside. This is so because only one of multiple veins may be involved, allowing adequate venous return through the remaining patent vessels. The most common complaint is calf pain. Examination may reveal posterior calf tenderness, warmth, increased tissue turgor or modest swelling, and rarely, a cord. Increased resistance or pain during dorsiflexion of the foot, Homan's sign, is an unreliable diagnostic sign.

Deep venous thrombosis occurs less frequently in the upper extremity than in the lower extremity, but the incidence is increasing because of greater utilization of subclavian catheters. The clinical features and complications are similar to those described for the leg.

Diagnosis Various noninvasive tests are used to diagnose deep venous thrombosis, including duplex venous ultrasonography (B-mode, i.e., two-dimensional, imaging and pulse-wave Doppler interrogation), plethysmographic techniques, and ^{125}I-fibrinogen scanning. By imaging the deep veins, the presence of thrombus can be detected by direct visualization or by inference when the vein does not collapse with compressive maneuvers. The Doppler ultrasound measures the velocity of blood flow in veins. This velocity is normally affected by respiration and by manual compression of the foot or calf. Flow abnormalities occur when deep venous obstruction is present. The positive predictive value of duplex venous ultrasonography approaches 95 percent for proximal deep vein thrombosis. Since it is more difficult to visualize calf veins than proximal veins, the sensitivity of this technique is only 50 to 75 percent, although the specificity of this technique for calf vein thrombosis is 95 percent.

Plethysmographic techniques used to measure changes in venous capacitance during physiologic maneuvers include impedance plethysmography (IPG) and phleborheography (PRG). IPG uses skin electrodes, and PRG uses a series of air-filled cuffs to detect changes in leg volume. Venous obstruction blunts the normal changes in venous capacitance that occur during respiration or following inflation and deflation of a thigh cuff. The predictive value of these tests for detecting occlusive thrombi in proximal veins is approximately 90 percent. However, these tests are much less sensitive in the detection of deep venous thrombosis of the calves.

^{125}I-fibrinogen scanning is occasionally used for the diagnosis of deep venous thrombosis. Since this isotope is actively taken up by the propagating venous thrombi, increases in radioactivity detected with a counter imply the presence of a thrombus. Fibrinogen scans detect more than 90 percent of calf vein thrombi but are less specific for proximal venous thrombi. A serious limitation of the technique is that it may take 48 to 72 h after administration of the isotope for a fibrinogen scan to become positive.

Deep venous thrombosis also can be diagnosed by venography. Contrast medium is injected into a superficial vein of the foot and

directed to the deep system by the application of tourniquets. The presence of a filling defect or absence of filling of the deep veins is required to make the diagnosis.

Deep vein thrombosis must be differentiated from a variety of disorders that cause unilateral leg pain or swelling, including muscle trauma or hemorrhage, a ruptured popliteal cyst, and lymphedema. It may be difficult to distinguish swelling caused by the postphlebitic syndrome from that due to acute recurrent deep venous thrombosis. Leg pain also may result from nerve compression syndrome, arthritis, tendinitis, fractures, and arterial occlusive disorders. A careful history and physical examination can usually determine the cause of these symptoms.

Management Prevention of pulmonary embolism is the most important reason for treating patients with deep vein thrombosis, since in the early stages the thrombus may be loose and poorly adherent to the vessel wall. Patients should be placed in bed, and the affected extremity should be elevated above the level of the heart until the edema and tenderness subside. Anticoagulants prevent thrombus propagation and allow the endogenous lytic system to operate. Heparin should be administered intravenously as an initial bolus of 5000 to 10,000 IU, followed by a continuous infusion of 1000 to 1500 IU/h. The rate of the heparin infusion should be adjusted so that the activated partial thromboplastin time (APTT) is approximately twice the control value. Intermittent intravenous and subcutaneous injections of heparin have been used as alternative forms of therapy. In less than 5 percent of patients, heparin therapy may cause thrombocytopenia. Infrequently, these patients develop arterial thrombosis and ischemia. Heparin treatment should be maintained for at least 7 to 10 days. Warfarin is administered during the first week of treatment with heparin and may be started as early as the first day of heparin treatment. It is important to overlap heparin treatment with oral anticoagulant therapy for at least 4 to 5 days because the full anticoagulant effect of warfarin is delayed. The dose of warfarin should be adjusted to maintain the prothrombin time by 4 to 7 s beyond control values, equivalent to an international normalized ratio (INR) of 2.0 to 3.0. The use of anticoagulants for isolated deep vein thrombosis of the calf is controversial because the incidence of pulmonary embolism is very low. However, approximately 20 percent of calf thrombi propagate to the thigh, thereby increasing the risk of pulmonary embolism.

The incidence of pulmonary embolism in patients presenting with deep calf vein thrombosis is 5 to 20 percent. Therefore, patients with calf vein thrombosis should either receive anticoagulants or be followed with serial noninvasive tests to determine whether proximal propagation has occurred. Anticoagulant treatment should be continued for 3 to 12 months for patients with acute proximal deep vein thrombosis to decrease the chance of recurrence. The duration of anticoagulant treatment for patients with calf vein thrombosis should be at least 6 weeks. The duration of treatment is indefinite for patients with recurrent deep vein thrombosis and for those in whom associated causes, such as malignancy or hypercoagulability, have not been eliminated. If treatment with anticoagulants is contraindicated because of a bleeding diathesis or risk of hemorrhage, protection from pulmonary embolism can be achieved by mechanically interrupting the flow of blood through the inferior vena cava. Inferior vena cava plication generally has been replaced by percutaneous insertion of a filter.

Thrombolytic drugs such as streptokinase, urokinase, and tissue plasminogen activator also may be used, but there is no evidence that thrombolytic therapy is more effective than anticoagulants in preventing pulmonary embolism. However, early administration of thrombolytic drugs may accelerate clot lysis, preserve venous valves, and decrease the potential for developing postphlebitic syndrome.

Prophylaxis should be considered in clinical situations where the risk of deep vein thrombosis is high. Low-dose heparin (5000 units 2 h prior to surgery and then 5000 units every 8 to 12 h postoperatively), warfarin, and external pneumatic compression are all useful. Low-dose heparin reduces the risk of deep vein thrombosis associated with thoracic and abdominal surgery and in patients placed at prolonged bedrest. Low-molecular-weight heparin (4000 to 5000 Da) has been shown to prevent deep vein thrombosis in patients undergoing abdominal or hip surgery. It is purported to have greater efficacy and a lower incidence of bleeding than conventional heparin. Warfarin, in doses that increase the prothrombin time, equivalent to an INR of 2.0 to 3.0, is effective in preventing deep vein thrombosis associated with bone fractures and orthopedic surgery. Warfarin is started the night before surgery and continued throughout the convalescent period. External pneumatic compression devices applied to the legs are used to prevent deep vein thrombosis when even low doses of heparin or warfarin may cause serious bleeding, such as during neurosurgery or transurethral resection of the prostate.

SUPERFICIAL VEIN THROMBOSIS   Thrombosis of the greater or lesser saphenous veins or their tributaries, i.e., superficial vein thrombosis, does not result in pulmonary embolism or chronic venous insufficiency. It is associated with intravenous catheters and infusions, occurs in varicose veins, and may develop in association with deep vein thrombosis. Migrating superficial vein thrombosis is often a marker for a carcinoma and also may occur in patients with vasculitides, such as thromboangiitis obliterans. The clinical features of superficial vein thrombosis are easily distinguishable from those of deep vein thrombosis. Patients complain of pain localized to the site of the thrombus. Examination reveals a reddened, warm, and tender cord extending along a superficial vein. The surrounding area may be red and edematous.

Therapy is primarily supportive. Initially, patients can be placed at bed rest with leg elevation and application of warm compresses. Nonsteroidal anti-inflammatory drugs may provide analgesia but also may obscure clinical evidence of thrombus propagation. If a thrombosis of the greater saphenous vein develops in the thigh and extends toward the saphenofemoral vein junction, it is reasonable to consider anticoagulant therapy to prevent extension of the thrombus into the deep system and a possible pulmonary embolism.

VARICOSE VEINS   These are dilated tortuous superficial veins that result from defective structure and function of the valves of the saphenous veins, from intrinsic weakness of the vein wall, from high intraluminal pressure, or rarely, from arteriovenous fistulas. Varicose veins can be categorized as primary or secondary. Primary varicose veins originate in the superficial system and occur two to three times as frequently in women as in men. Approximately half of patients have a family history of varicose veins. Secondary varicose veins result from deep venous insufficiency and incompetent perforating veins or from deep venous occlusion causing enlargement of superficial veins that are serving as collaterals.

Patients with venous varicosities are often concerned about the cosmetic appearance of their legs. Symptoms consist of a dull ache or pressure sensation in their legs after prolonged standing; it is relieved with leg elevation. The legs feel heavy, and occasionally, mild ankle edema develops. Extensive venous varicosities may cause skin ulcerations near the ankle. Superficial venous thrombosis may be a recurring problem, and rarely, a varicosity ruptures and bleeds. Visual inspection of the legs in the dependent position usually confirms the presence of varicose veins.

Varicose veins usually can be treated with conservative measures. Symptoms often decrease when the legs are elevated periodically, when prolonged standing is avoided, and when elastic support hose are worn. External compression stockings provide a counterbalance to the hydrostatic pressure within the veins. Small symptomatic varicose veins may be treated with sclerotherapy, in which a sclerosing solution is injected into the involved varicose vein and a compression bandage is applied. Surgical therapy usually involves extensive ligation and stripping of the greater and lesser saphenous veins and should be reserved for those patients who are very symptomatic, suffer recurrent superficial vein thrombosis, and/or develop skin ulceration. Surgical therapy may be indicated for cosmetic reasons.

CHRONIC VENOUS INSUFFICIENCY   This may result from deep vein thrombosis and/or valvular incompetence. Following deep vein

thrombosis, the delicate valve leaflets become thickened and contracted so that they are incapable of preventing retrograde flow of blood; the vein becomes rigid and thick-walled. Although most veins recanalize after an episode of thrombosis, the large proximal veins may remain occluded. Secondary incompetence develops in distal valves because high pressures distend the vein and separate the leaflets. Primary deep venous valvular dysfunction also may occur without previous thrombosis. Patients with venous insufficiency often complain of a dull ache in the leg that worsens with prolonged standing and resolves with leg elevation. Examination demonstrates increased leg circumference, edema, and superficial varicose veins. Erythema, dermatitis, and hyperpigmentation develop along the distal aspect of the leg, and skin ulceration may occur near the medial and lateral malleoli. Cellulitis may be a recurring problem. Patients should be advised to avoid prolonged standing or sitting; frequent leg elevation is helpful. Graduated compression stockings should be worn during the day. These efforts should be intensified if skin ulcers develop. Ulcers should be treated with applications of wet to dry dressings and occasionally dilute topical antibiotic solutions. Commercially available dressings comprising antiseptic solutions and compressive bandages may be applied and should be changed weekly until healing occurs. Recurrent ulceration and severe edema may be treated by surgical interruption of incompetent communicating veins. Rarely, surgical valvuloplasty and bypass of venous occlusions are employed.

LYMPHATIC DISORDERS

Lymphatic capillaries are blind-ended tubes formed by a single layer of endothelial cells. The absent or widely fenestrated basement membrane of lymphatic capillaries allows greater access to interstitial proteins and particles. Lymphatic capillaries merge to form larger vessels which contain smooth muscle and are capable of vasomotion. Small and medium-sized lymphatic vessels empty into progressively larger channels which drain into the thoracic duct. The lymphatic circulation is involved in the absorption of interstitial fluid and in the response to infection.

LYMPHEDEMA   Lymphedema may be categorized as primary or secondary (Table 211-3). The prevalence of primary lymphedema is approximately 1 per 10,000 individuals. Primary lymphedema may be secondary to agenesis, hypoplasia, or obstruction of the lymphatic vessels. It may be associated with the Turner syndrome, the Noonan syndrome, the yellow nail syndrome, the intestinal lymphangiectasia syndrome, and lymphangiomyomatosis. Women are affected more frequently than men. There are three clinical subtypes: congenital lymphedema, which appears shortly after birth; lymphedema praecox, which has its onset at the time of puberty; and lymphedema tarda, which usually begins after age 35. Familial forms of congenital lymphedema (Milroy's disease) and lymphedema praecox (Meige's disease) may be inherited in an autosomal dominant manner with variable penetrance; autosomal or sex-linked recessive forms are less common.

Secondary lymphedema is an acquired condition resulting from

TABLE 211-3   Causes of lymphedema

Primary
Congenital (includes Milroy's disease)
Lymphedema praecox (includes Meige's disease)
Lymphedema tarda
Secondary
Recurrent lymphangitis
Filariasis
Tuberculosis
Neoplasm
Surgery
Radiation therapy

damage to or obstruction of previously normal lymphatic channels (see Table 211-3). Recurrent episodes of bacterial lymphangitis, usually caused by streptococci, are a very common cause of lymphedema. The most common cause of secondary lymphedema worldwide is filariasis (Chap. 182). Tumors, such as prostate cancer and lymphoma, also can obstruct lymphatic vessels. Both surgery and radiation therapy for breast carcinoma may cause lymphedema of the upper extremity. Less common causes include tuberculosis, contact dermatitis, lymphogranuloma venereum, rheumatoid arthritis, pregnancy, and self-induced or factitious lymphedema following application of tourniquets.

Lymphedema is generally a painless condition, but patients may experience a chronic dull, heavy sensation in the leg, and most often patients are concerned about the appearance of the leg. Lymphedema of the lower extremity, initially involving the foot, gradually progresses up the leg so that the entire limb becomes edematous. In the early stages of lymphedema, the edema is soft and pits easily with pressure. In the chronic stages, the limb has a woody texture, and the tissues become indurated and fibrotic. At this stage, the edema may no longer be pitting. The limb loses its normal contour, and the toes appear square. Lymphedema should be distinguished from other disorders that cause unilateral leg swelling, such as deep vein thrombosis and chronic venous insufficiency. In the latter, edema is softer and there is often evidence of a stasis dermatitis, hyperpigmentation, and superficial venous varicosities.

The evaluation of patients with lymphedema should include diagnostic studies to clarify the cause. Abdominal and pelvic ultrasound and computed tomography can be used to detect obstructing lesions such as neoplasms. Lymphoscintigraphy and lymphangiography are rarely indicated, but either can be used to confirm the diagnosis or differentiate primary from secondary lymphedema. Lymphoscintigraphy involves the injection of radioactively labeled technetium-containing colloid into the distal subcutaneous tissue of the affected extremity. Lymphangiography requires the isolation and cannulation of a distal lymphatic vessel and subsequent injection of contrast material. In primary lymphedema, lymphatic channels are absent, hypoplastic, or ectatic. In secondary lymphedema, lymphatic channels usually are dilated, and the level of obstruction may be determined.

Management   Patients with lymphedema of the lower extremities must be instructed to take meticulous care of their feet to prevent recurrent lymphangitis. Skin hygiene is important, and emollients can be used to prevent drying. Prophylactic antibiotics are often helpful, and fungal infection should be treated aggressively. Patients should be encouraged to participate in physical activity; frequent leg elevation can reduce the amount of edema. Patients can be fitted with graduated compression hose to reduce the amount of lymphedema that develops with upright posture. Occasionally, intermittent pneumatic compression devices can be applied at home to facilitate reduction of the edema. Diuretics are contraindicated and may cause depletion of intravascular volume and metabolic abnormalities. Recently, microsurgical lymphovenous anastomotic procedures have been performed to rechannel lymph flow from obstructed lymphatic vessels into the venous system.

REFERENCES

ANDERSON FA JR et al: A population-based perspective of the incidence and case fatality rates of venous thrombosis and pulmonary embolism: The Worcester DVT study. Arch Intern Med 151:933, 1991

BLANKENHORN DH et al: Effects of colestipol-niacin therapy on human femoral atherosclerosis. Circulation 83:438, 1991

BROWSE NL: The diagnosis and management of primary lymphedema. J Vasc Surg 3:181, 1986

CAPEK P et al: Femoropopliteal angioplasty: Factors influencing long-term success. Circulation 83:170, 1991

CLEOPHAS TJ, NIEMEYER MG: Raynaud's syndrome, an enigma after 130 years. Angiology 44:196, 1993

COFFMAN JD: Intermittent claudication and rest pain: Physiologic concepts and therapeutic approaches. Prog Cardiovasc Dis 22:59, 1979

———: Raynaud's Phenomenon. New York, Oxford, 1989

CRIQUI MH et al: Mortality over a period of 10 years in patients with peripheral arterial disease. N Engl J Med 326:381, 1992

EUROPEAN WORKING GROUP ON CRITICAL LEG ISCHEMIA: Second European consensus document on chronic critical leg ischemia. Circulation 84:IV1, 1991

GOLDHABER SZ: Thrombolysis in venous thromboembolism: An international perspective. Chest 94:176S, 1990

GRESHAM CL: Deep venous thrombosis. South Med J 86:438, 1993

LOSCALZO J et al: The Textbook of Vascular Medicine and Biology. Boston, Little, Brown, 1992

OLIN JW et al: The changing clinical spectrum of thromboangiitis obliterans. Circulation 82:IV3, 1990

SMITH GD et al: Intermittent claudication, heart disease risk factors, and mortality: The Whitehall study. Circulation 82:1925, 1990

YOUNG JR et al: Peripheral Vascular Diseases. St. Louis, Mosby–Year Book, 1991

PART EIGHT   DISORDERS OF THE RESPIRATORY SYSTEM

212   APPROACH TO THE PATIENT WITH DISEASE OF THE RESPIRATORY SYSTEM

EUGENE BRAUNWALD

As in other branches of medicine, a careful and detailed history and physical examination are the cornerstones for establishing an accurate diagnosis in patients with disorders of the respiratory system. In addition, the roentgenographic examination occupies a particularly important role in the evaluation of patients with lung disease. Since abnormalities of the respiratory system are frequently a manifestation of a systemic process, a comprehensive evaluation of the patient's entire health status is essential. For example, the presence of a pulmonary lesion on x-ray may be due to metastatic disease with the primary tumor elsewhere, and hemoptysis may be due to a disorder of hemostasis. Diffuse pulmonary infiltrative disease may be secondary to diffuse scleroderma (Chap. 286), and multiple pulmonary cavities may be a manifestation of Wegener's granulomatosis (Chap. 291). All the so-called collagen vascular diseases may have prominent pulmonary manifestations. Carcinoma of the lung (Chap. 227) may be accompanied by prominent extrathoracic manifestations, which may overshadow the pulmonary lesion. These include myopathy, peripheral neuropathy, hypertrophic pulmonary osteoarthropathy, and a variety of endocrine and metabolic manifestations, including Cushing's syndrome, the carcinoid syndrome, a hyperparathyroid-like picture, inappropriate secretion of antidiuretic hormone, gonadotropin (Chap. 327), and increased frequency of pulmonary infections. Patients with AIDS frequently have pulmonary manifestations. These include pneumonia caused by *Pneumocystis carinii* (Chap. 178), commonly an "AIDS defining" illness. Other manifestations include Kaposi's sarcoma involving the tracheobronchial tree and pulmonary infection with a variety of organisms, including *Mycobacterium tuberculosis, Mycobacterium avium* complex, histoplasmosis, cryptococcosis, coccidioidomycosis, and cytomegalovirus.

HISTORY   In eliciting the history of patients with pulmonary disease, it must be appreciated that an increasing fraction of the population is exposed to materials which are potentially toxic to the lung (Chap. 219). The history must therefore contain a detailed *occupational and personal history* with a description of exposure to hazards such as asbestos, coal, silica, beryllium, bagasse, iron oxide, tin oxide, cotton dust, titanium oxide, silver, nitrogen dioxide, animals, moldy hay, air conditioners, and furnace humidifiers. It is useful to construct a work history, which includes the patient's duties, duration of exposure, use of protective devices, and the occurrence and nature of illness in fellow workers. The occupational history should include information on a job-by-job basis as well as the military service. Contact with both wild and domestic animals may result in pulmonary symptoms, such as bronchospasm in subjects allergic to pets or, less commonly, acute pneumonitis in patients with psittacosis, tularemia (Chap. 122), or Q fever. Because it is such an important risk factor for many forms of lung disease, a history of tobacco consumption, especially cigarette smoking, must be sought and should be quantified, generally in "pack-years." The habits of the patient with pulmonary disease must be explored. Aspiration pneumonia and pneumococcal and *Klebsiella* pneumonia are often seen in alcoholics; lung abscess occurs in intravenous drug abusers.

A history of intravenous drug abuse or of sexual relations with individuals at high risk for AIDS (Chap. 279) should be obtained, especially in patients with a pulmonary infiltrate and fever. A record of the patient's *previous residence* is of considerable importance in the diagnosis of histoplasmosis (the south and midwestern United States; Chap. 162), coccidioidomycosis (the southwestern United States; Chap. 163), tropical eosinophilia, and South American blastomycosis. For example, pulmonary mass lesions in patients in the Mediterranean Basin may be due to hydatid cysts, hemoptysis in patients from central China may be caused by paragonimiasis (Chap. 184), and in Egypt cor pulmonale frequently results from schistosomiasis (Chap. 183).

It is especially important to elicit a history of *drug exposure* in patients with unexplained pulmonary disease, since essentially every class of drugs can produce pulmonary toxicity (Chap. 218), and all parts of the respiratory apparatus can be affected, including the alveoli, tracheobronchial tree, mediastinum, pleural cavities, pulmonary vessels, respiratory muscles, and the medullary respiratory center. Examples include the interstitial infiltrative diseases caused by amiodarone, bleomycin, cyclophosphamide, methotrexate, nitrofurantoin, and sulfonamides; noncardiogenic pulmonary edema caused by heroin; bronchospasm caused by beta-adrenergic blockers, cholinergic drugs, and nonsteroidal anti-inflammatory drugs; pulmonary vasculitis from intravenous drug abuse; cough and pulmonary thromboembolism in women receiving oral contraceptives; (drug-induced) systemic lupus erythematosus with pleural involvement caused by hydralazine and procainamide; and respiratory depression caused by aminoglycoside antibiotics, opiates, and trimethaphan.

The *family history* should consider pulmonary diseases which may be genetic, such as cystic disease of the lung, pulmonary emphysema due to α_1-antitrypsin deficiency (Chap. 223), cystic fibrosis (Chap. 222), asthma (Chap. 217), hereditary telangiectasia, Kartagener's syndrome, and alveolar microlithiasis, as well as infections due to the tubercle bacilli and fungi where exposure to involved family members is important.

Dyspnea is a cardinal manifestation of diseases involving the respiratory and cardiovascular systems (Chap. 31). A detailed examination of both organ systems is therefore mandatory in every patient with this symptom. Dyspnea secondary to cardiac disease is often recognized by the presence of other evidence of heart failure, such as cardiac enlargement, gallop rhythms, and cardiac murmurs. It may be difficult to differentiate paroxysmal nocturnal dyspnea due to pulmonary edema of cardiac origin from nocturnal attacks of bronchial asthma and from chronic pulmonary disease with pooling of the secretions in the recumbent position, but a detailed description of the circumstances in which this symptom occurs is most useful. Dyspnea also is a common functional complaint, and an important clue in the identification of this form is the observation that shortness of breath often occurs at rest and is relieved during exertion; the opposite is the case in patients in whom this symptom is secondary to disease of the lungs or heart. Equally important in the differential diagnosis is a careful elucidation of the relationship of dyspnea to other symptoms such as angina pectoris (favoring ischemic heart disease) or cough with expectoration (favoring pulmonary disease).

Patients with diseases involving the respiratory system also may present with *chest pain* which is frequently caused by inflammation of the pleura, occurring in pneumonia, pulmonary thromboembolism, tuberculosis, and malignancy (Chap. 12). Pleuritic pain is usually localized to one side of the chest and is related to respiration and to movements of the thorax. Lesions confined to the pulmonary parenchyma do not produce pain, while diseases involving the organs in the mediastinum (Chap. 228) may cause local discomfort. Pain also may originate in or be referred to the chest wall; it may be due to intercostal neuritis, as in herpes zoster, or to compression of the intercostal nerves as they leave the spinal cord. Such pain is often superficial in character and may be intensified by coughing or straining. Thoracic pain also may be due to myositis, costochondral disturbances, myocardial ischemia, pericarditis, esophageal disease, and aortic dissection and aneurysm (Chap. 12). The most common causes of pain related to respiration are disorders of the chest wall, pleurisy, intercostal neuritis, and costochondral disease. The last condition characteristically causes chest pain intensified by palpation. A major task is to distinguish chest pain due to abnormalities of the bronchopulmonary system from that due to myocardial ischemia (see Chap. 12).

Cough and *expectoration* are also cardinal features of pulmonary disease (Chap. 30). Few patients can describe the severity of cough or quantity of expectoration reliably, and it is therefore desirable for the physician to inspect a 24-h collection of sputum. Cough is often precipitated by foreign materials irritating nerve endings in airways and is frequently caused by inflammation of the bronchi; the latter may be persistent (as in patients with a cigarette cough and chronic bronchitis) or acute (as in a variety of viral and bacterial infections). The time of occurrence of the cough and the character and quantity of expectorated material may point to the diagnosis. For example, bronchiectasis, lung abscess, and necrotizing pneumonia can produce purulent sputum which may have an offensive odor or be streaked with blood (Chaps. 220 and 221). In pulmonary edema, the sputum is pink, frothy, and watery (Chap. 31). Mucoid (translucent, viscid, shiny, white or gray) or mucopurulent (mucoid with flecks of yellow or green pus) sputum is characteristic of acute and chronic bronchitis. Sputum is bloody or rusty in pneumococcal pneumonia; it is thick, gelatinous, brick red, and laced with pus in *Klebsiella* pneumonia. Paroxysmal cough also may be the presenting feature in patients with bronchial asthma, in whom physical examination may or may not reveal wheezing respirations and squeaking musical sounds (Chap. 217); indeed unexplained cough may be caused by asthma. Paroxysmal cough occurs frequently in patients with left ventricular failure, in whom it generally occurs at night and in the recumbent position

(Chap. 195). Pulmonary tuberculosis (Chap. 130), though less common than previously, remains a common cause of chronic cough, as does primary neoplasm of the lung (Chap. 227). A change in the character of a chronic cough, unaccompanied by an acute infection, should alert the physician to the need to carry out a detailed examination.

Hemoptysis is often a frightening symptom (Chap. 30). Faint streaking of the sputum with blood may be observed in acute infections of the respiratory tract. However, many patients with bloody sputum have serious disease, such as pulmonary thromboembolism, tuberculosis, critical mitral stenosis, neoplasm of the lung, lung abscess, or bronchiectasis. In all instances it is necessary to exclude sources of blood in the nasopharynx and bleeding of gastric or esophageal origin. The character of the bloody expectorate should be defined, since it may be helpful in identifying the underlying disease process. Sputum which is frankly bloody without mucus or pus may be due to pulmonary thromboembolism (Chap. 226). When pus is present, pneumonia, bronchiectasis, or lung abscess should be considered. Dilute, pink, frothy sputum is observed in acute pulmonary edema (Chap. 31).

PHYSICAL EXAMINATION A careful examination of the thorax, including inspection, palpation, percussion, and auscultation, often provides the clue to the diagnosis of many common pulmonary disorders (Table 212-1). Abnormalities such as small or moderate amounts of fluid in the alveoli or in the mediastinum, bronchospasm, and pleural effusions can sometimes be detected more accurately by physical examination than by chest roentgenography or other imaging techniques. Tracheal deviation can be readily recognized on physical examination and may be observed in obstruction of a major bronchus and in atelectasis. A meticulous *general physical examination* is mandatory in patients with disorders of the respiratory system. Enlarged lymph nodes in the cervical and supraclavicular regions should be sought. Disturbances of mentation or even coma occurs in patients with acute carbon dioxide retention and hypoxemia. Telltale stains on the fingers point to heavy cigarette smoking; infected teeth and gums may occur in patients with aspiration pneumonitis and lung abscess; characteristic cutaneous lesions may point to sarcoidosis (Chap. 292), collagen vascular disease, Wegener's granulomatosis, Kaposi's sarcoma, and berylliosis, all of which may have prominent pulmonary manifestations. Clubbing of the fingers or, when advanced, osteoarthropathy (Chap. 299) may suggest carcinoma (Chap. 227) or suppurative disease (Chap. 220) of the lung, chronic hypoxemia, as occurs in patients with chronic bronchitis (Chap. 223), pulmonary arteriovenous fistula, or congenital heart disease with right-to-left shunt (Chap. 199). However, clubbing also occurs in some patients with biliary cirrhosis, regional enteritis, and ulcerative colitis. A careful search for infection in the teeth, gums, tonsils, or sinuses is

---

TABLE 212-1   Physical findings in some common pulmonary disorders

Disorder	Inspection	Palpation	Percussion	Auscultation
Bronchial asthma (acute attack)	Hyperinflation; use of accessory muscles	Impaired expansion; decreased fremitus	Hyperresonant; low diaphragm	Prolonged expiration; inspiratory and expiratory wheezes
Pneumothorax (complete)	Lag on affected side	Absent fremitus	Hyperresonant or tympanitic	Absent breath sounds
Pleural effusion (large)	Lag on affected side	Decreased fremitus; trachea and heart shifted away from affected side	Dullness or flatness	Absent breath sounds
Atelectasis (lobar obstruction)	Lag on affected side	Decreased fremitus; trachea and heart shifted toward affected side	Dullness or flatness	Absent breath sounds
Consolidation (pneumonia)	Possible lag or splinting on affected side	Increased fremitus	Dullness	Bronchial breath sounds; bronchophony; pectoriloquy; crackles

SOURCE: JF Murray, in *Textbook of Respiratory Medicine*, JF Murray, JA Nadel (eds), p 449.

recommended in patients suspected or known to have bronchiectasis or lung abscess.

Neurologic findings which may provide a clue to the presence of pulmonary disease include headache, drowsiness, papilledema, and other evidence of increased intracranial pressure which may occur in patients with pulmonary disease who have hypoxemia and hypercapnia. Vascular collapse is a late complication of carbon dioxide retention and is characterized by hypotension, flushed skin, sweating, and tachycardia. A detailed examination of the cardiovascular system (Chap. 187) is mandatory in patients suspected of having respiratory disease and in patients with unexplained dyspnea, cough, or cyanosis because of the frequent difficulty of differentiating disorders of the respiratory and cardiovascular systems.

DIAGNOSTIC TESTS The *roentgenographic examination* of the chest represents the cornerstone of the diagnostic workup of the patient with suspected pulmonary disease, and it is the integration of the information obtained from the clinical examination and the roentgenogram which often provides the key to diagnosis. Every effort must be made to obtain past chest x-rays. Unfortunately, physical examination of the chest has been deemphasized, largely because of the recognition of the enormous value of imaging techniques.

Chest roentgenograms obtained in the lateral decubitus position frequently reveal small pleural effusions not evident in the upright posture. A number of other potentially important abnormalities may be associated with normal roentgenograms. These include solitary lesions less than 6 mm in diameter, acute pulmonary thromboembolism without infarction, early interstitial pneumonia, diffuse granulomatous disease such as miliary tuberculosis, interstitial disease such as scleroderma and systemic lupus erythematosus, bronchiectasis, acute chronic bronchitis, mild to moderate emphysema, endobronchial masses only partially obstructing the airways, and the majority of instances of hypoventilation due to disorders of the central nervous system or neuromuscular disease. On the other hand, gross abnormalities of thoracic structure; pulmonary, mediastinal, and pleural masses; parenchymal consolidation; cysts; cavities; and abnormalities of the pulmonary vascular bed are all detected reliably by roentgenography.

An abnormal chest roentgenogram may be the presenting feature in an asymptomatic patient. In such circumstances, the physician must make every effort to obtain earlier films in order to determine whether the lesion is new or old. Computed tomography, magnetic resonance imaging, thoracic ultrasound, angiocardiography, and pulmonary scintigraphy (Chap. 215) are additional imaging modalities which may be helpful in establishing a diagnosis in a patient with an abnormality on the plain chest roentgenogram.

A variety of other diagnostic procedures are helpful in the workup of the patient with known or suspected pulmonary disease. These are discussed in Chap. 216 and include skin tests for tuberculosis, histoplasmosis, and a variety of other fungal infections, scratch or intradermal tests to detect atopic reactions, appropriate serum complement fixation tests, and examination and culture of the sputum, pleural fluid, and bronchial washings. Bronchoscopy, bronchial brushings, and bronchoscopic biopsy have been greatly facilitated by the development of the fiberoptic bronchoscope. Mediastinoscopy, scalene node and mediastinal node biopsy, and pleural and lung biopsy (open or via transcutaneous needle) also may be instrumental in establishing a diagnosis in an otherwise asymptomatic patient. Particularly important points which must be investigated in the history of the asymptomatic patient with an abnormality discovered on a routine chest roentgenogram include exposure to individuals with tuberculosis, a history of behavior placing the patient at high risk for developing AIDS, previous tuberculin and fungal skin tests, residence in or visits to areas where fungal disease is endemic, a history of smoking and of exposure to dusts, and symptoms of systemic disease such as fever, sweat, fatigue, and weight loss.

Physiologic (lung function) studies (Chap. 214) are of limited value in establishing an etiologic diagnosis in the patient with

pulmonary diseases but are occasionally diagnostic in the asthmatic with a normal examination who demonstrates reversible airflow obstruction or bronchial hyperresponsiveness. These studies are, however, very helpful in assessing the physiologic consequences of disorders of the respiratory system and chest wall, as well as in following the effects of their progression or remission and treatment. Simple functional tests, such as observing the patient climb a flight of stairs, may detect gross disablement.

In the approach to a patient with pulmonary disease, consideration must be given to the observation that substantial changes in the relative incidence of disease affecting the respiratory system have taken place in the United States during the past three decades. The prevalence of chronic infectious disorders such as lung abscess and bronchiectasis have decreased. Tuberculosis declined only to resurge when two susceptible populations, patients with AIDS and immigrants from Southeast Asia, increased. Patients with chronic bronchitis and with emphysema now survive longer and form an increasing fraction of patients with chronic respiratory disease, as do patients with environmental lung disease and with drug-induced pulmonary disease. Modern intercontinental travel has increased the appearance in the western world of parasitic infestations of the lung. Also, the reduction of immunologic competence which occurs in patients with AIDS and in diabetics as well as in the treatment of patients with a variety of malignancies and those receiving immunosuppressive drugs has led to an increasing incidence of opportunistic infections of the lungs with a variety of microorganisms rarely pathogenic in the past.

REFERENCES

Fishman AP (ed): *Update: Pulmonary Diseases and Disorders.* New York, McGraw-Hill, 1992

Holland WW: Chronic respiratory diseases. J Epidemiol Community Health 47:4, 1993

Jaakkola MS et al: Respiratory symptoms in young adults should not be overlooked. Am Rev Respir Dis 147:359, 1993

Murray JF: History and physical examination in *Textbook of Respiratory Medicine,* JF Murray, JA Nadel (eds). Philadelphia, Saunders, 1988, pp 431–451

Baum GL, Wolinsky E: *Textbook of Pulmonary Diseases,* 4th ed. Boston, Little, Brown, 1989

213 IMPACT OF CELL AND MOLECULAR BIOLOGY ON PULMONARY DISEASE

RONALD G. CRYSTAL

The major function of the lung is to exchange gases with the environment. As such, its essential role is mechanical—to bring the ambient air into close proximity to the output of the right heart, permitting efficient gas exchange at little energy cost. The traditional methods used to assess the lung in health and disease reflect this role, with chest x-rays used to evaluate lung anatomy and physiologic tests to assess lung function. These approaches define the type and extent of lung abnormalities associated with various categories of lung disease, but they give little insight into the pathogenic processes.

These traditional methods have now been supplemented with the disciplines of cell and molecular biology. For this to become a reality, it was first necessary to have access to sufficient numbers of purified cellular and extracellular components of the lung so that they could be evaluated in vitro. Two developments made this possible: (1) techniques permitting the purification and in vitro culture of lung inflammatory and parenchymal cells; and (2) the use of the fiberoptic bronchoscope to sample the components of the epithelial surface of the lung by bronchoalveolar lavage and epithelial brushing.

The adaptation of tissue culture techniques to lung cells made it possible to study purified human lung alveolar macrophages and T lymphocytes, as well as lung parenchymal cells including bronchial and alveolar epithelial cells, endothelial cells, and mesenchymal cells.

Bronchoalveolar lavage (BAL) is a simple extension of fiberoptic bronchoscopy and typically yields 1 to 3 mL of epithelial lining fluid containing 10 to 30 × 10^6 inflammatory cells from normal individuals and up to 200 × 10^6 cells from subjects with chronic inflammatory diseases. Both the extracellular and cellular components can be assessed by the techniques of cellular and molecular biology.

Epithelial brushing is also an extension of fiberoptic bronchoscopy and permits assessment of the surface epithelium of the large airways. Typically, 7 to 10 × 10^5 bronchial epithelial cells are recovered per brush, and several samples can be obtained from each individual, permitting ready assessment of gene expression in the airway epithelium.

Four disorders will be discussed to illustrate how these techniques have led to major advances in the understanding of human lung disease: idiopathic pulmonary fibrosis, chronic beryllium disease, alpha$_1$ antitrypsin deficiency, and cystic fibrosis.

IDIOPATHIC PULMONARY FIBROSIS (IPF)   IPF is a chronic inflammatory fibrotic disorder localized to the lower respiratory tract and characterized by an alveolitis dominated by alveolar macrophages and neutrophils and, to a lesser extent, lymphocytes and eosinophils (see Chap. 224). The disease usually presents as dyspnea on exertion, the chest x-ray shows diffuse reticulonodular infiltrates, and analysis of lung function reveals restrictive abnormalities. Evaluation of the inflammatory cells recovered by BAL led to the concept that the cell responsible for directing the process of scar formation is the alveolar macrophage, a cell that normally defends the alveolar structures by phagocytosing infectious agents and particulates. In IPF, for reasons not completely understood but likely related to immune complexes formed in the local milieu, the alveolar macrophages express several genes that code for potent polypeptide mediators capable of recruiting fibroblasts and signaling them to proliferate. The consequence is that fibroblasts are abundant in the milieu of chronic damage. Since fibroblasts secrete a collagenous extracellular matrix, more collagen, i.e., a scar, forms.

Among the polypeptide mediators released by alveolar macrophages of IPF patients is fibronectin, a 220-kDa dimeric glycoprotein that interacts with the connective tissue matrix and with specific receptors on fibroblasts. Studies of fibronectin gene expression in alveolar macrophages demonstrate that fibronectin mRNA levels correlate with fibronectin release. Indeed, alveolar macrophages recovered from IPF patients contain more fibronectin mRNA than do alveolar macrophages of normals (Fig. 213-1A and B).

Perhaps the most potent alveolar macrophage "growth factor" is platelet-derived growth factor (PDGF), a glycoprotein that in human alveolar macrophages is composed of dimers of A and B chains or homodimers of A or B chains. The genes for the A and B chains of PDGF are on different chromosomes and are modulated independently. Interestingly, the B chain is encoded by the c-*sis* gene, a cellular proto-oncogene on chromosome 22 with close homology to the v-*sis* gene, a transforming viral oncogene. Alveolar macrophages recovered from the lower respiratory tract of individuals with IPF express c-*sis* mRNA transcripts, and the PDGF protein product of the c-*sis* gene is released by these cells at a level fourfold greater than by normal macrophages (Fig. 213-1C). Thus, in this disease, a gene homologous to a viral oncogene is expressed in an exaggerated fashion in one site (the lower respiratory tract) and contributes to a localized proliferation of mesenchymal cells and eventual organ fibrosis. Importantly, glucocorticoid therapy (the conventional treatment) does not affect PDGF release by the macrophages. Consequently, it is no surprise that most IPF patients continue to deteriorate even when treated in this fashion.

CHRONIC BERYLLIUM DISEASE   Multiple exposures to airborne beryllium dusts, salts, or fumes can result, in susceptible individuals, in a chronic interstitial lung disorder characterized by the accumulation of lymphocytes and mononuclear phagocytes and the formation of noncaseating granulomas in the lower respiratory tract (see Chap. 219). The alveolitis is dominated by alveolar macrophages and T lymphocytes, activated CD4 + helper-inducer T cells, characteristic of the T cells in sites of chronic, delayed-type hypersensitivity reactions (Fig. 213-2A). Most noteworthy, the lung T cells proliferate in response to beryllium and do so to a greater extent than do blood T cells from the same individual, i.e., the antigen-specific T cells are compartmentalized to the site of the disease (Fig. 213-2B). Furthermore, the lung T cells proliferating in response to beryllium are confined to the helper-inducer subset and the extent of the proliferative response is modulated by subsets of the DP class of the MHC locus. The proliferative response of these lung T cells is truly beryllium-specific in that the cells do not proliferate in response to other metal salts or to typical recall antigens such as tetanus toxoid or streptokinase.

Together, these observations define chronic beryllium disease as a chronic hypersensitivity disease in which beryllium-primed lung CD4 + T cells play a central role in its pathogenesis. Beryllium presumably acts as an antigen by combining (as a hapten) with one or more proteins. However, since chronic beryllium disease develops in only a small proportion of those exposed to the agent, individual susceptibility must play a major role in determining who is at risk. Recent evidence suggests the HLA DP locus plays a major role in this process. The proliferative response of lung T cells to beryllium provides a diagnostic tool to identify individuals with this disorder, thus obviating the need for chemical analysis of the lung parenchyma.

ALPHA$_1$ ANTITRYPSIN DEFICIENCY   Alpha$_1$ antitrypsin (α1AT) deficiency is a hereditary disorder characterized by reduced serum levels of α1AT, an antiprotease that provides the major defense for the lower respiratory tract against the ravages of neutrophil elastase, a powerful destructive protease. The loss of this protective screen of the fragile alveolar walls results in emphysema (Chap. 223).

The emphysema is the result of a variety of mutations in the α1AT gene on chromosome 14 (Fig. 213-3A). The two parental α1AT genes are codominantly expressed and together define the α1AT level in serum. The gene is pleomorphic with approximately 75 known alleles, of which at least 20 can cause a clinically relevant deficiency state. Most normal α1AT alleles are classified as M-type. Most α1AT is synthesized by liver hepatocytes; the enzyme is a typical secretory glycoprotein that is translated on the rough endoplasmic reticulum (RER), glycosylated in the cisternae of the RER, translocated to the Golgi, and then secreted (Fig. 213-3B). The two most common "deficiency" mutations are Z (exon V, Glu^{342} GAG → Lys AAG) and S (exon III, Glu^{264} GAA → Val GTA).

The Z mutation, carried by 1 in 50 Caucasians of European descent, causes hepatocytes of homozygotes to secrete only 10 to 15 percent of the normal amount of α1AT. Because the Glu^{342} → Lys substitution reverses the charge at this residue, the Z-type α1AT molecules aggregate in the RER, less α1AT is translocated to the Golgi and subsequently secreted, and hence α1AT deficiency results.

The S mutation, carried by up to 1 in 25 persons, causes a different derangement of α1AT processing. The hepatocytes degrade an increased proportion of the newly synthesized α1AT, resulting in less α1AT for secretion and hence the deficiency state. However, the relative "deficiency" associated with the S allele is less than that associated with Z. Consequently, S homozygotes are not at risk for emphysema, but SZ heterozygotes are at mild risk.

Z homozygotes have reduced α1AT in the lung and hence have a deficient screen against proteolytic attack by neutrophil elastase (Fig. 213-3C). While S homozygotes also have reduced α1AT levels, the amount is sufficient to afford protection, i.e., the "threshold" protective level is between that of S and Z homozygotes. Based on this concept, strategies to prevent the emphysema associated with α1AT deficiency have focused on augmenting the protective screen of the lower respiratory tract with α1AT. In this regard, intravenous administration of 60 mg/kg body weight of α1AT once a week results in α1AT serum levels sufficient to maintain lung levels above that

FIGURE 213-1   Exaggerated expression of alveolar macrophage genes coding for polypeptide mediators that modulate fibroblast accumulation in the alveolar walls of patients with idiopathic pulmonary fibrosis. *A.* Example of in situ hybridization analysis of fibronectin mRNA transcripts in alveolar macrophages of a normal individual. The mRNA transcripts in macrophages recovered by bronchoalveolar lavage were assessed with a ^{35}S-labeled fibronectin antisense cRNA probe and autoradiography. The grains above the macrophage (arrow) indicate fibronectin mRNA transcripts ($\times 500$). *B.* Similar to panel *A*, but with alveolar macrophages of a patient with IPF. On the average, there are twofold more fibronectin mRNA transcripts per macrophage than in normals ($\times 500$). *C.* Spontaneous exaggerated release of PDGF by alveolar macrophages recovered from the lower respiratory tract of individuals with IPF. Macrophages recovered by bronchoalveolar lavage were cultured for 24 h. Supernatants were evaluated for the presence of PDGF using a specific immunoassay. Each symbol represents one individual. For the IPF patients, closed circles represent untreated patients and open circles represent those receiving prednisone. Note that therapy has no effect on the release of this potent mediator.

necessary to provide sufficient antielastase protection to the alveoli, i.e., augmentation therapy reverses the biochemical abnormalities at the site of the target organ and thus is a rational approach to prevent the emphysema. Based on these concepts, weekly augmentation therapy is now the standard treatment for α1AT deficiency.

CYSTIC FIBROSIS (CF)   CF is an autosomal recessive disorder of exocrine glands characterized in lung by accumulation of thick mucus, chronic bacterial infections, and chronic obstructive lung disease associated with severe bronchiectasis and parenchymal derangements (see Chap. 222). It is the most common lethal genetic disorder affecting Caucasian populations, with a heterozygote frequency of 1 in 20 to 25 individuals.

The gene causing CF, called the *cystic fibrosis transmembrane conductance regulator* (CFTR) gene, was localized to within approximately 300 kb in the q21-31 region of chromosome 7, using the technique of "chromosome walking" (Fig. 213-4*A*). Extensive analysis of the CFTR gene has led to the identification of more than 200 mutations, most in the 27 coding exons of the 250-kb gene. One mutation, an in-phase deletion of the codon for Phe^{508}, is responsible for 50 to 80 percent of all CF alleles.

The sequence of the CFTR gene predicts that it codes for a protein of 168 kDa that spans the plasma membrane and contains two domains capable of binding adenosine triphosphate and one domain that is phosphorylated. The CFTR protein has been clearly shown to function as a cAMP-regulated Cl$^-$ secretory channel on the apical surface of epithelial cells, although it may serve other functions as well. With mutations of the CFTR gene the cell has insufficient CFTR function, a fact relevant to the pathogenesis of the disease (Fig. 213-4*B*).

FIGURE 213-2   Beryllium-specific inflammatory processes in the lower respiratory tract of individuals with chronic beryllium disease. *A.* Inflammatory cells recovered by bronchoalveolar lavage of an individual with chronic beryllium disease. The alveolitis is dominated by lymphocytes (L) and alveolar macrophages (M) ($\times 500$). Flow cytometric analysis with appropriate monoclonal antibodies demonstrates that the lymphocytes are predominantly CD4+ helper-inducer T lymphocytes. *B.* In vitro proliferation of blood and lung T lymphocytes of patients with chronic beryllium disease and normals in response to beryllium. The data are presented as a stimulation index (values >1 represent proliferation above control) and each symbol represents one individual. Normal blood and lung T cells rarely proliferate in response to beryllium. In contrast, lung, but not blood, T cells from individuals with chronic beryllium disease respond briskly to beryllium, with the CD4+ helper-inducer T cells dominating the proliferative response.

Measurement of potential differences across the tracheal epithelium of CF homozygotes has demonstrated a higher voltage than in normals, consistent with the known abnormality in electrolyte transport. In CF

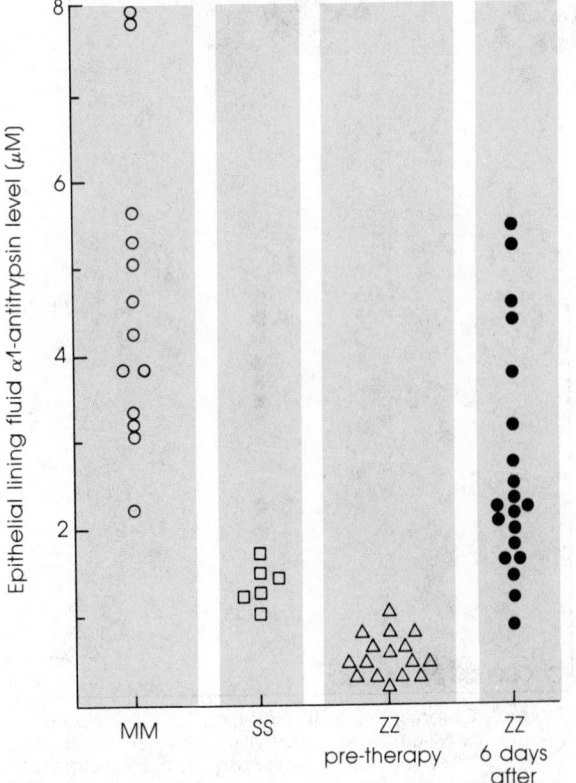

subjects who have received lung transplants the abnormal potential differences are no longer present. Cultured epithelial cells of CF patients exhibit abnormal potential differences similar to those observed in vivo. Importantly, the cultured epithelial cells are not capable of transporting Cl^- to the apical surfaces in a normal fashion. Together, these observations suggest that abnormalities of the CF gene are expressed in airway epithelial cells, causing a dysfunction in the regulation of airway epithelial apical Cl^- channels as the fundamental abnormality in CF. It is hypothesized that the defect in cAMP-mediated Cl^- channel function causes CF lung disease by modifying the quantity and composition of the airway epithelial fluid. Presumably, such changes alter the composition of mucus and thus interfere with mucociliary clearance mechanisms, resulting in chronic infection, inflammation, and derangement of the airways.

Based on this fundamental knowledge, there has been rapid progress in the development of strategies to treat the respiratory manifestations of CF by transferring the normal CFTR cDNA directly into the airway epithelium in vivo. This can be accomplished using a recombinant replication-deficient adenovirus vector to carry the normal cDNA into airway cells. Animal studies with brushing of the airway epithelium to recover the genetically modified cells have demonstrated the feasibility of this strategy and human studies will soon begin.

OTHER DISEASES   There are additional pulmonary disorders in which the application of cell and molecular biology methods has provided insight.

1   In the *pneumoconioses* (see Chap. 219), energy-dispersive x-ray analysis and electron diffraction methods permit identification and quantification of specific inorganic dusts in lung tissue and alveolar macrophages recovered by BAL. These methods provide new diagnostic techniques and new insights into the relationship of particle retention, host defense, and disease susceptibility associated with the chronic inhalation of inorganic dusts.

2   Despite the characteristic skin anergy in individuals with *sarcoidosis*, evaluation of T cells in the lower respiratory tract of patients with active disease has lead to the concept that sarcoid is a disease of heightened cellular immunity, with T cells responding to specific antigens in an exaggerated fashion at sites of disease (see Chap. 292).

3   The use of specific DNA probes now permits definitive diagnosis of *lung infection* previously very difficult to identify, including infection caused by various mycobacteria, fungi, and viruses. For example, in individuals seropositive for human immunodeficiency virus (HIV) infection (see Chap. 279), but without evidence of lung involvement, the HIV genome can be detected in lung inflammatory cells using HIV-specific DNA primers and the polymerase chain reaction.

4   *Pulmonary histiocytosis X* (eosinophilic granuloma of the lung) can be diagnosed using bronchoalveolar lavage and a monoclonal antibody (OKT6) specific for Langerhans cells (see Chap. 224).

FIGURE 213-3 Pathogenesis and therapy of alpha$_1$ antitrypsin (α1AT) deficiency. *A.* Schematic of the 12.2-kb, 7-exon (I_A-I_C, II-V) α1AT gene. The two most common mutations of the normal M gene are S and Z. *B.* Synthesis and secretion of α1AT by hepatocytes. The normal M α1AT mRNA protein is translated on the rough endoplasmic reticulum (RER), carbohydrates are added, the molecule is translocated to the Golgi and secreted. The Z mutation results in aggregation of newly synthesized α1AT in the RER while the S mutation results in degradation. *C.* Consequences of mutations in the α1AT gene at the level of the alveoli. Shown are α1AT levels in alveolar epithelial lining fluid recovered by bronchoalveolar lavage. Each symbol represents a single individual. S and Z homozygotes have "deficient" amounts of α1AT in the lung, with the level for Z homozygotes below the threshold levels necessary to protect the lung. With once-weekly intravenous augmentation therapy with purified human α1AT, the lung epithelial lining fluid α1AT level of Z homozygotes is restored above the protective threshold, thus protecting the lung from emphysema.

A

B

FIGURE 213-4 Current concepts of the molecular and biologic abnormalities associated with cystic fibrosis (CF). *A.* Localization of the cystic fibrosis transmembrane conductance regulator (CFTR) gene. Shown at the left is a representation of chromosome 7; the CF gene is localized to region q21-31. At the right is an expanded view of the region between the locus for the proto-oncogene MET and the genomic marker D7S8 (J3.11); XV2C, KM19, and MP6D9 are other marker regions of DNA containing polymorphisms useful in haplotype analysis. Chromosomal mapping localized the CFTR gene to a 250-kb region between the markers MP6D9 and D7S8. Even before the gene was identified with DNA probes, analysis of genomic DNA could accurately predict the inheritance of CF, permitting family planning. Now, specific probes have made accurate diagnosis rapid and simple. *B.* Schematic of the CFTR protein on the apical (air) membrane of an airway epithelial cell. In vivo measurements of electric potentials in the tracheal epithelium together with in vitro studies of cultured airway epithelial cells have shown that the CFTR protein functions as a cAMP-regulated Cl^- channel on the apical surface of the epithelial cell. The CFTR protein has three intracytoplasmic domains, nucleotide binding fold 1 (NBF1), a regulatory (R) region, and nucleotide-binding fold 2 (NBF2). Phosphokinase A (PKA), ATP, and cAMP play central roles in regulatory CFTR function. With mutations in the CFTR gene, the cells have insufficient CFTR function. This can be corrected by directed transfer of the normal CFTR cDNA to the epithelial cells of individuals with CF.

5 In the *respiratory distress syndrome of the newborn*, immature alveolar type II cells do not produce sufficient surfactant to maintain alveolar stability, leading to lung collapse. The control of surfactant biosynthesis in alveolar type II cells has been delineated using cell culture techniques, strategies have been developed to accelerate the expression of the surfactant system using pharmacologic agents, and the biochemical nature of surfactant has been fully defined. This definition has led to cloning of the apoproteins of surfactant, allowing in vitro reconstitution of an artificial surfactant for use in therapy.

6 In *asthma*, cell biology methodologies have led to the identification of a broad armamentarium of naturally occurring mediators that likely play a role in the pathogenesis of reversible airway disease, and several genes related to these mediators have been cloned and characterized (see Chap. 217).

7 Capitalizing on the identification, cloning, and in vitro production of a variety of potent "inflammatory" polypeptides, much attention has been given to the concept that mediators such as tumor necrosis factor play a role in modulating the parenchymal dysfunction characteristic of the respiratory failure of *adult respiratory distress syndrome*.

Finally, the recognition that it is the high concentration of DNA that gives purulent mucus its thick, sticky properties led to the cloning of human recombinant DNase I as a therapeutic agent. When given by aerosol to individuals with cystic fibrosis, there is improvement in lung function as the airways are opened and a decrease in the incidence of airway infections.

CONCLUSIONS The application of modern cell and biology methods to investigate human disease depends on the capacity to obtain appropriate biologic materials relevant to the pathogenesis of the disease. For most diseases, the relevant biologic material must be obtained directly from the target organ, and this is a difficult task for internal organs. Utilizing cell culture techniques and the fiberoptic bronchoscope to gain access to the epithelial surface of the lung, many pulmonary disorders can now be investigated by the techniques of cell and molecular biology. As a consequence there has been a remarkable advance in the understanding of the pathogenesis of a variety of lung disorders and for several new insights into therapy.

REFERENCES

ADACHI K et al: Evaluation of fibronectin gene expression by *in situ* hybridization: Differential expression of the fibronectin gene among populations of human alveolar macrophages. Am J Pathol 138:193, 1988

BOST T et al: Increased TNF-alpha and IL6 mRNA expression by alveolar macrophages in chronic beryllium disease. Chest 103:138S, 1993

COUTELLE C et al: Gene therapy for cystic fibrosis. Arch Dis Child 68:437, 1993

CRYSTAL RG: α1-Antitrypsin deficiency, in *Update: Pulmonary Disease and Disorders*, AP Fishman (ed). New York, McGraw-Hill, 1992, pp 19–35

——: Gene therapy strategies for pulmonary disease. Am J Med 1992:92 (suppl 6A):44 S–52 S

CRYSTAL RG et al: Interstitial lung disease of unknown cause: Disorders characterized by chronic inflammation of the lower respiratory tract. N Engl J Med 310:154, 235, 1984

HUBBARD RC, CRYSTAL RG: Vulnerability of the lung to proteolytic injury, in *The Lung: Scientific Foundations*, RG Crystal et al (eds). New York, Raven, 1991, pp 2059–2072

HUBBARD RC et al: A preliminary study of aerosolized recombinant human DNase therapy in the treatment of cystic fibrosis. N Engl J Med 326:812, 1992

MARTINET Y et al: Exaggerated spontaneous release of a platelet-derived growth factor by alveolar macrophages from patients with idiopathic pulmonary fibrosis. N Engl J Med 317(4):202, 1987

ROSENFELD MA et al: *In vivo* transfer of the human cystic fibrosis transmembrane conductance regulator gene to the airway epithelium. Cell 68:143, 1992

SALTINI C et al: Chronic pulmonary berylliosis: Maintenance of the alveolitis by proliferation of beryllium-specific helper T-cells. N Engl J Med 230:1103, 1989

SFERRA TJ, COLLINS FS: The molecular biology of cystic fibrosis. Annu Rev Med 44:133, 1993

WEWERS MD et al: Replacement therapy for alpha 1-antitrypsin deficiency associated with emphysema. N Engl J Med 316:1055, 1987

214 DISTURBANCES OF RESPIRATORY FUNCTION

STEVEN E. WEINBERGER / JEFFREY M. DRAZEN

The respiratory system includes the lungs, the central nervous system (CNS), the chest wall (with the diaphragm and intercostal muscles), and the pulmonary circulation. The CNS controls the activity of the muscles of the chest wall, which serve as the respiratory system pump. Because these components of the respiratory system act in concert to achieve gas exchange, malfunction of an individual component or alteration of the relationships among components can lead to disturbances in function. In this chapter we consider three major aspects of disturbed respiratory function: (1) disturbances in ventilatory function, (2) disturbances in the pulmonary circulation, and (3) disurbances in gas exchange. Disorders relating to CNS control of ventilation are discussed in Chap. 229.

DISTURBANCES IN VENTILATORY FUNCTION

Ventilation is the process whereby the lungs replenish the gas within the alveoli. Measurements of ventilatory function in common diagnostic use consist of quantification of the gas volume contained within the lungs under certain circumstances and the rate at which gas can be expelled from the lungs. Two measurements of lung volume commonly used for respiratory diagnosis are total lung capacity (TLC) and residual volume (RV). The former is the volume of gas contained within the lungs after a maximal inspiration, whereas the latter is the volume of gas remaining within the lungs at the end of a maximal expiration. The volume of gas that is exhaled from the lungs in going from TLC to RV is called the *vital capacity* (VC) (Fig. 214-1).

Common clinical measurements of airflow are obtained from maneuvers in which the subject inspires to TLC and then forcibly exhales to RV. Three measurements are commonly made from a volume-time recording, i.e., a spirogram, obtained during such a forced expiratory maneuver: (1) the volume of gas exhaled during the first second of expiration (forced expiratory volume in 1 s, or FEV_1), (2) the total volume exhaled (forced vital capacity, or FVC), and (3) the average expiratory flow rate during the middle 50 percent of the vital capacity (forced expiratory flow between 25 and 75 percent of the vital capacity, or $FEF_{25-75\%}$, also called maximal midexpiratory flow rate, or MMFR) (Fig. 214-2).

PHYSIOLOGIC FEATURES The lungs are elastic structures containing collagen and elastic fibers which resist expansion. In order

FIGURE 214-1 Lung volumes, shown by block diagrams (*left*) and by a spirographic tracing (*right*). TLC = total lung capacity; VC = vital capacity; RV = residual volume; IC = inspiratory capacity; ERV = expiratory reserve volume; FRC = functional residual capacity; V_T = tidal volume. (*From Weinberger.*)

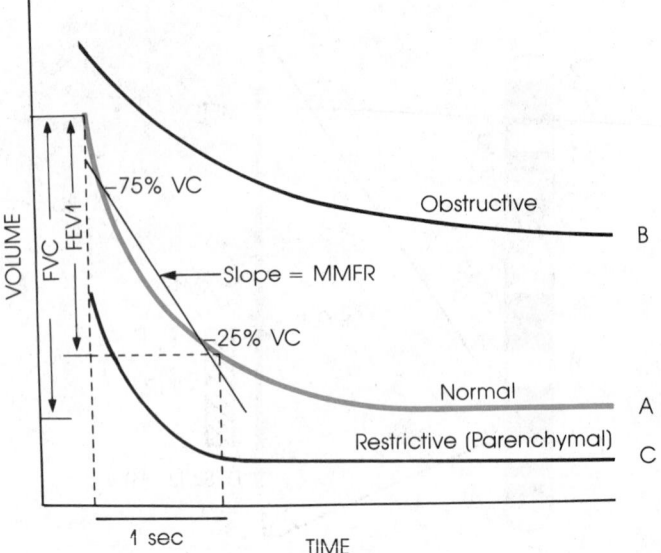

FIGURE 214-2 Spirographic tracings of forced expiration, comparing a normal tracing (*A*) and tracings in obstructive (*B*) and parenchymal restrictive (*C*) disease. Calculations of FVC, FEV_1, and $FEF_{25-75\%}$ are shown only for the normal tracing. Since there is no measure of absolute starting volume with spirometry, the curves are artificially positioned to show the relative starting lung volumes in the different conditions.

for normal lungs to contain air, they must be distended by either a positive internal pressure, i.e., within the airways and alveolar spaces, or a negative external pressure, i.e., outside the lung. The relationship between the volume of gas contained within the lungs and the distending pressure (transpulmonary pressure, or P_{TP}, defined as internal pressure minus external pressure) is described by the pressure-volume curve of the lungs (Fig. 214-3A).

The chest wall is also an elastic structure, with properties similar to that of an expandable and compressible spring. The relationship between the volume enclosed by the chest wall and the distending pressure for the chest wall is described by the pressure-volume curve of the chest wall (Fig. 214-3B). For the chest wall to assume a volume different from its resting volume, the internal or external pressures acting on it must be altered.

At functional residual capacity (FRC), defined as the volume of gas in the lungs at the end of a normal exhalation, the lungs are partially inflated, so their elastic recoil exerts a force tending to empty the lungs. At the same time, chest wall volume is such that its elastic recoil promotes outward expansion. Functional residual capacity occurs at the lung volume at which the tendency of the lungs to contract is opposed by the equal and opposite tendency of the chest wall to expand (Fig. 214-3C).

In order for the lungs and the chest wall to achieve a volume other than the resting volume or FRC, either the pressures acting on them can be changed passively, e.g., with a mechanical ventilator delivering positive pressure to the airways and alveoli, or the respiratory muscles can actively oppose the tendency of the lungs and the chest wall to return to FRC. During inhalation to volumes above FRC, the inspiratory muscles must actively overcome the tendency of the respiratory system to decrease volume back to FRC. During active exhalation below FRC, expiratory muscle activity must overcome the tendency of the respiratory system to increase volume back to FRC. At TLC, the maximal force applied by the inspiratory muscles to expand the lungs is primarily opposed by the inward recoil of the lungs. As a consequence, the major determinants of TLC are the stiffness of the lungs and inspiratory muscle strength. If the lungs become stiffer, i.e., less compliant, TLC is decreased. If the lungs become less stiff, i.e., more compliant, TLC is increased. If the inspiratory muscles are significantly weakened, they are less able to overcome the inward elastic recoil of the lungs, and TLC is lowered.

FIGURE 214-3 *A.* Pressure-volume curve of the lungs. *B.* Pressure-volume curve of the chest wall. *C.* Pressure-volume curve of the respiratory system, showing the superimposed component curves of the lungs and the chest wall. RV = residual volume; FRC = functional residual capacity; TLC = total lung capacity. (*From Weinberger.*)

At RV, the force exerted by the expiratory muscles to decrease lung volume further is balanced by the outward recoil of the chest wall, which becomes extremely stiff at low lung volumes. Two factors influence the volume of gas contained within the lungs at RV. The first is the ability of the subject to exert a prolonged expiratory effort, which is related to muscle strength and to the ability to overcome sensory stimuli from the chest wall. The second is the ability of the lungs to empty to a small volume. In normal lungs, as P_{TP} is lowered, lung volume decreases. In lungs with diseased airways, as P_{TP} is lowered, flow-limitation or airway closure can limit the amount of gas that is expired. Consequently, either weak chest wall muscles or intrinsic airways disease can result in an elevation in measured RV.

Dynamic measurements of ventilatory function are made by having the subject inhale to TLC and then perform a forced expiration to RV. If a subject performs a series of such expiratory maneuvers using increasing muscular intensity, expiratory flow rates will increase until a certain level of effort is reached. Beyond this level, additional effort will not result in an increment in forced expiratory flow rates; this phenomenon is known as the *effort independence* of forced expiratory flow. The physiologic mechanisms determining the flow rates during this effort-independent phase of forced expiratory flow have been shown to be the elastic recoil of the lung, the airflow resistance of the airways between the alveolar zone and the physical site of flow limitation, and the airway wall compliance at the site of flow limitation. Physical processes which decrease elastic recoil, increase airflow resistance, or increase airway wall compliance decrease the flow rate that can be achieved at any given lung volume. Conversely, processes that increase elastic recoil, decrease resistance, or stiffen airway walls increase the flow rate that can be achieved at any given lung volume.

MEASUREMENT OF VENTILATORY FUNCTION Ventilatory function is measured under static conditions for determination of lung volumes and under dynamic conditions for determination of forced expiratory flow rates. VC, expiratory reserve volume (ERV), and inspiratory capacity (IC) (see Fig. 214-1) are measured by having the patient breathe into and out of a spirometer, a device capable of

measuring expired or inspired gas volume while plotting volume as a function of time. Other volumes, specifically RV, FRC, and TLC, cannot be measured in this way because they include the volume of gas present within the lungs even after a maximal expiration. Two techniques are commonly used to measure these volumes: helium dilution or body plethysmography. In the helium-dilution method, the subject repeatedly breathes in and out from a reservoir with a known volume of gas containing a trace amount of helium. The helium is diluted by the gas previously present in the lungs and is not absorbed into the pulmonary circulation. From knowledge of reservoir volume and initial and final helium concentrations, the volume of gas present within the lungs can be calculated. With the helium-dilution method, the volume of gas present within the lungs may be underestimated if there are slowly communicating airspaces, such as bullae. In this situation, lung volumes can be more accurately measured with a body plethysmograph, a sealed box in which the patient sits while panting against a closed mouthpiece. Because there is no airflow into or out of the plethysmograph, pressure changes within the thorax during panting cause compression and rarefaction of gas within the lungs and simultaneous rarefaction and compression of gas within the plethysmograph. By measuring pressure changes in the plethysmograph and at the mouthpiece, the volume of gas present within the thorax can be calculated by using Boyle's law.

Lung volumes and measurements made during forced expiration are interpreted by comparing the values measured with the values expected based on the age, height, sex, and race of the patient (see Appendix). Regression curves have been constructed based on data obtained from large numbers of normal, nonsmoking individuals without any evidence of lung disease. Predicted values for a given patient can then be obtained by using the patient's age and height in the appropriate regression equation; different equations are used depending on the patient's race and gender. Because some variability among normal individuals is to be expected, values between 80 and 120 percent of predicted have traditionally been considered normal. Increasingly, calculated percentiles are used in determining normality. Specifically, values of individual measurements falling below the fifth percentile are considered below the lower limits of normal.

The normal ratio FEV_1/FVC is approximately 0.75 to 0.80, although this value does fall somewhat with advancing age. The $FEF_{25-75\%}$ is often considered a more sensitive measurement of early airflow obstruction, particularly in small airways. However, this measurement must be interpreted cautiously in the patient with abnormally small lungs (low TLC and VC). Then, less volume is exhaled during forced expiration, and the $FEF_{25-75\%}$ may appear abnormal when compared with the predicted value for the patient's age, height, race, and gender, even though it is normal relative to the size of the patient's lungs.

It is also a common practice to plot expiratory flow rates against lung volume (rather than against time); the close linkage of flow rates to lung volumes produces a typical *flow-volume curve* (Fig. 214-4). In addition, the spirometric values mentioned above can be calculated from the flow-volume curve. Commonly, flow rates during a maximal inspiratory effort performed as rapidly as possible are plotted as well, making the flow-volume curve into a *flow-volume loop*. At TLC, before expiratory flow starts, the flow rate is zero; once forced expiration has begun, a high peak flow rate is rapidly achieved. As expiration continues and lung volume approaches RV, the flow rate falls progressively, in a nearly linear fashion as a function of lung volume for a person with normal lung function. During maximal inspiration from RV to TLC, inspiratory flow is most rapid at the midpoint of inspiration, so the inspiratory portion of the loop is U-shaped or saddle-shaped. The flow rates achieved during maximal expiration can be analyzed quantitatively by comparing the flow rates at specified lung volumes with the predicted values or qualitatively by analyzing the shape of the descending limb of the expiratory curve.

Assessing the strength of respiratory muscles is an additional part of the overall evaluation of some patients with respiratory dysfunction. When a patient exhales completely to RV and then tries to inspire

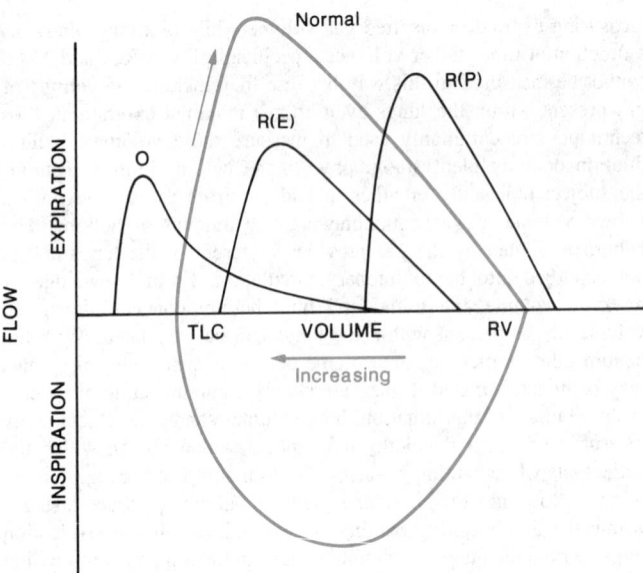

FIGURE 214-4 Flow-volume curves in different conditions: O = obstructive disease; R(P) = parenchymal restrictive disease; R(E) = extraparenchymal restrictive disease with limitation in inspiration and expiration. Forced expiration is plotted in all conditions; forced inspiration is shown only for the normal curve. TLC = total lung capacity; RV = residual volume. By convention, increasing lung volume is to the left on the abscissa. The arrow alongside the normal curve indicates the direction of expiration from TLC to RV.

maximally against an occluded airway, the pressure that can be generated is called the *maximal inspiratory pressure* (MIP). On the other hand, when a patient inhales to TLC and then tries to expire maximally against an occluded airway, the pressure generated is called the *maximal expiratory pressure* (MEP). In the proper clinical setting, these studies may provide useful information regarding the cause of abnormal lung volumes and the possibility that respiratory muscle weakness may be causally related to the lung volume abnormalities.

PATTERNS OF ABNORMAL FUNCTION The two major patterns of abnormal ventilatory function, as measured by static lung volumes and spirometry, are restrictive and obstructive patterns. In the *obstructive pattern*, the hallmark is a decrease in expiratory flow rates. With fully established disease, the ratio FEV_1/FVC is decreased, as is the $FEF_{25-75\%}$ (see Fig. 214-2, line *B*). The expiratory portion of the flow-volume loop demonstrates decreased flow rates for any given lung volume. Nonuniform emptying of airways is reflected by a coved (concave upward) configuration of the curve (see Fig. 214-4). With early obstructive disease, which originates in the small airways, FEV_1/FVC may be normal; the only abnormalities noted on routine testing of pulmonary function may be a depression in $FEF_{25-75\%}$ and

an abnormal configuration in the terminal portion of the forced expiratory flow-volume curve.

In obstructive disease, the TLC is normal or increased. When helium equilibration tests are used for measurement of lung volumes, the measured volume may be less than the actual volume if helium was not well distributed to all airways and to all regions of the lung. Residual volume is elevated due to trapping of air during expiration, and the ratio RV/TLC is increased. Vital capacity is frequently decreased in obstructive disease because of the striking elevations in RV with only minor changes in TLC.

A *restrictive pattern* can be broadly divided into subgroups, depending on the location of the pathology—pulmonary parenchymal versus extraparenchymal. For extraparenchymal disease, dysfunction can be predominantly in inspiration or in both inspiration and expiration (Table 214-1). The hallmark of a restrictive pattern, found in all these subcategories, is a decrease in lung volumes, primarily TLC and VC. In pulmonary parenchymal disease, RV is also generally decreased, and forced expiratory flow rates are preserved. In fact, when FEV_1 is considered as a percent of the FVC, the flow rates are often supranormal, i.e., disproportionately high relative to the size of the lungs (see Fig. 214-2, line *C*). The flow-volume curve may graphically demonstrate this disproportionate relationship between flow rates and lung volumes, since the expiratory portion of the curve appears relatively tall (preserved flow rates) but narrow (decreased lung volumes), as shown in Fig. 214-4.

In the extraparenchymal pattern characterized by *inspiratory dysfunction*, due to either inspiratory muscle weakness or a stiff chest wall, adequate distending forces are prevented from being exerted on an otherwise normal lung. As a result, achieved TLC values are less than predicted, RV is often not significantly affected, and expiratory flows are preserved. If inspiratory muscle weakness is the cause of this pattern, then MIP is decreased. In the extraparenchymal pattern characterized by *inspiratory and expiratory dysfunction*, the ability to expire to a normal RV is also limited, either because of expiratory muscle weakness or a deformed chest wall that is abnormally rigid at volumes below FRC. Consequently, RV is often elevated, unlike the pattern observed in the other restrictive subcategories. The ratio FEV_1/FVC is variable and depends on expiratory muscle strength. If expiratory muscle strength is significantly decreased, then MEP is decreased, the ability to expire rapidly is impaired, and FEV_1/FVC may be decreased even though there is no airflow obstruction. If expiratory muscle strength is normal but the chest wall is abnormally stiff below FRC, then FEV_1/FVC is normal or increased.

CLINICAL CORRELATIONS In Table 214-1, the expected alterations in ventilatory function as indicated by pulmonary function testing are summarized. One reason to establish a ventilatory diagnosis is to categorize the functional disorder. This in turn can provide diagnostic information as outlined in Table 214-2. Note that lung disease can be present without abnormal ventilatory function, but the presence of specific diagnostic findings is an aid in differential diagnosis.

TABLE 214-1 Alterations in ventilatory function

	TLC	RV	VC	FEV_1/FVC	MIP	MEP
Obstructive	N to ↑	↑	↓	↓*	N	N
Restrictive						
Pulmonary parenchymal	↓	↓	↓	N to ↑	N	N
Extraparenchymal—inspiratory	↓	N to ↓	↓	N	↓/N†	N
Extraparenchymal—inspiratory + expiratory	↓	↑	↓	Variable	↓/N†	↓/N†

* Mild obstructive (small airways) disease may have ↓$FEF_{25-75\%}$ with normal FEV_1/FVC.
† ↓ if due to respiratory muscle weakness; N if due to chest wall stiffness.
NOTE: N = normal; for other abbreviations, see text.

TABLE 214-2 Common respiratory diseases by diagnostic categories

OBSTRUCTIVE

Asthma
Chronic obstructive lung disease (chronic bronchitis, emphysema)
Bronchiectasis
Cystic fibrosis
Bronchiolitis

RESTRICTIVE—PARENCHYMAL

Sarcoidosis
Idiopathic pulmonary fibrosis
Pneumoconiosis
Drug- or radiation-induced interstitial lung disease

RESTRICTIVE—EXTRAPARENCHYMAL

Neuromuscular
   Diaphragmatic weakness/paralysis
   Myasthenia gravis*
   Guillain-Barré syndrome*
   Muscular dystrophies*
   Cervical spine injury*
Chest wall
   Kyphoscoliosis
   Obesity
   Ankylosing spondylitis*

* Can have inspiratory and expiratory limitation (see text).

DISTURBANCES IN THE PULMONARY CIRCULATION

PHYSIOLOGIC FEATURES The pulmonary vasculature must handle the entire output of the right ventricle, approximately 5 L/min in a normal adult at rest. The comparatively thin-walled vessels of the pulmonary arterial system provide relatively little resistance to flow and are capable of handling this large volume of blood at low perfusion pressures compared with those of the systemic circulation. The normal mean pulmonary artery pressure of 15 mmHg is much less than the normal mean aortic pressure of approximately 95 mmHg. Regional blood flow within the lung is dependent on hydrostatic forces. In the upright person, pulmonary arterial pressure is lowest at the apex of the lung and highest at the lung bases. As a result, in the upright position, perfusion is least at the apex and greatest at the lung bases. When cardiac output increases, as occurs during exercise, the pulmonary vasculature is capable of recruiting previously unperfused vessels and distending underperfused vessels. As a result, the pulmonary vascular system is capable of handling the increase in flow with a decrease in pulmonary vascular resistance, so the increment in mean pulmonary arterial pressure, even with a three- to four-fold increase in cardiac output, is small.

METHODS OF MEASUREMENT Assessment of circulatory function within the pulmonary vasculature depends on measuring pulmonary vascular pressures and cardiac output. Clinically, these measurements are commonly made in intensive care units capable of invasive monitoring and in cardiac catheterization laboratories. With a flow-directed pulmonary arterial (Swan-Ganz) catheter, pulmonary arterial and pulmonary capillary wedge pressures can be measured directly, and cardiac output can be obtained by the thermodilution method. Pulmonary vascular resistance can then be calculated according to the equation

$$PVR = 80(PAP - PCW)/CO$$

where PVR = pulmonary vascular resistance (dyn·s/cm⁵)
   PAP = mean pulmonary arterial pressure (mmHg)
   PCW = pulmonary capillary wedge pressure (mmHg)
   CO = cardiac output (L/min)

The normal value for pulmonary vascular resistance is approximately 50 to 150 dyn·s/cm⁵.

MECHANISMS OF ABNORMAL FUNCTION (See also Chap. 225) Pulmonary vascular resistance may increase by a variety of mechanisms. Pulmonary arterial and arteriolar vasoconstriction is a prominent response to alveolar hypoxia. Pulmonary vascular resistance also increases if intraluminal thrombi or proliferation of smooth muscle within vessel walls diminishes the luminal cross-sectional area. If small pulmonary vessels are destroyed, either by scarring or by loss of alveolar walls, the total cross-sectional area of the pulmonary vascular bed diminishes, and pulmonary vascular resistance increases. When pulmonary vascular resistance is elevated, pulmonary arterial pressure rises to maintain normal cardiac output or cardiac output falls if pulmonary arterial pressure does not increase.

CLINICAL CORRELATIONS Disturbances in function of the pulmonary vasculature as a result of primary cardiac disease, either congenital heart disease or conditions which elevate left atrial pressure such as mitral stenosis, are beyond the scope of this chapter and are discussed in Chaps. 191 and 201, respectively. Instead, the focus will be on the pulmonary vasculature as its function is affected by diseases primarily involving the respiratory system, including the pulmonary vessels themselves.

All diseases of the respiratory system causing hypoxemia are potentially capable of increasing pulmonary vascular resistance, since alveolar hypoxia is a very potent stimulus for pulmonary vasoconstriction. The more prolonged and intense the hypoxic stimulus, the more likely it is that a significant increase in pulmonary vascular resistance and pulmonary hypertension will result. In practice, patients with hypoxemia caused by chronic obstructive lung disease, interstitial lung disease, chest wall disease, and the obesity hypoventilation–sleep apnea syndrome are particularly prone to developing pulmonary hypertension. If there are additional structural changes in the pulmonary vasculature secondary to the underlying process, these will increase the likelihood of developing pulmonary hypertension.

With diseases directly affecting the pulmonary vessels, a decrease in the cross-sectional area of the pulmonary vascular bed is primarily responsible for increased pulmonary vascular resistance, while hypoxemia generally plays a lesser role. In the case of recurrent pulmonary emboli, parts of the pulmonary arterial system are occluded by intraluminal thrombi originating in the systemic venous system. With primary pulmonary hypertension (Chap. 225) or with pulmonary vascular disease secondary to scleroderma, the small pulmonary arteries and arterioles are affected by a generalized obliterative process that narrows and occludes these vessels. Pulmonary vascular resistance increases, and significant pulmonary hypertension often results.

DISTURBANCES IN GAS EXCHANGE

PHYSIOLOGIC FEATURES The primary functions of the respiratory system are to remove the appropriate amount of CO_2 from blood entering the pulmonary circulation and to provide adequate O_2 to blood leaving the pulmonary circulation. In order for these functions to be carried out properly, there must be adequate provision of fresh air to the alveoli for delivery of O_2 and removal of CO_2 (ventilation), adequate circulation of blood through the pulmonary vasculature (perfusion), adequate movement of gas between alveoli and pulmonary capillaries (diffusion), and appropriate contact between alveolar gas and pulmonary capillary blood (ventilation-perfusion matching).

A normal individual at rest inspires approximately 12 to 16 times per minute, each breath having a tidal volume of approximately 500 mL. A portion (approximately 30 percent) of the fresh air inspired with each breath does not reach the alveoli but remains in the conducting airways of the lung. This component of each breath, which is not generally available for gas exchange, is called the *anatomic dead space component*. The remaining 70 percent reaches and rapidly mixes with the gas resident in the alveolar zone and can participate in gas exchange. In this example, total ventilation each minute is approximately 7 L, composed of 2 L/min of dead space ventilation and 5 L/min of alveolar ventilation. In certain diseases, some alveoli are ventilated but not perfused so that additional ventilation beyond that portion related to the anatomic dead space is wasted. If total dead space ventilation is increased but total minute ventilation is unchanged, then alveolar ventilation must fall correspondingly.

Gas exchange is dependent on alveolar ventilation rather than total minute ventilation, as outlined below. The partial pressure of CO_2 in arterial blood (Pa_{CO_2}) is directly proportional to the amount of CO_2 produced per minute ($\dot{V}_{CO_2}$) and inversely proportional to alveolar ventilation ($\dot{V}_A$), according to the relationship

$$Pa_{CO_2} = 0.863 \times \dot{V}_{CO_2}/\dot{V}_A$$

where $\dot{V}_{CO_2}$ is expressed in mL/min, $\dot{V}_A$ in L/min, and Pa_{CO_2} in mmHg. At fixed $\dot{V}_{CO_2}$, when alveolar ventilation increases, Pa_{CO_2} falls, and when alveolar ventilation decreases, Pa_{CO_2} rises. Maintaining a normal level of O_2 in the alveoli (and consequently in arterial blood) also depends on provision of adequate alveolar ventilation to replenish alveolar O_2. This principle will become more apparent from consideration of the alveolar gas equation below.

Diffusion of O_2 and CO_2 Both O_2 and CO_2 diffuse readily down their respective concentration gradients through the alveolar wall and pulmonary capillary endothelium. Under normal circumstances, this process is rapid, and equilibration of both gases is complete within one-third of the transit time of erythrocytes through the pulmonary capillary bed. Even in disease states in which diffusion of gases is impaired, it is unlikely to be so severe that equilibration of the CO_2 and O_2 is not reached. Consequently, a diffusion abnormality rarely results in arterial hypoxemia at rest. If erythrocyte transit time in the pulmonary circulation is shortened, as occurs with exercise, and diffusion is impaired, then diffusion limitation may contribute to hypoxemia. Exercise testing can often demonstrate such physiologically significant abnormalities due to impaired diffusion. Even though diffusion limitation rarely makes a clinically significant contribution to resting hypoxemia, clinical measurements of what is known as *diffusing capacity* (see below) can be a useful measure of the integrity of the alveolar-capillary membrane.

Ventilation-perfusion matching In addition to the absolute levels of alveolar ventilation and perfusion, gas exchange is critically dependent on the proper matching of ventilation and perfusion. The spectrum of possible ventilation-perfusion ($\dot{V}/\dot{Q}$) ratios within an alveolar-capillary unit ranges from zero, in which ventilation is totally absent and the unit behaves as a shunt, to infinity, in which perfusion is totally absent and the unit behaves as dead space. The P_{O_2} and P_{CO_2} of blood leaving each alveolar-capillary unit depend on the gas tension (blood and air) entering that unit and on the $\dot{V}/\dot{Q}$ ratio of that particular unit. At one extreme, when an alveolar-capillary unit has a $\dot{V}/\dot{Q}$ ratio of 0 and behaves as a shunt, blood leaving the unit has the composition of mixed venous blood entering the pulmonary capillaries, i.e., $P\bar{v}_{O_2} \approx 40$ mmHg and $P\bar{v}_{CO_2} \approx 46$ mmHg. At the other extreme, when an alveolar-capillary unit has a high $\dot{V}/\dot{Q}$ ratio, it behaves almost like dead space, and the small amount of blood leaving the unit has partial pressures of O_2 and CO_2 ($P_{O_2} \approx 150$ mmHg, $P_{CO_2} \approx 0$ mmHg while breathing room air) approaching the composition of inspired gas.

In the ideal situation, all alveolar-capillary units have equal matching of ventilation and perfusion, i.e., with a ratio of approximately 1 when each is expressed in L/min. However, even in the normal individual, some $\dot{V}/\dot{Q}$ mismatching is present, since there is normally a gradient of blood flow from the apices to the bases of the lungs. Moreover, there is a similar gradient of ventilation from the apices to the bases, but the gradient is less marked for ventilation than for perfusion. As a result, ventilation-perfusion ratios are higher at the lung apices than at the lung bases. Therefore, blood coming from the apices has a higher P_{O_2} and lower P_{CO_2} than blood coming from the bases. The net P_{O_2} and P_{CO_2} of the resulting mixture of blood coming from all areas of the lung is a flow-weighted average of the individual components, which takes into account the relative amount

of blood from each unit and the O_2 and CO_2 *content* of blood coming from each unit. Because of the sigmoid shape of the oxyhemoglobin dissociation curve (see Fig. 302-4), it is important to distinguish between the partial pressure and the content of O_2 in blood. Hemoglobin is almost fully saturated at a P_{O_2} of 60 mmHg, and little additional O_2 is carried by hemoglobin even with substantial elevations of P_{O_2} above 60 mmHg. On the other hand, significant O_2 desaturation of hemoglobin occurs once P_{O_2} falls below 60 mmHg and onto the steep descending limb of the curve. As a result, blood coming from regions of the lung with a high $\dot{V}/\dot{Q}$ ratio, a high P_{O_2}, but only a small elevation in O_2 content cannot compensate for blood coming from regions with a low $\dot{V}/\dot{Q}$ ratio, a low P_{O_2}, and a significant decrease in O_2 content. Although $\dot{V}/\dot{Q}$ mismatching can influence P_{CO_2}, this effect is less marked and often is overcome by an increase in overall minute ventilation.

MEASUREMENT OF GAS EXCHANGE **Arterial blood gases** The most commonly used measures of gas exchange are the partial pressures of O_2 and CO_2 in arterial blood, i.e., Pa_{O_2} and Pa_{CO_2}, respectively. These partial pressures do not measure directly the quantity of O_2 and CO_2 in blood but rather the driving pressure for the gas in blood. The actual quantity or content of each of these gases in blood depends on the solubility of the gas in plasma and the ability of any component of blood to react with or to bind the gas of interest. Since hemoglobin is capable of binding large amounts of O_2, oxygenated hemoglobin is the primary form in which O_2 is transported in blood. The actual content of O_2 in blood therefore depends both on the hemoglobin concentration and on the Pa_{O_2}. The Pa_{O_2} determines what percentage of hemoglobin is saturated with O_2, based on the position on the oxyhemoglobin dissociation curve. Oxygen content in normal blood (at 37°C, pH 7.4) can be determined by adding the amount of O_2 dissolved in plasma to the amount bound to hemoglobin, according to the equation

$$O_2 \text{ content} = 1.34 \times [\text{hemoglobin}] \times \text{saturation} + 0.0031 \times P_{O_2}$$

since each gram of hemoglobin is capable of carrying 1.34 mL O_2 when fully saturated, and the amount of O_2 that can be dissolved in plasma is proportional to the P_{O_2}, with 0.0031 mL O_2 dissolved per deciliter of blood per mmHg P_{O_2}. In arterial blood, the amount of O_2 transported dissolved in plasma (approximately 0.3 mL O_2 per deciliter of blood) is trivial compared with the amount bound to hemoglobin (approximately 20 mL O_2 per deciliter of blood).

Most commonly, P_{O_2} is the measurement used to quantitate the adequacy of oxygenation of arterial blood. Direct measurement of O_2 saturation in arterial blood by oximetry is also important in selected clinical conditions. For example, in patients with carbon monoxide exposure, carbon monoxide preferentially displaces O_2 from hemoglobin, essentially making a portion of hemoglobin unavailable for binding to O_2. In this circumstance, carbon monoxide saturation is high and O_2 saturation is low, even though the driving pressure for O_2 to bind to hemoglobin, reflected by P_{O_2}, is normal. Measurement of O_2 saturation, in order to determine O_2 content, is also important when mixed venous blood is sampled from a pulmonary arterial catheter to calculate cardiac output by the Fick technique. In mixed venous blood, the P_{O_2} is normally about 40 mmHg, but small changes in P_{O_2} may reflect relatively large changes in O_2 saturation.

A useful calculation in the assessment of oxygenation is the alveolar-arterial O_2 difference ($PA_{O_2} - Pa_{O_2}$), commonly called the *alveolar-arterial O_2 gradient* (or A–a gradient). This calculation takes into account the fact that alveolar and, hence, arterial P_{O_2} can be expected to change depending on the level of alveolar ventilation, reflected by the arterial P_{CO_2}. When a patient hyperventilates and has a low P_{CO_2} in arterial blood and alveolar gas, alveolar and arterial P_{O_2} will rise; conversely, hypoventilation and a high P_{CO_2} are accompanied by a decrease in alveolar and arterial P_{O_2}. These changes in arterial P_{O_2} are independent of abnormalities in O_2 transfer at the alveolar-capillary level and reflect only the dependence of alveolar P_{O_2} on the level of alveolar ventilation.

In order to determine the alveolar-arterial O_2 difference, the alveolar P_{O_2} ($P_{A_{O_2}}$) must first be calculated. The equation most commonly used for this purpose, a simplified form of the alveolar gas equation, is

$$P_{A_{O_2}} = F_{I_{O_2}} \times (P_B - P_{H_2O}) - P_{a_{CO_2}}/R$$

where $F_{I_{O_2}}$ = fractional concentration of inspired O_2 (≈ 0.21 when breathing room air)

P_B = barometric pressure (approximately 760 mmHg at sea level)

P_{H_2O} = water vapor pressure (47 mmHg when air is fully saturated at 37°C)

R = respiratory quotient (the ratio of CO_2 production to O_2 consumption, usually assumed to be 0.8)

If the preceding values are substituted into the equation for the patient breathing air at sea level, the equation becomes

$$P_{A_{O_2}} = 150 - 1.25 \times P_{a_{CO_2}}$$

The alveolar-arterial O_2 difference can then be calculated by subtracting measured $P_{a_{O_2}}$ from calculated $P_{A_{O_2}}$. In a healthy young person breathing room air, the $P_{A_{O_2}} - P_{a_{O_2}}$ is normally less than 15 mmHg; this value increases with age and may be as high as 30 mmHg in elderly patients.

Adequacy of CO_2 elimination is measured by the partial pressure of CO_2 in arterial blood, i.e., $P_{a_{CO_2}}$. A more complete understanding of the mechanisms and chronicity of abnormal levels of P_{CO_2} also requires measurement of pH and/or bicarbonate (HCO_3^-), since P_{CO_2} and the patient's acid-base status are so closely intertwined (see Chap. 46).

Pulse oximetry Because measurement of $P_{a_{O_2}}$ requires arterial puncture and provides intermittent rather than continuous data about the patient's oxygenation, it is not ideal for close monitoring of unstable patients. Over the past several years, an alternative method for assessing oxygenation, pulse oximetry, has become readily available in many clinical settings. The pulse oximeter measures oxygen saturation (rather than $P_{a_{O_2}}$) using a probe usually clipped over a patient's finger. The device measures absorption of two wavelengths of light by hemoglobin in pulsatile, cutaneous arterial blood. Because of differential absorption of the two wavelengths of light by oxygenated and nonoxygenated hemoglobin, the percentage of hemoglobin that is saturated with oxygen, i.e., the $S_{a_{O_2}}$, can be calculated and displayed instantaneously.

Although the pulse oximeter has been a major advance in the noninvasive, continuous monitoring of oxygenation, there are several issues and potential problems that should be recognized when this device is used. First, the clinician must be aware of the relationship between oxygen saturation and tension as shown by the oxyhemoglobin dissociation curve (see Fig. 302-4). Because the curve becomes relatively flat above an arterial P_{O_2} of 60 mmHg (corresponding to $S_{a_{O_2}}$ = 90 percent), the oximeter is relatively insensitive to changes in $P_{a_{O_2}}$ above this level. In addition, the position of the curve and therefore the specific relationship between $P_{a_{O_2}}$ and $S_{a_{O_2}}$ may change depending on factors such as temperature, pH, and the erythrocyte concentration of 2,3-DPG. Second, when cutaneous perfusion is decreased, e.g., with low cardiac output or use of vasoconstrictors, the signal from the oximeter may be less reliable or even unobtainable. Third, other forms of hemoglobin, such as carboxyhemoglobin and methemoglobin, are not distinguishable when only two wavelengths of light are used. The reported values for $S_{a_{O_2}}$ by the pulse oximeter are not reliable in the presence of significant amounts of either of these forms of hemoglobin. In contrast, the device used to measure oxygen saturation in samples of arterial blood, called the CO-oximeter, uses at least four wavelengths of light and is capable of distinguishing oxyhemoglobin, reduced hemoglobin, carboxyhemoglobin, and methemoglobin. Finally, the clinician must remember that the often-used goal of $S_{a_{O_2}} \geq 90$ percent does not indicate anything about CO_2 elimination and therefore does not ensure a clinically acceptable P_{CO_2}.

Diffusing capacity The ability of gas to diffuse across the alveolar-capillary membrane is ordinarily assessed by the diffusing capacity of the lung for carbon monoxide (DL_{CO}). In this test, a small concentration of carbon monoxide (0.3%) is inhaled, usually in a single breath that is held for approximately 10 s. The carbon monoxide is diluted by the gas already present in the alveoli and is also taken up by hemoglobin as the erythrocytes course through the pulmonary capillary system. The concentration of carbon monoxide in exhaled gas is measured, and DL_{CO} is calculated as the quantity of carbon monoxide absorbed per minute per mmHg pressure gradient from the alveoli to the pulmonary capillaries. The value obtained for DL_{CO} depends on the alveolar-capillary surface area available for gas exchange and on the pulmonary capillary blood volume. In addition, the thickness of the alveolar-capillary membrane, the degree of $\dot{V}/\dot{Q}$ mismatching, and the patient's hemoglobin level will affect the measurement. Because of this effect of hemoglobin levels on DL_{CO}, the measured DL_{CO} is frequently corrected to take the patient's hemoglobin level into account. The value for DL_{CO}, ideally corrected for hemoglobin, can then be compared with a predicted value, based either on age, height, and gender or on the alveolar volume (V_A) at which the value was obtained. Alternatively, the DL_{CO} can be divided by V_A and the resulting value for DL_{CO}/V_A compared with a predicted value.

MECHANISMS OF HYPOXEMIA AND HYPERCAPNIA **Arterial blood gases** Hypoxemia is a common manifestation of a variety of diseases affecting the lungs or other parts of the respiratory system. The broad clinical problem of hypoxemia is often best characterized according to the underlying mechanism. The four basic mechanisms of hypoxemia are (1) decrease in inspired P_{O_2}, (2) hypoventilation, (3) shunt, and (4) $\dot{V}/\dot{Q}$ mismatching. Hypoxemia due to decreased diffusion occurs only under selected clinical circumstances and is not usually included among the general categories of hypoxemia. Determining the underlying mechanism for hypoxemia depends on measurement of the $P_{a_{CO_2}}$, calculation of $P_{A_{O_2}} - P_{a_{O_2}}$, and knowledge of the response to supplemental O_2. A flowchart summarizing the approach to the hypoxemic patient is found in Fig. 214-5.

Decrease in the inspired P_{O_2} and hypoventilation both cause hypoxemia by lowering $P_{A_{O_2}}$ and therefore $P_{a_{O_2}}$. In each case, gas exchange at the alveolar-capillary level occurs normally, and $P_{A_{O_2}} - P_{a_{O_2}}$ is not elevated. Hypoxemia due to decreased inspired P_{O_2} can be diagnosed by knowledge of the clinical situation. Inspired P_{O_2} is lowered either because the patient is at a high altitude, where barometric pressure is low, or, much less commonly, because the patient is breathing a gas mixture containing less than 21% O_2. The hallmark of hypoventilation as a cause of hypoxemia is an elevation in $P_{a_{CO_2}}$. This is associated with an increase in $P_{A_{CO_2}}$ and a fall in $P_{A_{O_2}}$. When hypoxemia is due purely to a low inspired P_{O_2} or to alveolar hypoventilation, $P_{A_{O_2}} - P_{a_{O_2}}$ is normal. If $P_{A_{O_2}} - P_{a_{O_2}}$ and $P_{a_{CO_2}}$ are both elevated, then an additional mechanism, such as $\dot{V}/\dot{Q}$ mismatching or shunt, is contributing to hypoxemia.

Shunting is a cause of hypoxemia when desaturated blood effectively bypasses oxygenation at the alveolar-capillary level. This occurs either because of a structural problem that allows desaturated blood to bypass the normal site of gas exchange or because perfused alveoli are not ventilated. Shunting is associated with an elevation in the $P_{A_{O_2}} - P_{a_{O_2}}$. When shunting is an important contributing factor to hypoxemia, the lowered $P_{a_{O_2}}$ is relatively refractory to improvement by supplemental O_2.

Finally, the largest clinical category of hypoxemia is $\dot{V}/\dot{Q}$ mismatching. With $\dot{V}/\dot{Q}$ mismatching, regions with low $\dot{V}/\dot{Q}$ ratios contribute blood with a low P_{O_2} and a low O_2 content. Corresponding regions with high $\dot{V}/\dot{Q}$ ratios contribute blood with a high P_{O_2}. However, because blood is already almost fully saturated with a normal P_{O_2}, elevation of the P_{O_2} to a high value does not significantly increase O_2 saturation or content and therefore cannot compensate for the reduction of O_2 saturation and content in blood coming from regions with a low $\dot{V}/\dot{Q}$ ratio. When $\dot{V}/\dot{Q}$ mismatch is the primary cause of hypoxemia, $P_{A_{O_2}} - P_{a_{O_2}}$ is elevated, and P_{CO_2} is generally

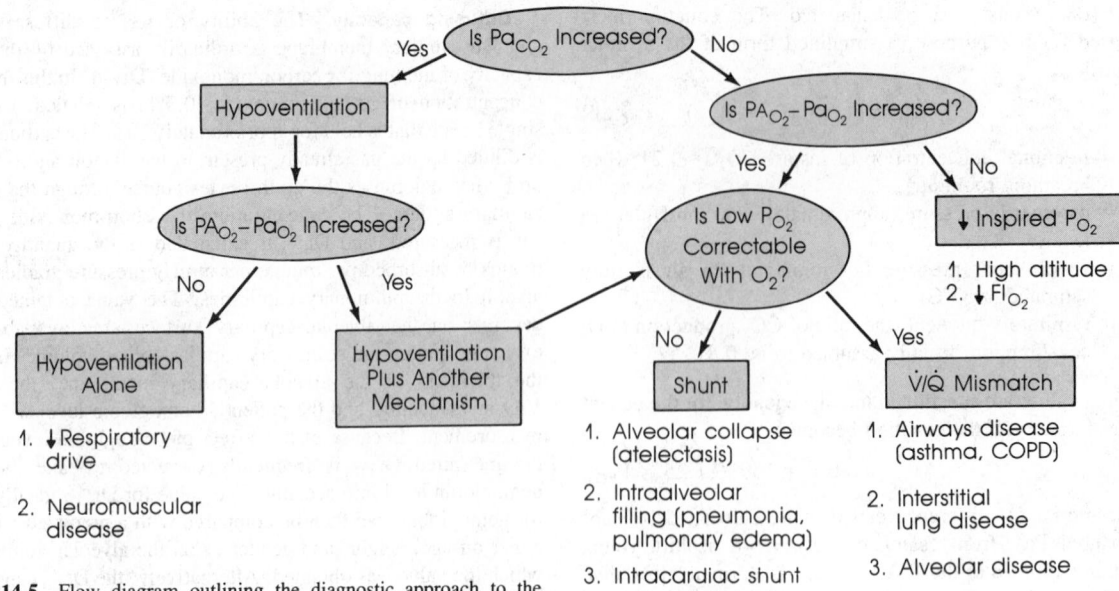

FIGURE 214-5 Flow diagram outlining the diagnostic approach to the patient with hypoxemia ($Pa_{O_2} < 80$ mmHg). $PA_{O_2} - Pa_{O_2}$ is usually < 15 mmHg for subjects ≤30 years old and increases ~3 mmHg per decade after age 30.

normal. Supplemental O_2 corrects the hypoxemia by raising the P_{O_2} in blood coming from regions with a low $\dot{V}/\dot{Q}$ ratio; this response distinguishes hypoxemia due to $\dot{V}/\dot{Q}$ mismatch from that due to true shunt.

The essential mechanism underlying all cases of hypercapnia is inadequate alveolar ventilation for the amount of CO_2 produced. It is conceptually useful to characterize CO_2 retention further, based on a more detailed examination of the potential contributing factors. These include (1) increased CO_2 production, (2) decreased ventilatory drive ("won't breathe"), (3) malfunction of the respiratory pump or increased airways resistance, making it more difficult to sustain adequate ventilation ("can't breathe"), and (4) inefficiency of gas exchange (increased dead space or $\dot{V}/\dot{Q}$ mismatch) necessitating a compensatory increase in overall minute ventilation. In practice, more than one of these mechanisms is commonly responsible for hypercapnia, since increased minute ventilation is capable of compensating for increased CO_2 production and for inefficiencies of gas exchange.

Diffusing capacity   Although abnormalities in diffusion are rarely responsible for hypoxemia, clinical measurement of diffusing capacity is frequently used to assess the functional integrity of the alveolar-capillary membrane, which includes the pulmonary capillary bed. Diseases solely affecting the airways generally do not lower DL_{CO}, whereas diseases affecting alveolar walls or the pulmonary capillary bed will have an effect on DL_{CO}. Even though DL_{CO} is a useful marker to assess whether disease affecting the alveolar-capillary bed is present, an abnormal DL_{CO} does not necessarily imply that diffusion limitation is responsible for hypoxemia in a particular patient.

CLINICAL CORRELATIONS   Useful clinical correlations can be made with the mechanisms underlying hypoxemia (see Fig. 214-5). A lowered inspired P_{O_2} contributes to hypoxemia either at high altitude or if the concentration of inspired O_2 is less than 21%. The latter problem occurs if a patient receiving anesthesia or ventilatory support is inadvertently given a gas mixture to breathe containing less than 21% O_2 or if O_2 is consumed from ambient gas, as can occur during smoke inhalation from a fire. The primary feature of hypoventilation as a cause of hypoxemia is an elevation in arterial P_{CO_2}. The clinical correlations with hypoventilation are discussed in Chap. 229.

Shunt as a cause of hypoxemia can reflect transfer of blood from the right to the left side of the heart without it ever entering the pulmonary circulation, as occurs with an intracardiac shunt. This problem occurs most commonly in the setting of cyanotic congenital

heart disease, when an interatrial or interventricular septal defect is associated with pulmonary hypertension, so that shunting is in the right-to-left rather than the left-to-right direction. Shunting of blood through the pulmonary parenchyma is most frequently due to disease causing absence of ventilation to perfused alveoli. This can occur if the alveoli are atelectatic or if they are filled with fluid, as in pulmonary edema (both cardiogenic and noncardiogenic) or with extensive intraalveolar exudation of fluid due to pneumonia. Less commonly, vascular anomalies with arteriovenous shunting in the lung can cause hypoxemia. These anomalies can be hereditary, as found with hereditary hemorrhagic telangiectasia (Osler-Rendu-Weber syndrome), or acquired, as in pulmonary vascular malformations secondary to hepatic cirrhosis, which are similar to the commonly recognized cutaneous vascular malformations ("spider hemangiomas").

Ventilation-perfusion mismatch is the most common cause of hypoxemia clinically. Most of the processes affecting either the airways or the pulmonary parenchyma are distributed unevenly throughout the lungs and do not necessarily affect ventilation and perfusion equally. Some areas of lung may have good perfusion and poor ventilation, whereas others may have poor perfusion and relatively good ventilation. Important examples of airways diseases in which $\dot{V}/\dot{Q}$ mismatch causes hypoxemia are asthma and chronic obstructive lung disease. Parenchymal lung diseases causing $\dot{V}/\dot{Q}$ mismatch and hypoxemia include interstitial lung disease and pneumonia.

Clinically important alterations in CO_2 elimination range from excessive ventilation and hypocapnia to inadequate CO_2 elimination and hypercapnia. These clinical problems are discussed in Chap. 229.

Diffusing capacity   Measurement of DL_{CO} may be useful for assessing disease affecting the alveolar-capillary bed or the pulmonary vasculature. In practice, three main categories of disease are associated with lowered DL_{CO}: interstitial lung disease, emphysema, and pulmonary vascular disease. With interstitial lung disease, scarring of alveolar-capillary units diminishes the area of the alveolar-capillary bed as well as pulmonary blood volume. With emphysema, alveolar walls are destroyed, so the surface area of the alveolar-capillary bed is again diminished. In patients with disease causing a decrease in the cross-sectional area and volume of the pulmonary vascular bed, such as recurrent pulmonary emboli or primary pulmonary hypertension, DL_{CO} is commonly diminished.

Diffusing capacity may be elevated if pulmonary blood volume is increased, as may be seen in congestive heart failure. However, once interstitial and alveolar edema ensue, the net $D_{L_{CO}}$ depends on the opposing influences of increased pulmonary capillary blood volume elevating $D_{L_{CO}}$ and pulmonary edema decreasing it. Finding an elevated $D_{L_{CO}}$ may be useful in the diagnosis of alveolar hemorrhage, such as in Goodpasture's syndrome. Hemoglobin contained in erythrocytes within the alveolar lumen is capable of binding carbon monoxide, so the exhaled carbon monoxide concentration is diminished and the measured $D_{L_{CO}}$ is increased.

REFERENCES

AMERICAN THORACIC SOCIETY: Lung function testing: Selection of reference values and interpretative strategies. Am Rev Respir Dis 144:1202, 1991

CLARK JS et al: Noninvasive assessment of blood gases. Am Rev Respir Dis 145:220, 1992

CRAPO RO, FORSTER RE II: Carbon monoxide diffusing capacity. Clin Chest Med 10:187, 1989

GIBSON GJ: Standardised lung function testing. Eur Respir J 6:155, 1993

QUANJER PH et al: Lung volumes and forced ventilatory flows. Report Working Party Standardization of Lung Function Tests, European Community for Steel and Coal. Official Statement of the European Respiratory Society. Eur Respir J Suppl 16:5, 1993

SOCIETY OF CRITICAL CARE MEDICINE: A model for technology assessment applied to pulse oximetry. Crit Care Med 21:615, 1993

WEINBERGER SE: *Principles of Pulmonary Medicine*, 2d ed. Philadelphia, Saunders, 1992

WEST JB: *Respiratory Physiology: The Essentials*, 4th ed. Baltimore, Williams & Wilkins, 1990

215 IMAGING IN PULMONARY DISEASE

PAUL J. FRIEDMAN

Radiologic examination of the lungs and pleura has grown beyond the capability—great as it is—of the plain chest radiograph and includes the imaging modalities of computed tomography, nuclear magnetic resonance, ultrasound, and nuclear medicine. This chapter will focus on their applications in relation to the traditional chest film.

THE BASIC PRINCIPLES OF CLINICAL IMAGING

Problem-based imaging The first step in ordering a radiologic examination is to define the problem clearly enough to indicate what new information needs to be provided by an imaging study.

Consultation The next step is to decide if a plain chest radiograph (CR) will suffice, whether special radiographic views are necessary, or if the problem demands more expensive and time-consuming techniques. In this era of growing specialization, rapidly changing technology, and cost consciousness, it is increasingly important to get radiologic consultation for this step.

Getting the results The value of a radiographic report often depends on whether the radiologist was aware of the question being asked. It has been shown that radiologic interpretation is far more accurate when an appropriate history is provided. Even with a relevant history, the false-negative error rate (the "misses") is 30 to 40 percent, on average, when measured in controlled situations. It is therefore important to (1) provide a history, (2) read the report carefully but skeptically, (3) look at the films yourself, and (4) review them with a radiologist.

Screening Ordering a routine posteroanterior (PA) and lateral CR is an exception to problem-based imaging, but admission films are needed only if there is suspicion of cardiac or pulmonary disease. Periodic health examinations do not require a CR unless there is a relevant history or physical finding.

OCCUPATIONAL HEALTH SCREENING Evaluating the extent of lung damage from exposure to coal or silica dust has been achieved by standardized CR, with an ingenious scoring system for pneumoconiosis. Health risks from exposure to asbestos dust are currently monitored by radiography, though with improved industrial hygiene the expected plaques are more rare and pulmonary fibrosis from asbestos is unusual. Occupational exposures to agents more likely to cause asthma than pneumoconiosis should not be monitored by CR.

APPLICATIONS OF IMAGING TECHNOLOGY, NEW AND OLD

Variations on chest radiography Chest radiologists uniformly agree that the technique of choice is high kilovoltage (>120 kVp), with a stationary scatter-absorbing grid, and a wide-latitude film-screen combination (more shades of gray, less black-and-white). Many new techniques are under development, from improved x-ray–sensitive fluorescent screens, to Xerox-like methods of transferring latent images from solid-state receivers, to electronic scanning, digitization, and storage of radiographic images. These new technologies allow computer manipulation of the images to compensate for exposure problems, speed image retrieval from archives, and allow their electronic transmission to other clinical sites. However, available displays lack the fine detail of the conventional chest radiograph.

Portable films Though necessary in many cases, the portable CR is deficient in detail resolution, latitude, and penetration and fails to show the normal gravitational gradient necessary for physiologic interpretation. It also has increased geometric distortion, more lung is obscured by heart or diaphragm, and it does not provide a lateral view. Because of these technical limitations, replacement of the conventional film-screen combination by photo-stimulable phosphor plates will be most acceptable and potentially useful at the bedside.

Lateral decubitus or prone positions may be useful in bedside radiography to show parts of the lung otherwise obscured by effusion; the lateral decubitus and other horizontal-beam films are good for demonstrating pneumothorax or fluid levels in the lung or pleural space. Portable radiographic examinations are also useful in assessing the positions of tubes and catheters commonly used in the intensive care unit.

Conventional tomography Essentially obsolete for chest work, tomography is rarely used even for studying the hilar regions; far more information can be obtained about the hilar structures and the adjacent mediastinum from computed tomography (CT) or magnetic resonance (MR) imaging. Screening the lungs for metastases, formerly a major application of conventional tomography, is better done with CT. Conventional tomography should be used only in facilities where more advanced technology is not available.

COMPUTED TOMOGRAPHY

The x-ray absorption of each point (pixel) in a cross section of the body can be calculated by measuring the absorption of many fine x-ray beams at many angles within the plane of the cross section. The calculated absorption coefficients are displayed as radiographic densities with far more shades of gray than possible with CR (Fig. 215-1). CT eliminates the superimposition of structures that makes CR anatomy so difficult, and though the images are "noisy," there is less problem with CT than with CR in detecting an abnormality because of obscuration by normal structures. However, a set of images is needed to encompass the chest, since each represents only the information in a 1-cm thick transverse cross section. Each set of data is collected during suspended respiration, taking 1 to 2 s, and requires patient cooperation in taking and holding a comparable breath each time for good results. The new generation of "spiral" CT scanners collect data for several serial sections continuously, greatly reducing the problem of missing parts of the lung because of inconsistent inspiratory efforts.

MEDIASTINAL CT After less than two decades of use in the chest, CT is well established as the diagnostic procedure of choice for studying the mediastinum (see Fig. 215-1*B*). The most common

A

B

FIGURE 215-1   Normal CT of the chest, supine, standard 1-cm section, after intravenous contrast material. *A*. Typical ''lung window'' settings, with normal pulmonary vessels and the top of the oblique fissure (F) of the left lung visible. The dark circle within the mediastinum is the tracheal air column (T). Note bulge (B) along left mediastinum. *B*. Mediastinal settings show a clear delineation between the enlarged lymphomatous nodes (LN) and the surrounding fat. The soft tissue structure dorsal to the trachea is the esophagus (E). The major vessels visible are the superior vena cava (V) and ascending (A) and descending (D) aorta; small veins are also seen in the fat in front of the spine behind the esophagus, and ventrally, behind the sternum, as well as in the generous layer of subcutaneous fat. The calcification (C) is a plaque in the aortic arch rather than a calcified lymph node. The mediastinal bulge (B) alongside the ascending aorta on the left is simply mediastinal fat, not an enlarged node.

use is the assessment of lymph node size in the staging of lung cancer (Chap. 227). Enlarged nodes require biopsy for diagnosis, since enlargement caused by acute inflammation cannot be confidently distinguished from that caused by metastasis on CT (or MR) images. The false-negative error rate of CT is significantly greater than that of mediastinoscopy, but CT is still useful in screening patients being considered for cancer surgery if mediastinoscopy is not planned.

Lumps and bumps of the mediastinum detected on CR are readily analyzed using CT. Mediastinal cysts, tumors, fat, and calcification are readily distinguished because of the good density resolution. CT is also excellent for distinguishing vascular from nonvascular structures and for recognizing vascular anatomic variants or aneurysms.

CONTRAST MATERIAL   There is no consensus about the indications for using intravenous contrast material in chest CT. Some institutions use contrast material universally and may even use the high dose–rapid infusion method known as *dynamic CT*. Others use contrast material regularly in studies of vessels or tumors but not for routine lung cancer staging. Injection of traditional hypertonic contrast material adds to the cost and risk of the study, since allergic and idiosyncratic reactions occur regularly. Serious reactions are uncommon, however, and death occurs no more than about once in every 40,000 intravenous injections. Newer low-osmolar agents are less toxic but are still several times as expensive.

CT OF THE PLEURA   CT imaging resolves complex abnormalities which might involve the lung or pleura or both. For example, the diagnosis of bronchopleural fistula requires distinguishing pleural pockets from lung abscesses or cysts. The solid and fluid components of a pleural collection, which are the same density on CR, can be usefully distinguished on CT.

Tumors of the pleura are demonstrated in the transverse plane much more clearly than on CR, where they are hard to distinguish from inflammatory pleural thickening. The true extent of malignant mesothelioma or metastatic adenocarcinoma is therefore best shown on CT. An asbestos-related application is the detection of pleural plaques and calcifications (Chap. 219). Though routine health screening of asbestos-exposed workers relies on the posteroanterior CR, sometimes it is necessary to use the much greater sensitivity of CT to detect pleural plaques or the characteristic small pleural calcifications.

HIGH-RESOLUTION CT OF THE LUNG AND AIRWAYS   Since CR has such excellent resolution and shows air/tissue density differences so well, this application of CT has been the slowest to develop. The geometric resolution of ordinary CT is nearly tenfold less than CR, but high-resolution (HRCT) technique brings it up to within a factor of two or three. HRCT uses a thin image plane, usually 1 to 2 mm instead of the conventional 10 mm, to reduce volume averaging of densities and a higher contrast or edge-enhancing image reconstruction. The result is comparable with a pathologist's naked-eye view of a slice of lung. The trade-off is that the number of these thin slices that can be made is limited by radiation exposure, which precludes covering the entire lung; HRCT is used to sample the lung, like a noninvasive biopsy.

The trachea and main bronchi are shown well in cross section (see Fig. 215-2), and CT shows the mediastinal extent of endobronchial lesions, though longitudinal images of the trachea would be more useful clinically. Intrinsic tumors or deformity from other mediastinal primary or secondary neoplasms are demonstrable but are not an indication for CT unless endoscopy is contraindicated. HRCT has much greater sensitivity for bronchial abnormality (thickening, dilation, mucoid impaction) than CR. HRCT has essentially replaced bronchography in screening for surgical bronchiectasis (Chap. 221), missing only minimal or localized cylindrical bronchiectasis.

Details of both airspace and interstitial lung diseases can be demonstrated well by HRCT. Characteristic changes have been described in many diffuse diseases such as carcinomatosis, interstitial fibrosis (see Fig. 215-3), eosinophilic granuloma, sarcoidosis, bronchiolitis, and emphysema. HRCT can reveal subtle interstitial fibrosis of asbestosis before it is evident on the chest film, and a delicate ground glass pattern of partial alveolar filling, such as in *Pneumocystis carinii* pneumonia, can be seen when the chest film still appears normal. The distribution and amount of emphysema can be assessed readily, and early destructive changes can be detected before pulmonary function tests become abnormal.

FIGURE 215-2 High-resolution CT, supine, 1.5-mm section, with edge-sharpening technique and standard "lung window." Patient has bronchiectasis in posterior segment of right upper lobe. The ring shadows and irregular patchy light regions just ventral to the major fissure (mf) represent, respectively, the dilated, thick-walled bronchi and patchy bronchopneumonia. An opacity was visible on the chest radiograph but the abnormal bronchi could not be perceived. Major vessels bulging the mediastinal shadow are the superior vena cava (SVC) and aortic arch (Arch). The left lung shows normal bronchi and vessels at this level.

The clinical indications for HRCT thus fall into two broad categories: first, to confirm the presence, extent, or activity of suspected interstitial, airspace, or airway disease, and second, to show the detailed pathology underlying an ambiguous radiographic pattern, enabling differential diagnosis of these several kinds of disease.

LIMITED CT STUDIES CT scans of the chest initially were complete, top to bottom, without and with contrast injection. With greater awareness of the capabilities of CT, studies of a limited part of the chest, using regular or HRCT technique and no contrast, should play an increasing role. Their cost can be substantially less than a full scan, hardly more than adding oblique views to a routine CR. Confusing CR findings can often be resolved rapidly using limited CT studies, in preference to waiting a few costly hospital days for the diagnosis to become clear. CT densitometry is useful in determining the presence or absence of calcification in solitary pulmonary nodules.

FIGURE 215-3 High-resolution CT, prone, 1.5 mm section, with edge-sharpening image processing, shown as a light "lung window." Chronic interstitial fibrosis with severe honeycombing: a graphic portrayal, comparable to looking directly at a lung specimen. HRCT can show detailed gross pathologic findings in many lung diseases, with great sensitivity for alveolar filling, for interstitial alterations of various kinds, and for emphysema. *(Courtesy of I. Feuerstein.)*

MAGNETIC RESONANCE IMAGING

Nuclear magnetic resonance is a property of atomic nuclei with an odd number of nucleons, of which the most abundant in the body is hydrogen. While in a strong magnetic field, the alignment of these spinning nuclei can be changed with a superimposed radio-frequency signal, and the rate at which they return to alignment with the field ("relaxation") can be measured by their emission of a faint signal. There are two kinds of relaxation rates, which are functions of the atomic and chemical environment of each nucleus, and therefore they differ in different tissues.

By ingenious use of gradients, relaxation rates can be measured simultaneously at many points within a three-dimensional volume, which allows them to be shown as a set of gray scale images, either in the transverse, coronal, or sagittal plane. The timing of the imposed radio-frequency signal determines which of the relaxation rates predominates, and therefore the constructed images have different shades of gray for the same tissue, though the underlying anatomic structure is unchanged. At this time, there is only limited standardization of technique, especially since optimal differentiation of specific abnormalities requires different machine settings.

Transverse MR images look much like CT images except for the different substitutions of light and dark for different tissues (Fig. 215-4). For example, fat is darker than water on CT but is the brightest tissue on "T_1-weighted" MR images. Water (e.g., cerebrospinal fluid) becomes as bright as fat on T_2-weighted MR images (see Fig. 215-4). The values T_1 and T_2 are the half-times of the relaxation rates mentioned above and are therefore a property of the tissue itself. The flexibility of eliciting and displaying the two relaxation rates provides MR images with even more effective tissue characterization contrast than CT.

Though the protons in blood have a strong MR signal because of the atomic environment of the iron and should therefore appear bright, flowing blood is seen as black, a signal void, on images. During the pause after the radio-frequency signal is triggered, while waiting to measure relaxation signals, the blood containing the altered protons has time to flow out of the plane of interest and is replaced by blood that is emitting no signal. Therefore, normal blood vessels as well as bronchi appear black on MR images (see Fig. 215-4), but the distinction between nodes and vessels in the hilar regions is greatly facilitated when compared with CT. There are artifactual signals from blood vessels, however, when blood flow is slow, notably on scans gated to diastole in the cardiac cycle (which are essential for studying the heart and hilar regions of the mediastinum) and on multisection simultaneous scans, when altered protons from one section may arrive at another level just in time for their signal to be detected. Newer methods of "fast scanning" result in images with flowing blood giving a bright image as in an angiogram.

MR scanning has important limitations compared with CT. A wide variety of artifacts complicate the interpretation of MR images, and the images are also noisier and less uniform than those of CT. The geometric resolution of whole-body scans is inferior to that of CT, though superficial small regions can be shown with superb detail using special surface antennae to detect the faint relaxation signals. The advantage of being able to display sections in any planar direction is weakened by the necessity (at present) of leaving a gap between the image slices. The collection of data (except with fast-scan techniques) requires several minutes, which means that there are breathing artifacts in addition to those from cardiac motion. The narrow magnet tunnel into which the patient is inserted promotes claustrophobia, and the changes in the magnetic field cause a distressing noise. Ferromagnetic materials, including those in the patient, cannot be brought into the magnet room safely, for they will fly toward the center of the magnet. Other metal in the patient will merely ruin the image in its vicinity. Finally, the cost of MR scanning is substantial, approximately twice that of a contrast CT.

MR APPLICATIONS Gated cardiac studies are of great interest (Chap. 191) but are outside the scope of this discussion. The spine

FIGURE 215-4 Magnetic resonance images of a patient with a bulky lower esophageal carcinoma (EC). Both bronchi and blood vessels show a signal void. *A.* The coronal plane image intersecting the tumor just ventral to the vertebral column. *B.* Transverse image at the level of the right pulmonary artery (rpa), where the wall of the esophagus (e) is only slightly thickened. *C.* At the level of the lower part of the left atrium (la), through the main tumor mass. Note the large azygos vein (av) on images *A* and *B* and the dilated chest wall veins (dv) on image *C*, raising a question of obstruction of the inferior vena cava. No distinct adenopathy is seen. Other anatomic structures seen include the ascending and descending aorta (aa, da), aortic root (ar) and arch (Arch), main and left pulmonary arteries (pa, lpa), bronchus intermedius (bi), left main bronchus (lb), and right atrium (ra).

can be displayed with the perspective of an anatomic diagram because of the availability of sagittal projections. This enables MR scanning to be particularly useful in questions of paraspinal, intraspinal, or intraosseous tumor. Tumors in the mediastinum can be analyzed by their T_1 and T_2 properties, but the ability to distinguish inflammatory enlargement of nodes from that of tumor has not been realized. As noted, MR imaging is more sensitive than CT for distinguishing nonvascular tissue in the complex hilar regions and in the central portions of the lung (see Fig. 215-4) but is probably less satisfactory in the mediastinum. Detection of intravascular pulmonary emboli or thrombi has been demonstrated experimentally, but clinical application is still limited.

Use of sagittal and coronal or oblique images of the mediastinum facilitates study of the arteries, so MR scanning of the aorta is the preferred noninvasive way to detect aortic dissection or aneurysm (Chap. 210). These projections should be ideal for studying the trachea, but the trachea and bronchi are poorly displayed, with an artifactual narrowing of the lumen. The staging of lung cancer by mediastinal scanning has about the same effectiveness using MR as CT.

SPECTROSCOPY When chemists use MR to analyze mixtures and determine chemical structure, they study many nuclei in addition to hydrogen. Only hydrogen is sufficiently abundant in the body to provide enough signal to form images, but other substances can be quantitated in a large volume that would be unsuitable for imaging. The most important is phosphorus, which has different resonant frequencies in its various molecular positions as part of ATP, AMP, creatine phosphate, inorganic phosphorus, etc. A limited number of relatively abundant cellular metabolites also can be measured by detecting protons with specific resonance values, if the strong proton signal from water is suppressed. Metabolic processes can therefore be monitored by in vivo MR spectroscopy, a research technique of potential future clinical application.

NUCLEAR MEDICINE IMAGING

Injected or inhaled radioisotopes (radionuclides) incorporated into carefully chosen substances can provide anatomic, physiologic, and pathologic information from their distribution and disposition, as revealed on gamma camera images. Nuclear medicine remains the primary technique for the clinical problem of pulmonary thromboembolism (Chaps. 216 and 226) and the regional functional assessment of obstructive lung diseases.

ULTRASOUND IN THE CHEST

Imaging with ultrasound requires the computerized reconstruction of series of echoes of high-frequency sound emitted at various angles from a piezoelectric crystal transducer. The echoes arise as the radiating sound encounters surfaces of different acoustic impedance at right angles to its path. Ultrasound does not pass through air or bone, so the lungs themselves and the ribs are major limitations on its usefulness in the chest. A fluid collection such as a cyst or abscess will be echo-free, or *sonolucent*, unless it has debris in it and will transmit sound to make deeper echoes without attenuation. In solid tissues, the signal is attenuated as the sound is absorbed, so the echoes become weaker as their depth in the tissue increases. Air-containing lung has no echo beyond the pleural interface at its surface, although consolidated lung may look like solid tissue.

APPLICATIONS The principal application of ultrasonography in the mediastinum is cardiac, discussed in detail in Chap. 190, including the detection of pericardial fluid and cysts. Bronchogenic cysts, in their most common subcarinal location, also may be confirmed to be fluid-containing by ultrasound. The most common pulmonary application is detection of fluid or pus in the pleural space. For diagnosis, ultrasound is convenient, since it can be performed with bedside apparatus, but it is not as accurate as CT (or MR) because it may confuse homogeneous pleural fibrosis or pulmonary consolidation with sonolucent pleural fluid. If the pleural fluid collection is loculated or small in amount, then localization by ultrasound enhances the safety and usefulness of thoracentesis.

INTERVENTIONAL RADIOLOGY

Advances in imaging with ultrasound and CT have brought with them a renaissance of percutaneous procedures for biopsy and drainage. Though fluoroscopically guided percutaneous needle biopsy of the lungs has been established for at least 30 years, CT has made it possible to pursue smaller targets and those close to vital structures.

Under CT control, needle biopsy of the mediastinum can replace mediastinoscopy, particularly when inoperability is being established by biopsy of enlarged nodes.

A more recent interventional innovation is drainage of pleural effusions, pneumothorax, and empyema in the thorax, and abscesses in the abdomen by catheters inserted over guidewires that have been introduced through percutaneous needles using techniques originally developed for angiography. The fluid or air pocket is localized and the needle position confirmed using ultrasound or CT, the specific technique depending on the ease with which the fluid can be delineated with ultrasound. Even lung abscesses can be drained percutaneously. Transcatheter embolization with particulate matter, coils, or detachable balloons has become widely used in the treatment of massive hemoptysis and arteriovenous malformations of the lung. Considerable savings are achieved in risk, pain, recovery time, and cost by avoiding major surgery with these methods.

REFERENCES

BERGIN CJ et al: Magnetic resonance imaging of lung parenchyma. J Thorac Imaging 8:12, 1993

DOBBINS JT et al: Threshold perception performance with computed and screen-film radiography: Implications for chest radiography. Radiology 183:179, 1992

FRIEDMAN PJ: Lung cancer staging: Efficacy of CT. Radiology 182:307, 1992

NAIDICH DP et al: Hemoptysis: CT-bronchoscopic correlations in 58 cases. Radiology 177:357, 1990

NAIDICH DP et al: *Computed Tomography and Magnetic Resonance of the Thorax.* New York, Raven, 1991

WEBB WR et al: *High-Resolution CT of the Lung.* New York, Raven, 1992

WHITE CS et al: Imaging in lung cancer. Semin Oncol 20:142, 1993

216 DIAGNOSTIC PROCEDURES IN RESPIRATORY DISEASES

KENNETH M. MOSER

In seeking a definitive diagnosis in the patient with respiratory disease, a wide choice of diagnostic procedures is available. These procedures vary considerably, not only in diagnostic reliability and specificity but also in terms of the discomfort, hazard, and cost to the patient. Hence, an orderly sequence of test selection is mandatory. This sequence should begin with procedures involving little risk and cost and, only if necessary, move on to those that entail greater expense as well as higher morbidity and potential mortality.

NONINVASIVE PROCEDURES

RADIOGRAPHIC PROCEDURES (See also Chap. 215) The *chest roentgenogram* serves two major roles in the search for a diagnosis in the patient with respiratory disease: *detector* and *guide*. Occasionally, in its role as a detector, the routine chest roentgenogram initiates the diagnostic search by disclosing an abnormality in an asymptomatic individual. However, routine chest roentgenography (e.g., as an element of all hospital admissions) is neither necessary nor cost-effective. Therefore, more commonly, it detects pulmonary involvement in someone already ill. Rarely, detection may coincide with diagnosis, e.g., in spontaneous pneumothorax or when a radiopaque foreign body has been aspirated.

Far more frequently, however, the roentgenogram, having detected potential disease, provides a guide to the selection of subsequent diagnostic procedures. Many radiographic findings are quite characteristic of certain diseases. A number of radiographic patterns are sufficiently repetitive to warrant descriptive names, such as bilateral hilar adenopathy, solitary pulmonary nodule, diffuse interstitial infiltrate, alveolar filling pattern, multinodular lesion, and honeycomb lung. Thus, a particular radiographic finding, combined with other pertinent data, often permits establishment of a reasonable list of possible diagnoses. For example, the radiographic detection of bilateral hilar adenopathy in an asymptomatic, 26-year-old black male immediately places sarcoidosis at the top of the list. A chest roentgenogram disclosing upper lobe cavities in a febrile male whose brother recently was admitted to a tuberculosis sanitarium would make tuberculosis the most likely entity. Or a "diffuse interstitial" infiltrate—for which more than 100 causes exist—may yield a prompt diagnosis of varicella pneumonia when combined with the classic skin lesions. A diffuse alveolar filling process in an HIV-positive patient suggests *Pneumocystis carinii* pneumonitis (PCP). Multinodular lesions, with some cavitating, in a patient with sinusitis and red cell casts on urinalysis makes Wegener's granulomatosis a primary diagnostic possibility. However, no radiographic pattern is sufficiently specific to *establish* a diagnosis. Lung cancer (primary and metastatic) can present many radiographic patterns, as can both infectious and noninfectious lung disorders. For example, cardiogenic pulmonary edema may present as a perihilar or diffuse alveolar filling pattern, as an interstitial process, and, rarely, as a lobar infiltrate or interlobar collection of fluid ("pseudotumor")—all with or without a pleural effusion.

In some instances, special radiographic techniques may provide valuable diagnostic insights.

Fluoroscopy allows visualization of the thoracic contents in a dynamic rather than static manner and also permits a wide range of special views. It also indicates whether a lesion is pulsatile, what its precise location in the thorax is, whether the hemidiaphragms move normally, i.e., whether they are fixed or move paradoxically, and how various zones of the lung behave during inspiration and expiration. Thus, fluoroscopy, a relatively inexpensive procedure, can define whether a radiographic density is actually in a rib or in the pleura rather than in the parenchyma; and may distinguish between a unilateral hyperlucent lung due to emphysema (mediastinum shifts toward the normal lung on expiration) or to unilateral pulmonary arterial obstruction (no shift).

Thoracic *computed tomography* (CT) has essentially replaced standard tomography (laminography, planigraphy). Both techniques provide a sequence of images, each representing a "slice of the lung" at a different depth. Ordinarily, "cuts" are made at 0.5- to 1.0-cm distances through the areas of interest. These procedures can identify a number of features that are not appreciated on the "routine" roentgenogram, including calcium in a solitary nodule (which if diffuse or in concentric rings signifies a benign etiology); a cavity within a mass lesion; and the presence of hilar, paratracheal, and subcarinal node enlargement. The CT scan is particularly useful in the definition of pleural disease (e.g., differentiating fluid from tumor; identifying calcium in asbestos-exposed individuals); with contrast injections, in differentiating tissue masses from vascular structures; and in identifying small parenchymal nodules. However, to some extent, the sensitivity of CT is a mixed blessing because it is still not known how many "normal" individuals have pleural or parenchymal abnormalities by CT and how these small, benign, hitherto undetected lesions can be distinguished from neoplastic lesions. The CT scan is also proving useful in the detection of interstitial lung disease not apparent (or equivocal) on routine chest roentgenogram and in quantifying emphysematous changes.

Magnetic resonance (MR) imaging remains, in terms of its value in pulmonary diseases, an investigational technique. It has potential value in achieving fine definition of mediastinal lesions, pleural lesions, and, perhaps, in defining embolic occlusion of major pulmonary arteries.

SKIN TESTS Having arrived at a tentative list of diagnostic possibilities based on the history, physical examination, and radiographic appearance, the physician should move to other procedures.

One of the simplest, least costly, and most commonly overlooked is the application of *skin tests* with specific antigens. Antigens are now available to assist in the diagnosis of tuberculosis, histoplasmosis, coccidioidomycosis, blastomycosis, trichinosis, toxoplasmosis, and aspergillosis. These tests vary with respect to sensitivity and cross-reactivity, and attention to scrupulous technique in performance and interpretation is vital. Also, some antigens (e.g., histoplasmosis) may confound serologic tests performed subsequently. A positive skin test indicates only that the antigen has been encountered previously by the host; it does not, regardless of reaction intensity, imply active disease. Furthermore, drugs or diseases that depress cell-mediated immunity (e.g., prednisone, cyclophosphamide, lymphomas, sarcoidosis, HIV infection, disseminated tuberculosis, or coccidioidomycosis) may cause skin anergy. Indeed, a negative battery of skin tests, if it incorporates antigens such as mumps, streptokinase-streptodornase, *Trichophyton*, and *Candida*, suggests that a cause of skin anergy should be sought.

SEROLOGIC TESTS These relatively inexpensive tests also may be useful in the diagnosis of histoplasmosis, blastomycosis, coccidioidomycosis, toxoplasmosis, *Mycoplasma* pneumonia, Legionnaires' disease, a variety of other infectious diseases involving the lungs, and certain immunologically mediated lung diseases (e.g., lupus erythematosus, Wegener's granulomatosis). Often, more extensive diagnostic procedures can be avoided if appropriate serologic tests are obtained. However, there is substantial interinstitutional variability with respect to the sensitivity, specificity, and types of serologic tests available. Therefore, their appropriate use requires close interaction with the responsible laboratory. Serologic testing for HIV status, of course, has become an important element in the evaluation of patients with a variety of pulmonary lesions.

SPUTUM EXAMINATION Another rapid, innocuous, and inexpensive diagnostic procedure is *sputum examination*. It is important that the specimen contain sputum, not saliva, the latter being identified by the presence of squamous (mouth) rather than epithelial (bronchial) cells. The gross nature of the sputum—color, odor, and the presence of blood—may provide valuable clues; e.g., foul sputum suggesting anaerobic pulmonary infection, and blood, in any amount, indicating an abnormality that mandates further investigation. Carefully stained smears of the sputum should be examined next, for these may disclose the causative organism in many bacterial pneumonias, tuberculosis, *Pneumocystis* pneumonia, and in some fungus infections. Sputum eosinophilia can suggest the presence of reversible airway disease responsive to glucocorticoids; hemosiderin-laden macrophages suggest the possibility of Goodpasture's syndrome. Often valuable time is lost because the sputum smear is not examined and results of culture are awaited instead. Sputum samples can be obtained from patients who are not coughing by having them inhale a heated mixture of a mildly irritative solution that induces cough. Such induced samples have been particularly useful in the diagnosis of *P. carinii* pneumonia and in obtaining cytologic specimens for the diagnosis of carcinoma of the lung (Chap. 227). Careful handling of such specimens and interpretive expertise heavily determine the diagnostic yield.

Culture of expectorated sputum (spontaneous or induced) has fallen into disrepute because of uncertain yield and, particularly, because of frequent and unavoidable contamination by the oropharyngeal bacterial flora. Although such cultures are invaluable for identification of organisms responsible for tuberculous and fungus infections, their utility in detection of other bacterial agents responsible for pulmonary infection is often uncertain and can be misleading, particularly in patients who are immunocompromised, intubated, or receiving antimicrobial therapy. Blood cultures may be useful in certain contexts, particularly in AIDS patients with *Mycobacterium avium-intracellulare* (MAI) infections in whom sputum examinations are often negative.

Beyond such standard approaches to obtaining material for culture, five procedures, described below, are now gaining wide acceptance because they limit oropharyngeal contamination and/or can be used to obtain representative samples of lung secretions from the area of lung involvement: (1) catheter-brush sampling, (2) bronchoalveolar lavage, (3) transtracheal aspiration, (4) transbronchial lung biopsy, and (5) percutaneous needle aspiration of the lung.

PULMONARY FUNCTION TESTS (See also Chap. 214)   Certain "patterns" of derangement in spirometric tests, arterial blood gases, diffusing capacity, and other functional parameters are particularly suggestive of certain pulmonary diseases. For example, diffuse interstitial fibrotic diseases of the lungs (Chap. 224) produce a "restrictive" spirometric defect, reduced pulmonary compliance, a reduced diffusing capacity, and an alveolar-arterial oxygen tension difference that is widened at rest and widens further with exercise. Emphysema (Chap. 223) characteristically causes expiratory obstruction, lung hyperinflation, decreased static elastic recoil (increased compliance), and a reduced diffusing capacity.

PULMONARY SCINTIPHOTOGRAPHY Scintiphotographs of intrathoracic structures are obtained by a variety of "scanning" devices that record the pattern of intrathoracic radioactivity after intravenous injection or inhalation of gamma-emitting radionuclides. Direct photographic or computer-derived images, or digital data, reflecting radionuclide distribution are used for diagnostic purposes. The most commonly used images are those that reflect the distribution of pulmonary blood flow (perfusion) and ventilation. Such scans have multiple diagnostic applications. For example, a normal perfusion scan excludes the diagnosis of acute pulmonary embolism (Chap. 226). When perfusion scans showing defects are combined with ventilation scans, ventilation-perfusion patterns are provided that assist in the diagnosis of parenchymal lung diseases and vascular occlusive disorders, including pulmonary embolism.

Another type of scan involves intravenous injection of radionuclides that have an affinity for intrathoracic inflammatory and neoplastic tissues. Gallium 67 is the most useful of such radionuclides now available. Concentration of such agents, defined by scanning, may permit detection of neoplastic or inflammatory disease in the lungs or mediastinal lymph nodes. Uptake by the lungs may, in some patients, reflect the intensity of inflammatory activity associated with diffuse interstitial pneumonitis, sarcoidosis, and granulomatous infections. Inapparent extrapulmonary foci of granulomatous or neoplastic diseases also may be detected by body scanning.

New radionuclides continue to emerge that, when complexed with such materials as platelets, white blood cells (e.g., indium 111), fibrinogen, and certain monoclonal antibodies, may allow imaging of intrathoracic vessels, thrombi, inflammation, and neoplasms. Tomographic and other image-processing methods are emerging that may further extend the value of these techniques.

All the above procedures involve minimal risks and discomfort to the patient. Where applicable, these approaches should be considered before the more invasive techniques discussed below are employed, unless the condition of the patient demands immediate diagnosis.

INVASIVE PROCEDURES

BRONCHOSCOPY The primary objectives of bronchoscopy include direct visualization of the tracheobronchial tree, including abnormalities such as tumors or granulomatous lesions; biopsy of suggestive or obvious endobronchial lesions; and lavage, brushing, or biopsy of lung regions for cultural and cytologic examinations. Both the *diagnostic reach of* and *accessibility to* bronchoscopy have been expanded by the flexible fiberoptic bronchoscope (FOB). This can be understood best by comparing the FOB with the "standard" rigid bronchoscope.

The rigid bronchoscope is a wide-bore metal tube that incorporates a lighted mirror-lens system. The FOB is composed of fiberoptic bundles that provide both illumination and visualization pathways. One or more small channels with a diameter of 1 to 3 mm traverse the FOB, through which instruments can be passed, fluids delivered, and suction applied. The rigid bronchoscope comes in various external diameters limited only by the feasibility of introducing the rigid device orally and through the larynx. Biopsy and other procedures can be carried out through the rather capacious interior of the rigid tube. The FOB also is available in various external diameters, but all are substantially smaller than rigid bronchoscopes (since no "wall" exists in the FOB). The distal tip of the FOB can be *flexed* easily to 90° and usually to 130° or more from the vertical.

Thus, the rigid bronchoscope permits visualization only of lobar bronchi and the orifices of some segmental bronchi. The flexible, smaller FOB extends the range of *view* to all segmental and subsegmental bronchi and the range for *biopsy and sampling* to the pulmonary parenchyma itself. A biopsy forceps, catheter, or brush passed through the FOB can be directed well beyond the tip of the bronchoscope itself, permitting *transbronchial lung biopsy*, *brushings*, or *aspiration of secretions* for culture and cytologic examination from the most distal regions of the lung. Indeed, both forceps and brush can reach and perforate the pleura, leading to pneumothorax. Therefore, when the lesion being approached is distal, fluoroscopic guidance is essential. Not only does this permit placement of the FOB, forceps, catheter, or brush directly into the area of interest but also it ensures that the pleura will not be inadvertently reached and punctured. The FOB also allows *regional* lung lavage to obtain materials for cytologic examination and culture. Specially designed catheters (see below) placed through the FOB are quite useful in obtaining representative, noncontaminated secretions for culture, thus avoiding the problems mentioned previously with expectorated sputum.

Thus, the FOB has sharply increased the limited diagnostic reach previously available with rigid bronchoscopy. Equally important, the FOB has made bronchoscopy more available to the physician and more acceptable to the patient. The performance of rigid bronchoscopy requires the supine position for peroral insertion of the device; can be performed safely by a relatively few trained physicians; and is often carried out under general anesthesia in an operating room. Therefore, it has been a procedure requiring significant preparation and hence delay. Fiberoptic bronchoscopy can be performed in the sitting or supine position, as the FOB is easily inserted transnasally; can be performed by a large number of trained pulmonary specialists as well as surgeons; usually requires only local anesthesia; and can be performed safely on the wards, in diagnostic rooms equipped with a "dentist-type" chair, and in intensive care units. The FOB can be used easily in intubated patients on ventilators with simple "side-arm" adapters attached to the endotracheal tube. Therefore, when bronchoscopy is indicated, it is not surprising that fiberoptic broncho-scopy is now commonly the first choice. The roomier rigid broncho-scope is now usually reserved for situations in which the small biopsy-suction channel in the FOB may be inadequate (e.g., for removal of large foreign bodies, for laser surgery). The FOB also has a widening range of therapeutic applications including aspiration or lavage of secretions in patients with airway obstruction or atelectasis due to retained secretions; obstruction of bleeding areas of the lung, with a wedged FOB itself or with a balloon catheter passed via the FOB, in patients who are poor surgical risks; removal of small foreign bodies; and placement of radionuclides in tumors. Transtracheal needle aspiration of paratracheal and subcarinal nodes also can be performed via the FOB, a procedure which is particularly useful in the staging of carcinoma of the lung.

FOB has assumed a particularly important role in diagnostic appraisal of patients with AIDS and pulmonary involvement. If induced sputa do not provide a diagnosis, bronchoalveolar lavage (BAL) specimens often do. For example, *Histoplasma capsulatum*, cryptococcal antigen, or cytomegalovirus may be recovered in BAL samples.

The hazards of bronchoscopy are modest but should be recognized. In addition to the risk of general anesthesia, which rigid bronchoscopy usually requires, they can include hypoxemia, laryngospasm, broncho-spasm, pneumothorax, and, of course, bleeding following biopsy. Proper management before, during, and after bronchoscopy should prevent most of these complications. There is no absolute contraindica-

tion to FOB. Even in the presence of massive hemoptysis, FOB with appropriate precautions can yield useful information. Patients with bronchospasm (or a history of bronchospasm) are at particular risk of acute enhancement of spasm and should be approached after good preparation and with resources for intubation-ventilation at hand. The primary contraindication to both rigid and fiberoptic bronchoscopy is the same: performance by inexperienced personnel. Lack of experience sharply reduces diagnostic and therapeutic yield while increasing risks.

BRONCHOGRAPHY In this method, radiopaque material is instilled into the tracheobronchial tree via a catheter or bronchoscope. In most situations in which bronchography was used in the past (e.g., for the diagnosis of bronchiectasis), it has been replaced by chest CT.

TRANSTRACHEAL, CATHETER-BRUSH, AND PERCUTANEOUS NEEDLE ASPIRATION OF THE LUNG All three of these procedures are used to obtain material for culture and microscopic examination. In the case of culture, all three techniques bypass the oropharyngeal flora, though transtracheal aspiration is the least certain in this regard.

Transtracheal aspiration involves needle puncture of the cricothy-roid membrane, insertion of a plastic cannula, and instillation of a saline solution, followed by suctioning of a sample. The procedure cannot be performed in intubated patients; contamination rates are high in previously intubated patients or those who have aspirated oropharyngeal contents. Because the procedure entails risks, although these are minimized by meticulous technique and experience, clear indications for its use should exist. These include apparent pulmonary infections in patients who are unable to cough, in whom cough is nonproductive, or in whom there has been a lack of response to therapy based on smears or cultures from expectorated sputum.

In these same contexts, *catheter-brush devices* specially designed with a distal plug to avoid oropharyngeal contamination can be used. These are manipulated (through an FOB or without it) under fluoroscopic guidance into the involved lung area. The distal absorba-ble plug is then ejected, and the inner brush or catheter advanced for sampling. Finally, an alternative procedure is direct percutaneous aspiration, which can be performed using a small (23- or 25-gauge), thin-walled, *noncutting* needle. The needle, connected to a syringe, is introduced percutaneously into the area of the lung of interest; 2 to 3 mL saline is injected and then aspirated into the syringe and the needle withdrawn. Both the catheter-brush and needle approaches are high-yield, low-contamination procedures. In experienced hands, the risks are low, consisting chiefly of pneumothorax and bleeding. Patients should be carefully monitored for both.

The presence of a hemorrhagic diathesis is a relative contraindica-tion to all three of the above procedures.

BRONCHOALVEOLAR LAVAGE This procedure is usually per-formed by lightly wedging a fiberoptic bronchoscope in distal airways, gently irrigating the air spaces beyond with saline, and analyzing the cells obtained. A "liquid biopsy" of the contents of the distal air spaces is obtained. The procedure has value in the diagnosis of *P. carinii* pneumonia and other infections, in alveolar proteinosis, and in some patients with interstitial pneumonitis of uncertain cause. Maximum diagnostic yield requires careful techniques and expert sample processing.

THORACENTESIS AND PLEURAL BIOPSY (See also Chap. 228) Thoracentesis should be performed to obtain pleural fluid in all pleural effusions of uncertain etiology and may be indicated for relief of symptoms in some patients with effusion of known cause. In effusions of uncertain cause, closed (needle) pleural biopsy should be performed as part of the same procedure.

When pleural fluid is small in amount or when its presence or location is uncertain from routine or lateral decubitus roentgenograms, performance of the thoracentesis and biopsy under fluoroscopic, ultrasound, or CT scan guidance enhances both yield and safety. Although utilizing such special procedures adds patient expense, the yield and/or safety gains justify their use in this context. Pleural fluid obtained should be examined for specific gravity, white blood cell count and differential, protein and glucose concentrations, lactic acid dehydrogenase (LDH), pH, P_{CO_2} (sample collected anaerobically), and amylase. Gram stain, cultures, and exfoliative cytologic specimens should be obtained, and, in some instances, rheumatoid factor and complement levels are measured. The gross appearance of the fluid, the quantity obtained, and the precise location of the thoracentesis should be recorded. A pleural fluid LDH above 200 IU, a pleural fluid/serum protein ratio greater than 0.5, and a pleural fluid/serum LDH ratio greater than 0.6 all indicate that an "exudative" rather than "transudative" process is present. A low pH (<7.20) often indicates that an empyema, probably requiring tube drainage, is present. Specific diagnostic findings in pleural fluid may include the opalescent, pearly fluid characteristic of chylothorax; positive smears or cultures for tuberculosis or other infections; a marked elevation of amylase indicative of effusion secondary to pancreatitis or a ruptured esophagus; and the very low glucose values often seen in effusions associated with rheumatoid arthritis.

As already noted, closed (needle) pleural biopsy should follow thoracentesis whenever the diagnosis is uncertain. It is important to leave some fluid in the pleural space as this makes biopsy easier and safer. Bleeding, pneumothorax, and bronchopleural fistula induced by cutting through the visceral pleura are all more likely in the absence of fluid, and a satisfactory biopsy specimen is less likely to be obtained. Several special needles are available for biopsy of the parietal pleura. All have a cutting edge and some device for retaining the biopsy. The needle is inserted into the pleural effusion, then withdrawn until it is seated on the parietal pleura, from which a biopsy is obtained with the cutting edge. Usually, three biopsies are taken from different sites at the same session. Care should be exercised to place the needle in a position least likely to impinge on the intercostal vessels. All fluid to be used for diagnosis should be removed before biopsy as postbiopsy bleeding may obscure the true character of the fluid.

Pleuroscopy   This is another procedure available for assisting in the diagnosis and management of pleural lesions. Insertion of rigid or flexible devices through intercostal trocars allows direct visualization of the pleural space. Aspiration of fluid, biopsy of pleural lesions or lung, and other types of intervention are possible.

Thoracoscopy   Although this procedure requires anesthesia and a degree of lung collapse, seems likely to replace alternative procedures for inspecting and sampling the pleura (e.g., open pleural biopsy through a limited thoracotomy and, in certain instances, closed needle biopsy). Use of miniaturized cameras allows excellent visualization of the pleural space and the lung. Rapid technical advances are likely to make this procedure widely applicable to the diagnosis and management of pleural and certain parenchymal diseases. Not only pleural biopsy but also lung biopsy can be performed, and in the hands of experienced physicians, such procedures as pleural abrasion or scarification and bullectomy are feasible in selected patients.

PULMONARY AND BRONCHIAL ANGIOGRAPHY   Visualization of the pulmonary arteries by *pulmonary angiography* is achieved by direct, rapid injection of radiopaque materials into the main pulmonary artery or its branches, preferably via cardiac catheterization. Nonionic radiopaque materials, although more expensive, reduce the frequency and severity of unwanted respiratory and hemodynamic responses (e.g., cough, elevation in pulmonary arterial pressure). Multiple, large films can be obtained by an automatic filmchanger, or motion picture or video film (cineangiography) can be used. If visualization of smaller pulmonary vessels is required, magnification techniques can be used. Digital subtraction pulmonary angiography, providing computer-derived images of digital data, may allow imaging of the larger pulmonary arteries with contrast injected more proximally (into superior or inferior vena cava or peripheral vein) or at lower concentrations; however, motion artifacts limit its sensitivity and specificity. Angiography is frequently used to detect pulmonary emboli and a variety of congenital and acquired lesions of the pulmonary vessels. The procedure carries some risk, particularly in

patients with pulmonary hypertension; but with appropriate precautions and experienced personnel that risk is extremely small.

Angioscopy, an experimental technique for direct visualization of the right cardiac chambers and pulmonary arterial system, can be accomplished by insertion of a fiberoptic device via a peripheral vein. The diagnostic role of this procedure in embolic and other disorders remains to be defined. To date it has been useful in defining which patients with chronic embolic pulmonary emboli may be candidates for thromboendarterectomy.

Bronchial arteriography is of value to identify and control (embolotherapy) otherwise obscure bleeding sites in the lungs. Transarterial placement of a catheter into the orifices or parent vessels of bronchial arteries can be accomplished by experienced operators. Radiopaque material is then injected so that these arteries can be visualized. If a bleeding site is identified, emboli can be injected via the catheter as a means for halting hemoptysis.

MEDIASTINOSCOPY AND MEDIASTINOTOMY   Another favored site for biopsy is the lymph nodes in the mediastinum. Because they receive lymphatic drainage from the lungs, these nodes often disclose intrathoracic diseases such as carcinoma, granulomatous infections, and sarcoidosis. As noted above, transtracheal needle aspiration of mediastinal nodes via the FOB is one approach to such nodes. Another is mediastinoscopy, which involves insertion of a lighted mirror-lens system, much like a bronchoscope, through an incision at the base of the neck anteriorly. The instrument is advanced under visual control into the mediastinum, where inspection and biopsy can be carried out. Because of its higher yield of diagnostic lymph nodes, mediastinoscopy has virtually replaced biopsy of the *scalene fat pad* for nodes of interest on the right side of the mediastinum. However, for anatomic reasons, mediastinoscopy on the left is less satisfactory and more hazardous. Nodes in this location are usually approached through a limited left anterior thoracotomy (mediastinotomy). Needle aspiration, mediastinoscopy, and mediastinotomy are low-risk, high-yield procedures. They are invaluable in the "staging" of patients with known or suspected pulmonary malignancy.

LUNG BIOPSY   Finally, if the diagnosis still remains unclear, biopsy of the lung may be required. Again, "closed" and "open" approaches are available. Closed biopsies are of three types: transbronchial, aspiration, and "cutting needle." Transbronchial biopsy, carried out through the fiberoptic bronchoscope, is a highly useful procedure, particularly since larger forceps have been introduced and the taking of multiple biopsies during one procedure has become routine.

However, when lesions are small and/or anatomically located beyond the reach of the FOB, direct aspiration needle biopsy is often more rewarding. *Aspiration* biopsy, mentioned previously, provides cytologic material but does not actually obtain a specimen of lung whose architecture can be examined, a feature that may be necessary to establish a diagnosis. Various "cutting" needles are available that do provide a "core" of the involved lung. However, this approach has waned in popularity because of the high incidence of pneumothorax and bleeding, occasional deaths due to air embolism, and the small size of the biopsy specimen, which may limit diagnostic interpretation. Fluoroscopic or CT guidance is essential in all these closed approaches, and they are contraindicated if pulmonary hypertension or a hemorrhagic diathesis is present.

Open-lung biopsy, requiring thoracotomy, is the final diagnostic resort. It is, however, a relatively safe procedure even in patients with respiratory failure, hemorrhagic diathesis, or pulmonary hypertension if meticulous surgical and anesthetic techniques are observed. Direct visualization allows selection of an optimum biopsy site, and of course, a specimen of adequate size is obtained. To what extent thoracoscopic lung biopsy may replace lung biopsy via thoracotomy remains to be identified. In selecting among these closed and open options, consideration of local expertise in their performance is a key factor.

All specimens obtained by biopsy should be both cultured and processed for pathologic examination.

REFERENCES

BORDOW RA, MOSER KM: *Manual of Clinical Problems in Pulmonary Medicine*. 3d ed. Boston, Little, Brown, 1991

DAVIS SD et al: MR imaging of pleural effusions. J Comp Assist Tomog 14:192, 1990

DURTSCHI MB: Use of thoracoscopy in clinical practice. Am J Surg 165:592, 1993

GIBSON SP: A prospective audit of the value of fibre optic bronchoscopy in adults admitted with community acquired pneumonia. Respir Med 87:105, 1993

HASLAM PL: Bronchoalveolar lavage. Semin Respir Med 6:55, 1984

HULL RD, RASKOB GE: Low probability lung scan findings: A need for change. Ann Intern Med 114:142, 1991

KUWANO K et al: The diagnosis of mild emphysema: Correlation of computed tomography and pathology scores. Am Rev Respir Dis 141:169, 1990

MILLER NL, MILLER RR: Computed tomography of chronic diffuse infiltrative lung disease. Am Rev Respir Dis 142:1205, 1440, 1990

PEARSON FG: Staging of the mediastinum. Role of mediastinoscopy and computed tomography. Chest 103:346S, 1993

PIOPED INVESTIGATORS: Value of the ventilation-perfusion scan in prospective investigations of pulmonary embolism diagnosis. JAMA 263:2753, 1990

SULAVIK SB et al: Recognition of distinctive patterns of 67-Ga distribution in sarcoidosis. J Nucl Med 31:1909, 1990

TURNER-WARWICK M, HASLAM PL: The value of serial bronchoalveolar lavage in assessing the clinical progress of patients with cryptogenic fibrosing alveolitis. Am Rev Respir Dis 135:26, 1987

217 ASTHMA

E. R. McFADDEN, JR.

DEFINITION Asthma is a disease of airways that is characterized by increased responsiveness of the tracheobronchial tree to a multiplicity of stimuli. Asthma is manifested physiologically by a widespread narrowing of the air passages, which may be relieved spontaneously or as a result of therapy, and clinically by paroxysms of dyspnea, cough, and wheezing. It is an episodic disease, acute exacerbations being interspersed with symptom-free periods. Typically, most attacks are short-lived, lasting minutes to hours, and after them the patient seems to recover completely clinically. However, there can be a phase in which the patient experiences some degree of airway obstruction daily. This phase can be mild, with or without superimposed severe episodes, or much more serious, with severe obstruction persisting for days or weeks, a condition known as *status asthmaticus*. In unusual circumstances, acute episodes can terminate fatally.

PREVALENCE AND ETIOLOGY Asthma is a very common disorder, and it is estimated that 4 to 5 percent of the population of the United States is affected. Similar figures have been reported from other countries. Bronchial asthma occurs at all ages but predominantly in early life. About one-half of the cases develop before age 10, and another third occur before age 40. In childhood, there is a 2:1 male/female preponderance, which equalizes by age 30.

From an etiologic standpoint, asthma is a heterogeneous disease. It is useful for epidemiologic and clinical purposes to classify asthma by the principal stimuli that incite or are associated with acute episodes. However, it is important to emphasize that this distinction may often be artificial, and the response of a given subclassification usually can be initiated by more than one type of stimulus. With this reservation in mind, one can describe two broad groups: allergic and idiosyncratic.

Allergic asthma is often associated with a personal and/or family history of allergic diseases such as rhinitis, urticaria, and eczema; positive wheal-and-flare skin reactions to intradermal injection of extracts of airborne antigens; increased levels of IgE in the serum; and/or positive response to provocation tests involving the inhalation of specific antigen.

A significant segment of the asthmatic population will present with negative family or personal histories of allergy, negative skin tests, and normal serum levels of IgE and therefore cannot be classified on the basis of defined immunologic mechanisms. These we term *idiosyncratic*. Many of these will develop a typical symptom complex upon contracting an upper respiratory illness. The initial insult may be little more than a common cold, but after several days the patient begins to develop paroxysms of wheezing and dyspnea that can last for days to months. These individuals should not be confused with persons in whom the symptoms of bronchospasm are superimposed on chronic bronchitis or bronchiectasis (see Chap. 223).

Unfortunately, many patients will not clearly fit into either of the preceding categories but will fall into a mixed group with features of each. In general, those patients whose onset of disease is in early life will tend to have a strong allergic component to their illness, while those who develop their asthma late tend to be nonallergic or to have mixed etiologies.

PATHOGENESIS OF ASTHMA The common denominator underlying the asthmatic diathesis is a nonspecific hyperirritability of the tracheobronchial tree. In asthmatics it correlates well with the clinical features of the illness. When airway reactivity is high, lung function becomes more unstable, symptoms are more severe and persistent, the acute response to bronchodilators is larger, and the amount of therapy required to control the patient's complaints increases. In addition, the magnitude of diurnal fluctuations in lung function becomes greater, and the patient tends to awaken at night or in the early morning with breathlessness.

In both normal and asthmatic subjects, airway reactivity is known to rise following viral infections of the respiratory tract and exposure to oxidant air pollutants such as ozone and nitrogen dioxide. Viruses have more profound consequences, and following a seemingly trivial upper respiratory tract infection, airway responsivity may remain elevated for many weeks. In contrast, with exposure to ozone, airway reactivity remains high for only a few days. Allergens can cause airway responsiveness to rise within minutes and to remain elevated for weeks. If the dose of antigen is high enough, acute episodes of obstruction may occur daily for a prolonged period of time following a single exposure.

A number of causes have been postulated for the increased airway reactivity of asthma; however, the basic mechanism remains unknown. The most popular hypothesis at present is that of airway inflammation. Following exposure to an initiating stimulus, mediator containing such cells as mast cells, basophils, and macrophages can be activated to release a variety of inflammatory compounds which produce direct effects on airway smooth muscle and capillary permeability, thereby evoking an intense local reaction which can then be followed by a more chronic one. The latter may be brought about by the release of chemotactic factors which recruit cellular elements to the site of injury. In addition, it is thought that the acute and chronic effects of mediator release and cellular infiltration may result in epithelial damage with involvement of neural endings within the airways and the activation of an axon reflex. In this fashion, an essentially local phenomenon can be amplified to have widespread effects throughout the tracheobronchial tree.

The stimuli that interact with airway responsiveness and incite acute episodes of asthma can be grouped into seven major categories: allergenic, pharmacologic, environmental, occupational, infectious, exercise-related, and emotional.

Allergens Allergic asthma is dependent on an IgE response controlled by T and B lymphocytes and activated by the interaction of antigen with mast cell–bound IgE molecules. Most of the allergens that provoke asthma are airborne, and in order to induce a state of sensitivity, they must be reasonably abundant for considerable periods of time. Once sensitization has occurred, however, the patient can then exhibit exquisite responsivity so that minute amounts of the offending agent can produce significant exacerbations of the disease. Immunologic mechanisms appear to be causally related to the development of asthma in 25 to 35 percent of all cases and contributory in perhaps another third. Higher prevalences have been suggested, but it is difficult to know how to interpret the data because of confounding factors. Allergic asthma is frequently seasonal, and it is most often observed in children and young adults. A nonseasonal form may result from allergy to feathers, animal danders, dust mites, molds, and other antigens present continuously in the environment. Exposure to antigen typically produces an immediate response in which airway obstruction develops in minutes and then resolves. In 30 to 50 percent of patients, a second wave of bronchoconstriction, the so-called late reaction, develops 6 to 10 h later. In a minority, only a late reaction occurs. It was formerly thought that the late reaction was essential to the development of the increase in airway reactivity that follows antigen exposure. Recent data show this not to be the case.

PATHOGENESIS The mechanism by which an inhaled antigen provokes an acute episode of asthma is unknown but seems to depend, in part, on antigen-antibody interactions on the surface of pulmonary mast cells with the subsequent generation and release of the mediators of immediate hypersensitivity. Current postulates hold that very small antigenic particles penetrate the lung's defenses and come in contact with mast cells that are interdigitating with the epithelium at the luminal surface of the central airways. (No mechanism has yet been proposed that explains how antigen can contact the mast cells in the submucosa.) The subsequent elaboration of mediators then produces the sequence outlined above. The mediators released—histamine; bradykinin; the leukotrienes C, D, and E; platelet-activating factor; prostaglandins PGE_2, $PGF_{2\alpha}$, and PGD_2, and thromboxane A_2— produce an intense inflammatory reaction with bronchoconstriction, vascular congestion, and edema formation. In addition to their ability to produce prolonged contraction of airway smooth muscle and mucosal edema, the leukotrienes also produce some of the other pathophysiologic features of asthma, such as increased mucus production and impaired mucociliary transport. The chemotactic factors elaborated (eosinophil and neutrophil chemotactic factors of anaphylaxis and leukotriene B_4) bring eosinophils, platelets, and polymorphonuclear leukocytes to the site of the reaction. One of the most important of these may be the eosinophil; when activated, these cells can produce leukotriene C_4 and platelet-activating factor and thereby contribute directly to airway narrowing and edema. They also can cause mast cells to release histamine and chemotactic factors which could set up a self-sustaining cycle in which additional secondary effector cells including more eosinophils are brought to the site of the reaction. Equally important, degranulation of eosinophils can release major basic protein and eosinophil cationic protein into the airways, thus causing cilia to stop beating and disrupting mucosal integrity with exfoliation of cells into the bronchial lumen in the form of Creola bodies.

While the preceding theories concerning pathogenesis are attractive, translation of the cellular events into precise pathophysiologic sequences is difficult and incomplete. For example, mediators per se cannot explain the whole picture, for they have been found in the blood of individuals with mast cell diseases such as cold-induced and cholinergic-induced urticaria and the airways of atopic nonasthmatics. Since these individuals were devoid of any lower respiratory illness or complaints, the alleged mediators of asthma appear to need a unique substrate upon which to exhibit their effects. Similarly, the inflammatory cells believed to be important in asthma are also found in the airways of atopic nonasthmatics, raising the possibility that they are merely nonspecific markers of atopy rather than specific indices of asthma.

Pharmacologic stimuli The drugs most commonly associated with the induction of acute episodes of asthma are aspirin, coloring agents such as tartrazine, beta-adrenergic antagonists, and sulfiting agents. The typical aspirin-sensitive respiratory syndrome primarily affects adults, although the condition may be seen in childhood. This problem usually begins with perennial vasomotor rhinitis that is followed by a hyperplastic rhinosinusitis with nasal polyps. Progressive asthma then appears. On exposure to even very small quantities of aspirin, affected individuals typically develop ocular and nasal congestion and acute, often severe episodes of airway obstruction. The prevalence of aspirin sensitivity in asthmatic subjects varies from

study to study, but many authorities feel that 10 percent is a reasonable figure. There is a great deal of cross reactivity between aspirin and other nonsteroidal anti-inflammatory compounds. Indomethacin, fenoprofen, naproxen, zomepirac sodium, ibuprofen, mefenamic acid, and phenylbutazone are particularly important in this regard. On the other hand, acetaminophen, sodium salicylate, choline salicylate, salicylamide, and propoxyphene are well tolerated. The exact frequency of cross reactivity to tartrazine and other dyes in aspirin-sensitive asthmatic subjects is also controversial, and again, 10 percent is the commonly accepted figure. This peculiar complication of aspirin-sensitive asthma is particularly insidious, however, in that tartrazine and other potentially troublesome dyes are widely present in the environment and may be unknowingly ingested by sensitive patients.

Patients with aspirin sensitivity can be desensitized by daily administration of the drug. Following this form of therapy, cross tolerance also develops to other nonsteroidal anti-inflammatory agents. The mechanism by which aspirin and other such drugs produce bronchospasm is unknown but may be related to aspirin-induced preferential generation of leukotrienes. Immediate hypersensitivity does not seem to be involved.

Beta-adrenergic antagonists regularly produce airway obstruction in asthmatics as well as in others with heightened airway reactivity and should be avoided in such individuals. Even the selective $beta_1$ agents have this propensity, particularly at higher doses. In fact, even the local use of $beta_1$ blockers in the eye for the treatment of glaucoma has been associated with worsening asthma.

Sulfiting agents, such as potassium metabisulfite, potassium and sodium bisulfite, sodium sulfite, and sulfur dioxide, which are widely used in the food and pharmaceutical industry as sanitizing and preservative agents, also can produce acute airway obstruction in sensitive individuals. Exposure usually follows ingestion of food or beverages containing these compounds, e.g., salads, fresh fruit, potatoes, shellfish, and wine. Exacerbation of asthma has been reported following the use of sulfite-containing topical ophthalmic solutions, intravenous glucocorticoids, and some inhalational bronchodilator solutions. The incidence and mechanism of action of this phenomenon are unknown. When suspected, the diagnosis can be confirmed by either oral or inhalational provocations.

Environment and air pollution (See Chap. 219) Environmental causes of asthma are usually related to climatic conditions that promote the concentration of atmospheric pollutants and antigens. These conditions tend to develop in heavy industrial or densely populated urban areas and are frequently associated with thermal inversions or other situations associated with stagnant air masses. In these circumstances, although the general population can develop respiratory symptoms, patients with asthma and other respiratory diseases tend to be more severely affected. The air pollutants known to have this effect are ozone, nitrogen dioxide, and sulfur dioxide. The last needs to be present in high concentrations and produces its greatest effects during periods of high ventilation.

Occupational factors (See Chap. 219) Occupation-related asthma is a significant health problem, and acute and chronic airway obstruction has been reported to follow exposure to a large number of compounds used in many types of industrial processes. Bronchoconstriction can result from working with, or exposure to, *metal salts* (e.g., platinum, chrome, and nickel), *wood and vegetable dusts* (e.g., oak, western red cedar, grain, flour, castor bean, green coffee bean, mako, gum acacia, karay gum, and tragacanth), *pharmaceutical agents* (e.g., antibiotics, piperazine, and cimetidine), *industrial chemicals and plastics* (e.g., toluene diisocyanate, phthalic acid anhydride, trimellitic anhydride, persulfates, ethylenediamine, para-phenylenediamine, and various dyes), *biologic enzymes* (e.g., laundry detergents and pancreatic enzymes), and *animal and insect dusts, serums, and secretions*. It is important to recognize that exposure to sensitizing chemicals, particularly those used in paints, solvents, and plastics, also can occur during leisure or non-work-related activities. The underlying mechanisms for this airway obstruction appear to be three in number: (1) in some cases the offending agent results in the formation of a specific IgE, and the cause seems immunologic (the immunologic reaction can be immediate, late, or dual); (2) materials being employed, in other cases, cause a direct liberation of bronchoconstrictor substances; and (3) work-related irritant substances, in still other cases, directly or reflexly stimulate the airways of either latent or frank asthmatics. With occupational exposures, other than those which give an immediate and dual immunologic reaction, the patients give a characteristic cyclic history. They are well when they arrive at work, and symptoms develop toward the end of the shift, progress after leaving the work site, and then regress. Absence from work during weekends or vacation periods brings about a remission. Frequently, there are similar symptoms in fellow employees.

Infections Respiratory infections are the most common of the stimuli that evoke acute exacerbations of asthma. Well-controlled investigations have demonstrated that respiratory viruses and not bacteria or allergy are the major etiologic factors. In young children, the most important infectious agents are respiratory syncytial virus and parainfluenza virus. In older children and adults, rhinovirus and influenza virus predominate as pathogens. Simple colonization of the tracheobronchial tree is insufficient to evoke acute episodes of bronchospasm, and attacks of asthma occur only when symptoms of an ongoing respiratory tract infection are, or have been, present. The mechanism by which viruses induce asthma is unknown, but it is probable that the resulting inflammatory changes in the airway mucosa alter host defenses and make the tracheobronchial tree more susceptible to exogenous stimuli. Supporting evidence for this concept is derived from the fact that the airway responsiveness of even normal (nonasthmatic) subjects to nonspecific stimuli is transiently increased after a viral infection. Increased airway responsiveness, associated with cough and rarely wheezing, can last from 2 to 8 weeks after the infection in both normal individuals and asthmatics.

Exercise Exercise is one of the most common precipitants of acute episodes of asthma. This stimulus differs from other naturally occurring provocations such as antigen or viral infections in that it does not evoke any long-term sequelae nor does it change airway reactivity. Initiation of bronchospasm by exercise is probably operative to some extent in every asthmatic patient, and in some it may be the only trigger mechanism that will produce symptoms. When such patients are followed for sufficient periods of time, they often develop recurring episodes of airway obstruction independent of exercise; thus the onset of this problem frequently can serve as the first manifestation of the full-blown asthmatic syndrome. There is a significant interaction among the ventilation achieved by the exercise task, the temperature, and water content of the inspired air and the magnitude of the postexertional obstruction. Thus, for the same inspired air conditions, running will produce a more severe attack of asthma than will walking. Conversely, for a given task, the inhalation of cold air during its performance will markedly enhance the response, while warm, humid air will blunt or abolish it. Consequently, activities such as ice hockey, cross-country skiing, or ice skating are more provocative than is swimming in an indoor heated pool. The mechanism by which exercise produces obstruction may be related to a thermally produced hyperemia and engorgement of the microvasculature of the bronchial wall and does not appear to involve smooth-muscle contraction.

Emotional stress Abundant objective data exist which demonstrate that psychological factors can interact with the asthmatic diathesis to worsen or ameliorate the disease process. The pathways and nature of the interactions are complex but have been shown to be operational to some extent in almost half the patients studied. Changes in airway caliber seem to be mediated through modification of vagal efferent activity, but endorphins also may play a role. The most frequently studied variable has been that of suggestion, and the weight of current evidence is that it can be quite an important influence in selected asthmatics. When psychically responsive individuals are given the appropriate suggestion, they can actually decrease or increase the pharmacologic effects of adrenergic and cholinergic

stimuli on their airways. The extent to which psychological factors participate in the induction and/or continuation of any given acute exacerbation is unknown but probably varies from patient to patient and in the same patient from episode to episode.

PATHOLOGY In a patient who has died of acute asthma, the most striking feature of the lungs at necropsy is their gross overdistention and failure to collapse when the pleural cavities are opened. When the lungs are cut, numerous gelatinous plugs of exudate are found in the majority of the bronchial branches down to the terminal bronchiole. Histologic examination shows hypertrophy of the bronchial smooth muscle, hyperplasia of mucosal and submucosal vessels, mucosal edema, denudation of the surface epithelium, pronounced thickening of the basement membrane, and eosinophilic infiltrates in the bronchial wall. In asthmatic patients who die from trauma and causes other than asthma itself, mucous casts, basement membrane thickening, and eosinophilic infiltrates are frequently observed. In both situations there is an absence of any of the well-recognized forms of destructive emphysema. It is now recognized that infiltration of the mucosa and submucosa with eosinophils and other inflammatory cells, as well as epithelial damage and denudation, exist in airway biopsies from asymptomatic asthmatics. These findings, in concert with those in airway mediator levels, have given rise to the construct that asthma is a chronic inflammatory disease.

PATHOPHYSIOLOGY The pathophysiologic hallmark of asthma is a reduction in airway diameter brought about by contraction of smooth muscle, vascular congestion, edema of the bronchial wall, and thick tenacious secretions. The net result is an increase in airway resistance, decreased forced expiratory volumes and flow rates, hyperinflation of the lungs and thorax, increased work of breathing, alterations in respiratory muscle function, changes in elastic recoil, abnormal distribution of both ventilation and pulmonary blood flow with mismatched ratios, and altered arterial blood gases. Thus, although asthma is considered to be primarily a disease of airways, virtually all aspects of pulmonary function are compromised during an acute attack. In addition, in very symptomatic patients there frequently is electrocardiographic evidence of right ventricular hypertrophy and pulmonary hypertension. When a patient presents for therapy, his or her forced vital capacity tends to be ≤50 percent of normal. The 1-s forced expiratory volume (FEV_1) averages 30 percent or less of predicted, while the maximum and minimum midexpiratory flow rates are reduced to 20 percent or less of expected. In keeping with the alterations in mechanics, the associated air trapping is substantial. In acutely ill patients, residual volume (RV) frequently approaches 400 percent of normal, while functional residual capacity doubles. The patients tend to report that their attacks have ended clinically when their RV has fallen to 200 percent of its predicted value and when the FEV_1 rises to 50 percent.

Hypoxia is a universal finding during acute exacerbations, but frank ventilatory failure is relatively uncommon, being observed in 10 to 15 percent of patients presenting for therapy. Most asthmatics have hypocapnia and a respiratory alkalosis. In acutely ill patients, the finding of a normal arterial carbon dioxide tension tends to be associated with quite severe levels of obstruction. Consequently, when found in a symptomatic individual, it should be viewed as impending respiratory failure and treated as such. Equally, the presence of metabolic acidosis in the setting of acute asthma heralds severe obstruction. Usually, there are no clinical counterparts to the derangements in blood gases. Cyanosis is a very late sign. Hence a dangerous level of hypoxia can go undetected. Likewise, the signs which are attributable to carbon dioxide retention, such as sweating, tachycardia, and wide pulse pressure, or to acidosis, such as tachypnea, do not tend to be of great value in predicting the presence of hypercapnia or hydrogen ion excess in individual patients, for they are too frequently seen in anxious patients with more moderate disease to be of much use. Thus trying to judge the state of an acutely ill patient's ventilatory status on clinical grounds alone can be extremely hazardous and should not be relied on with any confidence. Arterial blood gas tensions, therefore, must be measured.

may be dangerous. There is some evidence that addition of anticholinergics may enhance the bronchodilation achieved by sympathomimetics, but the effect is not large. The major disadvantages of the anticholinergics are that they are slow to act (60 to 90 min may be required before peak bronchodilation is achieved) and they are only of modest potency.

MISCELLANEOUS   It has been suggested that steroid-dependent patients might benefit from the use of immunosuppressant agents such as methotrexate or gold salts. The effects of these agents on steroid dosage and disease activity are minor, and side effects can be considerable. Consequently, this form of treatment can only be viewed as experimental. Opiates, sedatives, and tranquilizers should be absolutely avoided in the acutely ill asthmatic because the risk of depressing alveolar ventilation is great and respiratory arrest has been reported to occur shortly after their use. Admittedly most individuals are anxious and frightened, but experience has shown that they can be calmed equally well by the physician's presence and reassurances. Beta-adrenergic blockers and parasympathetic agonists are contraindicated because they can cause marked deterioration in lung function.

Expectorants and mucolytic agents have enjoyed great vogue in the past, but they do not add significantly to the treatment of the acute or chronic phases of this disease. Mucolytic agents such as acetylcysteine may actually produce bronchospasm when administered to susceptible asthmatics. This can be overcome by aerosolizing them in solution with a beta-adrenergic agent. The use of intravenous fluids in the treatment of acute asthma also has been advocated. There is little evidence to indicate that this adjunct hastens recovery.

SPECIAL INSTRUCTIONS   The treatment of patients with asthma who have coexisting conditions such as heart disease or pregnancy does not differ materially from that outlined above. Inhaled therapy with beta$_2$-selective and anti-inflammatory agents is the mainstay. The doses of adrenergics administered should be the lowest possible quantities required to produce the desired therapeutic effects.

FRAMEWORK FOR MANAGEMENT   Emergency situations
The most efficacious form of treatment for acute episodes of asthma are aerosolized beta$_2$ agonists. These drugs provide three to four times more relief than intravenous aminophylline. In emergency situations, they can be given every 20 minutes by hand-held nebulizer for three doses. Thereafter, the frequency can be reduced to every 2 h until the attack has subsided. Aminophylline can be added to the regimen after the first hour in an attempt to speed resolution.

Acute episodes of bronchial asthma represent one of the most common respiratory emergencies seen in the practice of medicine, and it is essential that the physician recognize which episodes of airway obstruction are life-threatening and which patients demand what level of care. This can be readily accomplished by assessing selected clinical parameters in combination with measures of expiratory flow and gas exchange. The presence of a paradoxical pulse, use of accessory muscles, and marked hyperinflation of the thorax signify severe airway obstruction, and failure of these signs to remit within short order following aggressive therapy mandates objective monitoring of the patient using arterial blood gases and the peak expiratory flow rate (PEFR) or FEV_1.

In general, there is a direct correlation between the severity of the obstruction with which the patient presents and the time that it takes to resolve it. Those individuals with the most impairment typically require the most extensive therapy for resolution. If the PEFR or FEV_1 is equal to or less than 20 percent of predicted on presentation and does not double within an hour of receiving the preceding therapy, the patient is likely to require extensive treatment including glucocorticoids before the obstruction dissipates. In such circumstances, if the clinical signs of a paradoxical pulse and accessory muscle use are diminishing, and/or if PEFR is increasing, there is no need to change medications or doses. One need only to continue to follow the patient. If, however, PEFR is falling or the magnitude of pulsus paradoxicus is increasing, serial measures of arterial blood gases are required as well as a reconsideration of the therapeutic modalities being employed. If the patient has hypocarbia, one can

afford to continue the current approaches a while longer. On the other hand, if the Pa_{CO_2} is within the normal range or is elevated, the patient should be monitored in an intensive care setting, and therapy should be intensified in order to reverse or arrest the patient's respiratory failure.

Chronic treatment   The goal of chronic therapy is to achieve a stable, asymptomatic state with the best pulmonary function possible. As in the acute situation, first-line therapy should be a beta$_2$ agonist by inhalation. In patients who have difficulty coordinating inhalation with activation of a metered-dose inhaler, a spacing device should be incorporated. If nocturnal complaints continue, a long-acting theophylline compound given at night may be included.

In patients with persistent symptoms and unstable lung function despite adequate bronchodilator therapy, treatment with inhaled steroids and/or mast cell stabilizing agents should be instituted. Since these agents frequently take weeks to lower airway reactivity, it may be efficacious to start a short but intense course of oral glucocorticoids to speed the remission. During this process, PEFR should be monitored and medication adjustments should be based on objective changes in lung function as well as the patient's symptoms. Once the asthma has stabilized, there should be a systematic reduction in medication, beginning with the most toxic, to find the minimum required to maintain the patient's well-being.

PROGNOSIS AND CLINICAL COURSE   The mortality from asthma is small. The most recent figures indicate less than 5000 deaths per year out of a population of approximately 10 million patients at risk. Death rates, however, appear to be rising in inner-city areas where there is limited availability of health care.

Information on the clinical course of asthma suggests a good prognosis for 50 to 80 percent of all patients, particularly those whose disease is mild and develops in childhood. The number of children still having asthma 7 to 10 years after the initial diagnosis varies from 26 to 78 percent, with an average of 46 percent; however, the percentage who continue to have severe disease is relatively low (6 to 19 percent).

Unlike other airway diseases such as chronic bronchitis, asthma is not progressive. Although there are reports of patients with asthma developing irreversible changes in lung function, these individuals frequently have comorbid stimuli such as cigarette smoking that could account for these findings. Even when untreated, asthmatics do not continuously move from mild to severe disease with time. Rather, their clinical course is characterized by exacerbations and remissions. Some studies suggest that spontaneous remissions occur in approximately 20 percent of those who develop the disease as adults and 40 percent or so can be expected to improve with less frequent and severe attacks as they grow older.

REFERENCES

AMERICAN THORACIC SOCIETY: Guidelines for the Evaluation of impairment/disability in patients with asthma. Am Rev Respir Dis 147:1056, 1993

BURR ML: Epidemiology of asthma. Monogr Allergy 31:80, 1993

HOLGATE S: Mediator and cytokine mechanisms in asthma. Thorax 48:103, 1993

KALINER MA, McFADDEN ER JR: Bronchial asthma, in Immunological Diseases, M Samter et al (eds). Boston, Little Brown, 1988, pp 1067–1118

KEMP JP: Approaches to asthma management. Realities and recommendations. Arch Intern Med 153:805, 1993

McFADDEN ER JR: Pulmonary structure, physiology and clinical correlates in asthma, in Allergy: Principles and Practice, E Middleton et al (eds). St Louis, Mosby, 1993

——, GILBERT IA: Asthma. N Engl J Med 327:1928, 1992

SHEFFER AL, TAGGART VS: The National Asthma Education Program. Expert panel report guidelines for the diagnosis and management of asthma. Med Care 31:MS20, 1993

SKORODIN MS: Pharmacotherapy for asthma and chronic obstructive pulmonary disease. Current thinking, practices, and controversies. Arch Intern Med 153:814, 1993

WARDLAW AJ: The role of air pollution in asthma. Clin Exp Allergy 23:81, 1993

218 HYPERSENSITIVITY PNEUMONITIS AND EOSINOPHILIC PNEUMONIAS

GARY W. HUNNINGHAKE / HAL B. RICHERSON

HYPERSENSITIVITY PNEUMONITIS

Hypersensitivity pneumonitis (HP), or extrinsic allergic alveolitis, is an immunologically induced inflammation of the lung parenchyma, involving alveolar walls and terminal airways, secondary to repeated inhalation of a variety of organic dusts and other agents by a susceptible host. In contrast to many of the other interstitial lung diseases, the cause of this interstitial and alveolar filling disease is known. The prevalence of HP is unknown but varies with the environmental exposure and the antigen involved. The prevalence of farmer's lung among Wisconsin dairy farmers has been reported as 42 per 100,000. The diagnosis of HP requires a constellation of clinical, radiographic, physiologic, pathologic, and immunologic criteria, each of which is rarely pathognomonic alone, and the preferred treatment is avoidance of the causative antigen when practical.

ETIOLOGY Agents implicated as causes of HP include those listed in Table 218-1. Many cases of HP occurring in various occupations involve exposure to similar agents, particularly the thermophilic actinomycetes. The common sources of causative antigens are "moldy" hay, silage, or grain; pet birds; and heating, cooling, and humidification systems. Simple chemicals, such as isocyanates, may also cause hypersensitivity pneumonitis.

PATHOGENESIS The finding that precipitating antibodies against extracts of moldy hay were demonstrable in most patients with farmer's lung led to the early conclusion that HP was an immune-complex-mediated reaction. Subsequent investigations of HP in human beings and animal models provided evidence for the importance of cell-mediated hypersensitivity. The very early (acute) reaction is characterized by an increase in polymorphonuclear leukocytes in the alveoli and small airways. This early lesion is followed by an influx of mononuclear cells into the lung and the formation of granulomas. The latter lesion appears to be a classic delayed hypersensitivity reaction to repeated inhalation of antigen and adjuvant-active materials.

Bronchoalveolar lavage (Chap. 216) in patients with HP consistently demonstrates an increase in T lymphocytes in lavage fluid (a finding that is also observed in patients with other granulomatous lung disorders). Patients with recent or continual exposure to antigen may also have an increase in polymorphonuclear leukocytes in lavage fluid. Increased numbers of mast cells have also been reported. In most patients examined during recovery from acute disease, the T lymphocytes in lavage fluid are predominantly the CD8+ T-cell subset. In patients with very recent exposure to antigen, however, the numbers of CD4+ T cells may increase in lavage fluid. Similar findings may be present in similarly exposed, asymptomatic individuals. These observations suggest that there is an active modulation of granuloma formation in the lung by immunoregulatory T cells in this disorder.

CLINICAL PRESENTATION The *clinical picture* is that of an interstitial pneumonitis, although it varies from patient to patient and is related to the frequency and intensity of exposure to the causative

TABLE 218-1 Selected examples of hypersensitivity pneumonitis (HP)

Disease	Antigen	Source of antigen
Bagassosis	Thermophilic actinomycetes	"Moldy" bagasse (sugar cane)
Bird fancier's, breeder's, or handler's lung	Parakeet, budgerigar, pigeon, chicken, turkey proteins	Avian droppings or feathers
Cephalosporium HP	Contaminated basement (sewage)	*Cephalosporium*
Cheese washer's lung	*Penicillium casei*	Moldy cheese
Chemical worker's lung	Isocyanates	Polyurethane foam, varnishes, lacquer, foundry casting
Coffee worker's lung	Coffee bean dust	Coffee beans
Compost lung	*Aspergillus*	Compost
Detergent worker's disease	*Bacillus subtilis* enzymes	Detergent
Familial HP	*Bacillus subtilis*	Contaminated wood dust in walls
Farmer's lung	Thermophilic actinomycetes*	"Moldy" hay, grain, silage
Fish meal worker's lung	Fish meal dust	Fish meal
Furrier's lung	Animal fur dust	Animal pelts
Hot tub lung	*Cladosporium* sp.	Mold on ceiling
Humidifier or air-conditioner lung (ventilation pneumonitis)	*Aureobasidium pullulans* or other microorganisms	Contaminated water in humidification and forced-air air-conditioning systems
Japanese summer house HP	*Trichosporon cutaneum*	House dust? Bird droppings
Laboratory worker's HP	Male rat urine	Laboratory rat
Lycoperdonosis	*Lycoperdon* puffballs	Puffball spores
Malt worker's lung	*Aspergillus fumigatus* or *A. clavatus*	Moldy barley
Maple bark disease	*Cryptostroma corticale*	Maple bark
Miller's lung	*Sitophilus granarius* (wheat weevil)	Infested wheat flour
Mushroom worker's lung	Thermophilic actinomycetes,* other	Mushroom compost
Paulis HP	Paulis reagent	Laboratory reagent
Pituitary snuff taker's lung	Animal proteins	Heterologous pituitary snuff
Potato riddler's lung	Thermophilic actinomycetes,* *Aspergillus*	"Moldy" hay around potatoes
Sauna taker's lung	*Auerobasidium* sp., other	Contaminated sauna water
Sequoiosis	*Aureobasidium, Graphium* sp.	Redwood sawdust
Streptomyces albus HP	*Streptomyces albus*	Contaminated fertilizer
Suberosis	Cork dust mold	Cork dust
Tap water lung	Unknown	Contaminated tap water
Thatched roof disease	*Saccharomonospora viridis*	Dried grasses and leaves
Tobacco worker's disease	*Aspergillus* sp.	Mold on tobacco
Winegrower's lung	*Botrytis cinerea*	Mold on grapes
Wood trimmer's disease	*Rhizopus* sp., *Mucor* sp.	Contaminated wood trimmings
Woodman's disease	*Pencillium* sp.	Oak and maple trees
Woodworker's lung	Wood dust; *Alternaria*	Oak, cedar, and mahogany dusts; pine and spruce pulp

* Thermophilic actinomycetes species include *Micropolyspora faeni, Thermoactinomyces vulgaris, T. saccharrii, T. viridis,* and *T. candidus.*

antigen and perhaps other host factors. The presentation can be *acute, subacute,* or *chronic.* In the *acute form,* symptoms such as cough, fever, chills, malaise, and dyspnea may occur 6 to 8 h after exposure to the antigen and usually clear within a few days if there is no further exposure to antigen. The *subacute form* often appears insidiously over a period of weeks marked by cough and dyspnea and may progress to cyanosis and severe dyspnea requiring hospitalization. In some patients, a subacute form of the disease may persist after an acute presentation of the disorder, especially if there is continued exposure to antigen. In most patients with the acute or subacute form of HP, the symptoms, signs, and other manifestations of HP disappear within days, weeks, or months if the causative agent is no longer inhaled. Transformation to a chronic form of the disease may occur in patients with continued antigen exposure, but the frequency of such progression is uncertain. The *chronic form* may also present as a gradually progressive interstitial disease associated with cough and exertional dyspnea without a prior history consistent with acute or subacute manifestations. Such a gradual onset frequently occurs with low-dose exposure to the antigen.

DIAGNOSIS Following acute exposure to antigen, neutrophilia and lymphopenia are frequently present. Eosinophilia is not a feature. All forms of the disease may be associated with elevations in erythrocyte sedimentation rate, C-reactive protein, rheumatoid factor, and serum immunoglobulins. Antinuclear antibodies are rarely present.

Examination for *serum precipitins* against suspected antigens, such as those listed in Table 218-1, is an important part of the diagnostic workup and should be performed on any patient with interstitial lung disease, especially if a suggestive exposure history is elicited. If found, precipitins indicate sufficient exposure to the causative agent for generation of an immunologic response. The diagnosis of HP is not established solely by the presence of precipitins, however, as precipitins are found in sera of many individuals exposed to appropriate antigens who demonstrate no other evidence of HP. False-negative results may occur because of poor-quality antigens or an inappropriate choice of antigens. Extraction of antigens from the patient's environment may at times be helpful.

No specific or distinctive *chest roentgenogram* occurs in HP. It can be normal even in symptomatic patients. The acute or subacute phase may be associated with poorly defined, patchy, or diffuse infiltrates or with discrete, nodular infiltrates. In the chronic phase, the chest x-ray usually shows a diffuse reticulonodular infiltrate. Honeycombing may eventually develop as the condition progresses. Abnormalities rarely seen in HP include pleural effusion or thickening, and hilar adenopathy. High-resolution chest computed tomography (CT) has been reported to show a characteristic constellation of abnormalities, providing support for an otherwise uncertain clinical diagnosis, although no pathognomonic CT features of HP have been described.

Pulmonary function studies in all forms of HP typically show a restrictive pattern with loss of lung volumes, impaired diffusion capacity, decreased compliance, and an exercise-induced hypoxemia. A resting hypoxemia may be found. Functional abnormalities may gradually increase in severity or may occur rapidly following acute or subacute exposure to antigen. As the chronic stage progresses, changes consistent with airway obstruction may become increasingly prominent.

Bronchoalveolar lavage is used in some centers to aid in diagnostic evaluation, and the characteristic features of the lavage fluid are described above.

Lung biopsy may be indicated in patients without sufficient other criteria to make a definitive diagnosis. The initial biopsy procedure is usually a transbronchial biopsy. In some patients, an open-lung biopsy may be necessary, as this procedure will provide adequate material for pathologic studies whereas transbronchial biopsy may not. Although the histopathology is distinctive, it may not be pathognomonic of HP. When the biopsy is taken during the active phase of disease, typical findings include an interstitial alveolar infiltrate consisting of plasma cells, lymphocytes, and occasional eosinophils and neutrophils, usually with accompanying granulomas. Interstitial fibrosis may be present but most often is mild in earlier stages of the disease. Some degree of bronchiolitis is found in about half the cases, whereas vasculitis is not a feature of the disorder. The triad of mononuclear bronchiolitis, interstitial infiltrates of lymphocytes and plasma cells, and single, nonnecrotizing, and randomly scattered parenchymal granulomas without mural vascular involvement is consistent with but not specific for HP.

The lack of standardized, nonirritating antigens and of proven controlled protocols makes *skin testing* and *inhalational challenge* useful only for research purposes. Similarly, *in vitro tests of cell-mediated (delayed) hypersensitivity* have not been shown to consistently correlate with clinical HP and have no place in the routine diagnostic workup.

In summary, the diagnosis in most cases is established by (1) consistent history, physical findings, pulmonary function tests, and chest x-ray; (2) exposure to a recognized antigen; and (3) finding an antibody to that antigen. In a few circumstances, bronchoalveolar lavage and/or lung biopsy may be needed. Provocation tests are research procedures and are not indicated.

DIFFERENTIAL DIAGNOSIS Chronic HP may often be difficult to distinguish from a number of other interstitial lung disorders such as idiopathic pulmonary fibrosis, interstitial lung disease associated with a collagen vascular disorder, and drug-induced lung diseases. A negative history for use of appropriate drugs and no evidence of a systemic disorder usually exclude the presence of drug-induced lung disease or a collagen vascular disorder. Bronchoalveolar lavage often shows predominance of neutrophils in idiopathic pulmonary fibrosis and a predominance of CD4+ lymphocytes in sarcoidosis. The diagnosis of sarcoidosis is also favored by hilar lymph node involvement or evidence of multisystem involvement. In some patients, a lung biopsy may be required to differentiate chronic HP from other interstitial diseases.

The lung disease associated with acute or subacute HP may clinically resemble other disorders that present with systemic symptoms and recurrent pulmonary infiltrates. These disorders include the collagen vascular disorders, drug-induced lung disease, allergic bronchopulmonary aspergillosis, and other eosinophilic pneumonias. Eosinophilic pneumonia is often associated with asthma and is typified by peripheral eosinophilia; neither of these is a feature of HP. Allergic bronchopulmonary aspergillosis is sometimes confused with HP because of the presence of precipitating antibodies to *Aspergillus fumigatus.* It is an obstructive rather than a restrictive lung disease, however, that is associated with allergic (atopic) asthma.

The term *inorganic dust toxic syndrome* has been applied to a condition often mistaken for HP; it follows heavy exposure to organic dusts and is characterized by transient fever and muscle aches, with or without respiratory symptoms. Serum precipitins are absent, and the chest x-ray is usually normal.

Massive exposure to moldy silage may result in a syndrome termed *pulmonary mycotoxicosis* or *atypical farmer's lung* with fever, chills, and cough and the presence of pulmonary infiltrates within a few hours of exposure. No previous sensitization is required, and precipitins are absent to *Aspergillus,* the suspected causative agent.

TREATMENT Because effective treatment depends largely on avoiding the antigen, identification of the causative agent and its source is essential. This is usually possible if the physician takes a careful environmental and occupational history or, if necessary, visits the patient's environment.

The simplest way to avoid the incriminated agent is to remove the patient from the environment or the source of the agent from the patient's environment. This recommendation cannot be taken lightly when it completely changes the life-style or livelihood of the patient. In many cases, however, the source of exposure (birds, humidifiers) can easily be removed. If occupational exposure is involved, an initial attempt can be made at antigen avoidance maneuvers least disruptive to the patient's livelihood, which usually means avoiding areas associated with heavy exposure and wearing an appropriate mask. This will not suffice for small-molecular-weight agents such as isocyanates, which require elaborate filtration devices. Pollen masks, personal dust respirators, airstream helmets, and ventilated helmets with a supply of fresh air are increasingly efficient means of purifying inhaled air. If symptoms recur or physiologic abnormalities progress in spite of these measures, then more effective measures to avoid antigen exposure must be pursued.

Compromises with environmental control pertain primarily to the acute, recurrent, transient clinical form of HP and must be accompanied by careful follow-up. Subacute forms are ordinarily the result of a heavy, sustained exposure. The chronic form typically results from low-grade or recurrent exposure over many months to years, and the lung disease may already be partially irreversible. These patients should be advised to avoid completely all possible contact with the offending agent, although follow-up studies of farmer's lung and bird fancier's lung have found resolution of the disease despite continued exposure in some patients.

Patients with the *acute*, recurrent form of HP usually recover without need for glucocorticoids. *Subacute* HP may be associated with severe symptoms and marked physiologic impairment and may continue to progress for several days despite hospitalization. Urgent establishment of the diagnosis and prompt institution of glucocorticoid treatment are indicated in such patients. Such therapy may also hasten recovery in patients with lesser involvement. Prednisone at a dosage of 1 mg/kg per day or its equivalent is continued for 7 to 14 days and then tapered over the ensuing 2 to 6 weeks at a rate that depends on the patient's clinical status.

Patients with *chronic* HP may gradually recover without therapy following environmental control. In many patients, however, a trial of prednisone may be useful to obtain maximal reversibility of the lung disease. Following initial prednisone therapy (1 mg/kg per day for 2 to 4 weeks), the drug is tapered to the lowest dosage that will maintain the functional status of the patient. Many patients will not require or benefit from long-term therapy if there is no further exposure to antigen. Available studies report no effect of glucocorticoid therapy on long-term prognosis of farmer's lung.

EOSINOPHILIC PNEUMONIAS

Eosinophilic pneumonias are composed of distinct individual syndromes characterized by eosinophilic pulmonary infiltrates and, commonly, peripheral blood eosinophilia. Since Loeffler's initial description of a transient, benign syndrome of migratory pulmonary infiltrates and peripheral blood eosinophilia of unknown cause, this group of disorders has been enlarged to include several diseases of both known and unknown etiology (Table 218-2). These diseases may be considered as examples of hypersensitivity lung disease but are not to be confused with hypersensitivity pneumonitis (extrinsic allergic alveolitis) in which eosinophilia is not a feature.

When an eosinophilic pneumonia is associated with bronchial asthma, it is important to determine if the patient has extrinsic (allergic, atopic) asthma and has wheal-and-flare skin reactivity to

TABLE 218-2 Eosinophilic pneumonias

ETIOLOGY KNOWN

Allergic bronchopulmonary aspergillosis
Parasitic infestations
Drug reactions

IDIOPATHIC

Loeffler's syndrome
Chronic eosinophilic pneumonia
Allergic granulomatosis of Churg and Strauss
Hypereosinophilic syndrome

TABLE 218-3 Diagnostic features of allergic bronchopulmonary aspergillosis (ABPA)

MAIN DIAGNOSTIC CRITERIA

1 Bronchial asthma
2 Pulmonary infiltrates
3 Peripheral eosinophilia ($> 1000/\mu$L)
4 Immediate wheal-and-flare response to *Aspergillus fumigatus*
5 Serum precipitins to *A. fumigatus*
6 Elevated serum IgE
7 Central bronchiectasis

OTHER DIAGNOSTIC FEATURES

1 History of brownish plugs in sputum
2 Culture of *A. fumigatus* from sputum
3 Elevated IgE (and IgG) class antibodies specific for *A. fumigatus*

Aspergillus allergens. If so, other criteria should be sought for diagnosis of *allergic bronchopulmonary aspergillosis* (ABPA) (Table 218-3). *A. fumigatus* is the most common cause, although other *Aspergillus* species have also been implicated. ABPA has been reported to complicate cystic fibrosis. The chest roentgenogram in ABPA may show transient, recurrent infiltrates or may suggest the presence of proximal bronchiectasis. High-resolution chest CT is a sensitive, noninvasive technique for the recognition of proximal bronchiectasis. The bronchial asthma of ABPA likely involves an IgE-mediated hypersensitivity, whereas the bronchiectasis associated with this disorder is thought to result from a deposition of immune complexes in proximal airways. Adequate treatment usually requires the long-term use of systemic glucocorticoids.

Tropical eosinophilia is usually caused by filarial infection; however, eosinophilic pneumonias also occur with other parasites such as *Ascaris, Ancyclostoma* species, *Toxocara* species, and *Strongyloides stercoralis*. Tropical eosinophilia due to *Wuchereria bancrofti* or *W. malayi* occurs most commonly in southern Asia, Africa, and South America, and is treated successfully with diethylcarbamazine.

Drug-induced eosinophilic pneumonias are typified by acute reactions to nitrofurantoin, which may begin 2 h to 10 days after nitrofurantoin is started, with symptoms of dry cough, fever, chills, and dyspnea; an eosinophilic pleural effusion accompanying patchy or diffuse pulmonary infiltrates may also occur. Other drugs associated with eosinophilic pneumonias include sulfonamides, penicillin, chlorpropamide, thiazides, tricyclic antidepressants, hydralazine, mephenesin, mecamylamine, nickel carbonyl vapor, gold salts, isoniazid, para-aminosalicylic acid, and others. Treatment consists of withdrawal of the incriminated drugs and the use of glucocorticoids, if necessary.

The idiopathic eosinophilic pneumonias consist of a group of diseases of varying severity. *Loeffler's syndrome* is a benign, acute eosinophilic pneumonia characterized by migrating pulmonary infiltrates and minimal clinical manifestations. *Acute eosinophilic pneumonia* has been described as an acute febrile illness of less than 7 days' duration, severe hypoxemia, pulmonary infiltrates, and no history of asthma. *Chronic eosinophilic pneumonia* presents with significant systemic symptoms including fever, chills, night sweats, cough, anorexia, and weight loss of several weeks to months' duration. The chest x-ray frequently shows peripheral infiltrates that have been described as a photographic negative of pulmonary edema. Some patients also have bronchial asthma, which is of the intrinsic or nonallergic type. Dramatic clearing of symptoms and chest x-rays is often noted within 48 h after initiation of glucocorticoid therapy.

Allergic angiitis and granulomatosis of Churg and Strauss is a multisystem vasculitic disorder that frequently involves the skin, kidney, and nervous system in addition to the lung (Chap. 291). The disorder may occur at any age and favors persons with a history of bronchial asthma. The asthma often is progressive until the onset of fever and exaggerated eosinophilia, at which time the symptoms of asthma may ease. The illness may be fulminating and the prognosis grave unless treated aggressively with glucocorticoids and immuno-suppressive therapy.

The hypereosinophilic syndrome is characterized by presence of over 1500 eosinophils per microliter of peripheral blood for 6 months or longer; lack of evidence for parasitic, allergic, or other known causes of eosinophilia; and signs or symptoms of multisystem organ dysfunction. Consistent features are blood and bone marrow eosinophilia with tissue infiltration by relatively mature eosinophils. The organs affected typically include the heart, lungs, liver, spleen, skin, and nervous system. Therapy of the disorder consists of glucocorticoids and/or hydroxyurea plus therapy as needed for cardiac dysfunction, which is frequently responsible for much of the morbidity and mortality in this syndrome.

REFERENCES

Hypersensitivity pneumonitis

GRAMMER LC, PATTERSON R: Occupational immunologic lung disease. Ann Allergy 58:151, 1987

HANSELL DM, MOSKOVIC E: High-resolution computed tomography in extrinsic allergic alveolitis. Clin Radiol 43:8, 1991

IMBEALT B. CORMIER Y: Usefulness of inhaled high-dose corticosteroids in allergic bronchopulmonary aspergillosis. Chest 103:1614, 1993

KOKKARINEN JI et al: Recovery of pulmonary function in farmer's lung. A five-year follow-up study. Am Rev Respir Dis 147:793, 1993

MARX JJ et al: Cohort studies of immunologic lung disease among Wisconsin dairy farmers. Am J Ind Med 18:263, 1990

PITCHER WD: Hypersensitivity pneumonitis. Am J Med Sci 300:251, 1990

RICHERSON HB: Unifying concepts underlying the effects of organic dust exposures. Am J Ind Med 17:139, 1990

——— et al: Guidelines for the clinical evaluation of hypersensitivity pneumonitis. J Allergy Clin Immunol 84:839, 1989

Eosinophilic pneumonias

ALLEN JN et al: Acute eosinophilic pneumonia as a reversible cause of noninfectious respiratory failure. N Engl J Med 321:569, 1989

GREENBERGER PA, PATTERSON R: Allergic bronchopulmonary aspergillosis: A model of bronchopulmonary disease with defined serologic, radiologic, pathologic and clinical findings from asthma to fatal destructive lung disease. Chest 91:165S, 1987

HUTCHESON PS et al: Variability in parameters of allergic bronchopulmonary aspergillosis in patients with cystic fibrosis. J Allergy Clin Immunol 88:390, 1991

ROSENOW EC III et al: Drug-induced pulmonary disease: An update. Chest 102:239, 1992

219   ENVIRONMENTAL LUNG DISEASES

FRANK E. SPEIZER

This chapter provides perspectives on ways to assess pulmonary diseases for which environmental causes are suspected. This assessment is important because removal of the patient from a harmful environment is often the only intervention that might prevent further significant deterioration or lead to improvement in a patient's condition. Furthermore, the identification of an environmentally associated disease in a single patient may lead to primary preventive strategies in other similarly exposed people who have not yet developed disease. Unless the physician specifically considers environmental exposures, these diseases and their causes will go undetected.

The exact magnitude of the problem is unknown, but there is no question that large numbers of people are at risk of developing serious respiratory disease as a result of occupational or environmental exposures. For example, recent estimates suggest that approximately 2.3 million workers have been exposed to crystalline silica or asbestos dust in mining and nonmining industries. If only 5 percent (a conservative estimate) of these workers are to suffer from respiratory disease as a result of their exposure, this represents more than 100,000 individuals in the United States.

Although industries are required to spend substantial amounts of capital in efforts to protect their workers, occupationally related respiratory diseases continue to occur. These diseases are often attributed to exposures in the distant past at a time when we were not aware of the risk incurred and the need for worker protection to the degree that we are today. We have, as a society, elected to pay compensation to affected individuals, and the physician is often called on to judge not only the physical condition of such a patient but also the degree to which the illness can be related to, or aggravated by, a particular occupational exposure.

HISTORY AND PHYSICAL EXAMINATION   The patient history is of paramount importance in assessing any potential occupational or environmental exposure. Often one is dealing with potential exposures in industries or environmental settings in which the physician has little personal experience. The physician must therefore ask the patient to describe a suspected environmental exposure in detail.

Inquiry into specific work practices should include questions about specific contaminants involved, the availability and use of personal respiratory protection devices, the size and ventilation of workspaces, the numbers of other workers potentially at risk of exposure, and whether other coworkers have similar complaints. In addition, the patient must be questioned about alternative sources for potentially toxic exposures, including hobbies or other environmental exposures at home. Short-term exposures to potential toxic agents in the distant past also must be considered. This information can be best elicited by a detailed occupational history which inquires about every job (beginning even with part-time jobs during schooling) and about the nature of the work, the materials handled, and the duration and chronologic years of employment (see Chap. 394).

Many people are aware of the potential hazards in their workplaces, and many states require that employees be informed about potentially hazardous exposures. These requirements include the provision of specific educational materials (including Material Safety Data Sheets), personal protective equipment and instructions in their use, and information on environmental control procedures. Reminders posted in the workplace may warn workers about hazardous substances. Protective clothing, lockers, and shower facilities may be considered necessary parts of the job. However, even in these more progressive industries, the introduction of new processes, particularly when related to the use of new chemical compounds, may change exposure significantly, and often only the employee on the production line is aware of the change. For the physician who regularly sees patients from a particular industry, a visit to the work site can be very instructive. Alternatively, physicians can request inspections by appropriate federal and/or state authorities through which clinically relevant exposure information can be obtained.

The physical examination of patients with environmentally related lung diseases may help to determine the nature and severity of the pulmonary condition. Unfortunately, the pulmonary response to most injurious agents is the development of a limited number of nonspecific physical signs. These findings do not point to the specific causative agent, and other types of information must be used to arrive at an etiologic diagnosis.

PULMONARY FUNCTION TESTS AND CHEST RADIOGRAPH The use of pulmonary function tests and radiographic examinations of the chest can provide insight into the nature of the exposures which have led to the current condition of the patient and the level of impairment. Many mineral dusts produce characteristic alterations in the mechanics of breathing and lung volumes which clearly indicate a restrictive pattern (Chaps. 214 and 224). Exposures to a number of organic dusts or chemical agents capable of producing occupational asthma result in pronounced obstructive patterns of pulmonary dysfunction that may be reversible (Chap. 217). Standardized approaches for measuring the mechanics of breathing and diffusion across the alveolar membrane (Chap. 214) have been proposed for screening large industrial groups. Measurement of change in forced expiratory volume (FEV$_1$) before and after a working shift can be used to detect an acute inflammatory or bronchoconstrictive response. An acute decrement of FEV$_1$ over the Monday work shift is a characteristic feature of cotton textile workers with byssinosis.

For many years the chest radiograph has been used to detect and monitor the pulmonary response to mineral dusts. To provide a standardized method of recording judgments about the kind and severity of radiographic abnormalities, the International Labour Organization (ILO) International Classification of Radiographs of Pneumoconioses was developed. The ILO scheme involves classifying chest radiographs according to the nature and size of opacities seen and the extent of involvement of the parenchyma. Although useful for screening large numbers of workers, the procedure lacks specificity and may over- or underestimate the functional impact of pneumoconiosis. With dusts causing rounded, regular opacities, such as in coal worker's pneumoconiosis, the degree of involvement on the chest radiograph may be extensive, while pulmonary function may be only minimally impaired. In contrast, in pneumoconiosis causing linear, irregular opacities, as seen in asbestosis, the radiograph may lead to underestimation of the severity of the impairment. It is possible to have a history of exposure, moderately reduced forced vital capacity (FVC), and a reduced diffusion in asbestosis with a relatively normal chest radiograph. The radiographic findings of irregular or linear opacities are simply more difficult to separate from normal markings until relatively late in the disease. When shadows become large (radiographic lesions greater than 1 cm in diameter), the condition is termed *complicated pneumoconiosis*, sometimes called *progressive massive fibrosis* (PMF). For the individual patient with a history of exposure, conventional computed tomography (CT) and high-resolution computed tomography (HRCT) have improved the sensitivity of identifying diffuse parenchymal abnormalities of the lung. The procedures have been shown to provide earlier detection of silicosis and asbestosis.

Other diagnostic procedures of use in identifying environmentally induced lung disease include evaluating heavy metal concentrations in urine (arsenic in smelter workers, cadmium in battery plant workers); bacteriologic studies (tuberculosis in medical care personnel, anthrax in wool sorters); fungal studies (coccidioidomycosis in southwestern farm workers, histoplasmosis in poultry or pigeon handlers); or serologic studies (psittacosis in pet shop workers or owners of sick birds, Q fever in tanners or slaughterhouse workers). Ultimately, a lung biopsy may be required both to make a morphologic diagnosis of the underlying pulmonary disease and to attempt to identify the specific etiologic agent.

MEASUREMENT OF EXPOSURE If reliable environmental sampling data are available, these sources of information should be used in assessing a patient's exposure. Since many of the chronic diseases result from exposure over many years, current environmental measurements should be combined with work histories to arrive at estimates of past exposure. However, the dose of any environmental agent is a complex interaction of chemical reaction, both at the emission source and in the ambient atmosphere, and physiologic factors, including ventilation rate and depth, which may affect transport and deposition of aerosols and gases in the lung. Even in acute conditions, when monitoring of exposure may be possible, little may be known about the actual dose received by the lung. Most of the research on health effects of air pollutants (discussed later in this chapter) has relied on fixed-station monitoring of outdoor air, often at locations somewhat distant from the residences of the people being studied. In addition, most people spend less than 20 percent of their time outdoors. Efforts to determine the penetration rate of outdoor contaminants into the indoors suggest that these penetration rates are highly pollutant specific. Therefore, outdoor measurements can be used only in a relative sense, and they cannot be relied on to estimate actual dose.

In situations where individual exposure to specific agents has been determined, either in a work setting or for ambient air pollutants, transport of these agents through the airways may be an important factor affecting dose. Highly soluble gases such as sulfur dioxide are absorbed in the upper airway and presumably produce their effects by reflex response to sensitive neural fibrils in the trachea or larger airways. In contrast, nitrogen dioxide, which is less soluble, may reach the bronchioles and alveoli in sufficient quantities to result in an acute life-threatening disease in farmers exposed even briefly to the gas evolved from moldy hay in silos (silo filler's disease).

Particle size and chemistry of air contaminants also must be considered. Particles above 10 to 15 μm, because of their settling velocities in air, do not penetrate beyond the upper airways. These larger particles are often referred to as "fugitive dusts" and include pollens, other windblown dusts, and dusts resulting from mechanical industrial processes. They have little or no role in chronic respiratory disease except as possibly related to cancer (see below).

Particles below 10 μm in size are created by the burning of fossil fuels or high-temperature industrial processes resulting in condensation products from gases, fumes, or vapors. These particles are divided into two size fractions on the basis of their chemical characteristics. Particles approximately 2.5 to 10 μm (coarse-mode fraction) contain crustal elements, such as silica, aluminum, and iron. These particles mostly deposit relatively high in the tracheobronchial tree. Particles less than approximately 2.5 μm (fine-mode fraction or accumulation mode) contain sulfates, nitrates, and organic compounds. The deposition of the fine-mode particles is more often in the terminal bronchioles and alveoli. The smallest particles, those less than 0.1 μm in size, remain in the airstream and deposit in the lung only on a random basis as they come into contact with the alveolar walls through thermal forces and/or Brownian movement.

Besides the size characteristics of particles and the solubility of gases, the actual chemical composition, mechanical properties, and immunogenicity or infectivity of inhaled material determine in large part the nature of the diseases found among exposed persons.

OCCUPATIONAL EXPOSURES AND PULMONARY DISEASE

INORGANIC DUSTS Asbestos exposure Except in localized regions with single industrial exposures, such as coal-mining or granite-quarrying regions, the most frequent inorganic dust–related chronic pulmonary diseases are associated with industries using *asbestiform fibers*. *Asbestos* is a generic term for several different mineral silicates, including chrysolite, amosite, anthophyllite, and crocidolite. Besides mining, milling, and manufacturing of asbestos products, the exceptional thermal and electric insulation properties of asbestos led to its widespread use in construction, leading to exposure of pipe fitters, boiler makers, and other workers in the building trades. In addition, asbestos was used in the manufacture of fire-smothering blankets and safety garments, as filler for plastic materials, in cement and floor tiles, and in friction materials, such as brake and clutch linings.

Exposure to asbestos is not limited to persons who directly handle the material. Cases of asbestos-related diseases have been encountered in individuals with only moderate exposure, such as the painter or electrician who works alongside the insulation worker in a shipyard or the housewife who does no more than shake out and wash her husband's work clothes. Community exposure has probably resulted from the use of asbestos-containing material sprayed on steel girders in many large buildings as a safety feature to prevent buckling in case of fire. Clusters of cases of mesothelioma have been noted in the neighborhood of an asbestos plant in London and in the communities near asbestos mines in South Africa.

Asbestos was first used extensively in the 1940s. Starting in 1975 it has been mostly replaced with man-made mineral fibers, such as fiberglass or slag wool. However, asbestos is still used in the manufacture of brake linings and remains as pipe and boiler insulation in hundreds of thousands of workplaces and homes. Despite current regulations mandating adequate training for any worker potentially exposed to asbestos, exposure probably continues among inexperienced demolition workers. The major health effects from exposure to asbestos are pulmonary fibrosis (asbestosis) and cancers of the respiratory tract and pleura and, rarely, peritoneum.

Asbestosis is a diffuse interstitial fibrosing disease of the lung which is directly related to the intensity and duration of exposure. Except for a history of exposure to asbestos (generally in a work setting), asbestosis resembles the other forms of diffuse interstitial fibrosis (Chap. 224). Usually at least 10 years of moderate to severe exposure has occurred before the disease becomes manifest.

Physiologic studies reveal a restrictive pattern with a decrease in lung volumes. Flow rates are commonly reduced less than would be predicted on the basis of the volume reduction. An early sign of severe disease may be a reduction in diffusing capacity.

Pulmonary fibrosis may occur following sufficient exposure to any of the asbestiform fiber types. The fibrotic lesions do not appear to relate to either shape or chemical composition of any fiber type. Recent studies indicate that during phagocytosis of the asbestos fiber, the membrane of the macrophage is damaged, which results in the release of lysosomes containing enzymes which may act to damage the lung parenchyma. The clinical manifestations are typical of those physical findings in any patient with pulmonary fibrosis (Chap. 224).

The chest radiograph can be used to determine a number of manifestations of asbestos exposure, as well as to identify specific lesions. Past exposure is specifically indicated by pleural plaques, which are characterized by either thickening or calcification along the parietal pleura, particularly along the lower lung fields, the diaphragm, and the cardiac border. Without additional manifestations, pleural plaques imply only exposure, not pulmonary impairment. Benign pleural effusions may occur, particularly in patients with asbestosis, but are not necessarily restricted to those with overt disease. The fluid is sterile but may be a serous or blood-stained exudate and may occur bilaterally. The effusion may be slowly progressive or may resolve spontaneously.

The radiographic diagnosis of asbestosis depends on the presence of irregular or linear opacities, usually first noted in the lower lung fields and spreading into the middle and upper lung fields as the disease progresses. An indistinct heart border or a ''ground glass'' appearance in the lung fields is seen in some cases. As the fibrotic changes in the parenchyma begin to coalesce, the patient develops obliteration of entire acinar units with eventual formation of the classical honeycombed lung, which appears on chest radiographs as coarse infiltrates with small (about 7- to 10-μm) air spaces. In cases in which the x-ray changes are less obvious, HRCT may show distinct changes of subpleural curvilinear lines 5 to 10 cm in length which appear to be parallel to the pleural surface. No specific therapy is available in the management of patients with asbestosis. The supportive care is that of any patient with diffuse interstitial fibrosis from any cause.

In general, newly diagnosed cases will have resulted from exposure levels that were present many years before and, in spite of the patients' having left the industry, are attributable to that former exposure. Since the patient may be eligible for compensation within a specific time frame after the diagnosis of an asbestos-related disease is made, the physician making the diagnosis should be certain to inform the patient promptly. On occasion, the physician may have reason to suspect ongoing exposure from a patient's current job description or actual monitoring data. In such cases, federal or state health authorities may need to be notified. Present-day occupational safety and health regulations, if followed properly, protect workers from exposure. Because the association of smoking and asbestos exposure increases the risk of developing lung cancer (see below), it is extremely important to advise patients with such exposure histories to stop smoking.

Lung cancer (Chap. 227), either squamous cell or adenocarcinoma, is the most frequent cancer associated with asbestos exposure. The excess frequency of lung cancer in asbestos workers is associated with a minimum lapse of 15 to 19 years between first exposure and development of the disease. Persons with more exposure are at greater risk of disease. In addition, there appears to be a significant multiplicative effect which leads to a far greater risk of lung cancer in persons who are cigarette smokers and have asbestos exposure than would be expected by taking the sum of both risks. Efforts to consider these high-risk individuals for special surveillance studies, including sputum cytologic examinations and repeated chest x-rays as frequently as every 4 to 6 months, suggest that cancers can be detected at an earlier stage and that the survival of these patients may be prolonged.

Mesotheliomas (Chap. 228), both pleural and peritoneal, also are associated with asbestos exposure. In contrast to lung cancer, there does not appear to be any association with smoking. Relatively short-term exposures of 1 to 2 years or less occurring some 20 to 25 years in the past have been associated with the development of mesotheliomas (which stresses the point of obtaining a complete environmental exposure history). The risk for this type of tumor peaks 30 to 35 years after initial exposure. Although approximately 50 percent of mesotheliomas metastasize, the tumor generally is locally invasive, and death usually results from local extension. Most patients present with effusions that may obscure the underlying pleural tumor. In contrast to other causes of effusion, because of the restriction placed on the chest wall, no shift of mediastinal structures toward the opposite chest will be seen. The major diagnostic problem is differentiation from peripherally spreading pulmonary adenocarcinoma or adenocarcinoma metastatic to pleura from an extrathoracic primary site. Although a needle biopsy may be diagnostic, an open biopsy is often necessary and even when performed may not provide a definitive diagnosis of the origin of the tumor.

One concern in making a definitive diagnosis of a mesothelioma relates to potential compensation to the survivors of a patient with this usually fatal disease. Since epidemiologic studies have shown that more than 80 percent of mesotheliomas may be associated with asbestos exposure, documented mesothelioma in a worker with occupational exposure to asbestos may be compensable in many parts of the United States.

Other naturally occurring asbestiform material (e.g., erionite, a fibrous zeolite) induces mesotheliomas in test animals and has been associated with an excess incidence of lung cancer and mesotheliomas in a population in central Turkey exposed to it in volcanic rock. Man-made mineral fibers (MMMF) have similar physiochemical properties to naturally occurring asbestiform fibers. However, recent studies of exposure suggest that if excess risks of lung cancer do occur, they are less than with naturally occurring fibers. To date, no cases of mesotheliomas from MMMF without exposure to asbestos have been reported. Part of the difficulty in assessing the effects of MMMF is that they have been used for relatively shorter periods and generally at lower exposure levels than for asbestos. Thus concern for worker protection needs to be maintained.

Silicosis   In spite of the technical adequacy of existing protective equipment, *free silica* (SiO_2), or crystalline quartz, is still a major occupational hazard. In the United States, estimates of potential numbers of exposed workers range between 1.2 to 3 million people. The major occupational exposures include mining, stone cutting, abrasive industries, foundry workers, packers of silica flour, and quarrying, particularly of granite. Most often the progressive pulmonary fibrosis (silicosis) occurs in a dose-response fashion after many years of exposure.

Workers exposed to sandblasting in confined spaces, tunneling through rock with high quartz content (15 to 25 percent), and engaged in the manufacture of abrasive soaps may develop acute silicosis with as little as 10 months' exposure. The disease may be rapidly fatal in less than 2 years despite the worker being removed from exposure. A radiographic picture of profuse miliary infiltration or consolidation is characteristic of acute silicosis.

In long-term, relatively less intense exposure, radiographic changes of rounded, small opacities in the upper lobes with retraction and hilar adenopathy classically appear after 15 to 20 years of exposure. Calcification of hilar nodes may occur in as many as 20 percent of cases and produces the characteristic "eggshell" pattern. These changes may be preceded by or be associated with a reticular pattern of irregular densities which are uniformly present throughout the upper lung zones.

The nodular fibrosis may be progressive in the absence of further exposure, with coalescence and formation of nonsegmental conglomerates of irregular masses in excess of 1 cm in diameter. These masses become quite large and are characteristic of progressive massive fibrosis (PMF). Significant functional impairment with both restrictive and obstructive components may be associated with this form of silicosis. In the late stages of the disease ventilatory failure may develop. In more subtle cases, CT may be helpful both in identifying nodules which are preferentially located in the posterior aspect of the upper lobes, as well as in identifying larger opacities and more coalescence than might be noted on regular chest x-rays. Patients with silicosis are at greater risk of acquiring *Mycobacterium tuberculosis* infections (silicotuberculosis), as well as atypical mycobacterial infections, although tuberculosis is not always involved in the progression of the disease to PMF. Because the frequency with which tuberculosis has been found at autopsy in patients with PMF exceeds considerably the frequency of premorbid diagnosis, treatment for tuberculosis is indicated in any patient with silicosis and a positive tuberculin test.

Other less hazardous silicates include fuller's earth, kaolin, mica, diatomaceous earths, silica gel, soapstone, carbonate dusts, and cement dusts. The production of fibrosis in workers exposed to these agents is believed to be related to either the free silica content of these dusts or, for substances which contain no free silica, to the potentially large dust loads to which these workers may be exposed.

Other silicates, including *talc dusts*, may be contaminated with asbestos and/or free silica. Accidental exposure to significant quantities of talc may result in an acute syndrome with cough, cyanosis, and labored breathing (acute talcosis). Severe progressive fibrosis with respiratory failure may ensue within a few years. Far more common is the fibrosis and/or pleural or lung cancer associated with chronic exposure in rubber workers who use commercial talc as a lubricant in tire molds. Pure talc does not produce fibrosis; thus it is difficult to sort out whether the effects are due to the contamination of commercial talc by asbestos or by free silica.

Coal worker's pneumoconiosis (CWP) *Coal dust* is associated with CWP, which has enormous social, economic, and medical significance in every nation in which coal mining is an important industry. Simple radiographically identified CWP is seen in 12 percent of all miners and in as many as 50 percent of anthracite miners with more than 20 years' work on the coal face. The prevalence of disease is lower in workers in bituminous coal mines. Since much of the western U.S. coal is bituminous, CWP is less prevalent in that region.

Much of the symptomatology associated with simple CWP appears to be similar and additive to the effects of cigarette smoking on the development of chronic bronchitis and obstructive lung disease (Chap. 223). In the early stages of simple CWP, radiographic abnormalities consist of small, irregular opacities (reticular pattern). With prolonged exposure, one sees small, rounded, regular opacities, 1 to 5 mm in diameter (nodular pattern). Calcification is generally not seen, although approximately 10 percent of older anthracite miners have calcified nodules.

Complicated CWP is manifested by the appearance on the chest radiograph of nodules ranging from 1 cm in diameter to the size of an entire lobe, generally confined to the upper half of the lungs. This condition, considered a form of PMF, is accompanied by a significant reduction in diffusing capacity and with premature mortality. In contrast to patients with silicosis, only a relatively small percentage of underground miners with simple CWP (5 to 15 percent, depending on the type of coal) develop PMF.

The mechanism whereby PMF occurs in CWP is not fully understood. Several hypotheses have been proposed, including (1) sufficient free silica is present in the dust, (2) normal clearance mechanisms are unable to clear the excessive dust loads, (3) an interplay occurs between an intrinsic immunologic mechanism and the dust and/or damaged lung tissue, and (4) atypical reactions to *Mycobacterium tuberculosis* occur. As previously described, PMF in silicosis is associated with prolonged duration and high intensity of exposure to free silica. Heavy exposure to carbon particles free of silica occurs in carbon black, graphite, and charcoal workers. The prolonged exposure of these workers may result in sufficient accumulation of carbon in the lung to produce PMF. The mechanism appears to relate to a breakdown of the clearance capacity of the airways.

Caplan's syndrome, which includes seropositive rheumatoid arthritis with characteristic PMF, is consistent with an immunopathologic mechanism. The syndrome was first described in coal miners but subsequently has been found in a number of pneumoconioses. Similarly, the high prevalence of antinuclear antibodies in sandblasting workers with silicosis and the elevation of gamma globulin levels in silicotic individuals suggest an immunologic mechanism. Although mycobacterial infections are found more often in coal miners than PMF is found in silicotic patients, tuberculosis does not appear to be associated with most of the cases of PMF in coal miners.

Berylliosis Beryllium may produce an acute pneumonitis or, far more commonly, a chronic interstitial pneumonitis. Unless one inquires specifically about occupational exposures to beryllium in the manufacture of alloys, ceramics, high-technology electronics, and, before the 1950s, the production of fluorescent lights, one may miss entirely the etiologic relationship to an occupational exposure. Nonspecific pulmonary function tests may be normal or may indicate evidence of restrictive disease. Between 2 and 15 years of exposure, depending on its intensity, is required for the disease to become manifest. On open lung biopsy, granulomatous formation similar to that seen in sarcoidosis (Chap. 292) may make differentiation impossible unless tissue levels of beryllium are measured.

Rarely, other hard metals, including aluminum powders, chromium, cobalt, titanium dioxide, and tungsten, may produce an interstitial pneumonitis.

Other inorganic dusts Other dusts are considered *nuisance dusts* because their major impact seems to be reduction in visibility and irritation of eyes, ears, nasal passages, and other mucous membranes. If they penetrate to the lower airways, they do not affect the architecture of the terminal bronchioles or acinar spaces or destroy collagen. Generally, clinical effects are reversible. Pulmonary function tests are usually normal unless another disease process coexists. If radiodense, macular collections of these dusts may produce striking radiographic pictures which are so characteristic that patients with a history of significant exposure are easily diagnosed as having the condition which bears the name reflecting the nature of the dust. Examples are iron and iron oxides from welding or silver finishing (*siderosis*); tin oxide used in metallurgy, color stabilization, printing, and the manufacture of porcelain, glass, and fabric (*stannosis*); and barium sulfate used as a catalyst for organic reactions, drilling mud components, and electroplating (*baritosis*). Other metal dusts producing similar radiodense pictures include *cerium dioxide* and *antimony salts*.

Most of the inorganic dusts discussed thus far are associated with the production of either dust macules or interstitial fibrotic changes in the lung. Another set of dusts (see Table 219-1), along with some of the dusts previously discussed, is associated with chronic mucous hypersecretion (chronic bronchitis), with or without reduction of expiratory flow rates. These conditions may be caused by cigarette smoking, and any effort to attribute some component of the disease to occupational and environmental exposures must take cigarette smoking into account. Most studies suggest an additive effect of dust exposure and smoking. The pattern of the effect is similar to that of cigarette smoking, suggesting that small airways may be the initial

TABLE 219-1   Selected occupational dusts believed to be associated with mucous hypersecretion and/or obstructive airway disease and other respiratory diseases*

Agent (exposure)	Mucous hyper-secretion	Obstruction	Other conditions[†]
INORGANIC DUSTS			
Antimony (storage batteries, solder, ceramics, glass, plastics)	X		P
Arsenic (manufacture of pesticides, pigments, glass, alloys)	X		C
Barium and compounds including BaO, $BaSO_4$, $BaCO_3$ (catalyst, drilling mud, electroplating)	X		P
Cadmium dust (electroplating, battery manufacture, welding, smelting, aluminum soldering)	X	X	P
Cement dust (construction trades, manufacture of cement blocks)	X	X	
Chromium and CrO_3, CrF_2 (corrosion inhibitor pigment, metallurgy, electroplating)	X		C
Coal dust (mining)	X		P
Coke oven emissions (retort house, coke ovens)	X	X	P, C
Graphite (steelmaking, lubricants, pencils, paints, stove polish)	X	X	P
Iron dust (steel and nonferrous foundry workers, welding)	X		P
Mica (insulation, roofing shingles, oil refining, rubber manufacturing)	X		P
Phosphorus, elemental chlorides, sulfides (manufacture of fireworks, agricultural chemicals, insecticides, pesticides)	X	X	
Rock dusts (miners, tunnelers, quarry workers)	X		P
Vanadium pentoxide (welding electrodes, additive to steel, by-product in ash from oil burning)	X	X	
ORGANIC DUSTS (see Chap. 218)			
Cotton dust, flax, hemp (manufacture of yarns for linen, rope, cotton; ginning, cottonseed crushing; waste fiber processing)	X	X	
Grain dusts (farmers, workers in grain elevators, barge and grain ship crewmembers)	X	X	
Moldy hay (farmers, other animal attendants)	X		HP

* The table excludes agents associated with asthma as the primary disease (see Chap. 217).
† Other conditions include hypersensitivity pneumonitis (HP), pneumoconiosis (P), and cancers (C).
NOTE: X indicates that mucous hypersecretion or obstruction are associated with exposure.

site of pathologic response to those cases associated with the development of obstructive lung disease. Cigarette smoke is usually the more noxious agent, and dust effects may be discernible only in nonsmokers.

ORGANIC DUSTS   Some of the specific diseases associated with organic dusts are discussed in detail in the chapters on asthma (Chap. 217) and hypersensitivity pneumonitis (Chap. 218). Many of these diseases are named for the specific setting in which the disease is

found, e.g., farmer's lung, malt worker's disease, or mushroom worker's disease. Occupational and other environmental exposures must be sought when these conditions are suspected. Often the temporal relation of symptoms to exposure furnishes the best evidence for the diagnosis. Three occupational groups are singled out for discussion because they represent the largest proportion of people affected by the diseases resulting from organic dusts.

Cotton dust (byssinosis)   Estimates of the number of exposed persons in the United States vary, but probably over 800,000 persons are exposed occupationally to cotton, flax, or hemp in the production of yarns for cotton, linen, and rope making. Although this discussion focuses on cotton, the same syndrome to a somewhat lesser degree has been reported in exposure to flax, hemp, and jute.

Although cotton dust–related disease was first described in the seventeenth century, it is only in the last 40 years that the disease has been recognized as a worldwide problem in the textile industry. Exposure occurs throughout the manufacturing process but is most pronounced in those portions of the factory involved with the treatment of the cotton prior to spinning—i.e., blowing, mixing, and carding (straightening of fibers). Cases reported from spinning rooms are believed to be due to secondary contamination from carding rooms. Recent attempts to control dust levels by use of exhaust hoods, general increases in ventilation, and wetting procedures in some settings have been highly successful. However, respiratory protective equipment appears to be required during certain operations to prevent workers from being exposed to levels of dust that exceed the current U.S. cotton dust standard.

Byssinosis is characterized clinically as occasional (early stage) and then regular (late stage) chest tightness toward the end of the first day of the workweek (Monday chest tightness). In epidemiologic studies, depending on the level of exposure in the carding room air, up to 80 percent of employees may show a significant drop in their FEV_1 over the course of a Monday shift.

Initially the symptoms do not recur on subsequent days of the week. However, in 10 to 25 percent of workers the disease may be progressive, with chest tightness recurring or persisting throughout the workweek. After more than 10 years of exposure, workers with recurrent symptoms are more likely to have an obstructive pattern on pulmonary function testing. These higher grades of impairment are seen in workers exposed both to high levels of dust and for greater durations. There is an additive effect of cotton dust exposure plus cigarette smoking. The highest grades of impairment are generally seen in smokers.

Treatment in the early stages of the disease is directed toward reversing the bronchospasm with bronchodilators; however, the chest tightness appears at least in part to relate to histamine release, and antihistamines have been shown to lessen the anticipated fall in FEV_1 the first day of the week. Clearly, reduction of dust exposure is of primary importance. All workers with persistent symptoms or significantly reduced levels of pulmonary function should be moved to areas of lower risk of exposure. Regular surveillance of pulmonary function in the industry has made it easier to identify affected persons. Persons with reduced pulmonary function, a personal history of respiratory allergy, and positive history of continued cigarette smoking should be considered at increased risk of developing byssinosis in association with working in the cotton industry.

Grain dust   Although the exact number of workers at risk in the United States is not known, at least 500,000 people work in grain elevators, and over 2 million farmers are potentially exposed. The presentation of disease in grain elevator employees or workers in flour or feed mills is virtually identical to the characteristic finding in cigarette smokers, i.e., persistent cough, mucus hypersecretion, wheeze and dyspnea on exertion, and reduced FEV_1 and FEV_1/FVC ratio (Chap. 214).

Dust concentrations in grain elevators vary greatly but appear to be in excess of 10,000 $\mu g/m^3$, with approximately one-third of the particles by weight being in the respirable range. The effect of grain dust exposure is additive to that of cigarette smoking, with approximately 50 percent of workers who smoke having symptoms. Among nonsmoking grain elevator operators, approximately one-quarter have mucus hypersecretion, about five times the number that would be expected in unexposed nonsmokers. However, evidence of obstruction on pulmonary function studies is observed only in workers who smoke. It is not clear if this results from an enhancement of cigarette smoking effect in exposed workers or if smokers are more susceptible to the effects of grain dust.

Farmer's lung This condition results from exposure to moldy hay containing spores of thermophilic actinomycetes that produce a hypersensitivity pneumonitis (Chap. 218). There are few good population-based estimates of the frequency of occurrence of this condition in the United States. However, among farmers in Great Britain, the rate of disease ranges from approximately 10 to 50 per 1000. The prevalence of disease varies in association with rainfall, which determines the amount of fungal growth, and with differences in agricultural practices related to turning and stacking hay.

The patient with acute farmer's lung presents 4 to 8 h after exposure with fever, chills, malaise, cough, and dyspnea without wheezing. The history of exposure is obviously essential to separate this disease from similar symptoms that might occur in influenza or pneumonia. In the chronic form of the disease, the history of repeated attacks after similar exposure is important to separate this syndrome from other causes of patchy fibrosis, e.g., sarcoidosis.

A wide variety of other organic dusts are associated with the occurrence of hypersensitivity pneumonitis (Chap. 218). For those patients who present with hypersensitivity pneumonitis, specific and careful inquiry about occupations, hobbies, or other home environmental exposures will, in most cases, reveal the source of the etiologic agent.

ASSESSMENT OF DISABILITY Significant reduction of dust levels in coal mines has resulted from federal legislation, enacted in the United States in 1969, which requires that respirable dust levels in underground mines be reduced to less than 2000 $\mu g/m^3$. This same legislation authorized payment to coal miners (or their survivors) totally disabled by CWP. The criteria for disability from CWP remain unclear and arbitrary. Much of the difficulty relates to the inability to determine in an individual with simple CWP what proportion of an observed respiratory impairment is related to coal dust and what proportion is due to cigarette smoking. The laws as currently interpreted suggest that to be eligible for payment of a claim, one need only show that an underlying condition (i.e., chronic bronchitis with obstruction, presumably due to cigarette smoking) is aggravated by CWP. Thus it becomes critical that physicians involved in occupational lung disease claim cases be aware of detailed exposure histories of their patients, in terms of both occupational exposures and other environmental exposures (cigarette smoking). In addition, these physicians must understand that the extent to which the level of physiologic impairment incapacitates an individual may not be the sole criterion for determining disability. To assess disability properly may require input not only from physicians but also from experts in ergonomics and vocational rehabilitation, lawyers, and employer and employee representatives.

TOXIC CHEMICALS Exposure to toxic chemicals affecting the lung generally occurs in the form of gases and vapors. A common accident is one in which the victim is trapped in a confined space where the chemicals have accumulated to toxic levels. In addition to the specific toxic effects of the chemical, the victim will often sustain considerable anoxia, which can play a dominant role in determining whether the individual survives.

Table 219-2 lists a variety of toxic agents which can produce acute and sometimes life-threatening reactions in the lung. All these agents in sufficient concentrations have been demonstrated, at least in animal studies, to affect the lower airways and disrupt alveolar architecture, either acutely or as a result of chronic exposure. Some of these agents may be generated acutely in the environment. For example, when plastics burn, a number of compounds, including hydrogen cyanide and hydrochloric acid, may be formed and released. The effects and

treatment of exposure to these toxic gases are discussed elsewhere (Chap. 395).

Firefighters and fire victims are at risk of *smoke inhalation*, a numerically important cause of acute cardiorespiratory failure. Smoke inhalation kills more fire victims than does thermal injury. Carbon monoxide poisoning with resulting significant hypoxemia can be life-threatening (Chap. 395). Firefighters may inappropriately use the "blackness" of the smoke to indicate the degree to which incomplete combustion and, thus, elevation of carbon monoxide levels are present. The use of synthetic materials (plastic, polyurethanes), which, when burned, may release a variety of other toxic agents, must be considered when evaluating smoke inhalation victims. Exposed victims may suffer some degree of lower respiratory tract inflammation, similar to that seen with exposure to other irritant gases, e.g., chlorine. Severe cases may develop pulmonary edema.

Firefighters and victims also may be exposed to large quantities of particulate smoke. Significant long-term effects are not clearly associated with this particulate exposure except as related to the production of irritating effects on the upper airways. Studies attempting to demonstrate either an increased risk of cardiovascular events, presumably from recurrent exposure to carbon monoxide, or excess incidence of chronic respiratory disease from repeated smoke inhalation are inconclusive, partly because of the difficulties in measuring exposure. Recent studies suggest increased airways responsiveness in firefighters with repeated episodes of smoke inhalation.

Some agents used in the manufacture of synthetic materials such as plastics, polyurethanes, and other polymers have resulted in some workers being sensitized to extremely low levels of *isocyanates, aromatic amines,* or *aldehydes*. Repeated exposure to these agents causes some workers to develop chronic cough and sputum production, asthma, or episodes of low-grade fever and malaise. Occasionally, as in byssinosis, these symptoms occur early in the workweek but usually recur without workweek periodicity. In the case of exposure to diisocyanate in the production of polyurethane, chronic and persistent asthma in selected individuals appears to result from exposure to concentrations well below the recognized industrial standard. Methods to identify susceptible individuals are needed. At present, challenge testing is being used to determine if a given patient is sensitive. These challenges can be carried out in special environmental chambers where the physician can simulate the work exposure. Alternatively, nonspecific challenges with either pharmacologic agents, such as methacholine and histamine, or isocapneic cold air breathing are being used to identify patients with hyperreactive airways. The usefulness of this nonspecific approach as a method to screen potential sensitive workers has yet to be established.

An unusual route of exposure occurs in *polymer fume fever*. Polymers, notably fluorocarbons, which at normal temperatures produce no reaction, may be transmitted from a worker's hands to his or her cigarettes. Upon burning the cigarette, the polymer is volatilized, and the inhaled agent causes a characteristic syndrome of fever, chills, malaise, and occasionally mild wheezing. The same condition occurs in workers exposed to heated polymers without cigarette use. The syndrome is obviously controlled by proper attention to hygiene in the workplace. A similar self-limited, influenza-like syndrome—*metal fume fever*—results from acute exposure to fumes or smoke of zinc, copper, magnesium, and other volatilized metals. The syndrome may begin several hours after work and resolves within 24 h, only to return on repeated exposure. A proper occupational history should make the diagnosis evident.

ENVIRONMENTAL RESPIRATORY CARCINOGENS Historically, it has been the astute clinician who has recognized a higher incidence of malignant tumors associated with certain environmental exposures. When these observations are linked to an occupational setting, they must be pursued by epidemiologic studies of relatively large groups of both current and former workers. Often the concentration and/or exact nature of the substances contained in the putative exposures cannot be determined. Rarely, the possibility that a substance can play an etiologic role in cancer is supported by observing

TABLE 219-2 Selected common toxic chemical agents

Agents	Selected exposures	Acute effects from high or accidental exposure	Chronic effects from relatively low exposure
Acid fumes; H_2SO_4, HNO_3	Manufacture of fertilizers, chlorinated organic compounds, dyes, explosives, rubber products, metal etching, plastics	Mucous membrane irritation, followed by chemical pneumonitis 2–3 days	No data
Ammonia	Refrigeration, petroleum refining, manufacture of fertilizers, explosives, plastics, and other chemicals	Same as for acid fumes	Chronic bronchitis
Cyanides	Electroplating, extraction of gold or silver, manufacture of mirrors, fumigants, photo supplies	Increase in respiratory rate followed by respiratory arrest, lactic acidosis, pulmonary edema, death	No data
Diazomethane	Methylating agent for acid compounds; laboratory workers	Violent coughing, dyspnea, wheezing, pulmonary edema	No data
Formaldehyde	Manufacture of resins, leathers, rubber, metals, and woods; laboratory workers, embalmers; emission from urethane foam insulation	Same as for acid fumes	Cancers in one species of animals; no data on humans
Halides (Cl, Br, F)	Bleaching in pulp, paper, textile industry; manufacture of chemical compounds; synthetic rubber, plastics, disinfectant, rocket fuel, gasoline	Mucous membrane irritation, pulmonary edema; possible reduced FVC 1–2 yrs after exposure	Dryness of mucous membrane, epistaxis, dental fluorosis, tracheobronchitis
Hydrogen sulfide	By-product of many industrial processes, oil, other petroleum processes and storage	Low exposure: conjunctival irritation; higher: respiratory paralysis similar to cyanides	Chronic bronchitis, recurrent pneumonitis
Isocyanates (TDI, HDI, MDI)	Production of polyurethane foams, plastics, adhesives, surface coatings	Mucous membrane irritation, dyspnea, cough, wheeze, pulmonary edema	Upper respiratory tract irritation, cough, asthma, allergic alveolitis
Nitrogen dioxide	Silage, metal etching, explosives, rocket fuels, welding, by-product of burning fossil fuels	Cough, dyspnea, pulmonary edema may be delayed 4–12 h; possible result from acute exposure: bronchiolitis obliterans in 2–6 wks	Emphysema in animals, ?chronic bronchitis
Ozone	Arc welding, flour bleaching, deodorizing, emissions from copying equipment, photochemical air pollutant	Mucous membrane irritant, pulmonary hemorrhage and edema, reduced pulmonary function transiently in children and adults exposed to summer haze	Chronic eye irritation
Phosgene	Organic compound, metallurgy, volatization of chlorine-containing compounds	Delayed onset of bronchiolitis and pulmonary edema	Chronic bronchitis
Phthalic anhydride	Manufacture of resin esters, polyester resins, thermoactivated adhesives	Nasal irritation, cough	Asthma, chronic bronchitis
Sulfur dioxide	Manufacture of sulfuric acid, bleaches, coating of nonferrous metals, food processing, refrigerant, burning of fossil fuels, wood pulp industry	Mucous membrane irritant, epistaxis	?Chronic bronchitis

that a few cases of a very rare tumor in a particular group represent "an epidemic." Examples of this are nasal sinus and lung cancer in nickel workers, angiosarcomas of the liver in vinyl chloride workers, and adenocarcinomas of the nose in woodworkers.

Only in those few cases in which animal studies have been carried out can one confirm that a given suspected agent is really a carcinogen. For example, bis(chloromethyl) ether (BCME) has been shown to produce tumors in animals and oat cell cancer of the lung in humans. In this particular case, BCME, used as a chemical intermediary in the manufacture of a number of organic compounds, was known to produce tumors in animals almost before the substance was introduced into industry. (This case is one of the prime examples of why federal legislation was enacted in the United States in the 1970s to control the release of toxic substances, particularly new chemicals.)

In addition to the asbestos trades, other occupational exposures associated with either proven or suspected respiratory carcinogens include acrylonitrile, arsenic compounds, beryllium (animal studies only), BCME, chromium, coke ovens (exposure to polycyclic hydrocarbons), iron oxide, isopropyl oil (nasal sinuses), mustard gas, the various ores used to produce pure nickel, talc (possible asbestos contamination in both mining and milling), vinyl chloride, welding, wood used in woodworking (nasal cancer only), and uranium. The occurrence of excess cancers in uranium miners raises the possibility that there exists a large number of workers at risk by virtue of exposure to similar radiation hazards. This includes not only workers involved in processing uranium, up to and including its use in nuclear power plants and in military nuclear hardware, but also workers exposed in underground mining operations where radon daughters may be emitted from rock formations. In the latter case, the levels of exposure are generally considered to be relatively low; however, specific consideration must be given to the possibility of excess exposure for any hard rock miner.

GENERAL ENVIRONMENTAL EXPOSURES

AIR POLLUTION Dramatic and disastrous episodes of air pollution inversion have been documented in many industrialized centers in the world. Each of these episodes has been associated with excess acute mortality in the very old, the very young, and those with chronic cardiopulmonary diseases. The most dramatic event was the London fog of 1952, in which approximately 4000 excess deaths occurred over a 2-week period following 5 days of severe cold and dense fog. Similar episodes in the United States, although less dramatic in terms of total deaths, occurred in Donora, Pennsylvania, in 1948, and in New York City in the 1960s. In these episodes, generally associated with cold temperature and air stagnation, patients with underlying cardiopulmonary disease were most severely affected.

In addition to significant excess mortality during these episodes, a large number of people required medical care for cardiorespiratory complaints. Subsequent follow-up studies failed to implicate these episodic disasters in the etiology of chronic respiratory disease in adults. On the other hand, many epidemiologic studies of both international and regional differences in the prevalences of chronic respiratory disease suggest that long-term exposures in polluted areas in the early to middle part of the twentieth century were associated with excess chronic respiratory disease.

In 1970, the U.S. government established air quality standards for several pollutants believed to be responsible for excess cardiorespiratory diseases. Primary standards regulated by the Environmental Protection Agency (EPA) designed to protect the public health with an adequate margin of safety exist for sulfur dioxide, particulates <10 μm in size, nitrogen dioxide, ozone, lead, and carbon monoxide. These standards were updated in 1990 based on additional health effects data. The standards vary in their averaging times and levels, in part related to the differences in the known physiologic responses and epidemiologic evidence for each pollutant.

Pollutants are generated from both stationary sources (power plants and industrial complexes) and mobile sources (automobiles), and none of the pollutants occur in isolation. Thus, except for the change in carboxyhemoglobin from carbon monoxide exposure, it becomes extremely difficult to relate any specific health effect to any single pollutant. Furthermore, pollutants may be changed by chemical reactions after being emitted. For example, reducing agents, such as sulfur dioxide and particulate matter from a power plant stack, may react in air to produce acid sulfates and aerosols, the precursors of acid rain, which can be transported long distances in the atmosphere. Oxidizing substances, such as oxides of nitrogen and oxidants from automobile exhaust, may react with sunlight to produce ozone. Although originally a problem confined to the southwestern part of the United States, in recent years, at least during the summertime, elevated ozone and acid aerosol levels can occur throughout the United States. Both acute and chronic effects of these exposures are currently under investigation.

The symptoms and diseases associated with air pollution are the same as the nononcogenic conditions commonly associated with cigarette smoking. In addition, respiratory illness in early childhood has been associated with chronic exposure to only modestly elevated levels of SO_2 and respirable particles. It is not known whether persistent chronic exposure to a relatively constant level of pollutant(s) and recurrent short-term peak exposures which average to the same mean level have different effects. One can only advise the individual with significant cardiopulmonary impairment to stay indoors during periods when pollution exceeds current standards.

INDOOR EXPOSURE Because of increased concern about energy costs, efforts to become energy efficient have led to reduced air exchange rates in indoor environments. The effects of these efforts have been to increase exposures to a variety of air contaminants heretofore not considered important.

Until relatively recently, little attention was given to the effects of *passive cigarette smoking*. Several studies have shown that the respirable particulate load in any household is directly proportional to the number of cigarette smokers living in the home. Increases in prevalence of respiratory illnesses and reduced levels of pulmonary function measured with simple spirometry have been found in children of smoking parents in a number of studies. Although a modest increase in the risk of lung cancer is found in the aggregate of studies,

the long-term consequences in terms of nononcogenic respiratory diseases are unknown.

A novel source of indoor exposure to *formaldehyde* results from the curing process involved in the placement of urea-formaldehyde insulating foam or in several wood products used in modern furniture and the construction of mobile homes. Natural "degassing" of formaldehyde occurs during the first few months after the foam has been blown into the walls, with concentrations of formaldehyde as high as 5 ppm rapidly dropping off to less than 0.1 ppm. Chronic exposure to low levels of urea-formaldehyde (generally less than 1 ppm) may result if the foam is improperly installed. Patients apparently sensitive to concentrations of formaldehyde generally well below 1 ppm will complain of upper airway irritation with occasional epistaxis and sore throats. Lower respiratory complaints, such as chest pain and wheeze, however, are uncommon, and often the most disturbing complaints are mild memory and mood disorders. Formaldehyde is a proven animal carcinogen. Whether it causes cancer in humans is not established.

Radon gas is believed to be a risk factor for lung cancer. The main radon product (radon 222) is a gas that results from the decay series of uranium 238, with the immediate precursor being radium 226. The amount of radium in earth materials determines how much radon gas will be emitted. Outdoors, the concentrations are trivial. Indoors, levels are dependent on the ventilation rate and the size of space into which the gas is emitted. Levels associated with excess lung cancer risk may be present in as many as 10 percent of the houses in the United States. Where smoking exists in the household, the problem is potentially greater, since the molecular size of radon particles allows them to readily attach to smoke particles that are inhaled. Fortunately, technology is available for assessing and reducing the level of exposure.

PORTAL OF ENTRY The lung is a primary source of entry into the body for a number of toxic agents that affect other organ systems. For example, the lung is a route of entry for benzene (bone marrow), carbon disulfide (cardiovascular and nervous systems), cadmium (kidney), and metallic mercury (kidney, central nervous system). Thus, in any disease state of obscure origin, it is important to consider possible inhaled environmental agents. Such consideration can sometimes furnish the clue needed to identify a specific external cause for a disorder that might otherwise be labeled "idiopathic."

REFERENCES

BALAAN MR et al: Clinical aspects of coal workers' penumononiosis and silicosis. Occup Med 8:19, 1993

BECKLAKE MR et al: The relationship between acute and chronic airway responses to occupational exposures. Curr Pulmonol 9:25, 1988

BERRY G: Prediction of mesothelioma, lung cancer, and asbestosis in former Wittenoom asbestos workers. Br J Ind Med 48:793-802, 1991

COCHRANE AL, MOORE FA: A 20-year follow-up of men aged 55–64 including coal miners and foundry workers in Stavley. Br J Ind Med 37:226, 1980

Guidelines for the Use of International Labour Office Classification of Radiographs of Pneumoconiosis. Occupational Safety and Health Sciences 22 (Revised 1980). Geneva, ILO, 1980

LAPP NL, CASTRANOVA V: How silicosis and coal workers' pneumoconioses develop—a cellular assessment. Occup Med 8:35, 1993

LARUNERYS RR: Occupational toxicology, in *Casarett and Doull's Toxicology, The Basic Science of Poison*, 3d ed, CD Kloassen, MD Amden, J Doull (eds). New York, MacMillan, 1986, chap 29

LEONARD JF, TEMPLETON PA: Pulmonary imaging techniques in the diagnosis of occupational interstitial lung disease, in *Occupational Medicine: State of the Art Reviews*, vol 7, no 2, WS Beckett, R Bascon (eds). Philadelphia, Hanley and Belfus, 1992, pp 241–260

MULLOY KB et al: Use of chest radiographs in epidemiological investigations of pneumoconioses. Br J Ind Med 50:273, 1993

PARKES WR: *Occupational Lung Disorders*, 2d ed. London, Butterworth, 1982

RAFFLE PAB: Occupational cancer and occupational asthma, in *Hunter's Diseases of Occupations*, PAB Raffle et al (eds). Boston, Little, Brown, 1987, chaps 24 and 25

ROGGLI VL et al: Asbestos fiber type in malignant mesothelioma: An analytical scanning electron microscopic study of 94 cases. Am J Ind Med 23:605, 1993

SAMET JM, SPENGLER JD: *Indoor Air Pollution: A Health Perspective*, Baltimore, Johns Hopkins, 1991, chaps 2 and 15

SHERSON D, LANDER F: Morbidity of pulmonary tuberculosis among silicotic and nonsilicotic foundry workers in Denmark. J Occup Med 32:110-113, 1990

220   PNEUMONIA, INCLUDING NECROTIZING PULMONARY INFECTIONS (LUNG ABSCESS)

MATTHEW E. LEVISON

Pneumonia is an infection of the pulmonary parenchyma. Various bacterial species, mycoplasmas, chlamydiae, rickettsiae, viruses, fungi, and parasites can cause pneumonia. Thus pneumonia is not a single disease, but a group of specific infections, each with a different epidemiology, pathogenesis, clinical presentation, and clinical course. Identification of the etiologic microorganism is of primary importance, since this is the key to appropriate antimicrobial therapy. However, because of the serious nature of the infection, patients generally need to be started on antimicrobial therapy immediately, often before laboratory confirmation of the causative agent. The specific microbial etiology remains elusive in about a third of patients, e.g., when no sputum is available for examination, the blood cultures are sterile, and there is no pleural fluid. Serologic confirmation, of necessity, requires weeks for formation of specific antibody.

The initial choice of antimicrobial therapy is often empirical, based on the setting in which the infection was acquired, the clinical presentation, patterns of abnormality on chest radiography, stains of sputum or other infected body fluids, and knowledge of current patterns of susceptibility to antimicrobial agents. After the etiologic agent is identified, specific antimicrobial therapy can be chosen.

DEFENSE MECHANISMS   The lung is a complex structure composed of aggregates of units that are formed by the progressive branching of the airways. Approximately 80 percent of the cells lining the central airways are ciliated, pseudostratified, columnar epithelial cells, with the percentage decreasing in peripheral airways. Each ciliated cell contains about 200 cilia that beat in coordinated waves about 1000 times per minute, with a fast forward stroke and a slower backward recovery. Ciliary motion is also coordinated between adjacent cells so that each wave is propagated toward the oropharynx. The cilia are covered by a liquid film, about 5 to 10 μm thick, that is composed of two layers. The outer, or gel, layer is viscous and traps deposited particles. The cilia beat in the less viscous inner, or sol, layer. During the forward stroke, the tips of the cilia just touch the viscous gel and propel it toward the oropharynx. During recovery, the cilia move entirely within the low-resistance sol layer. Ciliated cells are interspersed with mucus-secreting cells in the trachea and bronchi, but not in the bronchioles.

The alveolar walls, from blood to air, consist of the capillary endothelium that lines the network of anastomotic capillaries, the capillary basement membrane, the interstitial tissue, the alveolar basement membrane, the alveolar lining epithelial cells (which are either flattened type I pneumocytes that cover 95 percent of the alveolar surface or rounded, granular surfactant-producing type II pneumocytes), and epithelial lining fluid. The epithelial lining fluid contains surfactant, fibronectin, and immunoglobulin, which may opsonize or, in the presence of complement, lyse microbial pathogens that are deposited on the alveolar surface. Loosely attached to the lining cells or lying free within the lumen are the alveolar macrophages, lymphocytes, and a small number of polymorphonuclear leukocytes.

The normal lower respiratory tract is sterile, despite being adjacent to enormous numbers of microorganisms that reside in the oropharynx and being exposed to environmental microorganisms in the inhaled air. Sterility of the lower respiratory tract is the result of efficient filtering and clearance mechanisms.

Infectious particles deposited on the squamous epithelium of distal nasal surfaces normally are removed by sneezing, while those deposited on the more proximal ciliated surfaces are swept posteriorly in the mucus lining into the nasopharynx, where they are swallowed or expectorated. Reflex closure of the glottis and cough protect the lower respiratory tract. Those particles deposited on the tracheobronchial surface are swept by ciliary motion toward the oropharynx. Infectious particles that bypass defenses in the airways and are deposited on the alveolar surface are cleared by phagocytic cells and humoral factors. Alveolar macrophages are the major phagocytes in the lower respiratory tract. Some phagocytosed microorganisms are killed by the phagocyte's oxygen-dependent systems, lysosomal enzymes, and cationic proteins. Other microorganisms can evade microbicidal mechanisms and persist within the macrophage. For example, *Mycobacterium tuberculosis* persists within the lysosome, while *Legionella* resides within intracellular inclusions that fail to fuse with lysosomes. Intracellular pathogens can then be transported to the ciliated surfaces and into the oropharynx or via the lymphatics to regional lymph nodes. The alveolar macrophages process and present microbial antigens to the lymphocyte and also secrete cytokines (e.g., tumor necrosis factor and interleukin 1) that modulate the immune process in T and B lymphocytes. Cytokines facilitate the generation of an inflammatory response, activate alveolar macrophages, and recruit additional phagocytes and other immunologic factors from plasma. The inflammatory exudate is responsible for many of the local signs of pulmonary consolidation and systemic manifestations of pneumonia, such as fever, chills, myalgias, and malaise.

TRAMSMISSION   Microbial pathogens may enter the lung by one of several routes.

Aspiration of organisms that colonize the oropharynx   Most pulmonary pathogens originate in the oropharyngeal flora. Aspiration of these pathogens is the most common mechanism for production of pneumonia. Normal individuals transiently carry in the nasopharynx at various times during the year common pulmonary pathogens, including *Streptococcus pneumoniae*, *S. pyogenes*, *M. pneumoniae*, *Haemophilus influenzae*, and *Moraxella catarrhalis*. The sources of anaerobic pulmonary pathogens, such as *Porphyromonas gingivalis*, *Prevotella melaninogenica*, *Fusobacterium nucleatum*, *Actinomyces* spp., spirochetes, and anaerobic streptococci, are the gingival crevice and dental plaque, which contain more than 10^{11} colony-forming units (CFU) of microorganisms per gram. The frequency of aerobic gram-negative bacillary colonization of the oropharyngeal mucosa, which is unusual in normal patients (<2 percent), increases with hospitalization, worsening debility, severity of underlying illness, alcoholism, diabetes, and advanced age and may be a consequence of increased salivary proteolytic activity, which destroys fibronectin, a glycoprotein coating the surface of the mucosa. Fibronectin is the receptor for the normal gram-positive flora of the oropharynx. Loss of fibronectin exposes the receptors on the epithelial cell surface for aerobic gram-negative bacilli. The source of aerobic gram-negative bacilli may be either the patient's own stomach, which can become colonized with these organisms as a consequence of an increase in gastric pH with atrophic gastritis or following use of H-2 blocking agents or antacids, contaminated respiratory equipment, hands of health care workers, or contaminated food and water. Nasogastric tubes can facilitate transfer of gastric bacteria to the pharynx.

About 50 percent of normal adults aspirate oropharyngeal secretions into the lower respiratory tract during sleep. Aspiration occurs more frequently and may be more severe in individuals with an impaired level of consciousness (e.g., alcoholics, drug abusers, patients following seizures, strokes, or general anesthesia), neurologic dysfunction of the oropharynx, and swallowing disorders or mechanical impediments (e.g., nasogastric or endotracheal tubes). Pneumonia is a more likely outcome if the aspirated material is large in volume or contains virulent microbial flora or foreign bodies, such as aspirated food or necrotic tissue. The presence of an impaired cough reflex or mucociliary or alveolar macrophage dysfunction increases the risk of pneumonia.

Inhalation of infectious aerosols   Deposition of inhaled particles within the respiratory tract is primarily determined by particle size. Particles over 10 μm are deposited largely in the nose and upper airways. Particles less than 3 to 5 μm in diameter, also called *airborne* *droplet nuclei*, that contain one or perhaps two microorganisms fail to settle out by gravity and remain suspended in the atmosphere for long periods unless removed by ventilation or by filtration in the lungs of an individual breathing the contaminated air. These infectious aerosols are small enough to bypass host defenses in the upper respiratory tract and airways. More particles are deposited in small bronchioles and alveoli as particle size decreases below 5 μm. One inhaled particle of appropriate size may be sufficient to reach the alveolus and initiate infection. Examples of pneumonia typically acquired by inhalation of infectious aerosols include tuberculosis, influenza, legionellosis, psittacosis, histoplasmosis, and Q fever.

Hematogenous dissemination from an extrapulmonary site of infection   Hematogenous dissemination to the lung, usually with *Staphylococcus aureus*, occurs in patients, such as intravenous drug abusers, who have either right- or left-sided bacterial endocarditis or in patients with intravenous catheter infections. *Fusobacterium* infections of the retropharyngeal tissues (Lemierre's syndrome, i.e., retropharyngeal abscess and jugular venous thrombophlebitis) also disseminate to the lungs.

Two additional routes for transmission of bacteria to the lungs are direct inoculation as a result of either tracheal intubation or stab wounds of the chest and contiguous spread from an adjacent site of infection.

PATHOLOGY   The pneumonic process may involve primarily the interstitium or the alveoli. Involvement of an entire lobe is called *lobar pneumonia*. When the process is restricted to alveoli contiguous to bronchi, it is called *bronchopneumonia*. Confluent bronchopneumonia may be indistinguishable from lobar pneumonia. The classification of pneumonias is best based on the causative microorganism whenever possible rather than on these anatomic characteristics, as was formerly done.

EPIDEMIOLOGY   The patient's living circumstances, occupation, travel history, pet or animal exposure, disease in the patient's contacts, and knowledge of the epidemic curve of community outbreaks are useful clues to the microbial etiology of the infection (Table 220-1).

The relative frequency of various pulmonary pathogens varies with the setting in which the infection was acquired, e.g., community, nursing home, or hospital. In patients hospitalized with community-acquired pneumonia, the most frequent pathogens are *S. pneumoniae, H. influenzae, Chlamydia pneumoniae,* and *L. pneumophila. M. pneumoniae*, which usually causes mild illness, is common among nonhospitalized patients with community-acquired pneumonia. In contrast, enteric gram-negative bacilli and *Pseudomonas aeruginosa,* uncommon causes of community-acquired pneumonia, are estimated to account for over 50 percent and *S. aureus* over 10 percent of hospital-acquired pneumonia. The relative frequencies of pathogens in pneumonia acquired in nursing homes fall somewhere in between those of community- and hospital-acquired pneumonias, with enteric gram-negative bacilli and *P. aeruginosa* being more common among nursing home residents than among patients who acquire pneumonia in noninstitutional settings.

Oral anaerobes, frequently in combination with aerobic bacterial flora, such as viridans streptococci, are causes of community-acquired pneumonia and anaerobic lung abscess in patients who are prone to aspiration. Edentulous persons, who have lower numbers of oral anaerobes, are less likely to develop pneumonia due to anaerobes. When the etiology of the pneumonia has been studied in unselected patients hospitalized with community-acquired pneumonia by methods that use strict anaerobic bacteriology and that avoid contamination of lower respiratory tract secretions by oral flora, anaerobic bacteria have been found to account for as many as 20 to 30 percent of cases. In hospital-acquired pneumonia, anaerobes are the pathogens, with or without aerobic copathogens, in about a third of patients. However, in the case of hospital-acquired pneumonia, the aerobic copathogens are frequently virulent microorganisms in their own right, such as enteric gram-negative bacilli, *P. aeruginosa,* and *S. aureus.*

Age is another important predictor of the infecting agent in pneumonia—*Chlamydia trachomatis* and respiratory syncytial virus being common in infants under 6 months of age, *H. influenzae* in those between 6 months and 5 years, *M. pneumoniae* and *C. pneumoniae* in young adults, and *H. influenzae, L. pneumophila,* and *M. catarrhalis* in the elderly with chronic lung disease.

The season of the year and geographic location are other predictors. The frequency of influenza as a cause of both community-acquired and institutionally acquired pneumonia increases in the winter months. Influenza causes an increase in frequency of secondary bacterial pneumonias due to *S. pneumoniae, S. aureus,* and *H. influenzae.* Influenza outbreaks in a community tend to be explosive and widespread, with many secondary cases of influenza as a result of the short incubation period of several days and high communicability. Legionellosis also occurs in explosive outbreaks if large numbers of susceptible people are exposed to an infectious aerosol; however, no secondary cases occur, as a result of low communicability. *Mycoplasma* can cause outbreaks, usually in relatively closed populations, such as military bases, colleges, or households, but because of the long incubation period of 2 to 3 weeks and relatively low communicability, *Mycoplasma* infection moves through the community slowly, affecting another person as the first is recovering. In communities where human immunodeficiency virus type 1 (HIV-1) infection is endemic, *Pneumocystic carinii* and *M. tuberculosis* assume a more prominent role as causes of community-acquired pneumonia. Histoplasmosis, blastomycosis, and coccidioidomysis have specific geographic distributions, and *C. psittaci* produces illness in bird handlers.

CLINICAL MANIFESTATIONS   Community-acquired pneumonias   Traditionally these have been thought to present as two different syndromes, the typical and atypical presentations. Although recent data suggest that these two syndromes may be less distinct than was once thought, the characteristics of the clinical presentation may, nevertheless, have some diagnostic value.

The "typical" pneumonia syndrome is characterized by sudden onset of fever, cough productive of purulent sputum, and possibly pleuritic chest pain; signs of pulmonary consolidation (dullness, increased fremitus, egophony, bronchial breath sounds, and rales) may be found on physical examination in areas of radiographic abnormality. The typical pneumonia syndrome is usually caused by the most common bacterial pathogen of community-acquired pneumonia, *S. pneumoniae,* as well as other bacterial pathogens, such as *H. influenzae* and mixed oral anaerobes and aerobes.

The "atypical" pneumonia syndrome is characterized by a more gradual onset, dry cough, prominence of extrapulmonary symptoms (such as headache, myalgias, fatigue, sore throat, nausea, vomiting, and diarrhea), and abnormalities on chest radiographs despite minimal signs of pulmonary involvement on physical examination, other than rales. Atypical pneumonia is classically produced by *M. pneumoniae* but also can be caused by *L. pneumophila, C. pneumoniae,* oral anaerobes, and *P. carinii,* as well as *S. pneumoniae* and the less frequently encountered pathogens *C. psittaci, Coxiella burnetii, Francisella tularensis, Histoplasma capsulatum,* and *Coccidioides*

TABLE 220-1 Microbial pathogens that cause pneumonia	
Community-acquired	Hospital-acquired
Mycoplasma pneumoniae	Enteric gram-negative bacilli
Streptococcus pneumoniae	*Pseudomonas aeruginosa*
Haemophilus influenzae	*Staphylococcus aureus*
Chlamydia pneumoniae	Oral anerobes
Legionella pneumophila	
Oral anaerobes	
Moraxella catarrhalis	
Pneumocystis carinii	
Nocardia spp.	
Influenza virus, cytomegalovirus, respiratory syncytial virus, measles virus, herpes zoster virus	
Histoplasma, Coccidioides, Blastomyces	

immitis. Mycoplasma pneumonia (see Chap. 139) may be complicated by erythema multiforme, hemolytic anemia, bullous myringitis, encephalitis, and tranverse myelitis. *Legionella* (see Chap. 113) frequently produces deterioration in mental status, renal and hepatic abnormalities, and marked hyponatremia; the mycoses frequently produce erythema nodosum. In *C. pneumoniae* pneumonia (see Chap. 140), sore throat, hoarseness, and wheezing are relatively common. The atypical pneumonia syndrome in a patient with a history of behaviors that place them at risk of HIV infection suggests *Pneumocystis* infection. These patients may have concurrent infection with other opportunistic pathogens, such as oral thrush due to *Candida albicans* or extensive perineal ulcers due to herpes simplex virus.

Certain viruses also produce pneumonia that is usually characterized by an atypical presentation, i.e., chills, fever, dry, nonproductive cough, and predominance of extrapulmonary symptoms. Primary viral pneumonia can be caused by influenza, usually as part of a community outbreak in winter; respiratory syncytial virus infection in children or immunosuppressed individuals; measles and varicella, accompanied by their characteristic rashes; and cytomegalovirus infection in patients immunocompromised by HIV infection or therapy given for organ transplantation. Influenza, measles, and varicella can in addition predispose to secondary bacterial pneumonia as a result of destruction of the mucociliary barrier of the airways. Secondary bacterial infection may either follow the viral infection without interruption or be separated by several days of transient symptomatic relief. Bacterial infection may be heralded by sudden worsening of the patient's clinical course, with persisting or renewed chills, fever, and cough productive of purulent sputum, possibly accompanied by pleuritic chest pain.

The patient's underlying disease may be characterized by specific immunologic or inflammatory defects that predispose to pneumonia due to specific pathogens. For example, patients who have severe hypogammaglobulinemia (<200 mg/dL) are at risk of infection with encapsulated bacteria, such as *S. pneumoniae* and *H. influenzae*. HIV-infected patients also may have ineffective antibody formation, which predisposes to infection with these encapsulated bacteria. Severe neutropenia (<500 neutrophils per microliter) increases risks for infection due to *P. aeruginosa*, Enterobacteriaceae, *S. aureus*, and, if neutropenia is prolonged, *Aspergillus*. Those HIV-infected patients with circulating CD4+ lymphocyte counts of less than 500 per microliter are at risk of *M. tuberculosis;* with counts of less than 200 per microliter, *P. carinii*, *Histoplasma capsulatum*, and *Cryptococcus neoformans;* with counts of less than 50 per microliter, *Mycobacterium avium-intracellulare* and cytomegalovirus. Glucocorticoid therapy increases the risk of tuberculosis and nocardiosis. Nocardiosis (see Chap. 126) is frequently complicated by metastatic lesions to the skin and central nervous system. Signs of pulmonary consolidation, cough, and sputum production may be absent in patients unable to mount an inflammatory response, such as those with agranulocytosis. The major manifestations in these patients may be limited to fever, tachypnea, agitation, and altered mental status. Elderly or severely ill patients may fail to develop fever.

Nosocomial pneumonias Patients with nosocomial pneumonia often present a diagnostic challenge. The usual criteria, which include new or progressive pulmonary infiltrates, purulent tracheobronchial secretions, fever, and leukocytosis, are frequently unreliable in these patients who often have preexisting pulmonary disease, endotracheal tubes that irritate the tracheal mucosa, or multiple other problems likely to produce fever and leukocytosis. Patients with hematogenous *S. aureus* pneumonia may present with only fever and dyspnea. In these patients, the inflammatory response is initially confined to the pulmonary interstitium. Cough, sputum production, and signs of pulmonary consolidation occur only after infection extends into the bronchi. These patients are usually gravely ill, with intravascular infection as well as pneumonia, and may present with signs of endocarditis, e.g., cardiac murmurs, Janeway lesions, Osler nodes, and petechiae.

Anaerobic pneumonia and lung abscess Although aspirated oral anaerobes can initially produce an infiltrative process, ultimately they produce putrid sputum, tissue necrosis, and pulmonary cavities. The clinical course of an anaerobic, polymicrobial abscess in about three-quarters of patients is indolent and mimics that of a pulmonary tuberculosis, i.e., cough, shortness of breath, chills, fever, night sweats, weight loss, pleuritic chest pain, and blood-streaked sputum for several weeks or more. In other patients the disease may present more acutely. Patients with anaerobic abscesses are usually prone to aspiration of oropharyngeal contents and have periodontal disease. One of the oral anaerobes, *Actinomyces* spp., produces a chronic, fibrotic necrotizing process that crosses tissue planes and may involve the pleural space, ribs, vertebrae, and subcutaneous tissue with eventual discharge of sulfur granules (macroscopic bacterial masses) through the skin (empyema necessitatis).

DIAGNOSIS Radiography Chest radiographs can confirm the presence and location of the pulmonary infiltrate; assess the extent of the pulmonary infection; detect the presence of pleural involvement, pulmonary cavitation, or hilar lymphadenopathy; and gauge response to antimicrobial therapy. However, chest radiographs may be normal in patients who are unable to mount an inflammatory response (e.g., those with agranulocytosis) or early in an infiltrative process (e.g., hematogenous *S. aureus* pneumonia, *Pneumocystis* pneumonia in patients with AIDS).

Anatomic localization of the inflammatory process as visualized in chest radiographs occasionally has diagnostic implications. Most pulmonary pathogens produce focal lesions. Multicentric distribution suggests hematogenous infection, in which case remote infections, such as endocarditis or thrombophlebitis, should be sought. Hematogenous pneumonia, which results from septic embolization in patients with thrombophlebitis or right-sided endocarditis or from bacteremia in patients with left-sided endocarditis, appears on the chest radiograph as multiple areas of pulmonary infiltration that subsequently may cavitate. Diffuse distribution suggests *P. carinii*, cytomegalovirus, measles, or herpes zoster virus, the later two pathogens being diagnosed by the characteristic rash that always accompanies the pneumonia. Pleurisy and hilar nodal enlargement are unusual with *Pneumocystis* and cytomegalovirus pneumonia; their presence suggests another etiology. Diffuse lesions in immunocompromised patients also suggests possible legionellosis, tuberculosis, histoplasmosis, or *Mycoplasma* or disseminated *Strongyloides* infection.

Cavities occur when necrotic material is discharged into communicating airways, which results in either necrotizing pneumonia (multiple small cavities, each <2 cm in diameter in one or more bronchopulmonary segments or lobes) or lung abscess (one or more cavities >2 cm in diameter). Oral anaerobes, *S. aureus*, *S. pneumoniae* serotype III, aerobic gram-negative bacilli, *M. tuberculosis*, or fungi and certain noninfectious conditions can produce tissue necrosis and cavities (Table 220-2). In contrast, *H. influenzae*, *M. pneumoniae*, viruses, and most other serotypes of *S. pneumoniae* almost never cause cavities. Apical disease, with or without cavities, suggests reactivation tuberculosis. Anaerobic abscesses are located in dependent, poorly ventilated, and poorly draining bronchopulmonary segments, which characteristically have air-fluid levels, unlike the well-ventilated, well-drained upper lobe cavities caused by *M. tuberculosis*, an obligate aerobe. Air-fluid levels also may be present in cavities

---

TABLE 220-2 Causes of pulmonary cavities

INFECTIOUS

Bacteria: Oral anaerobes (*Bacteroides* spp., fusobacteria, *Actinomyces* spp., anaerobic and microaerophilic cocci), enteric aerobic gram-negative bacilli, *P. aeruginosa*, *Legionella* spp., *S. aureus*, type III *S. pneumoniae*, *M. tuberculosis*, *Nocardia* spp.
Fungi: *Histoplasma capsulatum*, *Coccidioides immitis Blastomyces* spp.

NONINFECTIOUS

Neoplasms, Wegener's granulomatosis, infarction, infected bullae and cysts due to other infectious causes of pulmonary necrosis. *Mucor* and *Aspergillus* invade blood vessels and cause pleural-based, wedge-shaped areas of pulmonary infarction; these infarcts may subsequently cavitate.

In the patient with an uncomplicated course, chest radiographs need not be repeated before discharge, since resolution of infiltrates may take up to 6 weeks after initial presentation. However, patients who do not respond clinically, who have a pleural effusion on admission, who are suspected of postobstructive pneumonia, or who are infected with certain pathogens (e.g., *S. aureus*, aerobic gram-negative bacilli, or oral anaerobes) need more intensive surveillance. At times, computed tomography (CT) may be especially helpful to distinguish different processes, e.g., pleural effusion versus underlying pulmonary consolidation, hilar adenopathy versus pulmonary mass, or pulmonary abscess versus empyema with an air-fluid level.

Sputum examination   Examination of the sputum remains the mainstay in evaluation of a patient with acute bacterial pneumonia. Unfortunately, expectorated material is frequently contaminated by potentially pathogenic bacteria that colonize the upper respiratory and, at times, the lower respiratory tract without actually causing disease. This contamination reduces the specificity of any lower respiratory tract specimen. In addition, it has been estimated that the usual laboratory processing methods yield the pulmonary pathogen in less than 50 percent of expectorated sputum samples in patients with bacteremic pneumonia. This loss of sensitivity may be due to misinterpretation of the alpha-hemolytic colonies of *S. pneumoniae* as nonpathogenic alpha-hemolytic streptococci ("normal flora"), overgrowth of the cultures by more hardy colonizing organisms, or loss of more fastidious organisms due to slow transport or improper processing. In addition, certain very common pulmonary pathogens, such as anaerobes, *Mycoplasma, Chlamydia, Pneumocystis*, mycobacteria, fungi, and *Legionella*, cannot be cultured by routine methods.

Since expectorated material is routinely contaminated by oral anaerobes, the diagnosis of anaerobic pulmonary infection is frequently putative. Confirmation requires culture of anaerobes from pulmonary secretions that are uncontaminated by oropharyngeal secretions, which in turn requires that pulmonary secretions be obtained by special techniques, such as transtracheal aspiration, transthoracic lung puncture, and protected brush via bronchoscopy. These procedures are invasive and usually are withheld, unless the patient fails to respond to empirical therapy.

Gram's stain of sputum specimens, screened initially under low-power magnification (10× objective and 10× eyepiece) to determine the degree of contamination with squamous epithelial cells, is of utmost diagnostic importance. In patients with the typical pneumonia syndrome who produce purulent sputum, the sensitivity and specificity of the Gram's stain of sputum minimally contaminated by upper respiratory tract secretions (>25 polymorphonuclear leukocytes and <10 epithelial cells per low power field) in identifying the pathogen as *S. pneumoniae* are 62 and 85 percent, respectively. The Gram's stain in this case is more specific and probably more sensitive than the accompanying sputum culture. The finding of mixed flora on Gram's stain of an uncontaminated sputum specimen suggests an anaerobic infection. Acid-fast stains of sputum should be done when mycobacterial infection is suspected. Examination of Giemsa-stained expectorated respiratory secretions from patients with AIDS has given satisfactory results for the diagnosis of *Pneumocystis* pneumonia when examined by experienced pathologists. The sensitivity of sputum examination has been increased by the use of monoclonal *Pneumocystis* antibodies and diminished by prior prophylactic use of inhaled pentamidine. Examination of wet preparations of sputum can be diagnostic for blastomycosis. Sputum can be examined for *Legionella* by staining directly with fluorescent antibody, but this test has a relatively high frequency of false-negative results. Sputum also should be cultured for *Legionella* on special media. A highly sensitive and specific urinary antigen test is available to detect *L. pneumophila* serogroup 1, which accounts for about 70 percent of *L. pneumophila* infection, in patients with pneumonia.

TABLE 220-3   Criteria for hospitalization of patients with pneumonia

1 Elderly (>65 years of age)
2 Significant comorbidity, e.g., renal, heart, or lung disease; diabetes mellitus; neoplasm; immunosuppression
3 Leukopenia (<5000 white blood cells per microliter) unattributable to a known condition
4 Suspected cause of pneumonia is *S. aureus*, gram-negative bacilli, or anaerobes
5 Suppurative complications, e.g., empyema, arthritis, meningitis, endocarditis
6 Failure of outpatient management
7 Inability to take oral medication
8 Tachypnea (>30 beats/min), tachycardia (>140 beats/min); hypotension (<90 mmHg systolic); hypoxemia (arterial P_{O_2} < 60 mmHg); acute alteration of mental status

---

In the initial evaluation of a patient with pneumonia, several blood cultures should be obtained, and if empyema is a clinical consideration, diagnostic thoracentesis is indicated. Bacteremia or positive pleural fluid cultures are generally considered diagnostic for the organisms causing the pneumonia. However, bacteremia and empyema each occur in fewer than 10 to 30 percent of patients with pneumonia. Serologic studies are sometimes helpful in defining the etiology of certain types of pneumonia, although serologic diagnosis, being delayed by the necessity to demonstrate at least a fourfold rise in convalescent phase antibody titer, is usually retrospective. A single elevated *Legionella* antibody titer of ≥1:128 suggests acute legionellosis.

Expectorated sputum is usually easily collected in patients with a vigorous cough but may be scant in those with an atypical syndrome, in the elderly, and in those with altered mental status. If the patient is not producing sputum and can cooperate, respiratory secretions should be induced with ultrasonic nebulization of 3% saline. An attempt to obtain lower respiratory secretions by passage of a catheter through the nose or mouth rarely achieves the desired results in an alert patient and is discouraged; usually the catheter can be found coiled in the oropharynx.

In some patients who do not require hospitalization (see Table 220-3), the need to establish an accurate microbial diagnosis may not be crucial, and empirical therapy can be started on clinical and epidemiologic evidence alone. This also may be the case with hospitalized patients who are not severely ill and who are unable to produce an induced sputum specimen. Use of more invasive procedures to establish a microbial diagnosis carries risks that must be weighed against potential benefits. However, the decision to initiate empirical therapy without evaluation of induced sputum should be undertaken with caution and always supplemented by several blood cultures in hospitalized patients. The ability to understand the cause (see Table 220-4) of a poor response to empirical antimicrobial therapy may be compromised by the lack of an initial sputum culture.

The sensitivities and specificities of invasive procedures described below for obtaining pulmonary material vary with different types of immunocompromised patients, different types of pulmonary lesions, and prior exposure to therapeutic or prophylactic antimicrobial agents.

TABLE 220-4   Factors involved in poor response to empirical antimicrobial therapy

Incorrect microbiologic diagnosis.
Inappropriate antimicrobial agent or dosing regimen.
Drug hypersensitivity or other adverse effect, e.g., *Clostridium difficile* colitis.
Infectious complication: empyema, metastatic spread, superinfection.
Atelectasis, parapneumonic effusion, phlebitis.
Poor host defenses, e.g., endobronchial obstruction, life-threatening comorbidity.

Transtracheal aspiration (TTA), popular several decades ago, is rarely performed today. Although the sensitivity of the procedure is high (approaching 90 percent), the specificity is low. Material, which is obtained from a catheter inserted through the cricothyroid cartilage and advanced toward the carina, is not contaminated by upper respiratory tract secretions but can contain organisms that colonize the tracheobronchial tree without necessarily being the cause of the pneumonia. Significant morbidity and even mortality have attended its use. TTA, which is contraindicated in patients with a bleeding diathesis, may cause infection at the puncture site and severe subcutaneous and mediastinal emphysema in patients who are coughing vigorously.

Percutaneous transthoracic lung puncture uses a skinny (small-gauge) needle that is advanced into the area of pulmonary consolidation with CT guidance. The procedure requires patient cooperation, good hemostasis, and the ability to tolerate pulmonary hemorrhage or pneumothorax that may be associated with the procedure. Patients on mechanical ventilation cannot undergo lung puncture because of the high incidence of complicating pneumothorax.

Fiberoptic bronchoscopy, safe and relatively well-tolerated, has become the standard invasive procedure to obtain lower respiratory tract secretions when indicated in seriously ill or immunocompromised patients with complex or progressive pneumonia. It allows direct vision of the lower airways. Specimens obtained by bronchoscopy should be stained with Gram's, acid-fast, *Legionella* direct fluorescent antibody, and Gomori's methenamine silver stains and cultured for routine aerobic and anaerobic bacteria, *Legionella*, mycobacteria, and fungi. Sampling is done with a protected double-sheathed brush (PSB), by bronchoalveolar lavage (BAL), or by transbronchial biopsy (TBB) at the site of pulmonary consolidation. The PSB sample is usually contaminated by oropharyngeal flora; quantitative cultures must be performed of the 1 mL of sterile culture medium in which the brush is placed after withdrawal from the inner catheter to differentiate contamination (<1000 CFU/mL) from infection (≥1000 CFU/mL). The results of PSB have shown high specificity and sensitivity, especially in patients who have not received antibiotics before culture. BAL is usually performed with 150 to 200 mL of sterile, nonbacteriostatic saline. Quantitative bacteriology of the BAL sample has given results similar to those of PSB. Gram's stain of the cytocentrifuged BAL specimen can serve as an immediate guide to antimicrobial therapy while awaiting results of cultures.

Open lung biopsy is needed most commonly in the immunocompromised patient with progressive pneumonia when bronchoscopically obtained specimens have been unrevealing. Limitations on performance of an open lung biopsy include hypoxemia and a bleeding diathesis, which may supervene while the physician is deciding whether to do this procedure. Results of an open lung biopsy are considered diagnostic because of the large tissue sample. Its diagnostic yield is highest in focal lesions, whereas bronchoscopic evaluation is most useful in diffuse lesions.

DECISION TO HOSPITALIZE   Use of hospital services is costly and at times hazardous to the patient (e.g., risk of nosocomial infections). Hospitalization should be justified by the patient's poor functional status or social support system that would compromise care at home, poor prognostic factors, unstable vital signs, or need for intensive nursing care or specialized diagnostic procedures. Guidelines for hospitalization are given in Table 220-3. Discharge from the hospital should be guided by similar considerations.

TREATMENT Community-acquired pneumonia: Outpatient management   Most community-acquired pneumonias in otherwise healthy adults do not require hospitalization. Since it is often not feasible to make a microbial diagnosis in an office setting, oral antimicrobial therapy frequently is empirical (see Table 220-5). The pathogen in such a situation is likely to be *Mycoplasma*, the pneumococcus, or *C. pneumoniae*. In older patients with chronic respiratory disease, *L. pneumophila*, *H. influenzae*, or *M. catarrhalis* also should be considered. In patients at risk of aspiration, oral anaerobes are an additional consideration. There is no oral therapy that has a reliable spectrum encompassing all these pathogens (see Table 220-5). Many experts still recommend penicillin V (500 mg every 6 h) or amoxicillin (500 mg every 8 h) for 7 to 10 days for community-acquired pneumonia with a "typical" presentation in younger outpatients without preexisting disease, since the pneumococcus is the most common pathogen. Second-generation cephalosporins (e.g., cefuroxime axetil, 500 mg every 8 h), doxycycline (100 mg every 12 h), and erythromycin (500 mg every 6 h) are alternative choices. Trimethoprim-sulfamethoxazole is not active against up to 10 percent of strains of *S. pneumoniae*, and ciprofloxacin has only borderline in vitro activity against pneumococci. For the past decade, pneumococcal isolates in other countries frequently have been reported to be erythromycin-resistant; recently, such resistance also has been reported in 10 to 20 percent of pneumococcal isolates from certain centers in the United States as well. These strains are resistant to other macrolides, such as clarithromycin and azithromycin, and are also more likely to be resistance to many other commonly used oral antibiotics. Pneumococcal strains resistant to multiple antibiotics, including penicillin, are not a problem in most of the United States at present. The Centers for Disease Control and Prevention (CDCP), Respiratory Diseases Branch, has reported that of 567 isolates of *S. pneumoniae* from normally sterile body sites submitted during the period for October 1991 through September 1992 in the national pneumococcal surveillance, 5.3 percent were resistant to erythromycin (MIC ≥ 2 μg/mL). The emergence of such strains, however, would require changes in antibiotic recommendations and deserves close scrutiny.

In older patients or adult outpatients with preexisting respiratory disease and "typical" presentation of community-acquired pneumonia and in whom ß-lactamase–producing pathogens, such as *H. influenzae* or *M. catarrhalis*, are common, amoxicillin plus clavulanate, a ß-lactamase inhibitor, doxycycline, or cefuroxime axetil can be used. Erythromycin has poor activity against *H. influenzae*. In comparison to erythromycin, two new oral antibiotics related to erythromycin, azithromycin (500 mg as a single dose on the first day and 250 mg once daily for 4 more days) and clarithromycin (500 mg twice daily for 7 to 10 days), have equal or greater potency against many lower respiratory pathogens and much less frequent gastrointestinal intolerance. Although more costly than erythromycin, these new macrolides may come to replace erythromycin for therapy of community-acquired pneumonia in outpatients if pneumococcal resistance to macrolides does not become a widespread problem.

TABLE 220-5   **Empirical oral antimicrobial therapy for outpatient management of community-acquired pneumonia**

Pathogen	Penicillin G	Amoxicillin/ clavulanate	Cefuroxime	Trimethoprim- sulfamethoxazole	Doxycycline	Erythromycin	Ciprofloxacin
S. pneumoniae	+	+	+	±	+	+*	±
H. influenzae	–	+	+	+	+	±	+
M. catarrhalis	±	+	+	–	+	+	+
Anaerobes	+	+	±	–	–	–	–
M. pneumoniae	–	–	–	–	+	+	+
C. pneumoniae	–	–	–	±	+	+	+
L. pneumophila	–	–	–	±	±	+	±

* 10 to 20 percent of strains recently have been reported to be resistant to macrolides in some locations in the United States (−, ineffective; +, effective).

Doxycycline, erythromycin, and ciprofloxacin are active against *M. pneumoniae* and *C. pneumoniae* and can be used in younger adults with an ''atypical'' presentation. Although erythromycin is the drug of choice for legionellosis, doxycycline, trimethoprim-sulfamethoxazole, and ciprofloxacin are alternative agents that have been used successfully according to anecdotal reports. Duration of therapy for *Mycoplasma* and *Legionella* infections is 2 to 3 weeks, the longer duration frequently recommended to prevent relapse. The optimal duration of therapy for *C. pneumoniae* infection is unknown but also probably is 2 to 3 weeks.

Pneumonia due to anaerobes can be treated with clindamycin (300 mg every 6 h or 450 mg every 8 h for 7 to 10 days), amoxicillin (500 mg every 8 h) combined with metronidazole (500 mg every 6 h), or amoxicillin/clavulanic acid (500 mg every 8 h). Metronidazole has inadequate activity against microaerophilic gram-positive cocci and must be supplemented by a ß-lactam agent that conpensates for this deficit in coverage.

Community-acquired pneumonia: Inpatient management Patients who have community-acquired pneumonia and are ill enough to be hospitalized (see Table 220-3) must have a prompt microbiologic evaluation, with the Gram's stained sputum and knowledge of the current antimicrobial sensitivities of the pulmonary pathogens in the local geographic area guiding empirical therapy, as outlined in Tables 220-6 and 220-7. Parenteral antimicrobial therapy in the hospitalized patient is usually mandatory. Lack of sputum production, an ''atypical'' clinical presentation, diffuse radiographic infiltrates in a patient with a rapidly progressive, downhill course, and poor response to prior empirical therapy are some of the reasons to use invasive procedures to detect the pulmonary pathogen, especially in the immunocompromised patient. Although broad-spectrum antibacterial therapy should be started while undertaking a full evaluation in severely ill patients with a rapidly progressing process, these empirical regimens cannot encompass all the possible pathogens without producing unnecessary toxicity and expense. Indeed, in immunocompromised patients, including those with neutropenia or HIV infection, the number of microbial as well as noninfectious causes of pulmonary disease is large and increasing. Since failure to specifically treat the causative agent can be rapidly fatal in these patients, a diagnosis should be sought aggressively so that optimal therapy can be started promptly.

Penicillin or ampicillin remains the drug of choice for suspected pneumococcal pneumonia in the United States. Penicillin resistance among pneumococci (screened with use of a 1-μg oxacillin disk) has become a worldwide problem; it is still unusual in most of the United States (4.1 percent nationwide for 1987–1988), although Alaska had a rate of 25.8 percent in 1987–1988. Data from the CDCP, Respiratory Diseases Branch, indicate that of 567 isolates from normally sterile body sites submitted during the period from October 1991 through September 1992 in the national pneumococcal surveillance, 6.9 percent had some level of resistance to penicillin (MIC > 0.1 μg/mL) and 1.2 percent had high-level resistance (MIC > 1.0 μg/mL). However, one study has reported an alarming increase in resistance (20.1 percent) in 1990–1991 in the United States, although most of

the 524 strains had minimal inhibitory concentrations (MICs) between 0.1 and 1.0 μg/mL penicillin. Penicillin-resistant stains also may be resistant to other groups of antimicrobial agents. Nevertheless, MICs of cefotaxime, ceftriaxone, imipenem, and vancomycin are lower than those of penicillin or ampicillin and most other ß-lactam antibiotics for penicillin-resistant strains. However, some strains with intermediate resistance to penicillin (MIC 0.25 to 1 μg/mL) have been reported recently to have high-level resistance to second- and third-generation cephalosporins. Although there are no good studies on the treatment of pneumonia due to penicillin-resistant strains, high-dose intravenous penicillin G (e.g., 10 to 20 million units daily) is probably adequate therapy for pneumonia due to strains exhibiting intermediate resistance to penicillin. High-level penicillin resistance (MIC 2 to 16 μg/mL) has been unusual in the United States, but the frequency of high-level penicillin resistance among the pencillin-resistant strains may approach 50 percent of isolates in some European countries. Effectiveness of high-dose intravenous penicillin for pneumonia due to these highly resistant strains is unknown, but anecdotal reports suggest that cefotaxime or ceftriaxone may be adequate. Since all penicillin-resistant strains are sensitive to vancomycin, initial therapy should include this antibiotic for patients with pneumococcal pneumonia who live in regions where penicillin resistance is common and are severely ill or have significant comorbidity.

If the sputum Gram's stain is not interpretable or not available, either a second- or third-generation cephalosporin plus metronidazole or ampicillin plus sulbactam is an adequate empirical regimen, unless *Legionella* or *Chlamydia* is the likely pathogen, in which case erythromycin should be added to the regimen. With rapid clinical improvement, therapy can be switched from intavenous to oral agents to complete a 7- to 10-day course if antimicrobial agents are available

---

TABLE 220-7 Dosage of antimicrobial agents for pneumonia in hospitalized patients*

Drug	Dosage
Ampicillin/sulbactam	3 g IV every 6 h
Aztreonam	2 g IV every 8 h
Cefazolin	1–2 g IV every 8 h
Cefotaxime, ceftizoxime	1–2 g IV every 8–12 h
Ceftazidime	2 g IV every 8 h
Ceftriaxone	1–2 g IV every 12–24 h
Cefuroxime	750 mg IV every 8 h
Ciprofloxacin	400 mg IV or 750 mg PO every 12 h
Clindamycin	600–900 mg IV every 8 h
Erythromycin	0.5–1.0 g IV every 6 h
Gentamicin (or tobramycin)	5 mg/kg in three equally divided dose IV every 8h
Imipenem	500 mg IV every 6 h
Metronidazole	500 mg IV or PO every 8 h
Nafcillin	2 g IV every 4 h
Penicillin G	1 million units IV every 4–6 h
Ticarcillin/Clavulanate	3.1 g IV every 4 h
Vancomycin	1 g IV every 12 h

* Dosage must be modified in patients with renal failure. Guidelines on duration of therapy for each pathogen are given in the text of this chapter and in individual chapters on infecting agents.

TABLE 220-6 Empirical antimicrobial therapy for the management of hospitalized patients with community-acquired pneumonia

Pathogen	Penicillin G	First-generation cephalosporin	Second- or third-generation cephalosporin	Metronidazole	Trimethoprim-sulfamethoxazole	Erythromycin	Ampicillin/ sulbactam
S. pneumoniae	+	+	+	−	±	+*	+
S. aureus	−	+	+	−	+	−	+
H. influenzae	−	−	+	−	+	±	+
M. catarrhalis	−	−	+	−	+	+	+
Anaerobic gram-positive cocci	+	+	+	+	−	−	+
Anaerobic gram-negative bacilli	−	−	−	+	−	−	+
C. pneumoniae	−	−	−	−	−	+	−
L. pneumophila	−	−	−	−	±	+	−

* 10 to 20 percent of strains recently have been reported to be resistant to macrolides in some locations in the United States (−, ineffective; +, effective).

that are readily absorbed after oral administration to achieve tissue levels above the MIC. The presence of *S. aureus*, aerobic gram-negative bacilli, or suppurative complications requires a more prolonged course of therapy. Legionellosis should be treated with 1 g erythromycin, IV, every 6 h for 3 weeks, to prevent relapses; rifampin should be added in critically ill patients with legionellosis. Anaerobic lung abscess should be treated with the regimens suggested for aspiration pneumonia until a chest radiograph (taken at 2-week intervals) is clear or shows only a small, stable scar. Therapy is prolonged for 6 weeks or more to prevent relapse, although shorter courses of therapy are probably sufficient for most patients. Surgery is rarely required for lung abscess; indications for surgery include massive hemoptysis and neoplasm. Supportive measures include supplemental oxygen, intravenous fluids, assistance in clearing secretions, fiberoptic bronchoscopy, and ventilatory support, if necessary. Caution should be exercised in bronchoscopic drainage of large, fluid-filled lung abscesses because of potential sudden, massive spillage of large collections of pus into the airways.

Patients with risk factors for HIV infection and an atypical pneumonia syndrome should be evaluated for *Pneumocystis* infections because of its frequency as an index diagnosis in HIV infection and its potential severity. Tuberculosis, as well as other causes of atypical pneumonia in these patients, must be excluded as part of the evaluation. Initial empirical therapy can be either trimethoprim-sulfamethoxazole (15 to 20 mg/kg of trimethoprim daily in four divided doses IV or PO) or pentamidine (3 to 4 mg/kg daily IV), and therapy is continued for 3 weeks in confirmed cases of *Pneumocystis* infection. Although some data suggest that trimethprim-sulfamethoxazole may be more effective than ·pentamidine, further studies directly comparing the two agents are needed. The frequency and severity of adverse effects of both drugs are thought by most to be equivalent. Addition of glucocorticoids (prednisone, 40 mg twice daily followed by a tapering dose) early in the course of *Pneumocystis* pneumonia in patients with an arterial $P_{O2} < 70$ mmHg decreases the need for mechanical ventilation and improves survival and functional status. Prophylaxis for recurrent *Pneumocystis* pneumonia must be started at the end of therapy.

Institutionally acquired pneumonia   Pneumonia acquired in institutions such as nursing homes or hospitals is frequently caused by enteric gram-negative bacilli, *P. aeruginosa*, or *S. aureus*, with or without oral anaerobes. Again, antimicrobial therapy should be guided by Gram's stain of sputum (see Tables 220-7 and 220-8) and knowledge of the prevalent nosocomial pathogens and curent in vitro antimicrobial sensitivity patterns of these nosocomial pathogens in the particular institution. An aggressive diagnostic approach is needed

in some circumstances, especially for the immunocompromised patient, as outlined above.

S. aureus acquired in some institutions is frequently methicillin-resistant. Such strains are resistant to all ß-lactam antibiotics and can be resistant to clindamycin, erythromycin, and the fluoroquinolones. Only vancomycin is predictably active against these organisms and should be added to an empirical regimen when methicillin-resistant organisms are possibly the cause of pneumonia.

Pneumonia due to gram-negative bacilli in the institutionalized patient when multiantibiotic resistance is not a problem can be treated initially with a ß-lactam active against *P. aeruginosa* (ceftazidime, ticarcillin/clavulanate, aztreonam, or imipenem) or a parenterally administered fluoroquinolone (ciprofloxacin or ofloxacin). Ticarcillin/clavulanate is preferred as an empirical antibiotic over other penicillins with activity against *P. aeruginosa*, such as piperacillin, which, although more potent against *P. aeruginosa*, is not sufficiently active against *Klebsiella pneumoniae*, a relatively common pathogen. Amipicillin/sulbactam, the other parenterally administered ß-lactam antibiotic/ß-lactamase inhibitor combination, does not have activity against many nosocomial pathogens, such as *P. aeruginosa*, *Enterobacter* spp., and *Serratia* spp., and therefore is inappropriate for empirical therapy of nosocomial pneumonia.

In seriously ill patients, especially those infected with *P. aeruginosa*, use of a ß-lactam/aminoglycoside combination for bactericidal synergy is prudent. Combinations of ß-lactam plus aminoglycoside are also used to broaden the spectrum of antibacterial activity for the possibility of infection with resistant pathogens, to treat polymicrobial infection, and to prevent emergence of antimicrobial resistance. Combinations of ß-lactams or aminoglycosides with a fluoroquinolone are not expected to exhibit an enhancement of the already rapid bactericidal activity of the fluoroquinolone alone; nevertheless, they are expected to broaden the spectrum and perhaps prevent the emergency of resistance. Fluoroquinolone plus either a ß-lactam or an aminoglycoside could be used in institutions where there is a greater expectation for infection with a fluoroquinolone-resistant nosocomial pathogen, e.g., *Acinetobacter calcoaceticus*, or with organisms that frequently exhibit emergence of resistance on therapy, e.g., *P. aeruginosa*.

Pneumonia due to possible coinfection with aerobic gram-negative bacilli and anaerobes, as reflected by a polymicrobial flora on Gram's stain of sputum, may usually be treated with any of the following regimens: (1) ceftazidime plus metronidazole or clindamycin, (2) aztreonam or a fluoroquinolone plus clindamycin, and (3) imipenem alone or ticarcillin/clavulanate. The regimens that contain a ß-lactam agent usually also should include an aminoglycoside (see Table 220-8).

Production of chromosomally encoded, inducible ß-lactamases by some aerobic gram-negative bacilli, including *Serratia marcescens*, *E. cloacae*, *Citrobacter freundii*, *Morganella morganii*, *P. aeruginosa*, and *Acinetobacter calcoaceticus*, has important implications for therapy of nosocomial pneumonia in institutions where these organisms are common nosocomial pathogens. Antibiotic resistance in these pathogens has been attributed to two related mechanisms: inducible production of chromosomally encoded ß-lactamases and selection of mutants that have lost a gene that controls expression of ß-lactamase production. The control gene represses ß-lactamase production in the absence of a ß-lactam agent and allows ß-lactamase production in the presence of a ß-lactam agent. This group of organisms has a relatively high mutation rate for loss of this control gene, and loss of the gene results in continuous production of large amounts of ß-lactamase (stable derepression). The derepressed mutants are resistant to third-generation cephalosporins, aztreonam, and broad-spectrum penicillins. These chromosomally encoded, inducible ß-lactamases are not inhibited by clavulanic acid or sulbactam.

Selection by the ß-lactam antibiotic of the derepressed mutants present in the dense bacterial populations of infected pulmonary tissue at the initiation of antibiotic therapy apparently accounts for emergence of resistance during therapy, which is especially a problem in severely

TABLE 220-8   Empirical antimicrobial therapy of institutionally acquired pneumonia based on Gram's stain of sputum

Presumptive *S. aureus*	Nafcillin or vancomycin*	
Presumptive	*1* Ceftazidime	±Aminoglycoside
Enteric gram-negative	2 Ticarcillin/clavulanate	±Aminoglycoside
bacilli or *P. aeruginosa*	3 Aztreonam	±Aminoglycoside
	4 Imipenem†	±Aminoglycoside
	5 Fluoroquinolone†	±Aminoglycoside or β-lactam
Mixed flora	*1* Ceftazidime + clindamycin (or metronidazole) ± aminoglycoside‡	
	2 Ticarcillin/clavulanate ± aminoglycoside‡	
	3 Aztreonam + clindamycin (or metronidazole§) ± Aminoglycoside‡	
	4 Imipenem† ± Aminoglycoside‡	
	5 Fluoroquinolone† + clindamycin (or metronidazole‡,§) ± aminoglycoside or β-lactam‡	

* If methicillin-resistant *S. aureus* is present in the institution, use vancomycin; otherwise, use an antistaphylococcal β-lactam, e.g., nafcillin or cefazolin.
† Use when chromosomal, inducible β-lactamase producers are endemic in the institution.
‡ Add vancomycin if methicillin-resistant *S. aureus* is present in the institution.
§ Metronidazole must be combined with vancomycin or another antimicrobial that covers microaerophilic and anaerobic gram-positive cocci.

compromised patients whose defective host defenses are unable to control the growth of at first few resistant mutants. The only ß-lactam agent that maintains activity against the derepressed mutants is imipenem. Ciprofloxacin and aminoglycosides may retain activity against these mutants. Trimethoprim-sulfamethoxazole also may remain active against these gram-negative bacilli, except *P. aeruginosa*, which is inherently resistant. Some clinicians have questioned the efficacy of aminoglycosides alone in the therapy of gram-negative bacillary pneumonia. The poor clinical efficacy has been attributed to low levels of aminoglycoside in bronchial secretions and loss of antimicrobial activity due to the relatively acidic purulent secretions, the anaerobic conditions in infected lung, and, in the case of *P. aeruginosa*, the presence of the divalent cations calcium and magnesium. The nephrotoxicity and ototoxicity of aminoglycosides lead to underdosing with these agents. These problems are compounded by unpredictable pharmacokinetics that necessitate measurement of serum levels of aminoglycosides. If multiantibiotic-resistant nosocomial organisms are likely to be pathogens in severely compromised patients, the only reliable empirical agents are fluoroquinolones and imipenem, unless resistance to these drugs is also endemic in the institution. Up-to-date knowledge of antimicrobial sensitivities of nosocomial pathogens and use of preventive practices are mandatory.

Amantidine (200 mg/d in most adults and 100 mg/d in persons over 65 years of age) is effective for prevention of influenza A infection in the unimmunized patients during an influenza A outbreak and for therapy (for 5 to 7 days) of early influenza A infection. Ribavirin is effective for respiratory syncytial virus infection. Intravenous acyclovir (5 to 10 mg/kg every 8 h for 7 to 14 days) is appropriate for varicella pneumonia. Relatively high doses of intravenous immunoglobulin combined with either ganciclovir (2.5 mg/kg every 12 h for 20 days, then 5 mg/kg once daily for 5 days a week for 20 more doses) may be effective for cytomegalovirus pneumonitis.

PREVENTION Prevention of pneumonia involves either decreasing the likelihood of encountering the pathogen or strengthening the host's response once the pathogen is encountered. The former method can include use of face masks by persons dealing with affected patients, use of negative-pressure isolation rooms for patients with contagious tuberculosis or with pneumonia spread by the aerosol route, prompt institution of effective chemotherapy for contagious patients, or use of therapy to correct conditions that facilitate aspiration. The latter method includes use of chemoprophylaxis or immunization of patients at risk. Chemoprophylaxis may be administered to patients who have encountered or are likely to encounter the pathogen before they become symptomatic (amantidine during a community outbreak of influenza A, INH for tuberculosis, trimethoprim-sulfamethoxazole for pneumocystosis) or administered to patients who are likely to have a recurrence following recovery from a symptomatic episode (trimethoprim-sulfamethoxazole for pneumocystosis in patients with HIV infection). Gastric acidity is a major factor that prevents colonization of the gastrointestinal tract by nosocomial gram-negative bacillary pathogens. To prevent stress ulceration, it is preferable to use sucralfate, which maintains gastric acidity, rather than H-2 blocking agents. Vaccines (see Chaps. 82, 101, and 112) are available for immunization against the following pulmonary pathogens: *S. pneumoniae, H. influenzae* type B, influenza viruses A and B, and measles virus. Influenza and pneumococcal vaccines are strongly recommended for those over 65 years of age and persons of any age who are at risk of adverse consequences of influenza or pneumonia because of underlying conditions. Pneumococcal, hemophilus, and influenza vaccines are recommended for HIV-infected patients who are still capable of responding to a vaccine challenge. The currently available 23-valent pneumococcal vaccine covers 88 percent of the serotypes causing systemic disease as well as 8 percent of related serotypes. The increasing prevalence of multiantibiotic resistance of pneumococci makes immunization of high-risk individuals with the pneumococcal vaccine of utmost importance. Immune serum globulin is available for replacement therapy in those patients with congenital or acquired hypogammaglob-

ulinemia. Prevention of nosocomial pneumonia requires good infecton-control practices, judicious use of broad-spectrum antimicrobial agents, and maintenance of patients' gastric acidity.

REFERENCES

CRAVEN DE et al: Nosocomial pneumonia in the 1990s: Update of epidemiology and risk factors: Semin Respir Infect 5:157, 1990

FANG GD et al: New and emerging etiologies for community-acquired pneumonia with implications for therapy. Medicine 69:307, 1990

FINE MJ: Pneumonia in the elderly: The hospital admission and discharge decisions. Semin Respir Infect 65:303,1990

HAHN DL et al: Association of *Chlamydia pneumoniae* (strain TWAR) infection with wheezing, asthmatic bronchitis and adult-onset asthma. JAMA 266:225, 1991

JACOBS MR: Treatment and diagnosis of infections caused by drug-resistant *Streptoccocus pneumoniae*. Clin Infect Dis 15:119, 1992

LEVISON ME, BUSH L: Pharmacodynamics of antimicrobial agents: Bactericidal and postantibiotic effects. Infect Dis Clin North Am 3:415, 1989

———— et al: Clindamycin compared with penicillin for the treatment of anaerobic lung abscess. Ann Intern Med 98:466, 1983

LEVISON, ME (ED): The pneumonias. Clinical approaches to infectious diseases of the lower respiratory tract. Boston, John Wright. PSG Inc, 1984.

LORBER B, SWENSON RM: Bacteriology of aspiration pneumonia: A prospective study of community and hospital acquired cases. Ann Intern Med 81:329, 1974

RIES K et al: Transtracheal aspiration in pulmonary infection. Arch Intern Med 133:453, 1974

RILEY RL: Airborne infection. Am J Med 57:466, 1974

SANDERS CC, SANDERS WE JR: Clinical significance of inducible beta-lactamase in gram-negative bacteria. Eur J Clin Microbiol 6:435, 1987

SHELHAMER JH et al: NIH conference: Respiratory disease in the immunosuppressed patient. Ann Intern Med 117:415, 1992

VERGHESE A, BERK SL: Bacterial pneumonia in the elderly. Medicine 62:271, 1982

WOODHEAD MA et al: Prospective study of the aetiology and outcome of pneumonia in the community. Lancet 1:671, 1987

221 BRONCHIECTASIS AND BRONCHOLITHIASIS

STEVEN E. WEINBERGER

BRONCHIECTASIS

DEFINITION Bronchiectasis is an abnormal and permanent dilatation of bronchi. It may be either focal, involving airways supplying a limited region of pulmonary parenchyma, or diffuse, involving airways in a more widespread distribution. Although this definition is based on pathologic changes in the bronchi, diagnosis is often suggested by the clinical consequences of chronic or recurrent infection in the dilated airways and the associated secretions that pool within these airways.

PATHOLOGY The bronchial dilatation of bronchiectasis is associated with destructive and inflammatory changes in the walls of medium-sized airways, often at the level of segmental or subsegmental bronchi. The normal structural components of the wall, including cartilage, muscle, and elastic tissue, are destroyed and may be replaced by fibrous tissue. The dilated airways frequently contain pools of thick, purulent material, while more peripheral airways are often occluded by secretions or obliterated and replaced by fibrous tissue. Additional microscopic features include bronchial and peribronchial inflammation and fibrosis, ulceration of the bronchial wall, squamous metaplasia, and mucous gland hyperplasia. The parenchyma normally supplied by the affected airways is abnormal, containing varying combinations of fibrosis, emphysema, bronchopneumonia, and atelectasis. As a result of the inflammation, vascularity of the bronchial wall increases, with associated enlargement of the bronchial arteries and anastomoses between the bronchial and pulmonary arterial circulations.

Three different patterns of bronchiectasis were described by Reid in 1950. In *cylindrical bronchiectasis* the bronchi appear as uniformly dilated tubes that end abruptly at the point that smaller airways are obstructed by secretions. In *varicose bronchiectasis* the affected bronchi have an irregular or beaded pattern of dilatation resembling varicose veins. In *saccular (cystic) bronchiectasis* the bronchi have a ballooned appearance at the periphery, ending in blind sacs without recognizable bronchial structures distal to the sacs.

ETIOLOGY AND PATHOGENESIS Bronchiectasis is a consequence of inflammation and destruction of the structural components of the bronchial wall. Infection is the usual cause of the inflammation, but on occasion airway injury is due to a toxin or an immune response. Secondary factors may perpetuate inflammation and impair mucociliary clearance, thereby promoting further infection. Microorganisms such as *Pseudomonas aeruginosa* and *Haemophilus influenzae* produce pigments, proteases, and other toxins that injure the respiratory epithelium and impair mucociliary clearance. The host inflammatory response, although protective on the one hand, also induces epithelial injury, largely as a result of mediators released from neutrophils. For example, serine proteases with elastolytic activity and oxygen-derived free radicals can produce additional damage to bronchial epithelium and further impair mucociliary clearance. As protection against infection is compromised, the dilated airways become more susceptible to colonization and growth of bacteria. Thus, a reinforcing cycle can result, with inflammation producing airway damage, impaired clearance of microorganisms, and further infection, which then completes the cycle by inciting more inflammation.

Infectious causes Infection, either as a single severe event or as a recurrent problem, is the trigger for bronchial wall inflammation and destruction in most cases. When a single episode of infection is responsible, the host usually does not have underlying compromise of local or systemic defense mechanisms. Rather, the characteristics of the infectious agent and the severity of the inflammatory response are presumably the important features.

A wide variety of infectious agents can initiate bronchiectasis. In the past, bronchiectasis during childhood was often a complication of measles or pertussis; these are now rare causes, the result of effective immunization. At present, adenovirus and influenza virus are the main viruses that cause bronchiectasis in association with lower respiratory tract involvement. Although not as common as in the preantibiotic era, virulent bacterial infections, especially with potentially necrotizing organisms such as *Staphylococcus aureus*, *Klebsiella*, and anaerobes, remain important causes of bronchiectasis when antibiotic treatment of a pneumonia is not given or is significantly delayed. Tuberculosis can produce bronchiectasis by a necrotizing effect on pulmonary parenchyma and airways and indirectly as a consequence of airway obstruction from bronchostenosis or extrinsic compression by lymph nodes. Nontuberculous mycobacteria are frequently associated with bronchiectasis, but usually as secondary infections or colonizing organisms rather than as primary pathogens. Mycoplasmal and necrotizing fungal infections are rare causes.

Impaired host defense mechanisms are often involved in the predisposition to recurrent infections. A localized structural defect may impair clearance of microorganisms and secretions from the affected airway(s), or a systemic defect may predispose to infection that potentially affects more than one region of lung.

The major cause of localized impairment of host defenses is endobronchial obstruction. Bacteria and secretions cannot be cleared adequately from the obstructed airway, which develops recurrent or chronic infection. Although primary lung cancer is the most common cause of endobronchial obstruction, it is an infrequent cause of bronchiectasis, since either the involved area is removed surgically or the disease progresses before bronchiectasis becomes an important problem. Slowly growing endobronchial neoplasms such as carcinoid tumors are more commonly associated with bronchiectasis. Foreign body aspiration is another important cause of endobronchial obstruction, particularly in children. Airway obstruction can also result from bronchostenosis, from impacted secretions, or from extrinsic compression by enlarged lymph nodes.

Generalized impairment of pulmonary defense mechanisms occurs with immunoglobulin deficiency, primary ciliary disorders, or cystic fibrosis. Infections and bronchiectasis are therefore often more diffuse. With panhypogammaglobulinemia, the best described of the immunoglobulin disorders associated with recurrent infection and bronchiectasis, patients often also have a history of sinus or skin infections. Selective IgA deficiency can be associated with bronchiectasis, frequently with coexisting deficiency of IgG subclasses (especially IgG2 or IgG4).

The primary disorders associated with ciliary dysfunction are termed *primary ciliary dyskinesia*. Numerous defects are encompassed under this category, including structural abnormalities of the dynein arms, radial spokes, and microtubules. The cilia become dyskinetic, their coordinated, propulsive action is diminished, and bacterial clearance is impaired. The clinical effects include recurrent upper and lower respiratory tract infections, such as sinusitis, otitis media, and bronchiectasis. Because normal sperm motility also depends on proper ciliary function, males are generally infertile (see also Chap. 48). Approximately half of patients with primary ciliary dyskinesia fall into the subgroup of *Kartagener's syndrome*, in which situs inversus accompanies bronchiectasis and sinusitis. It has been hypothesized that ciliary motility is necessary for proper rotation of the viscera during embryogenesis, so that visceral rotation is random when normal ciliary motion is lost.

In cystic fibrosis (see Chap. 222), the tenacious secretions in the bronchi are associated with impaired bacterial clearance, resulting in colonization and recurrent infection with a variety of organisms, particularly mucoid strains of *P. aeruginosa* but also *Staphylococcus aureus*, *H. influenzae*, *Escherichia coli*, and *P. cepacia*. Additional respiratory tract complications in cystic fibrosis include recurrent pneumothoraces, sinusitis, and nasal polyps. Males are generally infertile due to atresia of the vas deferens.

Noninfectious causes Some cases of bronchiectasis are associated with exposure to a toxic substance that incites a severe inflammatory response. Examples include inhalation of a toxic gas such as ammonia or aspiration of acidic gastric contents, though the latter problem is often also complicated by aspiration of bacteria. An immune response in the airway may also trigger inflammation, destructive changes, and bronchial dilatation. This mechanism is presumably responsible at least in part for bronchiectasis with allergic bronchopulmonary aspergillosis (ABPA), which is due to an immune response to *Aspergillus* organisms that have colonized the airway. Bronchiectasis accompanying ABPA often involves proximal airways and is associated with mucoid impaction. Bronchiectasis also occurs rarely in ulcerative colitis and rheumatoid arthritis, but it is not known whether an immune response triggers airway inflammation in these patients.

Bronchiectasis is a potential complication of uncommon disorders affecting airway cartilage. In *Williams-Campbell syndrome*, thought to be a congenital, perhaps inherited deficiency in bronchial cartilage of medium-sized airways, the affected airways may dilate. In *tracheobronchomegaly (Mounier-Kuhn syndrome)*, an acquired defect in components of the airway wall, including cartilage, elastic tissue, and muscle, is thought to be responsible for dilatation of the trachea and bronchi.

Other causes of bronchiectasis have also been described. In *Young's syndrome*, defined as obstructive azoospermia, men have normal spermatogenesis but obstruction of the epididymis by inspissated secretions. Approximately 20 to 30 percent of these patients also have bronchiectasis by an unknown mechanism. In *alpha₁-antitrypsin deficiency*, the usual respiratory complication is the early development of panacinar emphysema, but affected individuals may occasionally have bronchiectasis. In the *yellow nail syndrome*, which is due to hypoplastic lymphatics, the triad of lymphedema, pleural effusion, and yellow discoloration of the nails is accompanied by bronchiectasis in approximately 40 percent of patients. Finally, some cases of atelectasis and pulmonary fibrosis are associated with bronchial dilatation due to increased traction on the airways from the surrounding pulmonary parenchyma. Theoretically, the term bronchiectasis should not be used for the latter cases unless there is also destruction of components of the airway wall, which may be due to secondary infection in the involved airways.

CLINICAL MANIFESTATIONS Patients typically present with persistent or recurrent cough and purulent sputum production. Hemoptysis occurs in 50 to 70 percent of cases and can be due to bleeding from friable, inflamed airway mucosa. More significant, even massive bleeding is often a consequence of bleeding from hypertrophied bronchial arteries.

When a specific infectious episode initiates bronchiectasis, patients may describe a severe pneumonia followed by chronic cough and sputum production. Alternatively, patients without a dramatic initiating event often describe the insidious onset of symptoms. In some cases, patients are either asymptomatic or have a nonproductive cough, often associated with "dry" bronchiectasis in an upper lobe. Dyspnea or wheezing generally reflects either widespread bronchiectasis or underlying chronic obstructive pulmonary disease. With exacerbations of infection, the amount of sputum increases, the appearance becomes more purulent and often more bloody, and patients may become febrile. Such episodes may be due solely to exacerbations of the airway infection, but associated parenchymal infiltrates sometimes reflect an adjacent pneumonia.

Physical examination of the chest overlying an area of bronchiectasis is quite variable. Any combination of crackles, rhonchi, and wheezes may be heard, all of which reflect the damaged airways containing significant secretions. As with other types of chronic intrathoracic infection, clubbing may be present. Patients with severe, diffuse disease, particularly those with chronic hypoxemia, may have associated cor pulmonale and right ventricular failure.

Other nonpulmonary complications of bronchiectasis are now seen infrequently, largely because of better antibiotic control of the bacterial infections within the bronchiectatic airways. For example, brain abscess presumably results from septicemia, and amyloidosis can result from chronic infection and inflammation.

RADIOGRAPHIC AND LABORATORY FINDINGS Though the chest radiograph is important in the evaluation of suspected bronchiectasis, the findings are often nonspecific. At one extreme, the radiograph may be normal with mild disease. Alternatively, patients with saccular bronchiectasis may have prominent cystic spaces, either with or without air-liquid levels, corresponding to the dilated airways. These may be difficult to distinguish from enlarged airspaces due to bullous emphysema or from regions of honeycombing in patients with severe interstitial lung disease. Other findings are due to dilated airways with thickened walls, which result from peribronchial inflammation. Because of decreased aeration and atelectasis of the associated pulmonary parenchyma, these dilated airways are often crowded together in parallel. When seen longitudinally, the airways appear as "tram tracks"; when seen in cross-section, they produce "ring shadows." Because the dilated airways may be filled with secretions, the lumen may appear dense rather than radiolucent, producing an opaque tubular or branched tubular structure.

Bronchography, which involves coating the airways with a radio-opaque, iodinated lipid dye instilled through a catheter or bronchoscope, can provide excellent visualization of bronchiectatic airways. However, this technique has largely been replaced by computed tomography (CT), which also provides an excellent view of dilated airways as seen in cross-sectional images. With the advent of high-resolution CT scanning, in which the images are 1.5 mm thick, the sensitivity for detecting bronchiectasis has improved even further.

Examination of sputum often reveals an abundance of neutrophils and colonization or infection with a variety of possible organisms. Although common bacterial pathogens such as *Streptococcus pneumoniae* and *H. influenzae* may be present, a number of other organisms are seen frequently. *P. aeruginosa* is particularly common, and may be a clue to the presence of previously unsuspected bronchiectasis. Other organisms include *Staph. aureus*, anaerobes, and nontuberculous (atypical) mycobacteria. Appropriate staining and culturing of sputum often provides a guide to antibiotic therapy.

Additional evaluation is aimed at diagnosing the cause for the bronchiectasis. When bronchiectasis is focal, fiberoptic bronchoscopy may reveal an underlying endobronchial obstruction. In other cases, upper lobe involvement may be suggestive of either tuberculosis or ABPA. With more widespread disease, measurement of sweat chloride levels for cystic fibrosis, structural or functional assessment of nasal or bronchial cilia or sperm for primary ciliary dyskinesia, and quantitative assessment of immunoglobulins may explain recurrent airway infection. In an asthmatic person with proximal bronchiectasis or other historical features to suggest ABPA, skin testing, serology, and sputum culture for *Aspergillus* are helpful in confirming the diagnosis.

Pulmonary function tests may demonstrate airflow obstruction as a consequence of diffuse bronchiectasis or associated chronic obstructive lung disease. Bronchial hyperreactivity, e.g., to methacholine challenge, and some reversibility of the airflow obstruction with inhaled bronchodilators are relatively common for reasons not well defined. Other laboratory evaluation is often relatively nonspecific. For example, as a result of chronic infection within the thorax, patients may develop the normocytic, normochromic anemia of chronic disease.

TREATMENT Therapy has four major goals: (1) elimination of an identifiable underlying problem; (2) improved clearance of tracheobronchial secretions; (3) control of infection, particularly during acute exacerbations; and (4) reversal of airflow obstruction. Appropriate treatment should be instituted when a treatable cause is found, for example, treatment of hypogammaglobulinemia with immunoglobulin replacement, tuberculosis with antituberculous agents, and ABPA with glucocorticoids.

Secretions are typically copious and thick and contribute to the symptoms. Chest physical therapy with vibration, percussion, and postural drainage frequently helps patients with copious secretions. Mucolytic agents to thin secretions and allow better clearance are controversial. Data from a recent study utilizing iodinated glycerol in chronic obstructive lung disease have led to increasing interest in the use of mucolytics in the treatment of bronchiectasis.

Chronic or recurrent bacterial infections cause much of the morbidity of bronchiectasis. Antibiotics have an important role in management, but which antibiotic should be given and the frequency and duration of administration are not well established. For patients with infrequent exacerbations characterized by an increase in quantity and purulence of the sputum, antibiotics are commonly used only during acute episodes. Although choice of an antibiotic may be guided by Gram's stain and culture of sputum, empiric coverage (e.g., with ampicillin, amoxicillin, trimethoprim-sulfamethoxazole, or cefaclor) is often given initially. When *P. aeruginosa* is present, oral therapy with a quinolone or parenteral therapy with an aminoglycoside or third-generation cephalosporin may be appropriate. In patients with chronic purulent sputum despite short courses of antibiotics, more prolonged courses, e.g., with oral amoxicillin or inhaled aminoglycosides, or intermittent but regular courses of single or rotating antibiotics have been used.

Bronchodilators to improve obstruction and aid clearance of secretions are particularly useful in patients with airway hyperreactivity and reversible airflow obstruction. Although surgical therapy was common in the past, more effective antibiotic and supportive therapy has largely replaced surgery. However, when bronchiectasis is localized and the morbidity is substantial despite adequate medical therapy, surgical resection of the involved region of lung should be considered.

Complications present additional treatment issues. When massive hemoptysis, often originating from the hypertrophied bronchial circulation, does not resolve with conservative therapy, including rest and antibiotics, therapeutic options are either surgical resection or bronchial arterial embolization. Although resection may be successful if disease is localized, embolization is preferable with widespread disease. When embolization is performed by an experienced interventional radiologist, accidental embolization of a spinal artery with resulting spinal cord infarction, a serious complication of bronchial artery embolization, is rare. In patients with extensive disease, chronic hypoxemia and cor pulmonale may indicate the need for long-term supplemental oxygen. For selected patients who are disabled despite maximal therapy, lung transplantation is a therapeutic option.

BRONCHOLITHIASIS

Broncholithiasis is defined as the presence of one or more calcified stones within the tracheobronchial tree. These stones usually result from erosion of a calcified lymph node into an adjacent bronchus; less common causes are fragmentation and erosion of calcified tracheobronchial cartilage into the airway and calcification of aspirated foreign material. Eroding calcified lymph nodes are most frequently due to granulomatous infection, including histoplasmosis, tuberculosis, and coccidioidomycosis.

Manifestations include cough with expectoration of calcified material (lithoptysis), hemoptysis, and pneumonia or atelectasis secondary to obstruction of the airway with calcified material. Rarely, calcified material may also erode into the esophagus or the aorta, causing fistula formation between these structures and the airway.

Chest radiography often demonstrates one or more calcified densities representing calcified lymph nodes or the actual stone(s) within the airway lumen. Movement or disappearance of a calcified focus on chest radiograph is particularly suggestive of the diagnosis. Endobronchial obstruction may cause atelectasis, consolidation, or bronchiectasis involving the lung distal to the obstruction. The relationship between calcified material and an airway is best visualized noninvasively with CT scanning. Distortion and inflammatory changes of the airway may be demonstrated by fiberoptic bronchoscopy; calcified material within the lumen or adherent to the wall of the airway may also be seen.

Treatment is not always necessary, as symptoms may be minimal or the broncholiths may be spontaneously expectorated. Endoscopic removal of the calcified stones is sometimes possible with the rigid bronchoscope, which affords better airway control than does the fiberoptic bronchoscope and the use of larger instruments for retrieving stones. Surgical resection may be required for massive or recurrent hemoptysis, obstruction with recurrent infection, or fistula formation.

REFERENCES

Bronchiectasis

BARKER AF, BARDANA EJ JR: Bronchiectasis: Update of an orphan disease. Am Rev Respir Dis 137:969, 1988

COLE PJ: Inflammation: A two-edged sword—the model of bronchiectasis. Eur J Respir Dis 69(suppl 147):6, 1986

CURRIE DC, GARBETT ND et al: Double-blind randomized study of prolonged higher-dose oral amoxycillin in purulent bronchiectasis. Q J Med 76:799, 1990

DAVIS AL, SALZMAN SH: Bronchiectasis, in *Chronic Obstructive Pulmonary Disease*, NS Cherniack (ed). Philadelphia, Saunders, 1991, pp 316-338

GREENSTONE M, RUTMAN A et al: Primary ciliary dyskinesia: Cytological and clinical features. Q J Med 67:405, 1988

MURRAY JF: New presentations of bronchiectasis. Hosp Pract 26:55, 1991

PANG J, CHAN HS et al: Prevalence of asthma, atopy, and bronchial hyperreactivity in bronchiectasis: A controlled study. Thorax 44:948, 1989

TRUCKSIS M, SWARTZ MN: Bronchiectasis: A current view. Curr Clin Top Infect Dis 11:170, 1991

WESTCOTT JL: Bronchiectasis. Radiol Clin N Amer 29:1031, 1991

Broncholithiasis

CONCES DJ JR, TARVER RD et al: Broncholithiasis: CT features in 15 patients. Am J Radiol 157:249, 1991

DIXON GF, DONNERBERG RL et al: Advances in the diagnosis and treatment of broncholithiasis. Am Rev Respir Dis 129:1028, 1984

TRASTEK VF, PAIROLERO PC et al: Surgical management of broncholithiasis. J Thorac Cardiovasc Surg 90:842, 1985

222 CYSTIC FIBROSIS

RICHARD C. BOUCHER

Cystic fibrosis (CF) is a monogenetic disorder that presents as a multisystem disease. The first signs and symptoms typically occur in childhood, but nearly 3 percent of patients are diagnosed as adults. Due to improvements in therapy, more than 25 percent of patients reach adulthood and more than 9 percent live past the age of 30. Thus, CF is no longer only a pediatric disease, and internists must be prepared to recognize and treat its many complications. The disease is characterized by chronic airways infection that ultimately leads to bronchiectasis and bronchiolectasis, exocrine pancreatic insufficiency, abnormal sweat gland function, and urogenital dysfunction.

PATHOGENESIS   Genetic basis   CF is an autosomal recessive disease resulting from mutations in a gene located on chromosome 7. The prevalence of CF varies with the ethnic origin of a population. CF is detected in approximately 1 in 2500 live births in the Caucasian population of North America and northern Europe, 1 in 17,000 live births of African-Americans, and 1 in 90,000 live births of the Asian population of Hawaii. The most common mutation in the CF gene is a 3-base-pair deletion that results in an absence of phenylalanine at amino acid position 508 (ΔF_{508}) of the CF gene protein product, known as the CF transmembrane regulator (CFTR). The large number of other mutations identified in the CF gene (>200) makes it unfeasible to use DNA diagnostic technologies for identifying heterozygotes in populations at large, and no physiologic measurements allow heterozygote detection.

CFTR protein   (See Fig. 213-4, p. 1151)   The CFTR protein is a single polypeptide chain containing 1480 amino acids that appears to function as a cyclic AMP-regulated Cl^- channel. The fully processed form of CFTR is found in the plasma membrane in normal epithelia (Fig. 222-1). Biochemical studies indicate that the ΔF_{508} mutation leads to improper processing and intracellular degradation of the CFTR protein. Thus absence of CFTR protein at appropriate cellular sites may be a part of the pathophysiology of CF. However, other mutations in the CF gene produce CFTR proteins that are fully processed but are nonfunctional at the appropriate cellular sites.

Epithelial dysfunction   (See also Chap. 213)   The epithelia affected by CF exhibit different functions in their native state; i.e., some are volume-absorbing (airways and intestinal epithelia), some are salt-absorbing but not volume-absorbing (sweat duct), whereas others are volume-secretory (pancreas). Given this diverse array of native activities, it should not be surprising that CF produces very different effects on patterns of electrolyte and water transport. However, the unifying concept is that all affected tissues express abnormal cAMP-regulated Cl^- channel activity.

ORGAN-SPECIFIC PATHOPHYSIOLOGY   Lung   The diagnostic biophysical hallmark of CF is the raised transepithelial electric potential difference (PD) detected in airway epithelia. The transepithelial PD reflects components of both the rate of active ion transport and the resistance to ion flow of the superficial epithelium. CF airway epithelia exhibit both raised transport rates (Na^+) and decreased ion permeability (Cl^-) (Fig. 222-2). The Cl^- transport defect appears to be the result of abnormal regulation of Cl^- transport. CF epithelia do not respond to beta-adrenergic agonists or agonists that activate protein kinase C with Cl^- secretion as normal airway epithelia do. This failure to regulate cellular Cl^- transport is a direct consequence of mutations in the CFTR protein. An important observation is that there is an alternative Cl^- channel expressed in airway epithelia. This channel is different from CFTR and is regulated by intracellular Ca^{2+} levels or by extracellular triphosphate nucleotides, e.g., UTP. This channel can substitute for CFTR with regard to net Cl^- transport and may be a potential therapeutic target.

Raised Na^+ absorption is a feature of CF airway epithelia. Na^+ transport abnormalities in CF are not a widespread feature of the

FIGURE 222-1 Cellular metabolism of the CFTR protein. In a normal cell (*left*), CFTR is synthesized in the rough endoplasmic reticulum (RER), glycosylated in the Golgi apparatus, and functions as a Cl⁻ channel when located in the plasma membrane. Two possible outcomes of mutations in the CF gene are shown (*right*). (1) If a mutation disturbs protein folding, e.g., the ΔF_{508} mutation, CFTR is degraded intracellularly so that no protein is transported to the plasma membrane. (2) With other mutations, the abnormal protein is processed and traffics to the plasma membrane but functions abnormally at that site.

CF epithelial phenotype and appear confined to volume-absorbing epithelia. The mechanisms for Na⁺ hyperabsorption reflect in part an increase in apical cell membrane Na⁺ channel activity. It is not yet known how the abnormal CF gene product, CFTR, produces the Na⁺ transport defect.

The central hypothesis of CF airways pathophysiology has been that the abnormal Na⁺ and Cl⁻ transport rates produce secretions that are dehydrated and poorly cleared. The unique predisposition of CF airways to chronic infection by *Staphylococcus aureus* and *Pseudomonas aeruginosa* raises the issue that other as yet undefined abnormalities in airway surface liquids also may contribute to the failure of lung defense.

Gastrointestinal tract The gastrointestinal effects of CF are diverse. In the exocrine pancreas, it appears that the absence of the CFTR Cl⁻ channel in the apical membrane of pancreatic ductal epithelia impairs the function of an apical membrane Cl⁻-HCO₃⁻ exchanger to effect net secretion of bicarbonate and Na⁺ (by a passive process) into the duct. The failure to secrete Na⁺-HCO₃⁻ and water leads to retention of enzymes in the pancreas and ultimately destruction of virtually all pancreatic tissue. In CF the intestinal epithelium, because of the lack of Cl⁻ and water secretion, has an impaired ability to flush the secreted mucins and other macromolecules from intestinal crypts. Ultimately, this process can lead to obstruction of both the small and large intestines. In the hepatobiliary system, defective hepatic ductal salt (Cl⁻) and water secretion causes retention

of biliary secretions and focal biliary cirrhosis and bile duct proliferation in approximately 25 to 30 percent of CF patients. The inability of the CF gallbladder epithelium to secrete salt and water can lead to both chronic cholecystitis and cholelithiasis.

Sweat gland CF patients secrete nearly normal volumes of sweat into the sweat acinus but are unable to absorb NaCl from sweat as it moves through the sweat duct. The defect in ductal function represents the inability to absorb Cl⁻ across the Cl⁻-impermeable CF ductal epithelia.

DIAGNOSIS Because of the large number of CF mutations, DNA analysis is not used for primary diagnosis. The diagnosis of CF rests on a combination of clinical criteria and analyses of sweat Cl⁻ values. The values for the Na⁺ and Cl⁻ concentration in sweat vary with age, but typically in adults a Cl⁻ concentration of >70 mEq/L discriminates between CF patients and patients with other lung disease.

It is likely that DNA analyses will be performed increasingly in CF patients. Comprehensive genotype-phenotype relationships have not been established sufficiently for prognosis. A relationship between ΔF_{508} homozygosity and pancreatic insufficiency has been established, but no predictive relationship holds for ΔF_{508} homozygosity and lung disease. DNA diagnosis has not been used for newborn screening of CF patients.

Between 1 and 2 percent of patients with the clinical syndrome of CF have normal sweat Cl⁻ values. In most of these patients, the nasal

FIGURE 222-2 Comparison of ion transport properties of normal (*left*) and CF (*right*) airway epithelia. The vectors describe routes and magnitudes of Na⁺ and Cl⁻ transport. The normal basal pattern for ion transport is absorption of Na⁺ from the lumen via an amiloride-sensitive Na⁺ channel. This process is accelerated in CF. The capacity to initiate cAMP-mediated Cl⁻ secretion

is diminished in CF airway epithelia due to absence/dysfunction of the CFTR Cl⁻ channel. An alternative Cl⁻ channel (Cl_a^-), regulated by Ca²⁺ and extracellular nucleotides, is expressed in some but not all epithelia affected by CF. The Na⁺, K⁺-ATPase that provides the energy for both the Na⁺ and Cl⁻ transport is shown on the basolateral surface.

transepithelial PD is raised into the diagnostic range for CF and sweat acini do not secrete in response to injected beta-adrenergic agonists. A single mutation of the CFTR gene, 3789 + 10 kb G→T, is associated with approximately 50 percent of CF patients with normal sweat Cl⁻.

CLINICAL ASPECTS Most CF patients present with signs and symptoms of the disease in childhood. Approximately 10 percent of patients present within the first 24 h of life with gastrointestinal obstruction, termed *meconium ileus*. Other common presentations within the first year or two of life include respiratory tract symptoms, most prominently persistent cough and/or recurrent pulmonary infiltrates, and failure to thrive. A significant number of patients, however, are not diagnosed until their second decade of life.

Respiratory tract Upper respiratory tract disease is almost universal in CF patients. Chronic sinusitis is common in childhood and leads to nasal obstruction and rhinorrhea. The occurrence of nasal polyps approaches 15 to 20 percent and often requires surgery.

In the lower respiratory tract, the first symptom of CF is cough. With time the cough becomes continuous and produces viscous, purulent, often greenish colored sputum. Inevitably, periods of clinical stability are interrupted by "exacerbations," defined by increased cough, weight loss, increased sputum volume, and decrements in pulmonary function. Typically these exacerbations are treated with intravenous antibiotics (see below) with recovery of most lung function. Over the course of years, the exacerbations become more frequent and the recovery of lost lung function less complete, leading to respiratory failure.

CF patients exhibit a characteristic sputum microbiology. *Haemophilus influenzae* and *S. aureus* are often the first organisms recovered from samples of lung secretions in newly diagnosed CF patients. *P. aeruginosa* is typically cultured from lower respiratory tract secretions thereafter. After repetitive antibiotic exposure, *P. aeruginosa*, often in a mucoid form, is usually the predominant organism recovered from sputum and may be present as several strains with different antibiotic sensitivities. *P. cepacia* has been recovered from CF sputum and is pathogenic. Patient-to-patient spread of this organism indicates that infection control in the hospital should be practiced. Other gram-negative rods recovered from CF sputum include *Klebsiella*, *Proteus*, and *Escherichia coli*, also in mucoid forms. Up to 50 percent of CF patients have *Aspergillus fumigatus* in their sputum, and up to 10 percent of these patients exhibit the syndrome of allergic bronchopulmonary aspergillosis. *Mycobacterium tuberculosis* is rare in CF patients. However, 10 to 20 percent of adult CF patients have sputum cultures positive for nontuberculous mycobacteria, and in some patients these microorganisms are associated with disease.

The first lung function abnormalities observed in CF children, increased RV/TLC ratios, suggest that small airways disease is the first functional lung abnormality in CF. As the disease progresses, both reversible and irreversible changes in FVC and FEV₁ are noted. The reversible component reflects accumulation of intraluminal secretions and/or airway reactivity, which occurs in 40 to 60 percent of CF patients. The irreversible component reflects chronic destruction of the airway wall and bronchiolitis.

The earliest chest x-ray change in CF lungs is hyperinflation, reflecting small airways obstruction. Later, evidence of luminal mucus impaction, bronchial cuffing, and finally, bronchiectasis, e.g., ring shadows, is noted. For reasons that are still unknown, the right upper lobe displays the earliest and most severe changes. Neither CT nor MRI scanning are routinely performed on CF patients.

CF pulmonary disease is associated with many intermittent complications. Pneumothorax is common (>10 percent of patients). The production of small amounts of blood in sputum is common in CF patients with advanced pulmonary disease and appears to be associated with lung infection. Massive hemoptysis is life-threatening and difficult to localize bronchoscopically. With advanced lung disease, digital clubbing becomes evident in virtually all patients with CF. As late events, respiratory failure and cor pulmonale are prominent features of CF.

Gastrointestinal tract The syndrome of meconium ileus in infants presents with abdominal distention, failure to pass stool, and emesis. The abdominal flat plate can be diagnostic with small intestinal air fluid levels, a granular appearance representing meconium, and a small colon. In children and young adults, a syndrome termed *meconium ileus equivalent* or distal intestinal obstruction occurs. The syndrome presents with right lower quadrant pain, loss of appetite, emesis, and often a palpable mass. The syndrome can be confused with appendicitis, which occurs frequently in CF patients. The characteristic intestinal abnormalities are complicated by pancreatic insufficiency in more than 90 percent of CF patients. Insufficient pancreatic enzyme release yields the typical pattern of protein and fat malabsorption, with frequent, bulky, foul-smelling stools. Signs and symptoms of malabsorption of fat-soluble vitamins, including vitamins A, D, E, and K, are also noted. Because pancreatic beta cells are typically spared, the appearance of hyperglycemia and a requirement for insulin is a late finding in CF and occurs in only a small percentage of patients.

Genitourinary system Late onset of puberty is common in both males and females with CF. The delayed maturational pattern is likely secondary to the effects of chronic lung disease and inadequate nutrition on reproductive endocrine function. More than 95 percent of male patients with CF are azoospermic, reflecting obliteration of the vas deferens. Twenty percent of CF women are infertile due to effects of chronic lung disease on the menstrual cycle and thick, tenacious cervical mucus that blocks sperm migration. More than 90 percent of completed pregnancies produce viable infants, and CF women are generally able to breast-feed infants normally.

TREATMENT The major objectives of therapy for CF are to promote clearance of secretions and control infection in the lung, provide adequate nutrition, and prevent intestinal obstruction. Ultimately, gene therapy may be the treatment of choice.

Lung disease At present, the techniques for clearing pulmonary secretions are a combination of breathing exercises and chest percussion. A number of pharmacologic agents for increasing mucus clearance are being tested. *N*-Acetyl-cysteine has not been shown to have clinically significant effects on mucus clearance and/or lung function. However, agents that degrade the high concentrations of DNA in CF sputum, e.g., human recombinant DNAse, appear to be effective in decreasing sputum viscosity and increasing airflow during short-term administration. Experimental drugs aimed at restoring salt and water content of secretions, e.g., amiloride and triphosphate nucleotides, appear promising.

More than 95 percent of CF patients die of complications resulting from lung infection. Antibiotics are the principal agents available for treating lung infection, and their use should be guided by sputum culture results. Early intervention with antibiotics is useful, and long courses of treatment are the rule. Because of increased total-body clearance and volume of distribution of antibiotics in CF patients, the required doses are higher for CF patients than for non-CF patients with similar chest infections.

Increased cough and mucus production are treated with antibiotics given by the oral route. Typical oral agents used to treat *Staphylococcus* include a semisynthetic penicillin or a cephalosporin. Oral ciprofloxacin may reduce pseudomonal bacterial counts and control symptoms, but its clinical usefulness may be limited by rapid emergence of resistant organisms. More severe exacerbations require intravenous antibiotics. Traditionally, intravenous therapy is given in the hospital, but outpatient intravenous antibiotic administration is gaining acceptance. Usually, two drugs, often one of them an aminoglycoside, are used to treat *P. aeruginosa* to prevent emergence of resistant organisms. Drug dosage should be monitored so that levels for gentamicin or tobramycin peak at ranges of ~10 μg/mL and exhibit troughs of <2 μg/mL. Usually, a cephalosporin, e.g., ceftazadime, and/or a penicillin derivative is used as the second drug. Antibiotics directed at *Staphylococcus* and/or *H. influenzae* are added depending on the results of the culture. Aerosolization of antibiotics also may have an important role in treating CF lung infection. Large doses of aminoglycosides (600 mg tobramycin twice daily) via aerosol are optimal. Aerosol administration also permits other drugs, e.g., colistin, to be utilized that are ineffective by the intravenous route.

Inhaled beta-adrenergic agonists can be useful to control airways constriction. They achieve a short-term increase in airflow, but long-term benefit has not been shown. Inhaled anticholinergics provide an alternative. Oral steroids are not first-line agents for controlling airways constriction and are of no use in improving the nonreversible component of lung function. Steroids may be useful for treating allergic bronchopulmonary aspergillosis.

A number of pulmonary complications require acute interventions. Atelectasis is best treated with chest physiotherapy and antibiotic therapy. Pneumothoraces involving 10 percent or less of the lung can be observed. The use of chest tubes to expand collapsed, diseased lung often requires long periods of time, and sclerosing agents should be used with caution because of limitations for subsequent lung transplantation. Small-volume hemoptysis requires no specific therapy other than treatment of lung infection and assessment of coagulation and vitamin K status. If massive hemoptysis occurs, bronchial artery embolization can be successful. The most ominous complications of CF are respiratory failure and cor pulmonale. The most effective conventional therapy for these conditions is vigorous medical management of the lung disease. Ultimately, the only effective treatment for respiratory failure in CF is lung transplantation. The 2-year survival for lung transplantation exceeds 50 percent, and deaths in transplant patients result principally from graft rejection, often involving obliterative bronchiolitis. The transplanted lungs do not develop a CF-specific phenotype.

Gastrointestinal disease Maintenance of adequate nutrition is critical for the health of the CF patient. Most (>90 percent) of CF patients benefit from pancreatic enzyme replacement. Capsules generally contain between 4000 and 24,000 units of lipase. The dose of enzymes should be adjusted on the basis of weight gain, abdominal symptomatology, and character of stools. Replacement of fat-soluble vitamins is also required. Hyperglycemia most often becomes manifest in the adult. Principles for treating other causes of nonketotic hyperglycemia should be employed.

For treatment of acute obstruction due to meconium ileus equivalent, megalodiatrizoate or other hypertonic radiocontrast materials delivered by enema to the terminal ileum are utilized. For control of symptoms, adjustment of pancreatic enzymes and the supplementation of intake by salt solutions containing osmotically active agents, e.g., propyleneglycol, are utilized. Hepatic and gallbladder complications are treated as for non-CF patients. End-stage liver disease can be treated by transplantation, which has a 2-year survival rate exceeding 50 percent.

Psychosocial factors CF imposes a tremendous burden on patients. Health insurance, career options, family planning, and life expectancy become major issues, thus assisting patients with the psychosocial adjustments required by CF is critical.

REFERENCES

AITKEN ML et al: Recombinant human DNAse inhalation in normal subjects and patients with cystic fibrosis: A phase 1 study. JAMA 267:1947, 1992

AITKEN ML, FIEL SB: Cystic fibrosis. Dis Mon 39:1, 1993

BEAR CE et al: Purification and functional reconstitution of the cystic fibrosis transmembrane conductance regulator (CFTR). Cell 68:809, 1992

CHENG SH et al: Defective intracellular transport and processing of CFTR is the molecular basis of most cystic fibrosis. Cell 63:827, 1990

HARRIS A, ARGENT BE: The cystic fibrosis gene and its product CFTR. Semin Cell Biol 4:37, 1993

KNOWLES MR et al: Activation by extracellular nucleotides of chloride secretion in the airway epithelia of patients with cystic fibrosis. N Engl J Med 325:533, 1991

O'LOUGHLIN EV et al: Abnormal epithelial transport in cystic fibrosis jejunum. Am J Physiol 260:G758, 1991

SFERRA TJ, COLLINS FS: The molecular biology of cystic fibrosis. Annu Rev Med 44:133, 1993

WALTERS S et al: Demographic and social characteristics of adults with cystic fibrosis in the United Kingdom. Brit Med J 306:549, 1993

223 CHRONIC BRONCHITIS, EMPHYSEMA, AND AIRWAYS OBSTRUCTION

ROLAND H. INGRAM, JR.

Chronic bronchitis and emphysema are two distinct processes, most often present in combination in patients with chronic airways obstruction. The diagnosis of chronic bronchitis is made by history, chronic airways obstruction is assessed physiologically, and emphysema can be diagnosed with certainty in most instances only by histologic examination of sections of whole lung fixed at inflation. Although the relationships among clinical characteristics, physiologic derangements, and morphologic changes have been studied for many years, reasonably certain and uniform clinical criteria are still not available. Definitions and classifications have evolved, but these are not universally accepted. Nonetheless, the following definitions along with brief qualifications and descriptions are currently used by most persons involved in the diagnosis, treatment, and epidemiology of the chronic obstructive airways syndromes.

DEFINITIONS *Chronic bronchitis* is a condition associated with excessive tracheobronchial mucus production sufficient to cause cough with expectoration for at least 3 months of the year for more than 2 consecutive years. Several subclassifications have been proposed. *Simple chronic bronchitis* describes a condition characterized by mucoid sputum production. *Chronic mucopurulent bronchitis* is characterized by persistent or recurrent purulence of sputum in the absence of localized suppurative diseases such as bronchiectasis. Since there may or may not be obstruction as assessed by the use of the forced expiratory vital capacity maneuver, *chronic bronchitis with obstruction* deserves a separate classification. There is a further subset of patients with chronic bronchitis and obstruction who experience severe dyspnea and wheezing in association with inhaled irritants or during acute respiratory infections. Such patients are said to have *chronic infective asthma* or *chronic asthmatic bronchitis*. Since there is considerable but not complete reversibility of airflow obstruction with bronchodilator treatment and abatement of inflammation, and since hyperresponsiveness of airways to nonspecific stimuli is seen in this group of patients, confusion is possible between patients with this condition and those with asthma who may also have *chronic airways obstruction* (Chap. 217). The differentiation is based mainly on the history of the clinical illness. The patient with chronic asthmatic bronchitis has a long history of cough and sputum production with a later onset of wheezing, whereas the asthmatic with chronic obstruction gives a long history of wheezing with later onset of chronic productive cough.

Emphysema is defined as distention of the air spaces distal to the terminal bronchiole with destruction of alveolar septa. *Chronic obstructive lung disease* is defined as a condition in which there is chronic obstruction to airflow due to chronic bronchitis and/or emphysema (see below). Although the degree of obstruction may be less when the patient is free from respiratory infection and may improve somewhat with bronchodilator drugs, significant obstruction is always present.

PREVALENCE Approximately 20 percent of adult males have chronic bronchitis, yet only a minority of these are clinically disabled. According to all surveys, males are more often affected than females. With increased cigarette smoking in women, however, the prevalence of bronchitis in them is increasing. Although cigarette smoking is the single most important etiologic factor, occupational and environmental exposures are now receiving more attention, mainly as additive to the effects of cigarette smoking (Chap. 219).

Although CT scanning can detect emphysema, this tool cannot be used for population screening. Hence the incidence data are derived solely from postmortem surveys. It is rare to find adult lungs completely free of emphysema. There is a distinct increase in the extent of emphysema in the fifth decade, with further increases through the seventh decade and little increase after that. Approximately two-thirds of adult males and one-fourth of females (most without recognized dysfunction) will have well-defined emphysema, which is often limited in extent. Therefore, the majority of those with emphysema will not have had disability or even symptoms associated with it. The situation is analogous to atherosclerosis in that the morphologic changes are far more frequent than the clinical manifestations attributable to the changes.

PATHOLOGY *Chronic bronchitis* is associated with hyperplasia and hypertrophy of the mucus-producing glands found in the submucosa of large cartilaginous airways. Quantitation of this anatomic change, known as the *Reid index*, is based on the ratio of the thickness of the submucosal glands to that of the bronchial wall. In persons without a history of chronic bronchitis, the mean ratio is 0.44 with a standard deviation $\pm$ 0.09, whereas in those with such a history the mean ratio is 0.52 ± 0.08. Although a low index is *rarely* associated with symptoms and a high index is commonly associated with symptoms during life, there is a great deal of overlap. Therefore, many persons will have morphologic changes in large airways without having had chronic bronchitis.

Perhaps more important than the abnormalities in large airways are the changes often found in the small noncartilaginous airways. Goblet cell hyperplasia, mucosal and submucosal inflammatory cells, edema, peribronchial fibrosis, intraluminal mucus plugs, and increased smooth muscle are characteristic findings in small airways. The frequency of these latter findings in relation to premortem clinical and functional status has not been determined. However, in lungs from patients with chronic obstructive lung disease which have been studied at postmortem, the major site of airflow obstruction has been shown to be in the small airways.

Emphysema is classified according to the pattern of involvement of the gas-exchanging units (acini) of the lung distal to the terminal bronchiole. Although several morphologic patterns have been described, the two most important in the context of this discussion are those involving the respiratory bronchioles and alveolar ducts in the center of the acinus (centriacinar emphysema) and those involving the entire acinus (panacinar emphysema). Quite often both morphologic patterns are present in a single lung of a patient dying from chronic obstructive lung disease, although one type may predominate over the other.

With centriacinar emphysema the distention and destruction are mainly limited to the respiratory bronchiole and alveolar ducts, with relatively less change peripherally in the acinus. Because of the large functional reserve in the lung, many units must be involved in order for overall dysfunction to be detectable. The centrally destroyed regions of the acinus have a high ventilation/perfusion ratio because the capillaries are missing yet ventilation continues. This results in increased wasted ventilation (Vd/Vt), while the peripheral portions of the acinus have crowded and small alveoli with intact, perfused capillaries giving a low ventilation/perfusion ratio. This results in wasted blood flow to give a high alveolar-arterial P_{O_2} difference ($PA_{O_2} - Pa_{O_2}$) (Chap. 214). Mild degrees of centriacinar emphysema, often limited to the lung apices, are extremely common in lungs from persons above age 50 and are practically considered a normal finding.

Panacinar emphysema involves both the central and peripheral portions of the acinus, which results, if the process is extensive, in a reduction of the alveolar-capillary gas exchange surface and loss of elastic recoil properties. When emphysema is severe, it may be difficult to distinguish between the two types which most often coexist in the same lung.

CONTRIBUTORY FACTORS Smoking Cigarette smoking is the most commonly identified correlate with both chronic bronchitis during life and extent of emphysema at postmortem. Experimental studies have shown that prolonged cigarette smoking impairs ciliary movement, inhibits function of alveolar macrophages, and leads to hypertrophy and hyperplasia of mucus-secreting glands; massive

exposure in dogs can produce emphysematous changes. In addition to these chronic effects, it is probable that smoke inhibits antiproteases and causes polymorphonuclear leukocytes to release proteolytic enzymes acutely. Inhaled cigarette smoke can produce an acute increase in airways resistance due to vagally mediated smooth-muscle constriction, presumably by way of stimulating submucosal irritant receptors. The relationship of such recurrent episodes of acute bronchial constriction to the development and progression of chronic airways obstruction is uncertain. Recent studies, however, indicate that increased airways responsiveness is associated with more rapid progression in those with chronic airways obstruction.

It is now well established that some young asymptomatic smokers have anatomic and functional changes in small airways without there being a diminution in the forced expiratory volume in 1 s. However, flow rates at or below the mid-vital capacity range are often diminished in persons with mild small-airways obstruction. It has been shown that obstruction of small airways is the earliest demonstrable mechanical defect in young cigarette smokers and that the obstruction may disappear completely after cessation of smoking. Although smoking cessation does not result in complete reversal of more pronounced obstruction, there is a significant slowing of the decline in lung function in all smokers who give up cigarettes. In effect, it is never too late to quit smoking cigarettes.

Not only is cigarette smoking the most common single factor leading to chronic airways obstruction, it also adds to the effects of every other contributory factor to be discussed below.

Air pollution The incidence and mortality rates of both chronic bronchitis and emphysema may be higher in heavily industrialized urban areas. Exacerbations of bronchitis are clearly related to periods of heavy pollution with sulfur dioxide (SO_2) and particulate matter. While nitrogen dioxide (NO_2) can produce small-airways obstruction (bronchiolitis) in experimental animals exposed to high concentrations, there are no data convincingly implicating NO_2, at even the highest pollutant levels, in the pathogenesis or worsening of airways obstruction in humans (Chap. 219).

Occupation Chronic bronchitis is more prevalent in workers who engage in occupations exposing them to either inorganic or organic dusts or to noxious gases. Epidemiologic surveys have succeeded in demonstrating an accelerated decline in lung function in many such workers—e.g., workers in plastics plants exposed to toluene diisocyanate and carding room workers in cotton mills (Chap. 219)—suggesting that their occupational exposure contributes to their future disability.

Infection Morbidity, mortality, and frequency of acute respiratory illnesses are higher in patients with chronic bronchitis. Many attempts have been made to relate these illnesses to infection with viruses, mycoplasmas, and bacteria. However, only the rhinovirus is found more often during exacerbations; that is to say, pathogenic bacteria, mycoplasmas, and viruses other than rhinovirus are found just as often between as during exacerbations. It is intuitively appealing to assign some role to respiratory infections in the pathogenesis and progression of chronic obstructive lung disease, and although this question is under study, there has been no conclusion to date. Epidemiologic studies, however, implicate acute respiratory illness as one of the major factors associated with the etiology as well as the progression of chronic airways obstruction. It has been shown that cigarette smokers may either transitorily develop or worsen small-airways obstruction in association with even mild viral respiratory infections. There is also some evidence that severe viral pneumonia early in life may lead to chronic obstruction, predominantly in small airways.

Familial and genetic factors Familial aggregation of chronic bronchitis has been well demonstrated in the past. Recent surveys have shown that children of smoking parents may experience more frequent and severe respiratory illnesses and have a higher prevalence of chronic respiratory symptoms. In addition, nonsmokers who remain in the presence of cigarette smokers (passive smokers) have increased blood levels of carbon monoxide which indicate that they are significantly exposed to smoke. Another well-documented form of indoor air pollution relates to the use of natural gas for cooking. The role of such pollution, however, remains controversial. Thus a part of the familial aggregation may be related to home air pollution. However, some studies of monozygotic twins have suggested some genetic predisposition to the development of chronic bronchitis independent of personal or familial smoking habits and other indoor air pollution. The exact genetic mode of transmission, if it exists at all, is uncertain.

The protease inhibitor α_1-antitrypsin is an acute-phase reactant, and normally the serum levels rise in association with many inflammatory reactions and with estrogen administration. Either deficient or absent serum levels of α_1-antitrypsin are found in some patients with the early onset of emphysema. By use of the techniques of acid starch gel and immunoelectrophoresis, genetic typing of the protease inhibitor (Pi) types has been possible. Most members of the normal population have two M genes, designated as Pi type MM, and have serum α_1-antitrypsin levels in excess of 2.5 g/L. Several genes are associated with alterations in levels of serum α_1-antitrypsin, but the most common ones associated with emphysema are the Z and S genes. Individuals who are homozygous ZZ or SS have serum levels often near 0 but always less than 0.5 g/L and develop severe panacinar emphysema in the third and fourth decades of life. The panacinar process predominates at the lung bases. Progressive dyspnea with minimal cough characterizes the clinical presentation, although chronic bronchitis is prominent in smokers. Given that α_1-protease inhibitors can be chemically synthesized or biologically produced in significant quantities and can be shown with intravenous infusion to restore the protease-antiprotease balance in liquid lavaged from the lungs of ZZ patients, it has been suggested that replacement therapy with α_1-antitrypsin should be of value in preventing the development of emphysema in these patients. Since replacement therapy was available before efficacy had been assessed, a prospective, randomized trial has not been possible. Through a national registry, a natural history study is underway from which it might be possible to evaluate the effects of therapy if the treated and untreated groups turn out to be sufficiently comparable at entry.

The MZ and MS heterozygotes have intermediate levels of serum α_1-antitrypsin (i.e., between 0.5 and 2.5 g/L); hence the genetic expression is that of an autosomal codominant allele. It is a matter of some controversy whether the heterozygous state is associated with lung function abnormalities. Published studies are in direct conflict on this point, and further data are needed to be certain. The matter is of some importance, since the heterozygous state is common, with incidence estimates varying between 5 and 14 percent of the general population.

The precise way in which antitrypsin deficiency produces emphysema is unclear. In addition to inhibition of trypsin, α_1-antitrypsin is an effective inhibitor of elastase and several other proteolytic enzymes. There is experimental evidence that the structural integrity of lung elastin depends on this antienzyme, which protects the lung from proteases released from leukocytes. It is tempting to speculate that recurrent inflammatory reactions related to infection and pollutants play some role in pathogenesis by calling forth leukocytes whose released proteases are uninhibited and are free to cause the damage.

The role of proteolytic enzymes in the induction of emphysema is not restricted to patients with α_1-antitrypsin deficiency. Evidence is accumulating that proteolytic enzymes derived from neutrophilic leukocytes and alveolar macrophages can produce emphysema even in subjects with normal circulating levels of antiproteases. It is possible that local concentrations of proteolytic enzymes may exceed the inhibitory capacity of antiproteases, that some proteases present are not susceptible to the available antiproteases, or that some of the proteolytic enzymes may be physically inaccessible to the antiprotease activity. The ultimate clinical utility of exogenously produced protease inhibitors currently under development will undoubtedly depend on which of the protease-antiprotease interactions predominates in the production of emphysema. Reduction of endogenous elastase release

from leukocytes in the lung has been achieved by colchicine (0.6 mg/d orally) in a randomized, placebo-controlled trial in ex-smokers with chronic airways obstruction. Current smokers showed no such reductions. An assessment of the clinical efficacy of this inexpensive and nontoxic form of therapy in ex-smokers must await a large, prospective clinical trial.

PATHOPHYSIOLOGY   On the basis of the use of flow rates from forced expiratory vital capacity maneuvers and more sophisticated measures of airways resistance and elastic recoil properties of the lung, it has become clear that both chronic bronchitis and emphysema can exist without evidence of obstruction. However, by the time a patient begins to experience dyspnea as a result of these processes, obstruction is always demonstrable. Since chronic bronchitis and emphysema are usually combined, it might appear fruitless to determine the role of each in producing an individual patient's disability. However, one process may dominate over the other, and to the extent that inflammatory airways disease, secretions, and bronchospasm are present, there are therapeutic possibilities with some hope for improvement. Therefore, it is of value to understand the mechanisms of airways obstruction in order to guide therapy and anticipate results.

Both chronic bronchitis and emphysema result in airways narrowing. In addition to the primary airways processes of chronic bronchitis, loss of elastic recoil of the lung in emphysema accounts for a decrease in airways caliber through loss of radial traction on airways. Narrowing of airways is often associated with both an increase in airways resistance and a diminution in maximal expiratory flow rates.

There are occasions in which a normal or only slightly elevated airways resistance is accompanied by low maximal expiratory flow rates. Under such circumstances, an increase in the dynamic collapsibility of intrathoracic airways during forced exhalation is a possible explanation. Also in this context, the elastic recoil pressure of the lung must be considered in a slightly different way. In addition to providing radial support to airways during quiet breathing, the elastic recoil properties of the lung serve as a major determinant of maximal expiratory flow rates. The static recoil pressure of the lung is the difference between alveolar and intrapleural pressure. During forced exhalations, when alveolar and intrapleural pressures are high, there are points in the airway at which bronchial pressure equals pleural pressure. Flow does not increase with higher pleural pressure after these points become fixed so that the effective driving pressure between alveoli and such points is the elastic recoil pressure of the lung (Fig. 223-1). Hence maximal expiratory flow rates represent a complex and dynamic interplay between airways caliber, elastic recoil pressures, and collapsibility of airways. As a direct consequence of the altered pressure-airflow relationships, the work of breathing is increased in bronchitis and emphysema. Since flow-resistive work is flow rate–dependent, there is a disproportionate increase in the work of breathing with increased ventilation.

The designated subdivisions of the lung volume outlined in Chap. 214 are abnormal to varying degrees in both bronchitis and emphysema. The residual volume (RV) and functional residual capacity (FRC) are almost always higher than normal. Since the normal FRC is the volume at which the inward recoil of the lung is balanced by the outward recoil of the chest wall, loss of elastic recoil of the lung would clearly result in a higher static FRC. In addition, prolongation of expiration in association with obstruction would lead to a dynamic increase in FRC if inspiration is initiated before the respiratory system reaches its static balance point. Elevations of total lung capacity (TLC) are frequent. The exact cause is uncertain, but increases in TLC are often found in association with decreases in the elastic recoil of the lung. The vital capacity is frequently decreased, yet significant airways obstruction can be present with a normal to near-normal vital capacity.

The consequences of the airways and parenchymal processes are far more extensive than just the mechanical alterations discussed above. Maldistribution of inspired gas and blood flow is always

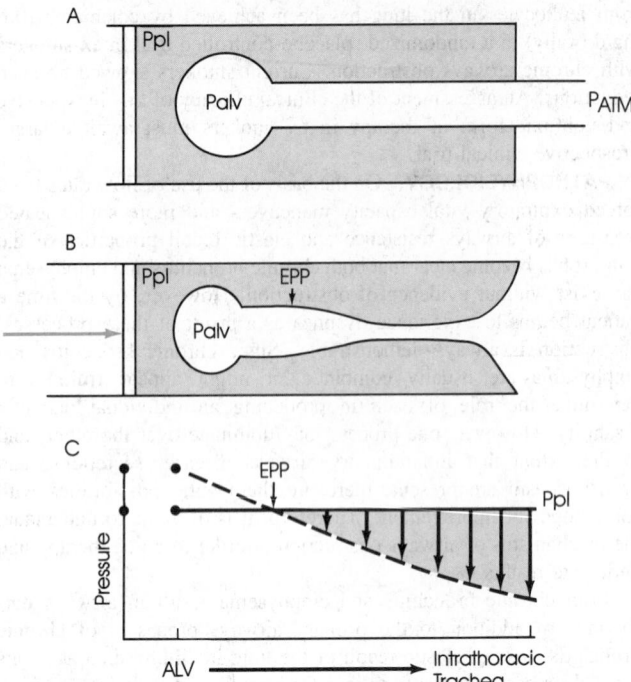

FIGURE 223-1 *A.* A schematic diagram of the lung and intrathoracic airways with no airflow. The alveolar pressure (Palv) is greater than pleural pressure (Ppl) by an amount equal to the elastic recoil pressure of the lung (Pel)—i.e., Palv is the algebraic sum of Ppl + Pel. With no airflow Palv = P atmospheric, and for all of the intrathoracic airways, pressure outside is less than the pressure inside due to the Pel. *B.* The same schematic lung during forced exhalation when pleural pressure becomes quite positive. Palv is still greater than Ppl by an amount equal to Pel. However, there is a pressure drop along the airway associated with flow, and at some point Ppl equals local bronchial pressure (so-called equal pressure point, EPP). Mouthward from this point, Ppl exceeds local bronchial pressure and hence acts to compress the airways. *C.* Pressure within the airways from alveoli to the intrathoracic trachea is shown as a dashed line (---) and Ppl is shown as a constant (———). Therefore, the driving pressure from alveoli to EPP is equal to Pel, and a decrease in Pel (i.e., loss of elastic recoil) would mean a smaller driving pressure and smaller flow rates.

present to some extent. When the mismatching is severe, impairment of gas exchange is reflected in abnormalities of arterial blood gases. There are regions of the lung with ventilation in excess of perfusion which increase the wasted ventilation ratio (that is, *Vd/Vt;* Chap. 214). At a normal resting CO_2 production, the net effective alveolar ventilation, as reflected by the arterial P_{CO_2}, may be excessive, normal, or insufficient depending on the relationship of the overall minute volume to the wasted ventilation ratio. The net contribution of regions with perfusion in excess of ventilation can be assessed by either estimating or measuring the alveolar-arterial P_{O_2} difference (that is, $P_{A_{O_2}} - P_{a_{O_2}}$; Chap. 214). In chronic bronchitis and emphysema, there are to some degree increases in both wasted ventilation and wasted blood flow.

The clinical manifestations depend, in large part, on the ventilatory response to the disordered lung function. Some patients, at the cost of extremely high effort of breathing and chronic dyspnea, will maintain a strikingly increased minute volume, which results both in a normal to low arterial P_{CO_2}, despite the high *Vd/Vt,* and a relatively high arterial P_{O_2}, despite the high difference, $P_{A_{O_2}} - P_{a_{O_2}}$. Other patients with only modest increases in effort of breathing and less dyspnea will maintain a normal to only moderately elevated minute volume at the cost of accepting a high arterial P_{CO_2} and a severely depressed arterial P_{O_2}.

Factors which account for clear differences in ventilatory responses between patients have been studied and debated for years. The bulk of available evidence suggests that those patients who maintain

relatively normal or low arterial P_{CO_2} levels are those with an increased ventilatory drive relative to their blood gas values and those who chronically maintain high arterial P_{CO_2} and lower P_{O_2} levels have a diminished ventilatory drive in relation to their more severely deranged blood gas values. It is not at all certain whether individual differences are accounted for by variations in peripheral or central chemoreceptor sensitivity or through other afferent pathways. Perhaps of more immediate value is the fact that patients with predominant emphysema are either normally or excessively responsive both to hypercapnia and to exercise, whereas those with predominant bronchitis are less responsive to both, despite similar degrees of airways obstruction by spirometry.

The pulmonary circulation malfunctions not only in terms of regional distribution of blood flow but in terms of abnormal overall pressure-flow relationships. There is often mild to severe pulmonary hypertension at rest with further increases disproportionate to cardiac output elevations during exercise. A reduction in the total cross-sectional area of the pulmonary vascular bed can be attributed to anatomic changes and constriction of vascular smooth muscle in pulmonary arteries and arterioles as well as destruction of alveolar septa with loss of capillaries. Rarely does loss of capillaries alone lead to severe pulmonary hypertension with cor pulmonale, except as a near-terminal event. Of more importance is the constriction of pulmonary vessels in response to alveolar hypoxia. The constriction is reversible upon increase in alveolar P_{O_2} with therapy. There is a synergism between hypoxia and acidosis which assumes importance during episodes of acute or chronic respiratory insufficiency. Chronic hypoxia leads not only to pulmonary vascular constriction but also to secondary erythrocytosis. The latter, although not proved to be a significant contributor to pulmonary hypertension, could add an unfavorable rheologic load. As discussed in Chap. 204, the chronic afterload on the right ventricle leads to hypertrophy and, in association with disordered blood gases, ultimately to failure.

CLINICAL-FUNCTIONAL CORRELATIONS Dyspnea and impairment of physical work capacity are characteristic only of severe to moderately severe airways obstruction. There is considerable variation among patients, and those with predominant emphysema have greater dyspnea and restriction of physical activity with lesser degrees of obstruction than those in whom chronic bronchitis predominates. The majority of patients have functionally mixed disease, will usually experience exertional dyspnea when the forced expiratory volume in 1 s (FEV_1) falls below 50 percent of that predicted, and will have dyspnea at rest when the FEV_1 is less than 25 percent of that predicted. In addition to dyspnea at rest, carbon dioxide retention and cor pulmonale frequently occur when the FEV_1 falls to 25 percent of that predicted. However, those with predominant bronchitis often have carbon dioxide retention and cor pulmonale with FEV_1 values above 25 percent of normal, in contrast to patients with predominant emphysema, whose FEV_1 usually falls well below that level before the onset of carbon dioxide retention and cor pulmonale. With a respiratory infection, small changes in the degree of obstruction can make a large difference in symptoms and gas exchange. Thus small therapeutic gains have rewarding results.

In general, the more severe the obstruction, the poorer the prognosis. Despite the general relationship, 20 to 30 percent of patients with severe obstruction and carbon dioxide retention will survive beyond 5 years.

CLINICAL SYNDROMES It is clear that the clinical presentation can vary in severity from simple chronic bronchitis without disability to the severely disabled state with chronic respiratory failure. From a practical standpoint, it is well to consider that any symptom or any measurable abnormality may foreshadow the development of severe disabling disease; hence cessation of smoking and avoidance of environmental irritants and toxins are to be advised. However, the advice to modify behavior and life patterns is rarely taken, and most physicians are called on to categorize and treat patients with fully developed, chronic airways obstruction. Thus the approach taken here is to describe two polar opposite types of fully developed, chronic

TABLE 223-1 Chronic obstructive lung disease: Salient features of the two types

	Predominant emphysema	Predominant bronchitis
Age at time of diagnosis, y	60±	50±
Dyspnea	Severe	Mild
Cough	After dyspnea starts	Before dyspnea starts
Sputum	Scanty, mucoid	Copious, purulent
Bronchial infections	Less frequent	More frequent
Respiratory insufficiency episodes	Often terminal	Repeated
Chest film	"Hyperinflation" ± bullous changes, small heart	Increased bronchovascular markings at bases, large heart
Chronic Pa_{CO_2}, mmHg	35–40	50–60
Chronic Pa_{O_2}, mmHg	65–75	45–60
Hematocrit, %	35–45	50–55
Pulmonary hypertension:		
Rest	None to mild	Moderate to severe
Exercise	Moderate	Worsens
Cor pulmonale	Rare, except terminally	Common
Elastic recoil	Severely decreased	Normal
Resistance	Normal to slight increase	High
Diffusing capacity	Decreased	Normal to slight decrease

obstructive pulmonary disease with the realization that the majority of patients will have some features of both types. The salient features of each type are outlined in Table 223-1.

Predominant emphysema These patients often give a long history of exertional dyspnea with minimal cough which is productive of only small amounts of mucoid sputum. Mucopurulent exacerbations in association with infections are not frequent. The body build is asthenic with evidence of weight loss. The patient appears distressed with obvious use of accessory muscles of respiration which serve to lift the sternum in an anterosuperior direction with each inspiration. There is tachypnea with a relatively prolonged expiration through pursed lips, or expiration is begun with a grunting sound. While sitting, these patients often lean forward, extending the arms to brace themselves. The neck veins may be distended during expiration, yet they collapse briskly with inspiration. The lower intercostal spaces retract with each inspiration, and by palpation the lower lateral chest wall can be felt to move inward. The percussion note is hyperresonant, and by auscultation the breath sounds are diminished, with faint, high-pitched rhonchi heard toward the end of expiration. The cardiac impulse, if at all visible, is seen only in the xiphoid and subxiphoid regions, and cardiac dullness is either absent or severely reduced. By palpation there is frequently a sustained forward and downward right ventricular impulse in the subxiphoid region, and a presystolic gallop accentuated during inspiration is commonly heard.

The arterial P_{O_2} is often in the mid-70s (mmHg), and the P_{CO_2} is low to normal. Because of the maintained increase in minute volume and the maintenance of arterial P_{O_2} sufficient to nearly saturate hemoglobin, these patients have been referred to as "pink puffers." Their increased ventilatory drive probably accounts for their relatively preserved oxygenation and lack of hypercapnia; however, this increased drive with attendant increases in ventilation undoubtedly contributes to the severity of their dyspnea.

The TLC and RV are invariably increased, the vital capacity is low, and the maximal expiratory flow rates are diminished. The elastic recoil properties of the lung are severely impaired, and in direct proportion to this impairment, the capacity of the lung to transfer carbon monoxide is lowered.

On radiographic examination the diaphragms are low and flattened, the bronchovascular shadows do not extend to the periphery of the lung, and the cardiac silhouette is lengthened and narrowed. These findings in association with a large retrosternal translucency on lateral

chest radiographs are interpreted as hyperinflation, which correlates well with increases in TLC and loss of elastic recoil. Peripheral attenuation of bronchovascular markings and increased retrosternal lucency correlate best with subsequent postmortem demonstration of extensive and severe emphysema which is predominantly of the panacinar type. Computed tomography (CT) has been shown to localize and quantitate emphysema. However, determining the localization of such regions most often is of little practical value, and the overall quantitative assessments from elastic recoil properties and carbon monoxide transfer are just as good. Hence CT scans are not ordinarily employed for this purpose.

It is fortunate that the patient with predominant emphysema is less prone to mucopurulent relapses than is the patient with predominant bronchitis, since such relapses frequently lead to severe respiratory failure and death. That is to say, right-sided heart failure and hypercapnic respiratory failure are often terminal events in those patients with predominant emphysema. In the absence of such relapses, the clinical course is characterized by severe and progressive dyspnea for which little can be done. The physician's role is to seek out and treat any factor that is possibly reversible and strive to avoid pollutants and infections.

Predominant bronchitis The patient with predominant bronchitis usually has an impressive history of cough and sputum production for many years with an immodest history of cigarette smoking. Initially the cough is present only in the winter months, and the patient is apt to seek medical attention, if at all, only during the more severe of the frequent mucopurulent relapses. Over the years the cough progresses from hibernal to perennial, and mucopurulent relapses increase in frequency, duration, and severity. After beginning to experience exertional dyspnea, the patient often seeks medical help and will be found to have a severe degree of obstruction. Occasionally, such a patient will seek out a physician only after the onset of peripheral edema secondary to overt right ventricular failure. More rarely the initial medical contact is made by family members who present the physician with a deeply cyanotic, edematous, and stuporous patient with acute respiratory insufficiency.

The patient with predominant bronchitis is often overweight and cyanotic. There is usually no apparent distress at rest, the respiratory rate is normal or only slightly increased, and there is no apparent usage of accessory muscles. The chest percussion note is normally resonant, and by auscultation, one can usually hear coarse rhonchi and wheezes which change in location and intensity after a deep and productive cough. There may be a sustained heave along the lower left sternal border which indicates right ventricular hypertrophy. In the presence of right ventricular failure there are often an early diastolic gallop and occasionally a holosystolic murmur, both of which are accentuated by inspiration. The latter finding is indicative of functional tricuspid regurgitation which is frequently accompanied by neck vein distention characterized by large *v* waves and brisk *y* descents. With right ventricular failure the cyanosis deepens and peripheral edema becomes prominent. Clubbing of the digits is unusual.

With or without right ventricular failure, the minute volume is only slightly increased due to an overall diminution in ventilatory drive which modulates the level of dyspnea. However, failure to increase minute volume greatly in the face of significant proportions of wasted ventilation and blood flow results in severely deranged arterial blood gases, with arterial P_{CO_2} values which are chronically increased to the range of the high 40s to low 50s (mmHg). The lowered P_{O_2} produces desaturation of hemoglobin, serves to stimulate erythropoiesis, and results in hypoxic pulmonary vasoconstriction. Desaturation and erythrocytosis combine to produce the cyanosis, and hypoxic pulmonary vasoconstriction accentuates the right-sided heart failure. Because of cyanosis and edema secondary to heart failure, such patients have been referred to as "blue bloaters." It has been proposed, with some supporting data, that one of the pathophysiologic events in blue bloaters is the occurrence of repeated episodes of severe nocturnal oxygen desaturation in association with episodes of sleep apnea or periods of worsening hypoventilation. Such sleep-related ventilatory events worsen the degree of pulmonary hypertension and secondary erythrocytosis.

The TLC is often normal, and there is a moderate elevation of RV. The vital capacity is mildly diminished, and maximal expiratory flow rates are invariably low. The elastic recoil properties of the lung are normal or only slightly impaired, and the capacity of the lung to transfer carbon monoxide is either normal or minimally decreased.

On radiographic examination the diaphragms are well rounded, the bronchovascular markings are increased in the lower lung fields, and the cardiac silhouette is somewhat enlarged. In association with right ventricular failure the cardiac silhouette enlarges further, pulmonary arteries become more prominent, and an antigravity distribution of perfusion is apparent.

Despite well-planned management (see below) the patient with predominant bronchitis may experience many episodes of respiratory failure from which recovery is frequent with proper therapy (see later). The ability to recover from such repeated episodes in these patients is in striking contrast to the frequently fatal outcome of such events in those with predominant emphysema. Ultimately, the lungs at postmortem will be found to have severe bronchitic changes in both large and small airways and only moderate emphysema, predominantly of the centriacinar variety.

It should be reemphasized that the preceding syndromes are described as polar ends of a continuous spectrum of clinical features. Hence most patients will have some characteristics of each syndrome. Recognizing and understanding the pathophysiologic bases for these aids in the planning of appropriate management strategies for each patient.

PRINCIPLES OF MANAGEMENT Intelligent management must be based on as complete knowledge as possible of the degree of obstruction, the extent of disability, and the relative reversibility of the patient's illness. To the extent that obstructive processes in the airways are contributory, there is a chance for treatment to be effective. Since emphysema is an irreversible process, prevention of progression and avoidance of acute insults constitute the main approach. History, physical examination, and chest radiographs should be supplemented by tests of lung function performed during a symptomatically stable period. Ideally, complete spirometry, plethysmographic lung volumes, transfer of carbon monoxide, arterial blood gases, and lung elastic recoil properties should be measured. Spirometry and lung volumes should be remeasured after the administration of bronchodilators in order to assess the degree of acutely reversible airways obstruction. Failure to see an acute change with bronchodilator drugs does not rule out the possibility of improvement with more prolonged administration of these agents. In instances in which the degree of exertional dyspnea appears to be disproportionately greater than the degree of obstruction, measurements of blood gases, minute volume, CO_2 production, and O_2 consumption during exercise are indicated in order to determine whether impaired lung function is sufficient to account for the symptoms. After the initial assessment, the physician has some idea of the relative emphasis to be placed on patient education, rehabilitative and preventive measures, and direct therapeutic interventions in management of the patient and the illness.

Smoking and the environment Cessation of smoking is the only certain means of influencing the progression of the chronic obstructive airways syndromes, and although such behavior modification is most effective at early stages of the disease processes, it is effective in slowing the rate of decline in lung function, even when such function is severely compromised. In the instances in which occupational or environmental exposures are thought to play a significant role, change of occupation or relocation of dwelling is advisable. The validity of such advice should be considered carefully, since the impact on both the patient and the family is likely to be great. A simpler environmental change is that of eliminating aerosol sprays such as deodorants, hair sprays, and insecticides from the household. Hair sprays have been shown to produce acute airways responses even in normal subjects.

Other preventive measures include yearly vaccination against the common or expected influenza virus strains. The patient need be given pneumococcal polysaccharide vaccine only once in a lifetime due to prolonged effectiveness of the immune response. However, if an earlier vaccine was used that contained only 14 capsular antigen types, revaccination with the current 23-valent vaccine is probably advisable.

Respiratory infections Infections cannot be totally avoided, and the patient should be made aware that increasing purulence, viscosity, or volume of secretions signals the onset of an infection which should be treated early. The most common pathogenic bacteria found are *Haemophilus influenzae* and *Streptococcus pneumoniae*. As mentioned above, however, the role of such bacteria is in question, since they are just as often isolated during periods of relative clinical quiescence. Nonetheless, a broad-spectrum antibiotic should be given for a 7- to 10-day course. It is practical to have the patient keep a 7- to 10-day supply of antibiotics at home and to begin treatment at the onset of symptoms. In Great Britain it is common practice to give continuous antibiotic therapy during winter months in order to prevent mucopurulent relapses. Although there is evidence that viruses are frequent causes of mucopurulent relapses, clinical studies have shown that the standard antibiotic regimens decrease the duration and severity of infective episodes unrelated to culturable bacterial pathogens. Microscopic examination and culture of sputum are indicated if there are chills, fever, or chest pain or if purulence fails to respond to usually administered antibiotics.

Exercise and nutrition It has been shown repeatedly that exercise programs, although not accompanied by measurable improvement in lung function, result in increased exercise tolerance and an improved sense of well-being. The improvement is usually task-specific, so most physicians advise walking in preference to the use of special apparatus, such as stationary bicycles. Arm exercise is poorly tolerated; the necessary muscles required for breathing are also recruited for the exercise task and hence are doing double duty.

If malnutrition (body weight less than 85 percent of ideal) is present, oral dietary supplements can result in improved muscle strength, less fatigability, and lessening of breathlessness. A carefully taken dietary history and elimination of other serious causes for low body weight and weight loss should precede the start of any major nutritional supplement effort. As with exercise programs, there is not a direct and measurable effect on lung function from treating malnutrition, yet subjective relief and objective improvement in strength and exercise performance have been of great benefit in such patients.

Bronchodilator drugs These are often quite helpful in alleviating symptoms, especially in those patients who respond to them acutely in the laboratory. These drugs form three categories: the methylxanthines, sympathomimetics with strong beta$_2$-adrenergic-stimulating properties, and anticholinergics. The ethylene diamine salt of theophylline (aminophylline), the most commonly used methylxanthine, can be given orally or parenterally; in addition to bronchodilatation, it stimulates respiration and has cardiotonic and diuretic properties. Oral theophylline preparations vary greatly in their intestinal release and rate of absorption. There is extreme variability in rates of absorption, degradation, and secretion among patients. In those patients who, with standard doses, either fail to benefit or show signs of toxicity, theophylline blood levels should be measured. Measurements at expected peak absorption and just before the subsequent dose will allow adjustment of dose. Blood levels between 10 and 20 mg/L should be maintained. Side effects such as insomnia and nervousness are frequent when levels are in the therapeutic range. Nausea, vomiting, tachyarrhythmias, and seizures are seen mainly when blood levels exceed 20 mg/L. Parenteral administration of theophylline is rarely indicated in the chronic obstructive syndromes, except during episodes of respiratory failure, when agents cannot be given orally. Selective beta$_2$-stimulating drugs such as albuterol and metaproterenol can be given both orally and by aerosol with fewer cardiac side effects than are experienced with isoproterenol. Orally and parenterally administered beta$_2$ agonists are effective but are associated with greater tremulousness and cardiovascular side effects than result from inhaled agents. The latter can be most conveniently given in metered-dose inhalers at two to four puffs four to six times a day. Collecting chambers or spacers may improve the reliability of deposition of these agents. Anticholinergic agents such as atropine have been avoided in the past because of their tendency to desiccate secretions; however, ipratropium bromide, an anticholinergic agent in metered-dose inhaler form, is an effective bronchodilator in chronic bronchitic patients. It is considered by many to be the bronchodilator of choice for these patients.

Corticosteroids The use of systemic glucocorticoids is, at our present state of knowledge, based on very little scientific data from properly controlled clinical trials. Since these agents have time- and dose-related side effects that vary from deleterious to catastrophic, the almost invariable subjective benefit must be supported by objective measurements. There is little room for doubt in the minds of physicians that some patients respond well, even dramatically, to these agents in both objective and subjective terms. The real problem is how to select those patients most likely to benefit. Eosinophilia in the sputum, rather than in the blood, appears in some instances to identify that subgroup in advance. However, the best guidelines are, first, to try these agents only after maximal bronchodilator and bronchopulmonary drainage measures have been tried without success; second, to begin prednisone 30 mg once per day; third, to confirm the objective change in terms of spirometry and gas exchange, stopping these agents if no objective benefit is seen; and fourth, to decrease to the smallest dose that will maintain the improved level of function. The role, if any, of inhaled glucocorticoid agents for these patients, in contrast to asthmatic patients, has not been established in the syndromes with chronic obstruction.

Bronchopulmonary drainage should be maintained in patients with hypersecretion. If the coughing mechanism is ineffective or if paroxysms of coughing are exhausting, postural drainage is often a useful adjunct. Although liquefaction of secretions by means of orally administered expectorants or aerosol delivery of mucolytic agents is an appealing idea, it has never been shown by properly designed trials to be more effective than simple maintenance of total-body hydration.

Intermittent positive pressure breathing (IPPB) devices were formerly advocated for home management. The various rationales included diminution in the work of breathing, promotion of bronchopulmonary drainage, and more efficient delivery of bronchodilator drugs. The first of the rationales has been shown to have no basis in fact, and the goals of the last two have been shown to be as well accomplished by postural drainage and use of less elaborate aerosol generators. Hence the use of IPPB for home management cannot be justified.

Treatment of hypoxia and erythrocytosis When arterial hypoxia is persistent and severe (Pa$_{O_2}$ of 55 to 60 mmHg) in association with cor pulmonale (see Chap. 204) and signs of right heart failure, continuous oxygen therapy is indicated. If the Pa$_{O_2}$ is persistently < 55 mmHg, with or without cor pulmonale, continuous oxygen supplementation also should be prescribed. The available data indicate that supplemental oxygen improves both exercise tolerance and neuropsychological function and alleviates pulmonary hypertension and right heart failure. In patients with severe hypoxemia, the need for hospitalization occurs less frequently and life span is lengthened by the use of supplemental oxygen.

Since most patients with chronic airways obstruction, especially those with features of predominant bronchitis, can be shown to decrease their Pa$_{O_2}$ values significantly during sleep, most prominently during the REM phase, nocturnal oxygen administration has been suggested. While the rationale is clear and the results quite good, a cooperative clinical trial that compared nocturnal with continuous O$_2$ supplementation in severely hypoxic patients found that continuous O$_2$ administration was associated with a significantly lower mortality rate. Patients in both treatment groups experienced neuropsychological

and hemodynamic benefits. Thus supplemental nocturnal oxygen is better than none, but continuous oxygen is better than nocturnal in such severely ill patients. Those patients not requiring continuous oxygen therapy may require supplementation during air travel. Even with modern pressurization, cabin altitudes may reach the equivalent of 8000 ft, at which the Pa$_{O_2}$ may fall by 25 mmHg below that found at sea level. Hence oxygen supplementation during prolonged flights should be considered for patients with sea level Pa$_{O_2}$ values in the mid-70s.

Secondary erythrocytosis with the hematocrit in excess of 50 percent is most easily viewed as a mechanism allowing greater oxygen delivery to compensate for the chronically lowered arterial P$_{O_2}$; hence improvement in oxygenation through improved lung function or by oxygen administration is the most physiologic means to reverse erythrocytosis. Since erythrocytosis results in elevation of blood viscosity at all shear rates, the proposal has been made that pulmonary vascular hypertension is aggravated by its presence. Although no study has demonstrated an objective improvement in hemodynamics, lung mechanics, or gas exchange at rest following phlebotomy, ventilatory and cardiovascular function during exercise improve. Some patients who complain of headaches and a sense of head fullness show a favorable subjective response to periodic phlebotomy when the hematocrit is in excess of 55 percent. In support of this subjective improvement is the demonstration that, following phlebotomy, cerebral blood flow, previously diminished, returns toward normal.

Other measures Despite employing all the foregoing measures, some patients remain severely incapacitated. For these patients, lung transplantation can return them to both a functional and comfortable state (see Chap. 232). Criteria for transplanting such patients are being evolved in the several centers performing this procedure. Medical directors of such programs should be consulted if the possibility of a lung transplant is being considered.

There are two therapeutic interventions well short of lung transplantation that have been proposed repeatedly by a few investigators and that remain extremely controversial. It cannot be denied that some supporting data exist; the counterintuitive nature of the interventions and the absence of controlled trials preclude their wide acceptance. These are (1) bilateral carotid body resection and (2) periodic use of negative pressure ventilation. The initial rationale for bilateral carotid body resection was to relieve dyspnea by diminishing the ventilatory responsiveness to hypoxemia and hypercapnia, which would present its own set of dangers. Several studies have shown improved lung mechanics and exercise performance after the procedure. Use of negative pressure ventilation for periods up to 8 h/d for 2 consecutive days has been shown to improve gas exchange, muscle strength, and ventilatory responsiveness for several subsequent days.

ACUTE RESPIRATORY FAILURE

DIAGNOSIS Although it may be strongly suspected on clinical grounds, the firm diagnosis of acute respiratory failure in chronic airways obstruction is based on measurements of arterial blood gas (Pa$_{O_2}$, Pa$_{CO_2}$) and pH values that must be interpreted in relation to the patient's chronic status. Since many patients will have chronically lowered Pa$_{O_2}$ levels and increased Pa$_{CO_2}$ values, the diagnosis is based on the degree of change from the usual state of the individual patient. With regard to oxygenation, an acute decrease in Pa$_{O_2}$ from a usual mid-70 range to the low 60s (mmHg) is just as indicative of acute respiratory failure as is an acute drop from a chronic mid-50 range to the mid-40s (mmHg). Thus a drop in Pa$_{O_2}$ equal to or greater than 10 to 15 mmHg indicates acute failure.

Since renal compensation for chronic hypercapnia results in adjustment of arterial pH to near-normal values, the acuteness of the increase in Pa$_{CO_2}$ can often be judged by the pH, unless there is a concomitant metabolic acidemia. As a practical guide, any level of hypercapnia associated with an arterial pH value less than 7.30 should be considered as acute respiratory failure.

PRECIPITATING FACTORS Increases in volume, viscosity, and/or purulence of secretions, presumably due to infection of the tracheobronchial tree, are the most common antecedents of acute respiratory failure in chronic obstructive lung disease. Increasing airways obstruction with airways inflammation and secretion, especially in association with a relatively blunted ventilatory drive, leads to worsening hypoxia and increasing CO_2 retention. Agitation, insomnia, and increasing dyspnea with impending respiratory failure are occasionally treated, mistakenly, with either sedatives or narcotics, and these, too, may precipitate frank respiratory failure. In fact, depressant drugs which impair ventilatory drive should be avoided at all times in patients with severe chronic obstructive lung disease. Major episodes of air pollution also can lead to respiratory failure, and the physicians responsible for patients with severe bronchitis and emphysema should be alert to these environmental events.

Pneumonia, thromboembolism, left ventricular failure, and pneumothorax occasionally precipitate acute respiratory failure and are extremely difficult to detect unless considered and specifically sought. As a minimum, chest radiographs, electrocardiograms, and sputum examinations should be obtained in addition to arterial blood gas measurements in all patients with respiratory failure.

TREATMENT OF RESPIRATORY FAILURE The treatment of respiratory failure consists of two simultaneous processes: (1) maintaining acceptable levels of oxygenation and ventilation and (2) treatment of infection, removal of secretions, and reversal of any airways constriction present.

Management of hypoxia These patients *need* oxygen when they are severely hypoxic, and while fears of respiratory depression due to the removal of the hypoxic respiratory stimulus are realistic, O_2 must be used, yet in the smallest concentration possible, to give a Pa_{O_2} in the mid-50 range while the patient's Pa_{CO_2}, pH, and clinical status are carefully monitored. It is best to begin with only modest increases in FI_{O_2} to approximately 0.24 (cf. air at 0.21), which can be accomplished using nasal prongs with O_2 flows at 1 to 2 L/min or, more precisely, with the use of a 0.24 Venturi mask. These latter masks, based on Bernoulli's principle, deliver a fixed concentration of O_2 irrespective of the O_2 flow rate by entraining air in direct proportion to O_2 flow rate. They are high-flow masks (oxygen plus air entrained from the room), each designed for a specific FI_{O_2} (0.24, 0.28, 0.35, 0.40). Even small increases in Pa_{O_2} when starting from low levels result in significant increases in arterial oxygen content due to the shape of the oxygen-hemoglobin saturation curve over this range (Chap. 302).

With improved oxygenation some patients will concomitantly increase their Pa_{CO_2} values. The standard explanation has been that this increase is due to the removal of the hypoxic drive to ventilation leading to further hypoventilation. While this is the most important mechanism, recent data indicate that worsening ventilation-perfusion relationships (Chap. 214) occur with O_2 treatment. This is attributed to reversal of hypoxic pulmonary arterial constriction in the more initially hypoxic, less well ventilated regions, which in turn leads to decreased perfusion of initially less hypoxic, better ventilated regions. The result is an increase in the wasted ventilation ratio (Vd/Vt; Chap. 214) leading to a smaller effective alveolar ventilation. In either case, the FI_{O_2} should be increased as little as possible to achieve a Pa_{O_2} in the mid-50 range. Some increase in Pa_{CO_2} can be expected and should not cause alarm if the patient is alert. The majority of patients can be managed in this conservative way with excellent results. However, occasionally, large increases in Pa_{CO_2} occur and lead to stupor and coma. This can be explained by CO_2-induced cerebral vascular dilatation with increased intracranial pressure, including the development of papilledema, combined with the effect of hypercapnia and hypoxia on cerebral function. It must be emphasized that if stupor and coma supervene, stopping the administration of oxygen is the *worst possible* course of action. When CO_2 narcosis is present, respirations are sufficiently depressed from the CO_2 itself that the patient will no longer respond to the rapidly worsening hypoxia, and fatal arrhythmias, generalized seizures, and death may ensue. The

only alternative is to intubate the trachea and provide mechanical ventilatory support. Mechanical ventilators are described in Chap. 231.

Once mechanical ventilation has been instituted, the tidal volume and frequency should be set to decrease gradually the Pa_{CO_2} only down to the chronically elevated level rather than attempt to decrease it to or below a normal value. Since such patients have renal compensation for their chronic hypercapnia, Pa_{CO_2} values at or below the normal level result in significant alkalemia which in turn can lead to severe tachyarrhythmias and generalized seizures.

Control of infection, bronchoconstriction, and secretions As mentioned above, maintaining oxygenation and ventilation serves to buy time while secretion removal, bronchial dilatation, and treatment of infection are instituted. Removal of secretions is accomplished by urging the patient to cough or by passing suction catheters into the trachea which, in addition to removing secretions that are present, stimulate cough that brings more secretions up to the region of the catheter tip. The advantage, if any, from the use of mucolytic agents in this process has yet to be demonstrated. However, beta$_2$-adrenergic bronchodilating agents have been shown to increase the rate of transport of particles by the mucociliary blanket, and, thus, in addition to bronchodilatation, such agents should improve the clearance of airway secretions. Postural drainage and chest percussion are other often-used adjuncts that have been shown, especially when secretions are voluminous, to improve tracheobronchial clearance, to increase sputum volume beyond that produced by cough, and to reduce airways obstruction.

Bronchodilatation with aminophylline given orally or by infusion and beta$_2$-adrenergic agonists and anticholinergics by inhalation has assumed a prominent role in treatment of acute respiratory failure in chronic airways obstruction. In addition to bronchodilatation these agents improve bronchopulmonary clearance and may help induce diuresis and hemodynamic improvement when there is cor pulmonale with heart failure (Chap. 204). Unless there is clearly an acute pneumonia, the use of antibiotics is more controversial in the setting of acute respiratory failure than in mucopurulent relapses without failure. Nonetheless, broad-spectrum antibiotics, if no single agent is suspected or isolated, or erythromycin, if legionellae or mycoplasmas are suspected, should be added to the regimen.

Management of complications Complications arising in the course of treatment for acute respiratory failure are cardiac arrhythmias, most often multifocal supraventricular tachycardias, left ventricular failure, pulmonary emboli, and gastrointestinal hemorrhage from stress ulceration. Cardiac arrhythmias resulting from rapid decreases in oxygenation or increases in pH due to overventilation can be readily avoided. However, when giving multiple drugs having cardiotonic properties, the question always arises as to whether the arrhythmias are related to these. Keeping serum theophylline levels in the 10 to 20 mg/L range and using relatively selective beta agonists, such as isoetharine or albuterol by inhalation, can minimize these effects.

Left ventricular failure, usually attributable to coronary atherosclerosis with acute myocardial infarction, systemic hypertension, or aortic valvular disease, is difficult to detect in the presence of cor pulmonale. Fortunately, improving lung function and oxygenation most often reverse the pulmonary hypertension and right ventricular failure (Chap. 204) and induce a brisk diuresis. If signs of congestive failure persist or worsen after providing adequate oxygenation, consideration must be given to left ventricular failure; an assessment in such patients is best made through echocardiography or radioventriculography, since the usual physical and radiographic findings are obscured in such patients. Only in the presence of adequate gas exchange and only with either the firm demonstration of, or strong clinical suspicion of, left ventricular failure should digitalis be used. Diuretic agents should also be reserved for left ventricular failure. They almost invariably produce hypokalemic, hypochloremic metabolic alkalemia that results in depression of ventilatory drive and interference with removal from mechanical ventilatory support.

Pulmonary emboli are suspected to be common in the setting of acute respiratory failure and are extremely difficult to detect since the lung scan is totally nonspecific and signs of cor pulmonale fluctuate in concert with the degree of lung dysfunction. Hence low-dose heparin prophylaxis should be used to prevent this complication. Gastrointestinal hemorrhage commonly complicates acute respiratory failure and is thought to be due to stress ulceration of the gastric mucosa. Awareness of this complication enhances the ability to detect it and act quickly. Antacids, coating agents such as sucralfate, nasogastric suction, and/or cimetidine have been used to diminish the frequency.

Weaning from mechanical ventilation For those patients who have required mechanical ventilatory support, the process of removal from that support is largely empirical. In general, improving gas exchange and lung mechanics along with alertness and responsiveness of the patient signal that the support can be removed. Data such as maximal voluntary inspiratory mouth pressures greater than 20 cmH$_2$O, vital capacity greater than 10 mL/kg of body weight, and spontaneous tidal volume greater than 5 mL/kg of body weight are reassuring. However, many patients can be removed from such support with lesser values than these.

Failure to maintain gas exchange after removal of mechanical ventilatory support can usually be explained. *First* on the list is the continued administration or persistence of sedative and tranquilizing drugs that may have been prescribed earlier for agitation. These should be discontinued and time allowed for their metabolism. *Second* is the possibility that the endotracheal tube is of small bore and imposes a resistive load. If so, it should be replaced by a larger one. *Third* is worsening airways obstruction and accumulation of secretions; continued bronchial dilatation and airway suctioning avoid these. *Fourth* is a metabolic alkalemia, with or without diuretic therapy, that should be treated with potassium chloride. *Fifth* is having maintained, while on mechanical ventilation, a Pa$_{O_2}$ and Pa$_{CO_2}$ that are too high and too low, respectively. This can be avoided by using an FI$_{O_2}$ just sufficient to keep the Pa$_{O_2}$ around 60 mmHg and using the assist mode with small enough tidal volumes to keep the Pa$_{CO_2}$ at the expected chronic level (i.e., that associated with a normal or slightly low arterial pH) before discontinuing mechanical support. *Sixth* is poor nutrition, hypokalemia, or neuromuscular disease, making the patient too weak to maintain breathing or resulting in fatigue of the respiratory muscles. Nutrition, of course, is a longer range problem that should be anticipated, while hypokalemia is often handled along with the metabolic alkalemia. Muscle fatigue, especially diaphragmatic, has received a great deal of attention. From a practical standpoint, paradoxical (inward) movement of the upper abdomen with inspiration is the key clinical finding. Experimental evidence suggests that therapeutic levels of aminophylline or beta$_2$ agonists, such as fenoterol, reverse the manifestations of fatigue, but the role of respiratory stimulants continues to be debated and the data to be inconclusive. In those patients with severely blunted ventilatory drive and improving lung function, stimulants may be tried cautiously. If there is severe metabolic alkalemia, acetazolamide can be tried as a stimulant while chloride replacement is being carried out. Medroxyprogesterone, a central stimulant, or almitrine, a peripheral chemoreceptor stimulant, appear to be safe and, in some instances, effective. Hypothyroidism is a metabolic condition with neuromuscular consequences and is difficult to detect in this clinical setting. Thus any prolonged and difficult weaning process should lead to the assessment of thyroid function.

PROGNOSIS On the average, data collected on large populations demonstrate a slow and relentless diminution in ventilatory function in patients with chronic airways obstruction. Although slow, the decrement in function with time far exceeds the rate of change seen with normal aging. In general, the likelihood of episodes of acute respiratory failure increases when the FEV$_1$ falls below 25 percent of predicted normal values. Although the in-hospital mortality rate averages 30 percent for a single episode and the 5-year survival rate after the initial episode of respiratory failure averages only 15 to 20 percent, the clinical syndrome is extremely important in determining both the short- and long-range prognosis. As noted above, those patients with predominant emphysema have a poorer prognosis after the onset of respiratory failure than do those with predominant bronchitis. In either case long-term oxygen treatment in those with severe hypoxemia results in prolongation of life and improvement in the quality of life.

BULLOUS EMPHYSEMA Confluent air spaces with diameters in excess of 1 cm are occasionally congenital but most often are found in association with generalized emphysema or progressive fibrotic processes. Gradual increases in size of such air spaces (or bullae) result from traction applied by regions with better elastic recoil properties, and such regions lose volume as the bullae become enlarged. If disability is severe, if the bulla is extremely large, and if either lobar gas sampling or ventilation and perfusion scans demonstrate that sufficient function remains in the nonbullous regions, surgical excision of the bulla may lead to functional improvement. Usually, however, improvement is relatively transitory because other emphysematous regions gradually enlarge into bullae after surgery.

VARIANTS OF EMPHYSEMA In addition to the centriacinar and panacinar forms of emphysema described above, other structural patterns have been described but are functionally less important. Often there is overdistention and alveolar septal destruction in lung regions surrounding scar tissue (paracicatricial or scar emphysema) or along the borders of the acinus (paraseptal emphysema). The latter form, when it occurs at the visceral pleural surface, may predispose to episodes of spontaneous pneumothorax (Chap. 228). Infants rarely develop a check valve mechanism in a lobar bronchus which leads to rapid and life-threatening overdistention (congenital lobar emphysema). Unilateral emphysema may be an incidental radiographic finding (Macleod's or Swyer-James's syndromes). Since, in this condition, the airways are normal in number and structure but the alveoli are reduced in number, this form of unilateral emphysema has been attributed to disease occurring before the age of 8 years when alveoli are normally increasing in number. Overdistention and alveolar septal destruction are not present, and so this condition does not fit the definition of true emphysema. Most often the pulmonary artery on the affected side is hypoplastic. Although usually an incidental finding, the affected lung may become repeatedly infected so that surgical excision may be indicated.

MISCELLANEOUS DIFFUSE OBSTRUCTIVE SYNDROMES *Bronchiolitis obliterans* is a term applied to widespread inflammatory and fibrotic obstruction of small airways. Initially this syndrome was thought to be restricted to those persons who had suffered severe viral infections in childhood, particularly those due to parainfluenza virus. However, recently this syndrome has also been described in adult patients with rheumatoid arthritis. The response to bronchodilator treatment is poor, as would be expected from the histopathologic findings, and fatal respiratory failure often ensues within 2 years. There have been reports suggesting a relationship between penicillamine therapy and the development of bronchiolitis obliterans in patients with rheumatoid arthritis; however, it is clear that this syndrome can develop in patients who have never received penicillamine.

A syndrome with similar histopathology has been described in recipients of autologous bone marrow transplants. Although most often interstitial pneumonitis and fibrosis are sequelae, it has been documented that some patients develop a bronchiolitis obliterans picture. It appears that the development of this process occurs most often in the setting of a chronic graft-versus-host syndrome; however, it is clear that diffuse airways obstruction has developed without evidence of this syndrome in bone marrow recipients.

Cystic fibrosis in the adult with chronic airways obstruction is discussed elsewhere (Chap. 222).

REFERENCES

BERG BW et al: Oxygen supplementation during air travel in patients with chronic obstructive lung disease. Chest 101:638, 1992

CAMPBELL EJ, SENIOR RM: Emphysema, in *Update: Pulmonary Diseases and Disorders*, AP Fishman (ed). New York, McGraw-Hill, 1992, pp 37–52

CRYSTAL RG: α₁-Antitrypsin deficiency, in *Update: Pulmonary Diseases and Disorders*, AP Fishman (ed). New York, McGraw-Hill, 1992, pp 19–36

DUNN WF et al: Oxygen-induced hypercarbia in obstructive pulmonary disease. Am Rev Respir Dis 144:526, 1991

FERNANDEZ E et al: Sustained improvement in gas exchange after negative pressure ventilation for 8 hours per day on 2 successive days in chronic airflow limitation. Am Rev Respir Dis 144:390, 1991

JOSEPHSON GD et al: Airway obstruction. New modalities in treatment. Med Clin North Am 77:539, 1993

KIM WD et al: Centrilobular and panlobular emphysema in smokers. Am Rev Respir Dis 144:1385, 1991

KING TE JR: Bronchiolitis obliterans. Lung 169:S159, 1991

ORR PH et al: Randomized placebo-controlled trials of antibiotics for acute bronchitis: A critical review of the literature. J FAM Pract 36:507, 1993

REID LM: Chronic obstructive pulmonary diseases, in *Pulmonary Diseases and Disorders*, 2d ed, AP Fishman (ed). New York, McGraw-Hill Book Co, 1988, pp 1247–1272

SKWARSKI K et al: Predictors of survival in patients with chronic obstructive pulmonary disease treated with long-term oxygen therapy. Chest 100:1522, 1991

STOCKLEY RA: Alpha-1-antitrypsin and the pathogenesis of emphysema. Lung 169:S205, 1991

WHIPP BJ et al: Physiologic changes following bilateral carotid-body resection in patients with chronic obstructive pulmonary disease. Chest 101:656 1992.

YANAI M et al: Site of airway obstruction in pulmonary disease: Direct measurement of intrabronchial pressure. J Appl Physiol 72:1016 1992

224   INTERSTITIAL LUNG DISEASES

HERBERT Y. REYNOLDS

The interstitial lung diseases (ILDs) are a heterogeneous group of conditions that involve the alveolar walls and perialveolar tissue. The ILDs are nonmalignant and are not caused by any defined infectious agents. Although an acute phase of illness may occur, the onset is often insidious, and the disease is usually chronic in duration. The initial response of the host to the disease process is inflammation in the air spaces and alveolar walls, causing an acute phase of intraluminal and mural alveolitis. If the disease is chronic and smoldering, inflammation will spread to adjacent portions of the interstitium and vasculature and eventually produce interstitial fibrosis. The resultant scarring and distortion of lung tissue leads to significant derangement of gas exchange and ventilatory function. Inflammation also can involve the conducting airways, and bronchiolitis obliterans associated with an organizing pneumonia is probably part of the spectrum of an ILD.

This diverse group of diseases has many features in common, including similarity of symptoms, comparable appearance of chest radiographs, consistent alterations in pulmonary physiology, and typical histologic features. However, ILDs have been difficult to classify because approximately 180 known individual diseases are characterized by interstitial lung involvement, either as primary disease or as a significant part of a multiorgan process, as occurs in the collagen vascular diseases. The chest radiograph is of limited aid in classification because it can have a similar appearance in many of the ILDs as well as in other unrelated lung diseases. One useful approach for classification is to separate ILDs into two groups, those with known causes and those with unknown causes; each of these groups can be divided into subgroups according to the presence or absence of histologic evidence of granulomas in interstitial or vascular areas (Table 224-1). For each ILD there may be an acute phase, and there is usually a chronic one as well.

Among the ILDs of known cause, the largest group comprises occupational and environmental inhalant exposures; these include diseases due to inhalation of inorganic dusts (Chap. 219), organic dusts, and various irritative or noxious gases (Chap. 218). The number of ILDs of unknown cause is also very large. The major ones within

TABLE 224-1   Major categories of alveolar and interstitial inflammatory lung diseases (ILDs)

Known cause	Unknown cause
LUNG RESPONSE: ALVEOLITIS, INTERSTITIAL INFLAMMATION, AND FIBROSIS	
Asbestos	Idiopathic pulmonary fibrosis
Fumes, gases	Collagen vascular diseases
Drugs (antibiotics) and chemotherapy drugs	Systemic lupus erythematosus, rheumatoid arthritis, ankylosing spondylitis, systemic sclerosis, Sjögren's syndrome, polymyositis-dermatomyositis
Radiation	
Aspiration pneumonia	
Residual of adult respiratory distress syndrome	Pulmonary hemorrhage syndromes
	Goodpasture's syndrome, idiopathic pulmonary hemosiderosis
	Pulmonary alveolar proteinosis
	Lymphocytic infiltrative disorders (lymphocytic interstitial pneumonitis associated with collagen vascular diseases)
	Eosinophilic pneumonias
	Lymphangioleiomyomatosis
	Amyloidosis
	Inherited diseases
	Tuberous sclerosis, neurofibromatosis, Niemann-Pick disease, Gaucher's disease, Hermansky-Pudlak syndrome
	Gastrointestinal or liver diseases (Crohn's disease, primary biliary cirrhosis, chronic active hepatitis, ulcerative colitis)
	Graft vs. host disease (bone marrow transplantation)
LUNG RESPONSE: AS ABOVE BUT WITH GRANULOMA	
Hypersensitivity pneumonitis (organic dusts)	Sarcoidosis
Inorganic dusts: beryllium silica	Langerhans cell granulomatosis (eosinophilic granuloma)
	Granulomatous vasculitides
	Wegener's granulomatosis, allergic granulomatosis of Churg-Strauss, lymphomatoid granulomatosis
	Bronchocentric granulomatosis

this category are idiopathic pulmonary fibrosis (IPF), sarcoidosis, and the ILD often associated with collagen vascular disorders. ILD secondary to inorganic dust exposure usually can be recognized if the occupational history is pursued. For the myriad (see Table 224-1) of other diffuse ILDs, however, a precise diagnosis is obtained with difficulty, usually only after interpretation of an open-lung biopsy specimen; most of these diseases are relatively rare.

Although the initiating agent(s) or circumstances of the various ILDs may be diverse, and many are unknown, the immunopathogenic responses of lung tissue are limited, so the initial mechanisms of injury, the development of alveolitis, and the attempts at repair sometimes leading to fibrosis will have common features. Idiopathic pulmonary fibrosis is discussed as the prototype ILD, since it is encountered relatively frequently and much of the recent research on mechanisms of lung fibrosis has focused on this disease.

IDIOPATHIC PULMONARY FIBROSIS (IPF)

Many patients who present with nonproductive cough, progressive dyspnea, a chest radiograph showing lower lung zone reticulonodular shadows, and pulmonary function tests showing a restrictive pattern (Chap. 214) will be said to have IPF after the diagnostic evaluation is completed. This condition is also known as *cryptogenic fibrosing alveolitis*. Although the terms *idiopathic* and *cryptogenic* mean that the etiologic agent is unknown, this is not a nebulous "wastebasket" diagnosis or just a diagnosis of exclusion but rather a well-defined clinical entity.

IMMUNOPATHOGENESIS   Several parts of the alveolar structure are affected in IPF, including the alveolar walls lined with type I and type II pneumocytes and the interstitial supporting structure composed of mesenchymal cells, especially fibroblasts and myofibroblasts, collagen, and various adhesive proteoglycans. The capillary endothelium also may be involved. The disease process does not affect the upper or conducting airways, but bronchiolitis of respiratory bronchioles may be present and alveolar units are always involved.

Normally, overlying or interspersed in the alveoli are a variety of immune cells, including alveolar macrophages, dendritic macrophages, interstitial monocytes, lymphocytes, and inflammatory cells, such as polymorphonuclear leukocytes (PMNs) and eosinophils. The cellular content of normal bronchoalveolar lavage (BAL) fluid consists of approximately 80 percent alveolar macrophages, 10 percent lymphocytes (of which 70 percent are T lymphocytes), 1 to 5 percent B lymphocytes or plasma cells, 1 to 3 percent polymorphonuclear leukocytes, and 1 percent eosinophils. In the lymphocyte population, the ratio of CD4 T helper and CD8 T suppressor/cytotoxic cells is about 1.5.

In the earliest, reversible forms of alveolar injury, "leakiness" of the alveolar type I cells and the adjacent capillary endothelial cells occurs, causing alveolar and interstitial edema and the formation of intraalveolar hyaline membranes. With persistence of the disease, increased alveolar-capillary permeability and desquamation of intraalveolar cells (alveolitis), mural inflammation, and interstitial fibrosis are present on biopsy. This process is also reflected in the composition of cells and enzymes recovered in BAL fluid (Table 224-2) and in cellular components present in lung biopsy tissue. The presence and severity of the disease process are spotty in distribution; a continuum of inflammatory and fibrotic changes can be found throughout the affected lung. Fibrosis follows from an organization of inflammatory exudate within the airspaces in which fibroblasts beneath the type I epithelium proliferate and increase their production of fibronectin and collagen.

Depicted in Fig. 224-1 are immunopathogenic mechanisms that interconnect the intraalveolar (luminal) and alveolar mural tissue with the interstitial space and capillary vascular areas. Although the inciting agent or stimulus is unknown, it is likely an antigen that can initiate an immunoglobulin response. This is reflected by an increased ratio

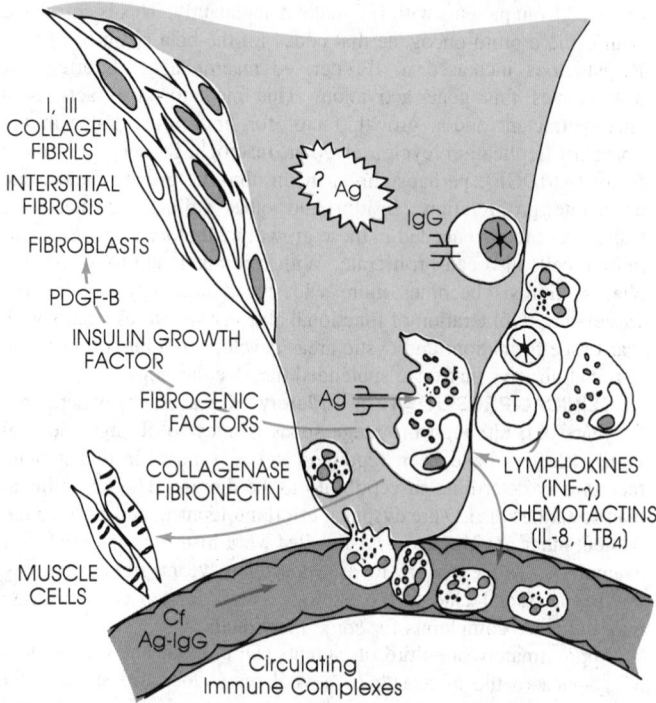

FIGURE 224-1 Immunologic mechanisms within the alveolar space, alveolar walls, and interstitium that can lead to inflammation and eventual fibrosis. The focus is the alveolar macrophage, which is activated, possibly by an immune complex and an as yet unidentified antigen (Ag). Through mediators such as chemotaxins, the macrophage attracts PMNs and other cells from the circulation to the alveolar space, or it can initiate fibrogenesis with various mediators that can stimulate fibroblasts and muscle cells to proliferate. Interstitial fibrosis may result. Abbreviations: IL-8 (interleukin 8), LTB₄ (leukotriene B₄), INF-γ (interferon γ), PDGF-B (platelet-derived growth factor). *(After Reynolds, HY: Idiopathic interstitial pulmonary fibrosis: Contribution of bronchoalveolar lavage analysis. Chest 89:139, 1986.)*

TABLE 224-2 Cellular and immunologic changes in various IPF specimens

BLOOD

IgG (IgG1,3) elevated, immune complexes, cryoglobulins
Serologic titers (low)
T lymphocytes (sensitized to type I collagen)

BRONCHOALVEOLAR FLUID

Alveolitis characterized by increased percentage of PMNs (20%) and eosinophils (2–4%), but lymphocytes may be increased also (20%)
Alveolar macrophages: activated macrophages and their secretory components are numerous:
  Chemotaxins to attract PMNs and muscle cells (IL-8, with mRNA for IL-8 expressed in macrophages, and leukotriene B₄)
  Plasminogen activator
  Macrophage-derived growth factor (or insulin-like growth factor)
  Fibronectin
  Platelet-derived growth factor B (expressed by c-*sis* oncogene)
Steroid receptors increased; mitotic index increased
Collagenase (PMN origin)
Antioxidant glutathione decreased
IgG increased (G3, G1 subclasses)
Immune complexes detectable
IgG-releasing cells present
Histamine elevated
Surfactant protein A reduced

LUNG TISSUE

Interstitial inflammation
Plasma cells, muscle cells, fibroblasts increased
Collagen synthesis increased
Fibrosis but no granuloma
Bronchiolitis obliterans can develop

of IgG subclasses IgG1 and G3, an increased number of IgG-releasing cells, and perhaps the formation of immune complexes. Recently, serum antibody against hepatitis C antigen was detected in about 20 percent of patients with IPF; most of these did not have antecedent hepatitis. Speculation continues that a viral etiology is probable for many cases of IPF.

An increased number of macrophages, which are activated phagocytes capable of producing many cytokines that affect other lung cells, is a hallmark of the alveolitis. These macrophage cytokines or mediators can operate in two directions. First, through the production of chemotaxins, which include leukotriene B₄ and interleukin 8, inflammatory cells such as PMNs and eosinophils are attracted into the alveoli. IPF lung macrophages express increased mRNA for IL-8, which correlates with the percent of PMNs in BAL fluid. An increased percentage of PMNs (20 percent or more) and eosinophils (1 to 4 percent) in the profile of BAL cells is usual in IPF. Lymphocytes are not usually increased, unless the IPF is part of a collagen vascular disease. Enzymes or oxidant radicals from inflammatory cells and histamine may cause local injury or alter the permeability of type I cells. Conversely, the antioxidant glutathione is deficient in the BAL fluid, further impairing neutralization of oxidants. Second, macrophages are also capable of secreting substances that stimulate mesenchymal cells. For fibroblasts to replicate in the interstitium and in the alveolar walls, they must be primed to enter the G₁ phase of a growth cycle to proliferate.

Several products from alveolar macrophages can participate in these steps. Platelet-derived growth factor B (PDGF-B) is a chemoattractant for mesenchymal cells and a stimulus for fibroblasts to change from resting cells to cells entering G₁. Although PDGF-B is not produced by normal monocytes or macrophages, alveolar macrophages obtained from patients with IPF make it abundantly. This is correlated with c-*sis*, a proto-oncogene that codes for the beta chain of PDGF-B, which is increased in IPF-derived macrophages. Interferon γ up-regulates this gene activation. This mediator also acts as a chemoattractant and a growth factor for fibroblasts. Later in the fibroblast replication cycle, alveolar macrophage–derived growth factor (AMDGF), perhaps similar to insulin-like growth factor, can accelerate proliferation. Insulin and other cellular or metabolic substances are also needed in these growth-regulatory steps. Smooth-muscle cells also can proliferate. With continued activity of macrophages, fibrosis becomes more widespread and may involve the vasculature. Obliteration of functional alveolar structures occurs with scar tissue formation, and cystic areas develop from retraction of the terminal airways that once subtended the alveolar unit.

CLINICAL PRESENTATION   History   On average, patients are 50 years old, although the range spans infancy to old age. Several family clusters have been reported, and it is possible that genetic factors may determine susceptibility to the disease. The first clinical manifestations of ILD are dyspnea, effort intolerance, and a dry cough without other obvious cause. A detailed work history is essential. For example, casual exposure to asbestos many years previously may provide a crucial clue to the etiology. Work-related compensation may influence complaints for some individuals.

Approximately one-third of patients can pinpoint their awareness of dyspnea to the aftermath of a viral respiratory illness. Usually months or years elapse between the onset of exertional dyspnea and its progression perhaps to the point of breathlessness at rest. Dyspnea and frequent coughing are often accompanied by other constitutional symptoms such as fatigue, anorexia, weight loss, and arthralgias.

Physical findings   Initially, the physical examination may not be revealing, and auscultation of the chest may be normal. As the disease advances, dry crackles, or coarse crackles on inspiration, are usually heard at the lung bases. There may be tachypnea at rest, cyanosis, and clubbing of the fingers and toes, usually without hypertrophic osteoarthropathy. In later stages, cor pulmonale (Chap. 204) is evident, with findings of pulmonary hypertension, such as an accentuated pulmonic second sound or a right-sided lift, and eventually signs of right-sided heart failure. The right ventricular ejection fraction determined by radionuclide ventriculography is often depressed in the face of normal left ventricular performance.

LABORATORY AND DIAGNOSTIC TESTS   Imaging studies The chest radiograph usually reveals a pattern of diffuse reticulonodular markings, prominent in the lower lung zones. Several radiographic patterns can be seen which correlate roughly with the duration of the disease. Early, a hazy "ground glass" appearance of the lower lung fields coincides with the stage of acute alveolitis. Later, curvilinear shadows predominate and may coalesce into nodular infiltrates. With end-stage disease, the linear opacities are seen in all lung fields, the lung fields appear contracted, and ring-shaped opacities resulting from cystic and bronchiectatic changes are obvious, creating the *honeycombed* or *swiss cheese* appearance of the lung. Biopsy-proven forms of diffuse IPF occur occasionally (about 14 percent) in patients with normal chest radiographs despite significant exercise intolerance, abnormal pulmonary function tests (including a reduced diffusing capacity), and dry crackles.

High-resolution computed tomographic (CT) scanning is a sensitive means of documenting tissue infiltration and the presence of bronchiectasis or pleural changes. It can distinguish between early cellular changes and more advanced fibrosis, emphasizing the inhomogeneous distribution of disease in IPF.

Laboratory examination   The erythrocyte sedimentation rate is usually elevated, circulating immune-complex titers and serum immunoglobulin levels may be increased, and cryoimmunoglobulins may be present. Serologic tests to screen for collagen vascular diseases are necessary to exclude these diagnoses. Although serum rheumatoid factor, antinuclear antibodies, depressed levels of complement, and other parameters of autoimmune diseases may be detected in approximately 10 percent of patients with IPF, the titers are generally quite low.

Lung function tests   In patients with advanced disease, reductions in total lung capacity, vital capacity, and residual volume are found (Chap. 214). Usually, evidence of airway obstruction is minimal and the FEV_1/FVC ratio is normal or increased. A restrictive respiratory functional pattern is usually present, reflecting the stiff, noncompliant lungs characteristic of IPF and its common aftermath, fibrosis. There is usually resting arterial hypoxemia, but the carbon dioxide tension is normal or decreased. Blood pH is normal. The alveolar-arterial oxygen gradient during exercise is elevated, and exercise tolerance is reduced. The carbon monoxide diffusing capacity is usually reduced by 30 to 50 percent. Changes in these variables are useful in monitoring the course of the illness and in assessing the effectiveness of treatment. However, current or former cigarette smoking in IPF patients can alter lung function to misrepresent the extent of restriction and/or obstruction if both emphysema and interstitial fibrosis are present; this has implications and raises caution for evaluating lung function in these patients. Diffusing capacity (DL_{CO}) becomes a more important test in this assessment.

Bronchoscopy   Direct investigation of the airways by fiberoptic bronchoscopy is part of the evaluation, and four to six transbronchial biopsies are taken to obtain lung tissue for diagnosis. These provide a sufficient quantity of tissue for a definitive pathologic diagnosis in approximately one-fourth of all cases of IPF. In some diffuse granulomatous interstitial diseases, such as sarcoidosis (Chap. 292), transbronchial biopsy will provide a tissue diagnosis in about 80 percent of cases. Bronchoscopy also permits bronchoalveolar lavage, which provides useful information about cells and proteins in the airways that generally correlates with histologic changes in the interstitial and alveolar tissues. An analysis of BAL fluid and cells can reveal a number of changes in IPF (see Table 224-2).

Lung biopsy   The importance of an adequate sample of lung tissue to permit a full histologic evaluation, good microbial cultures, immunofluorescence and electron-microscopic studies, and analysis of inorganic substances cannot be overemphasized. Therefore, if a transbronchial biopsy does not yield sufficient tissue for a confident diagnosis, open-lung biopsy should be considered. It is prudent to substantiate a tissue diagnosis before embarking on immunosuppressive therapy with its attendant complications.

DIAGNOSTIC APPROACH AND STAGING OF DISEASE ACTIVITY   Following the clinical examination, chest radiograph (or high-resolution chest CT scan), pulmonary function tests [lung volumes, FEV_1/FVC, and diffusing capacity (Chap. 214)], and arterial blood gas determination measuring desaturation under exercising conditions, the functional disability from the lung disease can be estimated. However, a histologic analysis of lung tissue should be made before the disease is diagnosed definitively. Fiberoptic bronchoscopy is usually the first invasive procedure and is important for ruling out infection, malignancy, and other specific diseases. Although transbronchial biopsy has a lower diagnostic yield in IPF than in sarcoidosis and other granulomatous diseases, it is nevertheless a useful, low-risk procedure with a 20 to 30 percent success rate for obtaining an adequate sample for a confident pathologic diagnosis. BAL for cellular and protein analysis may be useful in judging the nature of alveolar inflammation and immunologic activity (see Table 224-2). However, the value of the periodic use of BAL analysis to monitor disease activity or its response to therapy has not been established. Use of gallium 67 lung scanning does not add more diagnostic accuracy or help with monitoring activity.

If the diagnosis is still in doubt after the bronchoscopy and related procedures, an open-lung biopsy should be considered. The referring physician and the thoracic surgeon should cooperate in choosing the most representative area of the lung for biopsy, and the proper microbial cultures and immunologic studies should be obtained.

THERAPY   Treatment is usually offered to patients with IPF, even to patients with advanced fibrotic disease. About 2 weeks after the open-lung biopsy, a trial of oral prednisone can be instituted in a dose of 1 mg/kg daily and continued for 8 to 12 weeks. If lung disease shows objective improvement, the dose is tapered to a maintenance level. Should the disease not respond or be progressive, the dosage of prednisone can be increased, but immunosuppression with cyclophosphamide should be considered. Cyclophosphamide is given at a dose of about 1.0 mg/kg daily (50 to 75 mg) with the patient continuing on a daily maintenance dose of oral prednisone (0.25 mg/kg). The dosages of cyclophosphamide may be increased as necessary by 50-mg increments at 7- to 10-day intervals. The objective is to reduce the white blood cell count to approximately half the normal baseline value, causing a distinct drop in the total blood lymphocyte count. However, a minimum count of 1000 polymorphonuclear leukocytes per microliter should be maintained.

Use of high-dose, pulsed glucocorticoids does not offer special advantages over daily dosing. Azathioprine has been used in place of cyclophosphamide. Other agents such as colchicine, penicillamine, and cyclosporine have not been evaluated thoroughly.

Several other measures may help respiratory function. It is imperative that patients discontinue cigarette smoking. Since there is frequently a marked drop in Pa_{O_2} with exercise, supplemental oxygen therapy may be useful, sometimes using transtracheal catheter oxygen delivery, which can reduce oxygen requirements and help with the logistics of supplying high-flow therapy. As the pulmonary vascular bed is destroyed by progressive fibrosis, pulmonary hypertension and cor pulmonale can develop; right-sided congestive heart failure can be difficult to control. Judicious use of diuretics is advised. Adequate oxygenation is probably the best treatment for right-sided heart failure (Chap. 204). Some patients also may develop obstruction to airflow and wheezing and coughing which may respond to bronchodilators. Infection may occur during immunosuppressive therapy and should be treated promptly and aggressively. Prophylactic use of pneumococcal and influenza vaccines is indicated. If refractory disease limited to the chest is present, the possibility of lung transplantation should be considered. Success with single-lung transplantation for ILD makes this therapy a reality for some patients. Selection criteria, contraindications, and availability of organs must be discussed candidly with patients so as not to create unrealistic expectations.

INDIVIDUAL FORMS OF ILD

ILD ASSOCIATED WITH COLLAGEN VASCULAR DISORDERS
In these diseases, various pulmonary structures can be affected, especially the pleura, so that ILD is but one manifestation of intrathoracic involvement and often a minor part of the multiorgan process. Analysis of BAL fluid and cells from patients with ILD associated with rheumatoid arthritis and systemic sclerosis is similar to that found in IPF (see Table 224-2) and suggests similar pathogenetic mechanisms for fibrosis. A lymphocytic alveolitis may accompany some cases of ILD in rheumatoid disease and may predict a better response to immunosuppressive therapy.

Systemic lupus erythematosus (SLE) (See Chap. 284) About half of patients with SLE ultimately develop overt lung disease. Pleuritis, pleural effusion(s), and acute pneumonitis are the most frequent forms of lung disease, while a chronic, progressive ILD is uncommon. It is important to exclude pulmonary infection. Although pleuropulmonary involvement may not be evident clinically, pulmonary function testing, particularly the diffusing capacity for carbon monoxide, reveals abnormalities in many patients.

Rheumatoid arthritis (See Chap. 285) A variety of pulmonary manifestations can occur, including pleural disease (pleural effusion and subpleural nodules), parenchymal nodular infiltrates associated with pneumoconiosis in miners (Caplan's syndrome), and diffuse interstitial fibrosis. The ILD can develop before joint disease becomes evident, particularly in men, and is accompanied by high titers of rheumatoid factor. Rarely, upper airway obstruction can occur from arthritis of the cricoarytenoid joint. Patients with rheumatoid arthritis who are receiving treatment with methotrexate or gold may develop

ILD that represents a drug hypersensitivity, which must be differentiated from a preexisting or developing ILD associated with the underlying disease. Penicillamine therapy in patients with rheumatoid arthritis has been implicated as a cause of bronchiolitis obliterans.

Ankylosing spondylitis (See Chap. 289) Bilateral upper lobe fibrosis, which can be complicated by fibrocavitary disease, may develop late in the course.

Systemic sclerosis (See Chap. 286) Radiographic evidence of lung involvement develops in a majority of patients, but its severity or progression is variable. Because distal esophageal motor dysfunction is present in many patients, reflux with regurgitation and chronic aspiration is common. In addition, cutaneous scleroderma can involve the anterior chest wall and abdomen, causing restrictive lung function.

Sjögren's syndrome (See Chap. 288) General dryness and lack of airways secretions cause the major problems of hoarseness, cough, and bronchitis. Presence of an ILD in these patients may signify a lymphocytic infiltrate in lung tissue which can behave as a low-grade lymphoma.

Polymyositis and dermatomyositis (See Chap. 384) Although ILD is reported to occur in only 5 to 10 percent of patients, its presence is more common in the subgroup of patients with an anti-Jo-1 antibody that is directed to tRNA synthetase. Weakness of respiratory muscles contributing to aspiration pneumonitis is a common occurrence.

SYNDROMES OF ILD WITH PULMONARY HEMORRHAGE Recurrent hemoptysis, dyspnea, and hypoxemia in the presence of a chest radiographic pattern of diffuse alveolar opacities should raise the possibility of alveolar hemorrhage. An association between vasculitis involving the kidney (lung-renal syndromes) or other organ systems should be investigated. Alveolar hemorrhage occurs rarely in all collagen vascular disorders, but it is described most often with systemic lupus erythematosus. It can occur with systemic vasculitis and is described as an initial presentation of Wegener's granulomatosis; with Behçet's disease, in which aneurysm formation and rupture of small muscular arteries are manifestations of necrotizing vasculitis; in allergic Churg-Strauss granulomatosis; in Henoch-Schönlein purpura syndrome; and in essential (mixed) cryoimmunoglobulinemia. Exposure to the toxic aerosol trimellitic anhydride may cause alveolar hemorrhage. Serologic tests for antinuclear antibody, anti-glomerular basement membrane antibody, and complement to document a vasculitis and immunologic disorder are the first steps, but renal biopsy and possibly lung biopsy may be required for a definitive diagnosis. Some specific syndromes in this category will be discussed next.

Goodpasture's syndrome (See Chap. 241) Pulmonary hemorrhage and glomerulonephritis are the features of this disease in which most patients have antibodies to renal glomerular and lung alveolar basement membranes.

Idiopathic pulmonary hemosiderosis Diffuse alveolar hemorrhage can occur in the absence of other organ involvement or an obvious immunologic cause and is therefore a diagnosis of exclusion after considering the many causes of alveolar bleeding associated with collagen vascular and vasculitic diseases. A lung biopsy is usually necessary to document the lack of inflammatory injury in the lung tissues and to exclude other diseases with confidence. The clinical course can be variable, ranging from recurrent and fulminant with development of progressive interstitial fibrosis to minimal disease that may remit without sequelae. Children and young adults are usually affected. Glucocorticoid treatment is useful for control of bleeding acutely but is not a predictable long-term remedy for keeping the disease suppressed and preventing recurrence.

PULMONARY ALVEOLAR PROTEINOSIS Similar clinical symptoms and the general appearance of the chest radiograph, showing diffuse alveolar consolidation and/or nodular shadows typically radiating from the hilar regions, place pulmonary alveolar proteinosis (PAP) in the ILD category. Histologically, the alveoli are filled with granular material that stains with periodic acid Schiff reagent, but they exhibit no inflammation and have relatively normal septal structure. Strictly speaking, then, PAP is an intraalveolar process which resembles, but is not, an ILD. Because the proteinaceous response can be associated with inhaled dust exposure (silica and aluminum), malignancy, and chronic infection, termed *secondary PAP*, these disorders should be differentiated from primary PAP by lung biopsy. The intraalveolar material is a combination of surfactant phospholipid produced by type II pneumocytes and of other proteins and immunoglobulins found in alveolar lining fluid. The cytoplasm of alveolar macrophages appears engorged with inclusions (lamellar bodies). The "stuffed" macrophages with large phagolysosomes have diminished microbial killing capacity in vitro, but lung infections with unusual organisms are not frequent. Whole-lung lavage(s) will provide relief to many patients with dyspnea and progressive deterioration of arterial oxygenation and also may provide long-term benefit.

LYMPHOCYTIC INFILTRATIVE DISORDERS This is a group of disorders that feature lymphocyte and plasma cell infiltration of the lung parenchyma and either are benign or can behave as low-grade lymphomas. Within the spectrum of chronic interstitial pneumonias, a subset has been described with lung histology that shows diffuse interstitial infiltration with lymphocytes and plasma cells. In some of these patients, an autoimmune disease or dysproteinemia exists. However, lymphocytic interstitial pneumonia (LIP) is probably not a distinct entity, belongs within the IPF group, and can be associated with Sjögren's syndrome. LIP has been reported in patients, particularly children, with AIDS.

Included among these disorders is immunoblastic lymphadenopathy, also termed *angioimmunoblastic lymphadenopathy*, which usually is a fulminant lymphoma-like disease that may have an element of ILD in some cases. *Lymphomatoid granulomatosis* can be included, but its granulomatous response also places it with the granulomatous ILDs (see Table 224-1).

EOSINOPHILIC PNEUMONIAS (See Chap. 218) These pneumonias encompass a spectrum of diseases in which lung hypersensitivity plays a role and in which a specific cause may or may not be identified. For example, with extrinsic asthma and exposure to fungal antigens, allergic bronchopulmonary mycosis can develop; filarial and other parasitic infections can cause tropical pulmonary eosinophilia; many common drugs can induce eosinophilic pneumonia. Chronic eosinophilic pneumonia has features that make it difficult to distinguish from IPF and other forms of progressive ILD. The disease, which more commonly affects older females, has several radiologic characteristics that are helpful in diagnosis: (1) a peripheral pattern of dense lung infiltrates that appear to cross anatomic lobar boundaries with sparing of the central lung regions, (2) regression but reappearance of infiltrates in the same lung locations, and (3) extreme sensitivity of the infiltrates (and disease symptoms) to modest doses of oral glucocorticoids. The diagnosis can be established by lung biopsy, which shows an eosinophilic inflammatory process.

LYMPHANGIOLEIOMYOMATOSIS Immature smooth-muscle cells can proliferate in lung tissue around and throughout bronchial, vascular, and lymphatic structures, causing local obstruction or creating constricting lesions that develop into cysts. Lymphatics and lymph nodes in other organs are also usually affected. Because this disorder occurs predominantly in females of reproductive age, an association between estrogens and the disease is probable. Pulmonary symptoms consist of dyspnea, cough, and hemoptysis; a more overt presentation occurs with spontaneous pneumothorax, which can be recurrent, or with chylous effusion. In addition, the chest radiograph shows reticulonodular shadows and small cyst-like areas or honeycombing throughout the lung fields. In contrast to most forms of ILD, lung volumes are normal or increased, as is also the case with Langerhans cell granulomatosis (see below). Therapy for progressive lung disease has not been particularly effective. Pneumothoraces and effusions may require chemical or surgical pleurodesis. Treatment with progesterone combined with ovariectomy has been used. Lung transplantation may be considered for some patients.

AMYLOIDOSIS (See Chap. 281) Deposits of amyloid in the form of plaques or nodules can develop at all sites of the respiratory tract. Tracheal and endobronchial mucosal plaques or incidental parenchymal nodules can be difficult to diagnose clinically, but they usually coexist with extrapulmonary manifestations of primary or, less commonly, secondary amyloidosis. Lung biopsy is necessary for definitive diagnosis. As part of primary systemic amyloidosis or a plasma cell dyscrasia, an ILD may occur from amyloid deposits in alveolar septa and associated blood vessels, producing dyspnea, radiographic findings of diffuse reticulonodular shadows, and restrictive pulmonary function.

INHERITED DISORDERS ASSOCIATED WITH ILD Pulmonary infiltrates and respiratory symptoms typical of mild ILD can develop in related family members and in several inherited diseases. These include the phacomatoses (Chap. 378) tuberous sclerosis and neurofibromatosis and the lysosomal storage diseases (Chap. 349), such as Niemann-Pick disease and Gaucher's disease. The *Hermansky-Pudlak syndrome* is an autosomal recessive disorder in which granulomatous colitis and ILD may occur. It is characterized by oculocutaneous albinism, bleeding diathesis from platelet dysfunction, and the accumulation of a chromolipid, lipofuscin material in cells of the reticuloendothelial system. The pulmonary fibrosis is similar to IPF, but the alveolar macrophages may contain cytoplasmic ceroid-like inclusions.

GASTROINTESTINAL AND LIVER DISEASE Rarely, inflammatory bowel disease and chronic hepatitis may be associated with a mild form of ILD. Crohn's disease, which has a number of similarities with sarcoidosis, also may be accompanied by asymptomatic lymphocytic alveolitis.

GRAFT-VERSUS-HOST DISEASE (GVHD) (See Chap. 313) Some degree of GVHD occurs in all patients receiving bone marrow transplantation. However, in about 10 percent a chronic phase may ensue with the onset of dry cough, mucositis, dyspnea, and airflow obstruction in the small airways, as demonstrated by pulmonary function testing. Chest radiographs reveal peribronchiolar infiltrates, and lung biopsy shows focal areas of interstitial infiltration with a mixture of lymphocytes and PMNs. The lesions are consistent with bronchiolitis; no vasculitis is present. Some recipients of heart-lung transplants also develop bronchiolitis. Bronchiolitis in chronic GVHD may stabilize and disappear or may be progressive and fatal. Treatment includes increasing the doses of the immunosuppressive drugs together with bronchodilators and antibiotics. Infection, especially with viral agents, is a common complication.

ILD WITH A GRANULOMATOUS RESPONSE IN LUNG TISSUE OR VASCULAR STRUCTURES Inhalation of organic dusts, which causes hypersensitivity pneumonitis, or of inorganic particles such as silica, which causes alveolitis and elicits a granulomatous inflammatory reaction leading to ILD, produces diseases of known etiology (see Table 224-1) that are discussed in Chaps. 218 and 219. Sarcoidosis (Chap. 292) is prominent among granulomatous diseases of *unknown cause* in which ILD is an important feature.

Langerhans cell granulomatosis (eosinophilic granuloma or histiocytosis X) (See Chap. 58) This condition is being recognized with increasing frequency and may account for about 1 to 5 percent of ILD of unknown etiology. Previously, the proliferation of tissue macrophages (histiocytes) was thought to be characteristic of this disease that affects the lung, bones, and viscera. Now it is recognized that the precursor cell is the *dendritic cell*, which has potent stimulatory and accessory cell immune function, is normally found in the interstitium and alveolar septal areas, and is distinctly different from a tissue macrophage. The dendritic cell can evolve into the Langerhans cell, characterized by a specific CD1a surface antigen that reacts with a monoclonal antibody identified as T_6 and by intracytoplasmic organelles seen by electron microscopy that are called X bodies or Birbeck granules. Langerhans cells can be identified in skin and are present in bronchiolar epithelium of normal lung. Cigarette smoking or a similar irritant seems to be a stimulus for their proliferation. An increased number of these cells can be recovered in BAL from normal smokers, patients with bronchoalveolar carcinoma, and patients with IPF. However, in Langerhans cell granulomatosis of the lung, 3 percent or more of the BAL cells may be so identified, which greatly exceeds the percentage found in these other disorders. However, the Langerhans cells are not pathognomonic for this disease. The number of alveolar macrophages is also increased. Early in the disease a focus of Langerhans and surrounding inflammatory cells can be found adjacent to respiratory and terminal bronchioles, causing bronchiolitis. Later, alveolar structures are involved in progressive interstitial inflammation and fibrosis. In advanced disease, lung histology does *not* reveal the discrete typical granulomas that are found in sarcoidosis and hypersensitivity pneumonitis, nor are eosinophils greatly increased—two reasons that the prior appellation ''eosinophilic granuloma'' was really a misnomer.

The pulmonary form of this disease occurs in young and middle-aged adults, usually males, and in those who use tobacco heavily; it may remain focal or involve one or several bony sites (long bones, spine, skull, or jaw). Occasionally, multifocal disease can affect the posterior pituitary gland, causing diabetes insipidus, a condition that is termed *Hand-Schüller-Christian disease*. In infants, *Letterer-Siwe disease* is a more fulminant visceral form of this disorder that mimics a malignant lymphoma. In adults, the presenting symptoms and signs do not distinguish this disease from other forms of ILD unless signs of a bone lesion exist. A spontaneous pneumothorax may herald the disease. Chest radiographs will show diffuse micronodular shadows and cystic spaces, sparing the costophrenic angles and preserving lung volume, as occurs in lymphangioleiomyomatosis. Pulmonary function tests may disclose a combination of obstructive and restrictive defects. As the disease progresses, greater airway obstruction may develop, and the chest radiograph can resemble that in advanced chronic obstructive lung disease. Treatment involves a mandatory cessation of tobacco use, which may cause the pulmonary disease to stabilize or regress. Glucocorticoids usually are not helpful. Penicillamine has been used in an attempt to prevent fibrosis with variable success. Local bone lesions may require irradiation treatment. For patients with increasing symptoms of airway obstruction, supportive therapy and bronchodilators may be tried, but their success has been modest.

Granulomatous vasculitis (See Chap. 291) Certain forms of vasculitis, accompanied by a granulomatous response, can involve the respiratory tract as part of a multiorgan process or can occasionally be localized to the respiratory tract, as occurs with a predominantly pulmonary form of Wegener's granulomatosis in which glomerulonephritis may not be prominent. It is very important to differentiate these conditions from lymphomatoid granulomatosis. Allergic angiitis and the granulomatosis of Churg and Strauss are forms of granulomatous vasculitis affecting many organs but especially the lungs; a history of asthma and the presence of eosinophilia are distinguishing features.

Lymphomatoid granulomatosis (See Chaps. 58 and 291) This involves primarily the lungs and less frequently the skin, central and peripheral nervous systems, and kidneys with an infiltration of lymphocytoid, plasma-like cells and macrophages creating a necrotic granulomatous inflammatory reaction, especially in or near blood vessels. The disease can progress as a lymphoproliferative disorder and evolve into malignant lymphoma in as many as 50 percent of patients. Treatment of lymphomatoid granulomatosis with glucocorticoids and cyclophosphamide may induce a remission, and if this occurs, subsequent relapse and development of lymphoma are not likely.

BRONCHOCENTRIC GRANULOMATOSIS In contrast to the necrotizing granulomatous reaction in lung vessels, i.e., angiocentric vasculitis, granulomatous destruction of bronchioles occurs in this condition. There is usually associated parenchymal inflammation causing ILD. Eosinophils can be present if asthma and hypersensitivity to fungal antigens within the bronchi have occurred. In other cases without these associated conditions, hypersensitivity to other microbial antigens is postulated. Bronchocentric granulomatosis must be differentiated from hypersensitivity pneumonitis caused by inhalation of organic dusts (see Chaps. 218 and 219).

REFERENCES

Idiopathic pulmonary fibrosis

DU BOIS RM: Idiopathic pulmonary fibrosis. Annu Rev Med 44:441, 1993
CHERNIACK RM et al: Current concepts in idiopathic pulmonary fibrosis: A road map for the future. Am Rev Respir Dis 143:680, 1991
EPLER GR et al: Bronchiolitis obliterans with organizing pneumonia. N Engl J Med 312:152, 1985
LYNCH JP: Neutrophilic alveolitis in idiopathic pulmonary fibrosis. Am Rev Respir Dis 145:1433, 1992
PIQUET PF: Cytokines involved in pulmonary fibrosis. Int Rev Exp Pathol 34:173, 1993

Other interstitial lung diseases

ADAMSON D et al: Successful treatment of pulmonary lymphangiomyomatosis with oophorectomy and progesterone. Am Rev Respir Dis 132:916, 1985
CHAN CK et al: Small-airways disease in recipients of allogenic bone marrow transplants. Medicine 66:327, 1987
FAUCI AS et al: Lymphomatoid granulomatosis—prospective clinical and therapeutic experience over 10 years. N Engl J Med 306:68, 1982
HANCE AJ et al: Pulmonary and extrapulmonary manifestations of Langerhans cell granulomatosis (histiocytosis X). Semin Respir Med 9:349, 1988
HELMERS R et al: Pulmonary manifestations associated with rheumatoid arthritis. Chest 100:235, 1991
KARIMAN K et al: Pulmonary alveolar proteinosis: Prospective clinical experience in 23 patients for 15 years. Lung 162:223, 1984
MILLER KS et al: Lung disease associated with progressive systemic sclerosis. Am Rev Respir Dis 141:301, 1990
REYNOLDS HY: Bronchoalveolar lavage. Am Rev Respir Dis 135:250, 1987
———: Immunologic system in the respiratory tract. Physiol Rev 71:1117, 1991
SIBILLE Y et al: Macrophages and polymorphonuclear neutrophils in lung defence and injury. Am Rev Respir Dis 141:471, 1990
SPECKS U et al: Granulomatous vasculitis. Rheum Dis Clin North Am 16:377, 1990
TAZELAAR HD et al: Interstitial lung disease in polymyositis and dermatomyositis. Am Rev Respir Dis 141:727, 1990
TRULOCK EP et al: The Washington University–Barnes Hospital experience with lung transplantation. JAMA 266:1943, 1991

225 PRIMARY PULMONARY HYPERTENSION

STUART RICH

Primary pulmonary hypertension is an uncommon disease characterized by increased pulmonary artery pressure and pulmonary vascular resistance without an obvious cause. The diagnosis can be made only after all causes of pulmonary hypertension have been excluded. There is a female-to-male preponderance (1.7:1), with patients most commonly presenting in the third and fourth decades, although the age range is from infancy to greater than 60 years. Because the predominant symptom of primary pulmonary hypertension is dyspnea, which can have an insidious onset in an otherwise healthy person, the disease is typically diagnosed late in its course. By that time, the clinical and laboratory findings of severe pulmonary hypertension are usually present.

PATHOLOGY The histopathology of primary pulmonary hypertension is not pathognomonic for the disease but is observed in pulmonary hypertension from a variety of causes. The majority of patients have a primary pulmonary arteriopathy which incorporates the features of plexogenic and thrombotic arteriopathies.

Medial hypertrophy associated with concentric laminar intimal fibrosis and plexiform lesions (plexogenic arteriopathy) is characteristically found in younger women, whereas eccentric intimal fibrosis with medial hypertrophy, fibroelastic intimal pads in the arteries and arterioles, and scattered evidence of old recanalized thrombi appearing as fibrous webs (thrombotic arteriopathy) appear to affect men and women equally. In most patients, some features of both patterns of vascular changes can be found. The common pathogenetic denominator appears to be an undefined injury to the pulmonary vascular endothelium, which results in (1) an impaired ability to maintain a relaxed state of vasomotor tone and (2) a conversion to a procoagulant state within the pulmonary arteriolar bed that disposes to the development of in situ thrombosis. The types of vascular changes noted are likely determined by the nature of the injury to the pulmonary vascular endothelium and/or its duration, the patient's gender, and underlying genetic predisposition. The recent findings of primary pulmonary hypertension in patients infected with the human immunodeficiency virus (HIV), as well as the high frequency of antinuclear antibodies, implicates an abnormality of the immune system in the development of pulmonary hypertension in some patients. The association of primary pulmonary hypertension with cirrhosis and portal hypertension, while statistically significant, remains unexplained.

Pulmonary venoocclusive disease This is a distinct pathologic entity, found in less than 10 percent of patients with primary pulmonary hypertension. Histologically, it is manifest by widespread intimal proliferation and fibrosis of the intrapulmonary veins and venules, occasionally extending to the arteriolar bed. The pulmonary venous obstruction explains the increased pulmonary capillary wedge pressure observed in patients with advanced disease. These patients may develop orthopnea that can mimic left ventricular failure.

Pulmonary capillary hemangiomatosis This is a rare form of primary pulmonary hypertension. Histologically, it is characterized by infiltrating thin-walled blood vessels that are widespread throughout the pulmonary interstitium and walls of the pulmonary arteries and veins. These patients often have hemoptysis as a clinical feature.

CLINICOPATHOLOGIC CONSIDERATIONS It is difficult to distinguish the pathologic subsets of primary pulmonary hypertension on clinical grounds, since the symptoms are similar and the severity of pulmonary hypertension is comparable in all types. The perfusion lung scan is often abnormal, with a diffuse patchy pattern that seems to reflect widespread arteriolar thrombosis. Patients with pulmonary venoocclusive disease, along with abnormal perfusion scans, may have increased bronchovascular markings at the lung bases on chest radiograph. Patients with pulmonary capillary hemangiomatosis may have fluffy-appearing infiltrates in the lung fields, abnormal perfusion scans, and a uniquely abnormal appearance of the pulmonary angiogram revealing areas of increased vascularity at the lung periphery.

ETIOLOGY By definition, the underlying cause of primary pulmonary hypertension is unknown. Insight into possible mechanisms was provided from the experience in Europe in the late 1960s in which the number of patients with unexplained pulmonary hypertension increased with the introduction of aminorex fumarate, an amphetamine-like drug used for appetite suppression. Use by susceptible individuals caused development of chronic pulmonary hypertension, the mechanism possibly pulmonary vasoconstriction from endothelial injury. Histologically, features of plexogenic and thrombotic pulmonary arteriopathy have been described. The median survival of patients with pulmonary hypertension from aminorex was almost three times longer than that of patients with primary pulmonary hypertension. While some patients improved when the aminorex was discontinued, others had a progressive downhill course, even though the causative agent had been withdrawn.

Pregnancy and oral contraceptives had been proposed as etiologic factors, but this has not been substantiated by other studies. Their frequent association is more likely related to the prevalence of primary pulmonary hypertension in young women.

PATHOPHYSIOLOGY The underlying hemodynamic derangement in primary pulmonary hypertension is an increased resistance to pulmonary blood flow. Early in the disease there is a marked elevation in pulmonary artery pressure with relatively normal cardiac function. Over time the cardiac output becomes progressively reduced rather than the pulmonary artery pressure becoming progressively increased. Initially, the pulmonary arteries may respond to vasodilators, but as the disease progresses, the elevated pulmonary vascular resistance becomes fixed. The pulmonary capillary wedge pressure remains normal until the late stages, when it tends to rise in response to impaired diastolic filling of the left ventricle due to the altered configuration of the intraventricular septum. Eventually, as the right

ventricle fails, the right atrial and right ventricular end-diastolic pressures rise in an attempt to compensate for the myocardial depression that has developed in response to chronic severe right ventricular pressure overload.

Pulmonary function is usually normal in primary pulmonary hypertension, although a mild restrictive pattern (see Chap. 214) is sometimes seen. Hypoxemia is common and is believed to be due to a mismatch between pulmonary ventilation and perfusion, magnified by a low cardiac output. Occasional patients with a patent foramen ovale may develop right-to-left shunting, which also can contribute to systemic arterial desaturation.

DIAGNOSIS A thorough diagnostic evaluation to look for all potential causes should be undertaken (see Fig. 225-1 and Table 225-1). The history usually reveals the gradual onset of shortness of breath with effort, progressing until the patient is dyspneic with minimal activity. The average duration from symptom onset until diagnosis is 2.5 years. Other common symptoms are fatigue, angina pectoris which likely represents right ventricular ischemia, syncope, near syncope, and peripheral edema. Approximately 7 percent of the cases are familial with the features of an autosomal dominant defect with variable expression.

The physical examination is characteristic. Increased jugular venous pressure, a reduced carotid pulse, and an easily palpable right ventricular lift are typical. Most patients have an increased pulmonic component of the second heart sound and right-sided third and fourth heart sounds. Tricuspid and pulmonic regurgitation and peripheral cyanosis and edema may be noted. Clubbing is not a feature.

The chest x-ray generally shows enlarged central pulmonary arteries and clear lung fields. The electrocardiogram usually reveals right axis deviation and right ventricular hypertrophy. The echocardiogram demonstrates right ventricular enlargement, a reduction in left ventricular cavity size, and abnormal septal configuration consistent

FIGURE 225-1 An algorithm for the workup of a patient with unexplained pulmonary hypertension. (*Adapted with permission from S Rich.*)

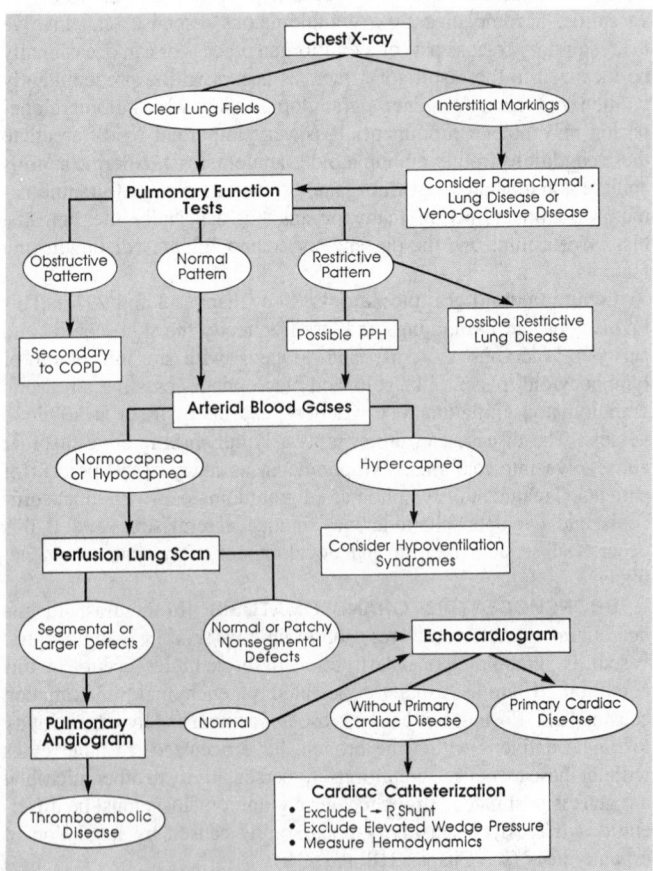

Persistent fetal circulation
Congenital heart disease
Valvular heart disease
Primary myocardial disease
Pulmonary thromboembolic disease
Obstructive lung disease
Interstitial lung disease
Arterial hypoxemia with hypercapnea
Collagen vascular disease
Parasitic disease involving the lung
Sickle cell anemia
Intravenous drug abuse
Granulomatous lung disease
Chronic liver disease
Pulmonary artery stenosis
Pulmonary venous hypertension
Aminorex fumarate ingestion

SOURCE: From S Rich, Prog Cardiovasc Dis 31:205, 1988; used with permission.

with right ventricular pressure overload. Doppler studies have revealed a marked dependence on atrial systole for ventricular filling. This would imply that atrial fibrillation could result in inadequate left ventricular filling and might be one cause for sudden death, since no patient with primary pulmonary hypertension and atrial fibrillation has been described. A mild restrictive pattern on pulmonary function tests is consistent with pulmonary hypertension and does not necessarily indicate restrictive lung disease. Hypoxemia, hypocapnia, and an abnormal diffusing capacity for carbon monoxide are almost invariable findings. Evidence of airways obstruction suggests a secondary etiology for the pulmonary hypertension. A perfusion lung scan may be normal or abnormal with multiple diffuse patchy filling defects of a nonsegmental nature and not suggestive of pulmonary thromboembolism. If the lung scan reveals perfusion defects of a segmental or subsegmental nature, a pulmonary angiogram must be done. Severe pulmonary hypertension in a patient with a high-probability lung scan should suggest a chronic process and not acute pulmonary embolism, since the nonconditioned right ventricle is unable to generate high systolic pressures acutely in the face of pulmonary thromboembolism. Chronic thromboembolic obstruction of the large pulmonary arteries (Chap. 226) can mimic primary pulmonary hypertension but can be amenable to treatment with surgical thromboendarterectomy. Defining the precise location and extent of the clots is imperative for surgical removal.

There is risk in performing pulmonary angiography in patients with primary pulmonary hypertension, particularly in the presence of right ventricular failure with elevated right ventricular end-diastolic pressure. In these patients it is recommended that selective or subselective injections with smaller amounts of contrast material be made to minimize the risks, and the use of low-osmolar, nonionic contrast material also may diminish risk. One mechanism for cardiac arrest in this setting is hypotension and bradycardia that may be vagally mediated; the pretreatment of selected patients with 1 mg atropine is also advocated.

Cardiac catheterization is mandatory to characterize the disease and exclude an underlying cardiac shunt as the cause. The use of balloon-flotation catheters, especially those with removable guidewires, can facilitate right heart catheterization, which can be technically difficult. A right-to-left shunt might be attributable to a patent foramen ovale, but any left-to-right shunting implies the presence of a congenital defect. Although it may be difficult to obtain an accurate pulmonary capillary wedge pressure tracing in some patients, the wedge pressure is not falsely elevated. If recordings suggest that the wedge pressure is increased, left heart catheterization also should be performed to exclude mitral stenosis or increased left ventricular end-diastolic pressures as the cause. Although the diagnostic evaluation of these patients can be hazardous, experience from a national multicenter study revealed no mortality or serious morbidity in more

than 300 patients whose evaluation included pulmonary angiography and cardiac catheterization. It is not necessary to perform an open lung biopsy in these patients to make an accurate diagnosis. If the diagnostic evaluation is undertaken as outlined, a correct diagnosis will almost always be made.

On occasion a patient may have marked elevations in pulmonary artery pressure and a relatively mild disease that is known to cause pulmonary hypertension. It would be a mistake to characterize these patients as having primary pulmonary hypertension on the belief that the pulmonary hypertension is out of proportion to the underlying associated condition. Since the pulmonary vascular bed has variable vasoreactivity, these cases probably reflect an exaggerated pulmonary vasoconstrictive response to the associated condition. Thus severe pulmonary hypertension can coexist with mild chronic obstructive pulmonary disease, small intracardiac shunts, mild mitral stenosis, and even ischemic heart disease. The distinction, however, is important because the treatment of pulmonary hypertension should always be focused toward the underlying cause.

NATURAL HISTORY The natural history of primary pulmonary hypertension is unknown because initially the disease is largely asymptomatic. Several series have reported a mean survival of 2 to 3 years for patients from the time of diagnosis. Few patients survive more than 10 years. Functional class is a strong predictor of survival, since patients who are functional class II and III have a mean survival of 3.5 years compared with those who are functional class IV, in whom the mean survival is 6 months. The cause of death is usually right ventricular failure or sudden death; sudden death appears to be a late feature of the disease. Increased right atrial pressure above 15 mmHg and reduced cardiac index below 2 (L/min)/m^2 are hemodynamic predictors of a poor prognosis.

MANAGEMENT The treatment of primary pulmonary hypertension, while still unsatisfactory, has improved considerably. Because the pulmonary vascular resistance increases dramatically with exercise, patients should be cautioned against participating in activities that demand increased physical stress. The use of digoxin remains controversial, since no studies have documented a benefit or detriment. Diuretic therapy may relieve dyspnea and peripheral edema and may be useful in reducing right ventricular volume overload in the presence of tricuspid regurgitation.

The main focus of therapy is vasodilator drugs. For vasodilators to have sustained beneficial effects, they must lower the pulmonary artery pressure along with the pulmonary vascular resistance while preserving systemic blood pressure. Calcium channel antagonists, when given in high doses (e.g., nifedipine 120 to 240 mg/d or diltiazem 540 to 900 mg/d*) that are titrated to the hemodynamic response, can produce dramatic reductions in pulmonary artery pressure and pulmonary vascular resistance associated with improvement in symptoms, regression of right ventricular hypertrophy, and improved survival. However, less than half the patients with primary pulmonary hypertension respond to this regimen. In addition, it is unknown whether the response depends on the histologic subtype, but the therapy appears to be more successful in patients who are diagnosed early and have less advanced disease. None of the other classes of vasodilator drugs that have been investigated, including beta-adrenergic agonists, alpha-adrenergic blockers, smooth-muscle vasodilators, nitrates, and angiotensin-converting enzyme inhibitors, has shown similar sustained effectiveness.

The administration of vasodilators can have serious acute and chronic adverse effects. The most common response is a reduction in pulmonary vascular resistance, manifest by an increased cardiac output, without a reduction in the mean pulmonary artery pressure. This results in increased stroke work of the right ventricle, which can result in worsening of ventricular function and precipitate right ventricular failure over time. In addition, maintenance of adequate systemic blood pressure is crucial, since right ventricular coronary

---

* These agents have not been approved for the treatment of primary pulmonary hypertension by the U.S. Food and Drug Administration.

blood flow is already compromised due to the loss of the normal gradient for myocardial perfusion between the aorta and right ventricle. Vasodilator drugs can provoke acute right ventricular ischemia, and deaths have been reported. For these reasons, the pharmacologic evaluation of primary pulmonary hypertension should always be undertaken with direct monitoring of systemic and pulmonary arterial pressures and cardiac output.

Prostacyclin† has been employed intravenously as a treatment of patients who fail to respond to calcium channel antagonists. Preliminary studies have shown that patients receiving prostacyclin have an improvement in exercise tolerance and a reduction in mortality. The mechanism by which prostacyclin exhibits its effects are unclear. The side effects of prostacyclin, which include flushing, jaw pain, bloating, and diarrhea, are generally tolerated by most patients. Whether the use of prostacyclin will be limited to patients with advanced disease who are waiting organ transplantation or as a chronic therapy remains to be determined.

Anticoagulant therapy also has been advocated based on the evidence that thrombosis in situ is common. One retrospective study and one prospective study have demonstrated that the anticoagulant warfarin increases the survival of patients with primary pulmonary hypertension, and thus consideration for its use should be given to all patients. The dose of warfarin is generally titrated to achieve an increase in INR of 1.5 to 2.5 of control. Anticoagulants should not be expected to cause regression of the disease and result in any substantial change in symptoms.

Patients who fail to respond to vasodilator drugs should be considered as possible candidates for heart-lung or lung transplantation (Chaps. 196 and 232). Single lung transplantation is the preferred operation, since it has been shown that patients with primary pulmonary hypertension who receive a single lung have a substantial reduction in the pulmonary artery pressure and a marked amelioration of symptoms, even in the face of preexisting right ventricular dysfunction and failure. It is also a simpler operation with a shorter waiting time than heart-lung transplantation. The operation is best reserved for patients who are in the advanced stages of the disease, in whom it may be predicted that survival is likely to be less than 1 year. Recurrence of disease has not been reported in any patient with primary pulmonary hypertension who has undergone single lung or heart-lung transplantation.

REFERENCES

D'ALONZO GE et al: Survival in patients with primary pulmonary hypertension: Results from a national prospective study. Ann Intern Med 115:343, 1991

FUSTER V et al: Primary pulmonary hypertension: Natural history and the importance of thrombosis. Circulation 70:580, 1984

PACKER M: Vasodilator therapy for primary pulmonary hypertension. Ann Intern Med 103:258, 1985

PASQUE MK et al: Single-lung transplantation for pulmonary hypertension: Three-month hemodynamic follow-up. Circulation 84:2275, 1991

PIETRA GG et al: Histopathology of primary pulmonary hypertension: A qualitative and quantitative study of pulmonary blood vessels from 58 patients in the National Heart, Lung and Blood Institute Primary Pulmonary Hypertension Registry. Circulation 80:1198, 1989

RICH S: Primary pulmonary hypertension. Prog Cardiovasc Dis 31:205, 1988

——— et al: High-dose calcium blocking therapy for primary pulmonary hypertension: Evidence for long-term reduction in pulmonary artery pressure and regression of right ventricular hypertrophy. Circulation 76:135, 1987

——— et al: Primary pulmonary hypertension: A national prospective study. Ann Intern Med 107:216, 1987

——— et al: The effect of high doses of calcium-channel blockers on survival in primary pulmonary hypertension. N Engl J Med 327:76, 1992

——— et al: Pulmonary hypertension from chronic pulmonary thromboembolism. Ann Intern Med 108:425, 1988

RUBIN LJ et al: Treatment of primary pulmonary hypertension with continuous intravenous prostacyclin (epoprosternol): Results of a randomized trial. Ann Intern Med 112:485, 1990

† This drug is currently available as an Investigational New Drug only.

226 PULMONARY THROMBOEMBOLISM

KENNETH M. MOSER

Pulmonary thromboembolism (PTE) is a leading cause of morbidity and mortality and can appear in many clinical contexts. Epidemiologic surveys indicate that PTE is responsible for more than 50,000 deaths in the United States annually. However, available data suggest that less than 10 percent of all pulmonary emboli result in death. Thus the incidence of fatal plus nonfatal emboli probably exceeds 500,000 annually. This overall incidence seems verified by autopsy statistics. Evidence of recent or old embolism is detected in 25 to 30 percent of routine autopsies; with special techniques, this figure exceeds 60 percent. Even these data underestimate incidence, since many emboli resolve without trace and are not found at postmortem examination. The high incidence of PTE at autopsy contrasts sharply with the incidence of antemortem diagnosis. Available information suggests that an antemortem diagnosis has been made in only 10 to 30 percent of all cases in which old or recent embolism is demonstrated at autopsy.

The incidence of embolism does not appear to be decreasing, despite advances in diagnosis and prophylaxis. This apparent paradox is likely explained by medical advances, e.g., higher survival in trauma patients, the increase in "open heart," orthopedic (e.g., hip replacement), and other medical and surgical procedures, particularly among patients in older age groups, and more widespread use of indwelling catheters. Thus there is an expanding population at high risk for developing venous thrombosis.

VENOUS THROMBOSIS

PATHOGENESIS Available data indicate that more than 95 percent of pulmonary emboli arise from thrombi in the deep venous system of the lower extremities. Furthermore, it appears that the larger leg veins (popliteal vein and above) are by far the most common source of those pulmonary emboli which reach clinical attention. Thrombi occurring in the right cardiac chambers or in other veins account for the remainder, but are uncommon unless some inciting factor is present, such as indwelling catheters or intracavitary pacing wires. In situ pulmonary arterial thrombosis is rare. Thus embolism should be viewed as a *complication* of deep venous thrombosis (DVT) in the lower extremity veins. Finally, some 90 percent of the deaths due to embolism occur within an hour or two—before a diagnostic-therapeutic plan can be implemented. These facts have several important implications with respect to PTE: (1) prevention of DVT is the most effective approach to prevention of, and death due to, embolism; (2) prompt treatment of DVT may limit the frequency of embolism; and (3) techniques which identify the patient at high risk of DVT and allow prompt diagnosis are the key to reduction of embolic risk.

The three factors which promote DVT (and, therefore, embolic risk), as defined by Virchow in the nineteenth century, are stasis, abnormalities of the vessel wall, and alterations in the blood coagulation system. Coagulation alterations have been studied extensively, but as yet there is no reliable test for a state of "hypercoagulability," i.e., a test which will predict the risk of DVT. However, there is a growing list of conditions in which thrombotic risk is increased: deficiencies of antithrombin III, protein C, protein S, and components of the fibrinolytic system; presence of a lupus anticoagulant; and homocystinuria. However, such discrete abnormalities are uncommon in the population that develops DVT and are usually discovered after the event. Therefore, the risk of DVT is best assessed by recognizing the presence of known "clinical" risk factors. Conditions associated with a high risk of venous thromboembolism include any surgical procedure requiring 30 min or more of general anesthesia, the postpartum period, left and right ventricular failure, fractures or injuries or surgical procedures involving the lower extremities, chronic deep venous insufficiency of the legs, prolonged bed rest, carcinoma, obesity, and the use of estrogens.

NATURAL HISTORY In the contexts noted above, deep venous thrombi usually develop in the region of a venous valve. Platelets aggregate, forming a nidus (white thrombus), followed by development of a large fibrin (red) thrombus. The process is apparently a rapid one; large, extensive thrombi can develop within minutes. Growth occurs by continued fibrin and platelet accretion. Beyond formation, two processes may contribute to resolution: fibrinolysis and organization. Fibrinolysis may result in complete resolution within hours to several days. Any remaining thrombus undergoes organization, leaving behind a fibrotic zone that becomes reendothelialized. Valves are often rendered incompetent by this process, and modest or extensive luminal narrowing may occur. Once thrombus growth has halted, available data indicate that fibrinolysis/organization reaches a stable state in 7 to 10 days. It is during the first few days after formation, therefore, that embolic risk is highest.

DETECTION The clinical diagnosis of DVT is difficult and, indeed, unreliable. DVT is frequently present in the absence of clinical signs (e.g., pain, heat, swelling), and it is absent in 50 percent of patients in whom clinical signs or symptoms suggest its presence. Therefore, a number of diagnostic tests have been developed. The gold standard is *ascending contrast venography*. The application of this test is often limited by technical and logistic considerations, however, and repetitive venography is impractical. Among available noninvasive techniques, two have been well-validated against venography: (1) impedance plethysmography (IPG), which detects venous outflow obstruction, is highly sensitive to acute above-knee thrombosis but fails to detect many below-knee thrombi, and (2) the radiofibrinogen method, which is very sensitive to thrombus formation in calf veins and lower thigh veins but not sensitive to thrombi which form in the upper thigh or above. Unfortunately, radiolabeled fibrinogen is no longer available for clinical use. Doppler ultrasound (''duplex'') studies are widely used. However, the criteria employed to interpret this test have not been standardized, the sensitivity and specificity of the technique have been poorly validated against venography, and the test is quite operator-dependent. Other methodologies employing radionuclides (attached to platelets, monoclonal antibodies directed against fibrin or platelet components) are under investigation.

PROPHYLAXIS Application of IPG and radiofibrinogen leg scanning has provided insights into the relative risks of DVT (and, therefore, PTE) in various patient populations. Such data, in turn, have led to recommendations for an escalating intensity of prophylaxis based on degree of risk. Four safe and effective prophylactic options have been validated: low-dose heparin, warfarin, intermittent venous compression devices, and combinations of either anticoagulant drug with the compression devices. Patients in the low- and or moderate-risk categories should receive either low-dose heparin (5000 units subcutaneously every 12 h) or intermittent venous compression (by devices which compress the calf, or calf and thigh, approximately once per minute). Patients in these categories include those undergoing major surgery (defined as any procedure requiring general anesthesia for 30 min or more), patients immobilized for any reason, patients with myocardial infarction and congestive heart failure, and women delivered by cesarean section. If heparin cannot be used (e.g., neurosurgery, spinal cord injury), compression devices alone can be applied. Patients at high risk include those with pelvic or lower extremity injury or surgery (e.g., hip/knee replacement). In these patients, combinations of compressive devices plus either heparin or warfarin are warranted. A prior history of DVT or PTE places any patient in the high-risk category. With these multiple options available, some prophylaxis is available for almost every patient at risk of DVT. In patients with severe trauma in whom no other option exists, prophylactic placement of an inferior vena caval filter can be considered.

NATURAL HISTORY OF PULMONARY EMBOLISM

THE ACUTE EVENTS The immediate result of thromboembolism is complete or partial obstruction of the pulmonary arterial blood flow to the distal lung. This obstruction leads to a series of pathophysiologic events which can be categorized as the ''respiratory'' and ''hemodynamic'' consequences of PTE.

Respiratory consequences Embolic obstruction produces a zone of the lung which is ventilated but not perfused—an intrapulmonary ''dead space'' (Chap. 214). Because it cannot participate in the process of gas exchange, ventilation of this nonperfused area is ''wasted,'' in the functional sense. A potential consequence of embolic obstruction is constriction of the air spaces and airways in the affected lung zone. This pneumoconstriction, which might be viewed as a homeostatic mechanism to reduce wasted ventilation, appears to be due to the marked bronchoalveolar hypocapnia that results from cessation of pulmonary capillary blood flow, because it is abolished by inhalation of carbon dioxide–enriched air. While it occurs in animal experiments in which a double-lumen tube separates the ventilation from each lung, it probably occurs very rarely in patients who inhale dead space air (rich in carbon dioxide) into embolized lung zones.

Another disturbance caused by embolic obstruction—loss of alveolar surfactant—does not occur immediately. This surface-active lipoprotein is required to maintain alveolar stability. In its absence, alveolar collapse occurs. Cessation of pulmonary capillary blood flow leads to reduction in surfactant within 2 or 3 h, which becomes severe at 12 to 15 h. Frank atelectasis—the morphologic expression of alveolar instability—can be detected 24 to 48 h after interruption of blood flow.

Arterial hypoxemia is a common, though by no means universal, consequence of PTE. Several mechanisms can contribute to hypoxemia: ventilation-perfusion disturbances, cardiac failure with a lowered mixed venous P_{O_2} (widened arteriovenous difference), and obligatory perfusion through hypoventilated lung zones. Such obligatory perfusion develops because elevation of pulmonary arterial pressure due to embolic obstruction can overcome the vasoconstriction normally present in hypoventilated lung zones.

Hemodynamic consequences The primary hemodynamic consequence of thromboembolic obstruction is a reduction in the cross-sectional area of the pulmonary arterial bed. This loss of vascular capacity increases the resistance to pulmonary blood flow, which, if marked, leads to pulmonary hypertension and acute failure of the right ventricle. Tachycardia and often a decline in cardiac output also occur.

The factors that determine the severity of these hemodynamic changes have been the subject of continued debate. There is agreement that the *extent of embolic obstruction* is a key factor. However, the reserve capacity of the pulmonary arteriocapillary bed is so extensive that more than 50 percent of the vascular area must be obstructed before significant elevation in pulmonary arterial pressure results. Because pulmonary hypertension occurs in some patients with occlusion of lesser extent, investigators have searched for reflex or humoral vasoconstrictor mechanisms associated with embolism. Despite a long and careful search for such mechanisms, their extent and frequency in human PTE remains unknown. Hence some workers maintain that the degree of embolic obstruction itself is the only determinant of hemodynamic impairment. They suggest that instances of apparent disparity between the extent of embolism and clinical response reflect only clinical underestimation of the magnitude of the embolism. Other investigators, however, have presented compelling evidence to support the occurrence of pulmonary vasoconstriction with embolism. Some have demonstrated that constriction is associated with obstruction of the smaller, but not the larger, pulmonary arterial vessels. According to another hypothesis, serotonin or thromboxane, known pulmonary vasoconstrictive-bronchoconstrictive substances, are released from platelets and coat fresh emboli as they lodge in the pulmonary tree. This thesis introduces the attractive concept that an embolus might be regarded, in part, as a packet with pharmacologic, as well as obstructive, potential. A consensus view is that while the extent of embolism is a key factor, humoral and/or reflex influences probably operate in certain patients and compromise the pulmonary circulation to a greater extent than might be expected on an anatomic basis alone.

The cardiopulmonary status of the patient prior to embolism is also critical in determining the clinical severity of embolism. A small embolus may have limited impact on an otherwise healthy individual but may have serious consequences in someone with advanced cardiac or pulmonary disease.

Both experimental and clinical studies have established that infarction—death of lung tissue—rarely accompanies embolic occlusion. It is likely that less than 10 percent of emboli in humans lead to infarction. That infarction rarely follows embolism should occasion little surprise. The lung has three avenues for obtaining oxygen: the pulmonary arterial circulation, the bronchial arterial circulation, and the airways. Thus infarction occurs infrequently, and its appearance usually is associated with compromise of bronchial arterial flow and/or airways to the involved area. Such compromise is promoted by the existence of other cardiac or pulmonary diseases, such as left ventricular failure, mitral stenosis, and chronic obstructive lung disease. Thus infarction may occur in 30 percent or more of such patients, while it is quite rare in individuals who are free of cardiopulmonary disease.

BEYOND THE ACUTE STATE The vast majority of pulmonary emboli resolve, and resolve rather quickly. Resolution of fresh emboli begins within the first few days and is well advanced in 10 to 14 days. As in DVT, two mechanisms promote restoration of vascular patency: the fibrinolytic system and the process of organization. However, the fibrinolytic system appears capable of more rapid dissolution of emboli than of venous thrombi.

The availability of these two efficient mechanisms raises the question why all emboli do not resolve. There may be some impairment of the intrinsic fibrinolytic system. The emboli may have been well organized prior to their lodgment in the lung so that they are subject to neither fibrinolytic attack nor further organization. Alternatively, some emboli may be recurrent, so their failure to resolve is more apparent than real.

Another important element of the natural history of thromboembolism is the development of bronchial arterial collateral circulation. If pulmonary arterial obstruction persists, bronchial arterial flow increases substantially over a period of several weeks, restoring flow to the capillary bed. With the return of flow, surfactant production is restored, so that alveolar stability is regained and atelectasis resolves.

DIAGNOSTIC FEATURES

Studies of patients with venous thrombosis of the thigh veins (popliteal and above) have demonstrated that *asymptomatic* embolism, often of substantial magnitude, occurs in some 40 to 60 percent. In those who do develop symptoms, and *sudden onset of unexplained dyspnea is the most common*, often the only, symptom of pulmonary embolism. *Pleuritic chest pain and hemoptysis are present only when infarction has occurred* and, because bland embolism rarely leads to infarction, are usually absent. With extensive embolism, severe substernal oppressive discomfort may be present, probably due to right ventricular ischemia. Patients also may present with syncope, suggesting a neurologic disorder. Other "occult" presentations in which embolism should be considered include repetitive bouts of otherwise unexplained supraventricular tachyarrhythmias, sudden onset or worsening of congestive heart failure (see Chap. 195); sudden deterioration in the patient with chronic obstructive lung disease, and as an alternative to the diagnosis of "psychic" (anxiety-associated) hyperventilation. The most reliable symptom, however, is breathlessness. Severe, persistent dyspnea is an ominous sign, for it usually indicates extensive embolic occlusion.

PHYSICAL EXAMINATION Findings on physical examination, like the history, may be deceptively normal. Examination of the lungs may disclose a few atelectatic rales; localized wheezes rarely are heard. A pleural friction rub or evidence of pleural effusion will not be present unless infarction has occurred.

On cardiac examination, the single consistent finding is tachycardia. Only in the rare cases of massive embolism will signs such as a right ventricular gallop, a palpable "lift" over the right ventricle (along the left sternal border), a loud pulmonary closure sound, or prominent *a* waves in the jugular venous pulse be found. A scratchy systolic ejection-type murmur may be heard in the pulmonic area. Also, a systolic or continuous murmur accentuated by inspiration may be audible over the lung fields. These murmurs appear to be generated by turbulence of flow in vessels partially obstructed by emboli, since they disappear after resection or resolution of emboli. They should be carefully sought in any patient suspected of having PTE. Wide, fixed splitting of the second heart sound may be present. This indicates extensive embolic obstruction and implies both severe pulmonary hypertension and right ventricular failure. As embolic resolution occurs, this finding disappears. Absence of an accentuated pulmonic closure sound is not a reliable guide to the severity of PTE, since when embolism is sufficiently massive to reduce cardiac output, pulmonary arterial pressure falls and the pulmonary closure sound may be normal or diminished.

The detection of *deep venous thrombosis* qualifies as an excellent clue to the diagnosis of embolism, but its absence does not exclude embolism, because the entire venous thrombus may embolize. Even when sought with diligence, *clinical* evidence of thrombophlebitis is found in less than half of patients with PTE. *Fever* in patients with pulmonary embolism is uncommon without complicating infection or infarction. With infarction, fever of 37.5 to 38.5°C (oral) is the rule, but temperature elevations to 39°C or above may occur, making the differentiation between pulmonary infarction and infection difficult.

On clinical grounds alone, then, a firm diagnosis of embolism cannot be made; the clinical *suspicion* of embolism requires confirmation by laboratory studies (Fig. 226-1).

LABORATORY STUDIES Routine laboratory studies contribute little toward the diagnosis. Leukocytosis and elevation of the sedimentation rate are rarely present in the absence of infarction. A variety of other blood tests, such as assay for specific fibrinopeptides, fibrin degradation products such as D-dimer, or enzymes, have been proposed; none has been shown to be diagnostically sensitive or specific.

Aside from tachycardia, the *electrocardiogram* is normal in most patients. With extensive embolization, there may be evidence of acute pulmonary hypertension (rightward shift of the QRS axis, a tall, peaked P wave), and ST-T changes indicative of right ventricular strain (Chap. 189). These changes are often transient, lasting minutes to hours, but when persistent, they suggest severe pulmonary vascular obstruction.

The *chest roentgenogram* may show a parenchymal infiltrate and evidence of a pleural effusion if *infarction* has occurred. Characteristically, the infiltrates caused by infarction abut against the pleura. However, their shape varies, and they do not usually appear until 12 to 36 h after the embolism has occurred. The effusion, which often precedes the infiltrate, is characteristically small. Thoracentesis usually, but by no means invariably, yields hemorrhagic fluid, with the characteristics of an exudate.

The radiographic findings with embolism alone are more subtle. Elevation of the hemidiaphragm may occur. *Differences in diameter between vessels that should be of equivalent size* should raise the suspicion of embolism. For example, embolic obstruction of the right main pulmonary artery can lead to dilation of the left main pulmonary artery because that vessel must accept the entire pulmonary flow. There may be abrupt "*cutoff*" of a vessel; i.e., as the vessel is traced distally, it suddenly disappears. Clot has the same radiodensity as blood, accounting for the proximal shadow; the absence of flow

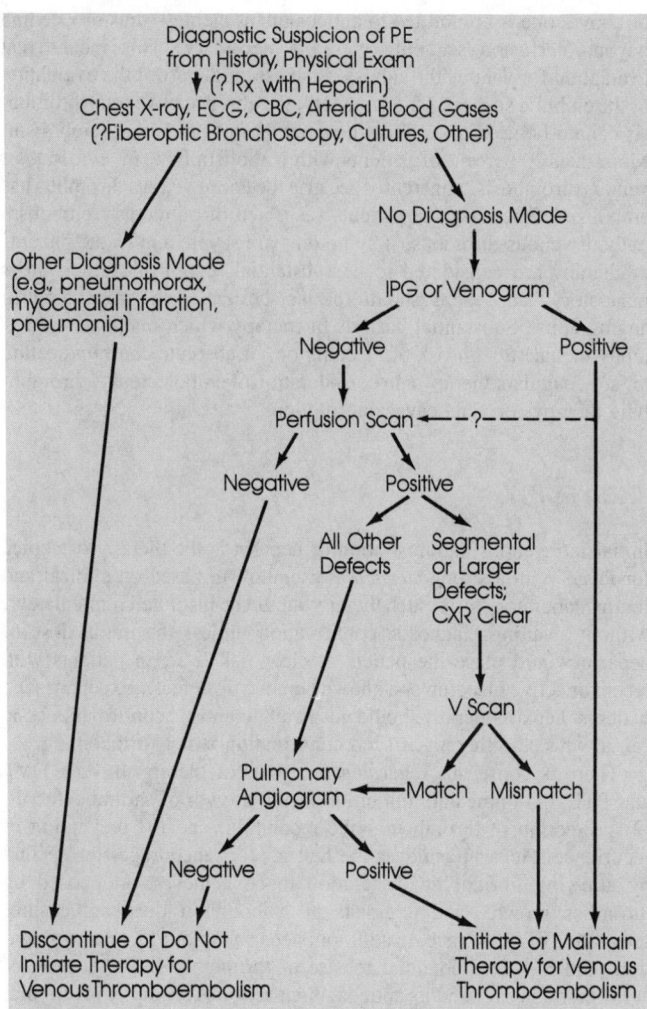

FIGURE 226-1 Flowchart used in diagnosis of pulmonary embolism (PE). IPG, impedance plethysmogram; V scan, ventilation scan.

beyond the clot explains the sudden radiographic "disappearance" of the vessel.

Organization of a clot within a pulmonary artery may lead to retraction of the vessel's walls and a so-called rattail configuration, in which the vessel is relatively normal proximally and suddenly tapers to a sharp point. Finally, there may be *abnormal radiolucency* in some lung zones due to absent or decreased flow. Such abnormally lucent areas (the "Westermark sign"), indicative of proximal arterial obstruction, are best appreciated by examining comparable areas in the two lung fields.

Even in embolization without infarction, the roentgenogram may show small infiltrates, which appear in about 24 h and reflect atelectasis secondary to surfactant depletion. They are not associated with effusion, may fail to touch a pleural surface, and disappear without the linear scarring characteristic of infarction. It should be emphasized that a *normal chest roentgenogram does not exclude the diagnosis of PTE.* Indeed, a *normal* chest roentgenogram is the *most common* finding in embolic disease.

Echo-Doppler studies Standard transthoracic echo-Doppler studies may suggest the diagnosis of embolism by demonstrating right ventricular enlargement, thrombi "trapped" in the right atrium or ventricle, an elevated pulmonary artery pressure, or echogenic densities in the right main pulmonary artery. Transesophageal echocardiography may provide a better view of embolic material in the right main, and rarely the proximal left main, pulmonary artery, but more distal emboli are not reliably detected.

CT with contrast and MRI CT "cuts" through the right and left main pulmonary arteries, with contrast injection, may identify

centrally placed emboli, but as with echo techniques, more distal emboli (which are the most common) cannot be reliably detected. The value of MRI techniques for embolic detection remains uncertain.

Arterial blood gases Massive embolism is commonly associated with arterial hypoxemia, hypocapnia, and respiratory alkalosis. In addition, the difference between alveolar P_{CO_2} and arterial P_{CO_2} ($PA_{CO_2} - Pa_{CO_2}$) may be widened owing to the increase in alveolar dead space (Chap. 214). However, a normal Pa_{O_2} does not exclude the diagnosis.

The laboratory tests discussed thus far are often negative in PTE, and most are relatively nonspecific. Therefore, it is usually necessary to proceed to two more definitive techniques: pulmonary perfusion and ventilation radiophotoscans and the pulmonary angiogram.

Pulmonary perfusion and ventilation scintigraphy Perfusion scintiphotographs (photoscans) are obtained by gamma-camera imaging of the distribution of intravenously injected gamma-emitting radionuclides. The most commonly used radionuclides are microspheres or macroaggregates of albumin (MAA), labeled with a gamma-emitting isotope such as technetium 99m. The radioactive particles, 50 to 100 μm in diameter, are trapped in the pulmonary capillary bed because the pulmonary capillaries approximate 10 μm in diameter. Alternatively, xenon 133 gas, dissolved in saline solution, may be used, but patients must hold their breath. The distribution of labeled particles entrapped in capillaries, or of xenon 133 evolved from them, accurately depicts the distribution of pulmonary blood flow.

The camera-generated perfusion image can be recorded on radiographic film, on special photographic film, on videotape, or projected on to a television screen. Normal scans exhibit homogeneous distribution of radioactivity, smooth margins, and a configuration which corresponds to the normal anatomy of the lungs. Any deviation from these characteristics requires explanation because it represents an abnormality in blood flow distribution.

The perfusion lung photoscan is quite valuable in the diagnosis of embolism. A properly performed perfusion scan which is *normal* excludes the diagnosis of clinically significant pulmonary embolism, as indicated by reports of the excellent outcomes of persons suspected of embolism, who had normal scans and who were not treated (so long as DVT also was absent). On the other hand, a scan demonstrating zones of absent or sharply decreased radioactivity in the patient whose other findings are compatible with PTE keeps the diagnosis of embolism among the possibilities. Scanning is simple, safe, and rapid. It can be repeated to define the resolution, or recurrence, of obstructive vascular phenomena. Like any laboratory test, however, the photoscan must be applied and interpreted with care. It is important, for example, to obtain multiple scan views because lesions not apparent in one view may be easily detected in others. Furthermore, the lung photoscan demonstrates only abnormalities of the *distribution of blood flow*. It does not provide anatomic information.

Many disorders other than PTE are associated with abnormalities in the distribution of pulmonary blood flow. Any disease process, such as pneumonia, atelectasis, or pneumothorax, which reduces the ventilation of a lung zone will decrease its perfusion. Parenchymal diseases, such as emphysema, sarcoidosis, bronchogenic carcinoma, and tuberculosis, can all produce scan defects. Therefore, an abnormal perfusion defect lacks specificity. One approach to enhancing specificity is the performance of a ventilation scan, best achieved by having patients breathe a radioactive gas such as xenon 127 or xenon 133.

To assist in deciding whether a ventilation scan may be useful and when pulmonary angiography is required, two factors should be considered: the size of the perfusion defect(s) and the chest roentgenographic findings. If all defects are subsegmental in size *or* if all defects (of any size) are limited to areas of roentgenographic infiltration, ventilation scanning will not be useful, and pulmonary angiography is required if a definitive diagnosis is necessary. If defect(s) are segmental or larger in size, and one or more are in areas clear by x-ray, a ventilation scan should be done. If the radioactive gas enters ("washes in") and is cleared ("washes out") from the

FIGURE 226-2   Perfusion scan (*left*), posterior view, shows multiple segmental and larger perfusion defects in right upper and lower lobes, left lower lobe, and lingula. Ventilation scan (*right*) is normal at equilibrium. Xenon 133 washed in and out normally. Multiple emboli were confirmed angiographically.

area(s) of perfusion defect(s), this "mismatch" of ventilation and perfusion is characteristic of vascular obstruction (Fig. 226-2). Pulmonary vascular obstruction is present in 90 percent or more of patients with this pattern. However, if ventilation is also abnormal (i.e., ventilation-perfusion "match" is present), no reliable diagnostic conclusion can be reached; pulmonary angiography is required. (It may not be required if DVT is present and already mandates therapy.) In some centers, ^{99m}Tc-DTPA particles are used for ventilation studies; this approach provides multiple views but does not allow "washout" evaluation.

In summary, three basic scan patterns emerge: normal, "diagnostic" (which others call "high probability"), and "nondiagnostic" (which others call "intermediate or low probability"). Patients in this last category require pulmonary angiography to establish or exclude the diagnosis of embolism.

Pulmonary angiography   This is the only established means for providing anatomic information about the pulmonary vasculature. Radiopaque material is injected, preferably through a cardiac catheter advanced into the pulmonary artery. Cardiac catheterization and angiography require specialized personnel and a reasonable period for preparation and performance, and they entail more risk than the procedures discussed above. However, angiography provides a visual image of the pulmonary vessels, and catheterization can provide potentially important hemodynamic data (pulmonary artery and wedge pressures, cardiac output). Interpretive limitations of angiography are of two types: (1) *Injection artifacts* may occur which suggest absence of flow to a vessel. Injection should be repeated whenever the question of such artifacts exists. (2) Interpretive errors also may be a consequence of *not looking for the proper type of defect*. There are only two findings diagnostic of acute embolism. One is the *abrupt "cutoff"* of a vessel at the point of embolic impaction. However, complete embolic obstruction is uncommon. Therefore, *filling defects* are the most frequent finding; i.e., the embolus creates a "negative" shadow as the radiopaque material flows around it. The major contraindication to angiography is the absence of personnel who are experienced in both performing the procedure and interpreting the results. Serious diagnostic errors are commonplace if optimal techniques are not used or the complexities of interpretation are not appreciated. However, the risks of angiography are low in experienced hands. Injection of large boluses of contrast medium into the main pulmonary artery should be avoided in favor of small injections into vessels supplying lung regions identified as abnormal on the perfusion scan.

How far one should proceed down the diagnostic pathway outlined above depends on many factors, the major ones being the presence or absence of documented venous thrombosis, the severity of the patient's symptoms, and the hazards of contemplated therapy. In each condition, there is a need for precise diagnosis. If IPG or venography already has documented deep venous thrombosis of the popliteal vein

or above, one is committed to anticoagulant therapy; thus proceeding beyond perfusion scanning is rarely necessary. This means that evaluation for venous thrombosis is an essential part of the evaluation of the embolic suspect. Unfortunately, the absence of venous thrombosis cannot be used to exclude the diagnosis of pulmonary embolism. More than 20 percent of patients with embolism have no evidence of venous thrombosis, apparently because the entire venous thrombus has embolized. Therefore, in patients suspected of pulmonary embolism without venous thrombus, if symptoms are severe and/or the hazards of therapy are considered to be substantial, diagnostic precision is mandatory, and there should be no hesitancy in proceeding to angiography. Substantial hazards of therapy which mandate angiography include a high risk of bleeding on, or absolute contraindication to, anticoagulant therapy and consideration of embolectomy, thrombolytic therapy, or vena caval interruption.

TREATMENT

Initial intravenous administration of heparin is the therapy of choice for PTE. With a strong *suspicion* of embolism based on clinical and routine laboratory tests, such therapy should be instituted immediately, without awaiting diagnostic confirmation, unless the initial dose of heparin would place the patient at clear risk (i.e., in patients with recent or active bleeding or a known hemostatic defect). Except in such patients, heparin therapy should not await diagnostic confirmation; one can always stop therapy if such confirmation is not forthcoming.

There is consensus regarding the goals of therapy in both DVT and PTE: (1) immediate inhibition of the growth of thromboemboli, (2) promotion of thromboembolic resolution, and (3) prevention of recurrence. Heparin achieves the first goal, it encourages the second by allowing fibrinolytic dissolution to be achieved unopposed by thrombus growth, and it assists in, although it does not ensure, prevention of recurrence. In addition, heparin inhibits platelet aggregation (and therefore potential release of thromboxane and serotonin) at the embolic site, and its anticoagulant action is promptly reversible.

There is *not* consensus, however, regarding (1) heparin regimens which best combine safety and efficacy, (2) the need for, and type of, tests for monitoring coagulation behavior during heparin therapy, (3) how long, and with what agents, antithrombotic therapy should be maintained, or (4) in which patients thrombolytic therapy should antedate antithrombotic therapy.

REGIMENS   In DVT, three methods of heparin administration have been advocated by various investigators: continuous intravenous, intermittent intravenous, and intermittent subcutaneous. Continuous intravenous heparin is usually given in a dose of approximately 1000 units per hour. Intermittent intravenous heparin is commonly given in a dose of approximately 5000 units every 4 h or 7500 units every 6 h. Subcutaneous heparin has been recommended at a dose of 5000 units every 4 h, 10,000 units every 8 h, or 20,000 units every 12 h. Studies exist which indicate that each of these regimens is more efficacious, safer, or both. Therefore, at this time, one can conclude only that *each* of these regimens (which approximate 30,000 to 40,000 units per 24 h) represents an acceptable treatment regimen. Despite such apparent comparability, the continuous intravenous regimen, delivered by an infusion pump, is by far the most popular in the United States. *Intramuscular* injection of heparin is to be avoided because hematomas will develop. (Indeed, *all* intramuscular injections should be avoided during anticoagulant therapy.)

It also should be recognized that there is a growing consensus that DVT that remains confined to the calf veins need *not* be treated with anticoagulant therapy. No increase in morbidity or mortality has been reported among patients in this category who are not treated. However, since 15 to 20 percent of calf-limited thrombi will extend to the popliteal veins and above during a 10- to 12-day period, such patients *must* be followed by serial IPG (or, perhaps, ultrasound) tests until this period has elapsed. If they cannot be followed in this manner, they should be treated.

In PTE, the same options for heparin therapy exist. The only additional question is whether an initial large intravenous bolus (10,000 to 20,000 units) should be given to inhibit the aggregation (and release reaction) of platelets adherent to the embolus. Most experts advocate such a dose, with one of the "standard" regimens being started 2 to 4 h later.

MONITORING The value of clotting times (CT), partial thromboplastin times (PTT), or other coagulation tests to monitor the safety and efficacy of heparin remains controversial. With regard to safety, the risk of hemorrhage (the principal complication of heparin therapy) is not clearly related to coagulation test alterations; rather, it appears related to such factors as the coexistence of other diseases associated with bleeding risk (gastric or duodenal ulcer, coagulopathies, uremia) and advanced age. Likewise, achievement of the desired effect of heparin (cessation of thrombus growth in vivo) has not been related consistently to coagulation tests. Therefore, it is questionable whether monitoring with such tests is superior to empiric use of one of the regimens described above. While animal investigations have disclosed that maintaining the PTT above 1.5 times control does prevent growth of venous thrombi, data are not available documenting this in human patients. If done improperly or poorly timed, the CT or PTT tests are worthless and may be misleading. Furthermore, even with continuous intravenous therapy, the CT and PTT may vary substantially during a 24-h period. Despite these vagaries, a majority of experts currently recommend attempting to keep the CT or PTT, measured *just prior* to the next intermittent dose, at or above 1.5 times the baseline CT or PTT and at 1.5 to 2.0 times control with continuous infusion.

DURATION OF THERAPY In DVT, full anticoagulant protection is usually maintained for 7 to 10 days, the rationale being that this is the period required for dissolution and/or organization of the thrombus. In PTE, for the same reasons, a similar duration of therapy is advised. Bed rest is indicated only until cardiopulmonary or leg symptoms subside. Carefully applied elastic support hose should be used (to encourage venous flow) as soon as leg pain, if present, subsides and the patient is ambulated.

During and beyond the acute phase there are several options for achieving proper anticoagulant protection. In deciding among these options, it should be recognized that the major question being addressed is: Does the patient need continued protection against the risk of *recurrent* DVT (and, therefore, PTE)? If the risk factor(s) that precipitated the acute episode of DVT-PTE is (are) no longer present, the patient is asymptomatic, and the IPG is normal, it is acceptable to reduce heparin to a lower dose starting on day 7, ambulate the patient, and, if no symptoms develop, discontinue heparin on day 9 or 10. If these criteria are not met, as is the case in most patients, prolonged prophylactic therapy is warranted. Two options exist for such prophylaxis. The most common one is to initiate a prothrombinopenic agent (e.g., warfarin) as soon as the decision for long-term protection is made. Often, this can be done on day 2 or 3 of heparin therapy. Prothrombinopenic drugs are not suitable for initial therapy in thromboembolism because their onset of action is too slow. Their only role is in maintaining anticoagulant protection for prolonged periods. If they are initiated early in the acute treatment course, the patient must be "in range," as defined by a prothrombin time of 1.5 to 1.8 times the control time for at least 3 days *before heparin is discontinued*. A second option for long-term protection is the use of self-injected subcutaneous heparin. Current data suggest that a dose of 7500 to 10,000 units every 12 h is adequate, is well-tolerated, and need not be monitored with coagulation tests.

There is no consensus regarding the period for which anticoagulant protection should be maintained beyond hospital discharge because firm data on this point are lacking. If *reversible* risk factors are present (e.g., immobilization after a leg fracture), therapy should be continued until the risk factors present have resolved. If the risk factors present are nonreversible (e.g., severe left and/or right ventricular failure), if the IPG remains positive, or if major lung scan defects persist at discharge, empiric decisions are made. At a minimum, 3 months of therapy seems wise, because recurrence is relatively common during this period. Beyond 3 months, however, continuation depends on the balance among specific risk factors exhibited by the patient, IPG results, lung scan results, and the risks of continued therapy. In some instances, this balance may warrant lifetime maintenance on anticoagulant drugs.

Thrombolytic therapy The place of thrombolytic (fibrinolytic) agents (Chap. 202) in the management of acute venous thromboembolism remains to be defined. There is no question that available first-generation agents (streptokinase, urokinase), the second-generation agents (tissue plasminogen activator, tPA), and potential third-generation agents can hasten the resolution of venous thrombi and pulmonary emboli. They do not replace antithrombotic therapy. When used, thrombolytic agents must be followed by a standard course of antithrombotic therapy. Despite extensive study, it has not been established that such agents alter short- or long-term morbidity, mortality, or recurrence rates among patients with DVT or PTE. These drugs, despite high fibrin specificity in the case of tPA, are associated with hemorrhagic risk in patients who have had, or require, any invasive procedure (e.g., vein puncture, arterial puncture, angiography, Swan-Ganz catheterization) and in patients with localized vascular lesions due to recent operation, trauma, or concomitant disease (e.g., peptic ulcer, stroke). If thrombolytic agents prove to have a therapeutic advantage, it would appear to be (1) in patients with extensive, large-vein DVT (e.g., iliofemoral) and (2) in patients with massive embolism and persistent systemic hypotension despite appropriate supportive measures (oxygen, pressor infusions).

Surgical therapy for DVT (thrombectomy) is now rarely considered because the results have not been encouraging. In PTE, surgical therapy should be reserved for those patients in whom heparin therapy is deemed inadequate or impractical. Anticoagulant therapy may be contraindicated by the presence of a bleeding diathesis, or the patient may be in such critical condition that it is felt unwise to await a response to medical therapy. In such instances, *venous interruption* and *pulmonary embolectomy* should be considered.

The objective of venous interruption is to prevent immediate recurrence of embolism from lower extremity venous thrombi. While multiple ligation and clipping procedures have been used in the past, these have been largely supplanted by the use of filters placed in the inferior vena cava by a transvenous approach (jugular, femoral veins). Ligation of the inferior vena cava has been abandoned because it requires surgery, obstructs venous return acutely, and encourages rapid collateral vein formation which bypasses the ligation. Clips require surgery for placement, may obstruct caval flow, and may thrombose. The filters, typified by the Greenfield filter, which has been the most widely used in recent years, are inserted transvenously, do not obstruct caval flow, protect against emboli greater than 2 mm in diameter, and are rarely subject to thrombosis.

There are two major indications for placement of a caval filter: (1) as a lifesaving procedure in patients with massive embolism who could not tolerate an embolic recurrence and (2) to prevent embolism in patients with documented venous thrombosis in whom anticoagulant therapy is contraindicated.

There is one instance, however, in which caval ligation may be the therapy of choice: septic thrombophlebitis of pelvic origin with multiple septic pulmonary emboli. If these patients do not respond promptly to a heparin-antibiotic regimen, they may die unless caval (and left ovarian vein) ligation is carried out.

Two criteria should be met before emergency pulmonary embolectomy is performed: (1) there must be evidence of severe hemodynamic compromise due to embolism, particularly sustained systemic hypotension, which is not responsive to supportive measures, and (2) the personnel and equipment required for embolectomy carried out with the aid of cardiopulmonary bypass must be available. Even with these criteria satisfied, it now appears likely that management of such patients by alternative approaches (e.g., placement of a caval filter plus heparin therapy, thrombolytic therapy) will be associated with lower mortality rates than is emergency embolectomy.

SPECIAL CONSIDERATIONS   Total resolution of emboli does not always occur. Why in some patients (perhaps 0.1 percent) emboli fail to resolve is not yet known. However, if residual vascular obstruction is substantial, the patient may present, months or years after the actual embolic events, with dyspnea and pulmonary hypertension of uncertain cause, often with right ventricular failure. Such patients commonly are misdiagnosed, for months or years, as having asthma, chronic lung disease, primary pulmonary hypertension, or cor pulmonale of unclear etiology, particularly if, as is commonly the case, the initial pulmonary embolic event went unrecognized.

Such patients should be studied by appropriate techniques, since emboli in the main or lobar arteries can be surgically removed (thromboendarterectomy), allowing cure of this otherwise fatal form of pulmonary hypertensive disease. This entity, once an autopsy curiosity, is more common than previously appreciated. More than 400 patients have been reported to have undergone thromboendarterectomy. Because surgical mortality is heavily conditioned by the severity of right ventricular dysfunction at the time of operation, early recognition is important. A follow-up lung scan after diagnosed massive embolism may help in this regard.

PROGNOSIS IN PULMONARY EMBOLISM   The prognosis of the patient with pulmonary embolism *in whom therapy is promptly instituted* is excellent. As stated at the outset of this chapter, less than 1 embolic event in 10 is lethal. The majority of these deaths occur suddenly and can be avoided only by prophylaxis (see above). The remainder appear to be due to embolic extension or recurrence, which therapy can moderate. Thus, for patients who survive long enough to reach medical attention and receive heparin, the outlook is quite good. Morbidity following embolism is uncommon, since embolic resolution is the rule, and very few patients develop the pulmonary hypertensive problem noted above.

Limited reliable data are available regarding recurrence rates in the months and years after a single embolic event (with or without prolonged postembolic anticoagulant therapy). In the absence of risk factors or a positive IPG, recurrence appears to be uncommon, but more precise data are needed.

Whether the therapeutic approaches discussed here will be altered by new agents, such as low-molecular-weight heparin, heparinoids, and newer thrombolytic agents, remains to be seen. However, in the case of low-molecular-weight heparin, data are appearing which suggest that once-daily subcutaneous injections of fixed doses, without monitoring, may someday become the "standard regimen" for both DVT and PTE.

NONTHROMBOTIC EMBOLISM

Because the lung vasculature serves as a filter of the venous circulation, it is the recipient of diverse materials which can gain entry into venous blood, including bone marrow, foreign bodies, parasites, and tumor cells. The most frequently encountered form of nonthrombotic embolism is *fat embolism*. This dramatic and controversial entity follows the introduction of neutral fat into the venous circulation, most commonly after bone trauma or fracture (marrow fat), but occasionally after trauma to adipose tissue or liver infiltrated by fat. The clinical sequence is characteristic. After a latent period of 12 to 36 h or more, during which the patient is asymptomatic, sudden cardiopulmonary and neurologic deterioration appears. Mental aberrations, delirium, and coma develop. Dyspnea, tachypnea, and tachycardia occur, and the chest roentgenographic and physiologic components of the "adult respiratory distress syndrome" appear (see Chap. 230). Anemia and thrombocytopenia are common, as are petechiae on the upper thorax and arms. The pathogenesis of the syndrome is not clear, but it seems likely that two events occur: release of free fatty acids (by action of lipases on the neutral fat), which induces a toxic vasculitis, followed by platelet-fibrin thrombosis, and actual obstruction of small pulmonary arteries by macroaggregates of fat. Several forms of therapy have been proposed (e.g., corticosteroids,

heparin, ethanol), but none has proved effective. Treatment remains supportive, and the mortality rate is high.

Another dramatic form of nonthrombotic embolism is *amniotic fluid embolism*. This occurs during both spontaneous delivery and cesarean section. Sudden and massive obstruction of the pulmonary microvasculature occurs, leading to shock and, often, death. With survival of the initial phase of the disease, the picture of disseminated intravascular coagulation appears. The syndrome is due to the entrance of a significant quantity of amniotic fluid into the venous circulation. This fluid is a potent thromboplastic agent which induces thrombosis in the pulmonary vasculature and elsewhere. The fluid also contains particulates which lodge in the lung. Treatment consists of supportive measures.

Nonembolic pulmonary arterial obstruction due to *vasculitis* has become a common problem among intravenous drug users. This vasculitis, caused by the drugs per se or materials (e.g., talc) mixed with the drugs, can induce thrombosis. This entity may be difficult to distinguish from PTE. Repetitive episodes may lead to irreversible and severe pulmonary hypertension. Other forms of vasculitis (e.g., Takayasu's arteritis) also may obstruct the large pulmonary arteries and mimic pulmonary embolism, as may primary pulmonary artery sarcomas and fibrosing mediastinitis.

REFERENCES

CARSON JL et al: The clinical course of pulmonary embolism. N Engl J Med 326:1240, 1992

HIRSH J: Oral anticoagulant drugs. N Engl J Med 324:1865, 1991

———: Heparin. N Engl J Med 324:1565, 1991

HOMMES DW et al: Subcutaneous heparin compared with continuous intravenous heparin administration in the initial treatment of deep vein thrombosis: A meta-analysis. Ann Intern Med 116:279, 1992

HUISMAN MV et al: Utility of impedance plethysmography in the diagnosis of recurrent deep vein thrombosis. Arch Intern Med 148:681, 1988

HULL RD, RASKOB GE: Low probability lung scan findings: A need for change. Ann Intern Med 114:142, 1991

——— et al: Subcutaneous low-molecular-weight heparin compared with continuous intravascular heparin in the treatment of proximal-vein thrombosis. N Engl J Med 326:975, 1992

——— et al: Pulmonary angiography, ventilation lung scanning and venography for clinically suspected pulmonary embolism in the abnormal perfusion scan. Ann Intern Med 98:891, 1983

KAKKAR VV et al: Prevention of post-operative embolism by low-dose heparin: An international multicenter trial. Lancet 2:45, 1975

LENSING AW et al: Detection of deep vein thrombosis by real-time B-mode ultrasonography. N Engl J Med 320:342, 1989

LINDBLAD B et al: Autopsy-verified pulmonary embolism in a surgical department: Analysis of the period from 1951 to 1988. Br J Surg 78:849, 1991

MERCANDETTI A et al: Influence of perfusion and ventilation scans on therapeutic decision-making and outcome among embolic suspects. West J Med 142:208, 1985

MOSER KM, FEDULLO PF: Venous thromboembolism: Three simple decisions. Chest 83:117, 256, 1983

——— et al: Chronic major vessel thromboembolic pulmonary hypertension. Circulation 81:1735, 1990

———: Venous thromboembolism: State of the art. Ann Rev Respir Dis 141:235, 1990

NIH CONSENSUS CONFERENCE: Prevention of venous thrombosis and pulmonary embolism. JAMA 256:744, 1986

PALEVSKI HI, FISHMAN AP: Diagnosis and treatment of pulmonary embolism and deep venous thrombosis, in *Update: Pulmonary Diseases and Disorders*, AP Fishman (ed). McGraw-Hill, New York, 1992, pp 451–464

PIOPED INVESTIGATIONS: Value of the ventilation/perfusion scan in acute pulmonary embolism: Results of the prospective investigation of pulmonary embolism diagnosis (PIOPED). JAMA 263:2753, 1990

RITTOO D et al: Role of transesophageal echocardiography in diagnosis and management of central pulmonary artery thromboembolism. Am J Cardiol 71:1115, 1993

SALZMAN EW et al: Intraoperative external pneumatic calf compression to afford long-term prophylaxis against deep vein thrombosis in urologic patients. Surgery 87:239, 1980

227 NEOPLASMS OF THE LUNG

JOHN D. MINNA

Each year, primary carcinoma of the lung affects more than 100,000 males and 50,000 females in the United States, most of whom die within 1 year of diagnosis, making it the leading cause of cancer death. The peak incidence of lung cancer occurs between ages 55 and 65 years. The overall incidence is increasing, causing the age-adjusted lung cancer death rate to double every 15 years. However, the effects of antismoking efforts begun 10 to 20 years ago have finally started to be seen in a flattening of the incidence rate of lung cancer in white males, while, unfortunately, the rate in females is still increasing. At the time of diagnosis, only 20 percent of all lung cancer patients will have local disease, while 25 percent will have disease spread to regional lymph nodes, and 55 percent will have distant metastatic cancer. Even in those patients with supposedly localized disease, overall 5-year survival is only 30 percent for males and 50 percent for females, and this survival rate has not changed significantly over the past 20 years. Thus primary carcinoma of the lung is a major health problem with a generally grim prognosis. However, an orderly approach to diagnosis, staging, and treatment based on knowledge of the clinical behavior of lung cancer allows selection of the best therapy for either potential cure or optimal palliation of individual patients. This approach should be multidisciplinary, involving interaction of internists, chest physicians, medical, radiation, and surgical oncologists, pathologists, and supportive care personnel.

PATHOLOGY

The histologic classification of primary lung neoplasms recommended by the World Health Organization in 1977 should be used. Four major cell types make up 95 percent of all primary lung neoplasms. These are *squamous* or *epidermoid carcinoma*, *small cell* (also called *oat cell*) *carcinoma*, *adenocarcinoma* (including bronchioloalveolar), and *large cell* (also called *large cell anaplastic*) *carcinoma*. The remainder include combined epidermoid and adenocarcinomas, carcinoids, bronchial gland tumors (including cylindromas and mucoepidermoid tumors), and mesotheliomas, as well as rarer tumor types. The various cell types have different natural histories and responses to therapy, and thus a correct histologic diagnosis by an experienced pathologist is the first step to correct treatment. In the past 10 years, for unknown reasons, the incidence of adenocarcinoma is rising, while that of epidermoid cancer is falling.

Major treatment decisions are made on the basis of the crucial distinction between histologic classification of a tumor as a small cell carcinoma or one of the non-small cell varieties (which include epidermoid, adenocarcinoma, large cell carcinoma, bronchioloalveolar carcinoma, and mixed versions of these). Some of these distinctions are summarized in Tables 227-1 and 227-2. In general, small cell carcinoma has spread beyond the bounds of resectional surgery at the time of presentation and is primarily managed with chemotherapy with or without radiotherapy. In contrast, non-small cell cancers found to be localized at the time of presentation should be considered for a curative attempt with either surgery or radiotherapy. Further, the response of non-small cell cancers to chemotherapy usually is not dramatic, making such therapy less important in metastatic disease than it is in nearly all small cell lung cancer patients.

Ninety percent of patients with lung cancer of all histologic types are cigarette smokers, while the rare nonsmoking patient who develops lung cancer usually has adenocarcinoma. However, in nonsmokers with adenocarcinoma involving the lung, the possibility of other primary sites should be considered. Epidermoid and small cell cancers

TABLE 227-1 Incidence, frequency of metastases, and surgical resectability of the major lung cancer histologic types

Cell type	Incidence, %*	Necropsy frequency of distant metastases when clinically localized, %[†]	Resectability rate (AJC study), %[‡]	5-Year survival after curative resection, %
Non-small cell carcinoma				
Epidermoid	17	17	60	37
Adenocarcinoma	40	40	38	27
Large cell carcinoma	15	14	38	27
Small cell carcinoma	25	63	11	<1

* Recent incidence figures reflect an increase in adenocarcinomas. In addition, 3 percent of tumors are mixtures of other types. The incidence of lung cancer with bronchioalveolar components is increasing (>5 percent) and is included in this 3 percent and with the adenocarcinomas.
[†] Determined from autopsy studies of patients dying of causes other than cancer within 30 days following an apparent curative surgical resection.
[‡] AJC = American Joint Committee Study for Cancer Staging and End Results Reporting, indicating percentage of cases thought to undergo a curative resection.
SOURCE: Adapted from DC Ihde et al, 1992.

usually present as central masses with endobronchial growth, while adenocarcinomas and large cell cancers tend to present as peripheral nodules or masses with pleural involvement. Epidermoid and large cell cancers cavitate in approximately 20 percent of cases. Bronchioloalveolar carcinoma can present as a single mass, a diffuse, multinodular lesion, or as a fluffy infiltrate.

ETIOLOGY

The large majority of lung cancers are caused by carcinogens and tumor promoters ingested via cigarette smoking. Overall, the relative risk of developing lung cancer is increased about 13-fold by active smoking and about 1.5-fold by long-term passive exposure to cigarette smoke. Probably there is a cocarcinogenic effect of smoking and industrial or environmental pollutants such as radon gas from natural sources in the ground. There is a dose-response relationship between the lung cancer death rate and the total amount (often expressed in "cigarette pack-years") of cigarettes smoked, such that the risk is increased 60- to 70-fold for the man smoking two packs a day for 20 years compared with the nonsmoker. Conversely, the chance of developing lung cancer decreases with cessation of smoking but may never return to the nonsmoker level. The increase in lung cancer in women is also associated with a rise in cigarette smoking. As a preventive measure, efforts to get persons to stop smoking are mandatory. However, this is extremely difficult because the smoking habit represents a powerful addiction to nicotine. Therefore, it is of vital importance to prevent people from starting to smoke. This requires new efforts targeted at children, since addiction to cigarettes has occurred by the late teen years.

The poor prognosis for most patients with lung cancer requires the continued performance of well-designed clinical trials to test new forms of therapy. These include further adjuvant and neoadjuvant trials combined with surgery and radiotherapy; prospective testing of tumor sensitivity in vitro to drugs, radiation therapy, and biologic response modifiers; tests of anti-growth factor therapy; and application of newer methods for early detection. The key intervention remains prevention, and broad antismoking efforts must continue. Recently, chemoprevention trials with agents such as retinoic acid have started. The detection of genetic lesions predisposing to malignancy in airway epithelial cells would be a major step forward in focusing preventive efforts, providing intermediate endpoints, molecular early diagnosis, and eventually targeting therapy at the products that make lung cancer cells malignant.

TABLE 227-2 Comparison between small cell and non-small cell lung cancers

	Small cell	Non-small cell
Histology	Scant cytoplasm; small hyperchromatic nuclei with fine chromatin pattern; nucleoli indistinct; diffuse sheets of cells	Abundant cytoplasm; pleomorphic nuclei with coarse chromatin pattern; nucleoli often prominent; glands or squamous architecture
General neuroendocrine properties:		
Dense core granules	Present	Absent*
L-Dopa decarboxylase activity	High	Absent
Chromogranin	Present	Absent
Synaptophysin	Present	Absent
Neuron-specific enolase	High	Low
Creatine kinase BB isozyme	High	Low
Leu-7, HNK-1 antigens	Present	Absent
Peptide hormone production:		
Gastrin-releasing peptide gene products	Present	Absent
Other neuropeptides	ACTH, AVP, calcitonin, ANF	PTH
Other markers:		
HLA, β_2-microglobulin	Absent/low	Present
Intermediate filament pattern	"SCLC"	"Non-SCLC"
Neurofilaments	Present	Absent
Opioid receptors	Present	Present
Nicotine receptors	Present	Present
EGF receptors	Low or absent	Present
Mucin	Absent	Present in adenocarcinomas
Surfactant associate proteins	Absent	Often present
Carcinoembryonic antigen	Present	Present
Cytogenetics and mutations:		
3p deletions	Present ~100%	Present in >90%
rb gene mutations	Present in ~100%	Present in >20%
p53 mutations	Present in >90%	Present in >50%
Other deletions (see text)	Present	Present
ras mutations	<1%	~30%
myc family overexpression	>50%	>50%
Response to radiotherapy	Objective shrinkage in 80–90%; often complete response	Objective shrinkage in 30–50%; uncommonly complete
Response to combination chemotherapy:		
Overall regression rate	90%	30–40%
Complete regression rate	50%	5%
Overall 5-year survival rates	5%	8%

* Ten percent of non-small cell lung cancers have populations of cells expressing neuroendocrine markers, and these are best demonstrated by immunohistochemical stains.

While human lung cancer is not thought of as a genetic disease, a variety of molecular genetic studies have shown that lung cancer cells have acquired a number of genetic lesions including activation of dominant oncogenes and inactivation of tumor suppressor or recessive oncogenes (Chap. 317). In fact, it appears that to become clinically evident, lung cancer cells have to accumulate a large number

(perhaps 10 or more) of such lesions. For the dominant oncogenes, these include point mutations in the coding regions of the *ras* family of oncogenes (particularly in the K-*ras* gene in adenocarcinoma of the lung) and amplification, rearrangement, and/or loss of transcriptional control of *myc* family oncogenes (c-, N-, and L-*myc*), with changes in c-*myc* found in non-small cell cancers while changes in all *myc* family members are found in small cell lung cancer. Tumor mutations in *ras* genes are associated with poor prognosis in non-small cell lung cancer, while tumor amplification of c-*myc* is associated with poor prognosis in small cell lung cancer.

For the recessive oncogenes (*tumor suppressor genes*), cytogenetic and restriction fragment length polymorphism (RFLP) analyses have shown deletions (allele loss) involving chromosome regions 1p, 1q, 3p14, 3p21, 3p24-25, 3q, 5q (familial polyposis gene cluster), 9p (interferon gene cluster), 11p, 13q14 (retinoblastoma, *rb*, gene), 16q, and 17p13 (*p53* gene), as well as other sites. There appear to be several candidate recessive oncogenes on chromosome 3p which are involved in nearly all lung cancers. The *p53* and *rb* genes are both mutated in more than 90 percent of small cell lung cancers, while *p53* is mutated in more than 50 percent and *rb* in more than 20 percent of non-small cell lung cancers. Mutations in the familial polyposis and interferon gene clusters are also common. The large number of genetic lesions in clinically evident cancer has prompted a search for these mutations in lung tissue before classic cytopathologic evidence of malignancy can be found, to provide for molecular early diagnosis and as intermediate endpoints in prevention efforts, including chemoprevention treatment.

The large number of lesions shows that lung cancer, like other common epithelial malignancies, is a multistep process likely to involve both carcinogens (causing initiation by mutagenesis) and tumor promoters (allowing the outgrowth of cells with genetic lesions). Prevention can be directed at both processes. Cell biologic studies have shown that lung cancer cells both produce a large number of peptide hormones and express receptors for these hormones, which thereby can act to stimulate tumor cell growth in an "autocrine" fashion. Nicotine potentially plays a very central role in lung cancer pathogenesis. Highly carcinogenic derivatives of nicotine are formed in cigarette smoke. Smoking is tied to nicotine addiction, and nicotine gum and patches are now widely used to help persons to stop smoking. Lung cancer cells of all histologic types express receptors for nicotine that are very similar to nicotinic acetylcholine receptors. Thus it is possible that nicotine itself could be directly involved in lung cancer pathogenesis.

While lung cancer does not have a clear pattern of Mendelian inheritance, there are several indications of a potential for familial association. These include inherited mutations in *rb* (patients with retinoblastomas living to adulthood) and *p53* (Li-Fraumeni syndrome) genes; studies that show that first-degree relatives of lung cancer probands have a significantly (two- to threefold) excess risk of lung cancer or other cancers, many of which are not smoking-related; and a strong risk of developing lung cancer has been shown to be linked with the development of chronic obstructive pulmonary disease. Finally, several studies have proposed an association between P450 enzyme phenotype or genotype with the development of lung cancer, the most prominent being inheritance of the high-debrisoquine metabolic phenotype [P450 enzyme 2D6 on chromosome 22 (see Chap. 66)] associated with a six- to tenfold increased risk of lung cancer.

CLINICAL MANIFESTATIONS AND MODE OF PRESENTATION

Lung cancer gives rise to signs and symptoms from local tumor growth, invasion or obstruction of adjacent structures, growth in regional nodes via lymphatic spread, growth in distant metastatic sites after hematogenous dissemination, or as a remote effect (paraneoplastic syndrome). The latter usually results from peptide hormone secretion by the tumor or immunologic cross reaction between tumor and normal tissue antigens. Appropriate identification of these signs and symptoms as tumor-related will guide further evaluation and therapy and be of prognostic importance.

If programs screening asymptomatic patients are excluded, 5 to 15 percent of patients are detected while asymptomatic, usually on a routine chest radiograph, while the vast majority of patients present with some sign or symptom. Signs and symptoms secondary to central or endobronchial growth of the primary tumor include cough, hemoptysis, wheeze and stridor, dyspnea, and pneumonitis (fever and productive cough) from obstruction. Signs and symptoms secondary to the peripheral growth of the primary tumor include pain from pleural or chest wall involvement, cough, dyspnea on a restrictive basis, and symptoms of lung abscess resulting from tumor cavitation. Signs and symptoms related to the regional spread of tumor in the thorax by contiguity or by metastasis to regional lymph nodes include tracheal obstruction, esophageal compression with dysphagia, recurrent laryngeal nerve paralysis with hoarseness, phrenic nerve paralysis with elevation of the hemidiaphragm and dyspnea, and sympathetic nerve paralysis with Horner's syndrome (enophthalmus, ptosis, miosis, and ipsilateral loss of sweat). *Pancoast's* (or *superior sulcus tumor) syndrome* results from local extension of a tumor (usually epidermoid) growing in the apex of the lung with involvement of the eighth cervical and first and second thoracic nerves, with shoulder pain which characteristically radiates in the ulnar distribution of the arm, often with radiologic destruction of the first and second ribs. Often Horner's syndrome and Pancoast's syndrome will coexist. Other problems of regional spread include *superior vena cava syndrome* from vascular obstruction; pericardial and cardiac extension with resultant tamponade, arrhythmia, or cardiac failure; lymphatic obstruction with resultant pleural effusion; and lymphangitic spread through the lungs with hypoxemia and dyspnea. In addition, bronchioloalveolar carcinoma can spread transbronchially, producing tumor growing along multiple alveolar surfaces with resultant impairment of oxygen transfer, respiratory insufficiency, dyspnea, hypoxemia, and production of large amounts of sputum.

Extrathoracic metastatic disease is found at autopsy in over 50 percent of patients with epidermoid carcinoma, 80 percent of patients with adeno- and large cell carcinoma, and over 95 percent of patients with small cell cancer. These autopsy studies have found lung cancer metastases in virtually every organ system. Thus the majority of lung cancer patients eventually need therapy to palliate symptoms. Common clinical problems related to extrathoracic metastatic lung cancer include brain metastases with neurologic deficits; bone metastases with pain and pathologic fractures; bone marrow invasion with cytopenias or leukoerythroblastosis; liver metastases causing biochemical liver dysfunction, biliary obstruction, and pain; lymph node metastases in the supraclavicular region and occasionally in the axilla and groin; and spinal cord compression syndromes from epidural or bone metastases.

Paraneoplastic syndromes are common in lung cancer patients and may be the presenting finding or first sign of recurrence. In addition, paraneoplastic syndromes may mimic metastatic disease and, unless detected, lead to inappropriate palliative rather than curative treatment. Often the paraneoplastic syndrome may be relieved with successful treatment of the tumor, and tumor treatment is the basis for correcting such syndromes. In some cases the pathophysiology of the paraneoplastic syndrome is known, particularly when a hormone with biologic activity is secreted by a tumor (Chap. 327). However, in many cases the pathophysiology is unknown. *Systemic symptoms* of anorexia, cachexia, weight loss (seen in 30 percent of patients), fever, and suppressed immunity are paraneoplastic syndromes of unknown etiology. *Endocrine syndromes* are seen in 12 percent of patients and have the best understood pathophysiology, including hypercalcemia and hypophosphatemia resulting from ectopic parathyroid hormone or PTH-related peptide production by epidermoid cancer, hyponatremia with the syndrome of inappropriate secretion of antidiuretic hormone or possibly atrial natriuretic factor by small cell cancer, and ectopic secretion of ACTH by small cell cancer,

which usually results in additional electrolyte disturbances, especially hypokalemia, rather than the changes in body habitus seen in Cushing's syndrome from a pituitary adenoma.

Skeletal–connective tissue syndromes include clubbing in 30 percent (usually non-small cell) and hypertrophic pulmonary osteoarthropathy in 1 to 10 percent (usually adenocarcinomas) with periostitis and clubbing giving pain, tenderness, and swelling over the affected bones and a positive bone scan. *Neurologic-myopathic syndromes* are seen in only 1 percent of patients but are dramatic and include the myasthenic *Eaton-Lambert syndrome* and retinal blindness with small cell cancer, while peripheral neuropathies, subacute cerebellar degeneration, cortical degeneration, and polymyositis are seen with all lung cancer types. Many of these are caused by autoimmune responses such as the development of antivoltagegated calcium channel antibodies in the Eaton-Lambert syndrome. *Coagulation and thrombotic and hematologic manifestations* occur in 1 to 8 percent of patients and include migratory venous thrombophlebitis (*Trousseau's syndrome*), nonbacterial thrombotic (marantic) endocarditis with arterial emboli, disseminated intravascular coagulation with hemorrhage, and anemia, granulocytosis, and leukoerythroblastosis. *Cutaneous manifestations* such as dermatomyositis and acanthosis nigracans are uncommon (1 percent or less), as are the *renal manifestations* of nephrotic syndrome or glomerulonephritis (1 percent or less).

DIAGNOSIS AND STAGING

EARLY DIAGNOSIS Screening persons at high risk (males over 45 years of age smoking 40 or more cigarettes per day) for lung cancer with sputum cytologies and chest radiographs every 4 months has shown a prevalence rate of lung cancer in asymptomatic patients of 4 to 8 cases per 1000 persons. With follow-up screening, 4 new cases of lung cancer are found per 1000 persons followed per year. These lung cancers are detected 72 percent of the time by radiographs alone and 20 percent by cytology alone, while 6 percent are detected by both methods. In contrast to nonscreened patients, 90 percent of these screened patients who develop lung cancer are asymptomatic, 62 percent have resectable lung cancer, and 53 percent of all the new cases are postoperative stage I (see below) with a 5-year survival probability of 45 percent. However, in a large, multi-institutional, prospective, randomized trial there was no difference in the survival rate between the screened and the nonscreened group of smoking males 45 years of age or older. This was because of the presence of clinically silent and undetected metastases in the majority of patients even when primary tumors were detected at a very early stage.

ESTABLISHING A TISSUE DIAGNOSIS OF LUNG CANCER Once signs, symptoms, or screening studies suggest lung cancer, it is necessary to establish a tissue diagnosis of malignancy, determine the histologic cell type, and stage the patient for appropriate treatment. In the initial evaluation of each patient, tumor tissue should be obtained so that a histologic diagnosis of cancer and tumor cell type can be firmly made. Distinction of small cell from non-small cell lung cancer is crucial and is often difficult in cytology preparations. Therefore, cytologic diagnoses from washings or needle aspirates should be reserved for very high risk patients or patients relapsing with cancer after initial treatment. Tumor tissue can be obtained from a bronchial biopsy or transbronchial forceps biopsy at fiberoptic bronchoscopy; from node biopsy at mediastinoscopy; from the operative specimen at the time of definitive surgical resection; from percutaneous biopsy of an enlarged lymph node, soft tissue mass, lytic bone lesion, bone marrow, or pleural lesion; or from an adequate cell block from a malignant pleural effusion.

STAGING PATIENTS WITH LUNG CANCER Lung cancer staging consists of two parts: first, a determination of the location of tumor (anatomic staging) and, second, an assessment of a patient's ability to withstand various antitumor treatments (physiologic staging). For example, in a patient with non-small cell lung cancer, it is crucial to

TABLE 227-3   TNM classification of lung cancer using the new International Staging System (ISS)

PRIMARY TUMOR (T)

T0	No evidence of a primary tumor.
TX	Occult cancer seen in bronchial washing cytologies but not seen on x-ray or fiberoptic bronchoscopy.
TIS	Carcinoma in situ.
T1	Tumor ≤3 cm in greatest dimension, surrounded by lung or visceral pleura, and without evidence of invasion proximal to a lobar bronchus at bronchoscopy. (Uncommon superficial tumors of any size with invasive components limited to the bronchial wall that extend proximal to the main bronchus are also classified as T1.)
T2	Tumor >3 cm in greatest dimension *or* a tumor of any size that either invades the visceral pleura or has associated atelectasis–obstructive pneumonitis extending to the hilar region. At bronchoscopy, the proximal extent of demonstrable tumor must be within a lobar bronchus or at least 2 cm distal to the carina. Any associated atelectasis or obstructive pneumonitis must involve less than an entire lung.
T3	A tumor of any size with direct extension into the chest wall (including superior sulcus tumors), diaphragm, mediastinal pleura, or pericardium without involving heart, great vessels, trachea, esophagus, or vertebral body *or* a tumor in the main bronchus within 2 cm of the carina without involving the carina.
T4	A tumor of any size with invasion of the mediastinum or involving heart, great vessels, trachea, esophagus, vertebral body, or carina *or* the presence of a malignant pleural effusion. (Pleural effusions that are not bloody and not exudative with several negative cytopathologic examinations are not scored as a malignant effusion for staging purposes.)

REGIONAL LYMPH NODES (N)

N0	No demonstrable metastasis to regional lymph nodes.
N1	Metastasis to lymph nodes in the peribronchial or ipsilateral hilar region, or both, including direct extension.
N2	Metastasis to ipsilateral mediastinal or subcarinal lymph nodes.
N3	Metastasis to contralateral mediastinal, contralateral hilar, ipsilateral or contralateral scalene, or supraclavicular lymph nodes.

DISTANT METASTASIS (M)

M0	No known distant metastasis.
M1	Distant metastasis present with site specified (e.g., brain).

STAGE GROUPING USING THE NEW ISS

Occult carcinoma	TX	N0	M0
Stage 0	TIS	Carcinoma in situ	
Stage I	T1	N0	M0
	T2	N0	M0
Stage II	T1	N1	M0
	T2	N1	M0
Stage IIIa	T3	N0	M0
	T3	N1	M0
	T1–3	N2	M0
Stage IIIb	Any T	N3	M0
	T4	Any N	M0
Stage IV	Any T	Any N	M1

SOURCE: Adapted from CF Mountain, 1988.

TABLE 227-4   Pretreatment staging procedures for lung cancer patients

ALL PATIENTS

Complete history & physical examination
  Determination of performance status and weight loss
  Ear, nose, and throat examination
Complete blood count with platelet determination
Serum electrolytes, glucose, calcium, phosphorus, renal and liver function tests
Electrocardiogram
Skin test for tuberculosis
Chest x-ray
Computed tomography scan of brain, chest, abdomen, and radionuclide scan of bone if any of the above studies suggest presence of tumor metastasis in these organs
X-rays of suspicious bony lesions detected by scan or symptom
Barium swallow radiographic examination if esophageal symptoms exist
Pulmonary function studies and arterial blood gas measurements if signs or symptoms of respiratory insufficiency are present
Biopsy of accessible lesions suspicious for cancer if a histologic diagnosis is not yet made or if treatment or staging decisions would be based on whether or not a lesion contained cancer

PATIENTS PRESENTING WITH NO OBVIOUS CONTRAINDICATION TO CURATIVE SURGERY OR RADIOTHERAPY

All above and:

Fiberoptic bronchoscopy with washings, brushings, and biopsy of suspicious areas
Pulmonary function tests and arterial blood gas measurements
Coagulation tests
Computed tomographic scans of brain, chest, and abdomen
If surgical resection is planned: surgical evaluation of the mediastinum at mediastinoscopy or at thoracotomy
If the patient is a poor surgical risk or a candidate for curative radiotherapy: Transthoracic fine-needle aspiration biopsy or transbronchial forceps biopsy of peripheral lesions if material from routine fiberoptic bronchoscopy is negative

PATIENTS PRESENTING WITH DISEASE THAT IS NOT CURABLE BY EITHER SURGERY OR RADIOTHERAPY*

For non-small cell lung cancer or unknown, all under ''All Patients'' and:

Fiberoptic bronchoscopy if indicated by hemoptysis, obstruction, pneumonitis, or no histologic diagnosis of cancer
Biopsy of accessible lesions suspicious for tumor to obtain a histologic diagnosis or if therapy would be altered by finding of tumor
Transthoracic fine-needle aspiration biopsy or transbronchial forceps biopsy of peripheral lesions if fiberoptic bronchoscopy is negative and no other material exists for a histologic diagnosis
Diagnostic and therapeutic thoracentesis if a pleural effusion is present

For proven small cell lung cancer, all under ''All Patients'' and:

Fiberoptic bronchoscopy with washings and biopsy
Chest, abdomen, and brain CT scans useful but not mandatory
Bone marrow aspiration and biopsy

* Patients with non-small cell lung cancer and extrathoracic metastatic disease, malignant pleural effusion, or intrathoracic disease beyond the bounds of a tolerable radiotherapy port.

---

determine if the tumor can be resected by a standard surgical procedure such as a lobectomy or pneumonectomy (determination of *resectability*) based on the anatomic stage of the tumor and whether the patient could tolerate such a surgical procedure (determination of *operability*) based on the cardiopulmonary condition of the patient.

Non-small cell lung cancer   The TNM international stage system (ISS) developed by the American Joint Committee (AJC) on End Results Reporting, and modified by an international commission, should be used in non-small cell lung cancer, particularly in preparing patients for curative attempts with surgery or radiotherapy (Table 227-3). The various T (tumor size), N (regional node involvement), and M (presence or absence of distant metastasis) factors are combined to form different stage groups, and in addition, there is a group covering occult carcinoma detected on screening cytology exam with no other evidence of tumor (Table 227-3).

Small cell lung cancer   A simple two-stage system adapted from the Veterans Administration Lung Cancer Study Group is used. In this two-stage system, *limited-stage disease* (about 30 percent of all small cell cancer patients) is defined as disease confined to one hemithorax and regional lymph nodes (including mediastinal, contralateral hilar, and usually ipsilateral supraclavicular nodes), while *extensive-stage disease* (about 70 percent of all patients) is defined as disease beyond this. Employed in staging are clinical studies such as physical examination, x-rays, scans, and bone marrow examination. In part, the definition of *limited stage* relates to whether the known tumor can be encompassed within a tolerable radiation therapy port. Thus contralateral supraclavicular nodes, recurrent laryngeal nerve involvement, and superior vena caval obstruction can all be limited-stage disease. However, cardiac tamponade, malignant pleural effusion, and bilateral pulmonary parenchymal involvement are generally scored as extensive-stage disease because of the size of the radiation therapy port required to cover all known disease.

GENERAL STAGING PROCEDURES (See Table 227-4)   All lung cancer patients should have a complete history and physical examination, with evaluation of all other medical problems and a determination of performance status and weight loss, both of which have great prognostic value. An ear, nose, and throat examination is also necessary because of the frequent occurrence of second cancers in this area. While not done in every patient, fiberoptic bronchoscopy remains a cornerstone of lung cancer staging and follow-up, providing material for pathologic examination and information on tumor size, location, degree of bronchial obstruction, and recurrence.

Chest roentgenograms are needed to evaluate tumor size and nodal involvement, and it is very useful to obtain old x-ray films for comparison. Computed tomography (CT) scans (chest and abdomen) are now widely used in the staging and follow-up of lung cancer patients. CT scans are of use in non-small cell lung cancer in preoperative staging to detect mediastinal nodes and pleural extension and occult abdominal disease (e.g., liver and adrenal glands), as well as in the planning of curative radiation therapy to allow design of fields to encompass all known tumor volume while avoiding as much normal tissue as possible. However, definitive characterization of mediastinal nodal involvement should depend on histologic proof when planning curative treatment. Likewise, unless the CT-detected abnormalities are unequivocal, malignancy of suspicious abdominal lesions should be confirmed by procedures such as fine-needle aspiration if the patient would otherwise be considered for curative treatment. In small cell lung cancer, CT scans are used for chest radiation treatment planning and assessing the response to chemotherapy and radiation therapy. In following patients after surgery or radiotherapy, procedures which can make interpretation of conventional chest x-rays difficult, CT scans can provide good evidence of tumor recurrence.

If signs or symptoms suggest organ involvement by tumor, appropriate CT or radionuclide scans (e.g., brain, liver, or bone) are performed, as well as radiographs of any suspicious bony lesions. Any accessible lesions suspicious for cancer should be biopsied if a histologic diagnosis has not already been made or if treatment decisions would be based on whether or not the lesion contained cancer.

In patients presenting with a mass lesion on chest x-ray and no obvious contraindications to a curative approach with surgery or radiotherapy after the initial evaluation, the mediastinum must be investigated. Approaches vary between different centers and include performing chest CT scan and mediastinoscopy (right-sided tumors) or lateral mediastinotomy (left-sided lesions) on all patients and proceeding directly to thoracotomy with staging of the mediastinum. In patients presenting with disease confined to the chest but not resectable, thus making them candidates for curative radiotherapy, other tests are done as indicated to evaluate specific symptoms. In patients presenting with non-small cell cancer that is not curable by either surgery, radiotherapy, or their combination, all the general procedures are done plus fiberoptic bronchoscopy as indicated to evaluate hemoptysis, obstruction, or pneumonitis, as well as diagnostic-therapeutic thoracentesis with cytologic examination if fluid is present.

STAGING OF SMALL CELL LUNG CANCER   Pretreatment staging for patients with histologically documented small cell lung cancer includes the initial general lung cancer evaluation as well as fiberoptic bronchoscopy with washings and biopsies to determine the tumor extent before therapy; brain CT scan, since 10 percent of patients have metastases; bone marrow biopsy and aspiration, since 20 to 30 percent of patients have tumor in the bone marrow; and CT (liver) and radionuclide scans (bone) if symptoms or other findings are suggestive of disease involvement in these areas. Chest and abdominal CT scans are very useful but not mandatory to evaluate and follow tumor response to therapy. CT-directed liver biopsy may be performed if other findings are suggestive but not diagnostic of the presence of tumor in the liver and if tumor involvement there would alter the planned therapy.

If signs or symptoms of spinal cord compression or leptomeningitis develop at any time in lung cancer patients of any histologic type, a myelogram or magnetic resonance scan and examination of the cerebrospinal fluid cytology are performed to determine the need for local therapy to the site of compression (usually with radiotherapy) and for intrathecal chemotherapy (usually with methotrexate) if malignant cells are detected. In addition, a brain CT scan is performed to search for brain metastases that are often associated with spinal cord or leptomeningeal metastases.

DETERMINATION OF RESECTABILITY AND OPERABILITY   In patients with non-small cell lung cancer, the following are major contraindications to curative attempts by surgery or radiotherapy alone using standard treatment methods: extrathoracic distant metastases, superior vena cava syndrome, vocal cord and, in most cases, phrenic nerve paralysis, malignant pleural effusion, cardiac tamponade, tumor within 2 cm of the carina (not curable by surgery but potentially curable by radiotherapy), metastasis to the contralateral lung, bilateral endobronchial tumor (potentially curable by radiotherapy), metastasis to the supraclavicular lymph nodes, lymph node metastasis in the contralateral mediastinum (potentially curable by radiotherapy), involvement of the main stem pulmonary artery. While a histologic diagnosis of small cell lung cancer is usually highly correlated with other findings of unresectability, if all other findings suggest the potential for resection, this option should be considered. This is usually encountered in small peripheral small cell lung cancer lesions (see below).

PHYSIOLOGIC STAGING   Patients with lung cancer often have cardiopulmonary and other problems related to chronic obstructive pulmonary disease as well as other medical problems. To improve their preoperative condition, correctable problems (e.g., anemia, electrolyte and fluid disorders, infections, and arrhythmias) should be addressed, smoking stopped, and appropriate chest therapy instituted. Since it is not always possible to predict whether a lobectomy or pneumonectomy will be required until the time of operation, a conservative approach is to restrict resectional surgery to patients who could potentially tolerate a pneumonectomy. In addition to nonambulatory performance status, a myocardial infarction within the past 3 months is a contraindication to thoracic surgery because 20 percent of patients will die of reinfarction alone, while an infarction in the past 6 months is a relative contraindication. Other major contraindications include uncontrolled major arrhythmias, maximum breathing capacities of less than 40 percent predicted, an FEV_1 of less than 1 L, CO_2 retention (which is more serious than hypoxemia), and severe pulmonary hypertension. Recommending surgery when the FEV_1 is 1.1 to 2.4 L requires careful judgment, while an FEV_1 of over 2.5 L will usually permit a pneumonectomy. In patients with borderline pulmonary status or a question of pulmonary hypertension, split pulmonary function testing by ventilation-perfusion lung scans can define physiologic operability. The activity from quantitative scans is summed for each lung in the anterior and posterior views, and the ratio of the normal to total lung activity is multiplied by the FEV_1. Pneumonectomy usually is physiologically tolerable if this predicted value is greater than 1 L.

TREATMENT

After a histologic diagnosis is obtained and appropriate anatomic and physiologic staging studies are completed, the overall treatment approach to patients with lung cancer may be formulated (Table 227-5).

NON-SMALL CELL LUNG CANCER: LOCALIZED DISEASE   In patients with non-small cell lung cancer of stages I and II (see Table 227-3) who can tolerate operation, the treatment of choice is pulmonary resection. In stage IIIa cases with favorable age, cardiopulmonary function, and anatomy, resection also should be considered. If a complete resection is possible, the 5-year survival rate for N1 disease is about 50 percent, while it is about 30 percent for N2 disease. However, only 20 percent of all patients who have N2 disease are technically resectable, and in most cases these resectable patients

TABLE 227-5   Summary of treatment approach to lung cancer patients

NON-SMALL CELL LUNG CANCER

Resectable (stages I, II, IIIa, and selected T3, N2 lesions)
 Surgery
 Radiotherapy for "nonoperable" patients
 Postoperative radiotherapy for N2 disease
Nonresectable (N2 and M1)
 Confined to chest: high-dose chest radiotherapy (RT) if possible
 Extrathoracic: RT to symptomatic local sites; chemotherapy (CT) (for
  good-performance-status patients, with evaluable lesions)

SMALL CELL LUNG CANCER

Limited stage (good performance status)
 Combination chemotherapy + chest RT
Extensive stage (good performance status)
 Combination chemotherapy
Complete tumor responders (all stages)
 Prophylactic cranial RT
Poor-performance-status patients (all stages)
 Modified-dose combination chemotherapy
 Palliative RT

ALL PATIENTS

Radiotherapy for brain metastases, spinal cord compression, weight-bearing
 lytic bony lesions, symptomatic local lesions (nerve paralyses, obstructed
 airway, hemoptysis in non-small cell lung cancer and in small cell cancer
 not responding to chemotherapy)
Appropriate diagnosis and treatment of other medical problems and
 supportive care during chemotherapy
Encouragement to stop smoking
Entrance into clinical trial, if eligible

are discovered to have N2 disease only at thoracotomy. Patients with contralateral or bilateral positive mediastinal (N3) nodes, extracapsular nodal involvement, or fixed nodes are not currently considered resectable. New approaches to convert patients from unresectable to resectable status include chest wall resections for direct extension of tumor, tracheal sleeve pneumonectomy, and sleeve lobectomy for lesions near the carina. Neoadjuvant (preoperative) chemotherapy, while experimental, gives tumor response rates of 50 to 60 percent and converts many responding patients to resectability. Video-assisted thoracic surgery (VATS) via thoracoscopy is being evaluated.

The extent of resection is a matter of surgical judgment based on findings at exploration. In general, conservative resection that encompasses all known tumor gives survival equal to that obtained with more extensive procedures. However, recent data from the Lung Cancer Study Group show that lobectomy is superior to wedge resection in terms of reducing local recurrences. Thus lobectomy is preferred to pneumonectomy and wedge resection, while wedge resections and segmentectomies are reserved for patients with poor pulmonary reserve and small peripheral lesions. Approximately 43 percent of all lung cancer patients will undergo thoracotomy. Of these, 76 percent will have a definitive resection, 12 percent will only be explored for disease extent, and 12 percent will have a palliative procedure with known disease left behind. The fraction of long-term survivors following definitive surgical therapy is remarkably consistent throughout major centers performing lung cancer surgery in the United States. Approximately 30 percent of all patients resected for cure survive 5 years, and 15 percent survive 10 years. The 30-day hospital mortality following pulmonary resection at major centers is also very consistent, 3 percent for lobectomy and 6 percent for pneumonectomy. As a function of postoperative treatment stage, the 5-year survival data are (1) epidermoid: stage I, 54 percent, stage II, 35 percent, stage IIIa N0–N1, 19 percent, stage IIIa N2, 13 percent, and (2) adenocarcinoma and large cell carcinoma: stage I, 51 percent, stage II, 18 percent, stage IIIa N0–N1, 10 percent, stage IIIa N2, 2 percent. Thus the majority of patients who were initially thought to have a "curative" resection ultimately died of metastatic disease (usually within 2 years of surgery).

MANAGEMENT OF OCCULT AND STAGE 0 CARCINOMAS
When sputum cytology screening indicates malignant cells but a normal chest radiograph is found (TX tumor stage), the lesion must be localized. Over 90 percent can be localized by meticulous examination of the bronchial tree with a fiberoptic bronchoscope under general anesthesia and collection of a series of differential brushings and biopsies. Often carcinoma in situ or multicentric lesions are found in these patients. Current recommendations are for the most conservative surgical resection, allowing removal of the cancer and conservation of lung parenchyma even if the bronchial margins are positive for carcinoma in situ. The 5-year overall survival for these occult cancers is approximately 60 percent. Close follow-up of these patients is indicated because of the high incidence of second primary lung cancers (approximately 5 percent per patient per year). A new approach to in situ or multicentric lesions uses systemically administered hematoporphyrin (which localizes to tumors and sensitizes them to light) followed by bronchoscopic phototherapy.

SOLITARY PULMONARY NODULE   When a patient presents with an asymptomatic, solitary pulmonary nodule (defined as an x-ray density completely surrounded by normal aerated lung, with circumscribed margins, of any shape, usually 1 to 6 cm in greatest diameter), a decision to resect or follow the nodule must be made. Approximately 35 percent of all such lesions in adults will be malignant, the majority being primary lung cancer, while less than 1 percent are malignant in nonsmoking patients under 35 years of age. A complete history, including a smoking history, physical examination, routine laboratory tests, fiberoptic bronchoscopy, and old chest x-rays are obtained. If no diagnosis is immediately apparent, the following risk factors would all argue strongly in favor of proceeding with resection to establish a histologic diagnosis: history of cigarette smoking; age 35 years or older; a relatively large-sized lesion; lack of calcification; chest symptoms; associated atelectasis, pneumonitis, or adenopathy; and growth of the lesion compared with old x-rays. At present, only two radiographic criteria are strongly reliable for benignity of a solitary pulmonary nodule: lack of growth over a period greater than 2 years and certain characteristic patterns of calcification. Calcification alone does not exclude malignancy. However, a dense central nidus, multiple punctate foci, and "bull's eye" (granuloma) and "popcorn ball" (hamartoma) calcifications are all highly suggestive of a benign lesion.

When old x-rays are not available and the characteristic calcification patterns are absent, the following approach is reasonable: Nonsmoking patients under 35 years can be followed with serial chest x-rays every 3 months for 1 year and then yearly. If any significant growth is found, a histologic diagnosis is needed. For patients over age 35 and all patients with a smoking history, a histologic diagnosis must be made. This can occur either at the time of nodule resection or, if the patient is a poor operative risk, via transthoracic fine-needle biopsy. Some institutions would use preoperative fine-needle aspiration on all such lesions; however, all positive lesions will have to proceed to resection, and negative cytologic findings will in most cases have to be confirmed by histology on a resected specimen. While much has been made of sparing patients an operation, the high probability of finding a malignancy (particularly in smokers over age 35) and the excellent chance for surgical cure when the tumor is small both suggest an aggressive approach to these lesions.

RADIOTHERAPY   Those patients who are stage III, as well as those with stages I and II disease who refuse surgery or appear not to be candidates for pulmonary resection for medical reasons, should be considered for radiation therapy with curative intent. The decision to administer high-dose and potentially curative radiotherapy is based on the extent of disease and the volume of the chest that requires irradiation. Patients with distant metastases, positive supraclavicular nodes, pleural effusion, or cardiac involvement are generally not considered for such curative radiation treatment. The median survival for unresectable patients with non-small cell lung cancer localized to the chest undergoing primary radiotherapy with curative intent is less than 1 year. However, 6 percent of these patients are alive at 5 years and cured when treated with radiotherapy alone. In addition to potential cure, radiotherapy, by controlling the primary tumor, may increase the quality and length of life of noncured patients. Treatment usually involves midplane doses of 55 to 60 Gy (5500 to 6000 rad), and the major concern is the amount of lung parenchyma and other organs in the thorax included within the treatment plan, including the spinal cord, heart, and esophagus. Patients with a major degree of underlying pulmonary disease may have to have the treatment plan compromised because of the deleterious effect of radiation on pulmonary function. Recent studies suggest that continuous fraction radiotherapy be given. The development of radiation pneumonitis is proportional to the dose of radiation and volume of lung incorporated within the radiation field. The full clinical syndrome (dyspnea, fever, and radiographic infiltrate corresponding to the treatment port) occurs in 5 percent of cases. Acute radiation esophagitis occurs during treatment but usually is self-limited, while spinal cord injury should be avoided by careful treatment planning. Twice-daily fractionated chest radiotherapy may achieve high doses and avoid toxicity.

COMBINED-MODALITY THERAPY Recent randomized trials have shown survival benefit for adjuvant chemotherapy given after surgical resection. However, this will have to be confirmed before adjuvant chemotherapy after surgery or radiotherapy is recommended for general use. While many centers give high-dose postoperative radiation if postoperative staging documents nodal disease, its efficacy has not been established. However, a randomized trial of postoperative radiotherapy, while showing improved local tumor control, did not show survival benefit.

Carcinomas of the superior pulmonary sulcus producing *Pancoast's syndrome* are often treated with combined radiotherapy and surgery. These patients should have the usual preoperative staging procedures, including mediastinoscopy and CT scans to determine tumor extent and neurologic examination with electromyography to document neurologic findings. Often a histologic diagnosis is not made, and with the constellation of tumor location and pain distribution, the diagnostic accuracy for cancer is better than 90 percent. If mediastinoscopy is negative, two curative approaches may be used in treating a Pancoast's syndrome tumor. In the first, preoperative irradiation [30 Gy (3000 rad) in 10 treatments] is given to the area followed by an en bloc resection of the tumor and involved chest wall 3 to 6 weeks later. At 3 years, survival figures of 42 percent for epidermoid and 21 percent for adeno- and large cell carcinomas have been reported. The second approach involves radiotherapy alone in curative doses and standard fractionation with similar survival to combined-modality therapy reported.

Data have now appeared suggesting a high frequency of brain metastases as isolated sites of relapse in patients with adenocarcinoma of the lung otherwise cured by surgery or radiotherapy. While there is no proven role for "prophylactic" cranial irradiation, it is not unreasonable to follow potentially cured, asymptomatic adenocarcinoma patients with frequent brain CT scans to detect such recurrence at the earliest possible time so that radiotherapy can be given.

DISSEMINATED NON-SMALL CELL LUNG CANCER The 70 percent of patients who have unresectable non-small cell cancer have a poor prognosis. For example, median survivals of 34, 25, 17, 8, and 4 weeks are seen for patients with performance status scores of 0 (asymptomatic), 1 (symptomatic, fully ambulatory), 2 (in bed < 50 percent of the time), 3 (in bed > 50 percent of the time), and 4 (bedridden), respectively. Standard medical management, the judicious use of pain medications, and the appropriate use of radiotherapy form the cornerstone of management. Patients whose primary tumors are causing symptoms such as bronchial obstruction with pneumonitis, hemoptysis, or upper airway or superior vena caval (SVC) obstruction should, in general, have radiotherapy to the primary tumor. The case for prophylactic treatment of the asymptomatic patient is to prevent major symptoms from occurring within the thorax. However, if the patient can be followed closely, deferring treatment until the development of symptoms is appropriate. Usually a course of 30 to 40 Gy (3000 to 4000 rad) over 2 to 4 weeks is given to the

tumor. The frequencies of relief by radiation therapy of intrathoracic symptoms are hemoptysis, 84 percent; SVC syndrome, 80 percent; dyspnea, 60 percent; cough, 60 percent; atelectasis, 23 percent; and vocal cord paralysis, 6 percent. Other symptoms of metastatic disease treated with radiotherapy include cardiac tamponade (treated with pericardiocentesis and radiation therapy to the entire cardiac silhouette), painful bony metastases (with relief in 66 percent of cases), brain or spinal cord compression, and brachial plexus involvement. Usually, with brain and cord compression, dexamethasone (25 to 100 mg total per day in four divided doses) is also given and then rapidly tapered to the lowest dosage which relieves neurologic symptoms.

The key to effective palliation is to detect the complication and begin radiotherapy at the earliest possible time. Pleural effusions are common and are usually treated with thoracentesis as needed, but without radiotherapy. If they recur and are symptomatic, chest tube drainage with a sclerosing agent such as intrapleural doxycycline is used. First, the chest cavity is completely drained. Xylocaine 1% is instilled (15 mL), followed by 50 mL normal saline. Then 500 to 750 mg doxycycline HCl is dissolved in 100 mL normal saline, and this is injected via the chest tube. The chest tube is clamped for 4 h if tolerated, and the patient is rotated onto different sides to distribute the sclerosing agent. Then 24 to 48 h later the chest tube is pulled when there is little drainage (usually less than 100 mL per 24 h). Recently, video-assisted thoracoscopy has been used to drain and treat large malignant effusions. Symptomatic intrabronchial lesions that recur after surgery or radiotherapy, or the development of such lesions in patients with severely compromised pulmonary function, are difficult to treat with conventional therapy. However, neodymium-YAG (yttrium-aluminum-garnet) laser therapy administered via a flexible fiberoptic bronchoscope (usually under general anesthesia) can provide palliation to 80 to 90 percent of patients even when the tumor has relapsed after radiotherapy. In addition, patients can be retreated with YAG laser therapy.

Chemotherapy The use of chemotherapy for non-small cell lung cancer requires careful judgment to balance potential benefits and toxicity. However, recent results suggest modest survival benefits from such combination chemotherapy. Approximately 30 to 40 percent of patients will have objective tumor response to combination chemotherapy. However, a complete clinical regression of tumor (a *complete response*) occurs in less than 5 percent of cases. Those patients whose tumors respond to chemotherapy have significantly longer survivals (around 30 to 40 weeks median survival) compared with those patients who do not respond to therapy (10 to 20 weeks median). The problem is that the responding patients also have better prognostic features (such as good performance status), and it is difficult to separate the effect of these on survival from that of chemotherapy. However, in patients with good performance status, response to chemotherapy is also associated with prolonged survival and, in some cases, relief of symptoms. Nevertheless, such combination chemotherapy can have severe side effects, including treatment-related mortality. Thus, in those patients with non-small cell lung cancer who desire chemotherapy, it is reasonable to give chemotherapy if the patient is fully ambulatory, has an evaluable tumor mass (to follow response to therapy), has not received prior chemotherapy, and is able to understand and accept the potential benefits and toxicities from such therapy. The chemotherapy should be delivered by an experienced physician or medical oncologist, who should use one of the published standard regimens, such as etoposide + cisplatin. Finally, all eligible patients should be encouraged to enter clinical trials.

SMALL CELL LUNG CANCER Untreated patients with small cell lung cancer have median survivals of only 6 to 17 weeks, while patients treated with combination chemotherapy have median survivals of 40 to 70 weeks. Thus the correct integration of chemotherapy with or without radiotherapy or surgery is the cornerstone of the treatment of small cell cancer. The goal of treatment is to obtain a complete clinical regression of tumor documented by repeating the initial positive staging procedures, particularly fiberoptic bronchoscopy with washings and biopsy. The initial response, determined 6 to 12 weeks after the start of therapy, predicts both median and long-term survival and potential cure. Patients obtaining a complete clinical regression of tumor survive longer than patients with only partial regression (tumor shrinkage of more than 50 percent of visible disease with no sign of tumor progression elsewhere), who in turn survive longer than patients with no response. In addition, all long-term (over 3 years) survivors come from the complete response group.

Following initial staging, patients are grouped into the limited or extensive disease stages and classified as being physiologically able or not able to tolerate combination chemotherapy or combined-modality chemoradiotherapy. The overall mortality rate from initial combination chemotherapy even in these selected patients is about 5 percent at major centers. This figure is comparable with the operative mortality rate for pulmonary resection and indicates the need for physiologic staging of patients before chemotherapy. Such therapy should be reserved for ambulatory patients with no prior chemotherapy or radiotherapy, no other major medical problems, and adequate heart, liver, renal, and bone marrow function. The arterial P_{O_2} on room air should be above 6.6 kPa (50 mmHg), and there should be no CO_2 retention. All patients with some or more of these limitations must have their initial chemoradio- or chemotherapy modified to prevent undue toxicity. In all patients the chemoradiotherapy must be coupled with supportive care for infectious, hemorrhagic, and other medical complications. This induction period is best supervised by a medical oncologist. Meticulous attention to the details of therapy and the day-to-day management of the patient through the initial 6 to 12 weeks of treatment is essential if therapy-related mortality is to be kept low.

Chemotherapy A variety of effective combination chemotherapy regimens have been reported for small cell lung cancer, including CAV (cyclophosphamide + doxorubicin + vincristine), CAVP-16 (cyclophosphamide + doxorubicin + VP-16), and VP-16 (etoposide) + cisplatin. At present, there is no evidence that any one regimen is better than another if adequate drug dosages and schedules are used. The initial combination chemotherapy often results in moderate to severe granulocytopenia (e.g., granulocyte counts less than 500 to 1500 per microliter) and thrombocytopenia (platelets less than 50,000 to 100,000 per microliter). Following the initial *induction* therapy, patients should be restaged to determine if they have entered a *complete clinical remission*, indicated by complete disappearance of all clinically evident lesions and paraneoplastic syndromes, or a *partial remission*, or have *no response* or tumor progression (seen in 10 percent of patients or less). Following this, *maintenance* chemotherapy is given to responding patients for periods of 6 to 12 months in 3-, 4-, or 6-week cycles, depending on the chemotherapy regimen used. Appropriate drug dose modifications are made to keep the white blood count above 2000 per microliter and the platelet count above 50,000 per microliter. The patients are restaged between 6 and 12 months, depending on the individual regimens; if they are still in a complete remission, chemotherapy is stopped. The value of more prolonged chemotherapy is not documented. Patients with a partial tumor regression are generally kept on chemotherapy until the time of objective tumor progression and then switched to new chemotherapy (either with known activity or on an experimental protocol). Patients not responding or with objective tumor progression should be switched to new chemotherapy, preferably with a non-cross-resistant combination in an attempt to get an objective tumor response.

Radiotherapy High-dose [40 Gy (4000 rad)] radiotherapy to the whole brain should be given to patients with documented brain metastases. Prophylactic cranial irradiation (PCI) may be given to patients with complete responses, since this will significantly decrease the development of brain metastases (occurring in 60 to 80 percent of patients living 2 or more years who do not receive such prophylactic radiotherapy), but such prophylactic therapy has not been shown to prolong survival. Because some studies indicate possible deficits in cognitive ability that could be related to PCI, long-term quality of life after PCI needs to be further studied. In the case of symptomatic,

progressive lesions in the chest or at other critical sites, if radiotherapy has not yet been given to these areas, it may be administered in full doses [e.g., 40 Gy (4000 rad) to the chest tumor mass].

There are definite toxicities of both an acute and chronic nature that should be expected with combined-modality chemoradiotherapy, particularly if chemo- and radiotherapy are given concurrently. However, retrospective analyses of long-term survivors and analyses of local failures in the chest following chemotherapy alone suggest that chest radiotherapy is of benefit, and thus it is currently recommended for limited-stage patients. Patients should be selected (limited-stage disease with PS 0–1 and initial good pulmonary function) such that radiotherapy can be given in full doses and in a manner that will not sacrifice too much lung. The radiation oncologist must be prepared to deliver tailored radiotherapy with shaping of fields during treatment, much the same as is done for Hodgkin's disease. Several centers employing twice-daily radiotherapy with concomitant etoposide + cisplatin chemotherapy have reported good results with respect to local tumor control and toxicity. In extensive-stage disease, the routine use of initial chest radiotherapy usually is not advocated. However, in favorable patients (e.g., those with PS 0–1, good pulmonary function, and only one site of extensive disease), radiotherapy can be considered. In all patients, if chemotherapy is inadequate to relieve local tumor symptoms, a course of radiotherapy can be added.

Several centers around the world have reported potential cure rates of 15 to 25 percent for limited-stage disease and 1 to 5 percent for extensive-stage disease. Overall, approximately 50 percent of patients with limited-stage and 30 percent with extensive-stage disease will enter a complete remission, and 90 to 95 percent of all patients will have some objective tumor shrinkage (complete or partial response). These responses increase the median survival from 2 to 4 months for untreated patients to 10 to 12 months for extensive-stage and 14 to 18 months for limited-stage patients. In addition, most patients have relief of their tumor-related symptoms and improvement of performance status. However, the maintenance of good performance status by the patient while receiving outpatient chemotherapy requires judgment and skill on the part of the medical oncologist delivering the chemotherapy so as to avoid undue therapeutic toxicity. New treatments such as new drug combinations, very intensive initial or "reinduction" therapy with autologous bone marrow infusion, as well as novel forms of combining chemo- and radiotherapy and surgery should all be reserved for approved clinical protocols.

While surgical resection is not routinely recommended for small cell lung cancer, occasional small cell cancer patients will either meet the usual AJC requirements for resectability (stage I or II with negative mediastinal nodes) or only have a histologic diagnosis made on review of the resected surgical specimen. Such patients have been reported to have high cure rates (above 25 percent) if adjuvant combination chemotherapy is used. Thus such uncommon, resectable small cell lung cancer patients are candidates for combined-modality surgery and chemotherapy.

BENIGN LUNG NEOPLASMS

The benign neoplasms of the lung, representing less than 5 percent of all primary tumors, include bronchial adenomas and hamartomas (90 percent of such lesions) and a group of very uncommon neoplasms (chondromas, fibromas, lipomas, hemangiomas, leiomyomas, teratomas, pseudolymphomas, and endometriosis). The diagnostic and primary treatment approach is basically the same for all these neoplasms. They can present as central masses causing airway obstruction, cough, hemoptysis, and pneumonitis with or without x-ray findings but be accessible to fiberoptic bronchoscopy. Alternatively, they can present without symptoms as solitary pulmonary nodules and thus will be evaluated as part of a solitary pulmonary nodule workup. In all cases, the extent of surgery must be determined at operation, and a conservative procedure with appropriate reconstructions is usually performed.

BRONCHIAL ADENOMAS Bronchial adenomas (80 percent of which are central) are slowly growing intrabronchial lesions that represent 50 percent of all benign pulmonary neoplasms. Eighty to ninety percent are carcinoids, 10 to 15 percent are adenocystic tumors (or cylindromas), and 2 to 3 percent are mucoepidermoid tumors. Adenomas present in patients 15 to 60 years old (average age 45) as intrabronchial lesions and are often symptomatic for several years. Patients may have chronic cough, recurrent hemoptysis, or obstruction with atelectasis, lobar collapse, or pneumonitis and abscess formation. Bronchial carcinoids, which usually follow a benign course, and small cell lung cancers, which are highly malignant, are both derived from the same normal bronchial epithelial component, the Kulchitsky cell. This cell is part of the amine precursor uptake and decarboxylation (APUD) system. Carcinoids, like small cell lung cancers, may secrete other hormones such as ACTH or arginine vasopressin and thus cause paraneoplastic syndromes which resolve with resection. In addition, bronchial carcinoids when metastatic (usually to the liver) may produce the carcinoid syndrome, with cutaneous flush, bronchoconstriction, diarrhea, and cardiac valvular lesions (see Chap. 276), which small cell lung cancer does not. Occasionally, pathologists may have difficulty in distinguishing carcinoids from small cell lung cancers. Carcinoid tumors appearing more aggressive histologically (referred to as *atypical carcinoids*) metastasize in 70 percent of cases to regional nodes, liver, or bone, compared with only a 5 percent metastasis rate of carcinoids with typical histology.

Bronchial adenomas of all types, because of their endobronchial and often central location, are usually visible via fiberoptic bronchoscopy, and tissue for histologic diagnosis is obtained in this manner. Because they are hypervascular, they can bleed profusely after bronchoscopic biopsy, and this should be anticipated. Bronchial adenomas must be dealt with as potentially malignant and thus require removal not only for symptom relief but also because they can be locally invasive or recurrent, potentially can metastasize, or may produce paraneoplastic syndromes. Surgical excision is the primary treatment for all types of bronchial adenomas. The extent of surgery is determined at operation and should be as conservative as possible. Often bronchotomy with local excision, sleeve resection, segmental resection, or lobectomy is sufficient. Five-year survival rates following surgical resection are 95 percent, decreasing to 70 percent if regional nodes are involved. The treatment of metastatic pulmonary carcinoids is currently unclear because they can either be indolent, growing slowly over several years, or behave more like small cell lung carcinoma. Assessment of the tempo and histology of the disease in the individual patient is necessary to determine if and when chemotherapy or radiotherapy is indicated.

HAMARTOMAS Pulmonary hamartomas have a peak incidence at age 60 and are more frequent in men than in women. Histologically, they contain normal pulmonary tissue components (smooth muscle and collagen) in a disorganized fashion. They are usually peripheral, clinically silent, and benign in their behavior. While it would be advantageous to avoid thoracotomy in these older patients, unless the radiographic findings are pathognomonic of hamartoma with "popcorn" calcification, the lesions will usually have to be resected for diagnosis, particularly if the patient is a smoker.

METASTATIC PULMONARY TUMORS

The lung is frequently the site of metastatic disease from primary cancers outside the lung. Usually such metastatic disease is considered incurable. However, two special situations may arise. First is the development of a solitary pulmonary shadow on chest x-ray in a patient known to have an extrathoracic neoplasm. This may represent a metastasis or a new primary lung cancer. Because the natural history of lung cancer is worse than for most other primary tumors, it is wise to approach the single pulmonary nodule in a patient with a known extrathoracic tumor as though the nodule were a primary lung cancer, particularly if the patient is over 35 years of age and a smoker. This means a vigorous evaluation looking for other sites of active cancer and, if none are found, surgical resection of the nodule. Second, multiple pulmonary nodules may be resected for cure as well. This is usually recommended if, after careful staging, (1) the patient can tolerate the contemplated pulmonary resection, (2) the primary tumor has been definitively and successfully treated, and (3) all known metastatic disease can be encompassed by the projected pulmonary resection. The key is selection and screening of patients to exclude patients with uncontrolled primary tumors and extrapulmonary metastases. Primary tumors whose pulmonary metastases have been successfully resected for cure include osteogenic and soft tissue sarcomas; colon, rectal, uterine, cervix, and corpus tumors; head and neck, breast, testis, and salivary gland cancer; melanoma; and bladder and kidney tumors. Five-year survival rates of 20 to 30 percent have been found in carefully selected patients, and the most dramatic results have been seen in osteogenic sarcomas, where resection of pulmonary metastases (sometimes requiring several thoracotomies) is becoming a standard curative treatment approach.

REFERENCES

BENOWITZ NL: Pharmacologic aspects of cigarette smoking and nicotine addiction. N Engl J Med 319:1318, 1988

CARBONE DP, MINNA JD: The molecular genetics of lung cancer. Adv Intern Med 37:145, 1991

GINSBERG RJ et al: Cancer of the lung: Non-small cell lung cancer, in *The Principles and Practice of Oncology*, 4th ed, VT DeVita et al (eds). Philadelphia, Lippincott, 1992

———, RUBENSTEIN L, FOR THE LCSG: Patients with T1N0 non-small cell lung cancer: Local recurrence increase with limited resection. Lung Cancer 7(suppl):83,1991

HENDERSON BE et al: Toward the primary prevention of cancer. Science 254:1131, 1991

IHDE DC, MINNA JD: Non-small cell lung cancer: I. Biology, diagnosis, and staging. Curr Probl Cancer 15:63, 1991

———, ———: Non-small cell lung cancer: II. Treatment. Curr Probl Cancer 15:107, 1991

——— et al: Cancer of the lung: Small cell lung cancer, in *The Principles and Practice of Oncology*, 4th ed, VT DeVita et al (eds). Philadelphia, Lippincott, 1992

LUNG CANCER STUDY GROUP: Effects of postoperative mediastinal radiation on completely resected stage II and stage III epidermoid cancer of the lung. N Engl J Med 315:1377, 1986

MACK M et al: The present role of thoracoscopy in the diagnosis and treatment of diseases of the chest. Ann Thorac Surg 54:403, 1992

MANSSON I: Treatment of malignant pleural effusion with doxycycline. Scand J Infect Dis Suppl 53:29, 1988

MOUNTAIN CF: Prognostic implications of the International Staging System for Lung Cancer: A new international staging system for lung cancer. Semin Oncol 15:236, 1988

———: Value of the new TNM staging system for lung cancer. Chest 96:475, 1989

THE HEALTH CONSEQUENCES OF SMOKING: Nicotine Addiction. A report of the Surgeon General. Washington, DC, Dept Health and Human Services, 1988

228 DISORDERS OF THE PLEURA, MEDIASTINUM, AND DIAPHRAGM

RICHARD W. LIGHT

DISORDERS OF THE PLEURA

STRUCTURE AND FUNCTION The pleural space lies between the lung and chest wall and normally contains a very thin layer of fluid. The pleural space with its thin layer of liquid serves as a coupling system between the lung and chest wall. The serous membrane covering the lung parenchyma is called the *visceral pleura*, while the serous membrane covering the chest wall, the diaphragm, and the mediastinum is called the *parietal pleura*.

PLEURAL EFFUSION A patient has a pleural effusion when there is an excess amount of fluid in the pleural space. More than 1 million cases of pleural effusion occur annually in the United States.

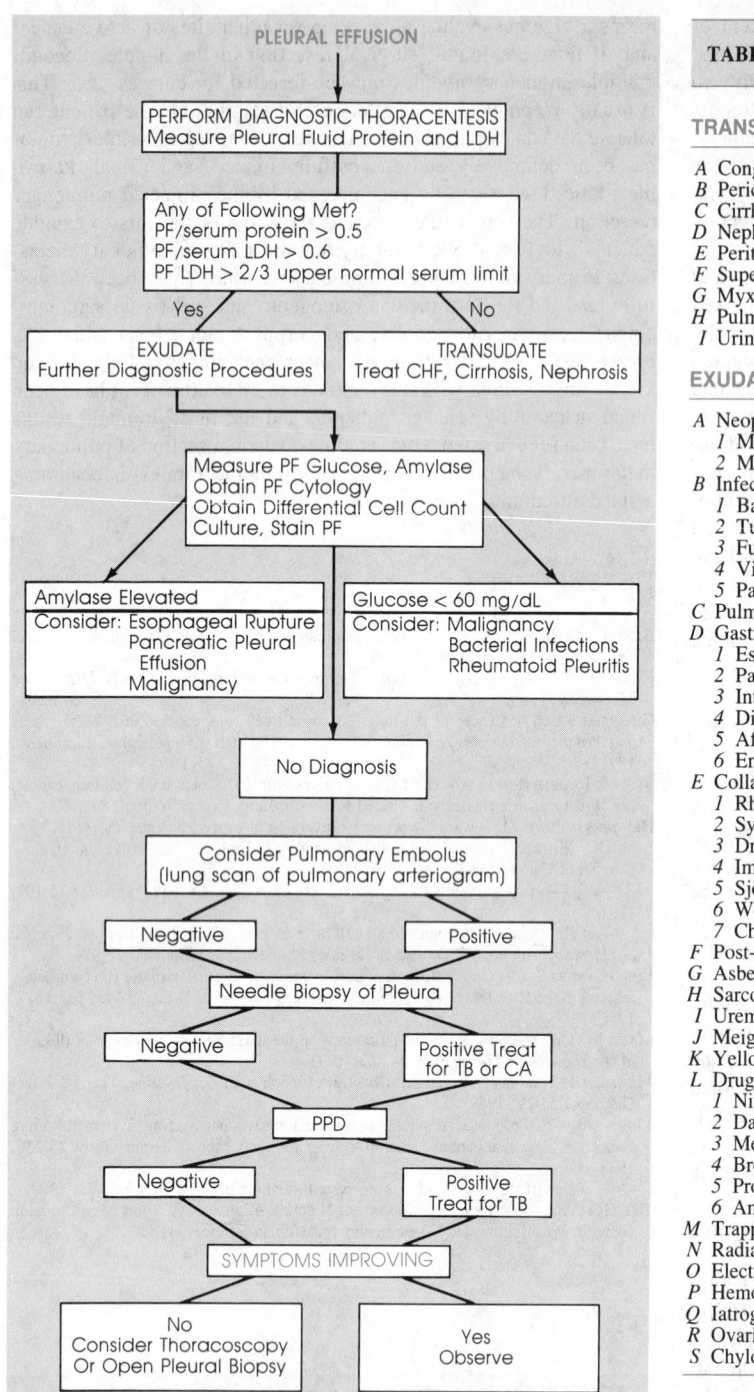

FIGURE 228-1   Approach to the diagnosis of pleural effusions.

TABLE 228-1   Differential diagnoses of pleural effusions

TRANSUDATIVE PLEURAL EFFUSIONS

A   Congestive heart failure
B   Pericardial disease
C   Cirrhosis
D   Nephrotic syndrome
E   Peritoneal dialysis
F   Superior vena cava obstruction
G   Myxedema
H   Pulmonary emboli
I   Urinothorax

EXUDATIVE PLEURAL EFFUSIONS

A   Neoplastic diseases
   1   Metastatic disease
   2   Mesothelioma
B   Infectious diseases
   1   Bacterial infections
   2   Tuberculosis
   3   Fungal infections
   4   Viral infections
   5   Parasitic infections
C   Pulmonary embolization
D   Gastrointestinal disease
   1   Esophageal perforation
   2   Pancreatic disease
   3   Intraabdominal abscesses
   4   Diaphragmatic hernia
   5   After abdominal surgery
   6   Endoscopic variceal sclerotherapy
E   Collagen-vascular diseases
   1   Rheumatoid pleuritis
   2   Systemic lupus erythematosus
   3   Drug-induced lupus
   4   Immunoblastic lymphadenopathy
   5   Sjögren's syndrome
   6   Wegener's granulomatosis
   7   Churg-Strauss syndrome
F   Post-cardiac injury syndrome
G   Asbestos exposure
H   Sarcoidosis
I   Uremia
J   Meigs' syndrome
K   Yellow nail syndrome
L   Drug-induced pleural disease
   1   Nitrofurantoin
   2   Dantrolene
   3   Methysergide
   4   Bromocriptine
   5   Procarbazine
   6   Amiodarone
M   Trapped lung
N   Radiation therapy
O   Electrical burns
P   Hemothorax
Q   Iatrogenic injury
R   Ovarian hyperstimulation syndrome
S   Chylothorax

Etiology   Pleural fluid accumulates when pleural fluid formation exceeds pleural fluid absorption. Normally, fluid enters the pleural space from the capillaries in the parietal pleura and is removed via the lymphatics situated in the parietal pleura. Fluid also can enter the pleural space from the interstitial spaces of the lung via the visceral pleura or from the peritoneal cavity via small holes in the diaphragm. The lymphatics have the capacity to absorb 20 times more fluid than is normally formed. Accordingly, a pleural effusion may develop when there is excess pleural fluid formation (from the parietal pleura, the interstitial spaces of the lung, or the peritoneal cavity) or when there is decreased fluid removal by the lymphatics.

Diagnostic approach   When a patient is found to have a pleural effusion, an effort should be made to determine the cause (Fig. 228-1). There are many different causes of pleural fluid accumulation (Table 228-1). The first step is to determine whether the patient has a transudative or an exudative pleural effusion. A *transudative* pleural effusion occurs when *systemic factors* that influence the formation and absorption of pleural fluid are altered. The leading causes of transudative pleural effusions in the United States are left ventricular failure (~500,000 per year), pulmonary embolism (~75,000 per year), and cirrhosis (~50,000 per year). An *exudative* pleural effusion occurs when *local factors* that influence the formation and absorption of pleural fluid are altered. The leading causes of exudative pleural effusions are bacterial pneumonia (~300,000 per year), malignancy (~200,000 per year), viral infection (~100,000 per year), and pulmonary embolism (~75,000 per year). The primary reason to make this differentiation is that additional diagnostic procedures are indicated only with exudative effusions to define the cause of the local disease.

Transudative and exudative pleural effusions are distinguished by measuring the lactate dehydrogenase (LDH) and protein levels in the pleural fluid. Exudative pleural effusions meet at least one of the following criteria, whereas transudative pleural effusions meet none:

1 Pleural fluid protein/serum protein >0.5
2 Pleural fluid LDH/serum LDH >0.6
3 Pleural fluid LDH more than two-thirds normal upper limit for serum

If a patient has an exudative pleural effusion, the following tests on the pleural fluid should be obtained: description of the fluid, glucose level, amylase level, differential cell count, microbiologic studies, and cytology.

Effusion due to heart failure The most common cause of a pleural effusion is congestive heart failure with left ventricular failure. The effusion occurs because the increased amounts of fluid in the lung interstitial spaces exit in part across the visceral pleura. This overwhelms the capacity of the lymphatics in the parietal pleura to remove fluid. The effusions are usually bilateral and roughly the same size. A diagnostic thoracentesis should be performed if the effusions are not bilateral and comparable in size, if the patient is febrile, or if the patient has pleuritic chest pain to verify that the patient has a transudative effusion. Otherwise the patient is best treated with diuretics. If the effusion persists despite diuretic therapy, a diagnostic thoracentesis should be performed. Diuretic therapy for a few days does not significantly change the biochemical characteristics of the pleural fluid.

Hepatic hydrothorax Pleural effusions occur in approximately 5 percent of patients with cirrhosis and ascites. The predominant mechanism is the direct movement of peritoneal fluid through small holes in the diaphragm into the pleural space. The effusion is usually right-sided and frequently is large enough to produce severe dyspnea. If medical management does not control the ascites and the effusion, there are no good alternatives. Consideration can be given to inserting a peritoneal-venous shunt, thoracotomy with surgical repair of the leak, or tube thoracostomy with the injection of a sclerosing agent.

Parapneumonic effusion A parapneumonic effusion is any pleural effusion associated with bacterial pneumonia, lung abscess, or bronchiectasis. These effusions are probably the most common exudative pleural effusion in the United States at this time. The term *complicated parapneumonic effusion* is used to refer to those effusions that require tube thoracostomy for their resolution. An *empyema* is pus in the pleural space, and this term is reserved for effusions on which the Gram stain of the pleural fluid is positive.

Patients with aerobic bacterial pneumonia and pleural effusion present with an acute febrile illness consisting of chest pain, sputum production, and leukocytosis. Patients with anaerobic infections present with a subacute illness with weight loss, a brisk leukocytosis, mild anemia, and a history of some factor that predisposes them to aspiration. Although aerobic bacteria are responsible for many more cases of pneumonia than are anaerobic bacteria, positive cultures on pleural fluid are roughly equally divided between the two different types of bacteria.

The possibility of a parapneumonic effusion should be considered whenever a patient with a bacterial pneumonia is initially evaluated. The presence of free pleural fluid can be demonstrated with a lateral decubitus radiograph. If the free fluid separates the lung from the chest wall by more than 10 mm on the decubitus radiograph, a diagnostic thoracentesis should be performed. The purpose of this diagnostic thoracentesis is to determine whether or not chest tubes should be inserted.

Any of the following is an indication for tube thoracostomy in patients with parapneumonic effusion:

1 The presence of gross pus in the pleural space
2 Organisms visible on Gram stain of the pleural fluid
3 Pleural fluid glucose level of less than 50 mg/dL
4 Pleural fluid pH below 7.00 and 0.15 units lower than arterial pH

There should be no delay in its performance because a free-flowing parapneumonic effusion can become loculated within a matter of hours.

If the pleural fluid is loculated and is not adequately drained with one chest tube, either streptokinase, 250,000 units, or urokinase, 100,000 units, should be injected intrapleurally to dissolve the fibrin membranes which create the loculations. If the pleural drainage is inadequate after the intrapleural thrombolytic therapy, a decortication should be performed. If the patient is too sick to tolerate a decortication, then an open drainage procedure can be done.

Effusion secondary to malignancy Malignant pleural effusions secondary to metastatic disease are the second most common type of exudative pleural effusion (~200,000 per year). The three tumors that cause approximately 75 percent of all malignant pleural effusions are lung carcinoma (30 percent), breast carcinoma (25 percent), and tumors of the lymphoma group (20 percent). Most patients complain of dyspnea which is frequently out of proportion to the size of the effusion. The pleural fluid is an exudate, and its glucose level may be reduced if the tumor burden in the pleural space is high.

The diagnosis is usually made via cytology of the pleural fluid. If the initial cytologic examination is negative, then a needle biopsy of the pleura with repeat cytology is indicated. If there is still no diagnosis, thoracoscopy is likely to provide the diagnosis if the patient has malignancy. At the time of thoracoscopy, talc or some similar agent should be instilled into the pleural space to effect a pleurodesis.

Patients with a malignant pleural effusion are treated symptomatically for the most part, since the presence of the effusion indicates disseminated disease and most malignancies associated with pleural effusion are not curable with chemotherapy. The only symptom that can be attributed to the effusion itself is dyspnea. If the patient's lifestyle is compromised by dyspnea, and if the dyspnea is relieved with a therapeutic thoracentesis, then one of the following procedures should be performed: (1) tube thoracostomy with the instillation of a sclerosing agent such as bleomycin, 60 IU, or minocycline, 5 to 10 mg/kg, (2) thoracoscopy with pleural abrasion or the insufflation of talc, or (3) insertion of a pleuroperitoneal shunt.

Mesothelioma Malignant mesotheliomas are primary tumors which arise from the mesothelial cells that line the pleural cavities. Most cases of malignant mesothelioma are related to asbestos exposure. Patients with mesothelioma present with chest pain and shortness of breath. The chest radiograph reveals a pleural effusion, generalized pleural thickening, and a shrunken hemothorax. Usually either thoracoscopy or open pleural biopsy is necessary to establish the diagnosis. Various treatment modalities, including radical surgery, chemotherapy, and radiation therapy, have been tried, but none has been proven to be more effective than symptomatic therapy. It is recommended that chest pain be treated with opiates and that shortness of breath be treated with oxygen and/or opiates.

Effusion secondary to pulmonary embolization The diagnosis most commonly overlooked in the differential diagnosis of a patient with an undiagnosed pleural effusion is pulmonary embolism. Dyspnea is reported by more than 80 percent of patients and is usually greater than one would expect from a similar-sized effusion with a different cause.

There is nothing characteristic about the pleural fluid associated with pulmonary embolization, and it can be either transudative or exudative. The diagnosis is suggested by lung scanning and/or pulmonary arteriography. Treatment of the patient with a pleural effusion secondary to pulmonary embolism is the same as for any patient with pulmonary emboli. If the pleural effusion increases in size with treatment, the patient probably has recurrent emboli or another complication such as a hemothorax or a pleural infection.

Tuberculous pleuritis In many parts of the world, the most common cause of an exudative pleural effusion is tuberculosis, but in the United States this is relatively uncommon. Tuberculous pleural effusions are thought to be due primarily to a hypersensitivity reaction to tuberculous protein in the pleural space. Patients with tuberculous pleuritis present with fever, weight loss, dyspnea, and/or pleuritic chest pain. The pleural fluid is an exudate with predominantly small lymphocytes. The diagnosis is usually established by the demonstration of granulomas on needle biopsy of the pleura. Adequate treatment consists of isoniazide, 300 mg/d, plus rifampin, 600 mg/d, for 6 months.

Effusion secondary to viral infection   Viral infections are probably responsible for a sizable percentage of undiagnosed exudative pleural effusions. In many series, no diagnosis is established for approximately 20 percent of exudative effusions, and these effusions resolve spontaneously with no long-term residua. The importance of these effusions is that one should not be too aggressive in trying to establish a diagnosis for the undiagnosed effusion, particularly if the patient is improving clinically.

AIDS   Pleural effusions are uncommon in such patients. The most common cause is Kaposi's sarcoma, followed by parapneumonic effusion. Other common causes are tuberculosis, cryptococcosis, and lymphoma. Pleural effusions are very uncommon with *Pneumocystis carinii* infection.

Chylothorax   A chylothorax occurs when the thoracic duct is disrupted and chyle accumulates in the pleural space. The most common cause of chylothorax is trauma, but it also may result from tumors in the mediastinum. Patients with chylothorax present with dyspnea, and the chest radiograph reveals a large pleural effusion. Thoracentesis reveals milky fluid, and biochemical analysis reveals a triglyceride level which is usually above 110 mg/dL. Patients with chylothorax and no obvious trauma should have a lymphangiogram and a mediastinal computed tomographic (CT) scan to assess the mediastinum for lymph nodes. The treatment of choice for most chylothoraces is implantation of a pleuroperitoneal shunt. Patients with chylothoraces should not undergo tube thoracostomy with prolonged chest tube drainage because this will lead to malnutrition and immunologic incompetence.

Hemothorax   When a diagnostic thoracentesis reveals bloody pleural fluid, a hematocrit should be obtained on the pleural fluid. If the hematocrit is greater than 50 percent that of the peripheral blood, the patient has a hemothorax. Most hemothoraces are the result of trauma; other causes include rupture of a blood vessel or tumor. Most patients with hemothorax should be treated with tube thoracostomy. Placing a chest tube allows continuous quantification of bleeding. If the bleeding emanates from a laceration of the pleura, apposition of the two pleural surfaces is likely to stop the bleeding. If the pleural hemorrhage exceeds 200 mL/h, consideration should be given to thoracotomy.

Miscellaneous causes of pleural effusion   There are many other causes of pleural effusion (see Table 228-1), and space precludes an in-depth discussion of these multiple entities. Key features of some of these conditions are as follows: If the pleural fluid amylase level is elevated, the diagnosis of esophageal rupture or pancreatic disease is likely. If the patient is febrile, has predominantly polymorphonuclear cells in the pleural fluid, and has no parenchymal abnormalities, an intraabdominal abscess should be considered. The diagnosis of lupus pleuritis is best made by demonstrating an elevated antinuclear antibody (ANA) level in the pleural fluid. The diagnosis of an asbestos pleural effusion is one of exclusion. Benign ovarian tumors can produce ascites and a pleural effusion (Meigs' syndrome). Several drugs can cause pleural effusion, and the associated fluid is usually eosinophilic. Many pleural effusions follow from medical manipulations such as abdominal surgery, coronary artery bypass surgery, endoscopic variceal sclerotherapy, radiation therapy, or the intravascular insertion of central lines.

PNEUMOTHORAX   Pneumothorax is the presence of gas in the pleural space. A *spontaneous* pneumothorax is one that occurs without antecedent trauma to the thorax. A *primary spontaneous* pneumothorax occurs in an individual without underlying lung disease, while a *secondary spontaneous* pneumothorax occurs in an individual with underlying lung disease. A *traumatic* pneumothorax results from penetrating or nonpenetrating chest injuries. A *tension* pneumothorax is a pneumothorax in which the pressure in the pleural space is positive throughout the respiratory cycle.

Primary spontaneous pneumothorax   Primary spontaneous pneumothoraces are usually due to rupture of apical pleural blebs. These are small cystic spaces, seldom exceeding 1 to 2 cm in diameter, which lie within or immediately under the visceral pleura. These pneumothoraces most commonly occur in tall, thin individuals. Primary spontaneous pneumothoraces occur almost exclusively in smokers, which suggests that the patients indeed do have subclinical lung disease. Approximately 50 percent of individuals who have an initial primary spontaneous pneumothorax will have a recurrence. The initial recommended treatment for primary spontaneous pneumothorax is simple aspiration. If the lung does not expand with aspiration, or if the patient has a recurrent pneumothorax, tube thoracostomy with instillation of a sclerosing agent such as minocycline is indicated. Thoracoscopy or thoracotomy with pleural abrasion is almost 100 percent successful in preventing recurrences.

Secondary spontaneous pneumothorax   Most secondary spontaneous pneumothoraces are due to chronic obstructive pulmonary disease, but pneumothoraces have been reported with virtually every lung disease. Pneumothorax in patients with lung disease is more life-threatening than it is in normal individuals because of the lack of pulmonary reserve in patients with lung disease. Nearly all patients with secondary spontaneous pneumothorax should be treated with tube thoracostomy and the instillation of a sclerosing agent. Patients with either primary or secondary spontaneous pneumothoraces who have a persistent air leak or an unexpanded lung after 6 days of tube thoracostomy should be subjected to open thoracotomy.

Traumatic pneumothorax   Traumatic pneumothoraces can result from both penetrating and nonpenetrating chest trauma. Traumatic pneumothoraces should be treated with tube thoracostomy. If a hemopneumothorax is present, one chest tube should be placed in the superior part of the hemithorax to evacuate the air, and another should be placed in the inferior part of the hemithorax to remove the blood. Iatrogenic pneumothorax is a type of traumatic pneumothorax which is becoming more common. The leading causes are transthoracic needle aspiration, thoracentesis, and the insertion of central intravenous catheters. The treatment differs according to the degree of distress and can be observation, supplemental oxygen, aspiration, or tube thoracostomy.

Tension pneumothorax   Tension pneumothorax usually occurs during mechanical ventilation or resuscitative efforts. The positive pleural pressure is life-threatening both because ventilation is severely compromised and because the positive pressure is transmitted to the mediastinum, which results in decreased venous return to the heart and reduced cardiac output.

Difficulty in ventilation during resuscitation or high peak inspiratory pressures during mechanical ventilation strongly suggest the diagnosis. The diagnosis is made by physical examination of the patient, which reveals an enlarged hemithorax with no breath sounds and shift of the mediastinum to the contralateral side. Tension pneumothorax must be treated as a medical emergency. If the tension in the pleural space is not relieved, the patient is likely to die from inadequate cardiac output or marked hypoxemia. A large-bore needle should be inserted into the pleural space through the second anterior intercostal space. If large amounts of gas escape from the needle after insertion, the diagnosis is confirmed. The needle should be left in place until a thoracostomy tube can be inserted.

DISORDERS OF THE MEDIASTINUM

The mediastinum is the region between the pleural sacs. It is separated into three compartments. The *anterior mediastinum* extends from the sternum anteriorly to the pericardium and brachiocephalic vessels posteriorly. It contains the thymus gland, the anterior mediastinal lymph nodes, and the internal mammary arteries and veins. The *middle mediastinum* lies between the anterior and posterior mediastina and contains the heart; the ascending and transverse arches of the aorta; the venae cavae; the brachiocephalic arteries and veins; the phrenic nerves; the trachea, main bronchi, and their contiguous lymph nodes; and the pulmonary arteries and veins. The *posterior mediastinum* is bounded by the pericardium and trachea anteriorly and the vertebral column posteriorly. It contains the descending thoracic aorta, esophagus, thoracic duct, azygos and hemiazygos veins, and the posterior group of mediastinal lymph nodes.

MEDIASTINAL MASSES The most common abnormality of the mediastinum is a mass. The first step in evaluating a mediastinal lesion is to place it in one of the three mediastinal compartments, since each compartment has different characteristic lesions. The most common lesions in the anterior mediastinum are thymomas, lymphomas, teratomatous neoplasms, and thyroid masses. The most common masses in the middle mediastinum are vascular masses, lymph node enlargement from metastases or granulomatous disease, and pleuropericardial and bronchogenic cysts. In the posterior mediastinum, neurogenic tumors, meningoceles, meningomyeloceles, gastroenteric cysts, and esophageal diverticula are commonly found.

The diagnostic approach to disorders of the mediastinum may be divided into imaging techniques (CT scans, magnetic resonance imaging, radionuclide studies, and intravenous contrast studies) and procedures for obtaining tissue samples (needle aspiration, mediastinoscopy, thoracoscopy, and open biopsy). CT scan of the mediastinum is the most valuable imaging technique and is probably the only imaging technique that should be done. Magnetic resonance imaging (MRI) appears to have no distinct advantages over CT in imaging the mediastinum. Barium studies of the gastrointestinal tract are indicated in many patients with posterior mediastinal lesions, since hernias, diverticula, and achalasia are readily diagnosed in this manner. A iodine 131 nuclear medicine scan can efficiently establish the diagnosis of intrathoracic goiter.

A definite diagnosis can be obtained with mediastinoscopy or anterior mediastinotomy in many patients with masses in the anterior or middle mediastinal compartments. A diagnosis can be established without thoracotomy via percutaneous fine needle aspiration biopsy of mediastinal masses in any of the mediastinal compartments. Video-assisted thoracoscopy will probably be used in the future to make the diagnosis in many instances.

ACUTE MEDIASTINITIS Most cases of acute mediastinitis are either due to esophageal perforation or occur after median sternotomy for cardiac surgery. Patients with esophageal rupture are acutely ill with chest pain and dyspnea due to the mediastinal infection. The esophageal rupture can occur spontaneously or as a complication of esophagoscopy or the insertion of a Blakemore tube. Appropriate treatment is exploration of the mediastinum with primary repair of the esophageal tear and drainage of the pleural space and the mediastinum.

The incidence of mediastinitis following median sternotomy is 0.4 to 5.0 percent. Patients most commonly present with wound drainage. Other presentations include sepsis or a widened mediastinum. The diagnosis is usually established with mediastinal needle aspiration. Treatment includes immediate drainage, debridement, and parenteral antibiotic therapy, but the mortality still exceeds 20 percent.

CHRONIC MEDIASTINITIS The spectrum of chronic mediastinitis ranges from granulomatous inflammation of the lymph nodes in the mediastinum to fibrosing mediastinitis. Most cases are due to tuberculosis or histoplasmosis, but sarcoidosis, silicosis, and other fungal diseases are at times causative. Patients with granulomatous mediastinitis are usually asymptomatic. Those with fibrosing mediastinitis usually have signs of compression of some mediastinal structure such as the superior vena caval syndrome, large airway obstruction, phrenic or recurrent laryngeal nerve paralysis, or obstruction of the pulmonary artery or proximal pulmonary veins. In most cases, mediastinal exploration is necessary to distinguish benign mediastinitis from malignant processes. No medical or surgical therapy has been demonstrated to be effective for mediastinal fibrosis, but the patient should be treated for tuberculosis if smears or cultures demonstrate tuberculous organisms.

PNEUMOMEDIASTINUM With this condition there is gas in the interstices of the mediastinum. The three main causes are (1) alveolar rupture with dissection of air into the mediastinum, (2) perforation or rupture of the esophagus, trachea, or main bronchi, and (3) dissection of air from the neck or the abdomen into the mediastinum. The symptoms associated with pneumomediastinum range from none to severe. Typically, there is severe substernal chest pain with or without radiation into the neck and arms. The physical examination usually reveals subcutaneous emphysema in the suprasternal notch and *Hamman's sign*, which is a crunching or clicking noise synchronous with the heartbeat and best heard in the left lateral decubitus position. The diagnosis is confirmed with the chest radiograph. Usually no treatment is required, but the mediastinal air will be absorbed faster if the patient inspires high concentrations of oxygen. If mediastinal structures are compressed, the compression can be relieved with needle aspiration.

DISORDERS OF THE DIAPHRAGM

The diaphragm is the principal muscle of breathing and moves like a piston within the cylinder of the thoracic cavity.

DIAPHRAGMATIC PARALYSIS The presence of bilateral diaphragmatic paralysis almost always causes severe morbidity in adults. The most common causes include high spinal cord injury, thoracic trauma (including cardiac surgery), multiple sclerosis, anterior horn disease, and muscular dystrophy. Most patients with severe diaphragmatic weakness will present with hypercapnic respiratory failure, frequently complicated by cor pulmonale and right ventricular failure, atelectasis, and pneumonia.

The degree of diaphragmatic weakness is best quantitated by measuring transdiaphragmatic pressures. Normally, this pressure is greater than $100 \, cmH_2O$. The treatment of choice is assisted ventilation for all or part of each day. This may be accomplished without tracheostomy using a rocking bed, corset-type positive-pressure wrap, nasal continuous positive pressure, or a negative-pressure ventilation. If the nerve to the diaphragm is intact, diaphragmatic pacing may be a viable alternative. If the paralysis occurs during open heart surgery, recovery frequently occurs, but it may take 6 months or more.

Unilateral paralysis of the diaphragm is much more common than is bilateral paralysis. The most common cause is nerve invasion from malignancy, usually a bronchogenic carcinoma. If the patient does not have malignancy, then usually no cause for the paralysis is found. The diagnosis is suggested by finding an elevated hemidiaphragm on the chest roentgenogram. Confirmation is best established with the "sniff test." When a patient is observed with fluoroscopy while sniffing, the paralyzed diaphragm will move paradoxically upward with the sniff due to the negative intrathoracic pressure. Patients with a unilateral paralyzed diaphragm are usually asymptomatic. Their vital capacity and total lung capacity are each reduced about 20 percent. If a patient has a mediastinal mass in conjunction with the diaphragmatic paralysis, further workup should be done. However, if the patient is asymptomatic with a normal chest radiograph, no invasive procedures are warranted.

HICCUP A hiccup is an involuntary spasm of the inspiratory muscles followed by an abrupt closure of the glottis. Hiccups are usually precipitated by irritation of the diaphragm, most commonly due to gastric distention or inflammation following rapid or excessive eating or drinking. Although hiccups usually are of short duration, if they persist, they may be very distressing. Patients with troublesome hiccups should first be asked to rapidly swallow 1 teaspoon of dry white granulated sugar. If this is ineffective, the stomach can be decompressed with a nasogastric tube, which also provides pharyngeal irritation. Pharmacologic agents that at times are curative are chlorpromazine, 10 to 20 mg every 4 to 6 h, or quinidine, 200 mg four times a day orally. As a last resort, a phrenic nerve can be blocked with bupivacaine or interrupted surgically.

REFERENCES

BERKMAN N, KRAMER MR: Diagnostic tests in pleural effusion—an update. Postgrad Med J 69:12, 1993

LIGHT RW: *Pleural Diseases*. Philadelphia, Lea & Febiger, 1990

MILES DW, KNIGHT RK: Diagnosis and management of malignant pleural effusion. Cancer Treat Rev 19:151, 1993

MULLER NL: Imaging of the pleura. Radiology 186:297, 1993

————: Pleural diseases. Dis Mon 28:266, 1992

PISTOLESI M et al: Pleural liquid and solute exchange. Am Rev Respir Dis 140:825, 1989

THOMAS CR JR, BONOMI PD: Mediastinal tumors. Curr Opin Oncol 3:335, 1991

229 DISORDERS OF VENTILATION

ELIOT A. PHILLIPSON

HYPOVENTILATION

DEFINITION AND ETIOLOGY   Alveolar hypoventilation exists by definition when arterial P_{CO_2} (Pa_{CO_2}) increases above the normal range of 37 to 43 mmHg, but in clinically important hypoventilation syndromes Pa_{CO_2} is generally in the range of 50 to 80 mmHg. Hypoventilation disorders can be acute or chronic. The acute disorders, which represent life-threatening emergencies, are discussed in Chap. 230; this chapter deals with chronic hypoventilation syndromes.

Chronic hypoventilation can result from numerous disease entities (Table 229-1), but in all cases the underlying mechanism involves a defect in either the metabolic respiratory control system, the respiratory neuromuscular system, or the ventilatory apparatus. Disorders associated with impaired respiratory drive, defects in the respiratory neuromuscular system, some chest wall disorders such as obesity, and upper airway obstruction produce an increase in Pa_{CO_2}, despite normal lungs, because of a reduction in overall minute volume of ventilation and hence in alveolar ventilation. In contrast, most disorders of the chest wall and disorders of the lower airways and lungs may produce an increase in Pa_{CO_2}, despite a normal or even increased minute volume of ventilation, because of severe ventilation-perfusion mismatching that results in net alveolar hypoventilation.

Several hypoventilation syndromes involve combined disturbances in two elements of the respiratory system. For example, patients with chronic obstructive pulmonary disease may hypoventilate not simply because of impaired ventilatory mechanics but also because of a reduced central respiratory drive, which can be inherent or secondary to a coexisting metabolic alkalosis (related to diuretic and steroid therapy).

PHYSIOLOGICAL AND CLINICAL FEATURES   Regardless of cause, the hallmark of all alveolar hypoventilation syndromes is an increase in alveolar P_{CO_2} (PA_{CO_2}) and therefore in Pa_{CO_2} (Fig. 229-1). The resulting respiratory acidosis eventually leads to a compensatory increase in plasma HCO_3^- concentration and a decrease in Cl^- concentration. The increase in PA_{CO_2} produces an obligatory decrease in PA_{O_2}, resulting in hypoxemia. If severe, the hypoxemia manifests clinically as cyanosis and can stimulate erythropoiesis and induce secondary polycythemia. The combination of chronic hypoxemia and hypercapnia also may induce pulmonary vasoconstriction, leading eventually to pulmonary hypertension, right ventricular hypertrophy, and congestive heart failure. The disturbances in arterial blood gases are typically magnified during sleep because of a further reduction in central respiratory drive. The resulting increased nocturnal hypercapnia may cause cerebral vasodilation leading to morning headache; sleep quality also may be severely impaired, resulting in morning fatigue, daytime somnolence, mental confusion, and intellectual impairment. Other clinical features associated with hypoventilation syndromes are related to the specific underlying disease (see Table 229-1).

DIAGNOSIS   Investigation of the patient with chronic hypoventilation involves several laboratory tests that will usually localize the disorder to either the metabolic respiratory control system, the neuromuscular system, or the ventilatory apparatus (Fig. 229-2). Defects in the control system impair responses to chemical stimuli, including ventilatory, occlusion pressure, and diaphragmatic electromyographic (EMGdi) responses. During sleep, hypoventilation is usually more marked, and central apneas and hypopneas are common. However, because the behavioral respiratory control system (which is anatomically distinct from the metabolic control system), the neuromuscular system, and the ventilatory apparatus are intact, such patients can usually hyperventilate voluntarily, generate normal

TABLE 229-1   Chronic hypoventilation syndromes

Mechanism	Site of defect	Disorder
Impaired respiratory drive	Peripheral and central chemoreceptors	Carotid body dysfunction, trauma Prolonged hypoxia Metabolic alkalosis
	Brainstem respiratory neurons	Bulbar poliomyelitis, encephalitis Brainstem infarction, hemorrhage, trauma Brainstem demyelination, degeneration Chronic drug administration Primary alveolar hypoventilation syndrome
Defective respiratory neuromuscular system	Spinal cord and peripheral nerves	High cervical trauma Poliomyelitis Motor neuron disease Peripheral neuropathy
	Respiratory muscles	Myasthenia gravis Muscular dystrophy Chronic myopathy
Impaired ventilatory apparatus	Chest wall	Kyphoscoliosis Fibrothorax Thoracoplasty Ankylosing spondylitis Obesity-hypoventilation
	Airways and lungs	Laryngeal and tracheal stenosis Obstructive sleep apnea Cystic fibrosis Chronic obstructive pulmonary disease

SOURCE: Phillipson, in Murray and Nadel (eds), pp. 1831–1840, with permission.

FIGURE 229-1   Physiologic and clinical features of alveolar hypoventilation. (*After Phillipson.*)

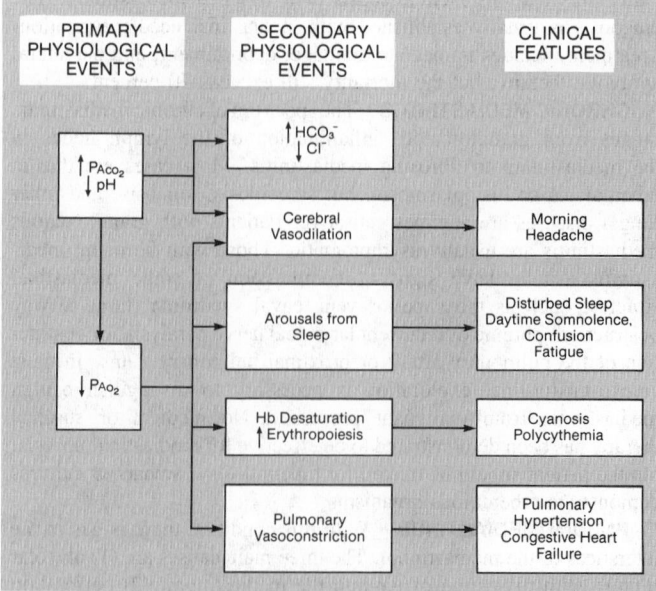

PRIMARY PHYSIOLOGICAL EVENTS	SECONDARY PHYSIOLOGICAL EVENTS	CLINICAL FEATURES
↑PA_{CO_2} ↓pH	↑HCO_3^- ↓Cl^-	
	Cerebral Vasodilation	Morning Headache
	Arousals from Sleep	Disturbed Sleep Daytime Somnolence, Confusion Fatigue
↓PA_{O_2}	Hb Desaturation ↑Erythropoiesis	Cyanosis Polycythemia
	Pulmonary Vasoconstriction	Pulmonary Hypertension Congestive Heart Failure

SITE OF DEFECT	Responses to CO₂, Hypoxia			Sleep Studies	Voluntary Hyperventil.	PImax, PEmax	Volumes Flow Rates	Resistance, Compliance	$(A-a) P_{O_2}$
	Ventil.	P.1	EMG di						
Metabolic Control System (chemoreceptors, brainstem integrating neurons)	↓	↓	↓	↑ hypoventil, central apneas	N	N	N	N	N
Respiratory Neuromuscular System (brainstem motoneurons, spinal cord, respiratory nerves and muscles)	↓	↓	↓	↑ hypoventil, central apneas	↓	↓	↓	N	N
Ventilatory Apparatus (chest wall, lungs, airways)	↓	N	N	variable	↓	N	abnormal	abnormal	↑

FIGURE 229-2 Pattern of laboratory test results in alveolar hypoventilation syndromes, based on the site of defect. Ventil = ventilation; P.1 = mouth pressure generated after 0.1 s of inspiration against an occluded airway; EMGdi = diaphragmatic EMG; PI_{max}, PE_{max} = maximum inspiratory or expiratory pressure that can be generated against an occluded airway; $(A - a) P_{O_2}$ = alveolar-arterial P_{O_2} difference; N = normal. Defects in the metabolic control system impair central respiratory drive in response to chemical stimuli (CO_2 or hypoxia); therefore responses of EMGdi, P.1, and minute volume of ventilation are reduced and hypoventilation during sleep is aggravated. In contrast, tests of voluntary respiratory control, muscle strength, lung mechanics, and gas exchange [$(A - a)P_{O_2}$] are normal. Defects in the respiratory neuromuscular system impair muscle strength; therefore all tests dependent on muscular activity (voluntary or in response to metabolic stimuli) are abnormal, but lung resistance, lung compliance, and gas exchange are normal. Defects in the ventilatory apparatus usually impair gas exchange. Because resistance and compliance are also impaired, all tests dependent on ventilation (whether voluntary or in response to chemical stimuli) are abnormal; in contrast, tests of muscle activity or strength that do not involve airflow (that is, P.1, EMGdi, PI_{max}, PE_{max}) are normal. (*After Phillipson.*)

inspiratory and expiratory muscle pressures (PI_{max}, PE_{max}, respectively) against an occluded airway, generate normal lung volumes and flow rates on routine spirometry, and have normal respiratory system resistance and compliance and a normal alveolar-arterial P_{O_2} [$(A - a) P_{O_2}$] difference. Patients with defects in the respiratory neuromuscular system also have impaired responses to chemical stimuli but in addition are unable to hyperventilate voluntarily or to generate normal static respiratory muscle pressures, lung volumes, and flow rates. However, at least in the early stages of the disease the resistance and compliance of the respiratory system and the alveolar-arterial oxygen difference are normal.

In contrast to patients with disorders of the respiratory control or neuromuscular systems, patients with disorders of the chest wall, lungs, and airways typically demonstrate abnormalities of respiratory system resistance and compliance and have a widened $(A - a)P_{O_2}$. Because of the impaired mechanics of breathing, routine spirometric tests are abnormal, as is the ventilatory response to chemical stimuli. However, because the neuromuscular system is intact, tests that are independent of resistance and compliance are usually normal, including tests of respiratory muscle strength and of respiratory control that do not involve airflow.

TREATMENT The management of chronic hypoventilation must be individualized to the patient's particular disorder, circumstances, and needs and should include measures directed toward the underlying disease. Coexistent metabolic alkalosis should be corrected, including elevations of HCO_3^- that are inappropriately high for the degree of chronic hypercapnia. Administration of supplemental oxygen is effective in attenuating hypoxemia, polycythemia, and pulmonary hypertension but can aggravate CO_2 retention and the associated neurologic symptoms. For this reason, supplemental oxygen must be prescribed judiciously and the results monitored carefully. Pharmacologic agents that stimulate respiration (particularly progesterone) are of benefit in some patients, but generally, results are disappointing.

Most patients with chronic hypoventilation related to impairment of respiratory drive or neuromuscular disease eventually require mechanical ventilatory assistance for effective management. When hypoventilation is severe, treatment may be required on a 24-h basis, but in most patients ventilatory assistance only during sleep produces dramatic clinical improvement and lowering of daytime Pa_{CO_2}. In patients with reduced respiratory drive but intact respiratory lower motor neurons, phrenic nerves, and respiratory muscles, diaphragmatic pacing through an implanted phrenic electrode can be very effective. However, for patients with defects in the respiratory nerves and muscles, electrophrenic pacing is contraindicated. Such patients can usually be managed effectively with either intermittent negative-pressure ventilation in a cuirass or intermittent positive-pressure ventilation delivered through a tracheostomy or nose mask. For patients who require ventilatory assistance only during sleep, positive-pressure ventilation through a nose mask is the preferred method because it obviates a tracheostomy and avoids the problem of upper airway occlusion that can arise in a negative-pressure ventilator.

Hypoventilation related to restrictive disorders of the chest wall (see Table 229-1) also can be managed effectively with nocturnal intermittent positive-pressure ventilation through a nose mask or tracheostomy. Nocturnal ventilatory assistance also has been advocated for patients with hypercapnic chronic obstructive lung disease as a means of alleviating possible chronic respiratory muscle fatigue, but the efficacy of such an approach has yet to be confirmed.

HYPOVENTILATION SYNDROMES

PRIMARY ALVEOLAR HYPOVENTILATION Primary alveolar hypoventilation (PAH) is a disorder of unknown cause characterized by chronic hypercapnia and hypoxemia in the absence of identifiable neuromuscular disease or mechanical ventilatory impairment. The disorder is thought to arise from a defect in the metabolic respiratory control system, but few neuropathologic studies have been reported in such patients. Isolated PAH is relatively rare, and although it occurs in all age groups, the majority of reported cases have been in males aged 20 to 50 years. The disorder typically develops insidiously and often first comes to attention when severe respiratory depression follows administration of standard doses of sedatives or anesthetics. As the degree of hypoventilation increases, patients typically develop lethargy, fatigue, daytime somnolence, disturbed sleep, and morning headaches, and eventually cyanosis, polycythemia, pulmonary hypertension, and congestive heart failure occur (see Fig. 229-1). Despite severe arterial blood gas derangements, dyspnea is uncommon, presumably because of impaired chemoreception and ventilatory drive. If left untreated, PAH is usually progressive over a period of months to years and ultimately fatal.

The key diagnostic finding in PAH is a chronic respiratory acidosis in the absence of respiratory muscle weakness or impaired ventilatory mechanics (see Fig. 229-2). Because patients can hyperventilate voluntarily and reduce Pa_{CO_2} to normal or even hypocapnic levels, hypercapnia may not be demonstrable in a single arterial blood sample, but the presence of an elevated plasma HCO_3^- level should draw attention to the underlying chronic disturbance. Despite normal ventilatory mechanics and respiratory muscle strength, ventilatory responses to chemical stimuli are reduced or absent (see Fig. 229-2), and breath-holding time may be markedly prolonged without any sensation of dyspnea.

Patients with PAH maintain rhythmic respiration when awake, although the level of ventilation is below normal. However, during sleep there is typically a further deterioration in ventilation with frequent episodes of central hypopnea or apnea, a disturbance that has been termed *Ondine's curse*.

PAH must be distinguished from other central hypoventilation syndromes that are secondary to underlying neurologic disease of the brainstem or chemoreceptors (see Table 229-1). This distinction requires a careful neurologic investigation for evidence of brainstem or autonomic disturbances. Unrecognized respiratory neuromuscular disorders, particularly those which produce diaphragmatic weakness, are often misdiagnosed as PAH. However, such disorders can usually be suspected on clinical grounds (see below) and can be confirmed by the finding of reduced voluntary hyperventilation, as well as Pi_{max} and Pe_{max}.

Some patients with PAH respond favorably to respiratory stimulant medications and to supplemental oxygen. However, the majority eventually require mechanical ventilatory assistance. Excellent long-term benefits can be achieved with diaphragmatic pacing by electrophrenic stimulation or with negative- or positive-pressure mechanical ventilation. The administration of such treatment only during sleep is sufficient in most patients.

RESPIRATORY NEUROMUSCULAR DISORDERS   Several primary disorders of the spinal cord, peripheral respiratory nerves, and respiratory muscles produce a chronic hypoventilation syndrome (see Table 229-1). Hypoventilation usually develops gradually over a period of months to years and often first comes to attention when a relatively trivial increase in mechanical ventilatory load (such as mild airways obstruction) produces severe respiratory failure. In some of the disorders (such as motor neuron disease, myasthenia gravis, and muscular dystrophy), involvement of the respiratory nerves or muscles is usually a later feature of a more widespread disease. In other disorders, respiratory involvement can be an early or even isolated feature, and hence the underlying problem is often not suspected. Included in this category are the postpolio syndrome [a form of chronic respiratory insufficiency that develops 20 to 30 years following recovery from poliomyelitis (Chap. 375)], the myopathy associated with adult acid maltase deficiency, and idiopathic diaphragmatic paralysis.

Generally, respiratory neuromuscular disorders do not result in chronic hypoventilation unless there is significant weakness of the diaphragm. Distinguishing features of bilateral diaphragmatic weakness include orthopnea, paradoxical movement of the abdomen in the supine posture, and paradoxical diaphragmatic movement under fluoroscopy. However, the absence of these features does not exclude diaphragmatic weakness. Important laboratory features are a rapid deterioration of ventilation during a maximum voluntary ventilation maneuver and reduced Pi_{max} and Pe_{max} (see Fig. 229-2). More sophisticated investigations reveal reduced or absent transdiaphragmatic pressures, calculated from simultaneous measurement of esophageal and gastric pressures; reduced diaphragmatic EMG responses (recorded from an esophageal electrode) to transcutaneous phrenic nerve stimulation; and marked hypopnea and arterial oxygen desaturation during rapid eye movement (REM) sleep, when there is normally a physiologic inhibition of all nondiaphragmatic respiratory muscles and breathing becomes critically dependent on diaphragmatic activity.

The management of chronic alveolar hypoventilation due to respiratory neuromuscular disease involves treatment of the underlying disorder, where feasible, and mechanical ventilatory assistance, as described for the primary alveolar hypoventilation syndrome. However, electrophrenic diaphragmatic pacing is contraindicated in these disorders, except for high cervical spinal cord lesions in which the phrenic lower motor neurons and nerves are intact.

OBESITY-HYPOVENTILATION SYNDROME   Massive obesity represents a mechanical load to the respiratory system because the added weight on the rib cage and abdomen serves to reduce the compliance of the chest wall. As a result, the functional residual capacity (i.e., end-expiratory lung volume) is reduced, particularly in the recumbent posture. An important consequence of breathing at a low lung volume is that some airways, particularly those in the lung bases, may be closed throughout part or even all of each tidal breath, resulting in underventilation of the lung bases and widening of the $(A - a)P_{O_2}$. Nevertheless, in the majority of obese subjects, central respiratory drive is increased sufficiently to maintain a normal Pa_{CO_2}. However, a small proportion of obese subjects develop chronic hypercapnia, hypoxemia, and eventually polycythemia, pulmonary hypertension, and right-sided heart failure. Those patients who also develop daytime somnolence have been designated as having the *Pickwickian syndrome* (see Chap. 29). In many such patients, obstructive sleep apnea is a prominent feature, and even in those patients without sleep apnea, sleep-induced hypoventilation is an important element of the disorder and contributes to its progression. Most patients demonstrate a decrease in central respiratory drive which may be inherent or acquired, and many have mild to moderate degrees of airflow obstruction, usually related to smoking. Based on these considerations, several therapeutic measures can be of considerable benefit, including weight loss, cessation of smoking, elimination of obstructive sleep apnea, and enhancement of respiratory drive by medications such as progesterone.

SLEEP APNEA   *Sleep apnea* is defined as an intermittent cessation of airflow at the nose and mouth during sleep. By convention, apneas of at least 10 s duration have been considered important, but in most patients the apneas are 20 to 30 s in duration and may be as long as 2 to 3 min. There is uncertainty as to the minimum number of apneas that should be considered clinically important, although by the time most patients come to attention they have at least 10 to 15 events per hour of sleep.

Sleep apneas have been classified into three types: central, obstructive, and mixed. In central sleep apnea (CSA) the neural drive to all the respiratory muscles is transiently abolished. In contrast, in obstructive sleep apnea (OSA) airflow ceases despite continuing respiratory drive because of occlusion of the oropharyngeal airway. Mixed apneas, which consist of a central apnea followed by an obstructive component, are a variant of OSA.

OBSTRUCTIVE SLEEP APNEA   Pathogenesis   The definitive event in OSA is occlusion of the upper airway usually at the level of the oropharynx (Fig. 229-3). The resulting apnea leads to progressive asphyxia until there is a brief arousal from sleep, whereupon airway patency is restored and airflow resumes. The patient then returns to sleep, and the sequence of events is repeated, often up to 400 to 500 times per night.

The immediate factor leading to collapse of the upper airway in

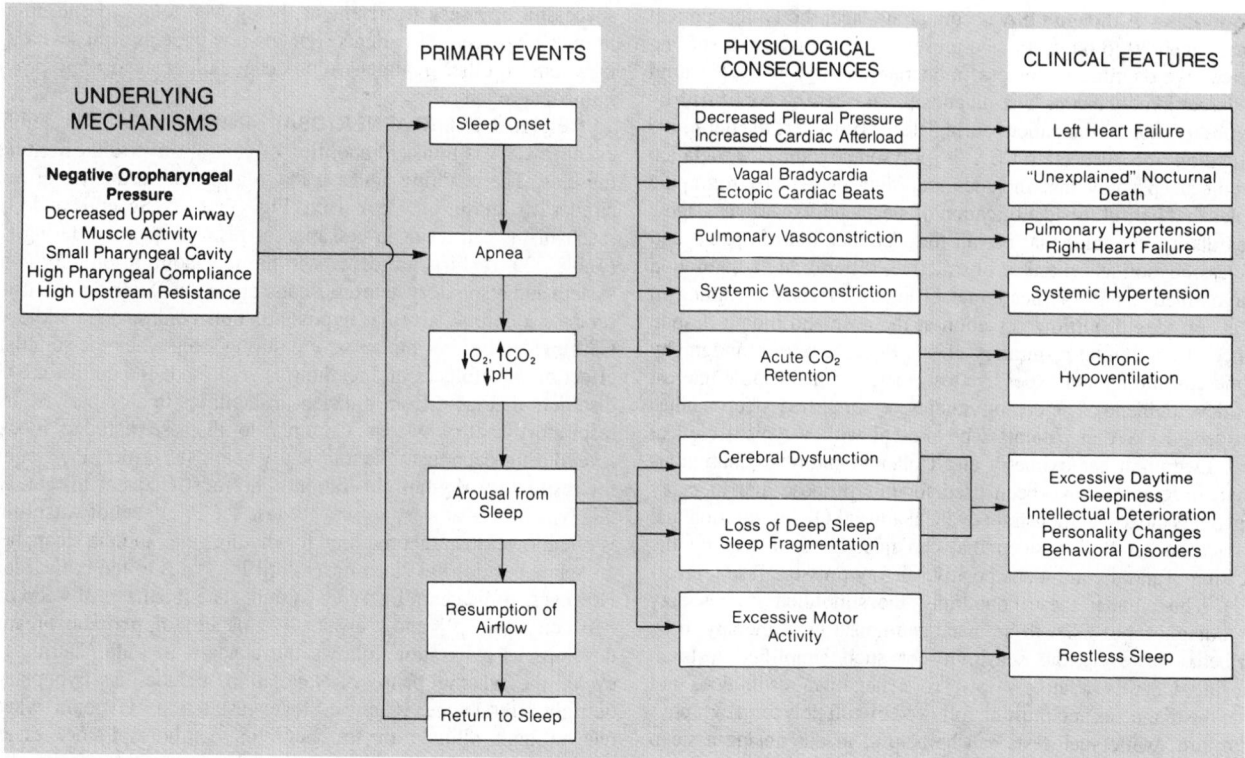

FIGURE 229-3 The primary sequence of events, underlying mechanisms, physiologic responses, and clinical features of obstructive sleep apnea. *(From EA Phillipson, Med North Am 23: 2314, 1982.)*

OSA is the generation of a critical subatmospheric pressure during inspiration that exceeds the ability of the airway dilator and abductor muscles to maintain airway stability (see Fig. 229-3). Sleep plays a permissive but crucial role by reducing the activity of the muscles of the upper airways. Alcohol is frequently an important cofactor because of its selective depressant influence on these muscles. In most patients the patency of the airway is also compromised structurally and therefore predisposed to occlusion. In a minority of patients the structural compromise is due to obvious anatomic disturbances, such as adenotonsillar hypertrophy, retrognathia, and macroglossia. However, in the majority of patients the structural defect is simply a subtle reduction in airway size that can often be appreciated clinically as "pharyngeal crowding" and that can usually be demonstrated by imaging and acoustic reflection techniques. Obesity frequently contributes to the reduction in size of the upper airways. Snoring, a high-frequency vibration of the palatal and pharyngeal soft tissues that results from the decrease in size of the upper airway lumen, may aggravate the narrowing by producing edema of the soft tissues. More sophisticated studies also demonstrate a high airway compliance—i.e., the airway is "floppy" and therefore prone to collapse. In some patients, a high upstream (i.e., nasal) resistance contributes to collapse of the upper airway by increasing the subatmospheric pressure generated in the pharynx during inspiration.

Pathophysiologic and clinical features The narrowing of the upper airways during sleep, which predisposes to OSA, inevitably results in snoring. In most patients, snoring antedates the development of obstructive events by many years. However, the majority of snoring individuals do not have an OSA disorder; hence, in the absence of other symptoms, snoring alone does not warrant an investigation for OSA.

The recurrent episodes of nocturnal asphyxia and of arousal from sleep that characterize OSA lead to a series of secondary physiologic events, which in turn give rise to the clinical complications of the syndrome (see Fig. 229-3). The most common manifestations are neuropsychiatric and behavioral disturbances that are thought to arise from the fragmentation of sleep and loss of slow-wave sleep induced by the recurrent arousal responses. Nocturnal cerebral hypoxia also

may play an important role. The most pervasive manifestation is excessive daytime sleepiness. OSA is now recognized as a leading cause of daytime sleepiness and has been implicated as an important risk factor for motor vehicle accidents. Indeed, several studies have demonstrated two to three times more automobile accidents in patients with OSA compared with other drivers. Other related symptoms include intellectual impairment, memory loss, personality disturbances, and impotence.

The other major manifestations are cardiorespiratory in nature and are thought to arise from the recurrent episodes of nocturnal asphyxia (see Fig. 229-3). Most patients demonstrate a cyclical slowing of the heart during the apneas to 30 to 50 beats per minute, followed by a tachycardia of 90 to 120 beats per minute during the ventilatory phase. A small number of patients develop severe bradycardia with asystoles of 8 to 12 s duration or dangerous tachyarrhythmias, including unsustained ventricular tachycardia. The presence of such arrhythmias has led to the notion that OSA may result in sudden death during sleep, but firm corroborative data are lacking. Several epidemiologic studies have implicated OSA as a risk factor for the development of systemic hypertension, myocardial ischemia and infarction, stroke, and premature death. However, because these studies were cross-sectional or retrospective in design, the natural history of OSA remains largely undefined. OSA also markedly aggravates left ventricular failure in patients with underlying heart disease. This complication is probably due to the combined effects of increased left ventricular afterload during each obstructive event, secondary to increased negative intrathoracic pressure (see Fig. 229-3), recurrent nocturnal hypoxemia, and chronically elevated sympathoadrenal activity. Treatment of OSA in such patients often results in dramatic improvement in left ventricular function. Finally, a small proportion of patients with OSA (10 to 15 percent) develop pulmonary hypertension, right ventricular failure, polycythemia, and chronic hypercapnia and hypoxemia. All such patients have evidence of sustained daytime hypoxemia in addition to the nocturnal ventilatory disturbance, usually as a result of reduced ventilatory drive and/or diffuse airways obstruction. Most of these patients are obese and sleepy and are therefore said to have the *Pickwickian syndrome*.

Diagnosis   Although OSA occurs at any age, the typical patient is a male aged 30 to 60 years who presents with a history of snoring and excessive daytime sleepiness, moderate obesity, and often mild to moderate hypertension. The diagnosis can often be confirmed by direct observation of the patient during sleep. However, the definitive investigation for suspected OSA is polysomnography, a detailed overnight sleep study that includes recording of (1) electrographic variables that permit the identification of sleep and its various stages, (2) ventilatory variables that permit the identification of apneas and their classification as central or obstructive, (3) arterial O_2 saturation by ear oximetry, and (4) heart rate. The key diagnostic finding in OSA is episodes of airflow cessation at the nose and mouth despite evidence of continuing respiratory effort. Because polysomnography is a time-consuming and expensive test, there is considerable interest in the development of screening studies or simplified sleep studies for suspected OSA in patients who present with a typical clinical picture. Overnight ear oximetry and Holter monitoring (continuous electrocardiography) have been used for this purpose and in many such patients clearly demonstrate cyclical arterial O_2 desaturation and brady/tachycardia during sleep that can then be abolished by the application of nasal continuous positive airway pressure (see "Treatment"). Thus, under these conditions, the simplified studies may allow a diagnosis of OSA to be made and nonsurgical therapy to be prescribed. However, the sensitivity of such simplified tests in diagnosing OSA is relatively low, so a negative result does not exclude the diagnosis and must be followed by full polysomnography. Furthermore, while such tests can be helpful in diagnosing a sleep apnea disorder, they are not useful in identifying or excluding other possible causes of daytime sleepiness (narcolepsy, periodic leg movements during sleep, nonrestorative sleep syndromes, phase-shift disorders) that may coexist with sleep apnea.

Treatment   Several approaches to treatment of OSA have been advocated, based on an understanding of the mechanisms underlying the disorder (Table 229-2). The specific choice of treatment depends largely on the severity of OSA. Mild to moderate OSA can often be managed effectively by modest weight reduction, avoidance of alcohol, improvement of nasal patency, and avoidance of sleeping in the supine posture. In some patients with more severe OSA, tricyclic medications, particularly protriptyline (20 to 30 mg at bedtime), have been beneficial. The role of nocturnal supplemental oxygen in managing OSA is uncertain but is generally not satisfactory. The most widely used treatments in moderate to severe OSA are uvulopalatopharyngoplasty and nasal continuous positive airway pressure (CPAP) during sleep. Uvulopalatopharyngoplasty is a surgical procedure designed to increase the pharyngeal lumen by resecting redundant soft tissue. When applied to unselected patients with OSA, it produces long-term benefits in only about 50 percent. More recent attempts to select patients based on the specific site of upper airway occlusion have yielded a higher success rate. Nasal CPAP, which prevents upper airway occlusion by splinting the pharyngeal airway with a positive pressure delivered through a nose mask, is currently the most

successful approach to treatment, being well-tolerated and effective in over 80 percent of patients. For the few patients with severe OSA in whom all other treatment approaches fail, tracheostomy provides immediate relief.

CENTRAL SLEEP APNEA (CSA)   Pathogenesis   The definitive event in CSA is transient abolition of central drive to the ventilatory muscles. The resulting apnea leads to a primary sequence of events similar to those of OSA (see Fig. 229-3). Several underlying mechanisms can result in cessation of respiratory drive during sleep (Table 229-3). First are defects in the metabolic respiratory control system and respiratory neuromuscular apparatus. Such defects usually produce a chronic alveolar hypoventilation syndrome (in addition to CSA) which becomes more severe during sleep when the stimulatory effect of wakefulness on breathing is abolished. In contrast are CSA disorders that arise from transient instabilities in an otherwise intact respiratory control system. Common to all these disorders is a P_{CO_2} level during sleep that falls transiently below the critical P_{CO_2} required for respiratory rhythm generation. The most frequent instability of this type occurs at sleep onset, because the P_{CO_2} level of wakefulness is often lower than that required for rhythm generation in sleep; hence an apnea develops at sleep onset until P_{CO_2} rises to the critical level. However, if the central nervous system state fluctuates at sleep onset between "asleep" and "awake," a pattern of periodic breathing develops as respiration follows the changes in state. During each cycle, the waning phase of ventilation includes an hypopnea or outright central apnea (Cheyne-Stokes respiration). Hypoxia, whether due to high altitude or to underlying cardiorespiratory disease, enhances the tendency to periodic breathing and CSA because of the associated hyperventilation that may drive P_{CO_2} levels during wakefulness well below the critical value required for respiratory rhythm generation during sleep. Hyperventilation due to CNS disease or to lung congestion secondary to heart failure produces periodic breathing and CSA by a similar mechanism. Circulatory slowing secondary to cardiac failure also may induce ventilatory instability by prolonging the time lag between changes in blood gas values by ventilation and the detection of those changes by the peripheral and central chemoreceptors (Chap. 195). Consequently, the ventilatory system overshoots the mark before reversing direction, resulting in periodic breathing that frequently includes central apneas.

Pathophysiologic and clinical features   Many healthy individuals demonstrate a small number of central apneas during sleep, particularly at sleep onset and in REM sleep. These apneas are not associated with any physiologic or clinical disturbances. In patients with clinically important CSA, the primary sequence of events that characterizes the disorder leads to prominent physiologic and clinical consequences (see Fig. 229-3). In those patients whose CSA is a component of an alveolar hypoventilation syndrome, daytime hypercapnia and hypoxemia are usually evident, and the clinical picture is dominated by a history of recurrent respiratory failure,

---

TABLE 229-2   Management of obstructive sleep apnea (OSA)

Mechanism	Mild to moderate OSA	Severe OSA
↑ Upper airway muscle tone	Avoidance of alcohol, sedatives	Tricyclics
↑ Upper airway lumen size	Weight reduction Avoidance of supine posture Oral prosthesis	Uvulopalatopharyngoplasty
↓ Upper airway subatmospheric pressure	Improved nasal patency	Nasal continuous positive airway pressure
Bypass occlusion		Tracheostomy

SOURCE: Phillipson, in Murray and Nadel (eds), pp. 1841–1860, with permission.

TABLE 229-3   Mechanisms underlying central sleep apnea

Underlying mechanism	Clinical example
Defects in metabolic control system or respiratory muscles	Primary and secondary central alveolar hypoventilation syndromes Respiratory muscle weakness
Transient instabilities in central respiratory drive	Sleep onset Hyperventilation-induced hypocapnia Hypoxia (high altitude, pulmonary disease) Cardiovascular disease, pulmonary congestion CNS disease Prolonged circulation time
Inhibition of central respiratory drive by upper airway reflexes	Esophageal reflux Aspiration Upper airway collapse

SOURCE: Phillipson, in Murray and Nadel (eds), pp 1841–1860, with permission.

polycythemia, pulmonary hypertension, and right-sided heart failure. Complaints of sleeping poorly, morning headache, and daytime fatigue and sleepiness are also prominent. In contrast, in patients whose CSA results from an instability in respiratory drive, the clinical picture is dominated by features related to sleep disturbance, including recurrent nocturnal awakenings, morning fatigue, and daytime sleepiness.

Diagnosis Initially, many patients with CSA are suspected clinically of having OSA because of a history of snoring, sleep disturbance, and daytime sleepiness. However, obesity and hypertension are less prominent in CSA than in OSA. Definitive diagnosis of CSA requires a polysomnographic study, with the *key observation being recurrent apneas that are not accompanied by respiratory effort*. Measurements of transcutaneous P_{CO_2} are particularly useful in CSA. Those patients with a defect in respiratory control or neuromuscular function typically demonstrate an elevated P_{CO_2} that tends to increase progressively during the night, particularly during REM sleep. In contrast, patients with instabilities in the respiratory control system often demonstrate a mild degree of hypocapnia, which is an integral pathogenetic feature of their disorder (see above).

Treatment The management of patients whose CSA is a component of an alveolar hypoventilation syndrome is essentially the same as management of the underlying hypoventilation disorder. Management of patients whose CSA arises from an instability of respiratory drive is more problematic. Patients with hypoxemia usually respond favorably to nocturnal supplemental oxygen. Others have responded to acidification with acetazolamide, and recent reports indicate a good response to nasal CPAP (as for OSA). The precise mechanism by which CPAP abolishes central apneas is not clear but probably involves a small increase in Pa_{CO_2} as a result of the added expiratory mechanical load.

HYPERVENTILATION AND ITS SYNDROMES

DEFINITION AND ETIOLOGY Alveolar hyperventilation exists when Pa_{CO_2} decreases below the normal range of 37 to 43 mmHg. *Hyperventilation* is not synonymous with *hyperpnea*, which refers to an increased minute volume of ventilation without reference to Pa_{CO_2}. Although hyperventilation is frequently associated with dyspnea, patients who are hyperventilating do not necessarily complain of shortness of breath; and conversely, patients with dyspnea need not be hyperventilating.

Numerous disease entities can be associated with alveolar hyperventilation (Table 229-4), but in all cases the underlying mechanism involves an increase in respiratory drive. Thus hypoxemia drives ventilation by stimulating the peripheral chemoreceptors, and several pulmonary disorders and congestive heart failure drive ventilation by stimulating afferent vagal receptors in the lungs and airways. Low cardiac output and hypotension stimulate the peripheral chemoreceptors and inhibit the baroreceptors, both of which increase ventilation. Metabolic acidosis, a potent respiratory stimulant, excites both the peripheral and central chemoreceptors and increases the sensitivity of the peripheral chemoreceptors to coexistent hypoxemia. Hepatic failure also can produce hyperventilation, presumably as a result of metabolic stimuli acting on the peripheral and central chemoreceptors.

Several neurologic disorders are thought to drive ventilation through the behavioral respiratory control system. Included in this category are psychogenic or anxiety hyperventilation and severe cerebrovascular insufficiency, which may interfere with the inhibitory influence normally exerted by cortical structures on the brainstem respiratory neurons. Rarely, disorders of the midbrain and hypothalamus induce hyperventilation, and it is conceivable that fever and sepsis also cause hyperventilation through effects on these structures. Several drugs cause hyperventilation by stimulating the central or peripheral chemoreceptors or by direct action on the brainstem respiratory neurons. Chronic hyperventilation is a normal feature of pregnancy and results from the effects of progesterone and other hormones acting on the respiratory neurons.

TABLE 229-4 Hyperventilation syndromes

Hypoxemia
A High altitude
B Pulmonary disease

Pulmonary disorders
A Pneumonia
B Interstitial pneumonitis, fibrosis, edema
C Pulmonary emboli, vascular disease
D Bronchial asthma
E Pneumothorax

Cardiovascular disorders
A Congestive heart failure
B Hypotension

Metabolic disorders
A Acidosis (diabetic, renal, lactic)
B Hepatic failure

Neurologic disorders
A Psychogenic or anxiety hyperventilation
B Central nervous system infection, tumors

Drug-induced
A Salicylates
B Methylxanthine derivatives
C Beta-adrenergic agonists
D Progesterone

Miscellaneous
A Fever, sepsis
B Pain
C Pregnancy

PHYSIOLOGIC AND CLINICAL FEATURES Because hyperventilation is associated with increased respiratory drive, muscle effort, and minute volume of ventilation, the most frequent symptom associated with hyperventilation is dyspnea. However, there is considerable discrepancy between the degree of hyperventilation, as measured by Pa_{CO_2}, and the degree of associated dyspnea. In patients whose hypocapnia is associated with alkalemia, neurologic symptoms may be present, including dizziness, visual impairment, syncope, and seizure activity (secondary to cerebral vasoconstriction); parasthesias, carpopedal spasm, and tetany (secondary to decreased free serum calcium); and muscle weakness (secondary to hypophosphatemia). Severe alkalemia also can induce cardiac arrhythmias and evidence of myocardial ischemia. Patients with a primary respiratory alkalosis are also prone to periodic breathing and central sleep apnea (see "Central Sleep Apnea").

DIAGNOSIS In most patients with a hyperventilation syndrome, the cause is readily apparent on the basis of history, physical examination, and knowledge of coexisting medical disorders (see Table 229-4). In patients in whom the cause is not clinically apparent, investigation begins with arterial blood gas analysis, which establishes the presence of alveolar hyperventilation (decreased PA_{CO_2}) and its severity. Equally important is the arterial pH, which generally allows the disorder to be classified as either a primary respiratory alkalosis (elevated pH) or a primary metabolic acidosis (decreased pH). Also of importance is the Pa_{O_2} and calculation of the $(A - a)P_{O_2}$, since a widened alveolar-arterial oxygen difference suggests a pulmonary disorder as the underlying cause. The finding of a reduced plasma HCO_3^- level establishes the chronic nature of the disorder and points toward an organic cause. Measurements of ventilation and arterial or transcutaneous P_{CO_2} during sleep are very useful in suspected psychogenic hyperventilation, since such patients do not maintain the hyperventilation during sleep.

The disorders that most frequently give rise to unexplained hyperventilation are pulmonary vascular disease (particularly chronic or recurrent thromboembolism) and psychogenic or anxiety hyperventilation. Hyperventilation due to pulmonary vascular disease is associated with exertional dyspnea, a widened $(A - a)P_{O_2}$ and maintenance of hyperventilation during exercise. In contrast, patients with psychogenic hyperventilation typically complain of dyspnea at rest and not during mild exercise and of the need to sigh frequently.

They are also more likely to complain of dizziness, sweating, palpitations, and paresthesias. During mild to moderate exercise, their hyperventilation tends to disappear and $(A - a)P_{O_2}$ is normal, but heart rate and cardiac output may be increased relative to metabolic rate.

TREATMENT Alveolar hyperventilation is usually of relatively minor clinical consequence and therefore is generally managed by appropriate treatment of the underlying cause. In the few patients in whom alkalemia is thought to be inducing significant cerebral vasoconstriction, parasthesias, tetany, or cardiac disturbances, inhalation of a low concentration of CO_2 can be very beneficial. For patients with disabling psychogenic hyperventilation, careful explanation of the basis of their symptoms can be reassuring and is often sufficient. Others have benefited from beta-adrenergic antagonists or an exercise program. Specific treatment for anxiety may also be indicated.

REFERENCES

CHERNIACK NS, LONGOBARDO GS: Abnormalities in respiratory rhythm, in *Handbook of Physiology*, section 3: *The Respiratory System*, vol 2, *Control of Breathing*, NS Cherniack, JG Widdicombe (eds). Bethesda, Md, Am Physiol Soc, 1986, pp 729–749

FAIRBANKS DN: Uvulopalatopharyngoplasty: Strategies for success and safety. Ear Nose Throat J 72:46, 1993

FUJITA S: Obstructive sleep apnea syndrome: Pathophysiology, upper airway evaluation and surgical treatment. Ear Nose Throat J 72:77, 1993

HUDGEL DW, CHERNIACK NS: Sleep and breathing, in *Update: Pulmonary Diseases and Disorders*, AP Fishman (ed). New York, McGraw-Hill, 1992, pp 249–262

PHILLIPSON EA: Hypoventilation syndromes, in *Textbook of Respiratory Medicine*, JF Murray, JA Nadel (eds). Philadelphia, Saunders, 1988, chap 84, pp. 1831–1840

———: Sleep disorders, in *Textbook of Respiratory Medicine*, JF Murray, JA Nadel (eds). Philadelphia, Saunders, 1988, chap 85, pp 1841–1860

———, BRADLEY TD (eds): Breathing disorders in sleep. *Clin Chest Med* 13:(3)383, 1992

230 ADULT RESPIRATORY DISTRESS SYNDROME

ROLAND H. INGRAM, JR.

Adult respiratory distress syndrome (ARDS) is a descriptive term that has been applied to many acute, diffuse infiltrative lung lesions of diverse etiologies when they are accompanied by severe arterial hypoxemia. The term was chosen because of several clinical and pathologic similarities between such acute illnesses in adults and the neonatal respiratory distress syndrome. However, in the neonatal form, immaturity of alveolar surfactant production and a highly compliant chest wall are primarily involved in the pathophysiology, whereas in the adult form, alveolar surfactant changes are secondary to the primary process and the chest wall is not compliant. Despite the large number of causes (Table 230-1), the clinical characteristics, respiratory pathophysiologic derangement, and current techniques for supportive management of these acute abnormalities are remarkably similar. It has been argued that the "lumping" of such processes of different etiologies obscures the unique features of each in terms of pathogenesis, prevention, and specificity of treatment. However, irrespective of cause, there are many common features at the onset of respiratory failure. The conditions listed do not always lead to respiratory failure, and specific treatment of the underlying processes will often be different. The most common cause of ARDS is sepsis; therefore, that etiology and its pathogenesis will be the focus of this chapter. The reader is urged to refer to the appropriate sections of this text for the special characteristics of other causes. Several causative factors can come into play during the course of ARDS; for example, respiratory failure in association with acute pancreatitis can

TABLE 230-1 Conditions which may lead to the adult respiratory distress syndrome

1 Diffuse pulmonary infections (e.g., viral, bacterial, fungal, *Pneumocystis*)
2 Aspiration (e.g., gastric contents with Mendelson's syndrome, water with near drowning)
3 Inhalation of toxins and irritants (e.g., chlorine gas, NO_2, smoke, ozone, high concentrations of oxygen)
4 Narcotic overdose pulmonary edema (e.g., heroin, methadone, morphine, dextropropoxyphene)
5 Nonnarcotic drug effects (e.g., nitrofurantoin)
6 Immunologic response to host antigens (e.g., Goodpasture's syndrome, systemic lupus erythematosus)
7 Effects of nonthoracic trauma with hypotension
8 In association with systemic reactions to processes initiated outside the lung (e.g., gram-negative septicemia, hemorrhagic pancreatitis, amniotic fluid embolism, fat embolism)
9 After cardiopulmonary bypass ("pump lung," "postperfusion lung")

be complicated by a bacterial pneumonia, which, in turn, can lead to a sepsis syndrome (see below). ARDS then becomes the pulmonary manifestation of a systemic disorder associated with diffuse endothelial injury and increased capillary permeability in multiple organ systems.

PATHOPHYSIOLOGY Regardless of the initiating process, ARDS is invariably associated with increased liquid in the lungs. It is a form of pulmonary edema, although distinct from cardiogenic pulmonary edema because pulmonary capillary pressure is not elevated (Chap. 31). Since hydrostatic pressures are not elevated, there is increased permeability of the alveolocapillary membranes that occurs via direct chemical injury in the case of inhaled toxic gases or aspirated acid or indirectly through activation and aggregation of formed elements of the blood within pulmonary capillaries. In association with sepsis, bacterial endotoxins (gram-negative bacteria) or exotoxins (gram-positive bacteria) stimulate monocytic phagocytes and polymorphonuclear leukocytes to adhere to endothelial surfaces and undergo a respiratory burst to inflict oxidant injury and release mediators of inflammation such as leukotrienes, thromboxanes, and prostaglandins. The monocytic phagocytes, mainly macrophages in the alveoli and those lining the vasculature, also release oxidants, mediators, cytokines, and a series of degradative enzymes and peptides that directly damage endothelial and alveolar surfaces and cause polymorphonuclear leukocytes to release their lysosomal enzymes. Initially, the injury to the alveolocapillary membrane results in leakage of liquid, macromolecules, and cellular components from the blood vessels into the interstitial space and, with increasing severity, into the alveoli.

The increasing vascular permeability to proteins (decreased reflection coefficient σ, discussed in Chap. 31) leaves the hydrostatic gradient unopposed so that even mild elevations in capillary pressures (due to increased intravenous fluid loads and cardiac dysfunction characteristic of sepsis) greatly increase interstitial and alveolar edema. Alveolar collapse occurs secondary to the effect of the alveolar liquid, especially its fibrinogen, that interferes with normal surfactant activity and the possible impairment of further surfactant production by injury to the granular pneumocytes. Fibrinolytic mechanisms that would normally clear the alveoli are inhibited, and their deficiency can lead to hyaline membranes that may act as a matrix for fibrogenesis. Though radiographically diffuse, the regional dysfunction is nonhomogeneous; it leads to severe ventilation-perfusion imbalance and the shunting of blood through regions in which alveoli are collapsed or filled with liquid and fibrin. The lungs become less compliant—i.e., stiffen because of interstitial edema, alveolar collapse, and increase in surface forces. Because of the decreased compliance, large inspiratory pressures must be generated by the respiratory muscles, so the work of breathing is elevated. The large mechanical load may lead to fatigue of the muscles of breathing with resulting diminution in tidal volumes and worsening gas exchange. Both hypoxemia and the stimulation of receptors in the stiff lung parenchyma cause an increase in respiratory frequency, decrease in tidal volume, and deterioration in gas exchange.

PATHOLOGY In the absence of specific demonstrable pathogens, the pathology is remarkably similar among the various conditions leading to ARDS, since the lung has a limited number of ways in which it reacts to a large number of injuries. Grossly, the lungs are heavy, edematous, and nearly airless with regions of hemorrhage, atelectasis, and consolidation. By light microscopy, there is edema and cellular infiltration of interalveolar septa and interstitial spaces surrounding airways and blood vessels, atelectasis and hyaline membranes in many regions, engorgement of vessels with red blood cells, and aggregates of platelets and polymorphonuclear leukocytes along with interstitial and alveolar hemorrhage. In addition to loss of alveolar type I pneumocytes, both hyperplasia and dysplasia of the granular (type II) pneumocytes are often present.

If the illness has been prolonged beyond 10 days, there is often a surprising amount of fibrosis in addition to the acute changes. In instances of recovery and subsequent death from another cause, significant interstitial fibrosis and emphysematous changes may be found in the lung. Many patients, however, will recover completely and have normal pulmonary function with no respiratory symptoms. Hence aggressive clinical management is both indicated and often rewarding.

CLINICAL CHARACTERISTICS At the time of initial injury and for several hours thereafter, the patient may be free of respiratory symptoms or signs. The earliest sign often is an increase in respiratory frequency followed shortly by dyspnea. Arterial blood gas measurement in the earlier period will disclose a depressed P_{O_2} despite a decreased P_{CO_2} so that the alveolar-arterial difference for oxygen (Chap. 214) is increased. At this early stage, administration of oxygen results in a significant increase in the arterial P_{O_2}. The brisk rise in P_{O_2} indicates that ventilation-perfusion mismatching and, possibly, diffusion impairment account for the widened alveolar-arterial P_{O_2} difference [$(A - a)P_{O_2}$] initially. Physical examination may be unremarkable, although a few fine inspiratory rales may be audible. Radiographically, the lung fields may be clear or demonstrate only minimal and scattered interstitial infiltrates. With progression, the patient becomes cyanotic and increasingly dyspneic and tachypneic. Rales may become more prominent and easily heard throughout both lung fields along with regions of tubular breath sounds; the chest radiograph demonstrates diffuse, extensive bilateral interstitial and alveolar infiltrates (Fig. 230-1). At this point, hypoxemia cannot be corrected simply by increasing the oxygen concentration of the inspired gas, and mechanical ventilatory support must be started. Right-to-left shunting of blood through collapsed or filled alveoli becomes the major mechanism for arterial hypoxemia at this more advanced stage. In contrast to ventilation-perfusion mismatching and diffusion impairment, with right-to-left shunts, $(A - a)P_{O_2}$ remains high with breathing of pure oxygen. Positive end-expiratory pressure (PEEP) serves to increase lung volume, which in turn opens collapsed alveoli and decreases shunting. With further progression, and if mechanical ventilator and PEEP therapy are delayed, the combination of increasing tachypnea and decreasing tidal volumes results in alveolar hypoventilation, a rising P_{CO_2}, and worsening hypoxemia; these represent an ominous constellation of findings.

When there is evidence of infection, most commonly intraabdominal, renal, or lung; the presence of tachycardia (>90 beats per minute), tachypnea (>20 breaths per minute), either fever (>38.3°C) or hypothermia (<35.5°C), and some combination of alteration in mental status, lactic acidemia, oliguria (<0.5 mL/kg for more than 1 h); and an elevated alveolar-arterial P_{O_2}, the criteria for the sepsis syndrome are met. It is at this point that many immunologic and pharmacologic interventions directed against bacterial products, cytokines, oxidants, and arachidonic acid metabolites are being tried.

If the syndrome progresses to frank ARDS with hypotension and multiorgan failure, which occurs in a large percentage of cases of the sepsis syndrome, the mortality rate is exceedingly high despite supportive measures.

SUPPORTIVE MANAGEMENT OF HYPOXEMIC RESPIRATORY FAILURE The brief description given above contains the salient

FIGURE 230-1 A standard posteroanterior chest radiograph from a patient with the adult respiratory distress syndrome secondary to a severe viral pneumonitis. Such a diffuse radiographic change is typical of all conditions listed in Table 230-1 when they are severe enough to cause acute hypoxemic respiratory failure. A similar radiographic picture is also seen in pulmonary edema due to left ventricular failure (Chap. 31). Often in such acutely ill patients, the radiograph must be taken with a portable unit and the film exposed from the anterior direction. Both the anteroposterior exposure and the failure to take a deep inspiration result in an apparent enlargement of the cardiac silhouette which further obscures the reliable detection of left ventricular failure.

principles of management, integrated with the clinical events that lead to escalation of therapeutic interventions. Implicit in that description is that the simplest method and the lowest inspired fraction of oxygen (FI_{O_2}) should be used to give the desired result. The oxyhemoglobin dissociation curve gives some guide to the most desirable level of Pa_{O_2}. At a P_{O_2} of 60 mmHg, hemoglobin is approximately 90 percent saturated. Therefore, a reasonable objective is to achieve that Pa_{O_2}, since higher levels add little to oxygenation and introduce the risk of oxygen toxicity to the lung. In contrast to respiratory failure complicating chronic airways obstruction (Chap. 223), depression of ventilation is not an important factor in hypoxemic respiratory failure.

There are multiple means for delivering O_2, in order of increasing effectiveness: soft nasal prongs, simple face masks, and face masks with inspiratory reservoir bags. The effective FI_{O_2} (that is actually entering the trachea) will be determined by the concentration of O_2 delivered from the tank or wall device, its flow rate, and the minute ventilation of the patient. In the hypoxemic form of respiratory failure, it is reasonable to start with moderate flow rates (5 to 10 L/min of 100% O_2) and monitor arterial blood gases, adjusting flow rates and O_2 concentrations depending on results.

Mechanical ventilatory support If adequate oxygenation cannot be maintained with these less invasive measures, endotracheal intubation is needed and mechanical ventilatory support should be instituted (see Chap. 231). The rationale behind mechanical ventilatory support in a patient who is hyperventilating is *not* to increase ventilation but to increase mean lung volume, thereby opening previously closed airways and improving oxygenation. This is accomplished by using large tidal volumes (approximately 10 to 15 mL/kg of lean body weight) at a slower breathing rate (12 to 15 breaths per minute) than the spontaneous one of the patient. Most often, at this juncture, the respiratory system is sufficiently stiff that high inflation pressures are required and a volume-cycled ventilator (in contrast to the pressure-cycled ones) is needed. If the patient makes expiratory efforts during the inflation cycle, peak inspiratory pressures will increase, possibly enough to activate the high-pressure pop-off valve, which results in delivery to the patient of a smaller tidal volume than selected. Under these circumstances during controlled ventilation, consideration is often given to sedation and/or neuromuscular paralysis. However, an alternative is to institute synchronized intermittent mandatory ventilation (SIMV). In the SIMV mode, the patient is allowed to breathe spontaneously with periodic delivery of mandatory breaths that are synchronized with spontaneous inspiratory efforts. If the spontaneous breathing rate is so rapid that expiratory efforts occur before the mandatory breath is fully delivered, sedation and/or paralysis should be used with controlled ventilation.

Use of PEEP Should the Pa_{O_2} be greater than 60 mmHg, the next step is to lower the Fi_{O_2}. If the Fi_{O_2} can be lowered to 0.6 or less with a Pa_{O_2} equal to or greater than 60 mmHg, the mechanical ventilation should proceed at that Fi_{O_2} as long as necessary. There are two indications for the addition of PEEP, the rationale for which is to increase lung volume further, thereby opening previously closed alveoli. First, if the Fi_{O_2} cannot be lowered to or below 0.6, then PEEP should be added to allow a decrease of the Fi_{O_2} below the toxic range. Second, if the Pa_{O_2} cannot be increased to or above 60 mmHg with an Fi_{O_2} of 1.0, PEEP should be added. The optimal magnitude of the PEEP is determined by the response of the Pa_{O_2} and the extent of the cardiovascular alterations resulting from the higher pressure. The major alteration is a decrease in cardiac output due to two mechanisms. First, increased intrapleural pressures serve to impede venous return directly, an effect which is, to a variable extent, offset by peripheral venoconstriction. Second, increases in lung volume may increase pulmonary vascular resistance, leading to increased pressure and dilatation of the right ventricle, which in turn displaces the interventricular septum toward the left. This displacement decreases left ventricular diastolic compliance; hence less filling leads to smaller stroke volumes. An additional mechanism for decreased diastolic filling of the ventricles is direct compression of the heart by the stiffened lung. The optimal levels of PEEP are those associated with the greatest delivery of O_2 to the body; the latter is the product of cardiac output and arterial oxygen content.

Patients who are critically ill may simultaneously develop both deterioration of arterial oxygenation, due to increased lung fluid and/or a fall in mixed venous oxygen levels, and precarious hemodynamics, due to the pressure effects of mechanical ventilation and/or cardiac dysfunction with either a contracted or an expanded intravascular volume. Ventilator adjustments (see Chap. 231) are not often helpful because higher inflation pressures reflect worsening lung function. In this situation of falling blood pressure, urinary output, and arterial oxygenation, the decision to expand intravascular volume by infusion or to decrease it by diuresis is difficult. Body-weight change is rarely a reliable indicator of blood volume, since there is often fluid retention from positive intrathoracic pressures produced by the ventilator (see Chap. 231) plus "third space" fluid sequestration, especially with sepsis. Nor is physical examination of much help, since rales are usual in any case and portable anteroposterior chest radiographs do not allow accurate assessment of subtle changes in cardiac size. Therefore, a flow-directed right heart balloon-tipped (Swan-Ganz) catheter is often used for monitoring pulmonary arterial and capillary wedge pressures and measuring changes in cardiac output by the thermodilution technique. Recognition of overdamping and accelerative artifacts in the pulmonary arterial pressure signal and learning the criteria for true wedging are essential if serious misinterpretations are to be avoided. Even with accurate pressure measurements, there is an additional precaution that must be taken with regard to interpretation of intrathoracic vascular pressures referenced to atmosphere when PEEP is being used. If pleural pressure is greater than atmospheric pressure, as is most often the case with PEEP, the transmural (i.e., intravascular minus pleural) pressure will be overestimated and could lead to errors in both assessment and management. Since the lungs are stiff, only a portion of the applied PEEP is transmitted to the pleural space. A reasonable estimate of the transmural pressure is gained by examining vascular pressures just before inflation and subtracting from these pressures an amount equal to one-half the value of PEEP. In view of the leaky alveolocapillary membrane, it is best to keep the pulmonary capillary wedge pressure

as low as is compatible with a reasonable cardiac output, arterial pressure, and urinary output. Inotropic and selective vasoactive agents (e.g., dopamine) have been used with some success to achieve this but require careful monitoring to assess effects and adjust doses.

Mixed venous blood P_{O_2} values have long been considered to indicate the adequacy of oxygen delivery relative to demand. A low value (e.g., <20 mmHg) surely indicates that there is tissue hypoxemia irrespective of measured cardiac output and Pa_{O_2}. However, a high value does not exclude serious tissue hypoxia, especially in gram-negative septicemia, in which systemic low-resistance shunts can develop and leave several capillary beds underperfused.

Body position also may affect the degree of arterial oxygenation. Although patients with ARDS have diffuse lung disease, there may be some regional variation in the extent of disease such that one side is more severely involved than the other. In this instance, the less involved lung should be the more dependent one when the patient is in a lateral position. Since the distribution of pulmonary blood flow is so heavily determined by gravity (Chap. 214), having the more involved lung, with its minimal ventilation, in the more dependent position results in a measurable increase in intrapulmonary shunting which may be manifested by a striking fall in Pa_{O_2}. The possible contribution of a positional effect on arterial oxygenation should always be considered before escalating therapeutic interventions.

Occasionally, PEEP must be gradually increased to levels in excess of 20 cmH$_2$O in an attempt to maintain arterial oxygenation. At these high levels of PEEP there may be a paradoxic decrease in Pa_{O_2}. The explanation for this paradox is as follows: High levels of PEEP may not open some of the closed airways but will overdistend those alveolar units already open. Overdistention of units increases the vascular resistance in these regions and results in more blood perfusing regions with closed airways, thereby increasing the degree of shunt. The only alternative is to decrease PEEP to a level associated with the greatest delivery of oxygen to the body (product of cardiac output and arterial oxygen content).

High inflation pressures, the necessity of which indicate severe lung dysfunction, have been shown to directly damage the alveolar capillary membrane in the experimental setting. Based on the clinical suspicion that high inflation pressures also might compound the lung injury in ARDS, attempts have been made to remove CO_2 by extracorporeal perfusion techniques, thereby allowing the use of smaller tidal volumes and pressures from the ventilator. The clinical value of this approach has not yet been established.

In the situations where maximal PEEP with an Fi_{O_2} of 1.0 does not supply sufficient oxygen, the possibility of utilizing extracorporeal membrane oxygenators (ECMO) has been both considered and tried. Despite the logical appeal of this form of supportive therapy, a randomized, large prospective study of ECMO therapy has demonstrated that while it can support gas exchange, there is no effect on survival in acute hypoxemic respiratory failure.

Inactivation and decreased production of surfactant undoubtedly contribute to the gas exchange and mechanical abnormalities of the lung. Replacement of surfactant in ARDS, using either bovine sources or a synthetic phospholipid in combination with a recombinant human protein, is being assessed in clinical trials. Given the unresolved issues of optimal delivery systems, doses, intervals of administration, and appropriateness of end points, an early and clear answer is not likely.

Strategies in the management of sepsis causing ARDS (See also Chap. 83) Identification of the source of infection and the organism(s) responsible is necessary for proper antibiotic therapy. If there is a localized source of sepsis requiring surgical drainage, this must be accomplished quickly. Although the surgical mortality is high, failure to drain a purulent focus leads to an almost uniformly fatal outcome.

The range of implicated bacterial products, endogenously produced mediators, cytokines, peptides, enzymes, and oxidants gives a rationale for many interventions designed to interrupt the injurious processes. Most strategies only represent reasonable postulates, others are backed by limited experiments, several are subjects of current trials, and very few, if any, have been tested clinically and found to be both practical and useful. A major problem is that the sequence of events and the relative role of each participant are not clear. The most logical intervention, in the case of gram-negative sepsis, is the administration of antibodies to endotoxin, since endotoxin release appears to initiate the cascade of tissue injury. The human monoclonal IgM antibody, HA-1A, which binds to endotoxin, prevents death in laboratory animals and appears to modify the clinical outcome only in the bacteremic subset of patients with sepsis. Given the delay in establishing the presence of bacteremia and the apparent need for early treatment, most patients with sepsis would be treated needlessly and at great expense. Guidelines for the use of this expensive therapy are in the process of being established.

COMPLICATIONS Increasing severity of the clinical illness and continued radiographic progression in association with the primary process often obscure complications that arise during the course of acute hypoxemic respiratory failure. The development of *left ventricular failure* is a good example of a common, easily missed complication. This is so because all patients are likely to have diffuse rales and rhonchi, even without left ventricular failure, and these sounds also serve to make it difficult to detect gallop rhythms. An additional difficulty is that portable chest films are taken in the anteroposterior direction, often at less than full lung inflation, so the cardiac silhouette appears enlarged. As a consequence, the ordinary physical and radiographic assessments are not always reliable. With deterioration, therefore, left ventricular failure should be suspected; it is helpful to insert a Swan-Ganz catheter (see above) which can be used to monitor pulmonary arterial pressure continuously and intermittently to assess pulmonary capillary wedge pressure and oxygen content of mixed venous blood.

With a diffuse radiographic pattern, a secondary bacterial infection is easily overlooked; therefore, frequent sputum smears and cultures should be obtained, especially when there is fever. With many conditions—e.g., gram-negative septicemia, acute hemorrhagic pancreatitis, and "shock lung"—there may be associated *disseminated intravascular coagulation*, which leads to gastrointestinal and intrapulmonary hemorrhage. Frequent monitoring of platelet count, fibrinogen level, and partial thromboplastin and prothrombin times is helpful in the early detection of this complication and in guiding treatment.

Bronchial obstruction by endotracheal or tracheostomy tubes is common. When these tubes are too long or poorly anchored, they may slide into one main bronchus, usually the right one because of its less angulated origin from the trachea. The tube then blocks ventilation of the other main bronchus, and atelectasis may ensue. This event usually causes abrupt deterioration in the patient with respiratory failure. It is detected readily by physical examination, which reveals the absence of breath sounds over the occluded lung. The tube should immediately be pulled back slowly if this complication is suspected. In the course of treating ARDS with mechanical ventilators and high inflation pressures, *pneumothorax* or *pneumomediastinum* may develop and may be impossible to detect except radiologically. Occasionally, the presence of subcutaneous emphysema provides a clinical clue. Any deterioration should lead to consideration of this complication, repetition of the chest radiograph, and immediate institution of treatment of pneumothorax, if present. If deterioration is sudden, *tension pneumothorax* should be suspected; if physical signs are present, a pleural catheter should be inserted immediately without radiographic confirmation. High oxygen concentrations (>0.60) for prolonged periods can produce both the lesions and the clinical picture of ARDS. Therefore, the *minimal* oxygen concentration associated with acceptable arterial oxygenation should always be used.

Discontinuation of mechanical ventilatory support The ability of the patient to maintain adequate gas exchange without the support of a mechanical ventilator is most often heralded by a decreasing FI_{O_2} requirement, smaller inflation pressures for mandatory or assisted breathing, and a fall in spontaneous respiratory rate (see Chap. 231).

PROGNOSIS Given the diversity of the etiologies and the frequency of associated diseases, it is difficult, if not impossible, to give meaningful prognostic figures for ARDS. If all recently published series are taken together, the mortality rate is between 50 and 60 percent. This represents an improved survival rate over the nearly 100 percent mortality rate of a few years ago and is a result of the application of modern treatment techniques described above. If ARDS is due to drug overdose, the mortality rate is low; if associated with shock, the chances of a fatal outcome are much greater. Multiple organ system failure (e.g., renal, hepatic) supervenes when there is an extrapulmonic source of sepsis in need of surgical drainage, and almost all such patients die despite maximal support of the respiratory and cardiovascular systems. Other etiologies and associated diseases fall between these two extremes. The following factors appear to be associated with a poor outcome: an increase in $(A - a)Pa_{O_2}$, requiring increasing inspired O_2 concentrations and PEEP; decreasing compliance, requiring greater inflation pressures; either low or falling colloid osmotic pressures; and the onset of systemic arterial hypotension not responding to intravascular volume replacement.

In survivors with previously normal lung function, the long-term prognosis for recovery appears to be remarkably good. Lung volumes and arterial blood gases have been shown to return to normal levels within 4 to 6 months after respiratory failure. There are instances, however, when the fibrotic residua are sufficiently great that complete recovery is unlikely.

REFERENCES

ALBELDA SM: The alveolar-capillary barrier in adult respiratory distress syndrome, in *Update: Pulmonary Diseases and Disorders*, AP Fishman (ed). New York, McGraw-Hill, 1992, pp 197–212

BERNARD GR: *N*-Acetylcysteine in experimental and clinical acute lung injury. Am J Med Suppl 30:54S, 1991

BONE RC et al: Adult respiratory distress syndrome: Sequence and importance of development of multiple organ failure. Chest 101:320, 1992

———: Gram-negative sepsis: Background, clinical features, and intervention. Chest 100:802, 1991

FISER DH: Adult respiratory distress syndrome. Pediatr Rev 14:163, 1993

GREGORY TJ et al: Surfactant chemical composition and biophysical activity in acute respiratory distress syndrome. J Clin Invest 88:1976, 1991

HYERS TM et al: Tumor necrosis factor levels in serum and bronchoalveolar lavage fluid of patients with the adult respiratory distress syndrome. Am Rev Respir Dis 144:268, 1991

INGRAM RH, BRAUNWALD E: Pulmonary edema: Cardiogenic and noncardiogenic, in *Heart Disease*, E Braunwald (ed). Philadelphia, Saunders, 1992, p 551

MARINI JJ: Recent advances in mechanical ventilation, in *Update: Pulmonary Diseases and Disorders*, AP Fishman (ed). New York, McGraw-Hill, 1992, pp 401–418

MARTIN TR et al: The function of lung and blood neutrophils in patients with the adult respiratory distress syndrome: Implications for the pathogenesis of lung infections. Am Rev Respir Dis 144:254, 1991

METZ C, SIBBALD WJ: Anti-inflammatory therapy for acute lung injury: A review of animal and clinical studies. Chest 100:1110, 1991

MORRIS P, BERNARD GR: Adult respiratory distress syndrome: Strategies to provide support and enhance oxygen delivery. Postgrad Med 90:163, 1991

PATTISHALL EN, LONG WA: Surfactant treatment of adult respiratory distress syndrome, in *Update: Pulmonary Diseases and Disorders*, AP Fishman (ed). New York, McGraw-Hill, 1992, pp 225–236

PETTY TL et al: Contemporary clinical trials in acute respiratory distress syndrome. Chest 101:550, 1992

RANIERI VM et al: Effects of positive end-expiratory pressure on alveolar recruitment and gas exchange in patients with the adult respiratory distress syndrome. Am Rev Respir Dis 144:544, 1991

SEEGER W et al: Alveolar surfactant and adult respiratory distress syndrome. Pathogenetic role and therapeutic prospects. Clin Investig 71:177, 1993

WEST JB, MATHIEU-COSTELLO O: Stress failure of pulmonary capillaries: Role in lung and heart disease. J Appl Physiol 70:1731, 1991

ZIEGLER EJ et al: Treatment of gram-negative bacteremia and septic shock with HA-1A human monoclonal antibody against endotoxin. N Engl J Med 324:429, 1991

231 MECHANICAL VENTILATORY SUPPORT

EDWARD P. INGENITO / JEFFREY M. DRAZEN

Ventilators are medical devices that provide external mechanical support of the ventilatory function of the respiratory system. They are considered a mainstay of physiologic supportive care; they provide ventilatory support to patients through episodes of respiratory failure as the underlying disease process is definitively treated.

INDICATIONS FOR MECHANICAL VENTILATION

Respiratory failure is the primary indication for initiation of mechanical ventilation. It is important to distinguish among the various forms of respiratory failure because the therapeutic goals of mechanical ventilation differ depending on which form is present.

Hypoxemic respiratory failure most commonly results from pulmonary conditions such as severe pneumonia, pulmonary edema, pulmonary hemorrhage, and respiratory distress syndrome causing ventilation-perfusion ($\dot{V}/Q$) mismatch. Hypoxemic respiratory failure is present when arterial oxygen saturations of less than 90 percent are observed despite an inspired oxygen fraction of greater than 0.6. The goal of ventilator treatment in this setting is to provide adequate arterial oxygen saturation.

Hypercarbic respiratory failure results from disease states causing either a decrease in minute ventilation or an increase in physiologic dead space such that, despite adequate total minute ventilation, alveolar ventilation is inadequate to meet metabolic demands. Common clinical conditions associated with hypercarbic respiratory failure include neuromuscular diseases, such as myasthenia gravis, ascending polyradiculopathy, and myopathies, as well as diseases that cause respiratory muscle fatigue due to increased workload, such as asthma, chronic obstructive pulmonary disease, and restrictive lung disease. *Acute* hypercarbic respiratory failure is present when arterial P_{CO_2} values exceed 50 mmHg and the arterial pH is below 7.30 (Chap. 46). *Chronic* hypercarbic respiratory failure is characterized by arterial P_{CO_2} values of greater than 50 mmHg and an arterial pH above 7.30.

Mechanical ventilation generally should be instituted in acute hypercarbic respiratory failure. In contrast, the decision to institute mechanical ventilation when components of both acute and chronic hypercarbic respiratory failure are present depends on blood gas parameters and clinical evaluation. In particular, if a patient is not in respiratory distress and is not mentally impaired by CO_2 accumulation, it is not mandatory to initiate mechanical ventilation while other forms of treatment are being administered. The goal of ventilator treatment in hypercarbic respiratory failure is to normalize arterial pH through changes in carbon dioxide tensions. Hypoxemic and hypercarbic respiratory failure may coexist in a given individual; in such cases, the indications for and goals of mechanical ventilation are similar to those in these two individual entities.

Accepted therapeutic applications of mechanical ventilation include controlled hyperventilation to reduce cerebral blood flow in patients with increased intracranial pressure or to improve pulmonary hemodynamics in patients with postoperative pulmonary hypertension. Mechanical ventilation also has been used to reduce the work of breathing in patients with congestive heart failure, especially in the presence of myocardial ischemia. In addition to being used in established respiratory failure, ventilator support is indicated in conjunction with endotracheal intubation to prevent aspiration of gastric contents in otherwise unstable patients during gastric lavage for suspected drug overdose or during upper gastrointestinal endoscopy. In the critically ill patient, intubation and mechanical ventilation are indicated before essential diagnostic or therapeutic studies if it appears that respiratory failure may occur during these maneuvers.

PHYSIOLOGIC ASPECTS OF MECHANICAL VENTILATION

Most modern mechanical ventilators function by providing warmed and humidified gas to the airway opening in conformance with various specific volume, pressure, and time patterns. The ventilator serves as the energy source for inspiration, replacing the muscles of the diaphragm and chest wall. Expiration is passive, driven by the recoil of the lungs and chest wall; at the completion of inspiration, internal ventilator circuitry vents the airway to atmospheric pressure or a specified level of positive end-expiratory pressure (PEEP).

PEEP helps maintain alveolar patency in the presence of destabilizing factors and therefore reverses hypoxemia and atelectasis by improving $\dot{V}/Q$ matching. PEEP levels between 0 and 5 cmH$_2$O are generally safe and effective; higher levels are recommended only in the management of significant refractory hypoxemia unresponsive to increments in inspired oxygen content up to an inspired oxygen content (FI$_{O_2}$) of 0.6.

ESTABLISHING AN AIRWAY A cuffed endotracheal tube must be inserted to allow positive-pressure ventilators to deliver conditioned gas, at pressures above atmospheric pressure, to the lungs in a controlled fashion. If neuromuscular paralysis is to be induced during intubation, the use of agents whose mechanism of action includes depolarization at the neuromuscular junction, such as succinylcholine chloride, should be avoided in patients with renal failure, tumor lysis syndrome, crush injuries, or medical conditions associated with elevated serum potassium levels because these agents may elevate the serum potassium to potentially lethal levels. Opiates and benzodiazepines can have a deleterious effect on hemodynamics in patients with depressed cardiac function or low systemic vascular resistance and should be used cautiously in this setting. Morphine can promote histamine release from tissue mast cells and may worsen bronchospasm in asthmatics; fentanyl, sufentanil, and alfentanil are acceptable alternatives to morphine. Ketamine may increase systemic arterial pressure as well as intracranial pressure and has been associated with dramatic hallucinatory responses; it should be used with caution in patients with hypertensive crisis, increased intracranial pressures, or a history of psychiatric disorders.

VENTILATOR MODE This setting specifies the manner in which ventilator breaths are triggered, cycled, and limited; commonly used modes of mechanical ventilation are given in Table 231-1. The *trigger,* either an inspiratory effect or a time-based signal, defines what the ventilator senses to initiate an assisted cycle. This trigger may be either an inspiratory effort or a time-based signal. *Cycle* refers to the factors that determine end inspiration. For example, in volume-cycled ventilation, inspiration ends when a specific tidal volume is delivered to the patient. Other types of cycling include pressure cycling, time cycling, and flow cycling. *Limiting factors* are operator-specified values, such as airway pressure, that are monitored by internal ventilator circuitry throughout the respiratory cycle; if the specified values are exceeded, inspiratory flow is immediately stopped and the ventilator circuit vented to atmospheric pressure or the specified PEEP.

Assist control mode ventilation (ACMV) This mode is patient/time triggered, volume cycled, and pressure limited. An inspiratory cycle is initiated either by the patient's inspiratory effort or, if no patient effort is detected within a specified time window, by a timer signal within the ventilator. Every breath delivered consists of the full operator-specified tidal volume. Ventilatory rate is determined either by the patient or by the operator-specified backup rate, whichever is of higher frequency (Fig. 231-1A). ACMV is the recommended mode for initiation of mechanical ventilation because it ensures a backup minute ventilation in the absence of an intact respiratory drive and allows for synchronization of the ventilator cycle with the patient's inspiratory effort.

TABLE 231-1   Clinical characteristics of commonly used modes of mechanical ventilation

Independent variables (set by user)	Dependent variables (monitored by user)	Trigger/cycle limit	Advantages	Disadvantages	Initial settings
ASSIST/CONTROL MODE VENTILATION (ACMV)					
FI_{O_2} Tidal volume Ventilator rate Level of PEEP Inspiratory flow pattern Peak inspiratory flow Pressure limit	Peak airway pressure, Pa_{O_2}, Pa_{CO_2} Mean airway pressure I/E ratio	Patient/timer Pressure limit	Timer backup Patient-vent synchrony Patient controls minute ventilation	Not useful for weaning Potential for dangerous respiratory alkalosis	$FI_{O_2} = 1.0*$ $V_t = 10-15$ mL/kg $f = 12-15$/min PEEP $= 0-5$ cmH$_2$O Inspiratory flow $= 60$ L/min
SYNCHRONIZED INTERMITTENT MANDATORY VENTILATION (SIMV)					
Same as for ACMV	Same as for ACMV	Same as for ACMV	Timer backup useful for weaning	Potential dysynchrony	Same as for ACMV
CONTINUOUS POSITIVE AIRWAY PRESSURE (CPAP)					
FI_{O_2} Level of CPAP	Tidal volume Rate, flow pattern Airway pressure Pa_{O_2}, Pa_{CO_2}, I/E ratio	No trigger Pressure limit	Allows assessment of spontaneous function Helps prevent atelectasis	No backup	$FI_{O_2} = 0.5-1.0*$ CPAP $= 5-15$ cmH$_2$O
PRESSURE-CONTROL VENTILATION (PCV)					
FI_{O_2} Inspiratory pressure level Ventilator rate Level of PEEP Pressure limit I/E ratio	Tidal volume Flow rate, pattern Minute ventilation; Pa_{O_2}, Pa_{CO_2}	Timer/patient Timer/pressure limit	System pressures regulated Useful for barotrauma treatment Timer backup	Requires heavy sedation Not useful for weaning	$FI_{O_2} = 1.0*$ PC $= 20-40$ cmH$_2$O PEEP $= 5-10$ cmH$_2$O $f = 12-15$/min I/E $= 0.7/1-4/1$
PRESSURE-SUPPORT VENTILATION (PSV)					
FI_{O_2} Inspiratory pressure level PEEP Pressure limit	Same as for PCV + I/E ratio	Inspiratory flow Pressure limit	Ensures synchrony Good for weaning	No timer backup	$FI_{O_2} = 0.5-1.0*$ PS $= 10-30$ cmH$_2$O 5 cmH$_2$O usually the level used PEEP $= 0-5$ cmH$_2$O

*FI_{O_2} is usually set to 1.0 initially, unless there is a specific clinical indication to minimize FI_{O_2}, such as history of chemotherapy with bleomycin. Once adequate oxygenation is documented by blood gas analysis, FI_{O_2} should be decreased in decrements of 0.1 to 0.2 as tolerated, until the lowest FI_{O_2} required for an Sa_{O_2} of greater than 90 percent is achieved.

A number of potential problems can arise when ACMV is used. In patients with tachypnea due to nonrespiratory, nonmetabolic factors such as anxiety, pain, or airway irritation, respiratory alkalemia may develop and may trigger myoclonus or seizures. Dynamic hyperinflation (so-called auto-PEEP) may occur if the patient's respiratory mechanics are such that inadequate time is available for complete exhalation between inspiratory cycles. Auto-PEEP can limit venous return and decrease cardiac output. ACMV is not effective for weaning patients from mechanical ventilation because it provides full ventilator assistance on each patient-initiated breath.

Synchronized intermittent mandatory ventilation (SIMV) This mode is similar to ACMV in that it is dually patient/time triggered, volume cycled, and pressure limited. The major difference between SIMV and ACMV is that in the former the patient is allowed to breathe spontaneously, i.e., without ventilator assist, between delivered ventilator breaths. However, at a frequency determined by the operator, mandatory breaths are delivered in synchrony with the patient's inspiratory efforts. If the patient fails to initiate a breath, the ventilator delivers a fixed-tidal-volume breath and resets the internal timer for the next inspiratory cycle (see Fig. 231-1*B*). SIMV differs from ACMV in that only the preset number of breaths is ventilator-assisted.

SIMV allows patients with an intact respiratory drive to exercise inspiratory muscles between assisted breaths. This characteristic makes SIMV a useful mode of ventilation for both supporting and weaning intubated patients. SIMV may be difficult to use in patients

with tachypnea because they may attempt to exhale during the ventilator-programmed inspiratory cycle. When this occurs, the airway pressure may exceed the inspiratory pressure limit, the ventilator-assisted breath will be aborted, and minute volume may drop below that programmed by the operator. In this setting, if the tachypnea is in response to respiratory or metabolic acidosis, a change to ACMV will increase minute ventilation and help normalize the pH while the underlying process is further evaluated. If the tachypnea is in response to a stimulus other than acidosis, the addition of sedative medications is appropriate while the underlying processes are further evaluated.

Continuous positive airway pressure (CPAP) This is not a true support-mode ventilation, since all ventilation occurs through the patient's spontaneous efforts. The ventilator provides fresh gas to the breathing circuit with each inspiration and charges the circuit to a constant, operator-specified pressure that can range from 0 to 20 cmH$_2$O (see Fig. 231-1*C*). CPAP is used to assess extubation potential in patients who have been effectively weaned and are requiring little ventilator support and in patients with intact respiratory system function who require an endotracheal tube for airway protection.

Pressure-control ventilation (PCV) This form of ventilation is time triggered, time cycled, and pressure limited. During the inspiratory phase, a given pressure is imposed at the airway opening, and the pressure remains at this user-specified level throughout inspiration (Fig. 231-2*A*). Since inspiratory airway pressure is specified by the operator, tidal volume and inspiratory flow rate are *dependent* rather than *independent* variables and are not user specified. PCV is

FIGURE 231-1 *A.* Airway pressure and lung volume versus time profile during ACMV. Assisted breaths are triggered by the patient's effort. Controlled breaths are triggered by the ventilator timer. Every breath, whether triggered by the patient or by the timer, is a complete volume-cycled breath, with airway pressure as a dependent variable. The pressure limit is set above the peak inspiratory pressure.

B. Airway pressure and lung volume versus time profiles during SIMV. Spontaneous breaths occur between patient-triggered assisted breaths and timer-triggered breaths. The tidal volume of the spontaneous breaths is determined by the patient's effort and lung impedance. Assisted and controlled breaths are volume cycled.

C. Airway pressure and lung volume versus time profiles during CPAP. Breathing is spontaneous, and no ventilator assist is provided. The spontaneous profile is superimposed on an elevated mean airway pressure that the user specifies.

the preferred mode of ventilation for patients with documented barotrauma, since airway pressures can be limited, and for postoperative thoracic surgical patients, in whom the shear forces across a fresh suture line should be limited. When using PCV, minute ventilation and tidal volume must be monitored; minute ventilation is altered through changes in rate or in the pressure-control value.

The major practical limitation of PCV is patient-ventilator asynchrony related to its time-cycled and time-triggered characteristics. Since PCV requires that the patient passively accept ventilator breaths, most patients require heavy sedation to be maintained on this ventilatory mode, which may be hazardous in the hemodynamically unstable patient.

Modified versions of PCV designed to improve patient-ventilator synchrony are available on some newer ventilators. The first type is patient/time-triggered, time-cycled, and pressure-limited PCV, where every breath initiated by the patient is pressure-assisted with concurrent time-cycled pressure-assist backup. In second type of PCV, a mandatory number of synchronized, patient-triggered, time-cycled, and pressure-limited PCV breaths are provided with time-cycled backup, and spontaneous breathing can occur between mandatory breaths. These two modified versions of PCV are the pressure-assisted equivalents of ACMV and SIMV. Because they are dually patient and timer triggered, these modified versions of PCV are better tolerated than standard PCV and can be employed safely without heavy sedation.

Pressure-support ventilation (PSV)   This form of ventilation is patient triggered, flow cycled, and pressure limited; it is specifically designed for use in the weaning process. During PSV, the inspiratory phase is terminated when inspiratory airflow falls below a certain level; in most ventilators this flow rate cannot be adjusted by the operator. When PSV is used, patients receive ventilator assist only when the ventilator detects an inspiratory effort (see Fig. 231-2*B*). PSV also can be used in combination with SIMV to ensure volume-cycled backup for patients whose respiratory drive is depressed either spontaneously or as a result of various therapeutic maneuvers. However, when backup ventilation is provided, the usefulness of PSV as a weaning aid is partially vitiated.

PSV is well tolerated by most patients who are being weaned: PSV parameters can be set in such a way as to provide full or nearly full ventilatory support and can be withdrawn slowly over a period of days in a systematic fashion to gradually load the respiratory muscles.

COMPLICATIONS OF MECHANICAL VENTILATION

Endotracheal intubation and positive-pressure mechanical ventilation have direct and indirect effects on several organ systems, including the lung and upper airways, the cardiovascular system, and the gastrointestinal system. Pulmonary complications include barotrauma, nosocomial pneumonia, oxygen toxicity, tracheal stenosis, and deconditioning of respiratory muscles. *Barotrauma,* which occurs when high pressures (i.e., greater than 50 cmH$_2$O) disrupt lung tissue, is clinically manifest by interstitial emphysema, pneumomediastinum, subcutaneous emphysema, or pneumothorax. Although the former conditions may resolve simply by reducing airway pressures, clinically significant pneumothorax, as indicated by hypoxemia, decreased lung compliance, and hemodynamic compromise, requires tube thoracostomy.

Patients intubated for longer than 72 h are at high risk for *nosocomial pneumonia* as a result of aspiration from the upper airways via small leaks around the endotracheal tube cuff; the most common organisms responsible for this condition are enteric gram-negative rods, *Staphylococcus aureus,* and anaerobic bacteria. Because the endotracheal tube and upper airways of patients on mechanical ventilation are commonly colonized with bacteria, the diagnosis of nosocomial pneumonia requires "protected brush" bronchoscopic sampling of airway secretions coupled with quantitative microbiologic techniques to differentiate colonization from infection.

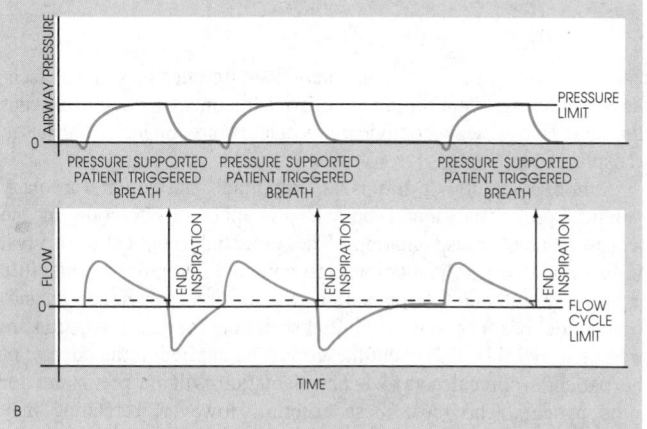

FIGURE 231-2 *A.* Airway pressure and lung volume versus time profiles during PCV. All breaths are timer triggered, timer cycled, and pressure limited. Peak airway pressure is set by the operator, and tidal volume is a dependent variable. The profiles shown here display the pressure limit as slightly higher than pressure-control level. This need not be the case, but it is appropriate to set the pressure limit only slightly above the pressure-control level when using this mode of ventilation for management of the patient with barotrauma.

B. Airway pressure and airway flow versus time profiles during PSV. All breaths are patient triggered and flow cycled. Inspiration is cycled off when the inspiratory flow drops below a predetermined threshold internally set in the ventilator circuit. In the example shown, the pressure limit is slightly greater than the pressure-support level. Since each can be set independently, this need not be the case.

Oxygen toxicity is a potential complication when an F_{IO_2} of 0.6 or greater is required for more than 72 h. The condition can be prevented in some cases through the use of PEEP to allow for F_{IO_2} values to go below 0.6 while primary therapy for the underlying condition is instituted. Although oxygen toxicity is thought to result from the effects of oxygen free radicals on the lung interstitium, the therapeutic use of antioxidants such as superoxide dismutase, catalase, selenium, and vitamin E remains experimental.

Hypotension resulting from elevated intrathoracic pressures with decreased venous return is almost always responsive to intravascular volume repletion. In patients judged to have hypotension or respiratory failure on the basis of alveolar edema, hemodynamic monitoring with a pulmonary arterial catheter may be of value in optimizing oxygen delivery via manipulation of intravascular volume, F_{IO_2}, and PEEP levels.

Gastrointestinal effects of positive-pressure ventilation include *stress ulceration* and *mild to moderate cholestasis*. It is common practice to provide prophylaxis with H-2 receptor antagonists or sucralfate for stress-related ulcers. Mild cholestasis (i.e., total bilirubin values ≤ 4.0) attributable to the effects of increased intrathoracic

pressures on portal vein pressures is common and generally self-limited. Cholestasis of a more severe degree should not be attributed to a positive-pressure ventilation response and is more likely due to a primary hepatic process. Additional complications, including malnutrition, decubitus ulcers, muscle deconditioning, venous thrombosis, and depression, are common and require appropriate treatment.

WEANING FROM MECHANICAL VENTILATION

Removal of mechanical ventilator support requires that a number of criteria be met. Upper airway function must be intact for a patient to remain extubated but is difficult to assess in the intubated patient. Therefore, if a patient can breathe on his or her own through an endotracheal tube but develops stridor or recurrent aspiration once the tube is removed, upper airway dysfunction or an abnormal swallowing mechanism should be suspected and plans for achieving a stable airway developed. An intact cough when respiratory secretions are suctioned is a good indicator of a patient's ability to mobilize secretions. Respiratory drive and chest wall function are assessed by observation of respiratory rate, tidal volume, inspiratory pressure, and vital capacity. The weaning index, defined as the ratio of breathing frequency to tidal volume (breaths per minute per liter), has been shown to be both sensitive and specific for predicting the likelihood of successful extubation. When this ratio is less than 105 with the patient breathing without mechanical assistance through an endotracheal tube, successful extubation is likely. An inspiratory pressure of more than -30 cmH$_2$O and a vital capacity of greater than 10 mL/kg are considered indicators of acceptable chest wall and diaphragm function. Alveolar ventilation is generally adequate when systemic arterial P_{CO_2} is less than or equal to 45 mmHg, and arterial oxygen saturations greater than 90 percent can be achieved with an F_{IO_2} of less than 0.5 and a PEEP of 5 cmH$_2$O or less. Although many patients may not meet all criteria for weaning, the likelihood that a patient will tolerate extubation without difficulty increases as more criteria are met.

Many approaches to weaning patients from ventilator support have been advocated. T-piece and CPAP weaning are best tolerated by patients who have undergone ventilation for brief periods and require little respiratory muscle reconditioning, while SIMV and PSV are best for patients who have been intubated for extended periods and require gradual respiratory-muscle reconditioning.

T-piece weaning involves brief spontaneous breathing trials with supplemental oxygen. These trials are usually initiated for 5 min/h followed by a 1-h interval of rest. T-piece trials are increased in 5- to 10-min increments until the patient can remain ventilator independent for periods of several hours. Extubation can then be attempted. CPAP weaning is similar to T-piece weaning except that trials of spontaneous breathing are conducted on the ventilator in CPAP mode.

Weaning by means of SIMV/IMV involves gradually tapering the mandatory backup rate in increments of 2 to 4 breaths per minute while monitoring blood gas parameters and respiratory rates. Rates of greater than 25 breaths per minute upon withdrawal of mandatory ventilator breaths generally indicate respiratory muscle fatigue and the need to combine periods of exercise with periods of rest. Exercise periods are gradually increased until a patient remains stable on SIMV at 4 breaths per minute or less without needing rest at higher SIMV rates. A CPAP or T-piece trial can then be attempted before planned extubation.

PSV, as described in detail above, is used primarily for weaning from mechanical ventilation. PSV is usually initiated at a level adequate for full ventilator support (PSV$_{max}$); i.e., PSV is set slightly below the peak inspiratory pressures the patient requires during volume-cycled ventilation. The level of pressure support is then gradually withdrawn in increments of 5 cmH$_2$O until a level is reached at which the respiratory rate increases to 25 breaths per minute. At this point, intermittent periods of higher-pressure support are alternated with periods of lower-pressure support to provide muscle reconditioning without causing diaphragmatic fatigue. Gradual withdrawal of PSV continues until the level of support is just adequate to overcome the resistance of the endotracheal tube (approximately 5 cmH₂O). At that point, support can be discontinued and the patient extubated.

REFERENCES

COHEN IL et al: Mechanical ventilation for the elderly patient in intensive care. Incremental changes and benefits. JAMA 269:1025, 1993

HINSON JR, MARINI JJ: Principles of mechanical ventilator use in respiratory failure. Annu Rev Med 43:341, 1992

INGENITO EP, DRAZEN JM: Mechanical ventilators, in *Principles of Critical Care*, JB Hall, GA Schmidt, LDH Wood (eds). New York, McGraw-Hill, 1992, pp 142–154

PHAM LH et al: Diagnosis of nonsocomial pneumonia in mechanically ventilated patients: Comparison of a plugged telescoping catheter with the protected specimen brush. Am Rev Respir Dis 143:1055, 1991

RANIERI VM et al: Physiologic effects of positive end-expiratory pressure in patients with chronic obstructive pulmonary disease during acute ventilatory failure and controlled mechanical ventilation. Am Rev Respir Dis 147:5, 1993

YANG KL, TOBIN MJ: A prospective study of indexes predicting the outcome of trials of weaning from mechanical ventilation. N Engl J Med 324:1445, 1991

---

232 LUNG TRANSPLANTATION

E. P. TRULOCK / JOEL D. COOPER

During the last decade transplantation became a therapeutic option for patients with end-stage lung disease, and activity in lung transplantation has increased exponentially since 1989. Worldwide, more than 1800 lung transplants had been reported through March 1993, and in the United States 534 lung transplants were recorded in 1992 alone. The number of patients awaiting lung transplantation has also been increasing rapidly, and by the end of 1992 the U.S. waiting list had almost 1000 registrants. The 1-year and 2-year actuarial survival rates are 68 percent and 60 percent respectively, for the cumulative experience in the St. Louis International Lung Transplant Registry, but these results have been exceeded at some centers.

INDICATIONS Patients with a variety of end-stage lung diseases have undergone transplantation. The most common diagnoses have been chronic obstructive pulmonary disease, antitrypsin deficiency emphysema, idiopathic pulmonary fibrosis, cystic fibrosis, and primary pulmonary hypertension, but a smaller number of patients with other diseases have also received lung transplants. Controversial indications include systemic diseases with predominantly pulmonary involvement and interstitial lung diseases caused by chemotherapy or radiotherapy for a previous neoplasm.

Recipient selection Potential recipients should have clinically and physiologically severe lung disease with a poor prognosis for survival in spite of optimal medical management, but should have no other health problems that would either jeopardize the success of the operation or limit life expectancy after transplantation. Specific recipient selection criteria vary somewhat among centers. In general, candidates should have normal left ventricular function without significant coronary artery disease and no significant dysfunction of other vital organs. They should be ambulatory and in acceptable nutritional condition, and they should have a satisfactory psychosocial profile and history of compliance with medical management.

Other considerations include the patient's age, prior thoracic surgical history, and glucocorticoid therapy. Typical age limits are ~50 to 55 years for bilateral lung transplantation and ~60 to 65 years for single lung transplantation. The technical difficulties and operative risks of lung transplantation in patients with prior thoracic procedures are variable; however, diagnostic open lung biopsy, tube thoracostomy with or without chemical pleurodesis for pneumothorax, or lobectomy

TABLE 232-1 Physiologic guidelines for timing the initial screening for lung transplantation

Chronic obstructive pulmonary disease
  Postbronchodilator $FEV_1 < 30$ percent predicted
  Resting hypoxia ($Pa_{O_2} < 55$–60 mmHg) or hypercapnia
  Significant secondary pulmonary hypertension
Cystic fibrosis
  Postbronchodilator $FEV_1 < 30$ percent predicted
  Resting hypoxia ($Pa_{O_2} < 55$ mmHg) or hypercapnia ($Pa_{CO_2} > 50$ mmHg)
Idiopathic pulmonary fibrosis
  Vital capacity or total lung capacity < 60 percent predicted
  Resting hypoxia
  Significant secondary pulmonary hypertension
Primary pulmonary hypertension
  New York Heart Association functional class III or IV
  Mean right atrial pressure > 10 mmHg
  Mean pulmonary arterial pressure > 50 mmHg
  Cardiac index < 2.5 (L/min)m²

usually do not preclude transplantation. With current surgical techniques pretransplantation glucocorticoid treatment in low doses has not increased airway complications and is no longer a barrier to transplantation.

Although quality of life is an important motivation for many patients, prognosis should be the principal consideration in the decision about transplantation. The potential recipient's survival probability after transplantation must compare favorably with the life expectancy without transplantation. Some disease-specific, physiologic guidelines for timing the initial screening for transplantation are presented in Table 232-1, but these must be applied in the context of the patient's clinical course. Transplantation will be premature for some patients who meet these criteria. However, screening may help identify patients who are likely to become candidates for transplantation in the future.

Donor-recipient matching Blood group compatibility and lung size, within reasonable tolerance, are the only factors that are routinely matched between the donor and recipient. When possible, cytomegalovirus (CMV) seronegative recipients should be transplanted with lungs from a CMV seronegative donor to prevent serious posttransplant CMV infection, but this strategy is often impractical because of the shortage of donor organs. Prospective histocompatibility matching has not been used in lung transplantation, and its impact on graft and patient survival have yet to be studied thoroughly.

PROCEDURES AND RESULTS Both combined heart-lung and isolated lung transplantation have been performed for many end-stage lung diseases. Heart-lung transplantation should be reserved for those situations which require cardiac replacement, e.g., Eisenmenger's syndrome with a surgically uncorrectable cardiac abnormality (Chap. 196). Cor pulmonale alone does not necessitate cardiac transplantation because right ventricular function can recover when the afterload is normalized by lung transplantation. Bilateral lung transplantation is mandatory for patients with generalized bronchiectasis and chronic pulmonary infection. Either bilateral or single lung transplantation can be utilized for most other diseases, but single lung transplantation maximizes the use of the limited supply of donor lungs.

Regardless of the type of operation, lung transplantation improves lung function in patients with restrictive or obstructive disease and alleviates pulmonary hypertension in patients with pulmonary vascular disease. Exercise performance and quality of life are enhanced; supplemental oxygen is unnecessary; and normal daily activities, including most occupations, can be resumed.

POSTTRANSPLANT MANAGEMENT AND COMPLICATIONS As an allograft the lung has been vulnerable to three major complications: bronchial anastomotic dehiscence and stenosis, acute and chronic rejection, and infection. Deaths soon after lung transplantation have been caused primarily by technical and cardiac complications of the operation, but mortality beyond the first postoperative month has been related to rejection and infection.

Anastomotic dehiscence and stenosis The bronchial circulation to the donor lung is severed during extraction, and after implantation the donor bronchus is dependent on retrograde blood flow from the pulmonary circulation until other collaterals develop. Although surgically reestablishing the bronchial supply to the donor lung is possible, the technique is complex and has not been widely used.

Endoscopically visible signs of airway ischemia or small defects in the anastomosis are not unusual, but the majority of these require no intervention and resolve without sequelae. Significant stenosis or dehiscence still occurs in ~10 to 20 percent of cases but can be managed by dilation and/or stent placement. Fatal airway complications are very rare with current surgical techniques.

Rejection Most recipients have early episodes of acute rejection, and 25 percent or more develop late, chronic rejection. Acute rejection can occur as early as three days and as late as several years after transplantation. Clinical features include cough, dyspnea, fever, adventitious lung sounds, radiographic infiltrates, and deterioration in oxygenation and pulmonary function. The chest radiograph, however, is normal or unchanged in three-fourths of episodes occurring more than 1 month after transplantation. Because the presentation of acute pulmonary rejection is nonspecific, bronchoscopy with transbronchial lung biopsy is useful to distinguish rejection from infection. The clinical utility of bronchoalveolar lavage is limited to the diagnosis of infection.

Standard treatment for acute rejection is high-dose methylprednisolone. Glucocorticoid therapy is sufficient to reverse most episodes, but refractory acute rejection can be treated with antilymphocyte globulin, antithymocyte globulin, or OKT3 monoclonal antibody.

Chronic rejection is a clinicopathologic syndrome characterized physiologically by airflow limitation and histologically by obliterative bronchiolitis and a variable degree of vascular sclerosis. Both antecedent acute rejection and CMV pneumonia appear to be risk factors. It is the most problematic late complication and the leading cause of late mortality and morbidity. With current immunosuppressive drug regimens and surveillance protocols, approximately 25 to 40 percent of long-term survivors are affected by chronic rejection.

Chronic rejection may develop as early as 2 months and as late as several years after transplantation, but the mean time to onset is 8 to 12 months. The most frequent presentation mimics an upper respiratory tract infection or bronchitis, but the onset may be more insidious. The diagnosis is based on the clinical, physiological, and pathologic features. The evolution of new or worsening airflow limitation is strongly suggestive of rejection. Transbronchial lung biopsy is less sensitive and less specific for chronic rejection than for acute rejection.

Chronic rejection is treated by augmenting the immunosuppressive therapy with glucocorticoids or the antilymphocyte agents. Beneficial results have been achieved with these, but the relapse rate has been high.

Infection The lung as an allograft is particularly vulnerable to infection. The lower respiratory tract of brain-dead, ventilator-dependent donors is often colonized with nosocomial organisms, and these potential pathogens are transmitted with the donor lung. After transplantation the normal pulmonary defense mechanisms are breached at many levels. Mucociliary clearance is diminished, and, because the transplanted lung is denervated, the cough reflex is depressed. Moreover, some of the antimicrobial functions of alveolar macrophages may be impaired. Bacterial, fungal, viral, and protozoal infections have all occurred, but the most common problems have been bacterial pneumonia and CMV pneumonia.

Purulent bacterial bronchitis and bronchopneumonia occur frequently in the early posttransplant period; gram negative, nosocomial bacteria and staphylococci are the predominant organisms. Because of the high risk of bacterial pneumonia in the perioperative period, antibiotic therapy should be directed at any potential pathogens isolated from respiratory specimens. Bacterial pneumonia is also a significant problem during long-term follow-up. Gram-negative organisms are responsible for most cases, but other community-acquired pathogens also contribute.

CMV pneumonia is the most frequent opportunistic pulmonary infection after lung transplantation. The risk and severity of infection are related to the CMV serologic status of the donor and recipient. First episodes of CMV pneumonia usually occur between 3 weeks and 4 months after lung transplantation. The clinical presentation is almost indistinguishable from allograft rejection, and the diagnosis should be confirmed by histology and virology. Most episodes respond to treatment with ganciclovir, but relapses are not uncommon.

Herpes simplex tracheobronchitis and pneumonitis occur occasionally, and other respiratory viruses are sometimes isolated and may be important depending on the clinical circumstances. Colonization with *Candida* species is common, particularly in the early posttransplant period, but invasive infection is infrequent. Subsequently, *Aspergillus* is the principal fungal pathogen. Pneumonias caused by other agents are unusual after lung transplantation. *Pneumocystis carinii* infection has been almost eliminated by prophylaxis, and *Nocardia* has not been problematic. Only a few cases of tuberculous or nontuberculous mycobacterial infections have been recorded.

Recurrence of the original disease The native disease has recurred in the allograft in some recipients with sarcoidosis. Other diseases have not recurred; however, the posttransplant follow-up of most recipients is relatively short compared to the natural history of their underlying diseases.

REFERENCES

AMERICAN THORACIC SOCIETY: Lung transplantation. Report of the ATS workshop on lung transplantation. Am Rev Respir Dis 147:772, 1993

GROSSMAN RF, MAURER JR (eds): Pulmonary considerations in transplantation. Clinics Chest Med 11(2):195, 1990

PATTERSON GA, COOPER JD (eds): *Lung Transplantation*. Chest Surgery Clin North Amer 3(1):1, 1993

TRULOCK EP: Management of lung transplant rejection. Chest 103:1566, 1993

233 APPROACH TO THE PATIENT WITH DISEASES OF THE KIDNEYS AND URINARY TRACT

FREDRIC L. COE / BARRY M. BRENNER

Diseases of the kidneys and urinary tract frequently give rise to consistent arrays or clusters of clinical signs, symptoms, and laboratory findings called *syndromes*. Syndromes are useful diagnostically because each has fewer causes than the individual clinical signs and symptoms it contains. For example, any injured capillary bed from glomerulus to urethral meatus can cause hematuria, but only glomerular injury also can cause heavy albuminuria and erythrocyte casts (Chap. 44), and only a few of the diseases that injure the glomerular capillaries enough to cause hematuria and proteinuria also cause a rapid fall in glomerular filtration rate. Routine clinical evaluation is often sufficient to suggest that a particular syndrome may be present (Table 233-1), but additional laboratory measurements beyond the routine, as well as radiologic and/or urologic evaluation and sequential clinical observations, are usually required to establish the diagnosis. This chapter presents the general features of the syndromes, lists the clinical and laboratory data required for their recognition, and outlines the diseases that cause them. Succeeding chapters describe the diseases and their treatment in detail.

ACUTE (ARF) AND RAPIDLY PROGRESSIVE RENAL FAILURE (RPRF) Whether the glomerular filtration rate falls over days (acute renal failure) or weeks (rapidly progressive renal failure) is a useful distinction, because the causes of these two syndromes are somewhat different (Tables 233-1 and 233-2). For example, acute tubular

TABLE 233-1 Initial clinical and laboratory data base for defining major syndromes in nephrology

Syndromes	Important clues to diagnosis	Findings which are common but not of diagnostic value	Location of discussion of diseases causing syndrome
Acute or rapidly progressive renal failure	Anuria Oliguria Documented recent decline in GFR	Hypertension, hematuria Proteinuria, pyuria Casts, edema	Chaps. 236, 240, 242, 243, 246
Acute nephritis	Hematuria, RBC casts Azotemia, oliguria Edema, hypertension	Proteinuria Pyuria Circulatory congestion	Chaps. 239, 240, 241
Chronic renal failure	Azotemia for > 3 months Prolonged symptoms or signs of uremia Symptoms or signs of renal osteodystrophy Kidneys reduced in size bilaterally Broad casts in urinary sediment	Hematuria, proteinuria Casts, oliguria Polyuria, nocturia Edema, hypertension Electrolyte disorders	Chaps. 235, 237
Nephrotic syndrome	Proteinuria > 3.5 g per 1.73 m² per 24 h Hypoalbuminemia Hyperlipidemia Lipiduria	Casts Edema	Chaps. 236, 241
Asymptomatic urinary abnormalities	Hematuria Proteinuria (below nephrotic range) Sterile pyuria, casts		Chap. 240
Urinary tract infection	Bacteriuria > 10⁵ colonies per milliliter Other infectious agent documented in urine Pyuria, leukocyte casts Frequency, urgency Bladder tenderness, flank tenderness	Hematuria Mild azotemia Mild proteinuria Fever	Chap. 90
Renal tubule defects	Electrolyte disorders Polyuria, nocturia Symptoms or signs of renal osteodystrophy Large kidneys Renal transport defects	Hematuria "Tubular" proteinuria Enuresis	Chaps. 242, 244
Hypertension	Systolic/diastolic hypertension	Proteinuria Casts Azotemia	Chaps. 34, 209, 243
Nephrolithiasis	Previous history of stone passage or removal Previous history of stone seen by x-ray Renal colic	Hematuria Pyuria Frequency, urgency	Chap. 245
Urinary tract obstruction	Azotemia, oliguria, anuria Polyuria, nocturia, urinary retention Slowing of urinary stream Large prostate, large kidneys Flank tenderness, full bladder after voiding	Hematuria Pyuria Enuresis, dysuria	Chap. 246

TABLE 233-2   Syndromes produced by diseases of the kidneys and urinary tract

Diseases (Chap.)	Syndromes					
	ARF	RPRF	AN	CRF	NS	AUA
Bilateral arterial occlusion (243)	T					
Acute tubular necrosis (236)	T					
Bilateral acute renal vein thrombosis (243)	T					
Acute uric acid nephropathy (242)	T					
Hypovolemia (236)	T					
Cardiovascular collapse (236)	T					
Acute bilateral upper tract obstruction (206)	T					
Hypercalcemic nephropathy (242)	T			O		
Hemolytic uremic syndrome (243)	T	O	O			
Acute urinary retention (246)	T					
Malignant nephrosclerosis (243)	T	O				
Essential mixed cyroimmunoglobulinemia (241)	T	O	O	O	O	
Nephrotoxic drugs and chemicals (236, 242)	T			O		
Oxalate nephropathy (242)	T			O		
Cortical necrosis (236)	T			O		
Postpartum glomerulosclerosis (236)	T			O		
Hypersensitivity nephropathy (242)	T		O			P,H,L
Scleroderma (243)	T					P
Idiopathic rapidly progressive GN (240)	O	T	T		R	
Goodpasture's syndrome (240)	O	T	T	O		P,H
Non-Goodpasture's anti-GBM disease (240)	O	T	T	O		P,H
Acute bacterial endocarditis or visceral sepsis (240)		T	T	O	O	
Microscopic polyarteritis nodosa (241, 243)		T	T			
Wegener's granulomatosis (241, 243)		T	T			
Allergic granulomatosis (291)		T	T			
Acute radiation nephritis (242)		T	T			P
Poststreptococcal glomerulonephritis (240)		R	T	O	R	P,H
Nonstreptococcal postinfectious GN (240)		R	T	R	R	P,H
Macroscopic polyarteritis nodosa (275, 241, 243)				T		P,H
Diffuse proliferative lupus nephritis (241)	R	O	R	T	O	P,H,L
Chronic radiation nephritis (242)				T	O	
Balkan nephropathy (242)				T		P*,H
Analgesic nephropathy (242)				T		L,H
Heavy metals (lead, cadmium, mercury) (242, 396)				T		P*
Cystinosis (242)				T		P*
Chronic obstructive uropathy (246)				T		H
Adult polycystic renal disease (244)				T		H,P
Medullary cystic renal disease (244)				T		
Gouty nephropathy (242)				T		
Minimal change disease (240)					T	
Idiopathic membranous nephropathy (240)				O	T	P,H
Membranoproliferative glomerulonephritis (240)		R	O	O	T	P,H
Renal amyloidosis (241)				O	T	P
Membranous lupus nephropathy (241)				O	T	P
Renal vein thrombosis (243)	O			O	T	
Rheumatoid arthritis (241)				O	T	
Congenital nephrotic syndrome (241)				O	T	
Dermatomyositis (240)					T	
Dermatitis herpetiformis (240)				O	T	P
Medullary sponge kidney (244)						T:H
Nephrolithiasis (239)						T:H
Neoplasms (247)						T:H
Arteriolar nephrosclerosis (243)				O		T:P
Waldenström's macroglobulinemia (241)	O					T:P
Multiple myeloma (241)	O	O		O	O	T:P
Reflux nephropathy (90, 243)				O	O	T:P
Diabetic nephropathy (241, 337)				O	O	T:P
Toxemia of pregnancy (6, 243)						T:P
Orthostatic proteinuria (240)						T:P
Sarcoid nephropathy (241)						T:P
Hypokalemic nephropathy (242)						T:P
Berger's (IgA) nephropathy (240)	R	R	O	O	O	T:H,P
Henoch-Schönlein purpura (241)		O	O	R	O	T:H,P
Fabry's disease (241)				O		T:H,P
Alport's syndrome (241)				O		T:H,P
Sickle cell nephropathy (241)				O	R	T:H,P
Subacute bacterial endocarditis (85)						T:H,P
Minimal and mesangial lupus nephritis (241)						T:P,H
Mesangial proliferative GN (240)				R	O	T:P,H
Mixed connective tissue disease (241)					R	T:P,H
Chronic glomerulonephritis (237)				O		T:P,H
Nail patella syndrome (241)				R		T:P,H
Focal glomerulosclerosis (240)		R	O	O	O	T:P,H,L
Focal and segmental lupus nephritis (241)				O	O	T:P,H,L
Sjögren's syndrome (241)						T:L,P
Urinary and renal infection (90)						T:L,H

NOTE: T, typical presentation; O, occurs frequently, but not invariably; R, occurs rarely; P*, tubular proteinuria; P, proteinuria; H, hematuria; L, leukocyturia; ARF, acute renal failure; RPRF, rapidly progressive renal failure; AN, acute nephritis; CRF, chronic renal failure; NS, nephrotic syndrome; AUA, asymptomatic urinary abnormality.

necrosis, from sepsis, nephrotoxic materials, shock, or other cause (see Chap. 236), is the usual cause of acute renal failure, whereas extracapillary proliferative (crescentic) glomerulonephritis, due to immunologic injury or to vasculitis, is an important cause of rapidly progressive, but not acute, renal failure (Chap. 240).

Proof for the existence of either syndrome requires serial determination of the glomerular filtration rate (GFR), blood urea nitrogen, or serum creatinine level. Anuria or oliguria (Chap. 44) strongly suggest acute renal failure, since life cannot be sustained for long with such inadequate renal function. Symptoms and signs of uremia of recent onset suggest rapidly progressive or acute renal failure but also could result from chronic renal failure that has only recently become life-threatening. Although edema, hypertension, and abnormalities of electrolytes and the urine sediment (Table 233-1) are frequent in acute and rapidly progressive renal failure, they occur in other syndromes as well and are not specific.

The causes of these two important syndromes number about 36, but only 18 (indicated by T, Table 233-2) typically cause acute renal failure, and 8 cause rapidly progressive renal failure. Urinary obstruction, acute tubular necrosis, some forms of vasculitis, major renal vascular accidents, and endogenous and exogenous nephrotoxins are the usual causes of acute renal failure. Vasculitis and crescentic glomerulonephritis are the main causes of rapidly progressive renal failure. Hemolytic-uremic syndrome, malignant nephrosclerosis, and essential mixed cryoimmunoglobulinemia occasionally present as rapidly progressive renal failure. Idiopathic rapidly progressive glomerulonephritis—the prototype of a disease that produces rapidly progressive renal failure—sometimes causes acute renal failure. Chronic renal failure may occur in some patients with diseases that typically cause acute renal failure. Nevertheless, despite some variability of disease presentations, the finding of acute or rapidly progressive renal failure narrows the range of causes.

ACUTE NEPHRITIS (AN) A number of diseases involve the glomeruli and, to a generally lesser extent, the tubules in an acute but transient inflammatory process, manifested clinically by acute reduction in GFR, rapidly progressive renal failure, and salt and water retention. Expansion of the extracellular volume, if marked, causes hypertension, pulmonary vascular congestion, and facial and peripheral edema (Chap. 240). Since the causes of this syndrome all can damage the glomerular wall enough to permit red blood cells and plasma proteins to enter the urinary space and appear in the urine, gross or microscopic hematuria, red blood cell casts, and proteinuria are necessary for the diagnosis of acute nephritis, and their absence suggests other diagnoses. Acute nephritis is a transient inflammatory process, so its clinical and laboratory manifestations wax and wane over days to weeks. Many of the diseases that cause acute nephritis also cause acute or rapidly progressive renal failure (see Table 233-2).

The fact that many diseases produce both acute nephritis and acute or rapidly progressive renal failure, some produce only acute nephritis, and some produce acute or chronic renal failure without acute nephritis is useful in diagnosis. Only two diseases, poststreptococcal glomerulonephritis and nonstreptococcal postinfectious glomerulonephritis, typically cause acute nephritis alone, and only three of the diseases that typically cause acute renal failure, idiopathic rapidly progressive glomerulonephritis, Goodpasture's syndrome, and non-Goodpasture's anti-glomerular basement membrane (anti-GBM) disease, also cause acute nephritis (see Table 233-2). On the other hand, most of the diseases that cause acute nephritis also cause rapidly progressive renal failure.

Acute glomerulonephritis following infection with group A streptococci is the prototype of a disease that causes acute nephritis alone (Chap. 240). Immune complexes deposit in the subepithelial region of the glomerular capillary wall, between the basement membrane and the visceral epithelial cells that separate the membrane from the urinary space, and provoke an intense but transient inflammatory process. GFR falls but returns to normal within weeks to months in most patients. Deposition of immune complexes is also believed to

be the cause of acute nephritis following other bacterial and viral infections and of lupus nephritis, membranoproliferative glomerulonephritis, Henoch-Schönlein purpura, and Berger's disease, i.e., IgA nephropathy. That the typical presentations of the last four diseases are chronic renal failure, nephrotic syndrome, and asymptomatic urinary abnormalities illustrates the weakness of relationships between pathogenesis and final clinical manifestations.

Renal biopsy is usually required for the evaluation of patients with acute nephritis, whether or not acute or rapidly progressive renal failure is also present. The usual histologic picture is proliferative glomerulonephritis, often with extracapillary crescent formation, but prognosis and treatment are influenced strongly by the precise histologic and ultrastructural pattern, as well as the types of immune complexes and immunoglobulins deposited in the renal tissues.

CHRONIC RENAL FAILURE (CRF) Chronic renal failure results from progressive and irreversible destruction of nephrons, regardless of cause (Chap. 237). This diagnosis implies that GFR is known to have been reduced for at least 3 to 6 months (see Table 233-1). Often a gradual decline in GFR occurs over a period of years. Proof of chronicity is also provided by the demonstration of bilateral reduction of kidney size by scout film, ultrasonography, intravenous pyelography, or tomography. Other findings of long-standing renal failure, such as renal osteodystrophy or symptoms of uremia, also help to establish this syndrome. Several laboratory abnormalities are often regarded as reliable indicators of chronicity of renal disease, such as anemia, hyperphosphatemia, or hypocalcemia, but these are not specific (Chap. 235). In contrast, the finding of broad casts in the urinary sediment (Chap. 44) is specific for chronic renal failure, the wide diameters of these casts reflecting the compensatory dilatation and hypertrophy of surviving nephrons. Proteinuria is a frequent but nonspecific finding, as is hematuria. Chronic obstructive uropathy, polycystic and medullary cystic diseases, analgesic nephropathy, and the inactive end stage of any chronic tubulointerstitial nephropathy are conditions in which the urine often contains little or no protein, cells, or casts even though nephron destruction has progressed to chronic renal failure.

When ARF occurs in the presence of CRF, the acute component must be evaluated as if CRF were not present, because the acute component is potentially reversible. In most instances, depletion of extracellular fluid volume is the cause of acute deterioration of renal function, but urinary tract obstruction, drug-induced nephrotoxicity, or exacerbation of underlying renal disease also may be responsible (Chap. 237).

NEPHROTIC SYNDROME (NS) This diagnosis previously implied that a patient excretes more than 3.5 g protein per 1.73 m^2 surface area per 24 h, the proteinuria consists mainly of albumin, and that the patient has reduced serum albumin, edema, and hyperlipidemia (Table 233-1). Massive proteinuria alone has now come to define the syndrome, since this finding connotes serious renal disease whether or not the protein losses lead to hypoalbuminemia, lipid disturbances, or edema (Chap. 44). Provided the proteins in the urine are not paraproteins readily excreted by the normal kidney (e.g., immunoglobulin light chains in multiple myeloma), massive proteinuria is invariably a sign of injury to the glomeruli.

Common causes of the nephrotic syndrome include minimal change disease, idiopathic membranous glomerulopathy, focal glomerulosclerosis, and diabetic glomerulosclerosis (Chaps. 240 and 241). Because these diseases typically cause less inflammation than those that cause acute nephritis, the urine contains fewer cellular elements, and acute changes in GFR and urine volume are uncommon. Hematuria may occur in some forms of nephrotic syndrome, however, especially chronic membranoproliferative glomerulonephritis (Chap. 240). The presence of cellular or granular casts should suggest lupus nephritis (Chap. 241) or acute nephritis associated with massive proteinuria, such as essential mixed cryoimmunoglobulinemia, acute bacterial endocarditis, visceral sepsis, and Henoch-Schönlein purpura (see Table 233-2).

ASYMPTOMATIC URINARY ABNORMALITIES (AUA)

As indicated in Table 233-2, mild microscopic hematuria, pyuria, and casts or less than 3.5 g protein per 1.73 m² surface area per 24 h may be present in the urine of a patient with no evidence of other nephrologic syndromes. By exclusion, these patients belong to the syndrome of asymptomatic urinary abnormalities. Isolated hematuria or proteinuria, or unexplained pyuria, are the most frequent abnormalities in this syndrome.

Isolated hematuria, without proteinuria or casts, may be the sole clue to the presence of neoplasm, stone, or infection (e.g., tuberculosis) in any part of the urinary tract (Chaps. 44, 239, 245, and 247). Isolated hematuria also may arise from renal papillae in analgesic and sickle cell nephropathies (Chaps. 242 and 243). Persistent isolated hematuria often requires intravenous pyelography, cystoscopy, and, occasionally, renal arteriography to identify the source of bleeding. *Nephronal hematuria*, in which casts contain red blood cells or hemoglobin pigment, indicates damage to the nephron (Chap. 44). It occurs without proteinuria, mainly in benign recurrent hematuria and Berger's disease (Chap. 240). *Nephronal hematuria and proteinuria* occur together in many renal diseases that may lead to chronic renal failure (Chap. 237). In general, the combination of nephronal hematuria and proteinuria suggests a worse prognosis than either alone.

Isolated proteinuria, without red blood cells or other formed elements in the urinary sediment, is characteristic of many renal diseases which manifest little or no inflammatory reaction within the glomeruli (e.g., diabetes mellitus, amyloidosis). Less than nephrotic-range proteinuria is common in mild forms of all the diseases that can cause overt nephrotic syndrome (Chaps. 240 and 241). "Tubular" proteinuria (Chap. 44) is the rule in cystinosis; in intoxication from cadmium, lead, or mercury; and in the peculiar Balkan nephropathy localized to a small region along the Danube River (Chap. 242).

Pyuria (leukocyturia) also may be a sole urinary abnormality and may reflect infection or inflammation of the lower urinary tract rather than parenchymal renal disease. Nevertheless, prominent pyuria can occur in any inflammatory disease of the kidneys, especially tubulointerstitial nephritis, lupus nephritis, pyelonephritis, and renal transplant rejection, but usually in association with mild proteinuria or hematuria. The finding of leukocyte casts (Chap. 44) establishes the kidney as the site of the inflammatory reaction.

Pyuria associated with urine that is sterile on routine bacteriologic culture presents a special problem. Causes of "sterile pyuria" include (1) recent bacterial urinary infection being treated with antibiotics, (2) glucocorticoid therapy, (3) acute febrile episodes, (4) cyclophosphamide administration, (5) pregnancy, (6) renal transplant rejection, (7) genitourinary trauma, and (8) prostatitis and cystourethritis. Leukocytes from vaginal secretions may contaminate the urine, so a midstream, clean-catch urine sample should be collected to substantiate a urinary origin. Pyuria associated with proteinuria, nephronal hematuria (Chap. 44), or casts usually signifies inflammatory disease of the renal glomeruli, tubules, interstitium, or microcirculation, and evaluation should focus not on the pyuria but on the nature of the renal disease.

Persistent sterile pyuria that cannot be ascribed to any of the foregoing causes has a narrow differential diagnosis. Unusual infections, such as tuberculosis, fungi, atypical mycobacteria, *Haemophilus influenzae*, anaerobic bacteria, fastidious bacteria that grow only on enriched media, and L forms, all must be sought. Intravenous pyelography may be needed to detect causes such as urinary tract calculi, papillary necrosis, and renal infiltration by lymphoma or myeloma cells. The latter is usually suspected because of other evidence of myeloma or lymphoma, for both rarely involve only the kidneys. If all tests are negative, cystoscopy may reveal cystitis or trigone inflammation.

URINARY TRACT INFECTION (UTI)

This syndrome is defined by the demonstration in urine of pathogenic organisms, either bacteria, tubercle bacilli, or fungi (Chap. 90). When urine is obtained for culture, the condition under which the urine is collected must minimize contamination from external surfaces. Women should void into a wide-mouthed sterile container after preliminary cleansing of the vulva with a moist, sterile gauze pledget. In men, midstream collection is usually adequate. Bacterial colony counts of 10^5 organisms per milliliter or greater in urine generally indicate urinary tract colonization and infection. Levels above 10^2 colonies per milliliter are sufficient to indicate infection in symptomatic patients (Table 233-1) and in urine samples obtained by suprapubic aspiration or bladder catheter (Chap. 242). When the urinary tract is anatomically normal, *Escherichia coli* is the usual pathogen. After prolonged antibiotic treatment of persistent infections, particularly when urinary drainage is impaired or stones are present, *Klebsiella*, *Enterobacter*, and *Proteus* species predominate.

As discussed in Chap. 90, a positive urine culture need not imply that an organism is producing tissue inflammation or injury. In some patients, tissue effects may be trivial; in others, injury may occur even though symptoms or urinary abnormalities are not present at the time of evaluation. When bacteriuria is associated with tissue inflammation or injury, clinical manifestations usually depend on the site(s) involved. Dysuria, frequency, urgency, and suprapubic tenderness are common symptoms of bladder and urethral inflammation (Chap. 44 and Table 233-1). Prostatitis also leads to frequency, dysuria, and urgency, and the prostate may be boggy and tender on rectal examination. Flank pain, chills, fever, nausea and vomiting, hypotension from sepsis, and leukocyte casts all suggest true renal parenchymal infection, i.e., pyelonephritis; their absence, however, does not exclude pyelonephritis.

RENAL TUBULE DEFECTS (RTD)

This syndrome encompasses a large number of acquired and hereditary disorders, all of which tend to affect tubules more than glomeruli. Hereditary anatomic defects, including polycystic renal disease, medullary cystic disease, and medullary sponge kidney, are readily detected by intravenous pyelography, which is usually performed because of hematuria, bacteriuria, flank pain, or unexplained azotemia (Chap. 244).

Defects in tubule transport functions, on the other hand, tend not to be associated with prominent renal anatomic defects and arise either as inherited traits (Chap. 244) or during the course of acquired renal disease (Chap. 242). In general, these functional defects impair secretion and/or reabsorption of electrolytes and organic solutes or limit urinary concentrating and diluting ability (see Table 233-1). Typical manifestations of such functional disturbances include polyuria and nocturia (Chap. 44), metabolic acidosis (Chap. 46), and various disorders of fluid and electrolyte balance (Chap. 45). Such defects are defined by direct physiologic measurements; their elucidation requires a sound understanding of normal renal physiology.

HYPERTENSION (H)

Hypertension implies that the average of a series of reliable blood pressure measurements exceeds 140 mmHg systolic or 90 mmHg diastolic (see Table 233-1). The pathogenetic mechanisms, clinical and laboratory manifestations, and therapeutic approaches are discussed in detail elsewhere (Chaps. 34 and 209). In addition, a number of renal complications of hypertension are reviewed in Chap. 243, as is the entity of renal artery stenosis, an infrequent but potentially curable cause of hypertension.

NEPHROLITHIASIS (N)

This syndrome is recognized with certainty when a stone is passed, visualized by x-ray, or removed at surgery or cystoscopy (see Table 233-1 and Chap. 245). Less certain, but suggestive, evidences of nephrolithiasis include renal colic, painful hematuria, or unexplained pyuria, dysuria, and urinary frequency (Chap. 44). Colic varies in its symptomatology but usually begins suddenly in one flank, radiates downward toward the groin, and is excruciatingly painful.

Most renal stones are composed of calcium, uric acid, cystine, or struvite (magnesium ammonium phosphate). All are radiopaque except for uric acid stones and are therefore visible by routine abdominal radiography. Uric acid stones appear as radiolucent filling defects and can be mistaken for tumor or blood clot.

URINARY TRACT OBSTRUCTION (UTO)

Documentation of the various structural or functional causes of urinary tract obstruction usually requires radiologic or surgical visualization. The manifestations of obstruction, which initiate the search for its causes, are numerous (see Table 233-1) and are reviewed in Chap. 246. Anuria in an adult is almost always due to obstruction of bladder outflow. Less commonly, blockage of upper urinary drainage from both kidneys or from a solitary functioning kidney accounts for total or near-total cessation of urine flow. A large bladder after voiding is a sign of outflow obstruction, usually due to urethral stricture, tumor, stone, neurogenic causes, or prostatic hypertrophy. Nocturia, frequency and overflow incontinence, and slowing or hesitancy of micturition also suggest outflow obstruction (Chap. 44). Upper tract obstruction often produces few manifestations. When it is incomplete or unilateral, urine volume may be normal or even elevated because of a loss of renal concentrating ability. Urinary stasis secondary to obstruction predisposes to recurrent urinary tract infection or chronic obstruction to progressive loss of renal function (Table 233-2).

REFERENCES

Coe FL, Bushinsky DA: Clinical and laboratory assessment of patients with renal and urinary tract disease, in *Clinical Nephrology*, BM Brenner, F Coe, FC Rector Jr (eds). Philadelphia, Saunders, 1987, p 1

Levey AS et al: Laboratory assessment of renal disease: Clearance, urinalysis and renal biopsy, in *The Kidney*, BM Brenner, FC Rector Jr (eds). Philadelphia, Saunders, 1991, p 919

Rosenberg ME, Hostetter TH: Proteinuria, in *The Kidney*, DW Seldin, G Giebisch (eds). New York, Raven, 1992, p 3039

234 IMPACT OF CELLULAR AND MOLECULAR BIOLOGY ON NEPHROLOGY

KARL L. SKORECKI / DANIEL G. BICHET / BARRY M. BRENNER

Like other branches of medicine, nephrology is being transformed by advances in molecular cell biology and recombinant DNA technology. Molecular cloning strategies now provide clinicians and investigators with erythropoietin, atrial natriuretic peptides, and endothelins—potent gene products whose availability (indeed, whose existence, in the case of the endothelins) was not imagined a decade ago. Advances also have been made in the cloning and sequencing of DNA constructs that encode various transport proteins; in unraveling the interplay of second messengers, G proteins, and intracellular calcium transients; in linking abnormalities of genotype with phenotype, as in autosomal dominant polycystic kidney disease and various oncogene-associated renal neoplasms; and in understanding the regulatory elements governing the immune response. This chapter will address several of these issues to illustrate the advances in nephrology made possible by these technologies.

MOLECULAR DETERMINANTS OF NEPHRON DEVELOPMENT AND FUNCTION Normal renal function depends on the axial organization of individual nephron segments. Beyond the glomerulus, the filtrate is processed by as many as 20 functional tubule segments, each containing distinct cells and each characterized by distinct functions. Key processes in the development and maintenance of coordinated function of nephron segments include (1) expression of the polarized epithelial cell phenotype, (2) epithelial cell migration and branching, (3) orderly segregation of the specialized cell types comprising each nephron segment, and (4) apposition at the proximal nephron of a highly specialized microcirculatory element (the glomerular capillary tuft) capable of generating large volumes of a nearly ideal (protein-free) ultrafiltrate. Many disorders of kidney function can now be understood in terms of disruptions of the molecular determinants of these processes either during renal development or in the response to nephron injury.

Molecular determinants of the polarized epithelial cell phenotype and epithelial morphogenesis Vectorial transport of solute is characteristic of all tubule segments and reflects cell polarity, the signature feature of epithelial cells. The polarized epithelial cell is characterized by distribution of plasma membrane proteins into distinct apical and basolateral domains and the polarized distribution of cytoplasmic organelles and structural proteins comprising the cellular cytoskeleton. In general, apical membrane proteins subserve functions of regulated solute and water transport to and from the tubule lumen, while basolateral membrane proteins facilitate cell-cell contact and adhesion and participate in generation of ion gradients and signal reception and transduction (Fig. 234-1).

In the developing kidney, a key step in the differentiation of precursor cells of the metanephros to an epithelial lineage capable of expressing the polarized epithelial phenotype involves induction as the result of cell contact with the ureteric bud. This process is analogous to induction of mesoderm by ectoderm and endoderm in *Xenopus*; fibroblast growth factor, members of the *wnt* gene family, and *activins* (relatives of TGF-β) are possible candidates in the induction process. Once induced, expression of the polarized epithelial phenotype depends either on cell-cell or cell-substratum (e.g., tubule basement membrane) contact. Cell surface molecules that are expressed with development of the polarized epithelial phenotype and that mediate such contact include the calcium-dependent cell adhesion molecule *E-cadherin* (cell-cell contact) and the matrix protein *laminin* (cell-substratum contact). Cell-cell contact promotes the formation of highly developed junctional complexes that link the cytoskeletons of adjacent cells to facilitate cell-cell communication. Soon after cell-cell or cell-substratum contact, the component of the cell membrane exposed to the lumen adopts distinctive characteristics in terms of lipid composition (rich in glycosphingolipids and depleted in phosphatidylcholine) relative to the basolateral membrane and serves as a site for insertion of specialized apical transport proteins. This targeting is a function of both the epithelial phenotype and sorting signals intrinsic to the targeted proteins. The formation of tight junctions segregates the proteins of the apical from the basolateral membrane and serves as a barrier to lateral diffusion of phospholipids of the outer leaflet of the apical membrane.

Another characteristic of the polarized epithelial phenotype is that no transport protein resides in both the apical and basolateral membranes at the same time within the same cell. Indeed, it is the coordinated expression and function of proteins in the basolateral membrane (e.g., Na^+, K^+-ATPase) with proteins on the apical membrane (e.g., Na^+ channels and Na^+-H^+ antiporter of the proximal tubule) that allow vectorial transepithelial transport (e.g., reabsorption of sodium and water) to occur. Acquired loss of epithelial polarity occurs in at least two kidney diseases, namely acute tubular necrosis (ATN) and autosomal dominant polycystic kidney disease. The disturbances in fluid and solute reabsorption in these disorders highlight the importance of the polarized epithelial phenotype to nephron function.

Some molecules of mesenchymal origin that appear to be responsible for cell migration, branching tubulogenesis, and other components of epithelial morphogenesis necessary for nephron organization have been identified. Three such factors are *hepatocyte growth factor* (and its receptor the *met* oncogene), *nerve growth factor*, and *epimorphin*. Interruption of the expression or function of these factors disrupts epithelial morphogenesis. Expression of these or related factors is believed to contribute to orderly repair following acute tubule cell injury.

Molecular determinants of specialized function of nephron segments Segmentation of nephrons depends on establishing demarcated boundaries for expression of genes that define a given cellular phenotype. This orderly segmental pattern of gene expression

Functions

Apical plasma membrane
- *regulation of nutrient and water uptake*
- *regulated secretion (pathway A)*
- *protection*

Lateral plasma membrane
- *cell contact and adhesion*
- *cell communication*

Basal-lateral membrane
- *signal reception and transduction*
- *generation of ion gradients*
- *constitutive secretion (pathway B)*

Basal membrane
- *cell-substratum contact*

Components

Apical plasma membrane
- *Hydrolases*
- *Amiloride - sensitive Na$^+$ Channel*
- *Na$^+$-dependent Transporters*
- *Cl$^-$ channel*
- *H$^+$-ATPase*
- *Proteins linked via glycosyl - phosphatidylinositol*
- *Glycolipids*

Lateral plasma membrane
- *Cell Adhesion Molecules*
- *Junctional Complex:*
  Zonula occludens (ZO)
  Zonula adherens (ZA)
  Desmosomes (D)
  Gap junctions (GJ)

Basal-lateral membrane
- *Anion Channel (Cl$^-$/HCO$_3^-$exchanger)*
- *Na$^+$,K$^+$-ATPase*
- *Growth factor receptors*
- *Hormone and Neurotransmitter receptors*
- *Transduction systems associated with receptors*

Basal membrane
- *Basement Membrane Receptors*

Basement membrane
- *Laminin, Type IV Collagen, Proteoglycans*

FIGURE 234-1 In polarized epithelial cells, the apical plasma membrane faces the lumen and is responsible for the absorption of ions and nutrients via ion channels and transporters. In secretory epithelial cells, the apical plasma membrane is also the site of regulated secretion (pathway A). The lateral plasma membrane participates in cell-cell contact, mediated by specialized components of the junctional complex. Tight junctions [zonula occludens (ZO)] serve as a paracellular barrier between lumen and interstitium. Cell-cell contact is initially influenced by cell adhesion molecules and maintained by belt [zonula adherens (ZA)] and spot desmosomes (D). Intercellular communication is facilitated by gap junctions (GJ), specialized channels that make possible the exchange of small solutes. The basal plasma membrane is attached to the basement membrane via specific receptors for laminin, type IV collagen, and proteoglycans. Proteins and receptors localized to the basolateral plasma membrane are involved in solute transport and signal transduction and participate in constitutive secretion (pathway B). (*After E Rodriguez-Boulan and WJ Nelson, Science 245:719, 1989. Copyright 1989 by the AAAS.*)

is reminiscent of the expression of homeobox genes that determine body segmentation in *Drosophila* and other species. Indeed, analogues of homeobox genes (including the *pax-2* member of the paired-box gene family) may play a causal role in mammalian kidney development.

The specialization of nephron segments in the mature kidney is well characterized at the functional level, and efforts have been made to isolate and identify genes encoding the proteins that subserve these specialized functions. *Expression cloning* has been a powerful tool to identify several of these genes and characterize their protein products. This technique involves the introduction (e.g., microinjection) of fractionated messenger RNA (mRNA) into an expression system (e.g., *Xenopus* oocyte), followed by screening of the test system for the new appearance of the function of interest (e.g., sodium-dependent glucose transport). This approach allows the isolation of a gene or genes on the basis of a given specialized functional activity prior to identification of the protein that subserves the function.

Another strategy to clone specific genes of interest to nephron function takes advantage of patterns of homology of conserved sequences (consensus motifs) for molecules that share common functions or interactions and are therefore part of a large gene family. With this approach, genes have been cloned that encode novel receptor tyrosine kinases, such as members of the fibroblast growth factor family, that appear to be of importance in tubulogenesis. The genes encoding several receptors that act by coupling to G proteins and novel members of the G-protein family itself also have been cloned in this way.

As a result of these and other strategies, functional differentiation of distinct renal cells can be defined in terms of the expression of identified or candidate genes that provide the molecular basis for nephron segment specialization. Table 234-1 provides a number of examples in which the isolation of cDNAs has yielded insight into the physiology or pathobiology of individual nephron segments.

GLOMERULUS In vivo micropuncture and cell physiologic studies of cultured cells of glomerular origin (endothelial, epithelial, mesangial) suggest that circulating and locally produced vasoactive hormones and growth factors regulate glomerular hemodynamics on a moment-to-moment basis and control cell growth and matrix elaboration long term. Alterations in this system occur in both acute and chronic forms of glomerular injury. For example, the basis for an autocrine loop of mesangial cell origin has been identified in which platelet-derived growth factor (PDGF) interacts with its receptor during normal glomerulogenesis. Reactivation of this autocrine loop in experimental glomerular injury promotes mesangial cell proliferation and glomerular vasoconstriction. Indeed, the infusion of a blocking antibody to PDGF in an animal model of mesangial proliferative glomerulonephritis

TABLE 234-1 Examples of nephron proteins whose cDNAs have been cloned

Nephron segment	Protein
Glomerulus	Endothelins
	Nitric oxide synthase (type I)
	Receptors for angiotensin (vascular subtype), parathormone, vasopressin (vascular subtype), endothelins, thromboxane A_2, prostaglandin E_2, prostacyclin, catecholamines, PDGF-β chain, epidermal growth factor, and fibroblast growth factor
Proximal tubule	Vasopressin-insensitive water channel
	Nonvascular type angiotensin receptor
	Sodium-dependent glucose cotransporters (SGLT-1 and SGLT-2)
	Sodium-hydrogen exchanger
	Sodium-phosphate cotransporter
	Amino acid transport protein (D-2)
Loop of Henle	Epidermal growth factor
	Sodium-potassium-chloride cotransporter
	Chloride channel
	K_{ATP} channel
	Tamm-Horsfall protein
Distal nephron, and collecting tubule	Vasopressin receptor (antidiuretic subtype)
	Vasopressin sensitive water channel
	Bradykinin
	Thiazide-sensitive Na-Cl cotransporter
	H-ATPase (32-kDa subunit)
	Dihydropyridine-sensitive calcium channel (CaCh4)
	Sodium-calcium exchanger
	K_{ATP} channel
	Sodium channel
	Urodilatin
	Insulin-like growth factor I
	Aldose reductase

inhibits mesangial cell proliferation, suggesting a potential therapy for glomerulonephritis. Similarly, identification by expression cloning of the cDNA clones encoding the vascular type vasopressin (V_1) and angiotensin II (AT_1) receptors and the thromboxane A_2 receptor extend the tools needed to clarify the role of these vasoactive mediators in glomerular disease states. Of particular interest in the case of angiotensin II, molecular probes (e.g., cDNAs encoding renin, angiotensin-converting enzyme, and the angiotensin II receptor) have been utilized to confirm the existence of a self-contained intrarenal renin-angiotensin system capable of modulating glomerular hemodynamics. Molecular identification of endothelin and its receptor antedated functional characterization. The latter revealed that interaction of this peptide of endothelial origin and its mesangial cell receptor results in glomerular vasoconstriction and glomerular cell proliferation in normal and disease states. An example of the latter includes the contribution of augmented endothelin release to acute cyclosporine nephrotoxicity.

Signals downstream from these vasoconstrictor and growth promoting receptors (endothelin, angiotensin II, and V_1 vasopressin) are transduced by several intracellular proteins whose cDNAs or genes have been cloned. These include the G_q member of the G-protein family, phospholipase-C β, protein kinase C isozymes, and the inositol trisphosphate receptor. The concerted actions of these signaling proteins mediate calcium- and protein kinase–mediated responses that eventuate in glomerular response to these hormones. Although the glomerulus is not usually considered in terms of ion transport or channel properties, membrane depolarization and calcium influx control glomerular hemodynamics by contractile mesangial cells of the glomerular microcirculation.

Three vasodilator systems have been identified in the glomerular microcirculation. The first involved identification of cDNAs encoding the phospholipase A_2 and cyclooxygenase proteins involved in the elaboration of vasodilatory eicosanoids and their receptors. The second was identification of cDNA clones encoding components of the synthetic pathway for production of nitric oxide from its precursor L-arginine in glomerular endothelial cells. The third was elucidation

of subclasses of receptors for atrial natriuretic peptides (ANP) and of ANP degradative enzymes, which provide a molecular basis for understanding heterogeneous pharmacologic responses to atrial natriuretic peptides in different sodium-retaining states. In all cases, elucidation of the molecules involved in synthesis, action, or degradation of vasodilator components provides the basis for development of therapeutic strategies to treat renal vasoconstriction (e.g., hypertension, cyclosporine toxicity).

Several approaches, including development of transgenic mice, have been applied to elucidate the basis of various forms of glomerular injury. Expression of *Thy-1*, a member of the immunoglobulin gene superfamily, in transgenic mice causes proteinuric glomerular disease characterized by mesangial cell proliferation and dense subendothelial deposits. The pathogenetic role of PDGF was elucidated, as noted above in the rodent counterpart of this form of immune-mediated glomerular injury. A reverse approach has involved insertional inactivation of native genes, which in the case of one transgenic mouse line, caused the nephrotic syndrome. It will now be possible to clone and identify the gene whose inactivation caused the disease. Glomerular cells from transgenic mice have been perpetuated as immortalized cell lines in culture, thereby facilitating their functional and molecular characterization.

Several candidate genes involved in glomerular cell hypertrophy and genes responsible for the production and degradation of extracellular matrix components have been identified and characterized. These include the genes encoding TGF-β and its receptor, specific collagen subtypes, a tissue inhibitor of metalloproteinase, and others. In the case of the TGF-β receptor, cloning of the cDNA revealed its function as a receptor serine/threonine kinase. The availability of probes for the mRNAs encoding these proteins and cytokines, which mediate glomerular injury, will make possible new approaches to the interpretation of information obtained from renal biopsy specimens. In particular, in situ hybridization and quantitative PCR processing of biopsy specimens with appropriate probes will allow more accurate diagnosis, improve understanding of pathogenesis, and suggest therapies for the management of glomerular disease.

PROXIMAL TUBULE Physiologic studies in isolated, perfused, proximal tubule segments led to the identification of apical and basolateral transporters that account for the functional characteristics of each segment. Perhaps the best characterized are the apical sodium-dependent glucose transporter and sodium-hydrogen antiporter. Together, these transporters are responsible for most transcellular transport of sodium in the earliest portions of the proximal tubule. The cDNA encoding the sodium-hydrogen antiporter was first cloned on the basis of the importance of this protein in the regulation of intracellular pH in all cells of the body, and the formation gleaned from this expression cloning was applied to the corresponding protein that mediates transcellular sodium and bicarbonate reabsorption in the proximal tubule. Expression cloning also was used to identify the cDNA encoding a family of sodium-dependent glucose transporters in a variety of epithelial cell systems. Lessons learned from cloning of the sodium-hydrogen antiporter and the sodium-dependent glucose transporter are enabling investigators to clone cDNAs for other sodium gradient–dependent transport systems in the renal proximal tubule (e.g., other sugars, amino acids, phosphate, sulfate, and organic metabolites). It is probable that molecular probes derived from other systems (e.g., red blood cell water channel; muscle and hepatic sodium-independent glucose carrier, red cell band 3 anion exchanger) will clarify some of the ambiguities as to the nature of the transport systems that contribute to overall transcellular solute and water uptake in the proximal tubule.

Identification of one of the members of the *multidrug resistance gene family* (*MDR1*) in the apical membrane of the proximal tubule utilized the reverse approach, in which molecular investigation antedated and motivated physiologic and pathophysiologic studies. The 170-kDa glycoprotein product of this gene mediates resistance to a wide variety of cationic hydrophobic cytotoxic drugs in cancer cells, presumably through an ATP-dependent drug-pumping efflux mechanism. Localization of this protein in the apical membrane of the proximal tubule implies a role in the transport of a naturally occurring substrate whose identification may shed light on the physiologic role of the pump.

The activity of transporters in each of the proximal tubule segments is regulated by input from a number of receptors in the basolateral membrane, such as the angiotensin II receptor and the parathyroid hormone receptor. cDNA clones encoding both receptors have been isolated. Transmembrane signal-transduction systems (G proteins coupled to the regulation of ion channels via lipoxygenase product intermediates) are also present on the apical membrane.

LOOP OF HENLE The countercurrent mechanism responsible for production of urine of varying osmolality depends on the differential axial expression of solute transporters and membrane permeabilities to water, urea, and ions. This pattern of expression of transporters and permeabilities defines each of the limbs of the loop of Henle. Several aspects of the function of the loop of Henle await clarification. For example, the thin ascending limb of Henle has the highest chloride permeability reported in the nephron. Physiologic studies have not been able to distinguish whether this permeability reflects predominantly a paracellular or transcellular route of chloride movement. Similarly, the principal, if not only, conductance in the basolateral membrane of cells of the thick ascending limb of Henle is a chloride conductance. It is likely that analysis of the characteristics of proteins that mediate chloride channel conductance in other systems will provide the clues or probes to enhance our understanding of chloride movement in the thin and thick ascending limb of Henle and in other nephron segments. Identification of the cystic fibrosis gene product as a chloride channel has increased interest in identification of genes encoding chloride channels in the nephron. However, to date, no cystic fibrosis gene homologues have been identified in the nephron.

Attempts are also underway to identify the proteins of the apical Na-K-2Cl cotransporter of the thick ascending limb of Henle. The cloning of the vasopressin V_2 receptor gene (see below) will make it possible to define the regulatory role of vasopressin in modulating activity of this transporter in the medullary thick ascending limb of Henle. The ascending limb of Henle is also a major site for production of epidermal growth factor (EGF). The precursor molecule (pre-pro-EGF) is inserted as an integral transmembrane glycoprotein into the apical membrane. The mature EGF is sheared off the luminal side and excreted into the urine. Excretion of EGF in the urine is decreased in acute renal failure. Furthermore, infusion of EGF accelerates recovery of injured cells in experimental models of ATN. EGF and its receptors are also present in vascular and glomerular sites in the kidney, where they are thought to regulate eicosanoid production. It is of interest that the most abundant normally secreted urinary protein, Tamm-Horsfall protein, which is also produced in the ascending limb of Henle, shows a high degree of structural homology with pre-pro-EGF. Although the Tamm-Horsfall protein cDNA has been cloned, the physiologic function of the protein and the significance of its urinary excretion remain to be delineated.

DISTAL AND COLLECTING TUBULE SEGMENTS The portion of the nephron beyond the macula densa contains at least 5 cell types (distal cell proper, connecting tubule cell, principal cell, and two configurations of intercalated cells) and at least 11 segments (4 in the distal tubule and 7 in the collecting tubule), as defined by morphologic and functional markers. It is at the connecting tubule that the demarcation of cells of ureteric bud (mesonephric) origin from cells of metanephric origin occurs, and beyond this demarcation the nephron displays branching tubulogenesis.

In a few instances genes and their proteins have been isolated whose differential expression defines the characteristics for a given segment or cell type. These include, among others, receptors for mineralocorticoid, ANP, and vasopressin. The vasopressin receptor in this case is the V_2 receptor coupled to adenylate cyclase and to the antidiuretic response. An unique cloning strategy based on the expression of adenylate cyclase responsiveness was used to identify V_2 receptor genomic DNA. Since the expression of the V_2 receptor

is relatively restricted to the kidney, the gene encoding this molecule is a candidate for the potential identification of kidney-specific transcription activating factors. In addition, isolation of the V_2 receptor gene has permitted the molecular examination of hereditary disorders of water conservation (see below). V_1 receptors coupled to calcium signaling and prostaglandin production are also present in the collecting tubule, but the functional role remains to be determined.

The unique transport properties of the collecting tubule segments reflect the expression of highly specialized channels and/or transport proteins coupled with tight junctions capable of sustaining the highest transtubular solute gradients and epithelial resistances found along the nephron. Much attention is now focused on cloning the genes encoding these highly specialized transport elements, with the greatest emphasis on those proteins whose functional characteristics have been best defined, e.g., vasopressin-sensitive water and urea channels (principal cell of cortical and medullary collecting tubule), apical sodium and potassium channels (principal cell of cortical collecting tubule), and H^+-ATPase and chloride-bicarbonate exchanger of intercalated cells. Progress has been made in the case of the water channel, utilizing strategies based on homology with the erythrocyte water channel. This approach, combined with expression cloning, has made it possible to identify the vasopressin-insensitive water channel in the proximal tubule of the nephron and may make it possible to identify the collecting tubule water channel responsible for the antidiuretic response to vasopressin.

MOLECULAR GENETICS OF SELECTED DISORDERS OF KIDNEY FUNCTION (See Table 234-2) The strategies involved in the characterization of the genetic defects responsible for hereditary renal disease will probably also find application in defining other renal illnesses.

Alport's syndrome In X-linked Alport's syndrome, ultrastructural and immunostaining defects in the glomerular basement membrane implicated an alteration in a structural protein, type IV collagen, as the cause of the glomerular defect. The product of the human *COL4A5* gene is the a5 (IV) collagen chain, which is a specific component of glomerular basement membrane. This gene, which maps to the same region of the X chromosome long arm as does

TABLE 234-2 Hereditary diseases of renal function and their chromosomal loci

Disease	Gene product	Locus
Renal cell carcinoma/ von Hippel–Lindau syndrome		3p25–p26
Osteopetrosis–renal tubular acidosis–cerebral calcification syndrome	Carbonic anhydrase II	8q22
Tuberous sclerosis		9q11–q22
Fructose intolerance	Fructose-1-phosphate aldolase B	9q22
Nail-patella syndrome		9q34
Wilms' tumor		11p13
Vitamin D–dependent rickets, type 2	1,25(OH)$_2$ vitamin D receptor	12
Hemodialysis-related amyloidosis		15q21–q22
Adult dominant polycystic kidney disease		16p13.3
Urolithiasis (2,8-dihydroxyadenine)	Adenosine phosphoribosyl-transferase	16q24
Diabetes insipidus		20
Hypophosphatemia		Xp22
Hypomagnesemia		Xp22
Fabry's disease		Xq22
Alport's syndrome		Xq22–q25
Lowe oculocerebrorenal syndrome		Xq25
Lesch-Nyhan syndrome	Hypoxanthine-guanine phosphoribosyl-transferase	Xq26–q27.2
Congenital nephrogenic diabetes insipidus		Xq28–qter
Proximal renal tubular acidosis		X
Pseudohypoparathyroidism		X

Alport's syndrome (q22–q25), has 51 coding exons spread over 100 kilobases of genomic DNA. Since the first *COL4A5* mutations were described in 1990, additional mutations have been identified, and attempts have been made to correlate phenotypes with the various point mutations, deletions, and insertions. To date, no clear genetic differences have been identified between juvenile-onset and adult-onset end-stage Alport's syndrome.

X-linked nephrogenic diabetes insipidus As noted above, the antidiuretic hormone arginine vasopressin (AVP) activates specific V_2 receptors on basolateral surfaces of renal collecting tubule cells. Subsequent stimulation of the Gs-protein/adenylate cyclase system promotes insertion of water channels into the luminal membrane and thereby facilitates reabsorption of water and excretion of concentrated urine. In congenital nephrogenic diabetes insipidus, the kidneys fail to respond to vasopressin, and physiologic studies implicated a defect in the V_2 receptor. The gene for nephrogenic diabetes insipidus has been assigned to the q28–qter portion of the X chromosome long arm by linkage and functional studies. Furthermore, the V_2 receptor gene colocalizes to the same region. A deletion and two separate point mutations in the V_2 receptor gene have been detected in three independent families with the disease, and it is likely that defects in the V_2 receptor gene are responsible for abnormal water conservation in most. In both Alport's syndrome and nephrogenic diabetes insipidus, prenatal diagnosis and detection of carrier females at risk are now possible. Also, understanding of the relation between the nature of these molecular defects and phenotypic expression may lead to the design of appropriate therapies.

Autosomal dominant polycystic kidney disease (ADPKD) and molecular mechanisms of cyst formation ADPKD is a single-gene disorder that affects approximately 1 in 100 whites and leads to end-stage renal disease. Affected individuals also have an increased incidence of subarachnoid hemorrhage, due to berry aneurysms, and cystic manifestations in other organs, especially liver and pancreas. Up to 10 percent of patients who undergo renal replacement therapy in North America have this disorder. The biochemical defect has not been identified. Demonstration of linkage with the α chain of hemoglobin and more than 10 other genetic markers made it possible to assign the principal (>95 percent) locus for ADPKD mutations (designated PDK_1) to chromosome 16 (16p13.3). Twenty-three genes, each larger than 65 kilobases have been identified in the PDK_1 region.

Mutations at other loci also can produce renal cystic disease. Accordingly, information concerning the molecular basis of cyst formation will facilitate screening of candidate mutations. One possibility is a defect in the molecular determinants of epithelial cell polarity; Na^+, K^+-ATPase is localized to the apical membranes of cells in the epithelial lining of cysts form ADPKD kidneys, in contrast to the typical location in the basolateral membrane of renal cells in adjacent normal tubules in the same kidney. The reversal of polarity is not specific to Na^+, K^+-ATPase, since several other basolateral proteins, including EGF receptor, ankyrin, fodrin, and E-cadherin, are also mis-sorted to the apical surface. By contrast, other proteins, including the band 3 anion transporter, gp 330 antigen, laminin, and type IV collagen, are located normally in cystic epithelia.

Wilms' tumor and other renal malignancy syndromes Wilms' tumor, an embryonal malignancy of the kidney, affects approximately 1 in 10,000 infants and children. In 1971, Knudson proposed a mechanism to account for both the sporadic and hereditary forms of retinoblastoma and the relative occurrence of multiple, bilateral tumors in the two groups, a unifying hypothesis that also applies to Wilms' tumors. It is based on the concept of the tumor suppressor gene: Somatic cells homozygous for mutations that interfere with a tumor gene product have proliferative advantages that lead to clonal overgrowth. Cells heterozygous for such a mutation behave normally because tumor suppressor activity encoded by the "normal" gene is sufficient to suppress proliferation. In other words, since tumor suppressor mutations are recessive, two mutations at the same locus are required for tumor formation—the "two hit" hypothesis. The Wilms' tumor gene (*wt1*) has been characterized. All or part of *wt1*

polypeptides have features characteristic of transcription regulatory factors (including zinc finger domains). The tumor suppressor gene *wt1* on chromosome 11 (p13) is expressed at high levels in the glomeruli of the kidney, the gonadal ridge of the developing gonad, Sertoli cells of the testes, and the epithelial and granulosa cells of the ovary, suggesting a developmental role in the genital system in addition to the kidney. Such a role might explain the 10-fold higher incidence of hypospadias and cryptorchidism among patients with bilateral Wilms' tumor compared with the general population. In the WAGR syndrome, Wilms' tumor (W), congenital aniridia (A), genitourinary malformations (G), and mental retardation (R) often coexist. This constellation of anomalies defines a cluster of genes within 11p13 that appears to be important in the development of the iris, kidney, urogenital tract, and brain. Of these, *wt1* is a recessive oncogene. A consistent chromosome 3p deletion and loss of heterozygosity has been reported in sporadic cases of renal cell carcinoma and in renal carcinoma associated with the von Hippel–Lindau syndrome. A candidate tumor suppressor gene responsible for the renal malignancies in the Von Hippel-Lindau syndrome has been identified by positional cloning. Characterization of the product of this gene will provide insight into the mechanisms for the regulation of growth and differentiation of the renal epithelium.

REFERENCES

ALPER SL, LODISH HF: Molecular biology of renal function, in *The Kidney*, 4th ed, BM Brenner, FC Rector Jr (eds). Philadelphia, Saunders, 1991, pp 132–163

BARKER DF et al: Identification of mutations in the COL4A5 collagen gene in Alport syndrome. Science 248:1224, 1990

BRENNER BM: Determinants of epithelial differentiation and early nephrogenesis in the developing kidney. J Am Soc Nephrol 1:127, 1990

KOVACS G et al: Consistent chromosome 3p deletion and loss of heterozygosity in renal cell carcinoma. Proc Natl Acad Sci USA 85:1571, 1988

LATIF F et al: Identification of the Von Hippel-Lindau disease tumor suppressor gene. Science 260:1317, 1993

PELLETIER J et al: Germline mutations in the Wilms' tumor suppressor gene are associated with abnormal urogenital development in Denys-Drash syndrome. Cell 67:437, 1991

REEDERS S: Multilocus polycystic disease. Genetics 1:235, 1992

ROSENTHAL W et al: Molecular identification of the gene responsible for congenital nephrogenic diabetes insipidus. Nature 359 (6392):233, 1992

235 DISTURBANCES OF RENAL FUNCTION

BARRY M. BRENNER / STEVEN C. HEBERT

Near constancy of the composition of the internal environment, including the volume, tonicity, and compartmental distribution of the body fluids, is essential to survival. With day-to-day variations in amount and composition of food and fluids, preservation of the internal environment requires the excretion of these substances (and/or their by-products) in amounts that balance the quantities ingested. Although losses from skin, lungs, and intestine contribute to this excretory capacity, the greatest responsibility for solute and water excretion is borne by the kidneys.

The kidneys operate primarily to maintain the composition and volume of the *extracellular* fluid compartment. The continuous exchange of water and solutes across all cell membranes, however, permits the kidneys to contribute indirectly to the regulation of the volume, composition, and tonicity of the *intracellular* fluids as well. To accomplish these tasks, physiologic mechanisms enable the individual to excrete excesses of water and nonmetabolized solute contained in the diet, as well as the nonvolatile end products of nitrogen metabolism, such as urea and creatinine. By contrast, when faced with deficits of water and/or any of the other major constituents of the body fluids, renal excretion of these substances can be curtailed, reducing the likelihood of volume or solute depletion. The purpose of this chapter is to review the excretory functions of the kidney and to examine the way these functions are affected by disease.

MECHANISMS OF RENAL EXCRETORY FUNCTION WITH NORMAL AND REDUCED NEPHRON MASS

The volume of urine excreted per day (about 1.5 L, or roughly 1 mL/min) is the small residuum of two large, and in many ways opposing, processes—namely, *ultrafiltration* of 180 L or more fluid per day (approximately 125 mL/min) across glomerular capillaries on the one hand and, on the other, *reclamation* (or *reabsorption*) of more than 99 percent of this ultrafiltrate by transport processes in the renal tubules. Under resting conditions, about 20 percent of the cardiac output passes through the kidneys, which comprise less than 1 percent of body weight. Hence, per unit weight of tissue, the rate of blood flow to the kidneys is greater than that to heart, brain, or liver.

GLOMERULAR ULTRAFILTRATION Urine formation begins with the elaboration of a protein-free ultrafiltrate of plasma across the walls of the glomerular capillaries. The rate of ultrafiltration (glomerular filtration rate, GFR) is determined by three factors: (1) the balance of pressures acting across the capillary wall (the glomerular capillary hydrostatic and Bowman's space oncotic pressures tend to favor filtration, while glomerular capillary oncotic and Bowman's space hydrostatic pressures tend to retard it), (2) the rate at which plasma flows through the glomeruli, and (3) the permeability and the total surface area of the filtering capillaries. A decrease in GFR can be expected when (1) glomerular hydrostatic pressure is reduced (as in hypotension), (2) tubule (hence Bowman's space) hydrostatic pressure is increased (ureteral or bladder neck obstruction), (3) plasma oncotic pressure rises to high levels (hemoconcentration due to dehydration, multiple myeloma, or other dysproteinemias), (4) renal (hence glomerular) blood and plasma flow are decreased (circulatory collapse, heart failure), and (5) permeability and/or total filtering surface area is reduced (acute or chronic glomerulonephritis).

Despite the high rate of water movement across the glomerular capillary wall, all but the smallest of plasma proteins are normally excluded from passage through this barrier. Molecules the size of inulin (approximately 5200 mol wt) or smaller normally appear in glomerular urine in the same concentrations as in plasma water, whereas the transport of substances of increasingly greater size diminishes progressively, approaching very low values as the size of albumin is approached. The *glomerular capillary basement membrane* and the *slitlike diaphragms* that connect adjacent epithelial cell foot processes on the glomerular capillary wall (see Fig. 44-1) serve as major barriers to protein filtration. In addition, *electrostatic factors* also retard the filtration of plasma proteins, especially albumin. The albumin molecule behaves as a polyanion in physiologic solution and is therefore retarded by the anionic glycoproteins in the glomerular wall. With disruption of these mechanical and electrostatic barriers, as in many forms of glomerular injury (see Chaps. 239 to 241), large quantities of plasma proteins gain access to the urine.

BIOLOGIC CONSEQUENCES OF SUSTAINED REDUCTIONS IN GFR Measurement of total GFR of both kidneys is a sensitive index of overall renal excretory function. When renal excretory function is impaired, either acutely or chronically, one or more determinants of GFR in affected nephrons is altered unfavorably so that total GFR declines. The magnitude of decline is determined by the sum of the impairments of function of individual glomeruli. Initially, the effect of such impairments in single-nephron GFR (SNGFR), no matter how small, is to reduce the total rate of excretion of water and solutes in the glomerular ultrafiltrate. In the steady state, these reduced rates of filtration, when accompanied by comparably reduced rates of excretion, lead to *retention* and *accumulation* of the unexcreted substances in the body fluids. Further reduction in GFR augments the degree to which these substances are retained.

Figure 235-1 depicts the major response to these impairments in

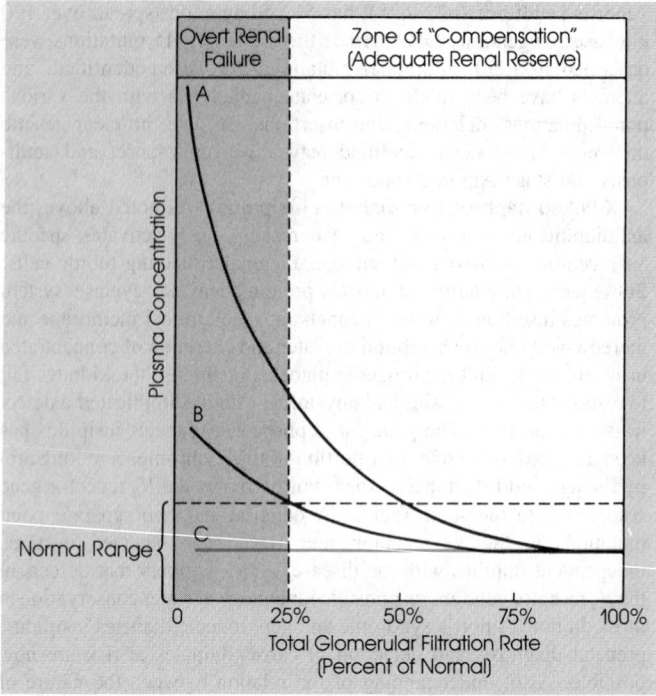

FIGURE 235-1 Representative patterns of adaptation for different types of solutes in body fluids in chronic renal failure. (*After NS Bricker et al, in Brenner and Rector, 4th ed.*)

filtration. The degree of reduction in total GFR is plotted on the abscissa, expressed as a percentage of normal (100 percent). For the various solutes normally contained in glomerular filtrate, three general types of response are common. Curve *A* describes the pattern with substances such as creatinine and urea which normally depend largely on glomerular filtration for excretion into the urine; i.e., urinary excretion is not appreciably influenced by secretion. Therefore, as GFR falls, plasma levels of creatinine, urea, and other substances normally excreted largely by filtration rise progressively, albeit in the nonlinear manner illustrated.

The clinical course of chronic renal failure (CRF) usually also conforms to the pattern described by curve *A*. Patients with CRF usually pass from a long asymptomatic period of "compensation" to a more accelerated and clinically symptomatic terminal phase. In other words, chronic forms of renal injury that lead to inexorable destruction of nephron mass usually lead to progressive but modest elevations in creatinine and urea levels in plasma but not to levels beyond the range of normal, despite loss of as much as 50 percent of total GFR. With further loss of nephron mass and further reduction in GFR, however (even though the rate of nephron destruction may not be accelerated), the limits of renal reserve are exceeded, and continued accumulation of curve *A*–type solutes leads to elevated plasma concentrations (see Fig. 235-1). Because these retained solutes are believed to exert "toxic" effects on all organ systems, manifestations of CRF now become overt. As a result, for patients with reduced renal mass, even small additional decrements in total GFR may spell the difference between "compensation" and overt uremia.

The accumulation of curve *A*–type solutes with progressive renal failure continues until external balance is achieved, i.e., until acquisition and/or production rates and excretion rates are exactly matched. In the case of creatinine, for example, assuming a constant rate of creatinine production, a 50 percent reduction in GFR results in an approximate doubling of the plasma creatinine concentration. The latter restores the filtered load of creatinine (i.e., GFR × plasma creatinine concentration) to normal, and the urinary excretion rate again is equivalent to creatinine production. Unfortunately, since no mechanism exists for augmenting creatinine excretion beyond this level, elimination of retained creatinine is not possible, and plasma concentration remains twice normal. With progressive reduction in GFR, plasma creatinine levels continue to rise, due both to the recent loss of nephron excretory function and to the retention associated with earlier nephron destruction (see Fig. 235-1). *In practice, so long as the net rates of acquisition and production (i.e., liver function and muscle mass) remain reasonably constant, the inverse relationship between plasma concentrations of solutes such as creatinine and urea and GFR is sufficiently reliable and predictable to allow plasma levels of the solutes to serve as clinical indexes of GFR.*

In contrast to solutes of the curve A type, plasma levels of phosphate, urate, and potassium (K^+) and hydrogen (H^+) ions usually do not rise until GFR falls to a small percentage of normal. With progressive renal failure this pattern of response (curve B in Fig. 235-1) reflects the participation of tubule transport mechanisms in the excretion of these substances. In other words, *as GFR declines, the tubules facilitate the excretion of greater fractions of the filtered load of these solutes, either by enhancing net secretion and/or by diminishing net reabsorption.* Plasma levels of curve B–type solutes, therefore, rise less than those of curve A because, with progressive reduction in GFR, *excretion rate per nephron* and, therefore, *fractional excretion* both increase. Eventually, however, enhanced fractional excretion can no longer offset the reduction in the filtered load of these solutes caused by a diminished GFR, and plasma levels rise (see Fig. 235-1). For urate, phosphate, and K^+, at least, increased fractional excretion serves to maintain normal plasma levels until GFR falls to less than one-fourth of normal.

Finally, for certain solutes, such as sodium chloride (NaCl), concentrations in plasma remain normal throughout the course of CRF, despite continued ingestion of these substances in normal amounts (curve C in Fig. 235-1). The compensation represents a fundamental adaptation to renal injury. To illustrate the magnitude of the adaptation involved, it is useful to compare the excretion of Na^+ in a normal individual (GFR of 125 mL/min) with that in advanced renal insufficiency (GFR of 2 mL/min). Both subjects are allowed to ingest a diet containing 7 g salt per day (120 mmol Na^+). With a normal serum Na^+ concentration of 140 mmol/L, external Na^+ balance is normally achieved by excreting approximately 0.5 percent of the filtered load. By contrast, for external balance to be maintained in the patient with CRF, fractional excretion of Na^+ must rise to 30 percent. *In other words, external balance for Na^+ demands that the same quantity of Na^+ (120 mmol) be excreted into the urine each day in the subject with CRF as in the normal subject.* Given the drastic reduction in GFR in CRF, external balance can be achieved only by transformation of the Na^+ reabsorptive processes in surviving tubules so that a progressively larger fraction of the filtered load of Na^+ escapes reabsorption and appears in final urine. In short, *the rate of excretion of Na^+ per surviving nephron increases in inverse proportion to the composite GFR of surviving nephrons.*

MECHANISMS OF TUBULE TRANSPORT WITH NORMAL AND REDUCED NEPHRON MASS   Loss of renal function with progressive renal disease is usually attended by distortion of renal morphology and architecture. Despite this structural disarray, glomerular and tubule functions often remain as closely integrated (i.e., *glomerulotubular balance*) as in the normal organ, at least until the final stages of CRF. A fundamental feature of this *intact nephron hypothesis* is that following loss of nephron mass, renal function is due primarily to the operation of surviving healthy nephrons, while the diseased nephrons cease functioning. Despite progressive nephron destruction, many of the mechanisms that control solute and water balance differ only quantitatively, and not qualitatively, from those that operate normally. The most important of these are considered below.

Tubule transport of sodium chloride and water   Most of the filtered water and Na^+ salts are reabsorbed by the tubules, leaving small and variable amounts, equivalent on average to the quantities ingested, to reach the final urine. About two-thirds of the glomerular ultrafiltrate is reabsorbed in the *proximal tubule* with little change in

the osmolality or Na^+ concentration of the unreabsorbed fraction (Fig. 235-2). In other words, fluid reabsorption in the proximal tubule is nearly *isosmotic* and is coupled to the active transport of Na^+. Since Cl^- and HCO_3^- are the primary anions in the extracellular fluid, most of the filtered Na^+ is reabsorbed with these anions. In the early convoluted portion of the proximal tubule, bicarbonate is the principal anion accompanying the reabsorption of sodium. This process occurs via a Na^+/H^+ exchange mechanism at the luminal brush border and is dependent on carbonic anhydrase. Glucose, amino acids, and other organic solutes (e.g., lactate) are also extensively reabsorbed in the proximal convoluted tubule by a cotransport process that links the cellular entry of these organic substrates with Na^+. Three processes appear to operate in parallel to couple water (i.e., volume) absorption with solute absorption. First, given the remarkably high water permeability of this nephron segment, very small transepithelial osmolality differences, i.e., *luminal hypotonicity* on the order of 2 to 3 mosmol, produced by solute absorption, could drive volume absorption. Second, due to the *preferential* absorption of HCO_3^- and organic solutes in the early portions of the proximal tubule, the concentrations of these substances decrease while that of Cl^- increases along the proximal tubule. Volume absorption would occur if the rate of Na^+ and Cl^- diffusion down their respective electrochemical gradients were more rapid than the back diffusion of sodium bicarbonate into the lumen. Finally, an *effective osmotic gradient* would be established (despite equal macroscopic osmolalities of luminal and peritubular fluids) if the effective osmolality of Cl^- in the lumen were greater than that for bicarbonate in the peritubular fluid.

The rate of reabsorption of fluid from proximal convoluted tubules and peritubular interstitium is sensitive to *physical factors*, i.e., the hydrostatic and colloid osmotic (or oncotic) pressures across the walls of the peritubular capillaries. Because the plasma proteins in glomerular capillaries are concentrated by ultrafiltration, there is a marked rise in the oncotic pressure along the glomerular capillary network. This step-up in plasma oncotic pressure is transmitted largely unchanged to the peritubular capillaries, via the efferent arterioles. These resistance vessels cause a substantial drop in hydrostatic pressure, however, so that when the plasma reaches the peritubular capillaries, oncotic pressure greatly exceeds hydrostatic pressure. These *Starling forces* are therefore oriented in an *uptake mode*, in contrast to the *filtration mode* at the glomerulus, where hydrostatic pressure exceeds oncotic pressure. The extent to which oncotic pressure exceeds hydrostatic pressure in the peritubular capillary network modulates the overall rate of reabsorption of fluid by the proximal tubules. Therefore, when peritubular oncotic pressure falls or hydrostatic pressure rises, uptake of fluid by these capillaries is reduced. As a result, fluid is retained in the interstitial space, altering the hydrostatic pressure in the space and ultimately retarding the egress of fluid from the lateral intercellular channels. Without an adequate route of drainage, fluid in the channels leaks back into the tubule lumen and diminishes *net fluid reabsorption* by this tubule segment. The opposite occurs in states in which peritubular oncotic pressure increases (increased filtration fraction) or hydrostatic pressure decreases (enhanced efferent arteriolar tone). Under these circumstances, peritubular capillary uptake of reabsorbate is augmented, leading ultimately to *enhanced net fluid reabsorption* by the proximal tubule.

In contrast to the proximal tubule, active outward transport of NaCl from tubule lumen to peritubular blood has not been established for the *thin ascending limb of Henle's loop*. However, passive outward salt transport does occur, as indicated in Fig. 235-2. In the next segment of the nephron, the *medullary thick ascending limb of Henle*, the concentration of NaCl is reduced below that at the beginning of this segment. Here Cl^- absorption occurs by an active process involving a furosemide-sensitive $Na^+:K^+:2Cl^-$ cotransport mechanism in the luminal membrane, with one-half of Na^+ absorption proceeding passively, driven by the lumen-positive transepithelial voltage. Since the ascending limb of Henle is impermeable to water, net NaCl reabsorption generates hypotonic tubule fluid and gives rise

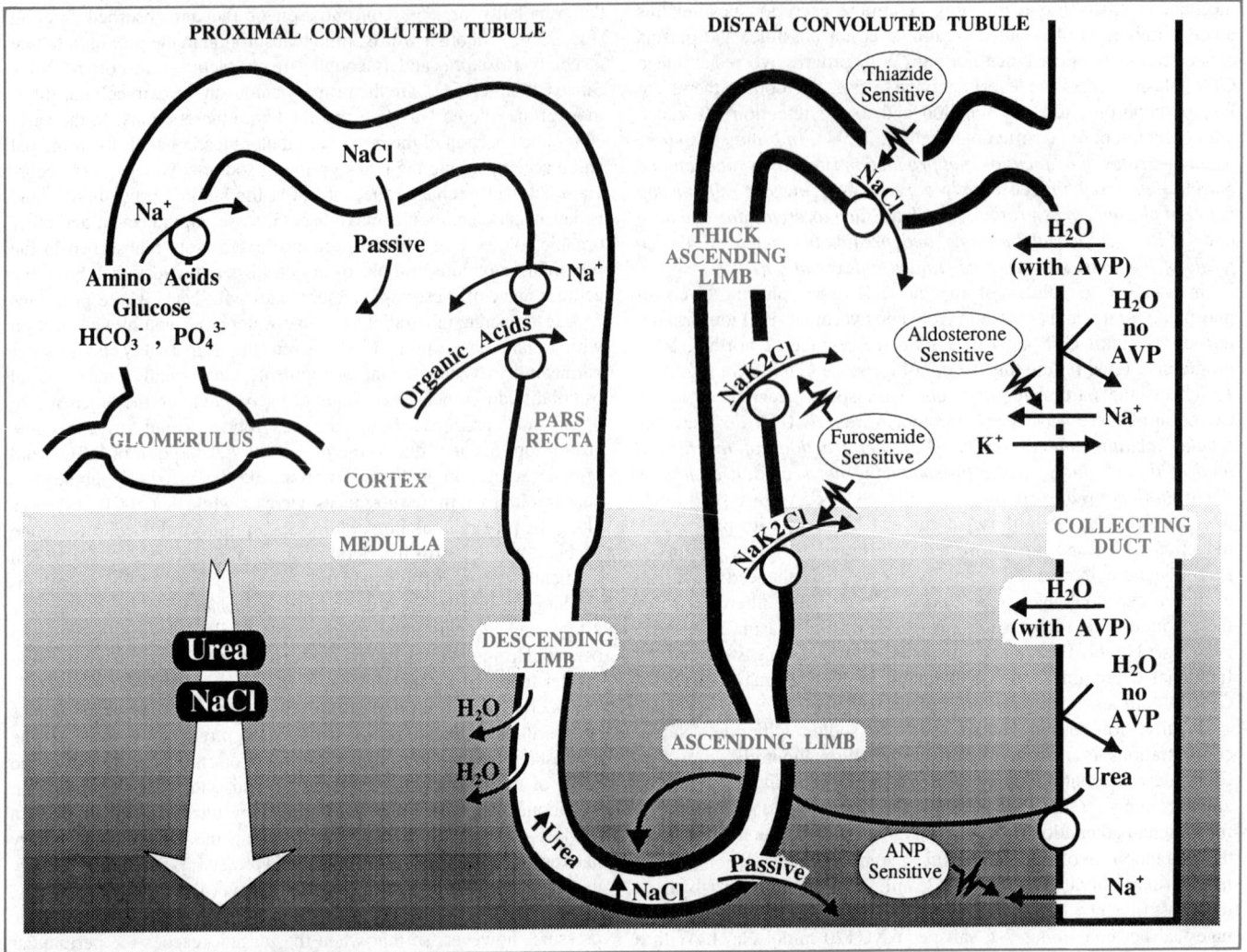

FIGURE 235-2 Transport functions of the various anatomic segments of the mammalian nephron. Fluid reabsorption across the proximal tubule is isosmotic and accounts for reabsorption of approximately two-thirds of the filtered Na^+ and H_2O. The major portions of the filtered HCO_3^-, amino acids, glucose, and phosphate are reabsorbed in the early proximal convoluted tubule. Reabsorption of glucose and amino acids is coupled to Na^+ transport and thereby generates a negative potential difference within the tubule lumen. At the same time, HCO_3^- is reabsorbed by a nonelectrogenic mechanism, via H^+ secretion. The active transport of these solutes results in transepithelial concentration and effective osmotic pressure gradients promoting H_2O flow across the proximal tubule, into the peritubular capillaries. The rise in tubule fluid Cl^- concentration is a necessary reciprocal consequence of the decreased luminal HCO_3^- concentration. The resultant high concentration of Cl^- becomes an important force for the outward passive transport of Cl^- down its concentration gradient, resulting in a lumen-positive potential difference in the late proximal convoluted tubule. The pars recta of the proximal tubule is capable of active electrogenic transport of Na^+ independent of organic solute transport. Under normal conditions, approximately one-third of the glomerular filtrate enters the descending limb of Henle's loop. Because the thin descending limb is incapable of active outward NaCl transport and is characterized by low permeability to Na^+ but high H_2O permeability, H_2O is abstracted passively as the fluid approaches the bend of Henle's loop. Hypertonic fluid with a greater NaCl concentration but lower urea concentration than the

surrounding medullary interstitium thus enters the thin ascending limb of Henle. This segment differs from the descending limb in that it is largely impermeable to H_2O and urea but highly permeable to NaCl. These characteristics allow for passive diffusion of NaCl out of the ascending limb. Active NaK_2Cl transport across the water-impermeable thick ascending limb of Henle allows for separation of solute and water. In consequence, tubule fluid becomes dilute and the medullary interstitium hypertonic.

Irrespective of the final osmolality of the urine, the fluid that enters the distal convoluted tubule is always hypoosmotic. This segment exhibits active Na^+ reabsorption. All but the terminal portion of the distal convoluted tubule is water-impermeable, even in the presence of ADH. Aldosterone exerts its effect in this segment by enhancing Na^+ reabsorption, which is variably coupled to K^+ and H^+ secretion. The cortical and papillary portions of the collecting duct are sites where ADH exerts its principal effect. The permeability of these segments to H_2O in the absence of ADH is very low but can be greatly enhanced in the presence of ADH. These segments are also characterized by active Na^+ reabsorption, which appears to depend on the presence of mineralocorticoid. In the absence of ADH, the collecting tubule is water impermeable so that hypotonic tubule fluid courses through it. However, in the presence of ADH, water is avidly reabsorbed here, resulting in hypertonic final urine. Sites of action of furosemide and thiazide diuretics and of aldosterone and atrial natriuretic peptide (ANP) are shown.

to the high NaCl concentration of the outer medullary interstitium (see Fig. 235-2). In certain animals, vasopressin (AVP or ADH) enhances NaCl absorption but not water permeability in the medullary portion of the thick ascending limb, but whether this occurs in human beings is uncertain.

The fluid leaving the thick ascending limb of Henle is normally low in NaCl concentration, a condition largely independent of the

organism's diet or state of hydration. In the *distal convoluted tubule*, water reabsorption is variable, depending on the state of hydration or, more specifically, on the presence or absence of AVP in plasma. In the absence of AVP, this and more distal nephron segments are impermeable to water, so the hypotonic fluid entering this segment is excreted as *dilute urine*. Indeed, continued salt reabsorption along the distal convoluted tubule, a process that can be initiated by thiazide diuretics, results in further dilution of the urine. In the presence of AVP, the permeability of the late portion of this segment to water increases, and as a result, the osmolality of the tubule fluid rises to a value close to that of plasma. NaCl continues to be reabsorbed from the tubule lumen, against moderately steep chemical and electrical gradients. The reabsorption of NaCl at this site is enhanced by *aldosterone*.

The *cortical collecting tubule* possesses a low permeability to water in the absence of AVP, whereas permeability increases in the presence of the hormone. The sensitivity of this segment to AVP appears to be more pronounced than that of the distal convoluted tubule. As with the distal convoluted tubule, the cortical collecting tubule is capable of active reabsorption of NaCl.

The terminal segment of the distal nephron is the highly branched *papillary collecting duct*. Continued electrolyte transport in this segment results in the large ion concentration differences that normally exist between urine and plasma. As in the cortical collecting tubule, Na^+ transport appears to be active, since reabsorption proceeds against sizable electrochemical gradients. The rate of Na^+ transport in this segment depends on the load of Na^+ delivered from more proximal segments and is affected by aldosterone. The permeability to water also increases markedly in the presence of AVP.

Effects of reduced nephron mass on sodium chloride transport in surviving nephrons With reductions in nephron mass, the remaining healthy or less damaged nephrons may hypertrophy so that GFR is increased toward normal. For example, a patient with a unilateral nephrectomy loses one-half of the nephron mass, and GFR is reduced by 50 percent at the time of surgery. However, within several months, GFR may return to 80 percent of the preoperative value for two kidneys. This requires that the blood flow, GFR, and transport functions of individual remaining nephrons increase above normal. This "compensatory hypertrophy" is evident by the large glomeruli and tubules observed on histologic sections and by increases in many of the biochemical processes associated with tubule transport (e.g., Na^+,K^+-ATPase). Similar hypertrophic changes occur in nephrons from kidneys damaged by other processes (e.g., glomerulonephritis); however, as nephron damage progresses, the hypertrophy of single nephrons can no longer make up for the magnitude of nephron loss, and GFR falls.

With progressive destruction, *maintenance of external balance for NaCl requires that fractional salt excretion increase as GFR decreases*. Several mechanisms contribute to this adaptive increase in fractional excretion. With losses of functioning nephron units, peritubular capillary hydrostatic and oncotic pressures are probably altered in directions that serve to suppress proximal tubule reabsorption of NaCl and water. For example, a rise in peritubular capillary hydrostatic pressure, which tends to inhibit net proximal fluid reabsorption, might be anticipated with hypertension, a common feature of renal insufficiency. Similarly, peritubular oncotic pressure probably declines with renal injury, owing both to reductions in filtration fraction and to hypoalbuminemia. Aldosterone, normally an important determinant of Na^+ reabsorption in distal portions of the nephron, is probably not a major factor responsible for reducing fractional Na^+ reabsorption, since levels in plasma are rarely reduced in CRF. Furthermore, external Na^+ balance is preserved in bilaterally adrenalectomized, uremic dogs maintained on fixed doses of mineralocorticoid. Yet another factor contributing to the suppression of fractional NaCl reabsorption in CRF may relate to the retention of solutes as GFR declines. In addition to urea and creatinine, *organic acids* (including *hippurates*) also accumulate. These substances are normally excreted by both filtration and tubule secretion; the latter process involves a carrier-mediated organic acid transport system in proximal tubule epithelia. When GFR is reduced and plasma levels of these organic acids increase, sufficient fluid may accompany their secretion into the proximal tubule lumen (by osmosis) to diminish net fluid reabsorption and even favor net fluid secretion. Evidence for this mechanism derives from studies in which uremic sera induced net fluid secretion in isolated proximal tubules of rabbits in vitro.

Several factors that regulate NaCl transport across the tubules also may participate in the enhanced fractional excretion of salt in renal insufficiency. Atrial natriuretic peptide is released from the cardiac atria in response to plasma volume expansion and atrial distention. This hormone effects a natriuresis by reducing net sodium reabsorption through complementary actions on active collecting duct Na^+ transport and on physical factors within the adjacent vasa recta. In addition, prostaglandin E reduces NaCl reabsorption from the thick ascending limb. Since prostaglandin E production per nephron appears to rise in renal insufficiency, the local action of this prostaglandin also may contribute to natriuresis in the setting of reduced renal mass. Finally, other inhibitors of ion transport appear in uremic serum, including an inhibitor(s) of the Na^+,K^+-ATPase. This factor(s) has not been fully characterized, and whether it represents an adaptation for maintenance of homeostasis or an unregulated accumulation of a toxin is also uncertain.

Serum and urine from patients with uremia contain factors capable of inhibiting NaCl transport across frog skin, toad bladder, and rat renal tubule. Accumulation of natriuretic factors in uremia may not be without cost; the "trade-off" for maintenance of external Na^+ balance is the possibility of abnormalities occurring in Na^+ transport across cell membranes, which often occurs in advanced renal insufficiency (see Chap. 237).

The obligatory high rate of solute excretion per surviving nephron (so-called osmotic diuresis due to urea and other retained solutes) also contributes to enhancing fractional NaCl excretion, much as occurs in normal subjects following administration of nonreabsorbable solutes such as mannitol. Finally, certain forms of CRF tend to be associated with unusually large salt losses in urine. These *salt-wasting nephropathies* include chronic pyelonephritis and other tubulointerstitial diseases (see Chap. 242) as well as polycystic and medullary cystic diseases. These disorders have in common greater destruction of medullary and interstitial than cortical and glomerular portions of the renal parenchyma. Preferential impairment of tubule reabsorptive function, rather than a primary reduction in GFR, may, therefore, underlie the salt-losing tendency in these disorders. Clinical derangements that alter renal handling of NaCl in CRF (including hypo- and hypervolemia, hypertension, etc.) are considered in Chap. 237.

Effects of reduced nephron mass on water reabsorption in surviving nephrons As with NaCl, there is a progressive increase in the fractional excretion of water with advancing renal insufficiency so that external water balance can be maintained even with a total GFR of 5 mL/min or less. The adaptations in the handling of water by the diseased kidney are of importance in the urinary concentrating defect and, hence, the polyuria and nocturia seen commonly in CRF (see Chap. 44). To appreciate the mechanisms involved, the responses of a normal and a uremic subject in maintaining external water balance need to be compared. Assuming that both subjects ingest the same diet and the same amount of fluid, total solute and volume excretion in each subject should be identical as well. If the *obligatory solute load* to be excreted in each is 600 mmol/d (600 mosmol/d), and urine osmolality is 300 mmol/kg water (300 mosmol/kg), a urine volume of 2 L/d will be required to excrete the total solute. If GFR in normal and uremic subjects is 180 and 4 L/d, respectively, urinary volume excretion of 2 L/d represents excretion of slightly more than 1 percent of the filtered water in the normal individual, compared with 50 percent in the uremic subject. Since the range of urine osmolalities that the diseased kidney can achieve [250 to 350 mmol/kg (250 to 350 mosmol/kg)] is narrower than in the normal [40 to 1200 mmol/kg (40 to 1200 mosmol/kg)], the individual with normal function is able to excrete the obligatory daily solute load of 600 mmol (600 mosmol) in as little as 500 mL urine per day or as much as 15 L/d, compared with the narrower range in renal insufficiency, from about 1.7 to 2.4 L/d.

In CRF, the limited ability to concentrate the urine usually correlates with other measures of impaired renal function. Isosthenuria is therefore a nearly universal finding when GFR falls below 25 mL/min. At this level of GFR and below, urine osmolality does not rise even with supraphysiologic doses of vasopressin, suggesting that the concentrating defect is related both to loss of diseased nephrons and to impaired concentrating ability in surviving nephrons. As has been discussed, with diminution in functioning nephron mass, there is a concurrent increase in fractional excretion of a number of solutes. As a consequence, solute diuresis per nephron obligates a nearly isosmotic amount of water and prevents the elaboration of either hypotonic or hypertonic urine. Disease-induced abnormalities of the architecture of the renal medulla (loops of Henle, vasa recta), aberrations in renal medullary blood flow, and defective transport of NaCl in the ascending limb of Henle also contribute to this defect in urine concentration. Finally, uremia per se may impair the responsiveness of terminal nephron segments to vasopressin.

Since patients with renal insufficiency are unable to excrete concentrated urine, they must have access to adequate amounts of water to ensure the excretion of total daily solute loads. For this reason, restriction of fluid intake may be hazardous in patients with CRF. Likewise, impairment of diluting capacity may prevent many patients from excreting large amounts of ingested fluids. The consequences of the abnormal water excretion patterns in CRF, including the tendencies to development of hypo- and hypernatremia, are considered in Chaps. 45 and 237.

Tubule transport of phosphate with normal and reduced nephron mass Under normal physiologic conditions, about 80 to 90 percent of the filtered load of phosphate is reabsorbed, mainly in the proximal tubule. *Parathyroid hormone (PTH)*, by augmenting phosphate excretion via inhibition of this proximal reabsorptive process (Chap. 356), plays a key role in phosphate homeostasis. When dietary phosphate intake increases, a *transient* rise in plasma phosphate concentration is usually observed. This results in a similarly transient reduction in the plasma ionized calcium concentration (due largely to calcium phosphate deposition in bone), which, in turn, stimulates PTH secretion. By enhancing fractional phosphate excretion, PTH restores external phosphate balance and normophosphatemia. This then enables plasma ionized calcium levels to return to normal, thereby removing the stimulus to PTH release and restoring the phosphate control system to the original steady state.

With advancing renal disease and constant dietary intake of phosphate, external phosphate balance is achieved by progressive reduction in fractional phosphate reabsorption. Enhanced PTH secretion is an important determinant of this phosphaturic response. With each succeeding decrement in GFR, the total amount of phosphate filtered by surviving glomeruli is reduced, leading to transient retention of phosphate and, therefore, a rise (albeit small) in the phosphate concentration in extracellular fluid, including plasma. This rise in plasma phosphate concentration leads to a reciprocal small decline in plasma ionized calcium concentration and a corresponding increase in PTH secretion. Although the phosphaturic response of surviving tubules to this elevation in circulating PTH restores plasma phosphate and, therefore, calcium levels to normal (at least in the "compensated" stage of CRF described by the relatively flat portion of curve *B* in Fig. 235-1), the biologic cost of this return to normophosphatemia and normocalcemia is a *persistent elevation in the plasma PTH level*. With successive decrements in GFR, each stage in this overall process is repeated, but at an ever-increasing cost, namely, *progressive elevation in the circulating level of PTH*.

Alterations in vitamin D metabolism also contribute to the elevated PTH levels in renal failure. The kidneys are normally the major site of *metabolic conversion of vitamin D to its active metabolites*. As discussed in Chap. 356, vitamin D, synthesized in skin or acquired from foods, undergoes initial hydroxylation in the liver to form 25-hydroxyvitamin D [25(OH)D]. The kidney is the site of a second important hydroxylation, formation of 1,25-dihydroxyvitamin D [1,25(OH)$_2$D]. This activated form of vitamin D acts directly on the parathyroid gland to suppress PTH secretion as well as to enhance intestinal calcium and phosphate absorption and promote resorption of these ions from bone. In addition, 1,25(OH)$_2$D probably opposes the phosphaturic action of PTH in the renal tubule by augmenting,

rather than diminishing, phosphate reabsorption. With advancing renal disease, reduction in renal mass causes vitamin D hydroxylation to be impaired; phosphate retention also suppresses this reaction. Not only are the circulating levels of 1,25(OH)$_2$D diminished in uremia, but the receptors that mediate its action within the parathyroid cells are also diminished. These two effects disinhibit parathyroid hormone secretion and thereby increase circulating PTH levels. Reduction in circulating 1,25(OH)$_2$D levels, by suppressing calcium absorption from gut, contributes to the development of the hypocalcemia and PTH excess of CRF (see Chap. 237).

At least two additional processes are thought to contribute to elevated PTH levels in renal failure. One relates to the skeletal resistance to the calcemic effect of PTH in uremia. This resistance necessitates a higher level of circulating PTH to effect an increment in serum calcium concentration. The other derives from the finding that reductions in renal mass impair the ability of the kidneys to degrade circulating PTH. The fact that phosphate conforms more to a curve *B*– than curve *C*–type solute in Fig. 235-1 indicates that these forms of adaptation are limited; ultimately, phosphate retention occurs when GFR falls below about 25 mL/min.

Since PTH exerts major biologic effects on bone, as well as renal tubules, the external balance of phosphate in CRF is achieved at the expense of elevated PTH levels, which, in turn, account for many of the bone changes of renal osteodystrophy (i.e., *secondary hyperparathyroidism*; see Fig. 237-1). In support of this *trade-off hypothesis*, when dietary phosphate intake is reduced in proportion to the reduction in GFR in animals with CRF, external balance of phosphate no longer requires augmentation of fractional phosphate excretion in surviving nephrons. Accordingly, circulating PTH levels no longer rise, and the bone changes of secondary hyperparathyroidism are diminished, if not prevented.

Hydrogen and bicarbonate transport with normal and reduced nephron mass As discussed in Chap. 46, the pH of extracellular fluid is normally maintained within a narrow range (7.36 to 7.44) despite day-to-day variations in the quantity of acids entering the body fluids from dietary and metabolic sources (approximately 1 mmol H$^+$ per kilogram of body weight per day). These acids consume both intracellular and extracellular buffers, of which bicarbonate (HCO$_3^-$) is the most important in the intracellular compartment. Such buffering minimizes the changes in pH. The HCO$_3^-$ buffer system would be of little long-term benefit were it not for homeostatic mechanisms, however, since with unrelenting acquisition of nonvolatile acids from dietary and metabolic sources, buffering capacity would ultimately be exhausted, culminating in fatal acidosis. The kidneys normally function to prevent this possibility by *regenerating* HCO$_3^-$ and, thereby, maintaining the concentration of HCO$_3^-$ in the plasma. In addition to generating HCO$_3^-$, the kidneys also *reclaim* the HCO$_3^-$ in the glomerular ultrafiltrate. This reabsorptive process takes place largely in the proximal tubule and is virtually complete below a critical serum HCO$_3^-$ concentration—the threshold concentration—which in humans is normally about 26 mmol/L, identical to the concentration of HCO$_3^-$ in plasma. As a consequence, urinary wastage of HCO$_3^-$ is prevented. Alternatively, when plasma HCO$_3^-$ rises above this threshold, reabsorption becomes less complete, and the excess HCO$_3^-$ escapes into the final urine, returning the plasma HCO$_3^-$ to the threshold level. Despite reabsorption of all the filtered HCO$_3^-$, metabolic acidosis would still ensue if HCO$_3^-$ consumed in buffering nonvolatile strong acids were not constantly regenerated.

The *reabsorption* of filtered HCO$_3^-$ in the proximal tubule occurs by the following mechanism. In proximal tubule cells, H$^+$, formed by the splitting of water into H$^+$ and OH$^-$, is secreted into the tubule lumen, very likely in exchange for Na$^+$. The OH$^-$ ion, under the influence of *carbonic anhydrase*, combines with CO$_2$ to form HCO$_3^-$, which moves across the peritubular cell membrane via an electrogenic Na(HCO$_3$)$_2$ cotransporter to enter the extracellular HCO$_3^-$ pool. The H$^+$ secreted into the tubule lumen combines with a filtered HCO$_3^-$, forming H$_2$CO$_3$. Dehydration of the latter in the proximal tubule lumen leads to the formation of CO$_2$, which also diffuses from lumen to peritubular blood. As a result, *a filtered HCO_3^- ion is reclaimed*. Secreted H^+ ions are also free to combine with non-HCO_3^- buffers (e.g., phosphate or ammonia) in the tubule fluid and are excreted in these forms in the final urine. HCO_3^-, the other original product of the breakdown of H_2CO_3, formed within the tubule cell, enters the peritubular blood, and *an HCO_3^- ion is regenerated*.

Hydrogen ions in the urine are bound primarily to filtered buffers (e.g., phosphate) in an amount (the so-called titratable acid) equivalent to the amount of alkali required to titrate the pH of the urine to the pH of blood. It is usually not possible, however, to excrete all the daily acid load as titratable acid alone. Metabolism of glutamine by proximal tubule cells to form ammonium (i.e., ammoniagenesis) serves as an additional mechanism for bicarbonate regeneration. Glutamine metabolism forms not only NH_4^+ (i.e., NH_3 plus H^+) but also HCO_3^- which is transported across the proximal tubule (HCO_3^- regeneration). The generated NH_4^+ must be excreted in urine for this process to be effective in bicarbonate regeneration. The excretion of ammonium involves secretion by proximal tubule cells (possibly on the Na:H exchanger as Na^+:NH_4^+), generation of high medullary interstitial NH_4^+ concentration by an elaborate countercurrent multiplication/exchange system, and finally, secretion of the interstitial NH_4^+ by the collecting duct by a combination of H^+ secretion and passive NH_3 diffusion. *Ammoniagenesis* is responsive to the acid-base needs of the individual. When faced with an acute acid burden and an increased need for HCO_3^-- regeneration, the rate of renal ammonia synthesis increases sharply.

The quantity of hydrogen ions excreted as titratable acid and NH_4^+ is equal to the quantity of HCO_3^- regenerated in tubule cells and added to the plasma. Under steady state conditions, the quantity of net acid excreted into the urine (the sum of titratable acid and NH_4^+ minus HCO_3^-) must equal the quantity of acid gained by the extracellular fluid from all sources. Metabolic acidosis and alkalosis result when this delicate balance is perturbed, the former the result of *insufficient* net acid excretion and the latter due to *excessive* acid excretion.

Progressive loss of renal function usually causes little or no change in arterial pH, plasma bicarbonate concentration, or arterial carbon dioxide tension (P_{CO_2}) until GFR falls below 50 percent of normal. Thereafter, all three quantities tend to decline as *metabolic acidosis* ensues. In general, the metabolic acidosis of CRF is not due to overproduction of endogenous acids but is largely a reflection of the reduction in renal mass, which limits the amount of NH_3 (and therefore HCO_3^-) that can be generated. Although surviving nephrons are probably capable of generating supernormal quantities of NH_3 *per nephron*, the diminished nephron population causes overall NH_3 production to be reduced to an extent inadequate to permit sufficient buffering of H^+ in urine. Although patients with CRF may acidify the urine normally (i.e., urine pH as low as 4.5), the defect in NH_3 production limits total daily acid excretion to 30 to 40 mmol, or one-half to two-thirds the quantity of nonvolatile acid formed in the same time period. Metabolic acidosis is the inevitable consequence of this positive balance for H^+, which in most patients with stable CRF is relatively mild and nonprogressive (arterial pH of approximately 7.33 to 7.37).

Given this substantial daily accumulation of H^+ and the typically stable and nonprogressive nature of the resulting acidosis, including the observed relative constancy of the plasma HCO_3^- concentration (albeit at reduced levels of 14 to 20 mmol/L), it follows that some large tissue source of buffering must account for the stability of the acidosis in CRF. Bone is the likely candidate, in view of its large reservoir of alkaline salts (calcium phosphate and calcium carbonate). Dissolution of this buffer source probably contributes to the osteodystrophy of CRF (see Fig. 237-1).

Although the acidosis of CRF is due to the reduction in total renal mass and is therefore tubular in origin, it nevertheless depends to a large extent on the level of GFR. When GFR is reduced to only a moderate extent (i.e., to about 50 percent of normal), retention of

anions, principally sulfates and phosphates, is not pronounced, so as the plasma HCO_3^- level falls owing to tubule dysfunction, retention of Cl^- by the kidneys leads to the development of *hyperchloremic acidosis*. At this stage, therefore, *the anion gap is normal*. With further reduction in GFR and more pronounced azotemia, however, retention of phosphates, sulfates, and other *unmeasured* anions is the rule, and plasma Cl^- concentration falls to normal levels despite the reduction in plasma HCO_3^- concentration. *A moderate to large anion gap therefore develops*.

Tubule potassium transport with normal and reduced nephron mass As with H^+, the concentration of K^+ in extracellular fluid is normally maintained within a relatively narrow range, 4 to 5 mmol/L. Ninety-five percent or more of total-body K^+ is in the intracellular fluid compartment, where the intracellular concentration is approximately 160 mmol/L. Normal individuals maintain external K^+ balance by excreting into the urine an amount of K^+ per day equivalent to the amount ingested, minus the relatively small amounts lost in stool and sweat. K^+ is freely filtered at the glomerulus, although the amount excreted usually represents no more than about 20 percent of the quantity filtered. The great bulk of the filtered K^+ is *reabsorbed* in the early portions of the nephron, about two-thirds in the proximal tubule, and an additional 20 to 25 percent in the loop of Henle. A K^+ *secretory process* operates in the distal tubule and terminal nephron segments. This process is largely dependent on Na^+ reabsorption and the accompanying lumen-negative voltage creating an electrical gradient across the tubule wall, favoring K^+ secretion into the lumen of distal tubule and collecting duct.

The ability to maintain external K^+ balance and normal plasma K^+ concentration until relatively late in the course of CRF is a consequence primarily of a progressive increase in fractional excretion of K^+. Greatly enhanced rates of K^+ secretion occur in distal portions of surviving tubules. The augmented secretion rate of aldosterone contributes to enhanced tubule secretion of K^+. In addition, both the increased distal tubule flow rates in residual functioning nephrons due to the osmotic diuresis and the enhanced luminal electronegativity created by the increased concentration of highly impermeable anions such as phosphate and sulfate enhance K^+ excretion. Aldosterone also stimulates net entry of K^+ into the lumen of the colon, a mechanism known to be enhanced in CRF. More detailed discussions of the abnormalities in K^+ homeostasis in acute and chronic forms of renal failure are given in Chaps. 236 and 237.

REFERENCES

BRENNER BM: Nephron adaptation to renal injury or ablation. Am J Physiol 249:F324, 1985

————— et al: Diverse biological actions of atrial natriuretic peptide. Physiol Rev 70:665, 1990

—————, RECTOR FC JR (eds): *The Kidney*, 4th ed. Philadelphia, Saunders, 1991

FEINFELD DA, SHERWOOD LM: Parathyroid hormone and 1,25(OH)$_2$D$_3$ in chronic renal failure. Kidney Int 33:1049, 1988

KAJI D, KAHN T: Na$^+$-K$^+$ pump in chronic renal failure. Am J Physiol 252:F785, 1987

MAXWELL MH et al: *Clinical Disorders of Fluid and Electrolyte Metabolism*, 4th ed. New York, McGraw-Hill, 1987

WARNOCK DG: Uremic acidosis. Kidney Int 34:278, 1988

236 ACUTE RENAL FAILURE

HUGH R. BRADY / BARRY M. BRENNER

Acute renal failure (ARF) is characterized by rapid decline in glomerular filtration rate (hours to weeks) and retention of nitrogenous waste products. This syndrome occurs in approximately 5 percent of all hospital admissions and up to 30 percent of admissions to intensive care units. Oliguria (urine output <400 mL/d) is frequent (~50 percent) but not invariable. ARF is usually asymptomatic and is diagnosed when screening of hospitalized patients reveals a recent increase in serum blood urea nitrogen (BUN) and creatinine. ARF may complicate a wide range of diseases which for purposes of diagnosis and management are conveniently divided into three categories: (1) disorders of renal hypoperfusion in which the kidney is intrinsically normal (*prerenal azotemia, prerenal ARF*) (~55 percent), (2) diseases of the renal parenchyma (*renal azotemia, intrinsic renal ARF*) (~40 percent), and (3) acute obstruction of the urinary tract (*postrenal azotemia, postrenal ARF*) (~5 percent). Although usually reversible, ARF is a major cause of in-hospital morbidity and mortality due to the serious nature of the underlying illnesses and the high incidence of complications.

ETIOLOGY AND PATHOPHYSIOLOGY   Prerenal azotemia (prerenal ARF)

This is responsible for half of cases. This syndrome is due to a functional response to renal hypoperfusion and is rapidly reversible upon restoration of renal blood flow and glomerular ultrafiltration pressure. Renal parenchymal tissue is not damaged; indeed, kidneys from individuals with prerenal azotemia function well when transplanted into recipients with normal cardiovascular function. However, severe or prolonged hypoperfusion may lead to ischemic renal parenchymal injury and intrinsic renal azotemia. Prerenal azotemia can complicate a variety of hemodynamic disturbances, including hypovolemia, low cardiac output, systemic vasodilatation, and selective renal vasoconstriction (Table 236-1).

Intravascular volume depletion sufficient to cause ARF may result from hemorrhage (e.g., surgical, traumatic, gastrointestinal), burns, dehydration, gastrointestinal fluid losses (e.g., vomiting, diarrhea, surgical drainage), urinary tract fluid losses (e.g., drug-induced or osmotic diuresis), or sequestration of fluid in extravascular compartments (e.g., peritonitis, pancreatitis, trauma, burns, or severe hypoalbuminemia). Prerenal azotemia also may occur when *"effective" arterial blood volume* is decreased despite normal or expanded intravascular volume. "Effective" hypovolemia may complicate *low cardiac output states* (e.g., myocardial, valvular, or pericardial disease, complicated arrhythmias) and diseases characterized by *systemic vasodilatation* (e.g., sepsis, vasodilator therapy, anesthesia, anaphylaxis).

True or "effective" hypovolemia leads to a fall in mean arterial pressure that is detected as reduced stretch by arterial (e.g., carotid sinus) and cardiac baroreceptors. The latter trigger a series of neurohumoral responses designed to maintain arterial pressure. These include activation of the sympathetic nervous system and renin-angiotensin-aldosterone system and release of vasopressin (AVP; ADH) and endothelin. Norepinephrine, angiotensin II, AVP, and endothelin cause vasoconstriction in musculocutaneous and splanchnic vascular beds, reduce salt loss through sweat glands, stimulate thirst and salt appetite, and promote renal salt and water retention. As a result, cardiac and cerebral perfusion is preserved relative to that of other "less essential" organs. Several renal responses combine to maintain glomerular perfusion and filtration in this setting. Stretch receptors in afferent arterioles, in response to a reduction in perfusion pressure, trigger relaxation of arteriolar smooth-muscle cells and vasodilatation (autoregulation). Biosynthesis of vasodilator renal prostaglandins (e.g., prostacyclin, prostaglandin E_2) and nitric oxide is also enhanced, and these compounds preferentially dilate afferent arterioles. In addition, angiotensin II induces preferential constriction of efferent arterioles, probably by virtue of the increased density of angiotensin II receptors at this location. As a result, intraglomerular pressure is preserved, and the fraction of renal plasma filtered by glomeruli (filtration fraction) is increased. During severe hypoperfusion, however, these responses prove inadequate, and ARF ensues.

Drugs that interfere with the adaptive responses may convert compensated renal hypoperfusion into overt prerenal azotemia or trigger progression of prerenal azotemia to intrinsic renal azotemia (see below). Consequently, inhibitors of renal prostaglandin biosynthesis (*cyclooxygenase inhibitors*) or of angiotensin-converting enzyme activity (*ACE inhibitors*) should be used with caution in high-renin

---

TABLE 236-1   Classification and major causes of acute renal failure

PRERENAL FAILURE

Hypovolemia
   Hemorrhage, burns, dehydration
   Gastrointestinal fluid loss: vomiting, surgical drainage, diarrhea
   Renal fluid loss: diuretics, osmotic diuresis (e.g., diabetes mellitus), adrenal
      insufficiency
   Sequestration of fluid in extravascular space: pancreatitis, peritonitis,
      trauma, burns, hypoalbuminemia
Low cardiac output
   Diseases of myocardium, valves, and pericardium, arrhythmias, tamponade
   Other: pulmonary hypertension, pulmonary embolus, positive pressure
      mechanical ventilation
Increased renal systemic vascular resistance ratio
   Systemic vasodilatation: sepsis, antihypertensives, afterload reducers, anes-
      thesia, anaphylaxis
   Renal vasoconstriction: hypercalcemia, norepinephrine, epinephrine,
      cyclosporine, amphotericin B
   Cirrhosis with ascites
Renal hypoperfusion with impairment of renal autoregulatory responses
   Cyclooxygenase inhibitors, angiotensin-converting enzyme inhibitors
Hyperviscosity syndrome (rare)
   Multiple myeloma, macroglobulinemia, polycythemia

INTRINSIC ACUTE RENAL FAILURE

Renovascular obstruction (bilateral or unilateral: one functioning kidney)
   Renal artery obstruction: atherosclerotic plaque, thrombosis, embolism,
      dissecting aneurysm, vasculitis
   Renal vein obstruction: thrombosis, compression
Diseases of glomeruli or renal microvasculature
   Glomerulonephritis and vasculitis
   Hemolytic uremic syndrome, thrombotic thrombocytopenic purpura, dissem-
      inated intravascular coagulation, toxemia of pregnancy, accelerated hyper-
      tension, radiation nephritis, scleroderma, systemic lupus erythematosus
Acute tubular necrosis
   Ischemia: as for prerenal azotemia (hypovolemia, low cardiac output,
      renal vasoconstriction, systemic vasodilatation), obstetrical complications
      (abruptio placentae, postpartum hemorrhage)
   Toxins: exogenous—contrast, cyclosporine, antibiotics (e.g., aminoglyco-
      sides, amphotericin B), chemotherapeutic agents (e.g., cisplatin), organic
      solvents (e.g., ethylene glycol), acetaminophen, illegal abortifacients;
      endogenous—rhabdomyolysis, hemolysis, uric acid, oxalate, plasma cell
      dyscrasia (e.g. myeloma)
Interstitial nephritis
   Allergic: antibiotics (e.g., beta-lactams, sulfonamides, trimethoprim, rifam-
      pin), cyclooxygenase inhibitors, diuretics, captopril
   Infection: bacterial (e.g., acute pyelonephritis, leptospirosis), viral (e.g.,
      CMV), fungal (e.g., candidiasis)
   Infiltration: lymphoma, leukemia, sarcoidosis
   Idiopathic
Intratubular deposition and obstruction
   Myeloma proteins, uric acid, oxalate, acyclovir, methotrexate, sulfonamides
Renal allograft rejection

POSTRENAL FAILURE (OBSTRUCTION)

Ureteric
   Calculi, blood clot, sloughed papillae, cancer, external compression (e.g.
      retroperitoneal fibrosis)
Bladder neck
   Neurogenic bladder, prostatic hyperplasia, calculi, cancer, blood clot
Urethra
   Stricture, congenital valve, phimosis

---

states associated with renal vasoconstriction and hypoperfusion. ACE inhibitors should be used with special caution in patients with bilateral renal artery stenosis or unilateral stenosis in a solitary functioning kidney. Under these circumstances, glomerular perfusion and filtration may be exquisitely dependent on the actions of angiotensin II. Angiotensin II preserves glomerular filtration pressure distal to stenoses by increasing systemic arterial pressure and by triggering selective constriction of efferent arterioles. ACE inhibitors blunt these responses and precipitate ARF, usually reversible, in approximately 30 percent of such patients. Indeed, while patients with renal artery stenosis are particularly prone to develop ARF following therapy with ACE inhibitors, severe systemic hypotension from any cause can compromise glomerular filtration in this setting.

Other pharmacologic agents that can induce *primary intrarenal vasoconstriction* and ARF, particularly in the setting of mild hypovolemia, include radiocontrast agents, cyclosporine, amphotericin B, epinephrine, norepinephrine, and high doses of dopamine. Hypercalcemia may compromise glomerular filtration in a similar manner. *Sepsis* due to gram-negative endotoxin-producing organisms can cause systemic vasodilatation in the presence of intense intrarenal vasoconstriction.

ARF may complicate hepatic failure (hepatorenal syndrome) due to cirrhosis or other *liver diseases*, including malignancy, hepatic resection, and biliary obstruction. Intrarenal vasoconstriction and avid sodium retention are early responses under these circumstances and may precede alterations in systemic hemodyamics. In addition, patients with liver disease complicated by portal hypertension and ascites usually have increased plasma volume but "effective" hypovolemia due to systemic vasodilatation and pooling of blood in the portal circulation. Azotemia may develop slowly as hepatic failure progresses or may be precipitated in compensated patients by hemodynamic insults such as hemorrhage, paracentesis, or administration of diuretics, vasodilators, or cyclooxygenase inhibitors. ARF may progress relentlessly in hepatic failure even in the presence of satisfactory plasma volume and blood pressure, possibly as a result of ongoing intrarenal vasoconstriction, hypoperfusion, and ischemia. It must be remembered, however, that patients with liver disease also can develop other forms of ARF (e.g., sepsis, nephrotoxic medications) and that a diagnosis of hepatorenal syndrome should be made only after exclusion of other causes.

Intrinsic renal azotemia (intrinsic renal ARF) This can complicate many disorders that affect the renal parenchyma (see Table 236-1). Most cases are caused either by ischemia secondary to renal hypoperfusion (ischemic ARF) or toxins (nephrotoxic ARF). Since ischemic and nephrotoxic ARF are frequently associated with necrosis of tubule epithelial cells, this syndrome is often referred to as *acute tubular necrosis* (ATN). Unfortunately, the terms *intrinsic renal ARF* and *ATN* are often used interchangeably, but this is inappropriate because some parenchymal diseases (e.g., vasculitis, glomerulonephritis, interstitial nephritis) can cause ARF without tubule cell necrosis. Furthermore, the pathologic term *ATN* is frequently inaccurate even in ischemic or nephrotoxic ARF because tubule cell necrosis may not be present in >20 to 30 percent of cases.

ISCHEMIC ARF   As noted above, prerenal azotemia and ischemic ARF can represent a spectrum of the same disease. They differ in that ischemic ARF, in contrast to prerenal azotemia, does not resolve rapidly upon restoration of normal renal perfusion. Renal hypoperfusion from any cause (see Table 236-1) may lead to ischemic ARF if severe enough to overwhelm renal autoregulatory and neurohumoral defense mechanisms (see above). Ischemic ARF occurs most frequently after cardiovascular surgery, trauma, hemorrhage, sepsis, or dehydration. This syndrome also may complicate mild forms of true or "effective" hypovolemia, particularly in patients receiving cyclooxygenase or ACE inhibitors or with renovascular disease.

Postulated mechanisms by which renal hypoperfusion and ischemia impair glomerular filtration include (1) reduction in glomerular perfusion and filtration (previously called *vasomotor nephropathy*), (2) obstruction of urine flow in tubules by cells and debris (including casts) derived from ischemic tubule epithelium, and (3) backleak of glomerular filtrate through ischemic tubule epithelium (Fig. 236-1). In addition, neutrophil activation within the renal vasculature and neutrophil-mediated cell injury may contribute.

Glomerular filtration is flow-dependent, and intrarenal vasoconstriction impairs GFR and compromises renal oxygenation. Ischemia of renal endothelial cells may cause a sustained fall in renal blood flow, glomerular ultrafiltration pressure, and surface area by blocking production of endothelial cell–derived vasodilators (e.g., nitric oxide, prostacyclin) and/or release of endothelial cell–derived vasoconstric-

FIGURE 236-1 Proposed pathophysiology of ischemic acute renal failure.

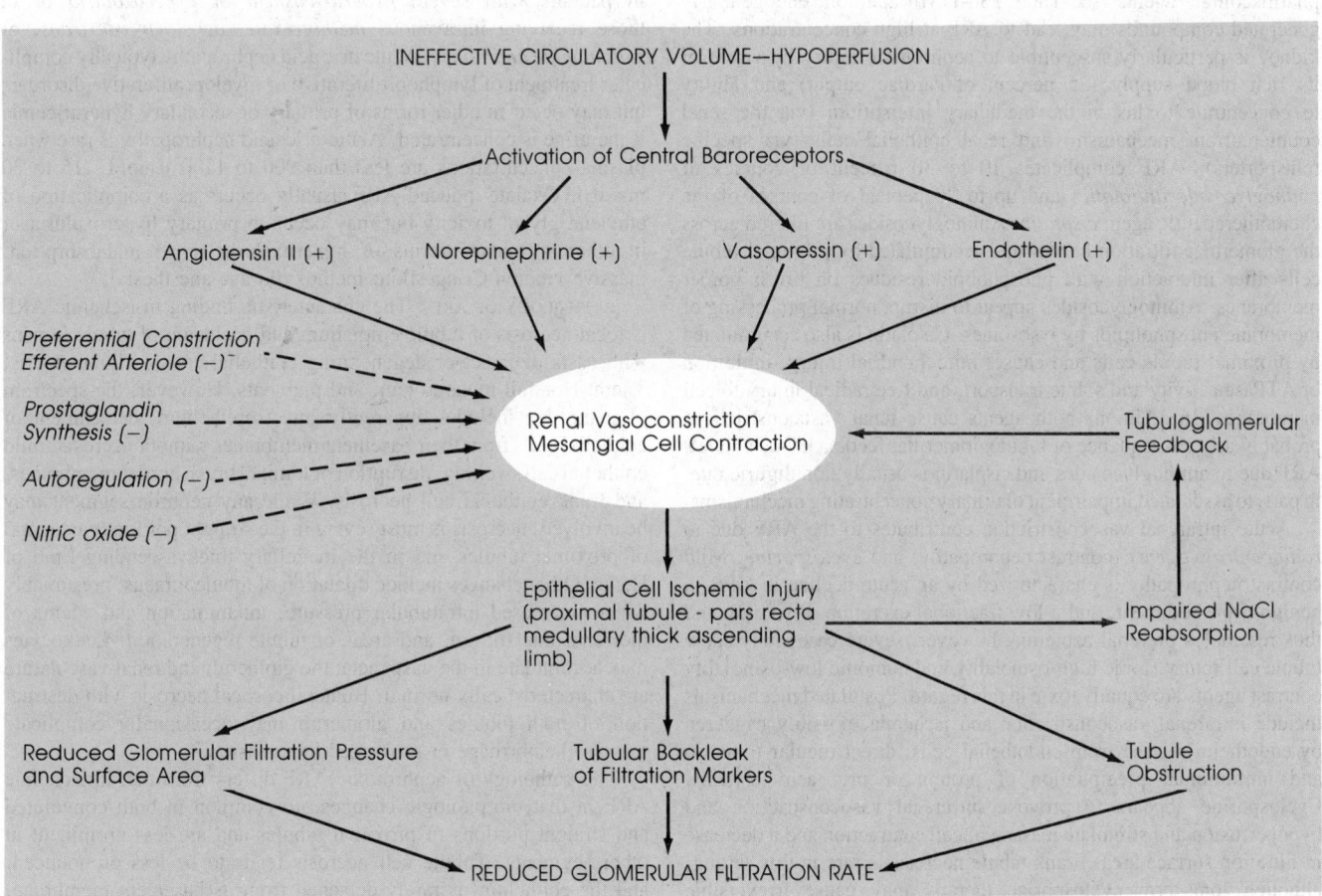

tors (e.g., endothelin). Renal hypoperfusion leads to ischemia of renal tubule cells, particularly the terminal straight portion of proximal tubules (pars recta) and the thick ascending limb of the loop of Henle. These segments traverse the corticomedullary junction and outer medulla, regions of the kidney that are relatively hypoxic compared with the renal cortex, even in health, because of the unique countercurrent arrangement of the vasculature. Furthermore, proximal tubules and thick ascending limb cells have greater oxygen requirements than other renal cells because of high rates of active (ATP-dependent) sodium transport. Proximal tubule cells may be prone to ischemic injury because they rely exclusively on mitochondrial oxidative phosphorylation (oxygen-dependent) for ATP synthesis and cannot generate ATP from anerobic glycolysis. Cellular ischemia causes alterations in energetics, ion transport, and membrane integrity that ultimately lead to cell necrosis. These include depletion of ATP, inhibition of active transport of sodium and other solutes, impairment of cell volume regulation and cell swelling, cytoskeletal disruption, accumulation of intracellular calcium, altered phospholipid metabolism, free radical formation, and peroxidation of membrane lipids. While epithelial cell function is impaired during ischemia, free radical–mediated injury may be most severe during reperfusion and reoxygenation. Necrotic tubule epithelium may permit backleak of filtered solutes, including creatinine, urea, and other nitrogenous waste products, thus rendering glomerular filtration ineffective. In addition, necrotic tubule cells may slough into tubule lumens, obstruct urine flow, increase intratubular pressure, and impair further formation of glomerular filtrate.

Epithelial cell injury per se causes secondary intrarenal vasoconstriction by a process termed *tubuloglomerular feedback*. Specialized epithelial cells in the macula densa region of distal tubules detect increases in distal salt (probably chloride) delivery due to impaired reabsorption by proximal nephron segments and in turn stimulate constriction of adjacent afferent arterioles and further compromise glomerular perfusion and filtration.

NEPHROTOXIC ARF   This may complicate administration of diverse pharmacologic agents (see Table 236-1). In addition, endogenously generated compounds may lead to ARF at high concentrations. The kidney is particularly susceptible to nephrotoxic injury by virtue of its rich blood supply (25 percent of cardiac output) and ability to concentrate toxins in the medullary interstitium (via the renal countercurrent mechanism) and renal epithelial cells (via specific transporters). ARF complicates 10 to 30 percent of courses of *aminoglycoside antibiotics* and up to 70 percent of courses of the chemotherapeutic agent *cisplatin*. Aminoglycosides are filtered across the glomerular filtration barrier and accumulated by proximal tubule cells after interaction with phospholipid residues on brush border membranes. Aminoglycosides appear to disrupt normal processing of membrane phospholipids by lysosomes. Cisplatin is also accumulated by proximal tubule cells and causes mitochondrial injury, inhibition of ATPase activity and solute transport, and free radical injury to cell membranes. In addition, both agents cause renal vasoconstriction, probably as a consequence of tubuloglomerular feedback (see above). ARF due to aminoglycosides and cisplatin is usually nonoliguric due, in part, to associated impairment of urinary concentrating mechanisms.

Acute intrarenal vasoconstriction contributes to the ARF due to *radiocontrast agents* (contrast nephropathy) and *cyclosporine*. Mild contrast nephropathy is characterized by an acute decline in GFR, a benign urine sediment, and a low fractional excretion of sodium and thus resembles prerenal azotemia; however, severe cases may show tubule cell injury. Ionic high-osmolality and nonionic low-osmolality contrast agents are equally toxic in this regard. Postulated mechanisms include intrarenal vasoconstriction and ischemia, possibly triggered by endothelin release from endothelial cells, direct tubular toxicity, and intraluminal precipitation of protein or uric acid crystals. Cyclosporine appears to provoke intrarenal vasoconstriction and hypoperfusion and stimulate mesangial cell contraction and a decrease in filtration surface area. Frank tubule necrosis is rare in this setting, although long-term cyclosporine therapy may cause irreversible

renal impairment as a consequence of chronic medullary ischemia. *Amphotericin* causes dose-related ARF by inducing intense renal vasoconstriction and via direct toxicity to proximal and distal tubule cells. Chronic renal failure, hypovolemia, concomitant exposure to other toxins, and old age predispose patients to most forms of nephrotoxic injury. In addition, diabetes mellitus and multiple myeloma are risk factors for acute contrast agent nephropathy.

Rhabdomyolysis and *hemolysis* can cause ARF, particularly in hypovolemic or acidotic individuals. Rhabdomyolysis and myoglobinuric ARF may occur with traumatic crush injury, muscle ischemia (e.g., arterial insufficiency, muscle compression, cocaine overdose), seizures, excessive exercise, heat stroke or malignant hyperthermia, alcoholism, and infectious (e.g., influenza, legionella) or metabolic disorders (e.g., hypokalemia, hypophosphatemia, or myophosphorylase or phosphofructokinase deficiency). ARF due to hemolysis is seen most commonly following blood transfusion reactions. The mechanisms by which rhabdomyolysis and hemolysis impair GFR are unclear, since neither hemoglobin nor myoglobin is nephrotoxic when injected into laboratory animals. Myoglobin and hemoglobin or other compounds released from muscle or red blood cells may cause ARF via direct toxic effects on tubule epithelial cells or by inducing intratubular cast formation. Hypovolemia or acidosis may contribute to ARF in this setting by promoting intranephronal cast formation. In addition, hemoglobin and myoglobin inhibit nitric oxide and may trigger intrarenal vasoconstriction and ischemia in patients with borderline renal hypoperfusion.

Intratubular obstruction may play an important role in ARF in several diseases. Casts containing filtered immunoglobulin light chains and other urine proteins, including Tamm-Horsfall protein produced by thick ascending limb cells, may cause ARF in patients with plasma cell dyscrasias (myeloma-cast nephropathy). High urine salt concentrations and low urine pH appear to promote this process. However, the correlation between cast formation and renal insufficiency is poor in myeloma, suggesting that light chains may be toxic to tubule epithelial cells. Intratubular obstruction also may cause ARF in patients with severe *hyperuricosuria* or *hyperoxaluria* or in those receiving intravenous *methotrexate*, *acyclovir*, *dextrans*, or *sulfonamide antibiotics*. Acute uric acid nephropathy typically complicates treatment of lymphoproliferative or myeloproliferative disorders but may occur in other forms of primary or secondary hyperuricemia if the urine is concentrated. Acute uric acid nephropathy is rare when plasma concentrations are less than 900 to 1200 μmol/L (15 to 20 mg/dL). Oxalate-induced ARF usually occurs as a complication of ethylene glycol toxicity but may occur in primary hyperoxaluria or in other secondary forms of hyperoxaluria (e.g., malabsorption, massive vitamin C ingestion, methoxyflurane anesthesia).

PATHOLOGY OF ARF   The characteristic finding in ischemic ARF is focal necrosis of tubule epithelium and occlusion of tubule lumens with casts of intact or degenerating epithelial cells, cellular debris, Tamm-Horsfall mucoprotein, and pigments. However, the spectrum of pathology includes apparently intact epithelium, detachment of epithelial cells from their basement membranes without necrosis, mild epithelial cell swelling, disruption of luminal brush border membranes, and frank epithelial cell necrosis. While any nephron segment may be involved, necrosis is most severe in the straight portion (pars recta) of proximal tubules and in the medullary thick ascending limb of Henle. Other changes include dilatation of tubule lumens, presumably due to increased intratubular pressure, inflammation and edema of the renal interstitium, and areas of tubule regeneration. Leukocytes may accumulate in the vasa recta; the glomeruli and renal vasculature are characteristically normal. Bilateral cortical necrosis with destruction of both tubules and glomeruli may occasionally complicate massive hemorrhage or prolonged hypotension.

The pathology of nephrotoxic ARF differs from that in ischemic ARF in that morphologic changes are common in both convoluted and straight portions of proximal tubules and are less prominent in other segments. Tubule cell necrosis tends to be less pronounced, and the epithelium is rarely detached from its basement membrane.

Indeed, renal biopsy specimens may be normal in nephrotoxic ARF even in the presence of epithelial cell dysfunction. Proximal tubule myeloid bodies, characteristic, albeit nonspecific, findings in aminoglycoside-induced ARF, are electron-dense lamellar structures that reflect accumulation of cell membrane phospholipids in lysosomes and likely result from abnormal intracellular phospholipid processing. Their role in the pathogenesis of aminoglycoside nephrotoxicity is uncertain.

COURSE OF ISCHEMIC AND NEPHROTOXIC ARF Most cases of ischemic or nephrotoxic ARF are characterized by three distinct phases. The *initiation phase* is the period from initial exposure to the causative insult to development of established ARF. Restoration of renal perfusion or elimination of nephrotoxins during this phase may reverse or limit the renal injury. The early initiation phase is usually identified retrospectively, since serum creatinine does not rise until GFR is reduced by 40 percent or more. In milder renal injury, the decline in GFR is counterbalanced by an increase in creatinine secretion into the tubule lumen. During the *maintenance phase* (average 7 to 14 days), the GFR is depressed, and metabolic consequences of ARF may develop. A *recovery phase* in most patients is characterized by tubule cell regeneration and a gradual return of GFR to or toward normal. The recovery phase may be complicated by diuresis (*diuretic phase*) due to excretion of retained salt and water and other solutes, continued use of diuretics, and/or delayed recovery of epithelial cell function (solute and water reabsorption) relative to glomerular filtration.

INTRINSIC RENAL AZOTEMIA FROM OTHER CAUSES Other diseases of the renal vasculature, glomeruli, and interstitium may lead to ARF (see Table 236-1). Acute obstruction of renal arteries or veins (e.g., thrombosis) may cause an abrupt decline in GFR if bilateral or if unilateral in patients with a solitary functioning kidney. Patients with advanced atherosclerosis may develop ARF spontaneously, following trauma, or after manipulation of the aorta or renal arteries due to embolization of cholesterol crystals to the renal vasculature. Cholesterol crystals lodge in small and medium-sized arteries and incite a giant cell and fibrotic reaction in the vessel wall with narrowing or obstruction of the lumen. Atheroembolic ARF is usually irreversible. Other diseases of the renal microvasculature that may cause intrinsic renal azotemia include acute glomerulonephritis and vasculitis, hemolytic-uremic syndrome (HUS), thrombotic thrombocytopenic purpura (TTP), disseminated intravascular coagulation (DIC), malignant hypertension, toxemia of pregnancy, scleroderma, and radiation injury. These disorders are characterized by either immune or physical injury to vessel walls, thrombotic microangiopathy, or both. Occlusion of renal arteries, arterioles, or glomerular capillaries leads to glomerular hypoperfusion and a fall in GFR. Pharmacologic agents may cause ARF by triggering allergic interstitial nephritis, characterized by infiltration of the interstitial space by macrophages, lymphocytes, plasma cells, polymorphonuclear leukocytes, and other inflammatory cells and interstitial edema. Common causes of allergic interstitial nephritis include antibiotics (e.g., penicillins, cephalosporins, trimethoprim, sulfonamides, rifampicin), nonsteroidal anti-inflammatory drugs, captopril, and diuretics (see Table 236-1). Occasionally, ARF may complicate interstitial nephritis due to infections, neoplasia, or infiltrative processes.

Pregnancy is associated with an increased risk of ARF, although the incidence has decreased with improvements in obstetric care. Azotemia is usually triggered by ischemic (e.g., abruptio placentae, postpartum hemorrhage) or nephrotoxic (illegal abortifacients) renal injury or toxemia of pregnancy. In addition, the postpartum period may be complicated by ARF and thrombotic microangiopathy.

Postrenal azotemia Urinary tract obstruction accounts for approximately 5 percent of ARF. Since one kidney has sufficient clearance capacity to excrete nitrogenous waste products, ARF from obstruction either requires obstruction between the external urethral meatus and bladder neck, bilateral ureter obstruction, or unilateral ureter obstruction in a patient with one functioning kidney. Bladder neck obstruction is the most common cause and may be due to

prostatic disease (e.g., hyperplasia, neoplasia, or infection), neurogenic bladder, or anticholinergic drugs. Less common causes include blood clots, calculi, and urethritis with spasm. Ureteric obstruction may result from intraluminal obstruction (e.g., calculi, blood clots, sloughed renal papillae), infiltration of the ureteric wall (e.g., neoplasia), or external compression (e.g., retroperitoneal fibrosis, neoplasia or abscess, inadvertent surgical ligature). During the early stages of obstruction (hours to days), continued glomerular filtration leads to increased intraluminal pressure upstream to the obstruction, eventuating in gradual distension of proximal ureter, renal pelvis, and calyces and a fall in GFR. While acute obstruction may cause an initial increase in renal blood flow, arteriolar vasoconstriction supervenes and leads to a further decline in glomerular filtration.

CLINICAL FEATURES AND DIFFERENTIAL DIAGNOSIS Patients with azotemia should be assessed to determine if renal failure is acute or chronic. An acute process is established if review of laboratory records reveals a recent rise in BUN and serum creatinine, but previous measurements are usually not available. Findings that suggest chronic renal failure include anemia, neuropathy, and radiologic evidence of renal osteodystrophy or small scarred kidneys (see Chap. 237). However, anemia also may complicate ARF (see below), and renal size may be normal or increased in chronic renal disease (e.g., diabetic nephropathy, amyloid, polycystic kidney disease). Once a diagnosis of ARF is established, appropriate management relies on elucidation of the cause of ARF and requires careful clinical assessment, including review of presenting symptoms, drug history and hospital course, physical examination and urinalysis, appropriate laboratory tests and renal imaging techniques, and occasional renal biopsy.

Clinical assessment *Prerenal azotemia* should be suspected in patients suffering an elevation in serum creatinine following hemorrhage, excessive gastrointestinal or urinary fluid loss, or extensive burns, particularly if access to fluids is restricted (e.g., as in comatose or obtunded patients or those on mechanical ventilation). Supportive evidence includes thirst, orthostatic hypotension and tachycardia, reduced jugular venous pressure, decreased skin turgor, dry mucous membranes, and reduced axillary sweating. Nursing and pharmacy records should be reviewed for evidence of a decline in urine output and body weight and recent use of cyclooxygenase or ACE inhibitors. Clinical examination may reveal stigmata of chronic liver disease and portal hypertension (e.g., palmar erythema, jaundice, telangiectasia, caput medusae, splenomegaly, ascites), cardiac failure (e.g., peripheral edema, hepatic congestion, elevated jugular venous pressure, bibasilar lung crackles, gallop rhythm, cold extremities), or other causes of "effective" hypovolemia (see Table 236-1). Invasive hemodynamic monitoring (central venous and/or Swan-Ganz catheterization) may be necessary in complicated cases. Definitive diagnosis of prerenal azotemia can only be made when restoration of renal perfusion results in prompt resolution of ARF.

Intrinsic renal azotemia due to ischemia is likely in patients with ARF following prolonged or severe renal hypoperfusion complicating hypovolemic or septic shock or major surgery. However, a significant fall in arterial blood pressure occurs in the latter setting in less than half of patients with clinical and biochemical features of ischemic ARF. The likelihood of ischemic ARF is increased further if ARF persists despite restoration of renal perfusion. Diagnosis of nephrotoxic ARF requires review of the history and of pharmacy, nursing, and radiology records for nephrotoxic medications or radiocontrast agents. ARF after cancer chemotherapy suggests a diagnosis of tumor lysis syndrome and acute urate nephropathy, although other considerations include prerenal azotemia due to emesis or diarrhea and direct nephrotoxicity of chemotherapeutic or antimicrobial agents. Rhabdomyolysis is suggested by a recent history of seizures, excessive exercise, alcohol or drug abuse, or muscle tenderness or limb ischemia on physical examination.

While ischemic and nephrotoxic ARF account for most intrinsic renal azotemia, patients should be assessed for other renal parenchymal diseases. Flank pain may be prominant following acute renal artery or vein occlusion and in acute pyelonephritis and acute necrotizing glomerulonephritis. Subcutaneous nodules, livedo reticularis, bright orange retinal arteriolar plaques, and digital ischemia despite palpable pedal pulses suggest atheroembolization. ARF in association with oliguria, edema, hypertension, and an "active" urine sediment (nephritic syndrome) suggests acute glomerulonephritis or vasculitis and should prompt a search for secondary causes (e.g., systemic lupus erythematosus, bacterial endocarditis, cryoglobulinemia). However, this constellation of findings may occur in patients with other diseases of the renal microvasculature (e.g., HUS, TTP, hypertensive nephrosclerosis, toxemia of pregnancy). HUS and TTP are considerations in patients with a history of infective diarrhea or upper respiratory tract infection and physical evidence of easy bruising, anemia, or neurologic deficit. Malignant hypertension is a likely cause in patients with moderate or severe hypertension and evidence of hypertensive injury to other organs (e.g., left ventricular hypertrophy and failure, hypertensive retinopathy and papilledema, neurologic dysfunction). Fever, arthralgias, and a pruritic erythematous rash suggest allergic interstitial nephritis, although systemic features of hypersensitivity are frequently absent.

Postrenal azotemia may be asymptomatic if obstruction develops slowly. Alternatively, suprapubic or flank pain may be present if there is acute distension of the bladder, renal collecting system, and capsule, respectively. Colicky flank pain radiating to the groin suggests acute ureteric obstruction. Prostatic disease should be suspected in men with a history of nocturia, frequency, and hesitancy and an enlarged or indurated prostate on rectal examination. Neurogenic bladder is likely in patients receiving anticholinergic medications (e.g., tricyclic antidepressants) or with physical evidence of neurologic disease and autonomic insufficiency (e.g., paralysis, abnormal rectal sphincter tone). Bladder distension may be evident on abdominal percussion and palpation. Definitive diagnosis of postrenal azotemia usually relies on judicious use of radiologic investigations and rapid improvement in renal function following relief of obstruction.

Urinalysis Assessment of urine volume is relatively unhelpful in evaluating ARF. Complete anuria suggests complete urinary tract obstruction but may complicate prerenal or intrinsic renal azotemia (e.g., renal artery occlusion, proliferative glomerulonephritis, bilateral cortical necrosis). Wide fluctuations in urine output suggest intermittent obstruction, and patients with partial urinary tract obstruction may have polyuria due to secondary impairment of urine concentrating mechanisms.

In contrast, examination of the sediment and supernatant of a centrifuged urine specimen is valuable in distinguishing among prerenal, intrinsic renal, and postrenal azotemia and in elucidating the etiology of intrinsic renal azotemia. Urine sediment should be inspected for casts, hematuria, pyuria, and crystals. In prerenal azotemia, the sediment is characteristically acellular and may contain transparent hyaline casts ("bland," "benign," "inactive" urine sediment). Hyaline casts are formed in concentrated urine from normal constituents of urine, principally Tamm-Horsfall protein that is normally secreted by epithelial cells of the loop of Henle. Postrenal azotemia also may have an inactive sediment, although hematuria and pyuria are common with intraluminal obstruction and prostatic disease. Pigmented "muddy brown" granular casts and casts containing tubule epithelial cells are characteristic of tubule necrosis and suggest ischemic or nephrotoxic ARF. They are usually found in association with microscopic hematuria and mild "tubular" proteinuria (<1 g/d); the latter reflects impaired reabsorption and processing of filtered proteins by injured proximal tubule cells. Casts may be absent in 20 to 30 percent of patients with ischemic or nephrotoxic ARF and are not requisite for diagnosis. Indeed, there is a poor correlation between the functional renal impairment and the urinalysis in these conditions. Red blood cell casts indicate acute glomerular injury. Dysmorphic red blood cells are more common in the urine of patients with glomerular injury but are less specific than red cell casts. Urine sediment abnormalities are variable in diseases involving preglomerular blood vessels (e.g., HUS, TTP, atheroembolic disease, vasculitis

involving medium-sized or large vessels) and range from benign to frankly nephritic. White cell casts and nonpigmented granular casts suggest interstitial nephritis, and the broad granular casts of chronic renal disease are probably due to interstitial fibrosis and dilatation of tubules. Eosinophiluria (between 1 and 50 percent of urine leukocytes) is common (~90 percent) in drug-induced allergic interstitial nephritis when studied using Hansel's stain. Wright's stain is less sensitive (~20 percent) in this regard. Eosinophiluria is, however, only 85 percent specific for allergic interstitial nephritis, and similar eosinophiluria can occur in atheroembolization, ischemic and nephrotoxic ARF, proliferative glomerulonephritis, pyelonephritis, cystitis, and prostatitis. Uric acid crystals (pleomorphic in shape) may be seen in urine in prerenal azotemia but suggest acute urate nephropathy if present in abundance. Oxalate (envelope-shaped) and hippurate (needle-shaped) crystals suggest ethylene glycol toxicity.

Increased urine protein excretion, characteristically <1 g/d, is common in ischemic or nephrotoxic ARF and reflects both failure of reabsorption of filtered protein and excretion of cellular debris ("tubular" proteinuria). Proteinuria of >1 g/d suggests injury to the glomerular ultrafiltration barrier ("glomerular" proteinuria) or excretion of myeloma light chains. The latter are not detected by conventional dipsticks (which detect albumin) and must be sought by other means (e.g., sulfosalicylic acid test, immunoelectrophoresis). Marked proteinuria is also frequent (~80 percent) with allergic interstitial nephritis triggered by cyclooxygenase inhibitors. These patients have interstitial inflammation and a glomerular lesion almost identical to minimal change glomerulonephritis. A similar syndrome has occurred with other agents, including ampicillin, rifampicin, and interferon-α. Hemoglobinuria or myoglobinuria should be suspected if urine is strongly positive for hemoglobin by dipstick but contains few red cells and if the supernatant of centrifuged urine is also positive for free hemoglobin. Hemolysis and rhabdomyolysis can usually be differentiated by inspection of plasma. The latter is pink in hemolysis but usually not in rhabdomyolysis, since free hemoglobin is a larger molecule than myoglobin, is protein-bound, and is filtered slowly by the kidney. Bilirubinuria may provide a clue to the presence of hepatorenal syndrome.

Renal failure indices Analysis of urine and blood biochemistry are useful in distinguishing prerenal from intrinsic renal azotemia (Table 236-2). Estimation of the fractional excretion of sodium (FeNa) relates sodium clearance to creatinine clearance. Sodium is reabsorbed avidly from glomerular filtrate in prerenal azotemia in an attempt to restore intravascular volume but not in ARF because of tubular

TABLE 236-2 Urine diagnostic indices in separation of prerenal from intrinsic renal azotemia

Diagnostic index	Prerenal azotemia	Intrinsic renal azotemia
Fractional excretion of sodium (%)* $$\frac{U_{Na} P_{Cr}}{P_{Na} U_{Cr}} \times 100$$	<1	>1
Urine sodium concentration (mmol/L)	<10	>20
Urine creatinine to plasma creatinine ratio	>40	<20
Urine urea nitrogen to plasma urea nitrogen ratio	>8	<3
Urine specific gravity	>1.018	<1.012
Urine osmolality (mmol/kg H$_2$O)	>500	<250
Plasma BUN/creatinine ratio (mg/dL)	>20	<10–15
Renal failure index* $$\frac{U_{Na}}{U_{Cr}/P_{Cr}}$$	<1	>1
Urinary sediment	Hyaline casts	Muddy brown granular casts

* Most sensitive indices

epithelial cell injury. In contrast, creatinine is reabsorbed less efficiently than sodium in both conditions. Consequently, patients with prerenal azotemia typically have an FeNa concentration of <1.0 percent (frequently <0.01 percent), while in patients with ischemic or nephrotoxic ARF the FeNa is usually >1.0 percent. The renal failure index (RFI) (see Table 236-2) provides similar information, since variations in serum sodium concentration are relatively small. Urine sodium concentration is a less sensitive index for distinguishing prerenal azotemia from ischemic and nephrotoxic ARF. Similarly, indices of urinary concentrating ability such as urine specific gravity, urine osmolality, urine to plasma creatinine or urea ratios, and serum urea nitrogen to creatinine ratio are of limited value, particularly in elderly subjects, in whom urine concentrating mechanisms are frequently impaired, while sodium reabsorption is preserved.

FeNa may occasionally be >1.0 percent in prerenal azotemia in patients receiving diuretics or with bicarbonaturia (accompanied by sodium to maintain electroneutrality), underlying chronic renal failure complicated by salt wasting, or adrenal insufficiency. In contrast, approximately 15 percent of patients with nonoliguric ischemic or nephrotoxic ARF have an FeNa concentration of <1.0 percent, which likely reflects a milder form of renal injury (intermediate syndrome). This syndrome has been described in patients with ARF from a variety of causes, including ischemia, aminoglycosides, radiocontrast agents, rhabdomyolysis, hemolysis, burns, sepsis, and hepatorenal syndrome. Under these circumstances, epithelial cell damage is probably localized to the corticomedullary junction and outer medulla with relative preservation of function in other sodium-transporting segments. The FeNa concentration is usually <1.0 percent in ARF due to urinary tract obstruction, glomerulonephritis, and diseases of the renal vasculature; other parameters must therefore be used to distinguish these conditions from prerenal azotemia.

Laboratory investigations Analysis of serial measurements of serum creatinine may be useful in differential diagnosis. Prerenal azotemia is frequently characterized by rapid fluctuations in creatinine that parallel changes in hemodynamic function. Serum creatinine rises rapidly (apparent within 24 to 48 h) in ARF following renal ischemia, atheroembolization, and radiocontrast exposure, three possibilities in patients undergoing emergency cardiac or aortic angiography and surgery. Peak creatinine levels in contrast nephropathy are usually observed after 3 to 5 days and return to normal within 5 to 7 days. In contrast, creatinine levels typically peak later (7 to 10 days) in ischemic ARF and atheroembolic disease. ARF usually resolves over the next 7 to 14 days in ischemic ARF but may be irreversible in atheroembolic disease. With many tubule epithelial cell toxins (e.g., aminoglycosides, cisplatin) the initial elevation of serum creatinine levels is characteristically delayed until the second week of therapy and probably reflects the need for accumulation of these agents within cells before overt injury is apparent biochemically.

Hyperkalemia, hyperphosphatemia, hypocalcemia, and elevations in serum uric acid and creatine kinase (MM isoenzyme) levels suggest rhabdomyolysis. Hyperuricemia of >900 μmol/L (>15 mg/dL) in association with hyperkalemia, hyperphosphatemia, and increased circulating levels of lactate dehydrogenase (LDH) may indicate acute urate nephropathy. Severe hypercalcemia from any cause can induce ARF. Elevated serum anion and osmolal gaps (measured serum osmolality minus calculated osmolality) suggest ethylene glycol toxicity, and severe anemia in the absence of hemorrhage suggests hemolysis, multiple myeloma, or thrombotic microangiopathy (e.g., HUS, TTP, toxemia, DIC, accelerated hypertension, SLE, scleroderma, radiation injury). Other laboratory findings of thrombotic microangiopathy include thrombocytopenia, dysmorphic red blood cells on peripheral blood smear, and elevated circulating levels of LDH. Systemic eosinophilia suggests allergic interstitial nephritis, atheroembolic disease, or polyarteritis nodosa. Depressed complement levels and high titers of anti-glomerular basement membrane antibodies, antineutrophil cytoplasmic antibodies, antinuclear antibodies, circulating immune complexes, or cryoglobulins are helpful with suspected glomerulonephritis or vasculitis.

Radiology Imaging of the urinary tract by ultrasonography, computed tomography (CT), or magnetic resonance (MR) imaging is recommended in most patients with ARF to exclude obstructive uropathy. While pelvicalyceal dilatation is usual with urinary tract obstruction (98 percent sensitivity), dilatation may not be observed during the initial period of obstruction or with obstruction due to ureteric encasement (e.g., retroperitoneal fibrosis, neoplasia). Retrograde or anterograde pyelography should be used for definitive diagnosis when these possibilities are considered likely and may be employed for precise localization of obstruction in other cases. Ultrasonography, CT, and MR imaging also provide a measure of renal size and cortical thickness that is useful in distinguishing ARF from chronic renal disease. A plain film of the abdomen is useful with suspected nephrolithiasis. Doppler ultrasonography and MR flow imaging appear promising for assessment of patency of renal arteries and veins in suspected vascular obstruction, but contrast angiography is required for definitive diagnosis.

Renal biopsy This is usually performed when prerenal and postrenal failure have been excluded and the cause of intrinsic renal azotemia is unclear. Biopsy is particularly useful when clinical assessment, urinalysis, and laboratory investigation suggest diagnoses other than ischemic or nephrotoxic injury that may respond to specific therapy. Examples include anti-glomerular basement membrane disease and other forms of necrotizing glomerulonephritis, vasculitis, HUS and TTP, and allergic interstitial nephritis.

COMPLICATIONS ARF impairs renal excretion of sodium, potassium, and water; divalent cation homeostasis; and urinary acidification mechanisms. As a result, ARF is frequently complicated by intravascular volume overload, hyponatremia, hyperkalemia, hyperphosphatemia, hypocalcemia, hypermagnesemia, and metabolic acidosis. In addition, patients are unable to excrete nitrogenous waste products and may develop the uremic syndrome (see Chap. 237). In general, the severity of complications mirrors the degree of renal impairment and the catabolic state.

Intravascular volume overload is a consequence of diminished salt and water excretion, especially in oliguric or anuric individuals. While milder forms are characterized by rales, increased venous pressure, peripheral edema, and increased body weight, severe volume expansion may precipitate life-threatening pulmonary edema. Volume overload is a particular problem in patients receiving multiple intravenous medications, sodium bicarbonate for correction of acidosis, or enteral or parenteral nutrition. *Hypertension* is uncommon (~15 percent) and usually mild in ischemic or nephrotoxic ARF. Moderate or severe hypertension suggests hypertensive nephrosclerosis, glomerulonephritis, renal artery stenosis, or other diseases of the renal vasculature. Excessive fluid ingestion or inappropriate administration of water can cause *hyponatremia*, which, if severe, can lead to cerebral edema.

Hyperkalemia is common. Serum potassium typically rises by 0.5 mmol/L per day in oliguric and anuric patients due to impaired excretion. Metabolic acidosis may exacerbate hyperkalemia by promoting potassium efflux from cells. Hyperkalemia may be particularly severe in patients with rhabdomyolysis, hemolysis, and tumor lysis syndrome. Mild hyperkalemia (<6.0 mmol/L) is usually asymptomatic. Higher levels are associated with ECG abnormalities, including peaked T waves, prolongation of PR intervals, P-wave flattening, widening of the QRS complex, and left axis deviation. These ECG changes may herald the onset of life-threatening cardiac arrhythmias, including bradycardia, heart block, ventricular tachycardia or fibrillation, and asystole. In addition, hyperkalemia may cause neuromuscular dysfunction, including paresthesias, hyporeflexia, weakness, ascending flaccid paralysis, and respiratory failure. *Hypokalemia* is rare in ARF by may complicate nonoliguric aminoglycoside, cisplatin, or amphotericin B nephrotoxicity, presumably reflecting profound epithelial cell injury.

Metabolism of dietary protein yields between 50 and 100 mmol/d of fixed nonvolatile acids that are normally excreted by the kidneys. Consequently, ARF is often complicated by *metabolic acidosis* and an increased serum anion gap. Acidosis may be particularly severe when endogenous acid production is increased by other mechanisms (e.g., diabetic or fasting ketoacidosis; lactic acidosis complicating generalized tissue hypoperfusion, liver disease, or sepsis; metabolism of ethylene glycol). *Metabolic alkalosis* is infrequent in ARF but may occur following overzealous correction of acidosis with bicarbonate or loss of gastric acid by vomiting or therapeutic aspiration. Mild asymptomatic *hyperuricemia* 700 to 900 mmol/L (12 to 15 mg/dL) is common since uric acid is cleared from blood by glomerular filtration and secretion by proximal tubule cells. Higher levels suggest increased uric acid production, such as after treatment of myeloproliferative or lymphoproliferative disorders (see above).

Mild *hyperphosphatemia* is almost invariable in ARF. Severe hyperphosphatemia occurs in highly catabolic patients or following rhabdomyolysis, hemolysis, or tumor lysis. Metastatic deposition of calcium phosphate can lead to *hypocalcemia*, particularly when the product of serum calcium (mg/dL) and phosphate (mg/dL) concentrations exceeds 70. Other factors that contribute to hypocalcemia include tissue resistance to the actions of PTH and reduced levels of 1,25-dihydroxyvitamin D. Hypocalcemia is usually asymptomatic, possibly due to the counterbalancing effects of acidosis on neuromuscular excitability. However, hypocalcemia can be symptomatic with rhabdomyolysis or acute pancreatitis or following treatment of acidosis with bicarbonate. Manifestations of hypocalcemia include perioral paresthesias, muscle cramps, seizures, hallucinations and confusion, and prolongation of the QT interval and nonspecific T-wave changes on ECG (also see Chap. 357). Chvostek's sign (contraction of facial muscles upon tapping of jaw over facial nerve) and Trousseau's sign (carpopedal spasm following occlusion of arterial blood supply to the arm for 3 min by a blood pressure cuff) are indices of latent tetany in high-risk patients. Mild asymptomatic *hypermagnesemia* is usual in oliguric ARF due to impaired excretion of ingested magnesium (dietary magnesium, magnesium-containing laxatives or antacids). *Hypomagnesemia* occasionally complicates nonoliguric cisplatin and amphotericin B nephrotoxicity and likely reflects injury to the thick ascending limb of loop of Henle, the principal site for magnesium reabsorption. Manifestations of magnesium deficiency include neuromuscular instability, cramps, seizures, and cardiac arrhythmias; most cases are asymptomatic.

Anemia develops rapidly in ARF and is usually mild and multifactorial in origin. Contributing factors include impaired erythropoiesis, hemolysis, bleeding, hemodilution, and reduced red cell survival time. Prolongation of the *bleeding time* and *leukocytosis* are also common. The former may result from thrombocytopenia, platelet dysfunction, and/or clotting factor abnormalities (e.g., factor VIII dysfunction), and leukocytosis usually reflects sepsis, stress response, or other concurrent illness. *Infection* is the dread complication, occurring in 50 to 90 percent of ARF and accounting for up to 75 percent of deaths. It is unclear if ARF causes a defect in host immune responses or whether the high incidence of infection reflects repeated breaches of mucocutaneous barriers (e.g., intravenous cannulae, mechanical ventilation, bladder catheterization). *Cardiac complications* include arrhythmias, myocardial infarction, and pulmonary embolism. While these events may reflect primary cardiac disease, abnormalities in myocardial contractility and excitability may be triggered or aggravated by intravascular volume overload, acidosis, hyperkalemia, and other complications of azotemia. The increased incidence of pulmonary embolism probably reflects immobilization. Mild *gastrointestinal bleeding* (10 to 30 percent) is usually due to stress ulceration of gastric or small intestinal mucosa. Alterations in *neurologic* function may be due to the uremic syndrome, metabolic complications, impaired excretion of psychotropic medications, or primary neurologic disease.

Protracted ARF is associated with development of the *uremic syndrome* (see Chap. 237). Manifestations of the uremic syndrome include pericarditis, pericardial effusion, and cardiac tamponade; gastrointestinal complications such as anorexia, nausea, vomiting, and ileus; and neuropsychiatric disturbances such as lethargy, confusion,

stupor, coma, agitation, psychosis, asterixis, myoclonus, hyperreflexia, restless leg syndrome, focal neurologic deficit, and seizures.

A vigorous diuresis during the *recovery phase* may lead to intravascular volume depletion and delayed recovery of renal function. *Hypernatremia* also may complicate recovery if water losses via hypotonic urine are not replaced. *Hypokalemia*, *hypomagnesemia*, *hypophosphatemia*, and *hypocalcemia* occur rarely during this period. Mild hypercalcemia during recovery may be a consequence of transient hyperparathyroidism or may be due to mobilization of sequestered calcium from injured muscle.

MANAGEMENT   Prevention   Many cases of ARF can be prevented if cardiovascular function and intravascular volume are protected and exposure to nephrotoxic drugs is minimized in high-risk situations. Renal function may be protected in patients receiving aminoglycoside antibiotics or cyclosporine if serum drug concentrations are monitored and drug doses adjusted accordingly. Diuretics, cyclooxygenase, ACE inhibitors, and other vasodilators should be used with caution in patients with suspected true or "effective" hypovolemia or renovascular disease. Hypovolemia also should be avoided in patients receiving nephrotoxic medications, since renal hypoperfusion potentiates the toxicity of most of these agents. Allopurinol limits uric acid generation in patients at high risk for acute urate nephropathy, while forced diuresis and alkalinization of urine may attenuate renal injury due to uric acid, methotrexate, or rhabdomyolysis. *N*-acetylcysteine limits acetaminophen-induced renal injury if given within 24 h of ingestion, and dimercaprol, a chelating agent, may prevent heavy metal nephrotoxicity. Ethanol inhibits ethylene glycol metabolism to oxalic acid and other toxic metabolites and is an important adjunct to hemodialysis in the emergency management of this intoxication.

Specific therapies   By definition, *prerenal azotemia* is rapidly reversible upon correction of the primary hemodynamic abnormality, and *postrenal azotemia* resolves upon relief of obstruction. There are no specific therapies for established *intrinsic renal ARF* due to ischemia or nephrotoxicity. Management of these disorders should focus on elimination of the causative hemodynamic abnormality or toxin, avoidance of additional insults, and prevention and treatment of complications. Treatment of other causes of intrinsic renal azotemia varies according to the underlying pathology.

Treatment of *prerenal azotemia* due to hypovolemia varies depending on the fluid lost. Hypovolemia due to hemorrhage should be corrected with packed red blood cells in saline, while isotonic saline is usually appropriate replacement for plasma loss (e.g., burns, pancreatitis). Urinary and gastrointestinal fluid losses vary in composition but are usually hypotonic. Accordingly, initial replacement is with hypotonic solutions (e.g., 0.45% saline), and subsequent therapy should be based on measurements of the volume and ionic content of excreted or drained fluids. Serum potassium and acid-base status should be monitored. Potassium replacement is rarely required unless sodium bicarbonate is administered for moderate or severe metabolic acidosis. Cardiac failure may require aggressive management with antiarrhythmic drugs, inotropic agents, preload- and afterload-reducing agents, and/or mechanical aids such as intraaortic balloon pumps. Invasive hemodynamic monitoring may be required to guide therapy when clinical assessment of cardiovascular function and intravascular volume may be unreliable.

Fluid management may be particularly difficult in patients with ARF and cirrhosis with ascites. While ARF in this context usually results from combined intrarenal vasoconstriction and systemic vasodilation, systemic arterial hypovolemia may be a contributory factor in patients taking diuretics for control of ascites. The role of hypovolemia in this setting must be assessed by administration of a fluid challenge. Fluids should be administered slowly, and patients must be monitored closely because ascites formation may worsen and/or pulmonary edema may develop in nonresponders. Paracentesis usually can be used to drain large volumes of ascitic fluid without deterioration in renal function if albumin is administered simultaneously. Indeed, large-volume paracentesis may afford an increase in GFR possibly by lowering intraabdominal pressure and improving flow in renal veins. Shunting of ascitic fluid from the peritoneum to a central vein (peritoneojugular shunt, LeVeen or Denver shunts) is an alternative approach in refractory cases. This maneuver also may cause a transient improvement in GFR and sodium excretion, probably because the increase in central blood volume stimulates release of atrial natriuretic peptides and inhibits secretion of aldosterone and norepinephrine.

A variety of therapeutic agents have been tried in *ischemic* and *nephrotoxic ARF*. These include strategies to increase renal blood flow and urine flow (e.g., low-dose dopamine, atrial natriuretic peptide, mannitol, loop-blocking diuretics), relieve tubule obstruction (e.g., mannitol, loop-blocking diuretics), reduce epithelial cell swelling (e.g., mannitol), reduce epithelial cell ATP and oxygen requirements by inhibiting ion transport (e.g., loop-blocking diuretics), replenish cellular ATP levels (MgATP), scavenge oxygen free radicals (e.g., superoxide dismutase, catalase, mannitol), prevent accumulation of intracellular calcium (e.g., calcium channel blockers), and stimulate cellular regeneration (e.g., amino acid infusions). While many of these and other agents (e.g., glycine infusion, epidermal growth factor, growth hormone) afford some benefit in experimental models of ischemic or nephrotoxic ARF, they have been either ineffective or too toxic for use in humans.

Acute renal failure due to *other intrinsic renal diseases* such as acute glomerulonephritis or vasculitis may respond to glucocorticoids, alkylating agents, and/or plasmapheresis depending on the primary pathology. Glucocorticoids appear to hasten remission in some cases of allergic interstitial nephritis. Antiplatelet agents, plasma exchange, and plasma infusion are useful in treatment of HUS and TTP. Aggressive control of systemic arterial pressure is of paramount importance in limiting renal injury in the nephrosclerosis of malignant hypertension, toxemia of pregnancy, and other vascular diseases. Hypertension and ARF due to scleroderma may be exquisitely sensitive to treatment with ACE inhibitors.

Management of *postrenal azotemia* requires close collaboration among nephrologist, urologist, and radiologist. Obstruction of the urethra or bladder neck usually can be relieved temporarily by transurethral or suprapubic placement of a bladder catheter while the obstructing lesion is identified and treated. Similarly, ureteric obstruction may be treated initially by percutaneous catheterization of the dilated ureteric pelvis or ureter; indeed, obstructing lesions (e.g., calculus, sloughed papilla) often can be removed percutaneously or bypassed (e.g., carcinoma) by insertion of a ureteric stent. Most patients experience an appropriate diuresis for several days following relief of obstruction; approximately 5 percent develop a transient salt-wasting syndrome that may require administration of intravenous saline to maintain blood pressure.

Supportive measures Since intravascular volume overload, hyperkalemia, hyperphosphatemia, and metabolic acidosis are almost invariable in oliguric ARF, preventive measures should be taken from the time of diagnosis (Table 236-3). Prescription of nutrition should be designed to maintain caloric balance and minimize catabolism. In addition, doses of drugs excreted via the kidney must be adjusted for the degree of renal impairment.

Following correction of intravascular volume deficits, salt and water intake should be adjusted to match losses (urinary, gastrointestinal, drainage sites, insensible losses). *Intravascular volume overload* usually can be managed by restriction of salt and water intake and by use of diuretics. Indeed, there is no rationale for administration of diuretics in ARF other than to treat this complication. High doses of loop-blocking diuretics such as furosemide (up to 400 mg IV) or bumetanide (up to 10 mg IV) may be required in patients who fail to respond to conventional doses. Diuretic therapy should be discontinued in resistant patients to avoid complications such as deafness. Continuous intravenous infusion of low doses of dopamine (2 to 5 μg/kg per min) may promote salt and water excretion by increasing renal blood flow and GFR and by inhibiting sodium reabsorption in the proximal tubule. However, the role of dopamine remains to be established, since renal responses are variable under these circumstances. Ultrafil-

---

TABLE 236-3 Supportive treatment of intrinsic acute renal failure

Complication	Therapy
Intravascular volume overload	Salt (1–2 g/d) and water (usually <1 L/d) restriction Diuretics (usually loop blockers) Ultrafiltration or dialysis
Hyponatremia	Restriction of water intake
Hyperkalemia	Restriction of dietary K^+ Eliminate K^+ supplements and K^+-sparing diuretics Potassium-binding ion-exchange resins Glucose (50 mL of 50% dextrose) and insulin (10 units regular) Sodium bicarbonate (usually 50–100 mmol) Calcium gluconate (10 mL of 10% solution over 5 min) Dialysis
Metabolic acidosis	Restriction of dietary protein Sodium bicarbonate (maintain serum bicarbonate >15 mmol/L) Dialysis
Hyperphosphatemia	Restriction of dietary phosphate intake Phosphate binding agents (calcium carbonate, aluminum hydroxide)
Hypocalcemia	Calcium carbonate (if symptomatic or if sodium bicarbonate to be administered) Calcium gluconate (10–20 mL of 10% solution)
Hypermagnesemia	Discontinue Mg^{2+}-containing antacids
Hyperuricemia	Treatment usually not necessary if < 900 mmol/L (<15 mg/dL)
Nutrition	Restriction of dietary protein (− 0.5 g/kg/d) Carbohydrate (− 100 g/d) Enteral or parenteral nutrition (if recovery prolonged)
Drug dosage	Adjust doses for degree of renal impairment
Indications for dialysis	Clinical evidence (symptoms or signs) of uremia Intractable intravascular volume overload Hyperkalemia or severe acidosis resistant to conservative measures

---

tration or dialysis may be employed for volume reduction when conservative measures fail. *Hyponatremia* usually can be corrected by restriction of water intake. Conversely, *hypernatremia* is treated by administration of water or hypotonic saline solutions.

Mild *hyperkalemia* (<5.5 mmol/L) should be managed initially by restriction of dietary potassium intake and elimination of potassium supplements and potassium-sparing diuretics. Moderate hyperkalemia (5.5 to 6.5 mmol/L) in patients without clinical or electrocardiographic evidence of hyperkalemia usually can be controlled by administration of potassium-binding ion exchange resins such as sodium polystyrene sulfonate (15 to 30 g q 3–4 h) together with sorbitol (50 to 100 mL of 20% solution) by mouth or as a retention enema. Loop diuretics also increase potassium excretion in diuretic-responsive patients. Emergency measures should be employed in patients with serum potassium values of greater than 6.5 mmol/L and in all patients with ECG abnormalities or clinical features of hyperkalemia. Intravenous insulin (10 units of regular insulin) and glucose (50 mL of 50% dextrose) promote potassium shift into cells within 30 to 60 min, a benefit that lasts for several hours. Sodium bicarbonate (1 ampule, 44.6 mmol IV over 5 min) also promotes rapid (onset <15 min, duration 1 to 2 h) shift of potassium into the intracellular space. Since sodium polysterene sulfonate and sodium bicarbonate carry an obligatory sodium load, these compounds should be used judiciously in oliguric patients to avoid intravascular volume overload. Calcium gluconate (10 mL of 10% solution IV over 5 min) antagonizes the cardiac and neuromuscular effects of hyperkalemia and is a valuable emergency measure while other agents reduce serum potassium concentration. Dialysis is indicated if hyperkalemia is resistant to these measures.

Metabolic acidosis does not require treatment unless serum bicarbonate concentration falls below 15 mmol/L. More severe acidosis can be corrected by either oral or intravenous bicarbonate administration. Initial rates of replacement should be based on estimates of bicarbonate deficit and adjusted thereafter according to serum levels. Patients should be monitored for complications of bicarbonate administration, including metabolic alkalosis, hypocalcemia, hypokalemia, volume overload, and pulmonary edema. *Hyperphosphatemia* usually can be controlled by restriction of dietary phosphate intake and oral administration of agents (e.g., aluminum hydroxide or calcium carbonate) which reduce absorption of phosphate from the gastrointestinal tract. *Hypocalcemia* does not usually require treatment unless severe, such as with rhabdomyolysis or pancreatitis or following administration of bicarbonate. *Hyperuricemia* is usually mild in ARF [<900 mmol/L (<15 mg/dL)] and does not require intervention.

Nutritional management requires collaboration among physicians, nurses, and dieticians. The objective during the maintenance phase of ARF is to provide sufficient calories to avoid catabolism and starvation ketoacidosis while minimizing production of nitrogenous waste. This is best achieved by restricting dietary protein intake to approximately 0.5 g/kg of body weight per day of protein of high biologic value (i.e., rich in essential amino acids) and to provide most calories in the form of carbohydrate (approximately 100 g/d). Management of nutrition is easier in nonoliguric patients and after institution of dialysis. Parenteral alimentation has been claimed to improve prognosis, but a consistent benefit has not been demonstrated.

Anemia may neccessitate blood transfusion or administration of erythropoietin. Uremic bleeding usually responds to desmopressin, correction of anemia, estrogens, or dialysis. *Doses of drugs* which are excreted by the kidney must be adjusted for the degree of renal impairment. Antacids appear to reduce the incidence of *gastrointestinal hemorrhage* and may be more potent than H-2 blockers in this regard. Febrile patients must be investigated aggressively for *infection* and may be given broad-spectrum antibiotics while awaiting identification of specific organisms. Meticulous care of intravenous cannulas, catheters, and other invasive devices is mandatory. Unfortunately, prophylactic antibiotics do not appear to reduce the incidence of infection in these high-risk patients.

Dialysis Dialysis does not appear to hasten recovery in ARF. Early studies which suggested that early dialysis therapy improved prognosis have not been confirmed. Indeed, hemodialysis may potentially exacerbate renal hypoperfusion, since transient hypotension is a common complication. Accordingly, dialysis is reserved for treatment of symptoms or signs of uremia and management of volume overload, hyperkalemia, or acidosis refractory to conservative therapy. The type of dialysis (peritoneal dialysis, hemodialysis) and prescription depend on individual requirements. Peritoneal dialysis is effected through a temporary intraperitoneal catheter, and vascular access for short-term hemodialysis is usually achieved using a double-lumen catheter inserted into the subclavian, internal jugular, or femoral vein. Slow continuous arteriovenous hemofiltration and dialysis are alternative modalities for patients who do not tolerate conventional short-term dialysis and in whom peritoneal dialysis is not possible (e.g., after abdominal surgery). Ultrafiltration of plasma, without dialysis, may be used for intractable volume overload in patients without symptomatic uremia. Although many patients recover from ARF, a few (<5 percent) require long-term renal replacement therapy. With this in mind, every effort should be made to preserve veins (i.e., avoid venepuncture) on the nondominant arm of patients with severe ARF, since these may be required for chronic hemodialysis access (arteriovenous fistula) at a later date.

OUTCOME AND LONG-TERM PROGNOSIS The mortality rate from ARF approximates 50 percent and has changed little over the last 30 years. However, mortality rates vary depending on the cause: ~15 percent in obstetrical patients, ~30 percent in toxin-related

ARF, and ~60 percent following trauma or major surgery. Oliguria (<400 mL/d) at presentation and a rise in serum creatinine of greater than 260 μmol/L (3 mg/dL) are associated with a poor prognosis and probably reflect the extent of renal parenchymal damage and severity of the underlying disease. Mortality rates are higher in older, debilitated patients and those with multiple organ failure. With proper management, death usually results from primary diseases and rarely from uremia per se. Most patients who survive an episode of ARF recover sufficient renal function to live normal lives. However, half have subclinical impairment of glomerular filtration and urinary concentrating or acidification mechanisms or residual scarring on renal biopsy. Approximately 5 percent never recover function, presumably due to complete cortical necrosis, and require therapy with long-term dialysis or transplantation. An additional 5 percent have progressive decline in renal function following an initial recovery phase, probably due to hyperfiltration and subsequent sclerosis of remnant glomeruli (see Chap. 237). Progression to chronic renal failure may be observed more often following ARF as life-expectancy increases.

REFERENCES

ANDERSON RJ, SCHRIER RW: Acute tubular necrosis, in *Diseases of the Kidney*, RW Schrier, CW Gottschalk (eds). Boston, Little, Brown, 1988, p 1413

BRENNER BM, LAZARUS JM (eds). *Acute Renal Failure*, 3d ed. New York, Churchill Livingstone, 1993

BREZIS M et al: Acute renal failure, in *The Kidney*, 4th ed, BM Brenner, FC Rector Jr (eds). Philadelphia, Saunders, 1991, p 993

LIEBERTHAL W, LEVINSKY NG: Acute clinical renal failure, in *The Kidney, Physiology and Pathophysiology*, 2d ed, DW Seldin, G Giebisch (eds). New York, Raven, 1992, p 3181

OLSEN S: Acute tubular necrosis and toxic renal injury, in *Renal Pathology with Clinical and Functional Correlations*, CC Tisher, BM Brenner (eds). Philadelphia, Lippincott, 1989, p 656

---

237 CHRONIC RENAL FAILURE

BARRY M. BRENNER / J. MICHAEL LAZARUS

In contrast to the capacity of the kidney to regain function following acute renal injury, discussed in the preceding chapter, renal injury of a more sustained nature is often not reversible but leads to progressive destruction of nephron mass. Despite successful treatment of hypertension, urinary tract obstruction and infection, and systemic disease, many forms of renal injury progress inexorably to chronic renal failure (CRF). Reduction of renal mass causes structural and functional hypertrophy of remaining nephrons. This "compensatory" hypertrophy is due to adaptive hyperfiltration mediated by increases in glomerular capillary pressures and flows. Eventually, these adaptations prove "maladaptive" in that they predispose to glomerular sclerosis, an enhanced functional burden on less affected glomeruli, leading in turn to their ultimate destruction.

Glomerulonephritis, in its several forms, was the most common initiating cause of chronic renal failure in the past. Possibly because of more aggressive treatment of glomerulonephritis and because of changing practices in patient acceptance of end-stage renal disease programs, diabetes mellitus and hypertension are now the leading causes of chronic renal failure (see Fig. 237-1). These and other progressive forms of renal disease are considered in detail in the remaining chapters of this section. Irrespective of cause, the eventual impact of severe reduction in nephron mass is an alteration in function of virtually every organ system in the body. *Uremia* is the term generally applied to the clinical syndrome that results from profound loss of renal function. Although the cause(s) of the syndrome remain unknown, the term *uremia* was adopted originally because of the

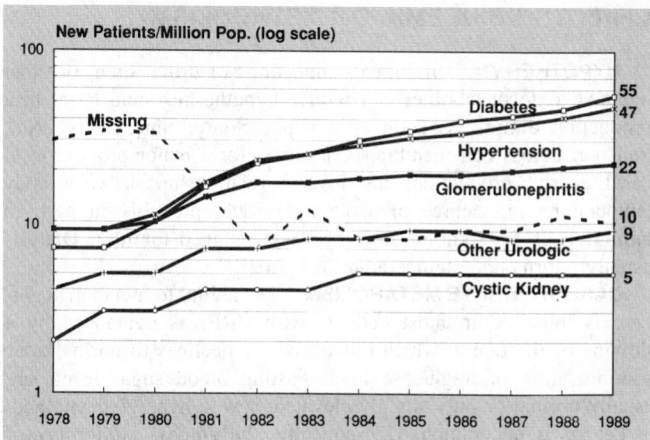

FIGURE 237-1 Incidence rates per million population of treated chronic renal failure by five major primary disease groups (diabetes mellitus, hypertension, glomerulonephritis, cystic kidney, other urologic), 1978–1989. Unadjusted, semilog scale; Medicare patients only.

presumption that the abnormalities result from retention in the blood of urea and other end products of metabolism normally excreted in the urine. But the term *uremia* represents more than renal excretory failure alone. A host of metabolic and endocrine functions normally subserved by the kidney are also impaired, and the inexorable course to renal failure is often accompanied by malnutrition; impaired metabolism of carbohydrates, fats, and proteins; and defective utilization of energy. Therefore, *uremia* refers generally to the constellation of signs and symptoms associated with CRF, regardless of cause.

The presentation and severity of signs and symptoms of uremia vary from patient to patient, depending, at least in part, on the magnitude of the reduction in functioning renal mass and the rapidity with which renal function is lost. As discussed in Chap. 235, in the relatively early stage of CRF [i.e., when total glomerular filtration rate (GFR) is reduced to levels about 35 to 50 percent of normal], overall renal function is sufficient to maintain the patient symptom-free, although renal reserve is diminished. At this stage, biosynthetic, excretory, and other regulatory functions of the kidney are generally well maintained. At a somewhat later stage in the course of CRF (GFR about 20 to 35 percent of normal), *azotemia* occurs, and initial manifestations of renal insufficiency usually appear. Although patients are relatively asymptomatic at this stage, renal reserve is diminished sufficiently that sudden stress, such as intercurrent infection, urinary tract obstruction, dehydration, or administration of a nephrotoxic drug, may compromise renal function still further, often leading to signs and symptoms of overt uremia. With further loss of nephron mass (GFR below 20 to 25 percent of normal), the patient develops *overt renal failure*. Uremia may be viewed as the final stage in this inexorable process, when many of or all the untoward manifestations of CRF become evident clinically. In this chapter the causes and characteristics of the disturbances of the various organ systems in CRF will be considered.

PATHOPHYSIOLOGY AND BIOCHEMISTRY OF UREMIA

The finding that sera from patients with uremia exert toxic effects in a variety of biologic test systems has motivated a diligent search to identify the responsible toxin(s). The most likely candidates as toxins in uremia are the *by-products of protein and amino acid metabolism.* Unlike fats and carbohydrates, which are eventually metabolized to carbon dioxide and water, substances that are easily excreted even in uremic subjects via lungs and skin, the products of protein and amino acid metabolism depend largely on the kidneys for excretion. A vast number of such products have been identified, with urea being

quantitatively the most important. *Urea* represents some 80 percent or more of the total nitrogen excreted into the urine. The *guanidino compounds* are the next most abundant of the nitrogenous end products of protein metabolism and include substances such as guanidine, methyl- and dimethylguanidine, creatinine, creatine, and guanidino-succinic acid. As with urea, guanidines are derived, at least in part, from urea cycle amino acids. Other metabolic products that are possible uremic toxins include *urates and other end products of nucleic acid metabolism, aliphatic amines,* a variety of *peptides,* and finally, several *derivatives of the aromatic amino acids tryptophan, tyrosine, and phenylalanine.* The role of these various substances in the pathogenesis of the uremic syndrome is unclear. Uremic symptoms correlate only in a rough and inconsistent way with concentrations of urea in blood. Nevertheless, although probably not a major cause of overt uremic toxicity, urea may account for some of the clinical abnormalities, including anorexia, malaise, vomiting, and headache. On the other hand, elevated levels of plasma *guanidinosuccinic acid,* by interfering with activation of platelet factor III by adenosine diphosphate (ADP), contribute to the impaired platelet function in CRF. *Creatinine,* generally regarded as a nontoxic substance, may cause adverse effects following conversion to metabolites such as sarcosine and methylguanidine. The extent to which these substances, as well as *creatine,* a metabolic precursor of creatinine, and the other compounds cited above, are of importance in the pathogenesis of uremic toxicity remains to be established.

Nitrogenous compounds of larger molecular weight are also retained in CRF. A toxic role for these substances has been suggested because of the impression that patients treated with intermittent peritoneal dialysis are less troubled with neuropathy than patients maintained on chronic hemodialysis, despite higher levels of urea and creatinine in blood in the former group. Since the clearance of small molecules depends mainly on blood and dialysate flow rates, which are higher with hemodialysis, whereas clearance of larger molecules depends more on membrane surface area and time, which are greater with peritoneal dialysis, this latter therapy may be a more effective means of removing substances of larger molecular weight. However, a multicenter study examining clearance of small versus middle-sized molecular substances, dialysis time, and morbidity indicated that urea or other small-molecular-weight substances play a more important role in determining uremic symptoms. The role of "middle" molecules in the uremic syndrome remains speculative.

Not all middle-sized molecules accumulate in uremic plasma because of decreased renal excretion alone. The kidney normally *catabolizes* a number of circulating plasma proteins and polypeptides; with reduced renal mass, this capacity may be impaired greatly. Furthermore, plasma levels of many polypeptide hormones [including parathyroid hormone (PTH), insulin, glucagon, growth hormone, luteinizing hormone, and prolactin] rise with renal failure, often markedly so, not only because of impaired renal catabolism but also because of enhanced secretion. Of these, excessive PTH may be an important uremic "toxin" because of its adverse effect on several organ systems. The consequences of high circulating levels of PTH and other hormones in chronic renal failure are considered below and in Chap. 235.

EFFECTS OF UREMIA ON CELLULAR FUNCTIONS

Alterations in the composition of intracellular and extracellular fluids in CRF are believed to be a consequence, at least in part, of *defective ion transport* across cell membranes generally, with retained uremic toxins possibly mediating these alterations in transmembrane ion transport. Integrity of cellular volume and composition depends to a large extent on the active outward transport of Na^+ from cell interior to exterior, the resulting intracellular fluid being relatively low in Na^+ and high in K^+, whereas the reverse is true for extracellular fluid. Active Na^+ transport is metabolically costly, accounting for a major fraction of basal energy utilization and oxygen consumption.

The consequences of this efflux of Na^+ from cells include (1) the generation of a resting electrical potential difference across the cell membrane (with this transcellular voltage oriented so that cell interior is electronegative to cell exterior) and (2) a mechanism for enhancing the influx of K^+ into cells.

In animals, partial inhibition of this active efflux mechanism for Na^+ across cell membranes leads to alterations in body composition and cell functions similar to those in erythrocytes, leukocytes, skeletal muscle, and other tissues of uremic subjects. These include increased and decreased intracellular concentrations of Na^+ and K^+, respectively, and reduction in magnitude of the transcellular voltage. These alterations are largely reversed by efficient hemodialysis and, for erythrocytes at least, are recreated when cells from normal subjects are incubated in uremic serum. Other derangements also have been implicated as causes for altered body composition in uremia. For example, *Na^+- and K^+-stimulated ATPase activity* is decreased in erythrocytes and brain from uremic patients and animals, respectively. Whether the uremic "toxins" that account for these derangements in cellular function represent abnormally retained products of metabolism that fail to be excreted or normal substances present in increased quantities in response to reduced renal mass remains unknown. *Parathyroid and natriuretic hormones*, examples of this category of substances, are discussed in this context in Chap. 235.

EFFECTS OF UREMIA ON WHOLE-BODY COMPOSITION

What is the impact of these disturbances in active transcellular Na^+ transport on the organism? From the pathophysiologic considerations already discussed, CRF is likely to lead to abnormally high intracellular Na^+ concentrations and hence to osmotically induced overhydration of cells, whereas these same cells are relatively deficient in K^+. With the development of malaise, anorexia, nausea, vomiting, and diarrhea, patients with CRF may eventually develop protein-calorie malnutrition and negative nitrogen balance, often with profound losses of lean body mass and fat deposits. Owing to the concomitant tendency for salt and water retention, these losses often go unnoticed until the late stages of CRF. Whereas a large fraction of the increase in total-body water in uremia is the result of expansion of intracellular volume, extracellular volume expansion also occurs. With initiation of intermittent hemodialysis or renal transplantation, there is often an immediate loss of body weight, due primarily to correction of this overhydration. With successful transplantation, the initial diuresis is followed by a period of weight gain, due to restoration of lean body mass and fat deposits to preillness levels. For patients on chronic dialysis, the anabolic response is less dramatic, even when therapy is regarded as optimal, involving mainly reaccumulation of fat deposits. The failure to restore lean body mass to normal with chronic dialysis may reflect insufficient intake of calories and protein, which, in adequately dialyzed patients, should be maintained at levels of 150 kJ/kg (35 kcal/kg) and 1.0 to 1.4 g/kg of body weight per day, respectively.

Deficits in intracellular K^+ concentration in CRF may result from inadequate intake (poor diet or overzealous K^+ restriction by the physician), excessive losses (vomiting, diarrhea, diuretics), reduction of Na^+- and K^+-stimulated ATPase, or a combination of these. In addition to promoting losses of K^+ into urine (which may be substantial if urine volume remains relatively normal in uremic subjects), the high levels of plasma aldosterone often seen in CRF also may augment net secretion of K^+ into the colon, thereby contributing to K^+ losses in stool or diarrheal fluids. Despite deficits in intracellular K^+, serum K^+ is usually normal or high in CRF, owing most often to metabolic acidosis, which induces an efflux of K^+ from cells. Uremic patients are also relatively resistant to the action of insulin (see below), which normally enhances K^+ uptake by skeletal muscle.

EFFECTS OF UREMIA ON METABOLISM

HYPOTHERMIA   In animals, injections of urine, urea, or other retained toxic metabolites can induce hypothermia, and basal heat production diminishes soon after nephrectomy. Since active Na^+ transport across cell membranes accounts for a major proportion of basal energy production, the inverse relationship between body temperature and degree of azotemia is due, probably in part, to inhibition of the sodium pump by some retained toxin(s). Dialysis usually returns body temperature to normal.

CARBOHYDRATE METABOLISM   The ability to metabolize glucose is impaired in most patients with CRF, as evidenced by a slowing of the rate at which blood glucose declines to normal after administration of a glucose load. Fasting blood sugar levels are usually normal or only slightly elevated; severe hyperglycemia and/or ketosis is uncommon. Consequently, the *glucose intolerance of CRF* usually does not require specific therapy (hence the term *azotemic pseudodiabetes*). Because insulin depends to a large extent on the kidney for its removal from plasma and degradation, circulating insulin levels in plasma are slightly to moderately increased in most fasting uremic subjects, and levels in excess of normal are usually demonstrable after a glucose load. The response to intravenous insulin in patients with CRF is also impaired, and the rate of utilization of glucose by peripheral tissues is diminished. The glucose intolerance of uremia results largely from this peripheral resistance to the action of insulin. Other possible factors contributing to glucose intolerance include intracellular deficits of potassium, metabolic acidosis, increased levels of glucagon, catecholamines, growth hormone, and prolactin, as well as the myriad of potentially toxic metabolites retained in CRF. In true insulin-dependent diabetics, there is often a decrease in insulin requirement with progressive azotemia, a phenomenon not related solely to decreased caloric intake.

NITROGEN AND LIPID METABOLISM   Since the capacity to eliminate the nitrogenous end products of protein catabolism is reduced, CRF may be regarded as a state of *protein intolerance*. As discussed above, retention of the end products of nitrogen metabolism is a dominant cause of the signs and symptoms of uremic toxicity.

Hypertriglyceridemia and decreased high-density lipoprotein cholesterol are common in uremia, whereas cholesterol levels in plasma are usually normal. Whether uremia accelerates triglyceride production by the liver and intestine is unknown. The enhancement of lipogenesis by insulin may contribute to increased triglyceride synthesis. In addition, the rate of removal of triglycerides from the circulation, which depends in large part on the enzyme *lipoprotein lipase*, is depressed in uremia, an effect not corrected appreciably by hemodialysis. The high incidence of premature atherosclerosis in patients on chronic dialysis (see "Cardiovascular and Pulmonary Abnormalities" below) may be related in part to these abnormalities in lipid metabolism.

CLINICAL ABNORMALITIES IN UREMIA

Chronic renal failure is associated with a constellation of signs and symptoms with or without reduced urine output but always with elevation in serum urea nitrogen and creatinine concentrations. As pointed out in Chap. 235, elevations of serum urea nitrogen and creatinine occur late in the course of renal failure. Differentiation between acute and chronic renal failure can be difficult. The history is often most helpful, particularly if normal renal function existed prior to a sudden recent insult. The laboratory findings and physical examination may not be helpful in the differentiation. The usual hallmark of chronic renal failure is reduced kidney size on ultrasound, abdominal scout film, or pyelogram. In the absence of small kidneys, renal biopsy may be necessary for diagnosis.

As noted earlier, CRF leads to disturbances in function of every organ system. With the application of chronic dialysis, the incidence and severity of these disturbances are modified so that where modern medicine is practiced, the overt and florid manifestations of uremia have largely disappeared. Unfortunately, however, even optimal dialysis therapy is not a panacea, because, as indicated in Table 237-1, some disturbances resulting from impaired renal function fail to respond fully, while others progress despite dialysis treatment. Furthermore, as with many complex therapeutic modalities, dialysis may cause unique abnormalities not seen prior to initiation of therapy; these abnormalities should be viewed as complications of dialysis.

FLUID, ELECTROLYTE, AND ACID-BASE DISORDERS (See also Chaps. 45 and 46) **Sodium and volume homeostasis** In most patients with stable CRF, total-body Na$^+$ and water content are increased modestly, although extracellular fluid (ECF) volume expansion may not be apparent. With ingestion of excessive amounts of salt and water, however, control of excess volume becomes an important consideration. In general, excessive *salt* ingestion contributes to, or aggravates, congestive heart failure, hypertension, ascites, and edema. On the other hand, hyponatremia and weight gain are the consequence of excessive ingestion of *water*, abnormalities that in most patients are relatively mild or asymptomatic. In most patients, daily intake of fluid equal in volume to urine volume per day plus about 500 mL usually maintains the serum Na$^+$ concentration at normal levels. Hypernatremia is relatively infrequent in CRF. In the edematous patient with CRF not on dialysis, diuretics and modest restriction of salt and water intake are the mainstays of therapy.

In volume-expanded dialysis patients, management should include ultrafiltration and restriction of salt and water intake between dialyses.

Patients with CRF have impaired renal mechanisms for conserving Na$^+$ and water (see Chap. 235). When an *extrarenal* cause for increased fluid loss is present (e.g., vomiting, diarrhea, fever), these patients are prone to develop ECF volume depletion, with dryness of mouth and other mucous membranes, dizziness, syncope, tachycardia, decreased filling of jugular veins, orthostatic hypotension, and vascular collapse. Depletion of extracellular fluid volume typically results in deterioration of residual renal function and, in the previously stable and asymptomatic patient with mild CRF, signs and symptoms of overt uremia. Cautious fluid repletion usually restores extracellular and intravascular volumes to normal and often returns renal function to stable levels.

Potassium homeostasis Derangements in K$^+$ balance (see Chaps. 45 and 235) are occasionally documented by laboratory analysis in patients with CRF but are rarely responsible for clinical symptoms unless GFR is below 5 mL/min or unless an endogenous (hemolysis, trauma, infection) or exogenous (stored blood, K$^+$-containing medications) K$^+$ load is administered. Despite progression of renal failure, most patients maintain normal serum K$^+$ concentrations until the final stages of uremia. This ability to sustain K$^+$ balance with advancing renal failure is due to adaptations in the renal distal tubules and colon, sites where aldosterone and other factors serve to enhance K$^+$ secretion (see Chap. 235). Not surprisingly,

---

TABLE 237-1 Clinical abnormalities in uremia*

FLUID AND ELECTROLYTE DISTURBANCES

Volume expansion and contraction (I)
Hypernatremia and hyponatremia (I)
Hyperkalemia and hypokalemia (I)
Metabolic acidosis (I)
Hyperphosphatemia (I)
Hypocalcemia (I)

ENDOCRINE-METABOLIC DISTURBANCES

Renal osteodystrophy (I or P)
Osteomalacia (D)
Aluminum-induced
Vitamin D–deficient osteomalacia (I)
Secondary hyperparathyroidism (I or P)
Carbohydrate intolerance (I)
Hyperuricemia (I or P)
Hypothermia (I)
Hypertriglyceridemia (P)
Protein-calorie malnutrition (I or P)
Impaired growth and development (P)
Infertility and sexual dysfunction (P)
Amenorrhea (P)
Dialysis (beta$_2$-microglobulin, amyloid) arthropathy (D)

GASTROINTESTINAL DISTURBANCES

Anorexia (I)
Nausea and vomiting (I)
Uremic fetor (I)
Gastroenteritis (I)
Peptic ulcer (I or P)
Gastrointestinal bleeding (I, P, or D)
Hepatitis (D)
Refractory ascites on hemodialysis (D)
Peritonitis (D)

CARDIOVASCULAR AND PULMONARY DISTURBANCES

Arterial hypertension (I or P)
Congestive heart failure or pulmonary edema (I)
Pericarditis (I)

Cardiomyopathy (I or P)
Uremic lung (I)
Accelerated atherosclerosis (P or D)
Hypotension and arrhythmias (D)

DERMATOLOGIC DISTURBANCES

Pallor (I)†
Hyperpigmentation (I, P, or D)
Pruritus (P)
Ecchymoses (I or P)
Uremic frost (I)

NEUROMUSCULAR DISTURBANCES

Fatigue (I)†
Sleep disorders (P)
Headache (I or P)
Impaired mentation (I)†
Lethargy (I)†
Asterixis (I)
Muscular irritability (I)
Peripheral neuropathy (I or P)
Restless legs syndrome (I or P)
Paralysis (I or P)
Myoclonus (I)
Seizures (I or P)
Coma (I)
Muscle cramps (D)
Dialysis disequilibrium syndrome (D)
Dialysis dementia (D)
Myopathy (P or D)

HEMATOLOGIC AND IMMUNOLOGIC DISTURBANCES

Normocytic, normochromic anemia (I)†
Microcytic (aluminum-induced) anemia (D)
Lymphocytopenia (D)
Bleeding diathesis (I or D)
Increased susceptibility to infection (I or P)
Splenomegaly and hypersplenism (P)
Leukopenia (D)
Hypocomplementemia (D)

---

* Virtually all abnormalities in this table are completely reversed in time by successful renal transplantation. The response of these abnormalities to hemo- or peritoneal dialysis therapy is more variable. (I) denotes an abnormality that usually improves with an optimal program of dialysis and related therapy. (P) denotes an abnormality that tends to persist or even progress, despite an optimal program. (D) denotes an abnormality that develops only after initiation of dialysis therapy.
† Improves with dialysis and erythropoietin (EPO) therapy.

oliguria, or disruption of key adaptive mechanisms, can lead to *hyperkalemia* and its potentially ominous effects on cardiac function. Antikaliuretic drugs such as spironolactone, triamterene, or amiloride should be used with extreme caution in chronic renal failure. Likewise, angiotensin-converting enzyme inhibitors and beta blockers may cause hyperkalemia. In the transplanted patient, cyclosporine is another common cause of increased serum potassium. Hyperkalemia in CRF also may be induced by abrupt lowering of arterial blood pH, since acidosis is associated with efflux of K^+ from intracellular to extracellular fluids. A useful index of the magnitude of this hydrogen-potassium exchange is that for every 0.1-unit change in blood pH, there will be a reciprocal change in serum K^+ concentration of approximately 0.6 mmol/L. Correction of acidosis-induced hyperkalemia with sodium bicarbonate is the treatment of choice. Intravenous insulin and dextrose are useful in lowering serum potassium acutely, while the ion exchange resin sodium polystyrene sulfonate is useful in longer-term control of hyperkalemia. When hyperkalemia persists in the absence of excessive K^+ intake, oliguria, or acute acidosis, the possibility of *hyporeninemic hypoaldosteronism* should be considered. Patients with this syndrome have reduced circulating levels of renin and aldosterone in the plasma and often have diabetes mellitus.

Hypokalemia due to diminished ability of the kidneys to conserve K^+ is uncommon in most forms of CRF. When hypokalemia occurs in these patients, poor dietary K^+ intake, usually in association with excessive diuretic therapy or gastrointestinal losses, is likely to be the underlying cause. When hypokalemia occurs as a result of primary K^+ wasting in urine, it may represent a solitary renal reabsorptive defect or, more commonly, may be associated with other solute transport abnormalities, as in Fanconi's syndrome, renal tubular acidosis, or other forms of hereditary or acquired tubulointerstitial diseases (see Chaps. 242 and 244). The clinical consequences and

management of hypokalemia and hyperkalemia are discussed in Chap. 45.

Metabolic acidosis   With advancing renal failure, total daily acid excretion and buffer production fall below the level needed to maintain external balance of hydrogen ions. Metabolic acidosis is the inevitable result, and the mechanisms involved are considered in Chap. 235. In most patients with stable renal insufficiency, administration of 20 to 30 mmol/d sodium bicarbonate or sodium citrate corrects the acidosis. In response to a sudden acid challenge (whether from an endogenous or exogenous source), however, patients with CRF are susceptible to acidosis, which requires more substantial quantities of alkali for correction. Administration of sodium must be carried out with careful attention to volume status.

Phosphate, calcium, and bone   As discussed in Chap. 235, hypocalcemia in chronic renal failure results from the impaired ability of the diseased kidney to synthesize 1,25-dihydroxyvitamin D [1,25(OH$_2$)D], the active metabolite of vitamin D (Fig. 237-2). Absorption of calcium in the gut is impaired when circulating levels of this active metabolite are low. Also, serum phosphate concentration begins to rise when GFR falls below about 25 percent of normal. Calcium deposition in bone is dependent on the availability of phosphate; retention of phosphate in plasma, therefore, facilitates calcium entry into bone and contributes to the hypocalcemia and elevation of plasma PTH levels in CRF. Finally, in advanced CRF, the ability of PTH to mobilize calcium salts from bone may be altered. Despite hypocalcemia, tetany is rare unless patients are treated with large amounts of alkali.

Overproduction of parathyroid hormone, disordered vitamin D metabolism, chronic metabolic acidosis, and excessive fecal losses of calcium all contribute to the bone diseases in uremia (see Fig. 237-2). *Renal* and *metabolic osteodystrophy* are terms that

FIGURE 237-2   Pathogenesis of bone diseases in chronic renal failure.

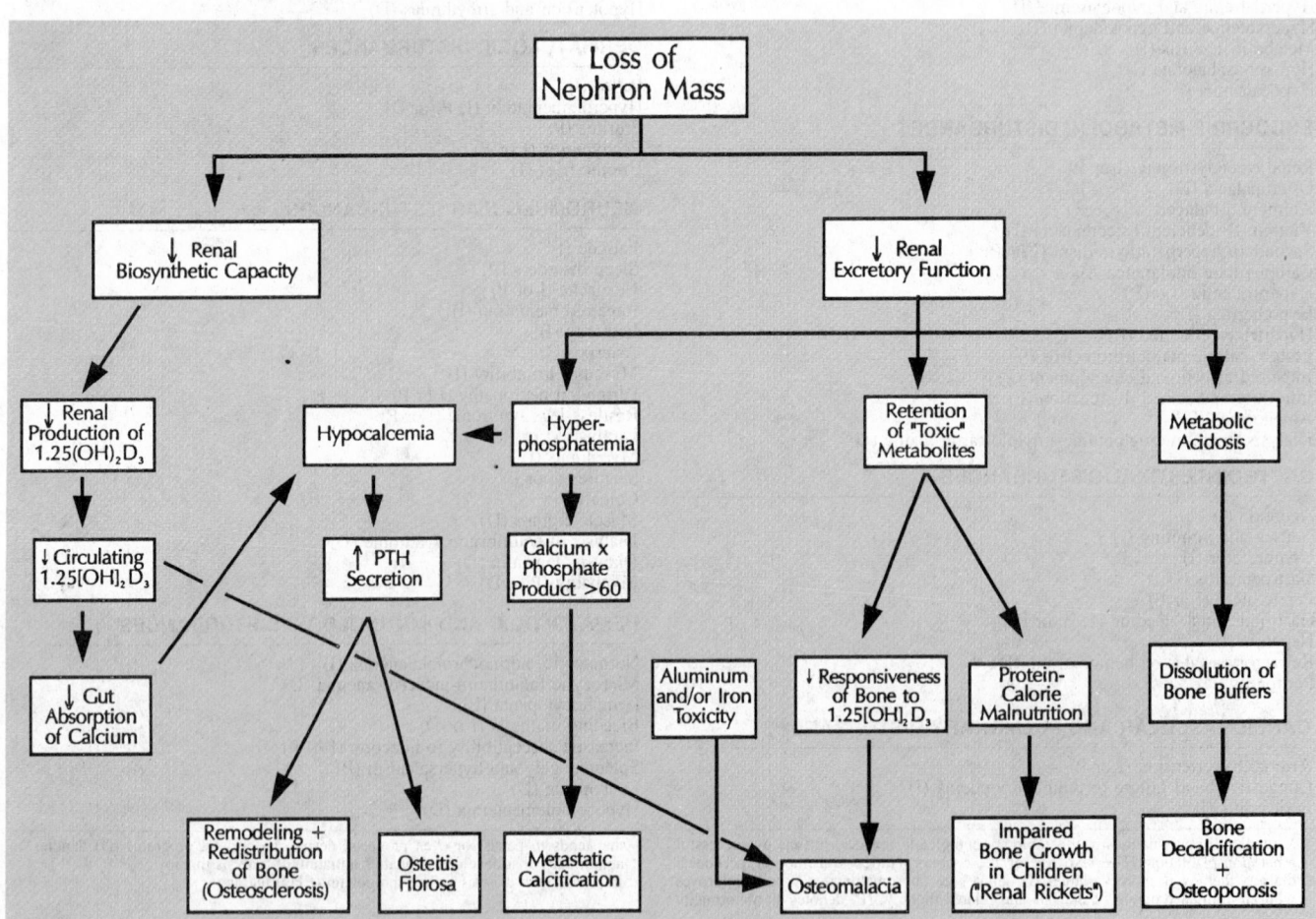

encompass a number of skeletal abnormalities, including osteomalacia, osteitis fibrosa cystica, osteosclerosis, and, in children especially, impaired bone growth. Although clinical symptoms of bone disease are present in less than 10 percent of predialysis patients with advanced renal failure, radiologic and histologic abnormalities are observed in, respectively, about 35 and 90 percent. In patients treated by dialysis for several years, bone disease is a major cause of morbidity. Renal osteodystrophy is more common in children than in adults, and especially in patients with slowly progressive renal insufficiency. On radiologic examination, three types of lesions can be identified: (1) changes analogous to those of nutritional rickets, namely, widened osteoid seams at the growth margin of bones (so-called renal rickets), (2) the bone changes of *secondary hyperparathyroidism (osteitis fibrosa cystica)*, characterized by osteoclastic bone resorption and subperiosteal erosions, especially of the phalanges, long bones, and distal ends of the clavicles, and (3) *osteosclerosis*, often best evidenced by enhanced bone density in the upper and lower margins of vertebrae, producing the so-called rugger jersey spine.

Osteomalacia can be secondary to decreased availability of $1,25(OH_2)D$ or to deposition of aluminum in the calcification fronts. The sources are aluminum in dialysate and aluminum-containing phosphate-binding agents. In aluminum-induced osteomalacia, the serum level of parathyroid hormone is usually low and that of calcium is often high. With osteitis fibrosa cystica and osteomalacia, there is a tendency to spontaneous fractures which are often slow to heal. The ribs are most commonly involved. Painful joints may occur due to calcium deposition in bursa and other periarticular structures. Bone pain may occur in the absence of fractures. When bone pain is severe, a proximal *myopathy* often coexists, giving rise to gait abnormalities and to impairment of ambulation. The incidence of *aseptic necrosis of the hip* is increased in renal transplant recipients, probably related to chronic glucocorticoid therapy, secondary hyperparathyroidism, and altered vitamin D metabolism. In CRF there is a tendency to *extraosseous*, or *metastatic, calcification* when the calcium-phosphate product is very high. Medium-sized blood vessels; subcutaneous, articular, and periarticular tissues; myocardium; eyes; and lungs are common sites of metastatic calcification. An arthropathy is associated with deposition of amyloid or beta$_2$ microglobulin. The cause is unknown but may be related to elevated levels of cytokines in chronic dialysis patients.

Management of renal osteodystrophy includes reduction in dietary phosphate through the use of a restricted phosphate diet as well as phosphate-binding agents. Calcium carbonate is the preferred phosphate-binding agent, but in some circumstances a combination of aluminum hydroxide and calcium carbonate is necessary. Dialysate calcium, oral calcium, aluminum hydroxide, and calcitriol must be properly balanced to maintain the serum phosporus at approximately 1.4 mmol/L (4.5 mg/dL) and the serum calcium at approximately 2.5 mmol/L (10 mg/dL) in an attempt to improve osteitis fibrosa cystica, osteomalacia, and myopathy. Treatment should be initiated early in chronic renal failure so that secondary hyperparathyroidism and bone disease may be prevented. It is particularly important to keep the calcium-phosphorous product in the normal range to avoid metastatic calcification or any possible role of these substances in progressive renal failure.

Other solutes   Other derangements in CRF include *hyperuricemia* and *hypermagnesemia*. Uric acid retention is a common feature of CRF but rarely leads to symptomatic gout. Hypophosphatemia is usually a consequence of overzealous oral administration of phosphate-binding gels. Because serum magnesium levels tend to rise in CRF, magnesium-containing antacids and cathartics should be avoided.

CARDIOVASCULAR AND PULMONARY ABNORMALITIES
Fluid retention in uremia often results in congestive heart failure and/or pulmonary edema. A unique form of pulmonary congestion and edema may occur even in the absence of volume overload and is associated with normal or mildly elevated intracardiac and pulmonary wedge pressures. This entity, characterized radiologically by perihilar vascular congestion giving rise to a ''butterfly wing'' distribution, is

due to increased permeability of the alveolar capillary membrane. This low-pressure pulmonary edema, as well as cardiopulmonary abnormalities associated with circulatory overload, usually responds promptly to vigorous dialysis.

Hypertension is the most common complication of end-stage renal disease. When it is not present, the patient either has a salt-wasting form of renal disease (e.g., polycystic or medullary cystic disease or chronic pyelonephritis), is receiving antihypertensive therapy, or is volume-depleted, the last condition usually being due to excessive gastrointestinal fluid losses or overzealous diuretic therapy. Since fluid overload is the major cause of hypertension in uremia, the normotensive state can usually be restored by dialysis. Nevertheless, some patients remain hypertensive despite rigorous salt and water restriction and ultrafiltration because of hyperreninemia. In approximately 30 percent of patients on chronic erythropoietin therapy, the severity of hypertension is increased. In most cases, routine antihypertensive drug therapy is effective. A minority develop *accelerated or malignant hypertension*, manifested by markedly elevated systolic and diastolic pressures, severe hyperreninemia, encephalopathy, seizures, retinal changes, and papilledema. Drugs such as diazoxide, minoxidil, captopril, enalapril, and nitroprusside, along with control of extracellular volume, generally control such hypertension.

Pericarditis, once a common complication of CRF, is now infrequent because of early initiation of dialysis. Retained metabolic toxins are thought to be the cause of *pericarditis*. The unusual occurrence of pericarditis in the well-dialyzed patient is usually due to viral infection or systemic disease.

The clinical presentation of pericarditis in uremic subjects is generally similar to that of other etiologies (Chap. 206), except that effusions are usually hemorrhagic. Treatment with intensive dialysis is recommended, and systemic anticoagulation should be avoided to minimize the occurrence of hemorrhagic tamponade. In some patients, pericardiocentesis with intrapericardial instillation of air or glucocorticoids is effective for pericardial tamponade. Pericardiectomy should be considered if more conservative treatment fails.

Chronically dialyzed patients have a high incidence of *accelerated atherosclerosis*, leading to coronary, cerebral, and peripheral vascular manifestations. Causes for these complications include hypertension, hyperlipidemia, glucose intolerance, chronic high cardiac output, and metastatic vascular and myocardial calcification.

HEMATOLOGIC ABNORMALITIES   *Normochromic, normocytic anemia* occurs regularly and contributes to the symptomology in CRF. Erythropoiesis is depressed in CRF, due both to the effects of retained toxins on bone marrow and to diminished biosynthesis of erythropoietin by the diseased kidney or to the presence of erythropoietin inhibitors. The administration of recombinant human erythropoietin (EPO) results in a dramatic increase in hematocrit and hemoglobin, suggesting that reduced serum erythropoietin is perhaps the more important of these factors. The anemia of chronic uremia also may be due in part to aluminum intoxication, which causes a microcytic anemia, fibrosis of the bone marrow due to hyperparathyroidism, and occasionally, inadequate replacement of folic acid. *Hemolysis* is due to an extracorpuscular defect, since survival of erythrocytes from normal subjects is reduced when these cells are transfused into uremic patients and erythrocytes from patients with CRF have relatively normal survival times when transfused into normal individuals. Gastrointestinal and chronic dialyzer *blood loss* contributes to anemia, as does *hypersplenism* in the occasional patient. Blood loss is exaggerated in hemodialysis patients because of the need for heparin during dialysis.

EPO is available for patients with advanced renal insufficiency and those on maintenance dialysis. Hematocrits of 30 to 36 vol% are attained in a high percentage of patients. In patients on dialysis, improved cardiovascular function, mental status, and energy level associated with the increased hematocrit enhanced the quality of life. The administration of 25 to 50 U/kg body weight three times per week is a reasonable starting dose. Dosage increases after 8 to 12 weeks may be warranted with careful monitoring of hematocrit.

Transfusions may contribute to suppression of erythropoiesis in CRF and, due to increased risk of hepatitis and hemosiderosis, should be avoided unless anemia fails to respond to EPO. Failure to respond to EPO is usually related to iron deficiency but may in part be due to aluminum-induced microcytosis or marrow fibrosis. Parenteral or oral iron therapy is indicated in patients with documented iron deficiency. Folic and ascorbic acids and the soluble B vitamins should be given to offset chronic losses of these substances via dialysis. Hemochromatosis is an uncommon complication since the introduction of EPO therapy.

Abnormal hemostasis is also common in CRF, characterized by a tendency to abnormal bleeding and bruising. Bleeding from the surgical wounds or spontaneously into the gastrointestinal tract, pericardial sac, and intracranial vault, in the form of subdural hematoma or intracerebral hemorrhage, is of greatest concern. Prolongation of bleeding time, decreased platelet factor III activity, abnormal platelet aggregation and adhesiveness, and impaired prothrombin consumption contribute to the clotting defects. The abnormality in factor III correlates with increased plasma levels of guanidinosuccinic acid and can largely be corrected by dialysis. Prolongation of the bleeding time is common even in the well-dialyzed patient. Abnormal bleeding times and coagulopathy in renal failure may be reversed with desmopressin, cryoprecipitate, conjugated estrogens, and blood transfusions, as well as by use of EPO.

Changes in leukocyte formation and function in uremia lead to *enhanced susceptibility to infection*. Lymphocytopenia and atrophy of lymphoid structures occur, whereas neutrophil production is relatively unimpaired. Nevertheless, function of all leukocyte cell types may be affected adversely by uremic serum. Decreased chemotaxis causes impairment of acute inflammatory response and decreased delayed hypersensitivity. There is a tendency for uremic patients to have less fever in response to infection. Leukocyte function also may be impaired in patients with CRF because of coexisting acidosis, hyperglycemia, protein-calorie malnutrition, and serum and tissue hyperosmolarity (due to azotemia). Mucosal barriers to infection also may be defective, and in dialysis patients, vascular access devices are common portals of entry for pathogens, particularly staphylococci. Glucocorticoids and immunosuppressive drugs add further to the risk of infection. Leukopenia is a common transient finding in patients exposed to cellophane-derived membranes during dialysis (Chap. 238).

NEUROMUSCULAR ABNORMALITIES   Subtle disturbances of central nervous system function, including inability to concentrate, drowsiness, and insomnia, are among early symptoms of uremia. Mild behavioral changes, loss of memory, and errors in judgment soon follow and may be associated with neuromuscular irritability, including hiccups, cramps, and fasciculations and twitching of muscles. Asterixis, myoclonus, and chorea are common in terminal uremia, as are stupor, seizures, and coma. Many of these neuromuscular complications of severe uremia resolve with dialysis, although nonspecific EEG abnormalities may persist.

Peripheral neuropathy is common in advanced CRF. Initially, sensory nerve involvement exceeds motor, lower extremities are involved more than the upper, and the distal portions of the extremities more than proximal. The "restless legs syndrome" is characterized by ill-defined sensations of discomfort in the feet and lower legs and frequent leg movement. If dialysis is not instituted soon after onset of sensory abnormalities, motor involvement follows, including loss of deep tendon reflexes, weakness, peroneal nerve palsy (foot drop), and eventually, flaccid quadriplegia. Accordingly, evidence of peripheral neuropathy is a firm indication to initiate dialysis or transplantation.

Two types of neurologic disturbances appear to be unique to patients on chronic dialysis. *Dialysis dementia* is seen in patients who have been on dialysis for a number of years and is characterized by speech dyspraxia, myoclonus, dementia, and eventually seizures and death. Aluminum intoxication is probably a major contributor to this syndrome. Other factors (viral infection?) probably play a role, since only a small percent of patients with aluminum exposure develop the syndrome. *Dialysis disequilibrium*, occurs during the first few dialyses, in association with rapid reduction of blood urea levels. Nausea, vomiting, drowsiness, headache, and even convulsions have been attributed to the more rapid (dialysis-induced) pH change and reduction in osmolality of extracellular than intracellular fluids within the cranium, leading to cerebral edema and raised intracranial pressure.

GASTROINTESTINAL ABNORMALITIES   Anorexia, hiccups, nausea, and vomiting are common, early manifestations of uremia. Carefully monitored protein restriction in the diet may be useful to slow progression of renal insufficiency if initiated early. Protein restriction is also useful in diminishing nausea and vomiting late in the course. Protein restriction should not, of course, be implemented in those patients with protein-calorie malnutrition. *Uremic fetor*, a uriniferous odor to the breath, derives from the breakdown of urea in saliva to ammonia and is often associated with unpleasant taste sensation. Mucosal ulcerations leading to blood loss can occur at any level of the gastrointestinal tract in very late stages of CRF—so-called uremic gastroenteritis. Peptic ulcer disease occurs in as many as one-fourth of uremic subjects. Whether this incidence is related to increased gastric acidity, hypersecretion of gastrin, or secondary hyperparathyroidism is unknown. Most gastrointestinal symptoms, except those related to peptic ulcer disease, improve with dialysis. Idiopathic ascites is seen rarely in patients on chronic dialysis, presumably secondary to fluid overload and/or chronic passive hepatic congestion. Patients with chronic renal failure, particularly those with polycystic kidney disease, have an increased incidence of diverticulosis. Viral hepatitis is more common in patients on chronic dialysis (see Chap. 238).

ENDOCRINE-METABOLIC DISTURBANCES   The disturbances in parathyroid function, glucose tolerance, and insulin metabolism, as well as the lipid, protein-calorie, and other nutritional abnormalities of uremia, have already been considered. Pituitary, thyroid, and adrenal functions are relatively normal, often despite abnormalities in circulating thyroxine, growth hormone, aldosterone, and cortisol levels. In women, estrogen levels are low, and amenorrhea and inability to carry pregnancies to term are early manifestations of uremia. While menses frequently reappear after chronic dialysis is initiated, successful pregnancies are rare. In men with CRF, including those on chronic dialysis, impotence, oligospermia, and germinal cell dysplasia are common, as are reduced plasma testosterone levels. As with growth, sexual maturation is often impaired in adolescent children, even among those on chronic dialysis.

DERMATOLOGIC ABNORMALITIES   The skin shows many abnormalities. This is not surprising in view of anemia (pallor), defective hemostasis (ecchymoses and hematomas), calcium deposition and secondary hyperparathyroidism (pruritus, excoriations), dehydration (poor skin turgor, dry mucous membranes), and the general cutaneous consequences of protein-calorie malnutrition. A sallow, yellow cast may reflect the combined influences of anemia and retention of a variety of pigmented metabolites, or *urochromes*. In advanced uremia, urea concentrations in sweat may reach sufficiently high levels that, after evaporation, a fine white powder can be found on the skin surface—so-called uremic (urea) frost. Although many of these cutaneous abnormalities improve with dialysis, *uremic pruritus* is usually resistant to most systemic and topical therapies. Hemochromatosis causes a slate-gray–bronze discoloration of the skin and is common in the dialysis patient who has received multiple transfusions.

CONSERVATIVE MANAGEMENT OF PROGRESSIVE RENAL FAILURE

Treatment directed to specific organ system abnormalities has been discussed in the preceding paragraphs. Principles of dialysis and transplant therapy are discussed in Chap. 238. Conservative (nondialytic, nontransplant) therapy is instituted early to control symptoms, minimize complications, prevent long-term sequelae, and slow the progression of renal insufficiency. The level of renal function should be ascertained at periodic intervals, and any reversible component that may be present should be corrected. In patients with slowly progressive renal failure, urine output is usually well maintained. Blood urea nitrogen and serum creatinine levels correlate only roughly with symptoms and are poor measures of glomerular filtration rate (GFR) (see Chap. 235). The inverse of serum creatinine (1/CR) was previously considered to be a more accurate measure of renal function and to be useful in comparing the effects of treatments that may affect renal failure progression. However, 1/CR is no more accurate than serum creatinine determination alone. Creatinine clearance (urine to plasma creatinine concentration ratio × volume of urine per minute) tends to overestimate GFR, while calculated urea clearance often underestimates GFR. By averaging simultaneously determined creatinine and urea clearances, a reasonably accurate estimation of GFR can therefore be obtained. More exact measures of GFR by isotope clearance techniques require injection of radioisotope and accurate collection of urine specimens at timed intervals over a 2- to 4-h period, usually by an experienced technician. Of those available, the iothalamate clearance (Glofil) is the most useful clinically.

Prerenal factors, such as volume depletion, decreased cardiac output, and renal artery stenosis, and postrenal components, such as urethral or ureteric obstruction, may exacerbate chronic renal insufficiency and must be identified and corrected. Hypertension, urinary tract infections, nephrolithiasis, structural abnormalities of the urinary tract, or those forms of glomerulonephritis that respond to immunosuppressive therapy also should be treated aggressively. Preventive aspects include avoidance of nephrotoxic drugs and radiopaque agents in the patient with compromised renal function.

Modification of diet is an important aspect of conservative therapy. Early restriction of sodium may be important in the treatment of hypertension. As renal insufficiency progresses, foods high in phosphate and potassium content should be restricted. Reduction of dietary protein content reduces anorexia, nausea, and vomiting and, if initiated early (GFR > 40 to 50 mL/min), may retard progression of renal disease. Adults should receive no less than 0.6 g protein per kilogram of body weight per day to avoid negative nitrogen balance. Protein diets of 0.28 to 0.60 g protein per kilogram per day must be supplemented with essential ketoamino acid therapy, allowing utilization of urea as a source of nonessential nitrogen. Preliminary results from a multicenter study (modification of diet in renal disease) sponsored by the U.S. National Institutes of Health/Health Care Financing Administration suggest that control of hypertension may be as important as control of the protein content of the diet. Completion of this study should make it possible to define the usefulness of protein restriction and aggressive treatment of hypertension in slowing progression. Preliminary data from other studies suggest a particularly beneficial role for angiotensin-converting enzyme (ACE) inhibitors. Hyperkalemia and compromised renal function (in the presence of renal artery stenosis) are not uncommon complications of these drugs. Combination therapy of ACE inhibitors with diuretics, calcium channel blockers, or beta-adrenergic blockers may be necessary to control hypertension.

Correction of electrolyte imbalance, e.g., use of sodium bicarbonate or calcium carbonate to correct metabolic acidosis and bicarbonate, dextrose-insulin combinations, or sodium-potassium exchange resins for treatment of hyperkalemia, may be necessary in more advanced uremia. Hypermagnesemia, hyperamylasemia, hypertriglyceridemia, and mild carbohydrate intolerance generally do not require or are not amenable to treatment. Hyperuricemia should be treated if gout develops. Mild hyperuricemia alone does not require therapy. Treatment of anemia has been discussed above. Secondary hyperparathyroidism may accentuate progression of renal failure. Whether this is due to hyperphosphatemia, an elevated calcium-phosphorus product, or parathyroid hormone itself is not clear. Nonetheless, vigorous efforts using phosphate-binding agents, calcium supplements, and vitamin D (dihydrotachysterol or calcitriol) to maintain appropriate serum calcium and phosphorous levels are often effective in sup-

pressing parathyroid levels, preventing severe bone disease, and perhaps even in slowing the progression of renal insufficiency. To avoid visceral and vascular calcification, the calcium-phosphorus product (conventional laboratory units) should be kept at less than 60. Dietary restrictions of sodium, potassium, phosphate, and protein often prove unacceptable to patients. Consequently, when the complications of uremia worsen despite conservative management, dialysis and/or transplantation are the remaining options for long-term life support.

REFERENCES

ANDERSON S, BRENNER BM: Progressive renal disease: A disorder of adaptation. Q J Med 70:185, 1989

ANDRESS DL et al: Intravenous calcitriol in the treatment of refractory osteitis fibrosa of chronic renal failure. N Engl J Med 321:274, 1989

ATTMAN PO, ALAUPOVIC P: Lipid abnormalities in chronic renal insufficiency. Kidney Int 39(suppl 31):S16, 1991

ESCHBACH JW et al: Recombinant human erythropoietin in anemic patients with end-stage renal disease: Results of phase III multicenter clinical trial. Ann Intern Med 111:992, 1989

FRASER CL, ARIEFF AI: Nervous system complications in uremia. Ann Intern Med 109:143, 1988

GLASSOCK RJ: Nutrition, immunology and renal disease. Kidney Int 24(suppl 16):S194, 1983

HAKIM RM, LAZARUS JM: Biochemical parameters in chronic renal failure. Am J Kidney Dis 11:238, 1988

KLEINMAN KS et al: The use of recombinant human erythropoietin in the correction of anemia in predialysis patients and its effect on renal function: a double-blind, placebo-controlled trial. Am J Kidney Dis 14:486, 1989

PERRONE RD et al: Utility of radioisotope filtration markers in chronic renal insufficiency: Simultaneous comparison of ^{125}I-iothalamate, ^{99m}Tc-DPTA, and insulin. Am J Kidney Dis 16:224, 1990

POWELL D et al: Toxins and inhibitors in chronic renal failure. Am J Kidney Dis 7:292, 1986

WALSER M et al: Reciprocal creatinine slopes often give erroneous estimates of progression of chronic renal failure. Kidney Int Suppl. 27:S81, 1989

---

238 DIALYSIS AND TRANSPLANTATION IN THE TREATMENT OF RENAL FAILURE

CHARLES B. CARPENTER / J. MICHAEL LAZARUS

Dialysis and transplantation prolong the lives of patients with renal insufficiency. The approach to treatment in acute renal failure is different than in chronic renal failure because of the irreversible nature of the latter. Conservative medical management and dialysis are the mainstays of therapy for acute renal failure. Obviously, transplantation is not a treatment for this group of patients.

The term *end-stage renal disease* (ESRD) is used by government agents such as HCFA and has come to be synonymous with the late stages of chronic renal failure. Initially, patients with ESRD are managed with conservative therapy, but eventually they require hemodialysis, peritoneal dialysis, or transplantation. Because of limited success with each of these modalities, chronic renal failure should be approached with the concept of moving from one form of therapy to another as indicated by the degree of success and incidence of complications with each.

Therapy for renal failure should be initiated when serious complications, as noted in Chaps. 235 and 237, will be prevented, but not when the patient is completely asymptomatic. The advanced complications of uremia should be avoided by early treatment. Early dialysis is appropriate in patients with acute renal failure in whom resumption of renal function can be expected and in patients with chronic renal failure who have a good immunologic match with a related donor and are to be transplanted without prior long-term dialysis. In the remainder of patients, the clinical judgment to move from conservative treatment to dialysis or transplantation is determined by the patient's quality of life and whether or not the benefits of treatment outweigh the risks. The correlation of uremic symptoms with renal function varies from patient to patient depending on the cause of renal disease (earlier onset of symptoms in subjects with diabetes mellitus), muscle mass (large, muscular patients tolerate high levels of azotemia), diet, nutritional status, and coexisting conditions. Therefore, it is ill-advised to assign a certain "usual" level of blood urea nitrogen, serum creatinine, or glomerular filtration rate to the need to start dialysis. Treatment with dietary protein restriction and aggressive control of hypertension, as described in Chap. 237, may prolong the time before dialysis and/or transplantation are required but should be carried out only if complications of such therapy do not worsen morbidity and mortality. For example, malnutrition is a major factor in mortality in dialysis patients.

Selection of patients to receive dialysis and/or transplantation is a matter of some debate. Because of the reversible nature of acute renal failure, *all* patients with this diagnosis should be supported with dialysis, at least for some period of time, to allow return of renal function. In patients with irreversible or chronic renal failure, criteria for selection for transplantation are generally more stringent than those for dialysis and are guided by the possibility of complications related to immunosuppressive therapy. Table 238-1 lists considerations in the selection of a recipient for a human renal allograft. Transplantation should be undertaken only when conservative treatment has failed, when there are no reversible elements in the renal failure, and when the patient is too ill to be maintained comfortably with the usual methods of treatment. However, morbidity is less if transplantation is performed before the patient is critically ill. Transplantation should not be utilized in an attempt to salvage patients from failure to thrive on dialysis.

The recipient should be free of life-threatening extrarenal complications such as cancer, severe coronary artery disease, and cerebrovascular disease. Provided that diffuse vascular involvement is not present, diabetes mellitus is not a contraindication. Oxalosis may recur in relatively short order in a transplanted kidney and is generally a contraindication for transplantation. Although advanced age may be a limiting factor, it is advanced "physiologic" rather than chronologic age that contraindicates transplantation. In general, patients reach a "physiologic" limit at approximately age 60 to 65 years, when the incidence of complications due to glucocorticoids becomes much higher. Although abnormalities of the bladder and urethra present additional hazards, successful renal allografts have been placed in individuals with these abnormalities by prior constitution of an artificial bladder (i.e., ileal conduit) into which the donor ureter is placed. Patients with any disease process that may be aggravated by glucocorticoids, cyclosporine, azathioprine, or other immunosup-

pressive agents or any patient with coexisting medical conditions so severe that the risks of operation and drug therapy are high should not be offered transplantation.

Criteria for treatment with hemodialysis or peritoneal dialysis are more liberal because dialysis has less morbidity than transplantation in older patients in those with the aforementioned medical complications. Because of the cost of these programs, some have suggested that entry be restricted in those of advanced age. Such decisions, based on moral, social, and economic issues, continue to generate debate. In general, nearly all patients are accepted if they or their families desire prolongation of life. The physician should inform the patient of the likelihood of success and review the complications and untoward effects. The patient and family should be given an estimate of prognosis and expected quality of life. In most areas of the world, the cost of medical care for chronic renal failure is borne by government. In the United States, the mechanism of coverage is by Medicare, with all patients eligible regardless of age.

PREPARATION FOR THERAPY OF ESRD

While conservative measures as described in Chap. 237 are being carried out, it is important to prepare the patient with an intensive educational program, explaining the likelihood and timing of complete renal failure and the various forms of therapy available. The more knowledgeable patients are concerning hemodialysis, peritoneal dialysis, and transplantation, the easier and more appropriate will be their decisions at a later time. With hemodialysis, the major method of obtaining blood for treatment is from an arteriovenous fistula. Since these devices often take months to develop, prophylactic placement of a fistula in a patient planning for hemodialysis is important in minimizing future complications of circulatory access. For those who select peritoneal dialysis (continuous ambulatory peritoneal dialysis—CAPD; or continuous cyclic peritoneal dialysis—CCPD), placement of the peritoneal catheter does not require preparation, and therapy can be instituted when uremic signs and symptoms develop. In those who may perform home dialysis or undergo transplantation, early education of family members for selection and preparation as a home dialysis helper or a related donor for transplantation should occur before the onset of symptomatic renal failure. In those patients who have a good antigenic match with a willing donor, transplantation without intervening hemodialysis or peritoneal dialysis should be considered. Approximately 25 percent of patients receiving renal transplants at our institution do so without having had prior dialysis. In considering related-donor transplantation, the risk of unilateral nephrectomy, including development of proteinuria and hypertension, should be considered. As discussed below, the success rate of cadaver-donor transplantation has improved sufficiently that this form of therapy should be considered both by the patient and by potential donors. Early referral of patients to ESRD programs will allow education of the patient and family and preparation for an appropriate therapy. Table 238-2 illustrates the distribution of treatment modalities based on age, sex, race, and disease etiology in the United States.

DIALYSIS Hemodialysis   Hemodialysis employs the process of diffusion across a semipermeable membrane to remove unwanted substances from the blood while adding desirable components. A constant flow of blood on one side of the membrane and a cleansing solution dialysate on the other allow removal of waste products in a fashion similar to that of glomerular filtration. By altering the composition of the dialysate, the method of exposure of blood and dialysate (geometry of the dialyzer), the type and surface area of dialysis membrane, and the frequency and duration of exposure (the dialysis prescription), patients without renal function can be maintained in a relatively healthy state. Hemodialysis equipment consists of three components—the blood delivery system, the composition and delivery system of the dialysate, and the dialyzer itself (Fig. 238-1). Blood is pumped to the dialyzer by a roller pump

---

TABLE 238-1   **Contraindications to kidney transplantation**

ABSOLUTE CONTRAINDICATIONS

Reversible renal involvement
Ability of conservative measures to maintain useful life
Advanced forms of major extrarenal complications (cerebrovascular or coronary disease, neoplasia)
Active infection
Active glomerulonephritis
Previous sensitization to donor tissue

RELATIVE CONTRAINDICATIONS

Age
Presence of vesical or urethral abnormalities
Iliofemoral occlusive disease
Psychiatric problems
Oxalosis

TABLE 238-2 Treatment Modality Summary by age,* sex, race, and primary diagnosis, December 31, 1989

Patient characteristics	Percent†			
	With a functioning transplant	Receiving center hemodialysis	Receiving home hemodialysis	Receiving CAPD/ CCPD
Total	25.0	58.0	1.6	9.0
Age 20	55.5	19.0	0.6	12.8
20–44	44.0	39.1	1.5	8.3
45–64	23.3	59.0	1.9	9.2
65 +	2.7	81.8	1.4	9.1
Male	28.0	55.3	1.7	8.6
Female	21.3	61.2	1.5	9.5
Native American	23.2	61.3	3.2	9.8
Asian	27.7	61.5	0.9	7.0
Black	13.3	74.1	1.0	6.8
White	30.4	51.0	1.8	10.1
Diabetes mellitus	18.9	66.1	1.0	10.5
Hypertension	12.2	75.2	1.2	8.5
Glomerulonephritis	35.8	47.4	1.9	9.9

* Age on December 31, 1989.
† Percents add to almost 100; the remainder includes other and unknown dialysis.
SOURCE: U.S. Renal Data System, *USRDS 1991 Annual Data Report*, The National Institutes of Health, National Institute of Diabetes and Digestive and Kidney Diseases, Bethesda, Md., August 1991.

through lines with appropriate equipment to measure flow and pressures within the system; blood flow should be approximately 300 to 450 mL/min. Negative hydrostatic pressure on the dialysate side of the system can be manipulated to achieve desirable fluid removal, so-called ultrafiltration. Dialysis membranes have differing ultrafiltration coefficients (i.e., fluid removed per millimeters of mercury pressure per minute), the selection of which, along with the hydrostatic pressure changes, determines fluid removal. The dialysate is delivered to the dialyzer from a storage tank or proportioning system which manufactures dialysate on-line. In most systems, dialysate passes once across the membrane, countercurrent to blood flow at a rate of 500 mL/min. The composition of the dialysate is similar to plasma water but may be altered depending on need. The dialysate potassium is varied most often, but the sodium, calcium, and acetate or bicarbonate are usually decided in each dialysis unit. Table 238-3 outlines the range of formulas available. The principal dialyzer in use in the United States is the hollow fiber or capillary dialyzer, in which membrane material is spun into fine capillaries, thousands of which are packed into bundles with blood flowing through the capillaries while dialysate is circulated on the outside of the fiber bundle.

With current dialysis techniques, most patients require between 9 and 12 h of dialysis per week, equally divided into several sessions. The time depends on body size, residual renal function, dietary intake, complicating illnesses, and degree of anabolism or catabolism. The time, frequency of treatments, type and size of dialyzer, and dialysate composition, blood, or dialysate flow may all be altered to accomplish

FIGURE 238-1 Schema for hemodialysis.

TABLE 238-3   Range of dialysis components available

Component	mmol/L
Sodium	138–145
Potassium	0–4.0
Calcium	2.0–3.5
Magnesium	0.4–1.0
Bicarbonate	30–37
Chloride	100–107

specific needs (see Fig. 238-2). The type of membrane and surface area (size) are determinants of ultrafiltration and clearance and are important in the immunologic (i.e., biocompatible) response by the patient. Cuprahane (Cupra-ammonium cellophase) and cellulose acetate are "tighter" membranes with less diffusive and ultrafiltration capabilities and less biocompatibility. Polyacrylnitrile (PAN), poly-methylmethacrylate (PMNA), and polysulphone are porous (high flux), biocompatible, and more expensive. Kinetic modeling, utilizing urea generation and protein catabolic rates, provides a more definite dialysis prescription. Urea kinetic modeling is based on the assumption that the body is a single pool. The term KT/V (K = clearance, T = dialysis time, and V = volume of distribution of the patient) is a dimensionless measure of treatment used in urea kinetic modeling. By determining each of these components, one can measure the adequacy of treatment as well as determine the protein catabolic rate (PCR), which is a measure of catabolism and, by inference, nutrition. An acceptable KT/V is 1.0 to 1.2, while the PCR should be approximately 1.2 g/kg per day. A simpler measure—the percent reduction of urea during each treatment (URR or PRU)—correlates well with KT/V. Based on these studies, an acceptable PRU or URR during each treatment is approximately 65 percent. The development of bicarbonate dialysis, variable sodium delivery, high-flux or ultraef-ficient membranes, and urea kinetic modeling has resulted in reductions in dialysis time. Clinical trials of this so-called high-flux, short-time dialysis are underway. Reduction of dialysis time without documentation of adequacy of treatment is associated with an increased morbidity and mortality. In addition to hemodialysis, a new method of treatment has been developed for the patient with acute renal failure. Slow continuous ultrafiltration (SCUF) or continuous arteriovenous hemodialysis (CAVHD) are techniques that employ high-efficiency dialyzers with cardiac-generated blood flow (via a cannulated femoral artery) along with very slow dialysate flow rates. This therapy is useful in the unstable, acute renal failure patient, has essentially replaced acute peritoneal dialysis in the ICU, and is often preferable to intermittent hemodialysis.

FIGURE 238-2 Factors in the development of the uremic syndrome and considerations in its treatment.

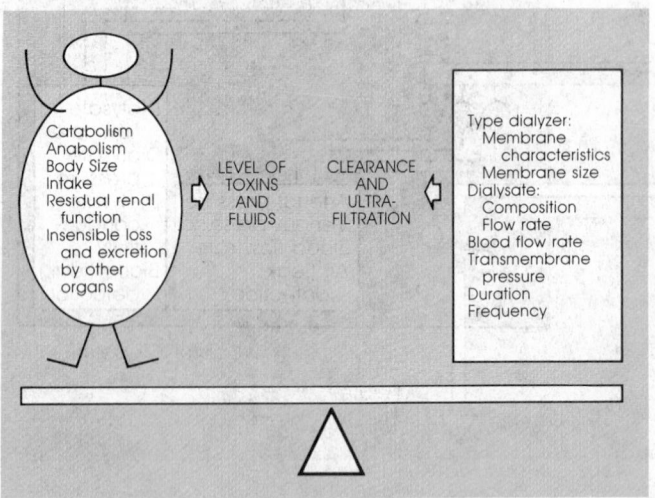

COMPLICATIONS OF HEMODIALYSIS Many complications of chronic dialysis are related to underlying disease or those uremic conditions not reversed by dialytic therapy. These and other related problems of hemodialysis are discussed in Chap. 237. The Achilles' heel of hemodialysis is access to the circulation. The development of the arteriovenous shunt made chronic dialysis possible. This device had a high failure rate because of infection and thrombosis and led in 1966 to the development of the arteriovenous (AV) fistula. The fistula is preferably created from a native vein, but a prosthetic conduit (extended polytetrafluoroethylene) subcutaneously placed between an artery and a nearby vein may be utilized. Cannulation of arteriovenous fistulas with 15- to 16-gauge needles allows blood flow sufficient to carry out hemodialysis. Unfortunately, infection, thrombosis, and aneurysm formation also occur in the arteriovenous fistula, particularly in prosthetic devices. There is a relatively high incidence of septicemia and septic embolization associated with shunt and fistula infection; the most common infecting agent is *Staphylococcus aureus*.

Depression and altered self-image are common psychiatric problems. The rapid flux in osmolality may cause a dialysis disequilibrium syndrome consisting of confusion, clouding of consciousness, and seizures. In addition, rapid changes in electrolytes (particularly potassium) may lead to arrhythmia during dialysis. Hypotension during hemodialysis is due to many factors—the size of the extracorporeal circulation, degree of ultrafiltration, change in serum osmolality, presence of autonomic neuropathy, concomitant use of antihypertensive agents, removal of catecholamines, or infusion of acetate (used as the dialysate buffer), which is a cardiac depressant and vasodilator. Careful estimation of the extracellular fluid to be removed and use of isolated ultrafiltration and higher-sodium dialysate are helpful in preventing hypotension. In addition, many dialysis units now use bicarbonate as the dialysate buffer rather than acetate. Syndromes of dialysis dementia and osteomalacia may be secondary to aluminum contamination of dialysate water or result from oral intake of aluminum hydroxide. An increased incidence of HBsAg (hepatitis B surface antigen) antigenemia is related to decreased immunologic integrity and an increased transfusion rate. Patients with chronic antigenemia are usually asymptomatic and have little derangement of liver function. There is a higher rate of non-A, non-B hepatitis and cytomegalovirus infection, but these, too, are usually of mild degree. As mentioned in Chap. 237, use of recombinant human erythropoietin (EPO) has reduced or eliminated the need for blood transfusion in hemodialysis patients, thus reducing the risk of hepatitis. In addition, use of hepatitis vaccine has decreased the incidence of hepatitis B. Occurrence of non-A, non-B hepatitis (hepatitis C) is of unknown signficance in dialysis patients; however, evidence of hepatic disease secondary to hepatitis C is important in the consideration for renal transplantation. Patients with AIDS may have a rapidly progressive nephropathy and have poor prognosis with or without dialysis. Because of this and because of the high incidence of AIDS in IV drug abusers who also have heroin nephropathy, the presence of HIV-positive patients is common in dialysis units. Based on clinical experience and recommendations from the Centers for Disease Control, these patients are treated in dialysis units as are other patients with no special precautions. It is extremely important however, that all patients receive universal precautions for infection control. Mechanical and/or iatrogenic complications, such as hemolysis, air embolus, blood leaks, and contaminated dialysate, are less common with improved equipment. Membrane-induced adverse reactions may occur, as exemplified by complement-mediated leukopenia and hypoxemia. More prominent symptoms, such as back and chest pain, broncho-spasm, and anaphylaxis, rarely occur in this reaction. Elaboration of cytokines, specifically IL-1, IL-6, and tumor necrosis factor (TNF), occurs with exposure of blood to some dialysis membranes. Simulation of the complement and cytokine systems likely plays a role in anorexia and hypercatabolism in hemodialysis patients. These cytokines also contribute to the development of dialysis-induced amyloid arthropathy—consisting of carpal tunnel syndrome, cystic degeneration of the cervical spine and femoral head and neck, and an infiltrating shoulder lesion. Use of the more biocompatible synthetic membranes—PAN, PMMA, and polysulphone—may have a beneficial effect in this regard. These membranes, as mentioned earlier, are expensive, however. Reuse of dialyzers, which occurs in approximately 68 percent of dialysis patients, will make their use feasible. Heparin, necessary during the hemodialysis procedure to prevent clotting in the lines and dialyzer, may lead to complications such as subdural hematoma and retroperitoneal, gastrointestinal, pericardial, and pleural hemorrhage. Recognition of the risks and modification of the dose of heparin reduce these complications. One of the major concerns in long-term dialysis patients is mortality related to myocardial infarction and cerebral vascular accidents. This is likely due to the preexistence and continuation of common risk factors in the uremic patient, such as hypertension, hyperlipidemia, vascular calcification due to hyperparathyroidism, and high cardiac output due to anemia or other factors. Control of hypertension is essential and can be accomplished in about 80 percent of dialysis patients with ultrafiltration and reduction of extracellular volume to the point of mild hypotension—so-called dry weight. For those in whom this is not possible because of cardiac or cerebral disease or who do not respond to ultrafiltration, use of hypertensive medications is warranted. Peripheral dilator agents and beta-adrenergic blockers seem to aggravate hypotension and must be used with care in the dialysis patient. ACE inhibitors and calcium channel blocking drugs cause less hypotension but in any case should be administered after the dialysis procedure. Hypercholesterolemia is uncommon in dialysis patients, while hypertriglyceridemia and decreased high-density lipoproteins are often seen. Hypocholesterolemic agents, such as lovastatin or gemfibrozil, are indicated when hypertriglyceridemia is accompanied by hypercholesterolemia. Hyperparathyroidism can often be controlled by binding phosphate with calcium carbonate along with use of calcitriol. Prevention of a calcium-phosphorous product greater than 60 will prevent vascular calcification. As mentioned earlier, EPO has virtually eliminated anemia.

The potential for complications should cause the physician to evaluate the risk/benefit ratio with dialysis before proceeding. Advantages of hemodialysis are the relatively short treatment time and minimal interruption of life-style between treatments. It is more efficient than peritoneal dialysis, allowing rapid changes in abnormal serum values. Hemodialysis can be performed in the home, but the patient requires an assistant during treatment. Hemodialysis is the most widely utilized form of dialysis.

Peritoneal dialysis Peritoneal dialysis, like hemodialysis, may be performed in various settings and with several techniques. In patients with acute renal failure, intermittent peritoneal dialysis has largely been replaced by intermittent hemodialysis or CAVHD. Chronic peritoneal dialysis was attempted in the late 1940s but was impractical until development of a permanent peritoneal catheter—the Tenckhoff catheter. Use of this indwelling catheter and closed continuous-cycle dialysate delivery equipment led to treatment protocols with which patients were treated two to three times per week for a total of 30 to 40 h (intermittent peritoneal dialysis—IPD) to achieve clearances and fluid removal similar to those of hemodialysis. In 1978, the concept of continuous peritoneal lavage with prolonged dwell times led to the development of CAPD, which differs from intermittent peritoneal dialysis in that patients instill fluid into the peritoneal cavity, seal the catheter, continue in an ambulatory mode, and every 4 to 6 h empty the peritoneal cavity and replace the dialysate. This technique generally utilizes 2-L containers of dialysate and obviates the need for dialysis equipment. Modification using a cyclic dialysate delivery device to exchange dialysate during the night and chronic dwelling of fluid during the waking hours (CCPD) is acceptable to some patients.

IPD or CCPD may be performed in a center or at home (usually overnight), while CAPD can be performed anywhere. As with hemodialysis, the composition of the dialysate can be modified for individual needs. The major difference in peritoneal dialysate formulas is in the amount of dextrose used as an osmotic agent (1.5, 2.5, or 4.25 g/dL). Advantages of peritoneal dialysis are avoidance of heparinization and vascular surgery and a slower clearance rate (helpful for some cardiovascular patients). It is more amenable to self-treatment. Disadvantages include the longer treatment time (intermittent or continuous involvement). It should not be used in patients with extensive abdominal surgery or pulmonary disease. Inadequate clearance may occur in patients with scleroderma, vasculitis, malignant hypertension, or peritoneal disease. Complications include catheter tunnel infection, peritonitis, protein loss with malnutrition, hypertriglyceridemia, hypercholesterolemia, obesity, and inguinal and abdominal hernias. Determination of adequacy of treatment by CAPD or CCPD is not as easy as with hemodialysis (see Table 238-2).

RESULTS Of new patients with ESRD, approximately 35 to 50 percent are physically and psychologically suitable for transplantation. Many are on hemodialysis and peritoneal dialysis awaiting availability of a kidney. An acutely ill or medically complicated patient will likely undergo dialysis in a hospital dialysis unit or intensive care unit, while stable patients may be dialyzed as outpatients or at home. Most centers attempt to have patients participate in their own care, so-called self-dialysis. Home dialysis (either hemodialysis or peritoneal) is preferable for many because of self-reliance and freedom from hospital or center schedules. Patient motivation is the primary factor in selection of home or in-center self-dialysis. Dialysis in the hospital setting is most expensive, while home dialysis with a nonpaid family assistant or alone (peritoneal dialysis only) is less expensive than in-center dialysis. Despite absence of equipment, peritoneal dialysis is as expensive as home hemodialysis because of the cost of dialysate and of hospitalization related to peritonitis. The total amount of Medicare payments for ESRD (covering hemodialysis, peritoneal dialysis, and transplantation) in the year 1991 was $3 billion, substantially greater than anticipated at the initiation of the ESRD program in 1973. This cost reflects an increasing number of recipients, not an increasing cost per patient, which, in fact, has been reduced over the past 20 years.

The mean age for patients on dialysis is 62 years. This number continues to rise also, partly because nephrosclerosis and eventual renal failure from other parenchymal diseases occur in older patients but more likely because the selection process favors transplantation in younger patients.

Approximately 10 to 20 percent of patients with chronic renal failure are totally rehabilitated by dialysis, and another 30 to 40 percent of nondiabetic patients may be rehabilitated to a functional status even if they are not employed. Twenty percent of patients will be returned to a level of function not considered rehabilitated but able to care for themselves. The remainder (approximately 20 percent) are dependent on support from others. Diabetics, who have rehabilitation and survival rates lower than those of nondiabetic patients, make up much of the latter two groups. Mortality rates vary, depending on the age of the patient and the disease process(es) involved. Yearly gross mortality rates of patients in the ESRD program in the United States have increased from 20 percent in 1982 to approximately 24 percent in 1990. This increase in mortality may be due to case-mix factors, i.e., acceptance in recent years of older patients with a higher incidence of comorbid conditions such as diabetes mellitus, nephrosclerosis, coronary artery disease, peripheral vascular disease, and pulmonary and hepatic disease. Others have suggested that treatment has become inadequate for a number of reasons. Clinical studies are underway to determine the causes of this increased mortality and to improve rehabilitation and quality of life. In patients less than 45 years of age and with no complicating medical illnesses, mortality with hemodialysis, peritoneal dialysis, or transplantation is below 5 percent per year.

TRANSPLANTATION

Transplantation of the human kidney is frequently appropriate for the treatment of advanced chronic renal failure. Worldwide, tens of thousands of such procedures have been performed. When azathioprine and prednisone are used as immunosuppressive drugs, the results with properly matched familial donors are superior to those with organs from cadaveric donors, namely, 75 to 90 percent compared with 50 to 60 percent graft survival rates at 1 year. When antilymphocyte globulins (ALG) are added to the treatment regimens in some centers, the results with cadaveric donors approach those with living related donors, at least for the first 2 years after transplantation. Cyclosporine has also improved 1-year cadaveric survival rates to the 80 percent range when used along with prednisone in place of azathioprine and ALG. With all therapies, the rate of graft loss from rejection is much slower after the first year, although occasionally acute irreversible rejection may occur after many months of good function. This is especially likely if the patient neglects to take the immunosuppressive drugs. Results in recent years have improved with regard to patient morbidity and mortality rates, the latter declining to less than 5 percent in a number of centers. This improvement is the result of a tendency on the part of transplant teams to decrease immunosuppressive therapy so that in the case of severe rejection the kidney rather than the patient is lost. Second and even third transplants can be performed, and the overall results show a 10 to 20 percent reduction in expected survival compared with first transplants; cyclosporine therapy does not erase the increased risk of rejecting subsequent transplants, however. Overall, transplantation returns the majority of patients to a near-normal life-style.

DONOR SELECTION   Donors can be cadavers or volunteer blood-related living donors. Living volunteer donors should be normal on physical examination and of the same major ABO blood group, because crossing major blood group barriers prejudices survival of the allograft. It is possible, however, to transplant a kidney of a type O donor into an A, B, or AB recipient. Selective renal arteriography should be performed on donors to rule out the presence of multiple or abnormal renal arteries, because the surgical procedure is difficult and the ischemic time of the transplanted kidney long when vascular abnormalities exist. Cadaveric donors should be free of malignant neoplastic disease because of possible transmission to the recipient.

In the United States, a coordinated national system (United Network for Organ Sharing) of computerized information about and logistic support for the transportation of cadaver kidneys to suitable recipients is under development. It is now possible to remove cadaver kidneys and to maintain them for over 48 h on cold pulsatile perfusion or simple flushing and cooling. This permits adequate time for typing, cross-matching, transportation, and selection problems to be solved.

TISSUE TYPING AND CLINICAL IMMUNOGENETICS   Matching for antigens of the HLA major histocompatibility gene complex (Chap. 64) is the ideal criterion for selection of donors for renal allografts. Each mammalian species has a single chromosomal region that encodes the strong, or major, transplantation antigens, and this region on the human sixth chromosome is called *HLA*. Other antigens, called "minor," may nevertheless play crucial roles, especially the ABH(O) blood groups and endothelial antigens that are not shared with lymphocytes. Evidence for designation of HLA as the genetic region encoding major transplantation antigens comes from the success rate in living related donor renal and bone marrow transplantation, with superior results in HLA-identical sibling pairs. Nevertheless, 5 to 10 percent of HLA-identical renal allografts are rejected, often within the first weeks after transplantation. These failures probably represent states of prior sensitization to non-HLA antigens. Non-HLA antigens are relatively weak and therefore suppressible by conventional immunosuppressive therapy. Once priming has occurred, however, secondary responses are much more refractory to treatment. In fact, ABH incompatibilities are hazardous because of the presence of natural anti-A and anti-B antibodies in recipients and the normal expression of A and B blood group substances on endothelium.

Living related donors   From 1962 to 1982 when azathioprine was the main immunosuppressive drug, living related donors provided superior graft survivals. Among first-degree relatives, the general level of expected graft success was in direct proportion to matching

for 2, 1, or no HLA haplotypes, as defined by HLA serologic typing and the presence or absence of a proliferative response in the mixed-lymphocyte response (MLR) (Chap. 64). HLA-incompatible siblings did slightly better than the overall average with cadaveric donors (50 to 60 percent at 1 year), while HLA semi-identicals (haploidentical) were in the 70 to 75 percent range. Intrafamilial MLRs among haploidenticals were found to be a measure of responsiveness. Low-responder donor-recipient pairs had a 1-year graft survival rate of 90 percent, while vigorous responders were at the level of 55 percent unless donor-specific blood transfusions were given to eliminate this disadvantage. The MLR is a relatively imprecise technique, but MLR reactivity with a specific donor was more predictive of graft outcome than serologic typing for HLA-A, -B, -C, or -DR antigens. Improvements in serologic and DNA-based techniques (Chap. 64) have made the MLR test unnecessary for most related-donor cases.

Cyclosporine has altered the assumption that living related donors are generally superior to cadaveric donors, because in most series cadaveric results now rival the 80 percent 1-year result attained with haploidentical relatives. One must now weigh the choices in light of the availability of organs and waiting times on dialysis rather than on the initial rate of graft success. Long-term survival rates, however, are not improved. With either azathioprine or cyclosporine, the half-life estimated after the first year is 25 to 30 years with HLA-identical donors, 11 to 12 years with haploidentical donors, and 7 to 9 years with cadaveric donors. The major advantage of cyclosporine over azathioprine, therefore, is in the initial results at 1 to 2 years for cadaveric transplantation and not in the rate of graft loss thereafter.

Concern has been expressed regarding the potential risk to a volunteer kidney donor of premature renal failure after several years of increased blood flow and hyperfiltration per nephron in the remaining kidney. There are a few reports of the development of hypertension, proteinuria, and even lesions of focal segmental sclerosis in donors under long-term follow-up. Difficulties in donors followed for 15 or more years are unusual, however, and it may be that having a single kidney becomes significant only when another condition, such as hypertension, is superimposed. In this regard, it is desirable to consider the risk of development of type I diabetes mellitus in a family member who is a potential donor to a diabetic renal failure patient. Anti-insulin and anti-islet antibodies should be measured, and glucose tolerance tests should be performed in such cases to rule out a prediabetic state. The acceptance of living unrelated donors (spouses, distant relatives, close friends) has been debated as a means to improve the supply of organs and to shorten the waiting period on dialysis. Since volunteer donors who are not matched for one or both HLA haplotypes present as strong a tissue barrier as randomly matched cadaveric donors, they cannot be expected to provide, on average, as reliable a source for long-functioning grafts as a well-matched cadaveric organ. Actual data on this matter are conflicting. It is illegal in the United States to purchase organs for transplantation.

HLA matching and cadaveric donors   The question of whether matching of HLA antigens in unrelated donor-recipient pairs would approximate the high initial success rates and slow rates of subsequent graft loss with HLA-identical sib pairs could not be answered until the late 1980s when reliable class II histocompatibility (DR) typing became widely available. With the 1-year success rate now at 80 to 85 percent for first cadaveric grafts, it is difficult to see an early improvement related to matching when small series of cases are compiled, especially, as is often the case, when the reporting centers have a very small fraction of well-matched cases. Now that pooled data on several thousands of cadaveric renal transplants from all over the world are available, the HLA-matching effect can be clearly seen, especially in the long-term survival figures. It is shown in Fig. 238-3 that there is an overall beneficial effect of HLA matching in first cadaveric grafts. When compared with HLA-identical transplants, where the 1-year graft survival rate is 95 percent and the subsequent half-life is 25 years, one-HLA-haplotype–matched family donor transplants and no-antigen–mismatched cadaveric cases have 1-year survival rates of 85 percent with an 11- to 12-year half-life. With

FIGURE 238-3 Survival of over 30,000 first cadaveric renal transplants over 5 years after transplantation. The transplants were performed in more than 200 centers around the world between 1982 and 1989. Cyclosporine was used in virtually all cases. The curves for each HLA matching grade are shown, according to the number of mismatches (MM) for HLA-A, -B, and -DR antigens. Since each individual has two genes for each locus, there is a potential for up to six mismatches. The overall effect of matching in this international Collaborative Transplant Study stratifies according to the mismatch grade (weighted regression, $p < 0.0001$) *(From Opelz.)*

increasing numbers of mismatches for cadaveric donors, the 1-year survival rate declines from 80 to 70 percent, and the half-life decreases from 9 to 7 years. The survival rates at the 10-year mark are projected to range from 50 (zero mismatches) to 30 percent (six mismatches). Many centers report 1-year graft survival rates in the 85 to 90 percent range for all renal transplants, possibly the result of heavy initial immunosuppression, but the subsequent half-lives are similar to those above. The contribution of the HLA locus to the matching effect is strongest for DR, moderate for B, and weak for A. Repeat transplants, following rejection of first grafts, do less well by about 15 to 20 percent; in these cases, the benefits of HLA matching are even more striking, while cyclosporine adds relatively little. The United Network for Organ Sharing requires that donor-recipient pairs with a "six-antigen match" for HLA-A, -B, and -DR be matched on a nationwide basis, while sharing for lesser degrees of match is voluntary. A 20 to 30 percent rate of DR-compatible cadaveric transplants has been achieved by some organ-sharing systems. With the waiting list in the United States having some 18,000 potential recipients and 8000 donors each year, matching grades approaching these rates and higher are possible if transplant centers are willing to share organs on this basis.

Presensitization A positive cross match of recipient serum with donor T lymphocytes representing anti-HLA class I is usually predictive of an acute vasculitic event termed *hyperacute* rejection. Patients making such antibodies, detected by testing against a surrogate panel of normal lymphocytes, were previously thought to be at high risk for accelerated, if not hyperacute, rejection, even when the donor-specific cross match was negative. That this is no longer so can be attributed to greater efforts in monitoring patients on dialysis and in defining not only the presence or absence of antibodies but also the HLA antigens to which they are directed. Patients with anti-HLA antibodies can be safely transplanted if careful cross matching is performed. Patients sustained by hemodialysis often show fluctuating antibody titers and specificity patterns, sometimes, but not always, temporally related to receipt of blood transfusions. At the time of assignment of a cadaveric kidney, cross matches are performed with more than one highly reactive serum, and the previously analyzed antibody specificities are also taken into account. Anti-HLA antibody responses do not necessarily recur several months later when the incompatible antigen is given in a blood-product transfusion. Indeed, it seems relatively safe to ignore positive cross matches with sera kept in storage for several months as long as recent sera are negative. Data on this point are conflicting, showing either no risk or a 15 percent increased risk of early graft loss if only the stored serum samples older than 6 months are reactive with donor cells. The loss of anamnesis to HLA by chronic dialysis patients may result from development of specific unresponsiveness due to suppressor cell activation or from anti-idiotypic immunity. Low-titer presensitization

to antigens expressed on B lymphocytes, but not T lymphocytes, is not a contraindication to transplantation. Some of these antibodies are anti-DR, while others are non-HLA IgM antibodies active in the cold and at room temperature but apparently not relevant to graft survival. High-titer (>1:4) anti-DR antibodies have been related to early graft rejection in a few reported cases. A cross match performed by fluorescence techniques on a flow cytometer may be useful in sensitized patients.

Endothelial-monocyte system In some cases of unexpected accelerated rejection, antibodies with reactivity to renal endothelium and blood monocytes have been found, both in the circulation and in eluates from rejected grafts. Practical aspects of typing and cross matching for this non-HLA system are difficult. Second transplants following rapid loss of the first graft seem to be particularly at risk.

Overview of transplantation immunogenetics In addition to the ABH(O) blood groups, the important histocompatibility antigens presently known are HLA-A, -B, -C, -DR, and the endothelial-monocyte system (Table 238-4). Major primary immunogenicity lies in the DR antigens, while A, B, C, and endothelial-monocyte antigens provide the major targets for effector IgG and, in the case of A, B, and C, at least, for killer T lymphocytes. Hence the current emphasis is on A, B, and C cross matching and DR matching, although HLA-B compatibility adds to the DR-matching effect. The predictive accuracy of class I typing is improved by defining HLA-A and -B antigens using the best-quality serologic typing, while for class II antigens studies of polymorphisms at the level of DNA sequences are most reliable (Chap. 64).

Blood transfusions At a time when it appeared that transfusion-induced sensitization against a random lymphocyte panel was predictive of a high graft failure rate, a number of transplantation units undertook a policy of withholding blood from as many dialysis patients as possible. The clinical need for blood was found to be less than originally thought, especially in nonnephrectomized patients, and avoidance of possible exposure to hepatitis also was a consideration. The overall experience with the nontransfused patients was the opposite to what had been predicted: Such patients were at the *highest*

TABLE 238-4 Histocompatibility in renal transplantation

Relative importance of typing and cross matching for serologically defined antigens

Antigens	Typing (antigen matching)	Cross matching
Class I (HLA-A, -B, -C)	+ +	+ + +
Class II (HLA-DR)	+ + +	−
Endothelial-monocyte (non-HLA)	? −	+ + +

risk for graft failure. Since the early 1980s, however, there has been a progressive loss of the transfusion effect, with little or no detriment now remaining in the nontransfused patients. The loss of the transfusion effect cannot be directly attributed to the introduction of cyclosporine, since the transfusion effect had declined before large numbers of patients received this agent. It seems unlikely that worldwide changes in blood bank processing practices are involved. It is most likely that the overall level of clinical management, particularly in recognition and prompt treatment of rejection, has played a role. Indeed, when looked at carefully, some centers withholding transfusions have noted increased rejection activity in their nontransfused patients but have not had difficulty in treating them. One study shows, however, that graft survival is still decreased in that subset of nontransfused patients who also have an early clinically apparent rejection episode. The current practice to use little or no blood in preparation for transplantation comes at a propitious time because of concerns regarding HIV transmission. The efficacy of recombinant erythropoietin in sustaining red blood cell mass in chronic renal failure patients further reduces the clinical need for blood transfusions.

IMMUNOLOGY OF REJECTION   Knowledge of the immunology of tissue transplantation stems largely from animal experimentation. However, enough evidence has accumulated in humans, particularly in kidney transplantation, to indicate that the evidence is similar, though not identical, for the different species. The immunologic mechanisms are not qualitatively different from those found in other areas of immunology (Chap. 277). Early rejection is associated with T lymphocytes having direct specificity against donor antigens. These may be cytotoxic cells (CD8+ or CD4+) or cells that mediate delayed hypersensitivity (CD4+); however, significant numbers of B lymphocytes, null cells, natural killer (NK) cells, and macrophages appear in the early infiltrate, and cells capable of mediating antibody-dependent cell-mediated cytotoxicity (ADCC) are also present (Fig. 238-4). Many of the B lymphocytes produce immunoglobulins. The spectrum of cellular and humoral response and graft injury is quite varied, depending on specific genetic differences between donor and recipient and states of presensitization. The greater the degree of presensitization, the more likely it is that one will find antibody-mediated vascular lesions. All the processes shown in Fig. 238-4 are possible, but their relative contribution varies from case to case. Further dissection of the heterogeneity of the human allograft response utilizing techniques for the identification of lymphocyte subsets is adding to the value of graft biopsy as a guide to therapy and prognosis. Monitoring of peripheral blood lymphocyte subsets utilizing monoclonal antibodies to functionally related surface molecules, such as CD4 (T helper cells) and CD8 (T suppressor/cytotoxic cells), has been related to the degree of rejection activity in some surveys, but the CD4/CD8 ratio has not always been meaningful. Part of the problem may lie in the fact that these subsets are not as uniquely related to function as originally believed. Indeed, the principal role of the CD4 molecule is to promote interaction of T cells with class II HLA molecules on antigen-presenting cells, and similarly, CD8 interacts with class I HLA (see Chap. 277). Finally, the cytokine mediators of the cellular immune response IL-1 to IL-4, IL-6, TNF, and IFN γ) are involved in the control and expression of the alloimmune rejection response. For example, T cell production of IFN γ causes increased expression of HLA antigens on endothelial cells. In normal immunobiology this effect may be to promote more efficient presentation of foreign antigen, while in transplantation it enhances the immunogenicity of the vascularized transplant. Also, IL-2, the major growth factor for expansion of effector T cells, is the product of a major subset of CD4 cells, while other CD4 cells produce B cell growth factors, such as IL-4.

The failure of transplanted kidneys after several years of adequate function is said to be due to "chronic rejection." In such kidneys, the development of nephrosclerosis, with proliferation of the vascular intima of renal vessels, and intimal fibrosis, with marked decrease in the lumen of the vessels, takes place (Fig. 238-5). The result is renal ischemia, hypertension, tubular atrophy, interstitial fibrosis, and glomerular atrophy with eventual renal failure. It is not established, however, whether slow deterioration of graft function over years is due to the same mechanisms in all cases. Except for the established influence of HLA incompatibility, little is known about the pathogenesis of progressive renal failure in transplanted patients.

IMMUNOSUPPRESSIVE TREATMENT   When histocompatibility differences exist between donor and recipient, it is necessary to modify or suppress the immune response to enable the recipient to accept a graft. Immunosuppressive therapy, in general, suppresses all immune responses, including those to bacteria, fungi, and even malignant tumors. In the 1950s when clinical renal transplantation began, sublethal total-body irradiation was employed. Currently, pharmacologic immunosuppression is safer. Agents to suppress the immune response are discussed in the following paragraphs.

Drugs   *Azathioprine*, an analogue of mercaptopurine, was for two decades the keystone to immunosuppressive therapy in humans. This agent can inhibit synthesis of DNA, RNA, or both. Because cell division and proliferation are a necessary part of the immune response to antigenic stimulation, suppression by this agent may be mediated by the inhibition of mitosis of immunologically competent lymphoid cells, interfering with synthesis of DNA. Alternatively, immunosuppression may be brought about by blocking the synthesis of RNA (possibly messenger RNA), inhibiting processing of antigens prior to lymphocyte stimulation. This drug has little effect in suppressing a secondary immune response, however. Therapy with azathioprine is generally instituted 2 days prior to transplantation in the recipient of a living-donor kidney and on the day of transplantation in the case of a cadaveric-donor kidney recipient at a level of 4 mg/kg per day. The drug is later tapered to levels of 1.5 to 3 mg/kg per day as long as the allograft functions. Because the drug is rapidly metabolized by the liver, its dosage need not be varied directly in relation to renal function, even though renal failure results in retention of the metabolites of azathioprine. Some patients are unusually sensitive to this drug, particularly when renal function is compromised, and reduction in dosage is required because of leukopenia and occasionally thrombocytopenia. Excessive amounts of azathioprine also may cause jaundice, anemia, and alopecia. If it is essential to administer allopurinol concurrently, the azathioprine dose must be reduced, since inhibition of xanthine oxidase delays degradation. This combination is best avoided.

Glucocorticoids are important adjuncts to immunosuppressive therapy. Of all the agents employed, prednisone has effects that are easiest to assess, and in large doses it is effective for the reversal of rejection. In general, 30 to 40 mg prednisone is given immediately prior to or at the time of transplantation, and the dosage is gradually reduced. The side effects of the glucocorticoids, particularly impairment of wound healing and predisposition to infection, make it desirable to taper the dose as rapidly as possible in the immediate postoperative period. Customarily, methylprednisolone, 0.5 to 1.0 g intravenously, is administered immediately upon diagnosis of beginning rejection and continued once daily for 3 days. When the drug is effective, the results are usually apparent within 96 h. Such "pulse" doses are less effective in chronic rejection. Most patients whose renal function is stable after 6 months or a year do not require large doses of prednisone; maintenance doses of 10 to 20 mg/d are the rule. Many patients tolerate an alternate-day course of steroids without an increased risk of rejection.

A major effect of steroids is on the monocyte-macrophage system, preventing the release of IL-6 and IL-1. Lymphopenia after large doses of glucocorticoids is primarily due to sequestration of recirculating blood lymphocytes to lymphoid tissue.

Cyclosporine is a fungal peptide with potent immunosuppressive activity. It appears to have a preferential effect on early activation of helper-inducer T lymphocytes, thereby sparing suppressor T cell responses. Although it works alone, cyclosporine is more effective in conjunction with glucocorticoids. Since cyclosporine blocks production of IL-2 by helper-inducer (CD4+) T cells, its combination with

FIGURE 238-4 Overall scheme of the development of effector mechanisms in graft rejection. A set of bone marrow precursor stem cells is selected in the thymus gland to become mature thymus-derived (T) lymphocytes which are clonally determined to recognize non-self antigens (Δ) presented as fragments bound to self major histocompatibility molecules. These antigen-presenting structures are on the surfaces of macrophages, dendritic cells, and B lymphocytes. In transplantation, major histocompatibility antigens, such as HLA, may be recognized directly as the antigen-presenting molecules present in the grafted tissues or as fragments of donor HLA presented by recipient antigen-presenting cells. In avian species, but not in mammals, an anatomic site called the *bursa of Fabricius* provides the differentiating stimuli for maturation of B lymphocytes from bone marrow precursors. B lymphocytes with immunoglubulin receptors for a given antigen (Δ) proliferate and differentiate by a process of somatic mutation of immunoglobulin genes and selection by antigen for further growth. They begin to secrete IgM and, subsequently, IgG, IgE, and IgA. The response matures with help from T lymphocytes, which includes elaboration of the cytokines IL-4, IL-5, and IL-2. The proliferative phases of T and B lymphocyte response are illustrated by the lymphoblast.

Humoral immunity produces tissue injury following binding of immunoglobulins to tissue and, in particular, to the endothelium of a transplanted organ. Complement activation and chemotaxis of polymorphonuclear cells (PMN) are common in "hyperacute" rejection lesions when recipients have antidonor antibodies. Cell-mediated immunity is principally mediated by T lymphocytes bearing receptors for tissue antigens. These cells receive a major degree of help initially from macrophages that secrete the cytokines IL-6 and IL-1. Expanded populations of graft-specific T lymphocytes exert tissue damage by a delayed type hypersensitivity mechanism or by direct cytotoxic "killer" mechanisms. As noted in text, the T lymphocyte CD4 or CD8 phenotypes indicate whether the target antigens are HLA class II or class I, respectively.

The principal growth factor for T lymphocytes is an autocrine product, IL-2. Other T cell products include cytokines, such as interferon γ and tumor necrosis factor, which increase the pace of tissue injury. Activated macrophages can add nonspecifically to the inflammatory process. Natural killer cells (NK) play a minor role; however, they, along with other cells that bear receptors for the Fc portion of immunoglobulin, can provide cell-mediated target damage after fixation to IgG molecules previously bound to grafted cells (antibody-dependent cell-mediated cytotoxicity—ADCC). Any of these mechanisms can result in vascular occlusion by platelet aggregation and thrombosis (see also Fig. 64-5).

steroids is expected to produce a double block in the macrophage → IL-1 → T cell → IL-2 sequence. As noted, clinical results with several thousands of renal transplants have been impressive. Of its toxic effects (nephrotoxicity, hepatotoxicity, hirsutism, tremor, gingival hyperplasia), only nephrotoxicity presents a serious management problem and is discussed further below.

Antibodies to lymphocytes When serum from animals made immune to host lymphocytes is injected into the recipient, a marked suppression of cellular immunity to the tissue graft results. The action on cell-mediated immunity is greater than on humoral immunity. A globulin fraction of serum (antilymphocyte globulin—ALG) is the agent generally employed. For use in humans, peripheral human lymphocytes, thymocytes, or lymphocytes from spleens or thoracic duct fistulas have been injected into horses, rabbits, or goats to produce antilymphocyte serum, from which the globulin fraction is then separated. Although ALG or ATG (antithymocyte globulin) is unquestionably effective in prolonging grafts in animals, its efficacy in the transplantation of human tissue is less clear, since it varies from source to source. Heterologous antibody against defined T lymphocyte subsets, in the form of mouse antihuman monoclonal antibody, may offer a more precise form of therapy. OKT3, in common clinical use, is such an antibody. It is directed to the CD3 molecules which form a portion of the T cell antigen-receptor complex; hence CD3 is expressed on all mature T cells. CD4 or CD8 molecules also form part of the fully activated cluster of molecules, and monoclonal antibodies to these offer the potential for more selective

FIGURE 238-5 Biopsy of the renal cadaveric allograft illustrating oblitera-tive endarteritis. Loss of the media is associated with intimal thickening. The elastic tissue shows dissolution of the elastica. The evidence for arteritis with subsequent thrombosis is typically the gaps in the elastica and media. The intimal thickening probably represents organization of a thrombus formed in response to the arteritis. (*From GJ Dammin, JP Merrill, in Structural Basis for Renal Disease, EL Becker (ed), New York, Hoeber-Harper, 1968.*)

targeting of T cell subsets. Another approach to more selective therapy is to target the 55-kDa beta chain of the IL-2 receptor, expressed only on T cells that have been recently activated. When the antibody is administered during the first 10 days after transplantation, a temporary protection from rejection is obtained. Clinical trials of genetically engineered ''humanized'' monoclonal antibodies are in progress. This approach offers the possibility of improved clearance and destruction of the targeted lymphocytes and reduced potential for development of human antimouse antibodies (HAMA). The latter response limits the efficacy of monoclonal antibody therapy. The destruction of targeted cells also can be improved by conjugation of antibodies with a cellular toxin, such as ricin.

Other techniques Thoracic duct lymph drainage, removal of thymus or spleen, and local irradiation of the transplanted kidney have been abandoned. Fractional total-lymph-node irradiation (TLI), as employed in the therapy of Hodgkin's disease, is under investigation.

CLINICAL COURSE AND MANAGEMENT OF THE RECIPIENT
Bilateral nephrectomy at some point prior to transplantation is performed for a specific cause but not as a routine. Hypertension which is difficult to control or infection involving the end-stage kidneys are the two most common indications. Nephrectomized patients maintain a much lower hematocrit, but this is no longer considered a disadvantage because of the availability of recombinant EPO. Nephrectomy per se does not appear to affect the survival of subsequent renal allografts.

Adequate hemodialysis should be performed within 48 h of surgery, and care should be taken that the serum potassium level is not markedly elevated so that intraoperative cardiac arrhythmias can be averted. The diuresis that commonly occurs postoperatively must be carefully monitored; in some instances it may be massive, reflecting the inability of ischemic tubules to regulate sodium and water excretion; with large diureses, massive potassium losses may occur. Most chronically uremic patients have some excess of extracellular fluid, and some degree of diuresis should be promoted, provided hemodynamics remain stable. Acute tubular necrosis (ATN) may cause immediate oliguria or may follow an initial short period of graft function. ATN is most likely when cadaveric donors have been hypotensive or if the interval between cessation of blood flow and organ harvest (warm ischemic time) is more than a few minutes. Recovery usually occurs within 3 weeks, although periods as long as 6 weeks have been reported. Superimposition of rejection on ATN is common, and the differential diagnosis may be difficult. Cyclosporine therapy prolongs ATN, and some patients do not diurese until they are switched to azathioprine. Many centers avoid starting cyclosporine for the first several days, using ALG or a monoclonal antibody along with azathioprine and prednisone until renal function is established.

The rejection episode Early diagnosis of rejection allows prompt institution of therapy to preserve renal function and prevent irreversible damage due to fibrosis. Clinical evidence of rejection may be characterized by fever, swelling, and tenderness over the allograft and by significant reduction in urine volume. The use of cyclosporine blunts such inflammatory signs. In patients whose renal function is good initially, oliguria may be accompanied by decreased urinary sodium concentration and increased osmolarity. These changes may not be present in the more chronic stages of rejection or when renal function is impaired at the onset of rejection.

Arteriography and radioactive iodohippurate sodium renograms of the transplanted kidney may be useful in ascertaining changes in the renal vasculature and in renal blood flow, even in the absence of urinary flow. Diagnostic ultrasound is the procedure of choice to rule out urinary obstruction or to confirm the presence of perirenal collections of urine, blood, or lymph. When renal function has been good initially, a rise in the serum creatinine level and a decrease in the creatinine clearance is the most sensitive and reliable indicator of possible rejection and may be the only sign.

Cyclosporine may cause deterioration in renal function in a manner similar to a rejection episode. In fact, rejection processes tend to be more indolent with cyclosporine, and the only way to make a diagnosis may be by renal biopsy. Cyclosporine has an afferent arteriolar constrictor effect on the kidney and, in addition, may produce permanent vascular and interstitial injury after sustained high-dose therapy. There is no universally accepted lesion(s) which makes a diagnosis of cyclosporine toxicity, although interstitial fibrosis and thickening of arteriolar walls have been noted by some. Basically, if the biopsy does not reveal moderate and active cellular rejection activity, the serum creatinine will most likely respond to a reduction in cyclosporine dose. Blood levels of drug can be useful if very high or very low but do not correlate precisely with renal function. If rejection activity is present in the biopsy, appropriate therapy is indicated.

OKT3 monoclonal antibody, given intravenously for 10 to 14 days, is effective in more than 90 percent of first rejections, although it is less effective if methylprednisolone pulses have failed and in cases of severe recurrent rejection activity. A major problem with OKT3 is that severe systemic reactions may be produced during the first day or two of therapy. Chills, fever, hypotension, and headache are the direct result of the antibody effects on the targeted T cells, most likely related to the known potential of OKT3 to activate T cells nonspecifically. If the antibody is administered to overhydrated oliguric patients, pulmonary edema may be induced. These reactions are not characteristic of other monoclonal antibodies, such as those to the IL-2 receptor. Recurrent or rebound rejection activity may require additional therapy. In such circumstances, methylprednisolone may be effective even though it failed initially. Second courses of OKT3 may be given in spite of antimouse antibodies generated in response to the first course if the titers are low and the human antibodies are not directed to the combining-site region (idiotype) of the OKT3.

Management problems Modification of the usual clinical manifestations of infection by immunosuppressive therapy is a major problem in the posttransplant period. The major toxic effect of azathioprine is bone marrow suppression, while cyclosporine has no marrow effects. They both may predispose to unusual opportunistic infections, however. The signs and symptoms of infection may be masked and distorted, and fever without obvious cause is common. Only after days or weeks will it become apparent that it has a viral or fungal origin. Bacterial infections are most common during the first month after transplantation. The importance of blood cultures in such patients cannot be overemphasized, because systemic infection without obvious foci is frequent, although wound infections with or without urinary fistulas are most common. Particularly ominous are rapidly occurring pulmonary lesions, which may result in death within 5 days of onset. When these become apparent, immunosuppressive agents should be discontinued, except for maintenance doses of prednisone. Aggressive diagnostic procedures, including transbronchial and open lung biopsy, are frequently indicated. In the case of *Pneumocystis carinii* (Chap. 178) infection, trimethoprim-sulfamethoxazole is the treatment of choice; amphotericin B has been used effectively in systemic fungal infections. Prophylaxis against *P. carinii* with daily low-dose trimethoprim-sulfamethoxazole is very effective. Involvement of the oropharynx with *Candida* (Chap. 166) may be treated with local nystatin. Small doses (a total of 300 mg) of amphotericin given over a period of 2 weeks may be effective in refractory oral candidiasis. *Aspergillus* (Chap. 167), *Nocardia* (Chap. 126), and cytomegalovirus (CMV) (Chap. 146) infections also occur. CMV is a common and dangerous infection in transplant recipients. It does not generally appear until the end of the first posttransplant month. Active CMV infection is sometimes associated, or occasionally confused, with rejection episodes. Patients at highest risk for severe CMV disease are those without anti-CMV antibodies who receive a graft from a CMV antibody–positive donor (15 percent mortality). Serial intravenous administration of high-titer CMV immune globulin is effective in reducing this risk. Prophylactic use of acyclovir and other antiviral agents is under study. Treatment of active CMV disease with ganciclovir is generally effective. Severe CMV disease is common after treatment with OKT3, and concurrent treatment with ganciclovir during OKT3 administration appears to be effective for prophylaxis of CMV activation. The complications of glucocorticoid therapy are well known and include gastrointestinal bleeding, impairment of wound healing, osteoporosis, diabetes mellitus, cataract formation, and hemorrhagic pancreatitis. The treatment of jaundice in transplant patients should include cessation of azathioprine or cyclosporine if hepatitis or drug toxicity is suspected. It is surprising that cessation of azathioprine or cyclosporine therapy in such circumstances often does not result in rejection of a graft, at least for several weeks. Antiplatelet agents and anticoagulants, although effective in theory, have not been successful in the prevention of the chronic vascular lesion. Persistent elevation of serum creatinine levels above 220 μmol/L (2.5 mg/dL) in patients on cyclosporine is an indication for dose reduction, particularly if cyclosporine blood levels are elevated. Some centers convert patients from cyclosporine to azathioprine after 6 to 12 months, but some patients have rejection episodes, and some of those lose their grafts. The alternative to conversion is to use lower doses of cyclosporine indefinitely. The risk of long-term cumulative toxicity to the kidney now seems to be low. Reduction of cyclosporine is best accomplished by routine use of "triple therapy," in which the following dose levels are used for maintenance after 6 to 8 months: cyclosporine, 3 to 5 mg/kg of body weight per day; azathioprine, 1.0 to 1.5 mg/kg per day; prednisone, 0.15 to 0.20 mg/kg per day. Many patients do well on cyclosporine and prednisone in these dose ranges, without azathioprine. In general, minimal or no

rejection during the first 6 months after transplantation is a predictor of safety in reducing immunosuppression therapy over subsequent months to years.

Despite the potential teratogenic effects of immunosuppressive agents, both women and men have become parents after transplantation. The incidence of congenital abnormalities in the offspring is not increased.

Glomerular lesions Even identical twins, who do not require immunosuppression, may develop glomerular lesions after transplantation. Glomerular lesions occur in 10 to 15 percent of allografts, even when the original disease was accidental removal of a solitary kidney. The pathogenesis is related to a chronic rejection process. In other cases the lesions resemble those of the original disease. The recurrence of the nephrotic syndrome with "nil disease" in transplanted kidneys whose recipient's original nil disease had progressed to renal failure with focal sclerosis, and the recurrence in renal allografts of the classic lesions of IgA nephropathy and of membranoproliferative glomerulonephritis with electron-dense deposit disease are examples. In the last of these, the incidence of recurrence has been reported to be as high as 30 to 40 percent. In most instances, the recurrence of the original renal lesions represents no threat to the immediate prognosis, and a primary diagnosis of glomerulonephritis is rarely a contraindication to transplantation.

Malignancy The incidence of tumors in patients on immunosuppressive therapy is 5 to 6 percent, or approximately 100 times greater than that in the general population of the same age range. The most common lesions are cancer of the skin and lips and carcinoma in situ of the cervix, as well as lymphomas, such as non-Hodgkin's lymphomas. The risks are increased in proportion to the total immunosuppressive load administered.

Other complications *Hypercalcemia* after transplantation may indicate failure of hyperplastic parathyroid glands to regress. Aseptic necrosis of the head of the femur is probably due to preexisting hyperparathyroidism, with aggravation by glucocorticoid treatment. With improved management of calcium and phosphorus metabolism during chronic dialysis, the incidence of parathyroid-related complications has fallen dramatically.

Hypertension may be caused by (1) native kidneys, (2) rejection activity in the transplant, (3) renal artery stenosis, if an end-to-end anastomosis was constructed with an iliac artery branch, and (4) renal cyclosporine toxicity. The latter may improve with reduction in cyclosporine dose. Whereas angiotensin-converting enzyme inhibitors may be useful, calcium channel blockers are frequently more effective in cyclosporine-treated patients.

Chronic hepatitis, particularly when due to hepatitis B virus, can be a progressive, fatal disease over a decade or so. Patients who are persistently HBsAg-positive are at higher risk, according to some studies, but the presence of hepatitis C is also a concern when one embarks on a course of immunosuppression in a transplant recipient.

Both chronic dialysis and renal transplant patients have a higher incidence of death from myocardial infarction and stroke than in the population at large, and this is particularly true in diabetics. Contributing factors are hypertension and hypertriglyceridemia. Increased low-density lipoprotein cholesterol and depressed high-density lipoprotein cholesterol concentrations may be exaggerated after transplantation and require treatment.

REFERENCES

BARTLETT RH et al: Continuous arteriovenous hemofiltration: Improved survival in surgical acute renal failure? Surgery 100:400, 1986

DAUGIRDAS JT: Dialysis hypotension: A hemodynamic analysis. Kidney Int 39:233, 1991

HERBELIN A et al: Influence of uremia and hemodialysis on circulating interleukin-1 and tumor necrosis factor α. Kidney Int 37:116, 1990

INSTITUTE OF MEDICINE SPECIAL REPORT: The Medicare end-stage renal disease program. N Engl J Med 324:1143, 1991

LOWRIE EG et al: Effect of the hemodialysis prescription on patient morbidity. N Engl J Med 305:1176, 1981

Lowrie EG, Lew NL: Death risk in hemodialysis patients: The predictive value of commonly measured variables and an evaluation of death rate differences between facilities. Am J Kidney Dis 15:458, 1990

Nolph KD: Continuous ambulatory peritoneal dialysis as long-term treatment for end-stage renal disease. Am J Kidney Dis 17:154, 1991

Novello AC: Ethical, social, and financial aspects of end stage renal disease, in *The Kidney*, 4th ed, B Brenner, F Rector (eds). Philadelphia, Saunders, 1991, p 2424

Opelz G: HLA matching should be utilized for improving kidney transplant success rates. Transplant Proc 23:46, 1991

Palder SB et al: Vascular access for hemodialysis: Patency rates and results of revision. Ann Surg 202:235, 1985

Ramos EL et al: Clinical aspects of renal transplantation, in *The Kidney*, 4th ed, B Brenner, F Rector (eds). Philadelphia, Saunders, 1991, p 2361

Strom TB, Carpenter CB: Immunobiology of kidney transplantation, in *The Kidney*, 4th ed, B Brenner, F Rector (eds). Philadelphia, Saunders, 1991, p 2336

Teehan BP et al: A quantitative approach to the CAPD prescription. Peritoneal Dialysis Bulletin, July-September 1985, p 152

Teraska PI (ed): *Clinical Transplants 1991*. Los Angeles, UCLA Tissue Typing Laboratory, 1991

239   IMMUNOPATHOGENIC MECHANISMS OF RENAL INJURY

RICHARD J. GLASSOCK / BARRY M. BRENNER

Immunologic events play an important role in many forms of renal injury, especially those involving the glomerular circulation. While investigation of animal models of disease has provided insight into these immunologic processes, the specific etiologic factors and pathogenetic pathways in human disease are incompletely understood.

Immune renal injury may be broadly divided into the initiating events and the processes that mediate tissue injury. The initiating events can be further categorized according to the site of the immune interaction (e.g., within the tissue or organ affected or within the general circulation) or according to the nature of the aberrant immune response (e.g., humoral or cell-mediated immunity).

The mechanisms for development of autoreactivity to self-antigens (autoimmunity) have been only partially elucidated but involve a failure of processes that maintain self-tolerance. Environmental factors, such as drugs and microbial organisms, interact with a predisposing genetic milieu in the pathogenesis of autoimmune disorders. Many conditions associated with the development of autoreactivity are associated with specific genes within the major histocompatability (HLA) complex on chromosome 6. Circulating antibody derived from an expanded B cell clone may react with its respective glomerular antigen in situ to initiate a cascade of events ultimately leading to structural and/or functional alterations in the glomerular circulation. The antigen may be an intrinsic constituent of the kidney or one that has been bound or "planted" in the renal tissue by virtue of a particular biochemical or immunologic affinity. Depending on the nature of the antigen, this category of injury is often referred to as an *antitissue antibody–mediated* or an *in situ immune-complex–mediated disease*. The intrinsic (native) antigens may be either insoluble, slowly renewable components of the extracellular matrix (e.g., basement membrane) or a soluble component of the cell intimately associated with the matrix components. On the other hand, bound or "planted" antigens can be derived from diverse sources, both endogenous and exogenous. The reaction of circulating antibody with an intrinsic or planted antigen can give rise to a variety of structural alterations and immunohistochemical features, as discussed below.

Antibody also may react with soluble intrinsic or extrinsic antigens in the general circulation, giving rise to macromolecular aggregates of antigen and antibody of varying size (i.e., circulating immune complexes). These immune complexes may localize and deposit in a variety of organs and tissues, including the kidney, and thereby invoke injury. This mechanism is often referred to as *circulating immune-complex disease*. Unlike antitissue antibody disease, the pathogenetic immune complexes need not bear any special immunochemical relationship with renal structures; indeed, the kidney is best viewed as passively damaged by immune events occurring outside the kidney. Immune-complex–induced disease can give rise to a variety of structural and immunohistochemical defects.

Cell-mediated processes independent of humoral immunity were originally believed to play only minor roles in renal injury. However, based on animal experiments, several disorders not readily explainable by an antibody-dependent mechanism may be caused by aberrant T cell–dependent events. Furthermore, even in disorders believed to be primarily due to antibody-dependent mechanisms, T cell–mediated renal injury may be an important component. In distinction to antibody-dependent mechanisms, the precise nature of the antigen and the details of the cellular interactions responsible for tissue injury still remain to be resolved in cell-mediated processes. Both antibody-dependent and cell-mediated reactions to the same antigen may occur simultaneously, since both reactions are activated concomitantly in most immune events.

Although antibodies, immune complexes, and activated cells can injure tissue independently, the outcome of immune-mediated renal injury is to a great extent conditioned by the secondary mediator systems called into play. These mediator systems also can be broadly divided into humoral and cellular categories (Table 239-1). Humoral mediators are derived from circulating precursor proteins or through the *de novo* synthesis of peptides or lipids. Complement and coagulation proteins are examples of the former, and vasoactive peptides, cytokines, growth factors, and eicosanoids are examples of the latter. Polymorphonuclear leukocytes, eosinophils, monocytes, macrophages, and platelets constitute the cellular mediators of injury. Through interaction with humoral mediators (e.g., complement, cytokines, platelet-activating factor), they are activated and release local factors that enhance tissue injury (e.g., toxic oxygen radicals, membrane-bound procoagulants, cationic proteins, enzymes, growth factors, and interleukins). The activation of cells also induces the expression on the cell surface of molecules that enhance their adhesion to vascular endothelium, thus promoting their migration and localization within sites of tissue injury. Both humoral and cell mediators can directly influence renal hemodynamics, capillary wall permeability, and tubular function. Complement activation can lead to the release of chemoattractant peptides and permeability factors and result in cytolysis or functional alterations of glomerular cells. Localized coagulation can further interfere with cell or organ function. Infiltrating leukocytes, called forth by complement-dependent or complement-independent mechanisms, can foster the local production of toxic oxygen radicals and promote the release of cytokines, growth factors, and degradative enzymes. Platelet activation and aggregation promote thrombosis and release mitogenic and growth factors locally. Monocytes and macrophages release interleukins, eicosanoids, and

TABLE 239-1   Mediators of glomerular injury

Soluble	Cellular
Complement components (C3, C5b-C9)	Polymorphonuclear leukocytes
Coagulation proteins (fibrinogen)	Monocytes (macrophages)
Cytokines (IL-1, IL-2, IL-6), tumor necrosis factor, interferon	Lymphocytes (T cells), platelets
Growth factors (transforming growth factor, platelet-derived growth factor)	
Platelet-activating factor	
Eicosanoids (prostaglandins, thromboxane, leukotrienes, lipoxins)	
Vasoactive peptides and amines (angiotensin, histamine)	
Reactive oxygen species	

procoagulant factors. Many of these mediator systems are held in check by naturally occurring inhibitors, e.g., toxic oxygen radical scavengers or enzyme inhibitors.

The mediators utilized for injury vary according to the nature of the immunologic attack and the site of the immune interaction. The final outcome of disease, i.e., complete healing or progressive disease, depends both on the initiating events and on the nature, intensity, and degree of the mediator response. Thus a single initiating event can lead to a self-limited injury that heals without defect or a relentlessly progressive disease that eventually destroys the tissue or organ. T cells and/or macrophages, either or both, are major participants in cell-mediated immune injury. T cells can be involved in the direct cytolysis of glomerular cells or, by virtue of the release of cytokines, may call forth a cascade of supporting cells or molecules. Immunologic specificity is conferred by the ability of T cell receptors to react with an antigenic peptide presented by the major histocompatibility complex molecule on other cells such as macrophages. Because all the elements necessary for a cell-mediated immune response are present within the kidney, indeed within the glomerulus itself, there is no requirement for delivery of sensitized, activated T cells from the circulation, although such activation is likely in many renal diseases. Finally, even with subsidence of the initiating immune events and quiescence of the inflammatory process, ongoing damage can be perpetuated by nonimmune, noninflammatory factors such as hypertension, vascular disease, atherosclerotic events at the microvascular level, or maladaptive processes arising from attempts to compensate for the loss of functioning nephron mass. These nonimmune factors may constitute an important determinant of the outcome of an immune-mediated renal injury.

ANTITISSUE ANTIBODY–INDUCED GLOMERULAR INJURY

Anti-basement membrane antibody disease The classic prototype of an antitissue antibody–mediated renal disease is that produced by reaction of a circulating autoantibody (usually of the IgG isotype) with a fixed, native, insoluble basement membrane antigen, often called *anti-basement membrane antibody disease*. The antigen involved in the classic variety involving the glomerulus is a product of a gene on chromosome 2 that encodes a noncollagenous lobular domain on the alpha-3 chain of type IV collagen. This domain is involved in the cross-linking of type IV basement membrane collagen and is in glomerular and tubular basement membranes and in other organs, such as the lung. Reaction of antibody with lung basement membrane antigens may give rise to pulmonary hemorrhage. *Goodpasture's disease* is defined by the presence of anti-basement membrane autoantibody to the noncollagenous domain of type IV collagen, pulmonary hemorrhage, and often glomerulonephritis. *Goodpasture's syndrome*, on the other hand, may be more broadly defined as any circumstance where pulmonary hemorrhage and glomerular injury are found concomitantly. The production of autoantibodies to particular basement membrane epitopes is the characteristic that defines Goodpasture's disease. Immunohistochemically, this disorder is characterized by linear deposits of IgG along the glomerular capillary wall. Ready access of this site to inflammatory mediators both of a cellular and humoral nature explains the participation of leukocytes, platelets, complement, and coagulation in the resultant immune injury. Other basement membrane constituents, such as laminin, intactin, and heparan sulfate proteoglycan, also could be targets of an antitissue antibody response, but such reactions provoking disease are rare in humans.

Antibody to non-basement membrane antigens The glomerulus is a complex structure composed of cellular (endothelial, mesangial, and epithelial cells) and matrix elements. Cell-surface antigens of the cellular elements can serve as targets for antitissue antibody responses. One of these, the so-called Heymann antigen, evokes a particular form of renal disease. The reaction of a circulating autoantibody with a high-molecular-weight glycoprotein (Gp330) in the clatherin-coated endocytotic pits of visceral epithelial cells results in the formation of immune complexes in situ. Presumably, IgG autoantibodies percolate through the glomerular basement membrane,

where they encounter their respective antigen on the surface of the visceral epithelial cells. An in situ immune complex is formed and shed into the surrounding subepithelial space. Newly synthesized antigen continually reacts with newly arriving antibody, and the immune complexes eventually grow to an ultrastructurally visible size, forming the subepithelial, electron-dense immune deposits characteristic of the disorder. Eventually, new basement membrane synthesis leads to thickening of the capillary wall. In this instance, the location of the immune reaction diminishes the opportunity for cellular mediators to participate, but soluble mediators, such as complement, cause functional alterations in the capillary wall, particularly enhanced permeability.

Mesangial cells also may be damaged by antibody- and complement-dependent processes, but because of the location of the immune events, greater involvement of other cells, such as monocytes and platelets, may occur.

Antibodies reacting with planted glomerular antigens Circulating endogenous or environmental substances with special affinity for glomerular structures, including the glomerular capillary wall or mesangium, may deposit in these structures and thus act as a "planted" antigen. An antibody or cellular response to these planted nonglomerular or extrinsic antigens could result in disease as a result of the formation of antigen-antibody complexes in situ. The pattern of disease produced depends on the sites of the planted antigen and the nature of the immune response. Examples of such planted antigens thus far described include certain drugs, plant lectins, cationized plasma proteins, aggregated immunoglobulins, and deoxyribonucleic acid. Experimental models of this sequence have been described, but there is little definitive information regarding comparable mechanisms in humans.

CIRCULATING IMMUNE-COMPLEX DISEASE (See Chap. 283)

The deposition in the kidney of immune complexes formed in the circulation accounts for many diseases of the kidney for which there is clear evidence of participation of some immunologic process. In this category, an immunogenic replicating or nonreplicating substance arises in the circulation either from an endogenous (autologous) or exogenous (environmental) source. An antibody response to the antigen while the antigen remains in the circulation leads to the formation of an aggregate of antigen and antibody known as a *circulating immune complex*. The complement system plays an important role in the transport and removal of circulating immune complexes, and defects in the complement system may predispose to the deposition and accumulation of immune complexes at various tissue sites, including the glomerulus. Activated complement components, particularly C1q and C3b, interfere with the precipitation of immune complexes or solubilize preformed immune complexes, thus preventing their deposition as insoluble aggregates. Circulating immune complexes containing bound C3b are transported to the mononuclear phagocyte system (liver, spleen) via the erythrocyte CR1 receptor. Such transport and delivery favor uptake and degradation of immune complexes by the mononuclear phagocyte system. A small fraction of circulating immune complexes may escape removal by the mononuclear phagocyte system and instead be trapped by vascular structures, including the glomeruli. Circulating immune complexes trapped in these sites have the capability of evoking inflammation utilizing many of the mediator systems described above. One of the best-studied examples of this circulating immune-complex disease involving a nonreplicating antigen is serum sickness, which results from the acute or chronic administration of an immunogenic, soluble, heterologous, foreign serum protein (see Fig. 283-1). A small portion of the immune complexes localize within the glomerular mesangium; in the walls of peripheral capillaries; and in joints, heart valves, choroid plexus, splenic sinusoids, and larger blood vessels, particularly at sites of turbulent flow. Once deposited, these complexes evoke an inflammatory response at the site of deposition.

Although this formulation presupposes that immune complexes form within the circulation and then are deposited in vascular structures, immune complexes may form in the extravascular (intersti-

FIGURE 239-1 *A.* Immunofluorescence photomicrograph of a portion of a glomerulus from a patient with anti-glomerular basement membrane antibody–mediated glomerular injury. Note the linear deposits (fluorescein-labeled antihuman IgG). *B.* Immunofluorescence photomicrograph of a portion of a glomerulus from a patient with immune-complex–mediated (in situ or circulating) glomerular injury. Note the irregular, granular deposits (fluorescein-labeled antihuman IgG). *C.* Electron micrograph of a portion of a glomerular capillary from a patient with immune-complex–mediated glomerular injury. Note the electron-dense deposits, *D.*

tial) compartment by virtue of diffusion into this fluid compartment of cell-derived antigens and circulating antibody. Such a phenomenon may explain the deposition of immune complexes in the interstitial areas of the kidney, with relative sparing of the glomerular circulation. Regardless of the nature of the antibody or antigen or the particular circumstances surrounding the immunologic events, a clue to the presence of immune-complex deposition or in situ formation is the morphologic pattern found when tissues are examined by immunofluorescence or electron-microscopic techniques. Granular, discontinuous, and irregular deposits of Ig, often in conjunction with complement components, are found by immunofluorescence (Fig. 239-1*B*), whereas electron-dense deposits are seen by electron microscopy (Fig. 239-1*C*). As indicated above, such deposits are not proof of origin in the circulation, since the formation of immune complexes in situ may produce similar deposits, particularly on the subepithelial aspect of the glomerular capillary wall. Sometimes these deposits acquire a definite substructure, but for the most part they are rather homogeneous. The deposits may develop in several locations within the glomerulus: beneath the epithelial cells (subepithelial), within the basement membrane (intramembranous), beneath the endothelium (subendothelial), and within the mesangial matrix. Immune complexes also may localize in the peritubular capillary network. The reason for localization at these different sites may involve factors such as size or charge of the complexes, receptors for the Fc or complement components within glomerular structures, or local hemodynamic events. The deposits appear to increase in size by cross-linking and aggregation, and glomerular cells may participate in their removal. The persistence of deposits is related to the rate of formation balanced by the activity of removal systems. Ig itself in a circulating immune complex trapped in the glomerular circulation may behave as a planted antigen, either via the idiotypic determinants in the antigen-binding sites of antibody or via the Fc portions evoking an anti-immunoglobulin (rheumatoid factor) response. The roles played by anti-idiotype antibody or rheumatoid factor in the evolution of glomerular lesions in immune-complex–mediated disease is not clear. Once deposited in glomeruli, circulating immune complexes evoke local inflammatory and functional changes, which at least for the glomerular circulation may be relatively independent of complement or polymorphonuclear leukocytes. Infiltrating monocytes may play a critical role in mediating glomerular injury. In situ formation of an immune complex in the subepithelial space may not be associated with the accumulation of inflammatory cells. The morphologic lesions which result from immune-complex deposition may vary considerably from diffuse proliferative to nonproliferative membranous or sclerosing lesions. Coagulation, platelet aggregation, cellular infiltration with cytokine and growth factor release, and release of vasoactive amines may participate in determining the pattern of morphologic response.

The *exogenous* antigens involved in circulating immune-complex–mediated disease are derived chiefly from infectious agents such as bacteria, viruses, or parasites. Replication of the organism provides a continuing source of antigen. The best-studied examples of these in humans are *infective endocarditis, leprosy, syphilis, hepatitis B,* and *malaria.* The *endogenous* antigens involved in human disease vary considerably and include *DNA, thyroglobulin, autologous immunoglobulins, erythrocyte stroma, renal tubule antigens,* and *tumor-specific* or *tumor-associated* antigens.

CELL-MEDIATED IMMUNITY IN GLOMERULAR AND TUBULOINTERSTITIAL DISEASES Monocytes (macrophages) and T cells participate actively in both the initiation and mediation of glomerular and tubulointerstitial injury. These cells are present in large numbers in the glomerulus and interstitium in many forms of glomerulonephritis and tubulointerstitial nephritis. Interference with the accumulation of these cells within the kidney may ameliorate the clinical and morphologic manifestations of disease. Recruitment of these cells to the sites of injury involves complement components, various cytokines, chemoattractant lipids, and adhesion molecules. The mechanisms by which these cells induce injury is not clear. Macrophages probably exert their deleterious effect in an immunologically nonspecific fashion by releasing cytokines (e.g., interleukin 1, tumor necrosis factor, interleukin 6), growth factors (transforming growth factor, platelet-derived growth factor), proteolytic enzymes, and reactive oxygen species. T cells may exert a damaging effect in an immunologically specific fashion by recognizing foreign antigens presented in association with class II major histocompatibility complex molecules and subsequently by direct cytolysis. In addition, T cells may participate in injury by elaborating factors that promote the infiltration of tissue by other damaging cells, such as macrophages. T cells also may promote fibrogenesis directly. Little is known about the specific nature of the T cell effector and the autoantigens that cause cell-mediated immunity in human disease. Glomerular diseases that lack the typical hallmarks of antibody-mediated disease, such as immunoglobulin deposits, are candidates for cell-mediated mechanisms. Minimal change disease associated with idiopathic nephrotic syndrome is such a candidate disease, and T cells may play a role in this disorder. The rejection of renal allografts and several forms of hypersensitivity interstitial nephritis are probably dependent on cell-mediated immunity.

COMPLEMENT-ASSOCIATED GLOMERULAR INJURY Although there is little evidence that complement activation, independent of antitissue antibody or circulating immune complexes, can bring about glomerular injury, there are certain associations between complement and renal disease. The clinicopathologic entity known as *idiopathic membranoproliferative glomerulonephritis* (see also Chap. 240) may be associated with serum complement deposition within glomeruli suggestive of involvement of the alternative pathway of complement activation, perhaps independent of immune-complex deposition. These patterns are not necessarily unique to this group of disorders, since they also may be observed in postinfectious glomerulonephritides and in certain collagen-vascular diseases.

In *idiopathic membranoproliferative glomerulonephritis*, particularly the subset known as *dense deposit disease*, serum C3 levels are depressed; C4, C1, and C2 levels tend to be normal; and C3 may be deposited in glomeruli without Ig (see also Chap. 240). In addition, an autoantibody (an immunoconglutinin) to alternative pathway C3 convertase is frequently found in the circulation. This autoantibody reacts with a conformational neoantigen of the alternative pathway C3 convertase and stabilizes this enzyme from the influence of C3b inactivator and the inhibitor protein β_1H in a fashion similar to properdin. As a result, sera containing this autoantibody are capable of inducing C3 cleavage in vitro by permitting the assembly of a stable fluid-phase C3 convertase. This antibody is also known as *C3 nephritic factor* (C3NeF) and was first described in patients with glomerulonephritis and persistent depression of C3 levels.

The relationship between these aberrations in the complement pathway and glomerular injury is uncertain. No experimental models of persistent activation of the alternative pathway are associated with glomerulonephritis; thus glomerular injury may be a closely associated but unrelated phenomenon, perhaps genetically determined. The recognition that certain structural genes for complement components (C2, C4) are closely associated with the major histocompatibility complex provides a potential explanation for the association of disease susceptibility with defects in biosynthesis of complement proteins. On the other hand, persistent hypocomplementemia may interfere with the normal removal processes for environmental antigens such as viruses. Such a defect might favor the persistence of these antigens in the circulation and enhance the likelihood of formation of circulating immune complexes. The discovery that C3 and its degradation products (primarily C3b) are able to solubilize aggregates of antigen and antibody may provide an additional explanation for the occurrence of immune-complex disease in association with defects of complement synthesis or activation.

REFERENCES

COUSER WG: Mechanisms of glomerular injury in immune complex disease. Kidney Int 28:569, 1985

GLASSOCK RJ (ed): A primer in renal immunology. Semin Nephrol 12:377, 1992

GLOTZ D, DRUET P: Immune mechanisms of glomerular damage, in *Oxford Textbook of Clinical Nephrology*, S Cameron et al (eds). Oxford, Oxford University Press, 1991, pp 240–262

WILSON CB: The renal response to immunological injury, in *The Kidney*, 4th ed, BM Brenner, FC Rector Jr (eds). Philadelphia, Saunders, 1991, pp 1062–1181

WILSON CB (ed): Immunopathology of renal disease, in *Contemporary Issues in Nephrology*, vol 18. New York, Churchill Livingstone, 1988, pp 1–297

240 THE MAJOR GLOMERULOPATHIES

RICHARD J. GLASSOCK / BARRY M. BRENNER

Alterations of the structural and functional integrity of the glomerular capillary circulation are often associated with hematuria, proteinuria, reduced glomerular filtration rate (GFR), and hypertension. Five major glomerulopathic syndromes are recognized: *acute glomerulonephritis*, *rapidly progressive glomerulonephritis*, *chronic glomerulonephritis*, the *nephrotic syndrome*, and *asymptomatic urinary abnormalities*. This chapter deals with diseases in which the kidney is either the sole or the predominant organ involved (i.e., the primary glomerulopathies) or is involved as a complication of infection or drug exposure. Glomerular injury associated with multisystem disorders is discussed in Chap. 241.

ACUTE GLOMERULONEPHRITIS

The causes of acute glomerulonephritis (AGN) are given in Table 240-1. The "acute nephritic syndrome" consists of the abrupt onset of *hematuria* and *proteinuria*, often accompanied by *azotemia* (i.e., reduced GFR) and renal *salt and water retention*. If GFR is reduced markedly, oligoanuria may be present (see also Chap. 236). Salt and water retention leads to circulatory congestion, hypertension, and edema. Hematuria is likely the consequence of migration of erythrocytes across damaged glomerular and/or peritubular capillary walls leading to the presence of erythrocytes in tubule fluid in the early part of the nephron. Proteinuria is the consequence of a loss of anionic charges of the capillary wall (charge-selective defect) or the appearance of glomerular capillaries with larger-than-normal pore radius, permitting large plasma protein molecules to traverse the glomerular filter. Glomerular filtration rate is reduced because of infiltration of the capillaries by inflammatory cells or by expansion of the number of intrinsic glomerular cells, which thereby reduce filtering surface area. Alternatively, the filtering surface area could be functionally decreased due to the local elaboration of vasoactive compounds capable of

---

TABLE 240-1 Causes of acute glomerulonephritis

Infectious diseases
  A Poststreptococcal glomerulonephritis*
  B Nonstreptococcal postinfectious glomerulonephritis
    1 Bacterial: infective endocarditis,* "shunt nephritis," sepsis,* pneumococcal pneumonia, typhoid fever, secondary syphilis, meningococcemia
    2 Viral: hepatitis B, infectious mononucleosis, mumps, measles, varicella, vaccinia, echovirus, and coxsackievirus
    3 Parasitic: malaria, toxoplasmosis
Multisystem diseases: systemic lupus erythematosus,* vasculitis,* Henoch-Schönlein purpura,* Goodpasture's disease
Primary glomerular diseases: membranoproliferative glomerulonephritis, Berger's disease (IgA nephropathy),* "pure" mesangial proliferative glomerulonephritis
Miscellaneous: Guillain-Barré syndrome, radiation of Wilms's tumor, diphtheria-pertussis-tetanus vaccine, serum sickness

* Most common causes.

reversibly contracting mesangial cells (e.g., angiotensin II, leuko-trienes), thereby leading to a reduction in the number of perfused glomerular capillaries. Proliferation of visceral or parietal cells admixed with infiltrating cells (monocytes) and polymerized fibrin may obliterate Bowman's space, further impeding filtration. Fluid retention is due both to decreased glomerular filtration rate and to persistence of avid distal nephron salt and water reabsorption. Extracellular and intravascular fluid volumes are expanded by salt and fluid retention.

The edema of acute glomerulonephritis tends to appear initially in areas of low tissue pressure, such as the *periorbital* areas, but may subsequently progress to involve dependent portions of the body and lead to *ascites* and/or *pleural effusions*. *Circulatory congestion* is manifested by an increase in systemic and pulmonary vascular pressures, and a normal or increased cardiac output. If pulmonary capillary pressure rises above the opposing plasma oncotic pressure pulmonary edema may ensue. *Arterial diastolic hypertension* is the consequence of extracellular fluid volume expansion, enhanced cardiac output, and modest increases in peripheral vascular resistance. Plasma renin activity, aldosterone, and the sympathetic nervous system are relatively suppressed. Hypertension may be accompanied by encephalopathy, particularly in young children.

The extent and severity of urinary abnormalities in AGN vary. Gross (macroscopic) *hematuria* is the most common and is often described as smoky-, coffee-, or cola-colored urine. Lesser degrees of hematuria may go unrecognized by the patient or parent; for this reason, the features of fluid retention and hypertension may be ascribed erroneously to other illnesses if examination of the urine sediment is omitted from the initial evaluation. Hematuria is often, but not invariably, accompanied by the excretion of *red cell casts*. The erythrocytes in the urinary sediment are characteristically small, distorted, fragmented, and hypochromic (dysmorphic hematuria). Leukocyturia and leukocyte casts may indicate the presence of inflammation in the glomerulus and interstitium. The degree of *proteinuria* varies according to the nature and severity of the underlying glomerular lesions. Rarely, protein excretion rates are within the normal range, but generally they are between 0.5 and 3 g/d. If proteinuria is marked and sustained, the nephrotic syndrome may appear (see below).

The short-term evolution of acute glomerulonephritis depends upon the underlying glomerular lesions and their treatment. For example, in infective endocarditis resolution of urinary findings and improved renal function may occur rapidly after control of the bacteremia by antimicrobials. Within a week or so of onset, most patients with poststreptococcal acute glomerulonephritis begin to experience spontaneous resolution of fluid retention and hypertension. Urinary abnormalities often take longer to resolve. A few patients with the acute nephritic syndrome will develop a rapidly progressive form of renal failure (i.e., rapidly progressive glomerulonephritis, discussed below). The long-term outlook for patients with AGN is also considered below. Renal biopsy is useful in characterizing the nature of the underlying lesion but need not be done in every case.

ACUTE POSTSTREPTOCOCCAL GLOMERULONEPHRITIS

Clinical features and diagnosis　This disorder is the archetype of AGN. Poststreptococcal glomerulonephritis (PSGN) follows in the wake of *pharyngeal* or *cutaneous infection* with one of a limited number of strains of *group A β-hemolytic streptococci*. These "nephritogenic" streptococci may be identified by serotyping of a cell wall antigen (M protein). Among outbreaks of infection with proved "nephritogenic" strains of streptococci the PSGN attack rate is relatively uniform. Among families, asymptomatic episodes of PSGN exceed symptomatic episodes by a factor of 3 or 4 to 1. Immunity to M protein is type-specific, long-lasting, and protective. Repeated episodes of PSGN are therefore unusual. Outbreaks of pharyngeal infection–associated PSGN are commonest in children aged 6 to 10. AGN following cutaneous streptococcal infection is commonly associated with poor personal hygiene, overcrowding, and concomitant cutaneous disease, such as scabies infestation. Seasonal

and geographic variations in prevalence of PSGN are more marked for pharyngeal- than for cutaneous-associated disease.

An important feature is the existence of a *latent period* between the earliest manifestations of infection and the onset of signs and symptoms of nephritis. Following pharyngeal infections the latent period usually is 6 to 10 days. Cutaneous infections are associated with longer latent periods, averaging about 2 weeks. Signs of glomerular inflammation occurring at the same time as, or shortly after, infection usually indicate *exacerbation* of a preexisting glomerular disease such as Berger's disease (IgA nephropathy).

The diagnosis of PSGN rests upon the demonstration of at least two of the following three features: (1) A group A β-hemolytic streptococcus of a potentially nephritogenic strain is found in a throat or skin lesion. (2) An immune response to one or more of the streptococcal *exoenzymes*, including antistreptolysin O (ASO), anti-streptokinase (ASK), anti-deoxyribonuclease B (ADNAase B), anti-nicotinyl adenine dinucleotidase (ANADase), or antihyaluronidase (AH). ASO responses are typically brisk in pharyngeal infections but often absent in cutaneous infection, whereas AH, ADNAase, and ANADase responses occur after the latter. Testing for multiple antibody responses and serial determinations are necessary to achieve a diagnostic accuracy of 90 percent. Early antimicrobial therapy may prevent the antibody response to exoenzymes and render throat cultures negative but may not prevent the development of PSGN; this makes accurate serologic diagnosis difficult or impossible; (3) A transient decline in the serum concentration of the C3 component of complement, with a return to normal within 8 weeks after the first signs of renal disease. Other complement components (i.e., C1q and C4) are less frequently depressed. In addition to these laboratory features it is desirable to document a latent period appropriate to the infection. Furthermore, the patient should not have any known preexisting renal disease.

The erythrocyte sedimentation rate is usually elevated, while C-reactive protein and rheumatoid factor are generally normal or undetectable. Cryoglobulinemia may be transiently detected. Mild anemia and hypoalbuminemia, both largely dilutional in origin, may occur. Severe hypoalbuminemia may develop if heavy proteinuria is prolonged. Excretion rates of urinary protein in excess of 3.5 g/d occur in less than 20 percent of hospitalized patients. Proteinuria is of a nonselective character and frequently contains high concentrations of fibrin-degradation products and C3 protein, particularly during the diuretic phase. Hyponatremia, hyperchloremia, hyperkalemia, and metabolic acidosis may be seen in azotemic or oliguric patients, especially those with free access to water or potassium. Plasma renin activity and aldosterone secretion rates are low, reflecting suppression secondary to expanded plasma volume and/or hyperkalemia with elevated levels of atrial natriuretic peptide. Urinary sodium concentration is usually low, reflecting avid salt reabsorption in the distal nephron. Abdominal films reveal normal or enlarged kidneys. The chest x-ray may be normal or reveal a slightly enlarged heart, often accompanied by pulmonary congestion. The electrocardiogram may reveal nonspecific T-wave abnormalities. Rheumatic fever rarely coexists with acute PSGN.

The differential diagnosis of PSGN includes other infectious or primary renal diseases which may produce an identical acute nephritic syndrome (Table 240-1). Multisystem diseases such as systemic lupus erythematosus, Henoch-Schönlein purpura, and vasculitis may present initially as acute nephritis (Chap. 241). Predominantly nonglomerular diseases, including thrombotic thrombocytopenic purpura, hemolytic-uremic syndrome, atheroembolic renal disease, and acute hypersensitivity interstitial nephritis may also present the features of the acute nephritic syndrome (Chaps. 242 and 243).

Pathology and pathogenesis　Renal biopsies early in the course reveal *diffuse, endocapillary proliferative glomerulonephritis*. Infiltration of glomeruli with polymorphonuclear leukocytes and mono-cytes is common. The glomerular capillary walls are usually thin and delicate and free of necrosis. Occasional discrete proteinaceous deposits projecting from the outer aspects of the capillary wall toward the urinary space (humps) may be recognized by light microscopy and coincide with the electron-dense deposits seen by electron microscopy. Segmental extracapillary proliferation (crescents) may involve a few glomeruli, but diffuse and extensive circumferential crescent formation is uncommon except among a subset presenting with severe and rapidly progressive acute renal failure (see section below on rapidly progressive glomerulonephritis). Extraglomerular vessels and tubulointerstitial areas are usually normal. Red blood cells are frequent in the lumens of distal tubules, where they form red blood cell casts.

By immunofluorescence microscopy, granular deposits of IgG are seen in peripheral capillary loops and mesangium, nearly always accompanied by C3 and less commonly by C1q and C4 (Chap. 239). Several patterns of Ig and/or C3 deposition have been described. Extensive involvement of the peripheral capillary loops with deposits may be associated with a poorer prognosis, while deposits exclusively involving the mesangium usually indicate a more benign outcome. The precise nature of the antigen-antibody systems involved remains unknown. Most likely the antigen is derived from the streptococcal organism. The profile of altered serum complement components described above, and the prominent C3 deposition in glomeruli are suggestive of involvement of the alternative pathway of complement activation (Chap. 239).

Course and treatment   The ultimate *prognosis* for PSGN differs between sporadic and epidemic forms and between adults and children. *Epidemic* forms of the disease in *children* have a favorable short- and long-term prognosis. Few patients die of complications of renal failure, and nearly all experience a spontaneous resolution of signs within a week after the onset of illness. Abnormalities in the urinary sediment and protein excretion subside slowly in the ensuing months; in a few cases, several years elapse before the urinary sediment is consistently normal. Among children with PSGN during epidemics of streptococcal infection, and in whom preexisting chronic glomerular disease was absent, long-term follow-up has revealed little or no evidence of progression to chronic renal disease. A small percentage may develop extensive crescentic glomerulonephritis with its progressive course. The site of the streptococcal infection, the type of M protein, the severity of abnormalities of complement or urinary sediment, or the extent of the rise in antibody response to exoenzymes have little bearing on the prognosis. Prolonged and persistent heavy proteinuria and/or abnormal GFR imply unfavorable outcome. *Sporadic* cases of PSGN among *children* may have more serious long-term consequences. After the subsidence of the acute disease, some children develop slowly progressive glomerular capillary obliteration (glomerulosclerosis), reduced GFR, and hypertension; after several decades, end-stage renal failure from chronic glomerulonephritis may result. The persistence of proteinuria is the rule in such cases.

The prognosis for *adults* with PSGN is less favorable than for children. The reason for this difference is poorly understood. Although the overall prognosis for PSGN in *epidemics* seems good, *sporadic* PSGN in adults is associated with lasting and/or progressive deterioration in renal function in one-third to one-half of cases. This may take the form of persistent proteinuria and/or hematuria or of slowly progressive glomerulosclerosis and renal failure, often accompanied by hypertension. This evolution is more likely when the initial disease is unusually severe. Whether milder forms of sporadic PSGN can lead to chronic disease is an unresolved issue (see ''Chronic Glomerulonephritis'' below).

The *treatment* of acute PSGN is supportive. It is reasonable to recommend bed rest until the signs of glomerular inflammation and circulatory congestion (primarily hypertension) subside, but prolonged inactivity is of no benefit in the healing process. Fluid retention, circulatory congestion, and edema may be treated with sodium and fluid restriction or loop diuretics. Diuresis alone often ameliorates mild to moderate hypertension. If severe hypertension is present, vasodilator drugs such as nitroprusside, nifedipine, hydralazine, or diazoxide may be useful. Encephalopathy and pulmonary congestion generally improve with lowering of blood pressure and the relief of circulatory overload. Digitalis should be avoided except in well-documented organic heart disease with congestive failure. Treatment with ion exchange resins and/or dialysis may be required for severe oliguria, fluid overload, and hyperkalemia. Mild protein restriction is desirable for azotemic patients. A 7- to 10-day course of antimicrobials (e.g., penicillin or erythromycin) should be given if streptococcal infection is documented. Long-term chemoprophylaxis is not indicated. Glucocorticoids and cytotoxic drugs are not of value.

NONSTREPTOCOCCAL ACUTE POSTINFECTIOUS GLOMERULONEPHRITIS   Clinical features and diagnosis   A wide variety of infectious illnesses other than those caused by group A β-hemolytic streptococci may also be associated with AGN (Table 240-1). These include *bacteremic states* and various *viral* and *parasitic* diseases. Ordinarily these diseases can be diagnosed by the presence of typical extrarenal clinical features or by bacteriologic or serologic findings. Infective endocarditis, sepsis of other types, typhoid fever, infectious mononucleosis, acute viral hepatitis (hepatitis B), falciparum malaria, and toxoplasmosis are infectious diseases capable of evoking AGN. Circulating immune complexes play an important role in the pathogenesis of AGN in these diseases. Chronic or subacute bacteremic states are frequently associated with depression of serum complement components C1q, C4, and C3, elevated levels of rheumatoid factor, circulating cryoimmunoglobulins, and positive tests for circulating immune complexes. Control of infection usually results in the resolution of glomerular inflammation, although rapidly progressive or chronic glomerulonephritis may ensue.

RAPIDLY PROGRESSIVE GLOMERULONEPHRITIS

Transient azotemia, often associated with oliguria, is common in AGN. A diuresis usually follows within days or a few weeks, and GFR returns to normal. On the other hand, some cases of AGN are characterized by a rapidly progressive form of renal failure, which often develops abruptly and displays little tendency for spontaneous or complete recovery. The clinical term *rapidly progressive glomerulonephritis* (*RPGN*) is often applied to this group to connote the development of renal failure in weeks to months, rather than years or decades, as is typical of chronic glomerulonephritis (see below). Extensive *extracapillary* (*crescentic*) *glomerulonephritis* is the pathologic lesion are often found in RPGN, but other lesions may include segmental or diffuse necrotizing glomerulonephritis.

RPGN can arise in one of four clinical settings (Table 240-2): (1) as a complication of an acute or subacute infectious disease, (2) as a renal complication of multisystem diseases, (3) in association with the use of certain drugs, and (4) as a primary glomerular disease in which the kidney is the sole organ affected by the disease process and in which extrarenal manifestations are the result of disturbances of renal function. In the latter circumstance RPGN can arise de novo or be superimposed on another primary glomerular disease process. RPGN occurring as a primary glomerular disease will be discussed here, while that arising secondary to infectious diseases, multisystem diseases, or drugs will be considered in Chap. 241. The term ''idiopathic'' RPGN is also applied to this latter group of disorders, by some despite the fact that the pathogenesis is understood.

IDIOPATHIC RAPIDLY PROGRESSIVE GLOMERULONEPHRITIS   Clinical features and diagnosis   This group of disorders affects individuals in a broad age distribution and has a predilection for males. Wide geographic differences in prevalence have been noted, and outbreaks (''miniepidemics'') may occur. Some patients have had exposure to volatile hydrocarbons, but there is little evidence to support a cause-and-effect relationship. While a flulike or viral prodrome may occur, frank arthritis, sinusitis, otitis, skin rash, neuritis, or encephalopathy are uncommon and are more in keeping with a multisystem disease. Symptoms of weakness, nausea, and vomiting (indicative of azotemia) usually dominate the clinical picture. Oliguria, abdominal or flank pain, and hemoptysis may also be present (see ''Goodpasture's Disease,'' Chap. 241). The blood pressure is

TABLE 240-2 Causes of rapidly progressive glomerulonephritis

INFECTIOUS DISEASES

A Poststreptococcal glomerulonephritis*
B Infective endocarditis*
C Occult visceral sepsis
D Hepatitis B infection (with vasculitis and/or cryoimmunoglobulinemia)

MULTISYSTEM DISEASES

A Systemic lupus erythematosus*
B Henoch-Schönlein purpura*
C Systemic necrotizing vasculitis (including Wegener's granulomatosis) and microscopic polyarteritis*
D Goodpasture's disease*
E Essential mixed (IgG/IgM) cryoimmunoglobulinemia
F Malignancy
G Relapsing polychondritis
H Rheumatoid arthritis (with vasculitis)

DRUGS

A Penicillamine*
B Hydralazine
C Allopurinol (with vasculitis)
D Rifampin

PRIMARY GLOMERULAR DISEASE

A Idiopathic or primary crescentic glomerulonephritis*
  1 Type I—with linear deposits of Ig .
    (anti-glomerular basement membrane antibody–mediated)
  2 Type II—with granular deposits of Ig (immune-complex–mediated)
  3 Type III—with few or no immune deposits of Ig ("pauci-immune")
    a Antineutrophil-cytoplasmic-antibody–associated (renal-limited microscopic polyarteritis)
    b Antineutrophil-antibody–negative
  4 Type IV—combinations of types I and IIIa
B Superimposed on another primary glomerular disease
  1 Mesangiocapillary (membranoproliferative glomerulonephritis)* (especially type II)
  2 Membranous glomerulonephritis*
    Berger's disease (IgA nephropathy)*

* Most common.

---

normal or modestly elevated. Urinalysis typically reveals dysmorphic hematuria and red cell casts, but relatively benign urine sediment rarely may be present. Proteinuria is always present and may be massive. Other biochemical features of the nephrotic syndrome are uncommon, probably because of the rapidity of disease development and concomitant reduction in GFR. Proteinuria is typically nonselective, and fibrin degradation products are found in urine. Azotemia develops early and tends to progress at a rapid rate. Other clinical and laboratory features relate to the underlying pathology and pathogenesis.

Pathology and pathogenesis Idiopathic or primary RPGN is not a homogeneous disease. By light microscopy the characteristic abnormality in the kidneys is *extensive extracapillary proliferation*, i.e., *crescents* often associated with segmental or diffuse necrotizing lesions of the glomerular capillaries. The extent and degree of glomerular involvement vary; however, among patients with rapid deterioration of renal function it is usual for more than 70 percent of glomeruli to be involved with circumferential crescents. Endocapillary proliferation, if prominent, suggests the presence of infection. Segmental or diffuse endocapillary necrosis suggests underlying vasculitis. Fibrin-related antigens are nearly always demonstrable within the crescents by special stains or by immunofluorescence. Gaps or focal discontinuities in the glomerular basement membrane (GBM) and/or Bowman's capsule are observed in association with crescents.

Variations in the underlying pathogenetic mechanisms responsible for RPGN are illustrated by immunofluorescence studies of renal biopsies and by serologic studies for the presence of varius autoantibodies. In approximately 5 to 20 percent of cases, *linear deposits* of IgG indicate involvement of *anti-GBM antibodies*. Circulating anti-

GBM antibodies can be demonstrated by indirect immunofluorescence, hemagglutination, or radioimmunoassay techniques. Patients in this subgroup tend to have normal serum complement levels and a tendency to develop hemoptysis (see also "Goodpasture's Disease," Chap. 241). These patients frequently are HLA-DR2 antigen–positive. About 15 to 30 percent of cases have findings of *immune-complex–mediated disease*, namely, *granular deposits* of immunoglobulin by immunofluorescence microscopy and electron-dense deposits by electron microscopy. This mechanism of RPGN tends to occur in older individuals, to produce more constitutional symptoms, and to result in more disturbances of the complement pathways than does anti-GBM antibody–mediated disease. Hemoptysis may also occur, but circulating anti-GBM antibodies are absent. C3 levels may be decreased. The remainder of cases of RPGN reveal scanty or no immunoglobulins or complement by immunofluorescence ("pauci-immune"); their pathogenesis is unknown. However, circulating autoantibodies to neutrophil (and monocyte) cytoplasmic antigens can frequently (about 70 to 80 percent) be demonstrated (see also Chap. 243). Because similar autoantibodies are also found in various systemic vasculitides, primarily microscopic polyarteritis, this group of disorders may be a renal form of vasculitis limited to the kidney. On rare occasions, antiglomerular basement membrane and antineutrophil cytoplasmic autoantibodies develop simultaneously or sequentially in patients with crescentic glomerulonephritis.

Uncommonly, other idiopathic (primary) glomerular diseases may be complicated by a rapidly progressive glomerulonephritis accompanied by extensive crescent formation. These glomerular diseases include mesangiocapillary (membranoproliferative) glomerulonephritis, Berger's disease (IgA nephropathy), and membranous glomerulonephritis (Table 240-2). The pathogenetic mechanisms underlying this complication vary. Lung hemorrhage may be observed in RPGN. This subject is covered in greater detail in the section on Goodpasture's Disease in Chap. 241.

Course and treatment The prognosis for preservation of renal function is poor. Patients with crescent formation in 70 percent or more of glomeruli or oliguria or severe reduction in GFR (less than 5 mL/min) at the time of presentation and those with an anti-GBM antibody–mediated process have the worst prognosis. Although advances in treatment are changing the outlook, as many as one-half require maintenance hemodialysis within 6 months of onset. Exceptional patients with crescentic glomerulonephritis have a more protracted illness. Spontaneous resolution is uncommon, except among patients with infection as the basis for formation of antigen-antibody complexes, where removal of antigen can take place.

Glucocorticoids, in the form of "pulses" of parenteral methylprednisolone in high doses, and daily oral prednisone, often combined with *cytotoxic agents* (azathioprine or cyclophosphamide), have yielded varying success, particularly in the patients with granular or minimal Ig deposits in glomeruli, especially in association with vasculitis. Since few controlled studies have yet been conducted, however, it is difficult to ascertain the value of these regimens. Nonetheless, more than two-thirds of patients treated with several "pulses" of intravenous methylprednisolone have experienced improvement in renal function often sufficient to avoid the necessity of dialysis. The addition of *anticoagulants* (heparin or warfarin sodium) and antithrombotic agents (dipyridamole, sulfinpyrazone) seems rational on the basis of evidence for involvement of the coagulation process in the genesis of crescent formation. However, evidence of benefit from such therapies in animals with experimentally induced crescentic glomerulonephritis is inconsistent, in part because of variations in the severity of the disease models, the timing of treatment, and the nature of the anticoagulant or antithrombotic agent used. Anticoagulants may be hazardous in advanced renal failure or with pulmonary hemorrhage. *Intensive plasma exchange* (plasmapheresis—2 to 4 L of plasma daily or three times weekly), combined with glucocorticoids and cytotoxic agents, has been employed. Encouraging long-term results have been obtained in patients revealing linear Ig deposits in glomeruli (anti-GBM antibody–mediated disease), providing therapy is begun *before* renal failure has progressed to require dialysis support. A beneficial effect of intensive plasma exchange combined with immunosuppressive agents has also been claimed in patients with RPGN who do not demonstrate evidence of anti-GBM antibody production. Such benefit has been observed primarily in patients who have progressed to dialysis-dependent renal failure. High dose glucocorticoids and immunosuppressive therapy seem to be sufficient for the majority of patients in this category who have not progressed to dialysis-dependent renal failure.

Renal biopsy assessment of the nature, severity, and potential reversibility of disease is a vital aspect of evaluation of patients suspected of having rapidly progressive glomerulonephritis. Such biopsies should be performed early in the course. Despite aggressive therapy, many patients with oliguria do poorly. Treatment must be individualized, and because dialysis therapy and/or transplantation are available to most patients, one should probably err on the side of a conservative approach, unless compelling evidence of potential reversibility is present.

RPGN may recur after renal transplant. At present it seems prudent to recommend that, after initiating dialysis, a period of 3 to 6 months be allowed to elapse before undertaking renal transplantation in patients who have circulating anti-GBM antibodies. There is no convincing evidence that bilateral nephrectomy in advance of transplantation reduces the risk of recurrent disease in the transplant.

THE NEPHROTIC SYNDROME

The nephrotic syndrome (NS) is characterized by *albuminuria, hypoalbuminemia, hyperlipidemia*, and *edema*. These abnormalities are consequences of excessive glomerular leakage of plasma proteins into the urine (see also Chaps. 33 and 44). The defects in the charge- or size-selective barriers of the glomerular capillary wall that underline the excessive filtration of plasma proteins can arise as a consequence of a variety of disease processes, including immunologic disorders, toxic injuries, metabolic abnormalities, biochemical defects, and vascular disorders. Thus, nephrotic syndrome is a common end point of a variety of disease processes that alter the permeability properties of the glomerular capillary wall. *Proteinuria* is the hallmark of the nephrotic state. Arbitrarily, total urinary protein excretion rates in excess of 3.5 g per 1.73 m² surface area per day [or urinary protein concentration of greater than 0.4 mg/mmol (3.5 mg/dL) creatinine] are considered to be in the nephrotic range, primarily because proteinuria of this magnitude is seldom observed in tubulointerstitial and vascular diseases of the kidney. Sustained heavy proteinuria is often, but not invariably, accompanied by *hypoalbuminemia*. Excessive urinary losses, increased renal catabolism, and inadequate hepatic synthesis of albumin all contribute to depression of plasma albumin. The resulting decrease in plasma oncotic pressure leads to a disturbance in the Starling forces across peripheral capillaries. Intravascular fluid migrates into the interstitial tissue (i.e., *edema*), particularly in areas of low tissue pressure. These disturbances are postulated to lead to "underfilling" of the circulation which in turn initiates a series of homeostatic adjustments designed to correct the deficit in effective plasma volume. These include activation of the renin-angiotensin-aldosterone system, enhanced vasopressin secretion, stimulation of the sympathetic nervous system, and perhaps an alteration in the secretion or renal response to atrial natriuretic peptide. These and other poorly understood adjustments lead to renal sodium and water retention, primarily because of avid reabsorption in distal nephron segments, resulting in unrelenting edema. In this formulation the kidney is viewed as responding maladaptively to a disturbance in effective arterial volume. However, the "underfilling" scenario may not be the complete explanation for salt and water retention in nephrotic syndrome. In fact, measurements of plasma volume, renin, and aldosterone, and determination of the events underlying renal salt and water reabsorption have documented heterogeneity in the pathophysiology of fluid volume homeostasis in nephrotic syndrome.

Some patients have expanded intravascular fluid volume and suppressed renin-aldosterone axis, presumably mediated by primary, non-aldosterone-dependent renal salt and fluid retention, resembling the pathophysiology of acute nephritis (see above). These patients often, but not invariably, have some decrease in GFR and structural glomerular lesions. At the other end of the spectrum are patients with overt hypovolemia, hyperreninemia, and avid secondary renal salt retention. Serum albumin levels are low, *extracellular* fluid volume is expanded, and edema is usually present in both groups. As expected, the magnitude of edema correlates with the degree of depression of plasma albumin (and thereby plasma oncotic pressure); however, the relationship is inexact, perhaps reflecting a component of primary renal sodium and water retention in many patients.

The diminished plasma oncotic pressure also appears to stimulate hepatic lipoprotein synthesis, and *hyperlipidemia* is a frequent accompaniment of the nephrotic state. Low-density lipoproteins and cholesterol are elevated most frequently, but as the plasma oncotic pressure falls further, very low density lipoproteins and triglycerides also increase. Excessive urinary losses of plasma protein factors regulating lipoprotein synthesis or disposal may also contribute to the hyperlipidemic state. Whether these lipid abnormalities contribute to accelerated atherosclerosis remains controversial. Lipid bodies (fatty casts, oval fat bodies) commonly appear in the urine.

Urine losses of plasma proteins other than albumin are also of importance. Loss of thyroxine-binding globulin may produce abnormalities in thyroid function tests, including a low thyroxine and an enhanced resin triiodothyronine uptake. Loss of cholecalciferol-binding protein may lead to vitamin D deficiency and secondary hyperparathyroidism and may contribute to the hypocalcemia and hypocalciuria seen commonly. Enhanced urinary excretion of transferrin may produce an iron-resistant microcytic, hypochromic anemia. Zinc and copper deficiency may result from urinary losses of metal-binding proteins. A hypercoagulable state frequently accompanies severe nephrotic syndrome [serum albumin less than 20 g/L (2 g/dL)]. A variety of factors contribute to the enhanced tendency to thrombosis in nephrotic patients including deficiencies in antithrombin III (due to urine losses), reduced levels or activity of protein C or protein S, hyperfibrinogenemia, impaired fibrinolysis, enhanced platelet aggregation, and hyperlipidemia.

Some patients develop severe IgG deficiency, in part due to urinary losses and hypercatabolism. Low-molecular-weight complement components may also be lost in the urine and contribute to defects in the opsonization of bacteria. Various drug-binding proteins (chiefly albumin) may be decreased, altering the pharmacokinetics and toxicity of many drugs. Electrophoresis of serum reveals, in addition to diminished albumin levels, increases of alpha and beta globulins.

COMPLICATIONS AND MANAGEMENT OF THE NEPHROTIC SYNDROME   *Edema* should be managed cautiously and conservatively. Overly vigorous diuresis with potent loop diuretics may result in an abrupt decline in effective plasma volume as the deficit in plasma oncotic pressure may preclude rapid mobilization of the extracellular fluid into the intravascular compartment. This is more likely to occur if plasma volume is diminished and may lead to further reduction in GFR, worsening azotemia, and postural hypotension. Severe extracellular volume depletion may predispose to the development of renal failure, but acute reversible renal failure may also develop even when plasma volume is normal or increased. Renal edema, intratubular obstruction from proteinaceous casts, and alterations in glomerular water permeability have been suggested to account for these episodes. The temptation to administer concentrated salt-poor albumin should be resisted, as nearly all the administered protein will be excreted in 24 to 48 h, so that any beneficial effect on plasma oncotic pressure will be transient. In addition, the increase in filtered protein may have adverse effects on the kidney or the response to therapy (e.g., diuretics). However, such treatment may be necessary in severely hypoalbuminemic patients suffering from profound postural symptoms or refractory anasarca.

The treatment of *hyperlipidemia* is frequently unsuccessful, and its influence on morbidity and mortality is uncertain. Colestipol, probucol, and lovastatin can all cause modest (25–40%) decrements in plasma total cholesterol in patients with nephrotic hyperlipidemia. Whether such treatment reduces risk for atherosclerosis and ischemic heart or cerebral disease is not proven. Nevertheless, most clinicians believe that an attempt should be made to lower cholesterol levels.

The *thromboembolic complications* of NS are reasonably common, including spontaneous peripheral venous and/or arterial, pulmonary arterial, and renal venous occlusions. *Renal vein thrombosis* (RVT), either unilateral or bilateral, is a particularly distressing complication. In the past, this was regarded as a cause rather than a consequence of NS, a conclusion no longer held. Certain glomerular lesions are more likely than others to be associated with RVT. These include membranous or membranoproliferative glomerulonephritis, and amyloidosis. Features suggestive of *acute* RVT include unilateral or bilateral flank or loin pain, gross hematuria, left-sided varicocele, widely fluctuating GFR and urinary protein excretion rates, and asymmetry of renal size and/or function. *Chronic* forms of RVT are commonly asymptomatic. Scalloping of the ureters (due to collateral circulation) and evidence of pulmonary emboli and/or infarction (Chap. 243) may occur in chronic RVT.

Some advocate an aggressive approach in nephrotic syndrome due to lesions associated with inherently high prevalence of RVT (e.g., membranous glomerulonephritis), routinely employing selective renal venous angiography. If RVT is detected, long-term (optimal duration unknown) anticoagulants are prescribed. Such an approach might prevent serious embolic complications, but since the risk of pulmonary embolism is not known, although probably low, the benefit-risk relationship of this approach cannot be determined. A more conservative approach has also been advocated in which renal venous angiography is performed only in those patients with a pulmonary embolism (e.g., symptoms, compatible laboratory findings, and a high-probability ventilation-perfusion scan or pulmonary angiogram) and who have no evidence of deep venous thrombosis in the lower extremities. Since such patients would receive anticoagulant therapy in any case, the value of localizing the site of thrombosis is not established. Intermediate probability ventilation-perfusion scans in asymptomatic nephrotic patients are likely to have limited value, since subsegmental defects in perfusion may be observed even in the absence of renal vein or lower extremity deep venous thrombosis. These changes could be due to in situ pulmonary arterial thrombosis. The risk of renal vein thrombosis or deep venous thrombosis is increased primarily in patients with a very low serum albumin level [e.g., less than 20 g/L (2 g/dL)]. The presence of a thromboembolic complication is usually regarded as a clear indication for long-term oral anticoagulation. The effectiveness of heparin may be impaired by concomitant antithrombin III deficiency, a factor required for the heparin-induced antithrombin effect.

High-protein diets are frequently prescribed; however, the main effect of increasing dietary protein is to increase urinary protein excretion, and the effect on serum albumin levels is modest. Furthermore, such diets are difficult to manage with concomitant salt restriction and, at least theoretically, could aggravate the progression of an underlying structural glomerular lesion. An alternative approach is to prescribe modest protein restriction (e.g., 0.6 g/kg body weight per day), particularly in azotemic patients; some also advocate adding a supplementary amount of dietary protein equal to urinary protein losses. Dietary protein should be of high biologic value and can be supplemented with amino acids. Plasma albumin and transferrin concentrations and urinary protein excretion rates should be monitored to evaluate the effect of diet on nutritional status. Correction of transport protein deficiencies is not feasible. Supplemental vitamin D might be desirable if deficiency is present. In rare circumstances, profound protein malnutrition or other complications of massive proteinuria may justify ablation of renal function by medical or surgical means.

A classification of the causes of nephrotic syndrome is provided in Table 240-3. The multisystemic, heredofamilial, neoplastic, and

---

TABLE 240-3   Causes of the nephrotic syndrome

PRIMARY GLOMERULAR DISEASES*

A   Minimal change disease*
B   Mesangial proliferative glomerulonephritis[†]
C   Focal and segmental glomerulosclerosis*
D   Membranous glomerulonephritis*
E   Membranoproliferative glomerulonephritis*
   1   Type I
   2   Type II
   3   Other variants
F   Other uncommon lesions
   1   Crescentic glomerulonephritis
   2   Focal and segmental proliferative glomerulonephritis[d]
   3   Fibrillary and/or immunotactoid glomerulonephritis

SECONDARY TO OTHER DISEASES

A   Infections: poststreptococcal glomerulonephritis,* endocarditis, "shunt nephritis," secondary syphilis, leprosy, hepatitis B,* HIV infection and AIDS, infectious mononucleosis, malaria, schistosomiasis, filariasis
B   Drugs: organic gold; inorganic, organic, and elemental mercury; penicillamine; "street" heroin, nonsteroidal anti-inflammatory agents,* probenecid; captopril; Tridione; mesantoin; perchlorate; antivenom; antitoxins; contrast media
C   Neoplasia: Hodgkin's disease, lymphomas, leukemia, carcinomas, melanoma, Wilms's tumor
D   Multisystem: systemic lupus erythematosus,* Henoch-Schönlein purpura,* vasculitis, Goodpasture's disease, dermatomyositis, dermatitis herpetiformis, amyloidosis,* sarcoidosis, Sjögren's syndrome, rheumatoid arthritis, mixed connective tissue disease
E   Heredofamilial: diabetes mellitus,* Alport's syndrome, sickle cell disease, Fabry's disease, nail-patella syndrome, lipodystrophy, lecithin-cholesterol acyltransferase deficiency, congenital nephrotic syndrome
F   Miscellaneous: preeclamptic toxemia, thyroiditis, myxedema, malignant obesity, renovascular hypertension, chronic interstitial nephritis with vesicoureteric reflux, chronic allograft rejection,* bee stings

*   Most common.
[†]   Includes Berger's disease (IgA nephropathy).

---

metabolic causes are discussed in Chap. 241. The primary (idiopathic) glomerular diseases associated with nephrotic syndrome, as well as the diseases secondary to infectious or drug causes, are considered below.

IDIOPATHIC NEPHROTIC SYNDROME   This diagnosis is arrived at by exclusion of known causes such as infections, drug exposure, malignancy, multisystem disease, or hereditary disorders. The exclusion of these disorders may, at times, prove difficult since they may exist in covert forms (especially cancer and hepatitis B). The idiopathic forms are further classified according to the morphologic features on renal biopsy (Table 240-4). Performance of a renal biopsy, at least among adults, is required for the accurate classification of idiopathic NS, for the formulation of a rational plan of treatment, and for the estimation of the likelihood of subsequent progressive to renal failure. Children need not always be subjected to renal biopsy since clinical study can often lead to accurate diagnosis.

Minimal change disease   In the past this lesion was called *lipoid nephrosis, nil lesion,* or *foot process disease.* In this form of idiopathic NS, although little or no alterations of the glomerular capillaries are demonstrable by light microscopy (hence the designation "minimal change"). Although mild degrees of hypercellularity of the glomerulus may be observed, the glomeruli are of normal size in contradistinction to focal sclerosis (see below). *Diffuse epithelial foot process effacement*[1] is evident by electron microscopy. Immunofluorescence microscopy reveals absent or irregular and nonspecific deposits of immunoglobulin and complement components (chiefly IgM and C3). Minimal change disease is the most frequently encountered form of idiopathic NS in children, accounting for more than 70 to 80 percent of cases diagnosed before the age of 16. Peak prevalence is between 6 and 8 years. This lesion is not rare in adults, representing 15 to 20 percent

---

[1] The term "fusion" is often used to describe these changes in foot processes, although true fusion of cell membranes does not occur.

TABLE 240-4   Idiopathic nephrotic syndrome: selected features of underlying primary glomerular lesions

Lesion	Morphology*			Approximate prevalence in children/ adults, %	Common clinical/ lab features	Response to therapy†	Likelihood of maintaining renal function‡
	LM	IFM	EM				
Minimal change disease	Normal or very mild proliferation	Negative–trace IgM	Foot process fusion, no deposits	70–80/15–20	Highly selective proteinuria,§ *normal* C3, decreased IgG, increased IgM	Steroids + + Cytotoxic drugs + (cyclophosphamide, chlorambucil) Cyclosporine + + Levamisole + Frequent relapses	95 +
Mesangial proliferative	Diffuse mesangial proliferation	Negative or variable mesangial IgM, IgG, C3¶	Mesangial deposits	15–20/5–10	Hematuria, *normal* C3	Steroids± Cytotoxic drugs (?)	80 (?)
Focal and segmental glomerulosclerosis (with hyalinosis)	Focal and segmental sclerosis and hyalinosis	Focal and segmental IgM, C3	Foot process fusion, sclerosis, hyalinosis, lipid deposits	10/10–20	Hematuria, leukocyturia, poorly selective proteinuria, *normal* C3	Steroids + Cytotoxic drugs + Cyclosporine +	45–50
Membranous glomerulonephritis	Thick capillary wall, spikes of BM material	Diffuse granular capillary wall IgG, ±C3	Subepithelial deposits	<5/30–40	Variable protein selectivity, *normal* C3, renal vein thrombosis	Steroids± Cytotoxic drugs + Intravenous IgG (?) Cyclosporine (?)	70 +
Membrano-proliferative glomerulonephritis							
Type I	Mesangial proliferation interposition, lobular change	Diffuse C3; variable IgG, IgM	Subendothelial deposits	8/<5	Hematuria, *reduced* C3 (intermittent)	Steroids (?) Anticoagulants (?) Cytotoxic drugs (?) Antithrombotics +	50
Type II	Mesangial proliferation interposition	C3 capillary wall and mesangial nodules	Intramembranous deposits	3/<5	Hematuria, *reduced* C3 (persistent), +C3NF	Steroids – Cytotoxic drugs –	40

* LM = light microscopy, IFM = immunofluorescence microscopy, EM = electron microscopy, BM = basement membrane.
† Response to therapy: + + = highly responsive, + = variably responsive, ± = occasionally responsive, – = unresponsive.
‡ Percent of patients maintaining sufficient renal function to obviate need for chronic dialysis or transplantation within 5 years.
§ Protein selectivity = differential protein clearance, e.g., IgG/transferrin clearance ratio. Highly selective = <0.1, moderately selective = 0.11 to 0.20, poorly selective = >0.20.
¶ IgA deposits are seen in Berger's disease, IgA nephropathy.
NOTE: C3NF = C3 nephritic factor.

of idiopathic NS in patients over age 16. There is a slight predilection for males. Typically patients present with overt NS, normal blood pressure, normal or slightly reduced GFR, and a "benign" urinary sediment. Varying degrees of microscopic hematuria are found in up to 20 percent of cases. Urinary protein is typically highly selective in children (e.g., it contains principally albumin and minimal amounts of high-molecular-weight plasma proteins such as IgG, alpha$_2$ macroglobulin, or C3) but is variable in adults. The pattern of protein excretion indicates a major "charge-selective" defect in permselectivity. Fibrin split products and C3 are absent in the urine. Serum levels of complement components are normal, except for a slight reduction in C1q. IgG concentrations are often depressed during relapse, whereas IgM levels are modestly increased, both during remission and relapse. Some cases may have associated allergic diathesis (e.g., to milk, pollens, etc.), a history of recent immunization, or upper respiratory infection. The histocompatibility antigen HLA-B12 is more prevalent when minimal change disease is associated with atopy, indicating a possible genetic predisposition to this disease. Thromboembolic manifestations occur, but renal vein thrombosis is uncommon.

Spontaneous remissions and relapses of heavy proteinuria may occur in 30 to 40 percent of untreated patients. Interestingly, an identical lesion is encountered in patients with Hodgkin's disease in whom NS develops, suggesting a role for lymphocytes in its pathogenesis. Except for patients who develop focal and segmental sclerosing lesions (see below), a progressive decline in GFR does not occur. Acute renal failure is rare. In the preantibiotic era infection

with encapsulated organisms (e.g., pneumococci) was a leading cause of death, but now the mortality rate is low, and most deaths are associated with complications of treatment rather than the disease itself. Rarely, acute renal failure may occur even without profound hypovolemia. The mechanism is obscure but could relate to tubular obstruction from heavy proteinuria or interstitial edema or severe glomerular epithelial cell effacement. The renal failure is often responsive to glucocorticoids and diuretics.

Since the etiology and pathogenesis are unknown, treatment is empirical and symptomatic. Glucocorticoids enhance the natural tendency for this disease to undergo spontaneous remission. Daily or alternate-day therapy seems to be equally effective; the latter is associated with fewer complications. Daily prednisone or prednisolone (60 mg/m² surface area in children, 1 to 1.5 mg/kg body weight in adults) for 4 weeks, followed by alternate-day prednisone (35 to 40 mg/m² in children, 1 mg/kg in adults) for 4 additional weeks is a regimen for initial treatment of this disorder. While initial therapy with high dose intravenous methylprednisolone (1.0 g/d for 3 to 6 doses) may accelerate the development of remission, a higher relapse rate also occurs.

Over 95 percent of children (less than age 16) with minimal change disease respond with a complete disappearance of proteinuria within 8 weeks of the institution of prednisone therapy. Because of the high probability of minimal change disease in children, many pediatricians treat without an initial renal biopsy. A complete steroid response in such circumstances is indicative of underlying minimal change disease in children.

On the other hand, only about 50 percent of adults with minimal change disease respond within 8 weeks of instituting prednisone therapy, with a maximum response often not attained until 20 to 24 weeks from initiation of treatment. Patients over the age of 40 seem to be less responsive than those under the age of 40. Ultimately the overall response rate in adults with minimal change disease is only slightly less than that in children. The delayed response to glucocorticoids in adults could be due, in part, to the lower doses of prednisone relative to the doses used in children. Because of the likelihood of a lesion other than minimal change disease and the fact that some other lesions (e.g., focal sclerosis) may also sometimes respond to glucocorticoids, a steroid-responsive adult patient with idiopathic nephrotic syndrome cannot be assumed to have minimal change disease.

Among both adults and children, 50 to 60 percent of patients with minimal change disease relapse during the tapering or after the cessation of therapy. Too rapid withdrawal of glucocorticoids seems to encourage relapse. Spontaneous remissions tend to be more stable with a low frequency of relapse. A relapse during the tapering phase of glucocorticoid therapy or shortly after the discontinuance of therapy defines the steroid-dependent state. Frequent relapses (more than three per year) may require repetitive treatment with steroids and may be associated with exogenous Cushing's syndrome. Such patients can ordinarily be identified within 12 to 18 months after steroid treatment. Relapses may be treated with the initial regimen but with more gradual withdrawal of prednisone and with low maintenance doses of 5 to 10 mg daily or on alternate days for 3 to 6 months.

A patient with multiple relapses may benefit by a brief course of cyclophosphamide 2 to 3 mg/kg body weight per day or chlorambucil 0.1 to 0.2 mg/kg body weight per day for 8 to 10 weeks preferably begun after a steroid-induced remission. The frequently relapsing patient has a lower likelihood of a prolonged relapse-free interval after such therapy. Such patients seem to have fewer relapses if therapy with cytotoxic drugs (e.g., cyclophosphamide or chlorambucil) is extended to 12 weeks. Overall, only about half of frequently relapsing patients with minimal change disease treated with cyclophosphamide or chlorambucil remain free of disease after 5 years. Among children with minimal change disease the frequency of relapses declines with age. However, cytotoxic agents have adverse effects on bone marrow, the gonads and urinary bladder. Careful monitoring of hematologic and urinary findings is mandatory. They may also be oncogenic. Since they may augment infectious diseases, particularly measles, varicella, tuberculosis, and fungal disease, appropriate precautions should be taken in patients at risk. Azathioprine, previously believed to be ineffective in minimal change disease, will require reevaluation because of anecdotal reports of slow but eventual disappearance of proteinuria in patients with minimal change disease and steroid-sensitive or steroid-dependent nephrotic syndrome treated for 6 months to 1 year with azathioprine 2 to 2.5 mg/kg body weight per day. Cyclosporine in doses of 4 to 6 mg/kg body weight per day induces remissions of nephrotic syndrome in about 70–80% of patients treated for 8 to 10 weeks; however, relapses upon discontinuance of this agent are common. Prolonged therapy (over 4 to 6 months) may be associated with nephrotoxicity. Further controlled trials are needed before this nephrotoxic agent can be recommended for routine use. Cyclosporine may prove to be valuable for steroid-dependent patients who continue to relapse despite cyclophosphamide or chlorambucil therapy or who become steroid unresponsive. Levamisole, an immuno-stimulatory agent, is also capable of inducing remissions in steroid-responsive or steroid-dependent minimal change disease but seldom results in a lasting cure of proteinuria.

The use of cytotoxic agents should be reserved for patients who develop complications of steroid therapy. The long-term prognosis of patients with the minimal change lesion is excellent; 15-year survival is in excess of 90 percent, but a few develop renal failure as a consequence of focal sclerosing glomerular lesions (see below) in association with acquired resistance to glucocorticoid therapy.

Mesangial proliferative glomerulonephritis   The lesion is characterized by a moderate diffuse increase in the cellularity of the glomerular capillary bed. The peripheral glomerular capillary walls are thin and delicate, and extracapillary proliferation is not seen. The precise nature of the proliferating cells is not clearly understood but may represent combinations of proliferating mesangial cells, endothelial cells, and infiltrating mononuclear cells. Glomerular involvement is usually reasonably uniform, although there may be segmental accentuation of hypercellularity. Necrosis of glomerular tufts is absent. Deposits of proteinaceous material, if seen, are confined to the mesangial areas. Interposition of mesangial cells and cytoplasm into the periphery of the glomerular capillary wall does not occur. By immunofluorescence, a variety of patterns are observed. If granular IgA deposits in the mesangium predominate, accompanied by C3 and fibrin-reactive antigens but not the early acting components of the complement cascade, then the lesion is categorized as IgA nephropathy, or Berger's disease (see below). Other patterns of immunofluorescence include a predominance of IgM deposits in a granular pattern diffusely throughout the mesangium, isolated mesangial C3 deposits, scattered mesangial IgG deposits, and no immunoglobulin or complement deposits. Thus, mesangial proliferative glomerulonephritis is a heterogeneous group of glomerular diseases. Some patients with this morphologic lesion may in fact represent resolving postinfectious glomerulonephritis, hereditary nephritis, or other multisystem diseases such as Henoch-Schönlein purpura, vasculitis, or systemic lupus erythematosus. Electron-microscopic findings are nonspecific. Occasionally small electron-dense paramesangial deposits may be observed. The findings of large electron-dense deposits in the mesangium in association with the morphologic appearance of mesangial proliferative glomerulonephritis should heighten the suspicion of a multisystem disease or IgA nephropathy.

This lesion accounts for approximately 5 percent of idiopathic nephrotic syndrome in adults and 5 to 10 percent in children. It is more common in older children and young adults. Males are affected slightly more often than females. Hematuria, either gross or microscopic, is common. Loin pain, bilateral or unilateral, may be seen in the idiopathic disorder but is more frequent in patients who have underlying IgA nephropathy. Laboratory features are not distinctive. Renal function may be modestly decreased or normal at diagnosis. Complement component levels are most often normal. IgG levels may be reduced, and IgA levels may be increased. Anti-streptolysin O titers are usually normal. Proteinuria is most often nonselective. The pathogenesis is almost certainly the result of diverse pathogenetic processes. The presence of mesangial immunoglobulin deposits and circulating immune complexes in some patients suggests an immune-complex pathogenesis, although the antigen(s) is unknown.

Among adult patients with nephrotic syndrome and moderate to severe diffuse mesangial proliferation, there is a tendency for persistence of proteinuria and progression to renal insufficiency. This is particularly true if lesions of focal and segmental glomerular sclerosis are superimposed on the mesangial proliferative lesion at the initial biopsy. Patients with milder forms of mesangial proliferative glomerulonephritis, particularly when unassociated with mesangial immunoglobulin deposition or superimposed focal and segmental glomerulosclerosis may follow a more benign course. Some patients, particularly children, behave in a fashion similar to those with the minimal change lesion. Since renal biopsies from patients with the minimal change lesion may display mild degrees of glomerular hypercellularity, the benign course may indicate that they have the minimal change lesion with more prominent mesangial proliferation rather than a separate disorder classifiable under the heading of mesangial proliferative glomerulonephritis. Well-developed mesangial proliferative lesions, particularly in association with mesangial IgM deposits, tend to be unresponsive to glucocorticoid therapy and to evolve over time into focal and segmental glomerular sclerosis. Patients with mesangial proliferative glomerulonephritis who have remission of proteinuria following treatment with glucocorticoids tend to do well, with little inclination toward progressive renal insufficiency. Exacerbations and remissions of proteinuria may occur. Steroid-unresponsive patients with persistent nephrotic syndrome progress at variable rates to renal insufficiency. The role of adjunctive cytotoxic therapy (cyclophosphamide, chlorambucil, or azathioprine) has not yet been established in this disorder.

Because of the variable pathogenesis and the relative rarity of this disorder, long-term prospective studies of natural history and therapy have not been conducted. Many patients, particularly those with mild degrees of proliferation and a remitting course following glucocorticoids, have a benign prognosis. Other patients, particularly those with steroid unresponsiveness and superimposed focal and segmental glomerulosclerosis on the initial biopsy, have a poor prognosis, often developing renal failure 5 to 10 years after diagnosis.

Focal and segmental glomerulosclerosis with hyalinosis (focal sclerosis) This lesion is characterized by sclerosis and hyalinosis of some, but not all, glomeruli (hence the term *focal*). Among affected glomeruli, only a portion of the glomerular tuft is abnormal (hence, *segmental*). Enlargement of the less-affected glomeruli is characteristic of the idiopathic lesion. There is a predilection for these lesions initially to affect the *juxtamedullary glomeruli* and to be associated with progressive tubulointerstitial damage. By immunofluorescence, granular and nodular deposits of IgM and C3 are found in the segmental sclerosing lesion. By electron microscopy, focal basement membrane collapse and denudation of epithelial surfaces are noted. All glomeruli, even those unaffected by sclerosis or hyalinosis, reveal diffuse epithelial foot process effacement. Visceral epithelial cell vacuolization is common. This lesion accounts for about 10 to 15 percent of cases of idiopathic NS among children and is more common in adults, particularly between the ages of 16 and 30. Males are affected more often than females. Focal sclerosis may represent a stage in the evolution of a subgroup of patients with minimal change disease or ''pure'' mesangial proliferative glomerulonephritis (see above). In more than two-thirds of cases of focal sclerosis overt NS is present at diagnosis; the remainder have proteinuria in the nonnephrotic range. Hypertension, reduced GFR, abnormal tubule function, and abnormal urinary sediment (leukocyturia, hematuria) occur commonly. Focal sclerosis may have clinical and laboratory features indistinguishable from either minimal change disease, mesangial proliferative glomerulonephritis, or membranous glomerulopathy (see below). Proteinuria is nearly always nonselective or becomes so on follow-up. Fibrin degradation products and C3 may be present in the urine. Serum levels of C3 are normal and IgG levels are reduced, but not as severely as in minimal change disease. Similar lesions may be seen in association with heroin abuse, vesicoureteral reflux, human immunodeficiency virus infection and acquired immunodeficiency syndrome, massive obesity, solitary kidney, and renal allograft rejection and may complicate other primary glomerular diseases in the late stages. The occurrence of focal and segmental glomerulosclerosis in remnant glomeruli after extensive renal ablation has led to the suggestion that glomerular hypertrophy hyperfiltration (or some hemodynamic determinant thereof) may play a causative role in pathogenesis. The attendant lipid abnormalities (e.g., hypercholesterolemia) may also contribute to the progressive nature of the underlying lesion. Abnormalities in the prevalence of HLA antigens have not been consistently described. Renal vein thrombosis is uncommon.

There is little tendency for spontaneous remission, except among children. GFR declines, albeit at variable rates. A subset of patients with focal sclerosis, heavy proteinuria (i.e., greater than 15 to 20 g/d), and profound hypoalbuminemia progress rapidly to end-stage renal failure, occasionally in a few months.

The cause and pathogenesis of focal sclerosis are unknown. A variety of mechanisms have been postulated including immunologic, toxic, biochemical, and hemodynamic disturbances. A systemic process is suggested by the high prevalence of recurrent disease in renal allografts (30 to 40 percent).

Although few prospective trials have been conducted, a decline

in proteinuria concomitant with glucocorticoid therapy and a lowered risk of progressive renal failure among patients with complete or partial remission of proteinuria suggest that steroids exert a beneficial effect on the disorder. Indeed, between 20 and 40 percent of patients treated with either alternate-day or daily prednisone in a fashion similar to that described for minimal change disease experience complete or partial remissions of proteinuria. If such remissions persist following reduction of steroid dosage, significant protection from progressive renal failure may be provided. The response of patients who have already developed renal insufficiency is less favorable. Cytotoxic drugs, such as cyclophosphamide, may be of value in patients who are fully or partially steroid responsive, but controlled trials have been disappointing. An aggressive approach with high-dose methylprednisolone given in reducing doses over many months combined with oral cyclophosphamide has given encouraging results, but prospective trials are needed. Cyclosporine, in doses of 4 to 6 mg/kg body weight per day combined with alternate-day oral prednisone will induce partial or complete remissions in 50 to 60 percent of steroid-responsive patients, but remissions are seen in only 15 to 20 percent of steroid-unresponsive patients. The effect seems to be dependent on continuous administration of the agent. Prolonged therapy, over 4 to 6 months, may be associated with nephrotoxicity, especially in patients with impaired renal function and those with tubular atrophy and/or interstitial fibrosis on initial renal biopsy. Further control trials are needed to determine the proper place of cyclosporine and related agents in the management of focal sclerosis. Angiotensin-converting enzyme inhibitors or other antihypertensive agents with antiproteinuric effects (e.g., diltiazem) may be useful in patients with heavy proteinuria and/or moderately impaired renal function even if hypertension is absent or mild. Such therapy may slow progression of the disease, but this has not yet been proven. Hyperlipidemia, often severe, is characteristic of focal sclerosis and probably deserves aggressive therapy with hypolipidemic agents such as lovastatin. At least half of patients with persistent heavy proteinuria develop end-stage renal failure or die of intercurrent illnesses within 10 years of diagnosis. The rate at which renal failure develops is inversely related to the magnitude of proteinuria. Patients who excrete more than 10 g/d develop end-stage renal failure in approximately 3 years. The prognosis is worse for those with azotemia or hypertension at diagnosis. This lesion commonly recurs in renal allografts, occasionally within a few hours of transplantation, suggesting as its cause a humoral factor. Repeated recurrence in subsequent transplants is the rule.

Membranous glomerulonephritis This lesion is characterized by irregular, discontinuous proteinaceous deposits along the outer (or subepithelial) aspect of the glomerular capillary wall. These deposits contain IgG and sometimes C3 and later-acting complement components (C5b–C9). The deposits also appear dense by electron microscopy. Unlike focal sclerosis, *all glomeruli are involved uniformly*. At an early stage all glomeruli may appear normal by light microscopy, but as the disease progresses, immune deposits coalesce, and new basement membrane-like material is produced, causing the capillary wall to thicken. Eventually, increased amounts of basement membrane material project toward the urinary space, giving the appearance of ''spikes.'' There is little proliferation of capillary endothelial or mesangial cells, although mesangial sclerosis may occur in advanced cases. Tubulointerstitial atrophy and vascular lesions are other late manifestations. The cause and pathogenesis of the idiopathic disorder are unknown, but the in situ formation of immune complexes in the subepithelial space is suggested by the similarity of the human disorder to experimental models.

This disorder accounts for 30 to 40 percent of cases of idiopathic NS in adults but is rare in children. In over 80 percent of cases the nephrotic syndrome is overt. In the remainder only isolated proteinuria is found. Men are affected more often than women. Blood pressure, GFR, and urinary sediment tend to be normal early in the course, making it difficult to distinguish membranous glomerulonephritis from minimal change disease on clinical grounds. Urinary protein selectivity is variable. The excretion of C5b–C9 antigens in the urine may indicate the formation of subepithelial immune deposits. Serum complement components are normal, but IgG levels are depressed. Membranous glomerulonephritis may develop in association with systemic lupus erythematosus (Chap. 241), certain chronic infections (e.g., malaria, hepatitis B), solid tumors (e.g., melanoma and cancer of the lung and colon), or exposure to heavy metals (gold, mercury) or drugs (penicillamine, captopril). Since these causes may be covert at the time of presentation a careful search for these causes is warranted in every case of membranous glomerulonephritis. Renal vein thrombosis is frequent (see above).

Spontaneous complete remissions of NS are common in children and occur in 20 to 40 percent of adults. Progressive renal failure is seen in only 20 to 30 percent of patients, usually 3 or more years after diagnosis and often in association with proteinuria over 5 g/d. Steroid treatment does not greatly influence the development of lasting complete remissions, but may temporarily reduce proteinuria to nonnephrotic levels. A long-term beneficial effect of steroids is unlikely since most prospective trials have not demonstrated benefit. On the other hand, randomized trials and case control studies have demonstrated a beneficial effect both on proteinuria and renal function of combinations of glucocorticoids and cytotoxic agents. The safest and most effective regimen is not known, but protocols involving daily oral prednisone and cyclophosphamide for 6 months to 1 year or sequential cycles of intravenous methylprednisolone, oral prednisone, and oral chlorambucil both appear to be effective. Nevertheless, since the overall long-term prognosis for patients with idiopathic membranous glomerulonephritis is favorable, a conservative approach to treatment is generally recommended. Parameters to identify patients likely to develop progressive renal insufficiency include male sex, older age at onset, hypertension, elevated serum creatinine at discovery, severe hyperlipidemia, proteinuria greater than 10 g/d. Renal biopsy findings often do not aid in the determination of prognosis, but advanced glomerular capillary wall alterations, segmental sclerosis, interstitial fibrosis, and tubular atrophy all indicate a poor prognosis. Patients with features associated with a poor prognosis may be candidates for an aggressive therapeutic approach. Delay of such an aggressive approach (e.g., combined cytotoxic agents and glucocorticoids) until *after* renal impairment is progressive is advocated by some investigators. Indeed, since one third or more of patients with membranous glomerulonephritis enter into a spontaneous remission, an initial aggressive approach may unnecessarily treat some patients destined to have a favorable course in the absence of intervention. On the other hand, if a delay to await progression prejudices against a response to therapy, then too long a delay of therapy may be inadvisable. Treating patients with adverse prognostic indicators initially makes sense, while a wait-and-see approach seems to be advisable for the majority with features compatible with a benign outcome. As indicated above, slowly progressive renal functional impairment occurs almost exclusively in patients with persistent proteinuria in the nephrotic range. Such renal failure seldom develops within 3 to 4 years of diagnosis. However, on occasion patients may have a more rapidly progressive course. The rapid decline of renal function in membranous glomerulonephritis suggests a complicating drug-induced interstitial nephritis, acute renal vein thrombosis, or superimposed crescentic glomerulonephritis. Within 10 years of diagnosis, however, 10 to 20 percent of patients die of intercurrent illness or end-stage renal failure. The majority of survivors have complete or partial remission of proteinuria. A few patients have developed superimposed RPGN. The lesion may recur or develop de novo in renal allografts.

Membranoproliferative glomerulonephritis This disorder is characterized by proliferation of mesangial cells, often with segmental or diffuse interposition of these cells or their cytoplasm into peripheral capillary loops. Mesangial matrix synthesis is increased as well. The glomerular capillary wall is irregularly thickened, by virtue of the mesangial extensions and the attendant synthesis of basement membrane–like material. This group of disorders is also known as *mesangiocapillary* or *lobular glomerulonephritis*. Immunofluorescence and electron-microscopic patterns reflect heterogeneous mechanisms of pathogenesis. In the *type I* lesion, subendothelial electron-dense deposits are present, C3 is deposited in a granular pattern indicative of immune-complex pathogenesis, and IgG and the early components of complement may or may not be present. In the *type II* lesion the lamina densa of the GBM is transformed into an electron-dense character, giving rise to the term *dense deposit disease*. Basement membranes in Bowman's capsules and in tubules are similarly affected. C3 is found irregularly in the GBM and in granules or rings in the mesangium. Small amounts of Ig (typically IgM) are present, but the early complement components are absent from the deposits. Properdin deposition is variable. Additional ultrastructural variants, based upon location of deposit and basement membrane changes, have been described.

Membranoproliferative glomerulonephritis, types I and II, is found in about 5 percent of idiopathic NS in children, particularly between the ages of 8 to 16 years, and somewhat less commonly in adults. Type I accounts for at least two-thirds of cases. Males and females are affected equally. In 50 to 75 percent of patients, a full-blown NS is present, often with features of AGN. In the remainder, proteinuria in the nonnephrotic range is nearly always accompanied by microscopic hematuria. Blood pressure and GFR are frequently abnormal, and the urinary sediment is active. Functional abnormalities of the renal tubules are common. Urinary protein selectivity is usually poor; fibrin degradation products and C3 are found in the urine. Serum C3 levels are reduced in the majority of cases. The early acting complement components C1q, C4, and C2 are often normal, especially in type II disease. This pattern may be indicative of activation of the alternate complement pathway (see Chap. 239). C3 nephritic factor (C3NF) is often found in the serum of patients with type II, especially if the C3 level is quite low. Circulating immune complexes are found in type I. Lesions similar to type I membranoproliferative glomerulonephritis may also be found in SLE, hemolytic-uremic syndrome, transplant rejection, chronic hepatitis B antigenemia, and "shunt" nephritis. Renal vein thrombosis may occur. Type II nephritis may be associated with partial lipodystrophy.

Spontaneous remissions are uncommon. Long-term, alternate-day prednisone therapy (0.3 to 0.5 mg/kg body weight every other day) may delay the progression of the disease. Treatment regimens that combine steroids and cytotoxic agents are not of proven value. Anticoagulants and inhibitors of platelet aggregation (acetylsalicylic acid plus dipyridamole) may have a long-term beneficial effect. The course is progressive, and approximately half of patients die or develop end-stage renal failure within 10 years of the diagnosis. The prognosis for type II lesions seems somewhat worse than for type I. Type II disease almost invariably recurs in the transplanted kidney but does not always result in the premature loss of the allograft.

Other forms of idiopathic nephrotic syndrome In a small percentage of adults and children with idiopathic NS other lesions are encountered on renal biopsy. These include *crescentic glomerulonephritis* and *focal* and *segmental proliferative glomerulonephritis*. The pathogenetic mechanisms for these lesions vary. For example, some cases of focal and segmental glomerulonephritis may have extensive mesangial IgA deposits and fit into the category of Berger's disease (see below). Serum C3 levels are usually normal. The clinical characteristics, natural history, and response to treatment of these lesions are not well defined. Hematuria is common and may be recurrent. Proteinuria tends to be nonselective. Spontaneous remissions of NS are uncommon. Since no controlled studies have been conducted, it is not possible to evaluate the effectiveness of treatment. *Crescentic glomerulonephritis* is likely to have a poor prognosis, whereas mesangial and focal and segmental proliferative glomerulonephritis have a more favorable long-term outlook. Another group of lesions may be encountered in older patients presenting with nephrotic syndrome often accompanied by hematuria and impaired renal function. These lesions, *fibrillary glomerulonephritis* and *immunotactoid* *glomerulopathy*, are characterized by fibrillary or microtubular deposits in the glomerular capillaries resembling amyloid. However, such deposits are Congo red negative and contain variable amounts of immunoglobulin, sometimes of restricted heavy chain isotype. These lesions may represent an unusual form of dysproteinemia or paraproteinemia, although as yet systemic abnormalities are rare and plasma cell or lymphocytic malignancies are not seen. Treatment is generally unsatisfactory, and many patients, particularly those with persisting heavy proteinuria, progress to renal failure.

NEPHROTIC SYNDROME CAUSED BY INFECTIOUS AGENTS, DRUGS, OR CHEMICALS   Table 240-3 lists the common infectious and drug-related causes of NS. In many instances, NS abates following cure of the infection or withdrawal of the offending medication. In patients receiving gold therapy for rheumatoid arthritis or in those exposed to inorganic, organic, or elemental mercury or to penicillamine, membranous glomerulonephritis is usually the lesion responsible for NS. Minimal lesions and interstitial nephritis are seen with *nonsteroidal anti-inflammatory agents.* Human immunodeficiency viral infection with or without full-blown AIDS may be associated with nephrotic syndrome and progressive renal failure. The renal lesion is quite distinctive and consists of focal sclerosis, interstitial nephritis, microscopic transformation of the proximal and distal tubules, and tubuloreticular inclusions (see Chap. 279). NS is known to follow immunization and antiserum treatment of tetanus or snakebite and to occur in situations associated with atopy.

ASYMPTOMATIC URINARY ABNORMALITIES

This group of patients has *proteinuria in the nonnephrotic range and/ or hematuria,* initially unaccompanied by edema, reduced GFR, or hypertension. Abnormalities are often discovered incidentally and may be persistent or recurrent. In some this syndrome is a phase in the natural history of other glomerulopathic syndromes, especially nephrotic syndrome or chronic glomerulonephritis. Common glomerular disorders that present as asymptomatic proteinuria and/or hematuria are listed in Table 240-5. The heredofamilial and multisystem diseases are discussed in Chap. 241. The presence of dysmorphic erythrocytes and/or red cell casts indicates a glomerular cause for the hematuria.

IDIOPATHIC RENAL HEMATURIA (See also Chap. 44)   **Berger's disease (IgA nephropathy)**   This disorder was first described by

---

TABLE 240-5   Glomerular causes of asymptomatic urinary abnormalities

Hematuria with or without proteinuria
A Primary glomerular diseases
  1 Berger's disease (IgA nephropathy)*
  2 Membranoproliferative glomerulonephritis
  3 Other primary glomerular hematurias accompanied by "pure" mesangial proliferation, focal and segmental proliferative glomerulonephritis, or other lesions
  4 "Thin basement membrane" disease*
B Associated with multisystem or heredofamilial diseases
  1 Alport's syndrome and other "benign" familial hematurias*
  2 Fabry's disease
  3 Sickle cell disease
C Associated with infections
  1 Resolving poststreptococcal glomerulonephritis*
  2 Other postinfectious glomerulonephritides*
Isolated nonnephrotic proteinuria
A Primary glomerular diseases
  1 "Orthostatic" proteinuria*
  2 Focal and segmental glomerulosclerosis*
  3 Membranous glomerulonephritis*
  4 Berger's disease (IgA nephropathy)
B Associated with multisystem or heredofamilial diseases
  1 Diabetes mellitus*
  2 Amyloidosis*
  3 Nail-patella syndrome
  4 Leaitin-cholesterol acyltransferase deficiency
  5 Von Gierke's disease

* Most common.

Berger and Hinglais in 1968 and is characterized by recurrent gross or microscopic hematuria. The diagnosis depends on the finding of prominent IgA deposits in the mesangium by immunofluorescence microscopy. Berger's disease is the most common cause of recurrent hematuria of glomerular origin. It most commonly affects older children and young adults, mostly males. It is common in certain Native American tribes. Typically, episodes of macroscopic hematuria are associated with minor flulike illnesses or vigorous exercise. Vague constitutional symptoms may be present, but skin rash, arthritis, and abdominal pain are absent. Urine protein excretion rates are usually less than 3.5 g/d; protein excretion is normal or mildly increased. The nephrotic syndrome develops occasionally. In some patients a self-limited and reversible form of acute renal failure may occur. Such episodes are frequently preceded by an upper respiratory infection and accompanied by bouts of macroscopic hematuria. Thus, these patients resemble those with acute poststreptococcal glomerulonephritis. On rare occasions, patients present with malignant hypertension. Blood pressure, GFR, and serum albumin are usually normal early in the disease. Serum IgA levels are increased in about 50 percent of cases, and serum complement component levels remain normal. IgA-fibronectin complexes, IgA rheumatoid factor, IgA antineutrophil cytoplasmic autoantibodies, and low-titer antinuclear antibodies may also be found. Biopsy of the skin of forearm sometimes reveals dermal capillary deposits of IgA, C3, and fibrin but not early acting complement components or IgA secretory fragments. Similar skin biopsy findings are encountered in Henoch-Schönlein purpura (Chap. 241). Indeed, Berger's disease may be a monosymptomatic form of Henoch-Schönlein purpura.

Renal biopsy reveals a spectrum of changes, but diffuse mesangial proliferative or focal and segmental proliferative glomerulonephritis is found most often. In some cases glomerular morphology may be normal by light microscopy; uncommonly, crescents are found particularly during episodes of macroscopic hematuria and impaired renal function. The distinguishing feature is the finding by immunofluorescence microscopy of *diffuse mesangial deposition of IgA,* often accompanied by lesser amounts of IgG, C3, and properdin, but not by C1q or C4. Fibrin reactive antigens are common in the mesangium or in association with crescents if the latter are present. The pathogenesis of IgA nephropathy is unknown, but the systemic character of the IgA deposits (skin and glomerular capillaries), the presence of circulating IgG and IgA complexes in the majority, and its similarity to Henoch-Schönlein purpura suggest that it is an immune-complex–mediated disease. The nature and source of the antigen are unknown.

The prognosis is variable, but the disease tends to progress slowly. Spontaneous remissions develop in less than 5 percent of adults but more commonly in children. Approximately 50 percent of patients develop end-stage renal failure within 25 years of diagnosis. Self-limited acute renal failure may develop, particularly following upper respiratory infections. Hematuria and biopsy findings of moderate crescent formation (less than 50 percent glomerular involvement and tubular abnormalities) are common in this setting. Azotemia, hypertension, or proteinuria in the nephrotic range are associated with a poor prognosis. At present, there is no evidence that therapy influences the natural history, although intermittent glucocorticoid therapy or broad-spectrum antibiotics may reduce the frequency of episodes of gross hematuria. Glucocorticoids may also result in remissions of proteinuria in those patients with mild glomerular abnormalities by light microscopy. High-dose intravenous methylprednisolone, cytotoxic drugs, and plasma exchange may be useful for patients with rapidly progressive glomerulonephritis with extensive crescents (greater than 50 percent glomerular involvement). IgA nephropathy recurs in the transplanted kidney in approximately 30 to 40 percent of cases. Such recurrences seldom result in loss of renal function but may be associated with hematuria.

Other primary renal hematurias   Some cases of recurrent hematuria do not exhibit the typical immunofluorescence seen in Berger's disease. This group is poorly defined, and the cause and pathogenesis are varied. Some may represent resolving acute glomerulonephritis or early examples of membranoproliferative or hereditary glomerulonephritis (Alport's syndrome, see Chap. 241). A common morphologic lesions is focal and segmental or diffuse mesangial proliferative glomerulonephritis, although mild and nonspecific changes may also be observed. Immunofluorescence studies reveal varying degrees of immunoglobulin and/or complement component deposition (principally IgM and/or C3) in the mesangium. Some show linear deposits of IgG, suggesting a possible anti-GBM antibody pathogenesis. Electron microscopy may reveal dense deposits in the mesangium. Overall, these patients have an excellent prognosis, with frequent spontaneous permanent remissions of recurrent hematuria. Progressive renal insufficiency is unusual. Because of the benign prognosis no treatment is indicated. In some cases, exceptionally thin basement membranes may be demonstrated by electron microscopy (thin basement membrane nephropathy). Such patients may have persistent microscopic hematuria and may have a family history of hematuria. The prognosis tends to be benign, but progression has been described.

ISOLATED NONNEPHROTIC PROTEINURIA OF GLOMERULAR ORIGIN (See also Chap. 44) Mild to moderate proteinuria (i.e., greater than 150 mg but less than 2.0 g/d), unaccompanied by abnormalities in the urinary sediment or evidence of hypertension or reduced renal function, is common. Such patients may display other features of heredofamilial or multisystem diseases, including diabetes mellitus, amyloidosis, rheumatoid arthritis, or cancer. The abnormality may be persistent or evanescent. Proteinuria may occur primarily in the upright posture (*orthostatic proteinuria*) or both in recumbent and erect positions (*constant proteinuria*). Fixed and reproducible orthostatic proteinuria has a benign prognosis and frequently disappears with time. Renal biopsies reveal normal glomeruli or trivial alterations of dubious significance. On the other hand, persistent and constant proteinuria may indicate more serious disease, and renal biopsies often reveal a structural lesion. Some of the lesions have been discussed in the context of idiopathic nephrotic syndrome. Other patients have an unsuspected disease such as amyloidosis or diabetes mellitus. In the remainder, the lesions are trivial and nonspecific, and the long-term significance is uncertain. In primary glomerular diseases, so long as urinary protein excretion remains modest (less than 2.0 g/d), the prognosis is excellent, and deterioration of renal function is relatively uncommon. Renal biopsy is not commonly undertaken in patients with persistent, isolated nonnephrotic proteinuria, as determining morphology seldom leads to specific therapy and adds information chiefly of a prognostic nature. Since patients with proteinuria more than 2.0 g/d are more likely to have lesions that progress, many nephrologists limit renal biopsies to this latter group of patients.

CHRONIC GLOMERULONEPHRITIS

The syndrome of chronic glomerulonephritis (CGN) is characterized chiefly by *persistent urinary abnormalities* (e.g., proteinuria and/or hematuria) and by *slowly progressive impairment of renal function*, eventuating in hypertension, contracted, granular kidneys, and end-stage renal failure. With the possible exception of the minimal change lesion associated with idiopathic nephrotic syndrome (see above) all the disorders described in this chapter and in Chap. 241 can lead eventually to CGN. The pathophysiology of CGN in the context of renal failure is described in Chaps. 235 and 237.

The structural alterations may be categorized as *proliferative* (including mesangial, endo- and/or extracapillary proliferative glomerulonephritis, and focal and segmental proliferative glomerulonephritis), *sclerosing* (including focal and diffuse glomerular sclerosis), and *membranous*. Such lesions are found in most patients with CGN. In the remainder, the lesions are not readily categorized morphologically and are often referred to as *chronic "nonspecific" glomerulonephritis*.

The clinical characteristics of the specific lesions are described in other sections of this chapter. The etiologic and pathogenetic origins of chronic nonspecific glomerulonephritis are heterogeneous. Complicating vascular disease contributes to the glomerular obliteration. Some patients with chronic nonspecific glomerulonephritis may have had an earlier unrecognized episode of acute PSGN.

The detection of CGN usually occurs in one of several ways: (1) the incidental finding of abnormal urine, impaired renal function, or hypertension during multiphasic screening of asymptomatic individuals; (2) the result of the insidious onset of symptoms or signs of renal disease, especially anemia and hypertension; or (3) after an exacerbation of glomerulonephritis, usually during the course of viral or bacterial illness. In advanced stages, the separation of CGN from other causes of renal failure may be difficult; however, the presence of symmetrically contracted kidneys, moderate to heavy proteinuria, abnormal urinary sediment (especially red blood cell casts), and x-ray evidence of normal pyelocalyceal systems suggest CGN.

The evolution of CGN varies, depending upon the underlying disease and the presence of complications, especially hypertension. Many years may elapse from the discovery of an abnormal urine sediment until the development of end-stage renal failure. Because hypertension is common and clinical and laboratory findings are nonspecific, many patients are diagnosed as having "essential hypertension" and secondary arteriolonephrosclerosis. Nevertheless, many, if not most, patients with essential "nonmalignant" hypertension who develop progressive renal insufficiency have an underlying renal parenchymal disease (including primary forms of glomerulonephritis such as IgA nephropathy). Renal biopsy is necessary to define the underlying glomerular lesion. The principal advantage of a morphologic evaluation is to determine prognosis rather than therapy.

Treatment is supportive and symptomatic. The management of specific lesions is discussed in greater detail in the relevant sections of this chapter. Hypertension and urinary tract infections should be treated vigorously, taking care to avoid nephrotoxic agents. Diuretics should be employed only as adjuncts to antihypertensive management or to deal with edema. Rigorous salt or potassium restriction is usually unnecessary and may be hazardous. In the absence of congestive heart failure or marked hypoalbuminemia, severe edema is rare until the terminal phases. Protein and phosphate restriction may slow the rate of progression of renal failure (see Chap. 237).

REFERENCES

D'AMICO G: The commonest glomerulonephritis in the world. IgA Nephropathy. Quart J Med 64:769, 1987

CAMERON JS, GLASSOCK RJ (eds): *The Nephrotic Syndrome*. New York, Marcel Dekker, 1988

DONADIO JV et al: Idiopathic membranous nephropathy. Kidney Int 33:708

GLASSOCK RJ et al: Primary glomerular disease, in *The Kidney*, 4th ed, BM Brenner, FC Rector Jr (eds). Philadelphia, Saunders, 1991, pp 1182–1279

REES AJ, CAMERON JS: Crescentic glomerulonephritis, in *Oxford Textbook of Clinical Nephrology*, J Cameron et al (eds). Oxford, Oxford University Press, 1992, pp 408–437

241 GLOMERULOPATHIES ASSOCIATED WITH MULTISYSTEM DISEASES

RICHARD J. GLASSOCK / BARRY M. BRENNER

Glomerular injury may be a prominent feature of diseases that affect multiple organs and systems. By and large, the etiologies of these diseases are unknown, but aberrant immunologic processes, neoplasia, metabolic disturbances, and biochemical abnormalities are believed to be dominant factors in their pathogenesis. These processes lead to alterations in glomerular structure and function. Some of the glomerular lesions are specific for the underlying disease (e.g., amyloidosis, Fabry's disease, nodular diabetic glomerulosclerosis); however, the majority are nonspecific. Proteinuria results from defects in the charge- and/or size-selective glomerular permeability barriers. Reductions in glomerular filtration rate develop because of loss of filtration surface area in individual nephrons or because of a decline in the total number of nephrons or both. Although extrarenal manifestations are often useful in establishing a diagnosis, some may present with predominant or exclusive renal involvement and only covert extrarenal manifestations.

IMMUNOLOGICALLY MEDIATED MULTISYSTEM DISEASES

SYSTEMIC LUPUS ERYTHEMATOSUS (See also Chap. 284) Systemic lupus erythematosus (SLE) is the archetype of an immunologically mediated multisystem disease and is representative of the multisystem diseases in which renal involvement is common. The cause of SLE is unknown; however, genetic factors and abnormal immune responsiveness probably interact to produce the disease. The principal mechanism for tissue injury in SLE appears to be the deposition of circulating immune complexes, although other mechanisms also play a role, including antitissue antibody and in situ immune-complex formation (see Chap. 239). The circulating immune complexes may be composed of a variety of endogenous antigens combined with autoantibodies. DNA (single-stranded and double-stranded) is a major antigenic component of immune complexes, but other nuclear or cytoplasmic antigens also may be involved. The prevalence of clinical renal involvement in SLE ranges from as low as 35 percent to more than 90 percent in different series. Manifestations of renal disease range from mild abnormalities of the urinary sediment (predominantly hematuria) to massive proteinuria and from chronic indolent glomerulonephritis to a fulminant inflammatory process leading to rapidly progressive renal failure.

The diagnosis and extrarenal manifestations of SLE are described in Chap. 284. This section will deal with the renal involvement. Although extrarenal features usually lead to the correct diagnosis, SLE may present initially with predominant renal manifestations. Morphologic evidence of renal involvement may exist with or without clinical manifestations of renal disease. If immunofluorescence and electron-microscopic studies of renal tissue are performed, abnormalities are present in virtually every patient with SLE. The abnormal glomerular morphologic lesions in SLE form a spectrum based on correlative light- and electron-microscopic and immunofluorescence studies of renal biopsies.

Minimal lupus glomerular lesion This pattern is characterized by few or no changes by light microscopy. Immunofluorescence

studies reveal moderate immunoglobulin and complement deposits exclusively in mesangium. Scattered electron-dense deposits are found in mesangium by electron microscopy. Clinical manifestations may include mild proteinuria and microscopic hematuria. Nephrotic syndrome is uncommon. Glomerular filtration rate (GFR) is almost always normal. Serologic manifestations vary depending on the activity of extrarenal disease. Antibodies to DNA are usually present in low titer, and levels of C3 and C4 may be decreased, especially if dermatitis is severe. Immune complexes also may be detected in skin lesions.

Mesangial lupus glomerulonephritis This pattern is characterized by mild to moderate diffuse mesangial cell proliferation and/or mesangial sclerosis. Immunofluorescence studies reveal immunoglobulins (IgG, IgM, and IgA) and complement components (C1q, C4, and C3) deposited in a granular pattern principally in the mesangium. By electron microscopy, electron-dense deposits are confined to the mesangium. This morphologic appearance present in the absence of clinical renal disease or associated with minor abnormalities in the urinary sediment and modest proteinuria. Nephrotic syndrome and hypertension occasionally may be present. GFR is almost always normal. Mesangial lupus glomerulonephritis may be the initial renal involvement in SLE, from which other patterns evolve. Associated serologic abnormalities depend on the degree of extrarenal activity. These include increased levels of antibody to native double-stranded DNA (dsDNA); depressed serum levels of C3, C4, and C1q; and detectable levels of circulating immune complexes (CIC) (Table 241-1).

Focal and segmental lupus glomerulonephritis This pattern is characterized by focal and segmental cellular proliferation, often associated with necrosis, superimposed on diffuse mesangial hypercellularity. Granular deposits of immunoglobulins and complement involve both the mesangium and occasional glomerular capillary loops. By electron microscopy, dense subendothelial deposits are found in the mesangium and in some peripheral capillary loops. Clinical and laboratory evidence of renal injury is more common than in mesangial lupus glomerulonephritis. Nephrotic syndrome may occur in 10 to 20 percent of patients, but in general, GFR is well preserved. This lesion may persist, resolve, or progress to diffuse proliferative lupus glomerulonephritis. Serologic features of active disease are often present in untreated patients.

Diffuse proliferative lupus glomerulonephritis This pattern is characterized by diffuse mesangial and endothelial cell proliferation that may include extensive peripheral capillary wall interposition of mesangial cells. In addition, focal cellular necrosis, hematoxylinophilic bodies, fibrinoid necrosis, and "wire loops" (capillaries with a thickened appearance owing to subendothelial deposits) may be present. Extensive extracapillary proliferative (crescentic) glomerulonephritis, vasculitis, and interstitial nephritis also may be found

---

TABLE 241-1 Serologic findings in selected multisystem diseases

Disease	C3	C4	FANA	Anti-dsDNA	Anti-GBM	ANCA	Cryo-Ig	CIC	Other
Systemic lupus erythematosus	↓ ↓	↓ ↓	+ + +	+ +	−	±	+ +	+ + +	↑ IgG, RF + +
Goodpasture's disease	−	−	−	−	+ + +	+	−	±	−
Henoch-Schönlein purpura	−	−	−	−	−	±	−	+ +	↑ IgA, IgA RF
Polyarteritis	↓ ↑	↓ ↑	+	±	+	+ + +	+ +	+ + +	↑ IgG
Wegener's granulomatosis	↓ ↑	−	−	−	−	+ + +	±	+ +	−
Cryoimmunoglobulinemia	↓	↓ ↓ ↓	−	−	−	−	+ + +	+ +	RF + + +
Multiple myeloma	−	−	−	−	−	−	±	−	↑ IgG, IgA, IgE, IgD, MC
Waldenström's macroglobulinemia	−	−	−	−	−	−	−	−	↑ IgM
Amyloidosis	−	−	−	−	−	−	−	−	Ig, MC

NOTE: C3 = C3 component of complement; Ig = immunoglobulin levels; FANA = fluorescent antinuclear antibody assay; anti-dsDNA = antibody to double-stranded (native) DNA; anti-GBM = antibody to glomerular basement membrane antigens; cryo-Ig = cryoimmunoglobulin; CIC = circulating immune complexes; ANCA = anti-neutrophil cytoplasmic antibody; RF = Rheumatoid factor; MC = monoclonal; − = normal; + = occasionally slightly abnormal; + + = often abnormal; + + + = severely abnormal.

occasionally. Varying chronic lesions include focal and segmental glomerulosclerosis, fibrocellular crescents, interstitial fibrosis, tubular atrophy, and nephroangiosclerosis. Granular deposits of immunoglobulins and complement components are extensive and involve the mesangium and nearly every capillary loop. Electron microscopy reveals widespread subendothelial and mesangial electron-dense deposits as well as occasional intramembranous or subepithelial deposits. Most patients have an active urinary sediment, heavy proteinuria, and progressive impairment of renal function; occasionally, clinical evidence of renal involvement is lacking. In the untreated patient, evidence of serologic activity is usually present, including depressed serum C3 and C4 concentrations, high levels of precipitating and complement-fixing antibody to dsDNA, cryoimmunoglobulinemia, and circulating immune complexes. This lesion is associated with an ominous prognosis, although vigorous treatment may modify the course (see below).

Membranous lupus glomerulonephritis   This pattern is nearly identical with that described for idiopathic membranous glomerulonephritis (Chap. 240), except that mesangial deposits and mesangial proliferation are more frequent. The glomerular capillary wall is thickened due to the presence of immunoglobulin and complement-containing electron-dense deposits in the subepithelial space, often associated with a spikelike basement membrane reaction. Nearly all patients have heavy proteinuria and the nephrotic syndrome. Although GFR may be normal initially, many patients ultimately develop progressive renal failure. A focal and segmental or diffuse proliferative lesion may be superimposed on the basic membranous lesions. These histologic findings confer a more ominous prognosis (see below). Serologic features of SLE may or may not be present at the time of diagnosis of this nephropathy. Antibody to dsDNA tends to be nonprecipitating and of low titer. Some patients with membranous lupus glomerulonephritis may be erroneously categorized as having idiopathic membranous glomerulopathy (see Chap. 240). Measurements of the level of antibody to dsDNA or of serum complement levels and biopsies of skin for dermal-epidermal deposits of Ig ("lupus band test") may be helpful for diagnosis in such cases.

Sclerosing or end-stage lupus glomerulonephritis   This pattern is characterized by obliterative and sclerosing lesions of the glomeruli and probably represents a late stage of proliferative lesions. Immunofluorescence studies may be only weakly positive for immunoglobulins; subendothelial deposits are infrequent. Hypertension and impaired renal function are common. Serologic parameters of activity of SLE may or may not be present.

Prognosis and treatment   The prognosis and treatment of SLE with renal involvement depend on the nature of the underlying renal lesion, the degree of renal functional impairment, and perhaps the activity and chronicity of renal lesions as disclosed by renal biopsy. Patients with milder forms of renal disease (e.g., minimal or mesangial lupus glomerulonephritis) tend to do well if treatment is directed toward control of the extrarenal manifestations of the disease. Glucocorticoids in modest doses, salicylates, or antimalarials are usually sufficient. Potent nonsteroidal, anti-inflammatory agents may cause functional depression of GFR and should be used with caution in patients with known renal involvement. Serologic parameters, including anti-dsDNA and complement components (C3, C4), should be followed serially. Fluorescent antinuclear antibody tests have little value in prognosis or in following the effectiveness of treatment. A return to normal values for antibody to dsDNA and/or complement components is a favorable sign; however, persistently abnormal serologic features do not necessarily indicate worsening or progressive renal involvement, especially in patients with active extrarenal manifestations. For patients with mild lesions, 85 percent or more can be expected to survive at least 10 years. Patients with membranous lupus glomerulonephritis uncomplicated by superimposed focal or diffuse proliferative lesions and who receive treatment directed primarily at the extrarenal features also have favorable long-term prognosis. On the other hand, patients with extensive focal or diffuse proliferative lupus glomerulonephritis or combined membranous and proliferative lesions do less well and, therefore, warrant a more aggressive approach toward ameliorating the renal disease. High-dose, long-term oral glucocorticoid therapy, although capable of improving extrarenal signs of active disease and reducing the acute inflammatory component of the renal lesions, is not an altogether satisfactory regimen for lupus nephritis. Such treatment is associated with a high prevalence of side effects and may not prevent progression of chronic lesions. High-dose, short-term intravenous methylprednisolone is effective in reducing signs of systemic and renal activity of the disease, especially in patients with recent deterioration. Adjunctive use of cytotoxic agents (azathioprine, cyclophosphamide, or chlorambucil) exerts a steroid-sparing effect and may prevent progression of chronic lesions, particularly among those with mild chronic lesions prior to therapy. The optimal regimen has not yet been established; however, intermittent intravenous cyclophosphamide (500 to 1000 mg/m² of surface area monthly for 6 to 12 months) plus low-dose oral prednisone (0.5 mg/kg of body weight per day) and combinations of azathioprine or cyclophosphamide with low-dose oral prednisone appear to be relatively safe and more effective than glucocorticoids alone in selected patients with severe proliferative lesions. Because prospective, randomized trials have involved only small numbers of patients, it is premature to adopt any particular regimen as the treatment of choice. Even combinations of azathioprine and low-dose prednisone may exert an overall beneficial effect in certain patients. Little is gained by using a combined steroid-cytotoxic approach in patients with advanced renal failure due to progressive glomerular capillary obliteration and sclerosis. These patients are best treated with dialysis and/or transplantation. Reports claiming efficacy of combined intensive plasma exchange and immunosuppressive therapy for severe glomerulonephritis have not been substantiated in a randomized, prospective trial. Such treatment therefore cannot be recommended for the *routine* management of patients with severe and progressive glomerular disease. However, anecdotal reports of dramatic recovery from extrarenal manifestations (e.g., central nervous system lupus) consequent to the use of intensive plasma exchange plus immunosuppression have appeared. Since, from time to time, patients with systemic lupus erythematosus may develop a syndrome closely resembling thrombotic thrombocytopenic purpura, the beneficial effect of intensive plasma exchange may be the consequence of an alteration in thrombotic microangiopathy rather than control of an active immunologically mediated process.

Serologic studies, especially serial measurements of antibody to dsDNA and complement components (C3, C4), may be useful in assessing patients under therapy. Return of these parameters to normal usually indicates satisfactory control of disease and that drug dosage can be safely diminished. These measurements also can be monitored to guide more aggressive therapy when appropriate. However, too heavy reliance on serologic parameters of activity should be discouraged. The correlation between clinical activity and serologic disturbances is poor, at least among patients receiving therapy with steroids and immunosuppressive agents.

Overall, long-term prognosis for patients with SLE and renal involvement has greatly improved. The degree to which changes in methods of diagnosis, serologic monitoring, or treatment are responsible is unknown. End-stage renal failure develops in 15 to 25 percent of patients with diffuse proliferative nephritis within 10 years of initiating therapy with aggressive regimens, such as low-dose alternate-day glucocorticoids combined with oral or intravenous cytotoxic agents. The degree of renal functional impairment and its response to therapy are the most powerful clinical predictors of outcome. Whether the information gleaned from renal biopsy adds to the prognosis is not clear. Cerebral involvement and infectious complications of therapy are now major causes of morbidity and mortality in SLE. Patients with SLE seem to do well on regular chronic dialysis; moreover, as uremia develops, some patients experience remissions of extrarenal activity. In transplanted patients, recurrence of SLE in the renal allograft is uncommon. Thus patients with SLE and nephritis are satisfactory candidates for both dialysis and transplantation.

GOODPASTURE'S SYNDROME The term *Goodpasture's syndrome* refers to the combination of alveolar hemorrhage and glomerular hemorrhage. Such clinical manifestations occur in a wide variety of disorders, including anti-basement membrane antibody–mediated nephritis (often referred to as *Goodpasture's disease*), systemic necrotizing vasculitis, microscopic polyarteritis, Wegener's granulomatosis, mixed essential cryoimmunoglobulinemia, Henoch-Schönlein purpura, and systemic lupus erythematosus. In addition, hemoptysis can occur with *Legionella* infection and interstitial nephritis, and renal vein thrombosis accompanying nephrotic syndrome can produce pulmonary emboli with infarction and hemoptysis. Thus two broad categories of this syndrome can be described: those in which production of an autoantibody to basement membrane antibodies can be documented (so-called Goodpasture's disease) and a heterogeneous group unassociated with anti-basement membrane antibody production. This section will deal with Goodpasture's disease as mediated by antibody to basement membrane antigens. The cause is unknown. Goodpasture's disease may appear at any age and typically affects young men. However, the frequency may be increasing in women.

Pulmonary hemorrhage may be covert and easily overlooked or severe and life-threatening. The initial manifestations of pulmonary involvement are cough, shortness of breath, and hemoptysis. Hilar pulmonary infiltrates may be seen by chest x-ray, and hypoxia is frequent. With marked intraalveolar hemorrhage, pulmonary carbon monoxide uptake is increased, and the pulmonary clearance of radioactive carbon monoxide is depressed. Pulmonary iron sequestration may be documented by scanning of the lungs with ^{59}Fe. Hemosiderin-laden macrophages may be seen in the sputum, but this is a nonspecific finding. Iron-deficiency anemia may result if pulmonary bleeding is prolonged and severe. A history of recent inhalation of volatile hydrocarbons or of viral influenza may be obtained. Cocaine inhalation also can provoke lung hemorrhage. Cigarette smoking increases the risk of alveolar bleeding in patients with anti-basement membrane antibody–mediated disease. Fever, arthralgias, and other systemic symptoms are mild or absent at the time of presentation. Other disorders in which renal disease is associated with pulmonary (alveolar) hemorrhage can ordinarily be differentiated from Goodpasture's disease by their extrarenal features and by typical serologic findings (see Table 241-1).

The glomeruli in Goodpasture's disease range from normal or nearly normal to focal proliferative and necrotizing glomerulonephritis; most often there is extensive extracapillary proliferation (crescents). Rapidly progressive renal failure is a common feature, although patients may initially have normal renal function and mild abnormalities in the urinary sediment. Immunofluorescence studies of renal biopsy material reveal the typical *linear deposits* of IgG (or rarely IgA) anti-basement membrane antibody, often but not necessarily always accompanied by C3 deposition. Electron-microscopic studies do not reveal electron-dense deposits.

Circulating antibody to glycopeptide antigens related to the noncollagenous domains on type IV (basement membrane) collagen are found in over 90 percent of cases if sera are examined early in the course by a sensitive immunoassay (see Table 241-1). The level of circulating antibody does not correlate well with the severity of the renal or pulmonary manifestations. Measurements of circulating antibody are of diagnostic value and have little or no prognostic significance. Serum complement components are nearly always normal, and circulating immune complexes and cryoimmunoglobulins are absent. On occasion, antineutrophil cytoplasmic autoantibodies may be found or develop subsequent to the initial diagnosis, often in association with systemic features of vasculitis. About 80 to 85 percent of patients are HLA-DR2 antigen–positive.

The course is variable. Patients surviving an initial bout of severe hemoptysis may undergo long-term remissions or may have repeated bouts of pulmonary hemorrhage. Mild forms of glomerular injury may not progress, and the principal clinical problems may be related to recurrent hemoptysis. The diagnosis in such patients may be confused with idiopathic pulmonary hemosiderosis. More commonly, the renal disease is progressive, sometimes fulminant, leading to oliguric renal failure in weeks or months (i.e., rapidly progressive glomerulonephritis).

Life-threatening pulmonary hemorrhage may respond temporarily to high doses of parenteral methylprednisolone (10 to 15 mg/kg of body weight) given over short periods. The effectiveness of such therapy in reversing extensive crescentic glomerular lesions is not established. Anticoagulants are contraindicated in the face of active pulmonary hemorrhage. Intensive plasma exchange in combination with cytotoxic drugs and modest doses of glucocorticoids has been associated with dramatic remissions of pulmonary hemorrhage and improvement of the glomerular lesions. This is particularly true if treatment is initiated early in patients with relatively acute disease in whom dialysis is not yet required for therapy of renal failure. The duration and frequency of plasma exchanges depend on the response of the patient and the changes in levels of circulating antibody to glomerular basement membrane antigens, but daily or every other day exchanges are recommended for the first week or two. Renal biopsy is helpful in guiding the management, but even in the presence of extensive crescent formation, responses may be satisfactory. If irreversible glomerular obliteration, extensive interstitial fibrosis, and tubular atrophy are found, especially in the oliguric patient requiring dialysis with long-standing disease, plasma exchange offers little hope for improving the renal lesion. Such patients are best managed by regular hemodialysis and/or transplantation. Although recurrences may develop, the diagnosis is not a contraindication to transplantation as long as the procedure is delayed until levels of circulating anti-basement membrane antibody decrease to undetectable levels. Long-term therapy is usually not required. Glucocorticoids and immunosuppressive agents may be withdrawn gradually after approximately 6 months of treatment with careful monitoring of clinical features and of anti-glomerular basement membrane and antineutrophil cytoplasmic autoantibody levels. Relapses are uncommon but may at times be due to the emergence of antineutrophil autoantibody–associated vasculitis. In patients with severe initial disease, persistent proteinuria and slowly progressive renal failure may ensue unrelated to anti-basement membrane antibody production (see below).

HENOCH-SCHÖNLEIN PURPURA (See also Chap. 315) This disorder is characterized by nonthrombocytopenic purpura, arthralgias, abdominal pain, and glomerulonephritis. Although usually a disease of children, typical disease may be seen in adults of any age. Renal involvement is common and is manifested chiefly by hematuria and proteinuria. In some instances, renal involvement is severe, leading to rapidly progressive glomerulonephritis or nephrotic syndrome. The onset of the disease may resemble acute postinfectious glomerulonephritis. Serum complement component levels are usually normal. Serum IgA levels are increased in about half the patients (see Table 241-1), and IgA rheumatoid factor, IgA-containing immune complexes, or IgA-fibronectin complexes can be detected in 50 to 80 percent. Renal biopsy reveals a spectrum of abnormalities. Mild diffuse mesangial cell proliferation and/or focal and segmental proliferative glomerulonephritis is most common when bouts of macroscopic hematuria and proteinuria are present. More severe and diffuse proliferative glomerulonephritis, sometimes accompanied by extracapillary proliferation (crescents), arises in patients with heavy proteinuria and/or rapidly diminishing GFR. Characteristically, immunofluorescence studies reveal mesangial and peripheral capillary granular deposits of IgA, IgG, C3, and fibrinogen but not C1q, C4, or IgA secretory piece. Similar immunofluorescence findings are present in the dermal capillaries of biopsies of involved and uninvolved skin. Electron microscopy reveals electron-dense deposits principally in the mesangium. These findings suggest that Henoch-Schönlein purpura is due to circulating IgA-containing immune complexes but that the nature of the antigen and the antibody reactivity of the IgA are unknown. Although food allergies and upper respiratory infections may be present, there is no clear-cut etiologic relationship. *Berger's disease* (IgA nephropathy, Chap. 240) may represent a monosymptomatic form of Henoch-Schönlein purpura.

The diagnosis is ordinarily not difficult when the typical clinical features are present. The differential diagnosis includes SLE, polyarteritis, infective endocarditis, postinfectious glomerulonephritis, and essential cryoimmunoglobulinemia.

The course is usually benign; however, progressive renal failure may occur. Renal biopsy is a useful prognostic tool. Patients with persistent urinary abnormalities may experience deterioration of renal function several years after diagnosis. Treatment is symptomatic. There is no convincing evidence that glucocorticoid or immunosuppressive therapy is beneficial for the renal lesion, although these treatments may ameliorate extrarenal features. Patients with rapidly progressive (crescentic) glomerulonephritis benefit from intensive plasma exchange combined with immunosuppressive drugs (see Chap. 240).

SYSTEMIC NECROTIZING VASCULITIS (See also Chap. 291) Glomerular involvement is common in the heterogeneous group of disorders that result from widespread inflammatory and necrotizing lesions of blood vessels. Several variations are recognized, including microscopic polyarteritis (hypersensitivity angiitis), macroscopic polyarteritis (periarteritis nodosa), Wegener's granulomatosis, allergic angiitis and granulomatosis (Churg-Strauss syndrome), rheumatoid vasculitis, temporal arteritis, and Takayasu's arteritis. Henoch-Schönlein purpura and SLE also can be considered examples of vasculitis. Many patients with glomerulonephritis accompanying systemic necrotizing vasculitis have characteristic extrarenal findings such as cutaneous palpable purpura, necrotizing skin lesions, pulmonary infiltrates, upper airway or sinus lesions, mononeuritis multiplex, fever, and wasting. Hypertension is frequent in polyarteritis nodosa but may be absent in hypersensitivity vasculitis and Wegener's granulomatosis. Necrotizing pulmonary infiltrates, upper airway disease, sinusitis, and otitis characterize the Wegener's granulomatosis variant. Laboratory findings, often nonspecific, include anemia, mild leukocytosis, eosinophilia, and markedly elevated erythrocyte sedimentation rate. Autoantibodies to cytoplasmic antigens present in polymorphonuclear leukocytes have been reported in a high percentage of patients with Wegener's granulomatosis and microscopic polyarteritis, as well as in some patients with polyarteritis nodosa and the Churg-Strauss syndrome. Because of the presence of these autoantibodies, many regard this latter disorder as a renal-limited form of microscopic polyarteritis. In addition, such autoantibodies also may coexist with anti-basement membrane autoantibodies (see "Goodpasture's syndrome" and Table 241-1). The detection of such autoantibodies is helpful in establishing the nature of the underlying disease in patients suspected of having vasculitis. Renal biopsies are a poor means of establishing the diagnosis, since they frequently reveal segmental or diffuse necrotizing glomerulonephritis with or without crescents in the absence of any extraglomerular vascular involvement. Lung biopsies more frequently reveal the typical granulomatous necrotizing vasculitis characteristic of Wegener's granulomatosis. Sural nerve biopsies may be useful in establishing the diagnosis of vasculitis in patients presenting with mononeuritis multiplex.

The prognosis is generally poor for patients with systemic necrotizing vasculitis, especially in the absence of treatment; however, aggressive management with glucocorticoids combined with oral cyclophosphamide has been associated with improvement in overall prognosis. Among the antineutrophil cytoplasmic autoantibody–positive subset of patients with vasculitis, a relapse may be predicted by rising titer or reappearance of autoantibody. Some patients with fulminant glomerulonephritis secondary to systemic necrotizing vasculitis in which severe glomerular involvement is accompanied by extensive crescent formation and rapidly progressive dialysis-dependent renal failure may benefit from combined therapy involving plasma exchange, glucocorticoids, and intravenous or oral cyclophosphamide. The long-term prognosis for such patients remains uncertain, since extrarenal involvement and/or complications of immunosuppressive treatment may ultimately be fatal. Late-onset renal failure associated with hypertension and persistent proteinuria may be due to nonimmune

processes and can be ameliorated with aggressive angiotensin converting enzyme inhibitor therapy.

MISCELLANEOUS IMMUNOLOGICALLY MEDIATED MULTISYSTEM DISEASES   Mixed connective tissue disease (MCTD)   In this disorder (see also Chap. 287) renal disease is uncommon and, if present, mild. Clinical manifestations include hematuria and proteinuria and occasionally nephrotic syndrome. Pathologically, membranous or membranoproliferative glomerulonephritis is seen. The prognosis is generally favorable. Glucocorticoid therapy often results in improvement of the glomerular lesions.

Rheumatoid arthritis   Several forms of glomerular injury may occur in rheumatoid arthritis (Chap. 285). Secondary amyloidosis is present in 5 to 10 percent of patients with long-standing arthritis. Nephrotic syndrome may arise as a complication of either gold or penicillamine therapy (see Chap. 240). In addition, the kidney may share in the vasculitis seen occasionally in severe rheumatoid arthritis. Finally, patients with rheumatoid arthritis (untreated with gold or penicillamine) may develop a mild proliferative or membranous glomerulonephritis which resembles lesions seen in SLE. Proteinuria, sometimes with nephrotic syndrome, is the principal clinical feature of such lesions. Prolonged and excessive use of analgesics may lead to renal papillary necrosis.

Other disorders   *Sjögren's syndrome* (Chap. 288) may be associated with nephrotic syndrome due to membranous or membranoproliferative glomerulonephritis (type I) or, more frequently, interstitial nephritis. *Sarcoidosis* is rarely complicated by membranous glomerulonephritis. *Partial or total lipodystrophy* may be associated with membranoproliferative glomerulonephritis (type II, dense deposit disease) (see Chap. 240). Complement abnormalities consist of depressed C3 levels, normal C1q and C4 levels, and circulating C3 nephritic factor.

Chronic liver disease may be complicated by glomerular disease. The nephrotic syndrome may appear in the course of *chronic active hepatitis* associated with persistent hepatitis B surface antigenemia (see below). Glomerular lesions include membranous membranoproliferative (type I) glomerulonephritis. Immunofluorescence studies in such patients reveal granular deposits of immunoglobulins, complement components, and hepatitis B viral antigens, indicating an immune-complex disease. Serum C3 levels are often reduced, and tests for circulating immune complexes and cryoimmunoglobulins are frequently positive. Occasionally, patients with little clinical evidence of liver disease develop distinct glomerular lesions secondary to chronic hepatitis B infection. *Acute viral hepatitis* may be associated with transient hematuria or proteinuria and may resemble other postinfectious glomerulonephritides (see Chap. 240). Severe *chronic liver disease* (cirrhosis) may be associated with diffuse glomerulosclerosis. Few clinical manifestations of glomerular disease are found. Prominent mesangial IgA deposits, of unknown pathogenic significance, have been noted in patients with cirrhosis.

MULTISYSTEM DISEASES ASSOCIATED WITH PARAPROTEINEMIA AND NEOPLASIA

ESSENTIAL (MIXED) CRYOIMMUNOGLOBULINEMIA   This disorder is associated with circulating cold-precipitable immunoglobulins (cryoimmunoglobulins), usually consisting of polyclonal IgG and monoclonal IgM; the latter possesses rheumatoid factor activity. Purpura, necrotizing skin lesions in cold-exposed areas, arthralgias, fever, and hepatosplenomegaly are common. Hepatitis B infection and other occult fungal, bacterial, or viral infections may be found to underlie this syndrome. Circulating cryoimmunoglobulins are also found in chronic infections and probably represent circulating immune complexes with unusual physical properties. Glomerular disease results from the precipitation of the polyclonal cryoimmunoglobulin in the glomerular capillaries and may result in acute renal failure, rapidly progressive (crescentic) glomerulonephritis, or the nephrotic syndrome. Serum complement, particularly the C4, components are depressed (see Table 241-1). Pathologically, a diffuse proliferative glomerulonephritis with extensive monocyte infiltration is seen with findings consistent with the deposition of the circulating cryoimmuno-globulin. Eradication of the underlying infection, if possible, is of value in treatment. Intermittent intravenous "pulses" of methylpred-nisolone and intensive plasma exchange, accompanied by the adminis-tration of oral glucocorticoids and cytotoxic agents, have been of some value in severe cases.

MONOCLONAL GAMMOPATHIES *Multiple myeloma* (Chap. 280) may be associated with several types of glomerular injury. Amyloidosis (Chap. 281) (see below) occurs in 10 to 15 percent of patients with multiple myeloma. Lesions resembling those in cryoimmunoglobulinemia also may develop. Proteinuria and the nephrotic syndrome are common. In addition, a tubulointerstitial lesion (myeloma kidney) consisting of large, laminated intratubular casts, tubule cell atrophy, interstitial fibrosis, and inflammation is common in patients with multiple myeloma and acute or chronic renal failure. *Light chain nephropathy* is characterized by deposits of monoclonal Ig light chains (usually the kappa chain) along the glomerular and tubular basement membranes and by lesions resem-bling nodular diabetic glomerulosclerosis. The urine typically contains large amounts of the monoclonal light chains, but serum electrophore-sis may reveal only hypogammaglobulinemia. Treatment with gluco-corticoids and alkylating agents may be beneficial. *Waldenström's macroglobulinemia* may cause acute renal failure when the IgM paraprotein precipitates in glomerular capillaries as "thrombi." Intensive plasma exchange and therapy with alkylating agents may be beneficial. Hyperviscosity may cause functional alterations in GFR. Renal amyloidosis is uncommon. *Benign monoclonal gammopa-thies* are seldom associated with glomerular complications, except for mild asymptomatic proteinuria and, rarely, nephrotic syndrome.

AMYLOIDOSIS (See also Chap. 281) This disorder may occur in the absence of systemic disease (primary amyloidosis), may be secondary to chronic inflammatory processes (e.g., rheumatoid arthritis, osteomyelitis, paraplegia), multiple myeloma, or other neoplastic diseases, or may occur in a hereditary form (e.g., in association with familial Mediterranean fever). All forms may affect the glomeruli.

Primary amyloidosis commonly affects the kidneys and usually occurs in older age groups. Proteinuria, often of nephrotic proportions, is the most common manifestation of renal involvement. The urine sediment tends to be benign. The degree of proteinuria is not necessarily related to the extent of glomerular deposition of amyloid. Enlarged kidneys may be present in patients with well-preserved renal function, but this is a nonspecific finding. The blood pressure is normal unless advanced uremia is present. Typical pathologic features include hypocellular glomeruli infiltrated with amorphous deposits that stain with Congo red and exhibit green birefringence under polarized light. The fibrillar nature of the amyloid deposits can be readily demonstrated by electron microscopy. Immunofluorescence studies reveal amorphous deposits of immunoglobulin and/or mono-clonal light chains and complement in glomeruli. Similar findings also may occur in another disorder discussed in Chap. 240, fibrillary or immunotactoid glomerulonephritis. In the latter disorder, the deposits are Congo red–negative, and the fibrils are larger. Renal vein thrombosis may complicate the course of amyloidosis.

Renal amyloidosis is a progressive disease for which there is no established treatment. Remissions may occur in secondary amyloidosis if the cause can be eliminated. Remissions in primary amyloidosis are exceedingly rare; a few reports describe remissions following the use of combinations of melphalan and glucocorticoids. Colchicine is of value in prevention of amyloidosis in familial Mediterranean fever. Overall, the 5-year survival for patients with primary amy-loidosis is less than 20 percent. Azotemia, persistent nephrotic syndrome, and myocardial involvement confer an even more ominous prognosis.

NEOPLASTIC DISEASE Glomerular alterations may develop with a variety of neoplastic diseases. *Carcinomas*, especially adenocar-cinoma of lung, colon, stomach, and breast, may be accompanied by glomerular lesions resembling idiopathic membranous glomerulone-phritis, although, on occasion, minimal change lesions, crescentic or focal and segmental proliferative glomerulonephritis, or even amyloidosis may be present. Nephrotic syndrome is the most common clinical renal manifestation, and approximately 5 to 10 percent of patients with idiopathic nephrotic syndrome associated with membra-nous glomerulonephritis harbor an underlying malignancy. However, among patients over age 60 at diagnosis of membranous glomerulone-phritis, as many as 20 percent may have underlying neoplastic disease. Successful treatment of the tumor, especially by surgical means, may lead to remission of the renal manifestation. Presumably the glomerular lesions arise because of the deposition of circulating immune com-plexes that are composed of tumor antigen and antitumor antibody.

Lymphomas and leukemias also may give rise to glomerular abnormalities. Hodgkin's disease is associated with the findings of idiopathic nephrotic syndrome (minimal change disease). Other glomerular lesions may include membranous glomerulonephritis, focal proliferative and sclerosing glomerulonephritis, and amyloidosis. The mechanism of the association of Hodgkin's disease with minimal change disease may involve an underlying T cell abnormality. Proteinuria may wax and wane with fluctuations in the clinical activity of the Hodgkin's disease. Remissions may be produced by local irradiation of involved lymph nodes or by systemic chemotherapy.

METABOLIC, BIOCHEMICAL, AND HEREDITARY DISORDERS

DIABETIC NEPHROPATHY (See also Chap. 337) Diabetes melli-tus affects the structure and function of the kidney in many ways. The term *diabetic nephropathy* encompasses all the lesions occurring in the kidneys of patients with diabetes mellitus. These lesions include *glomerulosclerosis* (diffuse or nodular), *arterionephrosclerosis, chronic interstitial nephritis, papillary necrosis,* and various tubular lesions. Diabetic nephropathy is associated with a variety of clinical syndromes, including mild asymptomatic proteinuria, nephrotic syn-drome, progressive renal failure (acute, rapidly progressive, or chronic), and hypertension. Glomerular lesions are particularly com-mon and account for the majority of abnormal clinical findings referable to the kidney. *Diffuse diabetic glomerulosclerosis* (diffuse intercapillary glomerulosclerosis) is the most common lesion and can be identified in the vast majority of diabetic patients regardless of the presence of abnormal clinical findings referable to the kidney. This lesion consists of a diffuse increase in the volume of mesangial matrix accompanied by an increased width of the glomerular basement membrane. Various exudative lesions, such as capsular drops and fibrin caps, also may be present. Hyaline arteriosclerosis, particularly of the efferent arteriole, is also common. Taken together, these lesions suggest the diagnosis of diabetes mellitus, but individually they are not specific. *Nodular glomerulosclerosis* (Kimmelstiel-Wilson lesion), on the other hand, is reasonably specific for diabetes mellitus. This lesion consists of PAS-positive, laminated, intercapillary nodules on a background of an increase in mesangial matrix. At the periphery of the nodules, open glomerular capillary loops are found. The nodules are relatively acellular, in contrast to the cellular lesions of membrano-proliferative glomerulonephritis. As noted above, *light chain nephrop-athy* may evoke a similar lesion. The pathogenesis of diffuse or nodular diabetic glomerulosclerosis is poorly understood but involves the deleterious effect of the diabetic milieu on matrix biosynthesis and turnover and hemodynamic alterations of the glomerular circulation.

The principal clinical manifestation of diabetic glomerular disease is proteinuria. Initially, only small amounts of albumin (15 to 40 µg/min) are excreted, particularly following exercise (microalbuminuria). This amount of albumin excretion is undetectable by routine screening methods. Under ordinary circumstances, microalbuminuria develops within 10 to 15 years of the onset of hyperglycemia and usually progresses within 3 to 7 years to overt proteinuria and clinical diabetic nephropathy. With "tight" control of hyperglycemia and/or rigorous control of elevated blood pressure, the development of microalbuminuria may be prevented or reversed. With time, the quantity of protein excreted usually increases and may progress to an overt nephrotic syndrome. Glomerular filtration rate is initially elevated and subsequently falls toward normal coincident with the onset of overt proteinuria. The urinary sediment is typically benign, although microhematuria and/or pyuria also may be present if a complicating urinary tract infection or papillary necrosis is present. Hypertension develops as microalbuminuria appears and as GFR falls from supernormal levels but is seldom of malignant proportions. When hypertension is severe or abrupt in onset, one should suspect a complicating atherosclerotic renal arterial stenosis. Typically, plasma renin activity is normal or decreased. Acquired hyporeninemic hypoaldosteronism with persistent hyperkalemia and mild hyperchloremic metabolic acidosis is common. Once azotemia develops, the disease progresses at variable rates, but GFR declines, on average, about 10 to 15 mL/min per year. End-stage renal failure usually develops within 5 to 7 years of the onset of overt proteinuria and clinical nephropathy depending on therapeutic intervention and compliance. Despite poor control of hyperglycemia, only about 50 to 60 percent of insulin-dependent diabetic patients develop clinical nephropathy. The factors that protect the remaining patients from renal failure are unknown but seem to be related to the propensity for the development of hypertension. Patients with non-insulin-dependent diabetes mellitus also may develop clinical nephropathy.

Until the cause of diabetes mellitus is established, prevention of the glomerulopathy will not be feasible. If the abnormal diabetic milieu is responsible for the vascular complications (including glomerular disease), as some have suggested, then very precise regulation of blood sugar (e.g., meticulous attention to diet, exercise, and insulin dosage and servofeedback devices for insulin administration) may be effective in reducing the development of nephropathy. During the microalbuminuric phase, tight metabolic control slows the rate of increase in albumin excretion, as does lowering the arterial blood pressure and dietary protein restriction. Once the nephropathy has reached the stage of overt proteinuria, aggressive management of hypertension will slow the rate of loss of renal function, but strict control of blood sugar does not seem to retard the rate of progression once overt nephropathy (proteinuria >500 mg/d) has emerged. Patients with end-stage renal failure due to diabetic nephropathy are not ideal candidates for long-term dialysis because of concomitant multiple organ dysfunction secondary to widespread arteriovascular disease. Mortality rates among diabetics on chronic dialysis are about three times higher than among similarly treated nondiabetics of comparable age. Renal transplantation may be successful in the younger diabetic, especially if a living related donor is available. The overall success rate is somewhat less than in the nondiabetic population owing to the adverse effects of extrarenal vascular involvement (e.g., coronary artery disease), but transplantation is a viable alternative to dialysis in selected patients. Recurrence of typical diabetic glomerular lesions has been documented in renal allografts, but thus far, progressive loss of GFR secondary to recurrent disease seems to be uncommon.

ALPORT'S SYNDROME   This disorder consists of sensorineural deafness associated with hereditary nephritis. Renal disease manifests itself at an early age, principally as recurrent hematuria. Men are more frequently and more severely affected than women. Slowly progressive renal insufficiency in men commonly terminates in end-stage renal disease in the second to third decade. There is no clear-cut relationship between the onset or severity of the hearing abnormality and the extent of renal disease. Other associated abnormalities include two related ophthalmologic complications, spherophakia and lenticonus, as well as thrombopenia, hyperprolinemia, and

cerebral dysfunction. Family studies have indicated autosomal dominant or X-linked modes of inheritance with variable expressivity. The pathogenesis may be due to defective synthesis of components of glomerular and tubular basement membranes. The gene responsible for the X-linked variety has been mapped to a particular site on the X chromosome (Xq21.2–q22.1) and appears to encode for the synthesis of a unique chain (alpha 5) in type IV collagen.

The pathologic features detected by light microscopy are nonspecific, and a diagnosis cannot be established by optical microscopy alone. Both glomerular and interstitial lesions are present. Focal and diffuse glomerular proliferation, with segmental sclerosis, is common. Interstitial foam cells are nonspecific findings. Electron microscopy reveals thinning, splitting, and delamination of both glomerular and tubular basement membranes, thought by some to be specific for the syndrome. Immunofluorescence studies fail to reveal deposits of immunoglobulins or complement components. The autoantibody to basement membrane antigens found in patients with Goodpasture's disease does not react with the glomeruli of some patients with Alport's syndrome. Treatment is supportive; glucocorticoids and cytotoxic agents are ineffective. The disease is not known to recur following transplantation. (See also Chap. 351).

FABRY'S DISEASE (See also Chap. 349)   This disorder, angiokeratoma corporus diffusum, is an X-linked inborn error of glycosphingolipid metabolism that leads to the accumulation of neutral glycosphingolipids in many tissues including the kidney. A milder disease may develop in heterozygous females. Manifestations are more frequent in hemizygous males and include angiokeratomas involving the lower trunk, scrotum, and buttocks; acroparesthesia; corneal opacities; tortuous retinal veins; and premature coronary and cerebral ischemic disease. Renal manifestations include hematuria and modest proteinuria, often associated with slowly progressive renal failure. Light-microscopic findings include foamy alterations of the epithelial cells of the glomerulus due to the accumulation of lipid. Electron microscopy reveals intracellular rounded laminated bodies ("myelin figures"). The disorder is untreatable unless replacement of the deficient enzyme can be ensured; successful renal transplantation may partially correct the enzyme deficiency.

NAIL-PATELLA SYNDROME   This autosomal dominant disease is characterized by dystrophic nails, absence of one or both patellae, iliac horns, and renal disease. The renal manifestations include isolated proteinuria and hematuria and occasionally the nephrotic syndrome. Progressive renal failure is uncommon. Glomerular lesions are nonspecific by light microscopy, but electron microscopy reveals a characteristic moth-eaten appearance of the glomerular basement membrane associated with intramembranous collagen fibrils. The prognosis is generally favorable. No treatment is known.

CONGENITAL NEPHROTIC SYNDROME   This autosomal recessive trait is characterized by the development of nephrotic syndrome at the time of or shortly after birth. It occurs with highest frequency in families of Finnish origin. Affected individuals have very large placentas, low birth weight, anasarca, polycythemia, and initially normal GFRs. Levels of alpha fetoprotein are increased in amniotic fluid and maternal serum. Proteinuria is marked and nonselective. Nephrotic syndrome appearing several months after birth is usually due to other causes, especially minimal change disease or focal glomerular sclerosis (Chap. 240). Congenital syphilis and congenital toxoplasmosis may produce similar syndromes and must be excluded. Pathologically, microcystic transformation of the cortical nephrons results from proximal tubular dilatation. Glomerular changes are nonspecific. The anionic charge density on glomerular basement membrane is reduced. Extensive effacement of the foot processes and sclerosis of the glomerular tufts are seen by electron microscopy. Immunofluorescence findings are nonspecific. The course is progressive, and few patients survive the first year of life. Treatment is ineffective. Death is usually due to inanition, infection, or renal failure. A few patients may survive long enough to be considered for renal transplantation.

SICKLE CELL DISEASE (See also Chap. 306) This disorder is an autosomal trait characterized by an abnormal hemoglobin (hemoglobin S). Glomerular lesions occur occasionally in homozygous disease. The medulla is affected, leading to impairment of concentrating ability and potassium and acid excretion and, occasionally, to papillary necrosis. Rarely, patients develop mainly glomerular lesions, either membranous or membranoproliferative glomerulonephritis, accompanied by proteinuria and a nephrotic syndrome. Immunofluorescence studies demonstrate glomerular deposition of immunoglobulin and complement in a granular pattern suggesting immune-complex–mediated disease. The course in patients with the glomerulopathy of sickle cell disease is often relentless, leading to end-stage renal disease. No treatment is known to be effective. Transplantation is occasionally successful.

LECITHIN:CHOLESTEROL ACYLTRANSFERASE DEFICIENCY (See also Chap. 344) This autosomal recessive trait leads to absence of the enzyme in plasma that catalyzes the conversion of lecithin and cholesterol to lysolecithin and cholesteryl ester. Multiple lipoprotein abnormalities develop, including absence of α and pre-β lipoproteins, hypertriglyceridemia, accumulation of abnormal lipoproteins, and increased plasma-esterified cholesterol. Corneal opacities, anemia, hyperuricemia, proteinuria, and progressive renal failure are characteristic. Foam cells are present in bone marrow and glomeruli, and a picture resembling focal and segmental glomerulosclerosis may evolve. Treatment is generally ineffective, but plasma or blood transfusions may transiently correct the disorder. Renal failure has been corrected by renal transplantation, but recurrence of disease in allografts may occur.

VON GIERKE'S DISEASE (See also Chap. 350) Glycogen storage disease secondary to glucose-6-phosphatase deficiency (Von Gierke's disease) causes renal manifestations. Patients with this autosomal recessive disorder are of short stature and have poorly developed skeletal muscles. Hypoglycemia may precipitate convulsions in childhood. The kidneys are enlarged, and a Fanconi-like syndrome with aminoaciduria, glycosuria, and phosphaturia may be present. Renal insufficiency is associated with moderate proteinuria and with focal and segmental glomulerulosclerosis. Hyperuricemia may cause gout. The kidneys and liver are uniformly enlarged.

DRUG-INDUCED GLOMERULAR DISEASE Many drugs have been associated with the development of glomerular-disease; however, it is usually difficult to establish a direct cause and effect relationship. In a few situations the association is clear-cut, and reexposure has led to recurrence of disease. A partial listing of these drugs is provided in Table 241-2. Certain *heavy metals* (Hg, Au) and their inorganic salts or organic compounds may produce membranous glomerulonephritis and nephrotic syndrome. Removal of the drug is not invariably associated with resolution. *Sulfhydryl compounds* (penicillamine, captopril) also may cause membranous or proliferative glomerulonephritis. The risk of developing a renal complication following penicillamine or gold therapy for rheumatoid arthritis is influenced by genes in the major histocompatibility complex. *Nonsteroidal anti-inflammatory agents* may produce nephrotic syndrome (minimal change disease), interstitial nephritis, and acute renal failure. *Probenecid, trimethadione,* or *paramethadione* may be associated with nephrotic syndrome and a variety of glomerular lesions, including minimal change disease and membranous glomerulonephritis. *Heroin* abuse may be associated with focal and segmental glomerulosclerosis that may progress to nephrotic syndrome and progressive renal failure. *Intravenous amphetamine abuse* may be associated with systemic necrotizing vasculitis. Chronic hepatitis B infection may be involved in the development of glomerular lesions in association with intravenous drug abuse. Allopurinol, hydralazine, and rifampin may cause vasculitis and/or crescentic glomerulonephritis.

INFECTION-RELATED GLOMERULAR DISEASES

As discussed in Chap. 240, a wide variety of infectious agents have been implicated in glomerular diseases, and a similarly broad array of clinical features and morphologic patterns of glomerular injury can complicate infectious disease. Acute glomerulonephritis, particularly that due to beta-hemolytic streptococcal infection is dealt with in detail in Chap. 240. *Infective endocarditis, visceral sepsis, salmonellosis, pneumococcal pneumonia, meningococcemia,* and *gonococcemia* have all been associated from time to time with glomerulonephritis, most typically a proliferative lesion associated with features of the acute nephritic syndrome. *Syphilis,* both congenital and secondary, may evoke the nephrotic syndrome with a proliferative or membranous lesion. Parasitic diseases such as *malaria, toxoplasmosis, schistosomiasis,* and *filariasis* also may produce proteinuria of the nephrotic syndrome or a picture resembling acute glomerulonephritis. Many acute viral diseases, including *hepatitis B, Epstein-Barr, measles,* and *varicella* infections, also may be associated with a transient glomerulonephritis. On the other hand, chronic viral diseases, such as *hepatitis B* and *human immunodeficiency virus* (HIV) infections, may evoke heavy proteinuria and nephrotic syndrome accompanied by progressive renal failure. Hepatitis B infection is most often associated with membranous glomerulonephritis. Serologic markers of chronic infection such as persistent hepatitis B surface or e antigen are present. Low C3 levels and cryoimmunoglobulins also may be present. Features of liver disease may be minimal. The long-term prognosis is poor. Glucocorticoids may worsen liver disease. Therapy with recombinant interferon-α and low doses of glucocorticoids may be beneficial. HIV infection seems to evoke a particular pattern of glomerular disease, most often in black men (see Chap. 279). Focal glomerulosclerosis, tubulointerstitial nephritis, microcystic changes in tubules, giant casts, and intracytoplasmic inclusions are commonly observed. Heavy proteinuria is associated with progressive renal failure. Kidney size is usually normal or increased. The renal lesion may be more severe than other manifestations of HIV infection. Therapy is usually ineffective, but treatment of the infection with antimetabolites, such as zidovudine or related agents, may retard the rate of progression of disease. Remissions are rare, and rapid development of end-stage renal failure is the rule.

TABLE 241-2 Drugs associated with glomerular lesions

Elemental, inorganic, or organic mercury compounds
Organic gold compounds
Penicillamine
Captopril
Heroin
Amphetamines
Probenecid
Oxazoladinedione derivatives (e.g., trimethadione)
Antivenoms and antitoxins
Sulfonamides
Vaccinations
Allopurinol
Hydralazine
Rifampin
Nonsteroidal anti-inflammatory agents

REFERENCES

Atkins CL et al: Alport syndrome, in *Disease of the Kidney*, 4th ed, RW Schrier, CW Gottschalk (eds). Boston, Little, Brown, 1988, pp 617–641
Austin HA et al: Therapy of lupus nephritis: Controlled trial of prednisone and cytotoxic drugs. N Engl J Med 314:1004, 1989
Glassock RJ et al: Secondary glomerular diseases, in *The Kidney*, 4th ed, BM Brenner, FC Rector Jr (eds). Philadelphia, Saunders, 1991, pp 1280–1368
Savage COS et al: Microscopic polyarteritis: Presentation, pathology and prognosis. Q J Med 56:467, 1985

242 TUBULOINTERSTITIAL DISEASES OF THE KIDNEY

THOMAS H. HOSTETTER / BARRY M. BRENNER

An etiologically diverse group of renal diseases can be distinguished from those considered in Chaps. 240 and 241 because the histologic and functional abnormalities involve the tubules and interstitium to a greater degree than the glomeruli and renal vasculature (see Table 242-1). Both clinically and histologically, these disorders can be divided into acute and chronic forms. The chronic group may be due to sustained insults by a factor or factors that initially cause acute disease or to a slower, progressive, cumulative insult without an identifiable acute episode. Morphologically, acute forms of these disorders are characterized by interstitial edema, often associated with cortical and medullary infiltration by polymorphonuclear leukocytes

and patchy areas of tubule cell necrosis. In more chronic forms, interstitial fibrosis predominates, inflammatory cells are typically mononuclear, and abnormalities of the tubules tend to be more widespread, as evidenced by atrophy, luminal dilatation, and thickening of tubule basement membranes. In the past, the diagnosis of chronic pyelonephritis (see Chap. 90) was almost universally applied when these chronic tubulointerstitial abnormalities were found. It is now apparent that only a small proportion of these lesions result from infection. Nonbacterial factors, including exogenous toxins and metabolic and immunologic derangements, constitute the major pathogenic mechanisms. Because of the nonspecific nature of the histology, particularly in chronic tubulointerstitial diseases, biopsy specimens rarely provide a specific diagnosis. The urine sediment is also unlikely to be diagnostic, except in allergic forms of acute tubulointerstitial disease, in which eosinophils may predominate in the urinary sediment.

Defects in renal function often accompany these alterations of tubule and interstitial structure (see Table 242-2). Proximal tubule dysfunction may be manifested as selective reabsorptive defects leading to hypokalemia, aminoaciduria, glycosuria, phosphaturia, uricosuria, or bicarbonaturia (proximal or type II renal tubular acidosis; see Chap. 244). In combination, these defects constitute the *Fanconi syndrome*. Protein excretion is usually modest, rarely exceeding 2 g/d. The excreted proteins are typically of low molecular weight and include $beta_2$ microglobulin, lysozyme, and immunoglobulin light chains. Defective proximal tubule reabsorption of these readily filtered small proteins accounts for their augmented excretion. Tubule sodium reabsorption also may be deranged in patients with advanced tubulointerstitial diseases, predisposing to salt wasting and hypovolemia. One or more of these reabsorptive defects are commonly encountered with heavy metal poisoning, multiple myeloma, and other diffuse tubulointerstitial processes.

Defects in urinary acidification and concentrating ability often represent the most troublesome of the tubule dysfunctions encountered in patients with tubulointerstitial disease. Hyperchloremic metabolic acidosis often develops at a relatively early stage in the course. Patients with this finding generally elaborate urine of maximal acidity (pH of 5.3 or less). In such patients the defect in acid excretion is usually caused by a reduced capacity to generate and excrete ammonia due to the reduction in renal mass. Preferential damage to the collecting ducts, as in amyloidosis or chronic obstructive uropathy, also may predispose to distal or type I renal tubular acidosis, characterized by high urine pH (>5.5) during spontaneous or NH_4Cl-induced metabolic acidosis. Patients with tubulointerstitial diseases affecting medullary and papillary structures predominantly also may evidence concentrating defects, with resultant nocturia and polyuria.

TABLE 242-1 Principal causes of tubulointerstitial disease of the kidney

TOXINS

Exogenous toxins
  Analgesic nephropathy*
  Lead nephropathy (see Chap. 396)
  Miscellaneous nephrotoxins (e.g., antibiotics, cyclosporine, radiographic contrast media, heavy metals)*[†]
Metabolic toxins
  Acute uric acid nephropathy (see Chap. 347)
  Gouty nephropathy (see Chap. 347)*
  Hypercalcemic nephropathy (see Chap. 357)
  Hypokalemic nephropathy (see Chap. 45)
  Miscellaneous metabolic toxins (e.g., hyperoxaluria, cystinosis, Fabry's disease)

NEOPLASIA

Lymphoma (see Chap. 34)
Leukemia (see Chap. 310)
Multiple myeloma (see Chap. 280)*

IMMUNE DISORDERS

Hypersensitivity nephropathy*[†]
Sjögren's syndrome (see Chap. 288)
Amyloidosis (see Chap. 281)
Transplant rejection (see Chap. 238)[†]
Tubulointerstitial abnormalities associated with glomerulonephritis
  (see Chaps. 240 and 241)
AIDS (see Chap. 279)

VASCULAR DISORDERS (see Chaps. 236 and 243)

Arteriolar nephrosclerosis*
Atheroembolic disease
Sickle cell nephropathy
Acute tubular necrosis*[†]

HEREDITARY RENAL DISEASES

Hereditary nephritis (Alport's syndrome) (see Chaps. 241 and 351)
Medullary cystic disease (see Chap. 244)
Medullary sponge kidney (see Chap. 244)
Polycystic kidney disease (see Chap. 244)

INFECTIOUS INJURY (see Chap. 90)

Acute pyelonephritis*[†]
Chronic pyelonephritis

MISCELLANEOUS DISORDERS

Chronic urinary tract obstruction (see Chap. 246)*
Vesicoureteral reflux*
Radiation nephritis

* Common.
[†] Typically acute.

TABLE 242-2 Transport dysfunctions of tubulointerstitial disease

Defect	Cause(s)
Reduced GFR*	Obliteration of vasculature and obstruction of tubules
Fanconi syndrome or competent defects	Damage to proximal tubular reabsorption of glucose, amino acids, phosphate, and bicarbonate
Hyperchloremic acidosis*	1. Reduced ammonia production 2. Inability to acidify the collecting duct fluid (distal renal tubular acidosis) 3. Proximal bicarbonate wasting
Tubular or small-molecular-weight proteinuria*	Failure of proximal tubule protein reabsorption
Polyuria, isothenuria*	Damage to medullary tubules and vasculature
Hyperkalemia*	Potassium secretory defects including aldosterone resistance
Salt wasting	Distal tubular damage with failure of sodium reabsorption

* Common

The impairment in maximal concentration is typically unresponsive to the administration of vasopressin and hence is a form of nephrogenic diabetes insipidus. Analgesic nephropathy and sickle cell disease are prototypes of this form of injury.

Although the major structural defects originate in the tubules and interstitium, progressive reduction in glomerular filtration rate (GFR) is a functional accompaniment of most, if not all, forms of tubulointerstitial damage, reflecting secondary injury to glomeruli and other elements of the renal microcirculation. Indeed, oliguric acute renal failure may be caused by acute forms of tubulointerstitial disease, and about a third of patients with chronic renal insufficiency suffer from a primary chronic tubulointerstitial disease.

TOXINS

The renal tubules and interstitium are prone to toxic injury. Although the kidneys constitute less than 1 percent of total body mass, they receive approximately 20 percent of the cardiac output, and 90 percent or more of renal blood flow is distributed to the renal cortex. Exposure of tubules and interstitium of the renal cortex to circulating toxins is therefore greater than is that of most other tissues. Transport processes in renal tubules contribute further to the intrarenal accumulation of toxins, enhancing local concentrations of noxious agents. The urinary concentrating mechanism also can establish high levels of toxins within medullary and papillary portions of the kidney, predisposing these regions to chemical injury. Finally, the relatively acid pH of the fluid within most nephron segments may affect the ionization characteristics of potentially toxic compounds and thereby influence local concentration and solubility. Although these processes render the kidney vulnerable to toxic injury, the role of nephrotoxins in renal damage often goes unrecognized because the manifestations of such injury are usually nonspecific in nature and insidious in onset. Diagnosis largely depends on a history of exposure to a certain toxin, a difficult matter because exposure may be occult. Particular attention should be paid to the occupational history, as well as to an assessment of exposure—current and remote—to drugs, especially antibiotics and analgesics. The recognition of a potential association between a patient's renal disease and exposure to a nephrotoxin is crucial, because, unlike many other forms of renal disease, progression of the functional and morphologic abnormalities associated with toxin-induced nephropathies may be prevented, and even reversed, by eliminating additional exposure.

EXOGENOUS TOXINS Analgesic nephropathy Individuals who ingest large quantities of analgesic drugs are prone to develop tubulointerstitial damage and papillary necrosis. Indeed, in Australia, Switzerland, and Sweden, analgesic abuse is one of the most common causes of chronic renal failure, and it is an important cause in the United States as well. While aspirin, phenacetin, and acetaminophen (the metabolite of phenacetin) may alone or in combination induce chronic renal disease, epidemiologic studies incriminate phenacetin and acetaminophen as the more injurious combination. Chronic ingestion of aspirin without these other compounds seems to be an uncommon cause of serious renal damage.

Morphologically, analgesic nephropathy is characterized by papillary necrosis and tubulointerstitial inflammation. At an early stage, damage to the vascular supply of the inner medulla (vasa recta) leads to a local interstitial inflammatory reaction and, eventually, to papillary ischemia, necrosis, fibrosis, and calcification. Destruction of papillae usually precedes extension of the tubulointerstitial abnormalities to the renal cortex and, therefore, occurs before renal size and GFR are reduced significantly. Although papillary necrosis is a common finding in patients with the nephropathy of analgesic abuse, necrosis of papillae also may occur in patients with chronic pyelonephritis, diabetes mellitus, sickle cell disease, and obstructive uropathy. The susceptibility of the renal papillae to damage by phenacetin is believed to be related to the establishment of a renal gradient for its acetaminophen metabolite, resulting in papillary tip concentrations tenfold higher than those in renal cortex. Hydration dissipates this gradient and may explain the protective effect of this maneuver in preventing phenacetin-induced papillary necrosis in animals. Aspirin in these analgesic compounds contributes to renal injury by uncoupling oxidative phosphorylation in renal mitochondria and by inhibiting the synthesis of renal prostaglandins, which are potent endogenous renal vasodilator hormones. Both effects of aspirin favor hypoxia in renal tissues and therefore enhance the susceptibility of the inner medulla to nephrotoxic injury.

Analgesic nephropathy occurs some three to five times more commonly in women than in men. A direct relationship exists between the total amount of analgesic compounds ingested and the degree of renal impairment. The intake of 1.0 g phenacetin per day for 1 to 3 years or the total ingestion of 2 kg phenacetin in combination with other analgesics appears to represent minimum requirements for the development of analgesic nephropathy. In such patients, renal function usually declines gradually, in association with chronic necrosis of papillae and diffuse tubulointerstitial damage to the renal cortex. Occasionally, papillary necrosis may be associated with hematuria and even renal colic owing to obstruction of a ureter by necrotic tissue. More than half of patients with analgesic nephropathy have pyuria, which, if persistently associated with sterile urine, provides an important clue to the diagnosis. Nonetheless, active pyelonephritis may coexist in patients with analgesic nephropathy. Proteinuria, if present, is typically mild (less than 1 g/d). Patients with analgesic nephropathy are usually unable to generate maximally concentrated urine, reflecting the underlying medullary and papillary damage. An acquired form of distal renal tubular acidosis may contribute to the development of *nephrocalcinosis*. The occurrence of anemia out of proportion to the degree of azotemia also may provide a clue to the diagnosis of analgesic nephropathy. Occult gastrointestinal bleeding (usually secondary to analgesic-induced gastritis) and, in an occasional patient, hemolysis (particularly in those with glucose-6-phosphate dehydrogenase deficiency) contribute to the anemia. Vague abdominal complaints, nonspecific headaches, and arthralgias are common. Moderate hypertension is also common and progresses to a malignant phase in only a small minority. When analgesic nephropathy has progressed to renal insufficiency, the kidneys usually appear bilaterally shrunken on intravenous pyelography, and the calyces are deformed. A "ring sign" on the pyelogram is pathognomonic of papillary necrosis and represents the radiolucent sloughed papilla surrounded by the radiodense contrast material in the calyx. Transitional cell carcinoma may develop in the urinary pelvis or ureters as a late complication of analgesic abuse.

Every effort must be made to convince the patient who ingests excessive analgesics to discontinue this hazardous practice. When renal damage is at an early stage, cessation of abuse usually arrests the progression of the nephrotoxic process; not infrequently, overall renal function improves with time. With continued abuse, however, progressive renal damage leads invariably to chronic renal failure.

Lead nephropathy (See also Chap. 396) Children and adults with lead intoxication often develop a chronic tubulointerstitial renal disease. In children, lead poisoning usually results from ingestion of lead-based paints (pica). The oxide of lead liberated from paint or present in the vapor arising from the welding of metals covered with lead-based paint may be inhaled in substantial quantities, thereby constituting an industrial form of exposure in adults. Alcohol, illegally distilled in an apparatus constructed from automobile radiators (so-called moonshine), is another cause of lead poisoning. Tubule transport processes enhance the accumulation of lead within renal cells, particularly in the proximal convoluted tubule, leading to cell degeneration, mitochondrial swelling, and eosinophilic intranuclear inclusion bodies rich in lead. In addition to tubule degeneration and atrophy, lead nephropathy is associated with ischemic changes in the glomeruli, fibrosis of the adventitia of small renal arterioles, and focal areas of cortical scarring. Eventually, the kidneys become atrophic. In addition to progressive azotemia, abnormalities of tubule function may occur, particularly *renal glycosuria* and *aminoaciduria*. Urinary excretion of lead, bile pigments, and porphyrin precursors, such as δ-aminolevulinic acid, coproporphyrin, and urobilinogen, may be increased. Patients with chronic lead nephropathy are characteristically *hyperuricemic*, a consequence of enhanced reabsorption of filtered urate. Acute gouty arthritis (so-called saturnine gout) occurs in about 50 percent of patients with lead nephropathy, in striking contrast to other forms of chronic renal failure in which gout is rare (also see Chap. 347). Hypertension is also a complication. Therefore, in any patient with slowly progressive renal failure, atrophic kidneys, gout, and hypertension, the diagnosis of lead intoxication should be considered. In addition, patients with chronic lead poisoning often complain of abdominal colic and have evidence of anemia, peripheral neuropathy, and encephalopathy. The diagnosis may be suspected by finding elevated serum levels of lead. However, because blood levels may not be elevated even in the presence of a toxic total-body burden of lead, the quantitation of lead excretion following infusion of the chelating agent calcium disodium edetate is a more reliable indicator of serious lead exposure. Urinary excretion of more than 0.6 mg/d of lead is indicative of overt or potential toxicity. Treatment includes removing the patient from the source of exposure and augmenting lead excretion with a chelating agent such as calcium disodium edetate.

Miscellaneous nephrotoxins Use of lithium salts for manic-depressive illness has been associated with tubulointerstitial disease. The most frequent clinical finding is a mild to moderate nephrogenic diabetes insipidus resulting in polyuria and polydipsia. It is unclear whether long-term lithium therapy produces irreversible chronic tubulointerstitial lesions and impairment of GFR. Though some patients develop histologic evidence of such injury, there are only rare reports of chronic renal insufficiency attributable to this agent. In any case, renal function should be followed in patients taking this drug, and caution should be exercised if lithium is employed in patients with underlying renal disease.

The immunosuppressant cyclosporine causes both acute and chronic renal injury. The acute injury and the use of cyclosporine in transplantation are discussed in Chap. 238. The chronic injury is a progressive decline in GFR with mild proteinuria and arterial hypertension. Hyperkalemia is a relatively common complication and results in part from tubule resistance to aldosterone. Hypomagnesemia due to urinary magnesium wasting is less common but can cause hypocalcemia. The histologic changes in renal tissue comprise patchy interstitial fibrosis and tubular atrophy. In addition, the intrarenal vasculature often demonstrates hyalinosis, and focal segmental glomerular sclerosis can be present as well. Indeed, renal vasoconstriction induced by the drug appears to be a major mechanism of the renal injury. In patients receiving this drug for renal transplantation, chronic rejection and recurrence of the primary disease may coincide with chronic cyclosporine injury, and on clinical grounds, distinction among these may be difficult. Whether the chronic injury can be prevented by dose reduction is uncertain. However, use of the lowest doses of cyclosporine consistent with adequate immunosuppression appears to mitigate nephrotoxicity. In addition, treatment of any associated arterial hypertension may lessen renal injury.

Many agents that commonly lead to acute renal failure are also capable of producing tubulointerstitial injury (see Chap. 236). These include antibiotics (e.g., aminoglycosides, amphotericin B), radiographic contrast agents, various hydrocarbons (e.g., carbon tetrachloride), and heavy metals (e.g., mercury, cadmium, and bismuth).

METABOLIC TOXINS Acute uric acid nephropathy (See also Chap. 347) Acute overproduction of uric acid and extreme hyperuricemia often lead to a rapidly progressive renal insufficiency, so-called acute uric acid nephropathy. This tubulointerstitial disease is usually seen in patients given cytotoxic drugs for the treatment of lymphoproliferative or myeloproliferative disorders but also may occur in these patients before such treatment is begun. The pathologic changes are largely the result of deposition of uric acid crystals in the kidneys and their collecting systems, leading to partial or complete obstruction of collecting ducts, renal pelvis, or ureter. Since obstruction is often

bilateral, patients typically show the clinical course of acute renal failure, characterized by oliguria and rapidly rising serum creatinine concentration. In the early phase uric acid crystals can be found in urine, usually in association with microscopic or gross hematuria. Peak serum uric acid levels vary but are almost always above 1200 μmol/L (20 mg/dL) and may even exceed 3500 μmol/L (60 mg/dL).

Prevention of hyperuricemia in patients at risk by treatment with allopurinol in doses of 200 to 800 mg/d prior to cytotoxic therapy reduces the danger of acute uric acid nephropathy. Once hyperuricemia develops, however, efforts should be directed to preventing deposition of uric acid within the urinary tract. Increasing urine volume with potent diuretics (furosemide or mannitol) effectively lowers intratubular uric acid concentrations, and alkalinization of the urine to pH 7 or greater with sodium bicarbonate and/or a carbonic anhydrase inhibitor (acetazolamide) enhances uric acid solubility. If these efforts, together with allopurinol therapy, are ineffective in preventing acute renal failure, dialysis should be instituted to lower the serum uric acid concentration as well as to treat the acute manifestations of uremia. The combination of conservative therapy and hemodialysis allows most patients with acute uric acid nephropathy to survive acute renal failure and ultimately recover renal function.

Gouty nephropathy (See also Chap. 347) Patients with less severe but prolonged forms of hyperuricemia are predisposed to a more chronic tubulointerstitial disorder, often referred to as *gouty nephropathy*. Since other conditions associated with hyperuricemia, such as hypertension, nephrolithiasis, pyelonephritis, and even lead poisoning, may contribute to renal damage, the effect of chronic hyperuricemia per se on renal function is unclear. Nevertheless, the severity of renal involvement correlates with the duration and magnitude of the elevation of the serum uric acid concentration. Histologically, the distinctive feature of gouty nephropathy is the presence of crystalline deposits of uric acid and monosodium urate salts in kidney parenchyma. These deposits are believed to represent the primary pathogenic process in gouty nephropathy, with intraluminal crystallization of uric acid taking place in distal tubules and collecting ducts where urine pH is generally quite low and where uric acid concentrations are considerably in excess of levels in plasma. These deposits not only cause intrarenal obstruction but also incite an inflammatory response, leading to lymphocytic infiltration, foreign-body giant cell reaction, and eventual fibrosis, especially of medullary and papillary regions of the kidney. Bacteriuria and pyelonephritis occur in about one-fourth of cases, presumably as complications of intrarenal urinary stasis. Since patients with gout frequently suffer from hypertension and hyperlipidemia, degenerative changes of the renal arterioles may constitute a striking feature of the histologic abnormality, often out of proportion to other morphologic defects. Clinically, gouty nephropathy is an insidious cause of renal insufficiency. Early in its course, GFR may be near normal, often despite focal morphologic changes in medullary and cortical interstitium, proteinuria, and diminished urinary concentrating ability. Whether reducing serum uric acid levels with allopurinol exerts a beneficial effect on the kidney remains to be demonstrated. Although such undesirable consequences of hyperuricemia as gout and uric acid stones respond well to allopurinol, use of this drug in asymptomatic hyperuricemia has not been shown to improve renal function consistently. On the other hand, uricosuric agents such as probenecid, which may increase uric acid stone production, clearly have no role in the treatment of renal disease associated with hyperuricemia.

Hypercalcemic nephropathy (See also Chap. 357) Chronic hypercalcemia, as occurs in primary hyperparathyroidism, sarcoidosis, multiple myeloma, vitamin D intoxication, or metastatic bone disease, can cause tubulointerstitial damage and progressive renal insufficiency. The earliest renal lesion induced by hypercalcemia is a focal degenerative change in renal epithelia, primarily in collecting ducts, distal convoluted tubules, and loops of Henle. Tubule cell necrosis leads to nephron obstruction and stasis of intrarenal urine, favoring local precipitation of calcium salts and infection. Dilatation and atrophy of tubules eventually occur, as do interstitial fibrosis, mononuclear leukocyte infiltration, and interstitial calcium deposition (nephrocalcinosis). Calcium deposition also may occur in glomeruli and the walls of renal arterioles. Clinically, the most striking defect is an inability to concentrate the urine maximally, resulting in polyuria and nocturia. Defective transport of chloride in the ascending limb of Henle's loop is responsible, at least in part, for this concentrating defect. Additionally, reduced collecting duct responsiveness to vasopressin may contribute to this abnormality. Reductions in GFR and renal blood flow also occur, both in acute severe hypercalcemia and with prolonged hypercalcemia of lesser severity. Distal renal tubular acidosis and sodium and potassium wasting also have been described in these chronic states. Eventually, uncontrolled hypercalcemia leads to severe tubulointerstitial damage and overt renal failure. Urinalysis is rarely a clue to the presence of hypercalcemic renal failure, but abdominal x-rays may demonstrate nephrocalcinosis as well as nephrolithiasis, the latter due to the hypercalciuria which often accompanies hypercalcemia. Treatment for hypercalcemic nephropathy consists of reducing the serum calcium concentration toward normal and correcting the primary abnormality of calcium metabolism. The management of hypercalcemia is discussed in Chap. 357. Prognosis for recovery of renal function depends on the severity of the renal lesion at the time hypercalcemia is corrected. Renal dysfunction of acute hypercalcemia may be completely reversible. Gradual, progressive renal insufficiency related to chronic hypercalcemia, however, may not improve with correction of the calcium disorder. Nonetheless, every effort should be made to return serum calcium concentration to normal to minimize further loss of renal function.

Hypokalemic nephropathy (See also Chap. 45)   Disturbances of renal structure and function occur commonly in patients with moderate to severe potassium depletion of at least several weeks' duration. Histologically, renal epithelial cells are often seen to contain numerous vacuoles, most marked in proximal and, to a lesser extent, distal convoluted tubules. These findings usually disappear with potassium repletion. Glomeruli are reduced in size and may become sclerotic, while larger blood vessels are usually uninvolved. Whether prolonged or recurrent potassium deficiency results in irreversible tubulointerstitial fibrosis, scarring, and atrophy is unresolved. Loss of urinary concentrating ability is the most commonly encountered functional defect. In animals this urinary concentrating abnormality is preceded by a period of primary polydipsia. The reduced concentrating capacity which eventually develops is due, at least in part, to defective operation of the countercurrent multiplier system. Elevated rates of intrarenal prostaglandin synthesis also may contribute to this concentrating defect, since prostaglandins antagonize the hydroosmotic action of antidiuretic hormone on collecting-duct epithelium. Nocturia, polyuria, and polydipsia are frequently encountered in patients with chronic potassium depletion, although, occasionally, patients with severe hypokalemia have no complaints referable to the urinary tract. Patients with hypokalemic nephropathy may have an enhanced susceptibility to pyelonephritis. The polydipsia is probably due to both the impaired renal concentrating ability and a primary disorder of the thirst mechanism, which is believed to be a common feature of chronic potassium depletion. Urinalysis often reveals no abnormalities except for mild proteinuria. Serum creatinine and urea nitrogen concentrations usually remain within normal limits. Treatment should be directed at repleting body potassium stores and correcting the primary process responsible for potassium loss. With correction of body potassium, functional and histologic abnormalities of the kidneys usually disappear, although maximal urinary concentrating ability may not return to normal for several months.

Miscellaneous metabolic toxins   Urinary oxalate, derived from the metabolism of glycine and, to a variable extent, from ingested oxalate, may deposit as insoluble intratubular calcium oxalate crystals and result in chronic tubulointerstitial damage in patients with hereditary or acquired forms of *hyperoxaluria*. *Cystinosis* and *Fabry's disease* are other hereditary depositional disorders affecting the renal tubules and interstitium (see Chaps. 241, 244, and 245).

RENAL PARENCHYMAL DISEASE ASSOCIATED WITH EXTRARENAL NEOPLASM

In addition to being the site of origin of several benign and malignant neoplasms (see Chap. 247), the kidneys are frequently affected by neoplasms arising outside the urinary tract. Except for the glomerulopathies associated with lymphomas and several solid tumors (see Chap. 241), the renal manifestations of primary extrarenal neoplastic processes are confined mainly to the interstitium and tubules. Although metastatic renal involvement by solid tumors is unusual, the kidneys are often invaded by neoplastic cells in various lymphomas and leukemias and in multiple myeloma. In postmortem studies of patients with *lymphoma*, renal involvement is found in approximately half. The involvement may be focal, in the form of multiple discrete nodules, or diffuse, with lymphomatous infiltration throughout the renal parenchyma. Diffuse infiltration is seen most commonly in lymphomas other than Hodgkin's disease. There may be flank pain related to massive renal infiltration, and x-rays may show enlargement of one or both kidneys. Renal insufficiency occurs in a minority of cases, and overt uremia is rare. Treatment of the primary disease may improve renal function in these cases.

The kidneys are also commonly involved in various forms of *leukemia*. At postmortem examination, bilateral renal involvement is present in approximately 50 percent of cases. As with lymphoma, uremia is rarely, if ever, a consequence of leukemic infiltration of the kidneys. The kidneys also can be involved in leukemias because of the associated high incidence of hyperuricemia, hypercalcemia, and lysozymuria. The myelogenous leukemias, particularly of the monocytic type, may be complicated by tubule defects involving potassium and magnesium wasting.

In contrast, infiltration of the kidneys with *myeloma* cells is infrequent (see also Chap. 280). When it occurs, the process is usually focal, so renal insufficiency from this cause is also uncommon. The more usual lesion is *myeloma kidney*, characterized histologically by atrophic tubules, many with eosinophilic intraluminal casts, and numerous multinucleated giant cells within tubule walls and in the interstitium. The frequent occurrence of myeloma kidney in patients with Bence Jones proteinuria has suggested a causal relation. Bence Jones proteins are thought to cause myeloma kidney through direct toxicity to renal tubule cells. In addition, Bence Jones proteins may precipitate within the distal nephron where the high concentrations of these proteins and the acid composition of the tubule fluid favor intraluminal cast formation and intrarenal obstruction. Indeed, positive immunofluorescence staining for immunoglobulin light chains can often be demonstrated in casts found in myeloma kidneys. Occasionally, acute renal failure occurs after intravenous pyelography in patients with multiple myeloma and is believed to result from the further precipitation of Bence Jones proteins induced by dehydration prior to radiographic study. Dehydration of the patient with myeloma in preparation for intravenous pyelography should therefore be avoided. Multiple myeloma also may affect the kidneys indirectly. Hypercalcemia or hyperuricemia may lead to the nephropathies described above. Proximal tubule disorders are also seen occasionally, including type II proximal renal tubular acidosis and the Fanconi syndrome. Additionally, intrarenal deposits of *amyloid* (see below) may contribute to impaired excretory function.

IMMUNE DISORDERS

HYPERSENSITIVITY NEPHROPATHY   An acute diffuse tubulointerstitial reaction may result from hypersensitivity to a number of drugs. First reported after the use of sulfonamides, acute tubulointerstitial damage is now seen most often with the antibiotic *methicillin*, although *ampicillin, penicillin, cephalothin, phenindione, thiazides, furosemide*, and nonsteroidal anti-inflammatory drugs also have been implicated. Of note, the tubulointerstitial nephropathy which develops in some patients taking nonsteroidal anti-inflammatory drugs may be associated with nephrotic-range proteinuria and histologic evidence of minimal change glomerulopathy. Grossly, the kidneys are usually enlarged. Histologically, the glomeruli appear normal. The principal pathologic abnormalities are in the interstitium of the kidney, which reveals pronounced edema and infiltration with polymorphonuclear leukocytes, lymphocytes, plasma cells, and, in some cases, large numbers of eosinophils. If the process is severe, tubule cell necrosis and regeneration also may be apparent. Immunofluorescence studies either have been unrevealing or have demonstrated a linear pattern of immunoglobin and complement deposition along tubule basement membranes. In a few cases of methicillin-induced acute tubulointerstitial disease, circulating anti-tubule basement membrane antibodies also have been found, suggesting that autoantibody formation may have been induced by the penicilloyl hapten of methicillin (by conjugation of hapten with tubule basement membrane proteins, thereby altering the native antigenicity of the basement membrane). In cases associated with nonsteroidal anti-inflammatory drugs, a role for cell-mediated immunity has been proposed, since renal infiltration by both T and B lymphocytes has been observed with a relative predominance of cytotoxic T cells. Evidence for an immunologic basis for these various drug-related nephropathies also derives from the facts that the onset of nephropathy does not appear to be dose-related, often follows a second exposure to the drug presumed to be responsible for the renal injury, and often is associated with increased levels of serum IgE. In the case of methicillin, the patients usually develop evidence of renal injury after about 2 weeks of drug administration. Hematuria, fever, skin rash, and eosinophilia are prominent. Many patients develop azotemia which typically resolves after withdrawal of the offending drug. Proteinuria and pyuria often accompany the hematuria, and occasionally eosinophils are found in the urine sediment. The clinical picture may be confused with acute glomerulonephritis, but when acute azotemia and hematuria are accompanied by eosinophilia, skin rash, and a history of drug exposure, a hypersensitivity reaction leading to acute tubulointerstitial nephritis should be regarded as the leading diagnostic possibility. Discontinuation of the drug usually results in complete reversal of the renal injury; rarely, renal damage may be irreversible. Glucocorticoids have been used, but their value has not been established.

SJÖGREN'S SYNDROME (See also Chap. 288)   Keratoconjunctivitis sicca, or Sjögren's syndrome, is an immunologic disorder characterized by dryness of mucous membranes and mononuclear cell infiltration of salivary and lacrimal glands; it is often seen in patients with rheumatoid arthritis. When the kidneys are involved, the predominant histologic findings are those of chronic tubulointerstitial disease. Interstitial infiltrates are composed primarily of lymphocytes, causing the histology of the renal parenchyma in these patients to resemble that of the salivary and lacrimal glands. Renal functional defects include diminished urinary concentrating ability and distal (type I) renal tubular acidosis. Urinalysis may show pyuria (predominantly lymphocyturia) and mild proteinuria.

AMYLOIDOSIS (See also Chaps. 241 and 281)   Glomerular pathology usually predominates and leads to heavy proteinuria and azotemia. However, tubule function also may be deranged, giving rise to a nephrogenic diabetes insipidus and to distal (type I) renal tubular acidosis. In several cases these functional abnormalities correlated with peritubular deposition of amyloid, particularly in areas surrounding vasa rectae, loops of Henle, and collecting ducts. Bilateral enlargement of the kidneys, especially in a patient with massive proteinuria and tubule dysfunction, should raise the possibility of amyloid renal disease.

HIV INFECTION (See also Chap. 279)   Chronic renal disease occurs in a fraction of patients infected with HIV. This complication usually presents with nephrotic proteinuria and a rapid decline in renal function and may precede overt AIDS. Glomerular abnormalities include focal and segmental glomerular sclerosis, and tubulointerstitial changes include tubular dilation with cystic change, epithelial cell vacuolization, and mononuclear cell infiltrates. Uncertainty exists whether direct infection of renal cells by the virus or some indirect immune reaction is responsible for the renal disease. Some renal abnormalities result from associated nephrotoxic insults including intravenous drug abuse and multiple exposure to nephrotoxic antibiotics. In addition, the accumulated effects of multiple septic episodes, such as infectious granulomatous cytomegalovirus inclusions, and Kaposi's sarcoma obviously are secondary to the compromised immune state and should not be considered HIV-specific renal disease. The prevalence of the specific HIV-related renal lesion appears to be variable. The reason for this disparity is uncertain. However, black patients with HIV are especially at risk for renal complications, and the variations in reported prevalence of renal disease in HIV infection may, in part, reflect different racial distributions among the HIV-infected populations studied.

TUBULOINTERSTITIAL ABNORMALITIES ASSOCIATED WITH GLOMERULONEPHRITIS   A number of primary glomerulopathies also may be associated with damage to tubules and interstitium. Pathogenically, the extraglomerular component in these renal disorders often involves the same mechanisms responsible for the more pronounced glomerular injury. For example, in more than half of patients with the nephropathy of systemic lupus erythematosus, deposits of immune complexes can be identified in tubule basement membranes, usually accompanied by an interstitial mononuclear inflammatory reaction. Similarly, in many patients with glomerulonephritis associated with anti-glomerular basement membrane antibody, the same antibody is reactive against tubule basement membranes as well.

MISCELLANEOUS DISORDERS

VESICOURETERAL REFLUX (See also Chaps. 90 and 246)   Normally, the junction of the terminal ureter with the urinary bladder provides a competent sphincter so that during micturition urine leaves the bladder only via the urethra. However, when the function of the ureterovesical junction is impaired, urine may reflux into the ureters due to the high intravesical pressure that develops during voiding. Clinically, reflux is often detected on the voiding and postvoiding films obtained during intravenous pyelography, although voiding cystourethrography may be required for definitive diagnosis. Bladder infection may ascend the urinary tract to the kidneys through incompetent ureterovesical sphincters. Not surprisingly, therefore, reflux is often discovered in patients with acute and/or chronic urinary tract infections. In children particularly, reflux of minor degree may disappear with standard therapy of intercurrent urinary infection. With more severe degrees of reflux, characterized by dilatation of ureters and renal pelves, progressive renal damage often appears, and although active infection also may be present, uncertainty exists as to the necessity of infection in producing the scarred kidney of reflux nephropathy. In contrast to those with other forms of chronic tubulointerstitial disease, patients with renal insufficiency and scarring due to reflux often demonstrate substantial proteinuria. Indeed, in such cases glomerular lesions similar to those of idiopathic focal glomerulosclerosis (Chap. 240) are often present in addition to the changes of chronic tubulointerstitial disease. Surgical correction of reflux is usually necessary only with the more severe degrees of reflux since renal damage correlates with the extent of reflux. Obviously, if extensive glomerulosclerosis already exists, urologic repair may no longer be warranted.

RADIATION NEPHRITIS   Renal dysfunction can be expected to occur if 23,000 Gy (2300 rad) or more of x-ray irradiation is administered to both kidneys during a period of 5 weeks or less. Histologic examination of the kidneys reveals hyalinized glomeruli, atrophic tubules, extensive interstitial fibrosis, and hyalinization of the media of renal arterioles. Radiation-induced renal ischemia is believed to be the main pathogenic factor responsible for the tubulointerstitial damage, which may not become evident clinically for months after completion of radiation. The presentation of acute radiation nephritis includes rapidly progressive azotemia, moderate to malignant hypertension, anemia, and proteinuria which may reach the nephrotic range. More than 50 percent progress to chronic renal failure. A more insidious form is characterized by slower development of azotemia, anemia, and nephrotic syndrome. Malignant hypertension may follow unilateral renal irradiation and resolve with ipsilateral nephrectomy. Radiation nephritis has all but vanished because of heightened awareness of its pathogenesis by radiotherapists.

REFERENCES

ADLER SG et al: Hypersensitivity phenomena and the kidney: Role of drugs and environmental agents. Am J Kidney Dis 5:75, 1985

ARANT BS: Reflux nephropathy. Kidney 21:19, 1989

BENNET WM: Lead nephropathy. Kidney Int 28:218, 1985

———, DEBROE ME: Analgesic nephropathy. A preventable renal disease. N Engl J Med 320, 1269, 1989

——— et al: Tubulointerstitial disease and toxic nephropathy, in *The Kidney*, 4th ed, BM Brenner, FC Rector Jr (eds). Philadelphia, Saunders 1991

BOTON R et al: Prevalence, pathogenesis, and treatment of renal dysfunction associated with chronic lithium therapy. Am J Kidney Dis 10:329, 1987

CAMERON JS: Immunologically mediated interstitial nephritis: Primary and secondary. Adv Nephrol 18:207, 1989

MURRAY T, GOLDBERG M: Chronic interstitial nephritis: Etiologic factors. Ann Intern Med 82:453, 1975

MYERS BD et al: The long-term course of cyclosporine-associated chronic nephropathy. Kidney Int 33:590, 1988

RAO TKS: Clinical features of human immunodeficiency virus associated nephropathy. Kidney Int 40(suppl 35):S-13, 1991

SANDLER DP et al: Analgesic use and chronic renal disease. N Engl J Med 320:1238, 1989

243 VASCULAR INJURY TO THE KIDNEY

KAMAL F. BADR / BARRY M. BRENNER

Adequate delivery of blood to the glomerular capillary network is crucial for glomerular filtration and overall salt and water balance. Thus, in addition to the threat to the viability of renal tissue, vascular injury to the kidney may compromise the maintenance of body fluid volume and composition. Involvement of the renal vessels by atherosclerotic, hypertensive, embolic, inflammatory, and hematologic disorders is usually a manifestation of generalized vascular pathology. The morphologic and clinical responses to these insults and the unique renal vasculopathy associated with the toxemias of pregnancy are considered in this chapter.

THROMBOEMBOLIC DISEASES OF THE RENAL ARTERIES

Thrombosis of the major renal arteries or their branches is an important cause of deterioration of renal function, especially in the elderly. It is often difficult to diagnose and therefore requires a high index of suspicion. Thrombosis may occur as a result of intrinsic pathology in the renal vessels (posttraumatic, atherosclerotic, or inflammatory) or as a result of emboli originating in distant vessels, most commonly fat emboli, emboli originating in the left heart (mural thrombi following myocardial infarction, bacterial endocarditis, or aseptic vegetations), or "paradoxical" emboli passing from the right side of the circulation via a patent foramen ovale or atrial septal defect. Emboli are bilateral in 15 to 30 percent of cases.

The clinical presentation is variable, depending on the time course and the extent of the occlusive event. Acute thrombosis and infarction, such as follows embolization, may result in sudden onset of flank pain and tenderness, fever, hematuria, leukocytosis, nausea, and vomiting. If infarction occurs, renal enzymes may be elevated, namely aspartate aminotransferase (AST), lactic dehydrogenase (LDH; most reliable), and alkaline phosphatase, which rise and fall in the order

---

TABLE 243-1 Clinical presentations of ischemic renal disease

1 Acute renal failure
2 Progressive azotemia in a patient with known renovascular hypertension (usually on medical therapy)
3 Unexplained progressive azotemia in an elderly patient with or without refractory hypertension
4 Hypertension and azotemia in a renal transplant patient

---

listed. Urinary LDH and alkaline phosphatase also may increase after infarction. Renal function deteriorates acutely, leading in bilateral thrombosis to acute oliguric renal failure. More gradual (i.e., atherosclerotic) occlusion of a single renal artery may go undetected. A spectrum of clinical presentations lies between these two extremes (Table 243-1). Hypertension usually follows renal infarction and results from renin release in the peri-infarction zone. Hypertension is usually transient but may be persistent. Diagnosis is established by renal arteriography.

Management of *acute* renal arterial thrombosis includes surgical intervention, anticoagulant therapy, conservative and supportive therapy, and control of hypertension. The choice of treatment depends mainly on (1) the condition of the patient, in particular the patient's ability to withstand major surgery, and (2) the extent of renovascular occlusion and amount of renal mass at risk of infarction. In general, supportive care and anticoagulant therapy are indicated in unilateral disease. In bilateral thrombosis, medical and surgical therapies yield comparable results. Twenty-five percent of patients die during the acute episode, usually from extrarenal complications. In *chronic* ischemic renal disease, surgical revascularization is more likely to preserve and improve renal function and to control the hypertension (see below).

ATHEROEMBOLIC DISEASE OF THE RENAL ARTERIES

Atheroembolic disease typically results from multiple showers of cholesterol-containing microemboli dislodged from atheromatous plaques in large arteries. Such emboli occlude small (150- to 200-μm diameter) vessels in the kidney and in other organs (retina, brain, pancreas, muscles, skin, and extremities). It usually occurs in an elderly individual with atherosclerotic disease elsewhere and usually follows aortic surgery or renal or coronary arteriography. Spontaneous atheroembolic disease has been reported. Manifestations include deterioration of renal function (sudden or gradual), mild proteinuria, microscopic hematuria, and leukocyturia. Urine volume may remain normal or fall to oliguric levels depending on severity. Renal ischemia can induce or exacerbate preexisting hypertension.

Antemortem diagnosis of atherosclerotic renal emboli is difficult. The demonstration of cholesterol emboli in the retina is helpful, but a firm diagnosis is established only by demonstration of cholesterol crystals in the smaller arteries and arterioles in renal biopsy or autopsy specimens. These also may be seen in asymptomatic skeletal muscle or skin. No specific treatment is available.

RENAL VEIN THROMBOSIS

Thrombosis of one or both main renal veins (RVT) occurs in a variety of settings (Table 243-2). The pathogenesis is not always clear, particularly when it occurs in so-called hypercoagulable states such as may develop in pregnant women, users of oral contraceptives, subjects with nephrotic syndrome, or

---

TABLE 243-2 Conditions associated with renal vein thrombosis

1 Trauma
2 Extrinsic compression (lymph nodes, aortic aneurysm, tumor)
3 Invasion by renal cell carcinoma
4 Dehydration (infants)
5 Nephrotic syndrome
6 Pregnancy or oral contraceptives

dehydrated infants. Nephrotic syndrome accompanying membranous glomerulopathy and certain carcinomas seems to predispose to the development of RVT, which occurs in 10 to 50 percent of patients with these disorders. RVT may exacerbate preexisting proteinuria but is infrequently the cause of the nephrotic syndrome.

The clinical manifestations depend on the severity and abruptness of its occurrence. Acute cases occur typically in children and are characterized by sudden loss of renal function, often accompanied by fever, chills, lumbar tenderness (with kidney enlargement), leukocytosis, and hematuria. Hemorrhagic infarction and renal rupture may lead to hypovolemic shock. In young adults RVT is usually suspected from an unexpected and relatively acute or subacute deterioration of renal function and/or exacerbation of proteinuria and hematuria in the appropriate clinical setting (underlying nephrotic syndrome, trauma, pregnancy, oral contraceptive use). In cases of gradual thrombosis, usually occurring in the elderly, the only manifestation may be recurrent pulmonary emboli or development of hypertension. A Fanconi-like syndrome and proximal renal tubular acidosis have been described.

The definitive diagnosis can only be established through selective renal venography with visualization of the occluding thrombus. Treatment consists of anticoagulation, the main purpose of which is prevention of pulmonary embolization, although some authors have also claimed improvement in renal function and proteinuria. Encouraging reports have appeared concerning the use of streptokinase. Spontaneous recanalization with clinical improvement also has been observed. Anticoagulant therapy is more rewarding in the acute thrombosis seen in younger individuals. Nephrectomy is advocated in infants with life-threatening renal infarction. Thrombectomy is effective in some cases.

RENAL ARTERY STENOSIS　Stenosis of the main renal artery and/or its major branches accounts for 2 to 5 percent of hypertension. The common cause in the middle-aged and elderly is an atheromatous plaque at the origin of the renal artery. In younger women, stenosis is due to intrinsic structural abnormalities of the arterial wall caused by a heterogeneous group of lesions termed *fibromuscular dysplasia*.

Renal artery stenosis should be suspected when hypertension develops in a previously normotensive individual over 50 years of age or in the young (under 30 years) with suggestive features: symptoms of vascular insufficiency to other organs, high-pitched epigastric bruit on physical examination, symptoms of hypokalemia secondary to hyperaldosteronism (muscle weakness, tetany, polyuria), and metabolic alkalosis. If renovascular hypertension is suspected, a positive captopril test, which has a sensitivity and specificity of greater than 95 percent, constitutes an excellent screening procedure to assess the need for more invasive radiographic evaluation. The test relies on the exaggerated increase in plasma renin activity (PRA) following administration of captopril to patients with renovascular hypertension as compared with those with essential hypertension. It is considered positive when all the following criteria are satisfied: stimulated PRA of 12 (μg/L)/h, absolute increase in PRA of 10 (μg/L)/h or more, and increase in PRA of greater than 150 percent [or 400 percent if baseline PRA is less than 3 (μg/L)/h]. In the appropriate clinical setting, particularly in the presence of a positive captopril test, digital subtraction renal arteriography should be performed. This procedure obviates the need for cannulation of the arterial system and has a low incidence of false-positive (5 percent) and false-negative (10 percent) results. The most definitive diagnostic procedure is bilateral arteriography with repeated bilateral renal vein and systemic renin determinations. If renal vein renin measurements from the two kidneys differ by a factor of 1.5:1 or more (higher value from the affected kidney) in a patient with radiographic unilateral renal artery stenosis, the chance of cure of hypertension by surgical reconstruction is almost 90 percent, particularly if renal vein renin level from the unaffected kidney is equal to or less than systemic levels (suppressible). A ratio of less than 1.5:1, however, does not exclude the diagnosis of renovascular hypertension, particularly in the presence of bilateral disease. Two diagnostic modalities for the noninvasive

evaluation of significant renal artery stenosis are duplex scanning (sensitivity 95 percent, specificity 90 percent) and magnetic resonance angiography (sensitivity 100 percent for lesions with $\geq$50 percent stenosis, specificity 92 percent).

The aims of treatment are control of the blood pressure and restoration of perfusion to the ischemic kidney. In general, it is now firmly established that interventional therapy (i.e., surgery or angioplasty) is superior to medical therapy, which, while controlling blood pressure, does little to salvage renal mass lost to ischemic injury. Success rates with percutaneous transluminal angioplasty in young patients with fibromuscular dysplasia are 50 percent cure and 30 percent improvement in blood pressure control. Angioplasty is best suited for noncalcified, segmental short lesions and is also useful in some elderly patients who are poor surgical risks. About half of elderly individuals with reduced renal function as a result of renal arterial stenosis improve following angioplasty or surgery, even when preintervention arteriography shows little evidence of cortical perfusion. Despite the risks associated with surgery, long-term follow-up studies demonstrate an advantage of surgery over angioplasty both with regard to the incidence of restenosis and to the preservation or improvement in GFR.

Renal artery stenosis, particularly if atherosclerotic, is a progressive disease that may lead to gradual and silent loss of renal functional tissue. Compensatory contralateral hypertrophy may maintain renal function until affected by superimposed pathologic processes, at which time azotemia supervenes. Even if angioplasty or surgery fail to return blood pressure to normal, these procedures usually render medical therapy easier.

HEMOLYTIC UREMIC SYNDROME (HUS) AND THROMBOTIC THROMBOCYTOPENIC PURPURA (TTP)　(See also Chap. 240) HUS and TTP, consumptive coagulopathies characterized by microangiopathic hemolytic anemia and thrombocytopenia, have a particular predilection for the kidney and the central nervous system, the latter especially in TTP. The kidneys of patients with HUS or TTP often exhibit a "flea-bitten" appearance, the result of multiple cortical hemorrhagic infarcts. The major sites of pathology are the small renal arteries and afferent arterioles, which are nearly occluded as a result of marked intimal hyperplasia (particularly in TTP) and fibrin deposits in the subintimal regions. When the vasoocclusive process is extensive, bilateral cortical necrosis may occur. In addition, arteriolar microaneurysms, glomerular infarction, or nonspecific focal changes may be seen. In keeping with the focal nature of the vascular lesions, patchy areas of interstitial edema, tubular necrosis, and, eventually, fibrosis occur. By immunofluorescence staining, complement components and immunoglobulins may be demonstrated in the arterioles, and fibrinogen deposits are present in arteries, arterioles, and glomerular capillary loops.

Several mechanisms have been implicated in the etiology of the intravascular coagulopathy seen in HUS and TTP, including induction of a generalized Shwartzman phenomenon by microorganisms or endotoxin, genetic predisposition, and deficiency of platelet antiaggregatory substance(s) (e.g., prostacyclin). Some patients improve following exchange transfusion or plasmapheresis, suggesting accumulation of an as yet unidentified toxin.

Renal failure is common in both HUS and TTP, usually manifested by oligoanuria (more severe in HUS), azotemia, mild proteinuria, microscopic and/or gross hematuria, and cylindruria. Patients with HUS have more severe renal failure, often marked by oligoanuria and hypertension and commonly progressing to chronic renal failure. The prognosis in HUS is better in children than in adults. In TTP, the course of which may span days to months, renal failure is usually less severe. The overall prognosis, however, remains poor in view of the severe central nervous system involvement.

In the management of TTP, high-dose glucocorticoids and plasma exchange often provide complete remission or cure. Plasma exchange should be initiated as early as possible, and the treatment cycles can be repeated if thrombocytopenia recurs. Splenectomy and antiplatelet therapy also have been used with varying degrees of success in TTP patients. The success of plasma exchange in adult HUS is less well established than in TTP.

ARTERIOLAR NEPHROSCLEROSIS Whether hypertension is "essential" or of known etiology, persistent exposure of the renal circulation to elevated intraluminal pressures results in development of intrinsic lesions of the renal arterioles (hyaline arteriolosclerosis) that eventually lead to loss of function (nephrosclerosis). Nephrosclerosis is divided into two distinct entities: "benign" and "malignant" (or accelerated).

Benign arteriolar nephrosclerosis Benign arteriolar nephrosclerosis is seen in patients who are hypertensive for an extended period of time (blood pressure more than 150/90 mmHg) but whose hypertension has not progressed to a malignant form (described below). Such patients, usually in the older age group, are often discovered to be hypertensive on routine physical examination or as a result of nonspecific symptomatology (e.g., headaches, weakness, palpitations).

Kidney size is normal to reduced, with loss of cortical mass leading to a fine granularity. Although the larger arteries may show atherosclerotic changes, the characteristic pathology is in the afferent arterioles, which have thickened walls due to deposition of homogeneous eosinophilic material (hyaline arteriolosclerosis). This material is composed of plasma proteins and fats that have been deposited in the arteriolar wall due to injury to the endothelium, probably secondary to the elevated intraluminal hydraulic pressure. Narrowing of vascular lumina results, with consequent ischemic injury to glomeruli and tubules.

Nephrosclerosis accompanying long-standing systemic arterial hypertension is only one manifestation of a generalized process affecting the cardiovascular system. Physical examination, therefore, may reveal changes in retinal vessels (arteriolar narrowing and/or flame-shaped hemorrhages), cardiac hypertrophy, and possibly signs of congestive heart failure. Renal disease may manifest as a mild to moderate elevation of serum creatinine concentration, microscopic hematuria, and/or mild proteinuria. In general, clinical evaluation does not reveal significant renal abnormalities. More specialized examination may disclose elevated urinary albumin excretion, tapering and loss of caliber of intrarenal vessels on arteriography, and an exaggerated natriuresis in response to a fluid challenge. Patients with benign nephrosclerosis maintain a near-normal GFR despite a reduction in renal blood flow.

Malignant arteriolar nephrosclerosis Patients with long-standing benign hypertension or patients not known to be hypertensive previously may develop malignant hypertension characterized by a sudden (accelerated) elevation of blood pressure (diastolic often above 130 mmHg) accompanied by papilledema, central nervous system manifestations, cardiac decompensation, and acute progressive deterioration of renal function. The absence of papilledema does not rule out the diagnosis in a patient with markedly elevated blood pressure and rapidly declining renal function. The kidneys are characterized by a flea-bitten appearance resulting from hemorrhages in surface capillaries. Histologically, two distinct vascular lesions can be seen. The first, affecting arterioles, is fibrinoid necrosis, i.e., infiltration of arteriolar walls with eosinophilic material including fibrin. There is thickening of vessel walls and, occasionally, an inflammatory infiltrate (necrotizing arteriolitis). The second lesion, involving the interlobular arteries, is a concentric hyperplastic proliferation of the cellular elements of the vascular wall with deposition of collagen to form a hyperplastic arteriolitis (onion-skin lesion). Fibrinoid necrosis occasionally extends into the glomeruli, which also may undergo proliferative changes or total necrosis. Most glomerular and tubular changes are secondary to ischemia and infarction. The sequence of events leading to the development of malignant hypertension is poorly defined. Two pathophysiologic alterations appear central in its initiation and/or perpetuation: (1) increased permeability of vessel walls to invasion by plasma components, particularly fibrin, which activates clotting mechanisms leading to a microangiopathic hemolytic anemia, thus perpetuating the vascular pathology, and (2) activation of the renin-angiotensin-aldosterone system at some point in the

disease process, which contributes to the acceleration and maintenance of blood pressure elevation and, in turn, to vascular injury.

Malignant hypertension is most likely to develop in a previously hypertensive individual, usually in the third or fourth decade of life. There is a higher incidence among men, particularly black men. The presenting symptoms are usually neurologic (dizziness, headache, blurring of vision, altered states of consciousness, and focal or generalized seizures). Cardiac decompensation and renal failure appear thereafter. Renal abnormalities include a rapid rise in serum creatinine, hematuria (at times macroscopic), proteinuria, and red and white blood cell casts in the sediment. Nephrotic syndrome may be present. Elevated plasma aldosterone levels cause hypokalemic metabolic alkalosis in the early phase. Uremic acidosis and hyperkalemia eventually obscure these early findings. Hematologic indices of microangiopathic hemolytic anemia (i.e., schistocytes) are often seen.

Control of hypertension is the principal goal of therapy for both benign and malignant forms. The time of initiation of therapy, its effectiveness, and patient compliance are crucial factors in arresting the progression of benign nephrosclerosis. Untreated, most of these patients succumb to the extrarenal complications of hypertension. In contrast, malignant hypertension is a medical emergency; its natural course includes a death rate of 80 to 90 percent within 1 year of onset, almost always due to uremia. Supportive measures should be instituted to control the neurologic, cardiac, and other complications of acute renal failure, but the mainstay of therapy is prompt and aggressive reduction of blood pressure, which, if successful, can reverse all complications in the majority of patients. Presently, 5-year survival is 50 percent, and some patients have evidence of partial reversal of the vascular lesions and a return of renal function to near-normal levels.

SCLERODERMA (PROGRESSIVE SYSTEMIC SCLEROSIS) Renal vascular involvement in scleroderma is characterized by a distinctive lesion of the small arteries (diameters of 150 to 500 μm) consisting of intimal proliferation, medial thinning, and increased collagen deposition in the adventitial layer. Fibrinoid changes in the walls of afferent arterioles and microinfarcts may occur. Glomerular changes are generally nonspecific and secondary to ischemic damage. Tubules are often atrophic. As part of a generalized increase in vasomotor tone, a vasospastic (Raynaud-like) phenomenon at the level of the renal vasculature contributes to the renal insufficiency. Reduction in renal blood flow is the major mechanism underlying the deterioration in kidney function, being present in 80 percent of patients, even in the absence of other clinical abnormalities. As vascular narrowing progresses, hypertension, azotemia, and proteinuria eventually develop. Plasma renin rises in response to sustained renal ischemia. The resulting hypertension causes further renal injury and may play a role in the intimate destruction of nephrons. As more and more nephrons are lost to the combined insults of ischemia and hypertension, development of azotemia heralds a particularly grim prognosis. Proteinuria, usually mild, is a consequence of ischemic and hypertensive glomerular injury.

Although the majority of patients with scleroderma present with extrarenal manifestations, renal involvement is eventually manifested in half of patients followed for up to 20 years. Renal involvement can present in one of two ways, depending on whether malignant hypertension is superimposed on the renal pathology: (1) *Persistent urinary abnormalities* with or without hypertension tend to follow an indolent course with mild proteinuria, occasional casts, cellular elements in the urinary sediment, and a propensity for development of hypertension. Azotemia is absent initially, but when it develops, dialysis is required within 1 year. (2) *Scleroderma renal crisis* is a rapid deterioration in renal function, usually accompanied by malignant hypertension, oliguria, fluid retention, microangiopathic hemolytic anemia, and central nervous system involvement. It may occur in patients with previously undemonstrable or slowly progressive renal disease. Untreated, it leads to chronic renal failure within days to months.

The prognosis of scleroderma renal disease is generally poor, particularly following the onset of azotemia. Aggressive antihypertensive therapy may be effective in delaying the progression of renal failure. In scleroderma renal crisis, prompt treatment with beta blockers, minoxidil, and particularly angiotensin I converting enzyme (ACE) inhibitors may reverse acute renal failure. The effect of these interventions on renal function over the long term is uncertain.

SICKLE CELL NEPHROPATHY (See also Chap. 241)   Sickle cell disease causes renal complications that arise mainly as a result of sickling of red blood cells in the microvasculature. The hypertonic and relatively hypoxic environment of the renal medulla, coupled with the slow blood flow in the vasa recta, favors the sickling of red blood cells, with resultant local infarction (papillary necrosis). Functional tubule defects in patients with sickle cell disease are likely the result of partial ischemic injury to the renal tubules.

In addition to the intrarenal microvascular pathology described above, young patients with sickle cell disease are characterized by renal hyperperfusion, glomerular hypertrophy, and hyperfiltration. Many of these individuals eventually develop a glomerulopathy leading to proteinuria (present in as many as 30 percent) and, in some, the nephrotic syndrome. Mild azotemia and hyperuricemia also can develop, but advanced renal failure and uremia are rare. Although an immunologic basis for the glomerulopathy of sickle cell disease has been proposed, hemodynamically mediated renal injury, resulting from intrarenal hyperperfusion and glomerular hyperfiltration, may be the major pathogenetic mechanism. Nephron loss secondary to ischemic injury also contributes to the development of azotemia in these patients.

The renal complications of sickle cell disease include the following: *Cortical infarcts* can cause loss of function, persistent hematuria, and perinephric hematomas. *Papillary infarcts*, demonstrated radiographically in 50 percent of patients with sickle trait, lead to an increased risk of bacterial infection in the scarred renal tissues and functional tubule abnormalities. Painless gross hematuria occurs with a higher frequency in sickle trait than in sickle cell disease and likely results from infarctive episodes in the renal medulla. *Functional tubule abnormalities* such as nephrogenic diabetes insipidus result from marked reduction in vasa recta blood flow, combined with ischemic tubule injury. This concentrating defect places these patients at increased risk of dehydration and, hence, sickling crises. The concentrating defect also occurs in individuals with sickle trait. Other tubule defects involve potassium and hydrogen ion excretion, occasionally leading to hyperkalemic metabolic acidosis and a defect in uric acid excretion which, combined with increased purine synthesis in the bone marrow, results in hyperuricemia. Glomerulopathy is an established consequence of sickle cell disease and is due to a combination of hemodynamically mediated glomerular injury referred to earlier and to an immune-complex glomerulonephritis in which tubule epithelial antigens, released into the circulation during episodes of ischemic injury, provoke an antibody response leading to immune-complex deposition in the glomeruli. Proteinuria is the chief manifestation of sickle cell glomerulopathy and may reach nephrotic proportions.

TOXEMIAS OF PREGNANCY (See also Chap. 6)   Renal function is "reset" at a higher level during normal pregnancy. Renal plasma flow (RPF) and glomerular filtration rate (GFR) both increase by 30 to 50 percent. Therefore, serum creatinine levels above 70 µmol/L (0.8 mg/dL) or blood urea nitrogen (BUN) levels above 4.6 mmol/L (13 mg/dL) are abnormal in pregnant women and should be investigated. Systolic and diastolic blood pressures decrease by an average of 10 to 15 mmHg below pregravid values. A diastolic pressure above 75 mmHg during the second trimester or above 85 mmHg during the third trimester is therefore abnormal. Vasodilation in the uterine, renal, and cutaneous beds, vasodilator prostaglandin release from the uteroplacental unit, and a decrease in arteriolar sensitivity to angiotensin II all play a role in the decline of blood pressure during pregnancy.

Preeclampsia-eclampsia   The toxemia syndrome, usually occurring in the third trimester of primigravidas, includes hypertension, proteinuria, edema, consumptive coagulopathy, sodium retention, hyperreflexia (preeclampsia), and, if uncontrolled, convulsions (eclampsia). In pure preeclampsia (i.e., not superimposed on previously existing hypertensive or renal disease), the primary sites of pathology are the glomerular endothelial cells. These cells show marked swelling due to an increase in cytoplasmic volume with vacuolization (endotheliosis) and encroach on the vascular lumen, rendering the enlarged glomeruli ischemic. The glomerular basement membrane and the extraglomerular blood vessels are intact. The pathogenesis is unknown. Coagulation abnormalities, hormonal factors, uteroplacental ischemia, and immune mechanisms have all been implicated. The mechanisms mediating the hypertension are also not understood. Despite sodium retention, intravascular volume is contracted as compared with pregravid values. An increased sensitivity to angiotensin II is the basis for the "roll-over test" (an increase in diastolic blood pressure of 20 mmHg or more upon changing the patient's position from lateral recumbent to supine, presumably due to alterations in circulating angiotensin levels). In the supine position, the reduction in venous return due to compression by the gravid uterus increases circulating levels of angiotensin II. This results in a hypertensive response in preeclamptic patients, who are hyperresponsive to angiotensin II, but not in normal women, in whom pregnancy leads to a relative resistance to the pressor effects of this hormone.

A diagnosis of preeclampsia-related hypertension can be made when repeated measurements over a 4- to 6-h period show a blood pressure of 140/85 mmHg or more. The rise in blood pressure tends to be more severe at night. When preeclampsia occurs in a previously hypertensive patient, a rapid acceleration of the blood pressure elevation is accompanied by an increase in proteinuria, oliguria, edema, and coagulopathy. This is a life-threatening syndrome and tends to recur with future pregnancies. In addition to proteinuria, which correlates with the severity of the renal lesion, GFR and RPF are depressed. In view of the preexisting high levels, however, GFR in preeclamptic women often remains above nonpregnant levels. Uric acid clearance also falls, resulting in hyperuricemia. In the postpartum period, these patients are particularly susceptible to the development of "postpartum renal failure," which is thought to be a form of adult HUS.

Management consists of bed rest in a quiet environment and control of neurologic manifestations and blood pressure, the former with magnesium sulfate and the latter usually with vasodilators such as hydralazine and methyldopa. Diuretics are avoided. The ultimate "treatment" is delivery, which should be induced if fetal maturity is adequate or if life-threatening coagulopathy or renal failure occur. The long-term prognosis is generally favorable.

Development of acute renal failure/preeclampsia in a pregnant woman should alert the physician to potential preexisting renal disease and/or hypertension. The latter is particularly likely if systolic blood pressure is greater than 200 mmHg. Hypertension and preexisting proteinuria tend to worsen in 50 percent of women during pregnancy. In addition, these abnormalities may be unmasked during pregnancy as the first manifestations of an underlying glomerulopathy. Conversely, patients with established underlying renal disease should be followed closely during pregnancy with monthly measurements of 24-h urinary protein excretion and GFR. Sudden deterioration should raise suspicion of superimposed preeclampsia. There is no convincing evidence that pregnancy has an adverse effect on the long-term outcome of immunologic glomerular diseases or diabetic nephropathy. In all situations, control of blood pressure should be the primary therapeutic goal in view of its established beneficial effects on the progression of renal injury.

Bilateral cortical necrosis   Acute bilateral cortical necrosis is associated with septic abortions, abruptio placentae, and preeclampsia. Coagulation in cortical vessels and arterioles leads to renal tissue necrosis. Anuria and renal failure ensue and may be irreversible. In other cases, renal function returns partially, but on long-term follow-up most patients slowly progress to uremia.

VASCULITIS (See also Chap. 241) The kidney is commonly involved in systemic disorders in which necrotizing inflammatory injury to vessels is a primary feature. Several lines of evidence point toward an immunologic pathogenesis for the vasculitides, the prototype of which is periarteritis nodosa (PAN).

Periarteritis nodosa In PAN, arcuate and intralobular arteries are primarily involved. Acute lesions are characterized by destruction of the internal elastic lamina, segmental fibrinoid necrosis of the intima and/or the entire vessel wall, intense intra- and periarterial leukocytic infiltration, and occasional aneurysmal dilatation of the vessel wall (demonstrable radiographically). Fibroblast proliferation leads eventually to occlusion and obliteration of vessel lumina. These vascular changes typically lead to glomerular ischemia, occasionally associated with proliferative changes in the glomerular tufts and juxtaglomerular apparatus. Progression to acute necrotizing crescentic glomerulonephritis may occur.

Clinically, renal involvement in PAN is often associated with hypertension (renin-mediated) which at times progresses to a severe or malignant form. Hematuria, microscopic or gross, also can occur as a result of ischemia, hypertensive renal injury, or glomerulonephritis. Proteinuria is usually mild, and the urinary sediment contains all the formed elements (red and white blood cells, renal epithelial cells, and their respective casts). Nephrotic syndrome is uncommon. Acute renal failure occurs in approximately 10 percent of cases and is usually the result of malignant hypertension and/or the development of rapidly progressive crescentic glomerulonephritis. The diagnosis of PAN can be established by documenting the typical arterial lesions in biopsy material from involved organs (testes, muscle, skin). Renal biopsy seldom shows the arterial lesions but may reveal focal or diffuse crescentic glomerulonephritis. Renal and celiac arteriography, however, frequently demonstrates characteristic aneurysmal dilatation of the involved arteries.

Untreated, PAN is generally progressive, causing death from renal failure, gastrointestinal bleeding, or other extrarenal catastrophes. Encouraging therapeutic results have been obtained with glucocorticoid therapy in combination with cytoxic agents (cyclophosphamide or azathioprine) and plasma exchange. In addition, hypertension should be controlled. Early initiation of antihypertensive therapy prolongs survival in more than 90 percent of patients and causes complete remission in 20 percent. Allergic granulomatosis (Churg-Strauss syndrome), a variant of PAN, is similar in its renal manifestations but also causes immediate-type hypersensitivity reactions, including primary pulmonary involvement, asthma, and eosinophilia.

Hypersensitivity angiitis (microscopic form of PAN) Hypersensitivity angiitis is an acute fulminant form of necrotizing vasculitis in which the characteristic pathologic finding is an intense leukocytic infiltration of the smaller renal vessels (arterioles, venules, capillaries) with or without fibrinoid necrosis. Thus the pathology is more often limited to the glomerular vessels (including the afferent and postglomerular arterioles). The infiltrating leukocytes fragment as they invade the vessel walls, giving rise to the term *leukocytoclastic angiitis*. Endothelial proliferative changes are also seen, and in severe cases the pathologic picture may be indistinguishable from crescentic (rapidly progressive) glomerulonephritis. Immunofluorescence staining may reveal IgG and IgM in the mesangium. In contrast to the subacute or chronic course of PAN, hypersensitivity angiitis is characterized by rapid onset of renal failure. Urinalysis reveals proteinuria (at times reaching nephrotic range), hematuria, and casts. Microangiopathic hemolytic anemia and systemic eosinophilia are often present. Hypertension, however, is characteristically absent or mild. Uremia leads to death in the majority. Treatment regimens are similar to those for PAN, but the response to glucocorticoids appears to be more favorable in this disease than in PAN.

Other vasculitides in which renal involvement is present include

Wegener's granulomatosis (in which the renal lesion is primarily in the form of a necrotizing glomerulitis) and Takayasu's arteritis, which may involve the main renal arteries and their branches (see Chap. 291).

REFERENCES

BARRÉ P et al: Successful treatment with streptokinase of renal vein thrombosis associated with oral contraceptive use. Am J Nephrol 6:316, 1986

BERLAND LL et al: Renal artery stenosis: Prospective evaluation of diagnosis with color duplex US compared with angiography. Radiology 174:421, 1990

EKNOYAN G, RIGGS SA: Renal involvement in patients with thrombotic thrombocytopenic purpura. Am J Nephrol 6:117, 1986

HAKIM RM et al: Successful management of thrombocytopenia, microangiopathic anemia, and acute renal failure by plasmapheresis. Am J Kidney Dis 3:170, 1985

HOFFMAN U et al: Role of duplex scanning for the detection of atheroslerotic renal artery disease. Kidney Int 39:1232, 1991

HOLLENBERG NK: The treatment of renovascular hypertension: Surgery, angioplasty, and medical therapy with converting enzyme inhibitors. Am J Kidney Dis 1(suppl):52, 1987

JACOBSON HR: Ischemic renal disease: An overlooked clinical entity? Kidney Int 34:729, 1988

KASHGARIAN M: Pathology of small blood vessels in hypertension. Am J Kidney Dis 5:A104, 1985

KIM D: Abdominal aorta and renal artery stenosis: Evaluation with MR angiography. Radiology 174:727, 1990

LINDHEIMER MD, BAYLIS C (eds): Renal function and disease in pregnancy: An international symposium. Am J Kidney Dis 9:243, 1987

LLACH F: *Renal Vein Thrombosis*. New York, Futura, 1983

MATERSON BJ: Special uses for captopril. Am J Kidney Dis 1(suppl):88, 1987

MULLER FB et al: The captopril test for identifying renovascular disease in hypertensive patients. Am J Med 80:6333, 1986

RATLIFFE N: Renal vascular disease: Pathology of large blood vessel disease. Am J Kidney Dis 5:A93, 1985

WORKING GROUP ON RENOVASCULAR HYPERTENSION: Final Report: Detection, evaluation, and treatment of renovascular hypertension. Arch Intern Med 147:820, 1987

244 HEREDITARY TUBULAR DISORDERS

FREDRIC L. COE / SATISH KATHPALIA

POLYCYSTIC RENAL DISEASE IN ADULTS

ETIOLOGY AND PATHOLOGY This disorder is found in 1 in 500 autopsies and 1 in 3000 hospital admissions and accounts for approximately 10 percent of end-stage renal failure. Inheritance is autosomal dominant and is linked in most families to the alpha-hemoglobin gene complex and the phosphoglycerate kinase genes on the short arm of chromosome 16. The cortex and medulla of both kidneys are usually filled with thin-walled, spherical cysts, ranging from millimeters to centimeters in diameter, that enlarge the organs and interfere with function, presumably by compressing the nephrons and causing localized obstruction. The cysts are lined by a low cuboidal epithelium and contain straw-colored fluid that becomes hemorrhagic with trauma or infection. The intervening renal parenchyma may be normal or show changes of nephrosclerosis or interstitial nephritis.

CLINICAL FEATURES Symptoms usually begin in the third or fourth decades. Common symptoms include flank pain, gross and microscopic hematuria, especially after trauma, and nocturia due to impaired concentrating ability. Ten percent of patients pass renal calculi whose composition and pathogenesis have not been well studied. Stones and blood clots can cause renal colic. The kidneys are usually palpable and asymmetric and have a knobby surface. Hypertension develops in 75 percent of patients, and progression to chronic renal failure is usual (Table 244-1).

TABLE 244-1 Renal tubule defects

Disease	Renal morphologic abnormalities	Functional abnormalities	Mode of Inheritance*	Associated abnormalities
Adult polycystic disease	Cortical and medullary cysts	Chronic renal failure	AD	Hepatic cysts, intracranial aneurysms
Infantile polycystic disease	Distal tubule and collecting duct cysts	Renal failure in the newborn	AR	Intrahepatic bile duct abnormalities
Childhood polycystic disease	Medullary ductal ectasia	Variable chronic renal failure	AR	Hepatic fibrosis and portal hypertension
Medullary sponge kidneys	Ectatic ducts of Bellini	Nephrocalcinosis	AD + S	None
Medullary cystic disease, recessive	Distal tubule and collecting duct cysts	Chronic renal failure, <20 yr salt wasting, polyuria	AR	Variable retinal degeneration (renal retinal dysplasia)
Medullary cystic disease, dominant	Same	Chronic renal failure, >20 yr salt wasting, polyuria	AD	None
Bartter's syndrome	Hyperplasia of juxtaglomerular and medullary interstitial cells	Hypokalemia, high renin and aldosterone levels, polyuria	AR	None
Liddle's syndrome	None	Hypokalemia, low aldosterone levels	AR	None
Familial nephrogenic diabetes insipidus	None	Vasopressin-resistant renal concentrating defect	XL	None
Renal tubular acidosis, type 1	Papillary nephrocalcinosis	Inability to lower urine pH normally, reduced acid excretion	AD	Periodic paralysis, hypokalemia, non-anion-gap metabolic acidosis, growth retardation, rickets
Renal tubular acidosis, type 2	None	Reduced bicarbonate reabsorption	AR AD XL	Non-anion-gap metabolic acidosis, growth retardation rickets, Fanconi syndrome
Renal tubular acidosis, type 4	Underlying renal disease	Reduced proton and potassium secretion	ACQ	Azotemia
X-linked hypophosphatemia	None	Reduced phosphate reabsorption, hypophosphatemia	XL	Rickets, osteomalacia, normal serum 1,25(OH)$_2$D
Vitamin D–dependent rickets, type 1	None	Defective renal 1,25(OH)$_2$D production	AR	Rickets, osteomalacia, low serum 1,25(OH)$_2$D
Vitamin D–dependent rickets, type 2	None	Defective cell, 1,25(OH)$_2$D receptors	AR	Rickets, osteomalacia, high serum 1,25(OH)$_2$D, variable alopecia
Oncogenic osteomalacia	None	Reduced phosphate reabsorptions, hypophosphatemia	ACQ	Osteomalacia; mesenchymal tumors; cancer of the prostate or lung
Renal glucosuria	None	Reduced glucose reabsorption	AD	None
Isolated hypouricemia	None	Reduced urate reabsorption	AR	Variable hypercalciuria, bone demineralization
Cystinuria	Cystine stones	Reduced reabsorption of dibasic amino acids	AR	Short stature
Hartnup disease	None	Reduced reabsorption of monoamino and carboxylic amino acids	AR	Pellagra-like rash, ataxia, delirium
Iminoglycinuria	None	Reduced reabsorption of proline, hydroxyproline, and glycine	AR	None
Adult Fanconi syndrome	Swan neck deformity of the proximal tubule	Reduced proximal tubule reabsorption of bicarbonate, glucose, uric acid, phosphate, and amino acids	AR	Rickets, osteomalacia, acidosis, dwarfism, low serum potassium
Lowe's syndrome (oculocerebrorenal syndrome)	Same	Same	XL	Ocular and cerebral malformations

* AR, autosomal recessive; AD, autosomal dominant; XL, X-linked; ACQ, acquired; S, sporadic.

Proteinuria rarely exceeds 2 g/d. Urinary infection occurs at some time in most patients, usually as a consequence of instrumentation and renal calculi; women are infected more frequently than men. Erythrocytosis may occur because of high erythropoietin levels; in other patients hematuria may cause blood loss anemia.

Acute renal failure can result from infection, ureteral obstruction due to clots or stone, or sudden angulation of a ureter by a cyst. Azotemia progresses slowly in the absence of these complications. Patients with end-stage renal failure tend to have higher hematocrits than patients with other renal diseases. Fluid overload is infrequent because of a tendency for renal salt wasting.

Hepatic cysts occur in about 30 percent of patients. Hepatic function is usually normal, and the liver cysts can be asymptomatic, cause epigastric discomfort or biliary colic, or become infected. Cysts also may occur in the spleen, pancreas, lungs, ovaries, testes, epididymis, thyroid, uterus, broad ligament, and bladder. Subarachnoid hemorrhage from intracranial aneurysm causes death or neurologic injury in about a tenth of patients, but routine cerebral arteriography is not warranted. Mitral valve prolapse (25 percent) and mitral, aortic, and tricuspid valve incompetence occur more often than in control groups.

DIAGNOSIS Palpable kidneys, hypertension, and abnormalities of urine in asymptomatic individuals may be the only manifestations. Excretory or retrograde urography typically shows large kidneys with elongated pelvises and flat calyces indented by cysts. Ultrasonography and radioisotopic renal scanning can both demonstrate the cysts quite well. Gray scale sonography is preferable to intravenous pyelography for screening individuals at risk, especially when genetic counseling is desired. Computed tomography may be useful.

TREATMENT Superimposed renal damage such as is produced by analgesics, obstruction, urinary infection, nephrotoxic antibiotics, and hypertension must be guarded against. Dehydration and inadequate intake of sodium chloride (less than 100 mmol/d) should be avoided. The management of chronic renal failure is simplified because fluid overload is not a usual problem and the hypertension usually responds to treatment, but the cysts can cause special problems, such as pain, bleeding, infection, or ureteral obstruction. Puncture of cysts, and in some instances even nephrectomy, may be necessary.

POLYCYSTIC RENAL DISEASE IN INFANTS AND CHILDREN

CLINICAL FEATURES The *infantile form* is manifest at birth by diffusely enlarged kidneys, renal failure, and maldevelopment of intrahepatic bile ducts. The *childhood form* consists of medullary ductal ectasia, which is usually asymptomatic, congenital hepatic fibrosis, and portal hypertension. Both conditions are rare, and both are inherited as autosomal recessive traits. Renal failure develops frequently in both forms, but death in the childhood form is usually due to hepatic disease.

MORPHOLOGY In the infantile form, the distal tubules and collecting ducts are dilated into elongated cysts that are arranged in a radial fashion, particularly in the cortex, and make the kidneys large and spongy. In the childhood form, cysts are fewer, cortical collecting ducts are less involved, and the kidneys are not as large. Small intrahepatic bile ducts are irregularly dilated, and large interconnecting spaces, lined by hyperplastic epithelium, fill the portal areas. There is portal fibrosis rather than dilatation and proliferation of small bile ducts, and portal hypertension is the rule by late childhood.

DIAGNOSIS AND TREATMENT Infantile polycystic kidneys may cause dystocia. At birth they do not function and cause oliguric renal failure, respiratory distress, hypertension, and congestive heart failure. Intravenous pyelography may reveal a mottled appearance with variable retention of contrast material in cysts that corresponds to dilated cortical and medullary collecting ducts. On rétrograde urography the calyces are blunted, and pyelotubular reflux may be seen. In the childhood type the intravenous pyelogram may suggest medullary sponge kidney, because medullary tubular ectasia is prominent. Renal failure and chronic infection are common.

MEDULLARY SPONGE KIDNEY

PATHOLOGY The ducts of Bellini, i.e., the terminal collecting ducts that reach the ends of the papillae and drain the urine into the renal pelvis, are dilated to cystic proportions and may contain calcium oxalate calculi. The kidneys are asymmetric, and the more abnormal kidney is usually the larger. One or more medullary cysts are found near the tip of each involved papilla, and calculi form in the terminal collecting ducts in or proximal to the cysts (Fig. 244-1). Parenchymal alterations are secondary to intrarenal obstruction. The cysts are lined by cuboidal and, sometimes, by pseudostratified and stratified squamous epithelium.

CLINICAL DIAGNOSIS AND TREATMENT Medullary sponge kidney is present in 1 in 200 unselected intravenous pyelograms. Although most cases are sporadic, autosomal dominant inheritance has been described. The disease has a bimodal pattern of appearance, the first in adolescence and the second during the third and fourth decades. Calculi, infection, and hematuria occur in 60, 35, and 30 percent of patients, respectively. Papillary nephrocalcinosis due to clusters of stones in cysts is common. Hypercalciuria occurs in about half of stone-forming patients but is equally common in other forms of calcium stone disease (Chap. 245). Hypertension is no more common than in the general population. Renal failure is rare, unless nephrolithiasis and/or renal infections are severe.

The diagnosis is made by intravenous urography. The magnitude of pyelotubular backflow varies from a simple papillary blush to tubular ectasia at the tips of the papillae. Small pyramidal cysts and nephrocalcinosis are frequent, and papillary concretions are obscured by the urographic contrast medium. Ectatic collecting ducts are difficult to fill during retrograde pyelography, and the contrast material remains separate from papillary concretions in the cysts.

Asymptomatic patients require no treatment except advice to avoid dehydration and thereby reduce the risk of stone formation. The cause of stones should be sought and treated conventionally, while infection and urologic consequences of stones should be treated as described in Chap. 245. Medullary sponge kidneys are vulnerable to infection, and urologic instrumentation should therefore be minimized.

MEDULLARY CYSTIC DISEASE (NEPHRONOPHTHISIS COMPLEX)

ETIOLOGY Several hereditary medullary cystic diseases have similar morphology but different patterns of inheritance. The recessive form is associated with renal failure before 20 years of age (early-

FIGURE 244-1 *A*. Radiographic appearance of medullary sponge kidney. Abdominal flat plate reveals multiple bilateral calcifications. *B*. Radiographic

contrast material accumulates in the dilated and cystic terminal collecting ducts and obscures the calcifications.

onset type), whereas the dominant form causes renal failure only after the second decade (adult-onset type). When renal disease is associated with retinal degeneration (renal retinal dysplasia), inheritance is recessive, and renal failure occurs during adult life.

PATHOLOGY In both forms, most of the cysts are in the medulla and corticomedullary region and involve the collecting ducts and distal convoluted tubules. Cysts have a low, frequently atrophic, epithelium and range in size from micrometers to millimeters. The kidneys usually are asymmetrically scarred and shrunken. Both tubular atrophy and periglomerular fibrosis are present, but the former is more severe. In advanced cases, glomeruli become sclerotic and hyalinized, cortical fibrosis and cellular interstitial infiltration appear, and the histology resembles that of chronic interstitial nephritis.

DIAGNOSIS AND TREATMENT Concentrating ability, acid excretion, and sodium conservation are defective as might be expected from a lesion that damages distal segments of the nephron. Polyuria, progressive renal failure, stunted growth, severe anemia, hyperchloremic metabolic acidosis, and poor sodium conservation are common. In adults, the inability to conserve sodium may cause salt-wasting that resembles adrenal insufficiency but is unresponsive to mineralocorticoids. Hypertension is a terminal event. The urinalysis is normal at first, but proteinuria may develop. On intravenous pyelography, the kidneys are small, scarred, and without calcification. The calyces are distorted by cysts in the corticomedullary area.

High sodium and water intake and alkali replacement for acidosis are needed. Treatment of infections, anemia, hypertension, and other aspects of end-stage renal failure are as discussed in Chap. 237. Genetic counseling may be helpful in family planning and in selection of an unaffected related donor for renal transplantation.

BARTTER'S SYNDROME

Bartter's syndrome consists of hypokalemia due to renal potassium wasting, elevated plasma renin activity and aldosterone secretion, normal blood pressure, hyporesponsiveness of blood pressure to infused angiotensin II, and hyperplasia of the granular cells of the juxtaglomerular apparatus of the kidney. Weakness or periodic paralysis and polyuria occur because of potassium depletion. Hypomagnesemia may be present. Hyperplasia of renal medullary interstitial cells, which produce prostaglandins PGE and PGF, and elevated PGF_2 production have been described. Inheritance is autosomal recessive, and manifestations commonly begin in childhood.

PATHOGENESIS The main defect seems to be reduced NaCl reabsorption by the thick ascending limb of Henle's loop (TAHL). Volume depletion stimulates aldosterone production and raises serum aldosterone levels, and the combination of high aldosterone levels and increased delivery of NaCl and water to the distal nephron causes kaliuresis and hypokalemia. Magnesuria and hypomagnesemia occur, perhaps because TAHL is a main site for magnesium reabsorption and because hypomagnesemia enhances kaliuresis. Hypokalemia further increases aldosterone production by stimulating release of prostaglandins E_2 and I_2, which promote increased secretion of renin. Both angiotensin II and aldosterone increase renal kallikrein, which increases plasma bradykinin. The normal blood pressure reflects an interaction between the vasodepressor actions of PGE_2 and bradykinin and elevated angiotensin II. Bartter's syndrome may be mimicked by magnesium deficiency, diuretic use, or vomiting. Magnesium depletion causes kaliuresis; diuretics cause potassium and volume depletion; vomiting causes renal potassium wasting and volume depletion.

Excessive production of PGE_2 resulting from hypokalemia, a stimulator of PGE_2 synthesis, may be a secondary consequence. In some cases blockade of PGE_2 production with indomethacin lowers renin levels and restores vascular response to angiotensin II infusion but does not reduce potassium wasting.

TREATMENT The dietary intake of sodium chloride and potassium should be liberal; potassium supplements may be required.

Aldosterone antagonists (spironolactone) can prevent potassium wasting, though sodium intake must be increased. Inhibition of prostaglandin synthesis with indomethacin, ibuprofen, or aspirin has varying success, as indicated above. Beta-adrenergic blockade may lower renin production.

LIDDLE'S SYNDROME (PSEUDOHYPERALDOSTERONISM)

This rare inherited disorder is characterized by hypertension, hypokalemic alkalosis, and negligible aldosterone secretion. It appears to be due to an unusual tendency of distal tubules or collecting ducts to conserve sodium and excrete potassium despite the virtual absence of aldosterone. No other biochemical abnormalities have been described. However, transport rates of sodium in red blood cells are altered. These patients respond to 100 mg/d of triamterene (Chap. 195), a diuretic agent that blocks sodium channels in the distal tubule.

X-LINKED NEPHROGENIC DIABETES INSIPIDUS (DI)

In affected males the distal tubules and collecting ducts are unresponsive to vasopressin because of an X-linked recessive disorder, and there is variable expressivity in heterozygous females. Affected individuals excrete large volumes of hypotonic urine even when plasma osmolality and vasopressin concentration are high. Polyuria, polydipsia, and hypertonic dehydration after restriction of fluid intake result from renal tubular insensitivity to vasopressin (AVP) (also see Chap. 333). Unresponsiveness to vasopressin in this disorder is due to mutations that impair the function of the vasopressin receptor (see Chap. 234). Other hereditary tubular defects such as juvenile nephronophthisis, medullary cystic and polycystic diseases, cystinosis, and congenital or acquired chronic urinary tract obstruction also can cause vasopressin-resistant (nephrogenic) DI, but in these syndromes the characteristic features of the underlying disorder are also present.

Affected infants easily become dehydrated, hypernatremic, and hyperthermic, and damage of the central nervous system, including mental retardation, may result. In the absence of dehydration, overall renal function is normal. On intravenous pyelography the renal pelvis, ureters, and bladder are dilated, as in all forms of DI, because of massive diuresis.

Oral hydration usually is adequate treatment except during early infancy, when hypotonic parenteral fluids may be required. Vasopressin and its synthetic analogues are ineffective, but diuretic agents such as hydrochlorothiazide reduce polyuria. This drug inhibits NaCl reabsorption in the distal convoluted tubule, thereby reducing production of free water. In addition, hydrocholorothiazide produces a diuresis, causes contraction of extracellular fluid volume, and in turn, stimulates reabsorption of NaCl and water in the proximal tubule and limits their delivery to the TAHL. Sodium restriction enhances its effect.

RENAL TUBULAR ACIDOSES (RTA)

In these disorders renal excretion of acid is reduced out of proportion to reduction of GFR. Metabolic acidosis results, but in contrast to renal failure the anions that accompany surplus hydrogen ions in the blood, such as sulfate and phosphate, are excreted normally and are unavailable to balance the fall in serum bicarbonate. Therefore, the kidneys reabsorb chloride in unusually large amounts, and serum chloride rises to preserve electroneutrality in the extracellular fluid. The result is *hyperchloremic acidosis*, and the unmeasured anion gap is normal. At least four types of RTA exist (Table 244-2). Types 1 and 2 are often hereditary. Type 3 is a rare mixture of types 1 and 2. Type 4 is acquired and is associated with either hyporeninemic

TABLE 244-2 Comparison of three types of renal tubular acidosis*

Finding	Type 1	Type 2	Type 4
Non-anion-gap acidosis	Yes	Yes	Yes
Minimum urine pH	>5.5	<5.5	<5.5
% filtered HCO_3 excreted	<10	>15	<10
Serum potassium	Low	Low	High
Fanconi syndrome	No	Yes	No
Stones/nephrocalcinosis	Yes	No	No
Daily acid excretion	Low	Normal	Low
Ammonium excretion	High for pH	Normal	Low for pH
Daily HCO_3 replacement needs	<4 mmol/kg	>4 mmol/kg	<4 mmol/kg

* HCO_3, bicarbonate. Type 3 renal tubular acidosis is a rare form of a mixture of types 1 and 2.

hypoaldosteronism or tubular hyporesponsiveness to mineralocorticoids.

TYPE 1 (DISTAL) RTA Sporadic cases occur, but autosomal dominant inheritance is usual. The kidney does not lower urine pH normally, either because the collecting ducts permit excessive back-diffusion of hydrogen ions from lumen to blood or because they fail to transport hydrogen ions against a steep pH gradient. Since titration of urine buffers and diffusion trapping of NH_4^+ in the tubules both depend on a low intraluminal pH, excretion of acid is deficient. However, urine ammonium excretion is as high or higher than in normal people whose urine is equally alkaline. Urinary concentration and potassium conservation also tend to be impaired.

Chronic acidosis lowers tubule reabsorption of calcium, causing renal hypercalciuria and mild secondary hyperparathyroidism. The hypercalciuria, alkaline urine, and low levels of urine citrate, which normally complexes about 40 percent of urine calcium, cause calcium phosphate stones and nephrocalcinosis. Growth in children is stunted because of rickets; this growth defect responds to amelioration of the acidosis with sodium bicarbonate or other alkali. In the adult, osteomalacia occurs. In both children and adults, bone disease may result, in part, from acidosis-induced loss of bone mineral and inadequate production of 1,25-dihydroxyvitamin D_3 [1,25$(OH)_2D_3$]. Since the kidney does not conserve potassium or concentrate the urine normally, polyuria and hypokalemia occur. With the stress of an intercurrent illness, acidosis and hypokalemia can be life-threatening.

The diagnosis is suggested by osteomalacia or rickets, hyperchloremic acidosis associated with alkaline urine, and calcium phosphate stones or nephrocalcinosis. To prove that the urine pH cannot be lowered normally, the oral ammonium chloride (NH_4Cl) loading test should be carried out: 0.1 g (1.9 mmol) NH_4Cl per kilogram of body weight is administered, and blood and urine pH are followed with time. Although systemic acidosis worsens, urine pH does not fall below 5.5. Urinary tract infection must not be present during this test because bacteria may possess urease, which hydrolyzes urea to ammonia and produces an alkaline urine. When hyperchloremic acidosis is severe and the urine is grossly alkaline, the test is unnecessary.

A confusing situation may occur when type 1 RTA results from nephrocalcinosis due to hereditary idiopathic hypercalciuria. In this circumstance, stones may be composed of calcium phosphate, but hypokalemia and metabolic acidosis are absent; urine pH is high and does not fall below 5.5 after NH_4Cl administration. *Incomplete RTA* is a common term for this circumstance. Other hereditary diseases that cause RTA, such as medullary sponge kidney, galactosemia, Ehler-Danlos syndrome, Fabry's disease, and hereditary elliptocytosis, can be excluded by clinical findings. The relatives of patients with type 1 RTA should be screened for this treatable disorder.

Treatment Sodium bicarbonate tablets (10 grains = 7.2 mmol base) and Shohl's solution (1 mmol base per milliliter, as Na and K citrate) are both convenient for treatment; the dose should be 0.5 to 2.0 mmol/kg of body weight in four or five divided doses daily. The

total dose of alkali should be raised until acidosis and hypercalciuria are both eliminated, and the patients should be followed by measurements of serum chloride and CO_2 content and of urine calcium excretion approximately twice yearly. Potassium supplementation is normally not required. Requirements for alkali usually rise during intercurrent illnesses but are usually below 4 mmol/kg of body weight per day. Incomplete RTA is best treated using thiazide diuretics as in ordinary idiopathic hypercalcemia (Chap. 245).

TYPE 2 (PROXIMAL) RTA Proximal RTA usually occurs as part of a generalized disorder of proximal tubule function. It can be a transient disorder of infancy that disappears in childhood. The pathophysiology is the same whether isolated or part of a generalized disorder. Bicarbonate reabsorption in the proximal tubule is defective, and renal bicarbonate wasting occurs at a normal concentration of plasma bicarbonate. As plasma bicarbonate falls, the filtered load drops to a level that the defective tubule can reabsorb. Then the urine is free of bicarbonate and has a low pH. Potassium wasting and hypokalemia occur, especially when supplementary alkali is given, because bicarbonate is excreted in the urine partly as the potassium salt. Hypercalciuria is moderate, and stone formation is rare. During the NH_4Cl loading test, urine pH falls below 5.5.

Treatment is often not required. When acidosis is severe, bicarbonate must be given in large amounts daily, often >4 mmol/kg of body weight, and even up to 10 mmol/kg per day, because bicarbonate is rapidly excreted in the urine. Another approach is to use a thiazide diuretic and a low-salt diet, which induce mild volume depletion and enhance proximal bicarbonate reabsorption, thereby reducing the required dose. Potassium supplements are needed during treatment because excessive sodium bicarbonate reaches the distal nephron, where much of the sodium is exchanged for potassium, which is then lost in the urine.

TYPE 4 RTA Some patients have a form of renal tubular acidosis that differs from types 1 and 2 and has been called type 4. They have metabolic acidosis without an elevation of the anion gap but differ from type 1 patients in having an acid urine during periods of severe acidosis (see Table 244-2) and from type 2 patients in having low urine excretion of bicarbonate and a daily alkali requirement of <4 mmol/kg of body weight. They differ from both types 1 and 2 in having a high serum potassium and a low urine ammonia excretion. They have neither Fanconi syndrome nor stone disease. Because potassium and hydrogen excretion are abnormal, such patients are considered to have generalized distal nephron dysfunction due either to intrinsic renal disease or to abnormal aldosterone levels. Hyperkalemia worsens acidosis by suppressing renal production of ammonia, which is the most important urinary buffer, and thereby limiting acid excretion.

Most patients with type 4 renal tubular acidosis have hyporeninemic hypoaldosteronism; plasma levels of renin and aldosterone are subnormal, even during extracellular volume depletion. Diabetic nephropathy, nephrosclerosis from hypertension, and chronic tubulointerstitial nephropathies are the usual causes. Hyperkalemia and acidosis can be treated with replacement doses of mineralocorticoid such as fludrocortisone, 0.1 to 0.2 mg/d; some require 0.3 to 0.5 mg/d, suggesting tubule unresponsiveness to the hormone. Furosemide also can improve the hyperkalemia and acidosis, provided salt intake is sufficient to prevent extracellular volume contraction.

A less common condition is *mineralocorticoid-resistant hyperkalemia;* hyperkalemia and acidosis do not improve despite mineralocorticoid treatment. This occurs in occasional patients with renal disease who also have severe salt wasting, as a consequence of distal nephron damage. Plasma renin and aldosterone levels are elevated, and extracellular fluid volume depletion may occur. Treatment requires salt and alkali, but mineralocorticoid supplements are not necessary. Other patients with mild acidosis have no evidence of renal disease and do not waste salt in the urine. Plasma renin and aldosterone levels are low, but hyperkalemia and acidosis do not respond to mineralocorticoid treatment. The cause is thought to be increased distal tubule permeability to chloride ion; sodium chloride reabsorption is elevated, the potential across the distal tubule epithelium is presumed to be below normal, potassium secretion is reduced because it is driven by the transepithelial voltage, hyperkalemia causes acidosis by suppressing ammonia production, and extracellular volume expansion from sodium chloride absorption suppresses renin and aldosterone levels and causes hypertension. The main evidence for this formulation is that infusion of sodium bicarbonate or sodium sulfate raises potassium excretion to normal or supranormal levels. Treatment is with thiazide diuretics or low-sodium diet.

Primary mineralocorticoid deficiency from diseases of the adrenals also causes hyperkalemia and acidosis. Evaluation and treatment of adrenal disorders is discussed in Chap. 335.

VITAMIN D DISORDERS

X-LINKED HYPOPHOSPHATEMIA (See also Chaps. 234 and 358) Reduced tubular reabsorption of phosphate by the proximal tubule and hypophosphatemia occur in this X-linked dominant disease, which is also termed *renal phosphate leak*. Patients may be asymptomatic but are usually short and have rachitic bones; the legs are particularly short and deformed, and osteomalacia develops in adult life. Bone age and dentition are retarded, and the teeth are poorly developed. The skull becomes deformed, and the maxillofacial region may be abnormal. Overgrowth of bone at sites of muscular attachment can limit movement or compress nerves. Bony abnormalities are less common in women. Serum alkaline phosphatase is elevated, serum parathyroid is normal or high, serum calcium is usually normal, and urinary calcium excretion is normal or low.

The hypophosphatemia arises in part from decreased tubular reabsorption of phosphate and increased fractional excretion of phosphate. Intestinal absorption of calcium and phosphate may be decreased in untreated patients and increased during treatment with vitamin D. Although glycinuria and mild glucosuria may occur, most patients exhibit only a defect in excretion of phosphate. Absence of hyperchloremic acidosis and a normal serum calcium concentration help to exclude RTA, malabsorption, and nutritional rickets.

Treatment requires oral neutral phosphate, 1 to 4 g/d, in divided doses, and either calcitriol or some other form of vitamin D. Bony deformities require orthopedic management, but corrective surgery, except for genu valgum, should be postponed until active growth is completed.

VITAMIN D–DEPENDENT RICKETS TYPE 1 (See also Chaps. 234 and 358) Also known as *hereditary pseudovitamin D–deficiency rickets*, this disease is inherited as an autosomal recessive trait. Defective production of $1,25(OH)_2D_3$ by the kidneys, perhaps because of a genetic defect in 25-hydroxycholecalciferol 1α-hydroxylase, is probably the basis for the disease. However, the dose of calcitriol required to heal rickets is higher than that for vitamin D–deficiency rickets, suggesting an attenuated response to, or excessive degradation of, $1,25(OH)_2D_3$.

Rickets usually begins before 2 years of age. Serum calcium is low, parathyroid hormone and alkaline phosphatase levels are high, and plasma phosphorus is variable. Urinary calcium is decreased, fecal calcium is increased, and tubular phosphate reabsorption is reduced. Serum levels of $1,25(OH)_2D$ are undetectable. Aminoaciduria and hyperchloremic acidosis can occur, but urinary cyclic AMP increases normally in response to PTH infusion.

The 1α-hydroxylated metabolites of vitamin D bypass the enzyme defect and produce a dramatic healing of rickets. Vitamin D is also effective, but oral calcium, 0.5 to 2.0 g/d, is needed as well. The need for vitamin D persists throughout life. Calcitriol is the drug of choice, but one must watch for hypercalcemia.

VITAMIN D–DEPENDENT RICKETS TYPE 2 Like type 1, this autosomal recessive disease causes rickets, hypocalcemia, hypophosphatemia, and secondary hyperparathyroidism. Serum levels of $1,25(OH)_2D$ are elevated, and treatment with additional $1,25(OH)_2D$ does not increase the serum calcium level or heal the bone disease

even though it can reduce serum levels of parathyroid hormone. Generalized alopecia is often present and may be either a linked defect or the result of the mineral disorder. The disorder is due to mutations that impair the function of the $1,25(OH)_2D_3$ receptor (also see Chaps. 234 and 329). Treatment with a high dose of calcitriol and mineral supplements may achieve healing of bone, but relapse may occur despite continued treatment.

ONCOGENIC OSTEOMALACIA Mesenchymal tumors, usually benign, can cause renal phosphate wasting similiar to that of X-linked hypophosphatemic rickets, with resulting osteomalacia. Carcinoma of the prostate and oat cell carcinoma of the lung also have caused this syndrome. The disease almost always occurs in adults and develops gradually, over years. The tumors occur mainly in the extremities, head, nose, and mandible, in close association with bone. Their removal cures the phosphate wasting and leads to healing of the osteomalacia.

RENAL GLUCOSURIA (See Chap. 353.)

ISOLATED HYPOURICEMIA (See also Chap. 353.)

There is a defect in proximal tubular reabsorption of sodium urate in this autosomal recessive trait. Hypouricemia also can occur in the Fanconi syndrome, Hartnup disease, and Wilson's disease. Uric acid clearance is high, and urine oxypurine levels are normal, excluding hereditary xanthinuria. Patients are asymptomatic except for occasional uric acid nephrolithiasis. No treatment is needed except the avoidance of dehydration. Coexistent hypercalciuria and decreased bone density have been described in a few patients, who may have a related disease.

SELECTED DISORDERS OF AMINO ACID TRANSPORT

HARTNUP DISEASE (See also Chap. 353) In this rare autosomal recessive disorder, renal and intestinal transport of monoamino-monocarboxylic amino acids is defective. An erythematous, scaly rash appears after exposure to sunlight, and episodic cerebellar ataxia, emotional instability, delirium, and aminoaciduria occur. The prevalence is 1 in 15,000 newborns.

Dietary monoamino-monocarboxylic amino acids undergo bacterial degradation in the intestinal lumen. At the same time, they are lost in the urine. Inadequate tryptophan availability limits nicotinamide synthesis and leads to secondary pellagra (see Chap. 77). Decreased absorption and urine loss of the other monoamino-monocarboxylic amino acids can cause generalized malnutrition.

The diagnosis is based on demonstration of massive urine losses of alanine, serine, threonine, asparagine, glutamine, valine, leucine, isoleucine, phenylalanine, tyrosine, tryptophan, histidine, glycine, and citrulline. Hypouricemia may occur. Renal function is otherwise normal. Most patients respond to treatment with oral nicotinamide, 40 to 200 mg/d, and a high-protein diet to compensate for amino acid malabsorption and loss. The ultimate prognosis is good, and the disease often improves with age.

FAMILIAL IMINOGLYCINURIA (See also Chap. 353) This autosomal recessive trait is characterized by excessive urinary excretion of proline, hydroxyproline, and glycine despite normal plasma levels of these amino acids, probably because of deletion or alteration of a membrane transport protein of the renal tubule cells. The patients are asymptomatic. Iminoglycinuria can occur in normal newborn infants up to 3 months of age.

FANCONI SYNDROME

Fanconi syndrome is a constellation of transport defects in the proximal tubule involving amino acids, monosaccharides, sodium, potassium, calcium, phosphate, bicarbonate, uric acid, and proteins. Generalized aminoaciduria, glucosuria, salt wasting, hypercalciuria, hypophosphatemia, proximal renal tubular acidosis, hypouricemia, and tubular proteinuria (Chap. 44) may result. Fanconi syndrome can be secondary to diseases such as cystinosis, tyrosinemia, galactosemia, fructose intolerance, glycogen storage disease (type 1), Wilson's disease, familial nephrosis, and hereditary amyloidosis. Lowe's (or oculocerebrorenal) syndrome is an X-linked recessive form of the Fanconi syndrome associated with ocular and cerebral abnormalities.

An autosomal recessive disease, *adult Fanconi syndrome*, occurs in the absence of any systemic disorder. The term *adult* is misleading because cases are recognized in childhood, but no abnormalities are apparent at birth. Dwarfism and hypophosphatemic rickets occur along with the laboratory abnormalities of Fanconi syndrome. Renal failure is rare, and the prognosis is good when the systemic manifestations are treated. Typically, there is a "swan-neck" deformity and cellular atrophy of the initial portion of the proximal tubule which is probably the anatomic basis of this tubular disorder. The associated defects in the transport of water, sodium, potassium, acid, and phosphate excretion often require treatment. Water, sodium, and potassium intake must be liberal, and phosphate supplements may be needed. Metabolic acidosis can be corrected by the administration of alkali. Vitamin D helps promote bone healing. Glucosuria, uricosuria, and tubular proteinuria do not require treatment.

CYSTINURIA (See Chap. 353.)

REFERENCES

BERGERON M, SCRIVER CR: Pathophysiology of renal hyperaminoacidurias and glycouria, in *The Kidney*, DW Seldin, G Giebisch (eds). New York, Raven, 1992, p 2947

BERNSTEIN J, KISSANE JM: Hereditary disorders of the kidney: Part 1. Parenchymal defects and malformations. Perspect Pediatr Pathol 1:117, 1973

BUCKALEW VM JR: Calcium nephrolithiasis and renal tubular acidosis, in *Disorders of Bone and Mineral Metabolism*, FL Coe, MJ Favus (eds). New York, Raven, 1992, p 729

CANTANI A et al: Familial juvenile nephronophthisis: A review and differential diagnosis. Clin Pediatr 25:90, 1986

COE FL, PARKS JH: Calcium phosphate stones and renal tubular acidosis, in *Nephrolithiasis: Pathogenesis and Treatment*. Chicago, Year Book, 1988, chap 5

ECONS MJ, DREZNER MK: Bone disease resulting from inherited disorders of renal tubule transport and vitamin D metabolism, in *Disorders of Bone and Mineral Metabolism*, FL Coe, MJ Favus (eds). New York, Raven, 1992, p 935

GABOW PA et al: Polycystic kidney disease: Prospective analysis of nonazulemic patients and family members. Ann Intern Med 101:238, 1984

GARRICK R et al: Bartter's syndrome: A unifying hypothesis. Am J Nephrol 5:379, 1985

HUSSACK KF et al: Echocardiographic findings in autosomal dominant polycystic kidney disease. N Engl J Med 319:907, 1988

LEVEY AS et al: Occult intracranial aneurisms in polycystic kidney disease. N Engl J Med 308:986, 1983

LEVY HL: Hartnup disorder, in *The Metabolic Basis of Inherited Disease*, 6th ed, CR Scriver et al (eds). New York, McGraw-Hill, 1989, chap 101, p 2515

LIBBER S et al: Treatment of nephrogenic diabetes insipidus with prostaglandin synthesis inhibitors. J Pediatr 108:35, 1986

LIDDLE GW et al: A familial renal disorder simulating primary aldosteronism but with negligible aldosterone secretion. Trans Assoc Am Phys 76:199, 1963

MORRIS RC, IVES HE: Inherited disorders of the renal tubule, in *The Kidney*, BM Brenner, FC Rector Jr (eds). Philadelphia, Saunders, 1991, p 1596

RASMUSSEN H, TENENHOUSE HT: Hypophosphatemias, in *The Metabolic Basis of Inherited Disease*, 6th ed, CR Scriver et al (eds). New York, McGraw-Hill, 1989, chap 105, p 2581

REEDERS ST: Genetic abnormalities of renal function, in *The Kidney*, DW Seldin, G Giebisch (eds). New York, Raven, 1992, p 3085

REEVES WB, ANDREOLI TE: Nephrogenic diabetes insipidus, in *The Metabolic Basis of Inherited Disease*, 6th ed, CR Scriver et al (eds). New York, McGraw-Hill, 1989, chap 78, p 1985

SCHWAB SJ et al: Renal infections in autosomal dominant polycystic kidney disease. Am J Med 82:714, 1987

SIRIS ES et al: Tumor-induced osteomalacia. Am J Med 82:307, 1987

TOFUKU Y et al: Hypouricemia due to renal urate wasting: Two types of tubular transport defects. Nephron 30:39, 1982

245   NEPHROLITHIASIS

FREDRIC L. COE / MURRAY J. FAVUS

TYPES OF STONES

Calcium salts, uric acid, cystine, and struvite ($MgNH_4PO_4$) are the basis of most kidney stones in the western hemisphere. Calcium oxalate and calcium phosphate stones make up 75 to 85 percent of the total (Table 245-1) and may be admixed in the same stone. Calcium phosphate in stones is usually hydroxyapatite [$Ca_5(PO_4)_3OH$] or, less commonly, brushite ($CaHPO_4 \cdot H_2O$).

Calcium stones are more common in men; the average age of onset is the third decade. Most persons who form a single calcium stone eventually form another, and the intervals between successive stones shorten or remain constant. The average rate of new stone formation in patients who have had a previous stone is about one stone every 2 or 3 years. Calcium stone disease is frequently familial.

In the urine, calcium oxalate monohydrate crystals (whewellite) usually grow as biconcave ovals that resemble red blood cells in shape and size but may occur in a larger, "dumbbell" form. In polarized light the crystals appear bright against a dark background with an intensity that is dependent on orientation, a property known as *birefringence*. Calcium oxalate dihydrate crystals (weddellite) are bipyramidal and only weakly birefringent. Apatite crystals do not exhibit birefringence and appear amorphous because the actual crystals are too small to be resolved by light microscopy. Brushite produces elongated lathlike (narrow, long, rectangular) crystals.

Uric acid stones (see Table 245-1) are radiolucent and are also more common in men. Half of patients with uric acid stones have gout; uric acid lithiasis is usually familial whether or not gout is present. In urine, uric acid crystals are red-orange in color because they adsorb the pigment uricine. Anhydrous uric acid produces small crystals that appear amorphous by light microscopy. They are indistinguishable from apatite crystals, except for their birefringence. Uric acid dihydrate tends to form teardrop-shaped crystals as well as flat, square plates; both are strongly birefringent. Uric acid gravel appears like red dust, and the stones are also orange or red on some occasions. *Cystine stones* are uncommon (see Table 245-1), are lemon yellow, and sparkle; radiopacity is due to the sulfur content. Cystine crystals appear in the urine as flat, hexagonal plates.

Struvite ($MgNH_4PO_4$) *stones* are common (see Table 245-1) and potentially dangerous. These stones occur mainly in women and result from urinary tract infection with urease-producing bacteria, usually *Proteus* species. The stones can grow to a large size and fill the renal pelvis and calyces to produce a "staghorn" appearance. They are radiopaque and have a variable internal density. In urine, struvite crystals are rectangular prisms said to resemble coffin lids.

MANIFESTATIONS OF STONES

As stones grow on the surfaces of the renal papillae or within the collecting system, they need not produce symptoms. Asymptomatic stones may be discovered during the course of radiographic studies undertaken for unrelated reasons. Stones rank, along with benign and malignant neoplasms, renal cysts, and genitourinary tuberculosis, among the common causes of isolated hematuria. Much of the time, however, stones break loose and enter the ureter or occlude the ureteropelvic junction, causing pain and obstruction.

STONE PASSAGE   A stone can traverse the ureter without symptoms, but passage usually produces pain and bleeding. The pain begins gradually, usually in the flank, but increases over the next 20 to 60 min to become so severe that narcotic drugs may be needed for its control. The pain may remain in the flank or spread downward and anteriorly toward the ipsilateral loin, testis, or vulva. Pain that

TABLE 245-1 Major causes of renal stones

Stone type and causes	Percent of all stones*	Percent occurrence of specific causes*	Ratio of men to women	Etiology	Diagnosis	Treatment
Calcium stones	75–85		2:1 to 3:1			
Idiopathic hypercalciuria		50–55	2:1	Hereditary (?)	Normocalcemia, unexplained hypercalciuria[†]	Thiazide diuretic agents
Hyperuricosuria		20	4:1	Diet	Urine uric acid >750 mg per 24 h (women), >800 mg per 24 h (men)	Allopurinol or diet
Primary hyperparathyroidism		5	3:10	Neoplasia	Unexplained hypercalcemia	Surgery
Distal renal tubular acidosis		Rare	1:1	Hereditary	Hyperchloremic acidosis, minimum urine pH >5.5	Alkali replacement
Intestinal hyperoxaluria		~1–2	1:1	Bowel surgery	Urine oxalate >50 mg per 24 h	Cholestyramine or oral calcium loading
Hereditary hyperoxaluria		Rare	1:1	Hereditary	Urine oxalate and glycolic or L-glyceric acid increased	Fluids and pyridoxine
Idiopathic stone disease		20	2:1	Unknown	None of the above present	Oral phosphate, fluids
Uric acid stones	5–8					
Gout		~50	3:1 to 4:1	Hereditary	Clinical diagnosis	Alkali to raise urine pH
Idiopathic		~50	1:1	Hereditary (?)	Uric acid stones, no gout	Allopurinol if daily urine uric acid above 1000 mg
Dehydration		?	1:1	Intestinal, habit	History, intestinal fluid loss	Alkali, fluids, reversal of cause
Lesch-Nyhan syndrome		Rare	Men	Hereditary	Reduced hypoxanthine-guanine phosphoribosyltransferase level	Allopurinol
Malignant tumors		Rare	1:1	Neoplasia	Clinical diagnosis	Allopurinol
Cystine stones	1		1:1	Hereditary	Stone type; elevated cystine excretion	Massive fluids, alkali, D-penicillamine if needed
Struvite stones	10–15		2:10	Infection	Stone type	Antimicrobial agents and judicious surgery

* Values are percent of patients who form a particular type of stone and who display each specific cause of stones.
† Urine calcium above 300 mg per 24 h (men), 250 mg per 24 h (women), or 4 mg/kg per 24 h either sex. Hyperthyroidism, Cushing syndrome, sarcoidosis, malignant tumors, immobilization, vitamin D intoxication, rapidly progressive bone disease, and Paget's disease all cause hypercalciuria and must be excluded in diagnosis of idiopathic hypercalciuria.

migrates downward indicates that the stone has passed to the lower third of the ureter, but if the pain does not migrate, the position of the stone cannot be predicted. A stone in the portion of the ureter within the bladder wall causes frequency, urgency, and dysuria that may be confused with urinary tract infection. Hematuria is usual with passage of a stone.

OTHER SYNDROMES Staghorn calculi Struvite, cystine, and uric acid stones often grow too large to enter the ureter. They gradually fill the renal pelvis and may extend outward through the infundibula to the calyces themselves.

Nephrocalcinosis Calcium stones grow on the renal papillae. Most break loose and cause colic, but they may remain in place so that multiple papillary calcifications are found by x-ray, a condition termed *nephrocalcinosis*. Papillary nephrocalcinosis is common in hereditary distal renal tubular acidosis and in other types of severe hypercalciuria. In medullary sponge kidney disease (see Chap. 244) calcification may occur in dilated distal collecting ducts.

Sludge Sufficient uric acid or cystine in the urine may plug both ureters with precipitate. Calcium oxalate crystals do not do this because less than 100 mg oxalate usually is excreted daily in the urine even in severe hyperoxaluric states, compared with 1000 mg uric acid in patients with hyperuricosuria and 400 to 800 mg cystine in patients with cystinuria. Calcium phosphate crystals can render the urine milky but do not plug the urinary tract.

INFECTION Although urinary tract infection is not a direct consequence of stone disease, it can occur after instrumentation and surgery of the urinary tract, which are frequent in the treatment of stone disease. Stone disease and urinary infection can enhance the seriousness of one another and interfere with treatment. Obstruction of an infected kidney by a stone may lead to sepsis and extensive damage of renal tissue, since it converts the urinary tract proximal to the obstruction into a closed, or partially closed, space that can

become an abscess. On the other hand, infection due to bacteria that possess the enzyme urease can cause stones composed of struvite.

ACTIVITY OF STONE DISEASE *Active disease* means that new stones are forming or that preformed stones are growing. Sequential radiographs of the renal areas are needed to document the growth or appearance of new stones and to ensure that passed stones are actually newly formed, not preexistent ones.

PATHOGENESIS OF STONES

Urinary stones usually arise because of the breakdown of a delicate balance. The kidneys must conserve water, but they also must excrete materials that have a low solubility. These two opposing requirements must be balanced during adaptation to diet, climate, and activity. The problem is mitigated to some extent by the fact that urine contains substances that inhibit crystallization of calcium salts and others that bind calcium in soluble complexes. These protective mechanisms are less than perfect. When the urine becomes supersaturated with insoluble materials, because excretion rates are excessive and/or because water conservation is extreme, crystals form and may grow and aggregate to form a stone.

SUPERSATURATION In a solution in equilibrium with crystals of calcium oxalate, the product of the chemical activities of the calcium and oxalate ions in the solution is termed the *equilibrium solubility product*. If the crystals are removed, and if either calcium or oxalate ions are added to the solution, the activity product increases, but the solution may remain clear; no new crystals form. Such a solution is *metastably supersaturated*. If new calcium oxalate seed crystals are now added, they will grow in size. Ultimately, the activity product reaches a critical value at which a solid phase begins to develop spontaneously. This value is called the *upper limit of* *metastability*, or the *formation product*. Stone growth in the urinary tract requires a urine that, on average, is above the equilibrium solubility product. Persistence of a stone requires an average activity product at least equal to the solubility product. Excessive supersaturation is common in stone formation.

Calcium, oxalate, and phosphate form many stable soluble complexes among themselves and with other substances in urine, such as citrate. As a result, their free ion activities are below their chemical concentrations and can be measured only by indirect techniques. Reduction in ligands such as citrate can increase ion activity without changing total urinary calcium. Urine supersaturation can be increased by dehydration or by overexcretion of calcium, oxalate, phosphate, cystine, or uric acid. Urine pH is also important; phosphate and uric acid are weak acids that dissociate readily over the physiologic range of urine pH. Alkaline urine contains more urate and dissociated phosphate, favoring deposits of sodium hydrogen urate, brushite, and apatite. Below a urine pH of 5.5, uric acid crystals (pK 5.47) predominate, whereas phosphate crystals are rare. The solubility of calcium oxalate, on the other hand, is not influenced by changes in urine pH. Measurements of supersaturation in a pooled 24-h urine sample probably underestimate the risk of precipitation. Transient dehydration or postprandial bursts of overexcretion may cause values considerably above average.

NUCLEATION   Homogeneous nucleation   In urine that is supersaturated with respect to calcium oxalate, these two ions form clusters. The higher the supersaturation, the larger and more numerous are the clusters. Most small clusters eventually disperse because the internal forces that hold them together are too weak to overcome the random tendency of ions to move away. Clusters of over 100 ions can remain stable because attractive forces balance surface losses. Once they are stable, nuclei can grow at levels of supersaturation below that needed for their creation. The formation product marks the point at which stable nuclei become frequent enough to create a permanent solid phase.

Heterogeneous nucleation   If a supersaturated urine is seeded with preformed nuclei of a crystal that is similar in structure to calcium oxalate, calcium and oxalate ions in solution will bind to the crystal's surface as they would on a seed crystal of calcium oxalate itself. The organized growth of one crystal on the surface of another is called *epitaxial growth*, and the seeding of a supersaturated solution by foreign nuclei is called *heterogeneous nucleation*. Sodium hydrogen urate, uric acid, and hydroxyapatite crystals can serve as heterogeneous nuclei that permit calcium oxalate stones to form even though urine calcium oxalate supersaturation never exceeds the metastable limit.

INHIBITORS OF CRYSTAL GROWTH AND AGGREGATION   Stable nuclei must grow and aggregate to produce a stone of clinical significance. Urine contains potent inhibitors of both these processes for calcium oxalate and calcium phosphate but not for uric acid, cystine, or struvite. Inorganic pyrophosphate is a potent inhibitor that appears to affect calcium phosphate more than calcium oxalate crystals. Other urine components that appear to be glycoproteins inhibit the growth of calcium oxalate crystals. Slowing of crystal growth increases the apparent upper limit of metastability because the critical growth of ion clusters into stable nuclei is hindered. As a consequence of the presence of these inhibitors, crystal growth in urine is slow compared with growth in simple salt solutions, and the upper limit of metastability is higher. Urine citrate also may inhibit crystal growth or nucleation.

EVALUATION AND TREATMENT OF PATIENTS WITH NEPHROLITHIASIS

Most patients with nephrolithiasis have remediable metabolic disorders that cause stones and can be detected by chemical analyses of serum and urine. A practical outpatient evaluation consists of three 24-h urine collections, each with a corresponding blood sample; measurements of serum and urine calcium, uric acid and creatinine, urine oxalate and

citrate, and serum electrolytes should be made. When possible, the composition of kidney stones should be determined because treatment depends on stone type (see Table 245-1). No matter what disorders are found, every patient should be counseled to avoid dehydration and to drink six to eight glasses of water daily. Since treatment is prolonged, the use of medications must be justified by the activity and severity of stone disease and the importance of protection against new stones.

The management of stones already present in the kidneys or urinary tract requires a combined medical and surgical approach. The specific treatment depends on the location of the stone, the extent of obstruction, the function of the affected and unaffected kidneys, the presence or absence of urinary tract infection, the progress of stone passage, and the risk of operation or anesthesia given the clinical state of the patient. In general, severe obstruction, infection, intractable pain, and serious bleeding are indications for removal of a stone.

In the past, stones were removed by operation or by passing a flexible basket retrograde up the ureter from the bladder during cystoscopy. There are now three alternatives. Extracorporeal lithotripsy causes the in situ fragmentation of stones in the kidney, renal pelvis, or proximal ureter by exposing them to shock waves. The patient is submerged in a water tank, the kidney with the stone is centered at the focal point of parabolic reflectors, and high-intensity shock waves are created by high-voltage discharge. The waves are focused by the reflectors so that they pass through the patient and fracture the stone as they pass. After multiple discharges, most stones are reduced to powder that moves through the ureter into the bladder. Larger fragments are removed by cystoscopy. Percutaneous ultrasonic lithotripsy requires the passage of a rigid cystoscope-like instrument into the renal pelvis through a small incision in the flank. Stones can be disrupted by a small ultrasound transducer, and fragments can be removed directly. The last method is endoscopic passage of an ultrasonic transducer into the ureter via a cystoscope; ureteral stones that are inaccessible to extracorporeal or percutaneous lithotripsy can be fragmented and removed. These various forms of lithotripsy have largely replaced pyelolithotomy and ureterolithotomy.

CALCIUM STONES   Idiopathic hypercalciuria   (See also Chap. 357)   This condition appears to be hereditary, and its diagnosis is straightforward (see Table 245-1). In some patients, primary intestinal hyperabsorption of calcium causes transient postprandial hypercalcemia that suppresses secretion of parathyroid hormone. The renal tubules are deprived of the normal stimulus to reabsorb calcium at the same time that the filtered load of calcium is increased. In other patients, reabsorption of calcium by the renal tubules appears to be defective, and secondary hyperparathyroidism is evoked by urinary losses of calcium. Renal synthesis of 1,25-dihydroxyvitamin D is increased, enhancing intestinal absorption of calcium. In the past, the separation of "absorptive" and "renal" forms of hypercalciuria was used to guide treatment. However, these may not be distinct entities but the extremes of a continuum of behavior. Hypercalciuria contributes to stone formation by raising urine saturation with respect to calcium oxalate and calcium phosphate.

Thiazide diuretics lower urine calcium in both types of hypercalciuria and are effective in preventing the formation of stones. The drug effect requires slight contraction of the extracellular fluid volume, and massive use of NaCl reduces its therapeutic effect. Potassium citrate is useful to prevent hypokalemia and raise urine citrate; the latter lowers urine calcium ion levels.

Hyperuricosuria   About 20 percent of calcium oxalate stone formers are hyperuricosuric, primarily because of an excessive intake of purine from meat, fish, and poultry. The mechanism of stone formation probably is heterogeneous nucleation of calcium oxalate by crystals of sodium hydrogen urate or uric acid. A low purine diet is desirable but difficult for many patients to achieve. The alternative is allopurinol, usually 100 mg bid.

Primary hyperparathyroidism   (See also Chap. 357)   The diagnosis of this condition is established by documenting that hypercalcemia that cannot be otherwise explained is accompanied by inappropriately elevated serum concentrations of parathyroid hormone. Hypercalciuria, usually present, raises the urine supersaturation of calcium phosphate and/or calcium oxalate (see Table 245-1). Prompt diagnosis is important because parathyroidectomy should be carried out before renal damage occurs.

Distal renal tubular acidosis (See also Chap. 244) The defect in this condition seems to reside in the distal nephron, which cannot establish a normal pH gradient between urine and blood, leading to hyperchloremic acidosis. The minimum urine pH in response to an oral challenge with NH_4Cl, 1.9 mmol/kg of body weight, is above 5.5. Hypercalciuria, an alkaline urine, and a low urine citrate level cause supersaturation with respect to calcium phosphate. Calcium phosphate stones form, nephrocalcinosis is common, and osteomalacia or rickets may occur. Renal damage is frequent, and glomerular filtration rate falls gradually. Treatment with supplemental alkali reverses hypercalciuria and limits the production of new stones. The usual dose of sodium bicarbonate is 0.5 to 2.0 mmol/kg of body weight per day in four to six divided doses. An alternative is Shohl's solution, which contains citrate and citric acid. In incomplete renal tubular acidosis (RTA), systemic acidosis is absent, but urine pH cannot be lowered below 5.5 after an exogenous acid load such as ammonium chloride. Incomplete RTA may develop in some patients who form calcium oxalate stones because of idiopathic hypercalciuria; the importance of the RTA in producing stones in this situation is uncertain, and thiazide treatment is a reasonable alternative. Some patients with incomplete RTA form calcium phosphate stones because of low urine citrate and an alkaline urine and are best treated with alkali as if RTA were complete.

Hyperoxaluria Overabsorption of dietary oxalate and consequent oxaluria, i.e., so-called intestinal oxaluria, is one consequence of fat malabsorption (Chap. 254). The latter can be caused by a variety of conditions, including bacterial overgrowth syndromes, chronic disease of the pancreas and biliary tract, jejunoileal bypass in treatment of obesity, or ileal resection for inflammatory bowel disease. With fat malabsorption, calcium in the bowel lumen is bound by fatty acids instead of oxalate, which is left free for absorption in the colon. Delivery of unabsorbed fatty acids and bile salts to the colon may injure the colonic mucosa and enhance oxalate absorption. Dietary excess of oxalate, ascorbic acid loading, and hereditary hyperoxaluric states are less common causes of hyperoxaluria. Ethylene glycol intoxication and methoxyflurane also can cause oxalate overproduction and hyperoxaluria. Hyperoxaluria from any cause can produce tubulointerstitial nephropathy (Chap. 242) and lead to stone formation.

The oxalate-binding resin cholestyramine at a dose of 8 to 16 g/d, correction of fat malabsorption, and a low-fat diet are effective treatments for oxaluria secondary to intestinal absorption. Calcium lactate, 8 to 14 g/d, which precipitates oxalate in the gut lumen, is an alternative form of therapy. There is no treatment for primary hyperoxaluria, the result of an enzymatic defect involving the metabolism of the precursor of oxalate that is inherited as an autosomal recessive (also see Chap. 352). A high fluid intake, phosphate, and pyridoxine (200 mg/d) are recommended, but irreversible renal failure secondary to recurrent stone formation usually occurs before age 20.

Idiopathic calcium lithiasis At least 20 percent of patients have no obvious cause for stones (see Table 245-1). The best treatment appears to be a high fluid intake so that the urine specific gravity remains at 1.005 or below throughout the day and night. Oral phosphate at a dose of 2 g phosphorus daily may lower urine calcium and increase urine pyrophosphate and thereby reduce the rate of recurrence. Orthophosphate causes mild nausea and diarrhea initially, but tolerance may improve with continued intake. Thiazide treatment to reduce calcium excretion and allopurinol to diminish uric acid output also may be helpful.

URIC ACID STONES These stones form because the urine becomes supersaturated with undissociated uric acid, uric acid that is protonated at its N-9 position. In gout, idiopathic uric acid lithiasis, and dehydration, the average pH is usually below 5.4 and often below 5.0. Undissociated uric acid therefore predominates and is soluble in

urine only in concentrations of 100 mg/L. Concentrations above this level represent supersaturation that causes crystals and stones to form. Hyperuricosuria, when present, increases supersaturation, but urine of low pH can be supersaturated with undissociated uric acid even though the daily excretion rate is normal. Myeloproliferative syndromes, chemotherapy of malignant tumors, and the Lesch-Nyhan syndrome cause such massive production of uric acid and consequent hyperuricosuria that stones and uric acid sludge form even at a normal urine pH. Plugging of the renal collecting tubules by uric acid crystals can cause acute renal failure.

The two goals of treatment are to raise urine pH and to lower excessive urine uric acid excretion to less than 1 g/d. Supplemental alkali, 1 to 3 mmol/kg of body weight per day, should be given in three or four evenly spaced, divided doses, one of which should be given at bedtime. The form of the alkali may be important. Potassium citrate may reduce the risk of calcium salts crystallizing when urine pH is increased, whereas sodium citrate or sodium bicarbonate may increase the risk. If the overnight urine pH is below 5.5, the evening dose of bicarbonate may be raised, or 250 mg acetazolamide added at bedtime. With massive overexcretion of uric acid, doses of allopurinol above 300 mg daily may be needed. Treatment with allopurinol should be instituted prior to chemotherapy of highly cellular tumors, since massive hyperuricosuria can be expected. Alkali treatment must be avoided if hypercalciuria is also present.

CYSTINURIA AND CYSTINE STONES (See also Chap. 352) In this disorder, proximal tubular and jejunal transport of the dibasic amino acids cystine, lysine, arginine, and ornithine are defective, and excessive amounts are lost in the urine. Clinical disease is due solely to the insolubility of cystine, which forms stones.

Pathogenesis Cystinuria probably occurs because of defective transport of amino acids by the brush borders of renal tubule and intestinal epithelial cells. Cystine, lysine, arginine, and ornithine appear to share a common renal transport pathway, since infusion of lysine decreases tubular reabsorption of the other three. However, cystine is also transported by a separate transport mechanism, because cystinuria and dibasic aminoaciduria can occur independently. The intestinal defects are not similar in all patients who are homozygous for cystinuria, and the extent of aminoaciduria in individuals who are heterozygous carriers of the defect varies from family to family. Three types of inheritance have been described (see Chap. 352).

Diagnosis and treatment Cystine stones are formed only by patients with cystinuria, but 10 percent of stones in cystinuric patients do not contain cystine; therefore, every stone former should be screened for the disease. The sediment from a first morning urine specimen in many patients with homozygous cystinuria reveals typical flat hexagonal platelike cystine crystals. Cystinuria also can be detected using the urine sodium nitroprusside test. The test is positive with 75 to 125 mg cystine per gram of creatinine, a concentration lower than that in the urine of patients with cystinuria but above the levels in normal urine. Because the test is sensitive, it is positive in many asymptomatic heterozygotes for cystinuria. A positive nitroprusside test or the finding of cystine crystals in the urine sediment should be evaluated by measurement of daily cystine excretion. Normal adults excrete 40 to 60 mg cystine per gram of creatinine, heterozygotes usually excrete less than 300 mg/g, and homozygotes almost always excrete above 250 mg/g.

Treatment consists of a high fluid intake, even at night. Daily urine volume should exceed 3 L. Raising urine pH with alkali is helpful, provided the urine pH exceeds 7.5. Because side effects are frequent, penicillamine, which forms the soluble disulfide cysteine-penicillamine, should be used only when fluid loading and alkali therapy are ineffective. Mercaptopropinylglycine has been used to dissolve renal calculi by perfusion of the renal pelvis and has been given by mouth to prevent stones. Low-methionine diets have not proved to be practical for clinical use.

STRUVITE STONES These stones are a result of urinary infection with bacteria, usually *Proteus* species, which possess urease, an enzyme that degrades urea to NH_3 and CO_2. The NH_3 hydrolyzes to

NH_4^+ and raises pH, usually to 8 or 9. The CO_2 hydrates to H_2CO_3 and then dissociates to CO_3^{2-} which precipitates with calcium as $CaCO_3$. The NH_4^+ precipitates PO_4^{3-} and Mg^{2+} to form $MgNH_4PO_4$. The result is a stone of calcium carbonate admixed with struvite. Struvite does not form in urine in the absence of infection, because NH_4^+ concentration is low in urine that is alkaline in response to physiologic stimuli. Chronic *Proteus* infection can occur because of impaired urinary drainage, urologic instrumentation or surgery, and especially with chronic antibiotic treatment, which can favor the dominance of *Proteus* in the urinary tract.

Treatment   Methenamine mandelate, which lowers urine pH and liberates formaldehyde, is used for chronic suppression of infection when a stone is present. More extreme lowering of urine pH with chronic administration of NH_4Cl may retard stone growth but also may raise urine calcium level and promote the formation of calcium oxalate stones. Antimicrobial treatment is best reserved for dealing with acute infection and for maintenance of a sterile urine after surgery, in the hope of preventing recurrence or minimizing stone growth. Surgery may be appropriate for severe obstruction, pain, bleeding, or intractable urinary infection. Since stones can regrow from any infected fragment which is left behind, recurrences following operation are quite common. In some centers it is possible to irrigate the renal pelvis and calyces with Renacidin, a solution that dissolves struvite, using a catheter passed through a cutaneous flank incision into the kidney.

REFERENCES

COE FL, PARKS JH: *Nephrolithiasis: Pathogenesis and treatment.* Chicago, Year Book, 1988

——————et al: Effect of low calcium diet on urine calcium excretion, parathyroid function, and serum 1,25(OH)₂D₃ levels in patients with idiopathic hypercalciuria and in normal subjects. Am J Med 72:25, 1982

COE FL, FAVUS MJ: Disorders of stone formation, in *The Kidney*, 4th ed, BM Brenner, FC Rector Jr (eds). Philadelphia, Saunders, 1991, p 1728

LEMANN J JR: Pathogenesis or idiopathic hypercalciuria and nephrolithiasis, in *Disorders of Bone and Mineral Metabolism*, FL Coe, MJ Favus (eds). New York, Raven, 1992, p 685

LINGEMAN JF: Mechanisms of stone disruption and dissolution, in *Disorders of Bone and Mineral Metabolism*, FL Coe, MJ Favus (eds). New York, Raven, 1992, p 625

NAKAGAWA Y et al: Purification and characterization of the principal inhibitors of calcium oxalate monohydrate crystal growth in human urine. J Biol Chem 258:12594, 1983

NEWMAN DM et al: Long-term follow-up of 1,900 ESWL treatments, in *Shock Wave Lithotripsy*, JE Lingeman, DM Newman (eds). New York, Plenum, 1988

RESNICK MI, PAK CYC: *Urolithiasis.* Philadelphia, Saunders, 1991

SMITH LH: Urolithiasis, in *Diseases of the Kidney*, 4th ed, RW Schrier, CW Gottschalk (eds). Boston, Little, Brown, 1988, p 785

STRAUSS AL et al: Factors that predict relapse of calcium nephrolithiasis during treatment. Am J Med 72:25, 1982

246   URINARY TRACT OBSTRUCTION

JULIAN L. SEIFTER / BARRY M. BRENNER

Obstruction to the flow of urine, with attendant stasis and elevation in urinary tract pressure, impairs renal and urinary conduit functions and is a common cause of acute and chronic renal failure. With early relief of obstruction, the defects in function usually disappear completely. However, chronic obstruction may produce permanent loss of renal mass (renal atrophy) and excretory capability, as well as enhanced susceptibility to local infection and stone formation. Early diagnosis and prompt therapy are therefore essential to minimize the otherwise devastating effects of obstruction on kidney structure and function.

ETIOLOGY   Obstruction to urine flow can result from *intrinsic* or *extrinsic mechanical blockade* as well as from *functional defects* not associated with fixed occlusion of the urinary drainage system.

Mechanical obstruction can occur at any level of the urinary tract, from the renal calyces to the external urethral meatus. Normal points of narrowing, such as the ureteropelvic and ureterovesical junctions, bladder neck, and urethral meatus, are common sites of obstruction. When blockage is above the level of the bladder, unilateral dilatation of the ureter (*hydroureter*) and renal pyelocalyceal system (*hydronephrosis*) occur; lesions at or below the level of the bladder cause bilateral involvement.

Common forms of obstruction are listed in Table 246-1. In childhood, *congenital malformations*, including marked narrowing of the ureteropelvic junction, anomalous (retrocaval) location of the ureter, and posterior urethral valves, predominate. The latter defect is the most common cause of bilateral hydronephrosis in boys. Children also may have bladder dysfunction secondary to congenital urethral stricture, urethral meatal stenosis, or bladder neck obstruction. In adults, urinary tract obstruction is due mainly to *acquired defects*. Pelvic tumors, calculi, and urethral stricture predominate. Ligation of, or injury to, the ureter during pelvic or colonic surgery can lead to hydronephrosis which, if unilateral, may remain relatively silent and undetected. *Schistosoma haematobium* and genitourinary tuberculosis are infectious causes of ureteral obstruction. Obstructive uropathy also may result from extrinsic neoplastic (carcinoma of cervix or colon, retroperitoneal lymphoma) or inflammatory disorders. One such inflammatory disorder is retroperitoneal fibrosis, a process of unknown cause seen most commonly in middle-aged men, which occasionally leads to bilateral ureteral obstruction. Retroperitoneal fibrosis must be distinguished from other retroperitoneal causes of ureteral obstruction, particularly lymphomas and pelvic neoplasms.

Functional impairment of urine flow usually results from disorders that involve both the ureter and bladder. Common functional lesions include neurogenic bladder, often with adynamic ureter, and vesicoureteral reflux. Reflux of urine from bladder to ureter(s) is more

TABLE 246-1   Common mechanical causes of urinary tract obstruction

Ureter	Bladder outlet	Urethra
CONGENITAL		
Ureteropelvic junction narrowing or obstruction	Bladder neck obstruction	Posterior urethral valves
Ureterovesical junction narrowing or obstruction	Ureterocele	Anterior urethral valves
Ureterocele		Stricture
Retrocaval ureter		Meatal stenosis
		Phimosis
ACQUIRED INTRINSIC DEFECTS		
Calculi	Benign prostatic hyperplasia	Stricture
Inflammation	Cancer of prostate	Tumor
Trauma	Cancer of bladder	Calculi
Sloughed papillae	Calculi	Trauma
Tumor	Diabetic neuropathy	Phimosis
Blood clots	Spinal cord disease	
Uric acid crystals	Anticholinergic drugs and alpha-adrenergic antagonists	
ACQUIRED EXTRINSIC DEFECTS		
Pregnant uterus	Carcinoma of cervix, colon	Trauma
Retroperitoneal fibrosis	Trauma	
Aortic aneurysm		
Uterine leiomyomata		
Carcinoma of uterus, prostate, bladder, colon, rectum		
Retroperitoneal lymphoma		
Accidental surgical ligation		

common in children than in adults and may result in severe unilateral or bilateral hydroureter and hydronephrosis. Abnormal insertion of the ureter into the bladder is the most common cause of vesicoureteral reflux in children. Reflux in the absence of urinary tract infection or bladder neck obstruction usually does not lead to renal parenchymal damage and often resolves spontaneously as the child matures. Surgical reinsertion of the ureter into the bladder is indicated if reflux is severe and unlikely to improve spontaneously if renal function deteriorates or if urinary tract infections recur despite chronic antimicrobial therapy. Hydronephrosis, usually more marked on the right than on the left, is common in pregnancy, due both to ureteral compression by the enlarged uterus and to functional effects of progesterone.

CLINICAL FEATURES   The pathophysiology and clinical features of urinary tract obstruction are summarized in Table 246-2. *Pain* is the symptom which most commonly provokes the need for medical attention. The pain of urinary tract obstruction is due to distention of the collecting system or renal capsule. The severity of the pain is influenced more by the rate at which distention develops than by the degree of distention. Acute supravesical obstruction, as from a stone lodged in a ureter (Chap. 245), is associated with excruciatingly severe pain, usually called *renal colic*. This pain is relatively steady and continuous, with little fluctuation in intensity, and often radiates to the lower abdomen, testes, or labia. By contrast, more insidious causes of obstruction, such as chronic narrowing of the ureteropelvic junction, may produce little or no pain yet result in total destruction of the affected kidney. Flank pain which occurs only with micturition is pathognomonic of vesicoureteral reflux.

Azotemia develops in urinary tract obstruction when overall excretory function is impaired. This may occur in the setting of bladder outlet obstruction, bilateral renal pelvic or ureteric obstruction, or unilateral disease in a patient with a solitary functioning kidney. Complete bilateral obstruction should be suspected when acute renal failure is accompanied by anuria. Any patient with renal failure otherwise unexplained or with a history of nephrolithiasis, hematuria, diabetes mellitus, prostatic enlargement, pelvic surgery, trauma, or tumor should be evaluated for urinary tract obstruction.

Symptoms of *polyuria* and *nocturia* commonly accompany chronic partial urinary tract obstruction and result from impaired renal concentrating ability. This defect usually does not improve with administration of vasopressin and is therefore a form of acquired nephrogenic diabetes insipidus. Disturbances in sodium chloride transport in the ascending limb of Henle and, in azotemic patients, the osmotic (urea) diuresis per nephron lead to decreased medullary hypertonicity and hence a concentrating defect. Partial obstruction, therefore, may be associated with increased rather than decreased urine output. Indeed, wide fluctuations in urine output in a patient with azotemia should always raise the possibility of intermittent or partial urinary tract obstruction. If fluid intake is inadequate, severe dehydration and hypernatremia may develop. Hesitancy and straining to initiate the urinary stream, postvoid dribbling, urinary frequency, and (overflow) incontinence are common with obstruction at or below the level of the bladder (see Chap. 44).

In addition to loss of urinary concentrating ability and azotemia, partial bilateral urinary tract obstruction often results in other derangements of renal function, including *acquired distal renal tubular acidosis, hyperkalemia,* and *renal salt wasting.* These defects in tubule function are often accompanied by renal tubulointerstitial damage. Morphologic abnormalities appear early in the course of obstruction; initially the interstitium becomes edematous and infiltrated with mononuclear inflammatory cells. With continued obstruction, the interstitium becomes fibrotic; scarring and atrophy of the papillae and medulla occur and precede these processes in the cortex.

The possibility of urinary tract obstruction must always be considered in patients with urinary tract infections or urolithiasis. Urinary stasis encourages the growth of organisms as well as the formation of crystals, especially magnesium ammonium phosphate (struvite). *Hypertension* is frequent in acute and subacute unilateral obstruction and is usually a consequence of increased release of renin by the involved kidney. Chronic unilateral or bilateral hydronephrosis, in the presence of extracellular volume expansion or other renal disease, may result in significant hypertension. *Polycythemia,* an infrequent complication of obstructive uropathy, is probably secondary to increased erythropoietin production by the obstructed kidney.

DIAGNOSIS   A history of difficulty in voiding, pain, infection, or changes in urinary volume is common. Evidence for distention of the kidney or urinary bladder often can be obtained by palpation and percussion of the abdomen. A careful rectal examination may reveal enlargement or nodularity of the prostate, abnormal rectal sphincter tone, or a rectal or pelvic mass. The penis should be inspected for evidence of meatal stenosis or phimosis. In the female, vaginal, uterine, and rectal lesions responsible for urinary tract obstruction are usually revealed by inspection and palpation.

Urinalysis and examination of the urine sediment may reveal hematuria, pyuria, and bacteriuria. Often, however, the urine sediment is normal, even when obstruction leads to marked azotemia and extensive structural damage. An abdominal scout film should be obtained to evaluate the possibility of nephrocalcinosis or a radiopaque stone at any level of the urinary collecting system. As indicated in Fig. 246-1, if urinary tract obstruction is suspected, abdominal ultrasonography should be performed to evaluate renal and bladder size, as well as pyelocalyceal contour. If these structures are not distended, functionally significant urinary tract obstruction can safely be excluded in differential diagnosis. Abdominal ultrasound also may detect an obstructing pelvic mass.

Intravenous pyelography is indicated if an obstructive abnormality is revealed by ultrasound. If the patient is not azotemic, a standard dose of contrast medium usually provides adequate information. With renal insufficiency, however, high-dose (drip-infusion) pyelography with nephrotomography is usually required for adequate visualization. In the presence of obstruction, the appearance time of the nephrogram is often delayed but eventually becomes more dense than normal because of slow tubular fluid flow rate which results in enhanced water reabsorption by the nephrons and greater concentration of contrast medium within tubules. The kidney involved by an acute

TABLE 246-2   Pathophysiology of bilateral ureteral obstruction

Hemodynamic effects	Tubule effects	Clinical features
ACUTE		
↑ Renal blood flow ↓ GFR ↓ Medullary blood flow ↑ Vasodilator prostaglandins	↑ Ureteral and tubule pressures ↑ Reabsorption of Na⁺, urea, water	Pain (capsule distention) Azotemia Oliguria
CHRONIC		
↓ Renal blood flow ↓ ↓ GFR ↑ Vasoconstrictor prostaglandins ↑ Renin-angiotensin production	↓ Medullary osmolarity ↓ Concentrating ability Structural damage; parenchymal atrophy ↓ Transport functions for Na⁺, K⁺, H⁺	Azotemia Hypertension ADH-insensitive polyuria Natriuresis Hyperkalemic, hyperchloremic acidosis
RELEASE OF OBSTRUCTION		
Slow ↑ in GFR (variable)	↓ Tubule pressure ↑ Solute load per nephron (urea, NaCl) Natriuretic factors present	Postobstructive diuresis Potential for volume depletion and electrolyte imbalance (Na⁺, K⁺, PO₄²⁻, Mg²⁺ excretion)

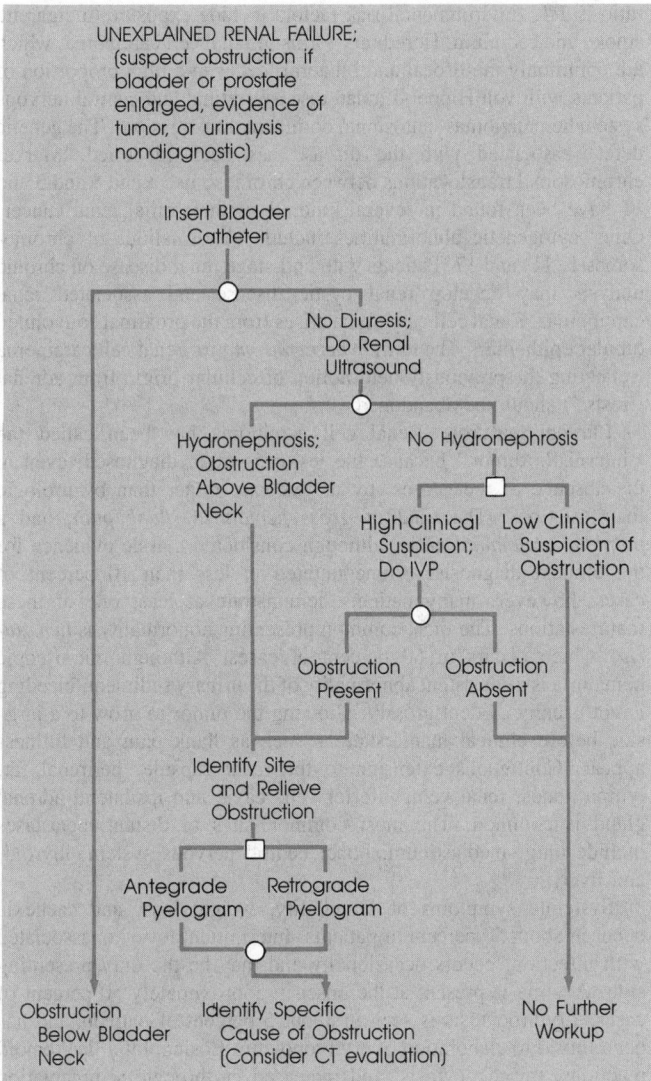

UNEXPLAINED RENAL FAILURE;
(suspect obstruction if
bladder or prostate
enlarged, evidence of
tumor, or urinalysis
nondiagnostic)

Insert Bladder
Catheter

No Diuresis;
Do Renal
Ultrasound

Hydronephrosis;
Obstruction
Above Bladder
Neck

No Hydronephrosis

High Clinical
Suspicion;
Do IVP

Low Clinical
Suspicion of
Obstruction

Obstruction
Present

Obstruction
Absent

Identify Site
and Relieve
Obstruction

Antegrade
Pyelogram

Retrograde
Pyelogram

Obstruction
Below Bladder
Neck

Identify Specific
Cause of Obstruction
(Consider CT evaluation)

No Further
Workup

FIGURE 246-1 Diagnostic approach for urinary tract obstruction in unexplained renal failure. Circles represent diagnostic procedures, and squares indicate clinical decisions based on available data. CT, computed tomography; IVP, intravenous pyelogram.

obstructive process is usually slightly enlarged, and there is dilatation of the calyces, renal pelvis, and ureter above the obstruction. The ureter, however, is not tortuous, as is the case when the obstruction is chronic. In comparison with the nephrogram, the pyelogram may be extremely faint, especially if the dilated renal pelvis is voluminous, causing dilution of the contrast medium. The radiographic study should be continued until the site of obstruction is determined or the contrast medium is excreted. Radionuclide scans define less anatomic detail than intravenous pyelography and, like the pyelogram, are of limited value when renal function is poor. Nonetheless, such scans are sensitive for the detection of obstruction and provide a substitute test in some patients at high risk for reaction to intravenous contrast dyes.

Patients suspected of having intermittent ureteropelvic obstruction (whether functional or mechanical) should have radiologic evaluation while they are in pain, since a normal pyelogram is commonly seen during asymptomatic periods. Hydration or mannitol infusion often helps to provoke a symptomatic attack. Voiding cystourethrography is of great value in the diagnosis of vesicoureteral reflux and bladder neck and urethral obstructions. Patients with obstruction at or below the level of the bladder exhibit thickening, trabeculation, and diverticula of the bladder wall. Postvoiding films reveal residual urine. If

these radiographic studies fail to provide adequate information for diagnosis, endoscopic visualization by the urologist often permits precise identification of lesions involving the urethra, prostate, bladder, and ureteral orifices. To facilitate visualization of a suspected lesion in a ureter or renal pelvis, *retrograde* or *antegrade pyelography* should be attempted. These diagnostic studies may be preferable to the intravenous pyelogram in the azotemic patient, in whom poor excretory function precludes adequate visualization of the collecting system. Furthermore, intravenous pyelography carries the risk of contrast-induced renal failure in patients with renal insufficiency, diabetes mellitus, and multiple myeloma, particularly when performed under conditions of dehydration. For these reasons, retrograde and antegrade pyelography may offer advantages over the intravenous approach in the diagnostic evaluation of the azotemic patient. The retrograde approach involves catheterization of the involved ureter under cystoscopic control, while the antegrade technique necessitates placement of a catheter into the renal pelvis via a needle inserted percutaneously under ultrasonic or fluoroscopic guidance. While the antegrade approach carries the added advantage of providing immediate decompression of a unilateral obstructing lesion, many urologists initially attempt the retrograde approach and resort to the antegrade method only when attempts at retrograde catheterization are unsuccessful or when cystoscopy or general anesthesia is contraindicated.

Computed tomography is useful in the diagnosis of specific intraabdominal and retroperitoneal causes of obstruction but is less practical as an initial test to establish the presence of obstruction. Magnetic resonance imaging also may be useful in the identification of specific obstructive causes.

TREATMENT AND PROGNOSIS An individual with any form of urinary tract obstruction complicated by infection requires relief of obstruction as soon as possible to prevent development of generalized sepsis and progressive renal damage. On a temporary basis, depending on the site of obstruction, drainage is often satisfactorily achieved by nephrostomy, ureterostomy, or ureteral, urethral, or suprapubic catheterization. The patient with acute urinary tract infection and obstruction should be given appropriate antibiotics based on in vitro bacterial sensitivity and ability of the drug to concentrate in the kidney and urine. Treatment may be required for 3 to 4 weeks. Chronic or recurrent infections in an obstructed kidney with poor intrinsic function may necessitate nephrectomy. When infection is not present, immediate surgery often is not required, even in the presence of complete obstruction and anuria (because of the availability of dialysis), at least until acid-base, fluid and electrolyte, and cardiovascular status are restored to normal. Nevertheless, the site of obstruction should be ascertained as soon as feasible, in part because of the possibility that sepsis may occur and necessitate prompt urologic intervention. Elective relief of obstruction is usually recommended in patients with urinary retention, recurrent urinary tract infections, persistent pain, or progressive loss of renal function. Infrequently, mechanical obstruction can be alleviated by nonsurgical means, as with radiation therapy for retroperitoneal lymphoma. Likewise, functional obstruction secondary to neurogenic bladder may be decreased with the combination of frequent voiding and cholinergic drugs. The approach to obstruction secondary to renal stones is discussed in Chap. 245.

With relief of obstruction, the *prognosis* regarding return of renal function depends largely on whether irreversible renal damage has occurred. When obstruction is not relieved, the course will depend mainly on whether the obstruction is complete or incomplete, bilateral or unilateral, and whether urinary tract infection is also present. Complete obstruction with infection can lead to total destruction of the kidney within days. In dogs, relief of complete obstruction of 1 and 2 weeks' duration restores glomerular filtration rate to 60 and 30 percent of normal, respectively; after 8 weeks of obstruction, recovery does not occur. Nevertheless, in the absence of definitive evidence of irreversibility, every effort should be made to decompress in the hope of restoring renal function at least partially.

In patients undergoing cystectomy for bladder cancer, the ileal conduit is the currently preferred urinary diversionary procedure. This approach is preferable to ureterosigmoidostomy, a procedure complicated by a high incidence of ureteral obstruction, reflux, hypokalemic metabolic acidosis, pyelonephritis, and neoplasms developing at the ureteral anastomotic site.

POSTOBSTRUCTIVE DIURESIS   Relief of bilateral, but not unilateral, complete urinary tract obstruction commonly leads to a postobstructive diuresis, characterized by polyuria, which may be massive. The urine is usually hypotonic and may contain a large amount of sodium chloride. The natriuresis is due, at least in part, to the excretion of retained urea, which acts as a poorly reabsorbable solute and diminishes salt and water reabsorption in the tubules (osmotic diuresis). The increase in intratubular pressure very likely also contributes to the impairment in net sodium chloride reabsorption, especially in the terminal nephron segments. Natriuretic factors (other than urea) also may accumulate during uremia induced by obstruction and depress salt and water reabsorption when urine flow is reestablished. In the majority of patients this diuresis is physiologic, resulting in the *appropriate* excretion of the excesses of salt and water retained during the period of obstruction. When extracellular volume and composition return to normal, the diuresis usually abates spontaneously. Therefore, replacement of urinary losses should serve only to prevent hypovolemia, hypotension, or disturbances in serum electrolyte concentrations. Occasionally, iatrogenic expansion of extracellular volume, secondary to administration of excessive quantities of intravenous fluids, is responsible for, or sustains, the diuresis observed in the postobstructive period. Replacement of no more than two-thirds of urinary volume losses per day is usually effective in avoiding this complication. In a rare patient, however, relief of obstruction may be followed by urinary salt and water losses severe enough to provoke profound dehydration and vascular collapse. In these patients, an intrinsic defect in tubule reabsorptive function is probably responsible for the marked diuresis. Appropriate therapy in such patients includes intravenous administration of large quantities of salt-containing solutions to replace sodium and volume deficits.

REFERENCES

GILLENWATER JY: The pathophysiology of urinary obstruction, in *Campbell's Urology*, 6th ed, PC Walsh et al (eds). Philadelphia, Saunders, 1992, pp 499–532

HARRIS RH, YARGER WE: The pathogenesis of post-obstructive diuresis. J Clin Invest 56:880, 1975

KAYE AD, POLLACK HM: Diagnostic imaging approach to the patient with obstructive uropathy. Semin Nephrol 2:55, 1982

WILSON DR: Renal function during and following obstruction. Ann Rev Med 28:329, 1977

————: Urinary tract obstruction, in *Diseases of the Kidney*, 4th ed, RW Schrier, SW Gottschalk (eds). Boston, Little, Brown, 1988, p 715

YARGER WE: Urinary tract obstruction, in *The Kidney*, 4th ed, BM Brenner, FC Rector Jr (eds). Philadelphia, Saunders, 1991, p 1768

247   TUMORS OF THE URINARY TRACT

MARC B. GARNICK / BARRY M. BRENNER

TUMORS OF THE KIDNEY

RENAL CELL CARCINOMA   Renal cell carcinoma (renal adenocarcinoma, formerly "hypernephroma") accounts for 85 percent of all primary renal neoplasms. Approximately 25,000 new cases are diagnosed annually, with 10,000 deaths in the United States. The peak age incidence is between 55 and 60 years; the male-to-female ratio is 2:1. Environmental risk factors include exposure to cigarette smoke and cadmium. Hereditary forms of renal cell carcinoma, which are commonly multifocal and bilateral, occur in a high proportion of patients with von Hippel–Lindau disease (retinal and central nervous system hemangiomas, autosomal dominant transmission). The genetic defect associated with the disease has been identified. Marker chromosomal translocations between chromosomes 3 and 8 and 3 and 11 have been found in several kindreds with familial renal cancer. Other cytogenetic abnormalities include abnormalities of chromosomes 1, 11, and 17. Patients with end-stage renal disease on chronic dialysis may develop renal cystic disease and associated renal carcinomas. Renal cell carcinoma arises from the proximal convoluted tubular epithelium. The term *hypernephroma* for renal cell carcinoma (reflecting the previously held notion of cellular origin from adrenal "rests") should be abandoned.

Clinical features   Renal cell carcinoma has been called the "internist's tumor" because the lesion is often diagnosed, even in the absence of metastases, by its *systemic* rather than by urologic manifestations. The triad of *gross hematuria, flank pain*, and a *palpable abdominal mass*, although considered classic evidence for the clinical diagnosis, is encountered in less than 10 percent of cases; however, many patients demonstrate at least one of these manifestations. The most common presenting abnormality is *hematuria*, which occurs in 60 percent of cases. Although microscopic hematuria is a consistent abnormality of the urinary sediment, bleeding is not usually evident grossly, allowing the tumor to grow to a large size before clinical manifestations such as flank pain and fullness appear. Contiguous extension to the renal capsule, perirenal fat, lymph nodes, renal vein, inferior vena cava, and ipsilateral adrenal gland is common. The most common sites of distant metastases include lung, mediastinum, bone, central nervous system, thyroid, and liver.

Systemic symptoms of fatigability, weight loss, and cachexia occur in about 50 percent of patients. Intermittent fever, unassociated with infection, occurs occasionally and may be the only presenting sign. Anemia is present at the onset in approximately 50 percent of cases. Erythrocytosis is seen in about 5 percent of patients and has been linked to elaboration of erythropoietin. Eosinophilia, leukemoid reactions, thrombocytosis, and increased erythrocyte sedimentation rate also occur. Renal cell carcinomas may produce hormones or hormone-like substances, including parathyroid hormone and prostaglandins (which may lead to hypercalcemia), prolactin (galactorrhea), renin (hypertension), gonadotropins (feminization and masculinization), and glucocorticoids (Cushing's syndrome). In vascular tumors, intrarenal arteriovenous fistulas may predispose to high-output congestive heart failure. Tumor invasion of the renal vein and inferior vena cava may result in the development of abrupt, symptomatic left varicocele and lower extremity edema, respectively. Hepatic vein occlusion by tumor, with or without vena caval obstruction, may lead to hepatosplenomegaly and ascites. Disturbances in liver function (elevated alkaline phosphatase, hypoalbuminemia, and prolonged prothrombin time) are sometimes found in patients without demonstrable liver metastases and are often reversed following removal of the primary tumor.

Diagnosis (Fig. 247-1)   Although intrarenal calcifications and/or alterations in renal contours on the abdominal scout film may suggest the presence of a renal cell carcinoma, *intravenous pyelography* (IVP) with *nephrotomography* is the primary examination by which most renal masses are detected and evaluated. The major task is to differentiate cystic lesions from renal neoplasms. Splaying, distortion, or nonvisualization of the collecting system and distorted renal outlines suggest cancer. Nephrotomography provides clear delineation of renal borders and further aids in distinguishing cystic from solid lesions. *Ultrasonography* has improved the ability to distinguish cysts from renal neoplasms. When combined with nephrotomography, the accuracy of ultrasonography in diagnosing a benign cyst approaches 97 percent. If a cystic lesion on IVP, combined with a benign-appearing sonolucent cystic lesion on ultrasound, is found in an asymptomatic

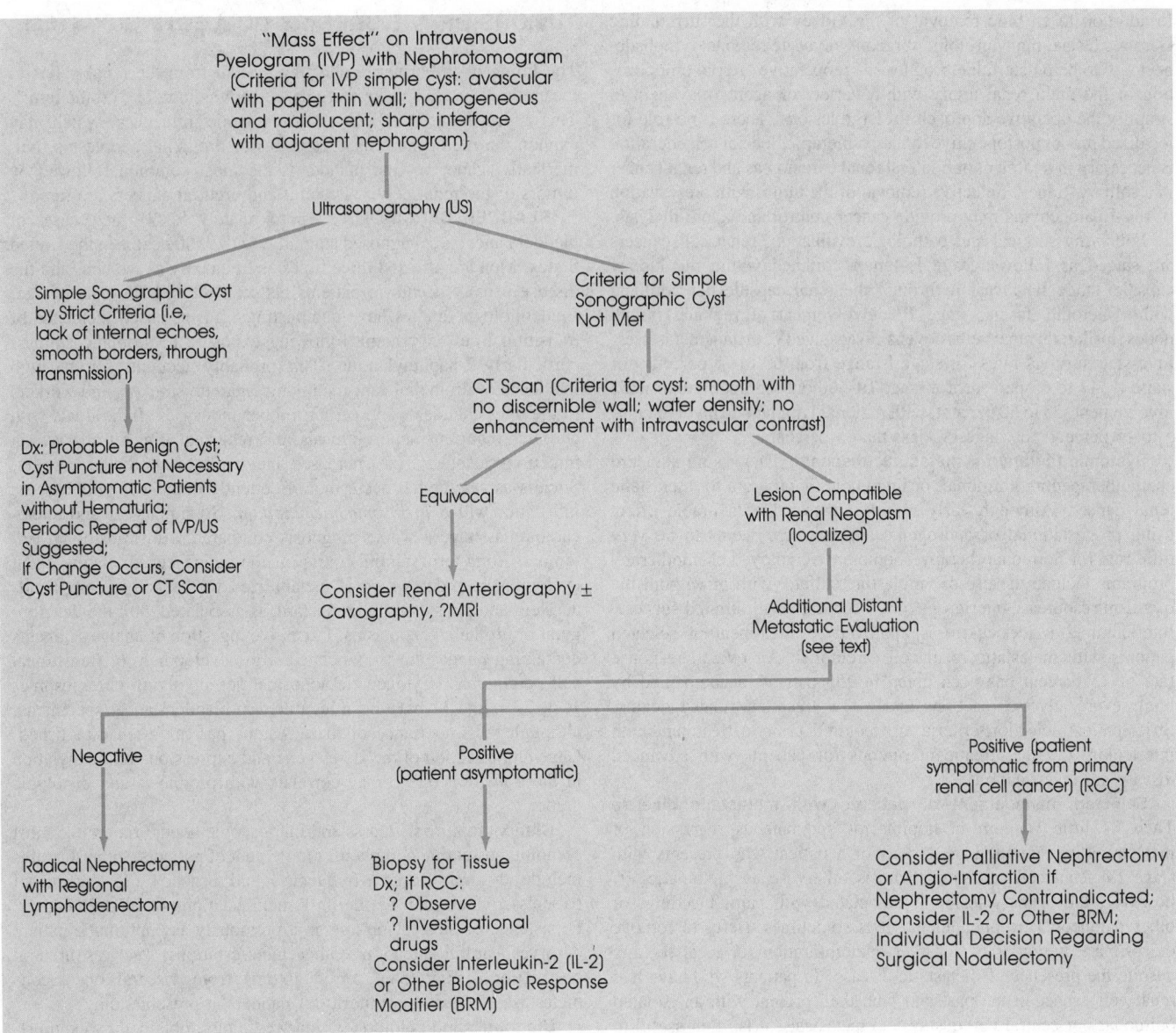

FIGURE 247-1 Diagnostic evaluation for renal mass.

patient without hematuria, cyst puncture is probably unnecessary. Repeat IVP or ultrasound should then be performed periodically, initially every year and then, if no change has occurred during the interval, less often.

If diagnostic accuracy beyond 97 percent is required, or if there are changes on repeat IVP or ultrasound, needle aspiration with evaluation of the aspirated fluid for cytology can be performed. The finding of clear yellow fluid or negative cytology usually supports the diagnosis of a simple cyst. Aspiration of cloudy or bloody fluid usually demands a surgical diagnosis, even though the cytology may be negative for cancer. A renal cystogram following aspiration can sometimes provide additional valuable information. Although renal cell carcinoma may coexist within a simple cyst, this is rare.

If the IVP or ultrasound examination demonstrates a lesion which does not satisfy the criteria for a benign, simple cyst, *computed tomography* (CT) is the next modality employed. CT is comparable and possibly superior to selective renal arteriography in both diagnosing and staging renal cell carcinoma. In addition, CT is equivalent to selective renal arteriography in the determination of renal vein involvement and superior to arteriography in determining whether regional nodes are enlarged (representing either tumor or hyperplasia) and/or the liver is involved. CT is the preferred modality for the diagnosis and staging of renal cell carcinoma. Thus selective renal

arteriography is not necessarily needed preoperatively. If, however, the findings on CT are equivocal or additional definition of vascular anatomy is required, renal arteriography should complement CT studies. Magnetic resonance imaging (MRI) also has been used extensively in the evaluation of renal masses. Its role compared to CT scanning is being defined; MRI may provide information for preoperative tumor staging, including nodal anatomy, perirenal fat involvement, adjacent organ extension, and renal vein involvement with thrombosis.

OTHER STUDIES   Evaluation of urinary cytology is not useful in the diagnosis of renal adenocarcinomas. Retrograde pyelography may be a useful adjunct for opacifying the collecting systems that are not filled by standard IVP and may suggest the diagnosis of transitional cell carcinoma of the renal pelvis. In patients who present with hematuria and a renal mass, cystoscopy is an important adjunct to exclude the coexistence of an unsuspected urothelial tumor, such as carcinoma of the bladder. If the diagnosis of renal cell carcinoma is likely, the patient should then undergo routine chest x-ray, bone scan, and liver function studies in addition to the abdominal CT to evaluate other potential sites of tumor spread.

Staging, primary treatment, and prognosis   If there is no evidence of metastatic disease following the preoperative evaluation, the treatment of choice for renal cell carcinoma is radical nephrectomy.

In addition to en bloc removal of the kidney with the surrounding Gerota's fascia, many urologic surgeons advocate regional lymphadenectomy to help determine prognosis. Preoperative arterial embolization of the main renal artery with a variety of agents may help to simplify the operative approach for large lesions. There is no role for localized pre- or postoperative radiation therapy. Special consideration is necessary in treatment of bilateral renal carcinomas and renal cancer in a solitary kidney. Selective removal of the tumor with preservation of renal parenchyma may provide cancer control and avoid dialysis.

Following surgical and pathologic evaluation, renal cell cancers are staged as follows: stage I, tumor confined within the kidney capsule; stage II, invasion through the renal capsule but confined within Gerota's fascia; stage III, involvement of regional lymph nodes, ipsilateral renal vein, or vena cava; stage IV, distant metastases. Five-year survival rates for stage I range from 60 to 75 percent; for stage II, 47 to 65 percent; for stage III without regional lymph node involvement, 25 to 50 percent; with regional lymph node involvement, 5 to 15 percent; for stage IV, less than 5 percent.

Systemic therapy for metastatic disease   There is no standard chemotherapeutic, hormonal, or immunologic program for metastatic renal cancer. Although early reports suggested a favorable effect using progestational or androgenic agents, there seems to be very little role for hormonal therapy. Commonly employed chemotherapy programs include the use of vinblastine sulfate, with or without the use of nitrosoureas. Interferons have been used with limited success. Interleukin 2 (Aldesleukin) is approved for treatment of selected patients with metastatic renal cell carcinoma. An overall response rate of 15 percent has been noted in 255 patients accompanied by both severe adverse reactions and a few treatment-related deaths. Strict patient selection criteria are required prior to treatment with interleukin 2. Other treatment options for patients with advanced disease are investigational.

Selected management of patients with metastatic disease   There is little wisdom in hoping for spontaneous regression of metastases by removing the kidney of a patient who presents with stage IV renal cell carcinoma who is otherwise asymptomatic. If, however, the primary lesion is associated with pain, bleeding, or other paraneoplastic phenomena, it is sometimes useful to remove the primary tumor or to consider angioinfarction for local therapy despite the presence of metastatic disease. In patients who have had renal cell cancer in the past and who then present with an isolated pulmonary or central nervous system metastasis, it is often useful to resect these metastases. Generally, patients selected for surgical nodulectomy have been disease-free for at least 1 year from the original diagnosis to the time of metastatic development and have tumors with a slow doubling time. On occasion, radiation therapy may offer palliation for painful bony lesions and may relieve an obstructed bronchus or ureter.

MISCELLANEOUS TUMORS OF THE KIDNEY   In children, Wilms' tumor (nephroblastoma) is the most common cancer of the kidney. These tumors respond well to multimodality therapy, including surgery, radiation, and combination chemotherapy, usually with dactinomycin and vincristine. Metastatic lesions to the kidney occur commonly in patients with lung and breast cancer and melanoma. Kidney involvement with malignant lymphoma, too, is common; however, functional renal abnormalities from parenchymal involvement are unusual.

Benign renal tumors are usually recognized as incidental findings at autopsy. CT scanning may suggest the presence of an angiomyolipoma, especially in patients with tuberous sclerosis. Surgery should always be considered when radiographic studies are equivocal. In addition, on occasion, benign lesions can cause persistent hematuria and, like the renal oncocytoma, can undergo malignant degeneration. These lesions are usually managed with nephrectomy when detected clinically. In newborns and infants, mesoblastic nephroma (fetal hamartoma) is the most common benign tumor and is successfully treated by simple nephrectomy.

TUMORS OF THE URINARY COLLECTING SYSTEM

The lining of the urinary collecting system from the renal pelvis to the urethra is made up of transitional cell epithelium, or "urothelium." This entire lining is subject to carcinogenic influences, which may explain the multicentric characteristics of urothelial neoplasms. Numerically, cancer of the bladder is the most common followed by tumors of the renal pelvis. Ureteral and urethral cancers are rare.

BLADDER CARCINOMA   Approximately 51,600 new cases of bladder cancer are diagnosed annually, with 9500 deaths in the United States. Men are affected three times as frequently as women, and the disease usually occurs in patients between 60 and 70 years of age. Epidemiologic studies have demonstrated an increased incidence of transitional cell carcinoma following exposure to aromatic amines, particularly 2-naphthylamine. This probably accounts for the high incidence of urothelial cancers among cigarette smokers and workers in the dye, chemical, and certain rubber industries. Individuals with chronic, recurrent nephrolithiasis and recurrent upper urinary tract infections also have an increased incidence of urothelial cancers. Squamous carcinomas occur more frequently in patients with chronic infestation with *Schistosoma haematobium*. Squamous cell and adenocarcinomas have a worse prognosis compared with transitional cell tumors. Long-term administration of the anticancer alkylating agent cyclophosphamide, which is metabolized to the active compounds acrolein and phosphoramide mustard, is associated with the development of urothelial neoplasms. Excessive ingestion of analgesic agents containing phenacetin is associated with development of transitional cell carcinomas. Cytogenetic abnormalities involving chromosomes 1, 5, 7, 9, and 11 have been identified in bladder cancer specimens, although the importance of these lesions has not been established. Gene amplification of the H-*ras* gene and expression and methylation in the c-*myc* oncogene may correlate with prognosis and histologic grade.

Clinical features   Gross and microscopic hematuria are the most common presenting complaints (75 percent of patients); other features include dysuria, urinary frequency, and urgency (25 percent of patients), which may be the only manifestations of bladder cancer. Persistence of these symptoms in a previously asymptomatic patient deserves careful attention. Other manifestations, such as ureteral obstruction, pelvic pain, or symptoms from visceral or osseous metastases, occur in a minority of patients at presentation.

Diagnosis and staging   Urinary cytology, obtained by examination of bladder washing, catheterized urine or voided urine, IVP, and cystoscopic evaluation with tumor biopsies and selected mucosal biopsies, as well as bimanual examination under anesthesia, are the mainstays for diagnosis of bladder cancer. Findings on IVP that suggest a bladder carcinoma include unilateral or bilateral ureteral obstruction with hydronephrosis, filling defect, or lack of distensibility of the bladder. Additional staging information may be obtained with abdominal or pelvic CT scanning. Following endoscopic resection of a bladder neoplasm, the depth of penetration into the bladder wall is assessed. If additional staging procedures, including physical examination, chest x-ray, and routine serum chemistries, are within normal limits, the patient is clinically staged, based on the cystoscopic biopsy, as having either *superficial* or *invasive* disease. Additional information about perivesical extension or nodal metastases can be obtained at the time of cystectomy and indicates the true pathologic stage of disease. A substantial number of patients who are clinically staged endoscopically as having muscle-invasive disease will have occult lymphatic or distant metastases if surgically staged at the time of cystectomy. Such occult micrometastatic disease indicates systemic involvement and accounts for the high percentage of patients who eventually develop distant metastatic disease despite treatment of the primary bladder lesion.

Treatment   Bladder cancer can be subdivided conceptually as being *superficial*, *invasive*, or *metastatic*. *Superficial carcinoma* of the bladder includes patients with carcinoma in situ, mucosal involvement (stage 0), or submucosal involvement (stage A). These patients are generally treated with endoscopic resection and selected bladder biopsies with repeat cystoscopic evaluations every 3 to 6 months. Approximately 50 to 70 percent of these patients have a superficial recurrence (limited to the mucosa or submucosa) within a period of 3 years following initial diagnosis. Patients with superficial recurrences are then often treated with intravesical therapies, including thiotepa, doxorubicin, mitomycin, bacillus Calmette-Guérin (BCG), or interferons, in addition to cystoscopic resection. BCG is most effective in treating carcinoma in situ of the urinary bladder. Other modalities include laser therapy applied directly to superficial lesions and photodynamic therapies in which hematoporphyrin derivatives, administered intravesically, can help localize superficial carcinomas. The use of intravesical therapy in selected instances may decrease the number of superficial recurrences and prolong relapse-free intervals.

An additional 12 percent with initial superficial disease eventually develop progressive disease into the bladder muscularis (stage B) and perivesical fat (stage C) or metastatic disease to lymph nodes (stage D1), bone, or other viscera (stage D2). Alternatively, patients may present initially with invasive or metastatic disease.

INVASIVE DISEASE These patients generally have extension of tumor into the muscle and/or perivesical fat. Traditional treatments are cystectomy (radical or simple) or radiation therapy. Preoperative radiation therapy followed by cystectomy does not provide survival benefit as compared with cystectomy alone. Five-year survival rates are approximately 50 percent with such treatments. The majority of these patients die of distant metastatic disease despite radical surgery or radiation rather than from local recurrences. In addition, the use of multimodality therapy, including chemotherapy with radiation therapy, may spare individuals with invasive disease radical cystectomy. Surgical techniques, utilizing portions of the small bowel as bladder reservoirs, have enhanced the quality of life in individuals undergoing radical cystectomy. Such procedures allow continent urinary diversion (e.g., Koch pouch, Indiana pouch, or Mainz pouch), thus eliminating the need for an external ostomy appliance. Many clinical studies today utilize systemic chemotherapy prior to definitive surgery or radiation therapy in attempts to ''control'' suspected systemic micrometastatic disease, as well as to improve control of the primary lesion. Preliminary data are encouraging.

METASTATIC DISEASE For patients who have distant metastatic disease in lymph nodes, viscera, or bone, the use of systemic chemotherapy has produced responses from 30 to 70 percent of patients but usually not lasting more than 6 months. Following the development of metastatic disease, most patients die within 2 years. The most active agents include cisplatin, methotrexate, doxorubicin, cyclophosphamide, and vinblastine, and combinations of these agents have on occasion produced meaningful and durable remissions. Myelosuppression, a common toxicity of chemotherapy programs, can be ameliorated with concurrent administration of erythropoietin.

TRANSITIONAL CELL CANCER OF THE RENAL PELVIS Renal pelvic tumors account for approximately 10 percent of all primary renal cancer. Nearly 90 percent are transitional cell carcinomas. In addition to the etiologic associations implicated for bladder carcinoma, renal pelvic tumors also occur with analgesic abuse nephropathy. These patients are usually middle-aged women with a psychiatric history or chronic headaches who ingest >3 kg of analgesics over years.

Most patients present with painless gross hematuria. Ureteral obstruction and pain secondary to clots are unusual. The diagnosis is suggested by IVP, which may demonstrate an obstructed, poorly functioning, or nonvisualized kidney or filling defects in a visualized kidney, and a positive urinary cytology. Cystoscopy and retrograde pyelography with brush biopsy generally establish the nature and location of the renal pelvic or ureteral tumor. For low-grade, low-stage tumors, conservative treatment with local excision and preservation of the kidney parenchyma is associated with favorable 5-year survival rates. For high-stage, high-grade lesions, the treatment of choice is radical nephroureterectomy and removal of the cuff of the bladder containing the ipsilateral ureteral orifice. This operative approach is dictated by the high likelihood of recurrence in the ureteral stump and orifice if not removed. In addition, routine follow-up with cystoscopies and urinary cytologies are mandatory to help detect the subsequent development of metachronous bladder carcinomas and/or contralateral ureteral and renal pelvic tumors. Five-year survival rates range from 10 to 50 percent. Although chemotherapy programs employed for bladder cancer have been used for patients with metastatic transitional cell carcinoma of the renal pelvis, the overall results are not as successful.

REFERENCES

BRODSKY G, GARNICK MG: Renal tumors in the adult patient, in *Renal Pathology*, CC Tisher, BM Brenner (eds). Philadelphia, Lippincott, 1989, p 1467

CHISHOLM GD, ROY RR: The systemic effects of malignant renal tumors. Br J Urol 43:687, 1971

CRONAN J, ZEMAN RK: Renal mass imaging: The internist's role. Am J Med 81:1026, 1986

CRONIN RE et al: Renal cell carcinoma: Unusual systemic manifestations. Medicine 55:291, 1976

GARNICK MB (ed): Genitourinary cancer, in *Contemporary Issues in Clinical Oncology*, vol 5. New York, Churchill Livingstone, 1985

HRICAK H: Detection and staging of renal neoplasms: A reassessment of MR imaging. Radiology 166:643, 1988

KALISH LA et al: A determination of appropriate endpoints in assessing efficacy of intravesical therapies in superficial bladder cancer. J Clin Oncol 5:2004, 1987

RAGHAVAN D et al: Biology and management of bladder cancer. N Engl J Med 322:1129, 1990

RIESELBACH RE, GARNICK MB (eds): *Cancer and the Kidney*. Philadelphia, Lea & Febiger, 1982

SAROSKY MF, LAMM DL: Long-term results of intravesical BCG therapy for superficial bladder cancer. J Urol 142:719, 1989

SEE WA, WILLIAMS RD: Tumors of the kidney, ureter and bladder. West J Med 156:523, 1992

STERNBERG CN et al: M-VAC (methotrexate, vinblastine, doxorubicin, and cisplatin) for advanced transitional cell carcinoma of urothelium. J Urol 139:461, 1988

WEST WH et al: Constant infusion recombinant interleukin-2 in adoptive immunotherapy of advanced cancer. N Engl J Med 316:898, 1987

section 1 Disorders of the alimentary tract

248 APPROACH TO THE PATIENT WITH GASTROINTESTINAL DISEASE

KURT J. ISSELBACHER / DANIEL K. PODOLSKY

BIOLOGIC CONSIDERATIONS The mucosal surface of the gastrointestinal tract is composed of a remarkably dynamic population of epithelial cells that are highly developed in their capacity for transmembrane absorption and secretion. These secretory and absorptive abilities facilitate the essential function of the digestive tract in digestion and nutrient uptake, which must be accomplished while maintaining the barrier between the host and potentially harmful pathogens and mutagens in the lumen. The latter is accomplished through both the physical integrity of the intact mucosal surface and the extensive population of resident immune cells.

The intestinal surface itself also contains the distinctive M cells that serve to sample the antigenic milieu of the lumen. The predominance of suppressor lymphocytes within the surface epithelial layer (intraepithelial lymphocytes) suggests that dampening of the body's response to the enormous number of potentially antigenic substances in the lumen is necessary to prevent the constant and unrestrained activation of immune and inflammatory processes. Conversely, the presence of large numbers of helper lymphocytes as well as other cellular effectors of immune response in the lamina propria and submucosa attests to a large armamentarium ready to respond when surface defenses have been breached. No doubt the concentration of so many immune cells capable of attracting and activating inflammatory cells predisposes to the numerous inflammatory conditions to which the gastrointestinal tract is subject.

The mucosal surface of the gastrointestinal tract is also remarkable for the very rapid turnover of the epithelial cell population. It is likely that the epithelium turns over in its entirety every 24 to 72 h. This may permit rapid restitution of a functional cell population following an acute insult and may reduce the risk of malignancy through loss of cells affected by the many potential and actual mutagens in the luminal contents. Nevertheless, this proliferative potential must inherently create the setting for neoplastic disorders, which are so common to the gastrointestinal tract. Another fundamental feature of gastrointestinal mucosa is the spatial segregation of the proliferative compartment from the terminally differentiated cells. This is true throughout the gastrointestinal tract but is most apparent in the small intestine where a gradient of differentiation exists from the depths of the crypts of Lieberkühn to the villus tip. This organization is important in understanding the histology and pathophysiology of many mucosal disorders, e.g., nontropical sprue.

In view of the important secretory and absorptive activities of mucosal surface, diseases of the gastrointestinal tract may result in clinical consequences secondary to the physical disruption of the mucosal layer (e.g., blood loss, fluid loss, pathogenic invasion) or nutritional derangements due to impaired digestion and nutrient absorption. In focal or localized disease processes the former predominate, whereas the latter may be especially prominent in disorders that affect extensive areas of the gastrointestinal tract in a diffuse manner.

While the essential role of the gastrointestinal tract is the absorption of nutrients and excretion of the products is in large part accomplished at the luminal surface, these processes are also dependent on the deeper muscular layers for the coordinated propulsion of food through the lumen. The complexity of both local and distant neural and endocrine factors that contribute to the regulation of intestinal motility is only now becoming fully appreciated. Disruption of normal motility is quite common, with functional bowel complaints affecting as many as 15 percent of adults. Alterations in frequency of bowel movements, abdominal distention, abdominal pain, and nausea, individually or in varying combinations, may result from dysmotility. In addition, structural lesions may also indirectly lead to symptoms through their impact on motility involving some or all regions of the gastrointestinal tract. These range from the *direct* effects of an obstructing lesion to the *indirect* actions of substances released by a primary mucosal disorder (e.g., inflammatory mediators such as arachidonic acid metabolites that also affect smooth-muscle activity).

Although valid unifying generalizations can be made about the gastrointestinal tract in its entirety, the spectrum of diseases affecting this system and their clinical manifestations are significantly related to the constituent organ(s) involved. Thus, esophageal disorders predominantly manifest through their relationship to swallowing, while gastric disorders are dominated by features relating to acid secretion, and disease of the small and large intestine by disruption of nutrition and alterations of bowel movements. Similarly, diseases of the related ancillary organs, the exocrine pancreas and the hepatobiliary system, present characteristic clinical challenges. Finally, it should be remembered that in addition to intrinsic disease, the gastrointestinal tract may be affected by systemic disorders. These include vascular, inflammatory, infectious, and neoplastic conditions leading to focal or diffuse structural lesions. Metabolic and endocrine abnormalities as well as drugs can disrupt normal bowel motility.

CLINICAL CONSIDERATIONS **History** A thorough clinical history is almost uniformly reliable in directing the clinician's attention to appropriate diagnostic considerations in the patient with gastrointestinal symptoms. The most common complaints resulting from disorders involving the gastrointestinal tract include pain, and alteration in bowel habit, especially diarrhea and constipation. Among these, *abdominal pain* is the most frequent and variable and may reflect a broad spectrum of problems from the least threatening to the most urgent. In conjunction with an estimation of its intensity, initial distinction should be made between pain of acute onset and more chronic discomfort. Pain of abrupt onset is often encountered in serious illness requiring urgent intervention, while a history of chronic discomfort may typically be related to an indolent disorder. However, change in the pattern or character of pain may be equally important, signifying progression of a problem of initial mild onset (either recent or chronic) to a more critical stage. Ascertaining the location (upper or lower, localized or diffuse), character (sharp, burning, cramping), and relationship of the pain to meals will often provide significant insight into the most important diagnostic considerations. If eating produces the symptom, the clinician should determine whether the discomfort occurs while eating (as in esophageal disorders and abdominal angina), shortly after the meal (as often occurs in biliary tract disease), or 30 to 90 min later (as typically seen in peptic disease). Pain that is not affected by eating suggests a process outside of the bowel lumen, such as an abscess, peritonitis, pancreatitis, and some malignancies. Conversely, identification of factors that relieve the symptom is also helpful, e.g., relief with eating or antacids is characteristic of peptic ulcer disease or gastritis. Relationship of the discomfort to bowel movement, especially in association with an altered bowel habit, should focus attention on a disorder of the small or large bowel such as inflammatory bowel disease.

Alterations in bowel habit can result from either disruption of normal intestinal motility or significant structural pathology. A thorough determination of the temporal evolution of the change and the nature of the alteration in conjunction with other constitutional symptoms such as weight loss, fever, or anorexia is important. Temporary variation in bowel habit in association with some life stress and in the absence of signs of systemic illness is suggestive of the common "irritable bowel syndrome," especially when the alteration varies between diarrhea and constipation. Small pellet-like stools are often described by the patient. Associated symptoms of bloating, nausea, and "gas" are also common. This diagnosis can essentially be made on the basis of a thorough history and physical examination and very limited laboratory testing, which exclude structural disease. In contrast, the onset of worsening constipation in an adult with previously regular habits, especially when accompanied by systemic symptoms such as weight loss, suggests the possible presence of an underlying obstructing process, particularly malignancy. If diarrhea is present, one should determine the average number of stools, their consistency, their pattern, and if any blood is present. Although *diarrhea* refers to an increased frequency of movements, patients will often use the term to describe loose or watery stools primarily. The occurrence of nocturnal or true bloody diarrhea almost always reflects structural rather than functional bowel disease. A pungent odor or the presence of undigested meat in the movement are suggestive of pancreatic insufficiency. An alteration in color can be seen in cholestasis or steatorrhea (light-colored) or hemorrhage (melenic to maroon or bright red). Mucus in the movement is usually a sign of functional bowel syndrome, while pus is more strongly suggestive of infectious or inflammatory disease. Less common but more dramatic are the symptoms of acute gastrointestinal bleeding, including hematemesis, melena, and hematochezia, which usually leads to prompt efforts to find medical attention but should always be solicited by the clinician.

In the evaluation of male patients, especially those with diarrhea, a tactful inquiry into sexual activity is essential. Homosexual males are at increased risk for a large variety of gastrointestinal disorders as well as AIDS, which may first manifest itself with gastrointestinal symptoms. Finally, careful attention must be given to a general medical history with an emphasis on any medications or nonprescription drugs that may have been used. Thyroid and other metabolic disorders, especially those affecting calcium metabolism, can cause a variety of gastrointestinal symptoms. Unless asked, patients may forget to mention that they take aspirin almost daily for headache, and this may account for occult blood found in the stool. The use of daily laxatives may explain chronic diarrhea.

Physical examination, endoscopy, and radiology All of the cardinal methods of examination are helpful in evaluating the patient with gastrointestinal symptoms. *Inspection* may disclose signs of cholestasis or nutritional deficiencies. An abnormal contour of the abdomen or inspection of the perianal region may manifest signs of a mass or a draining fistula. *Auscultation* is also important. A succussion splash can be elicited in the patients with symptoms of gastric outlet obstruction. The absence of bowel sounds or alteration in pitch can lead to recognition of an evolving ileus or an obstructing process. A bruit may also be appreciated where there are symptoms of ischemic bowel disease. Careful *palpation* of the abdomen is especially important in detecting tenderness and masses, which in the appropriate clinical setting will lead to the recognition of cholecystitis, regional enteritis, periappendiceal abscess, and many other disorders. Findings on abdominal palpation will often be complemented by *percussion*, which is essential to assessing liver and spleen size.

Elicitation of rebound tenderness, either direct or referred, after removal of the examining hand provides an important clue to localized or more generalized peritonitis characteristic of many abdominal emergencies, including a perforated viscus, intraabdominal abscess, or tissue infarction. The clinician should be particularly alert to these signs in patients with severe pain of abrupt onset. Typically, the patient will remain immobile to avoid the accentuation of pain that may follow even slight movement and jarring of the abdomen. This contrasts with the sometimes frantic efforts to find a position of comfort in patients with severe pain deriving from visceral disease, e.g., pancreatitis or intestinal ischemia. In these disorders, the absence of findings on palpation of the abdomen may be in striking contrast to the evident distress of the patient. Only with progression of the process to tissue destruction (e.g., necrotizing pancreatitis or intestinal infarction) and secondary peritonitis will the abdominal examination prove remarkable, often in concert with striking signs of systemic illness including hemodynamic instability. In addition to the examination of the abdomen, a carefully performed digital rectal examination is also essential. In the patient with complaints of incontinence the integrity of the sphincter can be assessed. Most importantly, masses intrinsic to the rectum as well as abnormalities in the pelvis or the pouch of Douglas may only be detected by this examination, and the presence or absence of frank or occult blood in the stool is always important diagnostic information. Sigmoidoscopy should be viewed as a routine extension of the physical examination in the patient with diarrhea or other alteration in bowel habit as well as in the patient with known or suspected blood loss from the lower bowel. This procedure, which can be performed with either the rigid sigmoidoscope or a flexible fiberoptic instrument, allows for direct inspection of the rectosigmoid mucosa permitting detection of cancers and polyps in this segment that may well be missed by barium x-rays. Inflammatory changes of the mucosa can help identify the patient with infectious dysentery or other forms of colitis, most notably ulcerative colitis. The findings of edema, granularity, and diffuse friability (easily induced mucosal bleeding) as well as superficial ulcerations are characteristic in the latter disorder. Fresh stool samples for microbiologic studies and superficial mucosal biopsies obtained at the time of sigmoidoscopy can also yield crucial diagnostic information.

Definitive demonstration or exclusion of structural lesions of the gastrointestinal tract, particularly the great majority of disorders that primarily affect mucosal surface, can often not be accomplished by physical examination alone. Many disorders of the upper or lower gastrointestinal tract are accessible to inspection through fiberoptic instruments. As a result, endoscopic studies are supplanting conventional contrast x-ray studies for many clinical problems, both because of the heightened precision of these diagnostic tools and the opportunity in many instances to accomplish a meaningful therapeutic intervention as an adjunct to the acquisition of diagnostic information. However, it should be emphasized that *no procedure should be considered routine* and used indiscriminately; there must be a rational basis for its use in the individual patient. These techniques are discussed in detail in Chap. 250. Upper gastrointestinal endoscopy permits evaluation of the esophagus, stomach, and duodenum and, with specially designed instruments, the proximal jejunum. When the clinical history warrants a diagnostic examination of the upper gastrointestinal tract for a structural lesion, endoscopic examination is preferable to radiologic study in most patients when the choice is available. Side-viewing scopes permit inspection and cannulation of the ampulla of Vater facilitating retrograde cholangiopancreatography. The colonoscope can be used to visualize the entire colon and often the terminal ileum, resulting in more accurate diagnosis of inflammatory bowel disease and mass lesions. Frequently colonic polyps can be removed at the time of initial colonoscopic identification.

Endoscopic techniques are relatively precise in defining many problems, but the limitations of these tools as well as the continued advantages of x-ray studies in some situations should be recognized. Endoscopic tools are not useful in assessing gastrointestinal (GI) motility, which may be more accurately gauged by barium studies. In addition, some areas, notably the small intestine, remain relatively inaccessible to fiberoptic instruments. In hospitals where endoscopy is not feasible, the upper GI series and barium enema remain good diagnostic modalities for the upper and lower GI tract especially when air-contrast techniques are employed. However, they should generally be avoided in the patient with GI bleeding or suspected bowel obstruction. In addition the physician must exercise judgment in preparing the patient for these studies, recognizing that cathartics may markedly worsen the condition of a patient with obstructing lesions or colitis.

Although endoscopy has obviated the need for many conventional GI x-rays, other radiologic imaging modalities have assumed a crucial role in the approach to the patient with gastrointestinal symptoms. These techniques include ultrasound (US), computed tomography (CT), and magnetic resonance imaging (MRI). The application of these tools to the liver and biliary tract is discussed in Chap. 262. Both US and CT are useful in the delineation of abdominal masses. CT, though more expensive, is often more effective in the evaluation of the lower abdomen, where inflammatory masses in patients with Crohn's disease or complications of diverticular disease may be accurately imaged. However, US is an effective and generally less expensive tool for the evaluation of the right upper quadrant including the gall bladder and biliary tract. These techniques are often complementary in the evaluation of pancreatic disease. In combination with Doppler analysis, US can be used to assess the patency and direction of blood flow in the portal vein in the patient with advanced liver disease. MRI may permit exquisitely accurate information on the anatomic extent of invasive rectal cancers and blood flow in patients with vascular disorders, but the full range of its uses in GI disorders remains to be delineated. More-sophisticated CT and MRI equipment can actually permit the performance of digital angiography without the invasive catheterization necessary in conventional visceral angiography.

Finally, one must emphasize that the optimal use of endoscopic and radiologic imaging techniques also depends on the recognition that each modality has inherent limitations. Only the clinician can determine whether the information is sufficient to establish or exclude a diagnosis in a patient with relevant historical and/or physical findings and a negative or nondiagnostic study. Was the preparation of the patient or the examination of sufficient quality to have detected an abnormality if present? Was the examiner aware of the important diagnostic considerations, and was the study adapted to address those concerns? Conversely only the physician can determine whether irregularities found in diagnostic studies are indeed causally related to the patient's symptoms. This judgment usually relies upon a sound understanding of the biologic basis of gastrointestinal disorders.

DIAGNOSTIC APPROACHES   Abdominal pain   Determination of the cause of abdominal pain remains an imposing clinical challenge. As noted above, a spectrum of disorders from the acute and catastrophic to the chronic and indolent causes abdominal pain. Furthermore, differential diagnostic considerations may encompass diseases extrinsic to the gastrointestinal tract per se including disorders of the genitourinary tract (e.g., pelvic inflammatory disease) and the peritoneum as well as alterations of the various constituents of the GI tract. The history and physical examination are essential guides to a sensible diagnostic approach to the broad potential array of disorders causing abdominal pain. The primary goal to be achieved through initial approaches to the patient is the distinction between an urgent problem requiring expeditious delineation and nonacute disorders. In the former, initial clinical impressions based on the history and physical examination can be further refined through routine laboratory tests such as a complete blood test and differential as well as plain films of the abdomen. Particular features will dictate the appropriateness of urgent US or CT examination or the need to proceed directly with emergency exploratory laparotomy. In the patient with a longstanding and relatively stable problem, diagnostic evaluation is undertaken in a more considered time frame. The clinician may be able to reasonably establish a functional basis for the complaint on the strength of the history and physical examination alone. Radiologic contrast studies, other imaging modalities (e.g., US, CT), or endoscopic examination may be appropriate to exclude or identify the gamut of disorders discussed above. If all these approaches prove inadequate to determine the cause of the patient's symptoms, more unusual causes of abdominal pain may have to be excluded through specific urine or blood tests (e.g., porphyrins).

Problems of swallowing   The approach should be as follows:

1 Thorough determination of the nature of dysphagia. Is the difficulty primarily in swallowing liquids, solids, or both? The location of the difficulty from the patient's perspective and presence or absence of accompanying odynophagia are important to ascertain. These historical clues are complemented by careful visual and neurologic examination of the oropharynx when appropriate.

2 Routine esophageal x-rays in the upright and lateral or Trendelenburg position. The horizontal views are essential for demonstration of the swallowing mechanism, unaided by gravity, and of the esophagogastric junction. For details of the pharyngoesophageal area cineradiography is necessary because of the rapidity with which the contrast medium passes through. Hiatus hernia is extremely common (in 15 to 35 percent of persons over 50) and often asymptomatic unless spontaneous reflux of gastric contents can be demonstrated to occur repeatedly. Careful attention is usually needed to detect lower esophageal rings or webs, which may be visible as indentations in the barium column only from a limited angle.

3 Esophagoscopy. This procedure is desirable to describe lesions suggested by x-ray or, if the lesion is unsuspected, to obtain biopsies from masses or abnormal mucosa and to obtain washings for exfoliative cytologic study. The diagnoses of peptic esophagitis and Barrett's esophagus are made endoscopically. Endoscopy is the most sensitive technique for identifying esophageal or gastric varices, although they are seldom important in the absence of hemorrhage. Fiberoptic instruments with US probes at their tip may ultimately become established as the most useful diagnostic tools for particular problems of the esophagus (and other sites of the GI tract), but instruments remain costly and continue to undergo significant technological evolution so that the ultimate role of so-called endosonography remains uncertain.

4 Manometric studies of the upper esophagus, particularly in conjunction with cineradiography. At present, this procedure offers the best differential between disorders primarily in the central nervous system, primary pharyngeal muscular disease, and cricopharyngeal dystonia. Manometry of the lower esophagus is useful in the diagnosis of diffuse esophageal spasm, achalasia, and infiltrative diseases that can alter esophageal motility.

Peptic or digestive disorders   The approaches to these disorders include:

1 Insertion of a nasogastric tube. This is used to establish whether significant gastric retention (more than 75 mL of gastric contents in the fasting state) exists and whether there is acid, bile, blood, or other material in these contents. If pyloric obstruction or gastric atony is present, the tube is used to maintain suction while the patient's electrolyte and fluid balance is restored to normal; the stomach is kept as clean as possible so that reliable diagnostic investigation may be carried out.

2 *Upper intestinal endoscopy.* This procedure is most helpful in identifying the diffuse mucosa in gastritis or, together with biopsy and brushings for cytology, in differentiating between peptic and neoplastic ulcerating lesions. It may identify a specific bleeding site in clinical situations where several potential bleeding sites could exist, such as in the patient with portal hypertension. In addition, it may be possible to cauterize or otherwise intervene to control hemorrhage with the endoscope (e.g., injections of vasoconstricting agents such as epinephrine). The frequent association of gastritis with *Helicobacter pylori* in patients with nonulcer dyspepsia, as well as in those with actual peptic ulceration, has been well documented, even if its true role in the pathogenesis of these disorders remains uncertain. Nevertheless, at this time, *H. pylori* infection can be most reliably documented in the individual patient by endoscopy and biopsy. Endoscopy can detect a number of potential sources of upper GI bleeding which are often missed by x-ray studies (e.g., erosive gastritis, Mallory-Weiss syndrome). Gastroscopy is particularly helpful in inspecting the postoperative stomach, especially in detecting stomal ulceration or so-called alkaline reflux gastritis. The first and second portions of the duodenum can also be routinely examined with the fiberoptic gastroscope, and important information about ulcers and other lesions can be obtained by this procedure. Radiologic studies may be useful when endoscopy is not readily available or in the assessment of suspected motility disorders (e.g., gastroparesis). In addition, radiologic examination may be preferred when there are contraindications to safe endoscopy.

3 *Gastric acid secretory studies.* Though not routinely necessary, these are useful in the diagnosis of the Zollinger-Ellison syndrome or atrophic gastritis and for determination of completeness of vagotomy. Suspected gastric carcinoma is better diagnosed directly through gastroscopy and biopsy than indirectly through acid secretory studies (achlorhydria). These studies should not be obtained for the routine diagnosis of uncomplicated duodenal ulcer. There is no convincing evidence that acid studies are useful in determining the type of surgery for duodenal ulcer.

Obstructive and vascular disorders of the small intestine When intestinal problems present as obstructive syndromes, the plain x-ray of the abdomen is the most important diagnostic adjunct to careful physical examination. Patterns of dilatation of individual loops of intestine may be characteristic, as in volvulus or acute pancreatitis; erect and decubitus views will often show fluid levels in the affected segments. Motility disorders of the small intestine (temporary ileus or chronic intestinal pseudoobstruction) may also present with obstructive symptoms and similar x-ray findings but must be managed medically without surgical intervention. Air under the diaphragm is diagnostic of a perforated viscus; air in the portal vein usually results from intestinal necrosis secondary to mesenteric vascular occlusion. The diagnostic accuracy of the plain x-ray in all types of intestinal obstruction is about 75 percent. In patients with symptoms of incomplete obstruction, the radiographic small-bowel series will often be diagnostic in defining the site and degree of obstruction. Infrequently, in this setting, all conventional x-ray studies are unremarkable. In such cases, the radiologist may perform a small-bowel enteroclysis study by passing a special tube into the proximal jejunum; the rapid instillation of barium through the tube will distend the intestine and often reveal subtle lesions missed by other tests.

Vascular diseases of the small intestine are among the most difficult diseases to diagnose. In chronic mesenteric ischemia, radiographic, endoscopic, and laboratory tests are usually normal. Early in the course of acute mesenteric ischemia, the plain film of the abdomen

may be unremarkable despite complaints of severe abdominal pain. In these settings, prompt mesenteric angiography is essential in confirming the diagnosis of vascular disease.

Inflammatory and neoplastic diseases of small and large intestine Patients with these conditions are usually identified by history, physical examination, and careful examination of the stools for exudate and blood. Examination of fresh stool samples for common bacterial pathogens and parasites by laboratories skilled in these techniques is important in identifying or excluding infectious causes of diarrhea, particularly in the patient with colitis. Sigmoidoscopy is valuable in identifying mucosal and neoplastic lesions of the lower 25 cm of the colon. The mucosal surface of the entire colon and terminal ileum can be examined directly and biopsied through the fiberoptic sigmoidoscope or colonoscope. The radiologic examination of the small intestine is highly reliable in identifying the prestenotic and stenotic lesions of Crohn's disease. In the colon a single barium enema examination in a well-prepared patient has a diagnostic accuracy of 80 to 85 percent; the addition of air-contrast technique brings the accuracy up over 90 percent, but none of these figures is meaningful if the patient is poorly prepared for the examination, and the cecal area is hard to examine adequately because of its anatomy. Colonoscopy may be preferable for its greater accuracy and the capability to remove the vast majority of polyps as well as to obtain preoperative tissue confirmation in the patient who probably has cancer. The immunologic assay for the carcinoembryonic antigen has not proved to be specific for colonic cancer; nevertheless, it does contribute to the detection of residual or recurrent disease in postoperative patients.

Peroral biopsy of the small intestine and forceps biopsy of the rectosigmoid are of considerable importance in revealing mucosal disease. Rectal biopsy is an excellent means of demonstrating amyloidosis, schistosomiasis, and amebiasis. Submucosal disease is not seen in these superficial biopsies. Hirschsprung's disease is histologically diagnosed by a deep surgical biopsy of the lower part of the rectum.

Malabsorption syndromes Malabsorption may be suspected on the basis of history and physical examination and is confirmed by examination of the stools. Radiologic examination is of general help in ruling out local lesions and suggesting motor and secretory dysfunction, but it is rarely diagnostic unless an abnormal small-bowel mucosa or fistulas between intestine and stomach are demonstrated.

The tests useful in the diagnosis of malabsorption are discussed in Chap. 254. A simple screening test for excessive fat in the stools can be accomplished by the microscopic examination of a stool specimen stained with Sudan. Chemical analysis of 3-day stool collection for fat, with the patient on a standard diet, is used to establish the diagnosis of steatorrhea. The D-xylose absorption test is about 90 percent accurate in separating mucosal disease from pancreatic insufficiency. Peroral biopsy of the small intestine via the endoscope or a specialized biopsy device is of value in the diagnosis of celiac disease, and it may show the less common infiltrations of the mucosa by amyloid or bacterial mucoproteins (Whipple's disease). Leakage of protein into the intestinal lumen may cause hypoproteinemia and can be demonstrated by the recovery in stools of the serum protein α_1-antitrypsin or intravenously administered markers such as albumin labeled with iodine or chromium isotopes.

Pancreas The pancreas is difficult to study directly because of its anatomic location and relative inaccessibility. Calcification of the pancreas on a plain abdominal film is highly suggestive of chronic pancreatitis and may be associated with fat malabsorption. Pancreatic exocrine insufficiency can be documented by intubation of the duodenum and collection of pancreatic juice after stimulation with secretin or a test meal. Abdominal US and CT are the best radiographic means of searching for pancreatic enlargement (see Chaps. 273 and 274). Both techniques may also be used to guide needle biopsies of the pancreas and may provide sufficient diagnostic information to obviate the need for exploratory surgery. The pancreatic duct can be cannulated via the fiberoptic duodenoscope and visualized by the

COLOR ATLASES

Atlas of Dermatology

Atlas of Dermatology

Stephen F. Templeton
Thomas J. Lawley

1 Common Skin Diseases and Lesions

A1-1 **Acne vulgaris** with inflammatory papules, pustules, and comedones.

A1-2 **Acne rosacea** with prominent facial erythema, telangiectasias, scattered papules, and small pustules.

A1-3 **Psoriasis** is characterized by small and large erythematous plaques with adherent silvery scale.

A1-4 **Atopic dermatitis** with excoriated, lichenified plaques in the popliteal fossa.

A1-5 **Dyshidrotic eczema,** characterized by deep-seated vesicles and scaling on palms and lateral fingers, is often associated with an atopic diathesis.

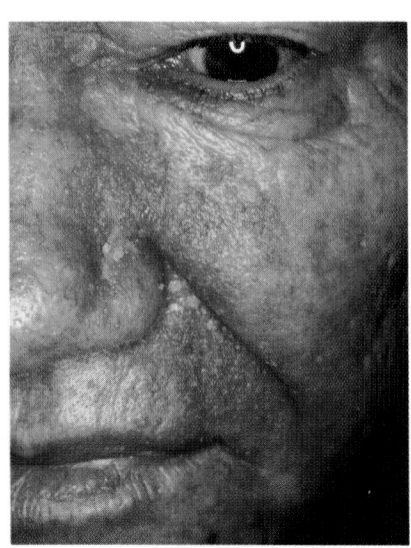

A1-6 **Seborrheic dermatitis** showing central facial erythema with overlying greasy, yellowish scale.

A1-7 **Stasis dermatitis** showing erythematous, scaly, and oozing patches over the lower leg. Several stasis ulcers are also seen in this patient.

A1-8 **Allergic contact dermatitis,** acute phase, with sharply demarcated, weeping, eczematous plaques in a perioral distribution.

A1-9 **Lichen planus** showing multiple flat-topped, violaceous papules and plaques. Nail dystrophy as seen in this patient's thumbnail may also be a feature.

A1-10 **Pityriasis rosea.** Multiple round to oval erythematous patches with fine central scale are distributed along the skin tension lines on the trunk.

A1-11 **Vitiligo** in a typical acral distribution demonstrating striking cutaneous depigmentation, as a result of loss of melanocytes.

A1-13 **Urticaria** showing characteristic discrete and confluent, edematous, erythematous papules and plaques.

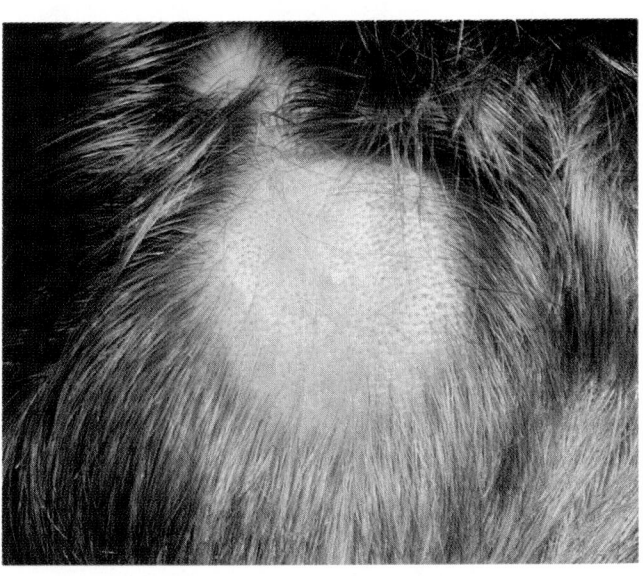

A1-12 **Alopecia areata** characterized by a sharply demarcated circular patch of scalp completely devoid of hairs. Follicular orifices are preserved, indicating a nonscarring alopecia.

A1-14 **Epidermoid cysts.** Several inflamed and noninflamed firm, cystic nodules are seen in this patient. Often a patulous follicular punctum is observed on the overlying epidermal surface.

A1-15 **Seborrheic keratoses** are seen as "stuck on," waxy, verrucous papules and plaques with a variety of colors ranging from light tan to black.

A1-16 **Keloids** resulting from ear piercing, with firm exophytic flesh-colored to erythematous nodules of scar tissue.

A1-17 **Cherry hemangiomas** are very common and arise in middle-aged to older adults. They are characterized by multiple erythematous to dark-purple papules usually located on the trunk.

2 Cutaneous Neoplasms

A2-18 **Actinic keratoses** consist of hyperkeratotic erythematous papules and patches on sun-exposed skin. They arise in middle-aged to older adults and have some potential for malignant transformation.

A2-19 **Keratoacanthoma** is a low-grade squamous neoplasm characterized by an exophytic nodule with central keratinous debris.

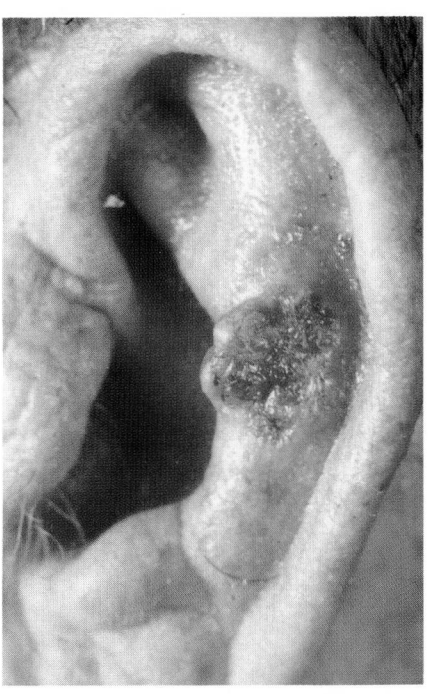

A2-20 **Basal cell carcinoma** showing central ulceration and a pearly, rolled, telangiectatic tumor border.

A2-21 **Squamous cell carcinoma** seen here as a hyperkeratotic crusted and somewhat eroded plaque on the lower lip. Sun-exposed skin such as the head, neck, hands, and arms are other typical sites of involvement.

A2-22 **Kaposi's sarcoma** in a patient with AIDS demonstrating patch, plaque, and tumor stages.

A2-23 **Mycosis fungoides** is a cutaneous T cell lymphoma, and plaque stage lesions are seen in this patient.

A2-24 **Non-Hodgkin's lymphoma** involving the skin with typical violaceous, "plum-colored" nodules.

A2-25 **Metastatic carcinoma** to the skin is characterized by inflammatory, often ulcerated dermal nodules.

3 Pigmented Lesions—Benign and Malignant

A3-26 **Nevus.** Nevi are benign proliferations of nevomelanocytes character-ized by regularly shaped hyperpigmented macules or papules of a uniform color.

A3-27 **Dysplastic nevi** are irregularly pigmented and shaped nevomelano-cytic lesions which may be associated with familial melanoma.

A3-28 **Superficial spreading melanoma** is the most common type of malignant melanoma and demonstrates color variegation (black, blue, brown, pink, and white) and irregular borders.

A3-29 **Lentigo maligna melanoma** occurs on sun-exposed skin as a large, hyperpigmented macule or plaque with irregular borders and variable pigmentation.

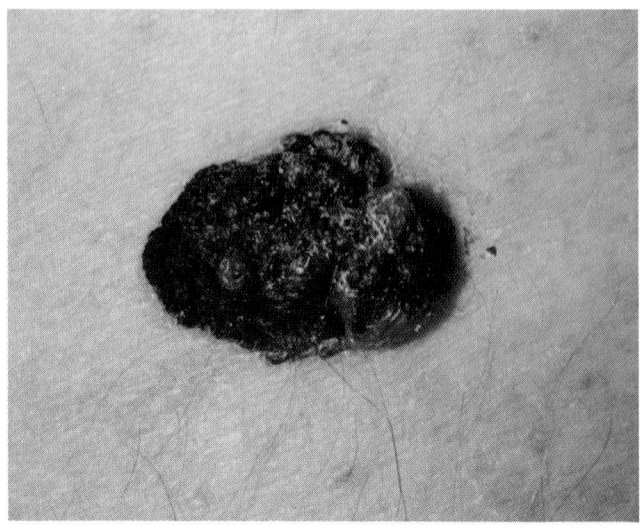

A3-30 **Nodular melanoma** most commonly manifests itself as a rapidly growing, often ulcerated or crusted black nodule.

A3-31 **Acral lentiginous melanoma** is more common in blacks, Orientals, and Hispanics and occurs as an enlarging hyperpigmented macule or plaque on the palms and soles. Lateral pigment diffusion is present.

4 Infectious Disease and the Skin

A4-32 **Impetigo contagiosa** is a superficial streptococcal or *Staph. aureus* infection consisting of honey-colored crusts and erythematous weeping erosions. Occasionally bullous lesions may be seen.

A4-33 **Folliculitis** is a bacterial infection of hair follicles and is seen as erythematous follicular papules and pustules.

A4-34 **Erysipelas** is a streptococcal infection of the superficial dermis and consists of well-demarcated, erythematous, edematous, warm plaques.

A4-35 **Herpes simplex.** Grouped vesiculopustules on an erythematous base characterize primary HSV infections.

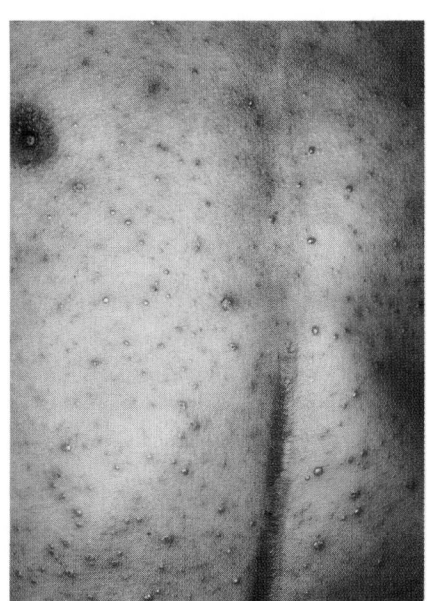

A4-36 **Varicella** showing numerous lesions in various stages of evolution: vesicles on an erythematous base, umbilicated vesicles, and crusts.

A4-37 **Herpes zoster** seen in this HIV-infected patient as hemorrhagic vesicles and pustules on an erythematous base grouped in a dermatomal distribution.

A4-38 **Verrucae** characterized as multiple hyperkeratotic, verrucous papules.

A4-39 **Molluscum contagiosum** is a cutaneous poxvirus infection characterized by multiple umbilicated flesh-colored or hypopigmented papules.

A4-40 **Oral hairy leukoplakia** often presents as white plaques on the lateral tongue and is associated with Epstein-Barr virus infection.

A4-41 **Pseudomembranous oral candidiasis.** Adherent white, mucoid plaques with an erythematous halo seen here on the palate often indicates an immunocompromised state.

A4-42 **Tinea corporis** is a superficial fungal infection seen here as an erythematous annular scaly plaque with central clearing.

A4-43 **Tinea cruris** is a superficial dermatophyte infection with bilateral scaly, erythematous, annular plaques extending from the inguinal crease to the upper thighs.

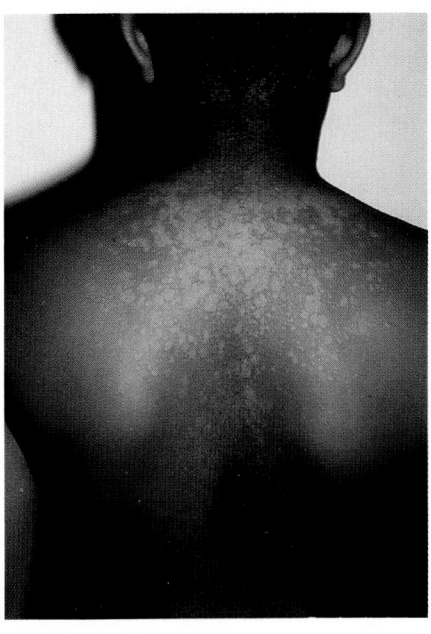

A4-44 **Tinea versicolor** is a superficial cutaneous fungal infection showing a wide variety of lesions. Finely scaling patches may be small or large, hyperpigmented or hypopigmented.

A4-45 **Scabies** showing typical scaling erythematous papules and few linear burrows.

A4-46 **Erythema chronicum migrans** is the early cutaneous manifestation of Lyme disease and is characterized by erythematous annular patches, often with a central erythematous papule at the tick bite site.

A4-47 **Rocky Mountain spotted fever** demonstrating faint erythematous palmar macules in the early phase of the disease. Lesions may become hemorrhagic (purpuric) as the disease progresses.

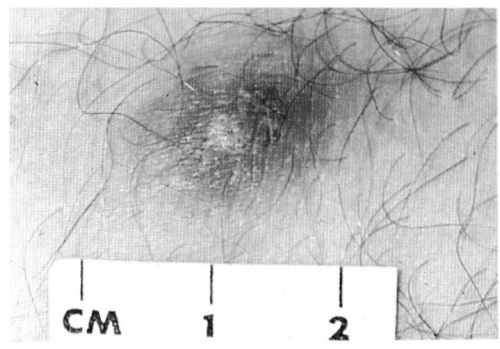

A4-48 **Disseminated gonococcemia** in the skin is seen as hemorrhagic papules and pustules with purpuric centers in an acral distribution.

A4-49 **Fulminant meningococcemia** with extensive angular purpuric patches.

A4-50 **Primary syphilis** with a firm, nontender chancre.

A4-51 **Secondary syphilis** demonstrating the papulosquamous truncal eruption.

A4-52 **Secondary syphilis** commonly affects the palms and soles with scaling, firm, red-brown papules.

A4-53 **Condylomata lata** are moist somewhat verrucous intertriginous plaques seen in secondary syphilis.

A4-54 **Chancroid** with characteristic penile ulcers and associated left inguinal adenitis (bubo).

A4-55 **Condylomata acuminata** are lesions induced by human papillomavirus (HPV) and in this patient are seen as multiple verrucous papules coalescing into plaques.

5 Immunologically Mediated Skin Disease

A5-56 **Systemic lupus erythematosus** showing prominent, scaly, malar erythema. Involvement of other sun-exposed sites is also common.

A5-57 **Discoid lupus erythematosus.** Violaceous, hyperpigmented, atrophic plaques, often with evidence of follicular plugging, which may result in scarring, are characteristic of this cutaneous form of lupus.

A5-58 **Dermatomyositis.** Periorbital violaceous erythema characterizes the classic heliotrope rash.

A5-59 **Dermatomyositis** often involves the hands as erythematous flat-topped papules over the knuckles (Gottron's sign) and periungal telangiectasias.

A5-60 **Scleroderma** showing acral sclerosis and focal digital ulcers.

A5-61 **Scleroderma** characterized by typical expressionless, mask-like facies.

A5-63 **Erythema nodosum** is a panniculitis characterized by tender deep-seated nodules and plaques usually located on the lower extremities.

A5-62 **Erythema multiforme** is characterized by multiple erythematous plaques with a target or iris morphology and usually represents a hypersensitivity reaction to drugs or infections (especially herpes simplex virus).

A5-64 **Vasculitis.** Palpable purpuric papules on the lower legs are seen in this patient with cutaneous small vessel vasculitis.

A5-65 **Pemphigus vulgaris** demonstrating flaccid bullae which are easily ruptured, resulting in multiple erosions and crusted plaques.

A5-66 **Dermatitis herpetiformis** manifested by pruritic, grouped vesicles in a typical location. The vesicles are often excoriated and may occur on knees, buttocks, and posterior scalp.

A5-67 **Bullous pemphigoid** with tense vesicles and bullae on an erythematous, urticarial base.

6 Skin Manifestations of Internal Disease

A6-68 Acanthosis nigricans demonstrating typical hyperpigmented axillary plaques with a velvet-like, verrucous surface.

A6-69 Pretibial myxedema manifesting as waxy, infiltrated plaques in a patient with Graves' disease.

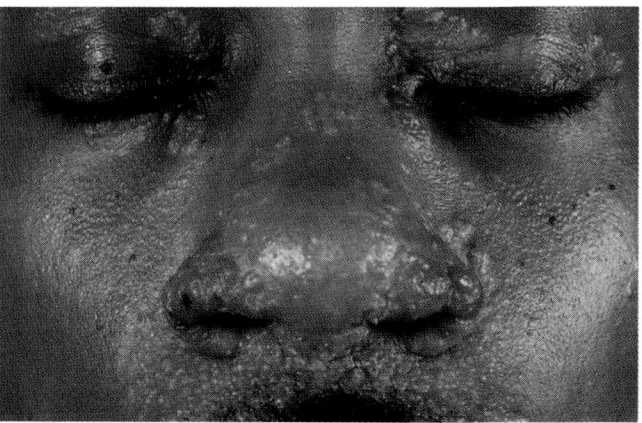

A6-70 Sarcoid. Infiltrated papules and plaques of variable color are seen in a typical paranasal and periorbital location.

A6-71 Neurofibromatosis demonstrating numerous flesh-colored cutaneous neurofibromas.

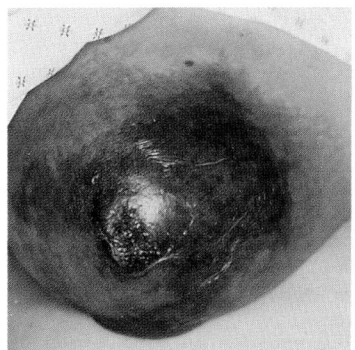

A6-72 Coumarin necrosis showing cutaneous and subcutaneous necrosis of a breast. Other fatty areas such as buttocks and thighs are also common sites of involvement.

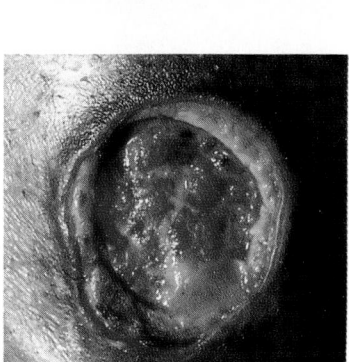

A6-73 Pyoderma gangrenosum showing a somewhat purulent ulcer with violaceous and undermined wound edges.

Sources of Photographs

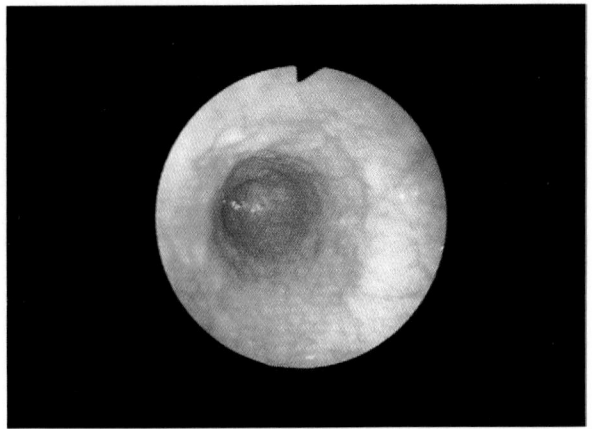

A7-1 **Normal esophagus;** fine vasculature can be seen.

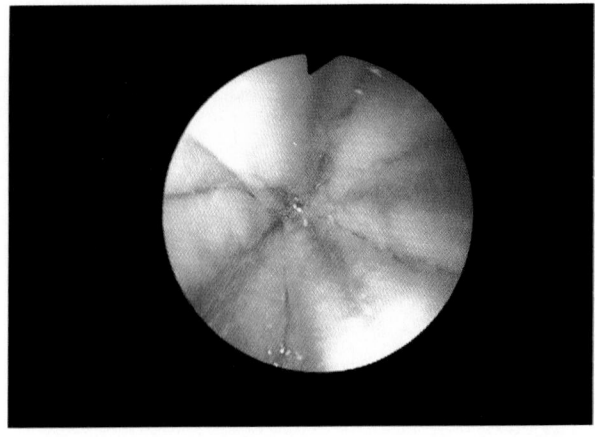

A7-2 **Peptic regurgitant esophagitis;** linear red streaks with a central white streak extend up the esophagus.

A7-3 **Ulcerated squamous cell carcinoma,** with a depressed center, involving one wall of the esophagus.

A7-4 **Moniliasis of the esophagus.** A white exudate is seen with underlying erythematous mucosa.

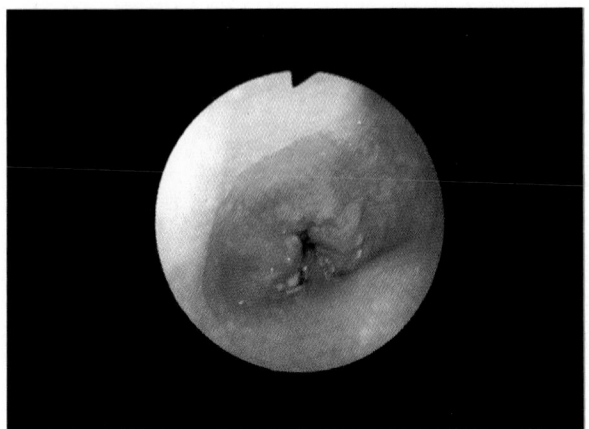

A7-5 **Barrett's metaplasia of the esophagus with an adenocarcinoma.** The squamocolumnar junction is noted in the proximal esophagus. A mucosal irregularity in the center of the photograph was an adenocarcinoma.

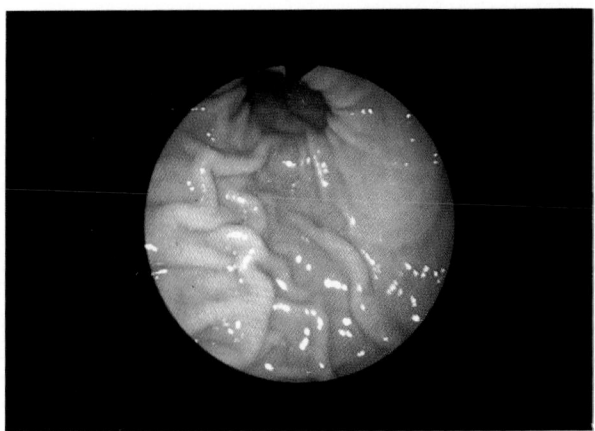

A7-6 **Normal body of the stomach with rugal folds.**

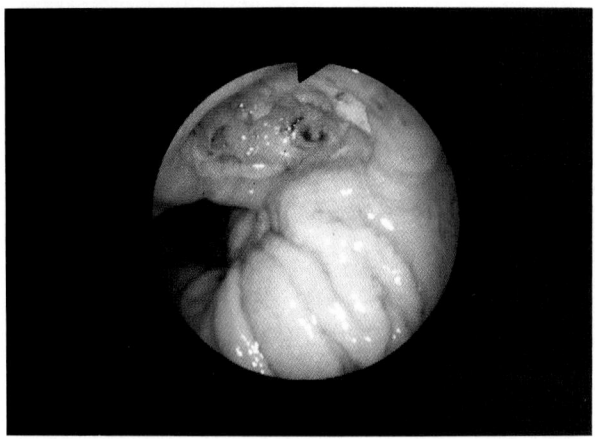

A7-7 **Large, benign, lesser curve gastric ulcer.** The folds end at the ulcer margin.

A7-8 **Gastric polyp.** The histologic type must be determined by excision and pathologic examination.

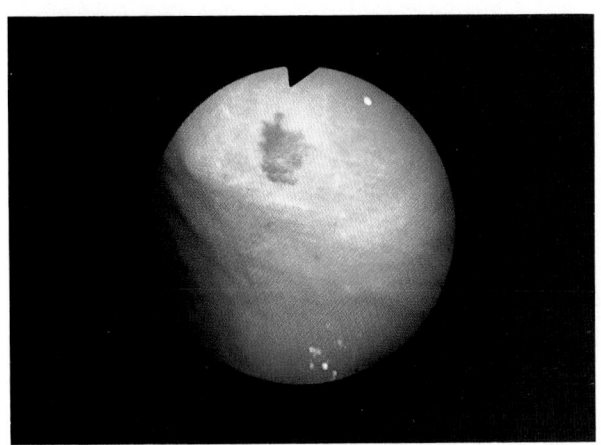

A7-9 **Arteriovenous malformation of the gastric mucosa.**

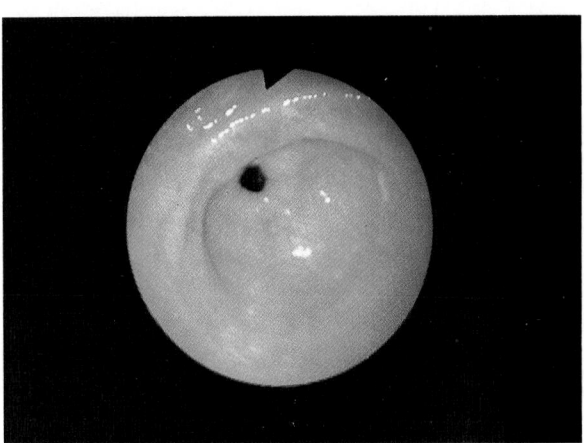

A7-10 **Normal pylorus.** Note the absence of gastric rugal folds in the antrum proximal to the pylorus.

A7-11 **Normal duodenal bulb.**

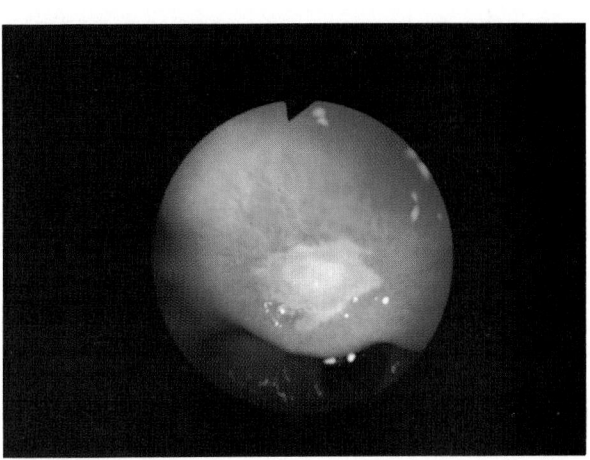

A7-12 **Duodenal ulcer.** A typical ulcer with a clean base is seen on the anterior surface of the duodenal bulb.

A7-13 **Normal papilla of Vater.** The fold pattern surrounding the papilla is normal; bile is seen adjacent to the papilla.

A7-14 **Periampullary carcinoma.** The mass at the papilla of Vater has been catheterized during ERCP.

A7-15 **Endoscopic papillotomy.** A papillotome has been passed into the papilla, the wire bowed, and an incision made, with electrosurgical current, in the superior aspect of the papilla.

A7-16 **Normal colon;** typical folds and vascular pattern can be seen.

A7-17 **Colonic adenomatous polyp.** The polyp is erythematous; a stalk is seen covered with normal mucosa.

A7-18 **Multiple, small, colonic adenomatous polyps** in a case of familial polyposis coli. This colon must be removed to prevent the development of cancer.

A7-19 **Colon adenocarcinoma.** The cancer is multilobed and growing into the lumen.

A7-20 **Crohn's colitis** with linear, serpiginous, white-based ulcers surrounded by colonic mucosa which is relatively normal.

A7-21 **Severe ulcerative colitis** with diffuse ulceration, bleeding, and exudation.

A7-22 **Kaposi's sarcoma involving the colon** in a patient with AIDS. The erythematous lesions involve most of the colonic mucosa in the photograph.

A7-23 **Colonic varices.** Multiple, serpiginous, subepithelial structures impinge on the colonic lumen.

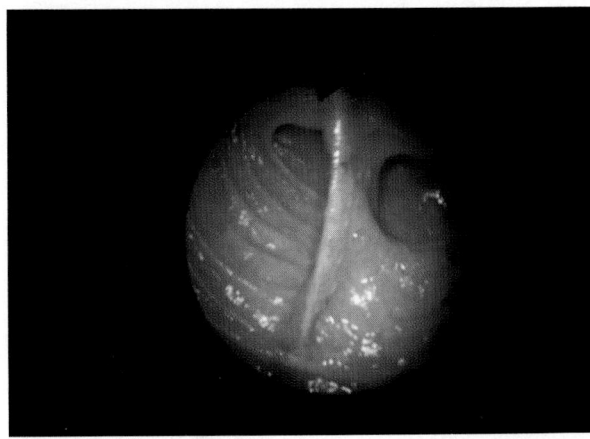

A7-24 **Ileal pouch.** The mucosa appears normal in this pouch reconstructed from ileum to provide a reservoir after total proctocolectomy and ileoanal anastomosis.

Source: All photographs except A7-12, A7-23, and A7-24 are courtesy of FE Silverstein and GN Tytgat: *Atlas of Gastrointestinal Endoscopy.* Gower Medical Publishing, New York, 1987. The three photographs listed above are courtesy of GN Tytgat.

A8-1 **Normal optic nerve and retina.**

A8-2 **Central retinal artery occlusion.**

A8-3 **Central retinal vein occlusion.**

A8-4 **Early papilledema.**

A8-5 **Drusen of the optic nerve head.**

A8-6 **Anterior ischemic optic neuropathy.**

A8-7 **Primary optic atrophy.**

A8-8 **Angioid streaks.**

A8-9 **Retinitis pigmentosa.**

A8-10 **Band keratopathy.**

A8-11 **Glaucomatous optic disk with secondary atrophy.**

A8-12 **Diabetic retinopathy with microaneurysms.**

A8-13 **Proliferative diabetic retinopathy.**

A8-14 **Cytomegalovirus retinitis in AIDS.**
(Courtesy of Donald J.D'Amico, M.D.)

A8-15 **Retinal arteriovenous malformation in the Wyburn-Mason syndrome.**

A8-16 **Kayser-Fleischer ring in Wilson's disease.**
(Note: The ring is the golden brown pigment at the periphery of the cornea and is characteristically broader superiorly and inferiorly than it is medially and laterally.)

A9-1 **Normal blood smear.** Normal red blood cells are round, possess an area of central pallor, appear slightly smaller than the nucleus of a mature lymphocyte, and vary little in size (anisocytosis) or in shape (poikilocytosis).

A9-2 **Megaloblastic anemia.** Oval macrocytes, well filled with hemoglobin, are admixed with lesser numbers of small teardrop-shaped red blood cells. Note also hypersegmented granulocyte.

A9-3 **Liver disease.** Round macrocytes of rather uniform size are seen. Many of the macrocytes are also target cells.

A9-4 **Iron-deficiency anemia.** In severe iron deficiency, the red blood cells are smaller than normal (microcytosis), and their central area of pallor is expanded (hypochromia) so that the cells appear to have only a thin rim of hemoglobin.

A9-5 **β Thalassemia intermedia.** Microcytic and hypochromic red blood cells are seen that resemble the red blood cells of severe iron deficiency anemia shown in Fig. A9-4. Many elliptical and teardrop-shaped red blood cells are noted.

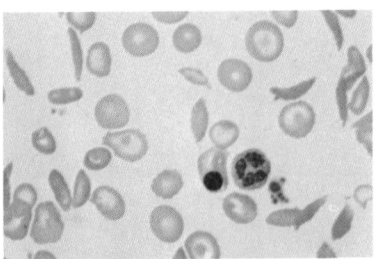

A9-6 **Sickle cell anemia.** The elongated and crescent-shaped red blood cells seen on this smear represent circulating irreversible sickled cells. Target cells and a nucleated red blood cell are also seen.

A9-7 **Traumatic hemolysis.** The helmet-shaped red blood cell and the small triangular-shaped red blood cells seen on this smear represent morphologic evidence of mechanical damage to red blood cells within the circulatory tree.

A9-8 **Spur cell anemia.** Spur cells are recognized as distorted red blood cells containing several irregularly distributed thornlike projections. Cells with this morphologic abnormality are also called acanthocytes.

A9-9 **Uremia.** The red blood cells in uremia may acquire numerous, regularly spaced, small spiny projections. Such cells, called burr cells or echinocytes, are readily distinguishable from the irregularly spiculated acanthocytes shown in Fig. A9-8.

A9-10 **Hereditary spherocytosis.** Small, densely staining red blood cells are seen that have lost their central area of pallor (microspherocytes). Microspherocytes may also be found in other hemolytic disorders (Fig. A9-11).

A9-11 **Immunohemolytic anemia.** Microspherocytes are seen on this blood smear along with several macrocytes with a slight purple tinge (polychromasia). The latter represent new red blood cells released early from the bone marrow. The microspherocytes seen in immunohemolytic anemia may be indistinguishable from the microspherocytes seen in hereditary spherocytosis (Fig. A9-10).

A9-12 **Myeloid metaplasia.** Teardrop-shaped red blood cells, a nucleated red blood cell, and immature myeloid cells are seen on this blood smear.

A **B**

A9-13 A. **Normal granulocyte.** The normal granulocyte has a segmented nucleus with heavy, clumped chromatin; fine neutrophilic granules are dispersed throughout its cytoplasm. *B.* **Normal monocyte and lymphocyte.** The normal monocyte is a large cell with an indented or folded nucleus containing loose, strandlike chromatin; the cytoplasm is a blue-gray color and usually contains fine azurophilic granules. The normal lymphocyte is a smaller cell. Its nucleus is usually round but may be indented, as in the cell shown in this plate. The nuclear chromatin has a smudgy appearance; the cytoplasm is a blue color.

A9-15 **Normal granulocyte precursors in marrow.** The earliest granulocytic precursor (myeloblast) possesses a round nucleus with fine, punctate chromatin and one or more nucleoli; the cytoplasm is blue. As nuclear differentiation proceeds, the nucleoli disappear, the chromatin coarsens, and the nucleus becomes increasingly indented and finally segmented. As cytoplasmic differentiation proceeds, azurophilic granules appear and the cytoplasm changes color from blue to the yellow-pink-gray hue of the mature granulocyte, and as this occurs the azurophilic granules become obscured by fine neutrophilic granules.

A **B**

A9-14 A. **Normal eosinophil.** The eosinophil contains large, bright-orange granules; the nucleus is bilobed. *B.* **Basophil.** The basophil contains large purple-black granules which fill the cell and obscure the nucleus.

A9-16 **Neutrophils with toxic granulation.** In infection and other toxic states, azurophilic granules may become visible in mature granulocytes as coarse, dark-staining cytoplasmic granules.

A9-17 **Band with Döhle body** (center). Döhle bodies are discrete, blue-staining nongranular areas found in the periphery of the cytoplasm of the neutrophil in infections and other toxic states. They represent aggregates of rough endoplasmic reticulum.

A9-18 **Hypersegmentation.** Frequent five-lobed granulocytes on a blood smear or granulocytes with more than five lobes are evidence of hypersegmentation, an important clue to the diagnosis of megaloblastic anemia.

A   **B**

A9-19 A. **Chédiak-Higashi anomaly.** In this ultimately fatal disorder, the granulocytes contain huge cytoplasmic granules, formed from aggregation and fusion of azurophilic and specific granules. Large, abnormal granules are found in other granule-containing cells throughout the body. *B.* **Pelger-Hüet anomaly.** In this benign disorder, the majority of granulocytes are bilobed. The nucleus frequently has a spectacle-like or "pince-nez" configuration.

A9-20 **Reactive lymphocytes** (infectious mononucleosis). Reactive lymphocytes are usually large, cytoplasmic lymphocytes. The nucleus may be eccentrically placed and may have irregular borders and indentations (not seen on this plate). The cytoplasm contains areas that stain a darker blue due to their increased content of RNA. The cytoplasm may be indented where it abuts against a red blood cell.

A9-21 **Chronic granulocytic leukemia.** The peripheral blood WBC count is high due to increased numbers of granulocytes and their precursors. The majority of the WBCs are segmented granulocytes or band forms, but as seen on this plate, myelocytes and promyeloblasts (not seen on this plate) may also be found on review of the blood smear.

A9-22 **Leukemic cell in acute promyelocytic leukemia.** Note multiple Auer rods.

A9-23 **Chronic lymphocytic leukemia.** The peripheral blood WBC count is high due to increased numbers of small, well-differentiated lymphocytes. However, the leukemic lymphocytes are fragile, and substantial numbers of broken, smudged cells are usually also present on the blood smear.

A9-24 **Leukemic cells in acute lympho-blastic leukemia** characterized by round or convoluted nuclei, high nuclear/cytoplasmic ratio and absence of cytoplasmic granules.

A9-25 **Hodgkin's disease:** Reed-Sternberg cell in marrow (center). The Reed-Sternberg cell is recognized by its bilobed, mirror-image nucleus, which contains in each lobe a giant, inclusion body-like nucleolus. The cytoplasmic borders of the cell cannot be identified on this plate.

A9-26 **Non-Hodgkin's nodular lymphoma** (lymph node). This low-power view illustrates that a proliferative process has caused the normal architecture of the lymph node to be replaced by multiple nodules of varying size that extend throughout the entire lymph node.

A9-27 **Multiple myeloma** (marrow). The cells bear the characteristic morphologic features of plasma cells, round or oval cells with an eccentric nucleus composed of coarsely clumped chromatin, a densely basophilic cytoplasm, and a perinuclear clear zone (hof) containing the Golgi apparatus. Binucleate and multinucleate malignant plasma cells also can be seen.

section 1 | Disorders of the alimentary tract

---

248 APPROACH TO THE PATIENT WITH GASTROINTESTINAL DISEASE

KURT J. ISSELBACHER / DANIEL K. PODOLSKY

BIOLOGIC CONSIDERATIONS The mucosal surface of the gastrointestinal tract is composed of a remarkably dynamic population of epithelial cells that are highly developed in their capacity for transmembrane absorption and secretion. These secretory and absorptive abilities facilitate the essential function of the digestive tract in digestion and nutrient uptake, which must be accomplished while maintaining the barrier between the host and potentially harmful pathogens and mutagens in the lumen. The latter is accomplished through both the physical integrity of the intact mucosal surface and the extensive population of resident immune cells.

The intestinal surface itself also contains the distinctive M cells that serve to sample the antigenic milieu of the lumen. The predominance of suppressor lymphocytes within the surface epithelial layer (intraepithelial lymphocytes) suggests that dampening of the body's response to the enormous number of potentially antigenic substances in the lumen is necessary to prevent the constant and unrestrained activation of immune and inflammatory processes. Conversely, the presence of large numbers of helper lymphocytes as well as other cellular effectors of immune response in the lamina propria and submucosa attests to a large armamentarium ready to respond when surface defenses have been breached. No doubt the concentration of so many immune cells capable of attracting and activating inflammatory cells predisposes to the numerous inflammatory conditions to which the gastrointestinal tract is subject.

The mucosal surface of the gastrointestinal tract is also remarkable for the very rapid turnover of the epithelial cell population. It is likely that the epithelium turns over in its entirety every 24 to 72 h. This may permit rapid restitution of a functional cell population following an acute insult and may reduce the risk of malignancy through loss of cells affected by the many potential and actual mutagens in the luminal contents. Nevertheless, this proliferative potential must inherently create the setting for neoplastic disorders, which are so common to the gastrointestinal tract. Another fundamental feature of gastrointestinal mucosa is the spatial segregation of the proliferative compartment from the terminally differentiated cells. This is true throughout the gastrointestinal tract but is most apparent in the small intestine where a gradient of differentiation exists from the depths of the crypts of Lieberkühn to the villus tip. This organization is important in understanding the histology and pathophysiology of many mucosal disorders, e.g., nontropical sprue.

In view of the important secretory and absorptive activities of mucosal surface, diseases of the gastrointestinal tract may result in clinical consequences secondary to the physical disruption of the mucosal layer (e.g., blood loss, fluid loss, pathogenic invasion) or nutritional derangements due to impaired digestion and nutrient absorption. In focal or localized disease processes the former predominate, whereas the latter may be especially prominent in disorders that affect extensive areas of the gastrointestinal tract in a diffuse manner.

While the essential role of the gastrointestinal tract is the absorption of nutrients and excretion of the products is in large part accomplished at the luminal surface, these processes are also dependent on the deeper muscular layers for the coordinated propulsion of food through the lumen. The complexity of both local and distant neural and endocrine factors that contribute to the regulation of intestinal motility is only now becoming fully appreciated. Disruption of normal motility is quite common, with functional bowel complaints affecting as many as 15 percent of adults. Alterations in frequency of bowel movements, abdominal distention, abdominal pain, and nausea, individually or in varying combinations, may result from dysmotility. In addition, structural lesions may also indirectly lead to symptoms through their impact on motility involving some or all regions of the gastrointestinal tract. These range from the *direct* effects of an obstructing lesion to the *indirect* actions of substances released by a primary mucosal disorder (e.g., inflammatory mediators such as arachidonic acid metabolites that also affect smooth-muscle activity).

Although valid unifying generalizations can be made about the gastrointestinal tract in its entirety, the spectrum of diseases affecting this system and their clinical manifestations are significantly related to the constituent organ(s) involved. Thus, esophageal disorders predominantly manifest through their relationship to swallowing, while gastric disorders are dominated by features relating to acid secretion, and disease of the small and large intestine by disruption of nutrition and alterations of bowel movements. Similarly, diseases of the related ancillary organs, the exocrine pancreas and the hepatobiliary system, present characteristic clinical challenges. Finally, it should be remembered that in addition to intrinsic disease, the gastrointestinal tract may be affected by systemic disorders. These include vascular, inflammatory, infectious, and neoplastic conditions leading to focal or diffuse structural lesions. Metabolic and endocrine abnormalities as well as drugs can disrupt normal bowel motility.

CLINICAL CONSIDERATIONS **History** A thorough clinical history is almost uniformly reliable in directing the clinician's attention to appropriate diagnostic considerations in the patient with gastrointestinal symptoms. The most common complaints resulting from disorders involving the gastrointestinal tract include pain, and alteration in bowel habit, especially diarrhea and constipation. Among these, *abdominal pain* is the most frequent and variable and may reflect a broad spectrum of problems from the least threatening to the most urgent. In conjunction with an estimation of its intensity, initial distinction should be made between pain of acute onset and more chronic discomfort. Pain of abrupt onset is often encountered in serious illness requiring urgent intervention, while a history of chronic discomfort may typically be related to an indolent disorder. However, change in the pattern or character of pain may be equally important, signifying progression of a problem of initial mild onset (either recent or chronic) to a more critical stage. Ascertaining the location (upper or lower, localized or diffuse), character (sharp, burning, cramping), and relationship of the pain to meals will often provide significant insight into the most important diagnostic considerations. If eating produces the symptom, the clinician should determine whether the discomfort occurs while eating (as in esophageal disorders and abdominal angina), shortly after the meal (as often occurs in biliary tract disease), or 30 to 90 min later (as typically seen in peptic disease). Pain that is not affected by eating suggests a process outside of the bowel lumen, such as an abscess, peritonitis, pancreatitis, and some malignancies. Conversely, identification of factors that relieve the symptom is also helpful, e.g., relief with eating or antacids is characteristic of peptic ulcer disease or gastritis. Relationship of the discomfort to bowel movement, especially in association with an altered bowel habit, should focus attention on a disorder of the small or large bowel such as inflammatory bowel disease.

Alterations in bowel habit can result from either disruption of normal intestinal motility or significant structural pathology. A thorough determination of the temporal evolution of the change and the nature of the alteration in conjunction with other constitutional symptoms such as weight loss, fever, or anorexia is important. Temporary variation in bowel habit in association with some life stress and in the absence of signs of systemic illness is suggestive of the common "irritable bowel syndrome," especially when the alteration varies between diarrhea and constipation. Small pellet-like stools are often described by the patient. Associated symptoms of bloating, nausea, and "gas" are also common. This diagnosis can essentially be made on the basis of a thorough history and physical examination and very limited laboratory testing, which exclude structural disease. In contrast, the onset of worsening constipation in an adult with previously regular habits, especially when accompanied by systemic symptoms such as weight loss, suggests the possible presence of an underlying obstructing process, particularly malignancy. If diarrhea is present, one should determine the average number of stools, their consistency, their pattern, and if any blood is present. Although *diarrhea* refers to an increased frequency of movements, patients will often use the term to describe loose or watery stools primarily. The occurrence of nocturnal or true bloody diarrhea almost always reflects structural rather than functional bowel disease. A pungent odor or the presence of undigested meat in the movement are suggestive of pancreatic insufficiency. An alteration in color can be seen in cholestasis or steatorrhea (light-colored) or hemorrhage (melenic to maroon or bright red). Mucus in the movement is usually a sign of functional bowel syndrome, while pus is more strongly suggestive of infectious or inflammatory disease. Less common but more dramatic are the symptoms of acute gastrointestinal bleeding, including hematemesis, melena, and hematochezia, which usually leads to prompt efforts to find medical attention but should always be solicited by the clinician.

In the evaluation of male patients, especially those with diarrhea, a tactful inquiry into sexual activity is essential. Homosexual males are at increased risk for a large variety of gastrointestinal disorders as well as AIDS, which may first manifest itself with gastrointestinal symptoms. Finally, careful attention must be given to a general medical history with an emphasis on any medications or nonprescription drugs that may have been used. Thyroid and other metabolic disorders, especially those affecting calcium metabolism, can cause a variety of gastrointestinal symptoms. Unless asked, patients may forget to mention that they take aspirin almost daily for headache, and this may account for occult blood found in the stool. The use of daily laxatives may explain chronic diarrhea.

Physical examination, endoscopy, and radiology All of the cardinal methods of examination are helpful in evaluating the patient with gastrointestinal symptoms. *Inspection* may disclose signs of cholestasis or nutritional deficiencies. An abnormal contour of the abdomen or inspection of the perianal region may manifest signs of a mass or a draining fistula. *Auscultation* is also important. A succussion splash can be elicited in the patients with symptoms of gastric outlet obstruction. The absence of bowel sounds or alteration in pitch can lead to recognition of an evolving ileus or an obstructing process. A bruit may also be appreciated where there are symptoms of ischemic bowel disease. Careful *palpation* of the abdomen is especially important in detecting tenderness and masses, which in the appropriate clinical setting will lead to the recognition of cholecystitis, regional enteritis, periappendiceal abscess, and many other disorders. Findings on abdominal palpation will often be complemented by *percussion*, which is essential to assessing liver and spleen size.

Elicitation of rebound tenderness, either direct or referred, after removal of the examining hand provides an important clue to localized or more generalized peritonitis characteristic of many abdominal emergencies, including a perforated viscus, intraabdominal abscess, or tissue infarction. The clinician should be particularly alert to these signs in patients with severe pain of abrupt onset. Typically, the patient will remain immobile to avoid the accentuation of pain that may follow even slight movement and jarring of the abdomen. This contrasts with the sometimes frantic efforts to find a position of comfort in patients with severe pain deriving from visceral disease, e.g., pancreatitis or intestinal ischemia. In these disorders, the absence of findings on palpation of the abdomen may be in striking contrast to the evident distress of the patient. Only with progression of the process to tissue destruction (e.g., necrotizing pancreatitis or intestinal infarction) and secondary peritonitis will the abdominal examination prove remarkable, often in concert with striking signs of systemic illness including hemodynamic instability. In addition to the examination of the abdomen, a carefully performed digital rectal examination is also essential. In the patient with complaints of incontinence the integrity of the sphincter can be assessed. Most importantly, masses intrinsic to the rectum as well as abnormalities in the pelvis or the pouch of Douglas may only be detected by this examination, and the presence or absence of frank or occult blood in the stool is always important diagnostic information. Sigmoidoscopy should be viewed as a routine extension of the physical examination in the patient with diarrhea or other alteration in bowel habit as well as in the patient with known or suspected blood loss from the lower bowel. This procedure, which can be performed with either the rigid sigmoidoscope or a flexible fiberoptic instrument, allows for direct inspection of the rectosigmoid mucosa permitting detection of cancers and polyps in this segment that may well be missed by barium x-rays. Inflammatory changes of the mucosa can help identify the patient with infectious dysentery or other forms of colitis, most notably ulcerative colitis. The findings of edema, granularity, and diffuse friability (easily induced mucosal bleeding) as well as superficial ulcerations are characteristic in the latter disorder. Fresh stool samples for microbiologic studies and superficial mucosal biopsies obtained at the time of sigmoidoscopy can also yield crucial diagnostic information.

Definitive demonstration or exclusion of structural lesions of the gastrointestinal tract, particularly the great majority of disorders that primarily affect mucosal surface, can often not be accomplished by physical examination alone. Many disorders of the upper or lower gastrointestinal tract are accessible to inspection through fiberoptic instruments. As a result, endoscopic studies are supplanting conventional contrast x-ray studies for many clinical problems, both because of the heightened precision of these diagnostic tools and the opportunity in many instances to accomplish a meaningful therapeutic intervention as an adjunct to the acquisition of diagnostic information. However, it should be emphasized that *no procedure should be considered routine* and used indiscriminately; there must be a rational basis for its use in the individual patient. These techniques are discussed in detail in Chap. 250. Upper gastrointestinal endoscopy permits evaluation of the esophagus, stomach, and duodenum and, with specially designed instruments, the proximal jejunum. When the clinical history warrants a diagnostic examination of the upper gastrointestinal tract for a structural lesion, endoscopic examination is preferable to radiologic study in most patients when the choice is available. Side-viewing scopes permit inspection and cannulation of the ampulla of Vater facilitating retrograde cholangiopancreatography. The colonoscope can be used to visualize the entire colon and often the terminal ileum, resulting in more accurate diagnosis of inflammatory bowel disease and mass lesions. Frequently colonic polyps can be removed at the time of initial colonoscopic identification.

Endoscopic techniques are relatively precise in defining many problems, but the limitations of these tools as well as the continued advantages of x-ray studies in some situations should be recognized. Endoscopic tools are not useful in assessing gastrointestinal (GI) motility, which may be more accurately gauged by barium studies. In addition, some areas, notably the small intestine, remain relatively inaccessible to fiberoptic instruments. In hospitals where endoscopy is not feasible, the upper GI series and barium enema remain good diagnostic modalities for the upper and lower GI tract especially when air-contrast techniques are employed. However, they should generally be avoided in the patient with GI bleeding or suspected bowel obstruction. In addition the physician must exercise judgment in preparing the patient for these studies, recognizing that cathartics may markedly worsen the condition of a patient with obstructing lesions or colitis.

Although endoscopy has obviated the need for many conventional GI x-rays, other radiologic imaging modalities have assumed a crucial role in the approach to the patient with gastrointestinal symptoms. These techniques include ultrasound (US), computed tomography (CT), and magnetic resonance imaging (MRI). The application of these tools to the liver and biliary tract is discussed in Chap. 262. Both US and CT are useful in the delineation of abdominal masses. CT, though more expensive, is often more effective in the evaluation of the lower abdomen, where inflammatory masses in patients with Crohn's disease or complications of diverticular disease may be accurately imaged. However, US is an effective and generally less expensive tool for the evaluation of the right upper quadrant including the gall bladder and biliary tract. These techniques are often complementary in the evaluation of pancreatic disease. In combination with Doppler analysis, US can be used to assess the patency and direction of blood flow in the portal vein in the patient with advanced liver disease. MRI may permit exquisitely accurate information on the anatomic extent of invasive rectal cancers and blood flow in patients with vascular disorders, but the full range of its uses in GI disorders remains to be delineated. More-sophisticated CT and MRI equipment can actually permit the performance of digital angiography without the invasive catheterization necessary in conventional visceral angiography.

Finally, one must emphasize that the optimal use of endoscopic and radiologic imaging techniques also depends on the recognition that each modality has inherent limitations. Only the clinician can determine whether the information is sufficient to establish or exclude a diagnosis in a patient with relevant historical and/or physical findings and a negative or nondiagnostic study. Was the preparation of the patient or the examination of sufficient quality to have detected an abnormality if present? Was the examiner aware of the important diagnostic considerations, and was the study adapted to address those concerns? Conversely only the physician can determine whether irregularities found in diagnostic studies are indeed causally related to the patient's symptoms. This judgment usually relies upon a sound understanding of the biologic basis of gastrointestinal disorders.

DIAGNOSTIC APPROACHES   Abdominal pain   Determination of the cause of abdominal pain remains an imposing clinical challenge. As noted above, a spectrum of disorders from the acute and catastrophic to the chronic and indolent causes abdominal pain. Furthermore, differential diagnostic considerations may encompass diseases extrinsic to the gastrointestinal tract per se including disorders

of the genitourinary tract (e.g., pelvic inflammatory disease) and the peritoneum as well as alterations of the various constituents of the GI tract. The history and physical examination are essential guides to a sensible diagnostic approach to the broad potential array of disorders causing abdominal pain. The primary goal to be achieved through initial approaches to the patient is the distinction between an urgent problem requiring expeditious delineation and nonacute disorders. In the former, initial clinical impressions based on the history and physical examination can be further refined through routine laboratory tests such as a complete blood test and differential as well as plain films of the abdomen. Particular features will dictate the appropriateness of urgent US or CT examination or the need to proceed directly with emergency exploratory laparotomy. In the patient with a longstanding and relatively stable problem, diagnostic evaluation is undertaken in a more considered time frame. The clinician may be able to reasonably establish a functional basis for the complaint on the strength of the history and physical examination alone. Radiologic contrast studies, other imaging modalities (e.g., US, CT), or endoscopic examination may be appropriate to exclude or identify the gamut of disorders discussed above. If all these approaches prove inadequate to determine the cause of the patient's symptoms, more unusual causes of abdominal pain may have to be excluded through specific urine or blood tests (e.g., porphyrins).

Problems of swallowing   The approach should be as follows:

1 *Thorough determination of the nature of dysphagia.* Is the difficulty primarily in swallowing liquids, solids, or both? The location of the difficulty from the patient's perspective and presence or absence of accompanying odynophagia are important to ascertain. These historical clues are complemented by careful visual and neurologic examination of the oropharynx when appropriate.

2 *Routine esophageal x-rays* in the upright and lateral or Trendelenburg position. The horizontal views are essential for demonstration of the swallowing mechanism, unaided by gravity, and of the esophagogastric junction. For details of the pharyngoesophageal area cineradiography is necessary because of the rapidity with which the contrast medium passes through. Hiatus hernia is extremely common (in 15 to 35 percent of persons over 50) and often asymptomatic unless spontaneous reflux of gastric contents can be demonstrated to occur repeatedly. Careful attention is usually needed to detect lower esophageal rings or webs, which may be visible as indentations in the barium column only from a limited angle.

3 *Esophagoscopy.* This procedure is desirable to describe lesions suggested by x-ray or, if the lesion is unsuspected, to obtain biopsies from masses or abnormal mucosa and to obtain washings for exfoliative cytologic study. The diagnoses of peptic esophagitis and Barrett's esophagus are made endoscopically. Endoscopy is the most sensitive technique for identifying esophageal or gastric varices, although they are seldom important in the absence of hemorrhage. Fiberoptic instruments with US probes at their tip may ultimately become established as the most useful diagnostic tools for particular problems of the esophagus (and other sites of the GI tract), but instruments remain costly and continue to undergo significant technological evolution so that the ultimate role of so-called endosonography remains uncertain.

4 *Manometric studies* of the upper esophagus, particularly in conjunction with cineradiography. At present, this procedure offers the best differential between disorders primarily in the central nervous system, primary pharyngeal muscular disease, and cricopharyngeal dystonia. Manometry of the lower esophagus is useful in the diagnosis of diffuse esophageal spasm, achalasia, and infiltrative diseases that can alter esophageal motility.

Peptic or digestive disorders   The approaches to these disorders include:

1 *Insertion of a nasogastric tube.* This is used to establish whether significant gastric retention (more than 75 mL of gastric contents

in the fasting state) exists and whether there is acid, bile, blood, or other material in these contents. If pyloric obstruction or gastric atony is present, the tube is used to maintain suction while the patient's electrolyte and fluid balance is restored to normal; the stomach is kept as clean as possible so that reliable diagnostic investigation may be carried out.

2 *Upper intestinal endoscopy.* This procedure is most helpful in identifying the diffuse mucosa in gastritis or, together with biopsy and brushings for cytology, in differentiating between peptic and neoplastic ulcerating lesions. It may identify a specific bleeding site in clinical situations where several potential bleeding sites could exist, such as in the patient with portal hypertension. In addition, it may be possible to cauterize or otherwise intervene to control hemorrhage with the endoscope (e.g., injections of vasoconstricting agents such as epinephrine). The frequent association of gastritis with *Helicobacter pylori* in patients with nonulcer dyspepsia, as well as in those with actual peptic ulceration, has been well documented, even if its true role in the pathogenesis of these disorders remains uncertain. Nevertheless, at this time, *H. pylori* infection can be most reliably documented in the individual patient by endoscopy and biopsy. Endoscopy can detect a number of potential sources of upper GI bleeding which are often missed by x-ray studies (e.g., erosive gastritis, Mallory-Weiss syndrome). Gastroscopy is particularly helpful in inspecting the postoperative stomach, especially in detecting stomal ulceration or so-called alkaline reflux gastritis. The first and second portions of the duodenum can also be routinely examined with the fiberoptic gastroscope, and important information about ulcers and other lesions can be obtained by this procedure. Radiologic studies may be useful when endoscopy is not readily available or in the assessment of suspected motility disorders (e.g., gastroparesis). In addition, radiologic examination may be preferred when there are contraindications to safe endoscopy.

3 *Gastric acid secretory studies.* Though not routinely necessary, these are useful in the diagnosis of the Zollinger-Ellison syndrome or atrophic gastritis and for determination of completeness of vagotomy. Suspected gastric carcinoma is better diagnosed directly through gastroscopy and biopsy than indirectly through acid secretory studies (achlorhydria). These studies should not be obtained for the routine diagnosis of uncomplicated duodenal ulcer. There is no convincing evidence that acid studies are useful in determining the type of surgery for duodenal ulcer.

Obstructive and vascular disorders of the small intestine When intestinal problems present as obstructive syndromes, the plain x-ray of the abdomen is the most important diagnostic adjunct to careful physical examination. Patterns of dilatation of individual loops of intestine may be characteristic, as in volvulus or acute pancreatitis; erect and decubitus views will often show fluid levels in the affected segments. Motility disorders of the small intestine (temporary ileus or chronic intestinal pseudoobstruction) may also present with obstructive symptoms and similar x-ray findings but must be managed medically without surgical intervention. Air under the diaphragm is diagnostic of a perforated viscus; air in the portal vein usually results from intestinal necrosis secondary to mesenteric vascular occlusion. The diagnostic accuracy of the plain x-ray in all types of intestinal obstruction is about 75 percent. In patients with symptoms of incomplete obstruction, the radiographic small-bowel series will often be diagnostic in defining the site and degree of obstruction. Infrequently, in this setting, all conventional x-ray studies are unremarkable. In such cases, the radiologist may perform a small-bowel enteroclysis study by passing a special tube into the proximal jejunum; the rapid instillation of barium through the tube will distend the intestine and often reveal subtle lesions missed by other tests.

Vascular diseases of the small intestine are among the most difficult diseases to diagnose. In chronic mesenteric ischemia, radiographic, endoscopic, and laboratory tests are usually normal. Early in the course of acute mesenteric ischemia, the plain film of the abdomen

may be unremarkable despite complaints of severe abdominal pain. In these settings, prompt mesenteric angiography is essential in confirming the diagnosis of vascular disease.

Inflammatory and neoplastic diseases of small and large intestine Patients with these conditions are usually identified by history, physical examination, and careful examination of the stools for exudate and blood. Examination of fresh stool samples for common bacterial pathogens and parasites by laboratories skilled in these techniques is important in identifying or excluding infectious causes of diarrhea, particularly in the patient with colitis. Sigmoidoscopy is valuable in identifying mucosal and neoplastic lesions of the lower 25 cm of the colon. The mucosal surface of the entire colon and terminal ileum can be examined directly and biopsied through the fiberoptic sigmoidoscope or colonoscope. The radiologic examination of the small intestine is highly reliable in identifying the prestenotic and stenotic lesions of Crohn's disease. In the colon a single barium enema examination in a well-prepared patient has a diagnostic accuracy of 80 to 85 percent; the addition of air-contrast technique brings the accuracy up over 90 percent, but none of these figures is meaningful if the patient is poorly prepared for the examination, and the cecal area is hard to examine adequately because of its anatomy. Colonoscopy may be preferable for its greater accuracy and the capability to remove the vast majority of polyps as well as to obtain preoperative tissue confirmation in the patient who probably has cancer. The immunologic assay for the carcinoembryonic antigen has not proved to be specific for colonic cancer; nevertheless, it does contribute to the detection of residual or recurrent disease in postoperative patients.

Peroral biopsy of the small intestine and forceps biopsy of the rectosigmoid are of considerable importance in revealing mucosal disease. Rectal biopsy is an excellent means of demonstrating amyloidosis, schistosomiasis, and amebiasis. Submucosal disease is not seen in these superficial biopsies. Hirschsprung's disease is histologically diagnosed by a deep surgical biopsy of the lower part of the rectum.

Malabsorption syndromes Malabsorption may be suspected on the basis of history and physical examination and is confirmed by examination of the stools. Radiologic examination is of general help in ruling out local lesions and suggesting motor and secretory dysfunction, but it is rarely diagnostic unless an abnormal small-bowel mucosa or fistulas between intestine and stomach are demonstrated.

The tests useful in the diagnosis of malabsorption are discussed in Chap. 254. A simple screening test for excessive fat in the stools can be accomplished by the microscopic examination of a stool specimen stained with Sudan. Chemical analysis of 3-day stool collection for fat, with the patient on a standard diet, is used to establish the diagnosis of steatorrhea. The D-xylose absorption test is about 90 percent accurate in separating mucosal disease from pancreatic insufficiency. Peroral biopsy of the small intestine via the endoscope or a specialized biopsy device is of value in the diagnosis of celiac disease, and it may show the less common infiltrations of the mucosa by amyloid or bacterial mucoproteins (Whipple's disease). Leakage of protein into the intestinal lumen may cause hypoproteinemia and can be demonstrated by the recovery in stools of the serum protein α_1-antitrypsin or intravenously administered markers such as albumin labeled with iodine or chromium isotopes.

Pancreas The pancreas is difficult to study directly because of its anatomic location and relative inaccessibility. Calcification of the pancreas on a plain abdominal film is highly suggestive of chronic pancreatitis and may be associated with fat malabsorption. Pancreatic exocrine insufficiency can be documented by intubation of the duodenum and collection of pancreatic juice after stimulation with secretin or a test meal. Abdominal US and CT are the best radiographic means of searching for pancreatic enlargement (see Chaps. 273 and 274). Both techniques may also be used to guide needle biopsies of the pancreas and may provide sufficient diagnostic information to obviate the need for exploratory surgery. The pancreatic duct can be cannulated via the fiberoptic duodenoscope and visualized by the injection of radiographic dye. Visualization of the duct may be helpful in the diagnosis of pancreatic pseudocysts, carcinoma, or chronic pancreatitis.

REFERENCES

JOHNSON LR et al: *Physiology of the Gastrointestinal Tract*, 2d ed. New York, Raven, 1987

SLEISENGER MH, FORDTRAN JS: *Gastrointestinal Disease*, 4th ed. Philadelphia, Saunders, 1989

YAMADA T et al: *Textbook of Gastroenterology*, Philadelphia, Lippincott, 1991

249 IMPACT OF CELLULAR AND MOLECULAR BIOLOGY ON GASTROINTESTINAL DISEASE

DANIEL K. PODOLSKY / KURT J. ISSELBACHER

In recent years, broad progress in biochemistry, cellular biology, and molecular biology has led to a better understanding of basic processes and in some instances their molecular alteration in gastrointestinal and liver diseases. This has been paralleled by newer approaches to diagnosis and treatment, increasingly dominated by medical rather than surgical interventions. While not attempting to describe all the recent advances in the cellular biology and molecular biology of the gastrointestinal tract, this chapter summarizes a number of those discoveries which are having an impact on the approach to the diagnosis and management of gastrointestinal disease.

CELL SURFACE RECEPTORS FOR SPECIFIC LIGANDS (NEUROTRANSMITTERS AND HORMONES) A seminal insight of the past two decades is the role of cell surface receptors in causing functional changes in response to diverse stimuli following binding of specific ligands. From this appreciation of receptor-ligand interaction has come the ability to develop agents that mimic ligands. If the agent binds and activates the receptor, agonist activity is observed; if it binds to but does not stimulate the receptor because it is structurally different from the natural ligand, antagonist activity results. The potential importance of this insight for the approach to disorders of the gastrointestinal tract is apparent when one considers how H-2 receptor antagonists have revolutionized the treatment of peptic ulcer disease.

The major functional properties of the gastrointestinal tract, including motility, secretion, absorption, growth, and proliferation, can be modulated by a variety of stimuli acting through cell surface receptors. The ligands capable of achieving important effects in this way include small amino acid derivatives (e.g., classical neurotransmitters), nucleotide derivatives (e.g., adenosine), and small to medium-sized peptides. While these regulatory ligands can be produced by any cell type, most are produced by neural and endocrine cellular elements.

As classically defined for endocrine hormone production and action, receptor-specific ligands may be released at a distance from the cellular targets expressing the receptor or close to its cellular targets, as in neural transmission. It is now recognized that some peptides, including many which modulate proliferation in the gastrointestinal tract, bind to receptors on the same cells as produce the growth factor (*autocrine* regulation) or to receptors on adjacent or nearby cells (*juxtacrine* and *paracrine* regulation, respectively).

The structural features of many important receptors in the gastrointestinal tract have been elucidated (Fig. 249-1). Most are members of a relatively small number of protein families. Within these families,

FIGURE 249-1 Cell surface receptors in the gastrointestinal tract. Three structurally distinct classes of cell surface receptors are especially important: (1) tyrosine kinase receptor, characterized by a single membrane-spanning domain of receptor in which the ligand binds to the extracellular domain and induces a tyrosine kinase activity present on either the intracellular portion of the same protein or present on another protein closely associated with the receptor (the latter kinase a member of the so-called nonreceptor tyrosine kinase family related to *src*); (2) ligand-gated ion channel receptors formed by the association of four or five separate subunits, each with approximately four membrane-spanning domains in which ligand binding alters the influx of specific ions through the channel formed by the subunits to result in a cellular response; and (3) single-chain receptors, which encompass seven membrane-spanning domains whose biologic activity following ligand binding is effected through interaction with a G protein complex. Examples of each class of receptor which play an important role in the gastrointestinal tract are indicated. (*After Logsdon.*)

RECEPTOR CLASS

Tyrosine Kinase (single membrane-spanning domain)

Ligand-Gated Ion Channel Receptor (4-5 subunits)

G Protein-Linked Receptor (7 membrane-spanning domains)

NH₂

COOH

LIGANDS IN GI TRACT

Epidermal Growth Factor
Transforming Growth Factor α
Fibroblast Growth Factors
Platelet-Derived Growth Factor

Catecholamines
Serotonin

Angiotensin
Gastrin-Releasing Peptide
Gastrin
Cholecystokinin
Histamine (H1 and H2)
Acetylcholine (muscarinic)
Neurotensin
Secretin
Somatostatin
VIP
Substance P
Peptide YY
Pancreastatin

individual members share significant structural similarities and mechanisms of signal transduction whereby ligand-receptor binding ultimately leads to changes in cellular function. Many receptors transmit an intracellular signal through association with guanosine triphosphate–binding proteins that possess GTPase activity. These *G protein–linked receptors* have seven membrane-spanning domains, and there is significant amino acid sequence similarity in the membrane-spanning domains of different receptors. This receptor class includes receptors for many nonpeptide neurotransmitters as well as many peptide ligands of the neuroendocrine network.

A second class of receptors in the gastrointestinal tract contains a single membrane-spanning domain and depends on tyrosine phosphorylation for signal transduction. Typically, these receptors are composed of a large extracytoplasmic domain and an intracellular cytoplasmic tail of varying length. In many instances, the cytoplasmic domain itself exhibits tyrosine kinase activity, generating an intracellular signal following ligand binding. In some receptor complexes, the tyrosine kinase activity may be present in a discrete cytoplasmic protein (nonreceptor tyrosine kinase) which associates with the receptor. In most instances, members of this class of receptor can phosphorylate specific residues within their own cytoplasmic domain, resulting in attenuation of receptor activity and thus a degree of autoregulation. Within the gastrointestinal tract, receptors of this class include those for various growth-regulatory peptides (e.g., epidermal growth factor, transforming growth factor α, insulin, and insulin-like growth factors). Other classes of receptors create an intracellular signal through either phosphokinase or phosphatase activities. Still other receptors are complexed to protein kinase C or enzymes which modulate the production of polyphosphinositides and related substances. The final effector steps in these pathways themselves may be quite diverse, including changes in membrane characteristics or the state of intramembrane proteins, changes in structural proteins, altered translation of mRNA, and/or, most important, changes in transcription of specific genes within the nucleus.

A third important class of surface receptors in the gastrointestinal tract encompasses ligand-gated ion channels. Interaction of a specific ligand with these receptors opens a channel that allows ions to enter the cell. In contrast to the G protein–linked and tyrosine kinase class of receptors, these receptors are composed of four or five separate, though homologous, subunits which form an aggregate that can create a central ion channel. Many neurotransmitters bind to ligand-gated ion channel receptors, e.g., nicotinic cholinergic receptors.

The recognition that there are families of receptors with structural homologies has allowed the identification of important receptors by molecular cloning without prior knowledge of their specific structural features. The type of signal-coupling mechanism involved in a particular cell response (e.g., G protein–coupled) can be ascertained by means of signal-pathway–specific analogues or inhibitors. The result allows a reasonable inference of the general structural class to which the receptor belongs. The presence of highly conserved segments among members of a particular class of receptor has made possible the molecular cloning of the receptors through the powerful polymerase chain reaction (PCR) technique utilizing oligonucleotide primers that correspond to the conserved sequences (Fig. 249-2A). This approach has led to the identification of receptors for a number of neurotransmitters in gastrointestinal tissues, including those for serotonin and histamine (notably the H-2 receptor, which is central to gastric acid secretion). The isolation of cDNA clones encoding these receptors provides the primary amino acid sequence from which structural characteristics can be inferred.

PCR in principle permits the identification within a given tissue mRNA of any member of a receptor family from which primers (e.g., "generic" for a class of receptor) have been prepared. It has led to the recognition that there are multiple receptor subtypes for many regulatory molecules, including at least three classes of muscarinic receptors and as many as five or more serotonin receptor subclasses within the neural and smooth-muscle components of the gastrointestinal tract. In some instances the isolation of multiple subclasses of structurally distinct receptors could be anticipated either from ligand-binding studies or by variability in the functional responses of different cells to different ligand congeners. In other instances the heterogeneity was unanticipated and has led to the appreciation of previously unrecognized distinctions in the functional effects of a ligand at different sites within the gastrointestinal tract. The importance of these insights into neurotransmitter and hormone receptors extends beyond giving us an expanded understanding of the physiology of these tissues, promising to help development of therapeutic agents that can selectively target one of the functional properties of a broadly important regulatory molecule such as acetylcholine or serotonin.

An alternative approach utilizing different molecular biologic techniques has allowed the characterization of other important receptors in the gastrointestinal tract (Fig. 249-2B). In these approaches, transfection of DNA-encoding genes expressed in a gastrointestinal tissue into a mammalian cell line capable of transcribing and translating that genetic information leads to the presence of the specific receptor on those cells which receive a segment of DNA encoding the receptor of interest. These cells can be identified by their acquired ability to bind the peptide of interest. The transfected DNA responsible for the appearance of specific peptide binding in the recipient cells can be reisolated and the features of the receptor evaluated by determination of its nucleotide sequence and in turn its amino acid sequence. This powerful approach has been effective in the study of receptors for diverse hormones, including gastrin and cholecystokinin.

It is likely that, by these approaches, the receptors of many or all of the known important regulatory peptides within the gastrointestinal tract will soon be identified and characterized. Most important, determination of the structural features of receptors, including those elements responsible for specific ligand binding, may facilitate rational design of agents that will either inhibit or augment the effects of regulatory hormones and other molecules.

SIGNAL TRANSDUCTION AND GENE REGULATION (See also Chap. 69) As knowledge of the structure of cell surface receptors has accumulated, considerable advances have been made in the identification and characterization of the intracellular mechanisms which couple the ligand-receptor binding to cellular response. Multiple pathways have been identified. In many instances there is significant overlap in the use of these pathways in association with different receptors; i.e., a single receptor may interact with more than one intracellular signaling pathway, and a given pathway may be activated (or inactivated) by association with different receptors in a single cell. Major signaling pathways include (1) those utilizing GTP-binding proteins, in which activation/inactivation of signal transduction is associated with hydrolysis of GTP to GDP; (2) those utilizing cAMP generated by an associated adenyl cyclase activity; (3) serine/threonine O-phosphorylation, which may be effected by the cytoplasmic portion of the receptor itself or a structurally discrete kinase; (4) tyrosine O-phosphorylation, which also may be found as an intrinsic activity of the receptor or reside in a nonreceptor tyrosine kinase (homologous to the first member of this family to be identified, c-*src*); (5) generation of polyphosphinositides resulting from the other protein kinase C and phospholipase; and (6) Ca^{2+}, whose intracellular concentration can be modulated directly or indirectly by a variety of factors, including the mediators generated by other signaling pathways.

The features of these various pathways have been elucidated in increasing detail, as exemplified by (1) the key role of ADP-ribosylation, which may be specifically inactivated by subunit B of pertussis toxin in modulating G protein–dependent signaling, and (2) the role of autophosphorylation of receptors by their intrinsic tyrosine kinase activity, leading to downregulation of the activated receptor's activity. The features of the G protein receptor-effector complex, seemingly the most prevalent receptor complex paradigm in the gastrointestinal tract, is illustrated in Fig. 249-3 (and also in Fig. 69-3). However, important details remain to be understood about each of these pathways; e.g., the full range of substrate proteins phosphorylated by a specific receptor kinase has not been delineated and in no instance has a complete sequence of events been determined

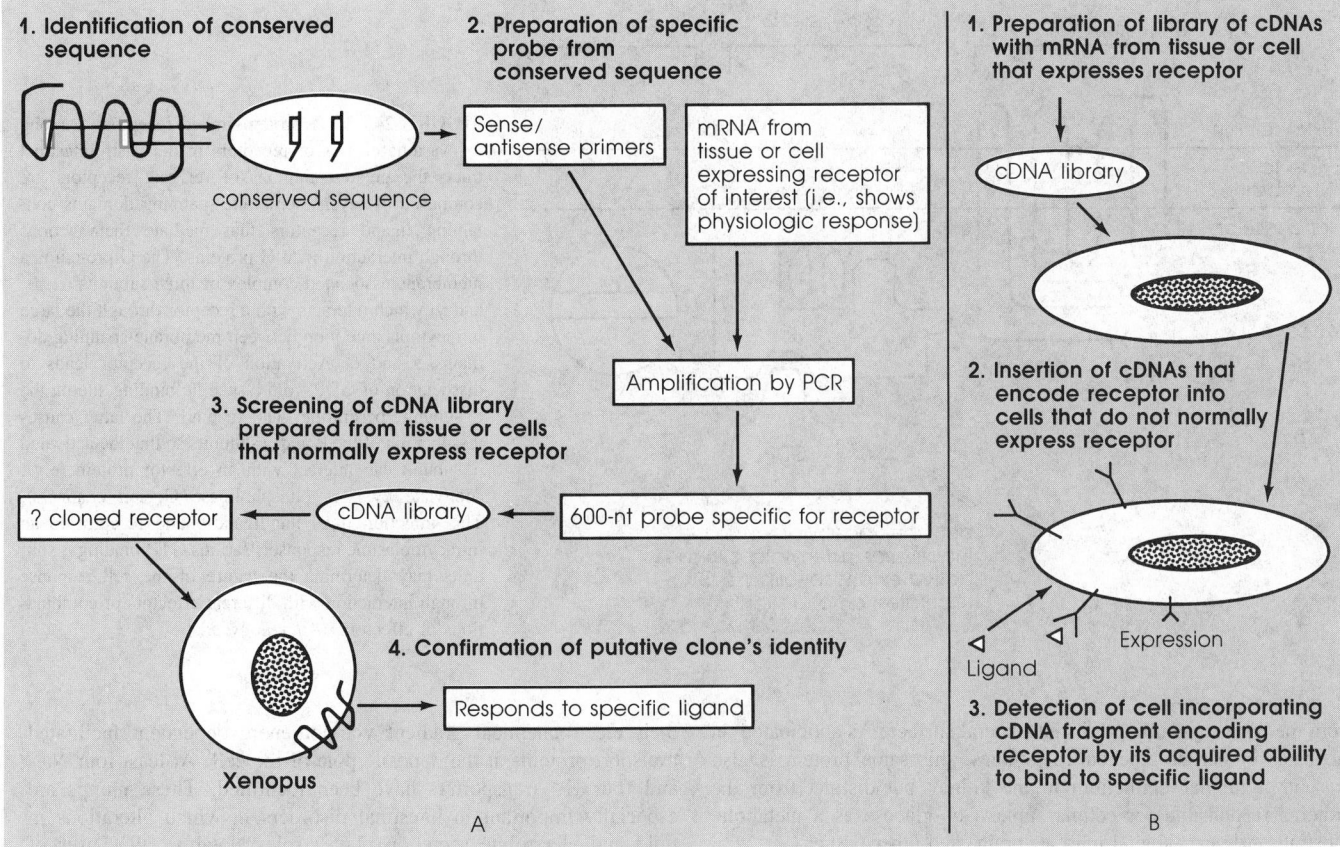

FIGURE 249-2 Experimental strategies for the isolation of specific receptors. *A.* Molecular cloning on the basis of structural conservation. Within receptor classes the amino acid sequence is highly similar in particular regions (e.g., within each corresponding membrane-spanning domain in the G-coupled receptor family). With a nucleotide primer based on these sequences and utilizing the polymerase chain reaction and mRNA from a tissue or cell known to express the receptor of interest, a nucleotide probe is obtained. The amplified probe, which will encompass sequences unique to the specific receptor, can then be used to identify clones within a cDNA library which encode the receptor protein. The validity of the isolated cDNA clones can be tested by introducing the DNA by a vector into a cell that does not bear the receptor and watching for responsiveness to the appropriate ligand. *B.* Molecular cloning on the basis of ligand binding. Complementary DNA is prepared from mRNA obtained from a tissue or cell known to express a specific receptor. The DNA is introduced (transfected) into mammalian cells capable of transcribing and translating introduced genetic material (designated an *expression cloning system*). The cells within this system that receive the DNA encoding the specific receptor can be identified by the specific binding of radioactively labeled ligand to their cell surface.

through which receptor activation leads to alteration in gene transcription in the nucleus. Nonetheless, it has been possible to determine the key signaling pathways involved in many cellular responses to important stimuli in the gastrointestinal tract through a variety of approaches, including the use of selective inhibitors to block cellular responses, e.g., pertussis toxin blockade of pancreatic response to secretin.

Progress in this area has been especially important in understanding the mechanism of toxin-mediated injury of many gastrointestinal tract pathogens, including cholera, *Clostridium difficile*, enterotoxigenic *E. coli*, and *Shigella*. These insights, in conjunction with studies of basic mechanisms of nutrient and electrolyte transport (see below), provide a rational basis for development of several important therapies, as exemplified by oral-based rehydration solutions. Studies of pathways involving receptors, signal transduction, and eventual alteration in gene transcription have served as a foundation for insights into the molecular basis of tumor formation in the gastrointestinal tract, particularly the colon (see below). This progress follows from the recognition that these pathways are utilized by various growth stimuli, including peptide growth factors, and the appreciation that alteration of any step in this pathway which converts one component to its growth-activating state will lead to a tonic growth stimulus with a high potential for promoting neoplasia. Thus corresponding oncogenes have been found for each component of these pathways.

CARRIER AND TRANSPORT PROTEINS/ION PUMPS   Absorption and secretion are the central functions of the gastrointestinal tract and its accessory organs. At the cellular level, these functions are accomplished through specialized proteins which transport nutrients, ions (and corresponding passive movement of water), and other special molecules across the epithelial cells which form the mucosal surface throughout the gastrointestinal tract. Over the past few years, molecular biologic approaches building on insights gained through earlier biochemical studies have finally led to identification and direct characterization of various transport proteins.

Molecular cloning of the genes encoding nutrient transport proteins has been accomplished by approaches similar to those useful in the molecular cloning of surface receptors. Injection of mRNA or a DNA copy from enterocytes or other cells into cells which normally do not express a given transporter (typically the large egg cells of the frog, *Xenopus laevis*) can be used to verify that the sample encodes the protein of interest by the appearance of the transport activity in the injected cells. These approaches, in conjunction with conventional biochemical techniques, have demonstrated active Na^+-coupled glucose uptake at the microvillar membrane in the initial process of concerted absorption of glucose. Five structurally distinct glucose transport proteins have been identified that are expressed by various tissues, including two proteins (designated GLUT2 and GLUT5) responsible for the efficient facilitated transport of this key nutrient

FIGURE 249-3 G protein–linked receptors. Among the various classes of receptors in the gastrointestinal tract, the greatest number of relevant receptors are composed of seven membrane-spanning domains containing ligand receptors that mediate their actions through interaction with G proteins. The G protein is a membrane-associated complex of three subunits (α, β, and γ) which interacts with a receptor through the large intracytoplasmic loop between membrane-spanning domains 5 and 6. Activation of the receptor leads to dissociation of GDP from a specific binding site on the α subunit, permitting GTP to bind. The latter causes dissociation of the β and γ subunits so that the activated α subunit can interact with an effector protein (e.g., adenylate cyclase, phospholipase C, ion channels). This infection links the ligand-bound receptor to an intracytoplasmic response. Various GTP-binding α subunits may determine the nature of the cell response through interaction with different effectors or combinations of effectors. (*After Logsdon.*)

from the enterocyte through its basolateral surface. As anticipated on the basis of earlier biochemical studies, this same protein is also present in tubular epithelium in the kidney but distinct from the proteins responsible for cellular uptake of glucose as a metabolic substrate in liver, skeletal muscle, brain, and other tissues.

With the molecular cloning of both types of glucose transporters, key structural features have become apparent, including the presence of 12 membrane-spanning domains which can form a channel through which the hexose traverses the lipid bilayer. This has provided a coherent view of the mechanisms responsible for glucose absorption through energy-dependent sodium-coupled glucose at the microvillar surface and the transfer of the absorbed glucose from the enterocyte by the non-energy-dependent facilitated transporters present at the basolateral surface. The transport proteins for other mono-, di-, and trisaccharides have been isolated by similar approaches, and it is likely these techniques also will allow characterization of amino acid transporters to yield a comprehensive understanding of the molecular basis of the absorption of the major nutrients.

Different approaches have led to an appreciation of the absorption of fatty acids liberated from dietary triglyceride by lipase from luminal micelles and their reesterification and association with apoprotein within the enterocyte prior to secretion as chylomicrons from the basolateral surface. Molecular cloning has identified the features of the fatty acid–binding protein present within enterocytes which is essential to this process as well as the nature of the apoproteins necessary for chylomicron formation. Interestingly, the intestinal form of the apoprotein (apoB48) is distinguished from its hepatocyte counterpart (apoB100) by the presence of a distinctive stop codon in the gene generating a protein truncated at its carboxy terminus. Molecular cloning techniques also have led to the identification and characterization of the binding and transport proteins which are necessary for the uptake of key vitamins such as vitamin B_{12} and folate.

Considerable progress has been made in understanding the fundamental basis of electrolyte uptake and secretion, which are essential functions throughout the gastrointestinal tract. Biochemical studies have provided kinetic characterization of the energy-dependent transport of the key cations Na^+, K^+, and H^+ as well as the important anions Cl^- and HCO_3^-. In general, active transport is accomplished against electrochemical concentration gradients through the hydrolysis of ATP by ion-coupled ATPases. Transport of ions across epithelial cells is completed by the passive movement of intracellular ions down their electrochemical gradient via non-energydependent facilitated transport proteins at the opposite pole of the cell. At least four Na^+ and four K^+ transporters have been identified. These pumps are especially important in intestinal disorders in which alterations in fluid and electrolyte secretion play a role. Notably, all causes of diarrhea may ultimately be related to excess net secretion of Cl^- and secondary net water movement. Conversely, an awareness that one of the most abundant pumps for Na^+ couples uptake of this cation with glucose forms the mechanistic rationale for fluid replacement in cholera and other so-called secretory diarrheal states (see Chaps. 39 and 254). Another indication of the therapeutic importance of understanding ion transport is made evident by the characterization of the H^+ pump (actually an H^+, K^+ ATPase) present at the parietal cell canalicular membrane in gastric mucosa which generates gastric acid secretion. Targeting of agents to block this pump (e.g., omeprazole) has proven an especially effective approach to control gastric acid secretion in the treatment of acid-dependent disorders, including reflux esophagitis and the Zollinger-Ellison syndrome (see Chaps. 251 and 252).

CELLULAR AND MOLECULAR BASIS OF DIGESTION AND SECRETION Extensive studies using both sophisticated morphologic and biochemical techniques have led to a detailed understanding of the structural basis of the highly specialized features of the enterocyte essential for its function in the digestion and absorption of nutrients and maintenance of mucosal integrity in the face of a complex mixture of potentially noxious substances in the lumen. These features include an extensive array of apical microvilli formed by several proteins (actin, myosin, fimbrin, talin, and others) which are coupled by a circumferential ring containing actomyosin linked to tight junctions at the lateral surface near the apical pole. These tight junctions between adjacent enterocytes provide the barrier necessary to maintain the integrity of the mucosa. The molecular details of most of the proteins which form these tight junctions have yet to be elucidated. It is possible that alterations in the structure and function of these tight junctions play a role in disorders of the gastrointestinal tract.

The enterocyte also makes an important contribution to mucosal immune function through the secretion of IgA into the lumen. Molecular approaches have clarified some features of the pathway responsible for secretion of IgA. These include uptake of dimeric IgA produced by plasma cells in the lamina propria by a specific receptor which is itself a member of the immunoglobulin protein superfamily on the basolateral surface of the enterocyte. Subsequently, the receptor-IgA complex is internalized and transported within the cell to the apical surface, where the dimer, in association with a fragment of the IgA receptor–designated secretory component resulting from proteolytic cleavage, is secreted into the lumen. These advances will undoubtedly serve as a foundation for understanding the mechanistic basis of the protective role of secretory IgA.

MOLECULAR CHARACTERIZATION OF VIRAL PATHOGENS Many of the most important disorders of the gastrointestinal tract and liver are the result of viral infection. Molecular biologic approaches have been especially productive in advancing understanding of common viral hepatitides, including infection resulting from hepatitis A, B, C, D, and E viruses. Molecular characterization has led to improved understanding of the pathogenesis of hepatitis B virus infection. The molecular sequence of the entire hepatitis B virus genome has been determined. Beyond the important information that molecular approaches have yielded in understanding the structure of HBV, these advances have facilitated the development of valuable vaccines by recombinant techniques. The impact of molecular biology on progress in the understanding, diagnosis, and treatment of viral hepatitis is considered in detail in Chap. 266.

BENIGN AND MALIGNANT NEOPLASIA Significant advances have been made in the understanding of tumorigenesis in the colon and liver using the tools of molecular biology. These observations include the detection of a variety of oncogenes among different colon tumors, both benign polyps and cancers, e.g., *ras* and *src*. However, additional insights have resulted from the study of the relatively rare familial adenomatous polyposis which have served to illuminate molecular mechanisms of neoplasia essential to the more common sporadic colon cancer. Using genetic markers scattered throughout the genome in combination with the technique of restriction-fragment length polymorphism, it was possible to assess whether a tumor contained both parenteral alleles for each genetic marker. This led to the demonstration that this familial disorder was associated with the germline loss of a copy of a presumptive tumor suppressor gene on the long arm of chromosome 5. Similar loss of allelic heterogeneity at other loci including chromosomes 17p and 18q also has been found in various sporadic tumors. The specific genes at these various sites whose loss is related to tumor formation have been identified and found to encode a variety of different types of protein products, including a presumptive cell adhesion molecule and a nuclear transcription factor (p53). Familial forms of colon cancer have been found to be associated with a germline mutation of a specific tumor suppressor gene (see Chap. 257).

While it is likely that other genetic alterations, including activation of oncogenes and inactivation of tumor suppressor genes, will be found to contribute to the development of some colonic neoplasia (and tumors at other sites of the gastrointestinal tract), important general concepts have already emerged from these observations. Malignant tumor formation appears to result from the accumulation of a critical aggregate number of genetic alterations rather than from a specific combination or order of genetic changes. The various genes which may be altered in different tumors encode diverse protein products. Variability in the biologic characteristics of tumors in different individuals (e.g., early invasion versus rapid local expansion) may be related to the profile of the genetic alterations. Many of these same genetic loci, especially those encoding oncogenes, have been implicated in the development of malignancies in the esophagus, stomach, pancreas, and liver. The interface between inherited genetic alterations and acquired mutations resulting from environmental factors has been highlighted by the study of hepatocellular carcinoma. In addition to the appreciation of the potential role of HBV acting as an insertional mutagen due to integration of the virus into the host genome, molecular analysis of hepatocellular carcinoma has shown mutation of a tumor suppressor gene with a chemical carcinogen. Thus aflatoxin, a chemical present in foodstuffs contaminated with *Aspergillus*, which has long been implicated by epidemiologic studies, has been demonstrated to be associated with a specific mutation of

the p53 tumor suppressor gene in some hepatocellular carcinomas in South Africa and China.

LABORATORY DIAGNOSIS AND FUTURE THERAPEUTIC APPROACHES The techniques of cellular and molecular biology in conjunction with new insights into specific diseases have already yielded powerful new diagnostic tools which aid the clinician. PCR, a technique which can detect even a single copy of a specific DNA molecule, has made possible a marked increase in the sensitivity and specificity of diagnostic detection of viral and other infectious agents. The development of monoclonal antibodies emerging from progress in cellular biologic studies has provided reagents for both serologic diagnosis and more precise morphologic analysis through immunohistochemistry and immunocytochemistry. The latter is occasionally essential in the determination of the origin of a seemingly undifferentiated tumor, particularly lymphomas of the gastrointestinal tract. In situ hybridization, a technique in which specific mRNA rather than protein can be localized within cells, promises to further enhance this capability. Finally, molecular probes encoding specific gene sequences or sequences linked with disease-associated loci are making possible genetic screening for inherited disorders (e.g., familial adenomatous polyposis) in members of affected kindreds. Although the HLA alleles which could be evaluated by specific antisera or monoclonal antibodies have been helpful in determining inheritance of disorders which are linked to these genes on chromosome 6 (e.g., hemochromatosis), disease-related genes elsewhere can only be assessed through markers scattered throughout the genome, which is feasible with collections of DNA probes.

One of the most profound outgrowths of recombinant DNA techniques is the identification and production of important regulatory proteins. A large network of cytokines, broadly defined as proteins that affect the functional characteristics of target cell populations, has been identified as the product of lymphocytes, monocytes, and other cell populations. Cytokines affect processes as diverse as immune activation, cell proliferation, fibrosis, and other functions. Recombinant interferons, a class of cytokines, have made these immunomodulatory proteins available for the treatment of chronic viral hepatitis. Recombinant forms of several other cytokines such as interleukin 1 receptor antagonist, macrophage inhibitory proteins, and transforming growth factor β are being explored for their effects on various inflammatory conditions of the gastrointestinal tract. In addition, considerable interest has focused on a number of growth factors, members of this cytokine network, for their potential importance in facilitating healing of mucosal ulceration and adaptation following resection or infarction of large segments of intestine. It is possible that growth factors may be employed to facilitate intestinal reconstitution following high-dose chemotherapy or radiation treatment for malignancy in a manner similar to the use of stem cell factors to restore hematopoietic function.

The most important impact of advances in molecular biology on gastrointestinal disease may ultimately lie in gene therapy, the introduction of DNA sequences with sustained function to correct an aberration or absence of a relevant gene. The liver will be an important target organ for these innovative approaches both because of its central role in the metabolic processes affected by many inherited disorders and because of the feasibility of targeting DNA to the hepatocytes. The use of DNA coupled to glycoproteins specifically taken up by hepatocyte has already demonstrated the feasibility of introducing DNA sequences with subsequent production of functional proteins (albumin, HMG CoA-reductase). While a number of significant hurdles remain, it is likely that the ability to introduce genetic information in a stable fashion into hepatocytes and other cells will lead to fundamentally new approaches to the treatment of disease of the liver and gastrointestinal tract as well as more systemic disorders.

REFERENCES

CADENA DL et al: Receptor tyrosine kinases. FASEB J 6:2332, 1992
ESCHER JC et al: Molecular basis of lactase levels in adult humans. J Clin Invest 89:480, 1992

GANTZ I et al: Molecular cloning of a gene encoding the histamine H2 receptor. Proc Natl Acad Sci USA 88:429, 1991

HIGUCHI K et al: Human apolipoprotein B (apoB) mRNA: Identification of two distinct apoB mRNAs, an mRNA with the apoB-100 sequence and an apoB mRNA containing a premature in-frame translational stop codon, in both liver and intestine. Proc Natl Acad Sci USA 85:1772, 1988

KOPIN AS et al: Expression cloning and characterization of the canine parietal cell gastrin receptor. Proc Natl Acad Sci USA 89:3605, 1992

LOGSDON CD: Receptors: Cell and molecular biology. Reg Peptide Lett 3:37, 1991

TAYLOR GR, FARMERY SM: Single gene disorders affecting the gastrointestinal tract. Gut 34:433, 1993

WILSON JM et al: Hepatocyte-directed gene transfer in vivo leads to transient improvement of hypercholesterolemia in low density lipoprotein receptor-deficient rabbits. J Biol Chem 267:963, 1992

250   GASTROINTESTINAL ENDOSCOPY

MICHAEL B. KIMMEY / FRED E. SILVERSTEIN

Fiberendoscopes have revolutionized the examination of the gastrointestinal tract. Because of the flexibility of the fiberoptic bundles and the controllability of the instrument tip, the operator can steer the instrument around multiple bends under visual control. A channel permits passage of a variety of endoscopic tools such as biopsy forceps, cytology brushes, wash tubes, and electrocautery snares. The viewing window and the light at the instrument's distal end can be washed free of obscuring material. Fluid can be aspirated from hollow organs, and air can be insufflated as needed to improve visualization. The videoendoscope is a modification of the fiberendoscope in which a charge-coupled device on the distal tip of the instrument transmits the image onto a TV screen. This system is being used increasingly because it permits storage, analysis, and transmission of the endoscopic images.

The usefulness of fiberendoscopy in diagnosing gastrointestinal disease is well established. Shallow lesions such as erosions or healing ulcers are missed by single-contrast x-ray but not by endoscopy. The brilliant success of polypectomy via the colonoscope has led to the development of other endoscopic therapeutic techniques such as endoscopic sphincterotomy; endoscopic therapy is now a recognized alternative to surgery in many situations.

Although esophagogastroduodenoscopy (EGD) is not a procedure for the occasional operator, it is widely available in both inpatient and outpatient settings. It is a relatively easy procedure to perform technically, but training and continued experience are necessary for optimal diagnostic accuracy. The more complex procedures such as colonoscopy and endoscopic retrograde cholangiopancreatography (ERCP) require special dexterity, a substantial investment of time for learning, and constant practice to maintain adequate skill; they are probably best accomplished by subspecialists. Complications are most frequent when the operator is inexperienced.

A history and physical examination should be done before any endoscopic procedure. Special care is taken in patients with significant cardiac or pulmonary disease; blood clotting parameters should be checked in those with a history of excessive bleeding. Patients with prosthetic heart valves and those with a history of bacterial endocarditis should receive antibiotic prophylaxis. Contraindications to endoscopy in most situations include the inability of the patient to cooperate or give informed consent, an unstable cardiac or pulmonary condition, and an unstable neck prior to upper endoscopy. Intestinal perforation is also a contraindication to any endoscopic procedure.

Most patients and endoscopists prefer to use conscious sedation for endoscopic procedures other than flexible sigmoidoscopy and some screening upper endoscopies. After insertion of an intravenous catheter, a benzodiazepine such as diazepam or midazolam is titrated to light sedation. Supplementation with a narcotic such as meperidine also may be useful. Adequate monitoring of vital signs and oxygen saturation is important, as is the availability of resuscitation equipment.

Topical pharyngeal anesthesia with a gargle or spray of lidocaine or similar anesthetic is useful prior to upper endoscopic procedures.

UPPER GASTROINTESTINAL ENDOSCOPY   The tip of a forward-viewing endoscope is placed at the cricopharyngeal sphincter of the esophagus, and the patient is encouraged to swallow while gentle pressure is exerted. Small amounts of air are passed through the endoscope to visualize the esophageal lumen. The endoscope is then passed under direct vision into the stomach. The gastric body and antrum are carefully examined. The instrument tip is retroflexed to view the gastric cardia, the fundus, and the whole lesser curvature. The pylorus is traversed, and the first and second portions of the duodenum are visualized. The examination is repeated as the instrument is withdrawn. Visualized lesions can be recorded on photographs or videotape. Biopsies and brush cytologic examinations can be obtained from suspicious areas.

EGD is a relatively safe procedure in experienced hands. Several large surveys suggest a risk of serious complications during diagnostic EGD of approximately 1 in 500 and a risk of death of approximately 1 in 10,000. The risks are higher in emergency procedures and in the elderly or seriously ill. In a survey of patients examined by endoscopy during bleeding, 1 in 200 had serious complications and 1 in 700 died from the procedure. The main causes of mortality were cardiopulmonary complications and perforations by the instrument. Endoscopy is preferred over x-ray in the urgent diagnosis of gastrointestinal illness in women who might be pregnant.

Gastroesophageal reflux disease   Esophagitis is one of the most common diseases of the upper gastrointestinal tract (see Chap. 251). Esophageal pain may be confused with cardiac disease, or esophagitis may present as painless blood loss. Because esophagitis usually involves only the superficial mucosa, it cannot be diagnosed by routine single-contrast radiography. At endoscopy, friable mucosa, linear erosions, and ulcerations are clearly visible. Not every patient with heartburn requires esophagoscopy, but the procedure is indicated if the patient complains of dysphagia; if an x-ray shows a stricture, a mass, or an ulcer; if symptoms persist despite therapy; or if antireflux surgery is contemplated. Patients over age 40 with significant complaints of heartburn for over 10 years should be considered for endoscopy to detect Barrett's esophagus.

The squamous mucosa of the esophagus is more vulnerable to peptic digestion than is the columnar epithelium of the stomach. Thus esophagitis is located on the squamous side of the esophagogastric junction and is most severe in the distal esophagus, where the squamous mucosa is most exposed to regurgitated acid and pepsin from the stomach. Discrete peptic ulceration of the esophagus is uncommon.

A short area of esophagitis or a stricture can be seen even in the upper esophagus. This is explained by progressive replacement of distal eroded squamous mucosa with metaplastic epithelium, which is more resistant to peptic digestion (Barrett's epithelium). This finding can be documented by biopsy. Such epithelium is more prone to malignant transformation and, therefore, may merit regular surveillance with esophagoscopy and biopsy every 12 to 24 months. Flow cytometry also may prove useful in the early detection of abnormal cell DNA populations (e.g., polyploidy). If dysplasia is present, more frequent surveillance may be indicated to detect early carcinoma.

Esophagitis may progress to scarring and stricture formation. The endoscopic appearance of a benign stricture is characteristic but not diagnostic; a malignancy should be ruled out by biopsy and cytologic brushing before medical treatment is undertaken with dilation and antacids. The whole length of the stricture should be sampled. Endoscopy is also indicated to biopsy the rim of an esophageal ulcer to rule out cancer.

Dilations of difficult strictures are best initiated by passing a flexible-tipped guidewire via the biopsy channel of the endoscope through the stricture under direct vision. The endoscope can then be withdrawn over the wire, which serves as a guide for passage of progressively larger polyvinyl dilators through the stricture under fluoroscopic control. An alternative technique utilizes balloon catheters passed via the endoscope channel or over a guidewire through the stricture. The balloon is inflated under endoscopic and/or fluoroscopic guidance to dilate the stricture.

Peptic ulcer Esophagogastroduodenoscopy is more accurate than upper gastrointestinal x-ray in detecting ulcers. It has been suggested that x-ray be abandoned entirely in favor of endoscopy for detecting ulcers. This makes sense when the source of acute upper gastrointestinal bleeding is sought and urgent surgical intervention is being considered. However, in the workup of the patient with less pressing ulcer complaints, a double-contrast upper gastrointestinal x-ray is still often used as the initial diagnostic test. The greater expense and discomfort of endoscopy are justified if the x-ray is equivocal or suggests that the ulcer is malignant, if the x-ray is negative but the clinical picture suggests peptic ulceration, or if the patient is about to be operated on for ulcer. Patients with duodenal ulcers shown by x-ray or with classic ulcer deformities of the duodenal bulb do not require endoscopy for diagnosis if the presenting symptoms are characteristic and if the symptomatic response to antiulcer treatment is good. Screening endoscopy using small-diameter endoscopes without sedation is a reasonable alternative to contrast x-rays as the initial diagnostic test in the symptomatic patient.

There are some situations in which x-ray reveals ulcers missed by endoscopy, e.g., ulcers in hourglass constrictions of the stomach or in small, incompletely visualized duodenal bulbs. Fiberendoscopy is especially useful in visualizing postbulbar ulcers, giant duodenal ulcers, and stomal ulceration after partial gastrectomy, all of which can be missed by x-ray. Endoscopy may be of use in determining the cause of gastric outlet obstruction.

In the enthusiasm for fiberendoscopy one must not forget that visual interpretation of gross pathology is subjective—one observer's ulcer is another's erosion. An erosion is confined to the mucosa and heals without a trace, whereas an ulcer is deeper and usually implies a chronic recurrent disease. Endoscopically, erosions are superficial, small, and multiple; ulcers are deeper and larger and tend to be solitary. As indicated above, visualized lesions can readily be recorded as photographs or on videotape.

Cancer The endoscopic appearance of upper gastrointestinal cancer may seem obvious, especially if there is a mass growing into the lumen. On the other hand, malignant ulcers, infiltrative carcinomas, or small early carcinomas are frequently impossible to diagnose by their gross appearance. Six to eight biopsies should be taken from the rim of a gastric ulcer to exclude malignancy. Experience and skill in choosing the biopsy site improves the accuracy. A cytologic examination of lavage or brush specimen adds to the diagnostic accuracy in all areas of the upper gastrointestinal tract (see Chap. 253).

In most patients, gastric ulcers should be assessed for healing by endoscopy after 12 weeks of antiulcer therapy. Persistent ulcers should be biopsied if they were not biopsied at the time of the initial diagnosis or they should be rebiopsied if they are not healing. Some patients with a low likelihood of malignancy, for example, a young person taking anti-inflammatory drugs, can be assessed for healing radiographically. Duodenal ulcers are rarely malignant and therefore do not need to be assessed for healing following therapy in most circumstances.

Primary gastric lymphoma can mimic benign gastric ulcer or adenocarcinoma on gastroscopy or x-ray. It can be diagnosed by biopsy or cytology, although the accuracy is not as high as in adenocarcinoma. The diagnosis of lymphoma is aided by special studies of fresh, unfixed biopsy specimens to detect a clonal population of lymphocytes.

If a polypoid lesion of the stomach is covered by mucosa that appears normal by gastroscopy, the likelihood of malignancy is very small. Such lesions are often intramural, subepithelial benign tumors such as leiomyomas or pancreatic rests. Biopsies of such lesions are usually not diagnostic. Lesions over 2 cm in diameter can be evaluated by endoscopic ultrasonography, a technique that combines diagnostic

ultrasound with endoscopy. Polyps covered by abnormal-appearing mucosa can be benign or malignant. Random biopsy can miss carcinoma within a polyp. If technically feasible, polyps should therefore be removed in their entirety by snare cautery for histologic examination. If over 2 cm in diameter, they are more likely to contain cancer (see Chap. 253). Large polyps may require surgical excision.

Ampullary carcinoma may be diagnosed by biopsy during duodenoscopy, although a prior endoscopic sphincterotomy may increase diagnostic yield. Other primary duodenal malignancies are very rare. Extensions from pancreatic or biliary tract cancer are difficult to diagnose because the tumor may not have extended into the mucosa and may therefore not be accessible for endoscopic biopsy or cytologic examination. In these secondary tumors, diagnosis must depend on some combination of echography, computed tomography, and ERCP with cytologic examination of ductal strictures.

Upper gastrointestinal bleeding (See also Chap. 41) Endoscopy within the first 12 to 24 h of an upper gastrointestinal hemorrhage can be very helpful in planning rational therapy by visualizing the bleeding source. Superficial lesions not visible by x-ray may be seen (esophagitis, Mallory-Weiss tear, erosive gastritis, stress ulcer, and telangiectasia). Lesions that are visible by x-ray may not be the source of bleeding. Endoscopy can determine the actual bleeding site and degree of bleeding. For example, visualization of a spurting artery which is flooding the stomach indicates massive ongoing bleeding requiring prompt therapeutic intervention. Several studies have shown that the demonstration at endoscopy of any bleeding whatsoever or a nonbleeding vessel or sentinel clot in the ulcer base makes rebleeding more likely. The diagnostic accuracy of emergency endoscopy in upper gastrointestinal bleeding approaches 90 percent.

Every patient having endoscopy for upper gastrointestinal bleeding merits a complete endoscopic examination of the esophagus, stomach, and duodenum. Finding a potential bleeding lesion is not proof that this is the source of hemorrhage unless active bleeding is seen. Up to 50 percent of patients with esophageal varices can be shown endoscopically to be bleeding from another source such as erosive gastritis, duodenal ulcer, or gastric ulcer. Occasionally it is not possible to diagnose the exact lesion that is bleeding, but localizing the area of bleeding can be very helpful; for example, bright red arterial blood may be seen pouring into the stomach from the duodenum when the esophagus and stomach are relatively free of blood.

There are three controversial areas. First, *do all bleeders need endoscopy?* Endoscopy is indicated in all patients who may require surgery because of continual bleeding or rebleeding because selection of the type of operation depends on what lesion is bleeding. Although 85 percent of upper gastrointestinal bleeders stop spontaneously, it is impossible to predict which ones will; therefore, endoscopy is recommended for most bleeders. Second, *how early should endoscopy be performed in the acutely bleeding patient?* Most studies suggest that the diagnostic accuracy of EGD remains high for the first 12 to 24 h after the bleeding episode. All would agree to delay endoscopy until vital signs have be blood replacement. Upper endoscopy i waking hours at a time during the fi patient's vital signs are stable and w available. Emergency endoscopy at n patients with continued massive ble immediate decision regarding surge is exsanguinating, endoscopy ca preceding surgery. Thus the endotracheal tube. Finally, do come? Earlier studies that did no that it does not. Recent studies of the lesions with heater probes and bipola methods are safe and reduce blood require and mortality in some patients with bleeding u

Injection therapy of bleeding lesions is another thera used to stop bleeding. Injection of a dilute solution of epi alone or followed by injection of either alcohol or a sclerosing agent often stops active bleeding from peptic ulcers. Injection of various sclerosing solutions into or next to esophageal varices is effective treatment for stopping active variceal bleeding. Alternatively, rubber band ligation of varices at endoscopy has been shown to stop bleeding. Repeated injection sclerotherapy or band ligation to achieve variceal eradication produces results comparable to portacaval shunting in terms of mortality, although rebleeding after endoscopic therapy may necessitate further endoscopic intervention or shunting.

Emergency and therapeutic endoscopy is not for the inexperienced. It requires considerable technical skill and interpretive experience and the best available instruments.

Percutaneous endoscopic gastrostomy   The placement of feeding or decompression gastrostomy tubes can be facilitated with the use of an endoscope. Under sedation, the endoscope's light within the stomach is used to identify a suitable location for a gastrostomy in the left upper quadrant of the abdomen. A needle is introduced into the stomach percutaneously, and then a snare passed through the endoscope is used to capture a wire or suture placed through the needle. A feeding tube is advanced over the wire into the stomach. Feedings are begun the following day. Hospitalization time and morbidity and mortality of operative gastrostomy are reduced.

Patients with transfer dysphagia secondary to strokes and degenerative neurologic disorders benefit the most from percutaneous endoscopic gastrostomy. Other indications include dysphagia produced by head and neck neoplasms and the inability to eat secondary to diffuse cerebral injury. Patients with severe gastroparesis can be fed through a jejunal feeding tube placed through the gastrostomy and then directed through the pylorus. Simultaneous gastric decompression is possible through a separate lumen in the gastrostomy.

Palliation of esophageal carcinoma   Patients with dysphagia caused by malignant esophageal strictures usually cannot be cured by esophagectomy. Surgical resection and radiation therapy are often chosen for palliation of dysphagia in this situation. The endoscopist also can help palliate these patients when radiation therapy has failed or when surgical risks are too great.

Dilation of malignant strictures is usually possible with polyvinyl dilators passed over an endoscopically placed guidewire. It may improve the patient's swallowing initially, but more definitive therapy is usually needed. This can be in the form of laser ablation or by placement of a prosthesis or stent. Tumor within the esophageal lumen can be destroyed by application of Nd:YAG laser energy using a laser waveguide placed through the biopsy channel of the endoscope. Alternatively, after stricture dilation, large-caliber stents can be placed over a dilator. When the dilator is removed, the stent lumen is available for the passage of food. Stenting is especially useful in the palliation of malignant tracheoesophageal fistulas.

Other indications   Upper endoscopy is usually substituted for x-ray in the urgent diagnosis of gastrointestinal illness in *pregnancy*. Pati___ ___ _ysphagia merit esophagoscopy because the cause is ___ ___ may be missed by x-ray. Dysphagia caused ___ ___ is best diagnosed by manometry or ___ ___ endoscopy. *Painful swallowing* (odyno-___ ___suppressed or diabetic patients, may ___ ___iopsy and brushings of the involved ___ ___ilial, herpetic, or cytomegalovirus ___ ___ a corrosive agent, if there is no ___ ___ gentle esophagoscopy is useful ___ ___ impacted foreign bodies ___ ___ch with a snare or ___ ___ually best removed by pulling ___ ___ tubular esophagoscope or into a ___ ___eroptic endoscope. Careful esophago-___ ___esophageal foreign body is important to ___ ___ is an underlying lesion which caused the ___ ___cer, benign stricture, peptic esophagitis). ___ ___operative stomach, gastroscopy is especially useful in ___ carcinoma, recurrent ulceration, retrograde intussusception,

and stomal stricture. Several European studies indicate a definite threat of carcinoma developing in the gastric stump 10 to 20 years after a Billroth II gastrectomy. The diagnosis of such postoperative carcinomas may require many biopsies of seemingly normal mucosa near the anastomosis. Studies of the natural history of this condition in the United States do not suggest a similar high incidence of postoperative carcinoma.

When the duodenal bulb shows reddening or nodularity, many endoscopists diagnose *duodenitis*. There is little evidence to suggest that this picture is of significance. On the other hand, diffuse and bleeding erosions of the duodenal bulb merit a diagnosis of *erosive duodenitis*, especially after ingestion of mucosal irritants such as aspirin. A nodular or narrow duodenum will occasionally yield granulomas on biopsy, indicative of Crohn's disease.

ENDOSCOPIC RETROGRADE CHOLANGIOPANCREATOGRA-PHY   ERCP involves placing a side-viewing instrument in the descending duodenum. The papilla of Vater is cannulated, contrast medium is injected, and the pancreatic ducts and hepatobiliary tree are visualized radiographically. Skilled operators can visualize 90 to 95 percent of pancreatic ducts and 90 percent of biliary ducts.

ERCP is performed on an x-ray table after sedation and induction of duodenal hypotonia with atropine or glucagon. The pancreatic duct is gently filled throughout its entire length with 2 to 5 mL of contrast material with constant fluoroscopic monitoring (Fig. 250-1A). Injection is continued until the first side branches are seen, and overfilling is avoided. By insertion of the cannula at a more acute cephalad angle, the common bile duct and the whole biliary tract including the gallbladder are visualized (Fig. 250-1B).

ERCP is a safe procedure when performed by an experienced operator. Asymptomatic amylase elevations occur in 30 to 40 percent of patients after pancreatography and are rarely of clinical significance. Pancreatitis occurs in less than 5 percent of patients but is usually benign and self-limited. In a nationwide survey of complications, the morbidity rate was 3 percent and mortality rate 0.2 percent. The main serious complication is retention of nonsterile contrast material proximal to an obstructed duct, causing cholangitis or pancreatic sepsis. Patients suspected of having bile duct obstruction are started on systemic antibiotics prior to the ERCP. Furthermore, if bile duct or pancreatic duct obstruction is first revealed by ERCP, antibiotic coverage is indicated to reduce the incidence of bacteremia; such patients should be drained, if possible, either with endoscopic therapy (papillotomy, stents, nasobiliary drains, etc.) or surgically within 36 h.

Retrograde cholangiography   This procedure is especially useful in patients with persistent jaundice the cause of which cannot be established by conventional diagnostic methods. The important differential diagnosis is between obstructive and nonobstructive jaundice. When the cause of jaundice is unclear, approximately 15 percent of patients thought to have nonobstructive jaundice prove to have extrahepatic biliary obstruction requiring surgery or endoscopic therapy, and conversely, the same percentage of patients thought to have obstructive jaundice prove to have an open ductal system by ERCP and can be spared unnecessary intervention.

Remediable causes of obstructive jaundice which can be diagnosed by retrograde cholangiography include common duct stones (Fig. 250-1C) and benign and malignant strictures. In jaundiced patients with suspected primary liver disease, such as primary biliary cirrhosis, ERCP can assure that no operable obstruction is being missed.

In addition to ERCP, other methods of visualizing the biliary tree in the jaundiced patient include *percutaneous transhepatic cholangiography* (PTC), in which contrast material is injected from the exterior via a needle into the intrahepatic bile ducts under fluoroscopic control, and the noninvasive methods of *ultrasound*, *computed tomography* (CT), and radionuclide biliary scintigraphy (see Chap. 262). Most physicians first use ultrasound or CT to see whether the biliary ducts are dilated and to seek the cause of the patient's jaundice (stones, pancreatic mass, etc.). The radionuclide scan will determine if the cystic duct and bile ducts are patent. Direct visualization is undertaken if the diagnosis is not established. PTC is

FIGURE 250-1 *A.* A tapering pancreatic duct of normal caliber is seen and may be compared to the endoscope (E) 1 cm in diameter. *B.* Normal cholangiogram. The diameter of the common duct (CBD) is normal. The intrahepatic ducts branch normally, and the gallbladder (GB) can be seen. The endoscope (E) is seen in the duodenum. *C.* Several stones (*arrows*) can be seen in an obstructed, dilated common duct. The gallbladder also contains several stones. Regurgitated contrast material is seen in the duodenum (D). *D.* The sharp cutoff (*arrow*) of the pancreatic duct is caused by a carcinoma of the body of the pancreas. (*Courtesy of Dr. Charles Rohrmann.*)

often attempted first if an intrahepatic or proximal bile duct obstruction is suggested by imaging tests. ERCP is used first if distal obstruction is suspected. Advantages of the endoscopic approach are that the papilla and the pancreatic duct are seen (in addition to the biliary ducts) and that therapy can be performed with endoscopic sphincterotomy or drainage when appropriate. In the event of a technical failure or incomplete information resulting from either ERCP or PTC, the other technique is tried. This approach detects most lesions requiring surgical intervention.

ERCP or PTC also can be useful in patients with biliary pain, cholangitis, or impaired liver function after previous biliary surgery. Remediable postoperative lesions such as strictures can be discovered and sometimes treated endoscopically. Should endoscopic therapy fail, their precise anatomy is outlined so that reoperation is less difficult. Biliary manometry also can be performed in this setting to

diagnose sphincter of Oddi dysfunction. A perfused catheter is placed into the sphincter via the endoscope, and pressures are recorded. A high basal sphincter pressure may predict a beneficial effect of sphincterotomy.

Retrograde pancreatography Patients with recurrent or chronic pancreatitis may merit retrograde pancreatography to seek a lesion which can be approached endoscopically or surgically, such as localized pancreatitis in the tail or ductal pathology amenable to endoscopic stenting or surgical drainage.

Patients with symptoms, signs, or laboratory findings suggesting pancreatic carcinoma may have pancreatograms suggesting malignancy with a narrowed, encased, or sharply ''cut off'' pancreatic duct (Fig. 250-1*D*). Differentiation of such pancreatic ductal findings from benign inflammatory disease can be difficult. Cytologic examination of pancreatic duct brushings obtained during ERCP may prove helpful.

Unfortunately, most patients with symptomatic pancreatic cancer diagnosed by ERCP are inoperable.

Patients presenting with painless steatorrhea of pancreatic origin may be shown to have a ductal pattern suggesting chronic pancreatitis or pancreatic carcinoma. Pancreatography has not been useful in the study of obscure upper abdominal pain. Pancreatic cysts can be better diagnosed by noninvasive techniques such as ultrasound, and pancreatography should be reserved for those cases where it is desirable to outline the anatomy immediately prior to surgery. Pancreatography alone is not a reliable method of screening for early pancreatic carcinoma.

Therapeutic ERCP Access to the pancreatic and biliary tree for the removal of stones and the placement of stents is made possible by endoscopic retrograde sphincterotomy (ERS). The pancreatic or biliary sphincter mechanism is cut using electrosurgical current passed through a wire attached to the ERCP catheter. Complications of bleeding, perforation, pancreatitis, and cholangitis occur in about 8 percent of patients with a resulting mortality rate of approximately 1 percent. The role of pancreatic sphincterotomy in the management of pancreatic stones and strictures is evolving; however, biliary sphincterotomy is now an established therapy for several conditions.

Common bile duct stones in patients with prior cholecystectomy are successfully removed from the bile duct after ERS by experienced operators 90 percent of the time. Small stones are pulled into the duodenum with a balloon catheter or after being captured by a basket. Stones larger than 1.5 cm in diameter may be difficult to extract without prior fragmentation by mechanical or other techniques. Common duct stones in younger patients with intact gallbladders have traditionally been removed at the time of cholecystectomy. However, with the increasing popularity of laparoscopic cholecystectomy, endoscopic stone removal is being utilized in this setting as well. Older patients with increased surgical risks can sometimes be managed with ERS and stone extraction alone; cholecystectomy can be delayed or avoided entirely. ERS is also assuming an increasing role in the initial treatment of patients with acute cholangitis and severe biliary pancreatitis. Early endoscopic stone removal in both these settings has been shown to reduce complications associated with these conditions.

Patients with benign and malignant bile duct strictures may benefit from the endoscopic placement of biliary stents after ERS. Benign strictures frequently remain dilated following removal of stents that have been left in place for several months. Patients with either pancreatic carcinoma or cholangiocarcinoma resulting in obstructive jaundice can be palliated effectively by placement of a plastic or metal biliary stent. Stents usually occlude after 3 to 6 months and must be exchanged if recurrent jaundice or cholangitis develops. Strictures involving the hilum of the liver (see Chap. 272) are difficult to palliate endoscopically; stents sometimes must be placed into both sides of the liver. These patients may require additional percutaneous radiologic procedures to achieve adequate biliary drainage.

COLONOSCOPY The interior of the entire length of the colon from anus to cecum can be visualized by the experienced colonoscopist. This is one of the most significant diagnostic and therapeutic applications of fiberoptic endoscopy because it can diagnose potentially curable colonic cancers missed by other techniques and remove potentially precancerous adenomatous polyps.

Most initial colonoscopies are performed to investigate findings on an abnormal barium enema or to elucidate the cause of gastrointestinal bleeding. The ability to examine the whole colon is also useful in the management of some patients with inflammatory bowel disease and in patients with a strong family history of colon polyps or cancer.

Patients are prepared for colonoscopy with laxatives and tap water enemas or by a total-gut lavage with a nonabsorbable electrolyte solution.

The main complications of colonoscopy are hemorrhage and perforation (morbidity rate is 0.5 to 1.3 percent; mortality rate is 0.02 percent). The complication rate for polypectomy is 1 to 2 percent. Diverticular or ischemic disease and prior irradiation make the procedure more difficult and hazardous. The risk of perforation is also increased in the patient with very active colitis, and colonoscopy should be avoided during the acute phase in most circumstances.

Polyps (See also Chap. 257) A polyp seen on barium enema merits colonoscopy for two reasons: It may be an artifact or a cancer, and a second polyp or cancer may have been missed. The polyp can usually be excised, with lower morbidity and mortality rates than with surgery. The best way to rule out cancer within a polyp is to remove it completely for histologic examination. Hyperplastic polyps do not become malignant; colonic polyps that show benign neoplasia histologically may become malignant (tubular and villous adenomas). The risk of neoplastic polyps being cancerous increases with their size. The risk is also higher in villous adenomas. Pedunculated polyps with cancer confined to the mucosa and with an uninvolved stalk can be cured by removal with an electrocautery snare during colonoscopy. Thus most colonoscopists will remove all polyps more than 0.5 cm in diameter. Polyps smaller than 0.5 cm in diameter should be biopsied or removed because more than 50 percent may be adenomatous, and the gross appearance of a polyp does not predict its histology. The wisdom of this course of action is suggested by a sigmoidoscopic study in which the removal of all polyps reduced the expected incidence and invasiveness of subsequent cancers in the anatomic area screened. Most agree that the patient with adenomatous polyps is more likely to develop another polyp or cancer and therefore merits a regular screening program. The optimal frequency of follow-up examinations after polypectomy is not yet established. The current recommendation is a digital examination and stool test for occult blood yearly. When a polyp is discovered, the entire colon should be examined for synchronous polyps or cancer. This should probably be repeated at 3- to 5-year intervals and more frequently in patients with a history of colon cancer or multiple polyps. If stools are positive for occult blood or symptoms develop, immediate evaluation is indicated.

Abnormal barium enema All filling defects on barium enema merit evaluation by colonoscopy. If the lesion is a pedunculated polyp, it can be removed for histologic examination; if its appearance suggests a cancer, it can be biopsied for histologic confirmation. When a polyp or a carcinoma is found, the remainder of the colon should be screened for additional polyps and synchronous carcinoma. This avoids multiple colotomies to search for a second lesion and reduces surgical morbidity. Some lesions diagnosed as a mass by x-ray may not be present on colonoscopy or are due to lesions such as a polyp rather than a cancer.

Narrowing by x-ray Determining the cause of segmental narrowing may be difficult by x-ray. Colonoscopy often permits this and also can help one differentiate adenocarcinoma from inflammation secondary to ischemia, irradiation, diverticular disease, or Crohn's colitis. Even the most classic "apple-core" lesion indicated by x-ray may be covered by normal mucosa at colonoscopy, suggesting an extrinsic inflammatory lesion. In 10 to 30 percent of patients, narrowed segments present on x-ray are not visualized during colonoscopy, probably because they are areas of temporary spasm. Such findings avoid unnecessary operations.

Chronic bleeding (x-ray and sigmoidoscopy negative) This is a common indication for colonoscopy. The x-ray is more likely to miss a lesion when single contrast is used rather than air contrast. The cause of bleeding is found in approximately 40 percent of such patients from such sources as adenomatous polyp, adenocarcinoma, and inflammatory bowel disease. If no bleeding source is found, a search may be appropriate for an upper gastrointestinal source with an upper gastrointestinal x-ray or upper endoscopy.

Inflammatory bowel disease Colonoscopy is not routinely indicated in patients with inflammatory bowel disease. Colonoscopy may help in the initial diagnosis, especially in differentiating Crohn's colitis from ulcerative colitis. It can aid the surgeon in assessing the activity and extent of the disease before surgery. Colonoscopy can help in the evaluation of radiographic abnormalities suggesting cancer, such as strictures, polyps, or masses. Colonoscopy may be indicated in patients with ulcerative colitis of more than 10 years' duration because of the increased risk of carcinoma; it is hoped that repeated colonoscopies will serve to detect these malignancies while the lesions are still curable. The optimal frequency of colonoscopy in such patients is not yet established. If an expert gastrointestinal pathologist finds high-grade dysplasia in colonic biopsies in a patient with long-standing ulcerative colitis, most would consider this to be an indication for colectomy. Colonoscopy is contraindicated in patients with toxic megacolon, very active disease, or a possible intestinal perforation.

Other indications The flexible sigmoidoscope is replacing the rigid 25-cm sigmoidoscope for routine screening because it can be passed to 40 to 60 cm with minimal preparation, less discomfort, and a higher diagnostic yield. After segmental colonic resection for carcinoma, colonoscopy may detect early mucosal recurrence and differentiate it from benign anastomotic strictures or bleeding suture granulomas. Colonoscopy is occasionally used during laparotomy to assist the surgeon in ruling out other lesions. The colonoscope can be advanced to the cecum rapidly with the surgeon's assistance and additional polyps removed without colotomy. Colonoscopy is useful in the management of selected patients with lower gastrointestinal bleeding. Patients with severe active bleeding are often managed with radionuclide-labeled red blood cell scans followed immediately, if active bleeding is present, by selective angiography. Colonoscopic visualization in this setting is difficult because of excessive luminal blood. If the labeled red blood cell scan is negative, colonic lavage with a balanced electrolyte solution followed in several hours by colonoscopy may identify the bleeding site. Bleeding polyps may be removed by snare electrocautery. Endoscopic hemostatic therapy may be useful in other bleeding lesions such as angiodysplasia.

Colonoscopy is usually not necessary for the diagnosis of familial polyposis because affected family members can be diagnosed by periodic flexible sigmoidoscopy. Carcinoma is a great threat in those familial polyposis syndromes which produce many adenomatous polyps (familial polyposis and Gardner's syndrome); in these conditions, polypectomy is useful for diagnosis, but colectomy is the only treatment which prevents development of carcinoma. These patients are also at risk of developing duodenal and periampullary cancer and should probably undergo periodic surveillance with a side-viewing duodenoscope.

CONSCIOUS DIAGNOSTIC LAPAROSCOPY The potentials for laparoscopy in conscious patients have not been as fully appreciated in North America as they have been in other countries, where it is used widely. This procedure has extremely low mortality and morbidity rates in experienced hands. The instrument usually used for laparoscopy is a rigid tube with a lens system that provides a superb view. Under local anesthesia, pneumoperitoneum is gradually induced with air or nitrous oxide.

Much of the exterior of the liver, gallbladder, spleen, peritoneum, diaphragm, and pelvic organs can be clearly visualized. Portions of the colon and small bowel also can be seen. Lesions can be biopsied under direct vision and any resultant bleeding controlled by electrocoagulation.

Laparoscopy may permit one to make a difficult diagnosis without resorting to laparotomy by biopsying localized hepatic disease under direct vision. Laparoscopy can often help differentiate nonobstructive from obstructive jaundice and also may enable staging of malignant disease without laparotomy.

REFERENCES

Cello JP et al: Endoscopic sclerotherapy versus portacaval shunt in patients with severe cirrhosis and acute variceal hemorrhage: Long-term follow-up. N Engl J Med 316:11, 1987

Cook DJ et al: Endoscopic therapy for acute nonvariceal upper gastrointestinal hemorrhage: A meta-analysis. Gastroenterology 102:139, 1992

Haggitt RC et al: Prognostic factors in colorectal carcinomas arising in adenomas: Implications for lesions removed by endoscopic polypectomy. Gastroenterology 89:328, 1985

Jensen DM, Machicado GA: Diagnosis and treatment of severe hematochezia: The role of urgent colonoscopy after purge. Gastroenterology 95:1569, 1988

Lai ECS et al: Endoscopic biliary drainage for severe acute cholangitis. N Engl J Med 326:1582, 1992

Laine L: Multipolar electrocoagulation in the treatment of active upper gastrointestinal tract hemorrhage. N Engl J Med 316:1613, 1987

Naveau S et al: Endoscopic Nd-YAG laser therapy as palliative treatment for esophageal and cardial cancer: Parameters affecting long-term outcome. Dig Dis Sci 35:294, 1990

Reid BJ etal: Flow cytometric and histologic progression to malignancy in Barrett's esophagus: Prospective endoscopic surveillance of a cohort. Gastroenterology 102: 1212, 1992

Silverstein FE, Tytgat GNJ: *Atlas of Gastrointestinal Endoscopy.* Philadelphia, Saunders, 1987

Sivak MV: *Gastroenterologic Endoscopy.* Philadelphia, Saunders, 1987

251 DISEASES OF THE ESOPHAGUS

RAJ K. GOYAL

The two major functions of the esophagus are the transport of the food bolus from the mouth to the stomach and the prevention of retrograde flow of gastrointestinal contents. The transport function is achieved by peristaltic contractions (see Chap. 37). Retrograde flow is prevented by the two esophageal sphincters, which remain closed between swallows. The upper esophageal sphincter remains closed by the elastic properties of its wall and by tonic contraction of the cricopharyngeus and inferior pharyngeal constrictor muscles due to continuous neural excitation of the lower motor neurons which innervate these muscles via motor end plates. The opening of the upper sphincter is due to inhibition of contraction of the cricopharyngeus and inferior pharyngeal constriction and forward displacement of the larynx by the suprahyoid muscles. In contrast, the lower esophageal sphincter remains closed largely because of its intrinsic myogenic tone. The lower esophageal sphincter is innervated by preganglionic parasympathetic fibers in the vagus nerve and postganglionic inhibitory and excitatory neurons in the wall of the esophagus that cause its relaxation and contraction, respectively. The neurotransmitters of the inhibitory nerves are vasoactive intestinal peptide (VIP) and nitric oxide. The antireflux function of the lower esophageal sphincter is supplemented by the diaphragmatic crura which surround the sphincter. A reflex decrease in the lower sphincter pressure occurs during the belching reflex and gastric distention. Fatty meals, smoking, and beverages with a high xanthine content (tea, coffee, cola) also cause a reduction in sphincter pressure. Many hormones and neurotransmitters can modify lower sphincter pressure. Cholinergic muscarinic (M-2 receptor) agonists, alpha-adrenergic agonists, gastrin, pancreatic polypeptide, substance P, and prostaglandin $F_{2\alpha}$ cause contraction; in contrast, nicotine, beta-adrenergic agonists, dopamine, cholecystokinin, secretin, VIP, calcitonin-gene–related peptide (CGRP), adenosine, and nitric oxide and nitric oxide donors such as nitrates cause relaxation of the sphincter. These effects are mediated by actions on the inhibitory intramural neurons or on the sphincter muscle directly. Effects of many of these agents are pharmacologic rather than physiologic.

SYMPTOMS

DYSPHAGIA See Chap. 37.

ESOPHAGEAL PAIN *Heartburn,* or pyrosis, is characterized by burning retrosternal discomfort that may move up and down the chest like a wave. When severe, it may radiate to the sides of the chest, neck, and angles of the jaw. Heartburn is a characteristic symptom of reflux esophagitis and may be associated with regurgitation or a feeling of warm fluid climbing up the throat. It is aggravated by bending forward, straining, or lying recumbent and is worse after meals. It is relieved by upright posture, by swallowing of saliva or water, or, more reliably, by antacids. Heartburn appears to be produced by heightened mucosal sensitivity and can be reproduced by infusion of dilute (0.1 *N*) hydrochloric acid (Bernstein test) or neutral hyperosmolar solutions into the esophagus.

Odynophagia, or painful swallowing, is characteristic of nonreflux esophagitis, particularly monilial and herpes esophagitis. Odynophagia also may occur with peptic ulcer of the esophagus (Barrett's ulcer), carcinoma with periesophageal involvement, caustic damage of the esophagus, and esophageal perforation. Odynophagia is unusual in uncomplicated reflux esophagitis. Crampy chest pain associated with impaction of a food bolus should be distinguished from odynophagia.

Atypical chest pain other than heartburn and odynophagia occurs in influx esophagitis or esophageal motility disorders such as diffuse esophageal spasm. This may occur spontaneously or during a meal. Chest pain due to periesophageal involvement caused by carcinoma or peptic ulcer may be constant and agonizing. Sometimes different types of esophageal pains exist together in the same patient, and frequently patients are not able to describe the pain accurately enough to allow its classification. Esophageal disease is a common cause of noncardiac atypical chest pain. However, many of these patients have nonspecific esophageal motor abnormalities. The cause-and-effect relationship of the nonspecific esophageal motor abnormalities and the atypical chest pain is unclear. Many of these patients have behavioral abnormalities, psychosomatic disorders, depression, anxiety, panic reactions, and other somatization disorders.

REGURGITATION   *Regurgitation* is the effortless appearance of gastric or esophageal contents in the mouth. In distal esophageal obstruction and stasis, as in achalasia or a large diverticulum, the regurgitated material consists of tasteless mucoid fluid or undigested food. Regurgitation of sour or bitter-tasting material occurs in severe gastroesophageal reflux and is associated with incompetence of both the upper and lower esophageal sphincters. Regurgitation may result in laryngeal aspiration, with spells of coughing and choking that awaken the patient from sleep, and aspiration pneumonia. Water brash is reflex salivary hypersecretion which occurs in response to peptic esophagitis; it should not be confused with regurgitation.

DIAGNOSTIC TESTS

RADIOLOGIC STUDIES   Barium swallow with fluoroscopy and esophagogram is the most widely used test for diagnosis of esophageal disease and can be used to evaluate both structural and motor disorders. The pharynx is examined to detect stasis of barium in the valleculae and piriform sinuses and regurgitation of barium into the nose and tracheobronchial tree. Since the oropharyngeal phase of swallowing lasts no more than a second, videofluoroscopy may be necessary to permit detection and analysis of abnormalities of oral and pharyngeal function. Spontaneous reflux of barium from the stomach into the esophagus should be sought in patients with suspected reflux esophagitis. Esophageal peristalsis is best studied in the recumbent position, since in the upright position the passage of most of the barium occurs by gravity alone. A double-contrast esophagogram, obtained by coating the esophageal mucosa with barium and distending the esophageal lumen with air using effervescent granules, is particularly useful in demonstrating mucosal ulcers and early cancers. Figures 251-1 and 251-2 illustrate the radiographic appearance of some esophageal disorders.

ESOPHAGOSCOPY   Fiberoptic esophagogastroduodenoscopy is described in Chap. 250. Esophagoscopy is the direct method of establishing the cause of mechanical dysphagia and of identifying mucosal lesions, such as superficial ulcers and esophagitis, which may not be identified by the usual barium swallow. In the presence of marked luminal narrowing, examination can be achieved by using a smaller-caliber endoscope, although on occasion a stricture must be dilated prior to a complete endoscopic examination. Transendoscopic biopsies are useful in diagnosing carcinoma, reflux esophagitis, or other mucosal diseases. Obtaining cells by scraping the mucosa with a Teflon brush during endoscopy may enable the cytologist to detect carcinoma.

ESOPHAGEAL MOTILITY   The study of esophageal motility entails simultaneous recording of pressures from different sites in the esophageal lumen. This is usually done with a train of three to four water-filled catheters connected to pressure transducers. The assembly is passed by mouth or nose through the esophagus into the stomach

FIGURE 251-1   Radiographic appearance of some motor disorders of the pharynx and esophagus. (1) Pharyngeal paralysis with tracheal aspiration (arrow). (2) Cricopharyngeal achalasia. Note the prominent cricopharyngeus, which is recognized by its smoothness and location in the posterior wall. (3) Diffuse esophageal spasm. Note typical corkscrew appearance of the lower part of the esophagus. (4) Achalasia showing dilated esophageal body with air-fluid level and closed lower esophageal sphincter. (5) Muscular (contractile) lower esophageal ring. Note a symmetric contraction in 5A that has disappeared in 5B, obtained during the same examination. (6) Scleroderma esophagus showing dilated esophagus with a stricture in 6A and reflux of barium from the stomach into the esophagus in 6B. *(Courtesy of Dr. Harvey Goldstein.)*

FIGURE 251-2 Selected structural lesions of the esophagus. (1) Carcinoma of the esophagus with typical annular narrowing with overhanging margins and destruction of the mucosa. (2) Leiomyoma of the esophagus with smooth filling defect and right angles of origin from the esophageal wall. (3) Esophageal ulcer in columnar-cell-lined esophagus (Barrett's esophagus). (4) Monilial esophagitis with irregular plaquelike filling defects. (5) Long stricture secondary to lye ingestion. (6) Peptic stricture, short and tubular, with associated hiatus hernia. (7) Mucosal lower esophageal mucosal (Schatzki) ring. Thin weblike annular constriction at the esophagogastric junction is associated with a small hiatal hernia. *(Courtesy of Dr. Harvey Goldstein.)*

and then gradually withdrawn 1 cm at a time until pressures from each centimeter of the esophagus and pharynx are recorded in between and during swallows. The upper and lower esophageal sphincters appear as zones of high pressure that relax on swallowing. The pharynx and esophageal body normally show peristaltic waves with each swallow.

Esophageal motility studies are very helpful in the diagnosis of achalasia, diffuse esophageal spasm and its variants, scleroderma, and other motor disorders of the esophagus, as well as neuromuscular disorders of the upper esophagus and pharynx (Fig. 251-3) but are of no value in the diagnosis of mechanical dysphagia. In patients with reflux esophagitis, esophageal manometry is useful in quantitating lower esophageal competence and providing information on the status of the esophageal body motor activity. The information obtained by manometry is quantitative and cannot be obtained by barium swallow or endoscopy.

Special tests for the evaluation of reflux esophagitis are described later.

MOTOR DISORDERS

STRIATED MUSCLE Pharyngeal paralysis Pharyngeal paralysis is characterized by dysphagia, nasal regurgitation, and tracheobronchial aspiration during swallowing. It occurs in a variety of neuromuscular disorders (see Table 37-2). Some of these disorders also may involve laryngeal and orofacial muscles. When the suprahyoid muscles are also paralyzed, the upper sphincter does not open with swallowing, leading to paralytic achalasia of the upper esophageal sphincter and severe dysphagia.

Barium swallow, oropharyngography, and cineradiography reveal stasis of barium in the valleculae and piriform sinuses, nasal and

FIGURE 251-3 Motility patterns in selected esophageal and pharyngeal disorders. In normal subjects, the upper and lower esophageal sphincters (UES and LES) appear as zones of high pressure. With a swallow (indicated by ↑), pressure in the sphincters falls and a contraction wave starts in the pharynx and progresses down the esophagus. In scleroderma, the lower part of the esophagus (smooth muscle) shows reduced amplitude of contractions, which may be peristaltic or simultaneous in onset, and hypotension of the lower sphincter. In achalasia, the lower part of the esophagus shows reduced amplitude of contractions that are simultaneous in onset. In contrast to scleroderma, the lower esophageal sphincter in achalasia is hypertensive and fails to relax in response to a swallow. In diffuse esophageal spasm, the lower part of the esophagus shows simultaneous onset, large amplitude, long duration, repetitive contractions. In polymyositis, the smooth-muscle part of the esophagus is normal. The skeletal muscle part shows reduced amplitude of contractions. The upper esophageal sphincter is hypotensive and may not relax normally on swallowing due to associated weakness of the suprahyoid muscles.

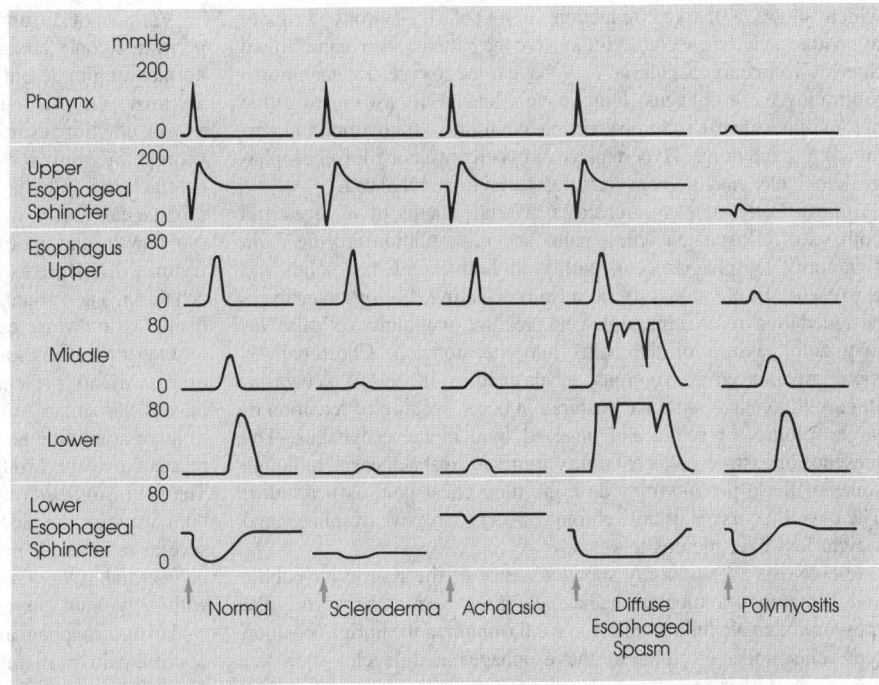

tracheobronchial aspiration, and closed upper sphincter (see Fig. 251-1). Pharyngeal motility studies demonstrate reduced amplitude of pharyngeal and upper esophageal contractions and reduced basal upper esophageal sphincter pressure without further relaxation on swallowing (see Fig. 251-3). Patients with myasthenia gravis and polymyositis respond to treatment for these diseases (see Chap. 386). Dysphagia in patients with cerebrovascular accident improves with time, although often not completely. Treatment consists of maneuvers to reduce pharyngeal stasis and enhance airway protection under the direction of a trained swallow therapist. Nasogastric tube feeding or endoscopically placed gastrostomy tube feeding may be needed for nutritional support. Cricopharyngeal myotomy is sometimes performed, but its usefulness is unproved. Extensive operative procedures to prevent aspiration are rarely needed. Death is often due to pulmonary complications.

Cricopharyngeal achalasia   Failure of the cricopharyngeus to relax on swallowing leads to a contracted cricopharyngeus, which appears as a prominent bar on the posterior wall of the pharynx on barium swallow (see Fig. 251-1). A transient cricopharyngeal bar is seen in up to 5 percent of subjects without dysphagia undergoing upper gastrointestinal studies; it can be produced in normal subjects during a Valsalva maneuver. When contraction is persistent, patients may complain of food sticking in their throats. Cricopharyngeal myotomy may be helpful, but it is contraindicated in the presence of gastroesophageal reflux because in such patients this procedure may lead to pharyngeal and pulmonary aspiration.

Globus pharyngeus   A sensation of a constant lump in the throat but with no difficulty during swallowing occurs especially in subjects with emotional disorders, particularly in women. Barium studies are normal, but manometry may show a hypertensive upper sphincter. Treatment is primarily one of reassurance.

SMOOTH MUSCLE   Achalasia   Achalasia is a motor disorder of the esophageal smooth muscle in which the lower esophageal sphincter is hypertensive and does not relax properly with swallowing, and the normal peristalsis of the esophageal body is replaced by abnormal contractions. Based on the changes in the esophageal body, achalasia can be of two types: In *classic achalasia* simultaneous contractions of small amplitude occur, while in *vigorous achalasia* contractions are simultaneous in onset, large in amplitude, and repetitive, resembling those seen in diffuse esophageal spasm.

PATHOPHYSIOLOGY   The underlying abnormality is defective innervation of the smooth-muscle portion of the esophageal body and the lower esophageal sphincter. Pathologically, vigorous achalasia is associated with less severe neural damage than classic achalasia, which shows a marked reduction in myenteric neurons. Primary idiopathic achalasia accounts for most of the patients seen in the United States. Secondary achalasia may be caused by gastric carcinoma infiltrating the esophagus, lymphoma, Chagas' disease, neuropathic chronic intestinal pseudo-obstruction syndrome, irradiation, and certain toxins and drugs. Hypertensive or hypercontracting lower esophageal sphincter may be considered as variants of achalasia.

CLINICAL FEATURES   Achalasia affects patients of all ages and both sexes. Dysphagia, chest pain, and regurgitation are the main symptoms. Dysphagia occurs early with both liquids and solids and is worsened by emotional stress and hurried eating. Various maneuvers designed to increase intraesophageal pressure, including the Valsalva, may help passage of the bolus into the stomach. Chest pain is more pronounced in vigorous achalasia than in classic achalasia. Regurgitation and pulmonary aspiration occur because of retention of large volumes of saliva and ingested food in the esophagus. The presence of gastroesophageal reflux argues against achalasia, although some of these patients may describe their chest pain as heartburn. The overall course is usually chronic, with progressive dysphagia and weight loss over months to years.

DIAGNOSIS   Chest x-ray shows absence of the gastric air bubble and sometimes a tubular mediastinal mass beside the aorta. The presence of an air-fluid level in the mediastinum in the upright position represents unpassed food in the esophagus and is characteristic.

Barium swallow shows esophageal dilatation, and in advanced cases the esophagus may become sigmoid. On fluoroscopy, normal peristalsis is lost in the lower two-thirds of the esophagus. The terminal part of the esophagus shows a persistent beaklike narrowing representing the nonrelaxing lower esophageal sphincter [see Fig. 251-1(2)]. In patients with vigorous achalasia, there may be pronounced nonperistaltic contractions without a dilated esophagus.

Manometry shows normal or elevated basal lower esophageal sphincter pressure and swallow-induced relaxation which is absent or reduced in degree, duration, and consistency (see Fig. 251-3). The esophageal body shows elevated resting pressure. In response to swallows, primary peristaltic waves are replaced by simultaneous-onset contractions. These contractions may be of poor amplitude (classic achalasia) or of large amplitude and long duration (vigorous achalasia). Administration of the cholinergic muscarinic agonist mecholyl causes a marked increase in baseline esophageal pressure, and administration of cholecystokinin (CCK), which normally causes a fall in the sphincter pressure, paradoxically causes contraction of the lower esophageal sphincter. This occurs because in achalasia the neurally transmitted inhibitory effect of CCK is absent due to the loss of inhibitory neurons. Endoscopy is helpful in excluding the secondary causes of achalasia, particularly gastric carcinoma.

TREATMENT   Medical treatment using soft foods, sedatives, nitrates, and anticholinergic drugs is usually unsatisfactory. Nitrates and calcium channel antagonists such as nifedipine have been used with some success. The best available therapy involves balloon dilation to reduce the basal lower esophageal sphincter pressure by tearing muscle fibers. In experienced hands this technique is effective in about 85 percent of patients. Perforation and bleeding are potential complications. Heller's extramucosal myotomy of the lower sphincter, in which the circular muscle layer is incised, is equally effective. Reflux esophagitis and peptic stricture (more often with myotomy than with balloon dilation) may follow successful treatment.

Diffuse esophageal spasm and related motor disorders   Diffuse esophageal spasm is a motor disorder of the esophageal smooth muscle characterized by multiple spontaneous contractions and by swallow-induced contractions that are of simultaneous onset, large amplitude, long duration, and repetitive occurrence. Variants show some but not all of these motor abnormalities.

PATHOPHYSIOLOGY   The pathogenesis of the various abnormalities of peristalsis in diffuse esophageal spasm is not known. Histopathologic studies show patchy neural degeneration localized to nerve processes rather than the prominent degeneration of nerve cell bodies seen in achalasia.

Variants of diffuse esophageal spasm, such as large amplitude but peristaltic contractions (sometimes called "nutcracker" esophagus) or normal amplitude but simultaneous contractions, frequently occur as a primary disease or in association with a variety of diseases as well as with emotional stress and aging. Collagen vascular disease, diabetic neuropathy, reflux esophagitis, irradiation esophagitis, esophageal obstruction, and cholinergic and anticholinergic drugs can cause esophageal motor abnormalities. The relationship between reflux esophagitis and motor abnormalities is controversial. Overlapping features of diffuse esophageal spasm and achalasia occur in vigorous achalasia. The variant syndromes are more frequent in clinical practice than classic diffuse esophageal spasm.

CLINICAL FEATURES   The symptomatic patient with diffuse spasm or its variants presents with chest pain, dysphagia, or both. Chest pain is particularly marked in patients with esophageal contractions of large amplitude and of long duration. Chest pain usually occurs at rest but may be brought on by swallowing or by emotional stress. The pain is retrosternal; it may radiate to the back, sides of the chest, both arms, or the sides of the jaw and may last for a few seconds to several minutes. It may be acute and severe, mimicking the pain of myocardial ischemia. Dysphagia for solids and liquids may occur with or without chest pain.

Diffuse esophageal spasm must be differentiated from other causes of chest pain, particularly ischemic heart disease with atypical angina.

Often a complete cardiac workup is done before the esophageal etiology is seriously considered. The presence of dysphagia in association with pain should point to the esophagus as the site of disease. Symptoms of esophageal spasm should be carefully distinguished from those of reflux esophagitis; the two may coexist.

DIAGNOSIS   Barium swallow shows that normal sequential peristalsis below the aortic arch is replaced by uncoordinated simultaneous contractions that produce the appearance of curling or multiple ripples in the wall, sacculations, and pseudodiverticula—the "corkscrew" esophagus [see Fig. 251-1(3)]. Sometimes an esophageal contraction obliterates the lumen, and barium is pushed away in both directions. The lower esophageal sphincter opens normally.

Manometry reveals the characteristic prolonged large amplitude and repetitive contractions of simultaneous onset in the lower part of the esophagus (see Fig. 251-3). Only one or two of these abnormalities may be present in variants of diffuse spasm. Because the abnormalities may be episodic, manometry may be normal at the time of the study; therefore, several techniques are used in attempts to provoke esophageal spasm. Cold swallows produce chest pain but do not produce spasm on manometric studies. Solid boluses and pharmacologic agents, particularly edrophonium, induce both chest pain and motor abnormalities. However, there is a poor correlation between induction of pain and motility changes. Ergonovine can induce motor abnormalities but also may cause coronary artery spasm and therefore should not be used. Overall, the usefulness of pharmacologic provocative tests is limited.

TREATMENT   Anticholinergics are usually of limited value. Agents that relax smooth muscle such as sublingual nitroglycerin (0.3 to 0.6 mg) or longer-acting agents such as isosorbide dinitrate (2.5 to 10 mg sublingually before meals) and nifedipine (10 to 20 mg before meals) may be helpful in some cases. Esophageal dilation with mercury-filled rubber dilators may produce symptomatic relief by distending the lower esophagus or by a placebo effect. Reassurance and tranquilizers are helpful in allaying patients' apprehension. Balloon dilation is sometimes attempted but can be hazardous in inexperienced hands. In severe cases resistant to all therapy, a longitudinal myotomy of esophageal circular muscle is performed; it relieves pain in up to two-thirds of patients.

Scleroderma involving the esophagus   The esophageal lesions in systemic sclerosis consist of atrophy of the smooth-muscle contraction, manifested by weakness in the lower two-thirds of the esophageal body and incompetence of the lower esophageal sphincter. The esophageal wall is thin and atrophic and may exhibit areas of patchy fibrosis. Patients usually present with dysphagia to solids. Liquids may cause dysphagia when the patient is in the recumbent position. Some patients present with heartburn and regurgitation due to gastroesophageal reflux and esophagitis, which in turn may lead to stricture formation and more pronounced dysphagia. Barium swallow shows dilation and loss of peristaltic contractions in the middle and distal portions of the esophagus. The lower esophageal sphincter is patulous, and gastroesophageal reflux may occur freely (see Fig. 251-1). Mucosal changes from esophageal ulceration may be detected, and esophageal stricture may be present. Motility studies show marked reduction in the amplitude of smooth-muscle contractions, which may be peristaltic or nonperistaltic. Lower esophageal sphincter resting pressure is subnormal, but sphincter relaxation is normal (see Fig. 251-3). Esophageal motor abnormalities are frequently found in patients with Raynaud's syndrome alone. Currently, there is no effective treatment for the motor difficulty. Reflux esophagitis and its complications should be treated aggressively, as described under reflux esophagitis.

INFLAMMATORY DISORDERS

GASTROESOPHAGEAL REFLUX AND ESOPHAGITIS   Reflux esophagitis consists of esophageal mucosal damage from reflux of gastric or intestinal contents into the esophagus. Depending on the causative agent, it is referred to as peptic, bile, or alkaline esophagitis.

Pathophysiology   Three considerations involved in the pathophysiology of reflux esophagitis are (1) the pathogenesis of the esophageal reflux episode, (2) the cumulative, or net, esophageal reflux, and (3) the pathogenesis of esophagitis.

Two conditions must be met for a *reflux episode* to occur: The gastrointestinal contents must be "ready" to reflux, and the antireflux mechanism at the lower end of the esophagus must be compromised. Gastrointestinal contents are most likely to reflux (1) when gastric volume is increased (after meals, with pyloric obstruction or gastric stasis syndrome, and in acid hypersecretory states), (2) when the gastric contents are located near the gastroesophageal junction (due to recumbency or bending), and (3) when gastric pressure is increased (with obesity, pregnancy, ascites, or tight binders or girdles).

The normal antireflux mechanisms consist of the lower esophageal sphincter (LES) and the anatomic configuration of the gastroesophageal junction. Reflux occurs only when the LES–gastric pressure gradient is lost. It can be caused by increased intragastric pressure or a transient or sustained decrease in the sphincter tone itself. The decrease in sphincter tone may be due to muscle weakness or possibly to neurally mediated inappropriate sphincter relaxation. The secondary causes of LES incompetence include scleroderma-like diseases, a myopathic type of chronic intestinal pseudo-obstruction syndrome, pregnancy, smoking, smooth-muscle relaxants (such as beta-adrenergics, aminophylline, nitrates, and calcium channel blockers), destruction of the sphincter by surgical resection, myotomy or balloon dilation, and esophagitis. Abnormal activity of the diaphragmatic crural muscle which surrounds the esophageal hiatus in the diaphragm and changes the anatomic configuration of the esophagogastric junction, as in hiatal hernia, also predisposes to gastroesophageal reflux.

The *net*, or *cumulative, esophageal reflux*, i.e., the amount and duration of refluxed noxious material remaining in the esophagus, is dependent on (1) the amount of refluxed material per episode, (2) the frequency of reflux episodes, (3) the rate of clearing of the esophagus by gravity and peristaltic contraction, and (4) neutralization of gastric acid by salivary secretion.

Esophagitis is a complication of reflux, and it develops when the mucosal defenses that normally counteract the effect of injurious agents on the esophageal mucosa succumb to the onslaught of the refluxed acid pepsin or bile. *Mild esophagitis* is manifested by microscopic changes of mucosal infiltration with granulocytes or eosinophils, hyperplasia of basal cells, and elongation of dermal pegs. It can occur with or without endoscopic abnormalities. *Erosive esophagitis* shows endoscopically visible damage to the mucosa in the form of marked redness, friability, bleeding, superficial linear ulcers, and exudates. *Peptic stricture* results from fibrosis that causes constriction of the esophageal lumen. The fibrosis is predominantly submucosal, but it may involve the whole wall. Peptic strictures occur in about 10 percent of patients with reflux esophagitis. Short peptic strictures caused by spontaneous reflux are usually 1 to 3 cm long and are present in the distal esophagus near the squamocolumnar junction (see Fig. 251-2). Long and tubular peptic strictures can result from persistent vomiting or prolonged nasogastric intubation. Replacement of the squamous epithelium of the esophagus by columnar epithelium *(Barrett's esophagus)* also may result from reflux esophagitis. Columnar cell–lined esophagus may be further complicated by peptic ulcer or peptic stricture high up in the lower or midesophagus, and by adenocarcinoma in 2 to 5 percent of cases. Adenocarcinoma frequently occurs in areas adjoining the squamous mucosa. Barrett's esophagitis also may occur as a result of esophageal mucosal damage due to chemotherapy.

Clinical features   Heartburn is the characteristic symptom and is produced by the contact of refluxed material with the inflamed esophageal mucosa. Angina-like or atypical chest pain may occur in some patients, while others may experience no heartburn or chest pain. Dysphagia suggests development of peptic stricture. In peptic strictures, the usual history is of several years of heartburn preceding dysphagia. However, in one-third of patients dysphagia may be the presenting symptom. Rapidly progressive dysphagia and weight loss may indicate development of adenocarcinoma in Barrett's esophagus. Bleeding occurs due to mucosal erosions or Barrett's ulcer. Reflux in the absence of esophagitis is usually asymptomatic. Severe reflux may reach the pharynx and mouth and result in laryngitis, morning hoarseness, and pulmonary aspiration. Recurrent pulmonary aspiration can cause aspiration pneumonia, pulmonary fibrosis, or chronic asthma.

Diagnosis Evaluation of reflux esophagitis is designed to assess the presence and severity of reflux, nature of refluxant, presence and severity of esophagitis, and pathophysiology of reflux. History, barium swallow, esophagoscopy, mucosal biopsy, esophageal motility, and a variety of special tests are utilized.

The *presence of reflux* is suggested by history. Spontaneous reflux from the stomach into the esophagus on barium examination suggests advanced reflux. Reflux of barium induced by stressful maneuvers is not very helpful, however, because of the high incidence of false-positive and false-negative results. Scintiscan using ^{99m}Tc-sulfur colloid has been used to quantitate gastroesophageal reflux. Several tests that utilize the recording of esophageal luminal pH with a small pH electrode have been proposed to detect and quantitate reflux of gastric acid. In these tests, the pH electrode is swallowed, positioned in the stomach, gradually withdrawn across the LES, and then fixed at 5 cm above the sphincter. In the standard acid reflux test, a diagnosis of reflux can be made by failure of the pH to rise as the electrode enters the esophagus and by a decrease in esophageal pH with straining maneuvers. Quantitative information on acid reflux is obtained by ambulatory long-term (24-h) esophageal pH recording. The pH recordings are helpful only in the evaluation of acid reflux. The presence of bile or alkaline reflux is suggested by the occurrence of reflux symptoms in the absence of gastric acid and by the demonstration of bile in the aspirate of esophageal reflux.

The *presence and complications of reflux esophagitis* are assessed by barium swallow, esophagoscopy, mucosal biopsy, and the Bernstein test. Barium swallow is usually normal in uncomplicated esophagitis but may reveal the complication of stricture or ulcer formation. A high esophageal peptic stricture, deep ulcer, and adenocarcinoma suggest complications of Barrett's esophagus. Uncomplicated Barrett's esophagus is not diagnosed reliably by barium studies. Esophagoscopy may reveal the presence of erosive esophagitis, distal peptic stricture, or columnar cell–lined lower esophagus with or without a proximally located peptic stricture, ulcer, or adenocarcinoma. Esophagoscopy may be normal in many patients with esophagitis; in such patients, mucosal biopsies and the Bernstein test are helpful. The mucosal biopsies should be obtained at least 5 cm above the LES because esophageal mucosal changes of chronic esophagitis are quite frequent in the most distal esophagus in otherwise normal subjects. False-positive and false-negative results occur in approximately 10 percent of biopsies. Patients with Barrett's esophagus will show columnar mucosa lining the esophagus which may be of gastric fundic, cardiac, or specialized type. The Bernstein test consists of an infusion of solutions of 0.1 N HCl and normal saline into the esophagus. It is useful in diagnosing reflux esophagitis which is not endoscopically obvious. In patients with reflux esophagitis, infusion of acid, but not of saline, reproduces the symptoms of heartburn. Infusion of acid in normal subjects usually produces no symptoms. Reflux esophagitis should be included in the differential diagnosis of chest pain, esophagitis, upper gastrointestinal bleeding, and dysphagia.

The *causative and predisposing factors* are assessed by history, esophageal motility, and esophageal clearance studies. Esophageal motility studies may provide useful quantitative information on the competence of the LES and of esophageal motor function. Barium swallow and scintiscans can be used to study esophageal clearance. An esophageal acid clearance test using a pH electrode quantifies the number of swallows necessary to clear the esophagus of 10 mL of instilled dilute 0.1 N HCl.

Full diagnostic evaluation is not necessary in every patient with reflux esophagitis. In transient and mild cases with a clear-cut history of reflux esophagitis, a therapeutic trial may be sufficient. In persistent cases and when the diagnosis is not clear, barium swallow, esophagoscopy, and esophageal motility with pH monitoring are indicated.

Patients with angina-like chest pain in whom coronary artery disease has been excluded may be investigated by the Bernstein test, 24-h ambulatory esophageal pH recording, and motility recording. Most of these patients are found to have reflux esophagitis, while a few have specific esophageal motor disorders. It also should be remembered that reflux esophagitis and nonspecific esophageal motility disorders may frequently coexist with coronary artery disease.

Treatment The goals of treatment are to decrease gastroesophageal reflux, renders the refluxate harmless, improve esophageal clearance, and protect the esophageal mucosa. These goals can be achieved by certain general measures and specific drug treatments. The management of uncomplicated cases generally includes weight reduction, sleeping with elevation of the head of the bed by about 4 to 6 in with blocks, and elimination of factors that increase abdominal pressure. Patients should avoid smoking, fatty foods, coffee, chocolate, alcohol, mint, orange juice, ingestion of large quantities of fluids with meals, and certain medications (such as anticholinergic drugs, calcium channel blockers, and other smooth-muscle relaxants). In mild cases, H-2 blocking agents (cimetidine 300 mg, ranitidine 150 mg, or famotidine 20 mg at bedtime) or antacids to neutralize acidity are usually successful.

In moderate to severe cases, the preceding measures are more strictly enforced. H-2 blockers are used in higher doses (cimetidine, 300 mg qid; ranitidine, 150 mg bid; famotidine, 20 mg bid). A protective agent such as sucralfate (1-g chewable tablet, 1 h before meals) is useful in some cases. If the patient does not respond fully, a prokinetic agent such as metoclopramide, 10 mg 30 min before meals and at bedtime, domperidone, or cisapride is prescribed to raise sphincter pressure, hasten gastric emptying, and improve esophageal clearance. (Domperidone and cisapride have not yet been approved for use in the United States.) Inhibition of H^+,K^+-ATPase, the parietal cell pump that is responsible for acid secretion, with omeprazole (20 to 40 mg tablet, daily) is very effective in resistant cases. If a complete response is not achieved, gastric juice pH should be checked to verify patient compliance or underlying acid hypersecretory state. Reflux esophagitis requires prolonged therapy for 3 to 6 months or longer if the disease recurs quickly. Patients with reflux esophagitis with complications such as Barrett's esophagus (with or without a deep ulcer) should be treated vigorously. Patients who have an associated peptic stricture are treated with dilators to relieve dysphagia in addition to vigorous treatment for reflux. To detect and treat high-grade dysplasia and early adenocarcinoma, close follow-up with periodic endoscopic biopsies is indicated every 2 years or so in patients without evidence of dysplasia; patients with dysplasia require more frequent surveillance.

Antireflux surgery, in which the gastric fundus is wrapped around the esophagus (fundoplication), increases the lower sphincter pressure and should be considered in resistant and complicated cases of reflux esophagitis that do not fully respond to medical therapy or in patients for whom long-term medical therapy is not desirable. In the ideal candidates for fundoplication, motility studies should show persistently inadequate lower sphincter pressure but normal peristaltic contractions in the esophageal body.

Patients with alkaline esophagitis are treated with general antireflux measures and neutralization of bile salts with cholestyramine, aluminum hydroxide, or sucralfate. Sucralfate is particularly useful in these cases, since it also serves as a surface protector.

INFECTIOUS ESOPHAGITIS With the recent increase in immunodeficiency states, infectious esophagitis has become increasingly important. Infectious esophagitis can be due to viral, bacterial, fungal, or parasitic organisms. In severely immunocompromised patients, multiple organisms may coexist.

Viral esophagitis (See also Chap. 143) *Herpes simplex virus* (HSV) type I may occasionally cause esophagitis in the immunocompetent person, but either type I or type II may afflict patients who are immunosuppressed. These patients complain of the acute onset of chest pain, odynophagia, and dysphagia. Bleeding may occur in severe cases, and systemic manifestations such as nausea, vomiting, fever, chills, and mild leukocytosis may be present. The persistent infection may lead to superinfection of denuded esophageal mucosa with fungi or bacteria. Herpes vesicles on the nose and lips sometimes provide a clue to the diagnosis. Barium swallow is inadequate to detect early lesions and cannot reliably distinguish HSV from other types of infections. Endoscopy shows vesicles and small, discrete, punched-out superficial ulcerations with or without fibrinous exudate. In later stages there is diffuse erosive esophagitis caused by enlargement and coalescence of the ulcers. Mucosal cells from biopsy of the edge of an ulcer or cytologic smear show ballooning degeneration, ground glass change in the nuclei with eosinophilic intranuclear inclusions (Cowdry type A), and giant cell formation on routine stains. Culture becomes positive within days and is helpful in diagnosis. For prophylaxis in a severely immunocompromised host, acyclovir, 800 mg orally twice daily or 250 mg/m² of body surface area every 12 h intravenously, is recommended. For treatment of esophagitis, intravenous therapy, 250 mg/m² every 8 h, is usually initiated. As swallowing improves, the therapy is changed to 200 to 400 mg orally five times daily. Symptoms usually resolve in 1 week, but large ulcerations may take longer to heal. Foscarnet may be useful if acyclovir resistance occurs. These patients also may have reflux esophagitis, which may worsen the symptoms and add to complications.

Varicella-zoster virus (VZV) sometimes produces esophagitis in children with chickenpox and adults with herpes zoster. Esophageal VZV also can be the source of disseminated VZV infection in the absence of skin involvement. In an immunocompromised host, VZV esophagitis causes vesicles and confluent ulcers and usually resolves spontaneously, but it may cause necrotizing esophagitis in a severely compromised host. On routine histology of mucosal biopsies or cytology specimens, VZV is difficult to distinguish from HSV, but the distinction can be made immunohistologically or on culture. Acyclovir is effective in prevention and treatment of esophagitis, but much higher doses are needed than those for HSV.

Cytomegalovirus (CMV) infections occur only in the immunocompromised patient. CMV is usually activated from a latent stage or may be acquired from blood product transfusions. CMV lesions initially appear as serpiginous ulcers in an otherwise normal mucosa. These may coalesce to form giant ulcers, particularly in the distal esophagus. The virus involves submucosal fibroblasts and endothelial cells of the blood vessels but not the epithelial cells.

Patients present with painful swallowing, chest pain, hematemesis, nausea, and vomiting. Barium swallow may show nonspecific abnormalities or large esophageal ulcers. Diagnosis requires endoscopy and biopsies of the center of the ulcer. Mucosal brushings are not useful. Routine histology shows intranuclear and small intracytoplasmic inclusions in large fibroblasts and endothelial cells of blood vessels. Immunohistology with monoclonal antibodies to CMV and in situ hybridization of CMV DNA can be performed on centrifugation culture and are useful for early diagnosis. Ganciclovir (DHPG), 5 mg/kg every 12 h intravenously, is the treatment of choice. Foscarnet can be used in resistant cases. Therapy is continued until healing, which may take weeks to months.

Human immunodeficiency virus (HIV) may be associated with a self-limited syndrome of acute esophageal ulceration associated with oral ulcers and a maculopapular skin rash. This syndrome occurs in homosexual men coincident with both HIV seroconversion and the inversion of the T lymphocyte helper/suppressor ratio. Electron microscopy of affected tissue reveals retrovirus-like particles that are different from CMV or HSV.

Bacterial esophagitis *Bacterial esophagitis* is unusual, but esophagitis caused by *Lactobacillus* and beta-hemolytic streptococci

has been described in the immunocompromised host. In profoundly granulocytopenic patients and in patients with cancer, bacterial esophagitis is often missed because it is commonly present with other organisms, including viruses and fungi, and because bacteria are difficult to identify on routine histology. In patients with AIDS, infection with *Cryptosporidium* and *Pneumocystis carinii* may cause nonspecific inflammation and *Mycobacterium tuberculosis* may cause deep ulcerations of the distal esophagus.

Candida esophagitis Many *Candida* species are normal commensals in the throat but become pathogenic and produce esophagitis in immunodeficiency states. These include HIV; malignant neoplasms (particularly lymphoma and leukemia); treatment with immunosuppressive agents, glucocorticoids, and broad-spectrum antibiotics; diabetes mellitus; hypoparathyroidism; systemic lupus erythematosus; hemoglobinopathy; corrosive esophageal injury; and esophageal stasis. Occasionally, monilial *Candida* esophagitis occurs in the absence of any of the above predisposing factors. Patients may be asymptomatic or complain of odynophagia and dysphagia. Oral thrush or other evidence of mucocutaneous candidiasis may be absent. Rarely, *Candida* esophagitis may be complicated by esophageal bleeding, perforation, and stricture or by systemic invasion. Barium swallow may be normal or may show multiple nodular filling defects of various sizes (see Fig. 251-2). Large nodular defects may resemble clusters of grapes. Endoscopy shows small yellow-white raised plaques with surrounding erythema in mild disease. In extensive disease, confluent linear and nodular plaques are seen. Diagnosis is made by demonstration of yeast or hyphae forms in the smear of plaques and exudate stained with Gram's, periodic acid–Schiff, or silver stains. Biopsies are usually not positive. Culture is not useful in diagnosis but may be helpful in confirming the species and, if needed, the drug sensitivities of the yeast (see Chap. 168). In normal or minimally immunocompromised patients, nystatin or clotrimazole is often successful. Nystatin is used as an oral suspension (100,000 units per milliliter) in doses of 10 to 20 mL every 6 h; clotrimazole (10-mg tablet) is to be sucked five times a day. Ketoconazole (200 to 400 mg in a single oral dose) is effective treatment; the higher dose is used in the severely immunocompromised host. The bioavailability of ketoconazole is severely reduced at increased gastric pH; therefore, it should not be used concurrently with gastric acid suppression therapy or in achlorhydric subjects. Fluconazole (200 mg on the first day, followed by 100 mg daily) is the preferred treatment because its absorption is not affected by high gastric pH. Poorly responsive patients are treated with amphotericin, 10 to 15 mg as an intravenous infusion for 6 h daily for a total dose of 300 to 500 mg. Miconazole and amphotericin lozenges are currently not available in the United States. The treatment is for 7 to 10 days followed by nystatin, clotrimazole, ketoconazole, or fluconazole for as long as the host resistance remains low.

OTHER TYPES OF ESOPHAGITIS *Radiation esophagitis* is a common occurrence during radiation treatment for lung, mediastinal, or esophageal carcinoma. The frequency and severity of esophagitis increase with the amount of radiation to the area and the subsequent use of certain chemotherapeutic agents such as doxorubicin, bleomycin, cyclophosphamide, and cisplatin. Dysphagia and odynophagia are the main symptoms and may last several weeks to several months after the conclusion of therapy. The esophageal mucosa becomes erythematous, edematous, and friable. Superficial erosions coalesce to form larger superficial ulcers. Submucosal fibrosis and degenerative changes in the blood vessels, muscles, and myenteric neurons may be present. The treatment is relief of pain with viscous lidocaine during the acute phase, while indomethacin may lessen the radiation damage. Esophageal stricture may develop and require dilation. *Corrosive esophagitis* occurs following ingestion of caustic agents, such as strong alkalies or acids. When severe, corrosive injury may lead to esophageal perforation, bleeding, and death. Steroids have not been shown to be useful in acute corrosive esophagitis. Healing is usually associated with stricture formation. Caustic strictures are usually long and rigid (see Fig. 251-2) and generally require dilation with dilators passed over a guidewire through the stricture. *Pill-induced esophagitis* is associated with the ingestion of certain pills and accounts for many cases of erosive esophagitis. Antibiotics such as doxycycline, tetracycline, and clindamycin account for over half the cases. Other commonly prescribed pills that cause esophageal injury include aspirin, potassium chloride, ferrous sulfate, quinidine, alprenolol, and various steroidal and nonsteroidal anti-inflammatory agents. Pill esophagitis can be prevented by washing pills down with copious amounts of fluids. *Sclerotherapy* for bleeding esophageal varices usually produces transient retrosternal chest pain and dysphagia due to edema, inflammation, and deranged motility. Esophageal ulcer, stricture, hematoma, or perforation may occur. *Esophagitis associated with mucocutaneous and systemic diseases* is usually associated with blister and bulla formation, epithelial desquamation, and thin, weblike or dense esophageal strictures. Esophageal involvement is indicated by development of odynophagia and dysphagia. Pemphigus vulgaris and bullous pemphigoid form intraepithelial and subepithelial bullae, respectively, and can be distinguished by a specific immunohistology. They are both characterized by sloughing of epithelium or esophageal casts. Glucocorticoid treatment is usually effective. Dystrophic epidermolysis bullosa is an inherited disease that presents in childhood in which local trauma is associated with bulla formation and scarring. Cicatricial pemphigoid, Stevens-Johnson syndrome, and toxic epidermolysis bullosa can produce esophageal bullous lesions and strictures requiring gentle dilation. Graft-versus-host disease occurs in patients who have received allogeneic bone marrow transplants and is associated with generalized desquamation and esophageal strictures. Behçet's disease and eosinophilic gastroenteritis may involve the esophagus and may respond to steroid therapy. Crohn's disease and an erosive lichen planus also can involve the esophagus, and Crohn's disease may cause inflammatory strictures, sinus tract, filiform polyps, and fistulas in the esophagus.

OTHER ESOPHAGEAL DISORDERS

DIVERTICULA Diverticula are outpouchings of the wall of the esophagus. *Zenker's diverticula* appear in the natural weakness in the posterior hypopharyngeal wall and cause halitosis and regurgitation of saliva and food particles consumed several days previously. When they become large and filled with food, they can compress the esophagus and cause dysphagia or complete obstruction. Nasogastric intubation and endoscopy should be performed with utmost care in these patients, since the two may cause perforation of the diverticulum. *Midesophageal diverticula* may be caused by traction from old adhesions or by propulsion associated with esophageal motor abnormalities. *Epiphrenic diverticula* may be associated with achalasia. Small or medium-sized diverticula and midesophageal and epiphrenic diverticula are usually asymptomatic. *Diffuse intramural diverticulosis* of the esophagus is due to dilation of the deep esophageal glands. This may lead to chronic candidiasis or a stricture high up in the esophagus. These patients may present with dysphagia. Symptomatic Zenker's diverticula are treated by cricopharyngeal myotomy with or without diverticulectomy. Very large symptomatic esophageal diverticula are removed surgically. When they are associated with motor abnormalities, distal myotomy is performed. Strictures associated with diffuse intramural diverticulosis are treated with rubber dilators.

WEBS AND RINGS Weblike constrictions of the esophagus are usually congenital or inflammatory in origin. Asymptomatic hypopharyngeal webs are demonstrated in up to 10 percent of normal individuals. When concentric, they cause intermittent dysphagia to solids. Symptomatic hypopharyngeal webs with iron-deficiency anemia in middle-aged women constitute *Plummer-Vinson syndrome*. The clinical importance of this syndrome is uncertain. Midesophageal webs are rare. *Lower esophageal mucosal ring* (Schatzki ring) is a thin, weblike constriction located at the squamocolumnar mucosal junction at or near the border of the lower esophageal sphincter (see

Fig. 251-2). It invariably produces dysphagia when the diameter is less than 1.3 cm. The dysphagia to solids is the only symptom, and it is usually episodic. Asymptomatic rings may be present in about 10 percent of normal individuals. Lower esophageal ring is one of the common causes of dysphagia. Symptomatic webs and mucosal lower esophageal ring are easily treated by dilation. *Lower esophageal muscular ring* (contractile ring) is located proximal to the site of mucosal rings and may represent the abnormal uppermost segment of the lower esophageal sphincter. These rings are characterized by a change in size and shape from one time to another (see Fig. 251-1). They also may cause dysphagia and should be differentiated from peptic strictures, achalasia, and lower esophageal mucosal ring. They are treated by dilation.

HIATAL HERNIA *Hiatal hernia* is a herniation of a part of the stomach into the thoracic cavity through the esophageal hiatus in the diaphragm. *Sliding hiatal hernia* is one in which the gastroesophageal junction and fundus of the stomach slide upward. A sliding hernia may result from weakening of the anchors of the gastroesophageal junction to the diaphragm, longitudinal contraction of the esophagus, or increased intraabdominal pressure. Small sliding hernias can be demonstrated commonly during barium studies if intraabdominal pressure is increased. Their incidence increases with age; in the sixth decade of life the prevalence of such hernias is around 60 percent. It is unlikely that a small sliding hiatal hernia by itself produces any clinical symptoms, but it plays a role in the pathogenesis of reflux esophagitis. *Paraesophageal hernia* is one in which the esophagogastric junction remains fixed in its normal location and a pouch of stomach is herniated beside the gastroesophageal junction through the esophageal hiatus. A paraesophageal or mixed paraesophageal and sliding hernia may become incarcerated and strangulate. This situation is manifested by acute chest pain, dysphagia, and a mediastinal mass and requires prompt operative treatment. A herniated gastric pouch may cause dysphagia and may be the site of gastritis and ulceration causing chronic blood loss. A large paraesophageal hernia should be surgically repaired because of a high rate of complications.

MECHANICAL TRAUMA *Esophageal rupture* may be caused by (1) iatrogenic damage from instrumentation of the esophagus or external trauma, (2) increased intraesophageal pressure associated with forceful vomiting or retching (this is also called *spontaneous rupture* or *Boerhaave's syndrome*), or (3) diseases of the esophagus such as corrosive esophagitis, esophageal ulcer, and neoplasm. The site of perforation is variable and depends on the cause. Instrumental perforation usually occurs in the pharynx or in the lower esophagus. The esophageal perforation often occurs just above the diaphragm in the posterolateral wall. Esophageal perforation causes severe retrosternal chest pain that may be worsened by swallowing and breathing. Free air enters the mediastinum and spreads to neighboring structures and causes palpable subcutaneous emphysema in the neck, mediastinal crackling sounds on auscultation, and pneumothorax. With time, secondary infection supervenes, and mediastinal abscess and pleuropulmonary suppurative complications may develop. Esophageal perforation associated with vomiting usually deposits gastric contents in the mediastinum and causes severe mediastinal complications. On the other hand, instrumental perforation may be clinically mild and free of severe complications. Spontaneous rupture of the esophagus may mimic myocardial infarction, pancreatitis, or ruptured abdominal viscus. Symptoms of chest pain may be mild, particularly in the elderly. Mediastinal emphysema may develop late. X-ray of the chest shows abnormalities in the majority of patients but computed tomographic scan of the chest is more sensitive in detecting mediastinal air. Diagnosis is confirmed by swallow of radiopaque contrast material. Treatment includes esophageal and gastric suction and parenteral broad-spectrum antibiotics. Surgical drainage and repair of the laceration should be performed as soon as possible. In patients with terminal carcinoma, surgical repair may not be feasible, and those with minor instrumental perforation can be treated conservatively. Extensive corrosive damage may require esophageal diversion and subsequent excision of the damaged portion of the esophagus.

Mucosal tear (Mallory-Weiss syndrome)   This is usually caused by vomiting and retching, and it usually involves the gastric mucosa near the squamocolumnar mucosal junction but also may involve the esophageal mucosa. Patients present with upper gastrointestinal bleeding that may be severe. In most patients bleeding ceases spontaneously; continued bleeding may respond to vasopressin therapy or angiographic embolization. Surgery is rarely needed.

Intramural hematoma   Emetogenic injury, particularly in patients with bleeding abnormalities, can cause bleeding between the mucosa and muscle layers of the esophagus. The patients develop sudden dysphagia. Diagnosis is made by barium swallow and computed tomographic scan. Spontaneous resolution usually occurs.

FOREIGN BODIES   Foreign bodies may lodge in the cervical esophagus just beyond the upper esophageal sphincter, around the aortic arch, or above the lower esophageal sphincter. Impaction of a bolus of food, particularly a piece of meat or bread, may occur when the esophageal lumen is narrowed due to stricture, carcinoma, or a lower esophageal ring. Acute impaction causes complete inability to swallow and severe chest pain. Both foreign bodies and food boluses may be removed endoscopically. Use of meat tenderizer to facilitate passage of an obstructed meat bolus is to be discouraged because of potential esophageal perforation and aspiration pneumonia.

REFERENCES

ANDERSON KD et al: A controlled trial of corticosteroids in children with corrosive injury of the esophagus. N Engl J Med 323:637, 1990

BOTT S et al: Medication-induced esophageal injury: Survey of the literature. Am J Gastroenterol 82:758, 1987

CONNOLLY GM: Oesophageal symptoms, their causes, treatment, and prognosis in patients with acquired immune deficiency syndrome. Gut 30:1033, 1989

DODDS WJ: The pathogenesis of gastroesophageal reflux disease. AJR 151:49, 1988

GOYAL RK, CRIST JR: Chest pain of esophageal etiology. Hosp Prac 23:15, 1988

HETZEL DJ et al: Healing and relapse of severe peptic esophagitis after treatment with omeprazole. Gastroenterology 95:903, 1988

McDONALD GB et al: Esophageal infections in immunosuppressed patients after marrow transplantation. Gastroenterology 88:1111, 1985

ORLANDO RC: Esophageal epithelial defense against acid injury. J Clin Gastroenterol 13:51, 1991

RICHTER JE et al: Esophageal chest pain: Current controversies in pathogenesis, diagnosis, and therapy. Ann Intern Med 110:66, 1989

SARTON S et al: Barrett's esophagus after chemotherapy with cyclophosphamide, methotrexate, and S-fluorouracil (CMF): An iatrogenic injury. Ann Intern Med 114:210, 1991

SHAPIRO J, GOYAL RK: Disorders of the upper esophageal sphincter, in *The Larynx: A Multidisciplinary Approach*, M Fried (ed). Boston, Little, Brown, 1988, pp 293–317

SIMON D et al: Treatment options for AIDS-related esophageal and diarrheal disorders. Am J Gastroenterol 87:274, 1992

SPECHLER SJ, GOYAL RK: Barrett's esophagus. N Engl J Med 315:362, 1986

——— et al: Comparison of medical and surgical therapy for complicated gastroesophageal disease in veterans. N Engl J Med 326:786, 1992

252   PEPTIC ULCER AND GASTRITIS

JAMES E. McGUIGAN

Peptic ulcer is a term used to refer to a group of ulcerative disorders of the upper gastrointestinal tract involving principally the most proximal portion of the duodenum and the stomach, which have in common the participation of acid-pepsin in their pathogenesis. The major forms of common peptic ulcer are duodenal ulcer and gastric ulcer, both of which are chronic diseases. Ulcer associated with the Zollinger-Ellison syndrome, caused by gastrin-releasing islet cell tumors (gastrinomas), is also considered a form of peptic ulcer. The term has also been used in reference to gastric or duodenal ulcers associated with stress or drug ingestion.

Although our present knowledge of the cause of peptic ulcer is incomplete, available information supports a crucial role for acid-

pepsin. Ulcer development or resistance to ulceration depends on the balance between *aggressive factors* (principally secreted gastric acid and pepsin) and factors that comprise *mucosal defense* or *mucosal resistance* to ulceration. Peptic ulcer results when the aggressive effects of acid-pepsin outweigh the protective effects of gastric or duodenal mucosal defense. Considering the extraordinarily corrosive character of acid-pepsin, why do not all humans develop peptic ulcer? The normal capacity of gastric and proximal duodenal mucosa to resist the corrosive effects of acid and pepsin is unique in the body. It is not shared by other tissues—hence the susceptibility of the esophageal mucosa to injury from refluxed gastric juice, the frequent ulceration of the small intestine when attached surgically to actively secreting gastric mucosa, and corrosion of the skin predictably produced with gastrocutaneous fistulas.

Much has been learned about mechanisms regulating gastric acid secretion and factors which appear important in development of peptic ulcer. Consideration of gastric physiology provides an understanding of some etiologic elements as well as a rational basis for treatment and prevention of peptic ulcer.

GASTRIC PHYSIOLOGY RELATED TO PEPTIC ULCER

AGGRESSIVE FACTORS: ACID AND PEPSINS   The gastric mucosa possesses an extraordinary capacity to secrete acid. Parietal cells (oxyntic cells), interspersed along the course of mucosal glands of the body and fundus of the stomach, secrete hydrochloric acid by a process involving oxidative phosphorylation. Parietal cells secrete hydrogen ions at a concentration about 3 million times that found in blood. The estimated concentration of HCl secreted directly by parietal cells is approximately 160 mM. Each secreted hydrogen ion (H$^+$) is accompanied by a chloride ion (Cl$^-$). With each increase in hydrogen ion secretion, there is a reciprocal decrease in sodium ion secretion. For each hydrogen ion secreted into the gastric lumen, one bicarbonate ion (HCO$_3^-$) is released into the gastric venous circulation, accounting for the *alkaline tide*, a direct reflection of the magnitude of gastric H$^+$ secretion. Bicarbonate is released from carbonic acid generated from carbon dioxide by parietal cell carbonic anhydrase. The final step in hydrogen ion secretion is accomplished by a proton pump mechanism involving a specific hydrogen-potassium adenosine triphosphatase (H$^+$,K$^+$-ATPase) located in the apical microvillus membrane and tubovesicular apparatus of the parietal cell. This H$^+$,K$^+$-ATPase exchanges hydrogen for potassium across the microvillus membrane.

Multiple *chemical*, *neural*, and *hormonal* factors participate in regulation of gastric acid secretion. *Acid secretion is stimulated* by gastrin and by postganglionic vagal fibers via muscarinic cholinergic receptors on parietal cells. Gastrin, the most potent known stimulant of gastric acid secretion, is contained in and released into the circulation from cytoplasmic secretory granules of gastrin cells (G cells) which are scattered singly or in small clusters among the epithelial lining cells of the middle and deeper portions of the antral pyloric glands. Gastrin release is inhibited by somatostatin and stimulated by the neuropeptide gastrin-releasing peptide. Gastrin in tissues and in the circulation exists in several molecular forms (Fig. 252-1). The principal form of gastrin in gastric antral mucosa (and in gastrinoma) is heptadecapeptide gastrin (G-17), which contains 17 amino acid residues, the active site region being the carboxyl-terminal tetrapeptide amide (Try-Met-Asp-Phe-NH$_2$). Gastrin II is the form in which the tyrosyl residue at position 12 is sulfated, and gastrin I is the nonsulfated form. G-17 accounts for more than 90 percent of gastrin in antral mucosa. Approximately two-thirds of serum gastrin is a larger molecular species of gastrin, which contains 34 amino acids (G-34). Although G-17 has a shorter half-life than G-34, circulating G-17 is approximately as potent as G-34 in stimulating gastric acid secretion.

Gastrin is also present in duodenal mucosa, with its highest

Big Gastrin (G34)	┌Glu-Leu-Gly-Pro-Gln-Gly-Pro-Pro-His-Leu-Val-Ala-Asp-Pro-Ser-Lys-Lys- -Gln-Gly-Pro-Trp-Leu-Glu-Glu-Glu-Glu-Glu-Ala-Tyr*-Gly-Trp-Met-Asp-Phe-NH₂
Heptadecapeptide Gastrin (G 17)	┌Glu-Gly-Pro-Trp-Leu-Glu-Glu-Glu-Glu-Glu-Ala-Tyr*-Gly-Trp-Met-Asp-Phe-NH₂
Minigastrin (G 14)	Trp-Leu-Glu-Glu-Glu-Glu-Ala-Tyr*-Gly-Trp-Met-Asp-Phe-NH₂
C-Terminal Pentapeptide	Gly-Trp-Met-Asp-Phe-NH₂

FIGURE 252-1 Amino acid sequences of selected gastrin peptides, all of which contain the common C-terminal penta-peptide amide. (*Tyrosyl is sulfated in gastrin II and nonsulfated in gastrin I molecules.)

concentration in the most proximal duodenum (approximately 10 percent of antral concentration). The mucosal concentration of gastrin and the proportion of G-17 decrease with progression down the duodenum. The effects of gastrin and vagal stimulation on gastric acid secretion are intimately interrelated. Vagal stimulation increases gastric acid secretion by cholinergic stimulation of parietal cell secretion, by stimulating release of gastrin into the circulation, and by lowering the parietal cell threshold for response to circulating gastrin concentrations. Certain vagal branches or fibers also inhibit gastrin release.

The gastric mucosa contains large amounts of histamine. Histamine is contained in cytoplasmic granules of mast cells, which are nonepithelial (interstitial) in location, and enterochromaffin-like (ECL) cells, epithelial endocrine cells distributed singly in the oxyntic glands, often in direct contact with parietal cells. For many years, views differed on the importance of histamine in stimulating gastric acid secretion; some suggested that histamine was the ''final common pathway'' for cholinergic and gastrin stimulation of parietal cell acid secretion. Others were skeptical about any role for histamine in the acid secretory process. Interest in the role of histamine in acid secretion was renewed by discovery of H-2 receptor antagonists which inhibit competitively the action of histamine on H-2 receptors (located on gastric parietal, cardiac atrial, and uterine smooth-muscle cells). These drugs exert negligible effects on H-1 receptors, which are inhibited readily by conventional antihistamines (H-1 receptor antagonists). H-2 receptor antagonists (e.g., cimetidine, ranitidine, famotidine, nizatidine) inhibit basal acid secretion as well as secretion in response to feeding, gastrin, histamine, hypoglycemia, or vagal stimulation. Most data support the conclusions that (1) histamine plays an important role in stimulating gastric acid secretion and (2) histamine acts in concert with gastrin and cholinergic activity on parietal cells, but that (3) there is still uncertainty as to whether histamine is the final common effector molecule in stimulation of parietal cell secretion. The basolateral membranes of parietal cells contain receptors for histamine, gastrin, and acetylcholine, which stimulate acid secretion, and for prostaglandins and somatostatin, which inhibit acid secretion. Parietal cell histamine, gastrin, and somatostatin receptors are members of the seven-membrane spanning class of G protein–coupled receptors. Gastrin stimulates gastric acid secretion by direct stimulation of parietal cells and by stimulating histamine release by ECL cells. Histamine stimulates gastric acid secretion by increasing parietal cell cyclic adenosine monophosphate (AMP), thereby activating cyclic AMP–dependent protein kinase(s). Gastrin and acetylcholine, which do not stimulate cyclic AMP production, stimulate acid secretion by increasing parietal cell cytosolic calcium.

The major physiologic stimulus for gastric acid secretion is ingestion of food. Traditionally, regulation of gastric acid secretion has been classified into three phases—cephalic, gastric, and intestinal. This classification is of some value in analyzing factors that participate in regulation of gastric acid secretion. The *cephalic phase* encompasses the gastric acid secretory response to the sight, smell, taste, and anticipation of food. The *gastric phase* is induced by food in the stomach. The *intestinal phase* is due to the entry or presence of food within the lumen of the small intestine. Although these three phases are convenient for considering the diverse contributions to gastric

acid secretion, each phase is complex and not due necessarily to a single stimulatory control mechanism.

The cephalic phase, which includes cortical and hypothalamic components, is mediated primarily by vagal activation, which increases gastric acid secretion principally by direct stimulation of parietal cells and to a lesser extent by promoting gastrin release. The gastric phase results from stimulation of chemical and mechanical receptors in the gastric wall by luminal contents. Mechanical distention of the stomach stimulates gastric acid secretion but results in little, if any, gastrin release; this mechanical effect is inhibited by atropine and appears to be mediated by vagal reflexes. Food in the stomach promotes gastric acid secretion by increasing gastrin release. It is principally the *protein* and especially the *products of protein digestion* contained in the meal that have this effect; oral glucose and fat cause slight increases in serum gastrin but do not stimulate gastric acid secretion. Food in the proximal small intestine stimulates the intestinal phase of gastric acid secretion. A peptone meal (partially hydrolyzed meat protein) in the small intestine stimulates gastric acid secretion but not gastrin release. Food in the small intestine may induce release of an intestinal hormone(s) (distinct from gastrin) that stimulates gastric acid secretion. Increases in circulating amino acids, absorbed from the small intestine, also may contribute to the intestinal phase of gastric acid secretion. *Basal* or *interdigestive gastric acid secretion* can be considered to be a *fourth phase* of acid secretion. This phase is unrelated to feeding, reaches its peak around midnight and its lowest point about 7 A.M., and neural pathways are probably most important in its regulation.

Ingestion of both caffeine-containing and caffeine-free *coffee* stimulates gastric acid secretion, and both stimulate gastrin release. Ingestion of *ethanol* and ethanol-containing beverages stimulates gastric acid secretion. Intravenous ethanol stimulates gastric acid secretion, suggesting that both systemic and local mechanisms are involved.

Intravenous *calcium* stimulates gastric acid secretion and produces minimal increases in serum gastrin levels. Oral calcium has been reported to stimulate gastric acid secretion directly, i.e., without an increase in serum calcium or gastrin concentrations. Except in patients who harbor gastrinomas, hypercalcemia is not usually associated with gastric acid hypersecretion or with increases in serum gastrin.

Inhibition of gastric acid secretion can be produced by several mechanisms. Acid secretion may be inhibited by acid in the stomach or duodenum, by hyperglycemia, or by hypertonic fluids or fat in the duodenum. Reduction of the intragastric pH to 3.0 produces partial inhibition of gastrin release; further reduction to pH 1.5 or below blocks completely release of gastrin to almost all stimuli. *Somatostatin* appears to play an important role in this acid-induced feedback-control inhibition of gastrin release. Somatostatin inhibits gastrin release by its local (paracrine) effects on gastrin cells. Somatostatin-containing antral mucosal endocrine cells (D cells) have cytoplasmic processes which extend to neighboring gastrin cells. In addition, cytoplasmic processes of somatostatin cells in oxyntic glands extend to direct intimate contact with parietal cells and other cells. Somatostatin reduces gastric acid secretion by inhibiting gastrin release and by directly inhibiting parietal cell secretion. Acid in the duodenum decreases gastric acid secretion by the stomach, most likely by stimulating release into the circulation of intestinal peptides that inhibit gastric acid secretion. *Secretin*, a linear polypeptide (27 amino acids) related structurally to glucagon, is capable of inhibiting gastric acid secretion. Secretin is released from endocrine cells (S cells) in the mucosa of the proximal small intestine in response to mucosal acidification. Fat in the duodenum also inhibits gastric acid secretion; gastric inhibitory peptide (GIP) has been proposed as a candidate for this enterogastrone action; however, this effect of GIP remains to be proven. The mechanisms by which hyperglycemia or intraduodenal hyperosmolality inhibit gastric acid secretion are not known. Additional small intestinal mucosal peptides possessing the capacity to inhibit gastric acid secretion include vasoactive intestinal peptide (VIP), enteroglucagon, neurotensin, peptide YY, and urogastrone. *Vasoactive intestinal peptide*, a neuropeptide and putative neurotransmitter, is unlikely to inhibit gastric acid secretion as a circulating hormone since, although released in response to feeding, it is inactivated during its portal passage through the liver. *Enteroglucagon* is composed of oxyntomodulin (glucagon with an 8 amino acid carboxyl-terminal extension) and glicentin (oxyntomodulin with a 32 amino acid amino-terminal extension). *Neurotensin*, oxyntomodulin, and *peptide YY* are released from the small intestine in response to luminal lipid perfusion. *Urogastrone* is structurally and functionally identical to epidermal growth factor. The extent to which these peptides contribute to the physiologic regulation of gastric acid secretion has not been defined.

The proteolytic effects of *pepsins* in concert with the corrosive properties of secreted gastric acid are the integral components which account for the tissue injury that produces peptic ulcer. Gastric acid catalyzes the cleavage of inactive pepsinogen molecules, converting them to proteolytically active pepsins, and also provides the appropriate low pH required for pepsin activity. Activity of pepsins is maximal at pH approximately 2.0 and is reduced substantially above pH 4.0. Pepsins are denatured and irreversibly inactivated at neutral or alkaline pH. A variety of pepsinogens and their respective pepsins are present in gastric juice. Pepsinogens (and their corresponding active pepsins) have been classified by immunochemical techniques as either PG I (pepsinogens 1 through 5) or PG II (pepsinogens 6 and 7). Pepsinogen I is found in chief and mucous cells in the body and fundus of the stomach. Pepsinogen II is located in cells of the pyloric glands, Brunner's glands of the duodenum, mucous cells of the gastric cardiac glands, and the same cells in which PG I is found. Both PG I and PG II are present in plasma, whereas only PG I is detected in urine. In general, there is a direct correlation between PG I serum concentrations and maximal gastric acid secretion. Most agents which stimulate gastric acid secretion also stimulate pepsinogen secretion. Cholinergic action is particularly potent in promoting pepsinogen secretion. Although it inhibits gastric acid secretion, secretin stimulates pepsinogen secretion.

In addition to secretion of hydrochloric acid, parietal cells also secrete *intrinsic factor*. Agents which stimulate gastric acid secretion also lead to secretion of intrinsic factor.

MUCOSAL DEFENSE The mechanisms whereby the normal stomach and duodenum resist the corrosive effects of acid-pepsin (i.e., *mucosal resistance* to injury or *mucosal defense*) have not been defined completely. However, a variety of factors have been identified which contribute to and are considered to comprise mucosal defense.

Gastric mucus is important in mucosal defense and in preventing peptic ulceration. Gastric mucus is secreted by mucous cells of the gastric mucosal epithelium and gastric glands. Mucus secretion is stimulated by mechanical or chemical irritation and by cholinergic stimulation. Gastric mucus is present in two phases: in gastric juice in a soluble phase and as an insoluble mucus gel layer, approximately 0.2 mm in thickness, which coats the mucosal surface of the stomach. Normally the mucus gel is secreted constantly by gastric mucous epithelial cells and is continuously solubilized by pepsins secreted into the gastric lumen. Gastric mucus is a large polymeric glycoprotein (2×10^6 mol wt) containing four subunits connected by disulfide bridges. Depolymerization of the glycoprotein subunits of mucus, by peptic digestion or disruption of disulfide bonds, renders the glycoprotein incapable of forming or maintaining the gel. When intact, this mucus gel serves as an unstirred water layer which slows ionic diffusion but is much more impermeable to penetration by macromolecules such as pepsins (34,000 mol wt). Pepsin molecules secreted into the gastric lumen are denied reentry by the intact mucus gel, thereby potentially protecting mucosal cells from proteolytic injury. Gel thickness is increased by prostaglandins of the E series and reduced by nonsteroidal anti-inflammatory drugs (NSAIDs), including aspirin. Gastric mucus glycoproteins also contain antigenic determinants used to classify AB(H) blood group substances. Approximately three-fourths of the population secrete gastric juice containing these AB(H) substances, and such individuals are referred to as *secretors*.

Bicarbonate ions, secreted by nonparietal gastric epithelial cells, enter the mucus gel, contributing to the development of a microenvironment in the gel with a substantial hydrogen ion gradient between the zone of the gel facing the gastric lumen (pH 1 to 2) and the zone in contact with the gastric mucosal cells (pH 6 to 7). As an unstirred water layer, the mucus gel slows hydrogen ion diffusion back toward the gastric mucosal surface, allowing buffering by bicarbonate within the gel. Gastric bicarbonate secretion is stimulated by calcium, certain prostaglandins of the E and F series, cholinergic agents, and dibutyryl cyclic guanosine monophosphate. It is inhibited by NSAIDs, including aspirin, and by acetazolamide, alpha-adrenergic agents, and ethanol.

Normally, the gastric epithelial cell luminal surfaces and intercellular tight junctions provide an almost completely impermeable *gastric mucosal barrier* to back-diffusion of hydrogen ions from the lumen; this barrier appears to be an important component of mucosal resistance to acid-peptic injury. The barrier can be interrupted by bile acids, salicylates, ethanol, and weak organic acids, thereby permitting back-diffusion of hydrogen ions from lumen into gastric tissues. This may cause cell injury, release of histamine from mast cells, further stimulation of acid secretion, damage to small blood vessels, mucosal hemorrhage, and erosion or ulceration. Interruption of the gastric mucosal barrier appears to contribute to the hemorrhagic erosive gastritis associated with salicylate or ethanol ingestion and with other forms of gastric mucosal injury. Because of its high rate of metabolic activity and substantial oxygen requirements, maintenance of normal *blood flow* to the gastric mucosa is an essential component of mucosal resistance to injury. Decreased mucosal blood flow, accompanied by back-diffusion of luminal hydrogen ions, is important in producing gastric mucosal damage.

Prostaglandins are abundant in the gastric mucosa. Various prostaglandins, particularly those of the E series, have been shown to inhibit gastric mucosal injury caused by a wide variety of agents. Endogenous prostaglandins are important elements constituting mucosal defense. They stimulate secretion of gastric mucus and gastric and duodenal mucosal bicarbonate, which buffer a substantial portion of secreted gastric acid. Prostaglandins participate in the maintenance of gastric mucosal blood flow and in the integrity of the gastric mucosal barrier. Prostaglandins promote epithelial cell renewal in response to mucosal injury.

MEASUREMENT OF GASTRIC ACID SECRETION Since HCl secretion by the stomach is important in producing peptic ulcer, measurement of basal and stimulated gastric acid secretion may be of value in the clinical assessment of some patients with peptic ulcer. The range of values for normal subjects is extremely broad and overlaps substantially with those for patients with duodenal ulcer, gastric ulcer, and even the Zollinger-Ellison syndrome. Mean basal acid output (BAO) in normal males without known ulcer disease is about 1.5 to 2.0 mmol/h. In general, basal and stimulated acid outputs in females are approximately two-thirds to three-fourths those found in males. In duodenal ulcer patients, mean basal acid output average from 4 to 6 mmol/h, again with wide variation. Patients with gastric ulcer tend to have acid secretory rates that are normal or often slightly less than those for normal subjects.

Measurement of gastric acid output is not helpful in the diagnosis or exclusion of peptic ulcer and clearly is not necessary in most ulcer patients. However, it is of value in selected clinical situations. Detection of gastric acid hypersecretion is important when the Zollinger-Ellison syndrome is suspected. Measurement of gastric output is useful to detect achlorhydria, as in patients with pernicious anemia. Since patients with benign gastric ulcer virtually always secrete some acid, pentagastrin-fast achlorhydria in a patient with a gastric ulcer is almost always associated with malignancy. Measurement of gastric acid secretion is indicated in the search for the cause of ulcer recurrence after peptic ulcer surgery. It is also of value in patients in whom hypergastrinemia has been identified, in order to distinguish between clinical conditions characterized by gastric acid hypersecretion or achlorhydria.

To measure gastric acid output, a radiopaque gastric tube is passed so that its tip is located in the most dependent portion of the stomach. With the patient reclining or semirecumbent on the left side, the tube position is verified by fluoroscopy. Gastric contents are aspirated and discarded. Secretions are then collected in four consecutive 15-min intervals to determine the 1-h basal acid output. Secretion volume and acid concentration (titrated with sodium hydroxide to pH 7.0 or calculated by formula from the pH of the aspirated gastric juice) are measured, and acid output is expressed in millimoles per hour.

A variety of substances have been used to stimulate maximal acid output (MAO) by the stomach. These include *histamine*; *betazole* (Histalog), a structural analogue of histamine; and *pentagastrin* (Peptavlon). Histamine, the first standard stimulant used for gastric acid secretory testing, requires simultaneous administration of an antihistamine (H-1 receptor antagonist) to inhibit systemic side effects. Betazole possesses fewer undesirable side effects than histamine and does not require concomitant administration of an antihistamine. Pentagastrin (*N-tert*-butyloxycarbonyl-β-Ala-Trp-Met-Asp-Phe-NH$_2$) contains the biologically active carboxyl-terminal tetrapeptide amide portion of gastrin and is the preferred agent to stimulate maximal acid secretion. Following collection of basal acid secretion, gastric juice is collected for four additional consecutive 15-min periods after the subcutaneous injection of pentagastrin (6 μg/kg). MAO is expressed as millimoles of acid aspirated during the 1 h after pentagastrin administration. Peak acid output (PAO) is calculated by combining the two highest consecutive 15-min acid outputs following pentagastrin injection and multiplying by 2.

DUODENAL ULCER

Duodenal ulcer is characteristically a chronic and recurrent disease. These ulcers are usually deep and sharply demarcated. They penetrate through the mucosa and submucosa, often into the muscularis propria. This is in contrast to erosions, which are superficial and limited to the mucosa. The ulcer floor contains no intact epithelium and usually consists of a zone of eosinophilic necrosis resting on a base of granulation tissue surrounded by variable amounts of fibrosis. The ulcer bed may be clear or may contain blood or a proteinaceous exudate with entrapped erythrocytes and acute and chronic inflammatory cells. More than 95 percent of duodenal ulcers occur in the first portion of the duodenum, and approximately 90 percent of those are located within 3 cm of the junction of the pyloric and duodenal mucosa. Duodenal ulcers are usually round or oval, but they may be irregular or elliptic. They are usually less than 1 cm in diameter. Rarely, duodenal ulcers are extremely large (3 to 6 cm in diameter) and may be mistaken radiographically for the entire duodenal bulb. These giant ulcers often escape radiologic detection and are usually identified by endoscopy, at surgery, or at postmortem examination.

The absolute prevalence of duodenal ulcer is not known. It is estimated to occur in from 6 to 15 percent of the population. This variation in estimates may be explained by differences in populations examined, study designs, diagnostic methods (e.g., endoscopy versus radiologic examination), and actual changes occurring in the frequency of duodenal ulcer. During the past 40 years, the frequency of duodenal ulcer (and its complications) has been decreasing in the United States

and England, especially in males. The reasons for this reduction are not known. Duodenal ulcers now appear to be approximately as common in males as in females. Best current estimates suggest that approximately 10 percent of the population has clinical evidence of duodenal ulcer at some time in their lives. The natural history of duodenal ulcer is that of spontaneous healing and recurrence; about 60 percent of healed duodenal ulcers recur within 1 year, and 80 to 90 percent recur within 2 years.

ETIOLOGY AND PATHOGENESIS Much is now known concerning factors that contribute to the development of duodenal ulcer, but we do not completely understand all aspects of its pathogenesis. It is clear that acid secretion by the stomach is required for production of a duodenal ulcer. However, all the factors which render the acid-secreting subject susceptible to duodenal ulceration have not been defined completely. Though as a group duodenal ulcer patients secrete more acid than normal, from one-half to two-thirds of them have acid secretory rates (BAO and MAO) within the normal range. Duodenal ulcer patients have approximately 1.9 billion parietal cells, with a maximum capacity of approximately 42 mmol gastric acid secreted per hour; this is in contrast to 1.0 billion parietal cells and 22 mmol/h secretion rate for nonduodenal ulcer subjects (mean approximate values). However, variations in both groups are so large that most duodenal ulcer patients fall within the normal range. As a group, in response to stimulation duodenal ulcer patients also have comparable increases in gastric secretion of pepsin and in serum PG I levels. Peptic ulcer develops when there is an unfavorable balance between acid-pepsin secretion and mucosal defense; in the pathogenesis of duodenal ulcer, evidence favors the importance of absolute or, in most instances, relative gastric hypersecretion. In contrast, for gastric ulcer, defective mucosal defense appears to be the major contributing factor.

Fasting *serum gastrin* concentrations are normal in duodenal ulcer patients. However, in many duodenal ulcer patients more gastrin is released into the circulation in response to a protein-containing meal than by normal subjects. Duodenal ulcer patients also have greater gastric acid secretory responses to administered gastrin than do nonulcer subjects. In duodenal ulcer patients, intragastric acid may be less effective in inhibiting gastrin release and further gastric acid secretion. Duodenal ulcer patients tend to empty their stomachs more rapidly than do nonduodenal ulcer patients. This phenomenon, when coupled with relative gastric acid hypersecretion, may contribute to a greater rate of acid delivery to the first part of the duodenum (the primary location of ulceration) in patients with duodenal ulcer. Acidification of the proximal duodenum in patients with duodenal ulcer results in less secretion of bicarbonate into the lumen by duodenal mucosal cells than in nonulcer subjects.

Genetic factors appear to be important. Duodenal ulcers are approximately three times as common in first-degree relatives of duodenal ulcer patients as in the general population. Patients with duodenal ulcers have an increased frequency of blood group O and of the nonsecretor status [those who do not secrete AB(H) blood group antigens in their gastric juice], but these associations are weak. An increased incidence of HLA-B5 antigen has been reported in white male subjects with duodenal ulcer.

Cigarette smoking has been associated with increased duodenal ulcer frequency, decreased response to therapy, and increased duodenal ulcer mortality. Cigarette smoking does not increase gastric acid secretion. It has been suggested that the increased incidence of duodenal ulcer among cigarette smokers may be due to inhibition of pancreatic bicarbonate secretion (an endogenous neutralizer of secreted gastric acid) by nicotine or cigarette smoke and/or by accelerated emptying of gastric acid into the duodenum.

The incidence of duodenal ulcer also has been reported to be increased in patients with chronic renal failure, alcoholic cirrhosis, renal transplantation, hyperparathyroidism, systemic mastocytosis, and chronic obstructive pulmonary disease. Antibodies to herpes simplex have been reported to be higher in titer and more frequent in sera of patients with duodenal ulcer than in normals.

The importance of *psychological factors* in the pathogenesis of duodenal ulcer remains controversial. Contrary to earlier views, there is no single, characteristic duodenal ulcer personality. Chronic anxiety and psychological stress may, however, be factors in exacerbation of ulcer activity. There is some evidence that patients with duodenal ulcer may view stress more negatively than nonulcer subjects. No differences have been identified in the frequency of duodenal ulcer among different socioeconomic classes or occupation groups.

HELICOBACTER PYLORI Gastric colonization with *Helicobacter pylori* has been reported in 90 to 95 percent of patients with duodenal ulcer and in 60 to 70 percent of patients with gastric ulcer. Healthy persons less than 30 years of age have prevalence rates of gastric colonization with *H. pylori* of approximately 10 percent. Gastric colonization increases with age, with those over age 60 having colonization rates approximating their age. Most patients with gastric colonization by *H. pylori* never develop ulceration and remain asymptomatic. Rates are increased with deprived socioeconomic circumstances as well as in custodial institutions and have been reported to be increased in black and Hispanic Americans. *H. pylori* is a spiral, gram-negative bacillus with multiple flagella with preference for a microaerophilic environment. *H. pylori* does not invade tissues. The organism resides in the mucus gel coating the epithelial cells, with a minor proportion of *H. pylori* directly adherent to the epithelial cells. Most *H. pylori*–infected persons have neutrophils in the lamina propria and epithelial glands and an increase in chronic inflammatory cells in the lamina propria. Colonization of *H. pylori* in the duodenum is restricted to areas of gastric metaplasia and is found in metaplastic gastric epithelium in the duodenal bulb of most patients with duodenal ulcer. *H. pylori* has been shown to be the cause of several forms of acute and chronic gastritis (see "Gastritis," below). *H. pylori* has been proposed as an important factor in the pathogenesis of duodenal ulcer. Evidence is mounting in support of this proposal. However, it remains to be established whether *H. pylori* is an important cause of duodenal ulcer, a potential contributing or modifying factor, or, and less likely, its presence reflects an extremely frequent commensal association.

CLINICAL FEATURES Epigastric pain is by far the most frequent symptom of duodenal ulcer. The pain is often described as sharp, burning, or gnawing. Alternatively, the pain may be ill-defined, boring, or aching or may be perceived as abdominal pressure or fullness or as a hunger sensation. In approximately 10 percent of patients the pain is located to the right of the epigastrium. The pain of duodenal ulcer characteristically occurs from 90 min to 3 h after eating. It frequently awakens the patient at night. Pain on awakening before breakfast is sufficiently rare in patients with duodenal ulcer as to challenge the diagnosis. The pain is usually relieved within a few minutes by food or antacids. Symptoms tend to be recurrent and episodic. The severity of pain varies widely from patient to patient. Duodenal ulcers recur often in the absence of pain. Episodes of pain may persist for periods of several days to weeks or months. Periods of remission usually last from weeks to years and are almost always longer than the episodes of pain. In some patients the disease is more aggressive, with frequent and persistent symptoms and/or development of complications. Pain relief with antacids or food is believed to result from acid neutralization. Ingestion of food leads to transient partial neutralization of gastric acid, which is followed by gastrin release and resultant stimulation of acid secretion. With subsequent gastric emptying and increasing gastric acid secretion, a sufficiently low pH is achieved in the stomach and first portion of the duodenum that pain results. Acid-induced pain in patients with duodenal ulcer is believed to be due to (1) acid stimulation of chemical receptors and/or (2) alterations in gastric motility.

Changes in the character of ulcer pain may signal the development of complications. For example, ulcer pain which becomes constant, is no longer relieved by food or antacids, or radiates to the back or to either upper quadrant may herald *penetration* of the ulcer (often posteriorly into the pancreas). Pain associated with duodenal ulcer which is accentuated, rather than relieved, by food and/or is accompanied by vomiting often indicates *gastric outlet obstruction*. Abrupt, severe, or generalized abdominal pain is characteristic of free ulcer *perforation* into the peritoneal cavity. Weight loss, in the absence of some degree of gastric outlet obstruction, is unusual. Duodenal ulcer may cause acute gastrointestinal *hemorrhage*, with vomiting of blood or "coffee grounds" material or with the passage of black, tarry stools or even frankly red blood, if the bleeding is massive. More commonly, blood loss with duodenal ulcer is more subtle, with occult blood loss detected by stool examination or by variable degrees of anemia which may be accompanied by iron deficiency.

It is important to emphasize that *many patients with active duodenal ulcer have no ulcer symptoms*. This leads to a significant, although not precisely quantifiable, underestimate of duodenal ulcer frequency in the population. Prospective studies using upper gastrointestinal endoscopy suggest that approximately half of duodenal ulcer recurrences are without symptoms. Endoscopic studies also show a lack of good correlation among ulcer activity, symptom resolution, and ulcer healing. The absence of ulcer-type pain does not exclude duodenal ulcer as a potential cause for acute or chronic gastrointestinal hemorrhage, gastric outlet obstruction, or abrupt ulcer perforation.

On *physical examination*, epigastric tenderness is by far the most frequent abnormal finding. The area of tenderness is usually in the midline, often midway between the umbilicus and the xiphoid process. In approximately 20 percent of patients the tender area is to the right of the midline. Acute free ulcer perforation into the peritoneal cavity often produces a rigid, boardlike abdomen, usually with generalized rebound tenderness. Initially, auscultation of the abdomen may reveal hyperactive bowel sounds which, with clinical progression, may diminish or disappear. Patients with gastric outlet obstruction caused by a duodenal or pyloric channel ulcer may have a "succussion splash" produced by fluid and air in the distended stomach. Tachycardia and/or hypotension, in some instances demonstrable only by orthostatic maneuvers, may result from acute duodenal ulcer hemorrhage. Cutaneous and mucosal pallor may reflect anemia from acute or chronic blood loss.

Only 5 percent of duodenal ulcers are located distal to the duodenal bulb, and most of those are in the immediate postbulbar portion of the first part of the duodenum. Postbulbar ulcer pain may be located in the right upper quadrant and may radiate to the back. Obstruction and hemorrhage are more frequent with postbulbar ulcers than with those in the duodenal bulb. Most immediate postbulbar ulcers, i.e., within 2 cm of the duodenal bulb, are of the common duodenal ulcer variety. Ulceration located in or beyond the second portion of the duodenum suggests the Zollinger-Ellison syndrome.

The pyloric channel, which is 1 to 2 cm in length, is the narrowest portion of the gastric outlet. Because of their gastric acid secretory characteristics and clinical features, pyloric channel ulcers are classified with duodenal rather than with gastric ulcers. Ulcers in this location often produce symptoms similar to those of a duodenal ulcer; however, symptoms tend to be less responsive to food and antacids. In patients with pyloric channel ulcers, food may accentuate rather than relieve ulcer pain and may produce vomiting due to partial gastric outlet obstruction. In general, surgery is required more frequently for pyloric channel ulcers than for those in the duodenal bulb.

DIAGNOSIS Barium examination of the upper gastrointestinal tract is of value in identifying duodenal ulcer and is still the most common initial method used to establish the diagnosis. The proportion of ulcers identified radiographically depends on the skill, persistence, enthusiasm, and diagnostic criteria of the radiologist. Using conventional single-contrast barium techniques, 70 to 80 percent of duodenal ulcers found at endoscopy can be identified by x-ray examination. With double-contrast barium examinations, it is possible to detect about 90 percent of duodenal ulcers. On x-ray, the typical duodenal ulcer appears as a discrete crater in the proximal portion of the duodenal bulb. Marked deformity of the duodenal bulb, common in patients with chronic recurrent duodenal ulcer, may make radiographic identification of the ulcer difficult or impossible (Figs. 252-2 and 252-3).

FIGURE 252-2   Deformed duodenal bulb with ulcer crater.

Endoscopic examination of the upper gastrointestinal tract has facilitated accurate diagnosis of duodenal ulcer. Endoscopy is not required for diagnosis of duodenal ulcer when it has been identified by barium radiographic examination. Endoscopy may be of greatest value, however, (1) in detecting duodenal ulcer suspected in the absence of a radiographically demonstrable ulcer, (2) in patients with

FIGURE 252-3   Distortion of the duodenal bulb with "cloverleaf" deformity.

radiographic deformity and uncertainty regarding ulcer activity, (3) in identifying ulcers too small or too superficial to be recognized by x-ray, and (4) in identifying (or excluding) an ulcer as the source of active gastrointestinal hemorrhage. Endoscopy permits direct visualization and photographic documentation of the character of the ulcer—its size, shape, and location—and may provide a reference base for assessment of ulcer healing.

Measurement of gastric acid secretion is not necessary in the assessment of most patients with suspected or confirmed duodenal ulcer. Determination of the serum gastrin level is recommended in those patients in whom surgery is planned or gastrinoma is considered. Epigastric pain readily relieved by food or antacids strongly suggests duodenal ulcer. However, even after careful radiographic and endoscopic examination many patients with these ulcer-like symptoms have no evidence of ulcer; this has led to the term *nonulcer dyspepsia*. Although symptoms are similar, it is uncertain whether this entity is related to peptic ulcer.

MEDICAL TREATMENT   Major objectives of duodenal ulcer therapy are relief of pain and acceleration of ulcer healing. Prevention of ulcer recurrence and complications is an additional important objective. In the past, enthusiasm has been expressed for virtually every kind of treatment ever tried for duodenal ulcer. Conclusions regarding the effectiveness of therapy were obscured by spontaneous healing of duodenal ulcer, an intrinsic component of the natural history of the disease, and by imprecise methods used to assess ulcer activity. Therapeutic agents shown to be effective which are currently available and recommended for consideration in treatment of duodenal ulcer are discussed below.

Antacids   For many decades, antacids have been a major form of treatment for duodenal ulcer. Prospective endoscopic studies conducted only relatively recently verified the effectiveness of antacids in accelerating duodenal ulcer healing. Many types of antacids are available for use in treatment of duodenal ulcer. The ideal antacid should be potent in neutralizing gastric acid, inexpensive, not adsorbed from the gastrointestinal tract, and contain negligible amounts of sodium. It should be sufficiently palatable to be tolerated with repeated dosage and should be free from side effects. Individual antacids differ substantially in their capacities to neutralize acid, their sodium contents, their absorption properties, and their potential adverse effects. Although the ideal antacid is yet to be developed, a number of preparations are available that can be used effectively in treatment of patients with duodenal ulcer.

The most widely used antacid preparations are mixtures of aluminum hydroxide and magnesium hydroxide, in some instances with additional agents. *Aluminum hydroxide* neutralizes hydrochloric acid with the production of aluminum chloride and water. Use of aluminum hydroxide tends to produce constipation. Aluminum binds phosphate within the gut lumen, thereby facilitating phosphate excretion. As a consequence, prolonged and regular use of aluminum hydroxide may induce systemic phosphate depletion with resultant weakness, malaise, and anorexia. Phosphate depletion is probably restricted to, and should be considered in, those patients with phosphate-poor diets, e.g., dietary deficiency with chronic alcoholism or other states of reduced dietary protein intake. *Magnesium hydroxide* is a potent antacid which neutralizes hydrochloric acid, producing magnesium chloride and water. Magnesium hydroxide may produce loose stools. This laxative effect and the constipating effects of aluminum hydroxide can be overcome by using antacids which contain these agents in combination. From 5 to 10 percent of magnesium in magnesium hydroxide is absorbed by the small intestine. Magnesium is excreted by the kidney, and hypermagnesemia, which is not a problem with normal renal function, develops in a small number of patients with renal insufficiency who are treated with magnesium-containing antacids. *Magnesium trisilicate*, which is included in various antacid mixtures, is a slow-acting weak antacid.

Calcium carbonate is a potent and inexpensive antacid. In neutralizing acid, it is converted to calcium chloride in the stomach. Approximately 10 percent of calcium ingested as calcium carbonate is absorbed from the proximal small intestine. Calcium carbonate is unique among antacids in that its ingestion is followed by stimulation of gastrin acid secretion (''acid rebound''). This is due to the direct action of calcium in stimulating parietal cell acid secretion and, perhaps to a lesser extent, to calcium-mediated stimulation of gastrin release. Chronic excessive calcium carbonate administration may be associated with the milk-alkali syndrome, producing elevations of serum calcium, phosphate, urea nitrogen, creatinine, and bicarbonate levels. These patients may develop renal calcinosis and progressive renal insufficiency. Because of its potential adverse effects, calcium carbonate is not recommended for use as an antacid for primary treatment of patients with peptic ulcer.

Sodium bicarbonate is a potent, rapidly acting, inexpensive antacid. However, because of its tendency to induce systemic alkalosis and its high sodium content, it should not be used as an antacid in the treatment of peptic ulcer.

Acceptance of the crucial role of acid in the pathogenesis of duodenal ulcer has provided a rational basis for the use of antacids in the treatment of patients with duodenal ulcer. In a controlled endoscopic study, 4 weeks of treatment with a potent magnesium and aluminum hydroxide antacid mixture increased the rate of duodenal ulcer healing. Ulcer healing occurred in 45 percent of patients receiving placebo and in 78 percent of those treated with 30 mL antacid (144 mmol) given 1 and 3 h after meals and at bedtime. It has been proposed that variably smaller and less frequent doses also may achieve satisfactory ulcer healing.

H-2 receptor antagonists It had been known for many years that conventional antihistamines, which block the actions of histamine on smooth muscle of blood vessels, gut, or bronchi, do not inhibit histamine-stimulated gastric acid secretion. This observation led to the development of specific classes of histamine antagonists for different types of histamine receptors. The gastric parietal cell receptor for histamine has been classifed as an H-2 receptor and that blocked by classic antihistamines as an H-1 receptor. H-2 receptor antagonists are potent inhibitors of basal (unstimulated) and stimulated gastric acid secretion. H-2 receptor antagonists exhibit some structural similarities to histamine and to each other, with variations in ring structures and side chains (see Fig. 252-4). H-2 receptor antagonists are safe and effective in accelerating healing and reducing recurrence of duodenal ulcer. Healing rates for H-2 receptor antagonists are similar to those described above for antacids. Compliance appears superior. Daily maintenance doses of H-2 receptor antagonists (one-half the therapeutic dose) reduce duodenal ulcer recurrence by 50 to 70 percent. At the present time, H-2 receptor antagonists are the therapeutic agents used most frequently in the management of patients with duodenal ulcer.

Cimetidine was the first H-2 receptor antagonist developed and has been used extensively in the treatment of duodenal ulcer. Cimetidine is related structurally to histamine (Fig. 252-4), sharing the same imidazole ring, but bearing an extended side chain containing a cyanoguanidine group. Much information regarding the actions of H-2 receptor antagonists was obtained in the detailed characterization of the actions of cimetidine. Cimetidine (300 mg) was shown to inhibit basal acid secretion by more than 80 percent and meal-stimulated acid secretion by approximately 70 percent. It strikingly reduced acid secretory responses to histamine, caffeine, insulin, hypoglycemia, and gastrin. Cimetidine was shown to be effective in promoting endoscopically verified duodenal ulcer healing. Initially, the oral dose of cimetidine recommended and used in treatment of duodenal ulcer was 300 mg four times daily, with meals and at bedtime. More recently, 400 mg cimetidine twice each day (morning and bedtime) or 800 mg once daily (at bedtime) has been shown to be equally effective. The 800-mg bedtime dose is recommended. Treatment of active duodenal ulcer with cimetidine is continued for periods from 4 to 8 weeks. In patients with healed duodenal ulcer, prolonged administration of cimetidine (400 mg at bedtime) has been shown to reduce substantially the frequency of duodenal ulcer recurrence.

FIGURE 252-4 Chemical structures of histamine and the H-2 receptor antagonists cimetidine, rantidine, famotidine, and nizatidine. Note the similarities and differences in the ring structures, including the imidazole ring shared by histamine and cimetidine, the furan ring in ranitidine, and the thiazole ring in famotidine and nizatidine.

Considering the enormous number of patients who have been treated with cimetidine, few serious adverse effects have been experienced. Slight and reversible increases in serum aminotransferase and creatinine levels may occur. Reversible confusional states have been reported in a small number of severely ill patients with preexisting hepatic-renal functional impairment. Brief increases in serum prolactin have been found after intravenous and oral cimetidine. Cimetidine has been shown to inhibit some cytochrome P450 hepatic microsomal enzyme systems and therefore may increase blood levels, duration of action, and pharmacologic effects of drugs metabolized by those systems. Tender gynecomastia due to the weak antiandrogenic effect of cimetidine has been reported in patients with the Zollinger-Ellison syndrome requiring and treated with extremely large doses for months to years.

Ranitidine, the second H-2 receptor antagonist made available for use, is prescribed frequently in the treatment of patients with duodenal ulcer. Ranitidine does not share the imidazole ring of histamine but rather is a substituted aminomethylfuran (see Fig. 252-4). On a molar basis, ranitidine is about six times as potent as cimetidine in inhibiting gastric acid secretion. Cimetidine and ranitidine have similar half-lives, approximately 1.5 to 2 h. They both appear to be effective in accelerating healing of duodenal ulcer and in reducing duodenal ulcer recurrence. The initial recommended dose of ranitidine for treatment of duodenal ulcer was 150 mg twice each day; 300 mg at bedtime has been found to be equally effective. The maintenance dose for reducing duodenal ulcer recurrence is 150 mg once a day at bedtime. Ranitidine may increase levels of serum AST and ALT (previously designated SGOT and SGPT). There have been occasional reports of reversible hepatitis with ranitidine administration. It appears to have no antiandrogen properties and exhibits less inhibitory effect on cytochrome P450 mixed oxygenase enzyme systems.

The most recently introduced H-2 receptor antagonists are famotidine and nizatidine. *Famotidine* is an extraordinarily potent H-2 receptor antagonist, being approximately 8 to 10 times as potent as ranitidine in inhibiting gastric acid secretion. Famotidine contains a thiazole ring (see Fig. 252-4). The recommended daily dose of famotidine is 40 mg once daily at bedtime. The maintenance dose for prevention of duodenal ulcer recurrence is 20 mg/d at bedtime. *Nizatidine* is another recently introduced H-2 receptor antagonist and has been shown to be comparable with other agents in this class in the treatment of patients with duodenal ulcer and in reduction of duodenal ulcer recurrence. Nizatidine, similar to famotidine, contains a thiazole ring. The recommended dose for treatment of duodenal ulcer is 300 mg once daily at bedtime. The maintenance dose for reduction of duodenal ulcer recurrence is 150 mg at bedtime. Associated blood dyscrasias have been noted rarely, and hepatotoxicity, similar to that with ranitidine and cimetidine, also has been reported.

Anticholinergic agents   Anticholinergic agents, such as atropine, act by blocking parietal cell muscarinic acetylcholine receptors. These agents decrease gastric acid secretion but are not nearly as effective as H-2 receptor antagonists. They also delay gastric emptying. Most studies have *not* shown that anticholinergic agents hasten healing or improve symptoms of duodenal ulcer; therefore, they are not recommended as primary agents for the treatment of duodenal ulcer. Side effects include dryness of mouth, blurring of vision, cardiac arrhythmias, and urinary retention. They should not be used in patients with glaucoma, impaired gastric emptying, or history or symptoms of urinary retention. There are several classes of muscarinic cholinergic receptors. *Pirenzepine* is a relatively selective anticholinergic agent which is more specific in inhibiting gastric acid secretion with fewer side effects than other anticholinergic agents. Pirenzepine, not yet available for prescribing in the United States, has been reported to be effective in treatment of duodenal ulcer. It may prove useful as primary therapy or as adjunctive therapy in duodenal ulcer patients.

Coating agents   Several drugs that act neither by neutralization nor by inhibition of gastric acid secretion have been used in treatment of duodenal ulcer. Among these is *sucralfate*, a complex polyaluminum hydroxide salt of sucrose sulfate. Sucralfate becomes highly polar at acid pH and binds to the ulcer bed for up to 12 h, whereas relatively little binds to intact gastric or duodenal mucosa. It is believed that adherence of sucralfate to granulation tissue impedes diffusion of H^+ to the base of the ulcer. In addition, sucralfate binds bile acids and pepsins and may therefore reduce their injurious effects. Sucralfate may increase endogenous tissue prostaglandins and thereby increase mucosal defense. It is only minimally absorbed, with less than 5 percent appearing in the urine. Sucralfate appears to be similar to antacids and H-2 receptor antagonists in its effectiveness in the treatment of duodenal ulcer and in prevention of duodenal ulcer recurrence. The recommended dose of sucralfate is 1 g 1 h before each meal and at bedtime. *Colloidal bismuth* compounds also aid ulcer healing. They form (in an acid medium) a bismuth-protein coagulant which is believed to protect the ulcer from acid-pepsin digestion. Colloidal bismuth compounds have little acid-neutralizing effect and do not reduce gastric acid secretion. These compounds inhibit pepsin activity, bind to the gastric mucus gel layer, and may prevent diffusion of hydrogen ions. They stimulate gastric mucosal secretion of prostaglandins, bicarbonate, and glycoprotein mucus. Bismuth-containing compounds also may be of value in the treatment of duodenal ulcer because of their effects on *H. pylori*, a bacterium which is responsible for some forms of gastritis (see ''Gastritis,'' below) and which, as noted previously, has been proposed as a potential pathogenetic factor in the etiology of duodenal ulcer. Colloidal bismuth compounds are the only class of antiulcer drugs that eradicate *H. pylori* and the gastritis associated with its colonization. Several duodenal ulcer clinical trials have shown good healing rates of duodenal ulcer in patients treated with colloidal bismuth subcitrate

as well as with various triple-therapy combinations of colloidal bismuth compounds, metronidazole, and other antibiotics, e.g., tetracycline or amoxicillin. In those therapeutic trials, eradication of *H. pylori* was associated with ulcer healing and recolonization with ulcer recurrence. Triple therapy results in 80 to 90 percent *H. pylori* eradication at 1 month. Several studies have shown greatly reduced rates of recurrence of duodenal ulcer following ulcer healing by treatment with colloidal bismuth or colloidal bismuth and antibiotic combinations when compared with treatment with H-2 receptor antagonists. When ulcers recurred, they were associated with gastric recolonization with *H. pylori*.

Prostaglandins   A variety of *prostaglandins*, particularly those of the E series (PGE_1 and PGE_2), have been shown to be effective in clinical trials in the treatment of duodenal ulcer, with healing rates approximately comparable to those achieved with antacid therapy and H-2 receptor antagonists. Their mechanism of action is believed to be twofold: (1) they reduce basal and stimulated gastric acid secretion, and (2) they enhance mucosal resistance to tissue injury. Exogenous prostaglandins exert the following actions important in enhancing mucosal defense: PGEs (1) stimulate gastric mucus secretion, (2) stimulate gastric and duodenal bicarbonate secretion, (3) maintain or increase gastric mucosal blood flow, (4) maintain the gastric mucosal barrier to back-diffusion of H^+, and (5) stimulate mucosal cell restitution. Although comparable with weaker H-2 receptor antagonists in inhibiting gastric acid secretion and in ulcer healing, PGEs are not approved in the United States for treatment of duodenal ulcer. Misoprostol, a PGE_1 analogue, is effective in preventing ulcers caused by nonsteroidal anti-inflammatory drugs (NSAIDs).

Proton pump inhibition   The final phase of hydrogen ion secretion by parietal cells is accomplished by an enzyme (H^+,K^+-ATPase) which serves as a proton pump, exchanging hydrogen for potassium. The H^+,K^+-ATPase is located in the apical membrane and tubulovesicular apparatus of parietal cells. The luminal surface of the transmembrane enzyme is exposed ot the gastric luminal acid pH. *Omeprazole*, a specific inhibitor of parietal cell H^+,K^+-ATPase, has been shown to be extraordinarily potent in decreasing gastric acid secretion. Omeprazole, a substituted benzimidazole (Fig. 252-5) binds to the H^+,K^+-ATPase, irreversibly inactivating the enzyme. Omeprazole, a weak base, is a prodrug that becomes concentrated in an acid environment (below pH 4) generating an active sulfur group which forms a covalent disulfide bond with the H^+,K^+-ATPase, thereby denaturing and inactivating the enzyme. Omeprazole completely blocks basal and stimulated acid secretion. It produces prolonged inhibition of gastric acid secretion, with acid secretory recovery requiring synthesis of new enzyme. The maximum effect of omeprazole occurs within 2 h, with 50 percent of maximum inhibition at 24 h and the duration of inhibition persisting for up to 72 h. With once-daily dosing a plateau is reached after 4 days, and after discontinuance, gastric acid secretory activity returns gradually over 3 to 5 days.

Omeprazole is approved and effective for treatment of duodenal ulcer, erosive esophagitis, and gastric acid hypersecretory states, including the Zollinger-Ellison syndrome. Omeprazole is recommended for treatment of duodenal ulcer at a dose of 20 mg daily in the morning before breakfast for periods from 4 to 8 weeks.

FIGURE 252-5   Chemical structure of omeprazole, a substituted benzimidazole which inhibits gastric acid secretion by inhibition of H^+,K^+-ATPase located on the tubovesicular apparatus and apical membranes of parietal cells.

Omeprazole

Omeprazole administration is associated with small to moderate increases in serum gastrin secondary to its effect on gastric acid secretion. Serum gastrin levels return to pretreatment levels within 2 weeks after drug discontinuance. Hyperplasia of gastric mucosal ECL cells and carcinoid tumors due to striking hypergastrinemia in rats receiving omeprazole have not been reported in humans.

DIET   With little or no justification, many different diet programs have been used for treatment of patients with duodenal ulcer. There is no evidence that bland diets reduce gastric acid secretion, promote healing, or relieve symptoms of duodenal ulcer. Similarly, soft diets or diet free of spices or fruit juices have not been proven of benefit. Although traditionally milk and cream were prescribed in the treatment of ulcer patients, there is no evidence that they benefit ulcer healing. They may contribute to development of the milk-alkali syndrome and may accelerate atherogenesis. Many physicians recommend that patients with duodenal ulcer avoid coffee, with or without caffeine, and other caffeine-containing beverages because of their effects on gastric secretion. It also may be desirable to restrict alcohol intake in these patients. It is reasonable to suggest that if patients experience symptoms after ingestion of certain foods, these foods should be avoided.

GENERAL THERAPEUTIC CONSIDERATIONS   How does one integrate the large amount of available information concerning treatment of duodenal ulcer in selecting a therapeutic program for individual patients? There are several reasonable alternatives: Effective therapy may be based on neutralization of gastric acid by antacids, on inhibition of gastric acid secretion by antisecretory agents, or on local actions of some other agents. There is no evidence that combinations of these drugs are required in the treatment of duodenal ulcer. The various classes of agents appear to be comparably effective in accelerating duodenal ulcer healing. In general, although side effects differ from group to group, these are all safe and effective drugs. Most duodenal ulcers will heal within 4 to 6 weeks of treatment with each of these groups of agents. It is seldom necessary to continue treatment of active duodenal ulcer for more than 8 weeks.

There is not yet general agreement concerning which patients should receive prolonged maintenance therapy to reduce the frequency of duodenal ulcer recurrence. Most physicians do not initiate maintenance treatment after the first (uncomplicated) episode of duodenal ulcer activity. Maintenance therapy is often recommended in patients with frequent, especially severe, duodenal ulcer recurrences; in those with previous, especially recurrent, duodenal ulcer complications; and perhaps in those with troublesome ulcer disease and other medical conditions which would make ulcer complications or surgery particularly hazardous. Maintenance therapy, when recommended, is usually continued for at least 1 year. Elimination of cigarette smoking, in most studies, appears to facilitate ulcer healing and may reduce duodenal ulcer recurrence. There is no evidence that dietary manipulation plays an important role in duodenal ulcer treatment.

GASTRIC ULCER

The peak incidence for gastric ulcer is in the sixth decade, approximately 10 years later than for duodenal ulcer. Slightly more than half of gastric ulcers occur in males. Although clinically recognized duodenal ulcer is decreasing, hospitalization for gastric ulcer has stabilized and may be increasing. Gastric ulcers are deep, penetrating beyond the mucosa of the stomach, and are similar histologically to duodenal ulcer, but usually with more extensive gastritis surrounding the ulcer. Almost all benign gastric ulcers are found immediately distal to the junction of the antral mucosa with the acid-secreting mucosa of the body of the stomach. The location of this junction is variable, especially on the lesser gastric curvature. In general, antral mucosa extends approximately two-thirds of the way up the lesser curvature and one-third of the way up the greater curvature of the stomach. Benign gastric ulcers are rare in the fundus of the stomach. Benign gastric ulcers are virtually always accompanied by antral

gastritis with variable amounts of mucosal atrophy. Gastritis may be present or absent with gastric ulcers associated with aspirin and other nonsteroidal anti-inflammatory drugs; they are usually located in the antrum, but they are not confined to the junction of the antral and parietal cell mucosa.

ETIOLOGY AND PATHOGENESIS   Acid-pepsin appears to be important in the pathogenesis of gastric ulcer; however, in contrast to duodenal ulcer, gastric ulcer patients generally have acid secretory rates that are normal or reduced compared with nonulcer subjects. True achlorhydria (in response to pentagastrin stimulation) almost never occurs in patients with benign gastric ulcer. Ten to twenty percent of patients with gastric ulcers also have duodenal ulcers. Patients with both duodenal and gastric ulcers tend to have acid secretory patterns that parallel those of duodenal ulcer. Patients with pyloric channel ulcers have acid secretory rates and clinical patterns similar to those found with common duodenal ulcer.

Most evidence supports the primary importance of defective gastric mucosal resistance and/or direct gastric mucosal injury in the pathogenesis of gastric ulcer. Unlike duodenal ulcer, serum gastrin levels are increased in a significant proportion of gastric ulcer patients, but increases are limited to those with gastric acid hyposecretion. Gastric emptying has been shown to be delayed in gastric ulcer. Regurgitation of duodenal contents, especially those containing bile, may induce gastric mucosal injury and subsequent gastric ulceration by interruption of the gastric mucosal barrier with resultant back-diffusion of secreted hydrogen ions. Nonsteroidal anti-inflammatory drugs (NSAIDs) are responsible for a large proportion of gastric ulcers. This is believed to be due primarily to reduced mucosal defense produced by inhibition of synthesis of gastric mucosal prostaglandins.

CLINICAL FEATURES   As with duodenal ulcer, epigastric pain is the most common symptom; however, it is less typical than in patients with duodenal ulcer. Some gastric ulcer patients experience no relief of pain with eating. Pain may actually be precipitated or accentuated by food, and symptom relief with antacids is less consistent than with duodenal ulcers. Gastric ulcers tend to heal but then recur, often in the same location. Recognizable episodes of recurrent gastric ulcer activity are, in general, less frequent than those of duodenal ulcer. The precise incidence of gastric ulcer is not known, since many gastric ulcer patients are asymptomatic. Although duodenal ulcer is identified clinically more frequently than gastric ulcer, most autopsy studies show an equal or greater proportion of gastric ulcers. This may be due in part to acute preterminal events but also may reflect the often asymptomatic clinical course of gastric ulcer. Whereas in duodenal ulcer patients nausea and vomiting almost always indicate gastric outlet obstruction, in patients with gastric ulcer they may occur in the absence of mechanical obstruction. Weight loss may occur due to anorexia or aversion of food due to discomfort produced by eating.

Hemorrhage is a common complication, occurring in approximately 25 percent. Mortality is greater in patients with gastric ulcer than in those with duodenal ulcer. Gastric perforation occurs less frequently than hemorrhage. Mortality with gastric ulcer perforation is approximately three times that with duodenal ulcers. Increased mortality is due in part to the increased age of gastric ulcer patients but also may result from uncertainty and delay in diagnosis and from greater soilage of the peritoneum with gastric ulcer perforation. Gastric outlet obstruction may develop when ulcers are in the pyloric channel or in the most distal antrum but is rare with ulcer in other parts of the stomach.

DIAGNOSIS   The history is of value in suspecting gastric ulcer, but it is not as characteristic as in duodenal ulcer. The two major methods for diagnosis are barium examination and endoscopy. Gastric ulcer usually can be identified by barium examination, with an accuracy approximating 80 percent. NSAID-associated gastric ulcers are frequently more superficial and are less often identified radiographically. Both benign and malignant gastric ulcers are more common on the lesser than on the greater curvature (Fig. 252-6). Radiation of

FIGURE 252-6 Benign lesser curvature gastric ulcer. Note ulceration beyond the projected margins of the stomach and the collar of edema.

gastric mucosal folds from the margin of the ulcer crater suggests a benign lesion. Large gastric ulcers, i.e., those greater than 3 cm in diameter, are more often malignant than smaller ones. An ulcer within a mass, as defined radiographically, also suggests malignancy. Approximately 4 percent of gastric ulcers which appear benign radiographically prove to be malignant (by endoscopic biopsy or at surgery). Because of false-positive and false-negative errors, radiographic appearance cannot be used as the sole criterion for the benign or malignant nature of a gastric ulcer.

Endoscopic visualization of the ulcer allows definition of its size, location, and, by biopsy, its histologic characteristics. To exclude malignancy at gastroscopy, a total of at least six biopsies are obtained from the inner margin of the ulcer and from the ulcer bed. If accurate cytology is available, brushings of the ulcer should be obtained prior to biopsy. By application of combined radiographic, endoscopic, and histologic techniques, distinguishing malignant from benign gastric ulcers should be possible with more than 95 percent confidence.

Gastric ulcer with pentagastrin-fast achlorhydria is rare. When it occurs, it almost always indicates gastric carcinoma. However, most patients with gastric carcinoma (about two-thirds to three-fourths) are capable of secreting gastric acid, but usually less than normal.

MEDICAL TREATMENT   In general, with whatever medical treatment modality is selected, gastric ulcers tend to heal more slowly than duodenal ulcers, and the healing response rates are somewhat less than those for duodenal ulcer. Larger gastric ulcers take longer to heal than smaller ones. *Antacids* are effective in gastric ulcer treatment. However, since acid hypersecretion is not characteristic of the disease, smaller doses of antacid may be required than for treatment of duodenal ulcer. *H-2 receptor antagonists* and *sucralfate* are approximately as effective as antacid therapy. The dosage schedules for these drugs are similar to those for duodenal ulcer.

Anticholinergic agents have been recommended by some physi-

cians. However, because of substantial side effects of anticholinergic drugs, their tendency to reduce gastric emptying (which is already impaired in these patients), the fact that gastric ulcer patients are often older and therefore more susceptible to the complications of these agents, and the lack of evidence for their benefit, the use of anticholinergic drugs in gastric ulcer treatment does not appear justified. Some studies have suggested that hospitalization and/or cessation of smoking are of benefit in gastric ulcer healing.

Since salicylates and other NSAIDs have been associated with the development of gastric ulcers, patients with gastric ulcer should not ingest these. Alcohol, because of its injurious effects on the gastric mucosa, probably also should be avoided. Milk and cream, as well as bland or homogenized diets, have not been shown to be of value in treatment. In general, it is probably sufficient to recommend that patients consume a diet of their own choice. Since coffee (caffeine-containing or caffeine-free) and other caffeine-containing liquids stimulate gastric acid secretion, it may be desirable to avoid these beverages.

Gastric ulcers are present in approximately 15 percent (10 to 30 percent) of patients receiving chronic NSAID treatment, with a smaller increase in the prevalence of duodenal ulcer. Patients at high risk for ulcer while on NSAIDs include patients of advanced age, females, those on high-dose and protracted-use NSAIDs, those undergoing simultaneous NSAID and glucocorticoid administration, and those with severe intercurrent disease. *Misoprostol*, a PGE_1 analogue, in doses of 100 μg or 200 μg four times a day, has been shown to reduce NSAID-associated gastric ulcer by approximately 75 and 95 percent, respectively. For ulcer prevention in high-risk patients requiring NSAID treatment, misoprostol is administered with gradual increases in dose, beginning at 100 μg/d and increasing, as tolerated, to the full dose of 200 μg four times a day. Gradual increments of 100 μg/d at 1- or 2-week intervals are suggested because of abdominal cramping and/or diarrhea which occasionally may be experienced with abrupt initiation of the full dose.

Carbenoxalone has been used in many countries (though not available in the United States) in the treatment of gastric ulcer. This drug, a hydrolytic product of glycyrrhizic acid (derived from licorice), has been shown to decrease symptoms and increase the rate of gastric ulcer healing. Carbenoxalone, which does not decrease gastric acid secretion, increases the life span of gastric mucosal epithelial cells as well as the secretion and viscosity of gastric mucus. Carbenoxalone possesses aldosterone-like effects, producing sodium and water retention. Its side effects and availability of effective alternatives have led to its decreased use.

Benign gastric ulcers should heal completely within 3 months of vigorous therapy. The failure of gastric ulcer to decrease satisfactorily in size and to heal with medical treatment has been used to suggest gastric malignancy. The following is suggested as one reasonable scheme to monitor gastric ulcer healing. Upper gastrointestinal barium examination or gastroscopy is suggested after 4 weeks of treatment, at which time definite healing of benign gastric ulcers should be demonstrable; i.e., the diameter of most ulcers should be reduced by more than 50 percent. If not, malignancy must be suspected, and endoscopy, exfoliative cytology, and biopsies of the ulcer should be performed. If no malignancy is identified, medical therapy should be continued. If the ulcer has not healed completely at 8 weeks, endoscopic examination should be repeated in another month, at which time most benign gastric ulcers should have healed. Apparently complete healing does not guarantee the benign nature of a gastric ulcer, since approximately 70 percent of gastric ulcers eventually found to be malignant will undergo significant (albeit usually incomplete) healing with medical treatment.

COMPLICATIONS AND SURGERY FOR PEPTIC ULCER

Surgery is reserved for patients with complications of peptic ulcer and for those who do not respond to vigorous and attentive medical treatment. Complications include hemorrhage, obstruction, and perforation.

Hemorrhage occurs in approximately 15 percent of patients with duodenal ulcers; a recurrence of bleeding is estimated to occur in about 40 percent of patients with an initial hemorrhage. Hemorrhage due to NSAID-associated ulcer occurs particularly frequently in the absence of prior peptic ulcer symptoms (approximately 50 percent). In most patients hemorrhage from peptic ulcer responds satisfactorily to medical management, including gastric suction and antacid or H-2 receptor antagonist administration.

Free *perforation* into the peritoneal cavity occurs in approximately 6 percent of patients with duodenal ulcer. Five to ten percent of these patients will have had no recognizable ulcer symptoms prior to perforation. Simultaneous hemorrhage occurs in approximately 10 percent of patients with duodenal ulcer perforation; mortality is greatly increased in this group. Duodenal ulcers, especially those located posteriorly, may penetrate into adjacent structures, most often the pancreas, frequently resulting in increased serum amylase levels. Less commonly, duodenal ulcers penetrate the liver, biliary tract, or colon.

Gastric outlet *obstruction* occurs in 2 to 4 percent of patients admitted to the hospital with duodenal or pyloric channel ulcers. Symptoms include abdominal bloating, nausea, vomiting, and weight loss. These patients usually have had ulcer symptoms for many years and often obstructive symptoms for several months.

Failure to respond satisfactorily to medical treatment requires consideration of surgery. The true incidence of lack of ulcer healing with vigorous medical programs is not known. It is clear that, especially with currently available drugs, the vast majority of patients with peptic ulcer can be treated successfully without surgery.

Decisions regarding surgery for patients with complications of peptic ulcer must be individualized. Risks of surgery must be balanced against risks of the disease. The patient's discomfort, costs of medical care and hospitalization, and time lost from work must be examined in relation to the morbidity and possible mortality associated with surgery and anesthesia, risks of recurrent ulcer, and long-term postoperative sequelae. The skill and experience of the surgeon must be weighed as major factors in considering operation.

SURGERY FOR DUODENAL ULCER   No single surgical procedure has been accepted universally as the most satisfactory duodenal ulcer operation. At present, the most commonly performed surgical procedures are *vagotomy with antrectomy, vagotomy with pyloroplasty*, and *parietal cell vagotomy* (also referred to as *proximal gastric* or *superselective vagotomy*) without a gastric drainage procedure.

With truncal vagotomy with antrectomy, the vagal trunks are transected, the antrum is removed, and gastrointestinal continuity is reestablished by anastomosis of the remaining stomach with the proximal duodenum (Billroth I anastomosis) or with a loop of the jejunum (Billroth II anastomosis). Vagotomy with antrectomy is an effective procedure with a low recurrence rate (approximately 1 percent). Morbidity and mortality with vagotomy with antrectomy are variable depending on patient selection and the skill of the surgeon but are probably slightly greater than with vagotomy with pyloroplasty.

When vagotomy with pyloroplasty is selected, pyloroplasty is performed to facilitate gastric drainage after truncal or selective vagotomy. Vagotomy is performed to inhibit vagal stimulation of gastric acid secretion. It does not inhibit gastrin release; in fact, release of gastrin is enhanced after vagal interruption. Three types of vagotomy are now used in the surgical treatment of duodenal or pyloric channel ulcer, namely *truncal vagotomy, selective vagotomy*, and *parietal cell vagotomy*. Pyloroplasty with truncal vagotomy is associated with approximately 1 percent mortality. Ulcer recurrence during the 5 years after surgery is about 5 to 8 percent. With selective vagotomy only the branches of the vagus that supply the stomach are transected, preserving the vagal innervation of other abdominal viscera. Selective vagotomy has been found by some surgeons to result in a more complete vagotomy, less ulcer recurrence, and fewer postvagotomy complications than truncal vagotomy. Parietal cell vagotomy denervates only the acid-secreting portion of the stomach,

sparing the branches of the vagus that innervate the antrum, which makes a gastric drainage procedure (e.g., pyloroplasty) unnecessary. Both immediate and late postoperative complications are less common with parietal cell vagotomy than with truncal vagotomy, and reductions in acid secretion are similar to those achieved with truncal or selective vagotomy. Mortality with parietal cell vagotomy is less than 1 percent. Most studies indicate that, with experience, recurrence is comparable to that of other forms of vagotomy with pyloroplasty. This procedure, which is being used with increasing frequency, appears to be a safe and effective surgical therapy.

SURGERY FOR GASTRIC ULCER   Surgical treatment is required for gastric ulcer patients who do not respond satisfactorily to medical therapy or who develop complications similar to those described for duodenal ulcer. With the available diagnostic accuracy of careful radiographic examination, endoscopy, biopsy of the ulcer margins, and exfoliative cytology, it is rarely necessary to operate because of uncertainty regarding the malignant or benign nature of the ulcer. The recommended surgical procedure for the treatment of gastric ulcer is antrectomy with gastroduodenal (Billroth I) anastomosis. It is not necessary to perform a vagotomy when antrectomy is performed for gastric ulcer (not located in the pyloric channel).

CONDITIONS AFTER PEPTIC ULCER SURGERY

Modern surgery for peptic ulcer is effective in the treatment of ulcer complications and in the prevention of ulcer recurrence. However, numerous postoperative sequelae and syndromes may occur.

RECURRENT ULCERATION   Recurrent ulceration has been reported in approximately 5 percent of all patients after surgery for peptic ulcer. Approximately 95 percent of these recurrences follow surgery for duodenal ulcer disease. The risk of recurrent ulcer is 3 to 10 percent after surgery for duodenal ulcer and approximately 2 percent after gastric ulcer surgery. Recurrence is more common after vagotomy with pyloroplasty and after parietal cell vagotomy than after vagotomy with antrectomy. When ulcers occur after partial gastric resection, the ulcer is usually located at the anastomosis (stomal or marginal ulcer) or immediately distal to it in the small intestine. Abdominal pain is the most common symptom in patients with a stomal ulcer. The pain is usually epigastric but is often not characteristic of common duodenal ulcer. It is usually, but not always, relieved by meals or antacids and, in general, tends to be more persistent and progressive than that observed with unoperated duodenal ulcer. Hemorrhage or anemia due to blood loss, nausea and vomiting from obstruction, weight loss, or symptoms from perforation may occur. The development of a stomal ulcer after duodenal ulcer surgery usually indicates that an incomplete vagotomy was performed. Inadequate gastric resection, when performed without vagotomy, also may result in stomal ulceration. Additional causes for recurrent ulcer include an excessively long jejunal afferent loop, an inadvertently performed gastroileal or gastrocolic anastomosis, poor gastric drainage, and ingestion of ulcerogenic drugs (especially NSAIDs). Less commonly, a marginal ulcer may be caused by acid hypersecretion secondary to gastrinoma or a retained antrum.

Radiographic examination with barium is of limited diagnostic value and identifies only from 50 to 60 percent of stomal ulcerations. Surgical deformity at the anastomotic site often may mimic stomal ulcer in its absence or conceal it when present. When suspected, endoscopic examination is required to identify stomal ulceration. Medical treatment with antacids is almost always unsatisfactory in patients with stomal ulcer. H-2 receptor antagonists have been reported to induce healing of stomal ulcers. The long-term effectiveness of these agents on stomal ulcers and prevention of their recurrence remain to be established. Surgery is usually necessary for treatment of ulcer recurrence, and it is usually successful. In patients with ulcer recurrent after surgery, provocative testing with measurement of serum gastrin is needed to identify or exclude gastrinoma (see below).

RECURRENT ULCER DUE TO RETAINED ANTRUM   Recurrent ulcers have been described in a small number of patients after antrectomy with gastrojejunostomy (Billroth II anastomosis) in which the antral resection was not complete. In these patients, the distal antrum, inadvertently not resected, remains in continuity with the duodenum after surgery. These patients usually develop or continue to have gastric acid hypersecretion due to gastrin release by the residual antral mucosa which is no longer is contact with gastric acid, the normal inhibitor of gastrin release. Fasting serum gastrin levels in these patients may be normal to moderately increased. Patients with retained antrum can be distinguished from those with gastrinoma by intravenous injection of secretin and measurements of serum gastrin levels. Gastrinoma patients exhibit substantial increases in serum gastrin (>200 pg/mL increase), whereas those with retained antrum exhibit decreased serum gastrin levels, stay the same, or show slight increases after secretin administration. These patients can be treated successfully by surgical removal of the remaining antrum.

AFFERENT LOOP SYNDROMES   Patients with partial gastric resection with gastrojejunostomy (Billroth II anastomosis) may experience abdominal bloating and pain 20 min to 1 h after eating, frequently followed by nausea and vomiting. The vomitus often contains large amounts of bile. Characteristically, the bloating and abdominal discomfort are relieved by vomiting. This type of afferent loop syndrome, which is uncommon, is believed to be caused by distention of an incompletely draining afferent intestinal loop by pancreatic and biliary secretions, which are stimulated by eating. Serum amylase levels may be mildly or moderately increased. Because of partial obstruction, it is often difficult to demonstrate the afferent loop by barium meal examination. Treatment is surgical correction of the incomplete afferent loop obstruction and, in some instances, revision to a gastroduodenal anastomosis.

A second form of afferent loop dysfunction is that due to stasis with bacterial overgrowth within the afferent loop. These patients may exhibit the same characteristics as those found with other forms of small intestinal bacterial overgrowth or blind loop syndromes (see Chap. 254) e.g., malabsorption, especially of fat and vitamin B_{12}. Correction of the afferent loop bacterial overgrowth syndrome can be accomplished by surgical revision of the afferent loop.

BILE REFLUX GASTRITIS   After peptic ulcer surgery, a small proportion of patients experience early satiety, abdominal discomfort, and vomiting, which is believed due to reflux of duodenal contents into the stomach. Endoscopic examination usually reveals regurgitated bile in the stomach and diffuse gastritis, often involving the entire gastric remnant. Various terms assigned to this entity include *alkaline reflux gastritis*, *bile reflux gastritis*, *duodenogastric reflux*, and *bilious vomiting*. The mechanisms or materials contained in the refluxed intestinal contents accounting for these symptoms have not been defined. Although the term *bile reflux gastritis* has been used, there is no certainty that regurgitated bile is responsible for the syndrome. Administration of cholestyramine, intended to bind bile acids and facilitate their excretion, has not been proven of benefit in this disorder. Some surgeons have reported successful treatment of bile reflux gastritis by diversion of duodenal contents from proximity to the stomach with a roux-en-Y anastomosis.

DUMPING SYNDROME   Following peptic ulcer surgery, some patients experience an assortment of vasomotor symptoms after eating. These include palpitation, tachycardia, light-headedness, diaphoresis, and, less frequently, postural hypotension. Abdominal discomfort and vomiting also may occur. The vasomotor symptoms, referred to as the *early dumping syndrome*, are usually experienced within 30 min after eating and are believed to result from rapid emptying of hyperosmolar gastric contents into the proximal small intestine. This leads to a shift of fluid into the gut lumen and produces intestinal distention and contraction of plasma volume. Additional proposed mechanisms for these symptoms include stimulation of autonomic reflexes secondary to small intestinal distention and/or release of hormones from the gut in response to rapid entry of gastric contents into the duodenum or jejunum.

The *late dumping syndrome* refers to a symptom complex comprising dizziness, light-headedness, palpitation, diaphoresis, confusion, and, in rare instances, syncope occurring 90 min to 3 h after eating. The symptoms can often be precipitated by meals rich in simple carbohydrates, especially sucrose. The syndrome appears to be caused by hypoglycemia due to insulin release stimulated by abrupt increases in blood glucose secondary to rapid emptying of sugar-containing meals into the proximal small intestine.

Both forms of the dumping syndrome are treated by dietary measures. These include limitation of simple sugar-continuing liquids and solids (sweets), elimination of liquids at mealtime, and frequent small meals. Most patients have not been benefited from surgical procedures such as creation of reversed jejunal loops and isoperistaltic jejunal interposition.

POSTVAGOTOMY DIARRHEA   A significant number of patients experience diarrhea after peptic ulcer surgery, especially with procedures including truncal vagotomy. Diarrhea has been estimated to occur in 20 to 30 percent of patients after truncal vagotomy with drainage, in 10 to 20 percent with selective vagotomy and drainage, and in only 1 to 8 percent of those with parietal cell vagotomy (without drainage). Diarrhea usually occurs within 2 h of eating. Although the mechanism is not clear, interruption of vagal fibers to the abdominal viscera appears important in production of the diarrhea. The surgical drainage procedure, pyloroplasty or antrectomy, removes the pyloric regulatory emptying mechanism. Rapid emptying of gastric contents into the small intestine, resulting in increased fluid volume within the intestinal lumen due to the osmotic action of the meal, also may contribute to the diarrhea.

HEMATOLOGIC COMPLICATIONS   Intrinsic factor secreted by gastric parietal cells is necessary for active absorption of vitamin B_{12} by the distal ileum. Patients after total gastrectomy invariably develop malabsorption of vitamin B_{12} and should receive monthly intramuscular injections of vitamin B_{12} (50 to 100 μg) indefinitely. Megaloblastic anemia due to vitamin B_{12} deficiency is rare after partial gastric resection; however, reduced serum vitamin B_{12} levels have been observed in about 14 percent of these patients. Even more rarely, vitamin B_{12} deficiency may be produced by bacterial overgrowth in a stagnant afferent loop following Billroth II anastomosis. Gastritis in the remaining stomach develops in more than 60 percent of duodenal ulcer patients after vagotomy with antrectomy or vagotomy with pyloroplasty. This may result in decreased vitamin B_{12} absorption. Inasmuch as the stomach secretes intrinsic factor approximately 100 times in excess of need, peptic ulcer patients treated with partial gastric resection do not develop vitamin B_{12} deficiency secondary to the amount of stomach resected. (In addition, the resected portion of the stomach is almost always principally antrum, which contains few parietal cells.) However, after peptic ulcer surgery, patients may develop decreased serum vitamin B_{12} levels as a result of reduced absorption of food-bound vitamin B_{12}; these patients will often have normal absorption of free vitamin B_{12}, as used in the Schilling test. The precise mechanism of the malabsorption of food-bound vitamin B_{12} is not known. It may be due in part to rapid emptying of gastric contents, with reduced efficiency of intrinsic factor binding of vitamin B_{12}. Anemia after peptic ulcer surgery also may result from deficiency produced by malabsorption of iron or folate. A combined deficiency of vitamin B_{12}, iron, and folate is common in patients with anemia following partial or subtotal gastric resection. Iron deficiency is the most common single hematologic defect after peptic ulcer surgery and may result from either blood loss (e.g., with persistent or recurrent ulcers) or iron malabsorption. Patients with gastric resection who malabsorb dietary iron have normal absorption of iron salts; therefore, they will respond favorable to treatment with therapeutic oral iron preparations. Folate deficiency may result from either reduced dietary intake or impaired folate absorption. Except for anemia from blood loss caused by early recurrent ulcer, development of anemia after peptic ulcer surgery is gradual, usually occurring over several years.

The nature of the anemia after ulcer surgery should be clarified by determination of the red blood cell morphology and by measurements of serum iron, folate, and vitamin B_{12}. Iron or folate deficiency should be treated by oral replacement. Vitamin B_{12} deficiency should be treated with monthly intramuscular injections of the vitamin.

OSTEOMALACIA AND OSTEOPOROSIS Osteoporosis and osteomalacia are common after partial or complete gastrectomy but occur rarely after vagotomy with pyloroplasty. Osteomalacia is extremely frequent following gastrojejunostomy or Billroth II anastomosis. These bone changes are believed to result from malabsorption of calcium and vitamin D. Patients may develop bone pain and have pathologic fractures. The incidence of bone fractures in men following gastric resection has been estimated to be almost twice that of control subjects of similar age. Reduced bone density identified by x-ray requires years to develop. Patients with osteomalacia usually have increased levels of serum alkaline phosphatase and may have reduced serum calcium concentrations. These patients should be treated by supplemental oral vitamin D and calcium. The frequency of osteoporosis and osteomalacia after partial or complete gastrectomy is sufficiently great to justify treatment with vitamin D and calcium indefinitely, especially in females, following gastric resection.

GENERAL MALABSORPTION (See also Chap. 254) Mild, chemically demonstable steatorrhea is common in patients after ulcer surgery. Weight loss is more common after partial gastric resection (approximately 60 percent of patients) than with vagotomy without resection. The major cause of weight loss is reduced food intake. On a 100-g fat diet, loss of stool fat seldom exceeds 15 g/d (normal individuals less than 7 g/d). The causes of maldigestion and malabsorption after peptic ulcer surgery include rapid gastric emptying, reduced dispersion of food in the stomach, reduced bile concentrations in the gut lumen, increased rate of transit of the meal through the small intestine, and reduced or delayed pancreatic secretory responses to feeding. Steatorrhea and weight loss, sometimes accompanied by vitamin B_{12} malabsorption, may develop as a result of bacterial overgrowth, especially in patients with afferent loop bacterial stasis. Overt symptoms and other manifestations of malabsorption appearing after surgery for peptic ulcer also may be due to other preexisting conditions, including latent celiac sprue and chronic pancreatitis.

CARCINOMA AFTER PARTIAL GASTRECTOMY Several studies have documented an increased incidence of adenocarcinoma of the stomach in duodenal ulcer patients following partial gastric resection and after vagotomy and drainage without resection. This usually develops 10 or more years after ulcer surgery. The possibility of carcinoma of the stomach should be considered when abdominal symptoms, which may be similar to or distinct from those due to the original ulcer, appear many years after apparently successful surgery.

ZOLLINGER-ELLISON SYNDROME (GASTRINOMA)

In 1955, Zollinger and Ellison described the syndrome that bears their names, which consists of ulcer disease of the upper gastrointestinal tract, marked increases in gastric acid secretion, and non-beta islet cell tumors of the pancreas.

ETIOLOGY AND PATHOGENESIS Zollinger and Ellison, in their original description of the syndrome, suggested that the ulcer disease in these patients resulted from release of a secretagogue from these tumors into the circulation which accounted for the often enormously increased rates of gastric acid secretion. Their proposal proved correct when in 1960 extracts of Zollinger-Ellison (Z-E) tumors were shown to stimulate gastric acid secretion. Subsequently, it was found that these pancreatic islet cell tumors contained gastrin and that there were large amounts of this hormone in the circulation producing the pathophysiologic characteristics of the syndrome. These gastrin-containing tumors are therefore now called *gastrinomas*.

Gastrinomas have been reported most often within the pancreas. Pancreatic gastrinomas may vary in size from 1 mm to more than 20 cm in diameter. Multiple primary tumors are common. From one-half to two-thirds of patients have multiple gastrinomas. Pancreatic gastrinomas are most common in the head of the pancreas. In more

than half of Zollinger-Ellison patients harboring gastrinomas the tumors cannot be identified at surgery. There is recent evidence that with careful search when gastrinomas are located they are found as frequently (or perhaps more frequently) in the wall of the duodenum as in the pancreas. Duodenal gastrinomas, approximately 50 percent of which are solitary, are usually found in the submucosa of the first or second parts of the duodenum. Gastrinomas also have been located less commonly in other sites, including the hilum of the spleen and rarely in the stomach. Gastrinomas have been found in lymph nodes in proximity to the pancreas, proximal duodenum, and spleen in the absence of demonstrated primary tumors. These probably represent local metastases from undiscovered duodenal wall gastrinomas. Approximately 90 percent of gastrinomas are found within an anatomic triangle (the gastrinoma triangle) which is comprised of the junction of the cystic and common bile ducts superiorly, the junction of the second and third portions of the duodenum inferiorly, and the junction of the pancreatic body and neck medially. In unusual instances, the Z-E syndrome has resulted from gastrinomas originating from remote organs, e.g., parathyroid and ovarian tumors. About two-thirds of gastrinomas are histologically or biologically malignant. Malignant gastrinomas usually grow slowly; however, a small portion may be rapidly invasive and may metastasize early and widely. Metastasis is most often to regional lymph nodes and liver; spread also may be to peritoneal surfaces, spleen, bone, skin, or mediastinum. Gastrinomas have light-microscopic similarities to carcinoid tumors and may be mistaken for these tumors, especially when gastrinomas arise from the mucosa of the small intestine or stomach. Pancreatic islet cell hyperplasia occurs in approximately 10 percent of patients with the Z-E syndrome. Hyperplasia of the islets, accompanying recognized or unidentified gastrinoma, appears to be an association or a consequence, rather than a cause, of excess gastrin release, since gastrin is not present in the hyperplastic tissue.

In an estimated 20 to 60 percent of patients with the Z-E syndrome the gastrinoma is a component of the multiple endocrine neoplasia type 1 (MEN 1) syndrome, an autosomal dominant disorder with a high degree of penetrance and great variability in expressivity. The MEN 1 locus is on chrosomome 11. Patients with MEN 1 may have clinically recognized hyperplasia, adenomas, or carcinoma involving, in order of frequency, the parathyroid glands, pancreatic islets, and pituitary. Hyperparathyroidism has been reported in 87 percent of patients with MEN 1 syndrome, and gastrinoma has been reported in approximately half of them (see Chap. 343). However, there is accumulating evidence that when carefully sought for there is probably involvement of all three organs in all patients with MEN 1, although it is frequently without overt clinical expression. Gastrinomas in non-MEN 1 patients are considered to be sporadic. Multiple gastrinomas are usually present in patients with MEN 1 and are usually smaller than sporadic gastrinomas. Gastrinomas with MEN 1 are located more frequently in the wall of the duodenum than in the pancreas. Patients, including those with duodenal gastrinomas, usually have multiple pancreatic islet cell tumors, most of which are not gastrinomas.

In most gastrinomas, approximately 80 to 95 percent of gastrin is in the form of heptadecapeptide gastrin (G-17), with most of the remainder being G-34. In contrast, approximately two-thirds of circulating gastrin in gastrinoma patients is G-34; most of the remainder is G-17. However, smaller amounts of even larger forms of gastrin and smaller gastrin fragments can be detected in the serum. When examined carefully, almost all gastrin-secreting islet cell tumors are found to contain multiple hormones that are usually clinically silent. These have included, among others, ACTH, glucagon, melanocyte-stimulating hormone, parathyroid hormone, growth hormone releasing factor (GRF), insulin, pancreatic polypeptide, and vasoactive intestinal peptide. Of these, ACTH is the most common; it is found in approximately 30 percent of gastrinomas. Cushing's syndrome with increased serum ACTH levels has been reported in 8 percent of 75 Z-E patients. ACTH-releasing gastrinomas are often aggressively malignant. In contrast, ACTH may be released by pituitary tumors in patients with MEN 1, in whom symptoms of Cushing's syndrome are generally mild and gastrinomas are usually not metastatic. Approximately one-third of patients with gastrinomas have increases in serum concentrations of *pancreatic polypeptide*.

The parietal cell mass is substantially expanded to from three to six times normal secondary to the trophic effects of circulating gastrin on parietal cells. Small, multicentric, noninvasive carcinoid tumors have been identified in the gastric mucosa of patients with the Z-E syndrome. These tumors and associated focal areas of enterochromaffin-like (ECL) cell hyperplasia are believed to result from substantial and sustained hypergastrinemia. They also have been found in the gastric mucosa of patients with pernicious anemia and achlorhydria, who have striking increases in serum gastrin in the range of those found with gastrinoma.

While the true incidence of the Z-E syndrome is not known, estimates are that it accounts for 0.1 to 1 percent of peptic ulcers. The Z-E syndrome may occur at any age, but initial manifestations occur most commonly between the ages 30 and 60.

CLINICAL FEATURES   From 90 to 95 percent of patients with gastrinomas develop ulceration of the gastrointestinal tract at some point during the course of their disease. Profound gastric acid hypersecretion is found in most, but not all, patients. Especially early in the course of the disease, symptoms are usually similar to those of patients with typical peptic ulcer. However, ulcer symptoms may be more fulminant, progressive, and persistent and, in general, respond poorly to usual medical and surgical peptic ulcer treatment programs. The anatomic site of the ulcers in patients with gastrinoma is similar, but not identical, to that of patients with common types of peptic ulcer. About 75 percent of gastrinoma patients have ulcers in the first portion of the duodenum or in the stomach; these are usually single but may be multiple. When multiple ulcers occur, they are frequently located not only in the first portion of the duodenum, the site of common duodenal ulcer, but also in the remainder of the duodenum or even the jejunum. In one large series, 14 percent of the ulcers were in the duodenum beyond its first portion and 11 percent in the jejunum.

Diarrhea occurs in about 40 percent of patients, and about 7 percent of patients with gastrinoma have diarrhea in the absence of ulcer disease. The diarrhea is due to the outpouring of large amounts of hydrochloric acid into the proximal duodenum and can be reduced or eliminated by aspiration of gastric juice. The excessive acid has been shown to reduce the pH of the contents of the proximal and distal jejunum to as low as 1 and 3.6, respectively. Inflammatory changes may be produced in the mucosa of the small intestine secondary to the injurious effect of large amounts of acid and pepsin. Steatorrhea, which is less common than diarrhea, results from inactivation of pancreatic lipase by large concentrations of acid in the proximal small intestine and from decreases in luminal bile acids. The decrease in intraluminal bile acid concentration is caused by precipitation of the major bile acids at low pH. This leads to impaired micelle formation, which, in turn, reduces intestinal absorption of fatty acids and monoglycerides (see Chap. 254). Vitamin B_{12} malabsorption, not correctable by addition of intrinsic factor, has been detected in some patients with the Z-E syndrome. Although gastric secretion of intrinsic factor appears normal, the reduced pH within the gut interferes with intrinsic factor–mediated vitamin B_{12} absorption. This can be corrected by neutralization of the intestinal contents. The mechanisms by which low pH in the gut interferes with intrinsic factor action is not known.

DIAGNOSIS   The presence of gastrinoma should be suspected in patients with a compatible clinical history, especially in those with marked acid hypersecretion. More than 90 percent of gastrinoma patients have basal gastric acid outputs (BAO) that exceed 15 mmol/h. In some instances, the basal output may be greater than 150 mmol/h. However, there is substantial overlap in rates of gastric acid secretion among patients with gastrinoma, those with duodenal ulcer, and normal subjects. Gastrinoma patients often have BAO rates that are greater than 60 percent of those induced by maximal stimulation (MAO). In most normal subjects and duodenal ulcer patients, basal

acid secretory rates are less than 60 percent of maximal secretion. However, because of frequent exceptions in patients with gastrinomas and common duodenal ulcers, the use of the BAO/MAO ratio is of no value in the certain identification of patients with gastrinoma.

Some radiographic features may suggest the diagnosis of the Z-E syndrome. Large mucosal folds may be demonstrated most prominently in the stomach but also in the duodenum and, in some instances, the jejunum. The lumen of the stomach and small intestine often contains large amounts of fluid. Radiographic features of most ulcers in these patients, except when they are distal in location, are similar to those of common peptic ulcer. Gastrinomas are difficult to localize. In almost half of patients with clinical and laboratory evidence, the tumors cannot be identified at surgery. Selective arteriography identifies gastrinomas in approximately one-third of patients with clinical and biochemical evidence of the Z-E syndrome. Computed tomography (CT) identifies gastrinomas in 30 percent and ultrasound in 15 percent of patients with the Z-E syndrome. Use of both selective arteriography and CT has been reported to identify 44 percent of gastrinomas in Z-E patients and 80 percent of those located at surgery. Endoscopic retrograde pancreaticoduodenography has not proved to be of assistance in the diagnosis or exclusion of pancreatic gastrinomas. A small number of duodenal wall gastrinomas have been identified and confirmed histologically by duodenoscopy.

The diagnosis in a patient with clinical features consistent with the Z-E syndrome depends on the demonstration of *increased serum gastrin levels* by radioimmunoassay. Fasting serum gastrin levels in normal subjects and patients with typical duodenal ulcer average approximately 20 to 50 pg/mL and usually do not exceed 150 pg/mL. Patients with gastrinoma almost always have fasting serum gastrin levels that are greater than 200 pg/mL and have been found as high as 450,000 pg/mL. Approximately half these patients have fasting serum gastrin levels that are less than 1000 pg/mL (an approximate mean value for serum gastrin for patients with gastrinoma).

Several provocative tests have been used to evaluate patients with possible gastrinoma, especially those who do not exhibit pronounced hypergastrinemia (i.e., serum gastrin > 1000 pg/mL). These tests utilize measurements of serum gastrin levels in response to intravenous secretin injection, calcium infusion, or ingestion of a standard test meal.

In the *secretin injection test*, secretin (Kabi secretin, 2 units per kilogram) is given intravenously over 30 to 60 s. Gastrin is measured in serum samples obtained immediately before injection of secretin, at 2 and 5 min after secretin, and at 5-min intervals thereafter for a total of 30 min. In normal individuals and patients with common duodenal ulcer, secretin produces no change, small reductions, or small increases in serum gastrin levels. In contrast, in gastrinoma patients, intravenous secretin induces substantial increases in serum gastrin. The serum gastrin levels increase promptly by at least 200 pg/mL, usually at 5 min (and virtually always by 10 min), and then gradually decrease toward or to preinjection levels by 30 min. In the *calcium infusion test*, serum samples for gastrin measurements are obtained before and at 30-min intervals for 4 h after initiation of a constant 3-h intravenous infusion of calcium gluconate (5 mg calcium per kilogram per hour). In gastrinoma patients, serum gastrin concentrations usually increase above the basal serum gastrin level by more than 400 pg/mL. The third provocative test involves the *feeding of a standard meal*: Gastrin is measured in serum samples obtained before the meal and at 15-min intervals after it for 90 min. This test has been used to attempt to distinguish between patients with gastrinoma and those with hypergastrinemia and gastric acid hypersecretion due to antral gastrin cell hypertrophy or hyperplasia.

The secretin injection test is by far the most valuable provocative test in identifying gastrinoma patients. Positive serum gastrin responses to intravenous secretin are found in more than 95 percent of patients with gastrinoma. Using the criteria suggested, substantial increases in serum gastrin following secretin injection have been detected only rarely in nongastrinoma patients. Reduced gastric acid secretion, achlorhydria or profound hypochlorhydria, is by far the most common cause of hypergastrinemia. For this reason, gastric acid secretion should be measured before consideration of the secretin injection test. Exaggerated release of gastrin in response to calcium infusion is found in more than 80 percent of gastrinoma patients; however, this exaggerated response to calcium infusion occurs in some nongastrinoma patients with hypergastrinemia (e.g., with achlorhydria). Enhanced gastrin release with calcium infusion is rarely observed in gastrinoma patients in the absence of the abnormally large gastrin release in response to secretin. Since the calcium infusion test does not add significantly to the sensitivity or specificity of the secretin injection test, and since calcium infusion is potentially more hazardous, it is usually not necessary or recommended.

In a very small proportion of duodenal ulcer patients (much less than 1 percent), gastric acid hypersecretion may be accompanied by increased serum gastrin levels due to hyperfunction and/or hyperplasia of antral gastrin cells (G cells). These patients can be distinguished from those with gastrinoma by the secretin injection and meal stimulation tests. In patients with this antral gastrin cell abnormality, intravenous secretin does not produce large increases in serum gastrin characteristic of gastrinoma. Some authors have reported increases in serum gastrin concentrations greater than 200 percent after test meals in patients with gastrin cell hypertrophy or hyperplasia, suggesting that this may be of value distinguishing these patients from those with gastrinoma. Other authors more recently have found similarly large amounts of gastrin released into the sera of patients with gastrinomas, suggesting that the meal-stimulated test is of limited value in distinguishing between patients with antral gastrin cell hyperplasia and those with gastrinoma.

TREATMENT In general, patients with Z-E syndrome are resistant to those medical therapies and surgical procedures designed for and usually effective in treating common peptic ulcer. Antacids may produce transient symptom relief but rarely, if ever, induce ulcer healing or sustained relief of symptoms. Incomplete gastric resection (with or without vagotomy) or pyloroplasty with vagotomy is frequently followed by prompt and often fulminant ulcer recurrence. In the past, many patients with gastrinoma had multiple surgical procedures, particularly in those instances in which the diagnosis was not established initially. Mortality was reported to be lowest in patients with the Z-E syndrome in whom gastrectomy was the initial gastric surgery. This led to the conclusion that when surgery was required in gastrinoma patients, total gastrectomy was the surgical procedure of choice.

Development of effective drugs to reduce acid secretion and more precise diagnostic techniques to locate gastrinomas have increased substantially the therapeutic options. The key to management in these patients is individualization of treatment, since patients with the Z-E syndrome are highly heterogeneous with respect to clinical manifestations and extent of disease. As with many other predominantly malignant tumors, the ideal treatment is removal of the gastrinoma.

H-2 receptor antagonists are effective in reducing gastric acid secretion, producing symptom relief, and inducing ulcer healing in patients with the Z-E syndrome. *Cimetidine* was the first H-2 receptor antagonist used successfully in the treatment of these patients. Improvement in clinical symptoms, decreases in gastric acid output, and ulcer healing were found in 80 to 85 percent. Administration of cimetidine was required at 4- to 6-h intervals, with total daily doses usually four to eight times those used in the treatment of common duodenal ulcer. More recently, *ranitidine, famotidine,* and *nizatidine* also have been shown effective in treatment of patients with the Z-E syndrome. These H-2 receptor antagonists require comparable increases in dosage when compared with doses used in treatment of common duodenal ulcer. When instituted, H-2 receptor antagonist therapy must be continued indefinitely, since even temporary discontinuance is usually followed by ulcer recurrence. Ulcers fail to respond or recur while on treatment with H-2 receptor antagonists in approximately 25 percent of patients with the Z-E syndrome. The dose of H-2 receptor antagonist required to maintain a satisfactory

reduction in gastric acid secretion can be assessed by measuring the basal gastric acid output during the hour immmediately prior to the next anticipated dose of the drug; the goal is to reduce gastric acid output to less than 10 mmol/h at that time.

Omeprazole, the parietal cell H^+,K^+-ATPase inhibitor, is the most effective drug and agent of choice in reducing gastric acid secretion and in healing ulcer in Z-E patients, including those with ulcers resistant to treatment with H-2 receptor antagonists. As a function of potency and dosage, the effectiveness of omeprazole can be prolonged and sustained. The usual initial daily recommended dose of omeprazole is 60 mg in a single dose administered in the morning before breakfast. The dose is adjusted to maintain gastric acid secretion to less than 10 mmol/h during the hour immediately before the next dose is due. Twice a day dosing is recommended if the patient requires 100 mg or more omeprazole per day. Some Z-E patients, in whom gastrinomas could not be identified or removed surgically, have been treated with parietal cell vagotomy, which has reduced or, in a few instances, eliminated the dose of H-2 receptor antagonist required in these patients.

Treatment for patients with the Z-E syndrome should be individualized. In selecting the best therapy, the biologic behavior of the tumor and the clinical manifestations in each patient must be taken into consideration. Early studies indicated that morbidity and mortality in patients with the Z-E syndrome were due principally to complications of severe ulcer disease. However, with earlier diagnosis, effective antiulcer treatment, and longer follow-up, more frequent consequences of the malignant properties of gastrinoma are now recognized. Approximately 50 percent of patients with the Z-E syndrome in whom the gastrinoma has not been removed will die from malignant invasion by the tumor. Complete *surgical resection of the tumors,* when possible, represents *optimal treatment in patients with gastrinoma.* Complete surgical removal of gastrinoma, with cure, has been achieved in approximately 25 percent of patients with the Z-E syndrome. Successful resection of tumor in Z-E patients with sporadic gastrinoma or with gastrinoma with MEN I requires thorough abdominal exploration and recognition and removal of multiple gastrinomas when found, including those in the wall of the duodenum and other extrapancreatic sites. Gastrinoma in lymph nodes and metastatic to the liver should be removed when safe and possible.

Treatment with omeprazole is indicated in the period during which the diagnosis is being established, while the location and extent of the tumor are being determined, and also as treatment prior to anticipated surgery. At present, omeprazole is certainly indicated for patients who are unsatisfactory candidates for surgery, in those who refuse surgery, and in those in whom surgical removal of the tumor is not possible. Patients with aggressively invasive gastrinoma have been treated with streptozotocin and 5-fluorouracil, in some instances combined with doxorubicin, in attempts to reduce tumor bulk and associated symptoms. Success with chemotherapy is limited, with only an initial response of approximately 40 percent and no complete responses. When metastatic and/or otherwise nonresectable gastrinoma is present, control of the ulcer disease may be achieved in most instances by treatment with omeprazole or, rarely, when required, by total gastric resection. There is no convincing evidence that tumor progression is usually influenced by gastrectomy.

STRESS ULCERS AND EROSIONS

A number of acute ulcerative lesions of the gastrointestinal tract are distinct clinically from chronic peptic ulcer. Among these are the acute upper gastrointestinal erosions and ulcers often observed in patients with shock, massive burns, sepsis, and severe trauma. These are often referred to as *stress erosions* and *ulcers.* These lesions, which are frequently multiple, are most common in the acid-secreting portion of the stomach, but they also may occur in the antrum and duodenum.

These erosions and superficial ulcers are extremely frequent and occur in about 80 to 90 percent of patients with massive injuries and burns. The most common clinical finding in these patients is painless gastrointestinal hemorrhage. Blood loss is usually minimal but may be substantial and life-threatening. Erosions develop most frequently approximately 24 h after trauma. Small amounts of blood loss may be detected in the first 24 to 48 h after trauma. However, when massive hemorrhage occurs, it is usually more than 2 or 3 days after the acute insult. Acute stress ulcers and erosions should be suspected when there is evidence of upper gastrointestinal bleeding in patients with severe injuries, burns, infections, and/or shock. The diagnosis is best established by upper gastrointestinal endoscopy. Erosions are usually too superficial to be recognized by barium examination of the upper gastrointestinal tract.

Many theories have been proposed to explain stress-associated acute mucosal ulceration. Mucosal ischemia and tissue injury from gastric acid appear to be important in their production. There is usually no evidence of acid hypersecretion; however, the lesions cannot be produced in experimental animals in the absence of acid. Most evidence supports the conclusion that ischemia of the gastric mucosa, which has enormous oxygen requirements, is the most important element in producing stress erosions and ulceration.

Treatment of acute stress ulcerations and erosions is principally preventive. In high-risk patients, the frequency of stress ulcerations can be diminished by vigorous use of antacids or H-2 receptor antagonists. When medical therapy fails to arrest bleeding, surgical approaches have included pyloroplasty with vagotomy and total gastrectomy.

The term *Cushing's ulcer* has been applied to acute ulcer of the upper gastrointestinal tract associated with intracranial injury or increases in intracranial pressure, e.g., with brain tumors or subdural hematoma. These ulcers may involve the stomach, proximal duodenum, or esophagus and frequently lead to hemorrhage or perforation. They do not differ histologically from acute stress ulceration. However, unlike stress ulcers, Cushing's ulcers are frequently associated with gastric acid hypersecretion. Treatment includes correction of increased intracranial pressure, when possible, and the usual measures for treatment of acute erosions and ulcerations, including vigorous therapy with antacids or H-2 receptor antagonists.

DRUG-ASSOCIATED ULCERS AND EROSIONS

Gastric and duodenal ulcers have been described following administration of many drugs. Aspirin is associated with an increased incidence of gastric ulcer and, to a lesser extent, duodenal ulcer and is a frequent cause of hemorrhagic erosive gastritis. Gastric mucosal injury, similar to that produced by aspirin, also has been observed in patients treated with a variety of other NSAIDs (e.g., indomethacin, ibuprofen, naproxen, tolmetin, sulindac, piroxicam, diflunisal, fenoprofen, and others). Several mechanisms by which salicylates and other NSAIDs induce gastric ulcer and erosions have been proposed. Aspirin and other NSAIDs are directly toxic to the gastric mucosa, and they deplete protective endogenous mucosal prostaglandins by inhibiting prostaglandin synthesis (see "Gastritis," below). Aspirin and other NSAIDs may contribute to development of gastric ulcer by interruption of the gastric mucosal barrier, permitting back-diffusion of hydrogen ions that may injure the gastric mucosa. They reduce gastric mucus secretion and gastric and duodenal bicarbonate secretion and may increase gastric acid secretion. Depletion of mucosal prostaglandins also impairs epithelial cell reconstitution after injury.

Administration of glucocorticoids has been reported and is commonly assumed to be associated with ulcer disease of the upper gastrointestinal tract. The association is controversial, supported by some data and rejected by other data.

GASTRITIS

Gastritis is *inflammation of the gastric mucosa*. Gastritis is not a single disease. Rather, it is a group of disorders that have inflammatory

changes in the gastric mucosa in common but that have different clinical features, histologic characteristics, and pathogeneses. Several classifications have been used for consideration of gastritis. In general, these classifications have been based on (1) the acuteness or chronicity of the clinical manifestations, (2) the histologic features characterizing the gastritis, (3) the anatomic distribution of the gastritis, or, in some instances, (4) the proposed pathogenesis of each of the two principal varieties of chronic gastritis. Based on the *clinical features* of the gastritis, the two principal forms, which constitute very different clinical entities, are *acute gastritis* and *chronic gastritis*. Different types of chronic gastritis exhibit histologic features which permit their classification according to the presence or absence of mucosal atrophy associated with the gastritis and the anatomic distribution of the gastritis or atrophy in the gastric mucosa.

In this section the major clinical forms of acute gastritis and chronic gastritis will be addressed, including reference to the histologic features of the major forms of gastritis. Attention also will be directed to additional specific forms of gastritis.

ACUTE GASTRITIS A principal, and certainly the most dramatic, form of acute gastritis is *acute hemorrhagic gastritis*, which is also referred to as *acute erosive gastritis*. These terms reflect the bleeding from the gastric mucosa almost invariably found in this form of gastritis and the characteristic loss of integrity of the gastric mucosa (erosion) that accompanies the inflammatory lesion. Gross examination in hemorrhagic gastritis shows edema, mucosal friability, erosions, and sites of bleeding with extravasation of blood into the mucosa and the lumen of the stomach. Gastric erosions and sites of hemorrhage may be distributed diffusely throughout the gastric mucosa or localized to the body or antrum of the stomach. They are often placed linearly on the crests of the gastric folds.

Histologic examination of the gastric mucosa reveals infiltration of the lamina propria with mononuclear cells and polymorphonuclear leukocytes with extravasation of blood in the mucosa, distorting the glandular structures. Proteinaceous exudate containing polymorphonuclear leukocytes may be present in gastric glands. Gastric erosions, by definition, are limited to the mucosa and do not extend beneath the muscularis mucosa. Acute erosive gastritis may accompany deeper, more focal lesions, which represent acute ulcers and may extend to and through all layers of the gastric wall.

Etiology and pathogenesis Acute erosive gastritis may develop without apparent explanation but is more likely to occur in several specific clinical circumstances. Erosive gastritis is usually associated with serious illness or with various drugs. Erosive gastritis has been estimated to occur in up to 80 to 90 percent of critically ill hospitalized patients. It is found most often in patients in medical or surgical intensive care units with severe trauma; major surgery; hepatic, renal, or respiratory failure; shock; massive burns; or severe infections with septicemia. Acute erosive gastritis associated with these severe illnesses is often referred to as *stress-induced gastritis*. The contributions of all mechanisms responsible for erosive gastritis in critically ill patients have not been defined completely. However, important factors appear to include ischemia of the gastric mucosa, acid diffusion from the gastric lumen into gastric mucosal tissues, and, perhaps in some forms, bile acids and/or other duodenal-pancreatic secretions refluxed into the gastric lumen. Mucosal ischemia and acid in the gastric lumen are clearly crucial elements in the etiopathogenesis of stress-induced gastritis. Septic shock with resulting mucosal ischemia produces gastric erosions in experimental animals. During such experimentally induced shock, the intramural pH of the gastric mucosa falls precipitously when the gastric lumen is irrigated with HCl; this produces severe hemorrhagic lesions. The decrease in intramural pH results from diffusion of luminal hydrogen ions, which damage the gastric mucosa. With neutral pH irrigation, the fall in intramural pH is much less, and gastric lesions are minimal. Counteracting the effects of acid by vigorous and continuous treatment with antacids or by inhibiting secretion with H-2 receptor antagonists has been effective in reducing the hemorrhagic complications of acute erosive gastritis in critically ill patients.

Various agents are known to injure the gastric mucosa. These include aspirin and other NSAIDs, bile acids, pancreatic enzymes, and ethanol. These agents disrupt the gastric mucosal barrier, which under normal conditions impedes the back-diffusion of hydrogen ions from the gastric lumen to the mucosa (despite and against an enormous H^+ concentration gradient). The most common and very important cause of drug-associated acute erosive gastritis is ingestion of aspirin or other NSAIDs. As indicated above, these drugs inhibit gastric mucosal cyclooxygenase activity, thereby reducing the synthesis and tissue levels of endogenous mucosal prostaglandins, which play important roles in mucosal defense. This reduction in tissue prostaglandins is thought to be a principal, but perhaps not the exclusive, mechanism by which aspirin and other NSAIDs damage the gastric mucosa. It is possible that aspirin may injure small vessels in the gastric mucosa by inhibition of prostacyclin in their walls or by inhibition of synthesis of thromboxane by platelets. An additional proposed mechanism for aspirin-induced gastrointestinal mucosal injury is via the effects of sodium salicylate, the product of aspirin metabolism found in the circulation, which is toxic to mitochondrial respiration and oxidative phosphorylation of cells. This may produce endothelial and epithelial cell injury with hemorrhage into the tissues or vascular thrombosis by endothelial cell disruption. Acid in the gastric lumen appears crucial to the production of salicylate-associated injury to the gastric mucosa.

Ethanol damage to the gastric mucosa is associated principally with subepithelial hemorrhages with surrounding edema and only slight to moderate increases in mucosal inflammatory cells. The mechanism by which alcohol injures the gastric mucosa is uncertain. Suggestions include cell injury due to its inherent lipophilic and lipolytic properties and/or interruption of the gastric mucosal barrier or direct damage to small mucosal blood vessels.

Clinical features Bleeding from the gastric mucosa with acute gastritis may range from abrupt and dramatic upper gastrointestinal hemorrhage to the most subtle blood loss, perhaps detected only by the presence of occult blood in the stool or development of mild, asymptomatic, and unexplained anemia. Except for possible consequences of blood loss, erosive gastritis is usually asymptomatic. However, less common symptoms may include epigastric or upper abdominal pain, nausea, and vomiting. Pain is much less common with erosive gastritis than with ulcer disease; in fact, painless gastrointestinal hemorrhage is frequently the only clinical manifestation. Physical examination is often normal in patients with acute hemorrhagic gastritis. However, they may have upper abdominal tenderness or evidence of blood loss such as pallor, tachycardia, and hypotension. When they occur, white blood cell count abnormalities, such as leukocytosis or leukopenia, more often reflect the associated serious illness than the gastritis.

Diagnosis The presence of erosive gastritis is usually first suspected by detection of blood in the stool or in the gastric aspirate. The diagnosis is best established by upper gastrointestinal endoscopy, which reveals mucosal hemorrhages, friability and congestion, erosions, and, in some instances, superficial or deep ulcerations which, when present, are usually in the fundus or body of the stomach. Radiographic examination is much less reliable than endoscopy in detecting acute hemorrhagic-erosive gastritis.

Treatment Treatment should be directed to prevention of erosive gastritis, treatment of the associated disease, withdrawal of the offending agent, and general supportive measures, as required, including maintenance of oxygen, blood volume, and fluid and electrolyte requirements. Hourly antacid administration (e.g., 30 mL of an aluminum-magnesium hydroxide liquid preparation) and/or administration of an H-2 receptor antagonist (usually intravenously) have been shown to be effective in reducing the frequency of hemorrhagic gastritis in critically ill patients. These drugs should be used in doses and frequencies sufficient to maintain the pH of gastric contents constantly above 4. Although proven of value in prevention, it is less certain that they are effective in treatment of acute hemorrhagic gastritis. However, a similar therapeutic program with

antacids or H-2 receptor antagonists does seem reasonable and generally is advised. Sucralfate also has been used in treatment.

Most patients with acute hemorrhagic gastritis respond favorably during vigorous treatment by the measures indicated. Acute hemorrhagic gastritis tends to improve as the patient's clinical condition improves. Because of the rapid cell renewal and restitutive properties of the gastric mucosa, lesions of acute hemorrhagic gastritis may disappear, both endoscopically and histologically, within 48 h of an acute event. However, occasionally, further measures are required in attempts to arrest persistent life-threatening blood loss. These have included embolization or vasopressin infusion of the left gastric artery. Uncommonly, surgery is required for relentless hemorrhage. Vagotomy with pyloroplasty with oversewing of focal bleeding ulcerations has been used with limited success, and rarely, total gastrectomy is required. Morbidity and mortality with surgery are very great, usually reflecting the severity of their associated illnesses. Surgery should not be performed unless absolutely necessary.

ENTEROPATHIC EROSIVE GASTRITIS Enteropathic erosive gastritis is a rare clinical entity with multiple erosions of the gastric mucosa found in the absence of recognized precipitating factors. These patients may have anorexia, nausea, vomiting, or poorly defined upper abdominal discomfort. Less commonly they show evidence of gastrointestinal blood loss or weight loss. Endoscopic examination is usually required to establish the diagnosis. Erosions, which may be few or numerous, are usually located on the crests of the folds but may be found in any portion of the gastric mucosa. Gastric biopsies are performed primarily to exclude other abnormalities, e.g., gastric lymphoma, carcinoma, and Crohn's disease. Erosions usually heal completely and may or may not return. The cause is not known, nor are there accepted principles for specific recommendations for therapy.

ACUTE GASTRITIS ASSOCIATED WITH *H. PYLORI* *H. pylori* is a short (0.2 to 0.5 μm in length), spiral-shaped, microaerophilic gram-negative bacillus responsible for certain forms of acute and chronic gastritis. Gastric colonization also has been associated with duodenal and gastric ulcer (see "Peptic Ulcer," above). With gastric colonization, *H. pylori* are found in the deep portions of the mucus gel layer that coats the gastric mucosa and between the mucus gel layer and the apical surfaces of the gastric mucosal epithelial cells. They also may be located in the regions of the tight junctions between adjacent mucosal epithelial cells. *H. pylori* may adhere to the luminal surfaces of gastric epithelial cells, but they do not invade the gastric mucosa.

H. pylori is the cause, or at least the principal cause, of a form of gastritis that has been designated *active chronic gastritis*. *H. pylori* is associated with active chronic gastritis in virtually 100 percent of patients. Active chronic gastritis is characterized by dense infiltration of the lamina propria of the gastric mucosa with invasion of the epithelial cell layer by polymorphonuclear leukocytes. The mucosal surface is usually intact, without erosions or hemorrhagic lesions. When erosions do occur, they are usually small and limited to the superficial epithelial cell layer. There is poor correlation between the histologic abnormalities and the endoscopic appearance of the mucosa; endoscopy may reveal subtle abnormalities, or more often, the endoscopic appearance is totally normal. Histologic abnormalities are associated with positive culture for *H. pylori*, and the degree of histologic abnormality, in general, parallels the number of organisms that can be identified. The more active the gastritis, reflected by mucosal infiltration with polymorphonuclear leukocytes, the greater the likelihood that *H. pylori* will be found. Healing of the gastritis occurs when the organism is eradicated and cultures become negative. Spontaneous disappearance of *H. pylori* has not been noted. Active chronic gastritis with *H. pylori* colonization has been observed to persist in gastric mucosal biopsies of untreated patients for years.

H. pylori can be identified in gastric mucosal samples by histologic examination, culture, urease activity, and endonuclease analysis. On stained tissue sections, *H. pylori* is Giemsa-positive and faintly hematoxylin-positive. The organisms can be cultured successfully from biopsy material but usually not from gastric secretions. *H. pylori* produces large amounts of urease. The rapid urease test of gastric biopsy material is a relatively simple and reliable method for presumptive identification of *H. pylori*. The biopsy urease test involves use of a urea-containing broth in which the gastric biopsy is placed. A positive test results in an increase in pH, with the phenol red indicator turning from light orange to red within 5 min. The test is inexpensive, with sensitivity of at least 90 percent and specificity approaching 100 percent. A urea breath test using ^{13}C or ^{14}C also has been developed for identifying *H. pylori*. Antibodies (IgG and IgA) to *H. pylori* have been identified in sera of individuals with *H. pylori* colonization. There is a high degree of correlation between these serum antibodies and histologic gastritis.

H. pylori produces a variety of proteins which appear to mediate or facilitate its damaging effects on the gastric mucosa. The urease produced by *H. pylori* catalyzes the hydrolysis of urea to yield ammonia and carbon dioxide. This provides a more alkaline microenvironment that protects *H. pylori* from the effects of gastric acid, which prevents gastric colonization by other bacteria. The urease results in damage to gastric mucosal epithelial cells by the hydroxide ions generated by the equilibration of water with ammonia. *H. pylori* produces surface proteins that are chemotactic for human neutrophils and monocytes and secretes a proinflammatory platelet-activating factor, as well as urease, which is also proinflammatory. *H. pylori* activates monocytes which express HLA-DR and interleukin 2 receptors on their cell surfaces and produce superoxides, interleukin 1, and tumor necrosis factor α. *H. pylori* produces proteases and phospholipases which degrade the glycoprotein-lipid complex of the mucus gel layer. This reduces the thickness and viscosity of the gastric protective mucus gel overlying the gastric mucosal epithelial cells in spite of increased mucus synthesis and secretion. *H. pylori* also produces an adhesin which facilitates the attachment of the bacterium to gastric epithelial cells.

At initiation of infection by *H. pylori*, there may be transient increased gastric acid secretion; however, this is often followed by hypochlorhydria which lasts for several months, followed by return to approximate preinfection acid secretory rates within 1 year. By retrospective examination, *H. pylori* were demonstrated in gastric mucosal biopsy specimens obtained from volunteers participating in gastric secretory studies who developed epidemic gastritis, with reductions in rates of gastric acid secretion. *H. pylori* infection may be associated with increased serum gastrin levels and normal gastric acid secretion; with eradication of *H. pylori*, serum gastrin levels return to normal, implying interruption of the acid-mediated feedback control mechanism regulating gastrin release by *H. pylori*. In patients with *H. pylori* infection, gastric mucosal somatostatin levels are reduced and inversely correlated with gastric luminal ammonia. This suggests somatostatin deficiency as the mechanism responsible for enhanced gastrin release in patients with *H. pylori* infection. This probably also explains increased gastrin release in response to feeding and decreased gastric mucosal somotostatin reported in duodenal ulcer patients (see "Peptic Ulcer," above).

H. pylori has been cultured from antral biopsy specimens in 90 to 100 percent of patients with duodenal ulcer, 60 to 70 percent with gastric ulcer, and about 50 percent of patients with nonulcer dyspepsia. *H. pylori* is also frequent in asymptomatic individuals considered to be otherwise well. In such asymptomatic individuals endoscopic examination has usually appeared normal, in spite of the histologic evidence of gastritis and *H. pylori*. It has not been proven that *H. pylori* gastritis produces symptoms. Nor has it been proven that *H. pylori* is responsible for symptoms in patients with nonulcer dyspepsia.

Colloidal bismuth compounds have been shown to eradicate *H. pylori* from gastric mucosa. Eradication may be due to antibacterial effects or to binding or coating of the organism. However, bismuth alone results in only approximately 10 percent long-term eradication. Amoxicillin (or other antibiotics), bismuth subsalicylate, and metronidazole have each been used singly or in combination for periods of from 1 week to 2 months to eradicate *H. pylori*. Therapy with

metronidazole, 250 mg three times a day, and bismuth, 525 mg (in the form of Pepto-Bismol) four times a day, eradicates the organism in 75 percent of patients for up to 12 months. Eradication of *H. pylori* results in disappearance of inflammatory changes. When recolonization of the organism occurs after treatment, it is usually with the same bacterial subtype and is associated with recurrence of gastritis.

CHRONIC GASTRITIS   The inflammatory cell infiltrate in chronic gastritis consists predominantly of lymphocytes and plasma cells. Polymorphonuclear leukocytes and eosinophils may be present in small numbers but do not predominate. Chronic gastritis is often patchy and irregular in distribution.

Histologic classification   Chronic gastritis has been classified descriptively on the basis of several characteristic histologic abnormalities. In its evolution, chronic gastritis initially involves the superficial and glandular areas of the gastric mucosa and progresses to glandular destruction, which may be followed by a profound reduction in gland number (atrophy) and/or gland metaplasia.

Superficial gastritis is that form of gastritis with inflammatory changes in the lamina propria of the superficial mucosa, with cellular infiltration and edema separating the gastric glands. Superficial gastritis appears to represent the initial stage in the development of chronic gastritis. With superficial gastritis, the inflammatory cell infiltrate is limited to the lamina propria of the upper (epithelial) half of the gastric mucosa, and the glands are preserved. There may be a decrease in mucus in glandular mucous cells and in mitotic figures in cells of the glands.

Atrophic gastritis is the next stage in the developmental chronology of chronic gastritis. In atrophic gastritis, the inflammatory infiltrate extends to the deep portions of the mucosa. There is progressive distortion and destruction of the glands, which become separated by the inflammatory process. Atrophic gastritis usually begins in the antrum and extends proximally into the body and fundus of the stomach. Atrophic gastritis is followed by the development of the final stage of chronic gastritis, which is *gastric atrophy*. With gastric atrophy, there is a profound loss of the glandular structures, which are now separated widely by connective tissue, with a greatly reduced or absent inflammatory infiltrate. The mucosa is thin, often revealing the prominence of its underlying vessels by endoscopic examination.

As chronic gastritis progresses, there may be changes in the morphology of the gastric glandular elements. *Intestinal metaplasia* is the term used to describe the conversion of gastric glands to the appearance of small intestinal mucosal glands containing goblet cells. Intestinal metaplasia may be patchy or extensive in the gastric mucosa. With *pseudopyloric gland metaplasia* the glands of the body of the stomach assume the appearance of antral pyloric glands. Pseudopyloric metaplasia may occur with either atrophic gastritis or gastric atrophy.

Chronic gastritis: Types A and B   The two major forms of chronic gastritis have been classified as types A and B based on their distributions in the gastric mucosa coupled with implications regarding their pathogenesis.

Type A gastritis is the less common form of chronic gastritis; it characteristically involves the body and fundus of the stomach, with relative sparing of the antrum. This is the form of gastritis that may lead to pernicious anemia. The frequent presence of antibodies to parietal cells and to intrinsic factor in sera of patients with Type A gastritis and pernicious anemia has suggested an immune or autoimmune pathogenesis for this form of gastritis. Antibodies to parietal cells have been shown to be cytotoxic for gastric mucosal cells. Cell-mediated immune mechanisms also have been proposed to participate in gastric mucosal cell injury in pernicious anemia and related forms of type A gastritis. Antibodies to parietal cells have been found in sera of approximately 90 percent of patients with pernicious anemia and in more than half of other patients with type A gastritis. Relatives of patients with pernicious anemia have a higher than normal frequency of serum antibodies to parietal cells, atrophic gastritis, and reduced gastric acid secretion. In control populations, parietal cell antibodies may be found in up to 20 percent of individuals over age 60 and in approximately 20 percent of all patients with hypoparathyroidism, Addison's disease, and vitiligo. About 50 percent of patients with pernicious anemia have antibodies to thyroid antigens, and approximately 30 percent of patients with thyroid disease have circulating antibodies to parietal cells. Serum antibodies to intrinsic factor are more specific than parietal cell antibodies and are present in about 40 percent of patients with pernicious anemia.

In patients with pernicious anemia, the gastric parietal cell–containing glands are invariably destroyed, accounting for their inability to secrete hydrochloric acid. Since, in human beings, parietal cells also secrete intrinsic factor, there is failure to absorb vitamin B_{12} actively, with resulting hematologic and/or neurologic consequences characteristic of pernicious anemia.

Type B gastritis is much the more common form of chronic gastritis. In younger patients type B gastritis principally involves the antrum, whereas in older patients the entire stomach is affected. This transition is estimated to require about 15 to 20 years. The incidence of chronic gastritis, most of it type B gastritis, increases with age, reaching 78 percent in individuals over age 50 and virtually 100 percent after age 70.

A large number of studies from various parts of the world have established that *H. pylori* is the agent responsible for type B gastritis. Chronic gastritis with *H. pylori* infection and/or persistence is associated with reduced gastric acid secretion. Eradication of *H. pylori* produces improvement in histologic findings; when treatment is stopped, inflammatory changes recur, and organisms reappear. These observations have supported the conclusion that type B gastritis is caused by chronic bacterial infection by *H. pylori*. Gastric colonization with *H. pylori* is found in virtually all patients with chronic superficial gastritis, with fewer bacteria demonstrable with progress to atrophic gastritis. *H. pylori* are few in number or rarely demonstrated with severe gastric atrophy. Chronic reflux of pancreatic-biliary secretions, bile acids and lysolecithin in particular, also has been proposed as a potential contributing factor in the production of type B chronic gastritis.

Gastric acid secretion is reduced in both type A and type B chronic gastritis. In general, the reduction in gastric acid secretion, which is complete in patients with pernicious anemia, is proportionate to the severity of parietal cell destruction and mucosal atrophy in the body and fundus of the stomach. Serum gastrin levels are usually elevated substantially in patients with pernicious anemia and are in approximately the same range as those of patients with the Z-E syndrome (gastrinoma). Since the antral mucosa is relatively spared, the antral gastrin-containing cells, deprived of feedback control normally exercised by acid in the stomach, release gastrin continuously. Serum gastrin levels are also often similarly elevated in patients with type A gastritis with achlorhydria or profound hypochlorhydria who do not have pernicious anemia. Patients with type B gastritis have fasting serum gastrin levels that are highly variable, not consistently elevated, and often in the normal range. A small portion of patients with type B gastritis have serum antibodies to gastrin, leading some to propose an autoimmune mechanism for this form of gastritis. Alternatively, and probably more likely, these antibodies may represent responses to the inflammatory process rather than contributing factors.

There is no persuasive evidence that acute gastric mucosal injury associated with stress, with ethanol, or with aspirin or other NSAIDs progresses to chronic gastritis. Acute gastritis caused by *H. pylori* appears to be the form of acute gastritis in which there is sufficient information to support progression to a chronic form of gastritis, i.e., type B chronic gastritis.

Diagnosis Biopsy provides the most reliable means of identifying and classifying gastritis. Caution must be exercised in the interpretation of a single gastric mucosal biopsy. The patchy and irregular distribution of the gastritis may lead to substantial sampling error. Therefore, several biopsies of suspected areas, when safe and possible, are recommended.

Treatment No specific treatment is required for type A or type B chronic gastritis with or without mucosal atrophy. The only form that requires specific treatment is pernicious anemia, the most complete expression of type A gastritis. Vitamin B_{12} deficiency in these patients, resulting from malabsorption of vitamin B_{12} secondary to destruction of parietal cells in the body and fundus of the stomach, requires indefinite regular parenteral vitamin B_{12} administration.

MÉNÉTRIER'S DISEASE *Ménétrier's disease* is a clinical entity characterized by large tortuous gastric mucosal folds. The abnormalities in Ménétrier's disease may be localized or diffuse throughout the stomach. Prominent mucosal folds are often most conspicuous in the gastric body and fundus. Histologic inflammation is not a component of this disease. Therefore, it is not a form of gastritis. The primary pathologic feature is thickening of the gastric mucosa due to hyperplasia of surface and glandular mucous cells, which replace most of the chief and parietal cells. Pits of the gastric glands elongate and may become extremely tortuous. The lamina propria may contain an increased number of lymphocytes. Intestinal metaplasia may be present.

The most common symptom is epigastric pain. Anorexia, nausea, vomiting, and weight loss are less frequent. Gastric bleeding is unusual and, when present, is due to superficial mucosal erosions. Uncommonly, gastric ulcer or gastric carcinoma may develop in these patients. Patients often develop a protein-losing gastropathy resulting in hypoalbuminemia and edema. Gastric acid secretion is usually reduced or may be absent. Barium examination of the upper gastrointestinal tract reveals the large gastric folds, which are readily confirmed by endoscopic examination. The diagnosis is best established by deep mucosal biopsy (and cytology) to exclude gastric malignancy. The depth of these lesions and the disconcerting prominence of the folds may require a surgical full-thickness biopsy to exclude lymphoma or infiltrating carcinoma.

Anticholinergic agents and H-2 receptor antagonists have been reported to decrease protein loss in patients with Ménétrier's disease. Treatment includes a high-protein diet, when required, to replace protein losses. If present, ulcers should be treated as described previously for common gastric ulcer. Severe disease with persistent substantial protein loss may require total gastrectomy.

GASTRITIS DUE TO CORROSIVE AGENTS Ingestion of a variety of corrosive chemicals can cause severe damage to the gastric mucosa. Because of its anatomic location, the antrum is a frequent site for such injury. Ingested substances which are particularly injurious to the gastric mucosa include strong acids (e.g., hydrochloric acid, sulfuric acid) or strong alkali (e.g., sodium hydroxide). Depending on dose and concentration, these agents can cause injury ranging from mild inflammation to extensive tissue necrosis. With alkali ingestion (especially lye), the esophagus is particularly susceptible to severe injury, necrosis, and potential subsequent stricture. The stomach, especially the antrum, is more susceptible to acute injury from ingestion of strong acid. With ingestion of these corrosive substances, patients may describe burning of the mouth, throat, and retrosternal area. Epigastric pain and vomiting often signal gastric injury. Hemorrhage and/or perforation may occur. Treatment of strong acid ingestion includes dilution with water, followed by antacids and supportive therapy as required. Neutralization of ingested lye by administrated acid is not recommended.

INFECTIOUS GASTRITIS Infectious causes of gastritis, other than that associated with gastric *H. pylori* colonization, are unusual. *Phlegmonous gastritis*, a rare form of bacterial gastritis, is a life-threatening disease with extensive infiltration of the gastric wall, tissue necrosis, and manifestations of generalized sepsis. Responsible infectious agents include, among others, streptococci, staphylococci, *Proteus* species, and *Escherichia coli*. Treatment includes appropriate intravenous antibiotics and necessary supportive care with fluid and electrolyte replacement as required. Lack of response to therapy may require gastrectomy. Additional infectious causes of gastritis may be found in immunocompromised patients. Gastric erosions may be produced by herpes simplex virus. Typical intranuclear inclusions of cytomegalovirus, with positive cultures, have been found by endoscopic gastric biopsy in some immunocompromised patients.

This has been interpreted to represent disseminated cytomegalovirus infection.

EOSINOPHILIC GASTRITIS   *Eosinophilic gastritis* may occur as isolated involvement of the stomach or as a component of eosinophilic gastroenteritis. Eosinophilic gastritis is characterized by extensive eosinophilic infiltration of the wall of the stomach, usually with circulating eosinophilia. Biopsy reveals extensive eosinophilic infiltration which may involve all coats of the stomach or may be limited to mucosa, submucosa, or muscular regions of the gastric wall. The antrum is involved more frequently than the gastric body or fundus. There may be prominent antral mucosal folds with edema and mucosal thickening, uncommonly leading to gastric outlet obstruction. Epigastric pain, which may be accompanied by nausea and vomiting, is the most frequent symptom. These patients usually respond favorably to treatment with glucocorticoids. Rarely, surgery is required to establish the diagnosis or for relief of obstructive symptoms.

GRANULOMATOUS GASTRITIS   A number of generalized diseases, some of which are infectious, can involve the stomach, producing *granulomatous gastritis.* Crohn's disease, as in the small intestine, may produce gastric ulceration, granulomatous infiltration, and/or scarring with stricture formation. Its distinction from other gastric lesions requires biopsy at the time of endoscopic examination. Less common infectious causes of granulomatous disease of the stomach include, among others, histoplasmosis, candidiasis, syphilis, and tuberculosis. Rarely, idiopathic granulomatous gastritis and eosinophilic granulomas also involve the stomach. In patients with granulomatous disease of the stomach, multiple biopsies and cytology are usually required to establish the diagnosis and to exclude malignancy. If the diagnosis is not established by biopsy at endoscopy, surgical exploration may be required.

GASTRITIS AND PRIOR GASTRIC SURGERY   Variable amounts of gastritis almost always occur in the remaining stomachs of patients treated surgically by partial gastrectomy and, to a somewhat lesser extent, after vagotomy with pyloroplasty. Gastritis is especially common and often severe after gastrojejunal (Billroth II) anastomosis.

Gastric surgery appears to accelerate the development of gastritis, with progressive loss of parietal cells in the gastric remnant after surgery. Most patients are asymptomatic; however, a small proportion develop mild or severe symptoms, most commonly epigastric pain, nausea, and vomiting. This form of gastritis has been referred to as *alkaline gastritis* or *bile reflux gastritis.* It has been assumed, but not proven, that gastritis results from reflux of pancreaticobiliary secretions. Endoscopic examination often reveals a beefy red and sometimes friable gastric mucosa. Abnormalities may be limited to mucosa in the region of the anastomosis or may involve all remaining gastric mucosa. Bile is often seen in the gastric remnant. Biopsies of involved mucosa at endoscopy show variable degrees of acute and/or chronic gastritis. Gastric acid secretion is usually decreased.

Managing patients with severe symptoms is very difficult. Various therapeutic approaches have been used with limited, if any, success. These have included cholestyramine, H-2 receptor antagonists, sucralfate, antacids, and pancreatic enzyme replacement. Surgery, which is sometimes successful, is Roux-en-Y, which diverts pancreaticobiliary secretions away from the gastric remnant. Nonsurgical modalities should be exhausted before proceeding with attempts to treat this disease by surgery.

REFERENCES

Peptic ulcer

BARDHAN KD et al: Double-blind comparison of cimetidine and placebo in the maintenance and healing of chronic duodenal ulceration. Gut 20:158, 1979

CRYER B, FELDMAN M: Effects of nonsteroidal anti-inflammatory drugs on endogenous gastrointestinal prostaglandins and therapeutic strategies for prevention and treatment of nonsteroidal anti-inflammatory drug-induced damage. Arch Intern Med 152:1145, 1992

GRAHAM DY et al: Effect of treatment of *Helicobacter pylori* infection on the long-term

recurrence of gastric or duodenal ulcer: A randomized, controlled study. Ann Intern Med 116:705, 1992

GREGORY RA et al: Amino acid constitution of two gastrins isolated from Zollinger-Ellison variety. N Engl J Med 278:1308, 1968

MATON PN et al: Cushing's syndrome in patients with the Zollinger-Ellison syndrome. N Engl J Med 315:1, 1986

MCARTHUR KE et al: Treatment of acid-peptic diseases by inhibition of gastric H^+,K^+-ATPase. Annu Rev Med 37:97, 1986

MCGUIGAN JE, TRUDEAU WL: Differences in rates of gastrin release in normal persons and patients with duodenal ulcer. N Engl J Med 288:64, 1973

———, ———: Immunochemical measurement of elevated levels of gastrin in the serum of patients with pancreatic tumors of the Zollinger-Ellison variety. N Engl J Med 278:1308, 1968

PETERSON WL: *Helicobacter pylori* and peptic ulcer disease. Curr Concepts Nutr 324:1043, 1991

PIPELEERS-MARICHAL M et al: Gastrinomas in the duodenums of patients with multiple endocrine neoplasia type 1 and the Zollinger-Ellison syndrome. N Engl J Med 322:723, 1990

PISEGNA JR et al: Effects of curative gastrinoma resection on gastric secretory function and antisecretory drug requirement in the Zollinger-Ellison syndrome. Gastroenterology 102:767, 1992

PEURA DA, JOHNSON LF: Cimetidine for prevention and treatment of gastroduodenal lesions in patients in an intensive care unit. Ann Intern Med 103:173, 1985

RICHARDSON CT: Sucralfate. Ann Intern Med 97:269, 1982

VINAYEK R et al: Famotidine in the therapy of gastric hypersecretory states. Am J Med 81:49, 1986

——— et al: Zollinger-Ellison syndrome: Recent advances in the management of the gastrinoma. Gastroenterol Clin North Am 19:197, 1990

WOLFE MM, SOLL AH: The physiology of gastric acid secretion. N Engl J Med 319:1707, 1988

Gastritis

BLASER MJ: Hypotheses on the pathogenesis and natural history of *Helicobacter pylori*–induced inflammation. Gastroenterology 102:720, 1992

DOIG P et al: Production of a conserved adhesin by the human gastroduodenal pathogen *Helicobacter pylori*. J Bacteriol 174:2539, 1992

HENTSCHEL E et al: Effect of ranitidine and amoxicillin plus metronidazole on the eradication of *Helicobacter pylori* and the recurrence of duodenal ulcer. N Engl J Med 328:308, 1993

KANEKO H et al: *Helicobacter pylori* infection induces a decrease in immunoreactive somatostatin concentrations of human stomach. Dig Dis Sci 37:409, 1992

LEE SP: The mode of action of colloidal bismuth subcitrate. Scand J Gastroenterol 26(suppl 185):1, 1991

MAJ UEH et al: Surface proteins from *Helicobacter pylori* exhibit chemotactic activity for human leukocytes and are present in gastric mucosa. J Exp Med 175:517, 1992

ROBERT A: Cytoprotection by prostaglandins. Gastroenterology 77:761, 1979

SEARCY CM, MALAGELADA JR: Ménétrier's disease and idiopathic hypertrophic gastropathy. Ann Intern Med 100:565, 1984

TAKEUCHI KD: Role of pH gradient of mucus in protection of gastric mucosa. Gastroenterology 84:331, 1983

VANE JR: Inhibition of prostaglandin synthesis as a mechanism for aspirin-like drugs. Nature 23:232, 1971

253   NEOPLASMS OF THE ESOPHAGUS AND STOMACH

ROBERT J. MAYER

ESOPHAGEAL CANCER

INCIDENCE AND ETIOLOGY   In the United States, cancer of the esophagus is a relatively uncommon but extremely lethal malignant condition. It is estimated that the diagnosis was made in 11,300 Americans in 1993, leading to 10,200 deaths. Worldwide, the incidence of esophageal cancer varies strikingly. It occurs frequently within a so-called Asian esophageal cancer belt extending from the southern shore of the Caspian Sea on the west to northern China on the east and encompassing parts of Iran, Central Asia, Afghanistan, Siberia, and Mongolia. Additionally, high-incidence "pockets" of the disease are present in such disparate locations as Finland, Iceland, Curaçao, southeastern Africa, and northwestern France. In North America and western Europe, the disease is far more common in blacks than whites, greater in males than females, appearing most frequently after age 50, and appearing to be an illness associated with lower socioeconomic classes.

A variety of causative factors have been implicated in the

TABLE 253-1 Some etiologic factors believed to be associated with esophageal cancer

Excess alcohol consumption
Cigarette smoking
Other ingested carcinogens
   A Nitrates (converted to nitrites)
   B Smoked opiates
   C Fungal toxins in pickled vegetables
Mucosal damage from physical agents
   A Hot tea
   B Lye ingestion
   C Radiation-induced strictures
   D Chronic achalasia
Host susceptibility
   A Esophageal web with glossitis and iron deficiency (i.e., Plummer-Vinson or Paterson-Kelly syndrome)
   B Congenital hyperkeratosis and pitting of the palms and soles (i.e., tylosis palmaris et plantaris)
? Dietary deficiencies—molybdenum, zinc, vitamin A
? Celiac sprue
Chronic gastric reflux (i.e., Barrett's esophagus)—for adenocarcinoma

development of the disease (Table 253-1). In the United States, 80 to 90 percent of esophageal cancer cases are believed attributable to excess consumption of alcohol and/or a long-standing history of cigarette smoking. The relative risk increases with either the amount of tobacco smoked or alcohol consumed. The consumption of whiskey is seemingly linked to a higher incidence than the consumption of wine or beer. The development of esophageal cancer has also been associated with the ingestion of other carcinogens such as nitrites, smoked opiates, and fungal toxins in pickled vegetables, as well as with mucosal damage caused by such physical insults as long-term exposure to extremely hot tea, the ingestion of lye, radiation-induced strictures, and chronic achalasia. The presence of an esophageal web in association with glossitis and iron deficiency (i.e., Plummer-Vinson or Paterson-Kelly syndrome) and congenital hyperkeratosis and pitting of the palms and soles (i.e., tylosis palmaris et plantaris) have each been linked with esophageal cancer, as have dietary deficiencies of molybdenum, zinc, and vitamin A. The risk for esophageal cancer may be slightly greater in individuals with celiac sprue and is definitely increased in the presence of chronic gastric reflux (i.e., Barrett's esophagus). In contrast to other esophageal cancers, neoplasms arising from Barrett's esophagus afflict white individuals far more commonly than blacks.

CLINICAL FEATURES Approximately 15 percent of esophageal cancers occur in the upper third of the esophagus ("cervical esophagus"), 50 percent in the middle third, and 35 percent in the lower third. More than 85 percent of esophageal tumors are squamous cell carcinomas, arising from the squamous epithelium which lines the lumen of the esophagus. Adenocarcinomas, while far less frequent, develop more commonly from columnar epithelium which may appear dysplastic in the distal esophagus in association with chronic gastric reflux (i.e., Barrett's esophagus). These malignancies have the biologic behavior of gastric rather than esophageal cancers. Attempts at endoscopic and cytologic screening for carcinoma in patients with Barrett's esophagus, while effective as a means of detecting high-grade dysplasia, have not yet been proven beneficial in positively influencing the prognosis in individuals found to have a carcinoma. It should be noted that squamous cell carcinomas and adenocarcinomas of the esophagus cannot be distinguished radiographically or endoscopically.

Progressive dysphagia and weight loss of short duration are the initial symptoms in the vast majority of patients. Dysphagia initially occurs with solid foods and gradually progresses to include semisolids and liquids. By the time these symptoms develop, the disease is usually incurable since difficulty in swallowing does not occur until 60 percent or more of the esophageal circumference is infiltrated with cancer. Dysphagia may be associated with pain on swallowing (odynophagia), pain radiating to the chest and/or back, regurgitation

or vomiting, and aspiration pneumonia. The disease most commonly spreads to adjacent and supraclavicular lymph nodes, liver, lungs, and pleura. Tracheoesophageal fistulas may develop as the disease advances, leading to severe suffering. As with other squamous cell carcinomas, hypercalcemia occasionally may occur in the absence of osseous metastases. This is believed to result from a tumor-secreted protein structurally analogous to a portion of parathyroid hormone.

DIAGNOSIS Routine, contrast radiographs effectively identify esophageal lesions of sufficient size to cause symptoms. In contrast to benign esophageal leiomyomata which result in esophageal narrowing with preservation of a normal mucosal pattern, esophageal carcinomas characteristically cause ragged, ulcerating changes in the mucosa in association with deeper infiltration, producing a picture resembling achalasia. Smaller, potentially resectable tumors are often poorly visualized despite technically adequate esophagograms. Because of this, esophagoscopy should be performed in all patients suspected of having an esophageal abnormality in order to visualize the tumor and to obtain histopathologic confirmation of the diagnosis. Since the same population of patients at risk for esophageal carcinoma (i.e., smokers and drinkers) also has a high rate of cancers of the lung and head and neck region, endoscopic inspection of the larynx, trachea, and bronchi also should be considered. A thorough examination of the fundus of the stomach (by retroflexing the endoscope) is imperative as well. Endoscopic biopsies of esophageal tumors fail to recover malignant tissue in one-third of cases because the biopsy forceps cannot penetrate deeply enough through normal mucosa pushed in front of the carcinoma. Cytologic examination of tumor brushings frequently complements standard biopsies and should be performed routinely. The extent of tumor spread to the mediastinum and paraaortic lymph nodes should also be assessed by computed tomography (CT) scans of the chest and abdomen.

TREATMENT The prognosis for patients with esophageal carcinoma is poor. Less than 5 percent of patients are alive 5 years after the initial diagnosis, leading many physicians to focus management efforts solely on symptomatic control. Surgical resection of all gross tumor (i.e., total resection) is feasible in only 40 percent of cases, with residual tumor cells frequently present at the resection margins. Such esophagectomies have been associated in the past with a postoperative mortality rate in excess of 20 percent due to anastomotic fistulas, subphrenic abscesses, and respiratory complications; more recent reports suggest far better tolerance and diminished morbidity from these surgical procedures. Less than 20 percent of patients who survive a total resection can be expected to be alive after 5 years. The therapeutic outcome following the administration of primary radiation therapy (5500 to 6000 cGy) is not dissimilar to that of radical surgery, sparing patients perioperative morbidity but often resulting in less satisfactory palliation of obstructive symptoms. The evaluation of chemotherapeutic agents in patients with esophageal carcinoma has been hampered by ambiguity in the definition of "response" (i.e., benefit) and the debilitated physical condition of many treated individuals. Nonetheless, significant reductions in the size of measurable tumor masses have been reported in 15 to 25 percent of patients given single-agent treatment and in 30 to 60 percent of patients treated with drug combinations which include cisplatin. Recent therapeutic efforts have been directed at utilizing combination chemotherapy and radiation therapy as the initial therapeutic approach, either alone or followed by an attempt at operative resection. Although the preliminary results of these experiences have been encouraging, it remains to be determined whether such an intensive multimodality approach will increase the cure rate.

For the incurable, surgically unresectable patient with esophageal cancer, dysphagia, malnutrition, and the management of tracheoesophageal fistulas loom as major issues. Approaches to palliation of these cancer-related complications include repeated endoscopic dilatation, the surgical placement of a gastrostomy or jejunostomy for hydration and feeding, and the surgical insertion of a polyvinyl prosthesis to bypass the tumor. Endoscopic fulguration of the obstructing tumor with lasers appears to be the most promising of these techniques.

TUMORS OF THE STOMACH

GASTRIC ADENOCARCINOMA Incidence and epidemiology

For reasons which remain uncertain, the incidence and mortality rates for gastric cancer have decreased markedly during the past 60 years. In 1930, gastric cancer represented the leading cause of cancer-related deaths among American men by a factor of two, while the disease in women ranked just behind tumors of the uterine cervix and breast. During the ensuing years, the mortality rate from gastric cancer in the United States has dropped in men from 28 to 5.3 per 100,000 population, while in women, the rate has decreased from 27 to 2.3 per 100,000. Nonetheless, it was estimated in 1993 that 24,000 new cases of stomach cancer were diagnosed in the United States and that 13,600 Americans died of the disease. The decreased incidence in gastric cancer in the United States is also reflected worldwide. The incidence of gastric cancer varies widely among different countries, being comparatively high in Japan, China, Chile, and Ireland; however, a decrease in both incidence and mortality has occurred in these areas as well.

Epidemiologic surveys have suggested the risk of gastric cancer to be greater among lower socioeconomic classes. Furthermore, migrants from high- to low-incidence nations appear to maintain their susceptibility to gastric cancer while the risk for their offspring more closely approximates that of the new homeland. These findings suggest that an environmental exposure, probably beginning early in life, is related to the development of gastric cancer with dietary carcinogens considered the most likely factor(s).

Pathology Approximately 90 percent of stomach cancers are adenocarcinomas with 10 percent due to non-Hodgkin's lymphomas and leiomyosarcomas. Gastric adenocarcinomas may be subdivided into two categories: a *diffuse type* in which cell cohesion is absent, resulting in individual cells infiltrating and thickening the stomach wall without forming a discrete mass; and an *intestinal type* characterized by cohesive neoplastic cells forming glandlike tubular structures. The diffuse carcinomas occur more often in younger patients, develop throughout the stomach including the cardia, result in a loss of distensibility of the gastric wall (so-called linitis plastica or "leather bottle" appearance), and are associated with a far more ominous prognosis. Intestinal-type lesions are frequently ulcerative, more commonly appear in the antrum and lesser curvature of the stomach, and are often preceded by a prolonged precancerous process. While the incidence of diffuse carcinomas is similar in most populations, the intestinal type tends to predominate in the high-risk geographic regions mentioned earlier and is less likely to be found in areas where the frequency of gastric cancer is declining. Thus, different etiologic factor(s) may be involved in these two subtypes. In the United States, the distal stomach is the site of origin of about half of gastric cancers. Approximately 20 percent of these tumors arise in the lesser curvature, 25 percent in the cardia, and only 3 to 5 percent in the greater curvature. More than 10 percent of gastric carcinomas involve the entire stomach.

Etiology The relationship between dietary patterns and the development of gastric carcinoma has been extensively investigated. The long-term ingestion of high concentrations of nitrates in dried, smoked, and salted foods appears to be associated with a higher risk. The nitrates are thought to be converted to carcinogenic nitrites by bacteria (Table 253-2). Such bacteria may be introduced exogenously through the ingestion of the partially decayed foods which are consumed in abundance worldwide by the lower socioeconomic classes. Bacteria such as *helicobacter pylori* may also appear endogenously, possibly as a result of a lack or loss of gastric acidity. This may occur when acid-producing cells of the gastric antrum have been surgically removed 15 to 20 years previously at the time of a partial gastrectomy to control benign peptic ulcer disease or when achlorhydria, atrophic gastritis, and even pernicious anemia develop in the elderly. Serial endoscopic examinations of the stomach in patients with atrophic gastritis have documented replacement of the usual gastric mucosa by intestinal-type cells. This process of intestinal

TABLE 253-2 Dietary factors as a cause of gastric carcinoma*

Sources of nitrate-converting bacteria

Exogenous
  A Bacterially contaminated food
  B Frequent in lower socioeconomic classes who have higher incidence of the disease
  C Diminished by improved food preservation and refrigeration
  D ? *Helicobacter pylori* infection

Endogenous
  A Decreased gastric acidity
  B Prior gastric surgery (antrectomy)—15 to 20 year latency period
  C Atrophic gastritis and/or pernicious anemia
  D ? Prolonged exposure to histamine-2-receptor antagonists

*Hypothesis: Dietary nitrates are converted to carcinogenic nitrites by bacteria

metaplasia may lead to cellular atypia and eventual neoplasia. Since the declining incidence of gastric cancer in the United States is primarily a reflection of a decline in distal, ulcerating, intestinal-type lesions, it is conceivable that better food preservation and the availability to all socioeconomic classes of refrigeration for food storage have resulted in a decrease in the dietary ingestion of exogenous bacteria. It remains uncertain whether the iatrogenic achlorhydria induced by the widespread, prolonged use of parietal cell histamine antagonists will result in a future increase in intestinal-type gastric cancer.

Several additional etiologic factors have been associated with gastric carcinoma. Gastric ulcers and adenomatous polyps have occasionally been so linked, but data regarding a cause-and-effect relationship are unconvincing. The inadequate clinical distinction between benign gastric ulcers and small ulcerating carcinomas may, in part, account for this presumed association. The presence of extreme hypertrophy of gastric rugal folds (i.e., Ménétrier's disease), giving the impression of polypoid lesions, has been associated with a striking frequency of malignant transformation; such hypertrophy, however, does not represent the presence of true adenomatous polyps. Individuals with blood group A have been reported to have a higher incidence of gastric cancer than persons with blood group O; it is possible that this observation is related to differences in the mucous secretion of the various ABO blood groups, thereby leading to greater or lesser mucosal protection from carcinogens. No association has been identified between duodenal ulcers and gastric cancer.

Clinical features Gastric cancers, when superficial and surgically curable, usually produce no symptoms. As the tumor becomes more extensive, patients may complain of an insidious upper abdominal discomfort varying in intensity from a vague, postprandial fullness to a severe, steady pain. Anorexia, often with slight nausea, is very common but is not the usual presenting complaint. Weight loss may eventually be observed and nausea and vomiting are particularly prominent with tumors of the pylorus; dysphagia may be the major symptom caused by lesions of the cardia. There are no early physical signs of the disease, and the finding of a palpable abdominal mass generally indicates long-standing growth and, all too often, regional extension.

Gastric carcinomas spread by direct extension through the gastric wall to the perigastric tissues, occasionally adhering to adjacent organs such as the pancreas, colon, or liver. The disease also spreads via lymphatics or by seeding of peritoneal surfaces. Metastases to intraabdominal and supraclavicular lymph nodes may occur frequently as may metastatic nodules to the ovary (Krukenberg's tumor), periumbilical region ("Sister Mary Joseph node") or to the peritoneal cul-de-sac (Blumer's shelf); malignant ascites may also develop. The liver is the most common site for hematogenous spread of tumor.

The presence of iron-deficiency anemia in men and occult blood in the stool of both sexes should mandate a search for an occult lesion in the gastrointestinal tract. Such a careful assessment is of particular importance in patients having atrophic gastritis or pernicious anemia. Unusual clinical features associated with gastric adenocarcinomas include migratory thrombophlebitis, microangiopathic hemolytic anemia, and acanthosis nigricans.

Diagnosis A double-contrast radiographic examination is the simplest diagnostic procedure for the evaluation of a patient with epigastric complaints. The use of double-contrast techniques helps to detect small lesions by improving mucosal detail. The stomach should be distended at some time during every radiographic examination since decreased distensibility may be the only indication of a diffuse infiltrative carcinoma. Although gastric ulcers can be detected fairly early, it may be impossible to distinguish benign from malignant lesions. The anatomic location of an ulcer is not in itself an indication of the presence or absence of a cancer.

Radiographic demonstrations of benign-appearing gastric ulcers presents special problems. Some physicians believe that gastroscopy is not mandatory if the radiographic features are typically benign, if complete healing can be visualized by x-ray within 6 weeks, and if a follow-up contrast radiograph several months later is normal. However, many feel that gastroscopic biopsy and brush cytology are required for all patients with a gastric ulcer in order to exclude a malignancy. The identification of malignant gastric ulcers prior to their penetration into surrounding tissues is crucial since the curability of such early lesions when limited to the mucosa or submucosa, even in the United States, is greater than 80 percent. Since gastric carcinomas are difficult to distinguish clinically or radiographically from gastric lymphomas, endoscopic biopsies should be made as deeply as possible due to the submucosal location of lymphoid tumors.

Treatment Surgical removal of the complete tumor with resection of adjacent lymph nodes offers the only chance for cure. However, this is possible in less than one-third of patients. In general, a subtotal gastrectomy represents the treatment of choice for patients with distal carcinomas while total or near-total gastrectomies are required for more proximal tumors. The prognosis following complete surgical resection is adversely influenced by the degree of tumor penetration into the stomach wall, regional lymph node involvement, vascular invasion, and abnormal DNA content (i.e. aneuploidy), characteristics found in the vast majority of American patients. As a result, the probability of survival after 5 years for the 25 to 30 percent of patients in the United States able to undergo a complete resection of a gastric cancer is approximately 25 percent for distal tumors and less than 10 percent for proximal tumors, with continued tumor recurrences being observed for at least 8 years following surgery. In the absence of ascites or extensive hepatic or peritoneal metastases, however, even the patient who is believed to be surgically incurable should be offered an attempt at resecting the primary lesion since the reduction of residual tumor offers the best form of palliation and may enhance the probability of subsequent benefit if chemotherapy and/or radiation therapy are administered.

Gastric adenocarcinoma is a relatively radioresistant tumor, requiring doses of external beam irradiation in excess of the tolerance of surrounding structures such as bowel mucosa and spinal cord if adequate control of the primary tumor is to be achieved. As a result, the major role of radiation therapy in patients with gastric cancer has been limited to palliation of pain. Controlled trials have indicated that radiation therapy alone after a complete resection does not prolong survival. In the setting of surgically unresectable disease limited to the epigastrium, comparative studies have shown that patients treated with 3500 to 4000 cGy did not live longer than similar patients not receiving radiotherapy; however, survival was prolonged slightly when 5-fluorouracil (5-FU) was given concomitantly with radiation therapy. In this clinical setting, the 5-FU may well be functioning as a radiosensitizer.

The administration of combinations of cytotoxic drugs to patients with advanced gastric carcinoma has been associated with reductions of greater than 50 percent in measurable tumor masses ("partial responses") in 30 to 50 percent of cases, providing significant benefit to individuals who respond to treatment. Such drug combinations have generally included 5-FU and doxorubicin together with mitomycin-C, cisplatin, or high doses of methotrexate. Despite this encouraging

response rate for a malignant condition once thought untreatable, complete disappearances of tumor masses remain uncommon, the partial responses are transient, and the overall impact of such multidrug therapy on survival has been a source of debate. The use of prophylactic (i.e., adjuvant) chemotherapy following the complete resection of a gastric cancer as a means of eradicating clinically undetectable micrometastases and improving the potential for cure has generally proven to be unsuccessful. The role of such adjuvant treatment as well as preoperative ("neoadjuvant") chemotherapy should be considered investigational.

PRIMARY GASTRIC LYMPHOMA Primary lymphoma of the stomach is relatively uncommon, comprising about 7 percent of gastric malignancies and about 2 percent of all lymphomas. It is however, the most frequent extranodal location for lymphoma. The disease is difficult to distinguish clinically from gastric adenocarcinoma; both tumors are most often detected during the sixth decade of life, present with epigastric pain, early satiety, and generalized fatigue, and are usually characterized by ulcerations with a ragged, thickened mucosal pattern demonstrated by contrast radiographs. The diagnosis of lymphoma of the stomach may occasionally be made through cytologic brushings of the gastric mucosa, but usually requires a biopsy at the time of gastroscopy or laparotomy. The failure of gastroscopic biopsies to detect lymphoma should not be interpreted as being conclusive since superficial biopsies may miss the more deeply situated lymphoid infiltrate. The macroscopic pathology of gastric lymphoma may also mimic adenocarcinoma, either as a bulky ulcerated lesion localized in the corpus or antrum or as a diffuse process spreading throughout the entire gastric submucosa and even extending into the duodenum. Microscopically, the vast majority of gastric lymphoid tumors are non-Hodgkin's lymphomas of B-cell origin; Hodgkin's disease involving the stomach is extremely uncommon. Histologically, these tumors may range from well-differentiated, superficial processes (mucosa-associated lymphoid tissue, "MALT") to high-grade, large cell lymphomas. Gastric lymphomas spread initially to regional lymph nodes (often to Waldeyer's ring) and may then disseminate.

Primary gastric lymphoma is a far more treatable disease than adenocarcinoma of the stomach, underscoring the need for making the correct diagnosis. All detectable tumor can be removed in over two-thirds of patients by some type of a subtotal gastrectomy. The prognosis in such patients is encouraging with 5-year survival rates of 40 to 60 percent having been reported. The best prognosis seems to be associated with those gastric lymphomas having small, single lesions, more differentiated histologies, and absence of spread to adjacent lymph nodes. While postoperative radiation therapy to the abdomen has been employed in the past, even when all obvious disease has been resected, the value of such a practice is open to serious question since the majority of recurrences develop in anatomic sites distant from the epigastrium and outside the fields of radiation treatment. Combination chemotherapy, which has proved to be highly effective in the management of disseminated non-Hodgkin's lymphoma including the diffuse large cell subtype, has gained favor as an adjunct to surgery, particularly when regional lymph node involvement is present. In the past, such drug therapy was not considered to be a substitute for surgery, even if the lymphoma were localized, since the rapid destruction of lymphoma masses by chemotherapy occasionally led to life-threatening hemorrhage. The results of recent clinical trials, however, have suggested that the probability for such bleeding may be relatively small and that drug treatment alone may be adequate to eradicate the lymphoma. If widespread disease is discovered at the time of laparotomy, combination chemotherapy should be utilized.

GASTRIC (NONLYMPHOID) SARCOMA Leiomyosarcomas are the most common of this group of gastric malignancies and comprise approximately 1 to 3 percent of all gastric neoplasms. They most frequently involve the anterior and posterior walls of the gastric fundus and often ulcerate and bleed. Even those lesions which appear benign on histologic examination may behave in a malignant fashion.

Leiomyosarcomas rarely invade adjacent viscera and characteristically do not metastasize to lymph nodes but may spread to the liver and lungs. The treatment of choice is surgical resection. Combination chemotherapy should be reserved for patients with metastatic disease.

REFERENCES

Esophageal cancer

BLOT WJ et al: Rising incidence of adenocarcinoma of the esophagus and gastric cardia. JAMA 265:1287, 1991

BOYCE HW: Palliation of advanced esophageal cancer. Semin Oncol 11:186, 1984

FORASTIERE AA et al: Preoperative chemoradiation followed by transhiatal esophagectomy for carcinoma of the esophaghus. Final report. J Clin Oncol 11:1118, 1993

HAGIWARA A et al: Endoscopic local injection of a new drug delivery format of pleomycin for superficial esophageal cancer. A pilot study. Gastroenterology 104:1037, 1993

HERSKOVIC A et al: Combined chemotherapy and radiotherapy compared with radiotherapy alone in patients with cancer of the esophagus. N Engl J Med 326:1593, 1992

KELSEN D: Chemotherapy of esophageal cancer. Semin Oncol 11:159, 1984

LIGHTDALE CJ, WINAWER SJ: Screening diagnosis and staging of esophageal cancer. Semin Oncol 11:101, 1984

POPLIN E et al: Combined therapies for squamous-cell carcinoma of the esophagus, a Southwest Oncology Group Study (SWOG - 8037). J. Clin Oncol 5:622, 1987

REID BJ et al: Endoscopic biopsy can detect high-grade dysplasia or early adenocarcinoma in Barrett's esophagus with grossly recognizable neoplastic lesions. Gastroenterology 94:81, 1988

SCHOTTENFELD D: Epidemiology of cancer of the esophagus. Semin Oncol 11:92, 1984

SKINNER DB: Surgical treatment for esophageal carcinoma. Semin Oncol 11:136, 1984

Gastric tumors

BEDIKIAN AY et al: The natural history of gastric cancer and prognostic factors influencing survival. J Clin Oncol 2:305, 1984

CORREA P: Human gastric carcinogenesis: a multistep and multifactorial process—First American Cancer Society award lecture on cancer epidemiology and prevention. Cancer Res 52:6735, 1992

DOUGLASS HO, NAVA HR: Gastric adenocarcinoma—management of the primary disease. Semin Oncol 12:32, 1985

GOHMANN JJ, MACDONALD JS: Chemotherapy of gastric cancer. Cancer Invest 7:39, 1989

HABER DA, MAYER RJ: Primary gastrointestinal lymphoma. Semin Oncol 15:154, 1988

KELSEN D: Adjuvant therapy of upper gastrointestinal tract cancers. Semin Oncol 18:543, 1991

KURTZ RC, SHERLOCK P: The diagnosis of gastric cancer. Semin Oncol 12:11, 1985

LANGMAN MJS: Antisecretory drugs and gastric cancer. Br Med J 290:1850, 1985

LIGHT JD et al: Gastrointestinal sarcomas. Semin Oncol 15:181, 1988

NANUS DM et al: Flow cytometry as a predictive indication in patients with operable gastric cancer. J Clin Oncol 7:1105, 1989

PARSONETT J et al: Helicobacter pylori infection and the risk of gastric carcinoma. N Engl J Med 325:1127, 1991

POWELL J, MCCONKEY CC: Increasing incidence of adenocarcinoma of the gastric cardia and adjacent sites. Brit J Cancer 62:440, 1990

SEVERSON RK, DAVIS S: Increasing incidence of primary gastric lymphoma. Cancer 66:1283, 1990

TERSMETTE AC et al: Meta-analysis of the risk of gastric stump cancer: detection of high risk patient subsets for stomach cancer after remote partial gastrectomy for benign conditions. Cancer Res 50:6486, 1990

254   DISORDERS OF ABSORPTION

NORTON J. GREENBERGER / KURT J. ISSELBACHER

MECHANISMS OF ABSORPTION

Diseases of the small intestine are frequently accompanied by alterations in intestinal function, and clinically, this impaired function is seen as the malabsorption syndrome. In order to obtain a better appreciation of the derangements which occur in the many disorders of intestinal function, the processes of normal absorption will first be reviewed.

It is important to distinguish between digestion and absorption, since an increased loss of nutrients in the stool may be a reflection of a derangement of either process. Digestion involves the breakdown or hydrolysis of nutrients to smaller molecules in order to prepare the ingested substances for absorption, or transport across the intestinal cell. It will be recalled that most of the digestive process is initiated in the stomach by acid and pepsin and is continued in the upper small intestine primarily by the action of pancreatic enzymes such as lipase, amylase, and trypsin. As a result of these digestive actions carbohydrates are broken down to monosaccharides and disaccharides, proteins to peptides and amino acids, and fats to monoglycerides and fatty acids. In the adult it is in this form that nutrients are, to a large extent, transported across the epithelial surface of the intestinal cell.

ANATOMIC AND PHYSIOLOGIC FACTORS   The intestine has an enormous surface area. This can be attributed in large part to its length, which in the adult is more than 4 m, and to the foldings of the surface plicae. At the light-microscopic level, the villi of the small intestine provide additional surface area, which is further augmented by the presence of microvilli (approximately 2×10^8 per square centimeter) on the outer, or brush border, region of epithelial cells. Thus the total absorptive area of the small intestine is enormous.

Motility (contractility) of the bowel is an important process which permits nutrients to remain in intimate contact with the intestinal cells and possibly influences the continued movement of the nutrients *into* and along the absorbing channels, such as the lymphatics. Two types of motility aid in this process: the gross motility of the intestine itself and the motility of individual villi. Entrance of the nutrients into the general circulation is achieved via the capillaries into the portal system or via the lacteals into the intestinal lymphatics.

TYPES OF ABSORPTION (See also Chap. 39)   Four mechanisms have been considered to be important in the transport of substances across the intestinal cell membrane, namely, active transport, passive diffusion, facilitated diffusion, and endocytosis.

Active transport involves the transport of a substance across the cell against an electric or chemical gradient; this process requires energy, is carrier-mediated, and is subject to competitive inhibition. *Passive diffusion* is the opposite of this process; energy is not required, transport is with (rather than against) the electric or chemical gradient, the process is not carrier-mediated, and it does not show properties of competitive inhibition. Thus active transport may be viewed as "uphill" transport, whereas passive diffusion is equivalent to "downhill" transport. *Facilitated diffusion* is similar to passive diffusion except that such a process shows evidence of being carrier-mediated and frequently subject to competitive inhibition.

Endocytosis is a process akin to phagocytosis. By this mechanism, nutrients (soluble or particulate) upon entering the cell are surrounded by the components of the outer plasma cell membrane. In the intestinal tract, endocytosis occurs in the neonatal period and, contrary to earlier belief, also occurs to a limited extent in the adult. While quantitatively limited, it appears to account, at least in part, for uptake of antigens.

SITES OF ABSORPTION   While many substances are absorbed throughout the length of the small intestine, certain nutrients tend to be absorbed more in one region than in others. The proximal intestine is a major area for the absorption of iron, calcium, water-soluble vitamins, and fat (monoglycerides and fatty acids). Sugars are absorbed in the proximal intestine as well as the midintestine. While the amino acids appear to be absorbed primarily in the middle of the small intestine, or jejunum, some absorption also occurs in the upper and lower areas. The distal small intestine appears to be the *major* absorptive area for bile salts and vitamin B_{12}. As is emphasized below, this is of clinical significance in circumstances where there has been removal or disease of the ileum.

The colon is important for the absorption of water and electrolytes, a process which occurs predominantly in the cecum. Although the rectum is not a usual site for absorption of ingested nutrients, drugs introduced by rectum may be absorbed there. Thus drugs introduced by this route, such as salicylates or steroids, may have systemic as well as local effects.

ABSORPTION OF SPECIFIC NUTRIENTS   Carbohydrate absorption   Much of the carbohydrate we ingest is in the form of starch, a complex polysaccharide consisting of many hexose units (attached either in a 1,4 or 1,6 linkage). By the action of salivary and pancreatic amylase, starch is hydrolyzed to oligosaccharides and then to disaccharides (mostly maltose). While monosaccharides such as glucose are readily absorbed, disaccharides are not. Disaccharides are split enzymatically into their component sugars by disaccharidases (or oligosaccharidases) located in the microvilli of intestinal epithelial cells. The two types of disaccharidases are β-galactosidases (lactase) and α-glucosidases (sucrase, maltase). By the action of these enzymes, lactose is split into glucose and galactose, sucrose into glucose and fructose, and maltose into two molecules of glucose. The resultant monosaccharides are then transported through the cell into the portal circulation. Most disaccharides are hydrolyzed so rapidly by brush border enzymes that the capacity of the transport mechanism is exceeded and some monosaccharides diffuse back into the intestinal lumen. Lactose, however, is hydrolyzed at a slower rate, and thus lactose hydrolysis is the rate-limiting step in lactose absorption.

Sugars such as glucose and galactose are absorbed by an active transport mechanism. Glucose (and galactose) entry into the cell is largely coupled to sodium ions (so-called symport); both sodium and glucose appear to bind to the hexose carrier in the microvillus membrane. Energy is required for the movement of glucose into the cell, which seems largely to come from the sodium pump and the Na^+,K^+-ATPase of the basolateral membrane (see below).

Protein and amino acid absorption   Dietary proteins are initially subject to degradation in the stomach by pepsin. However, complete hydrolysis is largely achieved by the action of pancreatic trypsin and chymotrypsin, as well as by other endopeptidases and exopeptidases such as carboxypeptidase. By these enzymatic processes, oligopeptides, dipeptides, and amino acids are formed. Just as there are disaccharidases in mucosal cells to digest disaccharides, there are also oligopeptidases to split small peptides. Dipeptidases are located in the cytoplasm as well as on the microvilli. Dipeptides are absorbed more rapidly than amino acids, and presumably their uptake involves a separate mechanism. Thus digestion of proteins to amino acids occurs in three locations: intestinal lumen, brush border, and cytoplasm of mucosal cells. As indicated above, contrary to earlier beliefs, proteins also can be absorbed by the adult intestine. Although quantitatively limited, protein absorption can be immunologically significant.

Most naturally occurring amino acids are L-amino acids, and these are subject to a number of different transport processes. *Neutral* amino acids share a common carrier mechanism; thus amino acids such as tryptophan and alanine show competitive inhibition. Among the *dibasic* amino acids which appear to have a distinct transport mechanism are arginine, ornithine, and lysine. The neutral amino acid cystine shares this mechanism. There is a separate transport system for *glycine* and the *imino acids* proline and hydroxyproline. There is also a transport system for *dicarboxylic* acids such as glutamic and aspartic acids. Therefore, in genetic disorders such as cystinuria, one will find impaired absorption not only of cystine but also of arginine, ornithine, and lysine. Similarly, in Hartnup disease, a defect in the transport of neutral amino acids (especially of tryptophan, phenylalanine, histidine) is found. In these genetic disorders, uptake and absorption of dipeptides is normal (see Chap. 353).

Absorption of amino acids is rapid in the duodenum and jejunum but slow in the ileum. As in the case of carbohydrates, sodium ions are necessary for the entry of these acids and the energy needed for their concentration within the cell. Some amino acids have affinity for more than one mechanism. For example, glycine may be transported by both the neutral and imino acid transport systems.

Fat absorption (Fig. 254-1)   Most of the ingested dietary fats are in the form of long-chain triglycerides. These triglycerides contain both saturated fatty acids (such as palmitic and stearic) and unsaturated fatty acids (such as oleic and linoleic). The particle size of the fat is decreased largely by the churning action of the stomach. The entry of fat into the duodenum, plus the presence of acid, causes release of secretin and cholecystokinin, which in turn leads to a stimulation of the flow of bile and pancreatic juice.

ROLE OF PANCREATIC LIPASE   The hydrolysis of triglycerides by pancreatic lipase is a complex process involving lipase, colipase, and bile salts. Pancreatic lipase binds to the oil-water interface of an emulsified triglyceride substrate. The detergent properties of bile salts permit pancreatic lipase to gain access to water-insoluble lipids. One of the important functions of bile salts is to clear the oil-water interface of dietary fat from proteins of exogenous and endogenous origin, thus making it available for pancreatic lipolysis. Colipase, a protein present in pancreatic juice, is also essential for the action of lipase; its function is to anchor the lipase close to the surface of the triglyceride droplet. All three components, i.e., pancreatic lipase, colipase, and bile salts, form a *ternary complex* which generates lipolytic products that diffuse away from the complex and are absorbed. With colipase present, lipase remains at the interface and forms 2-monoglycerides and fatty acids, which are the major end products of triglyceride hydrolysis. Less than 5 percent of ingested fat remains in the form of diglycerides and triglycerides. Without colipase, bile acids would actually wash pancreatic lipase away from the interface, and the hydrolytic rate of triglycerides would be reduced.

FIGURE 254-1   Scheme of intestinal digestion, absorption, esterification, and transport of dietary triglycerides. TG = triglycerides; FA = fatty acids; MG = monoglycerides; BS = bile salts.

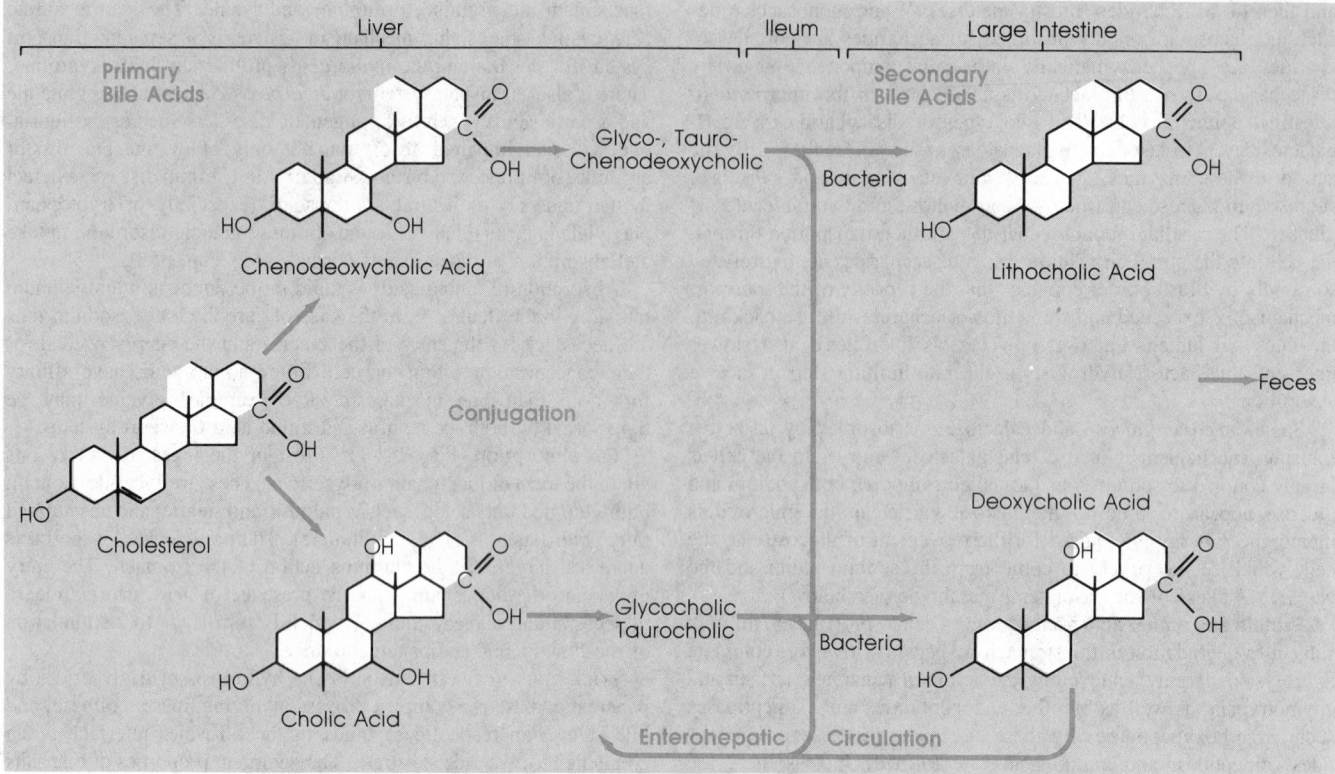

FIGURE 254-2   Scheme of hepatic and intestinal metabolism of bile salts and the enterohepatic circulation (from ileum to liver). Note that bacteria lead to the formation of secondary bile acids; of the latter, only deoxycholic acid is absorbed to any appreciable extent.

ROLE OF BILE SALTS (Fig. 254-2)   Bile salts play an important role in the digestion and absorption of fat. They are synthesized in the liver (approximately 200 to 600 mg daily) from cholesterol and excreted in the bile in the form of their glycine or taurine conjugates. In humans the principal bile acids excreted are conjugates of cholic and chenodeoxycholic acid. Bile salts are good detergents, because they have both polar (hydrophilic) and nonpolar (hydrophobic) groups. During digestion, the concentration of conjugated bile salts in the lumen is in the range of 5 to 15 μmol/mL, and at these concentrations the bile salts aggregate to form *micelles*. Fatty acids and monoglycerides enter these micelles, forming mixed micelles. An emulsion of triglyceride is turbid; mixed micelles containing bile salts, fatty acids, and monoglycerides are clear solutions. The formation of *mixed micelles*, and hence the solubilization of fatty acids and monoglycerides, is much more effectively achieved with *conjugated bile salts* at the pH which normally exists in the intestinal lumen (see Fig. 254-2).

Most conjugated bile salts are absorbed in the ileum and after entering the portal vein are subject to an enterohepatic circulation. By this process, about 90 percent of the conjugated bile salts reaching the ileum is reabsorbed. As a consequence, only about 200 to 600 mg bile salts is excreted in the feces per day, while, as part of the enterohepatic circulation, the 3- to 4-g bile salt pool circulates many times each day so that actually 20 to 30 g of bile salts may enter the duodenum each day. When the enterohepatic circulation is intact, the size of the bile salt pool is largely determined by the frequency of the enterohepatic circulation, i.e., the number of cycles per day (see also Chap. 272). If the ileum is diseased or removed, absorption of bile salts is impaired, and a significant fecal loss of bile salts will occur. As a consequence of this bile salt depletion, the concentration of bile salts in the intestinal lumen also will decrease, leading to further impairment of fat absorption. A similar result will occur if bile salt reabsorption is prevented by chelating agents, such as cholestyramine (see "Regional Enteritis," below). Diarrhea per se may result in increased fecal excretion of bile salts. This has been demonstrated both in normal subjects in whom diarrhea has been induced and in patients with chronic idiopathic diarrhea.

INTRAMUCOSAL ASPECTS OF FAT ABSORPTION (Fig. 254-1)   After the hydrolysis of fatty acids to monoglycerides and their interaction with bile salts to form mixed micelles, the lipids pass through an "unstirred" water layer covering the cell surface. The mixed micelles apparently do not enter the cell, but instead the component fatty acids and monoglycerides are released from the micellar phase and then enter the cell by diffusion. In aqueous duodenal contents, large bile salt mixed micelles saturated with products of lipolysis coexist with larger liquid crystal liposomes of the same lipids saturated with free fatty acids and mixed bile salts. These phases are interconvertible, and both may be important in fat digestion and absorption. Upon entry into the mucosal cell, fatty acids interact with specific binding proteins. The subsequent fate of the intracellular lipid is strongly influenced by the fatty acid chain length. Fatty acids and monoglycerides derived from long-chain triglycerides (i.e., containing C-16 to C-18 fatty acids) are promptly *reesterified to triglycerides* by enzymes of the endoplasmic reticulum. These triglycerides then interact with specific apolipoproteins plus cholesterol and phospholipid to form chylomicrons and very low density lipoproteins. These initially accumulate in the Golgi region of the cell and then are secreted into the lacteals and the intestinal lymph. There are thus four major steps in the absorption of long-chain fatty acids and monoglycerides: (1) mucosal uptake and interaction with binding proteins, (2) reesterification to triglycerides, (3) lipoprotein formation, and (4) secretion into lymph.

By contrast, fatty acids derived from medium-chain triglycerides (i.e., containing C-8 and C-12 fatty acids) are *not reesterified* to any significant extent within the cell and are not incorporated into lipoproteins. Instead, they rapidly enter the portal venous system, where they are transported as fatty acids bound to albumin. The major aspects of fat absorption are summarized in Fig. 254-1.

Absorption of cholesterol and fat-soluble vitamins (A, D, E, K)   In addition to contributing significantly to the total-body synthesis of cholesterol, the intestine also plays an active role in the absorption of cholesterol and its esters. Within the lumen, cholesterol esters from the bile and diet are hydrolyzed by a pancreatic esterase. There is also a separate cholesterol esterase in the intestinal microvilli which completes this hydrolysis. As a result, only free cholesterol enters the intestinal cell. However, just as in the case of long-chain fatty acids, much of the cholesterol is reesterified and is then secreted primarily into lymph.

The absorption mechanisms of the fat-soluble vitamins A, D, E, and K are not well understood. The intestine is able to convert β-carotene into vitamin A. The vitamin A thus formed or absorbed from the lumen is esterified in the mucosa primarily with palmitic acid, transported in the chylomicrons of the lymph, and stored as retinol palmitate in the liver. The other lipid-soluble vitamins also appear in lymph chylomicrons, but esterification with fatty acids does not appear to be necessary for their transport.

Water and sodium absorption (See also Chap. 39) The mechanisms responsible for fluid absorption differ in the jejunum, ileum, and colon. There are two pathways by which water and ions cross the intestinal mucosa: the paracellular and transcellular pathways. Individual intestinal mucosa cells are joined near their apex by a ''tight junction,'' and ions and water traverse this *paracellular* pathway during absorption and secretion. The tight junction pathway contains aqueous-filled channels or pores. Such intercellular spaces are closed in the resting state and dilated during absorption. Considerable evidence has accumulated indicating that pumps and carriers are involved in intestinal water and solute transport. For example, in the ileum, Na^+ enters in exchange for H^+, and Cl^- enters in exchange for HCO_3^-. Sodium entry into the cell also occurs coupled with glucose via the glucose-sodium carrier in the microvillus membrane. Inside the cell, the Na^+ pump located in the basolateral membrane actively transports Na^+ out of the mucosal cell and into the intercellular space. *Transcellular* transport requires passage of ions through two membrane barriers, i.e., the apical brush border plasma membrane and the basolateral membrane. After Na^+ and Cl^- are transported across the brush border membrane into the cell, Na^+ is pumped across the basolateral membrane and Cl^- either follows passively or is also pumped into the intercellular space. The Na^+,K^+-ATPase is present in the basolateral but not in the brush border membrane and is the biochemical mediator of this pump. Bulk water movement obviously influences the movement of Na^+, K^+, and Cl^-. This ''solvent drag'' effect is explained by two mechanisms: (1) solutes may be caught in a moving stream of water and transported across a membrane, and (2) water movement results in increased concentration of solute on the side of the membrane from which water was transported, which causes solute to diffuse through the direction of flow. Diarrhea can be simply defined as impaired net absorption of water and electrolytes by the small intestine or colon. Some mechanisms producing diarrhea are listed in Table 254-1.

Calcium absorption Calcium is actively transported by the small intestine, and this process is intimately linked to the active form of vitamin D_3, namely, 1,25-dihydroxycholecalciferol. The role of two other intestinal cell proteins, calcium-binding protein and calmodulin, in the absorption of calcium remains unclear. Recent studies indicate that calcium is absorbed to the same extent from various calcium salts (carbonate, citrate, gluconate, lactate, and acetate) and from milk in healthy subjects; an average of 32 percent of the ingested calcium was absorbed from the various sources.

Iron absorption The formation of soluble iron complexes is important for maintaining intraluminal iron in an absorbable form. Gastric acid facilitates the chelation of inorganic iron with substances such as ascorbic acid, sugars, amino acids, and bile; these macromolecular complexes then remain soluble in the more alkaline duodenum and jejunum. With the average western diet the iron intake averages 15 to 25 mg/d; iron absorption averages 0.5 to 1.0 mg/d in men and 1.0 to 2.0 mg/d in women during their reproductive years. Iron is actively transported by the small intestine, and the duodenum is the principal site of iron absorption. The transferrin receptor and also

---

TABLE 254-1 Some mechanisms in the production of diarrhea

SECRETORY DIARRHEA

A Secretory agents associated with adenylate cyclase system
  1 Enterotoxin-producing bacteria (*Vibrio cholerae, Escherichia coli*)
  2 Methylxanthines (caffeine, theophylline)
  3 Prostaglandins
  4 Vasoactive intestinal peptide (VIP)
  5 Dihydroxy bile acids (affect colon primarily; effects seen after ileal resection)
B Secretory agents *not associated* with adenylate cyclase system
  1 Glucagon, secretin, cholecystokinin-pancreozymin, serotonin, calcitonin, gastrin inhibitory polypeptide (GIP)
  2 Some laxatives* (ricinoleic acid, bisacodyl, phenolphthalein, dioctyl sodium sulfosuccinate)
  3 Bacterial enterotoxins (*Shigella, Staphylococcus aureus, Clostridium perfringens*)
C Mucosal injury, altered cell permeability
  1 Salmonella, Shigella, invasive *E. coli*, gastroenteritis viruses
  2 Celiac sprue
  3 Inflammatory bowel disease (ulcerative colitis, regional enteritis)
D Neoplasms with or without hormone production
  1 Gastrinoma (gastrin)
  2 Carcinoid syndrome (serotonin, prostaglandins)
  3 Medullary carcinoma of thyroid (calcitonin, prostaglandins)
  4 Pancreatic cholera syndrome (? VIP)
  5 Villous adenoma
E Medications
  1 Diuretics
  2 Theophylline
  3 Colchicine
  4 Prostaglandins (misoprostol)
  5 Azodisalicylate
F Congenital
  1 Microvillus inclusion disease
  2 Congenital chloridorrhea

OSMOTIC DIARRHEA

A Impaired carbohydrate absorption
  1 Disaccharidase deficiency (lactose or sucrose-isomaltose intolerance)
  2 Glucose-galactose malabsorption
B Nonabsorbable osmotically active agents (lactulose, sorbitol, mannitol, dietetic foods)
C Laxative ingestion or abuse
  1 Saline purgatives (magnesium phosphate, magnesium hydroxide–containing antacids)
D Postoperative disorders
  1 Vagotomy and pyloroplasty*
  2 Gastrojejunostomy* (Billroth I and II)

MOTILITY DISORDERS

A Laxative abuse*
B Irritable bowel syndrome
C Diverticular disease of the colon
D Diabetic diarrhea with visceral neuropathy
E Hyperthyroidism

* Multiple mechanisms involved in production of diarrhea.

---

duodenal ferritin in small intestinal mucosal cells appear to have a regulatory/inhibitory role in iron absorption. The absorption of elemental iron in humans and animals involves at least two distinct steps: (1) mucosal uptake of iron from the lumen and (2) mucosal transfer of iron to the plasma. Much of the iron entering the mucosal cell is not transferred to the plasma but remains trapped within the cell and is excreted into the lumen when the cell is shed. Iron lost by this mechanism seems to vary inversely with body iron stores. However, this mucosal regulatory mechanism can be overcome when pharmacologic doses of iron are ingested. Hemoglobin iron is also absorbed by human subjects depending on body requirements for iron; the heme is split from globin in the lumen and absorbed as an intact metalloporphyrin. Organic iron in the form of hemoglobin is absorbed more effectively than iron from cereals and vegetables. The absorption of inorganic iron is increased by ascorbic acid. Similarly, the presence of anemia, liver injury, pregnancy, idiopathic hemochromatosis, or a portacaval shunt may result in increased iron absorption.

Conversely, the prior ingestion of large doses of iron and the presence in the lumen of phosphates, carbonates, and phytates may lead to decreased absorption of inorganic iron. Impaired absorption of iron is frequent in disorders (such as celiac sprue) which involve the duodenal mucosa.

Water-soluble vitamins *Vitamin B_{12} absorption* is discussed in Chap. 304. In the case of *folic acid absorption*, it should be emphasized that folates exist in food conjugated with glutamyl peptides. These *polyglutamates* must be deconjugated (by folic deconjugase) to monoglutamates for absorption to occur. Certain drugs (such as oral contraceptives, sulfasalazine, diphenylhydantoin, trimethoprim, and pyrimethamine) inhibit the absorption of dietary folate and hence can cause folate deficiency. Sulfasalazine, for example, competitively inhibits three enzymes important in the intestinal metabolism of folate, i.e., dihydrofolate reductase, methylene tetrahydrofolate reductase, and serine transhydroxymethylase. Thiamine and riboflavin appear to be absorbed by passive diffusion.

TESTS USEFUL IN THE DIAGNOSIS OF MALABSORPTION

Most of the tests useful in the diagnosis of malabsorption indicate the presence of abnormal absorptive or digestive function, and only a few tests may suggest a specific diagnosis. Accordingly, it is frequently necessary to employ a combination of tests to establish a diagnosis. To illustrate the use of various tests, the characteristic findings in celiac sprue, an example of a primary malabsorptive disorder, and pancreatic insufficiency, an example of impaired digestion, are compared in Table 254-2.

Stool fat The qualitative examination of the stool for undigested muscle fibers, neutral fat, and split fat is a simple and reliable screening test for steatorrhea. The finding of an increased number of muscle fibers indicates impaired intraluminal digestion. Properly performed, the qualitative microscopic examination of a stool specimen with the Sudan III stain is of value and correlates well with the quantitative determination of fecal fat. The latter remains the most reliable measurement of steatorrhea. A normal fecal fat excretion is less than 6 g for 24 h, or greater than 94 percent coefficient of fat absorption. It has been demonstrated that diarrhea itself can induce mild secondary steatorrhea. When the quantitative fecal fat test is used in patients with diarrhea, mild abnormalities (up to 14 g/d) are not specific for a primary defect in fat digestion or absorption, i.e., they may represent false-positive results.

Although not used frequently, oral [^{14}C]triolein can be used as an effective test for fat absorption. During the digestive process, the triolein is hydrolyzed, and the labeled glycerol is absorbed and metabolized by the liver. The $^{14}CO_2$ produced is exhaled and can then be measured hourly (for 6 h) in the expired air. Normally, more than 3.5 percent of the administered label [0.185 MBq (5 μCi)] appears in the breath per hour.

Xylose absorption In the most commonly employed test of carbohydrate absorption, the patient ingests 25 g D-xylose. A 5-h urine xylose excretion of 26 mmol (4.0 g) or greater is considered normal. Low values may be obtained in patients with ascites, intestinal bacterial overgrowth, or renal insufficiency, after administration of certain drugs (e.g., aspirin, indomethacin), and most commonly if the urine collection is incomplete. To prevent difficulties in interpreting the test, it is advisable to determine the blood xylose level 2 h after ingestion of xylose. A blood xylose level of 2 mmol/L (30 mg/dL) or greater indicates normal absorption of D-xylose. An abnormal D-xylose absorption test is found most frequently in disorders affecting the mucosa of the proximal small intestine, such as celiac sprue and tropical sprue.

Gastrointestinal x-ray studies All patients with malabsorption should have radiographic examinations of the small intestine and, in many cases, of the esophagus, stomach, and colon as well. Occasionally, the latter two examinations may provide important clues to the presence of such disorders as celiac sprue, scleroderma, Zollinger-Ellison syndrome, regional enteritis, ulcerative colitis, and intestinal fistulas. Traditional radiographic findings suggesting a diagnosis of

malabsorption include flocculation of barium within fluid-filled loops causing fragmentation and segmentation of the barium column. However, these patterns are no longer demonstrated reliably in small-bowel series because of widespread use of barium products that contain a nonflocculating suspension of micropulverized barium sulfate. In celiac sprue, the most consistent abnormalities are thickened and nodular duodenal folds and dilatation of the small bowel. However, these findings are nonspecific and may be found in several of the disorders listed in Table 254-3. Some representative examples of abnormal small-bowel radiographs are shown in Fig. 254-3.

Small-intestinal biopsy The most commonly used instrument for obtaining peroral biopsy specimens from the small intestine is the upper gastrointestinal endoscope, which has largely superseded the use of the Crosby, Carey, and Ross-Moore capsules. Examination of small-bowel biopsy specimens has proved to be of considerable value in the differential diagnosis of malabsorptive disorders. Table 254-3 lists disorders associated with abnormalities in intestinal biopsies, and Fig. 254-4 depicts some illustrative lesions.

Schilling test for vitamin B_{12} absorption The Schilling test is valuable in the differential diagnosis of malabsorption and is frequently carried out in three stages: (1) without intrinsic factor, (2) with intrinsic factor, and (3) after a course of treatment with antibiotics or anti-inflammatory drugs. Since vitamin B_{12} is absorbed primarily in the distal ileum, an abnormal Schilling test may indicate a pathologic condition of the distal small bowel. In disorders affecting the terminal ileum, such as regional enteritis and lymphomas, the first- and second-stage Schilling tests are frequently abnormal. The ileal receptor site appears to be damaged in these disorders, and the impaired absorption of B_{12} is not corrected by the addition of intrinsic factor or the use of antibiotics. However, the Schilling test may normalize after treatment with prednisone or sulfasalazine. The Schilling test also may be useful in establishing a diagnosis of abnormal bacterial overgrowth of the small bowel, which may be present in disorders such as blind loop syndrome, scleroderma, and multiple small-bowel diverticula (see below). In the blind loop syndrome, for example, the bacteria can actually take up vitamin B_{12} with resultant impaired absorption of B_{12}. Under these conditions, the first-stage Schilling test is frequently abnormal, as is the second stage. After appropriate antibiotic treatment, the Schilling test usually returns to normal. Vitamin B_{12} absorption is frequently abnormal in patients with exocrine pancreatic insufficiency (see Chap. 274).

Secretin and other pancreatic tests The secretin test, secretin cholecystokinin test, intraduodenal perfusion with essential amino acids, and bentiromide test, which may be useful in establishing a diagnosis of pancreatic insufficiency, are discussed in detail in Chap. 273.

Serum calcium, albumin, cholesterol, magnesium, and iron Abnormal serum calcium, albumin, cholesterol, magnesium, and iron values may be found in several malabsorptive disorders. The primary value of such tests is to suggest that abnormal intestinal absorptive function may be present. These tests are usually of limited value in the *differential diagnosis* of malabsorption but, if abnormal, may be helpful in supporting this diagnosis.

Serum carotenes, vitamin A, and prothrombin time Absorption of the fat-soluble vitamins A, D, K, and E is frequently impaired in patients with steatorrhea. Measurements of serum carotene and vitamin A levels are useful as screening tests for malabsorption. However, other tests not only are more sensitive but often give more specific information than the serum carotene and vitamin A levels. The blood prothrombin time is an important test, since patients with malabsorption may present with abnormal bleeding due to vitamin K deficiency. If the decreased prothrombin activity is due to malabsorption, it should be readily correctable with parenteral vitamin K.

Breath tests The bile acid breath test utilizing [^{14}C]cholylglycine is a reasonably reliable screening test for bacterial overgrowth syndromes. Approximately two-thirds of patients with a positive small-bowel culture will have an abnormal bile acid breath test.

TABLE 254-2 Tests useful in the diagnosis of malabsorptive disorders

Test	Normal values	Typical findings Malabsorption (celiac sprue)	Typical findings Maldigestion (pancreatic insufficiency)	Comment
I Quantitative determination of stool fat	<6 g per 24 h: >95% coefficient of fat absorption	>6 g per 24 h	>6 g per 24 h	Best test for establishing presence of steatorrhea
II Carbohydrate absorption				
A D-Xylose absorption (25-g oral dose)	5-h urinary excretion >26 mmol (>4.5 g); peak blood level >2.0 mmol/L (>30 mg/dL)	↓	Normal	A good screening test for carbohydrate absorption
III Small-intestine x-rays		Malabsorption pattern	Normal or minimal malabsorption pattern; occasionally pancreatic calcification	
IV Blood tests				
A Serum calcium	2.2–2.7 mmol/L (9–11 mg/dL)	Frequently ↓	Usually normal	
B Serum albumin	35–55 g/L (3.5–5.5 g/dL)	Frequently ↓	Usually normal	Decreased levels of both serum albumin and globulins should raise the question of protein-losing enteropathy
C Serum cholesterol	3.90–6.45 mmol/L (150–250 mg/dL)	↓	Frequently ↓	Usually decreased in disorders associated with significant steatorrhea
D Serum iron	14–24 μmol/L (80–150 μg/dL)	Frequently ↓	Normal	Low values may reflect decreased body iron stores
E Serum magnesium	0.6–1.0 mmol/L (1.2–2.0 mEq/L)	Frequently ↓	Usually normal	
F Serum zinc	12–20 μmol/L	Frequently ↓	Usually normal	Decreased levels common in malnutrition, cirrhosis, and malabsorption
G Serum carotenes	>100 IU/dL	↓	Usually ↓	Fairly satisfactory screening tests for malabsorption
H Serum vitamin A	>100 IU/dL	↓		
I Prothrombin time	70–100%; 12–15 s	Frequently ↓	Frequently ↓	
V Small intestinal mucosal biopsy		Abnormal	Normal	A specific diagnosis can be established in a small number of disorders (see text)
VI Urine tests				
A Vitamin B$_{12}$ absorption	>8% urinary excretion in 48 h	Frequently ↓	Frequently ↓	Useful in determining whether vitamin B$_{12}$ malabsorption is due to gastric or small-intestinal disorders
B Urine 5-hydroxyindole-acetic acid (5-HIAA)	10–47 μmol per 24 h (2–9 mg per 24 h)	↑	Normal	Slightly increased level (12–16 mg per 24 h) characteristically found in celiac sprue
VII Breath tests				
A Breath H$_2$ (after 50 g lactose)	Minimal breath H$_2$	May be ↑	Normal	Secondary to lactase deficiency (see text)
B Breath H$_2$ (after 10 g lactulose)	Minimal breath H$_2$	May be normal or ↓	Normal	Early peak in bacterial overgrowth; can be used to determine intestinal transit time
C Breath $^{14}CO_2$ (after [^{14}C]xylose)	Minute amounts $^{14}CO_2$	May be ↓	Usually normal	Increased in bacterial overgrowth
D Glycocholic acid metabolism (oral glycine-1-[^{14}C]glycocholate)	<1% of dose excreted $^{14}CO_2$ in 4 h	Normal	Normal	Increased $^{14}CO_2$ excretion with bacterial overgrowth or bile acid malabsorption (due to ileal resection or inflammatory disease)
	<4% of dose excreted in stools	Normal	Normal	Increased fecal excretion of ^{14}C in bile acid malabsorption
E [^{14}C]Triolein absorption (breath test)	>3.5% of dose as breath $^{14}CO_2$ per hour	Decreased	Decreased	Correlates well with chemical stool fat; recently introduced test
VIII Miscellaneous				
A Bacteria (culture)	<10^3 organisms per milliliter	Normal	Normal	>10^5 organisms per milliliter indicates bacterial overgrowth
B Secretin test	Volume >1.8 (mL/kg)/h Bicarbonate concentration >80 mmol/L	Normal	Abnormal	See discussion of pancreatic insufficiency in Chaps. 273 and 274
C Bentiromide test	Urine excretion arylamines ≥50%	May be abnormal	Abnormal	See discussion of pancreatic disease in Chaps. 273 and 274

However, in patients with suspected malabsorption of bile acids, the test is rather insensitive without the additional determination of fecal bile acid excretion. The excretion of breath hydrogen after ingestion of lactose is a sensitive, specific, and noninvasive test for detecting lactase deficiency. Lactulose and [^{14}C]xylose breath tests for bacterial overgrowth also have been found helpful.

PATHOPHYSIOLOGIC BASIS FOR SYMPTOMS AND SIGNS IN MALABSORPTIVE DISORDERS The common symptoms and signs found in malabsorptive disorders are listed in Table 254-4. The most frequent symptoms are those of malnutrition, weight loss, and diarrhea. However, in each of the clinical settings listed in Table 254-4, it is important to consider the cause of the malabsorption.

A

B

C

FIGURE 254-3 *A.* X-ray of a normal small intestine showing good mucosal pattern. *B.* Intestinal x-ray of a patient with celiac sprue. Note dilatation of small bowel, lack of mucosal markings, and segmentation and clumping of barium. *C.* Intestinal x-ray of patient with obstructed lymphatics due to Köhlmeier-Degos disease, with "accordion-pleated" pattern (*lower edge*).

DISORDERS OF MALABSORPTION (See Table 254-5)

INADEQUATE DIGESTION   Liver and biliary tract disease It is not generally appreciated that patients with acute or chronic liver disease may develop malabsorption due to impaired intraluminal digestion. Steatorrhea has been described in acute viral hepatitis,

chronic extrahepatic biliary tract obstruction, primary biliary cirrhosis, and postnecrotic and nutritional cirrhosis. Absorption of D-xylose and vitamin B_{12} is usually normal, and small-intestinal mucosal biopsy specimens are generally unremarkable. The steatorrhea associated with liver and biliary tract disease is thought to be due to impaired

TABLE 254-3   Disorders associated with abnormalities in small-bowel biopsy specimens

BIOPSY HAS DIAGNOSTIC VALUE (DIFFUSE LESIONS)

A Whipple's disease: Lamina propria infiltrated with macrophages containing PAS-positive glycoproteins
B Abetalipoproteinemia: Villus structure normal; epithelial cells vacuolated due to excess fat
C Agammaglobuinemia: Flattened or absent villi; increased lymphocyte infiltration; absence of plasma cells

BIOPSY MAY HAVE DIAGNOSTIC VALUE (PATCHY LESIONS)

A Intestinal lymphoma: Infiltration of lamina propria and submucosa with malignant cells
B Intestinal lymphangiectasia: Dilated lacteals and lymphatics in lamina propria; clubbed villi
C Eosinophilic enteritis: Diffuse or patchy eosinophilic infiltration in lamina propria and mucosa
D Amyloidosis: Presence of amyloid confirmed by special stains
E Regional enteritis: Noncaseating granulomas
F Parasitic infestations: Parasitic invasion of mucosa; adherence of trophozoites to mucosal surface, as in giardiasis
G Systemic mastocytosis: Mast cell infiltration of lamina propria

BIOPSY IS ABNORMAL BUT NOT DIAGNOSTIC

A Celiac sprue: Shortened or absent villi; hypertrophied crypts; damaged surface epithelium; mononuclear infiltrate
B "Collagenous" sprue: Indistinguishable from celiac sprue; extensive subepithelial collagen deposition
C Tropical sprue: Lesion similar to celiac sprue with shortened or absent villi; lymphocyte infiltration
D Folate deficiency: Shortened villi; megalocytosis; decreased mitoses in crypts
E Vitamin B_{12} deficiency: Similar to folate deficiency
F Acute radiation enteritis: Similar to folate deficiency
G Systemic scleroderma: Fibrosis around Brunner's glands
H Bacterial overgrowth syndromes: Patchy damage to villi and increased lymphocyte infiltration

FIGURE 254-4 Typical peroral intestinal biopsies. *A*. Jejunal mucosa of patient with celiac sprue. Note virtual absence of villi, elongated crypts (some cut in cross section), mononuclear infiltrate, cuboidal instead of columnar epithelium on top of villi (300×). *B*. Biopsy from the same patient as in *A*, after 9 months on a gluten-free diet. Note reappearance of villi with normal-appearing columnar cells and reduction in infiltrate and crypt height (300×). *C*. Biopsy from patient with agammaglobulinemia. The features bear a striking resemblance to those of celiac sprue. There is a marked mononuclear infiltration, some of it in aggregates (200×). *D*. Close-up of villi of patient with protein-losing enteropathy. Note broadened and dilated tips, and lymphatic spaces (*arrows*). (450×). *E*. Intestinal biopsy from patient with abetalipoproteinemia. The villus tips have a "lacy" appearance (*arrow*) due to retained fat (300×). *F*. High-power micrograph of villus in *E*. Vacuoles are filled with lipid (750×). Insert shows dark-staining (osmium) lipid droplets in mucosal cells (osmium counterstained with Giemsa; 800×).

TABLE 254-4 Pathophysiologic basis for symptoms and signs in malabsorptive disorders

Symptom or sign	Pathophysiology
GASTROINTESTINAL	
Generalized malnutrition and weight loss	Malabsorption of fat, carbohydrate, and protein → loss of calories
Diarrhea	Impaired absorption or increased secretion of water and electrolytes; unabsorbed dihydroxy bile acids and fatty acids → decreased absorption of water and electrolytes; excess load of fluid and electrolytes presented to the colon may exceed its absorptive capacity
Flatus	Bacterial fermentation of unabsorbed carbohydrate
Glossitis, cheilosis, stomatitis	Deficiency of iron, vitamin B_{12}, folate, and other vitamins
Abdominal pain	Distention or inflammation of bowel
GENITOURINARY	
Nocturia	Delayed absorption of water, hypokalemia
Azotemia, hypotension	Fluid and electrolyte depletion
Amenorrhea, ↓ libido	Protein depletion and "caloric starvation" → secondary hypopituitarism
HEMATOPOIETIC	
Anemia	Impaired absorption of iron, vitamin B_{12}, and folic acid
Hemorrhagic phenomena	Vitamin K malabsorption → hypoprothrombinemia
MUSCULOSKELETAL	
Bone pain	Protein depletion → impaired bone formation → osteoporosis Calcium malabsorption → demineralization of bone → osteomalacia
Osteoarthropathy	Cause uncertain
Tetany, paresthesias	Calcium malabsorption → hypocalcemia; magnesium malabsorption → hypomagnesemia
Weakness	Anemia: electrolyte depletion (hypokalemia)
NERVOUS SYSTEM	
Night blindness	Impaired absorption vitamin A → vitamin A deficiency
Xerophthalmia	Vitamin A deficiency
Peripheral neuropathy	Vitamin B_{12}, thiamine deficiency
SKIN	
Eczema	Cause uncertain
Purpura	Vitamin K deficiency
Follicular hyperkeratosis and dermatitis	Deficiency of vitamin A, zinc, essential fatty acids, and other vitamins

TABLE 254-5 Classification of the malabsorption syndromes

Inadequate digestion
  A Postgastrectomy steatorrhea*
  B Deficiency or inactivation of pancreatic lipase
    1 Exocrine pancreatic insufficiency
      a Chronic pancreatitis
      b Pancreatic carcinoma
      c Cystic fibrosis
      d Pancreatic resection
    2 Ulcerogenic tumor of the pancreas (Zollinger-Ellison syndrome, gastrinoma)*
Reduced intestinal bile salt concentration (with impaired micelle formation)
  A Liver disease
    1 Parenchymal liver disease
    2 Cholestasis (intrahepatic or extrahepatic)
  B Abnormal bacterial proliferation in the small bowel
    1 Afferent loop stasis
    2 Strictures
    3 Fistulas
    4 Blind loops
    5 Multiple diverticula of the small bowel
    6 Hypomotility states (diabetes, scleroderma, intestinal pseudoobstruction)
  C Interrupted enterohepatic circulation of bile salts
    1 Ileal resection
    2 Ileal inflammatory disease (regional ileitis)
  D Drugs (by sequestration or precipitation of bile salts)
    1 Neomycin
    2 Calcium carbonate
    3 Cholestyramine
Inadequate absorptive surface
  A Intestinal resection or bypass
    1 Mesenteric vascular disease with massive intestinal resection
    2 Regional enteritis with multiple bowel resections
    3 Jejunoileal bypass
  B Gastroileostomy (inadvertent)
Lymphatic obstruction
  A Intestinal lymphangiectasia
  B Whipple's disease
  C Lymphoma
Cardiovascular disorders
  A Constrictive pericarditis
  B Congestive heart failure
  C Mesenteric vascular insufficiency
  D Vasculitis
Primary mucosal absorptive defects
  A Inflammatory or infiltrative disorders
    1 Regional enteritis*
    2 Amyloidosis
    3 Scleroderma*
    4 Lymphoma*
    5 Radiation enteritis
    6 Eosinophilic enteritis
    7 Tropical sprue
    8 Infective enteritis (e.g., salmonellosis)
    9 Collagenous sprue
    10 Nonspecific ulcerative jejunitis
    11 Mastocytosis
    12 Dermatologic disorders (e.g., dermatitis herpetiformis)
  B Biochemical or genetic abnormalities
    1 Celiac sprue (gluten-induced enteropathy)
    2 Disaccharidase deficiency
    3 Hypogammaglobulinemia
    4 Abetalipoproteinemia
    5 Hartnup disease
    6 Cystinuria
    7 Monosaccharide malabsorption
Endocrine and metabolic disorders
  A Diabetes mellitus*
  B Hypoparathyroidism
  C Adrenal insufficiency
  D Hyperthyroidism
  E Ulcerogenic tumor of the pancreas (Zollinger-Ellison syndrome, gastrinoma)*
  F Carcinoid syndrome

* Malabsorption caused by multiple defects.

hepatic synthesis or excretion of conjugated bile salts, resulting in impaired formation of micellar lipid. In addition to steatorrhea, patients with liver disease may have impaired absorption of vitamin D and calcium, resulting in severe metabolic bone disease. This is particularly common in patients with primary biliary cirrhosis. Skeletal roentgenograms may show increased porosity of bone, cortical thinning, vertebral compression, and spontaneous pathologic fractures. Patients with alcohol-induced liver disease also may have exocrine pancreatic insufficiency. Accordingly, pancreatic function should be evaluated in patients with liver disease and malabsorption.

Postgastrectomy malabsorption The presence of a malabsorption syndrome has been documented frequently in patients after subtotal gastrectomy. Steatorrhea is more common with a Billroth II than a Billroth I type of anastomosis. Usually the fat loss is minimal, ranging from 7 to 10 g per 24 h. Patients with gross steatorrhea usually have impaired intraluminal fat digestion due to several factors: (1) With a Billroth II anastomosis the duodenum is bypassed, and there is a decreased entry of stomach contents into the proximal duodenum (i.e., afferent loop). This leads to a decreased stimulus for the release of *secretin* and *cholecystokinin-pancreozymin* from the duodenum and may result in a depressed pancreatic enzyme response. (2) There may be *inadequate mixing* of the pancreatic enzymes and bile salts secreted into the proximal duodenum with the gastric contents entering the jejunum. (3) There may be *stasis* of intestinal contents in the afferent loop, resulting in abnormal bacterial proliferation in the proximal small bowel. This in turn may lead to abnormalities in bile salt metabolism (see "Malabsorption Due to Bacterial Overgrowth of the Small Bowel, Pathophysiology," below). (4) The presence of maldigestion may lead to *protein depletion*, which in turn may produce further impairment in pancreatic function. (5) The *loss of the reservoir function of the stomach* may result in decreased intestinal transit time. Perhaps the most important factor is rapid gastric emptying, which results in low luminal concentrations of digestive secretions for the first 60 to 80 min after a meal. Such a disorder has been described in patients with subtotal gastrectomy and duodenostomy (Billroth I), gastrojejunostomy (Billroth II), and truncal vagotomy and pyloroplasty (V&P). That gastric emptying rates are somewhat slower in patients with V&P may account for the overall less severe nutritional deficiencies in such patients. In some patients, treatment with pancreatic enzymes may lead to significant improvement. Specimens of duodenal or jejunal fluid should be obtained for culture of both aerobic and anaerobic organisms and appropriate antibiotic therapy instituted if there is evidence of abnormal bacterial overgrowth (colony count of greater than 10^7 per milliliter of jejunal fluid). Because the duodenum is the principal site of absorption of iron and calcium, in patients with a Billroth II anastomosis, impaired absorption of calcium and iron also may develop. Occult metabolic bone disease occurs frequently in this setting.

INADEQUATE ABSORPTIVE SURFACE (SHORT BOWEL SYNDROME)

Extensive intestinal resection often results in the short bowel syndrome. The most common disorders resulting in short bowel syndrome are (1) massive intestinal resection following a vascular insult to the small intestine, (2) regional enteritis with multiple bowel resections, and (3) jejunoileal bypass for morbid obesity. In general, the absorption of nutrients will be influenced by the extent and site of small bowel resected, the presence of the ileocecal valve, and adaptation of the remaining small bowel. Resection of 40 to 50 percent of the small bowel is usually well tolerated, provided the proximal duodenum, the distal half of the ileum, and the ileocecal valve are spared. By contrast, resection of the ileum and the ileocecal valve alone may induce severe diarrhea and malabsorption, even though less than 30 percent of the small intestine is resected.

Several measures are important in the management of short bowel syndrome: (1) The diet should contain at least 2500 kcal and consist primarily of carbohydrate and protein, with fat restricted to less than 40 g/d. A fat-restricted diet is effective in reducing diarrhea, presumably because there is decreased production of hydroxy fatty acids from long-chain fats. Such hydroxy fatty acids, in essence, are cathartics and increase net secretion of water and electrolytes by the colon as well as the small bowel. (2) It is often necessary to provide vitamin and mineral supplements, which usually include K^+, Cl^-, Mg^{2+}, Ca^{2+}, trace metals (Zn, Cd, Mn), iron, folate, vitamin B_{12}, other vitamins (A, D, E, K, B_1, B_2, B_6, biotin), and essential fatty acids. (3) Specific drugs (e.g., belladonna alkaloids, diphenoxylate, loperamide, and codeine) which decrease intestinal motility and prolong mucosal contact time are helpful in controlling diarrhea. These agents also decrease ileostomy outputs. (4) A bile salt–sequestering agent such as cholestyramine blunts the effects of bile salts, which stimulate net secretion of water and electrolytes by the colon. (5) Patients with short bowel syndrome may have gastric acid hypersecretion which is often transient and which results in dilution of pancreatic secretions as well as inactivation of pancreatic enzymes. Under these conditions, a histamine H-2 receptor antagonist is useful because it will suppress gastric acid secretion and decrease the volume of fluid entering the proximal small bowel, thus leading to an increased

concentration of pancreatic enzymes. In addition, supplemental pancreatic enzyme therapy may be required. (6) A bypassed colon can be used to receive infusions of fluid and electrolytes, since a portion of the colon can still absorb 1000 to 1500 mL fluid per day. (7) Octreotide, the long-acting somatostatin analogue, reduces digestive secretions (biliary, pancreatic, succus entericus) and thus may ameliorate diarrhea. Finally, (8) total parenteral nutrition is frequently required during the first 6 months after massive intestinal resection until some degree of adaptation has occurred. Such patients also may require long-term parenteral hyperalimentation with a silicone rubber catheter in the superior vena cava, and this can be done at home.

For a discussion of regional enteritis see Chap. 255.

MALABSORPTION DUE TO BACTERIAL OVERGROWTH OF THE SMALL BOWEL

The proximal small intestine is usually bacteriologically sterile because of three factors: (1) the acid milieu of the stomach, (2) intestinal peristalsis, which sweeps bacteria to the distal small bowel, and (3) secretion into the lumen of the intestine of immunoglobulins, which may serve as coproantibodies. When bacteria are isolated from the upper small bowel, they are frequently contaminants transported from the mouth and upper respiratory tract, and the colony count rarely exceeds 10^4 per milliliter of jejunal fluid. The major mechanism limiting the growth of bacteria in the small intestine is normal peristalsis. Any disorder leading to impaired intestinal motility may result in abnormal stasis of intestinal contents with ineffective mechanical cleansing of bacteria. This, in turn, may lead to abnormal bacterial proliferation and malabsorption. Several malabsorptive disorders have been associated with bacterial overgrowth of the small bowel, and these are listed in Table 254-6.

Pathophysiology Bacterial overgrowth may result in changes in bile salt metabolism, and these are believed directly and indirectly to account for the steatorrhea. First, bacteria (especially anaerobic gram-positive bacteria) may lead to the intraluminal deconjugation of bile salts with a consequent production of free bile acids. In contrast to conjugated bile salts, unconjugated bile salts may be absorbed in the proximal small bowel by nonionic diffusion, resulting in decreased intraluminal concentrations of bile salts in the jejunum. Second, the decreased bile salt concentrations, the increase of unconjugated bile salts, and the decrease of the conjugated salts all serve to contribute to impaired intraluminal micelle formation and hence fat malabsorption. In addition to abnormalities in bile salt metabolism, intestinal

---

TABLE 254-6   Causes of intestinal bacterial overgrowth (intestinal colonization)

Structural abnormalities producing stasis of intestinal contents
  A Multiple small-bowel diverticula
  B Strictures
    1 Regional enteritis*
    2 Radiation enteritis*
    3 Occlusive vascular disease: vasculitis
  C Billroth II subtotal gastrectomy with afferent loop stasis*
  D Multiple laparotomies resulting in adhesions and partial small-bowel obstruction
Fistulas
  A Gastrocolic, gastroileal, jejunoileal, jejunocolic
Motor abnormalities resulting in intestinal hypomotility
  A Scleroderma*
  B Amyloidosis*
  C Diabetes mellitus*
  D Hypothyroidism
  E Vagotomy
  F Intestinal pseudoobstruction (see Table 254-7)
Miscellaneous
  A Hypogammaglobulinemia*
  B Nodular lymphoid hyperplasia
  C Pancreatic insufficiency
  D Gastric hypochlorhydria/achlorhydria
    1 Subtotal gastrectomy
    2 Pernicious anemia
    3 Prolonged use of H-2 receptor antagonists

* No underlying disorder detected.

mucosal lesions have been demonstrated in patients with intestinal stasis. Such lesions are often patchy in distribution, and the histologic appearance ranges in severity from minimal changes in villous architecture to severe lesions with virtual absence of villi. The cause of these lesions is unclear; possible causes include damage caused by bacterial invasion, bacterial toxins, or metabolic products such as unconjugated bile salts. In this regard, certain bacteria such as *Bacteroides* elaborate proteases which solubilize brush border proteins and destroy disaccharidases such as sucrase and maltase. The impaired absorption of vitamin B_{12} is not related to the disturbed bile salt metabolism but appears to be due to uptake of vitamin B_{12} by microorganisms.

Many of the preceding abnormalities in bile salt metabolism may be reversed by appropriate antibiotic therapy. When such treatment is instituted, unconjugated bile salts in the jejunal fluid decrease, an increase in the micellar lipid phase occurs, and steatorrhea diminishes or disappears. In addition, significant improvement in the absorption of vitamin B_{12} occurs with broad-spectrum antibiotics such as tetracycline.

Clinical manifestations   Breath tests, i.e., tests with ^{14}C-labeled bile acid, [^{14}C]xylose, and lactulose, are useful screening tests for malabsorption syndrome due to abnormal bacterial overgrowth of the small intestine. The 2-h 50-g glucose breath hydrogen test reliably predicts the presence of bacterial overgrowth; a positive test is characterized by a rise in breath hydrogen of at least 12 parts per million (ppm) within 2 h of a 50-g glucose challenge *and* a high fasting breath hydrogen level of at least 15 ppm. A definitive diagnosis is established by demonstrating larger numbers of microorganisms (greater than 10^5 per milliliter) and a polymicrobial flora in cultures of duodenal or jejunal fluid. Other clinical features include the following: (1) steatorrhea of a moderate degree, usually in the range of 15 to 30 g fecal fat per 24 h, (2) macrocytic anemia with a megaloblastic bone marrow, (3) impaired absorption of vitamin B_{12} which is not corrected by intrinsic factor, and (4) correction of steatorrhea and impaired vitamin B_{12} absorption by antibiotic therapy. Absorption of D-xylose, peroral small-intestinal biopsy specimens, and other tests of absorptive function (see Table 254-2) may be normal in these patients. A single course or intermittent courses (2 to 3 weeks per month) of therapy with antibiotics such as tetracycline, ampicillin, metronidazole, or trimethoprim-sulfamethoxazole are usually given.

Chronic intestinal pseudoobstruction   (See also Chap. 257) Chronic intestinal pseudoobstruction is a heterogeneous syndrome with a variety of causes (Table 254-7). Primary or idiopathic intestinal

---

TABLE 254-7 Causes of chronic intestinal pseudoobstruction

PRIMARY: IDIOPATHIC

A Visceral myopathy
B Visceral neuropathy

SECONDARY

A Collagen vascular disease
 1 Scleroderma
 2 Dermatomyositis/polymyositis
 3 Systemic lupus erythematosus
B Amyloidosis
C Endocrine disorders
 1 Hypothyroidism
 2 Diabetes mellitus
D Neurologic diseases
 1 Chagas' disease
E Paraneoplastic visceral neuropathy
 1 Small cell lung carcinoma
F Drugs
 1 Chronic narcotic use (narcotic bowel syndrome)
 2 Tricyclic antidepressants
G Miscellaneous
 1 Jejunal diverticulosis
 2 Jejunoileal bypass

---

pseudoobstruction is a chronic illness characterized by recurrent episodes of intestinal obstruction in which all known causes of mechanical obstruction and other illnesses known to produce intestinal pseudoobstruction have been excluded. In addition to abnormalities in small-bowel motility, derangements in esophageal, gastric, and colonic motility also have been described. The primary clinical manifestations are nausea and vomiting, abdominal pain, distention, constipation, diarrhea, and urinary tract symptoms. Patients typically exhibit prolonged transit of chyme along the gastrointestinal tract, especially the small bowel, where pressure activity patterns are markedly disordered. Oral cisapride accelerates gastric emptying, normalizes intestinal transit, and improves propulsive small-bowel activity in patients with pseudoobstruction. Octreotide also may prove to be useful. Malabsorption secondary to stasis of intestinal contents with resultant abnormal bacterial proliferation in the small bowel is frequently present.

Tropical sprue   Tropical sprue is a malabsorptive disorder of unknown cause affecting residents of or visitors to tropical regions. Both epidemic and endemic forms of the disease have been recognized. Tropical sprue may have its onset months or even years after a patient has returned from the tropics. The etiology of the disorder has not been elucidated, but it might well result from one or more of the following: (1) a nutritional deficiency, (2) a transmissible infectious microorganism, and (3) a toxin elaborated by a microorganism or contained in the diet. It is of interest that coliform organisms, shown to produce an enterotoxin causing fluid secretion, have been isolated from the jejunum of tropical sprue patients but not from other patients with bacterial overgrowth of the proximal small bowel. Anorexia, diarrhea, weight loss, symptoms of anemia, sequelae of nutritional deficiency (see Table 254-4), and abdominal distention are common findings. Patients are frequently deficient in iron as well as vitamin B_{12} and folate. Laboratory studies usually reveal anemia (megaloblastic in 60 percent of cases) and impaired absorption of fat, xylose, and vitamin B_{12}. Malabsorption of at least two nutrients is considered essential for the diagnosis. Jejunal biopsy classically reveals shortened and thickened villi, increased crypt depth, and increased infiltration of mononuclear cells in the lamina propria and epithelium (see Table 254-3). However, these biopsy findings are not specific, and the lesion may be patchy; in addition, interpretation is difficult because "control" biopsies from asymptomatic residents in the same tropical region are often considered abnormal when compared with normal biopsies from patients in temperate zones. Such histologic findings have been termed *tropical jejunitis*. Treatment with vitamin B_{12}, folate, and antibiotics have all been effective in inducing a remission. A short course, i.e., 2 to 4 weeks, of combined therapy with a sulfonamide or tetracycline and folic acid is usually given. Occasional patients require more prolonged antibiotic therapy.

Scleroderma   Although there are numerous reports of small-intestinal involvement in scleroderma, frank malabsorption has been reported in only one-third of patients. Malabsorption is due to two key factors: (1) impaired intestinal motility and jejunal pseudodiverticulosis leading to relative stasis of intestinal contents and hence bacterial overgrowth and (2) involvement of the intestinal wall by the disease. In some cases, abnormal bacterial proliferation in the upper small bowel can be documented, and in these patients antibiotic therapy may result in decreased steatorrhea, gain in weight, and increased absorption of vitamin B_{12}. In the intestinal wall there also may be extensive deposition of collagen, especially in the muscular mucosa, submucosa, and muscularis externa, with significant muscle atrophy. Studies of duodenal myoelectric activity in scleroderma revealed absence of migrating motor complexes in the basal state and decreased excitability of the bowel to mechanical stimuli such as distention and humoral stimuli such as pentagastrin and secretin. This motor dysfunction is an important factor in the dilatation, atony, and stasis of intestinal contents in scleroderma. Therapy with the somatostatin analogue octreotide has stimulated intestinal motility, reduced bacterial overgrowth, and ameliorated obstructive gut symptoms.

Malabsorption in AIDS Diarrhea and weight loss occur frequently in patients with AIDS. These symptoms are often due to enteric infections or small-intestinal Kaposi's sarcoma. The jejunal mucosa is often abnormal in patients infected with HIV, and such abnormalities can be masked by an opportunistic infection. However, such symptoms can be due to malabsorption, which has been well documented in patients with AIDS in whom identifiable enteric infections and intestinal involvement with Kaposi's sarcoma have been excluded. The presence of malabsorption in these patients has been documented by steatorrhea and abnormal D-xylose absorption tests. Serum zinc levels may be decreased. In addition, small-bowel biopsy specimens have revealed dense infiltration of mononuclear cells and histiocytes. Microorganisms also have been identified in the mucosa.

DISORDERS ASSOCIATED WITH LYMPHATIC OBSTRUCTION

Whipple's disease This is a rare disorder characterized clinically by arthralgia, abdominal pain, diarrhea, progressive weight loss, dilated lacteals in the bowel wall, and impaired intestinal absorption. Wasting, low-grade fever, increased skin pigmentation, and peripheral lymphadenopathy are frequently present. In addition, central nervous system manifestations, including confusion, memory loss, focal cranial nerve signs, nystagmus, and ophthalmoplegia, may be present. Laboratory examination usually reveals the presence of steatorrhea, impaired xylose absorption, abnormal small-bowel x-rays, hypoalbuminemia, and anemia. Hypoalbuminemia is due to excessive loss of serum albumin into the gastrointestinal tract as well as impaired synthesis of albumin.

The diagnosis is established by demonstrating the presence in the mucosa of macrophages containing large cytoplasmic granules which give a brilliant magenta stain with the periodic acid Schiff reagent (PAS). Such macrophages also may be seen in other tissues such as lymph nodes, spleen, or liver. The finding of PAS-positive macrophages in the lamina propria is not specific for Whipple's disease, but virtual replacement of most cellular elements in the lamina propria by these macrophages has been seen only in this disorder. In addition to the PAS-positive macrophages, jejunal biopsies frequently show dilated lymphatics and some degree of blunting of the intestinal mucosal villi.

Electron-microscopic studies have revealed the presence of rod-shaped structures (or bacilliform bodies) 0.3 by 1.5 to 2.5 μm within and adjacent to the macrophages in the lamina propria as well as within epithelial cells and polymorphonuclear leukocytes. The bacterium has not been cultured but has been identified as a gram-negative actinomycete with distinct morphologic characteristics and thus named *Tropheryma whippelii*. It is of particular interest that after treatment of the patient with antibiotics the bacilliform bodies decrease or disappear together with a decrease in the number of PAS-positive macrophages. In addition, the reappearance of the bacteria often heralds the onset of a clinical relapse after antibiotics have been withdrawn.

Whipple's disease at one time was thought to be invariably fatal. However, it is now clear that therapy with antibiotics will usually induce a clinical remission. In a few cases there has been complete reversal of the histologic abnormalities in the jejunal mucosa, and some of these cases have been followed for more than 10 years. Patients with Whipple's disease should be treated with antibiotics such as trimethoprim-sulfamethoxazole for at least 1 year. Treatment with tetracycline alone or penicillin alone is not adequate initial therapy; relapse rates with these drugs are approximately 40 percent. The most important parameter for following the disease and predicting its course is the presence or absence of bacilli in sections of small-bowel biopsies.

Intestinal lymphoma Steatorrhea is a manifestation of *primary* intestinal lymphoma. The disease occurs predominantly in men, and the mean age of onset of symptoms is about 50 years. The diagnosis should be suspected in patients with malabsorption with the following findings: (1) a malabsorption syndrome in which clinical and biopsy features resemble those of celiac sprue but in which there is an incomplete response to a gluten-free diet, (2) the presence of

abdominal pain and *fever*, and (3) signs and symptoms of intestinal obstruction. The usual stigmata of generalized lymphoma are frequently absent. Hepatomegaly, splenomegaly, palpable abdominal masses, and peripheral adenopathy are usually not found. Lymphangiography and CT scanning may reveal abnormal intraabdominal nodes. The diagnosis can be established by laparotomy and often may be made by thorough examination of multiple mucosal biopsy specimens obtained perorally. There may be a total absence of villi or lesser degrees of blunting and shortening of the villi. In contrast to celiac sprue, the lamina propria is usually massively infiltrated with lymphoid cells. Malignancy may be diagnosed by demonstrating lymphoid cells with the cytologic features of malignancy, the presence of reticulum cells outside germinal centers, and infiltration and destruction of crypts by pleomorphic lymphoid cells. Some patients elaborate or secrete a fragment of the heavy chain of IgA immunoglobulins (α-*chain disease*). The latter is probably a variant of intestinal lymphoma.

The mechanism of malabsorption in intestinal lymphoma may be related to several factors: (1) diffuse involvement of the small-intestinal mucosa, (2) involvement of the bowel wall with lymphatic obstruction, and (3) localized stenosis with stasis of intestinal contents and bacterial overgrowth. It should be emphasized that it is often difficult, by clinical and morphologic features alone, to distinguish celiac sprue from intestinal lymphoma. Indeed, there is evidence to suggest that lymphoma may develop as a late complication of celiac sprue.

The course of intestinal lymphoma has ranged from 4 months to 4 years from the onset of symptoms. Perforation, bleeding, and intestinal obstruction are common terminal complications. There is insufficient evidence to determine whether radiation therapy, chemotherapy, or localized surgical resection modifies the natural course of the disease.

CARDIOVASCULAR DISORDERS
Steatorrhea has been described in patients with chronic congestive heart failure, superior mesenteric artery insufficiency, and constrictive pericarditis. Abnormal dilated mucosal lymphatics and excessive enteric loss of protein have been demonstrated in patients with constrictive pericarditis. The mechanism of steatorrhea in patients with chronic heart failure remains uncertain. It might be due to congestion and edema of the mucosa, mucosal hypoxia, or abnormalities in pancreatic function. Although pronounced steatorrhea is uncommon in congestive heart failure, these patients are frequently anorectic, and a low fat intake could mask a latent steatorrhea. Steatorrhea is quite infrequent in patients with vasculitis and is thought to be due to segmental infarction of the small bowel in addition to intestinal ischemia.

DEFECTS IN MUCOSAL FUNCTION

INFLAMMATORY OR INFILTRATIVE DISORDERS
Regional enteritis The clinical features of regional enteritis are described in Chap. 255. Malabsorption in regional enteritis may result from several factors: (1) interruption of the enterohepatic circulation of bile salts by ileal disease or resection, (2) deconjugation of bile salts due to bacterial overgrowth, in turn related to strictures and/or fistulas, (3) active inflammatory bowel disease causing impaired mucosal cell function, (4) inadequate absorptive surface resulting from intestinal resection or fistulas, and (5) severe protein depletion producing impaired exocrine pancreatic function. Active ileal disease and/or ileal resection resulting in an interrupted enterohepatic circulation of and deficiency of conjugated bile salts appears to be the major factor responsible for steatorrhea as well as impaired absorption of vitamin B_{12}. Small-bowel absorptive function has been correlated with the extent of ileal disease or resection. When the length of ileal dysfunction exceeds 90 to 100 cm, virtually all patients will have steatorrhea and vitamin B_{12} malabsorption. After intestinal resection, the functional capacity of the remaining small bowel will depend on the site and extent of resection as well as the presence of residual inflammatory disease. Massive intestinal resection usually results in impaired

absorption of all food constituents. When the malabsorption is due to strictures and blind loops as a result of previous surgical therapy, antibiotic therapy may be helpful, but surgical removal of these areas is usually necessary for long-term improvement. With diffuse inflammatory disease, a florid malabsorption syndrome may occur with steatorrhea, hypocalcemia, impaired vitamin B$_{12}$ absorption, and hypoalbuminemia due to increased enteric protein loss. Treatment with sulfasalazine, glucocorticoids, and other immunosuppressive drugs may be beneficial (see Chap. 255).

After *ileal resection*, patients frequently have bothersome diarrhea. This appears to be due to *interruption of the enterohepatic circulation* whereby increased amounts of bile salts reach the colon, where they interfere with water and electrolyte absorption and thus have a cathartic effect. The *bile salt–induced diarrhea* after ileal resection may respond to treatment with cholestyramine, an exchange resin which binds bile salts and causes them to lose their biochemical effect on the bowel. Patients with ileal resection of less than 100 cm and fecal fat excretion less than 20 g/d show the best symptomatic response to cholestyramine, usually at a dose of 4 g tid.

Chronic nongranulomatous ulcerative jejunoileitis This disorder is characterized by abdominal pain, weight loss, fever, diarrhea, steatorrhea, hypoalbuminemia, and protein-losing enteropathy. Clinical features mimic those found in both regional enteritis and celiac sprue. Indeed, the intestinal lesion may be indistinguishable from celiac sprue. However, exclusion of gluten from the diet does not result in any benefit. Glucocorticoid treatment has resulted in transient improvement, but long-term effects are unpredictable.

Amyloidosis This disorder is discussed in detail in Chap. 281.

Radiation injury to the small bowel Extensive morphologic damage of the small-intestinal mucosa often follows normal or excessive abdominal irradiation. These changes include a decrease in crypt mitoses, marked shortening of the villi, megalocytosis of epithelial cells, and inflammatory cell infiltration of the lamina propria. This may be associated with transient diarrhea and impaired intestinal absorption. However, restoration of normal intestinal architecture is usually complete within 2 weeks after cessation of therapy. Persistent diarrhea and malabsorption may develop shortly after x-ray therapy, or there may be a latent period of several years before the onset of diarrhea. Steatorrhea, ranging from 10 to 40 g/d, has been observed frequently, but impaired absorption of calcium, iron, D-xylose, or vitamin B$_{12}$ is less common. In some patients, intestinal strictures due to vasculopathy and ischemia may develop following irradiation, and thus stasis of intestinal contents and abnormal bacterial proliferation may occur. In others, intestinal lymphangiectasia, presumably due to lymphatic obstruction, has been documented. Diarrhea and malabsorption may be refractory to all methods of management. Treatment with antibiotics, pancreatic enzymes, gluten-free diet, adrenal glucocorticoids, and opiates has met with but limited success.

Eosinophilic enteritis Eosinophilic gastroenteritis is a disorder of the stomach, small bowel, and colon of unknown etiology characterized by peripheral blood eosinophilia and eosinophilic infiltration of the gut wall but without evidence of vasculitis. The clinical manifestations, usually recurrent, are protean and relate to the site of gastrointestinal tract involvement. Three main patterns have been identified: (1) Predominant mucosal disease manifested by iron-deficiency anemia, hypoalbuminemia due to protein-losing enteropathy, and mild steatorrhea. Patients in this group often present with a malabsorption syndrome and a history of intolerance to specific foods. (2) Predominant muscle layer disease characterized by marked thickening and rigidity of the stomach and proximal small bowel with obstructive symptoms and radiologic features of pyloric narrowing and obstruction. The obstructive form of eosinophilic gastroenteritis accounts for half the cases reported since 1970. Accordingly, eosinophilic enteritis should be considered in the differential diagnosis of gastric outlet obstruction, diffuse small-bowel disease, and ileocolitis. Indeed, eosinophilic enteritis often mimics regional enteritis. (3) Predominant subserosal disease in which the cardinal manifestation is ascites with marked eosinophilia in the ascitic fluid. Although the

preceding classification based on tissue layer of major involvement is useful in understanding the principal manifestations, it should be emphasized that multiple clinical forms, e.g., ascites (serosal involvement) and obstruction (muscular involvement), also occur.

Previous reports have emphasized food allergy and mucosal features of this disease. However, food sensitivity is related to symptoms in less than 20 percent of patients. In such patients, fasting serum IgE levels are often elevated, and challenge with offending foods frequently evokes symptoms of abdominal pain and diarrhea in addition to a marked increase in serum IgE levels. In most patients with eosinophilic enteritis, however, immunologic studies, including serum immunoglobulins, serum complement, lymphocyte quantitation, and lymphocyte response to nonspecific mitogens, reveal no abnormalities. Thus both IgE-mediated and IgE-dependent mechanisms may be operative in different patients with eosinophilic gastroenteritis. Several nonreaginic factors influence peripheral blood and tissue eosinophilia. It seems clear that evidence of allergy or food sensitivity is often absent and is not required for the diagnosis of eosinophilic enteritis. In addition, even in patients with food allergies, elimination diets are frequently ineffective, and such patients may require prolonged glucocorticoid therapy to remain well. Surgical treatment for relief of obstructive symptoms and glucocorticoids are the mainstays of therapy.

Dermatitis and malabsorption A malabsorption syndrome, usually mild, has been reported in patients with a variety of dermatologic disorders, including psoriasis, eczematoid dermatitis, and dermatitis herpetiformis. Proximal intestinal mucosal abnormalities are almost invariably found in patients with dermatitis herpetiformis. In one study, 21 of 22 patients had lesions ranging in severity from a completely "flat" to an almost normal intestinal mucosa. The mucosal lesions were often patchy in distribution. Clinical and laboratory evidence of significant malabsorption was infrequent, possibly due to the limited length of small intestine involved in this skin disorder. While the skin lesions of dermatitis herpetiformis respond to sulfone, the gut lesions do not. By contrast, in some patients with blunted and flattened intestinal mucosal lesions and steatorrhea, there may be a striking improvement in villous architecture and regression of steatorrhea after withdrawal of gluten from the diet without improvement in the skin lesions. Further, in patients with dermatitis herpetiformis and a morphologically normal small-intestinal mucosa, administration of a high-gluten diet may result in blunted and flattened mucosal lesions indistinguishable from those of celiac sprue. As in the latter disease, an increased frequency of HLA-A1 and HLA-B8 is also seen. These observations raise the interesting question as to whether certain patients with dermatitis herpetiformis and a malabsorption syndrome have latent celiac sprue.

BIOCHEMICAL OR GENETIC ABNORMALITIES   Celiac sprue
Celiac sprue is a disorder characterized by malabsorption, abnormal small-bowel structure, and intolerance to gluten, a protein found in wheat and wheat products. It has been appropriately referred to as *gluten-induced enteropathy*. Celiac disease in children and celiac sprue in adults are probably one and the same disorder with the same pathogenesis.

There are insufficient data to provide an accurate estimation of the incidence of celiac sprue in any population. This is largely because the severity of the disease varies greatly, and individuals may have typical mucosal change and yet have no overt symptoms. Seventy percent of the cases in most reported series are women. The incidence in siblings appears to be many times higher than that in the general population, and it has been suggested that sprue may be inherited through a dominant gene of incomplete penetrance. Celiac sprue patients have an increased frequency of serum histocompatibility antigens, particularly of the HLA-DR3 and HLA-DQw2 types. The HLA-DR3 phenotype has been found in 70 to 90 percent of sprue patients as compared with 20 to 25 percent in normal subjects. The HLA antigens may be linked to immune response genes which may determine the immunologic recognition of certain substances (see Chap. 64). It has been suggested that such genetic factors may predispose to immunologic tolerance of dietary proteins such as the peptides in gluten or to the production of pathogenic antigluten antibodies which could result in binding of gluten to epithelial cells with subsequent tissue damage. The discordance for celiac sprue among HLA-identical siblings and some identical twins raises the question of whether an additional susceptibility gene (or genes) not yet identified is required for the development of celiac sprue.

PATHOPHYSIOLOGY Gluten and the related substance gliadin are high-molecular-weight proteins found especially in wheat. The alcohol-soluble fraction of gluten consists of glutamine-rich gliadin polypeptides, which can be fractionated into γ, β, δ, and α subgroups; peptides from all four gliadin subgroups are toxic and induce the intestinal lesion when administered to celiac sprue patients in remission. The exact mechanism for this effect is not clear, but two theories have been proposed, namely, a "toxic" and an immunologic theory. One possible mechanism is that patients with celiac sprue lack a specific mucosal peptidase so that gluten or its larger glutamine-containing peptides are not effectively hydrolyzed to smaller peptides (i.e., dipeptides or amino acids). As a consequence, "toxic" peptides might accumulate in the mucosa. It has been demonstrated that patients with celiac sprue in remission will develop steatorrhea and typical mucosal changes when they are given gluten. Similar results will occur with the administration of peptide hydrolysates containing at least eight amino acids with a terminal glutamine residue. It has been shown that when gluten is instilled into the *ileum* of celiac sprue patients, histologic changes begin to occur within hours. This does not occur in the *upper jejunum*, suggesting that the effect is immediate and local rather than systemic. After noxious gluten fractions damage surface absorptive cells, the damaged cells are sloughed rapidly from the mucosal surface into the gut lumen. To compensate for this, cell proliferation increases, crypts undergo hypertrophy, and cell migration accelerates to replace the damaged and sloughed epithelial cells. This more rapid than normal epithelial cell renewal can be reversed by a gluten-free diet. The intestinal mucosa of patients with celiac sprue shows many enzyme alterations, including decreased levels of disaccharidases, alkaline phosphatase, and peptide hydrolases, as well as impaired ability to digest gluten peptides. However, these abnormalities usually revert toward normal after successful treatment with a gluten-free diet. There is additional evidence supporting the concept of toxicity of gluten and gluten breakdown products in celiac sprue. First, gliadin, especially the A-gliadin moiety, is toxic to sprue mucosa maintained in organ culture, causing ultrastructural changes and depression of disaccharidase activity. Second, sprue mucosa hydrolyzes a specific fraction of a gliadin digest (i.e., fraction 9) in a defective manner, and fraction 9 is selectively toxic to sprue mucosa. Third, specific fractions of gluten fed to celiac sprue patients cause transient alterations in mucosal histology and depression of disaccharidase activity, but full recovery is observed in 72 h. The rapid onset of these changes and prompt recovery are consistent with a direct toxic effect. Despite intensive study, however, no persistent, specific, or selective peptidase or other enzyme deficiency has been demonstrated.

It also has been suggested that gluten or gluten metabolites may initiate an *immunologic reaction* in the intestinal mucosa. Alternatively, the interaction of T lymphocytes with crypt epithelium may be a primary event in the pathogenesis of the intestinal lesion. The presence of a mononuclear inflammatory cell infiltrate in the lamina propria of the mucosa, the beneficial response to glucocorticoid drugs, the finding of abnormal antibodies to gliadin in the serum of celiac sprue patients, the synthesis of increased amounts of antigliadin antibody by sprue mucosa maintained in organ culture, and the elaboration of lymphokines such as migration inhibitory factor (MIF) by sprue mucosa incubated with gliadin have all been cited as evidence in support of this hypothesis. However, there is still no definitive evidence indicating that an abnormal (immune) mechanism is important in initiating or perpetuating this disease process.

A possible role for adenovirus serotype 12 (Ad12) in the pathogenesis of celiac sprue has been proposed based on two observations: (1) homology of amino acid sequences between a portion of A-gliadin and a viral-encoded protein (E16) produced by Ad12, and (2) patients with untreated celiac sprue have a much higher frequency of antibodies to Ad12 compared with treated celiac sprue patients and controls. Other studies, however, have not demonstrated a strikingly higher prevalence of previous infection with type 12 adenovirus among a cohort of celiac sprue patients compared with persons without the disease. Nonetheless, these observations are in accord with the hypothesis that there must be an *environmental* factor as well as a *genetic predisposition* to explain why only certain people develop celiac sprue. Despite intensive studies, there is not yet enough information to integrate the distinctive dietary, immunologic, and genetic features of celiac sprue into a clear understanding of the pathogenesis of the disease.

Jejunal biopsy specimens from patients with celiac sprue usually show a characteristic lesion. There is blunting and flattening of the mucosal surface, with villi either absent or broad and short. The crypts are elongated, and there is generally a dense infiltration of inflammatory cells in the lamina propria. The surface epithelium is altered with a sparse brush border, cuboidal rather than the normal columnar cells, and infiltration of inflammatory cells in the epithelial layer. These changes are usually most severe in the proximal small bowel, presumably because this area of the bowel is exposed to the highest gluten concentration. The typical morphologic changes illustrated in Fig. 254-4 are characteristic of celiac sprue but are not specific. Similar changes have been described in other conditions, including lymphoma, tropical sprue, and hypogammaglobulinemia associated with malabsorption. Many biochemical abnormalities have been demonstrated in mucosal biopsy specimens from celiac sprue patients. Impaired esterification of fatty acids to triglycerides, decreased uptake of amino acids, and decreased activity of intestinal disaccharidases (especially lactase) have been well documented. The latter observation may account for the high incidence of milk intolerance in untreated celiac sprue patients or those in relapse. However, the greater abundance of undifferentiated crypt cells may be important, since crypt cells normally have a lower capacity for nutrient uptake than do villus cells.

Since the mucosa is damaged and altered in patients with celiac sprue, there may be *decreased release of pancreatotropic hormones* (secretin and cholecystokinin, i.e., CCK). This results in decreased stimulation of the pancreas with lower than normal intraluminal levels of pancreatic enzymes in response to a meal. In addition, the gallbladder appears to be resistant to the action of cholecystokinin, resulting in absent or minimal contractions of the gallbladder, in turn leading to sequestration of bile salts in an inert gallbladder. These two defects may result in impaired intraluminal digestion of fat and protein, which will be superimposed on the defect in intestinal transport caused by a damaged mucosa.

Diarrhea is common in celiac sprue patients and is due to a number of factors, including *impaired absorption* of salt and water by duodenum and jejunum, net *secretion* of water and electrolytes by an abnormally permeable jejunal mucosa, and net colonic secretion of water and electrolytes induced by unabsorbed fatty acids and hydroxy fatty acids. However, the distal small intestine in celiac sprue has the ability to adapt to the damage and loss of absorptive capacity in the proximal small intestine. Indeed, increased ileal absorption of sodium, chloride, and water has been demonstrated in celiac sprue patients.

CLINICAL FEATURES Most patients with celiac sprue will have a typical malabsorption syndrome characterized by weight loss, abdominal distention and bloating, diarrhea, steatorrhea, and abnormal tests of absorptive function. The characteristic alterations in tests of intestinal absorption are outlined in Table 254-2. It should be emphasized, however, that some sprue patients may present with isolated abnormalities which initially do not suggest the diagnosis of celiac sprue. Thus a patient may be admitted for investigation of iron-deficiency anemia without apparent blood loss or of abnormal bleeding due to hypoprothrombinemia but may not have diarrhea or overt steatorrhea. Likewise, sprue patients may present with puzzling these patients when treated with the antiserotonin drug methysergide. Although side effects may occur, for control of diarrhea and steatorrhea, patients may be given a trial of 8 to 12 mg methysergide per day.

PROTEIN-LOSING ENTEROPATHY The gastrointestinal tract has been shown to play a significant role in the metabolism and physiologic degradation of plasma proteins. The exact magnitude of the normal gastrointestinal protein loss in human beings has remained unclear, but studies with labeled albumin have suggested that between 10 and 20 percent of the normal turnover of albumin may be accounted for by enteric protein loss. However, under certain pathologic conditions, excessive gastrointestinal protein loss may develop. An extensive number of disorders have been found to be associated with intestinal protein loss. Some of these are listed in Table 254-8.

Pathophysiology Several mechanisms have been proposed for the passage of plasma proteins across the gastrointestinal mucosa, both normally and in certain disease states. First, plasma proteins may pass into the gastrointestinal tract through an inflamed or ulcerated mucosa and account for the protein loss occasionally seen in regional enteritis and ulcerative colitis. Second, plasma protein loss may occur as a result of disordered mucosal cell structure. For example, patients with celiac sprue have abnormal villous structure and surface epithelium, and these changes could facilitate the diffusion of plasma protein between the cells. Third, in the presence of increased lymphatic pressure, there may be increased passage of plasma proteins into the lumen via the intercellular spaces of the mucosal epithelium. This might be expected to occur in disorders in which there is granulomatous or neoplastic involvement of lymphatics. Fourth, dilated lymph vessels in the mucosa may rupture through the surface epithelium, discharging their contents into the intestinal lumen. This is thought to be important in the pathogenesis of steatorrhea and hypoproteinemia.

TABLE 254-8   Disorders associated with protein-losing enteropathy

STOMACH

A Gastric carcinoma
B Giant hypertrophy of the gastric mucosa
C Atrophic gastritis
D Postgastrectomy syndrome

SMALL INTESTINE

A Intestinal lymphangiectasia
B Celiac sprue
C Tropical sprue
D Regional enteritis
E Whipple's disease
F Lymphoma
G Intestinal tuberculosis
H Acute infectious enteritis
I Scleroderma
J Jejunal diverticulosis
K Allergic gastroenteropathy

COLON

A Colonic neoplasm
B Ulcerative colitis
C Granulomatous colitis
D Megacolon

HEART

A Congestive heart failure
B Constrictive pericarditis
C Interatrial septal defect
D Primary cardiomyopathy

MISCELLANEOUS

A Esophageal carcinoma
B Gastrocolic fistula
C Agammaglobulinemia
D Nephrosis

---

in patients with idiopathic intestinal lymphangiectasia (see "Intestinal Lymphangiectasia," below).

Several techniques have been developed for the detection and quantitation of gastrointestinal protein loss. In the past these have primarily involved the use of intravenously administered radiolabeled macromolecules such as ^{125}I-labeled serum albumin, ^{51}CrCl$_3$, ^{51}Cr-labeled albumin, and indium 111. ^{111}In-labeled transferrin and ^{51}CrCl$_3$ (which rapidly become attached to circulating transferrin) are the compounds available commercially for clinical use. After the intravenous administration of 0.93 to 1.11 MBq (25 to 30 μCi) of the labeled compound to normal subjects, between 0.1 and 0.7 percent of the administered radioactivity is recovered in the stool over a 4-day period. Patients with excessive enteric protein loss may excrete from 2 to 40 percent of the injected radioactive label versus 0.1 to 0.7 percent in normal subjects. False-positive results may be obtained if the stool specimen is contaminated with urine. There is also a reliable and sensitive *nonisotopic* method to measure intestinal protein loss which involves the measurement of α_1-antitrypsin (AT). This serum enzyme, which has the same molecular weight as albumin (50,000), is resistant to proteolysis and when leaked into the intestinal lumen is not degraded. One can easily measure AT in serum and stool by radial immunodiffusion in order to obtain AT loss in stool (normal loss is less than 2.6 mg/g of stool) or intestinal clearance of AT (normal is less than 13 mL/d). Results using AT as a marker of intestinal protein loss correlate well with the more cumbersome and costly isotopic methods. Random fecal AT assays also can be used as a simple screening method for enteric protein loss.

The rate of albumin synthesis and degradation can be determined using intravenously administered radioiodinated albumin and measuring the decline in radioactivity in the serum. Such studies carried out in patients with protein-losing enteropathies have demonstrated a reduced circulating (intravascular) and total-body pool of albumin, a normal or increased rate of albumin synthesis, markedly shortened albumin survival, and increased fecal protein loss. Whereas normal subjects catabolize 5 to 10 percent of their intravascular albumin pool each day (the fractional catabolic rate), patients with excessive enteric protein loss may have fractional catabolic rates of 50 to 60 percent.

Studies utilizing radioiodinated immunoglobulins have demonstrated a decreased intravascular globulin pool and increased fractional catabolic rate. However, the synthesis of IgG is usually normal, suggesting that a decreased level of IgG and increased enteric protein loss are not potent stimuli for IgG synthesis. The increase in fractional catabolic rate is comparable for albumin, IgG, and IgM immunoglobulins, further suggesting that there is bulk loss of plasma proteins into the intestinal tract and not a selective loss of certain proteins. The finding of decreased globulins often is an ancillary aid in excluding renal, cardiac, and hepatic causes of hypoalbuminemia.

Abnormalities in albumin and globulin metabolism in patients with a protein-losing enteropathy may be reversed or diminished within a few months after the institution of appropriate therapy. It is obviously important that a specific etiologic diagnosis should be established in all patients with treatable disorders, who may be expected to have a remission induced by the appropriate therapy for the underlying disease. The intestinal protein loss in patients with celiac sprue, Whipple's disease, constrictive pericarditis, regional enteritis, ulcerative colitis, and Ménétrier's disease has been ameliorated by therapy appropriate to the underlying disorder.

Intestinal lymphangiectasia PATHOPHYSIOLOGY The disorder intestinal lymphangiectasia is characterized by increased enteric loss of protein, hypoproteinemia, edema, lymphocytopenia, malabsorption, and abnormal dilated lymphatic channels in the small intestine. The high incidence of chylous effusions and abnormal peripheral, retroperitoneal, and thoracic lymphatics indicates that intestinal lymphangiectasia is part of a generalized congenital disorder of the lymphatic system. It has been suggested that the hypoplastic visceral lymphatic channels result in obstruction to lymph flow, with the subsequent development of increased intestinal lymphatic pressure. This, in turn, may lead to dilated lymphatic vessels throughout the small-bowel wall and mesentery. Hypoproteinemia and steatorrhea are thought to be due to rupture of the dilated lymphatic vessels with discharge of lymph into the bowel lumen. In adults, approximately 1500 mL lymph, containing 70 g fat and 50 g albumin, passes through the thoracic duct each day. The leakage of a small amount of this lymph might be expected to result in considerable loss of protein and fat into the intestinal lumen. In addition, absorption of dietary long-chain triglycerides stimulates lymph flow, and this may increase further the retrograde leakage of intestinal lymph into the lumen. Three lines of evidence support the concept of intestinal leakage of lymph in intestinal lymphangiectasia: (1) chylous fluid has been recovered from the duodenum in these patients, (2) retrograde passage of contrast material from retroperitoneal lymphatics into the duodenum and jejunum has been documented, and (3) significant steatorrhea may persist in patients after institution of a completely fat-free diet, suggesting an increased enteric loss of endogenous fat present in lymph.

CLINICAL FEATURES   The disease affects primarily children and young adults. All patients have edema, which may be asymmetric because of hypoplastic peripheral lymphatics. Chylous effusions and diarrhea are common symptoms. The primary laboratory finding is hypoproteinemia with decreased serum levels of albumin, immunoglobulins IgG, IgA, and IgM, transferrin, and ceruloplasmin. Despite moderate to severe hypogammaglobulinemia, there does not appear to be an increased incidence of pyogenic bacterial infections. In addition, circulating antibody response to challenge with *Brucella* and typhoid antigens is normal. Steatorrhea is usually mild, although in some instances fat loss may be as much as 40 g/d. Some patients have hypocalcemia and impaired absorption of vitamin B_{12}. Lymphocytopenia (due to the loss of lymphocytes in lymph) is common, with lymphocyte counts ranging from 400 to 1000 per milliliter (normal: 1500 to 4000 per milliliter). This is associated with abnormal delayed hypersensitivity, as evidenced by prolonged homograft survival and impaired cutaneous responsiveness to antigens such as mumps and monilia.

Small-bowel roentgenograms are frequently abnormal, showing changes of mucosal edema and a malabsorption pattern. Lymphangiograms may demonstrate hypoplastic peripheral and visceral lymphatics with the absence of groups of retroperitoneal lymph nodes. Specimens of jejunal mucosa characteristically reveal dilated and telangiectatic lymphatic vessels in the lamina propria and submucosa. The villi may be club-shaped because of distortion from grossly dilated lymphatics (see Fig. 254-4). Such changes in the intestinal mucosa may be reversed after appropriate therapy. The diagnosis of intestinal lymphangiectasia is therefore established by (1) small-intestinal biopsy and (2) demonstration of increased enteric protein loss using radioactive macromolecules.

TREATMENT   A low-fat diet, by decreasing lymph flow, usually results in significant improvement with decreased fecal fat excretion, decreased enteric protein loss, increased serum calcium and albumin levels, and an increased half-life of injected ^{125}I-labeled albumin. Similar results may be obtained by the substitution of medium-chain triglycerides (MCT) for dietary long-chain triglycerides, since MCT are transported as medium-chain fatty acids by the portal vein rather than via the lymph.

REFERENCES

ARRANZ E, FERGUSON A: Intestinal antibody pattern in celiac disease: Occurrence in patients with normal jejunal biopsy histology. Gastroenterology 104:1263, 1993

CHERNER JA et al: Gastrointestinal dysfunction in systemic mastocytosis. A prospective study. Gastroenterology 95:657, 1988

CHIN JS et al: Paraneoplastic visceral neuropathy as a cause of severe gastrointestinal motor dysfunction. Gastroenterology 95:1279, 1988

CORAZZA G et al: Gliadin immune reactivity is associated with overt and latent enteropathy in relatives of celiac patients. Gastroenterology 102:1517, 1992

FERGUSON A et al: Clinical and pathological spectrum of coeliac disease—acitve, silent, latent, potential. Gut 34:150, 1993

FINE KD et al: Diagnosis of magnesium-induced diarrhea. N Engl J Med 324:1012, 1991

——, FORDTRAN JS: The effect of diarrhea on fecal fat excretion. Gastroenterology 102:1936, 1992

FLORENT C et al: Intestinal clearance of α_1-antitrypsin: A sensitive method for the detection of protein-losing enteropathy. Gastroenterology 81:777, 1981

GASKIN KJ et al: Colipase and maximally activated pancreatic lipase in normal subjects and patients with steatorrhea. J Clin Invest 69:368, 1982

GILLIN JS et al: Malabsorption and mucosal abnormalities of the small intestine in the acquired immunodeficiency syndrome. Ann Intern Med 102:619, 1985

HAMMER HF et al: Carbohydrate malabsorption: Its measurement and its contribution to diarrhea. J Clin Invest 86:1936, 1990

HARMS HK: Enzyme substitution therapy with the yeast saccharomyces cerevisial in congenital sucrase-isomaltase deficiency. N Engl J Med 316:1306, 1987

KAGNOFF M et al: Evidence for the role of human intestinal adenovirus in the pathogenesis of coeliac disease. Gut 28:5, 1987

KEINATH RD et al: Antibiotic treatment and relapse in Whipple's disease. Long term followup of 88 patients. Gastroenterology 88:1867, 1985

KERLIN P, WONG L: Breath hydrogen testing in bacterial overgrowth of the small intestine. Gastroenterology 95:982, 1988

KHOURI MR et al: Sudan stain of fecal fat: New insight into an old test. Gastroenterology 96: 421, 1989

KLIPSTEIN FA: Tropical sprue in travelers and expatriates living abroad. Gastroenterology 80:590, 1981

LOUGHRAN TP et al: T-cell intestinal lymphoma associated with celiac sprue. Ann Intern Med 104:44, 1986

LUBY LD et al: Lactulose/mannitol test: An ideal screen for celiac disease. Gastroenterology 96:79, 1989

MARSH M: Gluten: Major histocompatability complex, and the small intestine. Gastroenterology 102:330, 1992

PETERS TJ, BJARNASON I: Coeliac syndrome: Biochemical mechanisms and the missing peptidase hypothesis revisited. Gut 25:913, 1984

RELMAN DA et al: Identification of the uncultured bacillus of Whipple's disease. N Engl J Med 327:293, 1992

SCHILLER LR et al: Studies on the prevalence and significance of radiolabeled bile acid malabsorption in a group of patients with idiopathic chronic diarrhea. Gastroenterology 92:151, 1987

SLEIKH MS et al: Gastrointestinal absorption of calcium from milk and calcium salts. N Engl J Med 317:532, 1987

STANGHELLINI V: Chronic idiopathic intestinal pseudo-obstruction: Clinical and intestinal manometric findings. Gut 28:5, 1987

TRIER JS: Medical progress: Celiac sprue. N Engl J Med 325:1709, 1991

VAN ELBURG RM et al: Intestinal permeability in patients with coeliac disease and relatives of patients with coeliac disease. Gut 34:354, 1993

255 INFLAMMATORY BOWEL DISEASE (Ulcerative colitis and Crohn's disease)

ROBERT M. GLICKMAN

DEFINITION   *Inflammatory bowel disease* (IBD) is a general term for a group of chronic inflammatory disorders of unknown cause involving the gastrointestinal tract. Since there are no pathognomonic features or specific diagnostic tests, in a strict sense, these disorders remain diagnoses of exclusion. Their features are sufficiently characteristic, however, to permit accurate diagnosis in the majority of cases. Chronic IBD may be divided into two major groups, chronic nonspecific *ulcerative colitis* and *Crohn's disease*. The original description of the disease by Crohn, Ginzberg, and Oppenheimer in 1932 localized the disease to segments of ileum. However, the same process may involve the buccal mucosa, esophagus, stomach, and duodenum, as well as the jejunum and ileum. Crohn's disease of the small bowel is also known as *regional enteritis*. In addition, a similar inflammatory picture may occur in the colon, either alone or with accompanying small-intestinal involvement. In most instances, this form of colitis can be distinguished clinically and pathologically from ulcerative colitis and is also referred to as *Crohn's disease of the colon*. *Granulomatous colitis* is a less accurate term because only a portion of cases exhibit granulomas. Clinically these disorders are characterized by recurrent inflammatory involvement of intestinal segments with diverse clinical manifestations often resulting in a chronic, unpredictable course.

EPIDEMIOLOGY   The epidemiologic and etiologic considerations in ulcerative colitis and Crohn's disease share many features in common and will be discussed together. These diseases are more common in whites than in blacks and Orientals with an increased incidence (three- to sixfold) in Jews compared with non-Jews. Both sexes are equally affected.

The incidence and prevalence of the two diseases differ slightly, with most studies showing ulcerative colitis to be more common. When analyzed in western Europe and the United States, ulcerative colitis (including ulcerative proctitis) has an incidence of approximately 6 to 8 cases per 100,000 population and an estimated prevalence of approximately 70 to 150 cases per 100,000 population. Estimates of the incidence of Crohn's disease (colonic plus small bowel) are approximately 2 cases per 100,000 population; the prevalence is estimated at 20 to 40 per 100,000 population. Many believe the incidence of Crohn's disease (especially colonic) to be increasing. In western Europe and North America, the incidence and prevalence of Crohn's disease have been increasing five times faster than for ulcerative colitis.

While peak occurrence of both diseases is between the ages of 15 and 35, it has been reported in every decade of life. A familial incidence of IBD has been recorded with estimates that 2 to 5 percent of persons with Crohn's disease or ulcerative colitis will have one or more relatives affected. There is no specificity, however, for a given form of IBD within a given family. Such epidemiologic clustering of cases could argue for either genetic or common environmental influences on the development of these diseases (see below). It has been suggested that there is a probable hereditary basis for these disorders plus a strong environmental component.

ETIOLOGY AND PATHOGENESIS　　While the cause of ulcerative colitis and Crohn's disease remains unknown, certain features of these diseases have suggested several areas of possible importance. These include familial or genetic, infectious, immunologic, and psychological factors.

Inflammatory bowel disease is more common in whites, occurs with an increased frequency in Jews, and exhibits some familial clustering. This suggests that there may be a *genetic* predisposition to the development of the disease. An increased incidence of Crohn's disease in monozygotic twins provides strong evidence for a genetic component. A search for genetic markers which might be of value in identifying susceptible individuals has not identified any single marker (i.e., histocompatibility antigen) in patients with inflammatory bowel disease.

The chronic inflammatory nature of these diseases has prompted a continuing search for a possible *infectious* cause. Despite numerous attempts to find known bacterial, fungal, or viral agents, none has thus far been isolated. Preliminary reports of isolates of cell wall variants of *Pseudomonas* or of transmissible agents producing cytopathic effects in tissue culture have yet to be confirmed. Efforts to produce specific granulomatous tissue reactions with filtrates from Crohn's disease tissue have yielded conflicting and nonreproducible results. As discussed below, many infectious agents can produce *acute* colitis or ileitis; however, there is no evidence that these agents are involved in *chronic* inflammatory bowel disease.

The theory that an *immune* mechanism may be involved is based on the concept that the extraintestinal manifestations which may accompany these disorders (e.g., arthritis, pericholangitis) may represent autoimmune phenomena and that therapeutic agents, such as glucocorticoids and azathioprine, may exert their effects via immunosuppressive mechanisms. Patients with inflammatory bowel disease may have *humoral antibodies* to colon cells, bacterial antigens such as *Escherichia coli*, lipopolysaccharide, and foreign proteins such as cow's milk protein. In general, the presence and titer of these antibodies do not correlate with disease activity. It is likely that these antigens gain access to immunocompetent cells secondary to epithelial damage. In addition, IBD has been described in association with agammaglobulinemia as well as IgA deficiency, casting further doubt on the pathogenetic role of humoral antibodies. *Immune complexes* also have been invoked to explain extraintestinal manifestations of IBD. While there are well-defined examples of tissue injury resulting from immune complexes, studies utilizing specific detection tech-

niques have failed to demonstrate an increased frequency of immune complexes in patients with IBD.

Associated abnormalities of *cell-mediated immunity* include cutaneous anergy, diminished responsiveness to various mitogenic stimuli, and decreases in the number of peripheral T cells. Since many of these changes may revert to normal when the disease is quiescent, it is likely that they are secondary phenomena. Many associated abnormalities of cell-mediated immunity have been described in the mucosa of patients with IBD. They include increased mucosal IgG cells, as well as changes in subsets of T cells, suggesting antigenic stimulation. Activation of mucosal immune cells results in a complex expression of cytokines which may contribute to the mucosal inflammatory response. In addition, noncytokine inflammatory mediators such as prostaglandin and thromboxane products are elevated in the mucosa of patients with IBD and are further stimuli for the inflammatory response. Several recent animal models of IBD, including a transgenic rat model which expresses human HLA-B27, a mouse deficient in interleukin 2, and the spontaneous chronic colitis of the cotton-top tamarin, also may shed important insights into the pathogenesis of IBD. Thus far, however, none of the altered immunologic findings has been specific for either ulcerative colitis or Crohn's disease.

The *psychological* features of patients with inflammatory bowel disease also have been stressed. It is not uncommon for these diseases to present initially or to flare in association with major psychological stresses such as the loss of a family member. It has been suggested that patients with IBD have a characteristic personality which renders them susceptible to emotional stresses which in turn may precipitate or exacerbate their symptoms. While there is little evidence directly relating possible emotional factors to the etiology of inflammatory bowel disease, there is little doubt that a chronic disease of unknown cause affecting individuals in the prime of their life often results in feelings of anger, anxiety, and some degree of depression. These reactions are undoubtedly important factors in modifying the course of these diseases and in the response to therapy.

PATHOLOGY　　In ulcerative colitis there is an inflammatory reaction primarily involving the colonic mucosa. Grossly, the colon appears ulcerated, hyperemic, and usually hemorrhagic (Fig. 255-1). A striking feature of the inflammation is that it is *uniform* and *continuous* with no intervening areas of normal mucosa. The rectum is usually involved (95 percent of cases), and the inflammation extends proximally in a continuous fashion but for a variable distance. When

FIGURE 255-1　　Ulcerative colitis. Resected colon with portion of terminal ileum. The specimen showed uniform inflammation, erythema, and hemorrhage and a normal terminal ileum.

there is involvement of the entire colon, there may be minimal involvement of a few centimeters of the terminal ileum, referred to as "backwash ileitis." This involvement never leads to the thickening and narrowing characteristic of Crohn's disease. The surface mucosal cells as well as the crypt epithelium and submucosa are involved in an inflammatory reaction with neutrophilic infiltration (Fig. 255-2A). This progresses to epithelial damage with loss of surface epithelial cells resulting in multiple ulcerations. Infiltration of the crypts with neutrophils results in characteristic (but not specific) small crypt abscesses and their eventual destruction. There also may be loss of crypt epithelium with a loss of goblet (mucus-producing) cells and submucosal edema. With repetitive cycles of inflammation, mild submucosal fibrosis develops. Regenerative activity is evidenced by irregular crypt epithelium often showing bifurcation at the base of the crypts. It is important to stress that, unlike Crohn's disease, deeper layers of the bowel beneath the submucosa usually are not involved. In severe ulcerative colitis, as seen with toxic megacolon, the bowel wall may become extremely thin, the mucosa denuded, and inflammation extending to the serosa, leading to dilatation and subsequent perforation.

Recurrent inflammation may lead to characteristic features of chronicity. Fibrosis and longitudinal retraction result in shortening of the colon. Loss of the normal haustral pattern leads radiologically to a smooth, "lead-pipe" appearance of the colon. Regenerating islands of mucosa surrounded by areas of ulceration and denuded mucosa appear as "polyps" protruding into the lumen of the colon. However, these protrusions are inflammatory in nature and not neoplastic and are therefore called *pseudopolyps* (Fig. 255-2B).

With long-standing ulcerative colitis, the surface epithelium may show features of *dysplasia*. Changes of nuclear and cellular atypia are thought to represent a premalignant change occurring in the setting of long-standing ulcerative colitis. Marked dysplasia in colonic biopsies in the setting of long-standing colitis is associated with a significant risk of a coexistent carcinoma elsewhere in the colon and may influence the decision to advise colectomy.

Crohn's disease, in contrast to ulcerative colitis, is characterized by chronic inflammation extending through *all layers of the intestinal wall* and involving the mesentery as well as regional lymph nodes. Whether or not the small bowel or colon is involved, the basic pathologic process is the same.

The earliest pathologic changes in Crohn's disease are poorly defined, since surgery is usually not electively undertaken early in the course of the disease. At laparotomy, the terminal ileum appears hyperemic and boggy, with mesentery and mesenteric lymph nodes swollen and reddened. At this early stage, the bowel wall, although edematous, is usually pliable. While some patients with this initial presentation will subsequently develop typical regional enteritis, a significant number will recover completely. This acute form of ileitis will undoubtedly be shown to have diverse causes. Indeed, a significant number of patients with this presentation have been shown to be infected with *Yersinia enterocolitica*, an organism capable of producing a self-limited, acute inflammatory ileitis.

As the disease progresses, the gross appearance assumes a characteristic picture. The bowel appears greatly thickened and leathery with the lumen narrowed (Fig. 255-3). This characteristic stenosis can occur in any portion of the intestine and may be associated with varying degrees of intestinal obstruction. The mesentery appears greatly thickened, fatty, and often extends over the serosal surface of the bowel in characteristic finger-like projections. The appearance of the mucosa is variable, depending on the severity and stage of the disease, but it may appear relatively normal in sharp contrast to ulcerative colitis. In more advanced cases, the mucosa has a nodular, "cobblestoned" look. This is the result of submucosal thickening and mucosal ulceration, often linear in the long axis of the bowel at the base of mucosal folds. These ulcerations may penetrate into the submucosa and muscularis and coalesce to form intramural channels which become manifested as fistulas and fissures.

There are other morphologic features distinguishing Crohn's disease from ulcerative colitis. In Crohn's disease, the disease is often *discontinuous;* severely involved segments of bowel are separated from each other by "skip areas" of apparently normal bowel. In approximately 50 percent of Crohn's disease of the colon, the rectum may be spared. In sharp contrast, in ulcerative colitis the involvement is contiguous and the rectum is almost always involved. In addition, in Crohn's disease the transmural inflammatory process, involving serosa and mesentery, also accounts for the characteristic fistula and abscess formation. As a result of serosal inflammation, adjacent loops of small intestine may become adherent and matted together by a fibrinous peritoneal reaction, leading to a palpable mass, most often in the right lower quadrant. Fistula formation may occur between adherent loops of intestine, colon, or other adjacent organs such as the bladder or vagina. Fistulous tracts also may lead to the skin or end blindly within the peritoneum or retroperitoneum, surrounded by adherent loops of bowel and inflammatory tissue. Fistula formation is not seen in ulcerative colitis.

Microscopically, granulomas are most helpful in distinguishing Crohn's disease from other forms of inflammatory bowel disease; they do not occur in ulcerative colitis. They may be seen in rectal or colonoscopic biopsies (Fig. 255-2D). While granulomas are a helpful finding when present, it is the chronic inflammation involving all layers of the intestinal wall which is most characteristic.

In most series reporting the distribution of Crohn's disease, approximately 30 percent will involve the small intestine (usually the terminal ileum) without colonic disease, 30 percent with only colonic involvement, and 40 percent with ileocolic involvement usually of the ileum and right colon. In a small number of patients (mostly children and adolescents) there may be diffuse and extensive ulceration of the jejunum and ileum.

While there often are sufficient features to permit distinction between ulcerative colitis and Crohn's disease of the colon (Table 255-1), in 10 to 20 percent of cases this distinction may not be possible.

CLINICAL FEATURES

ULCERATIVE COLITIS The major symptoms of ulcerative colitis are bloody diarrhea and abdominal pain, often with fever and weight loss in more severe cases. With mild disease, there may be one or two semiformed stools containing little blood and with no systemic manifestations. In contrast, the patient with severe disease may have frequent liquid stools containing blood and pus, complain of severe cramps, and demonstrate symptoms and signs of dehydration, anemia, fever, and weight loss. With predominantly rectal involvement, constipation rather than diarrhea may be present, and tenesmus may be a major complaint. On occasion, intestinal symptoms may be overshadowed by fever, weight loss, or one of the extracolonic manifestations of the disease (see below).

The physical findings in ulcerative colitis are usually nonspecific; there may be some abdominal distention or tenderness along the course of the colon. In mild cases, the general physical examination will be normal. Extracolonic manifestations include arthritis, skin changes, or evidence of liver disease. Fever, tachycardia, and postural hypotension are usually associated with more severe disease. The laboratory findings are often nonspecific and usually reflect the degree and severity of bleeding and inflammation. There may be anemia which reflects chronic disease as well as iron deficiency from chronic blood loss. Leukocytosis with a left shift and an elevated sedimentation rate are often seen in the severely ill, febrile patient. Electrolyte abnormalities, especially hypokalemia, reflect the degree of diarrhea. Hypoalbuminemia is common with extensive disease and usually represents luminal protein loss through an ulcerated mucosa. An elevated alkaline phosphatase level may indicate associated hepatobiliary disease (see below).

A

B

C

D

The clinical course of ulcerative colitis is variable. The majority of patients will suffer a relapse within 1 year of the first attack, reflecting the recurrent nature of the disease. There may, however, be prolonged periods of remission with only minimal symptoms. In general, the severity of symptoms reflects the extent of colonic involvement and the intensity of the inflammation. At one end of the spectrum are patients who present with limited involvement of the rectum (ulcerative proctitis) or rectum and sigmoid (ulcerative proctosigmoiditis). Consistent with this limited colonic involvement, the disease is usually mild, with minimal systemic or extracolonic manifestations, although ulcerative proctitis may on occasion be therapeutically difficult, with protracted bleeding and tenesmus. The major symptoms are rectal bleeding and tenesmus. Most of these patients, especially those with only rectal involvement, will not develop more extensive disease. In the remainder, the disease may extend proximally with variable involvement. Perhaps 85 percent of patients with ulcerative colitis will have mild to moderate disease of an intermittent nature and can be managed without hospitalization. In approximately 15 percent of patients, the disease assumes a more fulminant course, involves the entire colon, and presents with severe bloody diarrhea and systemic signs and symptoms. The patients are at risk to develop toxic dilatation and perforation of the colon (described below) and represent a medical emergency.

CROHN'S DISEASE   As discussed above, the basic pathologic features of Crohn's disease are the same whether the disease involves the small bowel or colon. The clinical presentation, however, will largely reflect the anatomic location of the disease and to some degree will predict which complications of the disease may develop. The clinical features of ulcerative colitis and Crohn's disease are compared in Table 255-1.

The major clinical features of Crohn's disease are fever, abdominal pain, diarrhea often without blood, and generalized fatigability. There may be associated weight loss. With *colonic involvement*, diarrhea and pain are the most frequent symptoms. Rectal bleeding is distinctly less common than with ulcerative colitis and reflects (1) sparing of the rectum in many patients and (2) the transmural nature of the disease with only irregular mucosal involvement. There may be associated severe anorectal complications such as fistulas, fissures, and perirectal abscess. Such features may antedate the clinical onset of colitis and should always raise the suspicion of associated Crohn's disease. With recurrent perirectal inflammation, the anal canal may be thickened, and perianal fistulas or scarring may be present. With extensive colonic involvement, dilatation of the colon may occur. However, since Crohn's disease often results in a thickened colonic wall, this is less common with Crohn's disease than with ulcerative colitis. Extracolonic manifestations (discussed below), particularly arthritis, are seen more commonly with colonic than with small-bowel Crohn's disease (regional enteritis).

With involvement of the *small bowel*, there may be additional presenting signs and symptoms. Typically, the disease has its onset in a young adult with a history of fatigue, variable weight loss, right lower quadrant discomfort or pain, and diarrhea. Low-grade fever, anorexia, nausea, and vomiting also may be present. The abdominal pain may be steady and localized to the right lower quadrant or may assume a colicky or crampy pattern, reflecting variable degrees of intestinal stenosis. The diarrhea is often moderate, usually without gross blood; if there is no rectal involvement, tenesmus is absent. Physical examination at this time often reveals right lower quadrant

FIGURE 255-3   Regional enteritis. Resected specimen of terminal ileum demonstrates thickened bowel wall and chronically inflamed mucosa. Note the relatively sharp demarcation of the diseased segment with grossly normal mucosa on either side.

tenderness with an associated fullness or mass reflecting adherent loops of bowel. At this time the patient may have mild anemia, mild to moderate leukocytosis, and an elevated sedimentation rate.

Since acute ileitis may have an abrupt onset with fever, leukocytosis, and right lower quadrant pain, the clinical picture may be indistinguishable from acute appendicitis. The diagnosis can be made only at laparotomy, when the characteristic beefy red terminal ileum, boggy mesenteric fat, and succulent mesenteric lymph nodes indicate that appendicitis alone could not produce this picture.

While the symptoms of diarrhea and abdominal pain will usually alert the clinician to the possibility of regional enteritis, other symptoms may dominate the clinical presentation. In children and the aged, fever of undetermined origin and unexplained weight loss may be prominent and initially may cause one to suspect underlying

FIGURE 255-2   Colonic biopsies in inflammatory bowel disease. *A.* Ulcerative colitis. The surface mucosa is destroyed and the submucosa is diffusely infiltrated with polymorphonuclear leukocytes. Crypt abscesses are also present. *B.* Pseudopolyp. Regenerating island of mucosa with adjacent area of ulceration. *C.* Ulcerative colitis. Severe dysplasia occurring in long-standing chronic ulcerative colitis. Note atypical changes in the nuclei and marked palisading of nuclei of the crypt epithelium. *D.* Crohn's disease of the colon. Note the relatively intact mucosa with a solitary granuloma in the lamina propria.

TABLE 255-1   Pathologic and clinical features of IBD

	Ulcerative colitis	Crohn's disease
PATHOLOGIC		
Segmental	0	+ +
Transmural involvement	+/−	+ +
Granulomas	0	+/+ + (50%)
Fibrosis	+	+ +
Fissuring, fistulas	+/−	+ +
Mesenteric fat, lymph node involvement	0	+ +
CLINICAL		
Diarrhea	+ +	+ +
Rectal bleeding	+ +	+
Abdominal pain	+	+ +
Palpable mass	0	+ +
Fistulas	+/−	+ +
Strictures	+	+ +
Small bowel involvement	+/− ("backwash ileitis")	+ +
Rectal involvement	+ + (95%)	+/+ + (50%)
Extracolonic disease	+	+
Toxic megacolon	+	+/−
Recurrence after colectomy	0	+
Malignancy (with long-standing disease)	+	+/−

NOTE: 0 = never; +/− = rare; + = occasional; + + = frequent, common.

malignancy. In some patients, the first manifestation of the disease may be intestinal obstruction; in others, the disease may present with fistula formation in the form of perianal sepsis or urinary tract infection resulting from an enterovesical fistula. Similarly, right ureteral obstruction and hydronephrosis may occur due to external compression of the ureter by a right lower quadrant inflammatory mass. On occasion, often in the setting of extensive small-bowel involvement, features of malabsorption may be prominent. These features, along with anorexia and the catabolic effects of the chronic inflammatory process, may combine to produce striking degrees of weight loss.

The complications of the disease are often local, resulting from intestinal inflammation and involvement of adjacent structures.

Intestinal obstruction is a frequent complication, occurring in 20 to 30 percent of patients during the course of the disease. In the initial stages, the obstruction usually is due to the acute inflammation and edema of the involved intestinal segment, usually the terminal ileum. However, as the disease progresses and fibrosis develops, obstruction may be due to a fixed narrowing of the bowel.

Fistula formation is a frequent complication of chronic regional enteritis as well as Crohn's disease of the colon. Fistulas may occur between contiguous segments of intestine; they also may burrow into the retroperitoneal spaces and present as cutaneous fistulas or indolent abscesses. In a significant number of patients, the first indication of the disease may be the presence of persistent rectal fissures, a perirectal abscess, or a rectal fistula. Although uncommon, pneumaturia should raise the suspicion of enterovesical fistula and is often associated with a persistent urinary tract infection.

Since Crohn's disease is a transmural disease with the bowel wall greatly thickened, free *intestinal perforation* is uncommon. In a small number of cases, however, it may be the presenting feature, and the disease is first discovered at the time of laparotomy for a perforated viscus. The passage per rectum of bright red blood should alert one to the possible coexistence of rectal involvement (i.e., ileocolitis). Crohn's disease also may involve the *stomach* and *duodenum*. The involvement is usually of the antrum and/or the first and second portions of the duodenum. Symptoms may include pain mimicking peptic ulcer disease. Later in the course of the disease, chronic scarring may produce gastric outlet or duodenal obstruction.

There are increasing reports of *small-bowel* and *colonic malignancy* developing in the setting of long-standing Crohn's disease. Although the risk of developing malignancy is statistically increased, the complication is uncommon when compared with the frequency of malignancy in ulcerative colitis (see below). As in other chronic inflammatory diseases, patients with long-standing Crohn's disease may rarely develop secondary *amyloidosis*, which may manifest itself with hepatosplenomegaly or significant proteinuria. The presence of extensive ileal disease, resulting in *bile salt malabsorption*, is associated with a decreased bile salt pool and an increased lithogenicity of bile (see Chap. 254). Up to 30 percent of patients with extensive ileal disease will develop gallstones. Also, in the setting of ileal disease and an intact colon there is increased colonic absorption of dietary oxalate with resultant hyperoxaluria and the development of *urinary oxalate stones*. Dehydration due to diarrhea is an additional predisposing factor in renal stone formation.

DIAGNOSIS

The diagnosis of IBD should be entertained in all patients presenting with diarrhea or bloody diarrhea, persistent perianal sepsis, and abdominal pain. There may be atypical presentations such as fever of unexplained origin in the absence of bowel symptoms or with extracolonic manifestations such as arthritis or liver disease antedating or overshadowing the bowel involvement. Since Crohn's disease also may involve the small intestine, it should be considered in the differential diagnosis of all types of malabsorption syndromes, intermittent intestinal obstruction, and abdominal fistulas.

The laboratory examination is usually nonspecific and reflects the extent and severity of the inflammatory reaction. In addition, when Crohn's disease involves the small bowel, laboratory features of malabsorption may be present. There may be a variable degree of anemia, from occult blood loss or the effect of chronic inflammation on the bone marrow. Folate or vitamin B_{12} malabsorption also may contribute to the anemia. While the Schilling test may be abnormal in patients with extensive ileal disease, frank macrocytic anemia due to vitamin B_{12} malabsorption alone is unusual, attesting to the marked efficiency of ileal absorption of the vitamin. When there is significant diarrhea, electrolyte abnormalities (hypokalemia, hypomagnesemia) may be prominent. Hypocalcemia may reflect extensive mucosal involvement and malabsorption of vitamin D. Hypoalbuminemia may result from amino acid malabsorption as well as from protein-losing enteropathy. Variable degrees of steatorrhea may result from bile salt depletion and mucosal damage. Mild abnormalities of liver function (especially an increased serum alkaline phosphatase) may reflect the development of a fatty liver in the malnourished patient or a coexisting early sclerosing cholangitis. Significant jaundice is unusual. Proteinuria may reflect secondary amyloidosis, a rare complication.

Sigmoidoscopy and *radiologic* studies of the bowel are most important in establishing the diagnosis of inflammatory bowel disease. Sigmoidoscopy must be performed in all patients presenting with chronic diarrhea and in all instances of rectal bleeding. While meticulous air-contrast barium enema examination of the perfectly prepared colon may disclose the earliest mucosal changes in either ulcerative colitis or Crohn's disease (see below), a conventional barium enema examination is often ''normal'' in early disease. Direct visualization of the colonic mucosa combined with biopsy is the most sensitive way of determining whether rectal inflammation is present. It can often be performed without prior enema preparation in the patient actively having diarrhea. The goal of sigmoidoscopy is to establish *whether* mucosal inflammation is present and not necessarily to determine its full *extent* at the initial examination. Thus, if sigmoidoscopic changes are encountered within the first 8 to 10 cm, it is not necessary to pass the instrument to its full length, which may cause discomfort when the bowel is acutely inflamed. In ulcerative colitis, findings include a loss of mucosal vascularity, diffuse erythema, friability of the mucosa, and often an exudate consisting of mucus, blood, and pus. Mucosal friability and uniform involvement are characteristic. Once diseased mucosa is encountered (usually in the rectum), there are no areas of intervening normal mucosa before the proximal extent of the disease is reached. Ulceration is shallow, may be small or confluent, but invariably occurs in segments of active colitis. Full colonoscopic examination of the colon in ulcerative colitis is not indicated in the acutely ill patient. Rectal biopsy may corroborate mucosal inflammation. With more chronic disease, the mucosa may show a granular appearance, and pseudopolyps may be present.

Endoscopic examination of the colon is also of value in the diagnosis of colonic Crohn's disease. The findings are of ulcerations which may be tiny, aphthous erosions or deep, longitudinal fissures. They usually occur in segments of otherwise normal mucosa. Since the mucosa is not uniformly involved, friability and diffuse granularity, which are hallmarks of ulcerative colitis, are not characteristic of Crohn's colitis. Rather, a cobblestone appearance, which is a coarse irregularity of the mucosal surface, reflects submucosal inflammation and is characteristic of Crohn's disease. Pseudopolyps, edema, and strictures may be seen in Crohn's colitis as well as in ulcerative colitis. Colonic mucosal biopsy reveals granulomas in 30 to 50 percent of specimens taken from involved areas. Features such as crypt abscesses, infiltration with inflammatory cells, or ulcerations are nonspecific but compatible features. Since skip areas and rectal sparing are characteristic of Crohn's disease, colonoscopy may be superior to sigmoidoscopy in the evaluation of Crohn's disease. Colonoscopic examination is also indicated when Crohn's disease appears only to involve the small bowel. Ileal biopsy may be feasible, and coexisting colonic involvement occurs in a significant number of cases. Perianal inflammatory lesions as well as areas of rectal disease seen at endoscopy will often show granulomatous inflammation. Rectal biopsy of seemingly uninvolved areas also may show microscopic evidence of granulomatous inflammation in only 5 to 15 percent of patients.

The *radiologic evaluation* of the bowel provides essential information in the diagnosis of IBD. Barium enema, in ulcerative colitis, may reveal the extent of the disease and help define associated features such as stricture, pseudopolyposis, or carcinoma. The earliest features seen in ulcerative colitis are irritability and incomplete filling due to associated inflammation. Fine ulcerations may be seen at this time as serrations along the contour of the bowel producing a hazy margin (Fig. 255-4). The ulcerations may become deeper and with more fulminant disease produce a grossly ragged and irregular contour. Polypoid defects appear as a result of edematous mucosa between ulcerations. The diffuse pattern of ulceration is best seen on the evacuation film or on air-contrast barium enema. In the chronic stage of the disease (Fig. 255-5), the characteristic features are shortening of the bowel, depression of the flexures, narrowing of the bowel lumen, and rigidity. The bowel has a symmetric, ahaustral, tubular appearance with a decreased mucosal pattern. Although strictures are uncommon, when they occur, they have a concentric lumen with fusiform tapering margins. Eccentricity should raise the suspicion of an associated carcinoma.

Barium enema examination in Crohn's disease of the colon has features which usually distinguish it from ulcerative colitis. Features characteristic of Crohn's disease include rectal sparing, the presence of skip lesions, and the finding of small ulcerations occurring on small irregular nodules. The small ulcerations often extend to produce longitudinal ulcers (Fig. 255-6) and transverse fissures which in reality are limited sinus tracts. These may extend into adjacent tissues to produce fistulas. Irregular thickening and fibrosis may lead to stricture formation, which may be multiple. In 10 to 15 percent of cases the disease may uniformly involve the entire colon, making differentiation from ulcerative colitis more difficult. Reflux of barium into the

FIGURE 255-5 Chronic ulcerative colitis. Note the loss of haustrations and the fusiform stricture in the transverse colon. *(Courtesy of R Gold, Columbia Presbyterian Medical Center.)*

FIGURE 255-4 Acute ulcerative colitis, air-contrast study. Note the diffuse fine ulceration of the entire colon, producing serration along the contour of the bowel. *(Courtesy of R Gold, Columbia Presbyterian Medical Center.)*

terminal ileum during barium enema may reveal characteristic ileal changes of regional enteritis.

When Crohn's disease involves the small intestine, the terminal ileum is most characteristically involved with features similar to colonic involvement. Careful x-ray examination of the small bowel may demonstrate loss of mucosal detail and rigidity of involved segments resulting from submucosal edema or stenosis. The submucosal inflammation may lead to the characteristic radiologic cobblestoned appearance of the mucosa (Fig. 255-7), and fistulous tracts may be seen, especially in the ileocecal area (Fig. 255-8). Involvement of the stomach and duodenum usually appears radiologically as stiffening and infiltration of the mucosa and can mimic an infiltrative tumor. If such an appearance is due to regional enteritis, there is almost always coexistent involvement of either the jejunum or ileum. In Crohn's disease, computed tomographic (CT) imaging of the abdomen may be of value in the evaluation of thickened, separated bowel loops and to help distinguish thickened, matted loops (phlegmon) from intraabdominal abscess.

While barium studies often provide information on the pattern and extent of inflammatory bowel disease, caution must be exercised in obtaining these studies in the acutely ill patient with severe colitis, in whom barium study and the bowel cleansing which precedes it may result in a worsening of the disease and can precipitate toxic dilatation of the colon.

Fiberoptic colonoscopy has added greatly to the diagnosis of colonic inflammatory bowel disease. Areas formerly beyond the reach of the sigmoidoscope can now be directly visualized and biopsy material obtained. Early in the course of colonic inflammation, endoscopic examination and biopsy are the most sensitive techniques to demonstrate mucosal involvement. Polypoid lesions, strictures, and unclear x-ray features can usually be fully defined. Periodic colonoscopic examination and biopsy are being used increasingly in cancer surveillance in patients with long-standing inflammatory bowel disease (see below).

FIGURE 255-6   Crohn's colitis. Air-contrast study.

DIFFERENTIAL DIAGNOSIS

Many entities must be considered in the differential diagnosis in IBD. The focus of the differential diagnosis in large measure will be determined by the presenting features of the disease. When *rectal bleeding* is the presenting complaint, a colonic source should be considered. While *hemorrhoids* are commonly found, they must be considered a tentative source of bleeding until sigmoidoscopy and barium enema have eliminated other colonic lesions. Colonic *neoplasms* (carcinoma, adenomatous polyps) also may present with rectal bleeding and can usually be diagnosed by barium enema with subsequent sigmoidoscopic or colonoscopic biopsy. It should be remembered that carcinoma may complicate long-standing colitis. Rectal bleeding from *colonic diverticula* or *arteriovenous malformations* usually presents no problem in differential diagnosis, since radiologic and endoscopic features of inflammatory bowel disease are absent. *Radiation proctitis*, which may present as a localized area of colitis, is usually found in the setting of pelvic irradiation. The onset

may, however, occur at variable (months to years) periods of time after irradiation. Characteristic features on sigmoidoscopy include mucosal atrophy and telangiectasia along with friability and small ulcerations. A colitis sometimes indistinguishable from ulcerative colitis may occur in Behçet's syndrome and is associated with aphthous oral ulceration, uveitis, and urethritis.

Acute colitis may be caused by a variety of *infectious* agents (Chap. 87). Often presenting with bloody diarrhea, infectious colitis may be difficult to distinguish from IBD at initial presentation, and severe cases may present with colonic dilatation mimicking toxic megacolon. Rectal biopsy in infectious colitis shows marked polymorphonuclear infiltration with pronounced edema and relative sparing of the crypts, features which may distinguish it from idiopathic inflammatory bowel disease. A listing of these agents is given in Table 255-2.

Amebiasis may present with bloody diarrhea and at sigmoidoscopy may be indistinguishable from idiopathic ulcerative colitis. A history of recent foreign travel or homosexual exposure would be important. Amebic serologies may be of value, although initial positive titers may indicate prior infection of indeterminate age. Since specific amebicidal therapy is necessary to eradicate this infection and corticosteroids may be detrimental, every effort should be made to exclude this diagnosis in appropriate individuals via serologic titers and careful examination of colonic secretions and biopsies. Acute *bacillary dysentery* may be caused by *Shigella* and *Salmonella* or *Campylobacter*, all easily diagnosed by stool culture. *Yersinia enterocolitis*, which may present as acute ileitis, also can produce a self-limited colitis, sometimes with granulomatous reaction. Infectious agents may cause acute proctitis indistinguishable from idiopathic ulcerative proctitis. Such infections, often seen in homosexuals, may be due to herpes simplex virus, *gonorrhea*, *lymphogranuloma venereum* (LGV), cytomegalovirus, *Isospora*, or *Treponema pallidum*, as well as *amebiasis*. In homosexual men, non-LGV strains of *Chlamydia* have been shown to produce a granulomatous proctitis closely resembling Crohn's disease of the rectum.

Pseudomembranous colitis (antibiotic-associated colitis) is caused by a necrolytic toxin elaborated by *Clostridium difficile*, which under certain circumstances proliferates within the bowel. Most often the

FIGURE 255-7   Crohn's ileocolitis. Note the nodularity and ulceration of the terminal ileum and the deformity of the cecum.

FIGURE 255-8 Regional enteritis. X-ray showing fistulas between loops of bowel. Insert is a compression film of this area; note fistulas between adjacent loops of bowel.

disease is a result of antibiotic therapy which presumably upsets the normal ecologic balance of the bowel flora and permits *C. difficile* to proliferate. Almost every antibiotic has been implicated, although cases related to the use of vancomycin or aminoglycosides are rare. Most often diarrhea is profuse and watery, although bloody diarrhea occurs in 5 percent of cases. Characteristic lesions are seen on sigmoidoscopy and appear as multiple, discrete yellowish plaques which on biopsy show features of acute inflammation and ulceration with a pseudomembrane of fibrin and necrotic material. On occasion, lesions may be beyond reach of the sigmoidoscope and require colonoscopy. Diagnosis is best made by detecting *C. difficile* toxin in the stool. Treatment is initially directed at eradicating *C. difficile* organisms from the stool. Vancomycin (250 mg PO qid for 7 to 14 days) is the treatment of choice for more severely ill patients and should produce clinical improvement within 5 days. Since vancomycin therapy is expensive, alternative therapies have been proposed. The use of metronidazole (500 mg PO qid for 7 to 14 days) has been shown to be equally effective as vancomycin. Alternatively, bacitracin (20,000 units qid for 7 to 14 days) is also quite effective. With all forms of therapy, relapse rates (15 to 30 percent) have been observed and may require a subsequent course of therapy to eradicate the organism. On occasion, infectious causes of colitis will be superimposed on ulcerative colitis or Crohn's disease. In this case, once the acute infection has subsided, symptoms and inflammatory mucosal changes may persist, raising the possibility of associated idiopathic IBD. Similar considerations apply to the patient with IBD who uncommonly may develop associated *pseudomembranous* colitis. The finding of *C. difficile* toxin in the stool and subsequent treatment will serve to clarify this presentation.

Abdominal pain in association with rectal bleeding, especially in the older age group, may be due to *ischemic colitis* and be most difficult to distinguish from inflammatory bowel disease, especially Crohn's disease. Because of an excellent collateral circulation, the rectum is usually spared. Radiologic features are often characteristic, showing submucosal edema or hemorrhage (thumb printing) which typically resolves spontaneously over several weeks.

Inflammatory bowel disease may be difficult to distinguish from functional diarrhea early in the course of disease. The presence of constitutional symptoms such as fatigue, fever, weight loss, and nocturnal diarrhea, coupled with laboratory features of anemia, elevated erythrocyte sedimentation rate, or occult blood in the stool, should alert the clinician to the possibility of IBD. Similarly, finding leukocytes in a stained stool specimen points to an inflammatory basis for the diarrhea. In all cases, stool cultures and parasitologic examination of the stool are required to rule out enteric bacterial pathogens or amebiasis. In the *irritable bowel syndrome*, sigmoidoscopy, rectal biopsy, and barium enema examination are all normal.

Once the diagnosis of idiopathic IBD has been established, the distinction between ulcerative colitis and Crohn's disease of the colon is usually possible. Differential diagnostic features are shown in Table 255-1.

With small-intestinal involvement (regional enteritis), the differential diagnosis should include disorders presenting with intraabdominal abscesses, fistulas, intestinal obstruction, and malabsorption. The finding of associated colonic involvement in patients with ileal disease will often serve to distinguish Crohn's disease from other ileal disorders. With diffuse involvement of the jejunum and ileum, regional enteritis must be distinguished from *nongranulomatous ulcerative jejunoileitis*. Abdominal pain and diarrhea are prominent features of this disorder, and weight loss, malabsorption, and hypoproteinemia tend to be more prominent than in regional enteritis. Small-bowel biopsy shows a more diffuse lesion with flattened villi (similar to celiac sprue), infiltration of the lamina propria, and mucosal ulceration. *Abdominal lymphoma* may likewise present with clinical and radiologic features difficult to distinguish from regional enteritis.

TABLE 255-2 Microbiologic causes of colitis

Shigella
Salmonella
Amebiasis
Yersinia
Campylobacter
Lymphogranuloma venereum (LGV)
''Non-LGV'' *Chlamydia*
Gonorrhea
Pseudomembranous colitis (*Clostridium difficile* toxin)
Tuberculosis

Hepatosplenomegaly and peripheral adenopathy, when present, are helpful clues, but often disease is confined to the intestine. In such cases, laparotomy is usually required to make the definitive histologic diagnosis.

The advanced presentation of regional enteritis with areas of stenosis and draining fistulas also may be confused with *chronic fungal infection of the bowel*, including actinomycosis, aspergillosis, and blastomycosis. These infections often are seen in debilitated patients with impaired host defenses. Fungal skin tests and examination of fistula drainage and biopsy material for characteristic granules and fungi are helpful in making the diagnosis.

Intestinal tuberculosis characteristically produces stenotic lesions, usually in the terminal ileum, also often involving the contiguous cecum and ascending colon. Unlike regional enteritis, skip areas are unusual. Histologically, the granulomatous inflammation seen with *Mycobacterium tuberculosis* infection may be indistinguishable from regional enteritis; acid-fast stains and cultures are required. Fortunately, in western countries primary intestinal tuberculosis is now rare; when intestinal involvement does occur, it invariably is associated with pulmonary tuberculosis.

COMPLICATIONS OF INFLAMMATORY BOWEL DISEASE

The complications of IBD may be classified as local, which are a direct reflection of mucosal inflammation and its extension, or systemic (Table 255-3). Local complications of IBD such as fistulas, abscesses, and strictures have been described above. In addition, perforation, toxic dilatation, and the development of carcinoma may complicate both ulcerative colitis and Crohn's disease.

PERFORATION Intestinal perforation can occur in severe ulcerative colitis since with extensive ulceration the bowel wall may become extremely thin. The clinical features are those of acute peritonitis with signs of peritoneal inflammation and the demonstration of free air under the diaphragm on upright film of the abdomen. These are an indication for immediate colectomy.

Toxic dilatation of the colon may occur in Crohn's colitis but is more common in ulcerative colitis. This complication can best be considered as a severe form of ulcerative colitis with the additional

---

TABLE 255-3 Some systemic complications of inflammatory bowel disease

Nutritional and metabolic
Weight loss, ↓ muscle mass, growth retardation (children)
Electrolyte deficiency (K^+, Ca^{2+}, Mg^{2+})
Hypoalbuminemia (↓ nutrition, protein-losing enteropathy)
Anemia (chronic disease, iron deficiency; rarely folate or vitamin B_{12} deficiency in Crohn's disease)
Bile salt deficiency with ileal disease (steatorrhea and fat-soluble vitamin deficiency; ↑ colonic oxalate absorption → renal stones; ↑ lithogenicity of bile → gallstones)
Musculoskeletal
Peripheral arthralgia, arthritis
Ankylosing spondylitis, sacroiliitis
Granulomatous myositis (rare)
Hepatobiliary disease
Fatty liver
Cholelithiasis
Pericholangitis, biliary cirrhosis (rare)
Sclerosing cholangitis
Bile duct carcinoma
Chronic active hepatitis and cirrhosis
Skin and mucous membrane
Erythema nodosum
Pyoderma gangrenosum
Aphthous stomatitis
Crohn's disease of buccal mucosa, gingiva, vagina
Eye
Iritis, uveitis, episcleritis
Venous thrombosis and thromboembolism (hypercoagulability, dehydration, stasis)

---

feature of colonic dilatation. It is thought that the neuromuscular tone of the bowel is affected by the severe inflammation, resulting in dilatation. Injudicious use of hypomotility agents (codeine, diphenoxylate, loperamide, paregoric, anticholinergic agents) to treat diarrhea in the setting of acute colitis can precipitate this complication. Similarly, cathartic preparation and barium enema examination as well as superimposed hypokalemia may be contributing factors. Clinically, features of severe colitis are present with high fever, tachycardia, volume depletion, electrolyte imbalance, and abdominal pain. On examination, the patient appears toxic, and colonic dilatation may be evident. There is abdominal tenderness, and if perforation has already occurred, peritoneal signs are present. Diarrhea may actually decrease markedly due to colonic atony, creating the false impression that the colitis is clinically improved. Plain film of the abdomen will show colonic dilatation with the colonic diameter more than 6 cm. There may be air in the wall of the colon, and irregular, ulcerated islands of mucosa may be silhouetted against the air shadow. While the transverse colon is the most common site of dilatation, this is probably largely positional, since with the patient supine this is the highest portion of the colon. This presentation of colitis represents a true medical emergency and is associated with a mortality of greater than 30 percent if perforation has occurred. Appropriate therapy is discussed below.

CARCINOMA AND INFLAMMATORY BOWEL DISEASE There is an increased incidence of carcinoma in patients with chronic IBD when compared with the general population, especially in patients who have more extensive mucosal involvement (i.e., pancolitis) and those who have had their disease for extended periods of time. Cumulative risk of cancer begins to rise 10 years after the disease is diagnosed. While the incidence of cancer varies with the patient population studied, it is estimated that the overall incidence of cancer is 0.5 to 1 percent per year after 10 years. It has been estimated that with pancolitis there is a risk of cancer of 12 percent at 15 years, 23 percent at 20 years, and 42 percent at 24 years, although estimates in community-based practices have been lower, with the probability that colon cancer will develop in patients with pancolitis being 10 percent at 26 years. In children, the risk of cancer appears to rise more sharply after the first 10 years of disease, perhaps reflecting the higher incidence of pancolitis in children. Patients with ulcerative proctitis (disease limited to rectum) have no increased risk of cancer. Malignancy developing in Crohn's disease of the colon or small bowel is less well documented, but the incidence of both small- and large-bowel malignancy is increased compared with the general population. However, it is lower than in ulcerative colitis, perhaps because less mucosa is often chronically involved with Crohn's disease than with ulcerative colitis.

The development of colon carcinoma arising in the setting of IBD demonstrates important differences when compared with carcinoma arising in a noncolitic population. Clinically, many of the earlier warning signs of a colonic neoplasm (i.e., rectal bleeding, change in bowel habits) will be difficult to interpret in the setting of colitis. In colitic patients, the distribution of carcinomas is more uniform throughout the colon than in noncolitic patients; in the latter the majority of carcinomas are in the rectosigmoid, within reach of the sigmoidoscope. In colitis patients, the tumors are more often multiple, flat, and infiltrating and appear to have a higher grade of malignancy. There is some evidence to suggest that these features may reflect the younger age at which they occur rather than the associated colitis. Further adding to the difficulty in diagnosis is the frequent occurrence of mucosal irregularities, ulcerations, and pseudopolyps, making a small carcinoma difficult to diagnose radiologically or endoscopically.

Efforts have been directed toward devising effective screening procedures to detect carcinoma developing in the setting of IBD. Carcinoembryonic antigen (CEA) may be elevated nonspecifically in ulcerative colitis and therefore is of limited value. Periodic barium enemas and/or sigmoidoscopy or colonoscopy have been suggested, but interpretation is sometimes hampered by abnormalities related to the colitis itself. The addition of colonic mucosal biopsy may add a significant dimension. It was originally suggested that a generalized precancerous lesion may be present in high-risk patients with colitis who either harbor an occult malignancy or who will develop cancer. Subsequent studies in patients with long-standing colitis showed that if severe dysplasia was present, there was approximately a 50-percent chance that an associated malignancy was present in those patients who subsequently came to colectomy. Complicating these findings was the fact that dysplastic changes were found in rectal biopsies only 60 percent of the time, making colonoscopy with multiple biopsies desirable. In addition, in some patients not undergoing colectomy, dysplasia was not a consistent finding on subsequent biopsies. While more information is needed on the prognostic significance and reproducibility of finding dysplastic changes on mucosal biopsy, it seems prudent to examine patients with colonic IBD of greater than 8 to 10 years' duration with colonoscopy and multiple mucosal biopsies at regular intervals. The frequency of such examinations has not been established, with recommendations varying from 6 months to 2 years. If severe dysplasia is found, then confirmation at less than 6-month intervals seems prudent. While most authorities would not advise "prophylactic" colectomy in the patient with long-standing colitis with mild or moderate dysplasia, the finding of severe dysplasia may well identify a subgroup who already harbor an occult carcinoma or who are at high risk of its development. There can be no uniform recommendation for this small group of patients, but many physicians will advise colectomy in this setting.

EXTRAINTESTINAL MANIFESTATIONS OF INFLAMMATORY BOWEL DISEASE

There are a variety of nonintestinal symptoms and signs which may be associated with IBD and occur in both ulcerative colitis and Crohn's disease (see Table 255-3). Since some of these manifestations may not coincide with or may overshadow the underlying bowel disease, they may on occasion pose difficult diagnostic problems. Their cause is currently unknown.

Joint manifestations occur in 25 percent of patients with IBD. These may range from arthralgia only to an acute arthritis with painful, swollen joints.

The nondeforming arthritis is mono- or polyarticular and often migratory. Knees, ankles, and wrists are most commonly involved, but any joint may be affected. Joint fluid, if aspirated, reveals findings of an acute arthritis without crystals or evidence of infection. Tests for specific forms of arthritis (rheumatoid factor, antinuclear antibody, and LE factor) are negative. Typically, the arthritis correlates with activity of the underlying bowel disease. Rarely, peripheral arthritis may truly antecede clinical bowel symptoms. Arthritis is found more commonly in patients with colonic than with small-bowel involvement alone (regional enteritis).

In contrast, the central arthritis or ankylosing spondylitis associated with IBD is unrelated to the activity of the underlying bowel disease. It may antedate the bowel disease by years and persist after surgical or medical remission of the disease has been achieved. Symptoms are of low backache and stiffness with eventual limitation of motion. This may be associated with sacroiliitis as well. X-rays usually reveal characteristic changes. In contrast to the peripheral arthritis, there is a strong association of HLA-B27 with ankylosing spondylitis, whether or not IBD is present.

Like the peripheral arthritis, *skin manifestations* are more common with colonic disease. They occur in about 15 percent of patients, and when present, the severity correlates with activity of the bowel disease. *Erythema nodosum* may be seen and heals without scarring. *Pyoderma gangrenosum*, an ulcerating lesion often occurring on the trunk, is relatively painless and may heal with scarring. In the rare patient, the lesion may persist even after colectomy for ulcerative colitis. *Aphthous ulcers* resemble "canker sores" of the mouth, and in approximately 5 to 10 percent of patients they are present during periods of active disease and then resolve. Their cause is unknown, and they are treated symptomatically. *Ocular manifestations* such as episcleritis, recurrent iritis, and uveitis occur in approximately 5 percent of patients and may represent a severe manifestation of the disease. In general, their activity parallels the course of the bowel disease, and the lesions may respond dramatically when colectomy is done for other indications.

Abnormalities of *liver function* are common in IBD. In the severely ill, malnourished patient, mild abnormalities of serum aminotransferases and alkaline phosphatase are often seen and represent nonspecific focal hepatitis or fatty infiltration. Factors favoring fatty infiltration of the liver in the severely ill patient are poor nutrition and often concomitant steroid therapy. The lesion is not progressive and resolves with disease remission. *Pericholangitis* is characterized histologically by portal tract inflammation, some bile ductular proliferation, and concentric fibrosis around bile ductules. Some authorities feel that this lesion represents the intrahepatic form of sclerosing cholangitis. Most often, the lesion is clinically insignificant, and its sole manifestation is an elevated serum alkaline phosphatase level. It is usually nonprogressive and requires no therapy. Rarely, there may be an apparent progression to cirrhosis of either the postnecrotic or biliary type. Uncommonly, patients with IBD may develop *sclerosing cholangitis* (Chap. 272), a chronic inflammation of unknown cause involving the extrahepatic and intrahepatic bile ducts which may produce varying degrees of extrahepatic biliary obstruction. Corticosteroids and immunosuppressive therapy are not beneficial. Reversal of the disease after colectomy is an inconsistent result and should not form the sole indication for colectomy. Cholangiocarcinoma, arising in the extrahepatic biliary tree, has an increased incidence in patients with chronic ulcerative colitis. Such patients will present with extrahepatic biliary obstruction which must be distinguished from sclerosing cholangitis. Finally, *chronic active hepatitis* which may progress to *cirrhosis* may be seen in IBD, although the exact relationship between these disorders is unknown. The evaluation and therapy are similar to the disease occurring in noncolitic patients. There is no clear evidence that colectomy influences the course of this form of liver disease.

TREATMENT

In general, the treatment of ulcerative colitis and Crohn's disease shares certain common principles. Initial treatment of all forms of uncomplicated IBD is primarily medical, and the principles of medical therapy are similar. Surgery is reserved for (1) specific complications and (2) intractability of disease. There are certain important differences, however, between ulcerative colitis and Crohn's disease; namely, the response to drug therapy may differ, complications often differ, and the prognosis after surgical therapy is not the same.

ULCERATIVE COLITIS Medical therapy Once the diagnosis is established, the severity of the disease must be assessed. Mild ulcerative colitis, including ulcerative proctitis, can usually be treated on an ambulatory basis. It should be noted that on occasion, disease, although limited to the rectum, may be severe. More severe disease, especially at initial presentation, is best treated in a hospital setting. The disease can worsen rapidly, and the course of a given attack cannot be predicted at the outset. The aims of therapy are to control the inflammatory process and replace nutritional losses. A certain degree of improvement usually follows intravenous correction of fluid and electrolyte disturbances. Blood transfusions may be required in severe anemia, especially when there is continued active bleeding. Agents to control diarrhea (diphenoxylate, loperamide, codeine, anticholinergics) should be used with extreme caution for fear of precipitating colonic dilatation and toxic megacolon. The decision to institute specific nutritional replacement therapy will be determined by the nutritional status of the patient and whether a protracted clinical course can be anticipated. In the severely ill patient, even clear liquids orally may stimulate colonic activity, and it is often wise to give the patients nothing by mouth. In this setting, intravenous alimentation, either peripheral or central, has been used as interim nutritional replacement therapy (see Chap. 76). While there is no evidence that intravenous alimentation is effective as primary therapy, it is an important component of a treatment program. In the less severely ill patients able to tolerate fluids by mouth, the use of elemental oral diets may be beneficial, providing supplemental nutrition with low fecal volume. While milk is not contraindicated in ulcerative colitis, diarrhea will be exacerbated if there is an associated lactase deficiency.

The principal drugs used in the therapy of ulcerative colitis are the *anti-inflammatory agents, sulfasalazine* (Azulfidine), and *adrenal glucocorticoids.* Sulfasalazine consists of a sulfonamide (sulfapyridine) moiety chemically bound to a salicylate (5-aminosalicylate); it undergoes bacterial cleavage in the colon. The liberated sulfapyridine is efficiently absorbed and largely excreted in the urine; the liberated 5-aminosalicylate, believed to be the active component, remains largely in the colon and is excreted in the stool. The salicylate moiety is thought to exert its action through inhibition of prostaglandin synthesis. While most physicians are familiar with the use of sulfasalazine to prevent recurrences of ulcerative colitis, it is less well appreciated that this agent is effective in the therapy of acute ulcerative colitis of mild to moderate severity. Therapeutic doses of 4 to 6 g/d are required. The drug is usually started at a dose of 500 mg bid and then increased daily or every other day by 1 g until the therapeutic dose is achieved. Topical preparations of 5-aminosalicylate (mesalamine) given as an enema are effective in the control of distal proctocolitis. Several preparations of oral 5-aminosalicylate (encapsulated in a pH-sensitive slow-release form or as two molecules of 5-aminosalicylate conjugated to each other as a dimer) are also effective.

In the severely ill patient who may not tolerate oral medication and for whom a more rapid time frame of therapy is often desired, initial therapy is begun with glucocorticoids. While ACTH is equally effective when given in equivalent dosages and by comparable routes of administration, most physicians seldom use ACTH. The choice is one of individual preference; oral prednisone (45 to 60 mg/d) is usually employed initially. In the severely ill patient, parenteral administration of corticosteroids (i.e., intravenous prednisolone, 45 to 60 mg/d) is preferable to avoid the uncertainty of adequate oral absorption. Improvement is usually noted after 7 to 10 days of such therapy by a reduction in fever, decrease in bloody diarrhea, and improvement in appetite.

After initial improvement, low-roughage oral feedings can be resumed. At this point, the dose of steroids can be tapered. There is no specific schedule for tapering glucocorticoids. The guiding principle, however, is that once clinical remission is achieved, there is no evidence that chronic steroid administration favorably influences the long-term outlook of the disease or that recurrences can be prevented by chronic steroid therapy. In practice, steroid therapy can be tapered and discontinued over a 2- to 3-month period after discharge. In some patients (10 to 15 percent), efforts to completely eliminate steroids may be associated with a flare of the disease, and low to moderate steroids (10 to 15 mg prednisone daily) may be required to suppress disease activity. This should not be confused with the prophylactic administration of steroids to patients in remission but rather represents incompletely responsive disease. Once the acutely ill patient is taking oral feedings, sulfasalazine should be added as described above in a daily dose of 2 g. Controlled trials have shown that this dose of sulfasalazine, when administered chronically to patients with ulcerative colitis, is effective in decreasing the frequency of relapses and should be continued chronically after glucocorticoids have been discontinued. Patients with glucose phosphate dehydrogenase deficiency or those exhibiting severe allergic reactions to the drug unfortunately cannot be maintained on it. Patients who exhibit intolerance for the drug (headache, nausea) or mild skin allergic reactions can be treated with formulations of 5-aminosalicylate (see above), thus avoiding allergic reactions due to sulfa. Targeted systems for the delivery of the active moiety, 5-aminosalicylate (mesalamine), provide a number of options for the physician. Mesalamine enemas

are effective topical therapy for distal ulcerative colitis and are necessary to maintain remission. Oral formulations of 5-aminosalicylate (see above) also can be employed in patients intolerant of sulfasalazine who prefer oral to topical therapy.

The use of immunosuppressive therapy with drugs such as azathioprine is less well established in ulcerative colitis. As a single agent in the therapy of acute ulcerative colitis, the drug is ineffective. However, the drug may be added to the regimen at a dose of 1.5 to 2.0 mg/kg when glucocorticoids fail or when the steroid dose needed to reduce inflammation is too high. It is desirable to monitor the blood count and observe the patient carefully for infection. Azathioprine also may have a limited role as a "steroid-sparing agent" in the patient with chronic ulcerative colitis who must be maintained on corticosteroids to control disease activity. Cyclosporine, a potent immunosuppressive agent, also has been found to be beneficial in severely ill patients, with marked improvement in this group of patients otherwise requiring colectomy. In these patients, the limited use of cyclosporine may be indicated.

Toxic megacolon is a major complication of severe ulcerative colitis which requires rapid, intensive management, best carried out jointly by the internist or gastroenterologist and surgeon. Once the diagnosis is established, prompt and vigorous use of intravenous fluids, electrolyte replacement therapy, and blood transfusions are indicated. Because of the fear of perforation and high likelihood that bacteremia and occult perforation have occurred, many physicians institute broad-spectrum antibiotic coverage after appropriate cultures have been obtained. The patient is given nothing by mouth, and nasogastric suction is often instituted. Full intravenous corticosteroid therapy is also begun. Majority opinion favors an initial period of medical stabilization for the first 24 to 48 h. If significant objective improvement has not occurred, and if perforation seems imminent, emergency colectomy should be carried out. While it is certainly true that some patients, under maximal medical therapy, may slowly improve and thus avoid colectomy, the risk of this course of action must be considered carefully. If perforation occurs, mortality rates rise sharply, approaching 50 percent in those who subsequently go on to colectomy.

At the other end of the spectrum is the patient with mild ulcerative colitis, limited to the rectum or rectosigmoid, who is managed on an ambulatory basis. Therapy is started with sulfasalazine, 0.5 to 1.0 g four times a day with meals. Alternatively, in the sulfa-allergic patient, 5-aminosalicylate enemas or oral 5-aminosalicylate preparations can be substituted. If rectal symptoms such as tenesmus are prominent, topical steroids in the form of small enemas may produce marked improvement. The equivalent of 100 mg hydrocortisone (20 mg prednisone) in 60 to 100 mL saline is used as a bedtime enema. On occasion, the use of steroid foam preparations may be better tolerated in the patient with severe tenesmus. Retention enemas have been shown to deliver medication as far as the descending colon, and absorption of steroid is small (10 to 20 percent). If large doses of rectal steroids are required for control, it is preferable to use oral prednisone at a moderate dosage (20 mg/d).

Psychotherapy The elements of trust and mutual understanding combined with the compassion and expertise of the physician are essential in the therapy of any chronic disease and are particularly important in the long-term management of patients with inflammatory bowel disease. Often these patients are intelligent young adults who are frequently resentful of a disease affecting them during the most productive years. Through the vigorous participation of the physician, many patients are able to lead reasonably stable and productive lives. More formal psychiatric assistance may be required in the chronically ill patient, in particular children or adolescents, or in the elderly, in whom severe depressive reactions are common. This is particularly true when colectomy is being advised and in the emotional adjustment which must be made after colectomy.

Pregnancy and ulcerative colitis While many physicians are apprehensive about the management and prognosis of ulcerative colitis in the pregnant patient, the outcome for the patient and the fetus is excellent. In general, the pregnancy is not threatened by coexistent colitis, with no increase in stillbirths or premature deliveries when compared with the general population. When patients with inactive colitis become pregnant, approximately 50 percent may have an exacerbation of their disease, with some clustering of these flares during the first trimester and in the postpartum period. The therapy of ulcerative colitis during pregnancy is largely the same as in the nonpregnant patient. Sulfasalazine is used to treat mild to moderate disease, since there is no evidence that the drug is harmful to the fetus or leads to increased incidence of fetal malformations. Women with inactive colitis who enter a pregnancy on maintenance sulfasalazine should be continued on the drug to protect the mother during the postpartum period from a relapse of disease. Corticosteroids should be used in the same dosage and for the same indications as in the nonpregnant patient. Immunosuppressive agents should not be used during pregnancy.

Thus it is clear that the patient with colitis can realistically plan to have a family. It is prudent, however, to bring active disease under control before pregnancy is undertaken to ensure the most optimal physical and emotional setting for the pregnancy. Similar conclusions apply to the management of Crohn's disease during pregnancy.

Surgical therapy Approximately 20 to 25 percent of patients with ulcerative colitis will require colectomy during the course of their disease. A major indication for colectomy is failure to respond to intensive medical management. Such patients, although not showing colonic dilatation, may fail to improve after 7 to 10 days of optimal medical therapy. Fever, persistent bloody diarrhea, and severe fatigue may persist, and consideration should be given to semielective colectomy. Elective colectomy may be performed in patients whose disease remains chronically active and who require continuous corticosteroid administration. Such patients are at risk of developing the complications of chronic steroid therapy. After colectomy, these patients often feel more energetic and usually gain back weight to their preillness level. As discussed above, the patient with long-standing colitis is at high risk for colonic cancer. While most authorities do not advise "prophylactic" colectomy in the patient with quiescent disease, the finding of marked dysplasia on colonoscopic biopsies done as a part of a surveillance program should make the physician think seriously about advising colectomy.

The decision to advise colectomy in other than emergency circumstances is difficult for both patient and physician. Many patients have an understandable reluctance to undergo colectomy and have difficulty in conceptualizing life with an ileostomy. In most metropolitan centers there are ileostomy groups who visit patients preoperatively and can provide answers to many practical questions. It is also desirable for the patient to be visited by a nurse familiar with stoma care to instruct the patient on the practical aspects of handling the ileostomy.

While total proctocolectomy with permanent ileostomy has been the standard surgical procedure for almost all patients undergoing colectomy, several alternative approaches may be desirable. The *continent ileostomy* is an ileal loop reservoir fashioned under the skin with a nipple valve to prevent spilling of ileal contents. Ileal effluent collects in this reservoir, which must be emptied with a soft rubber catheter. Only a small stoma is externally visible, thus eliminating an external ileostomy appliance. Problems with leakage and frequent revisions have made this procedure less attractive. There is great enthusiasm for ileal-rectal anastomosis with an internal ileal pouch created to act as a reservoir. This often produces a highly satisfactory result, with continence and five to seven stools per day. Complications such as pouchitis or the need for surgical revision seem less frequent than with the continent ileostomy. The procedure is an excellent alternative for those patients who will not accept an ileostomy.

CROHN'S DISEASE The medical management of colonic Crohn's disease is similar in most respects to that of ulcerative colitis. In a multicenter study (National Cooperative Crohn's Disease Study), sulfasalazine was shown to be effective in the therapy of active colonic disease. Glucocorticoids also were efficacious but less so than

with small-bowel involvement. The indications and dosages of these medications are similar to those for ulcerative colitis. Since in Crohn's disease intraabdominal sepsis can result from fistula or abscess formation, corticosteroids must be used with caution, and constant attention is required to detect evidence of sepsis, which can be masked by these agents. In general, the disease is less explosive in onset, and although toxic dilatation and perforation can occur, they are less common than in ulcerative colitis. The principles of management are the same. Because of the indolent nature of the disease, the response to therapy is often less complete than in ulcerative colitis, and the disease tends to progress despite apparent clinical inactivity. It may be more difficult to achieve a clinical remission and to withdraw steroids completely. As in ulcerative colitis, controlled studies have shown no benefit to continuing steroids after remission, since the frequency of recurrence is not altered by prophylactic steroid therapy. Disappointingly, sulfasalazine did not decrease recurrence rates in Crohn's disease.

While response to therapy of the initial attack of Crohn's colitis may be satisfactory, many patients continue to have persistently active disease. This may express itself as progressive weight loss, diarrhea, and deterioration of general health. Perianal disease with predominantly left-sided colonic involvement (fistula formation and perirectal abscesses) may constitute a recurrent problem. In one controlled study, *metronidazole* (20 mg/kg per day in divided dosage) resulted in marked improvement in 10 of 18 patients with chronic perineal fistulas associated with Crohn's disease. It is not clear whether the drug is active because of its antibacterial properties or through another mechanism. It is possible that this drug may prove to be of value in the therapy of the perineal complications of Crohn's disease before surgical therapy is attempted. The role of immunosuppressive therapy in the treatment of Crohn's disease has become better established in recent years. The use of 6-mercaptopurine or azathioprine (1.5 to 2.0 mg/kg) has been shown to decrease activity, close or decrease the activity of fistulas, exert a steroid-sparing effect, and may decrease relapse rate if used as maintenance therapy. Often, adding these drugs to a maximal program in the nonresponding patient produces beneficial results. However, a beneficial response may take 3 to 4 months.

The management of Crohn's disease of the small intestine (regional enteritis) is similar to that for colonic Crohn's disease, and as noted, many patients have concomitant small- and large-bowel disease. Several additional considerations are pertinent, however. *Intestinal obstruction* is not uncommonly a presenting feature with ileal involvement. Initially, this may be secondary to acute inflammation and will respond to corticosteroids. With recurrent involvement and the development of fibrosis, steroid therapy is less effective, and surgical decompression is required. *Nutritional problems* often are more severe with involvement of the small intestine than with colonic involvement alone. Added to the general catabolic nature of the disease may be loss of absorptive surface, which may result from progressive involvement or because of surgical resection. Refinements in the technique of parenteral alimentation have made it possible to provide a patient's total daily caloric intake intravenously for a period of weeks or even months (see Chap. 76). Parenteral alimentation has been employed with increasing frequency in the severely ill patient as a means of placing the gastrointestinal tract "at rest" and in preparing the malnourished patient for surgery. With this approach, the disease may become quiescent, and the drainage from fistulas may decrease. However, disease activity frequently recurs when oral feedings are resumed. On occasion, prolonged intravenous alimentation, administered at home, may be required when oral feedings are not effective or in children exhibiting severe growth failure associated with Crohn's disease. Most often it is possible to design a dietary program of oral supplementation to nourish the patient adequately.

In patients with extensive small-bowel involvement or in those with a short bowel resulting from extensive intestinal resection, supplementation of electrolytes, minerals, and vitamins will be required. Extensive ileal disease or resection often results in diarrhea induced by bile salts and in malabsorption; cholestyramine may be needed to control the diarrhea, and medium-chain triglycerides may need to be added to reduce fat malabsorption (see Chap. 254). In patients with stenotic segments of intestine, a low-residue (low-fiber) diet should be recommended. A lactose-free diet should be instituted if there is an associated lactase deficiency. Other dietary modifications have not been shown to have any beneficial effect on the primary disease process. Patients should be encouraged to eat a nutritious, appealing diet of their own choosing. *Surgical therapy* is generally reserved for the complications of Crohn's disease rather than as a primary form of therapy. In contrast to ulcerative colitis, more patients with Crohn's disease will require surgery in the chronic management of the disease. Approximately 70 percent of patients will require at least one operation during the course of their disease. Although each case and situation must be individualized, in general, surgery may be required (1) for persistent or fixed bowel narrowing or obstruction, (2) for symptomatic fistula formation to the bladder, vagina, or skin, (3) for persistent anal fistulas or abscesses, and (4) for intraabdominal abscesses, toxic dilatation of the colon, or perforation. In contrast to ulcerative colitis, where colectomy is curative, in Crohn's disease surgical resection of the small or large intestine is followed by a high rate of recurrence. With resection of segments of small bowel or ileum and reanastomosis, a recurrence rate of 50 to 75 percent over a 5-year period is not unusual. Recurrence of disease is invariably proximal to the created anastomosis. When total colectomy and ileostomy are performed for Crohn's disease of the colon without significant small-intestinal involvement, recurrence rates are lower, varying from 10 to 30 percent. Despite these recurrences, most patients do not develop a short bowel syndrome and usually can expect significant improvement. Faced with the possibility of recurrent disease, many physicians are reluctant to advise surgery in Crohn's disease, except for the type of clear-cut complications described above. Alternatively, patients with persistently active disease may require chronic maintenance on unacceptably high levels of corticosteroids and with the appreciable risk of steroid side effects. Just as a failure of medical therapy should lead to colectomy in ulcerative colitis, it should be the conclusion in the patient with Crohn's colitis without major small-bowel involvement. While in this setting there is also a definite rate of recurrence, such recurrences are often not disabling. When extensive small-bowel disease is present, surgical therapy is often not feasible and should only be reserved for specific disease complications. In selected patients, limited surgical procedures (strictureplasty) can be employed to open highly strictured areas and avoid further resective surgery.

The therapy of Crohn's disease in children presents special problems, since normal growth and development may be retarded in the presence of active disease. In addition to conventional drug therapy, intensive nutritional therapy or the judicious use of surgery may be required.

PROGNOSIS

The overall prognosis of IBD has been favorably affected by the use of corticosteroids and sulfasalazine, as well as by supportive techniques such as intravenous alimentation. In *acute* ulcerative colitis, these therapeutic modalities can result in a remission in almost 90 percent of patients. The mortality of an initial acute attack is approximately 5 percent. Poor prognostic factors and an increased mortality rate are likely when there is total colonic involvement, when the onset occurs over age 60, and when toxic megacolon develops.

The long-term prognosis of *chronic* ulcerative colitis is more difficult to assess due to the variable and intermittent nature of the disease and improvements in therapy. Left-sided colitis and ulcerative proctitis have a very favorable prognosis and probably no increase in mortality; similarly, the long-term prognosis for extensive colitis has improved greatly. Older studies suggested a poor prognosis for extensive colitis, with less than 50 percent of patients surviving 15 years after onset. More recent observations (longest follow-up 11

years) show a 10-year mortality rate of between 5 and 10 percent for severe first attacks (excluding toxic megacolon). Approximately 75 percent of patients will experience relapses, and 20 to 25 percent will require colectomy. The problem of carcinoma developing in the setting of long-standing chronic ulcerative colitis is an important factor in determining the long-term prognosis of ulcerative colitis. As discussed above, periodic surveillance with colonoscopy and multiple biopsies to detect dysplastic changes are indicated to detect a high-risk group for which to advise colectomy.

The prognosis for Crohn's disease is not as favorable as for ulcerative colitis. An exception is *acute regional enteritis*, often discovered during laparotomy for suspected appendicitis; this has an excellent prognosis. More than two-thirds of such patients may show no subsequent evidence of regional enteritis, and this form of acute ileitis may well be due to *Yersinia* infection (see above). Prevailing surgical opinion favors a conservative approach in this situation, and in most instances operative resection is not advised.

In the majority of patients with Crohn's disease, the course is chronic and intermittent regardless of the site of involvement. The disease responds less well to medical therapy with time, and over two-thirds of patients develop complications requiring surgery at some point in their disease. In contrast to ulcerative colitis, where mortality appears greatest early in the disease, in Crohn's disease the mortality rate increases with the duration of the disease and probably ranges from 5 to 10 percent. Most deaths occur from peritonitis and sepsis. As indicated above, following surgery, patients with Crohn's disease often have recurrence and relapses. Nevertheless, the therapy of Crohn's disease will result in reasonably stable and productive lives for most Crohn's disease patients.

REFERENCES

General

KIRSNER JB, SHORTER RG (EDS): *Inflammatory Bowel Disease*, 3d ed. Philadelphia, Lea & Febiger, 1988
PODOLSKY DK: Inflammatory bowel disease. N Engl J Med 325:928, 1991
SLEISENGER MH, FORDTRAN JS (EDS): *Gastrointestinal Diseases*, 4th ed. Philadelphia, Saunders, 1989
STENSON WF, MACDERMOTT RP: Inflammatory bowel disease, in *Textbook of Gastroenterology*, T Yamada et al (eds). Philadephia, Lippincott, 1991

Etiology and diagnostic aspects

BLASER MJ, RELLER LB: *Campylobacter* enteritis. N Engl J Med 305:1444, 1981
GOLDBERG HI et al: Computed tomography in the evaluation of Crohn's disease. Am J Roent 140:277, 1983
GREENSTEIN AJ et al: The extraintestinal complications of ulcerative colitis and Crohn's disease: A study of 700 patients. Medicine 55:401, 1976
JESS P: Acute terminal ileitis: A review of recent literature on the relationship to Crohn's disease. Scand J Gastroenterol 16:321, 1981
MACDERMOTT RP, STENSON WF: Alterations of the immune system in ulcerative colitis and Crohn's disease. Adv Immunol 42:285, 1988
QUINN TC et al: *Chlamydia trachomatis* proctitis. N Engl J Med 305:195, 1981
SURAWICZ CM, BELIC L: Rectal biopsy helps to distinguish acute self limited colitis from idiopathic inflammatory bowel disease. Gastroenterology 86:104, 1984
VAN TRAPPEN G et al: *Yersinia* enteritis and enterocolitis: Gastroenterological aspects. Gastroenterology 72:220, 1977

Therapy of inflammatory bowel disease

AZAD KHAN AK et al: Optimum dose of sulphasalazine for maintenance treatment in ulcerative colitis. Gut 12:232, 1980
BRANDT LJ et al: Metronidazole therapy for perineal Crohn's disease: A follow-up study. Gastroenterology 83:383, 1982
COLLINS RH et al: Colon cancer in ulcerative colitis. Gastroenterology 94:1089, 1988
DONALDSON RM JR: Management of medical problems in pregnancy: Inflammatory bowel disease. N Engl J Med 312:1616, 1985
EKBOM A et al: Ulcerative colitis and colorectal cancer. N Engl J Med 323:1228, 1990
FABRICIUS PJ et al: Crohn's disease in the elderly. Gut 26:461, 1985
FARMER RG et al: Long-term follow-up of patients with Crohn's disease. Relationship between clinical pattern and prognosis. Gastroenterology 88:1818, 1985
GAGINELLA TS, WALSH RE: Sulfasalazine: Multiplicity of action. Dig Dis Sci 37:801, 1992
KELTS DG et al: Nutritional basis of growth failure in children and adolescents with Crohn's disease. Gastroenterology 76:720, 1979
LENNARD JONES JE et al: Cancer in colitis: Assessment of the individual risk by clinical and histological criteria. Gastroenterology 73:1280, 1977
PEMBERTON JH et al: Ileal pouch—Anal anastomosis for chronic ulcerative colitis. Long-term results. Ann Surg 206:504, 1987

PEPPERCORN MA: Advances in drug therapy for inflammatory bowel disease. Ann Intern Med 112:50, 1990

PRESENT DH et al: 6-Mercaptopurine in the management of inflammatory bowel disease: short- and long-term toxicity. Ann Intern Med 111:641, 1989

RANSOHOFF DF et al: Ulcerative colitis and colon cancer: Problems in analyzing the diagnostic usefulness of mucosal dysplasia. Dis Colon Rectum 28:383, 1985

RIDDELL RH et al: Dysplasia in inflammatory bowel disease. Hum Pathol 14:931, 1983

SANDBORN WJ et al: Ulcerative colitis disease activity following treatment of associated primary sclerosing cholangitis with cyclosporin. Gut 34:242, 1993

SCHROEDER KW et al: Coated oral 5-aminosalicylate acid therapy for mild to moderately active ulcerative colitis. A randomized study. N Engl J Med 317:1625, 1987

SUGITA A et al: Colorectal cancer in ulcerative colitis: Influence of anatomical extent and age at onset in colitis-cancer interval. Gut 32:169, 1991

URSING B et al: A comparative study of metronidazole and sulfasalazine for active Crohn's disease. The Cooperative Crohn's Disease Study in Sweden. Gastroenterology 83:550, 1982

256 DISEASES OF THE SMALL AND LARGE INTESTINE

J. THOMAS LaMONT / KURT J. ISSELBACHER

SYMPTOMS OF INTESTINAL DISEASE

SYMPTOMS OF SMALL-INTESTINAL DISEASE The major clinical manifestations of small-bowel disease are *motility disturbances*, abdominal *pain* and *distention*, gastrointestinal *bleeding*, and *malabsorption*.

Altered intestinal peristalsis is a common manifestation of a variety of diseases. The presentation may be one of decreased motility, such as paralytic ileus resulting from metabolic disturbance or peritonitis, or intestinal obstruction caused by tumors, adhesions, volvulus, or intussusception (Chap. 258). Diarrhea frequently accompanies small-bowel disease (Chap. 39) resulting from direct mucosal involvement by inflammatory or infiltrative lesions (sprue, regional enteritis). The associated malabsorption of fat and bile salts is an important factor in the pathogenesis of diarrhea in these conditions (Chaps. 39 and 254).

Abdominal pain due to small-intestinal disease is usually periumbilical or supraumbilical and often poorly localized. With obstruction, pain is classically described as intermittent or colicky. Visceral pain arises from distention or stretching of the intestinal wall or from inflammation of the overlying parietal peritoneum. As the intestine becomes progressively dilated with loss of muscular tone, the colicky nature of the pain may become less apparent. Acute inflammation of the small intestine which involves the visceral or parietal peritoneum is associated with steady, aching pain, usually located directly over the inflamed area, and may be accompanied by guarding and rebound tenderness if the parietal peritoneum is involved. *Gastrointestinal bleeding* due to small-bowel disease may be detected as occult bleeding or, less commonly, brisk hemorrhage. In general, bleeding from the stomach or small intestine causes black or tarry stool (melena), while bleeding from the colon causes passage of red blood or clots. Obviously, the appearance of blood in the stool depends not only on site of bleeding but also on the rate of the hemorrhage and the rapidity of transit; thus localization of the bleeding site by stool appearance alone may be misleading.

An important clue to the presence of small-bowel disease is the presence of fat malabsorption. With extensive mucosal damage or lymphatic obstruction, the presenting symptoms may relate to any of the features of a malabsorption syndrome or protein-losing enteropathy (Chap. 254) and should direct attention to the small intestine.

SYMPTOMS OF COLONIC DISEASE The major symptoms of colonic disease are *alteration in bowel habit*, *rectal bleeding*, and *pain*. Alteration in bowel habit implies a change from previous patterns of defecation; hence a detailed history is important. Most normal individuals have one to three movements of well-formed

stools each day. *Diarrhea* means the passage of watery or loose stools usually with increased frequency, while *constipation* implies infrequent passage of hard, dry stools; *obstipation* is the absence of spontaneous bowel movements. A persistent change in bowel habit, particularly in older individuals with no previous irregularity, is usually an important early symptom of organic disease of the colon and should never be labeled *functional* unless a thorough diagnostic evaluation is negative. The appearance of the stool also may provide important diagnostic clues. Blood coating the exterior of a formed stool implies a lesion in the anal canal or rectum, while blood admixed with the feces indicates a bleeding source higher in the colon. Brisk hemorrhage from the colon or distal small intestine results in passage of fresh blood, called *hematochezia*. This may appear as fresh blood and clots if the lesion is in the left colon or darker, maroon-colored blood if the bleeding source is in the right colon.

Pain resulting from colonic disease is usually localized to either of the lower abdominal quadrants, as opposed to pain of small-intestinal origin, which is localized to the periumbilical area or higher. Rectal pain is often felt deep in the pelvis, while pain in the anal canal is accurately localized to the perineum. The mechanisms of colonic pain are similar to those in other intestinal viscera (see Chap. 13). Distention from gas or fluid causes crampy or colicky pain from stretching of the muscle layers and resulting contraction or spasm. Pain of this type is often relieved by passage of flatus or stool. Pain also may result if the colonic wall is inflamed or infiltrated by tumor. Acute colonic inflammation which involves the visceral or parietal peritoneum produces sharply localized pain, which may be accompanied by abdominal guarding and rebound tenderness. An important symptom of rectal disease is *tenesmus*, or painful straining at stool, with a sensation of incomplete emptying after defecation. This symptom can be caused by retention of stool in the rectum, by tumors of the rectum which simulate retained stools, or by colonic inflammation.

DIAGNOSTIC PROCEDURES

PHYSICAL EXAMINATION Careful *examination* of the abdomen may disclose a mass or fistula associated with inflammatory or neoplastic disease, localized tenderness, or abdominal distention resulting from ileus or intestinal obstruction. The physical examination and findings in the patient with acute abdominal pain are discussed in Chap. 13.

Thorough examination also may reveal extraintestinal findings associated with small-intestinal diseases. Thus buccal pigmentation or telangiectasia may indicate coexistent small-bowel polyposis or intestinal telangiectasia and may clarify episodes of abdominal pain or chronic bleeding. Similarly, evidence of iritis, arthritis, or erythema nodosum may suggest the presence of inflammatory bowel disease.

Perhaps the most important part of the physical examination in the diagnosis of colonic diseases is the *digital rectal examination*. This procedure should never be omitted for reasons of modesty or fear of embarrassment because it is essential in the diagnosis of perianal, sphincteric, and ampullary lesions; prostatic and uterine abnormalities; and even small rectal masses. A metastatic tumor may be felt in the perirectal tissues as a shelflike deformity (Blumer's shelf), especially anteriorly above the prostate. The fecal material on the glove should be immediately tested with guaiac-impregnated cards for occult blood. Approximately one-half of all rectal carcinomas lie within reach of the index finger, and omission of the rectal examination may delay diagnosis and worsen the prognosis.

STOOL EXAMINATION Abnormal stools constitute important objective evidence of colonic disease. Stools should be examined by the physician as soon as possible after defecation for the presence of visible blood on the surface or within the specimen. A small sample should be tested for occult blood. Microscopic examination of fresh stool is important in the diagnosis of parasitic diseases, particularly in amebic colitis when motile trophozoites can be seen in fresh, warm stool suspensions. Stool suspensions also can be stained with a drop of methylene blue for polymorphonuclear leukocytes, which indicate the presence of an acute inflammatory exudate, such as occurs in ulcerative colitis, amebic colitis, and bacillary dysentery. Fixed and stained slides of stool also may reveal amebas and other parasites, while stool culture is essential for the diagnosis of bacillary dysentery. Sudan III stain of stool is a useful screening test for steatorrhea.

BARIUM STUDIES   The considerable length of the small intestine (some 4 to 7 m in the adult) makes *radiologic studies* of the small bowel of prime importance, and these studies usually form the basis for the diagnosis of small-bowel diseases. *Small-bowel x-rays* are not usually part of a routine upper gastrointestinal series and must be specifically requested. In view of the length of the small bowel and wide variations in transit time, it is essential to provide the radiologist with as much information as possible, since the precise nature of the problem may determine various technical aspects of the examination. Enteroclysis is a specialized small-bowel barium study during which barium is infused rapidly via a nasogastric tube into the jejunum. This technique allows distention of bowel loops and rapid filling of the entire small intestine, thus avoiding the problems of inadequate distention and poor transit sometimes encountered in routine small-bowel barium studies. Enteroclysis is indicated in patients with suspected small-bowel lesions not visualized by ordinary barium studies.

Barium enema is a useful diagnostic tool for the identification of certain colonic diseases, including diverticulosis and its complications, motility disturbances, and displacement of the colon by extrinsic lesions. Barium enema is also useful for detection of loss of haustral markings in chronic ulcerative colitis and for diagnosis of intestinal fistulas. Fiberoptic colonoscopy is more accurate for the diagnosis of early changes of inflammatory bowel disease or for detection of colonic neoplasms. Colonoscopy offers the additional advantage of allowing biopsy of suspicious lesions and removal of most polyps.

SIGMOIDOSCOPY   The technique of fiberoptic sigmoidoscopy is not difficult to master, and with practice, the discomfort to the patient is minimal. The availability of flexible fiberoptic sigmoidoscopes now makes it possible to examine the lower 40 to 60 cm of the colon, compared with the 25-cm limit of the rigid sigmoidoscope. Flexible sigmoidoscopy is generally less painful than rigid sigmoidoscopy. Because approximately half of all colorectal neoplasms lie in the distal 50 cm of the bowel, sigmoidoscopy is an important diagnostic tool. It should be stressed that a rectal carcinoma can be missed on routine barium enema yet easily visualized and biopsied through the sigmoidoscope. Furthermore, the earliest changes of ulcerative colitis may not be demonstrated radiographically but may be obvious through the sigmoidoscope. Rectal biopsy is easily and painlessly accomplished through the instrument and is associated with minimal morbidity except in the presence of bleeding disorders.

COLONOSCOPY   See Chap. 250.

MESENTERIC ANGIOGRAPHY   Angiography is helpful in the diagnosis of two conditions: intestinal ischemia and gastrointestinal hemorrhage. Patients suspected of having acute intestinal ischemia from arterial embolus as well as chronic ischemia (intestinal angina) should undergo angiography to locate the site of blockage. Angiography may be diagnostic in some patients with acute gastrointestinal blood loss, especially when bleeding exceeds 0.5 mL/min.

RADIONUCLIDE BLEEDING SCAN   Bleeding from the small or large bowel can be localized in certain circumstances by radionuclide scanning of the abdomen after intravenous injection of technetium 99m sulfur colloid or autologous red cells labeled with the same agent (Fig. 256-1). If the patient is bleeding at a rate of 0.1 to 0.5 mL/min or greater, the location of radioactivity in the abdomen may indicate the source of bleeding. This diagnostic approach usually requires confirmation by another diagnostic modality such as angiography or endoscopy. The radionuclide bleeding scan is noninvasive, a particular advantage in older patients with bleeding from the small bowel or colon. The bleeding scan is not recommended in patients with suspected bleeding from the esophagus, stomach, or duodenum, who are best studied by upper endoscopy.

DISORDERS OF INTESTINAL MOTILITY

A major function of the intestinal tract is to propel the intestinal contents (food, secretions, chyme, feces) from stomach toward anus. Abnormalities of motility comprise the most common intestinal diseases: diverticulosis, megacolon, constipation, and irritable bowel syndrome. Although these conditions share a common abnormality, i.e., dysmotility, their clinical features are quite diverse.

DIVERTICULOSIS   Diverticula may be either congenital or acquired and may affect either the small or large intestine. Congenital diverticula are herniations of the entire thickness of intestinal wall, while the more common acquired diverticula consist of herniations of the mucosa through the muscularis, generally at the site of a nutrient artery.

Small-intestinal diverticula   Diverticula may occur in any portion of the small intestine; however, with the exception of Meckel's diverticulum, the most common locations are in the duodenum and jejunum. Most often diverticula are asymptomatic and discovered incidentally on upper gastrointestinal x-rays. On occasion, however, they may cause symptoms either because of their anatomic proximity to other structures or rarely from inflammation or bleeding.

Duodenal diverticula arise singly from the medial surface of the second portion of the duodenum. In most patients, they cause no symptoms. Rarely, they may present as acute diverticulitis with abdominal pain, fever, gastrointestinal bleeding, or, most rarely, perforation. Periampullary diverticula are occasionally associated with cholangitis or pancreatitis. Jejunal diverticula, while less common,

10 min   **30 min**

FIGURE 256-1 Radionuclide bleeding scan using intravenous injection of technetium-labeled autologous red cells. Ten minutes after injection, a blush appears in the right abdomen over the cecum (*arrow*). Thirty minutes after injection, the blush has increased in intensity. The cardiac blood pool is noted at the top. Surgery revealed a bleeding diverticulum in the cecum.

also may be the site of acute inflammation, bleeding, or perforation with resulting abscess or peritonitis.

Multiple jejunal diverticula may be associated with a malabsorption syndrome related to bacterial overgrowth within the diverticula, similar to other situations where intestinal stasis (i.e., blind loops) permits bacterial proliferation. The consequences of bacterial proliferation with resultant mucosal damage, deconjugation of bile salts, and vitamin B_{12} malabsorption are discussed in Chap. 254.

Meckel's diverticulum, a persistent omphalomesenteric duct, is the most frequent congenital anomaly of the digestive tract, occurring in approximately 2 percent of autopsied adults. The diverticulum is wide-mouthed, about 5 cm long, and arises from the antimesenteric border of the ileum, usually within 100 cm of the ileocecal valve. The sac may be lined with normal ileal mucosa (approximately 50 percent) or contain gastric, duodenal, pancreatic, or colonic mucosa. While rarely symptomatic after age 5, Meckel's diverticulum may produce hemorrhage, inflammation, and obstruction in children and teenagers.

Hemorrhage occurs almost exclusively before age 10 and invariably results from peptic ulceration of ileal mucosa adjacent to a Meckel's diverticulum lined with gastric mucosa. The diagnosis may be established by isotope scanning of the abdomen after injection of technetium, which is taken up by the ectopic gastric mucosa in the diverticulum. False-negative and false-positive Meckel's scans are not uncommon; thus other clinical and laboratory features must be assessed carefully before recommending surgery. In older children and young adults, inflammation of the diverticulum may mimic acute appendicitis. Mechanical obstruction also may occur if the diverticulum intussuscepts into the lumen of the bowel or twists on a fibrous remnant of the omphalomesenteric duct which extends from the diverticulum to the abdominal wall. The treatment of any of these complications of Meckel's diverticulum is surgical excision.

Colonic diverticula Diverticula of the colon are herniations or saclike protrusions of the mucosa through the muscularis, at the point where a nutrient artery penetrates the muscularis. Diverticula occur most commonly in the sigmoid colon and decrease in frequency in the proximal colon. They increase with age, and the incidence ranges between 20 and 50 percent in western populations over age 50. The exact mechanism for their formation is unknown but may be related to an increase in intraluminal pressure. Thickening of the muscle coat of the colon in most patients with diverticula suggests that herniations of mucosa are caused by increased pressure produced by colonic muscle contractions. The rarity of colonic diverticula in underdeveloped nations in contrast to their frequent occurrence in western countries has led to the speculation that diverticula result from the highly refined western diet, which is deficient in dietary fiber or roughage. It is proposed that such diets result in decreased fecal bulk, narrowing of the colon, and an increase in intraluminal pressure in order to move the smaller fecal mass. The role of dietary fiber in the etiology and treatment of diverticular disease remains to be determined.

Colonic diverticula are usually asymptomatic and are an incidental finding on barium enema or colonoscopy. The major complications of inflammation, both acute and chronic, and hemorrhage occur in only a small percentage of individuals with diverticulosis. Since diverticulosis is quite common in older patients, one must avoid the temptation of attributing pain or bleeding to the diverticula unless other conditions, especially colonic neoplasm, have been excluded.

Diverticulitis Inflammation can occur in or around the diverticular sac. The cause of diverticulitis is probably mechanical, related to retention in the diverticula of undigested food residues and bacteria, which may form a hard mass called a *fecalith*. This compromises the blood supply to the thin-walled sac (made up solely of mucosa and serosa) and renders it susceptible to invasion by colonic bacteria. The inflammatory process may vary from a small intramural or pericolic abscess to generalized peritonitis. Some attacks are accompanied by minimal symptoms and seem to heal spontaneously. Studies of resected specimens indicate that most perforations of the diverticular sac are small and result in inflammation of the sac itself and the adjacent serosal surface. Diverticulitis occurs more often in men than in women and three times as often in the left as in the right colon. This suggests that diverticulitis may be related to the higher intraluminal pressures and the more solid fecal material in the sigmoid and descending colon.

Acute colonic diverticulitis is a disease of variable severity characterized by fever, left lower quadrant abdominal pain, and signs of peritoneal irritation—muscle spasm, guarding, rebound tenderness. Rectal examination may reveal a tender mass if the area of inflammation is close to the rectum. Although constipation may not have been noted prior to onset of the illness, the inflammation around the colon often results in some degree of acute constipation or obstipation. Rectal bleeding, usually microscopic, is noted in 25 percent of cases; it is rarely massive. Polymorphonuclear leukocytosis is common. Complications include free perforation, which results in acute peritonitis, sepsis, and shock, particularly in the elderly. The perforation may be walled off by adherent omentum or neighboring structures such as the bladder or small bowel. Abscess formation or fistulas then occur as the inflammatory mass burrows into other organs. Severe pericolitis may cause a fibrous stricture around the bowel which can be associated with colonic obstruction and may mimic a neoplasm.

DIAGNOSIS During the acute phase of diverticulitis, barium enema and sigmoidoscopy may be hazardous, since contrast material or air under pressure may lead to rupture of an inflamed diverticulum and convert a walled-off inflammatory lesion to a free perforation. These examinations are usually safe after adequate treatment and healing of the diverticulitis. The radiologic findings on barium enema suggestive of diverticulitis are leakage of barium from a diverticular sac, stricture formation, and the presence of a pericolic inflammatory mass. In many patients, the distortion caused by inflammation prevents a clear distinction between cancer and diverticulitis. In these cases, colonoscopy or surgical excision may be required for accurate diagnosis. Abdominal CT scan may be useful in demonstrating the presence of a pericolic abscess.

TREATMENT Most patients with acute diverticulitis should be hospitalized for bowel rest, intravenous fluids, and broad-spectrum antibiotics. Repeated attacks of diverticulitis in the same area generally require surgical resection. Severe attacks with acute peritoneal signs, suspected abscess, or perforation require intravenous antibiotics directed against gram-negative anaerobic bacteria, followed by surgical drainage or resection. The usual procedure is a diverting colostomy with resection of the involved colon; reanastomosis is then performed at a second operation.

Painful diverticular disease without diverticulitis Some patients with diverticulosis develop recurrent left lower quadrant colicky pain without clinical or pathologic evidence of acute diverticulitis. They often have bouts of alternating constipation and diarrhea, and the pain may be relieved by defecation or passage of flatus. These features suggest the coexistence of the irritable bowel syndrome (see below). Examination during a bout of pain reveals tenderness of the sigmoid colon, but signs of peritoneal inflammation such as rebound tenderness, muscle guarding, fever, and leukocytosis are absent. Barium enema shows typical diverticula without evidence of inflammation and stricture, plus a "sawtooth" irregularity of the lumen reflecting muscle hypertrophy and spasm. In some patients the pain is severe enough to warrant observation in a hospital and restriction of food, since feeding aggravates the pain by causing colonic contraction. Anticholinergics, which reduce sigmoid contractions, and mild sedation are usually all that is required. After recovery, the patient should be started on a high-residue diet or given a bulk laxative such as hemicellulose, unprocessed bran, or psyllium extract. Surgical excision is usually not indicated unless acute diverticulitis or its complications occur.

Hemorrhage from diverticula Massive hemorrhage from colonic diverticula is one of the most common causes of hematochezia in patients over age 60. This complication of diverticulosis is caused by erosion of a vessel by a fecalith within the diverticular sac. The bleeding is painless and not accompanied by signs or symptoms of diverticulitis. Most cases of mild or moderate hemorrhage stop spontaneously with bed rest and blood transfusion. Localization of bleeding can be obtained by bleeding scan or angiography. In patients with severe hemorrhage, mesenteric angiography can be both diagnostic in localizing the bleeding site and therapeutic, since vasoconstrictive drugs or artificial blood clot infused intraarterially can sometimes effectively control hemorrhage. Colonoscopy is also useful in evaluating acute hematochezia, and the endoscopist may be able to cauterize angiodysplasias (see Chap. 41). The location of bleeding diverticula demonstrated at angiography on several series has been more commonly in the right colon, particularly the ascending colon, in contrast to the sigmoid colon, where diverticula are more numerous.

MEGACOLON   Megacolon, or giant colon, is characterized by massive distention of the colon, usually accompanied by severe constipation or obstipation. This condition can be either congenital or acquired and is seen in all age groups. Acute toxic megacolon is a severe complication of chronic ulcerative colitis (see Chap. 255).

Aganglionic megacolon (Hirschsprung's disease)   This is a congenital disorder which becomes manifest in early infancy, occurring more frequently in males, and is often familial. These infants have massive abdominal distention, absent bowel movements, and impaired nutrition due to chronic obstruction of the colon. In some individuals with less severe symptoms the disease may not be diagnosed until adolescence or early adulthood. The inability to defecate is caused by the absence of ganglion cells (Meissner's and Auerbach's plexuses) in a small segment of the distal colon, usually near the anus. This aganglionic segment is unable to relax to permit passage of stool, causing the normal colon proximal to it to become greatly dilated. On rectal examination, the ampulla is empty of feces and the anal sphincter is normal. Barium enema reveals a narrowed segment in the rectosigmoid area, with massive dilatation above. Diagnosis is made by full-thickness surgical biopsy under anesthesia and demonstration of absent ganglion cells in the diseased segment. In most patients the aganglionic segment is in the rectosigmoid colon; in rare instances the lesion may involve more proximal bowel or even the entire colon. The treatment of choice is a pull-through procedure in which normally innervated colon is anastomosed to the distal rectum just above the internal sphincter, thus bypassing the contracted aganglionic segment and restoring normal defecation.

Chronic idiopathic megacolon   This condition, also called *psychogenic megacolon*, has its onset later in childhood, usually at the time toilet training begins. It is characterized by severe chronic constipation and distention, and in contrast to Hirschsprung's disease, digital examination reveals the rectal ampulla to be invariably distended with feces. Barium enema shows the entire colon to be distended with stools, no narrowed segment is seen, and rectal biopsy discloses the normal complement of ganglion cells in Auerbach's plexus. Treatment is based on education in normal bowel habits, but a long course of enemas or large doses of mineral oil may be required until the patient acquires more normal bowel movements.

Acquired megacolon   In Central and South America, infection with *Trypanosoma cruzi* (Chagas' disease) can result in destruction of the ganglion cells of the colon, producing a clinical picture similar to congenital megacolon, except that the onset is in adult life rather than childhood. A number of other diseases are associated with megacolon in adults. Patients with schizophrenia or depression, particularly institutionalized patients, may have obstipation and massive colonic dilatation. Severe neurologic disorders, including cerebral atrophy, spinal cord injury, and parkinsonism, also may cause megacolon. Myxedema, infiltrative diseases such as amyloidosis, and scleroderma also can reduce colonic motility and produce marked colonic distention. Narcotic drugs, particularly morphine and codeine, can cause severe constipation, especially when administered to bedridden patients. Digital rectal examination of adults with acquired megacolon reveals a rectum distended with feces, as opposed to the empty rectum in aganglionic megacolon. Treatment is aimed

at the underlying disease, as well as the careful use of enemas and cathartics.

INTESTINAL PSEUDOOBSTRUCTION   Intestinal pseudoobstruction is an acute or chronic motility disorder characterized by distention or dilatation of the small and large intestine. Abdominal pain, nausea, and vomiting may lead to diagnostic confusion with mechanical obstruction, but as the name of this condition implies, the underlying cause is not obstruction but rather a severe dysmotility resulting in distention. Pseudoobstruction may be primary or secondary and acute or chronic. In primary or idiopathic pseudoobstruction, no other contributing condition can be identified, and the motility disorder is attributed to abnormalities of sympathetic innervation or of the muscle layers of the intestine. Secondary pseudoobstruction may result from scleroderma, diabetes, amyloidosis, neurologic diseases, drugs, or sepsis.

Chronic or intermittent secondary pseudoobstruction   Numerous medical conditions can cause chronic dilatation of the large and small bowel. Some of these may involve the intestinal smooth muscle, such as scleroderma, dermatomyositis, amyloidosis, or muscular dystrophy. Endocrine disorders, including myxedema and diabetes mellitus, may result in chronic distention, which in the diabetic results from autonomic visceral neuropathy. Chronic neurologic diseases, including Parkinson's disease and stroke, may be complicated by chronic pseudoobstruction; in these patients drugs and relative immobility are contributing features. Finally, psychotic patients (especially those who are institutionalized) may suffer from prolonged megacolon.

The symptoms of chronic secondary pseudoobstruction are chronic or intermittent constipation, crampy abdominal pain, anorexia, and bloating. Gastric distention and disordered swallowing may be present. Abdominal x-rays reveal gaseous distention of the large and small bowel and occasionally of the stomach. Air fluid levels are unusual and should raise the possibility of mechanical obstruction. Upper gastrointestinal series and barium enema do not reveal specific abnormalities of the intestine such as tumor, stricture, or volvulus. The presence of an autoimmune disorder or endocrinopathy may require confirmation by serologic or blood tests; biopsy may be needed as in amyloidosis or muscular dystrophy.

The treatment of chronic intestinal pseudoobstruction is made difficult by the complexity and chronicity of the underlying systemic disease. Patients with scleroderma may respond to broad-spectrum antibiotics if intestinal bacterial overgrowth is suspected. Metoclopramide may benefit gastric dysmotility in the diabetic. Discontinuation of psychotropic or anti-Parkinson drugs occasionally may result in improvement. Cathartics and enemas may be required to relieve fecal impaction, and the regular use of stool softeners and a high-fiber diet may help prevent recurrences.

Idiopathic intestinal pseudoobstruction   This term encompasses patients with signs and symptoms of pseudoobstruction in whom no systemic disease can be identified. The typical patient has recurrent attacks of abdominal pain and distention with nausea and vomiting. The small intestine is primarily involved, and chronic constipation is much less frequent than in secondary pseudoobstruction. Steatorrhea secondary to bacterial overgrowth of the small intestine is common and may lead to chronic diarrhea and malnutrition. Many patients exhibit abnormalities of motility in the esophagus and urinary bladder, in addition to the small and large intestine. Neuromuscular defects have been described in patients with this syndrome, including abnormalities of the mesenteric plexus and myopathy of the intestinal and urinary bladder smooth muscle (so-called hollow visceral myopathy). Elevated prostaglandin E levels have been reported in some patients. Treatment of idiopathic pseudoobstruction is unsatisfactory. Surgery to relieve "obstruction" is to be avoided, since the condition is often worsened by abdominal surgery. Medical therapy with metoclopramide and cholinergic agents has been unsuccessful. Nutritional support in the form of low-residue elemental diets or parenteral hyperalimentation may be helpful. Unfortunately, the lack of effective therapy and the progressive nature of the illness make the prognosis of idiopathic pseudoobstruction rather unfavorable. Death from malnutrition and steatorrhea are common. The long-term impact of total parenteral nutrition on this disease is not yet clear.

Acute intestinal pseudoobstruction This entity, sometimes referred to as *Ogilvie's syndrome*, is characterized by acute intestinal dilatation involving primarily the colon but occasionally also the small intestine. As in other forms of pseudoobstruction, the clinical features are difficult to distinguish from mechanical obstruction. The patient may complain of colicky lower abdominal pain and acute constipation. Examination reveals a distended, tympanitic abdomen, with reduced or absent bowel sounds. Localized tenderness over the distended colon is common, but diffuse abdominal tenderness, rigidity, or rebound tenderness are unusual. Abdominal films reveal massive dilatation of the colon and small intestine, occasionally with the presence of air fluid levels. The cecum, being the most capacious part of the colon, is often massively dilated and tender. The onset of these symptoms usually occurs in patients who have recently undergone severe surgical or medical stress such as major surgery, myocardial infarction, sepsis, or respiratory failure. Patients with acute pseudoobstruction are frequently on respirators, have received narcotics or sedatives, and have metabolic and electrolyte disturbances.

Management of acute pseudoobstruction requires careful correction of fluid and electrolyte abnormalities, intubation of the stomach or small intestine for decompression, and avoidance of drugs which depress intestinal motility. Barium enema may be hazardous because of the risk of perforating the already dilated bowel. Decompressive colonoscopy is beneficial in some patients, and cecostomy may be required in some patients with massive cecal dilatation. The outcome depends in large part on the prognosis of the associated medical or surgical conditions. Patients who recover from the underlying medical or surgical conditions usually have a return of normal colonic function.

IRRITABLE BOWEL SYNDROME The irritable bowel syndrome (IBS) is the most common gastrointestinal disease in clinical practice, and although not a life-threatening illness, it causes great distress to those afflicted and feelings of helplessness and frustration for the physician attempting to treat it. The patient with IBS may present with one of *three clinical variants*. Patients with so-called spastic colitis complain primarily of chronic abdominal pain and constipation. A second group has chronic intermittent diarrhea, often without pain. Some patients have both features and complain of alternating constipation and diarrhea.

IBS is characterized by chronic intermittent symptoms, including recurrent abdominal pain, usually in the left lower quadrant; altered frequency of defecation with hard stools (constipation) or watery stools (diarrhea); stool urgency; a sense of incomplete evacuation; feeling of abdominal distention; and excess flatus.

Two pathophysiologic abnormalities appear to underlie these symptoms: altered intestinal motility and increased visceral perception. Patients with diarrhea have accelerated transit of fecal material through the ascending and transverse colon, while patients with constipation have overall delays in colonic transit. Small-bowel motility patterns are also abnormal in conscious IBS patients but not during sleep, suggesting that altered gut motility may result, in part, from central nervous system input.

Heightened visceral perception in IBS patients has been demonstrated by excessive sensitivity to balloon distention in the ileum, colon, and rectum. This increased sensitivity to distention is accompanied by development of increased reflex intestinal motor activity. It is thought that these findings may explain the frequent complaints of gaseous distention in IBS patients, even though the volume of intestinal gas in these patients does not differ from that in normal individuals.

Evidence of significant psychological disturbances may be seen in some patients with IBS. Depression, hysteria, and obsessive-compulsive traits are common, and psychological stress frequently triggers an exacerbation of symptoms. Some female patients give a history of childhood sexual abuse. It should be noted, however, that

increased intracolonic pressure has been observed in normal volunteers during acute stress. This suggests that psychological stress may be a nonspecific trigger of symptoms in IBS, as is the case in many other illnesses of diverse etiology.

Clinical features IBS is a disease of young or middle-aged adults; the female-to-male ratio is 4:1. The predominant feature is a history of chronic constipation, diarrhea, or both occurring *intermittently* for months or years. The diarrhea is usually worse in the morning upon arising or after breakfast. After the passage of three or four loose stools with excessive mucus, the patient may feel well for the remainder of the day. Diarrhea throughout the day or especially nocturnal diarrhea is most unusual. The diarrhea may last for weeks or months and then disappear spontaneously for variable periods of time. Some patients describe "pencil-like," pasty stools rather than diarrhea.

Another typical presentation is that of chronic abdominal pain with constipation or with alternating constipation and diarrhea. These patients describe intermittent crampy lower abdominal pain, often over the sigmoid colon, which is usually relieved by passage of flatus or stool. The patient may describe excessive bloating which is not discernible to the physician. A variety of other complaints, such as heartburn, excessive bloating, back pain, weakness, faintness, and palpitations, are frequent in patients with IBS. The pain may occasionally be in the right upper quadrant, or midepigastric pain may lead to diagnostic confusion with biliary tract or peptic ulcer disease.

Physical examination reveals these patients to be anxious, but significant abdominal tenderness or distention is unusual. A tender sigmoid full of feces may be palpated in the left lower quadrant. Sigmoidoscopy may reveal a prominent vascular pattern, muscle spasm, or excess mucus, but the mucosa itself is normal.

The *diagnosis* of IBS is suggested by the chronic intermittent nature of symptoms without obvious signs of physical deterioration, the relation of symptoms to environment or emotional stress, and the exclusion of other conditions. The evaluation should include a careful history, complete physical examination, and stool examination for occult blood, parasites, and pathogenic bacteria. In some patients, colonoscopy will be necessary to exclude inflammation or neoplasia. Barium enema may reveal spasticity of the sigmoid, accentuated haustra, and a tubular appearance to the descending colon. Lactase deficiency may masquerade as IBS and should be excluded by a trial of milk restriction, a lactose tolerance test, or a lactose breath hydrogen test (see Chap. 254). Thyrotoxicosis is easily confused with IBS and should be excluded by appropriate laboratory studies. Endometriosis also can cause altered bowel habit and pelvic pain.

Treatment of the IBS requires both skill and patience. It is important that the patient be reassured that this condition normally does not lead to the development of chronic inflammatory bowel disease (i.e., ulcerative colitis) or colonic malignancy. It is also important for both the patient and the physician to realize that the condition is chronic, and while it may be alleviated, it cannot be cured. The patient should be encouraged to adapt to the symptoms so as to minimize their impact on life-style. The physician should not imply that the symptoms are largely emotional or psychological in origin, since this is usually rejected by the patient. It is appropriate, however, to emphasize the relationship between psychological stress and the onset of severity of symptoms, since this may allow the patient to better deal with the disease. After the diagnosis is established, frequent x-rays and endoscopies are not necessary; general physical examinations, hemograms, and stool examinations for occult blood, however, should be carried out at regular intervals.

Drug treatment is aimed at altering the abnormal colonic motility in this disease. Patients with constipation may respond to an increase in dietary bulk in the form of unprocessed bran or psyllium bulk laxatives. Mild sedation with tranquilizers may be indicated, and anticholinergic drugs such as dicyclomine are useful in some patients. Troublesome diarrhea may respond to diphenoxylate or loperamide. Unfortunately, no specific drug or dietary regimen affords good relief in all patients, and thus a number of therapeutic maneuvers need to be tried.

CHRONIC CONSTIPATION The mechanism of defecation is discussed in Chap. 39. Chronic constipation is widespread in western society, with approximately 10 percent of the population taking laxatives on a regular basis. Most cases of chronic constipation arise from habitual neglect of afferent impulses, failure to initiate defecation, and accumulation of large, dry fecal masses in the rectum. This voluntary suppression of the call to stool may arise during the period of toilet training in childhood or later in life because of a sense of social impropriety, unaccustomed surroundings, uncomfortable toilet facilities, or illnesses which require confinement to bed. Chronic constipation is much more common in women, with onset typically in late adolescence or early adulthood. As constant distention of the rectum with feces becomes chronic, the patient grows less aware of rectal fullness. Bowel movements become progressively more difficult, and painful hemorrhoids or anal fissures reinforce suppression of the urge to defecate. To avoid these problems, the patient begins the chronic use of laxatives or enemas, without which defecation becomes impossible.

Treatment The physician should make every attempt to educate the patient about the chain of events which has led to chronic constipation. Attempts should be made to alter patterns of many years' duration, and the patient must recognize the importance of responding to, rather than suppressing, the urge to defecate. It is helpful to initiate a routine whereby defecation is attempted at a given time each day. In most individuals the call to stool occurs in the morning after breakfast. Physical exercise such as a brisk walk just before attempts at defecation may be helpful. Patients are instructed to increase dietary bulk with foods rich in fiber, such as green vegetables and unprocessed cereal grains, or by the regular use of bulk laxatives, such as hemicellulose, psyllium extract, and powdered unprocessed bran. The success of such a regimen depends to some extent on the duration of symptoms. Elderly patients with long-standing constipation and reliance on enemas or laxatives are more resistant to these measures than younger patients whose bowel patterns are less established. Moreover, poor muscle tone, reduced physical activity, and increased incidence of other medical conditions make the problem more difficult in the older age group. Bedridden elderly patients often develop severe constipation and even fecal impaction unless preventive measures are taken. This applies not only to patients with previous constipation but also to those with regular bowel movements prior to their confining illness. Regular administration of stool softeners, bulk laxatives, or mild cathartics is necessary until full ambulation and a normal diet are resumed. The onset of fecal impaction in bedridden patients is heralded by a feeling of rectal distention, urgency of defecation, or tenesmus. Occasionally, the fecal impaction will result in low-grade chronic obstruction with dilatation and increased fluid content proximal to the impaction; "paradoxical diarrhea" may thus occur as fluid moves past the obstructing fecal mass. This situation will be aggravated if antidiarrheal drugs are given because the underlying constipation will be worsened. The appropriate maneuver is to disimpact the rectum manually or to administer gentle enemas if the impaction is beyond the reach of the finger.

VASCULAR DISORDERS OF THE INTESTINE

Ischemia is the end result of interruption or reduction of the blood supply of the intestine. However, the clinical manifestations of intestinal ischemia range from mild chronic symptoms to catastrophic episodes, depending on the segment involved, the degree of involvement, and the rapidity of the process, and the clinician should be aware of this spectrum of manifestations (Table 256-1). The gut derives its arterial blood supply from the celiac axis and the superior and inferior mesenteric arteries. The small intestine is supplied by the celiac and superior mesenteric arteries; the colon is supplied by

TABLE 256-1 Patterns of intestinal ischemia

Condition	Etiology	Clinical features	Management
Mesenteric artery embolus	Arterial embolus associated with atrial fibrillation or rheumatic heart disease	Acute central abdominal pain, shock, peritonitis	Immediate angiography and embolectomy if possible
Abdominal angina	Atherosclerosis of celiac and superior mesenteric arteries	Chronic postprandial pain, weight loss	Angiography and surgery in selected cases
Ischemia colitis	Low-flow state	Acute lower abdominal pain, rectal bleeding	Sigmoidoscopy; surgery only for peritonitis

branches of the superior and inferior mesenteric arteries. A rich network of anastomotic vessels and the possible development of collateral circulation determine the clinical picture of acute or chronic intestinal arterial insufficiency.

MESENTERIC ISCHEMIA AND INFARCTION Acute small-intestinal ischemia may be classified as *occlusive* or *nonocclusive*. Occlusion may result from arterial thrombus or embolus of the celiac or superior mesenteric arteries or from venous occlusion in the same distribution. Arterial embolus occurs most commonly in patients with chronic or recurrent atrial fibrillation, artificial heart valves, or valvular heart disease, while arterial thrombosis is associated with extensive atherosclerosis or low cardiac output. Venous occlusion is quite rare and is occasionally seen in women taking oral contraceptives. Approximately one-half of patients with mesenteric ischemia do not have a definite occlusion of a major vessel, a condition referred to as *nonocclusive* ischemia. The exact cause of nonocclusive disease is obscure; systemic arterial hypotension, cardiac arrhythmias, prolonged heart failure, digitalis therapy, dehydration, and endotoxemia have been suggested as contributing factors.

The outstanding clinical feature of acute mesenteric ischemia is severe abdominal pain, often colicky and periumbilical at the onset, later becoming diffuse and constant. Vomiting, anorexia, diarrhea, and constipation are also frequent but of little diagnostic help. Examination of the abdomen may reveal tenderness and distention. Bowel sounds are often normal even in the face of severe infarction. Some patients have a surprisingly normal abdominal examination in spite of severe pain. Mild gastrointestinal bleeding is often detected by guaiac examination of stool, but gross hemorrhage is unusual except in ischemic colitis (see below). A typical laboratory finding is a pronounced polymorphonuclear leukocytosis. Late in the course of the disease (24 to 72 h), gangrene of the bowel occurs with diffuse peritonitis, sepsis, and shock. Abdominal plain films in patients with mesenteric ischemia may reveal air fluid levels and distention. Barium study of the small intestine reveal nonspecific dilatation, poor motility, and evidence of thick mucosal folds ("thumbprinting") (Fig. 256-2).

Acute mesenteric ischemia is a grave condition with a high morbidity and mortality. Patients suspected of having acute arterial embolus should undergo immediate celiac and mesenteric angiography to localize the embolus, followed by embolectomy. Restoration of normal circulation may allow complete recovery if performed before irreversible necrosis or gangrene has occurred. Unfortunately, infarction and transmural necrosis are frequently found at surgery, necessitating resection. Arterial or venous thrombosis is not generally amenable to surgical removal of the thrombus, and resection of the affected bowel is required. Similarly, patients with nonocclusive ischemia are not candidates for corrective vascular surgery (as major vessels are patent). These individuals often have extensive necrosis of the small or large intestine because of the widespread nature of the ischemic event. The decision to operate on patients with suspected mesenteric ischemia is a difficult one because the typical patient is a poor surgical risk owing to advanced age, dehydration, sepsis, and other serious medical conditions.

FIGURE 256-2 Barium enema showing "thumbprinting" or submucosal edema of the inferior margin of the transverse colon, in a patient with acute ischemic colitis.

Chronic arterial insufficiency may precede acute vascular insufficiency, producing so-called abdominal angina. As in angina pectoris, the pain of chronic mesenteric insufficiency occurs under conditions of increased demand for splanchnic blood flow. The patient complains of intermittent dull or cramping midabdominal pain 15 to 30 min after a meal, lasting for several hours postprandially. Significant weight loss is primarily due to a decreased food intake; however, chronic intestinal ischemia also may produce mucosal damage and malabsorption, which in turn aggravates the weight loss. Since abdominal angina may progress to bowel infarction, serious consideration should be given to performing arteriographic studies to confirm the diagnosis in those patients who are candidates for abdominal vascular surgery. The only definitive treatment is vascular surgery or balloon angioplasty to remove the thrombus or the construction of bypass arterial grafts to the ischemic bowel.

A number of systemic conditions are associated with *vasculitis* of the large and small arteries supplying the intestine. Most often these disorders can be recognized by the associated extraintestinal manifestations, as in polyarteritis nodosa, lupus erythematosus, dermatomyositis, Henoch-Schönlein purpura (allergic vasculitis), and rheumatoid vasculitis. When larger arteries are involved, as in polyarteritis nodosa, the picture of acute intestinal infarction is similar to that of embolic or atherosclerotic vascular occlusion. Often the involvement of smaller vessels leads to areas of intramural hemorrhage and edema resulting in abdominal pain, variable degrees of intestinal obstruction, and bleeding. Barium enema may show "thumbprinting" and "spiculation" due to localized edema, hemorrhage, and ulceration. In many instances, treatment of the underlying disorder may lead to regression of symptoms. If signs of an acute abdomen develop, surgical exploration is usually indicated.

Intramural small-intestinal hemorrhage may occur with vasculitis, trauma, or impaired coagulation, especially in patients receiving anticoagulants. The clinical and radiologic features resemble those seen with vasculitis and local mucosal hemorrhage.

ISCHEMIC COLITIS Ischemia of the colon most often affects the elderly population because of the greater frequency of vascular disease in that group. Ischemic colitis is almost always a nonocclusive disease, that is, obstruction of major arteries is not seen. Shunting of blood away from the mucosa may contribute to this condition, but the mechanism of ischemia is not known.

The clinical picture depends on the degree of ischemia and the rate of its development. In *acute fulminant ischemic* colitis, the major manifestations are severe lower abdominal pain, rectal bleeding, and hypotension. Dilatation of the colon and physical signs of peritonitis

are seen in severe cases. Plain abdominal films may reveal thumbprinting from submucosal hemorrhage and edema. Barium enema is hazardous in the acute situation because of the risk of perforation. Sigmoidoscopy or colonoscopy may detect ulcerations, friability, and bulging folds from submucosal hemorrhage. Angiography is not helpful in the management of patients with presumed ischemic colitis because a remediable occlusive lesion is very rarely found. Surgical resection may be required in some patients with fulminant ischemic colitis to remove gangrenous bowel; others with lesser degrees of ischemia may respond to conservative medical management.

Subacute ischemic colitis, the most common clinical variant of ischemic colonic disease, produces lesser degrees of pain and bleeding, often occurring over several days or weeks. The left colon may be involved, but the rectum is usually spared because of collateral blood flow, a distinguishing feature from acute ulcerative colitis. Barium enema reveals edema, cobblestoning, thumbprinting, and occasionally superficial ulceration. Angiography is not indicated because almost all cases are nonocclusive. Occasionally, *stricture formation* may follow a bout of ischemic colitis or may present de novo without a history of antecedent pain or bloody diarrhea. Most cases of nonocclusive ischemic colitis resolve in 2 to 4 weeks and do not recur. Surgery is not required except for obstruction secondary to postischemic stricture.

ANGIODYSPLASIA OF THE COLON These are vascular ectasias (not neoplasms) which occur in the right colon of many older individuals and may cause bleeding (see Chap. 41). Angiodysplasia is a degenerative lesion consisting of dilated, distorted, thin-walled vessels lined by vascular endothelium. Angiodysplasia may result from partial obstruction of the submucosal venous plexus by the tension generated in the cecal wall during muscular contraction. Aortic stenosis occurs in some patients and may cause chronic ischemia of the colon that leads to angiodysplasia. Grossly, angiodysplasias look similar to spider angiomas of the skin and appear as star-shaped branching vessels in the submucosa measuring from 2 mm to 1 cm in diameter. The lesions are usually multiple and are found primarily in the cecum and ascending colon, but in some patients they may be distributed from the stomach to rectum.

Cecal angiodysplasia is important because of the likelihood of bleeding, either massively or chronically. In patients over age 60, approximately one-quarter of colonic bleeding episodes are secondary to angiodysplasia. The diagnosis is easiest to establish by colonoscopy, which allows treatment by electrocautery or injection with sclerosant. Some patients with massive uncontrolled bleeding or multiple sites of angiodysplasia may require right hemicolectomy. Angiodysplasias also may respond to chronic estrogen-progesterone therapy.

ANORECTAL PROBLEMS

HEMORRHOIDS The internal hemorrhoidal plexus of veins is located in the submucosal space above the valves of Morgagni. The anal canal separates it from the external hemorrhoidal venous plexus, but the two spaces communicate under the anal canal, the submucosa of which is attached to underlying tissue to form the interhemorrhoidal depression. Whenever the internal hemorrhoidal plexus is enlarged, there is associated increase in supporting tissue mass, and the resultant venous swelling is called an *internal hemorrhoid*. When veins in the external hemorrhoidal plexus become enlarged or thrombosed, the resultant bluish mass is called an *external hemorrhoid*.

Both types of hemorrhoids are very common and are associated with increased hydrostatic pressure in the portal venous system, such as during pregnancy, straining at stool, or with cirrhosis. When internal hemorrhoids enlarge, pain is not a usual feature until the situation is complicated by thrombosis, infection, or erosion of the overlying mucosal surface. Most persons complain of bright red blood on the toilet tissue or coating the stool, with a feeling of vague anal discomfort. The discomfort is increased when the hemorrhoid enlarges or prolapses through the anus; prolapse is often accompanied by edema and sphincteric spasm. Prolapse, if not treated, usually becomes chronic as the muscularis stays stretched, and the patient complains of constant soiling of underclothing with very little pain. Prolapsed hemorrhoids may be infected or thrombosed; the overlying mucous membrane may bleed profusely from the trauma of defecation.

External hemorrhoids, because they lie under the skin, are quite often painful, particularly if there is a sudden increase in their mass. These episodes result in a tender blue swelling at the anal verge due to thrombosis of a vein in the external plexus and need not be associated with enlargement of the internal veins. Since the thrombus usually lies at the level of the sphincteric muscles, anal spasm often occurs.

The diagnosis of internal and external hemorrhoids is made by inspection, digital examination, and direct vision through the anoscope and proctoscope. Since such lesions are very common, they must not be regarded as the cause of rectal bleeding or chronic hypochromic anemia until a thorough investigation has been made of the more proximal gastrointestinal tract. Acute blood loss can occasionally be attributed to internal hemorrhoids. Chronic anemia or occult blood in the stool in the presence of large but not definitely bleeding hemorrhoids requires a search for a polyp, cancer, or ulcer.

Most hemorrhoids respond to conservative therapy such as sitz baths or other forms of moist heat, suppositories, stool softeners, and bed rest. Internal hemorrhoids which remain permanently prolapsed are best treated surgically; milder degrees of prolapse or enlargement with pruritus ani or intermittent bleeding can be handled successfully by banding or injection of sclerosing solutions. External hemorrhoids which become acutely thrombosed are treated by incision, extraction of the clot, and compression of the incised area following clot removal. No surgical procedure should be carried out in the presence of acute inflammation of the anus, ulcerative proctitis, or ulcerative colitis. Proctoscopy or colonoscopy should always be performed before a patient is subjected to hemorrhoidectomy.

ANAL INFLAMMATION   Perianal inflammatory lesions may be primary or may be associated with inflammatory bowel disease or diverticular disease, as mentioned above. Anal *fissures* are superficial erosions of the anal canal which usually heal rapidly with conservative therapy. Anal *ulcers* are more chronic and deep and give symptoms largely as the result of painful spasm of the external anal sphincter during and after defecation. Bleeding may occur with either fissure or ulcer; healing of the ulcer often is associated with a hypertrophied anal papilla and some degrees of anal contracture. *Fistula in ano*, a tract leading from the rectal lumen to the perianal skin, usually results from local crypt abscesses. The fistula is a chronically inflamed canal made up of fibrous tissue surrounding granulation tissue, the lumen of which may be difficult to demonstrate. Perirectal *abscesses* often represent the tracking down into the anal area of purulent material escaping from the rectosigmoid; diverticulitis, Crohn's disease, ulcerative colitis, or previous surgery may be the underlying cause. Fistulas between the rectum and vagina or the rectum and bladder represent serious complications of granulomatous, septic, or malignant disorders and require the patient to be hospitalized for definitive diagnostic and therapeutic procedures.

REFERENCES

Disorders of motility

COLEMONT LJ, CAMILLERI M: Chronic intestinal pseudo-obstruction: Diagnosis and treatment. Mayo Clin Proc 64:60, 1989

DROSSMAN DA, THOMPSON WG: The irritable bowel syndrome: Review and a graduated multicomponent treatment approach. Ann Intern Med 116:1009, 1992

PRESTON DM, LENNARD-JONES JE: Severe chronic constipation of young women: Idiopathic slow transit constipation. Gut 27:41, 1986

Diverticular diseases

BRIAN JE, STAIR JM: Non-colonic diverticular disease. Surg Gynecol Obstet 161:189, 1985

STEFANSSON T et al: Increased risk of left sided colon cancer in patients with diverticular disease. Gut 34:499, 1993

THOMPSON WG, PATEL DG: Clinical picture of diverticular disease of the colon. Clinics Gastrol 15:903, 1986

Intestinal ischemia and angiodysplasia

CLAVIEN PA: Diagnosis and management of mesenteric infarction. Br J Surg 77:601, 1990

NAVEAU S et al: Long-term results of treatment of vascular malformations of the gastrointestinal tract by neodynium YAG laser photocoagulation. Dig Dis Sci 35:821, 1990

SARGEANT IR et al: Laser ablation of upper gastrointestinal vascular ectasias: Long term results. Gut 34:470, 1993

VAN CUTSEM E et al: Treatment of bleeding gastrointestinal vascular malformations with oestrogen-progesterone. Lancet 1:953, 1990

257   TUMORS OF THE LARGE AND SMALL INTESTINE

ROBERT J. MAYER

COLORECTAL CANCER

INCIDENCE   Cancer of the large bowel is second only to lung cancer as a cause of cancer death in the United States. Approximately 152,000 new cases were anticipated in 1993, resulting in 57,000 deaths. The incidence and mortality rates for this extremely common malignant condition have not changed substantially in males during the past 40 years, although, for some reason, a slight decrease in the mortality rate has appeared in females. Colorectal cancer generally occurs in individuals 50 years of age or older.

ETIOLOGY AND RISK FACTORS (Table 257-1)   **Diet**   The etiology for most cases of large-bowel cancer appears to be related to environmental factors. The disease occurs more often in upper socioeconomic populations who live in urban areas. Epidemiologic studies in various countries have documented a direct correlation between mortality from colorectal cancer and per capita consumption of calories, meat protein, and dietary fat and oil as well as elevations in the serum cholesterol concentration and mortality from coronary artery disease. Any geographic variations in incidence do not appear to be related to genetic differences, since migrant groups tend to assume the large-bowel cancer incidence rates of their adopted countries. Furthermore, population groups such as Mormons and Seventh Day Adventists, whose lifestyle and dietary habits differ somewhat from those of their neighbors, have significantly lower-than-expected incidence and mortality rates for colorectal cancer, while the appearance of colorectal cancer has increased in Japan since that nation has adopted a more "western" diet. It is therefore assumed that dietary patterns influence the development of colorectal cancer. At least two hypotheses have been proposed to explain this relationship, neither of which is fully satisfactory.

ANIMAL FATS   Based on the association of colorectal cancer with hypercholesterolemia and coronary artery disease as well as the increased incidence of large-bowel tumors in geographic areas where meat is a dietary staple, it has been suggested that the ingestion of animal fats leads to an increased proportion of anaerobes in the gut microflora, resulting in the conversion of normal bile acids into

TABLE 257-1   Risk factors for the development of colorectal cancer

Diet
  ? Animal fat
  ? Fiber
Hereditary syndromes (autosomal dominant inheritance)
  Polyposis coli
  Non-polyposis syndrome
Inflammatory bowel disease
Streptococcus bovis bacteremia
Ureterosigmoidostomy

carcinogens. This provocative hypothesis is supported by several reports of increased amounts of fecal anaerobes in the stools of patients with colorectal cancer. However, there are conflicting data from population studies relating fat intake to the risk for colon cancer and from unsuccessful attempts at altering the profile of fecal microflora through short-term alterations in diet. Any definitive assessment of the animal fat concept must await a prospective survey of a defined population, correlating carefully obtained and periodically updated dietary histories with quantitative cultures of stool microflora, and determining the incidence of colorectal cancer in these individuals over a 10 to 20 year period of time.

FIBER   The observation that South African Bantus ingest a diet far higher in roughage, produce more frequent, bulkier stools, and have a lower incidence of large-bowel cancer than their American and European counterparts led to the proposal that the higher rate of colorectal cancer in western society is in large part the result of a low intake of dietary fiber. This theory suggests that dietary fiber accelerates intestinal transit time, thereby reducing the exposure of colonic mucosa to potential carcinogens and diluting these carcinogens because of enhanced fecal bulk. Such a proposition appears somewhat simplistic when subjected to careful scrutiny. Although an enhanced fiber intake increases fecal bulk, there has been no consistent evidence that a higher fiber intake actually shortens the transit time of stool. Additionally, despite the generally higher fiber intake in low-incidence countries, the environmental differences between developing and industrialized nations are myriad and include such other important dietary variables as meat and fat consumption. Finally, a diet low in fiber may lead to chronic constipation and such associated conditions as diverticulosis. If a low fiber diet alone were a significant factor in colorectal cancer, individuals having diverticulosis should be at higher risk for the development of large-bowel tumors; this does not appear to be the case.

OTHER   Emerging data suggest that the risk for the development of colorectal cancer may be diminished by calcium supplements or aspirin. It is thought that dietary calcium may inactivate bowel carcinogens through the formation of insoluble soaps. In support of this concept are (1) the finding that supplementary dietary calcium reduced the proliferation of colonic epithelial cells in familial colon cancer kindreds and (2) the results of a survey of the dietary habits of a cohort of about 2000 men over a 19-year period, suggesting that the risk of colonic cancer decreased with increased oral intake of calcium.

Aspirin, an inhibitor of arachidonic acid metabolism, inhibits the growth of chemically induced colon tumors in rodents. A recent survey suggested that human colon cancer mortality might be reduced by the regular use of aspirin although it remains uncertain whether such a reduction was the result of prevention or earlier detection. Confirmation of this observation through a prospective trial will be required before routine use of aspirin as a form of chemoprevention can be recommended.

Thus, while the weight of epidemiologic evidence implicates diet as being the major etiologic factor for colorectal cancer, no single foodstuff has been sufficiently identified as being a causative or protective agent to justify specific recommendations for widespread changes in eating habits.

Hereditary factors and syndromes   As many as 25 percent of patients with colorectal cancer may have a family history of the disease, suggesting a hereditary predisposition. Such inherited large-bowel cancers can be divided into two main groups: the well-studied but uncommon polyposis syndromes and the less well defined nonpolyposis syndromes (Table 257-2).

Polyposis coli (i.e., familial polyposis of the colon) is a rare condition characterized by the appearance of thousands of adenomatous polyps throughout the large bowel. The condition is transmitted in an autosomal dominant manner; the occasional patients with no family history are thought to have developed the polyposis due to a spontaneous mutation. Molecular studies have associated polyposis coli with a deletion in the long arm of chromosome 5 (*APC* gene). It has been hypothesized that the loss of this genetic material (i.e., allelic loss) results in the absence of tumor-suppressor genes whose protein products would normally inhibit neoplastic growth. The presence of soft tissue, bony tumors, and ampullary cancers in addition to the colonic polyps characterizes a subset of polyposis coli known as *Gardner's syndrome*, while the appearance of malignant tumors of the central nervous system accompanying polyposis coli defines *Turcot's syndrome*. The colonic polyps in all these conditions are rarely present prior to puberty but are generally evident in affected individuals by age 25. If left surgically untreated, colorectal cancer will develop in almost all patients prior to age 40. Polyposis coli has been studied intensively and appears to result from a defect in the colonic mucosa leading to an abnormal proliferative pattern and an impaired ability for cellular repair following exposure to radiation or ultraviolet light. Once the multiple polyps that constitute polyposis coli are detected, patients should have a total colectomy. It remained unclear in the past (*A*) whether the optimal operative approach in such a clinical setting was to resect the entire colon and rectum, requiring the young patient to have a permanent ileostomy, or to perform an ileoproctostomy. While the latter procedure retained the distal rectum and anal sphincter, it placed the patient at continued risk for the development of cancer in the rectal remnant and necessitated semiannual or annual proctoscopic surveillance. The development of the ileoanal anastomotic technique allows removal of the entire bowel while retaining the anal sphincter and appears to be the best treatment. (*B*) The offspring of patients with polyposis coli, who are often prepubertal when the diagnosis is made in the parent, have a 50 percent risk for the eventual development of this premalignant disorder and should be carefully screened by annual flexible sigmoidoscopy until age 35. Testing for occult blood in the stool is an inadequate screening maneuver. Unfortunately, no disease-specific screening technique is generally available for the children of polyposis coli patients, although radioautographic measurements of colonic mucosal proliferation have been utilized with apparent efficacy in a small number of patients at highly specialized medical centers. Conceivably, molecular probes for the *APC* gene will prove to be useful in this regard in the future.

The hereditary predisposition for colorectal cancer in families

---

TABLE 257-2   Hereditable (autosomal dominant) gastrointestinal polyp syndromes

Syndrome	Distribution of polyps	Histologic type	Malignant potential	Associated lesions
Familial colonic polyposis	Large intestine	Adenoma	Common	None
Gardner's syndrome	Large and small intestines	Adenoma	Common	Osteomas, fibromas, lipomas, epidermoid cysts, ampullary cancers
Turcot's syndrome	Large intestine	Adenoma	Common	Brain tumors
Non-polyposis syndrome	Large intestine	Adenoma	Common	Endometrial tumors
Peutz-Jeghers syndrome	Small and large intestines, stomach	Hamartoma	Rare	Mucocutaneous pigmentation; tumors of the ovary, breast, pancreas, endometrium
Juvenile polyposis	Large and small intestines, stomach	Hamartoma rarely progressing to adenoma	Rare	Various congenital abnormalities

having no history of polyposis coli, the so-called hereditary nonpolyposis colorectal cancer syndrome, has received increased attention since the identification of several kindreds who displayed risks as high as 50 percent for the development of a colonic malignancy. These lesions involved the proximal large bowel in an unusually high frequency. Such families frequently include patients having multiple primary cancers, with the association of colorectal and endometrial adenocarcinomas being especially prominent in women. The trait for cancer appears to be transmitted in an autosomal dominant manner, possibly involving an abnormality in chromosome 2, and the median age for the appearance of an adenocarcinoma is about age 45, 15 to 20 years below the usual age for the general population. The offspring of such predisposed patients should undergo intensive screening, consisting of triannual colonoscopies, from age 25.

Inflammatory bowel disease (See also Chap. 255) Large-bowel cancer represents a not infrequent complication in patients with long-standing inflammatory bowel disease. The development of a neoplasm appears to occur more commonly in patients with ulcerative colitis than in those with granulomatous colitis, but such an impression may result in part from the occasional difficulty in differentiating these two conditions. The risk of colorectal cancer in a patient with inflammatory bowel disease is relatively small during the initial 10 years following the onset of the disease, but then appears to increase at a rate of approximately 0.5 to 1.0 percent per year. Actuarially derived cumulative cancer rates in such symptomatic patients have ranged from 8 to 30 percent after 25 years. The risk is generally considered to be higher in younger patients with pancolitis.

Cancer surveillance in patients with inflammatory bowel disease is unsatisfactory. Symptoms such as bloody diarrhea, abdominal cramping, and obstruction, which may signal the appearance of a tumor, are similar to the complaints of patients whose underlying disease is flaring. In patients with a history of inflammatory bowel disease lasting 15 years or more who continue to experience exacerbations, the surgical removal of the colon can significantly reduce the risk for cancer and also eliminate the target organ for the underlying chronic gastrointestinal disorder. The value of such surveillance techniques as colonoscopy with mucosal biopsies and brushings for less symptomatic individuals with chronic inflammatory bowel disease is uncertain. The purpose of such procedures has been the identification of premalignant mucosal dysplasia, thereby justifying surgical intervention. The lack of uniformity regarding the pathologic criteria that characterize dysplasia and the absence of data that such surveillance reduces the development of lethal cancers, however, has made this costly practice an area of controversy.

Other high-risk conditions STREPTOCOCCUS BOVIS BACTEREMIA For unknown reasons, individuals who develop endocarditis or septicemia from this fecal bacteria seem to have a high incidence of occult colorectal tumors and, possibly, upper gastrointestinal cancers as well. Endoscopic or radiographic screening appears advisable.

URETEROSIGMOIDOSTOMY There is a 5 to 10 percent incidence of colon cancer 15 to 30 years after ureterosigmoidostomy to correct congenital extrophy of the bladder. Neoplasms characteristically are found at a site distal to the ureteral implant where colonic mucosa is chronically exposed to both urine and feces.

POLYPS The majority of colorectal cancers, regardless of etiology, are believed to arise from adenomatous polyps. A polyp is a grossly visible protrusion from the mucosal surface and may be classified pathologically as a nonneoplastic hamartoma (*juvenile polyp*), a hyperplastic mucosal proliferation (*hyperplastic polyp*), or an adenomatous polyp. Only adenomas are clearly premalignant and only a minority of such lesions ever develop into cancer. Population-screening studies and autopsy surveys have revealed that adenomatous polyps may be found in the colons of about 30 percent of middle-aged or elderly people. Based on this prevalence and the known incidence of colorectal cancers, it appears that less than 1 percent of polyps ever become malignant. Most polyps produce no symptoms and remain clinically undetected. Occult blood in the stool may be found in less than 5 percent of patients with such lesions.

A number of molecular changes have been described in the DNA obtained from adenomatous polyps, dysplastic lesions, and polyps containing microscopic foci of tumor cells (i.e., *carcinoma in situ*). Consistent with the multistep process leading to cancer, a series of alterations has been observed, often beginning with a specific mutation in the *ras* proto-oncogene followed by deletions in chromosomes 5, 18, and 17 (see Chap. 63, Fig. 63-9). The loss of genetic material on the short arm of chromosome 17 appears to be associated with activation of a gene leading to the production of transformation-associated protein p53. Thus, the altered proliferative pattern of the colonic mucosa (which results in the progression to a polyp and then to a carcinoma) may involve the mutational activation of an oncogene followed by and coupled with the loss of genes which normally suppress tumorigenesis. Based on this model, it is believed that neoplasia develops only in those polyps in which all of these mutational events take place.

Clinically, the probability of an adenomatous polyp becoming a cancer is dependent upon the gross appearance of the lesion, its histologic features, and its size. Adenomatous polyps may be pedunculated (i.e., extending from adjacent bowel on a stalk) or sessile (i.e., flat). Cancers develop more frequently in sessile polyps. Histologically, adenomatous polyps may be tubular, villous (i.e., papillary), or tubulovillous. Villous adenomas, which are predominantly sessile in appearance, become malignant more than three times as often as tubular adenomas. The likelihood that any polypoid lesion in the large bowel contains invasive cancer is related to the size of the polyp, being negligible (<2 percent) in lesions smaller than 1.5 cm, intermediate (2 to 10 percent) in lesions 1.5 to 2.5 cm in size, and substantial (>10 percent) in lesions larger than 2.5 cm.

Following the detection of an adenomatous polyp, the entire large bowel should be visualized endoscopically or radiographically since synchronous lesions are present in approximately one-third of cases. Colonoscopy should then be repeated periodically, even in the absence of a previously documented malignancy, since such patients have a 30 to 50 percent probability of developing another adenoma and are at a higher-than-average risk for developing a colorectal carcinoma. Adenomatous polyps are thought to require more than 5 years of growth before becoming clinically significant; therefore, colonoscopy need not be carried out more frequently than every 3 years.

SCREENING The rationale for colorectal cancer screening programs is that the earlier detection of localized, superficial neoplasms in asymptomatic individuals will increase the surgical cure rate. Screening strategies have been based on the assumption that more than 60 percent of such early lesions are located in the rectosigmoid, making them accessible to rigid proctosigmoidoscopy. For unexplained reasons, however, there has been a consistent decrease during the past several decades in the proportion of large-bowel cancers arising in the rectum with a corresponding increase in the more proximal descending colon. As such, the potential for rigid proctosigmoidoscopy to detect a sufficient number of occult neoplasms to make the procedure cost-effective has been questioned. Nonetheless in support of periodic rigid proctosigmoidoscopic examination is a case-control study reporting a reduction in mortality from a distal large bowel cancer in individuals who had undergone such screening. The availability of flexible, fiberoptic sigmoidoscopes, permitting trained operators to visualize the colon for up to 60 cm, should further enhance cancer detection and resolve this issue.

Most programs directed at the early detection of colorectal cancers have focused on digital rectal examinations and testing stool for the presence of occult blood. The digital examination should be part of any routine physical evaluation in adults older than age 40, serving as an effective screening test for prostate cancer in men, a component of the pelvic examination in women, and as an inexpensive maneuver for the detection of masses in the rectum. The development of the Hemoccult test has greatly facilitated the potential to detect occult fecal blood. Unfortunately, even when performed optimally, the Hemoccult test has major limitations as a screening technique. Approximately 50 percent of patients with documented colorectal cancers have a negative fecal Hemoccult test, consistent with the intermittent bleeding pattern of these tumors. When random cohorts of asymptomatic persons have been tested, 2 to 4 percent have Hemoccult-positive stools. Colorectal cancers have been found in only 5 to 10 percent of these "test-positive" cases, with benign polyps being detected in an additional 20 to 30 percent. Consequently, a colorectal neoplasm will *not* be found in the majority of asymptomatic individuals with occult blood in their stool. Nonetheless, persons found to have Hemoccult-positive stool routinely undergo further medical evaluation that includes sigmoidoscopy, barium enema, and/or colonoscopy—procedures that not only are uncomfortable and expensive, but also are associated with a low but finite risk for significant complications. The added cost of these studies would appear justifiable if the minority of patients found to have occult neoplasms because of Hemoccult screening could be shown to have an improved prognosis and prolonged survival. Prospectively controlled trials addressing this issue are ongoing. One of these studies, conducted at the University of Minnesota, involving more than 46,000 participants, reported a statistically significant reduction in mortality from colorectal cancer for individuals undergoing annual screening. However, this benefit only emerged after more than 13 years of follow-up and was extremely expensive to achieve since all positive tests (the majority of which were falsely positive) were followed by colonoscopy.

Screening techniques for large-bowel cancer in asymptomatic persons remain unsatisfactory. Recommendations from governmental and private agencies are conflicting. At present, the American Cancer Society suggests annual digital rectal examinations beginning at age 40, annual fecal Hemoccult screening beginning at age 50, and sigmoidoscopy (preferably flexible), every 3 to 5 years, beginning at age 50 for asymptomatic individuals having none of the high-risk factors for colorectal cancer. More effective techniques for screening are needed, perhaps taking advantage of the molecular changes which have been described in these tumors. An analysis for specific *ras* proto-oncogene mutations from DNA recovered from stool in patients with a history of colorectal cancer represents an initial step in this direction.

CLINICAL FEATURES **Presenting symptoms** Symptoms vary with the anatomic location of the tumor.

Since stool is relatively liquid as it passes through the ileocecal valve into the right colon, neoplasms arising in the cecum and ascending colon may become quite large, significantly narrowing the bowel lumen, without resulting in any obstructive symptoms or noticeable alterations in bowel habits. Lesions of the right colon commonly ulcerate, leading to chronic, insidious blood loss without a change in the appearance of the stool. Consequently, patients with tumors of the ascending colon often present with symptoms such as fatigue, palpitations, and even angina pectoris and are found to have a hypochromic, microcytic anemia indicative of iron deficiency. Since the cancer may bleed intermittently, however, a random test for the presence of occult blood in the stool may be negative. As a result, the unexplained presence of iron-deficiency anemia in any adult (with the possible exception of a premenopausal, multiparous woman) mandates a thorough endoscopic and/or radiographic visualization of the entire large bowel (Fig. 257-1).

Since stool becomes more concentrated as it passes into the transverse and descending colon, tumors arising there tend to impede the passage of stool, resulting in the development of abdominal cramping, occasional obstruction, and even perforation. Radiographs of the abdomen often reveal characteristic annular, constricting lesions ("apple-core" or "napkin-ring") (Fig. 257-2).

Neoplasms arising in the rectosigmoid often are associated with hematochezia, tenesmus, and narrowing in the caliber of stool; nonetheless, anemia is an infrequent finding. While these symptoms may lead patients and their physicians to suspect the presence of hemorrhoids, the development of rectal bleeding and/or altered bowel habits demands a prompt digital rectal examination and proctosigmoidoscopy.

Staging, prognostic factors, patterns of spread The prognosis

FIGURE 257-1 Double-contrast air-barium enema revealing a sessile tumor of the cecum in a patient with iron-deficiency anemia and guaiac-positive stool. The lesion at surgery was a stage B adenocarcinoma.

FIGURE 257-2 Annular, constricting adenocarcinoma of the descending colon. This radiographic appearance is referred to as an "apple-core" lesion and is always highly suggestive of malignancy.

TABLE 257-3   Modified Dukes classification of colorectal cancer

Stage	Pathologic description	Approximate 5-year survival, %
A	Cancer limited to mucosa and submucosa	>90
B_1	Cancer extends into muscularis	85
B_2	Cancer extends into or through serosa	70–85
C	Cancer involves regional lymph nodes	30–60
D	Distant metastases (i.e., liver, lung, etc.)	5

for individuals having colorectal cancer is closely related to the depth of tumor penetration into the bowel wall and the presence of both regional lymph node involvement and distant metastases. These variables are incorporated into the staging system introduced by Dukes (Table 257-3). Patients with superficial lesions not penetrating into the muscularis or involving regional lymph nodes are designated as having *stage A* disease; those individuals whose tumors penetrate more deeply but without spread to lymph nodes are said to have *stage B* disease (with lesions restricted to the muscularis termed *stage B_1* disease while lesions involving the serosa classified as *stage B_2* disease); regional lymph node involvement defines *stage C* disease; and metastatic spread to sites such as liver, lung, or bone indicates *stage D* disease. Unless gross evidence of metastatic disease is present, it is impossible to accurately determine disease stage prior to surgical resection and pathologic analysis of the operative specimens.

Most recurrences after a surgical resection of a large-bowel cancer occur within the first 4 postoperative years, making the 5-year mark a fairly reliable indicator of cure. The likelihood for 5-year survival in patients with colorectal cancer is closely associated with their Dukes stage (Table 257-3). That likelihood has appeared to improve during the past several decades when similar surgical stages have been compared. The most plausible explanation for this improvement appears to be more thorough intraoperative and pathologic staging. In particular, more exacting attention to pathologic detail has revealed that the prognosis following the resection of a colorectal cancer is not related merely to the presence or absence of regional lymph node involvement but may be more precisely assessed by the number of involved lymph nodes (i.e., 1 to 4 lymph nodes versus >5 lymph nodes). Other predictors of a poor prognosis after a total surgical resection include tumor penetration through the bowel wall into pericolic fat, poorly differentiated histology, perforation and/or tumor adherence to adjacent organs (increasing the risk for an anatomically adjacent recurrence), and venous invasion by tumor (Table 257-4). Regardless of the clinicopathologic stage, a preoperative elevation of the plasma carcinoembryonic antigen (CEA) titer is suggestive of eventual tumor recurrence. The presence of abnormal DNA content (i.e., aneuploidy) and specific chromosomal deletions (i.e., so-called allelic loss) in tumor cells, as determined by flow cytometry and

TABLE 257-4   Poor prognostic predictors following total surgical resection

Tumor spread to regional lymph nodes
Number of regional lymph nodes involved
Tumor penetration through the bowel wall
Poorly differentiated histology
Perforation
Tumor adherence to adjacent organs
Venous invasion
Preoperative elevation of CEA titer (>5.0 ng/mL)
Aneuploidy
Specific chromosomal deletion (allelic loss)

restriction fragment length polymorphism analysis respectively, appears to predict a higher risk for metastatic spread. In contrast to most other carcinomas and sarcomas, the prognosis in individuals with colorectal cancer is *not* influenced by the size of the primary lesion when adjusted for nodal involvement and histologic differentiation.

Cancers of the large bowel generally spread to regional lymph nodes or to the liver via the portal venous circulation. The liver represents the most frequent visceral site of metastatic dissemination; it is the initial site of distant spread in one-third of recurring colorectal cancers and eventually becomes involved in greater than two-thirds of such patients at the time of death. In general, colorectal cancer rarely metastasizes to the lungs, supraclavicular lymph nodes, bone, or brain without prior spread to the liver. A major exception to this rule occurs in patients having primary tumors in the distal rectum, from where tumor cells may spread through the paravertebral venous plexus, escaping the portal venous system and thereby reaching the lungs or supraclavicular lymph nodes without hepatic involvement. The median survival after the detection of distant metastases may range from 6 to 9 months (hepatomegaly, liver abnormalities) to 24 to 30 months (small liver nodule initially identified by elevated CEA level and subsequent CT scan).

TREATMENT   Total resection of tumor represents optimal management when a malignant lesion is endoscopically or radiographically detected in the large bowel. An evaluation for the presence of metastatic disease, including a thorough physical examination, a chest radiograph, biochemical assessment of liver function, and a plasma CEA level, should be performed prior to surgery. When possible, a colonoscopy of the entire large bowel should be performed to identify synchronous neoplasms and/or polyps. The detection of metastases should not preclude surgery in patients with tumor-related symptoms such as gastrointestinal bleeding or obstruction, but may often result in a less radical operative procedure being carried out. At the time of laparotomy, the entire peritoneal cavity should be examined with the liver, pelvis, and hemidiaphragm being thoroughly inspected and the full length of the large bowel being carefully palpated. Following recovery from a complete resection, patients should be carefully observed for 5 years by semiannual physical examinations and yearly blood chemistries. If a complete colonoscopy was not performed preoperatively, this should be carried out within the first several postoperative months. Some authorities favor obtaining plasma CEA levels at 3-month intervals because of the sensitivity of this test as a marker for otherwise undetectable tumor recurrence. Subsequent endoscopic or radiographic surveillance of the large bowel, probably at triannual intervals, is indicated, since patients who have been cured of one colorectal cancer have a 3 to 5 percent probability of developing an additional bowel cancer during their lifetime and a risk in excess of 15 percent for the development of adenomatous polyps. Anastomotic (i.e., "suture-line") recurrences are infrequent in colorectal cancer patients, if the surgical resection margins were adequate and free of tumor.

Radiation therapy to the pelvis is generally recommended for patients with rectal cancer because of the 30 to 40 percent probability of regional recurrences following complete surgical resection of stages B and C tumors, especially if they have penetrated through the serosa. This alarmingly high rate of local disease recurrence is believed to be due to the fact that the contained anatomic space within the pelvis limits the extent of the resection and because the rich lymphatic network of the pelvic side wall immediately adjacent to the rectum facilities the early spread of malignant cells into surgically inaccessible tissue. Prospectively randomized trials have indicated that the prophylactic use of radiation therapy, either pre- or postoperatively, reduces the likelihood of pelvis recurrences but does not appear to prolong survival. Preoperative radiotherapy is clearly indicated for patients with large, potentially unresectable rectal cancers, since such anatomically fixed lesions may shrink sufficiently to permit subsequent surgical removal.

Chemotherapy in patients with advanced colorectal cancer has proven to be of only marginal benefit. Since its introduction into clinical trials more than 25 years ago, 5-fluorouracil (5-FU) remains the most effective treatment for this disease. It is as useful when given alone as when combined with other drugs, but is associated with only a 15 to 20 percent likelihood of reducing measurable tumor masses by 50 percent or more (i.e., partial response). While the probability for tumor response appears to be somewhat greater for patients with liver metastases when such chemotherapy is infused directly into the hepatic artery as compared to a peripheral vein, intraarterial treatment is costly and toxic and does not appear to prolong survival. The results of recent studies have suggested that the concomitant administration of folinic acid (also known as leucovorin or citrovorum factor) will improve the efficacy of 5-FU in patients with advanced colorectal cancer, presumably by enhancing the binding of 5-FU to its target enzyme, thymidylate synthase, thereby increasing the suppression of DNA synthesis and accompanying cytotoxicity. The majority of randomized trials have indicated a threefold improvement in the likelihood of partial response when folinic acid is combined with 5-FU; however, the effect on survival appears marginal and the optimal dose-schedule remains to be defined.

The value of postoperative chemotherapy and/or radiation therapy has been assessed in patients with stages B and C cancers as a means of eradicating clinically undetectable micrometastases and thereby increasing the probability for cure. The weight of evidence from more than 12 prospectively randomized trials in patients who have undergone the resection of a colon cancer suggests that the use of such prophylactic chemotherapy (i.e., including 5-FU given alone or in combination with other cytotoxic drugs) does not reduce the recurrence rate or prolong survival. However, the results of two clinical studies have indicated that the administration of adjuvant 5-FU with an anthelmintic agent, levamisole, to patients with stage C cancers, leads to a decrease in the likelihood of recurrence and a modest improvement in survival. The levamisole is thought to act in this therapeutic setting as a nonspecific immunomodulator. In contrast, in patients who have undergone the resection of a rectal cancer, data from controlled studies indicate that postoperative radiation therapy when combined with chemotherapy appears to reduce the likelihood of regional recurrences and increase the potential for cure. It has been postulated that the chemotherapy, believed to be ineffective when given prophylactically for patients with colon lesions, acts as a radiation sensitizer when given to individuals who have been operated upon for rectal cancer, thereby enhancing the biologic effect of the radiotherapy.

TUMORS OF THE SMALL INTESTINE

Small-bowel tumors comprise only 3 to 6 percent of gastrointestinal neoplasms. Because of their rarity, a correct diagnosis is often delayed. Abdominal symptoms are usually vague and poorly defined, and conventional radiographic studies of the upper and lower intestinal tract are often normal. Small-bowel tumors should be considered in the following situations: (1) recurrent, unexplained episodes of crampy abdominal pain; (2) intermittent bouts of intestinal obstruction, especially in the absence of inflammatory bowel disease or prior abdominal surgery; (3) intussusception in the adult; and (4) evidence of chronic intestinal bleeding in the presence of negative conventional radiographs. A careful small-bowel barium study is the diagnostic procedure of choice; the diagnostic accuracy may be improved by infusing barium through a nasogastric tube placed into the duodenum (enteroclysis).

BENIGN TUMORS In general, the histology of benign small-bowel tumors is difficult to predict on clinical and radiologic grounds alone. The symptomatology of benign tumors is not distinctive, with pain, obstruction, and hemorrhage being the most frequent symptoms. These tumors are usually discovered during the fifth and sixth decades of life, more often in the distal rather than the proximal small intestine. The most common benign tumors are adenomas, leiomyomas, lipomas, and angiomas.

Adenomas These tumors include those of the islet cells and Brunner's glands as well as polypoid adenomas. *Islet cell adenomas* are occasionally located outside the pancreas; the associated syndromes are discussed in Chap. 338. *Brunner's gland adenomas* are not truly neoplastic but represent a hypertrophy or hyperplasia of submucosal duodenal glands. These appear as small nodules in the duodenal mucosa that secrete a highly viscous alkaline mucus. Most often this is an incidental radiographic finding not associated with any specific clinical disorder.

Polypoid adenomas (See Table 257-2) Approximately 25 percent of benign small-bowel tumors are polypoid adenomas. They may present as single polypoid lesions or, less commonly, as papillary villous adenomas. As in the colon, the sessile or papillary form of the tumor is sometimes associated with a coexistent carcinoma. Occasionally, patients with Gardner's syndrome (a variant of polyposis coli) may develop premalignant adenomas in the small bowel; such lesions are generally in the duodenum. Multiple polypoid tumors may occur throughout the small bowel (and occasionally the stomach and colorectum) in the Peutz-Jeghers syndrome. The polyps are usually hamartomas (juvenile polyps) having a low potential for malignant degeneration. Mucocutaneous melanin deposits as well as tumors of the ovary, breast, pancreas, and endometrium are also associated with this autosomal dominant condition.

Leiomyomas These neoplasms arise from smooth-muscle components of the intestine and are usually intramural, affecting the overlying mucosa. Ulceration of the mucosa may cause gastrointestinal hemorrhage of varying severity. Cramping, intermittent abdominal pain is frequently encountered.

Lipomas These tumors occur with greatest frequency in the distal ileum and at the ileocecal valve. They have a characteristic radiolucent appearance, are usually intramural and asymptomatic, but may on occasion be associated with bleeding.

Angiomas While not true neoplasms, these lesions are important because they frequently cause intestinal bleeding. They may take the form of telangiectasia or hemangiomas. Multiple intestinal telangiectasia occur in a nonhereditary form confined to the gastrointestinal tract or as part of the hereditary Osler-Rendu-Weber syndrome. Vascular tumors may also take the form of isolated hemangiomas, most commonly in the jejunum. Angiography, especially during bleeding, is the procedure of choice in evaluating these lesions.

MALIGNANT TUMORS While infrequent in appearance, small-bowel malignancies occur in patients with long-standing regional enteritis and celiac sprue as well as in individuals with AIDS. In contrast to benign tumors, malignant tumors of the small bowel are frequently associated with fever, weight loss, anorexia, bleeding, and a palpable abdominal mass. After ampullary carcinomas (many of which arise from biliary or pancreatic ducts), the most frequently occurring small-bowel malignancies are adenocarcinomas, lymphomas, carcinoid tumors, and leiomyosarcomas.

Adenocarcinomas The most common primary cancers of the small bowel are adenocarcinomas, which account for about 50 percent of the malignant tumors. These neoplasms occur with highest frequency in the distal duodenum and proximal jejunum, where they tend to ulcerate and cause hemorrhage or obstruction. Radiologically, they may be confused with chronic duodenal ulcer disease or with Crohn's disease if the patient has long-standing regional enteritis. The diagnosis is best made by endoscopy and biopsy under direct vision. Surgical resection is the treatment of choice.

Lymphomas Lymphomatous involvement of the small bowel may be primary or secondary. A diagnosis of a primary intestinal lymphoma requires histologic confirmation of a lymphoproliferative neoplasm in a clinical setting in which palpable adenopathy and hepatosplenomegaly are absent and there is no evidence of lymphoma on a chest radiograph, CT scan, peripheral blood smear, or on bone marrow aspiration and biopsy. In general, symptoms referable to the small bowel are present, usually accompanied by an anatomically discernible lesion. Secondary lymphoma of the small bowel refers to involvement of the intestine by a lymphoid malignancy extending from involved retroperitoneal lymph nodes and hence is a manifestation of a generalized systemic neoplasm (see Chap. 317).

Primary intestinal lymphoma comprises 25 percent of malignancies of the small bowel. Essentially all these neoplasms are non-Hodgkin's lymphomas, most frequently having a diffuse, large-cell (i.e., "high-grade") histology. Intestinal lymphoma involves the ileum more frequently than the jejunum, which, in turn, is more commonly affected than the duodenum, a pattern which mirrors the relative amount of normal lymphoid cells in these anatomic areas. The risk of small-bowel lymphoma is increased in patients with a prior history of malabsorptive conditions (e.g., celiac sprue), regional enteritis, and depressed immunologic function due to congenital immunodeficiency syndromes, prior organ transplantation, autoimmune disorders, or AIDS.

The development of localized or nodular masses that narrow the lumen results in periumbilical pain (made worse by eating) as well as weight loss, vomiting, and occasional intestinal obstruction. The diagnosis of small-bowel lymphoma may be suspected by the appearance on contrast radiographs of patterns such as infiltration and thickening of mucosal folds, mucosal nodules, areas of irregular ulceration, or stasis of contrast material. The diagnosis can be confirmed by surgical exploration and resection of involved segments. Intestinal lymphoma may occasionally be diagnosed by peroral intestinal mucosal biopsy, but since the disease mainly involves the lamina propria, full-thickness surgical biopsies are usually required.

Resection of the tumor constitutes the initial treatment modality. While postoperative radiation therapy has been offered to some patients following such a total resection, most authorities favor short-term systemic treatment with combination chemotherapy. The frequent presence of widespread intraabdominal disease at the time of diagnosis and the occasional multicentricity of the tumor often make a total resection impossible. Combination chemotherapy would appear to be appropriate management for these patients as well. The probability of sustained remission or cure is approximately 75 percent in patients with localized disease, but 25 percent or less in individuals with unresectable lymphoma.

A unique form of small-bowel lymphoma, diffusely involving the entire intestine, was first described in oriental Jews and Arabs and is referred to as immunoproliferative small intestinal disease (IPSID), Mediterranean lymphoma, or alpha-heavy chain disease. The typical presentation includes chronic diarrhea and steatorrhea associated with vomiting and abdominal cramps; clubbing of the digits may be observed as well. A curious feature in many patients with IPSID is the presence in the blood and intestinal secretions of an abnormal IgA which contains a shortened alpha-heavy chain and is devoid of light chains. It is suspected that the abnormal alpha chains are produced by plasma cells infiltrating the small bowel. The clinical course of patients with IPSID is generally one of exacerbations and remissions, with death frequently resulting from either progressive malnutrition and wasting or the development of an aggressive lymphoma. Chemotherapy and radiation therapy have been ineffective.

Carcinoid tumors   Among the more common epithelial tumors of the small intestine are carcinoid tumors. They arise from argentaffin cells of the crypts of Lieberkühn and are found from the distal duodenum to the ascending colon, areas embryologically derived from the midgut. More than 50 percent of intestinal carcinoids are found in the distal ileum, with the majority congregating in close proximity to the ileocecal valve. Most intestinal carcinoids are asymptomatic and of low malignant potential, but invasion and metastases may occur, leading to the carcinoid syndrome (Chap. 276).

Leiomyosarcomas   Large, bulky tumors, leiomyosarcomas often are greater than 5 cm in diameter and may be palpable on abdominal examination. Bleeding, obstruction, and perforation are common.

CANCERS OF THE ANUS

Cancers of the anus account for 1 to 2 percent of the malignant tumors of the large bowel. The majority of such lesions arise in the anal canal which is defined as the anatomic area extending from the anorectal ring to a zone approximately halfway between the pectinate (or dentate) line and the anal verge. Carcinomas arising proximal to the pectinate line (i.e., in the transitional zone between the glandular mucosa of the rectum and the squamous epithelium of the distal anus) are known as basaloid, cuboidal, or cloacogenic tumors; approximately one-third of anal cancers have this histologic pattern. Malignancies arising distal to the pectinate line have a squamous cell histology, ulcerate more frequently, and represent approximately 55 percent of anal cancers. The prognosis for patients with basaloid and squamous cell cancers of the anus is identical when corrected for tumor size and the presence or absence of nodal spread.

Anal cancers occur most commonly in individuals with a prior history of chronic anal irritation. Such irritation may result from condylomata accuminata (i.e., viral lesions thought to be caused by papilloma virus infection), perianal fissures and/or fistulas, chronic hemorrhoids, and leukoplakia. The risk for anal cancer appears to be increased among homosexual males, presumably due to trauma related to anal intercourse. There presently are no data to indicate that anal cancers are AIDS-related tumors associated with direct infection by the human immunodeficiency virus. Anal cancers occur most commonly in middle-aged individuals, develop more frequently in women than men, and are most often associated with bleeding, pain, the sensation of a perianal mass, and perianal pruritus at the time of diagnosis.

Until recently, radical surgery (abdominal-perineal resection with lymph node sampling and a permanent colostomy) was the treatment of choice for this tumor type. The probability of survival 5 years following such a procedure ranged from 55 to 70 percent in the absence of spread to regional lymph nodes and decreased to less than 20 percent if nodal involvement was present. However, an alternative therapeutic approach combining external beam radiation with concomitant chemotherapy has resulted in biopsy-proven disappearance of all tumor in more than 80 percent of patients whose initial lesion was less than 3 cm in size. Tumor recurrences have occurred in less than 10 percent of these patients. Thus, it appears that approximately 70 percent of patients with anal cancers can be cured with nonoperative treatment and that disfiguring surgery should be reserved for the minority of individuals who are found to have residual tumor after being managed initially with radiation combined with chemotherapy.

REFERENCES

Colorectal cancer
Etiology and risk factors

AALTONEN LA et al: Clues to the pathogenesis of familial colorectal cancer. Science 260:812, 1993

BELL SM et al: Prognostic value of p53 overexpression and c-Ki *ras* gene mutations in colorectal cancer. Gastroenterology 104:57, 1993

COLLINS RH JR et al: Colon cancer, dysplasia, and surveillance in patients with ulcerative colitis. N Engl J Med 316:1654, 1987

EKBOM A et al: Increased risk of large-bowel cancer in Crohn's disease with colonic involvement. Lancet 336:357, 1990

———: Ulcerative colitis and colorectal cancer. A population-based study. N Engl J Med 323:1228, 1990

HAGGITT RC, REID BJ: Hereditary gastrointestinal polyposis syndromes. Am J Surg Path 10:871, 1986

HAMILTON SR: The molecular genetics of colorectal neoplasia. Gastroenterology 105:3, 1993

KINZLER KW et al: Identification of a gene located at chromosome 5q21 that is mutated in colorectal cancers. Science 251:1366, 1991

LIPKIN M, NEWMARK H: Effect of added dietary calcium on colonic epithelial cell proliferation in subjects at high risk for familial colonic cancer. N Engl J Med 313:1381, 1985

LYNCH HT et al: Hereditary colorectal cancer. Semin Oncol 18:337, 1991

NEUGUT AI et al: Dietary risk factors for the incidence and recurrence of colorectal adenomatous polyps. A case-control study. Ann Intern Med 118:91, 1993

TALAMONTI MS et al: Increase in activity and level of pp60$^{c\text{-}src}$ in progressive stages of human colorectal cancer. J Clin Invest 91:53, 1993

THUN MJ et al: Aspirin use and reduced risk of fatal colon cancer. N Engl J Med 325:1593, 1991

VOGELSTEIN B et al: Genetic alterations during colorectal-tumor development. N Engl J Med 319:595, 1988

WANG L et al: Mutation in the *nm23* gene is associated with metastasis in colorectal cancer. Cancer Res 53:717, 1993

WILLETT WC et al: Relation of meat, fat, and fiber intake to the risk of colon cancer in a prospective study among women. N Engl J Med 323:1664, 1990

Polyps

CANNON-ALBRIGHT LA et al: Common inheritance of susceptibility to colonic adenomatous polyps and associated colorectal cancers. N Engl J Med 319:533, 1988

FENOGLIO-PREISER CM, HUTTER RVP: Colorectal polyps: Pathological diagnosis and clinical significance. Cancer 35:322, 1985

O'BRIEN MJ et al: the National Polyp Study. Patient and polyp characteristics associated with high-grade dysplasia in colorectal adenomas. Gastroenterology 98:371, 1990

Screening

AHLQUIST DA et al: Accuracy of fecal occult blood screening for colorectal neoplasia. A prospective study using hemoccult and hemoquant tests. JAMA 269:1262, 1993

ALLISON et al: Hemoccult screening in detecting colorectal neoplasm: sensitivity, specificity and predictive value. Ann Inter Med 112:328, 1990

DUDOUET B et al: Presence of villin tissue specific cytoskeletal protein in sera of patients and an initial clinical evaluation of its value for the diagnosis and follow-up of colorectal cancers. Cancer Res 50:438, 1990

KNIGHT KK et al: Occult blood screening for colorectal cancer. JAMA 261:586, 1989

MANDEL JS et al: Screening for fecal occult blood reduces mortality from colorectal cancer: Results from the Minnesota Colon Cancer Control Study. N Engl J Med, in press

NEUGUT AI, PITA S: Role of sigmoidoscopy in screening for colorectal cancer: A critical review. Gastroenterology 95:492, 1988

RANSOHOFF DF, LANG CA: Screening for colorectal cancer. N Engl J Med 325:37, 1991

RANSOHOFF DF, LANG CA: Sigmoidoscopic screening in the 1990's. JAMA 269:1278, 1993

SELBY JV et al: A case-control study of screening sigmoidoscopy and mortality from colorectal cancer. N Engl J Med 326:653, 1992

SIDRANSKY D et al: Identification of *ras* oncogene mutations in the stool of patients with curable colorectal tumors. Science 256:102, 1992

SIMON JB: Occult blood screening for colorectal carcinoma: A critical review. Gastroenterology 88:820, 1985

WINAWER SJ et al: Randomized comparison of surveillance intervals after colonoscopic removal of newly diagnosed adenomatous polyps. N Engl J Med 328:901, 1993

Clinical features

GASTROINTESTINAL TUMOR STUDY GROUP: Adjuvant therapy of colon cancer—results of a postoperatively randomized trial. N Engl J Med 310:737, 1984

KERN SE et al: Allelic loss in colorectal carcinoma. JAMA 261:3099, 1989

WANEBO JH et al: Preoperative carcinoembryonic antigen level as a prognostic indicator in colorectal cancer. N Engl J Med 229:448, 1978

WITZIG TE et al: DNA ploidy and cell kinetic measurements as predictors of recurrence and survival in stages B$_2$ and C colorectal adenocarcinoma. Cancer 68:879, 1991

Treatment

FUCHS CS, MAYER RJ: Adjuvant chemotherapy for colon and rectal cancer. Semin Rad Oncol 3:29, 1993

GASTROINTESTINAL TUMOR STUDY GROUP: Prolongation of the disease-free interval in surgically treated rectal carcinoma. N Engl J Med 312:1465, 1985

KROOK JE et al: Effective surgical adjuvant therapy for high risk rectal carcinoma. N Engl J Med 324:709, 1991

MAYER A et al: The prognostic significance of proliferating cell nuclear antigen, epidermal growth factor receptor and *mdr* gene expression in colorectal cancer. Cancer 71:2454, 1993

MAYER RJ: Chemotherapy for metastatic colorectal cancer. Cancer 70:1414, 1992

MOERTEL CG et al: Levamisole and fluorouracil for adjuvant therapy of resected colon carcinoma. N Engl J Med 322:352, 1990

NIH CONCENSUS CONFERENCE: Adjuvant therapy for patients with colon and rectal cancer. JAMA 264:1444, 1990

Tumors of the small intestine

HABER DA, MAYER RJ: Primary gastrointestinal lymphoma. Semin Oncol 15:154, 1988

SINDELAR WF: Cancer of the small intestine, in *Cancer: Principles and Practice of Oncology*, VT DeVita Jr et al (eds), 3d ed. Philadelphia, Lippincott, 1989, pp 875–894

Anal cancer

DALING JR et al: Sexual practices, sexually transmitted diseases, and the incidence of anal cancer. N Engl J Med 317:973, 1987

LEICHMAN L et al: Cancer of the anal canal: Model for preoperative adjuvant combined modality therapy. Am J Med 78:211, 1985

PALEFSKY JM et al: Anal intraepithelial neoplasia and anal papilloma virus infection among homosexual males with group IV HIV disease. JAMA 263:2911, 1990

SISCHY B et al: Definitive irradiation and chemotherapy for radiosensitization in management of anal carcinoma: Interim report in Radiation Therapy Oncology Group study no. 8314. J Natl Cancer Inst 81:850, 1989

258 ACUTE INTESTINAL OBSTRUCTION

WILLIAM SILEN

ETIOLOGY AND CLASSIFICATION   Intestinal obstruction may be *mechanical* or *nonmechanical* (resulting from neuromuscular disturbances which produce either *adynamic* or *dynamic ileus*). The causes of mechanical obstruction of the lumen are conveniently divided into (1) lesions *extrinsic* to the intestine, e.g., adhesive bands, internal and external hernias, (2) lesions *intrinsic* to the wall of the intestine, e.g., diverticulitis, carcinoma, regional enteritis, and (3) obturation of the lumen, e.g., gallstone obstruction, intussusception. Clinically, however, it is most useful to consider whether the obstructive mechanism involves the small or large intestine, because the causes, symptoms, and treatments are different (see below). Adhesions and external hernias are the most common causes of obstruction of the small intestine, constituting 70 to 75 percent of cases of this type. Adhesions, however, almost never produce obstruction of the colon, whereas carcinoma, sigmoid diverticulitis, and volvulus, in that order, are the most common causes and together account for about 90 percent of the cases.

Adynamic ileus is probably the most common overall cause of obstruction. The development of this condition is mediated via the hormonal component of the sympathoadrenal system. Adynamic ileus may occur after any peritoneal insult, and its severity and duration will be dependent to some degree on the type of peritoneal injury. Hydrochloric acid, colonic contents, and pancreatic enzymes are among the most irritating substances, whereas blood and urine are less so. Adynamic ileus occurs to some degree after any abdominal operation; it usually lasts 2 to 3 days after most operative procedures. Retroperitoneal hematomas, particularly associated with vertebral fracture, commonly cause severe adynamic ileus, and the latter may occur with other retroperitoneal conditions, such as ureteral calculus or severe pyelonephritis. Thoracic diseases, including lower-lobe pneumonia, fractured ribs, and myocardial infarction, frequently produce adynamic ileus, as do electrolyte disturbances, particularly potassium depletion. Finally, intestinal ischemia, whether the result of vascular occlusion or intestinal distention itself, may perpetuate an adynamic ileus. *Spastic* or *dynamic ileus* is very uncommon and results from extreme and prolonged contraction of the intestine. It has been observed in heavy metal poisoning, uremia, porphyria, and extensive intestinal ulcerations. Primary intestinal pseudoobstruction (see Chap. 256) is a chronic motility disorder which frequently mimics mechanical obstruction. Unnecessary operations in such patients should be avoided.

PATHOPHYSIOLOGY   Distention of the intestine is caused by the accumulation of gas and fluid proximal to and within the obstructed segment. Between 70 and 80 percent of intestinal gas consists of swallowed air, and because this is composed mainly of nitrogen, which is poorly absorbed from the intestinal lumen, removal of air by continuous gastric suction is a useful adjunct in the treatment of intestinal distention. The accumulation of fluid proximal to the obstructing mechanism results not only from ingested fluid, swallowed saliva, gastric juice, and biliary and pancreatic secretions but also from interference with normal sodium and water transport. During the first 12 to 24 h of obstruction, there is a marked depression of flux from lumen to blood of sodium and consequently water in the distended proximal intestine. After 24 h, there is movement of sodium and water into the lumen, contributing further to the distention and fluid losses. Intraluminal pressure rises from a normal of 2 to 4 cmH$_2$O to 8 to 10 cmH$_2$O. During peristalsis, when simple obstruction or a "closed loop" is present, pressures reach 30 to 60 cmH$_2$O. Closed-loop obstruction of the small intestine results when the lumen is occluded at two points by a single mechanism such as a hernial ring or adhesive band, thus producing a closed loop whose blood supply is often obstructed at the same time. Strangulation of the loop itself is thus common in association with marked distention proximal to the involved loop. A form of closed-loop obstruction is encountered when complete obstruction of the colon exists in the presence of a competent ileocecal valve (85 percent of individuals). Although the blood supply of the colon is not entrapped within the obstructing mechanism, distention of the cecum is extreme because of its greater diameter (LaPlace's law), and impairment of the intramural blood supply is considerable with consequent gangrene of the cecal wall, usually anteriorly. Necrosis of the small intestine may occur by the same mechanism of interference with intramural blood flow when distention is extreme, but this sequence is uncommon in the small intestine. Once impairment of blood supply occurs, bacterial invasion supervenes, and peritonitis develops. The systemic effects of extreme distention include elevation of the diaphragm with restricted ventilation and subsequent atelectasis. Venous return via the inferior vena cava also may be impaired.

The loss of fluids and electrolytes may be extreme and, unless replacement is prompt, leads to hemoconcentration, hypovolemia, renal insufficiency, shock, and death. Vomiting, accumulation of fluids within the lumen by the mechanisms described above, and the sequestration of fluid into the edematous intestinal wall and peritoneal cavity as a result of impairment of venous return from the intestine all contribute to massive loss of fluid and electrolytes, especially potassium. As soon as significant impedance to venous return is present, the intestine becomes severely congested, and blood begins to seep into the intestinal lumen. Blood loss may reach significant levels when long segments of intestine are involved.

SYMPTOMS *Mechanical small-intestinal obstruction* is characterized by cramping midabdominal pain which tends to be more severe the higher the obstruction. The pain occurs in paroxysms, and the patient is relatively comfortable in the intervals between the pains. Audible borborygmi are often noted by the patient simultaneously with the paroxysms of pain. The pain may become less severe as distention progresses, probably because motility is impaired in the edematous intestine. When strangulation is present, the pain is usually more localized and may be steady and severe without a colicky component, a fact that often causes delay in diagnosis of obstruction. Vomiting is almost invariable, and it is earlier and more profuse the higher the obstruction. The vomitus initially contains bile and mucus and remains as such if the obstruction is high in the intestine. With low ileal obstruction, the vomitus becomes feculent, i.e., orange-brown in color with a foul odor, which results from the overgrowth of bacteria proximal to the obstruction. Singultus is common. Obstipation and failure to pass gas by rectum are invariably present when the obstruction is complete, although some stool and gas may be passed spontaneously or after an enema shortly after onset of the complete obstruction. Diarrhea is occasionally observed in partial obstruction. Blood in the stool is rare but does occur in cases of intussusception. Other than some minor but inconsistent differences in pain patterns noted above, the symptoms of strangulating obstructions cannot be distinguished from those of nonstrangulating obstructions.

Mechanical colonic obstruction produces colicky abdominal pain similar in quality to that of small-intestinal obstruction but of much lower intensity. Complaints of pain are occasionally absent in stoic elderly patients. Vomiting occurs late, if at all, particularly if the ileocecal valve is competent. Paradoxically, feculent vomitus is very rare. A history of recent alterations in bowel habits and blood in the stool is common because carcinoma and diverticulitis are the most frequent causes. Constipation becomes progressive, and obstipation with failure to pass gas ensues. Acute symptoms may develop over a period of a week. Cecal volvulus more closely resembles obstruction of the small intestine clinically, whereas patients with sigmoid volvulus more typically have the picture of colonic obstruction in which marked distention predominates, with relatively less pain.

In *adynamic ileus*, colicky pain is absent, and only discomfort from distention is evident. Vomiting may be frequent but is rarely

profuse. It usually consists of gastric contents and bile and is almost never feculent. Complete obstipation may or may not occur. Singultus is common.

PHYSICAL FINDINGS *Abdominal distention* is the hallmark of all forms of intestinal obstruction. It is least marked in cases of obstruction high in the small intestine and most marked in colonic obstruction. Early, especially in closed-loop strangulating small-bowel obstruction, distention may be barely perceptible or absent. Tenderness and rigidity are usually minimal; the temperature is rarely above 37.8°C (100°F) in nonstrangulating obstruction of the small and large intestine. Contrary to popular belief, the same is true of strangulating obstruction until very late, a fact that has often resulted in unfortunate delay in treatment. Signs and symptoms of shock also occur *very late* in strangulating obstruction. The appearance of shock, tenderness, rigidity, and fever often means that there has been contamination of the peritoneum with infected intestinal content. The presence of a palpable abdominal mass usually signifies a closed-loop strangulating small-bowel obstruction because the tense fluid-filled loop is the palpable lesion. Auscultation may reveal loud, high-pitched borborygmi coincident with the colicky pain, but this finding is often absent late in strangulating or nonstrangulating obstruction. A quiet abdomen does not eliminate the possibility of obstruction, nor does it necessarily establish the diagnosis of adynamic ileus.

LABORATORY AND X-RAY FINDINGS Leukocytosis, with shift to the left, usually occurs when strangulation is present, but a normal white blood cell count does not exclude strangulation. Elevation of the serum amylase level is encountered occasionally in all forms of intestinal obstruction, especially the strangulating variety.

The x-ray is extremely valuable but under certain circumstances also may be misleading. In nonstrangulating complete small-bowel obstruction, x-rays are almost completely reliable. Distention of fluid- and gas-filled loops of small intestine usually arranged in a "stepladder" pattern with air-fluid levels and an absence or paucity of colonic gas are pathognomonic (Fig. 258-1). These findings, however, are absent in slightly over half the cases of strangulating small-bowel obstruction, especially early in the disease. A general haze due to peritoneal fluid and sometimes a "coffee bean"–shaped

FIGURE 258-1 Acute mechanical obstruction of small intestine (upright film). Note air-fluid levels, marked distention of bowel loops, and absence of colonic gas.

mass are seen in strangulating obstruction. Occasionally, the films are normal, but when symptoms are consistent with obstruction of the small intestine, a normal film should suggest strangulation. Roentgenographic differentiation of partial mechanical small-bowel obstruction from adynamic ileus may be impossible because gas is present in both the small and large intestines; however, colonic distention is usually more prominent in adynamic ileus. A radiopaque dye given by mouth is useful in making this distinction.

Colonic obstruction with a competent ileocecal valve is easily recognized because distention with gas is mainly confined to the colon. Barium enema, sigmoidoscopy, or colonoscopy, depending on the suspected site of obstruction, is usually advisable to determine the nature of the lesion, except when concomitant perforation is suspected, a rare occurrence. Sigmoidoscopy may be therapeutic in cases of sigmoid volvulus. When the ileocecal valve is incompetent, the films resemble those of partial small-bowel obstruction or adynamic ileus, and barium enema or colonoscopy is necessary to establish the correct diagnosis. Barium given by mouth is perfectly safe when obstruction is in the small intestine, since the barium sulfate does not become inspissated in this location. *Barium should never be given by mouth to a patient with possible colonic obstruction* until that possibility has been excluded by barium enema.

PROGNOSIS AND TREATMENT Small-intestinal obstruction
The overall mortality rate for obstruction of the small intestine is about 10 percent, even under the most optimal conditions. While the mortality rate for nonstrangulating obstruction is as low as 5 to 8 percent, that for strangulating obstruction has been reported to be between 20 and 75 percent. Well over half the deaths from small-bowel obstruction occur in those with strangulation; however, the latter constitute only one-fourth to one-third of the cases. Careful studies indicate that the clinical, laboratory, and x-ray findings are not reliable in distinguishing strangulating from nonstrangulating obstruction when obstruction is complete. Complete obstruction is suggested when there has been a total cessation in the passage of gas or stool per rectum and when gas is absent in the distal intestine by x-ray. Since strangulating small-bowel obstruction is always complete, operation should always be undertaken in such patients after suitable preparation. Prior to operation, fluid and electrolyte balance should be restored and decompression instituted by means of a nasogastric tube. Replacement of potassium is especially important because intake is nil and losses in vomitus are large. Six to eight hours of preparation may be necessary. During this period, broad-spectrum antibiotics are indicated if strangulation is felt to be likely, but operation should not be delayed unless there is unequivocal clinical and roentgenographic evidence of resolution of the obstruction during the period of preparation. Attempts to pass a long tube into the small intestine usually fail while putting the patient through uncomfortable, unproductive manipulations which delay appropriate fluid replacement and decompression. *There are probably few, if any, indications for the use of a long intestinal tube.* Procrastination of operation because of improvement in well-being of the patient during resuscitation and gastric decompression usually leads to unnecessary and hazardous delay in proper treatment. Purely nonoperative therapy is safe only in the presence of incomplete obstruction and is best utilized in patients with (1) repeated episodes of partial obstruction, (2) recent postoperative partial obstruction, and (3) partial obstruction following a recent episode of diffuse peritonitis.

Colonic obstruction The mortality rate for colonic obstruction is about 20 percent. As in small-bowel obstruction, nonoperative treatment is contraindicated unless the obstruction is incomplete. Occasionally, but not always, when the obstruction is incomplete, nonoperative therapy may result in sufficient decompression that a definitive operative procedure can be undertaken at a later date. This usually can be accomplished by discontinuation of all oral intake and perhaps by nasogastric suction, although attempts to decompress a *completely* obstructed colon by intubation are almost invariably futile. A long intestinal tube will not decompress an obstructed colon with a competent ileocecal valve. When obstruction is complete, early

operation is mandatory, especially when the ileocecal valve is competent; cecal gangrene is likely if the cecal diameter exceeds 10 cm on plain abdominal film. For obstruction on the left side of the colon, the most common site, preliminary operative decompression by cecostomy or transverse colostomy followed by definitive resection of the primary lesion has been the treatment of choice. Recently, primary resection of obstructing left-sided lesions with on-table washout of the colon has been accomplished safely. For a lesion of the right or transverse colon, primary resection and anastomosis can be performed safely because distention of the ileum with consequent discrepancy in size and hazard in suture are not present.

Adynamic ileus This type of ileus usually responds to nonoperative continuous decompression and adequate treatment of the primary disease. The prognosis is usually good. Recently, successful decompression of severe colonic ileus has been accomplished by colonoscopy, but this should be avoided if tenderness in the right lower quadrant suggests possible cecal gangrene. Rarely, adynamic colonic distention may become so great that cecostomy is required if cecal gangrene is feared. Spastic ileus usually responds to treatment of the primary disease.

REFERENCES

BECKER WF: Acute adhesive ileus: A study of 412 cases with particular reference to the abuse of tube decompression in treatment. Surg Gynecol Obstet 95:472, 1952

BULKLEY GB et al: Intraoperative determination of small intestinal viability following ischemic injury: Prospective controlled trial of two adjuvant methods (Doppler and fluorescein) compared with standard clinical judgement. Ann Surg 193:628, 1981

COHN I, ATIK M: Strangulation obstruction: Closed loop studies. Ann Surg 153:94, 1961

DUBOIS A et al: Postoperative ileus: Physiopathology, etiology and treatment. Ann Surg 178:781, 1973

GOUGH IR: Strangulating adhesive small bowel radiographs. Br J Surg 65:431, 1978

HOFSETTER SR: Acute adhesive obstruction of the small intestine. Surg Gynecol Obstet 152:141, 1981

JACKSON BR: The diagnosis of colonic obstruction. Dis Colon Rectum 25:603, 1982

NOLAN DJ: Barium examination of the small intestine. Gut 22:682, 1981

SHIELDS R: The absorption and secretion of fluid and electrolytes by the obstructed bowel. Br J Surg 52:774, 1965

SILEN W: *Cope's Early Diagnosis of the Acute Abdomen*, 18th ed. London, Oxford, 1991

259 ACUTE APPENDICITIS

WILLIAM SILEN

INCIDENCE AND EPIDEMIOLOGY The maximum incidence of acute appendicitis occurs in the second and third decades of life. While the disease may be encountered at any time of life, it is relatively rare at the extremes of age. Males and females are equally affected, except between puberty and age 25, when males predominate in a 3:2 ratio. Perforation is relatively much more common in infancy and in the aged, during which periods mortality rates are highest. The mortality rate has decreased steadily in Europe and the United States from 8.1 per 100,000 of the population in 1941 to less than 1 per 100,000 in 1970 and subsequently. The absolute incidence of the disease also decreased by about 40 percent between 1940 and 1960 but since then has remained unchanged. Although various factors such as changing dietary habits, altered intestinal flora, and better nutrition and intake of vitamins have been suggested to explain the reduced incidence, the exact reasons have not been elucidated. The overall incidence of appendicitis is much lower in underdeveloped countries, especially parts of Africa, and in lower socioeconomic groups.

PATHOGENESIS The primary pathogenetic hallmark has always been thought to be luminal obstruction. While obstruction can be identified in 30 to 40 percent of cases, recent studies have shown that ulceration of the mucosa is the initial event in the majority. The causation of the ulceration is unknown, although a viral etiology has been postulated. Recently, it has been suggested that infection with *Yersinia* organisms may cause the disease, since high complement fixation titers have been found in as many as 30 percent of cases of proven appendicitis 1 week after operation. Whether the inflammatory reaction attendant with ulceration is sufficient to obstruct the tiny appendiceal lumen even transiently is not clear. Obstruction, when present, is most commonly caused by a fecalith, which results from accumulation and inspissation of fecal matter around vegetable fibers. Enlarged lymphoid follicles associated with viral infections (e.g., measles), inspissated barium, worms (e.g., pinworms, *Ascaris*, and *Taenia*), and tumors (e.g., carcinoid or carcinoma) also may obstruct the lumen. Secretion of mucus distends the organ, which has a capacity of only 0.1 to 0.2 mL, and luminal pressures rise as high as 60 cmH$_2$O. Luminal bacteria multiply and invade the appendiceal wall as venous engorgement and subsequent arterial compromise result from the high intraluminal pressures. Finally, gangrene and perforation occur. If the process evolves slowly, adjacent organs such as the terminal ileum, cecum, and omentum may wall off the appendiceal area so that a localized abscess will develop, whereas rapid progression of vascular impairment may cause perforation with free access to the peritoneal cavity. Subsequent rupture of primary appendiceal abscesses may produce fistulas between the appendix and bladder, small intestine, sigmoid, or cecum. Occasionally, acute appendicitis may be the first manifestation of Crohn's disease. While chronic infection of the appendix with tuberculosis, amebiasis, and actinomycosis may occur, a useful clinical aphorism states that *chronic appendiceal inflammation is not usually the cause of prolonged abdominal pain of weeks' or months' duration*. In contrast, it is clear that recurrent acute appendicitis does occur, often with complete resolution of inflammation and symptoms between attacks. Recurrent acute appendicitis may become more frequent as antibiotics are dispensed more freely.

CLINICAL MANIFESTATIONS The history and sequence of symptoms are among the most important diagnostic features of appendicitis. The initial symptom is almost invariably *abdominal pain* of the visceral type, resulting from appendiceal contractions or distention of the lumen. It is usually poorly localized in the periumbilical or epigastric region. There is often an accompanying urge to defecate or pass flatus, neither of which relieves the distress. This visceral pain is mild, often cramping, and rarely catastrophic in nature, usually lasting 4 to 6 h, but it may not be noted by stoic individuals or by some patients during sleep. As inflammation spreads to the parietal peritoneal surfaces, the pain becomes somatic, steady, and more severe, aggravated by motion or cough, and usually located in the *right lower quadrant*. *Anorexia* is so frequent that the presence of hunger should arouse serious suspicion of the diagnosis of acute appendicitis. *Nausea* and *vomiting* occur in 50 to 60 percent of cases, but vomiting is rarely profuse and protracted. The development of nausea and vomiting before the onset of pain is extremely rare. Change in bowel habit is of little diagnostic value, since any or no alteration may be observed, although the presence of diarrhea caused by an inflamed appendix in juxtaposition to the sigmoid may cause serious diagnostic difficulties. Urinary frequency and dysuria occur if the appendix lies adjacent to the bladder. The typical sequence of symptoms (poorly localized periumbilical pain followed by nausea and vomiting with subsequent shift of pain to the right lower quadrant) occurs in only 50 to 60 percent of patients, and some variations are considered below.

Physical findings vary with time after onset of the illness and according to the location of the appendix, which may be situated deep in the pelvic cul-de-sac, in the right lower quadrant in any relation to the peritoneum, cecum, and small intestine, in the right upper quadrant (especially during pregnancy), or even in the left lower quadrant. *The diagnosis cannot be established unless tenderness can be elicited*. While tenderness is sometimes absent in the early visceral stage of the disease, it ultimately always develops and is found in any location corresponding to the position of the appendix. Abdominal tenderness may be completely absent if a retrocecal or pelvic appendix is present, in which case the sole physical finding may be tenderness in the flank or on rectal or pelvic examination. Percussion, rebound tenderness, and referred rebound tenderness are often, but not invariably, present; they are most likely to be absent early in the illness. Flexion of the right hip and guarded movement by the patient are due to parietal peritoneal involvement. Hyperesthesia of the skin of the right lower quadrant and a positive psoas or obturator sign are often late findings and are rarely of diagnostic value. When the inflamed appendix is in close proximity to the anterior parietal peritoneum, muscular rigidity is present yet is often minimal early. The temperature is usually normal or slightly elevated [37.2 to 38°C (99 to 100.5°F)], but a temperature above 38.3°C (101°F) should always suggest the presence of perforation. Tachycardia is commensurate with the elevation of the temperature. Rigidity and tenderness become more marked as the disease progresses to perforation and localized or diffuse peritonitis. Distention is rare unless severe diffuse peritonitis has developed. The alleged disappearance of pain and tenderness just prior to perforation is extremely unusual. A mass may develop if localized perforation has occurred but usually will not be detectable before 3 days after onset of the disease. Earlier presence of a mass suggests carcinoma of the cecum or Crohn's disease. Perforation is rare before 24 h after onset of symptoms, but the rate may be as high as 80 percent after 48 h.

Laboratory examination does not establish the diagnosis because the latter is based primarily on clinical grounds. Although moderate leukocytosis of 10,000 to 18,000 cells per microliter is frequent (with a concomitant shift to immature cells), the absence of leukocytosis does not eliminate the possibility of acute appendicitis. Leukocytosis of greater than 20,000 cells per microliter should alert the clinician to the probability of perforation. Anemia and blood in the stool suggest a primary diagnosis of carcinoma of the cecum, especially in elderly individuals. The urine may contain a few white or red blood cells without bacteria if the appendix lies close to the right ureter or bladder.

Urinalysis is most useful, however, in excluding genitourinary conditions which may mimic acute appendicitis. X-rays are rarely of value except when an opaque fecalith (5 percent of patients) is observed in the right lower quadrant (especially in children) together with other clinical findings consistent with appendicitis. Consequently, there is no routine need to obtain films of the abdomen unless there is a possibility of other conditions such as intestinal obstruction or ureteral calculus. In some patients in whom symptoms are either recurrent or more prolonged, a careful barium enema may disclose an extrinsic defect on the medial wall of the cecum or a calcified fecalith. The diagnosis also may be established by the ultrasonic demonstration of an enlarged and thick-walled appendix, but if the appendix cannot be seen, the diagnosis cannot be excluded. Ultrasound is most useful to exclude ovarian cysts, ectopic pregnancy, or tuboovarian abscess.

While the typical historical sequence and physical findings are present in 50 to 60 percent of cases, it is obvious that a wide variety of atypical patterns of disease are encountered, especially at the age extremes and during pregnancy. The 70 to 80 percent incidence of perforation and generalized peritonitis in infants under 2 years of age is dramatic testimony to the importance of the history in the early detection of the disease. Any infant or child with diarrhea, vomiting, and abdominal pain is highly suspect. Fever is much more common in this age group, and abdominal distention is often the only physical finding. In the elderly, pain and tenderness are often obtunded, and thus the diagnosis is frequently delayed. A 30 percent incidence of perforation in patients over 70 attests to the importance of this delay. Elderly patients often present themselves initially with a slightly painful mass (a primary appendiceal abscess) or sometimes appear with adhesive intestinal obstruction 5 or 6 days after a previously undetected perforated appendix. Appendicitis occurs about once in every 1000 pregnancies and is the most common extrauterine condition requiring abdominal operation. The diagnosis may be missed or delayed because of the frequent occurrence of mild abdominal discomfort and nausea and vomiting during pregnancy. During the last trimester, when the mortality rate from appendicitis is highest, uterine displacement of the appendix to the right upper quadrant and laterally leads to confusion in diagnosis because pain and tenderness are similarly displaced.

DIFFERENTIAL DIAGNOSIS A listing of the differential diagnoses of acute appendicitis would produce an encyclopedic compendium of all conditions which cause abdominal pain, since appendicitis may simulate any of these diseases. Diagnostic accuracy is about 75 to 80 percent for experienced clinicians and must be based solely on the clinical criteria outlined above. It is probably better to err slightly in the direction of overdiagnosis, since delay is associated with perforation and increased morbidity and mortality. In unperforated appendicitis, the mortality rate is 0.1 percent, little more than that associated with general anesthesia; for perforated appendicitis, there is an overall mortality of 3 percent, a figure that increases to 15 percent in the elderly. In doubtful cases, 4 to 6 h of observation is always more beneficial than harmful, however. The most common conditions discovered at operation when acute appendicitis is erroneously diagnosed are, in rough order of frequency, mesenteric lymphadenitis, no organic disease, acute pelvic inflammatory disease, ruptured graafian follicle or corpus luteum cyst, and acute gastroenteritis. In addition, acute cholecystitis, perforated ulcer, acute pancreatitis, acute diverticulitis, strangulating intestinal obstruction, ureteral calculus, and pyelonephritis frequently present diagnostic difficulties.

It is useful to consider separately some of the more common and difficult diagnostic possibilities, especially in the female. Differentiation of *pelvic inflammatory disease* from acute appendicitis may be virtually impossible. Gram-negative intracellular diplococci on cervical smear are not pathognomonic unless *Neisseria gonorrhoeae* can be cultured. Pain on movement of the cervix is not specific and may occur in appendicitis if perforation has occurred or if the appendix lies adjacent to the uterus or adnexa. *Rupture of a graafian follicle* (mittelschmerz) occurs at midcycle with spill of blood and fluid to produce pain and tenderness more diffuse and usually of a less severe degree than in appendicitis. Fever and leukocytosis are usually absent. *Rupture of a corpus luteum cyst* is identical clinically to rupture of a graafian follicle but develops about the time of menstruation. The presence of an adnexal mass, evidence of blood loss, and a positive pregnancy test help differentiate *ruptured tubal pregnancy*, but a negative pregnancy test is present when tubal abortion has occurred. *Twisted ovarian cyst* and *endometriosis* occasionally are difficult to distinguish from appendicitis. In all these female conditions, ultrasonic examination of the pelvis and laparoscopy may be of great value.

Acute mesenteric lymphadenitis is the appellation usually given when enlarged, slightly reddened lymph nodes at the root of the mesentery and a normal appendix are encountered at operation in a patient who usually has right lower quadrant tenderness and a somewhat higher temperature than most patients with acute appendicitis. Whether this is a single, discrete entity is unclear, since the causative factor is not known. It has been recognized recently that some of these patients have infection with *Yersinia pseudotuberculosis* or *Y. enterocolytica*, in which case the diagnosis can be established by culture of the mesenteric nodes or by serologic titers (see Chap. 123). The diagnosis is essentially impossible clinically, although retrospectively there often appears to have been more diffuse pain and tenderness. Children seem to be affected more frequently than adults. Operation should be undertaken unless there is rapid resolution of all symptoms and findings. *Acute gastroenteritis* usually causes profuse watery diarrhea, often with nausea and vomiting, but without localized findings. Between cramps, the abdomen is completely relaxed. In *Salmonella* gastroenteritis, the abdominal findings are similar, although the pain may be more severe and more localized, and fever and chills are common. The occurrence of similar symptoms among other members of the family may be helpful. When the diagnosis of acute pelvic appendicitis with perforation has been

missed, gastroenteritis is the most common previous working diagnosis. Persistent abdominal or rectal tenderness should eliminate the diagnosis of gastroenteritis. *Regional enteritis* (Crohn's disease) is usually associated with a more prolonged history, often with previous exacerbations regarded by the patient or physician as episodes of gastroenteritis unless the diagnosis has been established previously. *Meckel's diverticulitis* usually cannot be distinguished from acute appendicitis but is very rare.

TREATMENT Cathartics and enemas should be avoided if appendicitis is under consideration, and antibiotics should not be administered when the diagnosis is in question, since they will only mask the presence or development of perforation. The treatment is early operation and appendectomy as soon as the patient can be prepared. Appendectomy has been successfully accomplished laparoscopically, but the exact role of this treatment, especially in cases of rupture, has not been clarified. Preparation rarely takes more than 1 to 2 h in early appendicitis but may require 6 to 8 h in cases of severe sepsis and dehydration associated with late perforation. The *only* circumstance in which operation is *not* indicated is the presence of a palpable mass 3 to 5 days after the onset of symptoms. Should operation be undertaken at that time, a phlegmon rather than a definitive abscess will be found, and complications from dissection of such a phlegmon are frequent. Such patients treated with broad-spectrum antibiotics, parenteral fluids, and rest usually show resolution of the mass and symptoms within 1 week. *Interval appendectomy* can and should be done safely 3 months later. Should the mass enlarge or the patient become more toxic, drainage of the abscess is necessary. The complications of subphrenic, pelvic, or other intraabdominal abscesses usually follow perforation with generalized peritonitis and can be avoided by early diagnosis of the disease.

REFERENCES

BOLTON JP: Assessment of the value of the white cell count in management of suspected acute appendicitis. Br J Surg 62:906, 1975

BUTLER C: Surgical pathology of acute appendicitis. Hum Pathol 12:870, 1981

GUERRANT RL, BOBAK DA: Bacterial and protozoal gastroenteritis. N Engl J Med 32:327, 1991

HOFFMAN J, RASMUSSEN OO: Aids in the diagnosis of acute appendicitis. Br J Surg 76:774, 1989

KOEPSELL TD et al: Factors affecting perforation in acute appendicitis. Surg Gynecol Obstet 153:508, 1981

PUVLAERT JBCM: A prospective study of ultrasonography in the diagnosis of appendicitis. N Engl J Med 317:666, 1987

RAVAL B et al: Use of computed tomography in appendicitis: Technique, findings, and pitfalls. J Comput Tomogr 11:17, 1987

SCHWERK WB et al: Ultrasonography in the diagnosis of acute appendicitis: A retrospective study. Gastroenterology 97:630, 1989

260 DISEASES OF THE PERITONEUM AND MESENTERY

KURT J. ISSELBACHER / J. THOMAS LaMONT

ACUTE PERITONITIS Peritonitis is a localized or generalized inflammatory process of the peritoneum that may appear in both acute and chronic forms. In the acute form, the motor activity of the intestine is decreased, and the intestinal lumen becomes distended with gas and fluid. Fluid accumulates as a result of failure to reabsorb the 7 or 8 L normally secreted daily into the lumen and absorbed from the distal small bowel and colon. Because of accumulation of fluid in the peritoneal cavity as well as decreased oral intake, rapid depletion of the plasma volume with impaired cardiac and renal function may occur.

Etiology *Bacterial* peritonitis may be due to entry of bacteria into the peritoneal cavity from a perforation in the gastrointestinal tract or from an external penetrating wound. *Chemical* peritonitis results from spillage of pancreatic enzymes, gastric acid, or bile as a result of injury or perforation of the intestine or biliary tract. *Sterile* peritonitis occurs in patients with systemic lupus erythematosus, porphyria, and familial Mediterranean fever during attacks of their disease.

The most common causes of bacterial peritonitis are appendicitis, perforations associated with diverticulitis, peptic ulcer, gangrenous gallbladder, and gangrenous obstruction of the small bowel from adhesive bands, incarcerated hernia, or volvulus. Any lesion leading to the escape of intestinal bacteria may be a source, including a perforating carcinoma, foreign body, and ulcerative colitis. The peritoneal cavity is remarkably resistant to contamination, and unless continuing contamination occurs, the peritonitis remains localized. Patients with alcoholic cirrhosis and ascites have an increased susceptibility to *spontaneous* bacterial peritonitis, usually from enteric pathogens. This complication occurs in the absence of recognizable perforation of a viscus and may be due to leakage of bacteria through the intestinal wall (see Chap. 268).

Clinical features The cardinal manifestations of peritonitis are acute abdominal pain and tenderness. The location of the pain and tenderness depends on the underlying cause and whether the inflammation is localized or generalized. In *localized* peritonitis, as seen in uncomplicated appendicitis or diverticulitis, the physical findings are limited to the area of inflammation. With widespread peritoneal inflammation there is *generalized* peritonitis with diffuse abdominal tenderness and rebound. Rigidity of the abdominal wall is a common finding in peritonitis and may be localized or generalized.

Peristalsis may be present initially but usually disappears as the illness progresses and bowel sounds disappear. Hypotension, tachycardia, oliguria, and leukocytosis, with cell counts greater than 20,000 cells per microliter, are common, especially in generalized peritonitis. Plain abdominal films may reveal dilatation of the large and small bowel with edema of the small-bowel wall, as evidenced by the distance between adjacent loops of gas-filled small intestine. Diagnostic paracentesis is sometimes valuable in determining the nature of the exudate as well as whether bacteria can be demonstrated or cultured.

GONOCOCCAL PERITONITIS This usually involves an extension of gonococcal infection from a primary focus in the female reproductive tract. The signs of inflammation usually are limited to the pelvis, but there may be findings of a mild generalized peritonitis. Occasionally, the patient has right upper quadrant pain and tenderness caused by gonococcal perihepatitis involving the liver capsule and adjacent peritoneum (Fitz-Hugh–Curtis syndrome; see also Chap. 110).

STARCH PERITONITIS An acute granulomatous peritonitis can develop in some patients as a foreign-body reaction to cornstarch used to powder surgical gloves. The clinical picture is that of acute abdominal pain and fever 10 to 30 days after an abdominal operation. The diagnosis can be made by paracentesis and demonstration of starch granules in monocytes. However, most patients are reexplored because of the fear of abscess or bacterial peritonitis, with the finding of foreign-body granuloma studding the peritoneum.

PSEUDOMYXOMA PERITONEI This is a rare condition resulting from rupture of a mucocele of the appendix, a mucinous ovarian cyst, or mucin-secreting intestinal or ovarian adenocarcinoma. The abdomen becomes filled with masses of jelly-like mucus. Occasionally, with removal of the mucocele or the ovarian cyst and most of the myxomatous material, a cure may ensue. In other cases, however, the mucoid material recurs, leading to progressive wasting and eventual death. Colloid carcinoma arising from the stomach or colon with peritoneal implants may resemble pseudomyxoma at laparotomy. The course of this type of highly malignant tumor is one of rapid cachexia and early death. The diagnosis usually can be made by the appearance of many highly malignant cells in the peritoneal implants.

CANCER OF THE PERITONEUM Aside from mesothelioma, which in most patients is caused by previous exposure to asbestos, cancer of the peritoneum is usually secondary to a neoplasm within the abdomen, most commonly of the stomach and ovary. This type of metastatic malignancy is invariably associated with progressive ascites with a high specific gravity and high protein content, often with large numbers of red blood cells or even gross blood. The diagnosis is established by demonstrating malignant cells in the fluid. The clinical progress of this malignant spread can sometimes be arrested by installations of radioactive gold, nitrogen mustard, or chloroquine.

FAMILIAL MEDITERRANEAN FEVER See Chap. 293.

PNEUMATOSIS CYSTOIDES INTESTINALIS This is a condition in which multiple gas-filled blebs or cysts accumulate in the intestinal wall beneath the serosal surface of the bowel. The exact source of the gas has not been explained satisfactorily. In some instances, this disease is associated with specific ulceration of the intestinal mucosa, in particular peptic ulcer with outlet obstruction. Cysts in the wall of the small bowel are seen as an occasional complication of mesenteric vascular occlusion. In the large bowel, these cysts are usually benign, may be seen with a variety of other disorders, and usually disappear over time.

There are no specific physical findings secondary to the pneumatosis, and the diagnosis is made either by x-ray or at laparotomy. Occasionally, the subserosal cysts may rupture, resulting in pneumoperitoneum.

CHYLOUS ASCITES This term refers to the accumulation of chyle (intestinal lymph) in the peritoneal cavity. The condition is sometimes associated with chylothorax. The fluid in the peritoneal cavity appears milky or creamy because of the presence of chylomicrons. This fat may be demonstrated microscopically by staining with Sudan III and may be removed by acidification of the fluid followed by extraction with ether. The chyle (lipid) will then go into the ether phase. Many conditions may be associated with the cloudy or milky-appearing peritoneal fluid, so-called pseudochylous ascites. The milky or turbid appearance is usually due to the presence of protein and desquamated cells. The turbidity of this fluid will not be removed with the ether but will clear with addition of alkali.

The causes of chylous ascites include (1) penetrating or nonpenetrating trauma that damages the main duct in the lymphatic system within the abdomen, (2) intestinal obstruction if it is associated with rupture of a major lymphatic channel, (3) congenital lymphangiectasia, (4) malignant disease or tuberculous infection that obstructs the intestinal lymphatics, (5) filariasis, or (6) cirrhosis.

The sudden accumulation of chyle in the peritoneal cavity often results in abdominal pain, signs of peritoneal irritation, and leukocytosis. These symptoms gradually subside, leaving the patient with a distended but nontender, fluid-filled abdomen. Lymphangiography is of value in determining the location of the leak or site of obstruction to the lymphatic channels. The course depends upon the underlying etiologic factors.

MESENTERIC LIPODYSTROPHY This is a rare disorder usually affecting middle-aged women and characterized pathologically by infiltration of the mesentery with lipid-laden macrophages and fibrous tissue. These patients present with ill-defined abdominal pain and occasionally an abdominal mass. The diagnosis is made at laparotomy by demonstration of thick fibrofatty masses at the root of the mesentery with retraction and distortion of the bowel loops.

REFERENCES

KIPFER RE et al: Mesenteric lipodystrophy. Ann Intern Med 80:582, 1974

LIMBER GK et al: Pseudomyxoma peritonei. Ann Surg 1978:587, 1973

PRESS OW et al: Evaluation and management of chylous ascites. Ann Intern Med 96:358, 1982

SCHWARTZ SI et al: *Principles of Surgery*, 5th ed. New York, McGraw-Hill, 1989

TITO L et al: Spontaneous bacterial peritonitis. Hepatology 8:27, 1988

WARSHAW AL: Diagnosis of starch peritonitis by paracentesis. Lancet 2:1054, 1972

YAMADA T et al (eds): *Textbook of Gastroenterology*. Philadelphia, Lippincott, 1991

section 2   Liver and biliary tract disease

261   APPROACH TO THE PATIENT WITH LIVER DISEASE

KURT J. ISSELBACHER / DANIEL K. PODOLSKY

BIOLOGIC CONSIDERATIONS   An understanding of diseases of the liver and their clinical manifestations can be derived from a knowledge of fundamental normal hepatic structure and function. An appreciation of anatomic aspects of the liver and biliary tree from the gross level to that of the individual hepatocyte and other cellular constituents is needed to understand the spectrum of clinical manifestations of liver disease. The dual blood supply, unique to the liver and including the portal venous system, makes the liver an intermediate filter for most of the venous drainage of the abdominal viscera. This often leads to secondary hepatic involvement in a number of extrahepatic diseases and makes the liver a relatively common site of solid tumor metastases. Furthermore, an appreciation of the relevant anatomy, especially that of the portal venous system, is important in understanding clinically important manifestations of portal hypertension, a common complication of chronic liver disease when scarring and regeneration lead to distortion of the intrahepatic microvasculature. These anatomic considerations lead the clinician to look for evidence of splenic enlargement and hypersplenism, gastrointestinal bleeding, accumulation of ascites, and signs of portal-systemic encephalopathy. Certainly an understanding of the anatomy of the biliary tract from canaliculus to common bile duct is integral to understanding the basis and sequelae of obstructive jaundice. While inflammation of the gallbladder may lead to fever and pain, choledocholithiasis will cause biliary colic as well as jaundice. Diffuse processes affecting the intrahepatic ducts, such as primary sclerosing cholangitis, will lead to cholestasis and its attendant symptoms, while a focal process affecting a single branch of the biliary tree, such as a neoplasm, usually will not.

The structural organization at a level intermediate between the gross anatomic and the cellular also contributes to the clinical patterns seen with disorders of the liver. While various concepts have been offered, the most useful is that of the traditional liver lobule. Blood emanates from the portal venules at the periphery and passes through the hepatic sinusoids to the central vein. The portal venules, terminal bile ductules, and hepatic arterioles are arranged in a *triad*. Appreciation of this organization and the presence of concentric zones of function within the lobule explain distinct patterns of injury such as the centrilobular injury resulting from ischemia. These structural features no doubt also provide the basis for the relative preservation of hepatocellular function in many disorders that can lead to significant portal hypertension, such as schistosomiasis and biliary cirrhosis.

As important as the anatomic features are in understanding liver disease, many liver disorders and their manifestations can only be appreciated in the context of the functional complexity of the liver at the cellular level. As detailed in Chap. 264, the hepatocyte plays an important role in diverse general metabolic processes that may be deranged as a consequence of liver disease. In addition, this metabolic diversity leads to hepatic involvement in many inborn errors of metabolism, including a wide variety of storage diseases, and less

well-understood disorders of iron metabolism (hemosiderosis and hemochromatosis) and copper homeostasis (Wilson's disease).

Some other functional aspects also should be emphasized. The hepatocyte modifies numerous endogenous (e.g., bilirubin) and exogenous (e.g., alcohol, acetaminophen) potentially toxic compounds through oxidation, reduction, and conjugation carried out by several enzymes of the endoplasmic reticulum. Conjugation of substrates generally facilitates their hepatic excretion, converting water-insoluble substances to water-soluble derivatives. It is therefore not surprising that parenchymal liver disease may lead to either conjugated or unconjugated hyperbilirubinemia and jaundice. Metabolic modifications may significantly alter the pharmacologic activity of drugs through formation of derivatives with either decreased or enhanced activity. These metabolic processes may create intermediates which are toxic to the liver itself. This explains the selective susceptibility of the liver to the toxicity of carbon tetrachloride, acetaminophen, and, most important, alcohol, which is converted to acetaldehyde.

Additional functions of the hepatocyte that may have significant clinical ramifications include the production of a variety of soluble proteins for secretion into the circulation and the presence of receptors specific for various circulating ligands. The latter is a property shared with the Kupffer cell, which fulfills much of its function as a constituent of the reticuloendothelial system by clearing a number of serum glycoproteins through asialoglycoprotein receptor–mediated endocytosis. There is evidence to suggest that some of the substances taken up by this endocytotic mechanism may subsequently pass to and through the hepatocyte to complete an enterohepatic circulation. Carcinoembryonic antigen (CEA) is a glycoprotein and tumor-associated marker which is handled in this manner, leading to artifactual elevations in hepatobiliary disease. In contrast to the Kupffer cell, the spectrum of ligands taken up by hepatocytes via specific receptors is much broader. In addition to ligands targeted for lysosomal degradation, the hepatocyte possesses receptors for ligands which are metabolically active after their uptake and dissociation from their receptors. These include transferrin-bound iron and, most important, low-density lipoprotein (LDL), which contributes to regulation of overall body cholesterol metabolism. Disruption of lysosomal degradation of specific ligands in hereditary storage disease leads to hepatomegaly and a variety of infiltrative disorders. Disruption of the nonlysosomal endocytotic pathway ligands can lead to systemic disorders. It is not clear whether specific receptors or other hepatocyte membrane components play a role in the relative or absolute tropism of infectious agents (particularly the hepatitis viruses) which account for a large proportion of both acute and chronic liver disease. However, the relative selectivity of the hepatitis viruses (A, B, C, E, and indirectly D) for the hepatocyte is essential in understanding the clinical features of the illnesses caused by these agents, which derive from the extent of hepatocyte destruction, largely due to immune destruction rather than direct cytopathic effects of the virus. At the same time, the hepatocyte may be infected by less strictly organotropic agents including other viruses (e.g., Epstein-Barr virus) and a wide variety of bacterial and parasitic organisms. The vascular supply of the liver leads to its frequent involvement in disseminated infections.

A final feature of hepatocyte cell biology that contributes to the expression of liver disease is the potential for proliferation and regeneration. Although few mitotic figures are seen in normal hepatic parenchyma, rapid regeneration involving both proliferation and cellular hypertrophy occurs following hepatic resection in experimental animals and humans. The capacity for hepatocellular regeneration is evident in the complete recovery which usually occurs following fulminant hepatitis (due either to viral or toxic agents) if the patient can be sustained through the period of acute injury. Architecturally disordered regeneration in concert with fibrosis is an essential factor in the development of cirrhosis and leads both to disruption of blood flow through the hepatic parenchyma and to uneven hepatocellular function due to distortion of normal lobular structure. Although the mechanisms which control hepatocyte proliferation after hepatocellular loss are incompletely understood, evidence suggests that a complex balance of various peptide growth factors plays an important role.

CLINICAL CONSIDERATIONS   In approaching the patient with known or suspected liver disease, consideration of the patient's problem in the context of a few salient questions permits the clinician to focus on the most important diagnostic possibilities and the severity of the illness. Is the problem primarily hepatocellular or cholestatic? Was the onset of the illness abrupt or gradual? Has the problem led to clinically significant impairment of normal hepatocellular function, such as signs of altered mentation or coagulopathy? Are there signs or symptoms of portal hypertension? Important and reliable clues which address these questions often may be obtained from a careful history and physical examination.

Clinical history   A number of historic features may distinguish cholestatic and hepatocellular disease processes. A history of marked right upper quadrant pain or previous indigestion suggests cholelithiasis, cholecystitis, or choledocholithiasis, whereas vague, nagging discomfort suggests hepatocellular or infiltrative disease with hepatomegaly causing pain due to distention of Glisson's capsule. Additional important symptoms which should be elicited include pruritus, jaundice, anorexia, weight loss, and fever. Complaints of easy bruising or mental confusion by the patient (or family) should be regarded as ominous signs of either fulminant acute or advanced chronic liver disease.

Family history is important with respect to jaundice, anemia, splenectomy, or cholecystectomy; a positive history may be helpful in diagnosing hemolytic anemia, congenital or familial hyperbilirubinemia, or gallstones. In Wilson's disease (hepatolenticular degeneration), there may be a family history of tremor or neurologic abnormalities. *Occupation* should be reviewed in detail, and *environmental factors* need to be examined. Note should be made of the use of any medications or exposure to known or putative toxins such as carbon tetrachloride, beryllium, or vinyl chloride. The patient should be asked about travel to other countries, especially to areas where hepatitis may be endemic. Careful questioning regarding alcohol intake is important in most cases. Since the alcoholic often denies or understates the amounts consumed, it may be desirable to check the validity of the history with relatives or close friends.

Contact with jaundiced patients (especially intimate or sexual relations) should be noted. If the patient has had any *injections*, hepatitis B or C infection may be the underlying disease. Injections include blood tests, blood or plasma transfusions, tattooing, and dental treatment. Postoperative jaundice may be due to the anesthetic, especially after multiple uses of halothane, or to impaired hepatic excretory function resulting from relative hypoxemia of liver cells during the operative or postoperative period.

As suggested, the *onset of the illness* should be noted. The relatively abrupt onset of nausea, anorexia, and aversion to smoking followed by progressive jaundice suggests viral hepatitis. A gradual development of jaundice associated with pruritus suggests cholestasis. Intermittent right upper quadrant abdominal pain followed by cholestatic jaundice points to gallstone disease, while the gradual onset of painless jaundice with weight loss is suggestive of tumor, such as carcinoma of the head of the pancreas. Jaundice associated with fever and chills makes cholangitis and extrahepatic biliary obstruction likely possibilities. The awareness of progressive abdominal swelling,

perhaps first noticed because of tightness of clothing, suggests ascites, which may be due to malignancy or an insidious first manifestation of cirrhosis. The patient with hepatitis generally feels ill, and dark urine and light stools occur before the appearance of scleral or skin icterus. In cholestatic hepatitis, the patient may feel relatively well and complain only of symptoms due to the obstruction, such as pruritus.

Physical examination   Jaundice is looked for in the sclera as well as the skin. Pallor indicative of anemia may be a reflection of hemolysis, cirrhosis, or neoplasm. Significant cachexia, especially of the extremities, may be associated with cancer or cirrhosis. In the cirrhotic patient, one should look for stigmas of alcohol abuse such as parotid and lacrimal gland enlargement and Dupuytren's contracture, as well as other features of cirrhosis, such as gynecomastia, testicular atrophy, and diminished axillary or pubic hair.

The *skin examination* may reveal ecchymoses due to prothrombin deficiency or purpura due to thrombocytopenia. *Palmar erythema* or *spider angiomas* may reflect acute or chronic liver disease. Spider angiomas are usually found above the umbilicus and especially on the face, neck, shoulders, forearms, and dorsum of the hands. The presence of a few spider angiomas is not abnormal in women, especially during pregnancy. However, their appearance in men is always abnormal and should be carefully searched for. In chronic cholestasis, *scratch marks, finger clubbing*, and *xanthoma* of the eyelids and extensor surfaces of the tendons of the wrists and ankles may be found. A *slate color* to the skin due to increased iron or bronze discoloration resulting from melanin deposition should suggest the presence of hemochromatosis.

Evaluation of the *mental state* and *neurologic function* is important. Slight deterioration of the intellect and minimal personality changes may suggest hepatocellular disease or the presence of portal-systemic venous shunts, but care must be taken to exclude other causes such as neurologic disease. The presence of flapping tremor of the hands (asterixis) may be found in association with portal-systemic encephalopathy or impending hepatic coma.

Abdominal examination may reveal ascites, which, together with dilated periumbilical veins, suggests cirrhosis and extensive portal collateral circulation. If additional features of liver disease are lacking, malignancy must be considered more seriously. A very large, nodular, and rock-hard liver suggests the presence of hepatoma or hepatic metastases. Careful percussion is necessary to evaluate the size of a nonpalpable liver. A small liver may indicate cirrhosis (especially postnecrotic); a small liver which diminishes in size suggests severe hepatitis or massive hepatic necrosis. In the alcoholic, fatty infiltration and cirrhosis often produce a uniform enlargement of the liver. The liver edge is tender in hepatitis, in congestive heart failure, and occasionally in malignant disease and with alcoholism (especially "alcoholic hepatitis").

A palpable, enlarged gallbladder (Courvoisier's sign) suggests extrahepatic biliary obstruction, often due to pancreatic cancer. A tender gallbladder and positive Murphy's sign suggest cholelithiasis or choledocholithiasis. A palpable spleen may indicate hepatitis or cirrhosis; significant splenomegaly may be a reflection of portal hypertension.

Abdominal auscultation may reveal the presence of a venous hum over dilated collateral veins radiating from the umbilicus, the so-called caput medusae. In advanced cirrhosis this venous hum is virtually diagnostic of significant portal hypertension. A bruit may sometimes be heard over large regenerating nodules in cirrhosis and occasionally over hepatomas and metastatic nodules in the liver. A friction rub occasionally may be heard over hepatomas and metastatic liver nodules.

Serum assays for biochemical markers of liver disease are an integral part of the proper evaluation of liver and biliary tract disease. In general, the serum bilirubin level is measured to confirm the presence and severity of jaundice and determine the extent of bilirubin conjugation. Aminotransferase (transaminase) elevations reflect the severity of active hepatocellular damage, though not necessarily the

PARENCHYMAL

I Hepatitis (viral, drug-induced, toxic, ischemic)
  A Acute
  B Chronic (persistent or active)
II Cirrhosis
  A Alcoholic (portal, nutritional, Laennec's cirrhosis)
  B Postnecrotic
  C Biliary
  D Hemochromatosis
  E Rare types (e.g., Wilson's disease, galactosemia, cystic fibrosis of pancreas, alpha$_1$-antitrypsin deficiency)
III Infiltrations
  A Glycogen
  B Fat (neutral fat, cholesterol, gangliosides, cerebrosides)
  C Amyloid
  D Lymphoma, leukemia
  E Granuloma (e.g., sarcoidosis, tuberculosis, idiopathic)
IV Space-occupying lesions
  A Hepatoma, metastatic tumor
  B Abscess (pyogenic, amoebic)
  C Cysts (polycystic disease, *Echinococcus*)
  D Gummas
V Functional disorders associated with jaundice
  A Gilbert's syndrome
  B Crigler-Najjar syndrome
  C Dubin-Johnson and Rotor syndromes
  D Cholestasis of pregnancy and benign recurrent cholestasis

HEPATOBILIARY

I Extrahepatic biliary obstruction (by stone, stricture, or tumor)
II Cholangitis (septic, primary biliary cirrhosis, primary sclerosing cholangitis, drug, toxic)

VASCULAR

I Chronic passive congestion and cardiac cirrhosis
II Hepatic vein thrombosis (Budd-Chiari syndrome)
III Portal vein thrombosis
IV Pylephlebitis
V Arteriovenous malformations
VI Venocclusive disease

aggregate severity of liver injury (e.g., transaminase levels may actually decline with near-complete hepatic parenchymal destruction), while alkaline phosphatase elevations are found with cholestasis and hepatic infiltrates. Serum albumin level and the prothrombin time are used as indexes of hepatic synthetic function. These and other tests are reviewed in Chaps. 42 and 263.

The further evaluation of patients with hepatobiliary disease should be individualized depending on the history, physical findings, and initial screening laboratory tests. Hepatocellular disease such as hepatitis is often sufficiently clear that only serologic tests are needed. Nonetheless, in many patients, computed tomography (CT), ultrasound, scintiscans, magnetic resonance imaging (MRI), or liver biopsy may be needed to determine the nature of the liver disease. When hepatic tumors are suspected, CT, ultrasound, MRI, or scintiscan may be performed followed by liver biopsy or laparoscopy for a more specific diagnosis. When biliary obstruction is suspected, the first examination is usually an ultrasound study to determine the size of the bile ducts, whether gallstones are present, or whether there is the suggestion of a mass in the head of the pancreas. Frequently, more information is needed, and thus a cholangiogram, performed through the endoscope or through percutaneous puncture under ultrasound or CT guidance, should be obtained.

CLASSIFICATION OF LIVER DISEASE No single classification of the various types of liver disease is entirely satisfactory because in many instances the etiology and pathogenetic mechanism are obscure. As a consequence, one finds an abundance of labels and names applied to hepatic disorders. Some individuals use the term *hepatitis* to imply viral infection; others, simply to connote evidence of hepatic inflammation. The often used words *acute, subacute,* and

chronic are ambiguous. *Chronicity* should refer to continuing or recurrent disease (i.e., duration). *Activity* should refer to evidence of the presence of perpetuation of liver cell injury; this is most readily identified by serum transaminase elevations and by the degree of hepatocellular necrosis on biopsy.

Because of the difficulties involved in defining the etiology of many types of liver disease, in most instances the process is best defined and described by an examination of the morphologic character of the lesion. Therefore, a *morphologic classification* of liver disease, as outlined in Table 261-1, appears at present more practical than one based on etiology.

REFERENCES

MILLWARD-SADLER GH et al: *Wright's Liver and Biliary Disease*, 3d ed. London, Saunders, 1992
SHERLOCK S, DOOLEY J: *Diseases of the Liver and Biliary System*, 9th ed., Oxford, Blackwell, 1993
ZAKIM D, BOYER TD: *Hepatology: A Textbook of Liver Disease*, 2d ed. Philadelphia, Saunders, 1990

262 HEPATOBILIARY IMAGING

LAWRENCE S. FRIEDMAN / LAURENCE NEEDLEMAN

Selection of appropriate imaging techniques for the liver and biliary tract in a given patient depends on the particular clinical problem and on an understanding of the uses and limitations of each technique; in many situations, two or more imaging methods may provide complementary and useful information. In determining the optimal studies, communication between the clinician and the radiologist is essential.

PLAIN ABDOMINAL RADIOGRAPHS AND BARIUM STUDIES OF THE GASTROINTESTINAL TRACT Standard plain films of the abdomen provide little diagnostic information about the hepatobiliary system. They may permit a rough estimation of hepatic size and detection of splenic enlargement or gross ascites. Their major value is in demonstrating *calcified lesions*, including gallstones (about 15 percent are radiopaque) and intrahepatic lesions such as echinococcal cysts, calcified granulomas due to previous tuberculosis or histoplasmosis, or, rarely, tumors or vascular lesions. Plain abdominal x-rays may also demonstrate *air in the biliary tract*, as may occur after endoscopic papillotomy or with a biliary-enteric fistula, either surgical or as a result of inflammation or erosion of a stone from the gallbladder into the intestine. Emphysematous cholecystitis is associated with air in the wall of the gallbladder as a result of severe inflammation. Air seen in a branching pattern extending to the periphery of the liver is usually within portal venous branches and associated with serious inflammatory processes in the intestine.

A barium swallow may demonstrate large esophageal varices in patients with portal hypertension, but the sensitivity is only about 50 percent and endoscopy is more sensitive for the detection of varices.

ULTRASONOGRAPHY Ultrasonography has the advantages of relatively low cost, portability, and safety, as ionizing radiation is not required. Ultrasound imaging depends on small differences in the acoustic properties of soft tissue. Short pulses (1 μs) of high-frequency sound (3 to 10 million Hz) are transmitted into the patient; at each interface between tissues of different acoustic properties, a small portion of the energy is reflected back to the transducer, which also acts as a receiver. With *B-mode*, or *gray-scale*, ultrasound scanning, ultrasound reflections are displayed as shades of gray; cross-sectional, transverse, longitudinal, or oblique images of organs can be produced depending on the orientation of the transducer. With *real-time* ultrasonography, scanning is so rapid that a continuously changing ("real time") image is displayed, thus permitting a survey of the abdominal anatomy in a short period of time and demonstration of physiologic tissue movements, such as arterial pulsations. The major limitation of ultrasonography is its inability to penetrate bone or air, including bowel gas, which may limit complete examination of abdominal organs. In general, tissue penetration of ultrasound decreases as resolution increases.

Ultrasonography is the preferred initial method for imaging the gallbladder and biliary tree (Fig. 262-1). It is sensitive and specific (>95 percent) for the detection of *cholelithiasis*, and, unlike oral cholecystography, is not limited by the presence of jaundice or dye allergy in the patient. Ultrasonography is also highly sensitive for detecting a *dilated biliary tract* in patients with cholestasis and may indicate whether the site of obstruction is in the intra- or extrahepatic ducts. The cause of biliary obstruction, such as a mass lesion in the head of the pancreas or porta hepatis, may also be detected by ultrasonography, although the area around the distal common bile duct may be obscured by bowel gas.

Ultrasonography is also a primary screening examination for hepatic disease, which may be suspected because of symptoms, hepatomegaly, abnormal liver function tests, jaundice, or the suspicion of a mass lesion (Fig. 262-2). In general, *focal hepatic lesions* are better visualized than diffuse parenchymal disease such as fatty liver, hepatitis, or cirrhosis. Hepatic masses as small as 1 cm may be detected, and cystic lesions or abscesses can be distinguished from solid lesions, although the nature of a solid hepatic mass (adenoma, hepatocellular carcinoma, metastasis, hemangioma, etc.) may not be identified. Nevertheless, a specific diagnosis may be facilitated by percutaneous "thin"-needle biopsy of hepatic lesions under ultrasound guidance, and insertion of a catheter under ultrasound guidance may permit nonoperative drainage of an abscess. Other uses of ultrasonography include detection of ascites when the physical examination is equivocal, demonstration of portal vein thrombosis in patients with bleeding gastroesophageal varices, and evaluation of patency of portosystemic shunts in patients with recurrent variceal bleeding after shunt surgery. Ultrasonography is usually the first

FIGURE 262-2   Sonogram showing an echogenic mass which represents a hemangioma (H) in the posterior right lobe of the liver lateral to the right hepatic vein (V). R = right side of the patient.

imaging study performed in patients with hepatic dysfunction after liver transplantation to look for a biliary leak or vascular occlusion.

Doppler ultrasonography, which may be enhanced by color imaging, allows detection of the presence and direction of blood flow based on changes in the frequency of back-scattered ultrasound waves caused by the movement of blood and is useful in detecting vascular occlusions, such as portal or hepatic vein occlusion. *Intraoperative ultrasonography* involves the application of the ultrasound transducer to the exposed liver at surgery, thereby increasing the sensitivity of detecting occult hepatic metastases. *Endosonography* involves the attachment of an ultrasound transducer to the tip of an endoscope to permit ultrasonographic imaging from within the bowel lumen, thereby minimizing the obscuring effects of bowel gas. Compared to conventional imaging techniques, endosonography permits more precise determination of the depth of tumor invasion through the bowel wall and improved detection of gastroesophageal varices and early pancreatic lesions, especially pancreatic islet cell tumors.

COMPUTED TOMOGRAPHY   Because computed tomographic (CT) scans can detect very small differences in the attenuation of x-rays, structures not visible on conventional radiographs can be identified. With current CT scanning techniques, the radiation dose received by the patient is similar to that of diagnostic procedures such as barium enema. The identification of anatomic structures can be facilitated by the administration of an oral contrast agent to define the bowel lumen and an intravenous contrast agent to enhance blood vessels and tissues. In general, anatomic definition is more complete with CT scanning than with ultrasonography, and CT scanning has the additional advantage that obesity and intestinal gas do not reduce the quality of the examination. However, a paucity of fat in malnourished patients or children may limit the resolution of the CT image. The disadvantages of CT scanning are radiation exposure and cost. In many instances, CT scanning is reserved for patients in whom ultrasonography is technically difficult or inconclusive.

CT scanning before and after intravenous administration of a contrast agent is an excellent method of evaluating *hepatic masses*. Cystic lesions are readily identified, and abscesses can usually be distinguished from tumors (Fig. 262-3). Masses as small as 1 cm can usually be identified by CT scanning, and, as with ultrasonography, the lesions can be biopsied under CT guidance. Intravenous administra-

FIGURE 262-1   Sonogram showing dilated bile ducts due to pancreatic carcinoma. The diameter of the extrahepatic bile ducts is 1.2 cm measured anterior to the portal vein (between asterisks). The site of maximal dilatation is 2.0 cm in the distal common bile duct (between arrows).

FIGURE 262-3 CT scan with contrast showing a low attenuation mass (A) in the dome of the liver, which represents an amebic abscess. R = right side of the patient.

tion of a contrast agent may result in enhancement of a primary or secondary tumor relative to the surrounding liver, and certain lesions, such as a cavernous hemangioma, may show a pattern of enhancement that is characteristic enough to confirm the diagnosis. Invasion of blood vessels by tumor may also be demonstrated in this way. *CT portography*, in which CT scanning follows injection of contrast into an angiographic catheter placed directly into the superior mesenteric artery, further enhances the sensitivity of detecting mass lesions in the liver. CT scanning has had an increasing role in the evaluation of diffuse liver disease, such as cirrhosis, which may be suggested by shrinkage and nodularity of the liver and associated portosystemic collaterals. Characteristic CT findings may also be associated with *fatty infiltration* of the liver, in which the density of the liver is significantly reduced (Fig. 262-4), and *hemochromatosis* or *secondary iron overload*, in which the density of the liver is increased and an estimate of hepatic iron concentration may be made.

Although CT scanning is nearly as accurate as ultrasonography in detecting cholelithiasis or dilated bile ducts, ultrasonography is usually the preferred initial test because of its availability, lack of risk, and lower cost. However, CT scanning is more accurate than ultrasonography in identifying the level and cause of biliary obstruction. CT scanning may also be used to define the extent of carcinoma of the gallbladder or pancreas.

MAGNETIC RESONANCE IMAGING Magnetic resonance imaging (MRI) detects the density of protons in tissue water and lipids and their relaxation times. Because hydrogen nuclei (protons) have an odd number of particles, they behave like magnets when placed in a strong magnetic field. In MRI, protons aligned in a magnetic field are subjected to a brief pulse of weak radio waves, the frequency of which (termed the *resonant frequency*) is related mathematically to the externally applied magnetic field. The pulse of radio waves causes the protons to change their direction of spin and alignment. After the radio wave pulse, the protons return to their original orientation and emit energy with the same radio frequency as that absorbed. Imaging may be accomplished by the detection and analysis of proton density, the T1 relaxation time (a measure of the rate at which the nuclei realign themselves in the magnetic field), or the T2 relaxation time (a measure of the rate at which the emitted radio frequency energy decays). Each method produces a slightly different type of image. The choice of imaging technique depends on the contrast resolution needed for a particular organ. In general, because the magnetic environments of protons in fat, intracellular water, and extracellular water differ, MRI provides sharp contrast differentiation of tissues containing varying amounts of water or fat. MRI is also an excellent method of detecting blood flow.

In addition to excellent contrast resolution between normal and abnormal tissues, advantages of MRI include the lack of ionizing radiation and the ability to image in transverse, longitudinal, coronal, or even oblique planes. Its disadvantages include cost, slow imaging time that results in blurred images due to respiration and peristalsis, and limitations imposed by a strong magnetic field, such as the inability to study patients with pacemakers and other metallic devices.

The range of applications of MRI and its role relative to other imaging modalities are continually evolving. MRI of *mass lesions* of the liver appears to have greater sensitivity than CT scanning; however, like CT scanning, MRI cannot reliably distinguish primary from metastatic tumors (Fig. 262-5). Hepatic abscesses can be detected readily, although on occasion it may be difficult to distinguish abscesses from tumors with necrotic centers. MRI is the technique of choice in the detection of hemangiomas, which have an appearance sufficiently characteristic to permit differentiation from hepatic malignancy. Whereas its value in diffuse parenchymal liver disease such

FIGURE 262-4 CT scan showing fatty infiltration of the liver. Note that the attenuation of the liver is lower than that of the spleen (S). The more highly attenuated linear structures of the liver (arrows) are the intrahepatic vessels. St = stomach filled with orally administered barium contrast agent.

FIGURE 262-5 Magnetic resonance (MR) image of the liver showing three hepatic metastases (arrows) with higher signal than the surrounding liver. R = right side of the patient, K = kidney.

as hepatitis or cirrhosis is still under investigation, MRI can distinguish a regenerating nodule in a cirrhotic liver from a tumor. MRI can also serve as a useful noninvasive method for the diagnosis and monitoring of iron and copper deposition in hemochromatosis, secondary iron overload, or Wilson's disease. A modification of MRI *(proton spectroscopic imaging)*, in which the image of fat is subtracted from the image of water, can identify fatty liver and may be used to quantify hepatic fat content. Because rapidly flowing blood is often signal-free on MRI, blood vessels can be distinguished without the need for a contrast agent in most cases; thus, MRI may be useful in assessing the surgical resectability of vascular tumors or detecting hepatic vein occlusion (Budd-Chiari syndrome).

The gallbladder and bile ducts can be demonstrated by MRI, and cholelithiasis and cholecystitis can be detected; however, MRI currently offers no advantages over other imaging techniques. Although gallstones in the common bile duct are not detected by MRI, other causes of bile duct obstruction, such as pancreatitis or pancreatic carcinoma, may be identified.

Currently, MRI is based on hydrogen, which is the most abundant nucleus in the body and very sensitive to MR. *MR spectroscopy* also permits imaging based on other isotopes, such as phosphorus 31, with the ability to permit study of the metabolic state of normal and diseased organs.

RADIOISOTOPE SCANNING A variety of radioisotopes can be used to study the anatomy and function of the liver and biliary system. After injection into a peripheral vein, the radioisotope is extracted by the liver and excreted in the bile. A scintillation (gamma) camera produces an image by detecting the radiation emitted during the decay of the radioisotope. Depending on the information desired, radioisotopes can be chosen that are taken up by hepatic parenchymal cells, Kupffer cells, or neoplastic and inflammatory cells or that are rapidly excreted in bile. Many previously available radioisotopes such as [198]gold or [75]selenomethionine are no longer in use. Because radioisotope scanning of the liver seldom provides a precise diagnosis, it has largely been replaced by ultrasonography and CT scanning for first-line imaging. However, radioisotope scanning of the biliary tract is an important tool in the investigation of acute cholecystitis.

Technetium 99m–labeled sulfur colloid scanning The most commonly used radiopharmaceutical for anatomic evaluation of the liver is ^{99m}Tc-labeled sulfur colloid, which is taken up by reticuloendothelial (Kupffer) cells in the liver. Such scanning can be used to assess the size and shape of the liver. Any disease process that results in replacement of Kupffer cells, including *primary and metastatic tumors*, *cysts*, and *abscesses*, produces a ''cold'' area in the hepatic scintigram. Lesions greater than 2 to 3 cm in diameter can be reliably detected. Because of impaired blood flow and reticuloendothelial function, *diffuse hepatic disease*, such as hepatitis and cirrhosis, may result in decreased or patchy uptake of radiocolloid with preferential uptake by the bone marrow and spleen, particularly when portal hypertension is present. Occasionally, the irregular uptake of radiocolloid in cirrhosis results in the falsely positive appearance of hepatic filling defects. *Obstruction of the hepatic veins* (Budd-Chiari syndrome) may result in preferential uptake of radiocolloid by the caudate lobe of the liver.

Indium (^{111}In)-labeled colloids are also taken up by Kupffer cells and may be used to image the liver but are more expensive than ^{99m}Tc-sulfur colloid and expose the patient to a greater radiation dose. Newer scintigraphic techniques designed to improve the sensitivity of liver imaging include *single photon emission computed tomography* (SPECT), which permits visualization of the cross-sectional distribution of a radioisotope, and *positron emission tomography* (PET), which utilizes isotopes that decay by positron emission and provides information about regional blood flow and alterations in tissue metabolism. Scintigraphy following the injection of radioactively labeled antibody to tumor antigens has shown promise in distinguishing benign from malignant liver masses.

Gallium scanning [67]Gallium citrate accumulates in tissues actively synthesizing protein and is taken up by *tumors and abscesses*.

On scanning, the lesion appears as an area of increased activity, or ''hot spot.'' Imaging with this agent may be useful in detecting hepatocellular carcinomas, Hodgkin's disease, some non-Hodgkin's lymphomas, and melanomas, although nonspecific uptake of gallium by the liver, bone marrow, and gastrointestinal tract limits the reliability of gallium scanning.

Tagged blood cell scanning Intravenous injection of *autologous white blood cells* labeled with ^{111}In increases the specificity of radioisotope scanning for the detection of hepatic (and abdominal) *abscesses*. Similarly, *autologous red blood cells* or circulating proteins such as albumin or transferrin labeled with ^{111}In or ^{99m}Tc provide a sensitive method of identifying *hemangiomas* that are detected as mass lesions by ultrasonography or CT scanning (Fig. 262-6).

Biliary scanning A variety of radiopharmaceuticals are rapidly cleared by hepatocytes and excreted in the bile, thus permitting scintigraphic evaluation of the biliary tract. The first agent used for this purpose was ^{131}I-rose bengal, which, because of its high radiation dose, has been replaced by agents that can be labeled with [99m]Tc. The most widely used agents are *N*-substituted iminoacetic acids (HIDA, PIPIDA, DISIDA), which concentrate in the bile even when serum bilirubin levels are elevated. Biliary scanning is used most often in evaluating patients with suspected *acute cholecystitis*, in whom visualization of the gallbladder excludes obstruction of the cystic duct and hence acute cholecystitis (Fig. 262-7). Persistent nonvisualization of the gallbladder over several hours with normal visualization of the liver, bile ducts, and intestine indicates a diagnosis of acute cholecystitis with 95 percent accuracy. False-positive results may occur in patients receiving parenteral nutrition or narcotics and those with hepatitis. Biliary scanning is less accurate in patients with chronic cholecystitis, in whom delayed visualization of the gallbladder is frequent. However, biliary scanning may be useful in identifying *cholestasis, acute and chronic biliary obstruction, bile leaks, biliary-enteric fistulas*, and *choledochal cysts*.

ORAL CHOLECYSTOGRAPHY Although the use of oral cholecystography declined markedly with the advent of ultrasonography, the recent development of nonsurgical approaches to the treatment of cholelithiasis (e.g., extracorporeal shock wave lithotripsy and oral dissolution therapy with chenodeoxycholic or ursodeoxycholic acid) has led to a resurgence of interest in oral cholecystography. The test is simple and inexpensive. It involves radiographic assessment of gallbladder opacification 14 to 16 h after oral administration of iopanoic acid or 10 to 12 h after oral administration of sodium tyropanoate, both of which are concentrated in the gallbladder after intestinal absorption and hepatic excretion. A second dose of dye may need to be administered to as many as 15 to 25 percent of

FIGURE 262-6 ^{99m}Tc-labeled autologous red blood cell scan of the hemangioma shown in Fig. 262-2. S = spleen, K = kidney.

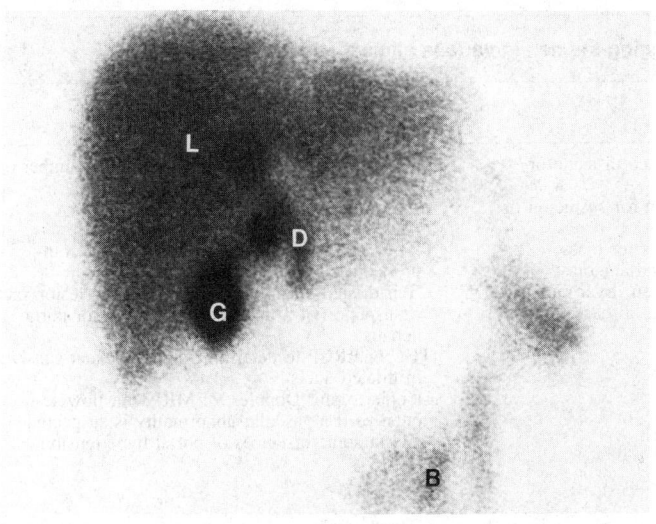

A

B

FIGURE 262-7 *A.* Hepatobiliary scan using ^{99m}Tc-DISIDA in a normal person showing uptake in the liver (L), gallbladder (G), bile ducts (D), and bowel (B) with patency of the cystic duct and biliary system. *B.* Abnormal hepatobiliary scan showing radioisotope in the liver (L), bile ducts (D), and bowel (B) but not in the gallbladder. This is due to an obstructed cystic duct (with a patent common bile duct) due to acute cholecystitis.

persons in whom gallbladder opacification is not achieved after a single dose.

Nonvisualization of the gallbladder indicates *gallbladder disease* with nearly 95 percent certainty, whereas normal visualization excludes gallbladder disease with 97 percent certainty. Failure of the gallbladder to opacify may also result from patient noncompliance, intestinal malabsorption, and liver disease; the gallbladder will not visualize when the serum direct bilirubin level is greater than 34 μmol/L (2 mg/dL). Oral cholecystography is as sensitive as ultrasonography in the overall detection of gallbladder disease (stones, polyps, adenomyomatosis, cholesterolosis, cholecystitis), although ultrasonography is more sensitive in detecting stones per se. However, oral cholecystography is more accurate in determining the *number and size of stones* and, unlike ultrasonography, can demonstrate *cystic duct patency*, factors that are important in determining a patient's suitability for nonoperative gallstone therapy.

CHOLANGIOGRAPHY In the past, *intravenous cholangiography*, in which contrast dye is administered as a bolus by peripheral vein, was the principal radiographic technique to visualize the bile ducts. Because of a high rate of serious reactions to the dye, the lack of bile duct visualization when the serum bilirubin level was above 42 μmol/L (2.5 mg/dL), and the development of more effective radiologic techniques to visualize the bile ducts, intravenous cholangiography has become obsolete.

Percutaneous transhepatic cholangiography (THC) This technique involves the direct percutaneous injection, via a "thin" (22-gauge) needle, of contrast dye into bile ducts in the liver under fluoroscopic guidance. When intrahepatic ducts are dilated, the success rate of duct opacification approaches 100 percent, but when the intrahepatic ducts are not dilated, as in primary sclerosing cholangitis, the success rate is around 90 percent and multiple attempts may be required. Serious complications occur in no more than 3 percent of cases and include hemorrhage, bile peritonitis, and sepsis.

THC may be used to determine the cause of *biliary obstruction* or *cholestasis* and is of particular value in evaluating the potential surgical resectability of proximal cholangiocarcinomas. In addition, biliary biopsies and cytologic brushings may be obtained and strictures may be balloon-dilated via a catheter inserted through the THC tract. In patients with biliary obstruction who are poor operative risks, an external drain may be left in place to permit biliary decompression or an internal stent (endoprosthesis) may be placed to relieve obstruction.

Endoscopic retrograde cholangiopancreatography (ERCP) (See Chap. 250) This technique uses fiberoptic endoscopy to visualize the ampulla of Vater and guide the insertion of a catheter through the ampulla for the selective injection of contrast material into the common bile and pancreatic ducts, which are then imaged radiologically (see Chap. 250). The success rate for cannulation depends on the experience of the endoscopist and can approach 95 percent or more; unlike THC, successful biliary cannulation does not depend on a dilated bile duct. Serious complications may occur in about 5 percent of cases and include pancreatitis and cholangitis.

Using THC, ERCP, or both, the biliary system can be visualized in nearly all patients. ERCP is preferable when the bile ducts are not dilated and when an *ampullary*, *pancreatic*, or *distal bile duct lesion* is suspected. In patients with *choledocholithiasis*, ERCP permits sphincterotomy and stone extraction. Additionally, ERCP may permit ampullary biopsy, pancreatic or biliary ductal brushings for cytologic examination, balloon dilation of a stricture, placement of a nasobiliary drain to decompress an obstructed biliary system, and insertion of a stent to relieve biliary obstruction caused by tumors. ERCP can also be used for *manometric measurements of the sphincter of Oddi*, a potentially valuable technique in the diagnosis of papillary stenosis and ampullary spasm.

ANGIOGRAPHY Angiography is required less often now than in the past for evaluating the hepatobiliary system. Nevertheless, newer contrast agents, improved techniques of vascular catheterization, and the development of therapeutic applications make angiography of value in certain situations. Selective cannulation of the hepatic artery or one of its branches may be helpful in distinguishing certain *vascular lesions* of the liver, including hemangiomas, adenomas, focal nodular hyperplasia, hemangioendotheliomas, and hepatocellular carcinomas (Fig. 262-8). Angiography may be particularly valuable in assessing the *surgical resectability* of an isolated hepatic lesion or in identifying a vascular occlusion after liver transplantation. In planning portosystemic shunt surgery, angiography is an excellent imaging technique to define portal venous anatomy and assess the patency of the vessels to be used. The portal venous system may be examined on the venous phase of celiac and superior mesenteric arteriography or after direct injection of contrast into the portal venous system via a splenic or transhepatic route. Hepatic venography and hemodynamic measurements, including wedged hepatic venous pressures, can be obtained concurrently (see Chap. 268). Therapeutic applications of angiography include *embolization* of bleeding vessels, arteriovenous fistulas, or certain highly vascular or inoperable tumors, and nonsurgical creation of a *portosystemic shunt* via a transjugular approach (transjugular intrahepatic portosystemic shunt, or TIPS).

Although no algorithm for hepatobiliary imaging tests will satisfy

TABLE 262-1 Suggested guidelines for ordering hepatobiliary imaging studies in various clinical situations

Clinical problem	Initial imaging study	Supplemental imaging studies (if necessary)
Suspected gallbladder disease	US to detect stones or evidence of acute or chronic cholecystitis Nuclear medicine biliary scan for suspicion of acute cholecystitis	OCG to assess gallbladder function and number of stones CT if abscess suspected
Suspected bile duct abnormalities	US to detect dilatation, stones, or mass THC or ERCP to define ductal anatomy	CT to detect stones or cause of extrinsic compression
Jaundice	US to detect biliary obstruction, liver masses, or obvious hepatic parenchymal disease	CT if dilated ducts to detect obstructing lesion or if suspicion of a mass in the pancreas or porta hepatis THC or ERCP to determine site and exact cause of dilated ducts
Hepatic parenchymal disease	US ^{99m}Tc-labeled sulfur colloid scan MRI	Doppler, color Doppler, or MRI with flow sequences if a vascular abnormality is suspected and in some instances of portal hypertension
Screening for liver mass	US ^{99m}Tc-labeled sulfur colloid scan	MRI
Characterizing known liver mass Suspicion of malignancy	US- or CT-directed biopsy	CT portogram MRI Intraoperative US Angiography
Suspicion of benign lesion (hemangioma, regenerative nodule, focal nodular hyperplasia, adenoma)	MRI (after detection on US or CT) Nuclear medicine scan (e.g., ^{99m}Tc-labeled red blood cell scan for suspected hemangioma)	US- or CT-directed biopsy
Suspicion of abscess	US or CT US- or CT-directed aspiration	Nuclear medicine abscess scan (gallium or ^{111}In-labeled white blood cell scan)

NOTE: US, ultrasound; OCG, oral cholecystogram; CT, computed tomography; THC, transhepatic cholangiography; ERCP, endoscopic retrograde cholangiopancreatography; MRI, magnetic resonance imaging; Tc, technetium; In, indium.

all clinical scenarios, broad guidelines for the sequential use of these tests are offered in Table 262-1. In general, techniques that are less invasive and less expensive should be considered before those that are more invasive and more expensive, but the choice of specific tests may depend as well on availability and local expertise.

FIGURE 262-8 Arterial phase of a selective hepatic angiogram showing a hepatocellular carcinoma as a hypervascular mass (outlined by arrows) with many irregular and corkscrew-shaped tumor vessels in the right lobe of the liver.

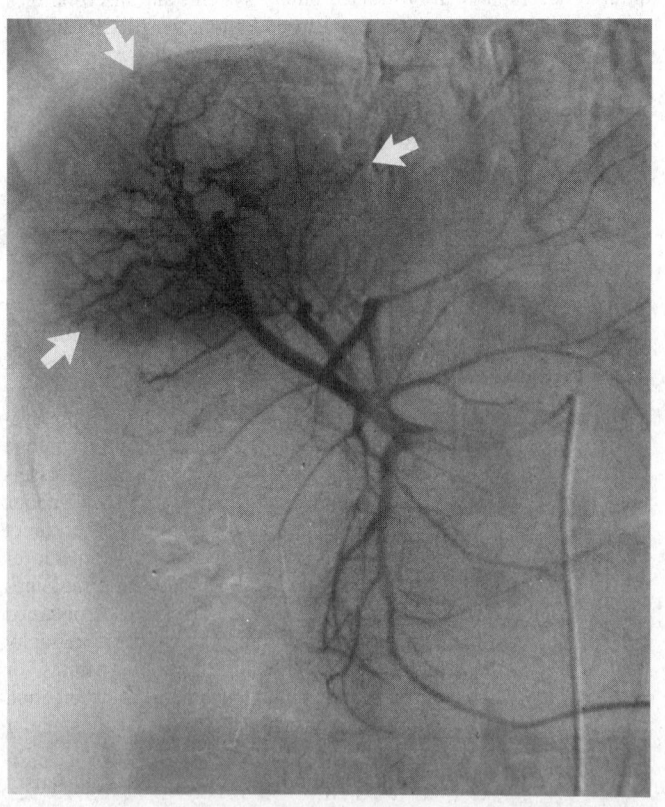

REFERENCES

BENNETT WF, BOVA JG: Review of hepatic imaging and a problem-oriented approach to liver masses. Hepatology 12:761, 1990

BERNARDINO ME (ed): Imaging of the liver and biliary tree. Rad Clin North Am 29:1129, 1991

COUNCIL ON SCIENTIFIC AFFAIRS, AMERICAN MEDICAL ASSOCIATION: Magnetic resonance imaging of the abdomen and pelvis. JAMA 261:420, 1989

FERRUCCI JT: Liver tumor imaging: Current concepts. AJR 155:473, 1990

——— et al: Advances in hepatobiliary radiology. Radiology 168:3198, 1988

MARTON KI, DOUBILET P: How to image the gallbladder in suspected cholecystitis. Ann Intern Med 109:722, 1988

MITCHELL DG: Focal manifestations of diffuse liver disease at MR imaging. Radiology 185:1, 1992

NABI HA, DOERR RJ: Radiolabeled monoclonal antibody imaging (immunoscintigraphy) of colorectal cancers: Current status and future perspectives. Am J Surg 163:448, 1992

ROTHSCHILD MA, ORATZ M: Hepatic imaging. Semin Liv Dis 9:1, 1989

SHERLOCK S, DOOLEY J: Diseases of the Liver and Biliary System, 9th ed. Oxford, Blackwell, 1993

STARK DD, BRADLEY WG: Magnetic Resonance Imaging. St Louis, Mosby Year Book, 1991

263 DIAGNOSTIC TESTS IN LIVER DISEASE

DANIEL K. PODOLSKY / KURT J. ISSELBACHER

The diversity of normal liver functions and the disruption of these functions by the spectrum of disorders which may affect the liver preclude the use of any single test as a reliable measure of overall liver function. Many disease processes may lead to severe impairment of some liver functions, while others remain entirely unaffected. Since no battery of tests is universally applicable, those most appropriate to a given clinical problem must be selected, their potential value and risks considered, and the results interpreted in relation to the clinical findings.

In assessing the severity and course of liver disease, the physician should be guided by several practical principles. The tests selected should (1) assess different parameters of liver function, (2) be used *serially* in order to evaluate the evolution or course of the disease, and (3) be interpreted within the total clinical context, with recognition that any single laboratory test may be fallible.

BLOOD TESTS OF LIVER FUNCTION   (See Table 263-1)

BILIRUBIN   Bilirubin metabolism and its assessment are discussed in detail in Chaps. 42 and 265. Spectrophotometric determinations of serum bilirubin in the clinical laboratory measure two pigment fractions: (1) the water-soluble conjugated fraction that gives a *direct reaction* with the diazo reagent and consists largely of conjugated bilirubin (as the mono- and diglucuronide) and (2) the lipid-soluble *indirect-reaction* fraction (total minus direct) that represents primarily unconjugated bilirubin. The serum of normal adults (when measured by the van den Bergh reaction) contains less than 4.2 µmol/L (0.25 mg/dL) direct-reacting bilirubin and 17 µmol/L (1 mg/dL) or less of total bilirubin. Studies with high-performance liquid chromatography (HPLC) suggest that even these levels may be artifactually high in normal persons (see Chap. 42).

Conjugated hyperbilirubinemia with elevated direct- and indirect-reacting material indicates impairment of secretion into the bile, while unconjugated hyperbilirubinemia reflects impaired conjugation. The latter is found in a limited number of processes, including such nonhepatic conditions as hemolytic anemia and ineffective erythropoiesis (increased pigment load) and a few hepatic disorders, principally Gilbert's syndrome or the relatively rare Crigler-Najjar syndrome. Although measurement of both the direct and total serum bilirubin will determine whether the patient has predominantly unconjugated or conjugated hyperbilirubinemia, this distinction is of limited usefulness, since the majority of hepatobiliary disorders lead to conjugated hyperbilirubinemia. In most instances, fractionation of serum bilirubin does not distinguish cholestasis due to parenchymal disease from that arising from biliary tract processes.

Bilirubin appears in the urine only after it is converted to a water-soluble form; generally this involves conjugation with polar glucuronide groups which enhance water solubility. Rapid assessment of bilirubinuria is possible using commercially available dipsticks and may be helpful as an initial screening measure. Bilirubinuria occurs with even minimal degrees of jaundice and may be detected before jaundice is evident. Its usefulness is otherwise quite limited. Urobilinogen, a product of luminal bacterial metabolism of bilirubin, is reabsorbed from the bowel and secreted in the urine. Complete bile duct obstruction blocks excretion of bilirubin into the gut and results in disappearance of urobilinogen from the urine. Assessment of urobilinogen in a freshly collected 2-h urine specimen by the Watson method (normal values 0.2 to 1.2 units) may distinguish biliary tract obstruction from parenchymal dysfunction, but this test has been largely superseded by newer methods.

SERUM ENZYME ASSAYS   A number of serum enzymes have been used to distinguish and assess hepatocellular injury and biliary tract dysfunction or obstruction. All have inherent limitations in sensitivity and specificity, and none truly distinguishes these processes definitively. Elevations in enzyme activities also may be seen in association with nonhepatic disorders. Nevertheless, with proper and careful interpretation, a number of serum enzymes provide important clinical tools.

Aminotransferases (transaminases)   Assays of many serum enzymes have been proposed as indicators of hepatocellular damage. Of these, aspartate aminotransferase (AST, SGOT) and alanine aminotransferase (ALT, SGPT) activities have proven most useful. These enzymes catalyze the transfer of the γ-amino groups of aspartate and alanine, respectively, to the γ-keto group of ketoglutarate, leading to the formation of oxaloacetic acid and pyruvic acid. In contrast to ALT, which is found primarily in the liver, AST is present in many tissues, including heart, skeletal muscle, kidney, and brain, and is thus somewhat less specific as an indicator of liver function. The source of serum AST and ALT in the normal person [less than 0.58 µkat/L (35 U/L)] is unclear, and the mechanism responsible for clearance of these enzymes is uncertain. In the hepatocyte, ALT is found exclusively in the cytosol, while different isoenzymes of AST exist in mitochondria and the cytosol. Although elevated serum levels of AST or ALT may be observed in a variety of nonhepatic diseases, notably in myocardial infarction and skeletal muscle disorders, these disorders can usually be distinguished clinically from liver disease. Conversely, uremia may lead to spuriously low aminotransferase values.

Serum AST and ALT are elevated to some extent in nearly all liver disorders. Highest levels are found in association with conditions causing extensive hepatic necrosis, such as severe viral hepatitis, toxin-induced liver injury, or prolonged circulatory collapse. Lesser elevations are encountered in mild acute viral hepatitis as well as in both diffuse and focal chronic liver diseases (e.g., chronic active hepatitis, cirrhosis, and hepatic metastases). However, the absolute levels of aminotransferases correlate poorly with severity of liver injury or prognosis, and serial determinations are usually most helpful. Thus, in the patient with massive hepatic necrosis, there may be marked elevations in the early phase (i.e., 24 to 48 h), but by the time the patient is tested 3 to 5 days later, the levels may be in the range of 3.34 to 5.8 µkat/L (200 to 350 U/L). It is noteworthy that in severe alcoholic hepatitis one commonly finds only modest increases in these enzymes (generally less than 5.0 µkat/L). Minimal elevations of AST and ALT (less than 1.67 µkat/L) also may be found in association with biliary tract obstruction; higher levels suggest the development of cholangitis with resultant hepatic cell necrosis.

In general AST and ALT levels parallel each other, with a couple of exceptions. In alcoholic hepatitis the AST/ALT ratio may be greater than 2; this appears to result from a reduction in hepatic ALT content due to a deficiency in the cofactor pyridoxine-5-phosphate. An increase in the ratio of AST/ALT (>1) also can be seen occasionally in patients with the fatty liver associated with pregnancy.

Alkaline phosphatase   Human serum contains several forms of alkaline phosphatase, a plasma membrane–derived enzyme of uncertain physiologic function which hydrolyzes synthetic phosphate esters at pH 9. These activities arise from bone, intestine, liver, and placenta. A number of different assays have been developed which utilize different substrates.

In the absence of bone disease or pregnancy, elevated levels of alkaline phosphatase activity usually reflect impaired biliary tract function. The increased levels reflect increased synthesis of the enzyme by hepatocytes and biliary tract epithelium rather than regurgitation of enzyme due to obstruction. Bile acids may play a role both by inducing synthesis and by promoting solubilization of the membrane-associated enzyme activity.

Slight to moderate increases in alkaline phosphatase (1 to 2 times normal) occur in many patients with parenchymal liver disorders such as hepatitis and cirrhosis; transient increases may occur in all types

TABLE 263-1   Abnormalities shown by tests of liver function

Test	Type of liver disease	
	Obstructive	Parenchymal
AST and ALT (SGOT and SGPT)	↑	↑ – ↑ ↑ ↑
Alkaline phosphatase	↑ ↑ ↑	↑
Albumin	N	↓ – ↓ ↓ ↓
Prothrombin time	N– ↑ *	↑ – ↑ ↑ ↑
Bilirubin	N– ↑ ↑ ↑	N– ↑ ↑ ↑
γ-Glutamyl transpeptidase (GGT)	↑ ↑ ↑	N– ↑ ↑ ↑
5′-Nucleotidase	↑ – ↑ ↑ ↑	N– ↑

* Correctable with parenteral vitamin K if elevated.
NOTE: N, normal: ↑, elevated; ↓, decreased.

of liver disease. However, the most striking increases in alkaline phosphatase (3 to 10 times normal) occur with extrahepatic biliary tract (mechanical) obstruction or with intrahepatic (functional) cholestasis, as in drug-induced cholestasis or primary biliary cirrhosis. Conversely, it is unusual for the serum alkaline phosphatase to remain normal when there is obstructive jaundice, and a normal enzyme level argues strongly against the presence of cholestasis. The alkaline phosphatase is usually mildly elevated in metastatic or infiltrative liver disease (e.g., leukemia, lymphoma, and sarcoid). The enzyme may be elevated in the presence of incomplete biliary obstruction or when there is obstruction of only one hepatic duct, conditions in which the serum bilirubin is often normal or only slightly elevated. Serum alkaline phosphatase is also elevated in nonhepatic disorders, most notably in some bone disorders (e.g., Paget's disease, osteomalacia, and metastases to bone) and sometimes with malignancy. Occasionally, tumors produce an alkaline phosphatase which is identical or similar to the placental form, the so-called Regan isoenzyme.

Although one can usually make a reasonable assessment as to whether an elevation of the alkaline phosphatase is of hepatic or nonhepatic origin, several methods can distinguish the different isoenzymes, facilitating resolution of any uncertainty. In contrast to that derived from bone, the hepatic isozyme is stable to treatment with heat (56°C for 15 min) or urea. These enzymes also can be separated by electrophoresis, but this is usually impractical. Parallel determination of serum 5′-nucleotidase activity is also helpful; an increase of both 5′-nucleotidase and alkaline phosphatase is consistent with an hepatobiliary source of the enzyme elevation. Even after correction for age and sex (higher levels being found in the young and in older women), isolated elevations in alkaline phosphatase may occasionally be encountered in adults with no apparent disease.

5′-Nucleotidase, leucine aminopeptidase, and γ-glutamyltranspeptidase *5′-Nucleotidase* catalyzes the hydrolysis of phosphate from the 5′ position of the pentose component of the nucleotide. Although tissue distribution is widespread, elevations are generally associated with hepatobiliary disease. The principal value of the 5′-nucleotidase measurement is to confirm the hepatic origin of an elevated alkaline phosphatase level in children or pregnant women or in those settings where coincident bone disease may be present. However, 5′-nucleotidase levels do not always parallel alkaline phosphatase in liver disease, and lack of elevation does not exclude an hepatic source of elevated serum alkaline phosphatase.

γ-Glutamyltranspeptidase GGT catalyzes the transfer of the γ-glutamyl group from peptides such as glutathione to other amino acids and may play a role in amino acid transport. It is found throughout the hepatobiliary system as well as in other tissues. In liver disease, GGT correlates with alkaline phosphatase levels and is the most sensitive indicator of biliary tract disease. However, elevations of GGT are nonspecific and may be associated with pancreatic, cardiac, renal, and pulmonary disorders as well as with diabetes and alcoholism. This enzyme may be increased by agents which induce microsomal enzymes, and it has been suggested as a potential marker of alcoholism. However, overall lack of specificity has limited its clinical usefulness.

Other enzymes Measurement of total serum lactic dehydrogenase (LDH) or its isoenzymes is usually not helpful in diagnosis of liver disease because of this enzyme's nearly ubiquitous body distribution. Moderate LDH elevations are common in acute viral hepatitis, cirrhosis, and metastatic carcinoma to the liver. Biliary tract disease also may produce slight elevations. Marked elevations of LDH in association with abnormal results of other liver function tests may reflect a hematologic malignancy such as lymphoma. Numerous other dehydrogenases (e.g., isocitrate dehydrogenase, sorbitol dehydrogenase, and glutamate dehydrogenase) have been used or proposed as markers of liver disease, but none appears to offer significant diagnostic improvement over standard aminotransferase determinations. Elevation of serum ornithine carbamyl transferase (OCT), a urea cycle enzyme present only in liver and intestine, occurs primarily

in liver disease, but its lack of association with any specific type of liver disease has limited its diagnostic usefulness.

SERUM PROTEINS Extensive liver injury may lead to *decreased* blood levels of albumin, prothrombin, fibrinogen, and other proteins synthesized exclusively by hepatocytes. In contrast to measurements of serum enzymes, serum protein levels reflect liver synthetic function rather than just cell injury. Three important caveats should be remembered regarding interpretation of serum protein levels: (1) they are neither early nor sensitive indicators of liver disease (because of the extent of hepatic reserve and their half-life, see below), (2) they are of little value in the differential diagnosis of liver disease, and (3) decreases in their serum levels are not specific for liver disease.

Albumin and globulin Albumin is quantitatively the most important serum protein synthesized by the liver; the normal serum value ranges from 35 to 55 g/L (see Chap. 264). Albumin has a fairly long half-life (14 to 20 days) with less than 5 percent turnover daily; it is therefore not a good indicator of acute or mild liver injury. Furthermore, there is a substantial reserve of hepatic albumin synthesis; thus adequate synthesis may continue until there is extensive hepatocellular injury. Serum levels are influenced by a variety of nonhepatic factors, most notably nutritional status, hormonal factors, and plasma oncotic pressure. Routes of degradation in health remain undefined, but nonhepatic conditions may lead to depressed serum albumin levels mainly due to excessive loss despite adequate synthetic function (e.g., nephrotic syndrome or protein-losing enteropathy). Nonetheless, reduction in the serum albumin levels provides an excellent indication of the severity of chronic liver disease. In the patient with ascites, an increased volume of distribution as well as an absolute reduction in protein synthesis may contribute to hypoalbuminemia.

Serum globulins are a heterogeneous group of proteins whose production in a variety of tissues is influenced by a number of factors. Serum globulins (normal 20 to 35 g/L) include alpha and beta globulins as well as serum immunoglobulins, the latter largely accounting for the gamma fraction. Serum globulins are often diffusely elevated in association with chronic liver disease and in other nonhepatic disorders. In cirrhosis, varying degrees of hyperglobulinemia may occur; this may reflect increased stimulation of the peripheral reticuloendothelial compartment due to shunting of antigens past the liver and impaired clearance by hepatic Kupffer cells. Although some have suggested that elevations in different globulin fractions as assessed by electrophoretic or other means may have a differential diagnostic value, this remains a largely unfulfilled promise. Similarly, the albumin/globulin ratio has no physiologic significance.

Clotting factors The liver synthesizes six coagulation factors: fibrinogen (factor I), prothrombin (factor II), and factors V, VII, IX, and X. With the exception of factor V, production of functional proteins requires the presence of the cofactor vitamin K. Because most of these factors are normally present in excess concentrations, impaired coagulation is usually seen only in severe liver disease. Abnormalities of these factors can be most efficiently determined by the one-stage *prothrombin time*, which measures the rate of prothrombin conversion to thrombin in the presence of thromboplastin and calcium and requires the integrity of most of the vitamin K–dependent clotting factors (see Chap. 57). Factor VII is the rate-limiting factor in this pathway and thus has the greatest influence on the prothrombin levels. The prothrombin time is dependent on normal hepatic synthesis of clotting factors and sufficient intestinal uptake of vitamin K. Absorption of this fat-soluble vitamin itself requires adequate dietary intake and normal function of intestinal mucosa and biliary secretion. Severe acute or chronic parenchymal liver injury may lead to prolongation of the prothrombin time due to impaired synthesis of the clotting proteins. Because these proteins have a shorter half-life than that of albumin, the prothrombin time may be an earlier indicator than serum albumin level of severe liver injury. In both acute and chronic hepatocellular injury, an increase in the prothrombin time serves as an ominous prognostic sign. Because vitamin K is a fat-soluble vitamin, prolongation of the prothrombin time can result from vitamin K malabsorption, which may occur with cholestasis due to biliary tract disease or due to fat malabsorption (steatorrhea) of any cause (e.g., pancreatic insufficiency). Poor dietary intake, antibiotic therapy, and use of warfarin-type anticoagulants are additional causes of a prolonged prothrombin time, owing to deficiencies of active vitamin K. These processes can be distinguished from hepatic synthetic failure by demonstrating normalization of the prothrombin time (within 24 to 48 h) after parenteral injections of vitamin K. The *partial thromboplastin time*, which reflects the activities of fibrinogen, prothrombin, and factors V, VIII, IX, X, XI, and XII, also may be prolonged in severe liver disease. Clotting functions should be assessed in all patients with liver disease prior to any surgical procedure, including liver biopsy (see Chaps. 57 and 315).

BLOOD AMMONIA Ammonia is elevated in the blood of some patients with either acute or chronic liver disease. Although influenced by a number of factors (summarized in Chap. 264), elevations in blood ammonia reflect disruption of the pathways of urea synthesis by which the liver detoxifies amine groups. A markedly elevated blood ammonia usually reflects severe hepatocellular necrosis. Cirrhotic patients, especially those with endogenous or surgically created portal-systemic shunting, often have varying degrees of hyperammonemia and hepatic encephalopathy. However, there is only a rough correlation between blood ammonia levels and the degree of hepatic encephalopathy; some patients will function normally with a twofold elevation, while others will be stuporous at the same concentration. Ammonia levels may increase before the onset of coma; similarly, they may return to normal some 48 to 72 h before improvement of the neurologic status.

SERUM LIPIDS AND LIPOPROTEINS AND BILE ACIDS Abnormalities in serum lipids and lipoproteins are sensitive but nonspecific indicators of liver diseases. Acute parenchymal liver disease is commonly associated with increased plasma triglycerides, decreased cholesterol esters, and abnormal lipoproteins. The absence of alpha and prebeta bands with a concomitant increase in the beta fraction is typical of acute viral hepatitis. Less marked but more persistent abnormalities are found in patients with chronic parenchymal disease reflecting deficiencies in lecithin:cholesterol acyltransferase (LCAT) and hepatic triglyceride lipase. Either intra- or extrahepatic cholestasis may lead to an increase in unesterified cholesterol and in serum phospholipids.

Removal of bile acids from portal blood is impaired in liver disease because of parenchymal damage and portal-systemic shunts; there also may be reentry of bile acids into blood from injured hepatocytes or an obstructed biliary tract. Although there are a variety of techniques for measuring serum bile acids, these determinations are not yet of proven value for routine clinical use.

IMMUNOLOGIC AND OTHER TESTS

A number of immunologic derangements may be seen in liver disease. Antimitochondrial antibodies are found in 85 to 90 percent of patients with primary biliary cirrhosis. These antibodies appear to be directed against components of the pyruvate dehydrogenase complex and other related mitochondrial enzyme complexes. In this test, serum is incubated with rabbit hepatocytes. The presence of antimitochondrial antibodies can then be assessed after subsequent staining with a fluorescein-tagged second antibody. However, this marker is not entirely specific and is occasionally found in patients with chronic active hepatitis and drug-induced hepatitis. Its primary value is in helping to distinguish primary biliary cirrhosis from extrahepatic biliary obstruction. In chronic active hepatitis, the *lupus erythematosus–cell test* (LE-cell test) may be positive, and *antinuclear antibodies* as well as *anti-smooth-muscle antibodies* may be present (see Chap. 284). Alpha fetoprotein is of value in the diagnosis of hepatocellular carcinoma (see Chap. 269). Measurements of serum alpha$_1$-antitrypsin and ceruloplasmin should be performed in infants with cirrhosis or

hepatitis since they may reflect alpha$_1$-antitrypsin deficiency or Wilson's disease, respectively (see Chaps. 270 and 348).

Studies assessing iron stores are essential in the evaluation of those patients suspected of hemochromatosis on clinical grounds, those exhibiting compatible nonspecific abnormal liver function tests results (e.g., unexplained mild to moderate elevation of aminotransferase), or those with evidence of liver disease, early or advanced, of uncertain cause. Routine tests include iron, total serum iron-binding capacity (TIBC), and ferritin. Hemochromatosis is associated with elevated levels of both iron and TIBC and an increased ratio of iron/TIBC, typically >90 percent, consistent with a high degree of saturation of iron-binding capacity. While elevated levels of saturation may be seen in many chronic systemic illnesses, the overall level of iron and TIBC will be diminished. Serum levels of ferritin, the intrahepatic ion storage protein, are typically markedly elevated in hemochromatosis. Somewhat less pronounced increases may be seen in other forms of liver injury, including alcoholic liver disease and other diseases (e.g., lymphoma). Particular confusion may arise in distinguishing secondary hemosiderosis, most commonly seen in alcoholics but also encountered in patients receiving numerous transfusions (e.g., sickle cell anemia), from primary idiopathic hemochromatosis by these initial serum determinations. Diagnosis often ultimately requires percutaneous liver biopy or other more specific tests (see Chap. 345).

OTHER DIAGNOSTIC PROCEDURES **Percutaneous needle biopsy of the liver** Percutaneous needle biopsy is a safe, simple, and valuable method for the diagnostic evaluation of liver disease. *Diffuse parenchymal disorders* such as cirrhosis, hepatitis, and drug reactions may be diagnosed with remarkable accuracy. In *disseminated focal diseases* (such as granulomas or tumor infiltrates), serial sections may demonstrate characteristic lesions.

Biopsy is performed under local anesthesia, usually with the Menghini (aspiration), Klatskin, or Vim-Silverman (cutting) needle, by either a transpleural or subcostal approach. If the operator is skillful and patients are carefully selected, morbidity should be quite low and limited to occasional postbiopsy pain or vasovagal reactions.

Some of the most frequent indications for needle biopsy are (1) unexplained hepatomegaly or hepatosplenomegaly, (2) cholestasis of uncertain cause, (3) persistently abnormal liver function tests, (4) suspected systemic or infiltrative diseases such as sarcoidosis, miliary tuberculosis, or fever of unknown origin, and (5) suspected primary or metastatic liver tumor. Percutaneous liver biopsy may be performed either for diagnostic purposes or to evaluate the extent and severity of a known disease process. However, other new and improved noninvasive diagnostic methods have obviated the need for biopsy in many circumstances, and thus biopsy should be performed only when information from these other techniques is inadequate.

Needle biopsy should not be performed if (1) the patient is unable to cooperate, (2) clinical or laboratory evidence indicates impaired hemostasis (prothrombin time prolonged by 3 s or more over control, thrombocytopenia less than 80 to 100 $\times$ 10^9 platelets per liter, or partial thromboplastin time or bleeding time prolonged), (3) there is infection of the right pleural space or septic cholangitis, (4) tense ascites is present, with risk of continued leakage of ascitic fluid, (5) compatible blood is not available for transfusion in case of hemorrhage, (6) high-grade biliary obstruction is suspected and there is an increased risk of bile peritonitis, or (7) a vascular lesion is suspected. In patients in whom a percutaneous biopsy cannot be performed safely due to impaired hemostasis or ascites, biopsy can sometimes be carried out by a transjugular approach, in which the tissue is obtained via the hepatic vein and any bleeding occurs directly into the vascular space. With the increasing use of CT scan and ultrasonography, it is possible to perform "directed" aspiration biopsies of isolated lesions with very thin needles. Aspirated material can be used for cytology (tumors) and culture (abscesses) but is often inadequate for assessment of liver architecture.

Laparoscopy and laparotomy (peritoneoscopy) See Chap. 250.

REFERENCES

FERRUCCI JT JR et al: Advances in hepatic radiology. Radiology 168:3198, 1988

Moss, AA et al Hepatic tumors: Magnetic resonance and CT appearance. Radiology 150:191, 1984

ROTHSCHILD MA et al: Serum albumin. Hepatology 8:385, 1988

SABESIN SM: Cholestatic lipoproteins. Their pathogenesis and significance. Gastroenterology 83:704, 1982

ZAKIM D, BOYER TD: *Hepatology, A Textbook of Liver Disease*, 2d ed. Philadelphia, Saunders, 1990

———, ORATZ M: Hepatic imaging. Semin Liv Dis 9:1, 1989

264   DERANGEMENTS OF HEPATIC METABOLISM

DANIEL K. PODOLSKY / KURT J. ISSELBACHER

The liver plays a central role in the maintenance of metabolic homeostasis. It is therefore not surprising that the development of clinically important liver disease is accompanied by diverse manifestations of disordered metabolism. Although some functions are more sensitive than others, the liver has considerable reserve capacity, so minimal or even moderate cell injury may not be reflected by measurable metabolic changes. However, a variety of defects may be seen, depending on the nature and extent of the initial insult.

The biochemical functions in which the liver plays a major role include (1) the intermediate metabolism of amino acids and carbohydrates, (2) synthesis and degradation of proteins and glycoproteins, (3) metabolism and degradation of drugs and hormones, and (4) regulation of lipid and cholesterol metabolism. The derangements of these functions are discussed in connection with their occurrence in various forms of parenchymal liver disease. Alterations of bilirubin, bile salt, and porphyrin metabolism are discussed elsewhere (Chaps. 41, 254, and 346).

Metabolic derangements are most evident in the patient with advanced liver disease, and the manifestations are similar regardless of the initial etiologic insult. To a varying degree, similar abnormalities are observed in patients with severe chronic hepatitis, micronodular cirrhosis, and postnecrotic cirrhosis. Since the many functions of the liver may be affected to varying degrees in individual patients, no single test effectively measures the overall state of liver function. The proper interpretation of liver function tests is discussed in Chap. 263.

CARBOHYDRATE METABOLISM   The liver functions to maintain normal levels of blood sugar by a combination of glycogenesis, glycogenolysis, glycolysis, and gluconeogenesis. These pathways are regulated by a number of hormones, including insulin, glucagon, growth hormone, and certain catecholamines. Although it has been presumed that exquisite sensitivity of the hepatocytes to insulin is responsible for the uptake of an oral glucose load by the liver, there are also data that have challenged the importance of insulin-mediated glucose uptake by the hepatocyte. In the fasting state, the liver contributes to glucose homeostasis by glycogenolysis and gluconeogenesis in response to hypoinsulinemia and hyperglucagonemia. Maintenance of normal blood glucose levels through gluconeogenesis is ultimately related to catabolism of muscle protein, which provides the necessary amino acid precursors, especially alanine. In a complementary fashion, in the postprandial state, the liver directs alanine and branched-chain amino acids to the peripheral tissues, where they are then incorporated into muscle protein. These reciprocal pathways form a glucose-alanine shuttle which is modulated by ambient changes in the hormones mentioned above (Fig. 264-1). While it has been presumed that synthesis of glycogen and fatty acid in the postprandial state arises from direct conversion of glucose, there are data to suggest that, in fact, these pathways are *indirect*, with products deriving from three-carbon metabolites of glucose or other gluconeogenic compounds such as lactate, fructose, and alanine.

Abnormalities of glucose homeostasis are common in cirrhosis (Table 264-1). Most frequently, hyperglycemia and glucose intolerance are observed. Glucose intolerance is associated with normal or increased levels of plasma insulin (except in patients with hemochromatosis), suggesting that insulin resistance rather than insulin deficiency may be responsible. One of the factors that may play a role in the apparent insulin resistance is an absolute decrease in the liver's ability to metabolize a glucose load because of a decrease in functioning hepatocellular mass. There is also evidence that response to insulin is diminished due to both receptor and postreceptor defects in hepatocytes of patients with cirrhosis. In addition, both hyperinsulinemia and hyperglucagonemia may be present due to decreased hepatic clearance of this hormone resulting from portal-systemic shunting. In patients with hemochromatosis, insulin levels, however, may indeed be low due to pancreatic iron deposition and sometimes concomitant diabetes mellitus. Patients with cirrhosis also may have elevated serum lactate levels, reflecting the decreased capacity of the liver to utilize lactate for gluconeogenesis.

Hypoglycemia, although more common in acute fulminant hepatitis, also may be seen with end-stage cirrhosis. Glycogen in the liver accounts for 5 to 7 percent of the normal tissue weight. Because the capacity of the liver to store glycogen is limited (approximately 70 g) and glucose consumption continues at a constant rate (approximately 150 g/d), hepatic glycogen stores are depleted after 1 day of fasting. Hypoglycemia in end-stage cirrhosis may be due to decreased hepatic glycogen stores, diminished glucagon responsiveness, or decreased capacity to synthesize glycogen due to extensive parenchymal destruction.

AMINO ACID AND AMMONIA METABOLISM   Through a variety of anabolic and catabolic processes, the liver is the major site of amino acid interconversion. Amino acids utilized for hepatic protein synthesis are derived from dietary protein, metabolic turnover of endogenous protein (primarily from muscle), and direct synthesis in the liver. Most of the amino acids entering the liver via the portal vein are catabolized to urea (except for the branched-chain amino acids leucine, isoleucine, and valine). A lesser amount is released into the general circulation as free amino acids, and these may play an important role in the glucose-alanine cycle mentioned above. In addition, amino acids are utilized for the synthesis of liver intracellular proteins, plasma proteins, and special compounds such as glutathione, glutamine, taurine, carnosine, and creatine. Disruption of normal amino acid metabolism may be reflected in altered plasma amino acid concentrations. In general, levels of aromatic amino acids normally metabolized by the liver (as well as methionine) are elevated, while those of the branched-chain amino acids, largely utilized by skeletal muscle, tend to be normal or depressed. It has been suggested that an alteration in the ratio of these two types of amino acids plays a role in the development of hepatic encephalopathy (see below), but there is not agreement on this concept.

Hepatic catabolism or degradation of amino acids involves two major reactions: transamination and oxidative deamination. In transamination, an amino group of an amino acid is transferred to a keto acid. This process is catalyzed by aminotransferases, which are found in very high amounts in liver but are also present in other tissues, such as kidney, muscle, heart, lung, and brain. Glutamic-oxaloacetic acid transaminase (aspartate aminotransferase, AST) has been studied most extensively, and increased levels are found in the serum secondary to various types of liver injury (e.g., acute viral and drug-induced hepatitis). As a result of transamination, amino acids can enter the citric acid cycle and then function in the intermediary metabolism of carbohydrates and lipids. Most of the nonessential amino acids are also synthesized in the liver by transamination. Oxidative deamination, which results in conversion of amino acids to keto acids (and ammonia), is catalyzed by L-amino acid oxidase with two exceptions: Glycine oxidation is catalyzed by glycine oxidase, and glutamic oxidation is catalyzed by glutamic dehydrogenase. With severe liver damage (e.g., massive hepatic necrosis), utilization of amino acids is impaired, free amino acids in the

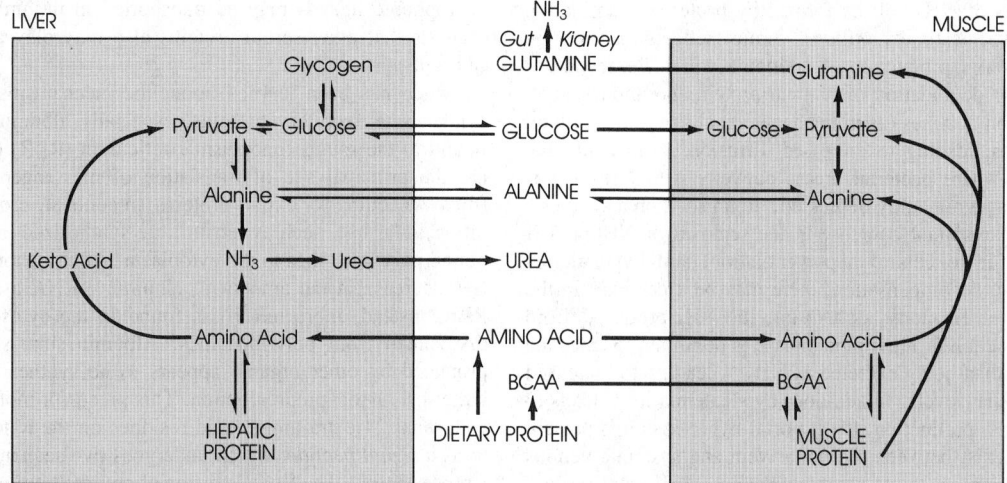

FIGURE 264-1 Carbohydrate-protein exchange between muscle and liver. After an overnight fast there is net release of amino acids by muscle (predominantly alanine and glutamine). These are derived from transamination of pyruvate, degraded amino acids, and glucose. Branched-chain amino acids (BCAA) are particularly important as a source of nitrogen for alanine synthesis. Alanine is utilized for gluconeogenesis by the liver, and urea is formed as a by-product. The main sites of glutamine uptake are the kidney and gut, where it is used for ammonia production and as a possible source of energy, respectively. Following ingestion of dietary protein, skeletal muscle goes into an anabolic phase; there is selective hepatic escape and muscle uptake of dietary BCAA, reduced muscle output of alanine and glutamine, and a reduced rate of hepatic gluconeogenesis. Hepatic tissue protein also goes into an anabolic phase following protein ingestion. (*Modified with permission from AS Tavill in Wright et al.*)

bloodstream increase, and an "overflow" type of aminoaciduria may occur.

Urea production is intimately related to the metabolic pathways outlined above, providing a means for disposal of ammonia, the toxic product of nitrogen metabolism. Disruption of this process is of particular clinical importance in the patient with severe acute and chronic liver disease. The fixation of amino acid–derived NH_3 in the form of urea is carried out via the Krebs-Henseleit cycle. The final step of this cycle, the formation of urea by arginase, is irreversible. In advanced liver disease, urea synthesis is often depressed, leading to an accumulation of NH_3, usually with a significant reduction in blood urea nitrogen (BUN), an ominous sign of liver failure. This finding may be obscured by superimposed renal impairment, which often develops in patients with severe hepatic failure. Urea is mostly excreted by the kidney, but approximately 25 percent will diffuse into the intestine, where it is converted to NH_3 by bacterial urease. The intestinal production of ammonia also occurs from the bacterial deamination of unabsorbed amino acids and of protein derived from the diet, exfoliated cells, or blood in the gastrointestinal tract.

Gut NH_3 is absorbed and transported to the liver via the portal vein, where it is again converted to urea. The kidney also produces varying amounts of NH_3, largely by the deamination of glutamine.

The contributions of the gut and kidney to ammonia synthesis have important implications for the management of the hyperammonemic state frequently seen in patients with advanced liver disease, usually in association with portal-systemic shunting of blood.

While the exact chemical mediators of hepatic encephalopathy remain unknown and may include endogenous benzodiazepine compounds, elevated levels of blood NH_3 generally correlate with the degree of encephalopathy, although approximately 10 percent of such patients have normal levels of blood ammonia. In addition, therapeutic measures that reduce serum NH_3 levels also usually lead to clinical improvement. The several mechanisms known to lead to increased blood NH_3 levels in patients with cirrhosis are illustrated in Fig. 264-2 and include the following: (1) If there is excessive nitrogenous material in the intestine (from bleeding or dietary protein),

FIGURE 264-2 Major factors (steps 1 to 4) influencing the level of blood ammonia. In cirrhosis with portal hypertension, venous collaterals allow ammonia to bypass the liver (step 5), permitting the entry of ammonia into the systemic circulation (portal-systemic shunting).

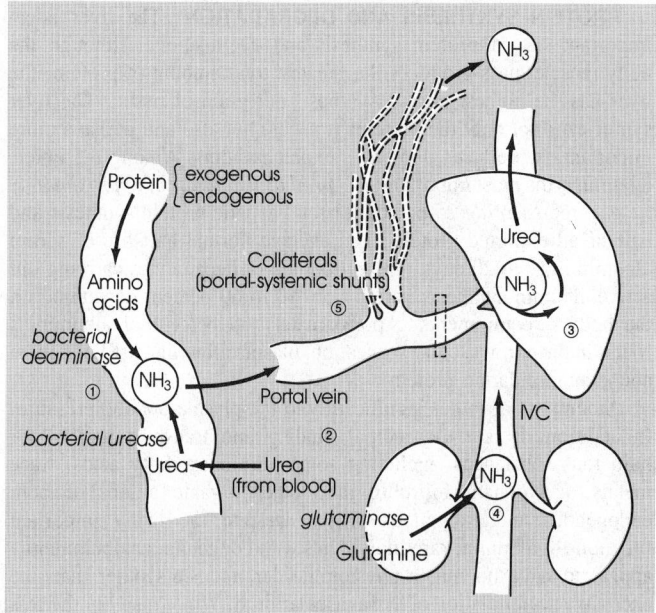

TABLE 264-1 Alteration of glucose metabolism in cirrhosis

FACTORS LEADING TO HYPERGLYCEMIA

Decreased hepatic glucose uptake
Decreased hepatic glycogen synthesis
Hepatic resistance to insulin
Portal-systemic glucose shunting
Peripheral insulin resistance
Hormonal abnormalities (serum)
  ↑ Glucagon
  ↑ Cortisol
  ↑ Insulin (↓ in hemochromatosis)

FACTORS LEADING TO HYPOGLYCEMIA

Decreased gluconeogenesis
Decreased hepatic glycogen content
Hepatic resistance to glucagon
Poor oral intake
Hyperinsulinemia secondary to portal-systemic shunting

excessive amounts of NH_3 will be formed by bacterial deamination of amino acids. If intestinal motility is diminished, as manifest by constipation, bacterial production of ammonia will increase due to prolonged time for degradation of luminal protein and amino acids. (2) If renal function declines (as in the hepatorenal syndrome), blood urea nitrogen rises, leading to increased diffusion of urea into the intestinal lumen, where bacterial urease converts it to NH_3. (3) If hepatic function is significantly depressed, diminished urea synthesis may occur with a resultant decrease in the removal of NH_3. (4) If alkalosis (often due to central hyperventilation) and hypokalemia accompany hepatic decompensation, there may be a decrease in the renal availability of H^+ ions; as a result, the NH_3 produced from glutamine by the action of renal glutaminase is permitted to enter the renal vein (rather than being excreted as NH_4^+), leading to increased peripheral blood NH_3 levels. In addition, hypokalemia itself leads to increased renal NH_3 production. (5) If portal hypertension is present and anastomoses exist between the portal vein and systemic venous channels, these portal-systemic shunts will allow NH_3 from the gut to bypass hepatic detoxification, leading to elevated blood NH_3 levels. Thus, with portal-systemic shunting of blood, elevated NH_3 levels may develop with relatively modest hepatocellular dysfunction. It is unclear what effects these same factors may have on other compounds which may play a role in the development of hepatic encephalopathy.

An additional factor important in determining whether a given NH_3 level in the blood will be detrimental to the central nervous system is the blood pH. The more alkaline the pH, the more toxic a given level of NH_3 is likely to be. At 37°C, the pK of NH_3 is 8.9; this is close enough to the pH· of blood that minor changes in pH can affect the NH_4^+/NH_3 ratio. Because un-ionized NH_3 crosses membranes more readily than NH_4^+ ions, alkalosis favors the entry of ammonia into the brain (with subsequent changes in cell metabolism) by shifting the equilibrium of the following reaction to the right

$$NH_4^+ + OH^- \rightleftharpoons NH_3 + HOH$$

As a result, alkalosis not only increases peripheral blood NH_3 levels by renal mechanisms but also increases tissue levels by influencing the diffusion of NH_3 across membranes. Similarly, alterations in the pH of intestinal luminal contents also will affect the equilibrium between NH_4^+ and NH_3; a more alkaline lumen will shift the balance in favor of NH_3, permitting increased absorption. In theory, laxatives that cause relative acidification of luminal contents (e.g., lactulose) may be more effective as agents for the treatment of hepatic encephalopathy. However, this theoretical effect on the equilibrium between NH_4^+ and NH_3 has never been convincingly demonstrated for available laxatives.

PROTEIN SYNTHESIS AND DEGRADATION The liver is an important site of protein synthesis and degradation. Although the body muscle mass produces the greatest total amount of protein, the liver has the highest rate of synthesis per gram of tissue. The liver synthesizes not only the proteins it needs, but also and perhaps more important, it produces numerous export proteins. Among the latter, albumin is the most important; *it is produced at a rate of approximately 12 g/d,* representing 25 percent of total hepatic protein synthesis and half of all exported protein. The average normal half-life of serum albumin is 17 to 20 days. The proportion of hepatocytes carrying out active albumin synthesis varies from 10 to 60 percent depending on the body's requirements. Approximately 60 percent of albumin is found in the extravascular spaces, but plasma albumin is still the most abundant circulating protein.

Albumin contributes significantly to the plasma oncotic pressure. In addition, it is the principal binding and transport protein for numerous substances, including some hormones, fatty acids, trace metals, tryptophan, bilirubin, and other organic anions of both endogenous and exogenous origin. Despite the many important functions of albumin, rare individuals with congenital analbuminemia appear to have no major physiologic derangements other than the excessive accumulation of extravascular fluid. While many of the less

hydrophobic ligands may be transported in the unbound form, this suggests that other serum proteins also may play a role in binding and transport.

Much has been learned about the mechanisms involved in the synthesis of secretory proteins, especially albumin. Polyribosomes bound to the rough endoplasmic reticulum (RER) of the hepatocyte are the principal site of translation of messenger ribonucleic acid (mRNA) coding for export proteins; in contrast, proteins destined for intracellular use, such as ferritin, are synthesized on free rather than bound polyribosomes in the cytoplasm. After a short-term fast, there is a decrease in the amount of albumin mRNA associated with the RER; instead, more mRNA is found in the cytosol and in a state dissociated from polyribosomes. Albumin, like secretory proteins produced by other organs, appears to be synthesized initially as a larger precursor, preproalbumin. This precursor molecule contains an additional 24 extra amino acid residues on the N terminus, referred to as a *signal peptide*, which undergoes two sequential cleavages (or "processing"). The "pre" portion of preproalbumin is cleaved within the RER even before protein synthesis is completed; the "pro" segment is removed within the lumen of the RER. The molecule is then transported to the Golgi apparatus prior to secretion. Once synthesis and processing are completed, albumin is transported from the Golgi vesicles to the hepatocyte surface by mechanisms which are unclear but almost certainly involve the microfilaments and microtubule apparatus of the cell. Although the hepatic lymph space of Disse provides a potential avenue for the newly released albumin, most secreted proteins enter the plasma.

Albumin synthesis is subject to a number of regulatory influences. These include the rate of transcription of specific mRNAs and the availability of the substrate tRNA (transfer RNA). At the translational level, the integrity of polyribosomes and their synthetic abilities are modified by factors affecting initiation, elongation, and release of peptides and proteins as well as by the availability of ATP, GTP, and magnesium ions. The rate of albumin synthesis is also influenced by the availability of amino acid precursors, especially tryptophan, the scarcest of the essential amino acids. Indeed, in patients with large carcinoid tumors, albumin synthesis may decrease precipitously when tryptophan is consumed by carcinoid cells in the production of 5-hydroxytryptophan (serotonin) (see Chap. 276). The rate of albumin synthesis is also affected by colloid oncotic pressure, with increased production occurring in response to falling oncotic pressure. Finally, influences of hormones such as insulin and glucagon on hepatic protein metabolism are closely integrated with the nutritional factors discussed above.

The liver also produces a wide variety of other secretory proteins, most of which have a synthetic pathway and processing procedure similar to that of albumin. The presence of a *signal peptide*, such as the "prepro" segment of albumin, which is subsequently removed during protein maturation appears to be a general mechanism for orienting proteins in the membranes of the endoplasmic reticulum and directing them for export rather than for intracellular use or degradation. Most proteins undergo even further modification in the form of sequential *glycosylation* in the RER and Golgi apparatus. The carbohydrate moieties of these glycoproteins appear to be important in determining their site of action and their rate of tissue uptake after secretion. Some of the clinically important secretory glycoproteins include ceruloplasmin, α_1-antitrypsin, and most other alpha and beta globulins. While the site of albumin catabolism is uncertain, the removal of terminal sialic acid residues after secretion and the resultant exposure of penultimate galactose or N-acetylglucosamine residues appears to result in receptor-mediated uptake of "aged" proteins by hepatocytes and Kupffer cells, followed by their subsequent degradation. Reduced amounts of the hepatic receptor for asialoglycoproteins appear to result in elevated serum concentrations of these glycoproteins in patients with severe and chronic liver disease.

One of the clinically most important derangements in protein metabolism is the development of hypoalbuminemia, which results largely from reduced synthetic activity. Decreased synthesis may be caused by a decrease in the number as well as the function of hepatocytes. A decrease in the dietary supply of amino acids also can contribute to deficient synthesis. To some extent the body attempts to compensate for decreased albumin synthesis by reducing the rate of degradation. Attempts to raise the serum albumin level by intravenous infusions are often futile because this compensatory mechanism can be blunted and the decrease in albumin degradation may not occur. The reduced degradation of albumin is not a general phenomenon in chronic liver disease because other proteins such as fibrinogen are degraded more rapidly than normal. In the patient with ascites, the degree of hypoalbuminemia is worsened by the loss of large amounts of the body's albumin into the ascitic fluid. When there is increased hepatic venous pressure (as in postsinusoidal or hepatic vein outflow block), there may be increased hepatic lymph production with extravasation into the peritoneal cavity. In contrast to intestinal lymph, the protein content of hepatic lymph appears to be relatively uninfluenced by ascitic oncotic pressure, most likely reflecting the lack of tight junctions between sinusoidal endothelial cells.

Other proteins produced by the liver include many of the blood-clotting factors: fibrinogen (factor I), prothrombin (factor II), and factors V, VII, IX, and X, as well as inhibitors of both coagulation and fibrinolysis. Factors II, VII, IX, and X are vitamin K–responsive and are dependent on normal intestinal fat absorption. Vitamin K activates an enzyme system in liver endoplasmic reticulum which catalyzes the γ carboxylation of selected glutamyl residues in clotting factor precursors. The γ carboxylation enhances the Ca^{2+} and phospholipid-binding capacity of prothrombin and permits its rapid conversion to thrombin in the presence of factors V and X (Chap. 315).

The liver is involved in the process of hemostasis by virtue of both anabolic and catabolic functions. As expected, severe liver disease leads to reduced synthesis of prothrombin, a vitamin K–dependent clotting factor. The presence of malnutrition, the use of broad-spectrum antibiotics, or concomitant impairment of fat absorption due to reduction in intestinal bile salt concentration (e.g., cholestasis) may accentuate hypoprothrombinemia by decreasing the amount of vitamin K that can be absorbed from the intestine. In these situations, prothrombin levels may be at least partially corrected by parenteral vitamin K administration. However, when the coagulopathy results from impaired hepatocellular function and not cholestasis or intestinal factors, exogenous vitamin K is unlikely to correct or improve prothrombin synthesis. The vitamin K–dependent clotting proteins have a substantially shorter serum half-life than albumin; therefore, hypoprothrombinemia usually precedes the development of hypoalbuminemia, especially in the patient with acute hepatocellular disease. In cirrhosis, coagulopathy may be further aggravated by the thrombocytopenia resulting from hypersplenism.

Since the liver is also the site of production of non-vitamin K–dependent clotting factors, severe liver disease injury may lead to decreased plasma concentrations of factor V in addition to factors II, VII, IX, and X. It is unusual for fibrinogen to be reduced significantly, unless there is an associated disseminated intravascular coagulation (DIC). For unclear reasons, the damaged liver may actually produce increased amounts of fibrinogen as well as other proteins collectively designated acute-phase reactants (C-reactive proteins, haptoglobin, ceruloplasmin, and transferrin). The latter are produced both in response to liver injury (e.g., severe chronic active hepatitis) and in association with systemic illnesses such as cancer, rheumatoid arthritis, bacterial infections, burns, and myocardial infarctions. Cytokines, including interleukins 1 and 6, appear to be major stimuli of hepatic synthesis of acute-phase reactants. However, while the diseased liver may produce normal or increased amounts of fibrinogen, the molecules themselves may be qualitatively abnormal (i.e., structurally and functionally), reflecting more subtle derangements in protein synthesis. These functionally abnormal fibrinogen molecules may contribute to the altered hemostasis frequently found in patients with chronic liver disease.

DETOXIFICATION MECHANISMS Water-soluble drugs and endogenous substances usually are excreted unchanged in the urine or bile. However, lipid-soluble compounds tend to accumulate in the body and affect cellular processes, unless they are converted to less active compounds or to more water-soluble metabolites which are more easily excreted. Hepatic blood flow, protein binding, and the intrinsic capacity of the liver to eliminate a drug are all primary determinants of hepatic drug clearance. The liver has an important role in the metabolism of many exogenous drugs and endogenous hormones by virtue of several enzyme systems involved in biochemical transformation as well as the "first-pass effect" of blood flow from virtually the entire gastrointestinal tract through the liver via the portal circulation. The relative importance of these various factors differs depending on how well a drug is extracted by the liver. There are two major types of reactions. The first, *phase I reactions*, result in chemical modification of reactive groups by oxidation, reduction, hydroxylation, sulfoxidation, deamination, dealkylation, or methylation. Such modifications usually involve one of several enzymatic systems, including the mixed-function oxidases, cytochromes b_5 and P-450 (microsomal), and the glutathione S-acyltransferases (cytoplasmic). These biochemical reactions usually lead to *inactivation* of drugs such as barbiturates and benzodiazepines. However, *activation* also may occur. For example, cortisone is activated to cortisol and prednisone to prednisolone (both products being more potent than the parent compounds); imipramine, a depressant, is converted to desmethylimipramine, an antidepressant. In the same manner, phase I reactions may even convert a nontoxic compound to a toxic one, as in the metabolism of isoniazid and acetaminophen. Similarly, some carcinogens may be activated by formation of highly reactive epoxide intermediates in the liver, while other carcinogens may be detoxified.

The enzymes responsible for phase I reactions, especially those involving the cytochrome P-450 system, can be induced by drugs such as ethanol, barbiturates, haloperidol, and glutethimide. Conversely, hepatic microsomal enzymes may be inhibited by agents such as chloramphenicol, cimetidine, disulfiram, dextropropoxyphene, allopurinol, and, paradoxically, ethanol. The concomitant administration of two drugs metabolized by the same microsomal enzyme may result in modification, potentiation, or diminution of the pharmacologic efficacy of either or both drugs. Activity of phase I reactions also may change with aging.

Phase II reactions may follow phase I reactions or proceed independently; these involve the conversion of substances to their glucuronide, sulfate, acetyl, taurine, or glycine derivatives, thereby converting lipophilic substances to water-soluble derivatives and permitting their excretion in bile or urine. Conjugation catalyzed by microsomal UDP (uridine diphosphate)-glucuronyltransferases to form glucuronide derivatives is one of the most common phase II reactions. In general, the conjugates are more soluble than the parent compound and are pharmacologically inactive.

An awareness that there may be varying degrees of impairment in the hepatic uptake, detoxification, and excretion of certain drugs is important in the clinical management of patients with chronic liver disease. Portal-systemic shunting of blood may decrease the "first-pass effect" of drugs absorbed from the gut. In cirrhosis, altered intrahepatic hemodynamics due to a disordered liver architecture also may reduce the rates of hepatic drug clearance. Hypoalbuminemia will permit drugs usually bound to albumin to be present in increased concentrations of their unbound form in the circulation and extracellular spaces; this may result in an increased activity of such drugs. Most important, a decrease in the amount of function of microsomal enzymes responsible for phase I and phase II reactions will result in slower rates of drug inactivation and elimination. Drugs for which there may be a decreased clearance in patients with liver disease include anticonvulsants (e.g., phenytoin, phenobarbital), anti-inflammatory agents (e.g., acetaminophen, phenylbutazone, glucocorticoids), minor tranquilizers, cardioactive drugs (e.g., lidocaine, quinidine, propranolol), and antibiotics (e.g., nafcillin, chloramphenicol, tetracyclines, clindamycin, trimethoprim, rifampin, pyrazinamide). This will lead to decreased dosage requirements and a narrowing of the range between therapeutic and toxic drug levels. Finally, the patient with chronic liver disease may demonstrate alterations in the pharmacologic effects of drugs in addition to or independent of changes in their pharmacokinetics, such as an increased central nervous system sensitivity to opiates and other sedatives.

The difficulties in safely administering pharmacologic agents to patients with both acute and chronic liver disease are underscored by the frequency with which administration of benzodiazepines is cited as precipitating hepatic coma. It may be very difficult clinically to determine whether agitation, confusion, and irrational behavior are due to early hepatic encephalopathy or are related to the concurrent use of benzodiazepines, opiates, barbiturates, and other depressants. It should be recognized that there is great variation of drug clearance in patients with liver disease; although data on average clearances may provide a reasonable estimate for initial dosages, subsequent adjustments in dose need to be individualized in order to attain the desired plasma drug concentration.

The mechanism by which some agents exert a hepatotoxic effect may involve the same metabolic pathways responsible for normal drug detoxification. The mechanism of acetaminophen toxicity is particularly illustrative. Acetaminophen is metabolized and detoxified by the hepatic mixed-function oxygenase system, but one of the intermediate products is a potent free radical (postulated metabolite N-acetylimidoquinone) which can inactivate many enzymes and proteins by binding irreversibly to their sulfhydryl groups. Normally, this interaction can be prevented by reduced glutathione. In the presence of excessive amounts of the acetaminophen free radical (e.g., from overdosage or underlying liver disease), the glutathione levels of the hepatocytes are readily exhausted, and the excess free radicals can lead to inactivation of cellular proteins and produce widespread hepatocellular necrosis. In the case of acetaminophen overdosage, the very early administration of sulfhydryl groups in the form of N-acetylcysteine can often prevent this drug-induced liver injury.

HORMONE METABOLISM In addition to its role in the metabolism of diverse pharmacologic agents, the liver is also responsible for inactivation or modification of several endogenous hormones; therefore, chronic liver disease may be accompanied by signs of apparent hormonal imbalance. Some hormones (e.g., insulin and glucagon) are inactivated in the liver by proteolysis or deamination. Thyroxine and triiodothyronine are metabolized in the liver by reactions involving deiodination. Steroid hormones, such as glucocorticoids and aldosterone, are first inactivated to their tetrahydro derivative (by reduction of the Δ^4 double bond and the 3-keto group), followed by conjugation, mostly with glucuronic acid. Testosterone is metabolized to the isomeric 17-ketosteroids androsterone and etiocholanolone and excreted in the urine mostly as sulfate conjugates. Estrogens, such as estradiol, may be converted to estriol and estrone and then conjugated with glucuronic acid or sulfate. Abnormalities in estrogen (and testosterone) metabolism are believed to be involved in the development of the spider angiomas, loss of axillary or pubic hair, and testicular atrophy frequently seen in patients with chronic liver disease. In addition, increased portal-systemic shunting of testosterone and androstenedione secondary to portal hypertension may lead to the development of gynecomastia in cirrhotic males due to increased peripheral conversion to estradiol and estrone, especially in patients with alcoholic cirrhosis. In patients with alcoholic liver disease, feminization also may be related to the direct toxic effects of alcohol on the gonadal-pituitary-hypothalamic axis which lead to the overall reduction in serum testosterone found in patients with cirrhosis. Similar effects are also seen in patients with hemochromatosis due to deposition of iron in these sites. However, gynecomastia is often lacking in the latter, apparently due to a coincident reduction in plasma concentration of androstenedione, a major precursor for estrogen synthesis.

Estrogens also act directly on the liver to impair hepatic secretory activity. Estradiol and related estrogens, such as those present in contraceptive pills, interfere with sodium sulfobromophthalein and bile salt excretion and worsen the preexisting defect in secretion of conjugated bilirubin in patients with Dubin-Johnson syndrome; they also may elevate plasma alkaline phosphatase levels (see Chap. 263). Related steroids such as etiocholanolone and pregnanediol have been shown to stimulate δ-aminolevulinic acid (ALA) synthetase activity, leading to increased porphobilinogen excretion. Since these steroids exert these effects only in their unconjugated form, the increased hepatic levels of δ-aminolevulinic acid synthetase in patients with alcoholic cirrhosis may be secondary to the action of gonadal steroids.

LIPID METABOLISM: FATTY ACIDS AND TRIGLYCERIDES
Under normal conditions, most of the fatty acids taken up by the liver and esterified to triglyceride are derived from adipose tissue or the diet. Some fatty acids (especially saturated ones) are synthesized in the liver from acetate. The fatty acids may then be converted enzymatically to triglyceride, esterified with cholesterol, incorporated into phospholipids, or oxidized to CO_2 or ketone bodies. Most of the triglyceride is produced for export, but in order to be secreted it must be converted to lipoproteins by combining with relatively specific apoprotein moieties. This emphasizes the importance of protein synthesis for the release and secretion of triglyceride from the liver. It should be noted that the liver plays a major role in regulating lipoprotein levels by virtue of both its degradative and synthetic functions. Thus the liver is quantitatively the major site of low-density lipoprotein (LDL) catabolism, with dual high- and low-affinity receptor-mediated pathways playing a role. In addition, chylomicron remnants are removed and degraded by the liver, where their constituents have a number of metabolic effects. The liver is not only the primary site of very low density lipoprotein (VLDL) secretion but also accounts for a major portion of its subsequent degradation by mechanisms similar to that of chylomicron remnant degradation and conversion to LDL via the action of hepatic lipase. The liver also may play a role in high-density lipoprotein (HDL) catabolism. It is noteworthy that with the exception of cholestatic disease (see below), clinically significant alterations in lipoprotein and cholesterol metabolism are usually not found in patients with chronic liver disease.

Studies on the production of fatty liver have shown that singly or in combination, one or more of the steps depicted in Fig. 264-3 may be involved. An increased influx of fatty acids mobilized from adipose tissue due to drugs (e.g., ethanol or glucocorticoids) or secondary to diabetic ketosis may lead to a fatty liver. Similarly, increased levels of fatty acids in the liver, either from enhanced fatty acid synthesis or from decreased fatty acid oxidation, may lead to increased triglyceride formation. In some instances (e.g., ethanol excess) there also may be increases in the carbohydrate backbone, α-glycerophosphate, involved in fatty acid esterification to triglyceride. Since release of triglyceride involves the formation of lipoproteins, lipid accumulation may occur because of decreased apoprotein synthesis. This appears to be the case in fatty livers seen in patients with protein-calorie malnutrition (kwashiorkor) and due to toxins such as carbon tetrachloride, phosphorus, or ethionine, as well as following excessive doses of antibiotics such as tetracycline that can inhibit protein synthesis. Finally, there may be impaired lipoprotein secretion from the liver. Different alterations disrupting hepatic fat metabolism may lead to different patterns of fat accumulation designated *macrovesicular* (most common) and *microvesicular*; these are reviewed in Chap. 270. Alcohol is perhaps the most common agent leading to a fatty liver, but the mechanism(s) whereby alcohol leads to increased liver triglyceride is not clear. Depending on factors such as dose or duration, alcohol ingestion may affect any of the seven steps shown in Fig. 264-3; however, the primary factor for the production of the alcohol-induced fatty liver remains to be determined. The alterations in the redox state due to excessive accumulation of NADH resulting from oxidation of alcohol also may contribute.

In addition to the changes leading to fatty liver, there are many metabolic alterations which may be found in the blood of patients following the ingestion of large amounts of alcohol. These include, among others, *increased* plasma levels of lactate, proline, urate, and

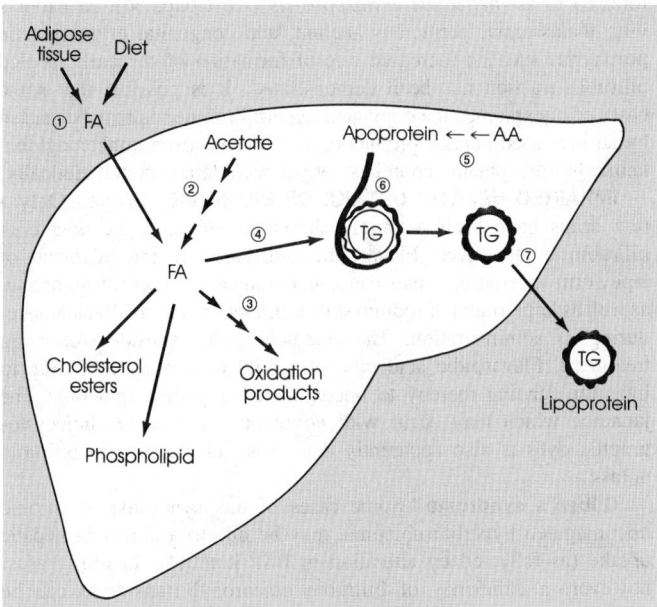

FIGURE 264-3 Factors in the uptake and esterification of fatty acids to triglyceride by the liver, including the formation and release of triglyceride as lipoprotein. The numbers refer to steps, which, if altered, may result in increased liver triglyceride (i.e., fatty liver).

triglycerides and *decreased* plasma levels of glucose, magnesium, phosphate, and triiodothyronine (T_3).

CHOLESTEROL   Cholesterol and bile acid synthesis is carried out primarily by the liver. Cholesterol synthesis is subject to a number of metabolic controls, most of them mediated via the rate-limiting biosynthetic enzyme 3-hydroxy-3-methylglutaryl coenzyme A reductase (HMG-CoA reductase). Cholesterol exists either free or combined with fatty acids in the form of cholesterol esters; in the plasma, both are found primarily in association with β-lipoproteins. The plasma and liver also contain lecithin–cholesterol acyltransferase (LCAT), an enzyme involved in the conversion of free cholesterol to its esterified form. Since there is exchange of free cholesterol between tissues, changes in plasma cholesterol levels reflect changes in total body cholesterol. However, decreases in plasma cholesterol esters may reflect hepatic damage and impaired hepatic cholesterol esterification.

Severe liver injury often leads to a decrease in *total* serum cholesterol levels, including both free and esterified fractions. This may be due to decreased synthesis of cholesterol and cholesterol esters, decreased apoprotein synthesis, or both. In cholestasis (either intra- or extrahepatic), total serum cholesterol often increases strikingly. Disorders of cholestasis are associated with marked abnormalities of lipoprotein metabolism. In primary biliary cirrhosis there are pronounced elevations in serum free cholesterol and LDL; conversely, serum HDL is reduced and may disappear from the serum in patients with long-standing disease. Similar but less marked changes are seen in other cholestatic conditions.

The increase in serum free cholesterol (and phospholipid) and the concomitant decrease in esterified cholesterol in cholestasis may be related to a decrease in the hepatic production of LCAT. Reduced levels of LCAT are also correlated with the appearance of an abnormal LDL, referred to as *lipoprotein X* (LP-X). Although LP-X, which has a high content of free cholesterol and triglyceride, was originally thought to be a specific indicator of biliary tract obstruction, it is evident that it appears in any cholestatic condition. While the depressed hepatic production of LCAT may be responsible for altered lipid content and composition of lipoproteins, the factors leading to the overall increase in total serum cholesterol are not clear. In experimental animals, bile duct ligation results in a net increase in hepatic cholesterol synthesis, and in "regurgitation" of bile salts, cholesterol, and LP-X into venous radicals. However, it is difficult

to translate these experimental findings to the patient with primary biliary cirrhosis unless any insult to cells lining the biliary canaliculi and ductules can impair the delicate balance of lipid synthesis and removal.

The alterations in cholesterol and related substances resulting from liver disease may lead to significant changes in the composition of erythrocyte membranes. Such changes in composition lead to altered morphology with the development of spur and burr cell forms. The presence of these altered erythrocytes is usually an ominous sign of advanced liver disease.

Most of the derangements of hepatic metabolism discussed above are evident only in patients with severe or long-standing liver disease. Indeed, in all but the most severe cases of acute viral hepatitis, hepatic metabolic functions are remarkably well preserved, and in most cases of mild to moderate acute viral hepatitis, it is uncommon to observe clinically important alterations in carbohydrate, protein, and lipid metabolism. However, in the patients with severe or fulminant hepatitis, whether from a viral or toxic agent, the metabolic derangements may be similar to those seen in more chronic disease. For example, in fulminant hepatitis there may be pronounced hypoprothrombinemia and impaired coagulation, hypoalbuminemia, and the relatively acute development of ascites, as well as hyperammonemia and encephalopathy. However, in contrast to patients with cirrhosis, abnormalities in carbohydrate metabolism are more likely to lead to profound hypoglycemia than to hyperglycemia. This hypoglycemia appears to reflect both a marked decrease in hepatic glycogen stores and a diminished glucagon responsiveness. There also may be poor oral intake due to nausea and anorexia together with increased glucose utilization secondary to hyperinsulinemia (due to portal-systemic shunting and decreased insulin degradation).

REFERENCES

ARIAS IM et al: *The Liver: Biology and Pathophysiology*, 2d ed. New York, Raven, 1988

BUTTERWORTH RF: Pathogenesis and treatment of portal-systemic encephalopathy: An update. Dig Dis Sci 37:321, 1992

CAVALLO-PERIN P et al: Mechanism of insulin resistance in human liver cirrhosis. Evidence of a combined receptor and post-receptor defect. J Clin Invest 75:1659, 1985

COOPER AD: Role of the liver in the degradation of lipoproteins. Gastroenterology 88:192, 1984

FLANNERY DB et al: Current status of hyperammonemic syndromes. Hepatology 2:495, 1982

HOYUMPA AM et al: Hepatic encephalopathy. Gastroenterology 77:803, 1979

KLEG HK et al: Conversion of androgens to estrogens in idiopathic hemochromatosis: Comparison with alcoholic liver disease. J Clin Endocrin Metab 61:1, 1985

MILLWARD-SADLER GH et al: *Wright's Liver and Biliary Disease*, 3d ed. London, Saunders, 1992

OWEN OE et al: Hepatic, gut and renal substrate flux rates in patients with hepatic cirrhosis. J Clin Invest 68:240, 1981

ROTHSCHILD MA et al: Serum albumin. Hepatology 8:355, 1988

SHERLOCK S, DOOLEY J: *Diseases of the Liver and Biliary System*, 9th ed. Oxford, Blackwell, 1993

SMITH AR et al: Alteration in plasma and CSF amino acids, amines and metabolites in hepatic coma. Ann Surg 187:343, 1978

WILLIAMS RC: Drug administration in hepatic disease. N Engl J Med 309:1616, 1983

ZAKIM D, BOYER TD: *Hepatology, A Textbook of Liver Disease*, 2d ed. Philadelphia, Saunders, 1990

265   BILIRUBIN METABOLISM AND HYPERBILIRUBINEMIA

KURT J. ISSELBACHER

The normal metabolism of bilirubin and the approach to the patient with jaundice have been presented in Chap. 42. With a consideration of these pathways, the disorders of bilirubin metabolism can be divided into four major categories, namely, those due to (1) increased pigment production, (2) reduced hepatic uptake of bilirubin, (3) impaired hepatic conjugation, and (4) decreased excretion of the conjugated pigment from the liver into bile. The first three of these disorders are associated with predominantly unconjugated hyperbilirubinemia. The fourth group, defective excretion, is associated with predominantly conjugated hyperbilirubinemia and bilirubinuria.

DISORDERS CAUSING PREDOMINANTLY UNCONJUGATED HYPERBILIRUBINEMIA

The plasma concentration of unconjugated bilirubin is determined by (1) the rate at which newly synthesized bilirubin enters the plasma (bilirubin turnover) and (2) the rate of removal of bilirubin by the liver (hepatic bilirubin clearance). Disturbances of the latter can result from derangements of hepatic bilirubin uptake, conjugation, or both. Measurements of these variables, although not routinely available, permit a classification of patients into those with *increased bilirubin turnover* (e.g., hemolysis), those with *decreased bilirubin clearance* (e.g., Gilbert's syndrome), and those in whom both mechanisms operate.

OVERPRODUCTION OF BILIRUBIN (INCREASED TURNOVER) Increased destruction of circulating erythrocytes (intravascular and extravascular hemolysis)   In disorders associated with hemolysis, most commonly the hemolytic anemias, the rate of bilirubin production is increased and may even exceed the amount that can be removed by a normal liver. The resulting jaundice is primarily an unconjugated hyperbilirubinemia. There is often also a small increase in the serum conjugated bilirubin. If significant anemia or other adverse factors are present (e.g., fever, sepsis, hypoxemia, or vascular collapse), the ability of the liver to handle the pigment load will be compromised, and the degree of jaundice will be greater.

The clinical and diagnostic features of the various hemolytic anemias are described in Chap. 307. The presence of reticulocytosis, shortened red blood cell survival, and increased fecal urobilinogen, in the absence of clinical and laboratory evidence of liver disease, strongly suggest hemolysis and overproduction of bilirubin as the cause of the jaundice. It is obvious, however, that in some cases (e.g., cirrhosis, tumors, and sepsis), hemolysis *plus* deranged liver function may be present. In most cases of uncomplicated hemolytic states, the mean serum bilirubin level will be in the range of 51 to 68 μmol/L (3 to 4 mg/dL); rarely, higher levels may be seen.

Jaundice due to increased pigment production also may be seen as a consequence of *tissue infarction* (e.g., pulmonary infarcts) and large *collections of blood in tissues* (e.g., leakage from blood vessels after catheterization studies, rupture of an aortic aneurysm). If hypotension and hypoxemia also supervene, jaundice is usually more pronounced, and the resulting impairment of liver function also may lead to a significant increase in the serum conjugated bilirubin level (see "Postoperative Jaundice," below).

Except in early infancy, elevations of serum unconjugated bilirubin levels are not harmful per se, and the prognosis is that of the hemolytic process itself. However, in the neonatal state and infancy, unconjugated bilirubin levels above 340 μmol/L (20 mg/dL) may lead to *kernicterus* due to bilirubin deposition in the lipid-rich basal ganglia (see Chap. 378). Chronic overproduction of bilirubin may result in the formation of gallstones composed predominantly of bilirubin ("pigment stones"). In this situation, all the potential complications of calculus disease of the biliary tract (Chap. 272) may be superimposed on the chronic hemolytic state which produced it.

Increased production of bilirubin from sources other than circulating erythrocytes   About 15 to 20 percent of the circulating bilirubin is normally derived from sources other than the destruction of circulating red blood cells. This represents the so-called early-labeled fraction; it includes the synthesis of bilirubin from nonhemoglobin heme in the liver and from hemoglobin heme in the marrow.

In some conditions, jaundice results from an increased destruction of red blood cells or their precursors in the marrow—a process

referred to as *ineffective erythropoiesis* (see Chap. 56). In patients with thalassemia, pernicious anemia, and congenital erythropoietic porphyria, such an increased rate of formation of the early-labeled bilirubin fraction has been demonstrated. It is possible that some cases of unexplained unconjugated hyperbilirubinemia may be caused by an increased hepatic production of bilirubin from nonhemoglobin heme, but this phenomenon has not yet been demonstrated clinically.

IMPAIRED HEPATIC UPTAKE OF BILIRUBIN   Drugs   Only a few drugs have been definitely shown to influence the uptake of bilirubin by the liver. Flavaspidic acid, used in the treatment of tapeworm infestation, may cause unconjugated hyperbilirubinemia, as well as impairment of sodium sulfobromophthalein (BSP) clearance, during its administration. The jaundice readily subsides following treatment. Flavaspidic acid competes with bilirubin for binding to ligandin, leading thereby to unconjugated hyperbilirubinemia. The jaundice which may occur with novobiocin and some cholecystographic dyes is also apparently due to an interference in bilirubin uptake.

Gilbert's syndrome   Some cases of this syndrome of chronic unconjugated hyperbilirubinemia may be due to a defect in hepatic uptake (as reflected by alteration in BSP kinetics). In most cases, however, a deficiency of bilirubin glucuronyl transferase can be demonstrated. Hence this syndrome is best considered as a defect in bilirubin conjugation (see below).

IMPAIRED BILIRUBIN CONJUGATION (DECREASED ACTIVITY OF BILIRUBIN GLUCURONOSYL TRANSFERASE)   Neonatal jaundice (physiologic jaundice of the newborn)   Almost every infant exhibits some transient unconjugated hyperbilirubinemia between the second and fifth days of life. While during gestation the placenta serves to clear bilirubin from the fetus, after birth infants must detoxify the pigments themselves. However, at this stage the hepatic enzyme glucuronosyl transferase is still "immature" and inadequate for the task. As a result, unconjugated bilirubinemia develops, usually not exceeding 86 μmol/L (5 mg/dL). The activity of glucuronosyl transferase increases within several days to 2 weeks after birth, and concomitantly, the serum bilirubin level returns to normal. In the premature infant, the glucuronosyl transferase activity is less, and the neonatal jaundice may be more pronounced. The "maturation" of the fetal and neonatal liver may be enhanced by treatment of the pregnant mother or the newborn infant with phenobarbital or related drugs. This results in a clear-cut reduction of the degree and duration of unconjugated hyperbilirubinemia in the newborn. In infants with a superimposed hemolytic process (e.g., erythroblastosis), the excessive pigment load leads to more pronounced jaundice, and bilirubin levels may exceed 340 μmol/L (20 mg/dL). It should be emphasized that neonatal jaundice is not present at the time of delivery; if jaundice is present at birth, other causes must be considered.

The cytoplasmic liver cell protein ligandin (glutathione-*S*-transferase B) binds bilirubin in the hepatocyte and may assist in the transfer of bilirubin to the endoplasmic reticulum for conjugation (Chap. 42). Deficiency of ligandin may contribute to neonatal jaundice.

An additional facet of the "immature" liver is a concomitant defect in the excretion of *conjugated* bilirubin. Rarely this defect persists beyond the time needed for the development of adequate glucuronide conjugation and may explain the occasional presence of conjugated hyperbilirubinemia in infants with erythroblastosis (*inspissated bile syndrome*).

When in the neonatal state unconjugated bilirubin levels approach or exceed 340 μmol/L (20 mg/dL), the infants may develop and die of *kernicterus* (bilirubin encephalopathy). This condition results from unconjugated bilirubin deposition in the lipid-rich basal ganglia. In the past, treatment consisted of exchange transfusions, and albumin infusions were used to increase binding of bilirubin in the circulation and diminish its entry into the brain. The current approach is *phototherapy;* intense illumination of these patients with strong white or blue light leads to the *photoisomerization* of bilirubin to water-soluble isomers that are rapidly excreted in the bile without the prior

TABLE 265-1 Hereditary unconjugated hyperbilirubinemias with deficiency of glucuronosyl transferase

Features	Mild (Gilbert's syndrome)	Moderate (Crigler-Najjar syndrome type II)	Severe (Crigler-Najjar syndrome type I)
Inheritance	Unclear*	Dominant†	Recessive
Serum bilirubin, μmol/L (mg/dL)	17–102 (1–6)	102–340 (6–20)	340–770 (20–45)
Kernicterus	No	Rare	Yes
Conjugated bilirubin in bile	Yes (↑ mo-noconjugates)	Yes (↑↑ mo-noconjugates)	No
Response to phenobarbital	Yes	Yes	No
Bilirubin conjugation	↓ ‡	↓↓	Absent

* Many cases have no familial incidence.
† Variable expressivity.
‡ Other defects such as occult hemolysis and decreased bilirubin uptake may coexist.

need of conjugation. Another novel approach involves decreasing bilirubin production from heme by inhibitors of the enzyme heme oxygenase. Synthetic protoporphyrins, such as tin protoporphyrin, have been administered successfully to patients with neonatal hyperbilirubinemia with marked reduction in the serum bilirubin and with no major side effects.

Hereditary glucuronosyl transferase deficiency There are currently three syndromes that fall into this category. As indicated in Table 265-1, they reflect progressive decreases in the activity of glucuronosyl transferase and thus may be part of a spectrum, i.e., from minimal deficiency to complete absence of bilirubin glucuronosyl transferase.

GILBERT'S SYNDROME Since the original report by Gilbert in 1907, there has been an increased recognition of this benign but chronic disorder characterized by mild, persistent, unconjugated hyperbilirubinemia. The patient usually does not manifest this disorder until after the second decade and is often unaware of the jaundice until it is detected by physical examination or routine laboratory testing. The total serum bilirubin level usually ranges and fluctuates from 21 to 51 μmol/L (1.2 to 3 mg/dL) and rarely exceeds 86 μmol/L (5 mg/dL). With the van den Bergh diazo reaction, less than 20 percent of bilirubin gives a direct reaction; however, studies using more accurate methods (such as high-pressure liquid chromatography) show that the serum bilirubin in patients with Gilbert's syndrome is almost all unconjugated. Typically, the jaundice fluctuates and is exacerbated following prolonged fasting (see below), surgery, fever or infection, and excessive exertion or alcohol ingestion. Liver function tests are normal, and the liver cells usually appear normal by light microscopy.

With the exception of hemolytic anemias, Gilbert's syndrome is probably the most common cause of mild unconjugated hyperbilirubinemia. Detailed studies show these patients to have a partial deficiency of bilirubin glucuronosyl transferase. Some patients also manifest decreased bilirubin uptake and increased hemolysis. Decreased glucuronosyl transferase alone or together with a decrease in bilirubin uptake appears to account for the observed *decrease in hepatic bilirubin clearance.* A decreased clearance and hepatic uptake of bile salts also have been shown.

Previously, Gilbert's syndrome was traditionally defined as mild, chronic, unconjugated hyperbilirubinemia occurring in the absence of hemolysis. However, with the use of radiobilirubin kinetics and erythrocyte half-life studies, at least two forms of Gilbert's syndrome have been described. One group includes patients with decreased bilirubin clearance and *no hemolysis.* A second group includes those who also have *evidence of hemolysis* (often occult) and hence increased bilirubin turnover. The simultaneous presence of both derangements appears to be a chance occurrence of two not uncommon disorders

in the same patient and does not imply a causal relationship. There is additional evidence of the heterogeneity of patients with Gilbert's syndrome. Thus, some patients have an increase in hepatocyte lipofuscin and an increase in the smooth endoplasmic reticulum (SER); others show an increase in hepatic lysosomal enzymes.

A feature of Gilbert's syndrome which can be useful diagnostically is the increase in serum bilirubin following prolonged fasting or calorie deprivation. Patients with this disorder, when placed on 1255 kJ (300 kcal) per day for 2 days, will increase their serum bilirubin by 25 μmol/L (1.5 mg/dL) or more, the major increase being in the unconjugated fraction. A decrease in glucuronosyl transferase activity is needed to obtain this effect. Patients with hemolysis do not show an increase in serum bilirubin with fasting. As a reflection of the mild decrease in glucuronosyl transferase in Gilbert's syndrome, (1) serum bilirubin levels will decrease when the enzyme activity is enhanced following phenobarbital administration, and (2) the bile shows a modest increase in monoconjugates of bilirubin (see Table 265-1).

In general, the diagnosis of this benign but not uncommon disorder is made by exclusion. The syndrome is suspected in a patient with low-grade unconjugated hyperbilirubinemia with (1) no systemic symptoms, (2) *no overt* or clinically recognizable hemolysis, (3) normal tests of routine liver function, and (4) a liver biopsy (although usually not necessary) that is normal by light microscopy.

CRIGLER-NAJJAR SYNDROME (TYPES I AND II) This disorder is known to exist in two forms. Type I is the clinically *severe* form (originally described by Crigler and Najjar) and is due to *absence of glucuronosyl transferase* (or lack of function of one or more isoenzymes of the transferase). Type II has more *moderate* clinical findings due to *partial deficiency of glucuronosyl transferase.* The major differences are summarized in Table 265-1.

Type I (Crigler-Najjar) is a rare disorder. Infants develop high unconjugated bilirubin levels in the serum [340 to 770 μmol/L (20 to 45 mg/dL)]. Absence of the enzyme can be demonstrated in the liver by enzymatic or molecular genetic techniques. Routine liver function tests are normal, as is liver histology. Because of the lack of glucuronosyl transferase activity, no conjugated bilirubin is formed by the liver; hence no bilirubin is secreted into the bile and liver, and the bile is colorless.

Phototherapy may temporarily and transiently reduce the unconjugated bilirubin level. Phenobarbital has no effect, since the enzyme defect is complete and no drug "induction" is therefore possible. Affected infants usually die within the first year of life, although some patients have survived to the second or third decade of life. Death is usually from kernicterus. A strain of rats (Gunn rat) with the type I defect exists and is widely used as an animal model of the Crigler-Najjar syndrome (type I).

Type II patients have a *partial deficiency* of glucuronosyl transferase (due to a mutation of the enzyme) and their disorder is less severe. Serum unconjugated bilirubin levels are lower [103 to 340 μmol/L (6 to 20 mg/dL)], jaundice may not appear until adolescence, and neurologic complications are uncommon. The bile contains variable amounts of conjugated bilirubin with a significant increase in monoconjugates. Phenobarbital is effective in lowering the serum bilirubin level in type II patients. However, the disorder is relatively benign in those patients whose bilirubin level is less than 308 to 340 μmol/L (18 to 20 mg/dL).

Acquired deficiency of glucuronosyl transferase As with any enzyme, glucuronosyl transferase is susceptible to inhibition by a variety of agents, and because of the decreased activity of the enzyme in the neonatal state, such inhibition may be more evident at that time. Neonatal jaundice may be aggravated or prolonged in infants treated with *drugs* such as chloramphenicol or novobiocin or with *vitamin K.* In some breast-fed infants, jaundice has been ascribed to the presence in *breast milk* of pregnane-3β,20α-diol, an inhibitor of glucuronosyl transferase. When the infant is removed from the breast, the "breast-milk jaundice" subsides.

Hypothyroidism delays the normal "maturation" of glucuronosyl transferase. In cretins, neonatal jaundice may be prolonged for weeks or months. In fact, the presence of prolonged unconjugated hyperbilirubinemia after birth may be a clue to an underlying hypothyroidism.

In the infant, as well as in the adult, *liver cell damage* leads to impairment in glucuronide conjugation as a result of decreased transferase activity. However, since excretion is probably the rate-limiting step in bilirubin metabolism, and since this step appears to be interfered with to a greater extent than conjugation in parenchymal liver disease, the pigment which accumulates in the blood is predominantly conjugated bilirubin.

DISORDERS CAUSING COMBINED CONJUGATED AND UNCONJUGATED HYPERBILIRUBINEMIA

In jaundice due to primary liver disease, the plasma usually exhibits elevated levels of both conjugated and unconjugated bilirubin, and *urine contains bilirubin*. The relative proportions of the two pigments are highly variable. In many familial hepatic abnormalities (described below) and in some forms of liver injury, the jaundice is largely due to increases in conjugated bilirubin. Such a serum pigment pattern is also seen with extrahepatic biliary obstruction. One *cannot differentiate* intrahepatic and extrahepatic causes of jaundice from either the levels or proportions of unconjugated and conjugated bilirubin in serum. Thus the main purpose of the initial fractionation of the serum bilirubin is to distinguish hepatic parenchymal and biliary obstructive disease from the disorders associated with predominantly unconjugated hyperbilirubinemia.

FAMILIAL DEFECTS IN HEPATIC EXCRETORY FUNCTION
Dubin-Johnson syndrome   This disorder, also called *chronic idiopathic jaundice*, is a benign, autosomally inherited hyperbilirubinemia characterized by the presence of a dark pigment in the centrilobular region of the liver cells. Functionally, there exists a *defect in biliary excretion* of bilirubin, cholephilic dyes, and porphyrins. Using the diazo method for measuring bilirubin, the serum pigment in these patients typically is in the range of 51 to 257 μmol/L (3 to 15 mg/dL) and predominantly of the conjugated type. However, with the newer and more accurate method (alkaline methanolysis and high-pressure liquid chromatography), homozygous patients with the Dubin-Johnson syndrome have been shown to have significant levels of serum *unconjugated bilirubin*. This finding may in part reflect pigment which, after conjugation by the liver, is deconjugated in the hepatobiliary system and refluxed into the plasma. Moreover, the serum contains more diconjugated than monoconjugated bilirubin, just the reverse of what is seen in acquired hepatobiliary disease and Rotor syndrome. This reversed ratio is believed to be characteristic and diagnostic for homozygous patients.

Patients with Dubin-Johnson syndrome may be asymptomatic or have vague constitutional or gastrointestinal symptoms. Not infrequently the liver is slightly enlarged; in about one-fourth of cases there is mild hepatic tenderness. Oral and intravenous cholangiography fails to visualize the biliary tract. There is typically and characteristically a late rise in the plasma BSP elimination curve at *90 min*. This is caused by the reflux from the liver of the conjugated dye and reflects the defect in the hepatic excretory transport maximum (T_m). It is noteworthy that there is no such secondary rise in plasma when dyes that are not conjugated by the liver are given, such as indocyanine green. When bile salts such as ursodeoxycholic acid are given, these patients show a decreased hepatic uptake and clearance. In the liver the striking feature is the presence of a *brown or black pigment in the hepatocytes*. Some findings suggest that this unique pigment is "melanin-like"; others indicate it to be a polymer of epinephrine metabolites.

These patients also show an abnormality in coproporphyrin excretion. Normal urine contains mostly coproporphyrin III and small amounts of coproporphyrin I; Dubin-Johnson patients show a reversal of this pattern; i.e., they excrete predominantly coproporphyrin I. Heterozygotes show an intermediate excretory pattern.

There is impaired excretion of many metabolites, including conjugated bilirubin, BSP, and iodinated dyes. Excretion of bile acids, however, is normal. Oral contraceptive agents may accentuate hyperbilirubinemia or may produce jaundice for the first time. Features of cholestasis such as pruritus or steatorrhea are usually lacking, and specifically, serum alkaline phosphatase levels are *not* elevated. The overall prognosis of the disorder is excellent.

Rotor syndrome   This is similar in many respects to the Dubin-Johnson syndrome. However, *there is no pigment in the liver cells*, and the serum conjugated bilirubin has more monoconjugates than diglucuronide conjugates. The gallbladder is usually visualized on cholecystography, and there is an increase in the *total* urinary coproporphyrins but *not* an increased percentage in excretion of coproporphyrin I. The BSP excretion pattern does *not* show a secondary rise at 90 min. The impairment in excretion which is typical of Dubin-Johnson syndrome is not present; instead, in most cases of the Rotor syndrome there is impairment of *hepatic storage capacity* (*S*). This rare syndrome is inherited as an autosomal recessive trait and is genetically distinct from Dubin-Johnson syndrome.

Benign familial recurrent cholestasis   This is a relatively rare syndrome characterized by recurrent attacks of pruritus and jaundice. During an attack, the serum alkaline phosphatase and bile acid levels are markedly elevated, and liver biopsy shows the morphologic features of cholestasis. However, there is no mechanical biliary obstruction, with cholangiography revealing a patent biliary tree. Remissions are the rule, and at such times hepatic function tests and liver morphologic features are usually normal. The cause of the disorder is unknown; cirrhosis does not develop, and the disorder is benign. A congenital origin has been postulated on the basis of the early age of onset and familial incidence.

Recurrent jaundice of pregnancy   This form of jaundice is also known as *intrahepatic cholestasis of pregnancy*. During a normal pregnancy, some derangements in liver function occur, especially during the last trimester. Usually these consist of slight increases in BSP retention and in serum alkaline phosphatase. This mild increase in alkaline phosphatase during pregnancy is normally of placental rather than of hepatic origin. With a normal pregnancy, elevations of serum bilirubin level either do not occur or are less than 34 μmol/L (2 mg/dL).

In a small number of pregnant women an intrahepatic cholestasis may appear. This usually occurs in the third trimester but may develop any time after the seventh week of gestation. The clinical features consist primarily of pruritus and jaundice. Serum bilirubin levels are usually less than 103 μmol/L (6 mg/dL). The serum alkaline phosphatase and cholesterol levels are elevated significantly, while other liver function tests are only mildly deranged. Histologically, the liver shows varying degrees of cholestasis but only a few parenchymal cell changes. The clinical and laboratory abnormalities subside promptly after delivery and are usually normal within 7 to 14 days.

This condition has been seen more frequently in Scandinavia and Europe than in the United States. Since steroid hormones and specifically estrogens can induce changes in hepatic excretory function in normal individuals (see Chap. 264), these patients probably have an increased susceptibility or sensitivity to the hepatic effects of estrogenic and progestational hormones. The intrahepatic cholestasis is usually termed *recurrent*, since the syndrome often (but not always) reappears in subsequent pregnancies. The process is benign and self-limited, and treatment is usually not needed, but cholestyramine administration will diminish the pruritus. This disorder must be distinguished from the many other causes of jaundice not unique to pregnancy, such as viral hepatitis. It also must be distinguished from the idiopathic *acute fatty liver of pregnancy* and the *tetracycline-induced fatty liver*. The latter two conditions are rare, occur in the last trimester, and have a high fatality rate; however, in these disorders there is evidence of diffuse parenchymal damage and not only cholestasis.

TABLE 265-2 Conditions causing or contributing to postoperative jaundice

Increased pigment load
 A Hemolytic anemia
 B Transfusions (especially of stored blood)
 C Resorption of hematomas, blood in extravascular spaces
Impaired hepatocellular function
 A Hepatitis-like picture
  1 Halothane anesthesia
  2 Drugs
  3 Shock
  4 Infection with hepatitis viruses
 B Cholestatic picture
  1 Hypotension, hypoxemia
  2 Drugs
  3 Sepsis
Extrahepatic obstruction
 A Bile duct injury
 B Choledocholithiasis

is relevant that one-third of the reported patients with jaundice due to oral contraceptives also have a history of recurrent intrahepatic cholestasis of pregnancy.

The nature of these changes produced by the natural and synthetic female sex hormones is very similar to those resulting from the administration of certain testosterone analogues, especially those with α substitutions at the 17 position of the steroid nucleus. These agents (such as methyltestosterone and norethandrolone) commonly cause BSP retention and less commonly cause jaundice or significant changes in other liver functions. However, unlike the female hormones, these agents have been implicated as a cause of chronic liver disease, especially biliary cirrhosis.

Because of these phenomena, synthetic steroid sex hormones should not be used in patients with liver disease. Conversely, in individuals using these agents, the appearance of jaundice or elevations in serum aminotransferase (transaminase) or alkaline phosphatase levels contraindicates their further use. However, mild to moderate increases in BSP retention alone are probably not of clinical significance, although liver function tests should be carried out periodically.

As is discussed in detail in Chap. 266, there are many drugs which may produce not only cholestasis but liver injury resembling acute hepatitis or cholestatic hepatitis. In contrast to the jaundice produced by the steroid hormones, the clinical features are those of fever, rash, arthralgia, and sometimes eosinophilia, with the liver showing a pronounced inflammatory reaction. These features suggest that such

ACQUIRED DEFECTS OF HEPATIC EXCRETORY FUNCTION

Drug-induced cholestasis A condition entirely analogous to the intrahepatic cholestasis of pregnancy may occur in some women following the use of oral contraceptive agents. In some, mild cholestatic jaundice may occur, liver function returns to normal when the drugs are withdrawn, and chronic liver disease does not result. It

TABLE 265-3 Laboratory features in icteric states

Bilirubin disorder	Serum bilirubin		Urine bilirubin	Comments
	Unconjugated	Conjugated		
OVERPRODUCTION				
A Hemolysis (intra- and extravascular)	↑	N	0	↑ Bilirubin turnover; serum bilirubin rarely exceeds 68 μmol/L (4 mg/dL)
B Ineffective erythropoiesis	↑	N	0	Splenomegaly; normal RBC survival; normoblasts in marrow
DEFECTIVE HEPATIC UPTAKE				
A Some drugs (e.g., flavaspidic acid, novobiocin)				
B Gilbert's syndrome (some cases)	↑	N	0	Normal liver biopsy
DEFECTIVE CONJUGATION				
A Neonatal jaundice	↑	Low	0	↓ Glucuronosyl transferase; ? ↓ ligandin
B Gilbert's syndrome	↑	Low	0	↓ Glucuronosyl transferase and ↓ bilirubin uptake; some may have ↑ hemolysis; bile contains ↑ monoconjugates
C Crigler-Najjar syndrome (types I and II)	↑	Low	0	Type I = absence of transferase Type II = deficiency of transferase; bile contains ↑↑ monoconjugates
DEFECTIVE EXCRETION				
A Intrahepatic obstruction				
1 Familial syndromes				
a Dubin-Johnson	↑	↑	+	Abnormal BSP curve, hepatic lipochrome pigment; ↑ urinary coproporphyrin type I
b Rotor	↑	↑	+	No liver pigment; ↑ total urinary coproporphyrin
2 Drugs (e.g., chloramphenicol, methyltestosterone)	↑	↑	+	↑ Alkaline phosphatase but other function tests usually normal
3 Benign recurrent cholestasis	↑	↑	+	↑ Alkaline phosphatase
4 Recurrent jaundice of pregnancy (third trimester)	↑	↑	+	↑ Alkaline phosphatase; may be reproduced in afflicted subjects by estrogens or progesterone
B Extrahepatic obstruction (tumors, stone, stricture of bile duct)				↑↑ Alkaline phosphatase (often > fourfold)
1 Partial	↑	↑	+	
2 Complete	↑	↑	+	
HEPATOCELLULAR DISEASE*				
A Hepatitis	↑	↑	+	Conjugated/total serum bilirubin >50–70%; liver biopsy important for diagnosis
B Cirrhosis: Same as hepatitis	↑	↑		

* Note that in hepatocellular disease there is generally an interference in all pathways of bilirubin metabolism (i.e., impaired uptake, conjugation, and excretion).

reactions are *allergic* or *toxic* in nature and therefore differ from the effects caused by the steroid hormones, which probably represent an exaggerated response by the liver to the normal action of these hormones.

Postoperative jaundice   The occurrence of postoperative jaundice is a problem of increasing importance. It is perhaps seen more frequently now than in earlier years because patients are able to undergo more major surgical procedures (i.e., cardiac surgery, repair of ruptured aneurysms) and survive. In approaching this problem, the possible pathogenic mechanisms listed in Table 265-2 need to be considered. The patient may have *pigment overload*, especially from blood transfusions (with hemolysis of stored blood), from resorption of blood in extravascular spaces, and less commonly, from hemolytic anemia. *Hepatocellular damage* and decreased liver cell function may occur due to concurrent use of hepatotoxic drugs (Chap. 266) or anesthetics such as halothane. Hepatocellular necrosis may follow profound shock; with lesser degrees of hypotension or hypoxemia, morphologic damage may be slight, but significant impairment of function may occur. Hence prior shock or hypotension plus pigment overload may produce significant jaundice. Extensive sepsis also can produce jaundice, often of a cholestatic type. Concurrent renal impairment due to hypotension and hypoxemia may enhance the degree of jaundice because the renal excretion of conjugated bilirubin is decreased. *Extrahepatic obstruction* due to surgical damage or stones needs to be considered and may be excluded by sonography.

A form of jaundice referred to as *benign postoperative intrahepatic cholestasis* may be seen. In the typical case, the patient has had major and prolonged surgery for a catastrophic event such as a ruptured aortic aneurysm complicated by hypotension and hypoxemia, extensive blood loss into tissues, and massive blood replacement. Jaundice may be noted on the second or third postoperative day, and the serum bilirubin, predominantly conjugated, may reach 340 to 680 μmol/L (20 to 40 mg/dL) by the eighth to tenth day. Serum alkaline phosphatase levels may be elevated three- to tenfold. Typically, the serum aspartate aminotransferase (AST, SGOT) is only mildly elevated. The liver morphology is striking in that necrosis is not seen, only cholestasis and erythrophagocytosis.

The cause of this type of postoperative cholestatic jaundice is uncertain. However, it probably reflects (1) increased pigment load, (2) decreased liver function due to hypoxemia and hypotension, and (3) decreased renal bilirubin excretion due to varying degrees of tubular necrosis as a result of shock. This diagnostic possibility must be considered in the postoperative patient with marked cholestatic jaundice. The course of the jaundice is self-limited and will subside if the other systemic complications do not predominate and lead to death.

Hepatitis and cirrhosis   These disorders, discussed in detail in Chaps. 266 to 268, constitute the *most common disorders associated with jaundice.* As has been stated previously, when the liver cell is damaged, as in viral hepatitis, there is often impairment in all three major hepatic phases of bilirubin metabolism, namely, uptake, conjugation, and excretion. Since the excretory step is the one which is rate-limiting and most readily affected by injury, significant amounts of conjugated bilirubin reenter the systemic circulation. There are also lesser increases in the serum unconjugated bilirubin. This phenomenon is probably a reflection of the impaired uptake and conjugation and is due in part to the shortened life span of red blood cells often found in liver disease. In most patients with hepatitis and cirrhosis, the total serum bilirubin levels tend not to exceed 860 μmol/L (50 mg/dL). (For a summary of laboratory features in icteric states, see Table 265-3.)

EXTRAHEPATIC BILIARY OBSTRUCTION   Anatomic or mechanical obstruction of the bile ducts is most commonly due to stones, tumors, or strictures. The clinical picture is quite similar to that of intrahepatic cholestasis, with pronounced elevations of the serum conjugated bilirubin and alkaline phosphatase levels. Usually, but not always, fever, pain, and chills may be present. In contrast to hepatitis and cirrhosis, the serum bilirubin level often tends to plateau and

rarely exceeds levels of 600 μmol/L (35 mg/dL). The reason for this plateau is not clear but may be related to renal excretion of conjugated bilirubin or alternative pathways of bilirubin catabolism in obstructive jaundice.

REFERENCES

Benign familial recurrent cholestasis

DePagter AGF et al: Familial benign intrahepatic cholestasis. Gastroenterology 71:202, 1976

Endo T et al: Bile acid metabolism in benign recurrent intrahepatic cholestasis. Gastroenterology 76:1002, 1979

Dubin-Johnson and Rotor syndromes

Rosenthal P et al: Homozygous Dubin-Johnson syndrome exhibits a characteristic serum bilirubin pattern. Hepatology 1:540, 1981

Swartz HM et al: On the nature and excretion of the hepatic pigment in the Dubin-Johnson syndrome. Gastroenterology 76:958, 1979

Wolkoff AW et al: Hereditary jaundice and disorders of bilirubin metabolism, in *The Metabolic Basis of Inherited Disease*, 6th ed. CR Scriver et al (eds). New York, McGraw, 1989, pp 1367–1408

Wolpert E et al: Abnormal sulfobromophthalein metabolism in Rotor's syndrome and obligate heterozygotes. N Engl J Med 206:1099, 1977

Glucuronosyl transferase deficiency states

Berthelot P, Dhumeaus D: New insights into the classification and mechanisms of hereditary, chronic, non-hemolytic hyperbilirubinemia. Gut 19:474, 1978

Bosma PJ et al: Mechanism of inherited deficiencies of multiple UDP-glucuronosyl transferase isoforms in two patients with Crigler-Najjar syndrome type I. FASEB J 6:2859, 1992

Chowdury JR, Chowdury NR: Unveiling the mysteries of inherited disorders of bilirubin glucuronidation. Gastroenterology 105:288, 1993

Dawson J et al: Gilbert's syndrome: Evidence of morphologic heterogeneity. Gut 20:848, 1979

Fevery J et al: Unconjugated bilirubin and an increased proportion of bilirubin monoconjugates in the bile of patients with Gilbert's syndrome and Crigler-Najjar disease. J Clin Invest 60:970, 1977

Ohkubo H et al: Ursodeoxycholic acid oral tolerance test in patients with constitutional hyperbilirubinemias and effect of phenobarbital. Gastroenterology 81:126, 1981

Olsson R et al: Gilbert's syndrome: does it exist? A study of the prevalence of symptoms in Gilbert's syndrome. Acta Med Scand 224:485, 1988

Ritter JK et al: Identification of a genetic alteration in the code for bilirubin UDP-glucuronosyl transferase in the UGT1 gene complex of a Crigler-Najjar type I patient. J Clin Invest 90:150, 1992

van ES HG et al: Immunochemical analysis of uridine diphosphate glucuronosyl transferase in four patients with the Crigler-Najjar syndrome type I. J Clin Invest 85:1199, 1990

Postoperative jaundice

Hootegem PV et al: Serum bilirubins in hepatobiliary disease: Comparison with other liver function tests and changes in the postobstructive period. Hepatology 5:112. 1985

LaMont JT, Isselbacher KJ: Postoperative jaundice. in *Wright's Liver and Biliary Disease*, 3d ed, GH Millward-Sadler et al (eds). Philadelphia, Saunders, 1992

---

266   ACUTE HEPATITIS

JULES L. DIENSTAG / KURT J. ISSELBACHER

ACUTE VIRAL HEPATITIS

Acute viral hepatitis is a systemic infection affecting the liver predominantly. Five categories of viral agents have been implicated: hepatitis A virus (HAV), hepatitis B virus (HBV), hepatitis C virus (HCV), the HBV-associated delta agent or hepatitis D virus (HDV), and hepatitis E virus (HEV). Although these agents can be distinguished by their antigenic properties, all five types produce clinically similar illnesses. These range from asymptomatic and inapparent to fulminant and fatal acute infections common to all five types, on the one hand, and from subclinical persistent infections to rapidly progressive chronic liver disease with cirrhosis and even hepatocellular carcinoma, common to the bloodborne types (HBV, HCV, and HDV), on the other.

FIGURE 266-1 *A.* Electron micrograph of 27-nm hepatitis A virus particles purified from stool of a patient with acute hepatitis A virus infection and aggregated by hepatitis A antibody. *B.* Electron micrograph of concentrated serum from a patient with acute hepatitis B infection, demonstrating the 42-nm virions, tubular forms, and spherical 22-nm particles of hepatitis B surface antigen. 132,000×. (Hepatitis D resembles 42-nm virions of hepatitis B but is smaller, 35 to 37 nm; hepatitis E resembles hepatitis A virus but is slightly larger, 32 to 34 nm; hepatitis C has not been visualized.)

A   B

VIROLOGY AND ETIOLOGY   Hepatitis A   Hepatitis A virus (HAV) is a nonenveloped 27-nm, heat-, acid-, and ether-resistant RNA virus in the picornavirus family; classified initially as enterovirus type 72, it is now classified within the heparnavirus genus of the picornavirus family (Fig. 266-1). Its virion contains four capsid polypeptides designated VP1 to VP4, which are cleaved posttranslationally from the polyprotein product of a 7500-nucleotide genome. Inactivation of viral activity can be achieved by boiling for 1 min, by contact with formaldehyde and chlorine, or by ultraviolet irradiation. Despite nucleotide sequence variation of up to 20 percent among isolates of HAV, all strains of this virus identified to date are immunologically indistinguishable and belong to one serotype. Hepatitis A has an incubation period of approximately 4 weeks. Its replication limited to the liver, the virus is present in the liver, bile, stools, and blood during the late incubation period and acute preicteric phase of illness. Despite persistence of virus in the liver, viral shedding in feces, viremia, and infectivity diminish rapidly once jaundice becomes apparent. Unlike other hepatitis viruses, hepatitis A virus will replicate in tissue culture but replicates poorly compared with other picornaviruses.

Antibodies to HAV (anti-HAV) can be detected during acute illness when serum aminotransferase activity is elevated and fecal HAV shedding is still occurring. This early antibody response is predominantly of the IgM class and persists for several months, only rarely for 6 to 12 months. During convalescence, however, anti-HAV of the IgG class becomes the predominant antibody (Fig. 266-2). Therefore, the diagnosis of hepatitis A is made during acute illness by demonstrating high-titer anti-HAV of the IgM class. Following acute illness, anti-HAV of the IgG class remains detectable indefinitely, and patients with serum anti-HAV are immune to reinfection. Indeed, neutralizing antibody activity parallels the appearance of anti-HAV, and the IgG anti-HAV present in immune globulin accounts for the protection it affords against HAV infection.

FIGURE 266-2 Scheme of typical clinical and laboratory features of viral hepatitis type A.

Hepatitis B   Hepatitis B virus is a DNA virus with a remarkably compact genomic structure; despite its small, circular, 3200-base-pair size, HBV DNA codes for four sets of viral products and has a complex, multiparticle structure. HBV achieves its genomic economy by relying on an efficient strategy of encoding proteins from four overlapping genes: S, C, P, and X, as detailed below. Once thought to be unique among viruses, HBV is now recognized as one of a family of animal viruses, hepadnaviruses (hepatotropic DNA viruses), and is classified as hepadnavirus type 1. Similar viruses infect certain species of woodchucks, ground and tree squirrels, and Pekin ducks, to mention the most carefully characterized. Like HBV, all have the same distinctive three morphologic forms, have counterparts to the envelope and nucleocapsid virus antigens of HBV, replicate within the liver but exist in extrahepatic sites, contain their own endogenous DNA polymerase, have partially double-stranded, partially single-stranded genomes, are associated with acute and chronic hepatitis and hepatocellular carcinoma, and rely on a replicative strategy unique among DNA viruses but typical of retroviruses. Instead of DNA replication directly from a DNA template, hepadnaviruses rely on reverse transcription (effected by the DNA polymerase) of minus-strand DNA from a "pregenomic" RNA intermediate. Then plus-strand DNA is transcribed from the minus-strand DNA template by the DNA-dependent DNA polymerase. Viral proteins are translated by the pregenomic RNA, and the proteins and genome are packaged into virions and secreted from the hepatocyte. Although HBV is difficult to cultivate in vitro in the conventional sense from clinical material, several cell lines have been transfected with HBV DNA. Such transfected cells support in vitro replication of the intact virus and its component proteins.

Three particulate forms of HBV (Table 266-1) can be demonstrated by electron microscopy (see Fig. 266-1). The most numerous are the 22-nm particles, which appear as spherical or long filamentous forms; these are antigenically indistinguishable from the outer surface or coat of HBV, and they are thought to represent excess viral coat protein. Outnumbered in serum by a factor of 100 or 1000 to 1 compared with the spheres and tubules are large, 42-nm, double-shelled spherical particles which represent the intact hepatitis B virion. The protein expressed on the outer surface of the virion and on the smaller spherical and tubular structures is referred to as *hepatitis B surface antigen* (HBsAg). Infection with HBV is unique in that the concentration of HBsAg and virus particles in the blood may reach 500 μg/mL and 10 trillion particles per milliliter, respectively. The envelope protein, HBsAg, is the product of the S gene of HBV.

HBsAg consists primarily of two major polypeptides, one of 24,000 mol wt and its glycosylated counterpart of 28,000 mol wt. A number of different HBsAg subdeterminants have been identified. There is a common group-reactive antigen, *a*, shared by all HBsAg isolates. In addition, HBsAg may contain one of several subtype-specific antigens, namely, *d* or *y*, *w* or *r*, as well as other more recently characterized specificities. These HBsAg subtypes provide additional epidemiologic markers in evaluating the transmission of hepatitis B infection in that subtypes "breed true." For example, studies of hepatitis outbreaks have shown that index cases and their

TABLE 266-1 Nomenclature and features of hepatitis viruses

Hepatitis type	Virus particle	Morphology	Genome*	Classification	Antigen(s)	Antibodies	Remarks
HAV	27 nm	Icosahedral nonenveloped	7.5-kb RNA, linear, ss, +	Heparnavirus	HAV	anti-HAV	Early fecal shedding Diagnosis: IgM anti-HAV Previous infection: IgG anti-HAV
HBV	42 nm	Double-shelled virion (surface and core) spherical	3.2-kb DNA, circular, ss/ds	Hepadnavirus	HBsAg HBcAg HBeAg	anti-HBs anti-HBc anti-HBe	Bloodborne virus; carrier state Acute diagnosis: HBsAg, IgM anti-HBc Chronic diagnosis: IgG anti-HBc, HBsAg Markers of replication: HBeAg, HBV DNA Liver, lymphocytes, other organs.
	27 nm	Nucleocapsid core			HBcAg HBeAg	anti-HBc anti-HBe	Nucleocapsid contains DNA and DNA polymerase; present in hepatocyte nucleus; HBcAg does not circulate; HBeAg (soluble, nonparticulate) and HBV DNA circulate—correlate with infectivity and complete virions.
	22 nm	Spherical and filamentous; represents excess virus coat material			HBsAg	anti-HBs	HBsAg detectable in >95% of patients with acute hepatitis B; found in serum, body fluids, hepatocyte cytoplasm; anti-HBs appears following infection—protective antibody.
HCV	Not visualized; approx. 30–60 nm	Enveloped	9.4-kb RNA, linear, ss, +	Flavivirus-like	HCV C100-3 C33c C22-3	anti-HCV	Bloodborne agent, formerly labeled non-A, non-B hepatitis Acute diagnosis: anti-HCV (C33c, C22-3), HCV RNA Chronic diagnosis: anti-HCV (C100-3, C33c, C22-3) and HCV RNA; cytoplasmic location in hepatocytes
HDV	35–37 nm	Enveloped hybrid particle with HBsAg coat and HDV core	1.7-kb RNA, circular, ss, −	Resembles viroids and plant satellite viruses	HBsAg HDVAg	anti-HBs anti-HDV	Defective RNA virus, requires helper function of HBV (hepadnaviruses); HDVAg present in hepatocyte nucleus Diagnosis: IgM/IgG anti-HDV, HDV RNA; HBV/HDV coinfection—IgM anti-HBc and anti-HDV; HDV superinfection—IgG anti-HBc and anti-HDV.
HEV	32–34 nm	Nonenveloped icosahedral	7.6-kb RNA, linear, ss, +	Alphavirus-like	HEVAg	anti-HEV	Agent of enterically transmitted non-A, non-B hepatitis; rare in USA; occurs in Asia, Mediterranean countries, Central America Diagnosis: IgM/IgG anti-HEV (assays being developed); virus in stool, bile, hepatocyte cytoplasm

* ss = single-stranded; ss/ds = partially single-stranded, partially double-stranded; − = minus-stranded; + = plus-stranded.

contacts have identical HBsAg subtypes. Clinical course and outcome, however, are independent of subtype.

Upstream of the S gene are the pre-S genes, which code for pre-S gene products, including receptors on the HBV surface of polymerized human serum albumin and for hepatocyte receptors. The pre-S region actually consists of both pre-S1 and pre-S2. Depending on where translation is initiated, three potential HBsAg gene products are synthesized. The protein product of the S gene is HBsAg (*major protein*), the product of the S region plus the adjacent pre-S2 region is the *middle protein*, and the product of the pre-S1 plus pre-S2 plus S regions is the *large protein*. Compared with the smaller spherical and tubular particles of HBV, complete 42-nm virions are enriched in the large protein. Both pre-S proteins and their respective antibodies can be detected during HBV infection, and the period of pre-S antigenemia appears to coincide with other markers of virus replication, as detailed below.

The intact 42-nm virion can be disrupted by mild detergents and the 27-nm nucleocapsid core particle isolated. Nucleocapsid proteins are coded for by the C gene. The antigen expressed on the surface of the nucleocapsid core is referred to as *hepatitis B core antigen* (HBcAg), and its corresponding antibody is anti-HBc. A third HBV antigen is *hepatitis B e antigen* (HBeAg), a soluble, nonparticulate, nucleocapsid protein that is immunologically distinct from intact HBcAg but is a product of the same C gene. The C gene has two initiation codons, a precore and a core region. If translation is initiated at the precore region, the protein product is HBeAg, which has a signal peptide that binds it to the smooth endoplasmic reticulum and leads to its secretion into the circulation. If translation begins with

the core region, HBcAg is the protein product; it has no signal peptide, it is not secreted, but it assembles into nucleocapsid particles which bind to and incorporate RNA and which, ultimately, contain HBV DNA. Also packaged within the nucleocapsid core is a DNA polymerase, which directs replication and repair of HBV DNA. In vitro, the polymerase can repair the single-stranded gap and render it double-stranded; it directs the synthesis of plus-strand DNA from a minus-strand template. When packaging within viral proteins is complete, synthesis of the incomplete plus strand stops; this accounts for the single-stranded gap and for differences in the size of the gap. HBcAg particles remain in the hepatocyte, where they are readily detectable by immunohistochemical staining, and are exported after encapsidation by an envelope of HBsAg. Therefore, naked core particles do not circulate in the serum. The secreted nucleocapsid protein, HBeAg, provides a convenient, readily detectable, qualitative marker of HBV replication and relative infectivity.

HBsAg-positive serum containing HBeAg is more likely to be highly infectious and to be associated with the presence of hepatitis B virions (and DNA polymerase and HBV DNA, see below) than HBeAg-negative or anti-HBe-positive serum. For example, HBsAg carrier mothers who are HBeAg-positive almost invariably (>90 percent) transmit hepatitis B infection to their offspring, while HBsAg carrier mothers with anti-HBe rarely (10 to 15 percent) infect their offspring.

In every individual with acute HBV infection, HBeAg develops transiently, early in the course of illness, but persistent HBeAg positivity correlates with ongoing viral replication and may be associated with continuing disease activity in chronic hepatitis; its disappearance may be a harbinger of biochemical improvement and potential resolution of infection. Unfortunately, HBeAg is not a sufficiently discriminating marker to support prognostic predictions or to substitute for morphologic evaluation of severity in patients with chronic hepatitis.

The third of the HBV genes is the largest, the P gene, which codes for the DNA polymerase; as noted above, this enzyme has both DNA-dependent DNA polymerase and RNA-dependent reverse transcriptase activities. The fourth gene, X, codes for a small, nonparticulate protein which has been shown to be capable of transactivating the transcription of both viral and cellular genes. Such transactivation may enhance the replication of HBV, leading to the clinical association observed between the expression of the product of the X gene, hepatitis B x antigen (HBxAg), and antibodies to it in patients with severe chronic active hepatitis and hepatocellular carcinoma. The transactivating activity can enhance the transcription of other viruses besides HBV, such as HIV. Therefore, HBV may be responsible for enhanced replication of other viruses. Cellular processes transactivated by X include the human interferon-β gene and class I major histocompatibility genes; potentially, these effects could contribute to enhanced susceptibility of HBV-infected hepatocytes to cytolytic T cells. The X gene and its protein product, however, are absent in nonmammalian hepadnaviruses; therefore, X is not essential for hepadnavirus replication.

After infection with HBV, the first virologic marker detectable in serum is HBsAg (Fig. 266-3). Circulating HBsAg precedes elevations of serum aminotransferase activity and clinical symptoms and remains detectable during the entire icteric or symptomatic phase of acute hepatitis B and beyond. In typical cases, HBsAg becomes undetectable 1 to 2 months following the onset of jaundice and rarely persists beyond 6 months. After HBsAg disappears, antibody to HBsAg (anti-HBs) becomes detectable in serum and remains detectable indefinitely thereafter. Because HBcAg is sequestered within an HBsAg coat, HBcAg is not detectable routinely in the serum of patients with HBV infection. On the other hand, antibody to HBcAg (anti-HBc) is readily demonstrable in serum, beginning within the first 1 to 2 weeks after the appearance of HBsAg and preceding detectable levels of anti-HBs by weeks to months. Because variability exists in the time of appearance of anti-HBs following HBV infection, occasionally a gap of several weeks or longer may separate the disappearance of HBsAg and the appearance of anti-HBs. During this "gap" or "window" period, anti-HBc may represent serologic evidence of current or recent HBV infection, and blood containing anti-HBc in the absence of HBsAg and anti-HBs has been implicated in the development of transfusion-associated hepatitis B. In part because the sensitivity of immunoassays for HBsAg and anti-HBs has increased, however, this

window period is rarely encountered. In some persons, years after HBV infection, anti-HBc may persist in the circulation longer than anti-HBs. Therefore, isolated anti-HBc does not necessarily indicate active virus replication; most instances of isolated anti-HBc represent hepatitis B infection in the remote past. Rarely, however, isolated anti-HBc represents low-level hepatitis B viremia, with HBsAg below the detection threshold; occasionally, isolated anti-HBc represents a cross-reacting or false-positive immunologic specificity. Distinction between recent and remote HBV infection can be accomplished by determination of the immunoglobulin class of anti-HBc. Anti-HBc of the IgM class (IgM anti-HBc) predominates during the first approximately 6 months after acute infection, whereas IgG anti-HBc is the predominant class of anti-HBc beyond 6 months. Therefore, patients with current or recent acute hepatitis B, including those in the anti-HBc window, have IgM anti-HBc in their serum. In patients who have recovered from hepatitis B in the remote past as well as those with chronic HBV infection, anti-HBc is predominantly of the IgG class. Infrequently, in no more than 1 to 5 percent of patients with acute HBV infection, levels of HBsAg are too low to be detected; in such cases, the presence of IgM anti-HBc establishes the diagnosis of acute hepatitis B. When isolated anti-HBc occurs in the rare patient with chronic hepatitis B whose HBsAg level is below the sensitivity threshold of contemporary immunoassays (a low-level carrier), the anti-HBc is of the IgG class. Generally, in persons who have recovered from hepatitis B, anti-HBs and anti-HBc persist indefinitely.

The temporal association between the appearance of anti-HBs and resolution of HBV infection as well as the observation that persons with anti-HBs in serum are protected against reinfection with HBV suggest that *anti-HBs is the protective antibody*. Therefore, strategies for prevention of HBV infection are based on providing susceptible persons with circulating anti-HBs (see below). Occasionally, in 10 to 20 percent of patients with chronic hepatitis B, low-level, low-affinity anti-HBs can be detected. This antibody is directed against a subtype determinant different from that represented by the patient's HBsAg; its presence is thought to reflect the stimulation of a related clone of antibody-forming cells, but it has no clinical relevance and does not signal imminent clearance of hepatitis B.

The other readily detectable serologic marker of HBV infection, HBeAg, appears concurrently with or shortly after HBsAg. Its appearance coincides temporally with high levels of virus replication and reflects the presence of circulating intact virions, DNA polymerase, and HBV DNA. Pre-S1 and pre-S2 proteins are also expressed during periods of peak replication, but assays for these gene products are not routinely available. In self-limited HBV infections, HBeAg becomes undetectable shortly after peak elevations in aminotransferase activity, before the disappearance of HBsAg, and anti-HBe then becomes detectable, coinciding with a period of relatively lower infectivity (see Fig. 266-3). Because markers of HBV replication appear transiently during acute infection, testing for such markers is of little clinical utility in typical cases of acute HBV infection. In contrast, markers of HBV replication provide valuable information in patients with protracted infections. Departing from the pattern typical of acute HBV infections, in chronic HBV infection, HBsAg remains detectable beyond 6 months, anti-HBc is primarily of the IgG class, and anti-HBs is either undetectable or detectable at low levels (see "Laboratory Features," below) (Fig. 266-4). During early chronic HBV infection, HBV DNA can be detected both in serum and in hepatocyte nuclei, where it is present in free or episomal form. This *replicative stage* of HBV infection is the time of maximal infectivity and liver injury; HBeAg is a qualitative marker and HBV DNA a quantitative marker of this replicative phase, during which all three forms of HBV circulate, including intact virions. Over time, the replicative phase of chronic HBV infection gives way to a relatively *nonreplicative phase*. This occurs at a rate of approximately 10 percent per year and is accompanied by seroconversion from HBeAg-positive to anti-HBe-positive. In most cases, this seroconversion coincides with a transient, acute hepatitis–like elevation in aminotransferase activity, believed to reflect cell-mediated clearance

FIGURE 266-3   Scheme of typical clinical and laboratory features of acute viral hepatitis type B.

Jaundice

↑ ALT

HBeAg   Anti-HBe

HBsAg

IgG Anti-HBc

IgM Anti-HBc

Anti-HBs

0 4 8 12 16 20 24 28 32 36   52   100

Weeks After Exposure

FIGURE 266-4 Scheme of typical laboratory features of chronic viral hepatitis type B. HBeAg and HBV DNA can be detected in serum during the *replicative phase* of chronic infection, which is associated with infectivity and liver injury. Seroconversion from the replicative phase to the *nonreplicative phase* occurs at a rate of approximately 10 to 15 percent per year and is heralded by an acute hepatitis–like elevation of ALT activity; during the nonreplicative phase, infectivity and liver injury are limited.

of virus-infected hepatocytes. In the nonreplicative phase of chronic infection, when HBV DNA is demonstrable in hepatocyte nuclei, it tends to be integrated into the host genome. In this phase, only spherical and tubular forms of HBV, *not intact virions*, circulate, and liver injury tends to subside. Most such patients would be characterized as asymptomatic HBV *carriers*. In reality, the designations *replicative* and *nonreplicative* are only relative; even in the so-called nonreplicative phase, HBV replication can be detected with highly sensitive amplification probes such as the polymerase chain reaction. Still, the distinctions are pathophysiologically and clinically meaningful. Occasionally, nonreplicative HBV infection converts back to replicative infection. Such spontaneous reactivations are accompanied by reexpression of HBeAg and HBV DNA as well as by exacerbations of liver injury.

Recently, attention has focused on molecular variants of HBV. Variation occurs throughout the HBV genome, and clinical isolates of HBV that do not express viral proteins have been attributed to mutations in individual or even multiple gene locations. For example, variants have been described which lack nucleocapsid proteins, envelope proteins, or both. Two categories of HBV have attracted the most attention. One of these was identified initially in Mediterranean countries among patients with an unusual serologic-clinical profile. They have severe chronic HBV infection and detectable HBV DNA but with anti-HBe instead of HBeAg. These patients were found to be infected with an HBV mutant that contained an alteration in the precore region rendering the virus incapable of encoding HBeAg. Although several potential mutation sites exist in the pre-C region, the region of the C gene necessary for the expression of HBeAg (see "Virology and Etiology," above), the most commonly encountered in such patients is a single base substitution, from G to A, which occurs in the second to last codon of the pre-C gene at nucleotide 1896. This substitution results in the replacement of the TGG tryptophan codon by a stop codon (TAG), which prevents the translation of HBeAg. Patients with such precore mutants that are unable to secrete HBeAg tend to have severe liver disease that progresses rapidly to cirrhosis and that does not respond readily to antiviral therapy. Both "wild-type" HBV and precore mutant HBV can coexist in the same patient, or mutant HBV may arise during wild-type HBV infection. In addition, clusters of fulminant hepatitis B in Israel and Japan have been attributed to common-source infection with a precore mutant. Fulminant hepatitis B in North America and western Europe, however, occurs in patients infected with wild-type

HBV, in the absence of precore mutants, and both precore mutants and other mutations throughout the HBV genome occur commonly even in patients with typical, self-limited, milder forms of HBV infection. Therefore, additional investigation will be necessary to define the effect of precore mutants on the pathogenicity and natural history of HBV infection.

The second important category of HBV mutants consists of *escape mutants*, in which a single amino acid substitution, from glycine to arginine, occurs at position 145 of the immunodominant *a* determinant common to all subtypes of HBsAg. This change in HBsAg leads to a critical conformational change that results in a loss of neutralizing activity by anti-HBs. This specific HBV/*a* mutant has been observed in two situations, active and passive immunization, in which humoral immunologic pressure may favor evolutionary change ("escape") in the virus—in a small number of hepatitis B vaccine recipients who acquired HBV infection despite the prior appearance of neutralizing anti-HBs and in liver transplant recipients who underwent the procedure for hepatitis B and who were treated with a high-potency human monoclonal anti-HBs preparation. Although such mutants have not been appreciated frequently, their existence raises a concern that may complicate vaccination strategies and serologic diagnosis.

Hepatitis B antigens and HBV DNA have been identified in extrahepatic sites, including lymph nodes, bone marrow, circulating lymphocytes, spleen, and pancreas. Although the virus does not appear to be associated with tissue injury in any of these extrahepatic sites, its presence in these "remote" reservoirs has been invoked to explain the recurrence of HBV infection after orthotopic liver transplantation. A more complete understanding of the clinical relevance of extrahepatic HBV remains to be defined.

Hepatitis D The delta hepatitis agent, or hepatitis D virus (HDV), is a defective RNA virus which coinfects with and requires the helper function of HBV (or other hepadnaviruses) for its replication and expression. Slightly smaller than HBV, delta is a formalin-sensitive, 35- to 37-nm virus with a hybrid structure. Its nucleocapsid expresses delta antigen, which bears no antigenic homology with any of the HBV antigens, and contains the virus genome. The delta core is "encapsidated" by an outer envelope of HBsAg, indistinguishable from that of HBV except in its relative compositions of major, middle, and large HBsAg component proteins. The genome is a small, 1700-nucleotide, circular, single-stranded RNA (minus strand) that is nonhomologous with HBV DNA (except for a small area of the polymerase gene) but that has features and the rolling circle model of replication common to genomes of plant satellite viruses or viroids. HDV RNA contains many areas of internal complementarity; therefore, it can fold on itself by internal base pairing to form an unusual, very stable, rodlike structure. HDV RNA replicates via RNA-directed RNA synthesis by transcription of genomic RNA to a complementary antigenomic (plus strand) RNA; the antigenomic RNA, in turn, serves as a template for subsequent genomic RNA synthesis. Between the genomic and antigenomic RNAs of HDV, there are coding regions for nine proteins. Delta antigen, which is a product of the antigenomic strand, exists in two forms, a small, 195-amino-acid species, which plays a role in facilitating HDV RNA replication, and a large, 214-amino-acid species, which appears to suppress replication but is required for assembly of the antigen into virions. Although complete hepatitis D virions and liver injury require the cooperative helper function of HBV, intracellular replication of HDV RNA can occur without HBV. Genomic heterogeneity among HDV isolates has been described; however, pathophysiologic and clinical consequences of this genetic diversity have not been recognized.

HDV can either infect a person simultaneously with HBV (*coinfection*) or superinfect a person already infected with HBV (*superinfection*); when HDV infection is transmitted from a donor with one HBsAg subtype to an HBsAg-positive recipient with a different subtype, the HDV agent assumes the HBsAg subtype of the recipient, rather than the donor. Because HDV relies absolutely on HBV, the duration of HDV infection is determined by the duration of (and cannot outlast) HBV infection. HDV antigen is expressed primarily in hepatocyte nuclei and is occasionally detectable in serum. During acute HDV infection, anti-HDV of the IgM class predominates, and 30 to 40 days may elapse after symptoms appear before anti-HDV can be detected. In self-limited infection, anti-HDV is low titer and transient, rarely remaining detectable beyond the clearance of HBsAg and HDV antigen. In chronic HDV infection, anti-HDV circulates in high titer, and both IgM and IgG anti-HDV can be detected. HDV antigen in the liver and HDV RNA in serum and liver can be detected during HDV replication.

Hepatitis C (formerly called non-A, non-B hepatitis) Sensitive serologic tests for identifying both types A and B hepatitis have led to the identification of hepatitis cases with incubation periods and modes of transmission consistent with an infectious disease but without serologic evidence of hepatitis A or B infection. Identified initially among recipients of transfused blood, these cases of so-called non-A, non-B hepatitis have not been associated serologically with Epstein-Barr virus or cytomegalovirus (except in rare instances) or with other viruses known to involve the liver.

An almost 15-year quest to identify an agent of non-A, non-B viral hepatitis ended in 1988 with the identification of an RNA virus with immunologic specificity for transfusion-associated non-A, non-B hepatitis. Among complementary DNA (cDNA) fragments cloned in *Escherichia coli* from the pellet of a chimpanzee plasma with unusually high infectivity, one clone, designated 5-1-1, expressed a protein that reacted with antibody in convalescent serum but not preillness serum from chimpanzees with experimentally induced non-A, non-B hepatitis. This viral clone hybridizes with the livers of infected, but not uninfected-control, chimpanzees. A protein product of this virus-specific clone was expressed in yeast, and this protein, designated C100-3, was used as an antigen in the first immunoassay to detect antibody in serum. Validation of the relationship between this agent and non-A, non-B hepatitis came most convincingly from the ability of the antibody immunoassay to distinguish, in panels of coded serum samples, between pedigreed non-A, non-B hepatitis cases and pedigreed negative, noninfectious samples as well as other-disease controls. Analysis of overlapping clones permitted identification of the entire genome, and the agent has been labeled *hepatitis C virus* (HCV). HCV is a linear, single-stranded, positive-polarity, 9400-nucleotide RNA virus with a single open reading frame (gene) that codes for a virus polyprotein of approximately 3000 amino acids. Five distinct genotypes have been identified by nucleotide mapping, although they all appear to be antigenically similar. The 5′ end of the genome consists of an untranslated region adjacent to the genes for structural proteins, the nucleocapsid core and the viral envelope. The 5′ untranslated and core genes are highly conserved among genotypes, but the envelope proteins are coded for by the hypervariable region, which varies from isolate to isolate and even within the same agent isolated over time from the same patient. This allows the virus to evade host immunologic mechanisms directed at virus-envelope proteins. The 3′ end of the genome contains the genes for nonstructural (NS) proteins 1 through 5. The original clone, 5-1-1, and the nucleotide sequence coding for C100-3 reside within the NS4 gene, and the RNA-dependent RNA polymerase through which HCV replicates is coded for by the NS5 region (Fig. 266-5). The genome of HCV has no homology with HBV, retroviruses, or other hepatitis viruses, and because it does not replicate via a DNA intermediate, HCV does not integrate into the host genome. Studies of its gene structure suggest that HCV is a distant relative of flaviviruses, animal pestiviruses, and plant potyviruses. Like other flaviviruses and pestiviruses, HCV will probable be included in the family Flaviviridae but will comprise a new genus. HCV tends to circulate in very low titer (100 to 1000 virions per milliliter); therefore, no virus particles have been visualized. Although in vitro HCV replication is difficult to accomplish convincingly, the chimpanzee has proven to be an invaluable animal model. Neutralizing antibodies have not been identified.

As noted above, the first assay introduced detected antibodies to C100-3, a recombinant polypeptide derived from the NS4 region of the genome. In most patients with transfusion-associated hepatitis C, antibody detected with this assay appears between 1 to 3 months after the onset of acute hepatitis but sometimes not for a year or longer. Second-generation assays incorporate recombinant proteins from the nucleocapsid core region, C22-3, and the NS3 region, C33c (expressed in combination with C100-3 as C200); these assays are more sensitive (by approximately 20 percent) and detect anti-HCV 30 to 90 days earlier, during the period of acute hepatitis. Because nonspecificity has been encountered in clinical samples tested for anti-HCV, a supplementary recombinant immunoblot assay (RIBA) was introduced. Reactivity in an immunoassay is "confirmed" by incubation with a nitrocellulose strip which contains individual bands for the proteins of the first-generation (the product of recombinant bacterial clone 5-1-1 and recombinant yeast polypeptide C100-3, both nonstructural proteins) and second-generation immunoassays (nonstructural polypeptide C33c and core polypeptide C22-3) as well as a superoxide dismutase (SOD, a fusion protein with which recombinant HCV proteins are expressed in yeast and to which some false-positive reactivity is directed) band. This approach allows the demonstration of individual antibodies to nonstructural and structural viral proteins and identifies false-positive reactivity associated with bacterial, yeast, or SOD immunologic specificities. Still, detection of anti-HCV is insufficient to identify all persons infected with HCV. The most sensitive indicator is the presence of HCV RNA, which requires molecular amplification by polymerase chain reaction (Fig. 266-6). HCV RNA can be detected within a few days of exposure to HCV, well before the appearance of anti-HCV, and tends to persist for the duration of HCV infection; however, in patients with chronic HCV infection, occasionally, HCV RNA may be detectable only intermit-

FIGURE 266-5 Organization of the hepatitis C virus genome and its associated proteins. Structural genes at the 5′ end include the nucleocapsid region, C, and the envelope regions, E1 and E2. The 5′ untranslated region and the C region are highly conserved among isolates, while the envelope domain E2/NS1 contains the hypervariable region. At the 3′ end are five nonstructural (NS) regions. Viral proteins included in the first-generation (c100-3) and second-generation (c200, a fusion protein of c100-3 and c33c, and c22-3) immunoassays and in the recombinant immunoblot assay (5-1-1, c100-3, c33c, c22-3) are presented below their corresponding genes (AA = amino acid).

FIGURE 266-6   Scheme of typical laboratory features during acute hepatitis type C progressing to chronicity. HCV RNA is the first detectable event, preceding ALT elevation and the appearance of anti-HCV. The appearance of antibody to C100, detectable with first-generation assays, is delayed from 1 to 3 months after the appearance of antibody to C22 and C33, antibodies which are included in second-generation immunoassays. Anti-HCV detectable with second-generation assays appears during acute hepatitis C.

tently. Application of sensitive molecular probes for HCV RNA has revealed the presence of replicative HCV in peripheral blood lymphocytes of infected persons; however, as is the case for HBV in lymphocytes, the clinical relevance of HCV lymphocyte infection is not known.

Long before HCV was identified as an agent of non-A, non-B hepatitis, cross-challenge studies in chimpanzees suggested that there are at least two bloodborne non-A, non-B hepatitis agents. One, isolated from clotting factor VIII concentrates and the agent of most cases of transfusion-associated hepatitis, is chloroform-sensitive and induces ultrastructural cytoplasmic tubular changes in hepatocytes. This agent is HCV. The other, isolated from clotting factor IX concentrates, is chloroform-resistant and does not induce cytoplasmic tubular changes in hepatocytes. Theoretically, the chloroform-resistant agent could be a "non-A, non-B, non-C" hepatitis agent. The fact that all serologic and molecular markers of HCV are absent in a substantial proportion of sporadic cases of non-A, non-B hepatitis, a small proportion of cases of transfusion-associated hepatitis and "cryptogenic" cirrhosis, and almost all cases of non-A, non-B fulminant hepatitis also lends support to the existence of another agent. On the other hand, exhaustive attempts to identify another such viral agent have failed, and reinterpretation of the original cross-challenge studies in chimpanzees with serologic and molecular assays for HCV infection indicates that what were thought to be new infections with a distinct agent actually represented infection with a different genotype of HCV or reinfection with the *same* HCV agent. Whether rechallenge was with the same inoculum or a different inoculum, the chimpanzees became reinfected, suggesting that neither *homologous* nor *heterologous* immunity develops after acute HCV infection. Although the potential that there are other non-A, non-B hepatitis agents cannot be dismissed entirely, cumulative observations indicate that if they exist, they play no more than a minor role. HCV is the predominant, if not exclusive, agent of what used to be labeled non-A, non-B hepatitis.

Hepatitis E   A distinct type of waterborne "non-A, non-B" hepatitis has been identified in India, Asia, Africa, and Central America (previously labeled *epidemic* or *enterically transmitted non-A, non-B hepatitis*). This agent, with epidemiologic features resembling those of hepatitis A, has been classified as hepatitis E virus (HEV). Hepatitis E virus is a 32- to 34-nm, nonenveloped, HAV-like virus with a 7600-nucleotide, single-stranded RNA genome. All HEV isolates appear to belong to a single serotype, despite genomic heterogeneity of up to 25 percent. There is no genomic or antigenic homology, however, between HEV and HAV or other

picornaviruses, and HEV, although resembling calciviruses, appears to be sufficiently distinct from any known agent to merit a new classification of its own within the alphavirus group. The virus has been detected in stool, bile, and liver from infected patients, as well from experimentally infected nonhuman primates, chimpanzees, and cynomolgus macaques. The entire virus genome has been characterized by molecular cloning of complementary DNA constructed from virus RNA extracted from bile obtained from an infected macaque. Studies in humans and experimental animals have shown that HEV is excreted in the stool during the late incubation period and that immune responses to viral antigens occur very early during the course of acute infection. Both IgM anti-HEV and IgG anti-HEV can be detected, but both fall rapidly after acute infection, reaching low levels within 9 to 12 months. Currently, serologic testing for HEV infection remains in the domain of research laboratories, but the availability of tests for routine clinical purposes is anticipated.

PATHOGENESIS   Under ordinary circumstances, none of the hepatitis viruses is known to be directly cytopathic to hepatocytes. Evidence suggests that the clinical manifestations and outcomes following acute liver injury associated with viral hepatitis are determined by the immunologic responses of the host. Studies of the pathogenesis of hepatitis A, C, D, and E have been limited, but the immunopathogenesis of hepatitis B has been studied extensively. Certainly for this agent, the existence of asymptomatic hepatitis B carriers with normal liver histology and function suggests that the virus is not directly cytopathic. The facts that lymphoid cells are juxtaposed with necrotic hepatocytes in the livers of patients with liver injury and that patients with defects in cellular immune competence are more likely to remain chronically infected rather than to clear the virus are cited to support the role of cellular immune responses in the pathogenesis of hepatitis B–related liver injury. To date, however, because adequate animal and laboratory models are lacking, support for this hypothesis remains circumstantial. Still, the model that has the most experimental support involves cytolytic T cells sensitized specifically to recognize host and hepatitis B viral antigens on the liver cell surface. Although HBsAg was initially thought to be the most likely viral target antigen on the hepatocyte surface, recent laboratory observations suggest that nucleocapsid proteins (HBcAg and possibly HBeAg), present on the cell membrane in minute quantities, are the viral target antigens that, with host antigens, invite cytolytic T cells to destroy HBV-infected hepatocytes. Still, this hypothesis is insufficient to explain differences in outcomes between those who recover after acute hepatitis and those who progress to chronic hepatitis or between those with mild and severe (fulminant) acute HBV infection. As convincing as are the cumulative data supporting nucleocapsid proteins as the target of cell-mediated immunologic injury, attention has been refocused on the envelope protein, HBsAg, by the demonstration that in transgenic mice with the gene for HBsAg inserted into their genomes, cytolytic T cells directed against HBsAg can be shown to destroy hepatocytes. Therefore, HBsAg cannot be dismissed as a potential immunologic target.

Moreover, debate continues over the relative importance of viral and host factors in the pathogenesis of HBV-associated liver injury and its outcome. As noted above, precore genetic mutants of HBV have been associated with the more severe outcomes of HBV infection (severe chronic and fulminant hepatitis), suggesting that, under certain circumstances, relative pathogenicity is a property of the virus, not the host. The fact that concomitant HDV and HBV infections are associated with more severe liver injury than HBV infection alone and the fact that cells transfected in vitro with the gene for HDV (delta) antigen express HDV antigen and then become necrotic in the absence of any immunologic influences are also consistent with a viral effect on pathogenicity. Similarly, in patients who undergo liver transplantation for end-stage chronic HBV infection, occasionally, rapidly progressive liver injury appears in the new liver. This clinical pattern is associated with an unusual histologic pattern in the new liver, *fibrosing cholestatic hepatitis*, which, ultrastructurally, appears to represent a choking of the cell with overwhelming quantities of HBsAg. This observation suggests that under the influence of the potent immunosuppressive agents required to prevent allograft rejection, HBV may have a direct cytopathic effect on liver cells, independent of the immune system.

Although the precise mechanism of liver injury in HBV infection remains elusive, studies of nucleocapsid proteins have shed light on the profound immunologic tolerance to HBV of babies born to mothers with highly replicative (HBeAg-positive), chronic HBV infection. In HBeAg-expressing transgenic mice, in utero exposure to HBeAg, which is sufficiently small to traverse the placenta, induces T cell tolerance to both nucleocapsid proteins. This, in turn, may explain why, when infection occurs so early in life, immunologic clearance does not occur, and protracted, lifelong infection ensues.

Although the mechanism of HBV-induced liver injury remains uncertain, immune complex–mediated tissue damage appears to play a major pathogenetic role in the extrahepatic manifestations of acute hepatitis B. The occasional prodromal serum sickness–like syndrome observed in acute hepatitis B appears to be related to the deposition in tissue blood vessel walls of circulating immune complexes leading to activation of the complement system. The clinical consequences are urticarial rash, angioedema, fever, and arthritis. During the early prodrome of HBV infection in these patients, HBsAg in high titer in association with small amounts of anti-HBs leads to the formation of soluble, circulating immune complexes (in antigen excess). Complement components in the serum are depressed during the arthritic phase of the illness and are also detectable in the circulating immune complexes. In addition to complement components, these complexes contain HBsAg, anti-HBs, IgG, IgM, IgA, and fibrin. After the patient recovers from the serum sickness–like syndrome, these immune complexes disappear.

In patients who become carriers of HBsAg following acute hepatitis, other types of immune-complex disease may be seen. Glomerulonephritis with the nephrotic syndrome is occasionally observed; HBsAg, immunoglobulin, and C3 deposition has been found in the glomerular basement membrane. While polyarteritis nodosa develops in considerably fewer than 1 percent of patients with HBV infection, 20 to 30 percent of patients with polyarteritis nodosa have HBsAg in serum. In these patients, the affected small and medium-sized arterioles have been shown to contain HBsAg, immunoglobulins, and complement components. Another extrahepatic manifestation of viral hepatitis, essential mixed cryoglobulinemia (EMC), was reported initially to be associated with hepatitis B. The disorder is characterized clinically by arthritis and cutaneous vasculitis (palpable purpura) and serologically by the presence of circulating cryoprecipitable immune complexes of more than one immunoglobulin class. Many patients with this syndrome have chronic liver disease, but the association with HBV infection has always been controversial. Recent reevaluation of patients with EMC suggests instead that a substantial proportion have chronic HCV infection. Their circulating immune complexes contain HCV RNA at a concentration that exceeds its serum concentration; this observation argues against secondary trapping of HCV in the immune complexes and favors a primary role for the virus in the pathogenesis of EMC.

PATHOLOGY   The typical morphologic lesions of hepatitis A, B, C, D, and E are often similar and consist of panlobular infiltration with mononuclear cells, hepatic cell necrosis, hyperplasia of Kupffer cells, and variable degrees of cholestasis. Hepatic cell regeneration is present, as evidenced by numerous mitotic figures, multinucleated cells, and "rosette" or "pseudoacinar" formation. The mononuclear infiltration consists primarily of small lymphocytes, although plasma cells and eosinophils are occasionally seen. Liver cell damage consists of hepatic cell degeneration and necrosis, cell dropout, ballooning of cells, and acidophilic degeneration of hepatocytes (forming so-called Councilman-like bodies). Large hepatocytes with a ground glass appearance of the cytoplasm may be seen in chronic but not in acute HBV infection; these cells have been shown to contain HBsAg and can be identified histochemically with orcein or aldehyde

fuchsin. In uncomplicated viral hepatitis, the reticulin framework is preserved.

In hepatitis C, the histologic lesion is often remarkable for a relative paucity of inflammation, a marked increase in activation of sinusoidal lining cells, the presence of fat, and occasionally, bile duct lesions in which biliary epithelial cells appear to be piled up without interruption of the basement membrane. Occasionally microvesicular steatosis occurs in hepatitis D. In hepatitis E, a common histologic feature is marked cholestasis. A cholestatic variant of slowly resolving acute hepatitis A also has been described.

A more severe histologic lesion, *bridging hepatic necrosis*, also termed *subacute* or *confluent necrosis*, is occasionally observed in some patients with acute hepatitis. "Bridging" between lobules results from large areas of hepatic cell dropout, with collapse of the reticulin framework. Characteristically, the bridge consists of condensed reticulum, inflammatory debris, and degenerating liver cells that span adjacent portal areas, portal to central veins, or central vein to central vein. This lesion has been thought to have prognostic significance; in many of the originally described patients with this lesion, a subacute course terminated in death within several weeks to months, or chronic active hepatitis and postnecrotic cirrhosis developed. More recent investigations have failed to uphold the association between bridging necrosis and such a poor prognosis in patients with acute hepatitis. Although the frequency of bridging may be higher among hospitalized patients with severe acute hepatitis, and although cirrhosis, chronic hepatitis, and even death have been observed in this group, the frequency of bridging necrosis in uncomplicated acute viral hepatitis is probably on the order of 1 to 5 percent. Prospective studies have failed to demonstrate a difference in prognosis between patients with acute hepatitis who have bridging necrosis and those who do not. Therefore, although demonstration of this lesion in patients with chronic hepatitis has prognostic significance (see Chap. 267), its demonstration during acute hepatitis is less meaningful, and liver biopsies to identify this lesion are no longer undertaken routinely in patients with acute hepatitis. In *massive hepatic necrosis* (fulminant hepatitis, acute yellow atrophy), the striking feature at postmortem examination is the finding of a small, shrunken, and soft liver. Histologic examination reveals massive necrosis and dropout of liver cells of most lobules with extensive collapse and condensation of the reticulin framework.

Immunofluorescence and immunoperoxidase antibody studies have been instrumental in localizing HBsAg to the cytoplasm and plasma membrane of infected liver cells. In contrast, HBcAg predominates in the nucleus, but occasionally, scant amounts are also seen in the cytoplasm and on the cell membrane. Electron-microscopic studies of liver biopsy material have demonstrated the presence of HBsAg particles in the cytoplasm and HBcAg particles in the nucleus of liver cells during hepatitis B infection. These morphologic observations suggest that DNA is synthesized and packaged within core particles in the nucleus, while the surface coat is assembled in the cytoplasm, resulting in the formation of intact hepatitis B virus. HDV antigen is localized to the hepatocyte nucleus, while HAV, HCV, and HEV antigens are localized to the cytoplasm.

EPIDEMIOLOGY   Prior to the availability of serologic tests for hepatitis viruses, all viral hepatitis cases were labeled either as "infectious" or "serum" hepatitis. Modes of transmission overlap, however, and *a clear distinction among the different types of viral hepatitis cannot be made solely on the basis of clinical or epidemiologic features* (Table 266-2). The most accurate means to distinguish the various types of viral hepatitis involves specific serologic testing.

Hepatitis A   *This agent is transmitted almost exclusively by the fecal-oral route.* Person-to-person spread of HAV is enhanced by poor personal hygiene and overcrowding, and large outbreaks as well as sporadic cases have been traced to contaminated food, water, milk, and shellfish. Intrafamily and intrainstitutional spread are also common. Early epidemiologic observations suggested that there is a predilection for hepatitis A to occur in late fall and early winter. In of acute viral hepatitis are systemic and quite variable. Constitutional symptoms of anorexia, nausea and vomiting, fatigue, malaise, arthralgias, myalgias, headache, photophobia, pharyngitis, cough, and coryza may precede the onset of jaundice by 1 to 2 weeks. The nausea, vomiting, and anorexia are frequently associated wth alterations in olfaction and taste. A low-grade fever between 38 and 39°C (100 to 102°F) is more often present in hepatitis A and E than in hepatitis B or C, except when hepatitis B is heralded by a serum sickness–like syndrome; rarely, a fever of 39.5 to 40°C (103 to 104°F) may accompany the constitutional symptoms. Dark urine and clay-colored stools may be noticed by the patient from 1 to 5 days prior to the onset of clinical jaundice.

With the onset of *clinical jaundice*, the constitutional prodromal symptoms usually diminish, but in some patients mild weight loss (2.5 to 5 kg) is common and may continue during the entire icteric phase. The liver becomes enlarged and tender and may be associated with right upper quadrant pain and discomfort. Infrequently, patients present with a cholestatic picture, suggesting extrahepatic biliary obstruction. Splenomegaly and cervical adenopathy are present in 10 to 20 percent of patients with acute hepatitis. Rarely, a few spider angiomas appear during the icteric phase and disappear during convalescence. During the *recovery phase*, constitutional symptoms disappear, but usually some liver enlargement and abnormalities in biochemical tests of hepatic function are still evident. The duration of the posticteric phase is variable, ranging from 2 to 12 weeks, and usually is more prolonged in acute hepatitis B and C. Complete clinical and biochemical recovery is to be expected 1 to 2 months after all cases of hepatitis A and E and 3 to 4 months after the onset of jaundice in three-quarters of uncomplicated cases of hepatitis B and C. In the remainder, biochemical recovery may be delayed. A substantial proportion of patients with viral hepatitis never become icteric.

Infection with HDV can occur in the presence of acute or chronic HBV infection; the duration of HBV infection determines the duration of HDV infection. When acute HDV and HBV infection occur simultaneously, clinical and biochemical features may be indistinguishable from those of HBV infection alone, although occasionally they are more severe. As opposed to patients with *acute* HBV infection, patients with *chronic* HBV infection can support HDV replication indefinitely. This can happen when acute HDV infection occurs in the presence of a nonresolving acute HBV infection. More commonly, acute HDV infection becomes chronic when it is superimposed on an underlying chronic HBV infection. In such cases, the HDV superinfection appears as a clinical exacerbation or an episode resembling acute viral hepatitis in someone already chronically infected with HBV. In the past, events resembling acute hepatitis in an HBV carrier or a patient with chronic hepatitis B were attributed to superimposed "non-A, non-B" hepatitis or to the natural history of the disease. A proportion of such episodes, however, represent acute superinfection with HDV. Superinfection with HDV in a patient with chronic hepatitis B often leads to clinical deterioration (see below).

In addition to superinfections with other hepatitis agents, acute hepatitis-like clinical events in persons with chronic hepatitis B may accompany spontaneous HBeAg–to–anti-HBe seroconversion or spontaneous reactivation, i.e., reversion from nonreplicative to replicative infection. Such reactivations can occur as well in therapeutically immunosuppressed patients with chronic HBV infection when cytotoxic-immunosuppressive drugs are withdrawn; in these cases, restoration of immune competence is thought to allow resumption of previously checked cell-mediated cytolysis of HBV-infected hepatocytes.

Laboratory features The serum aminotransferases AST and ALT (previously designated SGOT and SGPT) show a variable increase during the prodromal phase of acute viral hepatitis and precede the rise in bilirubin level (see Figs. 266-2 and 266-3). The acute level of these enzymes, however, does not correlate well with the degree of liver cell damage. Peak levels vary from 400 to 4000 IU or more; these levels are usually reached at the time the patient is clinically

icteric and diminish progressively during the recovery phase of acute hepatitis. The diagnosis of anicteric hepatitis is difficult and requires a high index of suspicion; it is based on clinical features and on aminotransferase elevations, although mild increases in conjugated bilirubin also may be found.

Jaundice is usually visible in the sclera or skin when the serum bilirubin value exceeds 43 µmol/L (2.5 mg/dL). When jaundice appears, the serum bilirubin typically rises to levels ranging from 85 to 340 µmol/L (5 to 20 mg/dL). The serum bilirubin may continue to rise despite falling serum aminotransferase levels. In most instances, the total bilirubin is equally divided between the conjugated and unconjugated fractions. Bilirubin levels above 340 µmol/L (20 mg/dL) extending and persisting late into the course of viral hepatitis are more likely to be associated with severe disease. In certain patients with underlying hemolytic anemia, however, such as glucose-6-phosphate dehydrogenase deficiency and sickle cell anemia, a high serum bilirubin level is common, resulting from superimposed hemolysis. In such patients, bilirubin levels greater than 513 µmol/L (30 mg/dL) have been observed and are not necessarily associated with a poor prognosis.

Neutropenia and lymphopenia are transient and are followed by a relative lymphocytosis. Atypical lymphocytes (varying between 2 and 20 percent) are common during the acute phase. These atypical lymphocytes are indistinguishable from those seen in infectious mononucleosis. Measurement of the prothrombin time (PT) is important in patients with acute viral hepatitis, for a prolonged value may reflect a severe synthetic defect, signify extensive hepatocellular necrosis, and indicate a worse prognosis. Occasionally, a prolonged PT may occur with only mild increases in the serum bilirubin and aminotransferase levels. Prolonged nausea and vomiting, inadequate carbohydrate intake, and poor hepatic glycogen reserves may contribute to hypoglycemia noted occasionally in patients with severe viral hepatitis. Serum alkaline phosphatase may be normal or only mildly elevated, while a fall in serum albumin is uncommon in uncomplicated acute viral hepatitis. In some patients, mild and transient steatorrhea has been noted as well as slight microscopic hematuria and minimal proteinuria.

A diffuse but mild elevation of the gamma globulin fraction is common during acute viral hepatitis. Serum IgG and IgM are elevated in about one-third of patients during the acute phase of viral hepatitis, but serum IgM elevation is seen more characteristically during acute hepatitis A. During the acute phase of viral hepatitis, antibodies to smooth muscle and other cell constituents may be present, and low titers of rheumatoid factor, antinuclear antibody, and heterophil antibody also can be found occasionally. In hepatitis C and D, antibodies to liver-kidney microsomes (LKM) occur; however, the species of LKM antibodies in the two types of hepatitis are different from each other as well as from the LKM antibody species characteristic of autoimmune chronic active hepatitis type 2 (see Chap. 267). The autoantibodies in viral hepatitis are nonspecific and also can be associated with other viral and systemic diseases. In contrast, virus-specific antibodies, which appear during and after hepatitis virus infection, are serologic markers of diagnostic importance.

As described above, serologic tests are available with which to establish a diagnosis of hepatitis A, B, D, and C. Tests for fecal or serum HAV are not routinely available. Therefore, a diagnosis of type A hepatitis is based on detection of IgM anti-HAV during acute illness (see Fig. 266-2). Rheumatoid factor can give rise to false-positive results in this test.

A diagnosis of HBV infection can usually be made by detection of HBsAg in serum. Infrequently, levels of HBsAg are too low to be detected during acute HBV infection even with the current generation of highly sensitive immunoassays. In such cases, the diagnosis can be established by the presence of IgM anti-HBc. Alternatively, de novo appearance of anti-HBc and anti-HBs during illness and convalescence may support the diagnostic impression.

The titer of HBsAg bears little relation to the severity of clinical disease. Indeed, there may be an inverse correlation between the serum concentration of HBsAg and the degree of liver cell damage. For example, titers are highest in immunosuppressed patients, lower in chronic liver disease (but higher in chronic persistent than in chronic active hepatitis), and very low in acute fulminant hepatitis. These observations suggest that in hepatitis B the degree of liver cell damage and the clinical course are probably related to variations in the patient's immune response to HBV rather than to the amount of circulating HBsAg. In immunocompetent persons, however, there is a correlation between markers of HBV *replication* and liver injury (see below).

Another serologic marker that may be of value in patients with hepatitis B is HBeAg. Its principal clinical usefulness is as an indicator of relative infectivity. Because HBeAg is invariably present during early acute hepatitis B, HBeAg testing is indicated primarily during follow-up of chronic infection.

In patients with hepatitis B surface antigenemia of unknown duration, e.g., blood donors whose blood is found to be HBsAg-positive and who are referred to a physician for evaluation, testing for IgM anti-HBc may be useful to distinguish between acute or recent infection (IgM anti-HBc-positive) and chronic HBV infection (IgM anti-HBc-negative, IgG anti-HBc-positive). A false-positive test for IgM anti-HBc may be encountered in patients with high-titer rheumatoid factor.

Anti-HBs is rarely detectable in the presence of HBsAg in patients with *acute* hepatitis B, but 10 to 20 percent of persons with *chronic* HBV infection may harbor low-level anti-HBs. This antibody is directed not against the common group determinant, *a*, but against the heterotypic subtype determinant (e.g., HBsAg of subtype *ad* with anti-HBs of subtype *y*). In most cases, this serologic pattern cannot be attributed to infection with two different HBV subtypes, and the presence of this antibody is not a harbinger of imminent HBsAg clearance. When such antibody is detected, its presence is of no recognized clinical significance.

After immunization with hepatitis B vaccine, which consists of HBsAg alone, anti-HBs is the only serologic marker to appear. A summary of the commonly encountered serologic patterns of hepatitis B and their interpretations appears in Table 266-3. Tests for the detection of HBV DNA in liver and serum are now available. Like HBeAg, serum HBV DNA is an indicator of HBV replication, but tests for HBV DNA are more sensitive and quantitative. These markers are useful in following the course of HBV replication in patients with chronic hepatitis B receiving antiviral chemotherapy, e.g., with interferon (see Chap. 267). In immunocompetent persons, a general correlation does appear to exist between the level of HBV replication, as reflected by the level of HBV DNA in serum, and the degree of liver injury. High serum HBV DNA levels, increased expression of viral antigens, and necroinflammatory activity in the liver go hand in hand unless immunosuppression interferes with cytolytic T cell responses to virus-infected cells; reduction of HBV replication with antiviral drugs, such as interferon, tends to be accompanied by an improvement in liver histology.

Before the availability of reliable serologic tests for hepatitis C, a diagnosis of non-A, non-B hepatitis was made by serologic exclusion of HAV and HBV infection in the setting of a compatible history. A helpful clinical clue is the episodic pattern of aminotransferase elevation seen frequently in non-A, non-B hepatitis. Currently, a specific serologic diagnosis of hepatitis C can be made by demonstrating the presence in serum of anti-HCV. When a second-generation immunoassay (that detects antibodies to nonstructural and nucleocapsid proteins) is used, anti-HCV can be detected in acute hepatitis C during the initial phase of elevated aminotransferase activity. This antibody may never become detectable in 20 to 30 percent of patients with acute hepatitis C, and levels of anti-HCV may become undetectable after recovery from acute hepatitis C. In patients with chronic hepatitis C, anti-HCV is detectable in >90 percent of cases. Because nonspecificity can confound immunoassays for anti-HCV, a supplementary recombinant immunoblot assay should be done to establish the specific viral proteins to which anti-HCV is directed (see "Virology and Etiology," above). Still a research tool, a polymerase chain reaction assay for HCV RNA is the most sensitive test for HCV infection. This test can detect HCV RNA even before acute elevation of aminotransferase activity and before the appearance of anti-HCV in patients with acute hepatitis C. In addition, HCV RNA remains detectable indefinitely, continuously in most but intermittently in some, in patients with chronic hepatitis C (even detectable in some persons with normal liver tests, i.e., asymptomatic carriers). Thus a diagnosis of hepatitis C can be supported by detection of anti-HCV and by exclusion of false-positive reactivity. In the small minority of patients with hepatitis C who lack anti-HCV, a diagnosis can be supported by detection of HCV RNA, if available. If all these tests are negative and the patient has a well-characterized case of hepatitis following percutaneous exposure to blood or blood products, a diagnosis of "non-A, non-B," perhaps caused by another agent, can be entertained. A proportion of patients with hepatitis C have isolated anti-HBc in their blood, a reflection of a common risk in certain populations to multiple bloodborne hepatitis agents. The anti-HBc in such cases is almost invariably of the IgG class and represents either HBV infection in the remote past or current HBV infection with low-level virus carriage.

The presence of HDV infection can be identified by demonstrating intrahepatic HDV antigen or, more practically, an anti-HDV seroconversion (a rise in titer of anti-HDV or de novo appearance of IgM

HBsAg	Anti-HBs	Anti-HBc	HBeAg	Anti-HBe	Interpretation
+	−	IgM	+	−	Acute HBV infection, high infectivity
+	−	IgG	+	−	Chronic HBV infection, high infectivity
+	−	IgG	−	+	Late-acute or chronic HBV infection, low infectivity
+	+	+	+/−	+/−	1 HBsAg of one subtype and heterotypic anti-HBs (common) 2 Process of seroconversion from HBsAg to anti-HBs (rare)
−	−	IgM	+/−	+/−	1 Acute HBV infection 2 Anti-HBc window
−	−	IgG		+/−	1 Low-level HBsAg carrier 2 Remote past infection
−	+	IgG	−	+/−	Recovery from HBV infection
−	+	−	−	−	1 Immunization with HBsAg (after vaccination) 2 Remote past infection (?) 3 False-positive

TABLE 266-3 Commonly encountered serologic patterns of hepatitis B infection

TABLE 266-4   Simplified diagnostic approach in patients presenting with acute hepatitis

Serologic tests of patient's serum

HBsAg	IgM anti-HAV	IgM anti-HBc	anti-HCV	Diagnostic interpretation
+	−	+	−	Acute hepatitis B
+	−	−	−	Chronic hepatitis B
+	+	−	−	Acute hepatitis A superimposed on chronic hepatitis B
+	+	+	−	Acute hepatitis A and B
−	+	−	−	Acute hepatitis A
−	+	+	−	Acute hepatitis A and B (HBsAg below detection threshold)
−	−	+	−	Acute hepatitis B (HBsAg below detection threshold)
−	−	−	+	Acute hepatitis C

anti-HDV). Circulating HDVAg, also diagnostic of acute infection, is detectable only briefly, if at all. Because IgM anti-HDV is transient and IgG anti-HDV is often undetectable once HBsAg disappears, retrospective serodiagnosis of acute self-limited, simultaneous HBV and HDV infection is difficult. Early diagnosis of acute infection may be hampered by a delay of up to 30 to 40 days in the appearance of anti-HDV.

When a patient presents with acute hepatitis and has HBsAg and anti-HDV in the serum, determination of the class of anti-HBc is helpful in establishing the relationship between infection with HBV and HDV. Although IgM anti-HBc does not distinguish *absolutely* between acute and chronic HBV infection, its presence is a reliable indicator of recent infection and its absence a reliable indicator of infection in the remote past. In simultaneous acute HBV and HDV infections, IgM anti-HBc will be detectable, while in acute HDV infection superimposed on chronic HBV infection, anti-HBc will be of the IgG class.

In the future, tests for the presence of HDV RNA will be useful for determining the presence of ongoing HDV replication and relative infectivity. Currently, probes for this marker are restricted to a limited number of research laboratories. Similarly, diagnostic tests for hepatitis E are cumbersome and remain limited to a small number of research laboratories. Routine diagnostic tests are being developed, however.

Liver biopsy is rarely necessary or indicated in acute viral hepatitis, except when there is a question about the diagnosis or when there is clinical evidence suggesting a diagnosis of chronic active hepatitis.

A diagnostic algorithm can be applied in the evaluation of cases of acute viral hepatitis. A patient with acute hepatitis should undergo four serologic tests, HBsAg, IgM anti-HAV, IgM anti-HBc, and anti-HCV (Table 266-4). The presence of HBsAg, with or without IgM anti-HBc, represents HBV infection. If IgM anti-HBc is present, the HBV infection is considered acute; if IgM anti-HBc is absent, the HBV infection is considered chronic. A diagnosis of acute hepatitis B can be made in the absence of HBsAg when IgM anti-HBc is detectable. A diagnosis of acute hepatitis A is based on the presence of IgM anti-HAV. If IgM anti-HAV coexists with HBsAg, a diagnosis of simultaneous HAV and HBV infections can be made; if IgM anti-HBc (with or without HBsAg) is detectable, the patient has simultaneous acute hepatitis A and B, and if IgM anti-HBc is undetectable, the patient has acute hepatitis A superimposed on chronic HBV infection. The presence of anti-HCV, if confirmable, supports a diagnosis of acute hepatitis C. Occasionally, repeat anti-HCV testing later during the illness is necessary to establish the diagnosis. Absence of all serologic markers is consistent with a diagnosis of "non-A, non-B" hepatitis, if the epidemiologic setting is appropriate.

In patients with chronic hepatitis, initial testing should consist of HBsAg and anti-HCV. Anti-HCV supports the diagnosis of chronic hepatitis C. If a serologic diagnosis of chronic hepatitis B is made, testing for HBeAg and anti-HBe is indicated to evaluate relative infectivity. Testing for HBV DNA in such patients provides a more quantitative and sensitive test for the level of virus replication and, therefore, is very helpful during antiviral therapy (see Chap. 267). In patients with hepatitis B, testing for anti-HDV is useful under the following circumstances: severe and fulminant cases, severe chronic cases, cases of acute hepatitis-like exacerbations in patients with chronic hepatitis B, persons with frequent percutaneous exposures, and persons from areas where HDV infection is endemic.

PROGNOSIS   Virtually all previously healthy patients with hepatitis A recover completely from their illness with no clinical sequelae. Similarly, in acute hepatitis B, 95 percent of patients have a favorable course and recover completely. There are, however, certain clinical and laboratory features which suggest a more complicated and protracted course. Patients of advanced age and with serious underlying medical disorders may have a prolonged course and are more likely to experience severe hepatitis. Initial presenting features such as ascites, peripheral edema, and symptoms of hepatic encephalopathy suggest a poorer prognosis. In addition, a prolonged prothrombin time, low serum albumin level, hypoglycemia, and very high serum bilirubin values suggest severe hepatocellular disease. Patients with these clinical and laboratory features deserve prompt hospital admission. The case-fatality rate in hepatitis A and B is very low (approximately 0.1 percent) but is increased by advanced age and underlying debilitating disorders. Among patients ill enough to be hospitalized for acute hepatitis B, the fatality rate is 1 percent. Hepatitis C occurring after transfusion is less severe during the acute phase than type B hepatitis and is more likely to be anicteric; fatalities are rare, but the precise case-fatality rate is not known. In outbreaks of waterborne hepatitis E in India and Asia, the case-fatality rate is 1 to 2 percent and up to 10 to 20 percent in pregnant women. Patients with simultaneous acute hepatitis B and hepatitis D do not necessarily experience a higher mortality rate than do patients with acute hepatitis B alone; however, in several recent outbreaks of acute simultaneous HBV and HDV infection among drug addicts, the case fatality rate has been approximately 5 percent. In the case of HDV superinfection of a person with chronic hepatitis B, the likelihood of fulminant hepatitis and death is increased substantially. Although the case-fatality rate for hepatitis D has not been defined adequately, in outbreaks of severe HDV superinfection in isolated populations with a high hepatitis B carrier rate, the mortality rate has been recorded in excess of 20 percent.

COMPLICATIONS AND SEQUELAE   A small proportion of patients with hepatitis A experience *relapsing hepatitis* weeks to months after apparent recovery from acute hepatitis. Relapses are characterized by recurrence of symptoms, aminotransferase elevations, occasionally jaundice, and fecal excretion of HAV. Another unusual variant of acute hepatitis A is *cholestatic hepatitis*, characterized by protracted cholestatic jaundice and pruritus. Rarely, liver test abnormalities persist for many months, even up to a year. Even when these complications occur, hepatitis A remains self-limited and does not progress to chronic liver disease. During the prodromal phase of acute hepatitis B, a serum sickness–like syndrome characterized by arthralgia or arthritis, rash, angioedema, and rarely hematuria and proteinuria may develop in some patients. This syndrome occurs prior to the onset of clinical jaundice, and these patients are often erroneously diagnosed as having rheumatoid arthritis or other rheumatologic diseases such as systemic lupus erythematosus. This syndrome occurs in about 5 to 10 percent of patients with acute hepatitis B. The diagnosis can be established by measuring serum aminotransferase levels, which are almost invariably elevated, and serum HBsAg.

The most feared complication of viral hepatitis is *fulminant hepatitis* (massive hepatic necrosis); fortunately, this is a rare event. This is primarily seen in hepatitis B and D, as well as hepatitis E, but rare fulminant cases of hepatitis A occur primarily in older adults and in persons with underlying chronic liver disease. Hepatitis B accounts for more than 50 percent of fulminant hepatitis cases, a sizable proportion of which are associated with HDV infection. Participation of HDV can be documented in approximately one-third of patients with acute fulminant hepatitis B and two-thirds of patients with fulminant hepatitis superimposed on chronic hepatitis B. Fulminant hepatitis is seen rarely in hepatitis C, but hepatitis E, as noted above, can be complicated by fatal fulminant hepatitis in 1 to 2 percent of all cases and in up to 20 percent of cases occurring in pregnant women. Patients usually present with signs and symptoms of encephalopathy that may evolve to deep coma. The liver is usually small and the prothrombin time excessively prolonged. The combination of rapidly shrinking liver size, rapidly rising bilirubin level, and marked prolongation of the prothrombin time, together with clinical signs of confusion, disorientation, somnolence, ascites, and edema, indicates that the patient has hepatic failure with encephalopathy. Cerebral edema is common; brainstem compression, gastrointestinal bleeding, sepsis, respiratory failure, cardiovascular collapse, and renal failure are terminal events. The mortality is exceedingly high (greater than 80 percent in patients with deep coma), but patients who survive may have a complete biochemical and histologic recovery.

It is particularly important to document the disappearance of HBsAg following apparent clinical recovery from acute hepatitis B. Before laboratory methods were available to distinguish between acute and acute hepatitis–like exacerbations (*spontaneous reactivations*) of chronic hepatitis B, observations suggested that approximately 10 percent of patients remained HBsAg-positive for longer than 6 months after the onset of clinically apparent acute hepatitis B. Half these persons were found to clear the antigen from their circulations during the next several years, but the other 5 percent remained chronically HBsAg-positive. More recent observations suggest that the true rate of chronic infection after clinically apparent acute hepatitis B is as low as 1 to 2 percent in normal, immunocompetent, young adults. Earlier, higher estimates may have been biased by inadvertent inclusion of acute exacerbations in chronically infected patients; these patients, chronically HBsAg-positive before exacerbation, were unlikely to seroconvert to HBsAg-negative thereafter. Whether the rate of chronicity is 10 or 1 percent, such patients have anti-HBc in serum; anti-HBs is either undetected or detected at low titer against the opposite subtype specificity of the antigen (see "Laboratory Features," above). These patients may (1) be asymptomatic carriers, (2) have low-grade chronic persistent hepatitis, or (3) have chronic active hepatitis with or without cirrhosis. The likelihood of becoming an HBsAg carrier after acute HBV infection is especially high among neonates, persons with Down's syndrome, chronically hemodialyzed patients, and immunosuppressed patients, including persons with human immunodeficiency virus infection.

Chronic active hepatitis is a major late complication of acute hepatitis B occurring in a small proportion of acute cases but more common in those who present with chronic infection without having experienced an acute illness (see Chap. 267). Certain clinical and laboratory features suggest progression of acute hepatitis to chronic active hepatitis: (1) lack of complete resolution of clinical symptoms of anorexia, weight loss, and fatigue and the persistence of hepatomegaly; (2) the presence of bridging or multilobular hepatic necrosis on liver biopsy during protracted, severe acute viral hepatitis; (3) failure of the serum aminotransferase, bilirubin, and globulin levels to return to normal within 6 to 12 months following the acute illness; and (4) the continued presence of HBsAg and HBeAg 6 months or more after acute hepatitis, suggesting chronic, replicative viral infection of the liver.

Although acute hepatitis D infection does not increase the likelihood of chronicity of simultaneous acute hepatitis B, hepatitis D has the potential for contributing to the severity of chronic hepatitis B. Hepatitis D superinfection can transform asymptomatic or mild chronic hepatitis B into severe, progressive chronic active hepatitis and cirrhosis; it also can accelerate the course of chronic active hepatitis B. Some HDV superinfections in patients with chronic hepatitis B lead to fulminant hepatitis. Although HDV and HBV infections are associated with severe liver disease, mild hepatitis and even asymptomatic carriage have been identified in some patients. After transfusion-associated acute hepatitis C, as many as 50 percent of patients have abnormal biochemical liver tests for more than a year. In a majority of such patients, liver histology is consistent with chronic active hepatitis. Although many of these patients have no symptoms and a nonprogressive course, ultimately, cirrhosis develops in as many as 20 percent of those with *chronic* posttransfusion hepatitis C within 10 years of acute illness. The likelihood of chronic hepatitis is also approximately 50 percent after sporadic hepatitis C occurring in the absence of identifiable percutaneous inoculation with blood products or contaminated needles. In contrast, neither HAV nor HEV causes chronic liver disease.

Rare complications of viral hepatitis include pancreatitis, myocarditis, atypical pneumonia, aplastic anemia, transverse myelitis, and peripheral neuropathy. *Carriers* of HBsAg, particularly those infected in infancy or early childhood, have an enhanced risk of hepatocellular carcinoma. The risk of hepatocellular carcinoma is increased as well in patients with cirrhosis associated with chronic hepatitis C (see Chap. 269). In children, hepatitis B may present rarely with anicteric hepatitis, a nonpruritic papular rash of the face, buttocks, and limbs, and lymphadenopathy (papular acrodermatitis of childhood or Gianotti-Crosti syndrome).

DIFFERENTIAL DIAGNOSIS Viral diseases such as infectious mononucleosis; those due to cytomegalovirus, herpes simplex, and coxsackieviruses; and toxoplasmosis may share certain clinical features with viral hepatitis and cause elevation in serum aminotransferase and less commonly in serum bilirubin levels. Tests such as the differential heterophil and serologic tests for these agents may be helpful in the differential diagnosis if HBsAg, anti-HBc, IgM anti-HAV, and anti-HCV determinations are negative. A complete drug history is particularly important, for many drugs and certain anesthetic agents can produce a picture of either acute hepatitis or cholestasis (see below). Equally important is a past history of unexplained "repeated episodes" of acute hepatitis. This should alert the physician to the possibility that the underlying disorder is chronic active hepatitis. Alcoholic hepatitis also must be considered, but usually the serum aminotransferase levels are not as markedly elevated and other stigmata of alcoholism may be present. The finding on liver biopsy of fatty infiltration, a neutrophilic inflammatory reaction, and "alcoholic hyaline" would be consistent with alcohol-induced rather than viral liver injury. Because acute hepatitis may present with right upper quadrant abdominal pain, nausea and vomiting, fever, and icterus, it is often confused with acute cholecystitis, common duct stone, or ascending cholangitis. Patients with acute viral hepatitis may tolerate surgery poorly; therefore, it is important to exclude this diagnosis, and in confusing cases, a percutaneous liver biopsy may be necessary prior to laparotomy. Viral hepatitis in the elderly is often misdiagnosed as obstructive jaundice resulting from a common duct stone or carcinoma of the pancreas. Because acute hepatitis in the elderly may be quite severe and the operative mortality high, a thorough evaluation including biochemical tests, radiographic studies of the biliary tree, and even liver biopsy may be necessary to exclude primary parenchymal liver disease. Another clinical constellation that may mimic acute hepatitis is right ventricular failure with passive hepatic congestion or hypoperfusion syndromes, such as those associated with shock, severe hypotension, and severe left ventricular failure. Clinical features are usually sufficient to distinguish between the two entities. Very rarely, malignancies metastatic to the liver can mimic acute or even fulminant viral hepatitis. Occasionally, genetic or metabolic liver disorders (e.g., Wilson's disease, α_1-antitrypsin deficiency) are confused with viral hepatitis.

MANAGEMENT **Treatment of acute attack** There is no specific treatment for *typical acute viral hepatitis*. Although hospitalization may be required for clinically severe illness, most patients do not require hospital care. Forced and prolonged bed rest is not essential

TABLE 266-5   Some features of toxic and drug-induced hepatic injury

Features	Direct toxic effect		Idiosyncratic			Other	
	(Carbon tetrachloride, e.g.)	(Acetaminophen, e.g.)	(Halothane, e.g.)	(Isoniazid, e.g.)	(Chlorpromazine, e.g.)	(Oral contraceptive agents, e.g.)
Predictable and dose-related toxicity	+	+	0	0	0	+
Latent period	Short	Short	Variable	Variable	Variable	Variable
Arthralgia, fever, rash, eosinophilia	0	0	+	0	+	0
Liver morphology	Necrosis, fatty infiltration	Centrilobular necrosis	Similar to viral hepatitis	Similar to viral hepatitis	Cholestasis *with* portal inflammation	Cholestasis *without* portal inflammation, vascular lesions

These include industrial toxins (e.g., carbon tetrachloride, trichloroethylene, and yellow phosphorus), the heat-stable toxic bicyclic octapeptides of certain species of *Amanita* and *Galerina* (hepatotoxic mushroom poisoning), and more commonly, pharmacologic agents used in medical therapy. It is essential that any patient presenting with jaundice or impaired liver function be questioned carefully about exposure to chemicals used in work or at home and drugs taken by prescription or bought "over the counter." In general, two major types of chemical hepatotoxicity have been recognized: (1) direct toxic type and (2) idiosyncratic type.

As shown in Table 266-5, direct toxic hepatitis occurs with predictable regularity in individuals exposed to the offending agent and is dose-dependent. The latent period between exposure and liver injury is usually short (often several hours), although clinical manifestations may be delayed for 24 to 48 h. Agents producing toxic hepatitis are generally systemic poisons or are converted in the liver to toxic metabolites. The direct hepatotoxins result in morphologic abnormalities which are reasonably characteristic and reproducible for each toxin. For example, carbon tetrachloride and trichloroethylene characteristically produce a centrilobular zonal necrosis, whereas yellow phosphorus poisoning typically results in periportal injury. The hepatotoxic octapeptides of *Amanita phalloides* usually produce massive hepatic necrosis. The lethal dose of the toxin is about 10 mg, the amount found in a single deathcap mushroom. Tetracycline, when administered in intravenous doses greater than 1.5 g daily, leads to microvesicular fat deposits in the liver. Liver injury, which is often only one facet of the toxicity produced by the direct hepatotoxins, may go unrecognized until jaundice appears.

In idiosyncratic drug reactions the occurrence of hepatitis is usually infrequent and unpredictable, the response is not dose-dependent, and it may occur at any time during or shortly after exposure to the drug. Extrahepatic manifestations of hypersensitivity, such as rash, arthralgias, fever, leukocytosis, and eosinophilia occur in about one-quarter of patients with idiosyncratic hepatotoxic drug reactions; this observation and the unpredictability of idiosyncratic drug hepatotoxicity contributed to the hypothesis that this category of drug reactions is immunologically mediated. More recent evidence, however, suggests that, in most cases, even idiosyncratic reactions represent direct hepatotoxicity but are caused by drug metabolites rather than by the intact compound. Even the prototype of idiosyncratic hepatoxicity reactions, halothane hepatitis, and isoniazid hepatotoxicity, associated frequently with hypersensitivity manifestations, are now recognized to be mediated by toxic metabolites which damage liver cells directly. Currently, most idiosyncratic reactions are thought to result from differences in metabolic reactivity to specific agents; host susceptibility is mediated by the kinetics of toxic metabolite generation, which differs among individuals. Occasionally, however, the clinical features of an allergic reaction (e.g., prominent tissue eosinophilia, autoantibodies, etc.) are difficult to ignore. In vitro models have been described in which lymphocyte cytotoxicity can be demonstrated against rabbit hepatocytes altered by incubation with the potential offending drug. Similarly, in selected cases, a drug or its metabolite

has been shown to bind to a host cellular component forming a hapten; the immune response to this "neoantigen" is postulated to play a role in the pathogenesis of liver injury. Therefore, some authorities subdivide idiosyncratic drug hepatotoxicity into hypersensitivity (allergic) and "metabolic" categories. Several unusual exceptions notwithstanding, true drug allergy is difficult to support in most cases of idiosyncratic drug-induced liver injury.

Idiosyncratic reactions lead to a morphologic pattern that is more variable than those produced by direct toxins; a single agent is often capable of causing a variety of lesions, although certain patterns tend to predominate. Depending on the agent involved, idiosyncratic hepatitis may result in a clinical and morphologic picture indistinguishable from viral hepatitis (e.g., halothane) or may simulate extrahepatic bile duct obstruction clinically with morphologic evidence of cholestasis and minimal hepatocellular damage (e.g., chlorpromazine). Morphologic alterations also may include bridging hepatic necrosis (e.g., methyldopa), or, infrequently, hepatic granulomas (e.g., sulfonamides).

Not all adverse hepatic drug reactions can be classified as either toxic or idiosyncratic in type. For example, oral contraceptives, which combine estrogenic and progestational compounds, may result in impairment of hepatic function and occasionally in jaundice. However, they do not produce necrosis or fatty change, manifestations of hypersensitivity are generally absent, and susceptibility to the development of oral contraceptive–induced cholestasis appears to be genetically determined.

Because drug-induced hepatitis is often a presumptive diagnosis and many other disorders produce a similar clinicopathologic picture, evidence of a causal relationship between the use of a drug and subsequent liver injury may be difficult to establish. The relationship is most convincing for the direct hepatotoxins, which lead to a high frequency of hepatic impairment after a short latent period. Idiosyncratic reactions may be reproduced, in some instances, when rechallenge, after an asymptomatic period, results in a recurrence of signs, symptoms, and morphologic and biochemical abnormalities. Rechallenge, however, is often ethically unfeasible, because severe reactions may occur.

Treatment of toxic and drug-induced hepatic disease is largely supportive, as in acute viral hepatitis. Withdrawal of the suspected agent is indicated at the first sign of an adverse reaction. In the case of the direct toxins, liver involvement should not divert attention from renal or other organ involvement which also may threaten survival.

In Table 266-6, several classes of chemical agents are listed, together with examples of the pattern of liver injury produced by them. Certain drugs appear to be responsible for the development of chronic as well as acute hepatic injury. For example, oxphenisatin, alpha methyldopa, and isoniazid have been associated with chronic active hepatitis, and halothane and methotrexate have been implicated in the development of cirrhosis. A syndrome resembling primary biliary cirrhosis has been described following treatment with chlorpromazine, methyl testosterone, tolbutamide, and other drugs. Portal

TABLE 266-6 Principal alterations of hepatic morphology produced by some commonly used drugs and chemicals*

Principal morphologic change	Class of agent	Example
Cholestasis	Anabolic steroid	Methyl testosterone[†]
	Antithyroid	Methimazole
	Antibiotic	Erythromycin estolate, nitrofurantoin
	Oral contraceptive	Norethynodrel with mestranol
	Oral hypoglycemic	Chlorpropamide[†]
	Tranquilizer	Chlorpromazine[†]
	Oncotherapeutic	Anabolic steroids, busulfan, tamoxifen
	Immunosuppressive	Cyclosporine
	Anticonvulsant	Carbamazine
	Calcium channel blocker	Nifedipine, verapamil
Fatty liver	Antibiotic	Tetracycline
	Anticonvulsant	Sodium valproate
	Antiarrhythmic	Amiodarone
	Oncotherapeutic	Asparaginase, methotrexate
Hepatitis	Anesthetic	Halothane[‡]
	Anticonvulsant	Phenytoin, carbamazine
	Antihypertensive	Methyldopa,[‡] captopril, enalapril
	Antibiotic	Isoniazid,[‡] rifampicin, nitrofurantoin
	Diuretic	Chlorothiazide
	Laxative	Oxyphenisatin[‡]
	Antidepressant	Iproniazid, amitriptyline, imipramine
	Anti-inflammatory	Ibuprofen, indomethacin
	Antifungal	Ketoconazole, fluconazole
	Antiviral	Zidovudine, dideoxyinosine
	Calcium-channel blocker	Nifedipine, verapamil, diltiazem
Mixed hepatitis/cholestatic	Immunosuppressive	Azathioprine
	Lipid-lowering	Nicotinic acid, lovastatin
Toxic (necrosis)	Hydrocarbon	Carbon tetrachloride
	Metal	Yellow phosphorus
	Mushroom	*Amanita phalloides*
	Analgesic	Acetaminophen
	Solvent	Dimethylformamide
Granulomas	Anti-inflammatory	Phenylbutazone
	Antibiotic	Sulfanomides
	Xanthine oxidase inhibitor	Allopurinol
	Antiarrhythmic	Quinidine
	Anticonvulsant	Carbamazine

* Several agents cause more than one type of liver lesion and appear under more than one category.
† Rarely associated with primary biliary cirrhosis–like lesion.
‡ Occasionally associated with chronic active hepatitis or bridging hepatic necrosis or cirrhosis.

hypertension in the absence of cirrhosis may result from alterations in hepatic architecture produced by vitamin A or arsenic intoxication, industrial exposure to vinyl chloride, or administration of thorium dioxide. The latter three agents also have been associated with angiosarcoma of the liver. Oral contraceptives have been implicated in the development of hepatic adenoma and, rarely, hepatocellular carcinoma and occlusion of the hepatic vein (Budd-Chiari syndrome). Another unusual lesion, peliosis hepatis (blood cysts of the liver), has been observed in some patients treated with anabolic steroids. The existence of these hepatic disorders expands the spectrum of liver injury induced by chemical agents and emphasizes the need for a thorough drug history in all patients with liver dysfunction.

The following are the patterns of adverse hepatic reactions for some prototypic agents.

ACETAMINOPHEN HEPATOTOXICITY (DIRECT TOXIN) Acetaminophen has caused severe centrolobular hepatic necrosis when ingested in large amounts in suicide attempts or accidentally by children. A single dose of 10 to 15 g, occasionally less, may produce

clinical evidence of liver injury. Fatal fulminant disease is usually (although not invariably) associated with ingestion of 25 g or more. Blood levels of acetaminophen correlate with the severity of hepatic injury (levels above 300 µg/mL 4 h after ingestion are predictive of the development of severe damage, while levels below 150 µg/mL suggest that hepatic injury is highly unlikely). Nausea, vomiting, diarrhea, abdominal pain, and shock are early manifestations occurring 4 to 12 h after ingestion. Then 24 to 48 h later, when these features are abating, hepatic injury becomes apparent. Maximal abnormalities and hepatic failure may not be evident until 4 to 6 days after ingestion. Renal failure and myocardial injury may be present.

Acetaminophen hepatotoxicity is mediated by a toxic reactive metabolite formed from the parent compound by the cytochrome P450 mixed-function oxidase system of the hepatocyte. This metabolite is detoxified by binding to glutathione. When excessive amounts of the metabolite are formed, glutathione levels in the liver fall, and the metabolite is covalently bound to nucleophilic hepatocyte macromolecules. This process is believed to lead to hepatocyte necrosis; the precise sequence and mechanism are unknown. Hepatic injury may be potentiated by prior administration of alcohol or other drugs, by conditions which stimulate the mixed-function oxidase system, or by conditions such as starvation which reduce hepatic glutathione levels. In chronic alcoholics, the toxic dose of acetaminophen may be as low as 2 g.

Treatment of acetaminophen overdosage includes gastric lavage, supportive measures, and oral administration of activated charcoal or cholestyramine to prevent absorption of residual drug. Neither of the latter agents appears to be effective if given more than 30 min after acetaminophen ingestion; if they are used, the stomach lavage should be done before other agents are administered orally. In patients with high acetaminophen blood levels (>200 µg/mL measured at 4 h or >100 µg/mL at 8 h after ingestion), the administration of sulfhydryl compounds (e.g., cysteamine, cysteine, or N-acetylcysteine) appears to reduce the severity of hepatic necrosis. These agents appear to act by providing a reservoir of sulfhydryl groups to bind the toxic metabolites or by stimulating synthesis and repletion of hepatic glutathione. Therapy should be begun within 8 h of ingestion but may be effective even if given as late as 24 to 36 h after overdose. Later administration of sulfhydryl compounds is of uncertain value.

Survivors of acute acetaminophen overdose usually have no evidence of hepatic sequelae. In a few patients, prolonged or repeated administration of acetaminophen in therapeutic doses appears to have led to the development of chronic active hepatitis and cirrhosis.

HALOTHANE HEPATOTOXICITY (IDIOSYNCRATIC REACTION)
Halothane, a nonexplosive fluorinated hydrocarbon anesthetic agent that is structurally similar to chloroform, has been reported to result in severe hepatic necrosis in a small number of individuals, many of whom have previously been exposed to this agent. The failure to produce similar hepatic lesions reliably in animals, the rarity of hepatic impairment in human beings, and the delayed appearance of hepatic injury suggest that halothane is not a direct hepatotoxin but may be a sensitizing agent. However, manifestations of hypersensitivity are seen in fewer than 25 percent of cases. A genetic predisposition leading to an idiosyncratic metabolic reactivity has been postulated and appears to be the most likely mechanism of halothane hepatotoxicity. Supporting this postulate is the demonstration in patients with halothane hepatitis and their family members of increased lymphocyte susceptibility to damage in vitro by electrophilic drug metabolites. Adults (rather than children), obese people, and women appear to be particularly susceptible. Fever, moderate leukocytosis, and eosinophilia may occur in the first week following halothane administration. Jaundice usually is noted 7 to 10 days after exposure but may occur earlier in previously exposed patients. Nausea and vomiting may precede the onset of jaundice. Hepatomegaly is often mild, but liver tenderness is common. The serum aminotransferase levels are elevated. The pathologic changes at autopsy are indistinguishable from massive hepatic necrosis resulting from viral hepatitis. The case-fatality rate of halothane hepatitis is not known but may vary from

20 to 40 percent in cases with severe liver involvement. With its increasing use, its occasional hepatotoxicity is being
instances, cirrhosis has been observed following repeated ed with growing frequency. Its likelihood is unpredictable,
halothane hepatitis; however, in most patients who recover, n it occurs, trimethoprim-sulfamethoxazole hepatotoxicity
returns to normal. It is strongly suggested that patients i relatively uniform latency period of several weeks and is
unexplained spiking fever, especially delayed fever, or companied by eosinophilia, rash, and other features of a
develops after halothane anesthesia not receive this age sitivity reaction. Biochemically and histologically, acute
Because cross-reactions between halothane and methoxyflu lular necrosis predominates, but cholestatic features are quite
been reported, the latter agent should not be used after l Occasionally, cholestasis without necrosis occurs, and very
reactions. Later-generation halogenated hydrocarbon anest severe cholangiolytic pattern of liver injury is observed. In
felt to be associated with a lower risk of hepatotoxicity; es, liver injury is self-limited, but rare fatalities have been
rare cases have been observed.

The hepatotoxicity is attributable to the sulfamethoxazole

METHYLDOPA HEPATOTOXICITY (TOXIC AND ht of the drug and is similar in features to that seen with
CRATIC REACTION) Minor alterations in liver tests are r onamides; tissue eosinophilia and granulomas may be seen.
about 5 percent of patients treated with this antihypertensi
These trivial abnormalities typically resolve despite contir
administration. In less than 1 percent of patients, acute li
resembling viral hepatitis, or chronic active hepatitis, or
cholestatic reaction is seen 1 to 20 weeks after methyldopa
In 50 percent of cases the interval is shorter than 4 weeks. A
of fever, anorexia, and malaise may be noted for a few d
the onset of jaundice. Rash, lymphadenopathy, arthra
eosinophilia are rare. Serologic markers of autoimmunity
quently detected, and fewer than 5 percent of patients have
positive hemolytic anemia. In about 15 percent of pat
methyldopa hepatotoxicity, the clinical, biochemical, and
features are those of chronic active hepatitis with or withou
necrosis and macronodular cirrhosis. With discontinuat
drug, the disorder usually resolves, although progression
seen in a few patients.

ISONIAZID HEPATOTOXICITY (TOXIC AND IDIOSYNC
ACTION) In approximately 10 percent of adults treated
antituberculosis agent isoniazid, elevated serum amino
levels develop during the first few weeks of therapy; this
represent an adaptive response to a toxic metabolite of
Whether or not isoniazid is continued, these values (usu
200 units) return to normal in a few weeks. In about 1
treated patients, an illness develops which is indistinguis
viral hepatitis; approximately half of these cases occur wit
2 months of treatment, while in the remainder, clinical c
be delayed for many months. Liver biopsy reveals n
changes similar to those of viral hepatitis or bridging hepat
The disease may be severe, with a case-fatality rate of
Important liver injury appears to be age-related, increasi
tially in frequency after age 35; the highest frequency is
over age 50, the lowest under the age of 20. Isoniazid he
is enhanced by alcohol and rifampicin. Fever, rash, eosin
other manifestations of drug allergy are distinctly unusual
metabolite of acetylhydrazine, a metabolite of isoniaz
responsible for liver injury. A picture resembling chr
hepatitis has been observed in a few patients.

SODIUM VALPROATE HEPATOTOXICITY (TOXIC
SYNCRATIC REACTION) Sodium valproate, an anticon
ful in the treatment of petit mal and other seizure disorde
associated with the development of severe hepatic toxicity
fatalities in both children and adults. Asymptomatic el
serum aminotransferase levels have been recognized in
45 percent of treated patients. These "adaptive" change
appear to have no clinical importance, for major hepatoto
seen in the majority of patients despite continuation of dr
In those rare patients in whom jaundice, encephalopathy, a
of hepatic failure are found, examination of liver tis
microvesicular fat and bridging hepatic necrosis predomir
centrolobular zone. Bile duct injury also may be apparer
likely that sodium valproate is not directly hepatotoxic
metabolite, 4-pentenoic acid, may be responsible for he

PHENYTOIN HEPATOTOXICITY (IDIOSYNCRATIC
Phenytoin, formerly diphenylhydantoin, a mainstay in th
of seizure disorders, has been associated in rare instanc

NCES

titis

al: Hepatitis C virus infection in post-transfusion hepatitis: An analysis with
econd-generation assays. N Engl J Med 325:1325, 1991
al: Detection of antibody to hepatitis C virus in prospectively followed
recipients with acute and chronic non-A, non-B hepatitis. N Engl J Med
1989
al: The clinical significance of molecular variation within the hepatitis B
me. Hepatology 15:144, 1992
THOMAS HC: Genetic variation in hepatitis B virus. Gastroenterology
92
DISEASE CONTROL: Protection against viral hepatitis: Recommendations of
ization Practices Advisory Committee (ACIP). Morb Mort Week Rep
2):1, 1990
al: Isolation of a cDNA clone derived from a blood-borne non-A, non-B
is genome. Science 244:359, 1989
patitis A virus: Insights from molecular biology. Hepatology 9:889, 1989
et al: The natural history of asymptomatic hepatitis B surface antigen
n Intern Med 118:191, 1993
AM et al: Long-term clinical and histologic follow-up of chronic
ion hepatitis. Hepatology 14:969, 1991
Non-A, non-B hepatitis: I. Recognition, epidemiology, and clinical
Experimental transmission, putative virus agents and markers, and
Gastroenterology 85:439, 743, 1983
iral hepatitis. Semin Liver Dis 11:73, 1991
et al: The declining risk of post-transfusion hepatitis C virus infection. N
327:369, 1992
al: High rate of infectivity and liver disease in blood donors with antibodies
virus. Ann Intern Med 115:443, 1991
long-term study of hepatitis C virus replication in non-A, non-B hepatitis.
d 325:98, 1991
et al (eds): Viral Hepatitis and Liver Disease. Baltimore, Williams &
1
: Type D (delta) hepatitis. JAMA 261:1321, 1989
et al: Molecular biology of the hepatitis C viruses: Implications for
velopment and control of viral disease. Hepatology 14:381, 1991
DIENSTAG JL: Prevention and therapy of viral hepatitis. Semin Liver Dis
pe A viral hepatitis: New developments in an old disease. N Engl J Med
85
al: Compact organization of the hepatitis B virus genome. Hepatology

Isolation of a cDNA from the virus responsible for enterically transmitted
B hepatitis. Science 247:1335, 1990
he delta agent. Hepatology 3:729, 1983
A serologic follow-up of the 1942 epidemic of post-vaccination hepatitis
States Army. N Engl J Med 316:965, 1987
(eds): Viral Hepatitis and Liver Disease. Orlando, Grune & Stratton,

et al: A controlled trial of formalin-inactivated hepatitis A vaccine in
en. N Engl J Med 327:453, 1992
(ed): Viral Hepatitis and Liver Disease. New York, Liss, 1988

d hepatitis

Isoniazid-associated hepatitis in 114 patients. Gastroenterology 69:389,

inophen hepatotoxicity. Annu Rev Med 35:577, 1984
l: Cholestatic hepatitis from erythromycin ethylsuccinate. Am J Med

al: Improved outcome of paracetamol-induced fulminant hepatic failure
istration of acetylcysteine. Lancet 335:1572, 1990
NS: Hepatic injury associated with the phenothiazines: Clinicopathologic
study of 36 patients. Arch Pathol 93:283, 1972
(ed): Recent advances in drug metabolism and hepatotoxicity. Semin
33, 1990
rug-induced hepatotoxicity. Ann Intern Med 104:826, 1986

ular hepati-
ation of the
iver lobule.
ly resolving
rtal fibrosis
progression
Thus chronic
ic persistent
tory features
ronic lobular
notransferase
and transient
qualifications
stent hepatitis

characterized
rtal and, to a
g in severity
nized to be a
re, and death.
include (1) a
re substantially
e, plasma cells
uction of the
of the limiting
lled piecemeal
rtal tracts and
g parenchymal
4) evidence of
kened liver cell
may be patchy,
fuse. Histologic
ilman or acido-
neal necrosis is
nosis of chronic
mild, relatively
A more severe
ubacute hepatic
e form of chronic
een occasionally
s no prognostic
n is associated
characterized by
between portal
rtal tracts and
Collapse of the
is, and bridging
reorganization by
sive and ominous
llapse, in which
ver and which is
even acute liver

to demonstrate in
solated piecemeal
patitis, progression
nic active hepatitis
rhosis, even early
es of "cryptogenic"
ic active hepatitis.
ere clinically than
a sizable proportion
omatic, the majority
nptoms, especially
vary depending on
will be discussed
with chronic liver
n, aminotransferase

levels tend to be higher, and jaundice and hyperbilirubinemia are more frequent in this form of chronic hepatitis.

CHRONIC VIRAL HEPATITIS Both the enterically transmitted forms of viral hepatitis, hepatitis A and E, are self-limited and do not cause chronic hepatitis (rare reports notwithstanding in which acute hepatitis A serves as a trigger for the onset of autoimmune chronic active hepatitis in genetically susceptible patients). In contrast, the entire clinicopathologic spectrum of chronic hepatitis occurs in patients with chronic viral hepatitis B and C as well as in patients with chronic hepatitis D superimposed on chronic hepatitis B.

Chronic hepatitis B The likelihood of chronicity after acute hepatitis B varies as a function of age. Infection at birth is associated with a clinically silent acute infection but a 90 percent chance of chronic infection, while infection in young adulthood is associated typically with clinically apparent acute hepatitis but a risk of chronicity of only 1 to 2 percent. Most cases of chronic hepatitis B among adults, however, occur in patients who never had a recognized episode of clinically apparent acute viral hepatitis. The degree of liver injury in patients with chronic hepatitis B is variable, ranging from none in asymptomatic carriers, to mild in chronic persistent hepatitis, to severe in chronic active hepatitis. Among adults with chronic hepatitis B, histologic features are of prognostic importance. In one long-term study of patients with chronic hepatitis B, investigators found a 5-year survival of 97 percent for patients with chronic persistent hepatitis, of 86 percent for patients with chronic active hepatitis, and of only 55 percent for patients with chronic active hepatitis and postnecrotic cirrhosis. On the other hand, more recent observations do not allow us to be so sanguine about the prognosis in patients with chronic persistent hepatitis; among patients with chronic persistent hepatitis followed for 1 to 13 years, progression to chronic active hepatitis and cirrhosis has been observed in more than a quarter of cases.

Probably more important to consider than histology alone in patients with chronic hepatitis B is the degree of hepatitis B virus (HBV) replication. As reviewed in Chap. 266, chronic hepatitis B can be divided into two phases based on the relative level of HBV replication. The relatively *replicative phase* is characterized by the presence in the serum of markers of HBV replication (HBeAg, HBV DNA), by the presence in the liver of detectable intrahepatocyte nucleocapsid antigens (primarily HBcAg), by high infectivity, and by accompanying liver injury; HBV DNA can be detected in the liver but is extrachromosomal. In contrast, the relatively *nonreplicative phase* is characterized by the absence of conventional markers of HBV replication (HBeAg and HBV DNA detectable by hybridization) but associated with anti-HBe, the absence of intrahepatocytic HBcAg, limited infectivity, and minimal liver injury; HBV DNA can be detected in the liver integrated into the host genome. Those in the replicative phase tend to have more severe chronic hepatitis (e.g., chronic active hepatitis), while those in the nonreplicative phase tend to have mild chronic hepatitis (chronic persistent hepatitis) or to be asymptomatic hepatitis B carriers; however, distinctions in HBV replication and in histologic category do not always coincide. The likelihood of converting spontaneously from relatively replicative to

nonreplicative chronic HBV infection is approximately 10 to 15 percent per year. As noted in Chap. 266, the conversion from replicative to nonreplicative chronic hepatitis B is associated with a transient elevation in aminotransferase activity resembling acute hepatitis; occasionally, spontaneous resumptions of replicative activity occur in nonreplicative infection; and rarely, HBV variants occur in which serologic markers of replication (HBeAg) are absent, despite the presence of replicative infection. As reviewed in Chap. 269, chronic HBV infection, especially when acquired at birth or in early childhood, is associated with an increased risk of hepatocellular carcinoma. A discussion of the pathogenesis of liver injury in patients with chronic hepatitis B appears in Chap. 266.

The spectrum of *clinical features* of chronic hepatitis B is broad, ranging from asymptomatic infection to debilitating disease or even end-stage, fatal hepatic failure. As noted above, the onset of the disease tends to be insidious in most patients, with the exception of the very few in whom chronic disease follows failure of resolution of clinically apparent acute hepatitis B. The clinical and laboratory features associated with progression from acute to chronic hepatitis B are discussed in Chap. 266. *Fatigue* is a common symptom, and persistent or intermittent *jaundice* is a common feature in severe or advanced cases. Intermittent deepening of jaundice and recurrence of malaise and anorexia, as well as worsening fatigue, are reminiscent of acute hepatitis; such exacerbations may occur spontaneously, often coinciding with evidence of virologic reactivation, may lead to progressive liver injury, and when superimposed on well-established cirrhosis, may cause hepatic decompensation. Complications of cirrhosis occur in end-stage chronic active hepatitis and include ascites, edema, bleeding gastroesophageal varices, hepatic encephalopathy, coagulopathy, or hypersplenism. Occasionally, these complications bring the patient to initial clinical attention. Extrahepatic complications of chronic hepatitis B, similar to those seen during the prodromal phase of acute hepatitis B, are associated with deposition of circulating hepatitis B antigen-antibody immune complexes. As reviewed in Chap. 266, these include arthralgias and arthritis, which are common, and the more rare purpuric cutaneous lesions (leukocytoclastic vasculitis), immune-complex glomerulonephritis, and generalized vasculitis (polyarteritis nodosa).

Laboratory features of chronic hepatitis B do not distinguish adequately between histologically mild and severe hepatitis. Aminotransferase elevations tend to be modest for chronic hepatitis B but may fluctuate in the range of 100 to 1000 units. As is true for acute viral hepatitis B, alanine aminotransferase (ALT or SGPT) tends to be more elevated than aspartate aminotransferase (AST or SGOT); however, once cirrhosis is established, AST tends to exceed ALT. Levels of alkaline phosphatase activity tend to be normal or only marginally elevated. In severe cases, moderate elevations in serum bilirubin (3 to 10 mg/dL or 51.3 to 171 µmol/L) occur. Hypoalbuminemia and prolongation of the prothrombin time occur in severe or end-stage cases. Hyperglobulinemia and detectable circulating autoantibodies are distinctly absent in chronic hepatitis B (in contrast to autoimmune chronic active hepatitis). Viral markers of chronic HBV infection are discussed in Chap. 266.

TABLE 267-1 Clinical and laboratory features of chronic hepatitis

Type of hepatitis	Diagnostic test(s)	Autoantibodies	Therapy
Chronic hepatitis B	HBsAg, IgG anti-HBc, HBeAg, HBV DNA	Uncommon	Interferon-α
Chronic hepatitis C	Anti-HCV (EIA* and RIBA‡), HCV RNA	Anti-LKM1†	Interferon-α
Chronic hepatitis D	Anti-HDV, HDV RNA, HBsAg, IgG anti-HBc	Anti-LKM3	Interferon-α (?)
Autoimmune chronic active hepatitis	ANA (homogeneous), anti-LKM1(±), hyperglobulinemia	ANA, anti-LKM1	Prednisone, azathioprine

* Enzyme immunoassay.
† Antibodies to liver-kidney microsomes type 1.
‡ Recombinant immunoblot assay.

Management of chronic hepatitis B depends on the level of virus replication. Although progression to cirrhosis is more likely in chronic active than in chronic persistent or lobular hepatitis B, all three forms of chronic viral hepatitis can be progressive. Randomized, prospective, controlled trials have established that patients with well-compensated chronic replicative hepatitis B, selected to have chronic hepatitis on liver biopsy and aminotransferase elevations, regardless of histologic features, respond to antiviral therapy with interferon-α. A 4-month (16-week) course of subcutaneous injections, daily at a dose of 5 million units or three times a week at a dose of 10 million units, is associated with an approximately 40 percent seroconversion from replicative (HBeAg and HBV DNA detectable in serum) to nonreplicative (anti-HBe detectable) HBV infection, with a concomitant improvement in liver histologic features and an approximately 10 percent chance of losing detectable HBsAg. In most cases, successful interferon therapy and seroconversion is accompanied by an acute hepatitis–like elevation in aminotransferase activity, which is believed to represent an immunostimulatory effect of interferon on the interaction between the cellular immune system and virus-infected hepatocytes. Relapse after successful therapy is rare indeed (1 to 2 percent). The likelihood of responding to interferon is higher in patients with moderate to low levels of HBV DNA (<200 pg/mL) and in patients with substantial elevations of aminotransferase activities (e.g., >100 to 200 units). The likelihood of losing HBsAg *during therapy* is increased in patients with brief-duration disease (mean duration 1½ years); followed sufficiently long after successful interferon-induced loss of replicative markers, approximately 70 percent of such patients have been observed to lose HBsAg, i.e., all serologic markers of infection, over a 5-year period. Immunosuppressed patients with chronic hepatitis B do not appear to be responsive to interferon therapy.

Complications of interferon therapy include systemic "flulike" symptoms, marrow suppression, emotional lability (irritability commonly, depression rarely), autoimmune reactions (especially autoimmune thyroiditis), and miscellaneous side effects such as alopecia, rashes, diarrhea, and numbness and tingling of the extremities. With the possible exception of autoimmune thyroiditis, all these side effects are reversible upon dose lowering or cessation of therapy.

In patients with chronic active hepatitis B, long-term therapy with glucocorticoids is not only ineffective but also detrimental. Under certain circumstances, however, the predicted impact of glucocorticoids on HBV and the immune system can be exploited for the patient's benefit. Glucocorticoids increase HBV replication and expression in hepatocytes and depress the activity of cytolytic T cells. Theoretically, then, if steroids are administered for a brief time and then withdrawn, cytolytic T cells, suppressed while HBV replication was being steroid-induced, could resume their presteroid function and be capable of attacking and destroying the new crop of HBV antigen–expressing hepatocytes. Such appears to be the case; an acute hepatitis–like elevation of aminotransferase activity follows and may be accompanied by a dramatic drop in, or even a loss of, HBV replication. A preliminary 6-week period of glucocorticoid therapy (prednisone at doses of 60 mg for 2 weeks, 40 mg for 2 weeks, and 20 mg for 2 weeks), followed by its abrupt withdrawal, has been shown to be of benefit in conjunction with interferon therapy (5 million units subcutaneously daily for 4 months) in patients with chronic hepatitis B, primarily those with near-normal or only modest elevations in aminotransferase levels.

No treatment is indicated or available for asymptomatic, nonreplicative hepatitis B carriers, and antiviral therapy should be withheld from patients with decompensated hepatitis B, in whom treatment may be associated with hepatic decompensation. Such patients should be referred to research centers involved in clinical trials. Other interferons and several nucleoside analogues active against HBV are being evaluated in experimental trials.

For patients with end-stage chronic hepatitis B, liver transplantation is the only potential lifesaving intervention. Reinfection of the new liver is almost universal; however, the likelihood of liver injury associated with hepatitis B in the new liver is variable. The majority of patients become high-level viremic carriers with minimal liver injury. Unfortunately, an unpredictable proportion experience severe hepatitis B–related liver injury, sometimes a fulminant-like hepatitis, sometimes a rapid recapitulation of the original severe chronic hepatitis B (see Chap. 271).

Chronic hepatitis D (delta hepatitis)   The clinical and laboratory features of chronic HDV infection are summarized in Chap. 266. Chronic hepatitis D may follow acute coinfection with HBV but at a rate no higher than the rate of chronicity of hepatitis B. That is, although HDV coinfection can increase the severity of acute hepatitis B, HDV does not increase the likelihood of progression to chronic hepatitis B. When, however, HDV superinfection occurs in a person who is already chronically infected with HBV, long-term HDV infection is the rule and a worsening of the liver disease the expected consequence. Except for severity, chronic hepatitis B plus D has similar clinical and laboratory features to those seen in chronic hepatitis B alone. Chronic active hepatitis, with or without cirrhosis, is the rule and chronic persistent hepatitis the exception. A distinguishing serologic feature of chronic hepatitis D is the presence in the circulation of antibodies to liver-kidney microsomes (anti-LKM); however, the anti-LKM seen in hepatitis D are designated anti-LKM3 and are distinct from anti-LKM1 seen in patients with autoimmune chronic active hepatitis and in a subset of patients with chronic hepatitis C.

Management is not well defined. Glucocorticoids are ineffective and are not used. Preliminary experimental trials of interferon-α suggested that conventional doses and durations of therapy lower levels of HDV RNA and aminotransferase activity only transiently during treatment but have no impact on the natural history of the disease. A more recent trial suggests that high-dose interferon-α (9 million units) three times a week for 12 months may be associated with a sustained loss of HDV replication and clinical improvement in up to 50 percent of patients. Antiviral therapy for chronic hepatitis D remains the subject of experimental trials. In patients with end-stage liver disease secondary to chronic hepatitis D, liver transplantation has been effective. If hepatitis D recurs in the new liver without the expression of hepatitis B (an unusual serologic profile in immunocompetent persons, but common in transplant patients), liver injury is limited. In fact, the outcome of transplantation for chronic hepatitis D is superior to that for chronic hepatitis B (see Chap. 271).

Chronic hepatitis C (non-A, non-B hepatitis)   Regardless of the epidemiologic mode of acquisition of HCV infection, chronicity follows acute hepatitis C in approximately 50 percent of cases. What is more, in patients with chronic transfusion-associated hepatitis followed for 10 years, progression to cirrhosis has been recorded in 20 percent. Such is the case even for patients with relatively clinically mild chronic hepatitis, including those without symptoms, with only modest elevations of aminotransferase activity, and with chronic persistent hepatitis on liver biopsy. Even in cohorts of well-compensated patients with chronic hepatitis C (no complications of chronic liver disease and with normal hepatic synthetic function), the prevalance of cirrhosis may be as high as 50 percent. Many cases of hepatitis C are identified in asymptomatic patients who have no history of acute hepatitis C, e.g., those discovered while attempting to donate blood or as a result of routine laboratory screening tests. The source of HCV infection in most of these cases remains a mystery, and the natural history of chronic hepatitis C identified under these circumstances is unknown. Among asymptomatic persons with anti-HCV, even when aminotransferase levels are normal, between a third and a half have been reported to have chronic hepatitis on liver biopsy. In these asymptomatic persons with normal aminotransferase levels, the presence of detectable circulating HCV RNA appears to distinguish those with chronic hepatitis on biopsy from those with normal liver histology.

Despite this substantial rate of progression of chronic hepatitis C, and despite the fact that liver failure can result from end-stage chronic hepatitis C, the long-term prognosis for chronic hepatitis C in a majority of patients is relatively benign. Mortality over 10 to 20 years among patients with transfusion-associated chronic hepatitis C (non-A, non-B hepatitis) has been shown not to differ from mortality in a matched population of transfused patients in whom non-A, non-B hepatitis did not develop. Although death in the hepatitis group is more likely to result from liver failure, and although hepatic decompensation may occur in approximately 15 percent of such patients over the course of a decade, the majority (almost 60 percent) of patients remain asymptomatic and well compensated, with no clinical sequelae of chronic liver disease. Overall, then, chronic hepatitis C tends to be very slowly and insidiously progressive. The impact of relative levels of HCV replication or of HCV genotype on long-term prognosis in patients with chronic hepatitis C has not been studied. On the other hand, severity of chronic hepatitis is greater and progression of chronic liver disease is more accelerated in patients who have chronic hepatitis C as well as other liver processes, including alcoholic liver disease, chronic hepatitis B, and α_1-antitrypsin deficiency. No other epidemiologic or clinical features of chronic hepatitis C (e.g., severity of acute hepatitis, level of aminotransferase activity, presence or absence of jaundice) are predictive of eventual outcome. Despite its relative benignity over time, cirrhosis following chronic hepatitis C has been associated with the late development, after several decades, of hepatocellular carcinoma (see Chap. 269).

Clinical features of chronic hepatitis C are similar to those described above for chronic hepatitis B. Generally, *fatigue* is the most common symptom; jaundice is rare. Extrahepatic complications of chronic hepatitis C are less common than they are in chronic hepatitis B, with the exception of essential mixed cryoglobulinemia (see Chap. 266). *Laboratory features* of chronic hepatitis C are similar to those in patients with chronic hepatitis B, but aminotransferase levels tend to fluctuate more (the characteristic episodic pattern of aminotransferase activity) and to be lower, especially in patients with long-standing disease. An interesting and occasionally confusing finding in patients with chronic hepatitis C is the presence of autoantibodies. Rarely, patients with autoimmune chronic active hepatitis (see below) and hyperglobulinemia have false-positive enzyme immunoassays for anti-HCV. On the other hand, a proportion of patients with serologically confirmable chronic hepatitis C have circulating autoantibodies to liver-kidney microsomes (anti-LKM). These antibodies are anti-KLM1, as seen in patients with autoimmune chronic active hepatitis *type 2* (see below), and are directed against a 33-amino-acid sequence of P450 IID6. The occurrence of anti-KLM1 in some patients with chronic hepatitis C may result from the partial sequence homology between the epitope recognized by anti-LKM1 and two segments of the HCV polyprotein. In addition, the finding of this autoantibody in some patients with chronic hepatitis C suggests that autoimmunity may be playing a role in the pathogenesis of chronic hepatitis C. Histopathologic features of chronic hepatitis C, especially those which distinguish hepatitis C from hepatitis B, are described in Chap. 266.

In the *management* of chronic hepatitis C, glucocorticoids are ineffective. Based on the outcome of prospective, randomized, controlled clinical trials, interferon-α has been approved for the treatment of chronic hepatitis C. Doses ranging from 2 to 5 million units three times a week have been shown to be effective in these trials, but the officially approved dose recommendation is 3 million units by subcutaneous injection three times a week for 6 months (24 weeks). This regimen is associated with a likelihood of biochemical response (return of ALT to normal or a 50 percent reduction of ALT to within 1.5 times the upper limit of normal) in approximately 50 percent of patients. Unlike hepatitis B, in chronic hepatitis C a successful response to interferon is not accompanied by an acute hepatitis–like elevation in aminotransferase activity; instead, ALT levels fall precipitously. Between 85 and 90 percent of responses occur within the first 3 months of therapy; responses thereafter are rare. In addition, histologic improvement in periportal and lobular inflammation has been demonstrated, primarily in biochemically responding patients, but also in biochemical nonresponders. After

completion of 6 months of therapy, at least 50 percent of responding patients experience a biochemical relapse. Thus the likelihood of a sustained response is no greater than 25 percent. In those who relapse after responding, however, retreatment with interferon leads invariably to response again. Neither longer initial therapy, e.g., for 12 months, nor higher-dose therapy lowers the frequency of relapse. Whether sustained, long-term even indefinite therapy will be necessary or effective in those who relapse remains to be determined. Similarly, the impact of short-term therapy on the long-term natural history of chronic hepatitis C continues to be studied.

Levels of HCV RNA fall in tandem with ALT levels during interferon therapy, but loss of detectable HCV RNA does not preclude relapse. In fact, no single clinical or laboratory feature of chronic hepatitis C has been found which is predictive of responsiveness to interferon. Responses occur in patients with established cirrhosis, although, some observers report, at a frequency lower than that seen in patients with chronic active hepatitis without cirrhosis. Some observers report that responsiveness in chronic persistent hepatitis exceeds that in chronic active hepatitis.

Although a consensus exists that patients with symptomatic chronic active hepatitis should be treated with interferon, treatment of asymptomatic patients and those with mild chronic persistent hepatitis remains controversial. Because progression to cirrhosis can occur in an unpredictable proportion of such cases, the potential benefit of therapy should not be dismissed out of hand in these patients. Additional study is needed. Currently, no authorities advocate treating asymptomatic hepatitis C "carriers" with normal aminotransferase levels or patients with decompensated cirrhosis secondary to chronic hepatitis C. For those with decompensated, end-stage disease, liver transplantation is an option. Although the likelihood of reexpressing detectable anti-HCV after transplantation is low, the likelihood of reinfection of the new liver is almost universal. Nevertheless, and the occasional exception notwithstanding, most patients who undergo liver transplantation for chronic hepatitis C experience little, if any, morbidity, allograft loss, or mortality associated with recurrent hepatitis C infection (see Chap. 271).

AUTOIMMUNE CHRONIC ACTIVE HEPATITIS **Definition** Autoimmune chronic active hepatitis is a chronic disorder characterized by continuing hepatocellular necrosis and inflammation, usually with fibrosis, which tends to progress to cirrhosis and liver failure. When fulfilling criteria of severity, this type of chronic active hepatitis may have a 6-month mortality of as high as 40 percent. The prominence of extrahepatic features of autoimmunity as well as seroimmunologic abnormalities in this disorder supports an autoimmune process in its pathogenesis, and this concept is reflected in the labels "lupoid," plasma cell, or autoimmune chronic active hepatitis. Because autoantibodies and other typical features of autoimmunity do not occur in all cases, however, a broader, more appropriate designation for this type of chronic active hepatitis is "idiopathic" or cryptogenic. Cases in which hepatotropic viruses, metabolic/genetic derangements, and hepatotoxic drugs have been excluded merit this designation and probably include a spectrum of heterogeneous liver disorders of unknown cause, a proportion of which have characteristic autoimmune features.

Immunopathogenesis The weight of evidence suggests that the progressive liver injury in patients with idiopathic/autoimmune chronic active hepatitis is the result of a cell-mediated immunologic attack directed against liver cells; in all likelihood, predisposition to autoimmunity is inherited, while the liver specificity of this injury is triggered by environmental (e.g., chemical or viral) factors. For example, patients have been described in whom apparently self-limited cases of acute hepatitis A or B led to autoimmune chronic active hepatitis, presumably because of genetic susceptibility or predisposition. Evidence to support an autoimmune pathogenesis in chronic active hepatitis includes the following: (1) In the liver, the histopathologic lesions are composed predominantly of cytotoxic T cells and plasma cells; (2) circulating autoantibodies (nuclear, smooth muscle, thyroid, etc.; see below), rheumatoid factor, and hyperglobulinemia are common; (3) other autoimmune disorders—such as thyroiditis, rheumatoid arthritis, autoimmune hemolytic anemia, ulcerative colitis, proliferative glomerulonephritis, juvenile diabetes mellitus, and Sjögren's syndrome—occur with increased frequency in patients who have chronic active hepatitis and in their relatives; (4) histocompatibility haplotypes associated with autoimmune diseases, such as HLA-B1, -B8, -DRw3, and -DRw4, are common in patients with autoimmune chronic active hepatitis; and (5) this type of chronic active hepatitis is responsive to glucocorticoid/immunosuppressive therapy, effective in a variety of autoimmune disorders.

Cellular immune mechanisms appear to be important in the pathogenesis of autoimmune chronic active hepatitis. In vitro studies have suggested that in patients with this disorder, lymphocytes are capable of becoming sensitized to hepatocyte membrane proteins and of destroying liver cells. Abnormalities of immunoregulatory control over cytotoxic lymphocytes (impaired suppressor cell influences) may play a role as well. Studies of genetic predisposition to autoimmune chronic active hepatitis demonstrate that certain haplotypes are associated with the disorder. These include HLA-B8, -DR3, -Dw3 and certain complement alleles, C2 and C4. The precise triggering factors, genetic influences, and cytotoxic and immunoregulatory mechanisms involved in this type of liver injury remain poorly defined.

Intriguing clues into the pathogenesis of chronic active hepatitis come from the observation that circulating autoantibodies are prevalent in patients with this disorder. Among the autoantibodies described in these patients are antibodies to nuclei (so-called antinuclear antibodies, ANA, primarily in a homogeneous pattern), smooth muscle (so-called anti-smooth-muscle antibodies, ASMA, directed at actin), antibodies to liver-kidney microsomes (anti-LKM; see below), antibodies to "soluble liver antigen" (anti-SLA, directed at cytokeratins), as well as antibodies to the liver-specific asialoglycoprotein receptor (or "hepatic lectin") and other hepatocyte membrane proteins. Although some of these provide helpful diagnostic markers, their involvement in the pathogenesis of autoimmune chronic active hepatitis has not been established.

Humoral immune mechanisms have been shown to play a role in the extrahepatic manifestations of chronic active hepatitis. Arthralgias, arthritis, cutaneous vasculitis, and glomerulonephritis occurring in patients with autoimmune (and viral) chronic active hepatitis appear to be mediated by the deposition in affected tissue vessels of circulating immune complexes, followed by complement activation, inflammation, and tissue injury. While specific viral antigen-antibody complexes can be identified in acute and chronic viral hepatitis, the nature of the immune complexes in autoimmune chronic active hepatitis has not been defined.

Many of the *clinical features* of autoimmune chronic active hepatitis are similar to those described for chronic viral hepatitis. The onset of disease may be insidious or abrupt; the disease may present initially like, and be confused with, acute viral hepatitis; and a history of recurrent bouts of what had been labeled acute hepatitis is not uncommon. A subset of patients with autoimmune chronic active hepatitis has distinct features. Such patients are predominantly young to middle-aged women with marked hyperglobulinemia and high-titer circulating ANA. This is the group with positive LE preparations (initially labeled "lupoid" hepatitis) in whom other autoimmune features are common. Fatigue, malaise, anorexia, amenorrhea, acne, arthralgias, and jaundice are common. Occasionally, arthritis, maculopapular eruptions (including cutaneous vasculitis), erythema nodosum, colitis, pleurisy, pericarditis, anemia, azotemia, and sicca syndrome (keratoconjunctivitis, xerostomia) occur. In some patients, complications of cirrhosis, such as ascites and edema (associated with hypoalbuminemia), encephalopathy, hypersplenism, coagulopathy, or variceal bleeding, may bring the patient to initial medical attention.

The course of chronic active hepatitis may be variable. In those with mild disease or limited histologic lesions (e.g., piecemeal necrosis without bridging), progression to cirrhosis is limited. In those with severe symptomatic chronic active hepatitis (aminotransfer-

ase levels >10 times normal, marked hyperglobulinemia, "aggressive" histologic lesions—bridging necrosis or multilobular collapse, cirrhosis), the 6-month mortality without therapy may be as high as 40 percent. Such severe disease accounts for only 20 percent of cases; the natural history of milder disease is variable, often accentuated by spontaneous remissions and exacerbations. Especially poor prognostic signs include multilobular collapse at the time of initial presentation and failure of the bilirubin to improve after 2 weeks of therapy. Death may result from hepatic failure, hepatic coma, other complications of cirrhosis (e.g., variceal hemorrhage), and intercurrent infection. In patients with established cirrhosis, hepatocellular carcinoma may be a late complication (see Chap. 269).

Laboratory features of autoimmune chronic active hepatitis are similar to those seen in chronic viral hepatitis. Liver biochemical tests are invariably abnormal but may not correlate with the clinical severity or histopathologic features in individual cases. Many patients with chronic active hepatitis have normal serum bilirubin, alkaline phosphatase, and globulin levels with only minimal aminotransferase elevations. Serum aspartate aminotransferase (AST or SGOT) and alanine aminotransferase (ALT or SGPT) levels are increased and fluctuate in the range of 100 to 1000 units. In severe cases, the serum bilirubin level is moderately elevated [51 to 171 μmol/L (3 to 10 mg/dL)]. Mild hypoalbuminemia occurs in patients with very active or advanced disease. Serum alkaline phosphatase levels may be moderately elevated or near normal. In a small proportion of patients, marked elevations of alkaline phosphatase activity occur; in such patients, clinical and laboratory features overlap with those of primary biliary cirrhosis (see Chap. 268). The prothrombin time is often prolonged, particularly late in the disease or during active phases.

Hypergammaglobulinemia (>2.5 g/dL) is common in autoimmune chronic active hepatitis. Rheumatoid factor is common as well. As noted above, circulating autoantibodies are also common. The most characteristic are antinuclear antibodies (ANA) in a homogeneous staining pattern. Smooth-muscle antibodies are less specific, seen just as frequently in chronic viral hepatitis. Because of the high levels of globulins achieved in the circulation of some patients with autoimmune chronic active hepatitis, occasionally the globulins may bind nonspecifically in solid-phase binding immunoassays for viral antibodies. This has been recognized most commonly in tests for antibodies to hepatitis C virus, as noted above. In fact, studies of autoantibodies in chronic active hepatitis have led to the recognition of new categories of autoimmune chronic active hepatitis. *Type I* autoimmune chronic active hepatitis is the classic syndrome occurring in young women, associated with marked hyperglobulinemia, lupoid features, and circulating ANA. *Type II* autoimmune chronic active hepatitis, often seen in children and more common in Mediterranean populations, is associated not with ANA but with antibodies to liver-kidney microsomal antigens (anti-LKM). Actually, anti-LKM represent a heterogeneous group of antibodies. In type II autoimmune chronic active hepatitis, the antibody is anti-LKM1, directed against P450 IID6. This is the same anti-LKM seen in some patients with chronic hepatitis C. Anti-LKM2 is seen in drug-induced hepatitis, and anti-LKM3 is seen in patients with chronic hepatitis D. Type II autoimmune chronic active hepatitis has been subdivided by some authorities into two categories, one more typically autoimmune and the other associated with viral hepatitis type C. Autoimmune chronic active hepatitis type 2a is felt to be autoimmune, is more likely to occur in young women, is associated with hyperglobulinemia, is associated with high-titer anti-LKM1, responds to glucocorticoid therapy, and is seen commonly in western Europe and the United Kingdom. Type 2b chronic active hepatitis is associated with hepatitis C virus infection, tends to occur in older men, is associated with normal globulin levels and low-titer anti-LKM1, responds to interferon, and occurs most commonly in Mediterranean countries.

The mainstay of *management* in autoimmune or idiopathic (nonviral) chronic active hepatitis is glucocorticoid therapy. Several controlled clinical trials have documented that such therapy leads to symptomatic, clinical, biochemical, and histologic improvement as well as increased survival. A therapeutic response can be expected in up to 80 percent of patients. Unfortunately, therapy has not been shown to prevent ultimate progression to cirrhosis. Although some advocate the use of prednisolone, the hepatic metabolite of prednisone, prednisone is just as effective and is favored by most authorities. Therapy may be initiated at 20 mg/d, but a popular regimen in the United States relies on an initiation dose of 60 mg/d. This high dose is tapered successively over the course of a month down to a maintenance level of 20 mg/d. An alternative, but equally effective, approach is to begin with half the prednisone dose (30 mg/d) along with azathioprine (50 mg/d). The advantage of the combination approach is a reduction, over the course of an 18-month course of therapy, in serious, life-threatening complications of steroid therapy from 66 percent down to under 20 percent. Azathioprine alone, however, is not effective in achieving remission, nor is alternate-day glucocorticoid therapy. Although therapy has been shown to be effective for severe chronic active hepatitis, therapy is not indicated for chronic persistent hepatitis or chronic lobular hepatitis, and the efficacy of therapy in mild or asymptomatic chronic active hepatitis has not been established.

Improvement of fatigue, anorexia, malaise, and jaundice tends to occur within days to several weeks; biochemical improvement occurs over the course of several weeks to months, with a fall in serum bilirubin and globulin levels and an increase in serum albumin. Serum aminotransferase levels usually drop promptly, but improvements in AST and ALT alone do not appear to be a reliable marker of recovery in individual patients; histologic improvement, characterized by a decrease in mononuclear infiltration and in hepatocellular necrosis— conversion from chronic active hepatitis to a less severe lesion, such as chronic persistent hepatitis—may be delayed for 6 to 24 months. Still, if interpreted cautiously, aminotransferase levels are valuable indicators of relative disease activity, and many authorities do *not* advocate serial liver biopsies to assess therapeutic success or to guide decisions to alter or stop therapy. Therapy must continue for at least 12 to 18 months. After tapering and cessation of therapy, the likelihood of relapse is at least 50 percent, even if posttreatment histology has improved to show chronic persistent hepatitis, and the majority of patients require therapy at maintenance doses indefinitely. Continuing azathioprine alone after cessation of prednisone therapy may reduce the frequency of relapse.

If medical therapy fails, or when chronic active hepatitis progresses to cirrhosis and is associated with life-threatening complications of liver decompensation, liver transplantation is the only recourse (see Chap. 271). Recurrence of autoimmune chronic active hepatitis in the new liver has not been documented to occur.

DIFFERENTIAL DIAGNOSIS Early during the course of chronic active hepatitis, the disease may resemble typical *acute viral hepatitis*. Without histologic assessment, chronic active hepatitis cannot be readily distinguished based on clinical or biochemical criteria from *chronic persistent hepatitis* and *chronic lobular hepatitis*. In adolescence, *Wilson's disease* may present with features of chronic active hepatitis long before neurologic manifestations become apparent and before the formation of Kayser-Fleischer rings; in this age group, serum ceruloplasmin and serum and urinary copper determinations and measurement of liver copper levels will establish the correct diagnosis. *Postnecrotic* or *cryptogenic cirrhosis* and *primary biliary cirrhosis* share clinical features with chronic active hepatitis; biochemical, serologic, and histologic assessments are usually sufficient to allow these entities to be distinguished from chronic active hepatitis. Of course, the distinction between autoimmune ("idiopathic") and viral chronic active hepatitis is not always straightforward, especially when viral antibodies occur in patients with autoimmune disease or when autoantibodies occur in patients with viral disease. Finally, the presence of extrahepatic features such as arthritis, cutaneous vasculitis, or pleuritis—not to mention the presence of circulating autoantibodies—may cause confusion with *rheumatologic disorders* such as rheumatoid arthritis and systemic lupus erythematosus. The existence of clinical and biochemical features of progressive necroinflammatory

liver disease distinguishes chronic active hepatitis from these other disorders, which are not associated with severe liver disease.

REFERENCES

CZAJA AJ et al: Laboratory assessment of severe chronic active liver disease during and after corticosteroid therapy: Correlation of serum transaminase and gamma globulin levels with histologic features. Gastroenterology 80:687, 1981

——— et al: Sustained remission after corticosteroid therapy of severe hepatitis B surface antigen-negative chronic active hepatitis. Gastroenterology 92:215, 1987

——— et al: Features reflective of early prognosis in corticosteroid-treated severe autoimmune chronic active hepatitis. Gastroenterology 95:448, 1988

——— et al: Frequency and significance of antibodies to liver/kidney microsome type 1 in adults with chronic active hepatitis. Gastroenterology 103:1290, 1992

DAVIS GL et al: Treatment of chronic hepatitis C with recombinant interferon alfa: A multicenter randomized, controlled trial. N Engl J Med 321:1501, 1989

DIENSTAG JL, ISSELBACHER KJ: Therapy for acute and chronic hepatitis. Arch Intern Med 141:1419, 1981

FATTOVICH G et al: Natural history and prognostic factors for chronic hepatitis type B. Gut 32:294, 1991

HOMBERG J-C et al: Chronic active hepatitis associated with antiliver/kidney microsome antibody type 1: A second type of "autoimmune" hepatitis. Hepatology 7:1333, 1987

KATKOV WN, DIENSTAG JL: Prevention and therapy of viral hepatitis. Semin Liver Dis 11:165, 1991

KRAWITT EL, WEISNER RH (eds): *Autoimmune Liver Diseases.* New York, Raven, 1991

LUNEL F et al: Liver/kidney microsome antibody type 1 and hepatitis C virus infection. Hepatology 16:630, 1992

MEYER ZUM BÜSCHENFELDE K-H (ed): Autoimmune hepatitis. Semin Liver Dis 11:183, 1991

PERRILLO RP et al: A randomized, controlled trial of interferon alpha-2b alone and after prednisone withdrawal for the treatment of chronic hepatitis B. N Engl J Med 323:295, 1990

SEEFF LB et al: Long-term mortality after transfusion-associated non-A, non-B hepatitis. N Engl J Med 327:1906, 1992

STELLON AJ et al: Maintenance of remission in autoimmune chronic active hepatitis with azathioprine after corticosteroid withdrawal. Hepatology 8:781, 1988

SUMMERSKILL WHJ et al: Prednisone for chronic active liver disease: Dose titration, standard dose, and combination with azathioprine compared. Gut 16:876, 1975

WEISSBERG JI et al: Survival in chronic hepatitis B: An analysis of 379 patients. Ann Intern Med 101:613, 1984

268 ALCOHOL-RELATED LIVER DISEASE AND CIRRHOSIS

DANIEL K. PODOLSKY / KURT J. ISSELBACHER

Cirrhosis is a pathologically defined entity which is associated with a spectrum of characteristic clinical manifestations. The cardinal pathologic features reflect irreversible chronic injury of the hepatic parenchyma and include extensive fibrosis in association with the formation of regenerative nodules. These features result from hepatocyte necrosis, collapse of the supporting reticulin network with subsequent connective tissue deposition, distortion of the vascular bed, and nodular regeneration of remaining liver parenchyma. The pathologic process should be viewed as a final common pathway of many types of chronic liver injury. Clinical features of cirrhosis derive from the morphologic alterations and often reflect the severity of hepatic damage rather than the etiology of the underlying liver disease. Loss of functioning hepatocellular mass may lead to jaundice, edema, coagulopathy, and a variety of metabolic abnormalities; fibrosis and distorted vasculature lead to portal hypertension and its sequelae, including gastroesophageal varices and splenomegaly. Ascites and hepatic encephalopathy result from both hepatocellular insufficiency and portal hypertension.

Classification of the various types of cirrhosis based solely on etiology or morphology is unsatisfactory. A single pathologic pattern may result from a variety of insults, while the same insult may produce several morphologic patterns. Nevertheless, most types of cirrhosis may be usefully classified by a mixture of etiologically and morphologically defined entities as follows: (1) alcoholic, (2) cryptogenic and postviral or postnecrotic, (3) biliary, (4) cardiac, (5) metabolic, inherited, and drug-related, and (6) miscellaneous. This chapter considers first the various types of cirrhosis and then the major clinical complications of chronic liver disease and cirrhosis.

ALCOHOLIC LIVER DISEASE AND CIRRHOSIS

Definition   *Alcoholic cirrhosis*, historically referred to as *Laennec's cirrhosis*, is the most common type of cirrhosis encountered in North America and many parts of western Europe and South America. It is usually characterized by diffuse fine scarring, fairly uniform loss of liver cells, and small regenerative nodules, and therefore, it is sometimes referred to as *micronodular cirrhosis*. However, micronodular cirrhosis also may result from other types of liver injury (e.g., following jejunoileal bypass), and thus *alcoholic cirrhosis* and *micronodular cirrhosis* are not necessarily synonymous. Conversely, alcoholic cirrhosis may progress to macronodular cirrhosis with time.

Alcoholic cirrhosis is only one of many consequences resulting from chronic alcohol ingestion, and it often accompanies other forms of alcohol-induced liver injury. The three principal alcohol-induced hepatic lesions are designated (1) *alcoholic fatty liver*, (2) *alcoholic hepatitis*, and (3) *alcoholic cirrhosis*. These morphologic categories are rarely found in a pure form, and features of each may be present to varying degrees in an individual patient.

Etiology   Although chronic alcoholism is the most common cause of cirrhosis, the quantity and duration of drinking necessary to cause cirrhosis remain unclear. The typical alcoholic patient with cirrhosis has had a daily consumption of a pint or more of whiskey, several quarts of wine, or an equivalent amount of beer for at least 10 years. The amount and duration of ethanol ingestion, rather than the type of alcoholic beverage or the pattern of ingestion, appear to be the important determinants of liver injury. In general, the latent period preceding the development of cirrhosis is inversely related to the level of daily alcohol intake. Rates of ethanol metabolism are under genetic control, but no metabolic defect has been identified in cirrhotic patients or their families to suggest a unique "susceptibility" to ethanol or its toxic effects. Although malnutrition per se does not appear to lead to cirrhosis, it is possible that nutritional factors may augment the detrimental effects of chronic alcohol ingestion on the liver. The finding that only 10 to 15 percent of alcoholics develop cirrhosis suggests that other factors may affect the impact of alcohol on the liver. Women, on average, appear to develop alcohol-induced liver injury at lesser levels of consumption than men, suggesting that hormonal factors may play a role in susceptibility.

Alcoholic fatty liver occurs in most heavy drinkers but is reversible on cessation of alcohol consumption and is not thought to be an inevitable precursor of alcoholic hepatitis or cirrhosis. In contrast, alcoholic hepatitis, an inflammatory lesion characterized by infiltration of the liver with leukocytes, liver cell necrosis, and alcoholic hyaline, is thought to be the major precursor of cirrhosis. Subsequent healing accompanied by fibrosis distorts the normal lobular architecture. Indeed, *deposition of collagen in perivenular spaces* may be the earliest manifestation of the process which ultimately leads to cirrhosis.

Pathology and pathogenesis   ALCOHOLIC FATTY LIVER   The liver is enlarged, yellow, greasy, and firm. Hepatocytes are distended by large macrovesicular cytoplasmic fat vacuoles which push the hepatocyte nucleus against the cell membrane. Accumulation of fat in the liver of the alcoholic results from the combination of impaired fatty acid oxidation, increased uptake and esterification of fatty acids to form triglycerides, and diminished lipoprotein biosynthesis and secretion.

ALCOHOLIC HEPATITIS   Morphologic features include hepatocyte degeneration and necrosis, often with ballooned cells, and an infiltrate of polymorphonuclear leukocytes and lymphocytes. The polymorphonuclear cells may encircle damaged hepatocytes which contain *Mallory bodies*, or *alcoholic hyaline*. These are clumps of perinuclear, deeply eosinophilic material believed to represent aggregated intermediate filaments. Mallory bodies are highly suggestive of, but *not specific* for, alcoholic hepatitis, since morphologically similar material has been seen in association with morbid obesity, jejunoileal bypass surgery, poorly controlled diabetes mellitus, and a variety of other disorders, including Wilson's disease and Indian childhood cirrhosis. Deposition of collagen around the central vein and in perisinusoidal areas, often termed *central hyaline sclerosis*, may be associated with an increased likelihood of progression to cirrhosis.

ALCOHOLIC CIRRHOSIS   With continued alcohol intake and destruction of hepatocytes, fibroblasts (including myofibroblasts with contractile properties) appear at the site of injury and stimulate collagen formation. Weblike septa of connective tissue appear in periportal and pericentral zones and eventually connect portal triads and central veins. This fine connective tissue network surrounds small masses of remaining liver cells which regenerate and form nodules. Although regeneration occurs within the small remnants of parenchyma, cell loss generally exceeds replacement. With continuing hepatocyte destruction and collagen deposition, the liver shrinks in size, acquires a nodular appearance, and becomes hard as "end-stage" cirrhosis develops. Although alcoholic cirrhosis is usually a progressive disease, appropriate therapy and strict avoidance of alcohol may arrest the disease at most stages and permit functional improvement.

Clinical features   SIGNS AND SYMPTOMS   Clinical manifestations of *alcoholic fatty liver* are often minimal or entirely absent, and the disorder may not be recognized unless another illness (frequently alcohol-related) brings the patient to medical attention. Hepatomegaly, at times accompanied by tenderness, may be the only finding. Jaundice, ascites, and edema are only seen with more serious liver injury.

The clinical severity of *alcoholic hepatitis* varies enormously, ranging from asymptomatic or mild illness to fatal hepatic insufficiency. Typically, the clinical features of alcoholic hepatitis resemble those of viral or toxic liver injury. Patients often experience anorexia, nausea and vomiting, malaise, weight loss, abdominal distress, and jaundice. Fever sometimes as high as 39.4°C (103°F) may be seen in about half of cases. On physical examination, tender hepatomegaly is common, and splenomegaly is found in about one-third of patients. The patient may have cutaneous arterial "spider" angiomas and jaundice. More severe cases may be complicated by ascites, edema, bleeding, and encephalopathy. At the time of initial presentation, the central nervous system findings may be difficult to distinguish from manifestations of concurrent alcohol intoxication or withdrawal (see below).

Although jaundice, ascites, and encephalopathy may subside with abstinence, continued alcohol excess and poor dietary habits usually lead to repeated acute episodes of hepatic decompensation. Some patients die during these acute exacerbations, but most recover after several weeks or months. Even after complete abstinence, clinical recovery may be protracted, and histologic abnormalities can persist up to 6 months or longer. Cholestatic jaundice mimicking biliary tract obstruction also may develop in some cases of acute alcoholic hepatitis.

Alcoholic cirrhosis also may be clinically silent; in fact, 10 percent of cases are discovered incidentally at laparotomy or autopsy. In many cases symptoms are insidious in onset, occurring usually after 10 or more years of excessive alcohol use and progressing slowly over subsequent weeks and months. Anorexia and malnutrition lead to weight loss and a reduction in skeletal muscle mass. The patient may experience easy bruising, increasing weakness, and fatigue. Eventually the clinical manifestations of hepatocellular dysfunction and portal hypertension ensue, including progressive jaundice, bleeding from gastroesophageal varices, ascites, and encephalopathy. The abrupt onset of one of these complications may be the first event prompting the patient to seek medical attention. In other cases, cirrhosis first becomes evident when the patient requires treatment of symptoms related to alcoholic hepatitis.

A firm, nodular liver may be an early sign of disease; the liver may be either enlarged, normal, or decreased in size. Other frequent findings include jaundice, palmar erythema, spider angiomas, parotid and lacrimal gland enlargement, clubbing of fingers, splenomegaly, muscle wasting, and ascites with or without peripheral edema. Men may have decreased body hair and/or gynecomastia and testicular atrophy, which, like the cutaneous findings, result from disturbances in hormonal metabolism, including increased peripheral formation of estrogren due to diminished hepatic clearance of the precursor androstenedione. Testicular atrophy may reflect hormonal abnormalities or the toxic effect of alcohol on the testes. In women, signs of virilization or menstrual irregularities may occasionally be encountered. Dupuytren's contractures resulting from fibrosis of the palmar fascia with resulting flexion contracture of the digits are associated with alcoholism but are not specifically related to cirrhosis.

Over a period of 3 to 5 years, the cirrhotic patient typically becomes emaciated, weak, and chronically jaundiced. Ascites and other signs of portal hypertension become increasingly prominent. Most patients with advanced cirrhosis die in hepatic coma, commonly precipitated by hemorrhage from esophageal varices or intercurrent infection. Progressive renal dysfunction often complicates the terminal phase of the illness.

LABORATORY FINDINGS   Routine hematologic and biochemical blood tests are usually normal in patients with alcoholic fatty liver, except for minimal elevations of the serum AST (aspartate aminotransferase); occasionally alkaline phosphatase and bilirubin levels are also elevated. In more advanced alcoholic liver disease, abnormalities of laboratory tests are more common. Anemia may result from acute and chronic gastrointestinal blood loss, coexistent nutritional deficiency (notably of folic acid and vitamin B_{12}), hypersplenism, and a direct suppressive effect of alcohol on the bone marrow. Hemolytic anemia, presumably due to effects of hypercholesterolemia on erythrocyte membranes resulting in unusual spurlike projections (acanthocytosis), has been described in some alcoholics with cirrhosis. Leukocytosis is often present in severe alcoholic hepatitis; however, some patients with this disorder may have leukopenia and thrombocytopenia due to hypersplenism or an inhibitory effect of alcohol on the bone marrow. Mild or pronounced hyperbilirubinemia may be found, usually in association with varying elevations of serum alkaline phosphatase levels. Levels of serum AST are frequently elevated, but levels greater than 5 μkat (300 units) are unusual and should prompt one to look for other coincident or complicating factors. In contrast to viral hepatitis, the serum AST is usually disproportionately elevated relative to ALT (alanine aminotransferase) i.e., AST/ALT ratio >2. This discrepancy may result from the proportionally greater inhibition of ALT synthesis by ethanol, which may be partially reversed by pyridoxal phosphate.

The serum prothrombin time is frequently prolonged, reflecting reduced synthesis of clotting proteins, most notably the vitamin K–dependent factors (see ''Coagulopathy'' below). The serum albumin level is usually depressed, while serum globulins are increased. Hypoalbuminemia reflects in part overall impairment in hepatic protein synthesis, while hyperglobulinemia is thought to result from nonspecific stimulation of the reticuloendothelial system. Elevated blood ammonia levels in patients with hepatic encephalopathy reflect diminished hepatic clearance because of impaired liver function and shunting of portal venous blood around the cirrhotic liver into the systemic circulation (see below and Chap. 264).

A variety of metabolic disturbances may be detected. Glucose intolerance due to endogenous insulin resistance may be present; however, clinical diabetes is uncommon. Central hyperventilation may lead to respiratory alkalosis in patients with cirrhosis. *Dietary deficiency* and *increased urinary losses* lead to hypomagnesemia and *hypophosphatemia*. In patients with ascites and dilutional hyponatremia, hypokalemia may occur from increased urinary potassium losses due in part to hyperaldosteronism. Prerenal azotemia is also observed in such patients.

Diagnosis   *Alcoholic fatty liver* should be suspected in alcoholic patients with hepatomegaly and normal or minimally deranged liver function tests. Alcoholic fatty liver may be seen in combination with alcoholic hepatitis or established cirrhosis. *Alcoholic hepatitis* should be considered in an alcoholic who has been drinking heavily and demonstrates jaundice, fever, an enlarged, tender liver, or ascites. The clinical impression is often supported by the deranged results of tests of liver function and other laboratory abnormalities described above. Alcoholic hepatitis or fatty liver may be present in association with alcoholic cirrhosis.

Alcoholic cirrhosis should be strongly suspected in patients with a history of prolonged or excessive alcohol intake and physical signs of chronic liver disease. The clinical features and laboratory findings are usually sufficient to provide reasonable indication of the presence and extent of hepatic injury. Although a percutaneous needle biopsy of the liver is not usually necessary to confirm the typical findings of alcoholic hepatitis or cirrhosis, it may be helpful in distinguishing patients with less advanced liver disease from those with cirrhosis and in excluding other forms of liver injury such as viral hepatitis. Biopsy also may be helpful as a diagnostic tool in evaluating patients with clinical findings suggestive of alcoholic liver disease who deny alcohol intake. In patients with features of cholestasis, ultrasonography may be appropriate to exclude the presence of extrahepatic biliary obstruction. When the clinical status of an otherwise stable cirrhotic patient deteriorates without an obvious explanation, complicating conditions, such as infection, portal vein thrombosis, and hepatocellular carcinoma, should be sought.

Prognosis   The patient with an alcoholic fatty liver and no complications has a good prognosis; rapid and complete resolution usually follows cessation of alcohol intake. In patients with alcoholic hepatitis, the presence of marked hyperbilirubinemia, rising serum creatinine, marked prolongation of the prothrombin time (>1.5 times control), ascites, and encephalopathy are associated with a poor short-term prognosis; the in-hospital mortality in these patients may exceed 50 percent. In milder cases, clinical recovery may be complete, but repeated bouts of alcoholic hepatitis usually lead to irreversible and progressive chronic liver injury. Abstinence from alcohol as well as early and appropriate medical care can decrease long-term morbidity and mortality and delay or prevent the appearance of further complications. Patients who have had a major complication of cirrhosis and who continue to drink have a 5-year survival of less than 50 percent. However, those patients who remain abstinent have a substantially better prognosis. In general, overall outlook in patients with advanced liver disease remains poor; most of these patients eventually die as a result of massive variceal hemorrhage and/or profound hepatic encephalopathy.

Treatment   Alcoholic hepatitis and cirrhosis are serious illnesses that require long-term medical supervision and careful management. Therapy of the underlying liver disease is largely supportive. Specific treatment is directed at particular complications such as variceal bleeding and ascites (see below). Some studies suggest that administration of prednisone or prednisolone in moderately large doses may be helpful in patients with severe alcoholic hepatitis and encephalopathy. However, the use of glucocorticoids in acute alcoholic hepatitis remains controversial and should probably be reserved for those with severe disease. Although a number of studies have supported the use of propylthiouracil in the management of acute alcoholic hepatitis, the way it works is as yet undefined, and its efficacy has not been unequivocally established. More recently, maintenance therapy with colchicine (0.6 mg PO bid) has been shown to slow disease progression and increase longevity of the patient with alcoholic liver disease in one long-term study. Other agents, such as penicillamine and intravenous infusion of insulin and glucagon, have been used experimentally, but their therapeutic efficacy and safety have not been demonstrated.

In the absence of signs of impending hepatic coma, the patient should be placed on a diet containing at least 1 g protein per kilogram of body weight and 8500 to 12,500 kJ (2000 to 3000 kcal) per day. Use of diets enriched in branched-chain amino acids has been advocated in patients predisposed to hepatic encephalopathy, but the value of these diets in patients with compensated cirrhosis is unproven. Daily multivitamin supplements should be prescribed, with the addition of large parenteral doses of thiamine in patients with Wernicke-Korsakoff disease (see Chap. 377). The patient should be made to realize that there is no medication that will protect the liver against the effects of further alcohol ingestion. Therefore, alcohol should be absolutely forbidden. An important component of the complete care of such patients is encouragement to become involved in an appropriate alcohol counseling program.

All medicines must be administered with caution in the patient with cirrhosis, especially those eliminated or modified through hepatic metabolism or biliary pathways. In particular, care must be taken to avoid overzealous use of drugs that may directly or indirectly precipitate complications of cirrhosis. For example, vigorous treatment of ascites with diuretics may result in electrolyte abnormalities or hypovolemia, which can lead to coma. Similarly, even modest doses of sedative can lead to deepening encephalopathy.

POSTNECROTIC CIRRHOSIS, POSTVIRAL CIRRHOSIS

Definition   Postnecrotic cirrhosis represents the final common pathway of many types of advanced liver injury. *Coarsely nodular*, *posthepatitic*, and *multilobular cirrhosis* are terms synonymous with *postnecrotic cirrhosis*. The term *cryptogenic cirrhosis* has been used interchangeably with *postnecrotic cirrhosis*, but this designation should be reserved for those cases in which the etiology of cirrhosis is unknown (approximately 10 percent of all patients with cirrhosis).

Postnecrotic cirrhosis is characterized morphologically by (1) extensive confluent loss of liver cells, (2) stromal collapse and fibrosis resulting in broad bands of connective tissue containing the remains of many portal triads, and (3) irregular nodules of regenerating hepatocytes, varying in size from microscopic to several centimeters in diameter.

Etiology   *Postnecrotic cirrhosis* is a morphologic term referring to a defined stage of advanced chronic liver injury of both specific and unknown (cryptogenic) causes. Epidemiologic and serologic evidence suggests that viral hepatitis (hepatitis B or hepatitis C) may be an antecedent factor in from one-fourth to three-fourths of cases of apparently cryptogenic postnecrotic cirrhosis. In areas where hepatitis B virus infection is endemic (e.g., Southeast Asia, sub-Saharan Africa), up to 15 percent of the population may acquire the infection in early childhood, and cirrhosis may ultimately develop in one-fourth of these chronic carriers. Although hepatitis B infection is much less prevalent in the United States, it is relatively common among certain high-risk groups (e.g., promiscuous homosexual men, intravenous drug abusers) and contributes to an increased incidence of cirrhosis. In the United States, hepatitis C appears to account for many cases of cirrhosis following blood transfusions. Before hepatitis C screening of blood donors was introduced, hepatitis C occurred in 5 to 10 percent of blood recipients. In as many as half of those surviving 20 years or more, cirrhosis may ultimately develop. Conversely, the recent identification of hepatitis C virus and the availability of specific serologic markers have led to the demonstration that more than half of patients with cryptogenic chronic liver disease have evidence of hepatitis C infection. Postnecrotic cirrhosis also may develop in patients with chronic active hepatitis of the autoimmune type (see Chaps. 266 and 267).

Other probable causes of postnecrotic cirrhosis, including drugs and toxins, are listed in Table 268-1. In some instances, advanced alcoholic liver disease and primary biliary cirrhosis may lead to postnecrotic cirrhosis.

Pathology   The postnecrotic liver is typically shrunken in size, distorted in shape, and composed of nodules of liver cells separated by dense and broad bands of fibrosis. The microscopic picture is consistent with the gross impression: Nodules are highly variable in

TABLE 268-1   Cirrhosis and/or liver disease associated with various disorders

INFECTIOUS DISEASES

Brucellosis (Chap. 121)
Echinococcus (Chap. 184)
Schistosomiasis (Chap. 183)
Toxoplasmosis (Chap. 177)
Viral hepatitis [hepatitis B, hepatitis C, hepatitis D, cytomegalovirus (Chaps. 146, 266, and 267)]

INHERITED AND METABOLIC DISORDERS (see also Chap. 270)

Alpha$_1$-antitrypsin deficiency (Chap. 270)
Fanconi's syndrome (Chap. 349)
Galactosemia (Chap. 354)
Gaucher's disease (Chap. 349)
Glycogen storage disease (Chap. 350)
Hemochromatosis (Chap. 345)
Hereditary fructose intolerance (Chap. 354)
Hereditary tyrosinemia (Chap. 352)
Wilson's disease (Chap. 348)

DRUGS AND TOXINS (Chap. 266)

Arsenicals
Isoniazid
Methotrexate
Methyldopa
Oral contraceptives (Budd-Chiari)
Oxyphenisatin
Perhexilene maleate
Pyrrolidizine alkaloids (venoocclusive disease)

OTHER OR UNPROVEN CAUSES

Chronic inflammatory bowel disease (Chap. 255)
Cystic fibrosis (Chap. 222)
Diabetes mellitus (Chap. 337)
Graft-versus-host disease (Chap. 313)
Jejunoileal bypass (Chap. 40)
Sarcoidosis (Chap. 266)

size, with large amounts of connective tissue separating the disorganized islands of regenerating parenchyma.

Clinical features   In patients with cirrhosis of known etiology in whom there is progression to a postnecrotic stage, the clinical manifestations are an extension of those resulting from the initial disease process. Usually clinical symptoms are related to portal hypertension and its sequelae, such as ascites, splenomegaly, hypersplenism, encephalopathy, and bleeding esophageal varices. The hematologic and liver function abnormalities resemble those seen with other types of cirrhosis. In a few patients with postnecrotic cirrhosis the diagnosis may be made incidentally at operation, at postmortem, or by a needle biopsy of the liver performed to investigate asymptomatic hepatosplenomegaly.

Diagnosis and prognosis   Postnecrotic cirrhosis should be suspected in patients with signs and symptoms of cirrhosis or portal hypertension. Needle or operative liver biopsies confirm the diagnosis, although nonuniformity of the pathologic process may result in sampling errors. The diagnosis of cryptogenic cirrhosis is reserved for those patients in whom no known etiology can be demonstrated. About 75 percent of patients have progressive disease despite supportive therapy and die within 1 to 5 years from complications, including exsanguinating variceal hemorrhage, hepatic encephalopathy, or superimposed hepatocellular carcinoma.

Treatment   Management is usually limited to treatment of the complications of portal hypertension, including control of ascites, avoidance of drugs or excessive protein intake that may induce hepatic coma, and prompt treatment of infections (see below). In patients with asymptomatic cirrhosis, expectant management alone is appropriate. In those patients in whom postnecrotic cirrhosis has developed as a result of a treatable condition, therapy directed at the primary disorder may limit further progression (e.g., Wilson's disease, hemochromatosis).

BILIARY CIRRHOSIS

Biliary cirrhosis results from injury to or prolonged obstruction of either the intrahepatic or extrahepatic biliary system. It is associated with impaired biliary excretion, destruction of hepatic parenchyma, and progressive fibrosis. Primary biliary cirrhosis is characterized by chronic inflammation and fibrous obliteration of intrahepatic bile ductules. Secondary biliary cirrhosis is the result of long-standing obstruction of the larger extrahepatic ducts. Although primary and secondary biliary cirrhosis are separate pathophysiologic entities with respect to the initial insult, many clinical features are similar.

PRIMARY BILIARY CIRRHOSIS   Etiology and pathogenesis The cause of primary biliary cirrhosis remains unknown. Several observations suggest that a disordered immune response may be involved. Primary biliary cirrhosis (PBC) is frequently associated with a variety of disorders presumed to be autoimmune in nature, such as the CRST syndrome (calcinosis, Raynaud's phenomenon, sclerodactyly, telangiectasia), the sicca syndrome (dry eyes and dry mouth), autoimmune thyroiditis, and renal tubular acidosis.

Most important, a circulating IgG antimitochondrial antibody (AMA) is detected in more than 90 percent of patients with primary biliary cirrhosis and only rarely in other forms of liver disease. In recent years, it has been demonstrated that these autoantibodies recognize three to five inner mitochondrial membrane proteins identified as enzymes of the pyruvate dehydrogenase complex (PDC), the branched chain α-ketoacid dehydrogenase complex (BCKDC), and the α-ketoglutarate dehydrogenase complex (KGDC). The major autoantigen in PBC (found in 90 percent of patients) has been identified as the 74-kDa E2 component of the PDC, dihydrolipoamide acetyltransferase. The antibodies are directed to a region essential for binding of a lipoic acid cofactor and inhibit the overall enzymatic activity of PDC. Other AMA autoantibodies in PBC patients are directed to similar constituents of BCKDC and KGDC and also inhibit their enzymatic function. Despite the demonstrated ability of autoantibodies found in PBC sera to inhibit key enzymatic activities, it is unclear whether these properties have a direct pathogenetic role in the development of PBC. In addition to AMA, elevated serum levels of IgM and cryoproteins consisting of immune complexes capable of activating the alternate complement pathway are found in 80 to 90 percent of patients. Lymphocytes are prominent in the portal regions and surround damaged bile ducts. These histologic findings resemble those noted in graft-versus-host disease following liver and bone marrow transplantation and suggest that damage to bile ducts may be immunologically mediated, perhaps reflecting a defect in a suppressor cell population.

Pathology Primary biliary cirrhosis is often divided into four stages based on morphologic findings. The earliest recognizable lesion (stage I), termed *chronic nonsuppurative destructive cholangitis*, is a necrotizing inflammatory process of the portal triads. It is characterized by destruction of medium and small bile ducts, a dense infiltrate of acute and chronic inflammatory cells, mild fibrosis, and occasionally, bile stasis. At times, periductal granulomas and lymph follicles are found adjacent to affected bile ducts. Subsequently, the inflammatory infiltrate becomes less prominent, the number of bile ducts is reduced, and smaller bile ductules proliferate (stage II). Progression over a period of months to years leads to a decrease in interlobular ducts, loss of liver cells, and expansion of periportal fibrosis into a network of connective tissue scars (stage III). Ultimately, cirrhosis, which may be micronodular or macronodular, develops (stage IV).

Clinical features SIGNS AND SYMPTOMS Many patients with primary biliary cirrhosis are asymptomatic, and the disease is initially detected on the basis of elevated serum alkaline phosphatase levels during routine screening. The majority of such patients remain asymptomatic for prolonged periods, although many may ultimately develop progressive liver injury.

Among patients with symptomatic disease, 90 percent are women aged 35 to 60. Often the earliest symptom is pruritus, which may be either generalized or limited initially to the palms and soles. In addition, fatigue is commonly a prominent early symptom. After several months or years, jaundice and gradual darkening of the exposed areas of the skin (melanosis) may ensue. Other early clinical manifestations of primary biliary cirrhosis reflect impaired bile excretion. These include steatorrhea and the malabsorption of lipid-soluble vitamins, often resulting in easy bruising (vitamin K deficiency), bone pain due to osteomalacia (vitamin D deficiency) which is typically present in conjunction with osteoporosis, occasionally night blindness (vitamin A deficiency), and dermatitis (possibly vitamin E and/or essential fatty acid deficiency). Protracted elevation of serum lipids, especially cholesterol, leads to subcutaneous lipid deposition around the eyes (xanthelasmas) and over joints and tendons (xanthomas). Over a period of months to years, the itching, jaundice, and hyperpigmentation slowly worsen. Eventually signs of hepatocellular failure and portal hypertension develop and ascites appears. Progression may be quite variable. Whereas a proportion of asymptomatic patients may show no signs of progression for a decade or longer, in others, death due to hepatic insufficiency may occur within 5 to 10 years after the first signs of the illness. Such decompensation is often precipitated by uncontrolled variceal hemorrhage or infection.

Physical examination may be entirely normal in the early phase of the disease, when patients are asymptomatic or pruritus is the sole complaint. Later, there may be jaundice of varying intensity, hyperpigmentation of the exposed skin areas, xanthelasmas and tendinous and planar xanthomas, moderate to striking hepatomegaly, splenomegaly, and clubbing of the fingers. Bone tenderness, signs of vertebral compression, ecchymoses, glossitis, and dermatitis may all be noted. Clinical evidence of the sicca syndrome can be found in as many as 75 percent of patients, and serologic evidence of autoimmune thyroid disease in 25 percent. Other conditions encountered with increased frequency include rheumatoid arthritis, CRST syndrome, scleroderma, pernicious anemia, and renal tubular acidosis. Bone disease is often a significant problem encountered over the course of the disease. While osteomalacia occurs due to diminished vitamin D absorption, accelerated osteoporosis in this patient population (the majority of whom are postmenopausal women) is even more common.

LABORATORY FINDINGS Primary biliary cirrhosis is increasingly diagnosed at a presymptomatic stage, prompted by the finding of a two- to fivefold elevation of the serum alkaline phosphatase during routine screening. Serum 5'-nucleotidase activity is also elevated. In this setting, serum bilirubin and aminotransferase levels are usually normal, but the diagnosis is supported by a positive antimitochondrial antibody test (titer > 1:40). The latter is both *relatively* specific and sensitive; a positive test is found in over 90 percent of symptomatic patients. As the disease evolves, the serum bilirubin level rises progressively and may reach 510 μmol/L (30 mg/dL) or more in the final stages. Serum aminotransferase values rarely exceed 2.5 to 3.3 μkat (150 to 200 units). Hyperlipidemia is common, and a striking increase of the serum unesterified cholesterol is often noted. An abnormal serum lipoprotein (lipoprotein X) may be present in primary biliary cirrhosis but is not specific and appears in other cholestatic conditions. A deficiency of bile salts in the intestine leads to moderate steatorrhea and impaired absorption of the fat-soluble vitamins and hypoprothrombinemia. Patients with primary biliary cirrhosis have elevated liver copper levels, but this finding is not specific and is found in all disorders in which there is prolonged cholestasis.

Diagnosis Primary biliary cirrhosis should be considered in middle-aged women with unexplained pruritus or an elevated serum alkaline phosphatase level and in whom there may be other clinical or laboratory features of protracted impairment of biliary excretion. Although a positive serum antimitochondrial antibody determination provides important diagnostic evidence, false-positive results do occur, and therefore, liver biopsy should be performed to confirm the diagnosis. In most cases the biliary tract should be evaluated to exclude remediable extrahepatic biliary tract obstruction, especially in view of the frequent presence of coexisting cholelithiasis.

Treatment There is no specific therapy for primary biliary cirrhosis. Glucocorticoids are ineffective and may actually worsen the bone disease. D-Penicillamine has been tried because of its ability to chelate copper and because of its possible antifibrotic and immunomodulating activities. However, the drug appears to be ineffective and has a high incidence of unacceptable side effects. While some have suggested that azathioprine may be helpful in slowing the progression of disease, this has not been established. Colchicine has been shown to have some limited effectiveness in slowing the progression of disease in symptomatic patients and should be tried (0.6 mg PO bid) unless gastrointestinal intolerance is limiting. Treatment with low-dose methotrexate has been reported to halt or reverse progression of primary biliary cirrhosis. Controlled trials may eventually settle the proper role of this agent in the management of symptomatic primary biliary cirrhosis. Cyclosporine has been suggested to slow disease progression in one relatively small trial. However, the benefit needs to be weighed against the relatively frequent nephrotoxicity caused by this agent before it can be advocated for a condition which will persist for the life of the individual. Recently, ursodiol treatment (13 to 15 mg/kg per day) also has been reported to achieve both symptomatic improvement and "improvement" in serum biochemical markers in patients with clinically overt primary biliary cirrhosis. The mechanism of action of ursodeoxycholic acid in achieving this benefit remains obscure. While further confirmation is needed, this agent is generally well tolerated and safe.

Treatment is generally directed toward the relief of symptoms. Although the mechanism of the protracted pruritus is not entirely clear, cholestyramine, an oral bile salt–sequestering resin, may be helpful in doses of 8 to 12 g/d to decrease both the pruritus and the hypercholesterolemia. Steatorrhea can be reduced by a low-fat diet and substituting medium-chain triglycerides for dietary long-chain triglycerides. Fat-soluble vitamins A and K should be given by parenteral injection at regular intervals to prevent or correct night blindness and hypoprothrombinemia, respectively. Zinc supplementation may be necessary if night blindness is refractory to vitamin A therapy. Osteomalacia and osteoporosis may be ameliorated by dietary calcium supplements in conjunction with oral vitamin D. In advanced disease, $25(OH)D_3$ or $1,25(OH_2)D_3$ may be preferred to vitamin D, since poor hepatic function may limit conversion of vitamin D to the active metabolites. Progression of primary biliary cirrhosis leads to the typical complications of advanced liver disease.

The management of ascites, variceal hemorrhage, and encephalopathy is described below. Over the past several years, it has been well documented that orthotopic liver transplantation is a highly effective treatment for patients with advanced primary biliary cirrhosis. Stratified analysis of patients with a wide variety of risk levels utilizing a validated prognostic model demonstrated enhanced survival for all. Hepatic transplantation, when available, is the treatment of choice for advanced primary biliary cirrhosis.

SECONDARY BILIARY CIRRHOSIS Etiology Secondary biliary cirrhosis results from prolonged partial or total obstruction of the common bile duct or its major branches. In adults, obstruction is most frequently caused by postoperative strictures or gallstones, usually with superimposed infectious cholangitis. Chronic pancreatitis may lead to biliary stricture and secondary cirrhosis. Secondary biliary cirrhosis also may develop in patients with pericholangitis or idiopathic sclerosing cholangitis. Patients with malignant tumors of the common bile duct or pancreas rarely survive long enough to develop secondary biliary cirrhosis. In children, congenital biliary atresia and cystic fibrosis are common causes of secondary biliary cirrhosis. Choledochal cysts, if unrecognized, also may be a rare cause of secondary biliary cirrhosis.

Pathology and pathogenesis Unrelieved obstruction of the extrahepatic bile ducts leads to (1) bile stasis and focal areas of centrilobular necrosis followed by periportal necrosis, (2) proliferation and dilatation of the portal bile ducts and ductules, (3) sterile or infected cholangitis with accumulation of polymorphonuclear infiltrates around bile ducts, and (4) progressive expansion of portal tracts by edema and fibrosis. Extravasation of bile from ruptured interlobular bile ducts into areas of periportal necrosis leads to the formation of "bile lakes" surrounded by cholesterol-rich pseudoxanthomatous cells. As in other forms of cirrhosis, injury is accompanied by regeneration in residual parenchyma. These changes gradually lead to a finely nodular cirrhosis. In general, at least 3 to 12 months is required for biliary obstruction to result in cirrhosis. Relief of the obstruction is frequently accompanied by biochemical and morphologic improvement.

Clinical features SIGNS AND SYMPTOMS The signs and symptoms of secondary biliary cirrhosis are similar to those of primary biliary cirrhosis. Jaundice and pruritus are usually the most prominent features. In addition, fever and/or right upper quadrant pain, reflecting bouts of cholangitis or biliary colic, are typical. The manifestations of portal hypertension are found only in advanced cases.

LABORATORY TESTS Elevations in serum alkaline phosphatase and 5'-nucleotidase as well as conjugated hyperbilirubinemia are nearly always present. There is a moderate increase in serum aminotransferases. When the disease is complicated by cholangitis, elevations in aminotransferase levels and leukocytosis are more pronounced. As in primary biliary cirrhosis, there are abnormalities in serum lipids (including the presence of lipoprotein X) and laboratory findings consistent with steatorrhea. However, the antimitochondrial antibody test is usually negative.

Diagnosis Secondary biliary cirrhosis should be considered in any patient with clinical and laboratory evidence of prolonged obstruction to bile flow, especially when there is a history of previous biliary tract surgery or gallstones, bouts of ascending cholangitis, or right upper quadrant pain. Cholangiography (either percutaneous or endoscopic) usually demonstrates the underlying pathologic process. Liver biopsy, although not always necessary from a clinical standpoint, can document the development of cirrhosis.

Treatment Relief of obstruction to bile flow, by either surgical or endoscopic means, is the most important step in the prevention and therapy of secondary biliary cirrhosis. Effective decompression of the biliary tract results in a significant improvement in both symptoms and survival, even in patients with established cirrhosis. When obstruction cannot be relieved, as in sclerosing cholangitis, antibiotics may be helpful acutely in controlling superimposed infection or, when administered on a chronic basis, as prophylactic therapy in suppressing recurring episodes of ascending cholangitis. Without relief of obstruction, there is a steady progression to end-stage cirrhosis and its terminal manifestations.

CARDIAC CIRRHOSIS

Definition Prolonged, severe right-sided congestive heart failure may lead to chronic liver injury and cardiac cirrhosis. The characteristic pathologic features of fibrosis and regenerative nodules distinguish cardiac cirrhosis from both reversible passive congestion of the liver due to acute heart failure and acute hepatocellular necrosis ("ischemic hepatitis" or "shock liver") resulting from systemic hypotension and hypoperfusion of the liver.

Etiology and pathology In right-sided heart failure, retrograde transmission of elevated venous pressure via the inferior vena cava and hepatic veins leads to congestion of the liver. Hepatic sinusoids become dilated and engorged with blood, and the liver becomes tensely swollen. With prolonged passive congestion and ischemia from poor perfusion secondary to reduced cardiac output, necrosis of centrilobular hepatocytes ensues and leads to fibrosis in these central areas. Ultimately, centrilobular fibrosis develops, with collagen extending outward in a characteristic stellate pattern from the central vein. Gross examination of the liver shows alternating red (congested) and pale (fibrotic) areas, a pattern often referred to as "nutmeg liver." Improvement in management of cardiac disorders, particularly advances in surgical treatment, has reduced the frequency of cardiac cirrhosis.

Clinical features   In acute passive congestion, the liver becomes enlarged and tender, and the patient may complain of severe right upper quadrant pain due to stretching of Glisson's capsule. The serum bilirubin is usually only mildly increased and may be predominantly either conjugated or unconjugated. The AST level is also typically mildly elevated but may be transiently very high following a period of marked systemic hypotension (shock liver), when the clinical picture can mimic acute viral or drug-induced hepatitis. The serum albumin and prothrombin are usually normal, but may become abnormal in shock liver or with the development of cirrhosis. In cases of tricuspid insufficiency the liver may be pulsatile, but this finding disappears as cirrhosis develops. With prolonged right-sided heart failure the liver is enlarged, firm, and usually nontender. The signs and symptoms of heart failure usually overshadow the liver disease. Bleeding from esophageal varices is rare, but chronic encephalopathy may be prominent with a waxing and waning course reflecting variations in the severity of right-sided heart failure. Ascites and peripheral edema, often primarily related to the underlying cardiac dysfunction, may be worsened by the superimposed liver disease.

Diagnosis   The presence of a firm, enlarged liver with signs of chronic liver disease in a patient with valvular heart disease, constrictive pericarditis, or cor pulmonale of long duration (>10 years) should suggest cardiac cirrhosis. Liver biopsy can confirm the diagnosis but is usually contraindicated because of coagulopathy or ascites. Coexistent chronic heart and liver disease should also raise the possibility of hemochromatosis, amyloidosis, or other infiltrative diseases.

Budd-Chiari syndrome resulting from the occlusion of the hepatic veins or inferior vena cava may be confused with acute congestive hepatomegaly. In this condition the liver is grossly enlarged and tender, and severe intractable ascites is present. However, signs and symptoms of heart failure are notably absent. The most common cause is thrombosis of the hepatic veins, often in the setting of polycythemia rubra vera, myeloproliferative syndromes, paroxysmal nocturnal hemoglobinuria, oral contraceptive use, or other hypercoagulable states; it also may result from invasion of the inferior vena cava by tumor, such as renal cell or primary hepatocellular carcinoma. Idiopathic membranous obstruction of the inferior vena cava is the most common cause of this syndrome in Japan. Hepatic venography or liver biopsy showing centrilobular congestion and sinusoidal dilatation in the absence of right-sided heart failure establishes the diagnosis of Budd-Chiari syndrome. Venoocclusive disease affecting the sublobular branches of the hepatic veins and the hepatic venules may result from hepatic irradiation, treatment with some antineoplastic agents, or ingestion of pyrrolidizine alkaloids present in some herbal teas ("bush tea disease") and can mimic congestive hepatomegaly.

Treatment   Prevention or treatment of cardiac cirrhosis depends on the diagnosis and therapy of the underlying cardiovascular disorder. Improvement in cardiac function frequently results in improvement of liver function and stabilization of the liver disease.

METABOLIC, HEREDITARY, DRUG-RELATED, AND OTHER TYPES OF CIRRHOSIS (See Table 268-1)   Cirrhosis or hepatitis may result from a wide variety of other processes encompassing the spectrum of etiologic factors listed in Table 268-2. Although some of these disorders have distinctive clinical or morphologic features, the manifestations of cirrhosis are largely independent of the underlying pathogenic mechanism.

NONCIRRHOTIC FIBROSIS OF THE LIVER   Several diseases, either congenital or acquired, may be associated with localized or generalized hepatic fibrosis. They are distinguished from cirrhosis by the absence of hepatocellular damage and the lack of nodular regenerative activity. The clinical manifestations in such cases are largely secondary to portal hypertension. The different types of

TABLE 268-2   Some causes of noncirrhotic hepatic fibrosis

Idiopathic portal hypertension (noncirrhotic portal fibrosis, Banti's syndrome); three variants:
   Intrahepatic phlebosclerosis and fibrosis
   Portal and splenic vein sclerosis
   Portal and splenic vein thrombosis
Schistosomiasis ("pipe-stem" fibrosis with presinusoidal portal hypertension)
Congenital hepatic fibrosis (may be associated with polycystic disease of liver and kidneys)

these disorders are indicated in Table 268-2; with the exception of schistosomiasis, all these conditions are relatively rare.

MAJOR SEQUELAE OF CIRRHOSIS

The clinical course of patients with advanced cirrhosis is usually complicated by a number of important sequelae which are independent of the etiology of the underlying liver disease. These include portal hypertension and its consequences (i.e., gastroesophageal varices and splenomegaly), ascites, hepatic encephalopathy, spontaneous bacterial peritonitis, hepatorenal syndrome, and hepatocellular carcinoma.

PORTAL HYPERTENSION   Definition and pathogenesis   Normal pressure in the portal vein is low (10 to 15 cm saline) because vascular resistance in the hepatic sinusoids is minimal. Portal hypertension (>30 cm saline) most commonly results from increased resistance to portal blood flow. Because the portal venous system lacks valves, resistance at any level between the right side of the heart and splanchnic vessels results in retrograde transmission of an elevated pressure. Increased resistance can occur at three levels relative to the hepatic sinusoids: (1) presinusoidal, (2) sinusoidal, and (3) postsinusoidal. Obstruction in the *presinusoidal* venous compartment may be anatomically outside the liver (e.g., portal vein thrombosis) or within the liver itself but at a functional level proximal to the hepatic sinusoids so that the liver parenchyma is not exposed to the elevated venous pressure (e.g., schistosomiasis). *Postsinusoidal* obstruction also may occur outside the liver at the level of the hepatic veins (e.g., Budd-Chiari syndrome), the inferior vena cava, or, less commonly, within the liver (e.g., venoocclusive disease in which the central hepatic venules are the primary site of injury). When cirrhosis is complicated by portal hypertension, the increased resistance is usually sinusoidal. While distinctions between pre-, post-, and sinusoidal processes are conceptually appealing, functional resistance to portal flow in a given patient may occur at more than one level. Portal hypertension also may arise from increased blood flow (e.g., massive splenomegaly or arteriovenous fistulas), but the low outflow resistance of the normal liver makes this a rare clinical problem.

Cirrhosis is the most common cause of portal hypertension in the United States. Clinically significant portal hypertension is present in greater than 60 percent of patients with cirrhosis. *Portal vein obstruction* is the second most common cause; it may be idiopathic or occur in association with cirrhosis, infection, pancreatitis, or abdominal trauma. *Hepatic vein thrombosis* (Budd-Chiari syndrome) and hepatic venoocclusive disease are relatively infrequent causes of portal hypertension (see above). Portal vein occlusion may result in massive hematemesis from gastroesophageal varices, but ascites is usually found only with cirrhosis. Noncirrhotic portal fibrosis accounts for only a few patients with portal hypertension.

Clinical features   The major clinical manifestations of portal hypertension include hemorrhage from gastroesophageal varices, splenomegaly with hypersplenism, ascites, and acute and chronic hepatic encephalopathy. All these features are related, at least in part, to the development of portal-systemic collateral channels. The absence of valves in the portal venous system facilitates retrograde (hepatofugal) blood flow from the high-pressure portal venous system to the lower-pressure systemic venous circulation. Major sites of collateral flow involve the veins around the rectum (hemorrhoids), cardioesophageal junction (esophagogastric varices), retroperitoneal space, and the falciform ligament of the liver (periumbilical or abdominal wall collaterals). Abdominal wall collaterals appear as tortuous epigastric vessels that radiate from the umbilicus toward the xiphoid and rib margins (caput medusae).

Diagnosis   In patients with known liver disease, the development of portal hypertension usually becomes evident by the appearance of splenomegaly, ascites, encephalopathy, and/or esophageal varices. Conversely, the finding of any of these features should lead one to evaluate the patient for the presence of underlying portal hypertension and liver disease. Varices are most reliably documented by fiberoptic esophagoscopy; their presence lends indirect support to the diagnosis of portal hypertension. Although rarely necessary, portal venous pressure may be measured directly by percutaneous transhepatic "skinny needle" catheterization or indirectly through transjugular cannulation of the hepatic veins. Both free and wedged hepatic vein pressure (WHVP) should be measured. While WHVP is elevated in sinusoidal and postsinusoidal portal hypertension, including cirrhosis, this measurement is usually normal in presinusoidal portal hypertension. In patients in whom additional information is necessary (e.g., preoperative evaluation before portal-systemic shunt surgery) or percutaneous catheterization is not feasible, mesenteric and hepatic angiography may be helpful. Particular attention should be directed to the venous phase to assess the patency of the portal vein and the direction of portal blood flow.

Treatment   Although treatment is usually directed toward a specific complication of portal hypertension, attempts are sometimes made to reduce the pressure in the portal venous system. Surgical decompression procedures have been used for many years to lower portal pressure in patients with bleeding esophageal varices (see below). However, portal-systemic shunt surgery does not result in improved survival rates in patients with cirrhosis. Beta-adrenergic blockade with propranolol or nadolol reduces portal pressure through vasodilatory effects on both the splanchnic arterial bed and the portal venous system in combination with reduced cardiac output. Such therapy has been shown to be effective in preventing both a first variceal bleed and subsequent episodes after an initial bleed. Treatment of patients with clinically significant sequelae of portal hypertension, especially variceal bleeding, with doses of propranolol titrated to reduce the resting pulse by 25 percent is reasonable if no contraindications exist.

Vigorous treatment of patients with alcoholic hepatitis and cirrhosis, chronic active hepatitis, and other liver diseases may lead to a fall in portal pressure and to a reduction in variceal size. In general, however, portal hypertension due to cirrhosis is not reversible. In appropriately selected patients hepatic transplantation will be beneficial.

VARICEAL BLEEDING   **Pathogenesis**   While vigorous hemorrhage may arise from any portal-systemic venous collaterals, bleeding is most common from varices in the region of the gastroesophageal junction. The factors contributing to bleeding from gastroesophageal varices are not entirely understood but include the degree of portal hypertension and the size of the varices. Esophagitis with erosion of underlying varices does not appear to play an important role.

Clinical features and diagnosis   Variceal bleeding often occurs without obvious precipitating factors and usually presents with painless but massive hematemesis with or without melena. Associated signs range from mild postural tachycardia to profound shock, depending on the extent of blood loss and degree of hypovolemia. Because patients with varices may bleed from other gastrointestinal lesions (e.g., peptic ulcer, gastritis), exclusion of other bleeding sources is important even in patients with prior variceal hemorrhage. Fiberoptic endoscopy is the best choice for evaluating upper gastrointestinal hemorrhage in patients with known or suspected portal hypertension.

Treatment   Variceal bleeding is a life-threatening emergency. Prompt estimation and vigorous replacement of blood losses to maintain intravascular volume are essential and take precedence over diagnostic studies and more specific intervention to stop the bleeding. Replacement of clotting factors with fresh frozen plasma is important in patients with coagulopathy. Patients are best managed in an intensive care unit and often require close monitoring of central venous or pulmonary capillary wedge pressures, urine output, and mental status. Only when the patient is hemodynamically stable should attention be directed toward specific diagnostic studies (especially endoscopy) and other therapeutic modalities to prevent further or recurrent bleeding.

About half of all episodes of variceal hemorrhage cease without intervention, although the risk of rebleeding is very high. The medical management of acute variceal hemorrhage includes the use of vasoconstrictors (vasopressin or somatostatin), balloon tamponade, and endoscopic sclerosis of varices (sclerotherapy) or endoscopic ligation of varices and beta-adrenergic blockade. Intravenous infusion of *vasopressin* at a rate of 0.1 to 0.5 units per minute results in generalized vasoconstriction leading to diminished blood flow in the portal venous system. Intravenous infusion of vasopressin has been shown to be as effective as selective intraarterial administration. Control of bleeding can be achieved in up to 80 percent of cases, but bleeding recurs in more than half after the vasopressin is tapered and discontinued. Furthermore, a number of serious side effects, including cardiac and gastrointestinal tract ischemia, acute renal failure, and hyponatremia, may be associated with vasopressin therapy. It appears that concurrent treatment with venodilators such as nitroglycerin as an intravenous infusion or isosorbide dinitrate sublingually may enhance the effectiveness of vasopressin and reduce complications. Somatostatin is also a direct splanchnic vasoconstrictor. In some studies this peptide, given as an initial 250-μg bolus followed by constant infusion (250 μg/h), has been found to be as effective as vasopressin. If bleeding is too vigorous or endoscopy is not available, *balloon tamponade* of the bleeding varices may be accomplished with a triple-lumen (Sengstaken-Blakemore) or four-lumen (Minnesota) tube with esophageal and gastric balloons. Because of the high risk of aspiration, endotracheal intubation should be performed prior to attempts to place one of these tubes. After the tube is introduced into the stomach, the gastric balloon is inflated and pulled back into the cardia of the stomach. If bleeding does not stop, the esophageal balloon is inflated for additional tamponade. Complications are common, occurring in 15 percent or more of patients, and include aspiration pneumonitis as well as esophageal rupture.

Where available, *endoscopic* intervention should be employed as the first line of treatment to control bleeding acutely. Over the past decade, endoscopic sclerosis of varices has been extensively employed. In this procedure, the varices are injected with one of several sclerosing agents (e.g., sodium morrhuate) via a needle-tipped catheter passed through the endoscope. After initial endoscopic identification of varices as the presumed source of bleeding, such "sclerotherapy" controls acute bleeding in up to 90 percent of cases. In addition, repeated sclerotherapy can be performed until obliteration of all varices is accomplished in an effort to prevent recurrent bleeding. While available data support the efficacy of sclerotherapy in controlling bleeding acutely, repeated sclerotherapy to obliterate varices has not been documented to consistently prolong survival. Mucosal ulceration resulting from injection of the caustic sclerosant is sometimes seen and may result in further hemorrhage or stenosis. More recently, endoscopic ligation of varices has proven to be equally effective in controlling bleeding with fewer treatment-related complications. In this technique, varices are ligated and strangled with small, elastic O-rings placed endoscopically. Prophylactic sclerosis of esophageal varices in the absence of proven bleeding is not indicated.

The effectiveness of beta-adrenergic blocking agents (e.g., propranolol) in the management of acute variceal bleeding is limited due to concomitant hypotension resulting from hypovolemia. However, a number of studies suggest they may be of value in reducing the risk of recurrent upper gastrointestinal hemorrhage in the patient with portal hypertension. Moreover, prophylactic treatment with propranolol or nadolol in patients with large varices that have never bled may decrease the incidence of bleeding and prolong survival. Patients with portal hypertension without specific contraindications should be given propranolol in doses to effect a 25 percent reduction in the resting heart rate. Propranolol also may prevent recurrent bleeding from severe portal hypertensive gastropathy in patients with cirrhosis.

Surgical therapy of portal hypertension and variceal bleeding involves the creation of a portal-systemic shunt to permit decompression of the portal system. Two types of portal systemic shunts have been used: *nonselective shunts* to decompress the entire portal system and *selective shunts* intended to decompress only the varices while maintaining blood flow to the liver itself. Nonselective shunts include end-to-side or side-to-side portacaval and proximal splenorenal anastomoses; selective shunts include the distal splenorenal shunt. Nonselective shunts are more likely to be complicated by encephalopathy than selective shunts. Emergency portal-systemic nonselective shunts may control acute hemorrhage, but such surgery is usually used only as a last resort because early operative mortality is greater than 30 percent. The role of portal-systemic shunt surgery after initial control of bleeding by nonoperative means is also uncertain. Surgically created shunts effectively reduce the risk of recurrent hemorrhage, but the overall mortality of patients undergoing such surgery is comparable with that of unoperated patients. Although patients who have undergone portal-system surgery succumb to recurrent bleeding less commonly than unoperated patients, this improvement is counterbalanced by increased morbidity from encephalopathy and death from progressive liver failure. Prophylactic shunt surgery should not be performed in patients with nonbleeding varices. Increasingly, therapeutic portal-systemic shunt has been reserved for patients who experience further bleeding despite serial endoscopic sclerotherapy. Recently, techniques have been developed to create a portal-systemic shunt by a percutaneous approach. In this technique, designated *transjugular intrahepatic portosystemic shunt* (TIPS), an expandable metal stent is advanced to the hepatic veins under angiographic guidance and then through the substance of the liver to create a direct portacaval channel. Although control trials are needed, this technique may prove to be an appropriate alternative to surgery for refractory bleeding due to portal hypertension. Other surgical procedures (e.g., esophageal transection) also have been advocated for the management of acute variceal bleeding, although their efficacy remains unproven. Even though recent trials found that esophageal transection was as effective as endoscopic sclerotherapy, transection is considered a last resort by most authorities.

Portal hypertensive gastropathy Although variceal hemorrhage is the most commonly encountered bleeding complication of portal hypertension, many patients will develop a congestive gastropathy due to the venous hypertension. In this condition, identified by endoscopic examination, the mucosa appears engorged and friable. Indolent mucosal bleeding rather than the brisk hemorrhage resulting from a variceal source is typical. Beta-adrenergic blockade with propranolol (which reduces splanchnic arterial pressure as well as portal pressure) is sometimes effective in ameliorating this condition. H-2 receptor antagonists or other agents useful in the treatment of peptic disease are usually not helpful.

SPLENOMEGALY Definition and pathogenesis Congestive splenomegaly is common in patients with severe portal hypertension. Rarely, massive splenomegaly from nonhepatic disease leads to portal hypertension due to increased blood flow in the splenic vein.

Clinical features Although usually asymptomatic, splenomegaly may be massive and contribute to the thrombocytopenia or pancytopenia of cirrhosis. In the absence of cirrhosis, splenomegaly in association with variceal hemorrhage should suggest the possibility of splenic vein thrombosis.

Treatment Splenomegaly usually requires no specific treatment, although massive enlargement of the spleen may occasionally necessitate splenectomy at the time of shunt surgery. Splenectomy also may be indicated if splenomegaly is the cause rather than the result of portal hypertension. Thrombocytopenia alone is rarely severe enough to necessitate removal of the spleen.

ASCITES Definition Ascites is the accumulation of excess fluid within the peritoneal cavity. It is most frequently encountered in patients with cirrhosis and other forms of severe liver disease, but a number of other disorders may lead to either transudative or exudative ascites (see Chap. 43).

Pathogenesis The accumulation of ascitic fluid represents a state of total-body sodium and water excess, but the event that initiates this imbalance is unclear. Three theories have been proposed (see Fig. 268-1). The "underfilling" theory suggests that the primary abnormality is inappropriate sequestration of fluid within the splanchnic vascular bed due to portal hypertension and a consequent decrease in effective circulating blood volume. According to this theory, an apparent decrease in intravascular volume (underfilling) is sensed by the kidney, which responds by retaining salt and water. The "overflow" theory suggests that the primary abnormality is inappropriate renal retention of salt and water in the absence of volume depletion. A third theory, the peripheral arterial vasodilation hypothesis, has been proposed to account for the constellation of arterial hypotension and increased cardiac output in association with high levels of vasoconstrictor substances which are routinely found in patients with cirrhosis and ascites. Again, sodium retention is considered secondary to arterial vascular underfilling, but the result of a disproportionate increase of the vascular compartment due to arteriolar vasodilation rather than decreased intravascular volume. According to this theory, portal hypertension results in splanchnic arteriolar vasodilation leading to underfilling of the arterial vascular space and baroreceptor-mediated stimulation of renin-angiotensin, sympathetic output, and antidiuretic hormone release.

Regardless of the initiating event, a number of factors contribute to accumulation of fluid in the abdominal cavity (see Fig. 268-1). Elevated levels of serum epinephrine and norepinephrine have been well documented. *Increased central sympathetic outflow* is found in patients with cirrhosis and ascites but not in those with cirrhosis alone. Increased sympathetic output results in diminished natriuresis by activation of the renin-angiotensin system and diminished sensitivity to atrial natriuretic peptide. *Portal hypertension* plays an important

FIGURE 268-1 Multiple factors involved in development of ascites. Current concepts suggest that initiating factor may be primary sodium retention ("overflow"), diminished effective intravascular volume ("underfilling"), or arteriolar vasodilation.

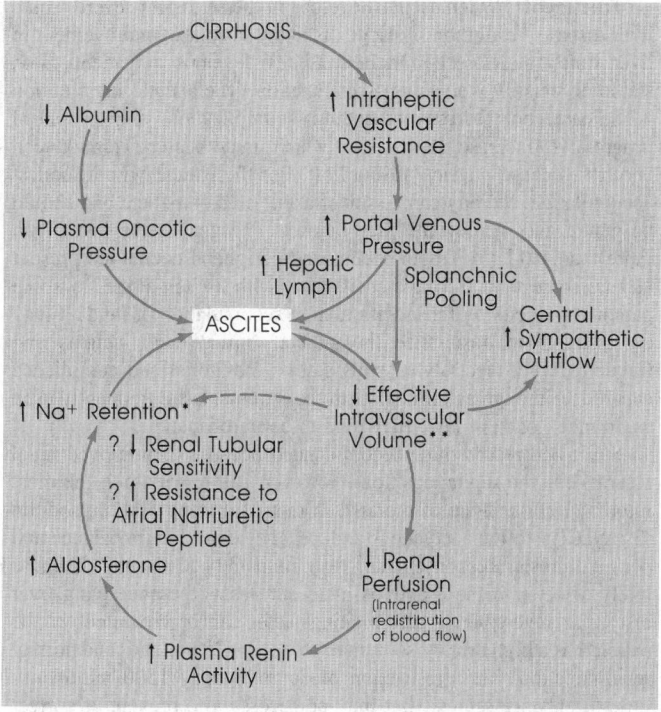

role in the formation of ascites by raising hydrostatic pressure within the splanchnic capillary bed. *Hypoalbuminemia* and *reduced plasma oncotic pressure* also favor the extravasation of fluid from plasma to the peritoneal cavity, and thus ascites is infrequent in patients with cirrhosis unless both portal hypertension and hypoalbuminemia are present. *Hepatic lymph* may weep freely from the surface of the cirrhotic liver due to distortion and obstruction of hepatic sinusoids and lymphatics and contribute to ascites formation. In contrast to the contribution of transudative fluid from the portal vascular bed, hepatic lymph may weep into the peritoneal cavity even in the absence of marked hypoproteinemia because the endothelial lining of the hepatic sinusoids is discontinuous. This mechanism may account for the high protein concentration present in the ascitic fluid of some patients with the Budd-Chiari syndrome.

Renal factors also play an important role in perpetuating ascites. Patients with ascites fail to excrete a water load in a normal fashion. They have increased renal sodium reabsorption by both proximal and distal tubules, the latter due largely to increased plasma renin activity and secondary hyperaldosteronism. Insensitivity to circulating atrial natriuretic peptide, often present in elevated concentrations in patients with cirrhosis and ascites, may be an important contributory factor in many patients. This insensitivity has been documented in those patients with the most severely impaired sodium excretion, who typically also exhibit low arterial pressure and marked overactivity of the renin-aldosterone axis. Renal vasoconstriction, perhaps resulting from increased serum prostaglandin or catecholamine levels, also may contribute to sodium retention.

Clinical features and diagnosis   Usually ascites is first noticed by the patient because of increasing abdominal girth. More pronounced accumulation of fluid may cause shortness of breath because of elevation of the diaphragm. When peritoneal fluid accumulation exceeds 500 mL, ascites may be demonstrated on physical examination by the presence of shifting dullness, a fluid wave, or bulging flanks. Ultrasound examination, preferably with a Doppler study, can detect smaller quantities of ascites and should be performed when physical examination is equivocal or when the cause of the recent onset of ascites is not clear (e.g., exclude Budd-Chiari syndrome or portal vein thrombosis). Paracentesis usually should be performed with a small-gauge needle at the time of initial evaluation or at the time of any clinical deterioration of a cirrhotic patient. A small amount of fluid (<200 mL) should be obtained and examined for evidence of infection, tumor, or other possible causes and complications of ascites.

Treatment   When ascites develops in the setting of severe, acute liver disease, resolution of ascites is likely to follow improvement in liver function. More commonly, ascites develops in patients with stable or steadily worsening liver function. Therapeutic intervention is indicated both to prevent potential complications and to control progressive increase in ascites, which may become pronounced enough to cause physical discomfort. For the patient with a modest accumulation, therapy can be undertaken as an outpatient and should be gentle and incremental (see below). The goal is the loss of no more than 1.0 kg/d if both ascites and peripheral edema are present and no more than 0.5 kg/d in patients with ascites alone. In some patients, particularly those with a large accumulation of fluid, it may be desirable to hospitalize the patient so that daily weights and frequent serum electrolyte levels can be monitored and compliance ensured. Although abdominal girth measurements are frequently used as an index of fluid loss, they tend to be unreliable.

Strict bed rest is often recommended because of improved renal clearance in the supine position. However, salt restriction is the most important cornerstone of therapy. A diet containing 800 mg sodium (2 g NaCl) is often adequate to induce a negative sodium balance and permit diuresis. Response to salt restriction and bed rest alone is more likely to occur if the ascites is of recent onset, the underlying liver disease is reversible, a precipitating factor can be corrected, or the patient has a high urinary sodium excretion (~25 mmol/d) and normal renal function. Fluid restriction of approximately 1500 mL/d does little to enhance diuresis but may be necessary to prevent or correct

hyponatremia. If sodium restriction alone fails to result in diuresis and weight loss, diuretic therapy should be instituted. Because of the role of hyperaldosteronism in sustaining salt retention, spironolactone or other distal tubule–acting diuretics (triamterene, amiloride) are the drugs of choice. These agents are also preferred because of their gentle action and specific potassium-sparing properties. Spironolactone is initially given in a dose of 25 mg four times a day and is increased as needed by 100 mg/d every several days up to a maximum dose, which rarely exceeds 400 mg/d. An indication of the minimum effective dose of spironolactone may be obtained by monitoring urinary electrolyte concentrations for a rise in sodium and fall in potassium levels reflecting effective competitive inhibition of aldosterone. Conversely, the development of azotemia or hyperkalemia may be dose-limiting or even warrant a reduction in the amount of this medication. In some patients, diuresis cannot be initiated despite maximal doses of distal tubule–acting agents (e.g., 400 mg spironolactone) because of avid proximal tubular sodium absorption. When this occurs, more potent and proximally acting diuretics (furosemide, thiazide, or ethacrynic acid) may be added cautiously to the regimen. Spironolactone plus furosemide, 20 or 80 mg/d, is usually sufficient to initiate a diuresis in most patients. However, such aggressive therapy must be used with great caution to avoid plasma volume depletion, azotemia, and hypokalemia, which may lead to encephalopathy.

In patients with a large accumulation of ascitic fluid, particularly those requiring hospitalization, large-volume paracentesis has proven to be an effective and less costly approach to initial management than prolonged bed rest and conventional diuretic treatment. In this approach, 4 to 6 L of fluid is removed by peritoneal cannula using strict aseptic techniques and monitoring hemodynamic and renal function. Albumin is infused intravenously, replacing that lost, to avoid depleting the intravascular space and precipitating hypotension. Paracentesis can be repeated daily or until all fluid has been removed. Maintenance diuretic therapy in conjunction with sodium restriction may then be instituted to avoid recurrent ascites.

A minority of patients with advanced cirrhosis have "refractory ascites" or rapidly reaccumulate fluid after control by paracentesis. In some patients, a side-to-side *portacaval shunt* may result in improvement in ascites, although generally these patients are extremely poor surgical risks. Intractable ascites also can be treated with the surgical implantation of a plastic *peritoneovenous shunt* which has a pressure-sensitive, one-way valve allowing ascitic fluid to flow from the abdominal cavity to the superior vena cava. However, the usefulness of this technique is limited by a high rate of such complications as infection, disseminated intravascular coagulation, and thrombosis of the shunt. Nonetheless, recent controlled studies have indicated equal effectiveness with medical therapies, although no benefit in survival could be documented.

SPONTANEOUS BACTERIAL PERITONITIS (SBP)   Patients with ascites and cirrhosis may develop acute bacterial peritonitis without an obvious primary source of infection. Patients with very advanced liver disease are particularly susceptible to SBP. The ascitic fluid in these patients typically has especially low concentrations of albumin and other so-called opsonic proteins which normally may provide some protection against bacteria. Typical features include abrupt onset of fever, chills, generalized abdominal pain, and rebound abdominal tenderness accompanied by cloudy ascitic fluid with a high white cell count and usually positive bacterial cultures. However, the clinical symptoms *may be minimal*, and some patients manifest only worsening jaundice or encephalopathy in the absence of localizing abdominal complaints. The diagnosis is based on careful examination of the ascitic fluid. An ascitic fluid leukocyte count of greater than 500 cells per cubic millimeter or more than 250 polymorphonuclear leukocytes should suggest the possibility of bacterial peritonitis while results of bacterial cultures of ascitic fluid are pending. Other measurements such as fluid pH or determination of gradients between serum and fluid pH or lactate are generally not necessary.

A variant of SBP, designated *monomicrobial nonneutrocytic*

bacterascites, is sometimes seen. In these patients, culture of ascitic fluid yields bacteria, but the neutrophil count is less than 250 cells per cubic millimeter. These patients often have less severe liver disease than those found initially to have typical SBP. While many patients with this variant have cleared the bacterascites at the time of a subsequent paracentesis, nearly 40 percent will develop typical SBP; thus follow-up paracentesis is usually warranted in this setting.

Empirical therapy with cefotoxanine or ampicillin and an aminoglycoside should be initiated when the diagnosis is first suspected because enteric gram-negative bacilli are found in the majority of cases; less frequently, the infection is caused by pneumococci and other gram-positive bacteria. Cefotaxime may be preferable due to the lower rate of renal toxicity. Specific antibiotic therapy can be selected once the specific organism is identified. Therapy is usually administered for 10 to 14 days, although one controlled study has suggested that a 5-day course of intravenous antibiotics may be as effective.

While appropriate antibiotic therapy is usually effective in the treatment of an episode of SBP, recurrent episodes are relatively common; as many as 70 percent of patients will experience at least one recurrence within a year of the first episode. The risk of recurrence likely reflects the predisposing role of the underlying advanced liver disease which contributed to the development of the first episode of SBP. Although the mechanism of SBP is still unclear, trials have suggested some benefit from prophylactic maintenance therapy with norfloxacin (400 mg/d) to prevent relapse or recurrence. This agent presumably causes selective decontamination of the intestine, eliminating many aerobic gram-negative bacilli.

HEPATORENAL SYNDROME Definition and pathogenesis
Hepatorenal syndrome is a serious complication in the patient with cirrhosis and ascites and is characterized by worsening azotemia with avid sodium retention and oliguria in the absence of identifiable specific causes of renal dysfunction. The exact basis for this syndrome is not clear, but altered renal hemodynamics appear to be involved. The kidneys are structurally intact; urinalysis and pyelography are usually normal. Renal biopsy, although rarely needed, is also normal, and in fact, kidneys from such patients have been used successfully for renal transplantation. There are indications that an imbalance in certain metabolites of arachidonic acid (prostaglandins and thromboxane) may play a pathogenetic role.

Clinical features and diagnosis Worsening azotemia, hyponatremia, progressive oliguria, and hypotension are the hallmarks of the hepatorenal syndrome. This syndrome, which is distinct from prerenal azotemia, may be precipitated by severe gastrointestinal bleeding, sepsis, or overly vigorous attempts at diuresis or paracentesis; it also may occur without an obvious cause. It is essential to exclude other causes of renal impairment often seen in these patients. These include prerenal azotemia or acute tubular necrosis due to hypovolemia (e.g., secondary to gastrointestinal bleeding or diuretic therapy) or an increased nitrogen load such as that seen as a result of bleeding. Drug nephrotoxicity is also often a consideration, particularly in the patient who has received agents such as aminoglycosides or contrast dye. The diagnosis is supported by the demonstration of avid urinary sodium retention. Typically, the urine sodium concentration is less than 5 mmol/L, a concentration lower than that generally found in uncomplicated prerenal azotemia. The urinary sediment is unremarkable.

Treatment Treatment is usually unsuccessful. Although some patients with hypotension and decreased plasma volume may respond to infusions of salt-poor albumin, volume expansion must be undertaken with caution to avoid precipitating variceal bleeding. Vasodilator therapy, including intravenous infusion of dopamine, is not effective.

HEPATIC ENCEPHALOPATHY Definition
Hepatic (portal-systemic) encephalopathy is a complex neuropsychiatric syndrome characterized by disturbances in consciousness and behavior, personality changes, fluctuating neurologic signs, asterixis or ''flapping tremor,'' and distinctive electroencephalographic changes. Encephalopathy may be *acute* and reversible or *chronic* and progressive. In severe cases, irreversible coma and death may occur. Acute episodes may recur with variable frequency.

Pathogenesis The specific cause of hepatic encephalopathy is unknown. The most important factors in the pathogenesis are severe hepatocellular dysfunction and/or intrahepatic and extrahepatic shunting of portal venous blood into the systemic circulation so that the liver is largely bypassed. As a result of these processes, various toxic substances absorbed from the intestine are not detoxified by the liver and lead to metabolic abnormalities in the central nervous system (CNS). Ammonia is the substance most often incriminated in the pathogenesis of encephalopathy. Many, but not all, patients with hepatic encephalopathy have elevated blood ammonia levels, and recovery from encephalopathy is often accompanied by declining blood ammonia levels. Other compounds and metabolites which may contribute to the development of encephalopathy include mercaptans (derived from intestinal metabolism of methionine), short-chain fatty acids, and phenol. Several observations suggest that excessive concentrations of γ-aminobutyric acid (GABA), an inhibitory neurotransmitter, in the CNS are important in the reduced levels of consciousness seen in hepatic encephalopathy. Increased CNS GABA may reflect failure of the liver to efficiently extract precursor amino acids or to remove GABA produced in the intestine. False neurochemical transmitters (e.g., octopamine), resulting in part from alterations in plasma levels of aromatic and branched-chain amino acids, also may play a role. An increase in the permeability of the blood-brain barrier to some of these substances may be an additional factor involved in the pathogenesis of hepatic encephalopathy. There is also evidence to suggest that endogenous benzodiazepines may contribute to the development of hepatic encephalopathy. This evidence includes isolation of 1,4-benzodiazepines from brain tissue of patients with fulminant hepatic failure as well as the partial response observed in some patients and experimental animals after administration of flumazenil, a benzodiazepine antagonist. The benzodiazepine receptor is closely associated with the GABA receptor and may facilitate GABA neurotransmission. However, the inconsistent effect of flumazenil in patients with encephalopathy, as well as potential methodologic pitfalls in the measurement of endogenous benzodiazepines, precludes definitive attribution of a role to these substances in the pathogenesis of hepatic encephalopathy.

In the patient with otherwise stable cirrhosis, hepatic encephalopathy often follows a clearly identifiable precipitating event (see Table 268-3). Perhaps the most common predisposing factor is *gastrointestinal bleeding*, which leads to an increase in the production

---

TABLE 268-3 Common precipitants of hepatic encephalopathy

INCREASED NITROGEN LOAD

Gastrointestinal bleeding
Excess dietary protein
Azotemia
Constipation

ELECTROLYTE IMBALANCE

Hypokalemia
Alkalosis
Hypoxia
Hypovolemia

DRUGS

Narcotics, tranquilizers, sedatives
Diuretics (see ''Electrolyte imbalance'')

MISCELLANEOUS

Infection
Surgery
Superimposed acute liver disease
Progressive liver disease

of ammonia and other nitrogenous substances which are then absorbed. Similarly, *increased dietary protein* may precipitate encephalopathy as a result of increased production of nitrogenous substances by colonic bacteria. *Electrolyte disturbances*, particularly hypokalemic alkalosis secondary to overzealous use of diuretics, vigorous paracentesis, or vomiting, may precipitate hepatic encephalopathy. Systemic alkalosis causes an increase in the amount of nonionic ammonia (NH_3) relative to ammonium ions (NH_4^+). Only nonionic (uncharged) ammonia readily crosses the blood-brain barrier and accumulates in the central nervous system. Hypokalemia also directly stimulates renal ammonia production. Hypoxia, injudicious use of CNS-depressing drugs (e.g., barbiturates, benzodiazepines) and acute infection may trigger or aggravate hepatic encephalopathy, although the mechanisms involved are not clear. Other potential precipitating factors include superimposed acute viral hepatitis, alcoholic hepatitis, extrahepatic bile duct obstruction, surgery, and other coincidental medical complications.

Clinical features and diagnosis Hepatic encephalopathy has protean manifestations, and any neurologic abnormality, including focal deficits, may be encountered. In patients with acute encephalopathy, neurologic deficits are completely reversible upon correction of underlying precipitating factors and/or improvement in liver function, but in patients with chronic encephalopathy, the deficits may be irreversible and progressive. Cerebral edema is frequently present and contributes to the clinical picture and overall mortality in patients with both acute and chronic encephalopathy.

The diagnosis of hepatic encephalopathy should be considered when four major factors are present: (1) acute or chronic hepatocellular disease and/or extensive portal-systemic collateral shunts (the latter may be either spontaneous, e.g., secondary to portal hypertension, or surgically created, e.g., portacaval anastomosis), (2) disturbances of awareness and mentation which may progress from forgetfulness and confusion to stupor and finally coma, (3) shifting combinations of neurologic signs, including asterixis, rigidity, hyperreflexia, extensor plantar signs, and rarely, seizures, and (4) a characteristic (but nonspecific) symmetric, high-voltage, slow-wave (2 to 5 per second) pattern on the electroencephalogram. Asterixis ("liver flap," "flapping tremor") is a nonrhythmic asymmetric lapse in voluntary sustained position of the extremities, head, and trunk. It is best demonstrated by having the patient extend the arms and dorsiflex the hands. Because elicitation of asterixis depends on sustained voluntary muscle contraction, it is not present in the comatose patient. Asterixis is nonspecific and also occurs in patients with other forms of metabolic brain disease. Alterations in personality, mood disturbances, confusion, deterioration in self-care and handwriting, and daytime somnolence are additional clinical features of encephalopathy. *Fetor hepaticus*, a unique musty odor of the breath and urine believed to be due to mercaptans, may be noted in patients with varying stages of hepatic encephalopathy. Some patients may develop spastic paraparesis or *chronic progressive hepatocerebral degeneration*, the latter a clinical variant of hepatic encephalopathy characterized by a slow decline in intellectual function, tremor, cerebellar ataxia, choreoathetosis, and psychiatric symptoms.

Grading or classifying the stages of hepatic encephalopathy is often helpful in following the course of the illness and assessing response to therapy. One useful classification is shown in Table 268-4.

The diagnosis of hepatic encephalopathy is usually one of exclusion. There are no diagnostic liver function test abnormalities, although an elevated serum ammonia level in the appropriate clinical setting is highly suggestive of the diagnosis. Examination of the cerebrospinal fluid is unremarkable, and computed tomography of the brain shows no characteristic abnormalities. A number of conditions, particularly disorders related to acute and chronic alcoholism, can mimic the clinical features of hepatic encephalopathy. These include acute alcohol intoxication, sedative overdose, delirium tremens, Wernicke's encephalopathy, and Korsakoff's psychosis (see Chap. 377). Subdural hematoma, meningitis, and hypoglycemia or other metabolic encephalopathies also must be considered, especially in

TABLE 268-4 Clinical stages of hepatic encephalopathy

Stage	Mental status	Asterixis	EEG
I	Euphoria or depression, mild confusion, slurred speech, disordered sleep	+/−	Usually normal
II	Lethargy, moderate confusion	+	Abnormal
III	Marked confusion, incoherent speech, sleeping but arousable	+	Abnormal
IV	Coma; initially responsive to noxious stimuli, later unresponsive	−	Abnormal

patients with alcoholic cirrhosis. In young patients with liver disease and neurologic abnormalities, Wilson's disease should be excluded.

Treatment Early recognition and prompt treatment of hepatic encephalopathy are essential. Patients with acute, severe hepatic encephalopathy (stage IV) require the usual supportive measures for the comatose patient. Specific treatment of hepatic encephalopathy is aimed at (1) elimination or treatment of precipitating factors and (2) lowering of blood ammonia (and other toxin) levels by decreasing the absorption of protein and nitrogenous products from the intestine. In the setting of acute gastrointestinal bleeding, blood in the bowel should be promptly evacuated with enemas and laxatives in order to reduce the nitrogen load. Protein should be excluded from the diet, and constipation should be avoided. Ammonia absorption can be decreased by the administration of lactulose, a nonabsorbable disaccharide that acts as an osmotic laxative. Metabolism of lactulose by colonic bacteria also may result in an acid pH that favors conversion of ammonia to the poorly absorbed ammonium ion. In addition, lactulose may actually diminish ammonia production through its direct effects on bacterial metabolism. Lactulose syrup can be administered in a dose of 30 to 50 mL every hour until diarrhea occurs; thereafter the dose is adjusted (usually 15 to 30 mL three times daily) so that the patient has two to four soft stools daily. Intestinal ammonia production by bacteria also can be decreased by oral administration of the antibiotic neomycin, at a dose of 0.5 to 1.0 g every 6 h. Although poorly absorbed, neomycin may reach sufficient concentrations in the bloodstream to cause renal toxicity. The use of agents such as levodopa, bromocriptine, keto analogues of essential amino acids, and intravenous amino acid formulations rich in branched-chain amino acids in the treatment of acute hepatic encephalopathy remains of unproven benefit. Flumazenil, a short-acting benzodiazepine antagonist, may have a role in management of hepatic encephalopathy precipitated by use of benzodiazepines, if there is a need for urgent therapy. Hemoperfusion to remove toxic substances and therapy directed primarily toward coincident cerebral edema in acute encephalopathy are also of unproven value.

Chronic encephalopathy may be effectively controlled by administration of lactulose. Management of patients with chronic encephalopathy should include dietary protein restriction, sometimes to levels as low as 40 g/d, in combination with low doses of lactulose or neomycin. Nephrotoxicity or ototoxicity may be limiting in prolonged usage of neomycin. There are suggestions that vegetable protein may be preferable to animal protein.

OTHER SEQUELAE OF CIRRHOSIS Coagulopathy Patients with cirrhosis often demonstrate a variety of abnormalities in both cellular and humoral clotting function. Thrombocytopenia may result from hypersplenism. In the alcoholic patient, there may be direct bone marrow suppression by ethanol. Diminished protein synthesis may lead to reduced production of fibrinogen (factor I), prothrombin (factor II), and factors V, VII, IX, and X. Reduction in levels of all factors except factor V may be worsened by the coincident malabsorption of the fat-soluble cofactor vitamin K due to cholestasis (see Chap. 254). Recent reports have documented the appearance of normal factor VIII levels following liver transplantation in patients with classical hemophilia, probably as a result of production by nonhepatocellular components of the donor organ.

Hepatocellular carcinoma See Chap. 269.

REFERENCES

Alcoholic and postnecrotic cirrhosis

ARROYO V, GINÉS P: Arteriolar vasodilation and the pathogenesis of the hyperdynamic circulation and renal sodium and water retention in cirrhosis. Gastroenterology 102:1077, 1992

BARRY RE, McGIVAN JD: Acetaldehyde alone may initiate hepatocellular damage in acute alcoholic liver disease. Gut 26:1065, 1985

BASKIN B et al: Ethanol and liver regeneration. Hepatology 8:408, 1988

BROWN J et al: Seroprevalence of hepatitis C virus nucleocapsid antibodies in patients with cryptogenic chronic liver disease. Hepatology 15:175, 1992

CARITHERS RL et al: Methylprednisolone therapy in patients with severe alcoholic hepatitis: A randomized multicenter trial. Ann Intern Med 110:685, 1989

GLUUD C et al: Prognostic indicators in alcoholic cirrhotic men. Hepatology 8:222, 1988

JEFFERS LJ et al: Prevalence of antibodies to hepatitis C virus among patients with cryptogenic chronic hepatitis and cirrhosis. Hepatology 15:187, 1992

KERSHENOBICH D et al: Colchicine in the treatment of cirrhosis of the liver. N Engl J Med 318:1709, 1988

ORREGO H et al: Long-term treatment of alcoholic liver disease with propylthiouracil. N Engl J Med 317:1421, 1987

RAMOND M-J et al: A randomized trial of prednisolone in patients with severe alcoholic hepatitis. N Engl J Med 326:507, 1992

Biliary cirrhosis

BESWICK DR et al: Asymptomatic primary biliary cirrhosis: A progress report on long-term follow-up and natural history. Gastroenterology 89:267, 1985

BODENHEIMER H JR et al: Evaluation of colchicine therapy in primary biliary cirrhosis. Gastroenterology 95:124, 1988

CHRISTENSEN E et al: Beneficial effects of azathioprine and predictor of prognosis in primary biliary cirrhosis: Final results of an international trial. Gastroenterology 89:1084, 1985

FREGEAU DR et al: Antimitochondrial antibodies of primary biliary cirrhosis recognize dihydrolipoamide acyltransferase and inhibit enzyme function of the branched chain α-ketoacid dehydrogenase complex. J Immunol 142:3815, 1989

——— et al: Inhibition of α-ketoglutarate dehydrogenase activity by a distinct population of autoantibodies recognizing dihydrolipoamide succinyltransferase in primary biliary cirrhosis. Hepatology 11:975, 1990

KAPLAN MM, KNOX TA: Treatment of primary biliary cirrhosis with low-dose weekly methotrexate. Gastroenterology 101:1332, 1991

MARKUS BH et al: Efficacy of liver transplantation in patients with primary biliary cirrhosis. N Engl J Med 320:1709, 1989

POUPON RE et al: A multicenter, controlled trial of ursodiol for the treatment of primary biliary cirrhosis. N Engl J Med 324:1548, 1991

WIESNER RH et al: A controlled trial of cyclosporine in the treatment of primary biliary cirrhosis. N Engl J Med 322:1419, 1990

YEAMAN SJ et al: Primary biliary cirrhosis: Identification of two major M2 mitochondrial autoantigens. Lancet 1:1067, 1988

Hepatic encephalopathy

BASILE AS et al: Elevated brain concentrations of 1,4-benzodiazepines in fulminant hepatic failure. N Engl J Med 325:473, 1991

BASSETT ML et al: Amelioration of hepatic encephalopathy by pharmacologic antagonism of the GABA-Benzodiazepene receptor complex in a rabbit model of fulminant hepatic failure. Gastroenterology 93:1069, 1987

BUTTERWORTH RF: Pathogenesis and treatment of portal-systemic encephalopathy: An update. Dig Dis Sci 37:321, 1992

DUDLEY FJ et al: Hepatorenal syndrome without avid sodium retention. Hepatology 6:248, 1986

FRASER CL, ARIEFF AI: Hepatic encephalopathy. N Engl J Med 313:865, 1985

JONES EA et al: The neurobiology of hepatic encephalopathy. Hepatology 4:1235, 1984

MORGAN MY, HAWLEY KE: Lactitol vs. lactulose in the treatment of acute hepatic encephalopathy in cirrhotic patients: A double blind randomized study. Hepatology 7:1278, 1987

SKOLNICK P: The γ-aminobutyric acid A (GABA$_A$)-benzodiazepine receptor complex, pp 534–536, in: Jones EA, moderator. The γ-aminobutyric A (GABA$_A$) receptor complex and hepatic encephalopathy: Some recent advances. Ann Intern Med 110:532, 1989

Portal hypertension and ascites

BURROUGHS AK et al: Randomized, double-blind, placebo-controlled trial of somatostatin for variceal bleeding. Gastroenterology 22:1388, 1990

CELLO JP et al: Endoscopic sclerotherapy versus portacaval shunt in patients with severe cirrhosis and variceal hemorrhage. N Engl J Med 311:1589, 1984

EPSTEIN M: The sodium retention of cirrhosis: A reappraisal. Hepatology 6:312, 1986

FLORAS JS et al: Increased sympathetic outflow in cirrhosis and ascites: Direct evidence from intraneural recordings. Ann Intern Med 114:373, 1991

GINÉS P et al: Comparison of paracentesis and diuretics in the treatment of cirrhotics with tense ascites: Results of a randomized study. Gastroenterology 93:234, 1987

——— et al: Paracentesis with intravenous infusion of albumin as compared with peritoneovenous shunting in cirrhosis with refractory ascites. N Engl J Med 325:829, 1991

MILLIKAN WJ et al: The Emory prospective randomized trial: Selective versus nonselective shunt to control variceal bleeding. Ann Surg 201:712, 1985

NICHOLLS KM et al: Sodium excretion in advanced cirrhosis: Effect of expansion of central blood volume and suppression of plasma aldosterone. Hepatology 6:235, 1986

PAGLIARO L et al: Prevention of first bleeding in cirrhosis: A meta-analysis of randomized trials of nonsurgical treatment. Ann Intern Med 117:59, 1992

PASTA L et al: Propranolol for prophylaxis of bleeding in cirrhotic patients with large varices: A multicenter randomized clinical trial. Hepatology 8:1, 1988

PINTO PC et al: Large-volume paracentesis in nonedematous patients with tense ascites: Its affect on intravascular volume. Hepatology 8: 207, 1988

PINZANI M et al: Altered furosemide pharmacokinetics in chronic alcoholic liver disease with ascites contributes to diuretic resistance. Gastroenterology 92:294, 1987

PYNARD T et al: Beta-adrenergic-antagonist drugs in the prevention of gastrointestinal bleeding in patients with cirrhosis and esophageal varices. N Engl J Med 324:1532, 1991

RING EJ et al: Using transjugular intrahepatic portosystemic shunts to control variceal bleeding before liver transplantation. Ann Intern Med 116:304, 1992

STIEGMANN GV et al: Endoscopic sclerotherapy as compared with endoscopic ligation for bleeding esophageal varices. N Engl J Med 326:1527, 1992

TERBLANCHE J et al: Controversies in the management of bleeding esophageal varices. N Engl J Med 320:1394, 1469, 1989

Spontaneous bacterial peritonitis

CROSSLEY JR, WILLIAMS R: Spontaneous bacterial peritonitis. Gut 26:325, 1985

DEPARTMENT OF MEDICINE, UNIVERSITY OF NEW MEXICO SCHOOL OF MEDICINE et al: Monomicrobial nonneutrocytic bacterascites: A variant of spontaneous bacterial peritonitis. Hepatology 12:710, 1990

GINÉS P et al: Norfloxacin prevents spontaneous bacterial peritonitis recurrence in cirrhosis: Results of a double-blind, placebo-controlled trial. Hepatology 12:716, 1990

RUNYON BA et al: Short-course versus long-course antibiotic treatment of spontaneous bacterial peritonitis: A randomized controlled study of 100 patients. Gastroenterology 100: 1737, 1991

TITÓ L et al: Recurrence of spontaneous bacterial peritonitis in cirrhosis: Frequency and predictive factors. Hepatology 8:27, 1988

---

269 TUMORS OF THE LIVER

KURT J. ISSELBACHER / JULES L. DIENSTAG*

BENIGN LIVER TUMORS

HEPATOCELLULAR ADENOMAS Hepatocellular adenomas are benign tumors of the liver found predominantly in women in their third and fourth decades. Their preponderance in women suggests a hormonal influence in their pathogenesis, and oral contraceptives have been implicated. There has been a striking increase in these adenomas since oral contraceptives were introduced, and the majority of patients in whom the tumors are found have been on these hormonal agents. Multiple hepatic adenomas have been associated with glycogen storage disease type I.

Hepatic adenomas occur predominantly in the right lobe of the liver, may be multiple, and are often quite large (i.e., >10 cm). Microscopically, they consist of normal or slightly atypical hepatocytes. They have an increase in glycogen, making them appear paler and larger than normal. Clinical features include pain and the presence of a palpable mass or features of intratumor hemorrhage (pain and circulatory collapse). The diagnosis is usually made by a combination of techniques: sonography, computed tomographic (CT) scan, selective hepatic arteriography, and radionuclide scans. The angiographic appearance is typically hypervascular but often also with hypovascular regions. Technetium 99m scans usually show a defect because phagocytosing Kupffer cells are absent. There is a risk of malignant change in the range of 10 percent; the risk is increased in large (>10 cm) and multiple adenomas.

As far as management is concerned, a patient taking oral contraceptives should stop doing so. If the lesion is large (i.e., 8 to 10 cm),

* The authors acknowledge Jack Wands' contribution to this chapter in the 12th edition.

near the surface, and resectable, surgery is appropriate. Because of the risk of rupture, pregnancy should be avoided.

FOCAL NODULAR HYPERPLASIA   Focal nodular hyperplasia is a benign tumor often picked up accidentally on CT scans or at laparoscopy done for other reasons. It also occurs predominantly in women, but in contrast to hepatic adenomas, oral contraceptives do not appear to be implicated, and hemorrhage and necrosis are rare. The risk of hemorrhage, however, appears to be increased in women taking oral contraceptives. Typically, it is a solid tumor, often in the right lobe, with a fibrous core and stellate projections. In the fibrous projections, one may find atypical hepatocytes, biliary epithelium, Kupffer cells, and inflammatory cells. A radionuclide technetium scan will usually show a hot spot because of the presence of Kupffer cells. The lesion appears vascular on angiography, and septations may be detectable. If the lesion is asymptomatic, surgery is not indicated.

HEMANGIOMA AND OTHER BENIGN TUMORS   *Hemangiomas* are probably the most common benign liver tumors, occurring predominantly in women and usually detected when abdominal imaging is done for unrelated symptoms or unexpectedly at surgery. The prevalence in the general population is in the range of 0.5 to 7.0 percent. These vascular lesions are usually asymptomatic and can be identified by magnetic resonance imaging (MRI), contrast-enhanced CT, labeled red blood cell nuclide scans, or hepatic angiography. They do not need to be removed unless they are large and are producing a mass effect. Hemorrhage is rare, and malignant change does not occur.

Nodular regenerative hyperplasia consists of multiple hepatic nodules resulting from periportal hepatocyte regeneration with surrounding atrophy. It may be associated with underlying conditions such as malignancy or connective tissue disease. Portal hypertension (in the absence of cirrhosis) is the most common clinical manifestation. Other less common benign hepatic lesions include *bile duct adenomas* and *cystadenomas*. *Juvenile hemangioendotheliomas* occur in children together with congestive heart failure and cutaneous hemangiomas.

CARCINOMAS OF THE LIVER

HEPATOCELLULAR CARCINOMA   **Epidemiology and etiology** Primary hepatocellular carcinoma is one of the most common tumors in the world. It is especially prevalent in regions of Asia and sub-Saharan Africa, where the annual incidence is up to 500 cases per 100,000 population. In the United States and western Europe, it is much less common, accounting for only 1 to 2 percent of malignant tumors at autopsy. Hepatocellular carcinoma is up to four times more common in men than in women and usually arises in a cirrhotic liver. The peak incidence occurs in the fifth to sixth decades of life in western countries but one to two decades earlier in regions of Asia and Africa with a high prevalence of liver carcinoma.

The principal reason for the high incidence of hepatocellular carcinoma in parts of Asia and Africa is the frequency of chronic infection with *hepatitis B virus* (HBV) and *hepatitis C virus* (HCV). These chronic infections frequently lead to cirrhosis, which itself is an important risk factor for hepatocellular carcinoma; 60 to 90 percent of these tumors occur in patients with macronodular cirrhosis. The role of HBV as a factor is fairly convincing. Studies in regions of Asia where hepatocellular carcinoma and HBV infection are prevalent have shown that the incidence over time of this cancer is about 100-fold higher in individuals with evidence of HBV infection than in noninfected controls. In patients with HBV infection and hepatocellular carcinoma, HBV DNA may be integrated into host genomic DNA, both in the tumor cells and in adjacent, uninvolved hepatocytes. In addition, there can be modifications of cellular gene expression by insertional mutagenesis, chromosomal rearrangements, or the transcriptional transactivating activity of the X and the pre-52/S regions of the HBV genome. These alterations probably occur during the process of liver cell injury and repair.

Since the discovery in 1989 of hepatitis C viruses as the agent responsible for most cases of non-A, non-B hepatitis, an increasing body of evidence has implicated HCV in hepatocellular carcinoma. In fact, studies of patients in Europe and Japan have shown HCV to be substantially more prevalent than HBV in cases of hepatocellular carcinoma. In some patients, both HBV and HCV can be demonstrated, but the clinical course of the liver malignancy does not appear to differ between patients with both infections and those in whom only one of the two viruses is implicated. One distinction in high-prevalence areas between hepatocellular carcinoma associated with HBV infection and that associated with HCV infection is in the timing of onset. In Asia, hepatitis B is acquired at birth via perinatal transmission, while HCV infection is acquired primarily during adulthood from transfused blood. As a reflection of this distinction in time of infection, the onset of liver carcinoma occurs one to two decades earlier in those with lifelong hepatitis B than it does in adult-acquired hepatitis C.

Any agent or factor that contributes to chronic, low-grade liver cell damage and mitosis makes hepatocyte DNA more susceptible to genetic alterations. Thus, as indicated above, *chronic liver disease* of any type is a risk factor and predisposes to the development of liver cell carcinoma. This includes alcoholic liver disease, α_1-antitrypsin deficiency, hemochromatosis, and tyrosinemia. In Africa and southern China, *aflatoxin B_1* is an important public health hazard. This mycotoxin appears to induce a very specific mutation at codon 249 in the tumor suppressor gene p53.

The loss, inactivation, or mutation of the p53 gene has been implicated in tumorigenesis and is the most common genetic derangement present in human cancers. Thus HBV and aflatoxin B_1 have been implicated in the pathogenesis of hepatocellular carcinoma in regions of Africa and southern China where both agents are prevalent.

In view of the male predominance in liver cancer, hormonal factors also may play a role. Hepatocellular tumors may occur with long-term androgenic steroid administration, with exposure to thorium dioxide or vinyl chloride (see below), and possibly with exposure to estrogens in the form of oral contraceptives.

Clinical and laboratory features   Cancers of the liver initially may escape clinical recognition because they often occur in patients with underlying cirrhosis, and the symptoms and signs may suggest progression of the underlying disease. The most common presenting features are abdominal *pain* with detection of an abdominal mass in the right upper quadrant. There may be a *friction rub* or *bruit* over the liver. Blood-tinged ascites occurs in about 20 percent of cases. Jaundice is rare, unless there is significant deterioration of liver function or mechanical obstruction of the bile ducts. Serum elevations of alkaline phosphatase and alpha fetoprotein (AFP) are common (see below). An abnormal type of prothrombin, des-γ-carboxy prothrombin, is also detectable and in general correlates with AFP elevations.

A small percentage of patients with hepatocellular carcinoma may have evidence of *paraneoplastic syndrome;* erythrocytosis may result from erythropoietin-like activity produced by the tumor, or hypercalcemia may result from secretion of a parathyroid-like hormone. Other manifestations may include hypercholesterolemia, hypoglycemia, acquired porphyria, dysfibrinogenemia, and cryofibrinogenemia.

Imaging procedures used to detect liver tumors include ultrasound, CT, MRI, hepatic artery angiography (see Chap. 248), and radionuclide scans with technetium 99m. Ultrasound is frequently used to screen high-risk populations and should be the first procedure if hepatocellular carcinoma is suspected; it is less costly than scanning procedures, is relatively sensitive, and can detect most tumors greater than 3 cm. MRI, however, is being used with increasing frequency.

Alpha fetoprotein (AFP) levels greater than 500 μg/L are found in about 70 to 80 percent of patients with hepatocellular carcinoma. Lower levels may be found in patients with large metastases from gastric or colonic tumors and in some patients with acute or chronic hepatitis. The presence and persistence of high levels of serum AFP (over 500 to 1000 μg/L) in an adult with liver disease and without an obvious gastrointestinal tumor strongly suggest hepatocellular carcinoma. Increasing levels with time suggest progression of the tumor or recurrence after hepatic resection or therapeutic approaches such as chemotherapy or chemoembolization (see below).

Percutaneous *liver biopsy* can be diagnostic if taken in an area localized by ultrasound or CT. The risk that tumor cells will migrate along the biopsy track exists, but it is small; because these tumors tend to be vascular, percutaneous biopsies should be done with caution. Cytologic examination of ascitic fluid is invariably negative for tumor cells. Occasionally, *laparoscopy* or *minilaparotomy* may be required, permitting liver cell biopsy under direct vision. This approach has the additional advantage of identifying the occasional patient with localized resectable tumor suitable for partial hepatectomy.

Course and management   The course of the disease is rapid; if untreated, most patients die within 3 to 6 months of diagnosis. In selected cases, therapy may prolong life. *Surgical resection* offers the only chance for cure; however, few patients have a resectable tumor at the time of presentation because of underlying cirrhosis, involvement of both hepatic lobes, or distant metastases (common sites are lung, brain, bone, and adrenal), and the 5-year survival is low. In patients at high risk for the development of hepatocellular carcinoma, such as HBsAg-positive patients and patients with cirrhosis, including that caused by chronic hepatitis C, screening programs have been initiated to identify small tumors when they are still resectable. Because 20 to 30 percent of patients with hepatocellular carcinoma do not have elevated levels of circulating AFP, ultrasonographic screening is recommended as well. In a study in the Far East, HBsAg-positive persons, with or without liver disease, were screened serially; a number of patients with small, subclinical tumors were identified and surgical resection undertaken. Follow-up observation revealed a 5-year survival rate in this group of 70 percent and a 10-year survival rate of 50 percent. These Asian patients, however, were unusual in that they had minimal or no liver disease and their tumors tended to be unifocal or encapsulated. The findings of this Asian study stand in contrast to a study in a large population of Italian patients with cirrhosis associated in most cases with chronic HBV and HCV infections; screening every 3 to 12 months permitted the detection of a 3 percent annual incidence of cancer in this cohort but in most cases failed to achieve the goal of early detection of surgically treatable disease.

Liver transplantation may be considered as a therapeutic option, but recurrence of tumor or metastases after transplantation have limited its usefulness (see Chap. 271). Other experimental approaches that are being evaluated include (1) hepatic artery embolization with chemotherapy (chemoembolization), (2) alcohol ablation via ultrasound-guided percutaneous injection, (3) ultrasound-guided cryoablation, (4) immunotherapy with monoclonal antibodies tagged with cytotoxic agents, and (5) gene therapy with retroviral vectors containing genes expressing cytotoxic agents.

OTHER MALIGNANT TUMORS

Fibrolamellar carcinoma differs from the typical hepatocellular carcinoma in that it tends to occur in young adults without underlying cirrhosis. This tumor is nonencapsulated but well circumscribed and contains fibrous lamellae; it grows slowly and is associated with a longer survival if treated. Surgical resection has resulted in 5-year survivals exceeding 50 percent; if the lesion is nonresectable, liver transplantation is an option, and the outcome far exceeds that observed in the nonfibrolamellar variety of liver cancer. *Hepatoblastoma* is a tumor of infancy typically with very high serum AFP levels. The lesions are usually solitary, may be resectable, and have a better 5-year survival than hepatocellular carcinoma. *Cholangiocarcinoma* is uncommon but has been associated with primary sclerosing cholangitis and in the Far East with clonorchiasis or opisthorchiasis. Often, the lesion occurs at the bifurcation of the common bile duct ("Klatskin

tumor"). These lesions are almost never resectable, and they invariably recur if liver transplantation is attempted. Biliary diversion, originally achieved surgically and nowadays accomplished by the insertion of stents, either percutaneously or endoscopically, can relieve biliary obstruction, but the prognosis remains poor. *Angiosarcoma* consists of vascular spaces lined by malignant endothelial cells. Etiologic factors include prior exposure to thorium dioxide (Thorotrast), polyvinyl chloride, arsenic, and androgenic anabolic steroids. *Epithelioid hemangioendothelioma* is of borderline malignancy; most are benign, but metastases occur. This tumor occurs in early adulthood, presents with right upper quadrant pain, is heterogeneous on sonography, hypodense on CT, and without neovascularity on angiography. Immunohistochemical staining reveals expression of factor VIII antigen. In the absence of extrahepatic metastases, these lesions can be treated by surgical resection or liver transplantation.

METASTATIC TUMORS   Metastatic malignant tumors of the liver are common in clinical practice, ranking second only to cirrhosis as a cause of fatal liver disease. In the United States, the incidence of clinically significant metastatic carcinoma is at least 20 times greater than that of primary carcinoma. Hepatic metastases have been reported at autopsy in 30 to 50 percent of patients dying from malignant disease.

Pathogenesis   The liver is uniquely vulnerable to invasion by tumor cells. Its size, high rate of blood flow, double perfusion by hepatic artery and portal vein, and its Kupffer cell filtration function combine to make it the most common site of metastases, except for the lymph nodes. In addition, local tissue factors or endothelial membrane characteristics appear to enhance metastatic implants. Virtually all types of neoplasms except those primary in the brain may metastasize to the liver. The most common primary tumors are those of the gastrointestinal tract, lung, breast, and melanomas. Less common are metastases from tumors of the thyroid, prostate, and skin.

Clinical features   Most patients with metastatic malignancy of the liver present with (1) symptoms usually referable only to the primary tumor, with asymptomatic hepatic involvement discovered in the course of clinical evaluation; (2) nonspecific symptoms of weakness, weight loss, fever, sweating, and loss of appetite, or rarely, (3) features indicating active hepatic disease, especially abdominal pain, hepatomegaly, or ascites.

Patients with widespread metastatic liver involvement usually have suggestive clinical signs of cancer and hepatic enlargement. Some have localized induration or tenderness, and occasionally, a friction rub may be found over tender areas of the liver.

Abdominal liver biochemical tests are frequent but often mildly elevated and nonspecific. They reflect the effects of fever and wasting, as well as those of the infiltrating neoplastic process itself. An increase in serum alkaline phosphatase is the most common and frequently the only abnormality noted. Hypoalbuminemia, anemia, and occasional mild elevation of aminotransferase levels also may be found with more widespread disease. Greatly elevated serum levels of carcinoembryonic antigen (CEA) are usually found when the metastases are from primary malignancies in the gastrointestinal tract, breast, or lung.

Diagnosis   Evidence of metastatic invasion of the liver should be sought actively in any patient with a primary malignancy, especially of the lung, gastrointestinal tract, or breast, before resection of the primary lesion is undertaken. Abnormal liver biochemical tests, particularly an elevated alkaline phosphatase, or demonstration of a mass by liver ultrasound, CT, or MRI may provide a presumptive diagnosis. Blind percutaneous needle biopsy of the liver will result in a positive diagnosis of metastatic disease in only 60 to 80 percent of cases with hepatomegaly and elevated alkaline phosphatase levels. Serial sectioning of specimens, two or three repeat biopsies, or cytologic examination of biopsy smears may increase the diagnostic yield by 10 to 15 percent. The yield is greatly increased when biopsies are directed by ultrasound or CT or obtained at laparoscopy.

Treatment   Most metastatic carcinomas respond poorly to all forms of treatment, which is usually only palliative. Surgical removal of a single, large metastasis is rarely feasible. Systemic chemotherapy with combinations of different chemotherapeutic agents may slow tumor growth briefly and reduce symptoms in some patients but does not significantly alter the prognosis. Chemoembolization, intrahepatic chemotherapy, and alcohol ablation may provide palliation. It remains to be determined whether newer drugs, combination chemotherapy, or novel strategies (including immunologic targeting) will eventually prove to be more effective.

REFERENCES

COLOMBO M et al: Hepatocellular carcinoma in Italian patients with cirrhosis. N Engl J Med 325:675, 1991

DiBisceglie AM: Hepatocellular carcinoma. Ann Intern Med 108:390, 1988

KERLIN P et al: Hepatic adenoma and focal nodular hyperplasia: Clinical pathologic and radiologic features. Gastroenterology 84:994, 1983

KEW MC: Hepatic tumors. Semin Liver Dis 4:89, 1984

OKUDA K: Hepatocellular carcinoma: Recent progress. Hepatology 15:948, 1992

OZTURK M: p53 mutation in hepatocellular carcinoma after aflatoxin exposure. Lancet 338:1356, 1991

SAITO I et al: Hepatitis C virus infection is associated with the development of hepatocellular carcinoma. Proc Natl Acad Sci USA 87:6547, 1990

TABOR E et al: *Etiology, Pathology, and Treatment of Hepatocellular Carcinoma in North America.* Houston, Gulf Publishing, 1991

TAO LC: Oral contraceptive–associated liver cell adenoma and hepatocellular carcinoma: Cytomorphology and malignant transformation. Cancer 68:341, 1991

VENOOK AP et al: Chemoembolization for hepatocellular carcinoma. J Clin Oncol 8:1108, 1990

270 INFILTRATIVE AND METABOLIC DISEASES AFFECTING THE LIVER

KURT J. ISSELBACHER / DANIEL K. PODOLSKY

Many disseminated, systemic, or metabolic diseases involve the liver in a diffuse manner by the infiltration of abnormal cells or the accumulation of chemical substances or metabolites. Chemical accumulation may be extracellular or intracellular and may involve hepatocytes, Kupffer cells, or other elements of the reticuloendothelial system. Although infiltrative diseases may vary widely in cause and extrahepatic manifestations, the findings in the liver may be quite similar. Generalized enlargement and firmness of the liver, gradual and nonspecific deterioration of liver function, and, less often, signs of portal hypertension or ascites are typical features of this group of diseases. Differential diagnosis by clinical means may be difficult on occasion, but in patients in whom ancillary clinical findings do not establish the diagnosis, the diffusely infiltrated liver provides an excellent source of tissue for diagnostic purposes.

FATTY LIVER (See also Chap. 264)

Slight to moderate enlargement of the liver due to a diffuse accumulation of neutral fat (triglycerides) in hepatocytes is an important clinical and pathologic finding. Imaging procedures such as computed tomography (CT), ultrasound, and magnetic resonance imaging (MRI) may each yield alterations suggesting increased fat in the liver. As discussed in Chap. 264, fatty liver can be due to increased amounts of fat reaching the liver via the bloodstream or lymphatics, increased synthesis or decreased oxidation of lipids in the liver, and/or decreased export of very low density lipoproteins (VLDL) from the liver. Fatty liver can be separated into two categories based on whether the fat droplets in the hepatocytes are macrovesicular or macrovesicular fat (Table 270-1).

TABLE 270-1 Causes of fatty liver

Macrovesicular (large fat droplets in hepatocytes)
  A Alcohol, alcoholic liver disease
  B Diabetes mellitus
  C Obesity
  D Protein-calorie malnutrition
  E Glucocorticoid therapy
  F Total parenteral nutrition
  G Drugs, e.g., methotrexate
Microvesicular (small fat droplets in hepatocytes)
  A Reye's syndrome
  B Acute fatty liver of pregnancy
  C Jamaican vomiting sickness
  D Valproic acid, tetracycline toxicity

MACROVESICULAR FATTY LIVER This is the most common type of fatty liver and is seen most frequently in alcoholism or alcoholic liver disease, diabetes mellitus, obesity, and prolonged parenteral nutrition. Hematoxylin and eosin–stained liver sections show hepatocytes with large, empty vacuoles with the nucleus "pushed" to the periphery of the cell. In general, fat in the liver is not damaging per se, and the fat will disappear with improvement or elimination of the predisposing condition.

Etiology The major causes of fatty liver with macrovesicular fat depend on the age, geographic location, and metabolic-nutritional status of the patient population. *Chronic alcoholism* is the most common cause of fatty liver in this country and in other countries with a high alcohol intake. The severity of fatty involvement is roughly proportional to the duration and degree of alcoholic excess. *Protein malnutrition*, especially in infancy and early childhood, accounts for most cases of severe fatty liver in the tropical zones of Africa, South America, and Asia. The hepatic changes may be associated with other clinical and pathologic features of kwashiorkor. Patients with adult-onset *diabetes mellitus*, especially those who are overweight and are poorly controlled, often have fatty livers. *Obesity* is commonly associated with fatty infiltration of the liver; this recedes as weight reduction occurs. However, *jejunoileal bypass* for surgical treatment of morbid obesity is sometimes associated with severe fatty liver and hepatic failure that may be fatal. In patients with Cushing's syndrome and in those receiving large doses of glucocorticoids, fatty infiltration of the liver may occur. In many *chronic illnesses*, especially those complicated by impaired nutrition or malabsorption, increased fat is found in liver cells. For example, patients with severe ulcerative colitis, chronic pancreatitis, or protracted heart failure frequently have moderately fatty livers at the time of death. Patients maintained on prolonged *total parenteral nutrition* also may develop fatty livers.

Acute fatty liver is caused by a number of hepatotoxins and is frequently accompanied by signs and symptoms of liver failure. Carbon tetrachloride intoxication, DDT poisoning, and ingestion of substances containing yellow phosphorus result in severe fatty liver. Acute and prolonged alcohol ingestion also may be considered in this category and may be associated with a rapidly enlarging and fat-laden liver.

Clinical features The signs and symptoms of fatty liver are related to the degree of fat infiltration, the time course of its accumulation, and the underlying cause. The obese or diabetic patient with chronic fatty liver is usually asymptomatic and has only mild tenderness over the enlarged liver. The liver function tests are normal or show mild elevations of alkaline phosphatase, transaminases, or aminotransferases. In contrast, the rapid accumulation of fat seen in the setting of hyperalimentation may lead to marked tenderness, presumably resulting from stretching of Glisson's capsule. Similarly, alcoholic patients with acute fatty liver following a bout of heavy drinking may have right upper quadrant pain and tenderness often with laboratory evidence of cholestasis. The clinical presentation of acute fatty liver of pregnancy or fatty liver from hepatotoxins is similar to that of fulminant hepatic failure arising from any cause, with evidence of hepatic encephalopathy, marked elevations of prothrombin time and transaminases, and variable degrees of jaundice.

Diagnosis The findings of a firm, nontender, and generally enlarged liver with minimal hepatic dysfunction in a patient with chronic alcoholism, malnutrition, poorly controlled diabetes mellitus, or obesity should suggest a fatty liver. This can usually be detected by CT scans, MRI, or ultrasound. When diagnostic uncertainty exists, needle biopsy of the liver will demonstrate the increased fatty content and possibly the underlying primary disorder.

Treatment Adequate nutritional intake, removal of alcohol or offending toxins, and correction of any associated metabolic disorders usually result in recovery. There is no clinical rationale for the use of lipotropic agents such as choline. When indicated, attention should be directed to abstinence from alcohol, careful control of diabetes, weight loss, or correction of intestinal absorptive defects. In the alcoholic fatty liver there is gradual disappearance of fat from the liver after 4 to 8 weeks of adequate diet and abstinence from alcohol. Similarly, fatty infiltration usually resolves within 2 weeks after discontinuation of parenteral hyperalimentation. However, patients with jejunoileal bypass may develop progressive liver inflammation and fibrosis in addition to fatty liver; hence restitution of intestinal continuity may not prevent progression of disease.

MICROVESICULAR FATTY LIVER This is the less common form of fatty liver. On microscopic examination, the fat is present in many small vacuoles. Although the droplets consist of triglycerides in both the macrovesicular and microvesicular forms, the reason for this difference in morphologic appearance is not clear.

REYE'S SYNDROME (FATTY LIVER WITH ENCEPHALOPATHY)
This acute illness is encountered exclusively in children below 15 years of age. It is characterized clinically by vomiting and signs of progressive central nervous system damage, signs of hepatic injury, and hypoglycemia. Morphologically, there is extensive fatty vacuolization of the liver and renal tubules. There is mitochondrial dysfunction with decreased activity of hepatic mitochondrial enzymes. The cause is unknown, although viral and toxic agents, especially salicylates, have been implicated. Increased aspirin use and much higher serum salicylate levels in children with this illness than in the general population have been described during outbreaks of Reye's syndrome. However, it seems clear that this illness also may occur in the absence of exposure to salicylates. In fatal cases, the liver is enlarged and yellow with striking diffuse fatty microvacuolization of cells. Peripheral zonal hepatic necrosis also has been present in some cases. Fatty changes of the renal tubular cells, cerebral edema, and neuronal degeneration of the brain are the major extrahepatic changes. Electron-microscopic studies show structural alterations of mitochondria in liver, brain, and muscle.

The onset usually follows an upper respiratory tract infection, especially influenza or chickenpox. Within 1 to 3 days, persistent vomiting occurs, together with stupor, which usually progresses rapidly to generalized convulsions and coma. The liver is enlarged, but *jaundice is characteristically absent or minimal*. Elevations in serum aminotransferases and prothrombin time, hypoglycemia, metabolic acidosis, and elevated serum ammonia levels are the major laboratory findings. The mortality rate in Reye's syndrome is approximately 50 percent. Therapy consists of infusions of glucose and fresh frozen plasma, as well as intravenous mannitol to reduce the cerebral edema. Chronic liver disease has not been reported in survivors.

Acute fatty liver of pregnancy is a syndrome that occurs late in pregnancy and is often associated with jaundice and hepatic failure. In half the cases it is associated with preeclampsia. If diagnosed in time, the disease usually resolves with termination of the pregnancy.

Microvesicular fat accumulation also may be seen as a toxic reaction to *valproic acid* and with excessive doses of *tetracycline*. It is a typical finding in *Jamaican vomiting sickness*, which is caused by hypoglycin A present in unripened ackee fruit.

STORAGE DISEASES

Lipid storage diseases include the hereditary disorders of Gaucher's and Niemann-Pick disease. Other rare disorders associated with increased fat in the liver include abetalipoproteinemia, Tangier disease, Fabry's disease, and types I and V hyperlipoproteinemia (see Chap. 344 for details). Hepatic enlargement caused by distention of liver cells with glycogen is present in some poorly controlled diabetics and frequently in juvenile diabetes. More often, however, hepatomegaly is due to fatty infiltration. Ketoacidosis and vigorous insulin therapy may further enhance hepatic enlargement. In the absence of cirrhosis, hepatomegaly usually decreases with control of the diabetes.

HEPATIC MINERAL ACCUMULATION

WILSON'S DISEASE (See Chap. 348) This rare disease, predominantly of young people, is characterized by cirrhosis, softening and degeneration of the basal ganglia, and pigmentation of the cornea (Kayser-Fleischer rings). Increased copper deposition in the tissues seems to be responsible for the liver and basal ganglia changes. Liver cells are ballooned and show increased glycogen with glycogen vacuolization in the nuclei. The liver shows all grades of changes, from minimal to severe periportal or macronodular cirrhosis.

HEMOCHROMATOSIS (See Chap. 345) This relatively common genetically determined disorder involves accumulation of abnormal amounts of iron due to inappropriate absorption in the intestine. The liver, as a primary site of iron storage, is affected most directly. There is diffuse deposition of excess iron in hepatocytes, in contrast to the characteristic accumulation of iron in the reticuloendothelial compartment typical of secondary iron overload and hemosiderosis. Hepatic iron overload commonly results in hepatomegaly. Although liver function is initially well preserved, if the disease is untreated, progressive impairment is followed by the development of cirrhosis.

OTHER INFILTRATIVE DISEASES

HURLER'S SYNDROME (See Chap. 349) This is an uncommon hereditary disease that is characterized by the widespread tissue deposition of mucopolysaccharide (chondroitin sulfate B and heparan sulfate) in many tissues. The liver is frequently enlarged and firm. Microscopically, Kupffer cells and other macrophages are enlarged and filled with metachromatic granular material. Cirrhosis may be a late complication.

α_1-ANTITRYPSIN DEFICIENCY (See also Chap. 223) Patients with homozygous deficiency of serum α_1-antitrypsin (α1AT) are prone to develop emphysema in adult life. The disease is suggested by the absence of alpha$_1$ globulin on serum electrophoresis (α1AT makes up 90 percent of this fraction normally) and confirmed by direct measurement of α1AT. The exact phenotype can then be determined by starch electrophoresis. Although there are 16 recognized alleles, only PiZ and PiS are associated with clinical disease. The molecular bases of these altered products have been related to single nucleic acid substitutions, e.g., PiZ is caused by a G (guanine) to A (adenine) transposition, which results in a substitution of a glutamic acid for lysine at residue 292 in the α1AT protein. Hepatocytes of some patients with this deficiency contain globules positive to the periodic acid Schiff (PAS) reaction. Approximately 10 percent of children with homozygous deficiency (PiZZ phenotype) of α1AT will develop significant liver disease, including neonatal hepatitis and progressive cirrhosis. It has been suggested that 15 to 20 percent of all chronic liver disease in infancy may be attributed to α1AT deficiency. In adults, the most common manifestation of α1AT deficiency is asymptomatic cirrhosis, which may progress from a micronodular to a macronodular state and may be complicated by the development of hepatocellular carcinoma. The occurrence of liver disease in these patients is not dependent on the development of lung disease.

RETICULOENDOTHELIAL DISORDERS (See also Chaps. 58 and 311)

Moderate to massive hepatomegaly and splenomegaly occur frequently in the various types of *leukemia* and *lymphoma*. Jaundice, when present, is usually slight and results from hemolysis. Deep and protracted jaundice is distinctly rare and is caused by obstruction of the intrahepatic or extrahepatic bile ducts by tumor. Liver biopsy specimens reveal portal and sinusoidal infiltrates in most cases of leukemia, but the cellular pattern may be mixed and nonspecific. Liver biopsy is diagnostic in only 5 percent of patients with *Hodgkin's disease*. This percentage is increased in those with advanced disease or splenomegaly. Directed biopsy at laparoscopy or laparotomy is more likely to be positive than "blind" needle biopsy. Nonspecific histologic changes in the liver have been described in patients with lymphoma and may contribute to the abnormal liver function tests.

Myeloid metaplasia and other myeloproliferative disorders associated with extramedullary hematopoiesis produce hepatomegaly which may reach huge proportions, especially following splenectomy. Serum alkaline phosphatase elevations are often found. Ascites and portal hypertension, resulting from diffuse involvement of portal venules and lymphatics, are rare complications.

GRANULOMATOUS INFILTRATIONS

Perhaps as a result of the large population of mononuclear phagocytes, a number of systemic granulomatous diseases involve the liver, including sarcoidosis, miliary tuberculosis, histoplasmosis, brucellosis, schistosomiasis, berylliosis, and drug reactions (Table 270-2). In addition, isolated granulomas of no diagnostic importance may be found occasionally in patients with various forms of cirrhosis and hepatitis. The liver infiltrated by granulomas may be slightly enlarged and firm, but hepatic dysfunction is usually limited and manifested

---

TABLE 270-2   Some causes of hepatic granulomas

Systemic disease
 A Sarcoidosis
 B Hodgkin's and non-Hodgkin's lymphoma
 C Primary biliary cirrhosis
 D Berylliosis
 E Crohn's disease
 F Wegener's granulomatosis
 G Granulomatous hepatitis, idiopathic
Infections
 A Bacterial
  1 Tuberculosis
  2 Mycobacterium avium intracellulare
  3 Brucellosis
  4 Leprosy
 B Viral
  1 Epstein-Barr virus
  2 Cytomegalovirus
  3 Chicken pox
 C Parasitic
  1 Schistosomiasis
 D Rickettsial
  1 Q fever
 E Spirochetes
  1 Syphilis
 F Drugs
  1 Sulfonamides
  2 Isoniazid
  3 Allopurinol

---

only by mild increases in serum alkaline phosphatase and occasionally aminotransferase levels. In a few patients with sarcoidosis or brucellosis, portal hypertension may develop, and extensive postnecrotic scarring or postnecrotic cirrhosis may follow healing of the granulomatous lesions, as in schistosomiasis.

In AIDS, evidence of liver disease is quite common but is usually mild with minimal morbidity. In these patients, hepatic granulomatous disease is often present and may be caused by opportunistic infections, with *Mycobacterium avium-intracellulare* being the most frequent pathogen. Cytomegalovirus hepatitis and hepatic mycoses are less common. These patients are frequently being treated for *Pneumocystis carinii* infections with sulfonamides, which also may cause hepatic granulomatous disease. AIDS cholangiopathy has been described with features of primary sclerosing cholangitis and infiltration of the biliary tree with cryptosporidia.

Needle biopsy of the liver often provides the first definite evidence of a systemic or disseminated granulomatous disease. In patients with sarcoidosis who have neither clinical nor laboratory evidence of hepatic involvement, needle biopsy is positive in about 80 percent of cases. In cases of suspected miliary tuberculosis, a portion of the biopsy should be cultured and stained for mycobacteria. The organism can be detected in the majority of cases, particularly when caseating granulomas are present. Serial sections of the biopsy specimen should be examined if granulomas are not apparent. Individual granulomas are rarely specific in their microscopic appearance, and final diagnosis usually requires other clinical, laboratory, or histologic data.

In approximately 20 percent of patients it is not possible to identify a cause for the granulomatous infiltration. When these infiltrates are accompanied by fever of unknown origin, the diagnosis of granulomatous hepatitis should be considered. This is an uncommon disorder of unknown cause and is diagnosed by exclusion. While granulomatous hepatitis invariably responds to moderate doses of corticosteroids, relapses are frequent, and such therapy should never be undertaken unless tuberculous disease or other causes of granulomatous infiltration have been excluded. This may include an initial empiric trial of antituberculous therapy.

AMYLOIDOSIS (See also Chap. 281)

Systemic amyloidosis, whether primary and idiopathic, familial, or secondary to chronic inflammatory or neoplastic diseases, often involves the liver. Grossly, the liver infiltrated with amyloid is enlarged and pale and rubbery in consistency. Microscopically, the birefringent amyloid deposits appear as homogeneous waxy material within the space of Disse, often being concentrated in the periportal areas and associated with atrophy of adjacent liver cell plates. Selective involvement of the walls of blood vessels, especially of the hepatic arterioles, may be a striking feature of primary amyloidosis. With this possible exception, however, the hepatic lesions are the same in all forms of amyloidosis and are present in 60 to 90 percent of cases.

An enlarged and firm liver is found in about 60 percent of patients, and ascites occurs in advanced stages of the disease in about 20 percent. Jaundice, portal hypertension, and other signs of chronic liver disease are usually absent. Liver function changes, although frequent, correlate poorly with the extent of liver infiltration. Hypoalbuminemia and elevated serum alkaline phosphatase are common. Hypoalbuminemia, however, may be related to the nephrotic syndrome owing to renal involvement; the prothrombin time is usually normal. The diagnosis is established by biopsy of rectum, skin, liver, or other involved organs and demonstration of the characteristic Congo red–staining deposits by polarizing microscopy.

REFERENCES

CRYSTAL RG: Alpha 1-antitrypsin deficiency, emphysema and liver disease: Genetic basis and strategy for therapy. J Clin Invest 85:1343, 1990

GISHAN FK, GREENE HL: Liver disease in children with PIZZ α₁-antitrypsin deficiency. Hepatology 8:307, 1988

HOFFMAN MS et al: Hepatic amyloidosis presenting as severe intrahepatic cholestasis: A case report and review of the literature. Am J Gastroenterol 83:783, 1988

HURWITZ ES et al: Public Health Service Study on Reye's syndrome and medications. N Engl J Med 313:842, 1985

HUTCHISON DC: Natural history of alpha 1-protease inhibitor deficiency. Am J Med 84:3, 1988

MINAKAMI H et al: Pre-eclampsia: A microvesicular fat disease of the liver. Am J Obstet Gynecol 159:1043, 1988

PERLMUTTER DH: The cellular basis for liver injury in alpha 1-antitrypsin deficiency. Hepatology 13:172, 1991

RILEY C et al: Acute fatty liver of pregnancy: A reassessment based on observations in nine patients. Ann Intern Med 106:703, 1987

RUSTGI VK: Liver disease in pregnancy. Med Clin North Am 73:1041, 1989

SCRIVER CR et al (eds): *The Metabolic Basis of Inherited Disease*, 6th ed. New York, McGraw-Hill, 1989

SHERLOCK S, DOOLEY J: *Diseases of the Liver and Biliary System*, 9th ed. Oxford, Blackwell, 1993

STERNLIEB I: Perspectives on Wilson's disease. Hepatology 12:1234, 1990

VAN COSTA RN et al: Adult Reye's syndrome: A review with new evidence for a generalized defect in intramitochondrial enzyme processing. Neurology 41:1815, 1991

271 LIVER TRANSPLANTATION

JULES DIENSTAG

Liver transplantation, the replacement of the native, diseased liver by a normal organ (allograft) recovered from a brain-dead donor, has matured from an experimental procedure reserved for desperately ill patients to an accepted, lifesaving operation applied much earlier in the natural history of end-stage liver disease. The preferred and technically most advanced approach is *orthotopic transplantation*, in which the native organ is removed and the donor organ is inserted in the same anatomic location. Pioneered in the 1960s by Starzl at the University of Colorado and, later, at the University of Pittsburgh and by Calne in Cambridge, England, liver transplantation is now performed routinely by dozens of centers throughout North America and western Europe. Success and survival have improved from approximately 30 percent in the 1970s to almost 60 percent today. These improved prospects for prolonged survival; dating back to the early 1980s, resulted from refinements in operative technique (including the introduction of venovenous bypass to allow venous return from the extremities and visceral circulation during clamping of the inferior vena cava), improvements in organ procurement and preservation, advances in immunosuppressive therapy, and, perhaps most influentially, more enlightened patient selection and timing. Despite the perioperative morbidity and mortality, the technical and management challenges of the procedure, and its costs, liver transplantation has become the approach of choice for selected patients whose chronic or acute liver disease is progressive, life-threatening, and unresponsive to medical therapy. Based on the current level of success, the number of liver transplants has continued to grow each year; in 1990, over 2500 patients received liver allografts in the United States

INDICATIONS Potential candidates for liver transplantation are children and adults who, in the absence of contraindications (see below), suffer from severe, irreversible liver disease for which alternative medical or surgical treatments have been exhausted or are unavailable. *Timing of the operation is of critical importance.* Indeed, improved timing and better patient selection are felt to have contributed more to the increased success of liver transplantation in the 1980s and beyond than all the impressive technical and immunologic advances combined. Although the disease should be advanced, and although opportunities for spontaneous or medically induced stabilization or recovery should be allowed, the procedure should be done sufficiently early to give the surgical procedure a fair chance for success. Ideally, transplantation should be considered in patients with end-stage liver disease who are experiencing or have experienced

a life-threatening complication of hepatic decompensation, whose quality of life has deteriorated to unacceptable levels, or whose liver disease will result predictably in irreversible damage to the central nervous system (CNS). If this is done sufficiently early, the patient will not have developed any contraindications or extrahepatic systemic deterioration. Although patients with well-compensated cirrhosis can survive for many years, many patients with quasi-stable chronic liver disease have much more advanced disease than may be apparent. As discussed below, the better the status of the patient prior to transplantation, the higher will be the anticipated success rate of transplantation. The decision about *when* to transplant is complex and requires the combined judgment of an experienced team of hepatologists, transplant surgeons, anesthesiologists, and specialists in support services, not to mention the well-informed consent of the patient and the patient's family.

Transplantation in children Indications for transplantation in children are listed in Table 271-1. The most common is *biliary atresia*. *Inherited or genetic disorders of metabolism* associated with liver failure constitute another major indication for transplantation in children and adolescents. In Crigler-Najjar disease type I and in certain hereditary disorders of the urea cycle and of amino acid or lactate-pyruvate metabolism, transplantation may be the only way to prevent impending deterioration of CNS function, despite the fact that the native liver is structurally normal. Combined heart and liver transplantation has yielded dramatic improvement in cardiac function and in cholesterol levels in children with homozygous familial hypercholesterolemia; combined liver and kidney transplantation has been successful in patients with hereditary oxalosis. In hemophiliacs with transfusion-associated hepatitis and liver failure, liver transplantation has been associated with recovery of normal factor VIII synthesis.

Transplantation in adults Liver transplantation is indicated for end-stage *cirrhosis* of all causes (see Table 271-1). In sclerosing cholangitis and *Caroli's disease* (multiple cystic dilatations of the intrahepatic biliary tree), recurrent infections and sepsis associated with inflammatory and fibrotic obstruction of the biliary tree may be an indication for transplantation. Because prior biliary surgery complicates, and is a relative contraindication for, liver transplantation, surgical diversion of the biliary tree has been all but abandoned for patients with sclerosing cholangitis. In patients who undergo transplantation for *hepatic vein thrombosis (Budd-Chiari syndrome)*, postoperative anticoagulation is essential; underlying myeloproliferative disorders may have to be treated but are not a contraindication to liver transplantation. If a donor organ can be located quickly, before life-threatening complications—including cerebral edema—set in, patients with *fulminant hepatitis* are candidates for liver

---

TABLE 271-1 Indications for liver transplantation

Children	Adults
Biliary atresia	Primary biliary cirrhosis
Neonatal hepatitis	Secondary biliary cirrhosis
Congenital hepatic fibrosis	Primary sclerosing cholangitis
Alagille's disease*	Caroli's disease‡
Byler's disease†	Cryptogenic cirrhosis
α₁-Antitrypsin deficiency	Chronic active hepatitis with cirrhosis
Inherited disorders of metabolism	Hepatic vein thrombosis
Wilson's disease	Fulminant hepatitis
Tyrosinemia	Alcoholic cirrhosis§
Glycogen storage diseases	Chronic viral hepatitis§
Lysosomal storage diseases	Primary hepatocellular malignancies§
Protoporphyria	Hepatic adenomas
Crigler-Najjar disease type I	
Familial hypercholesterolemia	
Hereditary oxalosis	
Hemophilia	

* Arteriohepatic dysplasia, with paucity of bile ducts, and congenital malformations, including pulmonary stenosis.
† Intrahepatic cholestasis, progressive liver failure, mental and growth retardation.
‡ Multiple cystic dilatations of the intrahepatic biliary tree.
§ Controversial indications (see text).

transplantation. More controversial as candidates for liver transplantation are patients with *alcoholic cirrhosis, chronic viral hepatitis,* and *primary hepatocellular malignancies.* Although all three of these categories are considered to be high risk, liver transplantation can be offered to carefully selected patients. Patients with alcoholic cirrhosis can be considered as candidates for transplantation if they meet strict criteria for abstinence and reform. Patients with chronic hepatitis C have done as well as any other subset of patients after transplantation, despite the fact that recurrent infection in the donor organ is the rule. In patients with chronic hepatitis B, the success of transplantation is reduced by approximately 10 to 20 percent; however, the majority of patients do well for at least several years. Issues of disease recurrence are discussed in more detail below. Patients with nonmetastatic primary hepatobiliary tumors—primary hepatocellular carcinoma, cholangiocarcinoma, hepatoblastoma, angiosarcoma, epithelioid hemangioendothelioma, and multiple or massive hepatic adenomata— have undergone liver transplantation; however, for hepatobiliary malignancies, overall survival is significantly lower than that for other categories of liver disease. To minimize the very high likelihood of recurrent tumor after transplantation, some centers are evaluating experimental adjuvant chemotherapy protocols. Because the likelihood of recurrent cholangiocarcinoma is almost universal, this tumor is no longer considered an indication for transplantation.

CONTRAINDICATIONS *Absolute contraindications* for transplantation include life-threatening systemic diseases, uncontrolled extrahepatic bacterial or fungal infections, preexisting advanced cardiovascular or pulmonary disease, multiple uncorrectable life-threatening congenital anomalies, metastatic malignancy, active drug or alcohol abuse, and human immunodeficiency virus (HIV) infection. Because carefully selected patients in their sixties and even seventies have undergone transplantation successfully, advanced age per se is no longer considered an absolute contraindication; however, in older patients, a more thorough preoperative evaluation should be undertaken to exclude ischemic cardiac disease. Advanced age (>60 years), however, may be considered a *relative contraindication,* that is, a factor to be taken into account with other relative contraindications. Other relative contraindications include highly replicative hepatitis B, portal vein thrombosis, preexisting renal disease not associated with liver disease, intrahepatic or biliary sepsis, severe hypoxemia resulting from right-to-left intrapulmonary shunts, previous extensive hepatobiliary surgery, and any uncontrolled serious psychiatric disorder. Any one of these relative contraindications is insufficient in and of itself to preclude transplantation. For example, the problem of portal vein thrombosis can be overcome by constructing a graft from the donor liver portal vein to the recipient's superior mesenteric vein.

TECHNICAL CONSIDERATIONS   Donor selection   Donor livers for transplantation are procured primarily from victims of head trauma. Organs from brain-dead donors up to age 60 are acceptable if the following criteria are met: hemodynamic stability, adequate oxygenation, absence of bacterial or fungal infection, serologic exclusion of hepatitis B and C viruses and HIV, absence of abdominal trauma, and absence of hepatic dysfunction. Cardiovascular and respiratory functions are maintained artificially until the liver can be removed. Compatibility in ABO blood group and organ size between donor and recipient are important considerations in donor selection; however, ABO-incompatible or reduced-donor-organ transplants can be performed in emergency or marked donor-scarcity situations. Tissue typing for HLA matching is not required, and preformed cytotoxic HLA antibodies do not preclude liver transplantation. Following perfusion with cold electrolyte solution, the donor liver is removed and packed in ice. The use of University of Wisconsin (UW) solution, rich in lactobionate and raffinose, has permitted the extension of cold ischemic time up to 20 h; however, 12 h may be a more reasonable limit. Improved techniques for harvesting multiple organs from the same donor have increased the availability of donor livers, but the availability of donor livers is far outstripped by the demand. Currently, in the United States, all donor livers are distributed through a nationwide organ-sharing network (United Network of Organ Sharing) designed to allocate available organs based on regional considerations and recipient acuity. Recipients who require the highest level of care (intensive care) have the highest priority.

Surgical technique   Removal of the recipient's native liver is technically difficult, particularly in the presence of portal hypertension with its associated collateral circulation and extensive varices, and even more so in the presence of scarring from previous abdominal operations. The combination of portal hypertension and coagulopathy (elevated prothrombin time and thrombocytopenia) translates into large blood product transfusion requirements. After the portal vein and infrahepatic and suprahepatic inferior vena cavae are dissected, a pump-driven venovenous bypass system is applied to reroute blood from the portal vein and inferior vena cava, preventing congestion of visceral organs. After the hepatic artery and common bile duct are dissected, the native liver is removed and the donor organ inserted. During the anhepatic phase, coagulopathy, hypoglycemia, hypocalcemia, and hypothermia are encountered and must be managed by the anesthesiology team. Caval, portal vein, hepatic artery, and bile duct anastomoses are performed in succession, the last by end-to-end suturing of the donor and recipient common bile ducts or by choledochojejunostomy to a Roux en Y loop if the recipient common bile duct cannot be used for reconstruction (e.g., in sclerosing cholangitis). A typical transplant operation lasts 8 h, with a range of 6 to 18 h. Because of excessive bleeding, large volumes of blood, blood products, and volume expanders may be required during surgery.

POSTOPERATIVE COURSE AND MANAGEMENT   Immunosuppressive therapy   The introduction in 1980 of cyclosporine as an immunosuppressive agent contributed substantially to the improvement in survival after liver transplantation. Cyclosporine depresses both humoral and cell-mediated immunity via inhibition of interleukin 2 production. This process occurs without affecting rapidly dividing cells in the bone marrow, which may account for the reduced frequency of posttransplantation systemic infections. The most common and important side effect of cyclosporine therapy is nephrotoxicity. Cyclosporine causes dose-dependent renal tubular injury and direct renal artery vasospasm. Following renal function, therefore, is important in monitoring cyclosporine therapy, perhaps even a more reliable indicator than blood levels of the drug. Nephrotoxicity is reversible and can be managed by dose reduction. Other adverse effects of cyclosporine therapy include hypertension, hyperkalemia, tremor, hirsutism, and gum hyperplasia. Like azathioprine, cyclosporine appears to be associated with a risk of lymphoproliferative malignancies (see below), which may occur earlier after cyclosporine than after azathioprine therapy. Because of these side effects, combinations of cyclosporine, prednisone, and azathioprine— all at reduced doses—are preferable regimens for immunosuppressive therapy.

In patients with pretransplant renal dysfunction or renal deterioration that occurs intraoperatively or immediately postoperatively, cyclosporine therapy may not be practical; under these circumstances, induction or maintenance of immunosuppression with monoclonal antibodies to T cells, OKT3, may be appropriate. Therapy with OKT3 has been especially effective in reversing acute rejection in the posttransplant period and is the standard treatment for acute rejection that fails to respond to methylprednisolone boluses. Intravenous infusions of OKT3 may be complicated by transient fever, chills, and diarrhea. When this drug is used to induce immunosuppression initially or to provide "rescue" in those who reject despite "conventional" therapy, the incidence of bacterial, fungal, and especially cytomegalovirus infections is increased during and after such therapy. In some centers, ganciclovir antiviral therapy is initiated prophylactically as a routine along with OKT3. A new, experimental drug, FK-506, is being introduced and is being tested primarily for "rescue" therapy in patients who fail to respond to other immunosuppressive agents. This drug is a macrolide antibiotic isolated from a Japanese soil fungus, *Streptomyces tsukubaensis,* with similar immunosuppressive effects and mechanisms to those of cyclosporine but with substantially higher potency. The use of FK-506 is still limited to research trials; unfortunately, it has similar nephrotoxicity to that of cyclosporine, and the nephrotoxicity is especially profound when the two drugs are used together. The important principle about immunosuppression is that the ideal approach strikes a balance between immunosuppression and immunological competence. Given sufficient immunosuppression, acute liver allograft rejection is always reversible; however, if the cumulative dose of immunosuppressive therapy is too large, the patient will succumb to opportunistic infection. Therefore, immunosuppressive drugs must be used judiciously, with strict attention to the infectious consequences of such therapy.

Postoperative complications Complications of liver transplantation can be divided into hepatic and nonhepatic categories. In addition, both immediately postoperative and late complications are encountered. Patients who undergo liver transplantation as a rule have been chronically ill for protracted periods and may be malnourished and wasted. The impact of such chronic illness and the multisystem failure that accompanies liver failure continues to require attention in the postoperative period. Because of the massive fluid losses and fluid shifts that occur during the operation, patients may remain fluid overloaded during the immediate postoperative period, straining cardiovascular reserve; this effect can be amplified in the face of transient renal dysfunction and pulmonary capillary vascular permeability. Continuous monitoring of cardiovascular and pulmonary function, measures to maintain the integrity of the intravascular compartment and to treat extravascular volume overload, and scrupulous attention to potential sources of and sites of infection are of paramount importance. Cardiovascular instability may result as well from the electrolyte imbalance that may accompany reperfusion of the donor liver. Pulmonary function may be compromised further by paralysis of the right hemidiaphragm associated with phrenic nerve injury. The hyperdynamic state with increased cardiac output that is characteristic of patients with liver failure reverses rapidly after successful liver transplantation.

Other immediate management issues include renal dysfunction; prerenal azotemia, acute kidney injury associate with hypoperfusion (acute tubular necrosis), and renal toxicity caused by antibiotics or cyclosporine are frequently encountered in the postoperative period, sometimes necessitating dialysis. Occasionally, postoperative intraperitoneal bleeding may be sufficient to increase intraabdominal pressure, which, in turn, may reduce renal blood flow—this effect is rapidly reversible when abdominal distention is relieved by exploratory laparotomy to identify and ligate the bleeding site and to remove intraperitoneal clot. Anemia also may result from acute upper gastrointestinal bleeding or from transient hemolytic anemia, which may be autoimmune, especially when blood group O livers are transplanted into blood group A or B recipients. This autoimmune hemolytic anemia is mediated by donor intrahepatic lymphocytes that recognize red blood cell A or B antigens on recipient erythrocytes. Transient in nature, this process resolves once the donor liver is repopulated by recipient bone marrow–derived lymphocytes; the hemolysis can be treated by transfusing blood group O red blood cells and/or by administering higher doses of glucocorticoids. Transient thrombocytopenia is encountered commonly as well. Aplastic anemia, a late occurrence, is rare but has been reported in almost 30 percent of patients who underwent liver transplantation for acute, severe hepatitis of unknown cause.

Bacterial, fungal, or viral infections are common and may be life-threatening postoperatively. Early after transplant surgery, common postoperative infections predominate—pneumonia, wound infections, infected intraabdominal collections, urinary tract infections, and intravenous line infections—rather than opportunistic infections; these infections may involve the biliary tree and liver as well. Beyond the first postoperative month, the toll of immunosuppression becomes evident, and opportunistic infections—cytomegalovirus, herpes viruses, fungal infections (*Aspergillus, Candida,* cryptococcal disease), mycobacterial infections, parasitic infections (*Pneumocystis, Tox-*

oplasma), bacterial infections (*Nocardia, Legionella,* and *Listeria*)—predominate. Rarely, early infections represent those transmitted with the donor liver, either infections present in the donor or infections acquired during procurement processing. De novo viral hepatitis infections acquired from the donor organ or from transfused blood products occur after typical incubation periods for these agents (well beyond the first month). Obviously, infections in an immunosuppressed host demand early recognition and prompt management; prophylactic antibiotic therapy is administered routinely in the immediate postoperative period. Use of sulfamethoxazole with trimethoprim reduces the incidence of postoperative *Pneumocystis carinii* pneumonia.

Neuropsychiatric complications include seizures, commonly associated with cyclosporine toxicity, encephalopathy, depression, and difficult psychosocial adjustment. Rarely, diseases are transmitted by the allograft from the donor to the recipient. In addition to viral and bacterial infections, malignancies of donor origin have occurred. Lymphoproliferative malignancies, especially B cell lymphoma, are a recognized complication associated with immunosuppressive drugs such as azathioprine and cyclosporine (see above). Epstein-Barr virus has been shown to play a contributory role in some of these tumors, which may regress when immunosuppressive therapy is reduced.

Hepatic complications Hepatic dysfunction after liver transplantation is similar to the hepatic complications encountered after major abdominal and cardiothoracic surgery; however, in addition, there may be complications such as primary graft failure, vascular compromise, failure or obstruction of the biliary anastomoses, and rejection. As in nontransplant surgery, postoperative jaundice may result from prehepatic, intrahepatic, and posthepatic sources. *Prehepatic* sources represent the massive hemoglobin pigment load from transfusions, hemolysis, hematomas, ecchymoses, and other collections of blood. *Early intrahepatic* liver injury includes effects of hepatotoxic drugs and anesthesia; hypoperfusion injury associated with hypotension, sepsis, and shock; and benign postoperative cholestasis. *Late intrahepatic* sources of liver injury include posttransfusion hepatitis and recurrent primary disease (see below). *Posthepatic* sources of hepatic dysfunction include biliary obstruction and reduced renal clearance of conjugated bilirubin. Hepatic complications unique to liver transplantation include primary graft failure associated with ischemic injury to the organ during harvesting; vascular compromise associated with thrombosis or stenosis of the portal vein or hepatic artery anastomoses; stenosis, obstruction, or leakage of the anastomosed common bile duct; and rejection.

Transplant rejection Despite the use of immunosuppressive drugs, rejection of the transplanted liver still occurs in a majority of patients, beginning 1 to 2 weeks after surgery. Clinical signs suggesting rejection are fever, right upper quadrant pain, and reduced bile pigment and volume. Leukocytosis may occur, but the most reliable indicators are increases in serum bilirubin and aminotransferase levels. Because these tests lack specificity, it may be difficult to distinguish among rejection and biliary obstruction, primary graft nonfunction, vascular compromise, viral hepatitis, cytomegalovirus infection, drug hepatotoxicity, and recurrent primary disease. Radiographic visualization of the biliary tree and/or percutaneous liver biopsy often help to establish the correct diagnosis. Morphologic features of acute rejection include portal infiltration, bile duct injury, and/or endothelial inflammation ("endothelialitis"); some of these findings are reminiscent of graft-versus-host disease and primary biliary cirrhosis. As soon as transplant rejection is suspected, treatment consists of intravenous methylprednisolone in repeated boluses; if this fails to abort rejection, many centers use antibodies to lymphocytes, such as OKT3, or polyclonal antilymphocyte globulin.

Chronic rejection is a relatively rare outcome that may follow repeated bouts of acute rejection or that occurs unrelated to preceding rejection episodes. Morphologically, chronic rejection is characterized by progressive cholestasis, focal parenchymal necrosis, mononuclear infiltration, vascular lesions (intimal fibrosis, subintimal foam cells, fibrinoid necrosis), and fibrosis. This process may be reflected as ductopenia—the vanishing bile duct syndrome. Some of the histologic hallmarks of chronic rejection may be so similar to those of chronic viral hepatitis that differentiation between the two may be difficult. Reversibility of chronic rejection is limited; in patients with therapy-resistant chronic rejection, retransplantation has yielded encouraging results.

OUTCOME Survival   The survival rate for patients undergoing liver transplantation has improved steadily since 1983. One-year survival rates have increased from approximately 70 percent in the early 1980s to 80 to 85 percent at the end of the decade. Currently, the 5-year survival rate approaches 60 percent. An important observation is the relation between clinical status before transplantation and outcome. For patients who undergo liver transplantation when their level of compensation is high (e.g., still working or only partially disabled), a 1-year survival rate of 85 percent is the rule. For those whose level of decompensation mandates continuous in-hospital care prior to transplantation, the 1-year survival rate is about 70 percent, while for those who are so decompensated that they require life support in an intensive care unit, the 1-year survival rate is approximately 50 percent. Indeed, the trend toward transplantation earlier in the natural history of end-stage liver disease is a major factor in the increased success of liver transplantation during the 1980s. Another important distinction in survival has been drawn between high-risk and low-risk patient categories. For patients who do not fit any "high risk" designations, 1-year and 4-year survival rates of 85 and 80 percent, respectively, have been recorded. In contrast, among patients in "high risk" categories—cancer, fulminant hepatitis, hepatitis B, age >60, concurrent renal failure, respirator dependence, portal vein thrombosis, and history of a portacaval shunt or multiple right upper quadrant operations—survival statistics fall into the range of 65 percent at 1 year and just above 50 percent at 4 years. Survival after retransplantation for primary graft nonfunction is approximately 50 percent. Causes of failure of liver transplantation vary with time. Failures within the first 3 months result primarily from technical complications, postoperative infections, and hemorrhage. Transplant failures after the first 3 months are more likely to result from infection, rejection, or recurrent disease (such as malignancy or viral hepatitis).

Recurrence of primary disease   The recurrence of autoimmune chronic active hepatitis or primary sclerosing cholangitis has not been reported. There have been reports of recurrent primary biliary cirrhosis after liver transplantation; however, the histologic features of primary biliary cirrhosis and acute rejection are virtually indistinguishable and occur as frequently in patients with primary biliary cirrhosis as in patients undergoing transplantation for other reasons. Hereditary disorders such as Wilson's disease and α_1-antitrypsin deficiency have not recurred after liver transplantation; however, recurrence of disordered iron metabolism has been observed in some patients with hemochromatosis. Hepatic vein thrombosis (Budd-Chiari syndrome) may recur; this can be minimized by treating underlying lymphoproliferative disorders and by anticoagulation. Cholangiocarcinoma recurs almost invariably; therefore, few centers now transplant such patients. In patients with hepatocellular carcinoma, tumor recurrence in the liver is common after approximately 1 year. Trials are underway to assess the benefit of adjuvant chemotherapy.

Hepatitis A can recur after transplantation for fulminant hepatitis A, but such acute reinfection has no serious clinical sequelae. In fulminant hepatitis B, recurrence is not the rule; however, hepatitis B recurs almost invariably after transplantation for end-stage chronic hepatitis B. With sufficient immunosuppressive therapy to prevent allograft rejection, levels of hepatitis B viremia increase markedly, regardless of pretransplantation values. A majority of patients undergoing transplantation for chronic hepatitis B become high-level HBV carriers without liver injury; however, some patients experience a rapid recapitulation of severe injury—chronic active hepatitis or even fulminant hepatitis—after transplantation. *Fibrosing cholestatic hepatitis* is a histologic feature linked to rapidly progressive liver injury in approximately 10 percent of patients transplanted for hepatitis B. These patients experience marked hyperbilirubinemia, substantial prolongation of the prothrombin time (both out of proportion to

relatively modest elevations of aminotransferase activity), and rapidly progressive liver failure. This lesion has been suggested to represent a "choking off" of the hepatocyte by an overwhelming density of HBV proteins. Complications such as sepsis and pancreatitis also have been observed more frequently in patients undergoing liver transplantation for hepatitis B. Thus the outcome of transplantation for hepatitis B is unpredictable. Some centers have relied on continuing infusions of hepatitis B immune globulin to prevent recurrent hepatitis B, but trials demonstrating an advantage over no therapy have not been done. Patients who undergo liver transplantation for chronic hepatitis B plus D have a better survival rate than patients transplanted for hepatitis B alone. Recurrence of hepatitis C virus (HCV) after liver transplantation can be documented in almost every patient, if sufficiently sensitive virus markers are used. Although, occasionally, patients have succumbed to HCV-associated liver injury, in the vast majority of patients the impact of recurrent hepatitis C on graft and patient survival appears to be negligible.

Posttransplantation quality of life   Full rehabilitation is achieved in the majority of patients who survive the early postoperative months and escape chronic rejection or unmanageable infection. Psychosocial maladjustment interferes with medical compliance in a small number of patients, but most manage to adhere to immunosuppressive regimens, which must be continued indefinitely. In one study, 85 percent of patients who survived their transplants returned to gainful activities. In fact, some women have conceived and carried pregnancies to term after transplantation without demonstrable injury to their infants.

REFERENCES

DAVIES SE et al: Hepatic histological findings after transplantation for chronic hepatitis B virus infection, including a unique pattern of fibrosing cholestatic hepatitis. Hepatology 13:150, 1991

FERAY C et al: Reinfection of liver graft by hepatitis C virus after liver transplantation. J Clin Invest 89:1361, 1992

LAU JYN et al: High-level expression of hepatitis B viral antigens in fibrosing cholestatic hepatitis. Gastroenterology 102:956, 1992

LUCEY MR et al: Selection for and outcome of liver transplantation in alcoholic liver disease. Gastroenterology 102:1736, 1992

MADDREY WC (ed): *Transplantation of the Liver.* New York, Elsevier, 1988

——, VAN THIEL DH: Liver transplantation: An overview. Hepatology 8:948, 1988

MARTIN P et al: Liver transplantation for viral hepatitis: Current status. Am J Gastroenterol 87:409, 1992

MUNOZ SJ, FRIEDMAN LS: Liver transplantation. Med Clin North Am 73:1011, 1989

SORRELL MF, SHAW BW JR (guest eds): A primer of liver transplantation for the referring physician. Semin Liver Dis 9:159, 1989

STARZL TE et al: Liver transplantation. N Engl J Med 321:1014, 1092, 1989

WEISNER RH (guest ed): Hepatic allograft rejection. Semin Liver Dis 12:1, 1992

——, et al: Hepatic allograft rejection: New developments in terminology, diagnosis, prevention, and treatment. Mayo Clin Proc 68:69, 1992

WRIGHT TL et al: Recurrent and acquired hepatitis C viral infection in liver transplant recipients. Gastroenterology 103:317, 1992

272   DISEASES OF THE GALLBLADDER AND BILE DUCTS

NORTON J. GREENBERGER / KURT J. ISSELBACHER

PHYSIOLOGY OF BILE PRODUCTION AND FLOW   Bile secretion and composition   Bile formed in the hepatic lobules is secreted into a complex network of canaliculi, small bile ductules, and larger bile ducts which run with lymphatics and branches of the portal vein and hepatic artery in portal tracts situated between hepatic lobules. These interlobular bile ducts coalesce to form larger septal bile ducts that join to form the right and left hepatic ducts, which in turn unite to form the common hepatic duct. The common hepatic duct is joined by the cystic duct of the gallbladder to form the common bile duct which enters the duodenum (often after joining the main pancreatic duct) through the ampulla of Vater.

Hepatic bile is a pigmented isotonic fluid with an electrolyte composition resembling blood plasma. The electrolyte composition of gallbladder bile differs from that of hepatic bile because most of the inorganic anions, chloride and bicarbonate, have been removed by reabsorption across the basement membrane.

Major components of bile by weight include water (82 percent), bile acids (12 percent), lecithin and other phospholipids (4 percent), and unesterified cholesterol (0.7 percent). Other constituents include conjugated bilirubin, proteins (IgA, by-products of hormones, and other proteins metabolized in the liver), electrolytes, mucus, and, often, drugs and their metabolic by-products.

The total daily basal secretion of hepatic bile is approximately 500 to 600 mL. The metabolic products of hepatocyte uptake and synthesis are secreted into the bile canaliculi, which are lined by microvillus membrane components associated with microfilaments of actin, microtubules, and other contractile elements. Within the hepatocyte, conjugation of many of the bile constituents may occur, while other components of bile, such as primary bile acids, lecithin, and some cholesterol, are synthesized de novo. Three mechanisms are important in regulating bile flow: (1) active transport of bile acids from hepatocytes into the canaliculi, (2) bile acid–independent ATPase-mediated transport of sodium, and (3) ductular secretion. The last is a secretin-mediated and cyclic AMP–dependent phenomenon which appears to result from the active transport of sodium and bicarbonate into the ductule with resulting passive movement of water across the cell membrane.

The bile acids The primary bile acids, cholic and chenodeoxycholic acids, are synthesized from cholesterol in the liver, conjugated with glycine or taurine, and excreted into the bile. Secondary bile acids, including deoxycholate and lithocholate, are formed in the colon as bacterial metabolites of the primary bile acids. However, lithocholic acid is much less efficiently absorbed from the colon than deoxycholic acid. Other secondary bile acids, found in trace amounts, which include ursodeoxycholic acid (a stereoisomer of chenodeoxycholate) and a variety of other unusual or "aberrant" bile acids, may be produced in increased amounts in patients with chronic cholestatic syndromes. In normal bile, the ratio of glycine to taurine conjugates is about 3:1, while in patients with cholestasis, increased concentrations of sulfate and glucuronide conjugates of bile acids are often found.

Bile acids are detergents which in aqueous solutions and above a critical concentration of about 2 mM form molecular aggregates called *micelles*. Cholesterol alone is poorly soluble in aqueous environments, and its solubility in bile depends on both the lipid concentration and the relative molar percentages of bile acids and lecithin. Normal ratios of these constituents favor the formation of solubilizing *mixed micelles*, while abnormal ratios promote the precipitation of cholesterol crystals in bile.

In addition to facilitating the biliary excretion of cholesterol, bile acids are necessary for the normal intestinal absorption of dietary fats via a micellar transport mechanism (see Chap. 254). Bile acids also serve as a major physiologic driving force for hepatic bile flow and aid in water and electrolyte transport in the small bowel and colon.

Enterohepatic circulation Bile acids are efficiently conserved under normal conditions. Conjugated and unconjugated bile acids are absorbed by *passive diffusion* along the entire gut. Quantitatively much more important for bile salt recirculation, however, is the *active transport* mechanism for conjugated bile acids in the distal ileum (see Chap. 254). The reabsorbed bile acids enter the portal bloodstream and are taken up rapidly by hepatocytes, reconjugated, and resecreted into bile (enterohepatic circulation).

The normal bile acid pool size is approximately 2 to 4 g. During digestion of a meal, the bile acid pool undergoes at least one or more enterohepatic cycles depending on the size and composition of the meal. Normally, the bile acid pool circulates approximately 5 to 10 times daily. Intestinal absorption of the pool is about 95 percent

efficient, so fecal loss of bile acids is in the range of 0.3 to 0.6 g/d. This fecal loss is compensated by an equal daily synthesis of bile acids by the liver, and thus the size of the bile salt pool is maintained. Bile acids returning to the liver suppress de novo hepatic synthesis of primary bile acids from cholesterol by inhibiting the rate-limiting enzyme 7α-hydroxylase. While the loss of bile salts in stool is usually matched by increased hepatic synthesis, the maximum rate of synthesis is approximately 5 g/d, which may be insufficient to replete the bile acid pool size when there is pronounced impairment of intestinal bile salt reabsorption.

Gallbladder and sphincteric functions In the fasting state, the sphincter of Oddi offers a high-pressure zone of resistance to bile flow from the common bile duct into the duodenum. This tonic contraction serves to (1) prevent reflux of duodenal contents into the pancreatic and bile ducts and (2) promote bile filling of the gallbladder. The major factor controlling the evacuation of the gallbladder is the peptide hormone cholecystokinin, which is released from the duodenal mucosa in response to the ingestion of fats and amino acids. Cholecystokinin produces (1) powerful contraction of the gallbladder, (2) decreased resistance of the sphincter of Oddi, (3) increased hepatic secretion of bile, and thus (4) enhanced flow of biliary contents into the duodenum.

Hepatic bile is "concentrated" within the gallbladder by energy-dependent transmucosal absorption of water and electrolytes. Almost the entire bile acid pool may be sequestered in the gallbladder following an overnight fast for delivery into the duodenum with the first meal of the day. The normal capacity of the gallbladder is 30 to 75 mL of bile.

DISEASES OF THE GALLBLADDER

CONGENITAL ANOMALIES Anomalies of the biliary tract may be found in 10 to 20 percent of the population, including abnormalities in number, size, and shape (e.g., agenesis of the gallbladder, duplications, rudimentary or oversized "giant" gallbladders, and diverticula). Phrygian cap is a clinically innocuous entity in which a partial or complete septum (or fold) separates the fundus from the body. Anomalies of position or suspension are not uncommon and include left-sided gallbladder, intrahepatic gallbladder, retrodisplacement of the gallbladder, and "floating" gallbladder. The latter condition predisposes to acute torsion, volvulus, or herniation of the gallbladder.

GALLSTONES **Pathogenesis of gallstones** Gallstones are quite prevalent in most western countries. In the United States, autopsy series have shown gallstones in at least 20 percent of women and in 8 percent of men over the age of 40. It is estimated that 16 to 20 million persons in the United States have gallstones and that approximately 1 million new cases of cholelithiasis develop each year.

Gallstones are crystalline structures formed by concretion or accretion of normal or abnormal bile constituents. These stones are divided into three major types; cholesterol and mixed stones account for 80 percent of the total, with pigment stones comprising the remaining 20 percent. Mixed and cholesterol gallstones usually contain more than 70 percent cholesterol monohydrate plus an admixture of calcium salts, bile acids and bile pigments, proteins, fatty acids, and phospholipids. Pigment stones are composed primarily of calcium bilirubinate; they contain less than 10 percent cholesterol.

CHOLESTEROL AND MIXED STONES AND BILIARY SLUDGE Cholesterol is relatively water insoluble and requires aqueous dispersion into either micelles or vesicles, both of which require the presence of a second lipid to "liquify" the cholesterol. When the cholesterol content of bile exceeds the amount which can be solubilized by bile salt and bile salt–lecithin micelles, the excess is dispersed in larger lipid vesicles (Fig. 272-1). Vesicles are spherical particles composed of lecithin and cholesterol and contain only traces of bile salts. Vesicles

FIGURE 272-1 Scheme showing pathogenesis of gallstone formation. Conditions or factors that increase the ratio of cholesterol to bile acids and lecithin favor gallstone formation (HMG-CoAR = hydroxymethylglutaryl–coenzyme A reductase; 7-α-OHase = 7α-hydroxylase).

and micelles are important cholesterol-solubilizing and -transport agents in bile supersaturated with cholesterol.

There are several important mechanisms in the formation of lithogenic (stone-forming) bile. The most important is increased biliary secretion of cholesterol. This may occur in association with obesity, high-caloric diets, or drugs (e.g., clofibrate) and may result from increased activity of hydroxymethylglutaryl–coenzyme A (HMG-CoA) reductase, the rate-limiting enzyme of hepatic cholesterol synthesis. In some patients, impaired hepatic conversion of cholesterol to bile acids also may occur, resulting in an increase of the lithogenic cholesterol/bile acid ratio. Lithogenic bile also results from decreased hepatic secretion of bile salts and phospholipids which may follow impaired hepatic synthesis (e.g., rare inborn errors of metabolism such as cerebrotendinous xanthomatosis) or conditions affecting

the enterohepatic circulation of these constituents (e.g., prolonged parenteral alimentation or ileal disease or resection). In addition, most patients with gallstones appear to have reduced activity of hepatic cholesterol 7α-hydroxylase, the rate-limiting enzyme for primary bile acid synthesis.

Thus an excess of biliary cholesterol in relation to bile acids and phospholipids may be due to hypersecretion of cholesterol, hyposecretion of bile acids, or both. While cholesterol saturation of bile is an important prerequisite for gallstone formation, it is not sufficient by itself to produce cholesterol precipitation in vivo. Most people with supersaturated bile do not develop stones because the time required for cholesterol crystals to nucleate and grow is longer than the time bile spends in the gallbladder. Two additional disturbances of bile acid metabolism which are likely to contribute to supersaturation of bile with cholesterol are (1) reduction of the bile acid pool and (2) enhanced conversion of cholic acid to deoxycholic acid with replacement of the cholic acid pool by an expanded deoxycholic acid pool. The first disorder may be caused by more rapid loss of primary bile acid from the small intestine into the colon. The second disturbance may result from enhanced dehydroxylation of cholic acid and increased absorption of newly formed deoxycholic acid.

A second important abnormality is defective vesicle formation. Ordinarily, cholesterol and phospholipid are secreted into bile as unilamellar bilayered vesicles which are unstable and are converted, along with bile acids, into other lipid aggregates such as micelles. During micellation of vesicles, more phospholipid than cholesterol is transferred to mixed micelles, leading to unstable cholesterol-rich vesicles which aggregate into larger multilamellar vesicles from which cholesterol crystals aggregate.

A third important mechanism is *nucleation* of cholesterol monohydrate crystals, which is greatly accelerated in human lithogenic bile; it is this feature rather than the degree of cholesterol supersaturation that distinguishes lithogenic from normal gallbladder bile. Accelerated nucleation of cholesterol monohydrate in bile may be due to either an *excess of pronucleating factors* or a *deficiency of antinucleating factors*. Nonmucin and mucin glycoproteins and lysine phosphatidyl-choline appear to be pronucleating factors, while apolipoproteins AI and AII and other glycoproteins appear to be antinucleating factors. However, the characterization of additional pronucleating and antinu-cleating factors remains incomplete. Cholesterol monohydrate crystal nucleation and crystal growth probably occur within the mucin gel layer. Vesicle fusion leads to liquid crystals, which, in turn, nucleate into solid cholesterol monohydrate crystals. Continued growth of the crystals occurs by direct nucleation of cholesterol molecules from supersaturated unilamellar or multilamellar biliary vesicles.

A fourth important mechanism in cholesterol gallstone formation concerns *biliary sludge*. Biliary sludge is a thick mucous material which upon microscopic examination reveals lecithin-cholesterol crystals, cholesterol monohydrate crystals, calcium bilirubinate, and mucin thread or mucous gels. Biliary sludge typically forms a crescent-like layer in the most dependent portion of the gallbladder and is recognized by characteristic echoes on ultrasonography (see below). In vitro, cholesterol monohydrate crystals (>50 μm) mixed with mucus produce echoes that are indistinguishable from gallbladder sludge observed in patients. The presence of biliary sludge implies two abnormalities: (1) the normal balance between gallbladder mucin secretion and elimination has become deranged; and (2) nucleation from biliary solutes has occurred. That biliary sludge is a precursor form of gallstone disease is evident from several observations. In one study, 96 patients with gallbladder sludge were followed prospectively by serial ultrasound studies. In 17 patients (18 percent), biliary sludge disappeared and did not recur for at least 2 years. In 58 patients (60 percent), biliary sludge disappeared and reappeared. Importantly, gallstones developed in 14 patients, in 8 of whom the gallstones were "silent." In 12 patients, cholecystectomies were performed, 6 for gallstone-associated biliary pain and 3 in symptomatic patients with sludge but without gallstones who had prior attacks of pancreatitis;

the latter did not recur after cholecystectomy. It should be emphasized that biliary sludge can develop with disorders that cause gallbladder hypomotility, i.e., surgery, burns, total parenteral nutrition, pregnancy, and oral contraceptives—all of which are associated with gallstone formation. Finally, biliary sludge can account for the observation that most cholesterol gallstones have a pigmented center.

To summarize, cholesterol gallstone disease occurs because of several defects, which include (1) bile supersaturation with cholesterol, (2) nucleation of cholesterol monohydrate with subsequent crystal retention and stone growth, and (3) abnormal gallbladder motor function with delayed emptying and stasis. Other important factors known to predispose to cholesterol stone formation are summarized in Table 272-1.

PIGMENT STONES Gallstones composed largely of calcium bilirubinate are much more common in the orient than in western countries. The presence of increased amounts of unconjugated, insoluble bilirubin in bile results in the precipitation of bilirubin which may aggregate to form pigment stones or may fuse to form the nidus for growth of mixed cholesterol gallstones. In western countries, chronic hemolytic states (with increased conjugated bilirubin in bile) or alcoholic liver disease are associated with an increased incidence of pigment stones. Deconjugation of soluble bilirubin mono- and diglucuronide may be mediated by the enzyme β-glucuronidase, which is sometimes produced when bile is chronically infected by bacteria. Pigment stone formation is especially prominent in Asians and is often associated with infections in the biliary tree (see Table 272-1).

Diagnosis of gallstones Procedures of potential use in the diagnosis of cholelithiasis and other diseases of the gallbladder are detailed in Table 272-2. The plain abdominal film may detect gallstones containing sufficient calcium to be radiopaque (10 to 15

percent of cholesterol and mixed stones and approximately 50 percent of pigment stones). Plain radiography also may be of use in the diagnosis of emphysematous cholecystitis, porcelain gallbladder, limey bile, and gallstone ileus.

Ultrasonography of the gallbladder is very accurate in the identification of cholelithiasis and has several advantages over oral cholecystography (see Fig. 272-2A). The gallbladder is easily visualized with the technique, and in fact, failure to image the gallbladder successfully in a fasting patient correlates well with the presence of underlying gallbladder disease. Stones as small as 2 mm in diameter may be confidently identified provided that firm criteria are used [e.g., acoustic "shadowing" of opacities that are within the gallbladder lumen and that change with the patient's position (by gravity)]. In major medical centers, the false-negative and false-positive rates for ultrasound in gallstone patients are about 2 to 4 percent. Biliary sludge is material of low echogenic activity that typically forms a layer in the most dependent position of the gallbladder. This layer shifts with postural changes but fails to produce acoustic shadowing; these two characteristics distinguish sludges from gallstones.

Oral cholecystography (OCG) is a useful procedure for the diagnosis of gallstones but has been largely replaced by ultrasound. False-positive results are rare, but the oral cholecystogram may be falsely negative (when good opacification is achieved) in approximately 5 to 10 percent of patients with gallstones. Factors which may produce nonvisualization of the OCG are summarized in Table 272-2. When these can be excluded, nonvisualization of the gallbladder following a second dose of oral contrast agent is highly correlated with underlying cystic duct obstruction or chronic inflammation of the gallbladder.

Radiopharmaceuticals such as ^{99m}Tc-labeled N-substituted iminodiacetic acids (HIDA, DIDA, DISIDA, etc.) are rapidly extracted from the blood and are excreted into the biliary tree in high concentration even in the presence of mild to moderate serum bilirubin elevations. Failure to image the gallbladder in the presence of biliary ductal visualization may indicate cystic duct obstruction, acute or chronic cholecystitis, or surgical absence of the organ. Such scans have their greatest application in the diagnosis of acute cholecystitis.

Symptoms of gallstone disease Gallstones usually produce symptoms by causing inflammation or obstruction following their migration into the cystic duct or common bile duct. The most specific and characteristic symptom of gallstone disease is biliary colic. Obstruction of the cystic duct or common bile duct by a stone produces increased intraluminal pressure and distention of the viscus which cannot be relieved by repetitive biliary contractions. The resultant visceral pain is characteristically a severe, steady ache or pressure in the epigastrium or right upper quadrant of the abdomen with frequent radiation to the interscapular area, right scapula, or shoulder.

Biliary colic begins quite suddenly and may persist with severe intensity for 1 to 4 h, subsiding gradually or rapidly. An episode of biliary pain is sometimes followed by a residual mild ache or soreness in the right upper quadrant which may persist for 24 h or so. Nausea and vomiting frequently accompany episodes of biliary colic, and mild elevations of serum bilirubin [not exceeding 85.5 μmol/L (5 mg/dL)] occur in 25 percent of patients. Persistence of a high serum bilirubin level suggests common duct stones. Fever or chills (rigors) with biliary colic usually imply an underlying complication, i.e., cholecystitis, pancreatitis, or cholangitis. Complaints of vague epigastric fullness, dyspepsia, eructation, or flatulence, especially following a fatty meal, should not be confused with biliary colic. Such symptoms are frequently elicited from patients with gallstone disease but are not specific for biliary calculi. Biliary colic may be precipitated by eating a fatty meal, by consumption of a large meal following a period of prolonged fasting, or by eating a normal meal.

Natural history of gallstones Gallstone disease discovered in an asymptomatic patient or in a patient whose symptoms are not referable to cholelithiasis is a common clinical problem. The natural history of "silent" or asymptomatic gallstones has occasioned much debate. In contrast to previous reports, a study of predominantly male silent

---

TABLE 272-1 Predisposing factors for cholesterol and pigment gallstone formation

CHOLESTEROL AND MIXED STONES

A Demography
   1 Northern Europe and North and South America greater than Asia, probable familial, hereditary aspects
B Obesity
   1 Normal bile acid pool and secretion but increased biliary secretion of cholesterol
C Weight loss
   1 Mobilization of tissue cholesterol leads to increased biliary cholesterol secretion while enterohepatic secretion of bile salt is decreased
D Female sex hormones
   1 Estrogens stimulate hepatic lipoprotein receptors, increase uptake of dietary cholesterol, and increase biliary cholesterol secretion
   2 Natural estrogens, other estrogens, and oral contraceptives lead to decreased bile salt secretion
E Ileal disease or resection
   1 Malabsorption of bile acids leads to decreased bile acid pool and decreased biliary secretion of bile salts
F Increasing age
   1 Increased biliary secretion of cholesterol, decreased size of bile acid pool, decreased biliary secretion of bile salts
G Gallbladder hypomotility leading to stasis and formation sludge/stools
   1 Prolonged parenteral nutrition
   2 Fasting
   3 Pregnancy
   4 Drugs such as octreotide
H Clofibrate therapy
   1 Increased biliary secretion of cholesterol
I Miscellaneous
   1 ? Diabetes mellitus
   2 High-calorie, high-fat diet

PIGMENT STONES

A Demographic/genetic factors: Asia, rural setting
B Chronic hemolysis
C Alcoholic cirrhosis
D Chronic biliary tract infection, parasite infestation
E Increasing age

TABLE 272-2   Diagnostic evaluation of the gallbladder

Diagnostic advantages	Diagnostic limitations	Comment
PLAIN ABDOMINAL X-RAY		

Low cost
Readily available
	Relatively low yield
	?Contraindicated in pregnancy
		Pathognomonic findings in:
		  Calcified gallstones
		  Limey bile, porcelain GB
		  Emphysematous cholecystitis
		  Gallstone ileus

ORAL CHOLECYSTOGRAM (OCG)		

Low cost
Readily available
Accurate identification of gallstones (90–95%)
Identification of GB anomalies, hyperplastic cholecystoses
Identification of chronic GB disease after non-visualization on double dose
	?Contraindicated in pregnancy
	?Contraindicated with history of reaction to iodinated contrast
	Nonvisualization with:
	  Serum bilirubin >34–68 μmol/L (2–4 mg/dL)
	  Failure to ingest or absorb tablets
	  Impaired hepatic excretion
	Very small stones may be undetected
	More time-consuming than GBUS
		A useful procedure in identification of gall-stones if diagnostic limitations prevent GBUS; largely superseded by GBUS

GALLBLADDER ULTRASOUND (GBUS)		
Rapid Accurate identification of gallstones (>95%) Simultaneous scanning of GB, liver, bile ducts, pancreas "Real-time" scanning allows assessment of GB volume, contractility Not limited by jaundice, pregnancy May detect very small stones	Bowel gas Massive obesity Ascites Recent barium study	Procedure of choice for detection of stones
RADIOISOTOPE SCANS (HIDA, DIDA, ETC.)		
Accurate identification of cystic duct obstruction Simultaneous assessment of bile ducts	?Contraindicated in pregnancy Serum bilirubin >103–205 μmol/L (6–12 mg/dL) Cholecystogram of low resolution	Indicated for confirmation of suspected chole-cystitis; useful in diagnosis of acalculous cholecystopathy, especially if given with CCK to assess gallbladder emptying

FIGURE 272-2   Examples of ultrasound and radiologic studies of the biliary tract. *A.* An ultrasound study showing a distended gallbladder containing a single large stone (*arrow*) which casts an acoustic shadow. *B.* Endoscopic retrograde cholangiopancreatogram (ERCP) showing normal biliary tract anatomy. In addition to the endoscope and large vertical gallbladder filled with contrast dye, the common hepatic duct (chd), common bile duct (cbd), and pancreatic duct (pd) are shown. The arrow points to the ampulla of Vater. *C.* Percutaneous transhepatic cholangiogram (PTHC) showing choledocholithiasis. The biliary tract is dilatated and contains multiple radiolucent calculi (*small arrows*). The dilatation is due to obstruction by a large stone in the distal portion of the duct (*large arrow*). *D.* ERCP showing sclerosing cholangitis. The common bile duct is to the right of the endoscope. Following retrograde cholangiography, the common bile duct shows thickening of the wall with a narrow, beaded lumen typical of sclerosing cholangitis.

gallstone patients suggests that the cumulative risk for the development of symptoms or complications requiring surgery is relatively low— 10 percent at 5 years, 15 percent at 10 years, and 18 percent at 15 years. Patients remaining asymptomatic for 15 years were found to be unlikely to develop symptoms during further follow-up, and most patients who did develop complications from their gallstones experienced *prior* warning symptoms. Similar conclusions apply to diabetics with silent gallstones. Decision analysis has suggested that (1) the cumulative risk of death due to gallstone disease while on expectant management is small, and (2) prophylactic cholecystectomy is not warranted.

Complications requiring cholecystectomy appear to be much more common in gallstone patients who have developed symptoms of biliary colic. Patients found to have gallstones at a young age are more likely to develop symptoms from cholelithiasis than are patients older than 60 years at the time of initial diagnosis. Patients with diabetes mellitus and gallstones may be somewhat more susceptible to septic complications, but the magnitude of risk of septic biliary complications in diabetic patients is incompletely defined. In addition, asymptomatic gallstone patients with nonvisualization of the gallbladder on OCG appear to have an increased tendency to develop symptoms and complications.

Treatment of gallstones SURGICAL THERAPY Although the management of silent gallstones remains controversial, the risk of developing symptoms or complications requiring surgery is quite small (in the range of 1 to 2 percent per year) in most asymptomatic gallstone patients. Thus a recommendation for prophylactic cholecystectomy in a patient with gallstones should probably be based on assessment of three factors: (1) the presence of symptoms which are frequent enough or severe enough to interfere with the patient's general routine, (2) the presence of a prior complication of gallstone disease, i.e., history of acute cholecystitis, pancreatitis, gallstone fistula, etc., or (3) the presence of an underlying condition predisposing the patient to increased risk of gallstone complications (e.g., calcified or porcelain gallbladder, cholesterolosis, adenomyomatosis, nonvisualizing gallbladder on OCG, and/or a previous attack of acute cholecystitis regardless of current symptomatic status). Patients with very large gallstones (over 2 cm in diameter) and patients having gallstones in a congenitally anomalous gallbladder also might be considered for prophylactic cholecystectomy. Although age under 50 years is a worrisome factor in asymptomatic gallstone patients, few authorities would now recommend routine cholecystectomy in all young patients with silent stones. Laparoscopic cholecystectomy is a minimal-access approach for the removal of the gallbladder together with its stones. Because of a markedly shortened hospital stay as well as decreased cost and a mortality rate of less than 1 percent, it is the procedure of choice for most patients referred for elective cholecystectomy; in only 4 to 5 percent of patients are surgeons compelled to convert to open cholecystectomy.

MEDICAL THERAPY—GALLSTONE DISSOLUTION Oral bile acid therapy is essentially ineffective in dissolving (1) pigment gallstones, which represent approximately 20 percent of radiolucent stones, (2) radiopaque or calcified gallstones, (3) gallstones greater than approximately 1.5 cm in diameter, and (4) gallstones in gallbladders poorly opacified following oral cholecystography. Treatment with oral chenodeoxycholic acid (CDCA, chenic acid) or its 7β-epimer ursodeoxycholic acid (UDCA) to dissolve cholesterol or mixed gallstones has resulted in complete or partial dissolution of such stones in approximately 50 to 60 percent of *selected* patients with radiolucent gallstones. The major therapeutic effect of CDCA is thought to be secondary to a decrease in HMG-CoA reductase activity, which, in turn, results in decreased hepatic cholesterol synthesis. UDCA administration appears to produce a lamellar liquid crystalline phase in bile which allows a dispersion of cholesterol from stones by physicochemical means. Ursodeoxycholic acid also may retard cholesterol crystal nucleation. UDCA is therapeutically more effective at lower doses (5 to 10 mg/kg per day) than CDCA and has not been associated with the relatively high incidence of diarrhea and serum aminotransferase elevations seen in CDCA-treated patients.

In *carefully selected* patients with radiolucent stones less than 15 mm in a functioning gallbladder, complete dissolution can be achieved within 2 years with UDCA or a combination of UDCA with CDCA in approximately 50 to 60 percent. The highest success rate, i.e., approximately 70 to 80 percent, occurs in patients with small (<5 mm), floating, radiolucent gallstones. If bile acid therapy is limited to patients with small, floating, radiolucent stones, probably no more than 10 percent of patients with symptomatic cholelithiasis are candidates for such treatment. However, in addition to the vexing problem of recurrence, there is also the factor of taking a costly drug for an indefinite period of time.

After complete dissolution of gallstones by either CDCA or UDCA and withdrawal of such treatment, there is a recurrence rate of 30 to 55 percent over 3 to 12 years of follow-up. There appears to be an approximately linear increase in gallstone recurrence of 10 to 15 percent per annum over the first 3 to 5 years, after which there may be a plateau with no further recurrence. The recurrence rate is lower in patients who had a single gallstone compared with those with multiple stones. In clinical trials designed to prevent recurrences, UDCA in doses of 3 mg/kg or 200 to 300 mg/d may delay and/or reduce recurrence.

Direct dissolution of gallstones within a period of hours using methyl tertiary butyl ether or other solvents through percutaneously placed biliary catheters also has been reported. Such solvent dissolution of gallbladder or ductal stones by continuous perfusion appears promising.

GALLSTONE LITHOTRIPSY Gallbladder stones may be fragmented by extracorporeal shock waves generated by the use of electrohydraulic, piezoceramic, or electromagnetic devices. Such shock-wave lithotripsy combined with medical litholytic therapy is a safe and effective treatment in carefully selected patients with gallbladder calculi. The usual criteria for selection of patients include (1) a history of biliary colic, (2) radiolucent stones, (3) a functioning gallbladder with opacification by oral cholecystography or normal emptying by cholecystokinin scintigraphy, (4) up to a maximum of three stones but preferably solitary stones ≤20 mm, and (5) absence of acute cholecystitis, cholangitis, biliary obstruction, acute pancreatitis, and pregnancy. The best results have been obtained in patients with solitary stones ≤20 mm; 60 to 70 percent of such patients remain stone- and fragment-free at 8 to 12 months. Results are less satisfactory for stones larger than 20 mm or for two or three stones. Side effects, caused mostly by passage of fragments after lithotripsy, include biliary colic (35 percent), pancreatitis (2 percent), and cholecystitis (1 percent). Approximately 5 percent of lithotripsy-treated patients have required cholecystectomy or urgent endoscopic sphincterotomy. If lithotripsy of gallstones is restricted to patients with symptomatic solitary gallstones ≤20 mm, only 10 to 15 percent of all patients with symptomatic gallstones will be eligible. There are still two problematic areas: (1) *recurrence* of gallstones in 10 to 15 percent of patients 2 years after lithotripsy combined with medical litholytic therapy, and (2) the *cost* of taking UDCA or UDCA plus CDCA for an indefinite period. Importantly, while the utilization of gallstone lithotripsy has decreased considerably since the emergence of laparoscopic cholecystectomy, lithotripsy does remain an option for carefully selected patients who wish to avoid surgery.

ACUTE AND CHRONIC CHOLECYSTITIS Acute cholecystitis Acute inflammation of the gallbladder wall usually follows obstruction of the cystic duct by a stone. Inflammatory response can be evoked by three factors: (1) *mechanical inflammation* produced by increased intraluminal pressure and distention with resulting ischemia of the gallbladder mucosa and wall, (2) *chemical inflammation* caused by the release of lysolecithin (due to the action of phospholipase on lecithin in bile) and other local tissue factors, and (3) *bacterial inflammation*, which may play a role in 50 to 85 percent of patients with acute cholecystitis. The organisms most frequently isolated by cystectomy syndromes may be due to (1) biliary strictures, (2) retained biliary calculi, (3) cystic duct stump syndrome, (4) stenosis or dyskinesia of the sphincter of Oddi, or (5) bile salt–induced diarrhea or gastritis.

CYSTIC DUCT STUMP SYNDROME   In the absence of cholangiographically demonstrable retained stones, symptoms resembling biliary colic or cholecystitis in the postcholecystectomy patient have frequently been attributed to disease in a long (>1 cm) cystic duct remnant (cystic duct stump syndrome). Careful analysis, however, reveals that postcholecystectomy complaints are attributable to other causes in almost all patients in whom the symptom complex was originally thought to result from the existence of a long cystic duct stump. Accordingly, considerable care should be taken to investigate the possible role of other factors in the production of postcholecystectomy symptoms before attributing them to cystic duct stump syndrome.

PAPILLARY DYSFUNCTION, PAPILLARY STENOSIS, SPASM OF THE SPHINCTER OF ODDI, AND BILIARY DYSKINESIA   Symptoms of biliary colic accompanied by signs of recurrent, intermittent biliary obstruction may be produced by papillary stenosis, papillary dysfunction, spasm of the sphincter of Oddi, and biliary dyskinesia. Papillary stenosis is thought to result from acute or chronic inflammation of the papilla of Vater or from glandular hyperplasia of the papillary segment. Five criteria have been used to define papillary stenosis: (1) upper abdominal pain, usually right upper quadrant or epigastric, (2) abnormal liver tests, (3) dilatation of the common bile duct upon endoscopic retrograde cholangiopancreatogram (ERCP) examination, (4) delayed (longer than 45 min) drainage of contrast material from the duct, and (5) increased basal pressure of the sphincter of Oddi, a finding that may be of only minor significance. A useful alternative to ERCP is hepatobiliary scintigraphy using ^{99m}Tc-diisopropyl iminodiacetic acid (DIDA), especially if ERCP and/or biliary manometry are either unavailable or not feasible. In patients with papillary stenosis, quantitative hepatobiliary scintigraphy has revealed delayed transit from the common bile duct to the bowel, ductal dilatation, and abnormal time-activity dynamics. This technique also can be used before and after sphincterotomy to document improvement in biliary emptying. Treatment consists of endoscopic or surgical sphincteroplasty to ensure wide patency of the distal portions of both the bile and pancreatic ducts. The greater the number of the preceding criteria present, the greater the likelihood that a patient does have a degree of papillary stenosis sufficient to justify correction. The factors usually considered as indications for sphincterotomy include (1) prolonged duration of symptoms, (2) lack of response to symptomatic treatment, (3) presence of severe disability, and (4) the patient's choice of sphincterotomy over surgery (given a clear understanding on his or her part of the risks involved in both procedures).

Criteria for diagnosing dyskinesia of the sphincter of Oddi are even more controversial than those for papillary stenosis. Proposed mechanisms include spasm of the sphincter, denervation sensitivity resulting in hypertonicity, and abnormalities of the sequencing or frequency rates of sphincteric contraction waves. When thorough evaluation has failed to demonstrate another cause for the pain, and when cholangiographic and manometric criteria suggest a diagnosis of biliary dyskinesia, medical treatment with nitrites or anticholinergics to attempt pharmacologic relaxation of the sphincter has been proposed. Endoscopic sphincterotomy or surgical sphincteroplasty may be indicated in patients who fail to respond to a 2- to 3-month trial of medical therapy, especially if basal sphincter of Oddi pressures are elevated.

BILE SALT–INDUCED CATHARSIS AND GASTRITIS   Postcholecystectomy patients may develop symptoms and signs of gastritis, which has been attributed to duodenogastric reflux of bile. However, firm data linking an increased incidence of bile gastritis with surgical removal of the gallbladder are lacking. Similarly, the occurrence of cholestyramine-responsive diarrhea in a small number of patients following cholecystectomy has been attributed to an alteration of the enterohepatic circulation of bile acids induced or unmasked by removal of the gallbladder.

THE HYPERPLASTIC CHOLECYSTOSES   The term *hyperplastic cholecystoses* is used to denote a group of disorders of the gallbladder characterized by excessive proliferation of normal tissue components.

Adenomyomatosis is characterized by a benign proliferation of gallbladder surface epithelium with glandlike formations, extramural sinuses, transverse strictures, and/or fundal nodule ("adenoma" or "adenomyoma") formation. Outpouchings of mucosa termed *Rokitansky-Aschoff sinuses* may be seen on oral cholecystography in conjunction with hyperconcentration of contrast medium. Characteristic dimpled filling defects also may be seen.

Cholesterolosis is characterized by abnormal deposition of lipid, especially cholesterol esters, in the lamina propria of the gallbladder wall. In its diffuse form ("strawberry gallbladder"), the gallbladder mucosa is brick red and speckled with bright yellow flecks of lipid. The localized form shows solitary or multiple "cholesterol polyps" studding the gallbladder wall. Cholesterol stones of the gallbladder are found in nearly half the cases. Cholecystectomy is indicated in both adenomyomatosis and cholesterolosis when symptomatic or when cholelithiasis is present.

CANCER OF THE GALLBLADDER   Most cancers of the gallbladder develop in conjunction with stones rather than polyps. In patients with gallstones, the risk for developing gallbladder cancer, while increased, is still quite low. In one study, gallbladder cancer developed in only 5 of 2583 patients with gallstones followed for a median of 13 years. In the United States, adenocarcinomas comprise the vast majority of the estimated 6500 new cases of gallbladder cancer diagnosed each year. The female/male ratio is 4:1, and the mean age at diagnosis is approximately 70 years. The clinical presentation is most often one of unremitting right upper quadrant pain associated with weight loss, jaundice, and a palpable right upper quadrant mass. Cholangitis may supervene. The preoperative diagnosis of the condition is difficult. Once symptoms have appeared, spread of the tumor outside the gallbladder by direct extension or by lymphatic or hematogenous routes is almost invariable. Over 75 percent of gallbladder carcinomas are unresectable at the time of surgery, the exceptions being tumors discovered incidentally at laparotomy. The 1-year mortality rate for unresectable disease is approximately 95 percent, and only 5 percent of patients survive 5 years or more from the time of diagnosis. Radical operative resection does not appear to improve survival. Results of trials with radiation and chemotherapy of primary gallbladder cancer also have been disappointing.

DISEASES OF THE BILE DUCTS

CONGENITAL ANOMALIES   Biliary atresia and hypoplasia   Atretic and hypoplastic lesions of the extrahepatic and major intrahepatic bile ducts are the most common biliary anomalies of clinical relevance encountered in infancy. The clinical picture is one of severe obstructive jaundice during the first month of life, with pale stools. The diagnosis is confirmed by surgical exploration with operative cholangiography. Approximately 10 percent of cases of biliary atresia are treatable with roux-en-Y choledochojejunostomy, with the Kasai procedure (hepatic portoenterostomy) being attempted in the remainder in an effort to restore some bile flow. Most patients, even those having successful biliary-enteric anastomoses, eventually develop chronic cholangitis, extensive hepatic fibrosis, and portal hypertension.

Choledochal cysts   Cystic dilatation may involve the free portion of the common bile duct, i.e., choledochal cyst, or may present as diverticulum formation in the intraduodenal segment. In the latter situation, chronic reflux of pancreatic juice into the biliary tree can produce inflammation and stenosis of the extrahepatic bile ducts leading to cholangitis or biliary obstruction. Because the process may be gradual, approximately 50 percent of patients present with onset of symptoms after age 10. The diagnosis may be made by ultrasound, abdominal CT, or cholangiography. Surgical treatment involves excision of the ''cyst'' and biliary-enteric anastomosis. Patients with choledochal cysts are at increased risk for the subsequent development of cholangiocarcinoma.

Congenital biliary ectasia Cystic dilatation of the intrahepatic bile ducts may involve either the major intrahepatic radicles (Caroli's disease) or the inter- and intralobular ducts (congenital hepatic fibrosis) or both. In Caroli's disease, clinical manifestations include recurrent cholangitis, abscess formation in and around the affected ducts, and sometimes, gallstone formation within portions of ectatic intrahepatic biliary radicles. The CT scan and cholangiographic patterns are usually diagnostic, and treatment with ongoing antibiotic therapy is usually undertaken in an effort to limit the frequency and severity of recurrent bouts of cholangitis. Progression to secondary biliary cirrhosis with portal hypertension, amyloidosis, extrahepatic biliary obstruction, cholangiocarcinoma, or recurrent episodes of sepsis with hepatic abscess formation is common.

CHOLEDOCHOLITHIASIS Pathophysiology and clinical manifestations Passage of gallstones into the common bile duct occurs in approximately 10 to 15 percent of patients with cholelithiasis. The incidence of common duct stones increases with increasing age of the patient so that up to 25 percent of elderly patients may have calculi in the common duct at the time of cholecystectomy. Undetected duct stones are left behind in approximately 1 to 5 percent of cholecystectomy patients. The overwhelming majority of bile duct stones are cholesterol or mixed stones formed in the gallbladder which then migrate into the extrahepatic biliary tree through the cystic duct. Primary calculi arising de novo in the ducts are usually pigment stones developing in patients with (1) chronic hemolytic diseases, (2) hepatobiliary parasitism or chronic, recurrent cholangitis, (3) congenital anomalies of the bile ducts (especially Caroli's disease), or (4) dilated, sclerosed, or strictured ducts. Common duct stones may remain asymptomatic for years, may pass spontaneously into the duodenum, or (most often) may present with biliary colic or a complication.

Complications CHOLANGITIS Cholangitis may be acute or chronic, and symptoms result from inflammation, which usually requires at least partial obstruction to the flow of bile. Bacteria are present on bile culture in approximately 75 percent of patients with acute cholangitis early in the symptomatic course. The characteristic presentation of acute cholangitis involves biliary colic, jaundice, and spiking fevers with chills (Charcot's triad). Blood cultures are frequently positive, and leukocytosis is typical. *Nonsuppurative* acute cholangitis is most common and may respond relatively rapidly to supportive measures and to treatment with antibiotics (see Chap. 98). In *suppurative* acute cholangitis, however, the presence of pus under pressure in a completely obstructed ductal system leads to symptoms of severe toxicity—mental confusion, bacteremia, and septic shock. Response to antibiotics alone in this setting is relatively poor, multiple hepatic abscesses are often present, and the mortality rate approaches 100 percent unless prompt surgical correction of the obstructing lesion and drainage of infected bile is carried out.

OBSTRUCTIVE JAUNDICE Gradual obstruction of the common bile duct over a period of weeks or months usually leads to initial manifestations of jaundice or pruritus without associated symptoms of biliary colic or cholangitis. Painless jaundice may occur in patients with choledocholithiasis, but this manifestation is much more characteristic of biliary obstruction secondary to malignancy of the head of pancreas, bile ducts, or ampulla of Vater.

In patients whose obstruction is secondary to choledocholithiasis, associated chronic calculous cholecystitis is very common, and the gallbladder in this setting may be relatively indistensible. The absence of a palpable gallbladder in most patients with biliary obstruction from duct stones is the basis for *Courvoisier's law*, i.e., that the presence of a palpably enlarged gallbladder suggests that the biliary obstruction is secondary to an underlying malignancy rather than to calculous disease. Biliary obstruction causes progressive dilatation of the intrahepatic bile ducts as intrabiliary pressures rise. Hepatic bile flow is suppressed, and regurgitation of conjugated bilirubin into the

bloodstream leads to jaundice accompanied by dark urine (bilirubinuria) and light-colored (acholic) stools.

Common bile duct stones should be suspected in any patient with cholecystitis whose serum bilirubin level exceeds 85.5 μmol/L (5 mg/dL). The maximum bilirubin level is seldom over 256.5 μmol/L (15.0 mg/dL) in patients with choledocholithiasis unless concomitant hepatic disease or another factor leading to marked hyperbilirubinemia exists. Serum bilirubin levels of 342.0 μmol/L (20mg/dL) or more should suggest the possibility of neoplastic obstruction. The serum alkaline phosphatase level is almost always elevated in biliary obstruction. A rise in alkaline phosphatase often precedes clinical jaundice and may be the only abnormality in routine liver function tests. There may be a two- to tenfold elevation of serum aminotransferases, especially in association with acute obstruction. Following relief of the obstructing process, serum aminotransferase elevations usually return rapidly to normal, while the serum bilirubin level may take 1 to 2 weeks to return to normal. The alkaline phosphatase level usually falls slowly, lagging behind the decrease in serum bilirubin.

PANCREATITIS The most common associated entity discovered in patients with nonalcoholic acute pancreatitis is biliary tract disease. Biochemical evidence of pancreatic inflammation complicates acute cholecystitis in 15 percent of cases and choledocholithiasis in over 30 percent, and the common factor appears to be the passage of gallstones through the common duct. Coexisting pancreatitis should be suspected in patients with symptoms of cholecystitis who develop (1) back pain or pain to the left of the abdominal midline, (2) prolonged vomiting with paralytic ileus, or (3) a pleural effusion, especially on the left side. Surgical treatment of gallstone disease is usually associated with resolution of the pancreatitis.

SECONDARY BILIARY CIRRHOSIS Secondary biliary cirrhosis may complicate prolonged or intermittent duct obstruction with or without recurrent cholangitis. Although this complication may be seen in patients with choledocholithiasis, it is more common in cases of prolonged obstruction from stricture or neoplasm. Once established, secondary biliary cirrhosis may be progressive even after correction of the obstructing process, and increasingly severe hepatic cirrhosis may lead to portal hypertension or to hepatic failure and death. Prolonged biliary obstruction also may be associated with clinically relevant deficiencies of the fat-soluble vitamins A, D, and K.

Diagnosis and treatment The diagnosis of choledocholithiasis is usually made by cholangiography (Table 272-3), either preoperatively or intraoperatively at the time of cholecystectomy. The incidence of coexisting common duct stones in patients with cholelithiasis is relatively high. Operative cholangiography should be performed routinely during surgical procedures on the biliary tract. Preoperative indications for common duct exploration include (1) cholangiographic demonstration of ductal stones, (2) jaundice or cholangitis preceding operation, (3) a history of gallstone-related pancreatitis, and (4) cholangiographic evidence of a markedly enlarged common bile duct. Operative indications for exploration of the duct include (1) manual palpation of stones in the common bile duct, (2) positive intraoperative cholangiogram, (3) enlargement of the common bile duct or cystic duct at operation, (4) multiple small stones or ''sand'' in the gallbladder, and (5) a gallbladder empty of stones at surgery in a patient with previously documented gallstones.

In most cases of choledocholithiasis, the treatment of choice is cholecystectomy with choledocholithotomy and T-tube drainage of the bile ducts. A T-tube cholangiogram is usually performed prior to T-tube removal on or before the tenth postoperative day. Retained calculi seen on T-tube cholangiography may be removed percutaneously by placement of a steerable basket catheter under radiographic guidance through the matured T-tube sinus tract. Endoscopic sphincterotomy followed by spontaneous or basket stone extraction is an additional nonoperative alternative in the management of patients with common duct stones, especially in elderly or poor-risk patients.

TRAUMA, STRICTURES, AND HEMOBILIA Benign strictures of the extrahepatic bile ducts result from surgical trauma in approximately 95 percent of cases and occur in about 1 in 500 cholecystectomies.

TABLE 272-3 Diagnostic evaluation of the bile ducts

Diagnostic advantages	Diagnostic limitations	Contraindications	Complications	Comment
HEPATOBILIARY ULTRASOUND (HBUS)				
Rapid Simultaneous scanning of GB, liver, bile ducts, pancreas Accurate identification of dilated bile ducts Not limited by jaundice, pregnancy Guidance for fine-needle biopsy	Bowel gas Massive obesity Ascites Barium Partial bile duct obstruction Poor visualization of distal CBD	None	None	Initial procedure of choice in investigating possible biliary obstruction
COMPUTED TOMOGRAPHY (CT)				
Simultaneous scanning of GB, liver, bile ducts, pancreas Accurate identification of dilated bile ducts, masses Not limited by jaundice, gas, obesity, ascites High-resolution image Guidance for fine-needle biopsy	Extreme cachexia Movement artifact Ileus Partial bile duct obstruction High cost May not be readily available	Pregnancy	Reaction to iodinated contrast, if used	Indicated for evaluation of hepatic or pancreatic masses Procedure of choice in investigating possible biliary obstruction if diagnostic limitations prevent HBUS
PERCUTANEOUS TRANSHEPATIC CHOLANGIOGRAM (PTHC)				
Extremely successful when bile ducts dilated Best visualization of proximal biliary tract Possible separate visualization of obstructed left ductal system Bile cytology/culture Percutaneous transhepatic drainage	Nondilated or sclerosed ducts	Pregnancy Uncorrectable coagulopathy Massive ascites ? Hepatic abscess	Bleeding Hemobilia Bile peritonitis Bacteremia, sepsis	Usually, initial cholangiogram of choice when bile ducts are dilated
ENDOSCOPIC RETROGRADE CHOLANGIOPANCREATOGRAM (ERCP)				
Simultaneous pancreatography Visualization/biopsy of ampulla and duodenum Best visualization of distal biliary tract Bile or pancreatic cytology Endoscopic sphincterotomy and stone removal Biliary manometry Not limited by ascites, coagulopathy, abscess	Gastroduodenal obstruction ? Roux en Y biliary-enteric anastomosis	Pregnancy ? Acute pancreatitis ? Severe cardiopulmonary disease	Pancreatitis Cholangitis, sepsis Infected pancreatic pseudocyst Perforation (rare) Hypoxemia, aspiration	Cholangiogram of choice in: Absence of dilated ducts ? Pancreatic, ampullary or gastroduodenal disease Prior biliary surgery PTHC contraindicated or failed Endoscopic sphincterotomy a treatment possibility

NOTE: Intravenous cholangiography (IVC) is an obsolete technique because 40 percent of common duct stones are missed and there is poor resolution even with tomography. There are few indications for its use especially since other cholangiographic techniques are usually available.

Strictures may present with bile leak or abscess formation in the immediate postoperative period or with biliary obstruction or cholangitis as long as 2 years or more following the inciting trauma. The diagnosis is established by percutaneous or endoscopic cholangiography. Successful operative correction by a skillful surgeon with duct-to-bowel anastomosis is usually possible, although mortality rates from surgical complications, recurrent cholangitis, or secondary biliary cirrhosis are high.

Hemobilia may follow traumatic or operative injury to the liver or bile ducts, intraductal rupture of a hepatic abscess or aneurysm of the hepatic artery, biliary or hepatic tumor hemorrhage, or mechanical complications of choledocholithiasis or hepatobiliary parasitism. Diagnostic procedures such as liver biopsy, percutaneous transhepatic cholangiography (PTHC), and transhepatic biliary drainage catheter placement also may be complicated by hemobilia. Patients often present with a classic triad of biliary colic, obstructive jaundice, and melena or occult blood in the stools. The diagnosis is sometimes made by cholangiographic evidence of blood clot in the biliary tree, but selective angiographic verification may be required. Although minor episodes of hemobilia may resolve without operative intervention, surgical ligation of the bleeding vessel is frequently required.

EXTRINSIC COMPRESSION OF THE BILE DUCTS Partial or complete biliary obstruction may sometimes be produced by extrinsic compression of the ducts. The most common cause of this form of obstructive jaundice is carcinoma of the head of the pancreas. Biliary obstruction also may occur as a complication of either acute or chronic pancreatitis or involvement of lymph nodes in the porta hepatis by lymphoma or metastatic carcinoma. The latter should be distinguished from cholestasis resulting from massive replacement of the liver by tumor.

HEPATOBILIARY PARASITISM Infestation of the biliary tract by adult helminths or their ova may produce a chronic, recurrent pyogenic cholangitis with or without multiple hepatic abscesses, ductal stones, or biliary obstruction. This condition is relatively rare but does occur in inhabitants of southern China and elsewhere in Southeast Asia. The organisms most commonly involved are trematodes or flukes, including *Clonorchis sinensis*, *Opisthorchis viverrini* or *felineus*, and *Fasciola hepatica*. The biliary tract also may be involved by intraductal migration of adult *Ascaris lumbricoides* from the duodenum or by intrabiliary rupture of hydatid cysts of the liver produced by *Echinococcus* species. The diagnosis is made by cholangiography and the presence of characteristic ova on stool examination. When obstruction is present, the treatment of choice is laparotomy under antibiotic coverage, with common duct exploration and a biliary drainage procedure. It should be emphasized that in the Orient, one also sees cholangiohepatitis associated with pigment lithiasis, which may, in fact, be more common than cholangitis due to parasites.

SCLEROSING CHOLANGITIS Primary or idiopathic sclerosing cholangitis is a disorder characterized by a progressive, inflammatory, sclerosing, and obliterative process affecting the extrahepatic and, often, the intrahepatic bile ducts. The lesion may appear as an isolated entity or may occur in association with inflammatory bowel disease, especially ulcerative colitis, or with multifocal fibrosclerosis syndromes such as retroperitoneal, mediastinal, and/or periureteral fibrosis, Riedel's struma, or pseudotumor of the orbit. Papillary stenosis and sclerosing cholangitis are also important complications of AIDS; cytomegalovirus and cryptosporidia infections have been observed frequently in such patients, raising the question whether these microbes may be a pathogenetic factor in primary sclerosing cholangitis. Secondary sclerosing cholangitis may occur as a long-term complication of choledocholithiasis, cholangiocarcinoma, operative or traumatic biliary injury, or contiguous inflammatory processes.

Patients with sclerosing cholangitis often present with signs and symptoms of chronic or intermittent biliary obstruction: jaundice, pruritus, right upper quadrant abdominal pain, or acute cholangitis. Late in the course, complete biliary obstruction, secondary biliary cirrhosis, hepatic failure, or portal hypertension with bleeding varices may occur. The diagnosis is usually established by finding thickened ducts with narrow, beaded lumina on cholangiography (see Fig. 272-2D). The cholangiographic technique of choice in suspected cases is probably ERCP, since intrahepatic ductal involvement may make PTHC difficult. When a diagnosis of sclerosing cholangitis has been established, a search for associated diseases, especially for chronic inflammatory bowel disease, should be carried out.

Therapy with cholestyramine may help control symptoms of pruritus, and antibiotics are useful when cholangitis complicates the clinical picture. Vitamin D and calcium supplementation may help prevent the loss of bone mass frequently seen in patients with chronic cholestasis. Glucocorticoids have not been shown to be efficacious. Preliminary studies have identified three promising drugs that appear to be of benefit, i.e., urodeoxycholic acid, methotrexate, and cyclosporine. In cases where complete or high-grade biliary obstruction has occurred, balloon dilatation or surgical intervention may be appropriate. Efforts at biliary-enteric anastomosis or stent placement may, however, be complicated by recurrent cholangitis and further progression of the stenosing process. The role of colectomy in patients with sclerosing cholangitis complicating chronic ulcerative colitis is uncertain. The prognosis is unfavorable, with a mean survival of 4 to 10 years following the diagnosis, regardless of therapy. Primary sclerosing cholangitis is one of the most common indications for liver transplantation. In one study, the mean follow-up time from the diagnosis of primary sclerosing cholangitis to the time of liver transplantation was 5.8 years.

CHOLANGIOCARCINOMA Benign tumors of the extrahepatic bile ducts are extremely rare causes of mechanical biliary obstruction. The majority of these are papillomas, adenomas, or cystadenomas which present with obstructive jaundice or hemobilia. Adenocarcinoma of the extrahepatic ducts is relatively more common. There is a slight male preponderance (60 percent), and the peak age incidence is in the fifth to seventh decades. Apparent predisposing factors include (1) some chronic hepatobiliary parasitic infestations, (2) congenital anomalies with ectactic ducts, (3) sclerosing cholangitis and chronic ulcerative colitis, and (4) occupational exposure to possible biliary tract carcinogens (workers in rubber or automotive plants). Cholelithiasis is not clearly associated with cholangiocarci-

noma as a predisposing factor. The lesions may be diffuse or nodular; the latter often arise at the confluence of the hepatic ducts (Klatskin tumors). This tumor is usually associated with a *collapsed* gallbladder, and such a finding mandates that the proximal hepatic ducts be optimally visualized by cholangiography.

Patients with cholangiocarcinoma usually present with biliary obstruction, painless jaundice, pruritus, weight loss, and acholic stools. A deep-seated, vaguely localized RUQ pain may be an associated complaint. Hepatomegaly and a palpable, distended gallbladder are frequent accompanying signs. Fever is unusual unless associated with ascending cholangitis. Because the obstructing process is gradual, the cholangiocarcinoma is often far advanced by the time it presents clinically. The diagnosis is most frequently made by cholangiography following ultrasound demonstration of dilated intrahepatic bile ducts. Any focal strictures of the bile ducts should probably be considered malignant until proved otherwise. Long-term palliation of the tumor is possible in some cases when radiation and/or chemotherapy are combined with palliative drainage of the biliary tree.

CARCINOMA OF THE PAPILLA OF VATER The ampulla of Vater may be involved by extension of tumor arising elsewhere in the duodenum or may itself be the primary site of origin of sarcomas, carcinoid tumors, or adenocarcinomas. Papillary adenocarcinomas are associated with slow growth and a more favorable clinical prognosis than diffuse, infiltrative cancers of the ampulla, which are more frequently widely invasive. The presenting clinical manifestation is usually obstructive jaundice. ERCP is probably the preferred diagnostic technique when ampullary carcinoma is suspected, because it allows for direct endoscopic inspection and biopsy of the ampulla as well as for performance of pancreatography to exclude a diagnosis of pancreatic malignancy. Cancer of the papilla is usually treated by wide, often radical, surgical excision. Lymph node or other metastases are present at the time of surgery in approximately 20 percent of cases, and the 5-year survival rate following surgical therapy in this group is only 5 to 10 percent. In the absence of metastases, however, radical pancreaticoduodenectomy (Whipple procedure) is associated with 5-year survival rates as high as 40 percent, and several long-term survivors have been reported.

REFERENCES

BARKUN JS et al: Randomised controlled trial of laparoscopic versus mini cholecystectomy. Lancet 340:1116, 1992

BARR F et al: Disorders of bile acid metabolism in cholesterol gallstone disease. J Clin Invest 90:589, 1992

CAREY MC et al: Whither biliary sludge? Gastroenterology 95:508, 1988

CELLO JP: Acquired immunodeficiency syndrome cholangiopathy: Spectrum of disease. Am J Med 86:539, 1989

DOWLING RH et al: Gallstone recurrence and post dissolution management, in *Enterohepatic Circulation of Bile Acids and Sterol Metabolism*, G Paumgartren, A Stichl, W Gersk (eds). Lancaster, PA, MTP Press, 1985, pp 361–369

GEENEN JE et al: The efficacy of endoscopic sphincterotomy after cholecystectomy in patients with sphincter-of-Oddi dysfunction. N Engl J Med 320:82, 1989

GRACIE WA, RANSOHOFF DF: The natural history of silent gallstones. The innocent gallstone is not a myth. N Engl J Med 307:798, 1982

HOLZBACH RT et al: Biliary proteins: Unique inhibitors of cholesterol crystal nucleation in human gallbladder bile. J Clin Invest 72:35, 1984

JOHNSTON DE, KAPLAN MM: Medical progress: Pathogenesis and treatment of gallstones. N Engl J Med 328:412, 1993

LEE SP et al: Origin and fate of biliary sludge. Gastroenterology 94:170, 1988

LEVY PF et al: Human gallbladder mucin accelerates nucleation of cholesterol in artifical bile. Gastroenterology 87:270, 1984

MARINGHINI A et al: Gallstones, gallbladder cancer, and other gastrointestinal malignancies: An epidemiologic study in Rochester, Minnesota. Ann Intern Med 107:30, 1987

MEYERS WC: A prospective analysis of 1518 laparoscopic cholecystectomies. N Engl J Med 324:1073, 1991

PAUMGARTNER G et al: Gallstones: Pathogenesis. Lancet 338:1117, 1991

PODDA M et al: Efficacy and safety of a combination of dienodeoxycholic acid and ursodeoxycholic acid for gallstone dissolution. Gastroenterology 96:222, 1989

PORAYKO MK et al: Patients with asymptomatic primary sclerosing cholangitis frequently have progressive disease. Gastroenterology 98:1594, 1990

RANSOHOFF DF: Assessment of prophylactic cholecystectomy and medical therapy for diabetics with silent gallstones. Gastroenterology 92:1588, 1987

SACKMAN M et al: The Munich gallbladder lithotripsy study: Results of the first five years with 711 patients. Ann Intern Med 114:290, 1991

SAUERBRUCH T et al: Fragmentation of bile duct stones by extracorporeal shock waves. Gastroenterology 96:222, 1989

———— et al: Gallbladder stones: Management. Lancet 338:1121, 1991

SHAFFER EA et al: Cholescintigraphic detection of functional obstruction of the sphincter of Oddi: Effect of papillotomy. Gastroenterology 90:728, 1986

SILVIS SE et al: What is the post-cholecystectomy pain syndrome? Gastrointestinal Endoscopy 31:401, 1985

SMITH BF, LAMONT JT: The central issue of cholesterol gallstones. Hepatology 6:529, 1986

THISTLE JL et al: Dissolution of cholesterol gallbladder stones by methyl-tert-butyl ether administered by percutaneous transhepatic catheter. N Engl J Med 320:633, 1989

WIESNER RH et al: Comparison of clinicopathologic features of primary sclerosing cholangitis and primary biliary cirrhosis. Gastroenterology 88:108, 1985

YAP L et al: Acalculous biliary pain: Cholecystectomy alleviates symptoms in patients with abnormal cholescintigraphy. Gastroenterology 101:786, 1991

section 3 Disorders of the pancreas

273 APPROACH TO THE PATIENT WITH PANCREATIC DISEASE

PHILLIP P. TOSKES / NORTON J. GREENBERGER

GENERAL CONSIDERATIONS

Inflammatory disease of the pancreas may be acute or chronic. Although good data exist concerning the frequency of acute pancreatitis (about 5000 new cases per year in the United States with a mortality rate of about 10 percent), the number of patients who suffer with recurrent acute pancreatitis or chronic pancreatitis is largely undefined. Only one prospective study on the incidence of chronic pancreatitis is available; this showed an incidence of 8.2 new cases per 100,000 per year and a prevalence of 26.4 cases per 100,000. These numbers probably underestimate considerably the true incidence and prevalence, since non-alcohol-induced pancreatitis was largely ignored. At autopsy, the prevalence of chronic pancreatitis ranges from 0.04 to 5 percent. The relative inaccessibility of the pancreas to direct examination and the nonspecificity of the abdominal pain associated with pancreatitis make the diagnosis of pancreatitis difficult and usually dependent on elevation of blood amylase levels. Many patients with chronic pancreatitis do not have elevated blood amylase levels. Some patients with chronic pancreatitis develop signs and symptoms of pancreatic exocrine insufficiency, and thus objective evidence for pancreatic disease can be demonstrated. However, there is a very large reservoir of pancreatic exocrine function. Greater than 90 percent of the pancreas must be damaged before maldigestion of fat and protein is manifested. Even the secretin stimulation test, which is the most sensitive method of assessing pancreatic exocrine function, is probably abnormal only when greater than 60 percent of exocrine function has been lost. Noninvasive, indirect tests of pancreatic exocrine function (bentiromide, serum trypsinogen) are much more likely to be abnormal in patients with obvious pancreatic disease, i.e., pancreatic calcification, steatorrhea, or diabetes mellitus, than in patients with occult disease. Thus the number of patients who have subclinical exocrine dysfunction (i.e., less than 90 percent loss of function) is unknown.

The clinical manifestations of acute and chronic pancreatitis and pancreatic insufficiency are protean. Thus patients may present with hypertriglyceridemia, vitamin B_{12} malabsorption, hypercalcemia, hypocalcemia, hyperglycemia, ascites, pleural effusions, and chronic abdominal pain with normal amylase levels. Indeed, if the clinician considers pancreatitis as a possible diagnosis only when presented with a patient having classic symptoms (i.e., severe, constant epigastric pain that radiates through to the back, along with an elevated blood amylase level), only a minority of the patients with pancreatitis will be diagnosed correctly.

As emphasized in Chap. 274, the etiologies as well as the clinical manifestations are quite varied. Although it is well appreciated that *pancreatitis* is frequently secondary to alcohol abuse and biliary tract disease, pancreatitis is also caused by drugs, trauma, and viral infections and is associated with metabolic and connective tissue disorders. In addition, in approximately 20 percent of patients with acute pancreatitis and 25 to 40 percent of patients with chronic pancreatitis, the etiology is obscure.

TESTS USEFUL IN THE DIAGNOSIS OF PANCREATIC DISEASE

Several tests have proved of value in the evaluation of pancreatic exocrine function. Examples of specific tests and usefulness in the diagnosis of acute and chronic pancreatitis are summarized in Table 273-1. At most institutions, pancreatic function tests are performed if the diagnosis of pancreatic disease remains a possibility after noninvasive tests (ultrasound, computed tomographic scan) and invasive tests (ERCP) are normal or inconclusive. In this regard, tests employing *direct* stimulation of the pancreas are the most sensitive.

PANCREATIC ENZYMES IN BODY FLUIDS   The serum amylase level is widely used as a screening test for acute pancreatitis in the patient with acute abdominal pain or back pain. A value greater than 150 Somogyi units per deciliter should raise the question of acute pancreatitis. Levels greater than 300 units make the diagnosis more likely, and values greater than three times normal virtually clinch the diagnosis if gut perforation or infarction is excluded. In acute pancreatitis the serum amylase is usually elevated within 24 h and remains so for 1 to 3 days. Levels return to normal within 3 to 5 days unless there is extensive pancreatic necrosis, incomplete ductal obstruction, or pseudocyst formation. Approximately 85 percent of patients with acute pancreatitis will have an elevated serum amylase. Normal values, however, may occur if (1) there is a delay (2 to 5 days) in obtaining blood samples, (2) the underlying disorder is chronic pancreatitis rather than acute pancreatitis, and (3) hypertriglyceridemia is present. Patients with hypertriglyceridemia and proven pancreatitis have been found to have spuriously low levels of amylase and lipase activity.

The serum amylase is often elevated in other conditions (Table 273-2), in part because the enzyme is found in many organs in addition to the pancreas (salivary glands, liver, small intestine, kidney, fallopian tube) and can be produced by various tumors (carcinoma of the lung, esophagus, breast, and ovary). Isoenzymes of amylase fall into two general categories, those arising from the pancreas (P isoamylases) and those from nonpancreatic sources (S isoamylases). The measurement of serum isoamylases is of clinical importance. Isoamylase analysis of normal serum shows that about

TABLE 273-1 Tests useful in the diagnosis of acute and chronic pancreatitis and pancreatic tumors

Test	Principle	Comment
PANCREATIC ENZYMES IN BODY FLUIDS		
Amylase		
1 Serum	Pancreatic inflammation leads to increased enzyme levels	Simple; 20–40% false-negatives and -positives; reliable if test results are three times the upper limit of normal
2 Urine	Renal clearance of amylase is increased in acute pancreatitis	May be abnormal when serum levels normal; false-negatives and -positives
3 Amylase/creatinine clearance ratio (C_{am}/C_{cr})	Renal clearance of amylase greater than clearance of creatinine	No more sensitive than the serum amylase; many false-positives
4 Ascitic fluid	Disruption of gland or main pancreatic duct leads to increased amylase concentration	Can establish diagnosis of pancreatitis; false-positives with intestinal obstruction and perforated ulcer
5 Pleural fluid	Exudative pleural effusion with pancreatitis	False-positives with carcinoma of the lung and esophageal perforation
6 Isoenzymes	P isoamylases arise from the pancreas; S isoamylases are from other sources	More sensitive than total serum amylase in diagnosis of acute pancreatitis; useful in identifying nonpancreatic causes of hyperamylasemia
Serum lipase	Pancreatic inflammation leads to increased enzyme levels	New methods of determination greatly simplified; positive in 70–85% of cases.
Serum trypsin-like immunoreactivity (TLI)	Pancreatic inflammation leads to increased levels	*Elevated* in acute pancreatitis; *decreased* in chronic pancreatitis *with* steatorrhea; normal in chronic pancreatitis *without* steatorrhea and steatorrhea with normal pancreatic function
Pancreatic polypeptide (PP)	PP confined almost totally to the pancreas; release stimulated by nutrients and hormones; such release parallels pancreatic enzyme secretion	Basal, meal-simulated, and hormone (secretin CCK)-stimulated PP levels *decreased* in chronic pancreatitis; fasting PP levels >125 pg/mL argues against chronic pancreatitis and pancreatic cancer
STUDIES PERTAINING TO PANCREATIC STRUCTURE		
Radiologic and radionuclide tests		
1 Plain film of the abdomen	Abnormal in acute and chronic pancreatitis	Simple; normal in >50% of both acute and chronic pancreatitis
2 Upper gastrointestinal x-rays	Abnormally thickened duodenal folds; displacement of stomach or widening of duodenal loop suggests a pancreatic mass (inflammatory, neoplastic, cystic)	Simple; frequently normal; largely superseded by US and CT scanning
3 Ultrasonography (US)	Can provide information on edema, inflammation, calcification, pseudocysts, and mass lesions	Simple, noninvasive; sequential studies quite feasible; useful in diagnosis of pseudocyst
4 CT scan	Permits detailed visualization of pancreas and surrounding structures	Useful in the diagnosis of pancreatic calcification, dilated pancreatic ducts, and pancreatic tumors; may not be able to distinguish between inflammatory and neoplastic mass lesions
5 Selective angiography	Can identify pancreatic neoplasms (1) by sheathing of celiac or superior mesenteric branches by tumor or (2) by tumor staining; displacement of vessels by tumor	Indicated (1) in suspected islet cell tumors and (2) prior to pancreatic or duodenal resection; most reliable features reflect nonresectable pancreatic cancer
6 Endoscopic retrograde cholangiopancreatography (ERCP)	Cannulation of pancreatic and common bile duct permits visualization of pancreatic-biliary ductal system	Provides diagnostic data in 60–85% of cases; differentiation of chronic pancreatitis from pancreatic carcinoma may be difficult
Pancreatic biopsy with US or CT guidance	Percutaneous biopsy with skinny needle and localization of lesion by US	High diagnostic yield; laparotomy avoided; requires special technical skills
TESTS OF EXOCRINE PANCREATIC FUNCTION		
Direct stimulation of the pancreas with analysis of duodenal contents		
1 Secretin-pancreozymin (CCK) test	Secretin leads to increased output of pancreatic juice and HCO_3^-; CCK leads to increased output of pancreatic enzymes; pancreatic secretory response related to functional mass of pancreatic tissue	Sensitive enough to detect occult disease; involves duodenal intubation and fluoroscopy; poorly defined normal enzyme response; overlap in chronic pancreatitis; large secretory reserve capacity of the pancreas
Indirect stimulation of pancreas with measurement of pancreatic enzymes		
1 Lundh test meal	Test meal (fat, carbohydrate, and protein) causes increased release of CCK, which causes increased enzyme output; trypsin concentration measured	Useful in pancreatic exocrine insufficiency; false-negatives with delayed gastric emptying; false-positives in primary mucosal disease of the gut and choledocholithiasis; does not measure secretory capacity
2 Benzoyl-tyrosyl-*p*-aminobenzoic (Bz-Ty-PABA, bentiromide) test	Synthetic peptide (Bz-Ty-PABA) specifically cleaved by chymotrypsin, liberating PABA which is absorbed and PABA metabolite excreted in the urine	Simple and reliable test of pancreatic exocrine function. Measurement of blood PABA level increases sensitivity.
3 Pancreolauryl test	Fluorescein dilaurate is hydrolyzed by pancreatic elastase which is absorbed and fluorescein measured in urine	Sensitivity and specificity similar to Bentiromide test

TABLE 273-1 Tests useful in the diagnosis of acute and chronic pancreatitis and pancreatic tumors *(continued)*

Test	Principle	Comment
Measurement of intraluminal digestion products		
1 Microscopic examination of stool for undigested meat fibers and fat	Lack of proteolytic and lipolytic enzymes causes decreased digestion of meat fibers and triglycerides	Simple, reliable; not sensitive enough to detect milder cases of pancreatic insufficiency
2 Quantitative stool fat determination	Lack of lipolytic enzymes brings about impaired fat digestion	Reliable, reference standard for defining severity of malabsorption; does not distinguish between maldigestion and malabsorption
3 Fecal nitrogen	Lack of proteolytic enzymes leads to impaired protein digestion, increase in stool nitrogen	Does not distinguish between maldigestion and malabsorption; low sensitivity
Measurement of pancreatic enzymes in feces		
1 Chymotrypsin	Pancreatic secretion of proteolytic enzymes	May be useful in cystic fibrosis; tedious; 10% false-positive and false-negative results
Miscellaneous tests		
1 Dual-labeled Schilling test	Intrinsic factor [^{57}Co]cobalamin and Hog R protein [^{58}Co]cobalamin are given together. Since proteases are necessary to cleave R protein, the ratio of labeled cobalamin excreted in urine is an index of exocrine dysfunction.	Time-consuming and expensive

35 to 45 percent of the amylase is of pancreatic origin. For example, in patients with acute pancreatitis, the total serum amylase level returns to normal more rapidly than pancreatic isoamylase. Thus, in patients seen after the first day, the pancreatic isoamylase level is a more sensitive indicator of pancreatitis than the total serum amylase level. In addition, in certain conditions, such as the postoperative state, acute alcohol intoxication, and diabetic ketoacidosis, it had been assumed that elevations in serum amylase indicated acute pancreatitis. However, the elevation of serum amylase in such conditions has been shown to actually be of the S type. Simple tests to distinguish pancreatic amylase from nonpancreatic amylase are no longer readily available, and such tests are often not reliable when the total amylase is minimally to moderately elevated. The serum trypsinogen (performed by several commercial laboratories) is quite helpful in this regard. Since this enzyme is secreted specifically by the pancreas, a normal serum trypsinogen level in a patient with minimal elevation of serum amylase essentially rules out acute pancreatitis. Urinary amylase measurements, including the amylase/ creatinine clearance ratio, offer no increased sensitivity or specificity over blood amylase levels.

Elevation of ascitic fluid amylase occurs in acute pancreatitis as well as (1) in pancreatogenous ascites due to disruption of the main pancreatic duct of a leaking pseudocyst and (2) in other abdominal disorders which simulate pancreatitis (e.g., intestinal obstruction, intestinal infarction, and perforated peptic ulcer). Elevation of pleural fluid amylase occurs in acute pancreatitis, chronic pancreatitis, carcinoma of the lung, and esophageal perforation.

Lipase may now be the single best enzyme to measure for the diagnosis of acute pancreatitis. Improvements in substrates and technology offer clinicians improved options, especially when a turbidometric assay is used. The newer lipase assays have colipase as a cofactor and are fully automated. Nevertheless, a word of caution is in order. Many hospital laboratories are now using the Ektachem technique because it is rapid and contains the appropriate substrates. However, at least two reports have demonstrated poor specificity with this technique, i.e., patients with nonpancreatic disorders having elevated lipase levels.

Assay for trypsinogen (or trypsin-like immunoreactivity) has a theoretical advantage over amylase and lipase determinations in that the pancreas is the only organ that contains this enzyme. The test appears to be useful in the diagnosis of both acute and chronic pancreatitis. Sensitivity and specificity are comparable to amylase and lipase determinations. Since trypsinogen is also excreted by the kidney, elevated values are found in renal failure, as is the case with serum amylase and lipase levels. No single blood test is reliable for the diagnosis of acute pancreatitis in patients with renal failure. Whether a patient with renal failure and abdominal pain has pancreatitis remains a difficult clinical problem. A recent study found that in patients with renal dysfunction, serum amylase levels were elevated only when creatinine clearance was less than 50 mL/min. In such patients, the serum amylase level was invariably less than 500 IU/L in the absence of objective evidence of acute pancreatitis. In that

TABLE 273-2 Causes of hyperamylasemia and hyperamylasuria

PANCREATIC DISEASE

A Pancreatitis
  1 Acute
  2 Chronic: ductal obstruction
  3 Complications of pancreatitis
    a Pancreatic pseudocyst
    b Pancreatogenous ascites
    c Pancreatic abscess
B Pancreatic trauma
C Pancreatic carcinoma

NONPANCREATIC DISORDERS

A Renal insufficiency
B Salivary gland lesions
  1 Mumps
  2 Calculus
  3 Irradiation sialadenitis
  4 Maxillofacial surgery
C "Tumor" hyperamylasemia
  1 Carcinoma of the lung
  2 Carcinoma of the esophagus
  3 Breast carcinoma, ovarian carcinoma
D Macroamylasemia
E Burns
F Diabetic ketoacidosis
G Pregnancy
H Renal transplantation
I Cerebral trauma
J Drugs: morphine

OTHER ABDOMINAL DISORDERS

A Biliary tract disease: cholecystitis, choledocholithiasis
B Intraabdominal disease
  1 Perforated or penetrating peptic ulcer
  2 Intestinal obstruction or infarction
  3 Ruptured ectopic pregnancy
  4 Peritonitis
  5 Aortic aneurysm
  6 Chronic liver disease
  7 Postoperative hyperamylasemia

SOURCE: After WB Salt II, S Schenker, Medicine 55:269, 1976.

study, serum lipase and trypsin levels paralleled serum amylase values.

A recent study evaluated the sensitivity and specificity of five assays used to diagnose acute pancreatitis: two amylase assays, one lipase, one trypsin-like immunoreactivity (TLI), and one pancreatic isoamylase. The data obtained show that (1) if the best cutoff level is used, all assays have similar specificities and suggest that (2) total serum amylase is as good an indicator of acute pancreatitis as any of the others. However, inherent in many such studies is the problem that the recognition and diagnosis of acute pancreatitis hinge on the finding of an elevated serum amylase level. The question arises as to whether any diagnostic test result can be proved superior to the total serum amylase level if hyperamylasemia is required for the diagnosis. In other studies, when "objective" confirmation of the clinical diagnosis of pancreatitis was required (ultrasonography, computed tomography, laparotomy), the sensitivity of the serum amylase has been as low as 68 percent. With these limitations in mind, the recommended screening tests for acute pancreatitis are *total serum amylase* and *serum lipase activities*. Serum amylase values greater than three times normal are highly specific.

STUDIES PERTAINING TO PANCREATIC STRUCTURE   Radiologic tests   Plain films of the abdomen provide useful information in 30 to 50 percent of patients with acute pancreatitis. The most frequent abnormalities include (1) a localized ileus usually involving the jejunum ("sentinel loop"), (2) a generalized ileus with air-fluid levels, (3) the "colon cutoff sign," which results from isolated distention of the transverse colon, (4) duodenal distention with air-fluid levels, and (5) a mass, which is frequently a pseudocyst. In chronic pancreatitis, an important radiographic finding is pancreatic calcification, which characteristically is localized adjacent to and superimposed on the second lumbar vertebra (see Fig. 274-3A).

Upper gastrointestinal x-rays may reveal displacement of the stomach by the retroperitoneal mass (see Fig. 274-2A) or widening and effacement of the duodenal C loop, which also suggest the presence of a pancreatic mass that could be an inflammatory, cystic, or neoplastic process. However, their use has been largely superseded by ultrasound.

Ultrasonography (echography) can provide important information in patients with acute pancreatitis, chronic pancreatitis, pancreatic calcification, pseudocyst, and pancreatic carcinoma. It is a useful procedure in the evaluation of the patient with acute pancreatitis. Echographic appearances can indicate the presence of edema, inflammation, and calcification (not obvious on plain films of the abdomen), as well as pseudocysts, mass lesions, and gallstones (see Figs. 274-2B and 274-3B). In acute pancreatitis, the pancreas is characteristically enlarged. In pancreatic pseudocyst, the usual appearance is that of an echo-free, smooth, round fluid collection. Pancreatic carcinoma distorts the usual landmarks, and mass lesions greater than 3.0 cm are usually detected as localized, echo-free solid lesions. Ultrasound is often the initial investigation for most patients with suspected pancreatic disease. However, obesity, excess small- and large-bowel gas, and recently performed barium contrast examinations can interfere with ultrasound studies, which are often technically unsatisfactory.

Computed tomography (CT) is the best imaging study for initial evaluation of a suspected chronic pancreatic disorder and for the complications of acute and chronic pancreatitis. It is especially useful in the detection of pancreatic tumors, fluid-containing lesions such as pseudocysts and abscesses, and calcium deposits (see Figs. 274-3C and 274-4A). Most lesions are characterized by (1) enlargement of the pancreatic outline, (2) distortion of the pancreatic contour, or (3) fluid-containing lesions that have different attenuation coefficients than normal pancreas. However, it is occasionally difficult to distinguish between inflammatory and neoplastic lesions. Oral water-soluble contrast agents may be used to opacify the stomach and duodenum during CT scans; this permits more precise delineation of various organs as well as mass lesions. Dynamic (rapid intravenously administered contrast) CT scans are useful in estimating the degree of pancreatic necrosis and in predicting morbidity and mortality.

Selective catheterization of the celiac and superior mesenteric arteries combined with superselective catheterization of others such as the hepatic, splenic, and gastroduodenal arteries permits visualization of the pancreas and detection of pancreatic neoplasms and pseudocysts. Pancreatic neoplasms can be identified by the sheathing of blood vessels by a mass lesion (see Fig. 274-1D). Hormone-producing pancreatic tumors are especially likely to exhibit increased vascularity and tumor staining. Angiographic abnormalities are noted in many patients with pancreatic carcinoma but are uncommon in patients without pancreatic disease. Angiography complements ultrasonography and endoscopic retrograde cholangiopancreatography (ERCP) in the study of a patient with a suspected pancreatic lesion and may be carried out if ERCP is either unsuccessful or nondiagnostic.

Endoscopic retrograde cholangiopancreatography   ERCP may provide useful information on the status of the pancreatic ductal system and thus aid in the differential diagnosis of pancreatic disease (see Figs. 274-1C, 274-3D, and 274-4B). Pancreatic carcinoma is characterized by stenosis or obstruction of either the pancreatic duct or the common bile duct; both ductal systems are often abnormal. In chronic pancreatitis, ERCP abnormalities include (1) luminal narrowing, (2) irregularities in the ductal system with stenosis, dilatation, sacculation, and ectasia, and (3) blockage of the pancreatic duct by calcium deposits. Differentiation from carcinoma may be difficult because of similar overlapping features, i.e., ductal stenosis and irregularity. Elevated serum and/or urine amylase levels following ERCP have been reported in 25 to 75 percent of patients, but clinical pancreatitis is uncommon. In a series of 300 patients, pancreatitis occurred in only 5 patients following ERCP. If no lesion is found within the biliary and/or pancreatic ducts in a patient with repeated attacks of acute pancreatitis, manometric studies of the sphincter of Oddi may be indicated. Such studies, however, do increase the risk of post-ERCP/manometry acute pancreatitis. Such pancreatitis appears to be more common in patients with a nondilated pancreatic duct.

Pancreatic biopsy with radiologic guidance   Percutaneous aspiration biopsy of a pancreatic mass often distinguishes a pancreatic inflammatory mass from a pancreatic neoplasm.

TESTS OF EXOCRINE PANCREATIC FUNCTION

Pancreatic function tests (see Table 273-1) can be divided into the following:

1 Direct stimulation of the pancreas by intravenous infusion of secretin or secretin plus cholecystokinin (CCK) followed by collection and measurement of duodenal contents

2 Indirect stimulation of the pancreas utilizing nutrients or amino acids, fatty acids, and synthetic peptides followed by assay of proteolytic, lipolytic, and amylolytic enzymes

3 Study of intraluminal digestion products such as undigested meat fibers, stool fat, and fecal nitrogen

4 Measurement of fecal pancreatic enzymes such as chymotrypsin

The secretin test, used to detect diffuse pancreatic disease, is based on the physiologic principle that the pancreatic secretory response is directly related to the functional mass of pancreatic tissue. In the standard assay, secretin is given intravenously in a dose of 1 clinical unit (CU) per kilogram, either as a bolus or continuous infusion. Obviously, results will vary with the secretin preparation used, dose, mode of administration, and completeness of collection of duodenal contents. Normal values for the standard secretin test are (1) volume output >2.0 mL/kg per hour, (2) bicarbonate (HCO_3^-) concentration >80 mmol/L, and (3) HCO_3^- output >10 mmol in 1 h. The most reproducible measurement having the highest level of discrimination between normal subjects and patients with chronic pancreatitis appears to be the maximal bicarbonate concentration.

The *combined secretin-CCK test* permits measurement of pancreatic amylase, lipase, trypsin, and chymotrypsin. Although there is overlap in the distribution of enzyme output in normal subjects and patients with pancreatitis, markedly decreased enzyme outputs suggest advanced damage and destruction of acinar cells. With frank exocrine pancreatic insufficiency there is usually an overall reduction in both HCO_3^- concentration and output of several enzymes. However, with lesser degrees of pancreatic damage there may be a dissociation between HCO_3^- concentration and enzyme output. There also may be a dissociation between the results of the secretin test and other tests of absorptive function. For example, patients with chronic pancreatitis often have abnormally low outputs of HCO_3^- after secretin but have normal fecal fat excretion. Thus the secretin test measures the secretory capacity of ductular epithelium, while fecal fat excretion indirectly reflects intraluminal lipolytic activity. Steatorrhea does not occur until intraluminal levels of lipase are markedly reduced, underscoring the fact that only small amounts of enzymes are necessary for intraluminal digestive activities. An abnormal secretin test should suggest only that chronic pancreatic damage is present; it will not consistently distinguish between chronic pancreatitis and pancreatic carcinoma.

Another test of exocrine pancreatic function, which indirectly reflects intraluminal chymotrypsin activity, has been evaluated in patients with pancreatic disease. This test (the *tripeptide hydrolysis* or *bentiromide test*) utilizes a synthetic peptide, *N*-benzoyl-L-tyrosyl-*p*-aminobenzoic acid (Bz-Ty-PABA), that is specifically cleaved by chymotrypsin to Bz-Ty and PABA. Normally, after oral administration, the peptide reaches the small intestine, where it is hydrolyzed by chymotrypsin with the liberation of PABA, which is rapidly absorbed and excreted in the urine. Results in several hundred patients with chronic pancreatitis and other disorders indicate that PABA excretion is significantly lower in chronic pancreatitis compared with controls. Depending on the severity of pancreatic exocrine impairment, the overall sensitivity is 60 percent (range 46 to 74 percent), and the specificity if coupled with a D-xylose test approximates 90 percent. Measurement of blood PABA levels increases sensitivity.

Measurement of *intraluminal digestion products,* i.e., undigested muscle fibers, stool fat, and fecal nitrogen, is discussed in Chap. 254. Measurement of chymotrypsin in stool reflects pancreatic output of this proteolytic enzyme. Decreased chymotrypsin activity in stool has been reported in patients with chronic pancreatitis and cystic fibrosis. However, normal values may occur in patients with pancreatic insufficiency, and false-positive results have been reported in up to 10 percent of normal individuals.

Tests useful in the diagnosis of exocrine pancreatic insufficiency and the differential diagnosis of malabsorption are also discussed in Chaps. 254 and 274.

274   ACUTE AND CHRONIC PANCREATITIS

NORTON J. GREENBERGER / PHILLIP P. TOSKES / KURT J. ISSELBACHER

BIOCHEMISTRY AND PHYSIOLOGY OF PANCREATIC EXOCRINE SECRETION

GENERAL CONSIDERATIONS   The pancreas secretes 1500 to 3000 mL isosmotic alkaline (pH >8.0) fluid per day containing about 20 enzymes and zymogens. The pancreatic secretions provide the enzymes needed to effect the major digestive activity of the gastrointestinal tract and provide an optimal pH for the function of these enzymes.

REGULATION OF PANCREATIC SECRETION   Hormonal and

neural mechanisms   The exocrine pancreas is under both hormonal and neural control, with hormonal control being of primary importance. *Gastric acid* is the stimulus for the release of secretin, a peptide with 27 amino acids. Sensitive radioimmunoassay studies for secretin suggest that the pH threshold for the release of secretin from the duodenum and jejunum is 4.5. Secretin stimulates the secretion of pancreatic juice rich in *water and electrolytes*. Release of cholecystokinin (CCK) from the duodenum and jejunum is largely produced by long-chain fatty acids, certain essential amino acids (tryptophan, phenylalanine, valine, methionine), and gastric acid itself. CCK evokes an *enzyme-rich secretion from the pancreas*. Gastrin, although it shares an identical terminal tetrapeptide with CCK, is a weak stimulus for pancreatic enzyme output. The *parasympathetic nervous system* (via the vagus) exerts some control over pancreatic secretion. Part of this is mediated by the release of gastrin, and part is secondary to a direct effect of acetylcholine on the pancreatic acinar cell. Also, vagal stimulation effects release of vasoactive intestinal peptide (VIP), a secretin agonist. Vagal control of pancreatic secretion seems to be most important following a truncal vagotomy, but even in such patients severe maldigestion does not ensue. Bile salts also stimulate pancreatic secretion, thereby integrating the functions of the biliary tract, pancreas, and small intestine.

Pancreatic secretion at the cellular level   There appear to be two functionally distinct pathways by which secretagogues can stimulate pancreatic secretion. Studies with isolated pancreatic acinar cells indicate that secretin, VIP, and cholera toxin interact with receptors on the acinar cell, leading to an increase in cellular cyclic adenosine monophosphate (cyclic AMP). CCK, acetylcholine, gastrin, and various other peptides (e.g., bombesin, caerulein) react with other receptors on the acinar cell to cause an increased turnover of phosphatidylinositol and the release of membrane calcium and induce changes in the electrical properties of the pancreatic acinar cell surface and junctional membranes. When a secretagogue that increases cyclic AMP is added to a secretagogue that increases calcium outflux, potentiation of enzyme secretion occurs.

WATER AND ELECTROLYTE SECRETION   Although sodium, potassium, chloride, calcium, zinc, phosphate, and sulfate are found within pancreatic secretion, *bicarbonate is the ion of primary physiologic importance*. In the acini and in the ducts, secretin causes the cells to add water and bicarbonate to the fluid. In the ducts, an exchange occurs between bicarbonate and chloride. There is a good correlation between the maximal bicarbonate output after stimulation with secretin and the pancreatic mass. The bicarbonate output of 120 to 300 mmol/d helps neutralize gastric acid production and creates the appropriate pH for the activity of the pancreatic enzymes.

ENZYME SECRETION   The pancreas secretes amylolytic, lipolytic, and proteolytic enzymes. Amylolytic enzymes such as amylase hydrolyze starch to oligosaccharides and to the disaccharide maltose. The *lipolytic enzymes* include lipase, phospholipase A, and cholesterol esterase. Bile salts *inhibit* lipase, but colipase, another constituent of pancreatic secretion, binds to lipase and prevents this inhibition. Bile salts *activate* phospholipase A and cholesterol esterase. *Proteolytic enzymes* include *endopeptidases* (trypsin, chymotrypsin), which act on the internal peptide bonds of proteins and polypeptides; *exopeptidases* (carboxypeptidases, aminopeptidases), which act on the free carboxyl-terminal end and free amino-terminal end of peptides, respectively; and elastase. The proteolytic enzymes are secreted as inactive precursors (zymogens). Ribonucleases (deoxyribonucleases, ribonuclease) are also secreted. While parallel secretion of pancreatic enzymes usually occurs, nonparallel secretion can occur as a result of exocytosis from heterogeneous sources within the pancreas. *Enterokinase*, an enzyme found within the duodenal mucosa, cleaves the lysine-isoleucine bond of trypsinogen to form trypsin. Trypsin then activates the other proteolytic zymogens in a cascade phenomenon. All pancreatic enzymes have pH optima in the alkaline range.

AUTOPROTECTION OF THE PANCREAS   Autodigestion of the pancreas is prevented by the packaging of proteases in precursor form and by the synthesis of protease inhibitors. These protease inhibitors are found within the acinar cell, the pancreatic secretions, and the alpha$_1$- and alpha$_2$-globulin fractions of plasma.

EXOCRINE-ENDOCRINE RELATIONSHIPS Pancreatic glucagon (29 amino acid residues) has a high degree of structural similarity to secretin. It decreases volume and enzyme secretion by the pancreas but not bicarbonate secretion. Glucose, in large concentrations, also may inhibit pancreatic exocrine secretion. The choleretic and insulinotropic effects of secretin are shared by glucagon.

ENTEROPANCREATIC AXIS AND FEEDBACK INHIBITION Pancreatic enzyme secretion in human beings is controlled, at least in part, by a negative feedback mechanism induced by the presence of active serine proteases in the duodenum. To illustrate, intraduodenal perfusion with phenylalanine causes a prompt increase in plasma CCK levels as well as increased secretion of chymotrypsin. However, simultaneous perfusion with trypsin blunts both responses. Conversely, duodenal perfusion with protease inhibitors actually leads to enzyme hypersecretion. It appears that serine proteases inhibit pancreatic secretion by acting on a CCK-releasing peptide found within the lumen of the small intestine.

ACUTE PANCREATITIS

GENERAL CONSIDERATIONS Pancreatic inflammatory disease may be classified as (1) acute pancreatitis and (2) chronic pancreatitis by primarily clinical criteria, the obvious difference between them being restoration of normal function in the former and permanent residual damage in the latter. The pathologic spectrum of acute pancreatitis varies from *edematous pancreatitis*, which is usually a mild and self-limited disorder, to *necrotizing pancreatitis*, in which the degree of pancreatic necrosis correlates with the severity of the attack and its systemic manifestations. The term *hemorrhagic pancreatitis* is less meaningful in a clinical sense because variable amounts of interstitial hemorrhage can be found in pancreatitis as well as in other disorders such as pancreatic trauma, pancreatic carcinoma, and severe congestive heart failure.

The incidence of pancreatitis varies in different countries and depends on cause, e.g., alcohol, gallstones, metabolic factors, and drugs (Table 274-1). In the United States, for example, acute pancreatitis is related to alcohol ingestion more commonly than to gallstones; in England, the opposite obtains. Epidemiologic data based on autopsy data indicate that in the United States the overall prevalence of acute pancreatitis is approximately 0.5 percent. An upward trend has been noted in the crude death rate.

ETIOLOGY AND PATHOGENESIS There are many causes of acute pancreatitis (see Table 274-1), but the mechanisms by which these conditions trigger pancreatic inflammation have not been identified. Alcoholic patients with pancreatitis may represent a special subset, since most alcoholics do not develop pancreatitis. The list of identifiable causes is growing, and it is likely that pancreatitis related to viral infections, drugs, and as yet undefined factors is more common than heretofore recognized.

Approximately 5 percent of cases of acute pancreatitis are drug related (see Table 274-1). The pancreatitis can be mild or severe; over 85 drugs have been implicated, but many of these reports involve single cases. Drugs cause pancreatitis either by a hypersensitivity reaction or generation of a toxic metabolite, although in some cases this differentiation is not clear. Conventional criteria for establishing that a drug definitely causes pancreatitis are as follows: (1) no other drugs are involved, (2) other causes are excluded, and (3) there is a positive rechallenge. However, in some instances in which a drug has been implicated in several dozen cases, the latter criterion has not been met.

Autodigestion is one pathogenetic theory which proposes that proteolytic enzymes (e.g., trypsinogen, chymotrypsinogen, proelastase, and phospholipase A) are activated within the pancreas rather than in the intestinal lumen. A number of factors (e.g., endotoxins, exotoxins, viral infections, ischemia, anoxia, and direct trauma) are

TABLE 274-1 Causes of acute pancreatitis

Alcohol ingestion (acute and chronic alcoholism)
Biliary tract disease (gallstones)
Postoperative (abdominal, nonabdominal)
Postendoscopic retrograde cholangiopancreatography (ERCP)
Trauma (especially blunt abdominal type)
Metabolic
  A Hypertriglyceridemia
  B Apolipoprotein CII deficiency syndrome
  C Hypercalcemia (e.g., hyperparathyroidism), drug-induced
  D Renal failure
  E After renal transplantation*
  F Acute fatty liver of pregnancy†
Hereditary pancreatitis
Infections
  A Mumps
  B Viral hepatitis
  C Other viral infections (coxsackievirus, echovirus)
  D Ascariasis
  E Mycoplasma
Drug-associated
  A Definite association
    1 Azathioprine, 6-mercaptopurine
    2 Sulfonamides
    3 Thiazide diuretics
    4 Furosemide
    5 Estrogens (oral contraceptives)
    6 Tetracycline
    7 Valproic acid
    8 Pentamidine
    9 Dideoxyinosine (ddI)
  B Probable association
    1 Acetaminophen
    2 Chlorthalidone
    3 Ethacrynic acid
    4 Procainamide
    5 Erythromycin
    6 L-Asparaginase
    7 Metronidazole
    8 Nonsteroidal anti-inflammatory drugs (NSAIDs)
    9 Angiotensin-converting enzyme (ACE) inhibitors
Connective tissue disorders with vasculitis
  A Systemic lupus erythematosus
  B Necrotizing angiitis
  C Thrombotic thrombocytopenic purpura
Penetrating peptic ulcer
Obstruction of the ampulla of Vater
  A Regional enteritis
  B Duodenal diverticulum
Pancreas divisum
Recurrent bouts of acute pancreatitis without obvious cause
  A Consider
    1 Occult disease of the biliary tree or pancreatic ducts, especially occult gallstones (microlithiasis, sludge)
    2 Drugs
    3 Hypertriglyceridemia
    4 Pancreas divisum
    5 Pancreatic cancer
    6 Sphincter of Oddi dysfunction
    7 Cystic fibrosis
    8 Truly idiopathic

* Pancreatitis occurs in 3 percent of renal transplant patients and is due to many factors including surgery, hypercalcemia, drugs (glucocorticoids, azathioprine, L-asparaginase, diuretics), and viral infections.
† Pancreatitis also occurs in otherwise uncomplicated pregnancy and is most often associated with cholelithiasis.

believed to activate these proenzymes. Activated proteolytic enzymes, especially trypsin, not only digest pancreatic and peripancreatic tissues but also can activate other enzymes such as elastase and phospholipase. The active enzymes then digest cellular membranes and cause proteolysis, edema, interstitial hemorrhage, vascular damage, coagulation necrosis, fat necrosis, and parenchymal cell necrosis. Cellular injury and death result in the liberation of activated enzymes. In addition, activation and release of bradykinin peptides and vasoactive substances (e.g., histamine) are believed to produce vasodilatation, increased vascular permeability, and edema. There is thus a cascade of events culminating in the development of acute necrotizing pancreatitis.

The autodigestion theory has largely eclipsed two older theories.

First, the "common channel" theory holds that such an anatomic arrangement facilitates reflux of bile into the pancreatic duct, and this results in activation of pancreatic enzymes. (Actually, a common channel with free communication between the common bile duct and main pancreatic duct is infrequently encountered.) The second theory is that obstruction and hypersecretion are pivotal in the development of pancreatitis. Obstruction of the main pancreatic duct, however, produces pancreatic edema but not pancreatitis.

A recent hypothesis to explain the intrapancreatic activation of zymogens is that they become activated by *lysosomal hydrolases* within the pancreatic acinar cell itself. In two different types of experimental pancreatitis, it has been demonstrated that digestive enzymes and lysosomal hydrolases become admixed; as a result, the former can be activated within the acinar cell by the latter. In vitro, lysosomal enzymes such as cathepsin B can activate trypsinogen, and trypsin can activate the other protease precursors. It is still not clear, however, whether the appropriate pH (i.e., about 3.0) occurs within the human acinar cell to allow activation of trypsinogen by lysosomal hydrolases.

CLINICAL FEATURES *Abdominal pain* is the major symptom of acute pancreatitis. Pain may vary from a mild and tolerable discomfort to severe, constant, and incapacitating distress. Characteristically, the pain, which is steady and boring in character, is located in the epigastrium and periumbilical region and often radiates to the back as well as to the chest, flanks, and lower abdomen. The pain is frequently more intense when the patient is supine, and patients often obtain relief by sitting with the trunk flexed and knees drawn up. Nausea, vomiting, and abdominal distention due to gastric and intestinal hypomotility and chemical peritonitis are also frequent complaints.

Physical examination frequently reveals a distressed and anxious patient. Low-grade fever, tachycardia, and hypotension are fairly common. Shock is not unusual and may result from (1) hypovolemia secondary to exudation of blood and plasma proteins into the retroperitoneal space (i.e., a "retroperitoneal burn"), (2) increased formation and release of kinin peptides which cause vasodilatation and increased vascular permeability, and (3) systemic effects of proteolytic and lipolytic enzymes released into the circulation. Jaundice occurs infrequently; when present, it usually is due to edema of the head of the pancreas with compression of the intrapancreatic portion of the common bile duct. Erythematous skin nodules due to subcutaneous fat necrosis may occur. In 10 to 20 percent of patients there are pulmonary findings, including basilar rales, atelectasis, and pleural effusion, the latter most frequently left-sided. Abdominal tenderness and muscle rigidity are present to a variable degree, but compared with the intense pain, these signs may be unimpressive. Bowel sounds are usually diminished or absent. A pancreatic pseudocyst may be palpable in the upper abdomen. A faint blue discoloration around the umbilicus (Cullen's sign) may occur as the result of hemoperitoneum, and a blue-red-purple or green-brown discoloration of the flanks (Turner's sign) reflects tissue catabolism of hemoglobin. The latter two findings, which are uncommon, indicate the presence of a severe necrotizing pancreatitis.

LABORATORY DATA The diagnosis of acute pancreatitis is usually established by the presence of an increased serum amylase. Values elevated threefold above normal virtually clinch the diagnosis if overt salivary gland disease and gut perforation or infarction are excluded. However, there appears to be no definite correlation between the severity of pancreatitis and the degree of serum amylase elevation. After 48 to 72 h, even with continuing evidence of pancreatitis, total serum amylase values tend to return to normal. However, pancreatic isoamylase and lipase levels may remain elevated for 7 to 14 days. It will be recalled that amylase elevations in serum and urine occur in many conditions other than pancreatitis (see Table 273-2). Importantly, patients with *acidemia* (arterial pH ≤ 7.32) may have spurious elevations in serum amylase. In one study, 12 of 33 acidemic patients had an elevated serum amylase, but only 1 had an elevated lipase value; 9 had salivary-type amylase as the predominant

serum isoamylase. This explains why patients with diabetic ketoacidosis may have marked elevations in serum amylase without any other evidence to support a diagnosis of acute pancreatitis. The urine amylase C_{am}/C_{cr} ratio is usually elevated in patients with severe pancreatitis; this ratio usually is not increased in patients with normal serum amylase. Serum lipase activity increases in parallel with amylase activity, and measurement of both enzymes increases the diagnostic yield. An elevated serum lipase or trypsin value is usually diagnostic of acute pancreatitis; these tests are especially helpful in patients with nonpancreatic causes of hyperamylasemia (see Table 273-4). Markedly increased levels of peritoneal or pleural fluid amylase [>1500 nmol/L (>5000 units per deciliter)] are also helpful, if present, in establishing the diagnosis.

Leukocytosis (15,000 to 20,000 leukocytes per microliter) occurs frequently. More severe cases may show hemoconcentration with hematocrit values exceeding 50 percent because of loss of plasma into the retroperitoneal space and peritoneal cavity. *Hyperglycemia* is common and is due to multiple factors that include decreased insulin release, increased glucagon release, and increased output of adrenal glucocorticoids and catecholamines. *Hypocalcemia* occurs in approximately 25 percent of cases, and its pathogenesis is incompletely understood. While earlier studies suggested that the parathyroid gland response to a decrease in serum calcium is impaired, subsequent observations have failed to confirm this. Intraperitoneal saponification of calcium by fatty acids in areas of fat necrosis occurs occasionally with large amounts (up to 6.0 g) dissolved or suspended in ascitic fluid. Such "soap formation" also may be significant in patients with pancreatitis, mild hypocalcemia, and little or no obvious ascites. *Hyperbilirubinemia* [serum bilirubin >68 μmol/L (>4.0 mg/dL)] occurs in approximately 10 percent of patients. However, jaundice is transient, and serum bilirubin levels return to normal in 4 to 7 days. Serum alkaline phosphatase and aspartate aminotransferase (AST) levels are also transiently elevated and parallel serum bilirubin values. When markedly elevated [i.e., >8.5 μmol/L (>500 units per deciliter)], serum lactic dehydrogenase (LDH) levels suggest a poor prognosis. Serum albumin is decreased to ≤ 30 g/L (≤ 3.0 g/dL) in about 10 percent of cases and is associated with more severe pancreatitis and an increased mortality rate (Table 274-2). *Hypertriglyceridemia* occurs in 15 to 20 percent of cases, and serum amylase levels in such patients are often spuriously normal (see Chap. 273). Most patients with hypertriglyceridemia and pancreatitis, when subsequently examined, show evidence of an underlying derangement in lipid metabolism which probably antedated the pancreatitis, and this is discussed below. Approximately 25 percent of patients have *hypoxemia* (arterial $P_{O_2} \leq 60$ mmHg), which may herald the onset of

---

TABLE 274-2   Factors adversely affecting survival in acute pancreatitis

Ranson/Imrie criteria
A At admission or diagnosis
  1 Age >55 years
  2 Leukocytosis >16,000 per cubic millimeter
  3 Hyperglycemia >11 mmol/L (>200 mg/dL)
  4 Serum LDH >400 IU/L
  5 Serum AST >250 IU/L
B During initial 48 h
  1 Hematocrit fall >10 percent
  2 Fluid sequestration >4000 mL
  3 Hypocalcemia <1.9 mmol/L (<8.0 mg/dL)
  4 Hypoxemia (P_{O_2} <60 mmHg)
  5 BUN rise >1.8 mmol/L (>5 mg/dL) after IV fluids
  6 Hypoalbuminemia <32 g/L (<3.2 g/dL)
Acute physiology and chronic health evaluation (APACHE II) score > 12
Hemorrhagic peritoneal fluid
Key indicators
A Hypotension (BP <90 mmHg) or tachycardia >130 beats per minute
B P_{O_2} <60 mmHg
C Oliguria (<50 mL/h) or increasing BUN, creatinine
D Metabolic [serum calcium <1.9 mmol/L (<8.0 mg/dL) or serum albumin <32 g/L (<3.2 g/dL)]

adult respiratory distress syndrome. Finally, the electrocardiogram is occasionally abnormal in acute pancreatitis with ST-segment and T-wave abnormalities simulating myocardial ischemia.

Radiologic studies useful in the diagnosis of acute pancreatitis are listed in Table 273-1 and discussed in Chap. 273. Although one or more of the abnormalities are found in over 50 percent of patients, the findings are inconstant and nonspecific. The chief value of conventional x-rays [chest; kidney, ureter, and bladder (KUB)] in acute pancreatitis is to help exclude other diagnoses, especially a perforated viscus. Upper gastrointestinal tract x-rays have been superseded by ultrasonography and computed tomographic scanning. A CT scan may confirm the clinical impression of acute pancreatitis even in the face of normal serum amylase levels. Importantly, CT is quite helpful in indicating the severity of acute pancreatitis and its expected morbidity and mortality (see below). Sonography and radionuclide scanning (PIPIDA, HIDA) are useful in acute pancreatitis to evaluate the gallbladder and biliary tree.

DIAGNOSIS Any severe acute pain in the abdomen or back should suggest acute pancreatitis. The diagnosis is usually entertained when a patient with a possible predisposition to pancreatitis presents with severe and constant abdominal pain, nausea, emesis, fever, tachycardia, and abnormal findings on abdominal examination. Laboratory studies frequently reveal leukocytosis, abnormal x-rays of the abdomen and chest, hypocalcemia, and hyperglycemia. The diagnosis is usually confirmed by finding an elevated serum amylase and/or lipase. Obviously, not all the above features have to be present for the diagnosis to be established.

The *differential diagnosis* should include consideration of the following disorders: (1) perforated viscus, especially peptic ulcer, (2) acute cholecystitis and biliary colic, (3) acute intestinal obstruction, (4) mesenteric vascular occlusion, (5) renal colic, (6) myocardial infarction, (7) dissecting aortic aneurysm, (8) connective tissue disorders with vasculitis, (9) pneumonia, and (10) diabetic ketoacidosis. A penetrating duodenal ulcer usually can be identified by upper gastrointestinal x-rays and/or endoscopy. A perforated duodenal ulcer is readily diagnosed by the presence of free intraperitoneal air. It may be difficult to differentiate acute cholecystitis from acute pancreatitis, since an elevated serum amylase may be found in both disorders. Pain of biliary tract origin is more right-sided and gradual in onset, and ileus is usually absent; sonography and radionuclide scanning are helpful in establishing the diagnosis of cholelithiasis and cholecystitis. Intestinal obstruction due to mechanical factors can be differentiated from pancreatitis by the history of colicky pain, findings on abdominal examination, and x-rays of the abdomen showing characteristic changes of mechanical obstruction. Acute mesenteric vascular occlusion is usually evident in elderly debilitated patients with brisk leukocytosis, abdominal distention, and bloody diarrhea, in whom paracentesis shows sanguineous fluid and arteriography shows vascular occlusion. Serum as well as peritoneal fluid amylase levels are increased, however, in patients with intestinal infarction. Systemic lupus erythematosus and polyarteritis nodosa may be confused with pancreatitis, especially since pancreatitis may develop as a complication of these diseases. Diabetic ketoacidosis is often accompanied by abdominal pain and elevated total serum amylase levels, thus closely mimicking acute pancreatitis. However, the serum lipase and pancreatic isoamylase are not elevated in diabetic ketoacidosis.

COURSE OF THE DISEASE AND COMPLICATIONS It is important to identify those patients with acute pancreatitis who have an increased risk of dying. Ranson and Imrie have utilized multiple prognostic criteria and have demonstrated that there is an increased mortality rate with three or more risk factors identifiable either at the time of admission to the hospital or during the initial 48 h of hospitalization (see Table 274-2). The acute physiology and chronic health evaluation scoring system (APACHE II) utilizes the worst values of 12 physiologic measurements, age, and previous health status and provides a good description of illness severity for a wide range of common diseases; this score also correlates with outcome. Prospective studies have compared APACHE II with multiple prognostic criteria, i.e., Ranson and Imrie scores, in predicting the severity of acute pancreatitis. On admission, APACHE II identified approximately two-thirds of severe attacks, and after 48 h, the prognostic accuracy of APACHE II is comparable with Ranson and Imrie's scoring system. The drawbacks of APACHE II are (1) complexity, (2) requirement of a computer for scoring, and (3) standardization regarding peak values and cutoff scores. McMahon and colleagues have shown that the presence of a "toxic broth" or dark (hemorrhagic) fluid in abdominal pancreatitis is also an important prognostic indicator in acute pancreatitis. These multiple-factor scoring systems are difficult to use and have not been embraced consistently by clinicians. There is a great need for a reliable simple biochemical test consistently capable of predicting outcome in patients with acute pancreatitis. Two candidate markers which show great promise are serum granulocyte elastase and urinary trypsinogen activation peptide (TAP). The key indicators of a severe attack of acute pancreatitis are also listed in Table 274-2. Importantly, the presence of any one of these factors is associated with an increased risk of complications and any two criteria with a 20 to 30 percent mortality rate. The high mortality rate of such severely ill patients is due in large part to infection and warrants intensive radiologic intervention and monitoring and/or a combination of radiologic and surgical means as discussed in detail below.

The local and systemic complications of acute pancreatitis are listed in Table 274-3. Patients frequently develop an inflammatory mass in the first 2 to 3 weeks after pancreatitis. These may be phlegmons, abscesses, or pseudocysts (see below). Systemic complications include pulmonary, cardiovascular, hematologic, renal, metabolic, and central nervous system abnormalities. Pancreatitis, hypertriglyceridemia, and alcoholism constitute a triad in which cause and effect remain incompletely understood. However, several reasonable conclusions can be drawn. First, hypertriglyceridemia can precede and apparently cause the development of pancreatitis. Second, the vast majority (>80 percent) of patients with acute pancreatitis do not have hypertriglyceridemia. Third, almost all patients with pancreatitis and hypertriglyceridemia are *either* alcoholics who have been drinking shortly before the onset of pancreatitis *or* patients with preexisting hypertriglyceridemia. Fourth, many of the patients with this triad have persistent hypertriglyceridemia after recovery from pancreatitis and abstention from alcohol and are prone to recurrent episodes of pancreatitis. Fifth, any factor (e.g., drugs, alcohol) that causes an abrupt increase in serum triglycerides to levels greater than 11 mmol/L (1000 mg/dL) can precipitate a bout of pancreatitis that can be associated with significant complications and even become fulminant. Finally, patients with a deficiency of apolipoprotein CII have an increased incidence of pancreatitis; apolipoprotein CII activates lipoprotein lipase, which is important in clearing chylomicrons from the bloodstream.

Purtscher's retinopathy, a relatively unusual complication, refers to the sudden and severe loss of vision in patients with acute pancreatitis. It is characterized by a peculiar funduscopic appearance with cotton-wool spots and hemorrhages confined to an area limited by the optic disk and macula; it is believed to be due to posterior retinal artery occlusion with aggregated granulocytes.

The two most common causes of acute pancreatitis are alcoholism and biliary tract disease; other causes are listed in Table 274-1. However, after a conventional workup, a specific cause will not be identified actually in 10 to 20 percent of patients. It is important to note that ultrasound examinations will not detect gallstones, especially microlithiasis and/or sludge, in 4 to 7 percent of patients. In one series of 31 patients initially diagnosed as having idiopathic acute pancreatitis, 23 were found to have occult gallstone disease. Thus approximately two-thirds of patients with recurrent acute pancreatitis without an obvious cause actually have occult gallstone disease. Other diseases of the biliary tree and pancreatic ducts that can cause acute pancreatitis include choledochocele, ampullary tumors, pancreas divisum, and pancreatic duct stones, stricture, and tumor. Approximately 2 percent of patients with pancreatic carcinoma present with acute pancreatitis.

TABLE 274-3 Complications of acute pancreatitis

LOCAL

A Pancreatic phlegmon
B Pancreatic abscess
C Pancreatic pseudocyst
  1 Pain
  2 Rupture
  3 Hemorrhage
  4 Infection
  5 Obstruction of gastrointestinal tract (stomach, duodenum, colon)
D Pancreatic ascites
  1 Disruption of main pancreatic duct
  2 Leaking pseudocyst
E Involvement of contiguous organs by necrotizing pancreatitis
  1 Massive intraperitoneal hemorrhage
  2 Thrombosis of blood vessels
  3 Bowel infarction
F Obstructive jaundice

SYSTEMIC

A Pulmonary
  1 Pleural effusion
  2 Atelectasis
  3 Mediastinal abscess
  4 Pneumonitis
  5 Adult respiratory distress syndrome
B Cardiovascular
  1 Hypotension
    a Hypovolemia
    b Hypoalbuminemia
  2 Sudden death
  3 Nonspecific ST-T changes in electrocardiogram simulating myocardial infarction
  4 Pericardial effusion
C Hematologic
  1 Disseminated intravascular coagulation (DIC)
D Gastrointestinal hemorrhage*
  1 Peptic ulcer disease
  2 Erosive gastritis
  3 Hemorrhagic pancreatic necrosis with erosion into major blood vessels
  4 Portal vein thrombosis, variceal hemorrhage
E Renal
  1 Oliguria
  2 Azotemia
  3 Renal artery and/or renal vein thrombosis
F Metabolic
  1 Hyperglycemia
  2 Hypertriglyceridemia
  3 Hypocalcemia
  4 Encephalopathy
  5 Sudden blindness (Purtscher's retinopathy)
G Central nervous system
  1 Psychosis
  2 Fat emboli
H Fat necrosis
  1 Subcutaneous tissues (erythematous nodules)
  2 Bone
  3 Miscellaneous (mediastinum, pleura, nervous system)

* Aggravated by coagulation abnormalities (DIC).

TREATMENT In most patients (approximately 85 to 90 percent) with acute pancreatitis, the disease is self-limited and subsides spontaneously, usually within 3 to 7 days after treatment is instituted. Medical therapy is aimed at reducing pancreatic secretion and, in essence, "putting the pancreas at rest." Conventional measures include (1) analgesics for pain, (2) intravenous fluids and colloids to maintain normal intravascular volume, (3) no oral alimentation, and (4) nasogastric suction to decrease gastrin release from the stomach and prevent gastric contents from entering the duodenum. Recent controlled trials, however, have shown that nasogastric suction offers no clear-cut advantages in the treatment of mild to moderately severe acute pancreatitis. Its use, therefore, must be considered elective rather than mandatory.

It has been demonstrated that CCK-stimulated pancreatic secretion is almost abolished in four different experimental models of acute pancreatitis. This probably explains why drugs to block pancreatic secretion in acute pancreatitis have failed to have any therapeutic benefit. For this and other reasons, anticholinergic drugs are not indicated in acute pancreatitis. Although antibiotics have been used in the treatment of acute pancreatitis, three recent randomized, prospective trials have shown no benefit from the use of antibiotics in acute pancreatitis of mild to moderate severity. However, because secondary infection of necrotic pancreatic tissue (phlegmon, abscess, pseudocyst) or obstructed biliary passages (ascending cholangitis, complicating choledocholithiasis) contributes to much of the late mortality, appropriate *antibiotic therapy of established infection* is obviously quite important. Several other drugs have been evaluated by prospective, controlled trials and found *ineffective* in the treatment of acute pancreatitis. The list, by no means complete, includes glucagon, H-2 blockers, protease inhibitors such as aprotinin, glucocorticoids, calcitonin, somatostatin analogues such as octreotide, and nonsteroidal anti-inflammatory drugs (NSAIDs).

A CT scan, especially a contrast-enhanced dynamic CT (CECT) scan, provides valuable information on the severity and prognosis of acute pancreatitis (Fig. 274-1 and Table 274-4). In particular, the CECT allows estimation of the presence and extent of pancreatic necrosis. Recent studies suggest that the likelihood of prolonged pancreatitis or a serious complication is negligible when the CT severity index is 1 or 2 and unlikely with scores of 3 to 6. However, patients with CT severity index scores of 7 to 10 had a 92 percent morbidity and 17 percent mortality. A CECT is indicated in patients with three or more of Ranson's signs, in all seriously ill patients, and in patients who show evidence of clinical deterioration. The patient with mild to moderate pancreatitis usually requires treatment with intravenous fluids, fasting, and possibly nasogastric suction for 2 to 4 days. A clear liquid diet is frequently started on the third to sixth day and a regular diet by the fifth to seventh day. The patient with unremitting *fulminant pancreatitis* usually requires inordinate amounts of fluid and close attention to complications such as cardiovascular collapse, respiratory insufficiency, and pancreatic infection. The latter should be managed by a combination of radiologic and surgical means (see below). While earlier uncontrolled studies suggested that *peritoneal lavage* via a percutaneous dialysis catheter is helpful in severe pancreatitis, recent studies indicate that such treatment does not influence the outcome of such attacks. Laparotomy with adequate drainage and removal of necrotic tissue should be considered if conventional therapy does not halt the patient's deterioration. The use of parenteral nutrition makes it possible to give nutritional support to patients with severe, acute, or protracted pancreatitis who are unable to eat normally. Patients with severe gallstone-induced pancreatitis may improve dramatically if papillotomy is carried out within the first 36 to 72 h of the attack. Recent studies indicate that only those patients with gallstone pancreatitis who are in the very severe group should be considered for urgent endoscopic retrograde cholangiopancreatography (ERCP). Finally, the treatment for patients with hypertriglyceridemia-associated pancreatitis include (1) weight loss to ideal weight, (2) lipid-restricted diet, (3) exercise, (4) avoidance of alcohol and drugs that can elevate serum triglycerides (i.e., estrogens, vitamin A, thiazides, and beta-blockers), and (5) control of diabetes.

PANCREATIC PHLEGMON, ABSCESS, AND PSEUDOCYST
The *phlegmon* is a solid mass of swollen, inflamed pancreas often containing patchy areas of necrosis; it may be present for 1 to 2 weeks. This prolonged inflammatory process should not be confused with a pseudocyst, a differentiation which is usually accomplished by sonography. A phlegmon should be suspected if abdominal pain, fever, leukocytosis, and hyperamylasemia persist for more than 5 days and especially if an abdominal mass is also present. Differentiation from an abscess may be difficult even with a CT scan. Occasionally, extensive areas of pancreatic necrosis develop in phlegmons and require incision and drainage, especially if infected. Phlegmons also may be secondarily infected, resulting in abscess formation. The latter occurs in 10 percent of patients with acute pancreatitis. The early diagnosis of pancreatic infection can be

A

B

FIGURE 274-1 Acute pancreatitis: CT evolution. *A*. Contrast-enhanced CT scan of the abdomen performed on admission of a patient with clinical evidence of acute pancreatitis. Note the mildly decreased density of the body of the pancreas to the left of the midline (*arrow*). There are a few linear strands in the peripancreatic fat, suggesting inflammation (*open arrows*). A small amount of fluid is seen in the anterior pararenal space (*arrowhead*). *B*. Nine days after

admission, there is a marked worsening with severe inflammation of the pancreas evidenced by anterior displacement of the posterior gastric wall (*arrows*), increased inflammation of the peripancreatic fat, and increased pancreatic effusion in the anterior perirenal space and around the splenic vein (*open arrows*). (*Courtesy of Dr. P.R. Ros, University of Florida College of Medicine.*)

accomplished by CT-guided needle aspiration. In one study, 60 patients, representing 5 percent of all admissions for acute pancreatitis, were suspected of harboring a pancreatic infection on the basis of fever, leukocytosis, and an abnormal CT scan (phlegmon, pseudocyst, or extrapancreatic fluid collection). Importantly, 36 of 60 patients (60 percent) had a pancreatic infection, with 20 of the 36 (55 percent) developing infection within the first 2 weeks. This study suggests that only guided aspiration can reliably distinguish sterile from infected pancreatic necrosis. The following are guidelines for patients meeting the above selection criteria: (1) pseudocysts and phlegmons should be aspirated promptly because more than half could be infected; (2) extrapancreatic fluid collections need not be aspirated promptly because most are sterile; (3) if a phlegmon is found initially to be sterile but fever and leukocytosis persist, allow several days of observation before considering reaspiration, since clinical improvement frequently occurs; and (4) if fever and leukocytosis recur after an interval of well-being, consider reaspiration.

Severe pancreatitis with the presence of three or more risk factors, postoperative pancreatitis, early oral feeding, early laparotomy, and perhaps injudicious use of antibiotics predispose to the development

of pancreatic abscess, which occurs in 3 to 4 percent of patients with acute pancreatitis. Pancreatic abscess also may develop because of communication of a pseudocyst with the colon, after inadequate surgical drainage of a pseudocyst, or after needling of a pseudocyst. The characteristic signs of abscess are fever, leukocytosis, ileus, and rapid deterioration in a patient initially recovering from pancreatitis. However, the only manifestations may be persistent fever and signs of continuing pancreatic inflammation. Drainage of pancreatic abscesses by nonsurgical percutaneous catheter techniques, using CT guidance, has been only moderately successful (resolution in 50 to 60 percent of patients). Accordingly, laparotomy with radical sump drainage and possibly resection of necrotic tissue is usually required because the mortality rate for undrained pancreatic abscess approaches 100 percent. Multiple abscesses are common and reoperation is frequently required.

Pseudocysts of the pancreas are collections of tissue, fluid, debris, pancreatic enzymes, and blood which develop over a period of 1 to 4 weeks after the onset of acute pancreatitis in approximately 15 percent of patients. In contrast to true cysts, pseudocysts do not have epithelial lining, and the walls consist of necrotic tissue, granulation tissue, and fibrous tissue. Disruption of the pancreatic ductal system is common. However, the subsequent course of this disruption varies widely, namely, from spontaneous healing to continuous leakage of pancreatic juice, causing tense ascites. Pseudocysts are preceded by pancreatitis in 90 percent of cases and by trauma in 10 percent. Approximately 85 percent are located in the body or tail of the pancreas and 15 percent in the head. Some patients have two or more pseudocysts. Abdominal pain, with or without radiation to the back, is the usual presenting complaint. A palpable, tender mass may be found in the middle or left upper abdomen. The serum amylase level is elevated in 75 percent of patients some time during their illness and may fluctuate markedly.

Pseudocysts often displace some portion of the gastrointestinal tract on x-ray examination in 75 percent of cases (Fig. 274-2). Sonography, however, is reliable in detecting pseudocysts. Sonography also permits differentiation between an edematous and an inflamed pancreas (pancreatic phlegmon), which can give rise to a palpable mass and an actual pseudocyst. Furthermore, serial ultrasound studies

TABLE 274-4 Severity index in acute pancreatitis

	Points
GRADE OF ACUTE PANCREATITIS	
A Normal pancreas	0
B Pancreatic enlargement alone	1
C Inflammation compared with pancreas and peripancreatic fat	2
D One peripancreatic fluid collection	3
E Two or more fluid collections	4
DEGREE OF PANCREATIC NECROSIS	
A No necrosis	0
B Necrosis of one-third of pancreas	2
C Necrosis of one-half of pancreas	4
D Necrosis of more than one-half of pancreas	6

A

B

C

FIGURE 274-2 Pseudocyst of pancreas. *A.* Upper gastrointestinal x-ray showing displacement of stomach by pseudocyst. *B.* Sonogram showing pseudocyst (*cyst*). GB = gallbladder; MVP = portal vein. Behind the large pseudocyst is seen the calcified head of the pancreas. A dilated common bile duct (*asterisk*) is noted. (*Courtesy of Dr. C. E. Forsmark, University of Florida College of Medicine.*) *C.* CT scan showing pseudocyst. Note the large lobulated fluid collection (*arrows*) surrounding the tail of the pancreas (*arrowheads*). Note the dense, thin rim in the periphery representing the fibrous capsule of the pseudocyst. (*Courtesy of Dr. P. R. Ros, University of Florida College of Medicine.*)

will indicate whether a pseudocyst has resolved. CT scanning complements the use of ultrasound in the diagnosis of pancreatic pseudocyst (see Fig. 274-2), especially when it is infected.

In studies utilizing sonography, pseudocysts resolved in 25 to 40 percent of patients. However, pseudocysts that are greater than 5 cm and that persist for longer than 6 weeks rarely disappear. In others, serious complications may occur such as (1) pain caused by expansion of the lesion and pressure on other viscera, (2) rupture, (3) hemorrhage, and (4) abscess. Rupture of a pancreatic pseudocyst is a particularly serious complication. Shock almost always supervenes, and mortality rates range from 14 percent if the rupture is not associated with hemorrhage to over 60 percent if hemorrhage has occurred. Rupture and hemorrhage are the prime causes of mortality in pancreatic

pseudocyst. A triad of findings, i.e., increase in size of the mass, localized bruit over the mass, and a sudden decrease in hemoglobin and hematocrit levels without obvious signs of external blood loss, should alert one to the diagnosis of hemorrhage from a pseudocyst. Thus, in pseudocyst patients who are stable and uncomplicated and in whom serial ultrasound studies show a decreasing pseudocyst, conservative therapy is indicated. Conversely, patients with a pseudocyst which is expanding and which is complicated by rupture, hemorrhage, and abscess should be operated on. Using ultrasound or CT guidance, sterile chronic pseudocysts can be treated safely with single or repeated needle aspiration or more prolonged catheter drainage with an expected success rate of 45 to 75 percent. The success rate with infected pseudocysts is considerably less, i.e., 40 to 50 percent. Patients not responding to drainage require surgical therapy. Therapy consists of internal or external drainage of the cyst. Prolonged observation of a nonresolving pancreatic pseudocyst exposes the patient to increased risks which exceed those of elective surgery.

Pseudoaneurysms develop in up to 10 percent of patients with acute pancreatitis at sites reflecting the distribution of pseudocysts and fluid collections. The splenic artery is most frequently involved, followed by the inferior and superior pancreatic duodenal arteries. The diagnosis should be suspected in patients with pancreatitis who develop either upper gastrointestinal bleeding without an obvious cause or in whom a contrast-enhanced lesion is demonstrated within or adjacent to a suspected pseudocyst as determined by thin-cut CT examination. Arteriography is necessary to confirm the diagnosis.

PANCREATIC ASCITES AND PANCREATIC PLEURAL EFFU-SIONS Pancreatic ascites is usually due to disruption of the main pancreatic duct, often associated with an internal fistula between the duct and the peritoneal cavity or a leaking pseudocyst (see also Chap. 43). The diagnosis of pancreatic ascites is suggested in a patient with an elevated serum amylase level who also has increased levels of albumin [>30 g/L (>3.0 g/dL)] and amylase in the ascitic fluid. In addition, ERCP will often demonstrate passage of contrast material from a major pancreatic duct or a pseudocyst into the peritoneal cavity. As many as 15 percent of patients with pseudocysts have concurrent pancreatic ascites. The differential diagnosis should include intraperitoneal carcinomatosis, tuberculous peritonitis, constrictive pericarditis, and Budd-Chiari syndrome.

If the pancreatic duct disruption is posterior, an internal fistula may develop between the pancreatic duct and pleural space producing a pleural effusion, which is usually left-sided and often massive. This often requires thoracentesis or chest tube drainage.

Treatment usually involves placing the patient on nasogastric suction and parenteral alimentation to decrease pancreatic secretion. In addition, paracentesis is performed to keep the peritoneal cavity free of fluid and, it is hoped, effect sealing of the leak. The long-acting somatostatin analogue (octreotide) which inhibits pancreatic secretion is also useful in pancreatic ascites and pleural effusion. If ascites continues to recur after 2 to 3 weeks of medical management, the patient should be operated on following pancreatography to define the anatomy of the abnormal duct. Two or more sites of extravasation on ERCP identify patients unlikely to respond to conservative management.

CHRONIC PANCREATITIS AND PANCREATIC EXOCRINE INSUFFICIENCY

GENERAL AND ETIOLOGIC CONSIDERATIONS Chronic inflammatory disease of the pancreas may present as episodes of acute inflammation superimposed on a previously injured pancreas or as chronic damage with persistent pain or malabsorption. The causes of relapsing chronic pancreatitis are similar to those of acute pancreatitis (see Table 274-1), except that frequently there is an appreciable incidence of cases of undetermined origin. In addition, the pancreatitis associated with gallstones is predominantly acute or relapsing acute in nature. A cholecystectomy is almost always performed in patients after the first or second attack of gallstone-associated pancreatitis. Patients with chronic pancreatitis may present with persistent abdominal pain, with or without steatorrhea, and some may present with steatorrhea and no pain.

Patients with chronic pancreatitis who develop extensive destruction of the pancreas (i.e., less than 10 percent of exocrine function remaining) will demonstrate steatorrhea and azotorrhea. In the adult in the United States, alcoholism is the most common cause of clinically apparent pancreatic exocrine insufficiency, while cystic fibrosis is the most frequent cause in children. In up to 25 percent of adults in the United States with chronic pancreatitis, the cause is not known; i.e., they have idiopathic chronic pancreatitis. In other parts of the world, severe protein-calorie malnutrition is a common cause. Table 274-5 lists other causes of pancreatic exocrine insufficiency, but they are relatively uncommon.

PATHOPHYSIOLOGY Unfortunately, the events that initiate an inflammatory process within the pancreas are still not well understood, and the many hypotheses will not be reviewed. In the case of alcohol-induced pancreatitis, however, it has been suggested that the primary defect may be the precipitation of protein (inspissated enzymes) within the ducts. The resulting ductal obstruction can lead to duct dilatation, diffuse atrophy of the acinar cells, fibrosis, and eventual calcification of some of the protein plugs. However, that some alcoholic patients with recurrent acute pancreatitis show no evidence of chronic pancreatitis does not support the intraductal protein precipitation hypothesis. In fact, experimental and clinical observations have shown the direct toxic effects of alcohol on the pancreas. While patients with alcohol-induced pancreatitis generally consume large amounts of alcohol, some consume very little (i.e., 50 g/d or less). Thus prolonged consumption of ''socially acceptable'' amounts of alcohol is compatible with the development of pancreatitis. In addition, the finding of extensive pancreatic fibrosis in patients who have expired during their first attack of clinical acute alcohol-induced pancreatitis supports the concept that such patients already have chronic pancreatitis.

CLINICAL FEATURES Patients with relapsing chronic pancreatitis may present with symptoms identical to those found in acute pancreatitis, but their pain may be continuous or intermittent, or pain may be absent. The pathogenesis of this pain is poorly understood. Although the classic description is that of epigastric pain radiating through the back, the pain pattern is often atypical. The pain may be maximal in the right or left upper quadrants in the back or diffuse throughout the upper abdomen; it may even be referred to the anterior chest or flank. Characteristically, the pain is persistent, deep-seated, and unresponsive to antacids. It often is increased by alcohol and ingestion of heavy meals (especially foods rich in fat). Often the pain is so severe as to require the frequent use of narcotics.

Weight loss, abnormal stools, and other signs or symptoms suggestive of malabsorption (see Table 254-5) are common in chronic pancreatitis. However, clinically apparent deficiencies of fat-soluble vitamins are surprisingly rare. The physical findings in these patients are usually not impressive, such that there is a disparity between the severity of the abdominal pain and the paucity of physical signs (save some abdominal tenderness and mild temperature elevation).

DIAGNOSTIC EVALUATION (See Chap. 273) In contrast to patients with relapsing acute pancreatitis, the serum amylase and lipase levels are usually not elevated. Elevations of the serum bilirubin and alkaline phosphatase may indicate cholestasis secondary to chronic inflammation around the common bile duct (Fig. 274-3). Many

---

TABLE 274-5 Causes of pancreatic exocrine insufficiency

Alcohol, chronic alcoholism
Cystic fibrosis
Severe protein-calorie malnutrition with hypoalbuminemia
Pancreatic and duodenal neoplasms
Pancreatic resection
Gastric surgery
  A Subtotal gastrectomy with Billroth I anastomosis
  B Subtotal gastrectomy with Billroth II anastomosis
  C Truncal vagotomy and pyloroplasty
Gastrinoma (Zollinger-Ellison syndrome)
Hereditary pancreatitis
Traumatic pancreatitis
Hemochromatosis
Shwachman's syndrome (pancreatic insufficiency and bone marrow dysfunction)
Trypsinogen deficiency
Enterokinase deficiency
Isolated deficiencies of amylase, lipase, or proteases
α_1-Antitrypsin deficiency
Idiopathic pancreatitis

A   B

C   D

FIGURE 274-3 Radiologic abnormalities in chronic pancreatitis. *A*. Pancreatic calcification (*arrows*) and stenosis (*tapering*) of the intrahepatic portion of the common bile duct demonstrated by percutaneous transhepatic cholangiography. *B*. Pancreatic calcification (*large white arrow*) demonstrated by sonography. Note dilated pancreatic duct (*thin white arrow*) and splenic vein (*clear arrow*). *C*. Pancreatic calcification (*vertical arrows*) and dilated pancreatic duct (*horizontal arrow*) demonstrated by CT scan. *D*. Endoscopic retrograde cholangiogram shows grossly dilated pancreatic ducts (*arrows*) in a patient with long-standing pancreatitis.

patients demonstrate impaired glucose tolerance, and some may have an elevated fasting blood glucose level.

The classic triad of pancreatic calcification, steatorrhea, and diabetes mellitus usually establishes the diagnosis of chronic pancreatitis and exocrine pancreatic insufficiency but is found in less than one-third of chronic pancreatitis patients. Accordingly, it is often necessary to perform an intubation test such as the *secretin stimulation test*, which usually becomes abnormal when 60 percent or more of pancreatic exocrine function has been lost. Approximately 40 percent of patients with chronic pancreatitis have *cobalamin (vitamin B$_{12}$) malabsorption* which is corrected by the administration of oral pancreatic enzymes. There is usually a marked excretion of fecal fat (see Chap. 254), which can be reduced with the administration of oral pancreatic enzymes. The bentiromide test (Chap. 273) and D-xylose urinary excretion test are useful in patients with "pancreatic steatorrhea," since the bentiromide test will be abnormal and the D-xylose excretion usually normal. A decreased serum trypsinogen level strongly suggests pancreatic exocrine insufficiency.

The radiographic hallmark of chronic pancreatitis is the presence of scattered calcification throughout the pancreas (see Fig. 274-3). Diffuse pancreatic calcification indicates that significant damage has occurred and obviates the need for a secretin test. Alcohol is by far the most common cause of pancreatic calcification, but it also may be seen in severe protein-calorie malnutrition, hereditary pancreatitis, posttraumatic pancreatitis, hyperparathyroidism, islet cell tumors, and idiopathic chronic pancreatitis. An ongoing prospective study of 107 patients has shown convincingly that pancreatic calcification may decrease or even disappear either following ductal decompression or spontaneously in one-third of patients with severe chronic pancreatitis. Pancreatic calcification is a dynamic process that is incompletely understood.

Special techniques such as sonography, CT scanning, and ERCP have added new dimensions to the diagnosis of pancreatic disease. In addition to excluding pseudocysts and pancreatic cancer, sonography may show calcification or dilated ducts associated with chronic pancreatitis (Fig. 274-4). Similar benefits can be derived from CT

A

FIGURE 274-4 Chronic pancreatitis and pancreatic calculi: CT scan and ERCP appearance. *A.* In this contrast-enhanced CT scan of the abdomen, there is evidence of an atrophic pancreas with multiple calcifications (*arrows*). Note a markedly dilated pancreatic duct seen in this section through the body and tail (*open arrows*). *B.* ERCP in the same patient demonstrates the dilated pancreatic duct as well as an intrapancreatic duct calculus (*arrows*). These findings correlate nicely with the CT scan appearance.

B

scans. ERCP is the only nonoperative technique which provides a direct view of the pancreatic duct. In patients with alcohol-induced pancreatitis, ERCP may reveal a pseudocyst missed by sonography or CT scan.

COMPLICATIONS OF CHRONIC PANCREATITIS The complications of chronic pancreatitis are protean. *Cobalamin (vitamin B_{12}) malabsorption* occurs in 40 percent of patients with alcohol-induced chronic pancreatitis and in virtually all with cystic fibrosis. The cobalamin malabsorption is consistently corrected by the administration of pancreatic enzymes (containing proteases). The cobalamin malabsorption may be due to excessive binding of cobalamin by nonintrinsic factor cobalamin-binding proteins. The latter are ordinarily destroyed by pancreatic proteases, but with pancreatic insufficiency the nonspecific binding proteins escape degradation and compete with intrinsic factor for cobalamin binding. Although the majority of patients show *impaired glucose tolerance*, the development of diabetic ketoacidosis and coma is uncommon. Similarly, end organ damage (retinopathy, neuropathy, nephropathy) is also uncommon, and the appearance of these complications should raise the question of concomitant genetic diabetes mellitus. A nondiabetic retinopathy, peripheral in location and secondary to vitamin A and/or zinc

deficiency, is common in these patients. High-amylase-containing *effusions* occur within the pleura, pericardium, or peritoneum. *Gastrointestinal bleeding* may occur from a peptic ulcer, gastritis, a pseudocyst eroding into the duodenum, or ruptured varices secondary to splenic vein thrombosis due to inflammation of the tail of the pancreas. *Icterus* may occur, owing to either edema of the head of the pancreas compressing the common bile duct or chronic cholestasis secondary to chronic inflammatory reaction around the intrapancreatic portion of the common bile duct (see Fig. 274-3). This chronic obstruction may lead to cholangitis and ultimately biliary cirrhosis. *Subcutaneous fat necrosis* may appear as tender red nodules on the lower extremities. *Bone pain* may be secondary to intramedullary fat necrosis. Inflammation of the large and small joints of the upper and lower extremities may occur. The incidence of pancreatic carcinoma is probably increased in patients with diffuse calcification. Perhaps the most common and troublesome complication is addiction to narcotics.

TREATMENT AND APPROACH TO MANAGEMENT Therapy for patients with chronic pancreatitis is directed toward two major problems, namely, pain and malabsorption. Patients with intermittent attacks of pain are essentially treated like those with acute pancreatitis (see above). Patients with severe and persistent pain should avoid alcohol completely and avoid large meals rich in fat. Since the pain is often severe enough to require frequent use of narcotics (and hence addiction), a number of surgical procedures have been developed for pain relief. ERCP allows the surgeon to plan the operative approach. If there is a stricture of the pancreatic duct, then a *local resection* may ameliorate the pain. Unfortunately, isolated localized strictures are not common. In most patients with alcohol-induced disease, the pancreas is diffusely involved, and surgically correctible localized ductal disease is rare. When there is primary ductal obstruction and dilatation, ductal decompression may provide effective pain palliation. Short-term pain relief may be achieved in up to 80 percent of patients, while long-term pain relief occurs in approximately 50 percent. In some of these patients, however, pain relief can be achieved only by resecting 50 to 95 percent of the gland. Although pain relief is achieved in three-quarters of these patients, they tend to develop pancreatic endocrine and exocrine insufficiency and must be on pancreatic enzyme replacement therapy. It is important to screen patients carefully, for such radical surgery is contraindicated in those who are severely depressed or suicidal or continue to drink. Procedures such as sphincteroplasty, splanchnicectomy and celiac ganglionectomy, and nerve blocks usually bring only temporary relief and are not recommended. Although there is current enthusiasm for treating the pain of chronic pancreatitis by endoscopic placement of stents into the pancreatic duct, adequate control studies have not been carried out. In addition, significant complications, i.e., acute pancreatitis, pancreatic abscess, damage to the pancreatic duct, and death, have occurred in up to 36 percent of patients following stent placement.

Three double-blind trials have demonstrated that pancreatic enzymes decrease the abdominal pain in selected patients with chronic pancreatitis. In these trials, pain relief was obtained in approximately 75 percent of the patients evaluated. The patients most likely to respond to such therapy with amelioration of pain are those with mild to moderate exocrine pancreatic dysfunction, as evidenced by an abnormal secretin test, normal fat absorption, and minimal abnormalities on ERCP examination. These clinical observations seem to fit in with data in human beings and experimental animals which demonstrate a negative feedback regulation for pancreatic exocrine secretion controlled by the amount of proteases within the lumen of the proximal small intestine. It seems reasonable to approach the patient with severe persistent or continuous abdominal pain thought to be secondary to chronic pancreatitis in the following manner: After other causes of abdominal pain (peptic ulcer, gallstones, etc.) have been appropriately excluded, a pancreatic *sonogram* should be done. If no mass is found, a *secretin test* may be performed, since with chronic pancreatitis and pain this test usually will be abnormal. If the secretin test is abnormal (i.e., decreased bicarbonate concentration or volume output), a 3- to 4-week *trial of pancreatic enzymes* is appropriate. Eight conventional tablets or three enteric-coated capsules are taken at meals and at bedtime. If no relief is obtained, and especially if the volume secreted during the secretin test is very low, ERCP should be performed. If a pseudocyst or a localized ductal obstruction is found, surgery should be considered. A provocative study from South Africa questions the significance of the relationship of dilated ducts and/or strictures to pain. The finding of an appreciable obstruction or stricture in 65 percent of the patients who were pain-free more than 1 year, compared with 79 percent of the group with pain, suggests that factors other than duct obstruction or narrowing may be important in the pathogenesis of pain. It may be that the most important factors in the relief of pain are abstinence from alcohol and progressive pancreatic dysfunction rather than the surgical procedure per se. If no surgically remedial lesion is found and severe pain continues despite abstinence from alcohol, subtotal pancreatic resection may be necessary.

The treatment of malabsorption rests on the use of pancreatic enzyme replacement therapy. Although diarrhea and steatorrhea are usually improved, the results are frequently less than satisfactory. The major problem is delivery of enough active enzyme into the duodenum. Steatorrhea can be abolished if 10 percent of the normal amount of lipase could be delivered into the duodenum at the proper time. This concentration of lipase cannot be achieved with the presently available preparations of pancreatic enzymes, even if the latter are given in large doses. These poor results may be due to inactivation of lipase by gastric acid, food emptying from the stomach more rapidly than the exogenously administered pancreatic enzymes, and variation in the enzyme activity of various batches of commercially available pancreatic extracts.

For the usual patient, three to eight tablets or capsules of a potent enzyme preparation should be administered with meals. Some patients on conventional tablets require adjuvant therapy to improve enzyme replacement treatment. Although initially cimetidine was considered an effective adjuvant, studies have failed to confirm this. Sodium bicarbonate (1.3 g with meals) is effective and inexpensive. Antacids containing calcium carbonate or magnesium hydroxide are not effective and may actually result in increased steatorrhea. Adjuvant therapy should not be given with enteric-coated microsphere preparations because such therapy may increase the gastric pH such that these preparations would release their enzymes into the stomach rather than the small intestine.

Patients with severe exocrine pancreatic insufficiency secondary to alcohol who continue to drink have a high mortality (in one series 50 percent were dead when followed for 5 to 12 years) and significant morbidity (weight loss, lassitude, vitamin deficiency, and narcotic addiction). Pain may abate if progressive severe exocrine insufficiency continues. If abstinence is pursued and vigorous replacement therapy is utilized for the maldigestion-malabsorption, the patients do reasonably well.

HEREDITARY PANCREATITIS   Hereditary pancreatitis is a rare disease similar to chronic pancreatitis except for an early age of onset and evidence of hereditary factors (involving an autosomal dominant gene with incomplete penetrance). These patients have recurring attacks of severe abdominal pain which may last from a few days to a few weeks. The serum amylase and lipase levels may be elevated during acute attacks but are usually normal. Patients frequently develop pancreatic calcification, diabetes mellitus, and steatorrhea, and in addition, they have an increased incidence of pancreatic carcinoma. Such patients often require ductal decompression to obtain pain relief. Abdominal complaints in relatives of patients with hereditary pancreatitis should raise the question of pancreatic disease.

PANCREATIC ENDOCRINE TUMORS

Pancreatic endocrine tumors are summarized in Table 274-6 and are discussed in Chap. 276.

OTHER CONDITIONS

ANNULAR PANCREAS   When there is a failure in communication of the ventral and dorsal anlage of the pancreas, a ring of pancreatic tissue encircles the duodenum. Such an annular pancreas may cause intestinal obstruction in the neonate or the adult. Symptoms of postprandial fullness, epigastric pain, nausea, and vomiting may be present for years before the diagnosis is entertained. The radiographic findings are symmetric dilatation of the proximal duodenum with bulging of the recesses on either side of the annular band, effacement of the duodenal mucosa without destruction of the mucosa, accentuation of the findings in the right anterior oblique position, and lack of change on repeated examinations. The differential diagnosis should include duodenal webs, tumors of the pancreas or duodenum, postbulbar peptic ulcer, regional enteritis, and adhesions. Patients with annular pancreas have an increased incidence of pancreatitis and peptic ulcer. Because of these and other potential complications, the treatment is surgical even though the condition has been present for years. Retrocolic duodenojejunostomy is the procedure of choice,

TABLE 274-6   Pancreatic endocrine tumors

Syndrome	Hormone(s) produced	Primary hormone effects	Pathologic features	Clinical features
Zollinger-Ellison	Gastrin	Gastric acid hypersecretion with basal acid outputs usually >15 mmol/h (>15 meq/h)	Delta cell islet tumors; 10% aberrant (duodenal); 60% malignant	Severe peptic ulcer disease often refractory to therapy; ectopic ulcers; diarrhea; multiple endocrine adenomas (parathyroid, pituitary, adrenal, thyroid)
Insulinoma	Insulin	Hypoglycemia with inappropriately increased serum insulin levels	Beta cell islet tumors; 80–90% benign	Hypoglycemic symptoms
Glucagonoma	Glucagon; pancreatic polypeptide	Hyperglucagonemia →glucose intolerance	Alpha cell islet tumors; 60% malignant	Slow-growing pancreatic tumor; hyperglycemia; bullous and eczematoid dermatitis, weight loss; anemia; gastric and intestinal motor abnormalities
Somatostatinoma	Somatostatin; pancreatic polypeptide	Somatostatin inhibits insulin, gastrin and pancreatic enzyme secretion; decreased bile flow	Delta cell islet tumor	Pancreatic tumor; diarrhea; steatorrhea; gallstones; diabetes mellitus; anemia
Pancreatic cholera	Vasoactive intestinal peptide (VIP) ? Gastric inhibitory polypeptide ? Prostaglandin E ? Pancreatic peptide	Net secretion of salt and water by gut	? Delta cell tumor; >50% malignant	Pancreatic tumor with severe watery diarrhea; flushing; weight loss; hypokalemia; hypercalcemia; hypochlorhydria; hyperglycemia; inordinate fecal water and electrolyte losses
Carcinoid	Serotonin; prostaglandins	Altered gut motility; diarrhea	Enterochromaffin cells; non-beta cell islet tumors	Carcinoid syndrome with flushing; wheezing; diarrhea; alcohol intolerance; hepatomegaly

A

B

C

FIGURE 274-5   Illustration of the pancreatic ducts and typical ERCP of pancreas divisum. *A.* Diagram of the ventral and dorsal structures of the pancreas: (1) duct of Santorini, (2) pancreatic duct from the dorsal anlage, (3) pancreatic duct from the ventral anlage, (4) duct of Wirsung, and (5) common bile duct. *B.* ERCP, through the major papilla, demonstrating the ventral duct which does not communicate with the dorsal duct. *C.* ERCP demonstrating that the dorsal duct cannulated through the minor papilla does not communicate with the major papilla. (*Courtesy of Dr. C. E. Forsmark, University of Florida College of Medicine.*)

although some surgeons advocate Billroth II gastrectomy, gastroenterostomy, and vagotomy.

PANCREAS DIVISUM   Pancreas divisum occurs when the embryologic ventral and dorsal parts of the pancreas fail to fuse so that pancreatic drainage is accomplished mainly through the accessory papilla. Pancreas divisum is the most common congenital anatomic variant of the human pancreas. Current evidence indicates that this anomaly is not a predisposing factor to the development of pancreatitis in the great majority of patients with the anomaly. However, the combination of pancreas divisum and a small accessory orifice could result in dorsal duct obstruction. The challenge is to identify this subset of patients with dorsal duct pathology. Cannulation of the dorsal duct by ERCP is not as easily done as is cannulation of the ventral duct (Fig. 274-5). Patients with pancreatitis and pancreas divisum demonstrated by ERCP should be treated with conservative measures, including pancreatic enzyme therapy. Many of these patients have idiopathic pancreatitis unrelated to the pancreas divisum and will respond well to pancreatic enzyme therapy. Endoscopic or surgical intervention is indicated only when the above methods fail. If marked dilation of the dorsal duct can be demonstrated, surgical ductal decompression should be performed. The appropriate therapy for those patients without dilation of the dorsal duct is not yet defined. It should be stressed that the ERCP appearance of pancreas divisum, i.e., a small-caliber ventral duct with an arborizing pattern, may be confused with an obstructed main pancreatic duct secondary to a mass lesion.

MACROAMYLASEMIA   In macroamylasemia amylase circulates in the blood in a polymer form too large to be easily excreted by the kidney. The patient with this condition will demonstrate an elevated serum amylase value, a low urinary amylase value, and a C_{am}/C_{cr} ratio of less than 1 percent. The presence of macroamylase can be documented by chromatography of the serum. The prevalence of macroamylasemia is 1.5 percent of the nonalcoholic general adult hospital population. Usually macroamylasemia is an incidental finding and is not related to disease of the pancreas or other organs. It is important to be aware of this condition so that patients with macroamylasemia will not be needlessly evaluated and treated for pancreatic disease.

Macrolipasemia has now been documented in a patient with non-Hodgkin's lymphoma and in a patient with cirrhosis. These patients had normal ultrasound and CT examinations of the pancreas. Lipase was shown to be complexed with immunoglobulin A. Thus the possibility of *both* macroamylasemia and macrolipasemia should be considered in patients with elevated blood levels of these enzymes.

REFERENCES

AGARWAL N et al: Assessment of severity in acute pancreatitis. Am J Gastroenterol 86:1385, 1991

AMMANN RW: A critical appraisal of interventional therapy in chronic pancreatitis. Endoscopy 23:191, 1991

———— et al: Evolution and regression of pancreatic calcification in chronic pancreatitis: A prospective long-term study of 10 patients. Gastroenterology 95:1018, 1988

BALTHAZAR EJ et al: Acute pancreatitis: Value of CT in establishing prognosis. Radiology 174:331, 1990

BANKS PA: Management of pancreatic pain. Pancreas 6(suppl 1):52, 1991

CARR-LOCKE DL: Pancreas divisum: The controversy goes on. Endoscopy 23:88, 1991

COPENHAGEN PANCREATIC STUDY: An interim report from a prospective epidemiological multicenter study. Scand J Gastroenterol 16:305, 1981

GERZOF SG et al: Early diagnosis of pancreatic infection by computed tomography guided aspiration. Gastroenterology 93:1315, 1987

JOHNSON CD et al: CT of acute pancreatitis: Correlation between lack of contrast enhancement and pancreatic necrosis. AJR 156:92, 1991

KOLARS JC et al: Comparison of serum amylase, pancreatic isoamylase and lipase in patients with hyperamylasemia. Dig Dis Sci 29:289, 1984

LEE SP et al: Biliary sludge as a cause of acute pancreatitis. N Engl J Med 326:589, 1992

McMAHON MJ et al: A comparative study of methods for reproduction of severity of attacks of acute pancreatitis. Br J Surg 67:22, 1985

MOOSSA AR: Surgical treatment of chronic pancreatitis: An overview. Br J Surg 74:661, 1987

NEOPTOLEMOS JP et al: Control trial of urgent endoscopic retrograde cholangiopancreatography and endoscopic sphincterotomy versus conservative treatment for acute pancreatitis due to gallstones. Lancet 2:979, 1988

NIEDERAU C, GRENDELL JH: Diagnosis of chronic pancreatitis. Gastroenterology 88:1973, 1985

SARLES H: Definitions and classifications of pancreatitis. Pancreas 6:470, 1991

SLAFF J et al: Protease specific suppression of pancreatic exocrine secretion. Gastroenterology 87:44, 1984

STEINBERG WM et al: Diagnostic assays in acute pancreatitis: A study of sensitivity and specificity. Ann Intern Med 102:576, 1985

TOSKES PP: Biochemical tests in pancreatic disease. Curr Opin Gastroenterol 8:814, 1992

————: Medical therapy of chronic pancreatitis. Semin Gastrointest Dis 2:188, 1991

————: Hyperlipidemic pancreatitis. Gastroenterol Clin North Am 19:783, 1990

WILSON C et al: Prediction of outcome in acute pancreatitis: A comparative study of APACHE II, clinical assessment, and multiple screening systems. Br J Surg 77:1260, 1990

275   PANCREATIC CANCER

ROBERT J. MAYER

INCIDENCE AND ETIOLOGY   The incidence of pancreatic carcinoma in the United States has increased significantly as the median life expectancy of the American population has been prolonged. The tumor results in the death of more than 95 percent of afflicted patients. Approximately 25,000 individuals died of pancreatic cancer in 1993, making it the fifth most common cause of cancer-related mortality. The disease appears to occur somewhat more frequently in males than in females and in blacks than in whites. It rarely develops prior to the age of 50.

Little is known about the causes of pancreatic cancer. Cigarette smoking represents the most consistently observed risk factor for the development of the tumor, with the disease being two to three times more common in heavy smokers than in nonsmokers. It is uncertain whether this apparent association reflects a direct carcinogenic effect of metabolites of cigarette smoke on the pancreas or whether an as yet undefined exposure occurring more frequently in cigarette smokers is responsible for the enhanced risk. A large case control study has also correlated chronic pancreatitis with an increased risk of pancreatic cancer. There are no convincing data to link such epidemiologic factors as alcohol abuse, cholelithiasis, or preexisting diabetes mellitus with the development of pancreatic cancer. Furthermore, the weight of clinical data has failed to support any association between coffee consumption and pancreatic cancer. Mutations in c-K-*ras* genes have frequently been found in specimens of human pancreatic cancer.

CLINICAL FEATURES   More than 90 percent of pancreatic cancers are ductal adenocarcinomas, with islet cell tumors constituting the remaining 5 to 10 percent. Pancreatic cancers occur twice as frequently in the pancreatic head (about 70 percent of cases) as in the body (about 20 percent) or tail (about 10 percent) of the gland.

With the exception of jaundice, the initial symptoms associated with pancreatic cancer are often insidious in nature and are usually present for longer than 2 months prior to the time the cancer is diagnosed (Table 275-1). Pain and weight loss are present in more than 75 percent of patients. The pain typically has a gnawing, visceral

TABLE 275-1   Presenting signs and symptoms of pancreatic carcinoma

Frequent
 Abdominal pain
 Weight loss
 Jaundice (lesions of pancreatic head only)
Infrequent
 Glucose intolerance
 Palpable gallbladder
 Migratory thrombophlebitis
 Gastrointestinal hemorrhage
 Splenomegaly

quality, occasionally radiating from the epigastrium to the back, and generally representing a more severe problem in lesions arising in the body or tail since such tumors may become quite large prior to being detected. Characteristically, the pain improves somewhat on bending forward. The development of significant pain is suggestive of retroperitoneal invasion and infiltration of the splanchnic nerves, indicating the primary lesion to be far advanced and surgically unresectable. Rarely, such pain may be transient and associated with hyperamylasemia, indicative of acute pancreatitis caused by ductal obstruction by tumor. The weight loss observed in the majority of patients having pancreatic carcinoma is primarily the result of anorexia, although in the initial period of the disease, subclinical malabsorption may also be a contributing factor.

Jaundice due to biliary obstruction is found in more than 80 percent of patients having tumors in the pancreatic head and is typically accompanied by darkening of urine, a claylike appearance of stool, and pruritus. In contrast to the "painless jaundice" sometimes observed in patients having carcinomas of the bile ducts, duodenum, or periampullary regions, the majority of icteric individuals having ductal carcinomas of the pancreatic head will complain of significant abdominal discomfort. Although the gallbladder is usually enlarged in patients with carcinoma of the head of the pancreas, it is palpable in less than 50 percent of cases (Courvoisier's sign). The presence, however, of an enlarged gallbladder in a jaundiced patient without biliary colic should suggest malignant obstruction of the extrahepatic biliary tree.

The vast majority of patients with pancreatic cancer do not develop clinical diabetes mellitus; in one study, glucose intolerance was found in only 6 percent of a group of 924 patients whose presenting symptoms were carefully analyzed. Other uncommon initial manifestations include venous thrombosis and migratory thrombophlebitis, gastrointestinal hemorrhage resulting from varices due to tumor compression of the portal venous system, and splenomegaly caused by cancerous encasement of the splenic vein.

DIAGNOSTIC PROCEDURES (Fig. 275-1) Despite the availability of serologic tests for tumor-associated antigens such as the carcinoembryonic antigen (CEA) and CA 19-9 and noninvasive imaging techniques such as CT scanning and ultrasonography, the early diagnosis of a potentially resectable pancreatic carcinoma remains extremely difficult. The nonspecificity of the initial symptoms and the poor sensitivity of both serologic assays and noninvasive techniques have frustrated the development of effective screening procedures. When the disease is clinically suspected in a patient having vague, persistent abdominal complaints, ultrasound should be performed to visualize the gallbladder and the pancreas, as well as upper GI contrast radiographs to rule out a hiatal hernia or a peptic ulcer. If these studies fail to provide an explanation for the symptoms, a CT scan should be considered. It should encompass not only the pancreas but also the liver, retroperitoneal lymph nodes, and pelvis, since pancreatic cancer frequently spreads within the abdomen. While more costly than ultrasonography, CT is technically simpler, more reproducible, provides better definition of the body and tail of the pancreas, and requires less interpretive skill. CT generally detects a malignant pancreatic lesion in over 80 percent of cases; in 5 to 15 percent of patients with proven pancreatic carcinoma, the CT scan shows only generalized pancreatic enlargment suggestive of pancreatitis rather than malignancy. False-positive results have also been reported in about 5 to 10 percent of cases where no tumor was found on laparotomy. At present, magnetic resonance imaging (MRI) has not been shown superior to CT in the evaluation of pancreatic lesions.

In selected situations where clinical circumstances dictate additional diagnostic evaluation, endoscopic retrograde cholangiopancreatography (ERCP) may clarify the cause of ambiguous CT or ultrasound findings. The characteristic findings are stenosis or obstruction of either the pancreatic or the common bile duct; both duct systems are abnormal in over half the cases. The differentiation between carcinoma and chronic pancreatitis by ERCP can be quite difficult, particularly if both diseases are present. False-negative results with ERCP are

quite infrequent (less than 5 percent) and usually occur in the setting of islet cell, rather than ductal, carcinomas.

Selective and superselective angiography may be of value in some patients. Angiography is an effective means of detecting carcinomas in the body and tail of the pancreas by demonstrating vascular narrowing, displacement, or occlusion by tumor. Angiography is also useful in assessing whether encasement of peripancreatic vessels is present; this is of importance in determining the potential for surgical resection.

Regardless of the results of the above diagnostic studies, a histologic confirmation of a presumed pancreatic cancer is mandatory to be absolutely certain that malignancy exists and to rule out the presence of such other neoplasms as an islet cell tumor or a lymphoma, for which the therapeutic approach and prognosis differ significantly from those for the usual ductal carcinoma. Such tissue confirmation may often be obtained through a percutaneous needle aspiration biopsy of the pancreas with CT or ultrasonographic guidance, thereby obviating surgical exploration.

It should be emphasized that patients with carcinoma of the pancreas may undergo several months of investigation before a diagnosis is established. In the past, this period of diagnostic delay and accompanying emotional uncertainty erroneously led to an impression that the pain and weight loss might not have had an organic cause, resulting in an association of pancreatic cancer and depression. The availability of CT scans has resulted in a prompter diagnosis and dispelled this incorrect notion. Unfortunately, however, even laparotomy may not provide a definitive diagnosis, because chronic pancreatitis may also produce a hard mass in the head of the pancreas, making it indistinguishable from carcinoma by palpation. Furthermore, a superficial biopsy of such a mass may not show neoplastic tissue, revealing only evidence of pancreatitis since the cancer itself is often surrounded by edematous, inflamed, and fibrotic tissue (i.e., changes associated with chronic pancreatitis).

TREATMENT Complete surgical resection of pancreatic tumors offers the only effective treatment for this disease. Unfortunately, such "curative" operations are only possible in 10 to 15 percent of patients with pancreatic cancer and are limited, for all practical purposes, to those individuals having tumors in the pancreatic head in whom jaundice was the initial symptom. Patients considered for such a procedure should have no evidence of metastatic spread on a chest radiogram and abdominal-pelvic CT scan, should undergo preoperative celiac angiography (to exclude evidence of surgical unresectability such as vascular invasion by tumor), and should receive their care from an experienced surgeon, since mortality rates of greater than 15 percent have been associated with this procedure. Although the potential for cure in patients with pancreatic cancer is restricted to those few who are able to undergo a complete surgical resection, the 5-year survival rate following such operations is only 10 percent. Nonetheless, an attempt at the procedure merits strong consideration, particularly for lesions in the pancreatic head, since ductal carcinomas often cannot be distinguished preoperatively from ampullary, duodenal, and distal bile duct tumors or pancreatic cyst adenocarcinomas, all of which have far higher resectability and cure rates. Furthermore, survival is prolonged three- to fourfold in patients who eventually experience disease recurrence following resection over those whose tumor is not excised, indicating that such operations have a palliative as well as curative potential. The risk for tumor recurrence is unaffected by the type of operative procedure [i.e., total pancreatectomy versus pancreaticoduodenectomy ("Whipple resection")] but is increased by the presence of lymph node metastases or tumor invasion into adjacent viscera. As a rule, pancreaticoduodenectomy or distal pancreatectomy seems preferable to total pancreatectomy because of the retention of exocrine function and avoidance of brittle diabetes.

The median survival for patients whose pancreatic cancers are surgically unresectable is approximately 5 months. Management of such individuals should be directed at symptomatic palliation. Ambulatory patients having tumors in the pancreatic head should be

FIGURE 275-1 Carcinoma of the pancreas. *A*. Sonogram showing pancreatic carcinoma (P), dilated intrahepatic bile ducts (d), dilated portal vein (pv), and inferior vena cava (IVC). *B*. CT scan showing pancreatic carcinoma (arrow).

C. ERCP showing abrupt cut off of the duct of Wirsung (arrow). *D*. Arteriogram showing sheathing of splenic artery by tumor encasement (arrow).

considered for surgical diversion of the biliary system. If jaundice has already developed, therapeutic options include either nonoperative biliary decompression by endoscopic or percutaneous, transhepatic biliary drainage or surgical biliary bypass. External beam radiation in patients with unresectable tumors which have not spread beyond the pancreas does not appear to prolong survival, although a sufficient reduction in tumor size may lead to palliation of pain. However, the addition of 5-fluorouracil (5-FU) chemotherapy to external beam irradiation has increased the survival time for these patients, perhaps by acting as a radiosensitizing agent. A similar combination of radiation therapy and 5-FU appears to have prolonged the survival and increased the cure rate when compared to a prospectively randomized nontreatment control group of patients who had a complete surgical resection of their pancreatic cancer. This observation has been made in a small patient population and thus demands confirmation prior to the general acceptance of the efficacy of postoperative (''adjuvant'') treatment. The application of such chemoradiation therapy at diagnosis prior to surgery (''neoadjuvant'') treatment) as a means of increasing the potential for resectability is under investigation.

The experience utilizing chemotherapy in the management of patients with widely metastatic pancreatic cancer has been disappointing. No presently available drug regimen can be considered as being ''standard.'' Newer forms of therapy must be developed and should constitute the initial treatment for consenting, ambulatory patients.

Pancreatic endocrine tumors are discussed in Chap. 276.

REFERENCES

BERG RJ, CONNELLY RR: Updating the epidemiologic data on pancreatic cancer. Semin Oncol 6:275, 1979

CANCER OF THE PANCREAS TASK FORCE: Staging of cancer of the pancreas. Cancer 47:1631, 1981

CONNOLLY MM et al: Survival in 1001 patients with carcinoma of the pancreas. Ann Surg 206:366, 1987

GASTROINTESTINAL TUMOR STUDY GROUP: Pancreatic cancer. Adjuvant combined radiation and chemotherapy following curative resection. Arch Surg 120:899, 1985

GUDJONSSON B et al: Cancer of the pancreas. Diagnostic accuracy and survival statistics. Cancer 42:2494, 1978

LIN A, FELLER ER: Pancreatic carcinoma as a cause of unexplained pancreatitis: Report of ten cases. Ann Intern Med 113:166, 1990

LOWENFELS AB et al: Pancreatitis and the risk of pancreatic cancer. N Engl J Med 328:1433, 1993

MOERTEL CT et al: Therapy of locally unresectable pancreatic adenocarcinoma: A randomized comparison of high dose (6,000 rads) radiation alone, moderate dose radiation (4,000 rads) + 5-fluorouracil, and high dose radiation + 5-fluorouracil. The Gastrointestinal Tumor Study Group. Cancer 48:1705, 1981

MOOSA AR, LEVIN B: The diagnosis of "early" pancreatic cancer: The University of Chicago experience. Cancer 47:1688, 1981

O'CONNELL MJ: Current status of chemotherapy for advanced pancreatic and gastric cancer. J Clin Oncol 3:1031, 1985

SPEER AG et al: Randomized trial of endoscopic versus percutaneous stent insertion in malignant obstructive jaundice. Lancet 2:57, 1987

STEINBERG WM et al: Comparison of the sensitivity and specificity of the CA 19-9 and carcinoembryonic antigen assays in detecting cancer of the pancreas. Gastroenterology 90:343, 1986

WARSHAW AL, FERNANDO-DEL CASTILLO C: Pancreatic carcinoma. N Engl J Med 326:455, 1992

TABLE 276-1 Distribution of APUD tumors

Origin	Tumors
Gastrointestinal tract	Carcinoid tumor
Pancreas	Islet cell carcinoma
Central nervous system	Ganglioneuroblastoma, neuroblastoma, chemodactoma, paraganglionoma
Thyroid	Medullary thyroid carcinoma
Skin	Melanoma
Adrenal medulla	Pheochromocytoma
Lung	Carcinoid tumor, small cell carcinoma

276 ENDOCRINE TUMORS OF THE GASTROINTESTINAL TRACT AND PANCREAS

LEE M. KAPLAN

Tumors arising from neuroendocrine cells of the gastrointestinal tract and pancreas present special challenges in diagnosis and therapy. Unlike other gastrointestinal neoplasms, these tumors often cause symptoms from excess hormone secretion rather than from growth, invasion, or local anatomic effects. Frequently slow growing, they may nonetheless be life-threatening because of uncontrolled release of specific hormones and neurotransmitters. These neoplasms arise from within the gastrointestinal mucosa and pancreatic islets in cells that normally secrete regulatory monoamines and peptide hormones. For example, gastrin-secreting G cells within the gastric and duodenal mucosa regulate gastric acid secretion, and insulin-secreting β cells within the pancreatic islets have a crucial role in the homeostatic control of glucose metabolism. Overall, more than 30 distinct secretory products have been identified within neuroendocrine cells of the gut.

BIOLOGIC CONSIDERATIONS

A striking feature of neuroendocrine tumors is the preservation of highly differentiated cell function. Tumor cells contain secretory granules and maintain the capacity for *a*mine *p*recursor *u*ptake and *d*ecarboxylation (APUD), a process essential for the production of monoamine neurotransmitters such as serotonin, dopamine, and histamine. This characteristic has fostered the term *APUDomas* for neoplasms derived from these cells, which can be located in the thyroid (C cells), adrenal medulla, lung (neuroendocrine cells), skin (melanocytes), and nervous system (glial cells and neuroblasts), as well as the gastrointestinal tract and pancreas. These cells also synthesize and secrete *peptide* hormones by a separate mechanism. Several of the known APUDomas are listed in Table 276-1. It was postulated that this specialized capability implies a common embryologic origin for these diverse cells, but in fact, cells of *varied* heritage can acquire the APUD phenotype during differentiation.

Studies of neuroendocrine cell physiology have revealed several important characteristics of secretory cells and the clinical syndromes caused by their humoral products:

1 Cellular phenotype does not predict the nature of the secreted product. Thus neurons may secrete peptide "hormones" into the synaptic cleft, and endocrine cells may secrete monoamines previously classified as "neurotransmitters." Individual cells have the capacity to synthesize and secrete both peptide and monoamine transmitters, which may coexist in individual secretory granules. Many symptoms of enterochromaffin cell tumors (carcinoid tumors) appear to arise from the combined actions of monoamine and peptide products.

2 Transmitter secretion by neuroendocrine cells is frequently episodic or pulsatile. Although the regulation of secretion is incompletely understood, the temporal pattern of hormone release may vary depending on the hormonal milieu, physiologic state, or stage of development. Thus symptoms produced by abnormal secretion of hormones from neuroendocrine tumors may be intermittent, especially in early stages when tumor cells may behave more like their normal counterparts.

3 Individual cells have the *potential* to secrete a wide array of transmitters. This feature is particularly evident for the peptide hormones. Depending on the stage of development, cellular environment, and other as yet unidentified factors, neuroendocrine cells can change secretory profiles dramatically. For example, in cell culture, clonal populations may suddenly change from the secretion of insulin to cholecystokinin, gastrin, or even glucagon. Endocrine tumors may contain heterogeneous populations of cells so that within individual tumors a single cell type may predominate, or there may be multiple cell types in varying proportions. In addition, the secretory profile of a tumor may vary with time, producing a dramatic alteration of symptoms. Individual metastatic implants also can display different phenotypes from the primary tumor and from each other.

4 Individual hormones and transmitters secreted by neuroendocrine cells may regulate physiologic activity (e.g., secretion, absorption, or contractility), stimulate or inhibit growth, or affect the development of target cells. Thus the humoral activity of gut neuroendocrine tumors can cause a wide variety of effects, including gastric acid hypersecretion, abnormal intestinal motility, gastric epithelial hyperplasia, gallstone formation, mesenteric and cardiac fibrosis, and necrosis of the skin.

5 Hormone production by neuroendocrine cells is tightly regulated at many levels, including RNA transcription, precursor peptide processing, and secretion. These cells, in addition, may be subject to control by neighboring secretory cells (*paracrine regulation*). Thus multiple cell types may act in concert to control the growth, secretory characteristics, and thus the clinical manifestations of individual tumors. Abnormal secretion by the tumors themselves may disrupt the normal regulated function of neighboring neuroendocrine cells, and neoplastic transformation may disturb hormone secretion by these cells. Cells may secrete partially processed hormone precursors, leading to unpredictable effects, or display altered susceptibility to regulation by exogenous stimuli. Occasionally, such characteristics can be exploited to permit specific diagnostic tests for individual tumors.

Neuroendocrine tumors of the gastrointestinal tract can be classified by cell type, major hormone secreted, and site of origin. These characteristics, alone or in combination, correlate well with the observed clinical syndromes. Table 276-2 lists the important tumors in this category, along with their clinical presentations, major secreted products, cells of origin, and biologic behavior.

TABLE 276-2 Gastrointestinal endocrine tumor syndromes

Syndrome	Cell type	Clinical features	Percentage malignant	Major products
Carcinoid syndrome	Enterochromaffin, enterochromaffin-like	Flushing, diarrhea, wheezing, hypotension	~100	Serotonin, histamine, miscellaneous peptides
Zollinger-Ellison, gastrinoma	Non-ß islet cell, duodenal G cell	Peptic ulcers, diarrhea	~70	Gastrin
Insulinoma	Islet ß cell	Hypoglycemia	~10	Insulin
VIPoma (Verner-Morrison, WDHA)	Islet D_1 cell	Diarrhea, hypokalemia, hypochlorhydria	~60	Vasoactive intestinal peptide
Glucagonoma	Islet A cell	Mild diabetes mellitus, erythema necrolytica migrans, glossitis	>75	Glucagon
Somatostatinoma	Islet D cell	Diabetes mellitus, diarrhea, steatorrhea, gallstones	~70	Somatostatin
GRFoma	Non-ß islet cell	Acromegaly	–	Growth hormone-releasing hormone (GRF)
CRFoma	Non-ß islet cell	Cushing's syndrome	–	Corticotropin-releasing hormone (CRF)
PPoma	Islet PP cell	Rare necrolytic erythema	–	Pancreatic polypeptide (PP)
Neurotensinoma	Non-ß islet cell	None	–	Neurotensin
Miscellaneous tumors	Non-ß islet cell	Hypercalcemia, inappropriate ADH, hyperpigmentation	–	Parathyroid hormone, vasopressin, melanocyte-stimulating hormone

DIAGNOSTIC CONSIDERATIONS

Several distinct syndromes of hormone excess have been described in which symptoms may suggest the presence of an endocrine tumor of the gastrointestinal tract or pancreas. Moreover, these tumors may present as part of the type 1 multiple endocrine neoplasia (MEN 1) syndrome (see Chap. 343). MEN 1 patients frequently develop parathyroid and pituitary adenomas that may produce symptoms of hypercalcemia, hyperprolactinemia, hyperthyroidism, or growth hormone excess. Diagnosis is suggested by history, physical findings, elevated blood levels of the relevant peptide hormone(s), or elevated urinary levels of the major metabolites of monoamine transmitters. Further confirmation of hormone-producing tumors may be provided by provocative tests that reveal abnormalities in the regulation of hormone secretion. For example, tolbutamide may enhance somatostatin secretion from somatostatinoma cells. Normal somatostatin-secreting D cells do not show this effect. Other examples of *abnormal* regulation in tumor cells include enhancement by secretin of gastrin secretion in gastrinomas and pentagastrin stimulation of calcitonin secretion in medullary thyroid (C cell) tumors.

Anatomic definition for pancreatic tumors should be sought by computed tomography (CT), and endoscopic visualization or barium contrast studies should be obtained for suspected mucosal and submucosal tumors. In cases where tumors are too small to be visualized by these noninvasive methods, angiography or selective venous sampling for hormone determination may provide anatomic localization. CT and magnetic resonance imaging (MRI) are the preferred means of assessing metastatic spread, since the liver and lymph nodes are the initial sites of tumor metastasis.

THERAPEUTIC CONSIDERATIONS

Therapy of endocrine tumors has two goals: (1) to decrease or reverse the growth and spread of the tumor and (2) to relieve the symptoms of hormone overproduction. When the tumor is localized, both goals may be accomplished by surgical excision. However, most of these tumors are malignant and have spread by the time of diagnosis, and control of growth in such malignant tumors has proven difficult. Thus far, the greatest benefit has been seen with chemotherapeutic regimens that include streptozocin, alone or in combination with fluorouracil or doxorubicin. Control of hepatic metastases has been achieved with hepatic artery embolization or direct injection with cytotoxic agents (e.g., ethanol), although these approaches are palliative rather than curative.

Several approaches are used to control the effects of excess hormone production by these tumors. The most common is to block the function of the target tissue. For example, gastric acid hypersecretion induced by gastrin-producing tumors may be reversed by medications that inhibit acid secretion (e.g., H-2 receptor blockers or proton pump blockers) or by surgical resection of the stomach. Diazoxide is used to help reverse the effects of hyperinsulinemia, and hypomotility agents may ameliorate the diarrhea caused by hypersecretion of vasoactive intestinal peptide (VIP), gastrin, somatostatin, neurotensin, or serotonin.

A second approach is to block release of the transmitter from the tumor cells. The success of this approach depends on the continued ability of the tumor cells to respond to such physiologic or pharmacologic stimuli. Initial trials used somatostatin, a peptide hormone that inhibits the release of numerous hormones and amine transmitters. While somatostatin controls the symptoms of many of these tumors, it has a short half-life and must be given intravenously. These limitations have been largely overcome by the use of octreotide, a longer-acting analogue of somatostatin with similar actions that can be administered subcutaneously. The chemical structures of somatostatin and octreotide are shown in Fig. 276-1 (see also Chap.

FIGURE 276-1 Structures of somatostatin-14 and octreotide. The double circle denotes the substitution of D-tryptophan for the naturally occurring L-tryptophan. This substitution inhibits peptide degradation and prolongs serum half-life.

TABLE 276-3   Clinical uses of octreotide in gastrointestinal disease

Hormone-secreting tumors

Carcinoid tumor	Inhibits cutaneous flushing, controls diarrhea, reverses hypotension, aids perioperative management, ?inhibits growth
VIPoma	Controls diarrhea
Insulinoma	Controls hypoglycemia acutely, aids perioperative management
Gastrinoma	Perioperative management, ?controls diarrhea
Glucagonoma	Controls necrolytic erythema
Dumping syndrome	Controls diarrhea, vasomotor symptoms
Diarrhea	Inhibits intestinal secretion, motility
Short-bowel syndrome	
Ileostomy	
Diabetic neuropathy	
AIDS	
Fistulas	Inhibits fluid and enzyme secretion, promotes healing
Pancreatic	
Enteric	
Crohn's disease	
Gastrointestinal bleeding	
Portal hypertensive gastropathy	Reduces portal pressure, splanchnic blood flow
Esophageal and gastric varices	Reduces portal pressure, splanchnic blood flow

331). Octreotide frequently relieves the symptoms of several endocrine tumors that are inadequately controlled by tumor resection or ablation. In addition, tumor regression has occurred in occasional patients, suggesting that the hormone agonist may have some growth-inhibiting effects. The major known side effects of octreotide are dose-dependent and are similar to symptoms of somatostatin excess, including steatorrhea, mild hyperglycemia, nausea, and abdominal pain. Patients on long-term therapy with this agent have an increased tendency to develop gallstones. The clinical disorders that respond to therapy with octreotide are summarized in Table 276-3.

CARCINOID TUMORS

Carcinoid tumors are the most protean and the most common gastrointestinal endocrine tumors, accounting for approximately 55 percent of such neoplasms. The incidence of carcinoid tumors in the United States is approximately 15 per 1 million population per year. They may present with gastrointestinal bleeding, abdominal pain, obstruction from tumor growth or tumor-induced mesenteric fibrosis, or symptoms arising from tumor-secreted hormones. The name *carcinoid* was applied to these tumors because slow growth and the homogeneous appearance of tumor cells led early investigators to underestimate their malignant potential. They pursue an indolent course, and the interval between onset of symptoms and diagnosis averages 4.5 years. Carcinoid tumors arise from neuroendocrine cells throughout the body but are most prevalent in the gastrointestinal tract, pancreas, and pulmonary bronchi. Ninety percent of these tumors arise in the enterochromaffin, or Kulchitsky, cells within the gastrointestinal tract. The tumors can be found anywhere from the stomach to the rectum and are most common in the appendix, ileum, and rectum. Gastrointestinal carcinoids frequently cause abdominal pain, bleeding, or intestinal obstruction. Although they are rarely large, the tumors may become the leading point for intussusception. In addition, mesenteric spread stimulates a local fibrous reaction, causing intestinal kinking, obstruction, and vascular compromise. Rare sites of carcinoid tumors include the thymus, esophagus, biliary duct, Meckel's diverticulum, breast, and ovary. No risk factors have been clearly defined for these tumors, although the incidence of gastric carcinoids may be increased in patients with pernicious anemia, achlorhydria, and Hashimoto's thyroiditis. Carcinoids of the bronchus, stomach, and duodenum may occur in association with MEN 1. Thymic carcinoids may be associated with hyperparathyroidism or Cushing's syndrome.

Appendiceal tumors comprise nearly half of all carcinoid tumors and are incidental findings in 0.3 to 0.7 percent of routine appendectomy specimens. They are usually small, solitary, and benign. Local invasion is common but metastatic spread is rare, and the presence of tumor does not appear to confer appreciable morbidity or mortality. Colorectal carcinoids have a similarly benign course and are usually asymptomatic. In contrast, small-bowel and bronchial carcinoids have a more malignant course. Local transmural invasion, early metastasis to lymph nodes and liver, and symptoms from hormone secretion are common. Other sites of metastatic spread include bone and, less commonly, heart, breast, and eye. The risk of metastatic spread is dependent on tumor size. Metastases are found in fewer than 2 percent of tumors less than 1 cm in diameter but in nearly 100 percent of tumors greater than 2 cm. Additional primary tumor implants within the gastrointestinal tract are found in 40 percent of patients.

CARCINOID SYNDROME Enterochromaffin cells secrete a variety of hormones and are embryologically related to thyroid C cells, adrenal medullary cells, and melanocytes. Tumors of each of these cell types may produce syndromes of hormone excess. Hormone secretion by carcinoid cells can cause distinctive and debilitating effects (carcinoid syndrome) long before local growth or metastatic spread is otherwise apparent. Manifestations of the carcinoid syndrome include the "classic" triad of cutaneous flushing, diarrhea, and valvular heart disease and, less commonly, telangiectasias, wheezing, and paroxysmal *hypo*tension. Flushing, which is present in approximately 85 percent of patients with carcinoid syndrome, is also seen with many other conditions, including menopause, autonomic nervous system dysfunction, ethanol ingestion, disulfiram treatment, drug withdrawal, and a variety of hormone-secreting tumors, including pheochromocytoma, medullary thyroid carcinoma, VIPoma, and mastocytosis. It is estimated that approximately 5 percent of individuals presenting with the new onset of flushing will be found to have the carcinoid syndrome. Early in the course, symptoms are usually episodic and may be provoked by stress, catecholamines, and ingestion of food or alcohol. During acute paroxysms, systolic blood pressure typically falls 20 to 30 mmHg. Diarrhea may result from several mechanisms. The most common type is mixed secretory and hypermotility-induced, producing watery stools unresponsive to fasting. Other causes include partial mechanical obstruction from tumor or fibrosis and mesenteric vascular insufficiency from local fibrosis. Endocardial fibrosis can cause valvular heart disease, usually affecting the proximal side of the tricuspid and pulmonary valves and leading to tricuspid insufficiency, pulmonary stenosis, and secondary right-sided heart failure. Left-sided valvular disease may occur in association with bronchial carcinoids, presumably because venous effluent from these tumors passes directly into the pulmonary veins, avoiding inactivation of the hormone mediators in the lung.

Approximately 5 percent of all patients with carcinoid tumors experience one or more symptoms of the carcinoid syndrome. The likelihood of developing symptoms is strongly dependent on the origin and behavior of the tumor. While 30 to 60 percent of small-bowel carcinoids are associated with systemic manifestations, only 3.5 percent of lung, 1 percent of appendix, and virtually no rectal carcinoids produce the syndrome. In patients with intestinal carcinoids, the humoral symptoms only develop in the setting of metastatic disease to the liver. Bronchial and other extraintestinal carcinoids, whose hormone products are not immediately cleared by the liver, may produce the carcinoid syndrome in the absence of metastasis.

Carcinoid tumors may be classified on the basis of embryonic origin (Table 276-4). Clinical features, secreted hormones, diagnostic evaluation, and prognosis vary according to whether a carcinoid arises in foregut, midgut, or hindgut structures. For example, carcinoid syndrome is less common in patients with foregut carcinoids than midgut tumors, but the syndrome, when it occurs, is more likely to include wheezing. Patients with foregut carcinoid syndrome more often have dramatic cutaneous flushing involving the whole body than those with tumors of midgut or hindgut organs. The flush of bronchial carcinoids may be prolonged (lasting hours to days); associated with

TABLE 276-4 Characteristics of carcinoid tumors

Embryonic origin	Site of primary tumor	Carcinoid syndrome		
		Frequency, %	Characteristics	Monoamines
Foregut	Bronchus	3.5	Intense flush, lasting up to several hours; associated lacrimation, salivation, facial edema; wheezing; diarrhea; left- and right-sided cardiac lesions	5-HT, ± histamine
	Stomach	~5	Intense, pathcy, whole body flush, with defined borders, wheals, usually lasting several minutes; pruritus; wheezing; diarrhea	5-HTP, histamine, ± 5-HT
	Duodenum, jejunum	~40	Diarrhea	5-HT
	Pancreas, gallbladder	Rare	Occasional necrolytic erythema	
		~40	Facial flush, usually lasting seconds to minutes; telangiectasias; cardiac lesions; peritoneal fibrosis; diarrhea	5-HT, ± histamine
	Illeum	~1		
Midgut	Appendix			
	Colon	Rare	Mild facial flush	5-HT
Hindgut	Rectum	0	Diarrhea	

NOTE: 5-HT = 5-hydroxytryptamine (serotonin); 5-HTP = 5-hydroxytryptophan.

excessive lacrimation, salivation, and facial edema; and occasionally producing significant hypotension. The cutaneous manifestations of gastric carcinoids, though lasting only minutes, are frequently well-circumscribed and associated with wheals, pruritus, and high levels of histamine secretion. Midgut carcinoids commonly cause the carcinoid syndrome. Acute episodes of flushing tend to be less severe than those associated with foregut tumors, but facial telangiectasias may develop late in the course. Midgut tumors are more frequently associated with cardiac manifestations and peritoneal fibrosis. Hindgut tumors rarely cause the carcinoid syndrome. A rare variant syndrome associated with ovarian carcinoids causes severe peritoneal fibrosis.

Serotonin (5-hydroxytryptamine, 5-HT) is the most common secretory product of carcinoid tumors. As shown in Fig. 276-2, carcinoid tumors synthesize serotonin by enzymatic modification of circulating tryptophan. Up to 50 percent of the dietary intake of tryptophan can be converted to serotonin by these cells, which may leave inadequate substrate for incorporation into proteins and conversion to niacin. As a result, patients with widely metastatic carcinoid tumors may suffer symptoms of protein malnutrition (see Chap. 72) or mild pellagra (see Chap. 77). Serotonin induces intestinal secretion, inhibits intestinal absorption, and stimulates intestinal motility. High serotonin levels are likely the cause of diarrhea in most cases of carcinoid syndrome. Serotonin also stimulates fibroblast growth and fibrogenesis and thus may mediate or accelerate the peritoneal and cardiac valvular fibrosis in this disease. Excess serotonin secretion alone does not account for cutaneous flushing. Multiple monoamine and peptide factors contribute to the vasomotor changes; the relative contributions of each mediator may vary from patient to patient.

Carcinoid tumors elaborate multiple monoamines and peptide hormones, including histamine, catecholamines, bradykinins, tachykinins, enkephalins and endorphins, vasopressin, gastrin, adrenocorticotrophin, and prostaglandins (Table 276-5). Many secrete somatostatin, neurotensin, substance P, neurokinin A, and motilin. The elevated circulating levels of these substances mediate many of the pathophysiologic changes of carcinoid syndrome, although the relative contributions of each remain to be identified.

DIAGNOSIS The diagnosis of carcinoid tumors is influenced by the presenting features of the tumor. Patients with nonfunctional tumors (i.e., without the carcinoid syndrome) usually present with symptoms due to the direct effects of the tumor in the gastrointestinal tract, including abdominal pain or tenderness, nausea, malaise, weight loss, intestinal or biliary obstruction, or gastrointestinal bleeding. Depending on the location of the tumor and whether metastases are present, endoscopy, barium studies, or CT may allow anatomic localization. Radiographic studies should include small-bowel follow-through or direct instillation of radiographic contrast material into the small bowel (enteroclysis) to identify tumors in the jejunum and ileum. Despite the improved detection of tumors, however, their

pathologic identity is usually not suspected before resection or liver biopsy.

Evaluation of patients with clinical features of carcinoid syndrome is based on the observation that serotonin is secreted by the large majority of functional carcinoid tumors. As shown in Fig. 276-2, serotonin is metabolized in the blood to 5-hydroxyindoleacetic acid (5-HIAA), which is cleared by the kidneys. Plasma and platelet serotonin and urinary 5-HIAA levels are usually elevated in the setting of carcinoid syndrome. Measurement of urinary 5-HIAA excretion is the most useful diagnostic test, and approximately 75 percent of patients excrete more than 80 μmol/d (15 mg/d). Specificity of this test approaches 100 percent after exclusion of ingested substances

FIGURE 276-2 Metabolic pathway of serotonin in the carcinoid syndrome.

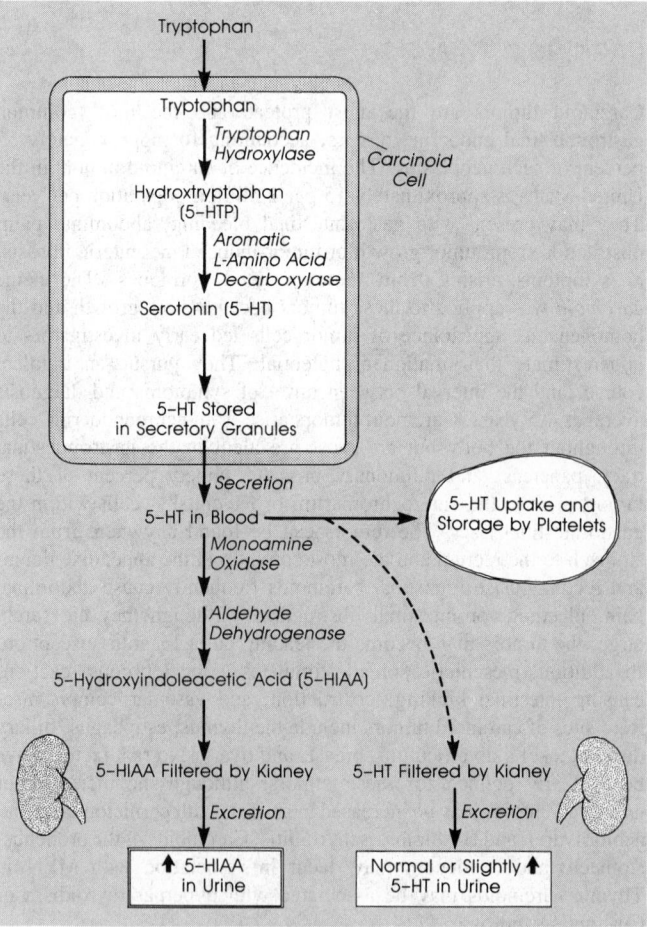

TABLE 276-5 Hormone mediators of carcinoid syndrome

Clinical feature	Frequency, %	Candidate mediators
Diarrhea	78	5-HT, histamine, prostaglandins, VIP, glucagon, gastrin, calcitonin
Cutaneous flushing	94	5-HT, 5-HTP, kallikrein, NKA, histamine, SK, SP, prostaglandins
Telangiectasia	25	Unknown
Wheezing	18	5-HT, histamine
Abdominal pain	51	Tumor, hepatic enlargment, bowel ischemia (fibrosis)
Heart disease		5-HT
Right-sided	40	
Left-sided	13	
Pellagra dermatosis	7	Tryptophan depletion (5-HT synthesis)

NOTE: 5-HT = 5-hydroxytryptamine (serotonin); 5-HTP = 5-hydroxytryptophan; NKA = neurokinin A; SK = substance K; SP = substance P; VIP = vasoactive intestinal peptide.
SOURCE: After W Creutzfeldt and F Stockmann, Am J Med 82(Suppl 5B):4, 1987.

known to elevate 5-HIAA levels; these include bananas, plantain, pineapple, kiwi fruit, walnuts, plums, pecans, avocados, guaifenesin, and acetaminophen. Conversely, aspirin and levodopa ingestion can cause a falsely depressed 5-HIAA level. In some patients with carcinoid syndrome and normal urinary 5-HIAA, documentation of elevated plasma or platelet serotonin concentrations may establish the diagnosis. However, many gastric carcinoid tumors lack the aromatic L-amino acid decarboxylase and convert 5-hydroxytryptophan (5-HTP) to serotonin with low efficiency. Since 5-HTP is not metabolized to 5-HIAA, urinary studies may be misleading. These patients may have elevated urinary serotonin levels, since renal cells contain aromatic L-amino acid decarboxylase. Diagnosis in these cases may be confirmed by demonstrating elevated plasma 5-HTP, histamine, or peptide hormone levels, although it frequently rests on the anatomic detection of the tumor itself. Attempts to provoke cutaneous flushing are helpful for documenting flushing in cases when the clinical history is equivocal. Ethanol, pentagastrin, or *micro*gram quantities of epinephrine can be used for this purpose. Abdominal ultrasonography, CT, and selective angiography are the most sensitive tests for detecting metastatic disease in the liver. Since most patients with the humoral syndrome have metastases, liver biopsy is the most common access to histologic diagnosis. Additional information about bone metastases and cardiac sequelae may be obtained with bone scans and echocardiography, respectively. In patients in whom a tumor cannot be detected, imaging with radiolabeled metaiodobenzyl guanidine (MIBG) or octreotide may be helpful. MIBG is concentrated by neuroendocrine cells and accumulates in many carcinoid tumors, and octreotide binds to somatostatin receptors, which are expressed in large numbers by many such tumors.

TREATMENT Effective treatment of the carcinoid syndrome may require more than one approach. Therapy should be selected according to the severity of symptoms. Since nearly all patients with carcinoid syndrome have metastatic disease, resection is rarely curative. Mild diarrhea may be controlled with hypomotility agents such as loperamide or diphenoxylate/atropine. In patients who have undergone ileal resection, diarrhea can be exacerbated by bile salt malabsorption and frequently responds to cholestyramine. Flushing, if rare and mild, may not require therapy. Combination therapy with histamine H-1 and H-2 receptor antagonists (e.g., diphenhydramine and ranitidine) can inhibit the cutaneous flush associated with foregut carcinoids. Phenoxybenzamine may provide additional benefit by inhibiting the release of bradykinin. Methylxanthine bronchodilators and glucocorticoids are helpful in relieving the dyspnea and wheezing associated with bronchial carcinoids. Beta-adrenergic agonists should be avoided because they may provoke acute exacerbations. Serotonin antagonists, including cyproheptadine and methysergide, have been used to provide

relief of diarrhea. Unfortunately, these agents have little effect on flushing and other vasomotor symptoms, and methysergide can induce fibrosis similar to that caused by the carcinoid itself.

Octreotide is a potent inhibitor of hormone secretion by carcinoid cells. Indeed, this agent provides effective control of diarrhea, flushing, and wheezing in more than 75 percent of cases. Octreotide is effective in the management of acute manifestations of the carcinoid syndrome such as hypotension or resulting angina, as well as the transient exacerbation caused by hepatic artery embolization or the induction of general anesthesia. However, octreotide must be administered in two or three subcutaneous injections each day. It is not yet known whether octreotide can prevent the observed cardiac (or mesenteric) fibrosis. Established valvular heart disease is not reversed by any form of medical therapy.

Surgery, hepatic artery embolization, and chemotherapy have been used to reduce the burden of tumor tissue. Surgery is the treatment of choice for small (<2 cm diameter) carcinoid tumors of the appendix or large bowel. Patients with carcinoid syndrome from isolated bronchial or other extraintestinal carcinoids also may be amenable to curative resection. Most patients with carcinoid syndrome, however, have gross metastatic disease. Hepatic resection generally provides only transient amelioration of symptoms and no improvement in survival. In isolated cases, however, long-term palliation has been achieved by resection of a *single* hepatic metastasis after removal of the primary tumor. Several less invasive approaches have been tried to limit the hepatic tumor burden and control humoral symptoms, including local irradiation, selective hepatic artery infusion of chemotherapy, CT-guided instillation of ethanol into metastatic implants, and hepatic arterial occlusion combined with chemoembolization. Unfortunately, carcinoid tumors are generally radioresistant and respond weakly to chemotherapy. Arterial occlusion by Gelfoam embolization provides transient relief of symptoms in approximately 90 percent of patients. Its success derives in part from the fact that the hepatic artery supplies less than half the blood supply of normal liver tissue but nearly all the blood supply of the tumor. Side effects of therapy include pain, fever, and occasional synthetic liver dysfunction. Effectiveness of therapy can be monitored with serum transaminase levels, which should rise substantially over the first 24 to 48 h after embolization. Patients undergoing embolization may experience acute exacerbation of carcinoid symptoms provoked by the sudden release of hormones from the tumor. Although such effects are rarely life-threatening, prophylactic treatment with histamine-receptor blockers and octreotide is recommended.

Several systemic chemotherapeutic protocols have been evaluated. Various combinations of streptozocin, fluorouracil, cyclophosphamide, and doxorubicin induce objective responses in approximately one-third of patients with metastatic disease, although the effect on survival is minimal. Leukocyte interferon decreases tumor size in approximately 20 percent and decreases urinary 5-HIAA excretion in about half of patients. Although octreotide has induced objective responses in a few cases, controlled trials have not yet demonstrated a significant effect.

The prognosis is highly dependent on the site and stage of the disease at diagnosis. As noted above, appendiceal and rectal carcinoids rarely affect survival. For other gastrointestinal carcinoids, 5-year survival is approximately 95 percent with local disease, 65 percent with lymph node involvement, and 18 percent with liver metastases. Median survival is $2\frac{1}{2}$ years after the first episode of flushing. Prognosis is inversely correlated with the degree of urinary 5-HIAA elevation. Despite attempts at therapy, patients excreting >800 μmol/d (>150 mg/d) have a median survival of only 1 year.

PANCREATIC ISLET-CELL TUMORS

GASTRINOMA (ZOLLINGER-ELLISON SYNDROME) (See also Chap. 252) In 1955, Zollinger and Ellison reported the association of severe peptic ulcer disease and gastrin-secreting tumors of the pancreas. These gastrinomas generate high serum gastrin levels, leading to hypersecretion of gastric acid and consequent duodenal and jejunal ulcers. Gastrinomas are the most common of the hormone-secreting tumors of the pancreatic islets, comprising nearly one-tenth of gastroenteropancreatic endocrine tumors and occurring with a frequency of approximately 4×10^{-7} in an unselected population in Ireland. Zollinger-Ellison syndrome may account for up to 0.1 percent of patients with duodenal ulcer disease in the United States. Ulcer disease develops in almost all patients with gastrinoma and is the presenting problem in approximately 70 percent. More than half of patients experience diarrhea (either watery stools or steatorrhea), and approximately 30 percent present with diarrhea alone. Radiologic and endoscopic examinations frequently reveal increased gastric fluid and thickened rugal folds. The age distribution of patients with gastrinoma is similar to that in ordinary acid peptic disease, with a broad peak in the fifth to eighth decades. Gastrinoma should be considered in all patients with recurrent or refractory ulcer disease, ulcers associated with gastric hypertrophy, ulcers in the distal duodenum or jejunum, ulcers in patients with diarrhea, kidney stones, hypercalcemia, or pituitary disease, or a strong family history of duodenal ulcer disease or endocrine tumors.

Between one-fourth and one-half of gastrinomas occur in association with the MEN 1 syndrome (see Chap. 343). Hyperparathyroidism is the most common component of MEN 1 and occurs in about 80 percent of patients with this form of Zollinger-Ellison syndrome. All gastrinoma patients should be screened for possible MEN 1 by measurement of serum calcium, phosphorus, cortisol, and prolactin levels and imaging of the sella turcica. First-degree relatives of patients with MEN 1 also should be similarly screened.

Approximately 80 percent of gastrin-secreting tumors arise in pancreatic islets, including nearly all those associated with MEN 1, and most are located in the pancreatic head. Another 10 to 15 percent arise from G cells in the duodenum, and the remainder are scattered in the distal small bowel, stomach, spleen, liver, lymph nodes, and ovary (mucinous cystadenoma). The tumors are usually small and are frequently multifocal, especially when associated with MEN 1. The biologic behavior may be variable. In most reported series, one-half to two-thirds of these tumors are malignant, with metastases in lymph nodes and liver and less frequently in bone. However, the prevalence of metastatic disease at the time of diagnosis appears to have decreased, perhaps owing to the more widespread consideration and earlier detection of these tumors. Such observations have important therapeutic implications, since isolated tumors are more likely to be cured by resection. Gastrinomas, like most other islet cell tumors, are generally slow-growing, but growth patterns vary widely and metastases may be more aggressive than the primary tumor itself.

Treatment of Zollinger-Ellison syndrome is directed at the sequelae of excess gastrin secretion and at the tumor itself. The availability of potent inhibitors of gastric acid secretion, including H-2 receptor blockers and the H^+,K^+-ATPase inhibitor omeprazole, has reduced the need for gastric surgery in these patients. The rare patient who fails to respond to medical therapy should be treated surgically. However, patients with coexistent hyperparathyroidism should undergo parathyroid resection before a decision is made about gastric surgery, since resolution of hypercalcemia may permit better medical control of gastric acid secretion.

Because of the effective control of hormone-mediated symptoms, morbidity and mortality from gastrinoma are increasingly related to the growth and spread of tumor itself. Curative resection of the gastrinoma is possible in 15 to 20 percent of cases and is favored by an extrapancreatic location and an inability to detect the tumor mass preoperatively. Gastrinomas in association with MEN 1 syndrome are not amenable to surgical cure, although these tumors generally have a benign natural history. Preoperative evaluation with CT and selective angiography is used to exclude multiple primary tumors and metastases. Treatment of unresectable gastrinoma includes chemotherapy, hormonal therapy, and hepatic artery embolization. Chemotherapeutic regimens including streptozocin and fluorouracil, with or without doxorubicin, commonly induce partial responses. Leukocyte interferon also may cause objective response, but octreotide does not appear to be effective. Hepatic artery embolization may decrease hepatic tumor burden and ameliorate pain. Unfortunately, none of these approaches prolongs survival of patients with metastatic disease, which approximates 25 percent at 10 years. For more information about the diagnosis and therapy of Zollinger-Ellison syndrome, refer to Chap. 252.

INSULINOMA (β CELL TUMOR)   The hallmark of pancreatic β cell tumors is the development of symptomatic hypoglycemia from unregulated insulin hypersecretion (see also Chap. 338). Insulinomas are the second most common functioning islet cell tumors and have a reported prevalence of approximately 8×10^{-7} in an unselected Irish population. They arise most frequently in the fifth to seventh decades, although cases have been reported at all ages. In infants and children, insulinoma must be distinguished from diffuse β cell adenomatosis and nesidioblastosis. Whipple's triad describes the classic presentation of insulinoma and includes fasting hypoglycemia, *symptoms* of hypoglycemia, and immediate relief after intravenous glucose administration. Weight gain may result from increased food ingested to combat symptoms of hypoglycemia. In the current era, the diagnosis of insulinoma is made by demonstrating fasting hypoglycemia in the presence of normal or elevated plasma insulin levels. Symptoms related to the hypoglycemia include headache, slurred speech, psychological alterations, visual disturbances, confusion, and, ultimately, coma and death. Hypoglycemia also induces the secondary release of catecholamines, leading to tremulousness, diaphoresis, pallor, palpitations, cardiac arrhythmias, and behavioral irritability. Because of the episodic release of insulin, symptoms early in the course may be intermittent or occur only after somewhat prolonged periods of fasting. However, symptoms do develop early so that tumors are usually small and solitary at the time of diagnosis. Multiple primary tumors are found in approximately 10 percent of patients. An additional 10 percent are malignant, with spread to the local lymph nodes and the liver. As with gastrinomas, insulinomas are frequently associated with MEN 1 (see Chaps. 338 and 343), and such tumors are more likely to be multifocal. Extrapancreatic insulin-secreting tumors are rare and usually arise in ectopic pancreatic tissue.

Diagnosis is made by demonstrating fasting hypoglycemia and an inadequate response of insulin to the hypoglycemia (see Chap. 338 for details). Patients are fasted under close supervision for up to 72 h, followed, if necessary, by an exercise tolerance test. The majority of patients with insulinoma develop hypoglycemia within 24 h, as evidenced by a serum glucose less than 2.8 mmol/L (50 mg/dL) in men or 2.5 mmol/L (45 mg/dL) in women. However, there is no absolute glucose level which defines hypoglycemia, so the diagnosis of insulinoma depends on demonstrating inadequate insulin suppression in the face of falling glucose levels. Documentation of rising cortisol levels excludes hypoglycemia secondary to hypothalamic-pituitary-adrenal dysfunction. It is also necessary to exclude other causes of fasting hypoglycemia, including administration of exogenous insulin, sulfonylurea ingestion, severe liver failure, and tumors that secrete insulinlike growth factors (e.g., fibrosarcoma, mesothelioma, and hemangiopericytoma). Exogenous insulin administration can be excluded by measuring levels of the C peptide of proinsulin, which normally vary in parallel with the plasma insulin concentrations. Since insulin administration suppresses endogenous insulin secretion, detection of normal or elevated C-peptide levels is inconsistent with insulin abuse. In addition, because insulinoma cells often process proinsulin incompletely, the serum often has an increased ratio of proinsulin to insulin. A ratio greater than 20 percent in the appropriate clinical setting is suggestive of insulinoma. Serum levels of sulfonylureas should be elevated if hyperinsulinemic hypoglycemia is caused by these agents. Normal glucose/insulin ratios exclude liver failure and tumors which secrete insulin-like growth factors. (Refer to Chap. 338 for a more complete discussion of hypoglycemia syndromes.)

Once a diagnosis of insulinemia is established, acute treatment is supportive with intravenous glucose infusion as required to maintain plasma levels within the normal range. Hyperglycemic agents, including diazoxide, beta-adrenergic receptor blockers, and phenytoin can be used to support serum glucose levels, but their effects are variable and may last only a short time. Octreotide frequently inhibits insulin secretion by these tumors and may be an effective agent for acute management. Definitive therapy is accomplished by surgical resection. Because insulinomas are usually small (most are <2 cm in diameter), only half are detected by CT. Angiography with selective venous sampling for insulin levels is about 80 percent sensitive, and palpation at laparotomy detects 80 to 90 percent of tumors. At surgery, detectable tumors should be resected. The effectiveness of intervention is monitored by determination of intraoperative blood glucose levels. If no detectable tumors are found, stepwise distal pancreatectomy is performed until frozen sections of resected specimens and/or blood glucose measurements indicate that all tumor has been removed. If no tumor is found, or if multiple tumors are present, pancreatectomy is limited to 70 to 80 percent to preserve digestive and endocrine pancreatic function.

Patients with metastatic disease and those whose insulinomas are not removed by partial pancreatectomy can frequently be managed with hyperglycemic agents such as diazoxide or octreotide. In one study, all seven patients with metastatic insulinoma showed a response to octreotide, although the degree of response was variable. However, hypoglycemia may be worsened by octreotide administration, perhaps owing to inhibition of glucagon or growth hormone by this agent. Diazoxide, though frequently effective, can cause troubling side effects, including salt and fluid retention, hypertrichosis, and gastrointestinal upset. The combination of streptozocin and doxorubicin is the mainstay of chemotherapy for metastatic disease; it is superior to streptozocin-fluorouracil. These agents induce objective remission in approximately half of patients and are associated with a modest but significant increase in survival. Patients with residual tumor should be followed carefully for changes in secretory profile which may affect therapy. Such changes may include development of hyperglycemia as a result of glucagon-secreting metastases.

VIPOMA [VERNER-MORRISON SYNDROME; WATERY DIARRHEA, HYPOKALEMIA, ACHLORHYDRIA (WDHA)] SYNDROME

Verner and Morrison described a syndrome of watery diarrhea, hypokalemia, and renal failure in association with non-β cell tumors of the pancreatic islets. The clinical features of this syndrome are caused by the high levels of vasoactive intestinal peptide (VIP) secreted by the tumors. VIPomas comprise approximately 2 percent of gastroenteropancreatic tumors and have a prevalence of approximately 1×10^{-7} in the Irish population studied. The manifestations of VIPoma include secretory diarrhea, profound weakness, hypokalemia, and hypochlorhydria. Stool volume is greater than 3 L/d in the majority of patients, and non-anion-gap acidosis usually occurs as a result of bicarbonate losses in the stool. Other electrolyte abnormalities include hypercalcemia in approximately two-thirds of patients and hypophosphatemia. Approximately half of patients develop hyperglycemia, which results from hypokalemia- and VIP-induced glycogenolysis in the liver, and a fifth of patients experience cutaneous flushing. Although most symptoms can be reproduced by infusion of exogenous VIP, these tumors also contain other peptide hormones, including the VIP-related peptide histidine-methionine (PHM), somatostatin, helodermin, and neurotensin, each of which may contribute to clinical features exhibited by individual patients. Diagnosis rests on the demonstration of high plasma VIP levels in the setting of a stool volume of at least 1 L/d. Lesser increases in VIP levels occur in patients with hepatic failure and intestinal ischemia.

VIPomas are most commonly pancreatic tumors. Unlike gastrinomas and insulinomas, however, VIPomas frequently grow to a large size before becoming clinically apparent. On average, the size of these tumors at the time of diagnosis is second only to that of nonfunctioning pancreatic islet cell tumors. Although they are slow-growing, these tumors are usually malignant. Approximately three-fifths are metastatic at the time of diagnosis. Most VIPomas are located in the body or tail of the pancreas. A few cases have been seen in association with MEN 1. However, there is no constant relation between the two syndromes. Between 10 and 15 percent of VIP-secreting tumors arise from neuroendocrine cells in the intestinal mucosa, and a few are ganglioneuroblastomas, mastocytomas, pheochromocytomas, or small cell carcinomas of the lung.

Treatment is surgical extirpation whenever possible. However, metastases may preclude this approach. Preoperative evaluation should include CT to localize the tumor and any metastases that may be present. In addition to supportive therapy with fluids and electrolytes, prednisone is frequently effective in reducing the volume of diarrhea, despite its inability to alter serum VIP levels. Octreotide inhibits the secretion of VIP and ameliorates symptoms in most patients. VIPomas often produce symptoms related to the large size of the tumor itself. Surgery may be indicated to relieve local effects or to remove a single large primary tumor. For patients with symptomatic metastatic disease, chemotherapy and hepatic artery embolization have the greatest benefit on tumor burden. Regimens combining streptozocin and doxorubicin or streptozocin-fluorouracil are the most effective chemotherapy, inducing objective partial remission in up to 90 percent of cases.

GLUCAGONOMA

In 1966, McGovern described a rare syndrome of diabetes mellitus and necrolytic migratory erythema in association with a pancreatic islet cell tumor. The observation that these tumors secrete high levels of glucagon suggested a cause for the diabetes and that the peptide may have a role in the other clinical features. Although these tumors frequently synthesize and secrete additional peptides, including pancreatic polypeptide, somatostatin, insulin, and gastrin, the common link is hyperglucagonemia. Glucagonomas are characteristically single, large, and slow-growing. More than 75 percent have metastasized at the time of diagnosis, most commonly to the liver and bones. Glucagonoma has been reported in association with MEN 1 (see Chap. 343). A fasting plasma glucagon of >1000 ng/L (>1000 pg/mL) establishes the diagnosis. More modest elevations of plasma glucagon levels may occur in diabetic ketoacidosis, renal failure, hepatic failure, sepsis, prolonged fasting, and gluten-sensitive enteropathy. Hypocholesterolemia and hypoaminoacidemia are common, with alanine, glycine, and serine levels usually less than 25 percent of normal. Glucagonoma may be distinguished from other hyperglucagonemic syndromes by the failure of glucose to suppress and the failure of arginine to enhance serum glucagon concentrations.

The characteristic glucagonoma skin rash is erythematous, raised, scaly, sometimes bullous, sometimes psoriatic, and ultimately crusted. It is located primarily on the face, abdomen, perineum, and distal extremities. After resolution, the regions of the acute eruption usually remain indurated and hyperpigmented. Patients also may experience glossitis, stomatitis, angular cheilitis, dystrophic nails, and hair thinning. The diabetes is usually mild or asymptomatic and may manifest only as an abnormality on an oral glucose tolerance test. Ketoacidosis has not been reported. Weight loss, hypoaminoacidemia, anemia, and thromboembolic disease also occur in association with this syndrome. A causal association between hyperglucagonemia and skin disease has been difficult to prove, leading to speculation that the rash may result from nutritional deficiency. In some patients, the rash responds to oral zinc or intravenous amino acid therapy. Octreotide therapy also has yielded good results. However, dermatologic symptoms frequently recur after each of these therapies.

Because the tumor is usually large and found only in the pancreas, it is easily identified by CT, ultrasound, or angiography. Surgical therapy is curative in approximately 30 percent of patients. Resection is more frequently aimed at decreasing tumor burden. Despite occasional objective responses, attempts at chemotherapy with combinations of streptozocin, fluorouracil, doxorubicin, and dacarbazine have little impact. Fortunately, the slow-growing nature of the tumor allows for prolonged survival even in many cases of metastatic disease.

SOMATOSTATINOMA

Somatostatin-secreting tumors are the most recent group to be identified with a defined clinical syndrome. The classic triad of somatostatinoma comprises diabetes mellitus,

TABLE 277-1 Disorders of the immune system

IMMUNODEFICIENCIES

Primary immunodeficiencies
Combined immunodeficiencies
  Severe combined immunodeficiency
    X-linked
    Autosomal recessive
  Adenosine deaminase (ADA) deficiency
  Purine nucleoside phosphorylase (PNP) deficiency
  MHC class II deficiency
  MHC class I deficiency (bare leukocyte syndrome)
  Reticular dysgenesis
Predominantly antibody deficiencies
  X-linked agammaglobulinemia
  X-linked hypogammaglobulinemia with growth hormone deficiency
  Ig deficiency with increased IgM (hyper-IgM syndrome)
  Ig heavy chain gene deletions
  κ chain deficiency
  IgA deficiency
  Selective deficiency of IgG subclasses
  Common variable immunodeficiency (CVID)
  Transient hypogammaglobulinemia of infancy
  Secretory component deficiency
Other well-defined immunodeficiency syndromes
  Wiskott-Aldrich syndrome
  Ataxia-telangiectasia
  Third and fourth pouch/arch syndrome (Di George)
Syndromes associated with immunodeficiency
  Chromosome abnormalities
    Bloom syndrome
    Fanconi syndrome
    Down syndrome
  Multiple organ system abnormalities
    Partial albinism
    Short-limbed dwarfism
    Cartilage hair hypoplasia
    Agenesis of corpus callosum
  Hereditary metabolic defects
    Transcobalamin II deficiency
    Acrodermatitis enteropathica (zinc deficiency)
    Type I orotic aciduria
    Biotin dependent carboxylase deficiency
  Hypercatabolism of Ig
    Familial hypercatabolism of Ig
    Myotonic dystrophy
    Intestinal lymphangiectasia
  Other
    Hyper-IgE syndrome
    Chronic mucocutaneous candidiasis
    Thymoma
    Immunodeficiency following hereditarily determined
      susceptibility to Epstein-Barr virus (Duncan's syndrome)
Acquired immunodeficiencies
Acquired immunodeficiency syndrome (AIDS)
Iatrogenic
Idiopathic CD4 + T lymphocytopenia

ALLERGIC DISEASES

Generalized
  Anaphylaxis
  Serum sickness
  Generalized drug reactions
  Food allergy
  Insect venom allergy
  Mastocytosis
Airways
  Allergic rhinitis
  Asthma
  Hypersensitivity pneumonitis
Skin
  Urticaria
  Angioedema
  Eczema
  Atopic dermatitis
  Allergic contact dermatitis
  Erythema multiforme and Stevens-Johnson syndrome
Ocular allergy
  Allergic conjunctivitis
  Atopic keratoconjunctivitis
  Venereal keratoconjunctivitis
  Giant papillary conjunctivitis
  Contact allergy

AUTOIMMUNITY

Organ specific
Endocrine system
  Thyroid gland
    Hashimoto's thyroiditis
    Graves' disease
    Thyroiditis with hyperthyroidism
  Type I autoimmune polyglandular syndrome
  Type II autoimmune polyglandular syndrome
  Insulin-dependent diabetes mellitus
  Immune-mediated infertility
  Autoimmune Addison's disease
Skin
  Pemphigus vulgaris
  Pemphigus foliaceus
  Bullus pemphigoid
  Dermatitis herpetiformis
  Linear IgA dermatosis
  Epidermolysis bullosa acquisita
  Autoimmune alopecia
  Erythema nodosa
  Contact dermatitis
  Herpes gestationis
  Cicatricial pemphigoid
  Chronic bullous disease of childhood
Hematologic system
  Autoimmune hemolytic anemia
  Autoimmune thrombocytopenic purpura
    Idiopathic
    Drug-related
  Autoimmune neutropenia
Neuromuscular system
  Myasthenia gravis
  Acute disseminated encephalomyelitis
  Multiple sclerosis
  Guillain-Barré syndrome
  Chronic inflammatory demyelinating polyradiculoneuropathy
Hepatobiliary system
  Autoimmune chronic active hepatitis
  Primary biliary sclerosis
  Sclerosing cholangitis
Gastrointestinal tract
  Gluten-sensitive enteropathy
  Pernicious anemia
  Inflammatory bowel disease

Organ nonspecific
Connective tissue diseases
  Systemic lupus erythematosus
  Rheumatoid arthritis
  Systemic sclerosis (scleroderma)
  Ankylosing spondylitis
  Reactive arthritides
  Polymyositis/dermatomyositis
  Sjögren's syndrome
  Mixed connective tissue disease
  Behçet's syndrome
  Psoriasis
Vasculitic syndromes
  Systemic necrotizing vasculitides
    Classic polyarteritis nodosa
    Allergic angiitis and granulomatosis (Churg-Strauss disease)
    Polyangiitis overlap syndrome
  Hypersensitivity vasculitis
  Wegener's granulomatosis
  Temporal arteritis
  Takayasu's arteritis
  Kawasaki's disease
  Isolated vasculitis of the central nervous system
  Thromboangiitis obliterans
  Miscellaneous vasculitides
Sarcoidosis
Graft-versus-host disease
Cryopathies

TABLE 277-1 Disorders of the immune system (*continued*)

NEOPLASMS

T cell neoplasms
  Adult T cell leukemia/lymphoma
  Acute lymphocytic leukemia
  Cutaneous T cell lymphoma
  Non-Hodgkin's lymphoma
  Hairy cell leukemia
  Acute lymphoblastic leukemia
  Chronic lymphocytic leukemia (rare)
B cell neoplasms
  Chronic lymphocytic leukemia
  Multiple myeloma
  Burkitt's lymphoma
  Hairy cell leukemia
  Acute lymphoblastic leukemia
  Non-Hodgkin's lymphoma
  Waldenström's macroglobulinemia
  Primary amyloidosis
  Heavy chain diseases
    gamma (Franklin's disease)
    alpha (Seligmann's disease)
    mu
Monocyte neoplasms
  Acute monocytic leukemia
  Hodgkin's disease
  Histiocytic lymphoma
  Histiocytosis X
    Eosinophilic granuloma
    Letterer-Siwe disease
    Hand-Schüller-Christian disease
  Malignant histiocytosis (histiocytic medullary reticulosis)
Other
  Proliferation of large granular lymphocytes

immunity, with subsets of T cells maturing into cytotoxic cells capable of lysis of virus-infected or foreign cells. T cells are also the primary regulatory cells of T and B lymphocyte and monocyte function by the production of lymphokines and by direct cell contact. In addition, T cells regulate erythroid cell maturation in bone marrow.

Human T cells express cell surface proteins that mark stages of intrathymic T cell maturation; many of these molecules mediate or augment specific T cell function (Table 277-2, Fig. 277-2).

A number of cytokines regulate the process of T cell proliferation and differentiation (Table 277-4). The earliest identifiable cells of T lineage are CD34+ pro-T cells (i.e., cells in which T cell receptor genes are neither rearranged nor expressed); they are found in fetal liver, yolk sac, and postnatal bone marrow. In the thymus, CD7+ T cell precursors begin cytoplasmic (c) synthesis of components of the CD3 complex of T cell receptor–associated molecules (see Fig. 277-2). Within CD7+, CD2+, and cCD3+ T cell precursors, T cell receptor (TCR) gene rearrangement begins and eventuates in two T cell lineages, expressing either TCRαβ chains or TCRγδ chains (see Chap. 278). T cells expressing the TCRαβ chains comprise the majority of peripheral T cells in blood, lymph node, and spleen and terminally differentiate into either CD4+ or CD8+ cells. Cells expressing TCRγδ chains circulate as a minor population in blood; their functions, although not fully known, have been postulated as immune surveillance at epithelial surfaces and in cellular defenses against mycobacterial organisms. CD1, CD4, and CD8 are expressed on immature cortical thymocytes; however, upon functional maturity, T cell expression of CD1 ceases and T cell subset antigens CD4 and CD8 are reciprocally expressed. Mature CD4+ TCRαβ+ cells induce B cell differentiation, induce CD8+ cytotoxic T cell proliferation, produce various lymphokines, and regulate certain stages of erythropoiesis. A subset of CD4+ cells also may function as cytotoxic effector cells, recognizing foreign peptide antigen fragments that are physically associated with MHC class II molecules on antigen-presenting cells. CD8+ TCRαβ+ cells function as suppressors of B cell antibody synthesis or as cytotoxic effector T cells, recognizing foreign peptide antigen fragments associated with MHC class I molecules (see Chap. 64).

T cell maturation stages are clinically relevant in that T cell acute lymphoblastic leukemia and lymphomas are malignancies of pro-T, pre-T, or immature T cells, while forms of cutaneous T cell lymphoma

expansion of virgin peripheral T cells into "memory" T cells that reside primarily in peripheral lymphoid organs. Mature T lymphocytes contribute 70 to 80 percent of normal peripheral blood lymphocytes, 90 percent of thoracic duct lymphocytes, 30 to 40 percent of lymph node cells, and 20 to 30 percent of spleen lymphoid cells. In lymph nodes, T cells occupy deep paracortical areas around B cell germinal centers, and in the spleen, they are in periarteriolar areas of white pulp (see Chap. 58). T cells are the primary effectors of cell-mediated

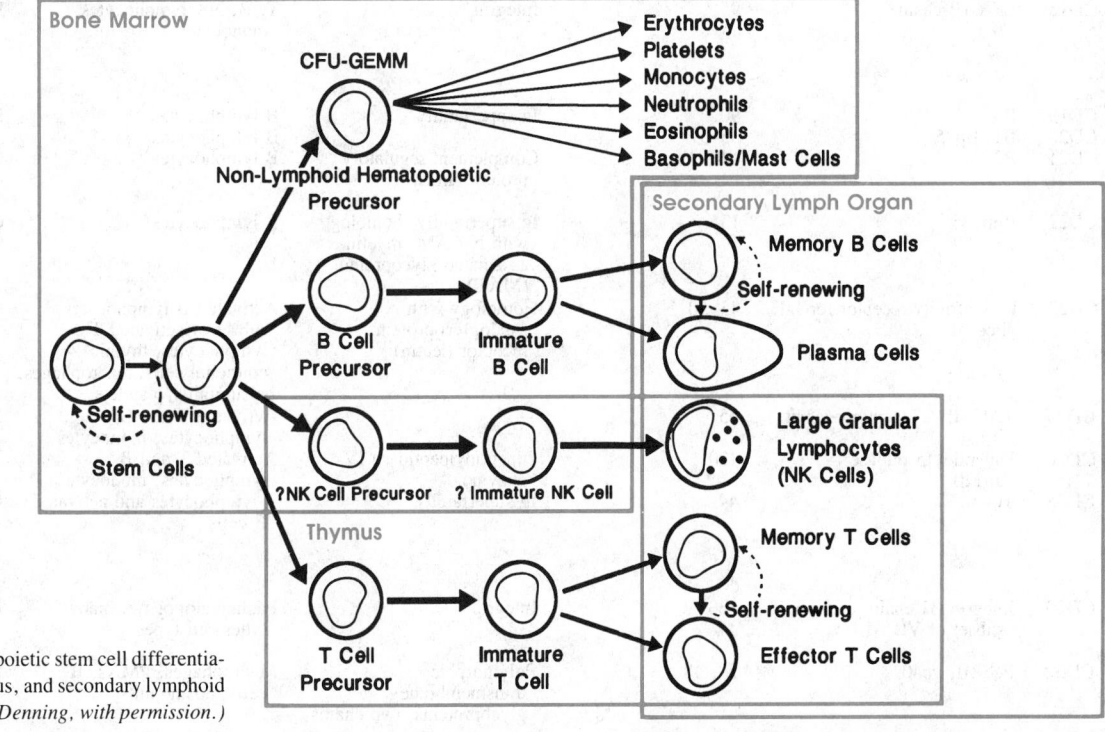

FIGURE 277-1 Hematopoietic stem cell differentiation in bone marrow, thymus, and secondary lymphoid organs. (*After Haynes and Denning, with permission.*)

TABLE 277-2   CD classification of human lymphocyte surface molecule

CD	Other names	Molecular mass, kDa	Molecular structure	Tissue/lineage	Function
CD1	T6	49,000	Ig superfamily associated with β2M	Cortical thymocytes, Langerhans cells, interdigitating cells	Antigen presentation to TCRγδ cells
CD2	T11, LFA-3 receptor, E-rosette receptor	50,000	Ig superfamily	T lymphocytes	Binds LFA-3 (CD58) on RBC, monocytes, thymic epithelial cells; alternative pathway of T cell activation
CD3	T3, CD3 complex, Leu4	CD3γ—26 CD3δ—20 CD3ε—20 CD3ζ—16 CD3η—28	CD3γ,δ,ε Ig superfamily; CD3 η, ζ; homologous to each other and with FcRε ζ chain comprise α family of signal transducers	CD3γ,δ,ε,ζ,η, T lymphocytes, cytoplasmic CD3ε, NK cells	T cell–associated molecules; transduce signals from T cell receptors
CD4	T4, Leu3a	59	Ig superfamily	T lymphocytes, monocytes, tissue macrophages, microglial cells, EBV-transformed B lymphocytes	Receptor for HIV env gp120; binds to HLA class II; associated with p56-lck tyrosine kinase
CD5	T1	67	Ig superfamily	T lymphocytes, B lymphocyte subset	Comitogenic for T lymphocytes; ligand for CD72
CD6	T12	100	Scavenger receptor type I superfamily	Subset of T and B lymphocytes	?
CD7	3A1, Leu9	40	Ig superfamily	T lymphocytes, NK cells; on subsets of T, B, and myeloid precursors	Comitogenic for T lymphocytes; Ca²⁺ inducible gene
CD8	T8, Leu2a	CD8α—38 CD8β—38	CD8 α, β, Ig superfamily	T cell subset	Receptor for MHC class I; associated with p56-lck tyrosine kinase
CD10	J5, CALLA, neutral endopeptidase	100	Endopeptidase enzyme	B lymphoid progenitor cells	Peptide cleavage
CD11a	LFA-1α chain	180	Integrin	T, B, NK lymphocytes, monocytes	With β2 integrin, ligand for ICAM-1 (CD54), ICAM-2, and ICAM-3; mediates leukocyte adhesion and leukocyte-endothelial adherence
CD11b	MAC-1, MO-1α chain, CR3	165	Integrin	NK cells, PMNs, monocytes	With β2 integrin, receptor for C3bi, fibrinogen, factor X
CD11c	gp150/95 α chain, CR4	150	Integrin	NK cells, PMNs, monocytes	With β2 integrin, mediates cell binding to C3bi
CD14	LeuM3, MO-2	55	Phosphoinositol-linked transmembrane glycoprotein	Monocytes	Endotoxin binding protein
CD15	Sialyl Lewis X (sLeˣ)	Carbohydrate	Neu Acα 2–3 Gal β1–4 (Fucα1–3) GlcNac	Granulocytes; cryptic form of CD15 is on T cells [Cutaneous lymphocyte antigen (CLA)]	Ligand for ELAM-1 on endothelial cells; CLA mediates T cell homing to skin
CD16	Fc receptor for IgG (low affinity) FcRγIII	50–65	Ig superfamily, PI and TM forms	NK cells, PMN, macrophages	FcR for IgG
CD18	LFA-1β chain	95	Integrin	T, B, NK lymphocytes, monocytes	Ligand for ICAM-1 (CD54), ICAM-2, and ICAM-3; mediates leukocyte-endothelial interactions
CD19	B4	90	Ig superfamily	B lymphocytes	Regulates B cell activation
CD20	B1, Bp35	35–37	—	B lymphocytes	Mediates B cell activation
CD21	B2	140	Complement regulatory protein family	B lymphocytes	C3d/EBV receptor, complement receptor 2 (CR2), ligand for CD23
CD22	Bgp135	135	Ig superfamily, homology with N-CAM, myelin-associated glycoprotein (MAG)	B lymphocytes	Comitogenic for B cell activation, interacts with CD45RO on T cells and CD75 on B cells
CD23	Low-affinity receptor for IgE FcεRII	45–50	Homology with asialoglycoprotein receptor (lectin)	Activated B lymphocytes, subset of activated T lymphocytes, thymic epithelial cells, macrophages, eosinophils, platelets	FcεRII, soluble CD23 activates immature T cells, ligand for CD21
CD25	TAC, IL-2 receptor α chain	55	—	Activated T and B lymphocytes, monocytes	Low-affinity receptor for IL-2
CD26	Dipeptidylpeptidase IV, gp120	120	Dipeptidylpeptidase IV enzyme	Activated T and B lymphocytes, monocytes	Serine exopeptidase; binds collagen
CD28	Tp44	44	Ig superfamily	T lymphocytes and activated B cells	Comitogenic for T lymphocytes, regulates T cell cytokine stability, Ligand for B7/BB1 molecules
CD29	Integrin β1 chain; common β subset of VLA-1-6	130	Integrin	Panhematopoietic, many other cell types	Ligand for many extracellular matrix molecules
CD32	FcδRII, gp40	39, 48	Polymorphic transmembrane glycoproteins, two chains	Macrophages, PMNs, B cells, eosinophils	Fc receptor for aggregated IgG, ligation leads to cell activation

TABLE 277-2   CD classification of human lymphocyte surface molecule (*continued*)

CD	Other names	Molecular mass, kDa	Molecular structure	Tissue/lineage	Function
CD34	MY10	105–120	Sialomucin with unique protein sequence	T lymphocyte, other hematopoietic precursors	?
CD35	CR1, C3b receptor	160–250	—	B cells, subset NK cells, PMNs, monocytes, RBC	Binds immune complexes
CD38	OKT10, T10	45	Single-chain glycoprotein	Activated lymphocytes, immature B cells	?
CD39	gp80	70–100	—	Activated B lymphocytes, T lymphocytes, and NK cells	Mediates homotypic adhesion of B cells
CD40	gp50	44–48	Homology with nerve growth factor receptor, fas(APO-1), and TNF receptor	B cells, follicular dendritic cells, macrophages	B cell activation, homotypic adhesion; binds to a TNF-like molecule, gp39, that is defective in X-linked hyper-IgM syndrome
CD43	Leukosialin, sialophorin, leukocyte sialoglycoprotein	95	Cell surface sialomucin	T, B, NK cells, monocytes	Involved in leukocyte activation, deficient in Wiskott-Aldrich syndrome, ligand for ICAM-1
CD44	Pgp-1, In(Lu)-related p80, Hermes, extracellular matrix receptor III	80–120	Cartilage link protein, core proteoglycan homology; multiple isoforms generated by alternative splicing	T, B, NK cells, monocytes, RBC	Transmembrane hyaluronate receptor, promotes leukocyte adhesion; comitogenic for T cells, mediates leukocyte-endothelial binding; promotes carcinoma metastasis
CD45	Leukocyte common antigen, T200	CD45RO—180 CD45RA—220 CD45RB—220, 205, 190	Multiple isoforms generated by alternative splicing	Leukocytes	Cytoplasmic domain is a tyrosine phosphatase, regulates lymphocyte activation, CD45RO in T cells is a ligand for CD22 on B cells
CD49b	VLA-2α chain	170	Integrin	Activated T cells, platelets	With β1 integrin, binds collagen
CD49d	VLA-4α chain	150	Integrin	T and B lymphocytes, monocytes	With β integrin, is the receptor for endothelial VCAM-1; mediates leukocyte–endothelial cell binding in Peyer's patches
CD54	ICAM-1	40	Ig superfamily	Endothelial cells, activated lymphocytes	Ligand for LFA-1, rhinoviruses, falciparum malaria, CD43
CD56	N-CAM, NKH-1	140	Ig superfamily, homology with N-CAM	NK cells	Mediates NK cell homotypic adhesion
CD57	HNK1, Leu7	110		NK cells, subset of T cells	?
CD58	LFA-3	40–65	Ig superfamily	Widespread, activated lymphocytes	Ligand for CD2
CD64	FcgRI, high-affinity receptor for IgG	75	Transmembrane glycoprotein	Monocytes, tissue macrophages	Binds monomeric IgG with high affinity, ligation leads to cell activation
CD69	Activation inducer molecule, EA-1, gp34/28	28, 34	Homodimer; type II membrane protein related to NK cell activation protein family	Activated B, T, NK cells, monocytes	Ligand binding to CD69 triggers cytolytic activity of NK and TCRγδ T cells
CD71	T9, transferrin receptor	95	Heterodimer	Activated T and B lymphocytes, monocytes, proliferating cells of many types	Binds transferrin
CD72	—	39, 43	Heterodimer	B cells	Ligand for CD5 molecule
CD73	Ecto-5′ nucleotidase	69	Nucleotidase enzyme	Subsets of B and T lymphocytes	Regulates uptake of nucleotides

(mycosis fungoides, Sézary syndrome) and the syndrome of adult T cell leukemia (associated with HTLV-I infection) share the phenotype of mature (usually CD4+) T cells.

Molecular basis of T cell recognition of antigen The T cell antigen receptor is a complex of molecules consisting of an antigen-binding heterodimer of either αβ or γδ chains noncovalently linked with five CD3 subunits (γ, δ, ε, ζ, and η) (Fig. 277-3). The CD3 ζ chains are either disulfide-linked homodimers (CD3-ζ₂) or disulfide-linked heterodimers composed of one ζ chain and one η chain. TCRαβ or TCRγδ molecules must be associated with CD3 molecules to be inserted into the T cell surface membrane, TCRα being paired with TCRβ and TCRγ being paired with TCRδ. Molecules of the

CD3 complex mediate transduction of T cell activation signals via T cell receptors, while TCRα and β or γ and δ molecules combine to form the TCR antigen-binding site.

The α, β, γ, and δ T cell antigen receptor molecules have amino acid sequence homology and structural similarities to immunoglobulin heavy and light chains, and like many functionally relevant molecules of immune cells (e.g., MHC class I or II, CD2, CD4, CD8), they are therefore members of the *immunoglobulin gene superfamily* of molecules. The TCRβ and δ chains contain four separately encoded regions, namely, the V (variable), D (diversity), J (joining), and C (constant) regions, and the TCRα and γ chains consist of V, J, and C regions. Thus molecules of the T cell antigen receptor have constant

TABLE 277-3 Cytokines that regulate multipotent or pluripotent hematopoietic stem cell (HSC) proliferation and differentiation

Cytokine	Other names/abbreviation	Effect on stem cells
Interleukin 1α,β	IL-1αβ	Indirectly stimulates HSC by inducing IL-6 production from BM stromal cells
Interleukin 3	IL-3	Promotes survival of HSC; synergizes with IL-11, LIF, and SCF for entry of HSC into cell cycle
Interleukin 4	IL-4, B cell differentiating factor (BCDF)	Synergizes with IL-11 for entry of HSC into cell cycle
Interleukin 6	IL-6	Synergizes with IL-3 for HSC differentiation into myeloid lineages
Interleukin 11	IL-11	Synergizes with IL-3 and SCF for entry of HSC into cell cycle
Stem cell factor	SCF, c-kit ligand, steel factor (SLF), mast cell differentiating factor	Synergizes with IL-3, IL-6, IL-11, G-CSF, and GM-CSF for HSC proliferation
Basic fibroblast growth Factor	BFGF	Synergizes with IL-3 and GM-CSF for HSC activation
Granulocyte colony stimulating factor	G-CSF	Stimulates HSC entry into cell cycle
Granulocyte/monocyte-macrophage colony stimulating factor	GM-CSF	Synergizes with SCF, IL-11, and IL-3 for HSC activation
Leukemia inhibitory factor	LIF, HILDA, DIA	Inhibits proliferation of HSC
Macrophage inflammatory protein 1α	MIP1α, stem cell inhibitor 1 (SCI-1)	Inhibits proliferation of embryonic stem cells but synergizes with SCF entry of HSC into cell cycle
Transforming growth factor β	TGF-β	Inhibits proliferation of HSC

SOURCE: Adapted with permission from Haynes and Denning.

and variable regions, and the genes encoding the α, β, γ, and δ chains of these molecules undergo rearrangement during T cell maturation, culminating in synthesis of the completed molecule.

The variable region elements of α, β, γ, and δ genes, which are separate in the germ line, are brought together by DNA rearrangement and deletion during intrathymic differentiation of the T lymphocyte.

Thus TCR diversity is due to the large numbers of V-J or V-D-J combinations formed during TCR gene rearrangement. As T cells mature in the thymus, the repertoire of antigen-reactive T cells is generated by selection processes that eliminate many autoreactive T cells, enhance the proliferation of needed antigen-reactive T cells, and allow T cells with nonuseful TCR to die (see below).

FIGURE 277-2 Human T cell maturation. sCD3 = surface CD3 expression, cCD3 = cytoplasmic CD3 expression.

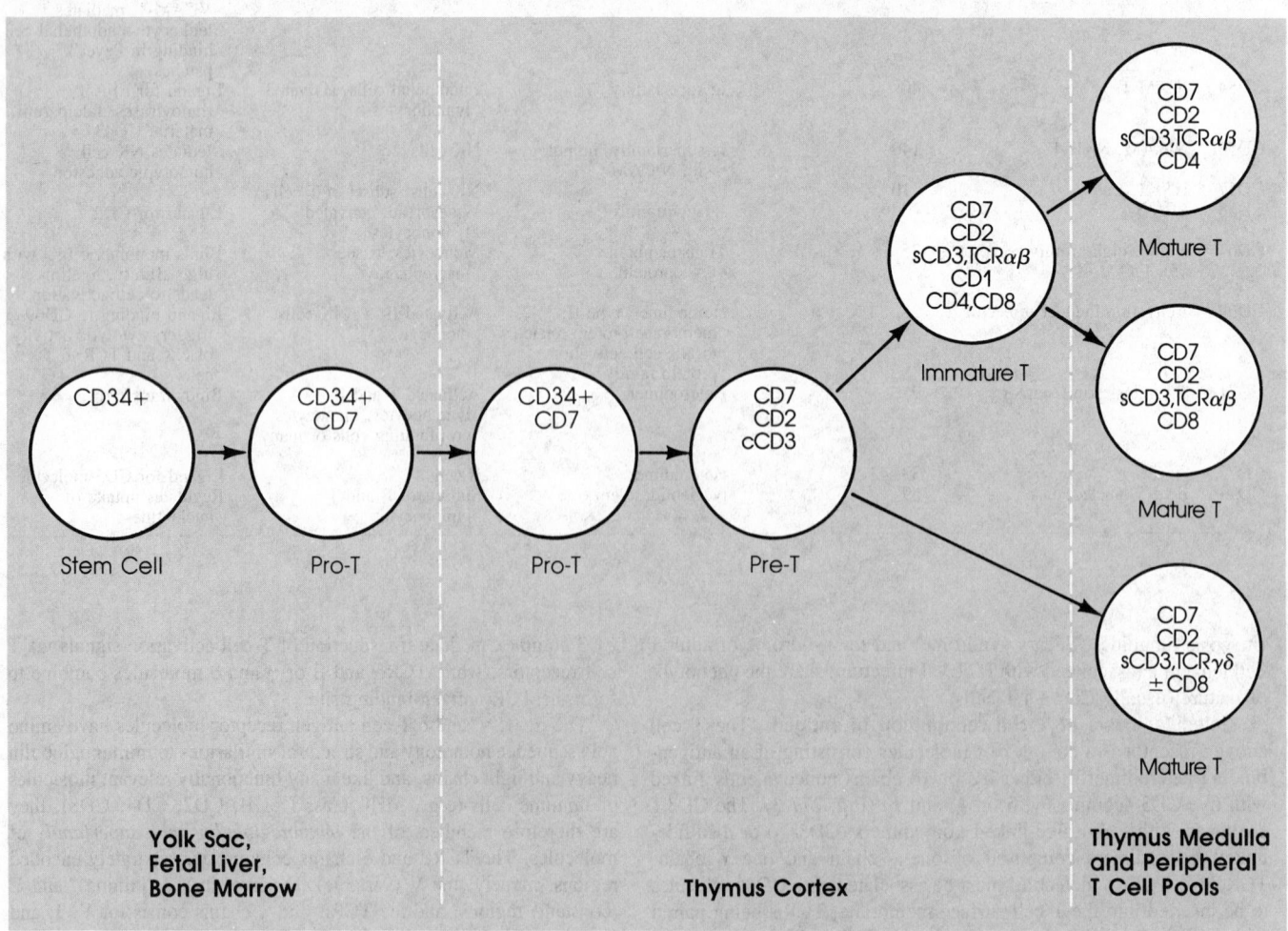

TABLE 277-4   Roles of cytokines in T cell proliferation and differentiation

Cytokine	Source within thymus	Function
IL-1α,β	Macrophages, TE cells, fibroblasts, endothelial cells, dendritic cells	Induces proliferation of thymocytes; induces production of other cytokines (i.e., IL-6, GM-CSF); with sCD23, induces TCRαβ maturation in T cell precursors
IL-2	Activated T cells	Induces proliferation of mature and immature thymocytes
IL-4	T cells	Induces proliferation of thymocytes; inhibits growth of TE cells
IL-5	Activated T cells	Induces cytotoxic T cell differentiation
IL-6	Activated T and B cells, macrophages, fibroblasts, TE cells, endothelial cells	Synergizes with mitogen or IL-1 for T cell/thymocyte proliferation
IL-7	Fibroblasts, BM stromal cell line	Comitogenic factor for thymocytes and T cells
IL-8	Monocytes-macrophages	Chemotactic for T cells
IL-10	Fetal and postnatal thymocytes, B cells	Costimulant for immature and mature thymocyte proliferation and maturation; inhibits cytokine production by mature T cells
Soluble CD23 (FcεRII)	TE cells, B cells	With IL-1, induces TCRαβ maturation in T cell precursors
GM-CSF	Activated T cells, fibroblasts, endothelial cells, T cells	Promotes growth of early T cell leukemias; promotes proliferation of immature thymocytes
G-CSF	TE cells, macrophages, fibroblasts	?Mitogenic for immature thymocytes
M-CSF	TE cells, monocytes, fibroblasts, endothelial cells	Supports differentiation of progenitors committed to the monocyte-macrophage lineages; ?mitogenic for immature thymocytes
LIF	TE cells, activated cells	?Prevents multilineage differentiation of intrathymic stem cells prior to signal to become T cell precursors
IFN-γ	Activated T cells, thymocytes	Up-regulates expression of TE, fibroblast, and macrophage CD54 (ICAM-1) and MHC class II; antiproliferative effect on thymocytes via adenylate cyclase pathway
TNF-α	Macrophages, activated T and B cells, thymocytes	IL-1–like effects
TGF-α	Activated macrophages, TE cells	Regulates production of other cytokines (IL-1 and IL-6) by TE cells; drives TE cell proliferation and/or differentiation via EGF receptor
TGF-β	?TE cells, T cells	Regulates expression of several oncogenes; suppresses lymphocyte responses to other cytokines; ?inhibits TE cell proliferation
EGF	?Monocytes-macrophages, ?fibroblasts, ?TE cells	Drives TE cell proliferation

NOTE: Unless otherwise stated, effect reported or postulated is in humans. TE = thymic epithelial; BM = bone marrow; EGF = epidermal growth factor; LIF = leukemia inhibitory factor; IFN-γ = γ-interferon; TNF = tumor necrosis factor; TGF = transforming growth factor; FcεRII = Fc receptor for IgE type II; IL = interleukin.
SOURCE: After Haynes et al.

T cells do not recognize native protein, carbohydrate or lipid antigens. Instead, T cells recognize only short (approximately 9 to 13 amino acids) peptide fragments that are derived from protein antigens taken up or produced in antigen-presenting cells. Foreign antigen is either taken up by endocytosis (exogenous antigen-presentation pathway) or arises exogenously (i.e., from an infectious agent) in antigen-presenting cells such as macrophages or dendritic cells (exogenous antigen-presentation pathway). Antigen-presenting cells proteolytically degrade foreign proteins and display peptide fragments embedded in the MHC class I or II antigen recognition site on the MHC molecule surface, where foreign peptide fragments bind to TCRαβ or TCRγδ chains of reactive T cells. CD4 molecules act as an adhesive and, by direct binding to MHC class II (DR, DQ, or DP) molecules, stabilize the interaction of TCR with peptide antigen (see Fig. 277-3). Similarly, CD8 molecules stabilize the TCR-antigen interaction by direct binding to MHC class I (A, B, or C) molecules.

Whereas it is generally agreed that the TCRαβ receptor recognizes peptide antigens in MHC class I or class II molecules, recent data suggest that the TCRγδ receptor may bind to other non-MHC molecules such as CD1.

Just as foreign antigens are degraded and their peptide fragments presented in the context of MHC class I or class II molecules on antigen-presenting cells, endogenous self-proteins are also degraded and self-peptide fragments are presented to T cells in the context of MHC class I or class II molecules on antigen-presenting cells. In peripheral lymphoid organs, T cells are present that are capable of recognizing self-protein fragments but normally are *anergic* and are nonresponsive to self-antigenic stimulation.

The specificity of reactivity of mature T cells is largely determined within the thymus during fetal and early postnatal development. In the thymus, the recognition of self-peptides on thymic epithelial cells and thymic macrophages is thought to play an important role in

shaping the T cell repertoire to recognize foreign antigen *(positive selection)* and in eliminating highly autoreactive T cells *(negative selection)*. As immature cortical thymocytes begin to express surface TCR, autoreactive thymocytes are destroyed *(negative selection)*, thymocytes with TCR capable of interacting with foreign antigen peptides in the context of self MHC antigens are activated and develop to maturity *(positive selection)*, and thymocytes with TCR that are incapable of binding to self MHC antigens die of attrition *(no selection)*. Mature thymocytes that are positively selected are either CD4 + helper T cells or MHC class II–restricted cytotoxic (killer) T cells, or they are CD8 + T cells destined to become MHC class I–restricted cytotoxic T cells. For T cells to be *MHC class I–* or *class II–restricted* means that T cells recognize antigen peptide fragments as immunogenic only when they are presented in the antigen recognition site of the same MHC antigens expressed by the thymic microenvironment during the time of T cell selection.

Once ligation of mature T cell TCR by foreign peptide occurs in the context of self MHC class I or class II molecules (see Fig. 277-3), binding of non-antigen-specific adhesion ligand pairs such as CD54-CD11/CD18 and CD58/CD2 is up-regulated to stabilize MHC peptide–TCR binding (see Fig. 277-3). Once TCR-MHC binding is stabilized, activation signals are transmitted to the T cell via tyrosine kinases associated with CD4 or CD8 molecules (p56-lck) and CD3 molecules (pp59-fyn), and ligation of CD28 by B7/BB1 molecules on antigen-presenting cells leads to T cell cytokine (IL-2, IL-4) mRNA stabilization. All these events lead to enhanced T cell activation. For control of T cell activation, the cytoplasmic tyrosine phosphatase domain of the CD45 family of molecules modulates the activation status of the triggered T cells by modifying the activity of intracellular tyrosine kinases p56-lck and pp59-fyn. Thus a concert of molecular and biochemical events is required for normal T cell recognition of antigen and subsequent T cell activation.

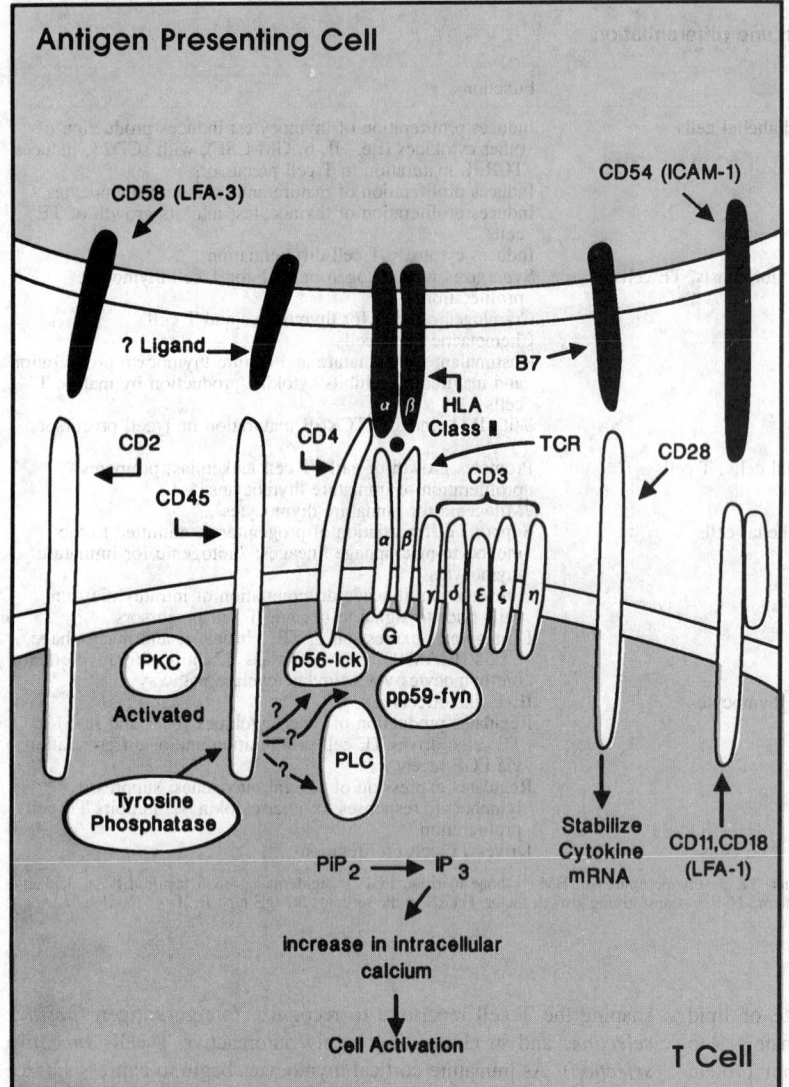

FIGURE 277-3 Molecules involved in human T cell recognition of antigen and in human T cell activation. The black circle at the tip of the αβ chains of HLA class II molecules represents a peptide fragment of "processed" protein antigen. TCRαβ and HLA (MHC) class II αβ + peptide interactions are stabilized by adhesion-ligand pairs such as LFA-1/ICAM-1 and CD2/LFA-3. Ligand binding to T cell CD28 induces stabilization of T cell–activating cytokines such as IL-2 and promotes T cell activation. Intracellular signals for T cell activation are mediated by the CD3 TCR-associated molecules and involve the activation of protein kinase C (PKC), the production of phospholipase C (PLC), and phosphorylation of proteins by the tyrosine kinases p56-lck and pp59-fyn. These events lead to production of phosphoinositol molecules (PIP2 and IP3) that mediate rises in intracellular calcium and eventually cell activation.

Superantigens in T cell development *Superantigens* are protein molecules capable of activating up to 20 percent of the peripheral T cell pool, whereas conventional antigens activate fewer than 1 in 10,000 T cells. T cell superantigens include staphylococcal enterotoxins, other bacterial products, and retroviral proteins. Conventional antigens bind to MHC class I or II molecules in the groove of the αβ heterodimer and bind to T cells via V regions of both TCRα and β chains. In contrast, superantigens bind directly to TCRβ chains and MHC class II β chains at sites that differ from conventional antigen peptides and stimulate T cells based solely on the Vβ gene utilized regardless of the D, J, and Vα chain present (Fig. 277-4). Superantigen stimulation of human peripheral T cells occurs in the clinical setting of the *staphylococcal toxic shock syndrome* leading to massive overproduction of T cell cytokines (see Chap. 102).

B CELLS Mature B cells comprise 10 to 15 percent of human peripheral blood lymphocytes, 50 percent of splenic lymphocytes, and approximately 10 percent of bone marrow lymphocytes. B cells express on their surface intramembrane immunoglobulin (Ig) molecules that function as B cell antigen receptors in a complex of Ig-associated α and β signaling molecules with intracellular signaling events similar to those in T cells (Fig. 277-5). B cells also express surface receptors for the Fc region of IgG molecules (CD32) as well as receptors for activated complement components (C3d or CD21, C3b or CD35). The primary function of B cells is to produce antibodies. Mature B cells are derived from bone marrow precursor cells that arise continuously throughout life (see Fig. 277-1).

B lymphocyte development can be separated into two phases: antigen-independent and antigen-dependent B cell development. Antigen-independent B cell development occurs in primary lymphoid organs, including fetal liver and bone marrow, and includes all stages of B cell maturation up to the surface (s) Ig + mature B cell. Antigen-dependent B cell maturation is driven by the interaction of antigen with B cell sIg leading to memory B cell induction and plasma cell formation. Antigen-dependent stages of B cell maturation occur in secondary lymphoid organs, including lymph node, spleen, and gut Peyer's patches. In contrast to the T cell repertoire that is generated intrathymically before contact with foreign antigen, the repertoire of B cells expressing diverse antigen-reactive sites is generated by further recombination of immunoglobulin genes after contact with antigen—a process called *somatic mutation*.

During B cell development, diversity of the antigen-binding variable region of Ig is generated by an ordered set of Ig gene rearrangements. First, the process brings diversity (D) segments to joining (J) segments and then brings a variable (V) gene segment and constant (C) segments to yield a functional Ig heavy chain gene (V-D-J-C). During later stages, a functional κ or λ light chain gene is generated by rearrangement of a V segment to a J segment, ultimately yielding an intact Ig molecule composed of heavy and light chains. The most immature B cell precursors (pro-B cells) express surface CD10 and CD34, lack B lineage–specific antigens CD19 and CD22, and also lack cytoplasmic (c) and surface (s) Ig (Fig. 277-6). The next stage in B cell development, the pre-pre-B cell, is marked

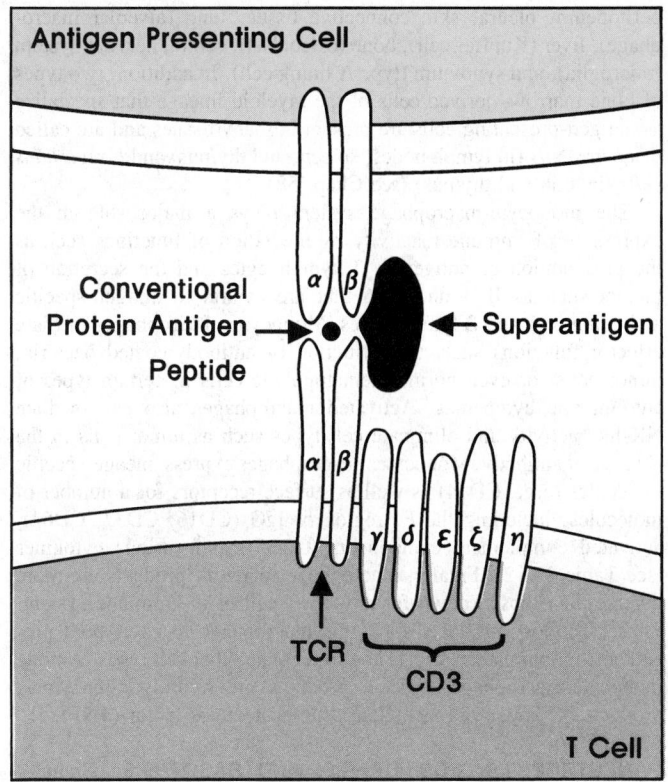

FIGURE 277-4 Comparison of site of superantigen binding to T cell receptor with the site of binding to T cell receptor of processed conventional antigen.

FIGURE 277-5 B cell antigen receptor for antigen-associated molecules. Immunoglobulin (Ig) associated α and β chains are disulfide-linked molecules that mediate the delivery of intracellular activation signals to B cells following interaction of membrane Ig with antigen. CD45 modulates the activation state of B cells by the tyrosine phosphatase activity of the cytoplasmic domain of CD45 molecules.

by the acquisition of CD19 and CD22 B cell antigens. Ig genes undergo rearrangement in pre-pre-B cells, but Ig heavy chain protein is not expressed. The hallmark of the next maturation stage, the pre-B cell, is expression of cμ heavy chain in association with expression of CD73 and CD21 surface proteins. Immature B cells have rearranged Ig light chain genes and express sIgM. As immature B cells develop into mature B cells, sIgD is expressed as well as sIgM and CD23. At this point, B lineage development in bone marrow is complete,

and B cells exit into the peripheral circulation and migrate to secondary lymphoid organs. There are approximately 300 VK genes and 5 JK genes, resulting in the pairing of VK and JK genes to create 1500 different light chain combinations. The number of distinct κ light chains that can be generated is increased by somatic mutations within the VK and JK genes, thus creating a large number of specificities from a limited amount of germ-line genetic information.

In heavy chain immunoglobulin gene rearrangement, the VH domain is created by the joining of three types of germ-line genes called VH, DH, and JH, thus allowing for even greater diversity in the variable region of heavy chains than for light chains (see Chap. 278).

A number of cytokines synergize to drive sequential stages of B cell maturation (Table 277-5). Bone marrow stromal cell– and T cell–derived IL-3 and IL-7 drive the earliest stages of B cell differentiation. Low-molecular-weight B cell growth factor (BCGF) binds to high-

FIGURE 277-6 Antigen-independent human B lymphocyte maturation. *(After Haynes and Denning, with permission.)*

	Stem Cell	Pro-B	Pre-Pre-B	Pre-Pre-B	Pre-B	Immature B	Mature B
	CD34	CD34	CD34	CD34	-	-	-
		CD10	CD10	CD10	-	-	-
			CD19	CD19	CD19	CD19	CD19
			CD40	CD40	CD40	CD40	CD40
				CD73	CD73	CD73	CD73
				CD22	CD22	CD22	CD22
				CD38	CD38	-	-
					CD21	CD21	CD21
							CD23
IL-7 Receptor	-	+	+	-	-	-	-
IL-3 Receptor	-	+	+	+	+	-	-
IL-4 Receptor	-	-	-	-	+	+	+
Immunoglobulin Gene Rearrangement	-	-	+	+	+	+	+
IgM Expression	-	-	-	-	cytoplasm	surface	surface
IgD Expression	-	-	-	-	-	-	surface

TABLE 277-5 Cytokines that regulate human B cell development

Cytokine	Source	Function
IL-7	T cells, bone marrow stromal cells	Drives pro-B and pre-pre-B cells to proliferate and differentiate
BCG-F (low-molecular-weight B cell growth factor)	Activated T cells	B cell precursor proliferation
IL-3	T cells, stromal cells	Induces B cell precursor proliferation
IL-1, IL-2, IL-4, IL-5, IL-6	T cells (IL-2, IL-4, IL-5), monocytes (IL-1, IL-6)	Drives mature B cells to proliferate and differentiate into Ig-secreting cells

affinity receptors expressed on all B cell precursors except pro-B cells and also triggers B cell differentiation. IL-1, IL-2, IL-4, IL-5, and IL-6 synergize to drive mature B cells to proliferate and differentiate into Ig-secreting cells.

LARGE GRANULAR LYMPHOCYTES Large granular lympho-cytes (LGL) (previously called "null cells") constitute approximately 5 to 10 percent of peripheral blood lymphocytes and are nonadherent, nonphagocytic cells with large azurophilic cytoplasmic granules. LGL express surface receptors for the Fc portion of IgG (CD16), and many LGL express some T lineage markers and proliferate in response to IL-2. LGL arise in both bone marrow and thymic microenvironments (see Fig. 277-1).

Functionally, LGL share features with both monocytes-macro-phages and neutrophils in that subsets of LGL mediate antibody-dependent cellular cytotoxicity (ADCC) and natural killer (NK) activity. ADCC is the binding of an opsonized (antibody-coated) target cell to an Fc receptor–bearing effector cell via the Fc region of antibody resulting in lysis of the target by the effector cell. Natural killer (NK) cell activity is the nonimmune (i.e., effector cell never having had previous contact with the target), non-antibody-mediated killing of target cells, which are usually malignant cell types or transplanted foreign cells. Thus LGL that mediate NK activity may play an important role in immune surveillance and destruction of cells that spontaneously undergo malignant transformation in vivo. Lymphokine-activated killer, or LAK, cells are NK lymphocytes that proliferate in vitro to high levels of IL-2 and develop the ability to kill tumor cells efficiently. LAK cells generated with IL-2 in vitro or in vivo from patients with solid tumors such as renal cell carcinomas have shown promising antitumor activity. Rare patients with complete absence of NK cells have been described who lack both NK activity and CD56+, CD16+ lymphocytes but have normal T and B cell function. NK cell hyporesponsiveness is also observed in patients with the *Chédiak-Higashi syndrome,* an autosomal recessive disease associated with fusion of cytoplasmic granules and defective degranu-lation of neutrophil lysosomes. Recently, a series of studies has suggested that NK cells can specifically recognize normal allogeneic cells in a clonal fashion. Studies of allogeneic target cells suggest that the genetic locus controlling NK alloantigen lysis is different from conventional MHC products, is inherited as an autosomal recessive trait, and is located on chromosome 6 in the same region as MHC class I genes.

MONOCYTES-MACROPHAGES Monocytes arise from precur-sor cells within bone marrow (see Fig. 277-1) and circulate with a half-life ranging from 1 to 3 days. Monocytes leave the peripheral circulation by marginating in capillaries and then migrating into a vast extravascular pool. Tissue macrophages arise by migration of monocytes from the circulation and by proliferation of macrophage precursors in tissue. Common locations of tissue macrophages (and some of their specialized names) are lymph node, spleen, bone marrow, perivascular connective tissue, serous cavities such as the

peritoneum, pleura, skin connective tissue, lung (alveolar macro-phage), liver (Kupffer cell), bone (osteoclast), central nervous system (microglia), and synovium (type A lining cell). In addition, two types of bone marrow–derived cells of the myeloid lineage that specialize as antigen-presenting cells are present in many tissues and are called *dendritic cells* (in lymph nodes, spleen, and thymus) and *Langerhans cells* (in skin and thymus) (see Chap. 58).

The monocyte-macrophage system plays a major role in the expression of immune reactivity by mediation of functions such as the presentation of antigen to T lymphocytes and the secretion of factors such as IL-1 and IL-6 that are central to antigen-specific activation of T and B lymphocytes. Monocytes-macrophages mediate effector functions such as destruction of antibody-coated bacteria, tumor cells, or even normal hematopoietic cells in certain types of autoimmune cytopenias. Activated macrophages also can mediate NK-like activity and eliminate cell types such as tumor cells in the absence of antibody. Monocytes-macrophages express lineage-specific molecules (e.g., CD14) as well as surface receptors for a number of molecules, including the Fc region of IgG (CD16, CD32, CD64), activated complement components (CD35), and various cytokines (see Table 277-2). Finally, macrophage secretory products are more diverse than those known for any other cell of the immune system. These secretory products allow the macrophage to exert both pro-and anti-inflammatory effects and to regulate other cell types. Among monocyte-macrophage–secreted products are hydrolytic enzymes, products of oxidative metabolism, tumor necrosis factor (TNF), IL-1, and IL-6.

NEUTROPHILS, EOSINOPHILS, AND BASOPHILS Granulo-cytes are present in nearly all forms of inflammation and are nonspecific amplifiers and effectors of specific immune responses. Unchecked accumulation and activation of granulocytes can lead to host tissue damage, as seen in neutrophil- and eosinophil-mediated *systemic necrotizing vasculitis.* Granulocytes are derived from stem cells in bone marrow (see Fig. 277-1). Each type of granulocyte (neutrophil, eosinophil, or basophil) is derived from a different subclass of progenitor cell which is stimulated to proliferate by colony stimulating factors. During terminal maturation of granulocytes, class-specific nuclear morphology and cytoplasmic granules appear that allow for histologic identification of granulocyte type.

Neutrophils express Fc receptors for IgG (CD16) and receptors for activated complement components (C3b or CD35) (see Table 277-2). Upon interaction of neutrophils with immune complexes, azurophilic granules (containing myeloperoxidase, lysozyme, elas-tase, and other enzymes) and specific granules (containing lactoferrin, lysozyme, collagenase, and other enzymes) are released, and microbi-cidal superoxide radicals (O_2) are generated at the neutrophil surface. The generation of superoxide leads to inflammation by direct injury to tissue and by alteration of macromolecules such as collagen and DNA.

Eosinophils express Fc receptors for IgG (CD32) and are potent cytotoxic effector cells for various parasitic organisms. Intracytoplas-mic contents of eosinophils, such as major basic protein, eosinophil cationic protein, and eosinophil-derived neurotoxin, are capable of directly damaging tissues and may be responsible in part for the organ system dysfunction in the *hypereosinophilic syndromes* (see Chap. 59). Since the eosinophil granule contains anti-inflammatory types of enzymes (histaminase, arylsulfatase, phospholipase D), eosinophils may down-regulate or terminate ongoing inflammatory responses in normal inflammation homeostasis.

The normal functions of basophils and tissue mast cells are not completely understood; the capacity of basophil mediators to increase local delivery of antibodies and complement by increasing vascular permeability is hypothetical. Thus the basophil is identified principally with allergic reactions and some delayed cutaneous hypersensitivity states. Certainly the promotion of increased vascular permeability by basophils is important in the genesis of inflammatory lesions in some vasculitis syndromes (see Chap. 291). Basophils express high affinity surface receptors for IgE (Fc RI) and, upon cross-linking of basophil-

TABLE 277-6   Mediators released from human mast cells and basophils

Mediator	Actions
Histamine	Smooth-muscle contraction, increased vascular permeability
Slow reacting substance of anaphylaxis (SRSA) (leukotriene C_4, D_4, E_4)	Smooth-muscle contraction
Eosinophil chemotactic factor of anaphylaxis (ECF-A)	Chemotactic attraction of eosinophils
Platelet-activating factor	Activates platelets to secrete serotonin and other mediators; smooth-muscle contraction; induces vascular permeability
Neutrophil chemotactic factor (NCF)	Chemotactic attraction of neutrophils
Leukotactic activity (leukotriene B_4)	Chemotactic attraction of neutrophils
Heparin	Anticoagulant
Basophil kallikrein of anaphylaxis (BK-A)	Cleaves kininogen to form bradykinin

FIGURE 277-7 Schematic structure of the immunoglobulin G (IgG) molecule.

bound IgE by antigen, release histamine, eosinophil chemotactic factor of anaphylaxis, and neutral protease—all mediators of immediate (anaphylaxis) hypersensitivity responses (Table 277-6). In addition, basophils express surface receptors for activated complement components (C3a, C5a), through which mediator release can be directly effected (see Chap. 282 for a discussion of tissue mast cells).

HUMORAL MEDIATORS OF SPECIFIC IMMUNITY: IMMUNOGLOBULINS

Immunoglobulins are the products of differentiated B cells and mediate the humoral arm of the immune response. The primary functions of antibodies are to bind specifically to antigen and bring about the inactivation or removal of the offending toxin, microbe, parasite, or other foreign substance from the body. The structural basis of immunoglobulin molecule function and immunoglobulin gene organization has provided insight into the role of antibodies in normal protective immunity and in pathologic immune-mediated damage by immune complexes and autoantibody formation against host determinants.

All immunoglobulins have the basic structure of two heavy and two light chains (Fig. 277-7). Immunoglobulin isotype (i.e., G, M, A, D, E) is determined by the type of Ig heavy chain present. IgG and IgA isotypes can be divided further into subclasses (G1, G2, G3,

G4, and A1, A2) based on specific antigenic determinants on Ig heavy chains. The characteristics of human immunoglobulins are outlined in Table 277-7. The four chains are covalently linked by disulfide bonds. Each chain is made up of a variable (V) region and constant (C) regions (also called *domains*), themselves made up of units of approximately 110 amino acids. Light chains have one variable (VL) and one constant (CL) unit; heavy chains have one variable unit (VH) and three or four constant (CH) units, depending on isotype. As the name suggests, the constant regions of immunoglobulin molecules are made up of homologous sequences and share the same primary structure as all other immunoglobulin chains of the same isotype and subclass. Constant regions are involved in biologic functions of immunoglobulin molecules. The CH2 domain of IgG and the CH4 units of IgM are involved with the binding of the C1q portion of C1. The CH region at the carboxy-terminal end of the IgG molecule, the Fc region (see Fig. 277-7), binds to surface Fc receptors (CD16, CD32, CD64) of macrophages, large granular lymphocytes, B cells, neutrophils, and eosinophils.

Variable regions (VL and VH) constitute the antibody-binding (Fab) region of the molecule. Within the VL and VH regions are hypervariable regions (extreme sequence variability) that constitute the antigen-binding site unique to each immunoglobulin molecule.

TABLE 277-7   Characteristics of human immunoglobulins

	IgG	IgM	IgA	IgD	IgE
Molecular mass, kDa	150	190 (950)*	160 (385)†	175	190
Heavy chain	γ1, γ2, γ3, γ4	μ	α1, α2	δ	ε
Light chain	κ or λ	κ or λ	κ or λ	κ or λ	κ or λ
Adult average serum level, mg/dL	1250 ± 300	125 ± 50	210 ± 50	4	0.03
Half-life, d	23.0	5.1	5.8	2.8	2.5
Classic pathway	IgG1, IgG2, IgG3 yes; IgG4 no	Yes	No	No	No
Alternative pathway	IgG1, IgG2, IgG3 no; IgG4 yes	No	Yes	Yes	Yes
Binding cells via Fc	Macrophages, neutrophils, eosinophils, large granular lymphocytes	Lymphocytes	Lymphocytes	None	Mast cells, basophils, B cells
Other biologic properties	Placental transfer	Primary antibody response, rheumatoid factor	Antibody in mucous secretions	Primary lymphocyte surface molecules	Mediates anaphylaxis, allergy

* IgM circulates as a pentameric molecule.
† Secretory IgA is a dimer.
SOURCE: Adapted with permission from CA Haseman and JD Capra, in *Fundamental Immunology*, WE Paul (ed), 2d ed. New York, Raven, 1989.

The idiotype is determined by the specific region of the Fab portion of the immunoglobulin molecule to which antigen binds. Antibodies against the idiotype portion of an antibody molecule are called *anti-idiotype antibodies*. The formation of such antibodies in vivo during a normal B cell antibody response may generate a negative (or "off") signal to B cells to terminate antibody production.

IgG comprises approximately 75 percent of total serum immunoglobulin. The four IgG subclasses are numbered in order of their level in serum, IgG1 being found in greatest amounts and IgG4 the least. IgG subclasses have clinical relevance in their varying ability to bind macrophage and neutrophil Fc receptors and to activate complement (see Table 277-7). Moreover, selective deficiencies of certain IgG subclasses give rise to clinical syndromes in which the patient is inordinately susceptible to bacterial infections. IgG antibodies are frequently the predominant antibody made after rechallenge of the host with antigen (secondary antibody response).

IgM antibodies normally circulate as a 950-kDa pentamer with 160-kDa monomers joined by a molecule called the *J chain*, a 15-kDa nonimmunoglobulin molecule that also effects polymerization of IgA molecules. IgM is the first immunoglobulin to appear in the immune response (primary antibody response) and is the initial type of antibody made by neonates. Membrane IgM in the monomeric form also functions as a major antigen receptor on the surface of mature B cells (see Fig. 277-5). IgM is an important component of immune complexes in autoimmune diseases. For instance, IgM antibodies against IgG molecules (rheumatoid factors) are present in high titers in *rheumatoid arthritis*, other collagen diseases, and some infectious diseases *(subacute bacterial endocarditis)*. IgM antibody binds the C1 component of complement via the CH4 domain and thus is a potent activator of complement.

IgA comprises only 10 to 15 percent of total serum immunoglobulin but is the predominant class of immunoglobulin in secretions. IgA in secretions (tears, saliva, nasal secretions, gastrointestinal tract fluid, and human milk) is in the form of secretory IgA (sIgA), a polymer consisting of two IgA monomers, a joining molecule called the *J chain*, and a glycoprotein called the *secretory protein*. Of the two IgA subclasses, IgA1 is primarily found in serum, whereas IgA2 is more prevalent in secretions. IgA fixes complement via the alternative complement pathway and has potent antiviral activity in humans by prevention of virus binding to respiratory and gastrointestinal epithelial cells.

IgD is found in minute quantities in serum (see Table 277-7) and along with IgM is a major receptor for antigen on the B cell surface. Present in serum is very low concentrations (see Table 277-7), IgE is the major class of immunoglobulin involved in arming mast cells and basophils by binding to these cells via the Fc region. Antigen cross-linking of IgE molecules on basophil and mast cell surfaces results in release of mediators of the immediate hypersensitivity response (see Table 277-6).

CELLULAR INTERACTIONS IN REGULATION OF THE NORMAL IMMUNE RESPONSE

The net result of activation of the humoral (B cell) and cellular (T cell) arms of the immune system by foreign antigen is the elimination of antigen directly by immune effector cells or in concert with specific antibody. In addition, a series of regulatory cells is activated which modulate T effector cell activation and B cell antibody production. Figure 277-8 is a simplified schematic diagram of the immune system outlining some of these cellular interactions.

T CELL–T CELL AND T CELL–B CELL INTERACTIONS The expression of immune cell function is the result of a complex series of immunoregulatory events that occur in phases. Both T and B lymphocytes mediate immune functions, and each of these cell types, when given appropriate signals, passes through stages, from activation and induction through proliferation, differentiation, and ultimately effector functions. The effector function expressed may be at the end

point of a response, such as secretion of antibody by a differentiated plasma cell, or it might serve a regulatory function that modulates other functions, such as is seen with CD4+ inducer or CD8+ regulatory T lymphocytes, which modulate both differentiation of B cells and activation of CD8+ or CD4+ cytotoxic T cells.

CD4 inducer (or helper) T cells can be subdivided on the basis of cytokines produced. Activated TH1-type inducer T cells secrete interferon-γ (IFN-γ) and IL-2, while activated TH2-type inducer T cells secrete IL-4, IL-5, IL-6, and IL-10. TH1 CD4+ T cells provide T cell help for generation of cytotoxic T cells and generally respond to antigens that lead to delayed hypersensitivity types of immune responses (such as *Mycobacterium tuberculosis*). In contrast, TH2 cells regulate the intensity of immune responses by the secretion of a cytokine, IL-10, that inhibits the production of other cytokines (see Table 277-4). In addition, TH2 CD4+ T cells provide help to B cells for specific Ig production and respond to antigens that require high antibody levels for foreign antigen elimination (such as in certain parasite infections).

As shown in Fig. 277-8, upon activation by antigen-presenting cells, regulatory T cell subsets that produce IL-2, IL-3, IFN-γ, and/or IL-4, IL-5, IL-6, and IL-10 are generated that exert positive and negative forces on effector T and B cells. For B cells, trophic effects are mediated by a variety of cytokines, particularly T cell–derived IL-3, IL-4, and IL-5, which act at sequential stages of B cell maturation, resulting in B cell proliferation, differentiation, and ultimately antibody secretion (see Table 277-5). For cytotoxic T cells, trophic factors include inducer T cell secretion of IL-2 and IFN-γ (see Table 277-4). In addition, B cells themselves are capable of serving as antigen-presenting cells, processing and presenting antigens to T cells, and secreting TNF-α and IL-6.

MONOCYTE–T CELL INTERACTIONS Many of the activation and regulatory effects of lymphocytes and monocytes occur via soluble mediators that regulate T and B cell maturation (see Tables 277-3, 277-4, and 277-5). Monocytes-macrophages are required for optimal activation of T cells by antigens or by mitogens (nonspecific activators of lymphocytes). A soluble macrophage product, IL-1, can substitute in some cases for intact macrophages for activation of lymphocytes. Upon contact with antigens or mitogens, macrophages secrete IL-1, IL-6, and TNF, two effects of which are (1) the induction of receptors for IL-2 on T cells and (2) the induction of T cell IL-2, IL-4, and other cytokine secretion. IL-2, IL-4, and other cytokines, in turn, activate other T cells, resulting in expansion of effector and regulatory T cells that also have been induced to express IL-2, IL-4, and IL-7 receptors (see Fig. 277-8). Effector T cells mediate a variety of functions, including the killing of virus-infected cells, graft rejection, graft-versus-host reaction, delayed-type hypersensitivity, and the release of a wide spectrum of immunoregulatory cytokines (see Tables 277-3, 277-4, and 277-5).

THE COMPLEMENT SYSTEM

The complement system is a cascading series of plasma enzymes, regulatory proteins, and proteins capable of cell lysis whose principal site of synthesis is the liver. There are two arms of the complement system (Fig. 277-9). Activation of the classic complement pathway via C1, C4, and C2 and activation of the alternative complement pathway via factor D, C3, and factor B both lead to cleavage and activation of C3. C3 is a protein whose activation fragments, when bound to target surfaces such as bacteria and other foreign antigens, are critical for opsonization (coating by antibody and complement) in preparation for phagocytosis.

The protein fragment C3b, split from C3, is necessary for activation of the terminal complement components C5–9. These form the membrane attack complex which, when inserted into cell membranes, brings about osmotic lysis of the cell.

C3b also joins with a cleavage product of factor B (called Bb) to form C3bBb, also known as the *alternative pathway C3 convertase*.

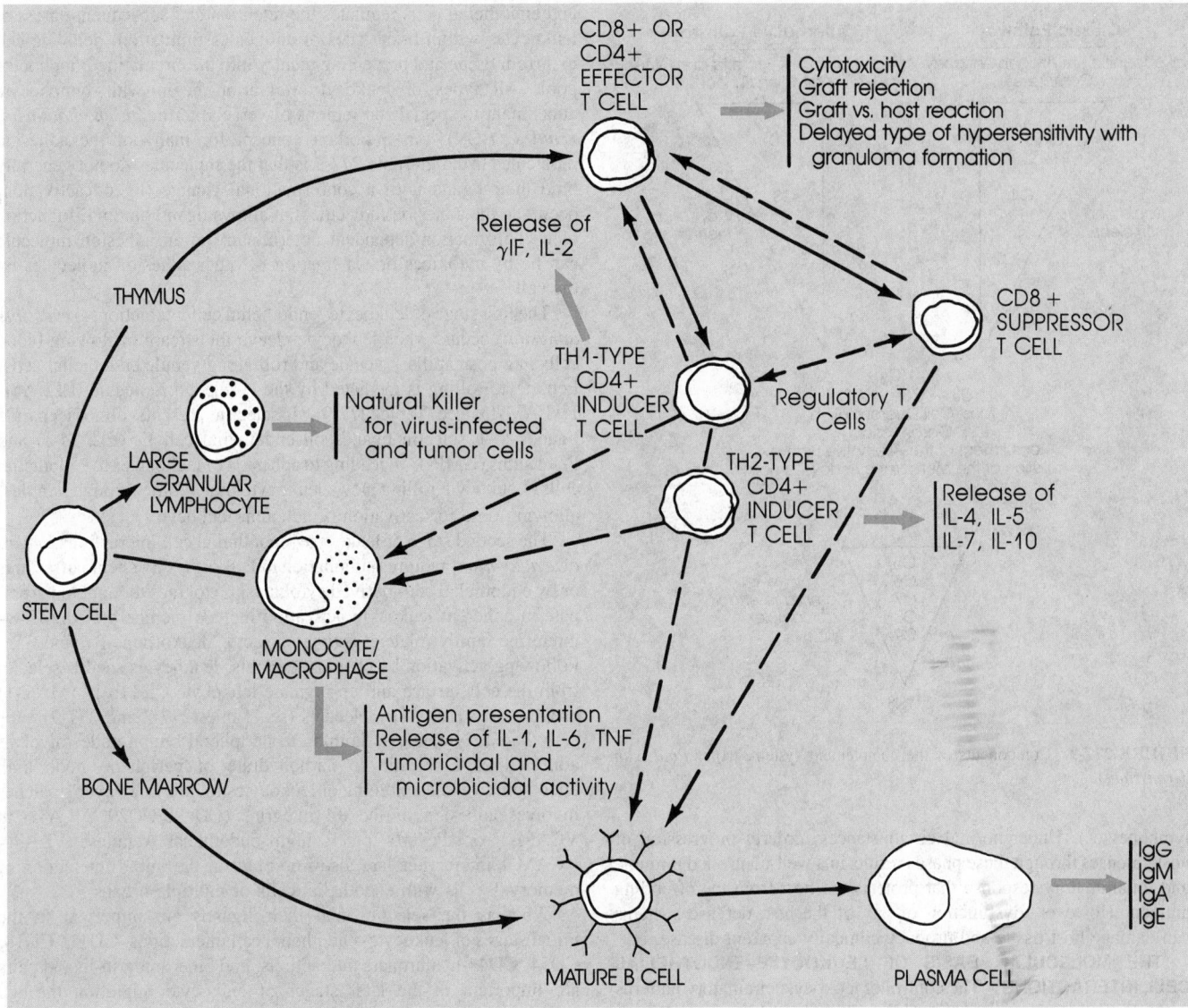

FIGURE 277-8 Schematic model of intercellular interactions of immune cells during the ontogeny and activation stages of immune responses.

Activation of the classic complement pathway results in cleavage of C4 and C2 with a resulting complex of fragments, C4b2a, also called the *classic pathway C3 convertase*. Both the classic pathway C3 convertase (C4b2a) and the alternative pathway C3 convertase (C3bBb) function to cleave C3 to form active C3b, thus driving activation of the C5–9 membrane attack complex. The fact that C3b can combine with Bb to form the alternative pathway C3 convertase gives rise to a potent positive feedback loop for production of C3b and thus continued activation of terminal complement components.

Activation of the classic complement pathway is by interaction of antigen and antibody to form immune complexes that bind C1q, a subunit of C1. Immunoglobulin isotypes that bind C1q and activate the classic pathway are IgM, IgG1, IgG2, and IgG3. In contrast, IgA1, IgA2, and IgD activate complement via the alternative pathway. Activation of the complement cascade via the classic pathway by IgG- or IgM-containing immune complexes is a rapid and efficient pathway to activation of terminal complement components. In contrast, activation of the alternative complement pathway via IgA-containing immune complexes or by bacterial endotoxin is a slower and less efficient pathway to terminal component activation. Thus the immunoglobulin isotype composition of immune complexes is a critical factor in determining complement activation and the efficiency of clearance of immune complexes by C3 receptor–bearing cells.

In addition to the role of complement in opsonization of bacteria and cell lysis, several complement component fragments are potent

mediators of immune cell activation. C3a and C5a bind to receptors on mast cells and basophils, resulting in release of histamine and other mediators of anaphylaxis. C5a is also a potent chemoattractant for neutrophils and monocytes-macrophages (Table 277-8).

MECHANISMS OF IMMUNE DAMAGE

Several responses by the host to foreign antigen culminate in the rapid and efficient elimination of nonself substances. In these scenarios, the classic weapons of the immune system (T cells, B cells, macrophages) interface with cells and soluble products that are mediators of inflammatory responses (neutrophils, eosinophils, basophils, kinin and coagulation systems, and complement cascade).

There are four general phases of host defenses: (1) migration of leukocytes to sites of antigen localization; (2) specific and nonspecific recognition of foreign antigens mediated by T and B lymphocytes, macrophages, and the alternative complement pathway; (3) amplification of the inflammatory response with recruitment of specific and nonspecific effector cells by complement components, lymphokines and monokines, kinins, arachidonic acid metabolites, and mast cell–basophil products; and (4) macrophage, neutrophil, and lymphocyte participation in antigen destruction with ultimate removal of antigen particles by phagocytosis (by macrophages or neutrophils) or by direct cytotoxic mechanisms (involving macrophages, neutrophils, and

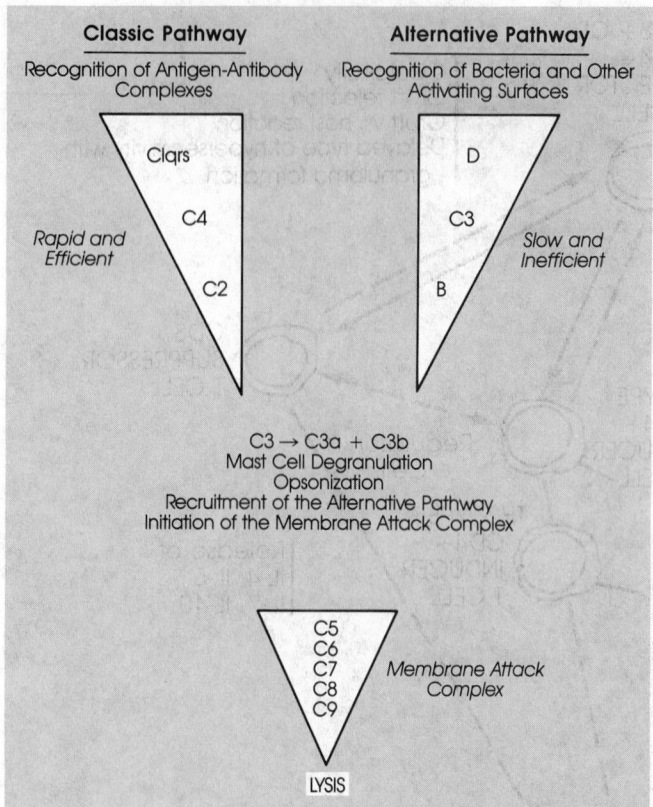

FIGURE 277-9 Components of the complement system. *(After Paul with permission.)*

lymphocytes). Under normal circumstances, orderly progression of host defenses through these phases results in a well-controlled immune and inflammatory response that protects the host from the offending antigen. However, dysfunction of any of the host defense systems can damage host tissue and produce clinically apparent disease.

THE MOLECULAR BASIS OF LEUKOCYTE–ENDOTHELIAL CELL INTERACTIONS

The control of leukocyte circulatory patterns between the bloodstream and peripheral lymphoid organs operates at the level of lymphocyte–endothelial cell interactions to control the specificity of lymphocyte subset entry into organs. Similarly, leukocyte–endothelial cell interactions regulate the entry of leukocytes into inflamed tissue. Adhesion molecule expression on leukocytes

and endothelial cells regulates the retention and subsequent egress of leukocytes within tissue sites of antigenic stimulation, delaying cell exit from tissue and preventing reentry into the circulating lymphocyte pool. All types of leukocyte migration begin with lymphocyte attachment to specialized regions of vessels, termed *high endothelial venules* (HEV). An important concept for many of the adhesion molecules listed in Table 277-9 is that the molecules do not generally bind their ligand until a conformational change (ligand activation) occurs in the adhesion molecule that allows ligand binding. Induction of a conformation-dependent determinant on an adhesion molecule can be by cytokines or via ligation of other adhesion molecules on the cell.

The first stage of leukocyte–endothelial cell interactions, *reversible adhesion,* occurs when leukocytes leave the stream of flowing blood cells in a postcapillary venule and roll along venule endothelial cells. Leukocyte rolling is mediated by the L-selectin molecule (LECAM-1, LAM-1) (see Table 277-9). L-selectin presents oligosaccharide ligands to L-selectin ligands on endothelial cell E- (ELAM-1) and P-selectins (GMP-140) leading to adhesion of leukocytes to endothelial cells. Leukocyte rolling slows leukocyte transit time through venules, allowing time for activation of adherent leukocytes.

The second stage of leukocyte–endothelial cell interactions, *leukocyte activation,* requires stimulation of leukocytes by chemoattractants or by endothelial cell–derived cytokines. Cytokines thought to participate in adherent leukocyte activation include members of the IL-8–intercrine family, platelet-activation factor, leukotriene B_4, and C5a. Following activation by chemoattractants, leukocytes shed L-selectin from the cell surface and up-regulate leukocyte CD11b/18 (MAC-1) or CD11a/18 (LFA 1) molecules (see Tables 277-2 and 277-9).

Whereas lymphocyte homing to peripheral lymph nodes involves adhesion of L-selectin to carbohydrate of peripheral node high endothelial venules, homing of leukocytes to intestine Peyer's patches involves adhesion of the $\alpha 4$ integrins (CD49d/CD29, VLA-4) to VCAM-1 on Peyer's patch high endothelial venules. VLA-4–VCAM-1 interactions are also important in the initial interaction of memory T cells with endothelial cells of multiple organs.

Whereas the selectins and their ligands are important in the initial stages of leukocyte–endothelial cell interactions, CD11a/CD18, CD54, CD44-hyaluronate interactions, and other integrin-ligand pairs are important in the later stages of leukocyte migration through endothelial cells into peripheral lymphoid organs or into inflamed tissue.

IMMUNE-COMPLEX FORMATION

Clearance of antigen by immune-complex formation between antigen and antibody is a highly effective mechanism of host defense. However, depending on the level of immune complexes formed and their physicochemical properties, immune complexes may or may not result in host and foreign cell damage. After antigen exposure, certain types of soluble antigen-antibody complexes freely circulate and, if not cleared by the reticuloendothelial system, can be deposited in blood vessel walls and in other tissues such as renal glomeruli. The precise mechanisms whereby immune complexes damage tissues, particularly blood vessels, are discussed in Chaps. 283 and 291.

IgE-MEDIATED ALLERGIC REACTIONS—ANAPHYLAXIS

T helper cells that drive antiallergen IgE responses are usually TH2-type inducer T cells that secrete IL-4, IL-5, IL-6, and IL-10. Mast cells and basophils have high affinity receptors for the Fc portion of IgE (Fc RI), and cell-bound antiallergen IgE effectively "arms" basophils and mast cells. Mediator release is triggered by antigen (allergen) interaction with Fc receptor–bound IgE; the mediators released are responsible for the pathophysiologic changes of allergic diseases (see Table 277-6). Mediators released from mast cells and basophils can be divided into three broad categories of action: (1) those which increase vascular permeability and contract smooth muscle (histamine, platelet-activating factor, SRS-A, BK-A); (2) those which are chemotactic for or activate other inflammatory cells (ECF-A, NCF, leukotriene B_4); and (3) those which modulate the release of other mediators (BK-A, platelet-activating factor) (see Chap. 282).

TABLE 277-8 Biologic activities of some complement components

Component	Activity
C4a weak anaphylatoxin	Evokes histamine release from basophils and mast cells
C3a	Anaphylatoxin; evokes histamine release from basophils and mast cells
C5a	Anaphylatoxin; evokes histamine release from basophils and mast cells; potent chemoattractant for monocytes and neutrophils
C3b, C3bi	Enhancement of phagocytosis by neutrophils and monocytes; promotes immune complex binding to cells within monocyte-macrophage system, as well as neutrophils; C3b with Bb forms alternative pathway C3 convertase and amplifies alternative pathway; promotes solubilization of immune complexes
C5–9	Membrane attack complex; forms transmembrane channels leading to cell destruction

SOURCE: Adapted with permission from S Ruddy, in Kelley et al.

TABLE 277-9   Leukocyte–endothelial cell adhesion molecules

Molecule	Distribution	Ligand	Functions
SELECTIN FAMILY			
L-selectin (LECAM-1, LAM-1)	Leukocyte	Lymph node addressin, sialylated oligosaccharides	Regulates leukocyte binding to inflamed endothelium; lymph node homing receptor
P-selectin (GMP-140)	Endothelial cells, alpha granules of platelets	Sialylated derivatives of Lewis X oligosaccharides	Involved in initial leukocyte–endothelial cell interactions
E-selectin (ELAM-1)	Endothelial cells	Sialylated derivatives of Lewis X oligosaccharides	Involved in initial leukocyte–endothelial cell interactions
INTEGRIN FAMILY			
$\alpha 1\beta 1$ (VLA-1, CD49a)	Activated T cells, monocytes, endothelial cells	Laminin, collagen	Activation-dependent adhesion receptor; marker for memory T cells
$\alpha 2\beta 1$ (VLA-2, CD49b)	Lymphocytes, endothelial cells, widespread	Collagen, laminin	Activation-dependen adhesion receptor
$\alpha 3\beta 1$ (VLA-3, CD49c)	Lymphocytes, endothelial cells, widespread	Fibronectin, collagen, laminin	Activation-dependent adhesion receptor
$\alpha 4\beta 1$ (VLA-4, CD49d)	Lymphocytes	VCAM-1, fibronectin fragment, vascular addressin	Involved in organ-specific homing; activation up-regulates adhesion
$\alpha 5\beta 1$ (VLA-5, CD49e)	Lymphocytes, endothelial cells, widespread	Fibronectin	Activation-dependent adhesion receptor; marker for memory T cells
$\alpha 6\beta 1$ (VLA-6, CD49f)	Widespread	Laminin	Adhesion to endothelial cells
$\alpha L\beta 2$ (LFA-1, CD11a)	Leukocytes	ICAM-1, ICAM-2, ICAM-3	Activation-dependent adhesion receptor
$\alpha M\beta 2$ (MAC-1, CD11b)	Myeloid, NK cells	ICAM-1, C3bi, factor X	Activation-dependent adhesion receptor; mediates adhesion of myeloid cells to endothelial cells
$\alpha X\beta 1$ (p150, 95, CD11c)	Myeloid cells, subset of lymphocyte	?	Activation-dependent adhesion receptor; mediates binding of myeloid cells to ligands derived from complement cascade
IMMUNOGLOBULIN GENE SUPERFAMILY			
CD2	T cells, NK cells	CD58 (LFA-3)	Activation-dependent adhesion receptor; can transmit proliferation signal
CD54 (ICAM-1)	Activated lymphocytes, thymic epithelium, cytokine (IL-1, TNF-α, IFN-γ)–stimulated endothelial cells	LFA-1, rhinoviruses, *P. falciparum*	Up-regulated expression on many tissues; mediates endothelial-leukocyte adherence
ICAM-2	Endothelial cells	LFA-1	Mediates leukocyte-endothelial adherence
ICAM-3	All resting leukocytes	LFA-1	Leukocyte-leukocyte interactions prior to leukocyte activation
CD58 (LFA-3)	Most tissue cell types	CD2	Up-regulated expression in lymphoid tissues; involved in CTL–target cell interactions
VCAM-1 (InCAM-110)	TNF-α– and IL-1–stimulated endothelial cells, follicular dendritic cells	VLA-4 ($\alpha 4\beta 1$)	Mediates homing of VLA-4 + leukocytes to Peyer's patches; mediates binding of B cells to germinal centers
CARTILAGE LINK PROTEIN FAMILY			
CD44 (Hermes, Pgpl, EcMRIII)	Leukocytes, widespread	Hyaluronan (hyaluronic acid)	Mediates leukocyte adhesion to endothelial cells, probably by activation-dependent adhesion; binds to various cytokines

SOURCE: Adapted with permission from Haynes and Denning.

CYTOTOXIC REACTIONS OF ANTIBODY   In this type of immunologic injury, complement-fixing (C1-binding) antibodies against normal or foreign cells or tissues (IgM, IgG1, IgG2, IgG3) bind complement via the classic pathway and initiate a sequence of events similar to that initiated by immune-complex deposition, resulting in cell lysis or tissue injury. Examples of antibody-mediated cytotoxic reactions include red cell lysis in *transfusion reactions, Goodpasture's syndrome* with anti-glomerular basement membrane antibody formation, and *pemiphigus vulgaris* with antiepidermal antibodies inducing blistering skin disease.

CLASSIC DELAYED-TYPE HYPERSENSITIVITY REACTIONS   Inflammatory reactions initiated by mononuclear leukocytes and not by antibody alone have been termed *delayed-type hypersensitivity reactions*. The term *delayed* has been used to contrast a secondary cellular response which appears 48 to 72 h after antigen exposure with an *immediate* hypersensitivity response generally seen within 12 h of antigen challenge and initiated by basophil mediator release or preformed antibody. For example, in an individual previously infected with *M. tuberculosis* (TB) organisms, intradermal placement of TB purified-protein derivative (PPD) as a skin test challenge results in an indurated area of skin at 48 to 72 h, indicating previous exposure to TB.

The cellular events that result in classic delayed-type hypersensitivity responses are centered around T cells (predominantly IFN-γ, IL-2, and lymphotoxin-secreting TH1-type helper T cells) and macrophages. First, local immune and inflammatory responses at the site of foreign antigen up-regulate endothelial cell adhesion molecule expression, promoting the accumulation of leukocytes at the tissue site. In the general scheme outlined in Fig. 277-8, antigen is processed by monocytes-macrophages and presented to T cells expressing a T cell receptor specific for the antigen. Macrophage-secreting IL-1 and IL-6 amplify the clonal expansion of antigen-specific T cells, and lymphokines (primarily IL-2, IFN-γ, and lymphotoxin) are secreted to recruit other T cells and macrophages to participate in the cellular inflammatory response. In particular, cytotoxic T cells are activated to become active killer cells by IL-2. Once recruited, macrophages frequently undergo epithelioid cell transformation and form giant cells in response to IL-4 and IFN-γ. This type of mononuclear cell infiltrate is termed *granulomatous inflammation*. Examples of diseases in which delayed-type hypersensitivity plays a major role are fungal infections *(histoplasmosis)*, mycobacterial infections *(TB, leprosy)*, chlamydial infections *(lymphogranuloma venereum)*, helminth infections *(schistosomiasis)*, reactions to toxins *(berylliosis)*, and hypersensitivity reactions to organic dusts *(hypersensitivity pneumonitis)*. In addition, delayed-type hypersensitivity responses may play a role in tissue damage in autoimmune diseases such as *rheumatoid arthritis* and *Wegener's granulomatosis* (see Chaps. 285 and 291).

AUTOIMMUNE DISEASE   Autoimmune disease is characterized by production of either antibodies that react with host tissue or immune effector T cells that are autoreactive to endogenous self peptides. Since B cell responses in humans generally require inducer T cells, a B cell autoantibody response directly implies disordered T cell immunoregulatory control. In some instances, autoantibodies may arise by a normal T and B cell response activated by foreign organisms or substances that contain antigens, particularly polysaccharides, that cross-react with similar self antigens in body tissues. This phenomenon is called *molecular mimicry*. Examples of clinically relevant autoantibodies are antibodies against acetylcholine receptors in *myasthenia gravis* and anti-DNA, antierythrocyte, and antiplatelet antibodies in *systemic lupus erythematosus*.

As mentioned above in the description of immunoglobulins, the unique portion of the variable region of the immunoglobulin molecule where antigen binds is called the *idiotype*, and an antibody that reacts specifically with that region is called an *anti-idiotype antibody*. Anti-idiotype antibodies may arise during the course of the normal immune response. For example, anti-idiotypes against antitetanus antibodies develop during normal immunization of humans to tetanus toxoid and serve to deliver "off" signals to B cells secreting antitetanus antibodies. Antibodies may be an important component of the normal immunoregulatory network. Anti-idiotype antibodies also may be relevant to two types of autoimmunity: (1) dysfunction of the idiotype–anti-idiotype antibody system could lead to B cell hyperreactivity by failure to generate "off" signals for B cell differentiation, and (2) some antireceptor antibodies produced in autoimmune diseases (anti-acetylcholine receptor antibodies in myasthenia gravis, anti-insulin receptor antibodies in forms of type I diabetes mellitus, and anti-thyrotropin receptor antibodies in autoimmune thyroid disease) may be anti-idiotype antibodies made against the antibody-combining site (idiotype) of an autoantibody.

Genetic factors likely play a role in the genesis of autoimmune disease, either by selecting for inherent B cell hyperreactivity and tendency toward autoantibody formation or, in the case of MHC antigen association with autoimmune diseases, via presentation of self or foreign peptides that stimulate an inappropriate antiself response. Myasthenia gravis, autoimmune thyroid disease, and pernicious anemia are all associated with HLA-B8 (MHC class I) and -DR3 (MHC class II) expression (see Chap. 64) and are also associated with certain immunoglobulin heavy chain markers. There is also a strong association of certain DR types with the development of rheumatoid arthritis.

Whereas organ-specific autoimmune diseases are likely the result of the combined effects of several factors that lead to inappropriate targeting of a particular organ or system to immune damage, generalized autoimmune diseases such as systemic lupus erythematosus can be thought of as diseases in which there is episodic breakdown of immunologic tolerance to self molecules. Recent studies have demonstrated that in a mouse model of autoimmunity (the MRL mouse), the cause of autoimmune disease is a defect in a cell surface molecule (fas/APO-1) on T cells that is required for the intrathymic death of autoreactive T lymphocytes. The defective fas/APO-1 molecule prevents negative selection of autoreactive T cells, leading to seeding of peripheral lymphoid organs with excessive numbers of autoreactive T cells. It is thought that rare serious multisystem lupus erythematosus–like syndromes in children may be the human homologues of murine MRL autoimmune disease. Instead of a defect in central (thymic) tolerance, adult acquired systemic lupus erythematosus is more likely to be a generalized defect in maintenance of peripheral tolerance in which the peripheral immune system lacks the ability to maintain anergy to self antigens. While the molecules involved in maintenance of peripheral tolerance/anergy to self antigens are not fully known, recent data suggest that T cell CD28 and B cell B7/BB1 molecules are involved in regulating this process.

CLINICAL EVALUATION OF IMMUNE FUNCTION

Clinical assessment of immunity requires investigation of the four major components of the immune system that participate in host defense and in pathogenesis of autoimmune diseases: (1) humoral immunity (B cells), (2) cell-mediated immunity (T cells, monocytes), (3) phagocytic cells of the reticuloendothelial system (macrophages), as well as polymorphonuclear leukocytes, and (4) complement. Clinical problems that require an evaluation of immunity include chronic infections, recurrent infection, unusual infecting agents, and certain autoimmune syndromes. The type of clinical syndrome under evaluation can provide information regarding possible immune defects (see Chap. 278). Defects in cellular immunity generally result in viral, mycobacterial, and fungal infections. An extreme example of deficiency in cellular immunity is the acquired immunodeficiency syndrome (AIDS) (see Chap. 279). Antibody deficiencies result in recurrent bacterial infections, frequently with organisms such as *Streptococcus pneumoniae* and *Haemophilus influenzae* (see Chap. 278). Disorders of phagocyte function frequently are manifested by recurrent skin infections, often due to *Staphylococcus aureus* (see Chap. 59). Finally, deficiencies of early and late complement components are associated with autoimmune phenomena and recurrent *Neisseria* infections (Table 277-10). Chapter 278 summarizes useful initial screening tests of immune function.

INTERVENTIONAL IMMUNOTHERAPY

Most current therapies for autoimmune and inflammatory diseases involve the use of nonspecific immune-modulating or immunosuppressive agents such as glucocorticoids or cytotoxic drugs. The goal of development of new treatments for immune-mediated diseases is to design ways to specifically interrupt pathologic immune responses, leaving nonpathologic immune responses intact. Novel ways to interrupt pathologic immune responses that are under investigation include the use of monoclonal antibodies against T lymphocytes as therapeutic agents, the use of toxin-labeled cytokines and/or specific cytokine inhibitors as anti-inflammatory agents, and the use of soluble adhesion molecules to interrupt inflammatory reactions associated with up-regulated adhesion molecule expression. For some animal models of organ-specific autoimmune disease, the TCR types of pathogenic T cells have been oligoclonal or monoclonal, giving hope

TABLE 277-10 **Complement deficiencies and associated diseases**

Component	Associated diseases
CLASSIC PATHWAY	
C1q, C1r, C1s, C4	Immune-complex syndromes,* pyogenic infections
C2	Immune-complex syndromes,* few with pyogenic infections
C1 inhibitor	Rare immune-complex disease, few with pyogenic infections
C3 AND ALTERNATIVE PATHWAY C3	
C3	Immune-complex syndromes,* pyogenic infections
D	Pyogenic infections
Properdin	*Neisseria* infections
I	Pyogenic infections
H	Hemolytic uremic syndrome
MEMBRANE ATTACK COMPLEX	
C5, C6, C7, C8	Recurrent *Neisseria* infections, immune-complex disease
C9	Rare *Neisseria* infections

* Immune-complex syndromes include SLE and SLE-like syndromes, glomerulonephritis, and vasculitis syndromes.
SOURCE: Adapted with permission from JA Schifferli and DK Peters, Lancet 88:957, 1983.

that anti-TCR therapy (TCR peptides, inducing anti-TCR antibodies or anti-TCR regulatory T cells) may be feasible. However, to date, pathologic T cells in human autoimmune disease have remained difficult to define, and specific TCR-directed therapy of T cell–mediated autoimmune diseases remains only a theoretical possibility.

REFERENCES

CLARK SC, KAMEN R: The human hematopoietic colony-stimulating factors. Science 236:1229, 1987

DAVIS MM: Molecular genetics of T cell antigen receptors. Hosp Pract 23:157, 1988

FINKEL TH et al: T-cell development and transmembrane signaling: Changing biological responses through an unchanging receptor. Immunol Today 12:79, 1991

FRANK MM: Complement in the pathophysiology of human disease. N Engl J Med 316:1525, 1987

GLEICH GJ: Eosinophils, basophils and mast cells. J Allergy Clin Immunol 84:1024, 1989

HAYNES BF, DENNING SM: Lymphopoiesis, in *The Molecular Basis of Blood Diseases,* 2d ed, G Stamatoyannopoulos et al (eds). Philadelphia, Saunders, 1993

——— et al: Intrathymic T cell maturation. Semin Immunol 2:67, 1990

HERMAN A et al: Superantigens: Mechanism of T-cell stimulation and the role in immune responses. Annu Rev Immunol 9:745, 1991

KELLEY WN et al (eds): *Textbook of Rheumatology,* 4th ed. Philadelphia, Saunders, 1993, chaps. 6, 7, 10, 13, 15, 16

PAUL WE (ed): *Fundamental Immunology,* 2d ed. New York, Raven, 1989

RETH M et al: The B-cell antigen receptor complex. Immunol Today 12:196, 1991

SPRINGER TA: Adhesion receptors of the immune system. Nature 346:425, 1990

278 PRIMARY IMMUNE DEFICIENCY DISEASES

MAX D. COOPER / ALEXANDER R. LAWTON III

Immunologic functions are mediated by two developmentally independent, but functionally interacting, families of lymphocytes. The activities of B and T lymphocytes and their products in host defense are closely integrated with the functions of other cells of the reticuloendothelial system. Macrophages, dendritic cells, and the Langerhans' cells in the skin play an important role in the trapping and presentation of antigens to T and B cells to initiate the immune response. Macrophages also become effector cells, especially when activated by cytokine products of lymphocytes. The scavenger activity of polymorphonuclear leukocytes is directed and made specific by antibodies in concert with cytokines and the complement system. Natural killer (NK) cells, a population of granular lymphocytes, may spontaneously kill tumor and virus-infected cells, activities that are enhanced by the cytokine products of immune and inflammatory cells. Killing by NK cells also can be targeted by IgG antibodies for which NK cells have cell-surface receptors. The interaction of basophils and tissue mast cells with IgE antibodies in causation of immediate-type hypersensitivity is discussed in Chap. 282. Consideration of these interrelationships is an important part of the analysis of patients with suspected immune deficiency.

CLINICAL DISEASE FEATURES COMMON TO IMMUNE DEFICIENCY Immunodeficiency syndromes, whether congenital, spontaneously acquired, or iatrogenic, are characterized by unusual susceptibility to infection and not infrequently to autoimmune disease and lymphoreticular malignancies. The types of infection often provide the first clue to the nature of the immunologic defect.

Patients with *defects in humoral immunity* have recurrent or chronic sinopulmonary infection, meningitis, and bacteremia, most commonly caused by pyogenic bacteria such as *Haemophilus influenzae, Streptococcus pneumoniae,* and staphylococci. These and other pyogenic organisms also cause frequent infections in individuals who have either neutropenia or a deficiency of the pivotal third component of complement (C3). The tripartite collaboration of antibody, complement, and phagocytes in host defense against pyogenic organisms makes it important to assess all three systems in individuals with unusual susceptibility to bacterial infections.

Antibody-deficient patients in whom cell-mediated immunity is intact have an interesting response to viral infections. The clinical course of primary infection with viruses such as varicella-zoster or rubeola, unless complicated by bacterial infection, does not differ significantly from that of the normal host. However, long-lasting immunity may not develop, and as a result, multiple bouts of chickenpox and measles may occur. Such observations suggest that intact T cells may be sufficient for control of established viral infections, while antibodies play an important role in limiting the initial dissemination of virus and in providing long-lasting protection. Exceptions to this generalization are becoming more widely recognized. Agammaglobulinemic patients fail to clear hepatitis B virus from their circulation and have a progressive, and often fatal, course. Poliomyelitis has occurred following live-virus vaccination in some patients. Chronic encephalitis, which may progress over a period of months to years, is a particular threat in congenitally agammaglobulinemic boys. Echoviruses and adenoviruses have been isolated from brain, spinal fluid, or other sites in such patients; in others no agent has been detected.

The occurrence of an unusually serious infection, for example, *H. influenzae* meningitis in an older child or adult, warrants consideration of humoral immune deficiency. Bacterial infections in certain sites also may suggest this possibility. Chronic otitis media occurs frequently in patients with hypogammaglobulinemia and is significant because of its relative rarity in normal adults. Pansinusitis, although almost invariably present in immunoglobulin deficiency, is a less helpful finding because it is not rare in apparently normal people. Bacterial infections of the skin or urinary tract are less frequent problems in hypogammaglobulinemic patients.

Infestation with the intestinal parasite *Giardia lamblia* is a frequent enough cause of diarrhea in antibody-deficient patients to warrant diagnostic duodenal aspiration and intestinal biopsy when the organism cannot be demonstrated in the stool.

Abnormalities of cell-mediated immunity predispose to disseminated virus infections, particularly with latent viruses such as herpes simplex (see Chap. 143), varicella zoster (see Chap. 144), and cytomegalovirus (see Chap. 146). In addition, patients so affected

FIGURE 278-1 Hypothetical model outlining the differentiation of hemopoietic stem cells along T and B cell lineages. Failure to develop T and B cells may result from defective stem cells or from inborn metabolic errors affecting both cell types. Rarely, other hemopoietic cell lines are also absent. Absence of either T or B cells suggests malfunction of central lymphoid tissues, including the thymus and the fetal liver–bone marrow complex. B cell deficiency may result from failure to generate pre-B cells from their stem cell precursors or from failure of pre-B cells to give rise to their B lymphocyte progeny. Similarly, differentiation may be arrested at several levels within the T cell lineage; arrests at the thymocyte level and failure to develop the helper subset have been observed in immunodeficient patients. Agammaglobulinemia and deficiencies of some T cell functions may occur despite the presence of normal numbers of B or T cells in the circulation. Failure of B lymphocytes to differentiate to plasma cells can be due to intrinsic cellular abnormalities or to faulty T cell regulation.

almost invariably develop mucocutaneous candidiasis and frequently acquire systemic fungal infections. Pneumonia caused by *Pneumocystis carinii* is also common (see Chap. 178).

T cell deficiency is always accompanied by some abnormality of antibody responses (see Fig. 278-1), although this may not be reflected by hypogammaglobulinemia. This explains in part why patients with primary T cell defects are also subject to overwhelming bacterial infection.

The most severe form of immune deficiency occurs in individuals, often infants, who lack both cell-mediated and humoral immune functions. Individuals with severe combined immunodeficiency are susceptible to the whole range of infectious agents including organisms not ordinarily considered pathogenic. Multiple infections with viruses, bacteria, and fungi occur, often simultaneously. Because donor lymphocytes cannot be rejected by these recipients, blood transfusions can produce fatal graft-versus-host disease.

DIFFERENTIATION OF T AND B CELLS   The functional deficits which occur in both congenital and acquired immunodeficiencies are usefully viewed as being caused by defects at various points along the differentiation pathways of immunocompetent cells. For this reason, certain features of the development and differentiation of T and B cells that are especially relevant to the analysis of immunodeficiency are briefly presented here; Chap. 277 provides a general account of their roles in cellular and humoral immunity.

A subpopulation of hematopoietic stem cells may become restricted to lymphoid differentiation prior to migration to the thymus, where T cells are generated, or to the fetal liver and adult bone marrow, where B cell development begins (see Fig. 278-1). A major function of these central lymphoid tissues is to generate the clonal diversity characteristic of the immune system. Each T or B lymphocyte is induced to express surface receptor molecules of a unique specificity for antigen. The receptors of B lymphocytes are immunoglobulin molecules which are formed by paired heavy and light chains of either κ or λ type. The heavy chain gene loci are on the long arm of chromosome 14; the 5'-3' order of these is V_H (variable), D (diversity), and J_H (joining) minigene families followed by the C_H (constant region) genes, C_μ, C_δ, $C_{\gamma3}$, $C_{\gamma1}$, $C_{\alpha1}$, $C_{\gamma2}$, $C_{\gamma4}$, C_ϵ, and $C_{\alpha2}$. The κ gene family, consisting of V_κ, J_κ, and C_κ genes, is located on chromosome 2 and the homologous λ gene loci on chromosome 22.

The T cell receptors are related cell surface molecules with antigen-binding specificity. The receptor on most T cells is composed of two polypeptide chains, called α and β. The β-chain family is located on chromosome 7 and consists of V$_β$, D$_β$, J$_β$, and C$_β$ minigene loci. The α-chain family on chromosome 14 similarly consists of a series of V$_α$, D$_α$, J$_α$, and C$_α$ genes. A smaller subpopulation of T cells express a T cell receptor composed of γ and δ polypeptide chains. The γ-chain gene family is located on chromosome 7, and the δ-chain family is located in the midst of the α gene locus on chromosome 14.

The genetic strategy for creating functional gene complexes encoding antigen receptors is similar for T and B cells. For example, a functional V region gene of the immunoglobulin heavy chain is formed by productive rearrangement of one each of the V$_H$, D, and J$_H$ genes and deletion of the intervening DNA to generate a contiguous coding structure which is then transcribed together with the nearest C$_H$ gene. Functional light chain genes are formed by a V-J rearrangement in either the κ or λ gene loci. The V$_β$ gene is similarly composed of a rearranged set of V$_β$, D$_β$, and J$_β$ genes forming a contiguous coding structure, which the T cell then transcribes along with the nearest C$_β$ gene. Because there are many different V, D, and J genes, they can be put together in various combinations to encode a large number of receptor molecules having different antigen-binding specificities.

Generation of clonal diversity requires cellular proliferation, such that each of the different receptor specificities encoded in the genome comes to be uniquely expressed by individual cells. A clone consists of all cells that express the identical antigen-binding receptors. Estimates for the total number of B cell clones usually vary between 10 and 100 million. T cell clonal diversity may be equally extensive. The initial step in clonal development is independent of antigen and reflects a genetically programmed sequence of differentiation analogous to that of primary erythropoiesis or myelopoiesis. This phase, termed *primary differentiation*, begins early in human fetal development and may continue into adult life.

The most primitive morphologically identifiable cell in the B lineage is called a *pro-B cell*. These cells are marked by the cell surface CD19 antigen and the nuclear expression of terminal deoxynucleotidyl transferase (Tdt). Pro-B cells undergo productive V$_H$DJ$_H$ rearrangement to express cytoplasmic μ chains (the heavy chain of IgM) and become pre-B cells. Since light chain gene rearrangement usually occurs later, pre-B cells lack the characteristic membrane-bound immunoglobulin receptors which characterize B lymphocytes but may express μ-chain/surrogate light chain receptors encoded by the nonrearranged V pre-B and 14.1 genes in the λ light chain gene locus. Pre-B cells are generated in the fetal liver and in bone marrow throughout life, dividing in response to growth factors made by neighboring stromal cells. After undergoing a productive rearrangement of light chain VJ genes, pre-B cells become immature B lymphocytes that express surface IgM receptors. These B lymphocytes differ from their more mature counterparts in an important physiologic characteristic; they are highly susceptible to inactivation when their receptors bind antigen. Consequently, immature B cells encountering self-antigens may be eliminated or rendered anergic. The antigen receptors on B cells are multichain units. In order for membrane-bound immunoglobulins to reach the B cell surface, they require association with Ig-α and Ig-β chains, which serve as signal transduction elements for the antigen receptor complex.

The developmental sequence for expression of diverse immunoglobulin classes by human B lymphocytes begins with expression of IgM. The expression of IgD- on IgM-bearing cells occurs later. Lymphocytes committed to synthesis of IgG, IgA, and IgE are derived from IgM-bearing precursors through a genetic switch mechanism. Each of the heavy chain constant region genes except C$_δ$ is preceded by a switch region composed of repetitive nucleotide sequences. The heavy chain class switch is initiated by splicing of the switch region of μ with the switch region in front of the downstream heavy chain gene to be expressed next and is completed by the terminal differentiation of plasma cells producing the new heavy chain class. Completion of the switch process thus involves antigenic stimulation

and the help of T cells which produce soluble switch factors, such as interleukin 4 and tumor growth factor β for IgA responses.

T lineage cells also undergo sequential rearrangements of the minigene families encoding their antigen receptors. On entering the epithelial thymus, lymphoid precursor cells may follow one of two T cell pathways. The first involves rearrangement of V$_γ$ and J$_γ$ genes to express γ chains and rearrangement of V$_δ$, D$_δ$, and J$_δ$ genes to express δ chains. These associate with the CD3 proteins to form the CD3/γδ T cell receptor (TCR) complex of γδ T cells. Pre-T cells beginning development along the second differentiation pathway in the thymus rearrange one each of the V$_β$, D$_β$, and J$_β$ genes prior to the expression of a complete β chain. At a later differentiation stage, similar rearrangements of V$_α$ and J$_α$ genes occur in the α-chain family, and then the completed antigen receptor molecule of one α chain and one β chain is expressed together with the CD3 protein complex on the cell surface of an immature αβ T cell. Initially, the αβ T cells express both the CD4 and CD8 accessory molecules on their surface. As these cells mature under the influence of a self-antigen selection process, they either down-regulate the CD8 molecule to become CD4+ T cells with helper cell potential or they cease to express the CD4 molecule to become CD8+ T cells with cytotoxic potential. The CD4+ αβ T cells leaving the thymus have been selected to recognize peptide fragments presented in the groove of class II major histocompatibility (MHC) molecules of antigen-presenting cells. The CD8+ αβ T cells migrating from the thymus have been selected to recognize peptide fragments in the cleft of class I MHC molecules expressed by virtually all types of nucleated cells. The CD4 and CD8 molecules are called *accessory receptors* because they have binding affinity for class II or class I MHC molecules, respectively, and are coupled to tyrosine kinase molecules that are active in signal transduction. While the γδ T cells express neither CD4 nor CD8 molecules during their intrathymic development, they may express CD8 molecules as mature T cells in the periphery. Expression of these and other cell surface molecules can be defined by specific monoclonal antibodies, thus providing a powerful tool for elucidating the developmental status of both T and B lymphocytes (see Fig. 278-1).

The αβ T cells bearing the CD4 markers constitute approximately 70 percent of circulating T cells and function as helper-inducer cells, necessary for expression of effector functions of both T and B cells. The αβ T cells expressing CD8 molecules constitute 20 to 30 percent of circulating T cells, mediate cytotoxic reactions, and may be responsible for suppression of immune responses. The γδ T cells constitute a minor population of T cells. While their function is still unclear, they may serve a protective role along epithelial surfaces and to eliminate damaged cells. Developmental arrests or failure of function of one or more of these T cell subsets may be responsible for immunodeficiency or autoimmune diseases.

The events designated *secondary differentiation* follow stimulation of specific clones of lymphocytes by antigen. These processes are synonymous with the immune response (see Chap. 277). Particularly important in consideration of immunodeficiencies are the collaborative interactions among macrophages, T cells, and B cells. While B lymphocytes may differentiate to IgM-secreting plasma cells when stimulated by thymus-independent antigens, such as lipopolysaccharides, most antibody responses, particularly those of the IgA and IgG classes, require intimate collaboration between T and B cells. Antigens bound to the antibody receptors on B cells are internalized, partially digested, and recycled to the cell surface, where they are presented on class II molecules to the T cell. The activated T cell in turn produces soluble factors that promote growth and differentiation of the B cell or inflammatory responses. These factors, which include interleukins IL-2, IL-4, IL-5, IL-6, and IL-10 and interferon-γ, may be differentially produced by individual T cells depending on their prior mode of activation.

Differentiation of T or B cells may be arrested at either the primary or secondary stages. Reflecting the complex cellular interactions involved in immune responses and the pivotal role played by T lymphocytes, immune deficiencies primarily involving T cells are usually also associated with abnormal B cell function. Conversely, immunodeficiencies manifested primarily by inability to produce antibodies may be caused by T cell defects not associated with abnormal cell-mediated immunity.

EVALUATION OF IMMUNODEFICIENT PATIENTS A careful history and physical examination will usually indicate whether the major problem involves the antibody-complement-phagocyte system or cell-mediated immunity. A history of a normal response to smallpox vaccination or of contact dermatitis due to poison ivy suggests intact cellular immunity. Persistent mucocutaneous candidiasis suggests deficient cell-mediated immunity. Lymphopenia and the absence of palpable lymph nodes may be important findings. However, patients with profound immunodeficiency may have diffuse lymphoid hyperplasia. Most immunodeficiencies may be diagnosed by thoughtful use of tests available in local or regional clinical laboratories. More precise evaluation of immunologic functions and treatment may require referral to specialized centers. Table 278-1 presents a résumé of widely available laboratory investigations.

Humoral immunity With rare exceptions, deficiency of humoral immunity is accompanied by diminished serum concentration of one or more classes of immunoglobulin. Normal values vary with age, and adult concentrations of IgM (1.0 g/L) are reached at about 1 year, of IgG (8.0 g/L) at 5 to 6 years, and of IgA (2.0 g/L) at puberty (see Chap. 277). Also, the wide range of values among normal adults creates difficulty in defining the lower limits of normal. Reasonable estimates for low normal values are 0.4 g/L for IgM, 5 g/L for IgG, and 0.5 g/L for IgA. In the presence of borderline hypogammaglobulinemia, assessing the patient's capacity to produce specific antibodies becomes particularly important. Isohemagglutinins, anti-streptolysin O, and "febrile agglutinins" are valuable standard assays, and measurements of pre- and postimmunization titers to tetanus toxoid, diphtheria toxoid, *H. influenzae* capsular polysaccharide, and *S.*

TABLE 278-1 Laboratory evaluation of host defense status

INITIAL SCREENING ASSAYS*

Complete blood count with differential smear
Serum immunoglobulin levels: IgM, IgG, IgA, IgD, IgE

OTHER READILY AVAILABLE ASSAYS

Quantification of blood mononuclear cell populations by immunofluorescence assays employing monoclonal antibody markers[†]
  T cells: CD3, CD4, CD8, TCRαβ, TCRγδ
  B cells: CD19, CD20, CD21, Ig(μ, δ, γ, α, κ, λ), Ig-associated molecules
       (α, β)
  NK cells: CD16
  Monocytes: CD15
  Activation markers: HLA-DR, CD25, B7/BB1 antigen (B cells)
T cell functional evaluation
  1 Delayed hypersensitivity skin tests (PPD, *Candida* histoplasmin, tetanus toxoid)
  2 Proliferative response to mitogens (anti-CD3 antibody, phytohemagglutinin, concanavalin A) and allogeneic cells (mixed lymphocyte response)
  3 Cytokine production
B cell functional evaluation
  1 Natural or commonly acquired antibodies: isohemagglutinins; antibodies to common viruses (influenza, rubella, rubeola) and bacterial toxins (diphtheria, tetanus)
  2 Response to immunization with protein (tetanus toxoid) and carbohydrate (pneumococcal vaccine, *H. influenza B* vaccine) antigens
  3 Quantitative IgG subclass determinations
Complement
  1 CH$_{50}$
  2 C3, C4
Phagocyte function
  1 Reduction of nitroblue tetrazolium
  2 Chemotaxis assays
  3 Bactericidal activity

---

* Together with a history and physical examination, these tests will identify more than 95 percent of patients with primary immunodeficiencies.
† The menu of monoclonal antibody markers may be expanded or contracted to focus on particular clinical questions.

pneumoniae serotypes provide a comprehensive assessment of humoral responsiveness.

Estimation of numbers of circulating B lymphocytes is of value in determining the pathogenesis of certain types of immune deficiency. B lymphocytes are identified by the presence of membrane-bound immunoglobulins, their associated α- and β-chain units, and other lineage-specific molecules on the B cell surface (Table 278-1), which can be identified and enumerated by specific monoclonal antibodies.

Since antibody deficiency may be mimicked clinically by deficiency of complement components, measurement of total hemolytic complement (CH$_{50}$) should be a part of the evaluation of host defense. Measurement of C3 alone is inadequate for screening, since deficiencies of both early and late complement components may predispose to bacterial infection (see Chap. 277).

Cellular immunity Human T lymphocytes may be enumerated by their expression of the TCR/CD3 complex of surface molecules. The CD2 antigenic molecule is also expressed by almost all the T cells and a few non-T lineage lymphocytes. The CD4 molecule serves as a marker for helper T cells, but macrophages also express this molecule in relatively low levels. Conversely, the CD8 molecule is expressed by cytotoxic T cells. This cell surface molecule also may be expressed by γδ T cells and by natural killer cells.

Normal levels of serum immunoglobulins and antibody responsiveness are reliable indices of intact helper T cell function. T lymphocyte function can be measured directly by delayed hypersensitivity skin testing using a variety of antigens to which the majority of older children and adults have been sensitized. The most generally useful skin test antigen is a 1:5 dilution of tetanus toxoid injected intradermally, since almost all individuals will have been sensitized. Purified protein derivative (PPD), histoplasmin, mumps antigen, and extracts of *Candida* or *Trichophyton* also may be used.

T lymphocyte function may be estimated in vitro by the capacity of cells to proliferate in response to antigens to which the patient has been sensitized, to lymphocytes from an unrelated donor, to antibodies that cross-link the CD3/TCR complex, or to the T cell mitogens, which include phytohemagglutinin, concanavalin A, and pokeweed mitogen. The response is usually quantified by measurement of incorporation of radioactive thymidine into newly synthesized DNA. It is also possible to measure the production of cytokines (or interleukins) by activated T cells. Finally, the ability of T cells activated in mixed lymphocyte culture to lyse target cells can be measured.

CLASSIFICATION Primary immunodeficiencies may be either congenital or acquired and are currently classified according to mode of inheritance and whether the defect involves T cells, B cells, or both (Table 278-2). The following discussion emphasizes three related concepts: (1) that immunodeficiencies are most logically viewed as defects of cellular differentiation, (2) that these defects may involve either primary development of T or B cells or the antigen-dependent phase of their differentiation, and (3) that defects of secondary B cell differentiation may in some instances reflect faulty T-B collaboration.

Secondary immunodeficiencies are those not caused by intrinsic abnormalities in development or function of T and B cells. The best known of these is AIDS, which may follow infection with the human immunodeficiency virus (see Chap. 279). Other examples are immune deficiency associated with malnutrition, protein-losing enteropathy, and intestinal lymphangiectasia. Also considered secondary are immunodeficiencies resulting from hypercatabolic states such as occur in myotonic dystrophy, immunodeficiency associated with lymphoreticular malignancy, and immunodeficiency resulting from treatment with x-rays, antilymphocyte serum, or cytotoxic drugs.

Incidence As a group, the primary immunodeficiencies are relatively common. The most frequent, isolated IgA deficiency, occurs in approximately 1 in 600 individuals in North America.

The more severe forms of primary immunodeficiency have their onset early in life and all too frequently result in death during childhood. Immunodeficiencies may become apparent at any age, however, and patients with congenital hypogammaglobulinemia may

TABLE 278-2 WHO classification of primary immunodeficiencies

COMBINED IMMUNODEFICIENCIES

Severe combined immunodeficiency (SCID):
  1 X-linked
  2 Autosomal recessive ("Swiss-type agammaglobulinemia")
Adenosine deaminase (ADA) deficiency
Purine nucleoside phosphorylase (PNP) deficiency
MHC class II deficiency
Reticular dysgenesis

PREDOMINANTLY ANTIBODY DEFICIENCIES

X-linked agammaglobulinemia
X-linked hypogammaglobulinemia with growth hormone deficiency
Ig deficiency with increased IgM ("hyper-IgM syndrome")
Ig heavy chain–gene deletions
κ-Chain deficiency
IgA deficiency
Selective deficiency of IgG subclasses (with or without IgA deficiency)
Common variable immunodeficiency (CVID)
Transient hypogammaglobulinemia of infancy

OTHER WELL-DEFINED IMMUNODEFICIENCY SYNDROMES

Wiskott-Aldrich syndrome
Ataxia telangiectasia
3d and 4th pouch/arch syndrome (DiGeorge)

SYNDROMES ASSOCIATED WITH IMMUNODEFICIENCY

Chromosome abnormalities:
  1 Bloom syndrome
  2 Fanconi anemia
  3 Down syndrome
Multiple organ system abnormalities:
  1 Partial albinism
  2 Short-limbed dwarfism
  3 Cartilage hair hypoplasia
  4 Agenesis of the corpus callosum
Hereditary metabolic defects:
  1 Transcobalamin II deficiency
  2 Acrodermatitis enteropathica (zinc deficiency)
  3 Type I orotic aciduria
  4 Biotin-dependent carboxylase deficiency
Hypercatabolism of Ig:
  1 Familial hypercatabolism of Ig
  2 Myotonic dystrophy
  3 Intestinal lymphagiectasia
Other:
  1 Hyper-IgE syndrome
  2 Chronic mucocutaneous candidiasis
  3 Thymoma
  4 Immunodeficiency following hereditarily determined susceptibility to Epstein-Barr virus

survive to middle age or beyond. In a referral center for patients with immunodeficiency diseases, approximately two-thirds of the immunodeficient patients will be adults. Improved methods of diagnosis and treatment may increase this ratio in the future.

Severe combined immunodeficiency (SCID) This syndrome is characterized by gross functional impairment of both humoral and cell-mediated immunity and by susceptibility to devastating fungal, bacterial, and viral infections. It is usually congenital, may be inherited either as an X-linked or autosomal recessive defect, or may occur sporadically. Affected infants rarely survive beyond 1 year without treatment. This syndrome has been associated with a diversity of defects in development of immunocompetent cells, some of which may be related to specific enzymatic abnormalities.

The classic example of SCID, *Swiss-type agammaglobulinemia*, is characterized by severe lymphopenia and is inherited with an autosomal recessive pattern. A genetic defect in the Ig and TCR recombination mechanism may underlie this failure in both T and B cell development. Rarely, other hematopoietic cell lines fail to develop in a variant form of SCID called *reticular dysgenesis*. About half of patients with autosomal recessive SCID are deficient in an enzyme involved in purine metabolism, adenosine deaminase (ADA), due to

deletions or point mutations in the ADA gene. Studies of the pathophysiologic relationship of ADA deficiency to abortive lymphoid differentiation suggest that intracellular accumulation of adenosine and deoxyadenosine nucleotides interferes with critical metabolic functions, including DNA synthesis. Improvement of both clinical status and immunologic function occurs in some patients treated with exogenous ADA conjugated to polyethylene glycol to prolong its half-life. The cellular defect in the lymphopenic forms of SCID logically rests with the precursor cells for both T and B lineages. The immunologic defects in all these types of SCID patients have been repaired following transplantation of bone marrow or fetal liver as a source of stem cells, confirming the hypothesis that the stromal microenvironments of the thymus and bone marrow of these patients are capable of supporting T and B cell differentiation of normal stem cells.

SCID also may occur with an X-linked inheritance pattern. Affected boys have normal numbers of B lymphocytes with few or no circulating T lymphocytes. This developmental disorder also can be repaired by transplantation of bone marrow stem cells from a histocompatible sibling. Transplants of haploidentical bone marrow, depleted of donor T cells to prevent graft-versus-host disease, also may correct the T cell deficit, but antibody deficiency requiring immunoglobulin therapy may persist for years in this instance.

Treatment of SCID patients should be performed in centers with a strong research interest in this problem. It is crucial that these patients be recognized early and not be given live viral vaccines or blood transfusions, which may cause fatal graft-versus-host disease.

T cell immunodeficiency Reflecting the diversity of T cell functions, abnormalities of T cell development may be responsible for a wide spectrum of immune deficiencies, including severe combined immunodeficiency, selective defects in cell-mediated immunity, and syndromes presenting as antibody deficiency with apparently normal cell-mediated immunity. These defects may be acquired (see Chap. 279) as well as congenital. Until recently, laboratory assays of T lymphocyte function were limited to correlates of cell-mediated immunity; no means were available for studying T cell regulatory functions. Improved assays of T cell subsets and their functional integrity are expanding the spectrum of immunodeficiencies primarily related to T cell abnormalities.

DI GEORGE'S SYNDROME This is the classic example of isolated T cell deficiency which results from maldevelopment of thymic epithelial elements derived from the third and fourth pharyngeal pouches. Defective development of organs dependent on cells of embryonic neural crest origin includes congenital cardiac defects, particularly those involving the great vessels; hypocalcemic tetany, due to failure of parathyroid development; and absence of a normal thymus. Associated abnormalities may include abnormal ears, shortened philtrum, micrognathia, and hypertelorism. Serum immunoglobulin concentrations are frequently normal, but antibody responses, particularly of IgG and IgA isotypes, are usually impaired. Lymphocyte levels are reduced, and most of the circulating lymphocytes are B cells. Affected individuals usually have a tiny, histologically normal thymus located near the base of the tongue or in the neck. With time, most patients develop functional T cells.

Children lacking the congenital anomalies associated with Di George's syndrome may present with severe impairment of cell-mediated immunity. Some patients have normal or even increased immunoglobulin levels, while others have selective deficiencies of one or more immunoglobulin classes. Specific antibody responses are usually impaired even in patients with normal concentrations of immunoglobulins. This ill-defined entity has been called the *Nezelof's syndrome*.

Inherited deficiency of the enzyme purine nucleoside phosphorylase (PNP) is associated with an often severe and selective deficiency of T lymphocyte function. This enzyme functions in the same purine salvage pathway as ADA; toxic effects of the *PNP deficiency* may be related to intracellular accumulation of deoxyguanosine triphosphate (GTP).

ATAXIA-TELANGIECTASIA This is an autosomal recessive genetic disorder characterized by cerebellar ataxia, oculocutaneous telangiectasia, and immunodeficiency. The responsible gene has been mapped to the q22–23 region on chromosome 11. Onset of truncal ataxia usually occurs in infancy and is progressive. Immunodeficiency may be clinically manifest by recurrent and chronic sinopulmonary infection leading to bronchiectasis. However, not all patients have immunodeficiency. The two most frequent causes of death are chronic pulmonary disease and malignancy. Lymphomas are most common, although carcinomas also have occurred.

The immunologic abnormalities seem to be related to maldevelopment of the thymus. The thymus is markedly hypoplastic and similar in appearance to an embryonic thymus. The peripheral T cell pool is frequently reduced in size, especially in lymphoid tissue compartments. Cutaneous anergy and delayed rejection of skin grafts are common. Although the number and class distribution of B lymphocytes are usually normal, most patients are deficient in serum IgE and IgA, and a smaller number have reduced serum levels of IgG, particularly of the IgG2, IgG4 subclasses. IgM and IgD are usually normal.

There is circumstantial evidence that ataxia-telangiectasia may involve a generalized defect in cellular differentiation related to the defects in DNA repair mechanisms which have been identified in these patients. Cultured cells from these patients are highly susceptible to radiation-induced chromosomal damage. Defective DNA repair mechanisms may account for the high incidence of malignancies in these patients. Ovarian agenesis also occurs frequently. Persistence of very high serum levels of oncofetal proteins, including alpha fetoprotein and carcinoembryonic antigen, may be of diagnostic value.

Only symptomatic treatment is available. Unless a severe IgG deficiency is present, therapy with immunoglobulin is not indicated. Unusual sensitivity to x-irradiation should be kept in mind in planning therapy for patients who develop cancer.

Immunoglobulin deficiency syndromes X-LINKED AGAMMA-GLOBULINEMIA Males with this syndrome often begin to have recurrent bacterial infections late in the first year of life, when maternally derived immunoglobulins have disappeared. Affected individuals have very few immunoglobulin-bearing B lymphocytes in their circulation and lack primary and secondary lymphoid follicles. However, B cell precursors are found in normal frequency in the bone marrow. This developmental block at the pre-B cell level contrasts with earlier and later arrests in B cell differentiation characterizing other immunodeficiencies (see below and Fig. 278-1). The defective kinase gene is located in the Xq 22 region. B cells from obligate carriers utilize the normal X chromosome exclusively, while T cells and myeloid cells express either X chromosome. *X-linked agammaglobulinemia with growth hormone deficiency* is a rare variant disorder that maps to the same region of the X chromosome.

Agammaglobulinemia is a misnomer, since most patients with this and other forms of severe panhypogammaglobulinemia synthesize some immunoglobulins. Within the same family, some affected males have had substantial levels of IgM, IgG, and IgA, while others have been nearly agammaglobulinemic. All these patients were markedly deficient in circulating B lymphocytes. This observation indicates that the few B lymphocytes that escape the block in differentiation are capable of plasma cell maturation and immunoglobulin synthesis. However, antibody replacement therapy is needed in all these patients because of the limited number of B cell clones that are generated.

Sinopulmonary infections constitute the most frequent clinical problem. A form of arthritis with some of the features of rheumatoid disease occurs in some of these patients. *Mycoplasma* organisms are sometimes the cause of the arthritis. Chronic encephalitis of viral etiology can be a fatal complication. Some of these patients have an associated dermatomyositis. The frequency with which these complications occur is reduced by adequate treatment with intravenous immunoglobulin.

TRANSIENT HYPOGAMMAGLOBULINEMIA OF INFANCY This is a reversible syndrome in which normal physiologic hypogammaglobulinemia of infancy is unusually prolonged and severe. IgG levels normally drop to 3.0 to 4.0 g/L between 3 and 6 months of age as maternally derived IgG is catabolized. The IgG levels subsequently rise, reflecting the infants' increased synthetic capacity. Periodic immunologic assessment is needed to differentiate transient hypogammaglobulinemia from other forms of antibody deficiency. Antibody replacement therapy is recommended only in rare instances of severe or recurrent infections.

ISOLATED DEFICIENCY OF IGA This immunodeficiency occurs with a frequency of approximately 1 in 600 individuals of European origin. IgA deficiency is much less common in people of Asian and African origin. In Japan, for example, the incidence is approximately 1 in 18,500. While the precise genetic basis for this difference in incidence is unknown, IgA deficiency is frequently associated with certain MHC haplotypes in Caucasians.

With rare exceptions, IgA1 and IgA2 subclasses are both deficient in serum and in mucous secretions. While most individuals with isolated IgA deficiency appear healthy, others have an increased number of respiratory infections of varying severity, and a few have severe pulmonary disease such as bronchiectasis. Chronic diarrheal disease also occurs. The incidence of asthma and other atopic diseases among IgA-deficient patients is high, and conversely, the incidence of IgA deficiency among atopic children has been found to be 20 to 40 times that in the normal population. IgA deficiency is also significantly associated with autoimmune diseases such as rheumatoid arthritis and systemic lupus erythematosus. Selective reductions in the IgG2 and IgG4 subclasses have been associated with the increased infections seen in some IgA-deficient individuals. Finally, IgA-deficient patients may develop significant levels of antibodies to IgA. These patients may have severe anaphylactic reactions when transfused with normal blood or blood products.

IgA deficiency is often familial. It also can occur in association with congenital intrauterine infections, such as toxoplasmosis, rubella, and cytomegalovirus infection, or following treatment with phenytoin, penicillamine, or other medications in genetically susceptible individuals.

The pathogenesis of IgA deficiency, whether genetic or induced by environmental insult, involves a block in terminal differentiation of B lymphocytes. The IgA-bearing lymphocytes in these patients also bear surface IgM. This immature phenotype, also prevalent in normal neonates, may reflect a primary defect in essential regulatory interactions between T and B cells.

Treatment of IgA deficiency is essentially symptomatic. IgA cannot be effectively replaced by exogenous immunoglobulin or plasma, and use of either can increase the risk of development of antibodies to IgA. IgA-deficient patients in need of transfusion should be screened for the presence of antibodies to IgA and ideally should be given blood only from IgA-deficient donors. Treatment with immunoglobulin may benefit the exceptional IgA-deficient person in whom IgG2 and IgG4 subclass deficiencies are associated with severe infections. The risk of anaphylactic reactions to contaminating IgA must always be considered in treating IgA-deficient patients.

IGG SUBCLASS DEFICIENCIES Selective deficiencies in one or more of the four IgG subclasses are seen in some patients with repeated infections. The IgG subclass deficiency may easily go undetected when the total serum IgG level is measured, because IgG2, IgG3, and IgG4 together account for only 30 to 40 percent of the IgG antibodies. Even a deficiency in IgG1 may be masked by increases in the remaining IgG isotypes. However, the availability of subclass-specific monoclonal antibodies allows precise measurement of IgG subclass levels.

Homozygous deletions of genes encoding the constant region of the different γ chains is the basis for the IgG subclass deficiency in some individuals. For example, deletion of the $C_{\alpha 1}$, $C_{\gamma 2}$, $C_{\gamma 4}$, and C_{ϵ} genes on both chromosomes 14 was responsible for one individual's inability to make IgA1, IgG2, IgG4, and IgE. Interestingly, individuals with this and other patterns of C_H-gene deletions may not have unusual infections.

Most of the IgG subclass–deficient individuals with repeated infections appear to have regulatory defects which prevent normal B cell differentiation. The defect may extend to other isotypes. IgA deficiency may accompany IgG2 and IgG4 subclass deficiencies (see "Isolated Deficiency of IgA," above), and an inability to produce IgM antibodies to polysaccharide antigens often reflects a broader defect in antibody responsiveness. While patients with IgG subclass deficiency may benefit from administration of immunoglobulin, a thorough immunologic assessment is needed to identify the relatively few who need this therapy.

COMMON VARIABLE IMMUNODEFICIENCY This diagnostic category includes a heterogeneous group of males and females, mostly adults, who have in common the clinical manifestations of deficient production of all major immunoglobulin classes. The majority of these panhypo-gammaglobulinemic patients have normal numbers of B lymphocytes which are clonally diverse but phenotypically immature. B lymphocytes in these patients are able to recognize antigens and can proliferate in response but fail to differentiate to become plasma cells. This abortive differentiation pattern leads to the frequent occurrence of nodular lymphoid hyperplasia, including splenomegaly and intestinal lymphoid hyperplasia. Three types of defects in B lymphocyte differentiation have been tentatively identified. First, an intrinsic abnormality of B lymphocytes may prevent their differentiation into immunoglobulin-secreting plasma cells even when provided with differentiation factors from normal T cells. Second, in some patients the T cells, or their products, may actively suppress the terminal differentiation of normal B lymphocytes. Third, the defective B cell response may reflect a deficiency of helper T cell function which may be associated with reduced numbers of CD+ T cells.

Common variable immunodeficiency and IgA deficiency may represent polar ends of a clinical spectrum due to the same underlying gene defect in a large subset of these patients. The two disorders feature similar B cell differentiation arrests, differing only in the numbers of immune globulin classes involved. Both disorders occur frequently within the same family, and the same MHC haplotypes are associated with both immunodeficiency patterns. The data suggest an underlying susceptibility gene in both disorders.

It is important to consider the diagnosis of common variable immunodeficiency in adults with chronic pulmonary infections, some of whom will present with unexplained bronchiectasis. Intestinal diseases, including chronic giardiasis, intestinal malabsorption, and atrophic gastritis with pernicious anemia, are common in this group of patients. Patients with common variable immunodeficiency also may present with signs and symptoms highly suggestive of lymphoid malignancy, including fever, weight loss, splenomegaly, generalized lymphadenopathy, and lymphocytosis. Routine histologic examination of lymphoid tissues usually reveals germinal center hyperplasia which may be difficult to distinguish from nodular lymphoma (see Chap. 311). Demonstration of a normal distribution of immunoglobulin isotypes and light chain classes on circulating and tissue B lymphocytes can serve to distinguish these patients from those having a monoclonal B cell malignancy with secondary hypogammaglobulinemia. The monthly administration of intravenous immunoglobulin in adequate doses (see below) is an essential part of the prevention and treatment of all these complications.

X-LINKED IMMUNODEFICIENCY WITH INCREASED LEVELS OF IGM In this syndrome, IgG and IgA levels are very low or undetectable, while IgD levels may be high. The normal development of B lymphocytes bearing IgM and IgD and the absence of IgG and IgA B lymphocytes indicate a defect in isotype switching. The defective gene in these patients may encode a transmembrane molecule on T cells that is the ligand for the CD40 molecule on B cells. The failure to express this CD40 ligand prevents normal T and B cell cooperation and isotype switching. The clinical patterns of infection are similar to those occurring with other hypogammaglobulinemic states. Lymphoid hyperplasia may be severe. Neutropenia often occurs in affected males and can increase their vulnerability to infections. Adequate antibody replacement by immunoglobulin administration may reverse the neutropenia and reduce the frequency of infections requiring antibiotic therapy.

ISOLATED DEFICIENCY OF IGM This syndrome has been reported rarely in the United States but was detected frequently in a British population. Approximately 60 percent of these patients had severe recurrent infections, often with bacteremia. Pneumococcal pneumonia and meningococcal meningitis have been noted in IgM-deficient patients. Other associated conditions included gastrointestinal disease, atopy, splenomegaly, and development of malignancy. The condition was frequently familial and was four times more common in males than in females. The number of circulating B lymphocytes has varied from very low to normal.

Miscellaneous immunodeficiency syndromes Infection with *Candida albicans* is the almost universal accompaniment of severe deficiencies in cell-mediated immunity. The syndrome of *chronic mucocutaneous candidiasis* is different because superficial candidiasis is usually the only major manifestation of immunodeficiency. These patients rarely develop systemic infection with *Candida* or other fungal agents and are not unusually susceptible to virus or bacterial disease. The syndrome is often congenital and may be associated with single or multiple endocrinopathies as well as iron deficiency. Treatment of associated conditions may lead to improvement or even cure of *Candida* infection.

No uniformity of immunologic defects has been identified in these patients, although defects of antibody formation have been detected occasionally. Humoral immunity, including ability to make specific anti-*Candida* antibodies, is usually normal. Many patients are anergic, some to a variety of antigens and some only to *Candida;* anergy in some patients has been related to inability of their lymphocytes to produce the cytokine called *migration inhibition factor*.

Results of treatment with antifungal agents, such as amphotericin B, have been variable. In some patients, intensive treatment with amphotericin B coupled with surgical removal of infected nails has led to sustained improvement. Ketoconazole, an oral antifungal agent, also may be effective, but long-term remissions are rarely achieved with therapeutic means that are presently available.

IMMUNODEFICIENCY WITH THYMOMA The association of hypo-gammaglobulinemia with spindle cell thymoma usually occurs relatively late in adult life. Bacterial infections and severe diarrhea often reflect the antibody deficiency, whereas fungal and viral infections are infrequent complications. T cell numbers and cell-mediated immunity are usually intact, but these patients are very deficient in circulating B lymphocytes and pre-B cells in the bone marrow. They also frequently have eosinopenia and may develop erythroid aplasia. Complete bone marrow failure has occurred in a few immunodeficient patients with thymoma. The relationship between the thymoma and apparent abnormalities of hematopoietic stem cells remains conjectural.

WISKOTT-ALDRICH SYNDROME This is an X-linked genetic disease characterized by eczema, thrombocytopenia, and repeated infections. The platelets are small and have a shortened half-life. Affected male infants often present with bleeding, and most do not survive childhood, dying of complications of bleeding, infection, or lymphoreticular malignancy. The immunologic defects are well characterized phenotypically but are poorly understood. Serum concentrations of IgM are usually decreased, while IgA and IgG are normal and IgE is frequently increased. Synthetic rates for all three classes may be elevated, indicating a significant element of hypercatabolism. The number and class distribution of B lymphocytes are usually normal. Functionally, these boys are consistently unable to make antibodies to polysaccharide antigens normally; responses to protein antigens are often impaired late in the course of the disease. While most patients acquire T cell deficiencies, serial appraisal suggests that the T cell defects are secondary. Affected boys frequently become anergic, and their T cells do not respond normally to challenge with ubiquitous antigens. The nature of the primary defect is still unknown.

Transplantation of histocompatible bone marrow from a sibling donor has corrected both hematologic and immunologic abnormalities in several patients. In patients lacking a suitable donor, splenectomy may improve platelet counts and reduce the risk of serious hemorrhage. Because of the increased risk of pneumococcal bacteremia, splenectomized patients should probably receive prophylactic penicillin.

X-LINKED LYMPHOPROLIFERATIVE SYNDROME   This is an X-linked recessive disease in which there appears to be a selective impairment in immune elimination of Epstein-Barr virus (EBV). Infectious mononucleosis in affected males may have a fulminant and fatal outcome, may be associated with development of B cell malignancies, or may result in acquired hypogammaglobulinemia, aplastic anemia, or agranulocytosis. Antibodies to EBV have been detected in some patients but are often absent in the face of infection. Generation of cytotoxic T cells appears to be the primary mechanism of control of EBV infection in normal persons, and natural killer cells also may play a role in eliminating EBV-infected B cells. While the gene defect has been mapped to the Xq 24–27 region, the nature of the cellular defect which prevents a normal response to EBV in patients with the X-linked lymphoproliferative syndrome has not been defined.

HYPER-IGE SYNDROME   The *hyper IgE syndrome* (see Chap. 54) is characterized by recurrent abscesses involving skin, lungs, and other organs and very high IgE levels. Staphylococcal infection is common to all patients, but most have infections with other pyogenic organisms as well. Males and females of all races are affected in an inheritance pattern suggesting an autosomal dominant defect with variable penetrance. A specific immunologic defect has not been identified. Abnormal neutrophil chemotaxis is an inconsistent finding, and diminished antibody responses to secondary immunization have been noted in some patients. Prophylaxis with penicillinase-resistant penicillins or cephalosporins is highly recommended to prevent staphylococcal infections. Pneumatocoeles, a frequent complication of penumonias, may require surgical excision.

Metabolic abnormalities associated with immunodeficiency The relation of deficiencies of the purine salvage enzymes adenosine deaminase and purine nucleoside phosphorylase to immunodeficiency was discussed earlier. The syndrome of *acrodermatitis enteropathica* includes severe desquamating skin lesions, intractable diarrhea, bizarre neurologic symptoms, variable combined immunodeficiency, and an often fatal outcome. This disease is apparently caused by an inborn error of metabolism resulting in malabsorption of dietary zinc and can be treated effectively by parenteral or large oral doses of zinc. Zinc deficiency might in part account for the immunodeficiency which accompanies severe malnutrition. Inherited *deficiency of transcobalamin II*, the serum carrier molecule responsible for transport of vitamin B_{12} to tissues, is associated with failure of immunoglobulin production as well as megaloblastic anemia, leukopenia, thrombocytopenia, and severe malabsorption. All abnormalities of this rare disorder are reversed by administration of vitamin B_{12}.

TREATMENT OF IMMUNODEFICIENCIES   Immunodeficiency diseases involving severe abnormalities of T cell function, with or without hypogammaglobulinemia, are often treatable with bone marrow transplants (see Fig. 278-1). Histocompatible marrow from a sibling donor is preferred, but haploidentical marrow may be used after removal of T cells. This therapy is complex and is best done by experienced research teams.

Replacement therapy with human immunoglobulin currently should be used in patients who have recurrent bacterial infections and are deficient in IgG. Maintenance of serum IgG levels above 5.0 g/L is sufficient to prevent most systemic infections and, together with antibiotic therapy, enhances reversal of chronic sinopulmonary infection. These serum levels usually can be achieved by intravenous administration of IgG, 400 mg/kg, at monthly intervals.

The advantage of intravenous immunoglobulin over intramuscular preparations is that higher amounts of antibodies can be given with less discomfort. Since higher levels of serum antibodies afford better protection from infections, intravenous antibody replacement is currently considered the treatment of choice for hypogammaglobulinemia. In patients with mild to moderate IgG deficiency (3.0 to 4.0

g/L), the decision to treat should be based on clinical symptoms and response to antigenic challenge.

Immunoglobulin treatment is of no value in patients with deficiencies of immunoglobulins other than IgG. This form of treatment is not benign. Some patients develop symptoms of diaphoresis, tachycardia, flank pain, and hypotension during or immediately following injections. This reaction may be mediated by aggregates of IgG or other biologically active substances, but it also may occur as a consequence of antibodies produced by the patient against donor immunoglobulins, particularly IgA (see Chap. 312).

Use of plasma or immunoglobulin selected on the basis of a high titer of antibodies to a particular agent may be indicated in certain situations. For example, antibodies to the causative virus may dramatically improve the chronic enteroviral encephalitis which occurs in some agammaglobulinemic patients.

Therapy with exogenous IgG may not suffice to eliminate the chronic sinopulmonary inflammation and its progression to pulmonary fibrosis and bronchiectasis. Therefore, maintenance of good pulmonary toilet with regular postural drainage can be an especially important part of patient management. The principles of antibiotic therapy are not different in these than in other patients, except that the index of suspicion of bacterial infection should remain very high.

The availability of purified interferon-γ and other biologically active cytokines promises to be important in the therapy of certain immunologic disorders. Gene therapy also holds great promise for therapy of defined genetic defects of the immune system.

REFERENCES

ARNAIR-VILLENA A et al: Human T cell activation deficiencies. Immunol Today 13:259, 1992

BLAESE RM, CULVER KW: Gene therapy for primary immunodeficiency disease. Immunodeficiency Rev 3:329, 1992

BUCKLEY RH, SHIFF RI: The use of intravenous immune globulin in immunodeficiency diseases. N Engl J Med 325:110, 1991

COOPER MD: B lymphocytes: Normal development and function. N Engl J Med 317:1452, 1987

FISCHER A: Severe combined immunodeficiencies. Immunodeficiency Rev 3:83, 1992

GOOD RA: Bone marrow transplantation for immunodeficiency diseases. Am J Med Sci 294:68, 1987

PAUL WE: *Fundamental Immunology*, 2d ed. New York, Raven, 1989

PREUD'HOMME JL, HANSON LA: IgG subclass deficiency. Immunodeficiency Rev 2:83, 1990

ROIFMAN CM, GELFAND EW: Replacement therapy with high dose intravenous gamma-globulin improves sinopulmonary disease in patients with hypogammaglobulinemia. Pediatr Infect Dis J 7:S92, 1988

ROSEN FS et al: Primary immunodeficiency diseases—Report of a WHO Scientific Group. Immunodeficiency Rev 3:195, 1992

ROYER HD, REINHERZ EL: T lymphocytes: Ontogeny, function, and relevance to clinical disorders. N Engl J Med 274:1171, 1987

SCHAFFER FM et al: IgA deficiency. Immunodeficiency Rev 3:15, 1991

279   HUMAN IMMUNODEFICIENCY VIRUS (HIV) DISEASE: AIDS AND RELATED DISORDERS

ANTHONY S. FAUCI / H. CLIFFORD LANE

The 1990s mark the second decade of the HIV/AIDS pandemic. The disease was first recognized in the United States in the summer of 1981 when the Centers for Disease Control (CDC) reported the unexplained occurrence of *Pneumocystis carinii* pneumonia in 5 previously healthy homosexual men in Los Angeles and Kaposi's sarcoma in 26 previously healthy homosexual men in New York and Los Angeles. Within months, the disease became recognized in male and female injection drug users (IDUs) and soon thereafter in recipients of blood transfusions and hemophiliacs who received plasma-derived coagulation factors. Early on in the epidemic, because of the disproportionate number of cases in Haitians, this group was incorrectly designated as a "risk" group. It soon because clear that the disease in Haitians was following a pattern of sexual transmission, both homosexual and heterosexual, the latter of which was virtually identical to the predominant mode of transmission in certain developing countries in Africa and elsewhere in the world (see below). As the epidemiologic pattern of the disease unfolded, it became clear that a microbe transmissible by sexual contact and blood or blood products was the most likely etiologic agent of the epidemic.

In 1983, HIV was isolated from a patient with lymphadenopathy and by 1984 it was clearly demonstrated to be the causative agent of AIDS. This retrovirus of the lentivirus family (see below) was formerly called *lymphadenopathy associated virus (LAV)*, *human T lymphotropic virus III (HTLV-III)*, and *AIDS-associated retrovirus (ARV)*. In 1985, a sensitive enzyme-linked immunosorbent assay (ELISA) blood test was developed which has led to an appreciation of the scope of HIV infection among cohorts of individuals who admittedly practice high-risk behavior (see below) as well as among selected populations which have been screened such as blood donors, military recruits and active duty military personnel, Job Corps applicants, and patients in various sentinel hospitals (see below). This surveillance approach together with monitoring of levels of CD4+ T cell counts as a parameter of immunosuppression has led to the clear appreciation that there is a broad spectrum of HIV disease ranging from the asymptomatic infected individual up to advanced clinical disease which has been referred to as *AIDS*.

In the 1980s, the care of AIDS patients in the United States was with few exceptions confined to relatively restricted groups of physicians and hospitals, mostly in urban areas particularly on the northeastern and western seaboards. Toward the end of the 1980s and certainly in the 1990s it has become evident that virtually every practicing physician in the country will be required to have some degree of familiarity with the workup, diagnosis, and treatment of HIV-infected individuals. HIV-infected patients are now and in increasing numbers will be presenting to their family practice physicians, internists, obstetrician/gynecologists, pediatricians, and surgeons with clinical problems that may be directly or indirectly related, or totally unrelated, to their HIV infection.

Scientific advances are occurring at an extremely rapid pace in the areas of molecular virology of HIV, pathogenesis (both virologic and immunopathogenic) and treatment of HIV, as well as the opportunistic diseases associated with HIV infection, prophylaxis of opportunistic infections, and vaccine development. Despite such advances the HIV pandemic is growing in magnitude worldwide and the cost in human life and suffering is staggering. Physicians and other health care providers are in the unusual position of caring for HIV-infected individuals within the framework of a rapidly evolving scientific and clinical discipline. The purpose of this chapter is to present the most current information available on the scope of the epidemic, on its pathogenesis, treatment, and prevention, and on prospects for vaccine development. Above all the aim is to provide the reader with a solid scientific basis and practical guidelines for a state of the art approach to the HIV-infected patient.

DEFINITION AIDS was originally defined for surveillance purposes by the CDC prior to the identification of HIV as the etiologic agent as the presence of a reliably diagnosed "opportunistic" disease that is at least moderately indicative of an underlying defect in cell-mediated immunity in the absence of known causes of underlying immune defects such as iatrogenic immunosuppression or malignant neoplasms. Upon the availability of sensitive and specific diagnostic tests for HIV, the case definition of AIDS has undergone several revisions with regard to inclusion and exclusion criteria. The current

TABLE 279-1 CDC surveillance case definition for AIDS (1993)

A Indicator diseases diagnosed definitively in the absence of other causes of immunodeficiency and without laboratory evidence of HIV infection
 1 Candidiasis of the esophagus, trachea, bronchi, or lungs
 2 Cryptococcosis, extrapulmonary
 3 Cryptosporidiosis with diarrhea persisting >1 month
 4 Cytomegalovirus disease of any organ excluding liver, spleen, and lymph nodes in a patient >1 month of age
 5 Herpes simplex virus infection causing a mucocutaneous ulcer persisting >1 month; or bronchitis, pneumonia, or esophagitis in a patient >1 month of age
 6 Kaposi's sarcoma in a patient <60 years old
 7 Lymphoma of the brain (primary) in a patient <60 years of age
 8 Lymphoid interstitial pneumonia and/or pulmonary lymphoid hyperplasia in a child <13 years of age.
 9 *Mycobacterium avium* complex or *M. kansasii* disease (disseminated)
 10 *Pneumocystis carinii* pneumonia
 11 Toxoplasmosis of the brain in a patient >1 month of age
B Indicator diseases diagnosed definitively regardless of the presence of other causes of immunodeficiency and in the presence of laboratory evidence of HIV infection
 1 Any disease listed in section A
 2 Bacterial infections (multiple or recurrent) in children <13 years of age caused by *Haemophilus*, *Streptococcus*, or other pyogenic bacteria.
 3 Coccidioidomycosis, disseminated
 4 HIV encephalopathy
 5 Histoplasmosis, disseminated
 6 Isosporiasis with diarrhea persisting >1 month
 7 Kaposi's sarcoma at any age
 8 Non-Hodgkin's lymphoma of B cell or unknown phenotype and having the histologic type of small noncleaved lymphoma or immunoblastic sarcoma
 9 Any mycobacterial disease, disseminated, excluding *M. tuberculosis*
 10 *M. tuberculosis*, extrapulmonary
 11 *Salmonella* (nontyphoid) septicemia, recurrent
 12 HIV wasting syndrome
C Indicator diseases diagnosed presumptively in the presence of laboratory evidence of HIV infection
 1 Candidiasis of the esophagus
 2 Cytomegalovirus retinitis with loss of vision
 3 Kaposi's sarcoma
 4 Lymphoid interstitial pneumonia and/or pulmonary lymphoid hyperplasia in a child <13 years of age
 5 Mycobacterial disease, disseminated
 6 *Pneumocystis carinii* pneumonia
 7 Toxoplasmosis of the brain in a patient >1 month of age
D Indicator diseases diagnosed definitively in the absence of other causes of immunodeficiency and in the presence of negative results for HIV infection
 1 *Pneumocystis carinii* pneumonia
 2 Other indicator diseases listed in section A and CD4+ T lymphocyte count <400 per microliter
E The 1993 expanded definition includes:
 1 All HIV-infected persons who have <200 CD4+ T lymphocyte counts per microliter, or a CD4+ T lymphocyte percentage of total lymphocytes of <14.
 2 Pulmonary tuberculosis
 3 Recurrent pneumonia
 4 Invasive cervical cancer

From: Morb Mort Week Rep (Suppl 1):1, 1987; Morb Mort Week Rep 41, no. RR-17, 1993.

surveillance case definition is shown in Table 279-1. In 1993, the case definition was further expanded to include any HIV-infected individual with a CD4+ T cell count less than 200 per microliter, even without symptoms, as well as HIV-infected individuals with pulmonary tuberculosis (TB), recurrent episodes of pneumonia, or invasive cervical carcinoma. This definition is complex and comprehensive; however, the clinician should view HIV disease simply as a broad spectrum ranging from the primary infection, with or without the acute HIV syndrome, to the asymptomatic infected state to advanced disease (see below), rather than focusing on the presence or absence of AIDS, a strict definition that was established not for the practical care of patients but for surveillance.

TABLE 279-2   The human retroviruses

Virus	Culture characteristics	Diseases
HTLV-I	Transforming	Leukemias/lymphomas of CD4+ T lymphocytes; tropical spastic paraparesis (TSP); HTLV-1–associated myelopathy (HAM)
HTLV-II	Transforming	None recognized
HIV-1	Cytopathic	HIV disease/AIDS
HIV-2	Cytopathic	HIV disease/AIDS; may be less virulent than HIV-1

ETIOLOGY

The etiologic agent of AIDS is HIV, which belongs to the family of human retroviruses and the subfamily of lentiviruses. Nononcogenic lentiviruses cause disease in other animal species including sheep, horses, goats, cattle, cats, and monkeys. The four recognized human retroviruses belong to two distinct groups: the human T lymphotropic viruses, HTLV-I and II, and the human immunodeficiency viruses, HIV-1 and -2 (Table 279-2). The reader is referred to Chap. 151 for a detailed description of the biology of the human retroviruses. The most common cause of HIV disease throughout the world and certainly in the United States is HIV-1. HIV-2 was first identified in 1986 in West African patients and was originally confined to West Africa. However, a number of cases of HIV-2 have been reported in Europe, South America, Canada, and the United States. Although HIV-2 has approximately 40 percent nucleotide sequence homology with HIV-1 it is much more closely related phylogenetically to the simian immunodeficiency virus (SIV) found in sooty mangabees. HIV-1 is more closely related to an SIV isolated from chimpanzees in 1990. The taxonomic relationship among primate lentiviruses is shown in Fig. 279-1.

MORPHOLOGY Electron microscopy illustrates that the HIV-1 virion is an icosahedral structure (Fig. 279-2A) containing numerous external spikes formed by the two major viral envelope proteins, the external gp120 and the transmembrane gp41. The virion buds from the surface of the infected cell and incorporates a variety of host proteins including major histocompatibility complex (MHC) class I and II antigens (see Chap. 64) into its lipid bilayer. The structure of HIV-1 is schematically diagrammed in Fig. 279-2B (see also Chap. 151).

FIGURE 279-1 Taxonomy of primate lentiviruses. Figure illustrates the various percents of nucleotide sequence homologies among the different viruses. *(From RC Desrosiers, A finger on the missing link. Nature 345:288, 1990.)*

A

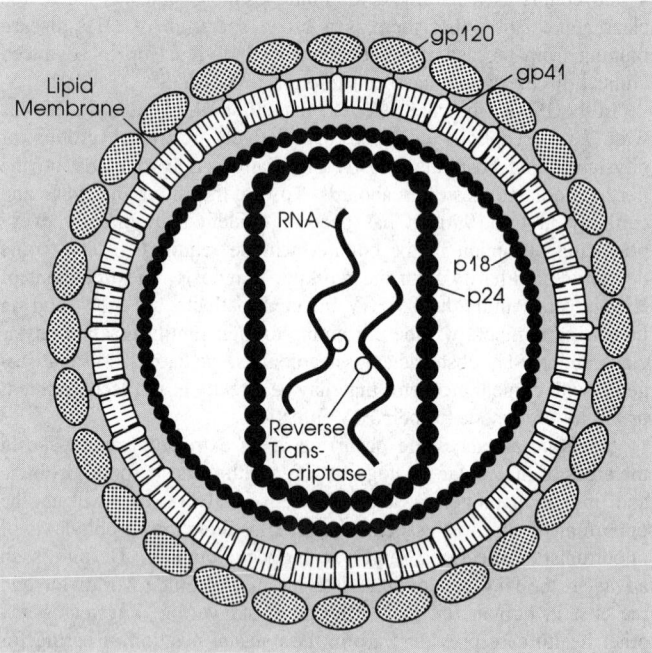

B

FIGURE 279-2 *A.* Electron micrograph of HIV. Figure illustrates a typical virion following budding from the surface of a CD4+ T lymphocyte together with two additional incomplete virions in the process of budding from the cell membrane. *B.* Structure of HIV-1, including the gp120 outer membrane, gp41 transmembrane components of the envelope, genomic RNA, enzyme reverse transcriptase, p18(17) inner membrane, and p24 core protein. *(Adapted from RC Gallo, The human immunodeficiency virus (HIV), Scientific American, January, 1987.)*

LIFE CYCLE The hallmark of the life cycle of HIV infection is the reverse transcription of genomic RNA to DNA by the enzyme called *reverse transcriptase*. The HIV life cycle begins with the high-affinity binding of the gp120 protein via a portion of its V1 region near the *N*-terminus to its receptor on the host cell surface, the CD4 molecule (Fig. 279-3). The CD4 molecule is a 55-kDa protein found

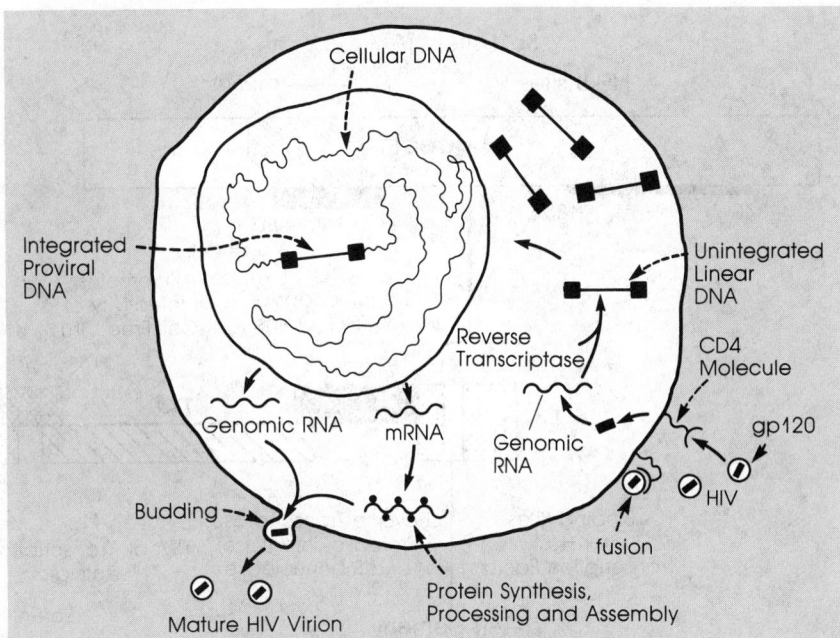

FIGURE 279-3 The life cycle of HIV. See text for description. *(From AS Fauci, The human immunodeficiency virus: Infectivity and mechanisms of pathogenesis. Science 239:617, 1988.)*

predominantly on a subset of T lymphocytes responsible for helper or inducer function in the immune response (see Chap. 277). It is also expressed on the surface of cells of the monocyte/macrophage lineage. Following binding, fusion with the host cell membrane occurs via the gp41 molecule, and the HIV genomic RNA is un-coated and internalized. The reverse transcriptase enzyme which was contained in the virion then catalyzes the reverse transcription of the genomic RNA into double-stranded DNA. The DNA migrates to the nucleus where it is integrated into the host cell chromosomes through the action of another virally encoded enzyme, *integrase*. The incorporation of this ''provirus'' into the cell genome is permanent. This provirus may remain transcriptionally inactive (latent) or manifest high levels of gene expression with active production of virus.

Cellular activation plays an important role in the life cycle of HIV. The activation of HIV expression from the latent state depends upon the interaction of a number of cellular and viral factors (see below). Incompletely reverse-transcribed DNA intermediates are labile in quiescent cells and will not be efficiently integrated into the host cell genome unless cellular activation occurs shortly after infection. Furthermore, activation of the host cell is required for the initiation of transcription of the integrated proviral DNA into either genomic or messenger RNA. Following transcription, HIV mRNA is translated into proteins which undergo modification through cleavage, glycosylation, myristilation, and phosphorylation. The viral core is formed by the assembly of HIV proteins, enzymes, and genomic RNA at the plasma membrane of the cells. Budding of the progeny virion occurs through the host cell membrane, where the core acquires its external envelope.

HIV GENOME A schematic diagram of the HIV-1 genome is shown in Fig. 279-4. Similar to other retroviruses, HIV-1 comprises genes which encode the structural proteins of the virus: *gag* encodes the proteins that form the virion core (including p24 antigen); *pol* encodes the enzymes responsible for reverse transcription and integration; and *env* encodes the envelope glycoproteins. However, HIV-1 is more complex than other retroviruses in that it also contains at least six other genes (*tat, rev, nef, vif, vpr,* and *vpu*) that encode for proteins which are involved in the regulation of HIV expression (see Chap. 151). Flanking these genes are the long terminal repeats (LTRs) which contain regulatory elements involved in gene expression (see below), such as the polyadenylation signal sequence, the TATA promoter sequence, the NF-κB and SP1 enhancer binding sites, the transactivating response (TAR) sequences where the *tat* protein binds,

and the negative regulatory element (NRE) whose deletion increases the level of gene expression (Fig. 279-4). The major difference in the genomes of HIV-1 and HIV-2 is the fact that HIV-2 lacks the *vpu* gene and HIV-2 has a *vpx* gene not contained in HIV-1.

TRANSMISSION

HIV is transmitted by sexual contact, homosexual and heterosexual; by blood or blood products; and by infected mother to infant intrapartum, perinatally, or via breast milk. Well into the second decade of the epidemic, there is absolutely no evidence that HIV is transmitted by casual contact or that the virus can be spread by insects such as by a mosquito bite.

SEXUAL TRANSMISSION Sexual contact is the major mode of transmission worldwide. Although transmission through homosexual contact has been the most common form of sexual transmission in the United States (see below), heterosexual transmission is the most common modality of transmission worldwide, particularly in developing countries; in addition, it is being seen with increasing frequency in the United States. HIV virus has been demonstrated in the semen both within infected mononuclear cells and in the cell-free seminal fluid. The virus appears to concentrate in the seminal fluid particularly in situations in which there are increased numbers of lymphocytes in the fluid, as in genital inflammatory states such as urethritis and epididymitis, conditions closely associated with other sexually transmitted diseases. The virus has also been demonstrated in cervical smears and vaginal fluid. There is a strong association of transmission of HIV with receptive anal intercourse, likely due to the fact that there is only a thin and fragile rectal mucosal membrane separating the deposited semen from potentially susceptible cells within and beneath the mucosa as well as the fact that there may be trauma associated with anal intercourse. The trauma associated with anal douching and receptive insertion of a clenched fist into the rectum (''fisting'') also increases the likelihood of infection during receptive anal intercourse. Although the vaginal mucosa is several layers thicker than the rectal mucosa and less likely to be traumatized during intercourse, it is clear that the virus can be transmitted to either partner through vaginal intercourse. There is approximately a twenty times greater chance of transmission of HIV from a man to a women than from a woman to a man through vaginal intercourse. This may be in part due to the prolonged exposure of the vaginal and cervical

FIGURE 279-4   *A*. The genome of HIV. *(From WC Greene, N Engl J Med, 324:308, 1991.) B*. The long terminal repeat of HIV. *(From ZF Rosenberg and AS Fauci, Immunol Today 11:176, 1990.)*

mucosa as well as the endometrium (which semen enters through the cervical os) to the infected semen. This is in comparison to the relatively brief period that the penis and urethral orifice are exposed to infected vaginal fluid. There is a close association of genital ulcerations and transmission, both from the standpoint of susceptibility to infection and infectivity. Infections with microorganisms such as *Treponema pallidum* (see Chap. 133), *Haemophilus ducreyi* (see Chap. 112), and herpes simplex virus (see Chap. 143) are important causes of genital ulcerations linked to transmission of HIV. Furthermore, there have been individual reports of associations of cervical ectopy as well as cervical erosions resulting from infection due to *Chlamydia trachomatis* (see Chap. 140) and *Neisseria gonorrhoeae* (see Chap. 110) with transmission of HIV infection. Thus, these phenomena in certain cases can be considered as *cofactors* for HIV transmission.

Oral sex appears to be a much less efficient mode of transmission of HIV; however, there have been rare individual reports of HIV transmission resulting from receptive fellatio and insertive cunnilingus.

BLOOD AND BLOOD PRODUCTS   The virus can be transmitted by blood and blood products both in individuals who share contaminated needles for intravenous drug use and in those who receive transfusions of blood or blood products. HIV infection and AIDS among IDUs continues to increase in the United States (see below). Infection occurs through the intravenous exposure to infected blood via contaminated needles and other drug paraphernalia. The risk of infection increases with the duration of injection drug use, the frequency of needle sharing, participation in the "shooting gallery" drug culture where several individuals share the same needle, and using injection drugs in a geographic area with a high prevalence of HIV infection such as in certain inner city areas particularly on the eastern seaboard.

From the late 1970s until the Spring of 1985 when mandatory testing of donated blood for HIV-1 was initiated, it has been estimated that over 10,000 individuals in the United States were infected through transfusions of blood or blood products (see Chap. 312). Approximately 5000 individuals who survived their primary illness for which the transfusion was administered have developed AIDS. It is estimated that 90 to 100 percent of those who were transfused with

HIV-infected blood became infected. Transfusion of whole blood, packed red blood cells, platelets, leukocytes, and plasma are all capable of transmitting HIV infection, while hyperimmune gamma-globulin, hepatitis B immune globulin, plasma-derived hepatitis B vaccine, and Rh_o (O) immune globulin have not been associated with transmission of HIV infection. The procedures involved in processing these products either inactivate or remove the virus.

In addition to the above, several thousand hemophiliacs were infected with HIV by receipt of HIV-infected fresh frozen plasma or concentrates of clotting factors. Approximately 2000 have developed AIDS. Currently, in the United States and in most developed countries, the combination of screening all blood for HIV antibody by ELISA and confirmatory western blot where applicable; the self-deferral of donors on the basis of risk behavior; the screening out of HIV-negative individuals with positive surrogate laboratory parameters for HIV infection such as hepatitis B and C; and serologic test for syphilis has made the risk of transmission of HIV infection by transfused blood or blood products extremely small. One study estmated that the risk of HIV-1 infection via transfused blood from an HIV-infected, but seronegative, donor ranged from 1 in 40,000 to 1 in 250,000, while in another study the estimate was 1 in 61,000. There have been no reported cases of transmission of HIV-2 in the United States via donated blood, and currently donated blood is screened for both HIV-1 and HIV-2 antibodies. The chance of infection of a hemophiliac via clotting factor concentrates has essentially been eliminated because of the added layer of safety resulting form heat treatment of the concentrates.

A small number of cases of transmission of HIV via semen used in artificial insemination and tissues used in organ transplantation have been well documented. Therefore, donors of such tissues are now screened for HIV infection prior to transplantation.

OCCUPATIONAL TRANSMISSION OF HIV: HEALTH CARE AND LABORATORY WORKERS   There is a small but definite occupational risk of HIV transmission among health care workers, laboratory personnel, and potentially others who work with HIV-infected specimens, particularly when sharp objects are involved. Large multi-institutional studies have indicated that the risk of HIV transmission following skin puncture from a needle or other sharp object that was contaminated with blood from a person with documented HIV infection is approximately 0.3 percent. The risk of a similar type of exposure to hepatitis B infection is 20 to 30 percent. There have been reports of health care workers who have become infected by exposure of mucous membranes or abraded skin to HIV-infected material.

However, the risk is much smaller than that for exposure via actual skin puncture with a contaminated object such as a needle (see "HIV and the Health Care Worker" below).

In 1990, the CDC reported that an HIV-infected dentist, by then deceased, had transmitted HIV infection to five of his patients on whom he had performed invasive dental procedures. Although the mechanisms of the transmission were never fully delineated, it was surmised that the infections occurred through instruments contaminated with HIV; the dentist supposedly used the same instruments on himself that he used in his practice and a breakdown in sterile procedures was suspected, but never proven. Subsequently, a number of epidemiologic studies were performed tracing the patients of several HIV-infected dentists, physicians, and surgeons and not a single case of HIV infection that could be linked to them was identified. Thus, the risk of transmission from an infected health care worker to his/her patient is extremely low and at this point too low to be measured. The very occurrence of HIV transmission as well as hepatitis B and C to and from health care workers underscores the importance of the use of universal precautions when caring for all patients (see below and Chap. 98).

MATERNAL-FETAL/INFANT TRANSMISSION HIV can be transmitted from an infected mother to her fetus during pregnancy or to her infant during delivery. Virologic analysis of aborted fetuses indicate that the fetus can be infected during pregnancy, as early as the first and second trimester. However, it is felt that maternal transmissions to the fetus/infant occur most commonly in the perinatal period. This is based on the time frame of identification of infection by culture or polymerase chain reaction (PCR) techniques in the infant following delivery (negative at birth and positive several months later) as well as the demonstration that the first born twin of an infected mother is more commonly infected than is the second born twin.

The rate of transmission of HIV from mother to fetus/infant averages approximately 30 percent with a low of 12.9 percent in a European collaborative study and a high of 45 percent in Nairobi, Kenya. These differences may relate to adequacy of prenatal care of the mother as well as to the stage of disease in the mother during pregnancy. Higher rates of transmission have been associated with a symptomatic mother and low maternal CD4+ T cell counts. In addition, it has been speculated that if the mother gets infected during pregnancy there is a higher rate of transmission to the fetus due to the high levels of viremia following primary infection.

Postnatal mother-to-infant transmission of HIV has been clearly documented, strongly implicating colostrum and breast milk as the vehicles of infection. Virus can be isolated from both. In rare cases, mothers have been infected by transfusions following delivery and have transmitted the infection to their infants with the only risk factor being breast feeding. Where possible, breast feeding by an infected mother should be avoided; however, this becomes problematic in certain developing countries where the only consistent source of adequate nutrition as well as immunity against potentially serious infections for the infant is breast milk.

OTHER BODY FLUIDS There is no convincing evidence that saliva can transmit HIV infection either by kissing or by other exposures such as occupationally to health care workers. Although HIV has been isolated from saliva, this has been successful in only a small percentage of infected individuals. Furthermore, saliva has been demonstrated to contain inhibitory activity to HIV. However, a most unusual form of HIV transmission from infected children to mothers in the former Soviet Union has been identified. In those cases, the children (infected through transfusion) were said to have bleeding sores in the mouth and the mothers were said to have lacerations and abrasions on and around the nipples of the breast resulting from trauma from the children's teeth. Breast feeding had been continued until the children were older than is usual in the United States and other developed countries.

There have been conflicting reports of the isolation of HIV from other body fluids such as tears, sweat, and urine. However, there is no evidence that HIV transmission can occur as a result of exposure to these fluids. Nonetheless, bodily wastes of patients should be handled according to universal precautions (see below).

EPIDEMIOLOGY

AIDS IN THE UNITED STATES By June 1, 1993, there were 302,000 cumulative cases of AIDS reported in adults and adolescents in the United States (Table 279-3) and approximately 60 percent of these have died thus far. The majority of these cases are among men who have had sex with men (56 percent), and there will continue to be large numbers of new cases of AIDS within this group in the future. However, over the past few years, the numbers of newly reported cases of AIDS among IDUs has surpassed those of men who have had sex with men in certain cities with a high IV drug usage.

TABLE 279-3 AIDS cases in adults/adolescents in the United States as of June 1, 1993

Exposure category	White, not Hispanic No. (%)	Black, not Hispanic No. (%)	Hispanic No. (%)	Asian/ Pacific Islander No. (%)	American Indian/ Alaskan Native No. (%)	Total* No. (%)
Men who have sex with men	115,988 (74)	30,786 (33)	19,406 (39)	1,395 (71)	329 (54)	168,249 (56)
Injecting drug use (IDU) (female and heterosexual male)	15,031 (10)	36,007 (39)	19,665 (39)	96 (5)	104 (17)	71,053 (24)
Men who have sex with men and inject drugs	10,864 (7)	5,297 (6)	2,743 (6)	49 (2)	85 (14)	19,054 (6)
Hemophilia/ coagulation disorder	2,206 (1)	237 (0)	206 (0)	33 (2)	11 (2)	2,699 (1)
Heterosexual contact	4,472 (3)	12,201 (13)	4,068 (8)	105 (5)	32 (5)	20,909 (7)
Receipt of transfusion of blood, blood components, or tissue	3,743 (2)	1,056 (1)	681 (1)	122 (6)	11 (2)	5,621 (2)
Other/undetermined	4,880 (3)	6,320 (7)	3,095 (6)	171 (9)	32 (5)	14,580 (5)
Adult/adolescent subtotal	157,184	91,904	49,864	1,971	604	302,165
Percent of total adult/ adolescent AIDS cases	(52)	(30)	(17)	(<1)	(<1)	(100)

* Includes 638 persons of unknown race/ethnicity.
SOURCE: Centers for Disease Control and Prevention, USPHS.

TABLE 279-4 Pediatric (<13 years) AIDS cases in

Exposure category	White, not Hispanic No. (%)
Hemophilia/coagulation disorder	134 (14)
Mother with/at risk for AIDS/ HIV infection:	616 (66)
IV drug related	369
Sex with bisexual male	37
Sex with person with hemophilia	12
Receipt of blood transfusion, blood components, or tissue	28
Other	143
Receipt of transfusion of blood, blood components, or tissue	164 (18)
Undetermined	15 (2)
Pediatric subtotal	929
Percent of total pediatric AIDS cases	(20)

* Includes 11 children of unknown race/ethnicity.
SOURCE: Centers for Disease Control and Prevention, USPHS.

In addition, the relative number of cases among women, and children have been increasing, reflectin indirectly the increase in numbers of cases among IDU By June 1, 1993, there were 4615 cumulative cases of children less than 13 years of age and greater than 50 died (Table 279-4). Greater than 80 percent of these infected mothers and in approximately 70 percent of t mother was either an IDU or the heterosexual partner of increasing prevalence of HIV infection and AIDS over t among infants and children directly reflects the increas of HIV infection among women who are IDUs heterosexual partners who are IDUs. The majority of among minorities (African-Americans and Hispani those who live in inner cities in the Northeast regions of the country. In this regard, HIV infection disproportionately affected minority populations in the African-Americans and Hispanics comprise only 12 percent of the population, respectively, yet they account and 17 percent of adult/adolescent AIDS cases, respec percent and 24 percent of AIDS cases in children, res majority of IDUs in these inner cities are African-A Hispanics and the above statistics reflect the high prev infection among IDUs in such areas. The relationship area of the country to the demography of HIV infecti particularly the interconnection among geography, IDU transmission, and HIV infection in women and co children is illustrated by the rate of reported cases 100,000 population by state comparing adolescent/a adolescent/adult women (Fig. 279-5). The more diffu of cases among men throughout the various states ref distribution of cases representing men who have had The concentrations on the East and West Coasts as w and Nevada further reflect the higher densities of men sex with men and to a lesser extent IDUs in those state the disproportionately high rate of AIDS cases amon Northeast and Florida, which have the highest rates and a relatively lower rate of AIDS, and in women on and Texas compellingly link IDU to heterosexual tra infection in women in the United States at the prese nine percent of women with AIDS have become in IDU compared to 20 percent of men with AIDS; 36 per with AIDS have become infected by heterosexual co to 3 percent of men with AIDS (Table 279-3). Onl

in a greater degree of high-risk be alence among IDUs in 61 treatr areas was 0 percent to 49 perce depending on the geographic loca l on the eastern seaboard and mu thwest. In this regard, in other st emale prostitutes also varied great ent, with the rates directly reflec ups surveyed as well as the pre geographic location at the tim e rates among 35 tuberculosis cli from 0 to 58 percent with the he overall range of HIV sero omen was 0 to 0.66 percent. M en from large metropolitan area manifesting higher rates than HIV national prevalence for percent or over 1 in every 70(to approximately 6000 infecte ng in approximately 2000 inf r end of the spectrum, screenin ure of national prevalence bec ferral among individuals pract 1985, 4 million blood donc Cross blood banks; the ove with a prevalence of 0.085 nparable survey was repeate was 0.0084 percent with a

AIDS as a leading cause of de 20 to 39, 1983–1990. (From N

y Males - Ages 20-39

seroprevalence of a certain segment n the United States comes from the 4-y. The Job Corps is a federal training onally disadvantaged young persons tates. Data from 1988 through 1990 evalence (0.36 percent) than that of . Rates were especially high among s, and seroprevalence was similar in underscores the seriousness of the sadvantaged adolescents, particularly

HIV seroprevalence among sexually from a serosurvey conducted at 19 ited States between April, 1988, and f 16,863 specimens (0.2 percent) were ositive specimens were found in 9 of e fact that all but 2 of the 30 infected marily reflecting infection of men who a seroprevalence rate for men of 0.5 men was 0.02 percent, a figure in sharp ocially and educationally disadvantaged rps survey (0.32 percent).

ucted at 38 sentinel hospitals throughout 88 through 1990 underscore the wide based largely on geographic location. patients hospitalized for diseases unlikely nfection. The median seroprevalence was 80-fold variation among hospitals (0.1 to ort, a serosurvey of a District of Columbia at 11.3 percent of white and 16.9 percent were HIV infected.

d AIDS is widespread in the United States among certain populations and stabilizing others. Similar to other STDs, it is highly on will spread homogeneously throughout ed States. However, it is clear that anyone behavior is at risk for HIV infection. In crease in infections and AIDS cases among partners, women, infants born of infected s, as well as the spread within certain inner nong underserved minority populations with lth care delivery testifies to the fact that the tion in the United States is a public health rtion.

FIGURE *Serosurveillance Summary, Results through 1990,* service, U and test d

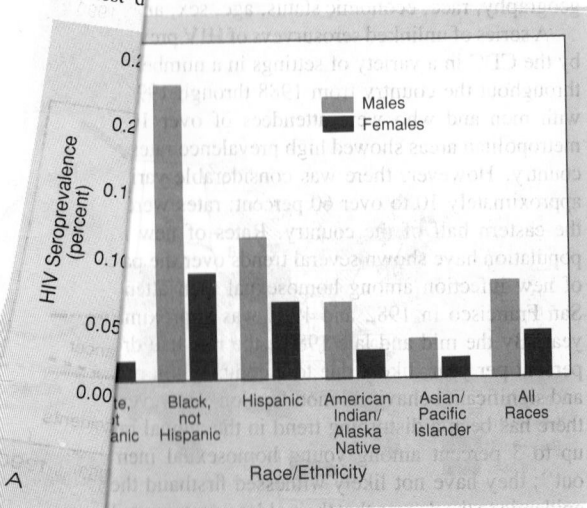

A

TABLE 279-6 Cumulative worldwide cases of AIDS reported to the World Health Organization as of July 1, 1993

Country/Region	Cases
Africa	247,577
Americas	371,086
Canada	7,770
Caribbean/Bahamas	9,250
Central America	4,436
Mexico	13,259
South America	47,051
United States of America	289,320
Asia	3,561
Europe	92,482
Oceania	4,188
Total	718,894

SOURCE: WHO, *Weekly Epidemiological Record*, No. 27, July 2, 1993.

HIV INFECTION AND AIDS WORLDWIDE HIV infection/AIDS is truly a global pandemic with cases reported from every continent. The reported cases of AIDS worldwide are a gross underestimate of the true incidence, mostly because of the incomplete reporting mechanisms available in certain developing countries. The reported cumulative cases of AIDS as of July 1, 1993, are shown in Table 279-6 and the estimated global distribution of adult HIV infections for the same time period is illustrated in Fig. 279-8. There is not and most likely will not be a uniform pandemic of AIDS worldwide. What is being witnessed are waves of epidemics with somewhat different characteristics in different regions of the world depending upon the demographics of the country or region in question and the timing of the introduction of HIV into the population. Considerable devastation has already been experienced in certain developing countries, particularly in sub-Saharan Africa, with respect to AIDS cases and deaths. This reflects the extensive spread of HIV which apparently began in the late 1970s and early 1980s. The major mode of transmission in this region is that of WHO Pattern II, which is heterosexual sex where the number of infected males and females are approximately equal. This is in contrast to North America and most of South America, Western Europe, Scandinavia, Australia, and New Zealand (Pattern I) where approximately 90 percent of cases are among men who have sex with men or among IDUs. Of note is the

fact that the annual incidence of HIV infections in sub-Saharan Africa is believed still to be on the increase, signaling even worse devastation through the 1990s. In South America and the Caribbean, the annual incidence of infection is also believed to be increasing, but at lower levels than sub-Saharan Africa. WHO estimates that 1 million HIV-infected children have been born since the start of the HIV pandemic and more than half of these have developed AIDS and have died. In addition, approximately 2 million uninfected children are currently or will become AIDS orphans; approximately 90 percent of children born to HIV-infected women are in sub-Saharan Africa. In certain sub-Saharan African countries such at Zaire and Uganda, available seroprevalence data indicate that 3 to 6% of the entire population may be infected.

Other Pattern II regions are the Caribbean and certain areas of South America. During the early phases of the epidemic in Haiti, the primary mode of transmission was via men who had sex with men but who were predominantly bisexual males. These infected bisexual men then began infecting their heterosexual partners and by the mid-1980s heterosexual spread emerged as the major mode of transmission, with increasing number of women becoming infected; accompanying this trend was an increase in infection rate among infants.

In certain developing countries, transmission of HIV by contaminated blood or blood products remains a major problem because of lack of facilities and/or resources for screening of blood donors and inadequare blood banking facilities. Significant outbreaks of HIV infection have occurred in Romania and the former Soviet Union by a breakdown or lack of sterile techniques involving needles and syringes as well as an inappropriate use of blood transfusions.

HIV-2 was first described in asymptomatic West Africans (see above) and remains a major cause of HIV disease in West Africa. However, a number of cases have now been reported in other regions of Africa, Western Europe, South America (particularly Brazil), Canada, and the United States. Infection is felt to cause a more indolent disease than HIV-1 with advanced disease evolving over a longer period of time than with HIV-1.

Substantial transmission of HIV was documented in only a few countries in South Asia and Southeast Asia in the late 1980s. However, the spread in certain countries in this region, particularly Thailand and India, has been rapid since then. The situation in Thailand is of particular note in that the epidemic began in earnest in 1988 and has subsequently emerged rapidly. During the early and mid 1980s,

FIGURE 279-8 Estimated distribution of adult HIV infections for late 1993. *(From WHO.)*

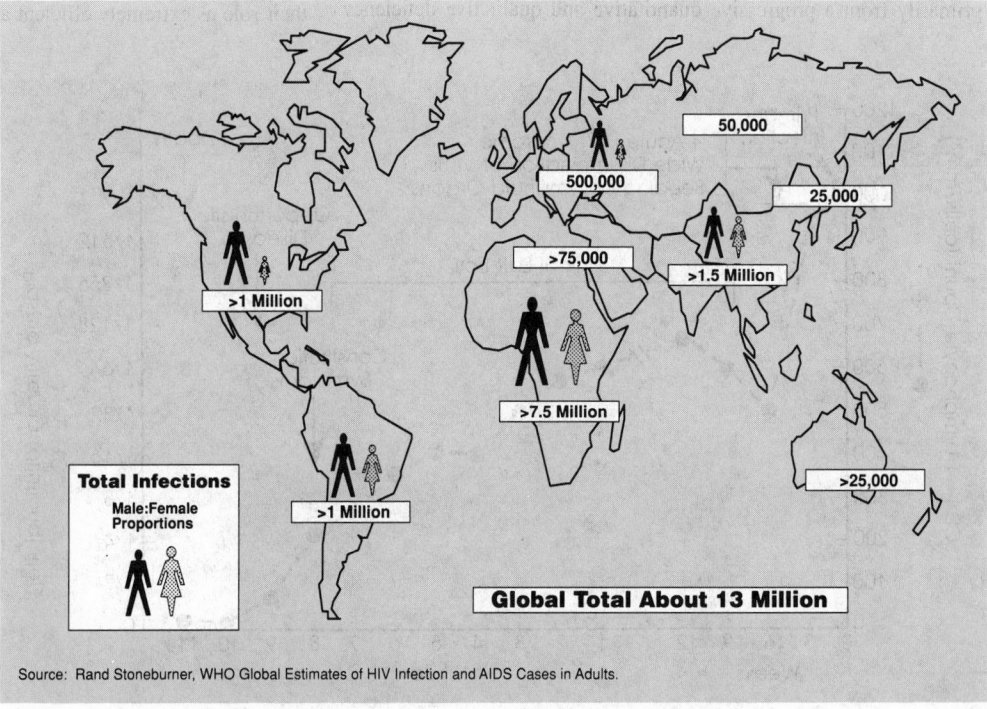

Source: Rand Stoneburner, WHO Global Estimates of HIV Infection and AIDS Cases in Adults.

Thailand was considered a Pattern III country, along with countries in Eastern Europe, North Africa, the Middle East, other Asian countries, and certain countries in the Pacific. Pattern III countries have relatively few cases of HIV infection/AIDS and most of these individuals have had contact with Pattern I and II countries. However, this paradigm was broken in Thailand. A single HIV-positive person was identified in Thailand among 101 male prostitutes in Bangkok in 1985, and it was expected that gay men would experience the first wave of rapid transmission. From 1985 through 1987 serosurveys among IDUs in Thailand revealed a prevalence of 0 to 1 percent, and similar surveys conducted among female prostitutes from 1985 through 1989 reported rates of less than 1 percent. There was not a wide appreciation of the potential for the epidemic to emerge into the general population. It was anticipated that it would remain confined to men who have sex with men and possibly to IDUs and would not substantially involve people who are generally considered to be at low risk. However, a remarkable pattern began to emerge in 1988. There was an extraordinary explosion of HIV prevalence among IDUs, from 1 percent at the beginning of 1988 to 32 to 43 percent by August-September of 1988. Thus unexpectedly, the first wave of HIV infection spread rapidly among IDUs. This was followed by successive waves of transmission to female prostitutes, then to their non-IDU male clients, and then ultimately into the low-risk, non-prostitute wives and girlfriends of these men in the general population. An indication of the extent of the HIV epidemic in Thailand is the prevalence among military recruits. Military service is mandatory for Thais at age 21. Serosurveys of conscripts indicate that in the northern provinces, including Chang Mai, the overall HIV prevalence among 21-year-old men is 10.3 percent. It is feared that such explosive patterns will also be seen in other Asian countries, particularly developing countries, such as India, which will equal and surpass sub-Saharan Africa as the most severely afflicted region in the remainder of the 20th century and into the 21st century.

WHO estimates that by the year 2000 there will be at least 40 million people worldwide infected with HIV. Other estimates are even higher ranging from 60 to 120 million. It is clear that the global impact of HIV infection and disease into the 21st century will be immense.

PATHOPHYSIOLOGY AND IMMUNOPATHOGENESIS

The hallmark of HIV disease is a profound immunodeficiency resulting primarily from a progressive quantitative and qualitative deficiency of the CD4+ subset of T lymphocytes referred to as the helper or inducer T cells. This subset of T cells is defined phenotypically by the presence on its surface of a CD4 molecule (see Chap. 277), which is the cellular receptor for HIV. Although the CD4+ T cell is the predominant cell type that is actually infected with HIV, virtually any human cell which expresses a CD4 molecule (written as CD4+) is capable of binding to and becoming infected with HIV. Although a number of mechanisms responsible for cytopathicity and immune dysfunction of CD4+ T cells have been demonstrated in vitro (see below), it is still unclear which mechanism or combination of mechanisms is primarily responsible for the progressive depletion and functional impairment of these cells in vivo. Nonetheless, when the CD4+ T cells decline beneath a certain level (see below) the patient is at high risk of developing a variety of opportunistic diseases, particularly infections and certain neoplasms which are AIDS-defining illnesses. Other features of AIDS such as Kaposi's sarcoma and neurologic abnormalities cannot be explained completely by the immunosuppressive effect of HIV since these complications may occur prior to the development of severe immunologic impairment.

The combination of viral pathogenic and immunopathogenic events which occur during the course of HIV disease from the moment of initial infection through the development of advanced disease are complex and heterogeneous. Although the precise sequence of events has not been fully delineated, there are reproducible in vivo and in vitro observations that have clarified certain of these real and potential mechanisms. It is highly likely that these mechanisms are quantitatively and qualitatively different at different stages of disease and so it is essential to consider the typical course of an HIV-infected individual in order to more fully appreciate these pathogenic events (Fig. 279-9).

PRIMARY INFECTION It is likely that the initial infection of susceptible cells varies somewhat with the route of infection. Virus that enters directly into the bloodstream via infected blood or blood products (i.e., transfusions, use of contaminated needles for IDU, sharp object injury, maternal to fetal transmission either intrapartum or perinatally, or in certain cases via sexual intercourse where there is trauma sufficient to cause bleeding) is likely cleared from the circulation to the lymphoid organs where it replicates to a critical level and then leads to a burst of viremia. It is uncertain which cell in the blood or lymphoid tissue is the first to actually become infected. It has been assumed that the CD4+ T cell or monocyte was the initial target. However, dendritic cells have been demonstrated to be efficient transporters or presenters of HIV to CD4+ T cells consistent with their role as extremely efficient antigen-presenting cells in the course

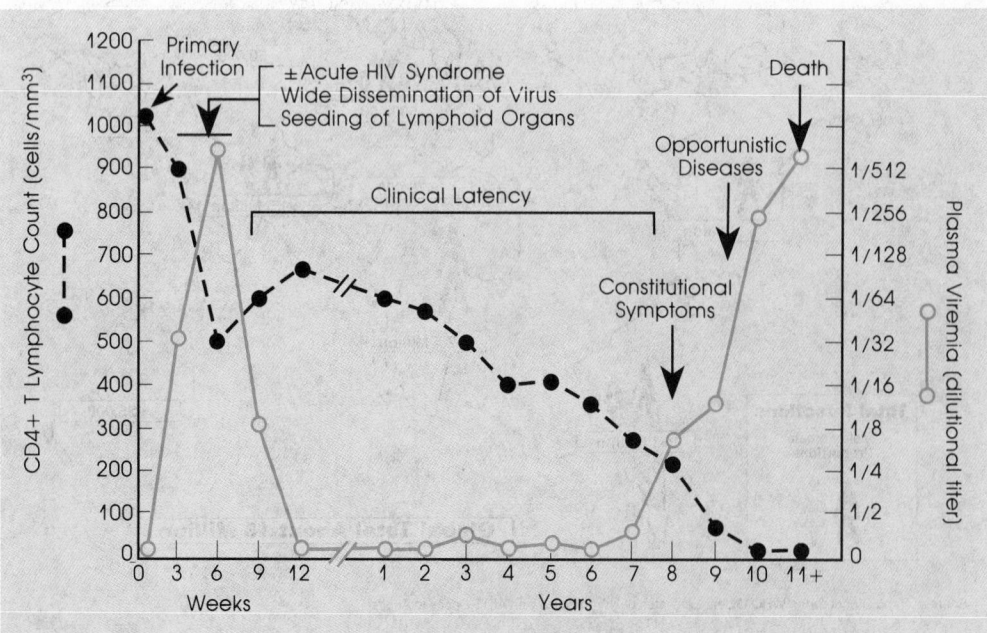

FIGURE 279-9 Typical course of an HIV-infected individual. See text for detailed description. (*From G Pantaleo et al, N Engl J Med 328:327, 1993.*)

of the normal immune response to antigen (see Chap. 277). One likely scenario is that dendritic cells carry virus to tissues, particularly lymph nodes, where they put the virus in contact with susceptible CD4+ T cells; this is somewhat different from the role of the follicular dendritic cells (FDC) residing in the germinal centers of the lymph nodes; these FDCs serve as traps or filters for the virus (see below). Dendritic cells have been reported to express low levels of CD4. However, there are conflicting reports as to whether the dendritic cells themselves can actually become infected with HIV. In circumstances where the virus enters "locally," such as via the rectum and the vagina in intercourse; the upper gastrointestinal tract via swallowed infected semen or vaginal fluid; or infected breast milk, it is likewise unclear which is the initial cell to become infected. Although infection of various mucosal cells of the gastrointestinal and genitourinary tract have been reported, it remains unclear whether they play a role in initial infection or whether CD4+ tissue macrophages and/or resident CD4+ T cells are the initial targets. Cells of dendritic cell lineage in the tissues could serve the same role as mentioned above by binding virus and "presenting" it to T cells. The common denominator of local infection would be a drainage to the regional lymph nodes with replication of virus and subsequent viremia which would then lead to more widespread infection of lymph nodes. A more detailed description of the role of lymphoid tissue in the immunopathogenesis of HIV infection is given below.

INITIAL VIREMIA AND DISSEMINATION OF VIRUS It has been well documented that patients who experience the "acute HIV syndrome" following primary infection have high levels of viremia which last for several weeks (see below). The acute mononucleosis-like symptoms are well correlated with the presence of viremia. It is highly likely that most patients develop some degree of viremia which contributes to virus dissemination even though they remain asymptomatic or do not recall experiencing symptoms. It is these early events which likely play a major role in the subsequent course of infection in that the degree of initial virus replication and seeding of organs such as lymph nodes establishes the magnitude of virus burden which the immune system will be required to contain and which will expose susceptible cells to infection. A combination of the development of an HIV-specific immune response (both humoral and cell-mediated) (see below) and the efficient trapping of virions in the FDC of the lymph node germinal centers leads to the curtailment of viremia, disappearance of symptoms, and the beginning of so-called clinical latency, which lasts for variable periods, with a median duration of approximately 10 years (Fig. 279-9).

IMMUNOPATHOGENIC EVENTS DURING CLINICAL LATENCY It has been the consistent observation of clinicians caring for AIDS patients that, with few exceptions, there is a gradual and progressive diminution over time of the level of CD4+ T cells. The slope of the decline is highly predictive of the pattern of the clinical course and the development of advanced disease. Most patients are entirely asymptomatic during this progressive decline of CD4+ T cells (see below), which has led to the term *clinical latency*. Culturable viremia and p24 antigenemia are uncommon during this period, and there are very few cells (usually 1:1000 to 1:10,000) which contain HIV provirus and at least 1 log less cells which are actively expressing HIV mRNA during this period. In most patients, it is extremely difficult to detect active virus replication in the peripheral blood mononuclear cells during this period. However, the progressive decline of CD4+ T cells belies true viral latency since both cytopathic effects and qualitative dysfunction of T cells that cannot be explained by mere lymphocyte depletion occur. It has been demonstrated that even during this prolonged clinically latent period, there is copious virus contained in the lymph nodes and active virus replication in the lymph nodes (see below). Therefore, it is essential to distinguish between clinical latency and true microbiologic latency.

ADVANCED HIV DISEASE After variable periods of time, usually measured in years, the CD4+ T cell count falls below a critical level (less than 200 cells per microliter) and the patient becomes highly susceptible to opportunistic disease. The patient may experience constitutional signs and symptoms or may develop an opportunistic disease without any prior symptoms. Even within this severely immunosuppressed state, the defect is progressive and unrelenting. It is not uncommon for CD4+ T cell counts to drop as low as 10 per microliter or even to zero, yet the patient may survive for months to more than 1 year. This is more common now that patients are more aggressively treated as well as given prophylaxis against the common life-threatening opportunistic infections such as *Pneumocystis carinii* pneumonia (see below). Ultimately, patients who progress to this severest form of immunosuppression will succumb to opportunistic diseases.

ROLE OF LYMPHOID ORGANS The lymph nodes are the major anatomic sites for the establishment as well as the acute and chronic propagation of HIV infection. Out of logistic necessity, most studies on the pathogenesis of HIV infection have focused on the peripheral blood mononuclear cells. However, the fact remains that lymphocytes in the peripheral blood at any given time represent only approximately 2 percent of the total body lymphocyte pool and so may not always accurately reflect the status of the entire immune system; the bulk of the body's lymphocytes reside in the lymphoid organs such as the lymph nodes, spleen, and gut-associated lymphoid tissue. Since HIV disease is an infectious disease of the immune system, it is critical to appreciate the pathogenic events that occur in the lymphoid tissue in HIV infection.

Certain patients will experience progressive generalized lymphadenopathy (see below) relatively early in the course of infection; others may experience varying degrees of transient lymphadenopathy. It has been suggested that progressive generalized lymphadenopathy represents an exaggerated immune response to HIV and carries a more favorable prognosis (see below); however, lymph node involvement is a common denominator of virtually all patients with HIV infection, even those without easily detectable lymphadenopathy. Simultaneous examination of lymph node and peripheral blood mononuclear cells in the same patients during various stages of HIV disease including the early asymptomatic stage (when CD4+ T cell levels generally are greater than 500 per microliter), the intermediate stage (when these levels are 200 to 500 per microliter), and the advanced stage of disease (when they are 0 to 200 per microliter) has led to substantial insight into the pathogenesis of HIV infection. By a combination of polymerase chain reaction (PCR) techniques for HIV DNA and RNA, in situ hybridization for HIV RNA, and electron microscopy, the following picture has emerged. In most patients, early in the course of infection prior to significant immunosuppression (CD4+ T cell levels of greater than 500 per microliter) culturable viremia or p24 antigenemia is uncommon, the viral burden in the peripheral blood mononuclear cells is extremely low, and expression of HIV in these cells in minimal or undetectable. Remarkably, at this time there are copious amounts of extracellular virions trapped within the germinal centers of the lymph nodes (Fig. 279-10A) and in situ hybridization reveals expression of virus in individual cells of the paracortical area and to a lesser extent the germinal center (Fig. 279-10B). The architecture of the germinal centers is preserved and may even be hyperplastic due to in situ proliferation of cells and recruitment of cells to the lymph nodes. Electron microscopy demonstrates a fine network of FDCs with interdigitating processes that envelop virtually every lymphocyte in the germinal center (Fig. 279-10C). Extracellular virions can be seen attached to the processes, yet the FDCs appear to be relatively healthy. It is difficult to demonstrate infection of the FDC at this point or even in advanced disease; however, rare examples of virus budding off FDCs have been reported. As the disease progresses, the architecture of the germinal centers begins to show disruption, and the trapping efficiency of the node diminishes. Electron microscopy reveals swollen organelles in the FDC and cell death. At this time, the relative burden of HIV as well as the expression of HIV in the peripheral blood mononuclear cells increase and begin to equilibrate with the relative viral burden per given number of cells in the lymph node. As the disease progresses to the advanced stage, there is complete disruption of the architecture of the germinal center.

FIGURE 279-10   HIV in the lymph nodes of HIV-infected individuals. *A.* Cervical lymph node from an asymptomatic individual with no culturable viremia or p24 antigenemia. In situ hybridization using a molecular probe for HIV RNA reveals copious virus demarcating the numerous germinal centers (bright areas) of the node. The virus was extracellular and bound to the processes of the follicular dendritic cells which interdigitate within the confines of the germinal centers. Original ×25. *(Courtesy of Dr. Cecil Fox.) B.* Individual cells infected with HIV. Two cells in the paracortical area of the lymph node are shown expressing HIV RNA by in situ hybridization using a radiolabeled molecular probe. Original × 250 *(Courtesy of Dr. Cecil Fox.) C.* Follicular dendritic cell in cervical lymph node of an asymptomatic HIV-infected individual. Electron microscopy reveals a follicular dendritic cell with a prominent nucleolus surrounded by several lymphocytes within the germinal center of the node. Higher magnification of several fields indicates that multiple processes of the follicular dendritic cell surround and are in contact with several lymphocytes. Original × 1920 *(Courtesy of Dr. Jan Orenstein.) D.* Dissolution of follicular dendritic cells in the germinal center of a cervical lymph node from a patient with advanced HIV disease. Widespread death of follicular dendritic cells is associated with a loss of ability of the lymph node to trap virus late in the course of HIV disease. Original × 3744. *(Courtesy of Dr. Jan Orenstein. Adapted from G Pantaleo et al, N Engl J Med 328:327, 1993.)*

This is accompanied by dissolution of the FDC network and massive dropout of FDCs (Fig. 279-10D). The trapping function of the lymph node is completely lost and virus freely spills over into the circulation. Simultaneous PCR analysis of lymph node and peripheral blood mononuclear cells indicates that the relative viral burden and expression of HIV in the blood versus the lymph node approach equilibrium at this stage. This advanced stage is accompanied by a burst of viremia which may represent a true increase in virus replication due in part to an escape from the immune system curtailment (see below) as well as a mechanical escape from the lymph node trapping function. At this point, the lymph nodes are characterized as "burnt out." It is unclear what the mechanism of FDC death is; there is no indication by electron microscopy of copious virus replication or budding of virions off the cell in great quantities. Thus, the lymphoid tissues play a major role in the pathogenesis of HIV disease. They serve as

an important reservoir of the virus, a filter or trapping apparatus of free virions, and a prominent milieu for the exposure of susceptible cells to large amounts of virus trapped among the processes of the FDC, which activate adjacent cells as well as present virus to these cells. Active virus replication occurs in individual cells within the lymph node throughout the entire course of HIV disease, even during the time of clinical latency when little, if any, virus or virus replication can be demonstrated in peripheral blood mononuclear cells. Understanding the pathogenic events that occur within the lymph node throughout the course of HIV disease adds considerably to our appreciation of how and why CD4 + T cells continue to progressively diminish in number during the time that the disease appears to be latent and so little viral burden and activity can be detected in peripheral blood. A schematic diagram of the role of lymphoid tissue in the pathogenesis of HIV disease is shown in Fig. 279-11.

FIGURE 279-11 The role of lymphoid organs in the pathogenesis of HIV infection. *(Adapted from G Pantaleo et al, N Engl J Med 328:327, 1993.)*

(IFN-γ) production in response to antigens, depressed HLA class I–restricted cytotoxic T lymphocyte responses against a number of viruses, decreased allogeneic responses, and decreased ability to help B cells to produce immunoglobulin.

HIV-specific CD8+ cytolytic T cells have been demonstrated in HIV-infected individuals early in the course of disease (see below). As the disease progresses, this functional capability is lost. The cause of this loss of cytolytic activity is unclear. However, it has been demonstrated that, as the disease progresses, CD8+ T cells assume an abnormal phenotype characterized by expression of activation markers such as HLA-DR with an absence of expression of the IL-2 receptor (CD25) and a loss of clonogenic potential. The levels of CD8+ T cells varies throughout the course of disease and may be normal, elevated, or decreased. It has been demonstrated in vitro that CD8+ T cells can suppress the induction of HIV expression, likely by secretion of a soluble factor.

B LYMPHOCYTE ABNORMALITIES B cells from HIV-infected individuals manifest abnormal activation reflected by increased spontaneous proliferation and immunoglobulin secretion, and by increased spontaneous secretion of tumor necrosis factor alpha (TNF-α) and IL-6. The enhanced spontaneous in vitro transformation of B cells with Epstein-Barr virus (EBV) is probably due to defective T cell immune surveillance and has as its in vivo counterpart an increase in incidence of EBV-related B cell lymphomas. Untransformed B cells cannot be infected with HIV. However, HIV or its products (particularly gp120) can directly activate B cells to secrete TNF-α and IL-6. It is likely that the in vivo activation of B cells by virus products accounts at least in part for the spontaneous activation of these cells noted in vitro. In vivo, this activated state manifests itself by hypergammaglobulinemia and by the presence of circulating immune complexes and autoantibodies. The B cells are also defective in that they respond poorly to in vitro stimulation with antigens and mitogens. HIV-infected individuals respond poorly to primary and secondary immunization with protein and polysaccharide antigens. These B cell defects are likely responsible in part for the increase in bacterial infections seen in advanced HIV disease in adults, as well as for the important role of bacterial infections in HIV-infected children who cannot mount an adequate humoral response to common bacterial pathogens.

MONOCYTE/MACROPHAGE   ABNORMALITIES Circulating monocytes are normal in number in HIV-infected individuals. Monocytes express the CD4 molecule on their surface and thus are targets for HIV infection. Certain strains of HIV have been demonstrated to have a selective tropism for CD4+ monocytes versus CD4+ T cells. Of note is the fact that the degree of cytopathicity of HIV for cells of the monocyte lineage is low and HIV can replicate extensively in cells of the monocyte lineage under certain circumstances with little cytopathic effect. Hence, monocyte lineage cells can serve as reservoirs of HIV infection and may play a role in the dissemination of HIV in the body. Infection of circulating monocytes occurs infrequently; however, infection of tissue macrophages and macrophage lineage cells in the brain and lung (pulmonary alveolar macrophages) can be easily demonstrated. Infection of monocyte precursors in the bone marrow may directly or indirectly be responsible for certain of the hematologic abnormalities in HIV-infected individuals. The predominant cells in the brain that are infected with HIV are cells of the monocyte lineage, infiltrating either macrophages or resident microglial cells (see below). A number of abnormalities of circulating monocytes have been reported in HIV-infected individuals, including defects in chemotaxis, secretion of IL-1, certain cytotoxic functions, and the ability to present antigen to T cells. The reported functional abnormalities of circulating monocytes are likely related in part to abnormal activation of these cells in vivo by cytokines.

NATURAL KILLER (NK) CELL ABNORMALITIES The presumed role of NK cells is to provide immunosurveillance against virus-infected cells, certain tumor cells, and allogeneic cells (see Chap. 277). HIV-infected individuals manifest functionally defective NK cell activity despite the fact that NK cells have been normal in

T LYMPHOCYTE ABNORMALITIES The range of T cell abnormalities in advanced HIV infection is broad. The defects are both quantitative and qualitative and impact every limb of the immune system (see below), bespeaking the critical dependence of the integrity of the immune system on the inducer/helper function of the CD4+ T cell. Virtually all the immune defects in advanced HIV disease can be explained by the quantitative depletion of CD4+ T cells. However, T cell dysfunction can be demonstrated in patients early in the course of infection even when the CD4+ T cell count is within the low-normal range. The degree of these dysfunctions increases as the disease progresses. One of the first abnormalities to be detected is a defect in response to soluble antigen at a time when mononuclear cells can still respond normally to mitogen stimulation. The mechanisms for this selective defect are unclear, but may involve abnormal antigen recognition as well as aberrant cell triggering (see below). In addition, the memory subset of T cells appears to be affected earlier and more profoundly than the naive subset. Essentially every T cell function has been reported to be abnormal at some stage of HIV infection. Certain of these abnormalities include defective T cell cloning and colony forming efficiencies, impaired expression of interleukin 2 receptors, defective IL-2 production, decreased interferon-gamma numbers and phenotype in most studies. The abnormality in NK cell function is thought to result from a defect in postbinding lysis. However, the lytic machinery does not appear to be impaired since NK cells from HIV-infected individuals mediate antibody dependent cellular cytotoxicity (ADCC) normally. It has been demonstrated that the addition of IL-2 enhanced the depressed NK cell activity in vitro. The in vivo mechanism for defective NK cell activity is unknown; however, it may be related to the lack of normal inductive signals from CD4+ T lymphocytes.

AUTOIMMUNE PHENOMENA Autoimmune phenomena are commonly noted in HIV-infected individuals. This usually occurs in the absence of autoimmune disease (see below). Autoimmune phenomena include antibodies to lymphocytes and less commonly to platelets and neutrophils. Antiplatelet antibodies have some clinical relevance in that they may contribute to the thrombocytopenia of HIV infection (see below). Antibodies to nuclear and cytoplasmic components of cells have been reported as have antibodies to cardiolipin. In addition, autoantibodies to a range of serum proteins including albumin, immunoglobulin, and thyroglobulin have been reported. Antibodies to MHC class II molecules may interfere with the antigen-presenting capabilities of certain cells or may contribute to their depletion via ADCC mechanisms.

OTHER CELL TYPES Although the CD4+ T lymphocyte and CD4+ cells of the monocyte lineage are the principal targets of HIV, virtually any cell that expresses the CD4 molecule can potentially be infected with the virus. Circulating dendritic cells have been reported to express low levels of CD4, and there have been conflicting reports of whether these cells can be infected with the virus. Epidermal Langerhans cells express CD4 and have been demonstrated to be infected in vivo with HIV. A variety of other cell types which express low levels of CD4, no detectable CD4, or only CD4 mRNA have been reported to be infected with HIV. These include megakaryocytes, astrocytes and oligodendrocytes, follicular dendritic cells, microglial cells, CD8+ T cells (under certain conditions), enterochromaffin cells, retinal cells, renal epithelial cells, cervical cells, rectal and colonic mucosal cells, trophoblastic cells, and cardiac myocytes. In certain of those studies in which in situ hybridization of tissue specimens was performed, it was not entirely clear whether monocytes in these tissues were the cells actually infected with HIV. In addition, a large number of established cell lines have been shown to be infected with HIV. However, the significance of these observations with regard to pathogenesis of HIV infection, including dysfunction of respective organs which contain such cells, is unclear. At present, the only cells that have unequivocally been shown to harbor HIV in vivo are CD4+ T lymphocytes and cells of monocyte/macrophage lineage.

Of potentially important clinical relevance is the demonstration that thymic precursor cells which were assumed to be negative for CD3, CD4, and CD8 molecules actually do express low levels of CD4 and can be infected with HIV in vitro. In addition, human thymic epithelial cells when transplanted into an immunodeficient mouse can be infected with HIV by direct inoculation of virus into the thymus. Since these cells likely play a role in the normal replenishment of CD4+ T cells, it is possible that their infection and depletion interferes with the replenishment of the CD4+ T cell pool in infected individuals, including those in whom antiretroviral therapy has at least temporarily suppressed virus replication (see below). In addition, CD34+ monocyte precursor cells residing in bone marrow are capable of being infected in vitro with HIV, and these cells may serve as a reservoir of HIV as well as play a role in the suppression of hematopoiesis. Furthermore, CD34+ bone marrow precursor cells have been shown to be infected in vivo in patients with advanced HIV disease. It is likely that these cells express low levels of CD4 and therefore it is not essential to invoke CD4-independent mechanisms to explain the infection. Other studies have demonstrated that the galactosyl ceramide molecule can serve as an alternative receptor for HIV in CD4-negative neural and colonic epithelial cells (see "Neuropathogenesis" below). CD4-independent infection of or

at least binding of HIV to certain neural cells via this receptor may play a role in the neuropathogenesis of HIV infection.

MECHANISMS OF CD4+ T LYMPHOCYTE DYSFUNCTION It is difficult to explain the profound immunosuppression noted in HIV-infected individuals only by the direct infection and quantitative depletion of CD4+ T cells. This is particularly apparent during the early course of infection when CD4+ T cell numbers may be only marginally depressed. Certainly, at the stage of advanced disease when CD4+ T cells are in the range of 0 to 50 cells per microliter, quantitative depletion alone can explain the immune defect. However, it is possible that CD4+ T cell dysfunction results from a combination of depletion of cells due to direct infection and a number of viral-related but indirect effects on the cell (Table 279-7).

Cell killing and syncytia formation have clearly been demonstrated in vitro and are directly related to virus infection of cells. Cytopathicity in an infected cell may result from a number of mechanisms, including accumulation of unintegrated viral DNA and interference with macro-molecular synthesis by the infected cell. Syncytia formation involves fusion of the cell membrane of an infected cell with the cell membrane of variable numbers of uninfected CD4+ cells. Although cell fusion has not been shown to be an important pathogenic process in vivo, a direct relationship between the presence of syncytia and the degree of cytopathic effect has been demonstrated in vitro, and a correlation has been reported between the presence of virus isolates which readily induce syncytia in vitro and a more aggressive clinical course in the patient. Syncytia formation depends on the leukocyte adhesion molecule LFA-1 (see Chap. 277) in human CD4+ T cells acutely infected with HIV in vitro.

Humoral and cellular immune responses to HIV may contribute to protective immunity by eliminating virus and viral infected cells (see below). However, since the targets of HIV infection are predominantly immune competent cells, these responses may contribute to the immune dysfunction by elimination of cells which are actually infected or "innocent bystander" cells. Soluble viral proteins, particularly gp120, can bind with high affinity to the CD4 molecules on uninfected T cells and monocytes; in addition, virus and/or viral protein can bind to dendritic cells or follicular dendritic cells. HIV-specific antibody can recognize these bound molecules and potentially collaborate in the elimination of the cells by ADCC.

Nonpolymorphic determinants of MHC class II products share a degree of homology with gp120 and gp41 proteins of HIV. Such similarities may lead to the generation of autoantibodies to self-MHC determinants. In fact, anti-HLA-DR antibodies have been demonstrated in the sera of HIV-infected individuals. These antibodies could contribute to the elimination of HLA-DR expressing cells by ADCC; in addition, it has been suggested that these antibodies may inhibit certain T cell functions which involve HLA-DR molecules.

Following binding of gp120/anti-gp120 complexes to the CD4 molecule, CD4+ T cells become refractory to further stimulation in vitro via the CD3 molecule. In addition, peripheral blood mononuclear cells acutely infected with HIV in vitro no longer respond to stimulation with anti-CD3 antibodies. Thus it has been hypothesized

TABLE 279-7 Potential mechanisms of CD4+ T lymphocyte dysfunction/depletion in HIV infection

HIV-mediated direct cytopathicity (single-cell killing)
HIV-mediated syncytia formation
Virus-specific immune responses:
  HIV specific cytolytic T lymphocytes
  Antibody dependent cellular cytotoxicity
  Natural killer cells
Autoimmune mechanisms
Anergy caused by inappropriate cell signalling via gp120/CD4 interaction
Superantigen-mediated pertubation of T cell subsets
Programmed cell death (apoptosis)

* From G Pantaleo et al., N Engl J Med 328:327, 1993.

that a negative or anergic signal is delivered to the cell upon interaction with gp120 or gp120/anti-gp120 complexes. Antibodies directed against gp120 have been detected on CD4+ T cells in HIV-infected individuals.

Conventional antigens bind in the groove of the MHC molecule of the antigen-presenting cell (see Chap. 277) and interact with the variable components of the T cell receptor alpha and beta chains in order to activate the T cell. Thus any given conventional antigenic peptide can stimulate only a very small fraction (<1/100,000) of total T cells. In contrast, certain microbial antigens are capable of binding to and activating entire subsets of T cells, not through true antigen receptor binding but by binding to another site on the variable (V) region of the beta (β) chain of the T cell receptor. This binding, to all members of a particular Vβ subset (1 to 10 percent of all T cells) can induce massive stimulation and expansion of T cells and/or, depending upon the state of activation of the T cell, result in deletion or anergy of the T cells bearing the specific Vβs. For this reason, these antigens have been referred to as *superantigens*. It has been hypothesized that superantigen(s), either retrovirally encoded or unrelated to HIV, may contribute to the immunopathogenesis of HIV infection. This hypothesis stems from the observations that endogenous or exogenous retroviral-encoded superantigens react with CD4+ T cells in the developing immune system of certain strains of mice, leading to anergy or deletion of the CD4+ T cells bearing specific Vβs. Certain studies have demonstrated that there are quantitative perturbations of certain Vβ subsets of CD4+ T cells in HIV-infected individuals, lending credence to the possibility that one or more superantigens may be involved in the nonrandom and preferential depletion of certain subsets of CD4+ T cells over others. It is unclear whether this process of direct superantigen-driven depletion actually occurs in vivo. However, it is certain that superantigens can activate CD4+ T cells, and so by simply increasing the susceptibility of certain T cell subsets to HIV infection they may contribute indirectly to their ultimate depletion.

Cells may die through one of two main mechanisms. The first of these, necrosis, is generally triggered by an exogenous injury. It is, for the most part random and accompanied by inflammation as cells spill their cytoplasmic contents into surrounding tissues. The other, programmed cell death, or apoptosis, is a more controlled process that serves a normal physiologic function in a variety of organ systems. It is part of the ontogeny of the immune system and is a mechanism for the clonal deletion of autoreactive T cells in the thymus. It depends on the process of cellular activation. It has been hypothesized that in HIV infection, sequential activation signals delivered to CD4+ T cells induce programmed cell death. Cross-linking of the CD4 molecule by gp120 or gp120/anti-gp120 complexes (see above) delivers the first of two signals to the cell which is required for apoptosis. The second signal, leading to cell death, is delivered via the T cell receptor upon activation by a conventional antigen or a superantigen. The latter would link the apoptosis and superantigen hypotheses of the depletion and/or functional impairment of CD4+ T cells in the absence of direct infection by HIV. Alternatively, HIV-induced alterations in tyrosine kinase activity may also trigger the cell to undergo programmed death.

INDUCTION OF HIV EXPRESSION Although HIV can initially infect both resting and activated CD4+ T cells in vitro with approximately the same efficiency, the ability of the virus to effectively reverse transcribe its genomic RNA and integrate its provirus into the cellular genome is heavily dependent on the state of activation of the cell. In addition, the process of expression of HIV in an infected cell followed by virion production and spread to other susceptible cells relies on a variety of inductive or activation signals. These inductive signals can derive from a wide range of sources and can be considered as cofactors for the spread of virus within a host. Coinfection or simultaneous cotransfection of cells with HIV and other heterologous viruses or viral genes has demonstrated that certain viruses such as cytomegalovirus (CMV), herpes simplex virus, human herpes virus

6, hepatitis B virus, and HTLV-I can up-regulate HIV expression. Furthermore, other microbes such as mycoplasma have been reported to contribute to the induction of HIV expression.

The immune system is homeostatically regulated by a complex network of immunoregulatory cytokines which are pleiotropic, redundant, and operate in a paracrine and autocrine manner. They are continuously being expressed even during periods of apparent quiescence of the immune system. Upon perturbation of the immune system by antigenic challenge, these cytokines are further expressed to varying degrees. Cytokines which are important components of this immunoregulatory network have been demonstrated to play a major role in the regulation of HIV expression in vitro. IL-1, IL-2, IL-3, IL-6, TNF-α and ß, IFN-γ, GM-CSF, and M-CSF may induce expression of HIV in chronically infected cells in vitro. IFN-α and -ß suppress whereas transforming growth factor (TGF)-ß and IL-4 both induce and suppress HIV expression. Several of these cytokines synergize in their inductive capabilities and others function in an autocrine and paracrine manner in the induction of HIV expression similar to their physiologic function in the regulation of the immune system. Molecular mechanisms of induction of virus expression range from stimulating new transcription via transcription-activating factors such as NF-κB, as is true with TNF-α, to predominantly posttranscriptional induction of virus as with IL6 and GM-CSF. TGF-ß interferes with both transcriptional and posttranscriptional induction of virus expression. Elevated levels of TNF-α and IL-6 have been reported in the plasma and cerebrospinal fluid of HIV-infected individuals, and increased expression of certain cytokines such as IFN-γ have been demonstrated in certain tissues such as lymph nodes of HIV-infected individuals. Thus, this complex network of immunoregulatory cytokines which is operable even during apparent immunologic quiescence likely contributes to the baseline induction of HIV expression, particularly in the lymph nodes.

NEUROPATHOGENESIS HIV infection can lead to a variety of neurologic abnormalities due to opportunistic infections and neoplasms as well as to direct effects of HIV or its products (see below). With regard to the latter, HIV has been demonstrated in the brains of infected individuals with neuropsychiatric abnormalities. In addition, the virus can be isolated from the cerebrospinal fluid of a high percentage of infected individuals without detectable neuropsychiatric findings. The predominant cells within the brain that are infected with HIV are of the monocyte/macrophage lineage such as microglial cells. It has been reported that virus isolates from brain are preferentially monocyte tropic as opposed to T cell tropic when cultured in vitro. There is no convincing evidence that neurons can be infected with HIV in vivo. However, galactosyl ceramide has been demonstrated to be an essential component of the neural receptor for HIV gp120 and antibodies to galactosyl ceramide inhibit enttry of HIV into neural cell lines in vitro.

HIV-infected individuals may manifest both white matter lesions as well as neuronal loss. The HIV-mediated effects on brain tissue are felt to be due to a combination of direct toxic or functional inhibitory influences of gp120 on neuronal cells as well as the toxic effects of a variety of cytokines released from infiltrating macrophages, resident microglial cells, and astrocytes. Neurotoxicity due to gp120 can be blocked in vitro in certain types of neurons by antagonists of L-type voltage-dependent calcium channels or by antagonists of *N*-methyl-D-aspartate (NMDA), which is a type of glutamate receptor. Factors which might be toxic or inhibitory to neurons include TNF-α, IL-1, IL-6, TGF-ß, and endothelin. Reactive gliosis has been demonstrated in the brains of HIV-infected individuals and TNF-α and IL-6 have been shown to induce astrocyte proliferation. Elevated TNF-α levels have been demonstrated in the cerebrospinal fluid of HIV-infected individuals. In addition, astrocyte-derived IL-6 can induce HIV expression in infected cells in vitro. The likelihood that HIV or its products are involved directly or indirectly in neuropathogenesis is supported by the observation that neuropsychiatric abnormalities may undergo remarkable and rapid improvement upon the initiation of zidovudine therapy, particularly in HIV-infected children.

PATHOGENESIS OF KAPOSI'S SARCOMA Kaposi's sarcoma does not result from a neoplastic transformation of cells and so is not truly a sarcoma. It is a manifestation of excessive proliferation of spindle cells which are believed to be of vascular origin with features in common with endothelial and smooth muscle cells. No chromosomal abnormalities nor evidence of viral infection have been identified in Kaposi's sarcoma cells cultured from HIV-infected individuals. It is a cytokine-mediated disease in which a number of factors including oncostatin M, basic fibroblast growth factor, IL-1ß, IL-6, and GM-CSF function in an autocrine and paracrine manner to sustain the growth and chemotaxis of the sarcoma cells (see Chap. 151). The pathogenic link between HIV infection and Kaposi's sarcoma is the fact that these inflammatory and angiogenic cytokines cooperate with the HIV-derived *tat* protein, which itself serves as a growth factor in the induction and progression of Kaposi's sarcoma in HIV-infected individuals. It remains unclear why there is a much greater incidence of Kaposi's sarcoma among HIV-infected homosexual men than among individuals with other risks for HIV infection. Theories which have been proposed include the presence in homosexual men of a chronically immune activated state and the possibility that another virus may be involved; neither of these have been substantiated by firm evidence (see below).

IMMUNE RESPONSE TO HIV

As detailed below, following an initial bout of viremia, individuals infected with HIV mount an immune response that appears to contribute to slowing the progression of infection and to delaying the ultimate development of clinically apparent disease for a median of 10 years. This immune response contains elements of both humoral and cell-mediated immunity (Table 279-8) and is directed toward multiple antigenic determinants of the HIV virion, as well as toward viral proteins produced within infected cells. Paradoxically, those CD4+ elements of the immune system with antigen receptors specific for HIV are theoretically those most likely to bind to infected cells and themselves become infected and destroyed. Thus, relatively early in the course of HIV infection there is destruction of the specific cellular components of host defense that are most important for the control of HIV infection.

Although a great deal of investigation has been directed toward attempting to dissect and understand the individual elements of this immune response, it remains unclear which of these phenomena are most important in delaying progression of infection and which, if any, may actually be playing a role in the pathogenic process.

THE HUMORAL IMMUNE RESPONSE As discussed below, antibodies to HIV usually appear within 2 weeks of the onset of the acute syndrome following primary infection and almost invariably within 8 weeks following initial infection (Fig. 279-12). It is the detection of these antibodies that forms the basis of most screening tests for HIV infection. Despite earlier claims to the contrary, there is currently no evidence to suggest that, apart from extremely rare exceptions, the period between initial infection and development of an antibody response is any longer than 3 months. The first antibodies detected are those directed toward the structural or *gag* proteins of HIV, p24 and p17 and the *gag* precursor, p55. The development of antibodies to p24 is associated with a decrease in the serum levels of free p24 antigen. Antibodies to the *gag* proteins are followed by the appearance of antibodies to the envelope proteins (gp160, gp120, p88, and gp41) and to the products of the *pol* gene (p31, p51, and p66). Additionally, one may see antibodies to low-molecular-weight proteins from HIV-infected cells corresponding to antibodies to the regulatory proteins produced by the HIV genes *vpr, vpu, vif, rev, tat,* and *nef*.

While antibodies are made to multiple antigens of HIV, the precise functional significance of these different antibodies is unclear. The best studied have been the antibodies directed toward the envelope proteins of the virus. As noted above, the envelope of HIV consists of an outer envelope glycoprotein, with a molecular weight of 120 kDa, and a transmembrane glycoprotein, with a molecular weight of 41kDa. These are initially synthesized as a 160 kDa precursor. The majority of the antienvelope antibodies are directed toward an epitope that lies within the gp41 region, from amino acid 579 to amino acid 613.

Antibodies directed toward the envelope proteins of HIV have been characterized as both protective and possibly contributing to the overall pathogenesis. Among the protective antibodies are those that function to directly neutralize HIV and prevent the infection of additional cells, as well as those that participate in ADCC. Neutralizing antibodies appear to be of two forms, type specific and group specific. Type-specific neutralizing antibodies are generally directed to a hypervariable region of the gp120 molecule known as the *V3 loop* (amino acids 303 to 338). These antibodies only neutralize viruses of a given strain and are present in low titer in most infected individuals. Group-specific antibodies, on the other hand, are capable of neutralizing a wide variety of HIV isolates. At least two forms of group-specific antibodies have been identified, those binding to amino acids 423 to 437 of gp120 and those binding to amino acids 728 to 745 of gp41. The other major class of protective antibodies are those that participate in ADCC. This is actually a form of cell-mediated immunity (see Chap. 277) in which Fc receptor–bearing natural killer cells, armed with specific anti-HIV antibodies via binding of the Fc portion of the antibodies to the cellular Fc receptors bind to and

FIGURE 279-12 Relationship between antigenemia and the development of antibodies to HIV. Antibodies to HIV proteins are generally seen 6 to 12 weeks following infection and to 3 to 6 weeks after the development of plasma viremia. Late in the course of illness, antibody levels to p24 decline, generally in association with a rising titer of p24 antigen.

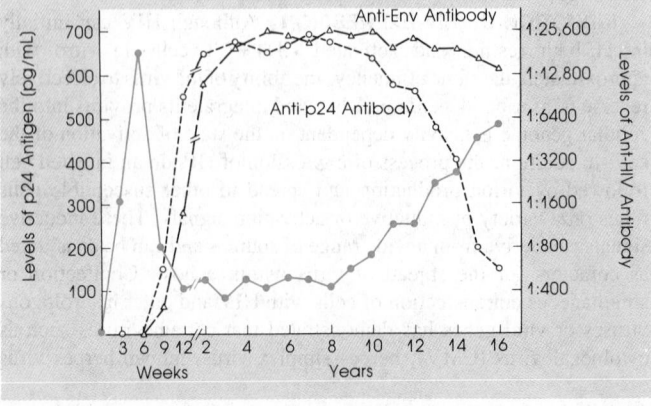

TABLE 279-8   Elements of the immune response to HIV

HUMORAL IMMUNITY

A Binding antibodies
B Neutralizing antibodies
  1 Type specific
  2 Group specific
C Antibodies participating in ADCC
  1 Protective
  2 Pathogenic (bystander killing)
D Enhancing antibodies

CELL MEDIATED IMMUNITY

A Helper CD4+ T lymphocytes
B Class I MHC-restricted cytotoxic CD8+ T lymphocytes
C CD8+ T cell-mediated inhibition (noncytolytic)
D Antibody-dependent cellular cytotoxicity
E Natural killer cell

destroy cells expressing HIV antigens (Fig. 279-13). Antibodies to both gp120 and gp41 have been shown to participate in ADCC-mediated killing of HIV infected cells. Levels of antienvelope antibodies capable of mediating ADCC are highest in patients at the earlier stages of HIV infection. ADCC-mediated killing can be augmented in vitro IL-2.

In addition to playing a role in host defense, HIV-specific antibodies also have been implicated in the pathogenesis of the disease. Antibodies directed to gp41, in low titer, have been shown

FIGURE 279-13 Schematic of the different immunologic effector mechanisms felt to be active in the setting of HIV infection. Detailed descriptions are given in the text.

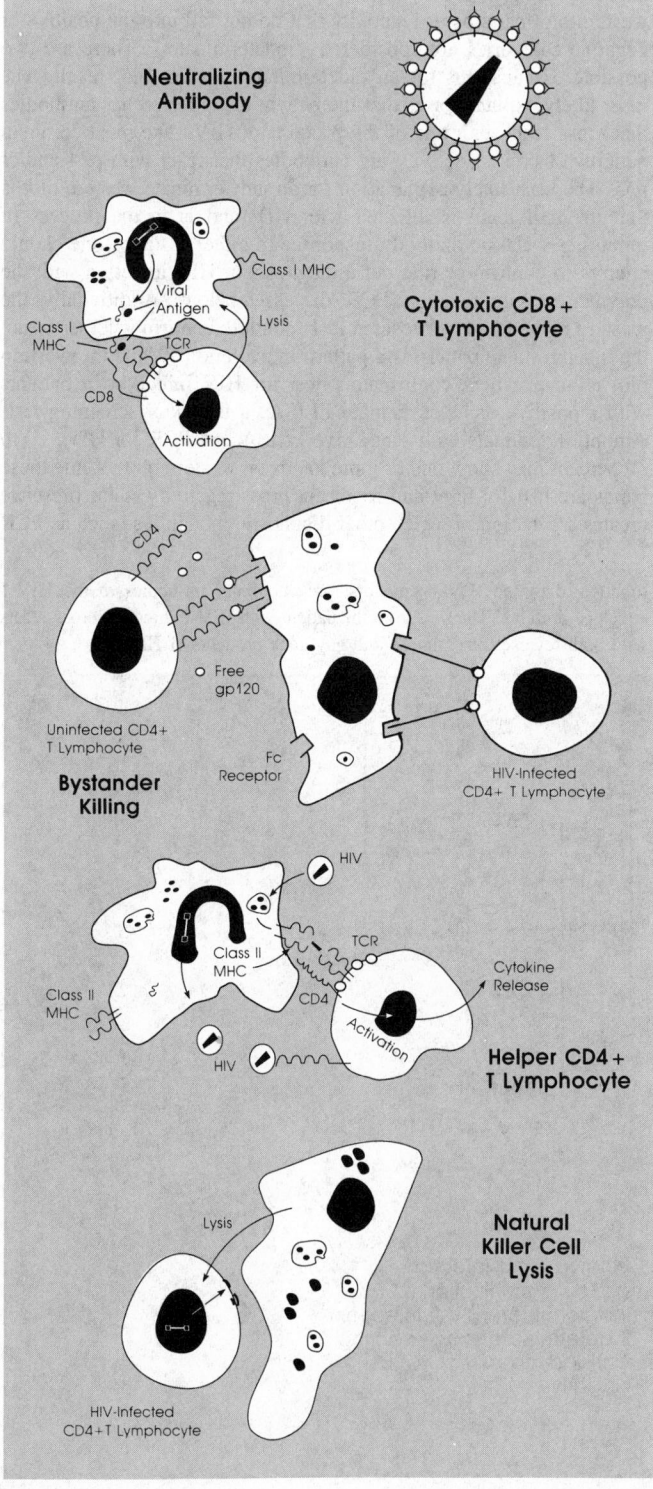

to be capable of facilitating infection of cells through an Fc receptor–mediated mechanism known as *antibody enhancement*. The same regions of the envelope protein of HIV that give rise to antibodies capable of mediating ADCC also elicit the production of antibodies that are capable of facilitating infection of uninfected cells. Additionally, it has been postulated that anti-gp120 antibodies participating in the ADCC killing of HIV-infected cells might also kill uninfected CD4+ T cells if the uninfected cells had bound free gp120 from the circulation, a phenomenon referred to as *bystander killing* (see above) (Fig. 279-13).

THE CELLULAR IMMUNE RESPONSE Given the fact that T cell–mediated immunity is known to play a major role in host defense against most viral infections (see Chap. 277), it is generally felt that this is an important component of the host immune response to HIV. T cell immunity can be divided into two major categories, that of the helper/inducer or CD4+ T cell and that of the cytotoxic/suppressor or CD8+ T cell. It has been very difficult to directly demonstrate the presence of HIV-specific CD4+ T cells in HIV-infected patients. This may be related to the fact that these cells, with their high affinity for binding to HIV-infected cells, may be among the first cells that are infected and destroyed during HIV infection. Nonetheless, through the use of computer modeling several regions of the HIV-1 envelope molecule have been identified that are structurally analogous to other known T cell epitopes by virtue of possessing structures known as *amphipathic helices*. Peptides from these envelope regions have been used to demonstrate the presence of T cells that are specific for these regions in the peripheral blood of HIV-infected individuals. Other studies have demonstrated that healthy, HIV-negative volunteers also possess T cells in their peripheral blood that react to the envelope proteins of HIV.

Classic, MHC class I–restricted, CD8+ cytotoxic T lymphocytes specific for HIV have been identified in the peripheral blood of HIV-infected patients. In this form of immunologic surveillance, CD8+ T lymphocytes, through their HIV-specific antigen receptors, bind to and cause the lytic destruction of HLA-identical cells expressing HIV antigens complexed with class I MHC molecules on the surface of the cell (Fig. 279-13). These cytotoxic T cells have been identified in the peripheral blood of HIV-infected individuals predominantly in the early stages of HIV infection with a relatively high precursor frequency of approximately 10 to 20 cytotoxic T cells per 10,000 peripheral blood mononuclear cells. Longitudinal studies have demonstrated that over time, paralleling the loss of CD4+ T lymphocytes, this element of specific host defense is lost, reinforcing the concept that the CD4+ T lymphocyte is an important element in maintaining antigen-specific cytotoxic T cell responses. Multiple HIV antigens appear capable of eliciting HIV-specific cytotoxic T cell responses and class I–restricted cytotoxic lymphocytes directed toward at least four of the HIV gene products, namely gag, envelope, polymerase, and nef have been identified.

In addition to classic, MHC-restricted cytotoxic T lymphocytes and the helper/inducer CD4+ T lymphocyte, at least three other forms of cell-mediated immunity to HIV have been described. These are CD8+ T cell–mediated inhibition, ADCC, and natural killer cell activity. CD8+ T cell–mediated inhibition refers to the ability of CD8+ T cells from an HIV-infected patient to inhibit the replication of HIV in tissue culture. This phenomenon requires that the T cells be from an HIV-infected individual; however, there is no requirement for HLA compatibility between the CD8+ T cells and the infected cells. It is likely that this effector mechanism is mediated by soluble factors expressed by activated CD8+ T lymphocytes. ADCC, as described above under humoral immunity, involves the killing of HIV-expressing cells by natural killer cells armed with specific antibody directed toward HIV antigens. Finally, natural killer cells alone have been shown capable of killing HIV-infected target cells in tissue culture systems. This primitive element of cytotoxic host defense, geared toward nonspecific surveillance of neoplastic transformation and viral infection, can also be enhanced by IL-2, similar to ADCC.

DIAGNOSIS AND LABORATORY MONITORING OF HIV INFECTION

Prior to the identification of HIV-1 as the causative agent of AIDS, a diagnosis of AIDS was made solely on clinical grounds. The establishment of HIV as the causative agent of AIDS and related syndromes early in 1984 was followed by the rapid development of sensitive screening tests for HIV infection and by March, 1985, blood donors in the United States were routinely being screened for antibodies to HIV (see above). At present a wide array of laboratory tests are available for both diagnosing and monitoring patients with HIV infection.

DIAGNOSIS OF HIV INFECTION The diagnosis of HIV infection is dependent upon the demonstration of antibodies to HIV and/or the direct detection of HIV or one of its components. As noted above, antibodies to HIV generally appear in the circulation 4 to 8 weeks following infection.

The standard screening test for HIV is the *enzyme-linked immunosorbent assay (ELISA)*. This solid-phase assay is an extremely good screening test, with a sensitivity of over 99.5 percent. Of note is the fact that the majority of diagnostic laboratories use a commercial ELISA kit that contains both HIV-1 and HIV-2 and thus either will be detected on routine screening. ELISA tests are generally scored as positive (highly reactive), negative (nonreactive), or indeterminate (partially reactive). While the ELISA is an extremely sensitive assay, it is not optimal with regard to specificity. In fact, in studies of low-risk individuals, such as volunteer blood donors, only 13 percent of ELISA-positive individuals actually had HIV infection. For this reason, anyone suspected of having HIV infection on the basis of an inconclusive or positive ELISA test must have that test result confirmed with a more specific assay.

The most commonly used confirmatory test is the *western blot* (Fig. 279-14). It takes advantage of the fact that multiple antigens of HIV, of different well-characterized molecular weights, elicit the production of specific antibodies. These antigens can be separated on the basis of molecular weight, and antibodies to each individual component can be detected as discrete bands on the western blot. A negative western blot is one in which no bands are present at molecular weights corresponding to HIV gene products. In a patient with a positive or indeterminate ELISA and a negative western blot, one can conclude with certainty that the ELISA reactivity was a false positive. On the other hand, a positive western blot, defined as one demonstrating antibodies to members of all three of the major gene products of HIV (*gag, pol,* and envelope proteins) is conclusive evidence of infection with HIV. In fact, according to most experts, as well as the criteria established by the Association of State and Territorial Public Health Laboratory Directors, a western blot can be considered positive for HIV-1 if it contains bands to at least two of the following gene products: p24, gp41, and gp120/160. By definition, western blot patterns of reactivity that do not fall into the positive or negative categories are considered "indeterminate." There are two possible explanations for an indeterminate western blot result. The most likely explanation is that the patient being tested has antibodies that cross react with one of the proteins of HIV. The most common patterns of cross reactivity are antibodies that react with p24 and/or p55. The least likely explanation for an indeterminate western blot is that the individual is infected with HIV and is in the process of mounting a classic antibody response. In either instance one should attempt to confirm or rule out a diagnosis of HIV infection with the polymerase chain reaction (PCR, discussed below). Additionally, the western blot should be repeated in 1 month to confirm whether or not the indeterminate pattern is a pattern in evolution. While the western blot is an excellent confirmatory test for HIV infection in patients with a positive or indeterminate ELISA, it is a poor screening test. Among individuals with a negative ELISA and PCR for HIV, 20 to 30 percent may show one or more bands on western blot. While these bands are usually faint and represent cross reactivity, their presence creates a situation in which other diagnostic modalities (such as PCR

FIGURE 279-14 *A.* Schematic representation of how a western blot is performed. *B.* Examples of patterns of western blot reactivity. In each instance the western blot strip contains antigens to HIV-1. The sera from the patient immunized to the HIV-1 envelope only contains antibodies to the HIV-1 envelope proteins. The sera from the patient with HIV-2 infection cross-reacts with both reverse transcriptase and *gag* gene products of HIV-1.

1. Virus digested; digest separated into components by molecular weight
2. Proteins transferred to filter paper; reaction with test serum
3. Enzyme-conjugated antihuman antibody added
4. Substrate added and color noted

1. Positive HIV-1 infection
2. gp160 immunization
3. Indeterminate HIV-2 infection
4. Indeterminate cross-reacting antibody to p24
5. Negative

A

B

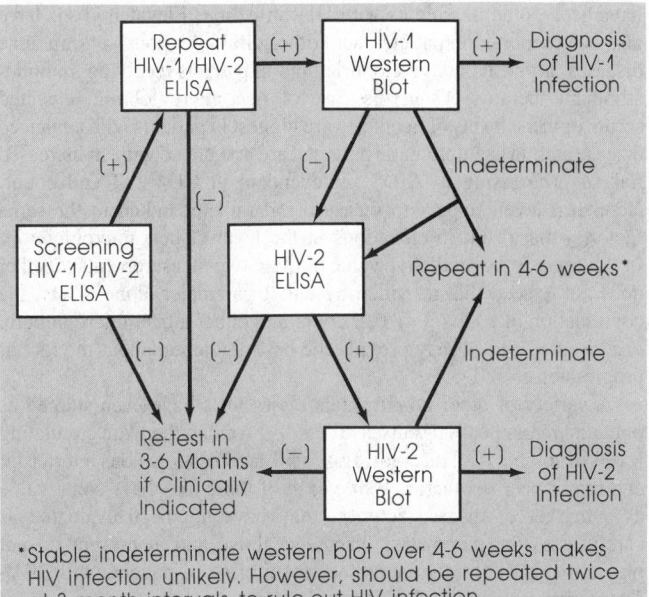

*Stable indeterminate western blot over 4-6 weeks makes HIV infection unlikely. However, should be repeated twice at 3 month intervals to rule-out HIV infection.

FIGURE 279-15 Algorithm for the use of serologic tests in the diagnosis of HIV-1 or HIV-2 infection.

or p24 antigen capture) must be employed to insure that the bands are not indicative of early HIV infection.

A guideline for the use of these serologic tests in attempting to make a diagnosis of HIV infection is depicted in Fig. 279-15. In a patient in whom HIV infection is suspected, the appropriate initial test is ELISA. If this is negative, unless one has a high suspicion of early HIV infection, such as an exposure within the previous 3 months, this result is sufficient to rule out the diagnosis and retesting should be performed only as clinically indicated. If the ELISA is indeterminate or positive, the test should be repeated. If the repeat is negative on two occasions, one can assume that the initial positive reading was due to a technical error in the performance of the assay and that the patient is negative. If the repeat is indeterminate or positive one should proceed to the western blot. If the western blot is positive, one has a diagnosis of HIV infection. If the western blot is negative, the ELISA can be assumed to have been a false positive and the diagnosis of HIV infection is ruled out. If the western blot is indeterminate one should proceed to the PCR with a repeat western blot in 1 month. If the PCR is negative and there is no progression in the western blot, a diagnosis of HIV is ruled out. If the PCR is positive and/or the western blot shows progression a diagnosis of HIV infection can be made.

A variety of other laboratory tests are available for the direct detection of HIV or its components. Although at present the ELISA and the western blot are the only licensed tests for making a diagnosis of HIV infection, many of these other tests are in common use in the research laboratory and are of considerable help when the western blot results are indeterminate. In addition, several of these direct measurements of HIV are currently being used to assess the antiviral activity of experimental therapies for HIV. The simplest of these is the *p24 antigen capture assay*. This is an ELISA-type assay in which the solid phase consists of antibodies to the p24 antigen of HIV. The viral protein p24 can be detected in the peripheral blood of HIV-infected individuals where it exists either as free antigen or complexed to anti-p24 antibodies. Overall, approximately 30 percent of individuals with HIV infection have detectable levels of free p24 antigen. This percentage increases to about 50 percent when samples are treated with a weak acid to dissociate antigen-antibody complexes prior to assay. Throughout the course of HIV infection an equilibrium appears to exist between p24 antigen and anti-p24 antibodies. During the first few weeks of infection, prior to the development of an

immune response, there is a brisk rise in p24 antigen levels. Following the development of anti-p24 antibodies these levels decline. Late in the course of infection, when circulating levels of free virus are high, p24 antigen levels also increase, particularly when detected by the use of techniques to dissociate antigen-antibody complexes. While the precise pathophysiologic significance of p24 antigenemia is unclear, it has been shown that for a group of asymptomatic patients with HIV infection and similar CD4+ T cell counts, those with detectable levels of p24 antigen are, on the average, three times more likely to show progression to AIDS than those in whom p24 antigen levels cannot be detected. Additionally, multiple clinical trials have demonstrated that patients receiving antiretroviral therapy will show a decline in their circulating levels of p24 antigen, and some have advocated the use of this assay for monitoring the effectiveness of such treatment. However, the validity of this recommendation has yet to be established. At present the p24 antigen capture assay seems to have its greatest utility as a screening test for HIV infection in patients suspected of having the acute HIV syndrome, and in whom high levels of p24 antigen are present prior to the development of antibodies.

The *direct cultivation of HIV* from plasma or peripheral blood mononuclear cells is a technique employed in many research laboratories and has proven very useful for monitoring the effects of experimental antiretroviral agents and generating isolates of HIV for studies of antiviral resistance and analysis of genomic drift. Most of the techniques employed involve cocultivation of patient material with an indicator cell line capable of supporting HIV replication, most commonly peripheral blood mononuclear cells that have been activated with phytohemagglutinin. When used as a clinical monitoring tool, the sample being studied (either cells or plasma) is serially diluted and an endpoint titration is determined. Cultures generally need to be maintained for up to 28 days, during which time they are periodically observed for the formation of syncytia or giant cells, and supernatants are sampled for the presence of HIV p24, using the antigen capture assays mentioned above. There is no role at present for HIV culture in the routine management of patients with HIV infection; however, such tests may become more common as one attempts to tailor antiretroviral therapy according to the sensitivities of patient-derived viral isolates.

The *polymerase chain reaction* is a diagnostic technique that has gained acceptance in many areas of clinical microbiology. Although the extreme sensitivity of this technique leads in many cases to false positives, in a well-controlled setting PCR has been of extraordinary value in furthering our understanding of the pathogenesis of HIV and has provided a true gold standard for the diagnosis of HIV infection. This is particularly true for the diagnosis of HIV infection in at-risk neonates. Two forms of PCR are used in the study of HIV infection, DNA PCR and RNA PCR. The DNA PCR is used for making a diagnosis of HIV infection by amplifying proviral DNA. In performing a DNA PCR test for HIV, peripheral blood mononuclear cells are lysed and the DNA region of interest is amplified utilizing primer pairs from relatively constant regions of the HIV genome. Primer pairs from both the *gag* and LTR regions are usually employed. The amplified DNA is then characterized utilizing nucleic acid hybridization techniques and, with the proper controls to check for contamination and success of amplification, it is possible to determine whether or not HIV proviral DNA is present at a frequency of one copy per 10,000 cells. Studies of this type have clearly documented that the interval between HIV infection and antibody positivity is on the order of 1 to 3 months.

In addition to being a diagnostic tool, DNA PCR is also useful for amplifying defined areas of proviral DNA for sequence analysis, and in this regard has become an important technique for studies of sequence diversity and microbial resistance to antiretroviral agents. RNA PCR has been used most frequently for monitoring changes in the level of the HIV genome present in plasma. In this technique, following DNAase treatment, a cDNA copy is made of all RNA species present in plasma. Insofar as HIV is an RNA virus (see above and Chap. 151), this will result in the production of DNA copies of HIV proportional to the amount of HIV present in plasma. This proviral cDNA is then amplified and characterized using the PCR technique employing primer pairs that can distinguish genomic cDNA from messenger cDNA. In the patient with a positive or indeterminate ELISA test and an indeterminate western blot and in the patient in whom serologic testing may be unreliable (such as in a patient with hypogammaglobulinemia), PCR is a valuable diagnostic tool for making a diagnosis of HIV infection. Given the cost and problems with contamination that can occur with PCR, however, its use as a diagnostic tool should be reserved for these instances where standard serologic testing has failed to give a definitive result.

LABORATORY MONITORING OF PATIENTS WITH HIV INFECTION   The epidemic of HIV infection and AIDS has provided the clinician with new challenges in the integration of clinical and laboratory data. The close relationship between clinical manifestations of HIV infection and CD4+ T cell count has made this immunologic test an essential part of routine evaluation of HIV-infected individuals. In addition, other tests such as the p24 antigen capture assay (described above), serum neopterin, and serum beta$_2$microglobulin levels may also provide information of value to the clinician.

At present, the CD4+ T cell count is the only laboratory test generally accepted as a reliable indicator of the progression of HIV infection. This measurement, which is the product of the percent of CD4+ T cells (determined by flow cytometry) and the total lymphocyte count (determined by the WBC and differential) has been shown to correlate very well with clinical progression. Patients with CD4+ T counts under 200 per microliter are at high risk of infection with *Pneumocystis carinii* while patients with CD4+ T cell counts under 100 per microliter are at high risk of infection with CMV and *Mycobacterium avium-intracellulare* (MAI). Patients with an initial diagnosis of HIV infection should have CD4+ T cell measurements performed approximately every 6 months and more frequently if a declining trend is noted. Antiretroviral therapy is indicated when the CD4+ T cell count falls below 500 per microliter, and a declining CD4 count may provide an indication for changing therapy. Once the CD4 count is under 200 per microliter patients should be placed on a regimen for *Pneumocystis carinii* pneumonia (PCP) prophylaxis. All effective forms of antiretroviral therapy to date have been associated with causing at least a transient increase in either CD4+ T cell count or CD4 percent.

Beta$_2$ microglobulin is an 11kDa protein that is expressed on the surface of most nucleated cells. It forms a heterodimer with the class I MHC molecules and exhibits amino acid homology with the constant region of immunoglobulin. Free beta$_2$microglobulin can be measured in both serum and urine. Levels of beta$_2$microglobulin are elevated in a variety of conditions characterized by lymphocyte activation and/or lymphocyte destruction, among them lymphoproliferative syndromes, autoimmune disease, and viral infections, including HIV infection. In addition, beta$_2$microglobulin is excreted by the renal tubule, and levels may be elevated in patients with renal disease. Levels of beta$_2$microglobulin correlate with the degree of disease progression in patients with HIV infection. The highest levels are seen in patients with AIDS, the lowest levels in patients with asymptomatic HIV infection. Levels of beta$_2$microglobulin have a predictive value for progression to AIDS that is independent of their inverse relationship to CD4+ T cell counts. In one large study the level of serum beta$_2$microglobulin was the single most important predictor of development of AIDS. In another study, 34 percent of patients with a beta$_2$microglobulin level over 3.8 µg/mL went on to develop AIDS over a 3-year period compared to only 7 percent of patients with a beta$_2$microglobulin level under 2.9 µg/mL. Levels of beta$_2$microglobulin have been shown to decrease in a dose-dependent fashion in patients treated with zidovudine (AZT).

Neopterin (6-D-erythro-trihydroxypropylpterin) is a low-molecular-weight compound derived from an intermediate product of the de novo biosynthesis of tetrahydrobiopterin from guanosine triphosphate (GTP). It is produced by activated monocytes and increased levels

have been noted in patients with HIV infection. Elevated levels have also been reported in patients with other viral infections, autoimmune diseases, atypical phenylketonuria, and in patients receiving immunostimulant therapy. As in the case of beta$_2$microglobulin, elevated serum or urine levels of neopterin are highest in patients with advanced disease and, in asymptomatic patients, are associated with an increased risk of progressing to AIDS, independent of CD4+ T cell count. Neopterin levels appear to measure a parameter linked to the same factor(s) that result in elevations in the level of beta$_2$microglobulin. In this regard, the predictive value of these two measurements together does not exceed that provided by either parameter alone. Thus, the combination of a CD4+ T cell count and either a beta$_2$microglobulin or a neopterin level may provide the best prediction about the risk of progression to AIDS.

A variety of other nonviral laboratory tests have been studied as potential markers of HIV disease activity. Among them are circulating levels of soluble IL-2 receptor, IgA, acid-labile endogenous interferon, and tumor necrosis factor. While each of these may have some value as a marker of disease activity, they have not been evaluated as carefully as the parameters discussed above and at present do not play a major role in the laboratory monitoring of patients with HIV-1 infection.

CLINICAL MANIFESTATIONS

The clinical consequences of HIV infection encompass a spectrum ranging from an acute syndrome associated with primary infection to a prolonged asymptomatic state to advanced disease. It is preferable to adopt the concept that HIV disease is manifested in various stages. As mentioned above, active virus replication and progressive immunologic impairment occur throughout the course of HIV infection, and so HIV disease actually progressses even during the clinically latent stage. HIV disease can be empirically divided on the basis of the degree of immunosuppression into an early stage (CD4+ T cell count greater than 500 per microliter), an intermediate stage (CD4+ T cell count between 200 and 500 per microliter), and an advanced stage (CD4+ T cell count less than 200 per microliter). Most AIDS-defining opportunistic infections and true malignancies occur within the advanced stage, while neurologic disease and Kaposi's sarcoma are not as strictly related to the level of immunosuppression. There are no recognized HLA associations with HIV infection or with the development of any particular manifestation of HIV disease. However, it has been reported that HLA-B35 is associated with an accelerated progression to AIDS (see Chap. 64). The two major classification systems for staging HIV infection are the CDC system (Table 279-9) and the Walter Reed Medical Center system (Table 279-10). Each has its own advantages and disadvantages, with the CDC system relying more on clinical condition for classification and the Walter Reed system relying more on immunologic status such as level of CD4+ T cell count and presence or absence of delayed cutaneous hypersensitivity. For the purposes of describing the clinical syndromes seen in patients with HIV infection, separate sections

---

TABLE 279-9   Centers for Disease Control classification system for HIV disease

Group I	Acute HIV syndrome
Group II	Asymptomatic infection
Group III	Persistent generalized lymphadenopathy
Group IV	Other diseases:
Subgroup A	Constitutional disease
Subgroup B	Neurologic disease
Subgroup C	Secondary infectious diseases
Subgroup D	Secondary neoplasms
Subgroup E	Other conditions

SOURCE: Modified from the Centers for Disease Control and Prevention, USPHS, 1986 and 1987.

TABLE 279-10   Walter Reed staging classification of HIV infection

Stage	HIV Antibody	Chronic lymphadenopathy	CD4 cells/mm³	DTH skin testing	Thrush	Opportunistic infections
WR0	–	–	>400	Normal (reactive to ≥2 skin test antigens)	–	–
WR1	+	–	>400	Normal	–	–
WR2	+	+	>400	Normal	–	–
WR3	+	+/–	<400	Normal	–	–
WR4	+	+/–	<400	Partial defect (reactive to 1 skin test antigen)	–	–
WR5	+	+/–	<400	Anergy and/or thrush (reactive to 0 skin test antigens)	–	
WR6	+	+/–	<400	Normal, partial defect or anergy	+/–	+

▢ absolute criteria required to be fulfilled for stage assignment

Abbreviations: + = present; – = absent; DTH = delayed type hypersensitivity
SOURCE: Modified from Redfield et al: The Walter Reed staging classification for HTLV-III/LAV infection. N Engl J Med 314:131, 1986.

will deal with the acute syndrome, the asymptomatic stage, early symptomatic disease, neurologic disease, secondary infections, neoplasms and organ-specific syndromes.

THE ACUTE HIV SYNDROME   It is estimated that approximately 50 to 70 percent of individuals with HIV infection experience an acute syndrome approximately 3 to 6 weeks following primary infection (Fig. 279-16). Varying degrees of clinical severity have been reported, and it has been suggested that symptomatic seroconversion may be prognostic of an increased risk for a more accelerated course. The typical clinical findings are listed in Table 279-11 and are accompanied by a burst of plasma viremia and p24 antigenemia. The syndrome is typical of an acute viral infection and has been likened to acute mononucleosis. Symptoms usually persist for 1 to 2 weeks and gradually subside as an immune response to HIV develops. Opportunistic infections have been reported during this stage of infection, presumably as a result of the transient immunosuppression. In this regard, a number of immunologic abnormalities accompany the acute HIV syndrome including multiphasic perturbations of the numbers of circulating lymphocyte subsets. Total lymphocyte and T cell subsets (CD4 and CD8) are initially reduced. An inversion of the

CD4+ to CD8+ T cell ratio occurs later because of a rise in the number of CD8+ T cells. The CD8+ T cell levels return to normal, but the CD4+ T cell levels remain somewhat depressed, resulting in the persistence of an abnormal ratio. Lymphadenopathy occurs in approximately 70 percent of people with symptomatic primary HIV infection. Lymph node biopsies show a reduction of extrafollicular B cells, CD8+ T cell follicular infiltration, and relatively little activation and proliferation of the germinal center cells. From 1 week to 3 months following the onset of symptoms, humoral and cellular immune responses are detected and coincide with the disappearance of symptoms and the decrease and/or disappearance of plasma viremia and p24 antigenemia. As mentioned above, the decrease in viremia is likely due to a combination of an immune clearance of virus and the sequestration of virus in the lymph nodes. Most patients recover spontaneously from this syndrome and are left with mild degrees of decrease in CD4+ T lymphocyte counts that may still remain within the normal range. However, an occasional patient will manifest a fulminant course of immunologic deterioration following primary infection even after disappearance of symptoms. In the vast majority of patients, primary infection, with or without the acute syndrome, is followed by a prolonged period of clinical latency.

THE ASYMPTOMATIC STAGE—CLINICAL LATENCY   Although the length of time from initial infection to the development of clinical disease (Table 279-9; Group IV) varies greatly from individual to

FIGURE 279-16   The acute HIV syndrome. See text for detailed description. *(From G Pantaleo et al, N Engl J Med 328:327, 1993.)*

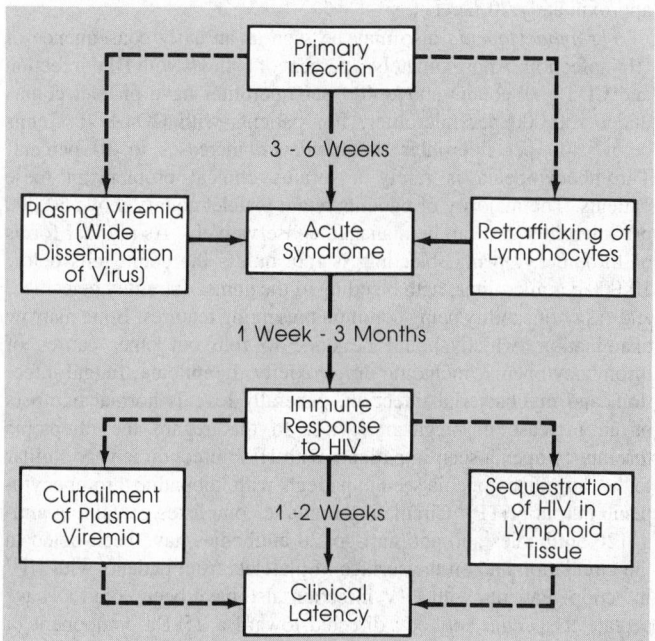

TABLE 279-11   Clinical findings in the acute HIV syndrome*

GENERAL

Fever
Pharyngitis
Lymphadenopathy
Headache/retro-orbital pain
Arthralgias/myalgias
Lethargy/malaise
Anorexia/weight loss
Nausea/vomiting/diarrhea

NEUROPATHIC

Meningitis
Encephalitis
Peripheral neuropathy
Myelopathy

DERMATOLOGIC

Erythematous maculopapular rash
Mucocutaneous ulceration

* From B Tindal and DA Cooper.

individual, the median time is approximately 10 years for homosexual or bisexual men. This median time varies somewhat with the mode of infection, with IDUs generally having a more aggressive course than homosexual men and hemophiliacs. As emphasized above, HIV disease with active virus replication progresses during this asymptomatic period. Certain patients will remain entirely asymptomatic despite the fact that their CD4+ T cell counts fall to extremely low levels. Initial symptoms may be associated with the first manifestations of an opportunistic disease. Other patients experience varying degrees of intermittent symptoms such as malaise, lethargy, weakness, and anorexia which are not persistent enough to be categorized as constitutional disease (Table 279-9; Group IVA). Certain patients, otherwise asymptomatic, develop persistent generalized lymphadenopathy (Table 279-9; Group III) (see below). With few exceptions, there is a progressive diminution of CD4+ T cell counts during this asymptomatic period which ultimately leads to a state of immunosuppression that is severe enough (CD4+ T cell count <200 per microliter) to place the patient at high risk for opportunistic, and hence clinically apparent, disease.

EARLY SYMPTOMATIC DISEASE   As noted above, viral replication continues and the immunologic function of the HIV-infected individual declines during the period of clinical latency. At some point in that decline, usually after the CD4+ T cell count has fallen below 500 cells per microliter, patients begin to develop signs and symptoms of clinical illness (Table 279-12). Many of these problems can be traced to minor opportunistic infections, not sufficiently indicative of a defect in cell mediated immunity to be considered an AIDS-defining illness, while some of them appear to be a direct effect of long-standing HIV infection. This stage of HIV infection has been given a variety of names in the past, among them *pre-AIDS* and *AIDS-related complex (ARC)*. These clinical findings, while indicative of a decline in immune function, are generally less predictive of the patient's overall status than are the data obtained from serial measurement of CD4+ T cell counts. At present antiretroviral therapy is indicated for patients in this group, particularly if their CD4+ T cell count is under 500 cells per microliter.

Generalized lymphadenopathy, defined as the presence of enlarged lymph nodes (>1 cm) in two or more extrainguinal sites for more than 3 months without an obvious cause, is often the earliest symptom of HIV infection following the acute syndrome. It is due to a marked follicular hyperplasia in response to HIV infection. In this condition the nodes are generally discrete and freely moveable. This feature of HIV disease, which may be seen at any point along the immunologic spectrum, is not associated with any increased likelihood of developing AIDS. Paradoxically, a loss in lymphadenopathy or a decrease in lymph node size may be a poor prognostic marker and indicative of disease progression. In the early and intermediate stages of HIV infection, as defined by CD4+ T cell counts above 200 per microliter, the main differential diagnosis is an adenopathic form of Kaposi's sarcoma. Late in the course of disease, one must extend the differential diagnosis to include mycobacterial infection, lymphoma, and bacillary angiomatosis. Lymph node biopsy is not indicated in early patients unless there are accompanying signs and symptoms of systemic illness such as fever and weight loss or if the nodes begin to enlarge, become fixed, or coalesce.

Oral lesions are particularly common during this phase of HIV infection. Among them are thrush, hairy leukoplakia, and aphthous

ulcers. Thrush, due to *Candida* infection, and oral hairy leukoplakia, presumed due to Epstein-Barr virus, are usually indicative of fairly advanced immunologic decline, generally occurring in patients with less than 300 CD4+ T cells per microliter. In one study, 59 percent of patients with oral candidiasis went on to develop AIDS over the next year. Thrush appears as a white, cheesy exudate, often on an erythematous mucosa (see Fig. A1-41). While most commonly seen on the soft palate, early lesions may be found along the gingival border. The diagnosis is made by direct examination of a scraping for pseudohyphal elements. Culturing is of no value insofar as the majority of patients with HIV infection will have a positive throat culture for *Candida* even in the absence of thrush. Oral hairy leukoplakia presents as a filamentous white lesion, generally along the lateral borders of the tongue (see Fig. A1-40). While usually more a sign of HIV-induced immunodeficiency than a clinical problem, severe cases have been noted to respond to therapy with acyclovir. Aphthous ulcers of the posterior oropharynx are also seen with regularity in patients with HIV infection. These lesions are of unknown etiology and can be quite painful and interfere with swallowing. Topical anesthetics are usually the best symptomatic treatment although the relief provided is of short duration. Recent reports that thalidomide may be of some help in this situation suggest that the pathophysiology may involve the action of tissue-destructive cytokines.

Reactivation herpes zoster or shingles (see Fig. A1-37) is seen in 10 to 20 percent of patients with HIV infection. This reactivation syndrome of varicella-zoster virus is an indication of modest decline in immune function and is often the first clnical indication of immunodeficiency. In one series, patients who developed shingles were noted to do so on the average of 5 years following HIV infection. In a cohort of patients with HIV infection, AIDS was noted to develop in 1 percent of the cohort per month following the diagnosis of localized zoster. In that study, AIDS was more likely to develop in those patients with severe pain, extensive disease, or disease involving cranial or cervical dermatomes. In patients who developed both shingles and oral hairy leukoplakia or thrush, shingles was noted to devleop approximately 1 year earlier. The clinical manifestations of reactivation zoster in HIV-infected patients, although indicative of immunologic compromise, are not as severe as that seen in other immunodeficient conditions. Thus, while lesions may extend over several dermatomes and frank cutaneous dissemination may be seen, visceral involvement has not been reported. In contrast to patients without a known underlying immunodeficiency, patients with HIV infection tend to have recurrences of zoster, with a relapse rate of approximately 20 percent.

Thrombocytopenia also may be seen as an early consequence of HIV infection. Approximately 3 percent of patients with HIV infection and CD4+ T counts above 400 per microliter have platelet counts under 150,000 per microliter. For patients with CD4+ T counts below 400 per microliter the incidence increases to 10 percent. Thrombocytopenia is rarely a serious clinical problem in these patients. The majority of patients retain platelet counts above 50,000 per microliter and can be managed conservatively. As in other forms of thrombocytopenia, bleeding is rare unless the count falls below 10,000 per microliter, with bleeding of the gums, extremity petechiae, and easy bruisability being common presenting features. Bone marrow examination, which should be done to rule out other causes of thrombocytopenia, including drug toxicity, lymphoma, fungal infection, and myobacterial infection, generally reveals normal numbers or an increase in megakaryocytes. In this regard the idiopathic thrombocytopenia seen in patients with HIV infection is very similar to the thrombocytopenia seen in patients with idiopathic thrombocytopenic purpura (ITP). Circulating immune complexes containing anti-gp120 antibodies and anti-anti-gp120 antibodies have been noted in the circulation and on the surface of platelets from patients with HIV infection. Patients with HIV infection also have been noted to have a platelet specific antibody directed toward a 25kDa component of the surface of the platelet. Consistent with the fact that these data

---

TABLE 279-12   Clinical characteristics of early symptomatic disease

Generalized lymphadenopathy
Thrush
Oral hairy leukoplakia
Shingles
Thrombocytopenia
Molluscum contagiosum

point to an immunologic basis for the thrombocytopenia seen in patients with AIDS, most of the therapeutic interventions that have been employed have been immune based. Either high dose intravenous immunoglobulin (IVIG) or glucocorticoids are capable of inducing transient increases in platelet counts; however, they do not generally provide long-term solutions. It has also been suggested that the thrombocytopenia in patients with HIV infection may be due to the direct effects of HIV on megakaryocytes, as evidenced by a decrease in platelet production. Consistent with this is the fact that the most effective medical approach to this problem has been the use of zidovudine. Even in patients without thrombocytopenia, therapy with zidovudine has been associated with a significant increase in platelet count and should be considered the treatment of choice for HIV-associated thrombocytopenia. Approximately 70 percent of patients with HIV-associated thrombocytopenia will have a satisfactory response to zidovudine. For patients with platelet counts below 20,000 per microliter the approach to therapy should be to initiate treatment with IVIG or glucocorticoids for an immediate response coupled with zidovudine for a more lasting response. Splenectomy is a viable option in patients refractory to medical management. The majority of patients with HIV-associated thrombocytopenia will respond to this surgical treatment. Because of the propensity to develop serious infections with encapsulated organisms, physicians should ensure that all patients with HIV infection, especially those about to undergo splenectomy, are immunized with pneumococcal polysaccharide. It should be noted that in addition to causing an increase in platelet count, removal of the spleen will result in an increase in total lymphocyte count, making determinations of total CD4+ T counts unreliable. In this situation one should rely on the CD4 percent for making diagnostic decisions with respect to the likelihood of opportunistic infections in the HIV-infected patient. Thrombocytopenia has also been reported in early HIV-infected patients as a consequence of classic thrombotic thrombocytopenic purpura (see Chap. 307). This clinical syndrome, consisting of fever, thrombocytopenia, hemolytic anemia, and neurologic and renal dysfunction is a rare complication of early HIV infection. As in other settings, the appropriate management is the use of salicylates and plasma exchange.

Miscellaneous clinical conditions frequently seen in patients with early stages of HIV infection include molluscum contagiosum, basal cell carcinomas of the skin, headache, condyloma acuminata, and recurrent bouts of oral or genital herpes simplex. In the past, unexplained fever, weight loss and diarrhea were included under the general heading of ARC. Many of these cases are now being diagnosed as specific opportunistic infections. In addition, this syndrome has been classified as an AIDS-defining illness in patients in whom no other diagnosis can be found, and is discussed below under generalized wasting.

NEUROLOGIC DISEASE Clinical disease of the nervous system accounts for a significant degere of morbidity in a high percentage of patients with HIV infection (Table 279-13). The neurologic problems that occur in the HIV-infected population may be primary to the overall pathogenic processes of HIV infection or may be secondary to opportunistic infections or neoplasms. Among the opportunistic infections and neoplasms that involve the central nervous system (CNS) are toxoplasmosis, cryptococcosis, progressive multifocal leukoencephalopathy, CMV, HTLV-I, mycobacterium tuberculosis, syphilis, and primary CNS lymphoma. These occur in about one-third of patients with AIDS and are discussed in more detail below under the various opportunistic infections and neoplasms. Primary processes related to HIV infection of the nervous system are somewhat similar to those seen with other lentiviruses such as the Visna-Maedi virus of sheep. Neurologic problems occur throughout the course of disease and may be inflammatory, demyelinating, or degenerative in nature. While only one of these, the AIDS dementia complex, is considered an AIDS-defining illness, most HIV-infected patients will have some neurologic problem during the course of their disease. As noted in the section on pathogenesis, damage to the CNS may be a direct result of viral infection of CNS macrophages or glial cells or

TABLE 279-13 Neurologic diseases in patients with HIV infection

OPPORTUNISTIC INFECTIONS

Toxoplasmosis
Cryptococcosis
Progressive multifocal leukoencephalopathy
Cytomegalovirus
Syphilis
Mycobacterium tuberculosis
HTLV-I

NEOPLASMS

Primary CNS lymphoma
Kaposi's sarcoma

PRIMARY HIV-1 INFECTION

Aseptic meningitis
AIDS dementia complex
Myelopathy
    Vacuolar myelopathy
    Pure sensory ataxia
    Paresthesia/dysesthesia
Peripheral neuropathy
    Acute demyelinating polyneuropathy
    Mononeuritis multiplex
    Distal symmetric polyneuropathy
Myopathy

secondary to the release of potentially toxic cytokines such as TNF and TGF-β. Virtually all patients with HIV infection have some degree of involvement of the nervous system with HIV. This is evidenced by the fact that cerebrospinal fluid (CSF) findings are abnormal in approximately 90 percent of patients, even at the asymptomatic stage of HIV infection. Included in these abnormalities are pleocytosis in 50 to 65 percent, isolation of virus in approximately 50 percent, elevated CSF protein in 35 percent, and evidence of intrathecal synthesis of anti-HIV antibodies in 89 percent. It should be pointed out, however, that evidence of CNS infection with HIV does not imply the presence of impairment of cognitive function, and while neurologic problems related to HIV infection can be seen at all stages of the illness, the mere presence of HIV infection in the CNS does not necessarily mean that the patient has a clinically relevant neurologic problem. In this regard the neurologic function of an HIV-infected individual should be considered normal unless clinical signs and symptoms suggest otherwise.

Aseptic meningitis may be seen throughout all but the very late stages of HIV infection. As noted above, in the setting of acute seroconversion patients may experience a syndrome of headache, photophobia, and, in some instances, frank encephalitis. CSF findings include a lymphocytic pleocytosis, elevated protein, and normal glucose. Cranial nerve involvement may be seen, predominantly cranial nerve VII, occasionally V, and/or VIII. This syndrome usually resolves spontaneously within 2 to 4 weeks; however, in some patients signs and symptoms may persist as a chronic problem. Such episodes may occur any time throughout the course of HIV infection; however, they become increasingly rare following the development of AIDS. This suggests that aseptic meningitis seen in the context of HIV infection is an immunologically mediated disease.

The AIDS dementia complex refers to a constellation of signs and symptoms of CNS disease that generally occurs late in the course of HIV infection (Table 279-14). As suggested by its name, a major feature of this entity is the development of dementia, which is defined as a decline in cognitive ability from a previously attained level. This may present as impaired ability to concentrate, increased forgetfulness, or increased difficulty performing complex tasks. Initially these symptoms may be indistinguishable from findings of situational depression or fatigue. In addition to dementia, patients with the AIDS dementia complex also may have motor and behavioral abnormalities.

TABLE 279-14 Clinical Staging of the AIDS Dementia Complex

Stage O (normal)	Normal mental and motor function.
Stage 0.5 (equivocal/subclinical)	Absent, minimal, or equivocal symptoms without impairment of work or capacity to perform activities of daily living (ADL). Mild signs (snout response, slowed ocular or extremity movements) may be present. Gait and strength are normal.
Stage 1 (mild)	Able to perform all but the more demanding aspects of work or ADL but with unequivocal evidence (signs or symptoms that may include performance on neuropsychological testing) of functional intellectual or motor impairment. Can walk without assistance.
Stage 2 (moderate)	Able to perform basic activities of self-care but cannot work or maintain the more demanding aspects of daily life. Ambulatory, but may require a single prop.
Stage 3 (severe)	Major intellectual incapacity (cannot follow news or personal events, cannot sustain complex conversation, considerable slowing of all output) or motor disability (cannot walk unassisted, usually with slowing and clumsiness of arms as well).
Stage 4 (end stage)	Nearly vegetative. Intellectual and social comprehension and output are at a rudimentary level. Nearly or absolutely mute. Paraparetic or paraplegic with urinary and fecal incontinence.

Adapted from JJ Sidtis and RW Price: Early HIV infection and the AIDS dementia complex. Neurology 40:197, 1990.

Among the motor problems are unsteady gait, poor balance, and difficulty with rapid alternating movements. Findings of increased tone and deep tendon reflexes may be present in patients with spinal cord involvement (see below). Late stages may be complicated by bowel and/or bladder incontinence. Behavioral problems include apathy and lack of initiative with progression to a vegetative state in some instances. In most instances these changes occur without significant changes in level of alertness, in contrast to the findings in patients with dementia due to toxic/metabolic encephalopathies.

The AIDS dementia complex is the initial AIDS-defining illness in approximately 10 percent of patients with HIV infection and thus rarely occurs prior to clinical evidence of immunodeficiency.

Clinically significant AIDS dementia complex eventually develops in approximately two-thirds of patients with HIV infection. As immunologic function declines, the risk and severity of the AIDS dementia complex increases. Autopsy series suggest that 80 to 90 percent of patients with HIV infection have histologic evidence of CNS involvement. Several classification schemes have been developed for grading AIDS dementia complex. The most commonly used clinical staging system is outlined in Table 279-14.

The precise cause of the AIDS dementia complex remains unclear although it is felt to represent the end result of the direct effects of HIV on the CNS. HIV has been demonstrated to be present in the brains of patients with AIDS dementia complex by Southern blot, in situ hybridization, and electron microscopy. Multinucleated giant cells, macrophages, and microglial cells appear to be the main cell types harboring virus in the CNS. Histologically, the major changes are seen in the subcortical areas of the brain and thus fit under the general category of subcortical dementia. In this regard AIDS dementia complex is similar to the dementia seen in patients with Parkinson's disease (see Chap. 371) and Huntington's chorea (see Chap. 370) and distinct from that seen in patients with Alzheimer's disease (see Chap. 370). Among the histopathologic changes are white matter pallor and gliosis, multinucleated giant cell encephalitis and vacuolar myelopathy. Less commonly, diffuse or focal spongiform changes in the white matter occur.

There are no specific criteria upon which a diagnosis of AIDS dementia complex rests, and thus this syndrome must be distinguished from a number of other diseases which affect the CNS of HIV-infected patients (Table 279-15). The diagnosis of dementia depends upon demonstrating a decline in cognitive function. This can be accomplished objectively with the use of the Mini-Mental Status Examination (Table 279-16) in patients for whom prior scores are available. For this reason it is advisable for all patients with a diagnosis of HIV infection to have a baseline Mini-Mental Status Examination. Imaging studies of the CNS, either computerized tomography (CT) or magnetic resonance imaging (MRI), often demonstrate evidence of cerebral atrophy (Fig. 279-17). MRI also may reveal small areas of increased density of T2-weighted images, often referred to as "unidentified bright objects." While a lumbar puncture is an important element of the evaluation of patients with HIV infection and neurologic abnormalities, it is generally most helpful in the diagnosis of opportunistic infections. In AIDS dementia complex, patients may have an increase in CSF cells and protein; however, these findings are nonspecific, and the diagnosis is truly one that can be made only after opportunistic pathogens and neoplasms have been ruled out. While HIV is often able to be isolated from the

TABLE 279-15 Characterization of the most common central nervous system diseases in patients with HIV infection

Disease	Approximate incidence, %	Clinical features	Characteristic CSF findings	Characteristic radiologic findings
AIDS dementia complex	67	Personality changes, dementia, unsteady gait, seizures	Nonspecific	Cortical atrophy, ventricular dilatation, bright spots on T2-weighted MRI
Toxoplasmosis	15	Fever, headache, focal neurologic deficits, seizure + antibodies in 85%	Nonspecific	Multiple ring-enhancing lesions in multiple locations
Cryptococcal meningitis	6–12	Fever, nausea, vomiting, confusion, headache	Elevated protein, low glucose, positive crypto Ag/culture	Nonspecific
Progressive multifocal leukoencephalopathy virus	4	Multiple focal deficits without changes in level of consciousness	Nonspecific	Multiple white matter lesions on T2-weighted images
Neurosyphilis	1	Meningitis, neuroretinitis, deafness, focal neurologic deficits	VDRL	Nonspecific
Central nervous system	1	Seizure, focal neurologic deficits, headache	Nonspecific in 1°CNS lymphoma; malignant cells in systemic lymphoma	Single or few ring-enhancing lesions
Tuberculous meningitis	1	Fever, headache, confusion, meningitis, cough	Elevated protein, low glucose, pleocytosis, positive AFB smear/culture	Mass lesions in approximately 50%, abnormal chest x-ray

TABLE 279-16 The Folstein Mini-Mental Status Examination

Question	Scoring	Maximum Score
1 Where are (state, county, city, hospital, clinic)?	1 point for each	5
2 What are the (day, date, month, season, year, time)?	1 point for each	5
3 "Say these three words after me: (yellow, apple, Ohio)"	1 point for each	3
4 Ask patient to begin with 100 and count backwards by 7's. Or, if patient refuses, ask to spell "world" backwards.	Stop after 5, score no. correct. Or, 1 point for each correct letter	5
5 Recall the three words given in question no. 3.	1 point for each	3
6 Ask the patient to name "watch" then "pencil."	1 point for each	2
7 Ask the patients to repeat "No ifs, ands, or buts."	1 point if correct	1
8 Three-stage command: Take this paper in your right hand, fold it in half, and put it on the floor.	1 point for each correct	3
9 Ask the patient to read silently and obey the command (print in block letters): CLOSE YOUR EYES.	1 point if correct	1
10 Ask the patient to write a sentence.	1 point if it contains a subject and verb and makes sense (ignore spelling and grammar)	1
11 "Draw a clock with numbers and hands showing the time to be 8:20"	2 points if correct	2
12 Have the patient copy this design:	1 point if all sides and angles are preserved and if intersecting sides form a quadrangle.	1

CSF of these patients, this finding is not specific for AIDS dementia complex and, in fact, there appears to be no correlation between the presence of HIV in the CSF and the presence of AIDS dementia complex. Elevated levels of beta$_2$microglobulin, neopterin, and quinolinic acid (a metabolite of tryptophan reported to cause CNS injury) have been noted in the CSF of patients with AIDS dementia complex. These findings suggest that cytokines may be involved in the pathogenesis of this syndrome; however, at this time definitive evidence is still lacking.

While there is no specific treatment for the AIDS dementia complex, multiple reports suggest that treatment with antiretroviral agents may be of benefit. Improvement in neuropsychiatric tests have been noted for both adult and pediatric patients treated with either zidovudine or didanosine. In fact, the rapid symptomatic improvement in cognitive function noted with the initiation of antiretroviral therapy suggests that at least some component of this problem is quickly reversible, again supporting at least a partial role of soluble mediators in the pathogenesis.

It should also be noted that these patients have an increased sensitivity to the side effects of neuroleptic drugs. The use of these drugs for symptomatic treatment is associated with an increased risk of extrapyramidal side effects, thus requiring that patients with AIDS dementia complex who receive these agents be monitored carefully.

Seizures are a relatively frequent complication of HIV infection and may be seen as a consequence of opportunistic infections, neoplasms, or AIDS dementia complex (Table 279-17). Seizures are seen in 15 to 40 percent of patients with cerebral toxoplasmosis, 15 to 35 percent of patients with primary CNS lymphoma, 8 percent of patients with cryptococcal meningitis, and 7 to 50 percent of patients with AIDS dementia complex. Seizures may also be seen in patients with CNS tuberculosis, aseptic meningitis, and progressive multifocal leukoencephalopathy. Seizures may be the presenting clinical symptom of HIV disease. In one study of 100 patients with HIV infection presenting with a first seizure, cerebral mass lesions were the most common cause, responsible for 32 of 100 new onset seizures. Of these 32, 28 were due to toxoplasmosis and 4 to lymphoma. AIDS dementia complex accounted for an additional 24 new-onset seizures. Cryptococcal meningitis was the third most common diagnosis, responsible for 13 of the 100 seizures. In 23 cases, no cause could be found and it is possible that these represent a subcategory of the AIDS dementia complex. Thus, the AIDS dementia complex may be the single leading cause of seizures in patients with HIV infection. Of these 23 cases, 16 (70 percent) had two or more seizures, suggesting that anticonvulsant therapy is indicated in all patients with HIV infection and seizure unless a rapidly correctable cause is noted. In this regard, while phenytoin remains the initial treatment of choice, hypersensitivity reactions to this drug have been reported in over 10 percent of patients with AIDS, and therefore the use of phenobarbital or valproic acid must be considered as alternatives.

FIGURE 279-17 Computed tomogram of the central nervous system of a patient with AIDS dementia complex. CT demonstrates cortical thinning and dilatation of the ventricles.

TABLE 279-17 Leading causes of seizures in patients with HIV infections

Disease	Overall contribution to seizures
AIDS dementia complex	24–47%
Cerebral toxoplasmosis	28%
Cryptococcal meningitis	13%
Primary central nervous system lymphoma	4%
Progressive multifocal leukoencephalopathy	1%

From DM Holtzman et al.

Spinal cord disease is present in approximately 20 percent of patients with AIDS, often as part of the AIDS dementia complex. In fact, 90 percent of the patients with HIV-associated myelopathy have some evidence of dementia, suggesting that similar pathologic processes may be responsible for both conditions. Three main types of spinal cord disease, or myelopathy, are seen in patients with AIDS. The first of these is a vacuolar myelopathy as discussed above under AIDS dementia complex. This is pathologically similar to subacute combined degeneration of the cord such as occurs with pernicious anemia. Although B_{12} deficiency is common in patients with AIDS, it does not appear to be responsible for the cord disease seen in these patients, given the fact that there is no response to treatment with parenteral B_{12}. Vacuolar myelopathy is characterized by a subacute onset and often presents with gait disturbances, predominantly ataxia and spasticity. This may progress to include bladder and bowel dysfunction. Physical findings include evidence of increased deep tendon reflexes and extensor plantar responses. The second form of spinal cord disease involves the dorsal columns and presents as a pure sensory ataxia. The third form is also sensory in nature and presents with paresthesias and dysesthesias of the lower extremities. In contrast to the cognitive problems seen in patients with the AIDS dementia complex these spinal cord syndromes do not generally respond to therapy with antivirals and therapy is mainly supportive. Other diseases involving the spinal cord in patients with HIV infection include HTLV-I–associated myelopathy (HAM) (see Chap. 151), neurosyphilis (see Chap. 133), herpesvirus infections (varicella-zoster, simplex, and CMV) (see Chaps. 143 and 144), tuberculosis (see Chap. 130), and lymphoma (see Chap. 311).

Peripheral neuropathies are common in patients with HIV infection; they occur at all stages of illness and take a variety of forms. Early in the course of HIV infection, an acute inflammatory demyelinating polyneuropathy resembling Guillain-Barré syndrome may occur (see Chap. 373). Patients commonly present with progressive weakness, areflexia, and minimal sensory changes. CSF examination reveals a pleocytosis, and peripheral nerve biopsy demonstrating a perivascular infiltrate suggesting an autoimmune etiology. Although generally a self-limited disease, in severe cases plasma exchange, intravenous immunoglobulin, or systemic glucocorticoids have been tried and have been reported to have variable degrees of success. Because of the immunosuppressive effect of glucocorticoids, they should be reserved for severe cases refractory to other measures. Another autoimmune peripheral neuropathy seen in patients with AIDS is mononeuritis multiplex (see Chap. 291). This necrotizing arteritis generally occurs in patients with moderate degrees of immunosuppression and may be managed as outlined above. However, the most common peripheral neuropathy in patients with HIV infection is a distal, symmetric, painful polyneuropathy generally seen only in patients with advanced HIV infection and AIDS. Although it is present clinically in only 30 to 40 percent of patients, two-thirds of patients with AIDS may be shown by electrophysiologic studies to have some evidence of peripheral nerve disease. This polyneuropathy, which is felt to be due to HIV-mediated axonal degeneration, most often presents as bilateral painful burning sensations in the feet and lower extremities. Antiretrovirals have been of little benefit in the management of this problem. Therapy is predominantly symptomatic through the use of tricyclics and analgesics. There are two important entities in the differential diagnosis of peripheral neuropathy in the HIV-infected patient. The first is CMV-associated progressive polyradiculopathy. This entity is generally fulminant in onset, with lower extremity and sacral paresthesias, difficulty in walking, areflexia, ascending sensory loss, and urinary retention. CSF examination reveals a predominantly neutrophilic pleocytosis. Therapy with ganciclovir or foscarnet can lead to rapid improvement. The second entity is dideoxynucleoside-associated peripheral neuropathy. This painful complication of either didanosine, zalcitabine, or stavudine therapy is most commonly seen at high doses and usually resolves following discontinuation of therapy. It is discussed in more detail below.

Myopathy may also complicate the course of HIV infection. Among the causes of myopathy in the setting of HIV infection are HIV itself, zidovudine, and the generalized wasting syndrome (see below). HIV-associated myopathy may range in severity from asymptomatic elevation in creatine kinase to a subacute syndrome characterized by proximal muscle weakness and myalgias. Quite pronounced elevations in creatine kinase may occur in asymptomatic patients, particularly following exercise. The clinical significance of this finding is unclear. A variety of both inflammatory and non-inflammatory pathologic processes have been noted in patients with more severe myopathy including myofiber necrosis with inflammatory cells, nemaline rod bodies, cytoplasmic bodies and mitochondrial abnormalities. Profound muscle wasting may be seen after prolonged zidovudine therapy. This toxic side effect of the drug appears to be related to its ability to interfere with the function of mitochondrial polymerases and is reversible following discontinuation of treatment.

SECONDARY INFECTIONS   Secondary infections are a late complication of HIV infection, for the most part occurring in patients with less than 200 CD4 cells per microliter. While characteristically caused by opportunistic organisms, such as *Pneumocystis carinii*, CMV, and other organisms that do not ordinarily cause disease in the absence of a compromised immune system, the spectrum of serious secondary infections that may be seen in patients with HIV infection also includes common bacterial and mycobacterial pathogens. Secondary infections are the leading cause of morbidity and mortality in patients with HIV infection. Approximately 80 percent of AIDS patients die as a direct result of an infection other than HIV, with infections due to opportunistic organisms heading the list. The clinical spectrum of diseases caused by secondary infections is constantly changing as patients live longer, and as new and better approaches to treatment and prophylaxis are developed.

Protozoal infections   *Pneumocystis carinii* (see Chap. 178) is one of the most common infections in patients with HIV infection; however, with the development of effective prophylactic regimens its incidence and relative contribution to morbidity and mortality have been decreasing. Approximately 70 to 80 percent of patients with HIV infection will experience at least one bout of *Pneumocystis carinii* pneumonia (PCP) at some time during the course of their disease and PCP is listed as the immediate cause of death in 15 to 20 percent of patients dying with AIDS. Depending upon the severity, the probability of death from a single episode of PCP varies from 10 to 50 percent. As a result of the AIDS epidemic PCP has become an increasing cause of community-acquired pneumonia. While the mode of transmission is unclear, infections with PCP probably represent reactivation of latent infection or failure of host defense mechanisms to combat a ubiquitous inhabitant of the environment. Nonetheless, in the hospital environment person-to-person spread of infection has been suggested anecdotally and it is prudent not to place a patient at risk for PCP (for example an HIV-infected patient with less than 200 CD4+ T cells per microliter) in the same room with someone suffering from an acute episode of PCP. The risk of infection with *Pneumocystis carinii* increases as the CD4+ T cell count declines. In this regard, in the patient with HIV infection, PCP is most commonly seen in patients who have experienced a previous bout of PCP and in patients who have under 200 CD4+ T cells per microliter. In the absence of PCP prophylaxis, following a primary bout of PCP, 31 percent will experience a second bout within 6 months, 66 percent within 12 months. For patients with over 200 CD4+ T cells per microliter, the attack rate for PCP is approximately 0.5 percent over a 6-month period. In contrast, for patients with under 200 CD4+ T cells per microliter the attack rate is 8 percent over 6 months and 18 percent over 12 months. For this reason, it is recommended that all patients with HIV infection who have either experienced a previous bout of PCP or who have a CD4+ T cell count under 200 per microliter (or CD4 percent under 15), receive some form of PCP prophylaxis (discussed below).

As suggested by its name, the most common manifestation of infection with *Pneumocystis carinii* is pneumonia. Patients generally present with fever and a cough that is usually nonproductive or productive of only scant amounts of white sputum. They may complain of a characteristic retrosternal chest pain that is usually worse on inspiration and described as either sharp or burning. In more severe cases, patients usually note dyspnea on exertion, fatigue, and weight loss. In stark contrast to PCP in the non-HIV setting, which is often a fulminant disease with patients usually presenting within 5 days of the onset of symptoms, HIV-associated PCP may have an indolent course characterized by weeks of vague symptoms prior to presentation or diagnosis. PCP should be included in the differential diagnosis of fever, pulmonary symptoms, or unexplained weight loss in any patient with HIV infection and less than 200 CD4+ T cells per microliter. Findings on physical examination are minimal. The usual findings for pneumonia are not present. Breath sounds are usually clear; however, they may be slightly diminished. While occasional rhonchi or wheezes may be heard, especially in patients with some other underlying pulmonary disease, findings of consolidation are usually absent. Chest x-ray may reveal a variety of patterns; however the most common finding is either a normal film, if the disease is suspected early, or a faint bilateral interstitial infiltrate. The classic finding of a dense, perihilar infiltrate described in patients with non-HIV–associated PCP is rarely seen in patients with AIDS. In patients with PCP who have been receiving aerosolized pentamidine for prophylaxis one may see a chest x-ray pattern with upper lobe cavitary disease, reminiscent of tuberculosis. Other less common findings on chest film include lobar infiltrates and pleural effusions.

PCP is complicated by pneumothorax in approximately 2 percent of cases. Pneumothorax is more common in patients with prior episodes of PCP and in patients who have received aerosolized pentamidine for prophylaxis, presumably due to the increased propensity for these patients to have apical cavitary disease. The mortality for patients with PCP-associated pneumothorax is approximately 10 percent and aggressive medical (sclerotherapy) and/or surgical intervention may be required.

The laboratory evaluation is usually of little help in the differential diagnosis of PCP. A mild leukocytosis is common; however, given the fact that HIV-infected patients generally have leukopenia with baseline WBC values in the range of 1500 to 3000 cells per microliter, a WBC on the order of 4000 to 6000 per microliter may represent an elevation. The serum LDH is often elevated, and arterial blood gases may indicate hypoxemia with a decline in Pa_{O_2} and an increase in the arterial-alveolar (a–A) gradient. Indeed, arterial blood gases not only aid in making the diagnosis of PCP but also provide important information for staging the severity of the disease and directing treatment (see below and Chap. 178).

A definitive diagnosis of PCP requires demonstration of the trophozoite or cyst forms of the organisms in samples obtained from induced sputum, bronchoalveolar lavage, transbronchial biopsy, or open lung biopsy (see Chap. 178). The diagnosis may be somewhat more difficult in patients who have been receiving aerosolized pentamidine for PCP prophylaxis insofar as the burden of organisms may be reduced. In this setting, the diagnostic yield from induced sputum decreases from 92 percent to 64 percent while the yield from bronchoalveolar lavage drops from 95 percent to 80 percent. More recently, PCR has been used in an attempt to identify specific DNA sequences for *Pneumocystis carinii* in clinical specimens. This technique may provide somewhat better sensitivity that that obtained through histologic staining. The differential diagnosis of PCP in patients with HIV infection includes CMV pneumonia, fungal pneumonia, nonspecific interstitial pneumonitis, tuberculosis and Kaposi's sarcoma (see below).

In addition to pneumonia, a number of other clinical problems have been reported in the HIV-infected patient as a result of infection with *Pneumocystis carinii*. Most of these reports, with the exception of otic disease, involve patients receiving aerosolized pentamidine as prophylaxis for PCP. This form of prophylaxis, while quite effective in preventing PCP, is ineffective in preventing disease outside the lung. *Pneumocystis carinii* appears capable of hematogenous spread and of seeding a variety of organ systems as well as causing a

primary infection of the ear (Table 279-18). These "extrapulmonary" manifestations of *Pneumocystis carinii* occur in approximately 2.5 to 5.0 percent of patients with HIV infection.

Otic involvement with *Pneumocystis carinii* is most commonly seen as a primary infection, i.e., in patients with no evidence of pulmonary disease. It usually presents as a unilateral polypoid mass that involves the external auditory canal. It may also involve the middle ear and may extend to the mastoid, resulting in radiographic abnormalities on plain films of the skull. Patients often complain of ear pain and decreased hearing. Perforation of the tympanic membrane has been reported in over half of the cases. In contrast, most of the other extrapulmonary forms of pneumocystis are seen in patients with a history of PCP. Most common in this group are ophthalmic lesions of the choroid that are usually noted on routine examination or in the context of evaluation for CMV retinitis. Multiple, bilateral lesions 0.5 to 2 disc diameters in size that appear as slightly elevated yellow-white plaques are generally seen. They are usually asymptomatic and are often confused with the cotton wool spots of the retina that are associated with HIV infection. *Pneumocystis carinii* has been reported to cause a necrotizing vasculitis that resembles Buerger's disease, bone marrow hypoplasia, and intestinal obstruction. Among the other organ systems involved have been the lymph nodes, spleen, liver, kidney, pancreas, pericardium, heart and adrenals. Of note has been the presentation of disease in either liver, kidney, or spleen which is generally asymptomatic; however, it can be associated with cystic lesions that appear calcified on CT or ultrasound.

A variety of therapeutic options are available for the patient with PCP or disseminated pneumocystis (Table 279-19) (see Chap. 178). The gold standard for therapy at present is trimethoprim/sulfamethoxazole which is effective in approximately 90 percent of patients. Trimethoprim/sulfamethoxazole is available in both intravenous and oral forms. The major disadvantage to this therapy is the relatively high incidence of side effects. In contrast to the non-HIV population where a 10 percent incidence of side effects is seen, there is a 50 to 65 percent incidence of side effects in the HIV-infected population. These include rash, fever, leukopenia, thrombocytopenia, and hepatitis, and although therapy need not be stopped when these occur, it is important to remain vigilant for more serious hypersensitivity reactions such as Stevens-Johnson syndrome. In addition, it is may be advisable to withhold other myelotoxic drugs such as zidovudine and ganciclovir during therapy with trimethoprim/sulfamethoxazole. In patients with mild disease, side effects may be minimized by slightly reducing dosage. Ideally, treatment with trimethoprim/sulfamethoxazole or the other agents mentioned below should be continued for 21 days. It should be noted that in contrast to many other infections in which one expects a stabilization, if not improvement, in clinical course wiithin 24 to 48 hours of initiation of appropriate antimicrobial therapy, patients with PCP often do not begin to improve until the end of the first week. In fact, during the first 5 days of treatment, particularly in moderate to severe cases, there is often a worsening of the patient's condition, presumably secondary to the inflammatory response resulting from the death of large numbers of organisms in the lung. This inflammatory response and its adverse clinical consequences can be markedly reduced by the adjunct use of

---

TABLE 279-18 Extrapulmonary manifestations of *Pneumocystis carinii* infection in patients with HIV infection

Acute otitis
Retinitis
Visceral cystic calcifications
Necrotizing vasculitis
Intestinal obstruction
Lymphadenopathy
Bone marrow involvement
Ascites
Thyroiditis

TABLE 279-19 Manifestations and treatment of secondary infections in patients with HIV disease

Infecting Agent	Manifestations	Treatment	Prophylaxis	Drug Toxicities	Comment
Pneumocystis carinii			TMP/SMX 1 DS daily Aerosolized pentamidine 300 mg/month	Rash, fever, neutropenia Bronchospasm	Begin once CD4+ T cell count <200/μL or CD4% <15
	Mild to moderate pneumonia [Pa$_{O_2}$≥70 mm Hg and (A-a)dO$_2$≤35] mmHg	TMP/SMX 15–20 mg/kg/d PO		Rash, fever, neutropenia	Treat for 21 d if possible, no less than 14 d
		TMP 20 mg/kg/d PO + dapsone 100 mg PO qd		Methemoglobinemia	Contraindicated in patients with G6PD deficiency
		Clindamycin 600 mg PO q6h + primaquine 15 mg PO qd		*C. difficile* colitis Rash, neutropenia	Contraindicated in patients with G6PD deficiency
		Intravenous pentamidine 3–4 mg/kg/d		Nephritis, pancreatitis, hypoglycemia, diabetes	
		Aerosolized pentamidine 300 mg/d		Bronchospasm	Provides no systemic effects. Not recommended but an option for multidrug allergic pt with mild pneumonia
	Severe pneumonia [Pa$_{O_2}$≤70mmHg or (A-a)dO$_2$≤35mmHg]	TMP/SMX 15–20 mg/kg/d IV initially (total course 14–21 d)		Rash, fever, leukopenia, thrombocytopenia, hepatitis	Prednisone, 40 mg bid for 2 d, then 40 mg/d for 5 d, then 20 mg/d to the end of therapy (21 d total) added to specific antimicrobial ASAP and no later than 36 h after diagnosis
		Pentamidine 3–4 mg/kg/d IV for 14–21 d		Nephritis, pancreatitis, hypoglycemia, diabetes	
		Clindamycin 900 mg IV q8h then 450 mg PO q6h + primaquine 30 mg PO qd for total of 14–21 d		*C. difficile* colitis Rash, neutropenia	Contraindicated in patients with G6PD deficiency
		Atovoquone 250 mg PO q6h for 14–21 d		Skin rash, neutropenia	For patients intolerant of other regimes. Less effective than standard therapy.
		Trimetrexate (dose from manufacturer)		Skin rash, neutropenia	Available only through treatment IND: call 1-800-TRIALSA. Bone marrow suppressive effects blunted by use of leucovorin
		Eflornithine (DFMO) 100 mg/kg IV q6h for 14 d followed by 75 mg/kg PO q6h for 4–6 weeks		Thrombocytopenia	1-800-TRIALSA for information
	Disseminated disease	Any of the systemic therapies outlined above			
Toxoplasma gondii			TMP/SMX 1 DS qd	Rash, fever neutropenia	More specific regimens under study
	Encephalitis, brain abscess, chorioretinitis, myocarditis	Sulfadiazine 1–2 g PO qid + pyrimethamine 25–100 mg qd		Crystalluria, rash Rash, fever, neutropenia	Treatment is generally for life. Leucovorin to minimize bone marrow suppression
		Clindamycin initially 200–400 mg IV q6h + pyrimethamine 25–100 mg qd followed by clindamycin 300–900 mg PO q8h + pyrimethamine 25–100 mg qd		*C. difficile* colitis Rash, fever, neutropenia	Leucovorin to minimize bone marrow suppression
		Atovoquone 250 mg PO q6h + pyrimethamine 25–100 mg qd		Rash, fever, neutropenia	Leucovorin to minimize bone marrow suppression
		Macrolides (clarithromycin or azithromycin)			Early results disappointing
Isospora belli	Diarrhea	TMP/SMX 10 mg/kg/d PO for 10 d then 1/2 dose for 3 months		Rash, fever, neutropenia	
Cryptosporidia/ Microsporidia	Diarrhea	No known specific therapy, supportive measures include somatostatin, parenteral nutrition			

TABLE 279-19   Manifestations and treatment of secondary infections in patients with HIV disease (Continued)

Infecting Agent	Manifestations	Treatment	Prophylaxis	Drug Toxicities	Comment
M. avium intracellulare			Rifabutin 300 mg PO qd		Begin prophylaxis once CD4+ T cell count <100/μL Treatment is generally for life
	Disseminated disease that may involve lung, bone marrow, liver	Ethambutol 15 mg/kg qd + clofazimine 100 mg PO qd + ciprofloxicin 750 mg PO qd + macrolide (azithromycin or clarithromycin)		Hepatitis, neuropathy (peripheral/optic) Darkening of skin, hepatitis	
Mycobacterium tuberculosis	Asymptomatic, PPD+	Isoniazid, 15 mg/kg up to 900 mg PO twice a week or 300 mg, PO daily for 1 y		Hepatitis	
	Active disease	Isoniazid, 300 mg PO × 1 y + rifampin 600 mg PO qd × 1 y + pyrazinamide 30 mg/kg/d in 2 doses		Hepatitis Hepatitis Hepatitis	Treat with 3 drugs for 2 months. If isolate is sensitive to isoniazid and rifampin then switch to those 2 drugs. Treat 9 months and at least 6 months after third negative culture.
	Active disease in a setting when there is a possibility of multidrug resistance	Add ethambutol 15–25 mg/kg/d and streptomycin or amikacin for active disease		Neuropathy (peripheral/optic) Nephrotoxicity, hearing loss	Quinolones may also be considered as a fifth drug
Candida albicans			Fluconazole 200 mg PO qd	Hepatotoxicity	Begin once CD4+ cell count <100/μL Treatment is generally prn (as needed)
	Thrush, vaginitis	Clotrimiazole troches, nystatin Fluconazole 200 mg PO qd		Hepatotoxicity	
	Esophagitis	Fluconazole 200 mg PO qd for 7–14 days Amphotericin B 0.25 mg/kg/d IV for 7–10 days		Hepatotoxicity Nephrotoxicity, fever/chills	
Crytoptococcus neoformans			Fluconazole 100–200 mg PO qd	Hepatotoxicity	Begin prophylaxis if CD4+ T cell count < 100/μL
	Meningitis, brain abscess, penumonia, disseminated disease	Amphotericin B 0.3 mg/kg/d IV + flucytosine 150 mg/kg/d PO for 6 weeks followed by fluconazole 100–200 mg PO qd indefinitely		Nephrotoxicity, fever/chills Bone marrow suppression Hepatotoxicity	Approximately 50% will need to have flucytosine held during therapy due to neutropenia. An alternative is amphotericin B alone at a dose of 0.8 mg/kg/d.
Histoplasma encapsulatum	Disseminated disease, pneumonia	Amphotericin B 0.6–1 mg/kg/d to a total 1 g then itraconazole 200 mg qd indefinitely		Nephrotoxicity, fever/chills Hepatitis	
Cytomegalovirus	Retinitis, esophagitis, colitis and pneumonia	Ganciclovir 5 mg/kg q12h for 14 d followed by 5 mg/kg qd IV indefinitely		Neutropenia	Neutropenia may be ameliorated by colony stimulating factors
		Foscarnet 60 mg/kg q8h for 14 d followed by 90–120 mg/kg qd IV indefinitely		Interstitial nephritis, seizure, hypocalcemia	Should be preceded by saline infusion
Herpes simplex	Recurrent perioral, perirectal, or genital ulcers	Acyclovir 200–400 mg PO 5id as needed			Foscarnet 60 mg/kg q8h × 14 d for patients with acyclovir-resistant herpes simplex or zoster
	Esophagitis; acute retinal necrosis	Acyclovir 5 mg/kg IV q8h for 10–14 days			
Herpes zoster	Cutaneous (local or disseminated); retinal necrosis	Acyclovir 800 mg PO 5id or 10 mg/kg IV q8h for 10–14 days or longer			
Treponema pallidum	Early syphilis	Benzathine penicillin G 2.4 million units IM weekly for 3 weeks			Approx 20% relapse, need retreatment. Immunologic abnormalities may cause inaccurate serology.
	Late or neurosyphilis	Aqueous penicillin G 2.4 million units IV daily for 10–14 d Procaine penicillin G, 1.2 million units IM daily for 10–14 d Ceftriaxone 1–2 g IM or IV qd 10–14 d			May be given with probnecid 500 mg PO qid

ficient individuals. Patients generally give a history of several months of intermittent diarrhea evolving to a several-month history of persistent diarrhea with copious watery stools, often up to several liters per day. In 75 percent of cases this is accompanied by crampy abdominal pain with approximately 25 percent of patients noting nausea and/or vomiting. This intestinal infection may be complicated by lactose intolerance and malabsorption. In addition to involving the intestinal tract, cryptosporidia may cause biliary tract disease in the HIV-infected population. Biliary disease may present as cholecystitis with or without accompanying cholangitis. Radiographic studies of the biliary tree reveal thickening of the gall bladder wall with luminal abnormalities accompanying bile duct dilatation and stricture. Cryptosporidia have also been noted in pulmonary specimens; however, the clinical significance in this setting is unclear. The diagnosis of cryptosporidial diarrhea is made by stool examination. The diarrhea is non-inflammatory and the characteristic finding is the presence of oocysts that stain with acid-fast dyes. Use of a sucrose flotation technique followed by concentration procedures to enrich for the cysts and to separate the cysts from other particles in the specimen may enhance detection. On electron microscopy of small bowel biopsy specimens, organisms may be seen adhering to the brush border of intestinal epithelial. Therapy is purely symptomatic at present.

Microsporidia are small unicellular organisms, obligate intracellular parasites that reside within the cytoplasm of enteric cells. The main species causing disease in man is *Enterocytozoon bieneusi*. The clinical manifestations are similar to those described for *Cryptosporidium* and include abdominal pain and diarrhea. The small size of the organism may make it difficult to detect; however, with the use of new chromotrope-based stains, organisms can be identified in stool samples by light microscopy. Definitive diagnosis generally depends upon electron microscopic examination of stool specimen, intestinal aspirate, or intestinal biopsy. In contrast to cryptosporidia, Microsporidia have been noted in a variety of extraintestinal locations, including the eye, muscle, and liver and have been associated with conjunctivitis and hepatitis. As in the case of *Cryptosporidium*, no effective therapies have been identified and treatment is purely symptomatic.

Isospora belli is a coccidian parasite, most commonly found as a cause of diarrhea in patients from the Caribbean and Africa. Its cysts appear in the stool as large acid-fast structures that can be differentiated from cryptosporidia by virtue of differences in size, shape, and number of sporocysts. Clinical syndromes caused by this organism appear identical to those caused by cryptosporidia; however, one important difference is that this infection can be treated with trimethoprim/sulfamethoxazole. While relapses are common, a three-times-a-week regimen, similar to that used to provide prophylaxis against PCP, appears adequate to prevent recurrence.

Entamoeba histolytica (see Chap. 173) and *Giardia lamblia* (see Chap. 179), although not opportunistic pathogens in that they can also cause disease in immunocompetent individuals, are seen with an increased frequency in patients with HIV infection. These treatable protozoa should be carefully looked for in any patient with HIV infection and persistent diarrhea. Other strains of *Entamoeba* and *Blastocystis hominis* are also seen with an increased frequency in homosexual men with HIV infection; however, these organisms are felt to be of little if any clinical significance.

Miscellaneous protozoal infections are being reported with increased frequency as the AIDS epidemic spreads in other regions of the world. In this regard visceral leishmaniasis (Chap. 175) is recognized with increasing frequency in patients who live in or travel to endemic areas. The clinical presentation is one of hepatosplenomegaly, fever, and hematologic abnormalities. Lymphadenopathy and other constitutional symptoms may be present. Organisms can be isolated from cultures of bone marrow aspirates, while histologic stains are often negative and antibody titers are of little help in diagnosis. Patients usually respond well initially to standard therapy although, as with most infections in HIV-infected individuals, eradication of the organisms is difficult and relapses are common. Among other protozoal infections that have been reported are severe and

recurrent babesiosis (Chap. 179), Chagas disease (Chap. 176) presenting as a CNS mass lesion, and meningoencephalitis due to *Acanthamoeba* or *Naegleria* (Chap. 173). No significant changes have been noted in the clinical manifestations of malaria in patients with HIV infection.

Bacterial infections   Atypical mycobacteria (see Chap. 132) account for a large number of opportunistic infections in patients with HIV infection although their overall contribution to mortality remains small. In the United States, disseminated infection with atypical mycobacteria, particularly *Mycobacterium avium* complex (MAC) is diagnosed in approximately 40 percent of HIV-infected patients antemortum and is seen in 80 percent of patients at autopsy. MAC accounts for 95 percent of the atypical mycobacterial infections seen in patients with AIDS in the United States; however, infections with at least 12 different mycobacteria, including *M. bovis* and representatives of all four Runyon groups, have been reported. Infections with MAC, which consists of *M. avium* and *M. intracellulare*, are predominantly seen in U.S. patients and are rare in Africa.

MAC infection probably represents an acute infection with organisms that are ubiquitous in the environment in both soil and water. The presumed portals of entry are the gastrointestinal and respiratory tract. MAC infection is a late complication of HIV infection, occurring in patients with CD4+ T cell counts under 100 cells per microliter. In one study the median CD4+ T cell count for patients with MAC was 60 cells per microliter. HIV-infected patients presenting with MAC infection have been reported to have a median survival of approximately 6 to 10 months, which likely reflects the late stage of HIV infection. While a variety of clinical syndromes have been attributed to MAC infections, the most common presentation is fever, weight loss, and night sweats, presumably due to disseminated disease. At least 85 percent of HIV-infected patients with MAC infection are mycobacteremic, and enormous numbers of organisms can often be demonstrated on bone marrow biopsy. Liver involvement is common and MAC infection should be suspected in any HIV-infected individual with a low CD4+ T cell count, unexplained fever, and an elevated alkaline phosphatase. The chest x-ray is abnormal in approximately 25 percent of patients. The most common radiographic pattern is a bilateral lower lobe interstitial infiltrate, suggestive of miliary spread. In addition, alveolar or nodular infiltrates and hilar and/or mediastinal adenopathy occur. Endobronchial lesions have also been reported. Other clinical findings include lymphadenopathy, abdominal pain, and diarrhea. Diagnosis is suspected by demonstration of long, slender acid-fast bacilli on bone marrow, lymph node, or liver biopsy or upon examination of stool specimens and confirmed by culture of blood or involved tissue. The finding of two consecutive sputum samples positive for MAC is highly suggestive of pulmonary infection. Cultures generally turn positive within 2 weeks. In earlier studies, treatment with various combination regimens that usually included ethambutol, clofazamine, and rifabutin, with or without an aminoglycoside, where shown to have little effect on mycobacteremia and to increase only marginally the median survival of patients with MAC infection from 6 months to 8 months. Given these data and the considerable toxicity encountered with these treatment regimens many clinicians chose not to treat MAC infection unless there was clear evidence of disease. However, both the macrolide and the fluoroquinolone classes of antibiotics now show considerable promise. Clarithromycin and azithromycin are two macrolide antibiotics that are licensed for the treatment of common respiratory tract infections. They are both characterized by broad spectrum antimicrobial activity, good tissue penetration, and good activity in vitro against MAC. Clarithromycin has been shown in a controlled trial to cause significant decreases in the titer of MAC organisms in the blood and to improve the patients' sense of well being. Similar encouraging data have been generated for azithromycin in open trials. Ciprofloxacin, ofloxacin, and sparfloxacin are fluorinated members of the quinoline family. While ciprofloxacin is the only one currently licensed, all three have shown activity against MAC in vitro, and clinical trials are currently underway to assess their efficacy in vivo. Given these data many physicians now choose to treat patients with MAC infection with a combination regimen consisting of ethambutol, clofazamine, ciprofloxacin, and a macrolide. As with all of the potentially life-threatening infections seen in patients with AIDS, prophylactic regimens when available should be employed. In this regard, the use of rifabutin in patients with advanced HIV infection has been shown to delay the onset of bacteremia and is now a recommend prophylaxis regimen for patients with under 100 CD4+ T cells per microliter.

A number of other atypical mycobacteria have been reported to cause infections in patients with HIV infection. Infection with *M. kansasii* generally presents as a pulmonary infection with 20 to 30 percent of patients showing evidence of disseminated disease. Patients usually present with fever, cough, and night sweats. Chest x-ray reveals upper lobe cavitation in approximately half of the patients, while a lower lobe interstitial pattern consistent with hematogenous spread may be seen in other patients. Organisms are usually identified easily in pulmonary secretions; evidence of disease is found in over 75 percent of the patients with a positive culture. *M. kansasii* infection is a particularly important diagnosis to make since it is relatively easy to treat with a combination regimen of isoniazid, rifampin, and ethambutol. *M. fortuitus, M. chelonia, M. marinum,* and *M. hemophilum* have all been reported to cause cutaneous lesions in patients with HIV infection; *M. hemophilum* is also reported to cause disseminated disease and septic arthritis. *M. gordonae,* generally a nonpathogen in humans, and *M. xenopi,* a colonizer of water storage tanks, have both been reported to cause disseminated disease. Therapy of these latter organisms is extremely difficult.

M. tuberculosis, while once thought to be on its way to extinction in the United States, has experienced a major resurgence in the context of the HIV epidemic (see Chap. 130). A 20-year decline in the number of new cases in the United States ended in 1986, and the number of new cases per year has since been on a steady increase. Approximately 5 percent of the patients with AIDS are reported to have active tuberculosis. While the prevalence and incidence of infection with *M. tuberculosis* as determined by Purified Protein Derivative (PPD) skin testing appears quite comparable among members of the same risk group regardless of HIV status, HIV infection increases the risk of developing active tuberculosis by a factor of 15 to 30. For the patient with HIV infection and a positive PPD skin test, the rate of reactivation is approximately 8 percent per year. Although the majority of tuberculosis cases in the HIV-infected population are felt to represent reactivation, acute infection and reinfection are being seen with an alarming frequency, especially in the context of the new outbreaks of multidrug resistant (MDR) tuberculosis. Active tuberculosis appears to be most common in patients of ages 25 to 44, in African-Americans and Hispanics, in patients in New York City and Miami, and in patients in developing countries. In these areas, 20 to 70 percent of the new cases of active tuberculosis are in patients with HIV infection. Given the fact that, in contrast to HIV infection, infection with *M. tuberculosis* can be spread through casual contact and respiratory droplets, this emerging second epidemic probably represents the greatest health risk to the general public and the health care profession to emerge from the HIV crisis. In contrast to infection with MAC, active tuberculosis often develops relatively early in the course of HIV infection and may be among the earliest clinical signs of HIV infection. In one study, the median CD4+ T cell count at presentation was 326 cells per microliter. The clinical manifestations of tuberculosis in the HIV-infected patients are quite varied and generally show different patterns as a function of the patient's CD4+ T cell count. In patients with relatively high CD4+ T cell counts, a typical pattern of pulmonary reactivation occurs in which patients present with fever, cough, dyspnea on exertion, weight loss, night sweats, and a chest x-ray revealing cavitary apical disease of the upper lobes. Disseminated disease is more common in patients with low CD4 counts. The chest x-ray in patients with disseminated disease may also reveal diffuse or lower lobe bilateral reticulonodular infiltrates consistent with miliary spread, pleural effusions, and hilar and/or mediastinal adenop-

athy. Infection may be present in bone, brain, meninges, gastrointestinal tract, lymph node (particularly cervical nodes), and viscera. Cases of visceral abscesses of the liver and prostate have been reported. Approximately 60 to 80 percent of patients will have pulmonary disease and 30 to 40 percent will have extrapulmonary disease.

Respiratory isolation and a negative-pressure room should be employed with patients in whom a diagnosis of pulmonary tuberculosis is being considered. This approach is critical in order to limit nosocomial and community spread of infection. A definitive diagnosis is made by culture of the organism from an involved site. Blood cultures are positive in 15 percent of cases. However, given the importance of making an early diagnosis and initiating treatment, especially given the emergence of MDR tuberculosis (see below), a presumptive diagnosis should be made based upon a positive acid fast stain and consistent clinical presentation while awaiting culture results. A positive PPD in a HIV-infected person is defined as any area of induration $\geq$ 5 mm. While this can be used to support the diagnosis and identify candidates for isoniazid prophylaxis, up to 50 percent of patients with HIV infection and active tuberculosis may be anergic, and thus a negative skin test does not rule out a diagnosis.

Standard therapy for tuberculosis is generally as successful in the HIV-infected patient as it is in the HIV-negative patient. In most cases, one initiates therapy with three drugs for a total course of at least 9 months and no less than 6 months beyond a third negative culture. Patients with HIV infection have a slightly higher incidence of adverse drug reactions. In one series, 18 percent of patients experienced a drug reaction, predominantly rash and hepatitis related to rifampin.

A major, emerging problem has been the increasing identification of strains of *M. tuberculosis* resistant to two or more first-line drugs, usually isoniazid and rifampin, so-called MDR tuberculosis (see Chap. 130). Outbreaks of MDR-tuberculosis have been reported from New York, Florida, Michigan, and Missouri. Of the initial 87 cases reported, 83 occurred in patients with HIV infection. Due to delays in obtaining antimicrobial sensitivities patients often received inadequate treatment regimens, and the initial mortality from MDR-tuberculosis has been as high as 72 to 89 percent. Thus therapy should be initiated with a five-drug regimen while awaiting formal sensitivity results for anyone contracting tuberculosis in an area where MDR-tuberculosis has become a problem.

Prevention of active tuberculosis can be a reality if the health care profession is aggressive in looking for evidence of latent tuberculosis by making sure that all patients at risk for tuberculosis and all patients with HIV infection receive a PPD skin test. As mentioned above, in the setting of HIV infection, an induration of $\geq$ 5 mm should be considered positive, and such patients should be treated for 1 year with isoniazid. Given the fact that 50 percent of patients will be anergic, some experts also recommend that any patient with HIV infection who is anergic and at high risk for TB be given a 1-year course of isoniazid.

Nonmycobacterial bacteria account for a high number of infections in patients with AIDS and are the second leading cause of death following opportunistic infections. Bacterial infections most frequently present clinically as respiratory tract infections, sepsis, and/or gastroenteritis. In addition, syphilis and bacillary angiomatosis may present with atypical features. Patients with HIV infection appear to be particularly prone to infections with encapsulated organisms, perhaps as a consequence of altered B cell activation and/or defects in neutrophil function that may be secondary to disease or drugs. *Streptococcus pneumonia* (see Chap. 101) and *Haemophilus influenzae* (see Chap. 112) are among the two most common bacterial infections seen in patients with HIV infection. These two organisms are responsible for the majority of cases of bacterial pneumonia in patients with AIDS and also contribute to the increased incidence of sinusitis that has been reported in this patient population. Patients with HIV infection have a 6-fold increase in the incidence of pneumoccal pneumonia and a 100-fold increase in the incidence of pneumococcal bacteremia. For these reasons, all patients with HIV infections should be receive immunization with pneumococcal polysaccharide. *Staphylococcus aureus* infections (see Chap. 102) are also seen with increased frequency in the setting of HIV infection. Carriage of staphylococcal organisms in HIV infected patients is approximately twice that seen in the general population. Staphylococcal infections are usually responsible for catheter-related sepsis with the risk increasing as the CD4+ T cell count declines. Pyomyositis is another complication of staphylococcal infection and is seen with increased frequency in the HIV-infected patient group. This disease, which was formerly rare in the United States, is generally seen in association with muscle injury; it has been postulated that the myopathy of HIV infection may be a predisposing factor.

Infections with enteric pathogens such as salmonella, shigella, and campylobacter are more common in homosexual men and are often more severe and more prone to relapse in patients with HIV infection. The latter patients have approximately a 20-fold increased risk of infection with *Salmonella typhimurium* (see Chap. 117). They may present with a variety of nonspecific symptoms, including fever, anorexia, fatigue, and malaise of several weeks' duration. Diarrhea, although common, may be absent. Diagnosis is made by culture of blood and stool. Although treatment is generally not indicated for salmonella gastroenteritis, because of the protracted course and high rate of recurrence in the HIV-infected population, long-term therapy is usually prescribed for them; the greatest degree of success has been reported with oral ciprofloxacin. Patients with HIV infection have an increased incidence of infection with *Salmonella typhi* in areas of the world where typhoid is a problem (see Chap. 117).

Shigella infections (see Chap. 118) cause particularly severe gastrointestinal disease in HIV-infected individuals, characterized by diarrhea and fever. *Shigella flexneri* is the most common species isolated, and up to 50 percent of patients with HIV infection and shigellosis are bacteremic in contrast to otherwise healthy hosts, where bacteremia is rare.

Campylobacter infections (see Chap. 119) occur with an increased frequency in HIV-infected patients. While *C. fetus* and *jejuni* are the strains most frequently isolated, infections with many other strains have been reported. Patients usually present with crampy abdominal pain, fever, and bloody diarrhea; infection may also present as proctitis. Stool examination reveals the presence of fecal leukocytes. Systemic infection may be seen with up to 10 percent of infected patients exhibiting bateremias. As in the case of the other enteric pathogens, infections with *Campylobacter* species are often persistent or recurrent, and prolonged therapy is usually needed. Most strains are sensitive to erythromycin; however, resistant strains have been reported.

Infections with *Treponema pallidum*, the etiologic agent of syphilis, play an important role in the HIV epidemic (see Chap. 133). In the HIV-negative individual, genital syphilitic ulcers rank with the ulcers of chancroid as major predisposing factors for heterosexual transmission of HIV (see above). While most HIV-infected individuals with syphilis will have a typical presentation, a variety of formerly rare clinical problems may be encountered. Among them are lues maligna, an ulcerating lesion of the skin due to a necrotizing vasculitis; unexplained fever; nephrotic syndrome; and neurosyphilis. Neurosyphilis may be asymptomatic or may present as acute meningitis, neuroretinitis, deafness, or stroke. In one series, 44 percent of all cases of neurosyphilis were found to occur in patients with HIV infection; the rate of neurosyphilis in this population may be as high as 1.5 percent. Given the immunologic abnormalities seen in patients with HIV infection, diagnosis through standard serologic testing may be challenging. On the one hand, a significant number of patients may have a false positive VDRL due to a polyclonal B cell activation. On the other hand, the development of a positive VDRL may be delayed in the patient with new infection and the anti-FTA antibody test may be negative due to immunodeficiency. Darkfield examination of appropriate specimens should be performed in any patient in whom a diagnosis of syphilis is suspected, even if the patient has a negative VDRL. Similarly, given the spinal fluid abnormalities seen with HIV infection alone, a diagnosis of neurosyphilis may be difficult to make. Any patient with a positive serum VDRL with neurologic findings who has an abnormal spinal fluid examination, with or without a positive CSF VDRL, should be considered a possible case of neurosyphilis. In the HIV infected patient with syphilis, treatment should follow standard guidelines. However, standard treatment may be inadequate and may need to be repeated in patients who fail to respond or who show evidene of relapse. In these patients, one also needs to have a high index of suspicion for neurosyphilis and treat accordingly with high-dose IV penicillin if this diagnosis is suspected.

Bacillary angiomatosis, a vascular proliferative disease felt to be due to the rickettsia-like organism *Rochalimaea henselae*, is seen with an increased frequency in patients with HIV infection (see Chap. 124). This disease usually presents with cutaneous erythematous papules that may appear similar to Kaposi's sarcoma. While 93 percent of patients have cutaneous manifestations, the disease may also involve lymph node, bone, and viscera. Fever, weight loss, and malaise are seen in the majority of patients. Mass lesions with abscess-like characteristics in spleen, liver, and CNS have been described. The disease may be associated with peliosis hepatica, a condition in which the liver contains multiple, cystic, blood-filled spaces resulting in hepatomegaly and abdominal pain. The diagnosis is made by demonstration of bacillary organisms on Warthin-Starry stain of appropriate clinical specimens. Patients usually respond well to treatment with erythromycin or tetracycline, although relapses occur in approximately 15 percent of cases.

Fungal infections *Candida* infections are the most common fungal infections occurring in patients with HIV infection; virtually all patients experience some candida infection over the course of their illness (see Chap. 166). Infections are often seen early in the course of HIV infection, heralding the onset of clinically apparent immunodeficiency. Although they are a significant cause of morbidity, *Candida* infections are generally easy to control and usually involve only the mucosal surfaces. Invasive disease is extremely rare and occurs predominantly as a consequence of iatrogenic measures such as indwelling catheters, broad spectrum antibiotics, and/or drug induced neutropenia.

Superficial infection of the oral cavity with *Candida* (thrush) generally presents as a white, cheesy exudative on the posterior oropharynx (Fig A1-41). Early lesions also may be detected along the gingival-labial margins. The exudate is easy to scrape, and branching pseudohyphae are readily detectable on wet-mount KOH preparations. In women with HIV infection, vaginal yeast infections are seen as an early sign of immunodeficiency.

Later in the course of HIV infection, generally in association with CD4+ T cell counts under 100 cells per microliter, candida infections of the esophagus, trachea, bronchi, or lungs may occur. These infections are felt to be indicative of a serious defect in cell-mediated immunity and are among the AIDS-defining conditions (Table 279-1). Perhaps the most common of these is esophagitis. While generally a late manifestation of HIV infection, *Candida* esophagitis has also been reported during the acute HIV syndrome. Esophagitis generally presents as odynophagia and retrosternal pain or burning. Oral thrush is often present as well, although it may be absent in patients who have been receiving topical oral medications. A definitive diagnosis is made through upper endoscopy and observation of characteristic white plaques shown by wet mount to contain pseudohyphae. However, a high index of suspicion based upon history and/or a barium swallow demonstrating a grossly irregular mucosa (Fig. 279-19) is sufficient to justify an empiric trial of antifungal therapy. If improvement does not occur within 4 to 6 days of therapy, upper endoscopy is needed to eliminate the other possible causes of esophagitis, namely CMV, herpes simplex virus, Kaposi's sarcoma, and lymphoma.

Oral and vaginal *Candida* infections may be treated with topical nystatin or clotrimazole troches; the frequency of administration should match the severity of disease. Nonetheless, many find it more convenient to use systemic therapy with either ketoconazole or

FIGURE 279-19 Barium swallow of a patient with *Candida* esophagitis. The flow of barium along the mucosal surface is grossly irregular.

fluconazole, both of which are effective in the majority of cases. Although fluconazole is more expensive, somewhat better results have been achieved, which may, at least in part, reflect the poor absorption of ketoconazole in patients with high gastric pH. A short course of intravenous therapy with amphotericin B followed by oral therapy with fluconazole may be indicated in particularly severe cases of candida infection.

Cryptococcus neoformans is the leading cause of meningitis in patients with AIDS (see Chap. 165). This ubiquitous, yeast-like fungus with a polysaccharide capsule causes serious, life-threatening infection in 6 to 12 percent of patients with AIDS. It is the initial AIDS-defining condition in 1.5 percent of patients, generally occurring in fairly advanced patients as defined by a CD4 + T cell count under 100 cells per microliter. The median survival of a patient with HIV infection following a diagnosis of cryptococcal infection is 9 months. Cryptococcal meningitis is particularly common in patients with AIDS in Africa, occurring in approximately 20 percent of individuals; it was the initial illness suggesting that a new epidemic of immunodeficiency was occurring in Africa. Although initial exposure is felt to occur via the respiratory route, the most common site of infection is the brain and meninges. CNS infection is seen in 67 to 85 percent of AIDS patients with cryptococcal disease; the majority of patients present with a picture of subacute meningoencephalitis. In addition to meningitis, patients may develop cryptococcomas which appear on MRI as multiple ring-enhancing lesions. Patients with CNS cryptococcal disease often display symptoms for weeks to months prior to diagnosis and, as is the case with many AIDS-associated

opportunistic infections, a high index of suspicion is essential in order to make an early diagnosis. Among the symptoms commonly seen are fever in virtually 100 percent of patients, nausea and vomiting in 40 percent, and altered mental status, headache, and meningeal signs in 25 percent. The incidence of seizures and focal neurologic defects is low. Pulmonary disease is seen in 40 percent of patients, 90 percent of whom will also have CNS infection. Patients with pulmonary disease present with fever, cough, dyspnea and, in some cases, hemoptysis. A focal or diffuse interstitial infiltrate is seen on chest x-ray in over 90 percent of patients. Chest x-ray may also reveal lobar disease, cavitary disease, pleural effusions, and hilar or mediastinal adenopathy. Over half the patients will be fungemic. In patients with fungemia fever, malaise and fatigue are common. While the majority of patients with cryptococcal disease present with CNS infection, 4 to 10 percent may present with pulmonary disease in the absence of other manifestations and 4 to 8 percent may present with fungemia as the only manifestation of infection. Uncommon manifestations of cryptoccocal infection in patients with HIV infection include skin lesions resembling molluscum contagiosum, lymphadenopathy, palatal and glossal ulcers, arthritis, gastroenteritis, myocarditis, and prostatitis. In fact, the prostate gland may serve as a reservoir for smoldering infection.

A presumptive diagnosis of cryptococcal infection can be made upon identification of organisms in spinal fluid on India ink examination, by measuring the presence of cryptococcal antigen in blood or spinal fluid, or by histologic evidence of cryptococcal infection in a biopsy specimen. A definitive diagnosis is made by culturing the organism from spinal fluid, blood, bone marrow, sputum, or tissue. A positive culture for *Cryptococcus neoformans,* regardless of site, should be considered significant and an indication for treatment. Cryptococcal antigen is present in the CSF of virtually all cases of cryptococcal meningitis, although in 15 percent of cases all other findings may be normal. In cryptococcal meningitis, the CSF WBC is over 20 cells per microliter in less than 50 percent of patients, the protein is elevated in 35 to 70 percent, and the glucose is low in about 50 percent. In patients with CNS cryptococcomas, both CSF antigen and culture may be negative and biopsy may be required to make the diagnosis.

Therapy with amphotericin B should be started immediately in any patient with evidence of cryptococcal infection, either by antigen or culture. Standard therapy in the HIV-infected patient consists of 6 weeks of amphotericin B at a daily dose of 0.3 mg/kg in combination with 150 mg/kg of flucytosine. Approximately 50 percent of patients will require that the flucytosine be omitted for at least part of the course of therapy due to neutropenia. Given the fact that with this therapy alone over 50 percent of patients will relapse, it is recommended that at the termination of amphotericin therapy patients be placed on fluconazole, 100 to 200 mg daily, indefinitely. Many physicians choose to place all patients with HIV infection on fluconazole, 100 to 200 mg daily, once the CD4 + T cell count falls below 100 cells per microliter as prophylaxis against both candida and cryptococcal infections.

Histoplasmosis is an opportunistic infection that is seen most frequently in patients in the Mississippi and Ohio River valleys, Puerto Rico, Dominican Republic, and South America; all of these are areas in which infection with *Histoplasma encapsulatum* is endemic (see Chap. 162). Because of this limited geographic distribution, the percentage of AIDS cases in the United States with histoplasmosis is only approximately 0.5 percent. In endemic areas, however, the incidence is much higher. The organism exists in the mycelial phase in soil, and large numbers of organisms are found in soil that contains droppings from birds or bats. The organism exists in the yeast phase at body temperature. Histoplasmosis is generally a late manifestation of HIV infection; however, it may be the initial AIDS-defining condition. The median CD4 + T cell count for patients with histoplasmosis was 33 cells per microliter in one study. While disease due to *H. encapsulatum* may present as a primary infection of the lung, disseminated disease, presumably due to reactivation, is to JC virus, indicative of prior infection, less than 10 percent show any evidence of ongoing viral replications. In contrast, close to 33 percent of HIV-infected individuals have evidence of active replication of JC virus. PML, the only known clinicial manifestation of JC virus infection is seen in 4 percent of HIV-infected individuals and is a late manifestation of AIDS. PML is a demyelinating disease that begins as small foci in subcortical white matter that eventually coalesce. The cerebral hemispheres, cerebellum, and brainstem may all be involved. Histologically, swollen oligodendritic nuclei with inclusions due to the nucleocapsid proteins of JC are seen. Death of the oligodendrocyte leads to demyelination without inflammation. Patients have a protracted clinical course, often developing multiple focal deficits without changes in mental status. Patients with PML may exhibit ataxia, hemiparesis, visual field cuts, aphasia, and sensory defects. The diagnosis is usually made by MRI, which reveals multiple white matter lesions on T2-weighted images. The clinical picture is generally much more impressive than the findings on MRI. Death usually occurs within 3 to 6 months of the onset of symptoms. Intrathecal cytosine arabinoside leads to improvement in some cases; however, no consistently effective therapy is currently available.

Evidence of infection with *human papilloma virus* is approximately twice as common in HIV-infected individuals (81 percent of patients in one series) as in the general population. The association of this virus with epidermal dysplasia suggests that both anal and cervical carcinomas will be seen in the HIV-infected population with increased frequency as survival is prolonged through the use of better antiretroviral regimens (see below).

Over 95 percent of HIV-infected patients have evidence of infection with *hepatitis B*: coinfection with *hepatitis C* and *hepatitis D* is also quite common. HIV infection has several effects on hepatitis virus infection. It is associated with approximately a threefold increase in the development of persistent hepatitis B surface antigenemia. However, patients with hepatitis B infection in the presence of HIV infection have decreased evidence of inflammatory liver disease, presumably due to the effects of HIV on the immune system. Hepatitis D is a defective RNA virus that requires concomitant infection with hepatitis B in order to replicate, and thus infection is only seen together with hepatitis B infection. Hepatitis D infection is more common in patients with HIV infection, is associated with higher levels of hepatitis B virus replication, and seems to be associated with slightly worse hepatic disease as evidenced by slightly higher levels of hepatic transaminases.

NEOPLASTIC DISEASES A variety of neoplastic and premalignant diseases occur with increased frequency in HIV-infected individuals. Among them are Kaposi's sarcoma, lymphoma, and intraepithelial dysplasia of the cervix and anus. These diseases are significant contributors to the morbidity and mortality of patients with HIV infection. The clinical manifestations of these complications as well as their epidemiologic profiles have undergone considerable change as new approaches to treatment develop and as the epidemic involves different demographic groups.

Kaposi's sarcoma is a multicentric neoplasm consisting of multiple vascular nodules appearing in the skin, mucous membranes, and viscera. The course ranges from indolent, with only minor skin or lymph node involvement, to fulminant, with extensive cutaneous and visceral involvement. In the initial period of the AIDS epidemic Kaposi's sarcoma was a prominent clinical feature of the first cases of AIDS, occurring in 79 percent of the patients diagnosed in 1981. By 1989 it was seen in only 25 percent of cases and by 1992 this number had decreased to 9 percent. Part of this decrease is a reflection of the fact that AIDS-related Kaposi's sarcoma, in contrast to classical or endemic forms, is a disease that occurs predominantly in homosexual men, with 96 percent of all cases occurring in that risk group. As the percentage of AIDS cases in other risk groups increases, the percentage of cases complicated by Kaposi's sarcoma decreases. This, however, is only a partial explanation for the observed decreased incidence in Kaposi's sarcoma in patients with AIDS. A growing body of epidemiologic data points to the possibility that a sexually

transmitted cofactor may play a role in the development of Kaposi's sarcoma. In this regard, Kaposi's sarcoma is four times more common in women who have had sexual contact with bisexual men, Kaposi's sarcoma has been seen in homosexual men without evidence of HIV infection, and homosexual men in New York and Los Angeles are more likely than homosexual men in the central states to have Kaposi's sarcoma. As safer sex practices are employed, especially in the homosexual community, the risk of transmission of this unknown cofactor and thus the risk of Kaposi's sarcoma decreases. Kaposi's sarcoma has been an early manifestation of HIV infection, at times occurring in patients with normal CD4 + T cell counts. Thus the rate of new cases of Kaposi's sarcoma may be influenced as much by the rate of new HIV infections as the total number of HIV infections. As the rate of new HIV infections among homosexual men decreases, a decrease in the overall incidence of new cases of Kaposi's sarcoma would be expected.

From a pathophysiologic perspective, Kaposi's sarcoma appears more like a consequence of disordered cytokine regulation of cell growth than a true cancer (see above and Chap. 151). Generally speaking, the tumor respects tissue planes and is rarely invasive.

Clinically, Kaposi's sarcoma may present in a variety of ways and may be seen at any stage of HIV infection, even in the presence of normal CD4 + T cell counts. The initial lesion may be a small, raised reddish purple nodule on the skin, a discoloration on the oral mucosa, or a swollen lymph node (see Fig. A1-22). Lesions often appear in sun-exposed areas, particularly the tip of the nose, and have a propensity to occur in areas of trauma (Kebner phenomenon). Because of the vascular nature of the tumors and the presence of extravasated red blood cells in the lesions, their color ranges from reddish to purple to brown and may often take on the appearance of a bruise with yellowish discoloration and tattooing. Lesions range in size from a few millimeters to several centimeters and may be either discrete or confluent. Kaposi's sarcoma lesions most commonly appear as raised macules; however, they also appear papular, particularly in patients with higher CD4 counts. Confluent lesions may give rise to surrounding lymphedema and may be quite disfiguring when they involve the face and disabling when they involve the lower extremities or the surfaces of joints. Lymph nodes, gastrointestinal tract, and lung are the organ systems most commonly affected by Kaposi's sarcoma; however, lesions have been reported in virtually every organ system including the heart and the CNS. In contrast to most malignancies where lymph node involvement implies metastatic spread and a poor prognosis, lymph node involvement may be seen very early in Kaposi's sarcoma and is of no special clinical significance. In fact, some patients may present with disease limited to the lymph nodes. These are generally patients with relatively intact immune function and thus have the best prognosis. Pulmonary involvement generally presents as shortness of breath. The chest x-ray characteristically shows bilateral lower lobe infiltrates that obscure the margins of the mediastinum and diaphragm (Fig. 279-21). Pleural effusions are seen in 70 percent of cases of pulmonary Kaposi's sarcoma, a fact that is often helpful in the differential diagnosis. Gastrointestinal involvement usually takes one of two forms. The first is mucosal involvement that may lead to bleeding that can be severe. These patients on occasion may also develop symptoms of gastrointestinal obstruction if large lesions develop. The second gastrointestinal manifestation is biliary tract involvement. Kaposi's sarcoma lesions may infiltrate the gallbladder and biliary tree leading to a clinical picture of obstructive jaundice similar to that seen with sclerosing cholangitis. In an effort to create a set of uniform parameters upon which to stage the extent of Kaposi's sarcoma, several systems have been proposed. Given the unique nature of this disorder, standard oncologic staging systems have not been useful. An excellent staging system has been developed by the National Institute of Allergy and Infectious Diseases AIDS Clinical Trials Group; it distinguishes patients on the basis of tumor extent, immunologic function, and presence or absence of systemic disease (Table 279-20).

A diagnosis of Kaposi's sarcoma is based upon biopsy of a

FIGURE 279-21 Chest x-ray of a patient with AIDS and pulmonary Kaposi's sarcoma. The characteristic findings include dense bilateral lower lobe infiltrates obscuring the heart borders and a pleural effusion.

suspicious lesion. Histologically one sees a proliferation of spindle cells, a proliferation of endothelial cells, and extravasation of red blood cells. Hemosiderin laden macrophages and, in early cases, an inflammatory cell infiltrate may be present. Included in the differential diagnoses are lymphoma (oral lesions), bacillary angiomatosis, and cutaneous mycobacterial infections.

Management of Kaposi's sarcoma (Table 279-21) should be carried out in consultation with an expert since definitive guidelines do not exist. In some cases lesions remain quite indolent and many patients can be managed with no specific treatment. Given the fact that less than 10 percent of AIDS patients with Kaposi's sarcoma die as a consequence of their malignancy and that death from opportunistic infections is much more common, whenever possible one should avoid treatment regimens that may further suppress the immune system and render the patients more susceptible to opportunistic infections. Treatment is indicated under two main circumstances. The first is when a single lesion or a limited number of lesions are causing significant discomfort or cosmetic problems. Examples of this would be prominent facial lesions, lesions overlying a joint, or lesions in the posterior oropharynx that interfere with swallowing. Under these circumstances treatment with localized radiation, intralesional vinblastine, or cryotherapy may be indicated. Patients with HIV infection are particularly sensitive to the side effects of radiation therapy. This is especially true with respect to the development of radiation-induced mucositis; doses of radiation directed at mucosal

surfaces, particularly in the head and neck region should be adjusted accordingly. The use of systemic single-agent chemotherapy should be considered in patients with a large number of lesions. Response rates varying from 26 to 80 percent have been seen with etoposide, vinblastine, doxorubicin, bleomycin, or IFN-α. The single most important determinant of response appears to be the CD4+ T cell count. It is ironic that the patients most likely to respond to therapy are those who need it the least and who generally should not be treated aggressively for fear of further compromising immune function. This relationship between response rate and baseline CD4+ T cell count is particularly true for IFN-α, where the response rate for patients with over 600 CD4+ T cells per microliter is approximately 80 percent, while for patients with under 150 CD4+ T cells it is under 10 percent. In contrast to the other single therapy agents, IFN-α provides an added advantage of having antiretroviral activity and thus may be considered an appropriate first choice for single-agent systemic therapy for the early patient with disseminated disease. Combination chemotherapy offers the best overall response rate for patients with life-threatening disease, with close to 90 percent of all patients responding to a low-dose combination regimen of doxorubicin, bleomycin, and vinblastine. As noted above, Kaposi's sarcoma is a radiation-sensitive tumor, and for patients with severe pulmonary involvement, one may also consider radiation therapy.

Lymphomas occur with an increased incidence in patients with either congenital or acquired T cell immunodeficiencies (see Chap. 278). AIDS is no exception to this general observation, with at least 3 percent of all patients developing lymphoma at some time during the course of their illness. This represents a 60-fold increased incidence compared to the general population. Lymphoma is seen in all risk groups, with the highest incidence (5.2 percent) in patients with hemophilia, and the lowest (1 percent), in patients from the Caribbean or Africa with heterosexually acquired infection. Lymphoma is a late manifestation of HIV infection, generally occurring in patients with under 200 CD4+ T cells per microliter. As HIV disease progresses, the risk of lymphoma increases. In contrast to Kaposi's sarcoma, which occurs at a relatively constant rate (2.4 percent per year) throughout the course of illness, the attack rate for lymphoma rises exponentially with increasing duration of HIV infection and decreasing level of immunologic function. At 3 years following infection, the risk of lymphoma is 0.8 percent per year. By 8 years following infection it has increased to 2.6 percent per year.

Three main categories of lymphoma are seen in patients with HIV infection. These are grade III or IV immunoblastic lymphoma, Burkitt's lymphoma, and primary CNS lymphoma (see Chap. 311). Approximately 90 percent of these lymphomas are B cell in phenotype and half contain Epstein-Barr virus DNA. These tumors may be either monoclonal or oligoclonal in origin and are probably in some way related to the pronounced polyclonal B cell activation seen in patients with AIDS (see "Pathophysiology and Immunopathogenesis" above).

Immunoblastic lymphomas account for approximately 60 percent of the cases of lymphoma in patients with AIDS. These are generally

TABLE 279-20 National Institute of Allergy and Infectious Diseases AIDS Clinical Trials Group TIS Staging System for Kaposi's sarcoma

Parameter	Good risk (stage 0): All of the following	Poor risk (stage 1): Any of the following
Tumor (T)	Confined to skin and/or lymph nodes and/or minimal oral disease	Tumor-associated edema or ulceration Extensive oral lesions Gastrointestinal lesions Nonnodal visceral lesions
Immune system (I) Systemic illness (S)	CD4+ T cell count ≥200 cells/µL No B symptoms* Karnofsky performance status >70 No history of opportunistic infection neurologic disease, lymphoma, or thrush	CD4+ T cell count < 200 cells/µL B symptoms* present Karnofsky performance status < 70 History of opportunistic infection neurologic disease, lymphoma, or thrush

* Defined as unexplained fever, night sweats, >10% involuntary weight loss, or diarrhea persisting for more than 2 weeks.

TABLE 279-21   Management of AIDS-associated Kaposi's sarcoma

Observation
Single or limited number of lesions
    Radiation
    Intralesional vinblastine
    Cryotherapy
Extensive, non-life-threatening disease
    Single-agent chemotherapy (etoposide; vinblastine; advanycin, or
    bleomycin)
    Interferon-α (if CD4+ T cell >150/μL)
Life-threatening disease
    Combination chemotherapy with low-dose, doxorubicin, bleomycin
    and vinblastine (ABV)
    Radiation

FIGURE 279-22   Diffuse histiocytic lymphoma involving the hard palate of a patient with AIDS.

high-grade and would have been classified as diffuse histiocytic lymphomas in earlier classification schemes. This tumor is more common in older patients, increasing from an incidence of 0 percent in HIV-infected individuals less than 1 year of age to over 3 percent in those over 50 years of age.

Small noncleaved cell or *Burkitt's lymphoma* accounts for approximately 20 percent of the cases of lymphoma in patients with AIDS. These are most frequent in patients 10 to 19 years of age and usually demonstrate characteristic *c-myc* translocations from chromosome 8 to chromosomes 14 or 22. Burkitt's lymphoma is not commonly seen in the setting of immunosuppression, and the incidence of this tumor in the setting of HIV infection is over 1000-fold higher than that seen in the general population. In contrast to African Burkitt's lymphoma, where 97 percent of cases contain an Epstein-Barr virus genome, less than 50 percent of HIV-associated Burkitt's lymphoma are Epstein-Barr positive.

Primary CNS lymphoma accounts for approximately 20 percent of the cases of lymphoma in patients with HIV infection. In contrast to the HIV-associated Burkitt's lymphoma, primary CNS lymphomas are more commonly Epstein-Barr virus positive; in one study, the incidence was 100 percent and the lymphomas did not appear to have a predilection for any particular age group. The median CD4+ T cell count at time of diagnosis for patients with primary CNS lymphoma is approximately 40 cells per microliter, compared to a mean of approximately 190 cells per microliter for patients with systemic lymphoma. This highlights the fact that CNS lymphoma generally presents at a later stage of HIV infection than does systemic lymphoma, and this may at least in part explain the poorer prognosis for this particular subset of patients (discussed below).

The clinical presentation of lymphoma in the patient with HIV infection is quite varied, ranging from focal seizures to rapidly growing mass lesions in the oral mucosa (Fig. 279-22) to persistent unexplained fever. At least 80 percent of patients will present with extranodal disease and a similar percentage will have B type symptoms of fever, night sweats, or weight loss. Virtually any site in the body may be involved. The most common extranodal site is the CNS, involved in approximately one-third of all patients with lymphoma; approximately 60 percent of these will be primary CNS lymphoma. Primary CNS lymphoma generally presents with focal neurologic deficits including cranial nerve findings, headaches, and/or seizures. MRI or CT generally reveals a limited number (one to three) of 3 to 5-cm lesions. The lesions are often ring enhancing with contrast and may occur in any location. The main differential diagnosis is cerebral toxoplasmosis, although cerebral Chagas disease may manifest a similar clinical picture. Prognosis is poor; the median survival following diagnosis is 2 to 3 months.

In addition to the 20 percent of all lymphomas in HIV-infected individuals that are primary CNS lymphomas, CNS disease unrelated to lymphoma is also seen in HIV-infected patients with systemic lymphoma, and approximately 20 percent of patients with systemic lymphoma will have CNS disease in the form of leptomeningeal

involvement. This fact underlines the importance of a lumbar puncture in the staging evaluation of patients with systemic lymphoma.

The second most common extranodal site is the GI tract, with involvement noted in 25 percent of patients. Any site in the GI tract may be involved, and patients may complain of difficulty swallowing or abdominal pain. The diagnosis is usually suspected based upon CT or MRI of the abdomen. Bone marrow involvement occurs in approximately 20 percent of patients and may be associated with a pancytopenia. Liver and lung involvement are each seen in approximately 10 percent of patients. Pulmonary disease may present as either a mass lesion, multiple nodules, or an interstitial infiltrate.

Both conventional and nonconventional approaches have been employed in an effort to treat HIV-related lymphomas. Initial attempts using standard intensive therapeutic regimens have largely been abandoned due to low response rate (20 to 30 percent) and a high incidence of fatal opportunistic infections. The median survival for patients treated with intensive regimens is approximately 4 to 6 months. These figures predominantly reflect results in patients with fairly advanced HIV infection and low CD4+ T cell counts. Patients with higher CD4+ T cell counts do better with intensive chemotherapy, and in these earlier-stage patients, response rates as high as 72 percent and disease-free intervals exceeding 15 months have been reported. Clinical trials are currently underway comparing standard chemotherapeutic approaches with low-dose modified regimens. At present, the median survival for patients with HIV-related systemic lymphoma is 10 months. Treatment of primary CNS lymphoma is almost uniformly unsuccessful. Palliative measures such as radiation therapy and/or glucocorticoids aimed at reducing the size of the lesion(s) and the accompanying cerebral edema may provide some symptomatic relief. The prognosis is poor for patients with primary CNS lymphoma; median survival is 2 to 4 months.

Intraepithelial dysplasia of either the cervix or the anus has been increasingly recognized as a complication of long-standing HIV infection. This human papilloma virus–associated condition correlates with the subsequent development of intraepithelial neoplasia and eventually invasive cancer. In two separate studies, HIV-infected men without anorectal symptoms were studied for evidence of dysplasia, and Papanicolaou smears were found to be abnormal in about 40 percent. These changes were persistent at 1-year follow-up, raising the possibility of a subsequent transition to a more malignant condition. While the incidence of an abnormal Papanicolaou smear of the cervix is approximately 5 percent in the otherwise healthy population, the incidence of abnormal smears in women with HIV infection is 60 percent, and invasive cervical carcinoma has been added to the list of AIDS-defining conditions. Thus far only small increases in the incidence of cervical or anal cancer have been seen as a consequence of HIV infection. However, given these findings, as patients with HIV infection live longer through the use of improved treatment strategies, it is likely that such conditions will begin to appear more frequently. For these reasons, all patients with HIV infection should have periodic rectal and/or pelvic examinations with Papanicolaou smears to look for evidence of cellular dysplasia.

A variety of other neoplastic conditions have been described in patients with HIV infection. While none of these other conditions have been reported to occur at a higher rate than that seen in the general population, these cancers may be more fulminant and difficult to treat in an HIV-infected patient. In this regard, Hodgkin's disease in the setting of HIV infection often presents as extensive disease with mixed cellular or lymphocyte depletion pathologic types. In contrast to the excellent results and high cure rates for Hodgkin's disease in the general population, the patient with HIV infection and Hodgkin's disease has a median survival of only 12 to 15 months. As the epidemic of HIV infection continues, additional neoplastic complications are to be expected.

ORGAN-SPECIFIC SYNDROMES Virtually every organ system in the body is vulnerable to disease either as a direct consequence of HIV infection or secondary to other infectious or neoplastic conditions. While the majority of these diseases are due to opportunistic infections or neoplasms (see above), there are also a variety of clinical problems for which no specific pathogens are clearly identified.

Pulmonary disease is seen in virtually every patient with HIV infection. Its evaluation is one of the most important components in management, given the importance of early diagnosis and initiation of specific therapy. The most common manifestation of pulmonary disease is pneumonia and the most common cause of pneumonia is *Pneumocystis carinii*. Other major causes of pneumonia include nonspecific interstitial pneumonitis, Kaposi's sarcoma, mycobacterial infections, and fungal infections. Although there are some distinguishing clinical and radiographic characteristics (Table 279-22), in most cases an accurate diagnosis is based upon histologic or microbiologic identification of the causative organism. Specimens for examination are derived from induced sputum, bronchoalveolar lavage, transbronchial biopsy, or open lung biopsy. In most of the conditions seen in HIV-infected patients, the chest x-ray reveals bilateral diffuse interstitial infiltrates. In patients with mycobacterial or fungal infections, hilar or mediastinal adenopathy may also be seen. In Kaposi's sarcoma the infiltrates are dense and often obliterate the borders of the heart and diaphragm; there is usually an accompanying pleural effusion. Upper-lobe cavitary disease is suggestive of reactivation TB or *Pneumocystis carinii* pneumonia in a patient receiving aerosolized pentamidine. The presence of a pneumothorax is most consistent with this latter condition. With the exception of bacterial pneumonias, sputum production is usually scant. Hemoptysis may be seen in the setting of cryptococcal pneumonia, tuberculosis, or Kaposi's sarcoma.

Two forms of idiopathic interstitial pneumonia have been described in patients with HIV infection; these are lymphoid interstitial pneumonitis (LIP) and nonspecific interstitial pneumonitis (NIP). LIP, while a common finding in children, is quite rare in adults, occurring in approximately 1 percent of patients. This disorder is characterized by a benign lymphocytic infiltrate of the lung and is felt to be part of the systemic polyclonal activation of lymphocytes seen in the context of HIV and EBV infections. Transbronchial biopsy is diagnostic in 50 percent of cases; an open lung biopsy is required for diagnosis in the remainder. This condition is generally self-limited and no specific treatment is necessary. Severe cases have been managed with a brief course of glucocorticoids. NIP is seen in up to half of all patients with AIDS and in some series is responsible for up to one-third of all pulmonary disease. Interstitial infiltrates with lymphocytes and plasma cells in a perivascular and peribronchial distribution are seen on histologic examination. Symptoms include fever and nonproductive cough occasionally accompanied by mild chest discomfort. Chest x-ray, which is normal in 50 percent of cases, may demonstrate a faint interstitial pattern. Similar to LIP, this is a self-limited process for which no therapy is indicated.

In addition to pneumonia, *sinusitis* is a common respiratory tract complication of HIV infection and is seen at all stages of infection. More severe cases are seen in patients with lower CD4+ T cell counts. Sinusitis presents as fever, nasal congestion, and headache; the diagnosis is best made by CT or MRI. Maxillary sinuses are most commonly involved; however, disease is frequently seen in ethmoid, sphenoid, and frontal sinuses as well. Although over 80 percent of patients show clinical improvement regardless of whether or not antibiotics are given, radiographic improvement is quicker and more pronounced in patients who have received antimicrobial therapy. It is postulated that this high incidence of sinusitis results from the increased frequency of infections with encapsulated organisms such as *Haemophilus influenzae* and *Streptococcus pneumoniae*, although this has not been formally proven.

Gastrointestinal disease is a common feature of HIV infection and is most frequently due to a secondary infection. The oral mucosa, in addition to being involved with thrush, oral hairy leukoplakia, and Kaposi's sarcoma also may be affected by large, shallow, painful aphthous ulcers. These lesions, which may be painful enough to result in a decrease in oral intake, are of unknown cause. While no specific therapy exists, some reports suggest that brief courses of high-dose glucocorticoids or thalidomide may be of help. Esophagitis (Fig. 279-19) generally presents with odynophagia and retrosternal pain and may be due to *Candida*, CMV, or HSV. In addition, the esophagus may be involved with Kaposi's sarcoma and lymphoma. The esophageal mucosa, similar to the oral mucosa, may have large, painful ulcers of unclear etiology. These lesions are somewhat similar in appearance to the ulcers of CMV esophagitis but do not respond to antiviral therapy and can pose a significant problem with regard to nutrition. Achlorhydria is a common problem in patients with HIV infection; however, gastric problems are otherwise rare. Kaposi's sarcoma as well as lymphoma may involve the stomach. Infections of the small and large intestine are among the most significant gastrointestinal problems in the HIV-infected patient. They usually present with diarrhea, abdominal pain, occasionally fever and, in severe cases, weight loss. In addition to specific secondary infections, patients with HIV infection may also experience a chronic diarrheal syndrome for which no etiologic agent other than HIV can be identified and which is generally referred to as *AIDS* or *HIV enteropathy*. This is a clinical condition resembling chronic gastroenteritis with diarrhea of more than 1 month duration for which no cause can be found. This condition is most likely a direct result of HIV infection within the gastrointestinal tract. Histologic examination of the small bowel in these patients reveals low-grade mucosal atrophy with a decrease in mitotic figures suggesting a hyporegenerative state. Patients often have decreased or absent small bowel lactase and malabsorption with accompanying weight loss.

TABLE 279-22 Characteristics of pneumonia in patients with HIV infection

Etiology	Sputum	Chest x-ray
Pneumocystis carinii	Scant	Normal/interstitial infiltrate
Pneumocystis carinii in setting of aerosolized pentamidine	Scant	Upper lobe cavitary lesions; pneumothorax
Bacterial	Neutrophils, organisms	Consolidation
Atypical mycobacteria	Scant	Interstitial infiltrate; hilar adenopathy
Reactivation *Mycobacterium tuberculosis*	White blood cells, organisms, occasional hemoptysis	Cavitary or miliary infiltrates; hilar adenopathy
Nonspecific interstitial pneumonitis (NIP)	Scant	Normal/interstitial infiltrate
Kaposi's sarcoma	Scant, occasional hemoptysis	Dense, bilateral lower lobe infiltrates; pleural effusions

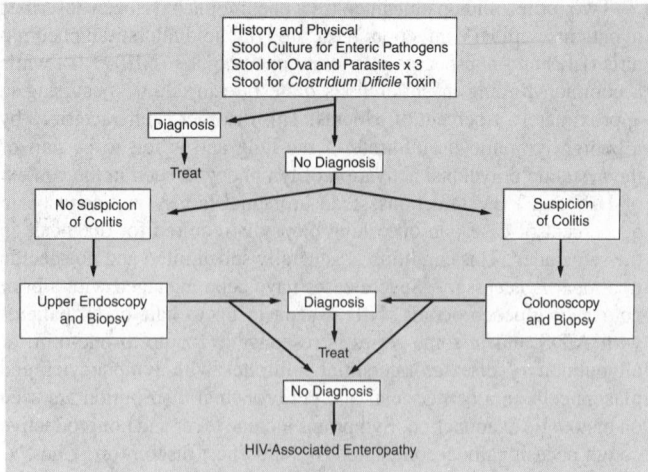

FIGURE 279-23 Algorithm for the evaluation of diarrhea in a patient with HIV infection. HIV-associated enteropathy is a diagnosis of exclusion and can be made only after other, generally treatable, forms of diarrheal illness have been ruled out.

TABLE 279-23   Causes of bone marrow suppression in patients with HIV infection

HIV infection
Mycobacterial infection
Fungal infections
B19 Parvovirus infection
Lymphoma
Medications
   Zidovudine
   Dapsone
   Trimethoprim/sulfamethoxazole
   Pyrimethamine
   5-Flucytosine
   Ganciclovir
   Interferon-α
   Trimetrexate
   Foscarnet

In working up a patient with HIV infection and gastrointestinal problems, a set of stool examinations, including culture, examination for ova and parasites, and examination for *Clostridium difficile* toxin should form the initial part of the evaluation. Approximately 50 percent of the time this work-up will demonstrate infection with pathogenic bacteria such as salmonella, shigella, campylobacter; mycobacteria (both atypical and *Mycobacterium tuberculosis*); protozoa such as giardia, *E. histolytica*, cryptosporidia, or *Isospora*; or *Clostridium difficile*. If these stool examinations are negative, additional evaluation, including upper and/or lower endoscopy with biopsy may establish a diagnosis of microsporidial or mycobacterial infection of the small intestine or CMV colitis in over half the patients. In patients for whom this diagnostic evaluation is nonrevealing and, if diarrhea has persisted for over 1 month, a presumptive diagnosis of HIV enteropathy can be made. An algorithm for the evaluation of diarrhea in patients with HIV infection is given in Fig. 279-23.

Rectal lesions are common in HIV-infected patients, particularly the perirectal ulcers and erosions due to the reactivation of HSV (Fig. 279-21). These may appear quite atypical, without vesicles, and respond well to treatment with acyclovir. Other rectal lesions more commonly seen in HIV-infected patients include condyloma acuminatum, Kaposi's sarcoma, and intraepithelial neoplasia.

Several different forms of hepatobiliary disease occur in patients with HIV infection. Biliary tract disease in the form of papillary stenosis or sclerosing cholangitis has been reported in the context of cryptosporidiosis, CMV infection, and Kaposi's sarcoma. Hepatic disease may take the form of hepatocellular injury due to hepatitis viruses, granulomatous hepatitis due to mycobacterial or fungal infections, or hepatic masses secondary to tuberculous abscess or peliosis hepatis. Fatty infiltration has also been reported, and it has been suggested that this may be related in some patients to nucleoside therapy.

Pancreatic injury is most commonly due to drug toxicity, notably that secondary to pentamidine or dideoxynucleosides. While up to 50 percent of patients with HIV infection may have biochemical evidence of pancreatic injury, and there is often evidence of pancreatic infection with CMV and MAC at autopsy, fewer than 5 percent of patients show any clinical evidence of pancreatitis that is not linked to a drug toxicity.

Hematologic problems are common throughout the course of HIV infection and occur as a direct consequence of HIV, as a manifestation of secondary infections and neoplasms, and as a side effect of therapy (Table 279-23). HIV has been shown to be present in the bone marrow, and there is evidence that it is capable of infecting early hematopoietic precursor cells. Bone marrow suppression may also

be associated with disseminated mycobacterial infections, fungal infections, and lymphoma. Direct histologic examination and culture of bone marrow in patients with HIV infection and unexplained hematologic abnormalities are often diagnostic. A significant precentage of bone marrow aspirates have been reported to contain lymphoid aggregates, the precise significance of which is unknown.

Anemia is the most common hematologic abnormality seen with HIV infection and is present in 18 percent of asymptomatic seropositive individuals, 50 percent of patients with early symptoms, and 75 percent of patients with AIDS. While generally mild, anemia can be quite severe and may require chronic blood transfusion. Among the specific reversible causes of anemia in HIV-infected individuals are drug toxicity, systemic fungal and mycobacterial infections, nutritional deficiences, and parvovirus B19 infections.

Zidovudine is a major contributor to the anemia seen in patients with advanced HIV infection. This nucleoside analogue (discussed below), has a somewhat selective ability to block erythroid maturation, an effect that is seen prior to effects on other marrow elements. A characteristic feature of zidovudine therapy is an elevated MCV. Another drug with selective effects on the erythroid series is dapsone. This agent can cause a serious hemolytic anemia in patients who are G6PD-deficient as well as create a functional anemia in others through induction of methemoglobemia.

Folate levels are usually normal in HIV-infected individuals; however, B_{12} levels may be depressed in patients with AIDS, presumably as a consequence of long-standing achlorhydria and malabsorption. Replacement therapy with B_{12} seems to have a minimal effect on HIV-associated anemia. True autoimmune hemolytic anemia is rare, although approximately 20 percent of patients with HIV infection may have a positive direct antiglobulin test, presumably as a consequence of polyclonal B cell activation. Some patients do develop a syndrome of increased peeripheral destruction or splenic sequestration of erythrocytes that in some instances has been reported in association with zidovudine treatment.

In addition to the more common secondary infections described above, patients with HIV infection have been reported to develop anemia secondary to infection with parvovirus B19. This is an important cause of anemia to be aware of, since it responds to treatment with intravenous immunoglobulin. Baseline erythropoietin levels in patients with HIV infection and anemia are generally less than expected, given the degree of anemia. The exception is zidovudine-associated anemia, where levels may be quite high. In fact, in patients with zidovudine-associated anemia and low erythropoietin levels, treatment with erythropoietin at a dose of 100 μg/kg three times a week may result in an increase in hemoglobulin levels. Erythropoietin seems to be of less benefit in patients with elevated erythropoietin levels and in patients with anemia due to causes other than zidovudine toxicity.

Neutropenia is seen in approximately half the patients with HIV infection. It is mild in most instances; however, it can be severe and place patients at risk of spontaneous bacterial infections. This is usually seen in patients receiving any of a number of myelosuppressive therapies used in the treatment of HIV infection and its complications. Zidovudine, ganciclovir, pyrimethamine, and trimethoprim/sulfamethoxazole are among the drugs that most commonly cause severe neutropenia in patients with HIV infection. Neutropenia is most severe in patients with more advanced disease. Folinic acid (leucovorin) may ameliorate the neutropenia induced by pyrimethamine. The role of colony stimulating factors in the management of patients with HIV infection and neutropenia has undergone extensive evaluation. Both G-CSF and GM-CSF have been shown to increase neutrophil counts in patients with HIV infection. These effects have been seen in both drug-induced and nondrug-induced neutropenias. While G-CSF is theoretically more attractive as a colony stimulating agent due to the fact that HIV replication is enhanced in vitro by GM-CSF, additional studies need to be performed to determine precisely the role of either of these factors in the management of patients with HIV infection and neutropenia.

Thrombocytopenia occurs in approximately 40 percent of patients with HIV infection and, in contrast to neutropenia and anemia, is often an early, primary manifestation of HIV infection (see above). The thrombocytopenia seen as direct result of HIV infection resembles that of idiopathic thrombocytopenic purpura (ITP) and responds not only to conventional strategies but, in a large number of cases, to therapy with antiretrovirals. Thrombocytopenia may also be seen as a side effect of medications; however, it is rarely a dose-limiting side effect. Other causes for thrombocytopenia in patients with HIV infection include bone marrow involvement with lymphoma, mycobacterial infection, or fungal infections.

Lymphadenopathy is also a common finding in patients with HIV infection, ranging from the generalized follicular hyperplasia seen early in disease to involvement secondary to opportunistic infections and neoplasms. Lymph node biopsy is not indicated in the lymphadenopathy seen early in disease unless it is associated with rapid enlargement, unusual consistency, or coalescence. While Kaposi's sarcoma may present in a lymphadenopathic form early in disease there are no data to suggest that early treatment is indicated. In contrast, new-onset lymphadenopathy in the setting of more advanced HIV infection, for example CD4+ T cell counts under 200 cells per microliter may be the first sign of a secondary infection or neoplasm and should be examined both histologically and with culture. Among the secondary infections commonly associated with lymphadenopathy are mycobacterial infections, fungal infections, and bacillary angiomatosis. In addition to Kaposi's sarcoma, lymphoma may also present as lymphadenopathy.

Renal disease may be associated with HIV infection (see Chaps. 241 and 242). Although renal disease is often the result of a drug-induced injury, a significant portion of patients with AIDS (up to 10 percent in some series) may develop renal disease as a direct consequence of HIV infection; this is designated as *AIDS*- or *HIV-associated nephropathy*. Secondary infections rarely result in significant renal impairment; however, one may see nephrocalcinosis as a result of infection with mycobacteria or *Pneumocystis carinii*.

Among the drugs commonly associated with renal damage in patients with AIDS are pentamidine, amphotericin, and foscarnet. In addition, trimethoprim/sulfamethoxazole may compete for tubular secretion of creatinine and cause an increase in the serum creatinine level, while sulfadiazine may crystallize in the kidney and result in an easily reversible form of renal shutdown.

HIV-associated nephropathy closely resembles heroin-associated nephropathy seen in IVDUs and initially was thought to be that condition in patients with HIV infection; however, it is now recognized as a true direct complication of HIV infection. HIV-associated nephropathy can be an early manifestation of HIV infection and is also seen in children. The severity of renal disease and propensity to develop end-stage renal failure appear to be a function of race and much more of a problem among blacks than whites, perhaps more so than any other manifestation of HIV infection. Given the fact that in

most series over 50 percent of patients with HIV-associated nephropathy were IVDUs, it was originally thought that this racial predilection was merely reflective of the increased portion of blacks in the IVDU group rather than a true race-related phenomenon. However, the incidence by race of HIV-associated end-stage renal failure in non-IVDU homosexual men suggests that race does play a major role and that end-stage renal failure occurs disproportionately among blacks.

The prototypic lesion of HIV-associated nephropathy is a focal segmental glomerulosclerosis, and is seen in approximately 80 percent of patients with this complication. Patients present with heavy proteinuria without edema or hypertension. Ultrasound examination usually reveals enlarged, hyperechogenic kidneys; a definitive diagnosis is obtained through renal biopsy. Progression to end-stage renal failure usually occurs within 1 year. The remainder of patients (approximately 20 percent) with HIV-associated nephropathy present with a mesangial hyperplasia with minimal glomerulosclerosis. It is believed that this may be the precursor lesion to focal segmental glomerulosclerosis.

There is no successful management for HIV-associated nephropathy. There seems to be little overall benefit of zidovudine on this complication of HIV infection, although temporary improvement following initiation of therapy has been noted by some investigators. In patients in whom renal disease is detected relatively early, at the stage of mesangial hyperplasia with minimal glomerulosclerosis, it has been proposed that a short course of glucocorticoids may be of value. While this seems a reasonable option it must be done with awareness of the potentially devastating effects of long-term glucocorticoid use in patients with HIV infection.

Dermatologic problems are common in patients with HIV infection (see Chap. 54). From the macular, roseola-like rash seen with the acute seroconversion syndrome to extensive end-stage Kaposi's sarcoma, cutaneous manifestations are present throughout the course of HIV infection. While many of these manifestations are covered elsewhere in this chapter under their respective causes and under the heading of early symptomatic disease, there are some additional dermatologic problems seen in the context of HIV infection that have not yet been discussed (see Chaps. 51, 52, and 54). Among these are seborrheic dermatitis, eosinophilic pustular folliculitis, and several minor cutaneous infections.

Seborrheic dermatitis occurs in 3 percent of the general population; however, it is seen in up to 50 percent of patients with HIV infection and is among the most common noninfectious manifestations of HIV infection. In fact, in the early days of the AIDS epidemic, patients with a community-acquired pneumonia and seborrheic dermatitis were often given a presumptive diagnosis of PCP. Seborrheic dermatitis increases in prevalence and severity as the CD4 count declines. Several reports have noted that in HIV-infected patients, seborrheic dermatitis may be aggravated by concomitant infection with *Pityrosporon*, a yeast-like fungus, and have recommended that topical antifungals may be of help in cases refractory to standard topical treatment.

Eosinophilic pustular folliculitis is a rare dermatologic condition seen with increased frequency in patients with HIV infection. It presents as multiple urticarial perifollicular papules that may coalesce to plaque-like lesions. Skin biopsy reveals an eosinophilic infiltrate of the hair follicle that in certain cases has been associated with the presence of a mite. Patients typically have an elevated IgE level and may respond to treatment with topical antihelminthics. There is at least one report of a patient with AIDS developing a severe form of Norwegian scabies with hyperkeratotic, psoriasiform skin lesions.

Although they are not reported to be increased in frequency, both psoriasis and icthyosis may be particularly severe when they occur in patients with HIV infection. Preexisting psoriasis may become guttae in appearance and more refractory to treatment.

As mentioned above there are a variety of secondary infections that present with cutaneous manifestations. Among them are HSV that causes severe erosive orolabial, genital, perirectal (Fig. 279-20), and whitlow lesions and VZ that causes both shingles and a forme clinically, and immunologically dissimilar to HIV infection and AIDS. Less than half of the ICL patients had risk factors for HIV infection, and there were wide geographic and age distributions. The fact that a significant proportion of patients did have risk factors is probably a reflection of selection bias in that physicians who take care of HIV-infected patients are more likely to monitor CD4 + T cells. Approximately one-third of the patients are women compared to 11 percent of women among HIV-infected individuals in the United States. Many patients with ICL remained clinically stable and their condition did not progressively deteriorate as is so commonly seen with seriously immunosuppressed HIV-infected patients. Certain patients with ICL even experienced spontaneous reversal of the CD4 + T lymphocytopenia. Immunologic abnormalities in ICL are somewhat different from those in HIV infection. ICL patients often have decreases in CD8 + T cells as well as B cells. Furthermore, immunoglobulin levels were either normal or, more commonly, decreased in ICL compared to the usually observed hypergammaglobulinemia of HIV-infected individuals. Finally, virologic studies revealed no evidence of HIV-1, HIV-2, HTLV-I, or HTLV-II or of any other mononuclear cell-tropic virus. Furthermore, there was no epidemiologic evidence to suggest that a transmissible microbe was involved. The cases of ICL were widely dispersed with no clustering. Close contacts and sexual partners who were studied were clinically well with negative serologic, immunologic, and virologic studies for HIV. ICL is a heterogeneous syndrome and it is highly likely that there is no common cause; however, there may be certain common causes among subgroups of patients that are currently unrecognized.

Patients who present with the laboratory data consistent with ICL should be worked up for underlying diseases which may be responsible for the immunosuppression. If no underlying cause is detected, no specific therapy should be initiated. However, if opportunistic disease occur, they should be treated appropriately (see below). Depending on the level of the CD4 + T cell count, patients should receive prophylaxis for the appropriate commonly encountered opportunistic infections.

TREATMENT OF HIV INFECTION AND ITS COMPLICATIONS

GENERAL PRINCIPLES OF PATIENT MANAGEMENT   The treatment of patients with HIV infection requires not only a comprehensive knowledge of the disease processes to be experienced but also the ability to deal with the problems of a chronic, life-threatening illness. Specific antiretroviral therapy and antimicrobial treatment and prophylaxis are critical measures in prolonging an acceptable quality of life; however, counseling and education are also of paramount importance in providing patients with optimal overall care. Patients must be educated about the infectious potential of their condition, with frank discussions about sexual practices and sharing of intravenous needles. The treating physician must not only be aware of the latest medications available for HIV infection and its complications but must also take the time to educate patients concerning the natural history of the illness and to listen to and be sensitive to their fears and concerns. As with other diseases, decisions about therapeutic maneuvers should be done in consultation with the patient when possible and with the patient's proxy if the patient is no longer capable of making decisions. In this regard, it is recommended that all patients with HIV infection and in particular those with under 200 CD4 + T cells per microliter give someone they trust durable power of attorney to make medical decisions on their behalf, if necessary.

No matter how well prepared patients may feel they are for adversity, initial awareness of a diagnosis of HIV infection is an invariably devastating event. For this reason it is recommend that anyone about to undergo testing have "pretest counseling" to at least partially prepare them should the results come back positive. Following a diagnosis of HIV infection the physician should be ready with immediate support systems for the newly diagnosed patient; these should include an experienced social worker or nurse who can spend time talking to the person and insuring that he/she is emotionally stable. Most communities have HIV crisis centers that can be of great help in these difficult situations.

Following an initial diagnosis of HIV infection there are several examinations and laboratory studies that should be performed to help stage the extent of disease and provide baseline standards for future reference. In addition to routine chemistry, hematology screening panels, and chest x-ray, one should also obtain a CD4 + T cell count and a VDRL. A PPD skin test should be done and a Mini-Mental Status Examination performed and recorded (Table 279-16). In addition, patients should be counseled with regard to sex practices and needle sharing, and counseling should be offered to others whom the patient knows or suspects may also be infected. Once these baseline activities are performed, short-term and long-term medical management strategies should be developed based on the information below.

ANTIRETROVIRAL THERAPY   The cornerstone of medical management of HIV infection is antiretroviral therapy. Suppression of HIV replication is an important component in prolonging life as well as improving the quality of life of patients with HIV infection. Many questions such as "When is the best time to start antiretroviral therapy?," "What is the best regimen to start with?," "When should therapy be changed?," and "What regimen should one change to?" currently lack definitive answers. Nonetheless, the physician and patient must come to a mutually agreeable plan based upon the best available data. At present an extensive clinical trials network involving both clinical investigators and patient advocates is in place attempting to develop improved approaches to therapy. As a result, new therapies and new therapeutic strategies are emerging and new drugs are often available through expanded access programs prior to official licensure. For these reasons, management of patients with HIV infection is best accomplished with the input of someone who is an expert in the field.

Zidovudine (AZT, 3'-azido-2',3'-dideoxythymidine) was the first approved drug for the treatment of HIV infection and is the prototype drug for the general class of compounds referred to as nucleoside analogues (Table 279-24). These compounds, in which the hydroxyl group in the 3' position of the ribose moiety is substituted with a hydrogen or other chemical group, act as DNA chain terminators due to their inability to form a 3'-5' phosphodiester linkage with another nucleoside. They bind much more avidly to the active site of the RNA-dependent DNA polymerase of HIV (reverse transcriptase) than they bind to the active site of mammalian cell DNA polymerases. This may, at least in part, explain their selective effect on HIV replication. Zidovudine also has a relatively high avidity for the DNA polymerase gamma of human mitochondria. This may contribute to the development of the myopathy sometimes seen in patients receiving zidovudine. The active form of zidovudine is the triphosphate, and the rate of phosphorylation, a thymidine kinase–dependent pathway, may be different in different cells. This may explain why zidovudine protects some cell types from HIV better than others. Zidovudine is well-absorbed orally, with a serum half-life of approximately 1 h. Hence, most recommended dosing regimens employ an every-4-h or five-times-a-day schedule. Given the fact that, as in the case of didanosine (see below), the intracellular half-life may be much longer, the rationale for this dosing schedule is unsubstantiated and a variety of more convenient schedules are often employed, particularly when zidovudine is given as part of a combination regimen.

The clinical efficacy of zidovudine was clearly established in a phase II, placebo-controlled trial in which 282 patients who had either experienced a single bout of PCP or who had a variety of AIDS-associated symptoms were randomized to receive either placebo or zidovudine at a dose of 200 mg every 4 h. The trial was stopped prematurely when it became clear that there were far fewer deaths and far fewer new opportunistic infections occurring in the patients receiving zidovudine (Fig. 279-24). In addition to this clinical benefit, patients treated with zidovudine were noted to have increases in total lymphocyte counts, including CD4 + T cell counts, declines in

TABLE 279-24 Currently licensed antiretroviral drugs

Drug	Structure	Standard dose	Other regimens	Toxicities	Special considerations
AZT, Zidovudine 3′ Azido-2′, 3′-dideoxythymidine		100 mg, 5 id	200 mg tid, 300 mg bid	Anemia, leukopenia, myopathy	
ddl, Didanosine 2′,3′ dideoxyinosine		200 mg bid, > 60 kg 100 mg bid, < 60 kg		Peripheral neuropathy, pancreatitis	Need at least 2 tablets dose
ddc, Zalcitabine 2′,3′ dideoxycytidine		0.75 mg tid		Peripheral neuropathy, pancreatitis	Only licensed in combination with AZT, 200 mg tid
d4T, Stavudine 2′,3′-didehydro-3′-deoxythymidine		10–40 mg bid		Peripheral neuropathy, hepatitis	

circulating levels of p24 antigen, and weight gain. In subsequent trials a beneficial effect was also noted in patients with neurologic disease and in earlier disease with higher CD4 + T cell counts. At the present time, zidovudine is indicated therapy for anyone with HIV infection and less than 500 CD4 + T cells per microliter. This recommendation is based upon the U.S. Food and Drug Administration approval and licensure process, which in turn is based solely upon the results of controlled clinical trials. Thus, the eventual indications

for zidovudine therapy may be even broader than those currently in place. Only controlled clinical trials will provide definitive guidelines whether to initiate antiretroviral therapy earlier than the currently recommended decision point.

Similarly, a great deal of effort has been directed toward defining the optimal dose of zidovudine. While the earliest trials, employing doses of 1200 mg/d showed benefit, there was also substantial toxicity. Subsequent trials have demonstrated that doses as low as 400 to 600 mg/d are equivalent in efficacy to higher-dose regimens and are significantly less toxic. At present the dose most frequently employed is 100 mg five times a day, although in patients taking other medications on a twice a day schedule or three times a day schedule, zidovudine regimens of 200 mg twice or three times a day may be used (Table 279-24).

While many patients experience fatigue, malaise, nausea, and headache upon the initiation of zidovudine therapy these side effects often subside over time. The major toxicities of zidovudine are on the bone marrow. Patients often develop a macrocytic anemia which, when seen in association with low serum erythropoietin levels, may be ameliorated somewhat with injections of recombinant erythropoietin beginning at a dose of 100 μ/kg three times a week. Although zidovudine-induced anemia is macrocytic, there is no evidence that deficiencies in B_{12} or folate play a role; exogenous administration of these vitamins is of no help. In addition to anemia, patients receiving zidovudine, especially advanced patients, may experience neutropenia and in some cases thrombocytopenia. Other common toxicities of zidovudine include a proximal myopathy characterized by weakness, muscle wasting, and in some patients an elevation in creatine kinase; and a bluish discoloration of the nails that is particulary noticeable in black patients. It has been suggested that some forms of HIV-associated cardiomyopathy may actually be a side effect of nucleosides; this is also true of some cases of fatty infiltration of the liver. Although an increased incidence of tumors of the vaginal epithelium

FIGURE 279-24 Comparison of number of events (deaths or new opportunistic infections) occurring in patients randomized to receive either oral palcebo or AZT (zidovudine). Following 6 weeks of therapy, fewer events were seen in the patients randomized to AZT. (*Courtesy of Burroughs Wellcome Co.*)

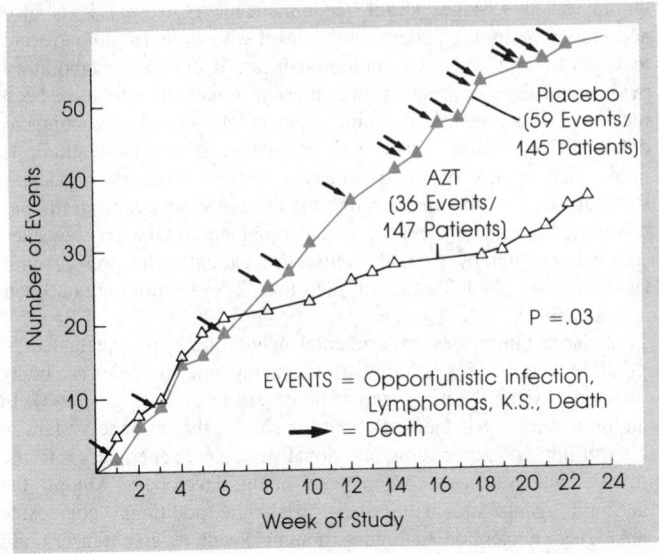

has been noted in rodents treated with extremely high doses of zidovudine, no increases in cancers in AIDS patients have thus far been attributed to zidovudine therapy. However, lymphomas are being seen with increased frequency as patients with AIDS live longer. Given these potential side effects, it is recommended that patients starting therapy with zidovudine be monitored for toxicity at least every other week for the first month and then monthly.

Considerable concern has been raised over the observation that strains of HIV resistant to zidovudine have been identified. This is usually seen in patients receiving zidovudine for periods of 6 months or longer, however, it has also been reported in isolates obtained at the time of seroconversion. Resistance is seen more quickly in late-stage patients where there is presumably a greater degree of viral replication and thus more chance for mutation. This resistance is secondary to mutations in the HIV reverse transcriptase and at least five different mutations have been identified that are associated with zidovudine resistance (codons 41, 67, 70, 215, and 219). Zidovudine resistance is not associated with resistance to either didanosine or zalcitabine. While the clinical significance of this observation has not been precisely defined, it does appear that this may be one factor limiting the long-term usefulness of zidovudine as monotherapy and provides a strong rationale for the early use of combination regimens.

Didanosine (ddI, 2',3'-dideoxyinosine) was the second drug licensed for the treatment of HIV infection. In a series of open trials, didanosine was shown to be capable of causing increases in CD4 + T cell counts and declines in p24 antigen levels. Licensure was based upon the demonstration in a controlled, randomized trial that patients who had received zidovudine for a minimum of 16 weeks and were switched to didanosine experienced increases in CD4 + T cell counts and fewer new opportunistic infections. Data are still being generated in a randomized trial comparing zidovudine to didanosine as initial therapy. At present, didanosine is an FDA-approved therapy for any patient with HIV infection who has received prolonged zidovudine therapy. Didanosine therapy is usually reserved for patients who have begun to show evidence of clinical or laboratory decline while receiving zidovudine. In this event, rather than switching patients to didanosine one may chose to merely add it to the zidovudine regimen. As in the case of zidovudine, patients receiving didanosine develop strains of HIV that are resistant to didanosine. At least some of these isolates, occurring in patients who had originally developed zidovudine-resistant isolates as a consequence of prior zidovudine therapy, have regained some degree of sensitivity to zidovudine. Strains of HIV resistant to didanosine are generally also resistant to zalcitabine.

The standard dose of didanosine is 200 mg twice a day for patients over 60 kg and 100 mg twice a day for patients under 60 kg. Didanosine is best absorbed on an empty stomach at a neutral pH. For this reason the current formulations of didanosine contain a buffer and each dose must be administered in no less than two tablets. Thus, a patient who requires 100 mg twice a day, should take two 50-mg tablets twice a day rather than one 100-mg tablet twice a day.

The toxicity profile of didanosine is quite different from that of zidovudine. The most frequent toxicity of didanosine is a painful sensory peripheral neuropathy that occurs in approximately 30 percent of patients receiving doses above 200 mg twice a day. This generally resolves with discontinuation of drug and may not recur when patients are retreated at a reduced dose. The other major toxicity is pancreatitis; it was reported to occur in 9 percent of patients in the early clinical trials, although the frequency was somewhat less in later studies using lower doses. Pancreatitis can be fatal, and for this reason all patients receiving didanosine should be monitored carefully. Didanosine should be discontinued if a patient experiences abdominal pain consistent with pancreatitis or elevated amylase and/or lipase and edematous pancreas on ultrasound. These patients should not be retreated and, as a general rule, didanosine is contraindicated for a patient with a prior history of pancreatitis, regardless of etiology. Didanosine has minimal effects on the bone marrow and can be given

in combination with bone marrow toxic drugs such as zidovudine, ganciclovir, or trimethoprim/sulfamethoxazole.

Zalcitabine (ddC, 2',3'-dideoxycytidine) is the third drug currently licensed for treatment of HIV infection. In contrast to zidovudine and didanosine, zalcitabine is not licensed for use as monotherapy and is only licensed as part of a combination regimen with zidovudine. This is a reflection of the results of the initial clinical trials designed to assess the efficacy of zalcitabine in the therapy of HIV infection. A direct comparison of zalcitabine to zidovudine was stopped prematurely when it was noted that there were significantly more deaths occurring in the zalcitabine-treated group (59 vs. 33). In a separate trial, however, the combination of zalcitabine with zidovudine was shown to cause greater and more sustained elevations in CD4 + T cell counts than zidovudine alone. Based upon these results, zalcitabine (0.75 mg/kg three times a day) was licensed as part of a combination regimen with zidovudine (200 mg three times a day) for patients with advanced HIV infection. Similar to didanosine, the main toxicity is a reversible peripheral neuropathy. While cases of pancreatitis have been reported in patients receiving zalcitabine, it has not been seen to the same degree as that reported with didanosine. Nonetheless, zalcitabine is also contraindicated in patients with a prior history of pancreatitis. The precise role of the zidovudine/zalcitabine combination regimen in the treatment of HIV infection has yet to be established, although some experts choose this regimen as initial therapy for patients with HIV infection who present with less than 200 CD4 + T cells per microliter, while others add zalcitabine to zidovudine monotherapy in patients showing an immunologic or clinical decline.

Stavudine (d4T,2',3'-didehydro-3'-deoxythymidine) is another nucleoside analogue. This agent is currently available for use under an expanded access program and thus formal approval is anticipated. Stavudine has an activity profile comparable to that of zidovudine in preclinical studies. Thus far, clinical trials have demonstrated that stavudine therapy is associated with increases in CD4 + T cell counts, declines in p24 antigen levels, and an improved sense of well being. In contrast to zidovudine, stavudine appears to have minimal myelosuppressive toxicity. Peripheral neuropathy and elevations in SGPT have been the primary toxicities observed to date. At present, stavudine is available only directly from the manufacturer (1-800-842-8036), and its use is limited to patients who are unable to take either zidovudine or didanosine because of intolerance or clinical failure.

One strategy for the institution of antiretroviral therapy is as follows: withhold therapy and follow patients with CD + T cell counts greater than 500 per microliter. As mentioned, active virus replication occurs throughout HIV infection, and theoretically it would be justifiable to begin therapy as soon as the diagnosis is made, as some clinicians do. However, given the toxicity of the available retroviral agents and the potential for the development of resistance to antivirals, therapy at this stage is not recommended. However, it is also acceptable to observe patients at this level who are asymptomatic and to begin therapy only if symptoms appear. If clinical or laboratory evidence of disease progression is present in patients who have been receiving single-agent zidovudine, the options include switching to didanosine or adding either it or zalcitabine to the zidovudine. If intolerance to any of these drugs or clinical progression occurs, stavudine can be obtained through the expanded access program and substituted for one of the drugs in the combination. One may consider combination therapy from the outset for patients who present with less than 200 CD4 + T cells per microliter. These options are outlined in Fig. 279-25.

A large number of experimental agents are being evaluated as possible therapies for HIV infection. Therapeutic strategies are being directed at virtually every step of the viral life cycle (Fig. 279-3). In addition, as more is learned about the role of the immune system in controlling viral replication, additional strategies, generically referred to as *immune-based therapies* are being developed. Among the antiviral agents in early clinical trials are additional nucleoside analogues, nucleotide analogues, nonnucleoside reverse transcriptase

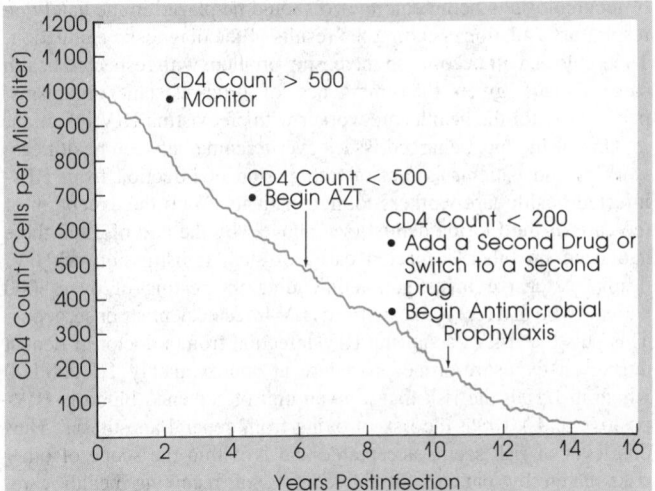

FIGURE 279-25 One possible strategy for the management of patients with HIV infection. In the early stages of illness, as long as the CD4 count is above 500 cells per cubic millimeter observation is the rule. Once the count falls below that level, therapy is initiated with a single agent, usually AZT. However, observation alone is acceptable if patients remain asymptomatic at this level of CD4 count. Combination therapy is given to the patient with more advanced disease, or the patient showing progression while on AZT alone.

inhibitors, *tat* inhibitors, protease inhibitors, and antisense nucleic acids. Among the immune-based therapies being tried are IFN-α, bone marrow transplantation with adoptive transfer of lymphocytes, active immunotherapy with subunit envelope vaccines or autologous cells genetically engineered to express viral proteins, passive immunotherapy with inactivated anti-HIV antisera or monoclonal antibodies, and IL-2. In addition, clinical trials are planned employing the techniques of molecular biology to combat HIV infection through the infusion of cells genetically modified to resist infection with HIV.

TREATMENT OF SECONDARY INFECTIONS, KAPOSI'S SARCOMA, AND LYMPHOMAS Treatment guidelines are outlined in Tables 279-19 and 279-21 and discussed in detail in the sections dealing with the secondary infections and neoplastic complications of HIV infection.

PROPHYLAXIS AGAINST SECONDARY INFECTIONS Enhanced survival and improved quality of life for patients with HIV infection can be traced not only to the introduction of zidovudine and related compounds but also to improved regimens for preventing secondary infections. As a result, the clinical profile of HIV-infected patients is continually evolving as immunodeficient patients live longer and at less risk of formerly inevitable problems such as PCP. Because certain secondary infections occur with predictability only when the competence of the immune system, as measured by the CD4+ T cell count, declines below a certain level, this knowledge can be used to help devise effective strategies for minimizing these risks.

PCP rarely occurs before the CD4+ T cell count drops below 200 cells per microliter or before the CD4 percent declines below 15 percent. At this point, patients should be started on a regimen of PCP prophylaxis. The preferred regimen, for patients able to tolerate it, is trimethoprim/sulfamethoxazole at a dose of 1 double-strength tablet twice a day. Another benefit of trimethoprim/sulfamethoxazole as a prophylaxis regimen is that it also provides protection against toxoplasmosis as well as certain bacterial infections. Alternate strategies for pneumocystis prophylaxis including atovoquone and clindamycin/pyrimethamine are currently being evaluated for patients who are sulfa intolerant. Aerosolized pentamidine remains an option for those unable to tolerate any systemic therapy.

Another opportunistic infection for which primary prophylaxis is clearly indicated is MAC. This infection is extremely common among

patients in the United States but is rarely seen with CD4+ T cell counts above 100 cells per microliter. Rifabutin, 100 mg/d, was effective in a clinical trial in delaying the onset of MAC bacteremia by an average of 6 months. Based upon these data, rifabutin has been licensed for use as a primary prophylaxis for MAC infection in patients with HIV infection and less than 100 CD4+ T cells per microliter.

Given the resurgence of tuberculosis in the HIV-infected population, any patient with HIV infection and at least 5 mm of induration on PPD skin testing should receive a 1-year course of isoniazid. In addition, any patient with HIV infection who is anergic and at high risk of tuberculosis should be given a year of isoniazid. These measures could be quite effective not only in helping the individual patient but also in curtailing the spread of tuberculosis in the community.

Patients with HIV infection are at increased risk for infection with encapsulated bacteria, particularly *H. influenzae* and *S. pneumoniae*. For this reason patients with HIV infection and especially patients in whom splenectomy is being considered should be vaccinated with the pneumococcal polysaccharide and *H. influenzae* type b vaccines.

While no generally accepted guidelines exist, many physicians recommend primary prophylaxis against cryptococcal and candidal infections with fluconazole; clinical trials of a candidate cryptococcal vaccine are underway. In addition, clinical trials are being conducted to evaluate the role of intermittent clindamycin/pyrimethamine as primary prophylaxis for toxoplasmosis in patients unable to tolerate trimethoprim/sulfamethoxazole and to evaluate the role of CMV IgG to prevent CMV reactivation syndromes.

Secondary prophylaxis, the prevention of second or subsequent episodes of a given infection, is indicated for virtually every opportunistic infection experienced by the patient with AIDS. These infections are usually impossible to eradicate and, with the exception of tuberculosis, life-long therapy or secondary prophylaxis is the rule (see Table 279-19). It is obvious that as the number of medications given to an individual patient increases, the chance for untoward drug reactions and interactions to occur increases. Thus, patients must be monitored carefully for such reactions. However, with the judicious use of prophylactic regimens a significant improvement in the quality of life for the patient with HIV infection and advanced immunodeficiency is clearly possible.

HIV AND THE HEALTH CARE WORKER

There is a small but definite risk that a health care worker, especially one who deals with large numbers of HIV-infected patients, may become infected with HIV in the course of his/her work (see "Occupational Transmission of HIV" above). By 1991, there had been a total of 27 well-documented seroconversions in health care workers that occurred as a direct result of exposure to contaminated blood or bloody body fluids. Twenty of these were due to a needle stick injury, two were due to cuts with contaminated objects, two were large mucous membrane exposures, two were felt to be the result of exposure of known open wounds to contaminated blood, and one was the the result of repeated and extensive cutaneous exposure to blood and body fluids. Twenty-four of these accidents involved blood, one involved bloody pleural fluid, and two involved concentrated virus stocks. In addition, another 109 HIV-infected health care workers had been identified with no identifiable risk for HIV infection other than occupational exposure. Taken together, the data from several large studies suggest that the risk of HIV infection following a percutaneous injury with an HIV-contaminated hollow-bore needle (in contrast to a solid bore, i.e., suture, needle) is approximately 0.3 percent. A seroprevalence survey conducted in May, 1991, of 3420 orthopedic surgeons, 75 percent of whom practiced in an area with a relatively high HIV infection rate and 39 percent of whom reported percutaneous exposure to patient blood, failed to reveal any cases of possible occupational infection, suggesting that the risk of infection with a suture needle may be considerably less than that with a blood-drawing needle.

The majority of cases of health care worker seroconversions occur as a result of needle stick injuries. When one considers the circumstances that result in needle stick injuries, it is immediately obvious that adhering to the standard guidelines for dealing with sharp objects would result in a significant decrease in this sort of accident. In this regard, in one study, 27 percent of needlestick injuries were the result of improper disposal of the needle (over half of these were due to recapping the needle), 23 percent occurred while attempting to start an intravenous line, 22 percent occurred during blood drawing, 16 percent were associated with an intramuscular or subcutaneous injection, and 12 percent were associated with giving an intravenous infusion.

The best management for a percutaneous injury with a needle contaminated with blood from a patient with HIV infection is a debated subject. While all agree that the wound should be immediately cleansed and antiseptic applied, the role of zidovudine prophylaxis is unclear. Among the arguments against the use of zidovudine are the fact that three separate SIV primate studies have failed to show any evidence of protection, that protection has been seen in the feline leukemia virus model only when the drug is given prior to exposure, that there are multiple anecdotes of health care workers who have serconverted despite immediately beginning zidovudine prophylaxis, and that the side effects of zidovudine are considerable. In one study, 70 percent of health care workers taking zidovudine for postexposure prophylaxis reported one or more side effects, particularly nausea, malaise, and headache. Arguments in favor of zidovudine prophylaxis are that the risk of a serious side effect is minimal while the potential benefit is great, and that if infection were to occur the patient would have started therapy at the earliest possible point in time. The ultimate decision must be individualized and reached after careful discussion between the injured health care worker and his/her physician. Since zidovudine prophylaxis, if it is going to be given, should probably be started as soon as possible (within 2 to 4 h) after the injury, health care workers at potential risk should think beforehand about what they would do if they were to be in this position.

There are several things health care workers can do to minimize their risk of an occupational HIV infection. These are listed in the July, 1991, CDC guidelines and include: adherence to universal precautions; refraining from direct patient care if one has exudative lesions or weeping dermatitis; and disinfecting and sterilizing reusable devices employed in invasive procedures. The premise of universal precautions is that each and every specimen should be handled as if it came from someone infected with a blood-borne pathogen. In this regard, all samples should be double bagged, gloves should be worn when drawing blood, and spills should be immediately disinfected with bleach.

In attempting to put this small but definite risk to the health care worker in perspective, it is important to point out that approximately 200 health care workers die each year as a result of occupationally acquired hepatitis B infection. The tragedy in this instance is that these infections and deaths due to hepatitis B could be greatly decreased by more extended use of the hepatitis B vaccine. The risk of hepatitis B infection following a needle stick injury from an antigen-positive patient is much higher than the risk of HIV infection (see "Transmission," above). There are multiple examples of needle stick injuries where the patient was positive for both hepatitis B and HIV and the health care worker became infected only with hepatitis B. For these reasons it is advisable, given the high prevalence of hepatitis B infection in patients with HIV infection, that all health care workers dealing with HIV-infected patients be immunized with the hepatitis B vaccine.

Tuberculosis is another infection common to patients with HIV infection that can be transmitted to the health care worker. For this reason, all health care workers should know their PPD status, have it checked yearly, and receive a year of isoniazid (INH) should their skin test become positive. In addition, all patients in whom a diagnosis

of tuberculosis is being entertained should be placed immediately on respiratory isolation, pending the results of the diagnostic evaluation. Tuberculosis will become an increasing problem with respect to health care workers given the emergence of drug-resistant organisms, particularly for the health care worker with preexisting HIV infection.

One of the most charged issues ever to come between health care workers and patients is that of tranmission of infection from HIV-infected health care workers to their patients. With the exception of the case of the Florida dentist (see above), by the end of 1992 there had been no other suspected cases of such transmission of HIV, despite extensive investigation inlcuding the testing of over 8000 patients who had received care from HIV-infected dentists or surgeons. This puts the risk of acquiring HIV infection from a doctor or dentist during an exposure-prone procedure at approximately 1/1,000,000 which is 1/10th the risk that a given unit of screened blood is HIV-positive and 1/100th the risk of dying from general anesthesia. Thus this level of risk seems acceptable and is within the scope of other risks taken by patients in the context of receiving health care. Theoretically, the same universal precautions that are being used to protect the health care worker from the patient with HIV infection will also protect the patient from the HIV-infected health care worker.

VACCINES

Given the fact that human behavior, especially human sexual behavior, is extremely difficult to change, the best hope for preventing the spread of HIV infection rests with the development of a safe and effective vaccine. This task is extremely problematic for a number of reasons, including the high degree of mutability of the virus, the fact that the infection can be transmitted by cell-free or cell-associated virus, and the likely need for the development of effective mucosal immunity. However, studies using animal models have been encouraging (see below). It should be pointed out that while the ideal goal of a vaccine for HIV is to prevent infection, a vaccine that does not necessarily prevent infection but significantly alters the course of disease after a person gets infected also may have a major impact on public health.

Preclinical work in the area of vaccine development has been greatly facilitated through the use of animal models of lentivirus infections. Perhaps the most useful model to date has been the simian immunodeficiency virus (SIV) infection of rhesus monkeys. SIV, a lentivirus that is closely related to HIV-2 and differs from HIV-1 in that it lacks the *vpu* gene and contains the *vpx* gene, causes an acute infection that leads to immunodeficiency, secondary injection, and death when administered to susceptible animals. Studies by several groups have clearly demonstrated that infection can be prevented by prior immunization of animals with either inactivated virus, recombinant vaccinia virus expressing the SIV envelope followed by a booster immunization with recombinant protein, or attenuated virus lacking the *nef* gene. Even in other studies using antigens that did not confer protection from infection, the clinical course following infection appeared to be delayed. Of note is the fact that in those studies demonstrating protection it has not always been obvious what components of the immune response were conferring the protection. In fact, in the studies of inactivated virus it has been shown that the protective elements of the immune response were not directed toward components of the virus at all but toward components of the cells used in growing up the viral stocks. These data suggest that antibodies to certain cell surface proteins that participate in SIV binding may provide excellent protection against infection, a hypothesis that have been supported in studies of CD4-immunized monkeys. While the protection studies carried out with envelope-expressing recombinant vaccinia virus and recombinant envelope boosting point to an immune response to the envelope as potentially protective there is still much to be learned with respect to the correlates of immunity involved in protection against infection and/or disease.

The only suitable animal model for HIV infection is the chimpanzee. However, this model has significant drawbacks in that chimpanzees are expensive, they are an endangered species, and although they can be infected with HIV, they do not develop disease. Thus unless a candidate vaccine prevents infection in this model, its overall impact on disease progression cannot be assessed. Most recently, however, immunization of chimps with either whole inactivated virus followed by protein or peptide boosting or with recombinant envelope proteins has been shown to confer protection against infection with HIV-1. These data from animal models suggest the feasibility of inducing at least partial protection against HIV infection in man by vaccination.

While awaiting clear signals from the preclinical animal work, clinical trials of candidate vaccines have nonetheless begun in man. In this regard both recombinant envelope proteins and recombinant vaccinia viruses expressing HIV envelope have been demonstrated to be safe and immunogenic in healthy uninfected volunteers. Certain of these vaccines are also being tested as forms of active immunotherapy in patients who are already infected. At present, one can state with a fair degree of certainty that humans can safely be immunized to several of the antigens of HIV and it is only a matter of time until one or more of these vaccine candidates will be tested in a vaccine efficacy trial. It is clear, however, that it will take several years of clinical trials to establish the efficacy or lack thereof of a candidate vaccine for HIV.

PREVENTION

Education, counseling, and behavior modification are the cornerstones of prevention of HIV infection. Widespread voluntary testing of individuals in whom there is any possibility that they had been or are in a high-risk behavior situation, together with counseling of infected individuals, should prove helpful in behavioral modification programs for infected individuals who might otherwise have been unaware of their HIV status and who could infect their sexual partners. In uninfected and infected individuals, the practice of safe sex is the most effective way to avoid contracting and spreading HIV infection. Abstinence from sexual relations is the only absolute way to prevent sexual transmission. However, this may not be feasible, and so there are a number of relatively safe practices that can markedly decrease the chances of transmission of HIV infection. Partners engaged in monogamous sexual relationships who wish to be assured of safety should both be tested for HIV antibody. It must be understood that any divergence from the monogamous nature of the relationship by either party puts both parties at risk; therefore, open discussions regarding the importance of honesty in such relationships should be encouraged by counseling parties. Where the HIV status of either of the partners is not known, there are a number of options. Use of condoms preferably together with the HIV-inhibiting spermatacide nonoxynol-9 can markedly decrease the chance of transmission of HIV. It should be remembered that condoms are not 100 percent effective in preventing transmission of HIV infection, and there is an approximately 10 percent failure rate of condoms used for contraceptive purposes. Most condom failures result from breakage or improper usage. Latex condoms are preferable as virus has been shown to leak through natural skin condoms. Petroleum-based gels should never be used for lubrication of the condom as they increase the likelihood of condom rupture. Nontraumatic mutual masturbation is considered safe provided there is no ingestion of semen, vaginal secretions, or other potentially infected body fluids. Kissing is considered safe although there remains the theoretical possibility of transmission via virus contained in saliva if saliva is exchanged.

The most effective way to prevent transmission of HIV infection among IVDUs is to stop the use of injecting drugs. Unfortunately, since addiction to injecting drugs is an illness, it is extremely difficult to accomplish this without entering the addict into a treatment program. For those who will not or cannot do so and who will continue to inject drugs, the avoidance of sharing of needles and other paraphernalia ("works") is the next best way to avoid transmission of infection. The cultural and social factors that contribute to the sharing

of paraphernalia are complex and difficult to overcome. In addition, needles and syringes may be in short supply, adding to the imperative to share. Under these curcumstances, works should be cleaned after each usage with a virucidal solution such as undiluted sodium hypochlorite (household bleach). Certain countries in Western Europe as well as certain communities in the United States have adopted programs of providing free needles and syringes in exchange for used paraphernalia. It is important for IVDUs to be tested for HIV infection and counseled in order to avoid transmission of HIV to their sexual partners. This form of transmission has increased greatly in the United States (see above).

Prevention of HIV transmission through tranfused blood or blood products has been dramatically decreased by a combination of screening of all blood donors for HIV infection as well as self-deferral of individuals who may be at risk for HIV infection. In addition, clotting factor concentrates are heat treated. Autologous tranfusions are preferable to transfusions from another individual. However, logistic contraints as well as the unpredictability of the need for most transfusions lessen the feasibility of this approach.

HIV can be transmitted via breast milk and colostrum. The avoidance of breast feeding may not be practical in developing countries where nutritional concerns override the risk of HIV transmission. However, in countries such as the United States where there is an option to breast feeding, bottled formula and milk should be used when a mother is HIV positive.

REFERENCES

AIDS in New York State. New York State Department of Health, 1991

ANDERSON RE et al: Use of ß2-microglobulin level and CD4 lymphocyte count to predict development of acquired immunodeficiency syndrome in persons with human immunodeficiency virus infection. Arch Intern Med 150:73, 1990

BERAL V et al: Kaposi's sarcoma among persons with AIDS: A sexually transmitted infection? Lancet 2:123, 1990

BHAT S et al: Galactosyl ceramide or a derivative is an essential component of the neural receptor for human immunodeficiency virus type 1 envelope glycoprotein gp120. Proc Natl Acad Sci USA 88:7131, 1991

BUSCH MP et al: Evaluation of screened blood donations for human immunodeficiency virus type I infection by culture and DNA amplification of pooled cells. N Engl J Med 325:1, 1991

CAMERON PU et al: Dendritic cells exposed to human immunodeficiency virus type-1 transmit a vigorous cytopathic effect to CD4+ T cells. Science 257:383, 1992

CEASE KB et al: Helper T cell antigenic site identification in the acquired immunodeficiency syndrome virus gp120 envelope protein and induction of immunity in mice to the native protein using a 16-residue synthetic peptide. Proc Natl Acad Sci USA 84:4249, 1987

CENTERS FOR DISEASE CONTROL: *National HIV Seroprevalence Surveys—Summary of Results: Data from seroprevalence activities through 1989.* DHHS publication # HIV/CID/9-90-006

———: *National HIV Serosurveillance Summary,* vol. 2. *Results through 1990.* DHHS publication # HIV/NCID/11-91/011

CHIN J: Global estimates of HIV infection and AIDS cases: 1991. AIDS 5 (suppl 2): S57, 1991

CIESIELSKI C et al: Transmission of human immunodeficiency virus in a dental practice. Ann Intern Med 116:798, 1992

CLERICI M et al: Interleukin-2 production used to detect antigenic peptide recognition by T-helper lymphocytes from asymptomatic HIV-seropositive individuals. Nature 339:383, 1989

COLLIER AC et al: Central nervous system manifestations in human immunodeficiency virus infection without AIDS. J Acquir Immune Defic Synd 5:229, 1992

COOMBS RW et al: Plasma viremia in human immunodeficiency virus infection. N Engl J Med 321:1626, 1989

DAGLEISH AG et al: Neutralization of diverse HIV-1 strains by monoclonal antibodies raised against a gp41 synthetic peptide. Virology 165:209, 1988

DAVEY RT, HC LANE: Laboratory methods in the diagnosis and prognostic staging of infection with human immunodeficiency virus type 1. Rev Inf Dis 12:912, 1990

ENSOLI B et al: Cytokines and growth factors in the pathogenesis of AIDS-associated Kaposi's sarcoma. Immunol Rev 127:147, 1992

EPSTEIN LG, GENDELMAN HE: Human immunodeficiency virus type 1 infection of the nervous system: Pathogenic mechanisms. Ann Neurol 33:429, 1993

EUROPEAN COLLABORATIVE STUDY: Children born to women with HIV-1 infection: Natural history and risk of infection. Lancet 337:253, 1991

FAUCI AS: CD4+ T lymphocytopenia without HIV infection—no lights, no camera, just facts. N Engl J Med 328:429, 1993

FISCHL MA et al: Safety and efficacy of sulfamethoxazole and trimethoprim chemoprophylaxis for *Pneumocystis carinii* pneumonia in AIDS. JAMA 259:1185, 1988

GAYLE HD et al: Prevalence of the human immunodeficiency virus among university students. N Engl J Med 323:1538, 1990

GELDERBLOM HR: Assembly and morphology of HIV: potential effect of structure on viral function. AIDS 5:617, 1991

GREENE WC: The molecular biology of human immunodeficiency virus type I infection. N Engl J Med 324:308, 1991

GREENSPAN D et al: Relation of oral hairy leukoplakia to infection with the human immunodeficiency virus and risk of developing AIDS. J Infect Dis 155:475, 1987

HAYNES BF: Scientific and social issues of human immunodeficiency virus vaccine development. Science 260:1279, 1993

HIRSCH MS, D'AQUILA RT: Therapy for human immunodeficiency virus infection. N Engl J Med 328:1686, 1993

HOLLANDER H, STRINGARI S: Human immunodeficiency virus associated meningitis. Am J Med 83:813, 1987

ITESCU S et al: A sicca syndrome in HIV infection: Association with HLA-DR5 and CD8 lymphocytosis. Lancet 466, 1989

JOHNSTON MI, HOTH DF: Present status and future prospects for HIV therapies. Science 260:1286, 1993

KARON JM et al: Projections of the number of persons diagnosed with AIDS and the number of immunosuppressed HIV-infected persons—United States. Morb Mort Wk Rep 41:1, 1993

KARZON DT et al: Development of a vaccine for the prevention of AIDS. A critical appraisal. Vaccine 10:1039, 1992

KAYE BR: Rheumatologic manifestations of infection with human immunodeficiency virus (HIV). Ann Intern Med 111:158, 1989

KLEIN RS et al: Oral candidiasis in high-risk patients as the initial manifestation of the acquired immunodeficiency syndrome. N Engl J Med 311:354, 1984

KRAMER A et al: Neopterin: A predictive marker of acquired immune deficiency syndrome in human immunodeficiency virus infection. J Acquir Immune Defic Synd 2:291, 1989

KROWN SE et al: Kaposi's sarcoma in the acquired immunodeficiency syndrome: A proposal for a uniform evaluation, response and staging criteria. J Clin Oncol 7:1201, 1989

LINDGREN S et al: HIV and child-bearing: Clinical outcome and aspects of mother-to-infant transmission. AIDS 5:1111, 1991

MASUR H et al: CD4 counts as predictors of opportunistic pneumonias in human immunodeficiency virus (HIV) infection. Ann Intern Med 111:223, 1989

MATSUSHITA S et al: Characterization of a human immunodeficiency virus neutralizing monoclonal antibody and mapping of the neutralizing epitope. J Virol 62:2107, 1988

McARTHUR JC: Neurologic manifestations of AIDS. Medicine 66:407, 1987

McNEIL JG et al: Trends of HIV seroconversion among young adults in the US Army, 1985 to 1989. JAMA 265:1709, 1991

MELBYE M et al: Risk of AIDS after herpes zoster. Lancet I:728, 1987

MILES SA et al: AIDS Kaposi sarcoma-derived cells produce and respond to interleukin 6. Proc Natl Acad Sci USA 87:4068, 1990

Monthly vital statistics report. Final data from the National Center for Health Statistics 40:1, 1992. DHHS publication # (PHS) 92-1120

MOSS AR et al: Seropositivity for HIV and the development of AIDS or AIDS related conditions: Three year follow-up of the San Francisco General cohort. Br Med J 296:745, 1988

MUSHER DM et al: Syphilis, the response to penicillin therapy, neurosyphilis and the effect of human immunodeficiency virus infection. Ann Intern Med 113:872, 1990

NAVI BA et al: Cerebral toxoplasmosis complicating the acquired immunodeficiency syndrome: Clinical and neuropathological findings in 27 patients. Ann Neurol 19:224, 1986

PADIAN NS et al: Female-to-male transmission of human immunodeficiency virus. JAMA 266:1664, 1991

PANTALEO G et al: HIV infection is active and progressive in lymphoid tissue during the clinically latent stage of disease. Nature 362:355, 1993

———: The immunopathogenesis of human immunodeficiency virus infection. N Engl J Med 328:327, 1993

PIZZO PA, BUTLER KM: In the vertical transmission of AIDS, timing is everything. N Engl J Med 325:652, 1991

PLATANIAS LC et al: Thrombotic thrombocytopenic purpura as the first manifestation of human immunodeficiency virus infection. Am J Med 87:699, 1989

POLI G, FAUCI AS: The effect of cytokines and pharmacologic agents on chronic HIV infection. AIDS Res Hum Retrovirus 8:191, 1992

POLK BF et al: Predictors of the acquired immunodeficiency syndrome developing in a cohort of seropositive homosexual men. N Engl J Med 316:61, 1987

RATNER L: Human immunodeficiency virus-associated autoimmune thrombocytopenic purpura: A review. Am J Med 86:194, 1989

RAVIGLIONE MC: Extrapulmonary pneumocystosis: The first 50 cases. Rev Inf Dis 12:1127, 1990

ROBINSON WE et al: Two immunodominant domains of gp41 bind antibodies which enhance human immunodeficiency virus type I infection in vitro. J Virol 65:4169, 1991

ROOK AH et al: Interleukin-2 enhances the depressed natural killer and cytomegalovirus specific activities of lymphocytes from patients with the acquired immune deficiency syndrome. J Clin Invest 72:398, 1982

ROSENBERG PS et al: Population-based monitoring of an urban HIV/AIDS epidemic. Magnitude and trends in the District of Columbia. JAMA 268:495, 1992

ROSENBERG ZF, FAUCI AS: Immunopathogenesis of human immunodeficiency virus infection. Adv Immunol 47:377, 1989

———, ———: Immunology of HIV infection, in *Immunology*, 2d ed, WE Paul (ed). New York, Raven, in press

SAFAI B et al: Spectrum of Kaposi's sarcoma in the epidemic of AIDS. Cancer Res 45:466s, 1985

SATTLER FR, FEINBERG J: New developments in the treatment of *Pneumocystis carinii* pneumonia. Chest 101:451, 1992

SCHRIER RD et al: B and T lymphocyte responses to an immunodominant epitope of human immunodeficiency virus. J Virol 62:2531, 1988

SCHWARTZ JS et al: Human immunodeficiency virus test: Evaluation, performance and use. JAMA 259:2574, 1988

SELIK RM et al: HIV infection as leading cause of death among young adults in US cities and states. JAMA 269:2991, 1993

SIMMS RW et al: Fibromyalgia syndrome in patients infected with human immunodeficiency virus. Am J Med 92:368, 1992

STEIN M et al: Causes of death in patients with human immunodeficiency virus infection. Am J Med 93:387, 1992

STEINMAN RM: The dendritic cell system and its role in immunogenicity. Ann Rev Immunol 9:271, 1991

ST. LOUIS ME et al: Human immunodeficiency virus infection in disadvantaged adolescents. Findings from the US Job Corps. JAMA 266:2387, 1991

TINDAL B, COOPER DA: Primary HIV infection: Host responses and intervention strategies. AIDS 5:1, 1991

WAKEFIELD AE et al: DNA amplification on induced sputum samples for diagnosis of *Pneumocystis carinii* pneumonia. Lancet 337:1378, 1991

WALKER BD et al: HIV specific cytotoxic T lymphocytes in seropositive individuals. Nature 328:345, 1987

WALKER CM et al: CD8 + lymphocytes can control HIV infection in vitro by suppressing virus replication. Science 234:1563, 1986

WEINHOLD KJ et al: Cellular anti-gp120 cytolytic reactivities in HIV-1 seropositive individuals. Lancet 1:902, 1988

WEISS RA: How does HIV cause AIDS? Science 260:1273, 1993

WENIGER BG et al: The epidemiology of HIV infection and AIDS in Thailand. AIDS 5 (suppl 2): S71, 1991

280 PLASMA CELL DISORDERS

DAN L. LONGO

GENERAL PRINCIPLES The *plasma cell disorders* are monoclonal neoplasms related to each other by virtue of their development from common progenitors in the B lymphocyte lineage. Multiple myeloma, Waldenström's macroglobulinemia, primary amyloidosis (see Chap. 281), and the heavy chain diseases comprise this group and may be designated by a variety of synonyms such as *monoclonal gammopathies*, *paraproteinemias*, *plasma cell dyscrasias*, and *dysproteinemias*. A schema for the normal development of B lymphocytes is depicted in Fig. 280-1. Mature B lymphocytes destined to produce IgG bear surface immunoglobulin molecules of both M and G heavy chain isotypes with both isotypes having identical idiotypes (variable regions). Under normal circumstances, maturation to antibody-secreting plasma cells is stimulated by exposure to the antigen for which the surface immunoglobulin is specific; however, in the plasma cell disorders the control over this process is lost. The clinical manifestations of all the plasma cell disorders relate to the expansion of the neoplastic cells, to the secretion of cell products (immunoglobulin molecules or subunits, lymphokines), and to some extent to the host's response to the tumor.

There are three categories of structural variation among immunoglobulin molecules that form antigenic determinants, and these are used to classify immunoglobulins (Chap. 277). *Isotypes* are those determinants that distinguish among the main classes of antibodies of a given species and are the same in all normal individuals of that species. Therefore, isotypic determinants are, by definition, recognized by antibodies from a distinct species (heterologous sera) but not by antibodies from the same species (homologous sera). There are five heavy chain isotypes (M, G, A, D, E) and two light chain isotypes (kappa, lambda). *Allotypes* are distinct determinants that reflect regular small differences between individuals of the same species in the amino acid sequences of otherwise similar immunoglobulins. These differences are determined by allelic genes, and by definition, they are detected by antibodies made in the same species. *Idiotypes* are the third category of antigenic determinants. They are unique to the molecules produced by a given clone of antibody-producing cells. Idiotypes are formed by the unique structure of the antigen-binding portion of the molecule.

Antibody molecules (see Fig. 280-2) are composed of two heavy chains (mol wt ~50,000) and two light chains (mol wt ~25,000). Each chain has a constant portion (limited amino acid sequence variability) and a variable region (extensive sequence variability).

Unclassified
ALL

Pre–B ALL

Burkitt's

Follicular/Diffuse Lymphomas

IgM ± IgG
or
IgG

TdT

TdT
HCR

TdT
HCR
κR or D

HCR
λ R or D

IgM

IgM

IgM

IgD

IgM

IgG

IgG

HLA–DR⁺
CD19⁺
CD20⁺
CD22⁺/–
CD21⁺/–

Follicular Center B Cells

HLA–DR⁺
CD19⁺

HLA–DR⁺
CD19⁺
CD10⁺

HLA–DR⁺
CD19⁺
CD10⁺
CD20⁺
CD22⁺

HLA–DR⁺
CD19⁺
CD20⁺
CD22⁺
CD21⁺

HLA–DR⁺
CD19⁺
CD20⁺
CD22⁺
CD21⁺

HLA–DR⁺
CD19⁺
CD20⁺
CD22⁺
CD21⁺

| Lymphoid Stem Cell | Early B Cells | Intermediate B Cells | Mature B Cell |

Waldenstrom's

IgM

Multiple Myeloma

CD19⁺/–
CD20⁺
CD38⁺

CD38⁺
PCA-1⁺

Secretory B Cells

DIDL

IgM

CLL
SL

IgM ± IgD

IgD

HLA–DR⁺
CD19⁺
CD10⁺/–
CD20⁺
CD22⁺
CD21⁺
CD5⁺

HLA–DR⁺
CD19⁺
CD20⁺
CD22⁺/–
CD21⁺
CD5⁺

Mantle Zone B Cells

Antigen-Independent Differentiation

Antigen-Driven Differentiation

FIGURE 280-1 Schematic representation of the pathway of differentiation of normal B cells. HLA-DR, CD10, CD19, CD20, CD21, CD22, CD5, and CD38 are cell markers used to distinguish stages of development. Terminal transferase (TdT) is a cellular enzyme. Immunoglobulin heavy chain gene rearrangement (HCR) and light chain gene rearrangement or deletion (kappa R or D, lambda R or D) occur early in B cell development. The approximate stage of differentiation arrest for each B cell lymphoproliferative disorder is shown. The following abbreviations are used: ALL, acute lymphoblastic leukemia; CLL, chronic lymphocytic leukemia; DIDL, diffuse intermediately differentiated lymphocytic lymphoma; SLL, small lymphocytic lymphoma. The mantle zone B cells give rise to CLL and DIDL, but the relationship between this lineage and follicular center B cells is not yet clear.

The light and heavy chains are linked by disulfide bonds and are aligned so that their variable regions are adjacent to one another. This variable region forms the antigen recognition site of the antibody molecule; its unique structural features form a particular set of determinants, or idiotypes, that are reliable markers for a particular clone of cells because each antibody is formed and secreted by a single clone. Each chain is specified by distinct genes, synthesized separately, and assembled into an intact antibody molecule after

FIGURE 280-2 Schematic depiction of an IgG molecule. Each molecule consists of two heavy and two light chains linked by disulfide bonds. There are two types of light chains, kappa (genes on chromosome 2) and lambda (chromosome 22), each containing two domains. There are 10 types of heavy chains: 4 types of G (G1 to G4), 2 of A (A1, A2), 2 of M (M1, M2), and 1 each of D and E (all on chromosome 14), each with four domains. A domain is 100 to 110 amino acids in length. Within each domain is an intrachain disulfide bond that produces a loop. V_H (variable domain of the heavy chain) and V_L (variable domain of the light chain) form an antigen binding site whose unique determinants form an idiotype. Immunoglobulins of the same isotype (e.g., IgG1κ) differ between individuals. The determinants that distinguish them are called allotypic determinants and are located on C_L (constant domain of the light chain) and C_{H2} (second constant domain of the heavy chain). C_{H2} is also the main site of glycosylation (CHO) and complement binding. Papain cleaves the molecule into antigen-binding (Fab) and crystallizable (Fc) components. The portion of the heavy chain in an Fab fragment is called the Fd piece. Fc receptors on cells bind to the C_{H3} domain. IgM and IgA occur as polymers and each unit of two heavy and two light chains is connected by a J (joining) chain. The heavy chain isotypes determine the function of the antibody.

Fab

V_L

C_L

V_H

C_{H1}

Antigen Binding Site
(idiotype)

S-S

S-S

PAPAIN
CLEAVAGE

HINGE
REGION

S-S
S-S

C_{H2}

C_{H3}

CHO

Determines biologic activity;
contains allotype and
heavy chain class and
subclass determinates

Fc

FIGURE 280-3 Immunoglobulin heavy chains are encoded by four distinct genetic elements, variable (Igh-V), diversity (Igh-D), joining (Igh-J), and constant (Igh-C) genes. The variable region of the immunoglobulin heavy chain is encoded by the V, D, and J genes. The same variable region may be associated with any of the 10 heavy chain constant region genes. In the germline genome (all cells except B cells) the V, D, and J genes are widely separated and exist in numerous forms. Once a cell becomes committed to B cell differentiation, a single V gene and a single D gene translocate to a single J gene, and the intervening genetic material is excised (VDJ joining). The newly formed VDJ gene is transcribed into a single message along with either an M or D isotype C gene. Upon exposure to antigen, another rearrangement may occur so that the VDJ gene may be associated with a G, A or E isotype C gene. In light chain genes there appear to be no D genes, and thus light chain variable regions are formed by VJ joining.

translation (see Fig. 280-3). Because of the mechanics of the gene rearrangements necessary to specify the immunoglobulin variable regions (VDJ joining for the heavy chain, VJ joining for the light chain; see Fig. 280-3), a particular clone rearranges only one of the two chromosomes to produce an immunoglobulin molecule of only one light chain isotype and only one allotype (allelic exclusion). After exposure to antigen, the variable region may become associated with a new heavy chain isotype (class switch). Each clone of cells performs these sequential gene arrangements in a unique way. This results in each clone producing a unique immunoglobulin molecule. In most cells, light chains are synthesized in slight excess, are secreted as free light chains by plasma cells, and are cleared by the kidney, but less than 10 mg of such light chains is excreted per day.

Electrophoretic analysis of components of the serum proteins permits determination of the amount of immunoglobulin in the serum (Fig. 280-4). The variety of immunoglobulins move heterogeneously in an electric field and form a broad peak in the gamma region. The gamma globulin region of the electrophoretic pattern is usually increased in the sera of patients and animals with plasma cell tumors. There is a sharp spike in this region called an *M component* (M for monoclonal). Less commonly, the M component may appear in the beta$_2$ or alpha$_2$ globulin region. The antibody must be present at a concentration of at least 5 g/L (0.5 g/dL) to be detectable by this method. This corresponds to approximately 10^9 cells producing the antibody. Confirmation that such an M component is truly monoclonal relies on the use of immunoelectrophoresis that shows a single light and heavy chain type. Hence immunoelectrophoresis and electrophoresis provide qualitative and quantitative assessment of the M component, respectively. Once the presence of an M component has been confirmed, electrophoresis provides the more practical information for managing patients with monoclonal gammopathies. In a given patient, the amount of M component in the serum is a reliable measure of the tumor burden. This makes the M component an excellent tumor marker, yet it is not specific enough to be used to screen asymptomatic patients. In addition to the plasma cell disorders, M components may be detected in other lymphoid neoplasms such as chronic lymphocytic leukemia and lymphomas of B or T cell origin; nonlymphoid neoplasms such as chronic myelogenous leukemia, breast and colon cancer; a variety of nonneoplastic conditions such as cirrhosis, sarcoidosis, parasitic diseases, Gaucher's disease, and pyoderma gangrenosum; and a number of autoimmune conditions, including rheumatoid arthritis, myasthenia gravis, and cold agglutinin disease. A very rare skin disease known as lichen myxedematosus or papular mucinosis is associated with a monoclonal gammopathy. Highly cationic IgGλ is deposited in the dermis of patients with this disease. It is unclear whether this organ specificity reflects the specificity of the antibody for some antigenic component of the dermis.

The nature of the M component is variable in plasma cell disorders. It may be an intact antibody molecule of any heavy chain subclass, or it may be an altered antibody or fragment. Isolated light or heavy chains may be produced. In some plasma cell tumors such as extramedullary or solitary bone plasmacytomas, less than a third of patients will have an M component. In about 20 percent of myelomas, only light chains are produced and in most cases are secreted in the urine as Bence Jones proteins. The frequency of myelomas of a

FIGURE 280-4 Representative electrophoretic patterns of serum and urine. The upper panel illustrates the normal pattern of serum and urine protein on electrophoresis. Since there are many different immunoglobulins in the serum, their differing mobilities in an electric field produce a broad peak. The lower panel illustrates the patterns of serum and urine proteins in a patient with myeloma. The predominance of a product of a single cell is reflected by a "church spire" sharp peak. The presence of free light chains in the urine is reflected in a peak, as well.

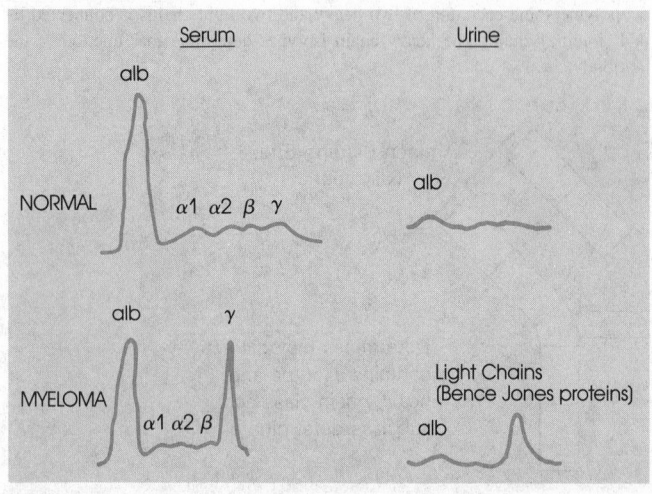

particular heavy chain class is roughly proportional to the serum concentration, and therefore IgG myelomas are more common than IgA and IgD myelomas.

MULTIPLE MYELOMA **Definition** Multiple myeloma represents a malignant proliferation of plasma cells. The terms *multiple myeloma* and *myeloma* may be used interchangeably. The disease results from the uncontrolled proliferation of plasma cells derived from a single clone. The tumor, its products, and the host response to it result in a number of organ dysfunctions and symptoms of bone pain or fracture, renal failure, susceptibility to infection, anemia, hypercalcemia, and occasionally clotting abnormalities, neurologic symptoms, and vascular manifestations of hyperviscosity.

Etiology The cause of myeloma is not known. Myeloma was found to occur with increased frequency in those exposed to the radiation of nuclear warheads in World War II after a 20-year latency. There is no direct evidence implicating oncogenes in human myeloma. In contrast to most other B cell tumors, consistent chromosomal alterations have not been found in patients with myeloma. Overexpression of *myc* or *ras* genes has been noted in some cases. The murine plasmacytoma models suggest that the induction of plasmacytomas (e.g., with mineral oil injection) may require exposure to foreign antigens as well as a cellular event. Thus chronic antigenic stimulation may play a role in the transformation of a particular B cell clone. There is also some evidence for a genetic predisposition to myeloma in humans. Myeloma has been seen more commonly than expected among farmers, wood workers, leather workers, and those exposed to petroleum products. The neoplastic event in myeloma may involve cells earlier in B cell differentiation than the plasma cell. Circulating B cells bearing surface immunoglobulin that share the idiotype of the M component are present in myeloma patients. It is possible that the malignant clone escapes normal control mechanisms at a pre-plasma cell stage of differentiation and the chronic exposure to a particular antigenic stimulus drives the cell to terminal differentiation. It remains difficult to distinguish benign from malignant plasma cells on the basis of morphologic criteria in all but a few cases.

Incidence and prevalence Myeloma increases in incidence with age. The median age at diagnosis is 68 years. It is rare under age 40. The yearly incidence is around 4 per 100,000 and remarkably similar in countries throughout the world. Males are slightly more commonly affected than females, and blacks have nearly twice the incidence of whites. In the age group over 25 the incidence is 30 per 100,000. Myeloma accounts for about 1 percent of all malignancies in whites and 2 percent in blacks; 13 percent of all hematologic cancers in whites and 33 percent in blacks.

Pathogenesis and clinical manifestations (Table 280-1) Bone pain is the most common symptom in myeloma, affecting nearly 70 percent of patients. The pain usually involves the back and ribs, and unlike the pain of metastatic carcinoma, which often is worse at night, the pain of myeloma is precipitated by movement. Persistent localized pain in a patient with myeloma usually signifies a pathologic fracture. The bone lesions of myeloma are caused by the proliferation of the tumor cells and the activation of osteoclasts which destroy the bone. The osteoclasts respond to osteoclast activating factors (OAF) made by the myeloma cells (OAF activity can be mediated by several cytokines, including interleukin 1, lymphotoxin, and tumor necrosis factor). However, production of these factors stops following administration of corticosteroids or interferon-γ. The bone lesions are lytic in nature and are rarely associated with osteoblastic new bone formation; therefore, radioisotopic bone scanning is less useful in diagnosis than plain radiography. The bony lysis results in substantial mobilization of calcium from bone, and serious acute and chronic complications of hypercalcemia may dominate the clinical picture (see below). Localized bone lesions may expand to the point that mass lesions may be palpated, especially on the skull (Fig. 280-5), clavicles, and sternum, and the collapse of vertebrae may lead to symptoms of spinal cord compression.

The next most common clinical problem in patients with myeloma is susceptibility to bacterial infections. The most common infections

TABLE 280-1 Pathogenesis and clinical manifestations of multiple myeloma

Clinical finding	Underlying cause	Pathogenic mechanism
Hypercalcemia, pathologic fractures, cord compression, lytic bone lesions, osteoporosis, bone pain	Skeletal destruction	Tumor expansion; production of osteoclast activating factors (OAF) by tumor cells
Renal failure	Light chain proteinuria, hypercalcemia, urate nephropathy, amyloid glomerulopathy (rare)	Toxic effects of tumor products, light chains, OAF, DNA breakdown products
	Pyelonephritis	Hypogammaglobulinemia
Anemia	Myelophthisis, decreased production, increased destruction	Tumor expansion; production of inhibitory factors and autoantibodies by tumor cells
Infection	Hypogammaglobulinemia, decreased neutrophil migration	Decreased production due to tumor-induced suppression; increased IgG catabolism
Neurologic symptoms	Hyperviscosity, cryoglobulins, amyloid deposits	Products of tumor; properties of M component; light chains
	Hypercalcemia, cord compression	OAF
Bleeding	Interference with clotting factors, amyloid damage of endothelium, platelet dysfunction	Products of tumor; antibodies to clotting factors; light chains; antibody coating of platelets
Mass lesions		Tumor expansion

are pneumonias and pyelonephritis, and the most frequent pathogens are *Streptococcus pneumoniae*, *Staphylococcus aureus*, and *Klebsiella pneumoniae* in the lungs and *Escherichia coli* and other gram-negative organisms in the urinary tract (Chap. 81). In about 25 percent of patients, recurrent infections are the presenting features, and over 75 percent of patients will have a serious infection at some time in their course. The susceptibility to infection has several contributing causes. First, patients with myeloma have diffuse hypogammaglobulinemia

FIGURE 280-5 Bony lesions in multiple myeloma. The skull demonstrates the typical "punched out" lesions characteristic of multiple myeloma. The lesion represents a purely osteolytic lesion with little or no osteoblastic activity. *(Courtesy of Dr. Geraldine Schechter.)*

if the M component is excluded. The hypogammaglobulinemia is related to both decreased production and increased destruction of normal antibodies. Moreover, some patients generate a population of circulating regulatory cells in response to their myeloma that can suppress normal antibody synthesis. In the case of IgG myeloma, normal IgG antibodies are broken down more rapidly than normal because the catabolic rate for IgG antibodies varies directly with the serum concentration. The large M component results in fractional catabolic rates of 8 to 16 percent instead of the normal 2 percent. These patients have very poor antibody responses, especially to polysaccharide antigens such as those on bacterial cell walls. Such responses are normally T cell–independent. Most measures of T cell function in myeloma are normal, but a subset of CD4+ cells may be decreased. Granulocyte lysozyme content is low, and granulocyte migration is not as rapid as normal in patients with myeloma, probably the result of a product of the tumor. There are also a variety of abnormalities in complement functions in myeloma patients. All these factors contribute to the immune deficiency of these patients.

Renal failure occurs in nearly 25 percent of myeloma patients, and some renal pathology is noted in over half. There are many contributing factors. Hypercalcemia is the most common cause of renal failure. Glomerular deposits of amyloid, hyperuricemia, recurrent infections, and occasional infiltration of the kidney by myeloma cells all may contribute to renal dysfunction. However, tubular damage associated with the excretion of light chains is almost always present. Normally, light chains are filtered, reabsorbed in the tubules, and catabolized. With the increase in amount of light chains presented to the tubule, the tubular cells become overloaded with these proteins, and tubular damage results either directly from light chain toxic effects or indirectly from the release of intracellular lysosomal enzymes. The earliest manifestation of this tubular damage is the adult Fanconi syndrome (a type 2 proximal renal tubular acidosis) with increased loss of glucose, amino acids, and defects in the ability of the kidney to acidify and concentrate the urine. The proteinuria is not accompanied by hypertension, and the protein is nearly all light chains. Generally, there is very little albumin in the urine because glomerular function is usually normal. When the glomeruli are involved, the proteinuria is nonselective. Patients with myeloma also have a decreased anion gap [i.e., sodium minus (chloride plus bicarbonate)] because the M component is cationic, resulting in retention of chloride. This is often accompanied by hyponatremia that is felt to be artificial (pseudohyponatremia) because each volume of serum has less water as a result of the increased protein.

Anemia occurs in about 80 percent of myeloma patients. It is usually normocytic and normochromic and related both to the replacement of normal marrow by expanding tumor cells and to the inhibition of hematopoiesis by factors made by the tumor. In addition, mild hemolysis may contribute to the anemia. A larger than expected fraction of patients may have megaloblastic anemia due to either folate or vitamin B_{12} deficiency. Granulocytopenia and thrombocytopenia are very rare. Clotting abnormalities may be seen due to the failure of antibody-coated platelets to function properly or to the interaction of the M component with clotting factors I, II, V, VII, or VIII. Raynaud's phenomenon and impaired circulation may result if the M component forms cryoglobulins, and hyperviscosity syndromes may develop depending on the physical properties of the M component (most common with IgM, IgG3, and IgA paraproteins). Hyperviscosity is defined on the basis of the relative viscosity of serum as compared with water. Normal relative serum viscosity is 1.8 (i.e., serum is normally almost twice as viscous as water). Symptoms of hyperviscosity occur at a level of 5 to 6, a level usually reached at paraprotein concentrations of around 40 g/L (4 g/dL) for IgM, 50 g/L (5 g/dL) for IgG3, and 70 g/L (7 g/dL) for IgA.

Although neurologic symptoms occur in a minority of patients, they may have many causes. Hypercalcemia may produce lethargy, weakness, depression, and confusion. Hyperviscosity may lead to headache, fatigue, visual disturbances, and retinopathy. Bony damage and collapse may lead to cord compression, radicular pain, and loss of bowel and bladder control. Infiltration of peripheral nerves by amyloid can be a cause of carpal tunnel syndrome and other sensorimotor mono- and polyneuropathies.

Many of the clinical features of myeloma, e.g., cord compression, pathologic fractures, hyperviscosity, sepsis, and hypercalcemia, can present as medical emergencies. Despite the widespread distribution of plasma cells in the body, tumor expansion is dominantly within bone and bone marrow and, for reasons unknown, rarely causes enlargement of spleen, lymph nodes, or gut-associated lymphatic tissue.

Diagnosis and staging The classic triad of myeloma is marrow plasmacytosis (>10 percent), lytic bone lesions, and a serum and/or urine M component. The diagnosis may be made in the absence of bone lesions if the plasmacytosis is associated with a progressive increase in the M component over time or if extramedullary mass lesions develop. There are two important variants of myeloma, solitary bone plasmacytoma and extramedullary plasmacytoma. These lesions are associated with an M component in less than 30 percent of the cases, they may affect younger individuals, and both are associated with median survivals of 10 or more years. Solitary bone plasmacytoma is a single lytic bone lesion without marrow plasmacytosis. Extramedullary plasmacytomas usually involve the submucosal lymphoid tissue of the nasopharynx or paranasal sinuses without marrow plasmacytosis. Both tumors are highly responsive to local radiation therapy. If an M component is present, it should disappear after treatment. Solitary bone plasmacytomas may recur in other bony sites or evolve into myeloma. Extramedullary plasmacytomas rarely recur or progress.

The most difficult differential diagnosis in patients with myeloma involves their separation from people with benign monoclonal gammopathies or monoclonal gammopathies of uncertain significance (MGUS). MGUS are vastly more common than myeloma, occurring in 1 percent of the population over age 50 and in up to 10 percent over age 75. Patients with MGUS usually have fewer than 20 g/L (2 g/dL) of M components, no urinary Bence Jones protein, less than 5 percent marrow plasmacytosis, and no anemia, renal failure, lytic bone lesions, or hypercalcemia. When bone marrow cells are exposed to radioactive thymidine in order to quantitate dividing cells, patients with MGUS always have a labeling index of less than 1 percent and patients with myeloma always have a labeling index of greater than 1 percent. Other discriminators include plasma cell acid phosphatase and β-glucuronidase, both of which are low in MGUS patients, and the salmon calcitonin stimulation test, which is positive only in patients with active ongoing bone destruction. Only about 11 percent of patients with MGUS go on to develop myeloma. Typically, patients with MGUS require no therapy.

The clinical evaluation of patients with myeloma includes a careful physical examination searching for tender bones and masses. It is paradoxic that only a small minority of patients have an enlargement of the spleen and lymph nodes, the physiologic sites of antibody production. Chest and bone radiographs may reveal lytic lesions or diffuse osteopenia. A complete blood count with differential may reveal anemia. Erythrocyte sedimentation rate is elevated. Very rare patients (~2 percent) may have plasma cell leukemia with more than 2000 plasma cells per microliter. This may be seen in disproportionate frequency in IgD (~12 percent) and IgE (~25 percent) myelomas. Serum calcium, urea nitrogen, creatinine, and uric acid may be elevated. Protein electrophoresis and measurement of serum immunoglobulins are useful for detecting and characterizing M spikes, supplemented by immunoelectrophoresis, which is especially sensitive for identifying low concentrations of M components not detectable by protein electrophoresis. A 24-h urine specimen is necessary to quantitate protein excretion, and a concentrated aliquot is used for electrophoresis and immunologic typing of any M component. Serum alkaline phosphatase is usually normal even with extensive bone involvement because of the absence of osteoblastic activity. It is also important to quantitate serum beta₂ microglobulin (see below).

The serum M component will be IgG in 53 percent of patients, IgA in 25 percent, and IgD in 1 percent, and 20 percent of patients will have only light chains in serum and urine. Dipsticks for detecting proteinuria are not reliable at identifying light chains, and the heat test for detecting Bence Jones protein is falsely negative in about 50 percent of patients with light chain myeloma. Fewer than 1 percent of patients have no identifiable M component, and these are usually light chain myelomas in which renal catabolism has made them undetectable in the urine. About two-thirds of patients with serum M components also have urinary light chains. The light chain isotype may have an impact on survival. Patients secreting lambda light chains have a significantly shorter overall survival than those secreting kappa light chains. It is not clear whether this is due to some genetically important determinant of cell proliferation or because lambda light chains are more likely to cause renal damage and form amyloid than are kappa light chains. The heavy chain isotype may have an impact on patient management as well. About half of patients with IgM paraproteins develop hyperviscosity compared with only 2 to 4 percent of patients with IgA and IgG M components. Among IgG myelomas, it is the IgG3 subclass that has the highest tendency to form both concentration- and temperature-dependent aggregates, leading to hyperviscosity and cold agglutination at lower serum concentrations.

The staging system for patients with myeloma is a functional system for predicting survival and is based on a variety of clinical and laboratory tests, unlike the anatomic staging systems for solid tumors. Details of the staging system are given in Table 280-2. Based on the hemoglobin, calcium, M component, and degree of skeletal involvement, the total-body tumor burden is estimated to be low (stage I, $<0.6 \times 10^{12}$ cells per square meter), intermediate (stage II, 0.6 to 1.2×10^{12} cells per square meter), or high (stage III, $>1.2 \times 10^{12}$ cells per square meter), and the stages are further subdivided on the basis of renal function (A if serum creatinine < 2 mg/dL, B if > 2). Patients in stage IA have a median survival of more than 5 years and those in stage IIIB about 15 months. Beta$_2$ microglobulin is a protein of 11,000 mol wt with homologies with the constant region of immunoglobulins that is the light chain of the class I major histocompatibility antigens (HLA-A, -B, -C) on the surface of every cell. Serum beta$_2$ microglobulin is the single most powerful predictor of survival and can substitute for staging. Patients with beta$_2$ microglobulin levels less than 0.004 g/L have a median survival of 43 months and those with levels higher than 0.004 g/L only 12 months. It is also felt that once the diagnosis of myeloma is firm, histologic features of atypia may also exert an influence on prognosis. Interleukin 6 may be an autocrine and/or paracrine growth factor for myeloma cells; elevated levels are associated with more aggressive disease. High labeling index and high levels of lactate dehydrogenase and thymidine kinase are also associated with poor prognosis.

Treatment and course About 10 percent of patients with myeloma will have an indolent course demonstrating only very slow progression of disease over many years. Such patients only require antitumor therapy when the serum myeloma protein rises above 50 g/L (5 g/dL) or progressive bone lesions develop. Patients with solitary bone plasmacytomas and extramedullary plasmacytomas may be expected to enjoy prolonged disease-free survival after local radiation therapy to a dose of around 40 Gy. There is a low incidence of occult marrow involvement in patients with solitary bone plasmacytoma. Such patients are usually detected because their serum M component falls slowly or disappears initially only to return after a few months. These patients respond well to systemic chemotherapy.

The vast majority of patients with myeloma require therapeutic intervention. In general, such therapy is of two sorts: systemic chemotherapy to control the progression of myeloma and symptomatic supportive care to prevent serious morbidity from the complications of the disease. All patients with stage II or III disease and stage I patients exhibiting Bence Jones proteinuria, progressive lytic bone lesions, vertebral compression fractures, recurrent infections, or rising serum M component should be treated with systemic combination chemotherapy. Therapy can prolong and improve the quality of life for myeloma patients.

TABLE 280-2 Myeloma staging system

Stage	Criteria	Estimated tumor burden ($\times 10^{12}$ cells/m^2)
I	All the following:	
	1 Hemoglobin >100 g/L (10 g/dL)	<0.6 (low)
	2 Serum calcium <12 mg/dL	
	3 Normal bone x-ray or solitary lesion	
	4 Low M-component production	
	a IgG level <50 g/L (<5 g/dL)	
	b IgA level <30 g/L (<3 g/dL)	
	c Urine light chain <4 g/24 h	
II	Fitting neither I nor III	0.6–1.20 (intermediate)
III	One or more of the following:	
	1 Hemoglobin <85 g/L (<8.5 g/dL)	>1.20 (high)
	2 Serum calcium (>12 mg/dL)	
	3 Advanced lytic bone lesions	
	4 High M-component production	
	a IgG level >70 g/L (>7 g/dL)	
	b IgA level >50 g/L (>5 g/dL)	
	c Urine light chains >12 g/24 h	

SUBCLASSIFICATION BASED ON SERUM CREATININE LEVELS

Level	Stage	Median survival, months
A < 2 mg/dL	IA	61
B > 2 mg/dL	IIA,B	55
	IIIA	30
	IIIB	15

STAGING BASED ON SERUM BETA$_2$ MICROGLOBULIN LEVELS

Level	Stage	Median survival, months
<4 μg/mL	I	43
>4 μg/mL	II	12

The standard treatment has consisted of intermittent pulses of an alkylating agent [L-phenylalanine mustard (L-PAM, melphalan), cyclophosphamide, or chlorambucil] and prednisone administered for 4 to 7 days every 4 to 6 weeks. The alkylating agents appear to be roughly equally active, but resistance to one agent is often accompanied by resistance to the others. The usual doses are as follows: melphalan, 8 mg/m^2 of body surface area per day; cyclophosphamide, 200 mg/m^2 per day; chlorambucil, 8 mg/m^2 per day; prednisone, 25 to 60 mg/m^2 per day. Because of their near equivalence in antitumor efficacy, we favor cyclophosphamide as the alkylating agent because it is less toxic to the marrow stem cell compartment and results in a lower incidence of acute myelodysplastic syndromes than do the other alkylating agents. Doses may need adjustment based on marrow tolerance. However, there are few constraints on the dose of the steroid pulse, and it appears that more is better. Recent evidence suggests that higher dose-intensity (i.e., mg/m^2 per week) of the steroid is associated with significantly longer survival. Patients responding to therapy generally have a prompt and gratifying reduction in bone pain, hypercalcemia, and anemia and often have fewer infections. The serum M component lags substantially behind the symptomatic improvement, often taking 4 to 6 weeks to fall. This fall depends on the rate of tumor kill and the fractional catabolic rate of immunoglobulin, which in turn depends on the serum concentration (for IgG). Light chain excretion, with a functional half-life of approximately 6 h, may fall within the first week of treatment. However, since urine light chain levels may relate to renal tubular function, they are not a reliable measure of tumor cell kill. Calculations of tumor cell kill are made by extrapolation of the serum M component level and rely heavily on the assumption that every tumor cell produces immunoglobulin at a constant rate. About 60 percent of patients will achieve at least a 75 percent reduction in serum M component level and tumor cell mass in response to an alkylating agent and prednisone.

Although this is a tumor reduction of less than one log, clinical responses may last many months. Efforts to improve the fraction of patients responding and the degree of response have involved adding other active chemotherapeutic agents to the treatment program. Patients with more advanced disease may benefit most from such an approach, but three- to five-drug therapy is experimental at this time. High-dose therapy with hematopoietic support is also being tested in younger patients.

The ideal duration of therapy has not been determined. Most physicians treat every 4 to 6 weeks for 1 or 2 years. Cessation of therapy is followed by relapse, usually within a year. Retreatment may be associated with a second response in up to 80 percent of patients. Maintenance therapy (e.g., with interferon-α) may prolong the duration of response, but no study has demonstrated this to result in prolonged survival. The regrowth rate of the tumor during relapse accelerates with each relapse. Patients primarily resistant to initial therapy have a median survival of less than a year. High-dose pulsed steroids used alone (200 mg prednisone every other day or 1 g/m^2 per day methylprednisolone for 5 days) or VAD combination chemotherapy (vincristine, 0.4 mg/d in a 4-day continuous infusion; doxorubicin, 9 mg/m^2 per day in a 4-day continuous infusion; dexamethasone, 40 mg/d for 4 days per week for 3 weeks) may offer useful palliation in patients resistant to primary therapy.

About 15 percent of patients die within the first 3 months after diagnosis, and subsequently, the death rate is about 15 percent per year. The disease usually follows a chronic course for 2 to 5 years before developing an acute terminal phase, usually marked by the development of pancytopenia with a cellular marrow that is refractory to treatment. Widespread organ infiltration by myeloma cells occurs, and survival is less than 6 months. About 46 percent of patients die in the chronic phase of disease from progressive myeloma (16 percent) and renal failure (10 percent), sepsis (14 percent), or both (6 percent). Death in the acute terminal phase (26 percent) is chiefly from progressive myeloma (13 percent) and sepsis (9 percent). Five percent of patients die of acute leukemia, myeloblastic or monocytic, and although it has been debated that this is related to the primary disease, it appears more likely to be the result of chronic therapy with alkylating agents. Nearly 23 percent of patients die of myocardial infarction, chronic lung disease, diabetes, or stroke, all intercurrent illnesses related more to the age of the patient group than to the tumor.

Supportive care directed at the anticipated complications of the disease may be as important as primary antitumor therapy. The hypercalcemia generally responds well to corticosteroid therapy, hydration, and natriuresis. Calcitonin may add to the inhibitory effects of steroids on bone resorption. Diphosphonates have also been shown to reduce osteoclastic bone resorption. Treatments aimed at strengthening the skeleton, such as fluorides, calcium, and vitamin D with or without androgens, have been suggested but are not of proven efficacy. Iatrogenic worsening of renal function may be prevented by the use of allopurinol during chemotherapy to avoid urate nephropathy and by maintaining a high fluid intake to help excrete light chains and calcium. In the event of acute renal failure, plasmapheresis is approximately 10 times more effective at clearing light chains than peritoneal dialysis, and acutely reducing the protein load may result in functional improvement. Urinary tract infections should be watched for and treated early. Chronic dialysis probably should not be initiated in patients who have failed to respond to antitumor therapy. Plasmapheresis may be the treatment of choice for hyperviscosity syndromes. Although the pneumococcus is a dreaded pathogen in myeloma patients, they do not respond to pneumococcal polysaccharide vaccines. The advent of intravenous gamma globulin preparations raises some hope that prophylactic administration may prevent some serious infections, but this has not been tested. Chronic oral antibiotic prophylaxis is probably not warranted. Patients developing neurologic symptoms in the lower extremities, severe localized back pain, or problems with bowel and bladder control may need emergency myelography and radiation therapy for palliation.

Most bone lesions respond to analgesics and chemotherapy, but certain painful lesions may respond most promptly to localized radiation. The chronic anemia may respond to hematinics (iron, folate, cobalamin), and some have responded to androgens. The pathogenesis of the anemia should be established and specific therapy instituted, where possible.

WALDENSTRÖM'S MACROGLOBULINEMIA In 1948, Waldenström described a malignancy of lymphoplasmacytoid cells that secreted IgM. In contrast to myeloma, the disease was associated with lymphadenopathy and hepatosplenomegaly, but the major clinical manifestation was the hyperviscosity syndrome. The disease resembles the related diseases chronic lymphocytic leukemia, myeloma, and lymphocytic lymphoma. Waldenström's macroglobulinemia and IgM myeloma both follow a similar clinical course. The diagnosis of IgM myeloma is usually reserved for patients with lytic bone lesions and is important only because of the hazard of pathologic fractures.

The cause of macroglobulinemia is unknown. The disease is similar to myeloma in being slightly more common in men and occurring with increased incidence with age (median 64 years). There have been reports that the IgM in some patients with macroglobulinemia may have specificity for myelin-associated glycoprotein (MAG), a protein that has been associated with demyelinating disease of the peripheral nervous system and may be lost earlier and to a greater extent than the better known myelin basic protein in patients with multiple sclerosis. There is a surface antigen on natural killer cells that is cross-reactive with the MAG, and coincidentally, natural killer cells are decreased in multiple sclerosis. Sometimes patients with macroglobulinemia develop a peripheral neuropathy before the appearance of the neoplasm. There is speculation that the whole process begins with a viral infection that may elicit an antibody response that cross-reacts with a normal tissue component.

Like myeloma, the disease involves the bone marrow, but unlike myeloma, it does not cause bone lesions or hypercalcemia. Like myeloma, a serum M component is present in the serum in excess of 30 g/L (3 g/dL), but unlike myeloma, the size of the IgM paraprotein results in little renal excretion and only around 20 percent of patients excrete light chains. Therefore, renal disease is not common. The light chain isotype is kappa in 80 percent of the cases. Patients present with weakness, fatigue, and recurrent infections, similar to myeloma patients, but epistaxis, visual disturbances, and neurologic symptoms such as peripheral neuropathy, dizziness, headache, and transient paresis are much more common in macroglobulinemia. Physical examination reveals adenopathy and hepatosplenomegaly, and ophthalmoscopic examination may reveal vascular segmentation and dilatation of the retinal veins characteristic of hyperviscosity states. Patients may have a normocytic, normochromic anemia, but rouleaux formation and a positive Coombs' test are much more common than in myeloma. Malignant lymphocytes are usually present in the peripheral blood. About 10 percent of macroglobulins are cryoglobulins. These are pure M components and are not the mixed cryoglobulins seen in rheumatoid arthritis and other autoimmune diseases. Mixed cryoglobulins are composed of IgM or IgA complexed with IgG, for which they are specific. In both cases, Raynaud's phenomenon and serious vascular symptoms precipitated by the cold may occur, but mixed cryoglobulins are not commonly associated with malignancy. Patients suspected of having a cryoglobulin based on history and physical examination should have their blood drawn into a warm syringe and delivered to the laboratory in a container of warm water to avoid errors in quantitating the cryoglobulin.

Control of serious hyperviscosity symptoms such as an altered state of consciousness or paresis can be achieved acutely by plasmapheresis because 80 percent of the IgM paraprotein is intravascular. Aside from this, management is identical to that of myeloma. About 80 percent of patients respond to chemotherapy, and their median survival is over 3 years. The absence of other serious organ toxicities results in a longer life span of patients with macroglobulinemia compared with those with myeloma.

HEAVY CHAIN DISEASES The heavy chain diseases are rare

lymphoplasmacytic malignancies. Their clinical manifestations vary with the heavy chain isotype. Patients secrete a defective heavy chain that usually has an intact Fc fragment and a deletion in the Fd region. Gamma, alpha, and mu heavy chain diseases have been described, but no reports of delta or epsilon heavy chain diseases have appeared. Molecular biologic analysis of these tumors has revealed structural genetic defects that may account for the aberrant chain secreted.

Gamma heavy chain disease (Franklin's disease) This disease affects people of widely different age groups and countries of origin. It is characterized by lymphadenopathy, fever, anemia, malaise, hepatosplenomegaly, and weakness. Its most distinctive symptom is palatal edema, resulting from node involvement of Waldeyer's ring, and this may progress to produce respiratory compromise. The diagnosis depends on the demonstration of an anomalous serum M component [often <20 g/L (<2 g/dL)] that reacts with anti-IgG but not anti-light chain reagents. The M component is typically present in *both serum* and *urine*. Most of the paraproteins have been of the gamma$_1$ subclass, but other subclasses have been seen. The patients may have thrombocytopenia, eosinophilia, and nondiagnostic bone marrow. Patients usually have a rapid downhill course and die of infection; however, some patients have survived 5 years with chemotherapy.

Alpha heavy chain disease (Seligmann's disease) This is the most common of the heavy chain diseases. It is closely related to a malignancy known as *Mediterranean lymphoma*, a disease that affects young people in parts of the world such as the Mediterranean, Asia, and South America in which intestinal parasites are common. The disease is characterized by an infiltration of the lamina propria of the small intestine with lymphoplasmacytoid cells that secrete truncated alpha chains. Demonstrating alpha heavy chains is difficult because the alpha chains tend to polymerize and appear as a smear instead of a sharp peak on electrophoretic profiles. Despite the polymerization, hyperviscosity is not a common problem in alpha heavy chain disease. Without J chain–facilitated dimerization, viscosity does not increase dramatically. Light chains are absent from serum and urine. The patients present with chronic diarrhea, weight loss, and malabsorption and have extensive mesenteric and paraaortic adenopathy. Respiratory tract involvement occurs rarely. Patients may vary widely in their clinical course. Some may develop diffuse aggressive histologies of malignant lymphoma. Chemotherapy may produce long-term remissions. Rare patients appear to have responded to antibiotic therapy, raising the question of the etiologic role of antigenic stimulation perhaps by some chronic intestinal infection.

Mu heavy chain disease The secretion of isolated mu heavy chains into the serum appears to occur in a very rare subset of patients with chronic lymphocytic leukemia. The only features that may distinguish patients with mu heavy chain disease are the presence of vacuoles in the malignant lymphocytes and the excretion of kappa light chains in the urine. The diagnosis requires ultracentrifugation or gel filtration to confirm the nonreactivity of the paraprotein with the light chain reagents because some intact macroglobulins fail to interact with these serums. The tumor cells seem to have a defect in the assembly of light and heavy chains because they appear to contain both in their cytoplasm. There is no evidence that such patients should be treated differently from other patients with chronic lymphocytic leukemia.

REFERENCES

ALEXANIAN R et al: Prognosis of asymptomatic multiple myeloma. Arch Intern Med 148: 1963, 1988

BARLOGIE B et al: Plasma cell myeloma—New biological insights and advances in therapy. Blood 73:865, 1989

———, ALEXANIAN R: Second International Workshop on Myeloma: Advances in biology and therapy of multiple myeloma. Cancer Res 49:7172, 1989

BATAILLE R et al: Serum levels of interleukin 6, a potent myeloma cell growth factor, as a reflection of disease severity in plasma cell dyscrasias. J Clin Invest 84:2008, 1989

CHAK LY et al: Solitary plasmacytoma of bone: Treatment, progression and survival. J Clin Oncol 5:1811, 1987

GREGORY WM et al: Combination chemotherapy versus melphalan and prednisone in the treatment of multiple myeloma: An overview of published trials. J Clin Oncol 10:334, 1992

GRIEPP PR et al: Value of beta-2-microglobulin level and plasma cell labeling indices as prognostic factors in patients with newly diagnosed myeloma. Blood 72:219, 1988

KYLE RA (ed): Myeloma and related disorders, in *Neoplastic Diseases of the Blood.* New York, Churchill Livingstone, 1991, pp 325–571

LOKHORST HM, DEKKER AW: Advances in the treatment of multiple myeloma. Cancer Treat Rev 19:113, 1993

MANDELLI F et al: Maintenance treatment with recombinant interferon-alpha-2b in patients with multiple myeloma responding to conventional induction chemotherapy. N Engl J Med 322:1430, 1990

PALMER M et al: Dose-intensity analysis of melphalan and prednisone in multiple myeloma. J Natl Cancer Inst 80:414, 1988

281 AMYLOIDOSIS

ALAN S. COHEN

DEFINITION AND CLASSIFICATION *Amyloidosis* may be defined as the extracellular deposition of the fibrous protein amyloid in one or more sites of the body. It was named by Virchow in 1854 on the basis of its color after staining with iodine and sulfuric acid. This protein has unique ultrastructural, x-ray diffraction, and biochemical characteristics. It can be deposited locally, where it has no clinical consequences, or it may involve virtually any organ system of the body, leading to severe pathophysiologic changes, or the disease may fall between these two extremes. The natural history of amyloidosis is poorly understood, and the clinical diagnosis is often not made until the disease is far advanced. It is now clear that there are multiple clinically and biochemically different forms of amyloid that are so classified because of the unique fibrous structure they all possess. The following classification is clinically the most useful: (1) primary (AL type) amyloidosis (no evidence for preexisting or coexisting disease), (2) amyloid associated with multiple myeloma (also AL type), (3) secondary or reactive (AA type) amyloidosis associated with chronic infectious diseases (e.g., osteomyelitis, tuberculosis, leprosy) or chronic inflammatory diseases (e.g., rheumatoid arthritis), (4) heredofamilial amyloidosis, a variety of neuropathic [AF transthyretin (prealbumin) type], renal, cardiovascular, and other syndromes, plus the amyloidosis associated with familial Mediterranean fever (AA type), (5) local amyloidosis (focal, often tumor-like, deposits which occur in isolated organs, often endocrine, without evidence of systemic involvement), (6) amyloidosis associated with aging, especially in the heart and in the brain, and (7) amyloid associated with long-term hemodialysis. These clinical forms and their current biochemical classification are listed in Table 281-1.

PATHOLOGY AND STRUCTURE Amyloid is amorphous, eosinophilic, extracellular, and ubiquitous in distribution. The involved organs may have a rubbery consistency and a waxy, pink or gray appearance. Organ enlargement, especially of the liver, kidney, spleen, and heart, may be prominent.

Microscopically, amyloid stains pink with the hematoxylin-eosin stain and shows metachromasia with crystal violet. The Congo red stain imparts a unique green birefringence when sections are viewed in the polarizing microscope. This is the single most useful procedure for establishing the presence of amyloid. Amyloid deposits may be focal in almost any area of the body but are most often perivascular.

The heart may show focal or diffuse interstitial deposits in the myocardium, endocardium, or pericardium. In the aged heart, the atrium is usually focally involved, or there may occur more diffuse lesions of the atria and ventricles. In the kidney, the glomerulus is primarily affected, although interstitial, peritubular, and vascular amyloid occur. In early lesions, small nodular or diffuse deposits appear near the basement membrane, and as the disease progresses, the glomerulus may be massively laden with amyloid and its capillary

TABLE 281-1 The 1990 guidelines for nomenclature and classification of amyloid and amyloidosis

Amyloid protein[a]	Protein precursor	Protein type of variant	Clinical
AA[b]	apoSSA		Reactive (secondary[b]) Familial Mediterranean fever Familial amyloid nephropathy with urticaria and deafness (Muckle-Wells syndrome)
AL	kappa, lambda (e.g., k III)	Ak, A, (e.g., A k III)	Idiopathic (primary), myeloma or macroglobulinemia-associated
AH	IgG 1(γ1)	Aγ1	
ATTR	Transthyretin	e.g., Met 30[c]	Familial amyloid polyneuropathy (Portuguese)
		e.g., Met 111	Familial amyloid cardiomyopathy (Danish)
		TTR or I1e 122	Systemic senile amyloidosis
AApoAI	apoAI	Arg 26	Familial amyloid polyneuropathy (Iowa)
AGel	Gelsolin	Asn 187[d] (15)	Familial amyloidosis (Finnish)
ACys	Cystatin C	Gln 68	Hereditary cerebral hemorrhage with amyloidosis (Icelandic)
AB	B protein precursor (e.g., BPP$_{695}$)[e]	Gln 618 (22)	Alzheimer's disease Down's syndrome Hereditary cerebral hemorrhage amyloidosis (Dutch)
AB$_2$M	Beta$_2$ microglobulin		Associated with chronic dialysis
AScr	Scrapie protein, precursor 33–35 kDa cellular form	Scrapie protein 27–30 kDa	Creutzfeldt-Jakob disease, etc.
		e.g., Leu 102	Gerstmann-Straussler-Scheinker syndrome
ACal	(Pro)calcitonin	(Pro)calcitonin	Medullary carcinoma of thyroid
AANF	Atrial natriuretic factor		Isolated atrial amyloid
AIAPP	Islet amyloid polypeptide		Islets of Langerhans Diabetes type II, Insulinoma

[a]Nonfibrillar proteins, e.g., protein AP (amyloid P component) excluded
[b]Abbreviation not explained in table: AA = amyloid A protein, SAA = serum amyloid A protein, apo = apolipoprotein, L = immunoglobulin light chain, H = immunoglobulin heavy chain
[c]ATTR Met 30 when used in text
[d]Amino acid positions in the mature precursor protein. The position in the amyloid fibril protein is given in parentheses
[e]Number of amino acid residues
SOURCE: Cohen, 1991.

bed occluded. In the gastrointestinal tract, there may be perivascular deposits only, or irregular or diffuse deposits may be found in the submucosa, the muscularis mucosa, or subserosa. The amyloid may appear at any level or portion of the gastrointestinal tract, including the gallbladder and pancreas. In the nervous system, amyloid has been described along peripheral nerves, in autonomic ganglia, and in senile plaques, neurofibrillary tangles, and blood vessels ("congophilic angiopathy") of the central nervous system. It may be found in any portion of the orbit, including the vitreous humor and cornea. In summary, there is virtually no area of the body that is spared. This ubiquitous distribution elicits a wide variety of clinical symptoms and signs.

All types of human amyloid consist of fine, nonbranching, rigid fibrils that in tissue sections measure approximately 10×10^{-9} m (100 Å) in diameter. Isolated amyloid fibrils have a delicate, thin, nonbranching fibrous character. The individual fibril (or filament) has a diameter of about 7×10^{-9} m (70 Å) and tends to aggregate laterally. Each fibril (filament) has subunit protofibrils of 3 to 3.5 $\times$ 10^{-9} m (30 to 35 Å) diameter. X-ray diffraction of isolated amyloid fibrils reveals a cross beta pattern, the "pleated sheet" of Pauling and Corey, indicating that the polypeptide chain runs transversely to the long axis of the fibril specimen.

A second component, the plasma component or pentagonal unit (P component or AP) with a different ultrastructure, x-ray diffraction pattern, and chemical characteristics, also has been isolated from amyloid and is identical with a serum alpha globulin (SAP). It has many similarities to C-reactive protein, but it does not behave in

humans as a classic acute-phase protein. It is not responsible for the characteristic tinctorial properties or ultrastructure of amyloid.

BIOCHEMISTRY OF AMYLOID FIBRILS The bulk of amyloid deposits consists of fibrils. Purified amyloid derived from the fibril is a protein. The chemical composition of the different clinical forms of amyloid are distinct and allow for more precise diagnosis (Table 281-1). The homology of the fibril of primary and myeloma amyloid to the N-terminal region of the variable fragment of an immunoglobulin light chain, and subsequently, in a limited number of cases, to a homogeneous light polypeptide chain, has been demonstrated. These light chain–related proteins range in size from about 5000 to 25,000 Da and are now termed amyloid light chain (AL) or AL$_\kappa$ or AL$_\lambda$ (Table 281-1). Amino acid sequence analysis indicates that most primary amyloid proteins contain the N-terminal amino acid residue identical to the variable regions of the light chain. Lambda chain class predominates over kappa in AL by a 2:1 ratio, whereas in multiple myeloma the reverse is true. Indeed, almost all lambda VI chains have been associated with amyloid. One heavy chain–related amyloid (AH) has been described recently.

Another protein, amyloid A (AA), unrelated to any known immunoglobulin, has been described in the secondary amyloid deposits. This protein can be isolated from the amyloid of patients with secondary amyloidosis and from that associated with familial Mediterranean fever. It is a unique protein with a molecular weight of about 8400 Da made up of approximately 76 amino acid residues arranged in a single chain. Some heterogeneity has been demonstrated (i.e., AAs of different molecular weights). AA is derived from serum

TABLE 281-2 Hereditary amyloid syndromes—1990

Clinical aspects*	Geographic or ethnic association	Protein and mutation
FAP—Distal limb peripheral neuropathy (sensory/motor); autonomic neuropathy with alternate constipation and diarrhea; nephropathy; cardiopathy with congestive failure (CHF) and arrhythmias; pupillary abnormalities in late disease (scalloped pupil); occasional vitreous opacities	Portuguese, Japanese, Swedish, Greek, Italian, Turkish	Transthyretin Met 30 (ATTR Met 30)
FAP—Peripheral neuropathy; autonomic neuropathy; cardiopathy, no renal (yet)	USA/German	ATTR Ala 30
FAP—Similar; few details known (neuropathy, diarrhea, vitreous opacities)	Israeli (Polish extraction)	ATTR Ile 33
FAP—Cardiomyopathy, vitreous opacities, mild neuropathy, renal (early report)	USA/Greek	ATTR Pro 36
FAP—Peripheral neuropathy; gastrointestinal (early report)	Japanese (Osaka)	ATTR Gly 42
FAP—Peripheral neuropathy; liver (early report)	Japanese	ATTR Arg 50
FAP—Cardiopathy; vitreous opacities	USA/Maryland/German extraction	ATTR His 58
FAP—Severe cardiopathy (often late in life); less peripheral neuropathy; occasional carpal tunnel syndrome	USA/West Virginia/Appalachia (English-Irish-German extraction	ATTR Ala 60
FAP—Neuropathy, diarrhea, nephropathy, cardiomyopathy	USA/Illinois/Texas (German extraction)	ATTR Tyr 77
FAP—Marked carpal tunnel syndrome; marked vitreous opacities, gastrointestinal symptoms	USA/Indiana (Swiss extraction)	ATTR Ser 84
FAC—Late-onset cardiopathy; vitreous opacities; no neuropathy as yet (early report)	USA/Italian	ATTR Asn 84
FAP—Severe cardiomyopathy; mild sensory neuropathy; vitreous opacities	USA/Italian	ATTR Asn 90
FAC—Primarily heart disease with congestive failure and arrhythmias	Danish	ATTR Met 111
FAP—Peripheral neuropathy; vitreous opacities; gastrointestinal; kidney (heart probable, early report)	Japanese (Osaka)	ATTR Cys 114
FAP—Lower limb neuropathy; nephropathy	USA/Iowa (Scottish-Irish-English)	Apolipoprotein AI Arg 26 (AApoAI Arg 26)
FAP—Cranial nerve neuropathy; skin changes; lattice corneal dystrophy; nephropathy	Finnish	Gelsolin Asn 187 (15) (AGel Asn 187 (15))
Hereditary cerebral hemorrhage with amyloidosis: cerebral angiopathy with spontaneous bleeds	Icelandic	Cystatin C Glh 68 (ACys Gln 68)
	Dutch	Beta protein
Familial(?) amyloid (senile, systemic) cardiopathy; heart disease in elderly patients; diagnosis at autopsy	Black	ATTR Ile 122
Familial Mediterranean fever—Fever; joint pain; polyserositis; skin rash; mostly autosomal recessive	Sephardic Jews, Armenians, Kurds	AA
Familial nephropathy with urticaria and deafness (Muckle-Wells syndrome)		AA

* FAP = familial amyloid polyneuropathy; FAC = familial amyloid cardiomyopathy.
SOURCE: Cohen, 1991.

amyloid A (SAA) by proteolysis. SAA is synthesized in the liver, migrates as an HDL complex, and is known as apoSAA. SAA is a polymorphic protein, expressed as SAA_1 and SAA_2, the former of which is the major component of tissue-extracted AA protein. To date, four human SAA genes have been described. Data from the mouse indicate that in that species only SAA_2 contributes to tissue amyloid deposits. These collective data suggest that minimal amino acid differences can affect amyloidogenicity, a concept supported by studies in other (i.e., hereditary) amyloidoses.

SAA behaves as an acute-phase reactant and is elevated in infection and inflammation. In addition, SAA is elevated in amyloid-resistant animals, suggesting that the appearance of amyloid is not solely determined by the level of SAA. An SAA inducing factor (now known to be interleukin 1) is released from stimulated macrophages and causes the release of SAA from hepatocytes, the site of SAA synthesis. The precise regulation of the conversion of SAA to the insoluble AA protein of amyloidosis is not understood.

Familial amyloid polyneuropathy (FAP) is a dominant hereditary disease affecting kinships originating in Portugal, Japan, Sweden,

and elsewhere. A 14,000-Da protein has been isolated from the tissues of patients from each of the above-noted geographically distributed kinships. Immunologic and amino acid sequence analyses have identified it as transthyretin (prealbumin), the first association of this molecule with a disease. It also has been shown that in many kinships there is a single amino acid substitution, methionine for valine at position 30, in the transthyretin isolated from the amyloid. Multiple other variants also have been shown to exist (Table 281-2).

A number of other amyloid proteins have been isolated and characterized. These include several from focal endocrine-related amyloid lesions such as precalcitonin from the amyloid of medullary carcinoma of the thyroid and insulinoma amyloid polypeptide (IAPP) of the pancreas found not only in association with insulinomas but with adult-onset diabetes mellitus as well. Transthyretin also has been isolated from senile cardiac amyloid, and atrial natriuretic peptide has been isolated as a distinct and separate protein from these lesions. Beta$_2$ microglobulin has been identified as the protein from the amyloid associated with chronic hemodialysis.

Of great interest is confirmation that the lesions known as senile plaques (which contain amyloid) and the meningeal vascular amyloid of Alzheimer's disease consist of a newly described protein, beta protein (or A4 protein), a 39 to 43 amino acid fragment of the large molecule known as beta protein precursor.

P component of amyloid In addition to the characteristic fibrils described above, a second component, the P component, has been noted in most amyloid deposits. P component (AP) has been recognized by electron microscopy as a pentagonal-shaped structured unit having an outside diameter of about 9×10^{-9} m (90 Å) and an inside diameter of about 4×10^{-9} m (40 Å). On immunoelectrophoresis it migrates as an alpha globulin, and it possesses antigenic identity with a constituent of normal human plasma (SAP). The amino acid sequence is distinct from that of the amyloid fibrils. Its pentagonal ultrastructure is similar to C-reactive protein (CRP), but the latter is one-half the molecular weight of AP and has other well-defined differences despite a 50 to 60 percent homology on amino acid sequence. AP binds to amyloid fibrils in a calcium-dependent fashion almost universally and has been used as a marker of amyloid.

IMMUNOBIOLOGY OF AMYLOID The precise etiology and pathogenesis of amyloidosis are unknown. Experimentally, the induction of AA amyloidosis has been shown to be a multifactorial process that is contributed to by the type of inflammatory stimulation, the nature of the SAA isotype, and the genetic background of the host. During inflammation, the mediator, interleukin 1, stimulates hepatic cells to produce increased SAA. SAA is partially degraded by monocyte or leukocyte surface enzymes to form AA. It is likely that macrophages play a role in the SAA degradation. Related abnormalities such as altered connective tissue glycosaminoglycans, altered macrophage enzymes, or enzyme inhibitors have all been postulated.

In AL amyloid, a monoclonal population of bone marrow plasma cells appears to be present and either consistently produces small lambda or kappa fragments or clones of immunoglobulins that are processed (cleaved) in an abnormal fashion by macrophage enzymes to produce the partially degraded light chains responsible for AL amyloidosis.

The formation of amyloid also may be determined in part by the intrinsic beta configuration of at least a portion of the polypeptide chain such as in transthyretin, beta$_2$ microglobulin, and other amyloidogenic proteins. Clearly, in the hereditary amyloidoses the substitution of a single amino acid variant contributes to the overall pathogenesis.

It also has been demonstrated that a substance known as amyloid enhancing factor (AEF), possibly a cytokine, contributes at least to the accelerated formation of secondary and probably other forms of amyloid.

CLINICAL MANIFESTATIONS The clinical manifestations of amyloidosis are varied and depend entirely on the area of the body which is involved.

Kidney Renal involvement may consist of mild proteinuria or frank nephrosis. In some cases, the urinary sediment may show only a few red blood cells. The renal lesion is usually not reversible and in time leads to progressive azotemia and death. The prognosis does not appear to be related to the degree of the proteinuria; when azotemia finally develops, the prognosis is grave. In one series, the mean survival of patients with renal amyloid from the time of biopsy was 29 months, but in a few cases there was presumptive evidence of regression of the renal amyloid. The utilization of chronic hemodialysis and of kidney transplantation has clearly improved the prognosis of renal amyloid. Hypertension is rare, except in long-standing amyloidosis. Renal tubular acidosis or renal vein thrombosis may occur. Localized accumulation of amyloid may be noted in the ureter, bladder, or other parts of the genitourinary tract. Renal pathology occurs in AA, AL, and many forms of heredofamilial disease and does not enable one to distinguish among the various types.

Liver While hepatic involvement is common, liver function abnormalities are minimal and occur late in the disease. The two tests most useful in indicating hepatic amyloid are the Bromsulphalein (BSP) extraction and serum alkaline phosphatase activity; however, no liver function tests are truly specific or sensitive for amyloid. Liver scans produce variable and nonspecific results. Portal hypertension occurs but is uncommon. Intrahepatic cholestasis has been noted in about 5 percent of patients with AL (primary) amyloidosis. In a series of 38 patients in whom liver tissue was available for examination, all 38 had some amyloid present, irrespective of the type of amyloidosis (primary or secondary), and contrary to previous notions, parenchymal amyloid was more extensive in the AL cases. Hepatomegaly is common, and AL hepatic amyloid is usually accompanied by the nephrotic syndrome and congestive heart failure. Prognosis is poor, and one group of 80 patients with proven AL hepatic amyloid had a median survival of 9 months. Amyloidosis of the spleen characteristically is not associated with leukopenia and anemia. Hepatic amyloid is uncommon and rarely of clinical importance in heredofamilial amyloidosis.

Heart Cardiac manifestations consist primarily of congestive failure and cardiomegaly (with or without murmurs) and a variety of arrhythmias. Cardiac amyloidosis is common in primary (AL) and heredofamilial amyloidosis and very rare in the secondary (AA) form. Although the cardiac manifestations predominantly reflect diffuse myocardial amyloid, the endocardium, valves, and pericardium may be involved as well. Pericarditis with effusion is rare, although the differential diagnosis of constrictive pericarditis versus restrictive cardiomyopathy frequently arises. Echocardiography has demonstrated symmetric thickening of the left ventricular wall, hypokinesia and decreased systolic contraction and thickening of the interventricular septum and left ventricular posterior wall, and left ventricular cavities of small to normal size. Two-dimensional echocardiography produces the characteristic findings of thickened right and left ventricles, a normal left ventricular cavity, and especially a diffuse hyperrefractile "granular sparkling" appearance. Hearts which are heavily infiltrated with amyloid may or may not show an enlarged silhouette. Fluoroscopy usually shows decreased mobility of the ventricular wall; angiographic studies usually demonstrate thickened ventricular wall, decreased ventricular mobility, and absence of rapid ventricular filling in early diastole. Cardiac amyloidosis can present as intractable heart failure. Electrocardiographic abnormalities include a low-voltage QRS complex and abnormalities in atrioventricular and intraventricular conduction, often resulting in varying degrees of heart block. Owing to their propensity to develop conduction defects and arrhythmias, patients with cardiac amyloidosis appear to be especially sensitive to digitalis, and this drug should be used with caution. Radionuclide techniques utilizing technetium 99m pyrophosphate for cardiac scanning are often positive, especially in patients with amyloid-related congestive heart failure.

Skin Involvement of the skin is one of the most characteristic manifestations of primary (AL) amyloidosis. The lesions may consist of slightly raised, waxy papules or plaques which usually are clustered in the folds of the axillae, anal, or inguinal regions, the face and neck, or mucosal areas such as ear or tongue. Periorbital ecchymoses ("black eye syndrome") have been reported. The lesions are seldom pruritic. Involvement of the skin or mucosa may not be apparent clinically but may be demonstrated by biopsy. Gentle rubbing of the skin may induce bleeding into the skin, leading to purpura. Cutaneous involvement also can occur in secondary amyloidosis; in one series it was found in 42 percent of such patients, in 55 percent of a group of patients with primary disease, and in all 11 patients with hereditary amyloid neuropathy.

Gastrointestinal tract Gastrointestinal symptoms are common in all systemic types of amyloidosis. They may result from direct involvement of the gastrointestinal tract at any level or from infiltration of the autonomic nervous system with amyloid. The symptoms include those of obstruction, ulceration, malabsorption, hemorrhage, protein loss, and diarrhea. Infiltration of the tongue occasionally leads to macroglossia. When not enlarged, the tongue may become stiffened and firm to palpation. While infiltration of the tongue is characteristic of primary amyloidosis (AL) or amyloidosis accompanying multiple myeloma, it is occasionally seen in the secondary (AA) form of the disease.

Gastrointestinal bleeding may occur from any of a number of sites, notably the esophagus, stomach, or large intestine, and may be severe. Amyloid infiltration of the esophagus may lead to an incompetent or nonrelaxing lower esophageal sphincter, nonspecific motility disorders of the esophageal body, or rarely achalasia. Small bowel lesions may lead to clinical and x-ray changes of obstruction. A malabsorption syndrome is seen at times. Amyloidosis may develop in association with other entities involving the gastrointestinal tract, especially tuberculosis, granulomatous enteritis, lymphoma, and Whipple's disease; differentiation of these conditions, which give rise to secondary amyloidosis, from diffuse primary amyloidosis of the small bowel may be difficult. Similarly, amyloidosis of the stomach may closely mimic gastric carcinoma, with obstruction, achlorhydria, and the radiologic appearance of tumor masses.

Nervous system Neurologic manifestations may include peripheral neuropathy, postural hypotension, inability to sweat, Adie's pupil, hoarseness, and sphincter incompetence. These manifestations are especially prominent in the heredofamilial amyloidoses. The cranial nerves are generally spared, except for those involving the pupillary reflexes. Carpal tunnel syndrome may be caused by several amyloidoses, especially primary (AL) and chronic hemodialysis (B$_2$M) amyloid. Peripheral neuropathy is frequent in the former type. Amyloid occurs in the central nervous system as a component of senile plaques, neurofibrillary tangles, and in blood vessels ("congophilic angiopathy"). The protein concentration in the cerebral spinal fluid may be increased. Infiltrates of the cornea or vitreous body may be present in hereditary amyloid syndromes. Certain of these syndromes are characterized by a bilateral scalloping appearance of the pupil.

Endocrine Amyloid may infiltrate the thyroid or other endocrine glands but rarely causes endocrine dysfunction. Local amyloid deposits almost invariably accompany medullary carcinoma of the thyroid. Amyloid is often found in the adrenal gland, pituitary gland, and pancreas. Little if any clinical dysfunction is present unless there is massive replacement of the gland by amyloid.

Joints Amyloid can directly involve articular structures by its presence in the synovial membrane and synovial fluid or in the articular cartilage. Amyloid arthritis can mimic a number of rheumatic diseases because it can present as a symmetric arthritis of small joints with nodules, morning stiffness, and fatigue. Most patients with amyloid arthropathy eventually are found to have multiple myeloma. The synovial fluid usually has a low white blood cell count, a good to fair mucin clot, a predominance of mononuclear cells, and no crystals. Studies of surgical specimens suggest a significant incidence of amyloid in cartilage, capsule, and synovium in osteoarthritis. Amyloid infiltration of muscle may lead to a pseudomyopathy.

Respiratory system The nasal sinuses, larynx, and trachea may be involved by accumulations of AL amyloid which block the ducts, in the case of the sinuses, or the air passages. Amyloidosis of the lung involves the bronchi and alveolar septa diffusely. The lower respiratory tract is affected most frequently in primary (AL) amyloidosis and in the disease associated with dysproteinemia. Pulmonary symptoms attributable to amyloid are present in about 30 percent of these patients and in some are the most serious manifestations of the disease. In secondary (AA) amyloidosis, pulmonary disease is a frequent histopathologic accompaniment but seldom gives rise to clinically significant symptoms. Amyloid also may be localized in the bronchi or pulmonary parenchyma and may resemble a neoplasm. In these cases, local excision should be attempted and, when successful, may be followed by prolonged remissions.

Hematopoietic system Hematologic changes may include fibrinogenopenia, increased fibrinolysis, and selective deficiency of clotting factors. Deficient factor X seems to be due to nonspecific calcium-dependent binding to the polyanionic amyloid fibrils. Splenectomy in the patient with such a factor X deficiency can relieve the deficiency and the associated bleeding disorder, since factor X has been shown to bind to the large masses of splenic amyloid.

HEREDOFAMILIAL AMYLOIDOSIS Until recently, there was no generally accepted nosology for the heredofamilial amyloid syndromes. Some reports emphasized the site of predominant organ involvement as neuropathic, nephropathic, or cardiopathic amyloidosis, while others stressed the genetic aspects. To date, virtually all analyses of pedigrees have shown that, with one major exception, the mode of inheritance is autosomal dominant. The exception is amyloidosis of familial Mediterranean fever (FMF), which is inherited as an autosomal recessive disorder and is an AA type of amyloid. Even in FMF amyloid, however, several kinships with autosomal dominant inheritance have been reported. While the recognizable clinical patterns can be used as the basis for classification, classification according to the specific point mutation is preferable (Table 281-2).

The heredofamilial amyloidoses include a group primarily involving the nervous system. The prototype is the lower limb neuropathy [familial amyloid polyneuropathy (FAP)], first described in Portugal, which has a poor prognosis and is characterized by progressively severe neuropathy, including marked autonomic nervous system involvement. This variety also has been described in Japan, Sweden, and in families of Greek, Swedish, and Italian origin. In some of these individuals, bilateral "scalloped" pupils are pathognomonic of the disease. The second type of neuropathy has been found in families of Swiss origin in Indiana and of German origin in Maryland. It is a milder disease and is often associated with a carpal tunnel syndrome and vitreous opacities. A more severe variety of generalized neuropathy associated with renal amyloidosis has been described in Iowa in a family of English-Irish-Scottish ancestry.

Several types of severe familial renal disease in association with amyloid have been described. Possibly the most remarkable is FMF, a disorder subdivided into phenotype I, with irregularly occurring fever and abdominal, chest, or joint pain, preceding or accompanying renal amyloid, and phenotype II, in which renal amyloidosis is the first or only manifestation of the disease. Colchicine treatment prevents attacks of FMF and appears to prevent subsequent deposition of amyloid as well. Sporadically, other hereditary forms of renal amyloidosis have been described, including the curious association of urticaria, deafness, and renal amyloid.

Severe familial amyloid heart disease has been described in a Danish family and familial persistent atrial standstill with amyloid in a family of Mexican-American origin. Hereditary cerebral amyloid with hemorrhage in an Icelandic family appears to be due to gamma trace protein (cystatin C) deposits and is associated with a decrease of these proteins in the cerebrospinal fluid. A similar disorder (but caused by beta protein) has been reported from the Netherlands. Miscellaneous hereditary amyloid syndromes include hereditary multiple endocrine neoplasms type II (including medullary carcinoma of the thyroid with amyloid) as well as others listed in Table 281-1.

DIAGNOSIS The specific diagnosis of amyloidosis depends on obtaining a tissue specimen by biopsy and the demonstration of amyloid with appropriate stains. First, of course, the disease must be suspected. When a patient with a chronic disorder predisposing to amyloid such as rheumatoid arthritis, tuberculosis, paraplegia, multiple myeloma, bronchiectasis, or leprosy develops hepatomegaly, splenomegaly, malabsorption, cardiac disease, or, most important, proteinuria, secondary (AA) amyloid should come to mind. In addition, in any heredofamilial syndromes, especially those which have a dominant autosomal mode of inheritance and are characterized by peripheral neuropathy, nephropathy, or cardiopathy, the diagnosis of amyloid should be considered. Finally, primary systemic (AL) amyloid should be considered in any individual with a diffuse noninflammatory infiltrative disease involving either mesenchymal tissues—blood vessels, heart, gastrointestinal tract—or parenchymal tissues—kidney, liver, spleen, adrenal.

When the diagnosis is suspected, it is good practice to perform an abdominal subcutaneous fat pad aspirate or rectal biopsy. If there is a specific reason for not carrying out these procedures, such other sites as skin, gums, or the suspected organ—kidney, liver—may be biopsied. All tissues obtained must be stained with Congo red and examined in the polarizing microscope for green birefringence. A modified potassium permanganate stain will allow reasonably accurate differentiation of the AA type from AL amyloid. In the former, pretreatment with permanganate, followed by the standard Congo red stain, abolishes the green birefringence (i.e., the tissue is permanganate-sensitive). Beta$_2$ microglobulin amyloid is also permanganate-sensitive. The AL and hereditary types are permanganate-resistant.

In order to establish the relationship of immunoglobulin-related amyloid to multiple myeloma, electrophoretic and immunoelectrophoretic studies on serum and urine should be performed when the biopsy reveals amyloid deposition. Most of these patients will have only relatively small paraprotein components, and only a few will have frank multiple myeloma.

PROGNOSIS AND TREATMENT   The course of amyloidosis is difficult to document, since dating the time of origin of the disease is rarely possible. When amyloidosis develops in patients with rheumatoid arthritis, it seldom becomes evident when the arthritis is less than 2 years in duration. The mean duration of arthritis before amyloidosis was detected was 16 years in one series. When amyloidosis develops in patients with multiple myeloma, manifestations leading to initial hospitalization are more apt to be related to amyloid disease than to myeloma. In these cases, prognosis is very poor, and life expectancy is usually less than 6 months.

Instances have been reported of amyloidosis accompanying treatable infections, such as osteomyelitis, in which at least partial remission has occurred following treatment of the primary disease. There have been similar experiences following successful treatment of tuberculosis or drainage of chronic empyema. However, many such reports are not substantiated by biopsy proof of resorption.

Generalized amyloidosis is usually a slowly progressive disease that leads to death in several years, but it may have a better prognosis than was suspected in the past. The average survival in most large series is 1 to 4 years, but a number of individuals with amyloid have been followed 5 to 10 years and longer.

The major causes of death are heart disease and renal failure. Sudden death, presumably due to arrhythmias, is common. Occasionally, gastrointestinal hemorrhage, respiratory failure, intractable heart failure, and superimposed infections are the terminal events.

There is no specific therapy for any variety of amyloidosis. Rational therapy should be directed at (1) decreasing chronic antigenic stimuli that produce amyloid, (2) inhibition of the synthesis and extracellular deposition of amyloid fibrils, and (3) promoting lysis or mobilization of existing amyloid deposits.

A variety of agents have been used to treat amyloidosis. Proof of their efficacy is not available. The finding that a portion of the immunoglobulin light chain is incorporated in the amyloid of patients with primary amyloidosis and its presumed synthesis by plasma cells has led to the use of alkylating agents. However, these agents cause bone marrow depression, and there are reports of acute leukemia developing in amyloidosis patients receiving melphalan. Recent trials have indicated that a prednisone/melphalan regimen or a prednisone/melphalan/colchicine program prolongs life. Studies in several centers are underway to compare these programs with each other and with colchicine alone (see below).

Patients with severe renal amyloidosis and azotemia have been treated by dialysis or kidney transplantation with very good outcomes. This has significantly improved the prognosis in patients whose major manifestations are renal. Heart transplantation also has been successful in a small number of carefully selected cases.

Colchicine has been shown to be effective in preventing acute attacks in patients with FMF, and two groups of investigators independently have reported the inhibition of amyloid deposition in the mouse model by colchicine. It is conceivable, therefore, that colchicine is effective in blocking amyloid deposition. One large study has shown it to be effective in prolonging life in primary (AL) amyloidosis using a life-table survivorship analysis. However, the exact mechanism of its action is unknown. The use of dimethylsulfoxide (DMSO) in the treatment of amyloid has had variable results.

REFERENCES

COHEN AS: Amyloidosis. N Engl J Med 277:522, 1967

———, JONES LA: Advances in amyloidosis. Curr Opin Rheumatol 5:62, 1993

———, SKINNER M: Diagnosis of amyloidosis, in *Laboratory Diagnostic Procedures in the Rheumatic Diseases*, 3d ed, AS Cohen (ed). Orlando, Fla, Grune & Stratton, 1985, pp 377–399

GLENNER GG et al: Amyloid fibril proteins: Proof of homology with immunoglobulin light chains by sequence analyses. Science 172:1150, 1971

HUSBY G et al: The 1990 guidelines for nomenclature and classification of amyloid and amyloidosis, in *Amyloid and Amyloidosis*, JB Natvig et al (eds). Dordrecht, Netherlands, Kluwer, 1990, pp 813–816

KYLE RA, GREIPP PR: Amyloidosis (AL): Clinical and laboratory features in 229 cases. Mayo Clin Proc 58:665, 1983

NATVIG JB et al (eds): *Amyloid and Amyloidosis*. Dordrecht, Netherlands, Kluwer, 1990

section 2   Disorders of immune-mediated injury

282   DISEASES OF IMMEDIATE TYPE HYPERSENSITIVITY

K. FRANK AUSTEN

The term *atopic allergy* implies a familial tendency to manifest alone or in combination such conditions as asthma, rhinitis, urticaria, and eczematous dermatitis (atopic dermatitis). However, individuals without an atopic background also may develop hypersensitivity reactions, particularly urticaria and anaphylaxis, associated with the same class of antibody, IgE, found in atopic individuals. The designation *diseases of immediate type hypersensitivity* presents a more suitable framework than the broad term *allergy* or the restrictive definition of atopy.

The fixation of IgE to human basophils has been demonstrated by radioautography and electron microscopy and to intraepithelial and perivenular mast cells in tonsils, adenoids, and nasal polyps of humans by immunofluorescence. IgE-dependent mediator generation and release also occur in the mast cells of human lung slices, nasal polyps, or skin and have been observed in those tissues most involved in diseases of immediate type hypersensitivity.

The high-affinity receptor for IgE, designated Fc$_\epsilon$RI, is composed of one α, one β, and two disulfide-linked γ chains, which together cross the plasma membrane seven times. The α chain is solely responsible for IgE binding, and the γ chains are responsible for signal transduction that results from the aggregation of the tetrameric receptors by polymeric antigen. The stereospecific receptor perturbation activates a polyphosphatidyl inositol–selective phospholipase C to elaborate 1,2-diacylglycerols (1,2-DAG) and inositol-1,4,5-*tris*-phosphate (IP$_3$), which in turn activate protein kinase C and mobilize intracellular calcium ions, respectively. These events may be augmented by the formation of calcium ion channels and attenuated by the activation of adenylate cyclase with formation of cyclic 3′,5′-adenosine monophosphate (cyclic AMP) and activation of cyclic AMP–dependent protein kinase. The calcium ion–dependent activation of phospholipases cleaves membrane phospholipids to generate lysophospholipids, which, like 1,2-DAG, are fusogenic and may facilitate the fusion of the secretory granule perigranular membrane with the cell membrane, a step that releases the membrane-free granule containing the preformed or primary mediators of mast cell effects. The arachidonic acid cleaved directly from phospholipids by phospholipase A$_2$ and secondarily from intermediates generated from phospholipase C– and D–activated pathways is processed to bioactive lipid mediators (Fig. 282-1). The lysophospholipid formed from release of arachidonic acid from 1-*O*-alkyl-2-acyl-*sn*-glyceryl-3-phosphorylcholine can be acetylated in the second position to form platelet-activating factor (PAF). The secretory granule of the human mast cell has a crystalline structure, unlike mast cells of lower species, and IgE-dependent cell activation can be characterized morphologically by solubilization and swelling of the granule contents within the first minute of receptor perturbation; this reaction is followed by the ordering of intermediate filaments about the swollen granule, movement toward the cell surface, and fusion of the perigranular membrane with that of other granules and with the plasmalemma to form extracellular channels for mediator release while maintaining cell viability.

Important insight into the diversity of mast cells within a species has been gained from studies of serosal mast cells considered to be connective tissue mast cell (CTMC) and mucosal mast cell (MMC)

populations from rats infected with *Nippostrongylus brasiliensis*. The CTMC secretory granules stain with alcian blue and counterstain with safranin; contain large amounts of histamine, heparin proteoglycan, chymotryptic protease termed *neutral protease I*, and carboxypeptidase A; generate prostaglandin D$_2$ upon IgE-Fc–dependent activation; and remain viable ex vivo in coculture with fibroblasts in the absence of added T cell factors. The MMC secretory granules stain with alcian blue but not safranin, synthesize chondroitin sulfate diB and E proteoglycan rather than heparin proteoglycan, contain small amounts of histamine and a distinct chymotryptic protease termed *neutral protease II*, generate leukotriene C$_4$ in preference to prostaglandin D$_2$ (PGD$_2$) during activation-secretion, and are T cell factor–dependent for appearance in vivo or generation from progenitors in vitro. The cloning of the cDNA and corresponding genes for four chymotryptic serine proteases of the mouse mast cell secretory granule has allowed demonstration of early expressed genes in the interleukin 3–dependent bone marrow–derived precursor population and subclass-specific, late expressed genes for CTMC and MMC, respectively.

The evidence for diversity of mast cells within the human is more subtle than in the rat but nonetheless is sufficient to suggest possible functional implications. Mast cells of human lung, intestine, and skin each stain with alcian blue but not safranin and have a similar histamine content. Dispersed partially purified human lung and intestinal mast cells respond to activation by IgE-Fc–dependent mechanisms with generation of LTC$_4$ and PGD$_2$, are not activated by various peptide agonists, are enriched for the secretory granule neutral protease tryptase but lack chymase and carboxypeptidase A, and exhibit secretory granules with a scroll and crystalline ultrastructure. In the lung they synthesize heparin proteoglycan in a 2:1 ratio to chondroitin sulfate E proteoglycan, and in the intestine they are T cell–dependent, as revealed by their absence from mucosal sites in patients with T cell deficiencies. The skin mast cells are readily stimulated for exocytosis by diverse peptides such as C5a anaphylatoxin, substance P, and f-Met-Leu-Phe; they elaborate PGD$_2$ with IgE-Fc receptor–dependent activation; they are much enriched for the secretory granule neutral proteases—tryptase, chymase, and carboxypeptidase A—and for heparin proteoglycan; they exhibit secretory granules with a lattice and crystalline ultrastructure; and they are present in the intestinal submucosa of patients with T cell deficiencies. Although there are, at least, two genes for human secretory granule mast cell tryptases, the homology of their expressed proteins is so great that they are not distinguished by immunohistochemical studies with monoclonal antibodies; hence it is likely that lung and mucosal mast cells contain a tryptase different from that in skin and submucosal mast cells. Whether mast cell diversity is determined entirely by the microenvironment or is dictated in part by different progenitors derived from a common marrow precursor is not established.

Mast cells bearing specific recognition units are distributed at cutaneous and mucosal surfaces and in deeper tissues about venules, are an expansile population during T cell stimulation, and could regulate the entry of foreign substances by their rapid response capability. Upon stimulus-specific activation in vitro, histamine and selected secretory granule–associated acid hydrolases are solubilized, whereas the neutral proteases, which are cationic, remain largely complexed to the anionic proteoglycans. It is speculated that the macromolecular complex serves to deliver the neutral proteases so that the endo- and exoproteases can function in concert at the substrate site to clear damaged tissue and facilitate repair. In addition to these preformed mediators, after activation, mast cells generate lipid mediators from membrane phospholipids and transcribe and translate a range of cytokines (Fig. 282-2). Histamine and the various lipid mediators alter venular permeability, thereby allowing influx of plasma proteins such as complement and immunoglobulins, and the cysteinyl leukotrienes constrict both vascular and nonvascular smooth muscle. Leukotrienes C$_4$ and D$_4$ (LTC$_4$ and LTD$_4$) are logs more potent than histamine in constricting human airway smooth muscle

FIGURE 282-1 Pathways for biosynthesis and release of membrane-derived lipid mediators from mast cells. In the 5-lipoxygenase pathway leukotriene A$_4$ (LTA$_4$) is the intermediate from which the terminal-pathway enzymes generate the distinct final products, leukotriene C$_4$ (LTC$_4$) and leukotriene B$_4$ (LTB$_4$), which leave the cell by separate saturable transport systems. Gamma glutamyl transpeptidase and a dipeptidase then cleave glutamic acid and glycine from LTC$_4$ to form LTD$_4$ and LTE$_4$, respectively, for which there appears to be a common receptor. The only mast cell product of the cyclooxygenase system is PGD$_2$.

FIGURE 282-2   Bioactive mediators of three categories generated by IgE-dependent activation of murine mast cells can elicit common but sequential target cell effects leading to acute and sustained inflammatory responses. *(Modified from Stevens and Austen.)*

when administered by aerosol, and leukotriene E$_4$ (LTE$_4$), the most stable member of the family, is also somewhat more potent than histamine. The 5-lipoxygenation of arachidonic acid to 5S-hydroperoxy-6-*trans*-8,11,14-*cis*-eicosatetraenoic acid (5-HPETE) and then to 5,6-*trans*-oxido-7,9-*trans*-11,14-*cis*-eicosatetraenoic acid (LTA$_4$) is followed by the adduction of glutathione via a microsomal LTC$_4$ synthase to yield 5S-hydroxy-6R-S-glutathionyl-7,9-*trans*-11,14-*cis*-eicosatetraenoic acid (LTC$_4$); upon transport across the membrane to the extracellular environment, LTC$_4$ undergoes sequential cleavage of the glutathione portion to yield the cysteinylglycyl (LTD$_4$) and cysteinyl (LTE$_4$) derivatives. Alternatively, a cytosolic LTA$_4$ epoxide hydrolase converts LTA$_4$ into 5S-12R-dihydroxy-6,14-*cis*-8,10-*trans*-eicosatetraenoic acid (LTB$_4$), which mediates leukocyte margination and directed (chemotactic) migration in human sites. This proinflammatory response would be sustained by a cytokine such as tumor necrosis factor alpha (TNF-α). Interleukin 4 is critical to the B cell switch for IgE biosynthesis, and IL-3 and IL-4 cause the proliferation of immature mast cells from bone marrow progenitors for tissue-directed differentiation. Thus there is the possibility of an autocrine mechanism for IgE/mast cell–mediated disease. There is even evolving evidence that mast cells, via their constituents, can regulate fibroblast proliferation and/or angiogenesis. Local and subclinical regulation of the tissue microenvironment would represent an initial and homeostatic physiologic response, whereas an intense or continuous stimulus would result in inflammation and tissue injury that could be either beneficial or detrimental (hypersensitivity) depending on the appropriateness of the immunologic specificity.

Consideration of the mechanism of immediate type hypersensitivity diseases in the human has focused largely on the IgE-dependent recognition of otherwise nontoxic substances. Support for this thesis has come from the finding that clinical atopic allergy is associated with elevated total levels of IgE and in some instances with an immune response that is specifically linked to the histocompatibility locus. Populations of allergic whites have a significantly higher total serum level of IgE than nonallergic individuals, and highly atopic persons with asthma have significantly higher serum levels of IgE than those with fewer allergic manifestations. IgE distribution in normal families is consistent with the dominant inheritance of the low-IgE phenotype. As a result of the action of a single IgE regulator gene, the majority of family members would have elevated IgE levels as a possible basis for their atopic state. The association between HLA histocompatibility type and the immediate hypersensitivity response has been noted in persons of the low-IgE phenotype who were studied with highly purified allergens, generally of small size. Such presumptive evidence of immune-response (Ir) genes by linkage sequilibrium, i.e., the association of the hypersensitivity response

with a particular histocompatibility haplotype, represents an additional element in the polygenic atopic allergic state. Nonetheless, all the studies taken together, both of families and of populations, seem to indicate that the genetically determined elevated IgE levels found in about three-fourths of atopic allergic subjects exert the predominant influence on most specific IgE responses. It is also likely that diseases of immediate type hypersensitivity may occur because of deficient intracellular controls of mediator generation or release, or both, or that the extracellular controls directed against mediator inactivation may be impaired.

ANAPHYLAXIS   **Definition**   The life-threatening anaphylactic response of a sensitized human appears within minutes after administration of specific antigen and is manifested by respiratory distress often followed by vascular collapse or by shock without antecedent respiratory difficulty. Cutaneous manifestations exemplified by pruritus and urticaria with or without angioedema are characteristic of such systemic anaphylactic reactions. Gastrointestinal manifestations include nausea, vomiting, crampy abdominal pain, and diarrhea.

Predisposing factors and etiology   There is no convincing evidence that age, sex, race, occupation, or geographic location predisposes a human to anaphylaxis except through exposure to some immunogen. According to most studies, atopy does not predispose individuals to anaphylaxis from penicillin therapy or venom of a stinging insect.

The materials capable of eliciting the systemic anaphylactic reaction in the human include the following: heterologous proteins in the form of hormones (insulin, vasopressin, parathormone), enzymes (trypsin, chymotrypsin, penicillinase), pollen extracts (ragweed, grass, trees), food (eggs, seafoods, nuts, grains, beans, cottonseed oil, chocolate), antiserum (antilymphocyte gamma globulin), occupational proteins (rubber products), and Hymenoptera venom (yellow jacket, yellow and baldfaced hornets, paper wasp, honey bee, imported fire ants); polysaccharides such as iron dextran; and most commonly drugs such as antibiotics (penicillins, cephalosporins, amphotericin B, nitrofurantoin), local anesthetics (procaine, lidocaine), vitamins (thiamine, folic acid), diagnostic agents (sodium dehydrocholate, sulfobromophthalein), and occupational chemicals (ethylene oxide), which are considered to function as haptens that form immunogenic conjugates with host proteins. The conjugating hapten may be the parent compound, a nonenzymatically derived storage product, or a metabolite formed in the host.

Pathophysiology and manifestations   Individuals differ in the time of appearance of perception of symptoms and signs, but the hallmark of the anaphylactic reaction is the onset of some manifestation within seconds to minutes after introduction of the antigen, generally by injection or less commonly by ingestion. There may be upper or lower airway obstruction or both. Laryngeal edema may be experienced as a "lump" in the throat, hoarseness, or stridor, while bronchial obstruction is associated with a feeling of tightness in the chest or audible wheezing. A particularly characteristic feature is the eruption of well-circumscribed, discrete cutaneous wheals with erythematous, raised, serpiginous borders and blanched centers. These urticarial eruptions are intensely pruritic and may be localized or distributed. They may coalesce to form giant hives, and they seldom persist beyond 48 h. A localized, nonpitting, deeper edematous cutaneous process, angioedema, also may be present. It may be asymptomatic or cause a burning or stinging sensation.

In fatal cases with clinical bronchial obstruction, the lungs show marked hyperinflation on gross and microscopic examination. The microscopic findings in the bronchi, however, are limited to luminal secretions, peribronchial congestion, submucosal edema, and eosinophilic infiltration, and the acute emphysema is attributed to intractable bronchospasm that subsides with death. The angioedema resulting in death by mechanical obstruction occurs in the epiglottis and larynx, but the process is also evident in the hypopharynx and to some extent the trachea; on microscopic examination there is wide separation of the collagen fibers and the glandular elements; vascular congestion and eosinophilic infiltration are also present. Patients dying of vascular collapse without antecedent hypoxia from respiratory insufficiency have visceral congestion with a presumptive loss of intravascular blood volume. The associated electrocardiographic abnormalities, with or without infarction, noted in some patients could reflect a primary cardiac event or be secondary to a critical reduction in plasma volume.

The angioedematous and urticarial manifestations of the anaphylactic syndrome have been attributed to release of endogenous histamine. A role for the cysteinyl leukotrienes in altering pulmonary mechanics by causing marked bronchiolar constriction seems likely. Vascular collapse without respiratory distress in response to experimental challenge with the sting of a hymenopteran was associated not only with marked and prolonged elevations in blood histamine but also with evidence of intravascular coagulation and kinin generation. Based on the findings that patients with systemic mastocytosis and episodic hypotension proceeding to vascular collapse excrete large amounts of PGD_2 in addition to histamine and are controlled by administration of a nonsteroidal agent but not by antihistamines alone, it may be that PGD_2 is also of importance in the hypotensive anaphylactic reactions. Because of the marked coronary arterial constrictor action of the cysteinyl leukotrienes upon administration to experimental animals, these substances may be involved in the disease process of patients with myocardial ischemia without or with infarction.

Diagnosis The diagnosis of an anaphylactic reaction depends largely on an accurate history revealing the onset of the appropriate symptoms and signs within minutes after the responsible material is encountered. When only a portion of the full syndrome is present, such as isolated urticaria, sudden bronchospasm in an asthmatic patient, or vascular collapse after intravenous administration of an agent, it is difficult to exclude a nonimmunologic, toxicologic, or idiosyncratic response. For example, intravenous administration of a chemical mast cell–degranulating agent may elicit generalized urticaria, angioedema, and a sensation of retrosternal oppression with or without clinically detectable bronchoconstriction or hypotension. Furthermore, nonsteroidal anti-inflammatory agents such as indomethacin, aminopyrine, mefenamic acid, and aspirin may precipitate a life-threatening episode of obstruction of upper or lower airways in asthmatic subjects that is clinically reminiscent of anaphylaxis but is not associated with a detectable IgE response. This syndrome may reflect a unique reactivity to an imbalance in the ratio of prostaglandin to leukotriene biosynthesis when cyclooxygenase is inhibited.

The presence of a labile reagin (IgE) in the heart blood of a patient dying of systemic anaphylaxis has been demonstrated at postmortem by passive transfer of the serum intradermally into a normal recipient, followed in 24 h by antigen challenge into the same site, with subsequent development of a wheal and flare, the Prausnitz-Küstner reaction. Indeed, such a reagin can be transiently identified in the serum of most patients who develop systemic anaphylaxis to a variety of different agents. In order to avoid the hazards of transferring hepatitis to the recipient in the Prausnitz-Küstner reaction, it is preferable to employ the less sensitive monkey recipient or a human leukocyte suspension enriched with basophils for subsequent antigen challenge. It is presumed that the activity responsible for most cases of systemic anaphylaxis resides with the IgE class, since the Prausnitz-Küstner activity in the sera of patients with systemic reactions to Hymenoptera venom or human seminal plasma protein can be removed by IgE immunosorbent columns. Furthermore, radioimmunoassays have demonstrated specific IgE antibodies in patients with anaphylactic reactions to insulin and to parathormone, but such approaches require purified antigens. In the transfusion anaphylactic reaction that occurs in patients with IgA deficiency, the responsible specificity resides in IgG anti-IgA rather than in IgE; the mechanism of the reaction is presumed to be complement activation with secondary mast cell participation.

Treatment and prevention Early recognition of an anaphylactic reaction is mandatory, since death occurs within minutes to hours after the first symptoms. Mild symptoms such as pruritus and urticaria can be controlled by administration of 0.2 to 0.5 mL of 1:1000 epinephrine subcutaneously, with repeated doses as required at 20-min intervals for a severe reaction. If the antigenic material was injected into an extremity, the rate of absorption may be reduced by prompt application of a tourniquet proximal to the reaction site, administration of 0.2 mL of 1:1000 epinephrine into the site, and removal without compression of an insect stinger, if present. An intravenous infusion should be initiated to provide a route for administration of 5.0 mL epinephrine, diluted 1:10,000, at 5- to 10-min intervals, volume expanders, and vasopressor agents such as dopamine if intractable hypotension occurs. Epinephrine provides both alpha- and beta-adrenergic effects, resulting in vasoconstriction, bronchial smooth-muscle relaxation, and attenuation of enhanced venular permeability. Beta blockers are relatively contraindicated in persons at risk for anaphylactic reactions, especially those sensitive to Hymenoptera venom or those undergoing immunotherapy for respiratory system allergy. When epinephrine fails to control the situation, hypoxia due to airway obstruction or related to a cardiac arrhythmia, or both, must be considered. Oxygen via a nasal catheter or intermittent positive-pressure breathing of oxygen with 0.5 mL isoproterenol diluted 1:200 in saline may be helpful, but either endotracheal intubation or a tracheostomy is mandatory for oxygen delivery if progressive hypoxia exists. Ancillary agents such as the antihistamine diphenhydramine, 50 to 80 mg intramuscularly or intravenously, and aminophylline, 0.25 to 0.5 g intravenously, are appropriate for urticaria-angioedema and bronchospasm, respectively. Intravenous corticosteroids are not effective for the acute event but may be considered for persistent bronchospasm and hypotension.

Prevention of anaphylaxis must take into account the sensitivity of the recipient, the dose and character of the diagnostic or therapeutic agent, and the effect of the route of administration on the rate of absorption. If there is a definite history of a past anaphylactic reaction, even though mild, it is advisable to select another agent or procedure. A knowledge of cross-reactivity among agents is critical since, for example, cephalosporins share a common β-lactam ring with the penicillins. A skin test should be performed before the administration of certain materials producing a high incidence of anaphylactic reactions, such as horse serum or allergenic extracts, or when the nature of the past adverse reaction is unknown. Since even a skin or conjunctival test can produce a serious reaction, a scratch test should precede these tests in a high-risk situation. With regard to penicillin, two-thirds of patients with a positive reaction history and positive intradermal skin tests to benzylpenicilloyl-polylysine (BPL) and/or the minor determinant mixture (MDM) of benzylpenicillin products experience allergic reactions with treatment, and these are almost uniformly of the anaphylactic type in those patients with minor determinant reactivity. Even patients without a history of previous clinical reactions have a 6 percent incidence of positive skin tests to the two test materials, and about 3 per 1000 with a negative history experience anaphylaxis with therapy, with a mortality of about 1 per 100,000. The value of skin testing is both to permit therapy with the agent in question when the risk does not exist and to emphasize the hazards where the sensitivity is confirmed. In the event that an agent must be used despite a positive history, a positive skin test, or both, the following precautionary measures should be taken: An intravenous infusion should be started, with intubation equipment and a tracheostomy set at hand; the material should be given intradermally, then subcutaneously, and then intramuscularly in increasing doses at 20- to 30-min intervals so that the initial dose by the next route does not exceed the final dose by the previous route. It is difficult to be certain that the mediator-containing cells have been exhausted, and therapeutic use of the agent may be accompanied by untoward consequences. It may be critical to give the therapeutic agent at regular intervals to prevent the reestablishment of a sensitized cell pool of large size.

A different form of protection involves the development of blocking antibody of the IgG class which is protective against Hymenoptera venom–induced anaphylaxis by interacting with antigen so that less reaches the sensitized tissue mast cells; to be effective, this immunotherapy requires the use of specific or cross-reacting Hymenoptera venom rather than whole-insect-body extracts.

Because sensitization can be transient, the maximal risk for systemic anaphylactic reactions in persons with Hymenoptera sensitivity occurs in association with a currently positive skin test. Although there is only low-grade cross-reactivity between honey bee and yellow jacket venoms, there is a high degree of cross-reactivity between yellow jacket venom and the rest of the vespid venoms (yellow or baldfaced hornets and wasps). Prevention involves modification of outside activities to exclude bare feet, wearing perfumed toiletries, eating in certain areas, clipping hedges or grass, and hauling away trash or fallen fruit. As with each anaphylactic sensitivity, the individual should wear an informational bracelet and have immediate access to an unexpired epinephrine kit located within the home, the vehicle, and/or carried. The limitations of lifestyle and the psychological duress can be addressed by venom immunotherapy to achieve a venom-specific IgG titer above 3.0 μg/mL of serum. Present knowledge favors indefinite continuation of venom therapy with a maintenance schedule or until the skin test becomes negative, with confirmation by immunochemical measurement of specific IgE in serum. For children with a systemic reaction limited to skin, the likelihood of progression to more serious respiratory or vascular manifestations is low, and thus immunotherapy is not recommended.

URTICARIA AND ANGIOEDEMA   Definition   Urticaria and angioedema may appear separately or together as cutaneous manifestations of localized nonpitting edema; a similar process may occur at mucosal surfaces of the upper respiratory or gastrointestinal tract. *Urticaria* involves only the superficial portion of the dermis, presenting as well-circumscribed wheals with erythematous raised serpiginous borders with blanched centers that may coalesce to become giant wheals. *Angioedema* is a well-demarcated localized edema involving the deeper layers of the skin, including the subcutaneous tissue. Recurrent episodes of urticaria and/or angioedema of less than 6 weeks' duration are considered acute, whereas attacks persisting beyond this period are designated chronic.

Predisposing factors and etiology   The occurrence of urticaria and angioedema is probably more frequent than usually described because of the evanescent, self-limited nature of such eruptions, which seldom require medical attention when limited to the skin. Although persons in any age group may experience acute or chronic urticaria and/or angioedema, these lesions increase in frequency after adolescence, with the highest incidence occurring in persons in the third decade of life; indeed, one survey of college students indicated that some 15 to 20 percent had experienced a pruritic wheal reaction.

The classification of urticaria-angioedema presented in Table 282-1 focuses on the different mechanisms for eliciting clinical disease.

TABLE 282-1   Classification of urticaria with angioedema

IgE-dependent
 A Atopic diathesis
 B Specific antigen sensitivity (pollens, foods, drugs, fungi, molds, Hymenoptera venom, helminths)
 C Physical: dermographism, cold, light, cholinergic, vibratory, exercise-related
Complement-mediated
 A Hereditary angioedema: type 1, type 2
 B Acquired angioedema: type 1, type 2
 C Necrotizing vasculitis
 D Serum sickness
 E Reactions to blood products
Nonimmunologic
 A Direct mast cell–releasing agents: opiates, antibiotics, curare, D-tubocurarine, radiocontrast media
 B Agents which presumably alter arachidonic acid metabolism: aspirin and nonsteroidal anti-inflammatory agents, azo dyes, and benzoates
Idiopathic

Only the IgE-dependent and the IgG-mediated reactions in IgA-deficient persons should be considered immediate hypersensitivity. However, the other mechanisms are important for differential diagnosis, and most cases of chronic urticaria are idiopathic. The appearance of urticaria and angioedema in atopic persons in the absence of a specific exposure is attributed to the atopic diathesis and implies an IgE mechanism. Urticaria and/or angioedema occurring during the appropriate season in patients with seasonal respiratory allergy or as a result of exposure to animals or molds is attributed to inhalation of pollens, animal dander, and mold spores, respectively. However, urticaria and angioedema secondary to inhalation are relatively uncommon compared with ingestion of fresh fruits, shellfish, chocolate, nuts, tomatoes, and various drugs, including penicillin-contaminated milk products, that may elicit not only the anaphylactic syndrome with prominent gastrointestinal complaints but also chronic urticaria.

Additional etiologies include physical stimuli such as cold, solar rays, exercise, and mechanical irritation. The physical urticarias can be distinguished by the precipitating event and other aspects of the clinical presentation. *Dermographism*, which occurs in 1 to 4 percent of the population, is defined by the appearance of a linear wheal at the site of a brisk stroke with a firm object or by any configuration appropriate to the eliciting event. Dermographism has a prevalence that peaks in the second to third decades. It is not influenced by an atopic diathesis and has a duration generally of less than 5 years. *Pressure urticaria*, which often accompanies dermographism or chronic idiopathic urticaria, presents in response to a sustained stimulus such as a shoulder strap or belt, running (feet), or manual labor (hands). *Cholinergic urticaria* is distinctive in that the pruritic wheals are of small size (1–2 mm) and are surrounded by a large area of erythema; attacks are precipitated by fever, a hot bath or shower, or exercise and are presumptively attributed to a rise in core body temperature. *Exercise-related anaphylaxis* begins with erythema and pruritic urticaria but progresses to angioedema of the face, oropharynx, larynx, or intestine or to vascular collapse; it is distinguished from cholinergic urticaria by presenting with wheals of conventional size and by not occurring with fever or a hot bath. *Cold urticaria*, either acquired or hereditary, is local at the exposed site (ice cube) or exposed body areas (ambient temperature) but can progress to vascular collapse with immersion in cold water (swimming). *Solar urticaria* is subdivided into three groups by the response to specific portions of the light spectrum. *Vibratory angioedema* may occur after years of occupational exposure or can be idiopathic; it may be accompanied by cholinergic urticaria. Other rare forms of physical allergy, always defined by stimulus-specific elicitation, include *local heat urticaria*, *aquagenic urticaria* from contact with water of any temperature, and *contact urticaria* from direct interaction with some chemical substance.

Angioedema without urticaria occurs with $C\bar{1}$ inhibitor ($C\bar{1}$INH) deficiency that can be inborn as an autosomal dominant characteristic or can be acquired. The urticaria and angioedema associated with classical serum sickness or with idiopathic cutaneous necrotizing angiitis are believed to be an immune-complex disease when hypocomplementemia is a concomitant. The idiosyncratic drug reactions to mast cell granule–releasing agents and to nonsteroidal anti-inflammatory drugs can be systemic, resembling anaphylaxis, or limited to cutaneous sites.

Pathophysiology and manifestations Urticarial eruptions are distinctly pruritic, involve any area of the body from the scalp to the soles of the feet, and appear in crops of 24- to 72-h duration, with old lesions fading as new ones appear. The most common sites are the extremities, external genitalia, and face, particularly the region of the eyes and lips. Although self-limited in duration, angioedema of the upper respiratory tract may be life-threatening due to laryngeal obstruction, while gastrointestinal involvement may present with abdominal colic, with or without nausea and vomiting, and may precipitate unnecessary surgical intervention. No residual discoloration occurs with either urticaria or angioedema unless there is an underlying process leading to superimposed extravasation of erythrocytes.

The pathology of urticaria and angioedema is usually characterized by massive edema of the dermis in urticaria and of the subcutaneous tissue as well as the dermis in angioedema. Collagen bundles in affected areas are widely separated, and the venules are sometimes dilated. The perivenular infiltrate may consist of lymphocytes, eosinophils, and neutrophils that are present in varying combination and number throughout the dermis. Allergen-induced wheal-and-flare reactions are characterized by mast cell degranulation and an accumulation of eosinophils over hours to days. The elicitation of a wheal-and-flare response upon injection of the relevant allergen into a patient with urticaria and/or angioedema or into a site in a normal recipient prepared with serum from the patient, the Prausnitz-Küstner reaction, indicates an IgE-dependent mast cell–mediated reaction.

Perhaps the best-studied example of mast cell–mediated urticaria and angioedema is *cold urticaria*. Cryoglobulins, cryofibrinogens, cold agglutinins, or hemolysins may be recognized, but not in the majority of patients. The finding in a number of patients of a serum factor, characterized as being of the IgE class, that is capable of transferring the cold urticaria reaction to a skin site of a normal recipient has focused attention on the mast cell in this condition. Immersion of an extremity in an ice bath precipitates angioedema of the distal portion with urticaria at the air interface within minutes of the challenge. Histologic studies reveal marked mast cell degranulation with associated edema of the dermis and subcutaneous tissues. The venous effluent of the cold-challenged and angioedematous extremity reveals a marked rise in plasma content of histamine, low-molecular-weight eosinophilotactic activity, and high-molecular-weight neutrophil chemotactic activity, which are presumably of mast cell origin, whereas the venous effluent of the contralateral normal extremity contains none of these mediators. Elevated levels of histamine have been found in the plasma content of venous effluent and in the fluid of suction blisters at experimentally induced lesional sites in patients with dermographism, pressure urticaria, vibratory angioedema, light urticaria, and heat urticaria. By ultrastructural analysis, the pattern of mast cell degranulation in cold urticaria resembles an IgE-mediated response with solubilization of granule contents, fusion of the perigranular and cell membranes, and discharge of granule contents, whereas in a dermographic lesion there is an additional superimposed zonal (piecemeal) degranulation. Elevations of plasma histamine with biopsy-proven mast cell degranulation also have been demonstrated with systemic attacks of *cholinergic urticaria* and *exercise-induced erythema-angioedema* precipitated experimentally by exercise on a treadmill while wearing a wet suit; however, only in cholinergic urticaria is there a concomitant decrease in pulmonary function.

Diagnosis The rapid onset and self-limited nature of urticarial and angioedematous eruptions are distinguishing features. Additional characteristics are the occurrence of the urticarial crops in various stages of evolution and the asymmetric distribution of the angioedema. Urticaria and/or angioedema involving IgE-dependent mechanisms are often appreciated by historical considerations implicating specific allergens or physical stimuli, by seasonal incidence, and by exposure to certain environments. Direct reproduction of the lesion with physical stimuli is particularly valuable because it so often establishes the cause of the lesion. The diagnosis of an environmental allergen can be sought by careful skin testing with the putative substance to determine if a local wheal and flare results. Passive transfer by the injection of serum from an affected individual of such a reaction into a skin site of a normal recipient followed by allergen challenge, the Prausnitz-Küstner phenomenon, is not appropriate because of the risks associated with any injection of donor serum. Passive transfer to the skin of a nonhuman primate or in vitro to human basophils may be attempted. IgE-mediated urticaria and/or angioedema may or may not be associated with an elevation of total IgE or with peripheral eosinophilia. Fever, leukocytosis, or an elevated sedimentation rate are characteristically absent.

The classification of urticarial and angioedematous states noted in Table 282-1 in terms of possible mechanisms necessarily includes some differential diagnostic points. Hypocomplementemia is not observed in IgE-mediated mast cell disease and can reflect either an acquired abnormality generally attributed to the formation of immune complexes or a genetic deficiency of C$\overline{1}$INH. Chronic recurrent urticaria, generally in females, associated with arthralgias, an elevated sedimentation rate, and normo- or hypocomplementemia suggests an underlying cutaneous necrotizing angiitis. Confirmation depends on a biopsy that reveals cellular infiltration, nuclear debris, and fibrinoid necrosis of the venules. The same pathobiologic process accounts for the urticaria in association with such diseases as systemic lupus erythematosus, Sjögren's syndrome, or viral hepatitis with or without an associated arteritis. Serum sickness per se or a similar clinical entity due to drugs includes not only urticaria but also pyrexia, lymphadenopathy, myalgia, and arthralgia or arthritis. Urticarial reactions to blood products or IgG treatment are defined by the event and generally are not progressive unless the recipient is IgA deficient in the former case or the reagent is aggregated in the latter.

Hereditary angioedema is an autosomal dominant state associated with the absence of functional C$\overline{1}$INH. The diagnosis is suggested not only by family history but also by the lack of urticarial lesions, the prominence of recurrent gastrointestinal attacks of colic, and episodes of laryngeal edema. Laboratory diagnosis depends on demonstrating the antigenic lack of C$\overline{1}$INH (type 1) in most kindreds, but some kindreds have an antigenically intact nonfunctional protein (type 2) and require a functional assay to establish the diagnosis. The natural substrates of uninhibited C$\overline{1}$, C4, and C2 are chronically depleted but fall further during attacks due to the activation of additional C1 to C$\overline{1}$. Because the C$\overline{1}$INH protein also regulates the Hageman factor–initiated activation of kallikrein and of plasmin, the vasoactive peptides responsible for the angioedema are likely some combination of bradykinin and a plasmin-derived fragment of C$\overline{1}$-cleaved C2. An acquired form of C$\overline{1}$INH deficiency, associated with lymphoproliferative disorders, has the same clinical manifestations and differs in the lack of a familial element; in the reduction of C1/C$\overline{1}$ as well as C$\overline{1}$INH, C4, and C2; and in the presence of an anti-idiotypic antibody to the monoclonal immunoglobulin expressed on the B cells (type 1). In a second acquired form of C$\overline{1}$INH deficiency with angioedema due to appearance of IgG anti-C$\overline{1}$INH (type 2) B cell malignancy has not been prominent.

Urticaria and angioedema must be differentiated from contact sensitivity, an acute vesicular eruption that progresses to chronic thickening of the skin with continued allergenic exposure. They must also be differentiated from atopic dermatitis, a condition that may present as erythema, edema, papules, vesiculation, and oozing proceeding to a subacute and chronic stage in which vesiculation is less marked or absent and scaling, fissuring, and lichenification predominate in a distribution that characteristically involves the flexor surfaces. In cutaneous mastocytosis, the reddish brown macules and papules, characteristic of urticaria pigmentosa, urticate with pruritus upon trauma; and in systemic mastocytosis, without or with urticaria pigmentosa, there is an episodic systemic flushing with or without urticaria but no angioedema.

Prevention and treatment Identification of the etiologic factor(s) and their elimination provide the most satisfactory therapeutic program; this approach is feasible to varying degrees with IgE-mediated reactions to allergens or physical stimuli. Topically applied steroids are of no benefit in the management of urticaria and/or angioedema; and while systemic steroids have no general value, they are helpful in an occasional patient with necrotizing cutaneous angiitis, pressure urticaria, or even ordinary urticaria and angioedema. Antihistamines of the H1 class and sympathomimetic agents often provide symptomatic relief; cyproheptadine, hydroxyzine, and a combination of H1 and H2 antihistamines are held to be even more beneficial. The therapy of inborn C$\overline{1}$INH deficiency has been simplified by the finding that attenuated androgens correct the biochemical defect and afford prophylactic protection. Since the affected individuals are heterozygous, with the depletion of C$\overline{1}$INH being due to a combination of deficient synthesis and excessive utilization of the normal gene product, the efficacy of the attenuated androgens is attributed to production by the normal gene of an amount of functional C$\overline{1}$INH sufficient to control the spontaneous activation of C1 to C$\overline{1}$. Since the use of such agents for children and pregnant women is not yet accepted, the antifibrinolytic agent ε-aminocaproic acid may be used occasionally to control spontaneous attacks or for preoperative prophylaxis in some patients.

SYSTEMIC MASTOCYTOSIS Definition *Systemic mastocytosis* is defined by mast cell hyperplasia that in most instances is indolent and nonneoplastic. Since human mast cells originate from pluripotent bone marrow cells (CD34 +) and disseminate as unrecognized progenitors for tissue-specific proliferation and maturation, the hyperplasia is generally recognized in bone marrow and such peripheral sites as skin, gastrointestinal mucosa, liver, and spleen. Mastocytosis occurs at any age and has a slight preponderance in males. The prevalence of systemic mastocytosis is not known, and a familial occurrence has not been established.

Classification, pathophysiology, and clinical manifestations A recent consensus classification for systemic mastocytosis recognizes four forms (Table 282-2). The form designated as *indolent* accounts for the majority of patients and is not known to alter life expectancy. When a patient is classified as having indolent systemic mastocytosis, the concomitant clinical findings must be carefully noted, since they define the complications and directions for management. In systemic mastocytosis *associated with hematologic disorders*, the prognosis is determined by the nature of that disorder, which can range from dysmyelopoiesis to frank leukemia. In *aggressive* systemic mastocytosis, mast cell proliferation in parenchymal organs such as liver, spleen, and lymph nodes is marked and in a subset of patients is associated with prominent eosinophilia; the prognosis is limited. *Mast cell leukemia* is the rarest form of the disease and is invariably fatal at present.

With the recognition from studies with mouse bone marrow–derived mast cells that some nine recombinant cytokines can regulate

proliferation and/or cellular phenotype, systemic mastocytosis of the human is viewed as a disorder of regulation in which the clinical manifestations are largely due to the chemical mediators provided by mast cells, with some contribution from the space occupancy of the mast cell load itself. The pharmacologically induced manifestations are pruritus, flushing, palpitations and vascular collapse, gastric distress, lower abdominal crampy pain, and recurrent headache. The increase in cell burden is evidenced by the small, reddish brown macules or papules, termed *urticaria pigmentosa*, at skin sites but also contributes to bone pain and malabsorption. The mast cell–mediated fibrotic changes are limited to liver, spleen, and bone marrow and presumably relate to the functional characteristics of mast cells developing at those sites, as opposed to those prominent at sites without fibrosis, such as the gastrointestinal tissue or skin. Immunofluorescent analysis of bone marrow and skin lesions in mastocytosis reveals only one mast cell phenotype with the epitopes of tryptase, chymase, and carboxypeptidase A.

The cutaneous lesions of urticaria pigmentosa respond to trauma with urtication and erythema (Darier's sign). Because of the difficulty in diagnosing systemic mastocytosis in the absence of skin lesions to biopsy, the apparent incidence of these lesions of 90 percent or greater in patients with indolent systemic mastocytosis may be an overestimation. Approximately 1 percent of patients with indolent mastocytosis have skin lesions that appear as tan-brown macules with striking patchy erythema and associated telangiectasia (telangiectasia macularis eruptive perstans). In the gastrointestinal tract, histamine-mediated hypersecretion is the most common problem, with resultant gastritis and peptic ulcer. The diarrhea and abdominal pain attributed to disease of the small intestine can be aggravated by malabsorption with nutritional insufficiency and osteomalacia. The periportal fibrosis associated with mast cell infiltration and a prominence of eosinophils can, on occasion, lead to portal hypertension and ascites. In some patients, flushing and recurrent vascular collapse are markedly aggravated by an idiosyncratic response to minimal dosage of nonsteroidal anti-inflammatory agents. The neuropsychiatric disturbances are clinically most evident as impaired recent memory and "migraine-like" headaches. Patients in every category of systemic mastocytosis can experience exacerbation of a specific clinical sign or symptom with alcohol ingestion, use of mast cell–interactive narcotics, and ingestion of nonsteroidal anti-inflammatory agents, to which the response is idiosyncratic.

Diagnosis Although the diagnosis is generally suspected on the basis of the clinical history and physical findings, the contention can be strengthened by certain laboratory procedures and established only by a tissue diagnosis. A 24-h urine collection for measurement of histamine, histamine metabolites, or metabolites of PGD$_2$ is currently the most common noninvasive approach. A convenient alternative, but with a lesser incidence of positivity, is to measure blood levels of histamine or the mast cell–derived neutral protease tryptase. Additional studies directed by the presentation include a bone scan or skeletal survey; contrast studies of the upper gastrointestinal tract with small bowel follow-through, CT scan, or endoscopy; and a neuropsychiatric evaluation, including an EEC. The tissue diagnosis is straightforward if there are lesions of urticaria pigmentosa, but the diagnosis of systemic mastocytosis requires involvement of other organs and is most frequently established by bone marrow biopsy and aspiration. The bone marrow lesions consist of focal and paratrabecular aggregates of mast cells, often mixed with eosinophils, lymphocytes, and, on occasion, plasma cells, histiocytes, and fibroblasts.

The differential diagnosis requires the exclusion of other flushing disorders. The 24-h urine assessment of 5-hydroxy-indoleacetic acid and metanephrines should exclude a carcinoid tumor or a pheochromocytoma. Most patients with recurrent anaphylaxis, including the idiopathic group, present with angioedema, which is not a manifestation of systemic mastocytosis.

Treatment The management of systemic mastocytosis uses a stepwise and symptom-sign–directed approach that includes an H1 antihistamine for flushing and pruritus, an H2 antihistamine or proton

---

TABLE 282-2 Classification of systemic mastocytosis

Type	Description
I	*Indolent* with cutaneous manifestations, vascular collapse, ulcer disease, malabsorption, skeletal disease, hepatosplenomegaly, or lymphadenopathy
II	*Concomitant hematologic disorder*, either myelodysplastic or myeloproliferative
III	*Aggressive* per se or lymphadenopathic mastocytosis with eosinophilia
IV	*Mastocytic leukemia*

pump inhibitor for gastric acid hypersecretion, oral cromolyn sodium for diarrhea and abdominal pain, and a nonsteroidal anti-inflammatory agent for severe flushing associated with vascular collapse despite use of H1 and H2 antihistamines to block biosynthesis of PGD_2. Although systemic glucocorticoids appear to alleviate the malabsorption, their use is complicated by disease of the upper gastrointestinal tract or bone. Chemotherapy is not appropriate for patients with indolent mastocytosis and apparently does not prolong survival in patients with mast cell leukemia. It is appropriate for associated hematologic disorders of other cell types and for the aggressive form of systemic mastocytosis.

ALLERGIC RHINITIS Definition Allergic rhinitis is characterized by sneezing; rhinorrhea; obstruction of the nasal passages; conjunctival, nasal, and pharyngeal itching; and lacrimation, all occurring in a temporal relationship to allergen exposure. Although commonly seasonal due to elicitation by airborne pollens, it can be perennial in an environment of chronic exposure. The incidence of allergic rhinitis in North America is about 7 percent, with the peak occurring in childhood and adolescence.

Predisposing factors and etiology Allergic rhinitis generally presents in atopic individuals, i.e., in persons with a family history of a similar or related symptom complex and a personal history of collateral allergy expressed as eczematous dermatitis, urticaria, and/ or asthma (see Chap. 217). Symptoms generally appear before the fourth decade of life and tend to diminish gradually with aging, although complete spontaneous remissions are uncommon. A relatively small number of weeds that depend on wind rather than insects for cross-pollination, as well as certain grasses and trees, produce sufficient quantities of pollen suitable for wide distribution by air currents to elicit seasonal allergic rhinitis. The dates of pollination of these species generally vary little from year to year in a particular locale but may be quite different in another climate. Molds, which are widespread in nature because they occur in soil or decaying organic matter, may propagate spores in a pattern dependent on climatic conditions. Perennial allergic rhinitis occurs in response to allergens that are present throughout the year such as in desquamating epithelium in animal dander, the processed materials or chemicals utilized in an industrial setting, or the dust accumulating at work or at home. Dust has a diverse content including mites, and many patients with perennial rhinitis are sensitive only to house dust. Moreover, in many patients with perennial rhinitis, no clear-cut allergen can be demonstrated. The ability of allergens to cause rhinitis rather than lower respiratory symptoms may be attributed to their size, 10 to 100 μm, and retention within the nose. However, even when the allergen penetrates to the lower respiratory tract, whether it elicits a bronchoconstrictor response resulting from mediator release depends on the presence of chronically hyperirritable airways.

Pathophysiology and manifestations Episodic rhinorrhea, sneezing, and obstruction of the nasal passages with lacrimation and pruritus of the conjunctiva, nasal mucosa, and oropharynx are the hallmarks of allergic rhinitis. The nasal mucosa is pale and boggy, but the nares are not reddened or excoriated. The conjunctiva may be congested and edematous; the pharynx is generally unremarkable but may appear injected. Swelling of the turbinates and mucous membranes with obstruction of the sinus ostia and eustachian tubes precipitates secondary infections of the sinuses and middle ear, respectively, commonly in perennial but rarely in seasonal disease. Nasal polyps often arise concurrently with edema and/or infection within the sinuses and increase obstructive symptoms.

The nose presents a large mucosal surface area through the folds of the turbinates and serves to adjust the temperature and moisture content of inhaled air and to filter out particulate materials. The convoluted nasal passages readily filter out particles above 10 μm in size by impingement in a mucous blanket at bends in their course; ciliary action then moves the entrapped particles toward the pharynx. Entrapment of pollen and digestion of the outer coat by mucosal enzymes such as lysozymes release protein allergens generally of 10,000 to 40,000 molecular weight. Although the initial interaction

occurs between the allergen and intraepithelial mast cells sensitized with specific IgE, the bulk of the mast cells are located beneath the mucosal surface and are recruited secondarily. During the symptomatic season when the mucosa are already swollen and hyperemic, there is enhanced adverse reactivity to the seasonal pollen as well as to antigenically unrelated pollens for which there is underlying hypersensitivity. This priming effect is attributed to improved penetration of the allergens to the deeper perivenular mast cells. Biopsy specimens of nasal mucosa during an episodic allergic reaction show profound submucosal edema with infiltration predominantly by eosinophils, although some neutrophil polymorphonuclear leukocytes are present. Polyps, a feature in perennial rhinitis, are mucosal protrusions containing chiefly edema fluid with variable degrees of eosinophilic infiltration.

The mucosal surface fluid contains not only IgA that is present preferentially because of its secretory piece but also IgE, which apparently arrives by diffusion from plasma cells distributed in proximity to mucosal surfaces. IgE fixes to mucosal and submucosal mast cells, and the intensity of the clinical response to inhaled allergens is quantitatively related to the naturally occurring or experimentally defined pollen dose. Specific IgE is distributed not only to tissue mast cells but also to circulating basophilic leukocytes; patients with more severe clinical disease have basophils that release histamine in response to lesser concentrations of allergen in vitro than do cells from patients with milder disease. Human nasal polyps from ragweed-sensitive patients release histamine, eosinophilotactic peptides, and spasmogenic leukotrienes upon challenge with ragweed allergen in vitro. In sensitive individuals, the introduction of allergen into the nose is associated with sneezing, "stuffiness," and discharge, and the fluid contains histamine, PGD_2, and leukotrienes. Thus the mast cells of nasal polyp tissue, and of the nasal mucosa and submucosa, generate and release mediators through IgE-dependent reactions which are capable of producing tissue edema and eosinophilic infiltration.

Diagnosis The diagnosis of seasonal allergic rhinitis depends largely on an accurate history of occurrence coincident with the pollination of the offending weeds, grasses, or trees. The continuous character of perennial allergic rhinitis due to contamination of the home or place of work makes historical analysis difficult, but there may be a variability in symptoms that can be related to animal exposure or work habits. Patients with perennial rhinitis commonly develop the problem in adult life, are more often women than men, and manifest nasal polyps and thickening of the sinus membranes by x-ray. The term *vasomotor rhinitis* designates a symptom complex resembling perennial allergic rhinitis without an established allergic basis. Other entities to be excluded are exposure to irritants, upper respiratory infection, pregnancy with prominent nasal mucosal edema, prolonged topical use of alpha-adrenergic agents in the form of nose drops, and the use of certain therapeutic agents such as rauwolfia. Nasal polyps are a characteristic of perennial allergic rhinitis and are often associated with sinus infection.

The nasal secretions of allergic patients are rich in eosinophils, and peripheral eosinophilia with elevations in relation to clinical exacerbations is a common feature. Local or systemic neutrophilia implies infection. Total serum IgE is frequently elevated, but the demonstration of immunologic specificity for IgE is critical to an etiologic diagnosis. Some normal individuals will exhibit a wheal-and-flare skin response to intracutaneous inoculation of high concentrations of common airborne allergens. The diagnosis rests not only on the skin test alone but also on the correlation of the clinical history with skin reactivity to concentrations of allergen selected by controlled testing. This provides the best balance of selectivity with specificity. Scratch tests with food allergens are unreliable, while intracutaneous testing may be dangerous, and elimination diets are the best approach to the diagnosis. Regardless of method of testing, food allergy is uncommon as a significant cause of allergic rhinitis.

Although standard radioimmunodiffusion techniques can be used to screen for patients with markedly elevated levels of IgE, their sensitivity of less than 1000 ng/mL is insufficient to detect the elevations in most atopic allergic patients. A commonly employed technique, sensitive to about 50 ng/mL, is known as the *competitive radioimmunosorbent test* (RIST). In this procedure, the IgE of the serum competes with radiolabeled IgE for solid-phase–bound anti-IgE; the displacement of radiolabeled IgE is compared with a standard curve to yield the IgE concentration of the serum. Other assays, such as the noncompetitive RIST, in which the anti-IgE immunosorbent is exposed to a series of standard IgE preparations before introducing the unknown, and double-antibody radioimmunoprecipitin test (RIP), have greater sensitivity and reproducibility, respectively, and, like the competitive RIST, establish a normal geometric mean serum IgE for nonallergic whites of less than 120 ng/mL. Even more useful is the measurement of specific anti-IgE in serum by its binding to a solid-phase allergen and quantitation by the subsequent uptake of radiolabeled anti-IgE. This radioallergosorbent technique (RAST) correlates satisfactorily with the bioassay of specific IgE by skin test or histamine release from peripheral blood leukocytes and is convenient for the patients; however, it requires defined allergens and full standardization. Further, neither the immunochemical nor bioassay detection of a previous immune response to a foreign material mandates a therapeutic intervention, unless there is relevant concomitant evidence of a significant clinical problem.

Prevention and treatment Avoidance of exposure to the offending allergen is the most effective means of controlling allergic diseases; removal of pets from the home to avoid animal danders, utilization of air filtration devices to minimize the concentrations of airborne pollens, travel to nonpollinating areas during the critical periods, and even a change of domicile to eliminate a mold spore problem may be necessary.

Management with pharmacologic agents represents the standard approach to seasonal or perennial allergic rhinitis. Antihistamines of the H1 class are effective for nasopharyngeal itching, sneezing, and watery rhinorrhea and for such ocular manifestations as itching, tearing, and erythema, but they are not efficacious for the nasal congestion. The older antihistamines are sedating, and their anticholinergic (muscarinic) effects include visual disturbance, urinary retention, and even arrhythmias. Because the newer H1 antihistaminics such as terfenadine or astemizole are less lipophilic, their ability to cross the blood-brain barrier is reduced, and therefore, their sedating and anticholinergic side effects are minimized. Alpha-adrenergic agents are generally used topically to alleviate nasal congestion and obstruction, but the duration of efficacy is limited because of rebound rhinitis and such systemic responses as insomnia, irritability, and hypertension. The latter are more frequent with use of oral alpha-adrenergic agonists. Cromolyn sodium, a liquid nasal metered-dose spray, is essentially without side effects and is the only intervention of a prophylactic nature; thus it is used to attenuate episodic allergen activation of nasal mast cells. Intranasal high-potency glucocorticoids such as beclamethasone or flunisolide are the most potent drugs available for the relief of established rhinitis, seasonal or perennial, and even vasomotor rhinitis; they provide efficacy with substantially reduced side effects as compared with this same class of agent administered orally. Their most frequent side effect is local irritation, with *Candida* overgrowth being a rare occurrence. Thus, for patients who do not benefit adequately from a full dosage of nonsedating H1 antihistamine and a maintenance dosage of cromolyn sodium, an alpha-adrenergic agent for short-term relief should be replaced by high-potency topical glucocorticoids.

Immunotherapy, often termed *hyposensitization*, consists of repeated subcutaneous injections of gradually increasing concentrations of the allergen(s) considered to be specifically responsible for the symptom complex. Controlled studies in ragweed and grass allergic rhinitis have established that patients are partially relieved of their symptoms by such treatments applied over a period of years. Improvement appears to be dose-related, and the end point is based either on severe adverse local or systemic reactions to the allergen injection or on satisfactory relief of symptoms. The immunologic

characteristics of a response include a rise in antibodies of the IgG class, a small increase in specific IgE early in the treatment course followed by a plateau or decline, and a decline in the percentage of histamine released from peripheral blood basophilic leukocytes challenged with a fixed concentration of the allergen. The antibodies of the IgG class might well reduce or neutralize the quantity of allergen available for interaction with the tissue mast cells but, more important, could modify the seasonal booster response in specific IgE synthesis. None of the individual parameters of the response to immunotherapy correlates well with the assessments of clinical efficacy, suggesting that benefit is derived from a complex of effects. Immunotherapy should be reserved for clearly documented seasonal diseases that cannot be managed with drugs because of their side effects.

REFERENCES

AUSTEN KF: The anaphylactic syndrome, in *Immunological Diseases*, 4th ed, M Samter et al (eds). Boston, Little, Brown, 1988

CRAIG SS et al: Ultrastructural analysis of human T and TC mast cells identified by immunoelectron microscopy. Lab Invest 58:682, 1988

GORDON JR et al: Mast cells as a source of multifunctional cytokines. Immunol Today 11:458, 1990

LEWIS RA et al: Leukotrienes and other products of the 5-lipoxygenase pathway: Biochemistry and relation to pathobiology in human diseases. N Engl J Med 323:645, 1990

METCALFE DD (ed): Clinical advances in mastocytosis: An interdisciplinary roundtable discussion. J Invest Dermatol 96:1S, 1991

NACLERIO RM: Allergic rhinitis. N Engl J Med 325:860, 1991

RAVETCH JV, KINET J-P: Fc receptors. Annu Rev Immunol 9:457, 1991

SOTER NA: Urticaria and angioedema, in *Dermatology In General Medicine*, 4th ed, TB Fitzpatrick et al (eds). New York, McGraw-Hill, 1993

STEVENS RL, AUSTEN KF: Recent advances in the cellular and molecular biology of mast cells. Immunol Today 10:381, 1989

VALENTINE MD, GOLDEN DBK: Insect venom allergy, in *Immunological Diseases*, 4th ed, M Samter et al (eds). Boston, Little, Brown, 1988

283 IMMUNE-COMPLEX DISEASES

MICHAEL M. FRANK / THOMAS J. LAWLEY

DEFINITION The term *immune-complex disease* refers to a group of diseases thought to be mediated by the deposition of immune complexes in specific organ or tissue sites including the glomerulus of the kidney and blood vessel walls. In general, these immune deposits are thought to arise from antigen-antibody complexes formed in the circulation. In some cases the antigens appear to be self- or autoantigens. In many cases these antigens are components of or are stimulated by infectious agents. Once deposited in tissues, the complexes activate a variety of potent soluble mediators of inflammation, such as the complement proteins, causing an influx of polymorphonuclear neutrophils and monocytes. They activate a variety of cells with surface membrane receptors for immunoglobulins, often directly inducing the release of cytokines. These activated cells release toxic products of oxygen and arginine metabolism as well as various proteases and other enzymes, ultimately causing tissue damage. While the specific etiology of these diseases is variable, they share a common pathophysiology. The clinical features of these diseases are quite diverse, ranging from mild cutaneous eruptions to severe organ involvement with pericarditis, glomerulonephritis, and vasculitis.

PATHOPHYSIOLOGY The introduction of foreign or noxious substances into an individual is often followed by an immune response. Specific antibody produced in the course of this response binds to antigen, forming immune complexes. In general, these complexes are phagocytosed and destroyed by neutrophils and macrophages locally in tissue sites. If formed or released into the circulation, they are cleared from the circulation by phagocytic cells of the reticuloendothelial system. However, at times these complexes are deposited in tissues, causing inflammation and tissue damage. In recent years there has been a concerted effort to understand the mechanisms underlying this damage.

The biologic activity of the complexes has been studied in detail. It has been shown that the isotype of antibody affects biologic activity. Thus IgG- and IgM-containing complexes activate the classic complement pathway, and IgA-containing complexes often activate the alternative complement pathway. In contrast, cell surface IgE complexes are capable of mediating the degranulation of mast cells by a noncytotoxic, complement-independent mechanism.

The size of the immune complexes in the circulation is an important parameter of toxicity. In general, the larger (>19 S) complexes cause more tissue damage than the smaller complexes. The size is related to the concentration and molar ratio of antibody and antigen, as well as to the avidity of the antibody for the antigen. The ratio of antigen to antibody may range from antibody excess through antigen-antibody equivalence to antigen excess. In marked antibody excess, antigen valences are saturated, and in general, the complexes are small. Under conditions of marked antigen excess, antibody-combining sites are saturated, chances for lattice formation are limited, and, again, the complexes are small. At equivalence or mild antigen excess, lattice formation is facilitated, and large complexes can form. Immune complexes formed at moderate antigen excess are thought to be most pathogenic, perhaps because they are most efficient at activating the various mediator systems such as the complement cascade.

Net charge of antigen and antibody also appears to be important in determining the pathophysiologic effect of the complexes. It has been shown that positively charged immune complexes or immune complexes containing antigens with patches of positive charged groups tend to deposit in renal glomeruli, while complexes containing similar antigen with neutral charge tend to penetrate glomeruli slowly. This is presumably due to the fact that the glomerulus presents a negatively charged surface to the circulation. Similarly, there is a relationship between the degree of binding of immune complexes to the basement membrane of skin, which is also negatively charged, and the degree of positive charge of the complexes.

The first human disease in which circulating immune complexes were thought to play a pathogenic role was serum sickness. In their classic monograph, "Die Serumkrankheit," Clemens von Pirquet and Bela Schick described in great detail their experiences with the use of horse antidiphtheria toxin in children. They found that a reproducible reaction pattern occurred 8 to 13 days following the subcutaneous injection of horse serum protein. The patients developed fever, malaise, cutaneous eruptions, arthralgias, leukopenia, lymphadenopathy, and albuminuria. The authors suggested that this reaction pattern was caused by the interaction of host antibody, formed in the 8 days following the injection of the horse serum, with horse serum protein circulating in the recipient. They believed that this interaction led to the deposition of antigen-antibody complexes in tissue with resulting tissue damage, but the technology necessary to pursue this hypothesis was not available.

Numerous large retrospective studies of human serum sickness confirmed the observations of von Pirquet and Schick, but it was not until the studies of Germuth and Dixon that evidence for the role of circulating immune complexes in serum sickness was obtained. These investigators utilized rabbit models of serum sickness.

In the acute serum sickness model, the injection of antigen is followed by a period of intravascular equilibration, then by intravascular-extravascular equilibration lasting several days, and then by a progressive decline in the level of antigen in the circulation, representing the normal degradation of the injected serum protein. Following this period of decay, there is a sudden acceleration in the clearance of the antigen from the circulation, usually beginning at about 7 to 8 days. The period of rapid decline in the level of antigen in the circulation is due to the development of an immune response in the recipient animal. This results in the formation of antigen-antibody

complexes and subsequent clearance of the complexes from the circulation by phagocytes of the reticuloendothelial system (RES) (Fig. 283-1). During the period in which the complexes are being formed in the circulation, there is a fall in the animal's serum complement levels. At this time, pathologic changes occur in large arteries, renal glomeruli, joints, and cardiac vessels. The glomerulonephritis noted during this period has been studied extensively. It is characterized by swelling of the endothelial cells and marked proteinuria with little hematuria; an infiltrate of monocytes but very few granulocytes is found in the renal glomeruli. Immunofluorescence studies have shown that antigen, host immunoglobulin, and C3 are deposited along the glomerular basement membrane in a typical granular pattern. On electron-microscopic examination of kidney sections, few abnormalities are seen except swelling of endothelial cells. Late in the reaction, subepithelial deposits of electron-dense material are noted in some animals; however, at this time fluorescent antibody examination is negative for immunoglobulin and complement in the glomeruli. The deposits may represent immunologically altered immunoglobulin or complement.

There is also a very high incidence of arteritis in the coronary artery outflow tract and at branching points of the aorta in the acute serum sickness model. The arteritis is characterized by marked intimal proliferation of endothelium. This is followed by degradation of the internal elastic lamina and adventitia with resulting fibrinoid necrosis of the vessel. On immunofluorescence microscopy, host immunoglobulin, antigen, and C3 are found roughly in the region of the internal elastic lamina, but these immunoreactive materials are rapidly removed and are gone in several days. It has been suggested that the polymorphonuclear neutrophils present in the lesions phagocytize these complexes. In contrast to the findings in glomerulonephritis, materials which decrease complement activity or inhibit the polymorphonuclear leukocytic response diminish or block the development of arteritis.

FIGURE 283-1 The rabbit model of acute serum sickness. Radiolabeled antigen is injected at day 0. After a period of equilibration of antigen between the intravascular and extravascular space, there is progressive elimination of antigen from the circulation. With the onset of the animal's immune response there is rapid elimination of antigen from the circulation. Coincident with the phase of rapid elimination is the appearance of antigen-antibody complexes in the circulation and a fall in serum complement. Complete antigen clearance is associated with the appearance of free antibody in the circulation. At the time when antigen-antibody complexes are seen in the circulation, immunopathologic findings are maximal.

At the time of the development of serum sickness in this animal model, there are high-molecular-weight immune complexes in the circulation; the animals that become sick regularly have complexes that are greater than 19 S in their sedimentation characteristics. Acute serum sickness is present only as long as these circulating immune complexes persist and resolves rapidly once the antigen is cleared from the circulation and the immune complexes are gone.

It is possible to induce chronic glomerulonephritis in animals by the repeated intravenous injection of the antigen. The dose of antigen injected is critical to the development of the disease. Antigen excess must be produced after each antigen administration, and immune complexes must circulate in the animals. These animals develop glomerulonephritis but not the arteritis characteristic of acute serum sickness.

Other animal models of immune-complex disease closely resemble systemic lupus erythematosus. The most widely studied and best characterized is the disease that occurs spontaneously in the F_1 hybrid of New Zealand Black (NZB) and New Zealand White (NZW) mice. These animals develop antibodies to nucleic acids including double-stranded DNA and have decreased numbers of suppressor T cells. They also develop circulating immune complexes and an immune-complex–mediated glomerulonephritis that eventuates in renal insufficiency and death. Direct immunofluorescence microscopy of the kidneys in these animals reveals deposits of DNA, antibodies to DNA, and C3 in the glomerular basement membrane. The female NZB-NZW mice develop these changes before the males, and this sex difference may be related to a switch in the class of antibodies to DNA from IgM to IgG that occurs much earlier in the females than in the males.

Over the years, a great deal of attention has been paid in animal models to the fate of immune complexes in an attempt to understand exactly why they are deposited in tissues in autoimmune diseases. Injection of antigens into immunized animals is followed by the deposition of the antigen in the liver, spleen, and lung, all elements of the RES. Detailed studies have examined the fate of preformed immune complexes of carefully determined size in a variety of animals. In general, the findings of these studies have paralleled those reported in the animal models of serum sickness. The very large insoluble complexes are rapidly removed from the circulation. Soluble complexes that are greater than 19 S in their sedimentation characteristics are removed by the liver and persist in the circulation for only a matter of minutes. The major factor appearing to govern the rate of clearance of these large, preformed complexes from the circulation is the rate of hepatic blood flow. In some studies, complement activation by complexes is also important in their metabolism, and injected complexes go through a complex series of processing steps. Large-lattice–sized complexes appear to be dissociated by complement into smaller entities. Following injection, complexes containing complement components become associated with cells with complement receptors. Human erythrocytes have complement receptors (CR1) on their surface membranes, and these cells bind complement-coated immune complexes, effectively removing them from the plasma. The complexes are stripped from these cells by the fixed phagocytes as they course through the sinusoids of the liver. They are then metabolized. Fc receptors for IgG also play a prominent role in the removal of IgG-containing immune complexes from the circulation, and any manipulation that affects the interaction of Fc receptors and the Fc fragment of IgG in the complexes predisposes to failure to clear the complexes and to tissue deposition. Studies have measured RES Fc-receptor functional activity in patients and normal individuals by intravenously injecting autologous radiolabeled erythrocytes sensitized with anti-Rh IgG antibody and then monitoring the rate of disappearance of these immune particles from the blood. Such antibody-sensitized cells are removed from the circulation as they traverse the sinusoids of the spleen. In those diseases with tissue deposition of immune complexes there tends to be an associated splenic RES Fc-receptor defect and delayed clearance of the antibody-sensitized cells from the circulation. Such findings suggest that there

may be a failure in adequate removal of the complexes from the circulation, allowing for their tissue deposition. Studies in animals support these conclusions and suggest that failure of normal clearance mechanisms precedes the development of immune-complex deposition. Recent work suggests that mechanisms that promote the degranulation of mast cells with histamine release (e.g., the formation of IgE antibody) facilitate immune-complex deposition by decreasing vascular endothelial cell contact.

Another form of immune-complex–mediated tissue damage follows local formation of immune complexes in tissues such as the kidney. Glomerular subepithelial immune-complex deposits are thought to form at times on an in situ basis. This may occur as a result of antibody binding to fixed glomerular antigens or antibody binding to "planted" nonglomerular antigens. In the latter instance it is believed that certain cationic antigens can bind to the laminae rarae of the capillary wall in a glomerulus through charge-dependent mechanisms. This "planted" antigen is then recognized by antibody, and local tissue damage results. The pathophysiologic events leading to tissue damage in immunologically mediated inflammation are under intense study. In order for circulating leukocytes to exit from blood vessels into tissue at sites of inflammation, they must first bind to the endothelial cells that line the postcapillary venules. This is accomplished by proteins or glycoproteins, known as *cell adhesion molecules*, on the surface of the leukocytes interacting with other cell adhesion molecules on the endothelial cells. The interaction of one cell adhesion molecule with another appears to be quite specific. The expression and/or affinity of many cell adhesion molecules can be induced or upregulated by exposure of endothelial cells to cytokines such as interleukin 1 or tumor necrosis factor-α. Thus an endothelial cell in a postcapillary venule, when exposed to tumor necrosis factor-α, will rapidly begin to express the cell adhesion molecule P-selectin and will begin to upregulate the expression of ICAM-1 on its surface. P-selectin will bind to sialyl Lewis X on leukocytes, and ICAM-1 will bind to leukocyte LFA-1. This cell-cell interaction will lead to binding of the leukocytes to the endothelium with subsequent transmigration to areas of immune-complex deposition.

DETECTION OF CIRCULATING IMMUNE COMPLEXES Many different assays are available for the detection of soluble immune complexes in various biologic fluids. Although these assays vary in their sensitivity and reproducibility, they have expanded our understanding of circulating immune complexes and their role in various disease states. In general, early tests for the detection of circulating immune complexes relied on physical characteristics of the immune complexes, such as their high molecular weight or cold insolubility. These rather insensitive techniques have been replaced by assays for immunologic components or biologic activities of immune complexes. Although there are now sensitive radioimmunoassays for the detection of circulating immune complexes containing IgG, IgM, and IgA, these tests are not antigen-specific. In fact, in most cases in which circulating immune complexes are demonstrable, the component antigen(s) is (are) unknown. As with most laboratory tests, immune-complex assays may be influenced by other factors. Anticoagulants, endotoxin, and free DNA as well as immunoglobulin aggregates formed after the sample is obtained may result in false-positive results. The impact of these factors can be reduced by the selection of immune-complex assays that are unaffected by these variables and by the use of two or more different assays in situations in which critical evaluation of circulating immune complexes is desired. Several of the most sensitive and commonly used immune-complex assays will be described briefly: (1) C1q binding, or solid-phase radioassays, (2) Raji cell assays, and (3) conglutinin assays. *C1q* is a subcomponent of the first component of complement and will bind to immune complexes containing IgG subclasses 1 to 3 or IgM via noncovalent attachment to a specific site on the Fc portion of immunoglobulin. *Raji cells* are a lymphoblastoid cell line with cell surface receptors for complement, especially C3. The assays are based on the ability of circulating immune complexes that contain bound complement components in their lattices to bind to the surface of the Raji cells via the complement receptors. The bound complexes are easily detected. *Conglutinin* is a 750-kDa nonimmunoglobulin protein found in certain bovine sera that will bind to a cleavage fragment of human C3 known as iC3b. Immune complexes containing iC3b will bind to conglutinin attached to a solid-phase substrate and can be detected.

SERUM SICKNESS Drug hypersensitivity reactions are the most common cause of serum sickness today. It is hypothesized that the drug acting as a hapten binds to a plasma protein. The drug-protein complex induces an immune response which in turn causes typical serum sickness. Commonly occurring signs and symptoms of serum sickness include fever, cutaneous eruptions (morbilliform and/or urticarial), arthralgias, lymphadenopathy, and albuminuria. Less common manifestations are arthritis, nephritis, neuropathy, and vasculitis. The time required for primary sensitization to an offending agent is approximately 1 to 3 weeks. However, clinical manifestations may develop within 12 to 36 h if there is a history of a previous immunizing exposure. Drug-induced serum sickness usually abates within days after withdrawal of the causative agent. Reactions may persist for longer intervals, particularly if repository or long-acting agents are responsible for the problem. Drugs responsible for serum sickness include penicillin, sulfonamides, thiouracils, hydantoins, *p*-aminosalicylic acid, phenylbutazone, thiazides, and streptomycin. Foreign antisera and blood products also may induce serum sickness reactions.

Studies of patients receiving intravenous infusions of horse antithymocyte globulin (ATG) as therapy for bone marrow failure have confirmed and expanded the immunologic findings in animal models of serum sickness in humans. The patients develop signs and symptoms of serum sickness 8 to 13 days after beginning therapy with ATG (Fig. 283-2). These include fever; malaise; cutaneous eruptions; arthralgias and arthritis, mainly of the large joints; gastrointestinal distress with nausea, vomiting, and melena; lymphadenopathy; and proteinuria. Clinical disease coincides with the development of very high levels of circulating immune complexes as measured by the ^{125}I-labeled C1q binding assay and marked decreases in serum C3, C4, and CH_{50} levels. The first cutaneous manifestation of serum sickness is a serpiginous band of erythema occurring along the sides of the hands, feet, fingers, and toes at the junction of palmar or plantar skin with the dorsolateral surface. Direct immunofluorescence of involved skin during serum sickness reveals deposits of immunoglobulins and C3 in the walls of small cutaneous blood vessels in most patients.

These studies provide strong support for a pathogenic role for circulating immune complexes in the pathophysiology of human serum sickness.

SYSTEMIC LUPUS ERYTHEMATOSUS Systemic lupus erythematosus (SLE) is a multisystem disease associated with a number of immunologic abnormalities, including the production of autoantibodies, hypergammaglobulinemia, suppressor T cell abnormalities, decreased levels of serum complement, and increased levels of circulating immune complexes (see Chap. 284). Immune complexes are thought to play a critical role in the pathophysiology of SLE. Early evidence for the role of circulating immune complexes in SLE included the finding by direct immunofluorescence of glomerular deposits of immunoglobulin, complement, and DNA in kidney biopsies. Mixed IgM-IgG cryoglobulins were found in the sera of a substantial number of SLE patients, and when the antibody specificity of these cryoprecipitates was examined, reactivity was found against single- and double-stranded DNA as well as ribonucleoprotein. Utilizing the newer, more sensitive assays, circulating immune complexes have been found in a high percentage of patients with SLE. Studies demonstrating a defect in the clearance by the spleen of autologous red cells sensitized with anti-Rh antibody have led to the suggestion that these patients have impaired function of RES Fc-IgG receptors. Such impaired function might allow complexes to circulate until they deposited in tissues. The prolonged RES clearance in patients with active SLE was found to be correlated with increased levels of circulating immune complexes as measured by the C1q binding assay and with clinical disease activity. Studies in the same patients after their disease improved with treatment revealed a significant correlation between clinical improvement, improvement of Fc-mediated clearance, and decreased levels of circulating immune complexes. Individuals with SLE also have decreased numbers of C3b receptors on their erythrocytes, which also may contribute to abnormalities in immune-complex clearance. Whether the decreased number of receptors is primary or secondary remains to be established. Nonetheless, abnormalities of both Fc-IgG and C3b receptors which are responsible for phagocytosis of circulating immune complexes are present in patients with SLE.

VASCULITIS There is strong circumstantial evidence for the role of circulating immune complexes in the various forms of hypersensitivity or necrotizing vasculitis (see Chap. 291). Features of the classic "palpable purpura" of cutaneous necrotizing vasculitis closely resemble the clinical, histopathologic, and immunopathologic

FIGURE 283-2 Serum sickness in human beings. Horse antithymocyte globulin was injected into patients with aplastic anemia daily for 10 days. After the fifth day of injection, C1q binding activity begins to rise (*A*). At the

same time there is a dramatic fall in plasma levels of C3 and C4 and onset of clinical symptoms (*B*).

features of the Arthus reaction. The Arthus reaction is a model for immune-complex–mediated vascular damage in which antigen is injected intradermally into an animal which possesses circulating antibody against that antigen. In both vasculitis and the Arthus reaction, deposits of immunoglobulin and complement are found in the walls of blood vessels in early lesions. The histopathology of both consists of infiltrates of polymorphonuclear neutrophils, leukocytoclasis, endothelial cell damage and necrosis, hemorrhage, and perivascular deposits of fibrin. Electron microscopy of lesions of cutaneous necrotizing vasculitis reveals subendothelial electron-dense deposits compatible with immune complexes. The available evidence indicates the presence of immune complexes at the site of tissue damage in necrotizing vasculitis. In accord with these findings is the demonstration of circulating immune complexes in a high percentage of patients with this disease.

LABORATORY FINDINGS In theory, the essential feature of immune-complex disease would be the finding of circulating immune complexes. In practice, there is great variability from disease to disease in the frequency of positive immune-complex assays. In some diseases, such as SLE, there is a high frequency of positive immune-complex assays. In others, such as membranoproliferative glomerulonephritis, the frequency of positive assays is much lower. Part of the reason for this has to do with the stage of disease under study. In some cases immunologic phenomena are responsible for the initiation of the disease and the initial tissue insult. However, subsequent injury is caused by scarring, inflammation, and repair mechanisms that result in more extensive tissue damage. Thus progression of disease may occur at a time when immunologic injury is no longer occurring. A second reason for the failure to detect circulating immune complexes in diseases thought to be mediated by them has to do with technical difficulties in the measurement of such complexes. There are many types of assays for immune complexes. Most are indirect and rely on a biologic or biochemical property of the complexes such as the binding of complement components. The pattern of positive reaction clearly varies from disease to disease. Clearly, each assay recognizes a different type of complex with maximal efficiency. Since multiple assays are rarely performed on one specimen, complexes, although present, may not be detected. Finally, although a disease is classified as immune-complex–related because of the finding of immune deposits in affected tissues or because of the similarity of its pathologic findings to those of animal models of immune-complex disease, the disease may not be actually caused by circulating immune complexes. For example, antibody may be formed to a tissue component, bind to it in a tissue site, and induce damage. Such is thought to be the case in Goodpasture's disease. For all these reasons, assays for the detection of circulating immune complex, while often useful, are rarely critical for diagnosis or patient management.

Examination of tissues using immunofluorescence techniques to detect immune deposits is also of great usefulness in establishing the diagnosis of immune-complex disease. Immune complexes deposited in tissues may be evanescent. In one animal model, subendothelial deposits of immune complexes, had a half-life of only 3.9 h. In cutaneous vasculitis, lesions must be biopsied within 12 h of their appearance. Although helpful in diagnosis and in establishing pathogenesis, testing for immune deposits in tissue is rarely required for diagnosis.

Another test commonly used to infer the presence of immune complexes is the measurement of serum complement. Decreased levels are taken to indicate the presence of complexes. In fact, it has been suggested that the levels of serum C4 and C3 and the appearance of complement protein cleavage fragments are the most sensitive indexes of disease activity in SLE. However, the correlation between disease activity and complement levels is rough at best, and some patients with active SLE may have relatively normal complement levels for several reasons. The normal range of complement component levels is wide, and a given patient may have depressed levels, with serum concentrations falling from high-normal levels to low-normal levels. In general, complement components act as acute-phase re-

actants, and the lowering of serum complement may be masked by increased synthesis. Moreover, activation of complement may mediate profound pathophysiologic effects, although relatively few molecules of complement are actually involved. For example, complement binding to red cells may be responsible for much of the red cell destruction that occurs with ABO-mismatched transfusions, yet serum complement levels may be unchanged because too few molecules are used in erythrocyte destruction to detect a fall in titer. Finally, all types of complexes do not activate complement in the same way. Massive antigen release from red cells occurring during the course of vivax malaria infection leads to the rapid formation of antigen-antibody complexes in the circulation. For unknown reasons, these complexes only interact with the early components of the classic complement pathway, while C3 and the later complement components are not recruited. Thus, if one measures levels of C3, no fall in titer is noted, although complexes are present and massive complement activation has taken place. The complexes formed in SLE activate optimally the classic pathway; presumably those involved in IgA glomerulonephritis activate the alternative pathway. Therefore, the complement test chosen for examination may be important.

Other tests may suggest indirectly the presence of immune-complex disease. For example, a finding of mixed IgG-IgM cryoprecipitates suggests the presence of immune complexes. The presence of antinuclear antibodies suggests autoimmunity, as does the presence of a number of tissue component–specific antibodies. Similarly, the presence of specific antigen such as hepatitis B surface antigen in the circulation together with appropriate clinical symptoms may suggest an immune-complex disease. Most patients with active immune-complex–mediated disease have an elevated erythrocyte sedimentation rate, although this is not invariably the case. Patients with Takayasu's arteritis may have a normal erythrocyte sedimentation rate during the later phases of the evolution of lesions, when most pathology is caused by scarring, fibrosis, and repair within vessel walls. Finally, specific laboratory test findings such as red cell casts in the urine in glomerulonephritis or mild cerebrospinal fluid pleocytosis in the presence of cerebritis are discussed in the chapters concerning those diseases.

TREATMENT The therapy of immune-complex–mediated disease relies on removal of the offending antigen and interruption of the inflammatory response. In general, serum sickness is a self-limited disease that is seldom life-threatening. In the case of drug-induced serum sickness, it is most important to discontinue the offending agent. In recent years, plasmapheresis (particularly in concert with cytotoxic agents) has been used to blunt the manifestations of acute immune-complex tissue injury. In many instances, supportive care combined with antihistamines for urticaria and acetaminophen for fever, myalgias, and arthralgias is adequate. If serious renal, vascular, or central nervous system involvement occurs, the use of systemic glucocorticoid therapy is indicated. These approaches to therapy are discussed elsewhere.

The therapy of SLE is discussed in Chap. 284, and the therapy of vasculitis is discussed in Chap. 291.

REFERENCES

COCHRANE CB, KOFFLER D: Immune complex disease in experimental animals and man. Adv Immunol 16:185, 1963

DIXON F: The role of antigen-antibody complexes in disease. Harvey Lect 52:21, 1963

FRANK MM et al: Immunoglobulin G–Fc receptor mediated clearance in autoimmune diseases. Ann Intern Med 98:206, 1983

GAUTHIER VJ, ABRASS CK: Circulating immune complexes in renal injury. Semin Nephrol 12:379, 1992

GERMUTH FC JR.: A comparative histologic and immunologic study in rabbits of induced hypersensitivity of the serum sickness type. J Exp Med 97:257, 1953

GLASSOCK RJ: Immune complex–induced glomerular injury in viral diseases. Kidney Int 40(suppl 35):55, 1991

KERJASCHKI D: Molecular pathogenesis of membranous nephropathy. Kidney Int 41:1090, 1992

LAWLEY TJ et al: A prospective clinical and immunologic analysis of patients with serum sickness. N Engl J Med 311:1407, 1984

MANNIK M, AREND WP: Fate of preformed immune complexes in rabbits and rhesus monkeys. J Exp Med 134:19s, 1971

MULLIGAN ME et al: Tissue injury caused by deposition of immune complexes is L-arginine–dependent. Proc Natl Acad Sci USA 88:6338, 1991

VON PIRQUET C, SCHICK B: *Serum Sickness.* Baltimore, Williams & Wilkins, 1951

THEOFILOPOULOS AN, DIXON FJ: The biology and detection of immune complexes. Adv Immunol 28:89, 1979

284 SYSTEMIC LUPUS ERYTHEMATOSUS

BEVRA HANNAHS HAHN

DEFINITION AND PREVALENCE Systemic lupus erythematosus (SLE) is a disease of unknown cause in which tissues and cells are damaged by pathogenic autoantibodies and immune complexes. Ninety percent of cases are in women, usually of childbearing age, but children, men, and the elderly can be affected. In the United States, the prevalence of SLE in urban areas varies from 15 to 50 per 100,000 population; it is more common in blacks than in whites. Hispanic and Asian populations are also susceptible.

PATHOGENESIS AND ETIOLOGY SLE probably results from interactions between susceptibility genes and the environment. This interaction results in abnormal immune responses with T and B lymphocyte hyperactivity which is not suppressed by the usual immunoregulatory circuits. Evidence for genetic predisposition includes increased concordance for disease in monozygotic compared with dizygotic twins, a 10 percent frequency of patients with more than one affected family member, and correlations of certain genes (especially MHC classes II and III) with disease and autoantibodies. C4AQO, a defective class III allele which fails to encode a functional C4A protein, is the most common genetic marker associated with SLE in many ethnic groups (found in 40 to 50 percent of patients compared with 15 percent of healthy controls). Certain extended haplotypes, such as B8.DR3.DQw2.C4AQO, predispose to SLE in some populations. The strongest single gene associations occur between HLA class II (especially DQ_{beta}) and autoantibodies which define clinical subsets of lupus. For example, high titers of IgG anti-DNA are associated with lupus nephritis and with DQB1*0201, *0602, and *0302 inherited with either DR2 or DR3. Antibodies to Ro/La (SS-A/SS-B) are associated with the dermatitis of subacute cutaneous lupus and with certain DQA and DQB genes inherited with DR3 (occasionally DR2). The lupus anticoagulant, correlated clinically with clotting, is associated with DQB*0301, *0302, *0303, and *0602 inherited with DR4 or DR7. The DQA or DQB susceptibility genes in each group share amino acid sequences that may determine the ability to make a particular autoantibody. Family studies suggest that genes unlinked to HLA also participate in susceptibility and that females are more likely than males to express the autoimmune manifestations of their genotypes. The more susceptibility genes one has, the higher is the relative risk for SLE; three or four different genes are probably required.

Environmental factors that flare SLE are largely unknown, with the exception of UV-B (and sometimes UV-A) light. As many as 70 percent of patients are photosensitive. Other factors such as ingested alfalfa sprouts and chemicals such as hydrazines and hair dye have been implicated. Searches for viral/retroviral disease inducers, currently in progress, are inconclusive. Although some drugs can induce lupus-like disease, there are notable clinical and autoantibody differences between drug-induced and spontaneous lupus. Femaleness is clearly a susceptibility factor, since the prevalence in women of childbearing years is seven to nine times higher than in men, whereas the female-to-male ratio is 3:1 in pre- and postmenopausal years. Metabolism of estrogenic and androgenic hormones may be abnormal in lupus patients. Sex hormones also influence immune tolerance.

Abnormal immune responses include sustained production of pathogenic subsets of autoantibodies and immune complexes (ICs). No immunoglobulin genes have been identified that exclusively encode harmful autoantibodies, although certain V-region genes (especially V_H) seem to be preferentially used, and there is probably clonal selection of B cells secreting high-avidity antibodies to autoantigens. In most murine lupus models, T cell help is critical to development of full-blown disease; there is active investigation of T cell suppression as a therapeutic intervention in patients. The abnormalities that permit hyperactivated self-reactive B and T cells to dominate immune repertoires in SLE are unclear. These cells escape normal tolerizing mechanisms; they are neither deleted nor anergized. Recent evidence in mice suggests that defective apoptosis, genetically encoded, may prevent elimination of self-reactive cells. There is some evidence that bone marrow stem cell precursors of B and, perhaps, of T lymphocytes are intrinsically abnormal. Alternatively, the microenvironment in which these stem cells develop may be abnormal. Perhaps genes, sex hormones, and exogenous antigens influence tolerance and cell activation. Alternatively, these cells could be altered by antilymphocyte antibodies. The structure of antigens that stimulate autoantibodies is under investigation. Some are clearly derived from self (histones, RNP, erythrocyte surface antigens); others may be from the external environment and mimic self (e.g., components of vesicular stomatitis virus mimic peptides in Ro antigen). Some autoantibodies induce disease by direct reaction with their antigens, such as those directed against surface antigens on erythrocytes or platelets. Others may attach to cell membranes (such as glomerular basement membrane, GBM) via cationic charge or because they cross-react with tissue constituents (e.g., some anti-DNA antibodies react with laminin in GBM). If these antibodies, when complexed with antigen, can fix complement, tissue damage occurs. Alteration of cell function after antibodies bind to membranes also occurs independent of complement activation. Autoantibodies characteristic of SLE are listed in Table 284-1.

Abnormalities of immune regulation are required to develop SLE. Immune complexes are cleared inadequately. CR1 receptors on erythrocytes are low in number (usually because they are stripped by high levels of IC, occasionally because of genetic control) so that many ICs are not transported to the mononuclear phagocyte system (MPS). The MPS is unable to process ICs normally. Idiotype–anti-idiotype networks fail to suppress hyperactivated T and B cells. T lymphocytes are heavily skewed toward help: CD4+CD8−, CD4−CD8+, CD4−CD8−, alpha/beta, and gamma/delta T cells have all been shown to help B cell production of autoantibodies in SLE. Therefore, the usual suppressor functions attributed to CD4−CD8+ cells and to the NK cells with which T cells interact are absent. Finally, normal tolerance mechanisms that eliminate or inactivate strongly autoreactive T and B lymphocytes are impaired.

In summary, some individuals are genetically predisposed to SLE. Under the influence of multiple genes, often triggered by environmental challenges and highly influenced by sex, they may develop a number of different clinical syndromes which fulfill diagnostic criteria for SLE. The cause of these syndromes is complex and probably differs between patients.

CLINICAL MANIFESTATIONS At onset, SLE may involve only one organ system (additional manifestations occur later) or may be multisystemic. Clinical manifestations are listed in Table 284-2; those which fulfill American Rheumatism Association criteria for a diagnosis of SLE are listed in Table 284-3. Autoantibodies are detectable at disease onset. Severity varies from mild and intermittent to persistent and fulminant. Most patients experience exacerbations interspersed with periods of relative quiescence. True remissions with no symptoms and requiring no therapy occur in less than 10 percent. Systemic symptoms are usually prominent and include fatigue, malaise, fever, anorexia, and weight loss.

Musculoskeletal Almost all patients experience arthralgias and myalgias; most develop intermittent arthritis. Pain is often out of proportion to physical findings of symmetric fusiform swelling in

TABLE 284-1 Autoantibodies in patients with SLE

	Incidence, %	Antigen detected	Clinical importance
Antinuclear antibodies	95	Multiple nuclear and cytoplasmic antigens	Human cell line substrates are more sensitive than standard murine tissues. A repeatedly negative test on both makes SLE diagnosis unlikely. Multiple antibodies are detected.
Anti-DNA	70	DNA	Anti-dsDNA is relatively disease specific; anti-ssDNA is not. Associated with nephritis and clinical activity.
Anti-Sm	30	Protein complexed to 6 species of small nuclear RNA	Specific for SLE.
Anti-RNP	40	Protein complexed to U1RNA	High titer seen in syndromes with features of polymyositis, scleroderma, lupus, and mixed connective tissue disease. If present in SLE without anti-DNA, risk for nephritis is low.
Anti-Ro (SSA)	30	Protein complexed to Y_1–Y_5 RNA	Associated with Sjögren's syndrome, DR3 haplotype, subacute cutaneous lupus, inherited complement deficiencies, ANA-negative lupus, lupus in the elderly, neonatal lupus, congenital heart block in infants. Can cause nephritis.
Anti-La (SSB)	10	Phosphoprotein complexed with RNA pol III transcripts	Always associated with anti-Ro; risk for nephritis is low if present in SLE. Associated with Sjögren's syndrome.
Antihistone	70	Histones	More frequent in drug-induced LE (95%) than in spontaneous SLE.
Anticardiolipin	50	Phospholipid	Increases risk for venous or arterial thrombosis, thrombocytopenia, valvular heart disease, and spontaneous abortion. Associated with prolonged PTT (lupus anticoagulant) and false-positive VDRL.
Antierythrocyte	60	Erythrocyte surface antigens	A small proportion of these patients develop overt hemolysis.
Antiplatelet	—	Platelet surface	Associated with thrombocytopenia.
Antilymphocyte	70	Lymphocyte surface antigens	Probably associated with leukopenia and abnormal T cell function.
Antineuronal	60	Neuronal and lymphocyte surface antigens	In CSF, high IgG titers correlate with diffuse CNS lupus.

joints [most frequently proximal interphalangeal (PIP) and metacarpophalangeal (MCP) joints of the hands, wrists, and knees], diffuse puffiness of hands and feet, and tenosynovitis. Joint deformities are unusual, with 10 percent of patients developing swan-neck deformities of fingers and ulnar drift at MCP joints. Erosions are rare; subcutaneous nodules occur. Myopathy can be inflammatory (during periods of active disease) or secondary to treatment (hypokalemia, glucocorticoid myopathy, hydroxychloroquine myopathy). Ischemic necrosis of bone is a common cause of hip, knee, or shoulder pain in patients receiving glucocorticoids.

Cutaneous The malar ("butterfly") rash is a fixed erythematous rash, flat or raised, over the cheeks and bridge of the nose, often involving the chin and ears. It is photosensitive. Scarring is absent; telangiectasias may develop. A more diffuse maculopapular rash, predominant in sun-exposed areas, is also common and usually indicates disease flare. Loss of scalp hair is usually patchy but can be extensive; hair often regrows in SLE lesions but not in discoid lupus lesions (DLE). DLE occurs in about 20 percent of patients with SLE and can be disfiguring, since the lesions have central atrophy and scarring, with permanent loss of appendages. DLE lesions are circular and characterized by an erythematous raised rim, scaliness, follicular plugging, and telangiectasia. They occur over the scalp, ears, face, and sun-exposed areas of the arms, back, and chest. Only 5 percent of patients with DLE subsequently develop SLE. Less frequent SLE skin lesions include urticaria, bullae, erythema multiforme, lichen planus–like lesions, and panniculitis ("lupus profundus").

Patients with subacute cutaneous lupus (SCLE) are a distinct subset with recurring extensive dermatitis. Arthritis and fatigue are frequent; central nervous system and renal involvement are not.

Some patients are antinuclear antibody (ANA)–negative. Most have antibodies to Ro (SS-A) or to single-stranded (ss) DNA and are HLA-DR3, -DQw1, or -DQw2. Skin lesions are photosensitive and may be annular or papulosquamous psoriasiform lesions over the arms, trunk and face; they become hypopigmented but do not scar.

Patients with SLE, DLE, or SCLE can develop vasculitic skin lesions. These include purpura, subcutaneous nodules, nail fold infarcts, ulcers, vasculitic urticaria, and gangrene of digits. Shallow, slightly painful ulcers in the mouth and nose are frequent in patients with SLE.

Renal Most patients with SLE have immunoglobulins deposited in glomeruli, but only one-half have clinical nephritis, defined by proteinuria. Early in the disease most are asymptomatic, although some develop the edema of nephrotic syndrome. Urinalysis shows hematuria, cylindruria, and proteinuria. Most patients with mesangial or mild focal proliferative nephritis (see discussion under "Pathology" below) maintain good renal function. Patients with diffuse proliferative nephritis develop renal failure if untreated. Since severe nephritis requires aggressive immunosuppression with high-dose glucocorticoids and cytotoxic drugs and mild lesions do not, renal biopsy may provide information that affects therapy. Patients with rapidly deteriorating renal function and active urine sediment require prompt, aggressive therapy; biopsy is not necessary unless such patients fail to respond to therapy. However, patients with a slow rise in creatinine to levels > 265 μmol/L (>3 mg/dL) may show a high proportion of sclerotic glomeruli on biopsy; they are unlikely to respond to immunosuppressive therapies and are candidates for dialysis or transplantation. Patients with persistently abnormal urinalyses, high titers of anti-dsDNA, and/or hypocomplementemia are at risk for severe nephritis; kidney biopsy may guide therapy.

TABLE 284-2 Clinical manifestations of SLE

	Percent of patients positive during course of disease
Systemic	95
Fatigue, malaise, fever, anorexia, nausea, weight loss	
Musculoskeletal	95
Arthralgias/myalgias	95
Nonerosive polyarthritis	60
Hand deformities	10
Myopathy/myositis	40/5
Ischemic necrosis of bone	15
Cutaneous	80
Malar rash	50
Discoid rash	15
Photosensitivity	70
Oral ulcers	40
Other rashes—maculopapular, urticarial, bullous, subacute cutaneous lupus	40
Alopecia	40
Vasculitis	20
Panniculitis	5
Hematologic	85
Anemia (of chronic disease)	70
Hemolytic anemia	10
Leukopenia ($<4000/mm^3$)	65
Lymphopenia ($<1500/mm^3$)	50
Thrombocytopenia ($<100,000/mm^3$)	15
Circulating anticoagulant	10–20
Splenomegaly	15
Lymphadenopathy	20
Neurologic	60
Cognitive dysfunction	50
Organic brain syndromes	35
Psychosis	10
Seizures	20
Other CNS (see text)	15
Peripheral neuropathy	15
Cardiopulmonary	60
Pleurisy	50
Pericarditis	30
Myocarditis	10
Endocarditis (Libman-Sachs)	10
Pleural effusions	30
Lupus pneumonitis	10
Interstitial fibrosis	5
Pulmonary hypertension	<5
ARDS/hemorrhage	<5
Renal	50
Proteinuria >500 mg/24 h	50
Cellular casts	50
Nephrotic syndrome	25
Renal failure	5–10
Gastrointestinal	45
Nonspecific (anorexia, nausea, mild pain, diarrhea)	30
Vasculitis with bleeding or perforation	5
Ascites	<5
Abnormal liver enzymes	40
Thrombosis	15
Venous	10
Arterial	5
Fetal loss	30 (of pregnancies)
Ocular	15
Retinal vasculitis	5
Conjunctivitis/episcleritis	10
Sicca syndrome	15

TABLE 284-3 The 1982 criteria for classification of systemic lupus erythematosus

1	Malar rash	Fixed erythema, flat or raised, over the malar eminences
2	Discoid rash	Erythematous raised patches with adherent keratotic scaling and follicular plugging; atrophic scarring may occur
3	Photosensitivity	
4	Oral ulcers	Includes oral and nasopharyngeal, observed by physician
5	Arthritis	Nonerosive arthritis involving two or more peripheral joints, characterized by tenderness, swelling, or effusion
6	Serositis	Pleuritis or pericarditis documented by ECG or rub or evidence of pericardial effusion
7	Renal disorder	Proteinuria greater than 0.5 g/d or greater than 3+, or cellular casts
8	Neurologic disorder	Seizures without other cause or psychosis without other cause
9	Hematologic disorder	Hemolytic anemia or leukopenia (less than $4000/mm^3$) or lymphopenia (less than $1500/mm^3$) or thrombocytopenia (less than $100,000/mm^3$) in the absence of offending drugs
10	Immunologic disorder	Positive LE cell preparation or anti-dsDNA or anti-Sm antibodies or false-positive VDRL
11	Antinuclear antibodies	An abnormal titer of ANAs by immunofluorescence or an equivalent assay at any point in time in the absence of drugs known to induce ANAs

If four of these criteria are present at any time during the course of disease, a diagnosis of systemic lupus can be made with 98 percent specificity and 97 percent sensitivity.

SOURCE: Criteria published by Tan EM et al: The 1982 revised criteria for the classification of systemic lupus erythematosus. Arthritis Rheum 25:1271, 1982.

psychosis, organic brain syndromes, headache (including migraine), focal infarcts, extrapyramidal disorders, cerebellar dysfunction, hypothalamic dysfunction with inappropriate antidiuretic hormone (ADH) secretion, pseudotumor cerebri, subarachnoid hemorrhage, aseptic meningitis, transverse myelitis, optic neuritis, cranial nerve palsies, and peripheral sensorimotor neuropathy. Depression and anxiety are frequent.

Laboratory diagnosis of CNS lupus can be difficult. Abnormal electroencephalograms occur in about 70 percent of patients and usually show diffuse slowing or focal abnormalities. Cerebrospinal fluid (CSF) shows elevated protein levels in 50 percent and increased mononuclear cells in 30 percent of patients; oligoclonal bands, increased Ig synthesis and antineuronal antibodies may be found. Lumbar puncture should be performed whenever CNS symptoms could result from infection, especially in immunosuppressed patients. CT scans and angiograms are most likely to be positive when focal neurologic deficits are present and are less helpful in cases with diffuse manifestations. Magnetic resonance imaging is the most sensitive radiographic technique to detect changes of SLE; changes are often nonspecific. Laboratory measures of disease activity (Table 284-4) often do not correlate with neurologic manifestations. Neurologic problems (with the exception of deficits resulting from large infarcts) usually improve with immunosuppressive therapy and/or time; recurrences are common.

Vascular Thrombosis in vessels of any size can be a major problem. Although vasculitis may underly thrombosis, there is increasing evidence that antibodies against phospholipids (lupus anticoagulant, anticardiolipin) are associated with clotting without inflammation. In addition, degenerative vascular changes after years of exposure of blood vessels to circulating immune complexes and hyperlipidemia from glucocorticoid therapy predispose to degenerative coronary artery disease in lupus patients. Therefore, anticoagulation is more appropriate than immunosuppression in some patients.

Hematologic Anemia of chronic disease occurs in most patients

Nervous system Any region of the brain can be involved in SLE, as can the meninges, spinal cord, and cranial and peripheral nerves. Central nervous system (CNS) events may be single or multiple and often occur when SLE is active in other organ systems. Mild cognitive dysfunction is the most frequent manifestation. Seizures of any type may occur. Less frequent manifestations include

TABLE 284-4 Laboratory manifestations of SLE

Tests that help *confirm the clinical diagnosis and predict severity*	Tests that may be helpful in *following the clinical course**
Relatively specific for SLE:	Titer of anti-dsDNA
Anti-dsDNA	Serum complement levels
Anti-Sm	Westergren erythrocyte sedimentation rate
Not specific:	Hematocrit
ANA (most sensitive)	Leukocyte count
THC, C3, C4	Platelet count
Anti-Ro	Urinalysis
Direct Coombs' test	Serum creatinine
VDRL	
PTT	
Anticardiolipin	
Hematocrit	
Leukocyte count	
Platelet count	
Urinalysis	
Serum creatinine	

* For each patient, the pattern of laboratory abnormalities (if any) associated with a disease flare should be established and only those tests used subsequently as adjuncts to clinical assessment.

when lupus is active. Hemolysis occurs in a small proportion of those with positive Coombs' tests; it is usually responsive to high-dose glucocorticoids; resistant cases may respond to splenectomy. Leukopenia (usually lymphopenia) is common but is rarely associated with recurrent infections and does not require treatment. Mild thrombocytopenia is common; severe thrombocytopenia with bleeding and purpura occurs in 5 percent of patients and should be treated with high-dose glucocorticoids. Short-term improvement can be achieved by administration of intravenous gamma globulin. If the platelet count fails to reach acceptable levels in 2 weeks, splenectomy should be considered.

The lupus anticoagulant (LA) belongs to a family of antiphospholipid antibodies. It is recognized by prolongation of the partial thromboplastin time and failure of added normal plasma to correct the prolongation. More sensitive tests include the Russell viper venom time and the rabbit brain neutral phospholipid test. Antibodies to cardiolipin (aCL) are detected in ELISA assays. Clinical manifestations of LA and aCL include thrombocytopenia, recurrent venous or arterial clotting, recurrent fetal loss, and valvular heart disease. If the LA is associated with hypoprothrombinemia or thrombocytopenia, bleeding may occur. Less commonly, antibodies to clotting factors (VIII, IX) arise; they cause bleeding. Bleeding syndromes usually respond to glucocorticoids; clotting syndromes do not.

Cardiopulmonary Pericarditis is the most frequent manifestation of cardiac lupus; effusions can occur and occasionally lead to tamponade; constrictive pericarditis is rare. Myocarditis can cause arrhythmias, sudden death, and/or heart failure. Valvular insufficiency (usually arotic or mitral) is an uncommon sequel of Libman Sachs endocarditis; it may be associated with antiphospholipids. Myocardial infarcts usually result from degenerative disease, although they can result from vasculitis.

Pleurisy and pleural effusions are common manifestations of SLE. Lupus pneumonitis causes fever, dyspnea, and cough; x-rays show fleeting infiltrates and/or areas of platelike atelectasis; this syndrome respond to glucocorticoids. However, the most common cause of pulmonary infiltrates in patients with SLE is infection. Interstitial pneumonitis leading to fibrosis occurs occasionally; the inflammatory phase may respond to treatment; the fibrosis does not. Pulmonary hypertension is an uncommon, grave manifestation of SLE. Infrequent pulmonary manifestations with high mortality include adult respiratory distress syndrome and massive intraalveolar hemorrhage.

Gastrointestinal Common gastrointestinal (GI) symptoms include nausea, diarrhea, and vague discomfort. Symptoms may result from lupus peritonitis. Vasculitis of the intestine is the most dangerous

manifestation, presenting with acute crampy abdominal pain, vomiting, and diarrhea. Intestinal perforation can occur and usually requires immediate surgery. Patients with pseudoobstruction have abdominal pain; x-rays show dilated loops of small bowel which may be edematous; surgery should be avoided unless frank obstruction is present. Glucocorticoid therapy is useful for all these GI syndromes. Some patients have GI motility disorders similar to those in scleroderma; they are not benefited by steroids. Acute pancreatitis occurs and can be severe, resulting from active SLE or from therapy with glucocorticoids or azathioprine. Elevated amylase levels may reflect pancreatitis, salivary gland inflammation, or macroamylasemia. Elevated serum transaminases are common in patients with active SLE but are not associated with significant hepatic damage; they return to normal as the disease is treated.

Ocular Retinal vasculitis is a serious manifestation; blindness can develop over a few days, and aggressive immunosuppression should be instituted. Examination shows areas of sheathed, narrow retinal arterioles and cytoid bodies (white exudates) adjacent to vessels. Other ocular abnormalities include conjunctivitis, episcleritis, optic neuritis, and the sicca syndrome.

PATHOLOGY Cutaneous lesions Lesions of acute SLE, discoid lupus (DLE), and subacute cutaneous LE (SCLE) show similar histopathology, with degeneration of the basal layer of the epidermis, disruption of the dermal-epidermal junction (DEJ), and mononuclear infiltrates around vessels and appendages in the upper dermis. In DLE, follicular plugging and hyperkeratosis are prominent. Deposits of immunoglobulins (Ig) and C' are seen in the DEJ in 80 to 100 percent of lesional and 50 percent of nonlesional skin in active SLE; the proportions are lower during remissions. Only 50 percent of SCLE lesions are positive for Ig and C' deposits. Ig deposition in the DEJ is not specific for LE. Vasculitis skin lesions usually show leukocytoclastic angiitis.

Renal lesions Glomerulonephritis (GN) is caused by deposition of circulating immune complexes or in situ complex formation in mesangium and glomerular basement membranes (GBM). Renal biopsy should be considered when results would affect therapy. Information regarding location of immune deposits, histologic pattern of renal damage, and activity and chronicity of lesions is all useful in predicting prognosis and selecting appropriate treatment. In mild GN unlikely to lead to renal failure, Ig deposits are confined to the mesangium, and histology shows no changes or mesangial proliferation. If Ig and C' are deposited outside the mesangium in capillary GBM, prognosis worsens. Histologic changes that should be treated with aggressive immunosuppression include focal proliferative, membranoproliferative, and diffuse proliferative GN (see Chap 241). Progression from focal to diffuse lesions can occur. Membranous changes without proliferation are uncommon but have a better prognosis than proliferative GN. Activity and chronicity scores indicate severity and reversibility of lesions. Reversible "active" lesions associated with high risk of progression to renal failure are glomerular necrosis, cellular epithelial crescents, hyaline thrombi, interstitial inflammatory infiltrates, and necrotizing vasculitis. Irreversible changes unlikely to respond to immunosuppression and highly associated with renal failure include glomerular sclerosis, fibrous crescents, interstitial fibrosis, and tubular atrophy. In patients with high chronicity scores, treatment of lupus should be determined by extrarenal disease.

LABORATORY MANIFESTATIONS The presence of characteristic antibodies (see Table 284-1) confirms the diagnosis of SLE. Antinuclear antibodies (ANAs) are the best screening test. If the test substrate contains human nuclei (WIL-2 or HEP-2 cells), more than 95 percent of lupus patients will be positive. A positive ANA test is not specific for SLE; ANAs occur in some normal individuals (usually in low titer); the frequency increases with aging. Other autoimmune diseases, viral infections, chronic inflammatory processes, and several drugs induce ANAs. Therefore, a positive ANA test supports the diagnosis of SLE but is not specific; a negative ANA test makes the diagnosis unlikely but not impossible. Antibodies to double-stranded

DNA (dsDNA) and to Sm are relatively specific for SLE; other autoantibodies listed in Table 284-1 are not. However, determining the complete autoantibody profile of each patient helps predict clinical subsets. High serum levels of ANAs and anti-dsDNA antibodies and low levels of complement usually reflect disease activity, especially in patients with nephritis. Total functional hemolytic complement (CH_{50}) levels are the most sensitive measure of complement activation but are also most subject to laboratory error. Quantitative levels of C2 and C4 are widely available. Very low levels of CH_{50} with normal levels of C3 suggest inherited deficiency of a complement component, which is highly associated with SLE and with ANA negativity.

Hematologic abnormalities include anemia (usually normochromic normocytic but occasionally hemolytic), leukopenia, lymphopenia, and thrombocytopenia. The Westergren erythrocyte sedimentation rate correlates with disease activity in some patients.

Urinalysis and serum creatinine determinations should be done periodically in patients with SLE. With active nephritis, the urinalysis usually shows proteinuria, hematuria, and cellular or granular casts. Urinary protein excretion measured over 24 h increases during periods of activity. See the discussion under "Pathology" for a description of renal biopsy.

PREGNANCY Fertility rates are normal in patients with SLE, but spontaneous abortion and stillbirths are frequent (30 to 50 percent), especially in women with lupus anticoagulant and/or antibodies to cardiolipin. Treatment of women with prior fetal loss and antiphospholipid antibodies is controversial. Options are no intervention, daily low-dose aspirin until the last month of pregnancy, low-dose aspirin plus daily high-dose glucocorticoids, and twice-daily subcutaneous heparin in full anticoagulating doses; there are data to support each approach.

Pregnancy has varied effects on SLE activity. Disease flares in a small proportion, especially during the 6 weeks postpartum. If severe renal or cardiac disease is absent and SLE activity is controlled, most patients complete pregnancy safely and deliver normal infants. Glucocorticoids (except dexamethasone and betamethasone) are inactivated by placental enzymes and do not cause fetal abnormalities; they should be used to suppress disease activity. Neonatal lupus, caused by transmission of maternal anti-Ro antibodies across the placenta, consists of transient skin rash and (rarely) permanent heart block. Transient thrombocytopenia from maternal antiplatelet antibodies also occurs.

DIFFERENTIAL DIAGNOSIS The American Rheumatism Association published diagnostic criteria for SLE (see Table 284-3). Any four of the manifestations listed establish a diagnosis of SLE. Early disease confined to a few systems is more difficult to classify; it may take several years for a patient to fulfill criteria. Disorders with which SLE can be confused include rheumatoid arthritis; various forms of dermatitis; neurologic disorders such as epilepsy, multiple sclerosis, and psychiatric disorders; and hematologic diseases such as idiopathic thrombocytopenic purpura. Many autoimmune disorders have overlapping features, so exact classification may be difficult. Mixed connective tissue disease has features of SLE, rheumatoid arthritis, polymyositis, and scleroderma, accompanied by high titers of anti-RNP antibodies (Chap 287); patients have a low incidence of nephritis and CNS disease and a high incidence of pulmonary manifestations and evolution into scleroderma. Therapy should be directed toward the dominant manifestations in each patient. The possibility of drug-induced lupus should always be considered.

DRUG-INDUCED LUPUS Several drugs can cause a syndrome resembling SLE, including procainamide, hydralazine, isoniazid, chlorpromazine, D-penicillamine, practolol, methyldopa, quinidine, alpha interferon, and possibly hydantoins, ethosuximide, and oral contraceptives. The syndrome is rare with all but procainamide, the most frequent offender, and hydralazine. There is genetic predisposition to drug-induced lupus, partly determined by drug acetylation rates. Procainamide induces ANAs in 50 to 75 percent of individuals within a few months; hydralazine induces ANAs in 25 to 30 percent. Ten to 20 percent of ANA-positive individuals develop lupus-like

symptoms. Most common are systemic complaints and arthralgias; polyarthritis and pleuropericarditis occur in 25 to 50 percent. Renal and CNS diseases are rare. All patients have ANAs, and most have antibodies to histones. Antibodies to dsDNA and hypocomplementemia are rare—a helpful point in distinguishing drug-induced from idiopathic lupus. Anemia, leukopenia, lupus anticoagulant, anticardiolipin antibodies, thrombocytopenia, cryoglobulins, rheumatoid factors, and false-positive VDRL and positive direct Coombs' tests can occur. The initial therapeutic approach is withdrawal of the offending drug; most patients improve in a few weeks. If symptoms are severe, a short course (2 to 10 weeks) of glucocorticoids is indicated. Symptoms rarely persist more than 6 months; ANAs may persist for years. Most lupus-inducing drugs can be used safely in patients with idiopathic SLE.

PROGNOSIS Survival in patients with SLE is approximately 70 percent over 10 years. Survival is lowest in nonwhite patients, low socioeconomic groups, and patients with severe involvement of kidneys, brain, lungs, or heart. Disability is common. Infection and renal failure are the leading causes of death.

TREATMENT There is no cure for SLE. Complete remissions are rare. Therefore, patient and physician should plan (1) to control acute, severe flares and (2) to develop maintenance strategies in which symptoms are suppressed to an acceptable level, usually at the cost of some drug side effects. Approximately 25 percent of LE patients have mild disease with no life-threatening manifestations, although pain and fatigue may be disabling. These patients should be managed without glucocorticoids. Arthralgias, arthritis, myalgias, fever, and mild serositis may improve on nonsteroidal anti-inflammatory drugs (NSAIDS) including salicylates. However, NSAID toxicities such as elevated liver enzymes, aseptic meningitis, and renal impairment are especially frequent in SLE. The dermatitides of SLE and, occasionally, lupus arthritis may respond to antimalarials. Doses of 400 mg hydroxychloroquine daily may improve skin lesions in a few weeks. Side effects are uncommon and include retinal toxicity, rash, myopathy, and neuropathy. Regular ophthalmologic examinations should be performed at least annually, since retinal toxicity is related to cumulative dose. Other therapies for rash include sunscreens (an SPF rating of 15 or higher is recommended), topical or intralesional glucocorticoids, quinacrine, retinoids, and dapsone. Systemic glucocorticoids should be reserved for patients with severe lesions unresponsive to other measures.

Life-threatening, severely disabling manifestations of SLE that are responsive to immunosuppression should be treated with high doses of *glucocorticoids* (1 to 2 mg/kg per day). When disease is active, glucocorticoids should be given in divided doses every 8 to 12 h. After the disease is controlled, therapy should be consolidated to one morning dose; thereafter, the daily dose should be tapered as rapidly as clinical disease permits. Ideally, patients should be slowly converted to alternate-day therapy with a single morning dose of short-acting glucocorticoid (prednisone, prednisolone, methylprednisolone) to minimize side effects. However, the disease may flare on the day off steroids, in which case the lowest single daily dose that suppresses disease should be used. Undesirable effects of chronic glucocorticoid therapy include cushingoid habitus, weight gain, hypertension, infection, capillary fragility, acne, hirsutism, accelerated osteoporosis, ischemic necrosis of bone, cataracts, glaucoma, diabetes mellitus, myopathy, hypokalemia, irregular menses, irritability, insomnia, and psychosis. Prednisone doses of 15 mg daily (or less) given before noon usually do not suppress the hypothalamic pituitary axis. Some side effects can be minimized; hyperglycemia, hypertension, edema, and hypokalemia should be treated; infections should be identified and treated early; immunizations with influenza and pneumococcal vaccines are safe and should be given if disease is stable. To minimize osteoporosis, supplemental calcium (1000 mg daily) should be added in most patients; in those with 24-h urinary calcium excretion < 120 mg, vitamin D 50,000 units one to three times weekly can be added (monitor for hypercalcemia), and estrogen replacement therapy should be considered at menopause. Calcitonin and bisphosphonates also express activation antigens such as HLA-DR. In addition, they express an increased density of molecules, such as leukocyte function associated antigen 1 (LFA-1, CD11a/CD18), that have been implicated in a variety of cell-to-cell interactions, including binding of circulating cells to postcapillary venules just prior to entry into sites of tissue inflammation. Finally, the T cells appear to have proliferated locally in the synovial tissue, perhaps in response to sequestered antigen, since they express determinants such as very late antigen-1 (VLA-1) that appears on T cells only after prolonged proliferation. Evidence of B cell activation also can be found in the inflamed synovium, and plasma cells producing immunoglobulin and rheumatoid factor are characteristic features of rheumatoid synovitis. Large numbers of macrophages with an activated phenotype are also found in rheumatoid synovium.

The rheumatoid synovium is characterized by the presence of a number of secreted products of activated lymphocytes, macrophages, and other cell types. The local production of these cytokines appears to account for many of the pathologic and clinical manifestations of RA. Table 285-2 lists cytokines that have been identified in rheumatoid synovial fluid and indicates their putative role in the rheumatoid inflammatory process. These cytokines include those that are derived from T lymphocytes such as interleukin 2 (IL-2), IL-6, granulocyte-macrophage colony stimulating factor (GM-CSF), tumor necrosis factor α, and transforming growth factor β; those originating from activated macrophages, including IL-1, tumor necrosis factor α, IL-6, IL-8, GM-CSF, macrophage CSF, platelet-derived growth factor, insulin-like growth factor, and transforming growth factor β; as well as those secreted by other cell types in the synovium, such as fibroblasts and endothelial cells, including IL-1, IL-6, IL-8, GM-CSF, and macrophage CSF. The activity of these cytokines appears to account for many of the features of rheumatoid synovitis, including the synovial tissue inflammation, synovial fluid inflammation, synovial proliferation, and cartilage and bone damage, as well as the systemic manifestations of RA. In addition to the production of cytokines that propagate the inflammatory process, local factors are produced that

tend to slow the inflammation, including specific inhibitors of cytokine action and additional cytokines, such as transforming growth factor β, which inhibits many of the features of rheumatoid synovitis including T cell activation and proliferation, B cell differentiation, and migration of cells into the inflammatory site.

These findings have suggested that the propagation of RA is an immunologically mediated event, although the original initiating stimulus has not been characterized. One view is that the inflammatory process in the tissue is driven by the CD4 + helper-inducer T cells infiltrating the synovium. Evidence for this includes (1) the predominance of CD4 + T cells in the synovium, (2) the increase in soluble IL-2 receptors, a product of activated T cells, in blood and synovial fluid of patients with active RA, and (3) amelioration of the disease by removal of T cells by thoracic duct drainage or peripheral lymphapheresis or suppression of their function by total lymphoid irradiation. In addition, administration of monoclonal antibodies directed at T cells or the CD4 + T cell subset has been shown to suppress rheumatoid inflammation in some patients. Finally, patients with established RA who become infected with the human immunodeficiency virus (HIV) also have been noted to improve. T lymphocytes produce a number of cytokines, including interferon-γ and GM-CSF, that can lead to activation of macrophages and also increased expression of HLA molecules. Moreover, T lymphocytes produce a variety of cytokines that promote B cell proliferation and differentiation into antibody-forming cells and therefore also may promote local B cell stimulation. The resultant production of immunoglobulin and rheumatoid factor can lead to immune-complex formation with consequent complement activation and exacerbation of the inflammatory process by the production of the anaphylatoxins, C3a and C5a, and the chemotactic factor C5a. The tissue inflammation is reminiscent of delayed-type hypersensitivity reactions occurring in response to soluble antigens or microorganisms. It is, however, unclear whether this represents a response to a persistent exogenous antigen or to altered autoantigens such as collagen, immunoglobulin, or one of the heat shock proteins. Alternatively, it could represent persistent responsiveness to activated autologous cells such as might occur as a result of Epstein-Barr virus infection or persistent response to a foreign antigen or superantigen in the synovial tissue. Finally, rheumatoid inflammation could reflect persistent stimulation of T cells by synovial-derived antigens that cross-react with determinants introduced during antecedent exposure to foreign antigens or infectious microorganisms.

Overriding the chronic inflammation in the synovial tissue is an acute inflammatory process in the synovial fluid. The exudative synovial fluid contains more polymorphonuclear leukocytes than mononuclear cells. A number of mechanisms play a role in stimulating the exudation of synovial fluid. Locally produced immune complexes can activate complement and generate anaphylatoxins and chemotactic factors. Local production by mononuclear phagocytes of factors such as IL-1, tumor necrosis factor α (TNF-α), and leukotriene B₄, as well as products of complement activation, can stimulate the endothelial cells of postcapillary venules to become more efficient at binding circulating cells, whereas TNF-α, IL-8, C5a, and leukotriene B₄ stimulate the migration of polymorphonuclear leukocytes into the synovial site. In addition, vasoactive mediators such as histamine produced by the mast cells that infiltrate the rheumatoid synovium also may facilitate the exudation of inflammatory cells into the synovial fluid. Finally, the vasodilatory effects of locally produced prostaglandin E₂ also may facilitate entry of inflammatory cells into the inflammatory site. Once in the synovial fluid, the polymorphonuclear leukocytes can ingest immune complexes, with the resultant production of reactive oxygen metabolites and other inflammatory mediators, further adding to the inflammatory milieu. Locally produced cytokines such as TNF-α, IL-8, and GM-CSF can additionally stimulate polymorphonuclear leukocytes. The production of large amounts of cyclooxygenase and lipoxygenase pathway products of arachidonic acid metabolism by cells in the synovial fluid and tissue further accentuates the signs and symptoms of inflammation.

TABLE 285-2 Cytokines in rheumatoid inflammation

Manifestation	Cytokine involved
1 Synovial tissue inflammation	
a Increased adherence of postcapillary venules	IL-1, TNF-α, IFN-γ
b Chemotaxis of T cells	IL-8
c T cell activation and proliferation	IL-1, TNF-α, IL-6, IL-2
d B cell differentiation and antibody formation	IL-1, TNF-α, IL-6, IL-2, IFN-γ
e Increased expression of HLA antigens	IFN-γ, TNF-α, GM-CSF
f Macrophage activation	IFN-γ, GM-CSF, M-CSF, IL-2
2 Synovial fluid inflammation	
a Increased adherence of postcapillary venules	IL-1, TNF-α, IFN-γ
b Chemotactic for PMN	TNF-α, IL-8
c Activation of PMN	TNF-α, GM-CSF, IL-8
3 Synovial proliferation	
a Fibroblast growth	PDGF, IL-1, IGF, FGF, TGF-β, EGF
b Neovascularization	TNF-α, FGF, TGF-β
4 Cartilage and bone damage	
a Activation of chondrocytes	IL-1, TNF-α
b Activation of fibroblasts	IL-1, TNF-α
c Activation of osteoblasts-osteoclasts	IL-1, TNF-α
5 Systemic manifestations	
a Fever, constitutional symptoms	IL-1, TNF-α
b Acute phase reactants	IL-1, TNF-α, IL-6

NOTE: IL-1, interleukin 1; IL-2, interleukin 2; IL-6, interleukin 6; TNF-α, tumor necrosis factor α; IFN-γ, interferon-γ; GM-CSF, granulocyte-macrophage colony stimulating factor; M-CSF, macrophage colony stimulating factor; PDGF, platelet-derived growth factor; PMN, polymorphonuclear cells; IGF, insulin-like growth factor; FGF, fibroblast growth factor; TGF-β, transforming growth factor β; EGF, epidermal growth factor.

The precise mechanism by which bone and cartilage destruction occurs has not been completely resolved. Although the synovial fluid contains a number of enzymes potentially able to degrade cartilage, the majority of destruction occurs in juxtaposition to the inflamed synovium, or pannus, that spreads to cover the articular cartilage. This vascular granulation tissue is composed of proliferating fibroblasts, small blood vessels, and a variable number of mononuclear cells and produces a large amount of degradative enzymes, including collagenase and stromelysin, that may facilitate tissue damage. The cytokines IL-1 and tumor necrosis factor α play an important role by stimulating the cells of the pannus to produce collagenase and other neutral proteases. These same two cytokines also activate chondrocytes in situ, stimulating them to produce proteolytic enzymes that can degrade cartilage locally. Finally, these two cytokines may contribute to the local demineralization of bone by activating osteoclasts. Prostaglandin E_2 produced by fibroblasts and macrophages also may contribute to bone demineralization. Systemic manifestations of RA can be accounted for by release of inflammatory effector molecules from the synovium. These include IL-1, TNF-α, and IL-6, which account for many of the manifestations of active RA, including malaise, fatigue, and elevation of serum acute phase reactants. In addition, immune complexes produced within the synovium and entering the circulation may account for other features of the disease, such as systemic vasculitis.

CLINICAL MANIFESTATIONS **Onset** Characteristically, RA is a chronic polyarthritis. In approximately two-thirds of patients, it begins insidiously with fatigue, anorexia, generalized weakness, and vague musculoskeletal symptoms until the appearance of synovitis becomes apparent. This prodrome may persist for weeks or months and defy diagnosis. Specific symptoms usually appear gradually as several joints, especially those of the hands, wrists, knees, and feet, become affected in a symmetric fashion. In approximately 10 percent of individuals, the onset is more acute, with a rapid development of polyarthritis, often accompanied by constitutional symptoms, including fever, lymphadenopathy, and splenomegaly. In approximately one-third of patients, symptoms may initially be confined to one or a few joints. Although the pattern of joint involvement may remain asymmetric in a few patients, a symmetric pattern is more typical.

Signs and symptoms of articular disease Pain, swelling, and tenderness may initially be poorly localized to the joints. Pain in affected joints, aggravated by movement, is the most common manifestation of established RA. It corresponds in pattern to the joint involvement but does not always correlate with the degree of apparent inflammation. Generalized stiffness is frequent and is usually greatest after periods of inactivity. Morning stiffness of greater than 1-h duration is an almost invariable feature of inflammatory arthritis and serves to distinguish it from various noninflammatory joint disorders. The length and intensity of the stiffness can be used as a crude assessment of disease activity. The majority of patients will experience constitutional symptoms such as weakness, easy fatigability, anorexia, and weight loss. Although fever to 40°C occurs on occasion, temperature elevation in excess of 38°C is unusual and suggests the presence of an intercurrent problem such as infection.

Clinically, synovial inflammation causes swelling, tenderness, and limitation of motion. Warmth is usually evident on examination, especially of large joints such as the knee, but erythema is infrequent. Pain originates predominantly from the joint capsule, which is abundantly supplied with pain fibers and is markedly sensitive to stretching or distention. Joint swelling results from accumulation of synovial fluid, hypertrophy of the synovium, and thickening of the joint capsule. Initially, motion is limited by pain. The inflamed joint is usually held in flexion to maximize joint volume and minimize distention of the capsule. Later, fibrous or bony ankylosis or soft tissue contractures lead to fixed deformities.

Although inflammation can affect any diarthrodial joint, RA most often causes symmetric arthritis with characteristic involvement of certain specific joints such as the proximal interphalangeal and metacarpophalangeal joints. The distal interphalangeal joints are rarely involved. Synovitis of the wrist joints is a nearly uniform feature of RA and may lead to limitation of motion, deformity, and median nerve entrapment (carpal tunnel syndrome). Synovitis of the elbow joint often leads to flexion contractures that may develop early in the disease. The knee joint is commonly involved with synovial hypertrophy, chronic effusion, and frequently ligamentous laxity. Pain and swelling behind the knee may be caused by extension of inflamed synovium into the popliteal space (Baker's cyst). Arthritis in the forefoot, ankles, and subtalar joints can produce severe pain with ambulation as well as a number of deformities. Axial involvement is usually limited to the upper cervical spine. Involvement of the lumbar spine is not seen, and lower back pain cannot be ascribed to rheumatoid inflammation. On occasion, inflammation from the synovial joints and bursae of the upper cervical spine leads to atlantoaxial subluxation. This usually presents as pain in the occiput but on rare occasions may lead to compression of the spinal cord.

With persistent inflammation, a variety of characteristic deformities develop. These can be attributed to a number of pathologic events, including laxity of supporting soft tissue structures; destruction or weakening of ligaments, tendons, and the joint capsule; cartilage destruction; muscle imbalance; and unopposed physical forces associated with the use of affected joints. Characteristic deformities of the hand include (1) radial deviation at the wrist with ulnar deviation of the digits often with palmar subluxation of the proximal phalanges ("Z" deformity), (2) hyperextension of the proximal interphalangeal joints, with compensatory flexion of the distal interphalangeal joints (swan-neck deformity), (3) flexion deformity of the proximal interphalangeal joints and extension of the distal interphalangeal joints (boutonnière deformity), and (4) hyperextension of the first interphalangeal joint and flexion of the first metacarpophalangeal joint with a consequent loss of thumb mobility and pinch. Typical deformities also may develop in the feet, including eversion at the hindfoot (subtalar joint), plantar subluxation of the metatarsal heads, widening of the forefoot, hallux valgus, and lateral deviation and dorsal subluxation of the toes.

Extraarticular manifestations RA is a systemic disease with a variety of extraarticular manifestations. Although these occur frequently, not all of them have clinical significance. However, on occasion, they may be the major evidence of disease activity and source of morbidity and require management per se. As a rule, these manifestations occur in individuals with high titers of autoantibodies to the Fc component of immunoglobulin G (rheumatoid factors).

Rheumatoid nodules develop in 20 to 30 percent of persons with RA. They are usually found on periarticular structures, extensor surfaces, or other areas subjected to mechanical pressure, but they can develop elsewhere, including the pleura and meninges. Common locations include the olecranon bursa, the proximal ulna, the Achilles tendon, and the occiput. Nodules vary in size and consistency and are rarely symptomatic, but on occasion they break down as a result of trauma or become infected. They are found almost invariably in individuals with circulating rheumatoid factor. Histologically, rheumatoid nodules consist of a central zone of necrotic material including collagen fibrils, noncollagenous filaments, and cellular debris, a midzone of palisading macrophages that express HLA-DR antigens, and an outer zone of granulation tissue. Examination of early nodules has suggested that the initial event may be a focal vasculitis.

Clinical weakness and atrophy of skeletal muscle are common. Muscle atrophy may be evident within weeks of the onset of RA and usually is most apparent in musculature approximating affected joints. Muscle biopsy may show type II fiber atrophy and muscle fiber necrosis with or without a mononuclear cell infiltrate.

Rheumatoid vasculitis (see Chap. 291) which can affect nearly any organ system is seen in patients with severe RA and high titers of circulating rheumatoid factor. Rheumatoid vasculitis is very uncommon in African Americans. In its most aggressive form, rheumatoid vasculitis can cause polyneuropathy and mononeuritis multiplex, cutaneous ulceration and dermal necrosis, digital gangrene, and visceral infarction. While such widespread vasculitis is very rare, more limited forms are not uncommon, especially in white patients with high titers of rheumatoid factor. Neurovascular disease presenting either as a mild distal sensory neuropathy or as mononeuritis multiplex may be the only sign of vasculitis. Cutaneous vasculitis usually presents as crops of small brown spots in the nail beds, nail folds, and digital pulp. Larger ischemic ulcers, especially in the lower extremity, also may develop. Myocardial infarction secondary to rheumatoid vasculitis has been reported, as has vasculitic involvement of lungs, bowel, liver, spleen, pancreas, lymph nodes, and testes. Renal vasculitis is rare.

Pleuropulmonary manifestations, which are more commonly observed in men, include pleural disease, interstitial fibrosis, pleuropulmonary nodules, pneumonitis, and arteritis. Evidence of pleuritis is found commonly at autopsy, but symptomatic disease during life is infrequent. Typically, the pleural fluid contains very low levels of glucose in the absence of infection. Pleural fluid complement is also low compared with the serum level when these are related to the total protein concentration. Pulmonary fibrosis can produce impairment of the diffusing capacity of the lung. Pulmonary nodules may appear singly or in clusters. When they appear in individuals with pneumoconiosis, a diffuse nodular fibrotic process (Caplan's syndrome) may develop. On occasion, pulmonary nodules may cavitate and produce a pneumothorax or bronchopleural fistula. Rarely, pulmonary hypertension secondary to obliteration of the pulmonary vasculature occurs. In addition to pleuropulmonary disease, upper airway obstruction from cricoarytenoid arthritis or laryngeal nodules may develop.

Clinically apparent heart disease attributed to the rheumatoid process is rare, but evidence of asymptomatic pericarditis is found at autopsy in 50 percent of cases. Pericardial fluid has a low glucose level and is frequently associated with the occurrence of pleural effusion. Although pericarditis is usually asymptomatic, on rare occasions death has occurred from tamponade. Chronic constrictive pericarditis also may occur.

RA tends to spare the central nervous system directly, although vasculitis can cause peripheral neuropathy. *Neurologic manifestations* also may result from atlantoaxial or midcervical spine subluxations. Nerve entrapment secondary to proliferative synovitis or joint deformities may produce neuropathies of median, ulnar, radial (interosseous branch), or anterior tibial nerves.

The rheumatoid process involves the *eye* in less than 1 percent of patients. Affected individuals usually have long-standing disease and nodules. The two principal manifestations are episcleritis, which is usually mild and transient, and scleritis, which involves the deeper layers of the eye and is a more serious inflammatory condition. Histologically, the lesion is similar to a rheumatoid nodule and may result in thinning and perforation of the globe (scleromalacia perforans). Fifteen to twenty percent of persons with RA may develop Sjögren's syndrome with attendant keratoconjunctivitis sicca.

Felty's syndrome consists of chronic RA, splenomegaly, neutropenia, and on occasion anemia and thrombocytopenia. It is most common in individuals with long-standing disease. These patients frequently have high titers of rheumatoid factor, subcutaneous nodules, and other manifestations of systemic rheumatoid disease. Felty's syndrome is very uncommon in African Americans. It may develop after joint inflammation has regressed. Circulating immune complexes are often present, and evidence of complement consumption may be seen. The leukopenia is a selective neutropenia with polymorphonuclear leukocyte counts of less than 1500 cells per microliter and sometimes less than 1000 cells per microliter. Bone marrow examination usually reveals moderate hypercellularity with a paucity of mature neutrophils. However, the bone marrow may be normal, hyperactive, or hypoactive; maturation arrest may be seen. Hypersplenism has been proposed as one of the causes of leukopenia, but splenomegaly is not invariably found and splenectomy does not always correct the abnormality. Excessive margination of granulocytes caused by antibodies to these cells, complement activation, or binding of immune complexes may contribute to granulocytopenia. Patients with Felty's syndrome have increased frequency of infections usually associated with neutropenia. The cause of the increased susceptibility to infection is related to the defective function of polymorphonuclear leukocytes as well as the decreased number of cells.

Osteoporosis secondary to rheumatoid involvement is common and may be aggravated by corticosteroid therapy. Corticosteroid treatment may cause significant loss of bone mass, especially early in the course of therapy, even when low doses are employed. Osteopenia involves both juxtaarticular bone and long bones distant from involved joints. RA is associated with a modest decrease in mean bone mass and a moderate increase in the risk of fracture. Bone mass appears to be adversely affected by functional impairment and active inflammation, especially early in the course of the disease.

LABORATORY FINDINGS No tests are specific for diagnosing RA. However, rheumatoid factors, which are autoantibodies reactive with the Fc portion of IgG, are found in more than two-thirds of adults with the disease. Widely utilized tests largely detect IgM rheumatoid factors. The presence of rheumatoid factor is not specific for RA. Rheumatoid factor is found in 5 percent of healthy persons. The frequency of rheumatoid factor in the general population increases with age, and 10 to 20 percent of individuals over 65 years old have a positive test. In addition, a number of conditions besides RA are associated with the presence of rheumatoid factor. These include systemic lupus erythematosus, Sjögren's syndrome, chronic liver disease, sarcoidosis, interstitial pulmonary fibrosis, infectious mononucleosis, hepatitis B, tuberculosis, leprosy, syphilis, subacute bacterial endocarditis, visceral leishmaniasis, schistosomiasis, and malaria. In addition, rheumatoid factor may appear transiently in normal individuals after vaccination or transfusion and also may be found in relatives of individuals with RA.

The presence of rheumatoid factor does not establish the diagnosis of RA but can be of prognostic significance because patients with high titers tend to have more severe and progressive disease with extraarticular manifestations. Rheumatoid factor is uniformly found in patients with nodules or vasculitis. The predictive value of the presence of rheumatoid factor in determining a diagnosis of RA is poor. Thus less than one-third of unselected patients with a positive test for rheumatoid factor will be found to have RA. The test is not useful as a screening procedure but can be employed to confirm a diagnosis in individuals with a suggestive clinical presentation and, if present in high titer, to designate patients at risk for severe systemic disease.

Normochromic, normocytic anemia is frequently present in active RA. It is thought to reflect ineffective erythropoiesis; large stores of iron are found in the bone marrow. In general, anemia and thrombocytosis correlate with disease activity. The white blood cell count is usually normal, but a mild leukocytosis may be present. Leukopenia also may exist without the full-blown picture of Felty's syndrome. Eosinophilia, when present, usually reflects severe systemic disease.

The erythrocyte sedimentation rate is increased in nearly all patients with active RA. A variety of other acute phase reactants including ceruloplasmin and C-reactive protein are also elevated, and generally such elevations correlate with disease activity and the likelihood of progressive joint damage.

Synovial fluid analysis confirms the presence of inflammatory arthritis, although none of the findings is specific. The fluid is usually turbid, with reduced viscosity, increased protein content, and a slightly decreased or normal glucose concentration. The white cell count varies between 5 and 50,000 cells per microliter; polymorphonuclear leukocytes predominate. Total hemolytic complement, C3, and C4 are markedly diminished in synovial fluid relative to total protein concentration as a result of activation of the classic complement pathway by locally produced immune complexes.

When monoclonal antibodies specific for T lymphocyte subsets are used to examine peripheral blood mononuclear cells of patients with RA, no specific changes in the numbers of circulating CD4+

(helper-inducer) or CD8 + (suppressor-cytotoxic) T cells are noted. However, an increased number of circulating T cells expressing HLA-DR, an indication of T cell activation, can be observed. This finding is most frequent in patients with active joint disease.

RADIOGRAPHIC EVALUATION Early in the disease, roentgenograms of the affected joints are usually not helpful in establishing a diagnosis. They reveal only that which is apparent from physical examination, namely, evidence of soft tissue swelling and joint effusion. As the disease progresses, abnormalities become more pronounced, but none of the radiographic findings is diagnostic of RA. The diagnosis, however, is supported by a characteristic pattern of abnormalities, including the tendency toward symmetric involvement. Juxtaarticular osteopenia may become apparent within weeks of onset. Loss of articular cartilage and bone erosions develop after months of sustained activity. The primary value of radiography is to determine the extent of cartilage destruction and bone erosion produced by the disease, particularly when one is considering therapy with disease-modifying drugs or surgical intervention. Other means of imaging bones and joints, including ^{99m}Tc bisphosphonate bone scanning and magnetic resonance imaging, may be capable of detecting early inflammatory changes but are rarely necessary in the routine evaluation of patients with RA.

CLINICAL COURSE AND PROGNOSIS The course of RA is quite variable and difficult to predict in an individual patient. Most patients experience persistent but fluctuating disease activity, accompanied by a variable degree of joint deformity. After 10 to 12 years, fewer than 20 percent of patients will have no evidence of disability or deformity. Features of patients that predict the development of disability include older age, female sex, more severe radiographic involvement, and the presence of rheumatoid nodules or elevated titers of rheumatoid factor. The pattern of disease onset does not appear to predict the development of disabilities. Approximately 15 percent of patients with RA will have a short-lived inflammatory process that remits without major deformity.

Several features of patients with RA appear to have prognostic significance. Remissions of disease activity are most likely to occur during the first year. White females tend to have more persistent synovitis and more progressively erosive disease than males. Persons who present with high titers of rheumatoid factor, C-reactive protein, and haptoglobin also have a worse prognosis, as do individuals with subcutaneous nodules or radiographic evidence of erosions at the time of initial evaluation. Although sustained disease activity of more than 1 year's duration portends a poor outcome, the rate of progression of joint abnormalities is not constant; the greatest progression takes place during the first 6 years of disease and at a much slower rate thereafter. Indeed, the rate of progression of joint damage is greater during the first year of observation compared with the second and third years. Within 3 years of disease, as many as 70 percent of patients will have some radiographic evidence of damage to joints. Foot joints are affected more frequently than hand joints. Despite the decrease in the rate of progressive joint damage with time, functional disability, which develops early in the course of the disease, continues to worsen at the same rate.

The median life expectancy of persons with RA is shortened by 3 to 7 years. Of the 2.5-fold increase in mortality rate, RA itself is a contributing feature in 15 to 30 percent. The increased mortality rate seems to be limited to patients with more severe articular disease and can be attributed largely to infection and gastrointestinal bleeding. Drug therapy also may play a role in the increased mortality rate seen in these individuals. Factors correlated with early death include disability, disease duration or severity, corticosteroid use, age, and male sex.

DIAGNOSIS The diagnosis of RA is easily made in persons with typical established disease. In a majority of patients, the disease assumes its characteristic clinical features within 1 to 2 years of onset. The typical picture of bilateral symmetric inflammatory polyarthritis involving small and large joints in both the upper and lower extremities with sparing of the axial skeleton except the cervical spine suggests

the diagnosis. Constitutional features indicative of the inflammatory nature of the disease, such as morning stiffness, support the diagnosis. Demonstration of subcutaneous nodules is a helpful diagnostic feature. Additionally, the presence of rheumatoid factor, inflammatory synovial fluid with increased numbers of polymorphonuclear leukocytes, and radiographic findings of juxtaarticular bone demineralization and erosions of the affected joints substantiate the diagnosis.

The diagnosis is somewhat more difficult early in the course when only constitutional symptoms or intermittent arthralgias or arthritis in an asymmetric distribution may be present. A period of observation may be necessary before the diagnosis can be established. A definitive diagnosis of RA depends predominantly on characteristic clinical features and the exclusion of other inflammatory processes. The isolated finding of a positive test for rheumatoid factor or an elevated erythrocyte sedimentation rate, especially in an older person with joint pains, should not itself be used as evidence of RA.

Recently, the American College of Rheumatology has developed revised criteria for the classification of rheumatoid arthritis (Table 285-3). The newer criteria are simpler to apply than the previous ones and demonstrate a sensitivity of 91 to 94 percent and a specificity of 89 percent when used to classify patients with RA compared with control subjects with rheumatic diseases other than RA. The major differences between the new and old criteria are that results of invasive procedures such as biopsies are not included, the classifications of probable, definite, and classic RA have been eliminated, and patients with more than a single diagnosis are not eliminated by exclusion criteria. Although these criteria were developed as a means of disease classification for epidemiologic purposes, they are useful as guidelines for establishing the diagnosis. Failure to meet these criteria, however, especially during the early stages of the disease, does not exclude the diagnosis.

TREATMENT General principles The goals of therapy of RA are (1) relief of pain, (2) reduction of inflammation, (3) preservation of functional capacity, (4) resolution of the etiopathogenic process, and (5) facilitation of healing. Currently available medications are capable of providing pain relief and some reduction in inflammation. Since the etiology of RA is unknown, the pathogenesis is speculative, and the mechanisms of action of many of the therapeutic agents employed are uncertain, therapy remain empirical. None of the therapeutic interventions are curative, and therefore, all must be viewed as palliative, aimed at relieving the signs and symptoms of

---

TABLE 285-3 The 1987 revised criteria for the classification of rheumatoid arthritis

1 Guidelines for classification
  a Four of seven criteria are required to classify a patient as having rheumatoid arthritis.
  b Patients with two or more clinical diagnoses are not excluded.
2 Criteria*
  a Morning stiffness: Stiffness in and around the joints lasting 1 h before maximal improvement.
  b Arthritis of three or more joint areas: At least three joint areas, observed by a physician simultaneously, have soft tissue swelling or joint effusions, not just bony overgrowth. The 14 possible joint areas involved are right or left proximal interphalangeal, metacarpophalangeal, wrist, elbow, knee, ankle, and metatarsophalangeal joints.
  c Arthritis of hand joints: Arthritis of wrist, metacarpophalangeal joint, or proximal interphalangeal joint.
  d Symmetric arthritis: Simultaneous involvement of the same joint areas on both sides of the body.
  e Rheumatoid nodules: Subcutaneous nodules over bony prominences, extensor surfaces, or juxtaarticular regions observed by a physician.
  f Serum rheumatoid factor: Demonstration of abnormal amounts of serum rheumatoid factor by any method for which the result has been positive in less than 5 percent of normal control subjects.
  g Radiographic changes: Typical changes of RA on posteroanterior hand and wrist radiographs which must include erosions or unequivocal bony decalcification localized in or most marked adjacent to the involved joints.

* Criteria *a–d* must be present for at least 6 weeks. Criteria *b–e* must be observed by a physician.

the disease. The various therapies employed are directed at nonspecific suppression of the inflammatory or immunologic process in the hope of ameliorating symptoms and preventing progressive damage to articular structures.

Management of patients with RA involves an interdisciplinary approach which attempts to deal with the various problems that these individuals encounter with functional as well as psychosocial interactions. A variety of physical therapy modalities may be useful in decreasing the symptoms of RA. Rest ameliorates symptoms and can be an important component of the total therapeutic program. In addition, splinting to reduce unwanted motion of inflamed joints may be useful. Exercise directed at maintaining muscle strength and joint mobility without exacerbating joint inflammation is also an important aspect of the therapeutic regimen. A variety of orthotic devices can be helpful in supporting and aligning deformed joints to reduce pain and improve function.

Medical management of RA involves three general approaches. The first is the use of aspirin and other nonsteroidal anti-inflammatory drugs, simple analgesics, and, if necessary, low-dose glucocorticoids to control the symptoms and signs of the local inflammatory process. These agents are rapidly effective at mitigating signs and symptoms, but they appear to exert minimal effect on the progression of the disease. The second line of therapy includes a variety of agents that have been classified as the disease-modifying or slow-acting antirheumatic drugs. These agents appear to have the capacity to decrease elevated levels of acute phase reactants in treated patients and, therefore, are thought to modify the destructive capacity of the disease. Other second-line agents are the immunosuppressive and cytotoxic drugs that have been shown to ameliorate the disease process in some patients. The third approach involves the use of a number of experimental modalities, such as total-lymphoid irradiation, lymph-oplasmapheresis, the administration of the immunosuppressive agent cyclosporine, and the administration of monoclonal antibodies to T cells and T cell subsets. Although some show potential for ameliorating disease, none has been shown to be a safe and cost-effective way to treat patients on a long-term basis. Recently, substitution of dietary omega-6 essential fatty acids with omega-3 fatty acids such as eicosapentaenoic acid found in certain fish oils also has been shown to provide symptomatic improvement in patients with RA. A variety of nontraditional approaches also have been claimed to be effective in treating RA, including diets, plant and animal extracts, vaccines, hormones, and topical preparations of various sorts. Many of these are costly, and none has been shown to be effective. However, belief in their efficacy ensures their continued use by some patients.

Nonsteroidal anti-inflammatory drugs Besides aspirin, there are now several additional nonsteroidal anti-inflammatory drugs (NSAIDs) available to treat RA. These include etodolac, fenoprofen, ibuprofen, indomethacin, ketoprofen, nabumetone, naproxen, meclofenamate, piroxicam, sulindac, tolmetin, diclofenac, oxaprozin, and flurbiprofen. As a result of the capacity of these agents to block the activity of the enzyme cyclooxygenase and therefore the production of prostaglandins, prostacyclin, and thromboxanes, they have analgesic, anti-inflammatory, and antipyretic properties. In addition, the agents may exert other anti-inflammatory effects. These agents are all associated with a wide spectrum of toxic side effects. Some, such as gastric irritation, azotemia, platelet dysfunction, and exacerbation of allergic rhinitis and asthma, are related to the inhibition of cyclooxygenase activity, while a variety of others, such as rash, liver function abnormalities, and bone marrow depression, may not be. Elderly patients on diuretics may be at higher risk for certain toxic effects. None of the NSAIDs has been shown to be more effective than aspirin in the treatment of RA. However, these nonaspirin drugs are associated with a lower incidence of gastrointestinal intolerance. None of the newer NSAIDs appears to show significant therapeutic advantages over the other available agents. In addition, there is no consistent advantage of any of these newer agents over the others with respect to the incidence or severity of toxic manifestations.

Disease-modifying antirheumatic drugs (DMARDs) Clinical ex-

perience has delineated a number of agents that appear to have the capacity to alter the course of RA. This group of agents includes gold compounds, D-penicillamine, the antimalarials, and sulfasalazine. Despite having no chemical or pharmacologic similarities, in practice, these agents share a number of characteristics. They exert minimal direct nonspecific anti-inflammatory or analgesic effects, and therefore, NSAIDs must be continued during their administration, except in a few cases when true remissions are induced with them. The appearance of benefit from DMARD therapy is usually delayed for weeks or months. As many as two-thirds of patients develop some clinical improvement as a result of therapy with any of these agents, although the induction of true remissions is unusual. In addition to clinical improvement, there is frequently an improvement in serologic evidence of disease activity, and titers of rheumatoid factor and C-reactive protein and the erythrocyte sedimentation rate frequently decline. Despite this, there is minimal evidence that DMARDs actually retard the development of bone erosions or facilitate their healing.

Each of these drugs is associated with considerable toxicity, and therefore, careful patient monitoring is necessary. Which DMARD should be the drug of first choice remains controversial, and trials have failed to demonstrate a consistent advantage of one over the other. Toxicity of the various agents thus becomes important in determining the drug of first choice. Failure to respond or development of toxicity to one agent does not preclude responsiveness to another. For example, a similar percentage of RA patients who have failed to respond to gold will respond to D-pencillamine when it is given as the second disease-modifying drug.

No characteristic features of patients have emerged that predict responsiveness to a DMARD. Moreover, the indications for the initiation of therapy with one of these agents are not well defined, although recently the trend has been to begin DMARD therapy early in the course of the disease. There is no convincing evidence that therapy with multiple DMARDs is more effective than treatment with a single agent.

Glucocorticoid therapy Although systemic glucocorticoid therapy can provide effective symptomatic therapy in patients with RA, these drugs should be avoided if possible because they do not alter the course of the disease and the potential toxicity of long-term therapy is substantial. Low-dose (less than 7.5 mg/d) prednisone has been advocated as useful additive therapy to control symptoms, but trials have not provided convincing evidence of efficacy. Monthly pulses with high-dose corticosteroids may be useful in some patients and may hasten the response when therapy with a DMARD is initiated.

Immunosuppressive therapy The immunosuppressive drugs azathioprine and cyclophosphamide have been shown to be effective in the treatment of RA and to exert therapeutic effects similar to those of the DMARDs. However, these agents appear to be no more effective than the DMARDs. Moreover, they cause a variety of toxic side effects, and cyclophosphamide appears to predispose the patient to the development of malignant neoplasms. Therefore, these drugs have been reserved for patients who have clearly failed therapy with DMARDs. On occasion, extraarticular disease such as rheumatoid vasculitis may require cytotoxic immunosuppressive therapy.

The folic acid antagonist methotrexate, given in an intermittent low dose (7.5 to 15 mg once weekly), also may be useful in the treatment of RA. Recent trials have documented the efficacy of methotrexate and have indicated that its onset of action is more rapid than other DMARDs, and patients tend to remain on therapy with methotrexate longer than they remain on other DMARDs because of better clinical responses and less toxicity. Long-term trials have indicated that methotrexate does not induce remission, but rather suppresses symptoms while it is being administered. Maximal improvement is observed after 6 months of therapy, with little additional improvement thereafter. Major toxicity includes gastrointestinal upset, oral ulceration, and liver function abnormalities that appear to be dose-related and reversible and hepatic fibrosis that can be quite insidious, requiring liver biopsy for detection in its early stages. Drug-induced pneumonitis also has been reported. Because of its therapeutic benefit and toxicity profile, methotrexate is used before other second-line drugs by many rheumatologists.

Recent trials have suggested that cyclosporine also may be effective in the treatment of RA. Although high-dose therapy may induce rapid improvement, it is associated with frequent renal and gastrointestinal toxicity. Lower doses of cyclosporine (<5 mg/kg per day), however, appear to cause slower but nonetheless significant improvement in disease activity with fewer toxic side effects that are reversed upon lowering the dose. Currently, cyclosporine has not been approved for use in RA.

Surgery Surgery plays a role in the management of patients with severely damaged joints. Although arthroplasties and total joint replacements can be done on a number of joints, the most successful procedures are carried out on hips and knees. Realistic goals of these procedures are relief of pain, correction of deformity, and modest functional improvement. Reconstructive hand surgery may lead to cosmetic improvement and some functional benefit. Open or arthroscopic synovectomy may be useful in some patients with persistent monarthritis, especially of the knee. Although synovectomy may offer short-term relief of symptoms, there is no evidence that it retards bone destruction or the natural history of the disease. In addition, early tenosynovectomy of the wrist may prevent tendon rupture.

Approach to the patient with RA At the onset of disease it is difficult to predict the natural history of an individual patient's illness. Therefore, the usual approach is to attempt to alleviate the patient's symptoms with NSAIDs. Some patients may have mild disease that requires no additional therapy. Since the DMARDs are potentially toxic and not universally effective, their use is usually delayed until it is apparent that symptoms cannot be controlled adequately with NSAIDs.

At some time during most patients' course, the possibility of initiating second-line therapy is entertained. With aggressive disease this might occur sooner, often within 1 to 3 months of diagnosis, whereas in patients with more indolent disease, smoldering activity may not require such therapy for many years. The development of bone erosions or radiographic evidence of cartilage loss is clear-cut evidence of the destructive potential of the inflammatory process and indicates the need for second-line drug therapy. The other indications, such as persistent pain, joint swelling, or functional impairment, are much more subjective, however. The decision to begin use of a second-line drug requires careful monitoring of joint swelling and functional activity, as well as an understanding of the patient's pain tolerance and expectation of therapy. In this setting, the fully informed patient must play an active role in the decision to begin second-line drug therapy, after careful review of the therapeutic and toxic potential of the various drugs.

If a patient responds to a second-line drug, therapy is continued with careful monitoring to avoid toxicity. All second-line drugs provide a suppressive effect and therefore require prolonged administration. Even with successful therapy, local injection of glucocorticoids may be necessary to diminish inflammation that may persist in a limited number of joints. In addition, NSAIDs may be necessary to mitigate symptoms. Even after inflammation has totally resolved, symptoms from loss of cartilage and supervening degenerative joint disease or deformities may require additional treatment. Surgery also may be necessary to relieve pain or diminish the functional impairment secondary to deformity. Only when patients have persistent inflammatory disease or severe extraarticular manifestations is the use of cytotoxic immunosuppressive drugs or experimental procedures justified. Recently an alternative approach to treat patients with RA has been suggested. This involves the initiation of therapy with multiple agents early in the course of disease in an attempt to control inflammation, followed by maintenance on one or more agents as necessary to control disease activity. The effectiveness of this therapeutic alternative has not been proven.

REFERENCES

ARNETT FC et al: The American Rheumatism Association 1987 revised criteria for the classification of rheumatoid arthritis. Arthritis Rheum 31:315, 1988

BOERS M, RAMSDEN M: Long-acting drug combinations in rheumatoid arthritis: A formal overview. J Rheumatol 18:316, 1991

BROOKS PM, DAY RO: Nonsteroidal anti-inflammatory drugs: Differences and similarities. N Engl J Med 324:1716, 1991

CUSH J, LIPSKY PE: Cellular basis for rheumatoid inflammation. Clin Orthop 265:9, 1991

FELSON DT et al: The comparative efficacy and toxicity of second-line drugs in rheumatoid arthritis. Arthritis Rheum 33:1449, 1990

GREGERSEN PK et al: The shared epitope hypothesis. Arthritis Rheum 30:1205, 1987

HARRIS ED JR: Rheumatoid arthritis: Pathophysiology and implications for therapy. N Engl J Med 322:1277, 1990

KAVANAUGH AF, LIPSKY PE: Gold, penicillamine, antimalarials and sulfasulazine, in Inflammation: Basic Principles and Clinical Correlates, 2d ed, JI Gallin et al (eds). New York, Raven, 1992, pp 1083–1101

KREMER JM, PHELPS CT: Long-term prospective study of the use of methotrexate in the treatment of rheumatoid arthritis. Arthritis Rheum 35:138, 1992

LAAN RFJM: Bone mass in patients with rheumatoid arthritis. Ann Rheum Dis 51:826, 1992

LEIGH JP, FRIES JF: Mortality predictors among 263 patients with rheumatoid arthritis. J Rheumatol 18:1307, 1991

NEPOM GT et al: The molecular basis for HLA class II associations with rheumatoid arthritis. J Clin Immunol 7:1, 1987

OCHI T et al: Effect of early synovectomy on the course of rheumatoid arthritis. J Rheumatol 18:1794, 1991

TUGWELL P et al: Low-dose cyclosporine versus placebo in patients with rheumatoid arthritis. Lancet 335:1051, 1990

VAN DER HEIJDE DMFM et al: Biannual radiographic assessments of hands and feet in a three-year prospective followup of patients with early rheumatoid arthritis. Arthritis Rheum 35:26, 1992

WEINBLATT ME et al: Long-term prospective study of methotrexate in the treatment of rheumatoid arthritis: 84-month update. Arthritis Rheum 35:129, 1992

WOLFE F, CATHEY MA: The assessment and prediction of functional disability in rheumatoid arthritis. J Rheumatol 18:1298, 1991

WORDSWORTH P, BELL J: Polygenic susceptibility in rheumatoid arthritis. Ann Rheum Dis 50:343, 1991

286 SYSTEMIC SCLEROSIS (SCLERODERMA)

BRUCE C. GILLILAND

DEFINITION Systemic sclerosis (SSc) is a multisystem disorder of unknown cause characterized by fibrosis of the skin, blood vessels, and visceral organs, including the gastrointestinal tract, lungs, heart, and kidneys. The degree and rate of skin and internal organ involvement vary among patients. Two subsets, however, can be identified, even though there is some overlap. One subset is referred to as *diffuse cutaneous scleroderma* and is characterized by the rapid development of symmetric skin thickening of proximal and distal extremity, face, and trunk. These patients are at greater risk for developing kidney and other visceral disease early in their course. The other subset is *limited cutaneous scleroderma*, which is defined by symmetric skin thickening limited to distal extremities and face. This subset frequently has features of CREST syndrome, an acronym standing for calcinosis, Raynaud's phenomenon, esophageal dysmotility, sclerodactyly, and telangiectasia. The prognosis in limited cutaneous scleroderma is better except for the occasional patient who, after many years, develops pulmonary arterial hypertension or biliary cirrhosis. Systemic sclerosis of visceral organs also may occur in the absence of any skin involvement, which is referred to as *systemic sclerosis without scleroderma*. Survival is determined by the severity of visceral disease, especially involving the heart, lungs, and/or kidneys.

Scleroderma also can occur in a localized form limited to the skin, subcutaneous tissue, and muscle and without systemic involvement. The two localized forms are morphea, which occurs as single or multiple plaques of skin induration, and linear scleroderma, which involves an extremity or face.

SSc also occurs in association with features of other connective tissue diseases. The term *overlap syndrome* has been used to describe such patients. *Undifferentiated connective tissue disease* has been suggested as a designation for patients who do not have diagnostic criteria for any one connective tissue disease. *Mixed connective tissue disease* is a syndrome involving features of systemic lupus erythematosus, systemic sclerosis, polymyositis, and rheumatoid arthritis and very high titers of circulating antibody to nuclear ribonucleoprotein antigen (see Chap. 287). *Eosinophilic fasciitis* and the *eosinophilia-myalgia syndrome* associated with L-tryptophan ingestion are scleroderma-like illnesses and will be discussed in this chapter.

EPIDEMIOLOGY   SSc has a worldwide distribution and affects all races. The onset of disease is usually in the third to fifth decade, and the incidence increases with age. Women are affected approximately three times as often as men, and even more often during the childbearing years. The onset of scleroderma in childhood is unusual. The annual incidence has been estimated to be 14.1 cases per million population based on a 20-year study performed in Allegheny County, Pennsylvania. The role of heredity has not been clarified. Several examples of familial SSc have been reported, and the finding of other connective tissue diseases and autoantibodies in relatives of involved patients suggests a hereditary predisposition. Some studies have shown an association of SSc with DR1, DR3, and DR5.

Several environmental factors have been associated with the development of SSc and scleroderma-like illnesses. SSc appears to be more common in coal and gold miners, especially in those with more extensive exposure, suggesting that silica dust may be a predisposing factor. Workers exposed to polyvinyl chloride may develop Raynaud's phenomenon, acroosteolysis, scleroderma-like skin lesions, and nailfold capillary abnormalities similar to those observed in SSc. These workers also may develop hepatic fibrosis and angiosarcoma. The development of scleroderma has been associated with exposure to vinyl chloride, epoxy resins, and aromatic hydrocarbons such as benzine and toluene. In 1981, in Spain, a multisystem disease resembling scleroderma occurred following the ingestion of adulterated cooking oil (rapeseed oil). Approximately 20,000 people were affected. The patients initially develop interstitial pneumonitis, eosinophilia, arthralgias, arthritis, and myositis, followed subsequently by joint contractures, skin thickening, Raynaud's phenomenon, pulmonary hypertension, sicca syndrome, and resorption of the distal fingertips. Extensive sclerosis of the dermis and subcutaneous tissue has been noted in patients receiving pentazocine, a nonnarcotic analgesic agent. Bleomycin, an anticancer agent, produces fibrotic skin nodules, linear hyperpigmentation, alopecia, gangrene of fingers, and pulmonary fibrosis affecting mainly the lower lobes. Scleroderma and other connective tissue diseases have been reported in women who have had silicone breast implants. At present, the evidence is not conclusive that women with these implants carry an increased risk for developing scleroderma or other connective tissue diseases. Localized fibrosis, however, can occur around the implant. The development of a scleroderma-like illness has been associated with the ingestion of products containing L-tryptophan and is referred to as the *eosinophilia-myalgia syndrome* (see Chap. 384).

PATHOGENESIS   The outstanding feature of SSc is overproduction and accumulation of collagen and other extracellular matrix proteins in skin and other organs. While the pathogenesis of SSC remains to be further elucidated, the disease process involves immunologic mechanisms, vascular damage, and activation of fibroblasts.

An early event in SSc that precedes fibrosis is vascular damage involving small arteries, arterioles, and capillaries in the skin, gastrointestinal tract, kidneys, heart, and lungs. Raynaud's phenomenon, the initial symptom of SSc in the majority of patients, is a clinical expression of this damage. Endothelial cell injury occurs early and is followed by thickening of the intima, narrowing of the lumen, and eventual obliteration of the vessel. As vascular damage progresses, the microvascular bed in the skin and other sites is diminished, producing a state of chronic ischemia. Vascular damage can be observed in the nailfolds by wide-field microscopy, which shows drop-out of capillaries with dilatation and tortuosity of remaining ones. In the skin, remaining capillaries may proliferate and dilate to become visible telangiectasia.

Several mechanisms for endothelial injury in SSc patients have been proposed. In the sera of some patients an endothelial cytotoxic factor has been found and identified as a serine protease present in granules of activated T cells. The sera of some patients mediate antibody-dependent cellular cytotoxicity directed against human endothelial cells. Circulating antiendothelial antibodies, present in some patients, may be yet another mechanism for cell injury. Tumor necrosis factor also can induce endothelial injury as well as stimulate fibrosis. Endothelial cell damage is reflected by elevated levels of factor VIII/von Willebrand factor in the sera of many but not all patients with SSc. The binding of von Willebrand factor to subendothelium mediates platelet activation with release of factors that alter vascular permeability, leading to edema. Activated platelets also release platelet-derived growth factor (PDGF), which is chemotactic and mitogenic for both smooth-muscle cells and fibroblasts, and transforming growth factor β (TGF-β), which stimulates fibroblast collagen synthesis. These and other cytokines stimulate intimal fibrosis and with their passage through the injured endothelium also could account for adventital and perivascular fibrosis. Endothelial damage along with a deficiency of tissue plasminogen activator factor enhances intravascular coagulation and, when extensive, can lead to microangiopathic hemolytic anemia observed in those patients at risk for developing acute renal failure.

Existing evidence indicates that cell-mediated immunity plays an important role in the development of fibrosis. Perivascular and diffuse mononuclear infiltrates consisting predominantly of T cells and monocytes are found in macroscopically normal appearing skin adjacent to areas of skin fibrosis. The T cells in these infiltrates are mostly helper T cells (CD4). Elevated levels of circulating interleukin 2 (IL-2), IL-2 receptors, and CD4 antigens are found in SSc patients, indicating activation of helper T cells. In early SSc, elevated levels of circulating IL-2 and IL-2 receptors have been shown to be associated with disease progression. The CD4+/CD8+ T cell ratio is increased in peripheral blood of SSc patients due usually to an increase number of CD4+ T cells and a decrease number of CD8+ T cells. Laminin and type IV collagen, components of the endothelial basement membrane, induce in vitro transformation of lymphocytes from SSc patients, suggesting that the target of cell-mediated immunity might be endothelium. Increased levels of circulating IL-1 and tumor necrosis factor in SSc patients indicate in vivo activation of monocytes. These two cytokines have been shown to stimulate fibroblasts. Additional support for involvement of cell-mediated immunity in the pathogenesis of SSc is the appearance of scleroderma-like lesions in patients with graft-versus-host disease (GVHD) after bone marrow transplantation and in a murine model of chronic GVHD, conditions known to be associated with activated T cells. Mast cells also may be involved in the development of fibrosis. Increased numbers of mast cells are found in the dermis in both involved and uninvolved skin. Mast cell degranulation has been noted in skin that subsequently became fibrosed. Interaction with T cells may be one mechanism for mast cell degranulation resulting in release of products that stimulate fibroblast collagen synthesis. Release of histamine from mast cells also may contribute to edema observed in early disease.

Humoral immune abnormalities are also present in patients with SSc. Antinuclear antibodies are found in approximately 95 percent of patients (see "Laboratory Findings," below), and antibodies to type IV collagen and laminin may be present. The role of these antibodies in the pathogenesis of SSc is not presently understood.

Regulatory mechanisms control fibroblast growth and synthesis of collagen, fibronectin, and glycosaminoglycans. Compared with fibroblasts from normal persons, the fibroblasts from SSc appear to have aberrant regulation of growth. When fibroblasts from affected SSc skin are removed and cultured in vitro, they continue to produce excessive quantities of collagen. The collagen is biochemically normal, and the proportion of type I to type III is the same as in normal skin. Fibroblasts from SSc patients appear to be in a state of permanent activation most likely as a result of stimulation by cytokines. These activated cells are thought to represent an expanded subpopulation of fibroblasts that inherently express increased matrix genes. Studies have revealed a subpopulation of SSc fibroblasts that produces two to three times more collagen than other cells from the same tissue. Fibroblasts expressing elevated levels of messenger RNA for types I and III collagen have been demonstrated by in situ hybridization particularly around dermal blood vessels in affected SSc skin. A small number of fibroblasts expressed increased levels of mRNA for type VI collagen. Platelet-derived growth factor receptors are expressed on SSc fibroblasts on cells not only from affected areas but also from macroscopically normal appearing skin. Fibroblasts from normal persons lack expression of these receptors. TGF-β has been shown to upregulate the expression of these receptors in SSc fibroblasts but not in normal cells and, in conjunction with PDGF, stimulates SSc fibroblast proliferation. Macrophages and fibroblasts are capable of secreting PDGF and TGF-β, and activated T cells release TGF-β.

Fibroblasts may activate T cells to release cytokines that stimulate fibrosis. Fibroblasts in SSc patients have been shown to have increased expression of an adhesion molecule which facilitates binding of T cells. This binding allows interaction between T cell antigen receptor and class II molecules and antigen on fibroblasts resulting in T cell activation and cytokine release. T cells also may be activated by their interaction with extracellular matrix molecules.

Chromosomal abnormalities have been noted in greater than 90 percent of SSc patients. These acquired abnormalities include chromatid breaks, acentric fragments, and ring chromosomes and are found in approximately 30 percent of mitotic cells. A chromosomal breakage factor has been found in the serum of SSc patients and their first-degree relatives. A recent study has shown that chromosome breaks are associated with the HLA haplotype A1, B8, and DR3. The significance of these chromosomal abnormalities is unknown.

PATHOLOGY   **Skin**   In the skin, a thin epidermis overlies compact bundles of collagen which lie parallel to the epidermis. Finger-like projections of collagen extend from the dermis into the subcutaneous tissue and bind the skin to the underlying tissue. Dermal appendages are atrophied, and rete pegs are lost. In early stages of disease, increased numbers of T cells, monocytes, plasma cells, and mast cells are found, particularly in the lower dermis of involved skin.

Gastrointestinal tract   In the lower two-thirds of the esophagus, the histologic findings consist of a thin mucosa and increased collagen in the lamina propria, submucosa, and serosa. The degree of fibrosis is less than in the skin. Atrophy of the muscularis in the esophagus and throughout the involved portions of the gastrointestinal tract is more prominent than the amount of fibrotic replacement of muscle. Ulceration of the mucosa is often present and may be due to either SSc or superimposed peptic esophagitis. Striated muscles in the upper third of the esophagus are relatively spared. Similar changes may be found throughout the gastrointestinal tract, especially in the second and third portions of the duodenum, in the jejunum, and large intestine. Atrophy of the muscularis of the large intestine may lead to the development of large-mouth diverticula. In the later stages of the disease, the involved portions of the gastrointestinal tract become dilated. Infiltration of lymphocytes and plasma cells in the lamina propria is also present.

Lung   With pulmonary involvement, diffuse interstitial fibrosis, thickening of the alveolar membrane, and peribronchial fibrosis are observed. Bronchiolar epithelial proliferation accompanies the pulmonary fibrosis. Rupture of septa produces small cysts and areas of bullous emphysema. Small pulmonary arteries and arterioles show intimal thickening, fragmentation of the elastica, and muscular hypertrophy; this may occur without interstitial pulmonary fibrosis and produce pulmonary hypertension.

Musculoskeletal system   The synovium in patients with arthritis is similar to that seen in early rheumatoid arthritis and shows edema with infiltration of lymphocytes and plasma cells. A characteristic finding is a thick layer of fibrin overlying and within the synovium. Later in the disease the synovium may become fibrotic. Fibrinous deposits appear on the surfaces of tendon sheaths and in the overlying fascia and may lead to audible creaking over moving tendons.

Histologic features of primary myopathy consist of interstitial and perivascular lymphocytic infiltrations, degeneration of muscle fibers, and interstitial fibrosis. Arterioles may be thickened, and capillaries may be decreased in number. Pathologic and electrophysiologic findings of polymyositis in proximal muscles are present in the few patients who are considered to have the overlap syndrome of SSc and polymyositis.

Heart   Cardiac involvement consists of degeneration of myocardial fibers and irregular areas of interstitial fibrosis that are most prominent around blood vessels. Fibrosis also involves the conduction system, leading to atrioventricular conduction defects and arrhythmias. The wall of smaller coronary arteries may be thickened. Fibrinous pericarditis and pericardial effusions are found in some patients.

Kidney   Renal involvement is found in over half the patients and consists of intimal hyperplasia of the interlobular arteries, fibrinoid necrosis of the afferent arterioles, including the glomerular tuft, and thickening of the glomerular basement membrane. Small cortical infarctions and glomerulosclerosis may be present. The renal pathologic change is often indistinguishable from that observed in malignant hypertension. Renal vascular lesions, however, may be present in the absence of hypertension. Immunofluorescence studies of kidney have shown IgM, complement components, and fibrinogen in the walls of affected vessels. Angiographic renal studies in patients with SSc may show constriction of the intralobular arteries, a finding that simulates the vasospasm of the digital arteries observed in Raynaud's phenomenon. Cold-induced Raynaud's phenomenon has been shown to decrease renal blood flow.

Other organs   Primary liver involvement is not common. Primary biliary cirrhosis occurs in some patients, particularly in those with the limited cutaneous form of SSc. Fibrosis of the thyroid gland may develop in the presence or absence of autoimmune thyroiditis.

Thickening of the periodontal membrane with replacement of the lamina dura is demonstrated radiographically as widening of the periodontal space and rarely causes loosening of the teeth.

CLINICAL MANIFESTATIONS   **Raynaud's phenomenon**   Systemic sclerosis usually begins insidiously; the first symptoms are frequently Raynaud's phenomenon and puffy fingers. Ninety-five percent of patients will experience Raynaud's phenomenon, which is defined as episodic vasoconstriction of small arteries and arterioles of fingers, toes, and sometimes the tip of the nose and earlobes. Episodes are brought on by cold exposure, vibration, or emotional stress. Patients experience pallor and/or cyanosis followed by rubor on rewarming. Pallor and/or cyanosis is usually associated with coldness and numbness of fingers and/or toes, and rubor with pain and tingling. Not all patients appreciate the three color phases. A history of digit pallor appears to be the most reliable symptom for the presence of Raynaud's phenomenon. Raynaud's phenomenon may precede skin changes by several months or even years in those patients who subsequently develop the limited cutaneous form of SSc. After 2 or more years of Raynaud's phenomenon, few patients who have this as their only symptom will subsequently develop SSc.

Skin features   In early disease, fingers and hands are swollen. Swelling also may involve forearms, feet, lower legs, and face. However, lower extremities are relatively spared. This edematous phase may last for a few weeks, months, or even longer. The edema may be pitting or nonpitting. The skin gradually becomes firm, thickened, and eventually tightly bound to underlying subcutaneous tissue (indurative phase). In patients with diffuse cutaneous scleroderma, skin changes will become generalized and involve the extremities, face, and trunk. Rapid progression of these changes over a 2- to 3-year period is associated with a greater risk of visceral disease, particularly of the lungs, heart, or kidneys. On the other hand, patients with limited cutaneous scleroderma will usually have a more gradual progression of skin changes which are restricted to fingers or distal extremity and face. After many years of disease, the skin may soften and return to normal thickness or become thin and atrophic.

In the extremities, the taut skin over fingers gradually limits full extension, and flexion contractures develop. Ulcers may appear on the volar pads of the fingertips and over bony prominences such as elbows, malleoli, and the extensor surface of the proximal interphalangeal joints of the hands. These ulcers may become secondarily infected. The volar pads of the fingertips develop pitting scars and lose soft tissue. In some instances, resorption of the terminal phalanges occurs. Skin over the extremities, face, and trunk may become darkly pigmented, even without exposure to the sun. Pigmentation of the skin may occur over superficial blood vessels and tendons. The skin loses hair, oil, and sweat glands and so becomes dry and coarse. Vaginal dryness occurs and may cause dyspareunia.

In some patients, particularly those with the limited cutaneous form of disease, calcific deposits develop in intracutaneous and subcutaneous tissue. The sites commonly involved are periarticular tissue, digital pads, olecranon and prepatellar bursae, and skin along the extensor surface of the forearms. The overlying skin may break down, with drainage of calcific material. Involvement of the face results in loss of skin wrinkles and facial expression, as well as microstomia, which may make eating and dental hygiene difficult. The capillary beds of nailfolds of the fingers may show enlargement of capillaries with little or no capillary loss, usually indicative of limited cutaneous scleroderma. In diffuse cutaneous scleroderma, there is disorganization of the capillary beds with dilated capillaries interspersed with areas where capillaries have disappeared. These capillary changes, which are observed by wide-angle microscopy or with an ophthalmoscope used as a magnifier, are not found in patients who have only Raynaud's phenomenon.

Musculoskeletal features   More than half the patients with SSc complain of pain, swelling, and stiffness of the fingers and knees. Symptoms of carpal tunnel syndrome may occur. A symmetric polyarthritis resembling rheumatoid arthritis may be seen. In more advanced stages of the disease, leathery crepitation can be palpated over moving joints, especially the knee. Extensive fibrotic thickening of the tendon sheaths in the wrist can produce a carpal tunnel syndrome. Muscle weakness usually is present in patients with severe skin involvement and, in most cases, is due to disuse atrophy. There is a distinctive histologic myopathy that accompanies SSc which is not associated with muscle enzyme abnormalities. A few patients develop a myositis characterized by proximal muscle weakness and muscle enzyme elevations that are identical to polymyositis (overlap syndrome). In addition to terminal phalanges, resorption of bone may involve ribs, clavicle, and angle of mandible.

Gastrointestinal features   Symptoms attributable to esophageal involvement are present in more than 50 percent of patients and include epigastric fullness, burning pain in the epigastric or retrosternal regions, and regurgitation of gastric contents. These symptoms, most noticeable when the patient is lying flat or bending over, are due to the reduced tone of the gastroesophageal sphincter and to dilatation of the distal esophagus. Peptic esophagitis frequently occurs and may lead to strictures and narrowing of the lower esophagus. However, it seldom results in bleeding. Dysphagia, particularly of solid foods, may occur independent of other esophageal symptoms and is caused by loss of esophageal motility due to neuromuscular dysfunction. Manometry or cineradiography reveals decreased amplitude or disappearance of peristaltic waves in the lower two-thirds of the esophagus.

Raynaud's phenomenon in the absence of a connective tissue disease is also associated with esophageal dysmotility. Later in the course of the illness, dilatation and atony of the lower portion of the esophagus as well as reflux are seen. With gastric involvement, barium studies show dilatation, atony, and delayed gastric emptying.

Hypomotility of the small intestine produces symptoms of bloating and abdominal pain and may suggest an intestinal obstruction or paralytic ileus (pseudoobstruction). Malabsorption syndrome with weight loss, diarrhea, and anemia is due to bacterial overgrowth in the atonic intestine or possibly to obliteration of lymphatics by fibrosis. Roentgenographic features of the second and third portions of the duodenum and of the jejunum include dilatation, loss of the usual feathery pattern, and delayed disappearance of barium. Pneumatosis intestinalis occasionally occurs and appears as radiolucent cysts or linear streaks within the wall of the small intestine. Benign pneumoperitoneum may result from the rupture of these cysts. Involvement of the large intestine may cause chronic constipation and fecal impaction with episodes of bowel obstruction. A segment of atonic bowel may act as a fulcrum for intussusception to occur. Barium studies of the large intestine may show dilatation, atony, and large-mouth diverticula. Some patients may have gastrointestinal features of SSc with little or no cutaneous or other organ involvement.

Pulmonary features   The lungs are affected in SSc in at least two-thirds of the patients. The most common symptom is exertional dyspnea, often accompanied by a dry, nonproductive cough. Symptoms may occur in the absence of pulmonary fibrosis, and patients with pulmonary fibrosis can be relatively asymptomatic. Bilateral basilar rales may be present. Restriction of chest movement caused by extensive skin involvement of the thorax rarely occurs. Aspiration pneumonia may result from gastric reflux due to lower esophageal atony. Superimposed bacterial or viral pneumonia can be a serious complication in patients with pulmonary fibrosis. There is an increased frequency of alveolar cell and bronchogenic carcinoma in patients with pulmonary fibrosis. Pulmonary function tests are frequently abnormal and show a reduction in vital capacity and decreased lung compliance. Impairment of gas exchange is reflected by a low diffusing capacity and low P_{O_2} with exercise. These abnormalities may be present even when the chest radiograph is normal. Chest film may show a pattern of linear densities, mottling, and honeycombing involving most prominently the lower two-thirds of the lung. Early pulmonary disease can be detected by high-resolution computed tomography (HRCT) and bronchoalveolar lavage (BAL). The recovery by BAL of increased number of cells, mostly alveolar macrophages accompanied by neutrophils and eosinophils, is evidence for alveolitis. Treatment of alveolitis with drugs such as cyclophosphamide conceivably may be more effective when alveolitis is detected early, although this is not proven. In the absence of significant interstitial fibrosis, a severe form of pulmonary arterial hypertension develops after many years of disease in patients with limited cutaneous scleroderma. Less than 10 percent of patients will develop this complication, which is caused by narrowing and obliteration of pulmonary arteries and arterioles by intimal fibrosis and medial hypertrophy. Pulmonary hypertension is manifested by progressive worsening of dyspnea and eventually by the appearance of right-sided heart failure. Electrocardiographic evidence of pulmonary hypertension is usually present. The prognosis is extremely poor with the development of pulmonary hypertension; the mean duration of survival is approximately 2 years.

Cardiac features   Primary cardiac involvement in SSc includes pericarditis with or without effusions, heart failure, and varying degrees of heart block or arrhythmias. The majority of patients with diffuse cutaneous SSc have cardiac abnormalities. Cardiomyopathy attributable to myocardial fibrosis appears in fewer than 10 percent of patients and involves primarily those patients with diffuse cutaneous scleroderma. Radionuclide studies have shown abnormalities of left ventricular function due to myocardial fibrosis. Cold-induced vasospasm of the hands produces defects in myocardial thallium perfusion. The characteristic pathologic feature of contraction band necrosis results from cardiac muscle damage caused by intermittent vasospasm of coronary vessels. Patients may experience angina pectoris even though coronary angiograms are normal. Patients also can develop left ventricular failure secondary to systemic hypertension or cor pulmonale secondary to pulmonary arterial hypertension.

Renal features Renal failure is the leading cause of death in SSc, accounting for almost half the deaths. Significant renal disease occurs mostly in those patients with diffuse cutaneous scleroderma. A high risk of renal crisis is present in those patients who have rapidly progressive widespread skin thickening in their first 2 to 3 years of disease. Renal crisis is characterized by malignant hypertension, which can rapidly progress to renal failure. These patients manifest hypertensive encephalopathy, severe headache, retinopathy, seizures, and left ventricular failure. Hematuria and proteinuria are followed by oliguria and renal failure. The mechanism for the hypertensive crisis is activation of the renin-angiotensin system. Before the advent of effective antihypertensive drugs, the majority of these patients died within 6 months. A small number of patients may develop renal crises in the absence of hypertension. Renal failure also can develop insidiously later in the course of disease in the setting of mild to moderate hypertension and proteinuria. In these patients or those with clinically unrecognized renal disease, reduction of renal plasma flow secondary to heart failure or volume depletion resulting from overdiuresis may precipitate renal crisis. An indicator of impending renal failure is microangiopathic anemia, which may occur in a normotensive patient. The presence of a chronic pericardial effusion may also herald subsequent renal failure.

Other features Symptoms of dry eyes and/or dry mouth are frequently present in patients with SSc. Lip biopsy may show lymphocytic infiltration of minor salivary glands characteristic of Sjögren's syndrome or intraglandular or periglandular fibrosis. Antibodies to SS-A (Ro) and/or SS-B (La) are found in those patients with lip biopsies consistent with Sjögren's syndrome and not in those with salivary gland fibrosis.

Hypothyroidism occurs in a significant number of patients and may be associated with high levels of antithyroid antibodies. Fibrosis of the thyroid gland may be present but also occurs in the absence of autoimmune thyroiditis. Other manifestations of SSc include trigeminal neuralgia and male impotence secondary to decreased penile tumescence. These men have normal serum levels of testosterone and gonadotropins. Pathogenesis of this abnormality has been considered to be vascular and/or autonomic nervous system abnormalities.

LABORATORY FINDINGS The erythrocyte sedimentation rate may be elevated. Hypoproliferative anemia related to chronic inflammation is the most common cause of anemia in SSc. Anemia also may be caused by iron deficiency secondary to gastrointestinal bleeding. Bacterial overgrowth due to atony of the small bowel may lead to vitamin B_{12} and/or folic acid–deficiency anemia. Microangiopathic hemolytic anemia is most often associated with renal involvement and is caused by the presence of intravascular fibrin in renal arterioles. Hypergammaglobulinemia, consisting mostly of IgG, is found in approximately half the patients. Rheumatoid factor, in low titer, is present in 25 percent of patients. Antinuclear antibodies detected by using a cultured human laryngeal carcinoma cell line (HEp-2) substrate are present in 95 percent of patients. Antinuclear antibodies that have a high specificity for SSc are antitopoisomerase 1 (Scl-70), antinucleolar, and anticentromere. Antitopoisomerase 1, originally called anti-Scl-70, recognizes the nuclear enzyme DNA topoisomerase 1. These antibodies are found in about 20 percent of patients and are associated with diffuse cutaneous involvement and interstitial pulmonary disease. They are seldom present in other disorders or in conjunction with anticentromere antibodies. Antinucleolar antibodies are relatively specific for SSc and are present in approximately 20 to 30 percent of patients. Anticentromere antibodies react with protein antigens located in the kinetochore region of chromosomes and are strongly associated with limited cutaneous scleroderma or CREST syndrome. Anticentromere antibodies are found in only about 10 percent of patients with diffuse cutaneous

scleroderma and rarely in other connective tissue diseases. They are found occasionally in patients with only Raynaud's phenomenon and may indicate subsequent development of limited cutaneous disease. Several antinucleolar antibodies have been associated with SSc: Anti-RNA polymerase 1 is found in patients with diffuse cutaneous SSc who have a higher prevalence of renal and cardiac involvement, anti-Th has been found in patients with limited cutaneous SSc, and anti-PM-Scl, formerly referred to as anti-PM1, may be found in SSc patients with polymyositis and renal involvement. *Anti-U3 nucleolar RNP is also highly specific for SSc, is more frequent in African Americans, and is associated with skeletal muscle disease and pulmonary arterial hypertension.* High titers of anti-RNP are present in those patients with features of mixed connective tissue disease. Anti-SS-A and/or anti-SS-B are present in those patients with overlap syndrome of SSc and Sjögren's syndrome.

DIAGNOSIS The diagnosis of SSc presents no difficulty in the presence of Raynaud's phenomenon, with typical skin lesions and visceral involvement. Although Raynaud's phenomenon may be the first symptom of SSc, most patients with Raynaud's phenomenon alone do not develop a connective tissue disease. Other causes of Raynaud's phenomenon include thoracic outlet (scalenus anticus and cervical rib) syndromes, shoulder-hand syndrome, trauma (jackhammer or vibratory machine operators), previous cold injury, vinyl chloride exposure, and circulating cryoglobulins or cold agglutinins. Linear scleroderma and morphea are localized forms of scleroderma that can usually be distinguished clinically. In early disease, SSc may initially be confused with rheumatoid arthritis, systemic lupus erythematosus, or polymyositis when articular or muscle involvement is prominent. SSc without cutaneous involvement should be considered in patients with unexplained pulmonary fibrosis, pulmonary hypertension, cardiomyopathies, heart block, dysphagia, or malabsorption syndrome. Several conditions have scleroderma-like features but lack the visceral involvement. Scleredema (scleredema adultorum of Buschke) occurs predominantly in children and is characterized by painless edematous induration involving the face, scalp, neck, trunk, and proximal portions of the extremities. Involvement of the hands and feet usually does not occur. Scleredema may be associated with previous streptococcal infection and is usually self-limited, resolving in 6 to 12 months. Histology reveals accumulation of mucopolysaccharides in the dermis and skeletal muscle. A rare entity, scleromyxedema (lichen myxedematosus), is manifested by yellowish or pale red papules in association with diffuse skin thickening which may involve the face and hands. Acid mucopolysaccharide deposits are found in the dermis. Monoclonal IgG may be detected in some of these patients. Primary amyloidosis may involve the skin of the extremities and face diffusely to give the appearance of scleroderma. Biopsy will clearly differentiate these entities.

COURSE AND PROGNOSIS The course of SSc is quite variable. Until disease differentiates into recognizable subsets, prognosis in early disease is difficult to predict. Patients with limited cutaneous scleroderma, especially those with anticentromere antibodies, have a good prognosis, with the notable exception of those few patients, less than 10 percent, who after 10 to 20 years or longer develop pulmonary arterial hypertension. Malabsorption syndrome and primary biliary cirrhosis are the causes of morbidity and mortality in some patients with limited cutaneous disease. On the other hand, the prognosis is generally worse in patients with diffuse cutaneous disease, particularly when the onset occurs at an older age. In addition, males have a worse prognosis. Renal and other visceral organ disease may develop early in the course of those patients with rapidly progressive generalized skin thickening. Death occurs most often from cardiac, renal, or pulmonary involvement. In one study the 10-year cumulative survival of patients with only renal involvement was 30 percent, and of patients with only lung involvement, 50 percent. In patients without heart, lung, or kidney involvement, survival was 71 percent.

Skin may spontaneously soften after years of disease. Softening occurs in the reverse order of original skin involvement, beginning with the trunk and followed by the proximal and then the distal extremities. Sclerodactyly may persist. Skin thickness may eventually approach normal.

TREATMENT Even though SSc cannot be cured, treatment of involved organ systems can relieve symptoms and improve function. The doctor-patient relationship is extremely important in caring for patients with this chronic debilitating illness. Once the diagnosis of SSc has been made, the patient and family should be instructed about this disorder. The patient will need repeated explanations and reassurances throughout his or her illness. Depending on the severity of illness, the patient will require monitoring of blood pressure, blood counts, urinalysis, and renal and pulmonary function on a regular basis.

Effectiveness of drug therapy in SSc is difficult to evaluate because of the variable course and severity of the disease. Many drugs have been used in the treatment of SSc without any consistent or prolonged benefit. In uncontrolled studies D-penicillamine has been reported to reduce skin thickening and prevent development of significant organ involvement. This drug interferes with inter- and intramolecular cross-linking of collagen and is also immunosuppressive. Its immunosuppressive activity also may lead to decreased collagen production. Penicillamine is better tolerated when started at a low dose, usually 250 mg/d, and then increased at 1- to 3-month intervals up to 1.5 g/d as tolerated. Although a few patients can tolerate higher doses, most patients are maintained on a dose between 0.5 and 1 g/d. For optimal absorption, it is important to give this drug 1 h before or 2 h after a meal. This drug can be quite toxic; its more serious complications include glomerulonephritis with nephrotic syndrome, aplastic anemia, leukopenia, thrombocytopenia, and myasthenia gravis. Other side effects are fever, rash, anorexia, nausea, and loss of taste. Patients should have monthly complete blood counts (including platelet count) and urinalyses. Azathioprine and other immunosuppressives also have been used in SSc and should be reserved for those patients with rapidly progressive and life-threatening disease. Control studies are lacking. Trials of treatment with recombinant interferon γ, 5-fluorouracil, and *extracorporeal photochemotherapy* have shown improvement in some disease parameters. No therapy, however, has been clearly demonstrated in a controlled, prospective study to suppress or reverse the disease process of SSc.

Antiplatelet therapy may play a role in the treatment of SSc, since the biologic products of platelets affect blood vessels. Low doses of aspirin block the formation of thromboxane A_2, a powerful vasoconstrictor and platelet aggregator. In addition, dipyridamole, 200 to 400 mg in divided daily doses, also decreases platelet adhesion to damaged vessel walls. While these drugs have a reasonable therapeutic rationale, a 2-year double-blind study did not show any benefit from their use. Reports of beneficial effects of colchicine or chlorambucil have not been documented in controlled studies.

Glucocorticoids are indicated in those patients with inflammatory myositis or pericarditis. The initial dose is 40 to 60 mg/d and is tapered based on clinical improvement. Prednisone 10 mg/d or less may be beneficial in treating arthritis refractory to nonsteroidal anti-inflammatory drugs and in reducing edema associated with the edematous phase of early skin involvement. Glucocorticoids are not otherwise indicated in the long-term treatment of SSc. High doses of glucocorticoids may play a role in precipitating acute renal failure. However, this association remains unclear.

The management of Raynaud's phenomenon is directed at control of vasospasm. Patients should be advised to dress warmly and wear mittens and socks, not to smoke, to remove causes of external stress, and to avoid drugs such as amphetamine and ergotamine. Beta blocking drugs may make Raynaud's phenomenon worse. Warmth of the central body induces peripheral vasodilatation. Drugs that block sympathetic vasoconstriction, such as reserpine, α-methyldopa, phenoxybenzamine, and prazosin, may be useful in the treatment of Raynaud's phenomenon, but their side effects often curtail extended use. The calcium channel blockers nifedipine and diltiazem can be effective in alleviating Raynaud's phenomenon, but side effects of light-headedness and palpitations may limit their use. The dose of nifedipine is 10 to 20 mg tid. Ketanserin, an oral serotonin antagonist, also has been shown to be effective. Studies with iloprost, a prostacyclin analogue, have shown a decrease in frequency and severity of Raynaud's phenomenon and healing of digital ulcers in some patients. Techniques of biofeedback also have been used with variable success for teaching patients to control the temperature of their hands. Surgical sympathectomy usually provides only temporary improvement, and it, along with other forms of therapy, does not prevent progression of the vascular lesion. The response to any therapy for Raynaud's phenomenon is limited by the degree of existing structural narrowing of digital arteries. Gangrene of distal digits may occur and require surgical amputation.

Numerous drugs have been claimed to soften the hidebound skin, but documentation in controlled studies is lacking. These drugs include D-penicillamine, colchicine, *p*-aminobenzoic acid, and vitamin E. Dryness of the skin may be reduced by avoiding frequent use of detergent soaps and by regularly applying hydrophilic ointments and bath oils. Regular exercise helps to maintain flexibility of extremities and pliability of skin. Massaging the skin several times a day also may be beneficial. Fingertip ulcerations can be protected by applying a guard or cage over the end of the finger. The use of an occlusive dressing over a noninfected ulcer may promote healing and protect the finger. Skin ulcers should be kept clean by soaking or by surgical or chemical debridement. Sympatholytic drugs or local nitroglycerine paste applied to the ulcer may be beneficial in promoting healing. Infected ulcers can usually be treated with topical antibiotics but may require systemic antibiotics, especially when there is a question of underlying osteomyelitis.

Patients with reflux esophagitis are treated with small, frequent meals, antacids between meals, and elevation of the head of the bed. Patients should be advised not to lie down for a few hours after a meal and to avoid coffee, tea, and chocolate, which reduce the pressure of the lower esophageal sphincter. Cimetidine or ranitidine may be beneficial. Omeprazole has been effective in treating erosive esophagitis in some patients. Metoclopramide, which increases esophageal motility and increases lower esophageal sphincter tone, also can be of help in some patients. Patients with dysphagia should be instructed to chew their food thoroughly and wash it down with fluids. Malabsorption syndrome due to duodenal hypomotility and bacterial overgrowth may improve with intermittent use of appropriate antibiotics. Patients with severe debilitating malabsorption may benefit from parenteral hyperalimentation. Stool softeners and mild laxatives are usually adequate for treating constipation caused by hypomotility of the colon.

Acute myositis is usually responsive to glucocorticoids; these drugs should not be used for the indolent primary form of muscle disease of SSc. Articular symptoms are treated with aspirin or other nonsteroidal anti-inflammatory agents.

Pulmonary fibrosis is not reversible, and therefore treatment is directed at symptoms or complications. Pulmonary infection requires prompt treatment with antibiotics. Hypoxia necessitates giving low concentrations of oxygen. The role of glucocorticoids in preventing progression of interstitial lung disease is not clear. Patients should receive Pneumovax and yearly influenza immunizations.

Recognition of early renal failure is important in order to preserve remaining function. Renal involvement is often accompanied by hypertension and mild to moderate proteinuria. An occasional patient may be normotensive. Antihypertensive agents are often effective in lowering blood pressure and stabilizing or reversing renal failure. These drugs include propranolol, clonidine, and minoxidil. Particularly effective are the angiotensin-converting enzyme inhibitors, which include captopril, enalapril, and lisinopril. Dialysis may be required in patients with progressive renal failure. Some patients, however, have a slow return of renal function after several months and may no longer require dialysis.

Patients with cardiac failure require careful monitoring of digitalis and diuretic administration. Pericardial effusions also may improve with diuretics. Care should be taken to avoid overdiuresis, which may lead to decreased renal blood flow, decreased cardiac output, and renal failure.

EOSINOPHILIC FASCIITIS Eosinophilic fasciitis is a scleroderma-like syndrome of unknown cause characterized by inflammation followed later by sclerosis of the dermis, subcutis, and deep fascia. The disease affects adults and often occurs after strenuous physical activity. Patients do not have Raynaud's phenomenon or internal organ involvement. Several immunologic abnormalities have been associated with eosinophilic fasciitis and include aplastic anemia, myelodysplastic syndrome, and thrombocytopenia. Patients usually have the abrupt onset of symmetric tenderness and swelling of the extremities which is rapidly followed by induration of the skin and subcutaneous tissue. The skin takes on a cobblestone or puckered appearance. Carpal tunnel syndrome appears early in the course, and flexion contractures develop later. A low-grade myositis is often present, but creatinine kinase levels are usually normal. A marked eosinophilia is found in the early stage of disease and subsequently decreases. Increased levels of polyclonal IgG and immune complexes are often present in the serum. A full-thickness biopsy consisting of skin, fascia, and superficial muscle shows perivascular infiltration of histiocytes, eosinophils, lymphocytes, and plasma cells. Biopsies later in the course show sclerosis. Spontaneous improvement and occasionally complete remission may occur after 2 to 5 years of disease. Some patients have persistent disease, while others are left with flexion contractures. Administration of glucocorticoids may provide symptomatic improvement and will decrease the eosinophilia. Improvement has been reported with the use of the H-2 blocker cimetidine.

EOSINOPHILIA-MYALGIA SYNDROME In 1989, reports of patients with scleroderma-like skin changes, myalgias, and eosinophilia dramatically increased. Most, but not all, of these cases were associated with ingestion of L-tryptophan manufactured by a single Japanese company. Batches of L-tryptophan implicated in eosinophilia-myalgia syndrome (EMS) were found to contain trace amounts of a contaminant identified as a dimer of L-tryptophan which appeared in 1988 after changes were made in the method of manufacturing this drug. It is not clear whether this chemical contaminant is the etiologic agent or another unidentified substance is responsible. *L-Tryptophan products were taken off the market in 1990.* The onset of EMS can be either abrupt or insidious. In the early phases of the disease, clinical manifestations include low-grade fever, fatigue, dyspnea, cough, arthralgias/arthritis, evanescent erythematous rashes, muscle cramping, and severe myalgias. Pulmonary infiltrates may be present. Over the next 2 to 3 months, scleroderma-like skin changes appear. Some patients develop a peripheral neuropathy which may persist. An ascending polyneuropathy may lead to paralysis and respiratory failure requiring ventilatory assistance. Cognitive dysfunction with impairment of memory and concentration has been recognized in this syndrome. Myocarditis and cardiac arrhythmias occur in some patients, and a few patients develop pulmonary hypertension. Approximately a third of patients have features of eosinophilic fasciitis. EMS most closely resembles toxic oil syndrome; however, Raynaud's phenomenon does not occur, and there is a lower prevalence of pulmonary hypertension and thromboembolic disease. The peripheral eosinophil count is greater than 1000 cells per cubic millimeter in most patients. The histologic findings on biopsy of skin, fascia, and superficial muscle are similar to that found in eosinophilic fasciitis. The clinical features of EMS may persist after L-tryptophan has been discontinued. EMS may run a chronic course, and response to therapy has been variable. Treatment has included glucocorticoids, antimalarial drugs, immunosuppressive drugs, and plasmapheresis. The pathogenesis and natural course of this disease are not yet known (see also Chap. 384).

REFERENCES

ABRAHAM D et al: Expression and function of surface antigens on scleroderma fibroblasts. Arthritis Rheum 34:1164, 1991

ALTMAN RD et al: Predictors of survival in systemic sclerosis (scleroderma). Arthritis Rheum 34:403, 1991

CARPENTIER PH, MARICQ HR: Microvasculature in systemic sclerosis. Rheum Dis Clin North Am 16:75, 1990

DEGIANNIS D et al: Soluble interleukin-2 receptors in patients with systemic sclerosis: Clinical and laboratory correlations. Arthritis Rheum 33:375, 1990

KAHALEH MB: Soluble immunologic products in scleroderma sera. Clin Immunol Immunopathol 58:139, 1991

——: Vascular disease in scleroderma: Endothelial T lymphocyte-fibroblast interactions. Rheum Dis Clin North Am 16:53, 1990

KAUFMAN LD: The eosinophilia-myalgia syndrome: Current concepts and future directions. Clin Exp Rheumatol 10:87, 1992

LAKHANPAL S et al: Eosinophilic fasciitis: Clinical spectrum and therapeutic response in 52 cases. Semin Arthritis Rheum 17:221, 1988

LEROY EC et al: Scleroderma (systemic sclerosis): Classification, subsets and pathogenesis. J Rheumatol 15:202, 1988

MEDSGER TA J: Systemic Sclerosis (Scleroderma), Localized forms of Scleroderma, and Calcinosis, in *Arthritis and Allied Conditions*, 12th ed, DJ McCarty (ed). Philadelphia, Lea & Febiger, 1993, p 1253

NEEDLEMAN BW et al: In vitro identification of subpopulation of fibroblasts that produces high levels of collagen in scleroderma patients. Arthritis Rheum 33:842, 1990

SEIBOLD J: Scleroderma, in *Textbook of Rheumatology*, 4th ed, WN Kelly et al (eds). Philadelphia, Saunders, Chap. 66, 1993

—— et al: Dermal mast cell degranulation in systemic sclerosis. Arthritis Rheum 33:1702, 1990

STEEN VD et al: Outcome of renal crisis in systemic sclerosis: Relation to availability of angiotensin converting enzyme (ACE) inhibitors. Ann Intern Med 113:352, 1990

YAMAKAGE A et al: Selective upregulation of platelet-derived growth factor α receptors by transforming growth factor β in scleroderma fibroblasts. J Exp Med 175:1227, 1992

287 MIXED CONNECTIVE TISSUE DISEASE

GORDON C. SHARP

DEFINITION Mixed connective tissue disease (MCTD) is an overlap syndrome characterized by a combination of clinical features similar to those of systemic lupus erythematosus (SLE) (see Chap. 284), scleroderma (see Chap. 286), polymyositis (see Chap. 384), and rheumatoid arthritis (see Chap. 285) and unusually high titers of circulating antibody to a nuclear ribonucleoprotein (RNP) antigen.

ETIOLOGY, PATHOGENESIS, AND PATHOLOGY The etiologic and pathogenic mechanisms of MCTD remain unknown, but characteristic immune findings include (1) immunoregulatory abnormalities with persistence of extremely high titers of antibody to nuclear RNP and a marked polyclonal hypergammaglobulinemia indicative of B cell hyperactivity, (2) circulating immune complexes during active disease but with normal clearance by the reticuloendothelial system in most patients, in contrast to SLE, (3) deposition of IgG, IgM, and complement within vascular walls and along sarcolemmal and glomerular basement membranes, and (4) widespread lymphocytic and plasma cell infiltration of numerous tissues. One of the chief underlying pathologic findings in some patients with MCTD is a vascular lesion with intimal proliferation and medial hypertrophy, resulting in narrowing of the lumen of large vessels (e.g., pulmonary, renal, and coronary arteries) and of small arterioles of many organs. Such lesions in the lungs in the absence of significant pulmonary fibrosis, in contrast to scleroderma, may contribute to pulmonary hypertension and abnormalities of pulmonary function.

CLINICAL MANIFESTATIONS The age range in published reports of MCTD is from 4 to 80 years, with a mean of 37 years. Approximately 80 percent of patients have been female. Typical clinical features include Raynaud phenomenon, polyarthritis, swollen hands or sclerodactyly, esophageal dysfunction, pulmonary involvement, and inflammatory myopathy. Malar rash, alopecia, lymphadenopathy, and cardiac and renal disease are less frequent.

Cutaneous features of MCTD include a swollen, sausage-like appearance of the fingers, nonscarring alopecia, lupus-like rashes, heliotrope eyelids, erythematous patches over the knuckles, periungual telangiectasia, and "squared" telangiectasia over the hands and face. Scleroderma-like changes may be present but rarely become extensive.

Musculoskeletal abnormalities occur in most patients. Arthritis is usually nondeforming but may resemble rheumatoid arthritis. Proximal muscle weakness is frequent and may be severe. Serum levels of creatine kinase and aldolase are often markedly elevated, electromyograms are typical of inflammatory myopathy, and biopsies show degeneration of muscle fibers and interstitial and perivascular infiltrates of lymphocytes and plasma cells.

Esophageal dysfunction has been demonstrated in 80 percent, including 70 percent who are asymptomatic. Abnormalities include reduced upper and lower esophageal sphincter pressures and decreased amplitude of peristalsis in the distal two-thirds of the esophagus.

Pulmonary involvement occurred in 85 percent of one series of MCTD patients and often was clinically silent until far advanced. Clinical findings include exertional dyspnea, pleuritic pain, and bibasilar rales. Reduced diffusing capacity for carbon monoxide is the most frequent functional abnormality. Pulmonary hypertension is the most frequent serious complication in MCTD.

Cardiac disease is less common than pulmonary involvement in adults but may be more frequent in children. Pericarditis is the most common finding; other findings have included mitral valve prolapse, myocarditis, congestive heart failure, and aortic insufficiency.

Renal disease in children and adults with MCTD has a combined prevalence of about 28 percent. Progressive renal failure is unusual; clinical and histologic findings suggest that vascular lesions may represent a more serious problem than immune-complex nephritis in MCTD.

Less frequent clinical manifestations include fever, lymphadenopathy, neurologic abnormalities, Sjögren's syndrome (see Chap. 288), hepatosplenomegaly, and intestinal involvement similar to that seen in scleroderma.

LABORATORY FINDINGS Almost all patients have positive fluorescent antinuclear antibody tests at high titers with a speckled pattern and very high titers of antibodies directed against the ribonuclease-sensitive nuclear RNP component of extractable nuclear antigen (ENA). Elevated anti–native DNA antibody titers and antibodies to the ribonuclease-resistant Sm component of ENA are uncommon in MCTD; their presence is usually associated with a severe flare-up of lupus-like features. High titers of circulating RNP antibodies usually persist for years, but antibody levels may decline significantly or become undetectable in patients in prolonged remission.

Recent studies have further elucidated the nature of the RNP and Sm antigens. Antibodies to RNP immunoprecipitate U1 snRNA-protein complexes and react with proteins designated 70K, A, and C, whereas Sm antibodies immunoprecipitate complexes containing U1, U2, U4, U5, and U6 snRNAs and react with proteins designated B/B' and D. Furthermore, these antigenic complexes have been shown to have important biologic roles in the processing of messenger RNA. Several reports indicate that antibodies to the 70K protein are associated with anti-U1 RNP antibodies in MCTD but rarely occur in SLE. Immunogenetic studies have revealed that U1 70K-positive MCTD patients have disease associated with the presence of either HLA-DR4 or HLA-DR2 but not with HLA-DR3, as is found in patients with SLE. A sequence of shared amino acids or a "shared epitope" within HLA-DR, which is common to both HLA-DR4 and HLA-DR2, may be the basis for this association.

Rheumatoid factor is found, often at very high titers, in half the patients. Less frequent findings include hypocomplementemia, leukopenia, anemia, and thrombocytopenia (mainly in children).

DIAGNOSIS The diagnosis of MCTD is based on a combination of typical overlapping clinical findings and high titers of circulating antibody to nuclear U1 RNP. In some, all the clinical manifestations may be present on initial evaluation. However, MCTD is now being recognized in an earlier phase in patients with minimal symptoms (e.g., Raynaud phenomenon, arthralgias, myalgias, and swollen hands). In some this mild "undifferentiated connective tissue disease"

syndrome may persist for years, but a prospective, long-term study showed that the majority of patients with high titers of U1 RNP antibodies and limited clinical manifestations ultimately developed signs and symptoms consistent with a diagnosis of MCTD.

TREATMENT AND PROGNOSIS Lacking controlled studies, specific treatment recommendations for MCTD are based on anecdotal information. Salicylates, other nonsteroidal anti-inflammatory agents, hydroxychloroquine, vasodilators, and/or low doses of glucocorticoids are used to treat mild disease. If the disease is more severe and significantly involves major organ systems, higher doses of glucocorticoids (e.g., 1 mg/kg per day of prednisone) are usually required. As with SLE, a cytotoxic agent may be added in steroid-resistant or -dependent cases. However, the efficacy of this latter therapeutic regimen has not been substantiated by controlled clinical trials. The prognosis for MCTD is generally similar to that of SLE and somewhat better than for scleroderma.

REFERENCES

KANEOKA H et al: Molecular genetic analysis of HLA-DR and HLA-DQ genes among anti-U1-70kD autoantibody-positive connective tissue disease patients. Arthritis Rheum 35:83, 1992

PETTERSSON I ET AL: The use of immunoblotting and immunoprecipitation of (U) small nuclear ribonucleoproteins in the analysis of sera of patients with mixed connective tissue disease and systemic lupus erythematosus. Arthritis Rheum 29:986, 1986

SHARP GC, SINGSEN BH: Mixed connective tissue disease, in *Arthritis and Allied Conditions*, 12th ed, DJ McCarty, W Koopman (eds). Philadelphia, Lea & Febiger, 1992, p 1213

TAKEDA Y ET AL: Enzyme-linked immunosorbent assay using isolated (U) small nuclear ribonucleoprotein polypeptides as antigens to investigate the clinical significance of autoantibodies to these polypeptides. Clin Immunol Immunopathol 50:213, 1989

288 SJÖGREN'S SYNDROME

HARALAMPOS M. MOUTSOPOULOS

DEFINITION Sjögren's syndrome is a chronic, slowly progressive autoimmune disease characterized by lymphocytic infiltration of the exocrine glands resulting in xerostomia and dry eyes. Approximately one-third of patients present with extraglandular (systemic) manifestations. A small but significant number of the patients may develop malignant lymphoma. The disease can be seen alone (primary Sjögren's syndrome) or in association with other autoimmune rheumatic diseases such as rheumatoid arthritis, systemic lupus erythematosus, or scleroderma (secondary Sjögren's syndrome).

INCIDENCE AND PREVALENCE The disease affects predominantly middle-aged women (female-to-male ratio 9:1), although it can be seen in all ages, including childhood. The incidence of the disease is still unknown, but it is considered to be very common since, in addition to the primary syndrome, 30 percent of patients with rheumatoid arthritis, systemic lupus erythematosus, and scleroderma suffer from secondary Sjögren's syndrome.

PATHOGENESIS The two main autoimmune phenomena observed in Sjögren's syndrome are lymphocytic infiltration of the exocrine glands and B lymphocyte hyperreactivity, as illustrated by circulating autoantibodies. The latter is accompanied by an oligo-monoclonal B cell process, which is characterized by serum and urine monoclonal light chains and cryoprecipitable monoclonal immunoglobulins.

Sera of patients with Sjögren's syndrome often contain a number of autoantibodies directed against non-organ-specific antigens such as immunoglobulins (rheumatoid factors) and extractable nuclear and cytoplasmic antigens (Ro/SSA, La/SSB) (Table 288-1). Molecular characterization and cloning have shown that Ro/SSA autoantigen consists of three polypeptide chains (52,000, 54,000, and 60,000 Da) in conjunction with HY_1, HY_3, HY_4, and HY_5 RNAs, whereas La/SSB protein of 48,000 Da is bound to RNA III polymerase transcripts. Autoantibodies to organ-specific antigens such as salivary duct cells, thyroid gland cells, and gastric mucosa also have been described. The presence of autoantibodies to Ro/SSA and La/SSB antigens in Sjögren's syndrome is associated with earlier disease onset, longer disease duration, salivary gland enlargement, severity of lymphocytic infiltration of minor salivary glands, and certain extraglandular manifestations such as lymphadenopathy, purpura, and vasculitis.

Phenotypic and functional studies have shown that the predominant cell infiltrating the affected exocrine glands is the helper/inducer T cell with characteristics of memory cells. Both B and T infiltrating lymphocytes are activated, as illustrated by production of immunoglobulins with autoantibody activity, spontaneous release of interleukin 2, as well as expression on the T cell surface of activation markers such as class II HLA molecules and LFA-1. Macrophages and NK cells are rarely detected in infiltrates, while epithelial cells of the affected glands inappropriately express class II molecules and possess messages for c-*myc* protooncogene and tranforming growth factor beta. All these phenomena suggest that the epithelial cell of the exocrine glands in Sjögren's syndrome may act as an antigen presenting cell, and recent studies indicate that a retrovirus may be the initiator of the autoimmune process.

Immunogenetic studies have demonstrated that HLA-B8, -DR3, and -DRw52 are prevalent in primary Sjögren's syndrome patients as compared with the normal control population. Further analysis of HLA class II genes by molecular techniques revealed that Sjögren's syndrome patients with anti-Ro/SSA and/or anti-La/SSB antibodies possess DQA_1/DQB_1 chains containing specific amino acid residues in their second hypervariable region.

CLINICAL MANIFESTATIONS The majority of the patients with Sjögren's syndrome have symptoms related to diminished lacrimal and salivary gland function. In most patients, the primary syndrome runs a slow and benign course. The initial manifestations can be nonspecific (such as arthralgias, fatigue, Raynaud's phenomenon), and usually 8 to 10 years elapse from the initial symptoms to full-blown development of the disease.

The principal oral symptom of Sjögren's syndrome is dryness (xerostomia). This is described as difficulty in swallowing dry food, inability to speak continuously, a burning sensation, increase in dental caries, and problems in wearing complete dentures. Physical examination shows a dry, erythematous, sticky oral mucosa. There is atrophy of the filiform papillae on the dorsum of the tongue, and saliva from the major glands is either not expressible or is cloudy. Enlargement of the parotid or other major salivary glands occurs in two-thirds of patients with primary Sjögren's syndrome but is uncommon in those with the secondary syndrome. Diagnostic tests include sialometry, sialography, and scintigraphy. All these techniques exhibit high sensitivity but not well established disease specificity. In contrast, the labial minor salivary gland biopsy exhibits higher specificity, permitting histopathologic confirmation of the focal lymphocytic infiltrates.

Ocular involvement is the other major manifestation of Sjögren's syndrome. Patients usually complain of dry eyes, with a sandy or gritty feeling under the eyelids. Other symptoms include burning,

accumulation of thick strands at the inner canthi, decreased tearing, redness, itching, eye fatigue, and increased photosensitivity. These symptoms are attributed to the destruction of corneal and bulbar conjunctival epithelium defined as keratoconjunctivitis sicca. Diagnostic evaluation of keratoconjunctivitis sicca includes measurement of tear flow by Schirmer's I test and tear composition as assessed by the tear breakup time or tear lysozyme content. The most specific diagnostic procedure, however, is slit-lamp examination of the cornea and conjunctiva after rose Bengal staining. This test reveals punctate corneal ulcerations and attached filaments of corneal epithelium.

Involvement of other exocrine glands occurs less frequently and includes a decrease in mucous gland secretions of the upper and lower respiratory tree resulting in dry nose, throat, and trachea (xerotrachea) and diminished secretion of the exocrine glands of the gastrointestinal tract leading to esophageal mucosal atrophy, atrophic gastritis, and subclinical pancreatitis. Dyspareunia due to dryness of the external genitalia and dry skin also may occur.

Extraglandular (systemic) manifestations are seen in one-third of patients with Sjögren's syndrome (Table 288-2), while they are very rare in patients with Sjögren's syndrome associated with rheumatoid arthritis. These patients complain more often of easy fatigability, low-grade fever, myalgias, and arthralgias. Most patients with primary Sjögren's syndrome experience at least one episode of nonerosive arthritis during the course of their disease. Manifestations of pulmonary involvement are frequent but rarely important clinically, with subclinical diffuse interstitial lung disease being the most common. Renal involvement includes interstitial nephritis, clinically manifested by hyposthenuria and renal tubular dysfunction with or without acidosis and Fanconi's syndrome. Untreated acidosis may lead to nephrocalcinosis. Glomerulonephritis is a rare finding that occurs in patients with systemic vasculitis, cryoglobulinemia, or systemic lupus erythematosus overlapping with Sjögren's syndrome. Renal biopsy reveals either membranous or membranoproliferative glomerulonephritis. Vasculitis affects small and medium-sized vessels. The most common clinical features are purpura, recurrent urticaria, skin ulcerations, and mononeuritis multiplex. Histologically, leukocytoclastic, lymphocytic, acute necrotizing angiitis, and endarteritis obliterans are seen.

It has been suggested that primary Sjögren's syndrome with vasculitis also may present with multifocal, recurrent, and progressive nervous system disease, such as hemiparesis, transverse myelopathy, hemisensory deficits, seizures, and movement disorders. Aseptic meningitis and multiple sclerosis also have been reported in these patients.

Lymphoma and Waldenström's macroglobulinemia are well-known manifestations of Sjögren's syndrome. Most lymphomas are of B cell origin. Pseudolymphoma or frank lymphoma should always be suspected when persistent major salivary gland enlargement, lymphadenopathy, lung nodules, or hilar or mediastinal lymphadenopathy is observed. Parenchymal organs, such as lungs and gastrointestinal tract can be affected. Lymphomas may appear in Sjögren's

TABLE 288-1 Incidence of non-organ-specific autoantibodies in Sjögren's syndrome (SS) compared with systemic lupus erythematosus (SLE)

	SS (% positive)	SLE (% positive)
Rheumatoid factor	80	25–30
Antibodies to double-stranded DNA	Absent	70–80
Antibodies to Ro/SSA	60	10–25
Antibodies to La/SSB	50	10

TABLE 288-2 Incidence of extraglandular manifestations in primary Sjögren's syndrome

Clinical manifestation	Percent
Arthralgias/arthritis	60
Raynaud's phenomenon	37
Lymphadenopathy	14
Lung involvement	14
Vasculitis	11
Kidney involvement	9
Liver involvement	6
Lymphoma	6
Splenomegaly	3
Peripheral neuropathy	2
Myositis	1

TABLE 288-3   Differential diagnosis of sicca symptoms

Xerostomia	Dry eye	Bilateral parotid gland enlargement
Viral infections	Inflammation	Viral infections
Drugs	Stevens-Johnson	Mumps
Psychotherapeutic	syndrome	Influenza
Parasympatholytic	Pemphigoid	Epstein-Barr
Antihypertensives	Chronic conjunctivitis	Coxsackievirus A
Psychogenic	Chronic blepharitis	Cytomegalovirus
Irradiation	Sjögren's syndrome	Human immunodefi-
Diabetes mellitus	Toxicity	ciency virus
Trauma	Burns	Sarcoidosis
Sjögren's	Drugs	Amyloidosis
syndrome	Neurologic conditions	Sjögren's syndrome
	Impaired lacrimal gland	Metabolic
	function	Diabetes mellitus
	Impaired eyelid function	Hyperlipoproteinemias
	Miscellaneous	Chronic pancreatitis
	Trauma	Hepatic cirrhosis
	Hypovitaminosis A	Endocrine
	Blink abnormality	Acromegaly
	Lid scarring	Gonadal hypofunction
	Anesthetic cornea	
	Epithelial irregularity	

syndrome patients after several years of an apparently benign course and are observed more often in patients with systemic disease.

Routine laboratory tests reveal mild normochromic, normocytic anemia. An elevated erythrocyte sedimentation rate is found in approximately 70 percent of patients.

DIAGNOSIS AND DIFFERENTIAL DIAGNOSIS   Diagnosis of Sjögren's syndrome is based on the presence of two of three of the following manifestations: keratoconjunctivitis sicca, xerostomia, and rheumatoid arthritis or another connective tissue syndrome. Salivary or lacrimal gland enlargement may or may not be present.

The differential diagnosis of Sjögren's syndrome includes other conditions which may cause dry mouth or eyes or parotid salivary gland enlargement (Table 288-3). HIV infection (see Chap. 279) also appears to produce a clinical picture indistinguishable from Sjögren's syndrome in certain patients (Table 288-4). Infiltrative processes such as sarcoidosis may cause parotid gland enlargement. This is distinguished from Sjögren's syndrome by minor salivary gland biopsy, which usually reveals noncaseating granulomas in sarcoidosis patients. These patients also lack autoantibodies.

TREATMENT   Sjögren's syndrome remains fundamentally an incurable disease, since no therapeutic modality has been identified that can alter the course of the disease. Hence treatment of Sjögren's syndrome is aimed at symptomatic relief and limiting the damaging local effects of chronic xerostomia and keratoconjunctivitis sicca by substitution of the missing secretions.

The sicca complex is treated with fluid replacement supplied as often as necessary. To replace deficient tears, there are several readily available ophthalmic preparations (Tearisol; Liquifilm; 0.5% methylcellulose; Hypo Tears). In severe cases, it may be necessary for patients to use these as often as every 30 min. If corneal ulceration

TABLE 288-4   Differential diagnosis of Sjögren's syndrome with HIV infection

HIV infection and sicca syndrome	Sjögren's syndrome
Predominant in young males	Predominant in middle-aged women
Lack of autoantibodies to Ro/SSA and/or La/SSB	Presence of autoantibodies
Lymphoid infiltrates of salivary glands by CD8-positive lymphocytes	Lymphoid infiltrates of salivary glands by CD4-positive lymphocytes
Association with HLA-DR5	Association with HLA-DR3 and -DRw52
Positive serologic tests for HIV	Negative serologic tests for HIV

is present, eye patching and boric acid ointments are recommended. Certain drugs which may increase lacrimal and salivary hypofunction such as diuretics, antihypertensive drugs, and antidepressants should be avoided. Propionic acid gels may be used to treat vaginal dryness.

Bromhexine given orally at high doses (48 mg/d) appears to improve sicca manifestations. However, frequent ingestion of fluids, particularly with meals, is often the best solution.

Preliminary studies suggest that hydroxychloroquine 200 mg/d partially corrects hypergammaglobulinemia and decreases IgG antibodies to La/SSB antigen and erythrocyte sedimentation rate while increasing the hemoglobin levels.

Glucocorticoids (1 mg/kg per day) or other immunosuppressive agents (i.e., cyclophosphamide) are indicated for the treatment of extraglandular manifestations, particularly when renal or severe pulmonary involvement and systemic vasculitis have been documented.

REFERENCES

MOUTSOPOULOS HM et al: Sjögren's syndrome (sicca syndrome): Current issues. Ann Intern Med 92:212, 1980

———, YOUINOU P: New developments in Sjögren's syndrome. Curr Opin Rheumatol 3:815, 1991

——— et al: Immunopathogenesis of Sjögren's syndrome: "Facts and fancy." Autoimmunity 5:17, 1989

——— et al: Nephrocalcinosis in Sjögren's syndrome: A late sequela of renal tubular acidosis. J Int Med 230:187, 1991

REVEILLE JD et al: Specific amino acid residues in the second hypervariable region of HLA-DQA1 and DQB1 chain genes promote the Ro (SS-A)/La (SS-B) autoantibody responses. J Immunol 146:3871, 1991

SKOPOULI FN et al: c-myc mRNA expression in minor salivary glands of patients with Sjögren's syndrome. J Rheumatol 19:693, 1992

TALAL N et al: Sjögren's syndrome: Clinical and immunological aspects. Berlin, Springer-Verlag, 1987

289   ANKYLOSING SPONDYLITIS, REACTIVE ARTHRITIS, AND UNDIFFERENTIATED SPONDYLOARTHROPATHY

JOEL D. TAUROG / PETER E. LIPSKY

The spondyloarthropathies are a group of disorders that share certain clinical features. In addition, each of these conditions is associated with expression of the HLA-B27 gene product. The similarity in clinical manifestations and in genetic predisposition suggest that the spondyloarthropathies may have a related pathogenic mechanism. These disorders include ankylosing spondylitis, Reiter's syndrome, reactive arthritis, psoriatic arthritis and spondylitis, enteropathic arthritis and spondylitis, juvenile-onset spondyloarthropathy, and the less clearly defined undifferentiated spondyloarthropathy.

ANKYLOSING SPONDYLITIS

Ankylosing spondylitis (AS) is an inflammatory disorder of unknown cause that primarily affects the axial skeleton; peripheral joints and extraarticular structures also may be involved. The disease usually begins in the second or third decade; the prevalence in men is approximately three times that in women. It is considered the prototype of the spondyloarthropathies. In Europe, AS is often referred to as *Marie-Strümpell disease* or *Bechterew's disease*.

EPIDEMIOLOGY   Ankylosing spondylitis shows a striking correlation with the histocompatibility antigen HLA-B27 and occurs worldwide roughly in proportion to the prevalence of this antigen (see Chap. 64). In North American Caucasians, the general prevalence of HLA-B27 is 7 percent, whereas over 90 percent of patients with AS have inherited this antigen. The association with HLA-B27 is independent of disease severity.

In population surveys, 1 to 2 percent of adults inheriting HLA-B27 have been found to have AS. In contrast, in families of patients with AS, 10 to 20 percent of adult first-degree relatives inheriting HLA-B27 have been found to have the disease. The concordance rate in identical twins is estimated to be 60 percent or less. These epidemiologic findings indicate that both genetic and environmental factors play a role in the pathogenesis of the disease and that the genetic factors may include allelic genes in addition to HLA-B27.

PATHOLOGY Sacroiliitis is usually one of the earliest manifestations of AS. The early lesion consists of subchondral granulation tissue-containing lymphocytes, plasma cells, mast cells, macrophages, and chondrocytes. Usually, the thinner iliac cartilage is eroded first, then the thicker sacral cartilage. The irregularly eroded, sclerotic margins of the joint are gradually replaced by fibrocartilage regeneration and then by ossification. Ultimately, the joint may be totally obliterated. Radiographically, this progression is evident as erosion of the cortical margins of the joint with subchondral bony sclerosis, followed by apparent widening of the joint space caused by extensive erosion of the cortical margins, bony bridging, and then fusion.

In the spine, the initial lesion consists of inflammatory granulation tissue at the junction of the annulus fibrosus of the disk cartilage and the margin of vertebral bone. The outer annular fibers are eroded and eventually replaced by bone, forming the beginning of a bony excrescence called a *syndesmophyte*, which then grows by continued enchondral ossification, ultimately bridging the adjacent vertebral bodies. Ascending progression of this process leads to the "bamboo spine" observed radiographically. Other lesions in the spine include diffuse osteoporosis, erosion of vertebral bodies at the disk margin (Romanus lesion), "squaring" of vertebrae, and inflammation and destruction of the disk-bone border. Inflammatory arthritis of the apophyseal joints is common; early, there is pannus eroding cartilage, often followed by bony ankylosis.

The pathology of peripheral joint arthritis in AS can show synovial hyperplasia, lymphoid infiltration, and pannus formation, but the process lacks the exuberant synovial villi, fibrin deposits, ulcers, and plaques of plasma cells seen in rheumatoid arthritis (see Chap. 285). Central cartilaginous erosions due to proliferation of subchondral granulation tissue are common in AS but rare in rheumatoid arthritis.

The enthesis, the site of tendinous or ligamentous attachment to bone, is another common site of pathology in AS, especially at sites localized around the spine and pelvis. Enthesitis is characterized by erosive, inflammatory lesions that may eventually undergo ossification.

Acute anterior uveitis occurs in approximately 20 percent of patients with AS. Few cases have been studied histologically, none at an early stage. After recurrent attacks, the iris shows nonspecific inflammatory changes, scarring, increased vascularity, and many macrophages laden with pigment.

Aortic insufficiency develops in a small percentage of cases. There is thickening of the aortic valve cusps and the aorta near the sinuses of Valsalva, with dense adventitial scar tissue and intimal fibrous proliferation, the scar tissue often extending into the ventricular septum with resultant heart block.

Microscopic inflammatory lesions of the colon and ileocecal valve have been found in a majority of patients with AS, even in those lacking any clinical evidence of inflammatory bowel disease. IgA nephropathy has been reported with increased frequency.

PATHOGENESIS The pathogenesis of AS is poorly understood. A number of features of the disease implicate immune-mediated mechanisms, including elevated serum levels of IgA and acute phase reactants, inflammatory histology, and close association with HLA-B27. No specific event or exogenous agent that triggers the onset of disease has been identified, although overlapping features with reactive arthritis and inflammatory bowel disease suggest that enteric bacteria may play a role. Evidence has been obtained suggesting antigenic interrelatedness between HLA-B27 and certain enteric bacteria, but it is not yet known whether this contributes to the pathogenesis of AS. Evidence that HLA-B27 plays a direct role is provided by the finding that rats transgenic for B27 spontaneously develop spondylitis.

CLINICAL MANIFESTATIONS The symptoms of the disease are usually first noticed in late adolescence or early adulthood; onset after age 40 is unusual. The initial symptom is usually dull pain, insidious in onset, felt deep in the lower lumbar or gluteal region, accompanied by low-back morning stiffness of up to a few hours' duration that improves with activity and returns following prolonged periods of inactivity. Within a few months of onset, the pain usually has become persistent and bilateral, and nocturnal exacerbation of the pain that forces the patient to get up and move around may be frequent.

In some patients bony tenderness may accompany back pain or stiffness, while in others it may be the predominant complaint. Common sites include the costosternal junctions, spinous processes, iliac crests, greater trochanters, ischial tuberosities, tibial tubercles, and heels. Occasionally, chest pain is the presenting complaint because of involvement of the thoracic spine and chest wall articulations. Arthritis in the hips and shoulders occurs in 25 to 35 percent of patients overall and can lead to early symptoms. Arthritis of peripheral joints other than the hips and shoulders has been reported in up to 30 percent of patients and can occur at any stage of the disease. Peripheral arthritis is usually asymmetric. Neck pain and stiffness, indicating involvement of the cervical spine, is usually a relatively late manifestation. Occasional patients, especially those with a juvenile onset, present with predominantly constitutional symptoms such as fatigue, anorexia, fever, weight loss, or night sweats.

The most common extraarticular manifestation is acute anterior uveitis, which can antedate the spondylitis. Attacks are typically unilateral and tend to recur, causing pain, photophobia, and increased lacrimation. Aortic insufficiency, sometimes producing the symptoms of congestive heart failure, occurs in a few percent of patients and occasionally occurs early in the course of the spinal disease. A high percentage of patients have inflammation in the colon or ileum, but this is usually asymptomatic.

Initially, physical findings reflect the manifestations of the inflammatory process. The most specific findings involve loss of spinal mobility, with limitation of anterior flexion, lateral flexion, and extension of the lumbar spine, and limitation of chest expansion. Limitation of motion is usually out of proportion to the degree of bony ankylosis, reflecting spasm secondary to pain and inflammation. Pain in the sacroiliac joints may be elicited either with direct pressure or with maneuvers that stress the joints. In addition, there is commonly tenderness upon palpation at the sites of symptomatic bony tenderness and paraspinous muscle spasm.

The Schober test is a useful measure of forward flexion of the lumbar spine. The patient stands erect, with heels together, and marks are made directly over the spine 5 cm below and 10 cm above the lumbosacral junction (identified by a horizontal line between the posterosuperior iliac spines.) The patient then bends forward maximally, and the distance between the two marks is measured. The distance between the two marks increases 5 cm or more in the case of normal lumbar mobility and less than 4 cm in the case of decreased lumbar mobility. Chest expansion is measured as the difference between maximal inspiration and maximal forced expiration in the fourth intercostal space in males or just below the breasts in females. Normal chest expansion is 5 cm or greater.

Limitation or pain with motion of the hips or shoulders is usually present if either of these joints is involved. Careful examination is also necessary to detect inflammatory disease of peripheral joints. It should be emphasized that early in the course of mild cases, symptoms may be mild and nonspecific, and the physical examination may be completely normal.

The course of the disease is extremely variable, ranging from the individual with mild stiffness and radiographically equivocal sacroiliitis to the patient with a totally fused spine, severe bilateral hip arthritis, and ankylosis, possibly accompanied by severe peripheral arthritis and extraarticular manifestations. Pain tends to be persistent early in the disease and then to become intermittent, with alternating exacerbations and quiescent periods. In a typical severe case with progression of the spondylitis to syndesmophyte formation, the patient's posture undergoes characteristic changes. The lumbar lordosis is obliterated with accompanying atrophy of the buttocks. The thoracic kyphosis is accentuated. If the cervical spine is involved, there may be a forward stoop of the neck. Hip involvement with ankylosis may lead to flexion contractures, compensated by flexion at the knees. The progression of the disease may be followed by measuring the patient's height, chest expansion, Schober test, and occiput-to-wall distance when the patient stands erect with the heels and back flat against the wall. Occasional individuals are encountered with advanced physical findings suggestive of long-standing AS who report having never had significant symptoms.

Onset of the disease in adolescence correlates both with a worse prognosis and more severe hip involvement. The disease in women tends to progress less frequently to total spinal ankylosis, although there is some evidence for an increased prevalence of isolated cervical ankylosis and of peripheral arthritis in women.

The most serious complication of the spinal disease is spinal fracture, which can occur with even minor trauma to the rigid, osteoporotic spine. The cervical spine is most commonly involved, and this can lead to quadriplegia. Cauda equina syndrome is another infrequent complication of long-standing spinal disease in AS. Pulmonary involvement, characterized by slowly progressive upper lobe fibrosis, is a rare complication of long-standing AS; eventually, the lesions can cavitate and become colonized by *Aspergillus*. Although cardiovascular involvement can occur early in the course of the disease, the prevalence of aortic insufficiency and of cardiac conduction disturbances, including third-degree heart block, increases with prolonged disease. Prostatitis has been reported to have an increased prevalence in men with AS. Amyloidosis is only rarely of clinical concern.

Despite the persistence of the disease, most patients with AS are able to remain gainfully employed. Only in uncommon instances does the disease appear to shorten life, these being largely the result of spinal trauma, complications of therapy such as upper gastrointestinal hemorrhage, aortic insufficiency, respiratory failure, or amyloid nephropathy. An excess mortality from leukemia was noted in patients treated with deep x-ray therapy to the spine, a common mode of therapy for AS until effective anti-inflammatory medications became available in the mid-1950s.

LABORATORY FINDINGS   There is no laboratory test that is diagnostic of AS. In most ethnic groups, the HLA-B27 gene is present in approximately 90 percent of patients with AS; American blacks appear to represent an exception, since the prevalence of B27 in this group has been reported to be only 50 percent. Most patients with active disease have an elevated erythrocyte sedimentation rate and an elevated C-reactive protein. A mild normochromic, normocytic anemia may be present. Patients with severe disease may show an elevated alkaline phosphatase. Elevated serum IgA levels are common. Rheumatoid factor and antinuclear antibodies are uniformly absent unless caused by a coexistent disease unrelated to AS. Synovial fluid from inflamed peripheral joints in AS is not distinctly different from that of other inflammatory joint diseases. In cases with restriction of chest wall motion, pulmonary function tests may demonstrate decreased vital capacity and increased functional residual capacity, but airflow measurements are normal and ventilatory function is usually well maintained.

RADIOGRAPHIC FINDINGS   Radiographically demonstrable sacroiliitis is usually present in AS. The earliest changes in the sacroiliac joints demonstrable by plain x-ray radiography show blurring of the cortical margins of the subchondral bone, followed by erosions and sclerosis. Progression of the erosions leads to "pseudowidening" of the joint space; as fibrous and then bony ankylosis supervene, the joints may become obliterated radiographically. The changes and progression of the lesions are usually symmetric.

In mild cases, years may elapse before unequivocal sacroiliac abnormalities are evident on plain radiographs. Although computed tomography and magnetic resonance imaging can detect abnormalities reliably at an earlier stage than plain radiography, these techniques are not generally used for routine diagnostic purposes.

Roentgenographic abnormalities generally appear in the sacroiliac joints before appearing elsewhere in the spine. In the lumbar spine, progression of the disease leads to straightening caused by loss of lordosis and reactive sclerosis caused by osteitis of the anterior corners of the vertebral bodies with subsequent erosion, leading to "squaring" of the vertebral bodies. Progressive ossification of the superficial layers of the annulus fibrosus leads to eventual formation of marginal syndesmophytes, visible on plain films as bony bridges connecting successive vertebral bodies on the anterior and lateral sides.

DIAGNOSIS   The diagnosis of early AS before the development of irreversible deformity can be difficult to establish. Currently, modified New York criteria (1984) are widely used for diagnosis. These consist of the following: (1) a history of inflammatory back pain (see below), (2) limitation of motion of the lumbar spine in both the sagittal and frontal planes, (3) limited chest expansion, relative to standard values for age and sex, and (4) definite radiographic sacroiliitis. Under these criteria, the presence of radiographic sacroiliitis plus any one of the other three criteria is sufficient for a diagnosis of definite AS. The increased sensitivity of these modified criteria is largely the result of the inclusion of earlier stages of radiographic sacroiliitis than are permitted under the original New York criteria.

Several studies have identified a sizable population of B27+ individuals with symptoms typical of AS who lack definite radiographic sacroiliitis. However, when followed over time, most of these patients eventually develop radiographic changes. These studies indicate that diagnostic criteria based on radiographic findings may in some cases be too insensitive for the diagnosis of early AS. The B27 test is useful only as a diagnostic adjunct, since the presence of B27 is neither necessary nor sufficient for the diagnosis, but it can be helpful in patients who have not yet developed radiographic sacroiliitis.

AS must be differentiated from numerous other causes of low-back pain. The inflammatory back pain of AS is usually distinguished by the following five features: (1) age of onset below 40, (2) insidious onset, (3) duration greater than 3 months before medical attention is sought, (4) morning stiffness, and (5) improvement with exercise or activity. The most common causes of back pain other than AS are primarily mechanical or degenerative rather than inflammatory and do not show these features. Less common metabolic, infectious, and malignant causes of back pain also must be differentiated from AS.

Marked calcification and ossification of paraspinous ligaments occur in *diffuse idiopathic skeletal hyperostosis* (DISH). Although DISH is often categorized as a variant of osteoarthritis, diarthrodial joints are not involved. Ligamentous calcification and ossification are usually most prominent in the anterior spinal ligaments and give the appearance of "flowing wax" on the anterior bodies of the vertebrae. However, a radiolucency may be seen between the newly deposited bone and the vertebral body, differentiating DISH from the marginal osteophytes in spondylosis. Intervertebral disk spaces are preserved, and sacroiliac and apophyseal joints appear normal, helping to differentiate DISH from spondylosis and from ankylosing spondylitis, respectively.

DISH occurs in the middle-aged and the elderly and is more common in men than in women. Patients are frequently asymptomatic but may have musculoskeletal stiffness. Radiographic changes are generally much more severe than might be predicted from the mild symptoms caused by DISH.

TREATMENT   There is no definitive treatment for AS. The principal goal of management is the conscientious participation by the patient in an exercise program designed to maintain functional posture and to preserve range of motion. Most patients require anti-inflammatory agents to achieve sufficient symptomatic relief to be able to remain functional and carry out the exercise program. It is not known whether drug treatment alone can alter the progression of the disease.

Worldwide, the most commonly used drug therapy for AS is indomethacin, although several other nonsteroidal anti-inflammatory drugs (NSAIDs) also have been proven to be effective in reducing pain and stiffness and are commonly used. Indomethacin is particularly effective as a 75-mg slow-release preparation taken once or twice daily. Although phenylbutazone, at doses of 200 to 400 mg/d, has been considered by several authorities to be the most effective agent in AS, because of its greater potential for serious side effects such as aplastic anemia and agranulocytosis, its use in the United States is confined to patients with severe disease whose symptoms do not respond well to other agents. Recent controlled trials suggest that sulfasalazine,* in doses of 2 to 3 g/d, may be useful in reducing peripheral joint symptoms as well as reversing laboratory evidence of inflammation. Its effects on axial arthritis and natural progression of the disease are unclear. The peripheral arthritis also may respond to the folic acid antagonist methotrexate.* No therapeutic role for gold, penicillamine, immunosuppressive drugs, or systemic glucocorticoids has been documented in AS. Occasionally, intralesional or intraarticular glucocorticoid injections may be beneficial in patients with persistent enthesopathy or synovitis unresponsive to anti-inflammatory agents.

The most common indication for surgery in patients with AS is severe hip joint arthritis, the pain and stiffness of which are often dramatically relieved by total hip arthroplasty. A small number of patients may benefit from surgical correction of extreme flexion deformities of the spine or of atlantoaxial subluxation.

Attacks of acute anterior uveitis are usually effectively managed with local glucocorticoid administration in conjunction with mydriatic agents. Coexistent cardiac disease may require pacemaker implantation or aortic valve replacement.

REACTIVE ARTHRITIS AND UNDIFFERENTIATED SPONDYLOARTHROPATHY

Reactive arthritis (ReA) refers to acute nonpurulent arthritis complicating an infection elsewhere in the body. In recent years, the term has been used primarily to refer to spondyloarthropathies following enteric or urogenital infections and occurring predominantly in individuals with the histocompatibility antigen HLA-B27. Included in this category is the constellation of clinical findings often referred to as *Reiter's syndrome*. Other forms of reactive arthritis not associated with HLA-B27 and showing a different spectrum of clinical features, such as rheumatic fever, are discussed elsewhere in this book (see Chap. 200).

HISTORICAL BACKGROUND In 1916, Reiter described a patient who, following an episode of bloody diarrhea, developed a systemic illness with polyarthritis, conjunctivitis, and nongonococcal urethritis. Although similar cases had been described previously, this report served to focus attention on the triad of arthritis, urethritis, and conjunctivitis, which subsequently was referred to as *Reiter's syndrome*. Additional clinical features, particularly mucocutaneous lesions, were later recognized to be frequent accompaniments of the syndrome.

The identification of bacterial species capable of triggering the clinical syndrome and the finding that three-fourths of the patients possess the HLA-B27 antigen have led to the unifying concept of reactive arthritis as a clinical syndrome triggered by a specific etiologic agent in a genetically susceptible host. A similar spectrum of clinical manifestations can be triggered by enteric infection with any of several

Shigella, *Salmonella*, *Yersinia*, and *Campylobacter* species, by genital infection with *Chlamydia trachomatis*, and possibly by other agents as well. Although Reiter's syndrome can be said to represent one part of the spectrum of the clinical manifestations of ReA, it can be reasonably argued that the term is now largely of historical interest. Undifferentiated spondyloarthropathy is a diagnosis given to patients with clinical findings suggestive of a spondyloarthropathy but whose disease does meet criteria for other diagnoses.

EPIDEMIOLOGY Like AS, ReA occurs predominantly in individuals who have inherited the HLA-B27 gene; in most series, 60 to 85 percent of patients are B27 +. In epidemics of arthritogenic bacterial infection, e.g., *S. flexneri*, it has been estimated that ReA develops in ~20 percent of exposed B27+ individuals. Some studies of families with multiple cases of AS or ReA have suggested that the two conditions tend to "breed true"; i.e., the two conditions are uncommonly found together within an individual family. Whether this is caused by genetic or environmental factors is not known. The disease is most common in individuals 18 to 40 years of age, but it is well recognized both in children over 5 years of age and in older adults.

The sex ratio in ReA following enteric infection is nearly 1:1, whereas venereally acquired ReA is predominantly a male disease. The overall prevalence and incidence of ReA are difficult to assess because of the variable prevalence of the triggering infections and genetic susceptibility factors in different populations. Certain populations, such as the Navajo Indians of the southwestern United States and the Inuit Eskimos of Greenland, show a very high occurrence of ReA, whereas the disease is quite uncommon in certain other populations such as the Haida Indians, with an equally high prevalence of HLA-B27. The reasons for these differences are not clear.

A particularly severe form of peripheral spondyloarthropathy has been described in patients with AIDS (see Chap. 279). Most of these patients are HLA-B27+. Whether B27+ individuals with HIV infection develop this syndrome at a higher than expected frequency is controversial.

PATHOLOGY Synovial histology is similar to that of other inflammatory arthropathies. Enthesitis is a common clinical finding in ReA; the histology of this lesion resembles that of AS. Microscopic histopathologic evidence of inflammation has been noted in the colon and ileum of patients with postvenereal as well as postenteric ReA. The skin lesions of keratoderma blenorrhagica are histologically indistinguishable from psoriatic lesions.

ETIOLOGY AND PATHOGENESIS The first bacterial infection to be causally related to ReA was *S. flexneri*. An outbreak of shigellosis among Finnish troops in 1944 resulted in numerous cases of ReA. Of the four species of *Shigella*, *sonnei*, *boydii*, *flexneri*, and *dysenteriae*, *S. flexneri* has most often been implicated in cases of ReA, both sporadic and epidemic. *S. sonnei*, although responsible for the majority of cases of shigellosis in the United States, has only rarely been implicated in cases of ReA.

Other bacteria that have been definitively identified as triggers of ReA include several *Salmonella* species, *Y. enterocolitica*, *C. jejuni*, and *C. trachomatis*. There is suggestive evidence implicating several other microorganisms, including *Y. pseudotuberculosis*, *Clostridium difficile*, *Neisseria gonorrhoeae*, *Ureaplasma urealyticum*, and *Streptococcus pyogenes*. There are also numerous isolated reports of acute arthritis preceded by other bacterial, viral, or parasitic infections, but whether the microorganisms involved are actual triggers of ReA remains to be determined.

It has not been determined whether ReA occurs by the same pathogenic mechanism following infection with each of these microorganisms, nor has the mechanism been fully elucidated in the case of any one of the known bacterial triggers. Most, if not all, of the triggering organisms share a capacity to invade host cells and survive intracellularly. Antigens from *Chlamydia*, *Yersinia*, and *Salmonella* have been shown to persist in the synovium of patients with ReA for long periods following the acute attack. CD4 + T cells that specifically

---

*This drug has not been approved for this purpose by the Food and Drug Administration at the time of publication.

inflammatory reactivity to any scratches or intradermal saline injection (pathergy test) is a common and specific manifestation in Japanese and eastern Mediterranean patients.

Eye involvement is the most dreaded complication, since it occasionally progresses rapidly to blindness. The eye disease is usually present at the onset but also may develop within the first few years. In addition to iritis, posterior uveitis, retinal vessel occlusions, and optic neuritis can be seen in some cases of the syndrome. Hypopyon uveitis, which is considered the hallmark of Behçet's syndrome, is in fact a rare manifestation.

The arthritis of Behçet's syndrome is not deforming and affects the knees and ankles.

Superficial or deep peripheral vein thrombosis is seen in one-fourth of the patients. Pulmonary emboli is a rare complication. The superior vena cava is obstructed occasionally, producing a dramatic clinical picture. Arterial involvement occurs infrequently and presents with aortitis or peripheral arterial aneurysm and arterial thrombosis. Pulmonary artery vasculitis presenting with dyspnea, cough, chest pain, hemoptysis, and infiltrates on chest roentgenograms has been reported recently in 5 percent of patients.

Central nervous system involvement is found more frequently in northern Europe and the United States. The most common lesions are benign intracranial hypertension, a multiple sclerosis–like picture, pyramidal involvement and psychiatric disturbances.

Gastrointestinal involvement is reported in patients from Japan and includes mucosal ulcerations of the gut.

Laboratory findings are mainly nonspecific indices of inflammation such as leukocytosis and elevated erythrocyte sedimentation rate as well as C-reactive protein levels; antibodies to human oral mucosa are also found.

PROGNOSIS AND TREATMENT   The severity of the syndrome usually abates with time. Apart from the cases with neurologic complications, the life expectancy seems to be normal, and the only serious complication is blindness.

Treatment of Behçet's syndrome is symptomatic and empirical. Mucous membrane involvement may respond to topical corticosteroids in the form of mouthwash or paste. The arthritis responds to rest and analgesics. Thrombophlebitis is treated with aspirin, 500 mg/d, and dipyridamole, 150 mg/d. Colchicine can be beneficial in the mild forms of the syndrome. Uveitis and central nervous system involvement require systemic corticosteroid therapy (prednisone, 1 mg/kg per day) and azathioprine, 2 to 3 mg/kg per day or cyclosporin A, 5 to 10 mg/kg per day.

REFERENCES

INTERNATIONAL STUDY GROUP FOR BEHÇET'S DISEASE: Criteria of diagnosis of Behçet's disease. Lancet 335:1078, 1990

NUSSENBLATT RB et al: Effectiveness of cyclosporin therapy for Behçet's disease. Arthritis Rheum 28:671, 1985

PLOTKIN GR et al: *Behçet's Disease: A Contemporary Synopsis.* New York, Futura, 1988

RAZ I et al: Pulmonary manifestations in Behçet's syndrome. Chest 95:585, 1989

YAZICI H, MOUTSOPOULOS HM: Behçet's disease, in *Current Therapy in Allergy and Immunology*, LM Lichtenstein, AS Fauci (eds). Philadelphia, Decker, 1985

———— et al: A controlled trial of azathioprine in Behçet's syndrome. N Engl J Med 322:281, 1990

291   THE VASCULITIS SYNDROMES

ANTHONY S. FAUCI

DEFINITION   *Vasculitis* is a clinicopathologic process characterized by inflammation of and damage to blood vessels. The vessel lumen is usually compromised, and this is associated with ischemia of the tissues supplied by the involved vessel. A broad and heterogeneous group of syndromes may result from this process, since any type, size, and location of blood vessel may be involved. Vasculitis and its consequences may be the primary or sole manifestation of a disease; alternatively, vasculitis may be a secondary component of another primary disease. Vasculitis may be confined to a single organ such as the skin, or it may simultaneously involve several organ systems.

PATHOPHYSIOLOGY AND PATHOGENESIS   Generally, most of the vasculitic syndromes are assumed to be mediated at least in part by immunopathogenic mechanisms (see Table 291-1). However, evidence to this effect is for the most part indirect and may reflect epiphenomena as opposed to true causality. Deposition of immune complexes in tissues (see Chap. 283) is the most widely accepted pathogenic mechanism of vasculitis. Nonetheless, the causal role of immune complexes has not been clearly established in most of the vasculitic syndromes. Circulating immune complexes need not result in deposition of the complexes in blood vessels with ensuing vasculitis, and many patients with active vasculitis do not have demonstrable circulating or deposited immune complexes. The actual antigen contained in the immune complex has only rarely been identified in vasculitic syndromes. In this regard, hepatitis B antigen has been identified in both the circulating and deposited immune complexes in a subset of patients with systemic vasculitis, most notably within the polyarteritis nodosa group (see below).

The mechanisms of tissue damage in immune-complex–mediated vasculitis resemble those described for serum sickness (Chap. 283). In this model, antigen-antibody complexes are formed in antigen excess and are deposited in vessel walls whose permeability has been increased by vasoactive amines such as histamine, bradykinin, and leukotrienes released from platelets or from mast cells as a result of IgE-triggered mechanisms. The deposition of complexes results in activation of complement components, particularly C5a, which is strongly chemotactic for neutrophils. These cells then infiltrate the vessel wall, phagocytose the immune complexes, and release their intracytoplasmic enzymes, which damage the vessel wall. As the process becomes subacute or chronic, mononuclear cells infiltrate the vessel wall. The common denominator of the resulting syndrome is compromise of the vessel lumen with ischemic changes in the tissues supplied by the involved vessel.

TABLE 291-1   Potential pathogenic mechanisms of blood vessel damage in the vasculitis syndromes

IMMUNOPATHOGENIC MECHANISMS

In situ formation or deposition of immune complexes in blood vessel wall
Direct antibody-mediated damage via antibodies directed at endothelial cells or other tissue components
Antibody-dependent cellular cytotoxicity directed against blood vessel tissue
Cytotoxic T lymphocytes directed at blood vessel components
Granuloma formation in blood vessel wall or adjacent to blood vessel
Cytokine-induced (i.e., interleukin 1, TNF-α), expression of adhesion molecules for leukocytes on endothelial cells

NONIMMUNOPATHOGENIC MECHANISMS

Infiltration of blood vessel wall or surrounding tissue by microbial agents
Direct invasion of blood vessel wall by neoplastic cells
Unidentified mechanisms

In addition to the classic immune-complex–mediated mechanisms of vasculitis, other immunopathogenic mechanisms may be involved in damage to vessels. The most prominent of these are delayed hypersensitivity and cell-mediated immune injury as reflected in the histopathologic feature of granulomatous vasculitis. However, immune complexes themselves may induce granulomatous responses. Vascular endothelial cells can express HLA class II molecules following activation by cytokines such as interferon-γ. This allows these cells to participate in immunologic reactions such as interaction with CD4 + T lymphocytes in a manner similar to antigen-presenting macrophages. Endothelial cells can secrete interleukin 1 (IL-1), which may activate T lymphocytes and initiate or propagate in situ immunologic processes within the blood vessel. In addition, IL-1 and tumor necrosis factor alpha are potent inducers of endothelial-leukocyte adhesion molecule 1 (ELAM-1) and vascular cell adhesion molecule 1 (VCAM-1), which may enhance the adhesion of leukocytes to endothelial cells in the blood vessel wall. Other mechanisms such as direct cellular cytotoxicity or antibody directed against vessel components or antibody-dependent cellular cytotoxicity have been suggested in certain types of vessel damage. However, there is no convincing evidence to support their causal contribution to the pathogenesis of any of the recognized vasculitic syndromes. Finally, antibodies to neutrophil cytoplasmic components have been described for certain of the vasculitis syndromes, particularly Wegener's granulomatosis (see below), but their pathogenic significance, if any, is unclear.

It is unknown why certain individuals develop vasculitis in response to certain antigenic stimuli, whereas others do not. However, it is likely that a number of factors are involved in the ultimate expression of a vasculitic syndrome. These include the genetic predisposition, the regulatory mechanisms associated with immune response to certain antigens, and the ability of the reticuloendothelial system to clear circulating complexes from the blood. The size and physicochemical properties of immune complexes, the relative degree of turbulence of blood flow, the intravascular hydrostatic pressure in different vessels, and the preexisting integrity of the vessel endothelium likely explain why only certain types of immune complexes cause vasculitis and why the vasculitic process is selective for only certain vessels in individual patients.

CLASSIFICATION OF VASCULITIC SYNDROMES A major feature of the vasculitic syndromes as a group is the fact that there is a great deal of heterogeneity at the same time as there is considerable overlap among them. This has led to both difficulty and confusion with regard to the categorization of these diseases. The classification scheme listed in Table 291-2 takes into account this heterogeneity and overlap and will serve as a matrix to emphasize the fact that certain syndromes are predominantly systemic in nature and almost invariably lead to irreversible organ system dysfunction and even death if untreated, while others are usually localized to the skin and rarely result in irreversible dysfunction of vital organs. The distinguishing and overlapping features of the diseases listed in Table 291-2, which justify this classification scheme, will be discussed below.

SYSTEMIC NECROTIZING VASCULITIS

CLASSIC POLYARTERITIS NODOSA **Definition** *Polyarteritis nodosa* (PAN) in its classic form was described in 1866 by Kussmaul and Maier. It is a multisystem, necrotizing vasculitis of small and medium-sized muscular arteries in which involvement of the renal and visceral arteries is characteristic. Classic PAN does not involve pulmonary arteries, although bronchial vessels may be involved; granulomas, significant eosinophilia, and an allergic diathesis are not part of the classic syndrome.

Incidence and prevalence It is difficult to establish an accurate incidence of this disease because of the fact that many reports of PAN actually have included diseases other than the classic syndrome.

TABLE 291-2 Classification of the vasculitic syndromes

Systemic necrotizing vasculitis
  Classic polyarteritis nodosa
  Allergic angiitis and granulomatosis of Churg-Strauss
  Polyangiitis overlap syndrome
Hypersensitivity vasculitis
  Exogenous stimuli proved or suspected
    Henoch-Schönlein purpura
    Serum sickness and serum sickness–like reactions
    Other drug-induced vasculitides
    Vasculitis associated with infectious diseases
  Endogenous antigens likely involved
    Vasculitis associated with neoplasms (particularly lymphoid malignacies)
    Vasculitis associated with connective-tissue diseases
    Vasculitis associated with other underlying diseases
    Vasculitis associated with congenital deficiencies of the complement system
Wegener's granulomatosis
Giant cell arteritis
  Temporal arteritis
  Takayasu's arteritis
Other vasculitic syndromes
  Kawasaki disease
  Isolated central nervous system vasculitis
  Thromboangiitis obliterans (Buerger's disease)
  Behçet's syndrome
  Miscellaneous vasculitides

It is clearly an uncommon, but not a rare, disease. The mean age at onset is 48 years, and the male-to-female ratio is 1.6:1.

Pathophysiology and pathogenesis The vascular lesion in classic PAN is a necrotizing inflammation of small and medium-sized muscular arteries. The lesions are segmental and tend to involve bifurcations and branchings of arteries. They may spread circumferentially to involve adjacent veins. However, involvement of venules is not seen in classic PAN and, if present, suggests the polyangiitis overlap syndrome (see below). In the acute stages of disease, polymorphonuclear neutrophils infiltrate all layers of the vessel wall and perivascular areas, which results in intimal proliferation and degeneration of the vessel wall. Mononuclear cells infiltrate the area as the lesions progress to the subacute and chronic stages. Fibrinoid necrosis of the vessels ensues with compromise of the lumen, thrombosis, infarction of the tissues supplied by the involved vessel, and, in some cases, hemorrhage. As the lesions heal, there is collagen deposition, which may lead to further occlusion of the vessel lumen. Aneurysmal dilatations up to 1 cm in size along the involved arteries are characteristic of classic PAN. Granulomas and substantial eosinophilia with eosinophilic tissue infiltrations are not characteristically found and suggest allergic angiitis and granulomatosis (see below).

Multiple organ systems are involved, and the clinicopathologic findings reflect the degree and location of vessel involvement and the resulting ischemic changes (Table 291-3). As mentioned above, pulmonary arteries are not involved in classic PAN, and bronchial artery involvement is uncommon. The pathology in the kidney is predominantly that of arteritis; however, glomerulitis occurs in up to 30 percent of patients. In patients with significant hypertension, typical pathologic features of glomerulosclerosis may be seen alone or superimposed on lesions of glomerulonephritis. In addition, pathologic sequelae of hypertension may be found elsewhere in the body.

The presence of hepatitis B antigenemia in approximately 20 to 30 percent of patients with systemic vasculitis, particularly of the classic PAN type, together with the isolation of circulating immune complexes composed of hepatitis B antigen and immunoglobulin, and the demonstration by immunofluorescence of hepatitis B antigen, IgM, and complement in the blood vessel walls, strongly suggest the role of immunologic phenomena in the pathogenesis of this disease. Hairy cell leukemia can be associated with classic PAN; the pathogenic mechanisms of this association are unclear.

TABLE 291-3 Classic PAN: Organ system involvement at autopsy

Organ system	Percent
Kidney	85
Heart	76
Liver	62
Gastrointestinal tract:	51
Jejunum	37
Ileum	27
Mesentery	24
Colon	20
Duodenum	10
Gallbladder	10
Rectosigmoid	10
Appendix	7
Muscle	39
Pancreas	35
Testes	33
Peripheral nerves	32
Central nervous system	27
Skin	20

SOURCE: Cupps and Fauci, 1981, p 32.

TABLE 291-4 Clinical manifestations related to organ system involvement in classic PAN

Organ system	Percent incidence	Clinical manifestations
Renal	60	Renal failure, hypertension
Musculoskeletal	64	Arthritis, arthralgia, myalgia
Peripheral nervous system	51	Peripheral neuropathy, mononeuritis multiplex
Gastrointestinal tract	44	Abdominal pain, nausea and vomiting, bleeding, bowel infarction and perforation, cholecystitis, hepatic infarction, pancreatic infarction
Skin	43	Rash, purpura, nodules, cutaneous infarcts, livedo reticularis, Raynaud's phenomenon
Cardiac	36	Congestive heart failure, myocardial infarction, pericarditis
Genitourinary	25	Testicular, ovarian, or epididymal pain
Central nervous system	23	Cerebral vascular accident, altered mental status, seizure

SOURCE: Cupps and Fauci, 1981, p 29.

Clinical and laboratory manifestations Nonspecific signs and symptoms are the hallmarks of classic PAN. Fever, weight loss, and malaise are present in over one-half of cases. Patients usually present with vague symptoms such as weakness, malaise, headache, abdominal pain, and myalgias. Specific complaints related to the vascular involvement within a particular organ system also may dominate the presenting clinical picture as well as the entire course of the illness (Table 291-4). Renal involvement most commonly manifests as ischemic changes in the glomeruli; however, glomerulonephritis is seen in approximately 30 percent of patients. Hypertension may be related to both the renal polyarteritis and the glomerulitis and may dominate the clinical picture. Classic PAN may involve any organ system; the clinical manifestations related to specific organ system involvement are listed in Table 291-4. No clinical features have been identified that discriminate PAN patients with or without hepatitis B antigenemia.

There are no diagnostic serologic tests for classic PAN. In over 75 percent of patients, the leukocyte count is elevated with a predominance of neutrophils. Eosinophilia is seen only rarely and, when present at high levels, suggests the diagnosis of allergic angiitis and granulomatosis. The anemia of chronic disease may be seen, and an elevated erythrocyte sedimentation rate (ESR) is almost always present. Other common laboratory findings reflect the particular organ involved. Hypergammaglobulinemia may be present, and up to 30 percent of patients have a positive test for hepatitis B surface antigen. Arteriograms may demonstrate characteristic abnormalities such as aneurysms in the small and medium-sized muscular arteries of the kidneys and abdominal viscera.

Diagnosis The diagnosis of classic PAN is based on the demonstration of characteristic findings of vasculitis on biopsy material of involved organs. In the absence of easily accessible tissue for biopsy, the angiographic demonstration of involved vessels, particularly in the form of aneurysms of small and medium-sized arteries in the renal, hepatic, and visceral vasculature, is sufficient to make the diagnosis. Aneurysms of vessels are not pathognomonic of classic PAN; furthermore, aneurysms need not always be present, and angiographic findings may be limited to stenotic segments and obliteration of vessels. Biopsy of symptomatic organs such as nodular skin lesions, painful testes, and muscle groups provides the highest diagnostic yields, while blind biopsy of asymptomatic organs is frequently negative.

Treatment and prognosis The prognosis of untreated classic PAN is extremely poor. The usual clinical course is characterized either by fulminant deterioration or by relentless progression associated with intermittent acute flare-ups. Death usually results from renal failure; from gastrointestinal complications, particularly bowel infarcts

and perforation; and from cardiovascular causes. Intractable hypertension often compounds dysfunction in other organ systems, such as the kidneys, heart, and central nervous system, leading to additional late morbidity and mortality. The 5-year survival rate of untreated patients has been reported to be 13 percent, while glucocorticoid treatment may increase this figure to over 40 percent. Extremely favorable therapeutic results have been reported in classic PAN with the combination of prednisone, 1 mg/kg per day, and cyclophosphamide, 2 mg/kg per day (see section on "Wegener's Granulomatosis" for a detailed description of this therapeutic regimen). This regimen has been reported to result in up to a 90 percent long-term remission rate even following the discontinuation of therapy. In addition, long-term remissions have been reported in PAN associated with hepatitis B virus antigenemia using the antiviral agent vidarabine in combination with plasma exchange with and without glucocorticoids. Careful attention to the treatment of hypertension can lessen the acute and late morbidity and mortality associated with renal, cardiac, and central nervous system complications of PAN.

ALLERGIC ANGIITIS AND GRANULOMATOSIS (CHURG-STRAUSS DISEASE) Definition *Allergic angiitis and granulomatosis* was described in 1951 by Churg and Strauss and is a disease characterized by granulomatous vasculitis of multiple organ systems, particularly the lung. It is similar in many respects to classic PAN, except that the former has a high frequency of lung involvement, vasculitis of blood vessels of various types or sizes (including veins and venules), intra- and extravascular granuloma formation together with eosinophilic tissue infiltration, and a strong association with severe asthma and peripheral eosinophilia.

Incidence and prevalence Allergic angiitis and granulomatosis is an uncommon disease whose exact incidence, similar to classic PAN, is difficult to determine due to the grouping of multiple types of vasculitic syndromes in many reported series. The disease can occur at any age with the possible exception of infants. The mean age of onset is 44 years, with a male-to-female ratio of 1.3:1.

Pathophysiology and pathogenesis The vasculitis which is characteristic of allergic angiitis and granulomatosis is similar to that of classic PAN (see above) with certain notable exceptions. In addition to small and medium-sized muscular arteries, capillaries, veins, and venules can be involved in the former disease. The characteristic histopathologic features of allergic angiitis and granulomatosis are granulomatous reactions that may be present in the tissues or even within the walls of the vessels themselves. These are usually associated with infiltration of the tissues with eosinophils. This process can occur in any organ in the body; however, in sharp contrast to classic PAN, lung involvement is predominant, with skin, cardiovascular system, kidney, peripheral nervous system, and gastrointestinal tract also commonly involved. Although the precise pathogenesis of this disease is uncertain, its strong association with asthma, its clinicopathologic manifestations which strongly suggest hypersensitivity phenomena, and its close similarity to classic PAN point to aberrant immunologic phenomena.

Clinical and laboratory manifestations Patients with allergic angiitis and granulomatosis exhibit nonspecific manifestations such as fever, malaise, anorexia, and weight loss similar to patients with classic PAN. In contrast to the latter disease, the pulmonary findings in allergic angiitis and granulomatosis clearly dominate the clinical picture with severe asthmatic attacks and the presence of pulmonary infiltrates. Skin lesions occur in approximately 70 percent of patients and include purpura in addition to cutaneous and subcutaneous nodules. Apart from the characteristic pulmonary findings, the multisystem involvement in this disease is quite similar to that of classic PAN (see above); an important exception is the fact that the renal disease in allergic angiitis and granulomatosis is less common and generally less severe than that of classic PAN.

The characteristic laboratory finding in virtually all patients with allergic angiitis and granulomatosis is a striking eosinophilia which reaches levels greater than 1000 cells per microliter in more than 80 percent of patients. The other laboratory findings are similar to those of classic PAN and reflect the organ systems involved.

Diagnosis Similar to classic PAN, the diagnosis of allergic angiitis and granulomatosis is made by biopsy, demonstrating vasculitis in a patient with the characteristic clinical manifestations. The biopsy findings are distinctive in the latter disease in that granulomatous vasculitis with eosinophilic tissue involvement together with peripheral eosinophilia are typical. Furthermore, pulmonary involvement is extremely common and is usually manifested by severe asthma associated with pulmonary infiltrates that may be fleeting in nature.

Treatment and prognosis The prognosis of untreated allergic angiitis and granulomatosis is poor, with a reported 5-year survival of 25 percent. Unlike classic PAN, the cause of death is more likely to be related to pulmonary and cardiac disease as opposed to renal or gastrointestinal involvement. Glucocorticoid therapy has been reported to increase the 5-year survival to more than 50 percent. In certain patients, the disease may be quite mild and may remit spontaneously or with short courses of glucocorticoids. In glucocorticoid failures or in patients who present with fulminant multisystem disease, the treatment of choice is a combined regimen of cyclophosphamide and alternate-day prednisone, which has resulted in a high rate of complete remission similar to the experience with classic PAN (see above).

POLYANGIITIS OVERLAP SYNDROME Many patients with systemic vasculitis manifest clinicopathologic characteristics which do not fit precisely into any classification but which have overlapping features of classic PAN, allergic angiitis and granulomatosis, Wegener's granulomatosis, Takayasu's arteritis, and the hypersensitivity group of vasculitides. This subgroup has been referred to as the *polyangiitis overlap syndrome* and is part of the major grouping of systemic necrotizing vasculitis. This entity has been designated with a distinct classification in order to avoid confusion in attempting to fit such overlap syndromes into one or other of the more classic vasculitic syndromes. This subgroup is truly a systemic vasculitis with the same potential for resulting in irreversible organ system dysfunction as the other systemic necrotizing vasculitides. The diagnostic and therapeutic considerations as well as the prognosis for this subgroup are the same as those for classic PAN and allergic angiitis and granulomatosis.

HYPERSENSITIVITY VASCULITIS

DEFINITION The term *hypersensitivity vasculitis* has been used to designate a heterogeneous group of disorders which are characterized by a vasculitic syndrome presumed to be associated with a hypersensitivity reaction following exposure to an antigen such as an infectious agent, a drug, or other foreign or endogenous substances. The terminology assigned to this particular group of vasculitis syndromes may be somewhat misleading, since most of the other groups of vasculitis syndromes are probably also associated with some form of hypersensitivity or aberrant immunologic reaction to as yet unidentified antigens.

The common denominator of this group of diseases is the involvement of small vessels. Although any organ can be involved with this type of vasculitis, skin involvement generally dominates the clinical picture, and the extracutaneous involvement is usually much less severe than that of the systemic vasculitides. There are multiple subgroups within the larger category of hypersensitivity vasculitis.

INCIDENCE AND PREVALENCE Although the exact incidence of this group of vasculitic syndromes is uncertain, it is clearly more common than the systemic necrotizing vasculitis group. The disease can occur at any age and in both sexes; however, different subgroups have a higher incidence in certain age groups, and some are more common in males than females, or vice versa.

PATHOPHYSIOLOGY AND PATHOGENESIS The typical histopathologic feature of the hypersensitivity vasculitides is the presence of vasculitis of small vessels. Postcapillary venules are the most commonly involved vessels; capillaries and arterioles may be involved less frequently. This vasculitis is characterized by a leukocytoclasis which refers to the nuclear debris remaining from the neutrophils that have infiltrated in and around the vessels during the acute stages. In the subacute or chronic stages, mononuclear cells predominate; in certain subgroups, eosinophilic infiltration is seen. Erythrocytes often extravasate from the involved vessels, leading to palpable purpura.

Immune-complex deposition is generally considered to be the immunopathogenic mechanism of this type of vasculitis; however, formal proof that this is the case has not been established for all subgroups (see above). The hypersensitivity vasculitides can be broken down empirically into two major categories depending on the type of putative antigen involved in the hypersensitivity reaction. In the originally described group, the antigen was foreign to the host, i.e., a drug, microbe, or foreign protein. In the second category, the antigen is felt to be endogenous to the host. Examples of these are the "self" proteins such as DNA or immunoglobulin which form immune complexes with their respective antibodies and lead to vasculitic complications in systemic lupus erythematosus and rheumatoid arthritis, respectively; other examples are the recognized and putative tumor antigens which form immune complexes with antibody and lead to vasculitis associated with certain neoplasms. Certain lymphoid malignancies also may secrete cytokines which contribute to the pathogenic process (see Table 291-1).

CLINICAL AND LABORATORY MANIFESTATIONS The hallmark of the broad group of hypersensitivity vasculitides is the predominance of skin involvement. Skin lesions may appear typically as palpable purpura; however, other cutaneous manifestations of the vasculitis may occur, including macules, papules, vesicles, bullae, subcutaneous nodules, ulcers, and recurrent or chronic urticaria. Despite the fact that skin lesions predominate, other organ systems may be involved to varying degrees, and the extent to which this occurs may define a relatively distinct subgroup. Even in patients with isolated cutaneous involvement, the disease may be characterized by systemic signs and symptoms such as fever, malaise, myalgia, and anorexia. The skin lesions may be pruritic or even quite painful, with a burning or stinging sensation. Lesions most commonly occur in the lower extremities in ambulatory patients or in the sacral area in bedridden patients due to the effects of hydrostatic forces on the postcapillary venules. Edema may accompany certain lesions, and hyperpigmentation often occurs in areas of recurrent or chronic lesions.

There are no specific laboratory tests which are diagnostic of hypersensitivity vasculitis. A mild leukocytosis with or without eosinophilia is characteristic, as is an elevated ESR. Cryoglobulins and rheumatoid factor may be seen in certain cases, and serum complement levels follow no definite pattern. Laboratory abnormalities related to specific organ dysfunction reflect the involvement of these organs in the particular syndrome in question.

Henoch-Schönlein purpura   The most distinctive subgroup of the hypersensitivity vasculitides is *Henoch-Schönlein purpura*, also referred to as *anaphylactoid purpura*, which is characterized by palpable purpura (most commonly distributed over the buttocks and lower extremities), arthralgias, gastrointestinal signs and symptoms, and glomerulonephritis. The disease is usually seen in children; however, individuals of any age may be affected. It has a remarkable tendency to resolve and recur several times over a period of weeks or months, usually ending in spontaneous resolution. A small percentage of patients progress to chronic disease. A number of antigens have been implicated in the immunopathogenesis of this disease, including infectious agents, drugs, certain foods, insect bites, and immunizations. IgA is the antibody class most often seen in the immune complexes of these patients. The typical palpable purpura is seen in virtually all patients; most patients develop polyarthralgias in the absence of frank arthritis. Gastrointestinal involvement, which is seen in almost 70 percent of pediatric patients, is characterized by colicky abdominal pain usually associated with nausea, vomiting, diarrhea, or constipation and which is frequently accompanied by the passage of blood and mucus per rectum; bowel intussusception may occur rarely. The renal involvement is usually characterized by a mild glomerulitis leading to hematuria with red blood cell casts (see also Chap. 241). Most patients recover completely, and some do not require therapy. When glucocorticoid therapy is required, it is usually administered as 1 mg/kg per day of prednisone and tapered according to the clinical response.

Serum sickness and serum sickness–like reactions   These reactions are characterized by the occurrence of fever, urticaria, polyarthralgias, and lymphadenopathy 7 to 10 days after primary exposure and 2 to 4 days after secondary exposure to a heterologous protein (classic serum sickness) or a nonprotein drug such as penicillin or sulfa (serum sickness–like reaction). Most of the manifestations are not due to a vasculitis; however, occasional patients will have typical cutaneous venulitis which may progress rarely to a systemic vasculitis. This disorder is discussed in detail in Chap. 283.

Vasculitis associated with other underlying primary diseases   A number of diseases have vasculitis as a secondary manifestation of the underlying primary process. Foremost among these are the connective tissue diseases, particularly *systemic lupus erythematosus* (Chap. 284), *rheumatoid arthritis* (Chap. 285), and *Sjögren's syndrome* (Chap. 288). The most common form of vasculitis in these conditions is the small-vessel venulitis isolated to the skin and clinically indistinguishable from the hypersensitivity vasculitides noted in response to an exogenous antigen. However, certain patients may develop a fulminant systemic necrotizing vasculitis indistinguishable from the PAN group.

Cryoglobulinemia may be seen in a number of the diverse vasculitic syndromes. *Essential mixed cryoglobulinemia* (see Chap. 241) may present as a typical hypersensitivity vasculitis confined to the skin. However, typically, it is associated with glomerulonephritis, arthralgias, hepatosplenomegaly, and lymphadenopathy in addition to skin involvement. The cryoglobulins usually consist of cryoprecipitable IgM rheumatoid factor directed against normal endogenous IgG.

Vasculitis can be associated with certain *malignancies*, particularly lymphoid or reticuloendothelial neoplasms. Leukocytoclastic venulitis confined to the skin is the most common finding; however, widespread systemic vasculitis may occur. Of particular note is the association of *hairy cell leukemia* (Chap. 310) with classic PAN.

A leukocytoclastic vasculitis predominantly involving the skin with occasional involvement of other organ systems may be a minor component of many other diseases. These include *subacute bacterial endocarditis*, *Epstein-Barr virus infection*, *chronic active hepatitis*, *ulcerative colitis*, *congenital deficiencies of various complement components*, *retroperitoneal fibrosis*, and *primary biliary cirrhosis*. Association of hypersensitivity vasculitis with *alpha$_1$-antitrypsin*

deficiency, *intestinal bypass surgery*, and *relapsing polychondritis* has been reported.

DIAGNOSIS   The diagnosis of hypersensitivity vasculitis is made by the demonstration of vasculitis on biopsy. Given the predominance of cutaneous involvement, biopsy material is generally readily available. Patients who present with what appears to be isolated cutaneous vasculitis should undergo a systemic (usually noninvasive) workup of other organ systems, since skin involvement is often the presenting feature of systemic vasculitis.

TREATMENT AND PROGNOSIS   Most cases of hypersensitivity vasculitis resolve spontaneously, and others, such as Henoch-Schönlein purpura, remit and relapse before finally remitting completely. In those patients in whom persistent cutaneous disease evolves or in whom extracutaneous organ system involvement occurs, a variety of therapeutic regimens have been tried with variable results. In general, the treatment of this type of vasculitis has not been satisfactory. This is in contrast to the systemic necrotizing vasculitis group (see above) and Wegener's granulomatosis (see below), which generally are much more serious diseases than hypersensitivity vasculitis but usually respond dramatically to the combination of prednisone and cyclophosphamide. Fortunately, since the disease is generally limited to the skin, this lack of consistent response to therapy usually does not lead to a life-threatening situation. When an antigenic stimulus is recognized as the precipitating factor in the vasculitis, it should be removed; if this is a microbe, appropriate antimicrobial therapy should be instituted. If the vasculitis is associated with another underlying disease, treatment of the latter often results in resolution of the former. In situations where disease is apparently self-limited, no therapy, except possibly symptomatic therapy, is indicated. When disease persists or results in progressive organ system dysfunction, such as renal failure in Henoch-Schönlein purpura, glucocorticoid therapy should be instituted, usually as prednisone, 1 mg/kg per day, in a regimen aimed at rapid tapering where possible, either directly to discontinuation or by conversion to an alternate-day regimen followed by ultimate discontinuation. In cases that prove refractory to glucocorticoids in which irreversible organ system dysfunction is likely, a trial of a cytotoxic agent such as cyclophosphamide in the regimen described above for systemic vasculitis is warranted. Patients with chronic vasculitis isolated to cutaneous venules rarely respond dramatically to any therapeutic regimen, and cytotoxic agents should be used only as a last resort in these patients. Plasmapheresis has been used with some success in fulminant cases. Dapsone has been tried in a number of patients with isolated cutaneous vasculitis with rare anecdotal reports of success. However, this drug has been consistently beneficial as therapy for cutaneous vasculitis only in patients with erythema elevatum diutinum (see below).

WEGENER'S GRANULOMATOSIS

DEFINITION   *Wegener's granulomatosis* is a distinct clinicopathologic entity characterized by granulomatous vasculitis of the upper and lower respiratory tracts together with glomerulonephritis. In addition, variable degrees of disseminated vasculitis involving both small arteries and veins may occur.

INCIDENCE AND PREVALENCE   Wegener's granulomatosis is an uncommon disease whose true incidence is difficult to determine. It is extremely rare in blacks compared with whites; the male-to-female ratio is 1:1. The disease can be seen at any age; approximately 15 percent of patients are less than 19 years of age, and only rarely does the disease occur before adolescence; the mean age of onset is approximately 40 years.

PATHOPHYSIOLOGY AND PATHOGENESIS   The histopathologic hallmarks of Wegener's granulomatosis are necrotizing vasculitis of small arteries and veins together with granuloma formation which may be either intravascular or extravascular. Lung involvement typically appears as multiple, bilateral, nodular cavitary infiltrates

FIGURE 291-1 CT scan of a patient with Wegener's granulomatosis. Patient developed multiple, bilateral, nodular, and cavitary infiltrates.

(Fig. 291-1) which on biopsy almost invariably reveal the typical necrotizing granulomatous vasculitis. Endobronchial disease, either in its active form or as a result of fibrous scarring, may lead to obstruction with atelectasis. Upper airway lesions, particularly those in the sinuses and nasopharynx, typically reveal inflammation, necrosis, and granuloma formation with or without vasculitis.

In its earliest form, renal involvement is characterized by a focal and segmental glomerulitis which may evolve into a rapidly progressive crescentic glomerulonephritis. Granuloma formation is only rarely seen on renal biopsy. In addition to the classic triad of upper and lower respiratory tracts and kidney disease, virtually any organ can be involved with vasculitis, granuloma, or both.

The immunopathogenesis of this disease is unclear, although the involvement of upper airways and lungs suggests an aberrant hypersensitivity response to an exogenous or even endogenous antigen that enters through or resides in the upper airway.

Although circulating and deposited immune complexes have been demonstrated in certain patients with Wegener's granulomatosis, there is no convincing evidence that immune complexes play a causal pathogenic role in this disease. The presence of granulomas with copious, well-defined multinucleated giant cells, particularly in involved pulmonary tissue, suggests delayed hypersensitivity and/or foreign-body reactions. However, direct evidence for either of these mechanisms is lacking.

A high percentage of patients with Wegener's granulomatosis develop antineutrophil cytoplasmic antibodies (ANCAs). The terminology of *cytoplasmic* or *c-ANCAs* refers to the coarse, granular pattern observed by immunofluorescence microscopy when serum antibodies bind to certain cytoplasmic components on indicator neutrophils. Proteinase-3, the 29-kDa neutral serine proteinase present in neutrophil azurophil granules, has been identified as the major c-ANCA antigen. Although ANCAs, particularly perinuclear or p-ANCAs (usually directed against myeloperoxidase or elastase), have been described in other vasculitic syndromes, c-ANCAs are a sensitive (88 percent) and specific (95 percent) marker for active Wegener's granulomatosis. There is no clear evidence that ANCAs plays a primary role in the pathogenesis of Wegener's granulomatosis.

The bronchoalveolar lavage fluid of patients with active Wegener's granulomatosis contains a high percentage of neutrophils compared with that of other granulomatous lung diseases such as sarcoidosis, in which increased numbers of lymphocytes are noted (see Chap. 292). The pathogenic significance of this difference is unclear.

CLINICAL AND LABORATORY MANIFESTATIONS A typical patient presents with severe upper respiratory tract findings such as paranasal sinus pain and drainage and purulent or bloody nasal discharge with or without nasal mucosal ulceration (Table 291-5). Nasal septal perforation may follow, leading to saddle nose deformity. Serous otitis media may occur as a result of eustachian tube blockage.

Pulmonary involvement may be manifested as asymptomatic infiltrates or may be clinically expressed as cough, hemoptysis, dyspnea, and chest discomfort. It is present in 85 to 90 percent of patients. Subglottic stenosis resulting from active disease or scarring occurs in approximately 15 percent of patients and may result in severe airway obstruction.

Eye involvement (52 percent of patients) may range from a mild conjunctivitis to dacryocystitis, episcleritis, scleritis, granulomatous sclerouveitis, ciliary vessel vasculitis, and retroorbital mass lesions leading to proptosis.

Skin lesions (46 percent of patients) appear as papules, vesicles, palpable purpura, ulcers, or subcutaneous nodules; biopsy reveals vasculitis, granuloma, or both. Cardiac involvement (8 percent of patients) manifests as pericarditis, coronary vasculitis, or, rarely, cardiomyopathy. Nervous system manifestations (23 percent of patients) include cranial neuritis, mononeuritis multiplex, or, rarely, cerebral vasculitis and/or granuloma.

Renal disease (77 percent of patients) generally dominates the clinical picture and, if left untreated, accounts directly or indirectly for most of the mortality in this disease. Although it may smolder in some cases as a mild glomerulitis with proteinuria, hematuria, and

TABLE 291-5 Wegener's granulomatosis: Frequency of clinical manifestations in 158 patients studied at the National Institutes of Health

Manifestation	Percent at disease onset	Percent throughout course of disease
Kidney		
Glomerulonephritis	18	77
Ear/nose/throat	73	92
Sinusitis	51	85
Nasal disease	36	68
Otitis media	25	44
Hearing loss	14	42
Subglottic stenosis	1	16
Ear pain	9	14
Oral lesions	3	10
Lung	45	85
Pulmonary infiltrates	25	66
Pulmonary nodules	24	58
Hemoptysis	12	30
Pleuritis	10	28
Eyes		
Conjunctivitis	5	18
Dacryocystitis	1	18
Scleritis	6	16
Proptosis	2	15
Eye pain	3	11
Visual loss	0	8
Retinal lesions	0	4
Corneal lesions	0	1
Iritis	0	2
Other*		
Arthralgias/arthritis	32	67
Fever	23	50
Cough	19	46
Skin abnormalities	13	46
Weight loss (greater than 10 percent body weight)	15	35
Peripheral neuropathy	1	15
Central nervous system disease	1	8
Pericarditis	2	6
Hyperthyroidism	1	3

*Less than 1 percent had parotid, pulmonary artery, breast, or lower genitourinary (urethra, cervix, vagina, testicular) involvement.
SOURCE: Hoffman et al, 1992.

red blood cell casts, it is clear that once clinically detectable renal functional impairment occurs, rapidly progressive renal failure usually ensues unless appropriate treatment is instituted.

While the disease is active, most patients have nonspecific symptoms and signs such as malaise, weakness, arthralgias, anorexia, and weight loss. Fever may indicate activity of the underlying disease but more often reflects secondary infection, usually of the upper airway.

Characteristic laboratory findings include a markedly elevated ESR, mild anemia and leukocytosis, mild hypergammaglobulinemia (particularly of the IgA class), and mildly elevated rheumatoid factor. Thrombocytosis may be seen as an acute-phase reactant; hypocomplementemia is not seen despite the presence of circulating immune complexes in some patients. Eighty-eight percent of patients with active disease and 43 percent of patients in remission are positive for c-ANCAs (see above).

DIAGNOSIS   The diagnosis of Wegener's granulomatosis is a clinicopathologic one made by the demonstration of necrotizing granulomatous vasculitis on biopsy of appropriate tissue in a patient with the clinical findings of upper and lower respiratory tract disease together with evidence of glomerulonephritis. Pulmonary tissue, preferably obtained by open thoracotomy, offers the highest diagnostic yield, almost invariably revealing granulomatous vasculitis. Biopsy of upper airway tissue usually reveals granulomatous inflammation with necrosis but may not show vasculitis. Renal biopsy confirms the presence of glomerulonephritis. The finding of elevated titers of c-ANCAs further supports the diagnosis.

In its typical presentation, the classic clinicopathologic complex of Wegener's granulomatosis usually provides ready differentiation from other disorders. However, if all the typical features are not present at once, it needs to be differentiated from the other vasculitides, particularly allergic angiitis and granulomatosis, Goodpasture's syndrome (see Chap. 241), tumors of the upper airway or lung, and infectious or noninfectious granulomatous diseases. Of particular note is the differentiation from idiopathic midline destructive disease (idiopathic midline granuloma; see Chap. 294) and upper airway neoplasms which may erode through the skin of the face, a feature very rarely seen in Wegener's granulomatosis.

Of particular importance in the differential diagnosis is a disease called *lymphomatoid granulomatosis*. It is characterized by lung, skin, central nervous system, and kidney involvement in which atypical lymphocytoid and plasmacytoid cells infiltrate tissue in an angioinvasive manner. In this regard, it clearly differs from Wegener's granulomatosis in that it is not an inflammatory vasculitis in the classic sense but an infiltration of vessels with atypical mononuclear cells; granuloma may be present in involved tissues. Approximately 50 percent of patients develop a true malignant lymphoma. The presence of c-ANCAs proves extremely helpful in the differentiation from all the preceding diseases.

TREATMENT AND PROGNOSIS   Wegener's granulomatosis was formerly universally fatal, usually within a few months after the onset of clinically apparent renal disease. Glucocorticoids alone led to some symptomatic improvement, with little effect on the ultimate course of the disease. It has been well established that the treatment of choice in this disease is cyclophosphamide given in doses of 2 mg/kg per day orally. The leukocyte count should be monitored closely during therapy, and the dosage should be adjusted in order to maintain the count above 3000 per cubic millimeter, which generally maintains the neutrophil count at approximately 1500 per microliter. With this approach, clinical remission can usually be induced and maintained without causing severe leukopenia with its associated risk of infection. Cyclophosphamide should be continued for 1 year following the induction of complete remission and gradually tapered and discontinued thereafter.

At the initiation of therapy, glucocorticoids should be administered together with cyclophosphamide. This can be given as prednisone, 1 mg/kg per day initially (for the first month of therapy) as a daily

regimen, with gradual conversion to an alternate-day schedule followed by tapering and discontinuation after approximately 6 months.

Using the above regimen, the prognosis of this disease is excellent; marked improvement is seen in more than 90 percent of patients, and complete remissions are achieved in 75 percent of patients. A number of patients who developed irreversible renal failure but who achieved subsequent remission on appropriate therapy have undergone successful renal transplantation.

Despite the dramatic remissions induced by the therapeutic regimen described above, long-term follow-up of patients has revealed that approximately 50 percent of remissions are later associated with one or more relapses. Reinduction of remission is almost always achieved; however, a high percentage of patients ultimately have some degree of morbidity from irreversible features of their disease, such as varying degrees of renal insufficiency, hearing loss, tracheal stenosis, saddle nose deformity, and chronically impaired sinus function.

Certain types of morbidity are related to toxic side effects of treatment. Since the preceding therapeutic regimen calls for conversion to alternate-day glucocorticoid therapy within 3 months and ultimate discontinuation within 6 to 12 months, glucocorticoid-related side effects such as diabetes mellitus, cataracts, life-threatening infectious disease complications, serious osteoporosis, and severe cushingoid features are infrequently encountered except in those patients requiring prolonged courses of daily glucocorticoids. However, cyclophosphamide-related toxicities are more frequent and severe. Cystitis to varying degrees occurs in 43 percent of patients, bladder cancer in 4 percent, and myelodysplasia in 2 percent.

Despite its life-saving effects in patients with Wegener's granulomatosis, cyclophosphamide cannot be tolerated by certain patients, such as those who develop severe neutropenia at low doses of drug or those who develop severe cystitis or bladder cancer. In these patients, alternative treatment regimens should be initiated. Azathioprine, in doses of 1 to 2 mg/kg per day, has proven effective in some patients, particularly in maintaining remission in those in whom remission was induced by cyclophosphamide. The drug should be administered together with the glucocorticoid regimen described above. Anecdotal reports have indicated therapeutic success with less frequent and severe toxic side effects using intermittent boluses of intravenous cyclophosphamide (1 g/m² per month) in place of daily drug administered orally. However, we have found that although 6 months of such a regimen induced improvement in approximately 90 percent of patients with remissions in 50 percent, 72 percent of patients were unable to maintain remission despite further treatment over 6 to 24 months. Although certain reports have indicated that trimethoprim-sulfamethoxazole may be of benefit in the treatment of Wegener's granulomatosis, there are no firm data to substantiate this, particularly in patients with serious renal and pulmonary disease. A regimen of methotrexate in doses up to 25 mg per week with alternate-day glucocorticoids has shown some promise in treatment of patients with moderate disease. Further studies over extended periods of time are needed to substantiate these early results.

TEMPORAL ARTERITIS

DEFINITION   *Temporal arteritis*, also referred to as *cranial* or *giant cell arteritis*, is an inflammation of medium- and large-sized arteries. It characteristically involves one or more branches of the carotid artery, particularly the temporal artery, hence the name *cranial* or *temporal arteritis*. However, it is a systemic disease that can involve arteries in multiple locations.

INCIDENCE AND PREVALENCE   Temporal arteritis is an uncommon disease, estimated to occur in 24 per 100,000 people. It is a disease of the elderly, occurring almost exclusively in individuals older than 55 years; however, well-documented cases have occurred in patients 40 years old or younger. It is more common in women than in men and is rare in blacks. Familial aggregation of this disease has been reported.

PATHOPHYSIOLOGY AND PATHOGENESIS Although the temporal artery is most frequently involved in this disease, patients often have a systemic vasculitis of multiple medium- and large-sized arteries which may go undetected. Histopathologically, the disease is a panarteritis with inflammatory mononuclear cell infiltrates within the vessel wall with frequent giant cell formation. There is proliferation of the intima and fragmentation of the internal elastic lamina. Pathophysiologic findings in organs result from the ischemia related to the involved vessels. Immunopathogenic mechanisms, particularly cell-mediated immunity, are felt to be involved in this disease, although the etiology is entirely unknown.

CLINICAL AND LABORATORY MANIFESTATIONS The disease is characterized clinically by the classic complex of fever, anemia, high ESR, and headaches in an elderly patient. Other manifestations include malaise, fatigue, anorexia, weight loss, sweats, and arthralgias. Temporal arteritis is closely associated with the polymyalgia rheumatica syndrome, which is characterized by stiffness, aching, and pain in the muscles of the neck, shoulders, lower back, hips, and thighs.

In patients with involvement of the temporal artery, headache is the predominant symptom and may be associated with a tender, thickened, or nodular artery which may pulsate early in the disease but may become occluded later. Scalp pain and claudication of the jaw and tongue may occur. A well-recognized and dreaded complication of temporal arteritis, particularly in untreated patients, is ocular involvement due primarily to ischemic optic neuritis, which may lead to serious visual symptoms, even sudden blindness in some patients. However, most patients have complaints relating to the head or eyes for months before objective eye involvement. Attention to such symptoms with institution of appropriate therapy (see below) will usually avoid this complication. Claudication of the extremities, strokes, myocardial infarctions, aortic aneurysms and dissections, and infarctions of visceral organs have been reported.

Characteristic laboratory findings in addition to the elevated ESR include a normochromic or slightly hypochromic anemia. Liver function abnormalities are common, particularly increased alkaline phosphatase levels. Increased levels of IgG and complement have been reported, as have increased levels of circulating immune complexes.

DIAGNOSIS The diagnosis of temporal arteritis and its associated clinicopathologic syndrome often can be made clinically by the demonstration of the classic picture of fever, anemia, and high ESR with or without symptoms of polymyalgia rheumatica in an elderly patient. The diagnosis is confirmed by biopsy of the temporal artery. Since involvement of the vessel may be segmental, the diagnosis may be missed on routine biopsy; serial sectioning of biopsy specimens is recommended. Dramatic response to a trial of glucocorticoid therapy can confirm the diagnosis.

TREATMENT AND PROGNOSIS Temporal arteritis and its associated symptoms are exquisitely sensitive to glucocorticoid therapy. Treatment should begin with prednisone, 40 to 60 mg per day, followed by a gradual tapering to a maintenance dose of 7.5 to 10 mg per day. In order to lessen glucocorticoid side effects in elderly individuals, conversion to alternate-day therapy may be attempted, but only after the disease has been put into remission with daily therapy. When ocular signs and symptoms occur, it is important that therapy be initiated or adjusted to control them. Because of the possibility of relapse, therapy should be continued for at least 1 to 2 years. The prognosis is generally good, and most patients achieve complete remission that is often maintained after withdrawal of therapy.

TAKAYASU'S ARTERITIS

DEFINITION *Takayasu's arteritis* is an inflammatory and stenotic disease of medium- and large-sized arteries characterized by a strong predilection for the aortic arch and its branches. For this reason, it is often referred to as the *aortic arch syndrome*.

INCIDENCE AND PREVALENCE Takayasu's arteritis is an uncommon disease, much less common than temporal arteritis. It is most prevalent in adolescent girls and young women. Although it is more common in the Orient, it is neither racially nor geographically restricted. An association of the disease has been described with HLA-DR2, MB1 in Japan and HLA-DR4, MB3 in the United States.

PATHOPHYSIOLOGY AND PATHOGENESIS The disease involves medium- and large-sized arteries, with a strong predilection for the aortic arch and its branches; the pulmonary artery also may be involved. The most commonly affected arteries seen by angiography are the subclavians, followed by the aortic arch, ascending aorta, carotids, and femorals. The involvement of the major branches of the aorta is much more marked at their origin than distally. Partial renal artery occlusion with resulting hypertension is common. The disease is a panarteritis with inflammatory mononuclear cell infiltrates and occasionally giant cells. There is marked intimal proliferation and fibrosis, scarring and vascularization of the media, and disruption and degeneration of the elastic lamina. Narrowing of the lumen occurs with or without thrombosis. The vasa vasorum are frequently involved. Pathologic changes in various organs reflect the compromise of blood flow through the involved vessels.

Immunopathogenic mechanisms, the precise nature of which is uncertain, are suspected in this disease. As with several of the vasculitis syndromes, circulating immune complexes have been demonstrated, but their pathogenic significance is unclear.

CLINICAL AND LABORATORY MANIFESTATIONS Takayasu's arteritis is a systemic disease with generalized as well as local symptoms. The generalized symptoms include malaise, fever, night sweats, arthralgias, anorexia, and weight loss which may occur months before vessel involvement is apparent. These symptoms may merge into those related to pain over the involved vessels followed by symptoms of ischemia in organs supplied by the compromised vessels. Pulses are commonly absent in the involved vessels, particularly the subclavian artery. Aortic regurgitation may occur; hypertension is seen in almost 50 percent of patients. Cardiomegaly and cardiac failure secondary to aortic or pulmonary hypertension occur commonly; the coronary arteries are uncommonly involved. Carotid artery involvement leads to a variety of central nervous system signs and symptoms with over half of patients experiencing syncopal episodes; stroke, which occurs in 15 percent of patients, may represent the first sign of disease; ocular signs and symptoms are present in 60 percent of patients.

The clinical course may be fulminant, may progress gradually, or may stabilize. Complications are related to the distribution of the involved vessels. Death usually occurs from congestive heart failure or cerebrovascular accidents.

Characteristic laboratory findings include an elevated ESR, mild anemia, and elevated immunoglobulin levels.

DIAGNOSIS The diagnosis of Takayasu's arteritis should be suspected strongly in a young woman who develops a decrease or absence of peripheral pulses, discrepancies in blood pressure, and arterial bruits. The diagnosis is confirmed by the characteristic pattern on arteriography which includes irregular vessel walls, stenosis, poststenotic dilatation, aneurysm formation, occlusion, and evidence of increased collateral circulation. Histopathologic demonstration of inflamed vessels adds confirmatory data; however, tissue is rarely readily available for examination.

TREATMENT AND PROGNOSIS The course of the disease is variable, and spontaneous remissions may occur. Reported mortality statistics range from less than 10 percent to 75 percent. Although glucocorticoid therapy in doses of 40 to 60 mg prednisone per day alleviates symptoms, there are no convincing studies which indicate that they alone increase survival. The combination of glucocorticoid therapy for acute signs and symptoms and an aggressive surgical and/or angioplastic approach to stenosed vessels has markedly improved survival and decreased morbidity by lessening the risk of stroke, correcting hypertension due to renal artery stenosis, and improving blood flow to ischemic viscera and limbs. Most recent mortality figures using this therapeutic approach are less than 10 percent. In individuals who are refractory to glucocorticoids, methotrexate in doses up to 25 mg per week has yielded encouraging results; however, long-term studies will be needed to confirm this.

KAWASAKI DISEASE

Kawasaki disease (mucocutaneous lymph node syndrome) is an acute, febrile, multisystem disease of children. It is characterized by unresponsiveness to antibiotics, nonsuppurative cervical adenitis, and changes in the skin and mucous membranes such as edema, congested conjunctivae, erythema of the oral cavity, lips, and palms, and desquamation of the skin of the fingertips. Although the disease is generally benign and self-limited, it is associated with coronary artery aneurysms in approximately 25 percent of cases, with an overall case fatality rate of 0.5 to 2.8 percent. These complications usually occur between the third and fourth weeks of illness during the convalescent stage. Vasculitis of the coronary arteries is seen in almost all the fatal cases which have been autopsied. There is typical intimal proliferation and infiltration of the vessel wall with mononuclear cells. Beadlike aneurysms and thromboses may be seen along the artery. Most investigators agree that many of the cases of PAN formerly reported in children were actually arteritic complications of unrecognized mucocutaneous lymph node syndrome. Other manifestations include pericarditis, myocarditis, myocardial ischemia and infarction, and cardiomegaly.

It is likely that immune-mediated injury to blood vessel endothelium is involved in the pathogenesis of this disease. Patients with Kawasaki disease have been demonstrated to have evidence of increased immune activation characterized by increased activated helper T cells and monocytes, elevated serum-soluble interleukin 2 receptor levels, elevated levels of spontaneous interleukin 1 production by peripheral blood mononuclear cells, anti-endothelial cell antibodies, and increased cytokine-inducible activation antigens on their vascular endothelium.

Apart from the up to 2.8 percent of patients who develop fatal complications, the prognosis of this disease for uneventful recovery is excellent. High-dose intravenous gamma globulin (2 g/kg as a single infusion over 10 h) together with aspirin (100 mg/kg per day for 14 days followed by 3 to 5 mg/kg per day for several weeks) have been shown to be effective in reducing the prevalence of coronary artery abnormalities when administered early in the course of the disease.

ISOLATED VASCULITIS OF THE CENTRAL NERVOUS SYSTEM

Isolated vasculitis of the central nervous system is an uncommon clinicopathologic entity characterized by vasculitis restricted to the vessels of the central nervous system without other apparent systemic vasculitis. Although the arteriole is most commonly affected, vessels of any size can be involved. The inflammatory process is usually composed of mononuclear cell infiltrates with or without granuloma formation. Cases have been associated with cytomegalovirus, syphilis, pyogenic bacterial, and varicella-zoster infections, as well as with Hodgkin's disease and amphetamine abuse; however, in most cases no underlying disease process has been identified.

Patients may present with severe headaches, altered mental function, and focal neurologic defects. Systemic symptoms are generally absent. Devastating neurologic abnormalities may occur depending on the extent of vessel involvement. The diagnosis is generally made by demonstration of characteristic vessel abnormalities on arteriography and confirmed by biopsy of the brain parenchyma

and leptomeninges. The prognosis of this disease is poor; however, in certain patients the disease may remit spontaneously, and some reports indicate that glucocorticoid therapy alone or together with cyclophosphamide in steroid-resistant patients administered as described above for the systemic vasculitides has induced sustained clinical remissions in a small number of patients.

THROMBOANGIITIS OBLITERANS (BUERGER'S DISEASE)

Thromboangiitis obliterans is an inflammatory occlusive peripheral vascular disease of unknown etiology which affects arteries and veins. Thrombosis of the vessels is likely the primary event, and so this disease is not a classic vasculitis. However, it is considered among the vasculitides because of the intense inflammatory response within the thrombus and the fact that there is often a vasculitis of the vasa vasorum in the arterial wall. The disease is discussed in detail in Chap. 211.

BEHÇET'S SYNDROME

Behçet's syndrome is a clinicopathologic entity characterized by recurrent episodes of oral and genital ulcers, iritis, and cutaneous lesions. The underlying pathologic process is a leukocytoclastic venulitis, although vessels of any size and in any organ can be involved. This disorder is described in detail in Chap. 290.

MISCELLANEOUS VASCULITIDES

A variety of disorders, many of which are uncommon, are characterized by varying degrees of inflammatory responses involving blood vessels. *Cogan's syndrome* is a disease characterized by nonsyphilitic interstitial keratitis together with vestibuloauditory symptoms. It may be associated with a systemic vasculitis involving vessels of different sizes as well as the aortic valve.

Erythema nodosum is a common disease which is recognized as a hypersensitivity manifestation of a number of other disorders. It is a painful nodular process of the dermis and subcutaneous tissues. However, histopathologically, there is a vasculitis of small venules (see Chap. 51).

Erythema elevatum diutinum is a rare chronic skin disorder of unknown etiology characterized by persistent red, purple, and yellowish papules, plaques, and nodules usually distributed symmetrically over the extensor surface of the limbs which on biopsy demonstrate a leukocytoclastic venulitis together with a marked dermal inflammatory infiltrate. The disease responds dramatically to dapsone therapy.

Certain *infections* may be associated with an inflammatory vasculitic process. For example, rickettsias can invade and proliferate in the endothelial cells of small blood vessels causing a vasculitis (see Chap. 138). In addition, the inflammatory response around blood vessels associated with certain systemic fungal diseases such as histoplasmosis (see Chap. 162) may mimic a primary vasculitic process.

Eales' disease is a retinal vasculitis which predominantly affects males in the second and third decades of life and which produces a syndrome of recurrent hemorrhages into the retina and vitreous.

APPROACH TO THE PATIENT WITH VASCULITIS

When a physician is presented with a patient in whom the diagnosis of vasculitis has been established clinically or pathologically, there are certain guidelines that may prove helpful to follow (Table 291-6). Each patient is unique and will require individual decision making; however, this framework should serve as a matrix. Expansion of each of the points in Table 291-6 is found in the text above.

TABLE 291-6   Guidelines to the approach to patients with vasculitis

1 Properly categorize the syndrome. Is it a specific syndrome (i.e., Wegener's granulomatosis, temporal arteritis, etc.)?

2 If syndrome is associated with an underlying disease or an offending antigen, treat underlying disease or remove offending antigen where possible.

3 Determine the extent of disease activity.

4 Institute therapy with appropriate agents in diseases in which therapy is essential and of proven benefit, such as with glucocorticoids in temporal arteritis and glucocorticoids and cyclophosphamide in Wegener's granulomatosis.

5 When feasible, avoid immunosuppressive therapy (glucocorticoids or cytotoxic agents) in diseases which rarely result in irreversible organ system dysfunction and which usually do not respond to such agents (i.e. chronic isolated cutaneous vasculitis).

6 Institute glucocorticoid therapy in patients with systemic vasculitis. Add a cytotoxic agent such as cyclophosphamide if an adequate response does not result or if a disease will historically respond only to cytotoxic agents, such as with Wegener's granulomatosis (see 4).

7 Be aware of the toxic side effects of therapeutic agents employed.

8 Continually attempt to taper glucocorticoids to an alternate-day regimen and discontinuation when possible. When using cytotoxic agents, taper and discontinue drug as soon as is feasible upon induction of remission according to established protocols.

9 Use alternative agents where the clinical situation dictates, such as with lack of responsiveness to or unacceptable toxic side effects with recommended agents.

REFERENCES

CUPPS TR, FAUCI AS: *The Vasculitides*. Philadelphia, Saunders, 1981

—— et al: Isolated angiitis of the central nervous system. Prospective diagnostic and therapeutic experience. Am J Med 74:97, 1983

FAUCI AS et al: The spectrum of vasculitis: Clinical, pathologic, immunologic, and therapeutic considerations. Ann Intern Med 89:660, 1978

—— et al: Wegener's granulomatosis: Prospective clinical and therapeutic experience with 85 patients for 21 years. Ann Intern Med 98:76, 1983

GIORDANO JM et al: Experience with surgical treatment of Takayasu's disease. Surgery 109:252, 1991

GROSS WL et al: ANCA and associated diseases: Immunodiagnostic and pathogenetic aspects. Clin Exp Immunol 91:1, 1993

HOFFMAN GS et al: Bronchoalveolar lavage analyses in Wegener's granulomatosis: A method to study disease pathogenesis. Am Rev Respir Dis 143:401, 1991

—— et al: Wegener's granulomatosis: An analysis of 158 patients. Ann Intern Med 116:488, 1992

KADISON P, HAYNES BF: Mechanisms of vessel damage, in *Inflammation: Basic Principles and Clinical Correlates*, JI Gallin et al (eds). New York, Raven Press, 1988, pp 703–717

KATZ P, FAUCI AS: Systemic vasculitis, in *Immunological Diseases*, M Sampter et al (eds). Boston, Little, Brown, 1988, pp 1417–1435

LEAVITT RY, FAUCI AS: Wegener's granulomatosis. Curr Opin Rheumatol 3:8, 1991

LEUNG DYM: New developments in Kawasaki disease. Curr Opin Rheumatol 3:46, 1990

NEWBURGER JW et al: A single intravenous infusion of gamma globulin as compared with four infusions in the treatment of acute Kawasaki disease. N Engl J Med 324:1633, 1991

SHELHAMER JH et al: Takayasu's arteritis and its therapy. Ann Intern Med 103:121, 1985

TREPO C et al: Superiority of a new curative etiopathogenic treatment of hepatitis B–related polyarteritis, using a short corticosteroid course, vidarabine, and plasma exchanges. Presse Med 17:1527, 1988

292   SARCOIDOSIS

RONALD G. CRYSTAL

DEFINITION   Sarcoidosis is a chronic, multisystem disorder of unknown cause characterized in affected organs by an accumulation of T lymphocytes and mononuclear phagocytes, noncaseating epithelioid granulomas, and derangements of the normal tissue architecture. Although there are usually skin anergy and depressed cellular immune processes in the blood, sarcoidosis is characterized at the sites of disease by exaggerated T helper lymphocyte immune processes. All parts of the body can be affected, but the organ most frequently affected is the lung. Involvement of the skin, eye, and lymph nodes is also common. The disease is often acute or subacute and self-limiting, but in many individuals it is chronic, waxing and waning over many years.

ETIOLOGY   The cause of sarcoidosis is unknown. A variety of infectious and noninfectious agents have been implicated, but there is no proof that any specific agent is responsible. However, all available evidence is consistent with the concept that the disease results from an exaggerated cellular immune response (acquired, inherited, or both) to a limited class of antigens or self-antigens.

INCIDENCE AND PREVALENCE   Sarcoidosis is a relatively common disease affecting individuals of both sexes and almost all ages, races, and geographic locations. Females appear to be slightly more susceptible than males. Cases of sarcoid have been described in all of the major races, and the disease is found throughout the world. It has been suggested that sarcoid is more common in certain geographic areas such as the southeastern part of the United States, but when case-matched controls have been used, these geographic differences are less convincing. There is a remarkable diversity of the prevalence of sarcoidosis among certain ethnic and racial groups. The prevalence of sarcoidosis is from 10 to 40 per 100,000 in the United States and Europe. In the United States, the majority of patients are black, with a ratio of blacks to whites ranging from 10:1 to 17:1. In Europe, however, the disease affects mostly whites. Furthermore, while the prevalence per 100,000 in Sweden is 64, in France it is 10, in Poland 3, yet for Irish females living in London it is 200. In contrast, the disease is very rare among Eskimos, Canadian Indians, New Zealand Maoris, and Southeast Asians.

Most patients present with sarcoidosis between the ages of 20 and 40, but it can occur in children and in the elderly. Several hundred kindred groups with familial sarcoidosis have been described, and the disease has been observed in twins, more commonly in monozygotic than in dizygotic pairs. There also have been several instances of husband-wife pairs identified, and geographic foci of sarcoid among unrelated individuals living closely within a community, arguing for some environmental factors in the pathogenesis of the disease. Although the disease is believed to result from exaggerated cellular immune responses to a limited class of antigens, no clear patterns in any HLA locus have emerged. Unlike many diseases in which the lung is involved, sarcoidosis favors nonsmokers.

PATHOPHYSIOLOGY AND IMMUNOPATHOGENESIS   The first manifestation of the disease is an accumulation of mononuclear inflammatory cells, mostly T helper lymphocytes and mononuclear phagocytes, in affected organs. This inflammatory process is followed by the formation of granulomas, aggregates of macrophages and their progeny, epithelioid cells, and multinucleated giant cells. The typical sarcoid granuloma is a compact structure composed of an aggregate of mononuclear phagocytes surrounded by a rim of T helper-inducer lymphocytes and, to a far lesser extent, B lymphocytes. The overall structure is relatively discrete and is interspersed with fine collagen fibrils, presumably remnants of the underlying connective tissue matrix. The giant cells within the granuloma can be of the Langhans' or foreign-body variety and often contain inclusions such as Schaumann bodies (conchlike structures), asteroid bodies (stellate-like structures), and residual bodies (refractile calcium-containing inclusions).

Together the accumulated T cells, mononuclear phagocytes, and granulomas represent the active disease. Other than the fact that they take up space and thus their bulk modifies the local architecture, there is no evidence that the mononuclear inflammatory cells dispersed in the tissue or in the granuloma injure the affected organ by releasing mediators that damage the normal parenchymal cells or the extracellular matrix. Rather, organ dysfunction in sarcoid results mostly from the accumulated inflammatory cells distorting the architecture of the affected tissue; if a sufficient number of structures vital to the function of the tissue are involved, the disease becomes clinically apparent in that organ. Thus, while autopsy series show that, to some extent, sarcoidosis involves most organs in the majority of patients, the disease manifests clinically only in organs where it affects function (such as the lung and eye) or in organs where it is readily observed

T lymphocytes   Macrophages

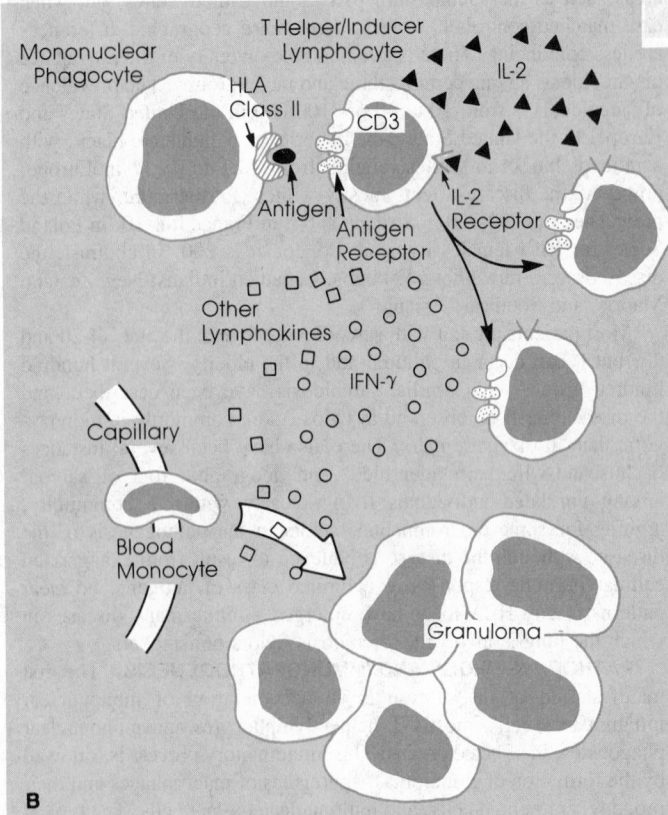

FIGURE 292-1 Pathogenesis of sarcoidosis. *A*. Histologic abnormalities. Normal alveoli *(left)* and alveoli in active sarcoidosis *(right)*. The latter are distorted by the accumulated T helper-inducer lymphocytes, alveolar macrophages, and macrophages aggregated into granulomas. There is mild damage to alveolar epithelial and endothelial cells. *B*. The exaggerated processes of T helper-inducer lymphocytes in affected organs result in the accumulation of these cells along with macrophages and macrophages aggregated into granulomas. The trigger for the T helper-inducer cells is unknown. It may be a limited class of antigens or self-antigens presented in the context of class II HLA surface molecules by mononuclear phagocytes to the T helper-inducer lymphocyte. The antigen class II HLA complex is identified by the T-cell antigen receptor, the CD3 signal transducing complex is triggered, and the T cell is activated. Consequent to this process the immune response is exaggerated and skewed to produce activated T helper-inducer cells that release interleukin 2, which drives the accumulation of more T helper cells. The activated T helper-inducer cells also release interferon-γ (IFN-γ) and other lymphokines, mediators that contribute to the recruitment and activation of blood monocytes and hence to granuloma formation.

(such as the skin or, by x-ray, the hilar nodes). For example, in the lung, the inflammatory cells and granulomas distort the walls of the alveoli, bronchi, and blood vessels (Fig. 292-1*A*), thus altering the intimate relationships between air and blood necessary for normal gas exchange. When a sufficient amount of pulmonary tissue is involved, it is sensed by the individual as dyspnea. In contrast, most individuals with sarcoidosis have granulomatous mononuclear cell inflammation in the liver but usually do not have symptoms or functional derangements referable to that organ, likely because the disease process does not modify the local structures sufficiently to affect function.

If the disease is suppressed, either spontaneously or with therapy, the mononuclear inflammation is reduced in intensity and the number of granulomas is reduced. The granulomas resolve either by dispersion of the cells or by centripetal proliferation of fibroblasts from the periphery of the granuloma inward, to form a small scar. In chronic cases, the mononuclear cell inflammation persists for years. If the intensity of the inflammation is sufficiently high for a sufficiently long period, the derangements to the affected tissues result in extensive damage, the development of fibrosis, and permanent loss of organ function.

All available evidence suggests that active sarcoidosis results from

an exaggerated cellular immune response to a variety of antigens or self-antigens, in which the process of T lymphocyte triggering, proliferation, and activation is skewed in the direction of helper-inducer T lymphocyte processes (Fig. 292-1*B*). The result is an exaggerated helper-inducer T cell response and thus the accumulation of large numbers of activated T cells in the affected organs. Since the activated helper-inducer T lymphocyte releases mediators that attract and activate mononuclear phagocytes, it is likely that the process of granuloma formation is a secondary phenomenon which is a consequence of the exaggerated helper-inducer T cell process. In this context, the current hypotheses of the cause of sarcoidosis, not mutually exclusive, include (1) the disease is caused by a class of antigens, nonself or self, that trigger only the helper-inducer T cell arm of the immune response, (2) the disease results from an inadequate suppressor arm of the immune response, such that helper-inducer T cell processes cannot be shut down in a normal fashion, or (3) the disease results from inherited (and/or acquired) differences in immune response genes, such that the response to a variety of antigens is an exaggerated, helper-inducer T cell process.

Independent of the inciting agent(s) or the reason why there is an exaggerated helper-inducer T cell response, there is a general understanding of the processes responsible for the maintenance of the inflammation and the development of the granuloma. The T helper-inducer lymphocytes accumulate at the sites of disease, at least in part, because they proliferate in these sites at an exaggerated rate. This T cell proliferation is maintained by the spontaneous release of interleukin 2 (IL-2), the T cell growth factor, by activated T helper-inducer cells in the local milieu. In this regard, sarcoidosis is a remarkable example of compartmentalization of the immune system and a dramatic illustration of why disease activity of sarcoidosis cannot be assessed by evaluating the immune system only in the blood. Whereas the T helper-inducer cells in the involved organs are releasing IL-2 and proliferating at an enhanced rate, the T cells in other sites, such as blood, are quiescent. Furthermore, while there is a marked enhancement of the number of T helper-inducer cells at the sites of disease, the numbers of T helper-inducer cells in the blood are normal or slightly reduced. In the involved organs, the ratio of helper-inducer to suppressor-cytotoxic T cells may be as high as 10:1 compared to the ratio of 2:1 found in normal tissues or in the blood of affected individuals.

In addition to driving other T helper-inducer cells in the affected organs to proliferate, the T helper-inducer cells at the sites of disease are activated and release mediators that both recruit and activate mononuclear phagocytes. The T helper-inducer cells accomplish this by releasing a variety of mediators (lymphokines) including proteins capable of recruiting blood monocytes to the local milieu of the activated T cells and interferon-γ, a protein that, among its many actions, activates mononuclear phagocytes. Together these mediators recruit blood monocytes to the affected organs and activate them, providing the building blocks for the formation of the granuloma.

In addition to these exaggerated cellular immune processes, active sarcoid is also characterized by hyperglobulinemia. Included among the immunoglobulins are antibodies against a variety of infectious agents as well as IgM anti-T cell antibodies. However, there is no evidence that any of these antibodies plays a role in the pathogenesis of the disease, and they are thought to result from the nonspecific polyclonal stimulation of B cells by the activated T cells at the site of disease.

If the damage in the affected organs is sufficiently extensive that the remaining parenchymal cells cannot reestablish the normal tissue architecture, the usual result is fibrosis, the proliferation of mesenchymal cells, and deposition of their connective tissue products. There is convincing evidence that the fibroblast proliferation is directed by tissue macrophages spontaneously releasing growth signals for fibroblasts, including platelet-derived growth factor, fibronectin, and insulin-like growth factor 1. It is not known, however, why this fibrotic process occurs only in a relatively small proportion of individuals with sarcoidosis.

CLINICAL MANIFESTATIONS Sarcoidosis is a systemic disease, and thus the clinical manifestations may be generalized or focused on one or more organs. However, because the lung is almost always involved, most patients have symptoms referable to the respiratory system. Independent of the site, the clinical manifestations of the disease relate directly to the exaggerated helper-inducer T cell–mononuclear phagocyte granulomatous inflammatory process itself or to the sequelae resulting from the permanent damage caused by this process.

Sarcoidosis is occasionally discovered in a completely asymptomatic individual, but more commonly it presents abruptly over 1 to 2 weeks or the affected individual develops symptoms insidiously over several months. Independent of the mode of presentation, about 75 percent of all cases present when the individual is less than 40 years of age.

The asymptomatic form is usually detected by a routine examination, such as a chest film. In the United States, this represents about 10 to 20 percent of all cases, but in countries where chest films are mandatory in preemployment screening programs, the proportion of asymptomatic patients is higher.

So-called acute or subacute sarcoidosis develops abruptly over a period of a few weeks and represents 20 to 40 percent of all cases. These individuals usually have constitutional symptoms such as fever, fatigue, malaise, anorexia, or weight loss. These symptoms are usually mild, but in approximately 25 percent of the acute cases the constitutional complaints are extensive. Many patients have respiratory symptoms, including cough, dyspnea, or a vague retrosternal chest discomfort. Two syndromes have been identified in the acute group. Löfgren's syndrome, frequent in Scandinavian, Irish, and Puerto Rican females, includes the complex of erythema nodosum and x-ray findings of bilateral hilar adenopathy, often accompanied by joint symptoms. The Heerfordt-Waldenstrom syndrome describes individuals with fever, parotid enlargement, anterior uveitis, and facial nerve palsy.

The insidious form of sarcoidosis develops over months and is associated usually with respiratory complaints without constitutional symptoms. In the United States, 40 to 70 percent of all sarcoid patients are in this category. About 10 percent of these individuals have symptoms referable to organs other than the lung. It is the individuals who present with the insidious form of sarcoidosis who most commonly go on to develop chronic sarcoidosis, with permanent damage to the lung and other organs.

Despite the fact that sarcoidosis is a systemic disease and some evidence of inflammation can be detected in most organs in the majority of patients, sarcoidosis is important clinically because of the pulmonary abnormalities and, to a lesser extent, lymph node, skin, and eye involvement. Far less commonly, other organs are involved significantly.

Lung Of individuals with sarcoidosis, 90 percent have an abnormal chest x-ray at some time during their course. Overall, approximately 50 percent develop permanent pulmonary abnormalities and 5 to 15 percent have progressive fibrosis of the lung parenchyma. Sarcoidosis of the lung is primarily an interstitial lung disease (see Chap. 224) in which the inflammatory process involves the alveoli, small bronchi, and small blood vessels. These individuals typically have symptoms of dyspnea, particularly with exercise, and a dry cough. In acute and subacute cases, physical examination usually reveals dry rales. Hemoptysis is rare, as is production of sputum. Occasionally, the large airways are involved to a degree sufficient to cause dysfunction. Distal atelectasis can result from endobronchial sarcoidosis or from external compression from enlarged intrathoracic nodes. Rarely, wheezing is heard, incorrectly suggesting asthma. Large-vessel pulmonary granulomatous arteritis is common, but it rarely causes major problems. If it dominates the pulmonary lesions, it is sometimes called *necrotizing sarcoidal granulomatosis*. The pleura is involved in 1 to 5 percent of cases, almost always manifesting as a unilateral pleural effusion with characteristics of an exudate containing lymphocytes. The effusions usually clear within a few weeks, but chronic pleural thickening can result. Pneumothorax is very rare.

Lymph nodes Lymphadenopathy is very common in sarcoidosis. Intrathoracic nodes are enlarged in 75 to 90 percent of all patients; usually this involves the hilar nodes, but the paratracheal nodes are commonly involved (Fig. 292-2A). Less frequently, there is enlargement of subcarinal, anterior mediastinal, or posterior mediastinal nodes. Peripheral lymphadenopathy is very common, particularly involving the cervical, axillary, epitrochlear, and inguinal nodes. The nodes in the retroperitoneal area and in the mesenteric chain also can enlarge. All these nodes are nonadherent, with a firm, rubbery texture. Palpation causes no pain. Unlike nodes in tuberculosis, the nodes do not ulcerate. The lymphadenopathy rarely causes a problem for the affected individual; however, if it is massive, it can be disfiguring and can impinge on other organs and lead to functional impairment.

Skin Sarcoidosis involves the skin in about 25 percent of cases. The most common lesions are erythema nodosum, plaques, maculopapular eruptions, subcutaneous nodules, and lupus pernio. Erythema nodosum, comprising bilateral, tender red nodules on the anterior surface of the legs, is not specific for sarcoidosis but is common, particularly in acute sarcoidosis, in combination with systemic symptoms and polyarthralgias. Treatment is not required, since the lesions resolve spontaneously in 2 to 4 weeks. Erythema nodosum is much more common among sarcoid patients in Europe than in the United States. Skin plaques associated with sarcoid are purple, indolent lesions, often raised, and usually occur on the face, buttocks, and extremities. The maculopapular eruptions occur on the face around the eyes and nose, on the back, and on the extremities. These are elevated lesions less than 1 cm in diameter with a flat, waxy top. Subcutaneous nodules are most common on the trunk and extremities. Lupus pernio is characterized by indurated blue-purple, swollen, shiny lesions on the nose, cheeks, lips, ears, fingers, and knees. The lesions on the tip of the nose cause a bulbous appearance, sometimes associated with varicosities. The nasal mucosa is usually involved, and underlying bone can be destroyed. Sarcoidosis also can involve old surgical scars and tattoos. Although it may be disfiguring, cutaneous sarcoidosis rarely causes major problems. Clubbing of the fingers is occasionally observed in sarcoidosis, usually in association with extensive pulmonary fibrosis.

Eye   Eye involvement occurs in approximately 25 percent of patients with sarcoidosis, and it can cause blindness. The usual lesions involve the uveal tract, iris, ciliary body, and choroid. Of those cases with eye involvement, approximately 75 percent have anterior uveitis and 25 to 35 percent have posterior uveitis. There is blurred vision, tearing, and photophobia. The uveitis can develop rapidly and may clear spontaneously over a 6- to 12-month period. It also can develop insidiously and be chronic. Conjunctival involvement is also common, usually with small, yellow nodules. When the lacrimal gland is involved, a keratoconjunctivitis sicca syndrome, with dry, sore eyes, can result.

Upper respiratory tract   The nasal mucosa is involved in up to 20 percent of patients, usually presenting with nasal stuffiness. Any of the structures of the mouth can be involved, particularly the tonsils. Sarcoidosis involves the larynx in about 5 percent of cases. The epiglottis and areas around the true vocal cords are usually involved, but the cords themselves are not. These individuals are usually hoarse, and they have dyspnea, wheezing, and stridor; complete obstruction can occur.

Bone marrow and spleen   Sarcoidosis of the marrow is reported in 15 to 40 percent of cases, but it rarely causes hematologic abnormalities other than a mild anemia, neutropenia, eosinophilia, and occasionally, thrombocytopenia. Although splenomegaly occurs in only 5 to 10 percent of patients, celiac angiography or splenic biopsy reveals involvement in 50 to 60 percent of cases. The presentation and complications of splenomegaly in sarcoidosis are similar to those of splenomegaly in general.

Liver   Although liver biopsy reveals liver involvement in 60 to 90 percent of cases, liver dysfunction is usually not important clinically. Sarcoidosis involves generally the periportal areas. Approximately 20 to 30 percent have hepatomegaly and/or biochemical evidence of liver involvement. Usually these changes reflect a cholestatic pattern and include an elevated alkaline phosphatase level; the bilirubin and aminotransferases are only mildly elevated, and jaundice is rare. Rarely, portal hypertension can occur, as can intrahepatic cholestasis with cirrhosis.

Kidney   Clinically apparent primary renal involvement in sarcoidosis is rare, although tubular, glomerular, and renal artery diseases have been reported. More commonly, but still in only 1 to 2 percent of all cases, there is a disorder of calcium metabolism with hypercalciuria, with or without hypercalcemia. If chronic, nephrocalcinosis and nephrolithiasis can result. It is believed that the calcium abnormalities are associated with enhanced calcium absorption in the gut, which is related to an abnormally high level of circulating 1,25-dihydroxyvitamin D produced by mononuclear phagocytes in the granulomas.

FIGURE 292-2   Common laboratory findings of sarcoidosis. *A.* Schematic view of the abnormal findings on the chest x-ray. Shown are changes observed with the average frequency of occurrence. *B.* Typical gallium 67 scan of an individual with active sarcoidosis. The isotope has accumulated in the lung parenchyma (LP), liver (L), spleen (S), parotid (P), hilar nodes (HN), and pelvic nodes (PN). *C.* Cells recovered by bronchoalveolar lavage of an individual with active pulmonary sarcoidosis. The lavage analysis reflects the inflammation in the tissue. Shown are alveolar macrophages (*large cells*) and lymphocytes (*small cells*). The cell population is dominated by lymphocytes, in contrast to normals, in whom lymphocytes represent <20 percent of the cell population.

Nervous system All components of the nervous system can be involved in sarcoidosis. Neurologic findings are observed in about 5 percent of patients. Seventh nerve involvement with unilateral facial paralysis is most common. It occurs suddenly and is usually transient. Other common manifestations of neurosarcoid include optic nerve dysfunction, papilledema, palate dysfunction, hearing abnormalities, hypothalamic and pituitary abnormalities, chronic meningitis, and occasionally, space-occupying lesions. Psychiatric disturbances have been described, and seizures can occur. Rarely, multiple lesions occur which mimic multiple sclerosis, spinal cord abnormalities, and peripheral neuropathy.

Musculoskeletal system The bones, joints, and/or muscles can be involved in sarcoidosis. Bone lesions are observed in 5 percent of patients and include variable-sized cysts in areas of expanded bone, well-defined, round, punched-out lesions, or lattice-like changes. Hand and foot bones are the common sites, but most bones can be involved. Occasionally, the bone lesions are tender and painful. Joint involvement is more common, with an incidence of 25 to 50 percent in known cases of sarcoidosis. Arthralgias and frank arthritis occur mostly in large joints; they can be migratory and are usually transient, but they can be chronic and result in deformities. Although muscle biopsy frequently demonstrates granulomatous inflammation, muscle dysfunction is rare. However, nodules, polymyositis, and chronic myopathy have been described.

Heart Approximately 5 percent of patients have significant heart involvement, with clinical evidence of cardiac dysfunction. Left ventricular wall involvement is common. Arrhythmias are frequent, and serious conduction disturbances, including complete heart block, can occur. Papillary muscle dysfunction, pericarditis, and congestive heart failure are also observed. Cor pulmonale secondary to chronic pulmonary fibrosis may occur but is uncommon.

Endocrine and reproductive system The hypothalamic-pituitary axis is the part of the endocrine system most commonly involved; this usually presents as diabetes insipidus. Anterior pituitary dysfunction is also seen, manifesting as a deficiency in one or more pituitary hormones. Complete hypopituitarism is rare. Much less frequently, sarcoidosis can cause primary dysfunction of other endocrine glands. Adrenal cortical involvement resulting in Addison's syndrome has been described. Involvement of the reproductive organs occurs, but infertility is rare. Pregnancy is not affected by sarcoidosis, and patients with sarcoidosis who become pregnant usually improve during pregnancy. However, the disease may flare post partum; presumably this variation results from fluctuations in endogenous glucocorticoid production.

Exocrine glands Parotid enlargement is a classic feature of sarcoidosis, but clinically apparent parotid involvement occurs in less than 10 percent of patients. Bilateral involvement is the rule. The gland is usually nontender, firm, and smooth. Xerostomia can occur; other exocrine glands are affected only rarely.

Gastrointestinal tract Although sarcoidosis involvement of the gastrointestinal tract is found occasionally at autopsy, it rarely has clinical importance. Occasionally, patients have esophageal or gastric symptoms.

COMPLICATIONS The respiratory tract abnormalities cause most of the morbidity and mortality associated with sarcoidosis. The major problems are those characteristic of interstitial lung disease (see Chap. 224), particularly dyspnea and insufficient oxygen delivery to vital organs. Respiratory failure with carbon dioxide retention is rare. In some patients, lung destruction results in formation of bullae that may harbor mycetomas, which are usually aspergillomas; erosion into the parenchyma can result in massive bleeding. The most common complications apart from the lung are associated with the eye; however, with therapy blindness is rare. Complications of other organs include a gamut of abnormalities. The most serious are CNS lesions or cardiac involvement leading to congestive heart failure or sudden death.

LABORATORY ABNORMALITIES Common abnormalities in the blood include lymphocytopenia, an occasional mild eosinophilia, an increased erythrocyte sedimentation rate, hyperglobulinemia, and an elevated level of angiotensin-converting enzyme. Hypercalcemia is rare. Other serum abnormalities relate to involvement of specific organs such as liver, kidney, or endocrine glands.

Because the lung is involved so commonly, the routine chest film is almost always abnormal (Fig. 292-2A). The three classic x-ray patterns of pulmonary sarcoidosis are type I—bilateral hilar adenopathy with no parenchymal abnormalities; type II—bilateral hilar adenopathy with diffuse parenchymal changes; and type III—diffuse parenchymal changes without hilar adenopathy. The type III pattern is sometimes split into two categories, with films that show fibrosis and upper lobe retraction classified separately. Although patients with type I x-rays tend to have the acute or subacute, reversible form of the disease while those with types II and III often have the chronic, progressive disease, these patterns do not represent consecutive "stages" of sarcoidosis. Thus, except for epidemiologic purposes, this x-ray categorization is mostly of historic interest. The hilar adenopathy is almost always bilateral, but unilateral node enlargement can be seen. Nodes are also common in the paratracheal region. The diffuse parenchymal changes are typically reticulonodular infiltrates, but an acinar pattern is observed occasionally. Large nodules, similar to those of metastatic disease, are unusual but can occur. When there is massive fibrosis, the hila are pulled upward and there are conglomerate masses in the midlung zones. Some of the unusual chest x-ray findings in sarcoidosis include "egg shell" calcification of hilar nodes, pleural effusions, cavitation, atelectasis, pulmonary hypertension, pneumothorax, and cardiomegaly.

The lung function abnormalities of sarcoidosis are typical for interstitial lung disease (see Chap. 224) and include decreased lung volumes and diffusing capacity with a normal or supernormal ratio of the forced expiratory volume in 1 s to the forced vital capacity. Occasionally there is evidence of airflow limitation. There is usually mild hypoxemia and a mild, compensated hypocarbia.

The gallium 67 lung scan is usually abnormal, showing a pattern of diffuse uptake. If present, enlarged nodes are detected in these scans, as is inflammation in a variety of extrathoracic sites that usually have no clinical importance (Fig. 292-2B). Bronchoalveolar lavage demonstrates typically an increased proportion of lymphocytes, most of which are activated helper-inducer T lymphocytes (Fig. 292-2C). The remainder of the cells are mostly alveolar macrophages. In patients with significant fibrosis, a small number of neutrophils are also found. Eosinophils are rare.

The other laboratory features of sarcoidosis depend on the specific organ involved.

DIAGNOSIS For a typical case, the diagnosis of sarcoidosis is made by a combination of clinical, radiographic, and histologic findings. In a young adult with constitutional complaints, respiratory symptoms, erythema nodosum, blurred vision, and bilateral hilar adenopathy, the diagnosis is almost always sarcoidosis. Commonly, however, the findings are more subtle. Furthermore, because sarcoidosis can occur in almost any place in the body, like tuberculosis or syphilis, it can be confused with many other disorders. In this context, the differential diagnosis of sarcoidosis must cover a wide range. However, it is confused most commonly with neoplastic diseases such as lymphoma or with disorders characterized also by a mononuclear cell granulomatous inflammatory process, such as the mycobacterial and fungal disorders.

The presence of skin anergy is typical but not diagnostic of sarcoidosis. The Kveim-Siltzbach skin test, the intradermal injection of a heat-treated suspension of a sarcoidosis spleen extract which is biopsied 4 to 6 weeks later, yields sarcoidosis-like lesions in 70 to 80 percent of individuals with sarcoidosis with less than 5 percent false-positive results. However, the material is not widely available, and with the use of the transbronchial biopsy to obtain lung parenchyma for diagnostic purposes, the Kveim-Siltzbach test is not in general use.

No blood findings are diagnostic of the disease. Angiotensin-converting enzyme is elevated in the serum in approximately two-thirds of patients with sarcoidosis, but false-positive and false-negative results are common. An elevated 24-h urine calcium level is consistent with the diagnosis but is not specific.

The chest x-ray cannot be used as the sole criterion for the diagnosis of sarcoidosis. While the finding of bilateral hilar adenopathy is the hallmark of this disease, a similar pattern is occasionally observed in lymphoma, tuberculosis, coccidioidomycosis, brucellosis, and bronchogenic carcinoma.

The pattern of the gallium 67 scan is not diagnostic for sarcoidosis, nor is the finding of an increased proportion of lymphocytes among the cells recovered by bronchoalveolar lavage. However, the typical patterns of these tests (Fig. 292-2*B* and *C*) put the diagnosis in the general category of granulomatous lung disorders.

Whether or not the presentation is "classic," biopsy evidence of a mononuclear cell granulomatous inflammatory process is mandatory in order to make a definitive diagnosis of sarcoidosis. Because the lung is involved so frequently, it is the most common site to be biopsied, usually through a fiberoptic bronchoscope. Less common, but acceptable, sites for biopsy are the hilar nodes (by mediastinoscopy), the skin, conjunctiva, or lip. Rarely, the spleen, intraabdominal nodes, muscle, parotid or other salivary glands, upper respiratory tract, or the heart is biopsied for diagnostic purposes. At any of these sites, the findings must include the typical noncaseating granulomas. However, although histologic evidence is mandatory for a definitive diagnosis of sarcoidosis, the histologic findings are not sufficiently specific to make the diagnosis by themselves, since noncaseating granulomas are found in a number of other diseases, including infections and malignancy. Furthermore, although the liver or scalene nodes often reveal "positive" biopsies in cases of sarcoidosis, noncaseating granulomas from other causes are so frequent in these sites that they are not considered acceptable sites for establishing the diagnosis. Thus the definitive diagnosis of sarcoidosis is based on the biopsy in the context of the history, physical examination, blood tests, x-ray, lung function, and, if available, gallium 67 scan and bronchoalveolar lavage. Patients with immunodeficiency virus (HIV) infection commonly have lymphocytopenia, chest x-ray abnormalities, positive gallium 67 chest scans, and increased proportions of lavage lymphocytes (early in the course of the disease), and they can have lung granulomas, and thus serologic testing for HIV infection should always be done in individuals suspected of having sarcoidosis.

PROGNOSIS   Overall, the prognosis in sarcoidosis is good. Most individuals who present with the acute disease are left with no significant sequelae. Approximately half of all patients have some permanent organ dysfunction, but for most this is mild, stable, and progresses rarely. In approximately 15 to 20 percent of cases, the disease remains active or recurs intermittently. Death is attributable directly to the disease in about 10 percent of all those affected.

TREATMENT   The therapy of choice for sarcoidosis is glucocorticoids. A variety of other drugs have been tried, including indomethacin, oxyphenbutazone, chloroquine, methotrexate, *p*-aminobenzoate, allopurinol, levamisole, and cyclophosphamide, but there is no evidence, apart from anecdotal, uncontrolled reports, to support their efficacy. Cyclosporine is ineffective for the pulmonary manifestations of the disease; anecdotal reports suggest that it may be useful in extrathoracic sarcoid not responding to glucocorticoids.

The major problem in treating sarcoidosis is in deciding when to treat. Because the disease clears spontaneously in about 50 percent of patients, and because the permanent organ derangements often do not improve with glucocorticoids, there is controversy among clinicians as to the criteria for treatment. However, there is no question that glucocorticoids suppress effectively the activated T helper-inducer cell processes occurring at the sites of disease. Thus the major problem in making decisions concerning therapy in sarcoidosis is to determine the extent and activity of the inflammatory process in the organs at greatest risk, such as the lung, eye, heart, and central nervous system.

For the lung, this is based on a combination of history, physical findings, chest x-ray, and pulmonary function tests. Centers that see

large numbers of these individuals also use criteria based on gallium 67 lung scans and bronchoalveolar lavage findings. The serum level of the angiotensin-converting enzyme has been suggested as a criterion for disease activity, but it is not specific for the lung. Unless the respiratory impairment is devastating, active pulmonary sarcoidosis is observed usually without therapy for 2 to 3 months; if the inflammation does not subside spontaneously, therapy is instituted. For the eye, decisions concerning therapy are based on slit-lamp examination and tests for visual acuity. For the heart and central nervous system, decisions are based on an estimate of the severity of the involvement; patients with minor dysfunction are usually observed, while patients with significant cardiac or neurologic abnormalities are treated. Usually, it is not necessary to treat the systemic symptoms, but occasionally the extent of the fevers, fatigue, and/or weight loss will necessitate therapy.

The usual therapy for sarcoidosis is prednisone, 1 mg/kg, for 4 to 6 weeks, followed by a slow taper over 2 to 3 months. This is repeated if the disease again becomes active. Alternate-day therapy is used by some clinicians, but there is no evidence that it is as effective. High-dose bolus intravenous glucocorticoids are used occasionally but are probably not as effective as oral therapy. Inhaled glucocorticoids are not efficacious. Mild ocular disease responds usually to local therapy, but suppression of the uveitis often requires systemic glucocorticoids.

REFERENCES

CRYSTAL RG Interstitial lung disease of unknown etiology: Disorders characterized by chronic inflammation of the lower respiratory tract. N Engl J Med 310:154, 235, 1984

FANBURG BL, PITT EA: Sarcoidosis, in *Textbook of Respiratory Medicine*, JF Murray, JA Nadel (eds). Philadelphia, Saunders, 1988, pp 1486–1500

GRASSI C et al: *Sarcoidosis and Other Granulomatous Disorders, Proceedings of the XI World Congress.* Amsterdam, Excerpta Medica, 1988

DUBOIS R et al: Granulomatous processes, in *The Lung: Scientific Foundations*, RG Crystal, JB West (eds). New York, Raven, 1991, pp 1925–1938

JOHNS CJ: Sarcoidosis, in *Pulmonary Diseases and Disorders*, AP Fishman (ed). New York, McGraw-Hill, 1988, pp 645–666

MOLLER DR et al: Bias toward use of a specific T-cell receptor β-chain variable region in a subgroup of individuals with sarcoidosis. J Clin Invest 82:1183, 1988

PINKSTON P et al: Spontaneous release of interleukin-2 by lung T-lymphocytes in active pulmonary sarcoidosis. N Engl J Med 208:793, 1983

ROBINSON BWS et al: Gamma interferon is spontaneously released by alveolar macrophages and lung T-lymphocytes in patients with pulmonary sarcoidosis. J Clin Invest 75:1488, 1985

SALTINI C et al: Spontaneous release of interleukin-2 by lung T-lymphocytes in active pulmonary sarcoidosis is primarily from the Leu3 + DR + T-cell subset. J Clin Invest 77:1962, 1986

SHARMA OP: Pulmonary sarcoidosis and corticosteroids. Am Rev Resp Dis 147:1598, 1993

VENET A et al: Enhanced alveolar macrophage-mediated antigen-induced T-lymphocyte proliferation in sarcoidosis. J Clin Invest 75:293, 1985

293   FAMILIAL MEDITERRANEAN FEVER (FAMILIAL PAROXYSMAL POLYSEROSITIS)

SHELDON M. WOLFF

DEFINITION   Familial Mediterranean fever (FMF) is an inherited disorder of unknown etiology, characterized by recurrent episodes of fever, peritonitis, and/or pleuritis. Arthritis, skin lesions, and amyloidosis are seen in some patients.

TERMINOLOGY   The variety of names given to FMF has led to confusion concerning its clinical features. None of the names, including FMF, is completely satisfactory. *Benign paroxysmal peritonitis* is inappropriate because many of the patients have involvement of serosal surfaces other than the peritoneum, and some die of amyloidosis. *Familial paroxysmal polyserositis* is an acceptable alternative for the term *familial Mediterranean fever*.

ETHNOLOGY AND GENETICS FMF occurs predominantly in patients of non-Ashkenazi (Sephardic) Jewish, Armenian, and Arabic ancestry. However, the disease is not restricted to these groups, and has been seen in patients of Italian, Ashkenazi Jewish, and Anglo-Saxon descent as well as others.

The earliest studies of the genetics of FMF were done in Israel, where the disease appears to be inherited as an autosomal recessive. Nevertheless, approximately 50 percent of patients give no family history of the disease. Consanguinity among the parents of FMF patients is as high as 20 percent, a figure which may be an underestimate. Approximately 60 percent of patients are male.

A recent paper in which 27 non-Ashkenasi Jewish families were studied reported that the gene that most likely causes FMF is located in the short arm of chromosome 16. Of great importance should be data derived from similar studies on FMF patients from other ethnic groups.

ETIOLOGY Although numerous pathogenetic mechanisms have been suggested, the cause of FMF is unknown. Fever and inflammation are such prominent signs that frequent attempts have been made to implicate infectious agents and/or their products. However, extensive studies have failed to implicate these or any other specific infectious agents. Others have suggested a deficiency in an inhibitor of C5a, thus implicating alterations in the immune system. Substantiation of such potential pathogenic mechanisms is awaited.

Because many FMF patients note that certain emotional or environmental changes may have profound effects on the frequency with which episodes of their disease occur, a psychosomatic basis has been suggested for the illness. There is no question that most patients eventually have transient or even permanent psychological alterations, which probably reflect their reaction to a chronic recurring illness that is forever threatening their social, economic, and personal well-being, but there is no evidence for a functional etiology for FMF.

The demonstration that FMF is inherited as an autosomal recessive disorder has led to the thesis that it is another inborn error of metabolism. Despite extensive studies, no such error has been found. Reported instances of excessive urinary excretion of porphyrins in FMF are probably examples of true porphyria and not FMF.

PATHOLOGY Despite the striking clinical manifestations during an acute attack of FMF, no specific pathologic alterations have been found. At laparotomy, only acute peritoneal inflammation in which the exudate contains a predominance of polymorphonuclear leukocytes is found to be present. A disproportionately large number of male patients develop gallbladder disease with and without cholelithiasis, but extensive histopathologic examination has failed to reveal any specific pathologic changes. Pleural and joint inflammation are also nonspecific.

In the amyloidosis which accompanies FMF, amyloid is deposited in the intima and media of the arterioles, the subendothelial region of venules, the glomeruli, and the spleen. Aside from their vessels, the heart and liver are uninvolved.

MANIFESTATIONS In the majority of patients, the symptoms of FMF begin between the ages of 5 and 15, although attacks sometimes commence during infancy, and onset has occurred as late as age 52. The duration and frequency of attacks vary greatly in the same patient, and there is no set rhythm or periodicity to their occurrence. The usual acute episode lasts 24 to 48 h, but some may be prolonged for 7 to 10 days. The attacks range in frequency from twice weekly to once a year, but 2 to 4 weeks is the commonest interval. Spontaneous remissions lasting years have been seen. In the majority of cases, pregnancy is associated with an absence of acute episodes, and many patients note less frequent attacks in the summer than in the winter. There may be a decrease in the severity and frequency of the attacks with age or with development of amyloidosis.

Fever Fever is a cardinal manifestation of FMF and is present during most but not all attacks. Rarely, fever may be present without

serositis. The temperature may be preceded by a chill and will peak in 12 to 24 h. Defervescence is often accompanied by diaphoresis. The fever ranges from 38.5 to 40°C but is quite variable.

Abdominal pain Abdominal pain occurs in more than 95 percent of patients, and may vary in severity in the same patient. Minor premonitory discomfort may precede an acute episode by 24 to 48 h. The pain usually starts in one quadrant and then spreads to involve the whole abdomen. The initial site is usually very tender. Tenderness may remain localized with referred pain in other areas, and there may be radiation to the back. There may be splinting of the chest and pain in one or both shoulders, typical of diaphragmatic irritation. Nausea and vomiting sometimes occur. The abdomen is usually distended, and may become rigid with decreased or absent bowel sounds. On x-ray, the wall of the small intestine may appear edematous, transit of barium is slowed, and fluid levels may be seen. An abdominal operation may precipitate an acute attack of FMF which may be confused with other postoperative complications.

Chest pain Most patients with abdominal attacks have referred chest pain at one time or another, and 75 percent also develop acute pleuritic pain with or without abdominal symptoms. In 30 percent, the attacks of pleuritis precede the onset of abdominal attacks by varying periods of time, and a small number of patients never develop abdominal attacks. Chest pain is usually unilateral and is associated with diminished breath sounds, a friction rub, or a transient pleural effusion.

Joint pain In Israel, 75 percent of patients report at least one episode of acute arthritis. Arthritis can be distinct from abdominal or pleural attacks, can be acute or, rarely, chronic, and may involve one or several joints. Effusions are common and the large joints are involved most frequently. Radiologic findings are nonspecific. Despite careful search, frank arthritis rarely has been seen in the United States. Some patients have a history of rheumatic fever–like illness in childhood, but in a large series of patients, including 30 from the Middle East, acute arthritis was not observed. Mild arthralgia is common during acute attacks but is nonspecific.

Skin manifestations Skin involvement is reported by 25 to 35 percent of patients. These lesions consist of painful, erythematous areas of swelling from 5 to 20 cm in diameter, usually located on the lower legs, the medial malleolus, or the dorsum of the foot. They may occur without abdominal or pleural pain and subside within 24 to 48 h.

Other signs and symptoms Involvement of other serosal membranes has been reported, but pericarditis and meningitis are rare. Hematuria, splenomegaly, and small white dots called *colloid bodies* in the ocular fundus are among the findings of questionable significance. Rarely migraine-like headaches accompany acute abdominal attacks, and some patients have become somewhat irrational or show extreme emotional lability during attacks. Whether these are primary manifestations of FMF or secondary effects of pain and fever is not known.

Complications A serious, but increasingly rare, complication of FMF is drug addiction or habituation. Obviously, efforts should be made to avoid use of narcotics. Depression and lack of motivation are common, and patients with FMF require considerable encouragement and support. A striking number of patients in one American series have developed gallbladder disease.

Amyloidosis has been reported in Israel, North Africa, and elsewhere in the Middle East, but there have been only rare reported instances of amyloidosis complicating FMF in the United States. These findings are even more striking because there are probably as many known FMF patients in the United States as in Israel. These differences are unexplained and suggest that environmental or nutritional, as well as genetic, factors may play a role in the development of amyloidosis in FMF.

LABORATORY FINDINGS Polymorphonuclear leukocytosis ranging from 10,000 to 30,000 cells per microliter is almost invariable during acute attacks. The erythrocyte sedimentation rate is elevated during attacks but returns to normal between attacks. Plasma fibrinogen, serum haptoglobin, ceruloplasmin, and C-reactive protein increase during the episodes. Plasma lipids are normal, and there are no consistent abnormalities of hepatic or renal function. When amyloidosis is present, laboratory findings are typical of a nephrotic syndrome followed by renal insufficiency. Electrocardiographic and electroencephalographic changes are inconstant and nonspecific.

DIAGNOSIS When the typical acute attacks of FMF occur in an individual of appropriate ethnic background who has a family history of FMF, the diagnosis is easy. When a patient is seen for the first time, a variety of other febrile illnesses must be excluded by appropriate study or observation. These include acute appendicitis, acute pancreatitis, porphyria, cholecystitis, intestinal obstruction, and other major abdominal catastrophes.

Some of the inherited forms of the hyperlipidemias may mimic the clinical picture of FMF, but lipid analysis will eliminate them from consideration. The patient with FMF is not immune to other diseases, and when an attack differs from the usual pattern or is more prolonged, consideration should be given to other diagnostic possibilities. The pleural form of the disease is sometimes difficult to differentiate from acute pulmonary infection or infarction, but the rapid disappearance of signs and symptoms resolves the problem. The joint manifestations may be more prolonged than other forms of FMF, and differentiation from septic arthritis, gout, and acute rheumatoid disease may be necessary. The erythema is sometimes difficult to differentiate from superficial thrombophlebitis or cellulitis.

Whether or not the patient is of the appropriate ethnic group, the most difficult diagnostic problem in FMF is the patient who presents with fever alone. In this situation, an extensive diagnostic workup for fever of unknown origin may be required. Fortunately, such patients are rare, and all eventually develop serosal involvement. Until specific diagnostic tests for FMF are available, patients with recurrent fever but without signs of inflammation of one of the serosal membranes should not be categorized as having FMF.

It has been reported that FMF patients have increased levels of plasma dopamine beta-hydroxylase (RHP) activity and that these levels returned to normal during colchicine treatment. Others have not confirmed these findings.

PROGNOSIS Despite the severity of the symptoms during some acute attacks, most patients are remarkably free of any debilitation during the intervals between attacks. With encouragement and an understanding of their disease, most FMF patients lead fairly normal lives. The greatest hazard to patients is prolonged periods of hospitalization due to erroneous diagnoses or failure to understand the disease. In the United States, the prognosis of patients with FMF does not seem to be different from that of patients with other chronic nonfatal illnesses. Death usually results from causes unrelated to the underlying disease.

In the past, the complication of amyloidosis in Israel, parts of North Africa, Turkey, and other parts of the Middle East made the prognosis quite different from that in America. In the past, approximately 25 percent of FMF patients in Israel were known to have amyloidosis, and this complication usually led to death. However, the widespread use of colchicine has resulted in dramatically decreasing the incidence of amyloidosis.

TREATMENT Among the therapies tried have been antibiotics, hormones (including estrogens and adrenal corticosteroids), antipyretic drugs, immunotherapy, psychotherapy, elimination and low-fat diets, chloroquine, and phenylbutazone. When carefully studied and followed up, none of these therapies proved effective.

During the past 20 years, the outlook of patients with FMF has been altered dramatically. Goldfinger reported in 1972 that the prophylactic use of colchicine in five patients dramatically reduced the number of attacks. Subsequently, controlled trials in the United States and Israel have shown that chronic administration of colchicine will greatly reduce the number of acute attacks of FMF. It is recommended that 0.6 mg colchicine be taken by mouth three times a day. Patients often develop gastrointestinal side effects with this dose, however, in which case the dose should be reduced to 0.6 mg

taken twice a day. Although an occasional patient will respond to 0.6 mg taken only once a day, this amount is less likely to be beneficial. Most FMF patients will respond favorably to colchicine prophylaxis.

REFERENCES

DINARELLO CA et al: Colchicine therapy for familial Mediterranean fever. A double-blind trial. N Engl J Med 291:934, 1974

MATZNER Y et al: C5a-Inhibitor deficiency in peritoneal fluids from patients with familial Mediterranean Fever. N Engl J Med 314:1001, 1986

MEYERHOFF J: Familial Mediterranean fever: Report of a large family, review of the literature, and discussion of the frequency of amyloidosis. Medicine 59:66, 1980

PRAS E et al: Mapping of a gene causing familial Mediterranean fever to the short arm of chromosome 16. N Engl J Med 326:1509, 1992

ZEMER D et al: Colchicine in the prevention and treatment of the amyloidosis of familial Mediterranean fever. N Engl J Med 314:1001, 1986

294 MIDLINE GRANULOMA

SHELDON M. WOLFF

DEFINITION Midline granuloma is an uncommon disease characterized by localized inflammation, destruction, and often mutilation of the tissues of the upper respiratory tract and face. This condition has also been referred to as *lethal midline granuloma, malignant granuloma*, and *granuloma gangrenescens*, none of which is an appropriate term.

ETIOLOGY The etiology of midline granuloma is unknown. In view of the intense granulomatous inflammation, the disease is thought to represent a localized hypersensitivity reaction which leads to tissue destruction and mutilation. However, the responsible antigen(s) is unknown, and there is no immunologic evidence supporting this hypothesis. A variety of microorganisms have been considered as possible causative agents, but detailed microbiologic investigations have failed to detect the consistent presence of pathogenic organisms. In view of the clinical and pathologic features of the illness as well as the fact that some tumors, in particular, lymphomas, can elicit a similar intense inflammatory response, some authors have suggested a neoplastic basis for midline granuloma. However, when malignant tissue is found in the lesions, the diagnosis of midline granuloma is no longer tenable.

It is possible that midline granuloma is part of the spectrum of what has been recently termed *angiocentric immunoproliferative lesions*. The latter are considered to represent a spectrum of postthymic T cell proliferative lesions. In fact, the association of malignant reticulosis and also of lymphomatoid granulomatosis with this group seems justified. Whether ''idiopathic'' midline granuloma is an early or arrested form of angiocentric immunoproliferative lesions awaits the kind of sophisticated immunocytologic studies that have been performed in patients with T cell lymphoproliferative diseases.

PATHOLOGY The most characteristic pathologic finding is acute or chronic inflammation with necrosis. Superimposed pyogenic infection of the involved tissues, including the sinuses, may contribute to nonspecific histologic findings. The pathologic hallmark, noncaseating granulomas, with or without giant cells, may be obscured by the inflammatory reaction, but when present this is strong evidence in favor of the diagnosis. Primary vasculitis is seen rarely; when it occurs, a search for other causes, most notably Wegener's granulomatosis, should be made (see Chap. 291). The presence of malignant cells makes the diagnosis of midline granuloma unacceptable. Until a cause is established, the diagnosis of midline granuloma will rest on the characteristic clinical features outlined below.

CLINICAL FEATURES The disease may occur at any age, but the majority of patients are in the fifth and sixth decades. It is more common in women than men and has been reported in all races. Many patients report recurrent "sinus" problems, and some have histories of allergic rhinitis, although the significance of these features is unknown.

The major symptoms are usually related to the nose. Patients frequently complain of nasal stuffiness and occasionally of discharge. The first symptom in a smaller percentage of patients relates to ulceration of the mucosa of the nose, the buccal mucosa, or the gums. This has led to loosening of the teeth, and dentists are often consulted first by these patients. Rarely, patients will present first with eye findings related to conjunctival inflammation or even ulceration. Although the progression of symptoms in some patients may be slow, all too often the disease steadily, and sometimes rapidly, progresses. The characteristic symptoms of nasal discharge, difficulty in breathing through the nose, and pain over the sinuses, nose, or eye become more prominent with time. Once ulceration begins, the disease often progresses rapidly. The ulcers frequently involve the nasal septum and will lead to the characteristic septal perforation and a saddlenose deformity. The majority of patients develop ulceration and eventually perforations of the soft and hard palates. Untreated, the disease can lead to massive destruction and mutilation of the tissues involved, including the skin of the face and the eyes. Frequently, the necrotic tissue becomes infected, and systemic symptoms such as fever and anorexia appear. The destructive lesions can become very malodorous. The disease extends to involve local tissues and does not progress below the neck; if this happens, other diseases should be considered. As the necrotic process progresses and involves vital organs, patients may lose sight in the affected eye, experience dysphagia, and have difficulty in speech. Although spontaneous temporary remissions have been reported, untreated midline granuloma is fatal. The progression of the disease can be rapidly accelerated by surgical procedures in the affected areas. The patient usually dies from secondary infection, although erosion by the process into a major blood vessel or penetration into the central nervous system with superimposed meningitis can also cause death.

Aside from the granulomatous inflammation, necrosis, and destruction, no other specific clinical or pathologic findings are associated with midline granuloma. Occasionally, with superimposed infection, local lymphadenopathy may be noted, but it is not characteristic of the disease per se.

LABORATORY FINDINGS With progression of the disease, a variety of nonspecific abnormalities may be noted. These changes are characteristic of inflammatory processes in general or of secondary infections. For example, mild anemia, leukocytosis, elevated sedimentation rate, and hyperglobulinemia are common in these patients. Radiographic examination reveals pansinusitis, and as the disease advances, destruction of bone in the involved areas is characteristic.

DIFFERENTIAL DIAGNOSIS The diagnosis of midline granuloma is made by finding the characteristic histologic lesions in biopsies of the affected tissues. When the specimens show only inflammatory tissue, a presumptive diagnosis of midline granuloma can be made only when the characteristic clinical picture is present and other diseases with similar presentation have been excluded. The diagnosis of Wegener's granulomatosis is ruled out by the absence of vasculitis in the biopsy specimens and the localized nature of midline granuloma (i.e., no pulmonary or renal involvement). In addition, Wegener's granulomatosis rarely, if ever, causes erosion through facial tissues. It is often difficult to differentiate true midline granuloma from neoplasms of the upper airways such as malignant reticulosis and certain lymphomas. These may be clinically similar to midline granuloma and are often associated with granulomatous inflammation. Careful examination of generous biopsy material as well as concomitant workup for disseminated neoplasm often provides the clinicopathologic distinction. Other diseases to be excluded by appropriate laboratory techniques are histoplasmosis, blastomycosis, coccidioidomycosis, leprosy, tuberculosis, syphilis, mucocutaneous leishmaniasis, rhinoscleroma, and pseudotumor of the orbit. Occasional patients who inhale cocaine develop septal perforations with inflammation that may be difficult to differentiate from midline granuloma (if the patients deny cocaine abuse).

TREATMENT The complications of midline granuloma such as superimposed infections can be treated specifically. Although adrenal glucocorticoids are often used in the therapy of midline granuloma, they are of no value and probably are contraindicated if infection is present. Sporadic reports of therapy with cytotoxic agents are difficult to interpret, since some of the patients reported clearly had lymphoma or Wegener's granulomatosis, diseases where such agents are of definite value. However, some patients appear to respond to cytotoxic chemotherapy. Surgical removal of the involved tissue has been attempted but is useless and may, in fact, cause rapid progression of the disease.

The treatment of choice is radiotherapy to the local lesion. Although low dosages [1000 cGy (1000 rad) and below] have been reported to be effective, many patients relapse after such therapy. Radiotherapy should be given in a dose of 5000 cGy (5000 rad) to the involved areas. Where such a regimen is employed, long-lasting remissions (more than 20 years) and probable cures have been achieved. Following irradiation and after an appropriate period to allow for tissue healing (usually 1 year), reconstructive and plastic surgery, which may be of enormous cosmetic and functional value, can be undertaken.

REFERENCES

Fauci AS et al: Radiation therapy of midline granuloma. Ann Intern Med 84:140, 1976

Fechner RE, Lamppin DW: Midline malignant reticulosis. Arch Otolaryngol 95:467, 1972

Grange C et al: Centrofacial malignant granulomas. Medicine 71:179, 1992

Lipford EH Jr: Angiocentric immunoproliferative lesions: A clinicopathologic spectrum of post-thymic T-cell proliferation. Blood 72:1674, 1988

section 3 Disorders of the joints

295 APPROACH TO ARTICULAR AND MUSCULOSKELETAL DISORDERS

JOHN J. CUSH / PETER E. LIPSKY

Musculoskeletal complaints account for more than 10 percent of all outpatient evaluations in general medical practice. Many of the musculoskeletal complaints that cause patients to seek medical attention are related to self-limited conditions requiring minimal evaluation and only symptomatic therapy and reassurance. However, some patients with similar symptoms may have a more serious condition that requires additional laboratory testing to confirm the suspected diagnosis or document the extent and nature of the pathologic process. The initial goal of the clinician is to diagnose accurately and provide timely therapy while avoiding excessive diagnostic testing and unnecessary treatment.

Individuals with musculoskeletal complaints should be evaluated in a uniform, logical manner with a thorough history, a comprehensive physical examination, and appropriate laboratory testing. With such an approach and an understanding of the pathophysiologic processes underlying musculoskeletal complaints, an adequate diagnosis can be made in the vast majority of individuals. However, some patients will not fit immediately into an established diagnostic category. Many musculoskeletal disorders resemble each other at the outset and may take months or even years to evolve fully into a specific, recognizable syndrome. Such knowledge should temper the desire to establish a definitive diagnosis at the first encounter. A logical approach to the evaluation of patients with musculoskeletal complaints is shown in Fig. 295-1.

A paramount objective during the initial encounter is to determine whether the condition requires additional evaluation or immediate therapy. To make this decision, a knowledge of the particular anatomic site(s) of involvement (articular, periarticular, or extraarticular) and the nature of the pathologic process (inflammatory or noninflammatory) is important (Table 295-1). In addition to the four cardinal signs of inflammation (erythema, warmth, pain, and swelling), inflammatory disorders may manifest morning stiffness, fever, systemic symptoms, and/or laboratory evidence of inflammation (i.e., elevated erythrocyte sedimentation rate, thrombocytosis, etc.). Information derived from the patient's symptoms and signs allows the clinician to narrow the diagnostic considerations and assess the need for immediate diagnostic testing, therapeutic intervention, or continued observation over a period of time.

CLINICAL HISTORY Historic features of the disorder are important in establishing the nature and extent of the pathologic process and also may provide important clues to the diagnosis. Aspects of the patient profile, including age, sex, race, and family history, can provide important information. Certain diagnoses are more frequent in different *age* groups. Systemic lupus erythematosus, rheumatic fever, and Reiter's syndrome occur more frequently in the young, whereas fibrositis is most frequent in middle age and osteoarthritis and polymyalgia rheumatica are more prevalent among the elderly. Diagnostic clustering is also evident when *sex* and *race* are considered. Gout and the spondyloarthropathies are more common in men, whereas rheumatoid arthritis and fibrositis are more frequent in women. Racial predilections are noted with disorders such as polymyalgia rheumatica and giant cell arteritis (whites) and sarcoidosis (blacks). *Familial aggregation* may be seen in disorders such as ankylosing spondylitis, gout, rheumatoid arthritis, and Heberden's nodes of osteoarthritis.

The type of clinical presentation also provides important diagnostic clues. The *mode of onset* is characteristically acute in septic arthritis or gout, whereas osteoarthritis, rheumatoid arthritis, and fibrositis may have more indolent presentations.

Precipitating events such as trauma, drug administration, or antecedent illnesses should be sought. The *number and pattern* of involved structures often provide useful information. Complaints secondary to trauma and gout are typically focal, whereas others, such as polymyositis, rheumatoid arthritis, and fibrositis, are more diffuse. Rheumatoid arthritis tends to be symmetric, whereas the spondyloarthropathies are asymmetric. The upper extremities are frequently involved in rheumatoid arthritis, whereas lower extremity arthritis is characteristic of Reiter's syndrome and gout at their onsets. Involvement of the axial skeleton is common in ankylosing spondylitis but is infrequent in rheumatoid arthritis, with the notable exception of the cervical spine. The *chronology and evolution* of the patient's complaints also may be useful in suggesting diagnostic possibilities. Chronic (osteoarthritis), intermittent (gout), migratory (rheumatic fever), and additive (Reiter's syndrome) patterns are suggestive of certain disease processes. The duration of signs and symptoms alters the diagnostic considerations. Thus the musculoskeletal signs and symptoms of hepatitis B virus infection may be identical with those of early rheumatoid arthritis, but they rarely persist beyond 2 to 3 weeks.

Associated features outside the musculoskeletal system also may provide useful diagnostic information. A variety of musculoskeletal disorders may be associated with systemic features such as fever (systemic lupus erythematosus, infection), rash (systemic lupus erythematosus, Reiter's syndrome, dermatomyositis), or morning stiffness (inflammatory arthritis). In addition, some are associated with involvement of other organs, including the eyes (Behçet's disease, sarcoid, Reiter's syndrome), the organs of the gastrointestinal tract (scleroderma, inflammatory bowel disease), the genitourinary tract (Reiter's syndrome, gonococcemia), or the nervous system (Lyme disease, vasculitis).

PHYSICAL EXAMINATION The goal of the physical examination is to ascertain the structures involved, the nature of the disorder, the extent and functional consequences of the process, and the presence of systemic manifestations. A knowledge of topographic anatomy is necessary to identify the primary site(s) of involvement and differentiate between articular, periarticular, and extraarticular disease. The musculoskeletal evaluation is largely dependent on careful inspection, palpation, and a variety of specific physical maneuvers to elicit diagnostic signs.

Examination of involved and uninvolved joints will determine the absence or presence of *warmth*, *erythema*, or *swelling*. The examination should distinguish true articular swelling caused by synovial effusion or synovial proliferation from periarticular involvement which usually extends beyond the normal joint margins. Synovial effusion can be distinguished from synovial hypertrophy or bony hypertrophy by palpation. Bursal effusions (i.e., olecranon, prepatellar) overlie bony prominences and are fluctuant with sharply defined borders. Joint *stability* can be assessed by palpation and by the

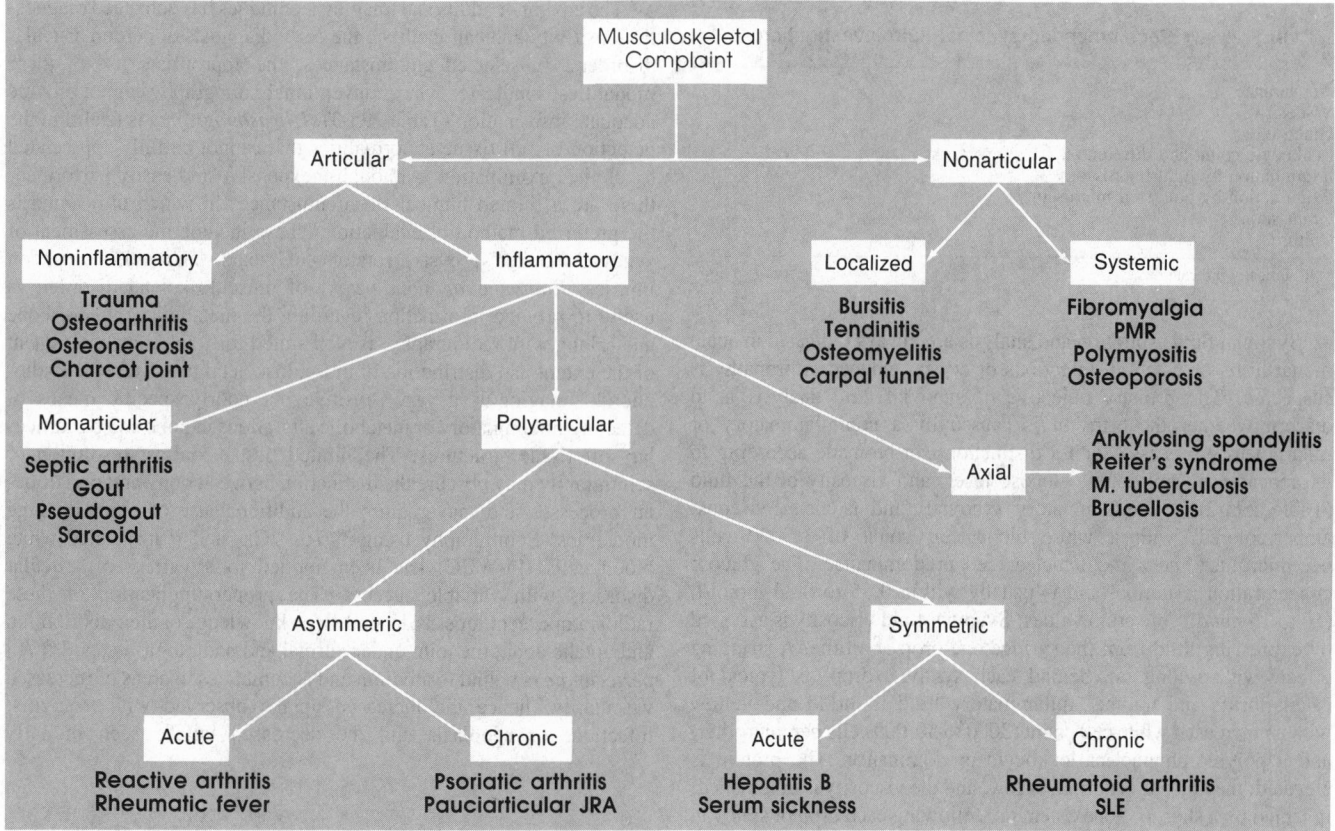

FIGURE 295-1 Approach to musculoskeletal disorders. An algorithm based on several rheumatologic symptoms and signs enables the physician to formulate a differential diagnosis (shown in italics) (PMR, polymyalgia rheumatica; SLE, systemic lupus erythematosus; JRA, juvenile rheumatoid arthritis).

application of manual stress. Subluxation or dislocation, which may be secondary to traumatic, mechanical, or inflammatory causes, can be assessed by inspection and palpation. Joint *volume* can be assessed by palpation. Distention of the articular capsule by various processes causes pain. The patient will attempt to minimize the pain by maintaining the joint in the position of greatest volume and least intraarticular pressure, usually partial flexion. Clinically, this may be reflected as obvious swelling, voluntary or eventually fixed flexion deformities, or diminished range of motion, especially on extension when joint volumes are decreased. Active and passive *range of motion* should be assessed in all planes and is best quantified by a goniometer with contralateral comparison. Joint *crepitus* may be felt during these maneuvers and may be prominent in degenerative disorders. Limitation of motion is frequently caused by effusion, pain, deformity, or

contracture. Contractures may be an indication of antecedent synovial inflammation or trauma. Joint *deformity* usually indicates a long-standing pathologic process. Deformities may result from ligament destruction, soft tissue contracture, bony enlargement, ankylosis, erosive disease, or subluxation. Examination of the musculature will document strength and the presence of atrophy and also will elicit pain or spasm. The examiner should assess carefully for periarticular involvement, especially when articular complaints are not supported by objective findings referable to the joint capsule. The identification of musculoskeletal pain of soft tissue origin (periarticular or extraarticular) will prevent unwarranted and often expensive further evaluations.

ADDITIONAL INVESTIGATIONS   The vast majority of musculoskeletal disorders can be easily diagnosed by a complete history and physical examination. However, in a number of circumstances, additional investigations may be required to establish the diagnosis or confirm a suspected etiology. A number of features indicate the need for additional evaluation. Patients with *acute monarticular* conditions require additional evaluation, as do those who present with *traumatic* or *inflammatory* conditions or those with *neurologic changes* or *systemic manifestations* of serious disease. Finally, individuals with *chronic (>6 weeks)* symptoms, even of minor severity, are candidates for additional evaluation. The extent and nature of the additional investigation should be dictated by the pattern of the involvement and suspected pathologic process. Broad batteries of diagnostic tests and radiographic procedures are rarely a useful or cost-effective means to establish a diagnosis.

Besides a complete blood count, including a white blood cell and differential count, the routine evaluation should include a determination of the erythrocyte sedimentation rate or C-reactive protein, which can be useful in discriminating inflammatory from noninflammatory musculoskeletal disorders. Serum uric acid determinations are only useful when clinically indicated.

TABLE 295-1   Characterizing musculoskeletal disorders

Anatomic sites of involvement	Pathologic processes
Articular	**Inflammatory**
Synovium	Infectious
Articular cartilage	Crystal-induced
Juxtaarticular bone	Immunologic
Other—menisci, capsule	Reactive
Periarticular	Idiopathic
Tendon	**Noninflammatory**
Bursa	Traumatic
Ligament	Mechanical or degenerative
Extraarticular	Functional
Bone	Neoplastic
Muscle	Other
Nerve	
Fascia	
Skin and subcutaneous tissue	

TABLE 295-2 Recommended synovial fluid investigation

Appearance
Viscosity
Glucose
Leukocyte count and differential
Examination by light microscopy
Examination by polarized microscopy
Gram stain*
Culture*

* If clinically indicated.

Synovial fluid aspiration and analysis are always indicated in acute monarthritis or when an infectious or crystal-induced arthropathy is suspected. The primary objective of synovial fluid analysis is to discern whether the effusion is caused by a noninflammatory or inflammatory process. Such a distinction can be made according to its appearance, cell count, glucose level, and viscosity of the fluid (Table 295-2). Noninflammatory synovial fluid is clear, viscous, amber-colored, with a white blood cell count of <3000 cells per microliter and a mononuclear cell predominance. The glucose concentration is normal and is usually within 0.55 to 0.83 mmol/L (10 to 15 mg/dL) of serum values. Synovial fluid viscosity is assessed by expressing fluid from the syringe one drop at a time. A stringing effect, with a long tail behind each synovial drop, is typical of osteoarthritis and trauma. Inflammatory fluid is turbid and yellow with an increased white cell count (3000 to 50,000 cells per microliter) and a polymorphonuclear leukocyte predominance. The protein is elevated, the glucose is normal or low, and the viscosity is diminished, reflected by a short or nonexistent tail following each drop of synovial fluid. Such effusions are found in rheumatoid arthritis, gout, other inflammatory arthritides, and occasionally septic arthritis. Infectious fluid is turbid and opaque, with a white cell count >50,000 cells per microliter and a polymorphonuclear leukocyte predominance. The protein is elevated, the glucose is often low, and viscosity is poor. Such effusions are typical of septic arthritis but may rarely occur with sterile inflammatory arthritides such as rheumatoid arthritis or gout. Additionally, hemorrhagic synovial fluid may be seen with hemarthrosis or trauma. Synovial fluid should be analyzed immediately for cellularity and crystals using a polarizing microscope. Monosodium urate, seen in gouty effusions, appears as long, needle-shaped, negatively birefringent, usually intracellular crystals, whereas calcium pyrophosphate dihydrate, found in chondrocalcinosis and pseudogout, is usually seen as short, rhomboid-shaped, positively birefringent crystals. Whenever infection is a possibility, synovial fluid should be Gram-stained and cultured appropriately. If gonococcal arthritis is suspected, immediate plating of the fluid on appropriate culture medium is indicated. It should be noted that on occasion both crystal-induced arthritis and infection may occur in the same joint.

Serologic tests for rheumatoid factor (antibodies to IgG), antinuclear antibodies, complement levels, or antistreptolysin O titers should be carried out only when there is clinical evidence to suggest a specific diagnosis, since these have poor predictive value as screening tests.

DIAGNOSTIC IMAGING IN JOINT DISEASES Historically, *conventional radiography* has played an integral part in the diagnosis and staging of articular disorders. Plain films are most appropriate when there is a history of prior trauma, suspected chronic infection, progressive disability, or monarticular involvement; when therapeutic alterations are considered; or when they are useful as a baseline assessment for what appears to be a chronic process. However, in most inflammatory disorders, early radiography is rarely helpful in establishing a diagnosis and often reveals only soft tissue swelling and juxtaarticular demineralization. As the disease progresses, calcification (soft tissue, cartilage, or bone), joint space narrowing, erosions, bony ankylosis, new bone formation (sclerosis, osteophytes, or periostitis), or subchondral cysts may develop and provide diagnostic information. The use of high-quality films and proper positioning can eliminate the need for further studies.

The advent of additional imaging techniques has enhanced diagnostic sensitivity and can facilitate the early diagnosis of certain articular disorders. In selected circumstances, the appropriate use of these modalities is indicated when conventional radiography cannot provide adequate information (Table 295-3). *Ultrasonography* is useful in the detection of soft tissue abnormalities that cannot be fully appreciated by clinical eximination. Although inexpensive and easily performed, there are a limited number of circumstances in which ultrasound is the preferred method of evaluation. These include the assessment of synovial (Baker's) cysts, rotator cuff tears, and various tendon injuries. *Radionuclide scintigraphy* of musculoskeletal disorders is useful to provide information regarding the metabolic status of bone and, along with radiography, is well suited for total-body assessment of the extent and distribution of musculoskeletal involvement. Radionuclide imaging is a very sensitive but poorly specific means of detecting inflammatory or metabolic alterations in bone and periarticular soft tissue structures. The limited tissue contrast resolution of scintigraphy may obscure the distinction between bony and periarticular processes and may require the additional use of other imaging modalities. Scintigraphy using ^{99m}Tc, ^{67}Ga, and ^{111}In-labeled white blood cells (In-WBC) has been applied to a variety of articular disorders with variable success. The proper application of these radioisotope techniques is dependent on knowledge of their distribution and uptake about the joint under normal and pathologic states. [^{99m}Tc] *pertechnate* is bound to albumin and accumulates in areas of increased vascularity, hence the increased uptake observed with synovitis, infection, or neoplasia and the decreased uptake seen in early

TABLE 295-3 Diagnostic imaging techniques for musculoskeletal disorders

	Imaging time (h)	Cost*	Imaging capacity	Indications
ULTRASOUND†				
	<1	+	Focal	Synovial cysts, rotator cuff tears, tendon injury
RADIONUCLIDE SCINTIGRAPHY				
^{99m}Tc	1–4	+ +	Diffuse	Metastatic bone survey, evaluation of Paget's disease, quantitative joint assessment, acute infection, acute and chronic osteomyelitis
^{111}In-WBC	24	+ + +	Diffuse	Acute infection, prosthetic infection, acute osteomyelitis
^{67}Ga	24–48	+ + + +	Diffuse	Acute and chronic infection, acute osteomyelitis
COMPUTED TOMOGRAPHY				
	<1	+ + +	Focal	Herniated intervertebral disk, sacroiliitis, spinal stenosis, spinal trauma, osteoid osteoma, tarsal coalition
MAGNETIC RESONANCE IMAGING				
	1/2–2	+ + + + +	Focal	Avascular necrosis, osteomyelitis, intraarticular derangement and soft tissue injury, derangments of axial skeleton and spinal cord, pigmented villonodular synovitis, inflammatory and metabolic muscle pathology

* Relative imaging cost.
† Operator dependent.

FIGURE 295-2 [^{99m}Tc] diphosphonate scintigraphy of the feet of a 33-year-old black male with Reiter's syndrome, manifested by sacroiliitis, urethritis, uveitis, asymmetric oligoarthritis, and enthesitis. This bone scan demonstrates increased uptake indicative of enthesitis involving the insertions of the left Achilles tendon, plantar aponeurosis, and the right tibialis posterior tendon and arthritis of the right first interphalangeal joint.

FIGURE 295-3 Superior sensitivity of magnetic resonance imaging in the diagnosis of osteonecrosis of the femoral head. A 25-year-old white male taking high-dose glucocorticoids for idiopathic thrombocytopenic purpura developed bilateral hip pain. Conventional x-ray films (*A*) demonstrated abnormalities only in the right hip consistent with stage II osteonecrosis (arrow). A bone scan (*B*) revealed increased uptake in the right hip only (arrow). MRI using spin-echo proton density images (*C* and *D*) demonstrated low-density signals from both femoral heads (arrows), indicative of bilateral osteonecrosis.

osteonecrosis. By contrast, [^{99m}Tc] *diphosphonate* is utilized as a bone-seeking radionuclide, whose distribution is dependent on blood flow and uptake during new bone formation. Increased uptake is seen with inflammation, increased blood flow, bone remodeling, and heterotopic bone formation (Fig. 295-2). The poor specificity of ^{99m}Tc scanning has limited its use to investigational and serial assessments of joint/bone involvement, inflammatory or infectious processes, and metastatic bone surveys. ^{67}Ga binds to serum and cellular transferrin and lactoferrin and is preferentially taken up by neutrophils, macrophages, bacteria, and tumor tissue (i.e., lymphoma) and is thus useful in the identification of infection and malignancies. Scanning with ^{111}In-WBC has been used to detect both infectious and inflammatory arthritis. Although both have been used with success, ^{111}In-WBC scanning is superior to ^{67}Ga in the early diagnosis of osteomyelitis and infected prosthetic joints. Prior treatment with antibiotics reduces the diagnostic sensitivities of both ^{67}Ga and ^{111}In-WBC scintigraphy. Other radionuclide conjugates (i.e., [^{111}In]chloride, ^{111}In- and ^{125}I-labeled polyclonal IgG, [^{99m}Tc]liposomes, and [^{99m}Tc]hexamethylpropyleneamine oxine) have been developed and used with variable success in the detection of infectious or inflammatory musculoskeletal disorders. Further comparative studies are needed to define the diagnostic indications for these modalities.

Computed tomography (CT) provides rapid reconstruction of sagittal, coronal, and axial images and spatial relationships among anatomic structures. It has proved to be most useful in the assessment of the axial skeleton because of its ability to visualize in the axial plane. Articulations previously considered difficult to visualize using conventional radiography, such as the zygoapophyseal, sacroiliac, sternoclavicular, and hip joints, can be evaluated effectively using CT. CT has been demonstrated to be useful in the diagnosis of low-back pain syndromes, sacroiliitis, avascular necrosis, osteoid osteoma, tarsal coalition, osteomyelitis, and intraarticular osteochondral fragments.

Magnetic resonance imaging (MRI) has emerged as a significant advancement in musculoskeletal imaging. MRI has the advantages of providing multiplanar images with fine anatomic detail and contrast resolution (Figs. 295-3 and 295-4). Moreover, the lack of ionizing radiation and adverse effects and the superior ability to visualize bone marrow and soft tissue periarticular structures have led to increased use of this modality. The advantages of MRI are counterbalanced by high costs and long procedural time, factors that have limited its use in the evaluation of musculoskeletal disorders. Therefore, it is recommended that MRI only be employed when less expensive and noninvasive modalities fail to provide necessary information that will affect the patient's clinical management.

MRI is capable of imaging fascia, vessels, nerve, muscle, cartilage, ligaments, tendons, pannus, synovial effusions, cortical bone, and bone marrow. Visualization of these structures can be enhanced by altering enumerable pulse sequences. In musculoskeletal imaging, the most frequently utilized techniques include T1-weighted and T2-weighted spin-echo, gradient-echo, and inversion recovery (including STIR) images. T1-weighted images usually demonstrate superior anatomic detail, whereas T2-weighted images enhance the visualization of soft tissues enriched in water molecules, thereby facilitating the visualization of fluid, edema, inflammation, and tumors. Structures containing few mobile hydrogen protons (cortical bone, fibrocartilage, tendons, and ligaments) will appear dark or black on T1- and T2-

FIGURE 295-4 Coronal magnetic resonance images of the wrist in a 54-year-old female with rheumatoid arthritis. *A*. T1-weighted image demonstrates an erosion of the triquetrum (arrow). *B*. Gadopentetate dimeglumine enhanced T1-weighted image demonstrates enhancement of the same erosion (arrow), indicating the presence of vascularized pannus. *C*. Inversion recovery (STIR) image demonstrates a fluid-dense, high-intensity signal near the triquetrum (arrow) and in the intercarpal spaces, suggesting widespread intercarpal inflammation.

TABLE 295-4 Musculoskeletal disorders in the elderly

INFLAMMATORY

Polymyalgia rheumatica/giant cell arteritis
Vasculitis (polyarteritis, cholesterol emboli syndrome)
Crystal arthropathies (gout, pseudogout)
Septic arthritis
Older-onset lupus

MECHANICAL

Osteoarthritis
Spinal stenosis
Low back pain
Trauma
Heel spurs

METABOLIC/ENDOCRINE

Osteoporosis
Paget's disease
Hypothyroidism/myxedema
Amyloid
Diabetes

NEOPLASIA-RELATED

Secondary gout
Carcinomatous arthropathy or neuromyopathy
Dermatomyositis
Sjögren's syndrome
Vasculitis (lymphoma, hairy cell leukemia)
Cryoglobulinemia
Panniculitis (pancreatic cancer, lymphoproliferative disorders)
Hypertrophic osteoarthropathy
Metastasis to bone
Atrial myxoma

DRUG-INDUCED

Gout (diuretics, low-dose salicylates, cytotoxics, alcohol)
Drug-induced lupus (procainamide, hydralazine, methyldopa, phenytoin, isoniazid, quinidine)
Myopathy (glucocorticoids, lovastatin, clofibrate, taxol, colchicine, penicillamine, hydroxychloroquine)
Osteonecrosis (glucocorticoids, ethanol, radiation, hip surgery)
Osteopenia (glucocorticoids, heparin, phenytoin)
Toxicity (salicylates, NSAIDs, narcotics)

EVALUATION OF THE ELDERLY FOR RHEUMATIC DISEASES

Musculoskeletal disorders in geriatric patients are often not diagnosed because signs and symptoms in the elderly may be insidious in onset and chronic in nature. In addition, older individuals frequently possess multiple interactive variables, including other medical conditions and therapies that may obscure the nature of the problem. This is compounded by the diminished reliability of laboratory testing in the elderly owing to the wider range of nonpathologic serologic variability, including elevated erythrocyte sedimentation rates and low titers of rheumatoid factor or antinuclear antibodies. Although nearly all rheumatic disorders can afflict the elderly, certain diseases and drug-induced disorders are more common in this age group (Table 295-4). The elderly should be approached in the same manner used for all patients with musculoskeletal complaints, with additional inquiry to exclude common geriatric musculoskeletal disorders. An emphasis on identifying the rheumatic consequences of intercurrent medical conditions and therapies is extremely important. Drug-induced lupus erythematosus, polymyalgia rheumatica, gout, and chronic salicylate toxicity are all more common in the elderly. The physical examination should emphasize coexistent disease that may influence subsequent diagnosis and treatment.

REFERENCES

Brower AC: Imaging techniques and modalities, in *Arthritis in Black and White*, AC Brower (ed). Philadelphia, Saunders, 1988, p 1

Calins E: Arthritis in the elderly. Bull Rheum Dis 40(3):1, 1991

Fries JF: Assessment of the patient with rheumatic disease, in *Textbook of Rheumatology*, 4th ed, WN Kelley et al (eds). Philadelphia, Saunders, 1993

Hasselbacher P: Arthrocentesis and synovial fluid analysis, in *Primer on the Rheumatic Diseases*, HR Schumacher Jr et al (eds). Atlanta, Arthritis Foundation, 1988, pp 55–60

Michet CJ, Hunder GG: Examination of the joints, in *Textbook of Rheumatology* 4th ed, WN Kelley et al (eds). Philadelphia, Saunders, 1993

Murakami DM et al: Advances in imaging of rheumatoid arthritis. Clin Orthop 265:83, 1991

Shmerling RH, Delbanco TL: The rheumatoid factor: An analysis of clinical utility. Am J Med 91:528, 1991

——— et al: Synovial fluid tests: What should be ordered? JAMA 264:1009, 1990

Stoller DW, Genant JK: Magnetic resonance imaging of the knee and hip. Arthritis Rheum 33:441, 1990

Tumeh SS, Tohmeh AG: Nuclear medicine techniques in septic arthritis and osteomyelitis. Rheum Dis Clin North Am 17:559, 1991

Wernick R: Avoiding laboratory test misinterpretation in geriatric rheumatology. Geriatrics 44:61, 1989

weighted images. The high fat content in bone marrow produces a bright signal on T1- and T2-weighted images and is nullified on STIR images. Whereas static fluid and fluid-dense structures appear dark to intermediate on T1-weighted images and bright on T2-weighted and STIR images, flowing blood does not generate a signal. As a result, vessels appear dark or black on most standard spin-echo sequences. Muscle, nerve, articular cartilage, and proliferative synovium demonstrate an intermediate signal on T1-weighted images and decreases on T2-weighted sequences.

Because of its sensitivity to changes in marrow fat, MRI has been shown to be a sensitive but nonspecific means of detecting osteonecrosis and osteomyelitis. The enhanced soft tissue contrast resolution of MRI is superior to arthrography and CT in the diagnosis of soft tissue injuries (i.e., meniscal and rotator cuff tears), intraarticular derangements, and spinal cord damage following vertebral injury, subluxation, and synovitis. MRI is also useful in the diagnosis of pigmented villonodular synovitis. In this condition, the synovial tissues are enriched in hemosiderin-laden macrophages, leading to a low signal intensity on T1- and T2-weighted images because of the paramagnetic effects of iron.

Newer imaging techniques such as gadopentetate dimeglumine–enhanced MRI, single-photon-emission computed tomography (SPECT), positron-emission tomography (PET), and magnetic resonance spectroscopy offer enhanced resolution and metabolic imaging of affected tissues. These modalities are currently investigational, and their clinical applicability remains to be determined.

296 OSTEOARTHRITIS

KENNETH D. BRANDT*

Osteoarthritis (OA), also termed *degenerative joint disease*, represents failure of the diarthrodial (movable, synovial-lined) joint. In idiopathic (primary) OA, the most common form of the disease, no predisposing factor is apparent. Secondary OA is pathologically indistinguishable from idiopathic OA but is attributable to an underlying cause (Table 296-1).

EPIDEMIOLOGY/RISK FACTORS   OA is the most common joint disease of mankind. Knee OA is the leading cause of chronic disability in developed countries; some 100,000 people in the United States are unable to walk independently from bed to the bathroom because of OA of the knee or hip.

Under the age of 55 years, the joint distribution of OA in men and women is similar; in older individuals, hip OA is more common in men, while OA of interphalangeal joints and the thumb base is

* The author acknowledges the contribution of Karen Kovalov-St. John to this chapter in the 12th edition.

TABLE 296-1 Classification of OA

IDIOPATHIC

Localized
  Hands: Heberden's and Bouchard's nodes (nodal), erosive interphalangeal arthritis (nonnodal), carpal-1st metacarpal
  Feet: hallux valgus, hallux rigidus, contracted toes (hammer/cock-up toes), talonavicular
  Knee:
    Medial compartment
    Lateral compartment
    Patellofemoral compartment
  Hip:
    Eccentric (superior)
    Concentric (axial, medial)
    Diffuse (coxae senilis)
  Spine:
    Apophyseal joints
    Intervertebral joints (disk)
    Spondylosis (osteophytes)
    Ligamentous (hyperostosis, Forestier's disease, diffuse idiopathic skeletal hyperostosis)
  Other single sites, e.g., glenohumeral, acromioclavicular, tibiotalar, sacroiliac, temporomandibular
Generalized (GOA): Includes three or more areas listed above (Kellgren-Moore)

SECONDARY

Trauma
  Acute
  Chronic (occupational, sports)
Congenital or developmental
  Localized diseases: Legg-Calvé-Perthes, congenital hip dislocation, slipped epiphysis
  Mechanical factors: unequal lower extremity length, valgus/varus deformity, hypermobility syndromes
  Bone dysplasias: epiphyseal dysplasia, spondyloapophyseal dysplasia, osteonychodystrophy
Metabolic
  Ochronosis (alkaptonuria)
  Hemochromatosis
  Wilson's disease
  Gaucher's disease
Endocrine
  Acromegaly
  Hyperparathyroidism
  Diabetes mellitus
  Obesity
  Hypothyroidism
Calcium deposition diseases
  Calcium pyrophosphate dihydrate deposition
  Apatite arthropathy
Other bone and joint diseases
  Localized: fracture, avascular necrosis, infection, gout
  Diffuse: rheumatoid (inflammatory) arthritis, Paget's disease, osteopetrosis, osteochondritis
Neuropathic (Charcot joints)
Endemic
  Kashin-Beck
  Mseleni
Miscellaneous
  Frostbite
  Caisson's disease
  Hemoglobinopathies

SOURCE: From Mankin et al.

TABLE 296-2 Risk factors for OA

Age
Female sex
Race
Genetic factors
Major joint trauma*
Repetitive stress, e.g., vocational*
Obesity*
Congenital/developmental defects*
Prior inflammatory joint disease
Metabolic/endocrine disorders

* Potentially modifiable
SOURCE: After Hochberg M, J Rheumatol 18:1438, 1991.

Thus the mother of a woman with distal interphalangeal joint OA (Heberden's nodes) is twice as likely to exhibit OA in these joints—and the proband's sister three times as likely—as the mother and sister of an unaffected woman. A point mutation in the cDNA coding for type II collagen was identified recently in several generations of a family with chondrodysplasia and polyarticular secondary OA. The prevalence of genetic abnormalities in matrix molecules will be a major focus of OA research in the coming years.

The most powerful risk factor for OA is age. A progressive increase in prevalence of OA is seen with increasing age. In a radiographic survey of women less than 45 years of age, only 2 percent had OA; between the ages of 45 to 64 years, however, the prevalence was 30 percent, while for those older than 65 years it was 68 percent. In males, the figures were similar but somewhat lower in the older age groups.

Major trauma and repetitive joint use both are risk factors for OA. In both humans and animal models, anterior cruciate ligament insufficiency and meniscus damage (and removal) lead to knee OA. Damage to the articular cartilage may occur at the time of injury or subsequently (during use of the affected joint), but even normal cartilage will degenerate when the joint is unstable.

The pattern of joint involvement is influenced by prior vocational or avocational overload. Thus ankle OA is common in ballet dancers and metacarpophalangeal joint OA in prize fighters, while OA is not common at either of these sites in the general population. The person with a trimalleolar fracture will almost certainly develop ankle OA.

In view of the growing participation of the population of this country in sports in general and in running in particular, it is important to note that there are no convincing data to support an association between specific athletic activities and arthritis if major trauma is excluded. This may, however, be due to the lack of good long-term studies and the difficulty of retrospective assessment of activities. Thus long-distance running and jogging have not been noted to cause OA, although selection bias, i.e., early discontinuation of the activity by those incurring joint damage, cannot be excluded.

In contrast, activities such as those performed by jackhammer operators, cotton mill workers, shipyard workers, coal miners, and others have been shown to lead to OA in those joints exposed to repetitive occupational use. In a study of three groups of textile workers, each of whom performed a different repetitive manual task, OA was more common in joints involved in repetitive usage than in other joints of the hand. Men whose jobs required knee bending and at least medium physical demand had higher rates of radiographic evidence of knee OA, and the radiographic changes were more likely to be more severe than those in men whose jobs required neither.

While the association between obesity and knee OA has been well documented, only recently has a causal relationship between the two been clearly shown. For those in the highest quintile for body mass index at baseline examination, the relative risk for developing knee OA in the ensuing 36 years was 1.5 for men and 2.1 for women. For *severe* knee OA, the relative risk rose to 1.9 for men and 3.2 for women, suggesting that obesity plays an even larger role in the etiology of the most serious cases of knee OA.

more common in women. Similarly, radiographic evidence of knee OA, especially *symptomatic* knee OA, appears to be more common in women than in men (Table 296-2).

Racial differences exist in both the prevalence of OA and the pattern of joint involvement. The Chinese in Hong Kong have a lower incidence of hip OA than whites; OA is more frequent in Native Americans than in whites. Interphalangeal joint OA and, especially, hip OA are much less common in South African blacks than in whites in the same population. Whether these differences are genetic or due to differences in joint usage related to life-style or occupation is unknown.

In other cases, the relationship of heredity to OA is less ambiguous.

While joint pain is the major feature leading the patient with OA to seek medical attention, the correlation between the pathologic severity of OA and symptoms is poor. Thus many individuals with radiographic changes of advanced OA are asymptomatic. The risk factors for *pain and disability* in affected individuals are poorly understood. Notably, for the same degree of pathologic severity, women are more likely to be symptomatic than men, those on welfare are more likely than those who are working, and divorced individuals are more likely than those who are married. In addition, for individuals with OA who had poor social support, a biweekly telephone call from a trained lay interviewer was as effective as a nonsteroidal anti-inflammatory drug (NSAID) in reducing joint pain, emphasizing the importance of psychosocial factors as determinants of pain in patients with OA.

PATHOLOGY The most striking changes in OA are usually seen in load-bearing areas of the articular cartilage. In the early stages the cartilage is thicker than normal, but with progression of OA the joint surface thins, the cartilage softens, the integrity of the surface is breached, and vertical clefts develop (fibrillation) (Fig. 296-1). Deep cartilage ulcers, extending to bone, may appear. Areas of fibrocartilaginous repair may develop, but the repair tissue is inferior to pristine hyaline articular cartilage in its ability to withstand mechanical stress. All the cartilage is metabolically active, and the chondrocytes replicate, forming clusters (clones). Later, however, the cartilage becomes hypocellular.

Remodeling and hypertrophy of bone are also major features. Appositional bone growth occurs in the subchondral region, leading to the "sclerosis" seen radiographically. The abraded bone under a cartilage ulcer may take on the appearance of ivory (eburnation). Growth of cartilage and bone at the joint margins leads to osteophytes (spurs), which alter the contour of the joint and may restrict movement. Soft tissue changes include a patchy chronic synovitis and thickening of the joint capsule, which may further restrict movement. Periarticular muscle wasting is common. These changes may play a major role in symptoms and disability.

PATHOGENESIS Articular cartilage, the major target organ in OA, serves two essential functions within the joint, both of which are mechanical. First, it provides a remarkably smooth bearing surface so that with joint movement one bone glides effortlessly over the other. (With synovial fluid as lubricant, the coefficient of friction for cartilage rubbed against cartilage, even with physiologic loading, is 15 times lower than that of two ice cubes passed across each other.) Second, articular cartilage prevents the concentration of stresses so that the bones do not shatter when the joint is loaded.

OA develops in either of two settings: (1) The biomaterial properties of the articular cartilage and subchondral bone are normal, but excessive loads applied to the joint cause the tissues to fail; or (2) the applied load is physiologically reasonable, but the material properties of the cartilage or bone are inferior.

Although articular cartilage is highly resistant to wear under conditions of repeated oscillation, repetitive impact loading soon leads to joint failure. This accounts for the high prevalence of OA at specific sites related to vocational or avocational overload (e.g., shoulders and elbows of baseball pitchers, ankles of ballet dancers, metacarpophalangeal joints of boxers, knees of basketball players). In general, the earliest progressive degenerative changes in OA occur at those sites within the joint which are subject to the greatest compressive loads. More than 80 percent of all cases of "idiopathic" OA of the hip may be due to subtle congenital or developmental defects, such as congenital subluxation/dislocation, acetabular dysplasia, Legg-Calvé-Perthes disease, or slipped capital femoral epiphysis, which increase joint congruity and concentrate dynamic loads. Notably, the institution in the 1940s of screening of newborns and infants for congenital hip disease has led to a marked decrease in the prevalence of hip OA in adults in Brittany.

Clinical conditions that reduce the ability of the cartilage or subchondral bone to deform are associated with development of OA. In ochronosis, for example, accumulation of homogentisic acid polymers leads to stiffening of the cartilage; in osteopetrosis, stiffness of the subchondral trabeculae occurs. In both conditions, severe

FIGURE 296-1 *A*. Normal articular cartilage. Note the intact surface and even distribution of chondrocytes. Mitotic figures are not present in normal adult articular cartilage. *B*. Osteoarthritic cartilage. Note the disruption of surface integrity, with vertical fissures (fibrillation) and irregular distribution of cells. Many of the chondrocytes have replicated and exist in clusters. Stained with safranin-O, which binds to the sulfated glycosaminoglycan chains of proteoglycans. Note patchy areas of diminished staining (pale extracellular matrix) due to proteoglycan depletion.

A

B

generalized OA is usually apparent by age 40. In the laboratory, if the subchondral bone is stiffened experimentally, repetitive impact loading leads rapidly to degeneration of the overlying cartilage. Conversely, osteoporosis, in which the bone is abnormally soft, may protect against OA. The elderly patient with a hip fracture rarely has hip OA.

The extracellular matrix of articular cartilage: Normal turnover Articular cartilage is composed of two major macromolecular species: proteoglycans (PGs), which are responsible for the stiffness of the tissue and its ability to withstand load, and collagen, which provides tensile strength and resistance to shear. Although lysomal proteases (cathepsins) have been demonstrated within the cells and matrix of normal articular cartilage, their low pH optimum makes it likely that the proteoglycanase activity of these enzymes will be confined to intracellular sites or to the immediate pericellular area. However, cartilage also contains a family of metalloproteinases, including stromelysin, collagenase, and gelatinase, which can degrade all the components of the extracellular matrix at neutral pH. Each is secreted by the chondrocyte as a proenzyme that must be activated by proteolytic cleavage of its *N*-terminal sequence. Net expression of neutral metalloproteinase activity represents the balance between activation of the latent forms and inhibition of the activity by tissue inhibitors.

The turnover of normal cartilage is effected through a degradative cascade, for which many investigators consider the driving force to be interleukin 1 (IL-1), a cytokine produced by mononuclear cells (including synovial lining cells) and synthesized by chondrocytes. IL-1 stimulates the synthesis and secretion of latent collagenase, latent stromelysin, latent gelatinase, and tissue plasminogen activator. Plasminogen, the substrate for the latter enzyme, may be synthesized by the chondrocyte or may enter the cartilage by diffusion from the synovial fluid. In addition to its catabolic effects, at concentrations even lower than those needed to stimulate cartilage degradation, IL-1 suppresses PG synthesis by the chondrocyte, inhibiting matrix repair (see below).

It is obvious that the preceding materials are potentially very destructive to cartilage. The balance of the system lies with at least two inhibitors: tissue inhibitor of metalloproteinase (TIMP) and plasminogen activator inhibitor 1 (PAI-1), both of which are synthesized by the chondrocyte and limit the degradative activity of active neutral metalloproteinases and plasminogen activator, respectively. If TIMP or PAI-1 are destroyed or present in insufficient concentrations relative to the active enzymes, stromelysin and plasmin are free to act on matrix substrates. Stromelysin can degrade the protein core of the PG and can activate latent collagenase. Conversion of latent stromelysin to an active, highly destructive protease by plasmin provides a second mechanism for matrix degradation.

Polypeptide mediators, e.g., insulin-like growth factor 1 (IGF-1) and transforming growth factor β (TGF-β), stimulate biosynthesis of PGs. They regulate matrix metabolism in normal cartilage and may play a role in matrix repair in OA. Notably, these growth factors modulate catabolic as well as anabolic pathways of chondrocyte metabolism; not only do they increase PG synthesis but, by downregulating chondrocyte receptors for IL-1, they also decrease PG degradation. Whether age-related changes occur in matrix concentrations of IGF-1 or TGF-β or in the responsiveness of the OA chondrocyte to these mediators is unknown.

In addition to its responsiveness to cytokines and a variety of other biologic mediators, chondrocyte metabolism in normal cartilage can be modulated directly by mechanical loading. Whereas static loading and prolonged cyclic loading inhibit synthesis of PGs and protein, loads of relatively brief duration may stimulate matrix biosynthesis.

Pathophysiology of cartilage changes in OA Most investigators feel that the primary changes in OA begin in the cartilage. Even though no alteration in collagen content occurs in OA, a change in the arrangement and size of the collagen fibers is apparent. The biochemical data are consistent with a defect in the collagen network of the cartilage, perhaps due to disruption of the "glue" that binds adjacent collagen fibers together in the matrix. This is among the earliest matrix changes observed and appears to be irreversible.

Although "wear" may be a factor in the loss of cartilage, strong evidence supports the concept that lysosomal and neutral metalloproteinases account for much of the loss of cartilage matrix in OA. Whether their synthesis and secretion are stimulated by IL-1 or by other factors (e.g., mechanical stimuli), neutral metalloproteinases, plasmin, and cathepsins all appear to be involved in the breakdown of articular cartilage in OA. TIMP and PAI-1 may work to stabilize the system, at least temporarily, and growth factors, such as IGF-1, TGF-β, and basic fibroblast growth factor (FGF), are implicated in repair processes that may heal the lesion or, at least, stabilize the process. A stoichiometric imbalance appears to exist between the levels of active enzyme, which may be several-fold higher than those in normal cartilage, and the level of TIMP, which may be only modestly increased.

The chondrocytes in OA cartilage undergo active cell division and are very active metabolically, producing increased quantities of collagen and PGs. Prior to the loss of cartilage and PG depletion, this marked biosynthetic activity may lead to an increase in PG concentration, which may be associated with thickening of the cartilage and "compensated," stabilized OA. (It is inaccurate to call OA "degenerative" joint disease.) These homeostatic mechanisms may maintain the joint in a reasonable functional state for years. The repair tissue, however, often does not hold up as well under mechanical stresses as normal hyaline cartilage. Eventually, at least in some cases, the rate of PG synthesis falls off and "end-stage" OA develops, with full-thickness loss of cartilage.

Is OA a focal joint disease or a systemic disorder? Several observations suggest that OA may be the result of a systemic abnormality of articular cartilage: First, although it may present in only a single joint, OA usually does not remain monarticular; in knees, hips, and small joints of the hand in particular, OA tends to become bilateral. Furthermore, knee OA is strongly associated with hand OA. The "monarthritis multiplex" pattern of OA, however, could as well be due to local mechanical factors as to a systemic cartilage abnormality.

CLINICAL FEATURES The joint pain of OA is often described as a deep ache, localized to the involved joint. Typically, the pain of OA is aggravated by joint use and relieved by rest, but as the disease progresses it may become persistent. Nocturnal pain, interfering with sleep, is seen particularly in advanced OA of the hip and may be enervating. Stiffness of the involved joint upon arising in the morning or after a period of inactivity (e.g., an automobile ride or an evening in a theater seat) may be prominent but usually lasts less than 20 minutes. Systemic manifestations are not a feature of primary OA.

Since articular cartilage is aneural, the joint pain in OA must arise from other structures (Table 296-3). In some patients it may be due to stretching of nerve endings in the periosteum covering osteophytes. In others it may arise from microfractures in subchondral bone or medullary hypertension caused by distortion of blood flow by thickened subchondral trabeculae. Muscle spasm and joint instability leading to stretching of the joint capsule also may be sources of pain.

In some patients with OA, joint pain may be due to synovitis. In advanced OA, histologic evidence of synovial inflammation may be as marked as that in the synovium of a patient with rheumatoid

---

TABLE 296-3 Causes of joint pain in patients with OA

Source	Mechanism
Synovium	Inflammation
Subchondral bone	Medullary hypertension, microfractures
Osteophyte	Stretching of periosteal nerve endings
Ligaments	Stretch
Capsule	Inflammation, distention
Muscle	Spasm

arthritis. Synovitis in OA may be due to phagocytosis of shards of cartilage and bone from the abraded joint surface (wear particles), release from the cartilage of soluble matrix macromolecules, (e.g., glycosaminoglycans or PGs), or the presence of crystals of calcium pyrophosphate or calcium hydroxyapatite. In other cases, immune complexes containing antigens derived from cartilage matrix may be sequestered in collagenous tissue of the joint, leading to low-grade chronic synovitis. In contrast, in the earlier stages of OA, even in the patient with chronic joint pain, synovial inflammation may be absent, suggesting that the pain is due to one of the other factors mentioned above. Notably, even in the absence of synovitis, joint pain in OA may be relieved by a nonsteroidal anti-inflammatory drug (NSAID), consistent with the fact that these drugs have analgesic actions independent of their anti-inflammatory effects.

Physical examination of the OA joint may reveal localized tenderness and bony or soft tissue swelling. Bony crepitus (the sensation of bone rubbing against bone, evoked by joint movement) is characteristic. Synovial effusions, when present, are usually not large. Palpation may reveal some warmth over the joint. Periarticular muscle atrophy may be due to disuse or to reflex inhibition of muscle contraction. In advanced stages of OA, gross deformity, bony hypertrophy, subluxation, and marked loss of joint motion may be striking. The notion that OA is inexorably progressive is incorrect. In many patients the disease stabilizes; in some, regression of joint pain, and even of radiographic changes, occurs.

LABORATORY AND RADIOGRAPHIC FEATURES   The diagnosis of OA is usually based on clinical and radiographic features. In the early stages, radiographs may be normal, but joint space narrowing becomes evident as articular cartilage is lost. Other characteristic radiographic findings include subchondral bone sclerosis, subchondral cysts, and marginal osteophytes. A change in the contour of the joint, due to bony remodeling, and subluxation may be seen. Although tibiofemoral joint space narrowing has been considered to be a radiographic surrogate for articular cartilage thinning, in patients with early OA who do not have radiographic evidence of bony changes (e.g., subchondral sclerosis or cysts, osteophytes), joint space narrowing alone does not accurately predict the status of the articular cartilage. Similarly, osteophytosis alone, in the absence of other radiographic features of OA, may be due to aging rather than to OA.

As indicated above, great disparity often exists between the severity of radiographic findings, severity of symptoms, and functional ability in OA. Thus, while more than 90 percent of people over age 40 have some radiographic changes of OA in weight-bearing joints, only 30 percent of these will have symptoms.

No laboratory studies are diagnostic of OA, but specific laboratory testing may help in identifying one of the underlying causes of secondary OA (see Table 296-1). Since primary OA is not systemic, the erythrocyte sedimentation rate, serum chemistry determinations, blood counts, and urinalysis are normal. Analysis of synovial fluid reveals mild leukocytosis (<2000 white blood cells per microliter), with a predominance of mononuclear cells.

Prior to the appearance of radiographic changes, the ability to clinically diagnose OA without an invasive procedure (e.g., arthroscopy) is limited. Approaches such as magnetic resonance imaging (MRI) and ultrasonography are expensive and not widely available, and the limits of resolution do not justify their routine clinical use for diagnosis of OA or for monitoring disease progression. Much effort is currently being devoted to evaluation of serologic tests for these purposes. The approach depends on detection in synovial fluid and/or serum of macromolecules (e.g., PGs, glycosaminoglycans) released from degenerating cartilage or bone. None of these tests has yet proved suitable for clinical use.

The Osteoarthritis Criteria Subcommittee of the American College of Rheumatology has recently developed sets of criteria that permit a diagnosis of OA of the hip, knee, or hand based on algorithms that utilize clinical data with or without radiographic and routine clinical laboratory data (e.g., synovial fluid analysis, erythrocyte sedimenta-

FIGURE 296-2   Nodal osteoarthritis. Note bony enlargement of distal and proximal interphalangeal joints (Heberden's nodes and Bouchard's nodes, respectively). *(From American College of Rheumatology.)*

tion rate). The sensitivity and specificity of these criteria for OA at each of the preceding sites are approximately 90 percent.

OA AT SPECIFIC JOINT SITES   **Interphalangeal joints**   Heberden's nodes, bony enlargements of the distal interphalangeal joints, represent the most common form of idiopathic OA (Fig. 296-2). A similar process at the proximal interphalangeal joints leads to Bouchard's nodes. Often, Heberden's nodes develop gradually, with little or no discomfort. However, they may present acutely with pain, redness, and swelling, sometimes triggered by minor trauma. Gelatinous dorsal cysts, filled with hyaluronic acid, may develop at the insertion of the digital extensor tendon into the base of the distal phalanx.

EROSIVE OA   In erosive OA (EOA), distal and/or proximal interphalangeal joints of the hands are most prominently affected. EOA tends to be more destructive than typical nodal OA. Radiographic evidence of collapse of the subchondral plate is characteristic, and bony ankylosis may occur. Joint deformity and functional impairment may be severe. Pain and tenderness are commonly episodic. The synovium is much more extensively infiltrated with mononuclear cells than in other forms of OA.

GENERALIZED OA   Generalized OA (GOA) is characterized by involvement of three or more joints or groups of joints (distal interphalangeal and proximal interphalangeal joints are counted as one group each). Heberden's and Bouchard's nodes are prominent. Symptoms may be episodic, with "flare-ups" of inflammation marked by soft tissue swelling, redness, and warmth. The erythrocyte sedimentation rate may be elevated, but serum rheumatoid factor tests are negative.

Thumb base   The second most frequent area of involvement in OA is the thumb base. Swelling, tenderness, and marked crepitus on movement of the joint are typical. Osteophytes may lead to a "squared" appearance of the thumb base (Fig. 296-3). In contrast to Heberden's nodes, which usually do not interfere significantly with function, OA at the base of the thumb frequently impairs function because of loss of motion and strength. Pain with pinch leads to adduction of the thumb and contracture of the first web space, often resulting in compensatory hyperextension of the first metacarpophalangeal joint and swan-neck deformity of the thumb.

The hip   Congenital or developmental defects (e.g., acetabular dysplasia, Legg-Calvé-Perthes disease, slipped capital epiphysis) may be implicated in as many as 80 percent of cases of hip OA. Twenty percent of patients will develop bilateral involvement. Pain from hip OA is generally referred to the inguinal area but may be referred to the buttock or proximal thigh. Less commonly, hip OA presents as knee pain. Pain can be evoked by putting the involved hip through

FIGURE 296-3 Osteoarthritis of the first carpometacarpal joint. Note the squared appearance of the thumb base due to bony enlargement and remodeling of the joint.

its range of motion initially; flexion may be painless, but internal rotation will exacerbate pain. Loss of internal rotation occurs early, followed by loss of extension, adduction, and flexion due to capsular fibrosis and/or buttressing osteophytes.

The knee OA of the knee may involve medial or lateral femorotibial compartments and/or the patellofemoral compartment. Palpation may reveal bony hypertrophy (osteophytes) and tenderness. Effusions, if present, are generally small. Joint movement commonly elicits bony crepitus. OA in the medial compartment may result in a varus (bow-legged) deformity; in the lateral compartment it produces a valgus (knock-knee) deformity. A positive "shrug" sign (pain when the patella is compressed manually against the femur during quadriceps contraction) may be a sign of OA in the patellofemoral joint.

Chondromalacia patellae, which also is characterized by knee pain and a positive shrug sign, is a syndrome of patellofemoral pain, often bilateral, occurring in teenagers and young adults. It is more common in females than in males. It may be caused by a variety of factors (e.g., abnormal quadriceps angle, patella alta, trauma). Although exploration of the knee may reveal softening and fibrillation of cartilage on the posterior aspect of the patella, this is usually not progressive, and in most cases, chondromalacia patellae is not a precursor of OA. Analgesics or NSAIDs and physical therapy are usually effective; in some, pain may be relieved by surgical correction of patellar malalignment.

The spine Degenerative disease of the spine can involve the apophyseal joint, intervertebral disks, and/or paraspinous ligaments. *Spondylosis* refers to degenerative *disk* disease. The term *OA of the spine* should be reserved for degeneration of the apophyseal joints (true diarthrodial joints). Symptoms of spinal OA include localized pain and stiffness. Nerve root compression by an osteophyte blocking a neural foramen, prolapse of a degenerated disk, or subluxation of an apophyseal joint may cause radicular pain and motor weakness. OA of the spine must be differentiated from diffuse idiopathic skeletal hyperostosis (DISH), which is characterized by marked calcification and ossification of the paraspinous ligaments (see Chap. 289).

TREATMENT No cure exists for OA. Treatment is aimed at reducing pain, maintaining mobility, and minimizing disability. The vigor of the therapeutic intervention should be dictated by the condition of the individual patient. For those with only mild disease, reassurance, instruction in joint protection, and an occasional analgesic may be all that is required.

Drug therapy Drug therapy in OA is symptomatic. Often the joint pain can be controlled with just a simple analgesic (e.g., acetaminophen). For more severe pain, dextrapropoxyphene hydrochloride may be used. Narcotics are rarely indicated in OA.

NSAIDs often decrease pain and improve mobility in OA. However, it is unclear whether this is due to their anti-inflammatory effect or to an analgesic action independent of their effect on inflammation. As indicated above, patients with OA may obtain symptomatic benefit from an NSAID even when evidence of synovitis is lacking. In a recent double-blind, controlled trial, an anti-inflammatory dose of ibuprofen (2400 mg/d) was no more effective than a chiefly analgesic dose of ibuprofen (1200 mg/d) or than acetaminophen in patients with symptomatic knee OA. Furthermore, the presence of clinical signs of inflammation (i.e., synovial swelling, tenderness) did not accurately predict that the response to anti-inflammatory therapy would be better than that to acetaminophen. Nonetheless, if simple analgesics are inadequate, it is reasonable to prescribe an NSAID for the patient with OA.

Claims have been made that some agents, such as polysulfated glycosaminoglycans, retard the progression of OA in human beings; it has been suggested that some NSAIDs also may have a "chondroprotective" effect. However, adequately controlled long-term clinical trials in human beings to support such claims are lacking.

Systemic glucocorticoids have no place in the treatment of OA. However, intra- or periarticular injection of a depot glucocorticoid preparation may provide marked symptomatic relief. The injection should not be repeated in a given joint more often than every 4 to 6 months, since too frequent injections may accelerate cartilage breakdown.

Capsaicin cream, which depletes local sensory nerve endings of substance P, a neuropeptide mediator of pain, may reduce joint pain and tenderness when applied topically by patients with hand or knee OA.

Reduction of joint loading OA may be caused or aggravated by poor body mechanics. Correction of poor posture and a support for excessive lumbar lordosis can be helpful. Excessive loading of the involved joint should be avoided. Overloading of the knee due to pronated feet or varus or valgus knee deformities may be corrected by orthotics or osteotomy. A wedged insole may decrease joint pain in patients with early medial OA of the knee. Running shoes also may be helpful in cushioning load.

Patients with OA of the knee or hip should avoid prolonged standing, kneeling, and squatting. Obese patients should be counseled to lose weight. In a strain of guinea pigs that develops spontaneous knee OA, dietary restrictions sufficient to result in a 28 percent decrease in body weight resulted in a 40 percent reduction in the severity of OA lesions. Moreover, while there are no data to show that it will decrease the prevalence of OA in obese humans, weight loss did reduce the risk of knee *symptoms* in obese women with radiographic evidence of knee OA.

Rest periods during the day also may be of benefit, but complete immobilization of the painful joint is rarely indicated. In patients with unilateral OA of the hip or knee, a cane, held in the contralateral hand, may reduce joint pain by reducing the joint contact force. Bilateral disease may necessitate the use of crutches or a walker.

Physical therapy Application of heat to the OA joint may reduce pain and stiffness. A variety of modalities are available. Often, the least expensive and most convenient is a hot shower or bath. Occasionally, better analgesia may be obtained with ice than with heat. Transcutaneous electrical nerve stimulation (TENS) may be helpful, especially for back pain due to OA of the lumbar spine.

Disuse of the OA joint and reflex inhibition of muscle contraction because of pain leads to muscle atrophy. Since they play a major role in protecting articular cartilage from stress, strengthening periarticular muscles is important. The atrophy of joint cartilage and bone which develops with disuse of a limb is due chiefly to reduction in loading of the joint by contraction of periarticular muscles (e.g., hamstrings and quadriceps for the knee). Exercises should be designed to maintain range of motion and strengthen muscles surrounding the joint. Isometric exercises are generally preferable to isotonic exercises, since they minimize joint stress. In a randomized trial in patients with prophylactic treatment with low doses of colchicine may be helpful. Unfortunately, effective treatment does not exist to remove CPPD deposits from cartilage and the joint capsule. As a result, CPPD tends to cause progressive forms of arthritis.

CALCIUM HA DEPOSITION DISEASE Pathogenesis Calcium hydroxyapatite is the primary mineral of bone and teeth. Abnormal accumulation can occur in areas of tissue damage (dystrophic calcification), in hypercalcemic or hyperparathyroid states (metastatic calcification), and in certain conditions of unknown cause (Table 297-2). In chronic renal failure, hyperphosphatemia enhances HA deposits within as well as around joints. It was not until 1976 that HA was clearly established as a cause of arthritis.

HA and other basic calcium phosphates may be released from exposed bone and cause the acute synovitis occasionally seen in chronic stable osteoarthritis (e.g., the ''hot'' Heberden's node). HA deposition is also an important factor in an extremely destructive chronic arthropathy of the elderly that occurs most often in knees and shoulders. Joint destruction is associated with attenuation or rupture of supporting structures, leading to instability and deformity. Progression tends to be indolent, and synovial fluid WBC counts are usually less than 1000 cells per milliliter. Symptoms range from minimal to severe pain and disability that may lead to joint replacement surgery. Whether severely affected patients merely represent an extreme synovial tissue response to HA crystals that are so common in osteoarthritis is uncertain. Observations that favor articular HA deposition and joint destruction being a unique entity rather than just a sequel of osteoarthritis include the following: (1) Primary osteoarthritis of the shoulders is infrequent. (2) High levels of activated collagenase and neutral protease, as well as fragments of collagen, have been found in the noninflammatory synovial fluids of patients with severe HA arthropathy; the concentration of these enzymes exceeded those for rheumatoid arthritis and uncomplicated osteoarthritis. (3) Synovial membrane tissue cultures exposed to HA crystals (or CPPD) markedly increased release of these enzymes, underscoring the destructive potential of abnormally stimulated synovial lining cells.

Clinical manifestations Periarticular and articular deposits may coexist and be associated with acute and/or chronic damage to the joint capsule, tendons, bursa, or articular surfaces. The most common sites of HA deposition include those in and/or around the knees, shoulders, hips, and fingers. Clinical manifestations include asymptomatic radiographic abnormalities, acute synovitis or tendinitis, and chronic destructive arthropathy. Most patients with HA arthropathy are elderly. Although the true incidence of HA arthritis is not known, 30 to 50 percent of patients with osteoarthritis have HA microcrystals in their synovial fluid. Such crystals can frequently be identified in clinically stable osteoarthritic joints but are more likely to come to attention in persons experiencing acute or subacute worsening of joint pain and swelling. The synovial fluid WBC count in HA arthritis is usually low (<2000 cells per milliliter) but may at times have as many as 50,000 cells per milliliter. Most synovial fluid analyses reveal a predominance of mononuclear cells. Occasionally, neutrophils may dominate.

Diagnosis Radiographic findings in HA arthropathy are not diagnostic. Intra- and/or periarticular calcifications with or without erosive, destructive, or hypertrophic changes may be present. X-ray films also may be normal.

Definitive diagnosis of HA arthropathy depends on identification of crystals from synovial fluid or tissue (Fig. 297-2). Individual crystals are very small, nonbirefringent, and can only be seen by electron microscopy. Clumps of crystals may appear as 1- to 20-μm shiny intra- or extracellular globules that stain purplish on Wright's stain and bright red with alizarin red S. Absolute identification depends on electron microscopy with energy dispersive elemental analysis, x-ray diffraction, or infrared spectroscopy.

Treatment of HA arthritis is nonspecific. Acute attacks of synovitis may be selflimiting within days to several weeks. Aspiration of effusions and the use of nonsteroidal anti-inflammatory agents for 2 weeks or intraarticular injection of glucocorticoid salts appear to

A

B

FIGURE 297-2 *A.* Cytoplasmic round inclusions inside synovial fluid cells represent aggregates of apatite crystals (fresh preparation, ordinary light microscopy; $\times$ 400). *B.* An electron micrograph demonstrates a cluster of dark apatite crystals within a synovial fluid mononuclear cell ($\times$ 30,000).

shorten the duration and intensity of symptoms. In patients with underlying severe destructive articular changes, response to medical therapy is usually less rewarding.

CaOx DEPOSITION DISEASE Pathogenesis *Primary oxalosis* is a rare hereditary metabolic disorder (Chap. 352). Enhanced production of oxalic acid may result from at least two different enzyme defects, leading to hyperoxalemia and deposition of calcium oxalate crystals in tissues. Nephrocalcinosis, renal failure, and death usually occur prior to 20 years of age. Acute and/or chronic CaOx arthritis and periarthritis may complicate primary oxalosis during later years of illness.

Secondary oxalosis is more common than the primary disorder. It is one of the many metabolic abnormalities that complicate end-stage renal disease (ESRD). In ESRD, calcium oxalate deposits have long been recognized in visceral organs, blood vessels, bones, and even cartilage. However, it was not until 1982 that such deposits were demonstrated to be one of the causes of arthritis in chronic renal failure. Thus far, reported patients have been dependent on long-term hemodialysis or peritoneal dialysis (see also Chap. 238), and many had received vitamin C (ascorbic acid) supplements. Ascorbic acid is metabolized to oxalate, which is inadequately cleared in uremia and by dialysis. Such supplements are now usually avoided in dialysis programs because of the risk of enhancing hyperoxalosis and its sequelae.

Clinical manifestations and diagnosis As was noted for the other calcium salts, CaOx aggregates can be found in bone, articular cartilage, synovium, and periarticular tissues. From these sites, crystals may be shed, causing acute synovitis. Persistent aggregates of CaOx may, like HA and CPPD, stimulate synovial proliferation and enzyme release, resulting in progressive articular destruction. Few well-studied cases have been reported. Deposits have been documented in fingers, wrists, elbows, knees, ankles, and feet. Any articular site could potentially be involved.

Each of the known microcrystalline arthropathies may be a complication of ESRD, and rare patients may have more than one type of crystal present in a joint effusion. The advent of crystallographic techniques has made it clear that most arthritic problems in ESRD are not, as was once believed, due to gout. Clinical features of acute CaOx arthritis may not be distinguishable from those due to sodium urate, CPPD, or HA. Radiographs may reveal chondrocalcinosis, a feature of either CPPD or CaOx deposition. CaOx-induced synovial effusions are usually noninflammatory, with less than 2000 leukocytes per milliliter. Predominant cell types have varied from being either neutrophils or mononuclear cells. In most instances, crystals are extracellular, although CaOx has been identified within neutrophils. Synovial membranes show modest signs of inflammation. CaOx has a variable shape and variable birefringence to polarized light. The most easily recognized forms are bipyramidal and strongly positively birefringent (Fig. 297-3).

Treatment of CaOx arthropathy with nonsteroidal anti-inflammatory agents, colchicine, intraarticular glucocorticoids, and increased frequency of dialysis has produced only slight improvement.

FIGURE 297-3 Bipyramidal and small polymorphic calcium oxalate crystals (ordinary light microscopy; × 400).

REFERENCES

ALVARELLOS A, SPILBERG I: Colchicine prophylaxis in pseudogout. J Rheumatol 13:804, 1986
BETH A et al: Articular cartilage vesicles generate calcium pyrophosphate dihydrate-like crystals in vitro. Arthritis Rheum 35:231, 1992
DIEPPE PA et al: Apatite deposition disease: A new arthropathy. Lancet 1:266, 1976
DOHERTY M et al: Inorganic pyrophosphate in metabolic diseases predisposing to calcium pyrophosphate dihydrate crystal deposition. Arthritis Rheum 34:1297, 1991
——— et al: Familial chondrocalcinosis due to calcium pyrophosphate dihydrate crystal deposition in English families. Br J Rheumatol 30:10, 1991
HALVERSON P, MCCARTY DJ: Basic calcium phosphate (apatite, octacalcium phosphate, tricalcium phosphate crystal deposition diseases), in *Arthritis and Allied Conditions*, 11th ed, DJ McCarty (ed). Philadelphia, Lea & Febiger, 1989
HOFFMAN GS et al: Calcium oxalate microcrystalline-associated arthritis in end-stage renal disease. Ann Intern Med 97:36, 1982
MCCARTY DJ et al: The significance of calcium phosphate crystals in the synovial fluid of arthritic patients: The "pseudogout syndrome." Ann Intern Med 56:711, 1962
REGINATO AJ, KURNIK B: Calcium oxalate and other crystals associated with kidney diseases and arthritis. Semin Arthritis Rheum 18:198, 1989
———, SCHUMACHER HR: Crystal associated arthropathies. Clin Geriatr Med 4:295, 1988
ROSENTHAL AK et al: Transforming growth factor beta 1 stimulates inorganic pyrophosphate elaboration by porcine cartilage. Arthritis Rheum 34:904, 1991
SCHUMACHER HR, REGINATO AJ: *Atlas of Synovial Fluid Analysis and Crystal Identification.* Philadelphia, Lea & Febiger, 1991, chaps 8, 9, and 10

298 PSORIATIC ARTHRITIS AND ARTHRITIS ASSOCIATED WITH GASTROINTESTINAL DISEASE

PETER H. SCHUR

PSORIATIC ARTHRITIS

Psoriatic arthritis is a chronic inflammatory arthritis that affects 5 to 8 percent of people with psoriasis.

ETIOLOGY AND PATHOGENESIS To date, the cause and pathogenesis are unknown. Indirect evidence has suggested that (viral) infections, trauma, increased cellular immunity to streptococci, decreased suppressor cell activation, immune complexes, and abnormal polymorphonuclear leukocyte (PMN) function may each play a role. Widespread severe psoriasis with rapidly progressive arthritis should make one suspect HIV infection (see Chap. 279). Familial aggregation suggests the influence of genetic factors. Although HLA-B13, B17, and CW6 are increased in frequency in patients with psoriasis, most studies have observed an increased frequency of HLA-B17, CW6, and/or B27 in patients with psoriatic spondylitis, while B27, B38, B39, and DR7a have been noted in association with peripheral arthritis in different studies.

CLINICAL MANIFESTATIONS Three major types of psoriatic arthritis have been identified: asymmetric inflammatory arthritis, symmetric arthritis, and psoriatic spondylitis. A mean of 47 percent of patients (range 16 to 70 percent) have an asymmetric inflammatory arthritis. Disease appears equally in men and women. Psoriasis tends to precede the arthritis by many years, although many complain of morning stiffness. The proximal and distal interphalangeal (PIP, DIP) joints are most frequently involved [with characteristic sausage-shaped digits (dactylitis)], while knees, hips, ankles, and wrists are less frequently involved. Most patients have onychodystrophy (onycholysis, ridging, pitting of nails), whose course does not parallel that of the synovitis. The prognosis is good, with only one-fourth of the patients developing progressive destructive disease; one-third develop inflammatory ocular complications (conjunctivitis, iritis, episcleritis).

A mean of 25 percent of patients (range 15 to 39 percent) develop symmetric arthritis resembling rheumatoid arthritis (see Chap. 285).

The disease occurs twice as frequently in women. Psoriasis and inflammatory arthritis usually develop simultaneously; again, most patients experience morning stiffness. The DIP, PIP, MCP, MTP, and, in particular, large peripheral joints are involved. Practically all have onychodystrophy, which helps distinguish these patients from those with rheumatoid arthritis. Over half this group goes on to develop destructive arthritis, including arthritis mutilans. Eye complications are uncommon. None have subcutaneous nodules, but one-fourth have rheumatoid factors.

A mean of 23 percent of the patients (range 5 to 33 percent) have psoriatic "spondylitis," with or without peripheral joint involvement. Psoriasis tends to precede the arthritis by a few years, and low-back pain with morning stiffness is common. Psoriatic spondylitis is more common in men. About half this group has spondylitis and the other sacroiliitis. The back disease is usually slowly progressive with little clinical deterioration as compared with ankylosing spondylitis; the peripheral disease also tends not to be destructive except for the occasional patient with arthritis mutilans. Enthesopathy, i.e., inflammation of tendons and ligamentous attachments to bone, is characteristic, viz., tendo Achillis, plantar fascia causing heel pain. Many have onychodystrophy, while few have inflammatory ocular complications.

Some authors have described additional subsets of psoriatic arthritis: predominant DIP joint involvement (6 percent of cases), arthritis mutilans (5 percent), juvenile psoriatic arthritis (2 percent), and SAPHO (sternoclavicular hyperostosis, chronic sterile multifocal osteomyelitis, hyperostosis of the spine, and a peripheral arthritis).

The pathology is similar to that seen in rheumatoid arthritis: synoviocytic hyperplasia, early PMN infiltration and later mononuclear cell infiltration, cartilage erosion, and pannus formation. Fibrosis of the joint capsule and marrow is prominent in many patients.

LABORATORY FINDINGS   There are a few laboratory abnormalities. Elevated erythrocyte sedimentation rates, C-reactive proteins, and complement levels reflect inflammation. Rheumatoid factors are uncommon and are more likely to be observed in those with symmetric arthritis. Immunoglobulin levels are normal. Uric acid levels may be elevated; sodium urate crystals in joint fluids suggest gout.

Radiologic investigation reveals findings quite similar to those of rheumatoid arthritis: soft tissue swelling, loss of the cartilage space, erosions, bony ankylosis, subluxations, subchondral cysts, but less demineralization. More unique and suggestive of psoriatic arthritis are erosions at DIP joints, expansion of the base of the terminal phalanx, tapering of the proximal phalanx and cuplike erosions of and bony proliferation of the distal terminal phalanx ("pencil-in-cup" appearance), proliferation of bone near osseous erosions, terminal phalangeal osteolysis, bone proliferation and periostitis (especially of phalanges), and telescoping of one bone into its neighbor, leading to the "opera-glass" deformity. The axial skeleton shows asymmetric or unilateral sacroiliitis and large asymmetric nonmarginal syndesmophytes.

DIAGNOSIS   The diagnosis of psoriatic arthritis should be considered in individuals with arthritis and psoriasis. Psoriasis should be distinguished from seborrheic dermatitis and eczema. Psoriatic lesions may be quite small peripherally or often hidden in the scalp, umbilicus, and gluteal folds. Fungal infection of nails can be distinguished from psoriasis, for the latter will demonstrate pitting and onycholysis. Furthermore, onychodystrophy is uncommon (20 percent) in uncomplicated psoriasis. Patients with ankylosing spondylitis (see Chap. 289) have more back symptoms and less (and less severe) peripheral arthritis than those with psoriatic arthritis. It is often difficult to distinguish Reiter's syndrome (see Chap. 289) from psoriatic arthritis, since both manifest dactylitis. Reiter's syndrome usually presents in younger individuals, especially males, is less frequently progressive or destructive, and more likely is associated with characteristic skin lesions (keratoderma blenorrhagica), urethritis, and conjunctivitis. Gout can be distinguished by the presence of intraarticular sodium urate crystals (see Chap. 347). Psoriasis in association with Heberden's nodes or Bouchard's nodes of the DIP and PIP joints, respectively, rather suggests osteoarthritis (see Chap. 296). Psoriatic arthritis differs from rheumatoid arthritis by the relative lack of rheumatoid factors; the tendency to asymmetry, dactylitis, iritis, enthesopathy, onychodystrophy; the high frequency of HLA-B27, especially in patients with axial skeletal involvement; and characteristic radiologic features.

TREATMENT   The treatment of psoriatic arthritis begins with patient education and physical and occupational therapy to maintain muscle strength and joint and muscle function. Orthotics and occasional intraarticular glucocorticoids for isolated acutely and severely inflamed joints may be added as needed. The mainstay, however, is the use of nonsteroidal anti-inflammatory drugs (NSAIDs), including salicylates, which reduce inflammation and alleviate pain for the majority of patients. Oral colchicine has been reported to be beneficial. For patients with more severe involvement, a disease-modifying antirheumatic drug should be utilized. While hydroxychloroquine is often successful in creating either amelioration or remission, it carries a significant risk of exacerbation of psoriasis. Sulfasalazine has been reported to be of benefit. Intramuscular gold salts have created remission in over 50 percent of patients, with few side effects. For more severe cases, especially with extensive skin involvement, methotrexate is recommended. A total of three doses of 2.5 to 5 mg given 12 h apart once a week is recommended. Most patients respond well with respect to both skin lesions and arthritis. Patients who are resistant to oral therapy may respond to intravenous therapy. Renal and liver function tests and a complete blood count should be monitored frequently, and any abnormalities should suggest withholding of the drug until tests normalize. Liver biopsies are recommended after a total of 1.5 g methotrexate and then every 2 years to identify patients with fibrosis and cirrhosis, which necessitate withdrawal of the drug. This occurrence is rare. However, patients are advised to avoid nephrotoxic and hepatotoxic (e.g., ethanol) drugs. If methotrexate cannot be tolerated, 6-mercaptopurine and azathioprine have proven successful. The arthritis of few patients responds to the psoriasis therapy known as PUVA (psoralen with UV-A radiation). Advanced forms of therapy such as cyclosporine should be provided only in consultation with or by persons expert in their use.

ARTHRITIS ASSOCIATED WITH GASTROINTESTINAL DISEASE

INFLAMMATORY BOWEL DISEASE (IBD)   Peripheral arthritis occurs in 9 to 20 percent of patients with IBD (e.g., ulcerative colitis, Crohn's disease; see Chap. 255). Arthritis is somewhat more likely to occur in patients with large bowel disease and in those patients with complications such as abscesses, pseudomembranous polyposis, perianal disease, massive hemorrhage, erythema nodosum, stomatitis, uveitis, and pyoderma gangrenosum. Males and females are affected equally. The arthritis tends to be acute, is associated with flares of the bowel disease, occurs early in the course of the bowel disease, is self-limiting (90 percent under 6 months), and does not result in destruction. Involved joints are swollen, erythematous, warm, and painful. The majority of patients (90 percent) have polyarticular disease with knees, ankles, elbows, and wrists more commonly affected than PIP, MCP, and MTP joints. Half of patients have migratory arthritis. Granulomas, associated with Crohn's disease, can cause an erosive arthritis. Rarely, a psoas abscess can result from bowel perforation, even resulting in (septic) hip arthritis. Rheumatoid factor tests are negative. In those persons who have only peripheral arthritis, there is no increase in frequency in HLA-B27. Synovial fluids have 5000 to 12,000 white blood cells per microliter, mostly PMNs. Radiographs demonstrate soft-tissue swelling and effusions without erosions or destruction. Pathologic examination of synovial biopsies reveals only nonspecific inflammation. The arthritis responds to successful treatment of the bowel disease such as colectomy (for ulcerative colitis), glucocorticoids, or sulfasalazine. NSAIDs relieve pain and inflammation but should be used with caution because of possible gastrointestinal side effects.

Spondylitis occurs in 1.1 to 26 percent of patients with IBD.

Males are somewhat more frequently affected. Patients will typically complain of stiffness in the back and/or buttocks in the morning or after rest. Stiffness and associated pain are often relieved by exercise. Back symptoms are unrelated to those of the gastrointestinal disease. Physical examination reveals limited spinal flexion and reduced chest expansion. Some patients may have peripheral arthritis, especially of the hips and/or shoulders. Iritis is a frequent complication. Radiographs of the back show the typical findings of ankylosing spondylitis and bilateral sacroiliitis. HLA-B27 is found in 53 to 75 percent of these patients. Treatment includes NSAIDs, gluococorticoids for the bowel disease, and physical therapy. The axial disease progresses in a slow manner akin to ankylosing spondylitis.

Asymptomatic sacroiliitis detected by radiography occurs in 4 to 25 percent of patients with IBD. By contrast, 52 percent of patients with IBD have abnormal technetium pyrophosphate bone scans of the sacroiliac joint. There is no increased frequency of HLA-B27. This "disease" does not necessarily progress to spondylitis.

Other complications of chronic IBD include (1) finger clubbing (observed in 4 to 13 percent of patients with Crohn's disease, especially those with small bowel involvement) which may regress after surgery, (2) development of amyloid, especially in association with Crohn's disease, and (3) osteoporosis resulting from inactivity, malabsorption, and/or treatment with glucocorticoids. Osteomalacia can result from malabsorption. In this setting, with acutely increased back pain, one should suspect compression fracture.

INTESTINAL BYPASS ARTHRITIS   Intestinal bypass surgery was developed for the treatment of obesity in 1952; 11 years later arthritis was recognized as a postoperative complication. Polyarthralgia and sometimes arthritis may occur weeks, even years, following surgery in 8 to 36 percent of patients. Pain and tenderness exceed objective findings in most cases; others have noted episodes of abrupt onset of pain and inflammation. Tenosynovitis is common, with episodes possibly lasting for days and even months; it tends to affect the knee, wrist, ankle, shoulder, and finger joints and cause pain in the neck and back. This syndrome occurs more likely after jejunocolic than after jejunoileal surgery and more in females than in males. There is often an associated urticarial, vesicular, pustular, macular, or nodular eruption. Raynaud's symptoms appear in one-third of patients. X-rays generally show no joint damage, except marginal erosions in patients with persistent arthritis. Synovial fluids generally have white blood cell counts of 500 to 27,000 cells per microliter, mostly PMNs. Synovial biopsies show chronic synovitis with lymphocytes but without lymphoid follicles. Tests for rheumatoid factors, antinuclear antibodies, and HLA-B27 are usually negative, while immune complexes (and cryoglobulins) are often present. They contain bacterial antigens, their antibodies, IgA secretory component, and various complement components. These observations suggest that the syndrome has the following pathogenesis: Bacteria proliferate in intestinal blind loops, bacterial antigens are absorbed, and antibodies to these antigens develop and combine with them to form immune complexes which deposit in synovial tissue to cause arthritis. NSAIDs and glucocorticoids can relieve the joint symptoms, but more lasting results can be achieved by tetracycline therapy to decrease bacteria; even better is reanastomosis of the bowel.

WHIPPLE'S DISEASE (INTESTINAL LIPODYSTROPHY)   Whipple's disease is rare and occurs mostly in middle-aged Caucasian males who develop arthritis, prolonged diarrhea, malabsorption, and weight loss. Up to 90 percent of patients develop arthritis, usually prior to other symptoms. Knees and ankles and, to a lesser extent, fingers, hips, shoulders, elbows, and wrists are involved. The arthritis is acute in onset and is characterized by tender, red, swollen joints. Symptoms are migratory, usually lasting just a few days, and are rarely chronic or cause permanent joint damage. Associated symptoms may include fever (54 percent), edema, serositis (pleurisy, pericarditis, endocarditis), pneumonia, hypotension, lymphadenopathy (54 percent), hyperpigmentation (54 percent), subcutaneous nodules, clubbing, and uveitis. Central nervous system involvement (43 percent) may develop, with loss of memory, confusion, depression, headache,

diplopia, and papilledema, and may be appreciated by abnormalities in magnetic resonance images of the brain. Laboratory abnormalities include anemia (75 percent), low serum carotene (95 percent) and albumin levels (93 percent), and HLA-B27 (8 to 30 percent) in those patients with axial arthritis. Synovial fluids have been reported to contain 450 to 36,000 white blood cells per microliter (30 to 95 percent neutrophils) or a mild monocytosis. Joint x-rays rarely show erosions but may show a sacroiliitis in those occasional patients who have axial skeletal symptoms; abdominal x-rays, computed tomographic scans, or ultrasound may reveal lymphadenopathy. The diagnosis is generally established by the detection of PAS-staining bacilliform structures in the lamina propria and/or in foamy macrophages in small intestine. These inclusion-containing foamy macrophages also have been detected in the synovium, synovial fluid, abdominal and peripheral lymph nodes, pericardium, myocardium, liver, spleen, kidney, brain, and other tissues. Electron microscopy reveals rod-shaped organisms in the lamina propria of the small intestine. Although bacteria have not been isolated or cultured from these patients, the syndrome responds well to long-term antibiotic therapy, e.g., penicillin, tetracyline, or erythromycin, 0.5 g qid for 1 year. Some have recommended an initial 2-week course of penicillin and streptomycin. Trimethoprim-sulfamethoxazole is beneficial in the event of central nervous system involvement.

REACTIVE ARTHRITIS   A Reiter's-like syndrome of arthritis 2 to 3 weeks following diarrhea caused by either *Shigella*, *Salmonella*, *Yersinia*, *Chlamydia trachomatis*, or *Campylobacter* organisms is described elsewhere (see Chap. 289).

REFERENCES

FLEMING JL et al: Whipple's disease: Clinical, biochemical and histopathologic features and assessment of treatment in 29 patients. Mayo Clin Proc 63:539, 1988
GLADMAN DD et al: Longitudinal study of clinical and radiological progression in psoriatic arthritis. J Rheumatol 17:809, 1990
GRAVELLESE EM, KANTROWITZ GF: Arthritic manifestations of inflammatory bowel disease. Am J Gastroenterol 83:703, 1988
HELLIWELL P et al: A re-evaluation of the osteoarticular manifestations of psoriasis. Br J Rheumatol 30:339, 1991
KAMMER GM et al: Psoriatic arthritis: A clinical, immunologic and HLA study of 100 patients. Semin Arthritis Rheum 9:75, 1979
KERR R, RESNICK D: Radiology of the seronegative spondyloarthropathies. Clin Rheum Dis 11:113, 1985
KHAN MA, VAN DER LINDEN SM: Ankylosing spondylitis and other spondyloarthropathies. Rheumatol Clin North Am 16:551, 1990
WOLHEIM FA: Enteropathic arthritis, in *Textbook of Rheumatology*, 4th ed, WN Kelley et al (eds). Philadelphia, Saunders, 1993
WOODROW JC: Genetic aspects of the spondyloarthropathies. Clin Rheum Dis 11:1, 1985

299   RELAPSING POLYCHONDRITIS AND MISCELLANEOUS ARTHRITIDES

BRUCE C. GILLILAND

RELAPSING POLYCHONDRITIS

Relapsing polychondritis is an episodic and often progressive inflammatory disorder of unknown cause affecting predominately the cartilage of the ears, nose, and tracheobronchial tree, as well as internal structures of the eyes and ears. Other manifestations include polyarthritis, vasculitis, cardiac abnormalities, skin lesions, and glomerulonephritis. It is most common between the ages of 40 to 60 years but may affect children and the elderly. Relapsing polychondritis progression of HOA tends to be more rapid when associated with malignancies, most notably bronchogenic carcinoma. Patients experience a burning or deep-seated aching pain in the distal extremities due to periostitis. The pain can be quite incapacitating and is aggravated by dependency and relieved by elevation of the affected limbs. Joint manifestations vary from arthralgias to very painful arthritis, most often affecting the metacarpophalangeal and metatarsophalangeal joints, wrists, ankles, and knees. The involved joints are warm, tender, and swollen. Joint effusions are usually small, and the fluid is noninflammatory, containing only a few white cells. The distal extremities may be swollen and the overlying skin warm and erythematous. Pressure applied over the distal end of the forearms and lower legs may be quite painful. Clubbing is usually asymptomatic, except for occasional warmth or burning of the fingertips. Clubbing usually evolves over months and often is first noted by the physician and not the patient. Patients, especially those with lung tumor, may experience severe skeletal pain prior to the appearance of clubbing. Clubbing is characterized by widening of the fingertips, enlargement of the distal volar pad, convexity of the nail contour, and the loss of the normal 15° angle between the proximal nail and cuticle. The thickness of the digit at the base of the nail is greater than the thickness at the distal interphalangeal joint. The base of the nail feels spongy when compressed, and the nail can be easily rocked on its bed. Marked periungual erythema is usually present. When clubbing is advanced, the finger may have a drumstick appearance. Excessive sweating, oiliness of the skin, and thickening of the facial skin are uncommon in secondary HOA.

HOA occurs in 5 to 10 percent of patients with intrathoracic malignancies, the most common being bronchogenic carcinoma and pleural tumors. Lung metastases infrequently cause HOA. HOA is also seen in patients with intrathoracic infections, including lung abscesses, empyema, bronchiectasis, chronic obstructive lung disease, and pulmonary tuberculosis. HOA also may accompany chronic interstitial pneumonitis, sarcoidosis, and cystic fibrosis. In the latter, clubbing is more common than the full syndrome of HOA. Other causes of clubbing include congenital heart disease with right-to-left shunts, Crohn's disease, ulcerative colitis, sprue, and neoplasms of the esophagus, liver, and small and large bowel. In patients with congenital heart disease with right-to-left shunts, clubbing alone occurs more often than the full syndrome of HOA.

Unilateral clubbing has been found in association with aneurysms of the aorta, subclavian, or innominate artery and with arteriovenous fistula of brachial vessels. Clubbing of the toes but not fingers has been associated with an infected abdominal aortic aneurysm. Clubbing of a single digit may follow trauma and has been reported in tophaceous gout and sarcoidosis.

Hyperthyroidism (Graves' disease), treated or untreated, may occasionally be associated with clubbing and periostitis of the bones of the hands and feet. This condition is referred to as *thyroid acropachy*. Periostitis is asymptomatic and occurs in the midshaft and diaphyseal portion of the metacarpal and phalangeal bones. The long bones of the extremities are seldom affected. Elevated levels of long-acting thyroid stimulator (LATS) are found in the serum of these patients.

Laboratory findings The laboratory abnormalities reflect the underlying disorder. The synovial fluid of involved joints has less than 500 white cells per microliter, and they are predominantly mononuclear. Radiographs show a faint radiolucent line beneath the new periosteal bone along the shaft of long bones at their distal end. These changes are observed most frequently at the ankles, wrists, and knees. The ends of the distal phalanges may show osseous resorption. Radionuclide studies show pericortical linear uptake along the cortical margins of long bones that may be present before any radiographic changes.

Treatment The treatment of hypertrophic osteoarthropathy is to identify the associated disorder and treat it appropriately. The symptoms and signs of hypertrophic osteoarthropathy may disappear completely with removal or effective chemotherapy of a tumor or with antibiotic therapy and drainage of a chronic pulmonary infection. Vagotomy or percutaneous block may lead to symptomatic relief in some patients. Aspirin, other nonsteroidal anti-inflammatory drugs, or analgesics may help control symptoms of hypertrophic osteoarthropathy.

FIBROMYALGIA Fibromyalgia, also termed *fibrositis*, is a commonly encountered disorder characterized by diffuse musculoskeletal pain, stiffness, paresthesia, nonrestorative sleep, and easy fatigability which affects predominantly women between the ages of 25 and 45 years. The term *fibrositis* is a misnomer, since this is not an inflammatory disorder of connective tissue; therefore, the term *fibromyalgia* is now preferred. Several causative mechanisms for fibromyalgia have been postulated. A disturbance of normal stage 4 (non-REM) sleep has been suggested as playing a role in its development. Symptoms of fibromyalgia were produced in normal subjects by disturbing stage 4 sleep with a buzzer without wakening them. Sleep studies in patients with fibromyalgia have shown more alpha-wave intrusion and less REM sleep, indicating disturbed and unrefreshed sleep; however, patients with chronic pain from other causes may have similar sleep patterns. Psychological factors, muscle abnormalities, and autonomic nervous system dysfunction also have been proposed to play a role in this disorder. Emotional stress, medical illness, surgery, thyroid disease, and trauma have been implicated in triggering fibromyalgia. Fibromyalgia has appeared in some patients with HIV infection, parvovirus B19 infection, or Lyme disease. In the last, fibromyalgia continued despite adequate antibiotic treatment for Lyme disease. A better understanding of fibromyalgia awaits further studies.

Symptoms are generalized aching and stiffness of the trunk, hip, and shoulder girdles. Other patients complain of generalized aching and muscle weakness. Patients perceive that their joints are swollen; however, joint examination is normal. Stiffness is usually present on arising in the morning and improves during the day but may last all day in some patients. Patients complain of exhaustion and wake up tired. They also awake frequently at night and have trouble falling back asleep. Symptoms are made worse by stress or anxiety, cold, damp weather, and overexertion. Patients often feel better during warmer weather and vacations. Disorders commonly associated with fibromyalgia include irritable bowel syndrome, irritable bladder, headaches (including migraine headaches), and dysmenorrhea. Symptoms of fibromyalgia also occur in patients who carry the diagnosis of chronic fatigue syndrome.

The characteristic physical feature is the demonstration of specific tender sites which are exquisitely more tender than adjacent areas. Tender sites should be distinguished from the trigger points found in myofascial pain syndromes. Pressure over trigger points causes pain to be referred to a nearby site, while pressure over tender sites causes pain only at that site. The patient may suddenly jump or withdraw when the tender site is palpated. The sites of tenderness are remarkably constant in location. Common sites of tenderness are bilaterally over the suboccipital muscle insertion at the base of the skull, the anterior aspect of the intertransverse process spaces at C5–C7, the midpoint of the upper border of the trapezius muscle, above the scapular spine near the medial border of the scapula, the second costochondral junction, the lateral epicondyle, the upper outer quadrant of the buttock, the posterior aspect of the trochanteric prominence, and the medial fat pad of the knee. Skinfold tenderness may be present, particularly over the upper scapular region. Subcutaneous nodules may be felt at sites of tenderness. Nodules in similar locations are present in normal persons but are not tender.

The diagnosis of fibromyalgia is made by recognizing the clinical manifestations. The joint and muscle examination is normal, and there are no laboratory abnormalities. The American College of Rheumatology in 1990 published uniform diagnostic criteria for fibromyalgia that required patients to have widespread pain in combination with 11 of the 18 tender sites described above. These criteria serve a useful purpose for enrolling patients in clinical studies; however, not all patients with fibromyalgia meet these criteria. Fibromyalgia may occur in patients with rheumatoid arthritis or other connective tissue diseases. A distinction is no longer made between primary and secondary fibromyalgia (concomitant with other disease).

Patients should be informed that they have a treatable condition which is not a crippling, deforming, or degenerative process. Salicylates or other nonsteroidal anti-inflammatory drugs only partially improve symptoms. Glucocorticoids have been of little benefit and should not be used in these patients. Local measures such as heat, massage, injection of tender sites with steroids or lidocaine, and acupuncture provide only temporary relief of symptoms. The use of tricyclics such as amitriptyline, 10 to 25 mg, doxepin, 10 to 25 mg, and cyclobenzaprine, 10 to 20 mg, at bedtime will give the patient restorative sleep resulting in clinical improvement. Higher doses of these medications may be necessary. A combination of alprazolam, 0.5 to 3 mg/d, and ibuprofen, 2.4 g/d, has been shown in a controlled study to be more effective than either drug alone. Patients also may benefit by regular aerobic exercises and by reducing the stress in their lives. While treatment of fibromyalgia may be effective in some patients, others continue to have chronic disease which may be only partially relieved, if at all.

PSYCHOGENIC RHEUMATISM Patients may experience severe joint pain involving a few to several joints without physical findings of arthritis. These patients are often convinced that they have rheumatoid arthritis, systemic lupus erythematosus, or another connective tissue disease. This disorder is recognized by the inconsistencies, exaggerations, and emotional lability of the patient during the history and physical examination. Laboratory studies are normal. Organic disease needs to be excluded, which requires seeing the patient at regular intervals. This condition also needs to be distinguished from fibromyalgia. Anti-inflammatory or other drugs are not helpful.

CARPAL TUNNEL SYNDROME Carpal tunnel syndrome is an entrapment neuropathy of the median nerve at the wrist producing paresthesias and weakness of the hands. The syndrome is caused by pressure on the median nerve where it passes in company with the flexor tendons of the fingers through the tunnel formed by carpal bones and the transverse carpal ligament.

Compression of the median nerve is produced by any process that encroaches on the carpal tunnel. Localized tenosynovitis of the flexor tendons of the fingers is a frequent cause of carpal tunnel syndrome, particularly in middle-aged women. Premenstrual edema or edema occurring in pregnancy also may cause these symptoms. Symptoms can be precipitated by activities which require repeated flexion, pronation, and supination of the wrist, e.g., sewing, driving, operating computers and cash registers, and playing squash or golf. Other causes of carpal tunnel syndrome, often bilateral, are rheumatoid arthritis, acromegaly, hypothyroidism, and amyloidosis. Unilateral carpal tunnel syndrome is more likely due to trauma, physical activities involving one wrist, tuberculosis, gout, or calcium pyrophosphate deposition disease.

Patients experience numbness or paresthesias of the palmar surface of the thumb, index and middle fingers, and radial half of the ring finger. Numbness or paresthesias of the whole hand may occur. Pain may be referred to the forearm and less commonly to the shoulder and neck regions. Pain or tingling of the fingers often occurs at night and is relieved by shaking or exercising the hand. Weakness and atrophy of the thenar muscles usually appear later and can occur without significant sensory symptoms.

Thenar muscle weakness is manifested by decreased strength of abduction, opposition, and flexion of the thumb. On examination, symptoms of paresthesia or pain in the fingers may be reproduced by percussion over the volar surface of the wrist (Tinel's sign) or by full flexion of the wrist for 1 min (Phalen's maneuver). A more sensitive and specific diagnostic maneuver to elicit symptoms of carpal tunnel syndrome is compressing the carpal tunnel with a modified sphygmomanometer set at 150 mmHg for up to 60 s. Decreased touch

or hyperpathia to pinprick and widening of two-point discrimination may be demonstrated over the sensory distribution of the median nerve. Nerve conduction studies of the median nerve show delayed latency across the wrist, confirming the diagnosis.

Treatment of patients with only sensory symptoms and minor nerve conduction abnormalities consists of a wrist splint to be worn mainly at night, anti-inflammatory drugs, and local injection with steroids. If symptoms persist or motor abnormalities are present, surgical decompression of the carpal tunnel with release of the transverse carpal ligament and debridement is indicated.

TARSAL TUNNEL SYNDROME Tarsal tunnel syndrome is an entrapment neuropathy of the posterior tibial nerve at the ankle producing aching, burning, tingling, and numbness of the plantar surface of the foot and toes. The syndrome is caused by compression of the posterior tibial nerve and its branches as they pass through the tunnel beneath the flexor retinaculum on the medial side of the ankle inferior and posterior to the medial malleolus. Also passing through this tunnel are the flexor tendons of the toes, vascular bundle, and the medial and lateral plantar branches of the posterior tibial nerve. Compression of the nerve in the tunnel may be caused by tenosynovitis or ganglia resulting from overuse or trauma and by inflammatory arthritis such as rheumatoid arthritis. A bony prominence from a talocalcaneal coalition also may compress the tunnel. Other causes include pregnancy, myxedema, and amyloidosis.

Patients experience paresthesias of the plantar surface of the foot and toes which may radiate up the calf. Symptoms often occur at night and after standing and may be relieved by movement of the foot and ankle. On examination, there may be loss of sensation over the plantar surface of the foot, but this is variable. Symptoms may be reproduced by percussion over the flexor retinaculum (Tinel's sign) or by applying firm pressure to this area. Diagnosis is confirmed by nerve conduction studies that show prolonged latency across the tunnel. Treatment consists of anti-inflammatory drugs and local injection of steroids. If symptoms persist, surgical decompression is indicated.

REFLEX SYMPATHETIC DYSTROPHY SYNDROME The reflex sympathetic dystrophy syndrome (RSDS) is characterized by pain and tenderness usually of a distal extremity accompanied by signs and symptoms of vasomotor instability, trophic skin changes, and the rapid development of bony demineralization. A precipitating event can be identified in two-thirds of cases. These include local trauma, myocardial infarction, strokes, peripheral nerve injuries, antituberculosis drugs, barbiturates, and recently, cylosporin A in patients undergoing renal transplantation. RSDS is observed most often in individuals over the age of 50, reflecting the frequency of the accompanying disorder. The sex distribution is equal. An entire hand or foot is usually affected. Occasionally, RSDS will involve an isolated site such as the patella, hip, or one or two rays of a foot or hand. The contralateral side may be affected in up to 50 percent of patients, and subclinical disease may be present in virtually all patients. The pathogenesis of RSDS is poorly understood. The vasomotor manifestations are thought to be caused by abnormal stimulation of the sympathetic nervous system.

RSDS evolves through three clinical phases. The clinical manifestations of the first phase are pain and swelling of a distal extremity, which develop weeks to months following the precipitating event. The pain has an intense, burning quality. The involved extremity is warm, edematous, and tender especially around joints. Increased sweating and hair growth occur. In 3 to 6 months, the skin gradually becomes thin, shiny, and cool (second phase). Clinical features of the first two phases overlap. In another 3 to 6 months, the skin and subcutaneous tissue become atrophic, and irreversible flexion contractures of the hand or foot develop (third phase). Motion of the shoulder on the affected side is frequently painful and greatly restricted, a condition referred to as *shoulder-hand syndrome* (see "Adhesive Capsulitis," below).

The laboratory abnormalities are those of the associated disorder.

Synovial chondromatosis is a disorder characterized by multiple focal metaplastic growths of normal-appearing cartilage in the synovium or tendon sheath. Segments of cartilage break loose and continue to grow as loose bodies. When calcification and ossification of loose bodies occur, the disorder is referred to as *synovial osteochondromatosis*. The disorder is usually monarticular and affects young to middle-aged individuals. The knee is most often involved, followed by hip, elbow, and shoulder. Symptoms are pain, swelling, and decreased motion of the joint. Radiographs may show several rounded calcifications within the joint cavity. Treatment is synovectomy; however, the tumor may recur.

Hemangiomas occur in synovium and in tendon sheaths. The knee is affected most commonly. Recurrent episodes of joint swelling and pain usually begin in childhood. The joint fluid is bloody. Treatment is excision of the lesion. *Lipomas* occur most often in the knee, originating in the subsynovial fat on either side of the patellar tendon. Lipomas also appear in tendon sheaths of the hands, wrists, feet, and ankles. In some instances, surgical removal is necessary.

Synovial sarcoma (malignant synovioma) is a neoplasm of connective origin arising from tissue adjacent to large joints and seldom from the joint itself. It occurs most often in young adults and is more common in men. The tumor presents as a slowly growing mass near a joint, without much pain. The tumor spreads along tissue planes. The most common site of visceral metastasis is lung. The diagnosis is made by biopsy. Treatment is wide resection of the tumor including adjacent muscle and regional lymph nodes. Amputation of the involved distal extremity may be required. Chemotherapy may be beneficial in some patients with metastatic disease.

Synovial chondrosarcoma may arise in the synovium, tendon sheath, or bursa and is very rare. Treatment is radical excision or amputation.

REFERENCES

ALTMAN RD, TENENBAUM J: Hypertrophic osteoarthropathy, in *Textbook of Rheumatology*, WN Kelley et al (eds). Philadelphia, Saunders, 1993

BENNETT RM, GOLDENBERG DL (eds): *Rheumatic Disease Clinics of North America: The Fibromyalgia Syndrome*. Philadelphia, Saunders, 1989

CHANG-MILLER A et al: Renal involvement in relapsing polychondritis. Medicine 66:202, 1987

DINERMAN H, STEERE AC: Lyme disease associated with fibromyalgia. Ann Intern Med 117:281, 1992

ELLMAN MH: Neuropathic joint disease (Charcot joints), in *Arthritis and Allied Conditions*, 13th ed, DJ McCarty, WJ Koopman (eds). Philadelphia, Lea & Febiger, 1993

GIURINI JM et al: Charcot's disease in diabetic patients. Postgrad Med 89:163, 1991

HERMAN JH: Polychondritis, in *Textbook of Rheumatology*, WN Kelley et al (eds). Philadelphia, Saunders, 1993

HUDSON JI et al: Comorbidity of fibromyalgia with medical and psychiatric disorders. Am J Med 92:363, 1992

KOZIN F: Painful shoulder and the reflex sympathetic dystrophy syndrome, in *Arthritis and Allied Conditions*, 13th ed, DJ McCarty, WJ Koopman (eds). Philadelphia, Lea & Febiger, 1993

MATSEN FA III, ARNTZ CT: Subacromial impingement, in *The Shoulder*, Lewis Reines (ed). Philadelphia, Saunders, 1990, p 623

MATUCCI-CERINIC M (ed): First International Workshop on Hypertrophic Osteoarthropathy. Clin Exp Rheumatol 10(suppl. 7):1, 1992

MICHET CJ: Vasculitis and relapsing polychondritis. Rheum Dis Clin North Am 16:441, 1990

MUÑOZ-GOMEZ J et al: Reflex sympathetic dystrophy syndrome of the lower limbs in renal transplant patients treated with Cyclosporin A. Arthritis Rheum 34:625, 1991

NEER CS II: Impingement lesions. Clin Orthop 173:70, 1983

PINEDA C et al: The spectrum of soft tissue and skeletal abnormalities of hypertrophic osteoarthropathy. J Rheumatol 17:626, 1990

SCHILLER AL: Tumors and tumor-like lesions involving joints, in *Textbook of Rheumatology*, WN Kelley et al (eds). Philadelphia, Saunders, 1993

UHTHOFF HK, SARKAR K: An algorithm for shoulder pain caused by soft-tissue disorders. Clin Orthop 254:121, 1990

WEISMAN MH: Arthritis associated with hematologic disorders, storage diseases, disorders of lipid metabolism, and dysproteinemias, in *Arthritis and Allied Conditions*, 13th ed, DJ McCarty, WJ Koopman (eds). Philadelphia, Lea & Febiger, 1993

WOLFE F et al: The American College of Rheumatology 1990 criteria for the classification of fibromyalgia: Report of the multicenter criteria committee. Arthritis Rheum 33:160, 1990

PART TWELVE

HEMATOLOGY AND ONCOLOGY

300 IMPACT OF MOLECULAR BIOLOGY ON HEMATOLOGY

STUART H. ORKIN

Phenotypic variation is the essence of genetics, whether reflected in normal polymorphism or inherited disease. Differences between individuals are encoded in cellular DNA (the *genome*), the reservoir of genetic information for the individual as well as the species. Until recently the precise relationship between a given phenotype (a trait or a disease) and a specific alteration in cellular DNA could only be inferred. For example, where a specific protein was known to be structurally abnormal in a clinical condition, demonstration of an amino acid replacement in the mutant product allowed one to predict a substitution in the DNA on the basis of the genetic code. Thus, the substitution of glutamic acid by valine at the sixth amino acid of the beta chain of sickle hemoglobin could be accounted for by a change in a single nucleotide in cellular DNA (Chap. 60).

During the past 15 years a revolution has occurred in the biomedical sciences with the introduction of the powerful methods of recombinant DNA that permit isolation of genes in pure form and their precise characterization. In many spheres of medicine recombinant DNA technology offers great promise, only one tangible consequence of which is the commercial production of new proteins such as growth factors, hormones, and enzymes. Nowhere has the impact of recombinant DNA been more immediate than in the understanding, diagnosis, and potential treatment of hematologic diseases.

IMMEDIATE IMPACT ON HEMATOLOGIC DISEASE

The application of recombinant DNA technology to the analysis of disease has expanded greatly since its introduction in about 1978; therefore discussion of its impact on hematologic disease must of necessity be selective. Consideration of the hemoglobinopathies, particularly thalassemia syndromes, is particularly instructive.

DETERMINING THE MOLECULAR BASIS OF DISEASE For nearly three decades it has been appreciated that thalassemia syndromes result from unbalanced synthesis of globin chains (Chap. 306). Prior to recombinant DNA methods, reduced (or absent) synthesis of specific globin polypeptides in various thalassemia syndromes was established, as was deficiency of specific messenger RNAs. Whether deficiency was secondary to mutations in globin genes per se or in genes that regulate their expression, and how specific mutations led to reduced mRNA synthesis or function, were largely unknown. This changed with the advent of procedures that permitted isolation of globin genes from patients with thalassemias, determination of their nucleotide sequences, and analysis of expression of the cloned genes upon their reintroduction into cells. It became possible to elucidate the precise molecular basis of these syndromes. Rather than representing a single type of mutation, thalassemia syndromes reflect the entire spectrum of molecular defects that might be predicted to interfere with gene expression. Lesions include gross gene deletions, but more commonly consist of *single base substitutions*

in globin genes that adversely affect gene transcription, proper removal of intervening sequences during RNA splicing, mRNA polyadenylation, translatability, or stability.

The thalassemia syndromes were the first genetic disorders to be described in detail at the molecular level. The comprehensive dissection of the thalassemia syndromes relied on combining gene cloning with RFLP haplotype analysis. The latter method takes advantage of RFLPs, or *restriction fragment length polymorphisms*, to characterize the chromosome vicinity of the globin genes. In a given chromosomal region, the pattern of restriction site differences constitutes a RFLP haplotype, much as differences at histocompatibility loci form a haplotype. It was reasoned that haplotype differences surrounding the human β-globin gene might provide a signature for different chromosomal backgrounds upon which mutations in the β-globin gene producing thalassemia might have arisen. It thus became possible to group potentially identical mutant alleles together and focus attention on those among them that differ from the others. Therefore, examination of cloned β-globin genes (representing different chromosome haplotypes) revealed a comprehensive picture of mutations in thalassemia with high efficiency and speed.

IMPACT ON DIAGNOSIS At the clinical level, the new genetic methods have had their greatest impact on diagnosis. This has resulted from the development of techniques for the detection of specific gene defects in uncloned DNA samples. The feasibility of identifying specific defects in small DNA samples permits examination of the distribution of mutations in populations, carrier detection in families at risk (or those possibly at risk), and prenatal diagnosis as early as the first trimester by chorionic villus biopsy sampling and later by amniocentesis.

Although extensive DNA deletion, insertion, or rearrangement may often be the molecular basis of an inherited disorder, most gene mutations in inherited disorders are single nucleotide changes that cannot be detected by gross examination of gene structure. To diagnose such defects, highly sensitive assays are required that distinguish mutant from normal DNA sequences in a specific region of a gene. With a catalogue of clinically relevant gene mutations for which individuals may be surveyed (as is available for the thalassemia syndromes), these procedures may be applied with great precision. The detection of the sickle cell mutation is already a classic demonstration of the application of recombinant DNA methods to diagnosis. A substitution of T for A in the sixth codon of the β-globin gene, which directs the replacement of valine for glutamic acid, is the underlying basis for sickle cell anemia. Quite fortuitously, this single change abolishes a recognition site in the gene for a restriction enzyme (Mst II) and, thereby, alters the fragments of the gene generated upon digestion of total DNA by this enzyme. With the procedure of Southern, in which DNA fragments are electrophoretically separated in gels and then probed for specific sequences by molecular hybridization (see Chap. 61), the relevant β-globin gene fragments may be visualized. In this manner a molecular diagnosis of normal, sickle trait, or sickle cell anemia can be achieved accurately and reliably with a small DNA sample from blood cells or fetal material. This approach has been used in the prenatal diagnosis of sickle cell anemia with considerable success (Chap. 306).

APPLICATIONS OF POLYMERASE CHAIN REACTION (PCR) The newer and simpler PCR method was also first applied in the analysis of the sickle cell mutation. With synthetic DNA primers flanking the sickle mutation, the critical DNA segment can be amplified in vitro more than a millionfold to provide material sufficient for analysis by restriction enzyme digestion, molecular hybridization, or even direct DNA sequencing. Since the method requires only minute samples, takes hours rather than days, and can be automated, PCR has rapidly found its way into clinical as well as research laboratories.

The extraordinary power of PCR methodology is perhaps best exemplified by its application to the analysis of minimal residual disease in hematologic malignancies. In many forms of cancer very specific cytogenetic alterations occur (Chap. 317). Often these involve breakage and union of ordinarily separate chromosomal regions; typical examples are the translocations found in chronic myelogenous leukemia (Chap. 310). To the extent that such translocations are found within a limited target region, these chromosomal abnormalities may be detected with PCR primers flanking the breakpoints. An especially informative example is follicular lymphoma, in which there is frequently a chromosome 14;18 translocation. The 14;18 breakpoints connect one of six immunoglobulin heavy chain joining (J_h) regions on chromosome 14 to a small breakpoint region on the *BCL2* gene on chromosome 18. With PCR (using primers flanking the junctures), a single abnormal cell is detectable among more than 10^6 normal cells. Therefore, PCR presents the means to identify the subclinical presence of residual neoplastic cells. Although the precise clinical significance of small numbers of residual leukemic cells in patients in apparent remission remains to be determined, it is highly likely that correlations of the residual neoplastic cell burden with clinical outcome and treatment will be important for management of hematologic malignancies.

DETECTION OF CLONALITY IN CELL POPULATIONS   A related application of recombinant DNA methods to hematologic malignancies is the detection of *clonality in cell populations*. The clonal expansion of lymphoid cells is generally taken to reflect proliferation of malignant cells, whereas polyclonal expansion is not. Rearrangements of immunoglobulin genes and T cell receptor loci normally accompany differentiation of B and T cells, respectively. In light of this, Southern blot analysis of lymphoid cell DNA with appropriate molecular probes can provide evidence regarding the clonality of cell populations. Taken together with other findings, such information can make clinical diagnoses more precise.

Using DNA probes that detect RFLPs, the cellular DNAs of virtually any two (or more) individuals can be distinguished, particularly if highly polymorphic probes (called *fingerprinting probes*) are employed. The capability of distinguishing the genotypes of cells has also found an application in the management of patients following bone marrow transplantation. Analysis of RFLPs following allogeneic transplantation enables assessment of the relative contribution of host and donor hematopoietic cells. Engraftment of donor marrow, reemergence of host elements, and mixed cell chimerism can be evaluated with RFLP analysis.

Selected applications of recombinant DNA methods in clinical diagnosis are summarized in Table 300-1.

IMPACT ON THE UNDERSTANDING OF DISEASE AND NORMAL BIOLOGY

Some diseases reflect a disturbance of normal cellular physiology. An understanding of their biochemical basis can often provide novel insights into normal biology. Until recently, the analysis of inherited human disorders required identification and characterization of specific proteins and their corresponding genes.

Many conditions, however, including those affecting the hematopoietic system, display phenotypes for which adequate biochemical explanations are lacking. In general, animal models that faithfully mimic human disorders are not available. However, using an approach that combines classic genetics and recombinant DNA methods, the gene affected in a disorder can now be identified without specific

TABLE 300-1   Recombinant DNA analysis in clinical diagnosis

Application	Examples
Detection of specific mutations in populations and families at risk	Carrier detection of sickle cell anemia Estimation of specific β-thalassemia mutations in populations
Prenatal diagnosis of disease	β Thalassemia, sickle cell anemia
Detection of minimal residual disease in malignancy	Chromosome 14;18 translocation in follicular lymphoma
Detection of clonality in cell populations	Rearrangement of Ig and T cell receptor gene loci in lymphomas
Distinguishing genotypes of hematopoietic cells	Assessment of host/donor cell contributions following allogeneic bone marrow transplantation

knowledge of the protein product. With DNA probes that recognize RFLPs within families at risk for an inherited condition, markers that are very closely linked to a particular disease locus may be identified. By a variety of methods, the region of the relevant gene may be further delimited by additional linkage mapping or by use of patient samples bearing DNA deletions or chromosomal translocations. Ultimately, a region of DNA that gives rise to an mRNA that is structurally or quantitatively deranged in the disease defines the gene itself. This approach to the identification and characterization of the affected gene and its product is now referred to as *positional cloning*.

IMPACT OF POSITIONAL CLONING OF DISEASE GENES   Examples of the impact of this approach to disease are rapidly emerging. One of the first involved the analysis of an inherited hematologic disorder, the X-linked variety of chronic granulomatous disease (X-CGD). In this disease activated phagocytic white blood cells of affected males fail to produce superoxide anion, an important chemical component of the host defense system against microorganisms (Chap. 79). The cellular biochemistry of superoxide generation and its derangement in X-CGD has been actively studied since the first description of this rare disorder more than 30 years ago. Nonetheless, considerable controversy existed regarding the nature of the essential cellular proteins and the X-chromosome-encoded locus in the disease. Although the details are beyond the scope of this chapter, the molecular cloning of the gene involved in X-CGD rapidly demonstrated the requirement for an unusual cytochrome molecule in white blood cell superoxide production. In addition, further work has provided useful biochemical and molecular reagents with which to pursue dissection of superoxide production in greater depth. Positional cloning has also elucidated the genetic defects in Duchenne muscular dystrophy and in retinoblastoma, neurofibromatosis, and fragile-X syndrome, among others.

The great promise of positional cloning to the understanding of inherited disorders relates to the power of recombinant DNA methods, where in rapid succession (1) the protein product of a gene can be determined from a DNA sequence; (2) specific reagents to that protein can be generated either by immunization with synthetic peptides deduced from the sequence or with material manufactured in bacteria; and (3) the normal versions of the involved genes can be introduced into mammalian cells to analyze protein function. This approach will facilitate understanding of normal cellular physiology as well as efforts to correct disease phenotypes.

NEW MODELS OF HEMATOLOGIC DISEASE   In addition to providing the relevant genes and the tools with which to study their encoded proteins and expression, recombinant DNA methods applied to mice allow for the generation of animal models of disease. For example, introduction of genes found at the sites of chromosomal translocations in various leukemias or lymphomas into the germline of mice ultimately leads to transgenic lines that develop malignancies which closely mimic those seen in humans. Furthermore, targeted gene mutation by homologous recombination provides the means to create mice with specific genetic deficiencies. In the coming years it is highly likely that mouse models for most of the inherited and acquired hematologic disorders will be developed.

IMPACT OF THE NEW GENETICS ON TREATMENT OF HEMATOLOGIC DISORDERS

In at least four areas recombinant DNA technology has had a major impact on clinical hematology (Tables 300-1 and 300-2). First, as noted above, identification of the specific gene mutations leading to thalassemia syndromes has led to effective and efficient prenatal diagnosis of disease. In geographic areas where these conditions are prevalent, programs for prenatal diagnosis, coupled with routine hematologic screening and genetic counseling, have dramatically reduced the incidence of births of newly affected individuals. This is a monumental achievement in public health management of a genetic disorder.

Second, as also noted above, the development of new methods for the detection of specific DNA abnormalities in only a few cells among many allows better assessment of residual disease in hematologic malignancies. Correlation of clinical outcome with residual disease status and treatment is likely to lead to improved therapy.

Third, the availability of new hematopoietic growth factors through molecular cloning and gene expression is beginning to change the clinical management of several conditions. For example, the introduction of erythropoietin into the clinic constitutes a major new approach to the treatment of the anemia of chronic renal disease. Abnormalities of white blood cell production, particularly the transient neutropenia accompanying cancer chemotherapy, is now more effectively managed by administration of growth factors (colony stimulating factors) for myelomonocytic cells.

Fourth, production of blood clotting factors by recombinant DNA methods provides a promising approach to the treatment of hemophilias.

Other applications of recombinant DNA technology in clinical hematology are more speculative, but two warrant discussion.

DRUG MANIPULATION OF GENE EXPRESSION   Since the production of fetal hemoglobin generally reduces the consequences of sickle cell anemia or thalassemia, studies have focused on the pharmacologic stimulation of fetal hemoglobin production in adults. Based on the observation that the modification of cellular DNA by methylation is often associated with gene inactivity, 5-azacytidine, a drug that causes widespread demethylation, has been tested for its effects on fetal hemoglobin production in patients with thalassemia or sickle cell anemia. While an augmentation in production was observed, the molecular basis for the effect has remained controversial. Nonetheless, this research has led to the testing of a variety of cytotoxic agents (such as hydroxyurea) and a variety of butyrate derivatives that appear to exert a similar effect on fetal hemoglobin production. Although the precise mechanisms by which such drugs exert their effect is unclear, increases in fetal hemoglobin production are often in the range predicted to be of clinical benefit. Hence, it is apparent that knowledge of the molecular biology of specific gene systems should generate novel therapies for the management of severe inherited hematologic disorders.

SOMATIC GENE THERAPY   A potential application of recombinant DNA technology to clinical hematology now being explored is *somatic gene therapy.* The ability to clone genes and reintroduce them into cells offers prospects for correcting inherited disease by genetic means. The intent of such an approach would be to treat only somatic cells of the affected individual (somatic gene therapy), rather than attempting to correct the germline. At present, somatic gene therapy is envisioned only for severe, life-threatening disorders for which conventional medical management is unsatisfactory. Many methods for the introduction of the normal version of a gene into a cell bearing defective versions have been considered. At present, the most promising avenue would appear to be the use of modified, recombinant RNA viruses (retroviruses) to achieve efficient transfer of new genetic material into hematopoietic stem cells. Recent attention has focused on modified adenoviruses as an alternative delivery vehicle.

In principle, the hematopoietic system is an attractive target for gene therapy because pluripotent stem cells self-renew and also give rise to cell progenitors and mature blood cells. Furthermore, extensive experience in bone marrow transplantation provides a strong base for management of the host, the handling of marrow cells, and the reconstitution of the hematopoietic system by infusion of donor cells. In somatic therapy, genetically modified cells of the affected patient, rather than stem cells from another individual, would be used for cellular reconstitution. The inherited disorders that seem most appropriate for this approach include immunodeficiencies, such as severe combined immunodeficiency due to lack of adenosine deaminase (Chap. 278), hemoglobinopathies (thalassemia and sickle cell anemia), storage disorders (such as Gaucher's disease), and coagulation factor deficiencies (such as hemophilia A). Although considerable progress in the methodologies required for somatic gene therapy has been made, efficient infection of sufficient numbers of stem cells by recombinant retroviruses and adequate expression of the introduced gene in hematopoietic stem cells and their progeny remain formidable problems retarding clinical use. Nonetheless, numerous research protocols are under study in many laboratories and should form the basis for attempts to cure various disorders by gene therapy. Preliminary attempts to manage adenosine deaminase deficiency by retroviral infection of host T cells and subsequent expansion of the cells in vitro appear promising. Because correction of a mutant gene in the chromosome (rather than introduction of a normal gene copy randomly into the host cell genome) would be preferable, since regulated expression would be guaranteed, attention is also being directed to the use of targeted gene insertion.

Current and potential applications of recombinant DNA methods in the management of hematologic disease are summarized in Table 300-2.

Disorders of the hematopoietic system have proved to be a fruitful arena for the application of recombinant DNA methods to clinical medicine. Progressively greater impact of these methods on diagnosis and on the understanding of pathophysiology is virtually assured. Sensitive diagnostic approaches to clonality and minimal residual disease are likely to guide future management of malignant disease. Finally, we can be cautiously optimistic about the potential of recombinant DNA technology to provide novel approaches to treatment, including pharmacologic manipulation of gene expression and somatic genetic therapy.

TABLE 300-2   Recombinant DNA and management of hematologic disease

Application	Examples
Current	
Prenatal diagnosis of inherited disorders	β Thalassemia and sickle cell anemia
Detection of minimal residual disease in malignancy	Translocation in follicular lymphoma
	Ig or T cell receptor gene rearrangements
Administration of hematopoietic growth factors	Erythropoietin for anemia of chronic renal disease
Administration of clotting factors	Factor VIII for hemophilia A
Under study	
Modulation of gene expression to ameliorate severity of clinical disease	Stimulation of fetal hemoglobin production in sickle cell anemia
	Use of γ-interferon in chronic granulomatous disease
Possible for future	
Somatic therapy for the correction of inherited disease	Candidates
	Hemoglobinopathies
	Adenosine deaminase deficiency
	Storage disorders
	Coagulation deficiencies

REFERENCES

ANDERSON WF: Human gene therapy. Science 256:808, 1992

COLLINS FS: Positional cloning: Let's not call it reverse anymore. Nature Genet 1:3, 1992

ERLICH HA (ed): *PCR Technology: Principles and Applications for DNA Amplification.* New York, Stockton Press, 1989

MULLIGAN RC: The basic science of gene therapy. Science 260:926, 1993

ORKIN SH: Molecular genetics and inherited human disease, in *The Metabolic Basis of Inherited Disease*, 6th ed, CR Scriver et al (eds). New York, McGraw-Hill, 1989

————, KAZAZIAN HH JR: Mutation and polymorphism of the human beta-globin gene and its surrounding DNA. Annu Rev Genet 18:131, 1984

ANDERSON WF: Human gene therapy. Science 256:808, 1992

COLLINS FS: Positional cloning: Let's not call it reverse anymore. Nature Genet 1:3, 1992

section 1 Disorders of the hematopoietic system

301 MOLECULAR AND CELLULAR HEMATOPOIESIS

MARK A. GOLDBERG / H. FRANKLIN BUNN

The understanding of blood cell formation, or hematopoiesis, has been greatly enhanced by recent advances in cell culture techniques and the application of recombinant DNA technology. The cloning and characterization of an array of hematopoietic growth factors have provided new insights into the regulation of production and the biologic function of hematopoietic cells. Several of these recombinant proteins have now been produced on a large scale and have made the transition from the laboratory bench to the bedside, where clinical applications are being investigated extensively.

HEMATOPOIETIC STEM CELLS   All the cells circulating in the blood are descendents of a very small number of pluripotent stem cells. These ancestral cells, which comprise less than 0.01 percent of the nucleated cells in the bone marrow, are capable of restoring normal hematopoiesis in irradiated animals and in patients with bone marrow aplasia. The pluripotent stem cell has the unique capacity for self-renewal and the potential for growth and differentiation along granulocytic, monocytic, erythroid, megakaryocytic, and lymphoid lineages. Some stem cells divide and give rise to progeny that lose their ability to differentiate along multiple pathways and become committed to a specific hematopoietic lineage. These committed progenitor cells continue to proliferate and differentiate into morphologically identifiable precursor cells which then undergo terminal maturation, thereby developing highly specialized functions and losing their ability to proliferate. Techniques have been developed which support the growth and differentiation of hematopoietic progenitor cells in vitro. Using these techniques, hematopoietic colonies of mixed and single lineages have been identified and characterized with respect to the factors required for their growth. These hematopoietic colonies are termed *colony forming units* (CFU) or *burst forming units* (BFU), with the specific type of colony designated by suffixes indicating the constituent cell types. Figure 301-1 depicts an outline of hematopoietic differentiation from the pluripotent stem cell to the highly specialized terminally matured blood cells.

CLONAL ORIGIN OF HEMATOPOIETIC MALIGNANCIES   Hematologic malignancies arise as a clonal proliferation of one of the progenitor cells depicted in Fig. 301-1. The clinical manifestations of a particular malignancy depend on the stage of differentiation and lineage of the affected cell as well as on the specific nature of the initial mutation and of subsequent mutations that may appear during clonal evolution. In order for the abnormal clone of cells to attain sufficient tumor mass to produce clinical symptoms and signs, it must possess a growth advantage over the normal cells.

Molecular techniques can be used to establish the clonal origin of known and suspected tumor cells. A monoclonal proliferation of cells in the blood, bone marrow, or lymph nodes can be distinguished from a polyclonal proliferation by morphologic examination of chromosomes in search of clonal karyotypic abnormalities. Alternatively, analysis of DNA by Southern blot hybridization or the polymerase chain reaction can be used to identify (1) clonal immunoglobulin gene rearrangements in suspected B lymphocyte malignancies, (2) clonal T cell receptor gene rearrangements in T lymphocyte malignancies, and (3) diagnostic gene translocations such as the *bcr-abl* translocation seen in chronic myelogenous leukemia. In females with the appropriate polymorphic loci on the X chromosome, clonality can be established by glucose-6-phosphate dehydrogenase isoenzyme patterns or analysis of DNA restriction fragments. This information is useful for several purposes: It may allow one to establish a definitive diagnosis of a malignancy; it may provide insight into the cell of origin and the steps in tumor progression; and it also may provide a sensitive tool for assessing remission or early relapse.

Clonal analysis of mature blood cells indicates that the myeloproliferative disorders generally arise in the pluripotent stem cell. Similarly, many of the myelodysplastic syndromes appear to be clonal stem cell disorders. The cell of origin in the acute leukemias and its effect on response to therapy and prognosis are currently being studied. Understanding the cell of origin in the various lymphoid malignancies has facilitated the classification of this complex group of disorders.

HEMATOPOIETIC GROWTH FACTORS   Also depicted in Fig. 301-1 are many of the known hematopoietic growth factors and cytokines necessary for growth and differentiation of cells in the various lineages. The biologic activities of most of these hematopoietic cytokines have been determined largely by in vitro cell culture experiments. Their in vivo regulation and physiologic roles are currently the object of intense study. As depicted in the diagram, some of the growth factors, such as stem cell factor (SCF; also known as *steel factor* or *c-kit ligand*), interleukin 3 (IL-3), and granulocyte-macrophage colony stimulating factor (GM-CSF), have the potential to influence the proliferation and differentiation of several hematopoietic lineages; in addition, they have overlapping and synergistic activities. Other growth factors, such as erythropoietin, granulocyte colony stimulating factor (G-CSF), and macrophage colony stimulating factor (M-CSF) act primarily on later progenitor cells committed to a single lineage. G-CSF also has been shown recently to play a synergistic role in stimulating early multilineage progenitors in hematopoietic cell culture experiments, though the in vivo importance of this observation is unknown. Furthermore, G-CSF, M-CSF, GM-CSF, and IL-3 have been shown not only to stimulate proliferation and differentiation of hematopoietic cells but also to modulate the function of mature granulocytes and mononuclear phagocytes.

The hematopoietic growth factors act by binding to specific receptors present on the surface of target cells. An increasing number of these growth factor receptors have been cloned; they share limited homologies with one another and appear to constitute a superfamily of growth factor receptor genes. The expression of a specific receptor

Pluripotent
Stem Cell

SCF   *IL-1*   *IL-1*
G-CSF   *IL-3*   *IL-6*
            IL-6   *SCF*

CFU-G, E, M, Mega   B Stem Cell   T Stem Cell

GM-CSF   *IL-1*   *IL-1*
IL-3   *IL-6*   *IL-2*
            IL-11   *GM-CSF*   *IL-7*   *IL-6*
                            IL-3   *IL-7*

Progenitor Cells

BFU-E   CFU-Mega   CFU-GM   CFU-Eo   CFU-Baso   Pre B Cell   Prothymocyte

GM-CSF   *GM-CSF*   *GM-CSF*   *GM-CSF*   *GM-CSF*   *IL-1*
IL-3   *IL-3*   *IL-3*   *IL-3*   *IL-3*   *IL-3* *IL-2*   *IL-2*
           IL-6   *IL-4*   *IL-4*
CFU-E   CFU-G   CFU-M   CFU-Eo   CFU-Baso   *IL-5*
                                                                    IL-6
Epo   *GM-CSF*   *GM-CSF*   *GM-CSF* *IL-3*
                      G-CSF   *M-CSF*   *IL-5*   *IL-4*

**Recognizable
Precursors**

Proerythroblast Mega-   Myeloblast Monoblast   Eosinophilic Basophilic   B   T
                 karyocyte   Myeloblast   Myeloblast   Lymphoblast Lymphoblast

Epo   *GM-CSF*   *GM-CSF*   *IL-3*   Antigen   Antigen
                            G-CSF   *M-CSF*   *IL-4*   Driven   Driven

Erythrocyte Platelet Neutrophil Monocyte   Eosinophil   Basophil   B Cell   T Cell

                                                                IL-3
                                                                IL-4

                              Macrophage   Mast Cell   Plasma Cell

FIGURE 301-1 A depiction of the stem cell model of hematopoiesis. Growth factors and cytokines influencing particular steps in the differentiation pathway are shown. Abbreviations not in the text: G, granulocyte; E, erythrocyte; M, monocyte; Mega, megakaryocyte; Eo, eosinophil; Baso, basophil; Epo, erythropoietin.

or combination of receptors on the cell surface may determine the cell's ultimate path of differentiation.

Erythropoietin This 30-kDa glycoprotein hormone is crucial to the regulation of erythropoiesis. The primary site of erythropoietin production after birth is the kidney, probably in peritubular interstitial cells located in the inner cortex and outer medulla. In the fetus, the liver is the major site of erythropoietin production. In response to the sensing of hypoxia in the kidney and liver, erythropoietin gene transcription increases, leading to increased erythropoietin mRNA and increased production and secretion of erythropoietin protein. The hormone travels to hematopoietic tissues, where it binds to its receptor on erythroid progenitor cells, stimulating proliferation and differentiation. This results in an increase in the oxygen-carrying capacity of the blood, thereby alleviating the hypoxic stimulus and providing a negative feedback loop. In patients with normal renal function, serum erythropoietin levels are inversely proportional to the hemoglobin concentration.

Myeloid growth factors G-CSF, M-CSF, GM-CSF, and IL-3 work together to stimulate granulocyte and monocyte/macrophage proliferation, differentiation, and function in vitro. Furthermore, GM-CSF and IL-3 contribute to in vitro stimulation of megakaryopoiesis and erythropoiesis (Fig. 301-1). Like erythropoietin, the myeloid cytokines are all relatively small glycoproteins. However, unlike erythropoietin, the recombinant proteins do not appear to require glycosylation for in vivo biologic activity. Many cell types can produce G-CSF, M-CSF, and GM-CSF in the setting of inflammation (Fig. 301-2), while IL-3 production appears to be limited to T lymphocytes and mast cells. The regulation of their production involves a complex network of signaling and feedback loops which are in large part influenced by inflammatory cytokines, including interleukin 1 (IL-1), tumor necrosis factor α (TNFα), interleukin 6 (IL-6), and interferon-γ (IFN-γ), as well as by foreign antigens. T

FIGURE 301-2 Network of signaling and feedback loops and sites of production of the hematopoietic growth factors and cytokines involved in the regulation of the inflammatory response.

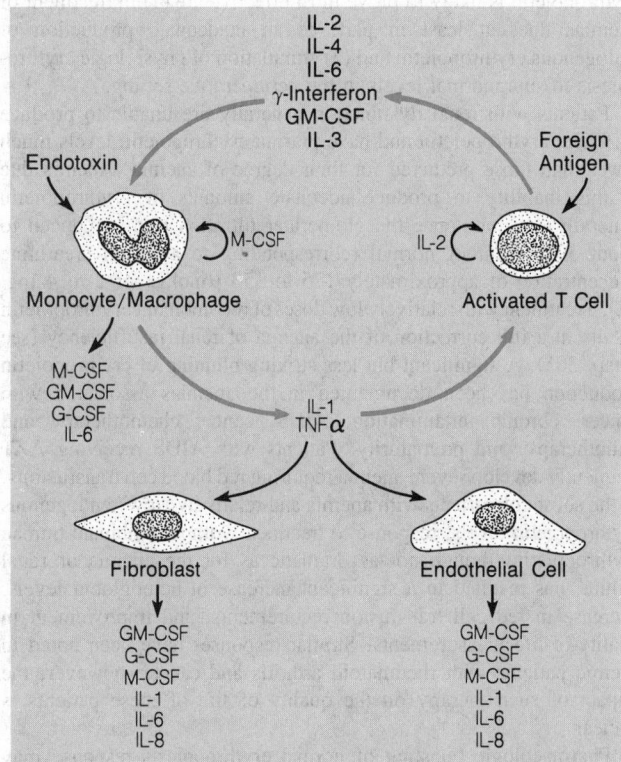

IL-2
IL-4
IL-6
γ-Interferon
GM-CSF
IL-3

Endotoxin   Foreign
                                             Antigen

            M-CSF   IL-2

Monocyte/Macrophage   Activated T Cell

M-CSF
GM-CSF   IL-1
G-CSF   TNFα
IL-6

Fibroblast   Endothelial Cell

GM-CSF   GM-CSF
G-CSF   G-CSF
M-CSF   M-CSF
IL-1   IL-1
IL-6   IL-6
IL-8   IL-8

lymphocytes are induced to produce IL-3, GM-CSF, IL-6, and IFN-γ as the result of activation by antigen or IL-1. These activated T cell products, in turn, stimulate monocytes/macrophages to release IL-1, TNFα, IL-6, and M-CSF. In response to endotoxin, mononuclear phagocytes secrete G-CSF and GM-CSF as well. Both TNFα and IL-1 also induce expression of GM-CSF, G-CSF, IL-6, and IL-1 in fibroblasts and endothelial cells. Additionally, fibroblasts and endothelial cells make M-CSF constitutively. The net result of these interactions is a dramatic increase in the production of G-CSF, M-CSF, GM-CSF, and IL-3 in response to inflammatory stimuli. These growth factors, in turn, both stimulate granulocyte and monocyte production in the bone marrow and enhance the function of granulocytes and macrophages at the site of inflammation. Hence these hematopoietic growth factors play a pivotal role in promoting leukocytosis and enhanced leukocyte function in response to infection and/or inflammation. However, their physiologic role in basal myelopoiesis is less clear.

GM-CSF is rarely present at concentrations sufficient to be detected in the plasma, suggesting that it either functions locally in the tissues that produce it or is rapidly cleared from the circulation. On the other hand, G-CSF is measurable in the plasma, and its concentration has been shown to correlate inversely with neutrophil concentrations in patients with aplastic anemia and cyclic neutropenia. However, in contrast to the deficiency of erythropoietin in renal disease which causes anemia, no G-CSF or GM-CSF deficiency states have been recognized.

CLINICAL APPLICATIONS   Numerous clinical trials have assessed the efficacy of recombinant hematopoietic growth factors, both alone and in combination, in a variety of disorders. Given the significant cost of these drugs, their efficacy and safety must be evaluated critically.

Erythropoietin   In patients with any type of anemia, intervention is generally warranted only to treat symptoms. Hence there is little need to correct a relatively mild anemia with few associated symptoms. Although it has been clearly demonstrated that recombinant human erythropoietin can increase the red cell mass in various patient groups as well as in normal individuals, the true utility of recombinant human erythropoietin depends on demonstrating that it can be used to decrease the need for homologous red blood cell transfusions and/or to improve the quality of life. The two general areas in which recombinant human erythropoietin is likely to prove most effective are (1) in treatment of anemias due, at least in part, to an inadequate production of endogenous erythropoietin and (2) stimulation of physiologic erythropoiesis to supranormal levels in the perioperative setting.

Patients with renal dysfunction generally are unable to produce sufficient erythropoietin and have plasma erythropoietin levels much lower than those predicted for their degree of anemia. Anemia due to this inability to produce adequate amounts of erythropoietin generally develops once the glomerular filtration rate is reduced to about 30 percent of normal (corresponding to a serum creatinine concentration of approximately 175 to 350 μmol/L, or 2 to 4 mg/dL). Treatment with relatively low doses of recombinant erythropoietin results in a full correction of the anemia of renal insufficiency (see Chap. 305). A significant but less striking blunting of erythropoietin production has been documented in the anemias associated with cancer, chronic inflammation, AIDS, cancer chemotherapy and radiotherapy, and prematurity. Patients with AIDS receiving AZT frequently develop severe anemia requiring red blood cell transfusions. In the subset of patients with anemia and relatively "low" endogenous erythropoietin levels, response to treatment with recombinant human erythropoietin, though not as dramatic as for the anemia of renal failure, has resulted in a significant increase in hemoglobin levels, decrease in red cell transfusion requirements, and improvement in quality-of-life measurements. Similar responses have been noted in anemic patients with rheumatoid arthritis and cancer; however, the impact of such therapy on the quality of life of these patients is unclear.

Pharmacologic boosting of normal erythropoiesis response may prove to be of benefit in the perioperative setting. Recombinant human erythropoietin may be used either as an adjunct to enhance autologous blood donation or to stimulate endogenous erythropoiesis without concomitant autologous donation. Such treatment has been shown to increase the number of units of blood that can safely be removed and preserved for autologous transfusion in the postoperative period. In addition, it is likely that recombinant human erythropoietin treatment would enable a reduction in the minimal interval between repeat phlebotomies for a normal blood donor, thereby enabling a recipient to receive multiple transfusions of blood from the same donor. Despite many potential applications of recombinant human erythropoietin in the perioperative setting, it is not yet clear which ones will prove more efficacious and more cost-effective than simply an aggressive preoperative autologous blood donation program.

Myeloid growth factors   The myeloid growth factors G-CSF and GM-CSF have been shown to stimulate neutrophil production in various clinical settings. However, demonstration of clinical efficacy demands more rigorous criteria. Initial studies in cancer patients undergoing intensive cytotoxic chemotherapy and/or radiotherapy suggested that stimulation of granulopoiesis translates into decreased periods of hospitalization and decreased incidence of neutropenia-associated fever and infection. In this regard, the efficacy of G-CSF has subsequently been borne out in multicenter, randomized, placebo-controlled studies. Based on these studies, G-CSF has been approved by the U.S. Food and Drug Administration to decrease the incidence of infection in patients with nonmyeloid malignancies receiving myelosuppressive anticancer medications. G-CSF also has been studied in nonrandomized clinical trials in patients with congenital neutropenia, cyclic neutropenia, myelodysplastic syndromes, AIDS, bone marrow infiltration, and aplastic anemia; it appears to increase the neutrophil count in many patients with these disorders. G-CSF often increases the neutrophil count sufficiently in patients with congenital and cyclic neutropenia and so decreases the frequency and severity of infection. In myelodysplastic syndromes, G-CSF also generally increases the neutrophil count. However, effects on the frequency of infection, progression to acute myelogenous leukemia, and survival are uncertain. G-CSF has been generally well tolerated with no apparent dose-limiting toxicity. The most frequent toxicity has been bone pain, which is usually responsive to mild analgesics.

GM-CSF has been used in settings similar to those in which G-CSF has been studied. Although GM-CSF has proliferative effects on a broader range of hematopoietic progenitors in vitro (see Fig. 301-1), its primary clinical benefit in vivo has been on granulopoiesis. On the basis of well-controlled clinical trials, it has been approved by the U.S. Food and Drug Administration for the acceleration of myeloid recovery following autologous bone marrow transplantation for lymphoid malignancies as well as for use in patients who have undergone allogeneic or autologous bone marrow transplantation in whom engraftment has failed or is delayed. The potential efficacy of GM-CSF in other settings is unclear. Unlike G-CSF, GM-CSF does not appear to be very effective in stimulating neutrophil production in patients with congenital and cyclic neutropenia. In myelodysplastic syndromes, GM-CSF frequently increases the neutrophil and eosinophil counts and occasionally may stimulate other hematopoietic lineages. However, as with G-CSF, its effects on the frequency of infection, progression to acute myelogenous leukemia, and survival in patients with myelodysplastic syndromes are uncertain. Likewise, neither G-CSF nor GM-CSF appears to be generally efficacious in treating severe aplastic anemia. In AIDS patients with neutropenia, the results of studies with GM-CSF have been similar to those with G-CSF. GM-CSF appears to be more toxic than G-CSF. In addition to bone pain, GM-CSF has been noted to cause rash, fevers, myalgias, fatigue, anorexia, phlebitis, thrombosis, eosinophilia, and, at high doses, capillary leak syndrome with pleural and pericardial effusions and edema. The side effects of GM-CSF, especially fever, can complicate the management of critically ill patients with severe neutropenia.

The use of G-CSF or GM-CSF in myeloid malignancies is still

experimental. The potential benefits of these growth factors in these conditions, including stimulating cells to differentiate or chemotherapy sensitization by putting resting cells into cycle, must be weighed against the possibility of enhancing proliferation of a malignant clone, thereby accelerating the pace of the disease.

Based on current information, definitive indications as to when to use G-CSF versus GM-CSF are unclear. Nonetheless, it is becoming evident that if stimulation of neutrophil production is the primary goal, this can be done more specifically, and with fewer potential side effects, with G-CSF. However, because of differences in the spectrum of activity of these cytokines, in situations other than the treatment of neutropenia, the relative utility of G-CSF versus GM-CSF remains to be determined.

Future applications Clinical trials are underway investigating the safety and efficacy of IL-3 and IL-6 in various clinical settings. Studies of many of the other hematopoietic growth factors and cytokines are sure to follow in short order. Many will focus on the potential synergy of combinations of these factors. A particularly exciting property shared by several of these growth factors, including G-CSF, GM-CSF, and IL-3, is the ability to increase markedly the concentration of progenitor cells and stem cells in the peripheral blood. These circulating progenitor cells can be collected by leukapheresis and reinfused along with hematopoietic growth factors following intensive myelosuppressive chemotherapy. In this setting, the combination of peripheral blood progenitor cells and growth factor has been shown to stimulate not only granulopoiesis but also megakaryopoiesis and erythropoiesis. Using combinations of peripheral blood progenitor cells and hematopoietic growth factors may allow further dose intensification of anticancer therapy with the hope of increasing response rates and survival. It also may allow peripheral blood stem cell transplantation to play an increasing role in clinical practice and, in selected patients, may supplant autologous bone marrow transplantation.

REFERENCES

BAGBY GC, SEGAL GM: Growth factors and the control of hematopoiesis, in *Hematology: Basic Principles and Practice*, R Hoffman et al (eds). New York, Churchill Livingstone, 1991, pp 97–121

CRAWFORD J et al: Reduction by granulocyte colony-stimulating factor of fever and neutropenia induced by chemotherapy in patients with small-cell lung cancer. N Engl J Med 325:164, 1991

EMERSON SG: The stem cell model of hematopoiesis, in *Hematology: Basic Principles and Practice*, R Hoffman et al (eds). New York, Churchill Livingstone, 1991, pp 72–81

ESCHBACH JW et al: Correction of the anemia of end-stage renal disease with recombinant human erythropoietin: Results of a combined phase I and II clinical trial. N Engl J Med 316:73, 1987

FLEISCHMAN RA: Southwestern Internal Medicine Conference: Clinical use of hematopoietic growth factors. Am J Med Sci 305:248, 1993

GARNICK MB (ed): *Erythropoietin in Clinical Applications: An International Perspective.* New York, Marcel Dekker, 1990

LIESCHKE GJ, BURGESS AW: Granulocyte colony stimulating factor and granulocyte-macrophage colony stimulating factor. N Engl J Med 327:28, 1992

OGAWA M: Differentiation and proliferation of hematopoietic stem cells. Blood 81:2844, 1993

SINGER JW: Use of recombinant hematopoietic growth factors in bone marrow transplantation. Am J Pediatr Hematol Oncol 15:175, 1993

302 PATHOPHYSIOLOGY OF THE ANEMIAS

H. FRANKLIN BUNN

There is a large and coherent body of information on the birth, life, and death of red cells. Familiarity with erythropoiesis and erythrocyte structure and function is necessary to understand the pathogenesis of the various anemias as well as to develop an orderly approach to diagnosis and management. Conversely, investigation of specific red cell disorders has provided unique insights into normal erythroid physiology.

RED CELL PRODUCTION Red cells are derived from an undifferentiated progenitor cell in the bone marrow called the *pluripotent stem cell* (Fig. 302-1). As explained in more detail in Chap. 301, a stem cell is one which is capable of both self-renewal and differentiation. Erythrocytes, as well as granulocytes, monocytes, platelets, and lymphocytes evolve from this ancestor cell. As Fig. 302-1 shows, the most primitive erythroid progenitor which has been cultured from both bone marrow and peripheral blood is called the *erythroid burst-forming unit* (BFU_e). After 10 to 15 days in tissue culture, it produces a large colony of recognizable red cell precursors. The BFU_e is responsive to high doses of the erythroid-promoting hormone erythropoietin, which acts synergistically with other hematopoietic growth factors (see Chap. 301). A more mature progenitor cell, the *erythroid colony forming unit* (CFU_e), is very sensitive to erythropoietin, producing a smaller clone of erythroid cells after 4 to 7 days in culture.

Erythropoietin is a glycoprotein hormone having a molecular weight of 30,400. Erythropoietin is produced, primarily by the kidneys, in response to hypoxia and is secreted into the plasma. Accordingly, anemic patients have increased plasma levels of this hormone, inversely proportional to their hemoglobin level. In contrast, patients with uremia usually have a marked impairment of erythropoietin production and therefore relatively low plasma levels.

Erythropoietin interacts with a specific receptor on the surface of committed erythroid progenitor cells, inducing them to differentiate into proerythroblasts, the earliest red cell precursor that can be recognized on examination of the bone marrow. Normally, the transition from the proerythroblast to the most mature normoblast involves three or four cell divisions over a 4-day period (see Fig. 302-1). During this time, the nucleus becomes smaller, and an increasing amount of hemoglobin is produced in the cytoplasm. Following the last division, the pyknotic nucleus is removed from the normoblast. What remains is the reticulocyte, which stays in the bone marrow for 2.5 to 3 days. The reticulocyte is then released into the general circulation, where it remains for another 24 h before it loses its mitochondria and ribosomes and assumes the morphologic appearance of a mature red cell.

Erythroid precursor cells ranging from the pronormoblast to the reticulocyte possess a specific surface receptor for the iron-transferrin complex, enabling them to incorporate sufficient iron for hemoglobin production (Fig. 302-2). The use of a radioactive iron label such as ^{59}Fe permits a quantitative assessment of erythropoiesis. From the rate at which injected ^{59}Fe-labeled transferrin disappears from the plasma, plasma iron turnover can be calculated. This parameter is generally proportional to the total developing erythroid cell mass. Normally, about 80 percent of ^{59}Fe bound to plasma transferrin goes to erythroid cells in the marrow. After 4 to 6 days, the labeled iron reappears in circulating erythrocytes. The extent to which circulating red cells acquire the label provides an index of the efficiency or effectiveness of erythropoiesis.

The normal marrow is capable of increasing its red cell production to about three to five times the normal rate within a week or two following stimulation by high levels of erythropoietin. In chronic hemolytic anemias, erythropoiesis may increase five- to sevenfold. As the erythroid marrow expands, fat is replaced by erythroid cells, and formerly inactive or "yellow" marrow becomes active or "red."

HEMOGLOBIN BIOSYNTHESIS Erythroid cell development involves the production of hemoglobin-containing cells. Hemoglobin is a tetramer composed of two pairs of polypeptides, e.g., $\alpha_2\beta_2$. The globin subunits, α, β, γ, and δ, are each covalently linked to a heme group. The synthesis of a particular globin subunit is directed by a corresponding gene inherited from each parent. As shown in Fig. 302-1, there is a marked amplification in the transcription of globin mRNA during the development of proerythroblasts. About 98 percent of the protein in the cytoplasm of circulating red cells is hemoglobin. In the red cells of normal adults, hemoglobin A ($\alpha_2\beta_2$) constitutes

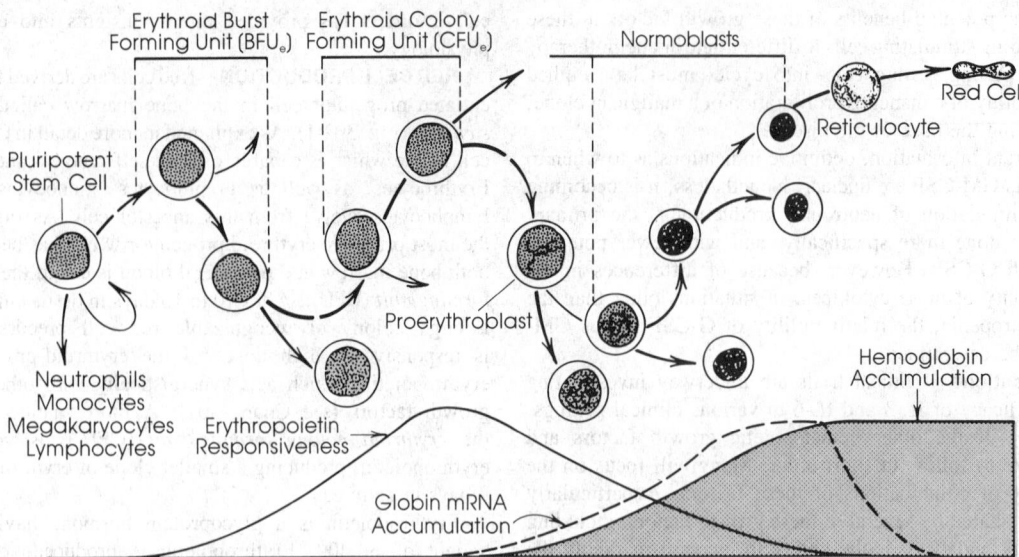

FIGURE 302-1 Differentiation and morphologic maturation of erythroid cells. Erythroid cells are derived from pluripotent stem cells (shown on left) which are also capable of differentiating into neutrophils, monocytes (macrophages), megakaryocytes, and lymphocytes. Under the influence of erythropoietin, erythroid progenitor cells ($BFU_e \rightarrow CFU_e$) differentiate into proerythroblasts, the earliest recognizable erythroid cells in the bone marrow. During further maturation, globin mRNA accumulates, directing the cell to synthesize hemoglobin.

about 97 percent of the total hemoglobin. The remaining 3 percent is primarily hemoglobin A_2 ($\alpha_2\delta_2$). As discussed in Chap. 306, this minor component is increased in patients with β thalassemia. Fetal hemoglobin (HbF or $\alpha_2\gamma_2$) usually accounts for less than 1 percent of total hemoglobin in normal adult red cells. HbF is localized to 1 to 7 percent of red cells. In contrast, it is the main hemoglobin component of fetal red cells. During the last 3 months of gestation, γ-chain synthesis switches to β-chain synthesis. However, in certain types of congenital hemolytic anemias such as the β thalassemias and sickle cell anemia, the production of γ chains (and therefore of HbF) persists. In addition, increased levels of HbF also may be encountered in certain acquired anemias in which there is disordered red cell proliferation.

Normally α- and β-chain synthesis in erythroid precursors is evenly balanced. In contrast, the thalassemias (Chap. 306) are characterized by imbalance in globin chain synthesis.

The synthesis of *heme* in red cell precursors is closely matched to globin chain production. As shown in Fig. 302-3, the initial and rate-limiting step is the condensation of succinyl coenzyme A (CoA) and glycine to form δ-aminolevulinic acid. This reaction, which takes place in mitochondria, requires that glycine be activated by pyridoxal phosphate. Accordingly, patients with sideroblastic anemia, in whom heme synthesis is usually defective, may sometimes respond to pyridoxine therapy (Chap. 303). The next steps of heme synthesis take place in the cytosol. Two molecules of δ-aminolevulinic acid condense to form a ring structure, porphobilinogen. This colorless pyrrole is elevated in acute intermittent porphyria and can be detected in urine by the Watson-Schwartz test. The subsequent steps in prophyrin synthesis are also shown in Fig. 302-3. The last three reactions take place in mitochondria. Iron is inserted into protoporphyrin IX to form heme. In iron deficiency, as well as in lead poisoning, increased levels of protoporphyrin can be detected in red cells.

FIGURE 302-2 Erythrocyte production, circulation, and destruction. Circulating iron-bound transferrin (TF) is bound to specific receptors on the surface of erythroid progenitors and precursors in the marrow. Most of this iron is incorporated into hemoglobin; the remainder is stored as ferritin. Following maturation of the erythroid precursor, the nucleus is shed and the red blood cell emerges from the marrow into the plasma where it circulates for approximately 120 days. The senescent red blood cell is taken up by the mononuclear phagocyte system and is destroyed. The heme iron is initially incorporated into ferritin. This storage iron is available for transport to the marrow via transferrin.

CYTOSOL

Porphobilinogen

Succinate + Glycine → Δ-ALA → Uroporphyrinogen III

Succinyl CoA Synthetase (Mg++, GTP + CoA·S-H ⇌ GDP + Pi)

Δ-ALA Synthetase (Pyridoxal Phosphate)

Δ-ALA-DH (GSH)

UIS, U III CoS

Heme ← (Fe++, GSH, HS) ← Protoporphyrin 9 ← Protoporphyrinogen 9 ← (CO) ← Coproporphyrinogen III

Uroporphyrinogen III → (UD) → Coproporphyrinogen III

Heme + Globin Subunits → Hemoglobin

MITOCHONDRION

FIGURE 302-3 The biosynthesis of heme. Enzymatic steps that occur in mitochondria are shown. The following abbreviations are used: CoA, coenzyme A; GTP, guanosine triphosphate; GDP, guanosine diphosphate; Pi, inorganic phosphorus; GSH, glutathione; δ-ALA-DH, δ-aminolevulinate dehydrase;

UIS, uroporphyrinogen I synthetase; UIII CoS, uroporphyrinogen III cosynthetase; UD, uroporphyrinogen decarboxylase; CO, coproporphyrinogen oxidase; HS, heme synthetase; A, acetate; P, proprionate; M, methyl; V, vinyl.

Disorders of porphyrin synthesis and metabolism are discussed in Chap. 346.

HEMOGLOBIN STRUCTURE AND FUNCTION The primary role of red cells is to transport oxygen from lungs to tissues and to transport carbon dioxide in the reverse direction. Both functions are assumed by hemoglobin. The three-dimensional structure of human hemoglobin has been determined from x-ray crystallographic analysis. The important functional properties of hemoglobin such as subunit cooperativity, the pH dependency of oxygen affinity (the Bohr effect), and the interaction with 2,3-bisphosphoglycerate can now be understood in stereochemical terms. This structural information also has been useful in explaining the abnormal functional properties of a number of human hemoglobin variants which are associated with clinical and hematologic manifestations (see Chap. 306).

During circulation through the lungs, hemoglobin becomes almost fully saturated with oxygen (1.34 mL O_2 per gram of hemoglobin). As red cells perfuse the capillary beds, oxygen is extracted. Efficient unloading of oxygen at relatively high oxygen tensions is possible because of the sigmoid shape of the oxygen dissociation curve (subunit cooperativity) (see Fig. 302-4). The affinity of hemoglobin for oxygen is modified by three intracellular cofactors: hydrogen ion, carbon dioxide, and 2,3-bisphosphoglycerate (2,3-BPG). Increasing the concentrations of each of these three effectors results in a "shift to the right" in the oxygen dissociation curve. In human red cells, 2,3-BPG is an important regulator of hemoglobin function. One molecule of 2,3-BPG binds to the β chains of deoxyhemoglobin, thereby decreasing oxygen affinity. Elevated levels of 2,3-BPG have been noted in various states of hypoxia. The resulting decrease in oxygen affinity permits enhanced oxygen release. The oxygenation of a particular organ or tissue depends on three main factors (depicted in

Fig. 302-5): blood flow, oxygen-carrying capacity of the blood (hemoglobin concentration), and the affinity of the hemoglobin for oxygen. Patients with a primary abnormality of one of these three

FIGURE 302-4 The oxyhemoglobin dissociation curve of normal blood. The major factors influencing the position of the curve are pH, temperature, and the intracellular concentration of 2,3-BPG. An increase in plasma pH or a decrease in temperature and 2,3-BPG causes an increase in oxygen affinity (shift to the left) and a relative decrease in oxygen unloading when going from an arterial P_{O_2} of 12.7 kPa (95 mmHg) to a venous P_{O_2} of 5.3 kPa (40 mmHg). Conversely, a decrease in pH or an increase in either temperature or 2,3-BPG causes a decrease in oxygen affinity (shift to the right) and a relative increase in oxygen unloading.

FIGURE 302-5 Oxygen delivered to an organ or tissue is directly proportional to (1) blood flow, (2) hemoglobin concentration, and (3) the difference in oxygen saturation of the arterial and venous blood. Patients with various types of hypoxia may compensate in the following ways: (1) The distribution of blood flow is altered to maintain oxygenation of vital organs; total cardiac output increases when hypoxia is severe. (2) Increased erythropoietin production stimulates erythropoiesis. (3) Oxygen unloading is enhanced by a shift to the right in the oxygen dissociation curve, mediated by an increase in red cell 2,3-BPG.

factors depend on adjustments in one or both of the other two in order to maintain optimal tissue oxygenation. For example, patients with anemia have two available modes of compensation: enhanced blood flow and decreased oxygen affinity, mediated by increased levels of 2,3-BPG. Conversely, individuals with a hemoglobin variant having increased oxygen affinity have a primary defect in oxygen unloading. As discussed in Chap. 306, such patients compensate by developing secondary erythrocytosis.

RED BLOOD CELL METABOLISM As the red cell emerges from the bone marrow, it loses its nucleus, ribosomes, and mitochondria and therefore all capability for cell division, protein synthesis, and oxidative phosphorylation. Compared with other cells, the erythrocyte has a rather simple scheme of intermediary metabolism. Glucose is virtually the only fuel utilized by the red cell. It readily enters the red cell by facilitated diffusion and is then converted to glucose-6-phosphate. There are two major pathways available for glucose-6-phosphate (see Fig. 307-2). About 80 to 90 percent of this intermediate is converted to lactate by means of the glycolytic (or Embden-Meyerhof) pathway. Two moles of adenosine triphosphate (ATP) are generated for every mole of glucose metabolized. The intracellular mediator of hemoglobin function, 2,3-bisphosphoglycerate, is synthe-

sized in a side reaction shown in Fig. 307-2. About 10 percent of intracellular glucose-6-phosphate undergoes oxidation by means of the hexose-monophosphate shunt. This pathway maintains glutathione in the reduced form, thereby protecting sulfhydryl groups in hemoglobin and the red cell membrane from oxidation by peroxides and superoxide as well as by certain drugs and toxins. Such oxidant stress can compromise red cell function and viability in patients with a deficiency in glucose-6-phosphate dehydrogenase, the first enzymatic step in the hexose-monophosphate shunt (see Chap. 307). Much less commonly, individuals may have a deficiency in one of the enzymes of the glycolytic pathway or in one of the other enzymes of the hexose-monophosphate shunt.

The red cell has rather modest metabolic obligations in keeping with its simplified structure. A significant portion of the ATP generated by glycolysis is spent in driving the sodium-potassium pump necessary to preserve the ionic milieu in the cytoplasm and prevent colloid osmotic lysis. In addition, some metabolic energy is expended on maintenance and repair of the red cell membrane. Certain proteins in the membrane become phosphorylated by means of ATP and protein kinases, but the physiologic significance of this process is not yet understood. Finally, a small amount of metabolic currency is spent on maintaining hemoglobin iron atoms in the reduced form (Fe^{2+}).

The 120-day survival of the circulating red cell is dependent on preservation of the pliability of its membrane. The red cell membrane is composed of 50 percent protein, 40 percent lipid, and 10 percent carbohydrate. It is a bilayer consisting of molecules of phospholipid and cholesterol in a 1.2:1 molar ratio assembled in a stacked array so that the hydrophobic portions of the molecules are oriented toward the interior while the polar side groups are either on the external surface of the cell (the plasma membrane) or on the inner cytoplasmic surface (Fig. 302-6). The distribution of phospholipids differs significantly in the two portions of the bilayer. The outer surface is relatively rich in lecithin and sphingomyelin, while the inner surface has relatively more phosphatidyl serine and phosphatidyl ethanolamine. The lipids on the outer surface exchange freely with plasma lipids.

The red cell membrane contains a limited number of major proteins depicted in Fig. 302-6 and a large number of minor components. These proteins can be divided into two groups. Among those that span the lipid bilayer are glycophorin, which contains a number of

FIGURE 302-6 Diagram of a cross section of the red blood cell membrane. Spectrin, actin, tropomyosin, and protein 4.1 form a meshwork which laminates the inner surface of the membrane. In contrast, other proteins such as the glycophorins (GP) and protein 3 (the anion transport channel) traverse the lipid bilayer. Long polysaccharide chains are covalently attached to these proteins on the outer surface of the cell and also to glycolipid. Ankyrin and

protein 4.2 form a bridge between spectrin and a fraction of the anion transport proteins. Protein 4.1 binds to GP. Phospholipids in the lipid bilayer include phosphatidylcholine (PC) and sphingomyelin (SM), which are located primarily on the outer surface of the membrane, and phosphatidyl serine (PS) and phosphatidyl ethanolamine (PE), which are located primarily on the inner surface of the membrane.

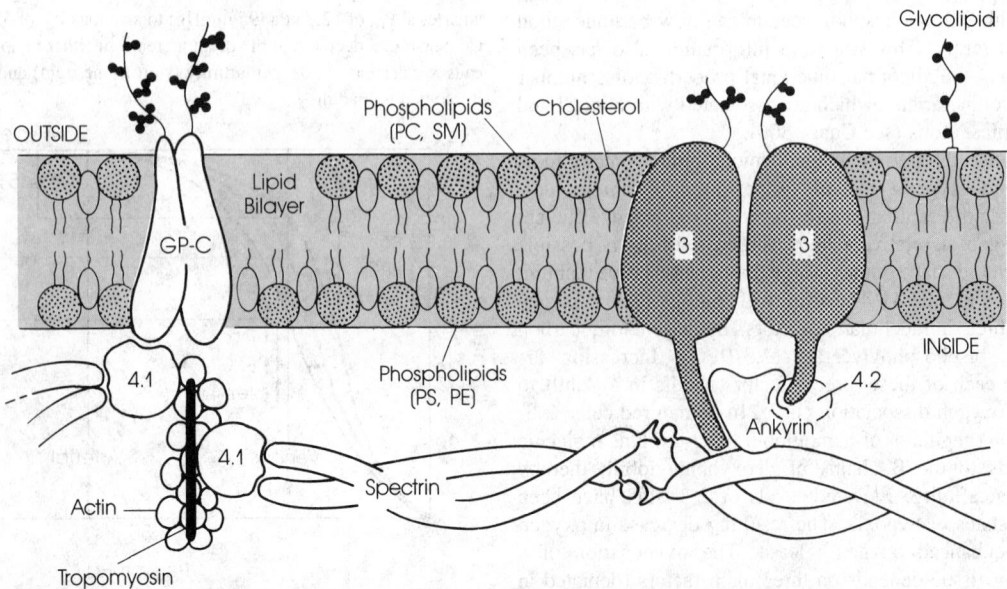

polysaccharide blood group antigens, and band 3, which serves as a channel for the passage of anions in and out of the red cell. Other proteins bind only to the inner surface of the red cell membrane. These include structural proteins such as spectrin and actin, which interact to form a meshwork that laminates the cytoplasmic surface of the membrane.

It is likely that the physiologic demise of 120-day-old red cells is due to a loss of membrane flexibility, preventing them from negotiating the narrow-bore channels of the microcirculation, including the sinusoids of the spleen. The factors responsible for red cell senescence are poorly understood. Experimental evidence indicates that deterioration of the red cell's metabolic machinery sufficient to deplete it of ATP can cause the cell to become spiculated (echinocytic) and lose its normal pliability. Depletion of ATP disrupts the spectrin and actin meshwork lining the inner membrane surface, resulting in aggregation of these proteins. Other factors such as coating with immunoglobulin also may contribute to the recognition of the senescent red cell by the mononuclear phagocyte system. In contrast to normal red cells, there is a large and well-documented body of information on the mechanisms responsible for red cell destruction in various hemolytic anemias. These are discussed in Chap. 307.

Once the senescent red cell is sequestered (see Fig. 302-2), hemoglobin is readily catabolized. Amino acids are released by proteolytic digestion and subsequently reutilized or metabolized. The heme group is catabolized by a microsomal oxidizing system. The porphyrin ring is converted to bile pigments which are excreted almost quantitatively by the liver. One mole of carbon monoxide is formed per mole of heme broken down. Endogenous carbon monoxide production correlates directly with erythroid cell destruction. As Fig. 302-2 shows, the iron released during heme catabolism is initially incorporated into the storage protein ferritin, but it is eventually transported to marrow erythroid precursors by transferrin, the plasma iron–binding protein.

If red cell production is disordered, there may be significant destruction of erythroid cells within the bone marrow. A number of anemias are characterized by *ineffective erythropoiesis*, particularly those in which erythroid maturation is morphologically abnormal and the circulating red cells are abnormal in size. Examples discussed in detail elsewhere include megaloblastic anemias, sideroblastic anemias, and β thalassemia major. Such disorders are characterized by erythroid hyperplasia in the bone marrow and rapid uptake of labeled iron into the marrow but a low recovery of the labeled iron in circulating red cells. Endogenous carbon monoxide production and plasma levels of unconjugated bilirubin are generally elevated in ineffective erythropoiesis.

REFERENCES

Babior BM, Stossel TP: *Hematology: A Pathophysiological Approach*, 2d ed. New York, Churchill Livingston, 1990

Beck WS (ed): *Hematology*, 5th ed. Boston, MIT Press, 1991

Bunn HF, Forget BG: *Hemoglobin: Molecular, Genetic and Clinical Aspects*. Philadelphia, Saunders, 1986

Jandl JH: *Blood Pathophysiology*. Boston, Blackwell, 1991

Jelkmann W: Erythropoietin: Structure, control of production and function. Physiol Rev 72:449, 1992

Palek J (ed): Cellular and molecular biology of the red cell membrane proteins in health and disease. Semin Hematol 29:229-239, 1992

303 ANEMIAS WITH DISTURBED IRON METABOLISM

KENNETH R. BRIDGES / H. FRANKLIN BUNN

Iron is involved in a broad repertoire of biochemical reactions, making it essential to all life. When complexed with porphyrin, iron forms heme, the prosthetic group for many proteins such as hemoglobin, where it binds oxygen reversibly, and cytochromes, where it is vital to oxidation-reduction reactions. Since the inorganic form of the element is highly toxic, specific processes have evolved for the assimilation, transport, and storage of iron. Under normal circumstances, iron homeostasis is precisely maintained, but it can go awry in a variety of clinical settings, leading either to iron deficiency or iron overload.

PHYSIOLOGY OF IRON

IRON ABSORPTION Iron absorption occurs predominantly in the duodenum and upper jejunum. Inorganic iron salts exist in either of two valence states, Fe^{2+} (ferrous) or Fe^{3+} (ferric). Most dietary iron consists of ferric salts, which form insoluble ferric oxyhydroxide complexes that precipitate at physiologic pH. Absorption is aided by gastric acidity, which maintains ferric iron in a soluble form. Normally, about 10 percent of the 10 to 20 mg of iron ingested per day in an average diet is absorbed by a poorly characterized mechanism. Heme is much more readily absorbed than inorganic iron. Unfortunately, a dearth of meat in the diets of many people throughout the world limits the availability of this excellent iron source.

The absorption of inorganic iron is greatly influenced by dietary compounds that may chelate the element. Citrate and ascorbate, for example, increase iron absorption by forming soluble complexes which readily enter the epithelial cells lining the upper gastrointestinal tract. Other compounds such as tannins, which are found in teas, plant phytates, and phosphates, form very tight complexes with iron and significantly inhibit absorption. The metabolic machinery involved in iron absorption is shared with several heavy metals, including lead, cadmium, and strontium. Increased iron absorption, as occurs, for instance, in iron deficiency, enhances the uptake of these elements.

TRANSPORT AND STORAGE Despite intense scrutiny, the precise mechanism by which iron is translocated across the epithelial barrier in the intestine is unknown. Once this task is accomplished, however, the element is coupled to transferrin, an 80-kDa serum glycoprotein that can bind two iron atoms and delivers iron to tissues throughout the body (Fig. 303-1). The aggregate binding sites of all the transferrin in the circulation comprise the total iron binding capacity (TIBC) of plasma. Normally, 20 to 45 percent of the iron binding sites of transferrin are filled. Specific receptors on the plasma membranes of cells recognize transferrin, leading to the internalization of the protein and the release of iron into the cell cytoplasm. As might be expected, erythroid precursor cells in the bone marrow, which have a high requirement for iron, have a correspondingly high density of transferrin receptors.

Excess iron is stored in the body as ferritin or hemosiderin. The iron in ferritin is enclosed within a protein shell, apoferritin, which can take up Fe^{2+} and oxidize it to Fe^{3+} that is deposited within the iron core. Iron stimulates the synthesis of apoferritin. With time, ferritin is engulfed by lysosomes and catabolized to hemosiderin, a nonspecific mixture of partially degraded protein, lipid, and iron. Iron enters and leaves the ferritin molecule in a metabolically controlled fashion, making it available for the normal physiologic functions of the cell. In contrast, the iron trapped in the hemosiderin meshwork returns to the metabolic mainstream of the cell in a slow and unregulated fashion. Small quantities of ferritin appear in serum.

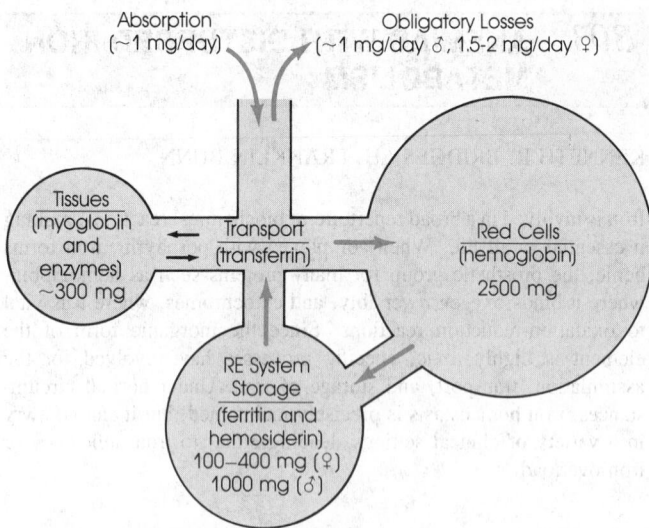

FIGURE 303-1 The distribution of iron in normal adults and internal iron kinetics. Bold arrows indicate major pathways of iron movement; RE = reticuloendothelial.

Normally, a close correlation exists between the serum ferritin concentration and body iron stores, with 1 μg/L serum ferritin equivalent to approximately 10 mg storage iron.

Body iron stores are assiduously conserved. In fact, no physiologic pathway of iron removal exists. About 1 mg of the element is lost daily from the shedding of senescent cells along the gastrointestinal and genitourinary tracts and from desquamation of skin (see Fig. 303-1). Menstruation results in the additional loss of about 1 mg/day of iron in women. Normally, these losses are closely balanced by daily absorption of about 10 percent of ingested iron. An increase in the demand for iron due to growth spurts, pregnancy, or pathologic hemorrhage can boost iron absorption to about 20 percent. Frank iron deficiency can increase the absorption of the element to between 30 and 40 percent of the amount ingested. With iron overload, absorption decreases.

Iron kinetics Between 80 and 90 percent of absorbed iron is delivered to the bone marrow for erythropoiesis. The dynamics of iron utilization by the peripheral tissues can be monitored by loading plasma transferrin with the radioisotope ^{59}Fe and injecting the labeled protein back into the circulation. Such ferrokinetic studies reveal an exponential loss of label from the plasma, with a half-life of about 75 min. The plasma iron turnover (PIT) is the absolute amount of iron released from transferrin per unit of time and is determined largely by the rate of erythropoiesis. Effective erythropoiesis results in the incorporation of 80 to 90 percent of iron into hemoglobin in circulating erythrocytes. A small fraction of developing normoblasts are destroyed by marrow macrophages in a process termed *ineffective erythropoiesis*. The normoblasts are ineffective at the task of producing mature circulating erythrocytes. With some anemias, such as the thalassemias, the megaloblastic anemias, and sideroblastic anemia, this medullary destruction is markedly exaggerated. The result is a high PIT, reflecting the increase in erythropoietic activity, but a diminished incorporation of the labeled iron into circulating erythrocytes. When erythropoiesis is diminished because of marrow hypoplasia, the PIT is correspondingly reduced.

LABORATORY INVESTIGATION OF IRON STORES   Direct assay This requires biopsy specimens. Most storage iron is found in the reticuloendothelial cells of the bone marrow, liver, and spleen or in hepatic parenchymal cells. The liver is a homogeneous tissue and therefore an excellent source by which to gauge iron stores. Prussian blue staining of liver biopsies, a commonly used technique, provides only a semiquantitative estimation of iron stores, whereas atomic absorption spectroscopy furnishes accurate quantitative data.

Formalin-fixed samples can be evaluated by this technique, allowing for transport and later testing. Liver biopsy with atomic absorption spectroscopic measurements is the touchstone for quantitative evaluation of iron overload. Bone marrow specimens are not reliable in the estimation of iron excess but are useful in the evaluation of iron deficiency. Because of the cellular heterogeneity of the marrow, histologic evaluation of iron deposits must focus on storage in macrophages. An absence of Prussian blue staining reliably indicates a deficiency in iron stores.

Indirect assay The simplest indirect assay is the ratio of serum iron to TIBC (Fig. 303-2). Iron deficiency depresses serum iron levels and boosts the TIBC. Therefore, the transferrin is generally less than 10 percent saturated. Iron loading increases the serum iron with little effect on the TIBC, leading to greater than 70 percent saturation of transferrin. The iron-to-TIBC ratio must be viewed with the patient's total clinical picture in mind. For example, serum iron and transferrin levels are depressed by conditions such as inflammation, cancer, and liver disease, leading at times to skewed ratios. These variables are particularly difficult to interpret in the elderly and in hospitalized patients. For these individuals the plasma ferritin reflects body iron stores most reliably.

Ferritin in the circulation is a secretory form of the protein which is glycosylated and differs in subunit composition from the storage form found in cells. The physiologic function of serum ferritin is presently unknown. The protein normally contains very little iron. The concentration of serum ferritin rises with iron loading and declines with depletion of tissue iron stores. The serum ferritin level also increases with inflammation, cancer, and liver disease. In addition, the normal ranges for serum ferritin vary with age and sex. Therefore, corrections for these factors should be made when values on a specific patient are interpreted. Using bone marrow biopsy as an absolute measure of iron stores, patients with values below about 14 μg/L are almost invariably iron deficient.

In patients with iron deficiency, protoporphyrin IX accumulates in the red cell because there is insufficient iron to convert it to heme (Fig. 302-3, p. 1719). The fluorometric assay of free erythrocyte protoporphyrin (FEP) is a reliable and cost-effective way of screening large groups of individuals such as school children for iron deficiency. Elevation of FEP occurs in other conditions that disrupt porphyrin metabolism, such as lead poisoning, therapy with isoniazid, and sideroblastic anemia. Exclusion of these conditions markedly enhances the specificity for iron deficiency of a high FEP.

Computed tomography (CT) of the liver provides an excellent assessment of body iron stores, particularly in patients with iron overload. The iron content of liver biopsy samples correlates well with determination by dual-energy CT scanning. Another sensitive

FIGURE 303-2 Serum iron and total iron binding capacity in various disorders.

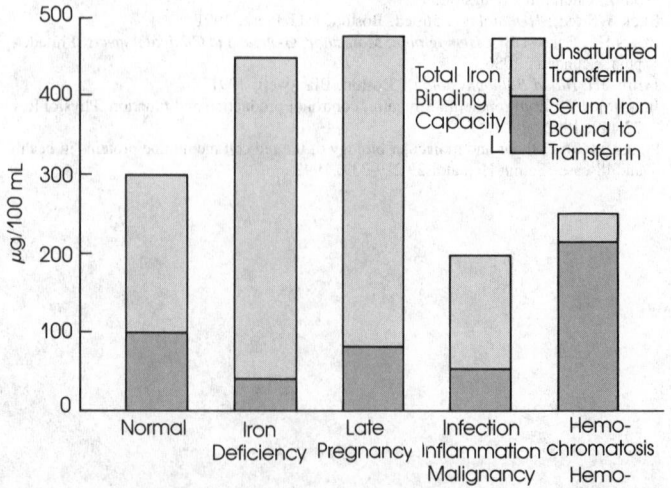

noninvasive technique for evaluating liver iron deposition is magnetic resonance imaging (MRI). Both instruments permit longitudinal evaluation and are valuable adjuncts in monitoring and treating patients with iron overload.

IRON-DEFICIENCY ANEMIA

ETIOLOGY Iron deficiency occurs when the rate of loss or utilization of the element exceeds its rate of assimilation. The stages of iron deficiency are shown in Table 303-1. Utilization is greatest during the rapid growth spurts of infancy and adolescence (Table 303-2). Depleted iron stores, if not frank anemia, are commonly seen in children in these two age groups. Neonates born to iron-deficient women are rarely anemic but do have low body iron stores. These infants lack the reserves needed for the swift growth that occurs after birth. Breast milk is a marginally adequate source of iron, whereas cow's milk has an even lower iron content. Iron deficiency during childhood has a number of deleterious consequences, including impaired cognition. Therefore, infants should receive iron supplementation.

In western countries, the increased demand for iron during adolescence is often accompanied by voluntary consumption of foods with low iron content. Among the elderly and the poor, financial constraints often produce a similar pattern of inadequate iron intake. Large numbers of people throughout the world have become inured to diets consisting of grains or cereals, which provide inadequate quantities of iron. The added burden of blood loss due to parasites such as hookworm makes iron deficiency a problem of staggering proportions.

Decreased absorption of iron This can occur in many clinical settings. After partial or total gastrectomy, the assimilation of dietary iron is impaired, owing primarily to increased motility and bypass of the proximal intestine, which is the primary site of iron absorption. Achlorhydria also contributes to decreased iron absorption. Patients with chronic diarrhea or intestinal malabsorption also can develop iron deficiency, particularly when the duodenum and proximal jejunum are involved. Sometimes iron-deficiency anemia is a harbinger of nontropical (celiac) sprue.

Iron loss This can be physiologic or pathologic. Examples of physiologic iron loss include menstruation and pregnancy. Menstrual blood loss doubles the daily iron requirement. With a term pregnancy, about 900 mg iron is lost by the mother to the fetus, the placenta, and to parturitional hemorrhage. Increased gastrointestinal absorption of the element by the mother compensates partially for these losses. In the absence of supplemental iron, however, the mother's stores will be depleted to meet the needs of the fetus. Currently, the vast majority of pregnant women who seek medical attention routinely receive prophylactic treatment with iron salts. Pregnant women who do not receive adequate antenatal care have a high incidence of clinically significant iron deficiency.

The gastrointestinal tract is most often responsible for pathologic blood loss and subsequent iron-deficiency anemia. The process is often insidious; the patient's presenting symptoms may be due solely

TABLE 303-2 Causes of iron deficiency

Increased iron utilization
  Postnatal growth spurt
  Adolescent growth spurt

Physiologic iron loss
  Menstruation
  Pregnancy

Pathologic iron loss
  Gastrointestinal bleeding
  Genitourinary bleeding
  Pulmonary hemosiderosis
  Intravascular hemolysis

Decreased iron intake
  Cereal-rich, meat-poor diets
  Pica
  Elderly and indigent
  Food faddists
  Malabsorption

to anemia. Common causes of chronic gastrointestinal blood loss include peptic ulcer disease, gastritis, hemorrhoids, angiodysplasia of the colon, and colonic adenocarcinoma. Salicylate ingestion often produces occult blood in the stool and occasionally causes significant blood loss. Gastrointestinal cancer is a specter haunting all patients with iron-deficiency anemia. Therefore, a complete gastrointestinal workup is necessary in men and postmenopausal women who are iron deficient. Stool guaiacs should be performed on six different occasions along with a digital rectal examination. Radiologic examination of the gastrointestinal tract, endoscopic procedures, or both are obligatory.

In about 15 percent of patients with documented gastrointestinal bleeding, no source is found, even after extensive radiologic and endoscopic investigation. In tropical areas, parasitic infestations, particularly hookworm, are a major cause of blood loss. Occasionally, as in patients with hereditary telangiectasia or in those with a bleeding diathesis, gastrointestinal bleeding arises from multiple sites. Thrombocytopenia, qualitative platelet disorders, and von Willebrand's disease are more apt to cause gastrointestinal bleeding than are deficiencies of the soluble coagulation factors.

Blood loss from other sources rarely produces iron-deficiency anemia. Bleeding in the genitourinary tract usually is sufficiently alarming that medical attention is sought early in the process. Intravascular hemolysis with hemoglobin loss in the urine, e.g., paroxysmal nocturnal hemoglobinuria, is very unusual. Pulmonary hemorrhage, secondary to bronchiectasis or idiopathic pulmonary hemosiderosis, also may cause iron-deficiency anemia.

CLINICAL CONSEQUENCES Iron deficiency impairs cell growth and proliferation. The production of red blood cells is in particular jeopardy owing to their high requirement for iron. Many symptoms of iron-deficiency anemia, including weakness, lassitude, palpitations, and sometimes exertional dyspnea, are common to all forms of chronic anemia. No definite link between these symptoms and tissue depletion of iron-dependent enzymes and cofactors has been established.

After the cells of the bone marrow, those of the gastrointestinal tract proliferate most actively. Consequently, many of the signs and symptoms of iron deficiency are localized to this organ system. Glossitis characterized by a reddened, swollen, smooth, shiny, and tender tongue occurs sporadically. Angular stomatitis involves erosion, tenderness, and swelling at the corners of the mouth. Gastric atrophy with achlorhydria occurs occasionally. A postcricoid web (Plummer-Vinson syndrome) may develop with long-standing iron deficiency. Koilonychia, or spoon-shaped nails, result from slowing in the rate of growth of the nail plate.

Menorrhagia is a common symptom in iron-deficient women. Both menorrhagia and gastric atrophy (mentioned above) may be a consequence as well as a cause of iron deficiency. In one study of

TABLE 303-1 Stages in the development of iron deficiency

	Normal	Mild	Moderate	Severe
Hemoglobin:	150 g/L	130 g/L	100 g/L	50 g/L
MCV	N	↓	↓	↓↓
MCHC	N	N	↓	↓↓
Marrow Fe stores	Present	Absent	Absent	Absent
Serum Fe/TIBC, μg/L	1000/3000	~750/3000	~500/4500	~250/6000

NOTE: MCV = mean corpuscular volume; MCHC = mean corpuscular hemoglobin concentration; TIBC = total iron-binding capacity; N = normal; ↓ = decreased.

600 female American blood donors, 13 percent were found to be iron deficient by FEP determinations. A recent evaluation of several thousand unselected women in Iceland revealed iron deficiency in 20 percent and iron-deficiency anemia in about 3 percent.

One peculiar symptom that is quite characteristic of iron deficiency is pica. Patients develop cravings for substances such as starch (amylophagia), ice (pagophagia), and clay (geophagia). Some of these materials, such as starch and clay, bind iron in the gastrointestinal tract, worsening the deficiency. The basis of this bizarre behavior is unknown.

A particularly invidious consequence of iron deficiency is increased intestinal absorption of lead. Children from impoverished families, who often have both iron deficiency and pica, are at greatest risk of developing lead poisoning. The toxicity of lead is due at least in part to a disruption of heme synthesis in neural tissues, a process abetted by iron deficiency. These unfortunate children are thereby placed in double jeopardy.

LABORATORY FINDINGS   The development of iron deficiency progresses in stages (see Table 303-1), each of which correlates with clinical laboratory abnormalities. *Storage iron depletion* occurs first, during which iron reserves are lost without compromise of the iron supply for erythropoiesis. At this stage, a bone marrow aspirate stained with Prussian blue shows markedly reduced or absent deposits of iron in macrophages. This condition is accompanied by a decrease in the level of serum ferritin. The next stage is *iron-deficient erythropoiesis*, during which the erythroid iron supply is reduced without the development of anemia. The iron binding capacity of the serum (TIBC) first rises, followed by a drop in serum iron. As a result, the fractional saturation of transferrin falls markedly. The level of transferrin saturation that is necessary to support erythropoiesis is about 15 percent. Iron-deficient erythropoiesis is inevitable below this value. The circulating red cells become microcytic and hypochromic. This is accompanied by an increase in FEP. The final stage is the development of frank *iron-deficiency anemia*, wherein the red cells become more severely hypochromic and microcytic (Plate A9-4). Often only a thin rim of cytoplasm appears at the periphery of the red cell. Small fragments and bizarre poikilocytes are also seen. The membranes of these iron-deficient erythrocytes are stiff, and these misshapen red cells have shortened survival in the circulation. Although the percentage of reticulocytes is usually normal, the absolute reticulocyte count, usually about 50,000 cells per cubic milliliter, is low. The white count is usually normal, while the platelet count is normal or increased. The bone marrow displays moderate erythroid hyperplasia. Many of the late normoblasts have scanty cytoplasm.

Transferrin receptors are shed from the plasma membranes of cells and can be detected in the plasma. The major source of plasma transferrin receptors is the hematopoietic cells of the bone marrow. The quantity of transferrin receptors in the plasma rises in patients with iron deficiency, providing another possible diagnostic test for this condition.

DIFFERENTIAL DIAGNOSIS   In a patient with hypochromic, microcytic anemia, the major diagnostic possibilities are iron deficiency, thalassemia, anemia of chronic inflammation, lead poisoning, and sideroblastic anemia. Several laboratory tests (Table 303-3) are useful in the differential diagnosis. Mild iron deficiency may be readily confused with β thalassemia trait or with the two-deletion forms of α thalassemia (α-/α- or --/αα) (see Chap. 322). In these mild forms of thalassemia, microcytosis is much more marked than hypochromia; accordingly, the mean corpuscular hemoglobin concentration (MCHC) is usually normal. The red cell size distribution is more uniform than that in iron deficiency. Target cells and basophilic stippling are usually more prominent in thalassemia than in iron deficiency. Hemoglobin A₂ is elevated in β thalassemia trait and decreased in iron deficiency and α thalassemia. If a patient with β thalassemia trait develops iron deficiency, the level of hemoglobin A₂ may fall to normal. The serum iron is normal or elevated in the thalassemias and decreased in both iron deficiency and the anemia of

TABLE 303-3   Differential diagnosis of microcytic, hypochromic anemia

	Iron-deficiency anemia	β Thalassemia trait	Anemia of chronic disease	Sideroblastic anemia
Serum iron	↓	N	↓	↑
TIBC	↑	N	↓	N
Serum ferritin	↓	N	↑	↑
Red cell protoprophyrin	↑	N	↑	↑ or N
Hb A₂	↓	↑	N	↓

NOTE: ↑ = increased; ↓ = decreased, N = normal; TIBC = total iron-binding capacity.

chronic disease. However, as Fig. 303-2 shows, the transferrin level is also decreased in the latter condition. The laboratory tests shown in Table 303-3 are not very helpful in determining whether a patient with a chronic inflammatory disease, such as rheumatoid arthritis, has become iron deficient. The finding of a low serum ferritin level or absent iron stores in a bone marrow aspirate would be diagnostic of iron deficiency in such patients. A trial of iron therapy may be necessary to settle the issue. The diagnosis of sideroblastic anemia rests on the demonstration of ringed sideroblasts in the bone marrow. These patients often have a population of hypochromic, microcytic red cells, even though the MCHC is usually normal.

THERAPY   Iron deficiency responds very well to the administration of oral agents such as iron salts (e.g., ferrous sulfate) or iron polysaccharide preparations (e.g., ferric polymaltose). Ferrous sulfate, which contains 50 mg elemental iron per 325-mg tablet, should be administered three times daily. Iron is best absorbed when taken between meals. Unfortunately, abdominal discomfort, characterized by bloating, fullness, and occasional pain, occurs commonly with this iron preparation. Ferrous gluconate and ferrous lactate often are better tolerated, particularly when taken at mealtime. Polysaccharide iron complex frequently fares better than any iron salt, despite the fact that each tablet contains 150 mg elemental iron. Iron-containing vitamin cocktails generally should be avoided, since these preparations are costly and contain suboptimal amounts of iron.

A reticulocytosis commences 3 to 4 days after the initiation of iron therapy, with a peak at about 10 days. Patients may not respond to iron replacement as a result of (1) an incorrect diagnosis, (2) noncompliance, (3) blood loss exceeding the rate of replacement, (4) bone marrow suppression by tumor, chronic inflammation, etc., or (5) malabsorption. Malabsorption of iron is an infrequent problem, but when it occurs, it requires parenteral iron replacement. Iron-dextran complex may be administered as intramuscular injections following a 25-mg dose to test for allergic reactions. A total of 100 mg iron-dextran per treatment session can be given in this fashion. Administration is repeated weekly until iron stores are replete. A Z-tract should be used for the injections to prevent oozing of the compound into the dermis, which can produce intractable skin discoloration. Iron-dextran can be given intravenously to patients who cannot tolerate the intramuscular injections or who require more rapid correction of iron deficiency. The most convenient approach is to dilute 500 mg of the compound into 100 mL sterile saline and to infuse a test dose of 1 mL. If no adverse reaction is noted, the remainder of the solution can be delivered over 2 h. The intravenous administration of up to 4 g iron at a single sitting allows the correction of iron deficiency at a single session. About 20 percent of patients experience arthralgias, chills, and fever which are dose-dependent and may persist for several days after the infusion. Iron-dextran should be used sparingly, if at all, in patients with rheumatoid arthritis since these symptoms are markedly enhanced with this disease. Nonsteroidal anti-inflammatory agents usually control these symptoms. Anaphylaxis, a serious complication of the administration of iron-dextran, occurs rarely. Intravenous administration of iron-dextran allows better control of this problem, since symptoms occur immediately with the beginning of the test dose. The infusion can be stopped, and correction of the condition with benadryl and epinephrine can be started. The 25-mg test dose used for the intramuscular injection cannot be retrieved should anaphylaxis develop, however. The amount of iron required for replacement can be calculated from the deficit in the red cell mass, with an additional 1000 mg to replace the body stores. Blood transfusions are rarely necessary except for patients in whom severe iron-deficiency anemia threatens cardiovascular or cerebrovascular function.

ANEMIAS WITH SECONDARY IRON LOADING

Iron overload in individuals with chronic anemias may result either from multiple transfusions or increased gastrointestinal absorption of the element owing to ineffective erythropoiesis.

SIDEROBLASTIC ANEMIAS   These comprise a group of disorders of diverse causes (Table 303-4) characterized by ringed sideroblasts in the nucleated erythroid precursors in the bone marrow. Greater than 10 percent of the normoblasts contain iron-laden mitochondria that surround the nucleus and appear as pathognomonic "rings" with Prussian blue staining. A number of metabolic abnormalities have been noted in the sideroblastic anemias, including defects in one or more of the steps in heme synthesis. Since the initial and final steps of heme synthesis are located in the mitochondrion (see Fig. 302-3), it is difficult to know whether such abnormalities are the cause or the result of iron loading. In addition to the presence of ringed sideroblasts, these disorders share certain other features: bone marrow erythroid hyperplasia with decreased red cell production (ineffective erythropoiesis); a population of hypochromic, microcytic red cells reflecting defective heme synthesis; and a marked increase in serum iron and transferrin saturation, sometimes accompanied by generalized iron overload.

Hereditary sideroblastic anemia is a rare X-linked disorder. Some cases have been associated with defective activity of δ-aminolevulinic acid synthetase, the initial and rate-limiting enzyme in heme biosynthesis. Affected males have anemia of variable severity that occasionally responds to treatment with large doses of pyridoxine.

Acquired sideroblastic anemias may be caused by a variety of insults, including ethanol and isoniazid, which disrupt heme metabolism, and lead, which inhibits several steps in the heme synthetic pathway (Table 303-4). Ringed sideroblasts are found in about 30 percent of patients hospitalized for alcohol abuse, particularly in the setting of coexistent folate deficiency and malnutrition. This morphologic abnormality disappears within several days following cessation of alcohol ingestion. Secondary sideroblastic anemia also has been observed in a variety of inflammatory and neoplastic states. A particularly intractable form of the disorder sometimes occurs following treatment of malignancy, especially multiple myeloma, with alkylating chemotherapeutic agents.

Most commonly, however, acquired sideroblastic anemia is idiopathic, appearing spontaneously in older individuals. Disturbed growth and maturation occur in all the lines that emanate from the hematopoietic stem cells. Chromosomal abnormalities involving bone marrow cells occur commonly. Neutropenia develops in a significant number of patients, as does thrombocytopenia. Some individuals have normal numbers of platelets that are, however, dysfunctional. A bleeding diathesis often results. About 10 percent of individuals with sideroblastic anemia will develop a particularly intractable form of acute myelogenous leukemia. This proportion appears to be higher in cases arising from therapy with alkylating agents.

The treatment of secondary sideroblastic anemia focuses primarily on withdrawal of the offending agent. No specific treatment is presently available for idiopathic cases. Since pyridoxine is innocuous and inexpensive, all patients should receive a trial of the vitamin at 200 mg/d for 2 to 3 months, despite the low probability of response in the acquired disorder. Occasionally, an improvement in hematocrit occurs with androgen therapy. This therapy should be used cautiously in patients with liver disease, diabetes, or benign prostatic hypertrophy. Ongoing clinical trials are attempting to define the role of cytokines such as granulocyte-monocyte colony stimulating factor (GM-CSF), interleukin 3, and erythropoietin in the treatment of sideroblastic anemia. Supportive therapy, including blood transfusions, is indicated in all patients.

TRANSFUSIONAL   HEMOCHROMATOSIS   Repeated blood transfusion is the most common cause of iron overload in patients with anemia. One unit of blood contains 200 to 250 mg iron. Therefore, a patient who requires 3 units of blood per month will accumulate about 8 g iron over the course of a year, enough to cause early clinical sequelae of iron loading. In order for the consequences of iron loading to play a major clinical role, a requirement for chronic transfusions must be coupled with a relatively long survival. The disorders that fulfill these criteria at present include (1) thalassemia major, (2) myeloproliferative and myelodysplastic syndromes (including sideroblastic anemia), (3) pure red cell aplasia, and (4) aplastic anemia of moderate severity. Patients with chronic renal failure on dialysis once fell into this category. The recent introduction of cloned erythropoietin has largely obviated this problem for these individuals.

Transfusional iron overload produces a spectrum of problems similar to those seen with idiopathic hemochromatosis. Of these, the most serious result from myocardial and hepatic iron deposition. Cardiac siderosis leads to arrhythmias, conduction defects, and a restrictive cardiomyopathy. Echocardiography (Chap. 190) is useful in detecting early myocardial dysfunction. Iron deposition in the liver injures hepatocytes, leading to necrosis, fibrosis, and ultimately cirrhosis. Since hepatic iron deposition produces very little inflammation as fibrosis progresses, serum transaminase levels are usually only modestly elevated. Disturbed glucose metabolism occurs commonly, although an oral glucose tolerance test is sometimes needed to demonstrate the defect. Gonadal dysfunction and ACTH deficiency are much less frequent. Hyperpigmentation reflects increased melanin production due to dermal iron deposition. Fair-skinned patients whose melanocytes are incapable of boosting melanin production (and who tan poorly) show little or no hyperpigmentation. In the assessment of these patients, liver biopsy provides the greatest yield of information, since iron content as well as the pathologic state of the organ can be determined. Liver CT scanning and MRI are the most reliable noninvasive methods of estimating iron deposition. The iron/TIBC ratio and serum ferritin level are both elevated with transfusional hemochromatosis but do not accurately establish the degree of iron overload.

The only treatment presently available for transfusional hemochromatosis is chelation. Desferrioxamine is the only agent that has been extensively evaluated and shown to prevent or reverse the complications of iron overload. The drug must be given parenterally over a period of 12 to 16 h by subcutaneous infusion with a portable syringe pump. No safe and effective oral iron chelating agent has been devised. Oral ascorbic acid supplementation markedly enhances iron excretion in patients on desferrioxamine therapy. The vitamin increases the availability of storage iron to the chelator by slowing the degradation of ferritin to hemosiderin. Cardiac toxicity has occurred in patients with hemochromatosis who consumed excessive

---

TABLE 303-4   The sideroblastic anemias

Hereditary or congenital sideroblastic anemias
Acquired sideroblastic anemias
    Associated with drugs and toxins (e.g., alcohol, lead, isoniazid, chloramphenicol)
    Associated with neoplastic and inflammatory disease (e.g., carcinoma, leukemia, lymphoma, rheumatoid arthritis)
    Alkylating agent chemotherapy (e.g., cyclophosphamide)

amounts of ascorbic acid, however. The generation of injurious free radicals by iron released from storage sites is the probable mechanism of this effect. Further investigation into the basis of cellular injury in patients with hemochromatosis treated with ascorbic acid is needed to clarify the possible therapeutic utility of this vitamin.

REFERENCES

BRIDGES KR: Transfusion hemochromatosis, in *Transfusion Medicine*, WH Churchill, S Kurtz (eds). Cambridge, Mass, Blackwell, 1988, p 129

BURNS ER et al: Clinical utility of serum tests for iron deficiency in hospitalized patients. Am J Clin Pathol 93:240, 1990

JANSEN BM et al: Screening with zinc protoporphyrin for iron deficiency in non-anemic female blood donors. Clin Chem 36:846, 1990

LANZKOWSKY P: Problems in diagnosis of iron deficiency anemia. Pediatr Ann 14:618, 1985

NATHAN DG (ed): Oral iron chelators. Semin Hematol 27:83, 1990

PIOMELLI S et al: Lead-induced abnormalities of porphyrin metabolism: The relationship with iron deficiency. Ann NY Acad Sci 514:278, 1987

SKIKNE BS et al: Serum transferrin receptor: A quantitative measure of tissue iron deficiency. Blood 75:1870, 1990

VANDERMOLEN L et al: Ringed sideroblasts in primary myelodysplasia: Leukemic propensity and prognostic factors. Arch Intern Med 148:653, 1988

YIP R, DALLMAN PR: Developmental changes in erythrocyte protoporphyrins: Roles of iron deficiency and lead toxicity. J Pediatr 104:710, 1984

304   MEGALOBLASTIC ANEMIAS

BERNARD M. BABIOR / H. FRANKLIN BUNN

The megaloblastic anemias are disorders caused by impaired DNA synthesis. Cells primarily affected are those having relatively rapid turnover, especially hematopoietic precursors and gastrointestinal epithelial cells. Cell division is sluggish, but cytoplasmic development progresses normally, so megaloblastic cells tend to be large, with an increased ratio of RNA to DNA. Megaloblastic erythroid cells tend to be destroyed in the marrow in excessive numbers, an abnormality termed *ineffective erythropoiesis* (Chaps. 56 and 302).

Most megaloblastic anemias are due to a deficiency of cobalamin (vitamin B_{12}) and/or folic acid. The various clinical entities associated with megaloblastic anemia are listed in Table 304-1. This classification is easier to comprehend if the physiologic and biochemical principles discussed below are kept in mind.

PHYSIOLOGIC CONSIDERATIONS

FOLIC ACID   Folic acid is the common name for pteroylmonoglutamic acid. It is synthesized by many different plants and bacteria. Fruits and vegetables constitute the primary dietary source of the vitamin. Some forms of dietary folic acid are labile and may be destroyed by cooking. The minimum daily requirement is normally about 50 μg, but this may be increased severalfold during periods of enhanced metabolic demand such as pregnancy.

The assimilation of adequate amounts of folic acid is dependent on the nature of the diet and its means of preparation. Folates in various foodstuffs are largely conjugated to polyglutamic acid. This highly polar side chain impairs the intestinal absorption of the vitamin. However, conjugases (γ-glutamyl carboxypeptidases) in the lumen of the gut convert polyglutamates to mono- and diglutamates, which are readily absorbed in the proximal jejunum.

There are binding proteins in plasma for folates, but their physiologic significance is unclear. Plasma folate is primarily in the form of N^5-methyltetrahydrofolate, a monoglutamate. N^5-Methyltetrahydrofolate is transported into cells by a carrier which is specific for the tetrahydro forms of the vitamin. Once in the cell, the N^5-

TABLE 304-1   Classification of the megaloblastic anemias

COBALAMIN DEFICIENCY

A Inadequate intake: vegetarians (rare)
B Malabsorption
  1 Inadequate production of intrinsic factor (IF)
    a Pernicious anemia
    b Gastrectomy
    c Congenital absence or functional abnormality of IF (rare)
  2 Disorders of terminal ileum
    a Tropical sprue
    b Nontropical sprue
    c Regional enteritis
    d Intestinal resection
    e Neoplasms and granulomatous disorders (rare)
    f Selective cobalamin malabsorption (Imerslund's syndrome) (rare)
  3 Competition for cobalamin
    a Fish tapeworm
    b Bacteria: blind loop syndrome
  4 Drugs: *p*-aminosalicylic acid, colchicine, neomycin
C Other
  1 Nitrous oxide
  2 Transcobalamin II deficiency (rare)

FOLIC ACID DEFICIENCY

A Inadequate intake: unbalanced diet (common in alcoholics, teenagers, some infants)
B Increased requirements
  1 Pregnancy
  2 Infancy
  3 Malignancy
  4 Increased hematopoiesis (chronic hemolytic anemias)
  5 Chronic exfoliative skin disorders
  6 Hemodialysis
C Malabsorption
  1 Tropical sprue
  2 Nontropical sprue
  3 Drugs: Phenytoin, barbiturates, (?) ethanol
D Impaired metabolism
  1 Inhibitors of dihydrofolate reductase: methotrexate, pyrimethamine, triamterene, pentamidine, etc.
  2 Alcohol
  3 Rare enzyme deficiencies: dihydrofolate reductase, others

OTHER CAUSES

A Drugs which impair DNA metabolism
  1 Purine antagonists: 6-mercaptopurine, azathioprine, etc.
  2 Pyrimidine antagonists: 5-fluorouracil, cytosine arabinoside, etc.
  3 Others: procarbazine, hydroxyurea, acyclovir, zidovudine
B Metabolic disorders (rare)
  1 Hereditary orotic aciduria
  2 Others
C Megaloblastic anemia of unknown etiology
  1 Refractory megaloblastic anemia
  2 Di Guglielmo's syndrome*
  3 Congenital dyserythropoietic anemia

* A form of acute nonlymphocytic leukemia with atypical, dysplastic changes in erythroid series.

methyl group is removed in a cobalamin-requiring reaction (see below), and the folate is then reconverted to the polyglutamate form. The polyglutamate form may be useful for retention of folate by the cell.

Normal individuals have about 5 to 20 mg folic acid in various body stores, half in the liver. In light of the minimum daily requirement, it is not surprising that a deficiency will occur within months if dietary intake or intestinal absorption is curtailed.

COBALAMIN   This vitamin is a complex organometallic compound in which a cobalt atom is situated within a corrin ring, a structure similar to the porphyrin from which heme is formed (see Fig. 302-3). Unlike heme, however, cobalamin cannot be synthesized in the human body and must be supplied in the diet. The only dietary source of cobalamin is animal products: meat and dairy foods. The minimum daily requirement for cobalamin is about 2.5 μg.

During gastric digestion, cobalamin in food is released and forms a stable complex with gastric R binder, one of a group of closely related glycoproteins of unknown function which are found in secretions (e.g., saliva, milk, gastric juice, bile), phagocytes, and plasma. On entering the duodenum, the cobalamin–R binder complex is digested, releasing the cobalamin, which then binds to intrinsic factor (IF). This glycoprotein of molecular weight 50,000 is produced by the parietal cells of the stomach. The secretion of intrinsic factor generally parallels that of hydrochloric acid. The cobalamin-IF complex is resistant to proteolytic digestion and travels to the distal ileum, where specific receptors on the mucosal brush border bind the cobalamin-IF complex, thereby enabling the vitamin to be absorbed. Thus intrinsic factor, like transferrin (see Chap. 303), serves as a cell-directed carrier protein. The receptor-bound cobalamin-IF complex is taken into the ileal mucosal cell, where over the course of several hours the IF is destroyed and the cobalamin is transferred to another transport protein, transcobalamin II (TC II). The cobalamin–TC II complex is then secreted into the circulation, from which it is rapidly taken up by the liver, bone marrow, and other cells. The pathway of cobalamin absorption is shown in Fig. 304-1. Normally, about 2 mg cobalamin is stored in the liver, and another 2 mg is stored elsewhere in the body. In view of the minimum daily requirement, about 3 to 6 years would be required for a normal individual to become deficient in cobalamin if absorption were to cease abruptly.

Although TC II is the acceptor for newly absorbed cobalamin,

most circulating cobalamin is bound to transcobalamin I (TC I), a glycoprotein closely related to gastric R binder. TC I appears to be derived in part from leukocytes. The paradox that most circulating cobalamin is bound to TC I rather than TC II, even though TC II initially carries all the cobalamin that is absorbed by the intestine, is explained by the fact that cobalamin bound to TC II is rapidly cleared from the blood ($t_{1/2}$ about 1 h), while clearance of cobalamin bound to TC I requires many days. The function of TC I is unknown.

BIOCHEMICAL CONSIDERATIONS

FOLATE The *prime function* of this vitamin is to transfer 1-carbon moieties such as methyl and formyl groups to various organic compounds (see Fig. 304-2). The source of these 1-carbon moieties is usually serine, which reacts with tetrahydrofolate to produce glycine and $N^{5,10}$-methylenetetrahydrofolate. An alternative source is formiminoglutamic acid, an intermediate in histidine catabolism, which gives up its formimino group to tetrahydrofolate to yield N^5-formiminotetrahydrofolate and glutamic acid. These derivatives provide entry into an interconvertible donor pool consisting of tetrahydrofolate derivatives carrying various 1-carbon moieties (see Fig. 304-2). The constituents of this pool can donate their 1-carbon moieties to appropriate acceptor compounds to form metabolic intermediates which are ultimately converted to building blocks used in the synthesis of biologic macromolecules. The most important building blocks are (1) purines, in which the C-2 and C-8 atoms are introduced in folate-dependent reactions, (2) deoxythymidylate monophosphate (dTMP), synthesized from $N^{5,10}$-methylenetetrahydrofolate and deoxyuridylate monophosphate (dUMP), and (3) methionine, formed by the transfer of a methyl group from N^5-methyltetrahydrofolate to homocysteine. Cobalamin is also required for the formation of methionine from homocysteine (see below).

In all but one of the 1-carbon transfer reactions, tetrahydrofolate is produced. It can immediately accept a 1-carbon moiety and reenter the donor pool. The single exception is the thymidylate synthetase reaction (dUMP → dTMP), in which dihydrofolate is the product (Fig. 304-2). This must be reduced to tetrahydrofolate by the enzyme dihydrofolate reductase before it can reenter the donor pool. A number of drugs are able to inhibit dihydrofolate reductase, thereby diverting folate from the donor pool and producing what amounts to a state of folate deficiency in the face of normal tissue folate concentrations.

COBALAMIN In humans there are two metabolically active forms of cobalamin, identified by the alkyl group attached to the sixth coordination position of the cobalt atom: methylcobalamin and adenosylcobalamin. The vitamin preparation which is used therapeutically is cyanocobalamin (also called vitamin B_{12}). Cyanocobalamin

FIGURE 304-1 The assimilation of cobalamin. On entering the stomach, dietary cobalamin (Cbl) forms a complex with R binding protein. As this protein is digested, cobalamin is transferred to intrinsic factor (IF). This complex passes through the intestine until it reaches specific receptors on the mucosa of the distal ileum. The internalized Cbl is then transferred to transcobalamin II (TC II), which circulates in the plasma until it binds to receptors on cells throughout the body and is internalized.

FIGURE 304-2 Scheme of folate metabolism.

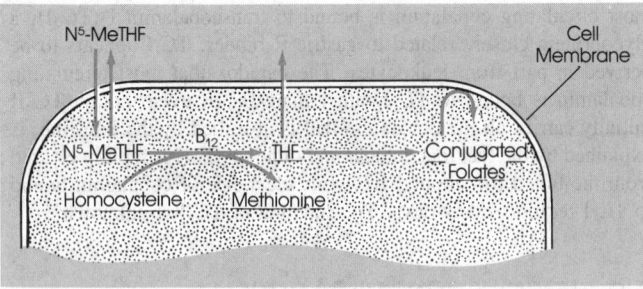

FIGURE 304-3 Diagram showing the interrelationship between cobalamin (methylcobalamin, B_{12}) and folate metabolism within the cell. N^5-MeTHF = N^5 methyltetrahydrofolate; THF = tetrahydrofolate.

has no known physiologic role and must be converted to a biologically active form before it can be used by tissues.

Methylcobalamin is an essential cofactor in the conversion of homocysteine to methionine (Fig. 304-3). When this reaction is impaired, folate metabolism is deranged, and it is this derangement which is thought to underlie the defect in DNA synthesis and the megaloblastic maturation pattern in patients who are deficient in cobalamin (see Fig. 304-3). In cobalamin deficiency, the unconjugated N^5-methyltetrahydrofolate newly taken from the bloodstream cannot be converted to other forms of tetrahydrofolate by methyl transfer. This is the so-called folate trap hypothesis. Since N^5-methyltetrahydrofolate is a poor substrate for the conjugating enzyme (this has been shown in rats and pigs but has not yet been demonstrated in humans), it largely remains in the unconjugated form and slowly leaks from the cell. Tissue folate deficiency therefore develops, and this results in megaloblastic hematopoiesis. This hypothesis explains why tissue folate stores in cobalamin deficiency are substantially reduced, with a disproportionate reduction in conjugated as compared with unconjugated folates, despite normal or supranormal serum folate levels. It also explains why large doses of folate can produce a partial hematologic remission in patients with cobalamin deficiency.

Impairment in the conversion of homocysteine to methionine also may be partly responsible for the neurologic complications of cobalamin deficiency (see below). The methionine formed in this reaction is needed for the production of choline and choline-containing phospholipids. Nervous system damage is postulated to result at least in part from interference with these processes due to decreased methionine production in cobalamin deficiency.

Adenosylcobalamin is required for the conversion of methylmalonyl coenzyme A (CoA) to succinyl CoA. Lack of this cofactor leads to large increases in the tissue levels of methylmalonyl CoA and its precursor, propionyl CoA. As a consequence, nonphysiologic fatty acids containing an odd number of carbon atoms are synthesized and incorporated into neuronal lipids. This biochemical abnormality also may contribute to the neurologic complications of cobalamin deficiency (see below).

CLINICAL DISORDERS

CLASSIFICATION OF MEGALOBLASTIC ANEMIAS (See Table 304-1)   The cause of megaloblastic anemia varies in different parts of the world. In temperate zones, folate deficiency in alcoholics and pernicious anemia are the common types of megaloblastic anemias. In certain areas close to the equator, tropical sprue is endemic and an important cause of megaloblastic anemia, while in Scandinavia, it is occasionally secondary to infestation by the fish tapeworm, *Diphyllobothrium latum*.

The dietary intake of cobalamin is more than adequate for the body's requirements, except in true vegetarians (individuals who live on a purely vegetable diet) and their breast-fed infants. Thus deficiency of cobalamin is almost always due to malabsorption. As explained in

the section above, the absorption of cobalamin depends on a specific binding protein produced in the stomach and uptake by a specific receptor in the mucosa of the distal ileum. Accordingly, several steps in this process can go awry and lead to malabsorption. In contrast, the dietary intake of folic acid is marginal in many parts of the world. Furthermore, since the body's stores of folate are relatively low, folic acid deficiency can arise rather suddenly during periods of decreased dietary intake or increased metabolic demand. Finally, folic acid deficiency may be due to malabsorption. Often two or more of these factors coexist in a given patient.

Combined deficiencies of cobalamin and folic acid are not uncommon. Patients with tropical sprue are often deficient in both vitamins. The biochemical lesion that results in megaloblastic maturation of bone marrow cells also causes structural and functional abnormalities of the rapidly proliferating epithelial cells of the intestinal mucosa. Thus severe deficiency of one vitamin can lead to malabsorption of the other. Furthermore, as discussed above, a deficiency of cobalamin causes a secondary reduction in cellular folic acid.

Finally, megaloblastic anemias may occasionally be induced by factors unrelated to a vitamin deficiency. Most such cases are caused by one or more of the many drugs which interfere with DNA synthesis. Less commonly, megaloblastic maturation is encountered in certain acquired defects of hematopoietic stem cells. Rarest of all are specific congenital enzyme deficiencies in which megaloblastic anemia is characteristically encountered.

COBALAMIN DEFICIENCY   There are many conditions in which cobalamin deficiency may develop. Although each has its own characteristic manifestations, certain clinical features are common to all. These clinical features involve the blood, the gastrointestinal tract, and the nervous system.

The hematologic manifestations are almost entirely the result of anemia, although very rarely purpura may appear, due to thrombocytopenia. Symptoms of anemia may include weakness, light-headedness, vertigo, and tinnitus, as well as palpitations, angina, and the symptoms of congestive failure. On physical examination, the patient with florid cobalamin deficiency is pale, with slightly icteric skin and eyes. The pulse is rapid, and the heart may be enlarged; auscultation will usually reveal a systolic flow murmur.

The gastrointestinal manifestations reflect the effect of cobalamin deficiency on the rapidly proliferating gastrointestinal epithelium. The patient sometimes complains of a sore tongue, which on inspection will be smooth and beefy red. Anorexia with moderate weight loss also may be evident, possibly accompanied by diarrhea and other gastrointestinal symptoms. These latter manifestations may be in part caused by megaloblastosis of the small-intestinal epithelium, which results in malabsorption.

The neurologic manifestations are the most worrisome of all, because they often fail to remit fully on treatment. They begin pathologically with demyelination, followed by axonal degeneration and eventual neuronal death; the final stage, of course, is irreversible. Sites of involvement include peripheral nerves; the spinal cord, where the posterior and lateral columns undergo demyelination; and the cerebrum itself. Signs and symptoms include numbness and paresthesias in the extremities (the earliest neurologic manifestations), weakness, and ataxia. There may be sphincter disturbances. Reflexes may be diminished or increased. The Romberg and Babinski signs may be positive, and position and vibration senses are usually diminished. Disturbances of mentation will vary from mild irritability and forgetfulness to severe dementia or frank psychosis. It should be emphasized that *neurologic disease may occur in a patient with a normal hematocrit* and normal red blood cell indexes.

In the usual patient, in whom hematologic problems predominate, the blood and bone marrow show characteristic megaloblastic changes which are described under "Diagnosis" below. The anemia may be very severe—hematocrits of 15 to 20 are not infrequent—but is surprisingly well tolerated by the patient because it develops so slowly.

Pernicious anemia The most common cause of cobalamin deficiency in temperate climates is pernicious anemia, in which intrinsic factor secretion ceases owing to atrophy of the gastric mucosa. It is most frequently seen in individuals of northern European descent and African-Americans and is much less common in southern Europeans and Asians. Men and women are equally affected. It is a disease of the elderly, the average patient presenting near age 60; it is rare under age 30, although typical pernicious anemia can be seen in children under age 10 (juvenile pernicious anemia). Inherited conditions in which a histologically normal stomach secretes either an abnormal intrinsic factor or none at all will induce cobalamin deficiency in infancy or early childhood.

There is considerable evidence for immunologic abnormalities in pernicious anemia. The incidence of pernicious anemia is substantially increased in patients with other diseases thought to be of immunologic origin, including Graves' disease, myxedema, thyroiditis, idiopathic adrenocortical insufficiency, vitiligo, and hypoparathyroidism. Patients with pernicious anemia also have abnormal circulating antibodies related to their disease: 90 percent have antiparietal cell antibody, while 60 percent have anti-intrinsic factor antibody. Antiparietal cell antibody is also found in 50 percent of patients with gastric atrophy without pernicious anemia, as well as in 10 to 15 percent of an unselected patient population, but anti-intrinsic factor antibody is usually absent from these patients. Relatives of patients with pernicious anemia have an increased incidence of the disease, and even clinically unaffected relatives may have anti-intrinsic factor antibody in their serum. Finally, treatment with corticosteroids has been reported to reverse the disease both pathologically and clinically.

The destruction of parietal cells in pernicious anemia is thought to be mediated by complement-fixing antibodies against the parietal cell surface. The observation that pernicious anemia is unusually common in patients with agammaglobulinemia, however, suggests that the cellular immune system also may play a role in its pathogenesis.

Pathologically, the most characteristic finding in pernicious anemia is gastric atrophy affecting the acid- and pepsin-secreting portion of the stomach; the antrum is spared. Other pathologic changes are secondary to the deficiency of cobalamin; these include megaloblastoid alterations in the gastric and intestinal epithelium and the neurologic changes described above. The abnormalities in the gastric epithelium appear as cellular atypia in gastric cytology specimens, a finding which must be carefully distinguished from the cytologic abnormalities seen in gastric malignancy.

The *clinical manifestations* are primarily those of cobalamin deficiency, as described above. The disease is of insidious onset and progresses slowly. Laboratory examination will reveal hypergastrinemia and pentagastrin-fast achlorhydria as well as the hematologic and other laboratory abnormalities discussed below under "Diagnosis."

Through appropriate replacement therapy, patients with pernicious anemia should experience complete and lifelong correction of all abnormalities which are due to cobalamin deficiency, except to the extent that irreversible changes in the nervous system may have occurred prior to treatment. These patients, however, are unusually subject to gastric polyps and have about twice the normal incidence of cancer of the stomach. In view of the latter complication, patients should be followed with frequent stool guaiac examinations together with further diagnostic studies when indicated.

Postgastrectomy Following total gastrectomy or extensive damage to gastric mucosa as, for example, by ingestion of corrosive agents, megaloblastic anemia may develop because the source of intrinsic factor has been removed. In such patients, the absorption of orally administered cobalamin is impaired. Megaloblastic anemia also may follow partial gastrectomy, but the incidence is lower than after total gastrectomy, in which cobalamin malabsorption occurs in 100 percent of patients. The cause of cobalamin deficiency after partial gastrectomy may be intestinal overgrowth of bacteria, but it does not always respond to antibiotics.

Intestinal organisms Megaloblastic anemia may occur with intestinal stasis due to anatomic lesions (strictures, diverticula, anastomoses, "blind loops") or pseudoobstruction (diabetes mellitus, scleroderma, amyloid). This anemia is caused by colonization of the small intestine by large masses of bacteria which divert cobalamin from the host. Steatorrhea also may be seen under these circumstances, because bile salt metabolism is disturbed when the intestine is heavily colonized with bacteria. Hematologic responses have been observed after administration of oral antibiotics such as tetracycline and ampicillin.

Megaloblastic anemia is seen, in Scandinavia especially, in persons harboring the fish tapeworm, *D. latum*. The anemia has been attributed to competition by the worm for cobalamin. Destruction of the worm eliminates the problem.

Ileal abnormalities Cobalamin deficiency is commonly found in tropical sprue, while it is an unusual complication of nontropical sprue (gluten-sensitive enteropathy; see Chap. 254). Virtually any disorder which compromises the absorptive capacity of the distal ileum can result in cobalamin deficiency. Specific entities include regional enteritis, Whipple's disease, and tuberculosis. Segmental involvement of the distal ileum by disease can cause megaloblastic anemia without any other manifestations of intestinal malabsorption such as steatorrhea. Cobalamin malabsorption is also seen after ileal resection. The Zollinger-Ellison syndrome (intense gastric hyperacidity due to a gastrin-secreting tumor) may cause cobalamin malabsorption by acidifying the small intestine. This will retard the transfer of the vitamin from R binder to intrinsic factor and will impair the binding of the cobalamin-IF complex to the ileal receptors. Chronic pancreatitis also may cause cobalamin malabsorption by impairing the transfer of the vitamin from R binder to intrinsic factor. This abnormality can be detected by tests of cobalamin absorption (see below, Schilling test), but it is invariably mild and never causes clinical cobalamin deficiency. Finally, there is a rare congenital disorder, Imerslund-Gräsbeck disease, in which a selective defect in cobalamin absorption is accompanied by proteinuria.

FOLIC ACID DEFICIENCY Patients with folic acid deficiency are more apt to be malnourished than those with cobalamin deficiency. Accordingly, they are likely to appear wasted. The gastrointestinal manifestations are similar to but may be more widespread and more severe than those of pernicious anemia. Diarrhea is often present, and cheilosis and glossitis are also encountered. However, in contrast to cobalamin deficiency, neurologic abnormalities do not occur.

The hematologic manifestations of folic acid deficiency are the same as those of cobalamin deficiency. Folic acid deficiency can generally be attributed to one or more of the following factors: inadequate intake, increased demand, and malabsorption.

Inadequate intake Folic acid malnutrition is commonly encountered among a number of groups. Alcoholics frequently become folate deficient because their main source of caloric intake is alcoholic beverages. Distilled spirits are virtually devoid of folic acid, while beer and wine do not contain enough of the vitamin to satisfy the daily requirement. In addition, alcohol may interfere with folate metabolism. Narcotic addicts are also prone to become folate deficient because of malnutrition. Many indigent and elderly individuals who subsist primarily on canned foods or "tea and toast" and occasional teenagers whose diet consists of "junk food" develop folate deficiency.

Increased demand Tissues with a relatively high rate of cell division such as the bone marrow or gut mucosa have a large requirement for folate. Therefore, patients with chronic hemolytic anemias or other causes of very active erythropoiesis may become deficient if their high folate requirement is not met by dietary intake. Likewise, a pregnant woman may become deficient in folic acid because of the high demand of the developing fetus. Deficiency in pregnancy can cause neural tube defects in newborns. Folate deficiency also may occur during the growth spurts of infancy and adolescence. Patients on chronic hemodialysis may require supplementary folate to replace that lost in the dialysate.

Malabsorption Folic acid deficiency is a common accompaniment of tropical sprue. Both the gastrointestinal symptoms and malabsorption are improved by the administration of either folic acid or antibiotics by mouth. Patients with nontropical sprue (gluten-sensitive enteropathy) also may develop significant folic acid deficiency which parallels other parameters of malabsorption. Similarly, folate deficiency in alcoholics may be due in part to malabsorption. In addition, other primary small-bowel disorders are sometimes associated with vitamin deficiency. These entities are all discussed in Chap. 254.

DRUGS Next to deficiency of folate or cobalamin, the most common cause of megaloblastic anemia is drug ingestion. Drugs which cause megaloblastic anemia do so by interfering with DNA synthesis, either directly or by antagonizing the action of folate. They can be classified as follows:

1 *Direct inhibitors of DNA synthesis.* The drugs in this category are used in the treatment of malignancy. Their efficacy depends on their ability to impair DNA synthesis. They include purine analogues (6-thioguanine, azathioprine, 6-mercaptopurine), pyrimidine analogues (5-fluorouracil, cytosine arabinoside), and other drugs which interfere with DNA synthesis by a variety of mechanisms (hydroxyurea, procarbazine).

   The antiviral agent zidovudine (AZT), used for treating the human immunodeficiency virus (HIV), often causes severe megaloblastic anemia, a problem not seen with acyclovir, which is used to treat herpes infections.
2 *Folate antagonists.* The most toxic of these is methotrexate, an exceedingly powerful inhibitor of dihydrofolate reductase which is used in the treatment of certain malignancies. Much less toxic but still capable of inducing a megaloblastic anemia are several weak dihydrofolate reductase inhibitors that are used to treat a variety of nonmalignant conditions. These include pentamidine, trimethoprim, triamterene, and pyrimethamine.

   The megaloblastic changes in methotrexate poisoning appear to result from a buildup of dUMP owing to impaired methylation to dTMP. The excess dUMP is partially phosphorylated to dUTP, which accumulates in the cell and is incorporated into newly synthesized DNA. As a result, defective strands of DNA are produced in which T is partly replaced by U.
3 *Nitrous oxide.* Nitrous oxide inhalation causes the destruction of endogenous cobalamin. As ordinarily used, this anesthetic does not destroy enough cobalamin to cause clinical manifestations. Repeated or protracted exposure, however, may lead to a megaloblastic anemia. Fatal megaloblastic anemia has been reported in patients with tetanus who were given nitrous oxide continuously for weeks.
4 *Others.* A number of drugs antagonize folate by mechanisms which are poorly understood but are thought to involve an effect on absorption of the vitamin by the intestine. In this category are the anticonvulsants phenytoin (Dilantin) and primidone (Mysoline) and phenobarbital (Luminal). Megaloblastic anemia induced by these agents is mild.

ACUTE MEGALOBLASTIC ANEMIA Occasionally, a full-blown megaloblastic state can develop over the course of just a few days. This is usually seen following nitrous oxide anesthesia but may occur in any patient with a serious illness requiring intensive care, especially a patient receiving multiple transfusions, dialysis, or total parenteral nutrition. An acute megaloblastic state also can be precipitated by the administration of a weak antifolate (e.g., trimethoprim) to a patient with marginal tissue folate stores.

The condition resembles an immune cytopenia, with a rapidly developing thrombocytopenia and/or leukopenia in the absence of anemia. The blood smear may be completely normal, but the marrow is always floridly megaloblastic. Acute megaloblastic anemia responds rapidly to treatment with folate plus cobalamin in the usual therapeutic doses.

OTHER Hereditary Megaloblastic anemia may be seen in several hereditary disorders. It is a regular feature of orotic aciduria, a deficiency of orotidylic decarboxylase and phosphorylase, leading to a defect in pyrimidine metabolism and characterized by retarded growth and development as well as by the excretion of large amounts of orotic acid. Megaloblastic anemia has been reported in a single case of the Lesch-Nyhan syndrome, a condition resulting from a deficiency of hypoxanthine-guanine phosphoribosyltransferase whose clinical manifestations include gout, mental retardation, and self-mutilation. It also has been described in methylmalonic aciduria due to a combined defect in the biosynthesis of methyl and adenosyl cobalamins, although it is not seen in methylmalonic aciduria due to methylmalonyl CoA mutase deficiency. Congenital folate malabsorption causes megaloblastic anemia, accompanied by ataxia and mental retardation. Megaloblastic anemia has been reported to accompany the congenital deficiency of two other folate-metabolizing enzymes: dihydrofolate reductase and N^5-methyltetrahydrofolate:homocysteine methyltransferase. These deficiencies are less well documented than is congenital folate malabsorption. A thiamine-responsive megaloblastic anemia accompanied by nerve deafness and diabetes mellitus has been reported in several children. Megaloblastic changes as well as multinuclearity of red blood cell precursors are seen in the marrow of certain patients with congenital dyserythropoietic anemia, a group of inherited disorders characterized by mild to moderate anemia presenting at any age and pursuing a benign course.

Transcobalamin II deficiency, like the congenital abnormalities in cobalamin absorption described previously, causes pronounced deficiency in cobalamin in infancy or early childhood, with all the accompanying manifestations. Megaloblastic anemia is not seen in hereditary transcobalamin I deficiency.

Refractory megaloblastic anemia This is a form of myelodysplasia in which megaloblastic erythropoiesis may sometimes be seen. Megaloblastic changes are restricted to the red blood cell series; large granulocyte precursors and giant metamyelocytes are not seen (see below). Like other forms of myelodysplasia, acquired sideroblastic anemia is associated with an increased incidence of acute leukemia.

Megaloblastic changes are seen in erythremic myelosis and acute erythroleukemia (di Guglielmo), where red blood cell precursors are prominently involved. Here, the marrow is characterized by bizarre erythroid maturation, with multinuclearity and multipolar mitotic figures in the red blood cell precursors. Erythremic myelosis is discussed further in Chap. 310.

DIAGNOSIS The finding of significant macrocytosis [mean corpuscular volume (MCV) > 100 fL] suggests the presence of a megaloblastic anemia. Other causes of macrocytosis include hemolysis, liver disease, alcoholism, hypothyroidism, and aplastic anemia. If the macrocytosis is marked (MCV > 110 fL), the patient is much more likely to have a megaloblastic anemia. Macrocytosis is less marked with concurrent iron deficiency or thalassemia. The reticulocyte count is low, and the leukocyte and platelet count also may be decreased, particularly in severely anemic patients. The blood smear (Fig. A9-2) demonstrates marked anisocytosis and poikilocytosis, together with macroovalocytes, which are large, oval, fully hemoglobinized erythrocytes typical of megaloblastic anemias. There is some basophilic stippling, and an occasional nucleated red blood cell may be seen. In the white blood cell series, the neutrophils show hypersegmentation of the nucleus. This is such a characteristic finding that a single cell with a nucleus of six lobes or more should raise the immediate suspicion of a megaloblastic anemia. A rare myelocyte also may be seen. Bizarre, misshapen platelets are also observed. The bone marrow examination is very helpful in the diagnosis of megaloblastic anemia. The marrow is hypercellular with a decreased myeloid/erythroid ratio and abundant stainable iron. Red blood cell precursors are abnormally large and have nuclei that appear much less mature than would be expected from the development of the cytoplasm (nuclear-cytoplasmic asynchrony). The nuclear chromatin is more dispersed than it should be and consequently stains less intensely than normal. To the extent that it is aggregated, it condenses in a peculiar fenestrated pattern which is very characteristic of megaloblastic erythropoiesis. Abnormal mitoses may be seen. Granulocyte precursors are also affected, many being larger than normal, including giant bands and metamyelocytes. Megakaryocytes are decreased and show abnormal morphology.

Megaloblastic anemias are characterized by ineffective erythropoiesis (Chap. 302). In a severely megaloblastic patient, as many as 90 percent of the red blood cell precursors may be destroyed before they are released into the bloodstream, compared with 10 to 15 percent in the normal subject. Enhanced intramedullary destruction of erythroblasts results in an increase in unconjugated bilirubin and lactic acid dehydrogenase (isoenzyme 1) in plasma. Abnormalities in iron kinetics also attest to the presence of ineffective erythropoiesis, with increased iron turnover but low incorporation of labeled iron into circulating red blood cells.

In evaluating a patient with megaloblastic anemia, it is important to determine whether there is a specific vitamin deficiency by measuring serum cobalamin and folate levels. The normal range of cobalamin in serum is 200 to 900 pg/mL; values less than 100 pg/mL indicate clinically significant deficiency. The normal serum concentration of folic acid ranges from 6 to 20 ng/mL; values of 4 ng/mL or less are generally considered to be diagnostic of folate deficiency. Unlike serum cobalamin, serum folate levels may reflect recent alterations in dietary intake. Measurement of red blood cell folate level occasionally provides useful information, since it is not subject to short-term fluctuations in folate intake and is, therefore, a better index of tissue folate stores than serum folate.

Once cobalamin deficiency has been established, its pathogenesis can be delineated by means of a Schilling test. A patient is given radioactive cobalamin by mouth, followed shortly thereafter by an intramuscular injection of unlabeled cobalamin. The proportion of the administered radioactivity excreted in the urine during the next 24 h provides an accurate measure of absorption of cobalamin, assuming that a complete urine sample has been collected. Since cobalamin deficiency is almost always due to malabsorption (see Table 304-1), this first stage of the Schilling test should be abnormal. The patient is then given labeled cobalamin bound to intrinsic factor. Absorption of the vitamin will now approach normal if the patient has pernicious anemia or some other type of intrinsic factor deficiency. If cobalamin absorption is still decreased, the patient may have bacterial overgrowth ("blind loop" syndrome) or ileal disease (including an ileal absorptive defect secondary to the cobalamin deficiency itself). Cobalamin malabsorption due to bacterial overgrowth can frequently be corrected by the administration of antibiotics. The Schilling test can provide equally reliable information after the patient has had adequate therapy with parenteral cobalamin.

Low serum cobalamin levels occur in some patients who are hematologically normal and have normal Schilling tests. Many of these patients absorb cobalamin poorly when the vitamin is mixed with food. Other patients show normal serum cobalamin levels but elevated levels of serum methylmalonic acid, a metabolic marker of cobalamin deficiency. Both these groups of patients are generally considered to have mild or "subtle" cobalamin deficiency. Poorly defined neuropsychiatric abnormalities occur in many of these patients, and it has been suggested that these abnormalities may be due to the patients' cobalamin-deficient state. Whether this is so remains to be conclusively demonstrated, but until the question is settled, the safest course is to treat these patients with cobalamin.

TREATMENT

COBALAMIN DEFICIENCY Apart from specific therapy related to the underlying disorder (e.g., antibiotics for intestinal overgrowth with bacteria), the mainstay of treatment for cobalamin deficiency is replacement therapy. Since the defect is one of absorption, replacement should be administered parenterally, specifically in the form of intramuscular cyanocobalamin. (If intramuscular administration is contraindicated or refused, cobalamin deficiency can be managed by oral replacement therapy, but at doses of 300 to 1000 μg daily, it is an expensive mode of treatment which requires very close medical supervision to avoid relapse.) Treatment should be started with 100 μg cobalamin per day for a week. The frequency of administration of the vitamin may then be decreased, the goal being to give a total of 2000 μg during the first 6 weeks. The patient may then be placed on 100 μg cyanocobalamin intramuscularly every month, a regimen that must be maintained for the rest of the patient's life. If necessary, larger doses may be given at less frequent intervals (e.g., 1 mg every 2 to 4 months), but the risk of relapse is substantially greater than if the vitamin is given monthly.

The response to treatment is gratifying. Shortly after treatment is begun, and several days before a hematologic response is evident in the peripheral blood, the patient will experience an increase in strength and an improved sense of well-being. Marrow morphology begins to revert toward normal within a few hours after treatment is initiated. Reticulocytosis begins 4 to 5 days after therapy is started and peaks at about day 7 (Fig. 304-4), with subsequent remission of the anemia over the next several weeks. If a reticulocytosis does not occur, or if it is less brisk than expected from the level of the hematocrit, a search should be made for other factors contributing to the anemia (e.g., infection, coexisting folate deficiency, or hypothyroidism). Hypokalemia and salt retention may occur early in the course of therapy.

In most cases, replacement therapy is all that is needed for the treatment of cobalamin deficiency. Occasionally, however, a patient with a severe anemia will have such a precarious cardiovascular status that emergency transfusion is necessary. This must be done with great care, since it is very easy to precipitate florid congestive failure in such patients by fluid overload. Blood must be administered slowly in the form of packed cells, with very close observation, giving as an initial dose no more than 100 mL. This small volume will frequently be enough to ameliorate the cardiovascular problems sufficiently that further therapy can be restricted to cobalamin replacement. If necessary, blood may be administered by exchanging patient blood (mostly plasma) for packed cells.

With lifelong treatment, patients should experience no further manifestations of cobalamin deficiency. As previously stated, neurologic symptoms may not be fully corrected even by optimal therapy. The potential for late development of gastric carcinoma in pernicious anemia necessitates careful follow-up of the patient.

FOLATE DEFICIENCY Like cobalamin deficiency, folate deficiency is treated by replacement therapy. The usual dose of folate is 1 mg/d, by mouth, but higher doses (up to 5 mg/d) may be required

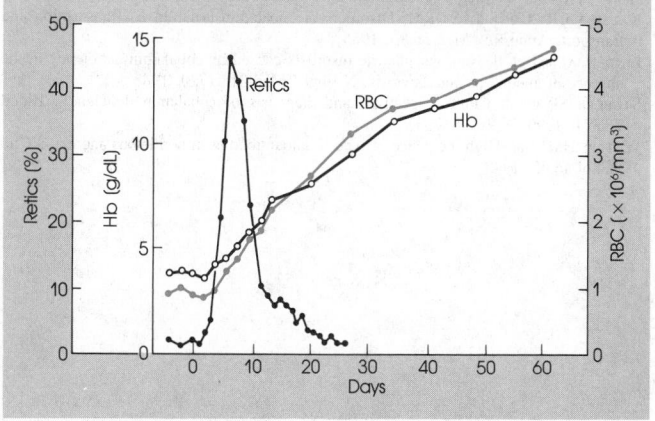

FIGURE 304-4 Hematologic response of a patient with pernicious anemia to an intramuscular injection of 100 μg cobalamin on day 0. *(From A Erslev, TG Gabuzda, Pathophysiology of Blood, Philadelphia, Saunders, 1975.)*

for folate deficiency due to malabsorption. Parenteral folate is rarely necessary. The hematologic response is similar to that seen after replacement therapy for cobalamin deficiency—that is, a brisk reticulocytosis after about 4 days, followed by correction of the anemia over the next 1 to 2 months. The duration of therapy depends on the basis of the deficiency state. Patients with a continuously increased requirement (such as patients with hemolytic anemia) or those with malabsorption or chronic malnutrition should continue to receive oral folic acid indefinitely. In addition, the patient should be encouraged to maintain an optimal diet containing adequate amounts of folate.

Folate, particularly in large doses, can correct the megaloblastic anemia of cobalamin deficiency without altering the neurologic abnormalities. The neurologic manifestations may even be aggravated by folate therapy. Cobalamin deficiency can thus be masked in patients who for one reason or another are taking large doses of folate. For this reason, a hematologic response to folate must never be used to rule out cobalamin deficiency in a given patient; cobalamin deficiency can be excluded only by appropriate laboratory evaluation.

OTHER CAUSES OF MEGALOBLASTIC ANEMIA Megaloblastic anemia due to drugs can be treated, if necessary, by reducing the dose of the drug or eliminating it altogether. The effects of folate antagonists which inhibit dihydrofolate reductase can be counteracted by folinic acid (citrovorum factor) in a dose of 100 to 200 mg/d. Since folinic acid is a derivative of tetrahydrofolate, it circumvents the block in folate metabolism imposed by dihydrofolate reductase inhibitors, replenishing the tissues with a form of folate which can directly enter the 1-carbon donor pool. Certain of the congenital megaloblastic anemia–producing enzyme deficiencies can be treated by appropriate specific therapeutic regimens. For the megaloblastic forms of sideroblastic anemia, pyridoxine in pharmacologic doses (as high as 300 mg/d) should be tried. A few patients will respond to this therapy. Simple supportive measures are all that appear to be in order for treatment of refractory megaloblastic anemia. Acute erythroleukemia (di Guglielmo's disease) is usually treated like other types of acute nonlymphocytic leukemia (see Chap. 310).

REFERENCES

BABIOR BM: The megaloblastic anemias, in *Hematology*, 4th ed, WJ Williams et al (eds). New York, McGraw-Hill, 1990

BECK WS: Diagnosis of megaloblastic anemia, in *Annual Review of Medicine, 1991*, WP Creger (ed). Stanford, Calif, Annual Reviews, Inc., 1991

———: Neuropsychiatric consequences of cobalamin deficiency. Adv Intern Med 36:33, 1991

BORCH K: Epidemiologic, clinicopathologic, and economic aspects of gastroscopic screening of patients with pernicious anemia. Scand J Gastroenterol 21:21, 1986

CHANARIN I et al: Cobalamin and folate: Recent developments. J Clin Pathol 45:227, 1992

COOPER BA, ROSENBLATT DS: Inherited defects of vitamin B_{12} metabolism. Annu Rev Nutr 7:291, 1987

HERBERT V: Don't ignore low serum cobalamin (vitamin B_{12}) levels. Arch Intern Med 148:1705, 1988

———: Nutritional anemias in the elderly, in *Nutrition and Aging*, DM Prinsley et al (eds). New York, Alan R. Liss, 1990

HSING AW et al: Pernicious anemia and subsequent cancer. Cancer 71:745, 1993

KAPADIA CR, DONALDSON RM: Disorders of cobalamin (vitamin B_{12}) absorption and transport. Annu Rev Med 36:93, 1985

LINDENBAUM J et al: Neuropsychiatric disorders caused by cobalamin deficiency in the absence of anemia or macrocytosis. N Engl J Med 318:1720, 1988

STABLER SP et al: Clinical spectrum and diagnosis of cobalamin deficiency. Blood 75:871, 1990

WATERS HM et al: High incidence of type II autoantibodies in pernicious anemia. J Clin Pathol 46:45, 1993

305 ANEMIA ASSOCIATED WITH CHRONIC DISORDERS

H. FRANKLIN BUNN

Among the most commonly encountered anemias are those which accompany a variety of chronic underlying diseases. They can be corrected only if the primary condition is reversible. As shown in Table 305-1, these anemias can be subdivided into several groups.

ANEMIA OF CHRONIC INFLAMMATION

CLINICAL FEATURES Patients who have a chronic systemic inflammatory disorder persisting more than a month usually develop a mild or moderate anemia. The extent of the anemia is roughly proportional to the duration and severity of the inflammatory process. These disorders include chronic infections such as subacute infective endocarditis, osteomyelitis, lung abscess, tuberculosis, and pyelonephritis. Noninfectious inflammatory disorders often associated with chronic anemia include rheumatoid arthritis, systemic lupus erythematosus, vasculitides (such as temporal arteritis), sarcoidosis, regional enteritis, and tissue injury such as fracture.

This kind of anemia is also commonly encountered in neoplastic disorders, including Hodgkin's disease and a variety of solid tumors such as carcinoma of the lung and breast. Other factors may contribute to the development of more severe anemia in cancer patients. In those with gastrointestinal or uterine cancer, blood loss can be the predominant factor. Chronic bleeding will lead to iron deficiency. Furthermore, cancer patients may develop progressive anemia if the bone marrow is invaded with tumor cells. Myelophthisic anemia is discussed in Chap. 308. Cancer patients are often malnourished and may be deficient in folate. Rarely, patients with disseminated malignancy develop severe traumatic hemolytic anemia (Chap. 307). Finally, suppression of hematopoiesis by chemotherapeutic agents or radiation therapy may aggravate anemia.

HEMATOLOGIC FEATURES Hemoglobin values generally range between 90 and 110 g/L. A hemoglobin level less than 80 g/L indicates the presence of one or more of the aggravating factors mentioned above. Although this group of anemias is generally classified as normocytic, normochromic, red blood cells are often slightly microcytic. The mean corpuscular hemoglobin concentration is about 320 g/L (normal $\cong$ 340 g/L). Examination of the bone marrow reveals normal erythroid maturation. However, the red blood cell precursors have less stainable iron than normal (i.e., fewer sideroblasts), while the macrophages in the marrow usually contain increased amounts of iron. Myeloid hyperplasia and an increase in plasma cells are often seen in chronic infections.

The corrected reticulocyte count is low. Careful measurement of red blood cell survival generally reveals moderately shortened erythrocyte life span. Cross-transfusion studies point to an extracorpuscular mechanism, probably hyperplasia of the mononuclear phagocyte system. There is seldom any other evidence of significant hemolysis. However, in certain chronic infections such as subacute

TABLE 305-1 Anemias secondary to chronic systemic diseases

1 Anemia of chronic inflammation
  a Infection
  b Connective tissue disorders, etc.
  c Malignancy
2 Anemia of uremia
3 Anemia due to endocrine failure
4 Anemia of liver disease

infective endocarditis and miliary tuberculosis, splenomegaly can contribute to further shortening of the red blood cell life span, thereby increasing the severity of the anemia. In this setting, spherocytes are often seen on the blood smear.

Serum iron is characteristically subnormal in this group of anemias, but in contrast to iron deficiency, the total transferrin level is also reduced (see Fig. 303-2). The fractional saturation of transferrin is lower than normal. The serum iron level falls within hours or days following the onset of the inflammation, whereas several weeks elapse before the transferrin level falls. Serum ferritin is increased in patients with inflammatory disorders. Certain other plasma proteins are characteristically elevated in chronic inflammation, probably under the stimulus of interleukin 1 (IL-1) and tumor necrosis factor, cytokines released by activated macrophages. These ''phase reactants'' include gamma globulin, the third component of complement, haptoglobin, α_1-antitrypsin, orosomucoid, and fibrinogen. The latter is usually not measured, since protein electrophoresis is routinely done on serum rather than plasma. Elevation of these proteins is responsible for the increased rate of red blood cell sedimentation which is so commonly observed.

It is often difficult to detect iron deficiency in a patient with chronic inflammation. The serum iron level is low, and red blood cell protoporphyrin is increased in both conditions. When iron deficiency is superimposed on a chronic inflammatory state, the serum ferritin level falls to less than 60 μg/L. The serum transferrin level rises, usually to within normal limits. Under such circumstances, the amount of storage iron in the bone marrow is unpredictable. This problem is commonly encountered in patients with rheumatoid arthritis who may have developed iron deficiency owing to gastrointestinal blood loss. Because of this diagnostic uncertainty, it is often prudent to give such a patient a trial of iron and ascertain whether the hemoglobin level increases. However, it is important to avoid prolonged administration of iron unless a true deficiency state persists.

PATHOGENESIS   The anemia of chronic inflammation is primarily due to defective red blood cell production and failure to compensate for the slightly decreased red blood cell life span. The subnormal amounts of iron in erythroblasts, despite an abundance of storage iron, suggest a defect in the transfer of iron to the developing erythroid cells. It is likely that inflammatory cytokines, such as IL-1, induce increased translation of ferritin in macrophages, thereby trapping iron and hindering release to transferrin. The cells that are formed are somewhat ''iron deficient'' and therefore tend to be small and pale. As in true iron deficiency, increased red blood cell protoporphyrin reflects the reduced availability of iron for heme synthesis. This block in iron utilization can be measured by iron kinetic studies. If radioactive iron bound to transferrin is administered, there is normal uptake into erythroblasts and incorporation into circulating red cells. In contrast, if hemoglobin labeled with radioactive iron is injected, the incorporation of label into circulating red cells is only half normal. The hyperplastic mononuclear phagocyte system which is responsible for decreased survival of circulating red cells probably traps the hemoglobin iron and prevents its transfer to the bone marrow. The macrophages' increased avidity for iron may be due to one of the actions of IL-1, i.e., release of lactoferrin from neutrophils. The iron binding protein lactoferrin captures free iron and rapidly transfers it to macrophages.

The modest suppression of red blood cell production is caused in part by decreased availability of iron. In addition, erythropoietin levels tend to be lower than expected for the degree of anemia. However, erythropoietin levels are not as low as in the anemia of renal failure (see below) and probably do not play a significant role in the pathogenesis of the anemia.

MANAGEMENT   The anemia of chronic inflammation is not responsive to hematinic agents such as iron, folic acid, or vitamin B_{12}. Since the anemia is seldom severe, blood transfusion is rarely indicated. Efforts should be directed toward correcting the underlying disorder. In addition, if the anemia is more severe than expected, it is essential to search for other factors such as blood loss or drug-induced myelosuppression that could contribute to the reduction of red blood cell mass. While erythropoietin therapy can increase the hematocrit, the improvement is modest and by itself does little to improve the patient's functional state.

ANEMIA OF UREMIA

Anemia almost always accompanies the uremic syndrome (Chap. 237). Although the hemoglobin level is highly variable among uremic patients, the severity of the anemia is roughly proportional to the degree of azotemia. The cause of the renal failure usually has little bearing on the extent of anemia. However, for any level of serum creatinine, patients with polycystic disease tend to be less anemic than those with other types of renal disease. In contrast to anemias associated with other chronic disorders discussed in this chapter, the anemia of uremia can be very severe, with hemoglobin levels as low as 40 g/L. However, patients often tolerate such marked anemia fairly well. This is largely due to compensatory adjustments such as redistribution of blood flow and a decrease in the oxygen affinity of the blood (see Chap. 302).

The anemia of uremia is normochromic and normocytic. Examination of the bone marrow seldom reveals any abnormalities. Red blood cell morphology is usually normal. In about one-third of patients, so-called burr cells are seen in the peripheral blood smear. These red blood cells have a characteristic evenly scalloped border (see Fig. A9-9). Neither the degree of anemia nor the red blood cell life span is influenced by the presence of burr cells. In most patients the corrected reticulocyte count is low, and the red blood cell survival is only modestly decreased. Thus the low red blood cell mass is due to decreased red blood cell production. The primary basis for this defect is that the diseased kidneys are unable to secrete adequate amounts of erythropoietin. Plasma erythropoietin levels are much lower than those of nonuremic patients with a comparable degree of anemia. Erythropoietin production is further impaired but not abolished in patients who have undergone bilateral nephrectomy. In addition, erythropoiesis may be somewhat suppressed by the accumulation of substances that are normally cleared by the kidneys. Iron kinetic measurements reveal impaired incorporation of iron into circulating red blood cells. Thus it is likely that the anemia is due in part to ineffective erythropoiesis (see Chap. 302). Improvement in the rate of utilization of iron by the bone marrow has been noted following hemodialysis.

A small minority of uremic patients, particularly those with advanced disease, have brisk hemolysis. Red blood cell survival studies indicate that the hemolysis is extracorpuscular. Either metabolic or mechanical factors may contribute to the hemolysis. Some patients may acquire a defect in the hexose monophosphate shunt which renders the red blood cell vulnerable to the formation of Heinz bodies (see Chap. 307). The hemolysis can be aggravated by oxidant drugs or oxidant compounds such as chloramine in the dialysis bath. If the renal failure is due to thrombotic thrombocytopenic purpura or hemolytic-uremic syndrome, patients will have a severe form of microangiopathic hemolytic anemia, with characteristic abnormalities of red blood cell morphology (see Chap. 307).

In some patients, aluminum salts that contaminate the tap water used in hemodialysis cause a worsening of anemia and the emergence of microcytosis and hypochromia.

Treatment of the anemia of uremia should focus on an attempt to reverse the renal failure. Red cell production may be modestly improved following hemodialysis. A prompt and dramatic correction of the anemia follows successful renal transplantation. Occasionally, polycythemia may be encountered following the renal engraftment and may be a harbinger of impending rejection.

The development of recombinant human erythropoietin has enabled definitive treatment of the anemia of uremia. Administration of this genetically engineered product either by intravenous infusion or by subcutaneous injection results in correction of anemia and gratifying symptomatic improvement. The agent is identical in structure to native erythropoietin and therefore safe and virtually free of side effects. However, overtreatment should be avoided, since it can aggravate hypertension and increase the likelihood of thromboses. Accordingly, sufficient recombinant erythropoietin should be given to maintain the patient's hematocrit between 0.32 and 0.37.

It is important to be aware of other factors that may aggravate the anemia of renal disease. Uremic patients have a propensity to hemorrhage, owing to a qualitative defect in platelet function. Thus gastrointestinal blood loss is commonly encountered. Furthermore, a small but significant amount of blood loss occurs during hemodialysis. For these reasons, some uremic patients become iron deficient. Folic acid deficiency also may occur owing to the poor nutrition of many patients or to the loss of this vitamin during dialysis.

ANEMIA SECONDARY TO ENDOCRINE FAILURE

A number of hormones, including thyroxine, glucocorticoids, testosterone, and growth hormone, are known to affect proliferation of human erythroid cells in vitro. Therefore, it is not surprising that a mild to moderate normochromic, normocytic anemia generally accompanies a number of endocrine deficiency states, including hypothyroidism, Addison's disease, hypogonadism, and panhypopituitarism. It is possible that the anemias associated with hypothyroidism and hypopituitarism are related to the decreased need for oxygen transport, since oxygen consumption is reduced when thyroid hormone or growth hormone is lacking.

The anemia of *myxedema* is usually normocytic. Red blood cell life span is normal, and erythropoiesis is effective. A minority of patients have macrocytic red blood cells which can usually be attributed to either folic acid or B_{12} deficiency. Patients with myxedema have an increased incidence of pernicious anemia. Hypothyroid patients, particularly females with menorrhagia, often develop iron deficiency and a microcytic anemia. Because the plasma volume may be reduced along with the red blood cell mass, the anemia of hypothyroidism may be masked. Since the signs and symptoms of myxedema are sometimes elusive, this diagnosis should be considered in the evaluation of any patient with unexplained anemia.

The anemia of *Addison's disease* is also masked by a decrease in plasma volume. Untreated patients have an average hemoglobin level of about 130 g/L. Upon hormone replacement, the plasma volume is rapidly reconstituted, and the hemoglobin level falls to 80 percent of its pretreatment value. With continued therapy, the red blood cell mass returns to normal.

Testosterone has a physiologic influence on red blood cell mass. During passage through adolescence, the mean hemoglobin level of males increases from 130 to 150 g/L. Eunuchoid males generally have a mean hemoglobin level averaging 130 g/L. Pituitary dysfunction or ablation is associated with a mild normochromic, normocytic anemia as well as occasional leukopenia.

The anemias secondary to endocrine failure are all readily corrected when adequate hormone replacement is given.

ANEMIA OF LIVER DISEASE

Patients with chronic liver disease, regardless of etiology, usually have a mild to moderate anemia which is normocytic or slightly macrocytic. An increased plasma volume may artificially lower the hematocrit and make the anemia seem worse than it is. Red blood cell morphology is normal, except for the presence of target cells (see Fig. A9-3) and occasional stomatocytes, which have increased membrane surface area owing to increased deposits of cholesterol and phospholipid. The bone marrow is usually normal. Erythropoiesis fails to compensate for a moderate shortening of red blood cell life span. The anemia persists as long as hepatic function is defective, but it may be corrected if normal hepatic function can be restored.

The situation is much more complex in patients with *alcoholic liver disease*. Many factors can contribute to the development of anemia. Alcohol is a direct suppressor of erythropoiesis. In alcoholics who have continued to drink up to the time of clinical evaluation, the bone marrow often reveals vacuoles in the cytoplasm of red and white blood cell precursors. In addition, ringed sideroblasts may be observed, particularly in patients who are malnourished. In alcoholics there is often suboptimal intake of dietary folic acid and impairment of folate utilization. Furthermore, anemia in alcoholics is commonly compounded by significant hemorrhage from gastritis, esophageal varices, or duodenal ulcer. The risk of gastrointestinal blood loss is further increased by the presence of thrombocytopenia or deficiencies in soluble clotting factors. Although alcoholics usually have increased iron stores, they may become iron deficient after prolonged gastrointestinal bleeding. Rarely, patients with alcoholic cirrhosis develop a severe hemolytic anemia accompanied by the appearance of rigid red blood cells with irregular borders called *acanthocytes*, or "spur" cells (see Fig. A9-8) (Chap. 307). In addition, alcoholics may acquire a defect in the erythrocyte hexose monophosphate shunt, similar to that encountered in patients with uremia.

REFERENCES

BUDMAN DR, STEINBERG AD: Hematologic aspects of systemic lupus erythematosus. Ann Intern Med 86:220, 1977

ESCHBACH JW, ADAMSON J: Anemia of end-stage renal disease. Kidney Int 28:1, 1985

—— et al: Correction of the anemia of end-stage renal disease with recombinant human erythropoietin. N Engl J Med 316:73, 1987

MEANS RT, KRANTZ SB: Progress in understanding the pathogenesis of the anemia of chronic disease. Blood 80:1639, 1992

MOWAT AG: Hematologic abnormalities in rheumatoid arthritis. Semin Arthritis Rheum 1:195, 1972

SAVAGE D, LINDENBAUM J: Anemia in alcoholics. Medicine 65:322, 1986

SEARS DA: Anemia of chronic disease. Med Clin North Am 76:567, 1992

306 DISORDERS OF HEMOGLOBIN

H. FRANKLIN BUNN

In 1910, Herrick wrote of a medical student from Jamaica who had a hemolytic anemia in conjunction with elongated, "sickled" red blood cells. Subsequently, sickle cell disease was shown to be associated with an electrophoretically abnormal hemoglobin (designated Hb S) which differed from normal Hb A by the substitution of valine for glutamic acid at the sixth position of the β chain. Since then, over 500 structurally different human hemoglobin variants have been discovered in widely scattered parts of the world. Generally, a new hemoglobin is named after the place where it is first encountered. No more than a third of these mutant hemoglobins are associated with significant clinical manifestations. The remainder have been discovered by serendipity or as a result of large population surveys.

This chapter focuses on the clinically significant hemoglobin variants. In addition, disorders of the biosynthesis of globin (the thalassemias) and methemoglobinemia are discussed.

GENETIC CONSIDERATIONS The synthesis of each of the subunits of hemoglobin (α, β, γ, δ, ε, ζ) is governed by separate genes. The ε and ζ subunits are found only in embryonic hemoglobin. Normal individuals inherit two β-chain genes (one from each parent), four α-chain genes, and four γ-chain genes. The ε-, γ-, δ-, and β-chain genes occupy adjacent loci on chromosome 11 (see Fig. 306-1). The ζ and α genes are located on chromosome 16. The structure and function of normal hemoglobin ($\alpha_2\beta_2$) are discussed in Chap. 302. The inheritance of abnormal hemoglobins follows classic mendelian genetics. If both parents are heterozygous for a hemoglobin variant

FIGURE 306-1 Diagram of human globin genes. (*Left*) The α-globin gene complex includes the embryonic ζ gene as well as two α genes. In the vast majority of individuals with α thalassemia 2 (α−) one α gene is deleted owing to a nonhomologous crossover between adjacent α genes. In α thalassemia 1 (− −) both α genes are deleted. (*Right*) The β-globin gene complex includes the embryonic ε gene, two fetal genes (Gγ and Aγ), the δ gene, and the β gene. Below is a diagram of the β gene showing the coding regions (■), the intervening segments (IVS), (□), and the flanking regions (▨) that are transcribed into mRNA below. Most cases of β+ thalassemia in Mediterranean individuals involve a base substitution causing partial impairment of splicing of an IVS. Most cases of β0 thalassemia in Mediterraneans involve a base substitution that creates either a stop codon or a frame shift.

such as Hb S, statistically one-quarter of their offspring will be SS homozygotes, another quarter will be normal (AA genotype), and half will have sickle trait (AS). The commonly encountered hemoglobinopathies such as S, C, and E are β-chain variants. Occasionally, an individual inherits two different β-chain variants, one from each parent. Hemoglobin SC disease is an example of such a compound heterozygous state. Genes for β thalassemia are located on the β-chain structural gene. Accordingly, an individual can inherit from one parent (and pass on to a child) either β thalassemia or a β-chain variant, but not both. Among the hemoglobinopathies associated with sickling (described below), only the homozygous state (Hb SS) or double heterozygous state (Sβ thalassemia or SC) has important clinical manifestations. In contrast, the unstable variants and those having abnormal oxygen-binding properties are encountered only in heterozygotes. In some cases, the homozygous state would be incompatible with life.

About 90 percent of these abnormal hemoglobins are single amino acid replacements due to a single base substitution in the corresponding triplet codon. The structural information accumulated on human mutant hemoglobins has provided ample verification of the fidelity of the genetic code. Other genetic mechanisms must be invoked to explain the structure of a few interesting hemoglobin variants. The Lepore hemoglobins have arisen because of nonhomologous crossover between the adjacent δ- and β-chain genes, giving rise to a fusion subunit in which the N-terminal end has the amino acid sequence of the δ chain and the C-terminal end has the sequence of the β chain (see Fig. 306-1). Some of the unstable hemoglobins have deletions

of one or more residues in sequence within a subunit. Finally, there are a few variants which have elongated subunits (e.g., Hb Constant Spring). These have arisen either because of a base substitution in the termination codon or because of a frame shift which puts the termination codon out of phase.

CLINICAL CLASSIFICATION The clinically significant hemoglobin variants are classified in Table 306-1. By far the most important and prevalent type of hemoglobinopathy is due to the presence of sickle hemoglobin, either in the homozygous state or in conjunction with another type of hemoglobin abnormality. The inheritance of an unstable hemoglobin variant may give rise to congenital hemolytic anemia associated with the presence of inclusions of precipitated hemoglobin within the red blood cells (Heinz bodies). Finally, hemoglobin variants may have abnormal functional or spectral properties, resulting in familial erythrocytosis or familial cyanosis.

SICKLE SYNDROMES

SICKLE CELL TRAIT About 8 percent of black Americans are heterozygous for Hb S. The gene frequency is highest in central Africa, particularly in regions where malaria is endemic. In some parts of Nigeria, over 30 percent of the population has sickle trait. The gene has persisted because heterozygotes gain slight protection against falciparum malaria. This is an example of balanced polymorphism.

The diagnosis of sickle trait or any of the other sickle syndromes depends on the demonstration of sickling under reduced oxygen tension. In the widely used sickle preparation, sickled cells can be visualized microscopically after the addition of an oxygen-consuming reagent such as metabisulfite. Many clinical laboratories prefer a solubility test which depends on the fact that deoxyhemoglobin S has a low solubility at high ionic strength. These tests are reasonably specific for Hb S, although some of the unstable variants may give a false-positive solubility test. Therefore, if one of these screening tests is positive, hemoglobin electrophoresis should be performed. Individuals with sickle trait usually have about 35 to 40 percent Hb S and 55 to 60 percent Hb A.

Hemoglobin S heterozygotes have minimal clinical problems. Their overall life expectancy and frequency of hospitalization are no

---

TABLE 306-1 Clinically important hemoglobin variants

I **Sickle syndromes**
  A Sickle cell trait (AS)
  B Sickle cell anemia (SS)
  C Compound heterozygous states: sickle β thalassemia, sickle C disease (SC), sickle D disease (SD)
II **Unstable hemoglobin variants: congenital Heinz body hemolytic anemia**
III **Variants with high oxygen affinity: familial erythrocytosis**
IV **M hemoglobins: familial cyanosis (see Table 306-3)**

different from those of a comparable group of individuals with hemoglobin A. AS red blood cells require a much lower oxygen tension for sickling than SS red cells. Accordingly, individuals with sickle trait may develop sickle cell crises only if they become severely hypoxic. They may occasionally sustain a splenic infarct. As discussed below, the renal medulla is particularly susceptible to sickling. Many AS individuals have impaired ability to form concentrated urine, and a few have recurrent episodes of painless hematuria as a result of medullary infarction. Infarction due to sickling has been encountered in other organs in sickle trait but is extremely rare. For these reasons, AS individuals should not be placed in any high-risk group for employment or insurance considerations.

SICKLE CELL ANEMIA   Sickle cell disease is a significant cause of morbidity and mortality among black individuals. About 0.15 percent of black children in the United States are SS homozygotes. The prevalence is lower among adults because patients with sickle cell anemia have a decreased life expectancy. The protean clinical manifestations of this disorder can all be attributed to a specific molecular lesion: the substitution of valine for glutamic acid at the sixth residue of the β chain.

Molecular pathogenesis   Upon deoxygenation, a red blood cell containing Hb S changes from a biconcave disk to an elongated crescent-shaped or "sickle"-shaped cell (see Fig. 306-2). Electron micrographs reveal the presence of fibers of stacked hemoglobin molecules. Each sickle fiber consists of a helical polymer with 14 strands. The polymer is stabilized by hydrophobic bonding between β6 valine and a complementary site on another portion of the β chain on an adjacent strand (Fig. 306-2). In addition, there are many other interactions between neighboring molecules. Sickling, both within the intact red blood cell and in free solution, is greatly affected by the presence of non-S hemoglobin. Hb A participates more readily than Hb F in copolymerization with Hb S.

Cellular pathogenesis   As discussed in Chap. 302, the ability of red blood cells to traverse the microcirculation depends in large part on their pliability. As sickle polymers are formed during deoxygenation, the red blood cell becomes rigid and, as a result, may obstruct capillary blood flow. The rate at which polymerization occurs depends primarily on the intracellular concentration of Hb S and the extent of deoxygenation. If polymerization occurs before the red cell escapes the narrow-bore capillary, obstruction may occur, resulting in local tissue hypoxia, further deoxygenation, and further sickling. This vicious cycle may result in the amplification of microscopic obstruction into a larger area of infarction. The oxygen-dependent sickle cycle is ordinarily reversible. However, the membrane of SS red blood cells may become sufficiently damaged that the cells lose potassium and water, leading to the formation of irreversibly sickled

forms. In these cells, the characteristic sickle shape persists even after they are exposed to ambient oxygen tension at room temperature and can readily be seen on examination of Wright-stained blood films (see Fig. A9-6).

The proportion of irreversibly sickled cells varies considerably among homozygous sicklers and is not correlated with clinical severity. Hemoglobin F is distributed unevenly among red blood cells of SS patients and composes between 2 and 20 percent of the total hemoglobin (the remainder is almost entirely Hb S). Since Hb F inhibits the polymerization of Hb S, those cells which contain Hb F are protected from sickling, whereas those cells which lack Hb F are at risk of becoming irreversibly sickled. It is not surprising that these rigid cells are readily culled from the circulation and destroyed. The continuous formation and destruction of irreversibly sickled cells contributes significantly to the severe hemolytic anemia shared by all patients with sickle cell anemia. Furthermore, these rigid cells may initiate small-vessel occlusions even if they lack sickle fibers.

Factors such as acidosis or increased erythrocyte 2,3-biphosphoglycerate, both of which lower the oxygen affinity of red blood cells, will enhance the formation of deoxyhemoglobin and, therefore, will promote intracellular polymerization and eventual sickling. In addition, sickling is highly dependent on hemoglobin concentration. Any pathophysiologic process which tends to pull water out of sickle red blood cells will greatly increase their tendency to sickle. Thus the hypertonic environment of the renal medulla can cause local sickling and the formation of papillary infarcts, even in individuals with sickle trait.

SS red blood cells have increased adherence to capillary endothelial cells. This interaction is likely to delay the transit time in the microcirculation, thereby increasing the extent of polymer formation.

Clinical manifestations   Patients with homozygous sickle cell anemia have a variety of clinical problems broadly outlined in Table 306-2. Signs and symptoms usually do not appear until after the sixth month of life, at which time most of the Hb F has been replaced by Hb S. Among the *constitutional* manifestations of sickle cell anemia are delay of growth and development. In addition, these patients have an increased tendency to develop serious infections, particularly due to pneumococcus. SS patients have marked impairment of splenic function, preventing effective clearance of circulating bacteria. With the passage of time, the organ sustains recurrent infarcts and eventually becomes a remnant of fibrous tissue.

ANEMIA   SS homozygotes have a severe hemolytic anemia with hematocrit values between 18 and 30 percent. The mean red blood cell survival is about 10 to 15 days. Those cells having relatively low levels of Hb F have a shorter life span, in part due to a greater chance of becoming irreversibly sickled. As a result of accelerated red blood

FIGURE 306-2   Polymerization of sickle hemoglobin. When the red cell (*A*) is deoxygenated, deoxyhemoglobin S aggregates to form domains of elongated rodlike polymers (*B*). In most cells these fibers align and distort the cell into the classic sickle shape (*C*). The individual Hb S molecules form a closely packed polymer consisting of 14 strands having a helical configuration (*D*). A close-up of the contacts between a pair of aligned strands (*E*) shows the abnormal β6 valine forming a hydrophobic contact with an acceptor site on the β chain of a molecule on the adjacent strand.

oxy   deoxy   O₂   β   α   β   ▪ = β6 Valine

TABLE 306-2 Clinical manifestations of sickle cell anemia

I **Constitutional**
  A Impaired growth and development
  B Increased susceptibility to infection

II **Vasoocclusive**
  A Microinfarcts → Painful crises
  B Macroinfarcts

               → Organ damage

III **Anemia**
  A Severe hemolysis
  B Aplastic crises

cell breakdown, patients with sickle cell disease have characteristic clinical and laboratory findings as discussed in Chap. 302. Even though hemolysis is primarily extravascular, plasma haptoglobin is generally low or absent, and plasma hemoglobin levels are moderately elevated.

The anemia becomes increasingly severe if erythropoiesis is suppressed. There are two main causes of "aplastic crises"—infection and folic acid deficiency. As discussed in Chap. 305, infection brings about a transient reduction in red blood cell production. In particular, parvovirus infection causes an abrupt suppression of erythropoiesis. In SS patients with severe ongoing hemolysis, this usually results in a rapid drop in hematocrit (see Table 306-2).

ACUTE PAIN CRISIS The morbidity and mortality of sickle cell disease are due primarily to recurrent vasoocclusive phenomena. As shown in Table 306-2, these can be divided into two groups. Throughout their lives, SS patients are plagued by recurrent *painful crises*. These episodes may appear with explosive suddenness and attack various parts of the body, particularly the abdomen, chest, back, and joints. About one quarter of painful crises are preceded by a viral or bacterial infection. The frequency of painful crises is highly variable. A given patient may have months or even years without a crisis and then have a cluster of frequent, severe attacks. In some individuals, crises occur more frequently in cold weather, perhaps precipitated by reflex vasospasm. In others, crises come more often in warm weather, during times when patients are likely to become dehydrated. It is often difficult to distinguish between painful sickle crisis and some other type of acute process such as biliary colic, appendicitis, or a perforated viscus. Many patients have been subjected to abdominal exploration because they were considered to have an acute surgical problem. Patients having abdominal sickle crises usually have normal bowel sounds and no rebound tenderness. If the abdominal pain is due to sickling, the surgeon usually finds no gross evidence of infarction or ischemia.

SS homozygotes frequently develop attacks of acute pleuritic chest pain with fever. Although the initial chest x-ray is often unremarkable, an infiltrate may evolve. The important differential diagnosis is between pneumonitis and pulmonary infarction. Culture and Gram's stain of the sputum will be helpful in establishing the presence of pneumonia. In these patients, pulmonary infarctions are much more likely due to thrombosis in situ than to emboli. Occasionally, pulmonary infarcts become secondarily infected.

When a sickle crisis is localized in the extremities, it may induce acute synovitis and joint effusion. Examination of the joint fluid is helpful in distinguishing sickle crisis from other causes of acute arthritis, such as sepsis, gout, or rheumatoid disease. If the effusion is due to sickling, the fluid will be clear and yellow, with a low white blood cell count (100 to 1000 mononuclear cells per cubic millimeter) and an absence of crystals or bacteria.

Sickle crises may occasionally involve the central nervous system. Patients can present with a seizure, stroke, or coma. Although such crises are frequently reversible, they may be fatal.

CHRONIC ORGAN DAMAGE By the time that patients reach adulthood, there is often objective evidence of anatomic or functional damage to various tissues due to the cumulative effects of recurrent

vasoocclusive episodes. Almost any organ may be involved, but the most common are the lungs, kidneys, liver, skeleton, and skin.

Cardiopulmonary Impairment of pulmonary function is a common complication of sickle cell disease. Resting arterial P_{O_2} is usually reduced in part because of intrapulmonary arterial-venous shunting. Since SS red blood cells have decreased oxygen affinity, arterial blood will be significantly undersaturated, leading to an increased tendency for red cells to sickle when they reach the peripheral circulation. SS homozygotes frequently develop congestive heart failure. The chronic severe anemia and hypoxemia impose a sustained burden on the heart. Most patients have a systolic ejection murmur as a result of their hyperdynamic circulation. Even though more oxygen is extracted by the myocardium than any other tissue, SS patients rarely develop vasoocclusive sickling in the myocardium, probably because of rapid transit through the microcirculation.

Genitourinary (See also Chaps. 241 and 243) The hypertonic and acidic environment of the renal medulla promotes sickling, resulting in microinfarcts. Virtually all patients have isosthenuria. The inability to form concentrated urine increases the risk of significant dehydration. In addition, like those with sickle trait, Sβ thalassemia, or SC disease, SS homozygotes may develop significant and prolonged painless hematuria as a result of papillary infarcts. Hematuria may be so extensive that iron deficiency develops. ε-Aminocaproic acid has proved to be effective in severe cases but must be used with caution because it may prevent the lysis of clots in the renal pelvis.

Mild nitrogen retention is commonly encountered, accompanied by moderate hyperuricemia. However, patients rarely have uric acid nephropathy or gout. As SS patients survive into the fourth and fifth decades, a substantial proportion develop progressive renal failure. The pathogenesis of the glomerular dysfunction is unclear. Male patients with sickle cell anemia occasionally develop priapism (spontaneous and painful engorgement of the penis). This distressing complication occurs with about equal frequency in prepubertal and postpubertal patients, although the latter are more difficult to treat and may develop impotence following the acute episode. Patients should be treated conservatively with sedation, analgesia, and intravenous fluids. The administration of packed red blood cells also may be effective. Surgical intervention is rarely indicated.

Hepatobiliary Like other patients with congenital hemolytic anemia, those with sickle cell anemia are icteric, owing to elevated nonconjugated bilirubin in the plasma, and have an increased tendency to form gallstones. As a rule, cholecystectomy is not recommended unless gallstones cause symptoms. It is often difficult to distinguish between the abdominal pain of acute cholecystitis and that due to a sickle crisis. Jaundice deepens markedly if a patient develops choledocholithiasis, and bilirubin levels as high as 855 μmol/L (50 mg/dL) have been reported. In addition, patients with sickle cell anemia may develop hepatic infarcts which occasionally become infected, resulting in abscess formation. If a significant portion of hepatic parenchyma becomes infarcted, fibrosis and deterioration of liver function may result, with deepening of jaundice.

Skeletal Like other patients with congenital hemolytic anemia, patients with sickle cell anemia demonstrate radiologic abnormalities due to the expansion of red marrow. However, the development of bony infarcts results in more characteristic x-ray abnormalities. The biconcave or "fishmouth" vertebrae are virtually pathognomonic of sickle cell disease. Skeletal infarction generally leads to increased bony trabeculation and sclerosis. Aseptic necrosis of the head of the femur is particularly common in patients with sickle cell disease and can lead to considerable disability. Selected patients benefit from surgical intervention, ranging from core decompression to total hip replacement. Like infarcts in other organs, bony infarctions are more likely to become infected. In patients who develop osteomyelitis, salmonella is a frequent pathogen.

Skin Chronic skin ulcers often occur in the distal lower extremities. The lesions appear to be more common in patients with more severe anemia. Ankle ulcers also have been encountered in rare patients with other types of congenital hemolytic anemia. This

TABLE 306-3   Differential diagnosis of cyanosis

I **Decreased oxygenation of hemoglobin (↑ deoxyhemoglobin)**
  A Reduced arterial oxygen tension (common)
    1 Pulmonary disease
    2 Cardiac right-to-left shunt
  B Hemoglobin variant having decreased oxygen affinity (rare)
II **Methemoglobinemia (rare)**
  A Hereditary
    1 M hemoglobins
    2 Cytochrome b₅ reductase deficiency
  B Acquired
    1 Nitrites and nitrates: sodium nitrite, amyl nitrite, nitroglycerin, nitroprusside, silver nitrate
    2 Aniline dyes
    3 Acetanilid and phenacetin
    4 Sulfonamides
    5 Other: lidocaine, chlorate, phenazopyridine

behavior. As a result of the hemoglobin's increased oxygen affinity, oxygen unloading to tissues is decreased, and there is an erythropoietin-mediated stimulus to erythropoiesis. This disorder is manifested in the heterozygous state and follows an autosomal codominant pattern of inheritance. Hematocrit levels are rarely high enough to cause a significant increase in blood viscosity. Thus affected individuals are generally asymptomatic and lack any pertinent physical findings other than a ruddy complexion. The diagnosis should be suspected in all patients with unexplained erythrocytosis, particularly when other family members are similarly affected, and can be established by the demonstration of increased oxygen affinity of the whole blood. About two-thirds of the high-affinity variants can be readily separated from Hb A by electrophoresis. No treatment is indicated. The patient should be reassured that the disorder is benign.

Hemoglobin variants having a marked decrease in oxygen affinity cause one form of familial cyanosis (Table 306-3). Because of the abnormality of hemoglobin function, arterial blood is partially unsaturated despite normal oxygen tension. Thus the cyanosis is due to increased levels of deoxyhemoglobin in the blood. Except for this cosmetic problem, affected individuals have no other clinical manifestations. Blood values are otherwise normal.

METHEMOGLOBINEMIA

Oxygen transport depends on the maintenance of intracellular hemoglobin in the reduced (Fe^{2+}) state. When hemoglobin is oxidized to methemoglobin, the heme iron becomes Fe^{3+} and is now incapable of binding oxygen. Normal red cells contain less than 1 percent methemoglobin. A small amount of hemoglobin autoxidizes as red cells circulate. This process probably occurs by the dissociation of the superoxide anion from oxyhemoglobin:

$$Hb^{2+}O_2 \rightarrow Hb^{3+} + O_2^-$$

Normally, the methemoglobin that is formed is reduced by the following reaction:

$$Hb^{3+} + RedCyt\ b_5 \rightarrow Hb^{2+} + OxCyt\ b_5$$

Reduced cytochrome b₅ (RedCyt b₅) is regenerated by the enzyme cytochrome b₅ reductase (methemoglobin reductase):

$$OxCyt\ b_5 + NADH \xrightarrow[\text{reductase}]{\text{Cytochrome b}_5} RedCyt\ b_5 + NAD$$

Hereditary methemoglobinemia is due either to the presence of one of the M hemoglobins (see below) or to the deficiency of the enzyme cytochrome b₅ reductase (Table 306-3). These inherited disorders are clinically mild, while the induction of methemoglobinemia by drugs or toxins can be life-threatening.

If methemoglobin exceeds 15 g/L (1.5 g/dL) (10 percent of the total hemoglobin), affected individuals will have clinically obvious cyanosis. The color of the skin is indistinguishable from the much

more common cyanosis due to impairment of oxygen saturation that may occur in pulmonary and cardiac disorders (see Table 306-3). With higher amounts of methemoglobin, patients become symptomatic. At a methemoglobin level of about 35 percent, the affected individual experiences headache, weakness, and breathlessness. Levels in excess of 80 percent are usually incompatible with life.

The toxicity of methemoglobinemia can be readily explained in terms of hemoglobin function. The fact that a certain proportion of the heme moieties is no longer able to bind oxygen is not a serious physiologic handicap per se. A proportion of 30 percent methemoglobin is much more deleterious than a 30 percent decrement in red cell mass, because the oxidized hemes have a marked effect on the remaining functional hemes in the hemoglobin tetramer. The conformation of methemoglobin (like that of carboxyhemoglobin) is very similar to that of oxyhemoglobin. Thus a partially oxidized hemoglobin tetramer has the same tertiary and quaternary structures as a molecule that is comparably oxygenated. In each case, the affinity of the remaining hemes for oxygen is increased. For this reason, methemoglobinemia [as well as carbon monoxide (Chap. 395)] causes a "shift to the left" of the oxyhemoglobin dissociation curve and, consequently, impaired unloading of oxygen to tissues.

CYTOCHROME b₅ REDUCTASE (METHEMOGLOBIN REDUCTASE) DEFICIENCY   This condition is inherited in an autosomal recessive pattern. The enzyme is a flavoprotein having properties similar to those of liver microsomal cytochrome b₅ reductase. The soluble erythrocyte enzyme is formed by cleavage of a hydrophobic tail from the microsomal enzyme.

Individuals with cytochrome b₅ reductase deficiency have lifelong cyanosis of variable degree, depending on the level of methemoglobin, but usually have no associated symptoms or other physical findings. Some may have mild polycythemia owing to increased oxygen affinity. Others have been noted to be mentally retarded. Untreated individuals usually have 15 to 30 percent methemoglobin. Methemoglobin levels are higher in the older population of red cells because the activity of the abnormal enzyme declines markedly with red cell age. There appears to be considerable heterogeneity in the variant enzymes from different families, as shown by differences in their electrophoretic mobility and kinetic parameters. In these ways, cytochrome b₅ reductase deficiency resembles glucose-6-phosphate dehydrogenase deficiency (Chap. 307).

ACQUIRED METHEMOGLOBINEMIA   This disorder is generally due to exposure to certain drugs or toxins. Compounds which can cause clinically significant methemoglobinemia are listed in Table 306-3. Some agents such as nitrite and chlorate oxidize the heme iron directly. Others such as sulfa drugs and aniline must undergo biochemical transformation before they cause methemoglobinemia. Few drugs currently in use cause significant methemoglobinemia, unless the individual is unusually susceptible. Exposure to local anesthetics such as procaine and to nitroprusside occasionally causes severe methemoglobinemia. As might be expected, individuals heterozygous for methemoglobin reductase deficiency are much more likely than normal individuals to develop clinically apparent methemoglobinemia after exposure to an oxidant stress. Thus the extent of methemoglobinemia depends not only on the dose of the toxic agent but also on the susceptibility of the exposed individual.

M HEMOGLOBINS   Five hemoglobin variants have abnormal absorbance spectra, owing to the oxidation of the heme iron in the affected subunit. They involve substitutions of amino acid residues responsible for the binding of the heme iron to the globin. These so-called M hemoglobins (Table 306-3) result in a rare form of congenital and familial cyanosis. Individuals with the α-chain variants Hb M Boston and Hb M Iwate are cyanotic at birth, while cyanosis does not appear in those with the β-chain variants (Hb M Saskatoon, Hb M Hyde Park, and Hb M Milwaukee) until about 4 to 6 months of age, when fetal hemoglobin has been replaced by adult hemoglobin. As with the unstable and high-affinity variants, an autosomal codominant inheritance pattern is found. Except for cyanosis, patients are asymptomatic.

DIAGNOSIS Methemoglobinemia should be considered in any cyanotic patient with no evidence of heart or lung disease. If the cyanosis is due to decreased oxygen saturation, a blood specimen will change from a purple to a red color upon mixing with air. In contrast, a blood specimen from a methemoglobinemic individual remains a chocolate brown color irrespective of exposure to air. Methemoglobinemia can be documented by spectroscopic examination of the hemolysate. Individuals with hereditary methemoglobinemia will have lower levels than patients symptomatic from acquired methemoglobinemia. Patients who have ingested an oxidant drug may have an additional hemoglobin derivative called *sulfhemoglobin* in which the protoporphyrin has been chemically modified. Sulfhemoglobinemia tends to cause cyanosis even more readily than methemoglobinemia. Unlike methemoglobin, the absorbance of sulfhemoglobin at 620 to 630 nm is not decreased by the addition of cyanide. The M hemoglobins have characteristic spectral abnormalities which differ from those obtained when normal Hb A is partially oxidized. Furthermore, these hemoglobin variants can be detected by hemoglobin electrophoresis.

TREATMENT In individuals with methemoglobin reductase deficiency, the oral administration of methylene blue (100 to 300 mg/d) or ascorbic acid (300 to 500 mg/d) will result in a marked reduction in the level of methemoglobin. The purpose of treatment is primarily cosmetic. Severe toxic methemoglobinemia is treated by the intravenous administration of methylene blue (2 mg/kg; repeat if needed). Within an hour, the methemoglobin level is usually reduced by at least 50 percent. Treatment is neither possible nor necessary in individuals having Hb M.

THALASSEMIAS

The thalassemias are a diverse group of congenital disorders in which there is a defect in the synthesis of one (or more) of the subunits of hemoglobin. As a result of decreased production of hemoglobin, the red blood cells are microcytic and hypochromic (see Table 56-2). The thalassemias involve a spectrum ranging from subtle morphologic abnormalities to life-threatening disease. In contrast to the qualitative hemoglobin abnormalities listed in Table 306-1, the thalassemias are quantitative abnormalities of subunit synthesis. Thus the β chains of patients with β thalassemia have normal structure but are produced in reduced and sometimes undetectable amounts. Conversely, patients with α thalassemia have impaired production of α chains. The reduction in globin chain synthesis can be demonstrated in vitro by incubating reticulocytes with labeled amino acids and determining the incorporation of radioactivity into globin subunits (Table 306-4). Most forms of thalassemia can be identified from the information summarized in Table 306-4. Establishing a definitive diagnosis requires analysis of globin gene structure.

α THALASSEMIA As mentioned at the beginning of this chapter, normal individuals inherit two α-chain genes from each parent. The great majority of cases of α thalassemia can be explained by deletions of α-chain genes owing to nonhomologous crossover (see Fig. 306-1). Specific gene deletions can be identified by analysis of patients' DNA following digestion by restriction endonucleases. The clinical manifestations of α thalassemia depend on the number of genes deleted (see Table 306-4). In the silent carrier state, heterozygous α thalassemia 2 (α−/αα), one of the four genes is deleted. Affected individuals have no hematologic abnormalities. Individuals with deletion of two of the four α-chain genes (α-thalassemia trait) have either homozygous α thalassemia 2 (α−/α−) or heterozygous α thalassemia 1 (−−/αα). They have microcytic and slightly hypochromic red blood cells but no significant hemolysis or anemia. Hemoglobin electrophoresis is normal except for a decreased amount of Hb A$_2$. Deletion of three α-chain genes (−−/α−) produces a well-compensated hemolytic state with microcytic hypochromic red blood cells including many target cells. Intracellular inclusions or Heinz bodies are formed by the precipitation of Hb H, a tetramer composed of β chains which accumulates because of the marked impairment of α-chain synthesis. The most severe form of α thalassemia, hydrops fetalis, is usually due to deletion of all four α-chain genes. The affected fetus has red blood cells containing only Hb Barts, a tetramer composed of γ chains. This condition is incompatible with life, since oxygen transport depends on the presence of heterotetramers such as α$_2$β$_2$ and α$_2$γ$_2$. In Southeast Asians, both the α− and the −− haplotypes are relatively common; thus both Hb H disease and hydrops fetalis are frequently encountered. In contrast, blacks and individuals from the Mediterranean and the Middle East commonly have the α− haplotype (gene frequency in blacks ≅ 0.15) but rarely have the −− haplotype. Therefore, Hb H disease is uncommon among them, and hydrops fetalis is extremely rare. Homozygous α thalassemia 2 is encountered in about 2 percent of blacks and is therefore a relatively common cause of microcytosis in an individual who is otherwise healthy and not iron-deficient.

The elongated α-chain variant Hb Constant Spring, often encountered among Southeast Asians, also has an α-thalassemia phenotype and, when inherited with the −− haplotype, can cause Hb H disease.

β THALASSEMIA Since individuals inherit only one β-chain gene from each parent, affected individuals are either heterozygotes, homozygotes, or compound heterozygotes. The gene frequency for β thalassemia approaches 0.1 in southern Italy and certain Mediterranean islands. β Thalassemia is also encountered quite commonly in central Africa, the Middle East, Southeast Asia, including certain parts of India, and the south Pacific. Statistically, one-quarter of the offspring of two heterozygotes (β-thalassemia trait) will have the homozygous state: β thalassemia major or Cooley's anemia. An individual may inherit a β-thalassemia gene from one parent and a β-chain structural variant from the other. Sickle β

TABLE 306-4 Classification of the thalassemias

Diagnosis	Globin chain synthesis in reticulocytes	RBC morphology	Hb electrophoresis	Clinical severity
α Thalassemia:	α/β*			
Silent carrier (α−/αα)	0.9	Normal	Normal, ↓ Hb A$_2$	0
α-thalassemia trait [(α−/α−) or (−−/αα)]	0.7	↓ MCV† ↓ MCV	Normal, ↓ Hb A$_2$	0
Hb H disease (−−/α−)	0.3	Heinz bodies, targets	↑ Hb H (β$_4$) (10–15%)	2+
Hydrops fetalis (−−/−−)	0	↑↑ Nucleated RBC	↑↑ Hb Barts (γ$_4$)	4+
β Thalassemia:	β/α*			
Heterozygous	0.5	↓ MCV, stippling ↓ MCV, hypochromic	↑ Hb A$_2$ (± ↑ Hb F)	0 to +
Homozygous (or compound heterozygous)	0–0.3	Nucleated RBC, targets bizarre shapes	↑↑ Hb F	4+ (major) 2–3+ (intermedia)

* Normal = 1.
† MCV = mean corpuscular volume.

thalassemia (discussed above) is a commonly encou
of such a compound heterozygous state.

The molecular pathogenesis of the β thalassemias is
and heterogeneous than that of α thalassemia. In
thalassemia, gene deletion is an uncommon cause of
Among the recognized types of β-gene deletion, an e
"hereditary persistence of fetal hemoglobin" has m
manifestations owing to efficient synthesis of γ
chromosome in which the β and δ genes are delete
majority of cases of β thalassemia, restriction endor
reveal no gross abnormalities of the β-globin gene comp
less, there are several steps in β-globin synthesis that
and lead to a thalassemic phenotype. A number of
mutations in or near one of the intervening sequences o
gene, leading to errors in the splicing of mRNA. Ofte
made but in reduced amounts (β+ thalassemia) (se
Other cases have nonsense mutations in the coding re
premature termination of β-globin chains. This is the
cause of β⁰ thalassemia (Fig. 306-1).

Cellular pathogenesis As a result of imbalance i
synthesis, the β thalassemias have varying degrees
erythropoiesis (see Chap. 302) and hemolysis. In β thal
there is a marked relative excess of α-chain production.
have decreased solubility and will form insoluble
inclusions within red blood cell precursors in the bone
congenital Heinz body hemolytic anemia due to unstab
variants, the inclusion bodies in thalassemia bring about
in membrane permeability as well as entrapment and
red blood cells by the macrophages in the mononucle
system. As a result, β thalassemia is characterized by bo
lary erythroid destruction and a shortening of the
circulating red blood cells that emerge from the bone
these patients have the characteristic parameters of bo
erythropoiesis (increased plasma iron turnover, decrease
tion of iron into red blood cells) and peripheral hemoly
these red blood cells are under double jeopardy, there is
compensatory stimulus to erythropoiesis, resulting both
of the red marrow and in extramedullary hematopoiesi
and spleen. Chain imbalance in β thalassemia is atte
variable degree by the "compensatory" synthesis of γ
are able to combine with excess free α chains and f
tetramer (Hb F). Patients with β thalassemia major
relatively high rate of γ-chain production have a less se
course. Individuals with β thalassemia minor have ab
mild ineffective erythropoiesis and hemolysis, detecta
patients by a slight elevation in fecal urobilinogen an
shortening of the red blood cell life span.

β Thalassemia minor This common entity, also re
β-thalassemia trait, is rarely associated with signific
manifestations. The diagnosis is generally made in pa
evaluated for mild anemia or in follow-up of abnormaliti
routine blood studies. Most individuals with β-thalassemia
diagnosis. About one-fifth of affected individuals ha
splenomegaly. Icterus is occasionally noted, particular
individuals who also have Gilbert's disease, another c
benign congenital disorder (see Chap. 265).

In otherwise healthy individuals with β-thalassemia tra
hemoglobin level is about 15 percent lower than in nor
of the same age and sex; the red blood cell count is usua
and the cells are microcytic. Indeed, at any level of
patients with β thalassemia minor have more marked m
than those with iron deficiency. In contrast, the mean
hemoglobin concentration is normal. In addition to m
examination of the blood film reveals occasional target
shaped cells, and a moderate amount of basophilic sti
reticulocyte count is normal. Special isotope techniques a
to demonstrate a slightly reduced red blood cell life spa
blood cells have decreased osmotic fragility. Serum iro

red cells. In this chapter we will describe the
of this important group of anemias, the diagnostic
in identifying the causes of the accelerated red
and the pathogenesis and management of specific
ers.

ents with hemolytic anemia, the diagnosis can be
careful history and physical examination. The patient
of fatigue and other symptoms of anemia (see
commonly, jaundice and even red-brown urine
are reported. A complete drug history is often
nily history is especially helpful in the diagnosis of
molytic anemia. The patient's physical examination
useful information. Icterus and splenomegaly are
variety of hemolytic anemias. As discussed in detail
a wide array of other historical and physical findings
th specific hemolytic anemias.
ests may be used initially to demonstrate the presence
Table 307-1) and then to demonstrate the cause of
ration of the reticulocyte count in the anemic patient
st useful indicator of hemolysis, reflecting erythroid
the bone marrow. Accordingly, biopsy of the bone
n unnecessary. Reticulocytes are also elevated in
tive blood loss, those with myelophthisis, and those
ering from suppression of erythropoiesis (see Chap.

logy of the red cells as seen on the peripheral blood
normal and may provide evidence both of hemolysis
the characteristic abnormalities and their associated
dromes are listed in Table 307-2. While in no case
al blood smear be totally diagnostic by itself, in many
w-cost, important clue to the presence of hemolysis
s.

ells may be lysed by their removal from the circulation
particularly those of the spleen and liver (extravascu-
ss commonly by disruption of the membrane during
(intravascular hemolysis). In intravascular hemolysis,
hemoglobin may result in hemoglobinuria. Both
sult in increased heme catabolism and enhanced
tetrapyrrole unconjugated bilirubin, which is normally
the liver by conjugation and subsequent excretion.
above, the plasma level of unconjugated bilirubin
enough to produce readily apparent jaundice. The
indirect) bilirubin level can be further elevated by a
countered defect in transport of bilirubin (Gilbert's

Laboratory evaluation of hemolysis

	Moderate hemolysis (RBC life span 20–40 days)	Severe hemolysis (RBC life span 5–20 days)
lm nt amination	Polychromatophilia ↑ Erythroid hyperplasia	Polychromatophilia ↑ Erythroid hyperplasia
SERUM		
	↑ Unconjugated ↓, absent	↑ Unconjugated Absent
bin	↑	↑↑
genase	↑ (variable)	↑↑ (variable)
	0	0
	0, +	+
	0	+ *

molysis.

ic anemias

d blood   } **Hereditary**

es
brane
ytosis
al

} **Acquired**

c.

There are four types
membrane: hereditary
ary pyropoikilocytosis,
y of information has
hisms underlying these

iduals have congenital
roteins in the red cell
ce area to volume and
n autosomal dominant
imately 1:4500. In 20
logic abnormalities in
ssive inheritance or a
es clinically apparent
il adult life.

cal features of heredi-
and jaundice. The
ts prior designation
increased concentra-
in plasma. Jaundice
d in early childhood.
ction, gallstones of
Compensatory nor-
s with the extension
nd occasionally with
to the formation of
Because the bone
y six- to eightfold
e, anemia is usually
otherwise healthy
rrupted by episodes
articularly parvovi-
reditary spherocyto-
y during systemic
ment. Chronic leg
ell anemia, occur

e spherocyte (Fig.
usually normal or
oglobin concentra-
eroidicity may be
lity (Fig. 307-1).
per unit volume,
ions of low salt

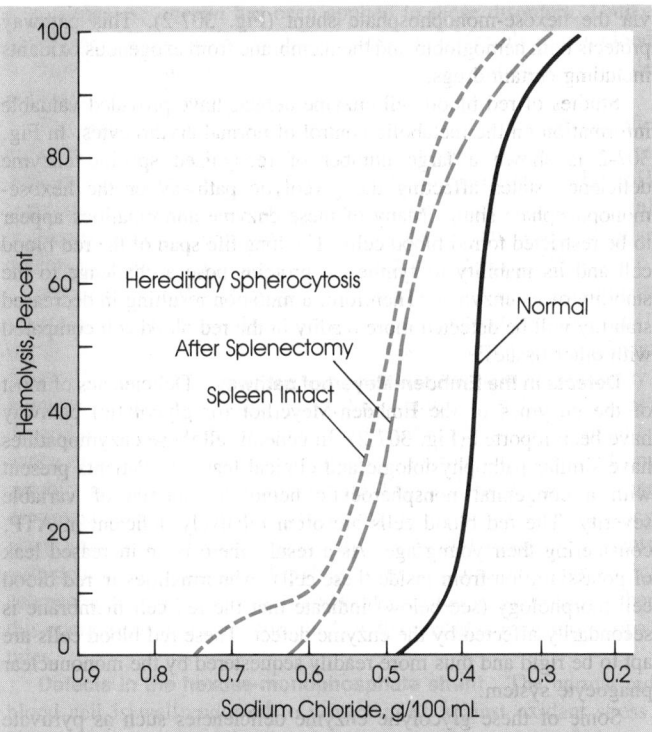

FIGURE 307-1 Osmotic fragility of red blood cells in hereditary spherocytosis. When the spleen is present, a small subpopulation of cells which are "conditioned" in the spleen form the fragile "tail" of the osmotic fragility curve. After splenectomy a single population exists which is more osmotically fragile than normal.

concentration. On microscopic examination, spherocytes are usually detected even when present in very small numbers. However, they will ordinarily not influence the osmotic fragility test unless they constitute more than 1 or 2 percent of the total cell population. A prominent increase in the osmotic fragility of red blood cells following sterile incubation of whole blood for 24 h at 37°C is also characteristic of hereditary spherocytosis. The autohemolysis test is an extension of this latter procedure and measures the amount of spontaneous hemolysis occurring after 48 h of sterile incubation. In hereditary spherocytosis, about 10 to 50 percent of the red blood cells are lysed (versus less than 4 percent of normal red blood cells). Autohemolysis of these red blood cells is largely prevented by the addition of glucose prior to incubation.

PATHOGENESIS The molecular abnormality in hereditary spherocytosis involves the proteins of the cytoskeleton. Nearly all patients have a significant deficiency of spectrin which is often secondary to the inherited molecular defect and correlates with the severity of the anemia. Many patients have a decrease and/or a structural abnormality in ankyrin, the protein that links spectrin to protein 3 (see Fig. 302-6). Other molecular defects include decreased production of spectrin and impaired assembly of spectrin with protein 4.1. The spheroidal contour and rigid structure of the red blood cells impede their passage through the spleen. There, the red blood cells are exposed to an environment in which their increased metabolic rate cannot be sustained. The first injury imposed on them by the spleen is a further loss of surface membrane. This "conditioning" produces a subpopulation of hyperspheroidal red blood cells in the peripheral blood. These are subsequently destroyed in the spleen.

DIAGNOSIS Hereditary spherocytosis must be distinguished from the spherocytic hemolytic anemias associated with red blood cell antibodies. The family history is helpful, when present. The diagnosis of immune spherocytosis is usually readily established by a positive direct Coombs test. Spherocytes, often in considerable numbers, are seen in association with hemolysis induced by splenomegaly in

patients with cirrhosis or chronic infections, and a few spherocytes are seen in the course of a wide variety of hemolytic disorders, particularly glucose-6-phosphate dehydrogenase (G6PD) deficiency.

TREATMENT AND PROGNOSIS Splenectomy reliably corrects the anemia, although the red blood cell defect persists. The operative risk is low. Red blood cell survival after splenectomy is normal or nearly so. Rare relapses have been reported and are probably attributable to postoperative growth of splenic autotransplants or to hyperplasia of secondary spleens which were overlooked at operation. Because of the potential for gallstones and for episodes of bone marrow hypoplasia or hemolytic crises, splenectomy should be performed in individuals in whom the disease causes symptoms. Splenectomy in children should be postponed until age 4, if possible. Beyond age 3, severe infections following splenectomy in hereditary spherocytosis are rare. Nonetheless, polyvalent pneumococcal vaccine should be administered to all patients who are to undergo splenectomy. Because of the increased requirement for folic acid in patients with hemolysis, they sometimes become deficient in this vitamin. Therapy with folic acid may result in an increased hemoglobin level.

Hereditary elliptocytosis and hereditary pyropoikilocytosis Red blood cells of oval or elliptic shape are normally found in birds, reptiles, camels, and llamas; however, they occur in appreciable numbers in humans only in *hereditary elliptocytosis*, a disorder which is transmitted as an autosomal dominant and affects 1 per 4000 to 5000 of the population, a frequency similar to that of hereditary spherocytosis. In most affected individuals, a structural abnormality of erythrocyte spectrin leads to impaired assembly. Others often have a deficiency of erythrocyte membrane protein 4.1, which is important in stabilizing the interaction of spectrin and actin in the cytoskeleton (see Fig. 302-6). Homozygotes with total absence of this protein have more marked hemolysis. In Southeast Asia there is a high incidence of hereditary ovalocytosis, in which a partial deletion of protein 3 confers resistance against malaria.

The great majority of patients manifest only mild hemolysis, with hemoglobin levels above 120 g/L, reticulocytes less than 4 percent, depressed haptoglobin levels, and red blood cell survivals just under the normal range. In 10 to 15 percent of patients, the rate of hemolysis is substantially increased, with chromium half-survival times of red blood cells as short as 5 days and reticulocytes ranging to 20 percent. Hemoglobin levels rarely fall below 90 to 100 g/L. Red blood cell destruction occurs predominantly in the spleen, which is enlarged in patients with overt hemolysis, and hemolysis is corrected by splenectomy.

In both the anemic and nonanemic varieties of this disorder the red blood cells are normochromic and normocytic. At least 25 percent and, more commonly, greater than 75 percent of red blood cells are elliptic, with an axial ratio (width/length) of less than 0.78. Patients with hemolysis frequently have microovalocytes, bizarre-shaped red blood cells, and red cell fragments, all of which increase in number following splenectomy. The degree of hemolysis does not correlate with the percentage of elliptocytes. Osmotic fragility is usually normal but may be increased in patients with overt hemolysis.

Hereditary pyropoikilocytosis (HPP) is related to hereditary elliptocytosis, since both have been encountered in the same family. HPP is a rare disorder characterized by bizarre-shaped, microcytic red cells which undergo disruption at temperatures of 44 to 45°C (in contrast to the normal thermal instability at 49°C). This results from an abnormality of spectrin self-assembly. Hemolysis, which is usually severe, is recognized in childhood and is partially responsive to splenectomy.

Hereditary stomatocytosis Stomatocytes are red blood cells having a slitlike central zone of pallor on dried smears. The syndrome of hereditary hemolytic anemia and stomatocytic red blood cells is inherited in an autosomal dominant pattern. Two major red blood cell defects have been delineated in this syndrome. First, the red blood cells have an increased permeability to sodium and potassium, which is compensated for by an increased active transport of these cations. Second, red cells have an increased surface area associated with an develops a severe hemolytic episode with hemoglobinuria, maintaining adequate urine output is important.

Attention should be directed toward the *prevention* of hemolytic episodes. Infections ought to be treated promptly. Subjects deficient in G6PD should be warned about risks posed by oxidant drugs and fava beans. Any black patient about to be given an oxidant drug should be screened for G6PD deficiency.

OTHER DEFECTS OF THE HEXOSE-MONOPHOSPHATE SHUNT   A few kindreds have been found to have congenital deficiency in red blood cell glutathione due to a defect in either of the two enzymes responsible for the synthesis of this tripeptide. Affected individuals have a hemolytic anemia with Heinz bodies that is aggravated by oxidant drugs. Deficiency of glutathione reductase has been reported, but its relationship to clinically significant hemolysis is not well established. Sometimes the deficiency state can be corrected by the administration of riboflavin (5 mg/d). There are also isolated reports of deficiencies of glutathione peroxidase and 6-phosphogluconate dehydrogenase, but again, their association with hemolysis is uncertain.

Other enzyme defects   Hemolytic anemia may sometimes be caused by abnormalities in enzymes of nucleotide metabolism. A growing number of individuals with pyrimidine 5'-nucleotidase deficiency have been encountered. Their red cells have marked basophilic stippling. Hemolytic anemia also has been noted in individuals whose red blood cells have supranormal levels of adenosine deaminase and relatively low levels of ATP.

HEMOGLOBINOPATHIES   The sickling disorders constitute an important form of congenital hemolytic anemia. Less commonly, hemolysis may be due to the inheritance of an unstable hemoglobin variant. These disorders of hemoglobin are discussed in Chap. 306.

ACQUIRED HEMOLYTIC ANEMIAS

In patients with acquired hemolytic anemia, red cells are made normally but are prematurely destroyed because of damage acquired in the circulation; the single exception is rare disorders characterized by acquired dysplasia of the cells of the bone marrow and the production of structurally and functionally abnormal red cells. The damage that occurs may be mediated by antibodies or toxins that mark the cell for premature death or may be due to vicissitudes encountered during the circulation, including an overactive reticuloendothelial system or traumatic lysis by natural or artificial impediments to smooth circulation.

SPLENOMEGALY AND HYPERSPLENISM   The spleen is particularly efficient in trapping and destroying red blood cells which have minimal defects, often so mild as to be undetectable by in vitro techniques. This unique ability of the spleen to filter mildly damaged red blood cells results from its unusual vascular anatomy. Almost all the blood circulating through the spleen flows rapidly from arterioles in the white pulp to sinuses in the spleen's red pulp and then into the venous system. In contrast, a small portion of splenic blood flow (normally 1 to 2 percent) leaves the arterioles of the white pulp to enter a nonendothelial portion of the spleen. In this sense, it is extravascular, although the entire spleen may be considered as a specialized part of the vascular system. This blood passes into the "marginal zone" of the lymphatic white pulp. Although the cells which occupy this zone are not phagocytic, they serve as a mechanical filter that hinders the progress of severely damaged blood cells. As red blood cells leave this zone and enter the red pulp, they flow into narrow cords which end blindly but which communicate with sinuses through small openings between the lining cells of the sinuses. These openings, averaging 3 μm in diameter, test the ability of red blood cells to undergo a deformation of shape. Red blood cells which do not pass the stringent test imposed on them by the spleen filter are engulfed by phagocytic cells and destroyed.

The normal spleen poses no threat to normal red blood cells until they become senescent. However, splenomegaly exaggerates the adverse conditions to which red blood cells are exposed. Splenic

enlargement may be considered in three broad categories. In the first are infiltrative diseases (such as myeloproliferative disorders; Chap. 309), lymphomas (Chap. 311), and storage diseases such as Gaucher's disease; (Chap. 349). In the second are systemic inflammatory diseases leading to splenic hypertrophy. In the third are diseases which cause congestive splenomegaly, particularly cirrhosis of the liver and thrombosis of the splenic, portal, or hepatic veins. Hemolysis may occur whenever the spleen is enlarged. Its occurrence is least predictable in infiltrative diseases of the spleen, where substantial splenomegaly may exist with no apparent hemolysis. Inflammatory and congestive splenomegaly is commonly associated with mild to moderate shortening of red blood cell survival, along with granulocytopenia and thrombocytopenia (hypersplenism). Patients with cytopenia(s) sufficient to produce symptoms generally benefit from splenectomy.

IMMUNOLOGIC CAUSES OF HEMOLYSIS   Immune hemolysis in the adult may be induced by three general types of antibodies:

1 Alloantibodies acquired by blood transfusions or pregnancies and directed against transfused red blood cells (Chap. 312).
2 Antibodies (usually IgG) reactive at body temperature and directed against the patient's own red blood cells (Table 307-5).
3 Antibodies (usually IgM) reactive in cold and directed against the patient's own red blood cells (Table 307-5).

The Coombs antiglobulin test is the major tool for diagnosing these disorders. This test relies on the ability of antibodies prepared in animals or by hybridomas and directed against specific human serum proteins to agglutinate red blood cells if these human serum proteins are present on the red blood cell surface. The serum proteins of particular interest are IgG and C3. The ability of anti-IgG or anti-C3 antisera to agglutinate the patient's red blood cells is referred to as the *direct Coombs test*. The presence or absence of IgG or C3 may give important information about the origin of the immune hemolytic anemia (see Table 307-5). Rarely, neither IgG nor complement may be found on the red cells of the patient (Coombs-negative immune hemolytic anemia).

At times, it may be important to demonstrate antibody in the serum of the patient by reacting the serum with normal red cells. IgM antibodies (usually cold-reacting) may be detected by agglutination of normal or fetal red cells. IgG antibodies may be directed by the *indirect Coombs test*, in which the serum of the patient is incubated with normal red cells and antibody is detected with anti-IgG as in the direct Coombs test.

"Warm" antibodies   Antibodies that react with protein antigens usually are IgG and react at body temperature; occasionally, they are IgA. This acquired syndrome is frequently designated *autoimmune hemolytic anemia, warm antibody type*. In recent years, as a number of drugs which induce this clinical syndrome have become recognized, attention has focused on the exogenous factors which may underlie the formation of these red blood cell antibodies, and the expression *immunohemolytic anemia* is preferred.

Clinical manifestations   Immunohemolytic anemia induced by warm-reacting IgG antibody occurs at all ages but is more common

TABLE 307-5   Use of the direct Coombs test in diagnosing the cause of autoimmune hemolytic anemia

Reaction with:		
Anti-IgG	Anti-C3	Causes
Yes	No	Antibodies to Rh protein, hemolysis caused by α-methyldopa or penicillin; not seen in SLE
Yes	No	Antibodies to glycoprotein antigens, SLE
No	Yes	Cold-reacting antibodies (agglutinins or Donath-Landsteiner antibody), most drug-related antibodies, IgM antibodies, IgG antibodies of low affinity, activation of complement by immune complexes

in adults, particularly women and older individuals. In approximately one-fourth of patients this disorder occurs as a complication of an underlying disease affecting the immune system, especially chronic lymphocytic leukemia, non-Hodgkin's lymphoma, and systemic lupus erythematosus (SLE) (Table 307-6). Occasionally, immunohemolytic anemia is seen in patients with advanced, active Hodgkin's disease. Case reports link it to a variety of nonlymphoid neoplasms.

The presentation and course of IgG immunohemolytic anemia are quite variable. In its mildest form, the only manifestation is a positive direct Coombs test. In this instance, insufficient antibody is present on the red blood cell surface to permit the reticuloendothelial system to recognize the cell as abnormal. This is particularly common in SLE. A large fraction of patients with immunohemolytic anemia have a chronic mild anemia and splenomegaly. In other cases this disorder may be more severe, with hemoglobin levels less than 70 g/L and reticulocyte counts of 30 percent and higher. Spherocytosis is usually marked (Fig. A9-11). Both the direct and indirect Coombs tests may be positive. In its most severe form, immunohemolytic anemia presents with fulminant, overwhelming hemolysis associated with hemoglobinemia, hemoglobinuria, and shock, a syndrome which may be fatal.

Associated findings include hyperbilirubinemia, decreased or absent haptoglobin levels, splenomegaly, and occasionally hepatomegaly. Thrombocytopenia also may be present. The coexistence of immune destruction of red blood cells and platelets is referred to as *Evans' syndrome*, a disorder in which separate antibodies are directed against platelets and red blood cells. Occasionally, venous thrombosis occurs.

Pathogenesis IgG antibodies bring about the destruction of the cells by two mechanisms: (1) immune adherence of red cells to destructive cells of the immune system mediated by the antibody itself and by complement components that become fixed to the membrane and (2) completion of the complement sequence, resulting in rupture of the membrane. In IgG-mediated immune adherence, the affixed antibody reacts with Fc receptors on macrophages; this binds the target to the destroyer and activates phagocytic processes that internalize the target, destroying it. Complement-mediated immune adherence is mediated by C3b and C4b interacting with a series of receptors on the macrophage; this is much less likely to lead to destruction of the target by itself but markedly increases the immune adherence due to IgG. Immune adherence is also enhanced by the peculiar circulation of the spleen, which brings cells into intimate contact with phagocytic cells. If internalization is only partial, membrane is preferentially removed; this results in the formation of spherocytes. These spherocytes are not able to pass through the fenestrations in the wall of the splenic sinus and thus accumulate in the spleen, where they are destroyed.

TABLE 307-6 Hemolysis due to antibodies

WARM-ANTIBODY IMMUNOHEMOLYTIC ANEMIA

A Idiopathic
B Lymphomas: Chronic lymphocytic leukemia, non-Hodgkin's lymphomas, Hodgkin's disease (infrequent)
C Systemic lupus erythematosus and other collagen-vascular diseases
D Drugs
   1 α-Methyldopa type
   2 Penicillin type (stable hapten)
   3 Quinidine type (unstable hapten)
E Post-viral infections
F Other tumors (rare)

COLD-ANTIBODY IMMUNOHEMOLYTIC ANEMIA

A Cold agglutinin disease
   1 Acute: *Mycoplasma* infection, infectious mononucleosis
   2 Chronic: Idiopathic, lymphoma
B Paroxysmal cold hemoglobinuria

Lysis by the direct lytic action of complement does not commonly occur because the mechanisms for the down-regulation of its activation are so effective that insufficient sequences are completed to breach the cell membrane.

Therapy and prognosis In the initial evaluation of the patient, it is important to be sure that drugs which are known to cause immunohemolytic anemia are not involved. This topic is discussed below.

Patients having a mild degree of hemolysis usually do not require therapy. In those with clinically significant hemolysis, initial therapy consists of glucocorticoids (e.g., prednisone, 1.0 mg/kg per day). A rise in hemoglobin is frequently noted within 3 or 4 days and occurs in most patients within 1 week. Prednisone is continued until the hemoglobin level has risen to normal values, and thereafter it is tapered slowly over the course of several months. More than 75 percent of patients will achieve an initial significant and sustained reduction in hemolysis; however, in half these patients the disease will relapse either during the period of steroid tapering or following the cessation of steroid therapy. Steroids appear to have two modes of action: an immediate effect due to inhibition of the clearance of IgG-coated red blood cells by the mononuclear phagocyte system and a later effect due to steroid-induced inhibition of antibody synthesis.

Patients with severe anemia may require blood transfusions. Because the antibody in this disease is a "panagglutinin," reacting with nearly all normal donor cells, the usual cross matching is impossible. The goal in selecting blood for transfusion is to avoid administering red cells with antigens to which patients have previously been sensitized and which are known to be associated with complement lysis and intravascular hemolysis. In addition to A and B, Kell, Kidd (Jk^a), and Duffy (Fy) account for almost all examples of this type of hemolysis. A common procedure is to adsorb the panagglutinin present in patient's serum using the patient's own red cells from which antibody has been eluted previously. Serum freed of autoantibody in this way can then be tested for the presence of alloantibody to specific donor blood groups. ABO-compatible red cells matched in this fashion are administered slowly, with attention paid to the possibility of an immediate-type transfusion reaction.

Splenectomy is the second line of therapy in immune hemolytic anemia due to IgG. It is recommended for patients who cannot tolerate or fail to respond to steroid therapy. To provide prophylaxis against pneumococcal infection, a risk in splenectomized individuals, patients should be immunized with polyvalent pneumococcal antiserum.

Patients who have been refractory to steroid therapy and to splenectomy have been treated with immunosuppressive drugs. The greatest experience is with azathioprine and cyclophosphamide. A variable success rate has been reported with each. Intravenous gamma globulin may be used when rapid cessation of hemolysis is required. However, it is not nearly as effective in this disorder as it is in immune thrombocytopenia.

In the majority of patients, this disease is controlled by steroid therapy alone, by splenectomy, or by a combination. In most of the remaining patients, a partial degree of control is achieved. Fatalities occur among three categories: (1) rare patients with overwhelming hemolysis in whom death is directly attributable to anemia, (2) those with major thrombotic events coincident with active hemolysis, and (3) those whose host defenses are impaired by glucocorticoids, splenectomy, and/or immunosuppressives. In patients in whom immunohemolysis develops as a complication of an underlying disorder, the prognosis is dominated by that of the primary disease.

Immunohemolytic anemia secondary to drugs Drugs which have been directly implicated in immunohemolytic anemia are of two kinds, as distinguished by their mechanisms of action: (1) drugs, such as α-methyldopa, an antihypertensive (Chap. 209), that induce a disorder identical almost in every respect to the warm-antibody immunohemolytic anemia described above, and (2) drugs that can become associated with the red blood cell surface and induce the formation of an antibody directed against the red blood cell–drug complex. The association of drug and glycoprotein may be relatively tight, as in the case of penicillin, or relatively loose, as in the case of quinidine.

A positive direct Coombs test is observed in up to 10 percent of patients receiving α-methyldopa therapy in a dose of 2.0 g/d. A small minority of these patients develop spherocytosis and hemolysis, often of severe degree. This "autoimmune" disorder is probably due to the fact that α-methyldopa alters the protein(s) bearing the Rh antigens so that the drug becomes immunogenic; the resulting antibodies cross-react with the normal Rh protein. Thus the antibody does not react with the drug, and the indirect Coombs test is positive even when the drug is not added to the test. Two distinctive features are that the indirect Coombs test is positive in almost all patients with hemolysis and that the red cells are coated with IgG but not C3. Hemolysis decreases over the course of several weeks after cessation of drug therapy, although the direct Coombs test may remain positive for more than 1 year.

In most other cases when a drug induces an immune hemolytic reaction, the antibody is directed against the combination of the drug and the membrane glycoprotein to which it is attached. Therefore, the indirect Coombs test is not positive unless the drug is added to reaction mixture. Further, the hemolytic reaction in vivo is also dependent on the presence of the drug and usually ceases shortly after the drug has been discontinued. Penicillin and its congeners may cause this type of reaction if the drug is given in very high doses (10 million units per day or more). The drug adheres relatively firmly to the glycoprotein of the red cell membrane. The hemolysis in vivo is usually not severe. Since the antibody is usually IgG, spherocytosis and splenic destruction may occur. Most other drugs do not adhere as tightly to their glycoprotein, and they and the antibodies that they have generated are removed during the washing steps of the Coombs reaction. Most of these antibodies are able to fix complement (especially those which are IgM), and these components remain on the red cell surface; thus the direct Coombs test is positive with anti-C3 but not anti-IgG. Again, the antibody is detected in the *indirect* Coombs test only when the drug is added to the incubation mixture. Hemolysis may be quite severe, sometimes resulting in signs of intravascular hemolysis; resolution is usually prompt after the drug is discontinued. In addition to quinine and quinidine, a number of drugs, including sulfonamides, sulfonureas, phenacetin, stibophen, and dipyrone, have been shown to cause this reaction.

Immune hemolysis due to cold-reactive antibodies Antibodies that react with polysaccharide antigens are usually IgM and react better at lower temperatures, hence the name *cold-reactive antibodies*. The clinical manifestations associated with IgM antibodies (the more common cold agglutinins) differ from those associated with IgG antibodies, the relatively uncommon Donath-Landsteiner antibody of paroxysmal cold hemoglobinuria.

Cold agglutinins arise in two clinical settings: (1) monoclonal antibodies as the product of lymphocytic neoplasia and (2) polyclonal antibodies in a response to infection. In many elderly patients, the "neoplasm" is benign monoclonal gammopathy, and although chronic, it does not progress and the protein product remains its only manifestation. In a few patients, the lymphoma may be aggressive. Occasionally, cold agglutinins are found in patients with nonlymphocytic neoplasms.

Transient cold agglutinins occur commonly in two infections: *Mycoplasma pneumoniae* infection and infectious mononucleosis. In both, the titer of antibody is usually too low to cause clinical symptoms, but its presence is of diagnostic value; only occasionally is hemolysis present. Cold agglutinins are less frequently encountered in a number of other viral infections. Their manifestations are usually benign.

The specificity of the antibody may be of diagnostic value. Cold agglutinins reacting more strongly with adult cells than fetal (cord) cells are called *anti-I*; these antibodies are seen in benign lymphoproliferation (chronic cold agglutinin monoclonal gammopathy) and in *Mycoplasma* infections. Those reacting more strongly with cord cells are called *anti-i*; these antibodies are seen in aggressive lymphomas

and in infectious mononucleosis. Rarely, the antibody may react with other antigens that are equally expressed on adult and cord cells.

The clinical manifestations elicited by the antibody are of two sorts: acrocyanosis and hemolysis. Acrocyanosis is the marked purpling of the extremities, ears, and nose when the blood becomes cold enough to agglutinate in the veins; it clears on warming and does not have the vasospastic characteristics of Raynaud's phenomenon (see Chap. 211).

The hemolysis is usually not severe and is manifest by a mild reticulocytosis, agglutination on the blood film, and agglutination during analysis of the blood by particle analysis (giving rise to a falsely high mean corpuscular volume). The degree of hemolysis depends on several variables.

1 *Antibody titer.* In general, the titer in symptomatic patients is above 1:2000 dilution of serum and may range to as high as 1:50,000. When collecting samples for testing the titer, great care must be taken that the serum is separated from the cells while maintaining the sample at 37°C so that the antibody will not adsorb onto the patient's own cells.
2 *Thermal amplitude of the antibody* (the highest temperature at which the antibody will react with the red cell). For most antibodies, this is 23 to 30°C. Those with a higher thermal amplitude (up to 37°C) will be more hemolytic, since it is more likely that these temperatures will be reached during the circulation of the cells.
3 *Environmental temperature.* Since the reaction can only occur at temperatures below body temperature, frequency and degree of exposure to cold are major determinants of the rate of hemolysis.

The hemolysis that occurs is due primarily to the hemolytic action of complement, since there are no functional Fc receptors for the IgM antibody. Complement is readily fixed, since a single molecule of antibody is enough to effect binding of C1 and initiate the sequence of reactions. However, the normal human red cell is remarkably resistant to the hemolytic action of complement because of several defense mechanisms. Therefore, severe hemolysis with hemoglobinuria will occur only with massive activation of the antibody, such as by sudden chilling. The activation of complement is always marked by the accumulation of a degradation product of C3, C3dg, on the surface; this is what is detected with appropriate antisera in the direct Coombs test in all patients with significant cold agglutinin disease.

THERAPY The cutaneous manifestations of this disorder are best treated by maintaining the patient in a warm environment. Because transfusion of normal blood presents to the patient a large number of red blood cells which have not been exposed previously to the cold agglutinin and are therefore not "protected," transfusion may be associated with an acceleration of the hemolytic process. Splenectomy is usually not of value in this disorder. Glucocorticoids are of limited value, although patients with the panthermal variety of cold agglutinin disease may respond favorably to this therapy. Chlorambucil and cyclophosphamide are the most commonly employed agents in those patients in whom therapy is indicated. Although some patients have experienced a dramatic improvement, the effectiveness of this therapy is usually marginal.

Cold agglutinin disease tends to be chronic and unremitting. The overall prognosis is dominated by the underlying lymphoproliferative disease, if present. In those patients in whom cold agglutinin disease appears to arise spontaneously, lymphoproliferative disease may become apparent after several years.

Paroxysmal cold hemoglobinuria (PCH) Now a rare disorder, PCH was more frequent at a time when tertiary syphilis was more prevalent. It results from the formation of the Donath-Landsteiner antibody, an IgG antibody which is directed against the P antigen complex and which can induce complement-mediated lysis. Attacks are precipitated by exposure to cold and are associated with hemoglobinemia and hemoglobinuria; chills and fever; back, leg, and abdominal pain; headache; and malaise. Recovery from the acute episode is prompt, and between episodes patients are asymptomatic. When this syndrome accompanies acute viral infections (e.g., measles and

TABLE 307-7 Disturbances of the formed elements of blood secondary to intravascular trauma

Etiology	Fragments	Hemolysis	Thrombo-cytopenia
Impact: march hemoglo-binuria, etc.	0	+	0
Cardiac (turbulence):			
Aortic valve prosthesis	+ + + +	+ + + +	0
Mitral valve prosthesis	+ +	+ +	0
Calcific aortic stenoses	+	±	0
Vessel disease*	+ + +	+	+
Thrombotic thrombo-cytopenic purpura	+ + + +	+ + + +	+ + + +
Hemolytic uremic syndrome	+ + + +	+ + + +	+ + + +
Adenocarcinoma	+ + + +	+ + + +	+ + + +
Disseminated intravas-cular coagulation	+ +	±	+ + + +

* Malignant hypertension, eclampsia, renal graft rejection, hemangiomas, immune disease (scleroderma).

mumps), it is self-limited. Although the direct Coombs test may show complement to be present (seldom IgG), this test may be completely negative. The diagnosis is made by demonstrating cold-reacting IgG antibodies either by lytic tests (when the titer is very high) or by special antiglobulin tests. When PCH is secondary to syphilis, it responds favorably to specific therapy for this disorder. Chronic autoimmune PCH may respond to prednisone or cytotoxic therapy (azathioprine or cyclophosphamide) but does not respond to splenectomy. Despite the severity of individual episodes, the natural history of this disease extends over many years.

TRAUMA IN THE CIRCULATION Mechanical trauma can cause hemolysis in three ways: (1) when red blood cells flow through small vessels over the surface of bony prominences and are subject to external impact during various physical activities, (2) when they flow across a pressure gradient created by an abnormal heart valve or valve prosthesis and are disrupted by a shear stress, and (3) when the deposition of fibrin in the microvasculature exposes them to a physical impediment that fragments them (Table 307-7).

External impact Hemoglobinemia and hemoglobinuria have been observed in individuals who have undergone a prolonged march or a prolonged jog, most typically on a hard surface and while wearing thin-soled shoes. The role of direct external trauma in this process has been demonstrated by the fact that hemolysis can be prevented by the insertion of a soft inner sole in the runner's shoes. Similar types of hemolysis have been described following karate and the playing of bongo drums. No abnormality of red blood cell morphology has been demonstrated, even during the acute episode, and no underlying red blood cell abnormality has been uncovered. A large percentage of individuals will develop hemoglobinemia and hemoglobinuria when exposed to the conditions described above. As a result of muscle damage during some of these activities, myoglobinuria also may occur, but renal function is preserved. No specific therapy is required.

Cardiac hemolysis Hemolysis associated with fragmented red blood cells (Fig. A9-7) occurs in approximately 10 percent of patients with artificial aortic valve prostheses. This incidence is somewhat greater with valves having stellite rather than Silastic occluders, greater with small valves as compared with larger valves, and greater when valves are cloth-covered or when there is a paravalvular leak. Traumatic hemolysis is much less common in recipients of porcine valves. Severe hemolysis may occur after repair of ostium primum or endocardial cushion defects with a prosthetic patch. Mitral valve prostheses also have been associated with hemolysis, but since the pressure gradient across these values is lower than across aortic prostheses, the incidence is lower. A moderately shortened red blood cell survival with little or no anemia occurs in some patients with severe calcific aortic stenosis. Indeed, almost any intracardiac lesion that alters hemodynamics may lead to some shortening of red blood

cell survival. In addition, traumatic hemolysis has been observed in patients who have undergone aortofemoral bypass.

CLINICAL MANIFESTATIONS In severe cases, hemoglobin levels fall to 50 to 70 g/L with reticulocytosis, fragmented red blood cells in the peripheral blood, depressed haptoglobin, elevated serum lactate dehydrogenase (LDH), and hemoglobinemia and hemoglobinuria. Iron loss (as hemoglobin or hemosiderin) in the urine may lead to iron deficiency. The direct Coombs test may rarely become positive.

PATHOGENESIS A number of factors combine to cause the fragmentation and destruction of red blood cells in this disorder. Direct mechanical trauma of red blood cells at the time of seating of the occluder of the prosthetic valve, the deposition of fibrin across disrupted attachment points, and, probably most important, the shear stress resulting from turbulent blood flow may all result in the fragmentation of red blood cells. The turbulence explains the higher incidence of hemolysis in patients who have a paravalvular leak and therefore greater velocity of blood flow across the aortic orifice during systole.

THERAPY AND PROGNOSIS Iron deficiency should be corrected by the administration of oral iron. The elevated hemoglobin which results may permit a decrease in the cardiac output and a slowing of the hemolytic rate. Limitation in physical activity also lessens the hemolytic rate. When these measures fail, any paravalvular leak must be repaired or the prosthetic valve replaced.

Deposition of fibrin in the microvasculature Fibrin deposition in the microvasculature fragments red blood cells and traps platelets under three general conditions: (1) abnormalities of the vessel wall in recognized disorders, such as malignant hypertension, eclampsia, rejection of a renal allograft, disseminated cancer, and hemangiomas, (2) two potentially fatal syndromes of unknown etiology, thrombotic thrombocytopenic purpura and the hemolytic uremic syndrome, and (3) disseminated intravascular coagulation.

ABNORMALITIES OF THE VESSEL WALL The degree of hemolysis induced by this family of disorders is usually quite mild, although the number of fragments in the peripheral blood may be striking. In some patients, thrombocytopenia may be severe. In each case, therapy is best directed at the primary disease. Thus reversal of renal graft rejection, treatment of malignant hypertension and eclampsia, control of cancer, etc. lead to a cessation of the hemolytic process. The relative importance of the primary vascular abnormality and of the deposition of fibrin in causing hemolysis is unclear.

Thrombotic thrombocytopenic purpura (TTP) This disease of unknown etiology affects individuals of all ages but primarily young adults, more often women.

CLINICAL MANIFESTATIONS Hemolysis is a striking feature of this disease. Anemia occurs in association with fragmented red blood cells, nucleated red cells in the peripheral blood, an elevated reticulocyte count, and thrombocytopenia of varying degree. Platelet counts range from 5000 to 100,000 per cubic millimeter. Mild jaundice can occur, and petechiae may be present, although usually to a less striking degree than in idiopathic thrombocytopenic purpura (ITP). Typically, the LDH level is very elevated, indicating the intravascular hemolysis. Tests of coagulation, such as the prothrombin time, partial thromboplastin time, fibrinogen concentration, and the level of fibrinogen split products, are usually normal or only mildly abnormal. If the coagulation tests indicate a major consumption of procoagulants, the diagnosis of TTP is doubtful. Erythroid hyperplasia and an increased number of megakaryocytes are present in the bone marrow. A positive antinuclear antibody (ANA) determination is obtained in approximately 20 percent of patients. Some patients experience significant, although not severe, bleeding of uterine, gastrointestinal, or other origin. Fever is present in many patients, and many experience nonspecific constitutional symptoms such as nausea, abdominal pain, and arthralgias. The spleen and liver usually are not palpable.

The course of TTP spans days to weeks in most patients but occasionally continues for months. As the disease progresses, the brain and kidneys can become involved, and their dysfunction is the dyserythropoietic anemia which can be readily distinguished on clinical grounds. The sucrose lysis test, in which complement is activated by reduction of the ionic strength of the incubation medium, is more sensitive but less specific. The most sensitive and specific test is determination of the absence of the GPI-linked proteins on granulocytes and platelets by flow cytometry; this test is not generally available.

Treatment Transfusion therapy is useful in PNH not only for raising the hemoglobin level but also for suppressing the marrow production of red blood cells during episodes of sustained hemoglobinuria or of sustained painful crisis. Whole blood transfusions infrequently cause an exacerbation of the hemolytic process. This can be prevented by using washed red blood cells rather than whole blood.

Therapy with androgens frequently results in a rise in hemoglobin level. Adrenocortical steroids also may be effective in reducing the rate of hemolysis but should be given in moderate doses (25 to 30 mg prednisone) only on alternate days.

Because of iron loss in the urine, iron deficiency is common. An exacerbation of hemolysis often follows the administration of iron because of the formation of a large number of young red blood cells, many of which are sensitive to complement. This may be minimized by giving prednisone (60 mg/d) or by suppressing the bone marrow with transfusions.

Acute thrombosis in PNH, particularly the Budd-Chiari syndrome and cerebral thrombosis, should be treated aggressively with thrombolytic agents. Heparin therapy should be instituted rapidly and maintained for several days before changing to coumadin therapy.

Antithymocyte globulin (ATG) is often of use in treating marrow hypoplasia, as it is in the related disease, aplastic anemia. A total dose of 150 mg/kg is given over 4 to 10 days; large doses of prednisone are usually needed to counteract the immune-complex disease that results from the administration of this foreign protein.

In patients, especially the younger ones, with either hypoplasia or thrombosis who have an appropriate sibling donor, marrow transplantation should be considered early in the course of the disease. The usual conditioning programs are sufficient to eradicate the aberrant clone.

REFERENCES

Amidon TM et al: Mitral and aortic paravalvular leaks with hemolytic anemia. Am Heart J 125:266, 1993

Becker PS, Lux SE: Disorders of the red cell membrane, in *Hematology of Infancy and Childhood*, DG Nathan, FA Oski (eds). Philadelphia, Saunders, 1992

Beutler E: Study of glucose-6-phosphate dehydrogenase: History and molecular biology. Am J Hematol 42:53, 1993

Beutler E: Glucose-6-phosphate deficiency. N Engl J Med 329:169, 1991

Cooper RA: Hemolytic syndromes and red cell membrane abnormalities in liver disease. Semin Hematol 17:103, 1980

Hirono A et al: Enzymatic diagnosis in non-spherocytic hemolytic anemia. Medicine 67:110, 1988

Kelton JG et al: The platelet aggregating factors of thrombotic thrombocytopenic purpura. Prog Clin Biol Rev 337:141, 1990

Moake JL: The role of von Willebrand factor (vWF) in thrombotic thrombocytopenic purpura. Prog Clin Biol Rev 337:135, 1990

Palek J, Sahr SE: Mutations of the red blood cell membrane proteins: From clinical evaluation to detection of the underlying genetic defect. Blood 80:308, 1992

Rosse WF: Autoimmune hemolytic anemia. Hosp Prac 20:105, 1985

———: *Clinical Immunohematology*. Cambridge, Blackwell Scientific, 1989

Robson WL et al: Hemolytic-uremic syndrome. Curr Probl Pediatr 23:16, 1993

Thompson CE: Thrombotic microangiopathies in the 1980s: Clinical features. Blood 80:1890, 1992

308 BONE MARROW FAILURE: APLASTIC ANEMIA AND OTHER PRIMARY BONE MARROW DISORDERS

JOEL M. RAPPEPORT / H. FRANKLIN BUNN

An important group of anemias is caused by primary disorders of the bone marrow in which the formation of erythropoietic precursors is impaired. The term *aplastic anemia* should be restricted to conditions in which a markedly hypocellular bone marrow results in pancytopenia (anemia, neutropenia, and thrombocytopenia). Rare patients develop selective aplasia of only erythroid cells (*pure red cell aplasia*). Alternatively, in *myelophthisic anemia*, erythropoiesis is suppressed because the marrow is infiltrated with tumor, granulomas, or fibrosis. The dysmyelopoietic or myelodysplastic anemias are associated with variable neutropenia and thrombocytopenia resulting from an acquired disorder of the hematopoietic pluripotent stem cell.

APLASTIC ANEMIA

ETIOLOGY Aplastic anemia is thought to be due to injury or destruction of a common pluripotential stem cell affecting all subsequent cell populations. Table 308-1 classifies aplastic anemia by cause. In approximately half the cases of aplastic anemia in the United States, no cause can be identified. In areas of the world where a larger percentage of the population may be exposed to toxins such as insecticides and benzenes in uncontrolled dose, the percentage of idiopathic cases is smaller. In some cases, disordered hematopoiesis results from an abnormal stem cell clone. In others, a damaged marrow microenvironment may contribute to marrow failure. In a substantial subset of patients, immune mechanisms appear to contribute to the pathogenesis of aplasia.

Congenital causes Fanconi's anemia, the most common type of constitutional aplastic anemia, is an autosomal recessively inherited disease usually appearing in childhood. This disorder is often associated with multiple congenital anomalies, including short stature, renal malformations, hyperpigmentation of the skin, and bony abnormalities, particularly hypoplastic or absent thumbs or radii. Most patients

TABLE 308-1 Causes of pancytopenia

Aplastic anemia
A Idiopathic anemias
B Constitutional anemias (Fanconi's anemia)
C Chemical and physical agents
  1 Dose-related: benzene, ionizing irradiation, alkylating agents, antimetabolites (folic acid antagonists, purine and pyrimidine analogues), mitotic inhibitors, anthracyclines, inorganic arsenicals
  2 Idiosyncratic: chloramphenicol, phenylbutazone, sulfa drugs, methylphenylethylhydantoin, gold compounds, organic arsenicals, insecticides
D Immunologically mediated aplasia
E Other associations: hepatitis, other viral infections, systemic lupus erythematosus, diffuse eosinophilic fasciitis, transfusion-associated graft-versus-host disease, pregnancy

Pancytopenia with normal or increased bone marrow cellularity
A Myelodysplastic syndromes
B Hypersplenism (Chap. 58)
C Vitamin B_{12} and folate deficiencies (Chap. 304)
D AIDS (Chap. 279)

Paroxysmal nocturnal hemoglobinuria (Chap. 307)

Bone marrow replacement
A Hematologic malignancies (Chaps. 151, 310, 311)
B Nonhematologic metastatic tumor
C Storage cell disorders (Chap. 349)
D Osteopetrosis (Chap. 362)
E Myelofibrosis (Chap. 309)

have chromosomal abnormalities owing to defective DNA repair. Patients who survive the complications of progressive marrow failure are at high risk of developing leukemia or other malignancies. Other congenital disorders have been associated with bone marrow failure, including dyskeratosis congenita.

Immune causes   A number of clinical observations have led to the concept that a significant proportion of cases of aplastic anemia may be mediated by immunologic mechanisms. These include recovery following immunosuppressive preparation for autologous marrow grafting and, in some patients, the necessity of immunosuppression for hematopoietic reconstitution following marrow transplantation from identical twin donors. A variety of in vitro culture techniques also have supported a humoral or cellular immune process in some patients with aplasia. However, in any given case, the identification of an immune mechanism may be difficult.

Drugs and toxins   Multiple and seemingly unrelated drugs and chemical agents have been incriminated as causes of aplastic anemia. The association varies from a predictable dose-related aplasia to idiosyncratic reactions unrelated to dose.

Agents which in an adequate dose will predictably produce bone marrow depression include the antineoplastic and immunosuppressive drugs along with ionizing radiation. These drugs include folic acid antagonists, alkylating agents, the anthracyclines, and the nitrosoureas, as well as purine and pyrimidine analogues. The degree of aplasia is dose related but may vary from individual to individual. The effects of combination chemotherapy may be additive. Withdrawal of the drug usually permits recovery of the marrow elements, although aplasia is occasionally irreversible. Marrow aplasia also may be induced by x-ray therapy, by chronic low-dose x-ray exposure, or, less commonly, by acute exposure from a laboratory or industrial accident. The severity of aplasia is dependent on the dose and rate of the exposure as well as the extent of marrow irradiated.

Benzene derivatives and other hydrocarbons have been associated with multiple hematologic abnormalities, including aplastic anemia. Benzene-induced aplasia may result from both industrial and domestic use of benzene-containing products. This aplasia may be reversible, although mild abnormalities such as macrocytosis may persist.

Chloramphenicol, a broad-spectrum antibiotic, is associated with two forms of bone marrow toxicity. The more common effect on the bone marrow is a reversible dose-related suppression of erythroid and, on occasion, granulocytic and megakaryocytic precursors. This condition is characterized by a transient anemia, associated with a drop in reticulocytes and elevation of serum iron. This bone marrow suppression is related to the dose and duration of administration of chloramphenicol. The bone marrow reveals vacuoles in the cytoplasm of early erythroid and granulocytic precursors. Similar morphologic features are seen much more commonly in patients who have ingested large amounts of alcohol.

The more serious form of bone marrow failure associated with chloramphenicol is an ''idiosyncratic'' reaction. This nitrobenzene compound has been the single most commonly incriminated drug in cases of aplastic anemia. These patients develop severe pancytopenia and often irreversible, fatal marrow aplasia. This complication is estimated to occur in approximately 1 in 50,000 patients who take the drug. The development of aplastic anemia seems to be unrelated to dose or duration of administration. Marrow aplasia cannot be anticipated or prevented by hematologic monitoring, since it may appear after cessation of the drug. Unfortunately, many cases of fatal aplastic anemia have occurred in patients who received chloramphenicol for trivial or dubious reasons. Therefore, this antibiotic should not be used when there are reasonable alternatives.

Other unrelated chemicals and drugs may be responsible for the development of aplastic anemia. These agents can be placed into two classes: those in which a number of associations have been reported and, therefore, a definite toxic potential has been established, and those in which only a few reported cases exist and, therefore, only a possibility of toxic potential exists at present. The establishment of these relationships is often confounded by the fact that many of the

patients have taken multiple drugs. Agents in which a definite potential toxicity exists are shown in Table 308-1.

Infections   A number of cases of aplastic anemia have been reported following infectious hepatitis. The antecedent hepatitis is not distinguished by its severity, and the aplastic anemia commonly appears as the hepatitis resolves. Aplasia has usually followed non-A, non-B hepatitis, including hepatitis C, but on occasion has been associated with types A and B. The aplasia tends to be severe and frequently has a fatal outcome. Other viruses, including Epstein-Barr virus, have been implicated in aplastic anemia. Many cases of so-called idiopathic aplastic anemia are preceded by a benign-appearing viral respiratory illness. Parvovirus selectively infects erythroblasts and therefore acutely aggravates anemia in patients with hemolysis (Chap. 307).

Some patients infected with human immunodeficiency virus will develop pancytopenia and a hypoplastic bone marrow. Contributing factors include direct suppression of hematopoietic cells by the virus, opportunistic infections such as cytomegalovirus or *Mycobacterium avium intracellulare*, and myelotoxic drugs such as trimethoprim-sulfamethoxazole and azidothymidine.

Aplastic anemia also has been reported in association with a number of other illnesses (see Table 308-1). The clinical and laboratory findings associated with paroxysmal nocturnal hemoglobinuria may accompany or precede the development of aplasia. Aplastic anemia that develops during pregnancy may remit following delivery of the fetus.

CLINICAL MANIFESTATIONS   The onset of aplastic anemia is usually insidious. Initial presenting symptoms include mild progressive weakness and fatigue attributable to the anemia and/or hemorrhage from the skin, nose, gums, vagina, or gastrointestinal tract due to the thrombocytopenia. The bleeding is usually mild, but occasionally retinal or central nervous system hemorrhage may be the initial mode of presentation. Although the patient may be severely neutropenic, it is less common for the initial presentation to be a bacterial infection.

Physical examination generally reveals pallor. Petechiae or ecchymoses may be noted in the skin, mucous membranes, conjunctivae, and fundi. Lymphadenopathy and hepatosplenomegaly are notably absent. Fever may be present, but despite the presence of an infection, the usual signs of inflammation may be absent because of neutropenia.

The *course* of the disease is generally determined by the severity of the aplasia, rather than by the etiology. Mild disease can progress to a more severe disorder. Conversely, complete recovery or partial recovery of one or more cell lines may develop. It is important to obtain an accurate assessment of the degree of aplasia. *Severe aplasia* is defined as marked pancytopenia with at least two of the following criteria: granulocytes fewer than 500 per microliter, platelets fewer than 20,000 per microliter, or anemia with corrected reticulocyte count less than 1 percent. The bone marrow is markedly hypoplastic and depleted of hematopoietic cells. Patients with severe disease have a high risk of dying from bleeding and/or infections in a matter of months, while patients with a milder form of the disease may live for years. The clinical course of the disease is affected primarily by infections and by the nature and location of bleeding. Although infections may not dominate the clinical picture initially, they assume greater importance with the passage of time. Because of the need for multiple red blood cell and platelet transfusions, over a period of time one may encounter the sequelae of hemosiderosis and/or hepatitis. Even those patients who recover may have mild thrombocytopenia and persistent macrocytosis for many years. Long-term survivors are at increased risk of developing acute leukemia, the myelodysplastic syndrome, or paroxysmal nocturnal hemoglobinuria.

LABORATORY DIAGNOSIS   The diagnosis of aplastic anemia and the assessment of its relative severity depend on a thorough laboratory evaluation. The peripheral blood usually shows pancytopenia. The absolute granulocyte count is low or becomes progressively depressed during the illness. The red blood cells are normochromic and usually somewhat macrocytic, reflecting stress erythropoiesis, and the corrected reticulocyte count is inappropriately low. Since serious bleeding and/or infection correlates with the degree of thrombocytopenia or neutropenia, these values must be determined initially and followed serially. A bone marrow aspirate may yield a "dry tap," but a bone marrow biopsy will reveal a severely hypocellular or aplastic marrow with replacement by fat. There is usually a severe depression of megakaryocytes and myeloid cells and a marked but relatively less severe depression of the erythroid precursors.

Elevated serum iron level coupled with a normal level of transferrin results in elevated transferrin saturation. Because of the reduction in erythroid precursors, plasma iron clearance is prolonged, and incorporation of iron into red blood cells is markedly decreased. There is no evidence of increased red blood cell destruction.

DIFFERENTIAL DIAGNOSIS The diagnosis of aplastic anemia implies the exclusion of the other causes of pancytopenia that are listed in Table 308-1. Splenomegaly and/or lymphadenopathy argue strongly against aplastic anemia. Malignant and nonmalignant invasion of the bone marrow must be excluded by microscopic examination of the marrow. Paroxysmal nocturnal hemoglobinuria and systemic lupus erythematosus should be ruled out by appropriate tests, including the sugar water and acid hemolysis tests. Vitamin B_{12} and folate deficiencies can be excluded by serum assays and morphologic changes. Pancytopenia rarely may be secondary to various infections, including AIDS. Before aplastic anemia can be classified as idiopathic, a careful history must exclude exposure to all known and suspected agents. In our complex society, all patients are exposed to potentially toxic agents in the environment. Nevertheless, this difficulty should not discourage a careful and extensive search for a cause.

TREATMENT The management of aplastic anemia has become one of the most challenging aspects of modern medicine, requiring a diligent multidisciplinary team of caregivers in a well-equipped tertiary care center. For patients with mild aplasia, every effort should be made to do as little as possible except to remove possible etiologic agents in expectation of spontaneous recovery. As noted below, androgens may be of value in mild aplasia. Patients with severe aplasia should be considered for an immediate bone marrow transplantation, if a suitable donor is available. As discussed in detail in Chap. 313, the great majority of patients who undergo marrow transplantation have complete correction of the hematopoietic defect.

Supportive care Regardless of the therapy chosen, the mainstay of treatment is good supportive care. The first and most immediate step is the removal of any suspected cause. If the disease is mild at presentation, no further supportive care need be instituted, unless there is subsequent deterioration. If a severe neutropenia exists (polymorphonuclear leukocytes fewer than 500 per microliter), the patient should be shielded from potential infections. Prophylactic systemic antibiotics should not be utilized. Intramuscular injections should be avoided. Established infections should be treated vigorously with specific antibiotics, and fever of undetermined etiology may, after appropriate bacteriologic evaluation, call for broad-spectrum antibiotic coverage until a specific diagnosis is established. Menstruating females should be placed on suppressive doses of birth control pills.

Transfusions Blood products should be used *judiciously* and restricted to appropriate component therapy, since future therapy and ultimate survival may be affected by transfusions. Red blood cells should be administered to maintain the well-being of the patient rather than to establish a certain hemoglobin level. Transfusions pose significant risks, such as development of hepatitis or hemosiderosis, as well as sensitization to both red blood cell antigens and transplantation antigens. Platelet transfusions should be administered in the face of serious hemorrhage. Some groups employ prophylactic transfusions when the platelet count is lower than 20,000 per microliter. Others, fearful of the development of resistance to future transfusions, administer platelets only when faced with hemorrhage. Responses to platelet transfusions may be blunted by the presence of infection. If a patient develops immune resistance to platelet transfusions, HLA-compatible platelet transfusions may be useful (Chap. 312). Should

a bone marrow transplant be considered, family members should be avoided as a source of blood products, since the patient may develop antibodies to minor transplantation antigens. Leukocyte transfusions are not administered prophylactically. However, white blood cell infusions may be of value in patients with documented gram-negative infections and severe neutropenia who have failed to respond to antimicrobial therapy.

Marrow-stimulating agents Although patients with mild aplasia sometimes respond to androgens, and a few appear to be androgen-dependent, those with severe aplasia are usually unresponsive. Patients with mild aplasia should be treated with adequate doses of androgens as the initial mode of therapy. The most widely used drugs at present are oxymetholone, fluoxymesterone, and nandrolone decanoate. Responses may occur as long as 3 to 6 months after the initiation of therapy. The administration of recombinant hematopoietic growth factors, either alone or in combination, is under active investigation. To date, granulocyte-macrophage colony stimulating factor is somewhat effective in boosting neutrophil, eosinophil, and monocyte counts but has little effect on platelets or red cell production.

Immunosuppressive agents Increasing clinical and laboratory evidence suggests that 40 to 50 percent of patients will have a complete or, more likely, partial response to a variety of immunosuppressive agents. The specificity and mechanism of this therapy are as yet undefined. The most commonly administered therapy is animal antisera directed against human lymphocytes and thymocytes. The effectiveness, as well as the dose and duration of administration, of these heterogeneous sera is variable from batch to batch. Serious side effects may accompany the administration of these heteroantisera. Very high doses of glucocorticoids or the immunosuppressive agent cyclosporine may yield similar responses.

In general, splenectomy has no role in the management of aplastic anemia.

Bone marrow transplantation (See Chap. 313)

OTHER PRIMARY BONE MARROW DISORDERS

PURE RED CELL APLASIA Pure red cell aplasia involves a selective failure in the production of erythroid elements in the bone marrow. Granulopoiesis and megakaryocytopoiesis remain normal. Patients have a normochromic, normocytic anemia with normal granulocyte count and platelet count. Severe reticulocytopenia exists, and the bone marrow is characterized by a virtual absence of any erythroid precursors in the face of otherwise normal cellular elements. An increase in lymphocytes may be seen in the marrow.

Constitutional red cell aplasia Blackfan-Diamond syndrome, a rare chronic constitutional red blood cell aplasia, may appear in infants from the time of birth to the age of 2 years. Twenty-five percent of patients have minor congenital anomalies. The disorder is of unknown etiology but has been corrected by both glucocorticoids and marrow transplantation.

Acquired red cell aplasia The rare acquired form of pure red cell aplasia is seen predominantly in middle-aged adults. About one-third of patients have thymomas. Five percent of all patients with thymomas have pure red cell aplasia. The association between thymoma and myasthenia gravis is somewhat stronger. In many patients, both with and without thymomas, erythropoiesis is inhibited by a complement-fixing IgG immunoglobulin which has selective cytotoxicity for marrow erythroblasts. A much smaller group of patients has been noted to have an inhibitor against erythropoietin. Occasionally, pure red cell aplasia is encountered in patients with T cell chronic lymphatic leukemia. The circulating T cells are distinguished by the presence of receptors for the Fc portion of IgG. Other disorders sometimes associated with pure red cell aplasia include acquired hypogammaglobulinemia, systemic lupus erythematosus, T-gamma lymphocytosis, and AIDS.

TREATMENT Since these patients have virtually no endogenous red blood cell production, they are totally dependent on red blood cell transfusion. If thymic enlargement is noted, a thymectomy may induce a remission in approximately 50 percent of patients. If the thymus is normal, thymectomy is of no benefit. Patients without thymoma or those with an unsuccessful thymectomy should receive glucocorticoids, alone or in combination with immunosuppressive agents such as cyclophosphamide, azathioprine, cyclosporine, or antithymocyte globulin. Treatment often results in both prolonged clinical remission and disappearance of the inhibitor.

MYELODYSPLASTIC SYNDROMES Also known as the *refractory dysmyelopoietic anemias*, these anemias are a heterogeneous group of normocytic anemias often associated with neutropenia, thrombocytopenia, and/or monocytosis. The bone marrow varies in cellularity and usually reveals disordered maturation of erythroid, myeloid, and megakaryocytic cells. In some patients, bilobed neutrophils (Pelger-Huet cells) can be detected on blood films. In others, erythroid cells accumulate large amounts of iron in mitochondria (ringed sideroblasts) (Chap. 303). The FAB (French, American, British) classification of the myelodysplastic syndrome includes five categories: refractory anemia (RA), refractory anemia with ringed sideroblasts (RARS), refractory anemia with excess of blasts (RAEB), chronic myelomonocytic leukemia (CMML), and refractory anemia with excess of blasts in transformation (RAEB-T). This intrinsic disorder of the hematopoietic pluripotential stem cell is most frequently noted in older people. Although the etiology of these disorders is unclear, some patients appear to develop the syndrome secondary to chemotherapy, particularly alkylating agents with or without accompanying radiation therapy. The most common cytogenetic abnormalities noted include the deletion of the long arm of chromosome 5 (5q−), deletion of chromosome 7 or 5 (−7, −5), or trisomy 8. Over time, a variety of additional cytogenetic changes may be observed. Survival is variable among the subtypes, with longer median survivals of 76 months noted in RARS and short median survivals of 3 to 6 months noted in RAEB-T. Patients frequently succumb to infections and hemorrhage because of the associated neutropenia and thrombocytopenia. These clonal disorders are frequently preleukemic, with subsequent conversion to frank leukemia in 5 to 20 percent of patients with RARS and greater than 50 percent of patients with RAEB-T.

The mainstay of treatment is supportive: appropriate transfusion therapy and antibiotics for febrile episodes. Occasional long-term survivors may require therapy for iron overload. Rarely, patients with sideroblastic anemia will respond to pyridoxine or pyridoxal phosphate. Although differentiation agents such as vitamin D, retinoic acid, and low-dose cytosine arabinoside are effective in vitro, their therapeutic efficacy has been disappointing. Bone marrow transplantation in the appropriate setting has been curative for the myelodysplastic syndromes, as it has for de novo leukemias. Stimulation of the bone marrow by a variety of agents has been studied. Androgen therapy has in some cases resulted in moderate improvement. Recombinant human hematopoietic growth factors, including GM-CSF (granulocyte-macrophage colony stimulating factor), G-CSF (granulocyte colony stimulating factor), IL-3 (interleukin 3), erythropoietin, and combinations thereof, are currently under investigation and offer the potential for stimulating blood cell production. Both their long-term therapeutic effect and the possibility of accelerating the development of leukemia are still to be determined. The treatment of leukemia evolving from the myelodysplastic syndrome is discussed in Chap. 310.

MYELOPHTHISIC ANEMIA Infiltration of the bone marrow with tumor, fibrosis, or granulomas can result in the development of a severe anemia. Tumor may be derived from cell lines indigenous to the bone marrow, as in leukemia, lymphoma, or myeloma, or the marrow may be invaded by metastatic deposits of solid tumor, usually carcinoma. Among the solid tumors most frequently associated with myelophthisic anemia are carcinoma of the breast, stomach, prostate, lung, and thyroid. Hepatomegaly and splenomegaly may develop in this setting, along with marrow fibrosis.

Fibrosis in the bone marrow, usually in association with myeloid metaplasia (see Chap. 309), can cause myelophthisic anemia. Granu-lomatous involvement of the bone marrow is usually due to advanced tuberculosis. Primary lipid storage disorders, such as Gaucher's disease and Niemann-Pick disease, occasionally produce a myelophthisic anemia, and the rare disorder osteopetrosis, or marble bone disease, also may give a similar hematologic picture.

The invasion of the bone marrow by tumor or granulomas impairs both erythropoiesis and thrombopoiesis. In contrast, neutrophil production is generally normal or increased. It is unlikely that the anemia and thrombocytopenia are due merely to "crowding" of the bone marrow space by extrinsic cells. Myelophthisis also causes a distortion of the microcirculation of the marrow, with premature release of immature cells.

Myelophthisis usually results in a severe normochromic, normocytic anemia. A variety of misshapen erythrocytes are noted, particularly teardrop cells and fragmented cells with some basophilic stippling. In addition, normoblasts are usually seen in the peripheral blood. The reticulocyte percentage is often slightly increased (3 to 6 percent). However, when corrected for the anemia and the premature release from the bone marrow, the absolute reticulocyte count is actually reduced and reflects a decrease in red blood cell production. While thrombocytopenia is usually present, the white blood cell count is often elevated, with a marked shift to the left in the differential count. The combination of immature myeloid cells and normoblasts in the peripheral blood constitutes the "leukoerythroblastic" morphology so characteristic of myelophthisic anemia. Striking abnormalities are usually seen on examination of the bone marrow. Often an aspirate yields a "dry tap" owing to the infiltration of the marrow with abnormal tissue, although, on occasion, tumor cells will be identified. Marrow biopsy is more likely to be diagnostic, revealing leukemia, lymphoma, or foci of metastatic tumor or granuloma. However, marrow involvement is often segmental, so the primary pathologic process may be missed on a single biopsy.

Treatment Treatment consists of attempts to reverse the primary pathologic process. It is particularly important to search for the presence of tuberculosis, since this disease is readily treatable. More often, however, the underlying disease is not amenable to therapy and requires supportive measures, such as blood transfusions.

REFERENCES

BACIGALUPO A et al: Bone marrow transplantation (BMT) versus immunosuppression for the treatment of severe aplastic amenia (SAA): A report of the EBMT SAA writing party. Br J Haematol 70:177, 1988

ESTEY EH: Prognosis and therapy of myelodysplastic syndromes. Cancer Treat Res 64:233, 1993

GORDON-SMITH EC: Fanconi anemia: Constitutional aplastic anemia. Semin Hematol 28(2):104, 1992

HAMBLIN T: Recent advances in the management of myelodysplastic syndromes. Hematol Oncol 11 (suppl I):27, 1993

NISSEN C: The pathophysiology of aplastic anemia. Semin Hematol 28(4):313, 1991

ROBINSON BE, QUESENBERY PJ: Hematopoietic growth factors: Overview and clinical applications. Am J Med Sci 300:163, 1990

ROSSE WF: Evolution of clinical understanding: Paroxysmal nocturnal hemoglobinuria as a paradigm. Am J Hematol 42:122, 1993

SPIVAK J: Pure red cell aplasia. Curr Issues Anemia 4(1): 2, 1992

STEWART FM: Hypoplastic/aplastic anemia: Role of bone marrow transplantation. Med Clin North Am 76(3):683, 1992

YOUNG N: The problem of clonality in aplastic anemia. Blood 79:1385, 1992

309 THE MYELOPROLIFERATIVE DISEASES

DAVID W. GOLDE / SUBHASH C. GULATI

DEFINITION The myeloproliferative diseases are a family of disorders characterized by increased blood cell production which arise in a clonal manner from abnormalities at the level of the hematopoietic stem cell. Specific syndromes in this family include chronic myelogenous leukemia (CML), polycythemia vera (PV), agnogenic myeloid metaplasia with myelofibrosis (MF, also called *idiopathic myelofibrosis*), and essential thrombocytosis (ET). While there is commonality in the pathologic and clinical manifestations, distinct transitions from one disease to another are unusual. The myeloproliferative disorders usually have a chronic course but also may transform to an aggressive phase or acute leukemia.

CHRONIC MYELOGENOUS LEUKEMIA (CML)

DEFINITION AND ETIOLOGY   CML is a clonal stem cell disorder characterized by markedly increased myelopoiesis and the presence of the Philadelphia (Ph) chromosome. The Philadelphia chromosome involves a translocation of the Abelson (*abl*) proto-oncogene on chromosome 9 to the breakpoint cluster region (*bcr*) of chromosome 22 with formation of a fusion gene called *bcr-abl*. CML is an acquired disorder. Although no specific etiologic agent has been identified, an increased incidence of CML was observed in survivors of the atomic bomb in Japan. The peak incidence of CML was seen 5 to 12 years after radiation exposure and appeared to be dose related.

PATHOPHYSIOLOGY   The Ph chromosome results from an exchange of DNA on the long arms of chromosomes 9 and 22 forming the translocation (9;22) (q34;q11). This rearrangement creates the *bcr-abl* fusion gene and leads to expression of a novel bcr-abl protein product (Fig. 309-1). The common translocations result in bcr-abl proteins of 210 (p210) and 190 (p190) kDa which differ in the amount of bcr amino acid residues included. The p190 protein is mainly associated with Ph-positive acute lymphoblastic leukemia (ALL), whereas p210 is found both in Ph-positive ALL and in CML. Retroviral constructs incorporating the p210 and p190 *bcr-abl* genes have been introduced into mouse bone marrow cells and transplanted into lethally irradiated mice. A variety of hematopoietic malignancies developed, including a CML-like disorder, lymphoblastic leukemia, histiocytosis, and erythroleukemia. Transgenic mice have been created where every cell had a p190 *bcr-abl* gene and the leukemias that developed were mainly of B lymphoblasts.

Transcription of the *bcr-abl* fusion gene results in a hybrid messenger RNA that is subsequently translated into a 210- or 190-kDa protein. The tyrosine kinase activity of the 190-kDa protein is greater than that of the 210-kDa protein, which, in turn, is greater than that of the normal 145-kDa c-*abl* gene product. It is likely that the bcr-abl protein provides a growth advantage to the CML cells by virtue of increased protein kinase activity which may amplify normal proliferative signals. Thus in CML there is expansion of committed myeloid precursor compartments associated with overproduction of mature myeloid elements. Genetic instability in the CML clone apparently leads to subsequent transformation into an acute leukemic phase with further chromosomal abnormalities, including a double Ph chromosome.

Using the polymerase chain reaction (PCR), minimal residual disease can be detected in CML by amplifying *bcr-abl* fusion RNA. Use of this technique also can confirm the diagnosis in patients who do not have a visible Ph chromosome. Rare patients with the CML syndrome have no Ph chromosome or evidence for the *bcr-abl* rearrangement. Even though Ph chromosome–containing cells predominate in the bone marrow in CML, normal stem cells remain but are suppressed by the Ph-positive clone. These normal diploid cells may be observed after long-term bone marrow culture in vitro and following treatment with interferon or high-dose chemotherapy.

SYMPTOMS AND SIGNS   The usual course of CML involves a chronic phase of variable duration, followed by blastic transformation, with some patients experiencing a distinct intermediate accelerated phase. Most patients are diagnosed in the chronic phase when an elevated white blood cell count is found in association with splenomegaly. At diagnosis, the white blood cell count can exceed 200,000 cells per microliter. Patients may present without symptoms after the incidental finding of an elevated white blood cell count or may complain of left upper quadrant discomfort from splenomegaly.

FIGURE 309-1   Formation of the Ph chromosome.

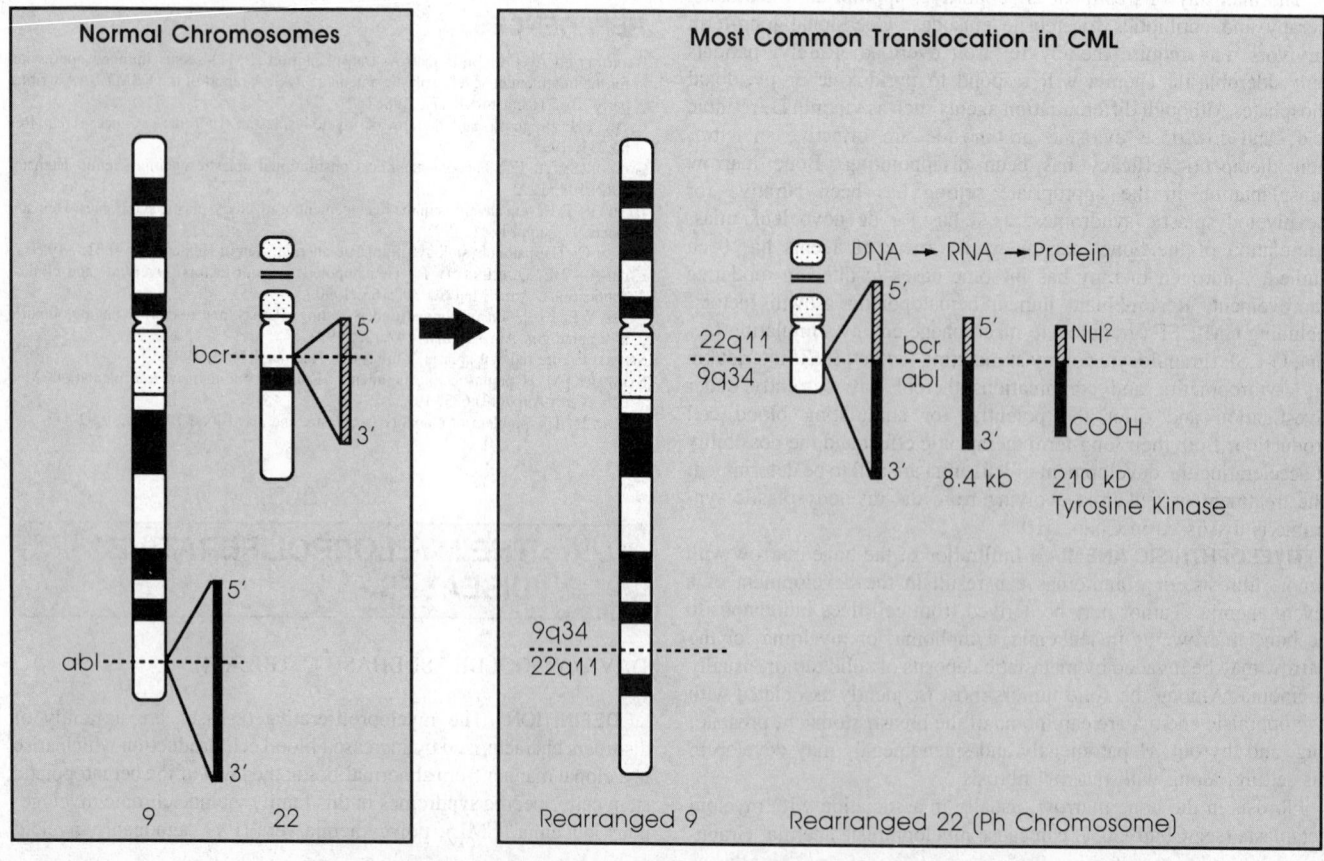

Other presenting symptoms relate to anemia or hypermetabolism with consequent weight loss, fatigue, fever, and elevated uric acid levels. The most consistent physical sign in CML is splenomegaly. An enlarged spleen is found in more than 90 percent of the patients. Hepatomegaly or, in rare instances, lymphadenopathy is observed and may suggest the transition to acute leukemia.

Bone pain and pain from splenic infarction are uncommon in the early stages of CML but are observed with disease progression. The accelerated phase is characterized by increasing resistance to therapy, progressive organomegaly, worsening anemia, thrombocytosis or thrombocytopenia, myelofibrosis, and fever. Blast crisis is associated with signs and symptoms of acute leukemia, often with extramedullary disease.

LABORATORY FINDINGS   Table 309-1 summarizes the distinguishing laboratory features of the myeloproliferative disorders. A white blood cell count over 100,000 cells per microliter is common at presentation in patients with CML, but with the increased use of laboratory screening, CML may be discovered at an early stage. The peripheral blood smear shows a marked increase in granulocytes with a left shift in differentiation, including increase in promyelocytes, myelocytes, and metamyelocytes. Eosinophilia and basophilia may be prominent. The neutrophil (leukocyte) alkaline phosphatase score is low or zero, in contrast to the high score seen in leukemoid reactions. Platelet function and morphology are usually normal in CML. A prominent elevation of serum vitamin B_{12} level, as well as an increased serum vitamin B_{12}–binding capacity, is noted because of increased granulocyte production of transcobalamin I.

A hemoglobin concentration of less than 11 g/dL is observed in one-third of the patients, and half of patients have a platelet count over 450,000 cells per microliter. The bone marrow is hypercellular with a marked increase in the myeloid-to-erythroid ratio. Occasionally, increased reticulin or collagen fibrosis is observed. In CML the marrow as well as the spleen may contain glycolipid-laden phagocytes, which resemble Gaucher cells or sea-blue histiocytes, due to the increased turnover of glucocerebrosides and sphingolipids. Hyperuricemia is often observed due to increased cell turnover in CML and can be exacerbated by cytotoxic treatment. The granulocytes in CML have near-normal phagocytic and bactericidal activity.

Features indicative of progression into blastic phase include bone lesions, pancytopenia, enlarging liver and spleen, and increase in the percentage of blasts in the bone marrow and blood. Blast crisis is usually of the myeloid type. About 30 percent of patients have lymphoblastic transformation, which needs to be distinguished from the myeloid blast crisis, since it is treated differently. Lymphoid characteristics include lymphoblast morphology, presence of the enzyme terminal deoxynucleotidyl transferase (TdT), and expression of the common acute lymphoblastic leukemia antigen (CALLA). Lymphoid transformation is associated with a lower-molecular-weight p190 *bcr-abl* translocation product. Blast crisis of erythroid, basophilic, and megakaryoblastic type is also seen.

DIAGNOSIS   The diagnosis of CML depends on the association of markedly increased myelopoiesis, splenomegaly, and the presence of the Ph chromosome. Examination of the peripheral blood smear and bone marrow usually leads to accurate diagnosis in the proper clinical setting. Cytogenetic studies are confirmatory. In some patients with the CML syndrome, the Ph chromosome is not observed. In 50 percent of such patients the *bcr-abl* abnormality can be detected by polymerase chain reaction, thus confirming the diagnosis of CML. A few patients with otherwise characteristic disease have no detectable *bcr-abl* translocation (Ph-negative CML). A rare form of myeloproliferative disease, called *juvenile CML*, is seen in patients less than 4 years of age. It is distinguished from adult-type CML by the absence of the Ph chromosome, elevated fetal hemoglobin, thrombocytopenia, and prominent monocytosis. Usually, moderate leukocytosis and a normal cytogenetic karyotype are observed. Patients with juvenile CML rarely undergo blastic transformation and usually die of infection or organ failure from monocyte and macrophage infiltration. Typically, CML can be differentiated from a leukemoid reaction associated with infection or neoplasm by the presence of the Ph chromosome, eosinophilia, basophilia, and a low neutrophil alkaline phosphatase score. Agnogenic myeloid metaplasia usually presents with marked myelofibrosis and splenomegaly with absence of the Ph chromosome.

THERAPY AND PROGNOSIS   Allogeneic bone marrow transplantation is the only curative treatment presently available for patients with CML. Early identification of possible histocompatible bone marrow donors is important, and all siblings should be HLA typed. Long-term disease-free survival is obtained in 50 to 70 percent of patients in the chronic phase who are treated by HLA-matched sibling bone marrow transplantation. Patients transplanted in an accelerated phase have a poorer prognosis, and transplantation in the blastic phase is curative in less than 10 percent of patients. After transplantation, patients may have reappearance of some cells containing the Ph chromosome or *bcr-abl* positivity by PCR. The long-term clinical significance of this mixed chimeric state in the early stages after bone marrow transplantation is not known.

Young patients who do not have an HLA-compatible sibling donor should be considered for HLA-matched unrelated bone marrow transplantation if a trial of interferon-α (IFN-α) therapy has not resulted in a major cytogenetic response. The search for a potential donor should be initiated at diagnosis. Unrelated, allogeneic bone marrow transplantation presents special hazard and should be performed in centers with sophisticated programs in the prevention and management of graft-versus-host disease. Patients who relapse after bone marrow transplantation often benefit from IFN-α therapy. The timing of bone marrow transplantation in patients with sibling histocompatible donors is controversial. Some clinicians prefer a trial of IFN-α prior to accepting the immediate risk of morbidity and mortality associated with bone marrow transplantation. Most centers, however, recommend bone marrow transplantation within the first year of diagnosis. Unfortunately, two-thirds of patients with CML do not have HLA-compatible siblings or are too old to tolerate the transplant conditioning regimen.

Emergency treatment of CML is usually not necessary unless the patient has evidence of leukostasis, painful splenomegaly, or a dangerously high white blood cell count. Hyperuricemia is common at presentation and can be managed with allopurinol and hydration. Patients with white blood cell counts in the 30,000 cells per microliter range with no symptoms can be observed until a definitive plan of therapy is determined.

The general goal of treatment for patients in chronic phase CML is to decrease myelopoiesis, thereby controlling the disease and its symptoms. Many chemotherapeutic drugs can accomplish this aim, but none are selective for the Ph-positive clone or are capable of delaying the development of blast crisis. IFN-α, which has not yet been approved for the treatment of CML in the United States, appears to be partially selective in inhibiting the neoplastic clone and therefore is often the first therapeutic option. The chemotherapeutic drug of choice for managing chronic-phase CML is hydroxyurea, which is

TABLE 309-1	The myeloproliferative diseases			
	CML	PV	MF	ET
Hematocrit	Normal or ↓	↑ ↑	↓	Normal
White blood cell count	↑ ↑ ↑	↑	↑ to ↓	Normal
Platelet count	↑ to ↓	↑	↑ to ↓	↑ ↑ ↑
Splenomegaly	+ + +	+	+ + +	+
Ph chromosome or *bcr/abl*	+	0	0	0
Marrow fibrosis	±	± or ↓	+ + +	±
Neutrophil alkaline phosphatase	↓ to 0	↑ ↑	↑ or normal	↑ or normal

preferred over busulfan because of ease of use and lower incidence of side effects. Hydroxyurea is usually given in doses of 1 to 3 g/d orally, with adjustments to keep the white blood cell count between 10,000 and 20,000 cells per microliter. Hydroxyurea can cause diarrhea, mucositis, or rash but is usually well tolerated. Serious side effects of busulfan include sterility, amenorrhea after prolonged use, pulmonary and retroperitoneal fibrosis, marrow fibrosis and aplasia, and hyperpigmentation of the skin. Busulfan can be given intermittently by mouth, but the dosage may be difficult to regulate. Other alkylating agents, such as cyclophosphamide, can control excess myelopoiesis and may be used if hydroxyurea is not tolerated or becomes ineffective in controlling blood counts.

Although still experimental in the treatment of CML, IFN-α is an effective agent in reducing the white blood cell and platelet counts. IFN-α appears to have preferential antiproliferative effects on CML progenitor cells. Durable complete cytogenetic responses may occur but are rare. Responding patients, however, show reemergence of normal hematopoietic precursors and a relative decrease in Ph-positive cells. It is not yet clear whether the development of blast crisis is delayed in these patients, although the observation of long-term disease control in cytogenetically responding patients supports the concept. IFN-α is usually started at 3 to 5 million units daily, intramuscularly or subcutaneously, and the dosage is adjusted to maintain the white blood cell count above 5000 cells per microliter. Patients can be maintained on a' 3- to 5-day per week treatment schedule. Some clinicians use IFN-α in conjunction with hydroxyurea or low-dose cytosine arabinoside. Liver function tests and blood counts should be monitored during interferon therapy, and cytogenetic analyses are needed to assess response. During interferon therapy, patients often experience a flulike syndrome associated with fever and myalgias. These side effects may be severe and lead to discontinuation of interferon, but symptoms usually respond to acetaminophen

and interferon dose adjustment. Leukopenia and thrombocytopenia also may occur. IFN-α is relatively contraindicated in patients with depression or preexisting psychiatric disorders and should be used with caution in patients with liver, thyroid, or cardiac disease.

Age, spleen size, high platelet count, presence of circulating blasts, marked basophilia or eosinophilia, and the presence of additional chromosomal abnormalities (double Ph, 8+, 17q+) are all associated with poor prognosis. Death seldom occurs during the chronic phase of CML. The risk of transformation from the chronic to the blastic phase is approximately 20 percent per year after the first year. Eighty-five percent of patients die while in the blastic phase. The overall median survival of patients in chronic phase of CML is 4 to 5 years. Patients in the accelerated phase have a median survival of 85 weeks, whereas patients in the blastic phase of CML have a median survival of only 15 to 20 weeks.

The optimal treatment strategy for chronic phase CML has not been determined. Young patients with HLA-matched sibling or unrelated donors should be offered bone marrow transplantation as the only known curative option. For older patients and those without a matched sibling bone marrow donor, an initial trial of IFN-α is warranted. Hydroxyurea is the chemotherapeutic drug of choice for controlling the excessive myelopoiesis in chronic phase disease.

Myeloid blast crisis is difficult to treat. A course of induction therapy for acute myeloblastic leukemia is usually warranted and can lead to reversion to chronic-phase disease or, rarely, cytogenetic remission. It is important to diagnose the lymphoid type of blast crisis accurately, since it may be treated effectively with aggressive acute lymphoblastic leukemia regimens that include vincristine and prednisone. Once remission is attained with the induction regimen, allogeneic bone marrow transplantation is an option for a few patients with HLA-matched siblings. Splenectomy or irradiation of the spleen is rarely used today, although elderly patients or those with splenic infarcts may be palliated by these procedures.

POLYCYTHEMIA VERA

DEFINITION AND ETIOLOGY   Polycythemia vera (PV) is a myeloproliferative disorder resulting from clonal expansion of a transformed hematopoietic stem cell associated with prominent overproduction of erythrocytes and, to a lesser extent, expansion of granulocytic and megakaryocytic elements. PV is gradual in onset and has a slowly progressive course. The disease generally begins in late middle life, and there is a slight male predominance. PV is relatively uncommon in blacks and occurs with increased frequency in Jews of European ancestry. Rare cases of PV in monozygotic twins and a minimal increased incidence in first-degree relatives of affected patients suggest a genetic role in rare cases. The cause of PV is unknown, and there is no known link to radiation exposure. A PV-like disease is seen in mice infected with certain strains of Friend erythroleukemia virus, but no viral relationship has been found for the human disease.

PATHOPHYSIOLOGY AND SYMPTOMATOLOGY   Polycythemia vera is a neoplastic stem cell disorder associated with excessive proliferation of erythroid, granulocytic, and megakaryocytic precursors. Since erythrocytosis is the primary manifestation of PV, it must be differentiated from secondary causes of erythrocytosis which usually are associated with syndromes of increased elaboration of erythropoietin (Table 309-2). The serum concentration of erythropoietin is low in PV but is not absent. While initially it was believed that PV erythropoiesis was autonomous, it is now known that the erythroid precursors in PV patients respond to erythropoietin and may be hypersensitive to its action. Bone marrow cells from patients with PV form colonies of erythroid precursors in culture in the absence of added erythropoietin. This phenomenon is rarely seen in other conditions. Much of this ''endogenous'' erythroid colony formation in PV is abrogated by the addition of antibodies to erythropoietin, suggesting increased sensitivity to erythropoietin. Some red cell

---

TABLE 309-2   **Classification of polycythemia**

PRIMARY (AUTONOMOUS)

Polycythemia vera
"Pure" erythrocytosis ("erythremia")
   Familial
   Sporadic

SECONDARY

Physiologically appropriate (decreased tissue oxygenation)
   High altitude
   Chronic lung disease
   Alveolar hypoventilation
   Cardiovascular right-to-left shunt
   High-oxygen-affinity hemoglobinopathy
   Carboxyhemoglobinemia ("smoker's erythrocytosis")
   Congenitally decreased erythrocyte 2,3,-DPG
Physiologically inappropriate (normal tissue oxygenation)
   Tumors producing erythropoietin or other erythropoietic stimuli
      Renal cell carcinoma
      Hepatocellular carcinoma
      Cerebellar hemangioblastoma
      Uterine leiomyoma
      Ovarian carcinoma
      Pheochromocytoma
   Renal diseases
      Cysts
      Hydronephrosis
      Diffuse parenchymal disease
      Bartter's syndrome
      Renal transplantation
      Nephrotic syndrome
      Long-term hemodialysis
   Adrenal cortical hypersecretion
   Exogenous androgens, erythropoietin, cobalt
   Unexplained ("essential")

RELATIVE POLYCYTHEMIA (SPURIOUS OR STRESS ERYTHRO-CYTOSIS, GAISBÖCK'S SYNDROME)

SOURCE: Hocking and Golde.

production in PV, however, may be autonomous with respect to erythropoietin. As with chronic myelogenous leukemia, there are increased myeloid and megakaryocytic progenitors in the bone marrow, indicating that the panmyelosis in PV is characterized by expansion of the committed precursor cell pools.

Patients with PV usually present with symptoms referable to an expanded blood volume. They may complain of headaches, vertigo, tinnitus, or blurred vision. Occasionally, patients present with thrombotic complications or hemostatic defects manifested by easy bruisability, epistaxis, or gastrointestinal hemorrhage. Other symptoms include weight loss, sweating, pain in the feet, peptic ulceration, or severe pruritus, which is often aggravated by bathing in warm water. These symptoms relate to hypermetabolism, hyperhistaminemia, hypervolemia, and abnormal platelet function. Approximately one-third of the patients have hypertension. An occasional patient will present with symptoms referable to splenomegaly or hyperuricemia. Asymptomatic patients are often identified by routine blood count determinations.

Physical examination typically shows plethora and, occasionally, dusky cyanosis. There is often venous prominence with engorgement of the retinal veins, and splenomegaly is present in approximately 75 percent of patients. Splenomegaly is a key physical finding in terms of differentiating PV from secondary polycythemia.

LABORATORY FINDINGS The diagnostic criteria of the Polycythemia Study Group are presented in Table 309-3. These criteria were developed to help ensure uniformity with regard to the diagnosis of PV, but they are stringent and may exclude early stages of the disease. Typically, patients present with an elevated hemoglobin concentration and hematocrit associated with thrombocytosis, leukocytosis, and splenomegaly. In these cases, diagnosis is straightforward. Patients presenting only with erythrocytosis need a systematic evaluation to establish a firm diagnosis. The confirmation of true polycythemia requires determination of a chromium 51 red cell mass and a plasma volume study. If the red cell mass is normal and the plasma volume low-normal or reduced, the patient does not have true polycythemia but, rather, a relative increase in hemoglobin concentration. This circumstance can be seen in patients receiving diuretic therapy or in those who fall in a heterogeneous group of patients previously referred to as having *Gaisböck's syndrome*, now known as *spurious* or *stress erythrocytosis*. If true polycythemia is documented by an increased red cell mass, PV needs to be distinguished from secondary causes of erythrocytosis (see Table 309-2). Signs of panmyelosis, including leukocytosis, basophilia, thrombocytosis, and splenomegaly, strongly point to the diagnosis of PV. In obvious cases, no elaborate testing is required. Bone marrow examination is usually not needed, but iron deposits may be absent and mild reticulin fibrosis may be present at the time of diagnosis. Cytogenetic studies in PV may show clonal markers ($+1$, $+8$, $+9$, 20q-) in up to 30 percent of the patients.

In the absence of clear-cut signs of PV, additional laboratory testing is necessary. Determination of the serum erythropoietin concentration is important in distinguishing primary from secondary causes of polycythemia. An elevated erythropoietin concentration suggests secondary erythrocytosis, while a low level is compatible with PV. An oxygen saturation of less than 92 percent suggests hypoxemia as the cause for erythrocytosis. Direct measurement of carboxyhemoglobin and arterial oxygen saturation can be helpful. Measurement of the P_{50} of the oxyhemoglobin dissociation curve is useful in detecting high-oxygen-affinity hemoglobins. Radiographic evaluation of the kidneys may be necessary to rule out a renal lesion secreting erythropoietin. In some patients, examination of the liver or the posterior fossa of the brain may be indicated to exclude hepatic lesions or cerebellar hemangioblastoma associated with abnormal erythropoietin production.

In PV, the neutrophil alkaline phosphatase score is frequently increased, as is the serum vitamin B_{12} level and serum vitamin B_{12}–binding capacity. Although they are included as part of the Polycythemia Vera Study Group criteria, these laboratory findings are seldom helpful in differential diagnosis.

COURSE AND PROGNOSIS The use of ^{32}P and myelosuppressive therapy with alkylating agents, while providing disease control, has led to an increased incidence of acute leukemia, and these therapies are rarely used today. The so-called spent or burnt-out phase of PV is characterized by marked splenomegaly and anemia associated with bone marrow fibrosis. Modern therapy may lead to an altered disease course, and survival in excess of 12 years is now common. The majority of patients in the past have died of vascular complications of the disease. Acute leukemia may occur in 2 percent of patients who have not been exposed to alkylating agents or radiotherapy.

TREATMENT While treatment for the patient with polycythemia vera needs to be individualized, phlebotomy is indicated initially in all patients to reduce the hematocrit to less than 46 percent. In young patients with normal cardiac function, a 1-unit phlebotomy can often be performed on alternating days or every third day until a safe hematocrit is achieved. Patients with cardiovascular disease and older patients should have smaller-volume phlebotomies performed twice weekly. Therapy should be directed toward maintaining the hematocrit between 42 and 44 percent. With continued phlebotomy, there is the inevitable development of iron deficiency, which will impair red cell production and permit phlebotomy at widely spaced intervals. Iron deficiency itself, however, may cause unwanted side effects, and secondary microcytosis may increase whole blood viscosity. Some iron supplementation may be required and necessitate phlebotomy at more frequent intervals. Patients who are managed by phlebotomy alone have a measurably high risk of thrombotic complications over a 5- to 7-year period after diagnosis. Thrombosis in patients treated with phlebotomy alone is more common in older patients, but hematocrit and platelet count do not have a significant impact on the risk of thrombosis.

The results of the Polycythemia Vera Study Group experience indicated that patients treated with ^{32}P or chlorambucil had a greater than 10 percent incidence of acute leukemia. Therefore, chlorambucil is now contraindicated in the treatment of PV. ^{32}P can only be recommended for the very elderly or for unusual circumstances where the patient cannot have regular medical supervision. Hydroxyurea has been shown to be highly effective in controlling the polycythemic syndrome, and approximately three-quarters of patients can achieve long-term disease control with this drug. While the lack of mutagenicity of hydroxyurea has been called into question, it appears to be one of the safest myelosuppressants available. Other alkylating agents are also effective in controlling the disease but appear to have leukemogenic potential equivalent to that of chlorambucil. IFN-α, an experimental agent in the treatment of PV that decreases panmyelosis and can control the erythrocytosis, has considerable promise. While the role of IFN-α in the treatment of PV is not yet determined, it is an active and useful agent without apparent leukemogenic potential. It also may be combined with intermittent phlebotomy or with hydroxyurea in difficult to manage patients. At present, it is not known if interferon has a selective effect on the neoplastic clone in PV as it does in CML.

TABLE 309-3 Diagnostic criteria for polycythemia vera

Category A
  1 Significantly elevated red cell mass
  2 Arterial blood oxygen saturation ≥ 92%
  3 Splenomegaly
Category B
  1 Thrombocytosis >400,000 per microliter
  2 Leukocytosis >12,000 per microliter
  3 Increased leukocyte alkaline phosphatase score in absence of fever or infection
  4 Serum vitamin B_{12} level greater than 900 pg/mL or vitamin B_{12}–binding capacity greater than 2200 pg/mL

Diagnosis of polycythemia vera if: A1 + A2 + A3 or A1 + A2 + any two factors from category B

SOURCE: Adapted from the Polycythemia Vera Study Group criteria.

Special problems arise in the management of patients with PV. Elective surgery should not be performed in uncontrolled PV, since hemorrhagic and thrombotic complications lead to a markedly increased perioperative mortality. Generally, such surgery should be postponed until the disease has been under control for 2 months. In emergency situations, isovolemic phlebotomy should be performed prior to surgery.

Severe pruritus may be an important problem, and attempts to treat it with agents such as hydroxyzine, cyproheptadine, or cimetadine are warranted, but inhibition of hematopoiesis with hydroxyurea or IFN-α may be required for symptom control. The use of antiplatelet agents in PV is controversial, particularly since they may increase the risk of hemorrhage. Small doses of aspirin (baby aspirin) may be indicated in patients with a thrombotic tendency. Where the platelet count cannot be controlled with hydroxyurea, IFN-α or anagrelide can be used. Hyperuricemia should be treated with allopurinol, and hemorrhagic complications may rarely require platelet transfusion.

AGNOGENIC MYELOID METAPLASIA WITH MYELOFIBROSIS (MF)

DEFINITION AND ETIOLOGY Agnogenic myeloid metaplasia with myelofibrosis (MF), also called *idiopathic myelofibrosis*, is a clonal disorder of the hematopoietic stem cell characterized by bone marrow fibrosis and extramedullary hematopoiesis. Gradual fibrosis of the bone marrow and hyperplasia of myeloid elements result in progressive anemia and variable changes in granulocyte and platelet counts associated with increasing splenomegaly. The disease begins in late middle life and is gradual in onset, chronic, and progressive. Males and females are equally affected, and there is a rare reported familial occurrence.

PATHOPHYSIOLOGY AND SYMPTOMATOLOGY Idiopathic MF is a clonal hematopoietic disorder in which fibroblastic proliferation is thought to be due to release of growth factors such as platelet-derived growth factor or tumor growth factor from platelets and megakaryocytes. Type III collagen is usually the cause of myelofibrosis. Bone marrow fibroblasts have been demonstrated not to be part of the neoplastic clone. MF commonly presents with symptoms related to anemia and splenomegaly. Splenomegaly is present in all patients, and in some, splenic enlargement may be massive. The splenomegaly may be present for years prior to diagnosis and can cause pain, abdominal fullness, and early satiety. Hepatomegaly is seen in approximately 50 to 75 percent of patients but is not observed in the absence of splenomegaly. As the disease progresses, patients may experience weight loss, skin and mucous membrane bleeding, and, less commonly, bone pain, jaundice, and lymphadenopathy.

LABORATORY FINDINGS Anemia is observed in over half of patients at diagnosis and ultimately develops in all patients. Initially, the anemia is due to ineffective erythropoiesis, but subsequently, there is increased pooling of red blood cells in the spleen and decreased red cell survival. Folate deficiency and, rarely, autoimmune hemolytic anemia or acquired hemoglobin H disease may develop. Examination of the peripheral blood smear reveals poikilocytosis with prominent teardrop forms. Fragmented red cells and nucleated red blood cells are commonly observed. An increase in platelet count is seen in half of patients, and giant platelets or megakaryocytes may be seen in the peripheral blood. A moderate elevation in neutrophil count is observed in most patients, but neutropenia is seen in up to 25 percent of the cases. Often there is a left shift toward early granulocytic forms, and occasionally, circulating blasts may be found. Some patients have an increase in absolute basophil count. The neutrophil alkaline phosphatase score is elevated in about half of patients, but others have a lower than normal value. Platelet function studies often show defective platelet adhesiveness and impaired secondary release of ADP in response to epinephrine.

Radiographically demonstrable bone sclerosis is seen in about 50 percent of patients, particularly in the proximal long bones and the vertebral bodies. Rarely, osteolytic lesions are demonstrable. Routine radiographic studies usually show splenomegaly and dense bones.

Bone marrow aspiration is almost always unsuccessful in patients with MF and results in a "dry tap." Bone marrow biopsy should be performed and reveals fibrosis of marrow spaces and often osteosclerosis. MF may be extensive or focal, and megakaryocytic hyperplasia is usually observed. Pathologically, the spleen shows features of extramedullary hematopoiesis in the red pulp.

DIAGNOSIS The diagnosis of idiopathic MF is usually not difficult, nor is it hard to distinguish it from other myeloproliferative disorders. The presence of the Ph chromosome and a low neutrophil alkaline phosphatase score distinguish CML from idiopathic MF. While MF and PV can present with a similar pathologic picture, the history of PV is usually distinctive. Rarely, myelodysplasia with MF may create confusion. Megakaryoblastic leukemia (acute MF) normally presents with fever and pancytopenia and should be differentiated from idiopathic MF.

THERAPY There is no definitive therapy for idiopathic MF. Bone marrow transplantation offers the only potential curative therapeutic option. Marrow fibrosis may be reversible after bone marrow transplantation, but few patients are of an appropriate age or have an HLA-matched sibling donor. Normally when therapy is required for idiopathic MF, it is because of anemia. Since the anemia may be multifactorial, a search for folate or iron deficiency and/or autoimmune hemolytic anemia is indicated, since specific therapy in these circumstances is effective. Treatment with androgens will lead to responses in approximately 30 to 40 percent of anemic patients. Danazol, 200 mg three times daily, orally, or testosterone enanthate, 400 mg weekly, intramuscularly, in men has been employed with some success, although the precise mechanism of androgen action is unknown. Androgen side effects may be serious, particularly in older men with occult prostate cancer. Measurement of the serum erythropoietin level can be helpful in guiding potential therapy with erythropoietin, although there are little controlled data regarding the utility of erythropoietin in this disease. Transfusions are necessary for unresponsive anemia.

In the face of marked splenomegaly, the issue of splenectomy must be addressed. Splenectomy performed under appropriate conditions offers an important opportunity to enhance the quality of life for patients with idiopathic MF. In the older literature, however, splenectomy was associated with unacceptable perioperative morbidity and mortality. While splenectomy does not affect the overall survival of patients with idiopathic MF, it can be a useful therapeutic approach to manage hemolytic anemia, thrombocytopenia, and painful splenic infarction, as well as portal hypertension. Splenectomy, however, is contraindicated in the face of increased platelet counts, and it is important to achieve optimal disease control beforehand.

Chemotherapy can be useful in the management of symptomatic patients with idiopathic MF. The drug of choice in these situations is hydroxyurea, which can reduce the leukocytosis and constitutional symptoms associated with the disease and may reduce spleen size and splenic discomfort. Hydroxyurea should be initiated at doses of approximately 0.5 to 1.0 g/d, but higher doses may be required to reduce platelet counts. The effect of hydroxyurea on marrow fibrosis is uncertain. Alkylating agents are now contraindicated, but IFN-α may be useful in selective patients with marked thrombocytosis. Overall experience with IFN-α is currently too limited to decide on its role. Glucocorticoids may be useful if autoimmune hemolytic anemia is associated with the MF and to reduce constitutional symptoms, but side effects limit its chronic use. Radiation therapy for massive splenomegaly has limited application in the palliation of debilitated and elderly patients.

ESSENTIAL THROMBOCYTOSIS

DEFINITION AND ETIOLOGY Essential thrombocytosis (ET) is a myeloproliferative disorder characterized by markedly elevated platelet production, with blood platelet counts above 600,000 cells

TABLE 309-4 Differential diagnosis of thrombocytosis

MYELOPROLIFERATIVE DISORDERS

Essential thrombocythemia
Polycythemia vera
Chronic myelogenous leukemia
Myelofibrosis

SECONDARY THROMBOCYTOSIS

Recovery from acute infection
Malignant disease
    Carcinoma
    Hodgkin's disease
    Lymphoma
Hemolytic anemia
Postoperative
    Splenectomy
    Other surgical procedures
Acute hemorrhage
Iron deficiency
Response to drugs
    Epinephrine
    Vincristine
Chronic inflammatory disorders
    Rheumatoid arthritis
    Ulcerative colitis
    Hepatic cirrhosis
    Sarcoidosis
Response to exercise, stress
Recovery from myelosuppresive drugs
Therapy of vitamin B_{12} deficiency
Others: Osteoporosis, 5q− syndrome

per microliter. Clinical involvement of hematopoietic lineages other than the megakaryocytic line is unusual. The disease must be distinguished from secondary thrombocytosis in response to inflammation, acute bleeding, iron deficiency, or neoplasia (Table 309-4). The cause of ET is unknown.

PATHOPHYSIOLOGY AND SYMPTOMATOLOGY ET is likely a disorder of the pluripotent hematopoietic stem cell, based on the demonstration of monoclonality in the bone marrow in about 90 percent of females determined using X chromosome–linked gene probes. "Autonomous" in vitro megakaryocytic colony formation is observed in this disease, and "autonomous" erythroid colony formation also has been reported. Clinically, however, evidence of polycythemia or granulocytosis is rare.

The symptoms of ET are related to the increased platelet count and platelet dysfunction. Two-thirds of patients are asymptomatic at diagnosis, and younger patients can remain asymptomatic for long periods. Vascular occlusion may be found in 20 to 50 percent of patients at diagnosis and involves both arteries and veins. Platelet emboli or local platelet aggregation can lead to microvascular occlusion associated with transient cerebral ischemic symptoms, stroke, or digital ischemia. Occlusion of the coronary or mesenteric vessels also may occur. Erythromelalgia is a syndrome of redness and burning in the extremities, which is probably due to arteriolar occlusion. Venous thrombosis is also observed in ET and may involve the portal, hepatic, or splenic veins. Hemorrhagic manifestations are found in up to 50 percent of patients, usually involving the mucous membranes or skin, but occasionally severe gastrointestinal hemorrhage can occur. Patients may complain of easy bruisability or prolonged bleeding after minor surgery or dental procedures. Usually there is a correlation between the platelet count and symptoms, but younger patients, especially women, may have high platelet counts and may be asymptomatic for prolonged periods.

LABORATORY FINDINGS An elevated platelet count is the most prominent abnormality in ET. The peripheral blood smear shows platelets of different size and shape, often with giant forms and hypogranularity. Functional abnormalities include impaired platelet aggregation in response to epinephrine, collagen, or adenosine diphosphate (ADP). The epinephrine defect is most characteristic.

No correlation is observed between bleeding and in vitro platelet aggregation abnormalities. Splenic enlargement is seen in two-thirds of patients and is usually modest. Anemia or granulocytosis is uncommon. Bone marrow examination reveals increased numbers of megakaryocytes which may show morphologic abnormalities, and modest reticulin fibrosis is seen in patients with advanced disease.

DIAGNOSIS A markedly elevated platelet count in the absence of an identifiable cause of secondary thrombocytosis is usually sufficient for a diagnosis of ET. Support for the diagnosis may be obtained by in vitro platelet aggregation studies and the documentation of splenomegaly. Cytogenetic abnormalities are uncommon. Secondary thrombocytosis is usually associated with increased numbers of megakaryocytes of small diameter and low ploidy. In ET, the megakaryocytes are large and hyperploid.

The Polycythemia Vera Study Group has proposed the following diagnostic criteria for ET: (1) platelet count persistently greater than 1 million per microliter in the absence of any identifiable cause, (2) normal red cell volume or hemoglobin less than 13 g/dL, (3) presence of iron in the bone marrow, (4) absence of collagen fibrosis in the bone marrow biopsy, and (5) absence of the Philadelphia chromosome.

COURSE AND PROGNOSIS Survival in older patients is similar to that of patients with PV. Patients usually die of hemorrhagic or thrombotic complications. ET can progress into MF in perhaps a quarter of patients and in about 5 percent transforms into an acute leukemia. The disease seems to follow a much more benign course in some young patients in whom there may not be an associated high risk of hemorrhage or thrombosis.

THERAPY Asymptomatic younger patients often can simply be observed, even if their platelet counts are over 1 million per microliter. Such asymptomatic patients may have stable disease for many years. All patients with thrombocytosis should be strongly encouraged not to smoke. Symptomatic disease should be treated, and older patients with platelet counts approaching 1 million per microliter also should receive therapy. Radioactive phosphorus and busulfan are no longer used because of significant toxicity and mutagenicity. Hydroxyurea is generally considered to be the initial treatment of choice to lower the platelet count to 500,000 per microliter or less. Hydroxyurea is usually given in doses of 500 to 2000 mg/d orally, with few side effects. IFN-α is an experimental agent with distinct activity in ET. The dose of IFN-α must be adjusted with respect to acute toxicity and the development of neutropenia. The tolerance for IFN-α varies considerably from patient to patient, but a frequent starting point is 3 million units subcutaneously daily. IFN-α is effective in controlling the platelet count and may partially reverse platelet function defects. Little is known of the possible long-term advantages or disadvantages of IFN-α as compared with hydroxyurea. Anagrelide is a novel compound with powerful antiaggregating effects on platelets which also significantly inhibits platelet production. Anagrelide has a specific effect on thrombopoiesis and does not appear to influence other hematopoietic lineages. Control of the platelet count with anagrelide is seen in over 90 percent of patients. The major side effects are neurologic, gastrointestinal, and cardiac and lead to discontinuation of the treatment in about 15 percent of patients. Fluid retention and peripheral edema are common.

The use of antiplatelet function agents such as aspirin or dipyridamole is controversial. These agents can lead to serious hemorrhage, yet they may protect against thrombosis in other patients. Control of the platelet count seems to be of primary importance, but in those rare patients in whom good control cannot be achieved or who develop thrombotic complications despite adequate lowering of the platelet count, the addition of low-dose aspirin seems warranted. Patients who hemorrhage despite control of the platelet count may rarely require platelet transfusion as a lifesaving measure.

REFERENCES

ANAGRELIDE STUDY GROUP: Anagrelide, a therapy for thrombocythemic states: Experience in 577 patients. Am J Med 69:76, 1992

BIGGS JC et al: Treatment of chronic myeloid leukemia with allogeneic bone marrow transplantation after preparation with Bu-Cy 2. Blood 5:1352, 1992

CUNNINGHAM I: Bone marrow transplantation for chronic myelogenous leukemia. Oncology 4:101, 1990

DALEY GQ et al: Induction of chronic myelogenous leukemia in mice by the P210[bcr/abl] gene of the Philadelphia chromosome. Science 247:824, 1990

DHINGRA K et al: Minimal residual disease in interferon-treated chronic myelogenous leukemia: Results and pitfalls of analysis based on polymerase chain reaction. Leukemia 6:754, 1992

GUILHOT F et al: Cytogenetic remissions in chronic myelogenous leukemia using interferon alpha-2a and hydroxyurea with or without low-dose cytosine arabinoside. Leuk Lymph 4:49, 1991

HEHLMANN R et al: Chronic myelogenous leukemia: Recent developments in prognostic evaluation and chemotherapy. Leukemia 6(suppl 3):110S, 1992

HOCKING WG, GOLDE DW: Polycythemia: Evaluation and management. Blood Rev 3:59, 1989

KOLB HJ et al: Donor leukocyte transfusions for treatment of recurrent chronic myelogenous leukemia in marrow transplant patients. Blood 76:2462, 1990

PEARSON TC: Primary thrombocythaemia: Diagnosis and management. Br J Haematol 78:145, 1991

SILVER RT: A new treatment for polycythemia vera: Recombinant interferon alpha. Blood 76:664, 1990

————: Chronic myeloid leukemia. Curr Opin Oncol 4:66, 1992

TALPAZ M et al: Interferon-alpha produces sustained cytogenetic responses in chronic myelogenous leukemia: Philadelphia chromosome-positive patients. Ann Intern Med 114:532, 1991

———— et al: Recombinant interferon-alpha therapy of Philadelphia chromosome-negative myeloproliferative disorders with thrombocytosis. Am J Med 86:554, 1989

WEINSTEIN IM: Idiopathic myelofibrosis: Historical review, diagnosis and management Blood Rev 5:98, 1991

310   THE LEUKEMIAS

DAVID A. SCHEINBERG / DAVID W. GOLDE

Leukemias are neoplasms derived from hematopoietic cells that proliferate initially in the bone marrow before disseminating to the peripheral blood, spleen, lymph nodes, and ultimately, other tissues. As such, they are distinguished from the lymphomas, which arise primarily in the lymph nodes but also may spread (in "leukemic phase") to the blood and marrow. Classification of leukemia is broadly related to the cell of origin (e.g., lymphoid or myeloid) as well as to the rapidity of the clinical course (e.g., acute or chronic), but modern categorizations have identified specific leukemias on the basis of biologic, antigenic, and molecular characteristics of these diseases. This chapter reviews acute myelogenous leukemia (AML), the acute and chronic lymphocytic leukemias (ALL and CLL), and hairy cell leukemia. Chronic myelogenous leukemia (CML) is covered in Chap. 309.

ETIOLOGY   The cause of leukemia is not known in most patients, although both genetic and environmental factors are important. There is a high concordance rate among identical twins if acute leukemia develops in the first year of life, and families with an excessive incidence of leukemia have been identified. Acute leukemia occurs with an increased frequency in a variety of congenital disorders, including the Down, Bloom, Klinefelter, Fanconi, and Wiskott-Aldrich syndromes.

Environmental factors are also known to play a role in the etiology of leukemia. Ionizing radiation causes leukemia in experimental animals, and there is a clear relationship between such exposure and the development of leukemia in humans. For example, individuals with occupational radiation exposure, patients receiving radiation therapy, and Japanese survivors of the atomic bomb explosions have a predictable and dose-related increased incidence of leukemia. Radiation exposure increases the risk of developing CML, AML, and possibly ALL, but there is no known relationship to CLL or to hairy cell leukemia. Exposure to chemicals such as benzene and other aromatic hydrocarbons or treatment with alkylating agents and other chemotherapeutic drugs also leads to an increased incidence of AML. The combination of radiation and chemotherapeutic agents, such

as in patients treated for Hodgkin's disease, results in additive leukemogenic effects. A role for electromagnetic energy in leukemogenesis remains unproven.

Although RNA-based retroviruses cause a number of leukemias in animals, a viral cause for a human leukemia has been established only for adult T cell leukemia (ATL), which is caused by the human T cell leukemia virus type I (HTLV-I). This virus can be transmitted horizontally by sexual contact or blood products as well as from mother to child (see Chap. 151). ATL is endemic in southwestern Japan and parts of the Caribbean and central Africa. The other known human leukemia virus, HTLV-II, has not yet been firmly linked to a specific leukemia. Epstein-Barr virus (EBV) has been associated with a form of ALL (L3 subtype) as well as certain aggressive lymphomas. The common forms of acute and chronic leukemia, however, are not contagious, and the incidence of leukemia is not increased among close contacts such as marital partners or in the offspring of women who develop leukemia during pregnancy.

INCIDENCE AND PREVALENCE   The incidence of all leukemias is approximately 13 per 100,000 people per year, and the age-related incidence of both acute and chronic leukemias is somewhat higher in men than in women. ALL is primarily a disease of children and young adults, whereas AML, CLL, and hairy cell leukemia increase in incidence with increasing age, peaking in the sixth and seventh decades.

PATHOPHYSIOLOGY   Acute leukemia is characterized by the clonal proliferation of immature hematopoietic cells. The leukemia arises following malignant transformation of a single hematopoietic progenitor, followed by cellular replication and expansion of the transformed clone. The most prominent characteristic of the neoplastic cells in acute leukemia is a defect in maturation beyond the myeloblast or promyelocyte level in AML and the lymphoblast level in ALL. The proliferating leukemia cells accumulate in the bone marrow, suppressing normal hematopoiesis and ultimately resulting in the replacement of normal elements. The consequent paucity of normal progenitors leads to the anemia, infections, and bleeding complications that characterize the disease. Leukemic cells proliferate primarily in the bone marrow, circulate in the blood, and may infiltrate into other tissues such as lymph nodes, liver, spleen, skin, gums, viscera, and the central nervous system (CNS). Although the diagnosis of leukemia is often first made by observation of large numbers of blasts in the blood, the majority of the leukemic cells are found in the marrow.

The cellular blood elements are derived from pluripotent and committed hematopoietic stem cells which reside in the bone marrow (Chap. 301). Leukemic transformation may occur in cells at several levels of differentiation. In some patients with AML who are heterozygous for glucose-6-phosphate dehydrogenase (G6PD) isoenzymes, the granulocytes, macrophages, erythrocytes, and megakaryocytes all contain the single G6PD isoenzyme present in the leukemic cells, suggesting that these cells are derived from the malignant clone and that leukemic transformation involved a multipotent stem cell. In other AML patients, only granulocytes and/or macrophages appear clonal, and in these patients, transformation may have occurred at the level of the committed granulocytic-macrophage progenitor. Clonality in different lineages also has been confirmed by fluorescence in situ hybridization studies.

The mechanism of neoplastic transformation producing leukemia is poorly understood but involves a fundamental alteration of DNA conferring hereditable malignant characteristics to the transformed cell and its progeny. In animals, leukemias can be induced by retroviruses which either carry a transforming gene (viral oncogene) or integrate into specific sites in DNA causing activation of cellular proto-oncogenes (insertional mutagenesis). The role of oncogenes in the pathogenesis of neoplasia is discussed in Chap. 63. With sensitive techniques, clonal cytogenetic abnormalities can be detected in most patients with acute and chronic leukemias. A wide range of cytogenetic abnormalities is associated with the various forms of leukemias, and distinctive nonrandom chromosomal abnormalities are found, as shown in Table 310-1. Chromosomal rearrangement in leukemic cells

TABLE 310-1   Common chromosomal abnormalities associated with leukemias

Abnormality	Associated disease	Comment
MYELOGENOUS LEUKEMIA		
t(8;21)	AML—M2	Better prognosis
t(15;17)	AML—M3	Retinoic acid receptor gene rearranged; better prognosis
inv (16); del (16q)	AML—M4 with eosinophils	Better prognosis
+8	AML—all subtypes	Poor prognosis
+21	AML—M1, M7	
+13	AML—biphenotypic	
5q−, −5, −7	AML—especially secondary AML	Poor prognosis
t(9;11)	AML—M5A	Poor prognosis
t(9;22)	CML	Poor prognosis; tyrosine kinase *bcr-abl* oncogene product created
t(4;11)	Biphenotypic leukemia	Poor prognosis
ACUTE LYMPHOCYTIC LEUKEMIA		
t(4;11)	ALL—L2	Poor prognosis
t(1;19)	ALL—L1; with clg expression	DNA binding fusion protein created
t(8;14)	ALL—L3	Poor prognosis; *myc* oncogene upregulated
Hyperdiploidy	ALL—L1, L2	Better prognosis
t(9;22)	ALL	Poor prognosis
t(10;14)	ALL—T cell	T cell receptor gene rearranged
9p−, 6q−, or 12p−	ALL	Most frequent abnormalities seen; up to 10% each in ALL
CHRONIC LYMPHOCYTIC LEUKEMIA		
+12	CLL	
14q+ Abnormalities	Any B lineage leukemias	

may alter the structure or regulation of cellular oncogenes, producing quantitative or qualitative changes in their gene products that may play a role in initiating or maintaining the leukemic state. For example, the t(15;17) translocation of acute promyelocytic leukemia (APL) results in the production of a new oncogenic protein that has retinoic acid–binding properties. Treatment of patients with APL with large doses of retinoic acid results in maturation of the cells and the induction of remission. The t(9;22) translocation results in an aberrant tyrosine kinase protein; the t(8;14) translocation yields an overexpression of the growth regulatory protein myc; and the t(1;19) translocation forms a new DNA-binding protein. Most data suggest that the development of leukemia is a multistep process, and in many cases, acute leukemia develops in patients with a preexisting myelodysplastic or myeloproliferative disorder.

The pathophysiology of bone marrow failure in leukemia is complex. Pancytopenia is typically present and results at least in part from physical replacement of the normal precursor cells by leukemic cells. Some patients with acute leukemia and pancytopenia have a hypocellular bone marrow, indicating that the marrow failure is not simply due to overcrowding by leukemic cells. Leukemic cells may directly inhibit normal hematopoiesis via cell-mediated or humoral mechanisms. Normal hematopoietic stem cells do remain in the bone marrow and are capable of proliferating and restoring hematopoiesis following effective antileukemic treatment.

Some patients develop AML after a preleukemic or myelodysplastic syndrome. The myelodysplastic syndromes are a heterogeneous group of disorders typically found in middle-aged or older patients and have been subclassified into the categories of refractory anemia (RA),

refractory anemia with ringed sideroblasts (RARS), refractory anemia with excess blasts (RAEB), refractory anemia with excess blasts in transformation (RAEB-T), and chronic myelomonocytic leukemia (CMMOL) (see Chap. 308). The term *preleukemia* should be reserved for a recognizable syndrome of hematopoietic dysfunction that typically precedes the classic findings of AML. This syndrome is usually characterized by a picture of ineffective hematopoiesis with anemia, thrombocytopenia, and sometimes granulocytopenia associated with a hypercellular, dysplastic bone marrow. In preleukemia, the leukemic clone is already established, and usually there is progressive impairment of hematopoiesis and accumulation of blasts. Megaloblastic hematopoiesis is common, and folate or vitamin B_{12} deficiency must be ruled out. Cytogenetic abnormalities are frequent; the most common chromosomal abnormalities are 5q−, −5, −7, and trisomy 8. When 5q− exists as the sole abnormality, the patient usually presents with refractory anemia associated with mild thrombocytosis. This disorder, referred to as the *5q − syndrome*, only progresses to acute leukemia in a minority of patients. Many patients with preleukemic or myelodysplastic syndromes never develop overt AML but die from complications of bone marrow failure. *Smoldering AML* refers to a syndrome in which the diagnostic features of acute leukemia are present, but the disease follows an indolent or subacute course. This disorder also tends to occur in elderly patients.

ACUTE LEUKEMIAS: ALL AND AML

PATHOLOGY AND CLASSIFICATION   The diagnosis of acute leukemia requires the demonstration of leukemic cells in the bone marrow, peripheral blood, or extramedullary tissues. The bone marrow is typically hypercellular with a monomorphic infiltration of leukemic blasts and a marked reduction in normal bone marrow elements. The diagnosis of the type of leukemia is currently based on a combination of morphologic, immunophenotypic, and cytochemical characteristics, as well as evidence of specific genetic translocations, when present. It is critical to distinguish ALL from AML, since these two diseases differ in natural history, prognosis, and response to various therapeutic agents. As many as one-third of adult ALL cases bear the t(9;22) translocation, with incidence increasing with age. It is important to identify these patients because prognosis is much poorer.

Acute lymphocytic leukemia can be identified and classified on the basis of morphology and immunologic phenotype related to the stage of lymphoid differentiation. The leukemic lymphoblasts in ALL are generally smaller (10 to 15 μm in diameter) than myeloblasts and typically have only a thin rim of agranular cytoplasm. The nucleus may be round or convoluted (see Fig. A9-24). Three morphologic subtypes are included in the French-American-British (FAB) classification: L1 cells are small and homogeneous with a regular nuclear membrane and a small nucleolus. L2 cells are larger, have a lower nucleus-to-cytoplasm ratio with more pleomorphism and typically have one or more prominent nucleoli. The L3 form of ALL is uncommon, occurring in less than 5 percent of cases; the leukemic cells in this variant contain large vesicular nuclei with basophilic, often vacuolated cytoplasm. L3 cells have a high mitotic index and represent the leukemic form of Burkitt's lymphoma.

Leukemic lymphoblasts in more than 90 percent of patients with ALL contain a nuclear enzyme terminal, deoxynucleotidyl transferase (Tdt), which is less commonly present in AML cells (about 20 percent). L3 ALL, a more mature subtype, is typically negative for Tdt, as are mature hematopoietic cells, CLL, and hairy cell leukemias. The leukemic cells from approximately half of patients with ALL react with the periodic acid Schiff stain, showing blocklike inclusions of glycogen. Lymphoblasts do not contain granulocytic or monocytic lysosomal enzymes and therefore do not react with cytochemical stains for peroxidase, Sudan black, and nonspecific esterase.

A large number of cell surface protein antigens on leukemia cells have now been identified by monoclonal antibodies. These antigens and antibodies are grouped according to cluster of differentiation

TABLE 310-2   Morphologic subtypes of acute leukemias

Subtype	Percent of cases	Morphology	Reactivity with special stains or markers			
			Peroxidase or Sudan black	Nonspecific esterase	Periodic acid-Schiff	Typical protein markers
M0, undifferentiated	3	Primitive cells; absence of cytochemical stains	−	−	−	CD34, 33, 13
M1, AML without maturation	20	Few if any azurophilic granules	+/−	+/−	−	CD34, 33, 13
M2, AML with maturation	25	Blasts with promyelocytic granules, Auer rods may be present	+ + +	+/−	−	CD34, 33, 15, 13
M3, promyelocytic leukemia	10	Hypergranular promyelocytes often with multiple Auer rods per cell	+ + +	+	+/−	CD33, 13, (HLA-Dr −)
M4, acute myelomonocytic leukemia	20	Monocytoid-appearing cells in peripheral blood; M4 with eosinophilia is subtype	+/−	+ + +	−	CD34, 33, 15, 14, 13
M5, acute monocytic leukemia	20	Two subtypes identified: (a) undifferentiated; (b) differentiated with 80% promonocytes and monocytes	−	+ + +	+/−	CD33, 15, 14, 13
M6, acute erythroleukemia	5	Predominance of erythroblasts and markedly dysplastic erythroid precursors	+/−	−	+ + +	CD33, glycophorin
M7, acute megakaryocytic leukemia	5	Undifferentiated blasts react with antiplatelet antibodies and contain platelet peroxidase	−	+/−	+ +	CD33, CD41
L1 ALL	75	Small round blasts with scanty cytoplasm	−	−	+ + +	CD10, 19, 34, Tdt
L2 ALL	20	Pleomorphic larger blasts with more cytoplasm and prominent nucleoli	−	−	+ + +	CD10, 19, 34, Tdt
L3 ALL	5	Large blasts with basophilic vacuolated cytoplasm and vesicular nuclei	−	−	+ + +	CD19, CD20, sIg

(CD) numbers. Certain antigens are preferentially expressed on cells of specific lineage and at different stages of maturation (Tables 310-2 and 310-3). Identification of these antigens is often useful in diagnosis. Virtually all lymphocytic leukemias of B cell origin express CD19, whereas most myeloid leukemias express CD33. Acute leukemias of both lineages often express CD34, a marker of hematopoietic stem cells. T-ALL cells express markers of the T cell lineage such as CD2, CD5, or CD7. Use of an appropriate panel of antigen markers and histochemical stains allows the diagnostic classification of nearly all leukemias, even in situations where the morphology is ambiguous.

Several forms of ALL can be defined based on immunologic phenotype. Approximately 60 percent of cases are termed *common ALL*; the cells are typically Tdt+, CD34+, and CD19+ and have the common ALL antigen (CALLA) CD10. They do not express surface membrane immunoglobulin or T cell antigens. These cells are derived from precursors of the B cell lineage and have immunoglobulin gene rearrangements. About 20 percent of cases of ALL are of the *T cell type*, where the T lymphoblasts express the E-rosette receptor CD2 or other T lymphocyte–related antigens, such as CD5, CD7, or CD1. T-ALL cells are Tdt+, usually CALLA-negative, and stain positively for acid phosphatase. T cell ALL typically occurs in adolescent males and is frequently associated with a high leukocyte count and an anterior mediastinal mass. Less than 5 percent of cases of ALL are of the *B cell type* (expressing Ig). The cells in this variant produce a monoclonal immunoglobulin that is bound to the surface membrane and has L3 morphology. In B cell ALL, the cells typically contain the t(8;14) chromosomal abnormality that is also characteristic of Burkitt's lymphoma.

The leukemic cells in AML are 12 to 20 μm in diameter, larger than lymphoblasts, and have a lower nucleus-to-cytoplasm ratio. The

TABLE 310-3   Cell surface markers used in diagnosing leukemias

Marker name	Normal cell distribution	Leukemia distribution
HLA-Dr	Early myeloid, monocytoid, B lineage	ALL, AML, CLL, HCL, not APL
CD34	Stem cells	ALL, AML (early subtypes)
CD19	B Lineage	ALL (B lineage), CLL, HCL
CD20	B Lineage	ALL (B lineage), CLL, HCL
CD21	Intermediate B	CLL
Surface Ig	Intermediate and maturing B	L3-ALL, CLL, HCL
CD13	Myeloid and monocytoid	AML (all subtypes)
CD14	Myeloid and monocytoid	AML (often M4, M5)
CD15	Myeloid and monocytoid	AML (later subtypes)
CD33	Early myeloid; monocytoid	AML (all subtypes)
CD1	Early (thymic) T cells	T-ALL
CD2	T lineage	T-ALL
CD3	Mature T cells	T-CLL, ATL
CD5	T lineage	T-ALL, B-CLL
CD7	T lineage	T-ALL, 20% of AML
CD16	NK, granulocytes	NK leukemia, Tγ leukemia
CD25	Activated T and B	HCL, ATL

leukemic myeloblasts usually have discrete nuclear chromatin and multiple nucleoli. Auer rods are sticklike abnormal primary granules present in the cytoplasm of leukemic cells. Such Auer rods are diagnostic of AML and are seen in 10 to 20 percent of patients with AML, particularly the M3 form (see Fig. A9-22). Dysplastic morphologic abnormalities may be prominent in granulocytic, erythroid, and megakaryocytic cells. Cytochemical stains are often helpful in classifying the pathologic subtypes of AML and in confirming the diagnosis. Myeloperoxidase, α-naphthyl-ASD-chloracetate esterase, and Sudan black are primarily present in cells undergoing granulocytic differentiation. Nonspecific esterase (α-naphthyl butyrate esterase) stains cells of the monocyte-macrophage lineage. A number of myeloid and monocytic cell surface antigens on AML cells also have been described and are useful in confirming a diagnosis in situations where the morphology and cytochemical stains are unclear (Table 310-3).

A collaborative French-American-British group divided AML into pathologic subtypes based on the degree of differentiation and maturation of the predominant cells toward granulocytes, monocytes, erythrocytes, or megakaryocytes. The characteristics of each subtype are summarized in Table 310-2. There are differences in the clinical features of some subtypes. The acute promyelocytic subtype (M3) is frequently associated with disseminated intravascular coagulation (DIC) induced by thromboplastic material released by the leukemic cells; DIC is usually present at the time of diagnosis and may be exacerbated during chemotherapy. It is important to immediately recognize the M3 APL variant because of the complications of DIC (see p. 1770) but also because remissions may be induced safely with *trans*-retinoic acid, rather than chemotherapy, as described above (p. 1765). Acute myelomonocytic leukemia (M4) and acute monocytic leukemia (M5) are more likely than other subtypes to involve extramedullary tissues, including skin, gingiva, and the nervous system. A recently defined subtype, M4EO, is characterized by increased abnormal eosinophils in the marrow, frequent CNS involvement, and an inv(16) chromosomal abnormality. There are several other specific disease syndromes associated with chromosomal abnormalities: t(4;11) is associated with a biphenotypic leukemia, splenomegaly, and poor prognosis; t(8;21) is associated with a good-prognosis AML-M2 in younger adults who often have splenomegaly or chloromas; t(9;11) is found with AML-M5; t(6;9) is seen with M2 and basophilia; and inv(3) or t(3;3) is found with increased platelets.

It may be difficult to distinguish AML without maturation (M1) from the L2 form of ALL by morphology alone. In these cases, cell surface markers and histochemistry usually define the leukemia type. Some patients have a biphenotypic or mixed-lineage acute leukemia in which the malignant cells express both myeloid and lymphoid markers. These cells may represent leukemias of primitive pluripotent stem cells, or the phenotype results from aberrant gene expression in a transformed myeloid or lymphoid progenitor.

Sensitive molecular methods for the detection of the t(9;22) translocation are now available using the polymerase chain reaction (PCR) with probes specific to the chromosomal breakpoints. These methods are capable of detecting as few as 1 leukemia cell in 1 million other cells. PCR is now available in a number of centers to document the t(15;17) translocation of APL and the immunoglobulin rearrangements seen in ALL and CLL. Less sensitive but useful fluorescence in situ hybridization (FISH) techniques also allow the identification of individual leukemia cells.

CLINICAL AND LABORATORY FEATURES ALL and AML share many clinical features. In the majority of patients, the initial symptoms of acute leukemia are present for less than 3 months. A preleukemic syndrome can be identified in approximately 25 percent of patients with AML; in these patients, anemia and other cytopenias are usually present for months to years preceding the development of overt leukemia. Patients with ALL and AML may present with pancytopenia without circulating blasts, with a normal leukocyte count, or with marked leukocytosis. Leukostasis due to occlusion of the microcirculation by leukemic blast cells can lead to hypoperfusion

of vital tissues, most commonly lung and brain. Leukostasis becomes increasingly common when the number of circulating blasts exceeds 100×10^9 per liter and is seen more often with the larger blast cells in AML than in ALL. Patients may complain of manifestations of anemia such as pallor, easy fatigability, and dyspnea on mild exertion.

Bleeding is a major problem in patients with acute leukemia and is primarily related to thrombocytopenia. In some patients, megakaryocytes are derived from the leukemic clone and produce platelets with abnormal functions. Petechiae and easy bruisability are common. Hemorrhage becomes increasingly common when the platelet count is less than 20×10^9 per liter, particularly in the setting of infection or coagulapathy, typically occurring from oral (particularly gingiva) and gastrointestinal mucous membranes. Spontaneous bleeding involving the CNS, lungs, or other viscera also may occur. Patients with APL, but also with other subtypes of AML, whose cells contain granules with procoagulant activity, often present with DIC with elevated prothrombin and partial thromboplastin times, low fibrinogen levels, and plasma fibrinogen split products.

Infection is a nearly universal complication of acute leukemia. The incidence of infection is inversely related to the number of circulating neutrophils and becomes a major risk in patients with neutrophil counts less than 0.5×10^9 per liter. Neutrophils derived from leukemic progenitors also may function abnormally, further compromising host defense. The leukemia and its treatment cause a breakdown of mucosal barriers, and systemic infections usually develop from organisms colonizing the skin, throat, and gastrointestinal tract. Common sites of infections in patients with acute leukemia include the blood, skin, gingiva, perirectal tissues, lung, and urinary tract. Septicemia often occurs without an apparent source. Gram-negative bacteria, gram-positive cocci, and *Candida* species are frequent pathogens, but often no positive cultures are obtained. Patients with ALL being treated with prednisone may harbor infection despite a lack of fever.

Hepatomegaly and splenomegaly due to leukemic infiltration are present in a majority of patients with ALL and a minority of patients with AML. Visceral involvement can produce symptoms of nausea, abdominal fullness, or early satiety. Lymphadenopathy is usually found in ALL and not commonly in AML. An anterior mediastinal mass is often present in patients with the T cell variant of ALL. Acute leukemia may infiltrate into extramedullary tissues such as the skin, lung, eye, gums, nasopharynx, kidneys, or nervous system, particularly with AML-M5 or ALL but in any patient at end stage. Testicular involvement at diagnosis or relapse is seen in males with ALL. Soft tissue masses of leukemic cells (*chloromas*) can develop in any location. Occasionally, extramedullary leukemia can precede detectable involvement in the bone marrow.

Symptoms related to the expanding malignant cell mass, such as bone pain and sternal tenderness, occur in approximately half of patients with acute leukemia; osteolytic lesions are rare. Renal abnormalities can develop as a result of leukemic infiltration, ureteral obstruction by uric acid stones or enlarged lymph nodes, urate nephropathy, or from infectious or hemorrhagic complications. Because of the rapid turnover of cells, especially during treatment, allopurinol and vigorous hydration with diuresis are usually instituted as soon as possible after diagnosis to prevent urate nephropathy and other manifestations of the "tumor lysis" syndrome. Alkalinization of the urine and careful monitoring for hyperphosphatemia, hypocalcemia, and hyperkalemia are indicated. The risk of metabolic complications with rapid tumor lysis after chemotherapy increases with the size of the tumor burden as well as in particular types of leukemia such as the ALL-L3, Burkitt's type.

The neoplastic cells may infiltrate into the subarachnoid space, causing leukemic meningitis or direct involvement of the brain or spinal cord parenchyma. Neurologic involvement is unusual at the time of diagnosis, but the CNS is a frequent site of relapse, particularly in patients with ALL. The first symptoms of leukemic meningitis may be headache, nausea, or cranial nerve palsies (especially cranial nerves III through VII). Papilledema, seizures, and altered mentation develop with disease progression. Cytocentrifuge preparations of cerebrospinal fluid (CSF) characteristically reveal leukemic blast cells; elevated CSF protein and reduced CSF glucose concentrations are seen.

Patients with acute leukemia often develop metabolic abnormalities. Hyponatremia and hypokalemia are possible due to renal tubular abnormalities induced by lysozyme or other products of the leukemic cells. The serum lactate dehydrogenase (LDH) level may be increased. The metabolic activity of large numbers of blasts can lead to artifactual reductions in results of laboratory tests, especially glucose and potassium concentrations and arterial blood oxygen levels. Hyperuricemia may be present due to accelerated turnover of cells with increased purine release; lactic acidosis occurs rarely in patients with a large burden of leukemic cells.

TREATMENT OF ACUTE LEUKEMIA   General considerations
The expansion of leukemic cells follows a Gompertzian growth curve with near exponential growth at a lower cell mass and progressive slowing of the growth rate at higher leukemic cell burdens. The leukemic mass is usually near 10^{12} cells at the time of diagnosis. Chemotherapeutic agents produce a fractional cell kill; that is, a percentage of tumor cells (not an absolute number) is killed with each course of treatment. Most chemotherapeutic regimens employed for acute leukemias are probably capable of a 3 to 5 log cell kill, resulting in the elimination of 99.9 to 99.999 percent of the leukemia cells.

The treatment of acute leukemia is classically divided into phases. *Remission induction chemotherapy* involving intensive systemic chemotherapy is administered with the goal of reducing the leukemic cell mass below the level of clinical detection. When the leukemic cell mass is reduced below approximately 10^9 to 10^{10} cells, leukemia can no longer be detected in the blood or bone marrow, and the patient appears to be in complete remission. The clinical criteria for complete remission include (1) less than 5 percent blasts in the bone marrow and absence of leukemic cells in the peripheral blood, (2) the restoration of normal peripheral blood counts, and (3) the absence of physical findings attributable to extramedullary involvement of the leukemia. If no further treatment is given, however, the residual leukemic cells will expand, leading to relapse. After remission is achieved, additional systemic chemotherapy must be given to further reduce the leukemic cell mass and, ideally, eradicate the leukemia. Intensive chemotherapy administered immediately following remission induction has been referred to as *consolidation* or *early intensification treatment*. Lower-dose chemotherapy that is generally continued over several years is referred to *maintenance treatment*. Local chemotherapy or radiation may be necessary to sites of frequent relapse (''sanctuary'' sites), such as the CNS, since systemic treatment may fail to eradicate disease in these areas.

Supportive care   The supportive care of patients with pancytopenia is a critical aspect of the treatment of acute leukemia, and this primarily involves the appropriate administration of blood products and management of infections. Newer approaches to supportive care involve the use of hematopoietic growth factors and hematopoietic stem cell support.

Adequate levels of hemoglobin can usually be maintained with transfusions of packed red blood cells. An adequate number of circulating platelets can initially be attained by transfusions of platelets from unselected donors, but many transfused patients eventually develop antiplatelet antibodies which shorten platelet survival and render the patient unresponsive to further platelet transfusions. Patients who fail to respond to transfusions of platelets from unselected donors may respond to platelets from an HLA-identical donor. The risk of spontaneous hemorrhage is directly related to the degree of thrombocytopenia. It is generally advisable to transfuse platelets to maintain the platelet count above 20×10^9 per liter, especially in the setting of fever, infections, or coagulapathy. Uterine bleeding should be minimized in menstruating women with thrombocytopenia by administering an anovulatory agent.

Previous data have indicated that survival is not improved by granulocyte transfusions either to prevent infections or to treat documented infections because of technical difficulty in collecting sufficient numbers of granulocytes from normal donors and the adverse effects associated with their transfusion, such as fever, leukoagglutination, pulmonary infiltrates, and transmission of cytomegalovirus (CMV) and other infections. Newer techniques for obtaining large numbers of granulocytes will allow a reexamination of their role in infection control in leukemia. Blood products given to patients with leukemia should be irradiated with 3000 cGy to prevent potential donor stem cell engraftment and graft-versus-host effects of live lymphocytes contaminating the transfusions. White cell filtering of platelet and red cell transfusions may reduce alloimmunization as well.

The prevention and treatment of infections are of critical importance in the management of patients with acute leukemia. Since most infections are caused by organisms colonizing the skin and gastrointestinal tract, a variety of approaches have been evaluated to suppress the endogenous flora in these sites. Most centers recommend the use of face masks, careful hand washing, and isolation for visitors of granulocytopenic patients. Oral absorbable and nonabsorbable antibiotics are widely used prophylactically. They have proven useful in the reduction of febrile episodes, but it has been argued that the marginal advantage is overbalanced by the development of resistant strains. The development of bacterial and fungal infections may be delayed or avoided by these measures.

Granulocytopenic patients who develop fever or other signs of infection require prompt evaluation and immediate treatment. Fever is usually due to a bacterial, fungal, or viral infection. Gram-negative sepsis is common in this setting and may be rapidly fatal. Granulocytopenic patients with unexplained fever or overt infections should receive empirical treatment for a presumed bacterial infection until a definitive diagnosis can be established. A combination of broad-spectrum antibiotics, such as an aminoglycoside or a third-generation cephalosporin, and a semisynthetic antipseudomonal penicillin should be employed and the antibiotic program modified when the results of bacterial and fungal cultures are available. Systemic fungal infections are also common in granulocytopenic patients with leukemia and should be suspected in patients after several days of fever or in those who fail to respond to antibiotics or who respond and develop recurrent fever. Definitive diagnosis of fungal infections may be difficult, and a therapeutic trial of amphotericin B is often indicated. The problem of infections in the immunocompromised host is discussed in Chap. 81.

TREATMENT OF ACUTE LYMPHOBLASTIC LEUKEMIA   Forty-five years ago ALL was uniformly fatal, and patients had a median survival of only 2 months. Therapy developed in the 1950s through the 1970s enabled more than 50 percent of children with ALL to achieve long-term remissions and probable cure. Adults and certain high-risk subgroups of children with ALL have a poorer prognosis, and long-term remissions are still only achieved in a minority of patients. Therapy for ALL consists of four parts: (1) remission induction chemotherapy, (2) CNS prophylaxis, (3) consolidation, and (4) maintenance therapy.

The combination of vincristine and prednisone with either L-asparaginase or daunorubicin induces complete remissions in over 90 percent of children with ALL within 4 weeks. Some patients with persistent leukemia may achieve remission with 2 to 4 additional weeks of treatment with the same or alternate drugs. Failure to achieve remission can be attributed primarily to the development of drug resistance, severe infections, or CNS leukemia.

In patients who achieve remission, prophylactic treatment to the CNS is required to prevent leukemic meningitis. Since the drugs used in remission induction in ALL generally penetrate poorly into the CSF, circulating leukemic cells that infiltrated into the CNS and CSF early in the course of the disease are sheltered from the effects of systemic chemotherapy. Over the ensuing months, these cells may proliferate, producing overt leukemic meningitis. Leukemic meningitis is the initial site of relapse in up to two-thirds of patients with ALL who do not receive prophylactic therapy. Prophylactic treatment to the CNS, instituted during or immediately after remission induction, has been successful in dramatically reducing the incidence of CNS relapse. Some centers employ 18- to 24-Gy whole-brain radiation in combination with intrathecal methotrexate. Cranial irradiation does produce subtle abnormalities in neurologic function and sometimes subacute necrotizing leukoencephalopathy, particularly in the youngest children, and there is considerable interest in evaluating chemotherapy-only regimens as alternative methods of CNS treatment. Preliminary data suggest that the combination of intrathecal and high-dose systemic methotrexate may provide adequate prophylactic treatment to the CNS.

Since patients in remission still harbor leukemia cells, further systemic treatment is required to prevent or delay leukemic relapse. The optimal approach to continuation therapy involves the administration of combination chemotherapy given in doses approaching maximal tolerance using 6-thioguanine, mercaptopurine, cytarabine, methotrexate, cyclophosphamide, doxorubicin, or etoposide. The combination of 6-mercaptopurine and methotrexate is the most frequently employed maintenance regimen, but more intensive consolidation and maintenance regimens with anthracyclines and cytosine arabinoside are used for adult patients and children with poor prognostic features.

The optimal duration of maintenance chemotherapy is unknown. Many patients can discontinue chemotherapy after 2 to 3 years and remain in long-term remission. Up to one-quarter of patients will relapse, however, after maintenance therapy is discontinued. It is not known whether maintenance therapy given for more than 3 years will further reduce the likelihood of relapse. Until widespread use of methods, such as PCR, to reliably detect small numbers of residual leukemic cells is available, there is no objective means to determine when therapy can be discontinued safely.

Complications of therapy for ALL Chemotherapy-induced myelosuppression and immunosuppression are inevitable immediate side effects of the treatment of ALL. The chemotherapy directed toward the leukemic lymphoblasts also affects normal T and B lymphocytes, resulting in lymphocytopenia and immunodeficiency. Peripheral blood B cells generally recover to normal levels within several months after treatment is discontinued, but T cell numbers and function may remain depressed for up to 1 year. *Pneumocystis carinii* pneumonia can occur while patients are in remission, and trimethoprim-sulfamethoxazole prophylaxis is effective in preventing this complication. Viral infections such as herpes simplex and zoster, measles, and cytomegalovirus are common. Growth in children is somewhat retarded during the administration of chemotherapy. Catch-up growth generally occurs once therapy is discontinued, and most children ultimately attain near-normal height and weight. Sterility may result from treatment with most chemotherapeutic agents and irradiation. Gonadal function may recover after a prolonged interval. The gonads in prepubertal patients are relatively resistant to the effects of chemotherapy, and most patients undergo normal puberty after therapy is discontinued. Late complications also include CNS and neuroendocrinologic disorders that can result from cranial irradiation, secondary cancers and myeloid leukemias that may occur after both irradiation and chemotherapy, and cardiac problems from toxic drugs.

Prognosis in ALL A number of characteristics of ALL have been identified as having a prognostic impact; as therapies are tailored to specific subgroups of patients, though, these characteristics may lose their importance. The factors most affecting prognosis are age, leukemic cell DNA content (ploidy), immunophenotype, the leukocyte count at the time of diagnosis, and specific cytogenetic abnormalities. Children between the ages of 3 and 9 years with white blood counts less than 10×10^9 per liter have the best prognosis; 50 to 70 percent achieve long-term survival and probable cure with current treatment. Older patients and those with higher leukocyte counts have a poorer prognosis. Fewer than 30 percent of adults with ALL are long-term survivors in most series, and it is uncertain whether the maintenance therapy that is effective in children is of benefit in adults. Males have a worse prognosis than females; L1 subtype, which is less often seen

in adults, gives a better prognosis than the L2 form. With regard to immunophenotype, patients with cells marking for CD10 (CALLA-positive) have the best prognosis; the T cell phenotype is a better prognostic indicator in adults but not children, whereas the B cell (L3) variant of ALL has the worst prognosis.

Chromosomal abnormalities provide independent prognostic information. Approximately one-half the patients with ALL have detectable cytogenetic abnormalities, including hypodiploidy, pseudodiploidy, or hyperdiploidy. A number of nonrandom chromosomal abnormalities are associated with ALL. Between 10 and 40 percent of patients with ALL have the Philadelphia (Ph) chromosome t(9;22), with the incidence rising with age. Patients with certain translocations, such as t(8;14), t(4;11), and t(9;22) have a poor prognosis; patients with hyperdiploidy have a better prognosis.

Remission and survival rates in adult patients with ALL (those over 15 years of age) are significantly lower than for children with the same disease. Remission induction rates in adults and high-risk children are generally between 50 and 70 percent following treatment with vincristine, prednisone, and daunorubicin; the median duration of remission is 10 to 20 months, and the 5-year survival rate is 20 to 30 percent with standard chemotherapy. Several centers have reported improved results in high-risk children and in adults with more intensive, multiple-drug consolidation and maintenance programs and allogeneic bone marrow transplant, but the optimal therapy for high-risk forms of ALL is uncertain.

Treatment of recurrent ALL Leukemia may recur either in the bone marrow or in extramedullary sites. Patients who relapse while receiving maintenance therapy have a very poor prognosis with little possibility of a long-term second remission. Combination chemotherapy with a three- or four-drug regimen including vincristine, prednisone, L-asparaginase, and/or daunorubicin results in a second remission in 50 to 70 percent of these patients, and these patients should be considered for bone marrow transplantation. Remission duration, however, is usually brief, and subsequent relapse is inevitable. Patients who relapse after discontinuation of maintenance therapy have a better prognosis. Second remissions can be induced in about 90 percent of these patients. Although most will relapse again, some have achieved long-term survival. These patients should probably have chemotherapeutic CNS prophylaxis repeated to prevent recurrent disease in this extramedullary site.

Meningeal leukemia is the most common site of extramedullary relapse in patients with ALL. Cranial irradiation plus intrathecal methotrexate alone or in combination with cytarabine is the standard therapy for CNS leukemia. Ommaya reservoirs to deliver chemotherapy into ventricular CSF are usually placed surgically in patients with ALL. Testicular relapse is common in male patients with ALL and may occur during or after cessation of maintenance therapy. The treatment of choice is irradiation of the affected testicle. Patients with extramedullary relapse involving the CNS, testes, or other tissues are at very high risk for subsequent relapse in the bone marrow. Systemic reinduction therapy is indicated and may prevent generalized relapse of ALL.

TREATMENT OF ACUTE MYELOGENOUS LEUKEMIA AML cells derive from early hematopoietic progenitors, and the drugs active in AML have marginal selectivity for leukemic cells over their normal bone marrow counterparts. Induction of severe myelosuppression is necessary in order to achieve a complete remission. The combination of cytarabine with anthracyclines such as daunorubicin or demethoxy-daunorubicin results in a complete remission rate of 60 to 80 percent in patients under 60 years of age who have not had a myelodysplastic preleukemic state. Mitoxantrone or amsacrine may be substituted for the anthracycline. If residual leukemia is present 2 to 4 weeks after chemotherapy, the same treatment is often repeated. Patients who fail to enter remission with this approach have a poor prognosis.

Patients with AML who achieve complete remission still have substantial residual leukemia. Further therapy is required therefore to treat the occult disease. The benefits of available forms of consolidation and maintenance treatment are controversial. The best results have been achieved in patients receiving two to three intensive cycles of consolidation chemotherapy similar to the induction regimen. Median remission duration varies from 9 months to 2 years in most series. Between 10 and 30 percent of patients survive over 5 years free of disease, and most of these patients are probably cured. Somewhat better results have been reported in preliminary studies using very intensive consolidation regimens, including high-dose cytarabine alone or in combination with other drugs. Prospective, controlled studies have reported no benefit for patients receiving maintenance treatments. Current data suggest that the major benefit in therapy is achieved with intensive induction and consolidation treatment.

Most patients who achieve complete remission will ultimately relapse, usually in the first 2 years. At that point, the disease is less responsive to therapy, and median survival is 3 to 6 months.

CNS leukemia in AML occurs in 10 to 20 percent of patients at some point in their disease and most commonly develops in patients with monocytic (M5) or myelomonocytic (M4) subtypes or at terminal stages. Unlike ALL, the CNS is rarely an isolated site of relapse in AML. CNS involvement usually occurs in the setting of systemic relapse, and prophylactic treatment to the CNS has not improved remission duration or survival. Patients who develop meningeal leukemia are treated with cranial irradiation and/or intrathecal chemotherapy with cytarabine and/or methotrexate.

Prognostic factors in AML Chromosomal abnormalities in AML are of prognostic value; patients with abnormalities such as t(8;21), t(15;17), or inv(16) tend to have a better prognosis than average, while −5, −7, t(9;22), and complex chromosomal abnormalities are associated with a poor prognosis.

Age is a major prognostic factor in many series; unfortunately, half of patients with AML are over 60 years of age. Patients over 60 years of age are less likely to achieve complete remission or to tolerate intensive therapy well and may be more difficult to support through the complications of pancytopenia. In addition, elderly patients are more likely to have leukemic cells with poor-risk chromosomal abnormalities such as −7 and −5 and often have a prior myelodysplastic or preleukemic syndrome. Elderly patients who do achieve remission, however, have a similar remission duration and survival as younger patients. Since the major factor influencing survival is the achievement of complete remission, intensive chemotherapy should be administered to most elderly patients, with careful attention to supportive care.

The AML leukemic subtype is of modest prognostic significance. Acute promyelocytic leukemia (M3) is typically associated with DIC; fatal CNS hemorrhage may complicate remission induction chemotherapy for this type of leukemia. *trans*-Retinoic acid differentiation therapy can induce complete remissions in this subtype and is rapidly replacing chemotherapy as the initial induction treatment. DIC is best treated with frequent platelet transfusions, as many as 6 to 12 units per day, and 2 to 4 units of fresh plasma daily, to replace lost coagulation factors and inhibitors until the fibrinogen is normalized and the white blood cell count reduced. Heparin and ε-amino caproic acid therapy remain controversial, but heparin is often used in conjunction with the preceding supportive measures. Patients with promyelocytic leukemia who do achieve remission appear to have a greater chance of long-term survival than other subgroups. Patients with erythroleukemia or monocytic or myelomonocytic leukemia, with the exception of the M4 eosinophilic variant associated with inv(16), may have a poorer prognosis than the M1 to M3 subgroups.

Patients with preleukemia or myelodysplastic syndromes evolving into AML or therapy-related leukemias respond poorly to chemotherapy; less than half of these patients achieve complete remission. Such patients also tend to have prolonged bone marrow aplasia following treatment and often succumb to complications of pancytopenia. Patients who do achieve remission have a remission duration similar to patients with de novo AML, and intensive induction therapy is usually indicated. No treatment has been consistently effective during the preleukemic phase, and intensive chemotherapy should be withheld until progressive overt leukemia develops. Efforts to treat preleuke-

mias with low doses of cytarabine, 5-azacytidine, and differentiating agents such as hexamethylene bisacetamide or retinoic acid occasionally lead to clinical improvement, but improvement in survival has not yet been documented. Studies with hematopoietic hormones such as granulocyte-macrophage or granulocyte colony stimulating factor (G-CSF, GM-CSF) suggest utility for this class of agents to improve granulopoiesis in myelodysplastic syndromes, and high-dose erythropoietin may stimulate increased red cell production. Patients who develop acute leukemia after a preexisting myeloproliferative disorder or paroxysmal nocturnal hemoglobinuria usually have a poor prognosis.

Patients who receive cytotoxic chemotherapy with or without concomitant radiation therapy have an increased risk of developing AML. Secondary or treatment-related leukemia is most commonly associated with prolonged therapy with alkylating agents, nitrosoureas, or procarbazine and has been seen primarily in patients with Hodgkin's disease, myeloma, and ovarian carcinoma. Almost all patients with treatment-related AML have chromosomal abnormalities, usually hypodiploidy with −5 and/or −7. These patients typically develop a preleukemic syndrome with pancytopenia several months before overt AML is recognized. They respond poorly to chemotherapy, and despite treatment, few survive more than 1 year.

BONE MARROW TRANSPLANTATION FOR ACUTE LEUKEMIA

Bone marrow transplantation from an identical twin or an HLA-identical sibling donor after intensive therapy is effective treatment for both ALL and AML. The objective of this approach is to administer very high doses of chemotherapy alone or with total-body irradiation and then to rescue the patient from severe myelosuppression by the transplantation of bone marrow from a normal donor. In addition, the transplantation of allogeneic bone marrow may confer an immune-mediated graft-versus-leukemia effect. Hence syngeneic (twin-donated) and T cell–depleted allogeneic marrow transplants generally result in a higher rate of relapse. The current results with bone marrow transplantation are summarized in Table 310-4. The principles of bone marrow transplantation are discussed in detail in Chap. 313.

Allogeneic bone marrow transplantation is associated with substantial risks. Approximately one-third of patients conventionally transplanted for leukemia will die from transplant-related complications, including graft-versus-host disease (GVHD), interstitial pneumonitis, and opportunistic infections. By depleting T cells from the donor marrow graft, these complications can be markedly reduced, but the relapse and graft failure rates climb so that long-term survival is largely unchanged. Most centers limit the use of bone marrow transplantation to patients under 60 years of age, since older patients generally have a poor outcome largely due to complications of GVHD and infection. Reports from several centers indicate that up to 30 percent of otherwise end-stage patients with refractory acute leukemia or patients with secondary leukemias have achieved long-term disease-

TABLE 310-4   Representative results of bone marrow transplantation (BMT) compared with conventional chemotherapy for AML and ALL

	Survival >3 years, %		
	Allo-BMT	Auto-BMT	Chemotherapy
ACUTE MYELOGENOUS LEUKEMIA			
First remission	30–70	30–60	20–50
Second remission or early relapse	30–50	20–40	<10
Third remission or relapse	10–30	20	0
ACUTE LYMPHOCYTIC LEUKEMIA			
First remission	40–60	20–40	10–50
Second remission or early relapse	20–40	20–30	<10
Third remission or relapse	10–20		0

free survival and probable cure following bone marrow transplantation. Although only a small proportion of patients in this category benefit, the results compare favorably with those obtained with other forms of treatment.

Survival figures are improved substantially when bone marrow transplantation is performed during remission, the burden of leukemic cells is low, and the patients are in relatively good general condition (see Table 310-4). In young patients with AML, transplantation in first remission is often recommended, but overall results are not consistently superior to intensive chemotherapy. Transplantation in *early first relapse* or *second remission* may be equally effective, but patients may be in poorer overall condition. Because many children with ALL can achieve a prolonged initial remission with chemotherapy, bone marrow transplantation has generally been reserved for patients in *second remission*; in this group, 30 to 60 percent have achieved prolonged survival with marrow transplantation. It is not clear that transplantation of most adults in *first remission* of ALL is more advantageous than intensive chemotherapy. Discussions regarding the time of bone marrow transplant in ALL relate to the likelihood of relapse.

Approximately 30 percent of patients with AML transplanted in *early relapse* or *second remission* have achieved long-term survival. There is controversy, though, as to whether patients with AML should receive allogeneic bone marrow transplantation or postremission chemotherapy while in *first* complete remission. Patients at high risk for relapse after chemotherapy, such as those with certain poor-risk karyotypes or with secondary leukemias, should probably be transplanted. For other patients, it is clear that the risk of recurrent leukemia is lower following bone marrow transplantation than with postremission chemotherapy; however, the transplanted patients usually represent a highly selected group. In addition, bone marrow transplantation is more likely to be associated with fatal treatment complications. In all patients, 3- or 5-year survival is 40 to 60 percent with bone marrow transplantation compared with 10 to 50 percent survival achieved with optimal chemotherapy. Patient age is a major prognostic factor with bone marrow transplantation, and the better results have been reported in children and young adults. Although young patients have better results with allogeneic bone marrow transplantation than with chemotherapy, this is less true for patients over 30 years of age. Of note is that the median age of patients with AML is 60. One major limitation of bone marrow transplantation as a general therapeutic approach is that only a minority of patients are eligible; most patients are either too old to be considered or lack an HLA-identical related donor. Recently, several large registries of potential unrelated donors have been formed, and bone marrow transplants from unrelated histocompatible donors are under active evaluation.

Autologous bone marrow transplantation also has been evaluated in patients with acute leukemia. With this approach, remission bone marrow is collected and cryopreserved. The patient may then receive intensive chemoradiotherapy followed by reinfusion of the cryopreserved bone marrow. Since remission bone marrow is likely to contain small numbers of residual leukemic cells, many centers have treated the collected marrow with antileukemic monoclonal antibodies or chemotherapy prior to cryopreservation in an attempt to "purge" residual leukemic cells. Autologous transplantation has the advantage of not requiring a matched donor and the lack of GVHD complications; thus a much larger group of patients is eligible for treatment by this approach. A disadvantage is the far higher rate of relapse. Selected patients with AML transplanted in first or second remission have achieved prolonged survival, but further studies are required to critically assess the efficacy of autologous versus allogeneic marrow transplantation for acute leukemia. Furthermore, neither the efficacy nor best methods of ex vivo treatment of the collected bone marrow to eradicate contaminating malignant cells have been demonstrated conclusively.

Because of the pace of advances in supportive care, methods of manipulating or modifying the graft-versus-leukemia effect and GVHD, newer purging methods in autologous transplantation, as well as more intensive nontransplant approaches with growth factor rescue, recommendations for the optimal therapy of acute leukemia are changing.

IMMUNOTHERAPY FOR ACUTE LEUKEMIAS Immunotherapy for acute leukemia has included the use of monoclonal antibodies that react with cell surface antigens on leukemia blasts, cytokine activation of cellular immunity, and nonspecific immunostimulatory agents. Clinical trials with nonspecific immune potentiating agents such as bacillus Calmette-Guerin (BCG), *Corynebacterium parvum*, or levamisole have not shown a benefit in prolonging the duration of remission. Interleukin 2–activated natural killer cells (LAK cells) have shown activity in reducing residual disease but not large leukemia burdens. Monoclonal antibodies to myeloid antigens have been apparently as effective at purging AML cells from autologous marrow ex vivo before reinfusion as ex vivo chemotherapy. Similar approaches to ALL therapy using antibodies to B cell antigens are also under investigation. Radiolabeled monoclonal antibodies to AML also have shown considerable antileukemic activity in vivo. At this time, the value of specific immunotherapy for acute leukemia remains to be proven in large trials.

SUMMARY AND FUTURE DIRECTIONS IN ACUTE LEUKEMIA Effective induction chemotherapy capable of inducing remission in most patients with ALL and AML is now available, but long-term survival is still achieved in only a minority of patients owing to the presence of residual leukemia. In the next decade, a focus of clinical research will be directed toward measures to prolong the duration of remission by use of innovative methods of consolidation treatment. This may include intensive chemotherapy or high-dose chemoradiotherapy with growth factor rescue, stem cell support, or bone marrow transplantation. It also will be important to develop effective, selective immunologic approaches that are capable of eliminating residual leukemic cells, such as antibody-based strategies, or vaccines against leukemia-associated oncogenic proteins, which may promote long-term active immunosuppression of relapse. For the success of these newer approaches, sensitive methods to detect and follow the presence of residual leukemia are needed in order to guide therapy. Already such PCR methods are available for the translocations causing CML and APL and for the immunoglobulin rearrangements seen in certain cases of ALL. Another aim of research will be the use of specific treatments tailored to individual types of leukemias stratified according to their genotype and immunophenotype.

CHRONIC LYMPHOCYTIC LEUKEMIA

Chronic lymphocytic leukemia (CLL) is a neoplasm of activated B lymphocytes. The CLL cells, which morphologically resemble mature, small lymphocytes of the peripheral blood, accumulate in the bone marrow, blood, lymph nodes, and spleen in large numbers. The disease is usually seen in patients over 50 years of age, but improved diagnosis has identified many younger patients. CLL is the most common form of leukemia in the United States and is more frequent in males than females. The CLL cells commonly have trisomy 12 alone or with additional chromosomal abnormalities. Clonality also can be demonstrated by expression of a single light chain (κ or λ) or immunoglobulin idiotype specificity. Rarely, cells that appear to be chronic lymphoid leukemias may be of T cell or NK cell origin. These less common varieties include diseases formerly known as T-CLL but are actually large granular lymphocytic leukemias, T suppressor leukemia, adult T cell leukemia, and T prolymphocytic leukemias. An unusual type of T cell CLL is seen in patients with ataxia-telangiectasia and is often associated with a translocation of genetic material between the number 14 chromosomes (t14;14).

The diagnosis of CLL usually can be made on the basis of physical examination and a review of the peripheral blood smear. Lymphocytosis is usually present, and the malignant cells characteristically appear as morphologically normal small lymphocytes (see Fig.

A9-23). The dual expression of B cell antigens (CD19, CD20, CD21, CD24) with a T cell antigen (CD5) on the cells is usually diagnostic of CLL. In most cases, a monoclonal immunoglobulin can be demonstrated on the cell surface, although immunofluorescent staining is relatively weak. Monoclonal surface IgM with or without IgD and occasionally IgG is characteristically present, and a small amount of this IgM paraprotein can often be detected in the serum with sensitive techniques. CLL cells have Fc receptors and the second complement receptor (CD21). Most patients develop some degree of hypogammaglobulinemia. Approximately 3 percent of patients with lymphoproliferative disorders have a T cell or, rarely, NK cell neoplasm. The neoplastic T cells form rosettes with sheep erythrocytes, in contrast to the mouse red cell rosettes formed by the more common B cell CLL. T cell CLL usually cannot be distinguished from B cell CLL morphologically, but expression of T cell markers is easily detected by flow cytometry. NK cell leukemias stain for CD16, and the neoplastic lymphocytes are usually granular.

DIFFERENTIAL DIAGNOSIS   It is important to distinguish early CLL from reactive lymphocytosis in asymptomatic patients. In reactive lymphocytosis, the cells are polyclonal and predominantly T lymphocytes, whereas in CLL they are always B cells. The demonstration of monoclonal surface membrane immunoglobulin unambiguously defines a B cell lymphocytosis as neoplastic. Chronic T cell leukemias must be distinguished from Sézary syndrome, where the cells have a characteristic lobulated nucleus and there usually is extensive skin involvement. Chronic T cell leukemias also must be distinguished from adult T cell leukemia (ATL) associated with HTLV-I. Prolymphocytic and prolymphocytoid leukemias are CLL variants seen in older people and are characterized by massive splenomegaly, often in the absence of lymphadenopathy. The neoplastic cell in these prolymphocytic leukemias is also usually of B cell origin, and it is larger than that seen in CLL, with prominent nucleolus. Prolymphocytic leukemia is typically associated with very high white blood cell counts (in excess of 200×10^9 per liter) and a poor response to therapy. Occasionally, diffuse or follicular lymphomas involving the marrow or spleen can spill out into the blood and mimic CLL morphologically. However, the cells often have a clefted nucleus, brightly staining cell surface monoclonal immunoglobulin, and the absence of CD5 staining. Lymphomas at this stage are typically far more aggressive. Splenic villous lymphomas typically cause splenomegaly, a plasma protein monoclonal band, and lower white blood cell counts than CLL. The cells have a small nucleolus and short villi. Unlike hairy cell leukemia, these cells are negative for tartrate-resistant acid phosphatase (TRAP) and CD25. Hairy cell leukemia is distinguished from CLL on the basis of the typical cellular morphology, markers such as CD25, and the presence of tartrate-resistant acid phosphatase in the hairy cells. Waldenström's macroglobulinemia is differentiated from CLL on the basis of bone marrow morphology and lower white blood cell counts, CD38 positivity, cytoplasmic Ig, and the secretion of a large amount of a monoclonal IgM paraprotein. Small lymphocytic lymphomas (diffuse well-differentiated lymphomas) are morphologically and immunophenotypically the same as CLL and appear to represent a different clinical variant of the same neoplasm.

CLINICAL FEATURES   The diagnosis of B-CLL is usually made when there is a minimum of 5×10^9 mature-appearing lymphocytes per liter of blood and 30 percent infiltration of the marrow with B cell phenotype cells bearing CD5. In more than 25 percent of patients with CLL, the disorder is discovered as an incidental finding. The common practice of ordering routine complete blood counts in adults has led to an earlier diagnosis of CLL in asymptomatic patients. The signs and symptoms of CLL usually relate to tissue infiltration, peripheral blood cytopenias, or immunosuppression. Patients may present with symptoms of anemia, lymph node enlargement, or intercurrent infection. Splenomegaly seldom leads to symptoms, and the liver is minimally enlarged in only about half of patients. The clinical course is quite variable, and prognosis is correlated directly with stage (see Table 310-4).

In CLL, the white blood cell count ranges between 5×10^9 and 200×10^9 per liter, with a preponderance of mature-appearing lymphocytes. There is little correlation between the leukocyte count and symptoms except at very high tumor burdens. Patients with advanced disease may present with anemia, granulocytopenia, and thrombocytopenia resulting from bone marrow infiltration by the leukemic cells. About 20 percent of patients develop a Coombs-positive autoimmune hemolytic anemia during the course of their disease. Occasionally, autoimmune thrombocytopenia or pure red cell aplasia occurs. CLL may evolve into an aggressive lymphocytic lymphoma (diffuse large cell lymphoma) referred to as *Richter's syndrome*, which may be due to a clonal evolution of the original leukemia.

TREATMENT   Because of the indolent nature of CLL, few attempts have been made at curative therapy. Typically, agents are given for disease control, although a number of centers are exploring strategies with curative intent. Experimental regimens have not yet prolonged survival significantly. Among a number of prognostic classifications of CLL that have been employed, the international classification is quite useful (Table 310-5). Patients with early-stage disease, limited to lymphocytosis alone or lymphocytosis plus limited lymphadenopathy, have a good prognosis. Patients with A(0) disease, characterized only by lymphocytosis without other poor prognostic signs, are unlikely to need therapy or die of CLL. Median survival exceeds 10 years; these patients usually require no treatment, and treatment may even be detrimental. Patients with more substantial lymphadenopathy and hepatosplenomegaly have an intermediate prognosis with a median survival of approximately 5 years. Patients with anemia or thrombocytopenia have a worse prognosis, with a median survival of less than 3 years. The value of these prognostic groups is changing as better therapies are used increasingly. In addition to the clinical staging classification, several other features have been proposed as prognostic indicators. Poorer prognosis is associated with an initial blood lymphocyte count of 50,000 per microliter or more, a lymphocyte count doubling time of under 12 months, complex chromosomal abnormalities, and a diffuse marrow infiltration pattern.

The indications for therapy in CLL include hemolytic anemia, important cytopenias, disfiguring lymphadenopathy, symptomatic organomegaly, or marked systemic symptoms. When treatment is required, the cornerstone of therapy is usually an alkylating agent. Chlorambucil is the most frequently prescribed drug for CLL, utilizing either small daily doses or a larger pulse every 3 to 6 weeks. Daily or pulse cyclophosphamide appears to be as effective as chlorambucil in the treatment of CLL. Maintenance therapy has no definite value, and continuing alkylating agent therapy may increase the risk of

TABLE 310-5   International workshop on CLL staging classification*

Stage	Description	Median survival, years
A	Lymphocytosis with clinical involvement of fewer than 3 lymph node groups[†]; no anemia or thrombocytopenia	8–10 or more
	A(0) No nodes enlarged	
	A(I) Nodes enlarged	
	A(II) Hepatomegaly or splenomegaly	
B	More than 3 lymph node groups[†] involved. No anemia or thrombocytopenia	5–6
	B(I) Nodes enlarged	
	B(II) Hepatomegaly or splenomegaly	
C	Anemia or thrombocytopenia regardless of number of lymph node groups involved	2.5
	C(III) Anemia	
	C(IV) Thrombocytopenia	

* This represents a combination of the Binet classification (A,B,C) with the Rai classification (0,I,II,III,IV).
† Lymph node groups—cervical, axillary, inguinal, liver, spleen.

future development of AML. Three newer drugs useful in the treatment of CLL include deoxycoformycin, 2-chlorodeoxyadenosine, and fludarabine monophosphate. These agents have considerable antileukemia activity, even in prior-treated patients. Fludarabine is now approved for therapy of CLL and is as effective as alkylating agent therapy in both treated and untreated patients, with response rates of 50 to 80 percent. Similarly, 2-chlorodeoxyadenosine is sometimes effective in fludarabine-resistant disease.

Glucocorticoids are useful for CLL in special circumstances, such as in the treatment of associated Coombs-positive hemolytic anemia or immune thrombocytopenia, and may be transiently effective in treating patients with pancytopenia and the "packed marrow" syndrome. Glucocorticoids have important side effects, including a predisposition to opportunistic infection, and should not routinely be used in CLL. In advanced CLL unresponsive to fludarabine and 2-chlorodeoxyadenosine, combination chemotherapy as used in lymphoma may be useful. Regimens that include an alkylating agent, vincristine, doxorubicin, and prednisone are often employed. Splenectomy may be indicated in patients with hypersplenism, refractory hemolytic anemia, or thrombocytopenia. Radiation therapy occasionally may be useful for palliating localized disease or hypersplenism in the aged. Experimental therapies such as allogeneic bone marrow transplantation, interferon α, interleukin 2, and monoclonal antibodies to cell surface antigens such as CD5, CD19, CD20, CD52, and CD25 used alone or conjugated to isotopes or toxins are currently under study with occasionally encouraging results. Hypogammaglobulinemia is common in patients with CLL, and life-threatening infectious complications may occur. Intravenous Ig preparations are effective in prophylaxis against recurrent infections, but the cost is high.

HAIRY CELL LEUKEMIA

Hairy cell leukemia is a rare lymphoid neoplasm characterized by peripheral blood cytopenias, splenomegaly, and morphologically typical malignant cells in the blood and bone marrow. Hairy cell leukemia is usually seen in male patients over 40 years of age. The disease is now recognized with increased frequency, and many large series have been reported. Hairy cell leukemia has been reported to occur worldwide.

Although originally referred to as *leukemic reticuloendotheliosis*, the term *hairy cell leukemia* is now widely accepted because it is descriptive of the characteristic cytoplasmic projections seen on the leukemic cell. The disorder is nearly always due to expansion of neoplastic B lymphocytes which express and often produce monoclonal immunoglobulin. Rare T cell variants which may represent a related disorder, including one case associated with the human retrovirus HTLV-II, have been described.

CLINICAL FEATURES AND PATHOLOGY Patients with hairy cell leukemia usually present with symptoms due to splenomegaly, pancytopenia, infection caused by impaired host defense, or vasculitis. Many asymptomatic patients are detected on routine complete blood counts. More than three-quarters of patients will have palpable splenomegaly, and in some cases splenic involvement is massive. Lymphadenopathy is rare, and substantial hepatomegaly is uncommon at the time of diagnosis, although infiltration of the portal triads by hairy cells is often seen microscopically. Occasionally, bone lesions may cause hip pain. Approximately 30 percent of patients with hairy cell leukemia have an associated vasculitis-like disorder. Common manifestations include erythema nodosum and cutaneous nodules due to perivasculitis. Visceral involvement similar to polyarteritis nodosa may occur.

Moderate pancytopenia is usually present at diagnosis. The leukocyte count is normal or low, and characteristic hairy cells are seen in the peripheral blood. These cells are about 15 to 20 μm in diameter and have an eccentrically placed nucleus with foamy cytoplasm. Cytoplasmic projections (hairs) may be seen on smear, but they are best appreciated by phase microscopy. These cells are

TRAP-positive. The cells stain with antibodies to B cell antigens and often CD25, the interleukin 2 receptor, an activation antigen. Bone marrow aspiration is often unsuccessful because of reticulin fibrosis. The biopsy typically shows replacement of the normal architecture by mononuclear cells that are not packed together but maintain spaces between the intercellular contacts. Splenic histology is typical, consisting of mononuclear cell infiltration of the red pulp and engorgement of the sinuses.

Hairy cell leukemia must be distinguished from chronic lymphocytic leukemia, prolymphocytic leukemia, splenic villous lymphoma, and Waldenström's macroglobulinemia. Some patients with hairy cell leukemia present with a hypocellular bone marrow which may be misdiagnosed as aplastic anemia or with an inaspirable marrow leading to confusion with primary myelofibrosis. The diagnosis depends on identifying the characteristic cells in the bone marrow and peripheral blood.

TREATMENT OF HAIRY CELL LEUKEMIA The course of hairy cell leukemia can be quite indolent; however, there is a wide spectrum of severity and rate of progression of the disease among patients. Approximately one-quarter of patients present without significant symptoms or complications of the disease; these patients require no immediate treatment. They should be followed at intervals and observed closely for infections. Infection is the primary cause of death in patients with hairy cell leukemia. Common infections include *Legionella* pneumonitis, toxoplasmosis, tuberculosis, and atypical mycobacterial disease, nocardiosis, and pyogenic infections. Patients probably benefit from pneumonococcal vaccination. Any significant fever should be evaluated thoroughly and treated aggressively with antibiotics. Since *Legionella* pneumonitis is relatively common in these patients, high-dose erythromycin should be administered to patients with pulmonary infiltrates.

Therapy directed at the leukemia is indicated in patients with pancytopenia, recurrent infections, symptomatic splenomegaly, autoimmune complications, or disease progression. Formerly, the cornerstone of therapy was splenectomy, which appeared to ameliorate the disease in a majority of patients. Splenectomy is now rarely performed except in situations where life-threatening cytopenias must be corrected immediately. Three drugs that are highly active in inducing remissions are now available: interferon α, deoxycoformycin (Pentostatin), and 2-chlorodeoxyadenosine (2CDA). Virtually all treated patients respond to interferon α, with about 70 percent achieving major hematologic benefit. Complete remissions are rare, but retreatment of recurrent disease is often successful. Pentostatin is also highly active in hairy cell leukemia, even in patients who have failed interferon-α, and often induces complete remissions. The most important new agent is 2CDA. 2CDA has an extremely high complete response rate of over 80 percent and a very low rate of relapse. Although additional follow-up is needed, this latter agent may be curative in some patients after a single course of therapy. When approved for use by the U.S. Food and Drug Administration, 2CDA will probably be the treatment of choice.

Short courses of glucocorticoids may be useful in controlling the vasculitis or autoimmune manifestations that are often associated with the disease but are not indicated as primary therapy. G-CSF may be useful during neutropenic periods. The prognosis in hairy cell leukemia is excellent, and prognosis-based published series are outdated because of the rapid recent improvements in treatment, including the application of interferon, deoxycoformycin, and 2CDA and better supportive care.

REFERENCES

General

CLARKSON B: New pharmacologic approaches to treatment of leukemia. Semin Oncol 28:99, 1991

FOON K, TODD R: Immunologic classification of leukemia and lymphoma. Blood 68:1, 1986

GOLDE DW: The stem cell. Sci Am 265:86, 1991

MANDELLI F (ed): Therapy of actue leukemias. Leukemia 6(suppl 2):1 1992

SCHEINBERG DA: Current applications of monoclonal antibodies for the therapy of hematopoietic cancers. Curr Opin Immunol 3:679, 1991

SCHIFFER CA: Interferon studies in the treatment of patients with leukemia. Semin Oncol 18:1, 1991

ALL

CHAMPLIN R, GALE RP: Acute lymphoblastic leukemia: Recent advances in biology and therapy. Blood 73:2051, 1989

HOELZER D et al: Prognostic factors in a multicenter study for treatment of acute lymphoblastic leukemia in adults. Blood 71:123, 1988

HOROWITZ MM et al: Chemotherapy compared with bone marrow transplantation for adults with acute lymphoblastic leukemia in first remission. Ann Intern Med 115:13, 1991

LIPSHULTZ SE et al: Late cardiac effects of doxorubicin therapy for acute lymphoblastic leukemia in childhood. N Engl J Med 325:808, 1991

NEGLIA JP et al: Second neoplasms after acute lymphoblastic leukemia in childhood. N Engl J Med 325:1330, 1991

PUI C-H: Acute myeloid leukemia in children treated with epipodophyllotoxins for acute lymphoblastic leukemia. N Engl J Med 325:1682, 1991

——— et al: Biology and clinical significance of cytogenetic abnormalities in childhood acute lymphoblastic leukemia. Blood 76:1449, 1990

RIVERA GK, MAUER AM: Controversies in the management of childhood acute lymphoblastic leukemia: Treatment intensification, CNS leukemia, and prognostic factors. Semin Hematol 24:12, 1987

VAN DER PLAS DC et al: Prognostic significancer of karyotype at diagnosis in childhood acute lymphoblastic anemia. Leukemia 6:176, 1992

AML

APPELBAUM FR et al: Chemotherapy versus marrow transplantation for adults with acute nonlymphocytic leukemia: A five-year follow-up. Blood 72:179, 1988

BAGBY GC: The preleukemic syndrome (hematopoietic dysplasia). Blood Rev 2:194, 1988

BENNETT JM et al: Proposal for a recognition of minimally differentiated acute myeloid leukaemia (AML-MO). Br J Hematol 78:325, 1991

FOON KA, GALE RP: Therapy of acute myelogenous leukemia. Blood Rev 6:15, 1992

RODEGHIERO F et al: Early deaths and anti-hemorrhagic treatments in acute promyelocytic leukemia: A GIMEMA retrospective study in 286 consecutive patients. Blood 75:2112, 1990

WARRELL RP JR et al: Differentiation therapy of acute promyelocytic leukemia with tretinoin (all-*trans* retinoic acid). N Engl J Med 324:1385, 1991

CLL

BENNETT JM et al: Proposals for the classification of chronic (mature) B and T lymphoid leukaemias. J Clin Pathol 42:567, 1989

CHUN HG et al: Fludarabine phosphate: A synthetic purine antimetabolite with significant activity against lymphoid malignancies. J Clin Oncol 9:175, 1991

DIGHIERO G et al: B-cell chronic lymphocytic leukemia: Present status and future directions. Blood 78:1901, 1991

KEATING MJ et al: Fludarabine: A new agent with marked cytoreductive activity in untreated chronic lymphocytic leukemia. J Clin Oncol 9:44, 1991

TEFFERI A, PHYLIKY RL: A clinical update on chronic lymphocytic leukemia. II. Critical analysis of current chemotherapeutic modalities. Mayo Clin Proc 67:457, 1992

Hairy cell leukemia

DURRELMAN S et al: 2'-Deoxycoformycin after failure of alpha-interferon in hairy cell leukemia. Eur J Haematol 43:297, 1989

GOLOMB HM, ELLIS E: Treatment options for hairy-cell leukemia. Semin Oncol 18:7, 1991

LILL MCC, GOLDE DW: Treatment of hairy cell leukemia. Blood Rev 4:238, 1990

O'DWYER PJ et al: 2'-Deoxycoformycin (Pentostatin) for lymphoid malignancies. Ann Intern Med 108:733, 1988

PIRO LD et al: Lasting remissions in hairy-cell leukemia induced by a single infusion of 2-chlorodeoxyadenosine. N Engl J Med 322:1117, 1990

SAVEN A, PIRO LD: Treatment of hairy cell leukemia. Blood 79:1111, 1992

311　MALIGNANT LYMPHOMAS

ARNOLD S. FREEDMAN / LEE M. NADLER

DEFINITION　The malignant lymphomas, in contrast to leukemias, are neoplastic transformations of cells which reside predominantly in lymphoid tissues. The two major variants of malignant lymphoma are non-Hodgkin's lymphoma and Hodgkin's disease. Although both these tumors infiltrate reticuloendothelial organs, they are biologically and clinically distinct. Table 311-1 compares non-Hodgkin's and Hodgkin's lymphomas with regard to cellular deriva-

TABLE 311-1　The malignant lymphomas

	Non-Hodgkin's	Hodgkin's
Cellular derivation	90% B cell 10% T cell	Unresolved
Sites of disease:		
Localized	Uncommon	Common
Nodal spread	Discontiguous	Contiguous
Extranodal	Common	Uncommon
Mediastinal	Uncommon	Common
Abdominal	Common	Uncommon
Bone marrow	Common	Uncommon
B symptoms	Uncommon	Common
Chromosomal translocation	Common	Yet to be described
Curability	30–40%	>75%

tion, sites of disease, presence of systemic symptoms, chromosomal translocations, and curability. This comparison supports the notion that they are fundamentally different diseases.

CELLULAR AND DEVELOPMENTAL ASPECTS OF NON-HODGKIN'S AND HODGKIN'S LYMPHOMAS　To date, biologic studies have provided no clear-cut explanations for the differences demonstrated in Table 311-1. A large number of studies have examined the cellular origins of these tumors in an attempt to relate the neoplastic

TABLE 311-2　Histologic classification of non-Hodgkin's lymphoma

Working formulation, malignant lymphoma	Rappaport terminology	Cellular lineage, %		Chromosomal abnormalities
		B	T	
LOW GRADE				
A　Small lymphocytic cell	Diffuse-well-differentiated lymphocytic (DWDL)	98	2	Trisomy 12 t(11;14) t(14;19)
B　Follicular, predominantly small cleaved cell	Nodular poorly differentiated lymphocytic (NPDL)	100	0	t(14;18) del(6)
C　Follicular mixed, small cleaved and large cell	Nodular mixed lymphocytic histiocytic (NM)	100	0	t(14;18) Trisomy, 3, 7, 8
INTERMEDIATE GRADE				
D　Follicular, predominantly large cell	Nodular histiocytic (NH)	100	0	Trisomy 7, 10, 12, 21 t(14;18)
E　Diffuse small cleaved cell	Diffuse poorly differentiated lymphocytic (DPDL)	80	20	del(6)(q) t(3;9), t(14;18)
F　Diffuse mixed, small and large cell	Diffuse mixed lymphocytic-histiocytic (DM)	90	10	Trisomy 3 t(14;18)
G　Diffuse large cell	Diffuse histiocytic (DH)	80	20	Trisomy 7, 12 t(14;18), t(3;22) del(6)(q21)
HIGH GRADE				
H　Large cell immunoblastic	Diffuse histiocytic (DH)	80	20	t(14;18) del(6)(q21)
I　Lymphoblastic	Diffuse lymphoblastic (LL)	10	90	
J　Small noncleaved cell; Burkitt's	Diffuse undifferentiated (DUL)	95	5	t(8;14), t(2;8), t(8;22)

cell to its normal cellular counterpart. By understanding the lineage and corresponding normal stage of differentiation, it should be eventually possible to further subgroup these tumors biologically according to cellular origin, ability to localize within specific microenvironments, propensity to further differentiate in vivo, production of cytokines, and response to therapy.

Non-Hodgkin's and Hodgkin's lymphomas are morphologically classified (as shown in Tables 311-2 and 311-6). In an attempt to understand the lineage derivation of these histologically defined subtypes, it is necessary to examine the normal populations of cells which reside in lymphoid tissues. To this end, B and T cell ontogeny will be reviewed. It will be within this context that the neoplastic lymphoma cell will be related to its normal cellular counterpart.

Lymphocytes can be functionally subdivided into distinct populations by their expression of unique cell surface and molecular markers. In the past, human B cells were identified by their expression of cell surface or cytoplasmic immunoglobulin and their capacity to secrete immunoglobulin. In contrast, human T lymphocytes were classically defined by the expression of sheep red blood cell receptors and their functional ability to regulate immune responses. The characterization of monoclonal antibodies (MAbs) directed against cell surface molecules expressed on human lymphoid cells has led to very significant advances in both the phenotypic and functional characterization of these cells. Monoclonal antibodies have been useful in assigning cellular lineage, identifying normal stages of lymphoid differentiation, and identifying the function of many of these molecules. Similarly, molecular biologic techniques demonstrating gene rearrangements have been helpful in defining lineage, clonality, and, to a lesser extent, stage of differentiation.

Normal B cell ontogeny CELL SURFACE ANTIGENS Normal B cell ontogeny has been operationally divided into functional stages, namely, pre-B cell, mature (resting) B cell, activated/proliferating B cell, differentiating B cell, and secretory (plasma) cell (Fig. 311-1). Several antigens have been very useful in defining B lineage derivation, since within the hematopoietic system they are uniquely expressed on B lymphocytes and their expression spans B cell ontogeny (see Fig. 311-1). Two of the most useful antigens are CD19 and CD20.

The most immature pre-B cells have been defined by their coexpression of cell surface antigens including major histocompatibility complex (MHC) class II (Ia) and CD19. Individual stages of pre-B cell ontogeny have been delineated by the sequential expression of the pre-B cell antigen CD10 (common acute lymphoblastic leukemia antigen, CALLA, enkephalinase), CD20, and finally, cytoplasmic immunoglobulin mu (cμ) heavy chains without the expression of light chains. As pre-B cells mature, they are exported to the peripheral blood and lymphoid tissues, where they reside until activated by antigen (mature B cell; see Fig. 311-1). Mature resting B cells continue to express cell surface Ia, CD19, and CD20 but no longer express CD10. These cells also express cell surface immunoglobulins IgM and IgD (the B cell antigen receptor), CD21 (which is the receptor for the C3d cleavage fragment of complement and for Epstein-Barr virus), and several lymphocyte homing and adhesion receptors including CD44, L-selectin, and CD11a/CD18 (LFA-1). These molecules are involved in lymphocyte recirculation, localization in distinct microenvironments, and cell-cell interactions.

Following triggering with antigen or other signals of activation, mature resting B cells are activated and subsequently proliferate (activated/proliferating B cell; see Fig. 311-1). From in vitro, in vivo, and in situ studies, the activation of resting B cells is accompanied by a sequence of cell surface antigenic changes. Resting B cells begin to lose cell surface IgD and CD21. As these antigens are lost, a number of B cell–associated and –restricted antigens sequentially appear (activation antigens). Activation antigens are cell surface molecules which are likely to be involved in the regulation of cellular proliferation and/or differentiation or alternatively play a role in the localization and binding of activated B cells within a microenvironment. These activation antigens include CD71 (transferrin receptor), CD54 (ICAM-1, ligand for LFA-1), CD25 (low-affinity interleukin 2 receptor), CD5, and B7 (adhesion molecule for T cells).

With further differentiation there is a sequential loss of the B cell activation antigens as well as pan-B cell antigens including Ia, CD19, and CD20. This stage is also characterized by the appearance of several other antigens (CD38 and PCA-1) which are expressed on plasma cells (secretory B cell).

FIGURE 311-1 Correlation of B cell differentiation and B cell malignancies.

B Cell Malignancies

viral etiology. Epstein-Barr virus (EBV) has a strong association with the pathogenesis of Burkitt's lymphoma and high-grade lymphoma in immunodeficiency patients, including HIV-1 infected individuals. The human T cell leukemia virus (HTLV-1) is the causative agent in adult T cell lymphoma in endemic areas, which include southwestern Japan and the Caribbean.

Although limited progress has been made in identifying agents which might be involved in inducing non-Hodgkin's lymphomas, exciting advances have been made in identifying those genes which appear to be involved in lymphomatous transformation. Cytogenetic abnormalities have been well documented in a number of non-Hodgkin's lymphomas (see Table 311-2). DNA sequence analysis of several of these chromosomal translocations has demonstrated that genes which normally regulate heavy and light chain immunoglobulin synthesis have been juxtaposed to genes that regulate normal cellular activation and proliferation. It is postulated that these transforming genes, or *oncogenes,* have come under the control of those regulatory elements which normally control B cell proliferation and differentiation. The best-studied example is the t(8;14) or variant t(2;8) or t(8;22) translocations of Burkitt's lymphoma present in over 90 percent of Burkitt's lymphomas and a subgroup of acute lymphoblastic leukemias. In this disease, the c-*myc* oncogene on chromosome 8 is joined to either the immunoglobulin heavy chain locus on chromosome 14, the κ light chain locus on chromosome 2, or the λ light chain locus on chromosome 22, leading to activation and overexpression of the c-*myc* gene product. In contrast, the non-Burkitt's subtype lacks c-*myc* activation and expression. Another example is the t(14;18) translocation which is seen in approximately 85 percent of patients with follicular lymphomas and 35 percent of those with diffuse lymphomas. In t(14;18), the gene bcl-2 (chromosome 18) is juxtaposed to the immunoglobulin heavy chain locus (chromosome 14). The bcl-2 gene product prevents programmed cell death or apoptosis. It is hypothesized that the alteration is bcl-2 expression is involved in the pathogenesis of the indolent behaving low-grade lymphomas.

A number of primary diseases have an increased incidence of subsequently developing non-Hodgkin's lymphoma and to a lesser extent Hodgkin's lymphoma. As seen in Table 311-3, diseases of inherited and acquired immunodeficiency as well as autoimmune diseases are associated with an increased incidence of lymphoma. Non-Hodgkin's lymphomas which occur in the context of drug-induced immunosuppression, acquired or congenital immunodeficiency, and AIDS are frequently associated with EBV. The association between immunosuppression and induction of non-Hodgkin's lymphomas appears to be compelling, since if the immunosuppression can be reversed (e.g., discontinuing immunosuppressive agents following organ transplantation), a percentage of these lymphomas regress

spontaneously. The incidence of lymphoma in iatrogenic immune suppression, AIDS, and autoimmune disease argues strongly for immune dysregulation contributing to the development of lymphoma. Patients with certain environmental exposures have a higher incidence of lymphomas. Patients with Hodgkin's disease treated with combined-modality treatment of radiation therapy and chemotherapy exhibit an increased risk of developing secondary large cell lymphomas. Lymphoma-like syndromes also have been found in patients treated with phenytoin. Although in most cases this disease regresses when the drug is stopped, a significant number of patients still develop malignant lymphomas.

CLINICAL PRESENTATION AND DIFFERENTIAL DIAGNOSIS

More than two-thirds of patients with non-Hodgkin's lymphoma present with persistent painless peripheral lymphadenopathy. At the time of presentation, differential diagnosis includes infectious causes due to bacteria, viruses (e.g., infectious mononucleosis, cytomegalovirus, and human immunodeficiency virus), and parasites (toxoplasmosis). In young patients, Hodgkin's lymphoma must be excluded. In older patients, other neoplasms must be considered. It is generally agreed that in adults, a firm lymph node greater than 1 cm in size that is not associated with a documentable infection and that persists longer than 4 to 6 weeks should be considered for biopsy. Certain clinical features suggest the diagnosis of non-Hodgkin's lymphoma. Involvement of Waldeyer's ring, epitrochlear, and mesenteric nodes is more suggestive of non-Hodgkin's lymphoma than Hodgkin's. Unlike Hodgkin's, which can present with weight loss, fever, or night sweats (B symptoms), it is less common for patients with non-Hodgkin's lymphoma to present with systemic complaints.

Non-Hodgkin's lymphomas also present with chest, abdominal, or extranodal symptomatology. Although much less common than Hodgkin's disease, approximately 20 percent of patients with non-Hodgkin's lymphoma have mediastinal adenopathy. These patients most frequently present with persistent cough and chest discomfort or without symptoms but have an abnormal chest x-ray. Occasionally, a superior vena cava syndrome accompanies presentation, especially in patients with T cell lymphomas and to a lesser extent in those with B cell diffuse large cell lymphoma. Differential includes infectious causes (e.g., histoplasmosis, tuberculosis, or infectious mononucleosis), sarcoidosis, Hodgkin's disease, and other neoplasms. Involvement of retroperitoneal, mesenteric, and pelvic nodes is common in most histologic subtypes of non-Hodgkin's lymphoma. Unless massive or leading to obstruction, these nodes usually produce no symptoms. In contrast, patients who come to medical attention because of an abdominal mass, massive splenomegaly, or primary gastrointestinal lymphoma present with complaints similar to those associated with other abdominal space-occupying lesions. These include chronic pain, abdominal fullness, early satiety, symptoms associated with viscus obstruction, or even acute perforation and gastrointestinal hemorrhage. Symptoms due to extralymphatic disease are more common in some subtypes of diffuse non-Hodgkin's lymphoma but are uncommon in follicular lymphomas. Rarely, some patients present with symptoms of unexplained anemia and thrombocytopenia due to marrow infiltration with lymphoma or hypersplenism. Diffuse non-Hodgkin's lymphomas can present with cutaneous lesions, testicular masses, acute spinal cord compression, solitary bone lesions, and rarely, lymphomatous meningitis. Primary non-Hodgkin's lymphoma of the brain constitutes only 1 percent of all non-Hodgkin' lymphomas. However with HIV-1 infection and the increasing use of immunosuppressive therapy in organ transplant recipients, primary central nervous system (CNS) lymphoma is becoming one of the most common types of primary brain tumors.

PATHOLOGIC CLASSIFICATION   Rappaport and Working Formulation classification schemes   The pathologic classification of non-Hodgkin's lymphomas has been difficult for both pathologists and clinicians. Histologic classifications is crucial, since therapeutic options are based on histologic subtype and less frequently by stage. In 1966, Henry Rappaport presented the first clinically relevant classification scheme for non-Hodgkin's lymphomas. This classifica-

---

TABLE 311-3   Diseases or exposures associated with increase risk of development of malignant lymphoma

Inherited immunodeficiency disease
  Klinefelter's syndrome
  Chediak-Higashi syndrome
  Ataxia telangiectasia syndrome
  Wiscott-Aldrich syndrome
  Common variable immunodeficiency disease
Acquired immunodeficiency diseases
  Iatrogenic immunosuppression
  Human immunodeficiency virus-1 infection
  Acquired hypogammaglobulinemia
Autoimmune disease
  Sjögren's syndrome
  Celiac sprue
  Rheumatoid arthritis and systemic lupus erythematosus
Chemical or drug exposures
  Phenytoin
  Radiation
  Prior combination chemotherapy and radiation therapy
Viral association (other than HIV)
  Epstein-Barr virus
  Human T cell leukemia virus

tion was based on assessment of overall pattern of lymph node architecture (low-power microscopy) as well as the cytologic classification of the neoplastic cell (high-power microscopy). The Rappaport classification subdivides the non-Hodgkin's lymphomas into two major subtypes, namely, nodular (follicular) and diffuse. Nodular lymphomas retain some features of normal lymph node architecture in that the neoplastic cells appear to form "germinal centers" (nodules). In contrast, in diffuse lymphomas, the normal cortical and paracortical lymph node architecture is largely effaced. Rappaport also divided non-Hodgkin's lymphomas into subgroups according to cytologic appearance of the malignant cell: (1) well-differentiated, (2) poorly differentiated, and (3) histiocytic. This suggested that these tumors corresponded morphologically to distinct stages of lymphoid and monocytic differentiation. The importance of the Rappaport classification (see Table 311-2) was that each histologically defined subtype of non-Hodgkin's lymphoma exhibited a unique natural history and response to therapy. The nodular lymphomas generally behaved in an indolent manner, while most diffuse lymphomas had an aggressive behavior.

With the advent of modern immunology, the Rappaport classification proved to have several biologic defects. First, the term *histiocytic* was incorrect, since virtually all these tumors were of lymphoid origin. Second, certain clinical entities were not accounted for by this classification scheme. By the late 1970s, six independent pathologic schemes were in use throughout the world, and therefore, therapeutic trials could not be compared. Because of this confusion, a new classification scheme was proposed and has been termed the *Working Formulation* (see Table 311-2). The latter incorporates the best features of the various classification systems and, more important, retains clinical relevance. The Working Formulation subdivides non-Hodgkin's lymphomas into *low-, intermediate-,* and *high-grade* subgroups dependent on their natural history. Low-grade lymphomas are characterized by an indolent clinical course, with their natural history not significantly altered by therapy. Intermediate- and high-grade lymphomas historically were associated with very short survivals. With the advent of aggressive combination chemotherapeutic regimens, some of the patients with intermediate- and high-grade tumors demonstrate long-term disease-free survivals. It should be noted that the Working Formulation omits several important histologic subtypes, including diffuse intermediate lymphocytic lymphoma (a low-grade disease), adult T cell lymphoma associated with HTLV-1, lymphoma of mucosa associated lymphoid tissue (MALT), and cutaneous T cell lymphoma. Table 311-2 compares the Working Formulation and the Rappaport classifications. In clinical practice, these classification schemes are frequently used interchangeably.

STAGING AND DISEASE DETECTION Conventional staging The Ann Arbor staging system developed for Hodgkin's disease also has been used in staging non-Hodgkin's lymphomas. This staging system focuses on the number of tumor sites (nodal and extranodal), location, and the presence or absence of systemic symptoms. Table 311-4 summaries this staging system. In stages I and II, sites of disease are on the same side of the diaphragm. Stage III disease involves both sides of the diaphragm, whereas stage IV is defined as extranodal lymphomatous involvement, most frequently of the bone marrow and liver. Systemic symptoms (fever, weight loss of more than 10 percent of body weight, and night sweats, i.e., B symptoms)

are less common in non-Hodgkin's lymphomas (about 20 percent of cases) than in Hodgkin's disease and therefore are not as useful in predicting prognosis. It must be emphasized that this classification scheme was developed specifically for Hodgkin's disease, which disseminates by contiguous lymphatic extension and to a much lesser extent hematogenously. Since non-Hodgkin's lymphomas most frequently disseminate hematogenously, this staging system has proven to be less useful in this type of lymphoma.

The concept of staging has a smaller impact on treatment strategy in patients with non-Hodgkin's lymphomas than in those with Hodgkin's disease. Only 10 percent of patients with follicular lymphoma have localized disease and are candidates for local radiation therapy. For the diffuse lymphomas, even patients with localized disease and the majority of patients with advanced stage disease now receive systemic treatment. Therefore, staging is undertaken in non-Hodgkin's lymphomas to identify those small numbers of patients who can be treated with local therapy and to stratify within histologic subtypes with the view to prognosticate and to assess the impact of therapeutic regimens.

Staging procedures after biopsy diagnosis Staging must be undertaken in the context of the Working Formulation histologic grade. A suggested staging workup for patients with non-Hodgkin's lymphoma is summarized in Table 311-5. An organized approach to staging a patient with non-Hodgkin's lymphoma is mandatory. After the initial excisional biopsy and documentation of the pathologic and, when possible, immunologic subtype of disease, blood tests should be obtained, including a complete blood count, routine chemistries, liver function tests, and serum protein electrophoresis to document the presence of circulating monoclonal paraprotein. Waldeyer's ring involvement is often associated with intestinal involvement, and

---

TABLE 311-5 Staging evaluation for non-Hodgkin's lymphoma

ESSENTIAL

1 Pathologic documentation by hematopathologist
2 Physical examination
3 Documentation of B symptoms
4 Laboratory evaluation
  a Complete blood counts
  b Liver function tests
  c Renal function tests
  d Uric acid
  e Calcium
  f Serum protein electrophoresis
5 Chest radiograph
6 CT scan of abdomen and pelvis
7 Bone marrow biopsy

ESSENTIAL UNDER CERTAIN CIRCUMSTANCES

1 Chest CT scan
2 Head CT scan
3 Lumbar puncture
4 Barium studies of GI tract
5 Endoscopic examination
6 Cytologic examination of effusion
7 Gallium scan (planar or SPECT)

USEFUL BUT NOT ESSENTIAL TESTS

1 Cell surface marker phenotypic analysis
2 Cytogenetic analysis
3 Gene rearrangement analysis
4 Polymerase chain reaction analysis of minimal residual disease
5 Flow cytometry for DNA analysis
6 Liver scan
7 Liver biopsy
8 Bone scan
9 Thallium scan
10 Lymphangiography
11 Ultrasonography
12 Magnetic resonance imaging
13 Echocardiogram
14 Laparotomy

TABLE 311-4 Ann Arbor staging system

Stage I	Involvement in single lymph node region or single extralymphatic site
Stage II	Involvement of two or more lymph node regions on the same side of diaphragm; can also include localized involvement of extralymphatic site (stage IIE)
Stage III	Involvement of lymph node regions or extralymphatic sites on both sides of diaphragm
Stage IV	Disseminated involvement of one or more extralymphatic organs with or without lymph node involvement

gastrointestinal contrast studies or endoscopy is indicated if the patient appears to have localized disease. Chest radiography is used to exclude mediastinal and hilar adenopathy, pleural effusions, and pulmonary parenchymal infiltration. Chest computed tomographic (CT) scan is used to more precisely assess the extent of disease and is strongly recommended for patients with abnormal chest radiographs. However, abdominal/pelvic CT scan is essential for accurate staging to assess lymphadenopathy in retroperitoneal, mesenteric, and retrocrural areas. Lymphangiography in less useful than in Hodgkin's disease, since common sites of disease in non-Hodgkin's lymphoma include nodes in the mesentery, hilum of liver, spleen, or kidneys as well as nodes in the deep bony pelvis, none of which is detected by this procedure. However, lymphogram may be an accurate predictor of intraabdominal lymphoma, since the majority of patients with a positive lymphogram also have disease in the liver and in abdominal nodes. The major advantage of lymphangiography over abdominal/pelvic CT scan is its ability to detect infiltrated but normal-sized retroperitoneal nodes. The major indication for lymphangiography is non-Hodgkin's lymphoma is for patients with localized inguinal disease who may be candidates for local radiotherapy, where CT scanning for intraabdominal disease may be falsely negative. Unilateral percutaneous bone marrow biopsies must be performed, since the likelihood of lymphomatous involvement of the marrow is relatively high, especially in low-grade lymphoma, where marrow involvement occurs in up to 60 percent of cases. With any indication of hepatic abnormalities on blood tests or on liver scan, a percutaneous liver biopsy may be indicated in patients who would otherwise have stage I disease. In patients with aggressive lymphomas with marrow involvement, with paranasal sinus involvement, or if clinically indicated, examination of the cerebrospinal fluid by lumbar puncture should be performed.

More invasive tests are reserved for the uncommon presentation with stage I or II non-Hodgkin's lymphoma. While staging laparotomy may be performed routinely in Hodgkin's disease, this is not so in the non-Hodgkin's lymphomas. In the diffuse non-Hodgkin's lymphomas, stages II, III, and IV can all be considered reflective of disseminated disease and are therefore usually treated with chemotherapy. In contrast, only true stage I disease or, depending on the histologic subtype, stage II disease will be considered as localized and treated with radiation alone. Therefore, for most patients with non-Hodgkin's lymphoma, it is less critical to ascertain the precise pathologic stage of disease. Moreover, it is common for these patients to exhibit disseminated disease after routine staging tests (e.g., bone marrow or liver biopsy), thus obviating the need for laparotomy to prove dissemination. For example, within follicular lymphomas, the small cleaved cell and mixed small and large cell types, following clinical staging and bone marrow biopsy, greater than 85 percent of these patients will have stage III or stage IV disease. Thus *surgical staging should never be considered a routine procedure in patients with non-Hodgkin's lymphoma.*

A number of other tests are becoming more important in both staging and advancing our knowledge of the biology of non-Hodgkin's lymphoma. Radionuclide scans, especially with gallium, appear to have clinical utility. Gallium scans are positive in virtually all intermediate- and high-grade lymphomas and in about 50 percent of low-grade lymphomas. Gallium scans, with high doses of isotope which permit delayed imaging, combined with single photon emission computed tomography (SPECT), are very sensitive in detecting tumor infiltration. These tests are also very useful in monitoring response to therapy. The role of magnetic resonance imaging (MRI) in detecting non-Hodgkin's lymphoma is under active investigation. To date, MRI appears to be most valuable for detecting occult marrow involvement. Immunologic and molecular biologic studies are proving increasingly useful in confirming diagnosis. For example, in cases with difficult histopathologic patterns, cell surface markers can distinguish between non-Hodgkin's lymphoma and carcinoma [leukocyte common antigen (CD45) is specific for lymphoma]. Similarly, MAbs directed against lineage-restricted antigens and rearrangement of immunoglobulin or

T cell receptor genes are useful in identifying lymphoid tumors. The delineation of the cell surface phenotype is becoming important because an increasing number of salvage treatment programs employ high-dose chemoradiotherapy and monoclonal antibody–purged autologous bone marrow support (see below). Definition of a specific chromosomal abnormality also may have prognostic significance.

Sensitive techniques to detect minimal residual disease The development of molecular techniques to define immunoglobulin and T cell receptor gene rearrangements has provided very sensitive tools with which to more accurately assess tumor cell infiltration. The most common and accessible tissues to be tested include peripheral blood and bone marrow. Whereas conventional histologic analysis of the bone marrow can detect 1 lymphoma cell infiltrating 20 normal cells, immunologic flow cytometric and Southern blot analysis each improve this level of detection to approximately 1 lymphoma cell in approximately 100 normal cells. Similarly, flow cytometry has been used to detect "clonal excess" in the blood of patients with B cell non-Hodgkin's lymphoma. More recently, molecular biologic techniques demonstrate that minimal disease detection can be markedly improved. For those non-Hodgkin's lymphomas with a known chromosomal translocation, it is now possible to identify a unique chromosomal "breakpoint." This has been most elegantly accomplished for the t(14;18) translocation present in the majority of follicular lymphomas and in about 30 percent of diffuse lymphomas. Based on DNA sequence, it is possible to amplify this unique stretch of DNA using specific oligonucleotide primers and the polymerase chain reaction (PCR) (see Chap. 61). With this approach, 1 tumor cell in 10^6 normal cells can be detected. Thus, while other tests may be negative, PCR may demonstrate that the blood or bone marrow is contaminated by lymphoma cells. These biologic techniques are presently being compared with more conventional staging methods. Considering their sensitivity, they may be useful in more accurately assessing complete remission and, more important, in determining whether treatment should be prolonged, truncated, or intensified.

NATURAL HISTORY BY HISTOLOGIC SUBTYPE Considering the heterogeneity of non-Hodgkin's lymphomas and the unique clinical presentation and natural history within histologically defined subtypes, it is important to briefly review these subtypes.

Low grade SMALL LYMPHOCYTIC (DIFFUSE WELL-DIFFERENTIATED LYMPHOCYTIC) This disease is the lymphomatous presentation of chronic lymphocytic leukemia (CLL) and therefore occurs in middle-aged and older patients. Patients usually present with asymptomatic generalized lymphadenopathy. Unlike CLL, the peripheral blood may be normal or reveal only a mild lymphocytosis (60 percent will have absolute lymphocytosis of >4000 per cubic millimeter at diagnosis). In contrast, the bone marrow is involved in 75 to 95 percent of cases. Serum paraprotein is found in about 20 percent of cases, and hypogammaglobulinemia is common. These patients can often be observed without treatment for 3 to 4 years, with a median survival of 8 to 10 years. A small percentage of small lymphocytic lymphomas and CLLs will undergo histologic conversion to diffuse large cell lymphoma (Richter's syndrome). These patients usually present with extensive disease, abdominal masses, and B symptoms and experience short survival.

FOLLICULAR, PREDOMINANTLY SMALL CLEAVED CELL (NODULAR POORLY DIFFERENTIATED LYMPHOCYTIC) Follicular lymphomas account for approximately 50 percent of the non-Hodgkin's lymphomas; the small cleaved cell type is the most common subtype. Patients usually present with painless peripheral adenopathy in cervical, axillary, inguinal, and femoral regions. Patients frequently note that lymph node enlargement has been present for long periods of time and these nodes have "waxed and waned." Less typically, there is enlargement of Waldeyer's ring and epitrochlear nodes. Some patients present with asymptomatic large abdominal and retroperitoneal masses with or without evidence of gastrointestinal and/or renal obstruction. Although patients may present with one or more sites of nodal disease, noninvasive workup usually demonstrates widely disseminated disease with involvement of spleen, liver, and bone marrow in over 80 percent of patients. Bone marrow involvement in follicular lymphoma reveals a unique pattern of paratrabecular infiltration. Peripheral blood involvement is seen in about 10 percent of patients, and CNS disease is rare, although epidural disease can be seen. In contrast to diffuse lymphomas, about 10 percent of patients present with extramedullary extranodal disease and less than 10 percent present with B symptoms. The course of this disease is quite variable. The conventional approach for most patients is that they can be observed with waxing and waning disease for a median of 3 years without the need for therapy. Although in patients with stage I or limited stage II disease local radiation therapy may provide long-term remissions or cure, others demonstrate more disseminated and rapid growth and require treatment because massive nodal or organ enlargement leads to pain, lymphatic obstruction, organ obstruction, or more rarely, neurologic symptoms. At the time of increasing generalized disease or rapid growth at a single site, involved nodes should be considered for rebiopsy. At that time, a significant number of patients will demonstrate a "conversion" or "transformation" to a more aggressive histologic pattern, often diffuse large cell. This conversion occurs in up 60 percent of patients with follicular small cleaved cell lymphoma. Histologic conversion can be associated with infiltration of extranodal sites, the development of systemic symptoms, and a poor prognosis, since the tumor is much less responsive to treatment. Historically, both disease-free and overall survivals of patients with follicular lymphoma have not changed despite many different therapeutic approaches. Although 40 to 70 percent of patients achieve complete remissions (noninvasively staged) with conventional single-agent or aggressive combination chemotherapy, the median duration of remission is between 2 and 3 years. Following relapse, patients can be observed or retreated; however, the median survival after first relapse is 5 years. Patients with follicular non-Hodgkin's lymphoma survive long periods of time, with median survivals for patients with stage III and IV disease approaching 7 to 9 years.

FOLLICULAR, MIXED SMALL CLEAVED AND LARGE CELL (NODULAR MIXED)   This entity has similarities with both follicular small cleaved cell and follicular large cell lymphomas. Bone marrow infiltration at presentation is less common than in small cleaved cell lymphoma, but large abdominal masses are seen more commonly. Since some studies suggest that a subset of these patients may be cured with conventional therapy, these patients are generally not observed but are treated soon after diagnosis with combination chemotherapy.

Intermediate grade   FOLLICULAR, PREDOMINANTLY LARGE CELL (NODULAR HISTIOCYTIC)   Although the follicular architecture of these tumors is preserved, this disease behaves much more like diffuse large cell lymphoma. In contrast to other follicular lymphomas, this histologic variant has less frequent infiltration of the marrow and liver and presents with large masses and frequently extranodal disease. A finite cure rate has been reported in selected series. Most follicular large cell lymphomas which are not cured by treatment eventually convert to diffuse large cell lymphoma.

DIFFUSE SMALL CLEAVED CELL (DIFFUSE POORLY DIFFERENTIATED LYMPHOCYTIC)   This disease behaves like a follicular variant. Patients are middle-aged or older. At the time of presentation, most have stage IV disease with infiltration of the spleen, liver, and bone marrow, with marrow and liver infiltration occurring in over 50 percent of patients. Later in the course of the disease, infiltration of other parenchymal organs (e.g., lungs) is observed. The overall median survival is much shorter than observed in patients with low-grade lymphomas; however, like low-grade lymphoma, aggressive combination chemotherapy has had a minimal impact on the natural history of this disease.

DIFFUSE MIXED SMALL AND LARGE CELL (DIFFUSE MIXED)   This tumor behaves most like diffuse large cell lymphoma. Some investigators consider these two tumors to be a spectrum of a single entity. In several clinical trials where patients with diffuse mixed and diffuse large cell lymphoma were treated identically, survival rates were comparable. However, in other series, a higher relapse rate was observed.

DIFFUSE LARGE CELL (DIFFUSE HISTIOCYTIC)   Patients who are generally middle-aged or older present with either nodal enlargement (especially in the neck or abdomen) or extranodal disease (in the gastrointestinal tract, testes, bone, thyroid, salivary glands, skin, and brain). During the course of the disease, the liver, kidneys, and lungs may be involved. Diffuse large cell lymphoma is highly invasive, with local compression of vessels or airways, involvement of peripheral nerves, and destruction of bone. Although bone marrow involvement initially is found in only 10 to 20 percent of patients, its detection is important because of its strong correlation with later spread to the CNS. Later in the disease, some patients demonstrate both extensive bone marrow infiltration and peripheral blood involvement. Several large studies have identified a number of clinical features considered to be associated with inability to achieve a complete remission and poor prognosis. These features include poor performance status, bulk of disease (>10-cm tumor masses), bone marrow infiltration, multiple sites of extranodal disease, markedly elevated serum lactic dehydrogenase (LDH), and systemic B symptoms. Using these prognostic variables, alternative therapies are being investigated to improve the survival for poor-prognosis patients with diffuse large cell lymphoma.

High grade   LARGE CELL IMMUNOBLASTIC (DIFFUSE HISTIOCYTIC)   This variant of diffuse large cell lymphoma demonstrates a unique pathologic appearance. This disease usually occur in adults, commonly over age 50, and often in a setting of prior immune-mediated or lymphoproliferative disease (e.g., celiac disease, Hashimoto's thyroiditis, angioimmunoblastic lymphadenopathy, Sjögren's syndrome, Mediterranean lymphoma, cold agglutinin disease, or Waldenström's macroglobulinemia). Anemia, lymphopenia, diffuse hypergammaglobulinemia, B symptoms, and advanced stage are common at presentation. Most patients present with extranodal disease, and invasion of the bone marrow and CNS is common. Although histologically distinct within the Working Formulation, with aggressive combination chemotherapy, the prognosis for these patients is similar to that for patients with diffuse large cell lymphoma.

LYMPHOBLASTIC (DIFFUSE LYMPHOBLASTIC)   Although lymphoblastic lymphomas represent a major subgroup of childhood non-Hodgkin's lymphomas, they are much less common in adults (less than 5 percent of adult non-Hodgkin's lymphomas). Patients are usually males in their twenties to thirties who present with lymphadenopathy in cervical, supraclavicular, and axillary regions (50 percent) or with a mediastinal mass (50 to 70 percent). In most patients, the mediastinal mass is anterior, >10 cm, symptomatic often with superior vena cava syndrome, and associated with pleural effusions. Less commonly, patients present with extranodal disease (e.g., skin, testicular, or bony involvement). Greater than 90 percent of patients present with stage III or IV disease, and half have B symptoms. Although the bone marrow can be normal at presentation, approximately 60 percent of patients develop bone marrow infiltration and a subsequent leukemic phase indistinguishable from T cell acute lymphoblastic leukemia. Patients with bone marrow involvement have a very high incidence of CNS infiltration. Prior to current aggressive acute leukemia–like therapy, this disease was rapidly fatal.

SMALL NONCLEAVED, BURKITT'S AND NON-BURKITT'S (DIFFUSE UNDIFFERENTIATED)   Burkitt's lymphoma is a childhood tumor which has two major clinical presentations. The endemic (African) form presents as a jaw tumor which spreads to extranodal sites, especially to the bone marrow and meninges. The nonendemic (American) form has an abdominal presentation with massive disease, ascites, and skin, bone, peripheral node involvement and, like the African form, also spreads to the bone marrow and CNS (although less than in the African form). Prior to aggressive therapeutic programs, all children died rapidly. These tumors are now treated with very aggressive chemotherapeutic programs with more gratifying results. Burkitt's lymphoma is uncommon in adults but is occasionally seen in patients up to age 35. In contrast, small noncleaved non-Burkitt's lymphomas are observed and are very aggressive and frequently present like diffuse large cell lymphoma in extranodal prognosis, with some studies suggesting that non-Hodgkin's lymphomas of T cell origin have a worse prognosis than B cell–derived tumors. Within the B cell diffuse large cell lymphomas, patients with tumors with an aberrant immunophenotype (lacking HLA-DR, CD20, or CD22) had a significantly shorter survival. Expression of the homing receptor CD44 also has been associated with disseminated disease and poor survival. Although these findings are of great interest, large prospective studies will be needed to confirm these observations. Presently, the treatment of non-Hodgkin's lymphomas is not altered by immunophenotype of the tumor cells.

Salvage chemotherapy   The prognosis for patients with intermediate- and high-grade non-Hodgkin's lymphoma who fail to achieve a complete remission or relapse following aggressive therapy is very poor. Salvage chemotherapy employing drugs such as cytosine arabinoside, cisplatin, etoposide, and ifosfamide, given as single agents or in combination, has been used to induce remissions. Depending on the histology and regimen, approximately 20 to 30 percent of patients attain a complete remission, with partial remissions in another 30 percent. Unfortunately, these remissions tend to be short-lived (approximately 2 to 6 months), with less than 3 percent of patients in remission beyond 2 years.

Bone marrow transplantation (BMT)   Patients whose disease is resistant to conventional or salvage therapeutic regimens can still be induced into a complete remission with very high doses of chemotherapy or the combination of high-dose chemotherapy and radiotherapy. This occurs because a steep dose-response curve persists in non-Hodgkin's lymphomas even after relapse. This treatment approach is complicated by very significant and prolonged myelosuppression. To overcome the latter, bone marrow as a source of hematopoietic stem cells can be infused from an identical twin (syngeneic), an HLA-matched relative (allogeneic), or the patient (autologous). Alternatively, hematopoietic stem cells can be isolated from peripheral blood. The vast majority of transplants for patients with lymphoma employ autologous marrow. Bone marrow transplantation has become widespread in the treatment of patients with refractory or relapsed non-Hodgkin's lymphoma, and retrospective analysis clearly demonstrates that only a subgroup of patients benefits from this approach. Patients whose disease has never responded to primary therapy are presently not salvaged by this approach. Following relapse from remission, patients whose disease is resistant to all forms of salvage therapy have less than 15 percent long-term disease-free survival. In contrast, approximately 40 percent of those patients whose disease is still responsive to therapy have long-term disease-free survival with high-dose therapy and marrow transplantation. While the majority of patients undergoing BMT have intermediate- and high-grade non-Hodgkin's lymphoma, studies in patients with low-grade lymphomas suggest that some patients experience long-term disease-free survival. Early studies with BMT reported treatment-related deaths in the range of 20 to 30 percent; however, as patients with no associated comorbid disease have been treated, this mortality has significantly decreased (approximately 5 percent). The use of recombinant hematopoietic growth factors to hasten myeloid cell recovery also has significantly reduced morbidity and length of hospitalization following high-dose therapy and marrow transplantation.

Lower treatment-related mortality has led some groups to use BMT as consolidation therapy in patients with incurable non-Hodgkin's lymphomas in first remission. Selected studies have demonstrated that patients with less than a 20 percent long-term disease-free survival following conventional therapy have a disease-free survival of 80 percent following early BMT. Although this modality is capable of curing some patients with relapsed non-Hodgkin's lymphomas, many issues still remain, including optimal therapeutic regimen, timing of transplantation, source of hematopoietic stem cells, the need to purge autologous marrow, and methods to minimize morbidity and mortality.

Newer modalities   A number of new therapeutic approaches have resulted from the advances in immunology and molecular biology. Over 10 years ago, MAbs directed against surface antigens expressed on non-Hodgkin's lymphoma cells were first used clinically in an attempt to specifically treat these tumors. The results of these studies suggest that MAbs by themselves do not induce significant tumor regression. Although there was initial enthusiasm about using MAbs directed against unique idiotypes expressed on B cell follicular lymphomas, few significant clinical responses have been observed. Newer trials are evaluating MAbs coupled with radionuclides or toxins to specifically produce cytotoxic effects, whereas other trials are using soluble factors (cytokines) which are potentially cytotoxic to tumor cells. The major cytokines being studied include the interferons, tumor necrosis factor, and interleukin 2. Recombinant hematopoietic growth factors which are responsible for growth of myeloid, lymphoid, and erythroid cells are also being tested. Conceptually, these growth factors will limit myelosuppression, thereby permitting higher doses and more frequent administration of chemotherapeutic drugs. Early results are encouraging, and agents such as GM-CSF and G-CSF appear to hasten recovery of myeloid cells. The role of all these agents in improving the treatment of lymphomas is being evaluated in many research centers.

HODGKIN'S DISEASE

EPIDEMIOLOGY AND ETIOLOGY   Approximately 7500 new cases of Hodgkin's disease are diagnosed annually in the United States. The epidemiology of this disease has provided important information regarding the possible role of age and genetic and environmental factors associated with its development. In non-Hodgkin's lymphomas there is a linear increase in incidence with age. In contrast, in Hodgkin's disease in the United States and developed western nations, the age-specific incidence curve is characteristically bimodal, with an initial peak in young adults (15 to 35 years) and a second peak after age 50. However, in Japan, there is an absence of the early peak, and in some third-world countries, there is a shift of the first peak into childhood as well as a shift of histology from nodular sclerosis to mixed cellularity and lymphocyte predominance. Hodgkin's disease is more prevalent in males, and when the age-specific incidence curve is compared with the sex distribution of the patients, the increased male prevalence is most prominent in young adults. A disproportionate number of patients in the first modal peak exhibit nodular sclerosis histology. In childhood Hodgkin's disease, this male predominance is even more striking, with over 80 percent of patients being male. This has lead some investigators to hypothesize a sex-linked genetic or hormonally related increase in susceptibility.

Although controversial, clustering of patients with Hodgkin's has been reported. Increased risk has been associated with decreased number of siblings, single-family dwellings, decreased number of playmates, early birth order, sibling with Hodgkin's disease, tonsillectomy, and certain HLA antigens. These findings have been used to suggest that Hodgkin's disease is caused by a virus possessing an oncogenic potential which is low but increases with age from the time of infection. These observations suggest that genetic and environmental factors may be associated with the development of this disease. As in non-Hodgkin's lymphomas, there is an increased risk of Hodgkin's disease in patients with immunodeficiencies and autoimmune diseases (see Table 311-3). The major obstacle to determining the cause of Hodgkin's disease is our inability to isolate and study the neoplastic cell. Unlike non-Hodgkin's lymphomas, no chromosomal abnormalities have been consistently demonstrated.

CLINICAL FEATURES AND DIFFERENTIAL DIAGNOSIS   Hodgkin's disease usually presents as a localized disease and subsequently spreads to contiguous lymphoid structures and ultimately disseminates to nonlymphoid tissues with a potentially fatal outcome. Hodgkin's disease commonly presents with a newly detected mass or group of lymph nodes which are firm, freely movable, and usually nontender. Approximately half of patients present with adenopathy in the neck or supraclavicular area, and over 70 percent of patients present with superficial lymph node enlargement. Because these are frequently not painful, detection by the patient may be delayed until the lymph nodes are quite large. Approximately 60 percent of patients present with mediastinal adenopathy. This is sometimes first detected on a routine chest x-ray. Nodes involved by Hodgkin's disease tend to be centripetal or axial in contrast to those in non-Hodgkin's lymphomas, which have a tendency to be centrifugal, involving epitrochlear, Waldeyer's ring, and abdominal nodes. In 2 to 5 percent of patients, lymph nodes or other tissues involved with Hodgkin's disease can become painful after the ingestion of alcoholic beverages. The growth of lymph nodes may be quite variable; some lesions can remain stable for long periods of time, while spontaneous and temporary regression of some nodes also may occur.

The majority of patients presenting with Hodgkin's disease have few or no symptoms related to their disease. However, 25 to 30 percent of patients have some constitutional symptoms; the most common is low-grade fever which can be associated with recurrent night sweats. For some patients, night sweats may be the sole complaint. A small number of patients may have high fluctuating fevers accompanied by drenching night sweats (Pel-Epstein fevers). These fevers can persist for several weeks, followed by afebrile intervals. Fevers and night sweats are seen more commonly in older patients and in those with more advanced stage. Some patients with extensive abdominal but limited peripheral adenopathy are first evaluated for fever and night sweats. They undergo a workup for fever of unknown origin and usually are found to have mixed cellularity or lymphocyte-depleted Hodgkin's disease. Another important presenting symptom is unexplained weight loss of greater than 10 percent over 6 months or less. Other frequent symptoms include fatigue, malaise, and weakness. Pruritus occurs in approximately 10 percent of patients at initial diagnosis; it is usually generalized and may be associated with a skin rash and rarely may be the only disease manifestation. Mediastinal, pulmonary, pleural, or pericardial involvement may be associated with cough, chest pain, shortness of breath, or hypertrophic osteoarthropathy; bone involvement may be associated with bone pain. Occasionally, a patient will present with obstruction of the superior vena cava as the first symptom. Sudden spinal cord compression can be a presenting complaint but is usually a complication of advanced progressive disease. Headache or visual disturbances may be seen in the very rare patient with intracranial Hodgkin's disease, and abdominal involvement may result in abdominal pain, bowel disturbances, and even ascites.

The differential diagnosis is similar to that described for non-Hodgkin's lymphoma. In patients with cervical adenopathy, such infections as bacterial or viral pharyngitis, infectious mononucleosis, and toxoplasmosis must be excluded. Other malignancies, such as non-Hodgkin's lymphomas, nasopharyngeal cancers, and thyroid cancers, also can present with localized cervical adenopathy. Axillary adenopathy must be differentiated from non-Hodgkin's lymphoma and breast cancer. Mediastinal adenopathy must be distinguished from infections, sarcoid, and other tumors. In older patients, the differential diagnosis includes tumors of the lung and mediastinum, specifically small cell and non-small cell carcinomas. Reactive mediastinitis and hilar adenopathy from histoplasmosis can be confused with lymphoma, since it occurs in otherwise asymptomatic people. Primary abdominal disease with hepatomegaly, splenomegaly, and massive adenopathy is uncommon, and other neoplastic diseases, especially non-Hodgkin's lymphoma, must be excluded under these circumstances.

DIAGNOSIS AND PATHOLOGIC CLASSIFICATION   The diagnosis of Hodgkin's disease requires a biopsy which contains sufficient tissue to permit an accurate microscopic diagnosis. Biopsy specimens are usually from lymph nodes but may occasionally be from other tissues. Needle aspirations or needle biopsies are not adequate for the histologic diagnosis of Hodgkin's disease.

The criteria for the diagnosis and classification of Hodgkin's disease have remained unchanged since 1966 when the Rye classification was adopted (Table 311-6). As indicated above, central to the diagnosis is the presence of the *Reed-Sternberg* (RS) cell, a large cell with a bilobed or multilobulated nucleus with prominent inclusion-

TABLE 311-6   Rye classification of Hodgkin's disease

| Histologic subgroup | Incidence, % | Pathology | | Prognosis |
		RS*	Other	
Lymphocyte-predominant	2–10	Rare	Predominance of normal-appearing	Excellent
Nodular sclerosis	40–80	Frequent "lacunae"	Lymphoid nodules, collage bands	Very good
Mixed cellularity	20–40	Numerous	Pleomorphic infiltrate	Good
Lymphocyte-depleted	2–15	Numerous, often bizarre	Lymphocytes, pleomorphic fibrosis	Poor

* RS = Reed-Sternberg cell.

like nucleoli. There are several morphologic variants of Reed-Sternberg cells, and it is the frequency of these variants, as well as the cellular and fibrous background of the proliferation, that helps to establish the histologic subtypes of Hodgkin's disease. It is important to note that Reed-Sternberg cells may occasionally be found in other conditions such as infectious mononucleosis and non-Hodgkin's lymphomas. Thus an accurate diagnosis of Hodgkin's disease depends on additional cellular and architectural features of the tissue and optimally also with supportive immunologic studies.

In the Rye classification, Hodgkin's disease is subdivided into four types, including (1) lymphocyte predominant, (2) nodular sclerosis, (3) mixed cellularity, and (4) lymphocyte depleted. Table 311-6 summarizes the major clinical characteristics of these types associated with the Rye classification. It is very important to stress that *treatment and prognosis in Hodgkin's disease is dependent on stage of disease, whereas in non-Hodgkin's lymphoma treatment is largely based on histologic subtype.*

STAGING AND OTHER LABORATORY ABNORMALITIES   Ann Arbor classification   Following biopsy and histopathologic classification of Hodgkin's disease, one must define the extent of the disease (i.e., staging), which is essential for the selection of optimal therapy. In the Ann Arbor staging classification (see Table 311-4), the patient receives both a clinical and a pathologic stage. The clinical stage is defined by the extent of disease based on physical examination and other noninvasive studies. The pathologic stage is defined by data obtained from invasive tests, including biopsy specimens obtained from different sites, usually during a staging laparotomy. The presence of localized extralymphatic disease is designated by the suffix *E*. Such extralymphatic involvement may include solitary involvement of lung, pericardium, or bone. Multifocal involvement in these organs usually is defined as disseminated disease. Bone involvement must be separated from bone marrow involvement, since bone marrow and liver involvement is always defined as stage IV disseminated disease.

The presence of systemic symptoms that are of prognostic importance is designated by the suffix *B* and their absence by the suffix *A*. The presence of both fevers and weight loss results in a less favorable prognosis, while night sweats are currently felt to be of no prognostic importance. Patients with limited disease, such as pathologic stage IA or IIA, are effectively treated with radiotherapy alone, while patients with more disseminated disease, such as pathologic stage IIIB, IVA, or IVB, are most effectively treated with chemotherapy alone or combined with radiotherapy.

Staging procedures after biopsy diagnosis   The diagnostic studies recommended for complete staging are outlined in Table 311-7. There is general agreement on the studies which are considered to be essential. Detailed physical examination with attention to documentation of all sites of nodal involvement and splenomegaly is essential. The chest radiograph is usually sufficient to exclude mediastinal, hilar, pleural, and parenchymal involvement. However, in patients with demonstrable thoracic disease, chest CT scan more accurately defines extent of disease. CT scan of the abdomen and

TABLE 311-7 Staging evaluation for Hodgkin's lymphoma

ESSENTIAL

1 Pathologic documentation by hematopathologist
2 Physical examination
3 Documentation of B symptoms
4 Laboratory evaluation
  a Complete blood counts
  b Liver function tests
  c Renal function tests
  d Uric acid
  e Erythrocyte sedimentation rate
5 Chest radiograph
6 CT scan of chest, abdomen, and pelvis
7 Bone marrow biopsy

ESSENTIAL UNDER CERTAIN CIRCUMSTANCES

1 Liver biopsy
2 Bipedal lymphangiogram
3 Gallium scan
4 Staging laporatomy
5 Bone scan
6 Bone radiographs

USEFUL BUT NOT ESSENTIAL TESTS

1 Cell surface marker phenotypic analysis
2 Gene rearrangement analysis
3 Ultrasonography
4 Magnetic resonance imaging
5 Estimation of patients delayed hypersensitivity status

pelvis has a definite place in the staging of Hodgkin's disease for the assessment of nodal and hepatic disease, but much less for splenic disease. CT scanning can detect the exact location and extent of all enlarged nodes, including iliac, mesenteric, and retrocrural nodal areas, as compared with a lymphogram, which evaluates only the paraaortic and common internal and external iliac nodes. However, the abdominal/pelvic CT scan is limited because it requires nodal enlargement for detection and rarely can detect splenic or hepatic involvement.

A number of more invasive diagnostic tests are required if patients are clinically stage I, II, or IIIA. Lymphograms of the lower extremities are very useful to demonstrate paraaortic and iliac nodal enlargement, and they are more sensitive than abdominal/pelvic CT scans because they can detect disease in normal-sized nodes. Moreover, lymphograms are useful prior to staging laparotomy to direct the surgeon to the nodes to be biopsied. However, the safety and accuracy of this procedure are highly dependent on the experience of the radiologist. If a staging laparotomy is considered, patients should undergo a bone marrow biopsy to exclude stage IV disease. However, the frequency of a positive bone marrow biopsy in clinical stage IA or IIA disease is less than 1 percent. The role of staging laparotomy is still controversial. Staging laparotomy includes biopsy of selected lymph nodes in the retroperitoneum, splenectomy, and several needle and wedge biopsies of the liver. Traditionally, all patients without obvious stage IV disease underwent laparotomy, and nearly one-third had their initial clinical stage changed as a result of the procedure. For example, one-third of patients with normal-sized spleens had demonstrable tumor infiltration at laparotomy, whereas 35 percent of patients with clinical splenomegaly had no histologic evidence of disease. Liver involvement is more common in patients with positive lymphograms and enlarged spleens. Although very important, the routine use of staging laparotomy in all patients may not be appropriate. Laparotomy should be utilized in patients whose clinical stages make them candidates for treatment with radiation therapy alone and in whom evidence of unsuspected abdominal disease will significantly change treatment. A staging laparotomy should not be performed in patients who are to receive chemotherapy based on the presence of bulky chest disease, bulky abdominal involvement, or stage IV

disease. A staging laparotomy with splenectomy should be performed by a surgeon who is skilled in this procedure after careful review of clinical, laboratory, pathologic, and radiologic studies. Finally, a number of ancillary studies may be very useful in selected patients and are listed in Table 311-7. Gallium scintigraphy is useful in following response to treatment and in detecting early recurrences. A gallium scan is necessary at the time of initial staging to determine whether the lymphoma is gallium-avid.

Laboratory abnormalities   Routine blood counts, liver function tests, and renal function tests are all necessary parts of the medical workup but do not provide information about the extent of Hodgkin's disease or of specific organ involvement. A moderate normochromic, normocytic anemia associated with low serum iron level and low iron-binding capacity but with normal or increased iron stores in the bone marrow may be present in patients with Hodgkin's disease as well as in other neoplastic and chronic diseases. A moderate to marked leukemoid reaction is common, particularly in symptomatic patients, and usually disappears with treatment. Mild peripheral absolute eosinophilia is not uncommon, especially in patients with pruritus. Absolute monocytosis is also observed. Absolute lymphocytopenia (<1000 cells per cubic milliliter) usually occurs in patients with more advanced disease. Many tests have been evaluated as indicators of disease activity. To date, the erythrocyte sedimentation rate still is the best monitor, but it suffers from its lack of specificity and can return to normal when residual disease is still demonstrable. Other abnormal tests include increased serum levels of copper, calcium, lactic acid, alkaline phosphatase, lysozyme, globulins, C-reactive protein, and other acute phase reactants.

Immunologic abnormalities   Hodgkin's disease is associated with a well-described but poorly understood immunologic defect. Untreated patients, including those with limited disease, have defective cellular immunity characterized by anergy to routine skin tests. They also have a reversal of the CD4/CD8 ratio, suggesting that this anergy may be due to an increased number of suppressor T cells as well as a decreased number of CD4-positive cells. In several studies, decreased immune reactivity correlates both with advanced stages of disease and the presence of systemic symptoms. However, anergy to recall and neoantigens appears to have no prognostic significance. Following successful therapy, anergy reverses to recall antigens but is still present in some patients to neoantigens. In addition to anergy, other tests of T cell function, including responses to mitogens and suppressor cell function, suggest a defect in immune function prior to and following treatment. Humoral immunity with antibody production to soluble antigens is normal in untreated patients. Thus patients who undergo staging laparotomy and splenectomy will develop humoral immunity to pneumococcal antigens if immunized with the pneumococcal vaccine prior to therapy. The clinical impact of these immune defects is limited. Except for a higher than normal incidence of herpes zoster and development of warts, these patients are not plagued by opportunistic infections.

NATURAL HISTORY ACCORDING TO HISTOLOGIC SUBTYPE
Patients with lymphocyte-predominant Hodgkin's disease are usually asymptomatic at presentation and tend to have localized disease. These patients are usually young, rarely have systemic symptoms or mediastinal mass, and are predominantly males. Nodular sclerosis Hodgkin's disease is found most frequently in adolescents and young adults who usually have localized disease; a preponderance are young women who present with a large mediastinal mass. Lymphocyte-depleted Hodgkin's disease is usually disseminated at the time of diagnosis and occurs in older patients who frequently have systemic symptoms. The mixed cellularity type occurs in all age groups and stages and is only slightly more common in males. There is a tendency toward an older age peak (30 to 40 years) than with nodular sclerosis, and approximately half of these patients have advanced disease. Patients with lymphocyte-predominant and nodular sclerosis Hodgkin's disease, if untreated, have a more indolent disease associated with a longer survival and are more likely to be cured with radiotherapy.

There are several variables which adversely affect the prognosis of Hodgkin's disease. The number of involved sites and presence of bulky disease are the most important variables because extensive disease is often associated with high frequency of drug-resistant tumor cells. Large masses in the chest (greater than one-third the chest diameter) respond poorly to radiotherapy or chemotherapy alone but respond better to combined treatment. The prognosis is generally poor if a patient's disease is resistant to primary therapy or relapse occurs within 12 months. Age and systemic B symptoms are poor prognostic signs regardless of stage. Systemic B symptoms forbode a very poor prognosis, especially when both fevers and weight loss are present.

TREATMENT OF HODGKIN'S DISEASE Essentially all patients can and should be treated with curative intent. Radiotherapy may cure over 80 percent of patients with localized Hodgkin's disease and chemotherapy over 50 percent of those with disseminated disease. *The choice of treatment regimen is totally dependent on stage of disease.* As with all neoplasms, the therapy of Hodgkin's disease is constantly being reevaluated to improve disease-free survival and decrease toxicity.

Radiotherapy Radiation therapy alone has been evaluated in patients with pathologic stages IA, IIA, IB, and IIB. Although previously some patients with stage IIIA disease were treated with radiotherapy alone, more recent studies suggest that chemotherapy yields better results in patients with stage IIIA disease. While lower doses of radiation therapy will cause tumor regression, it was the recognition that 4000 cGy delivered at the rate of 1000 cGy per week could eradicate localized Hodgkin's disease that revolutionized treatment and led to substantial cure rates in patients with localized disease. With the knowledge that Hodgkin's spreads by lymphatic contiguity, three types of radiation fields were devised—namely, the mantle field, the paraaortic field, and pelvic irradiation. The *mantle field* includes the submandibular, cervical, supraclavicular, infraclavicular, axillary, mediastinal, and hilar lymph nodes. The *paraaortic field* covers the transverse processes of the abdominal vertebral bodies and the spleen, if it has not been removed. *Pelvic irradiation* includes the common iliac, hypogastric, external iliac, and inguinal nodes. When there is gross pelvic nodal involvement, the femoral nodes are also treated. Sometimes the pelvic and paraaortic fields are treated as one unit, which is then commonly called the *inverted-Y field*. The use of pelvic irradiation has recently been reduced, since stage I and II supradiaphragmatic Hodgkin's disease can be treated without pelvic irradiation and for stage III disease total nodal irradiation has only a limited role. Patients now receive mantle and paraaortic irradiation and only rarely total nodal irradiation. Patients receive doses of 3600 to 4000 cGy with an additional "cone down" dose for a total of 4000 to 4400 cGy to areas of bulk disease.

Patients with localized nodal Hodgkin's disease (pathologic stages IA and IIA) treated with mantle or paraaortic radiation therapy have nearly 80 percent long-term disease-free survival. Patients with stage IB and IIB disease have a slightly reduced disease-free survival (70 percent); however, most patients who relapse can be treated successfully with optimal combination chemotherapy. Early-stage patients with large mediastinal involvement appear to have a higher risk of relapse after radiation therapy alone (disease-free survival of 40 to 55 percent) compared with patients with minimal or no mediastinal disease and should be managed with combined-modality therapy.

Radiation therapy can lead to acute and late complications. Acute side effects of mantle irradiation include transient dry mouth, pharyngitis, fatigue, and weight loss. Approximately 15 percent of patients within several months of mantle irradiation develop paresthesias in the lower extremities upon flexion of the neck or thighs (Lhermitte's syndrome). This syndrome usually resolves spontaneously; there is no correlation between this syndrome and irreversible spinal injury. Other long-term side effects include radiation pneumonitis (severe in less than 5 percent of patients) and symptomatic pulmonary fibrosis (<1 percent). Late complications of mantle irradiation involve cardiac damage, including pericardial effusion and, very rarely, myocardial damage. Cardiac irradiation also may accelerate coronary artery disease and induce early myocardial infarctions, although recent controlled studies have reported only a borderline significant increased risk with modern techniques. Hypothyroidism may occur in up to 30 percent of patients following mantle irradiation. Paraaortic irradiation is rarely associated with significant side effects. Pelvic irradiation acutely induces transient diarrhea and bladder irritation associated with frequency. Chronic effects include potential long-term bone marrow suppression and sterility; therefore, pelvic irradiation is less frequently employed. Moreover, increasing numbers of secondary tumors are being observed. A recent study revealed a 2.8-fold observed to expected cumulative risk of development of second tumors in 15-year survivors with Hodgkin's disease treated with radiation. The most serious of these is the emergence of second malignancies, particularly acute nonlymphocytic leukemia and high-grade non-Hodgkin's lymphomas, often seen in patients who received combined-modality therapy.

Chemotherapy By 1963, five agents had been identified as effective in the treatment of Hodgkin's disease, namely, alkylating agents, vinca alkaloids, procarbazine, methotrexate, and prednisone. While disease regression occurred in 30 to 70 percent of patients, complete response occurred in only 10 percent. Based on the principles of dose, schedule, and combination chemotherapy, a four-drug combination regimen termed MOPP [mechlorethamine (nitrogen mustard), vincristine (Oncovin), procarbazine, and prednisone] was introduced. In a 14-year median follow-up of 188 patients, DeVita and colleagues found that 84 percent had achieved a complete remission and 48 percent were alive. MOPP therapy has been associated with significant toxicity. Nearly all patients experience some degree of nausea and vomiting, which can be minimized by antiemetic therapy. Bone marrow suppression with associated leukopenia and thrombocytopenia is frequently observed. Less commonly, absolute neutropenia occurs with increased susceptibility to infection. All males and nearly all females over age 35 become sterile following MOPP therapy. There is a 2 percent actuarial risk of developing secondary leukemia at 10 years following MOPP, which returns to baseline thereafter. The acute nonlymphocytic leukemia which occurs following MOPP differs from primary acute nonlymphocytic leukemia in that the former more commonly exhibits a preleukemic or myelodysplastic syndrome, a different cytogenetic profile with emphasis on partial or complete deletions of the fifth and seventh chromosomes, and a much lower response rate to antileukemia therapy. MOPP chemotherapy has not been associated with the development of second solid tumors.

Other multiple-drug regimens have been tested in the treatment of advanced Hodgkin's disease. However, none of the "MOPP-derived combinations" have been superior to the original MOPP administered at optimal dose and schedule. Regimens also have been developed to treat MOPP-resistant patients. The best known of these is ABVD (adriamycin, bleomycin, vinblastine, and dacarbazine). A series of controlled clinical trials has demonstrated that ABVD is equivalent to MOPP in the successful treatment of primary advanced Hodgkin's disease. ABVD also has led to a significant number of prolonged complete remissions in MOPP treatment failures. Although most ABVD toxicities are identical to MOPP, the ABVD regimen produces only transient germ cell toxicity in males, no drug-induced amenorrhea, and an apparent lower incidence of second tumors (although the data on this point are limited), but an increased risk of myocardial and pulmonary damage can be seen when compared with MOPP. Another regimen with similar effectiveness but less toxicity is ChlVPP (chlorambucil, vinblastine, procarbazine, and prednisone).

More recent studies have attempted to sequentially combine MOPP with ABVD to improve cure rate. In several studies, the use of MOPP alternating with ABVD appears to produce higher complete remissions and disease-free survivals compared with MOPP alone, but longer periods of observation and more patients are necessary to confirm this result.

Salvage therapy After proper restaging, further radiotherapy can be delivered (if technically feasible) to patients who have relapsed outside a radiation field or following combination chemotherapy. In patients not achieving a complete remission or relapsing after MOPP, second-line non-cross-resistant regimens are available. If patients relapse more than 12 months after the completion of MOPP therapy, they should be retreated with MOPP or an appropriate alternate regimen; if they relapse in less than 12 months, they should be treated with a salvage regimen (crossover, i.e., ABVD for MOPP and MOPP for ABVD). With ABVD as a salvage regimen, 30 to 50 percent of patients will achieve a complete remission and 10 to 30 percent will experience long-term disease-free survival. Poor prognostic variables for salvage include stage IV disease at diagnosis, B symptoms at relapse, or remission lasting <12 months. Selected chemotherapy patients who relapse in limited nodal sites, even when the first remission is less than 12 months, can be treated with salvage radiotherapy, preferably with combination chemotherapy. Finally, as with non-Hodgkin's lymphoma, autologous or allogeneic bone marrow transplantation is an effective salvage treatment for some patients. Unlike non-Hodgkin's lymphoma, total-body irradiation has minimal value, and virtually all regimens include high-dose chemotherapy. The acute lethal pulmonary and hepatic toxicity from these regimens, however, can be very high (5 to 25 percent). As with non-Hodgkin's lymphomas, patient's whose disease remains sensitive to chemotherapeutic agents are more likely to experience long-term disease-free survival in the range of 40 percent.

Therapeutic recommendations by stage STAGE IA AND IIA, NONBULKY DISEASE Following staging laparotomy in patients with supradiaphragmatic disease, subtotal nodal irradiation is the treatment of choice. Rarely, in patients with subdiaphragmatic lymphoma, radiotherapy is delivered by an inverted-Y field including the splenic pedicle in stage I disease and through total nodal irradiation in stage II disease. Some studies suggest that treatment with involved-field radiotherapy combined with chemotherapy produces comparable results, but most do not consider this accepted treatment of choice. For patients with subdiaphragmatic stage II disease of paraaortic nodes, chemotherapy is recommended.

STAGE IB AND IIB, NONBULKY DISEASE The therapy is the same as for stage IA and IIA Hodgkin's disease; however, the relapse rate is higher (30 percent). Relapse can usually be salvaged with chemotherapy. Subtotal or combination chemotherapy with involved-field irradiation remains an alternative treatment for these patients.

STAGE II, BULKY Stage II disease with bulky mediastinal/hilar adenopathy should be managed with combined-modality therapy, including chemotherapy and radiotherapy to sites of bulk disease.

STAGE IIIA Patients who present with minimal splenic disease appear to respond equally well to total lymphoid irradiation, combination chemotherapy with irradiation, or chemotherapy alone. However, randomized, prospective trials are needed to further determine the relative roles of radiation therapy and chemotherapy. For patients with enlarged paraaortic and pelvic nodes, the recommended treatment is combination chemotherapy with or without irradiation to involved sites. Alternative therapy includes combination chemotherapy alone.

STAGE IIIB, STAGE IV Combination chemotherapy is recommended. In uncontrolled studies, the addition of radiation therapy to involved sites may improved disease-free survival.

REFERENCES

ARMITAGE JO: Bone marrow transplantation in the treatment of patients with lymphoma. Blood 73:1749, 1989

————: Drug therapy: Treatment of non-Hodgkin's lymphoma. N Engl J Med 328:1023, 1993

CANELLOS GP et al.: Chemotherapy of advanced Hodgkin's disease with MOPP, ABVD, or MOPP alternating with ABVD. N Engl J Med 327:1478, 1992

CASTELLINO RA: Diagnostic imaging evaluation of Hodgkin's disease and non-Hodgkin's lymphoma. Cancer 67(suppl):1177, 1991

COLTMAN CA JR (ed): Hodgkin's disease. Semin Oncol 17:641, 1990

FREEDMAN AS, NADLER LM: Immunologic markers in non-Hodgkin's lymphomas. Hematol Oncol Clin North Am 5:871, 1991

GROSSBARD ML et al: Monoclonal antibody–based therapies of leukemia and lymphoma. Blood 80:863, 1992

KAPLAN HS: *Hodgkin's Disease,* 2d ed. Cambridge, Harvard University, 1990

LEVINE AM: Acquired immunodeficiency syndrome–related lymphomas. Blood 80:8, 1992

WILLIAMS SF, GOLUMB HM (eds.): Non-Hodgkin's lymphoma. Semin Oncol 17:1, 1990

URBA W, LONGO DL: Hodgkin's disease. N Engl J Med 326:678, 1992

312 BLOOD GROUPS AND BLOOD TRANSFUSION

HARVEY G. KLEIN

BLOOD GROUP ANTIGENS AND ANTIBODIES

Human red blood cell membranes contain hundreds of different antigenic determinants (epitopes), the molecular structure of which is determined by genes at various chromosomal loci. The term *blood group* refers to any well-defined system of red blood cell antigens controlled by a locus having a variable number of allelic genes, such as A, B, and O in the ABO system. More than 20 blood group systems are currently recognized. The term *blood type* refers to the antigen phenotype, which is the serologic expression of the inherited blood group genes.

Alloantibodies specific for the different blood group antigens may occur "naturally," in the absence of known exposure to the antigen, or in response to transfusion or pregnancy. Naturally occurring antibodies tend to be IgM molecules and probably result from a thymus-independent immune response to widely occurring carbohydrate antigens. Anti-A and anti-B are examples of such antibodies. Antibodies formed in response to transfusion initially belong to the IgM class but switch to the IgG isotype within a few weeks or months. Most alloantibodies, regardless of class, are not clinically significant. However, serologic testing detects a variety of agglutinating, hemolyzing, and coating antibodies that may affect transfusion. Serologic reactivity at 30°C or higher best predicts clinical significance.

CARBOHYDRATE BLOOD GROUP ANTIGENS **ABO system: Genes and antigens** The ABO blood group is the most important system for blood transfusion. There are four major allelic genes in this system, A1, A2, B, and O. The locus for these alleles is on the long arm of chromosome 9. The gene products of the first three genes are glycosyl transferases, which attach specific sugars by alpha linkage to oligosaccharide chains. These chains comprise the carbohydrate moiety of the glycolipids and glycoproteins on red blood cells. The A and B genes differ in a few single-base substitutions, resulting in differences in A and B transferase specificity. A single-base deletion in the O gene results in an inactive protein that cross-reacts with the A and B transferases but has no detectable enzyme activity. The A1 and A2 transferases perform the same function but have different rate constants. Red cells from subjects who inherit the A1 gene have more A-reactive sites than do those with an A2 gene.

Nearly all individuals possess naturally occurring isoagglutinins, antibodies directed against the A and B antigens not present on their own red blood cells. These isoagglutinins account for the major blood group incompatibilities. Most of the major phenotypes represent more than one genotype. In practice, the ABO type is determined by testing the red cells with anti-A and anti-B and by testing the serum against A, B, and O reagent cells. The frequencies of the major ABO phenotypes in selected populations are shown in Table 312-1.

Red blood cells of types O and A2 have large amounts of another antigen, called H, which is the immediate precursor of A and B. H specificity depends on the presence of the monosaccharide fucose, attached to the oligosaccharides by a transferase that is the product of the very common H gene. The H and ABO loci are not genetically linked. Very rare individuals who fail to inherit an H gene from either

TABLE 312-1 Percentage of ABO phenotypes in selected populations

Population*	Phenotypes					
	A$_1$	A$_2$	B	A$_1$B	A$_2$B	O
European-American	35	10	8	3	1	43
African-American	23	6	17	3	1	50
German	32.5	9.4	11	3.1	1.1	42.8
South American Indian	0	0	0	0	0	100
Australian Aborigine	55.6	0	0	0	0	44.4
Lapps	36.1	18.5	4.8	6.2	6.2	18.2

* Selected populations do not necessarily apply to racial group.

parent cannot produce this transferase. As a result, even if an A or B gene is inherited, these subjects cannot produce A, B, or H antigens, and their serum contains all three antibodies. Because patients with this rare phenotype (O$_h$, Bombay) are extremely difficult to transfuse, blood of the same type must be sought from rare-donor registries.

Antibodies in the ABO system Red blood cells of newborn infants have a decreased number of A, B, and H reactive sites, and their plasma normally contains very little anti-A or anti-B. Maternal anti-A and anti-B are primarily IgM and do not cross the placenta. However, some type O adults produce an IgG cross-reacting antibody termed anti-A,B which can cross the placenta and react with fetal cells. For this reason, ABO hemolytic disease of the newborn (HDN) usually occurs in type A or B infants of type O mothers.

Safe transfusion practice prohibits transfusing A, B, or AB blood to patients whose red cells lack the corresponding antigens, since the recipient's plasma contains incompatible antibodies. Most fatal hemolytic transfusion reactions result from patient and sample identification errors that end in such incompatible transfusions. Type A or B blood, preferably as packed red cells, may be transfused to AB recipients, since the passively infused antibody is rarely of clinical significance. Although type O red blood cells may be given to patients of type A, B, or AB when type-specific blood is not available, plasma from some type O individuals contains a potent hemolytic antibody; thus type O should not be given as whole blood except in an emergency.

Lewis system Antibodies to Lewis system antigens are the most common cause of incompatibility during pretransfusion compatibility testing. Antigens in the Lewis system are not integral components of red blood cell membranes but are glycosphingolipid molecules absorbed from the surrounding plasma. The two most common Lewis antigens, Le^a and Le^b, are carbohydrate antigens that are structurally related to the ABH antigens and result from the action of the Lewis gene product, a fucosyl transferase, on an oligosaccharide precursor.

Anti-Le^a and anti-Le^b are common, naturally occurring, complement-binding antibodies of the IgM class. Lewis antibodies rarely cross the placenta and do not result in HDN. While anti-Le^a has caused hemolytic transfusion reactions, the plasma of Le^a+ donors usually contains sufficient Lewis antigen to neutralize the patient's antibody when whole blood is transfused. Anti-Le^b rarely causes transfusion reactions.

I system The I and i antigenic determinants are heterogeneous oligosaccharides that are biochemically related to the H, A, B, Le, and P antigens. The i antigen is an unbranched oligosaccharide chain that is converted by the I gene product, a glycosyltransferase, to the I antigen branched structure. Fetal and cord red blood cells react very weakly with anti-I and strongly with anti-i, suggesting that glycosyltransferase production is developmentally regulated. Rare adult red blood cells lack I antigen.

Polyclonal anti-I is a weak, clinically unimportant cold agglutinin found in the sera of most normal adults. High-titer, monoclonal anti-I autoantibodies, on the other hand, can cause chronic red cell destruction in some patients with cold agglutinin disease and lymphoproliferative disorders. An occasional patient with mononucleosis or

Mycoplasma pneumonia will develop high-titered cold agglutinins with anti-i or anti-I specificity. These antibodies are generally monoclonal and may cause autoimmune hemolysis. The rare, genetically I-negative person may develop alloanti-I. Alloanti-i has not been reported.

When patients with anti-i autoantibodies require transfusion, compatible blood is readily available. The red blood cells of most adults lack i antigen. Because anti-I autoantibodies generally react only at low temperatures, even patients with strong cold-reacting anti-I autoantibodies can be transfused safely if the blood is kept warm during the infusion.

P system Three structurally related glycosphingolipid antigens, P, P^k, and P$_1$ are considered together under the P blood group system. As in the ABO and Lewis systems, the gene products are glycosyltransferases. P$_1$ and P, the major antigenic determinants, result from different synthetic pathways and likely represent independent genetic systems.

Anti-P$_1$ is usually a weak IgM cold agglutinin that almost never damages red blood cells. In contrast, rare individuals who lack P antigens (p phenotype) may possess potent high-titer antibodies directed against one or more of the P antigens. One such antibody, anti-P$_1$PP^k (anti-Tj^a), can cause severe hemolytic transfusion reactions and HDN and has been associated with recurrent spontaneous abortions, possibly related to the presence of P-like antigens on trophoblastic tissue. Finally, sera of patients with paroxysmal cold hemoglobinuria may contain a peculiar biphasic complement-fixing autoantibody with anti-P specificity known as the *Donath-Landsteiner antibody*. Donath-Landsteiner antibodies, which bind to red blood cells in the cold and fix complement when warmed, have been reported with hemolytic syndromes associated with syphilis and different viral infections.

PROTEIN BLOOD GROUP ANTIGENS Rh system The Rhesus or Rh system is second in importance only to the ABO system in transfusion practice. The Rh locus is on chromosome 1. Rh antigenic determinants depend on poorly understood interactions between a hydrophobic 30- to 32-kDa red cell membrane protein and the posttranslational addition of phospholipid molecules. More than 40 Rh phenotypes have been defined serologically. Recent evidence identifies at least three tandem Rh loci, somewhat analogous to the HLA complex. The Rh alleles describe the structure of a set of epitope pairs, C or c, E or e, and D, the last having a postulated silent allele, d. Epitopes are inherited as haplotypes, e.g., CDe or cde.

Because Rho(D) is the most immunogenic alloantigen, donated blood is tested and labeled for the presence or absence of this antigen. Approximately 15 percent of Caucasians lack the D antigen and are classified as Rh-negative. About 80 percent of Rh-negative persons who receive a single unit of Rh-positive red blood cells will develop anti-D, an antibody that may cause severe hemolytic transfusion reactions and HDN. For this reason, Rh-negative patients are always given Rh-negative cellular blood components, except during emergency circumstances. Anti-D can be induced by as few as 0.5 mL red blood cells or 0.04 mL red blood cells when given in repeated injections. Premenopausal Rh-negative women must not receive Rh-positive blood components unless adequate amounts of Rh immunoglobulin are given to prevent primary immunization; otherwise, subsequent pregnancy with an Rh-positive child almost always stimulates a secondary immune response, resulting in HDN.

The Rh antigens C, c, E, and e are considerably less immunogenic (less than 2 percent of susceptible recipients), and matching transfusion recipients for these antigens is impractical. Of course, previously sensitized patients must receive blood lacking the corresponding specific antigen. About 20 percent of donors lack the c antigen and are therefore compatible with recipients whose plasma contains anti-c. However, only 2 percent of donors lack e antigen, so patients who have developed anti-e are difficult to match. Blood banks often maintain computerized lists of phenotyped donors for such circumstances, and autologous blood remains an option for elective surgical procedures.

MNS system Studies of the biochemistry and molecular genetics of the MNS system have contributed more to understanding red blood cell membrane structure and function than to practical transfusion problems. Closely linked genes on chromosome 4 determine the MN and Ss antigens, which are inherited as haplotypes: MS, Ms, NS, and Ns. A transmembrane protein, glycophorin A, carries M and N specificity, while S and s are on glycophorin B. Absence of these sialoglycoproteins is associated with rare red blood cell phenotypes such as En(a-), S^u, and M^k, but there are no associated hematologic abnormalities. Anti-M and anti-N are naturally occurring IgM agglutinins directed against epitopes involving both the sugar and amino acid components of the protein. Formation of anti-S or anti-s usually requires the stimulus of transfusion or pregnancy, and unlike anti-M and anti-N, these IgG class antibodies may destroy red blood cells. A third hemolytic antibody, anti-U, is formed by sensitized black patients with the S^u phenotype. Since less than 1 percent of black patients and no white patients are U negative, compatible blood is almost impossible to find.

Kell, Duffy, and Kidd systems The Kell blood group system contains more than 20 different antigens with multiple alleles at different loci. The Kell (K) and Cellano (k) antigens are codominant autosomal alleles, and Kell is the most potent red blood cell immunogen outside of the ABO and Rh systems. An X-linked gene determines expression of the Kell precursor antigen K_x, and rare individuals of the "McLeod phenotype" lack K_x on their red blood cells. Red blood cells of the McLeod phenotype exhibit acanthocytosis, weakened Kell antigens, and in vivo hemolysis. Furthermore, genes for K_x and for type II chronic granulomatous disease (CGD) are closely linked. Type II CGD patients may display the McLeod phenotype if the deletion affects both genes. Patients with the McLeod phenotype should avoid transfusion, since a single unit of blood may elicit antibodies that react with all Kell system red cell antigens.

The Duffy and Kidd blood group systems are composed of equally prevalent codominant alleles, Fy^a and Fy^b in the former and Jk^a and Jk^b in the latter. Both blood groups are significantly more complex at the level of the gene. Duffy blood group antigens function as receptor sites for invasion of red blood cells by at least one species of malarial parasite, *Plasmodium vivax*. More than 70 percent of native West Africans lack these red cell antigens, a rare finding among Caucasians, suggesting malaria-induced selective pressure in West Africa.

Anti-K and anti-Fy^a are commonly encountered antibodies capable of marked alloimmune red cell destruction. The Kidd antibodies, anti-Jk^a and anti-Jk^b, are notoriously transient and difficult to detect. A delayed hemolytic transfusion reaction that occurs with blood that tested compatible suggests the delayed appearance of anti-Jk^a.

BLOOD TRANSFUSION

Blood components are biologic medications licensed by the Food and Drug Administration. Responsible medical practice obliges physicians to acquire knowledge of blood to make sound transfusion judgments and to advise their patients accordingly. Physicians who use blood must understand the benefits and risks of each component.

WHOLE BLOOD AND RED BLOOD CELLS A unit of whole blood consists of approximately 450 mL blood with about 65 g hemoglobin. When refrigerated, the red blood cells are viable for up to 6 weeks, depending on the anticoagulant-preservative solution used. Whole blood is not a reliable source of platelets or granulocytes, and the labile coagulation factors V and VIII begin to deteriorate within hours of collection. Most other plasma coagulation proteins are stable for the entire storage period.

Few clinical situations require whole blood transfusion. Whole blood should be reserved for catastrophic medical or surgical bleeding, e.g., during rapid gastrointestinal hemorrhage or with major trauma, when simultaneous restoration of oxygen carrying capacity, volume, and coagulation factors is desired. Even in hemorrhagic shock, a combination of red cells and crystalloid or colloid solution is usually effective. In emergencies, rapid volume replacement generally takes precedence over red cell replacement, and cell-free resuscitation fluids should be used while the recipient's blood type is being determined. When the red blood cell deficit is critical, uncrossmatched type-specific whole blood or type O red cells are indicated.

Fresh whole blood is a poorly defined component and is rarely advantageous. During refrigerated storage, whole blood oxygen affinity increases as red cell 2,3-diphosphoglycerate (2,3-DPG) falls. Both oxygen affinity and 2,3-DPG levels return to normal within hours of transfusion. Other storage changes include a rise in extracellular potassium and lactate concentrations and a decline in pH. The clinical importance of these observations remains controversial. Blood less than 7 days old is still recommended for neonatal exchange transfusions, and a recent study suggests that blood less than 24 h old may benefit children undergoing cardiopulmonary bypass.

Red blood cells or "packed" cells are prepared by centrifuging whole blood and expressing the plasma into a satellite bag. Red cells are concentrated to a hematocrit of 80 percent or more and to a volume of about 200 mL. The refrigerated storage period is the same as that for whole blood. Red cells permit restoration of oxygen carrying capacity with less risk of volume overload and limit the quantity of sodium, potassium, citrate, and ammonia infused. The appropriateness of red blood cell transfusion should be determined by clinical signs and symptoms and not by a preset hemoglobin level.

Red blood cells are supportive therapy for perioperative blood loss and for chronic anemia when no timely definitive therapy is available. Each unit of red cells elevates an adult's hemoglobin concentration by about 1 g/dL and the hematocrit by about 3 points. The advent of a lineage-specific growth factor, recombinant human erythropoietin (rHuEpo), has dramatically decreased the use of red cell transfusion in patients with chronic end-stage renal disease, in whom endogenous erythropoietin is deficient. rHuEpo also has replaced red blood cell transfusion for selected patients with cancer, AIDS, and transfusion-dependent myelodysplasia.

Patients with autoimmune hemolytic anemia do not ordinarily receive red blood cell transfusion. Unless the autoantibody is directed against a specific blood group antigen, the transfused red cells will be destroyed as rapidly as the patient's own cells. Serious hemolytic reactions may result from alloantibodies difficult to detect in the presence of an autoantibody. However, when anemia is severe enough to cause hypoxemia or cardiac decompensation, cautious transfusion may be lifesaving. Patients with some forms of ineffective erythropoiesis, e.g., nutritional deficiencies of vitamin B_{12}, folate, or iron, are candidates for transfusion only if they are symptomatic and only if the cause of anemia cannot be corrected expeditiously by specific replacement therapy. These conditions number among the few indications for the single-unit transfusion.

Red blood cells in a hypertonic cryoprotective glycerol solution may be stored frozen for as long as 10 years. Once thawed, the cells must be washed thoroughly, lest residual glycerol cause intravascular hemolysis. The resulting red blood cell concentrate contains almost no plasma proteins, which makes it ideal for patients who experience reactions to donor plasma proteins. The markedly reduced number of platelets and leukocytes also decreases febrile reactions, immunogenicity, and cytomegalovirus transmission. Cryopreserved red blood cells retain biochemical and posttransfusion survival characteristics similar to those present at the time of freezing. Frozen cells are generally reserved for providing blood to persons with rare phenotypes or for storing autologous units in unusual circumstances. Some institutions stockpile cryopreserved cells for inventory control, and the Department of Defense has deployed such stockpiles for military emergencies. However, the thaw and wash process is slow, logistically difficult, and expensive, and the thawed cells outdate within 24 h.

PLATELETS Platelet concentrates are prepared either by centrifugation of platelet-rich plasma from single units of blood to yield 6 × 10^{10} platelets or by automated plateletpheresis to yield approximately six such units from individual donors. When stored at room temperature in gas-permeable containers to maintain aerobic metabolism and pH, platelets remain viable for up to 5 days. A unit of platelets should raise an adult's platelet count by at least 5000 cells per microliter, and platelets circulate for about a week in stable, nonimmunized, thrombocytopenic patients.

Platelet transfusions are indicated when either severe thrombocytopenia or platelet dysfunction is associated with active or imminent bleeding. Platelet transfusions usually control bleeding in thrombocytopenic patients who have suppressed platelet production, such as occurs with leukemia, chemotherapy, or radiotherapy, or who develop the dilutional thrombocytopenia observed during massive transfusion. Platelet transfusions are less effective when there is peripheral destruction, such as consumption coagulopathy or immune thrombocytopenic purpura (ITP), and are not recommended except when life-threatening hemorrhage occurs; in these situations, platelet transfusions may prevent potentially fatal hemorrhage until the cause of platelet destruction can be reversed. The use of prophylactic platelet transfusions for stable thrombocytopenic patients remains controversial. The threshold platelet count at which spontaneous bleeding occurs will vary with the cause of the thrombocytopenia and with the degree of platelet dysfunction. Most patients with platelet counts about 10,000 cells per microliter do not develop spontaneous bleeding complications. Certain complicating clinical factors such as sepsis, rapidly falling counts, medications that interfere with platelet function, and mucositis increase the risk of hemorrhage in patients receiving myelosuppressive therapy. Prophylactic platelet transfusions are often used to maintain counts above 20,000 cells per microliter in these circumstances. Patients in the immediate postoperative period and those with a second defect in hemostasis may require a platelet count of 50,000 to 100,000 cells per microliter. Platelet transfusions should be monitored with 1- or 24-h posttransfusion platelet counts.

Ideally, transfused platelets should be of the same ABO and Rh type as the patient. ABO-mismatched platelets result in lower platelet increments and may contribute to the development of platelet refractoriness. When group O donors are used for A, B, or AB recipients, donor plasma may contain sufficient antibody to destroy some of the patient's red blood cells. Incompatible plasma may be reduced for pediatric infusions or when adults require large numbers of single-donor platelets. Although platelets do not express the Rh antigen, the red blood cells present can sensitize an Rh-negative recipient of Rh-positive platelet concentrates. Rh-negative patients should receive platelets from Rh-negative donors when possible. When this is not possible, Rh immunization can be prevented by injection of Rh immune globulin. This is especially important for Rh-negative women in childbearing years.

Patients who receive platelet transfusions frequently develop alloantibodies to the HLA antigens that are expressed on lymphocytes in the platelet concentrates. Alloimmunized patients may become resistant (refractory) to further platelet transfusions unless the platelets come from HLA-compatible donors. As many as a third of alloimmunized patients fail to respond even to HLA-identical platelets. Suboptimal response to fresh histocompatible platelets suggests platelet-specific antibodies, nonimmune platelet consumption, or hypersplenism.

LEUKOCYTE-REDUCED BLOOD COMPONENTS Red blood cell and platelet components contain variable numbers of residual leukocytes, predominantly lymphocytes. Febrile reactions are common in sensitized patients who receive components containing more than 5×10^8 leukocytes, and alloimmunization to the HLA antigens of residual lymphocytes may occur when more than 10^6 lymphocytes are transfused. Certain cell-associated viruses such as cytomegalovirus (CMV) and HTLV I and II are transmitted by small numbers of lymphocytes. Recent evidence indicates that allogeneic leukocytes may activate latent viruses in the recipient. These observations have stimulated efforts to develop leukocyte-reduced cellular blood components. Cell washing procedures remove most plasma but reduce the leukocytes by only about 1 log, enough to eliminate some febrile reactions but insufficient to prevent other complications. Specially constructed filters can reduce the leukocyte content in red blood cell components or platelet concentrates by more than 3 logs to levels difficult to count with standard techniques. Blood cell separators also collect leukocyte-reduced platelets. These leukocyte-reduced components virtually eliminate febrile reactions, reduce the risk of HLA alloimmunization and cell-associated virus transmission, and may reduce reactivation of latent viruses such as CMV and HIV-1. Since transfusion-associated graft-versus-host-disease (GVHD) can result from as few as 10^4 allogeneic lymphocytes transfused to a severely immunocompromised patient, and since the outcome is frequently lethal, current leukocyte reduction techniques do not reliably protect such patients. To prevent transfusion-associated GVHD, blood components should be treated with gamma irradiation at a dose of 25 Gy.

GRANULOCYTE TRANSFUSIONS Infection has replaced bleeding as the major cause of death in severely pancytopenic patients. The frequency of infection increases as the absolute neutrophil count falls below 500 cells per microliter. Improved antibiotic regimens and recombinant myeloid growth factors (G-CSF and GM-CSF) that reduce the duration of neutropenia have improved the management of such patients. However, selected patients with fewer than 500 granulocytes per microliter and persistent fever, despite appropriate antibiotic therapy for at least 48 h, may benefit from granulocyte transfusions. Other less well documented indications include progressive fungal infections, inherited defects of granulocyte function such as CGD, and neonatal sepsis. Prophylactic transfusion of granulocytes to neutropenic patients does not appear to reduce the incidence of infections. A course of therapy consists of at least four daily transfusions of 10 to 30 $\times$ 10^9 neutrophils, probably a marginally effective number that represents only about 10 percent of normal daily neutrophil production. Transfusions are complicated by severe rigors, pulmonary injury, alloimmunization, and transmission of cell-associated viruses, particularly CMV. Leukocyte concentrates present a substantial risk of GVHD for immunosuppressed patients and premature infants. Prophylactic gamma irradiation is recommended but may adversely affect granulocyte function.

PLASMA COMPONENT THERAPY Fresh frozen plasma (FFP) and cryoprecipitate are the major plasma components used for patients with clotting disorders. (Management of inherited factor deficiencies with blood derivatives is discussed in Chap. 315.) FFP contains all coagulation factors found in fresh plasma. Each 250-mL unit infusion raises most coagulation factor levels 3 to 5 percent. FFP is used for bleeding patients with multiple coagulation factor deficiencies, such as occur in severe liver disease or dilutional coagulopathy. Warfarin-induced deficiency of vitamin K–dependent factors may be rapidly reversed with FFP, but ordinarily vitamin K administration produces a smooth reversal in 6 to 12 h. FFP is rarely indicated for prolongations of prothrombin time less than 1.5 times normal. FFP should not be used for volume expansion or prophylactically for cardiopulmonary bypass. When colloid volume expanders are indicated, human albumin fraction is equally effective and has been heat treated to inactivate viruses. Using plasma to supplement nutrition or to improve wound healing is likewise inappropriate.

Cryoprecipitate is prepared from FFP by a freeze-thaw process that concentrates about 60 percent of the fibrinogen, factor VIII, von Willebrand factor, and factor XIII into 10 percent of the original volume. Currently, the major uses are for patients with von Willebrand disease and for hypofibrinogenemia, as may occur with disseminated intravascular coagulation. Cryoprecipitate transmits the same viruses as plasma, and standard doses pooled from 12 to 20 donors carry an additive risk. Commercial clotting factor concentrates, treated to eliminate infectious agents, and recombinant clotting proteins have replaced plasma and cryoprecipitate for many uses.

HEMAPHERESIS Automated blood cell separators have made therapeutic plasmapheresis and blood cell removal rapid, safe, and easy. Two plasma volumes can be exchanged in less than 3 h, and intravascular solutes such as antibodies, immune complexes, and a variety of protein-bound toxins can be reduced by more than 50 percent with each exchange. The most established indications for plasmapheresis include symptomatic hyperviscosity syndrome, Goodpasture's syndrome, Guillain-Barré syndrome, and thrombotic thrombocytopenic purpura. For a variety of other illnesses, the efficacy and the appropriate volume, frequency, and replacement solutions have yet to be established.

Blood cells also may be efficiently exchanged or removed. Cell separators are routinely used for red cell exchange to manage acute complications of sickle cell disease such as stroke, chest syndrome, and priapism. When blast cells increase rapidly in acute leukemia, therapeutic leukapheresis can prevent associated cerebrovascular, pulmonary, and renal complications. Therapeutic plateletpheresis has been used to treat symptomatic thrombocythemia.

Recently, blood cell separators have been used to process bone marrow and to collect peripheral blood progenitor cells to support autologous bone marrow transplantation. Peripheral blood mononuclear cells also have been used for cancer and AIDS immunotherapy, as well as for somatic cell gene therapy of immune-deficient patients who lack adenosine deaminase.

CUSTOMIZED COMPONENTS   Autologous transfusion   The patient's own (autologous) blood may be collected and stored for future elective surgery. Other autologous techniques include intraoperative phlebotomy with crystalloid replacement (hemodilution), intraoperative collection of shed blood, and postoperative collection of blood from closed spaces such as mediastinal drainage. Autologous transfusion avoids the risks of immunologic mismatch and disease transmission. Autologous blood is recommended for patients planning elective surgical procedures that require 1 to 4 units of blood. For some patients with unstable cardiac and vascular disease, the benefits of autologous blood must be weighed against the medical risks of phlebotomy and the risks of delaying surgery. Supplemental iron with recombinant erythropoietin increases the amount of blood that can be collected, but the usefulness of this strategy has not been confirmed.

Directed donations   Some patients solicit blood donations from friends and family members in order to reduce the risk of infection from routine volunteer blood. Ironically, the prevalence of laboratory markers of infectious disease in blood from these directed donors exceeds the prevalence found in unselected repeat volunteer donors. For the donor, loss of anonymity and confidentiality is a further disadvantage of directed donation. For certain medical circumstances, e.g., maternal platelets for neonates with alloimmune thrombocytopenia and rare red blood cell phenotypes from compatible family members, directed donations are the preferred therapy. In contrast, medical considerations specifically contraindicate directed donations from a prospective father to a spouse in childbearing years and from a bone marrow donor to the marrow recipient before the transplant. Finally, transfusion-associated GVHD may result if cellular components from a relative are not irradiated.

MASSIVE TRANSFUSION   *Massive transfusion* is generally defined as replacement of total blood volume in less than 24 h. Dilution of platelets and, less often, of plasma coagulation factors may result when more than one blood volume is rapidly replaced with stored blood. Metabolic changes during massive transfusion are complex and interrelated. Rapid infusions of citrate anticoagulant can cause symptomatic hypocalcemia, especially in the presence of liver disease. Transient hyperkalemia and acidosis may result when the transfusion rate exceeds 100 mL/min. These changes are often followed by a metabolic alkalosis and hypokalemia as citric acid is metabolized to pyruvate and bicarbonate. Expectant use of calcium, potassium, or bicarbonate infusions is treacherous at best, and under no circumstances should these solutions be added to the blood components. When refrigerated blood infuses rapidly through large central venous lines, profound hypothermia may further complicate these metabolic changes and predispose the patient to seizures and cardiac arrhythmias. Commercial instruments are available to warm the blood during massive infusion.

COMPLICATIONS OF BLOOD TRANSFUSION   Transfusion reactions are classifed as immune or nonimmune (Table 312-2).

TABLE 312-2   Complications of transfusion per unit transfused

Immune complications	Frequency*	Nonimmune complications	Frequency*
Acute hemolysis	1/6000	Hepatitis	1/3000
Delayed hemolysis	1/1000	HIV (AIDS)	1/225,000
Febrile nonhemolytic	1/200	Hypervolemia	Unknown
Allergic cutaneous	1/200	Iron overload	Unknown
Anaphylactic	1/150,000	Bacterial sepsis	Rare
Alloimmunization (RBC)	1/100	Hypothermia	Rare
Alloimmunization (HLA)	1/10		
Graft-versus-host disease	Rare		

* Estimated.

Antibody-mediated reactions are directed against red blood cells, white blood cells, platelets, and at least one class of immunoglobulin, IgA. Transfusion of viable lymphocytes can result in cell-mediated GVHD. The major nonimmune reactions are due to circulatory overload, transfusional siderosis, and transmission of infectious agents. Reports that transfusion-induced immunomodulation decreases survival of cancer patients and increases postoperative infections further emphasize the seriousness of blood transfusion.

Hemolytic transfusion reactions   Red blood cell alloantibodies may lyse cells within the circulation or coat red blood cells and accelerate cell removal by the reticuloendothelial system. Approximately 1 in 100,000 units transfused will result in a fatal hemolytic reaction, usually from ABO incompatibility arising from misidentification of the patient or the blood specimen. Rapid cell destruction commonly involves the ABO system, since both anti-A and anti-B fix complement. Other antibodies reported to cause intravascular hemolysis include anti-Jk^a, anti-Fy^a, and rarely, anti-Le^a. Patients with acute hemolytic reactions may complain of flushing, pain at the infusion site, chest or back pain, restlessness, anxiety, nausea, or diarrhea. Signs include fever or chills and the typical findings of shock and renal failure. In comatose or anesthetized patients, the first indication may be hemoglobinuria or generalized bleeding resulting from disseminated intravascular coagulation.

Extravascular hemolysis is most often caused by antibodies of the Rh system, but several other antibodies, including those of Kell, Duffy, and Kidd systems, are common offenders. Malaise, jaundice, and fever are seen in about 1 in 500 patients transfused, are usually mild, and occur 5 to 10 days after transfusion. Shock and renal complications are rare. About 1 in 150 asymptomatic patients develop a new antibody about a week after transfusion, reflecting the anamnestic rise in previously undetected antibodies stimulated by the transfusion. The rare patient is found to have destroyed all the transfused cells in the absence of demonstrable antibodies.

Laboratory investigation   The initial investigation of a hemolytic transfusion reaction involves a careful check of the identity of donor and recipient, since clerical errors, especially mistakes in specimen labeling, are frequently involved. The next steps involve documenting red blood cell destruction, investigating its cause, and managing the patient's clinical status.

With recent intravascular hemolysis, free hemoglobin may color both plasma and urine. The laboratory can confirm elevated free hemoglobin, presence of methemalbumin, or reduced serum haptoglobin if necessary. The best indicators of extravascular hemolysis include a rise in unconjugated bilirubin and a failure of the hematocrit to reach the expected posttransfusion level.

A pretransfusion of the patient's blood is usually retained so that determination of both donor and recipient blood types can be repeated along with the compatibility test. If antibodies are detected, the pretransfusion specimen is used to determine specificity, since alloantibodies are formed only against those antigens not present on the patient's own cells. The posttransfusion specimen may not contain the offending antibodies if they have been absorbed by the transfused incompatible red blood cells. However, the red cells can be examined to determine whether transfused cells have been removed or coated with antibody, as indicated by the direct antiglobulin (Coombs') test.

Management of patients with extravascular hemolysis should be conservative. Additional transfusions should be withheld until serology is adequately defined, unless the patient's life is otherwise threatened. Intravascular hemolysis poses a far greater hazard, but there is no specific therapy. Management of hypotension, bleeding, or renal failure is supportive.

Other immunologically related reactions In the absence of red blood cell destruction, most febrile reactions can be ascribed to immune destruction of leukocytes or platelets. Most of these are mild and can be prevented by using leukocyte-reduced components. An allergic pulmonary edema related to sequestration of antibody-coated leukocytes in the lung has been reported. These rare reactions occur when a donor's plasma contains a high-titer antibody that reacts with the recipient's leukocytes. Cutaneous allergic reactions such as urticaria can be managed by slowing the transfusion and administering antihistamines. Patients with antibodies against IgA molecules may develop hypotensive anaphylactic reactions when exposed to plasma-containing components. Such patients are best managed with IgA-deficient blood components from relatives or from rare-donor lists. When necessary, cellular components can be washed extensively to remove the offending plasma. Finally, transfusion commonly results in alloimmunization to blood cell antigens, which complicates subsequent transfusions and bone marrow or solid organ transplants.

Nonimmune transfusion reactions The most significant nonimmune transfusion reactions, aside from infectious complications, are circulatory overload and transfusional siderosis. Circulatory overload manifested by pulmonary edema is a particular risk to the elderly, the infant, the patient with cardiac or renal compromise, and the patient with chronic anemia in whom red cell mass is decreased while the plasma volume is increased. The average unit of whole blood contains about 60 mEq sodium, while the average unit of red blood cells contains between 10 and 20 mEq. Transfusion-induced iron overload is an often fatal consequence of chronic transfusion for refractory anemia. Children with thalassemia major are the single largest group affected, but a substantial number of children with congenital anemias and adults with intensely treated refractory anemia are likewise at risk. Every milliliter of red blood cells deposits 1.08 mg iron in tissues as the red blood cells age and die. Iron deposition begins to affect endocrine, hepatic, and cardiac function when the total body burden has risen to more than 20 g, the equivalent of about 100 units of red blood cells. Lethal cardiac complications occur at about 60 g, or about 300 units. Iron chelation therapy should be considered for all patients who are likely to require intensive red cell support.

Infection Numerous different viral, bacterial, and protozoal agents can be transmitted through blood transfusion. To decrease potential disease transmission, donors are screened for risk factors by medical history and tested with a battery of laboratory screening assays. Sterilization techniques have been developed for some plasma components and fractionation products, but as yet no method for sterilizing cellular blood components has been found.

Hepatitis Emphasis on voluntary blood donations, donor screening, and specific assays for hepatitis B virus (HBV) and antibody to hepatitis C have reduced the risk of posttransfusion hepatitis in the United States from rates as high as 20 percent to a current rate of about 1 percent. Hepatitis A is almost never transmitted by blood. The current incidence of transfusion-associated hepatitis B is extremely low, and an effective hepatitis B vaccine is available for susceptible patients who anticipate chronic transfusion therapy. Most transfusion-transmitted hepatitis is caused by hepatitis C virus (HCV). Hepatitis C generally presents with few signs or symptoms, but serologic and biochemical evidence of infection can be detected 2 to 26 weeks after transfusion. Despite its mild presentation and declining incidence, posttransfusion hepatitis C remains a serious health concern, since more than 50 percent of infected patients progress to chronic liver disease. Furthermore, persuasive statistical evidence links both HBV and HCV with hepatocellular carcinoma.

Retroviral infections Several human retroviruses are readily transmitted by blood transfusion. Human immunodeficiency virus type 1 (HIV-1), the agent implicated in AIDS, infects about 90 percent of patients who receive an infected blood component (see Chap. 279). Prior to routine testing of blood donors, transfusions were implicated in 2 to 3 percent of total AIDS cases. Improved donor selection criteria and specific screening tests appear to have significantly reduced this figure. The current risk of infection is estimated at about 1 case per 225,000 units transfused. A related agent, HIV-2, has been associated with AIDS, and although no transfusion-related cases have yet been reported in the United States, blood donors are being tested for this agent as well. Cellular blood components are also screened for the cell-associated retroviruses HTLV-I and II isolated from patients with tropical spastic paraparesis, T cell leukemia, and hairy cell leukemia (see Chap. 151).

Other infectious agents CMV, ordinarily a common and relatively innocuous herpesvirus, can be an important pathogen in pregnant women, premature infants, and immunosuppressed patients (see Chap. 146). These patients should receive components from seronegative donors or blood processed to remove leukocytes. Bacterial growth in refrigerated blood is unusual. However, units contaminated with *Staphylococcus aureus* or with certain gram-negative organisms such as *Yersinia enterocolitica* and *Citrobacter* species that grow well at 4°C and in citrated blood may cause shock and death. A wide variety of bacteria and spirochetes grow well in platelet concentrates stored at room temperature. Malaria and Chagas' disease are among the most important infectious causes of transfusion-related morbidity and mortality worldwide. The rare cases detected in the United States are usually found among immigrants or travelers to areas where these diseases are endemic.

REFERENCES

AGRE P, CARTRON JP: Molecular biology of the Rh antigens. Blood 78:551, 1991

ALTER HJ et al: Detection of antibody to hepatitis C virus in prospectively followed transfusion recipients with acute and chronic non-A, non-B, hepatitis. N Engl J Med 321:1494, 1989

ANDERSON KC: The role of the blood bank in hematopoietic stem cell transplantation. Transfusion 32:272, 1992

Blood, Blood Components, and Plasma Expanders (Drug Evaluations Annual 1992). Chicago, American Medical Association, 1992, chap. 94, pp 2069–2092

BLUMBERG N et al: Transfusion-induced immunomodulation and its clinical consequences. Transfusion Med Rev 4 (suppl):24, 1990

HEYMAN MR, SCHIFFER CA: Platelet transfusion therapy for the cancer patient. Semin Oncol 17:198, 1990

MOLLISON PL et al (eds): *Blood Transfusion in Clinical Medicine*, 9th ed. Oxford, Blackwell Scientific, 1993

NATIONAL BLOOD RESOURCES EDUCATION PROGRAM EXPERT PANEL: The use of autologous blood. JAMA 263:414, 1990

ROSSI EC et al (eds): *Principles of Transfusion Medicine*. Baltimore, Williams & Wilkins, 1991

WALKER R et al: *The Technical Manual*, 11th ed. Arlington, Va, American Association of Blood Banks, 1993

YAMAMOTO F et al: Molecular genetic basis of the histo-blood group ABO system. Nature 345:229, 1990

313 BONE MARROW TRANSPLANTATION

E. DONNALL THOMAS

SELECTION OF THE PATIENT Marrow transplantation is a rational therapeutic option only if the patient's disease involves the marrow or if hazard to the normal marrow is the limiting factor in aggressive treatment of a disease. A marrow transplant involves a transplant not only of the donor myeloid, erythroid, and megakaryocytic systems but also of the donor lymphoid and macrophage-monocyte systems. The rationale is illustrated by the three types of disease for which marrow transplantation has been widely utilized:

1 *Genetic disease*. For immunologic deficiency diseases, the objective is to replace the recipient's genetically defective lymphoid system with the normal lymphoid system of the donor. For genetic diseases such as thalassemia major, the abnormal marrow must be destroyed and replaced by normal marrow.

2 *Aplastic anemia*. Regardless of cause, the disease process results in loss of the marrow, and the objective is to replace the defective organ with a normal functioning organ.

3 *Malignant disease*. For leukemia and other hematologic malignancies, the objective is the complete destruction of the malignant cell population and, unavoidably, normal marrow cells by intensive chemoradiotherapy with restoration of normal marrow function by the transplanted marrow.

TYPES OF TRANSPLANTS   A *syngeneic* graft describes a graft in which donor and recipient are genetically identical, i.e., identical twins. An *allogeneic* graft is one in which donor and recipient are of different genetic origins. A *chimera* is an individual whose body contains living, proliferating cells of different genetic origin. An *autologous* marrow graft refers to the removal of a patient's marrow, administration of chemo- and/or radiotherapy, and then return of the patient's own marrow.

SELECTION OF THE DONOR   The donor must be in good health, and the donor, or an appropriate advocate, must be capable of giving informed consent. The principal risk is the anesthesia. Selection of the donor is largely determined by histocompatibility testing. Red blood cell incompatibility is not a barrier to marrow transplantation.

Histocompatibility typing (See Chap. 64)   The HLA region is composed of a series of closely linked genes on chromosome 6. The array of genes encoded on a single chromosome is known as a *haplotype*. Each individual has two haplotypes, one inherited from each parent. The antigens are encoded at loci designated HLA-A, -B, -C, -DP, -DQ, and -DR. Serologic or molecular biologic techniques are used to detect the antigens. These closely linked genetic loci, each with a large number of known alleles, make the HLA region the most complex genetic polymorphism yet described. Despite this complexity, within a family there can be only four haplotypes. Therefore, for a given patient, each sibling has one chance in four of being HLA-identical with the patient. The most widely used transplants are those between HLA-identical siblings. There is now an increasing use of other family members and volunteer unrelated donors who match the patient or differ by only one HLA antigen.

PREPARATION OF THE PATIENT   Infants with severe combined immunologic deficiency are conditioned to accept a transplant by the nature of their disease. All other patients are immunologically competent, to a greater or lesser degree, and are able to reject the marrow graft unless prepared with some form of immunosuppressive therapy. An immunosuppressive regimen commonly used for patients with aplastic anemia is large doses of cyclophosphamide. Preparation of the patient with leukemia involves high-dose chemoradiotherapy for immunosuppression and to kill leukemic cells. A commonly used regimen involves cyclophosphamide followed by total-body irradiation. Approximately 10 Gy must be used for immunosuppression sufficient to permit consistent engraftment of marrow even though only 4 to 5 Gy will cause lethal marrow injury. Patients with leukemia or with genetic disease of the marrow may be prepared with busulfan to destroy the abnormal marrow along with cyclophosphamide for immunosuppression.

Marrow aspiration and infusion   In the operating room and under general or spinal anesthesia, multiple marrow aspirations are performed on the iliac crests. For adult donors, the volume of the mixture of blood and marrow cells is from 0.5 to 1.0 L. As each aspiration is performed, the marrow is mixed with heparin and tissue culture medium. The marrow is passed through stainless steel screens

to break up particles. It is then given to the recipient by intravenous infusion. The marrow stem cells pass through the lungs, and subsequent growth and reconstitution of the marrow are confined almost exclusively to the medullary cavities.

Support for the patient without marrow function   Usually 2 to 4 weeks are required before the transplanted marrow starts to produce the critical formed elements of the peripheral blood. Recently, the use of hematopoietic growth factors G-CSF or GM-CSF has shortened the period of granulocytopenia to 7 to 12 days. The patient should be cared for using the most effective available isolation facilities. Platelet transfusions are usually unnecessary at levels above 20,000 per microliter (see Chap. 314). Below that level, they should be used until values above 20,000 are sustained. If the patient becomes refractory to random donor platelets, the use of platelets from HLA-matched family members or unrelated donors may be necessary. Aspirin and other drugs that depress platelet function should be avoided. Granulocyte transfusions may be indicated for therapy of refractory infection in a granulocytopenic patient. Packed red blood cells should be given as needed to control symptoms of anemia, usually to keep the hematocrit above 25 percent. All blood products should be irradiated with at least 1.5 Gy to inactivate lymphocytes that might cause a graft-versus-host reaction.

Since infection is an ever-present danger, bacteriologic cultures should be obtained frequently. Onset of significant fever (38.5°C) should arouse a strong suspicion of infection in the granulocytopenic patient. Fever with clinical signs of bacteremia or fever sustained more than 24 h is an indication for starting systemic antibacterial therapy even if cultures are negative. Initial therapy usually includes an aminoglycoside active against *Pseudomonas* and a second agent with broad-spectrum activity against gram-negative organisms, with additional antibiotics added as indicated by culture results (see Chap. 81). Subsequently, if cultures are negative but fever persists, the addition of vancomycin and/or amphotericin may be considered. Once broad-spectrum antibiotic therapy has been initiated, it should be continued until the granulocyte count rises above 500 cells per microliter even if clinical signs of infection disappear.

Many patients coming to marrow transplantation have had inadequate nutrition because of their disease or the efforts to treat it (see Chap. 76). The preparation for marrow grafting results in nausea, vomiting, and mucositis which results in poor oral intake for at least several weeks. A Hickman modification of the Broviac catheter is installed routinely. The catheter makes it possible to administer hyperalimentation, medications, and blood products and is also used for drawing blood samples. Although some catheters are removed because of infection or suspected infection, about 90 percent of the patients have the catheter in place for approximately 3 months, the period of time when it is needed.

ENGRAFTMENT AND PROOF OF ENGRAFTMENT   Engraftment is signaled by a rise in granulocytes and platelets and the reappearance of reticulocytes. Proof of engraftment depends on use of cytogenetics, blood genetic markers, and/or restriction enzyme fragment length polymorphisms to distinguish donor from host cells. The regenerating marrow is usually entirely of donor type. Occasional patients show persistence of some host cells.

COMPLICATIONS FOLLOWING ENGRAFTMENT   The complications that may follow successful marrow engraftment are (1) graft rejection, a problem primarily occurring in patients with aplastic anemia, (2) infection, including early bacterial infections or later opportunistic infections such as cytomegalovirus (CMV) interstitial pneumonia, (3) veno-occlusive liver disease, (4) acute graft-versus-host disease (GVHD), the result of the immunologic reaction of the engrafted lymphoid elements against tissues of the recipient, (5) chronic GVHD, (6) recurrence of leukemia, and (7) miscellaneous complications such as hemorrhagic cystitis, cardiomyopathy, cataract formation, leukoencephalopathy, and sterility.

Marrow graft recipients, whether allogeneic or autologous, suffer impaired immune competence in the first few months after grafting. Hematopoietic growth factors have shortened the period of susceptibility to bacterial infections. Acyclovir and ganciclovir have reduced the complications associated with herpes simplex and CMV infection. Trimethoprim-sulfamethoxazole has removed the risk of *Pneumocystis carinii* infection.

CLINICAL RESULTS OF MARROW TRANSPLANTATION **Immunodeficiency diseases** Despite the rarity of these disorders, these patients are unique in that immunosuppressive therapy is not necessary to condition the patient to accept a graft, and because some myeloid function is usually present, rapid marrow engraftment is not essential.

Genetically determined hematologic diseases Marrow grafts have now been reported for thalassemia major, sickle cell disease, Kostmann's syndrome, chronic granulomatous disease, Chédiak-Higashi syndrome, Blackfan-Diamond syndrome, congenital aplastic anemia, Fanconi's anemia, and several storage diseases due to enzyme deficiencies. Thalassemia major is a significant cause of death in children in many parts of the world. In developed countries, therapy with transfusions and chelating agents can prolong life for one to three decades but at great expense. Since the first transplant in 1981, more than 500 marrow transplants for thalassemia major have been done. Approximately 10 percent of the patients died of complications of marrow grafting, and 10 percent have regenerated their own marrow and again have thalassemia major. Eighty percent of the patients appear to be cured of the disease, although some 5 percent of the cured patients are under treatment for chronic GVHD. Good results are now being reported for older, multiply transfused patients.

Transplantation for severe aplastic anemia (See Chap. 308) HLA-IDENTICAL SIBLING DONORS Patients with severe aplastic anemia must be prepared for engraftment with immunosuppressive therapy. The most widely used regimen is cyclophosphamide (CY) 50 mg/kg on each of 4 days followed 36 h later by donor marrow. The first two successful transplants were reported in 1972, and these recipients are alive and well.

For ethical reasons, the initial marrow transplants were carried out in patients who had failed to benefit from conventional therapy after receiving multiple transfusions. One-third of the patients rejected the graft, and the long-term survival of these end-stage patients was 40 to 50 percent.

Since blood transfusions can sensitize an intended marrow transplant recipient, resulting in rejection of the marrow graft, patients with severe aplastic anemia were identified early in the course of the disease so that marrow transplantation could be carried out before blood transfusions were given. The long-term survival of these patients is more than 80 percent. Therefore, patients with severe aplastic anemia and their families should have tissue typing performed immediately upon diagnosis. If a suitable donor can be identified, marrow transplantation should be carried out promptly before transfusions become necessary.

However, many patients with severe aplastic anemia present to the physician with bleeding and/or infection, and transfusions must be given as an urgent medical necessity. Therefore, marrow transplant teams are investigating other preparative regimens designed to prevent graft rejection and to improve survival. These include regimens using various combinations of antithymocyte globulin (ATG), CY, and partial-body or total-nodal irradiation. A regimen involving the administration of 30 mg/kg of ATG between each dose of CY shows a survival of greater than 90 percent.

IDENTICAL TWIN DONORS Aplastic anemia is not a common disease, and to find a patient with it who has an identical twin is even more uncommon. Nevertheless, a number of such transplants have been carried out. In some patients the simple intravenous infusion of marrow without any immunosuppressive treatment resulted in recovery. These results reinforce the concept that aplastic anemia is due to an acquired abnormality of the stem cell which can be corrected by transplantation of normal syngeneic stem cells. However, some patients did not recover after marrow infusion. These patients were then treated with the CY and given a second infusion of marrow from the twin, which resulted in complete hematopoietic reconstitution.

The results suggest that some cases may be due to an immune mechanism or abnormal regulators of cell growth. Whatever the mechanism, the rare patient with aplastic anemia who has a genetically identical twin has a 90 percent chance of being cured with marrow transplantation.

Transplantation for acute leukemia Acute leukemia (see Chap. 310) has served as a prototype malignant disease of the marrow for treatment by intensive chemoradiotherapy and marrow transplantation. Until a decade ago, almost all regimens used for preparing leukemic patients for marrow transplantation employed supralethal total-body irradiation (TBI). CY, etoposide, cytosine arabinoside, or other antileukemic drugs are given with TBI to kill a greater fraction of leukemic cells. More recently, regimens using busulfan (BU) and CY (without TBI) are showing results equivalent to those with TBI.

ACUTE LEUKEMIA IN REFRACTORY RELAPSE USING HLA-IDENTICAL SIBLING DONORS For ethical reasons, marrow transplantation was initially attempted only in patients with acute leukemia in relapse after chemotherapy. These end-stage patients presented with a heavy body burden of leukemic cells, were usually granulocytopenic and thrombocytopenic, and often were already infected with antibiotic-resistant bacteria and fungi. There were many deaths related to advanced illness, GVHD, opportunistic infections, or recurrent leukemia. Approximately 10 percent of these patients became long-term survivors with no further antileukemic therapy. The longest surviving patients are now 20 years postgrafting. Despite the use of a variety of different preparative regimens, long-term survival for these end-stage patients remains at about 5 to 15 percent.

ACUTE LEUKEMIA BEYOND FIRST REMISSION USING HLA-IDENTICAL SIBLING DONORS Patients with acute leukemia who relapse have a high probability of dying of the disease even though additional remissions may be achieved. Transplantation in second or subsequent remission avoids the problems associated with a large body burden of leukemic cells. Marrow grafting for these patients has resulted in long-term disease-free survival of 40 to 60 percent.

Approximately one-half of patients with acute myeloid leukemia (AML) who relapse die without achieving a second remission. Transplantation in first relapse before additional chemotherapy also results in approximately 40 to 60 percent disease-free survival. Transplantation at the first sign of relapse may be the optimal timing, but relapse signaled by infection and the difficulty of quickly arranging for a transplant are obstacles.

ACUTE MYELOID LEUKEMIA IN FIRST REMISSION USING HLA-IDENTICAL DONORS Patients with AML in first remission are known to have a poor prognosis. With combination chemotherapy, the median duration of the first remission is approximately 12 to 18 months, and only 20 to 25 percent of the patients are alive at 5 years after initial chemotherapy. Therefore, a study of marrow transplantation in those patients in first remission was considered to be ethically acceptable. Hundreds of such transplants have now been carried out, with various marrow transplant teams reporting 45 to 70 percent long-term disease-free survival.

Since about 20 percent of patients with AML in first remission already have been cured by chemotherapy, transplantation means that these patients will be exposed needlessly to the risks of this procedure. Nevertheless, five different randomized, prospective studies have demonstrated a better survival for patients given a marrow graft in first remission as compared with those treated with chemotherapy. Until methods for identifying those destined to relapse are perfected, marrow grafting is the preferred treatment.

ACUTE LYMPHOID LEUKEMIA IN FIRST REMISSION USING HLA-IDENTICAL DONORS Patients with "good risk" characteristics of ALL at diagnosis have a 50 to 70 percent chance of being cured by chemotherapy and are not candidates for a marrow graft. Marrow grafts for patients with ALL in first remission generally have been restricted to patients who have characteristics indicating a poor prognosis with chemotherapy. Survival of such patients after marrow grafting has ranged from 10 to 60 percent, apparently depending on the criteria for selection.

CHRONIC MYELOID LEUKEMIA USING HLA-IDENTICAL DONORS
Marrow transplantation for patients with CML in blast crisis, like
other forms of advanced leukemia, has resulted in a cure rate of
approximately 15 percent.

Patients with the chronic phase of the disease are good candidates
for a marrow graft because they usually are in good condition without
infection or having had transfusions. Most CML patients have been
transplanted after preparation with CY and TBI. The disease-free
survival is approximately 60 percent, with the longest period exceeding
15 years. The absence of the Ph chromosome indicates cure of these
patients. Several more recent studies using TBI-containing regimens
or a BU-CY regimen show, on actuarial analysis, disease-free plateaus
of approximately 80 percent. The improvement in survival is probably
related to several advances in transplant technology, including the
prevention of viral infections and reduction in GVHD.

CML is a disease that can be controlled with BU or hydroxyurea
but is not cured by chemotherapy. The median survival is 30 to 50
months. Therapy with interferon-α may result in disappearance of
the Ph chromosome in some patients but, as yet, has not been
demonstrated to affect survival. Since the best results with marrow
grafting are seen when the transplant is carried out in the first 2 years
after diagnosis, all patients with CML should be considered for
marrow grafting and a donor sought.

OTHER MALIGNANT DISEASES TREATED BY MARROW GRAFTING
FROM HLA-IDENTICAL SIBLINGS   Lymphomas, Hodgkin's disease,
multiple myeloma, myelodysplastic syndromes, breast cancer, ovarian
cancer, testicular cancer, and small cell lung cancer have been treated
with intensive chemoradiotherapy and a marrow graft. The results
vary widely, but in almost every category some patients have
apparently been cured of otherwise fatal disease. Particular attention
is being focused on lymphoma and Hodgkin's disease, with marrow
grafting being considered as the first form of therapy after failure of
initial standard therapy.

USE OF DONORS OTHER THAN HLA-IDENTICAL SIBLINGS   Only
one-third of patients will have an HLA-identical sibling. Marrow
transplantation has been carried out between family member donor-
recipient pairs in which one of the HLA haplotypes was genetically
identical and the other haplotype phenotypically identical or differing
by only one locus. The results of these transplants are quite similar
to the results using an HLA-identical sibling donor. The outcome is
largely a function of the stage of the disease at the time of transplant.

HLA typing makes it technically possible to find a suitably matched
unrelated donor, at least for patients with the more common HLA
haplotypes. The National Marrow Donor Program has recruited more
than 600,000 donors, and more than 1400 transplants from unrelated
donors have been carried out. The recipients have more GVHD, but
disease-free survival seems almost as good as in recipients of matched
sibling grafts. The long-term results of these transplants are not yet
known.

Autologous marrow transplantation   The technique for procur-
ing and cryopreserving marrow has been established for more than
20 years. The presence in the circulating blood of hematopoietic
progenitor cells (stem cells) also has been known for a long time.
Recently, it has been shown that the administration of G-CSF or GM-
CSF can markedly increase the number of stem cells in the circulating
blood and that these cells can be used for autologous grafting. Marrow
and blood stem cells can be used together to shorten significantly the
period of pancytopenia after autologous grafting. The use of autologous stem cells avoids the risk of GVHD. The following points are
pertinent in considering autologous stem cell transplantation: (1) The
stem cells should not be contaminated with malignant cells; (2)
autologous stem cells are of value only in protecting the patient
against lethal hematopoietic toxicity; (3) the tumor being treated must
show a dose-response curve such that supralethal chemoradiotherapy
can be expected to result in a significantly enhanced antitumor
response; and (4) the protocol must be designed so that the role of
autologous marrow can be demonstrated. In animals it is feasible to
administer "supralethal" therapy and to demonstrate that animals

given syngeneic marrow will survive while those not given marrow
will die. For obvious reasons, this kind of controlled experiment
cannot be done in humans. Failure to recognize these four principles
accounts for much of the current uncertainty about the value of
autologous marrow transplantation in the treatment of patients with
malignant disease.

As for allogeneic transplants, the tumors that might be expected
to show a significant improvement in response to high-dose chemoradiotherapy include the leukemias, Hodgkin's disease, non-Hodgkin's
lymphoma, multiple myeloma, small cell cancer of the lung, breast
cancer, testicular tumors, and ovarian tumors. Techniques being
explored for removal of tumor cells from the marrow include physical
separation, destruction by chemotherapeutic agents, and positive
selections of stem cells by monoclonal antibodies. The use of
cryopreserved autologous stem cells leads to successful hematopoietic
reconstitution in most patients. For hematologic malignancies, autologous transplantation after high-dose chemoradiotherapy results in
apparent cure of a significant fraction of patients; such a transplant
therefore offers an alternative to patients who do not have an HLA-
matched allogeneic donor. Autologous stem cell grafts are used
increasingly for treatment of metastatic breast cancer or breast
cancer patients with more than 10 positive nodes. The high-dose
chemotherapy includes CY, cisplatin, and carmustine. These autologous grafts are producing long-term disease-free survival of some
patients with breast cancer with an otherwise grim prognosis.

IMMUNOLOGIC ASPECTS OF MARROW TRANSPLANTATION

Marrow graft rejection   *Marrow graft rejection* describes a phenomenon in which the transplanted marrow graft begins to function, but
after a few days or weeks, the peripheral blood counts suddenly drop
and marrow biopsy shows the marrow to be devoid of myeloid
elements. Immunologically mediated marrow graft rejection is usually
a consequence of sensitization by transfusions. In addition, inadequate
immunosuppressive therapy before grafting may facilitate marrow
graft rejection.

Marrow graft failure may be due to causes other than immunologic
mechanisms. With a solid organ, such as the kidney, histologic proof
of graft rejection is easily obtained, but such proof usually cannot be
obtained with a marrow graft because the myeloid marrow simply
disappears. Other possible mechanisms of graft failure include (1)
defective or inadequate numbers of stem cells in the donor marrow,
(2) defective microenvironment in the marrow recipient, (3) allogeneic
resistance not associated with HLA, and (4) susceptibility of the
donor marrow to the same etiologic mechanism(s) responsible for the
original disease process.

Acute graft-versus-host disease   A "wasting disease" or "runt
disease" was described many years ago in newborn mice or in rodents
exposed to lethal TBI and given infusions of allogeneic hematopoietic
cells. The disease was recognized to be due to an immunologic
reaction of engrafted lymphoid cells, presumably T cells, against the
tissues of the host. In patients given a marrow graft from an HLA-
identical sibling and postgrafting immunosuppression, approximately
one-half develop moderate to severe GVHD.

Acute GVHD in humans usually involves the skin, gastrointestinal
tract, and/or the liver. A skin rash is usually the first sign of GVHD.
Intestinal involvement results in diarrhea and may progress to
abdominal pain and ileus. Liver disease is characterized by rises of
bilirubin, SGOT, and alkaline phosphatase. Severe immunologic
deficiency accompanies GVHD, and death from infection is frequent.

Since GVHD is immunologically mediated, efforts to prevent its
development have involved the use of immunosuppressive therapy.
Of the many agents studied, methotrexate, glucocorticoids, and
cyclosporine were found to be useful. Cyclosporine is a potent
immunosuppressive agent that does not cause mucositis, as methotrexate does, and does not suppress the marrow graft, so effective marrow
function is evident earlier. Cyclosporine is nephrotoxic, and marrow
graft recipients often receive other nephrotoxic agents such as
amphotericin. Creatinine and serum cyclosporine levels must be
monitored carefully, with prompt reduction of dosage if renal function

is threatened. A regimen using a short course of methotrexate along with cyclosporine has proved highly effective in reducing the incidence and severity of acute GVHD.

A number of studies have been carried out in an effort to treat acute GVHD once it becomes established. Recipients of HLA-identical marrow have been treated with rabbit, goat, or horse ATG, high-dose methyl prednisolone, cyclosporine, and/or anti-T cell monoclonal antibodies. About two-thirds of patients will respond to one or another of these agents. However, about one-third of the patients who develop moderate to severe GVHD will die of it or its infectious complications.

Experiments are underway designed to eliminate from the marrow inoculum the T cells believed to be responsible for GVHD while retaining hematopoietic stem cells. One approach involves treatment of the donor marrow with lectins for agglutination and separation of the T cells. Monoclonal antibodies that react with human T cells or subsets of T cells are being used in conjunction with complement or are bound to toxins, such as the A chain of ricin, to create an immunotoxin. The preliminary results of these studies indicate a reduction in the incidence and severity of GVHD. However, the incidence of graft failure and of recurrence of leukemia is significantly increased. The explanation for these problems is unknown.

Chronic GVHD Chronic GVHD occurs in approximately one-fourth of those recipients of marrow from an HLA-identical sibling who survive beyond 100 days. The manifestations include skin disease, keratoconjunctivitis, buccal mucositis, esophageal strictures, small- and large-intestinal involvement, pulmonary insufficiency, chronic liver disease, and generalized wasting. Histologically, the disease resembles the systemic collagen vascular diseases, especially morphea and lupus erythematosus profundus. Chronic GVHD may be associated with recurrent and occasionally fatal bacterial infections.

Treatment of chronic GVHD with short courses of ATG or prolonged treatment with prednisone has been only partially effective. Twenty percent continue to have problems which may be disabling, and cyclosporine, intermittent steroids, thalidomide, or monoclonal antibodies alone or bound to a toxin are being tried for the refractory patients.

Recovery of immunologic function Despite recovery from pancytopenia, most allogeneic recipients are susceptible to a wide variety of opportunistic infections. Historically, approximately one-fifth of patients developed an interstitial pneumonia, and cytomegalovirus was demonstrated in more than one-half of these pneumonias. The mortality rate was approximately 80 percent. Use of blood products from donors who are serologically negative for CMV for those donor-recipient pairs also serologically negative and the use of prophylactic ganciclovir have almost eliminated CMV infection and pneumonia. Susceptibility to infection is the result of a very slow return of immunologic function, which may be made worse by GVHD and by efforts to prevent or treat GVHD. Fortunately, by the end of the first year after grafting, most patients have recovered immunologically and are able to lead normal lives without an increased incidence of infection.

Tolerance The long-term healthy human recipients of allogeneic marrow transplants are true chimeras. Their myeloid, lymphoid, and monocyte-macrophage systems are made up of cells of donor origin. Clearly, these donor cells in the recipient are "tolerant" of the host's tissues. Studies of tolerance constitute a fascinating story in immunobiology, but a clear understanding of the state of tolerance has not emerged. At least three mechanisms may be operative, including classical central tolerance due to clonal deletion, tolerance due to clonal anergy, and tolerance related to the presence of active "suppressor" cells.

The effect of age The success of allogeneic marrow grafting is inversely proportional to the age of the recipient. For example, for patients transplanted in first remission of AML, long-term survival for those under age 20 is approximately 75 percent, and for patients aged 30 to 50, 40 percent. The most apparent explanation for this difference is the increased incidence and severity of GVHD in older patients. Most marrow transplant centers do not transplant patients over age 50. These age restrictions do not apply to syngeneic or autologous transplants because these patients do not have GVHD, although patients over age 50 do not tolerate intensive treatment as well as younger patients.

RECURRENT LEUKEMIA AFTER GRAFTING Frequency For patients with leukemia transplanted in relapse or in second remission, actuarial analysis shows a rather constant rate of recurrence of leukemia in the first year, a decreasing rate in the second year, and few recurrences thereafter. If there were no other causes of death, 30 to 70 percent would be destined to relapse. However, the risk of relapse is only 15 to 20 percent for patients with AML transplanted in first remission or CML transplanted in the chronic phase. It is evident that recurrent leukemia after grafting is a major problem for patients transplanted in relapse or in second or subsequent remission.

Nature of recurrent leukemia Blood genetic markers, cytogenetic techniques, and restriction enzyme fragment length polymorphisms can be used to identify the donor or host origin of the leukemic cells in patients who relapse after marrow transplantation. In the vast majority of patients, the recurrent leukemia is in host-type cells, indicating that the preparative regimen and the graft did not eliminate all the leukemic cells. However, several cases have now been reported in which the recurrent leukemic cells were shown to be of donor origin. The mechanism of donor cell transformation is unknown. In more than a dozen cases a lymphoblastic lymphoma associated with Epstein-Barr virus genomes has occurred in donor cells. These highly fatal lymphomas have usually occurred in patients undergoing intensive treatment for GVHD.

Graft-versus-leukemia effect In recipients of allogeneic marrow grafts, evidence supporting the existence of a graft-versus-leukemia effect has been difficult to obtain because of the large number of deaths from other causes among patients with severe GVHD. Statistical methods have shown that the relative relapse rate for patients transplanted in relapse or for ALL in second remission was 2.5 times greater in recipients without GVHD than in those with GVHD. Recipients of allogeneic marrow who did not develop GVHD had approximately the same relapse rate as recipients of syngeneic marrow, indicating that subclinical GVHD did not reduce the relapse rate.

GENERALIZATIONS ABOUT MARROW TRANSPLANTATION Because of the complexity of the marrow grafting regimens, transplantation should be undertaken only by teams with all the resources needed to ensure an optimal result. The number of such teams has increased rapidly over the past few years.

Marrow transplantation is obviously an expensive undertaking, primarily because of hospital costs, but cost has been reduced appreciably by transplantation earlier in the course of the disease when the patient is in relatively good condition. The introduction of hematopoietic growth factors should further reduce cost by shortening the time in the hospital. Cost analysis studies comparing marrow transplantation with combination therapy have found marrow transplantation to be more cost-effective.

The ethical problems of exposing a patient and donor to the marrow transplant regimen and the risk of death in the first 1 to 3 months after grafting have limited the use of marrow transplantation. However, the demonstration of better long-term survival rates with marrow transplantation compared with conventional therapy for several diseases and the cure of some diseases not cured by conventional therapy should alleviate the ethical concern. Extension of this form of therapy to other malignant diseases and to a variety of genetic disorders is being reported, and the current rapid rate of progress and the availability of unrelated volunteer donors may soon make a much broader application of marrow grafting a reality.

REFERENCES

ARMITAGE JD: Drug therapy: Treatment of non-Hodgkin's lymphoma. N Engl J Med 328:1023, 1993

APPELBAUM FR et al: Chemotherapy v marrow transplantation for adults with acute nonlymphocytic leukemia: A five-year follow-up. Blood 72:179, 1988

BEATTY PG et al: Marrow transplantation from related donors other than HLA identical siblings. N Engl J Med 313:765, 1985

CLIFT RA et al: The treatment of acute non-lymphoblastic leukemia by allogeneic marrow transplantation. Bone Marrow Transplant 2:243, 1987

COPELAN JC et al: Radiation-free preparation for allogeneic bone marrow transplantation in adults with acute lymphoblastic leukemia. J Clin Oncol 10:237, 1992

GOLDMAN JM et al: Bone marrow transplantation for chronic myelogenous leukemia in chronic phase. Ann Intern Med 108:806, 1988

GOODRICH JM et al: Prevention of cytomegalovirus disease after allogeneic marrow transplant by ganciclovir prophylaxis. Ann Intern Med 118:173, 1993

KESSINGER A, ARMITAGE JO: The evolving role of autologous peripheral stem cell transplantation following high-dose therapy for malignancies. Blood 77:211, 1991

LUCARELLI G et al: Bone marrow transplantation in patients with thalassemia. N Engl J Med 322:417, 1990

MARTIN P et al: Effects of in vitro depletion of T cells in HLA-identical allogeneic marrow grafts. Blood 66:664, 1985

MEYERS JD, THOMAS ED: Infection complicating bone marrow transplantation, in *Clinical Approach to Infection in the Immunocompromised Host*, RH Rubin, LS Young (eds). New York, Plenum Press, 1981, p 507

NEMUNAITIS J et al: Recombinant granulocyte-macrophage colony-stimulating factor after autologous bone marrow transplantation for lymphoid cancer. N Engl J Med 324:1773, 1991

PHILIP T et al: High-dose therapy and autologous bone marrow transplantation after failure of conventional chemotherapy in adults with intermediate-grade or high-grade non-Hodgkin's lymphoma. N Engl J Med 316:1493, 1987

STORB R et al: Marrow transplantation for aplastic anemia. Semin Hematol 21:27, 1984

———— et al: Methotrexate and cyclosporine compared with cyclosporine alone for prophylaxis of acute graft versus host disease after marrow transplantation for leukemia. N Engl J Med 314:729, 1986

SULLIVAN KM et al: Chronic graft-versus-host disease in 52 patients: Adverse natural course and successful treatment with combination immunosuppression. Blood 57:267, 1981

THOMAS ED et al: Bone-marrow transplantation. N Engl J Med 292:832, 895, 1975

———— et al: Marrow transplantation for the treatment of chronic myelogenous leukemia. Ann Intern Med 104:155, 1986

WEIDEN PL et al: Antileukemic effect of graft-versus-host disease in human recipients of allogeneic-marrow grafts. N Engl J Med 300:1068, 1979

YEAGER AM et al: Autologous bone marrow transplantation in patients with acute nonlymphocytic leukemia, using ex vivo marrow treatment with 4-hydroperoxycyclophosphamide. N Engl J Med 315:141, 1986

ZUTTER MM et al: Epstein-Barr virus lymphoproliferation after bone marrow transplantation. Blood 72:520, 1988

section 2   Clotting disorders

314   DISORDERS OF THE PLATELET AND VESSEL WALL

ROBERT I. HANDIN

Patients with platelet or vessel wall disorders usually bleed into superficial sites such as the skin, mucous membranes, or genitourinary or gastrointestinal tract. Bleeding begins immediately after trauma and either responds to simple measures such as pressure and packing or requires systemic therapy with glucocorticoids, plasma fractions, or platelet concentrates. The most common platelet/vessel wall disorders are (1) various forms of thrombocytopenia, (2) von Willebrand's disease, and (3) drug-induced platelet dysfunction. This chapter reviews the diagnosis and treatment of quantitative and qualitative platelet disorders as well as vessel wall defects which cause bleeding. The physiology of normal hemostasis and the cardinal manifestations of bleeding arising from hemostatic disorders have been reviewed in Chap. 57.

PLATELET DISORDERS

Platelets arise from the fragmentation of megakaryocytes, which are very large, polyploid bone marrow cells produced by several cycles of chromosomal duplication without cytoplasmic division. After leaving the marrow space, approximately one-third of the platelets are sequestered in the spleen, while the other two-thirds circulate for 7 to 10 days. Normally, only a small fraction of the platelet mass is consumed in the process of hemostasis, so most platelets circulate until they become senescent and are removed by phagocytic cells. The normal blood platelet count is maintained between 150,000 and 450,000 per microliter. Although the regulatory signals are not well-defined, a decrease in platelet mass stimulates an increase in the number, size, and ploidy of megakaryocytes, releasing additional platelets into the circulation.

The platelet count varies during the menstrual cycle, rising following ovulation and falling at the onset of menses. It is also influenced by the patient's nutritional state and can be decreased in severe iron, folic acid, or vitamin B_{12} deficiency. Platelets are *acute phase reactants*, and patients with systemic inflammation, tumors, bleeding, and mild iron deficiency may have an increased platelet count, a benign condition called *secondary* or *reactive thrombocytosis*. In contrast, the increase in platelet count that is characteristic of the myeloproliferative disorders such as polycythemia vera, chronic myelogenous leukemia, myeloid metaplasia, and essential thrombocytosis can cause either severe bleeding or thrombosis.

MECHANISM OF THROMBOCYTOPENIA   Thrombocytopenia is caused by one of three mechanisms—decreased bone marrow production, increased splenic sequestration, or accelerated destruction of platelets. In order to determine the etiology of thrombocytopenia, each patient should have a careful examination of the peripheral blood film, an assessment of marrow morphology by examination of an aspirate or biopsy, and an estimate of splenic size by bedside palpation supplemented, if necessary, by ultrasonography or computed tomographic (CT) scan. Occasional patients have "pseudothrombocytopenia," a benign condition in which platelets agglutinate or adhere to leukocytes when blood is collected with EDTA as anticoagulant. This is a laboratory artifact, and the actual platelet count in vivo is normal. A scheme for classifying patients with thrombocytopenia based on these clinical observations and laboratory tests is outlined in Fig. 314-1.

Impaired production   Disorders that injure stem cells or prevent their proliferation in marrow frequently cause thrombocytopenia. They usually affect multiple hematopoietic cell lines so that thrombocytopenia is accompanied by varying degrees of anemia and leukopenia. Diagnosis of a platelet production defect is readily established by examination of a bone marrow aspirate or biopsy, which should show a reduced number of megakaryocytes. The most common causes of decreased platelet production are marrow aplasia, fibrosis, or infiltration with malignant cells, all of which produce highly characteristic marrow abnormalities. Occasionally, thrombocytopenia is the presenting laboratory abnormality in these disorders. Cytotoxic drugs, which are frequently used in cancer chemotherapy, impair megakaryocyte proliferation and maturation and frequently cause thrombocytopenia. There are also rare marrow disorders such as congenital amegakaryocytic hypoplasia and thrombocytopenia with absent radii

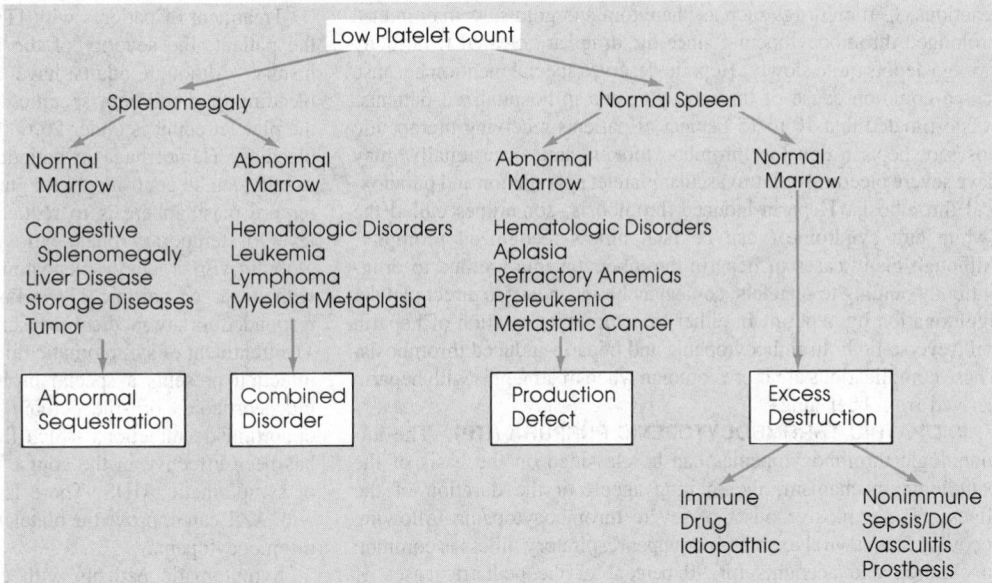

FIGURE 314-1 Clinical evaluation of patients with thrombocytopenia (*Modified from RI Handin, in W Beck (ed). Hematology, 4th ed, Cambridge, Mass, MIT Press, 1985.*)

(TAR syndrome), which selectively decrease megakaryocyte production.

Splenic sequestration Since one-third of the platelet mass is normally sequestered in the spleen, splenectomy will increase the platelet count by 30 percent. Postsplenectomy thrombocytosis is a benign self-limited condition which does not require specific therapy. In contrast, when the spleen enlarges, the fraction of sequestered platelets increases, lowering the platelet count. The most common causes of splenomegaly are portal hypertension secondary to liver disease and splenic infiltration with tumor cells in myeloproliferative or lymphoproliferative disorders or with macrophages in storage disorders such as Gaucher's disease. Isolated splenomegaly is rare, and in most patients, splenomegaly is accompanied by other clinical manifestations of the underlying disease. Many patients with leukemia, lymphoma, or a myeloproliferative syndrome have both marrow infiltration and splenomegaly and develop thrombocytopenia from a combination of impaired marrow production and splenic sequestration of platelets.

Accelerated destruction Abnormal vessels, fibrin thrombi, and intravascular prostheses can all shorten platelet survival and cause *nonimmunologic thrombocytopenia*. For example, thrombocytopenia is common in patients with vasculitis, the hemolytic uremic syndrome, thrombotic thrombocytopenic purpura (TTP), as one manifestation of disseminated intravascular coagulation (DIC), and in patients with prosthetic cardiac valves. In addition, platelets coated with antibody, immune complexes, or complement are rapidly cleared by mononuclear phagocytes in the spleen or other tissues inducing *immunologic thrombocytopenia*. The most common causes of immunologic thrombocytopenia are viral or bacterial infections, drugs, and a chronic autoimmune disorder referred to as *idiopathic thrombocytopenic purpura* (ITP). Patients with immunologic thrombocytopenia do not usually have splenomegaly and have an active bone marrow with an increased number of megakaryocytes.

DRUG-INDUCED THROMBOCYTOPENIA Many common drugs can cause thrombocytopenia (Table 314-1). As previously mentioned, many chemotherapeutic agents are cytotoxic and depress megakaryocyte production. Ingestion of large quantities of alcohol has a similar marrow-depressing effect leading to transient thrombocytopenia. The syndrome is particularly common in binge drinkers. Thiazide diuretics, which are used commonly to treat hypertension or congestive heart failure, impair megakaryocyte production and can produce mild thrombocytopenia (50,000 to 100,000 per microliter), which may persist for several months after the drug is discontinued.

Most drugs induce thrombocytopenia by eliciting an immune response in which the platelet is an innocent bystander. The platelet is damaged by complement activation following the formation of drug-antibody complexes. Current laboratory tests can identify the causative agent in 10 percent of patients with clinical evidence of drug-induced thrombocytopenia. The best proof of a drug-induced etiology is a prompt rise in the platelet count when the suspected drug is discontinued. Patients with drug-induced platelet destruction also may have a secondary increase in megakaryocyte number without other marrow abnormalities.

Although most patients recover within 7 to 10 days and do not require therapy, occasional patients with platelet counts below 10,000 to 20,000 per microliter have severe hemorrhage and may require temporary support with glucocorticoids, plasmapheresis, or platelet transfusions while waiting for the platelet count to rise. A patient who has recovered from drug-induced immunologic thrombocytopenia should be instructed to avoid the offending drug in the future, since only minute amounts of drug are needed to set up subsequent immune

---

TABLE 314-1 Drugs implicated in thrombocytopenia

SUPPRESSION OF PLATELET PRODUCTION

A Myelosuppressive drugs
  1 Severe: cytosine arabinoside, daunorubicin
  2 Moderate: cyclophosphamide, busulfan, methotrexate, 6-mercaptopurine
  3 Mild: vinca alkaloids
B Thiazide diuretics
C Ethanol
D Estrogens

IMMUNOLOGIC PLATELET DESTRUCTION

A Clinical suspicion plus convincing experimental evidence
  1 Antibiotics: sulfathiazole, novobiocin, *p*-aminosalicylate
  2 Cinchona alkaloids: quinidine, quinine
  3 Foods: beans
  4 Sedatives, hypnotics, anticonvulsants: apronalide, carbamazepine
  5 Arsenical drugs used to treat syphilis
  6 Digitoxin
  7 Methyldopa
  8 Stibophen
B Clinical suspicion (major drugs implicated)
  1 Aspirin
  2 Chlorpropamide
  3 Chloroquine
  4 Chlorothiazide and hydrochlorothiazide
  5 Gold salts
  6 Insecticides
  7 Sulfadiazine, sulfisoxazole, sulfamerazine, sulfamethazine, sulfamethoxypyridazine, sulfamethoxazole, sulfatolamide

reactions. Certain drugs such as phenytoin and gold salts may induce prolonged thrombocytopenia, since the drugs are cleared from body storage depots quite slowly. Heparin deserves special mention because it is a common cause of thrombocytopenia in hospitalized patients. It is estimated that 10 to 15 percent of patients receiving therapeutic doses of heparin develop thrombocytopenia and, occasionally, may have severe bleeding or intravascular platelet aggregation and paradoxical thrombosis. Heparin-induced thrombosis, sometimes called the "white clot syndrome," can be fatal unless recognized promptly. Although many cases of heparin thrombocytopenia are due to drug-antibody binding to platelets, some may be secondary to direct platelet agglutination by heparin. In either case, prompt cessation of heparin will reverse both thrombocytopenia and heparin-induced thrombosis. These complications are more common when treatment is with heparin derived from beef lung.

IDIOPATHIC THROMBOCYTOPENIC PURPURA (ITP) The immunologic thrombocytopenias can be classified on the basis of the pathologic mechanism, the inciting agent, or the duration of the illness. The explosive onset of severe thrombocytopenia following recovery from a viral exanthem or upper respiratory illness is common in children and accounts for 90 percent of the pediatric cases of immunologic thrombocytopenia. This syndrome is usually called *acute idiopathic thrombocytopenic purpura* (acute ITP). Of these patients, 60 percent recover in 4 to 6 weeks and over 90 percent recover within 3 to 6 months. Transient immunologic thrombocytopenia also complicates some cases of infectious mononucleosis, acute toxoplasmosis, or cytomegalovirus infection and can be part of the prodromal phase of viral hepatitis. Acute ITP is rare in adults and accounts for less than 10 percent of postpubertal patients with immune thrombocytopenia. Acute ITP is caused by immune complexes containing viral antigens which bind to platelet Fc receptors or by antibodies produced against viral antigens which cross-react with the platelet. In addition to the viral disorders described above, the differential diagnosis should include atypical presentations of aplastic anemia, acute leukemias, or metastatic tumor. A bone marrow examination is essential to exclude these disorders, which can occasionally mimic acute ITP.

Most adults present with a more indolent form of thrombocytopenia which may persist for many years and is referred to as *chronic ITP*. Women aged 20 to 40 are afflicted most commonly and outnumber men by a ratio of 3:1. They may present with an abrupt fall in platelet count and bleeding similar to patients with acute ITP. More often they have a prior history of easy bruising or menometrorrhagia. These patients have an autoimmune disorder with antibodies directed against target antigens on the glycoprotein IIb-IIIa or glycoprotein Ib-IX complex (see Fig. 57-2). Although most antibodies function as opsonins and accelerate platelet clearance by phagocytic cells, occasional antibodies bind to epitopes on critical regions of these glycoproteins and impair platelet function. A number of tests have been introduced to measure platelet-associated IgG. Although the tests are quite sensitive, their specificity is a problem. First, there is a high "background" level of IgG on normal platelets. Second, an elevation in plasma immunoglobulin levels or in circulating immune complexes will nonspecifically increase platelet-associated IgG.

Since a low platelet count may be the initial manifestation of systemic lupus erythematosus (SLE) or the first sign of a primary hematologic disorder, all patients with chronic ITP should have a bone marrow examination and an antinuclear antibody determination. In addition, patients with hepatic or splenic enlargement, lymphadenopathy, or atypical lymphocytes should have serologic studies for hepatitis, cytomegalovirus, Epstein-Barr virus, toxoplasma, and HIV. HIV infection has rapidly become a common cause of immunologic thrombocytopenia and should be considered in the differential diagnosis of thrombocytopenia, especially in high-risk groups—homosexuals, hemophiliacs, intravenous drug abusers, and heterosexual individuals with multiple partners. Thrombocytopenia can be the initial symptom of HIV infection or a complication of fully developed clinical AIDS.

Treatment of patients with ITP must take into account the age of the patient, the severity of the illness, and the anticipated natural history. Although adults have a higher incidence of intracranial bleeding than children, specific therapy may not be necessary unless the platelet count is under 20,000 per microliter or there is extensive bleeding. Hemorrhage in patients with either acute or chronic ITP usually can be controlled with glucocorticoids but, in rare cases, may require plasmapheresis to reduce the antibody or immune-complex level or temporary phagocytic blockade with intravenous gamma globulin. Emergency splenectomy is usually reserved for patients with acute or chronic ITP who are desperately ill and have not responded to any medical measures designed to improve hemostasis. The treatment of symptomatic thrombocytopenia in patients with HIV infection presents a special problem because the administration of glucocorticoids or splenectomy may increase susceptibility to the opportunistic infections which threaten these patients. Splenectomy has been effective in the course of HIV infection prior to the onset of symptomatic AIDS. There is increasing evidence that treatment with AZT can improve the platelet count in patients with HIV-induced thrombocytopenia.

Symptomatic patients with chronic ITP are usually placed on glucocorticoids. In one standard regimen, 60 mg prednisone is administered for 4 to 6 weeks and then decreased over another few weeks. Approximately 50 percent of patients with chronic ITP will normalize their platelet count on high doses of prednisone. However, the majority will have a fall in platelet count following steroid withdrawal. Patients with chronic ITP who fail to maintain a normal platelet count after a course of steroids are eligible for elective splenectomy. These steroid-responsive but steroid-dependent patients are very likely to respond to splenectomy, and 70 percent will have a normal platelet count within 1 week after surgery. Some patients who do not respond to glucocorticoids may still respond to splenectomy. Occasionally, patients may fail to respond to splenectomy because of the failure to remove an accessory spleen. In other patients, a small inactive accessory spleen may grow or new splenic foci may develop from splenic cells shed at the time of surgery and cause the late onset of thrombocytopenia. In either case, the presence of splenic tissue can be diagnosed by examination of the blood smear for Howell-Jolly bodies which appear in the red cells of asplenic individuals. This can be confirmed by a radionuclide scan.

Patients who are still thrombocytopenic after steroid therapy or splenectomy or who relapse months to years after initial therapy have received a variety of immunosuppressive drugs including azathioprine, cyclophosphamiade, vincristine, and vinblastine. More recently, danazol, an impeded androgen, has been used with some success. Although each of these drugs may be beneficial, it is important to use some restraint because they have serious side effects. Intravenous gamma globulin (IVIG) has become a popular therapy, although it is only transiently effective and is quite expensive. It should be used to temporarily raise the platelet count and to support patients prior to surgery or labor and delivery. Anti-RhD therapy appears to be equally effective, although a form suitable for intravenous administration must be obtained. If a patient is not bleeding and maintains a platelet count over 20,000 per microliter, consideration should be given to withholding therapy, since there are many patients with severe chronic thrombocytopenia who have lived with their disease for two or three decades.

VON WILLEBRAND'S DISEASE Von Willebrand's disease (vWD) is the most common inherited bleeding disorder and may occur in as many as 1 in 800 to 1000 individuals. The von Willebrand factor (vWF) is a heterogeneous multimeric plasma glycoprotein with two major functions. It facilitates platelet adhesion under conditions of high shear stress by linking platelet membrane receptors to vascular subendothelium; it also serves as the plasma carrier for factor VIII, the antihemophilic factor, a critical blood coagulation protein. Discrete domains in each vWF subunit mediate each of these important functions (Fig. 314-2). The normal plasma vWF level is 10 mg/L. The vWF activity is distributed among a series of plasma multimers

FIGURE 314-2 Domain structure of the von Willebrand protein (vWF) and its relation to the physical structure of the protein as determined by electron microscopy. The letters represent the repeated sequence elements that encode each vWF subunit. The propolypeptide, which is cleaved during multimer assembly, is encoded by the D1 and D2 repeats. The globular amino-terminal domain is encoded by the D2a and D3 repeats and the carboxy-terminal domain by the D4 repeat. The elongated filamentous region, which contains vWF binding sites for GpIb, heparin, and collagen, is encoded by the three A repeats. The amino acid residues that comprise the functional binding sites are shown at the top of the figure.

with estimated molecular weights ranging from 400,000 to over 20 million. A single large vWF precursor subunit is synthesized in endothelial cells and megakaryocytes, where it is cleaved and assembled into the disulfide-linked multimers present in plasma, platelets, and vascular subendothelium. A modest reduction in plasma vWF concentration or a selective loss in the high-molecular-weight multimers decreases platelet adhesion and causes clinical bleeding.

Although vWD is heterogeneous, there are certain clinical features which are common to all the syndromes. With one exception (type III disease), all forms are inherited as autosomal dominant traits and affected patients are heterozygous with one normal and one abnormal vWF allele. In mild cases, bleeding occurs only after surgery or trauma. More severely affected patients have spontaneous epistaxis or oral mucosal, gastrointestinal, or genitourinary bleeding. The laboratory findings are variable. The most diagnostic pattern is the combination of (1) a prolonged bleeding time, (2) a reduction in plasma vWF concentration, (3) a parallel reduction in ristocetin cofactor activity, and (4) reduced factor VIII activity. The variability in laboratory tests is related to both the heterogeneous nature of the defects in vWD and the fact that plasma levels are influenced by ABO blood group type, central nervous system disorders, systemic inflammation, and pregnancy. Since vWD is an autosomal dominant disorder, some vWF is produced by the remaining normal allele. Thus patients with mild defects may have laboratory values that fluctuate over time and may occasionally be within the normal range.

There are three major types of vWD. Patients with *type I disease*, the most common abnormality, have a mild to moderate decrease in plasma vWF. In the milder cases, although hemostasis is clearly impaired, the vWF level is just below the lower limit of normal (50 percent activity, or 5 mg/L). In type I disease, there is a parallel decrease in vWF antigen, factor VIII activity, and ristocetin cofactor activity, with a normal spectrum of multimers detected by sodium dodecyl sulfate–agarose (SDS-agarose) gel electrophoresis. Cultured endothelial cells derived from the umbilical cords of patients with vWD synthesize and secrete reduced quantities of vWF multimer and have a two- to fourfold reduction in vWF mRNA.

The variant forms of vWD (*type II disease*), which are much less common, are characterized by normal or near-normal levels of a dysfunctional protein. Patients with the *type IIa variant* of vWD have a deficiency in the high- and medium-molecular-weight forms of vWF multimer detected by SDS-agarose electrophoresis. This is due either to an inability to secrete the high-molecular-weight vWF multimers or to proteolysis of the multimers soon after they leave the endothelial cell and enter the circulation. Mutations in a localized region of the vWF A-2 domain have been identified in families with type IIa vWD. The quantity of vWF antigen and the amount of associated factor

VIII are usually normal. In the *type IIb variant*, there is also a loss in high-molecular-weight multimers. However, in type IIb disease, it is due to the inappropriate binding of vWF to platelets. This forms intravascular platelet aggregates which are rapidly cleared from the circulation, causing mild, cyclic thrombocytopenia. Mutations in a disulfide-bonded loop in the A-1 domain that binds to glycoprotein Ib-IX have been identified as the cause of the type IIb defect. A few patients have been described with a platelet membrane disorder which mimics type IIb vWD—*platelet-type vWD*. It is due to mutations in the portion of glycoprotein/IX which interacts with vWF. Levels of total vWF antigen and factor VIII are normal.

Approximately 1 in 1 million individuals have a very severe form of vWD that is phenotypically recessive (*type III disease*). Type III patients are usually the offspring of two parents with mild type I disease. However, in many cases, the parents are very mildly affected or are asymptomatic. Type III patients may inherit a different abnormality from each parent (a doubly heterozygous state) or be homozygous for a single defect. Type III patients have severe mucosal bleeding, no detectable vWF antigen or activity, and may have sufficiently low factor VIII levels to have occasional hemarthroses like mild hemophiliacs. Several type III families have been described with major deletions in the vWF gene that were detected by Southern blotting with vWF cDNA. In addition, families with nonsense mutations and a combination of a deleted and nonsense mutant allele have been described.

Appropriate therapy of vWD depends on the symptoms and the underlying type of disease. There are two therapeutic options. One involves the use of cryoprecipitate, a plasma fraction enriched in vWF, or factor VIII concentrates which retain high-molecular-weight vWF multimers (Humate-P, Koate HS). The factor VIII concentrates are highly purified and heat-treated to destroy HIV and are appropriate treatments for all the inherited forms of vWD. During surgery or after major trauma, patients should receive cryoprecipitate or factor VIII concentrate twice daily. This regimen should be continued twice daily for 48 to 72 h to ensure optimal hemostasis. Minor bleeding episodes such as prolonged epistaxis or severe menorrhagia may respond to a single transfusion. Recurrent menorrhagia, a major problem for women with severe vWD, can be treated effectively with oral contraceptive agents that suppress menses.

A second therapeutic option, which avoids the use of plasma, is the use of 1-desamino-8-D-arginine vasopressin (DDAVP), a vasopressin analogue which has minimal blood pressure-elevating and fluid-retaining properties and raises the plasma vWF level in normal individuals and patients with mild vWD. Patients with type I disease are the best candidates for DDAVP therapy. However, they must be tested for an adequate response prior to anticipated surgery, and vWF levels must be monitored closely during therapy, since the patient may develop tachyphylaxis when therapy is continued for more than 48 h. DDAVP should not be given to patients with variant forms of vWD without prior testing, since it may not improve multimer pattern or hemostasis in type IIa patients and it may actually worsen the defect by depleting high-molecular-weight multimers forming intravascular platelet aggregation and lowering the platelet count in type IIb patients. It is also ineffective therapy for most patients with the severe form (type III) of vWD.

Although most cases of vWD are inherited, there are also acquired forms of vWD caused by antibodies which inhibit vWF function or by lymphoid or other tumors which selectively adsorb vWF multimers onto their surfaces. Anti-vWF antibodies have developed in patients with severe vWD following multiple transfusions, as well as in patients with autoimmune and lymphoproliferative disorders. Adsorption of vWF to tumor surfaces has been documented in patients with Waldenström's macroglobulinemia and Wilm's tumor and inferred in other patients with lymphoma. Treatment of acquired vWD should focus on controlling the underlying disease, since plasma derivatives and DDAVP are often not effective and the disorder can be fatal.

PLATELET MEMBRANE DEFECTS Receptors which modulate platelet adhesion and aggregation are located on the two major platelet surface glycoproteins. As previously discussed (see Chap. 57), vWF facilitates platelet adhesion by binding to glycoprotein Ib-IX, while fibrinogen links platelets into aggregates via sites on the glycoprotein IIb-IIIa complex. There are two rare but well-defined platelet defects characterized by a loss of or a defect in these glycoprotein receptors. Patients with the *Bernard-Soulier syndrome* have markedly reduced platelet adhesion and cannot bind vWF to their platelets owing to deficiency or dysfunction of the glycoprotein Ib-IX complex. They also have reduced levels of several other membrane proteins, mild thrombocytopenia, and extremely large, lymphocytoid platelets. Platelets from patients with *Glanzmann's disease* or *thrombasthenia* are deficient in or have a defect in the glycoprotein IIb-IIIa complex. Their platelets do not bind fibrinogen and cannot form aggregates, although the platelets undergo shape change and secretion and are of normal size.

Both these disorders are inherited as autosomal recessive traits and are characterized by markedly impaired hemostasis and recurrent episodes of severe mucosal hemorrhage. In keeping with the selective nature of the defects, Bernard-Soulier platelets react normally to all stimuli except ristocetin. In contrast, thrombasthenic platelets adhere normally and will agglutinate with ristocetin but will not aggregate with any of the agonists which require fibrinogen binding, such as adenosine diphosphate (ADP), thrombin, or epinephrine.

The only effective therapy for hemorrhagic episodes in these two disorders is transfusion with normal platelets. This is usually effective, although alloimmunization will eventually limit the life span of infused platelets. In addition, a few patients have developed inhibitor antibodies with specificity for the missing protein. These antibodies bind to the protein which is expressed on the transfused normal platelets and impair their function.

PLATELET RELEASE DEFECTS   The most common mild bleeding disorders arise from the ingestion of aspirin and other nonsteroidal anti-inflammatory drugs (NSAIDs) which inhibit platelet production of thromboxane A_2, an important mediator of platelet secretion and aggregation (see Figs. 57-3 and 57-4). These drugs inhibit platelet cyclooxygenase, which converts arachidonic acid to a labile endoperoxide intermediate that is critical for thromboxane formation. Aspirin is the most potent agent, since it irreversibly acetylates the platelet enzyme so that a single dose impairs hemostasis for 5 to 7 days. The other agents are competitive and reversible inhibitors with more transient effects. Blocking thromboxane A_2 synthesis partially inhibits platelet release and aggregation with weak agonists such as ADP and epinephrine and produces a mild hemostatic defect. The administration of high doses of certain antibiotics, particularly penicillin, can coat the platelet surface, block platelet release, and impair hemostasis.

Patients generally have minimal symptoms such as easy bruising, and bleeding is usually confined to the skin. Occasional patients will have prolonged oozing after surgery, particularly with procedures involving mucous membranes such as periodontal, oral, or reconstructive plastic surgery. Not surprisingly, the antiplatelet effect of drugs such as aspirin is more dramatic when they are administered to patients with underlying defects like vWD or hemophilia. Patients with drug-induced cyclooxygenase deficiency often but not always have a mildly prolonged bleeding time, and their platelets fail to aggregate when incubated with arachidonic acid, epinephrine, or low doses of ADP. Since the bleeding time is not entirely reliable, if patients have taken aspirin, they should be treated as if they have a mild hemostatic defect for the next 5 to 7 days. Platelet responses to collagen and thrombin are impaired at low doses but normal at higher doses. Symptomatic patients should be encouraged to use drugs such as acetaminophen which do not impair platelet function. Although most cases of cyclooxygenase deficiency are drug-induced, occasional patients have inherited disorders in platelet cyclooxygenase activity which impair thromboxane production or receptor level defects which prevent platelets from responding to thromboxane A_2.

Although a number of metabolic disorders can perturb hemostasis, uremic platelet dysfunction is clinically the most important. The mechanism by which uremia impairs platelet function is not well understood, and retention of phenolic and guanidinosuccinic acids, excess prostacyclin production, or impaired vWF-platelet interactions have all been implicated. There is a good correlation between the degree of uremia and bleeding symptoms and the degree of anemia and bleeding. Bleeding can usually be reversed by dialysis and often improves after red cell transfusion or treatment with erythropoietin. In addition, the administration of cryoprecipitate or DDAVP, which raise plasma vWF levels, also can improve hemostasis. Conjugated estrogens improve hemostasis and can be used as long-term therapy.

STORAGE POOL DEFECTS   Platelet granules have considerable amounts of adenine nucleotides, calcium, and adhesive glycoproteins such as thrombospondin, fibronectin, and vWF, all of which promote platelet adhesion and aggregation. Thus, it is not surprising that patients with defective platelet granules have a mild bleeding disorder. Platelet storage pool defects may be inherited as an isolated disorder or be part of systemic granule packaging defects such as oculocutaneous albinism or the Hermansky-Pudlak or Chédiak-Higashi syndromes. Clinically, these patients cannot be distinguished from those with other functional platelet disorders, since they all have easy bruising, mucosal bleeding, and a prolonged bleeding time. They can be differentiated from patients with the cyclooxygenase defects because their platelets will usually aggregate in response to arachidonic acid. In addition, their platelets have decreased levels of specific granule constituents such as ADP and serotonin and abnormalities in granule morphology that are best visualized by electron microscopy.

Occasionally, patients with acute or chronic leukemia or one of the myeloproliferative disorders develop an acquired storage pool disorder due to dysplastic megakaryocyte development. In addition, patients with liver disease and some patients with systemic lupus erythematosus or other immune-complex-mediated disorders may have circulating platelets which have degranulated prematurely. Platelet degranulation and a transient storage pool disorder also have been described following prolonged cardiopulmonary bypass. Fortunately, most patients with storage pool defects have only mildly impaired hemostasis. They can be treated with platelet transfusions. Occasional patients have responded to DDAVP.

VESSEL WALL DISORDERS

Bleeding from vascular disorders (nonthrombocytopenic purpura) is usually mild and confined to the skin and mucous membranes. The pathogenesis of bleeding is poorly defined in many of the syndromes, and classical tests of hemostasis, including the bleeding time and tests of platelet function, are usually normal. Vascular purpura arises from damage to capillary endothelium, abnormalities in the vascular subendothelial matrix or extravascular connective tissues which support blood vessels, or from the formation of abnormal blood vessels. There are also several idiopathic disorders which involve the vessel wall and which can cause more severe bleeding and organ dysfunction.

THROMBOTIC THROMBOCYTOPENIC PURPURA   Thrombotic thrombocytopenic purpura (TTP) is a fulminant, often lethal disorder that may be initiated by endothelial injury and subsequent release of vWF and other procoagulant materials from the endothelial cell. In addition, some patients with TTP may have a unique circulating protein which induces platelet aggregation. Characteristic findings include the microvascular deposition of hyaline thrombi which stain for fibrin, thrombocytopenia, microangiopathic hemolytic anemia, fever, renal failure, fluctuating levels of consciousness, and evanescent focal neurologic deficits. The presence of hyaline thrombi in arterioles, capillaries, and venules without any inflammatory changes in the vessel wall is diagnostic. Gingival biopsies are positive in 30 to 40 percent of patients, and marrow biopsies are occasionally helpful. The presence of a severe Coombs-negative hemolytic anemia with schistocytes or fragmented red blood cells in the peripheral blood smear, coupled with thrombocytopenia, and minimal activation of the coagulation system help to confirm the clinical suspicion of TTP.

This disorder should be distinguished from vasculitis and systemic lupus erythematosus, which can predispose patients to TTP. Levels of platelet-associated IgG and complement are usually normal in TTP.

The treatment of acute TTP has changed radically in the past few years. Steroids and heparin or emergency splenectomy have been abandoned, and the enthusiasm for antiplatelet therapy has diminished. Increasingly, treatment has focused on the use of exchange transfusion or intensive plasmapheresis coupled with infusion of fresh frozen plasma. With this therapeutic approach, the overall mortality has been markedly reduced, and over half the patients with TTP are recovering from this formerly fatal disorder. Most patients surviving the acute illness recover completely with no residual renal or neurologic disease. Occasional patients with a chronic, relapsing form of TTP require maintenance plasmapheresis and plasma infusion, and a few patients are only controlled with glucocorticoids.

HEMOLYTIC-UREMIC SYNDROME Hemolytic-uremic syndrome (HUS) is a disease of infancy and early childhood which closely resembles TTP. Patients present with fever, thrombocytopenia, microangiopathic hemolytic anemia, hypertension, and varying degrees of acute renal failure. In many cases, onset is preceded by a minor febrile or viral illness, and an infectious or immune-complex–mediated cause has been proposed. As in TTP, there is no evidence of disseminated intravascular coagulation. In contrast to TTP, the disorder remains localized to the kidney, where hyaline thrombi are seen in the afferent arterioles and glomerular capillaries. Such thrombi are not present in other vessels, and neurologic symptoms, other than those associated with uremia, are uncommon. There is no effective therapy; however, with dialysis for acute renal failure, the initial mortality is only 5 percent. Between 10 and 50 percent of patients are left with some chronic renal impairment.

HENOCH-SCHÖNLEIN PURPURA Henoch-Schönlein or anaphylactoid purpura is a distinct, self-limited type of vasculitis which occurs in children and young adults. Patients have an acute inflammatory reaction in capillaries, mesangial tissues, and small arterioles which leads to increased vascular permeability, exudation, and hemorrhage. Vessel lesions contain IgA and complement components. The syndrome may be preceded by an upper respiratory infection or streptococcal pharyngitis or be associated with food or drug allergies. Patients develop a purpuric or urticarial rash on the extensor surfaces of the arms and legs and on the buttocks; they also have polyarthralgias or arthritis, colicky abdominal pain, and hematuria from focal glomerulonephritis. Despite the hemorrhagic features, all coagulation tests are normal. A small number of patients may develop fatal acute renal failure, and 5 to 10 percent develop chronic nephritis. Glucocorticoids provide symptomatic relief of the joint and abdominal pains but do not alter the course of the illness.

METABOLIC AND INFLAMMATORY DISORDERS A number of acute febrile illnesses cause capillary fragility and skin bleeding. Immune complexes containing viral antigens or the viruses themselves may damage endothelial cells. In addition, certain pathogens such as the rickettsiae which cause Rocky Mountain spotted fever replicate in endothelial cells and damage them. Thrombocytopenia is also a frequent finding in acute infectious disorders and may contribute to skin bleeding. In addition, whenever the platelet count falls below 10,000 per microliter, gaps which develop between endothelial cells allow the diapedesis of red cells into the dermis leading to the formation of petechiae. Drugs such as the sulfonamides, penicillin, and allopurinol may cause vascular inflammation resulting in maculopapular or urticarial rashes. Some of these mechanisms are additive, and drug reactions in thrombocytopenic individuals cause an intensely hemorrhagic rash.

Occasionally, patients with diffuse polyclonal hyperglobulinemia will develop purpuric lesions on the lower limbs—a benign condition referred to as *hyperglobulinemic purpura*. Vascular purpura may occur in patients with various monoclonal plasma protein abnormalities, including Waldenström's macroglobulinemia, multiple myeloma, and cryoglobulinemia. These proteins markedly increase serum viscosity and may impair blood flow through capillaries. Thus retinal hemorrhage, central nervous system dysfunction, and skin necrosis have all been described in these syndromes due to the marked elevation in viscosity. In addition, the globulins may impair platelet aggregation and adhesion and interfere with fibrin polymerization. Patients with mixed cryoglobulinemia develop a more extensive maculopapular lesion due to immune-complex–mediated damage to the vessel wall. The mixed cryoglobulinemia (usually IgG and anti-IgG) may be associated with arthralgias, diffuse weakness, and unexplained nephritis. Plasmapheresis will temporarily lower the level of globulins, remove immune complexes, and improve symptoms in these patients. However, long-term management must include control of the underlying disease which produces the abnormal globulins or immune complexes.

Patients with *scurvy* (vitamin C deficiency) develop painful episodes of perifollicular skin bleeding as well as bleeding into muscles and, occasionally, into the gastrointestinal and genitourinary tracts. The diagnosis is confirmed by the presence of hyperkeratosis of skin, gum swelling, and low levels of the vitamin in leukocytes. Vitamin C–deficient patients have markedly defective collagen synthesis, since ascorbic acid is needed to synthesize hydroxyproline, an essential constituent of collagen. Patients with *Cushing's syndrome*, which is characterized by excess production of glucocorticoids, or patients on large doses of glucocorticoids develop generalized protein wasting and may show skin bleeding or easy bruising due to atrophy of the supporting connective tissue around blood vessels. Aging causes a similar atrophy of perivascular connective tissue on the extensor surfaces of the hands and arms, leading to "senile purpura." These patients develop dark purple, irregularly shaped hemorrhagic areas due to abnormal skin mobility which tears small blood vessels.

Patients with inherited disorders of the connective tissue matrix such as *Marfan's syndrome*, *Ehlers-Danlos syndrome*, and *pseudoxanthoma elasticum* also have easy bruising. In addition to having fragile skin vessels and easy bruising, patients with Ehlers-Danlos syndrome may develop aneurysms in intraabdominal vessels and apoplectic rupture and hemorrhage due to defects in the vascular collagen network. Primary vascular abnormalities also can lead to bleeding. Patients with *Osler-Weber-Rendu disease* (hereditary hemorrhagic telangiectasia), an inherited autosomal dominant disorder, have frequent episodes of nasal and gastrointestinal bleeding from abnormal telangiectatic capillaries; patients with *angiodysplasia* of the colon have increased incidence of gastrointestinal bleeding. In the *Kasabach-Merritt syndrome*, patients may have very extensive and progressively enlarging vascular malformations which may involve large portions of their extremities. Bleeding is secondary to disseminated intravascular coagulation triggered by stagnant blood flow through the tortuous abnormal vessels.

REFERENCES

HANDIN RI, WAGNER DD: Molecular and cellular biology of von Willebrand factor, in *Progress in Hemostasis and Thrombosis*, vol 9, BS Coller (ed). Philadelphia, Saunders, 1989, pp 233–259

——— et al (eds): *Blood: Principles and Practice of Hematology and Hematologic Oncology*. Philadelphia, Lippincott, 1993

MAJERUS P: Platelets, in *The Molecular Basis of Blood Diseases*, G Stamatoyanopoulis et al (eds). Philadelphia, Saunders, 1987, pp 689–722

STUART MJ, KELTON JG: The platelet: Quantitative and qualitative abnormalities, in *Hematology of Infancy and Childhood*, 4th ed, DG Nathan, FA Oski (eds). Philadelphia, Saunders, 1992, p 1343–1479

WILLIAMS WJ: et al (eds): *Hematology*, 4th ed. New York, McGraw-Hill, 1990

315 DISORDERS OF COAGULATION AND THROMBOSIS

ROBERT I. HANDIN

Patients with congenital plasma coagulation defects characteristically bleed into muscles, joints, and body cavities hours or days after an injury. Most of the *inherited* plasma coagulation disorders are due to defects in single coagulation proteins, with the two X-linked disorders, factors VIII and IX deficiency, accounting for the majority of the congenital coagulation disorders. These patients merit special attention because they may have severe bleeding and chronic disability and require specialized medical therapy. With rare exceptions, the known disorders prolong either the prothrombin time (PT), partial thromboplastin time (PTT), or both these important laboratory screening tests. If they are abnormal, quantitative assays of specific coagulation proteins are then carried out using the PT or PTT tests with plasma from congenitally deficient individuals as substrate. The corrective effect of varying concentrations of patient plasma is measured and expressed as a percentage of a normal pooled plasma standard. The interval range for most coagulation factors is from 50 to 150 percent of this average value, and the minimal level of most individual factors needed for adequate hemostasis is 25 percent.

Acquired coagulation disorders are both more frequent and more complex, arising from deficiencies of multiple coagulation proteins and simultaneously affecting both primary and secondary hemostasis. The most common acquired hemorrhagic disorders are (1) disseminated intravascular coagulation, (2) the hemorrhagic diathesis of liver disease, and (3) vitamin K deficiency and complications of anticoagulant therapy.

Although congenital and acquired bleeding disorders are relatively rare, venous and arterial thrombosis and embolism are common medical disorders which have been recognized for over a hundred years. Although risk factors such as atherosclerotic vascular disease, congestive heart failure, malignancy, and immobility predispose patients to thrombosis, specific coagulation defects have not yet been identified in most patients with thromboembolism. Several inherited coagulation abnormalities have now been described which induce a hypercoagulable or prethrombotic state and predispose patients to thrombosis. These disorders merit special attention because they affect young people, cause recurrent episodes of thromboembolism, and may involve multiple members of a single family. An understanding of the biochemical basis of thromboembolism is also important because anticoagulant and antithrombotic regimes are based on the premise that modifying critical coagulation reactions will reduce the incidence of thrombosis. This chapter will review the diagnosis, natural history, and therapy of congenital and acquired plasma coagulation disorders, as well as the inherited prethrombotic disorders. The physiology of normal hemostasis and the cardinal manifestations of the hemorrhagic and thrombotic disorders are described in Chap. 57.

FACTOR VIII DEFICIENCY—HEMOPHILIA A Pathogenesis and clinical manifestations The antihemophilic factor (AHF) or factor VIII coagulant protein is a large (265-kDa), single-chain protein which regulates the activation of factor X by proteases generated in the intrinsic coagulation pathway (see Figs. 57-4 and 57-6). It is synthesized in liver parenchymal cells and circulates complexed to the von Willebrand protein (vWF). Previous efforts to purify and characterize the factor VIII molecule were limited by its low concentration (10 μg/L) and susceptibility to proteolysis. However, the cloning and sequencing of complementary DNA (cDNA) encoding the factor VIII molecule and the mapping of the factor VIII gene on the X chromosome have provided a detailed picture of its structure and have led to improved methods for carrier detection and prenatal diagnosis of hemophilia A.

One in 10,000 males is born with deficiency or dysfunction of the factor VIII molecule. The resulting disorder, hemophilia A, is characterized by bleeding into soft tissues, muscles, and weight-bearing joints. Although normal hemostasis requires at least 25 percent factor VIII activity, symptomatic patients usually have factor VIII levels below 5 percent, with a close correlation between the clinical severity of hemophilia and plasma AHF level. Patients with <1 percent factor VIII activity have *severe* disease; they bleed frequently even without discernible trauma. Patients with levels between 1 and 5 percent have *moderate* disease with less frequent bleeding episodes. Those with levels over 5 percent have *mild* disease with infrequent bleeding that is usually secondary to trauma. Occasional patients with factor VIII levels as high as 25 percent are discovered when they bleed after major trauma or surgery. The majority of patients with hemophilia A have factor VIII levels below 5 percent.

Hemophilic bleeding occurs hours or days after injury, can involve any organ, and, if untreated, may continue for days or weeks. This can result in large collections of partially clotted blood putting pressure on adjacent normal tissues and can cause necrosis of muscle (compartment syndromes), venous congestion (pseudophlebitis), or ischemic damage to nerves. For example, hemophiliacs often develop femoral neuropathy due to pressure from an unsuspected retroperitoneal hematoma. They also can develop large calcified masses of blood and inflammatory tissue that are mistaken for soft tissue sarcomas (pseudotumor syndrome).

Patients with severe hemophilia are usually diagnosed shortly after birth because of an extensive cephalhematoma or profuse bleeding at circumcision. However, patients with moderate disease may not bleed until they begin to walk or crawl, and mild hemophiliacs may not be diagnosed until they are adolescents or young adults. Typically, a hemophiliac patient presents with pain followed by swelling in a weight-bearing joint, such as the hip, knee, or ankle. The presence of blood in the joint (hemarthrosis) causes synovial inflammation, and repetitive bleeding erodes articular cartilage and causes osteoarthritis, articular fibrosis, joint ankylosis, and eventually muscle atrophy. Although bleeding may occur into any joint, after a joint has been damaged, it may become a site for subsequent bleeding episodes.

Hematuria, in the absence of any genitourinary pathology, is also common. It is usually self-limited and may not require specific therapy. The most feared complications of hemophilia are oropharyngeal and central nervous system bleeding. Patients with oropharyngeal bleeding may require emergency intubation to maintain an adequate airway. Central nervous system bleeding can occur without antecedent trauma or without evidence of a specific lesion.

Patients suspected of having hemophilia should have screening tests of hemostasis, including a platelet count, bleeding time, PT, and PTT. Typically, the patient will have a prolonged PTT with all other tests normal. Because of the clinical similarity of factor VIII deficiency and factor IX deficiency, any male with an appropriate bleeding history and a prolonged PTT should have specific assays for factor VIII and factor IX.

Therapy There are several tenets regarding the treatment of bleeding in hemophiliac patients: (1) Symptoms often precede objective evidence of bleeding. (2) Signs of bleeding may not appear until several days after well-documented trauma. Physicians caring for these patients have learned to rely on their patients to inform them of early symptoms, usually pain, and to begin treatment at that time. Early treatment is more effective, less costly, and can be lifesaving. (3) It is critical to avoid the use of aspirin or aspirin-containing drugs which impair platelet function and may cause severe hemorrhage.

Plasma products enriched in factor VIII have revolutionized the care of hemophilia patients, reduced the degree of orthopedic deformity, and permitted virtually any form of elective and emergency surgery. The widespread use of factor VIII concentrates also has produced serious complications, including viral hepatitis, chronic liver disease, and AIDS. The standard therapeutic products are cryoprecipitate and factor VIII concentrate. *Cryoprecipitate*, which contains about half the factor VIII activity of fresh frozen plasma in one-tenth the original volume, is simple to prepare and is produced in hospital or regional blood banks. It must be stored frozen and is thawed and pooled prior to administration. However, most patients utilize partially purified *factor VIII concentrate*, which is prepared from multiple donors and supplied as a lyophilized powder. It can be refrigerated and reconstituted just prior to use.

There are three recent developments which have increased the safety of factor VIII therapy. First, heating of lyophilized factor VIII concentrates under carefully controlled conditions can inactivate human immunodeficiency virus (HIV) without destroying factor VIII coagulant activity. Second, highly purified factor VIII can be produced by adsorbing and eluting factor VIII from monoclonal antibody columns. Third, recombinant factor VIII has just completed clinical trials and is being marketed. Patients with hemophilia should receive either monoclonal purified or recombinant factor VIII to minimize viral infections and exposure to irrelevant proteins.

It has been determined, empirically, that each unit of factor VIII infused, defined as the amount present in 1 mL normal plasma, will raise the plasma level of the recipient by 2 percent per kilogram of body weight. Factor VIII has a half-life of 8 to 12 h, making it necessary to infuse it continuously or at least twice daily to sustain a chosen factor VIII level. In patients with mild hemophilia, an alternative to the use of plasma products is desmopressin (DDAVP), which transiently increases the factor VIII level. DDAVP in general will increase the factor level two- to threefold. Although generally safe, it occasionally causes hyponatremia or may precipitate thrombosis in elderly patients.

An uncomplicated episode of soft tissue bleeding or an early hemarthrosis can be treated with one infusion of cryoprecipitate or factor VIII concentrate sufficient to raise the factor VIII level to 15 or 20 percent. A more extensive hemarthrosis or retroperitoneal bleeding requires twice-daily or continuous infusions in order to keep the factor VIII level between 25 and 50 percent for at least 72 h. Life-threatening bleeding into the central nervous system or major surgery may require therapy for 2 weeks with levels kept at a minimum of 50 percent of normal. In addition to the prompt infusion of factor VIII–enriched plasma products, patients need skilled orthopedic care with immobilization of inflamed joints to promote healing and to prevent contractures and physical therapy to strengthen muscles and maintain joint mobility. Prior to surgery, every patient should be screened for the presence of an inhibitor to factor VIII.

Patients with hemophilia who do not have an inhibitor should receive factor VIII infusions just prior to surgery and will require daily monitoring so that the factor VIII level is maintained above 50 percent for 10 to 14 days after surgery. When patients undergo joint replacement or other major orthopedic surgery, therapy should be continued for 3 weeks. This permits adequate wound healing and the institution of necessary joint mobilization and physical therapy.

Hemophiliacs also require treatment prior to dental procedures. Filling of a carious tooth can be managed by a single infusion of cryoprecipitate or factor VIII concentrate coupled with the administration of 4 to 6 g of ε-aminocaproic acid (EACA) four times daily for 72 to 96 h after the dental procedure. EACA is a potent antifibrinolytic agent which will inhibit plasminogen activators present in oral secretions and stabilize clot formation in oral tissue. Alternatives include tranexamic acid, a longer-acting antifibrinolytic. EACA is also effective when used as a mouthwash. For major oral and periodontal surgery and extractions of permanent teeth, patients should probably be hospitalized briefly and also treated with factor VIII concentrates. Therapy should begin just prior to surgery and be continued for a minimum of 48 to 72 h.

Many centers have organized home care programs so that patients can administer their own factor VIII infusions with the onset of symptoms. Occasional patients with very frequent bleeding receive regularly scheduled infusions. However, the expense and inconvenience usually limit the use of "prophylactic" infusions. Concern regarding transmission of AIDS has complicated therapy of hemophilia, and some patients are reluctant to treat themselves, despite the fact that current blood products carry a very low risk of transmitting HIV.

Complications Most hemophiliacs have had multiple episodes of hepatitis, and a majority have elevated hepatocellular enzyme levels and abnormalities on liver biopsy. Between 10 and 20 percent of hemophiliacs also have hepatosplenomegaly, and a small number develop chronic active or persistent hepatitis or cirrhosis. Recently, a few patients with hemophilia and end-stage liver disease have received liver transplants with cure of both diseases. Along with homosexuals and intravenous drug abusers, hemophiliacs are at high risk for AIDS because they frequently receive blood products. Hemophiliacs also can present with the full range of AIDS-related syndromes, including diffuse lymphadenopathy and immune thrombocytopenia. Although as many as 80 percent of multiply transfused hemophiliacs are HIV-positive and some have clinical AIDS, the advances in factor VIII concentrate technology discussed previously should prevent future HIV infection.

Despite frequent bleeding, severe iron-deficiency anemia is uncommon because most of the bleeding is internal and iron is effectively recycled. Mild iron deficiency from chronic epistaxis or gastrointestinal bleeding has been noted in some hemophiliacs. In addition, after receiving large doses of the older partially purified factor VIII concentrates, some patients have developed a mild Coombs-positive hemolytic anemia due to small amounts of anti-A and anti-B antibody that is present in commercial concentrates.

Following multiple transfusions, between 10 and 20 percent of patients with severe hemophilia develop inhibitors to factor VIII. Inhibitors are, generally, IgG antibodies which rapidly neutralize factor VIII activity and prevent effective transfusion therapy. There are two types of inhibitors which have different biologic characteristics and lead to different clinical presentations. Patients with type I inhibitors have a typical anamnestic response and raise their antibody titer following exposure to factor VIII. Patients with a type II inhibitor have a low antibody titer which cannot be stimulated by factor VIII infusion. Patients with the type I inhibitor should not receive factor VIII. In an emergency, control of bleeding may require intensive plasmapheresis or infusion of prothrombin complex concentrates which contain trace quantities of activated coagulation factors and can bypass the block in coagulation produced by the inhibitor. Patients with low-titer type II antibodies may respond to higher than normal doses of factor VIII.

Genetic counseling and carrier detection Until recently, carrier detection required biologic and immunologic assays which compared the ratio of factor VIII to vWF (von Willebrand factor) protein and were predictive in only 70 to 80 percent of cases. It is now possible to trace the defective allele in some families by examining the inheritance of restriction fragment length polymorphisms (RFLPs) linked to the factor VIII gene. In addition, in families in which a specific mutation has been defined in the factor VIII gene, it can be readily detected by gene amplification and allele-specific oligonucleotide hybridization. Previously, prenatal diagnosis required sampling fetal blood for coagulant activity. Now, in families with an identifiable RFLP linked to the gene or a known mutation, precise diagnosis is possible early in pregnancy from either chorionic villus biopsy or amniocentesis. The amount of material required has decreased, and the rapidity of diagnosis has increased with the introduction of the polymerase chain reaction to amplify desired segments of genomic DNA.

Female carriers of hemophilia, who are heterozygotes, usually produce sufficient factor VIII from the factor VIII allele on their normal X chromosome for normal hemostasis. However, occasional hemophilia carriers will have factor VIII levels far below 50 percent due to random inactivation of normal X chromosomes in tissue producing factor VIII. These symptomatic carriers may bleed with major surgery or bleed occasionally with menses. Rarely, true female hemophiliacs arise from consanguinity within families with hemophilia or from concomitant Turner's syndrome or XO mosaicism in a carrier female.

FACTOR IX DEFICIENCY—HEMOPHILIA B Factor IX is a single-chain, 55-kDa proenzyme which is converted to an active protease trates to correct thrombocytopenia. Those with acrocyanosis and incipient gangrene or other thrombotic problems need immediate anticoagulation with intravenous heparin. The use of heparin in the treatment of bleeding is still controversial. Although it is a logical way to reduce thrombin generation and prevent further consumption of clotting proteins, it should be reserved for patients with thrombosis or those who continue to bleed despite vigorous treatment with plasma and platelets.

Patients who initially have mild DIC and may not be symptomatic may begin to bleed following surgery or chemotherapy. For example, mild DIC, without clinical bleeding, has been documented during saline- or prostaglandin-induced midtrimester abortions. Prophylactic treatment of patients with heparin may prevent progression of a mild DIC syndrome and has been used in the treatment of patients with acute promyelocytic leukemia and in some patients with a retained dead fetus who require surgical extraction. However, most patients with low-grade DIC can be managed simply with plasma and platelet replacement and do not require heparin. Chronic DIC does not respond to oral warfarin anticoagulants, but it can be controlled with long-term heparin infusion. Occasional patients with indolent tumors and severe DIC have been maintained on heparin administered by intermittent subcutaneous injection or continuous infusion with portable pumps.

Despite our detailed understanding of the pathophysiology of DIC and a vigorous approach to therapy, there is little evidence that its treatment will change the natural history of the underlying disorder. Therapy will only stabilize the patient, prevent exsanguination or massive thrombosis, and permit institution of definitive therapy.

COAGULATION DISORDERS IN LIVER DISEASE   Since the liver plays a central role in the synthesis and metabolism of coagulation proteins, liver dysfunction is frequently accompanied by a hemostatic defect. The major causes of hemorrhage in patients with liver disease are outlined in Table 315-2. It is important to recognize that bleeding is usually due to an anatomic lesion, which can then be exacerbated by a hemostatic defect. Most patients bleed from complications of portal hypertension such as esophageal varices or from gastritis and peptic ulceration of the gastrointestinal tract. Portal hypertension also causes splenomegaly, with splenic sequestration of platelets and thrombocytopenia, which contributes to the hemostatic defect (see Chap. 268).

Patients with hepatocellular liver disease cannot store vitamin K optimally and may have some degree of vitamin K deficiency.

TABLE 315-2   Causes of bleeding in liver disease

ANATOMIC FACTORS

A Portal hypertension
   1 Varices
   2 Splenomegaly and secondary thrombocytopenia
B Peptic ulceration
C Gastritis

HEPATIC FUNCTION ABNORMALITIES

A Decreased synthesis of procoagulant proteins: fibrinogen, prothrombin, factors V, VII, IX, X, XI
B Decreased synthesis of coagulation inhibitors: protein C, protein S, antithrombin III
C Impaired absorption and metabolism of vitamin K
D Failure to clear activated coagulation proteins leading to
   1 Disseminated intravascular coagulation
   2 Systemic fibrinolysis

COMPLICATIONS OF THERAPY

A Dilution of platelets and coagulation proteins from massive transfusions
B Infusion of activated coagulation proteins in prothrombin complex concentrates
C Bleeding from heparin; thrombosis from ε-aminocaproic acid (EACA)

Cholestasis, which is a frequent feature of liver disease, impairs vitamin K absorption and further decreases liver vitamin K stores. Abnormalities in the gamma carboxylation of prothrombin complex proteins independent of vitamin K and the production of abnormal proteins also have been described. They also may have decreased production of other coagulation proteins, including fibrinogen and factor V. The liver also produces inhibitors of coagulation such as antithrombin III and proteins C and S and is the clearance site for activated coagulation factors and fibrinolytic enzymes. Thus patients with liver disease are also "hypercoagulable" and predisposed to developing DIC or systemic fibrinolysis. For these reasons, coagulation defects in advanced liver failure are often difficult to distinguish from those of DIC.

Each patient with hemorrhage and liver disease should have a PT, PTT, platelet count, and fibrinogen determination, although it is not always possible to determine the major hemostatic abnormality from a single set of laboratory values. It is helpful to have previous laboratory data available for patients with chronic liver disease who develop an acute complication. There is a good correlation between the degree of prolongation of the PT and the risk of bleeding. Most patients present with moderate prolongation of the PT and PTT, mild thrombocytopenia, and a normal fibrinogen level. However, they also may present with a more complex defect combining defective synthesis, abnormal clearance, and active consumption of coagulation proteins. Since vitamin K deficiency is so common, it is advisable to administer a single parenteral dose of vitamin K after initial laboratory studies have been obtained, even though this may only partially correct the laboratory abnormalities. The presence of severe thrombocytopenia or a low fibrinogen level suggests the additional complication of DIC and may require further studies and therapy.

The safest replacement therapy for a patient with liver disease is fresh frozen plasma, since it supplies all known coagulation factors. However, even this form of therapy has drawbacks, since large quantities of plasma may precipitate hepatic encephalopathy and cause fluid and sodium overload. Prothrombin complex concentrates should be avoided because they only replace the vitamin K–dependent factors, may be contaminated with hepatitis and AIDS virus, and contain trace quantities of activated coagulation proteins. Similarly, fibrinogen concentrates (or cryoprecipitate) which are rich in factor VIII and fibrinogen should not be used without additional fresh frozen plasma. Anticoagulation with heparin has been advocated to control DIC, but this is particularly hazardous and not recommended in cirrhosis because heparin is metabolized erratically and may thus lead to severe bleeding.

FIBRINOLYTIC DEFECTS   Bleeding also can occur from defects in the fibrinolytic system. Patients with alpha$_2$ plasmin inhibitor deficiency or plasminogen activator inhibitor-1 (PAI-1) have rapid fibrinolysis following fibrin deposition after trauma or surgery and so may experience recurrent hemorrhage. Similarly, patients with cirrhosis have an impaired clearance of tissue plasminogen activator and systemic fibrinolysis which may contribute to their hemorrhagic defect. Rarely, patients with tumors such as metastatic prostatic carcinoma may develop diffuse bleeding from primary fibrinolysis rather than DIC. Clues to the diagnosis include a disproportionately low fibrinogen level with a relatively normal PT and PTT and the presence of a normal or nearly normal platelet count. Although there are some exceptions, patients with primary fibrinolysis should have an elevated titer of fibrin degradation products (FPPs) but a normal D dimer level. However, at times it is difficult or impossible to differentiate primary fibrinolysis from the secondary fibrinolysis accompanying DIC. Patients with clearly established primary fibrinolysis should not receive heparin; they do require plasma therapy and, occasionally, fibrinolytic inhibitors such as EACA. However, EACA should not be given to patients suspected of having DIC unless they are also receiving heparin, since EACA can cause massive, often fatal, thrombosis in a patient with DIC.

CIRCULATING ANTICOAGULANTS   Circulating anticoagulants, or inhibitors, are usually IgG antibodies which interfere with coagulation reactions. Specific inhibitors inactivate individual coagulation proteins and may cause severe hemorrhage. As discussed above, they arise in 15 to 20 percent of patients with factor VIII or factor IX deficiency who have received plasma infusions. Specific inhibitors also occur in previously normal individuals. Although the most common target protein is factor VIII, inhibitors have been described with specificity for each of the coagulation proteins. In addition to hemophiliacs, anti-factor VIII antibodies are seen in postpartum females, in patients on various drugs, as part of the spectrum of autoantibodies in systemic lupus erythematosus patients, and in normal elderly individuals. Circulating anticoagulants also have been reported in patients with AIDS.

Nonspecific (lupus-like) inhibitors prolong coagulation tests by binding to phospholipids. They are assayed by their anticoagulant effect (LA activity) or their ability to bind to the complex phospholipid cardiolipin (ACLA activity). They do not perturb hemostasis in vivo, unless associated with thrombocytopenia or prothrombin deficiency. While they are most often encountered in patients with systemic lupus erythematosus, these nonspecific inhibitors have also been noted in patients with many other disorders and also in otherwise normal individuals.

The critical laboratory feature, which identifies the presence of either type of inhibitor, is the failure of normal plasma to correct a prolonged PT, PTT, or both. Plasma from patients with a specific inhibitor will progressively inactivate a coagulation protein and thus prolong whichever of these screening tests requires the participation of that clotting factor. This effect persists after dilution. Nonspecific inhibitors immediately prolong the PT and PTT and, at low dilution, block multiple coagulation reactions. However, these effects can be overcome by altering the quantity or type of phospholipid or by diluting the plasma.

Hemorrhage in patients with specific inhibitors may require treatment with massive plasma or concentrate infusion, the use of activated prothrombin complex concentrates to bypass the antibodies against factors VIII or IX, and plasmapheresis or exchange transfusion to lower antibody titer. Chronic immunosuppressive regimens have been sometimes employed and have been particularly useful in otherwise normal individuals with an acquired factor VIII antibody. Many patients lose their antibody and recover within 6 to 12 months, although the acute mortality rate from uncontrollable bleeding may approach 10 percent.

Patients with LA activity have normal hemostasis and will not bleed unless they have concomitant thrombocytopenia or prothrombin deficiency. Both thrombocytopenia and hypoprothrombinemia are secondary to autoantibodies which bind either to platelets or the prothrombin molecule. While these antibodies have no effect on function, they accelerate clearance of the coated platelets or the antibody-prothrombin complexes.

Although there is evidence that the presence of LA activity may predispose patients to thromboembolism and may cause midtrimester abortions, it is difficult to make firm predictions about the risk of thrombosis and the appropriate therapy for individual patients. First, tests for either LA or ACLA activity are not well standardized, and results vary among patients and can vary with serial measurements. The best predictor is a consistent prolongation of more than one coagulation test coupled with a high titer of ACLA activity. Second, the risk of thrombosis is increased in patients who have systemic lupus compared with those with idiopathic LA or ACLA activity. There is little evidence that prophylactic therapy is beneficial or that treatments aimed at reducing the titer of antibody are superior to conventional antithrombotic therapy.

Although therapy should be individualized, the following general guidelines may be helpful. They are based on personal experience and review of a rapidly expanding and changing literature. Patients with SLE and either LA or ACLA activity who have had a thrombotic episode are at high risk for a recurrence and should receive long-term anticoagulant therapy. Women who have had more than one midtrimester abortion, especially those with SLE, should have a trial

of anticoagulant therapy. Patients with a single thrombotic episode and no other risk factor except LA or ACLA activity may be treated, but the evidence for efficacy in this setting is minimal. Asymptomatic patients with laboratory abnormalities only should not be treated. Glucocorticoids should only be administered in conjunction with antithrombotic agents and are not of proven efficacy.

INHERITED PRETHROMBOTIC DISORDERS   As previously discussed (see Chap. 57), coagulation is carefully regulated by a series of inhibitors which limit thrombin generation and fibrin formation and by the fibrinolytic system which effectively removes fibrin thrombi (see Figs. 57-5 and 57-7). Inherited defects in the natural coagulation inhibitors (i.e., antithrombin, protein C, and protein S), abnormalities in the fibrinolytic system, and certain dysfibrinogenemias predispose patients to thrombosis (see Table 315-3). Although they are clearly important, defects in these proteins account for less than 10 percent of patients with recurrent thromboembolism. Antithrombin, protein C, and protein S defects are all autosomal dominant traits, so heterozygous individuals, who have a 50 percent reduction in protein concentration or a mixture of mutant and normal molecules, will have an increased risk of thrombosis. The patients all have similar clinical presentations with a strong family history of thrombosis, episodes of recurrent venous thromboembolism, and symptoms by their early twenties. Any patient with this distinctive history should be tested for the molecular abnormalities described below.

ANTITHROMBIN DEFICIENCY   Antithrombin complexes with activated coagulation proteins and blocks their biologic activity (see Fig. 57-5). The rate of this reaction is enhanced by heparin-like molecules within the vessel wall or on endothelial cells. Plasma antithrombin III content varies from 5 to 15 mg/L (50 to 150 percent), with values only slightly below normal increasing the risk of thrombosis. For optimal screening, it is important to assess both the antithrombin III concentration by immunoassay and the plasma antithrombin and heparin cofactor activity with functional assays. The most common defect is mild (heterozygous) antithrombin deficiency, which occurs in 1 in 2000 individuals. In addition, dysfunctional antithrombin molecules, with mutations affecting either the serine protease–binding site or the heparin-binding site, or activation of inhibitor by heparin have been described.

Patients with antithrombin deficiency who develop acute thrombosis or embolism can be treated with intravenous heparin, since there is usually sufficient normal antithrombin to act as a heparin cofactor. Following their first episode of thromboembolism, patients should be placed on oral anticoagulants for life to prevent recurrent thrombosis. Family studies should be conducted when an antithrombin-deficient individual is discovered, since up to half the members of a kindred may

---

TABLE 315-3   Prethrombotic disorders

INHERITED FORMS

Antithrombin III deficiency
Protein C deficiency
Protein S deficiency
Dysplasminogenemia
Dysfibrinogenemia
Defective release of plasminogen activator
Diminished venous content of plasminogen activator
Excessive release of plasminogen activator inhibitor (PAI-1)
Homocystinuria

ACQUIRED DISORDERS

Chronic congestive heart failure
Metastatic tumor
Metastatic malignancy
Extensive trauma or major surgery
Myeloproliferative disorders
Behçet's syndrome
Kawasaki's disease
Treatment with oral contraceptives or L-asparaginase GM-CSF

be affected. Asymptomatic individuals with antithrombin deficiency should receive prophylactic anticoagulation with heparin or plasma infusions to raise their antithrombin level prior to medical or surgical procedures which may increase their risk of thrombosis. Chronic oral anticoagulation is not recommended until individuals at risk have a clinical thrombotic episode.

DEFICIENCIES OF PROTEINS C AND S Protein C is a vitamin K–dependent hepatic protein which binds to the endothelial cell surface protein thrombomodulin and is converted to an active protease by thrombin (see Fig. 57-5). Activated protein C, in conjunction with protein S, proteolyzes factors Va and VIIIa, which shuts off fibrin formation. Activated protein C also may stimulate fibrinolysis and accelerate clot lysis. Deficiencies of proteins C and S are usually autosomal dominant disorders, and deficiencies in the two proteins cause an identical syndrome of recurrent venous thrombosis and pulmonary embolism. Dysfunctional molecules also have been definitely identified in some patients with thrombosis. In addition, rare patients with homozygous protein C deficiency have fulminant neonatal intravascular coagulation and require prompt diagnosis and treatment.

The correlation between protein C and S levels and the risk of thrombosis is not as precise as for antithrombin III deficiency. In fact, as large surveys have been completed, asymptomatic individuals with protein C "deficiency" have been discovered. Protein C levels in these individuals overlap those with recurrent thromboembolism. In addition, in some well-studied protein C–deficient kindreds, asymptomatic individuals may have protein C levels as low as or lower than relatives with recurrent thrombosis. These observations raise the possibility that an as yet undiscovered comorbid condition is present in symptomatic patients. Finally, since a fraction of the available protein S is bound to C4b-binding protein and is unavailable for coagulation reactions, it may be important to measure both free and total protein S or to have a concomitant measurement of C4b-binding protein for maximum accuracy.

Heterozygous patients with protein C or S deficiencies who develop acute thrombosis should be heparinized and then placed on oral anticoagulants. There are, however, two potential problems with the use of coumarin anticoagulants in these patients. First, these vitamin K antagonists (see Fig. 315-1 and Fig. 57-5), which lower the level of the procoagulant factors II, VII, IX, and X, also may reduce the concentration of proteins C and S sufficiently to nullify the desired antithrombotic effect. In addition, there are patients with coumarin-induced skin necrosis who are protein C–deficient, suggesting that this defect may predispose patients to a rare but serious complication of oral anticoagulants. Patients with homozygous protein C deficiency require periodic plasma infusions rather than oral anticoagulants to prevent recurrent intravascular coagulation and thrombosis.

DYSFIBRINOGENEMIAS AND FIBRINOLYTIC DEFECTS Several families have now been described with recurrent venous thrombosis and embolism due to defects in fibrinogen or plasminogen or with decreased synthesis or release of tissue plasminogen activator. While the majority of dysfibrinogenemias cause bleeding, several variants are characterized by excessively rapid release of fibrinopeptides and recurrent thromboembolism. Patients with this disorder as well as those with an abnormal plasminogen which resists activation by streptokinase and urokinase have been treated successfully with heparin and oral anticoagulants. Defects in tissue plasminogen activator content or release have not been completely characterized. One group of patients with recurrent venous thrombosis and embolism failed to increase venous blood fibrinolytic activity when challenged with local ischemia or physical exercise. The other group had impaired fibrinolytic activity in extracts prepared from biopsied veins. The cloning of cDNA for tissue plasminogen activator (tPA) coupled with the availability of immunoassays for tPA should facilitate more detailed studies of this class of defects. There is also recent evidence that young patients with acute myocardial infarction may have impaired fibrinolysis due to increased plasma levels of plasminogen

activator inhibitor (PAI), a serine protease inhibitor which binds to tPA and is derived from endothelial cells.

In addition to the inherited disorders which predispose patients to thromboembolism, many common illnesses are associated with an increased risk of thrombosis (see Table 315-3). These patients are said to have a "hypercoagulable" or "prethrombotic" state. This increased risk is seen in patients with chronic congestive heart failure and metastatic malignancy and in patients undergoing major surgery. In these patients, the generation of tissue factor activity in damaged or ischemic tissue or metastatic tumor, coupled with venous stasis and endothelial injury, induces the formation of venous and, more rarely, arterial thrombi. There are also several hematologic disorders including paroxysmal nocturnal hemoglobinuria, essential thrombocythemia, and polycythemia vera in which poorly defined abnormalities in circulating leukocytes and platelets or changes in blood flow and viscosity predispose patients to venous and arterial thrombosis. Diseases which affect the endothelial cell, such as Behçet's syndrome, Kawasaki's disease, and homocystinuria, or the administration of drugs such as the oral contraceptives, which lower antithrombin III levels, or L-asparaginase, which inhibits production of multiple coagulation factors, also may predispose patients to thrombosis. Infusion of GM-CSF has been associated with thrombosis as well.

REFERENCES

ANTONARAKIS SE: The molecular genetics of hemophilia A and B in man. Factor III and factor IX deficiency. Adv Hum Genet 17:17, 1988

FEINSTEIN DI: Lupus anticoagulant, anticardiolipin antibodies, fetal loss and systemic lupus erythematosus. Blood 80:859, 1992

GIDDINGS JC, PEAKE IR: Laboratory support in the diagnosis of coagulation disorders. Clin Haematol 14:571, 1985

GINSBURG KJ et al: Anticardiolipin antibodies and the risk for ischemic stroke and venous thrombosis. Ann Intern Med 117:997, 1992

KANE WH, DAVIE EW: Blood coagulation factors V and VIII: Structural and functional similarities and their relationship to hemorrhagic and thrombotic disorders. Blood 71:539, 1988

KASPER CK, DIETRICH SL: Comprehensive management of haemophilia. Clin Haematol 14:489, 1985

LAWN R: The molecular genetics of hemophilia. Sci Am 254:48, 1986

LUSHER JM et al: Recombinant factor VIII for the treatment of untreated patients with hemophilia A: Safety, efficacy and development of inhibitors. N Engl J Med 328:453, 1993

MAMMEN E: Congenital coagulation disorders. Semin Thromb Hemost 9:1, 1983

PIERCE GF et al: The use of purified clotting factor concentrates in hemophilia. Influence of viral safety, cost and supply on therapy. JAMA 261:3434, 1989

WHITE GC, SHOEMAKER CB: Factor VIII gene and hemophilia A. Blood 73:1, 1989

316 ANTICOAGULANT, FIBRINOLYTIC, AND ANTIPLATELET THERAPY

ROBERT I. HANDIN

ANTICOAGULANT AND FIBRINOLYTIC THERAPY

Anticoagulation with heparin, followed by treatment with oral vitamin K antagonists, is the standard treatment for acute venous thrombosis and pulmonary embolism. In addition, chronic oral anticoagulation is used to prevent cerebral arterial embolism from cardiac sources such as ventricular mural thrombi, atrial thrombi, or from an atherosclerotic, partially stenosed carotid or vertebral artery. Anticoagulants are also used, less successfully, to treat peripheral or mesenteric arterial thrombosis. These agents retard fibrin deposition on established thrombi and prevent the formation of new thrombi. The induction of a fibrinolytic state by the infusion of plasminogen activators like recombinant tissue plasminogen activator (rtPA), streptokinase (SK), or urokinase (UK) has become an accepted mode of therapy for some

TABLE 316-1 Anticoagulant therapy with heparin

Clinical indication	Dose, U.S.P. units	Route
Prophylaxis in general surgery	5000 q 12 h	SC
Prophylaxis in medical patients with congestive heart failure, cardiomyopathy, or myocardial infarction	10,000 q 12 h	SC
Venous thromboembolism (acute)	5000 (bolus) then 1000 qh	IV
Venous thromboembolism (prophylaxis in pregnancy, warfarin failures, or chronic DIC)	1000 qh	SQ pump

thromboembolic disorders. Fibrinolytic therapy has been advocated for patients with massive pulmonary embolism and systemic hypotension and to restore the patency of acutely occluded peripheral and coronary arteries. There is increasing evidence that prompt fibrinolytic therapy may reduce both myocardial damage and mortality following acute coronary occlusion (see Chap. 202).

ACUTE ANTICOAGULATION WITH HEPARIN Heparin is a naturally occurring mucopolysaccharide polymer with tetrasaccharide sequences that bind to and activate antithrombin III. It is an extremely potent anticoagulant that can dramatically reduce thrombin generation and fibrin formation in patients with acute venous and arterial thrombosis or embolism (Table 316-1). Heparin is administered to patients with acute thrombosis or embolism by continuous intravenous infusion at a rate sufficient to raise the activated partial thromboplastin time (APTT) to 1.5 to 2 times the patient's preheparin APTT. This requires infusion of approximately 1000 U.S.P. units per hour and is continued while patients are begun on oral anticoagulants and achieve appropriate prolongation of the prothrombin time. The usual duration of combined heparin-warfarin therapy is 5 to 7 days. Heparin is then discontinued, and the patient is maintained on warfarin. Alternatives to a continuous infusion include the administration of 5000 U.S.P. units of heparin four times a day either subcutaneously or intravenously. Long-term heparin administration via portable external or implantable pumps is occasionally needed for patients with recurrent thromboembolism that is refractory to oral anticoagulants, for pregnant women with thromboembolism, and for patients with chronic disseminated intravascular coagulation (DIC). Lower doses of heparin (5000 U.S.P. units every 12 h) have also been used to prevent deep venous thrombosis in high-risk surgical and medical patients. Patients with congestive heart failure, myocardial infarction, or cardiomyopathy may require 10,000 U.S.P. units every 12 h for similar protection.

The major complication of heparin therapy is bleeding—especially from surgical sites and into the retroperitoneum. Aspirin or aspirin-containing drugs impair platelet function. Thus, intramuscular injections in patients on both heparin and an antiplatelet drug may cause significant bleeding. Heparin's anticoagulant effect can be rapidly reversed by the administration of protamine sulfate. However, this is usually not necessary, since reduction or omission of heparin usually improves hemostasis and stops bleeding. Thrombocytopenia occurs in about 10 percent of heparin recipients, and is usually mild with the platelet count falling to 50,000 to 100,000 per milliliter. Thrombocytopenia is more common in patients receiving heparin derived from beef lung as opposed to porcine intestinal mucosa. Thus, porcine heparin is the preferred agent. Occasionally, thrombocytopenia can be severe and may be accompanied by intravascular platelet agglutination and arterial thrombosis. Recognition of the rare complication of thrombocytopenia and paradoxical thrombosis is critical, since discontinuing heparin can promptly reverse the syndrome and may be lifesaving. Heparin administration for longer than 2 months also carries a risk of osteoporosis.

Commercial heparin preparations are quite heterogeneous and only about 20 percent of the infused material has anticoagulant activity.

Low-molecular-weight heparin fractions, which retain anticoagulant activity, are being evaluated as an alternative to continued anticoagulation. These fractions do not interact with platelets and, thus, will not cause thrombocytopenia. However, low-molecular-weight heparin is not yet licensed for use in the United States.

CHRONIC ORAL ANTICOAGULATION The coumarin anticoagulants, which include warfarin and dicumarol (dicoumarol), prevent the reduction of vitamin K epoxides in liver microsomes and induce a state analogous to vitamin K deficiency (see Fig. 316-1). They slow thrombin generation and clot formation by impairing the biologic activity of the prothrombin complex proteins and are used to prevent the recurrence of venous thrombosis and pulmonary embolism. Although regimens employing loading doses of drug have been advocated, the simplest way to induce anticoagulation is to administer a single dose of a coumarin compound and monitor the prothrombin time (PT) until the desired prolongation is achieved. For example, treatment can be initiated with 5 to 10 mg/d of warfarin or equivalent, with the goal of prolonging the PT to 1.5 to 2 times the control value. Although the PT may reach this value after a few days of therapy, effective anticoagulation, with stable reduction of all the prothrombin complex proteins, requires at least 1 week of warfarin administration. Most patients require a daily maintenance dose of 2.5 to 7.5 mg of warfarin to remain anticoagulated. As discussed above, patients should remain on heparin until the appropriate dose of a coumarin anticoagulant, like warfarin, is established.

There is increasing concern that a more precise method is needed to assess the intensity of anticoagulation with warfarin. Commercial thromboplastins have different potencies and markedly affect the resulting PT. The International Normalized Ratio (INR) method is gradually being adopted by hospital laboratories and clinicians. In this reporting method, the ratio of the patient's PT is compared to the mean PT for a group of normal individuals. The ratio is adjusted for the sensitivity of the laboratory's thromboplastin determined by the International Sensitivity Index (ISI). Thus the INR $= (PT_{patient}/PT_{normal})^{ISI}$. Use of the INR permits physicians to obtain the appropriate level of anticoagulation independent of laboratory reagents and to follow published recommendations for intensity of anticoagulation.

Although warfarin anticoagulants reduce the recurrence of deep venous thrombosis and pulmonary or cerebral embolism, they may

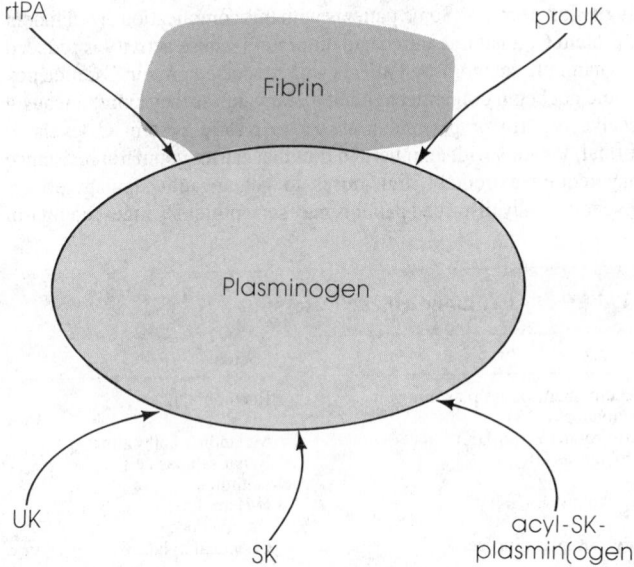

FIGURE 316-1 The mechanism of action of various plasminogen activators used for thrombolytic therapy. Recombinant tissue plasminogen activator (rtPA) and pro-urokinase (proUK) preferentially activate plasminogen bound to fibrin and are called "fibrin-specific" activators. Urokinase (UK), streptokinase (SK), and acylated streptokinase-plasminogen conjugates activate both free and fibrin-bound plasminogen.

TABLE 316-2   Effect of drugs and metabolic changes on oral anticoagulant potency

Factors leading to enhanced potency and increased prothrombin time
A Reduced coumarin clearance
  1 Disulfiram
  2 Metronidazole
  3 Trimethoprim-sulfamethoxazole
B Reduced albumin binding
  1 Phenylbutazone
C Additive hemostatic effect of certain drugs or disorders
  1 Aspirin
  2 Heparin
  3 Liver disease
  4 Thrombocytopenia
  5 Vitamin K deficiency
D Increased turnover of vitamin K
  1 Clofibrate
  2 Hypermetabolism (e.g., hyperthyroidism)

Factors leading to diminished potency and decreased prothrombin time
A Accelerated coumarin clearance—induction of hepatic metabolizing enzymes
  1 Barbiturates
  2 Rifampin
B Reduced absorption
  1 Cholestyramine
C Impaired metabolism
  1 Genetic coumarin resistance

also cause bleeding. Any patient who takes oral anticoagulants requires frequent monitoring of the PT. Despite the most careful management, fluctuations in PT can occur. Various drugs that alter liver microsomal metabolism of coumarins or compete for albumin binding sites can increase or decrease the potency of these drugs (Table 316-2).

There is a direct relation between the duration of anticoagulation and the risk of recurrent thrombosis. Although recommendations vary somewhat, most patients with a single uncomplicated thromboembolic event have maximal benefit after 3 to 6 months of anticoagulation. About 10 percent of patients on an oral anticoagulant for 1 year have a serious complication requiring medical supervision, and 0.5 to 1 percent have a fatal hemorrhagic event despite careful medical management. The anticoagulant effects of coumarins can be reversed by infusion of fresh frozen plasma or by the administration of vitamin K. In many cases, reduction or omission of several doses improves hemostasis and stops hemorrhage. Despite the risk of bleeding, patients with prosthetic heart valves, severe mitral stenosis, cardiomyopathy, chronic congestive heart failure, recurrent or persistent atrial fibrillation, or an inherited "prethrombotic" disorder may require lifelong anticoagulation.

One devastating complication of oral anticoagulation is hemorrhagic skin necrosis. Some patients with this complication are deficient in protein C, a natural anticoagulant protein whose activity is reduced by vitamin K antagonists. Patients with suspected protein C deficiency should not begin oral anticoagulant therapy unless they simultaneously receive heparin or plasma infusions to restore protein C levels to normal. Patients with an inherited trait that causes coumarin resistance may require extremely high doses to get an anticoagulant effect. Psychologically disturbed patients may surreptitiously ingest coumarin

and present with unexplained bleeding and a prolonged PT. Plasma coumarin levels can be measured to confirm such ingestion.

FIBRINOLYTIC THERAPY   Fibrinolysis, an important part of the normal hemostatic process, is initiated by the release of either tPA or pro-urokinase (proUK) from endothelial cells. These agents preferentially activate plasminogen, which is adsorbed onto fibrin clots. This serves to direct and localize the lytic process to sites that contain fibrin thrombi. Although fibrinolysis begins immediately after vascular injury, clot lysis and vessel recanalization may not be complete for 7 to 10 days. As previously discussed (see Chap. 57), the fibrinolytic pathway is important in normal hemostasis, as defects can predispose patients to either hemorrhage or recurrent thrombosis (see Chap. 315). Activators of the fibrinolytic system are now being used to accelerate clot lysis in patients with thromboembolism (see Fig. 316-1, Table 316-3).

The pharmacologic agents being used to accelerate clot lysis are either derived from natural products or are chemically modified derivatives. They differ with respect to fibrin specificity and some types of complications (see Table 319-3). For example, many individuals have antistreptococcal antibodies which react with streptokinase and reduce its potency and cause febrile reactions. All fibrinolytic agents cause hemorrhage. tPA, proUK, and several other agents are relatively "fibrin-specific" and preferentially activate plasminogen in the presence of fibrin. Although this makes it theoretically possible to achieve selective clot lysis, in practice there is little difference in either the efficacy or toxicity of the "specific" and "nonspecific" fibrinolytic agents. There is, however, a substantial difference in cost, with equivalent doses of rtPA costing ten times that of SK.

It is important to remember that there is always some systemic fibrinolysis after the infusion of clinically effective doses of fibrin-specific agents. In fact, the fibrinogen level falls approximately 25 percent after infusion of lytic doses of rtPA. In addition, both the fibrin-specific and -nonspecific agents can cause hemorrhage as they cannot differentiate between vital hemostatic plugs and pathologic thrombi. To minimize the risk of bleeding, systemic lytic therapy is not recommended for patients with recent surgery or a history of neurologic lesions, gastrointestinal bleeding, or hypertension.

The current indications for fibrinolytic therapy are listed in Table 316-4. Fibrinolytic agents have been given to patients with pulmonary embolism for over 30 years. Such therapy is currently recommended for patients with massive pulmonary embolism that is complicated by hypotension, hypoxemia, and right heart strain. It is also used for selected patients with peripheral arterial embolism or occlusion and for patients with extensive iliofemoral thrombophlebitis. While lytic therapy may hasten the resolution of venous thrombi, the long-term benefit still remains unproven, and there is no firm evidence that lytic therapy reduces postphlebitic complications. In contrast, fibrinolytic therapy may be of distinct benefit in patients with axillary vein thrombosis, a condition which does not usually respond to conventional anticoagulation. Fibrinolytic agents are also used to restore the patency of occluded venous catheters and dialysis shunts. For this indication the agents are instilled locally. The extensive literature on the use of fibrinolytic agents to treat patients with coronary artery disease and myocardial infarction is reviewed in Chap. 202. When

TABLE 316-3   Fibrinolytic activators

Product	Source	MW	Fibrin	Complications
Recombinant tissue plasminogen activator (rtPA)	Recombinant	70,000	+	Bleeding
Pro-urokinase (proUK)	Melanoma cell cultures	55,000	+	Bleeding
Urokinase (UK)	Renal tubular cell cultures	33,000	+	Bleeding
Streptokinase (SK)	β-Hemolytic streptococci	47,000	−	Immune reactions—hypotension, fever Bleeding
Acyl-SK-plasmin(ogen)	Chemical synthesis	139,000	+/−	Immune reactions—hypotension, fever Bleeding

TABLE 316-4 Indications for fibrinolytic therapy

Acute coronary occlusion/infarction
Acute peripheral arterial occlusion
Massive pulmonary embolism
Axillary vein thrombosis
Massive iliofemoral vein thrombosis
Occluded A-V shunt
Arterial or venous cannulae

given within a few hours of infarction it appears to reduce mortality and the extent of myocardial damage.

Although the doses and mode of administration may differ slightly, the general principles and complications are the same for all the fibrinolytic agents. SK and UK are the oldest and most extensively studied fibrinolytic agents. SK is a bacterial enzyme, and UK is a product of renal tubular epithelial cells. SK is an indirect plasminogen activator that interacts with circulating plasminogen to form an equimolar complex with proteolytic activity. The SK-plasminogen complex then activates additional plasminogen molecules that initiate fibrinolysis. In contrast, UK has intrinsic proteolytic activity and can activate plasminogen directly.

In the case of SK, one usually administers a loading dose of 250,000 units irrespective of body weight. Since patients may have antistreptococcal antibodies, the loading dose may need to be repeated. In addition, patients may develop acute allergic symptoms including urticaria and, occasionally, serum sickness reactions. With UK, a loading dose of 4400 units per kg body weight is administered over 10 to 30 min. Both regimens induce an intense lytic state as evidenced by a drop in fibrinogen, prolongation of the thrombin time, and a prolongation of the euglobulin lysis time—an in vitro measure of fibrinolytic activity. After the initial loading dose, 100,000 units of SK or 4400 units of UK per kg body weight are administered hourly for 24 to 72 h. At the desired time, the lytic state is reversed by discontinuing UK or SK and by administering heparin for 7 to 10 days. Heparin can be started at the same time as the fibrinolytic agent. To enhance the likelihood of success, fibrinolytic therapy should be initiated as soon as possible after the onset of thrombosis or embolism.

Fibrin-specific agents such as rtPA or proUK are also administered intravenously. For example, systemic infusion of 100 mg rtPA over 6 h restores coronary artery patency in approximately 75 percent of patients. Patients are then maintained on heparin for several days. ProUK given in a similar manner has almost identical effects.

ANTIPLATELET DRUG THERAPY

Antiplatelet drugs have a role to play in the management of patients with arterial vascular disease and thromboembolism (see Table 316-5). Aspirin is the most widely studied of these drugs because of its unique pharmacology. A single dose of aspirin irreversibly acetylates and inactivates the enzyme cyclooxygenase and thereby inhibits platelet

TABLE 316-5 Indications for antiplatelet drug therapy

Cerebrovascular disease
  Transient ischemic attacks
  Secondary prevention of cerebrovascular accidents
Cardiovascular disease
  Unstable angina pectoris
  Primary prevention of myocardial infarction
  Secondary prevention of myocardial infarction
  Following coronary bypass grafting
  Following insertion of a prosthetic valve
Renal disease
  To maintain the patency of A-V cannulas
  ? To slow the progression of glomerular disease

production of thromboxane A_2. Although aspirin may also inactivate cyclooxygenase in some tissues, including endothelial cells, such cells recover rapidly by synthesizing new enzyme. Platelets, which are anucleate, cannot synthesize new enzyme and remain inactive for the rest of their life span. As little as one 160 mg tablet of aspirin daily or a 325-mg tablet every other day inhibits platelet thromboxane production and aggregation.

Patients with coronary artery disease who have unstable angina are at high risk for myocardial infarction (Chap. 202). In two large clinical trials, the prompt administration of aspirin dramatically reduced progression to myocardial infarction in this group, although aspirin had no effect on the frequency, intensity, or duration of chronic angina. Aspirin also reduces the incidence of second infarction by 25 percent when administered to men who have had a myocardial infarct. In a large study of male physicians, daily aspirin therapy also reduced the incidence of first infarcts and is now widely used for prevention of myocardial infarction. The preliminary results of large-scale clinical and epidemiologic studies carried out in women suggest that the same beneficial effects of aspirin may be expected. The combination of aspirin and dipyridamole, when begun prior to surgery, may also increase the patency of coronary bypass grafts, and the same combination reduces the incidence of cerebral emboli in patients on warfarin who have prosthetic intracardiac valves. Although dipyridamole has been a popular antithrombotic agent, it has little efficacy when given alone. There is recent evidence that aspirin is probably the only active agent in the combination aspirin-dipyridamole trials. Thus, in most cases, dipyridamole could be eliminated in favor of aspirin alone.

Aspirin also reduces the frequency of transient ischemic attacks in patients with occlusive cerebrovascular disease. It has largely supplanted anticoagulation with the coumarin compounds in patients with transient ischemia. Aspirin also reduces the incidence of a second stroke by 25 percent when administered to men following the first cerebrovascular accident. Aspirin is also effective in maintaining the patency of arteriovenous cannulas inserted into patients with renal failure who require hemodialysis. Aspirin plus dipyridamole may also slow the progression of some forms of glomerulonephritis, although these drugs are not widely used in the treatment of renal disease. However, aspirin appears not to be effective in maintaining the patency of vessels following percutaneous angioplasty.

Although aspirin is clearly the most efficacious antiplatelet agent in clinical use today, there are a large number of new drugs being tested that may soon supplement aspirin therapy. Ticlopidine, which is a potent inhibitor of platelet function, has shown some efficacy in a limited number of clinical trials. In addition, analogues of the leech anticoagulant peptide hirudin, which are potent inhibitors of thrombin, may soon be available. Finally, there are a number of agents, including monoclonal antibodies and recombinant and chemically synthesized peptides, which block either platelet adhesion or aggregation, that are undergoing animal and early clinical trials.

REFERENCES

AMERICAN COLLEGE OF CHEST PHYSICIANS: Second Conference on Antithrombotic Therapy. Chest 95(supp), 1989

COLLEN D: Towards improved thrombolytic therapy. Lancet 342:34, 1993

COLLER BS: Platelets and thrombolytic therapy. N Engl J Med 322:33, 1990

LEE TH et al: Candidates for thrombolysis among Emergency Room patients with acute chest pain: Potential true- and false-positive rates. Ann Intern Med 110:957, 1989

LEVINE MN, HIRSH J: Hemorrhagic complications of anticoagulation therapy. Semin Thromb Hemost 12L:39, 1986

LOSCALZO J, BRAUNWALD E: Tissue plasminogen activator. N Engl J Med 319:925, 1988

MARDER VJ, SHERRY S: Thrombolytic therapy: Current status (parts 1 and 2). N Engl J Med 318:1512, 1988

SAOUR JN et al: Trial of different intensities of anticoagulation in patients with prosthetic heart valves. N Engl J Med 322:428, 1990

section 3   Neoplastic diseases

317   PRINCIPLES OF NEOPLASIA

JOHN MENDELSOHN

The past few years have witnessed remarkable progress in understanding the biologic and biochemical bases for cancer. Gains in the treatment of nonresectable cancer in adults have been gradual and have focused upon those malignancies characterized by unusual sensitivity to radiation and chemotherapy. These include primarily acute leukemia, the lymphoproliferative malignancies, testicular cancer, and breast cancer. New treatment modalities involving immunotherapy and agents that promote normal cell maturation remain experimental and are under intensive investigation. Meanwhile, the search has begun for compounds which can interact with oncogene products, gene regulators, and growth factors and their receptors. Research employing modern technology in molecular genetics and immunology promises to provide a new array of anticancer agents which could move rapidly into clinical trials. This is possible because understanding cancer as a pathologic process is buttressed by new knowledge of cancer as an acquired genetic derangement.

This chapter provides an overview of the biology, etiology, and clinical sequelae of the neoplastic process, followed by a description of the general methods for diagnosing cancer and determining its stage, or extent of spread. Oncogenes and the molecular genetics of malignant transformation are discussed in Chap. 63. Cancer treatment is presented in Chap. 318, and the details of managing patients with specific types of malignant disease will be found in the chapters devoted to disorders of various specific organs.

DEFINITION   The terms cancer, neoplasia, and malignancy are usually used interchangeably in both the technical and popular literature. The disease called *cancer* is best defined by four characteristics which describe how cancer cells act differently from their normal counterparts.

1 *Clonality:* Cancer originates from genetic changes in a single cell, which proliferates to form a clone of malignant cells.
2 *Autonomy:* Growth is not properly regulated by the normal biochemical and physical influences in the environment.
3 *Anaplasia:* There is a lack of normal, coordinated cell differentiation.
4 *Metastasis:* Cancer cells develop the capacity for discontinuous growth and dissemination to other parts of the body.

Properties similar to each of these characteristics *can* be expressed by normal, nonmalignant cells at certain appropriate times—for example, during embryogenesis and wound repair—but in cancer cells the characteristic is inappropriate or excessive. Benign tumors are clonal and have some degree of autonomy but remain differentiated and do not metastasize. The process by which a normal cell is converted into one which exhibits these four characteristic traits is termed *malignant transformation*.

THE CLINICAL PROBLEM   One-third of all individuals in the United States will develop cancer. The 5-year relative survival rate for these patients (the probability of escaping death from cancer for 5 years following diagnosis) has risen to 50 percent as a result of progress in the early diagnosis and therapy of this disease. Over 6 million living Americans have a history of cancer, and about 3 million were diagnosed 5 or more years ago. Cancer remains second only to cardiovascular disease as a cause of death in this country. More than

20 percent of Americans die from cancer, and this figure has been rising steadily as the population ages and deaths from heart disease decline. In the United States, malignancy accounted for 526,000 deaths in 1992. Half of the deaths were due to the three most common types of cancer: lung, breast, and colon-rectum. Lung cancer is more prevalent in males, while breast cancer is the most common form of malignancy in females. Cancer of the colon and rectum is equally common in males and females.

Information is provided yearly by the American Cancer Society, summarizing the incidence and mortality rates for the common types of cancer. Table 317-1 and Fig. 317-1 present just a small portion of the extensive data available. Of particular importance is the clear documentation in Fig. 317-1 that deaths from lung cancer are increasing in the face of stable or falling rates for a number of other types of malignant disease.

Cancer typically presents to the physician as an abnormal growth, or tumor, which causes illness by production of biochemically active molecules, by local expansion, or by invasion into adjacent or distant tissue sites. The symptoms of the illness depend upon the specific molecular products and the location(s) of the tumor. Each type of cancer has a relatively distinctive natural history that describes the likely clinical course of the particular neoplastic process. Designing a proper treatment plan for an individual patient with malignant disease depends upon determining the extent of disease spread, together with a knowledge of the natural history and the available therapeutic alternatives for the particular type of cancer.

TUMOR CELL BIOLOGY AND BIOCHEMISTRY   Since all cells in an organism originate from a single fertilized egg (zygote), all carry the identical genetic information. The proliferation and differentiation of this cell into an embryo, and eventually into a mature organism, involve selective and coordinated expression of the genomic repertoire. Control of gene expression is accomplished through incompletely understood molecular interactions which can be modulated, in part, by chemical influences in the environment. The genomic repertoire includes information which permits cells to expand clonally, to function with varying degrees of autonomy, to differentiate, and to move from one part of the organism to another

TABLE 317-1   Estimated new cases and deaths for major sites of cancer—1992

Site or type	Number of cases	Deaths
Lung	170,000	149,000
Colon-rectum	152,000	57,000
Breast	183,000	46,000
Prostate	106,000	30,000
Urinary tract	79,000	21,000
Uterus	45,000*	10,000
Lymphoma	43,000	21,000
Oral	30,000	8,000
Pancreas	28,000	25,000
Leukemia	29,000	19,000
Melanoma	32,000†	7,600
Stomach	24,000	14,000
Ovary	22,000	13,000
All sites‡	1,170,000	526,000

* Includes cervix. If carcinoma in situ is included, cases total about 100,000.
† Estimated new cases of skin cancer (nonmelanoma) = about 700,000.
‡ Includes additional sites.
NOTE: Estimates by the American Cancer Society are based on rates from the N.C.I. SEER program 1987–1989.

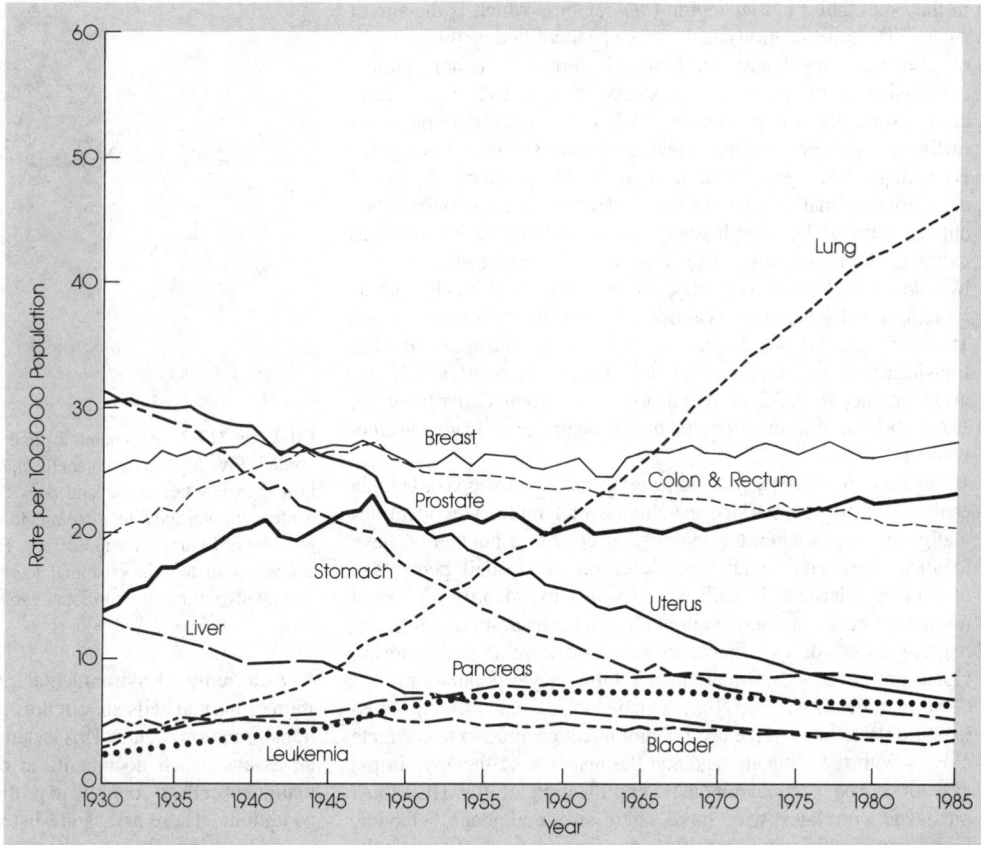

FIGURE 317-1 Cancer death rates by site in the United States, 1930 to 1985. *(Prepared by the American Cancer Society from data provided by the National Center for Health Statistics and the Bureau of the Census.)*

in a coordinated way. In the adult, the process of wound healing activates expression of these cellular characteristics in a more "embryo-like" fashion, but under well-coordinated control. In the case of malignancy, the normal control process is subverted or bypassed due to the anomalous activities of a select group of genes which have central importance to the regulation of cellular activities.

Clonality Careful cytogenetic analysis of metaphase chromosome preparations from cancer cells has yielded a wealth of information about the neoplastic process. It has become clear that virtually all solid tumors and a majority of hematopoietic malignancies display abnormalities in the chromosomal karyotype which are inherited by the population of tumor cells. These may involve translocations of chromosomal fragments into new positions, as well as additions or deletions of parts of chromosomes or whole chromosomes. A particular karyotypic alteration often occurs in a substantial fraction of all patients with a form of cancer. The first and most well known example of this is the Philadelphia chromosome (Ph) observed in 85 percent of patients with chronic myelogenous leukemia (CML), in which the long arm of chromosome 22 is translocated onto the long arm of chromosome 9. This alteration is so characteristic of CML that when analysis of some cases of acute lymphocytic leukemia demonstrated the identical translocation, it was inferred that the disease represented an unusual conversion from CML (which usually progresses to acute myelocytic leukemia). Characteristic chromosomal rearrangements have been described in a large number of other human cancers.

The observation of uniform karyotypic abnormalities in all cells within a tumor provides strong evidence for the clonal origin of the tumor. In turn, the chromosomal abnormalities serve as markers of a common malignant state in the individual cells.

A remarkable concordance between the chromosome locations of a number of human cellular oncogenes and the break points involved in chromosome translocations in human malignancies has been demonstrated. Furthermore, in many cases, these locations correlate with "fragile" sites in the chromosome. Treatment of cultured cells

with agents that inhibit the DNA repair process induces chromosomal breaks far more frequently at many of these loci. Accumulating data link these phenomena and suggest that chromosome rearrangements may result in unregulated activation of cellular oncogenes. For example, in Burkitt's lymphoma, the typical translocation between chromosomes 8 and 14 places the cellular *myc* gene adjacent to the immunoglobulin heavy chain locus, a site of gene activation in the normal lymphocyte.

The new techniques of molecular genetics permit direct assessment of genetic alterations in DNA extracts from tissues suspected of harboring malignancy, using the method of *Southern blotting*. This involves restriction endonuclease digestion, agarose gel electrophoresis, and identification of specific DNA molecular species by hybridization with labeled specific probes. Changes in gene expression can be detected by a similar technique with RNA extracts known as *northern blotting*. The new technology of molecular genetics is more powerful than cytogenetics because (1) clonal genetic abnormalities can be identified in nondividing cells, (2) genetic rearrangements are detectable even when few tumor cells exist in a population of predominantly normal cells, and (3) the sensitivity of detection is greatly enhanced by obviating assays dependent on visual identification of altered staining patterns of chromosomes. The polymerase chain reaction takes advantage of the availability of appropriate primers for certain recombinant genes to amplify abnormal genetic material present in rare cells within a population, thereby enabling detection of genetic abnormalities in these cells by Southern blotting. These approaches to the diagnosis of genetic abnormalities are presented in detail in Chap. 61.

Clonal abnormalities in the genetic makeup of cells that can be detected with molecular techniques include gene mutation, rearrangement, translocation, deletion, and amplification. Some examples will serve to demonstrate the utility of these methods.

1 CML: The Ph chromosome is formed by a translocation between chromosomes 9 and 22, with the break in chromosome 22 occurring in the break point cluster region (*bcr* region), which is the site of a gene. The translocation can therefore be identified by the presence of abnormal *bcr* bands on Southern blots. A fusion protein comprising portions of the products of *bcr* and *c-abl* (from chromosome 9) is expressed in CML cells, and detection of its mRNA by northern blotting is diagnostic (see Chaps. 63 and 310). By taking advantage of these techniques, the presence of residual cells from the malignant clone can be detected in bone marrow that appears normal by morphologic criteria as well as by standard cytogenetic criteria (e.g., 30 normal metaphase spreads).

2 Nodular lymphoma: The majority of patients with low-grade lymphomas display translocations between chromosomes 14 and 18, involving the *bcl*-2 gene located on chromosome 18. The translocation can be detected by identification of either re-arrangements in *bcl*-2 or the fusion gene product involving the *bcl*-2 and the immunoglobulin heavy chain gene from chromosome 14.

3 Monoclonal lymphocyte proliferation: Detection of kappa or lambda chain excess on the surface membranes of lymphocytes identifies malignant clones when the majority of cells in a population have identical light chain subtypes. Detection of a small percentage of clonally derived B cells is possible, by identifying clonal rearranagements of immunoglobulin genes. In a similar fashion, rearrangements of T cell receptor genes are of value in diagnosing clonal proliferation of a malignant T lymphocyte population.

4 Gene amplification: The N-*myc* oncogene is frequently amplified in neuroblastoma, and the level of amplification appears to correlate closely with the clinical stage and the response to therapy. In the case of breast adenocarcinoma, amplification of the HER2/*neu* oncogene correlates with more aggressive malignant behavior. Gene amplification in a clonally derived population of tumor cells is detected directly on Southern blots as increased intensity of labeling of the DNA bands derived from the amplified gene.

Studies of the selective expression of the X-linked isoenzymes of glucose-6-phosphate dehydrogenase (G6PD) in heterozygotic patients have provided further evidence for the clonal origin of cancer from a single progenitor cell. Examination of both G6PD isoenzymes and chromosomal karyotypes in CML patients has demonstrated clonal abnormalities in erythroid, myeloid, and megakaryocytic cells, as well as B lymphocytes, suggesting that this malignancy originates in a precursor cell common to all of these cell lineages.

While there is convincing evidence for the origin of cancer from genetic alterations in a single cell, further heritable alterations commonly occur, resulting in the presence of a heterogeneous mixture of subclones in a mature tumor cell population which has proliferated enough to be clinically detectable. This heterogeneity can be demonstrated by assaying a variety of characteristics in the subpopulations within a tumor; for example, further abnormalities in the chromosomal karyotype, varied drug sensitivities and metastatic capacities, difference in growth rates, and the presence or absence of hormone receptors or particular cell surface glycoproteins. With time, therefore, the progressive accumulation of heritable abnormalities in tumor subpopulations typically results in highly significant phenotypic changes which have their clinical counterpart in development of resistance to previously effective therapy or in increased metastatic spread. The appearance of new chromosomal abnormalities or other genetic alterations in patients with Ph positive CML heralds the onset of a rapidly progressive, fatal phase of the disease. A schematic model of this process of clonal progression, or clonal evolution, is shown in Fig. 317-2. It remains to be determined when in the life history of a typical malignancy the process of clonal progression occurs: genetic alterations may occur early, with later expansion of selected subpopulations from a heterogeneous mixture of cells as circumstances change; other genetic alterations may occur close to the time when they are detected by changes in the behavior of the tumor cells.

FIGURE 317-2 A schematic model of clonal progression. The N cell is normal. Five *hypothetical* genetic changes are noted. The first does not result in malignancy but the second does. The third adds invasiveness, the fourth confers the capacity to disseminate and produce metastases, and the fifth provides resistance to chemotherapy. Each may be accompanied by incremental alterations in the chromosomal karyotype, with an increasing tendency to aneuploidy during further clonal evolution.

Autonomy Environmental influences which regulate the proliferation of normal cells are circumvented when the process of malignant transformation occurs. This is demonstrable by a variety of experimental assays which document, in different ways, the capacity of the malignant cells to continue to proliferate under normally nonconducive conditions. These assays are listed in Table 317-2.

At least initially, the autonomy of human malignancies is relative rather than absolute. The well-known experiments of Huggins and associates in the 1950s led to a new form of cancer therapy which took advantage of the initial dependence of certain tumors upon the normal influences of sex hormones. The conversion of many prostatic and breast cancers from sensitivity to resistance to hormone therapy vividly demonstrates the further development of autonomy through clonal progression.

Many tumor cell lines can proliferate in culture medium without the usual requirement for serum, provided that a "cocktail" containing three to five essential growth factors and other growth-promoting agents is added. Examples of such factors are epidermal growth factor, platelet-derived growth factor, the carrier protein transferrin, and the hormone insulin. Malignant cells may find even these essential factors unnecessary. One mechanism, demonstrated experimentally and possibly of clinical significance, involves production of a growth

TABLE 317-2 Experimental detection of malignant transformation

Assay	Normal cell	Transformed cell
Capacity of single cells to form colonies in agar suspension	Unsuccessful	Successful
Density-dependent inhibition of cell proliferation in liquid culture	Yes	No
Generations obtained by continuous division in liquid culture	Limited to about 50	Unlimited
Requirements for serum or growth factors	Invariable	Reduced or absent
Capacity to grow as xenografts	Absent	Present

factor (or its analogue) by the tumor cells themselves, a process called *autocrine secretion*. In this situation a polypeptide secreted by the tumor cells may have the capacity to bind to a receptor on the surface of the cells, resulting in autostimulation (Fig. 317-3). The first growth factor to be described with the potential for autocrine stimulation of tumor cells was transforming growth factor alpha, an analogue of epidermal growth factor (EGF) which also binds to the EGF receptor.

A second mechanism by which tumor cells can reduce dependence on growth factors involves expression of increased numbers of receptors on the cell surface. Increased expression of EGF receptors is a common event in epithelial tumors, occurring in nearly all renal cell carcinomas and squamous lung carcinomas that have been examined, and in many other forms of malignancy. Tumor cells may develop a third mechanism for escaping regulation by a growth factor, by activating an internal biochemical process (e.g., the protein tyrosine kinase) ordinarily dependent upon binding of a specific growth factor to a cell surface receptor, thereby completely bypassing the need for exposure to the growth-promoting agent.

Many malignant cells also have the capacity to manipulate a key environmental element required for their growth, the development of an adequate blood supply. Angiogenesis factors produced by tumor cells, such as the fibroblast growth factors, can stimulate the entire series of events involved in the formation of capillaries and blood vessels. Recent data suggest that a high degree of tumor vascularization, observed microscopically on biopsy material, is correlated with a worse clinical prognosis. High levels of receptors for EGF or HER2 also are associated with a shorter survival in a number of malignancies.

Anaplasia Lack of normal differentiation is a most useful characteristic in the pathologic diagnosis of malignancy. While cancer cells usually bear some of the morphologic characteristics of their normal mature counterparts, they display cellular and histologic abnormalities readily detectable with the light microscope. The cells tend to have large nuclei, with more apparent chromatin and prominent nucleoli. There are increased mitoses, as well as abnormal mitoses and giant cells containing multiple nuclei, reflecting aneuploidy and/or a failure of karyokinesis. The degree of morphologic derangement typically correlates with the extent of disease spread or the metastatic potential of the tumor. The histologic appearance of malignancy is one of disarray, with partial or complete loss of normal tissue architecture. Partial formation of structures such as glands or villi may be suggested, even in poorly differentiated malignancies.

Although the term is not used this way, the process of anaplasia

FIGURE 317-3 A diagrammatic representation of autocrine, paracrine, and endocrine secretion. Peptide growth factors are shown in latent form within the cell. The thickened, semicircular regions of the cell membrane represent receptor sites. *(From MB Sporn, GJ Todaro, N Engl J Med 303:878, 1980, by permission.)*

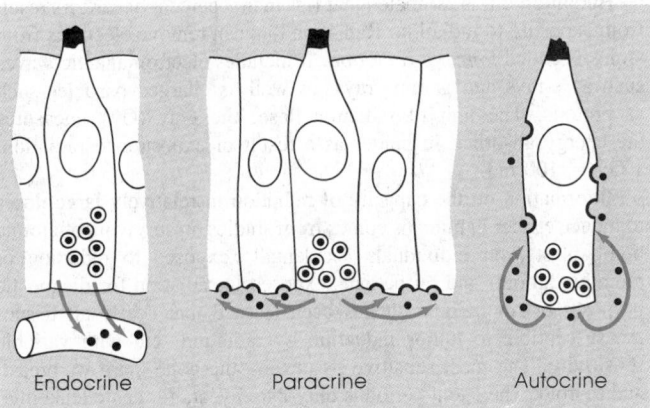

Endocrine   Paracrine   Autocrine

may be expressed at a biochemical level as production of hormones or hormone-related peptides that are either improperly regulated by normal feedback mechanisms (e.g., excessive steroid production by an adrenal carcinoma) or are not appropriate for the particular cell type if it were normally differentiated (e.g., ACTH production by a carcinoma of the lung). In such cases, the genomic repertoire of the malignant cell is expressed inappropriately. Another example is the unregulated production of immunoglobulin (partial or complete chains) by neoplastic derivatives of B lymphocytes.

Histologic features which are abnormal but do not meet the criteria of anaplasia (loss of differentiation) are designated *dysplastic*. Such changes may be seen in "premalignant" situations, for example, in the epithelial lining of the bronchi of cigarette smokers. These abnormalities are often reversible. Cessation of smoking can lead to normalization of the lung epithelium over a period of 5 years.

Metastasis This term encompasses a number of phenotypic traits which together result in the clinical problem that most often leads to death from cancer. The cells lose their adherence and restrained position within an organized tissue, move into adjacent sites, develop the capacity both to invade and to egress from blood vessels, and become capable of proliferating in unnatural locations or environments. These changes in growth patterns are accompanied by an accumulation of biochemical alterations which have the capacity to promote the metastatic process. In experimental situations where tumor cells show a propensity to select a particular organ as a preferred site of metastasis, surface molecules on the metastatic cells appear to have a high affinity for endothelial cells in the vasculature of the specific target organ. The tumor cells also may be dependent upon growth factors produced in the tissues at the preferred site.

The first step in tumor cell invasion probably involves attachment to the extracellular matrix, which is mediated by receptors on the plasma membrane that bind specifically to glycoproteins such as laminin and fibronectin. The second step involves secretion of a variety of tissue-degrading enzymes including collagenases and lysosomal hydrolases. Plasminogen activators which lead to promotion of fibrinolysis are also produced. The third step, which is less well understood, involves movement of tumor cells into the degraded zone of extracellular matrix.

Many biochemical alterations appear to be involved in the progression of a tumor from a homogeneous proliferating clone to a group of heterogeneous subpopulations of cells, some of which have progressively accumulated the entire array of enzymes and surface molecules required for metastasis. It may be for this reason that the rate of metastasis is low during early tumor growth, in spite of the well-documented fact that malignant cells are often released from a tumor into the circulation continuously and in large numbers. Agents which could block critical steps in the metastatic process would be of great value in the armamentarium of antineoplastic agents.

It appears that clonal progression of a tumor generates biochemical or physiologic alterations which confer greater autonomy, greater degrees of anaplasia, and a greater capacity to metastasize. Because there is progresive selection for cells with increased tumorigenic capacity, the process has been called clonal evolution and has been compared to Darwinian evolution, in this case at a cellular level.

ETIOLOGY Patterns of cancer incidence vary with sex, race, and geographic location. In addition, the types of tumors observed vary with age. Hereditary traits and variations in the internal environments around cells explain some of the differences in cancer incidence. It is clear from epidemiologic investigations that variations in diet and exposure to chemical and physical agents in the external environment contribute to the development of neoplasia. The environmental agents which have been linked to the incidence of cancer fall into three broad categories: radiation, a variety of chemicals, and viruses.

Genetic factors Genetic alterations play an essential role in oncogenesis. Several lines of evidence support this conclusion: (1) There are many examples of familial aggregation for specific histologic types of tumor (e.g., retinoblastoma). (2) Chromosomal abnormalities carried in the germ line confer increased risk of developing certain types of cancer (e.g., leukemia in trisomy 21). (3) Tumors often display specific somatic rearrangement of chromosomes or genes (e.g., CML). (4) Deficiency in the capacity to repair DNA damage by mutagens is accompanied by increased risk of malignancy (e.g., xeroderma pigmentosa). (5) The capacities for agents to mutate DNA and to act as carcinogens are closely correlated. (6) Mutations or unregulated expression of particular genes can convert cells that behave normally into cells that behave in a malignant fashion.

The molecular mechanisms underlying these genetic abnormalities are beginning to be understood (see Chap. 63). They appear to fall into two major categories:

1. *Oncogenes* are genes which can cause malignant transformation when inappropriately expressed, because of mutation, amplification, or rearrangements. In most cases, they code for growth factors, receptors, or other molecules involved in signal transduction pathways, or for transcription factors that regulate gene expression. Overexpression of these genes leads to constitutive activity of key regulatory molecules that normally are modulated during the cell cycle.
2. *Suppressor genes* act by inhibiting cell growth, and a related category of genes can act by inducing programmed cell death. These genes are involved in tumorigenesis when they are lost or inactivated. Malignant transformation due to suppressor genes is recessive, in that both alleles must be altered, as in the case of the retinoblastoma gene *Rb*-1. However, the genes may appear to have a dominant inheritance pattern because one allele may be constitutionally deleted or because the abnormal gene product may inactivate the normal one, as occurs in the case of p53.

Current models in this rapidly changing field suggest that suppressor genes may act normally by binding transcription factors required for cell-cycle progression, or by serving as transcription factors that activate genes which inhibit cell-cycle progression and proliferation. Gene deletions or loss of restriction fragment length polymorphisms, which identify potential site of suppressor genes, have been described in many types of malignancy.

Data from many sources have generated an interesting model of p53 function. Normal p53 may serve as a "molecular policeman," preventing cell-cycle progression when vital cellular machinery such as the DNA has been damaged by radiation, chemotherapy, or other agents. The cell can then repair the DNA, before resuming completion of the cell cycle. If repair fails in cells that are programmed to proliferate, p53 may trigger cellular suicide by apoptosis. However, in tumor cells with mutated or inactive p53, the capacity for cell-cycle arrest may be compromised. This could provide a genetic explanation for the high incidence of mutational events in malignant cells; such events create the possibility of clonal evolution and selection for more malignant properties. Inability to arrest the cell cycle could also explain why the mutated tumor cells have a high rate of cell death and why they may be more susceptible than normal cells to the lethal effects of chemotherapy and radiotherapy.

The genetic explanation for clonal evolution has been explored by Vogelstein and his collaborators, who carefully examined the molecular changes that occur in the entire spectrum of colorectal tumors, beginning with small adenomatous polyps and ending with invasive adenocarcinoma. These tumors appear to arise as a result of mutational activation of oncogenes, combined with mutational inactivation of suppressor genes. Mutations of at least four or five genes are required for the formation of a malignant tumor. Although the genetic alterations tend to occur in a preferred sequence, it is the total accumulation of changes rather than the order of occurrence that determines the malignant behavior of the tumor cells. The genetic changes that contribute to this process in colon cancer include: (1) mutations of the *ras* oncogene; (2) loss or mutation of three suppressor genes—the familial adenomatous polyposis (*FAP*) gene, the deleted in colon carcinoma (*DCC*) gene, and p53; and (3) DNA hypomethylation (see also Chap. 256).

There have been a number of reports of potential sites of suppressor genes, identified by chromosomal deletions and/or loss of restriction fragment length polymorphism alleles. These include Wilms' tumor (11p13), lung cancer (3p), renal cell carcinoma (3p), bladder cancer (11p), colorectal carcinoma (5q), and breast cancer (13). There are intensive efforts to discover cancer-related genes encoded in the genetic loci, shown above in parentheses. The gene at 11p13, which is involved in some forms of Wilms' tumor, has been found to encode a transcription factor that is believed to regulate the differentiation of nephroblasts.

The genetic changes that play a causal role in malignancy are described in detail in Chap. 63. Somatic mutations that lead to malignant transformation are acquired during the lifetime of the individual, whereas mutations in the germ cells are inherited and form the basis for hereditary neoplasms.

For many of the common malignancies, the incidence of cancer is higher (usually up to three-fold) among patients with positive family histories than among unselected patients. However, the risk can rise to as high as twenty-five- to thirtyfold in certain groups of patients with a familial history of breast cancer or bowel cancer. In addition, there are a number of uncommon inherited disorders involving either a high risk for the occurrence of a particular neoplasm or the presence of multiple preneoplastic lesions that can progress to frank malignancy.

The hereditary neoplasms (Table 317-3) may occur as the only manifestation of a gene defect, or as part of a generalized syndrome involving multiple developmental abnormalities. The inheritance patterns in these disorders are generally autosomal dominant, with varying penetrance. Half of the children of patients with these disorders will inherit the gene defect.

The preneoplastic states are grouped into four major categories (Table 317-3). Neurofibromatosis occurs in 1 of 3000 live births. The neurofibromas undergo sarcomatous changes in about 10 percent of patients, with development of gliomas in the brain or optic nerve, meningiomas, acoustic neuromas, or pheochromocytomas. Chromosome breakage disorders are characterized by the recessive inheritance of chromosomal instability and rearrangements of karyotypes; patients have an increased incidence of acute leukemia. The immune deficiency ataxia-telangiectasia is also characterized by chromosomal fragility. Patients with hereditary or acquired immunodeficiency states have an increased incidence of neoplasia, most commonly the lymphoproliferative malignancies.

Race is a genetic factor in the incidence of cancer, but interpretation of epidemiologic data is made difficult by the concurrent effects of environmental and socioeconomic influences. Both the incidence and the death rate from cancer are higher in American blacks than in American whites, with nearly all of the difference being accounted for by the higher cancer rate in black males. It is believed that later detection and less adequate treatment may account for part, but not all, of the difference in survival. The important effect of environmental factors is made clear by documented differences in cancer incidence for Asian families that have moved to Hawaii and California.

Radiation   It is estimated that less than 3 percent of cancers result from exposure to radiation. Radiation that can remove electrons from atoms is called *ionizing radiation*. It includes electromagnetic waves such as x-rays and gamma rays, as well as charged particles such as protons. The unit of radiation dose, the gray (Gy), measures the energy absorbed in matter as a result of exposure to radiation: 1 Gy = 100 rad.

Information on the capacity of radiation in relatively large doses to induce cancer in humans comes from studies on survivors of atomic bomb blasts, on individuals accidentally exposed to radiation or radiative fallout, and on patients exposed to radiation for diagnostic purposes or for therapy. It has been learned that nearly all tissues are susceptible to tumor induction by radiation, but with variable sensitivity. The most sensitive tissues are the bone marrow, breast, and thyroid. The latent period is only 2 to 5 years for acute leukemia, and 5 to 10 years for most solid tumors. There is a higher incidence

TABLE 317-3   Hereditary neoplasms and preneoplastic conditions

Disorder	Inheritance	Features
HEREDITARY NEOPLASMS		
Retinoblastoma	AD	Often bilateral; susceptibility to second tumors, especially osteosarcoma
Familial polyposis coli	AD	Multiple adenomatous polyps and adenocarcinomas of the colon; some families have osteomas, lipomas, and fibromas (Gardner's syndrome)
Multiple endocrine neoplasia I	AD	Adenomas of the pituitary, parathyroid, and pancreatic islet cells
Multiple endocrine neoplasia II	AD	Medullary carcinoma of the thyroid, pheochromocytoma, and parathyroid tumors
HEREDITARY PRENEOPLASTIC CONDITIONS		
Phakomatoses		
Neurofibromatosis (von Reckling hausen's disease)	AD	Gliomas of the brain and optic nerve, acoustic neuroma, meningioma, and pheochromocytoma
Tuberous sclerosis	AD	Glial tumors; hamartomatous growths in several organs
von Hippel-Lindau syndrome	AD	Hemangioblastomas of cerebellum and retina; renal cell carcinoma and pheochromocytoma
DNA-chromosomal instability		
Xeroderma pigmentosum	AR	Basal and squamous cell carcinoma of skin; malignant melanomas in patients exposed to UV light
Bloom's syndrome	AR	Acute leukemias, various carcinomas
Fanconi's anemia	AR	Acute leukemias, squamous cell carcinomas, and hepatomas
Ataxia-telangiectasia	AR	Acute leukemia, lymphoma, breast cancer in females
Immune deficiency syndrome		
X-linked agammaglobulinemia	XR	Lymphomas and leukemias
Wiskott-Aldrich-syndrome	XR	Acute leukemias and lymphomas
X-linked lymphoproliferative syndrome	XR	Abnormal response to EB virus; EBV-induced B cell immunoblastic lymphomas
Cancer family syndrome	AD	Cancers of multiple organs: colon, endometrium, breast, and lung

AD = autosomal dominant; AR = autosomal recessive; XR = X-linked recessive.
SOURCE: From RS Cotran et al, p. 267.

of leukemia in patients who have received radiation therapy for neoplastic diseases and for ankylosing spondylitis, and of thyroid cancer in children irradiated for thymic enlargement.

Solar radiation, resulting from exposure to electromagnetic radiation from the sun, is the primary risk factor in skin cancer. The evidence for this linkage comes from a variety of epidemiologic and experimental observations. Skin cancer is rare in blacks and the deeply pigmented racial groups, whereas it is especially common in fair-complexioned individuals. It occurs primarily on the parts of the body exposed to sunlight and has a higher incidence in outdoor workers. Patients with genetic diseases such as xeroderma pigmentosa and albinism, which are exacerbated by sunlight, have very high risks for the development of skin cancer.

The carcinogenic effect of solar radiation is greatest in the spectral range of 290 to 320 nm (UV-B radiation), which produces delayed erythema in human skin (sunburn). This range of wavelengths correlates with the action spectrum for UV-induced damage to DNA.

Exposure to solar ultraviolet radiation is also a risk factor in melanoma. As with skin cancer, there is a higher incidence of melanoma among populations living at a latitude nearer the equator, where exposure to UV is greatest.

Tobacco Numerous epidemiologic studies have demonstrated that the principal carcinogenic agent in our environment is inhaled tobacco smoke. The incidence of lung cancer is more than tenfold higher in male smokers than in nonsmokers. Furthermore, tobacco smoking is associated with increased rates of cancer of the oral cavity, esophagus, kidney, bladder, and pancreas. Particulate matter in tobacco smoke, known as "tar," contains a long list of chemicals, primarily polycyclic hydrocarbons, which have been shown experimentally to be contact carcinogens. In addition, the metabolic activation of tobacco components, for example, the cyclic *N*-nitrosamines, can produce carcinogens with the capacity to act upon the cells of internal organs. Tobacco-related malignancies account for one-third of all cancer deaths among men in the United States and for more than 10 percent of all female cancer deaths. Unfortunately, this figure is rising in females. As a result of increased use of tobacco by women in the period since World War II, the deaths from lung cancer in females exceeded deaths from breast cancer in 1988.

Consumption of alcoholic beverages has been shown to potentiate the incidence of malignancies due to tobacco smoke. Alcohol in the absence of smoking appears to play an etiologic role in hepatocellular carcinoma.

Clearly the single most effective action which could be taken against cancer at the present time involves not an application of molecular genetic research, but cessation of smoking. Fortunately, it appears that smoking cessation results in a gradual decrease in risk, so that after 10 to 15 years, exsmokers have nearly the same risk of lung cancer as nonsmokers. Because the habit of smoking is difficult to break, the physician's role in cessation of smoking is of critical importance. Doctors should deliver a *firm* antismoking message.

Occupational exposure to carcinogens The first report of cancer related to occupational hazards was Percival Pott's observation of an unusually high frequency of scrotal cancer among London chimney sweeps in 1775. It is now known that skin cancer (including scrotal) can be induced by a variety of coal tar products, such as the materials contacted in the London chimneys. Epidemiologic studies also have related lung cancer to exposure to coal by-products. Table 317-4 provides a partial listing of industrial agents which are known to cause cancer. Chemical carcinogens, including the components of tobacco smoke, may play two roles in carcinogenesis: as mediators of genetic mutations and as promoters of proliferation of cells bearing genetic mutations.

TABLE 317-4   Examples of occupational causes of cancer

Etiology	Site of malignancy
Arsenic (inorganic)	Lung, skin, liver
Asbestos	Mesothelium, lung
Benzene	Leukemia
Benzidine	Bladder
Chromium compounds	Lung
Radiation (mining, dial painting)	Numerous locations
Mustard gas	Lung
Polycyclic hydrocarbons (coal by-products)	Lung, skin
Vinyl chloride	Angiosarcoma of liver

Air pollution   It is clear that lung cancer incidence is increased by tobacco smoking and by certain industrial and occupational exposures (primarily related to coal tar and combustion by-products). Once the risks resulting from exposure to these factors are taken into account, the epidemiologic evidence that links ambient air pollution to lung cancer remains inconclusive. Studies correlating the incidence of lung cancer with increased levels of polycyclic hydrocarbons and benzo(a)pyrene in urban air are complicated by the difficulty of eliminating the contribution of exposure to these compounds through tobacco smoking as well as occupational exposure.

Medications   Certain drugs and hormones have been shown to be carcinogenic. The synthetic nonsteroidal estrogen diethylstilbestrol (DES), which was used for a period of time to reduce fetal wastage in pregnant women, caused an increased incidence of vaginal and cervical cancer in daughters who were exposed in utero. Conjugated estrogens have been shown to increase the incidence of endometrial cancer in patients treated for menopausal symptoms. The use of progesterone concomitantly, together with decreased estrogen dose, may obviate this problem.

Alkylating agents have been shown to cause an increased incidence of acute myelocytic leukemia and probably other malignancies. They are used in therapeutic situations in which the poor prognosis of malignancy far outweighs the increased risk of an additional cancer in the future. However, because of this risk, new drug regimens which avoid the use of alkylating agents are being explored in situations where substantial long-term benefits from chemotherapy have been demonstrated, for example, in Hodgkin's disease.

The recipients of organ transplants who are treated with immuno-suppressive agents, such as azathioprine and prednisone, have an increased incidence of histiocytic lymphoma as well as a variety of solid tumors. A similar increased incidence is observed in individuals with inherited and acquired immunodeficiency, for example, AIDS. This has been attributed to reduced immune surveillance, but a variety of other explanations are equally likely, such as activation of a latent oncogenic virus or chronic immunostimulation in conjunction with a compromised and malfunctioning immune system.

Diet   The role of diet and nutrition in carcinogenesis has been the subject of intensive investigation and equally intensive controversy. There are numerous nutritional hypotheses of carcinogenesis. Some of these have led to unconventional forms of cancer therapy that are based upon no scientific evidence. Unfortunately, these putative dietary therapies are propagated upon a patient population for which proven treatment modalities are often unsuccessful in achieving cure, and at a time when there is a popular emphasis on healthful nutrition.

Epidemiologic analyses of international variations in cancer incidence and comparisons of the types and frequencies of cancer in populations with different dietary habits have yielded a great deal of evidence that cancers of many major sites are influenced by diet. These studies were reviewed in an authoritative publication, *Diet, Nutrition, and Cancer.* Interim dietary guidelines are suggested which are both consistent with good nutritional practices and likely to reduce the risk of cancer: (1) Reduce the intake of fat, saturated and unsaturated, from its present average level (40 percent) to 30 percent of total energy value in the diet. (2) Include fruits (especially citrus), vegetables (especially carotene-rich and cruciferous), and whole cereal grain (fiber) in the daily diet; these provide amounts of vitamins A and C as well as fiber adequate to obviate dietary supplements. (3) Minimize consumption of salt-cured or smoked food. (4) Use alcoholic beverages in moderation, since they increase the risk of certain cancers, especially when combined with cigarette smoking.

Experimental data lend support to the inferences from epidemiologic studies, but additional research is necessary to understand how dietary factors influence carcinogenesis. For example, a number of epidemiologic studies have suggested that a high intake of fat is associated with increased risk of cancer at several sites, including breast and colon. Possible explanations for this observation include increased adiposity, leading to greater conversion of androstenedione to estrone, which could influence carcinogenesis in the breast; and stimulation of increased bile salt excretion which could alter gut flora and thereby augment the production of carcinogenic substances by the bacteria in the colon. Dietary fiber enhances the rapid transit of potential carcinogens through the colon, which could explain the low incidence of bowel cancer and rectal cancer in tropical Africa.

Vitamin C may act to prevent cancer by blocking endogenous formation of *N*-nitroso compounds in the gastrointestinal tract, but there are no data showing that taking vitamin C will prevent cancer in human beings. There is renewed interest in the possibility that increased intake of vitamins A and E may reduce the risk of malignancy. Retinoids have been shown to reduce the incidence of second malignancies, following treatment of head and neck cancers. Further clinical trials will be needed to determine the value of particular vitamins, minerals, or nutritional supplements in amounts greater than provided by a prudent diet. The physician must be alert to the scientifically unproven dietary treatments which patients with cancer may be urged to undertake. Of course the greatest tragedy occurs when patients whose malignancy could be cured by proven therapeutic modalities are misled into depending upon such dietary manipulations.

Viruses   Although there has been extensive research on viral oncogenesis with experimental murine tumors, viruses have been implicated as the direct cause of only a few human cancers. Infection with human T lymphotrophic virus I (HTLV-I) can lead to adult T cell leukemia, an aggressive malignancy of T lymphocytes, which has been reported in large series from Japan and the West Indies. The incidence of hepatocellular carcinoma in endemic regions of Asia and Africa is closely associated with previous infection with hepatitis B virus, followed by a carrier state, suggesting that a causal relationship is highly likely. Chronic hepatocyte infection by the virus might predispose to carcinogenesis in these cells. There may be a variety of contributing factors, including malaria, malnutrition, and exposure to aflatoxin. This is a serious health problem in Asia and Africa, where primary liver carcinomas represent as much as 30 percent of malignancies. There also is a strong statistical correlation between herpes simplex 2 viral infection, which is sexually transmitted, and the incidence of cervical cancer. The Epstein-Barr virus is closely associated with African Burkitt's lymphoma as well as nasopharyngeal carcinoma in Asia. Cofactors in the development of these malignancies might be holoendemic malaria in African Burkitt's lymphoma and a particular configuration of histocompatibility antigens in the case of nasopharyngeal carcinoma among Chinese. The capacity of Epstein-Barr virus to infect human B lymphocytes (infectious mononucleosis) and transform them in cell culture suggests a role for the virus in malignancy.

Risk of cancer   Knowledge of genetic and environmental factors that may contribute to cancer incidence can be utilized by the conscientious physician to identify patients who have an increased risk of malignancy. The presence of certain hereditary diseases in a patient's family may suggest procedures that can lead to early detection and prevention, for example, early surveillance by colonoscopy and prevention by prophylactic colectomy in persons who have familial polyposis of the colon. Environmental factors that increase cancer risks should be identified and avoided. It is evident, however, that changing an individual's life-style in order to avoid exposure to a carcinogen can require an extraordinary level of effort on the part of both the patient and the physician.

New methods are being discovered for detecting individuals at high risk for developing malignancies. These depend on the identification and sequencing of abnormal genes which have a causal role in cellular transformation. Polymerase chain reaction and in situ hybridization techniques can be used to identify the presence of such abnormal genes in cell specimens obtained from individuals with a positive family history. This approach will be extremely valuable in identifying high-risk individuals, who should either undergo frequent diagnostic procedures or consider prophylactic surgery, such as mastectomy. It is possible that within a decade every youngster will donate peripheral blood lymphocytes for a screening procedure that will predict susceptibility to the most common malignancies. The impact of this information on preventive versus therapeutic health care will be of major significance.

CLINICAL SEQUELAE The presence of a malignant lesion may not, in itself, cause symptoms in a patient with cancer. The primary lesion may, for a period of time, be unnoticed and unimportant for the normal maintenance of body functions, in which case its clinical significance is due to its potential for growth and spread. In addition, the presence of metastasis need not result in symptomatic illness. Patients with carcinoma of the bowel, whose disease may have spread beyond the limits of surgical curability, may live for many months or even years with easily detectable metastatic lesions in the lung or abdomen, yet remain free of symptoms until the function of a vital organ is compromised or obstructive problems appear.

Malignancies produce clinical symptoms in three general ways (Table 317-5): by direct effects resulting from invasion or compression of normal tissues; by release of cytokines, hormones, and other biologically active agents into the local and systemic environment; and by secondary psychological effects upon the patient. Each of these factors may contribute profoundly to the degree of illness experienced by the patient. Clinical symptoms resulting from released biologically active agents, as well as systemic problems caused by as yet undetermined mechanisms, are usually grouped under the category of "paraneoplastic syndromes."

Mass effects of malignancy In most cases tumors produce clinical problems as a result of local expansion, with obliteration of normal tissues, as the malignant cells proliferate within the confines of the involved organ: marrow replacement by leukemia results in reduced production of the normal cellular elements of the blood; lung cancer compromises oxygen exchange in involved alveoli; primary or metastatic cancer in bone causes weakened trabecular architecture, resulting in pathologic fractures; hepatomas replace normal hepatocytes and interfere with liver function. A second result of local expansion is compression of normal structures, with partial or complete obstruction of tubular organs, blood vessels, and lymphatics: colonic cancer may obstruct the gastrointestinal tract; lung cancer blocks airflow through bronchi and can obstruct pulmonary venous return; hepatic and biliary malignancies produce obstructive jaundice; a variety of intraabdominal neoplasms can encase the ureters, causing renal failure; in the extreme case, penetration of blood vessels can cause hemorrhage. A third result of local expansion is pain, due to pressure on or stretching of nerve fibers. When neoplasia causes increased pressure on nervous tissue within the confines of the skull, the symptoms include headache and vomiting as well as seizure disorders and brain dysfunction.

Paraneoplastic syndromes The malignant process is felt to develop as a result of the unregulated and/or inappropriate expression of certain genes crucial to cell proliferation and differentiation. The aggressiveness of the malignant process is increased by the subsequent uncovering of additional genetic information. In this evolutionary process, abnormal genetic information may be expressed which results in severe physiologic effects upon the patient. As noted above, there may be excessive synthesis of a gene product which is normally found in the particular cell type, or the malignant cell may produce a molecule which does not ordinarily originate from its normal counterpart.

A common type of molecule produced by malignant tumors falls into the category of polypeptide hormones. The synthesis of vasopressin or ACTH by small cell carcinoma of the lung or parathormone by some squamous cancers are examples. These can produce clinical illness by mediating normal physiologic functions to an excessive degree. Other active molecules have been detected which are homologous with or identical to known growth factors. The potential for autonomous stimulation of proliferation mediated by production of essential growth-promoting agents has been discussed.

From this brief introduction, it can be seen that biologically active agents produced by malignant cells can be clinically important for a number of reasons:

1 They may serve as markers for the presence of a type of tumor. Detection of such markers early in the course of the disease might increase chances for cure. They also may be used to follow the clinical progress of the disease and anticipate recurrence.

2 They may produce symptoms as a result of their intrinsic biologic activity. In some cases these can become the major clinical problems determining survival (e.g., hypercalcemia).

3 They may serve to promote the growth of the tumor directly. In turn, growth-promoting agents of this type may become the focus of new approaches to anticancer treatment.

The paraneoplastic sequelae of cancer which involve ectopic hormone production are described in Chap. 327, and the neurologic manifestations of neoplasia in Chap. 328. Cutaneous manifestations of internal malignancy are discussed in Chap. 54. The association of malignancy with certain metabolic disorders, hematologic abnormalities, and immunosuppression will be further described here.

Metabolic disorders One of the major and most characteristic problems seen with cancer is weight loss, usually associated with anorexia. The extensive wasting which results is known as cachexia. The cause for this commonly observed and often life-limiting disturbance remains to be determined in spite of the fact that many contributing factors have been identified. Abnormalities of taste and smell, physiologic malfunction of the gastrointestinal tract, excessive energy demands made by the tumor, and failure to adapt energy expenditure to the levels of nutrient intake have been implicated as causes of cachexia in patients with cancer. Biochemical abnormalities in energy metabolism have been well-characterized in these patients. Fatty acids are oxidized in preference to glucose, and anaerobic glucose metabolism is increased while oxidative phosphorylation is reduced. This results in an inefficient expenditure of ATP, which might lead to an energy deficit. However, none of these observations is felt to account for the magnitude of the problem.

Typically, the anorectic patient simply cannot ingest food, in spite of a clear understanding of the need for increased nourishment. The chief complaint is unpalatability. An aversion to meat has been clearly documented. While nausea may be a component of the syndrome, emesis occurs rarely. This may be because the patient feels so satiated that no food intake is tolerated.

Provision of alimentation through enteral tubes or by the intravenous route has the potential to provide total parenteral nutrition (TPN) to patients with cancer, and the techniques for performing these procedures have been well-described by investigators managing nonmalignant disease. At present there is no indication that the provision of nutritional support at this level can, by itself, affect the course of malignant disease. However, clinical trials have suggested a role for nutritional supplementation, including TPN, in preparing

---

TABLE 317-5 Symptoms caused by malignant diseases

Mass effects
  A Ablation by crowding or by invasion
  B Obstruction of vessels, tubes, and ducts
  C Rupture of blood vessels
Remote effects (paraneoplastic syndromes)
  A Ectopic hormone production
  B Neuropathies and CNS abnormalities
  C Dermatologic abnormalities
  D Metabolic disorders
    1 Anorexia, weight loss
    2 Fever
    3 Chronic inflammation
  E Hematologic disorders
  F Immunosuppression
  G Collagen vascular disorders
Psychosocial effects
  A Loss of control
  B Acceptance of personal finitude
  C Fear of pain and mutilation
  D Separation and loneliness

nutritionally deprived cancer patients for potentially beneficial surgical procedures or chemotherapy programs which otherwise might not have been tolerated due to the wasted state of the patient.

Tumor necrosis factor (TNF) is a polypeptide produced by macrophages. Administration of TNF can mimic the syndrome of cachexia in experimental animals, and it is therefore also known as cachectin. Cytokines released by inflammatory cells and tumor cells are likely candidates as etiologic agents for the debilitation and wasting that accompany aggressive malignancy.

Fever is another sign associated with malignancy, and it is usually attributable to infection. Because of the debility which often accompanies cancer, and the depression in circulating granulocytes and mononuclear cells resulting from aggressive therapeutic measures, the types of infection seen may be unusual. Infection by endogenous bacteria, fungi, viruses, and protozoa must be considered when evaluating fever of unknown etiology in patients with malignancy (see Chap. 16). There remain unusual instances when fever cannot be explained by infection and must be attributed to cytokines released by the patient's inflammatory cells or to a cause intrinsic to the neoplasm itself.

Hematologic abnormalities Anemia is found with increased incidence in advanced stages of malignant disease. The mechanisms accounting for anemia are, in nearly all cases, extrinsic to the tumor, and may be due to several causes. Increased destruction of erythrocytes can result from hypersplenism, microangiopathic hemolysis, and autoantibodies, seen especially in the lymphoproliferative malignancies. Anemia due to occult bleeding is one of the cardinal signs of malignancy in the gastrointestinal tract. Decreased production of erythrocytes may result from iron deficiency related to bleeding, vitamin B_{12} or folate deficiency, erythron depletion due to tumor crowding in the marrow, toxicity secondary to chemotherapy or radiotherapy, and the anemia associated with chronic inflammatory disease.

Granulocytopenia is commonly associated with marrow infiltration by hematologic malignancies, and also results from chemotherapy. The causes of thrombocytopenia are comparable to those associated with anemia. Depression in one or all of the circulating hematopoietic elements may result from one of the various forms of marrow failure or aplastic anemia which are known to be preleukemic.

An increase in the formed elements of the blood also may occur. Erythrocytosis resulting from inappropriate production of erythropoietin is observed not only in polycythemia vera, but also in renal cell carcinoma, hepatoma, and cerebellar hemangioma. An elevated granulocyte count may result from marrow infiltration by tumor cells or an inflammatory response to malignancy, and frank leukemoid reactions may be seen with nonhematopoietic tumors. Thrombocytosis unrelated to primary marrow disease is commonly associated with a systemic malignancy.

A hypercoagulable state is a rare clinical complication of malignancy, although it may be far more prevalent at a subclinical level. Mucin-producing tumors and adenocarcinomas, especially those of the pancreas and stomach, head the list of tumors reported to be associated with clinical disseminated intravascular coagulopathy (DIC). This may present as a migratory thrombophlebitis of unknown etiology, which can produce venous thrombosis as well as pulmonary embolism. Hypercoagulation also may be associated with marantic (nonbacterial) endocarditis and resultant thromboembolic episodes, which further complicate the clinical picture. The treatment of the primary malignancy is the only successful therapeutic attack on the problem. Anticoagulation, following the principles for treatment of DIC (Chaps. 57 and 316), may provide short-term benefits in acute situations, but with attendant risks.

Acute promyelocytic leukemia is often associated with abnormalities of hemostasis related to a hypercoagulable state. The malignant immature granulocytes can release procoagulant materials which initiate DIC.

Immunosuppression Advanced cancer is accompanied by abnormalities in immune function which can be demonstrated by skin testing against common antigens and by examination of lymphocyte responses to mitogenic stimulation in vitro. Morever, in general, the extent of malignant disease correlates well with the degree of immune dysfunction. In spite of a vast experimental literature on this subject, the two significant questions concerning immunosuppression in cancer patients continue to be unanswered: (1) What is the mechanism(s) of inhibition? (2) Is the immunosuppression merely secondary to the malignant state, or could it play an etiologic role (failure of "immune surveillance")?

Experimental data have implicated defects in both T and B cell function, as well as abnormalities of macrophages, in the etiology of the reduced immune competence in cancer patients. Primary malignancies of lymphocytes are accompanied by abnormalities in the functioning of the particular cell type involved. Some of the lymphoproliferative malignancies are characterized by an increase in autoimmune reactions, most notably in 25 percent of patients with chronic lymphocytic leukemia. In addition, both chemotherapy and radiotherapy can produce long-standing suppression of immune function.

One approach to cancer treatment involves attempts to stimulate an effective immune response with the hope that immune antitumor activity can act alone or in concert with the standard therapeutic modalities to eliminate the malignant cell population. Monoclonal antibodies against antigens present in relatively increased quantities on tumor cells may provide ways to reconstitute or hyperconstitute immune responses to malignancy. Treatment with high concentrations of cytokines such as the interferons has produced responses in a number of types of malignancy, and this is especially effective in the therapy of hairy cell leukemia and chronic myelocytic leukemia. Interleukin 2 (IL-2) is another cytokine which may produce antitumor responses in patients with renal carcinoma, when administered in pharmacologic doses alone or in combination with lymphokine-activated killer (LAK) cells.

Psychosocial effects The diagnosis of cancer immediately raises in the mind of the patient and his or her family a host of questions and fears which require the undivided attention of an empathetic, considerate, and skilled physician. This is especially true when the particular form of cancer has a poor chance for cure or when malignancy has recurred.

Of the variety of psychosocial problems experienced by patients, two which are particularly difficult to deal with are helplessness and loss of control. These involve both economic control and personal control of one's activity and one's future. Closely tied to these problems and adding to the feeling of helplessness is the difficulty of accepting personal finitude. A third major source of mental anguish is the fear of pain and mutilation. Finally, separation from loved ones, both anticipated and real, creates a void of loneliness and a fear of abandonment.

The reactions to the mental stresses which are produced by these problems can only be dealt with effectively by a professional who has become familiar with the patient's personality and his or her social and intellectual environment. Although one or another emotion may dominate at a particular time, the responses commonly observed include anger, denial, withdrawal, and depression. Added to these problems is the complexity resulting from the response of the patient's family to the illness and to the patient's own response to the illness. In spite of these stresses, some patients with incurable malignancies are able to adapt and reorient their lives in a creative and meaningful way. The intellectual and emotional challenge to the physician is obvious, and careful attention must be given to managing the patient's (and the family's) responses to malignancy in addition to providing specific treatment for the disease.

Does the patient's psychological attitude have a role in the cause or treatment of malignant disease? The question is a complex and controversial one. There is evidence, which is contested, that life stresses can predispose to systemic illness by producing anxiety or depression. One theory postulates that stress leads to a reduction in immunologic function, resulting in inadequate immune surveillance, but this explanation for the pathogenesis of cancer is not adequately supported by available clinical data. There are also reports that correction of emotional difficulties and development of positive attitudes can aid in prolonging the survival of patients with extensive malignancy. In favor of psychological support and counseling is the clear benefit to the quality of life which can be achieved by helping patients with cancer to develop positive attitudes and to gain some measure of control over *how* they are living. However, scientific evidence does not demonstrate that the patient's psyche can achieve regression or cure of the malignant process. The strongest and most responsible advocates of counseling and attitudinal approaches to cancer patient management also stress the need for concurrent treatment with standard anticancer therapies.

DIAGNOSIS AND STAGING   There are a number of general goals in evaluating a patient for the presence of malignancy. The first is to detect malignancy early, since the results of therapy of cancer are far better in this situation. Second, information must be gathered leading to biopsy of a candidate lesion, which alone can establish the pathologic diagnosis of neoplasia. The third goal is to determine as precisely as possible the extent of tumor spread, both at the site of origin and as metastases. The process of obtaining this information is known as *staging*. The fourth goal is to determine the growth rate and time course of the neoplasm in the particular patient undergoing diagnostic evaluation. The dictum that "every person is different" holds for cancers as well. Each malignancy is different, although there is a natural history which broadly characterizes each type of neoplasm. The rate of tumor growth can be determined by sequential assessment, using physical examinations or radiologic techniques, occasionally aided by the measurement of serum markers of tumor activity. The physician's ingenuity and persistence often come into play; an example is determining the existence of past radiologic studies, locating them, and obtaining them for review. The fifth goal in the evaluation is to determine the effects of the malignancy upon the health and performance of the patient. The importance of this in the design of a management plan is obvious, since control of symptoms and proper modification of activity levels will improve the well-being of the patient. In addition, it has become increasingly evident that the patient's performance status provides important data in predicting prognosis as well as response to anticancer therapy. The final goal in the diagnostic evaluation is the selection of appropriate anticancer therapy. The choice will depend on the information gathered as outlined, plus a knowledge of the treatment regimens which have the highest likelihood of producing cure, durable remission, or palliation. The principles of cancer therapy are presented in Chap. 318.

There are two widely used clinical scales of performance status, the Karnofsky scale and a modification developed by the Eastern Cooperative Oncology Group. The influence of performance status upon prognosis is demonstrated by a report correlating performance and medial survival in patients with inoperable lung cancer (Table 317-6).

Clinical evaluation   How does the clinician proceed to evaluate a patient for the presence of malignant disease? Early detection depends primarily on awareness of the hereditary and environmental factors contributing to the incidence of cancer, combined with thorough exploration for symptoms and signs which could lead to further diagnostic workup. The seven warning signals widely publicized by the American Cancer Society are useful to remember (Table 317-7) and are usually covered in a review of systems. A careful physical examination is especially useful in detecting early cancer of the breast, uterus, cervix, colon and rectum, prostate, mouth, skin, testes, thyroid, and lymph nodes. A number of diagnostic screening tests have proved of value in early detection: (1) the exfoliative cytology ("Pap smear") screen for cervical cancer, (2) fecal occult blood testing, accompanied by periodic sigmoidoscopy for colorectal cancer, and (3) mammograms for breast cancer. In addition, screening for elevated prostate specific antigen (PSA) is currently recommended for men over 50, although the potential benefits continue to be debated.

TABLE 317-6 Influence of pretreatment performance status on patients with inoperable lung cancer*

Performance status scale[†]			Median survival (weeks)	Patients in group (percent)
ECOG	Karnofsky	Definitions		
0	100	Asymptomatic, normal activity	34	2
1	80–90	Symptomatic, but ambulatory	24–27	32
2	60–70	Symptomatic, in bed less than 50% of day, needs minimal assistance	14–21	40
3	40–50	Symptomatic, in bed more than 50% of day, requires considerable assistance	7–9	22
4	20–30	100% bedridden, severely disabled	3–5	5

* N = 5022 males with inoperable lung cancer of all histologic types entered onto VA Lung Group protocols from 1968–1978.
† Eastern Cooperative Oncology Group (ECOG) performance status scale, and DA Karnofsky et al, Cancer 1:634, 1948.
SOURCE: Adapted from JD Minna et al, in VT DeVita, Jr et al., 1989.

The prudent guidelines for early cancer detection provided by the American Cancer Society are summarized in Tables 317-8 and 317-9.

The three most common malignancies involve bowel, lung, and breast, and it is significant that screening tests are suggested for only two of these. It has been estimated by the American Cancer Society that the 5-year survival rate for colorectal cancer could be increased from the curent level of 55 percent to as high as 85 percent, if the recommended early detection techniques were generally applied. When the recommended breast cancer detection techniques are applied, the proportion of cases found without lymph node involvement at the time of diagnosis rises from 53 percent to more than 75 percent. Unfortunately, trials of mass screening for lung cancer with chest x-rays and sputum cytology have not resulted in reduced mortality, even when subjects believed to be at high risk were followed. However, the physician who is evaluating a patient in order to attemp to detect cancer early must learn whether or not the patient smokes cigarettes and should attempt to intervene.

The approach to a patient who presents to the physician with a history of symptoms or with abnormal physical findings which could be attributed to cancer involves selection of appropriate diagnostic procedures from a wide variety of available radiologic tests and laboratory studies (Table 317-10). The choice of diagnostic procedures used in the evaluation of cancer patients is guided by the natural history of the various types of malignancy. For example, knowledge that distant spread of breast cancer most frequently occurs to the lung, liver, bone, brain, and contralateral breast leads to consideration of studies of each of these organs as part of the complete workup. The diagnostician must know the probability of spread to these various metastatic sites in the presence or absence of abnormal findings in

TABLE 317-7 Cancer's seven warning signals

Change in bowel or bladder habits
A sore that does not heal
Unusual bleeding or discharge
Thickening or lump in breast or elsewhere
Indigestion or difficulty in swallowing
Obvious change in wart or mole
Nagging cough or hoarseness

SOURCE: American Cancer Society.

TABLE 317-8 Recommended guidelines for early detection of cancer in asymptomatic average-risk women

Age	Recommendation
20–39	*Cancer-related checkup* every 3 years, to include counseling and examination of the oral cavity, thyroid, skin, lymph nodes, and ovaries, plus: – Breast self-examination, monthly – Clinical breast examination, every 3 years – Baseline mammography (35-39 years of age) – Pap test and pelvic examination every year; after 3 or more annual, consecutive satisfactory examinations, the Pap test may be performed less frequently at the discretion of the physician for women who are or have been sexually active or are age 18 or older.
40–49	*Cancer-related checkup* yearly, to include all the above plus: – Digital rectal examination, yearly – Breast self-examination, monthly – Clinical breast examination, yearly – Mammography, every 1 to 2 years – At menopause, endometrial tissue sample in high-risk women
50 and older	*Cancer-related checkup* yearly, to include all of the above, plus: – Stool blood test, yearly – Sigmoidoscopy, every 3 to 5 years – Mammography, yearly

SOURCE: From DJ Fink in Al Holleb et al, page 156.

the history, physical examination, and standard blood studies. For the asymptomatic patient with breast cancer who has no abnormal physical findings outside of a small palpable breast lesion, and normal hematologic and blood chemistry values, a chest x-ray and a mammogram are the tests typically performed to evaluate the extent of disease prior to a decision for definitive therapy. Similar considerations go into planning the diagnostic workup for patients with each of the various forms of malignancy. It is for this reason that a thorough familiarity with the natural history of malignancies of the various organs, as well as the efficacy of a wide variety of diagnostic procedures in detecting these cancers, is essential.

Pathologic diagnosis The diagnosis of cancer is made by pathologic examination. While there are definite limitations to histologic and cytologic examination of tumor specimens, this procedure is essential in order to exclude inflammatory processes as well as hyperplasia or benign tumors. In addition, the tissue of origin of a malignancy must be known in order to select the appropriate therapy. Specimens for pathologic examination are usually obtained by biopsy of a suspicious lesion. The procedure may involve a surgical operation under general anesthesia, but in many cases tissue specimens can be obtained through local incision (e.g., breast cancer) or by removal of a piece of tissue under direct visualization (bronchoscopy, colonoscopy). When direct visualization is not possible because of the internal location of a suspected lesion, it is often possible to obtain tissue

TABLE 317-9 Recommended guidelines for early detection of cancer in asymptomatic average-risk men

Age	Recommendation
20–39	Cancer-related checkup every 3 years, to include health counseling and examination of the oral cavity, thyroid, skin, lymph nodes, testes, and prostate
40–49	Cancer-related checkup yearly, to include all of the above, plus: – Digital rectal examination with palpation of the prostate, yearly
50 and older	Cancer-related checkup yearly, to include all of the above, plus: – Stool blood test, yearly – Sigmoidoscopy, every 3 to 5 years

SOURCE: From DJ Fink in Al Holleb et al, page 155.

TABLE 317-10 Methods for diagnosis and staging

History
Physical examination, including examination of oropharynx, Pap test, and proctoscopy
Radiologic studies
  A Roentgenogram
  B Ultrasound
  C Computed tomography
  D Angiography and lymphangiography
  E Nuclear medicine
  F Magnetic resonance imaging
  G Positron emission tomography
Laboratory studies
  A Hematologic evaluation
  B Chemical tests of internal organ function
  C Tumor markers
Pathologic examination of tissue
Cytogenetics and molecular genetics

fragments or clumps of cells by fine-needle biopsy aspiration, guided by computed tomography or fluoroscopy. In addition, suitable cytologic preparations can be obtained by washing or scraping surface lesions, as is commonly done to evaluate lesions on the cervix or in bronchi. Finally, in the case of malignancy involving the hematopoietic system or growing in body cavities (e.g., ascites), needle aspiration of tumor cells in suspension can be performed.

To make the diagnosis of cancer the pathologist looks for histologic and cytologic features characteristic of the disease. These include pleomorphism of cellular and nuclear structure, a high rate of mitosis and the presence of large or multiple nuclei, disordered tissue architecture, destruction or invasion of normal tissue boundaries, and the presence of cells in inappropriate locations (metastases). Special stains are useful for identifying chemical components characteristic of particular cell types and tissues. Additional evidence can be brought to bear upon the pathologic diagnosis, using the results of immunohistochemical studies, flow cytometry data on cellular DNA content, chromosomal karyotype analysis, Southern blotting for detection of diagnostic abnormalities in rearranged or amplified genes, and electron microscopy. However, in the overwhelming majority of cases, the diagnosis is made with the light microscope, on the basis of morphologic evaluation of the cells individually and as organized into tissue structures.

After the pathologic diagnosis of malignancy is established, the description usually includes three characteristics which classify the neoplasia:

1 The tissue of origin (e.g., adenocarcinoma, epidermoid carcinoma, sarcoma, leukemia)
2 Anatomic origin (e.g., colon, lung, breast)
3 Grade, or degree of differentiation (e.g., well-differentiated or poorly differentiated)

Each of these characteristics gives the therapist information relevant to the selection of treatment and to the prognosis. Although this terminology for classification is followed in general, there are many examples of exceptions based upon customary nomenclature involving particular tissues of origin or on the use of eponyms (e.g., Hodgkin's disease, glioblastoma multiforme).

Staging of cancer The staging of a cancer patient involves the detection of the anatomic extent of the tumor, both in its primary location and in metastatic sites. This process is of critical importance in the clinical management for a number of reasons:

1 The optimal treatment plan for an individual patient is selected on the basis of the stage of disease.
2 By determining the presence of early metastatic disease, treatment can often be designed which can increase the chance for cure, or delay the development of symptoms even if cure is not achievable.
3 Staging provides information from which the physician can better evaluate the prognosis.

4 Because half of the cases of cancer cannot be cured by the therapies available today and because rapid advances in the development of anticancer treatment are occurring, management of an individual patient often involves new drugs or experimental procedures which are in the process of being evaluated for toxicity and efficacy. Staging to determine the extent of disease accurately is essential for evaluating factors influencing the results of such new treatments.

The anatomic extent of disease is best described and communicated to other professionals by a standardized nomenclature known as the TNM system. The three elements characterized in this system are the primary *t*umor, the regional lymph *n*odes, and *m*etastases (Table 317-11). The details of classification were decided upon by the International Union against Cancer (UICC) and the American Joint Committee for Cancer Staging (AJCCS). There is a scale of subcategories with designations ranging from 0 to 4 for each of the three tumor characteristics listed in the table. These scales were chosen because they can provide useful predictions of the clinical course. The primary tumor is classified by its size and the extent of local involvement. The involvement of lymph nodes is typically stratified by the spread to locations at a varying distance from the primary lesion and by the number of involved nodes. The most relevant information regarding metastases is their presence or absence. The details of stratification within the TNM system vary for each type of malignancy and are highly individualized. They depend on the characteristic growth patterns and lymphatic drainage patterns of neoplasms of the various organs. There is not always agreement about the definitions of the TNM characteristics, which can create confusion.

The stage of the tumor is typically divided into three or four categories (e.g., I to IV). For each type of malignancy, the various T, N, and M designations are assigned to one of four stages, in order to develop separation into groupings which correlate with data on prognosis and clinical responses to therapy. This is best described by mentioning a specific example. For the neoplasm with the highest mortality rate, non-small cell carcinoma of the lung, the therapy which has the best chance for curing the patient is surgery. The staging system for lung cancer (Table 317-12) is designed in a way which stratifies patients into groups, for which different treatment protocols are indicated. For the stages I and II patients, and some stage III patients, surgery is the treatment of choice. The extent of the surgical procedure depends on the extent of disease designated by the T and N classification within these two stages. Total excision of all tumor is the therapeutic goal, with 5-year postresection survival rates of 50 percent for stage I, 30 percent for stage II, and 15 percent for stage IIIa.

Tumor markers A tumor marker is an abnormality which is specific for a particular type of malignancy. For example, the Ph chromosome abnormality in the karyotype is a marker for chronic myelogenous leukemia, and the exclusive presence of either κ or λ chains on the surface of a population of lymphocytes is a marker of the lymphoproliferative malignancies. Until recently there were no biochemical markers that were absolutely specific for and diagnostic of malignancy. However, utilization of molecular genetic technology has enabled detection of genetic alterations that are pathognomonic for particular malignancies (see discussion of ''Clonality'' above).

The term *marker* may also be used in a more restrictive sense,

TABLE 317-12 Stage Grouping of the New International Staging System for Lung Cancer*

Occult carcinoma	TX	N0	M0
Stage 0	TIS	Carcinoma in situ	
Stage I	T1	N0	M0
	T2	N0	M0
Stage II	T1	N1	M0
	T2	N1	M0
Stage IIIa	T3	N0	M0
	T3	N1	M0
	T1-3	N2	M0
Stage IIIb	Any T	N3	M0
	T4	Any N	M0
Stage IV	Any T	Any N	M1

* TX, positive cytology; TIS, carcinoma in situ; T1, less than or equal to 3 cm, no local invasion; T2, greater than 3 cm, more than 2 cm from carina; T3, direct extension to chest wall, diaphragm, pleura or pericardium; T4, invasion of mediastinum, intrathoracic organs, or vessels. N1, peribronchial or hilar nodes; N2, ipsilateral mediastinal nodes; N3, contralateral mediastinal nodes. M1, distant metastasis.
SOURCE: Mountain, CF: A new international staging system for lung cancer. Chest 89:225s–233s, 1986.

referring to molecules which are produced in abnormal amounts or under abnormal circumstances and are released into the circulation. The anaplasia and autonomy of the tumor cells permit production of molecules in greater than normal amounts or at inappropriate times in the life of the organism, and in this sense the abnormalities may become specific. Assays of such markers may be of great help to the clinician in a number of ways: (1) screening of high-risk individuals for the presence of malignancy, (2) diagnosis of malignancy, (3) monitoring of the effectiveness of therapy, (4) early detection of recurrence, and (5) immunodetection of metastatic sites, using radioactive-labeled antibodies against the markers.

The tumor marker of greatest use to the clinician is human chorionic gonadotropin (hCG), which has specificity because of its nearly exclusive production by the trophoblastic epithelium of the placenta under normal circumstances. The hCG levels rise during pregnancy. The hormone also may be secreted into the blood by trophoblastic tumors, as well as germ cell neoplasms of the testes and ovaries. Other neoplasms have been reported to be associated with elevated hCG levels, but the serum concentration rarely exceeds 10,000 ng/L (10 ng/mL) whereas trophoblastic tumors can produce concentrations over 100×10^6 ng/L (100,000 ng/mL). The usefulness of the assay for hCG is markedly enhanced by clinical data which show that changes in the serum hCG concentration in patients with secreting trophoblastic malignancies accurately reflect changes in the tumor burden. Therefore, decisions on the appropriate time to discontinue therapy can be based on the time course of serum levels, and decisions to reinstate therapy for recurrent disease are made on the basis of reappearance of hCG in the serum. The clinical test for hCG utilizes a radioimmunoassay for the beta subunit, to avoid cross reactivity with luteinizing hormone.

Two clinically useful tumor markers are products of genes which are expressed during the normal differentiation of fetal tissue but are partially or completely suppressed in the adult. These markers have been termed oncofetal antigens. Carcinoembryonic antigen (CEA) was originally thought to be specific for bowel cancer, but further studies have shown it to be a nonspecific tumor-associated antigen which also may be elevated in a variety of benign conditions. In the gastrointestinal tract, the molecule, a glycoprotein with a molecular weight of 180,000, is concentrated in the glycocalyx of epithelial cells, from which it is released into the lumen of the bowel. In the presence of malignancy, CEA concentrations may be elevated in the blood and other body fluids. Serum levels of CEA above the normal concentration of 2500 ng/L (2.5 ng/mL) are found in greater than 50 percent of neoplasms involving the colon, pancreas, stomach, lung, and breast. A variety of common nonmalignant conditions are associated with elevation of CEA, but typically not over 10,000 ng/L (10 ng/mL). These include cigarette smoking, chronic pulmonary disease, alcoholic cirrhosis, hepatitis, and inflammatory bowel dis-

TABLE 317-11 TNM system of anatomic staging

T: Primary tumor
   T0   No evidence of primary tumor
   T1–4   Ascending degrees of increase in tumor size and involvement
N: Regional lymph nodes
   N0   No evidence of disease in lymph nodes
   N1–4   Ascending degrees of nodal involvement
M: Distant metastasis
   M0   No evidence of metastasis
   M1–4   Ascending degrees of metastatic involvement

ease. CEA is not selective for cancer, and measurements of its levels should not be used in screening for the presence of malignant disease. However, serial measurements of CEA levels in patients with secreting malignancies can provide valuable information on the efficacy of treatment and the recurrence of disease. The possibility that early elevation of serum CEA can predict recurrence of bowel cancer soon enough to allow further surgical resection for cure is under study.

The second clinically useful oncofetal antigen is alpha fetoprotein (AFP), which is produced by the liver and gastrointestinal tract epithelium during gestation and which falls to levels less than 20,000 ng/L (20 ng/mL) after birth. Serum levels are elevated in 70 percent of patients with hepatocellular cancer, the majority of patients with nonseminomatous testicular cancer, and occasional patients with neoplasms of the gastrointestinal tract. As with CEA, the serum concentration of AFP may be elevated in benign conditions, especially in inflammatory disease of the liver. Its utility is in monitoring tumor activity, especially in the case of testicular tumors.

Elevation of either AFP or hCG is found in 80 to 90 percent of all nonseminomatous germ cell tumors of the testes. However, absence or normal levels of these biochemical markers of malignancy cannot be interpreted as proof that there is no tumor. Some tumors do not produce these marker molecules. Furthermore, because of tumor heterogeneity, it is possible for marker concentrations to fall in the presence of tumor, if a nonproducing subclone begins to grow preferentially. For this reason, recurrence of disease need not be accompanied by recurrence of elevated marker levels.

Other biochemical markers with clinical utility include calcitonin, with which familial medullary carcinoma of the thyroid can be detected in individuals who appear to be normal. As indicated above, elevation of serum prostate specific antigen is observed in patients with prostatic cancer, and is useful in monitoring the response to therapy.

There are many tumors which, because of increased cellular mass or loss of normal regulation, produce excessive quantities of polypeptides normally secreted into the circulation by the tissue of origin. Examples include the immunoglobulin molecules produced in multiple myeloma, and insulin or gastrin hypersecretion by islet cell tumors. In addition, tumors may secrete molecules which ordinarily are not produced in the tissue from which they are derived. This phenomenon has already been discussed in the description of the paraneoplastic syndromes, because in many cases these marker molecules have biologic activities which can produce clinical illness in the patient. In some cases of malignant disease, cultures of tumor cells have been found to secrete a variety of polypeptide hormones atypical of the tissue of origin. In addition, molecules related to normal hormones or to their precursor forms may be present in the patient's serum, in the absence of any demonstrable clinical effects. These observations provide evidence for the broad scope of genetic deregulation which may accompany the process of oncogene expression and carcinogenesis.

COST AND BENEFITS The problem of dealing with malignant disease raises many questions relevant to public health policy. It is likely that large numbers of individuals harbor genetic abnormalities which put them at high risk for developing certain types of malignancy. It is also clear that life-style issues such as smoking, dietary habits, and drinking have a major impact on cancer incidence. There will undoubtedly be increased efforts to allocate the funds and resources necessary to address cancer prevention in a more comprehensive and proactive way. However, in parallel, the expensive diagnostic equipment, procedures, and assays that are being developed, as well as the new biologic-based therapies on the horizon, make it likely that the cost of delivering care to patients with malignant disease will increase. With an increasing focus on controlling the costs of health care, it will be extremely important to carefully analyze the costs and benefits of procedures, tests, and treatment regimens, taking a critical look at the extent to which they contribute to a favorable outcome.

REFERENCES

BRUGGE J et al: *Origins of Human Cancer: A Comprehensive Review.* Cold Spring Harbor, Cold Spring Harbor Laboratory Press, 1991

COSSMAN J: *Molecular Genetics in Cancer Diagnosis.* New York, Elsevier, 1990

COTRAN RS et al: *Robbins Pathologic Basis of Disease,* 4th ed. Philadelphia, Saunders, 1989

DEVITA VT JR et al: *Cancer: Principles and Practices of Oncology,* 4th ed. Philadelphia, Lippincott, 1993

FRANKS LM et al: *Introduction to the Cellular and Molecular Biology of Cancer.* New York, Oxford University Press, 1991

GROBSTEIN C et al: *Diet, Nutrition, and Cancer.* Washington, D.C., National Academy Press, 1982

HOLLAND JF, FREI E: *Cancer Medicine,* 3d ed. Philadelphia, Lea and Febiger, 1993

HOLLEB AI et al: *American Cancer Society Textbook of Clinical Oncology.* Atlanta, American Cancer Society, Inc., 1991

VOGELSTEIN B, KINZLER KW: p53 function and dysfunction. Cell 70:523, 1992

WEINBERG RA: *Oncogenes and the Molecular Origins of Cancer.* Cold Spring Harbor, Cold Spring Harbor Laboratory Press, 1989

318 PRINCIPLES OF CANCER THERAPY

CHRISTOPHER A. SLAPAK / DONALD W. KUFE

The development of effective cancer therapy has been a major focus of biomedical research. As a direct result of fundamental and applied research efforts, some malignancies have been changed from highly lethal to often curable diseases. While progress in treating others has been frustratingly slow, advances in multiple disciplines will undoubtedly lead to improvements in these recalcitrant diseases as well.

The development of new cancer therapeutics has generated much attention and excitement. There has been a rapid increase in the discovery of biologic agents of potential clinical importance. New chemotherapeutic drugs, some of which represent novel classes of cytotoxic agents, are entering clinical trials. Differentiating agents, long a therapeutic goal, are being utilized in investigational approaches for the prevention and therapy of some malignancies.

The mainstay of cancer therapy is distributed among three interactive subspecialties. The role of the surgeon, the radiation oncologist, and the medical oncologist will continue to be reshaped as new agents become clinically available and a multimodality approach to cancer becomes the rule. The primary care physician will remain at the forefront of prevention and early detection of cancer. The further definition of cancer risk factors and the availability of more sensitive and specific screening procedures insures that the internist will influence cancer morbidity and mortality.

The approach to cancer therapy, whether it involves experimental therapeutics in a university hospital or standard state-of-the-art therapy in a community hospital, must begin with an adequate data base. Each patient requires a proper histologic diagnosis of cancer. Every patient needs adequate staging and an appropriate plan of management.

DIAGNOSIS The histologic diagnosis of cancer and the categorization of the proper tumor type is pivotal in planning further workup and in deciding on treatment options. Although a histologic diagnosis may frequently appear straightforward, the clinician must realize its limitations. Histologic subtyping with biochemical and immunologic tissue characterization has resulted in a level of distinction between diagnoses not previously possible. In addition to substantiating the diagnosis of malignancy, this subtyping provides information essential in guiding therapy. The distinction between histologically similar tumors is often critical as therapeutic options may differ. When histologic subtyping is not possible, the decision to obtain additional tissue must be made in consultation with an experienced oncologist to determine whether it will alter the approach to treatment.

STAGING   The extent of malignant disease is a prime determinant in planning appropriate therapy. Staging not only guides in selecting therapeutic modalities, but provides important prognostic information and may help the clinician minimize morbid complications. There is no routine set of tests appropriate for all patients. Understanding the natural history of the primary tumor, the pattern of spread to regional lymph nodes, and the possible sites of distant metastases assists in the selection of evaluations. The risks to the patient from any study must be balanced against the benefits gained by having additional staging information.

MANAGEMENT   After diagnosis and staging a plan of management must be derived. The plan must consider the biology and natural history of the tumor, the available treatment options and their appropriateness to the patient's clinical situation, and the wishes of the individual patient. The clinician must clearly establish the goals of any treatment plan and these goals should be explicitly communicated with the patient. Treatment with curative intent is clearly most desirable. The level of aggressiveness frequently required, often with attendant serious complications, requires the physician to evaluate realistically the potential for disease eradication. Treatment to improve longevity without long-term disease free survival requires the physician to consider carefully the risk-to-benefit ratios of each therapeutic option. The amount of additional time gained must be weighed against hospitalization time, potential complications, and side effects of therapy. Finally, treatment for palliation should not subject the patient to any unwarranted side effects, unnecessary complications, or other additional discomforts. The goal of palliation, relief of symptoms, prevention of complications, and maximization of quality of life, must always be kept in mind.

PRINCIPLES OF SURGICAL THERAPY

Surgery was the first modality used in the treatment of cancer dating back to the 19th century. After the development of ether anesthesia in 1840s and the principles of antisepsis in 1860s, advances in cancer surgery were pioneered by Billroth, Halsted, and others. For the first portion of this century, surgery was the only cancer treatment widely available that yielded significant disease-free survival. Surgery is still the only curative therapy in many of the most common solid tumors. However, advances in surgical techniques, as well as improved multimodality therapy, have dramatically altered the surgical approach to many cancers. More limited surgical resections that do not affect the outcome but minimize loss of normal organ function are now feasible for many tumor types. Present day surgical oncologists are an integral part of the multimodality approach to cancer therapy. Surgery has a primary role in the diagnosis, staging and treatment of many tumors.

DIAGNOSIS   A significant role for surgery in the treatment of patients with cancer is in obtaining adequate tissue samples for a histological diagnosis. Accurate diagnosis is a critical first step in planning appropriate cancer therapy. Once the diagnosis of cancer is entertained, it is essential to involve a surgeon experienced in the principles of oncologic diagnosis. An improperly performed biopsy may compromise subsequent surgical management and ultimately the outcome of the patient.

Several techniques are available for obtaining tissue specimens. An *aspiration biopsy* is generally performed by inserting a fine needle into the tissue of interest and aspirating material for cytologic examination. The availability of an experienced cytologist is essential for a proper interpretation. Superficial lesions are amenable to aspiration as are internal sites under sonographic or computed tomographic guidance. A definitive diagnosis of cancer may not be possible by cytology alone. A *needle biopsy* with radiologic guidance again may permit a percutaneous approach to internal structures. With

some tumors, however, particularly lymphomas and sarcomas, a larger amount of tissue is usually required for a definitive diagnosis. With either aspiration or needle biopsy, sampling errors are a significant problem. *Incisional biopsy,* removal of a section or a wedge of tissue from a larger tumor, is performed when removal of the entire tumor is impossible and is often performed prior to major surgical extirpation. An *excisional biopsy* removes the entire lesion and when possible is preferred to incisional biopsy. Excising the entire lesion ensures sufficient tissue for pathologic examination, lessens the risk of tumor dissemination, and eliminates sampling problems. The choice of the appropriate procedure is dictated by anatomic considerations, biology of the presumed tumor type, and by the requirements of the pathologist. For some tumors sufficient tissue for specialized studies such as immunophenotyping, cytogenetics, electron microscopy, or estrogen receptor status requires specialized handling and close interaction with the pathologist.

STAGING   Surgery is a principal means of staging many neoplastic diseases. Exploratory laparotomy to detect intraabdominal spread of Hodgkin's disease is usually indicated when planning conservative therapy. Axillary lymph node sampling in breast carcinoma provides important prognostic information that may guide further therapy. Intraoperative staging by the sampling of celiac lymph nodes will help establish the appropriateness of an esophagectomy in a patient with esophageal carcinoma.

TREATMENT   Surgery is an effective method to cure patients whose tumors are confined to particular anatomical sites. However, at presentation only about 25 percent of patients have tumors that are truly confined and amenable to surgical treatment alone. The challenge is to identify those patients who can be successfully treated by surgery alone, thus sparing unnecessary surgical morbidity for the majority of patients who will ultimately relapse. Careful clinical staging after a thorough history, physical examination, and appropriate imaging studies are often requisite to decide upon the appropriateness of surgery.

Removal of most solid tumors requires en bloc resections with adequate tumor free margins. Microscopic tumor invasion of surrounding normal tissue that is imperceptible to the surgeon may require multiple frozen biopsies to establish tumor free margins. Manipulation of the tumor should be minimized to decrease the risk of seeding distant metastases. Resection or sampling of the regional lymph node group is usually indicated; however extended resection of several involved nodal groups is generally not warranted since this has not resulted in improved survival due to the high probability of concurrent distant metastases when multiple lymph nodes are involved.

Another challenge in oncologic surgery is to identify patients for whom combined modality therapy will improve outcome and allow a decrease in the extent of surgery. The surgeon, the medical oncologist, and the radiation therapist should develop an integrated plan to deliver the most effective coordinated treatment. A dramatic example has been the impact of multimodality therapy in the treatment of early stage breast carcinoma. Radical mastectomy with extended axillary lymph node dissection has been replaced by lumpectomy with lymph node sampling together with local radiotherapy and, when indicated, systemic adjuvant chemotherapy.

Surgery has been used as means of cytoreduction when complete excision has not been possible. However, unless such surgical debulking is combined with additional therapy, such as chemotherapy for ovarian carcinoma or Burkitt's lymphoma, this approach has not yielded significant treatment benefit. A consideration of tumor cell biology demonstrates the futility of this approach: debulking a mass 10 cm in diameter containing approximately 1×10^{10} tumor cells to one 1 cm in diameter is a 1 logarithm reduction in tumor burden that will still leave the patient with 1×10^9 tumor cells.

Surgical resection of metastatic disease with intent to cure may be appropriate in special circumstances. Generally this approach is reserved for patients who have a localized metastasis occurring well after resection of the primary disease. The metastasis should be the only evidence of distant disease and it should be resectable with low morbidity. Examples include pulmonary metastases in patients with osteogenic sarcoma or solitary liver metastases in patients with colorectal carcinoma. In some patients, resection of these lesions can lead to long-term disease-free survival.

Finally, surgery is used for palliation. The selection of patients who will benefit from this approach requires considerable judgment and skill. Appropriate, judicious use of surgery in patients with metastatic disease may alleviate pain and improve the quality of life. An example is excision of an obstructing colon carcinoma in a patient with metastatic disease. However, overly aggressive surgical intervention in a palliative setting may lead to prolonged hospitalizations, unnecessary discomfort, and additional financial burden to the patient or family.

PRINCIPLES OF RADIATION THERAPY

Radiation therapy, like surgery, is a local modality used in the treatment of cancer. Its use depends to a large extent on the inherent radiosensitivity of the tumor and the adjacent normal tissues. Ideally radiation therapy should destroy cancerous tissue while causing minimal disruption to surrounding normal structures. Another consideration is the ability of the normal tissue to sustain and repair radiation-induced damage and for the patient to function adequately even if normal organ function is diminished.

PHYSICAL AND BIOLOGICAL CHARACTERISTICS   Radiation therapy is dependent on the application of ionizing electromagnetic radiation to a tumor site. The term *x-ray* denotes high-energy electromagnetic radiation produced by instruments such as linear accelerators. Gamma rays are also electromagnetic radiation but are produced by radioactive isotope decay. Both are used in radiation therapy and there is no inherent difference in their physical characteristics or biologic effects.

External beam radiation therapy refers to radiation delivered from a source outside the body. High-energy, megavolt electron beams are generated from linear accelerators or from radioisotope decay of cobalt 60 and are commonly used to irradiate internal, deep-seated lesions. Linear accelerators are the more widely used and produce a more focused beam with smaller penumbra. These high-energy, penetrating beams deliver a less intense superficial dose and thus spare the skin. Lesser energy, orthovoltage beams deliver a higher dose to superficial tissues and are used to treat lesions such as skin cancers. Radiation delivered by insertion of radioactive materials within the body near or at the tumor site is called *brachytherapy*. Brachytherapy may consist of intracavitary inserts, used in the treatment of gynecologic malignancies such as cervical or vaginal carcinomas, or interstitial implants, such as those used in prostate carcinoma. Brachytherapy may be used in conjunction with external beam therapy, e.g., in head and neck carcinoma, where the implants provide a high-intensity boost to the tumor bed.

Radiation dose is defined as the unit of absorbed energy (joules) per kilogram of tissue. The rad has been replaced by the Gray (Gy). One rad equals 0.01 Gy or 1 Gy equals 100 rad. A given dose of radiation kills a constant percentage of cells, not a constant number. At high doses of radiation, cell survival decreases with first-order kinetics in proportion to increasing radiation dose. At lower radiation doses a shoulder in the curve results from a decreased rate of cell death and may represent the presence of cellular repair mechanisms.

DNA is the target for radiation-induced cell death. Ionizing radiation generates free radicals and reactive oxygen intermediates that damage local cellular substituents including DNA. Cytotoxicity produced by clinically relevant doses of radiation is dependent upon cellular division and is called *mitotic cell death*. Rapidly proliferating normal tissues such as intestinal mucosa, bone marrow, and skin are particularly susceptible to radiation-induced cytotoxicity.

Cellular repair is normally complete within 4 to 6 h after radiation exposure. The capacity and extent of cellular repair mechanisms determine in part the radiosensitivity of a given tumor or normal tissue. Oxygen concentration is another important determinant of radiation sensitivity. Hypoxic tissues are relatively resistant to the effects of radiation. Thus, poorly vascularized central areas of larger tumor masses are likely to exhibit relative insensitivity to radiation. The presence of oxygen is important in generating and sustaining free radicals produced by radiation.

Particle beam therapy, which utilizes neutrons or charged particles such as protons, is currently available in specialized centers. Particle beams have the advantage of more precise tissue localization and are less dependent on the presence of oxygen for cytotoxicity as compared to conventional radiation therapy.

TREATMENT   Radiation therapy is performed by a team of nurses, dosimetrists, physicists, and radiation oncologists. A course of radiation therapy is preceded by simulation with appropriate radiographic tumor localization. Patient positioning during simulation must be exactly reproduced for each treatment to ensure maximal tumor delivery with minimal complications.

Radiation therapy is usually delivered in fractional doses, such as 180 to 300 cGy per day, five times per week. Clinical experience has demonstrated that fractional treatment schedules markedly improve the therapeutic index (see below) and result in better tumor control. This improved outcome may be related to several factors, including cellular repair of normal tissues, repopulation of destroyed tissues, and reoxygenation of relatively hypoxic tumor sites. Additionally, radiation therapy is often delivered from multiple external sites focusing on the tumor. This approach distributes the radiotherapy and lessens toxicity to the normal tissues.

Radiation therapy with curative intent as the sole treatment modality is employed in limited stage Hodgkin's disease, some non-Hodgkin's lymphomas, certain head and neck carcinomas such as laryngeal cancer, limited stage prostate carcinoma, gynecologic tumors including vaginal and cervical carcinomas, central nervous system neoplasms, such as medulloblastoma, and some skin cancers. Radiation therapy is often an integral part of curative multimodality approaches. For example, radiation therapy combined with chemotherapy has largely replaced surgery as a curative treatment for squamous cell carcinoma of the anus. Radiation therapy is a central component of breast conservation in the multimodality treatment of early stage breast carcinoma.

Radiation therapy is also used in the palliative management of many tumors. Irradiation of bony metastases may alleviate pain and stabilize weight-bearing structures in an attempt to prevent pathologic fractures. Brain metastases are often irradiated to provide symptomatic relief and prevent further neurologic complications. Palliative radiation therapy can also be employed to treat significant bleeding, refractory visceral pain, and vital organ obstruction. In general, doses employed for palliative management are lower than those used for curative therapy and result in less acute toxicity and discomfort to the patient.

Radiation therapy may be required on an urgent basis for the treatment of complications of malignant disease. An impending spinal cord compression in a patient with metastatic carcinoma is usually best treated with radiotherapy to the involved area. Alleviation of an obstructed airway or superior vena cava is generally treated effectively by radiotherapy.

COMPLICATIONS   Radiation therapy is associated with both acute toxicity and long-term sequelae. Acute reactions occur during or immediately following therapy. They are self-limited and usually do not determine the amount of radiation therapy that can be administered. Common manifestations include skin reactions with erythema and desquamation; gastrointestinal toxicity with nausea, vomiting, dysphagia, or diarrhea; and myelosuppression with leukopenia, thrombocytopenia, and anemia. If symptoms become a problem during therapy, fractional doses may need to be temporarily reduced to allow normal tissue repair.

Long-term sequelae are dose limiting and occur many months or years after the completion of therapy. Long-term complications occur rarely if known normal tissue tolerances are not exceeded. The

TABLE 318-1 Normal tissue tolerance of radiation therapy

Tissue	Dose, cGy	Complications
Brain	6000	Necrosis
Spinal cord	4500	Myelitis
Heart	4500	Pericarditis, myocardial damage
Intestine	4500	Stenosis, perforation
Liver	3000	Hepatitis, hepatic vein thrombosis
Lung	2000	Pneumonitis, fibrosis
Kidney	2000	Nephropathy, renal failure
Bone marrow	250	Aplasia

complications tend to be progressive rather than self-limited. Their occurrence does not correlate with appearance or severity of acute reactions. The mechanism behind late complications is incompletely understood but is believed to result from either the disruption of vascular endothelium or the depletion of normal tissue stem cells. Table 318-1 lists tissue tolerances of some common structures with late complications.

Radiation therapy is known to be mutagenic, carcinogenic, and teratogenic. Radiation therapy is associated with an increased risk of developing solid tumors in previously irradiated fields. The secondary tumors often appear more than 10 years after therapy is completed. The true incidence of this complication and other predisposing factors are areas of active investigation.

PRINCIPLES OF CHEMOTHERAPY

BACKGROUND Systemic chemotherapy is the primary treatment available for disseminated malignant disease. Progress in drug therapy has resulted in the development of curative chemotherapy regimens for several tumors (Table 318-2). Chemotherapy also has a significant role in palliation, often with improved survival, in a variety of other tumors. However, in several common solid tumors chemotherapy has only minor activity.

One of the most important and still evolving roles for systemic chemotherapy is its use in the adjuvant setting. *Adjuvant* therapy is administered after a definitive surgical resection to a patient who has no clinical, radiologic, or pathologic evidence of residual malignant disease. Its purpose is to eliminate undetectable micrometastatic disease. Table 318-2 lists tumors effectively treated with adjuvant chemotherapy. The term *neoadjuvant* refers to the administration of chemotherapy prior to surgery. This approach has been utilized in the treatment of head and neck carcinoma and bladder carcinoma. A patient who responds to neoadjuvant chemotherapy may benefit from more conservative local therapy.

Chemotherapy, whether given with curative or palliative intent, usually requires multiple cycles of treatment. Assessment of therapeutic efficacy prior to completing the entire course of treatment is often desirable. Discontinuation of ineffective treatments may allow institution of other salvage regimens, or in the absence of other effective regimens, the avoidance of unnecessary toxicity. Response to therapy can be measured directly by palpating superficial tumor masses or by imaging of internal lesions. Indirect measurements are possible but generally less desirable in the evaluation of tumor response.

Uniform criteria for describing a response to therapy are widely accepted and enable comparisons of the efficacy of alternative treatments. A complete response (or complete remission) is the disappearance of all detectable malignant disease. A partial response is a 50 percent decrease in the product of the greatest perpendicular diameters of one or more lesions. There can be no increase in size of any lesion or the appearance of new lesions. Stable disease means that there is no change in measurable tumor dimensions. Progressive disease means at least a 25 percent increase in the product of the greatest perpendicular diameter of one lesion or the appearance of new lesions.

TABLE 318-2 Response of tumors to chemotherapy

CURABLE BY CHEMOTHERAPY

Acute lymphocytic leukemia
Acute myelogenous leukemia
Ewing's sarcoma
Gestational trophoblastic carcinoma
Hodgkin's disease
Non-Hodgkin's lymphoma
    Burkitt's lymphoma
    Diffuse large cell lymphoma
    Follicular mixed lymphoma
Rhabdomyosarcoma
Testicular carcinoma
Wilms' tumor

CHEMOTHERAPY HAS SIGNIFICANT ACTIVITY

Anal carcinoma
Bladder carcinoma
Breast carcinoma
Cervix carcinoma
Chronic lymphocytic leukemia
Chronic myelogenous leukemia
Endometrial carcinoma
Hairy cell leukemia
Head and neck carcinoma
Lung (small cell) carcinoma
Multiple myeloma
Non-Hodgkin's lymphoma
    Follicular lymphoma
Ovarian carcinoma

CHEMOTHERAPY HAS MINOR ACTIVITY

Brain tumors (astrocytoma)
Colorectal carcinoma
Hepatocellular carcinoma
Kaposi's sarcoma
Lung (non-small cell carcinoma)
Melanoma
Pancreatic carcinoma
Prostate carcinoma
Renal cell carcinoma
Soft tissue sarcoma

ADJUVANT CHEMOTHERAPY IS EFFECTIVE

Breast carcinoma (axillary lymph node positive)
Colorectal carcinoma (Dukes B_2 or C)
Osteogenic sarcoma
Ovarian carcinoma (stage III)
Testicular carcinoma

The modern era of chemotherapy treatment for malignant disease began after the observation in World War II that exposure to mustard gas led to bone marrow and lymph node hypoplasia. The clinical use of nitrogen mustard was pioneered by Gilman at Yale in the 1940s in the treatment of lymphoma. Farber at Harvard, also in the 1940s, first induced remissions in childhood leukemia using aminopterin, a folate antagonist. In 1955, chemotherapy was first used to cure a solid tumor, gestational trophoblastic carcinoma. The subsequent development of multidrug regimens for childhood acute leukemia and Hodgkin's disease in the 1960s demonstrated that chemotherapy could consistently cure a high percentage of patients with certain chemoresponsive diseases. To appreciate more fully the development of modern chemotherapeutic regimens and their application to treatment of neoplastic diseases, it is necessary to understand principles of cytokinetics and pharmacodynamics.

CYTOKINETICS A primary determinant of malignant transformation is uncontrolled growth. All somatic cells, whether normal or malignant, multiply by cell division through the mitotic cell cycle (Fig. 318-1). The cell cycle is marked by two observable events; during *S-phase* (for synthesis) DNA replication occurs, and during *M-phase* (for mitosis) cellular division into two daughter cells occurs. G_1 (for gap) is the time between the end of mitosis and the start of the next S-phase; G_2 is the time between the completion of S and the

Pyrimidine-analogue antimetabolites The fluorinated pyrimidine 5-*fluorouracil* (5FU) was the result of rational drug design. For cytotoxicity, fluorouracil requires intracellular activation to one of several metabolites. Fluordeoxyuridine monophosphate (FdUMP) is a potent inhibitor of thymidylate synthase, an enzyme necessary for the synthesis of dTTP and ultimately DNA; fluorouridine triphosphate (FUTP) incorporates into RNA and interferes with its processing and function. Fluorodeoxyuridine triphosphate (FdUTP) is incorporated into DNA and eventually leads to DNA strand breakage. The importance of each of these mechanisms to fluorouracil-induced cytotoxicity has not been fully delineated. The interaction of the metabolite FdUMP with thymidylate synthase requires the presence of reduced folates. Studies suggest tumor cells may be deficient in reduced folates, so leucovorin has been administered with fluorouracil in an attempt to increase antitumor activity.

Extensive first-pass hepatic metabolism for fluorouracil has led to direct infusion into the hepatic artery for the treatment of hepatic metastases. The fluorouracil analogue *FUDR* (floxuridine), an inhibitor of thymidylate synthase with reportedly less effect on RNA synthesis than fluorouracil, is also available for intrahepatic infusion.

Like most antimetabolites, fluorouracil toxicity is schedule dependent. With bolus infusion, bone marrow suppression predominates whereas with continuous infusion therapy gastrointestinal toxicity may be more limiting. Fluorouracil has been infrequently associated with a myocardial ischemic syndrome characterized by chest pain, ECG, and isoenzyme changes. Neurologic symptoms, usually reversible, have been reported that include headaches, cerebellar ataxia, and somnolence. Dermatologic complaints are not uncommon and include dermatitis, hyperpigmentation, and skin atrophy. Fluorouracil is used predominantly in gastrointestinal malignancies including colorectal, stomach, esophageal, and pancreatic carcinomas and is widely used in combination therapy in the treatment of breast carcinoma.

Cytarabine is the 2′ epimer of cytidine. Cytarabine accumulates into cells by a carrier-mediated process using the deoxycytidine transport system. It is phosphorylated by a series of three enzymatic reactions to its active metabolite, ara-CTP. Ara-CTP incorporates into DNA and inhibits DNA replication by acting as a chain terminator. Cytarabine can be degraded intracellularly to an inactive compound (ara-U) by cytidine deaminase. The net effect of adequate cellular uptake and a balance between phosphorylation and deamination enzyme activities ultimately determines the cellular toxicity of cytarabine.

In the clinical setting cytarabine use is limited primarily to the treatment of acute myelogenous leukemia. It also has activity in acute lymphocytic leukemia and non-Hodgkin's lymphoma. Cytarabine is usually administered by a continuous 5- to 7-day infusion. High-dose cytarabine is often used in consolidation therapy or in drug refractory leukemia. When administered at low doses, cytarabine may promote myeloid cell differentiation. Intrathecal cytarabine administration is used to treat leukemic or carcinomatous meningitis but may cause chemical arachnoiditis.

When administered as a continuous infusion cytarabine causes profound myelosuppression lasting 14 to 21 days or longer. Gastrointestinal toxicity, including oral mucositis, is frequently observed. High-dose regimens are associated with a syndrome of cholestatic jaundice with elevation of liver transaminases. Cerebellar and cerebral toxicity manifested by ataxia, somnolence, and occasionally coma can be seen in patients on high-dose regimens. Patients with abnormal renal function, elevations of alkaline phosphatase (at least twofold), or age greater than 40 are at increased risk for cytarabine-induced neurotoxicity. Conjunctivitis, preventable by ophthalmic glucocorticoids, is also common with high-dose regimens.

Purine-analogue antimetabolites The thiopurine analogues 6-*mercaptopurine* (6MP) and 6-*thioguanine* (6TG) have a thiol substitution for a carbonyl group in the purine base. They are used in the treatment of acute leukemia and are essentially inactive against solid tumors. Both agents require modification by the enzyme hypoxanthine-

guanine phosphoribosyl transferase (HGPRT) before they can inhibit purine biosynthesis. Patients receiving allopurinol require a 75 percent decrease in mercaptopurine doses since elimination utilizes the enzyme xanthine oxidase, the target for allopurinol inhibition. Hepatotoxicity, consistent with cholestatic jaundice, has been observed with both agents, though it is more common with mercaptopurine. Both agents produce myelosuppression and gastrointestinal toxicity, although the latter is usually mild.

Fludarabine is a fluorinated/phosphorylated derivative of the antiviral agent vidarabine (ara-A) that, unlike vidarabine, is resistant to intracellular deamination. For cytotoxicity fludarabine requires intracellular phosphorylation by the enzyme deoxycytidine kinase to the triphosphate (F-ara-ATP) which incorporates into DNA and inhibits its synthesis. It is currently used in the treatment of chronic lymphocytic leukemia. Clinical studies suggest the drug may have activity in other lymphoid neoplasms. Neurotoxicity appears to be dose-limiting. Approximately 20 percent of patients experience mild, reversible neurotoxicity, although instances of severe irreversible toxicity including coma have been reported. In addition to myelosuppression, fludarabine causes immunosuppression with episodes of serious opportunistic infections documented in some patients. Administration of fludarabine is commonly associated with fevers and chills.

Pentostatin (2′-deoxycoformycin) is a natural product that is an irreversible inhibitor of the enzyme adenosine deaminase. Inhibition of this enzyme, found in particularly high levels in lymphocytes, results in the toxic accumulation of deoxyadenosine nucleotides. Pentostatin is used in treatment of hairy cell leukemia. Its use in other lymphoid malignancies is under investigation. Pentostatin causes profound immunosuppression, especially of T cell–mediated immunity. Myelosuppression otherwise is mild. Renal function impairment has been observed which may be minimized by adequate patient hydration. CNS toxicity including somnolence and coma as well as hepatoxicity with transaminase elevations also have been seen.

Chlorodeoxyadenosine is a purine analogue that inhibits DNA replication. It is used in the treatment of hairy cell leukemia but appears to have activity in other lymphoid and myeloid malignancies. Chlorodeoxyadenosine is both myelosuppressive and immunosuppressive. Other toxicities include mild gastrointestinal toxicity and hepatotoxicity.

Plant alkaloids The plant alkaloids currently comprise three groups: the vinca alkaloids, the taxanes, and the epipodophyllotoxins. The vinca alkaloids *vincristine* and *vinblastine* were originally isolated from the periwinkle plant (*Catharanthus roseus*). Both are active predominately during the M-phase. They exert cytotoxicity by binding to tubulin and inhibiting microtubule assembly. Microtubule assembly and disassembly are tightly controlled cellular processes; interfering with either leads to cytotoxicity. *Paclitaxel* (Taxol), a member of the taxane family, is derived from the Pacific yew (*Taxus brevifolia*). It functions by stabilizing microtubules and thereby preventing their disassembly. The epipodophyllotoxins *etoposide* and *teniposide* are semisynthetic derivatives of the natural product podophyllotoxin derived from the American mandrake plant. They also bind to tubulin but are believed to be cytotoxic through interaction with an enzyme topoisomerase II, capable of producing and repairing DNA-double stranded breaks. Etoposide and teniposide enhance DNA cleavage by inhibiting the reunion activity of topoisomerase II which leads to DNA fragmentation and ultimately cell death.

Neurotoxicity is dose limiting with vincristine. A peripheral sensory neuropathy characterized in its early stages by extremity paresthesias and decreased deep tendon reflexes is commonly observed. With continued use motor neuropathy may ensue and include cranial nerve palsies and extremity weakness. Autonomic neuropathy manifested by constipation is common and ileus can occur. Mild neuropathy generally improves with discontinuation of treatment. Vincristine has been associated with inappropriate secretion of vasopressin (antidiuretic hormone). Vincristine is essentially nonmyelosuppressive, but bone marrow hypoplasia is dose-limiting with vinblastine. Major neurotoxicity is less commonly observed with vinblastine. Mucositis can sometimes be severe, particularly at high doses. Vincristine is active in lymphocytic leukemia, Hodgkin's and non-Hodgkin's lymphomas, and Wilm's tumor. Vinblastine is active in testicular carcinoma, breast carcinoma, Hodgkin's and non-Hodgkin's lymphomas, and lung cancer.

Paclitaxel infusion is frequently associated with hypersensitivity reactions manifested initially by hypotension, bronchospasm, and urticaria. The vehicle in which paclitaxel is dissolved, cremophor EL (polyoxyethylated castor oil), may contribute to this high incidence. Prolonging the infusion time to 24 h and the use of extensive premedication have significantly abrogated this problem. Bradyarrhythmias, especially AV block, atypical chest pain, and rarely more severe cardiac problems have also been associated with paclitaxel infusion. Bone marrow suppression with neutropenia is the dose-limiting toxicity. Peripheral neuropathy with paresthesias in a glove-stocking distribution also is common; the ability to reverse this toxicity with cessation of therapy is unclear. Other toxicities include mucositis, myalgias, and alopecia. Paclitaxel has demonstrated activity in ovarian, breast, and head and neck carcinomas. The efficacy of paclitaxel in other malignancies is an area of intense investigation.

Leukopenia is the dose-limiting toxicity for etoposide and teniposide with white cell nadirs at approximately 14 days. Intravenous administration of either drug can be associated with fever, hypotension, bronchospasm, or rarely anaphylaxis. The incidence of these symptoms, possibly related to the drug vehicle, can be minimized by administering the drug over 1 h. A serious complication reported for both etoposide and teniposide treatment is the development of secondary leukemias. Epipodophyllotoxin-related acute myeloid leukemia appears to evolve within 3 years of receiving the drug and has been associated with cytogenetic abnormalities involving chromosome 11q23. The incidence may exceed 5 percent and appears dose and schedule dependent. The concomitant administration of cisplatin with etoposide also may increase the risk of developing secondary leukemias. Etoposide has activity in lung, testicular, and ovarian carcinomas and in refractory lymphomas and acute leukemias. Teniposide is approved for use as second-line therapy in childhood acute leukemia.

Antitumor antibiotics The antitumor antibiotics are a group of anticancer compounds isolated mainly from soil microorganisms. The anthracyclines have the widest spectrum of activity and are clinically the most important of these drugs.

The commercially available anthracyclines are *doxorubicin, daunorubicin,* and *idarubicin.* In addition, *Epirubicin* is available for clinical use outside of the United States. The anthracyclines are cell-cycle active and phase nonspecific but have pleiotropic actions upon the cell. Although they are classic DNA intercalating agents, their mechanism of cytotoxicity is likely related to interaction with the enzyme topoisomerase II with production of double-stranded DNA breaks. Other data suggest the anthracyclines undergo one- and two-electron reductions generating intracellular free radicals, particularly the hydroxyl radical, which is highly cytotoxic.

The anthracyclines are very myelosuppressive with white cell and platelet count nadirs at 10 to 14 days after treatment. The anthracyclines cause gastrointestinal toxicity including acute nausea and vomiting and mucositis later. These agents are severe vesicants. Extravasation during infusion can lead to local tissue necrosis. In extreme cases skin grafting may be required. The anthracyclines are cleared predominantly by liver metabolism; patients with elevations of serum bilirubin require dose modifications. Long-term administration is limited by cumulative dose-dependent cardiotoxicity. Irreversible cardiomyopathy with serious congestive heart failure is a significant risk in patients who have received doses in excess of 500 to 550 mg/m² of doxorubicin or daunorubicin. Previous chest radiotherapy or concomitant cyclophosphamide therapy may lower a patient's tolerable cumulative dose.

Doxorubicin is one of the most broadly active antitumor agents. It is used in the therapy of breast, bladder, lung, stomach, prostate, and thyroid carcinomas; Hodgkin's and non-Hodgkin's lymphomas;

and bony and soft tissue sarcomas. Daunorubicin has a much narrower range of activity and is used in the treatment of acute myeloid and lymphocytic leukemia. Idarubicin is approved for use in induction therapy for acute myeloid leukemia.

Mitoxantrone, an anthracenedione, is structurally related to the anthracyclines and was developed as a less cardiotoxic alternative to doxorubicin. The drug also appears to interact with topoisomerase II. While the incidence of cardiomyopathy is lower than for doxorubicin, it can still occur. Patients who have received lifetime doses greater than 125 mg/m² are at greatest risk. Complications from tissue extravasation are also less severe than with the anthracyclines. Mitoxantrone also causes marked myelosuppression. In clinical practice, mitoxantrone has not replaced the anthracyclines and is currently used as second-line therapy in breast carcinoma, acute leukemia, and non-Hodgkin's lymphomas.

Bleomycin is a mixture of cytotoxic glycopeptides. Bleomycin simultaneously interacts with the ferrous ion (Fe^{2+}) and DNA, resulting in single- and double-stranded DNA breaks through free radical generation. It is cytotoxic predominantly during the G_2–M phases of the cell cycle. Bleomycin has little myelosuppressive effect. Pulmonary toxicity manifested as a chronic interstitial pneumonitis is the most serious toxicity. Lung injury may initially present with cough, dyspnea, and infiltrates on chest radiograph, and it may ultimately progress to respiratory failure and death. Lifetime cumulative bleomycin dose is recommended not to exceed 200 U/m², less in patients with underlying pulmonary disease, previous chest radiotherapy, or of advanced age. Bleomycin is also associated with dermatologic toxicity characterized by hyperpigmentation and hyperkeratosis. Bleomycin infusion is associated with fever and less commonly hypotension, bronchospasm, and pulmonary edema. A test dose is often administered prior to full-dose therapy. Bleomycin is used in the treatment of Hodgkin's and non-Hodgkin's lymphoma and carcinoma of the testis and of the head and neck.

Mitomycin C is an agent used in the treatment of gastrointestinal malignancies. Mitomycin C is activated intracellularly where it is then capable of cross-linking DNA. Mitomycin C exhibits a delayed myelosuppression with leukocyte and platelet count nadirs at 4 to 6 weeks. Mitomycin C can precipitate progressive renal failure, often in association with microangiopathic anemia. The incidence of this hemolytic-uremic syndrome increases with cumulative mitomycin dose. Mitomycin C is also a severe vesicant.

Dactinomycin binds to DNA and inhibits RNA synthesis. It also appears to interact with the enzyme topoisomerase II. Its activity is limited to treatment of rhabdomyosarcoma, Ewing's sarcoma, and gestational trophoblastic carcinoma. It causes myelosuppressive and gastrointestinal toxicity.

Alkylating agents As a class, alkylating agents are among the most widely used antitumor agents. These drugs lead to inhibition of DNA synthesis by forming covalent bonds with nucleic acids. Most alkylating agents are bifunctional and are efficient at cross-linking DNA with subsequent strand breakage and ultimately cell death. These agents preferentially add alkyl groups to the N-7 of guanine in addition to other nitrogen or oxygen positions in adenine or cytidine. Although alkylation of DNA can occur at any phase of the cycle, cytotoxicity is greatest in those cells that are progressing through the cell cycle. It is most appropriate to regard these agents as cycle active, non-phase specific. The covalent alkylation of DNA is mutagenic and carcinogenic, resulting in long-term serious complications including detrimental effects on spermatogenesis and oogenesis, as well as predisposing to the development of secondary leukemias.

Azospermia resulting from alkylating agent treatment has been found in men receiving therapy for lymphoma and may persist for several years after completing therapy. The severity of gonadal injury appears to be dose dependent. In some men this complication is reversible since previously azospermic patients have subsequently fathered children. Amenorrhea and ovarian atrophy, sometimes permanent, have been associated with alkylating agent therapy in women. The possible resumption of normal menstrual cycles is inversely related to the age of the patient and the cumulative dose received.

Another serious long-term complication of alkylating agent chemotherapy is the development of secondary leukemias. In patients who have received an alkylating agent as part of combination chemotherapy for Hodgkin's or non-Hodgkin's lymphomas, the incidence of secondary acute myeloid leukemia may be as high as 5 to 10 percent. Secondary leukemias have also followed use of alkylating agent therapy for multiple myeloma and ovarian carcinoma. Not all the alkylating agents are equally leukemogenic. For example, melphalan appears to be associated with a higher incidence of secondary acute leukemia then cyclophosphamide when used in the treatment of ovarian carcinoma.

The most common dose-limiting toxicity of the alkylating agents is myelosuppression. The severity and duration varies with the individual drugs. Most of the alkyating agents are quite emetogenic and require extensive premedication. Gastrointestinal epithelial damage however is not prominent. Additional toxicities and activities of the individual agents are presented below.

Mechlorethamine (nitrogen mustard) was the first alkylating agent to receive widespread clinical use. Currently it is used almost exclusively in the therapy of Hodgkin's lymphoma. It has also been used in the treatment of malignant pleural effusions to obliterate the pleural space. Mechlorethamine is highly reactive in aqueous solution and is a severe vesicant. Administration is sometimes associated with minor cholinergic symptoms.

Cyclophosphamide is one of the most widely used broad-spectrum, antitumor agents. It is used in the treatment of carcinoma of the breast, lung, ovary, and bladder; non-Hodgkin's lymphoma; acute and chronic lymphocytic leukemias; soft tissue and bony sarcomas; and tumors of childhood including Wilms' and neuroblastoma. High doses are employed in myeloablative regimens prior to bone marrow transplantation. Cyclophosphamide is active only after microsomal liver metabolism to 4-hydroxycyclophosphamide. It is further metabolized in peripheral tissues to phosphoramide mustard and to acrolein. Cyclophosphamide therapy may be complicated by hemorrhagic cystitis, believed to be due to the metabolite acrolein, which is excreted unchanged in the urine. Adequate hydration with standard-dose therapy, and administration of the bladder protectant *mesna* with high-dose therapy, can help prevent this complication. Upon renal excretion, mesna (mercaptoethane sulfonate) is hydrolyzed to an active form which can complex with and inactivate toxic cyclophosphamide metabolites. Chronic bladder inflammation as a result of cyclophosphamide therapy has been associated with the development of malignant bladder tumors. Cyclophosphamide administration is associated with a syndrome of inappropriate antidiuresis due primarily to a distal renal tubular effect. Cyclophosphamide is also a potent immunosuppressive agent. In very high doses it has been rarely associated with acute myocardial necrosis.

Ifosfamide is a closely related analogue of cyclophosphamide that is less myelosuppressive but more urotoxic. It is usually administered with the uroprotectant agent mesna. Ifosfamide also requires hepatic metabolism for activation. A reversible neurotoxicity manifested as altered mental status can be seen in patients receiving ifosfamide. Currently ifosfamide is used in salvage therapy regimens for testicular carcinoma. Its use in other tumors including sarcoma, lymphoma, and lung carcinoma is under investigation.

Melphalan is a derivative of the amino acid phenylalanine. It has a broad antitumor activity but is used primarily in the treatment of multiple myeloma and ovarian carcinoma. Melphalan does not require hepatic activation and does not cause hemorrhagic cystitis. Melphalan appears to be one of the most leukemogenic alkylating agents. It has rarely been associated with the development of pulmonary fibrosis.

Chlorambucil is structurally related to mechlorethamine. It is available in oral form and is primarily used in the treatment of chronic lymphocytic leukemia and for indolent non-Hodgkin's lymphomas.

Busulfan is toxic to myeloid stem cells. As such it is primarily used in the treatment of myeloproliferative disorders including chronic

myelogenous leukemia and in high-dose myeloablative preparative regimens prior to bone marrow transplantation. Prolonged bone marrow hypoplasia may result even after standard-dose administration. Busulfan therapy is also rarely associated with interstitial pneumonitis and progressive pulmonary fibrosis. The initial clinical symptoms of dry cough and dyspnea on exertion may progress, even with cessation of therapy, to respiratory insufficiency and death. Busulfan treatment is also associated with skin hyperpigmentation.

Thiotepa is an trivalent alkylating agent that currently has a limited clinical role. It is used as second-line therapy in breast and ovarian carcinoma. Thiotepa has a toxicity profile typical of most alkylating agents, although it is generally less emetogenic.

Alkylating agents; nitrosoureas   The nitrosoureas *carmustine* and *lomustine* are a class of alkylating agents distinguished by high lipid solubility with excellent penetration into the central nervous system and activity against CNS neoplasms. The nitrosoureas are also used in salvage regimens for Hodgkin's and non-Hodgkin's lymphoma. The nitrosoureas produce a delayed myelosuppression lasting 4 to 6 weeks and appear to have a cumulative effect on the bone marrow. Patients heavily pretreated with chemotherapy may have protracted cytopenias with a few developing bone marrow aplasia. The nitrosoureas have also been associated with development of secondary leukemias. Moderate, but reversible, elevation of hepatic enzymes is common. A pulmonary fibrosis syndrome, similar to that seen with busulfan, has been reported. Prolonged treatment with the nitrosoureas can result in progressive renal insufficiency, even after cessation of therapy.

Alkylating agents; platinum compounds   The platinum compounds *cisplatin* and *carboplatin* are the only heavy metals approved for use as antitumor agents. Although they are not true alkylating agents, they do ultimately covalently cross-link DNA. Cytotoxicity is determined by the balance between cellular enzymatic repair of damaged DNA and the extent of the DNA cross-links.

Cisplatin produces nephrotoxicity and is toxic to both the proximal and distal tubular epithelial cells. Adequate intravenous hydration with saline diuresis, accompanied by furosemide or mannitol administration, can decrease the incidence of nephrotoxicity. Nausea and vomiting may at times be severe and protracted in patients receiving cisplatin. Sensory neuropathy and high-frequency hearing loss after several cycles of therapy are not uncommon. It produces modest myelosuppression. Cisplatin has significant activity in testicular, ovarian, bladder, head and neck, and lung carcinomas. Carboplatin is a cisplatin analogue that has less nephrotoxicity, is less emetogenic, less ototoxic, but is more myelosuppressive. It has a spectrum of activity similar to cisplatin.

Other agents   *Dacarbazine* appears to exert its cytotoxicity by acting as an alkylating agent and damaging DNA after activation by hepatic microsomal enzymes. Dacarbazine is used in the treatment of melanoma, Hodgkin's disease, and soft tissue sarcomas. It produces moderate myelosuppression. Nausea and vomiting are often severe and persistent.

Procarbazine, a monoamine oxidase inhibitor, was originally developed as an antidepressant and was later discovered to have antitumor activity. It requires oxidation by hepatic enzymes after which it functions like an alkylating agent, methylating nucleic acids. Myelosuppression is moderate but dose limiting. Procarbazine produces neurotoxicity manifested by peripheral sensory neuropathy in addition to changes in mood and mental status. Nausea and vomiting may also be severe. Due to its monoamine oxidase inhibitor activity, tyramine-rich foods and medication such as sympathomimetic amines or tricyclic antidepressants may precipitate a hypertensive crisis and should be avoided. A disulfiram-like effect is also common. Procarbazine can produce gonadal atrophy and may increase the risk for development of secondary leukemias. Procarbazine is used primarily in the treatment of brain tumors and Hodgkin's disease.

L-*Asparaginase* is the only enzyme utilized as an antitumor agent. Lymphocytes have a limited ability to synthesize the amino acid L-asparagine and are dependent on circulating pools to maintain protein synthesis. Asparaginase treatment results in depletion of extracellular pools of asparagine. While this effect is associated with cytotoxicity to lymphocytes, most normal tissues are largely unaffected since they are capable of de novo asparagine synthesis. Asparaginase is used in the treatment of acute lymphocytic leukemia. Asparaginase is associated with hypersensitivity reactions including anaphylaxis or serum sickness in a significant number of patients. Anaphylaxis may occur with the first dose. The effects of inhibiting protein synthesis may lead to hypoalbuminemia, hypoinsulinemia, hyperglycemia, and mental status changes. Thrombosis due to depletion of protein C and protein S and hemorrhage due to depletion of clotting factors have been observed. Hepatotoxicity and pancreatitis are also less commonly observed.

COMBINATION CHEMOTHERAPY Most cancers are treated with multiagent combination chemotherapy. While many regimens have been derived historically by empirical means, there are a series of principles which underlie most combinations of antitumor drugs. Each of the agents within a given regimen should have demonstrated independent activity against the specific tumor. Although unanticipated synergy with other drugs in the regimen may occur, adding an agent that alone produces no responses is likely to add toxicity without benefit. Each of the agents should usually have a different mechanism of action. It is in principle advantageous to target different points along a biochemical pathway. Drugs that either inhibit the same enzyme or damage the same target are less likely to yield additive antitumor activity. Likewise, agents should be non-cross resistant. A drug-resistant tumor subpopulation selected by one agent is unlikely to be cross resistant to an agent that produces cytotoxicity through a completely different mechanism. Finally, each of the drugs should have different dose-limiting toxicities. Administering two agents with the same toxicity profile at the maximal dose of each agent can produce unacceptable toxicity. As a result of these principles, carefully chosen combination regimens should result in an improved rate of tumor cell kill. In addition, the chances of emergence of a drug-resistant clone should decrease and each agent can likely be administered at full dose.

A drug regimen commonly used in the treatment of non-Hodgkin's lymphoma illustrates these points. Treatment with the regimen of cyclophosphamide, doxorubicin, vincristine, and prednisone, often referred to as CHOP [*c*yclophosphamide, *h*ydroxydaunorubicin (doxorubicin), *o*ncovin (vincristine), *p*rednisone] can lead to long-term disease free survival in about 50 percent of patients with diffuse large cell lymphoma. Each of the four agents produces cytotoxicity by a different mechanism in the cell cycle. Cyclophosphamide and doxorubicin are cycle active non-phase specific; vincristine is cycle active M-phase specific; while prednisone is non-cycle active. Each of the agents has independent activity in the treatment of diffuse large cell lymphoma and three of the agents are capable of inducing complete responses when given alone. None of the agents would be expected to exhibit cross resistance, although in reality it does happen (see below). Finally, except with cyclophosphamide and doxorubicin, dose-limiting toxicity is nonoverlapping. In the case of cyclophosphamide and doxorubicin, dose reduction is required to prevent an unacceptable degree of myelosuppression.

While these principles can in theory be used to design new, more effective regimens, there are often great difficulties in applying them in clinical practice. For example, in many of the common solid tumors, such as colorectal carcinoma, few agents demonstrate significant single-agent activity. Furthermore, the exact mechanism of action of many antitumor drugs is not precisely understood. Moreover, agents that are known to exert cytotoxicity by different mechanisms may still be susceptible to common mechanisms of acquired drug resistance. Finally, many of the most active agents have the same dose-limiting factor, myelosuppression, rendering it impossible to use them at their maximally tolerated doses.

High-dose chemotherapy or chemoradiotherapy followed by bone marrow transplantation has been used to overcome myelosuppression. The drugs most useful for transplantation are generally the alkylating agents, such as busulfan and cyclophosphamide, which exhibit a linear response between drug dose and cell kill in vitro. Administering these drugs in myeloablative combination regimens yields improved tumor cytotoxicity. In autologous transplantation, the patient's bone marrow is harvested, cryopreserved, and then reinfused after delivery of systemic high-dose therapy. In allogeneic transplantation, bone marrow from a suitable donor, usually an HLA-compatible sibling, is used to reconstitute the patient's hematopoietic system. Substantial evidence indicates that, in addition to the high-dose preparative regimens, immune effector mechanisms contribute to control of malignant disease after allogeneic bone marrow transplantation. The precise mediators of the so-called graft-versus-tumor effect remain to be elucidated. Transplantation has been most effective in treating tumors that are initially chemoresponsive such as acute leukemia, Hodgkin's and non-Hodgkin's lymphoma, breast carcinoma, and testicular carcinoma. This approach has been ineffective, however, in treating common epithelium-derived malignancies such as non-small cell lung carcinoma and colorectal carcinoma.

COMPLICATIONS Every chemotherapeutic regimen administered in adequate doses will have some deleterious side effect on normal host tissues. Most of the complications can be anticipated and considerable expertise has been gained in treating and if possible preventing these complications. Myelosuppression, nausea and vomiting, stomatitis, and alopecia are the most frequently observed complications associated with chemotherapy administration.

Myelosuppression Chemotherapy-induced bone marrow suppression is the most important complication of therapy and is most often the dose-limiting factor. Myelosuppression, manifested as leukopenia, thrombocytopenia, and anemia, occurs with most chemotherapeutic regimens. The blood counts usually reach their nadir between 10 and 14 days of treatment, with recovery noted by day 21 and a return to normal by day 28. Thus, most chemotherapeutic regimens are administered on 21- to 28-day cycles. However, regimens that contain drugs toxic to myeloid stem cells, such as a nitrosourea, require a longer period of bone marrow recovery and are usually administered every 6 weeks.

Leukopenia, and particularly neutropenia, increases the risk of infectious complications in patients receiving chemotherapy. Fever is the hallmark of infection. Any patient with neutropenia (absolute neutrophil count $<1.0 \times 10^9$ per liter) and fever requires a prompt medical evaluation and subsequent administration of empirical, broad-spectrum parenteral antibiotics. The use of recombinant hematopoietic growth factor support, particularly granulocyte colony stimulating factor and granulocyte-macrophage colony stimulating factor, can shorten the length of neutropenia associated with chemotherapy (see "Biologic therapy," below).

Thrombocytopenia may occur in patients receiving chemotherapy but is less often dose limiting than leukopenia. An increase in a patient's bleeding time can be detected when the platelet count falls below 100×10^9 per liter, but most patients are without symptoms with platelet counts $>50 \times 10^9$ per liter. The risk for a severe hemorrhagic complication, such as spontaneous intracranial bleeding, begins to increase when the platelet count falls below 20×10^9 per liter. Thrombocytopenia to this degree is usually only observed with very intense chemotherapeutic regimens such as those used in the treatment of acute leukemia.

Anemia to some degree is to be anticipated with chemotherapy. However, except with intense chemotherapeutic regimens transfusions are usually not required. In addition, there is no hemoglobin level below which all patients should receive transfusions for chemotherapy-induced anemia. Rather, transfusions should be administered only after considering the long-term goals of therapy and weighing the risk-to-benefit ratio for each patient.

Nausea and vomiting Nausea and vomiting are major side effects of cancer chemotherapy and previously were sufficiently severe that some patients would refuse further chemotherapy treatments. However, significant progress has been made in preventing and treating chemotherapy-induced nausea and vomiting. Progress has resulted from the development of newer and more effective antiemetics, the completion of multiple clinical trials that specifically address the problem, and the education of physicians regarding its prevention and management.

Chemotherapy appears to induce nausea and vomiting through several pathways. Vomiting is controlled by two medullary centers: the vomiting center and the chemoreceptor trigger zone (see Chap. 38). The vomiting center receives input from the chemoreceptor trigger zone and coordinates the process of vomiting through multiple efferent tracts. The chemoreceptor trigger zone is directly stimulated by various toxins or drugs to release neurotransmitters, such as dopamine, which then interact with the vomiting center. The vomiting center also directly receives input from the gastrointestinal tract where appropriate stimuli can induce emesis independent of the chemoreceptor trigger zone. Finally, cerebral input, especially from visual or olfactory stimuli can trigger the vomiting center.

The chemotherapeutic agents are not all equally emetogenic. Cisplatin consistently causes the most severe side effects. Dacarbazine, doxorubicin, and mechlorethamine are also highly emetogenic agents. However several chemotherapeutic drugs, particularly the antimetabolites such as methotrexate or fluorouracil, cause only minimal nausea and vomiting.

Prevention of nausea and vomiting should be a primary goal. Antiemetic regimens always should be given on a routine schedule. Treatment only as needed is generally inappropriate. Antiemetic regimens should err on the side of being too aggressive rather than insufficient, particularly in new patients. They can subsequently be modified if required. They should be commensurate with the emetogenic potential of the particular chemotherapy program. The commonly used antiemetic agents are briefly discussed below.

The phenothiazines such as *prochlorperazine* and *chlorpromazine* are the most widely used antiemetic agents and appear to be useful drugs due to their antidopaminergic and antiserotoninergic activities. They are available in several formulations, making them useful for outpatient regimens. As single agents they are effective for only mildly emetogenic drugs such as fluorouracil.

The benzamide *metoclopramide* appears to antagonize dopamine activity peripherally and centrally. When used parenterally in high doses (1 to 2 mg/kg every 2 to 4 h) it can effectively reduce nausea and vomiting associated with even the most potently emetogenic chemotherapeutic drugs. When used in high doses extrapyramidal side effects are not uncommon, and thus it is often administered with an antihistamine such as diphenhydramine or a benzodiazepine such as lorazepam.

Serotonin antagonists such as *ondansetron* are the newest and possibly the most effective antiemetic agents. Ondansetron appears to selectively block the serotonin receptor 5-HT$_3$ which is present peripherally on the vagus nerve and centrally in the chemoreceptor trigger zone. It is effective in the treatment of nausea and vomiting due to cisplatin but is without the dystonic reactions that may accompany metoclopramide.

The cannabinoid *dronabinol* contains the principal psychoactive agent in marijuana, Δ-9-THC. It is available only in oral formulation and appears to be most effective against mild or moderately emetogenic chemotherapeutic regimens. It produces significant mood alterations including dysphoria in a substantial number of patients and is thus generally reserved for patients not responding to other therapies.

Other miscellaneous agents are frequently employed in combination antiemetic regimens. High-dose glucocorticoids such as dexamethasone are often used for brief intervals, particularly with metoclopramide. Benzodiazepines are useful as sedatives for patients with anticipatory nausea and vomiting and as amnestic agents. Antihistamines have modest antinausea properties but are most useful to prevent dystonic reactions associated with phenothiazines or metoclopramide.

Stomatitis Stomatitis is an inflammation of the oral mucosa and a major complication of cancer chemotherapy. Early signs of stomatitis are erythema and edema which may progress to frank, painful ulcerations that persist for several days to a week or longer. The painful ulcers result in poor oral intake with subsequent dehydration and malnutrition. They also may become secondarily infected and further complicate patient management. Virtually all chemotherapeutic agents will cause stomatitis if given in sufficient dose intensity. With the antimetabolites, duration of exposure is probably a greater risk factor for developing stomatitis than peak drug level.

There currently is no known method to prevent stomatitis except for dose modification of the offending chemotherapeutic agents. Meticulous oral hygiene will help diminish pathogenic oral flora and decrease the risk of developing secondary infections. Treatment with topical oral anesthetics such as viscous xylocaine will relieve pain and help maintain adequate oral intake.

Alopecia Chemotherapy-induced hair loss is one of the most distressing aspects of cancer treatment for some patients and is due to the direct cytotoxic effects of antineoplastic agents on the hair follicle. Hair loss tends to be patchy and most severe on the scalp, usually becoming noticeable 1 to 2 weeks after beginning therapy. After cessation of chemotherapy, hair regrowth begins and should eventually return to pretreatment levels although it may differ in texture and color. Cyclophosphamide, dactinomycin, doxorubicin, paclitaxel, and vincristine generally cause the most profound alopecia. Scalp-cooling devices that apparently decrease scalp perfusion have been employed with mixed results.

DRUG RESISTANCE Tumor cell resistance to chemotherapeutic agents is a central problem in medical oncology. With improvements in supportive care such as a new generation of antimicrobials, multicomponent blood product and hematopoietic growth factor support, specialized oncology nursing, and high-technology intensive care units, drug resistance is probably the single most important obstacle to achieving high rates of curative cancer therapy.

The problem of drug resistance can be conveniently divided into two groups: de novo resistance and acquired resistance. In de novo resistance, tumor cells are initially unresponsive to chemotherapy. This situation unfortunately exists for many of the most common solid tumors. In acquired drug resistance, tumors are initially responsive to chemotherapy but resistance develops with continued therapy. Acquired resistance is a primary reason that only a small percentage of many responsive tumors are curable with chemotherapy.

The appearance of resistant clones within a larger population was addressed initially by Delbruck and Luria studying bacteria and later by Law and then Goldie and Coldman in tumor cells. Delbruck and Luria observed that populations of bacteria exhibited varying degrees of resistance to bacteriophage infection. They showed that resistant cells were present within the population due to spontaneous mutations that existed before exposure to the phage. Development of resistance was dependent on mutation frequency and population size.

The Delbruck-Luria principles were extended to tumor cell biology and treatment. An important property of tumor cells is genomic instability. As a tumor grows from a single transformed cell to a clinically detectable 1-mL mass of 1×10^9 cells, it undergoes spontaneous mutations and contains a heterogeneous population of cells, some of which have mutated to drug resistance purely by chance. Treatment with chemotherapy will eliminate the most sensitive cells, leaving the resistant subclones to grow. Clinically this situation occurs in patients who have responded to therapy, entered a complete remission, only later to relapse with drug-refractory tumors.

These concepts suggest some important principles to maximize chemotherapy effectiveness. Tumors are most likely to be responsive to chemotherapy when small in size prior to the development of multiple resistant subclones. Regimens that are not effective against bulky tumors may be curative when used in the adjuvant setting. Effective treatment should consist of combination chemotherapy containing non-cross resistant agents. The likelihood of two simultaneous mutations in the same cell affording resistance to two different classes of drugs is low, i.e., the product of two independent probabilities. Thus, the greater the number of truly non-cross resistant drugs administered at fully effective dose, the greater the chance of eliminating the entire tumor population.

While the combination chemotherapy concept provides useful predictions, several limitations must be understood. First, many of the antitumor agents, such as the alkylating agents, the anthracyclines, and the epipodophyllotoxins are mutagenic agents. Thus clinical drug refractoriness may result not only from prior spontaneous mutations but also from treatment with mutagenic drugs. Second, many of the antitumor drugs are cross resistant. Although the problem of multidrug resistance has gained increasing attention, much remains to be elucidated. It is clear that anticancer drug cross resistance cannot be anticipated from studies of cytotoxicity mechanisms alone.

Mechanisms of single-agent drug resistance Much of what is known about drug resistance is a result of in vitro studies. Cell lines have been made resistant to various chemotherapeutic agents by gradually selecting them in increasing concentrations of drug. By comparing resistant sublines to the parental cell lines, resistance mechanisms have been discerned. Determining the clinical importance of these in vitro mechanisms has been a slow and difficult process. Examples are given below of specific resistance mechanisms that have been determined for various agents.

DEFECTIVE TRANSPORT Several chemotherapeutic agents are transported into the cell by carrier-mediated uptake utilizing various physiologic transporters. Decreased expression or activity of a specific transporter will lead to decreased drug accumulation in the cell. For example, methotrexate resistance has been associated with loss of a folate transport protein, cytarabine resistance with loss of nucleoside transporter, and mechlorethamine resistance with loss of choline transporter.

DECREASED ACTIVATING ENZYME Some drugs require activation via intracellular biochemical pathways. A decrease in the activity of these pathways will lead to a decreased production of the cytotoxic metabolite. Decreased deoxycytidine kinase activity has been observed with cytarabine resistance, defective polyglutamylation with methotrexate resistance, and diminished HGPRT activity with thioguanine and mercaptopurine resistance.

INCREASED DRUG INACTIVATION Inactivation of cytotoxic drugs or their metabolites can also occur via intracellular biochemical pathways. Increased cytidine deaminase inactivates cytarabine, increased bleomycin hydrolase renders bleomycin inactive, and increased membrane alkaline phosphatase inactivates thioguanine and mercaptopurine.

INCREASE IN TARGET ENZYME When a chemotherapeutic drug targets a specific enzyme, increased expression of the target, often through gene amplification, can be observed. Methotrexate resistance can result from amplification of the dihydrofolate reductase gene, pentostatin resistance from amplification of the adenosine deaminase gene, and FUDR resistance from increased copy number of the thymidylate synthase gene.

ALTERATIONS IN TARGETS Rather than increasing expression of a target enzyme, the target can be structurally altered to diminish the cytotoxic effect of the drug. Tubulin alteration has been noted with vincristine resistance and paclitaxel resistance, thymidylate synthase change has been observed with decreased binding to the fluorouracil metabolite fluorodeoxyuridylate, and altered ribonucleotide reductase has been noted in resistance to hydroxyurea.

Mechanisms of multiple drug resistance The resistance mechanisms discussed above are relatively specific for a given drug. Clinical chemotherapy refractoriness, however, is often characterized by resistance to multiple drugs. The phenomenon of in vitro multidrug resistance was first described in the 1970s by Biedler and by Ling. Cells selected for resistance to one drug demonstrate cross resistance to other structurally and functionally unrelated compounds. The drugs that constitute the multidrug resistance family include the anthracyclines, the vinca alkaloids, the epipodophyllotoxins, and other agents such as dactinomycin and paclitaxel. Multidrug-resistant cells have energy-dependent decreased accumulation of cytotoxic drugs, due apparently to an outward efflux. The resistant cell lines overexpress a membrane glycoprotein of 150 to 180 kDa termed *P-glycoprotein*. The gene that codes for P-glycoprotein has been cloned

and is now recognized to belong to a family of ATP-binding cassette proteins. The human gene responsible for P-glycoprotein–mediated multidrug resistance is called *MDR1*.

P-glycoprotein–mediated efflux can be circumvented by any one of a series of ever-increasing number of reversing agents. These chemosensitizing agents, such as verapamil, quinine, and cyclosporine A, have entered clinical trials in an attempt to overcome multidrug resistance.

P-glycoprotein is expressed in normal tissues with the highest levels found on luminal surfaces such as renal tubules, small and large intestine, and bile canaliculi. The function and transport substrates of P-glycoprotein in these normal tissues remain elusive.

While P-glycoprotein expression is a well-defined mechanism of in vitro drug resistance, its role in clinical drug resistance has yet to be fully defined. Nonuniformity in assessing P-glycoprotein or *MDR1* expression in tumor specimens has led to conflicting results. Few studies compare expression in the same patients prior to therapy and after the acquisition of chemotherapeutic drug resistance. Additionally, studies that have added chemosensitizing agents to preexisting multiagent regimens have generally had marginal results or been inconclusive. In a few tumors, such as acute myeloid leukemia or childhood neuroblastoma, P-glycoprotein expression at presentation may portend a poor prognosis.

Additional mechanisms of in vitro multidrug resistance distinct from P-glycoprotein expression have been characterized. Altered activity and/or expression of the enzyme topoisomerase II has been shown to produce resistance to the anthracyclines, epipodophyllotoxins, and other drugs including dactinomycin and mitoxantrone. Altered topoisomerase activity may also exist in cells that simultaneously exhibit more than one mechanism of multidrug resistance. The clinical significance of topoisomerase II–mediated resistance is unknown.

An enhanced reducing environment with increased activity of glutathione detoxification pathways and elevated cellular pools of reduced glutathione also has been described. Resistance to alkylating agents including the nitrogen mustard derivatives and the nitrosoureas, as well as the anthracyclines, has been associated with increased glutathione detoxification. Buthionine sulfoximine, an agent that depletes cellular glutathione levels, has entered clinical trials as a chemosensitizing agent.

NEW DRUG DEVELOPMENT After the demonstration in the 1940s that some drugs have antitumor effects, the National Cancer Institute began a large-scale drug screening program. From 1955 through 1975 over 400,000 compounds were screened against murine leukemia models P388 and L1210. While many compounds were identified, the discovery of drugs with activity against rodent leukemias did not correlate well with drugs active in the treatment of the major human cancers. The drug screening protocol was then changed to include human tumors transplanted into athymic mice. It was subsequently further modified so that new compounds are now tested against a panel of about 60 human cancer cell lines representing many of the most common solid tumors. Compounds demonstrating in vitro antitumor activity are then tested against a panel of human tumor xenografts in nude mice. Compounds that are still promising then undergo further toxicology screening and formulation testing before beginning clinical trials.

Antitumor agents proceed through a series of clinical trials before they are accepted in widespread clinical use. There are currently three distinct phases of testing. From initial screening to approval by the Federal Drug Administration for a specific indication may take 10 years or longer. Table 318-3 lists some investigational anticancer agents currently in clinical trials.

Phase I trials are performed to determine drug toxicity in humans. To be eligible, patients must have a cancer not responsive to available therapies. An initial dose is chosen based on animal studies. Generally three patients are treated at a given dose before sequential dose escalation. Dose escalation proceeds until a dose-limiting toxicity is reached which defines the maximally tolerated dose. Since phase I trials are composed of relatively small numbers of often heavily

TABLE 318-3 Investigational anticancer drugs

Drug	Category	Mechanism of action
Amifostine (WR-2721)	Aminothiol; cisplatin: toxicity protectant	Scavenges free radicals
Dexrazoxane	Anthracycline: cardioprotectant	Chelates metal ions
Edatrexate	Antifolate	Inhibits dihydrofolate reductase
Irinotecan (CPT-11)	Camptothecin derivative	Inhibits topoisomerase I
Losoxantrone	Anthrapyrazole	Inhibits topoisomerase II
Ormaplatin	Platinum analogue	Cross-links DNA
Oxaliplatin	Platinum analogue	Cross-links DNA
Pirarubicin	Anthracycline	Inhibits topoisomerase II
Piritrexim	Antifolate	Inhibits dihydrofolate reductase
Rhizoxin	Macrocyclic lactone	Inhibits microtubule assembly
Suramin	Polyanion	Modulates growth factors (?)
Taxotere	Taxane	Promotes microtubule assembly
Topotecan	Camptothecin derivative	Inhibits topoisomerase I
Tretinoin (ATRA)	Retinoid	Promotes differentiation
Trimetrexate	Antifolate	Inhibits dihydrofolate reductase
Vinorelbine	Vinca alkaloid	Inhibits microtubule assembly

pretreated patients with diverse tumor types, the lack of tumor response does not preclude an agent from ultimate clinical usefulness.

Phase II trials are designed to determine if a drug has activity in a particular tumor type. Generally small groups of patients with advanced malignancies of a particular tumor type are treated according to a dose and schedule determined from the phase I study. Patients must have measurable tumor masses to assess the efficacy of therapy. A given compound generally undergoes several phase II studies against a broad array of tumor types. After the completion of phase II trials, a decision is made based on the available data whether to proceed to phase III or to abandon further testing.

Phase III studies are designed to test an agent against the standard, existing therapy for a particular tumor. This testing usually requires a randomized, two-arm study. The malignant diseases to be tested are determined from the phase II data. Patients generally have not received prior therapy at the time of treatment. Phase III trials require large numbers of patients and frequently are multi-institutional.

ENDOCRINE THERAPY Endocrine therapy for hormone-responsive malignancies has been utilized for many years. Hormonal therapy depends on the existence of underlying cellular growth control mechanisms derived from the normal tissues from which the tumor arose. Breast carcinoma and prostate carcinoma are the solid tumors most amenable to hormonal manipulation. The presence of estrogen and progesterone receptors in breast carcinoma predicts a response to endocrine therapy. In prostate carcinoma, androgen blockade is the most effective therapy for metastatic disease.

Most of the hormonal antitumor agents are functional agonists or antagonists of the steroid family. Steroid hormones bind to specific intracellular receptors and induce a conformational receptor change. The hormone-receptor complex interacts with DNA and thereby functions as a transcription factor which regulates gene expression.

Adrenocorticosteroids The adrenal steroids have activity in the treatment of lymphocytic leukemias and lymphomas. Because of nonoverlapping toxicities with many chemotherapeutic agents, particularly lack of myelosuppression, they are frequently employed in combination regimens. They function by binding to glucocorticoid-specific receptors present in lymphoid cells and apparently cause programmed cell death or apoptosis. While several synthetic glucocor-

ticoids are available, the most commonly used agents in cancer therapy are *prednisone, methylprednisolone,* and *dexamethasone.* These agents are generally employed in relatively high doses for short periods. The most common toxicities include CNS effects with alterations in mood and personality, and metabolic derangements such as hyperglycemia, hypokalemia, and fluid retention. Suppression of the adrenocortical axis is usually not a problem with short-term administration. Likewise the development of cushingoid features, osteoporosis, and cataract formation is also less of a concern. Glucocorticoids also have been employed for palliative treatment of breast carcinoma. Dexamethasone is commonly used to alleviate intracranial edema often associated with central nervous system neoplasms.

Androgens Androgens such as *fluoxymesterone* are occasionally used in the palliative treatment of breast carcinoma. These synthetic analogues of testosterone are somewhat less virilizing than the naturally occurring hormones. However, hirsutism, weight gain, and deepening of the voice are adverse effects that may not completely reverse themselves after discontinuing therapy. Amenorrhea occurs in many women during therapy. Synthetic androgens can cause hepatotoxicity with elevations of liver function tests.

Antiandrogens The antiandrogen *flutamide* effectively blocks androgen binding to its receptor in peripheral tissues. Although serum testosterone levels may rise, levels in the target tissues are decreased. Flutamide is used in the treatment of disseminated prostate carcinoma. It is often used after orchiectomy or with leuprolide. It has predictable antiandrogen side effects in men, including gynecomastia, decreased libido, and impotence. Elevation of liver function tests also has been reported.

Estrogens Estrogen therapy was once a mainstay in the palliative treatment of disseminated prostate carcinoma. Estrogens are occasionally used in the palliative treatment of breast carcinoma. In prostate carcinoma estrogens appear to function as potent antiandrogens; their mechanism of action in breast carcinoma is not entirely understood. Two commonly used preparations are *diethylstilbestrol* (DES) and *ethinyl estradiol.* Estrogen therapy may exacerbate underlying ischemic heart disease, predispose to thromboembolic phenomena, and lead to fluid retention. Gynecomastia and impotence in men are common.

Antiestrogens The antiestrogen *tamoxifen* is widely used in the therapy of breast carcinoma. It is employed both as an adjuvant in postmenopausal women and as palliative therapy for metastatic disease in both pre- and postmenopausal women. Tamoxifen binds directly to the estrogen receptor and appears to function as a weak agonist/antagonist. It has a long plasma half-life and requires 4 weeks or longer to achieve steady-state levels. Tamoxifen can cause amenorrhea, hot flashes, and occasionally nausea and vomiting. It has been reported to modestly increase the risk of thromboembolic phenomena. Changes in serum lipid profiles also have been noted.

Progestins Progestational agents such as *medroxyprogesterone* or *megestrol acetate* are used in the treatment of endometrial carcinoma and breast carcinoma. Their mechanism of action is unclear; however, studies suggest they may: (1) be directly cytotoxic to tumor cells; (2) disrupt the hypothalamic-pituitary-gonadal axis; (3) alter expression of estrogen receptors; and/or (4) have androgen-like effects. Progestins frequently cause menstrual irregularities. Fluid retention, hepatic enzyme elevations, and thromboembolic events all have been reported.

Aromatase inhibitor *Aminoglutethimide* inhibits several enzymes responsible for the conversion of androgens to estrogens in the peripheral tissues. It also inhibits the conversion of cholesterol to pregnenalone, a key step in steroid hormone biosynthesis. Aminoglutethimide treatment functions as a medical adrenalectomy, and patients receiving relatively high doses may need maintenance hydrocortisone to avoid adrenal insufficiency. It is used in the palliative treatment of metastatic breast carcinoma. Toxicity includes mild neurologic symptoms such as dizziness and ataxia. Lethargy is also frequent. A maculopapular skin rash, common during the first weeks of treatment, usually resolves and does not require discontinuing therapy. On rare occasions there are leukopenia and thrombocytopenia which quickly resolve with cessation of treatment.

Gonadotropin-releasing hormone agonists   The gonadotropin-releasing hormone (GnRH) agonist *leuprolide* is used in the treatment of disseminated prostate carcinoma. Continuous pituitary stimulation by GnRH, normally under pulsatile control, leads to an eventual downregulation of LH and FSH secretion with subsequent diminution of androgen levels. During the first weeks of therapy an initial LH and FSH release may precipitate a worsening of symptoms which may be avoided by instituting antiandrogen treatment. Peripheral edema with worsening of congestive heart failure also have been seen. Antiandrogen effects including gynecomastia, impotence, and hot flashes are seen to a varying degree.

Somatostatin analogues   The somatostatin analogue *octreotide* is used in the symptomatic treatment of patients with metastatic carcinoid or vasoactive intestinal peptide–secreting tumors. Somatostatin analogues suppress release of gastric and pancreatic peptides in addition to suppressing growth hormone release. Patients receiving octreotide experience a dramatic decrease in endocrine-related symptoms such as diarrhea, flushing, and hypoglycemia associated with tumor hormone secretion. The drug must be injected subcutaneously two or three times daily to maintain adequate relief of symptoms. Since somatostatin inhibits insulin secretion, patients must be monitored for hyperglycemia, particularly those with a prior history of impaired glucose tolerance. Other symptoms related to inhibition of normal gastric and pancreatic function such as indigestion, steatorrhea, abdominal pain, nausea, and vomiting also can be seen.

BIOLOGICAL THERAPY   The application of biological agents to the therapy of cancer has been eagerly anticipated by clinicians and investigators. The term *biologic response modifiers* is used to suggest that these agents function by altering the host response to cancer rather than by direct cytotoxicity. Despite much initial enthusiasm, the role of biologic agents in cancer therapy remains limited.

The availability of sufficient quantities of highly purified biologic agents has been possible only through the application of modern techniques in protein biochemistry and molecular biology. The identification and cloning of the genes coding the biologic response modifiers has allowed high-level in vitro expression of these proteins and their subsequent purification. Differences in posttranslational modification of proteins produced by nonhuman systems may result in biologic activity not identical to that of the naturally occurring products.

Assessing clinical usefulness of these agents has often been difficult since the paradigms for cytotoxic chemotherapy are generally inappropriate for biologic agents. The optimal biologic response often does not correlate with maximal tolerated dose. Biologic agents usually demonstrate peak activity within a range; concentrations higher or lower may result in suboptimal effect. Thus the optimal dose clinically is the one which produces the maximum effect, not the highest dose tolerated without unacceptable toxicity.

Monoclonal antibodies   With the development of hybridoma technology, the ability to produce monoclonal antibodies to a specific antigenic determinant led to high expectations for their widespread use in cancer therapy. While monoclonal antibodies have become important tools in cancer diagnostics, their use in cancer therapy has remained investigational. A major difficulty has been defining tumor-specific antigens serologically.

Immunophenotyping of leukemias and lymphomas utilizing monoclonal antibodies directed primarily against myeloid and lymphoid differentiation antigens has improved understanding of the natural history of these diseases and facilitated diagnostics. Immunophenotyping most often confirms the diagnosis determined by histopathology alone. Since it is impossible to determine prospectively which patients will have their diagnosis refined by immunophenotyping, however,

it is now common to immunophenotype all lymphoid and myeloid specimens.

Monoclonal antibodies do not yet have a proven role in cancer therapy, but they are being actively investigated. Antibodies directed against tumor-associated antigens have been conjugated to various drugs, radioisotopes, or toxins and administered to patients. Also, in autologous bone marrow transplantation studies, monoclonal antibodies have been used to purge harvested bone marrow of tumor cells prior to reinfusion.

Cytokines   Cytokines are a group of intercellular messenger proteins that are key immunoregulatory compounds. They comprise the largest group of biologic therapeutics in clinical trials and include the interferons, the interleukins, and the hematopoietic growth factors.

Interferons were the first biologic response modifiers to enter clinical trials. Interferons α and β share a common cellular receptor and are referred to as *type I interferons*. Interferon α is the product of a multigene family of at least 16 members, whereas interferon β is the product of a single gene. Both are produced by a variety of cell types. Type I interferons have immunoregulatory and antiproliferative effects. Recombinant interferon α is approved for use in the treatment of hairy cell leukemia and AIDS-related Kaposi's sarcoma. It also has activity in stable phase chronic myelogenous leukemia, low-grade non-Hodgkin's lymphoma, multiple myeloma, melanoma, and renal cell carcinoma. The potential clinical role of interferon β is under active investigation. Interferon γ, produced by lymphocytes, is referred to as *type II interferon* and has immunomodulatory properties distinct from type I interferons. It appears to have less single-agent antitumor activity than type I interferons. It is approved for use in chronic granulomatous disease but remains investigational as an antitumor agent. All the interferons produce a flu-like syndrome with fever, malaise, myalgias, and fatigue. Modest leukopenia is also common and hepatic transaminase elevations can also be seen.

Interleukins are cytokines that function predominantly as leukocyte messengers. Currently 12 interleukins have been identified, and several have entered clinical trials, but only recombinant interleukin 2 is an approved anticancer agent. Interleukin 2 (IL-2), previously known as T cell growth factor, is a key regulatory hormone in cell-mediated immunity. It stimulates the proliferation of T cells and natural killer (NK) cells and induces lymphokine-activated killer (LAK) cells. The latter, composed predominantly of activated NK cells, can directly lyse freshly isolated solid tumor cells. Studies at the National Cancer Institute demonstrated that infusion of high doses of IL-2 in conjunction with autologous LAK cells (expanded ex vivo) produced responses in metastatic melanoma and renal cell carcinoma. In subsequent trials, IL-2 administration produced a response in a minority of patients with metastatic renal cell carcinoma and melanoma, with a small percentage (5 to 10 percent) of patients achieving complete responses. However, cardiovascular complications were sufficient to warrant intensive care unit management. Multiple other organ system effects, generally reversible with cessation of therapy, including renal, hepatic, pulmonary, neurologic, hematopoietic and dermatologic toxicities, were noted. Subsequent studies have suggested that the use of ex vivo LAK cells may not contribute to the antitumor efficacy. The optimal dose and schedule of IL-2 administration have yet to be determined.

The other interleukins remain investigational agents for cancer therapy. Interleukin 1 activity is encoded by two proteins with minimal structural similarity, IL-1α and IL-1β. In addition a receptor antagonist, IL-1RA, has been identified. IL-1 is an important mediator of the inflammatory response and has pleiotropic biologic activities. Interleukin 3 is a hematopoietic growth factor which stimulates growth and differentiation of early myeloid progenitors and is under investigation in the treatment of myeloid malignancies. Interleukin 4 is a regulator of humoral and cell-mediated immunity, interleukin 5 is a regulator of eosinophilic growth and differentiation, and interleukin 6 has pleiotropic immunohematopoietic effects.

Tumor necrosis factor, composed of two related proteins TNF-α and TNF-β, appears to play a central role in the inflammatory response. In experimental systems, TNF administration causes direct tumor cytotoxicity, probably through the generation of free oxygen radicals. Its pronounced toxicity in humans has severely limited its clinical usefulness.

Hematopoietic growth factors Normal hematopoietic growth and differentiation is under the regulation of hematopoietic growth factors. The clinical use of these growth factors in cancer therapy has been limited mostly to ameliorating chemotherapy-induced myelosuppression. *Erythropoietin* is produced by the kidney and liver in response to hypoxia. It induces erythroid maturation in committed progenitor cells and increases the release of reticulocytes from bone marrow. The primary clinical use of recombinant erythropoietin is in treating deficiency states such as the anemia of chronic renal failure. Its role in supportive cancer therapy is limited.

Granulocyte-macrophage colony stimulating factor (GM-CSF) promotes the differentiation of the committed myeloid progenitor into mature granulocytes, monocytes, and eosinophils. It also stimulates growth of the multilineage hematopoietic stem cell. Recombinant GM-CSF hastens myeloid reconstitution after autologous bone marrow transplantation. GM-CSF administration is associated with fevers, chills, bone pain, myalgias, flushing, hypotension, anorexia, lethargy, and skin eruptions.

Granulocyte colony stimulating factor (G-CSF), stimulates the growth and differentiation of committed, neutrophilic progenitor cells. Administration to patients of recombinant G-CSF can shorten the period of neutropenia associated with chemotherapy-induced myeloid suppression. Preliminary clinical experience suggests G-CSF may be tolerated better than GM-CSF with fewer side effects. Bone pain is the most common complaint. The routine use of these agents in conjunction with chemotherapy regimens that produce significant neutropenia is under active investigation.

BIBLIOGRAPHY

CHABNER BA, COLLINS JM: *Cancer Chemotherapy: Principles and Practice.* Philadelphia, Lippincott, 1990

DEVITA VT et al (eds): *Cancer Principles and Practice of Oncology,* 4th ed. Philadelphia, Lippincott, 1993

HOLLAND JF et al (eds): *Cancer Medicine,* 3rd ed. Philadelphia, Lea and Febiger, 1993

MOOSSA AR et al (eds): *Comprehensive Textbook of Oncology,* 2d ed. Baltimore, Williams and Wilkins, 1991

PIZZO PH: Management of fever in patients with cancer and treatment-induced neutropenia. N Engl J Med 328:1323, 1993

WEISS RB (ed): New antitumor drugs in development. Semin Oncol 19(6):611, 1992

319   BREAST CANCER

I. CRAIG HENDERSON

Breast cancer is both one of the most common and one of the most treatable of all human malignancies. The incidence of this disease provides a poor estimate of the frequency with which breast problems are brought to the attention of physicians of all specialities. For each patient diagnosed with breast cancer, another 5 to 10 women are biopsied for suspicious symptoms, and for each patient biopsied, dozens seek consultation because of symptoms or concern. Breast cancer is one of the few tumors for which there is conclusive evidence that screening will substantially decrease mortality. In the treatment of breast cancer, radical surgical procedures have been almost entirely replaced by more limited forms of surgery, such as the modified radical mastectomy, and most breast cancer patients now have

the option of combining breast-sparing procedures (e.g., partial mastectomy or lumpectomy) with radiation therapy as an alternative to mastectomy. Medical therapies are now an important component of the treatment of almost all stages of invasive breast cancer, and medical interventions to prevent breast cancer are now being studied in randomized trials.

ETIOLOGY AND RISK FACTORS

Epidemiologic data suggest that genetic, endocrine, and environmental factors may be involved in the initiation and/or the promotion of breast cancer growth. Although the principal value of these studies is the identification of etiologic factors that may prove useful in primary prevention programs, epidemiologic data are often used to identify high-risk groups of women to be targeted for intensive surveillance or even prophylactic mastectomy. It has not been established, however, that these strategies will decrease breast cancer mortality in these high-risk groups, and an inappropriate emphasis on risk factors may obscure the fact that 70 to 80 percent of all breast cancers occur in patients without identifiable risk factors.

In the United States, the cumulative lifetime probability of developing breast cancer is 12 percent and of dying from breast cancer, 3.5 percent. Most of the risk of developing breast cancer is expressed after age 50, and the highest risk is after age 75 (Table 319-1). In counseling women regarding their risk of developing breast cancer, the use of 20- to 40-year interval probabilities may be more meaningful than the lifetime probability. For example, the probability of a woman without defined risk factors developing breast cancer between the ages of 50 and 70 is 4.67 percent; that of dying from breast cancer is 1.04 percent. A patient with a relative risk of 3 (e.g., a woman whose mother and sister have been diagnosed with breast cancer) would then have a 14 percent probability of developing breast cancer and a 3.1 percent probability of dying from breast cancer during this interval. This likely explains why no risk group with an observed cumulative incidence of breast cancer in excess of 30 to 40 percent or cumulative mortality in excess of 10 to 20 percent has been identified.

Genetic factors   Although all relatives of breast cancer patients are at some increased risk of developing breast cancer, first-degree relatives (siblings, parents, children) have a two- to threefold increase in risk compared with the general population. Thus the cumulative probability that a 30-year-old woman whose sister or mother had breast cancer will herself develop breast cancer by age 70 is somewhere between 8 and 18 percent. Some investigators have observed an even higher risk when two or more relatives are affected, when the affected patient is premenopausal, or when the patient has bilateral breast cancer, but these observations have not been consistent among epidemiologic studies.

TABLE 319-1   Probability of a white female developing and dying of breast cancer in specified time intervals (1985)

Age interval, years	Risk of developing breast cancer, %	Risk of dying of breast cancer, %
Birth to 110	10.20	3.60
20–30	0.04	0.00
20–40	0.49	0.09
35–45	0.88	0.14
35–55	2.53	0.56
50–60	1.95	0.33
50–70	4.67	1.04
65–75	3.17	0.43
65–85	5.48	1.01

SOURCE: From Seidman et al, CA 35:36, 1985.

As many as 5 percent of all breast cancer patients may have inherited a specific genetic abnormality contributing to the development of their breast cancer. Point mutations of the p53 tumor suppressor gene on chromosome 17 indicate which individuals in Li-Fraumeni families will develop one or more of six different cancers, including breast cancer. Linkage studies also have demonstrated an association between loss of heterozygosity on chromosome 17q and the breast-ovarian cancer syndrome. This gene, BRCA1, is less well characterized, but penetrance may be as high as 85 percent. Possibly as many as 1 in 200 to 400 American women may be carriers. Together these two gene abnormalities account for very few breast cancers, and routine screening for these genetic abnormalities in women without evidence of a very strong family history of breast cancers diagnosed at a very young age is not warranted. However, the recent identification of these genes gives promise that more prevalent genes will eventually be identified in ongoing linkage studies.

Endocrine factors Early age of menarche, late onset of menopause, nulliparity, and late age at first pregnancy appear to be independently associated with an increased incidence of breast cancer. Since both diet and exercise may affect both age of menarche and the regularity of menses, it has been suggested that this effect of diet and exercise may explain, at least in part, variations in breast cancer incidence among women with different life-styles. Age at first full-term pregnancy is a more important determinant of risk than the number of pregnancies. Compared to women with a first pregnancy before age 18, the relative risk of breast cancer is doubled if the first pregnancy is delayed until after age 24 and about quadrupled after age 30. The risk of breast cancer is actually higher among women with their first pregnancies after age 30 than among nulliparous women, suggesting that early pregnancy is protective while late pregnancy promotes development of the disease. These observations are consistent with the hypothesis that events between menarche and the first pregnancy are critical in determining the lifetime probability of developing breast cancer.

In light of the associations between endogenous endocrine factors and breast cancer, one might anticipate that hormone administration, such as estrogen replacement therapy (ERT) for postmenopausal symptoms or oral contraceptives (OC) for birth control, would either induce or promote the growth of breast cancer. Although the results of more than 50 case-control and cohort studies performed to study possible associations have been inconsistent, recently published meta-analyses suggest that any increased risk of breast cancer from using either of these treatments for durations of 5 to 10 years is nonexistent or extremely small. However, more prolonged use of estrogens to alleviate postmenopausal symptoms may be associated with a significant increase in relative risk to the range of 1.3 to 2.2, especially if ERT is begun while the woman is still premenopausal and if stilbestrol, rather than conjugated estrogens, is used. Unopposed estrogen use increases the risk of endometrial cancer, too, but this risk can be alleviated by the concomitant or sequential use of progestins with estrogen replacement therapy. Progestins have not been shown to have a similar beneficial effect in reducing breast cancer risk and may even augment that risk. Oral contraceptive use for periods in excess of 10 years may increase the chance that a woman will develop a cancer before the age of 45, and the use of OCs for durations in excess of 4 years prior to the first full-term pregnancy has been reported to increase the relative risk of breast cancer at an early age to as high as 1.7. The increased risk from the use of ERT or OCs may be greater in women with a history of breast cancer in a first-degree relative, but interactions with other underlying risk factors have not been demonstrated. Traditionally, women with a prior history of breast cancer have not been given estrogen replacement therapy. This policy is now being reexamined, especially among women with a low probability of recurrence from their breast cancer or a high probability of developing osteoporosis. In general, the net benefit from the proper use of either ERT or OCs substantially outweighs any increased risk of dying from cancer in most groups of women.

Environmental factors Studies of atomic bomb blast victims in Hiroshima and Nagasaki demonstrate a radiation dose effect in the induction of breast cancer after a latent period of about 20 years. The highest incidence was observed among women who were aged 10 to 14 at the time of the explosion, and there was almost no increase in breast cancer incidence among women who were aged 30 to 49 at the time.

Breast cancer incidence varies widely around the world, and the highest rates occur in affluent and westernized countries. The lowest incidence is among Asians, but both immigrant and second-generation Japanese women migrating to Hawaii and southern California have an increasing risk of developing breast cancer. The search for environmental factors that might explain this phenomenon has centered on diet, and especially dietary fat. There is an excellent correlation between international variation in dietary fat intake and breast cancer incidence, and rats fed high-fat diets have a greater tendency to develop mammary tumors. However, epidemiologic studies have thus far failed to reproducibly demonstrate an association between dietary fat and the development of breast cancer. Postmenopausal women who are obese have an increased risk of breast cancer. Moderate alcohol intake has been repeatedly shown to be associated with an increased risk of 40 to 60 percent, but the explanation for this is not readily apparent. While points of circumstantial evidence linking environmental factors and breast cancer risk are numerous, none is sufficiently well established to warrant strongly urging women to change their life-style in any particular way. Of course, recommendations to reduce dietary fat content and to maintain ideal body weight may be prudent because of their beneficial effects on other organ systems even if the benefits in reducing the risk of breast cancer are minimal.

BENIGN BREAST DISEASE In general, a woman's risk of subsequently developing breast cancer after a biopsy that demonstrates benign disease is increased relative to the total population of women. The most common histologic diagnosis assigned to these biopsy specimens is "fibrocystic disease," a poorly defined term that implies the presence of macroscopic, fluid-filled cysts and a nonspecific proliferation of epithelial and mesenchymal tissue. This has led many physicians to equate all lumps and irregularities detected on physical examination or mammography with "fibrocystic disease," suggesting that the women examined are at increased risk of developing breast cancer. It has not been demonstrated that women with lumpy breasts who have *not* had a biopsy have an increased risk of breast cancer, and it is estimated that most women (probably more than 80 percent) have at least some irregular tissue densities on examination and/or mammography. For these reasons, the diagnosis of "fibrocystic disease" should not be based on nonhistologic findings, and the term probably should be abandoned by pathologists as well because of its lack of specificity.

The increased risk of breast cancer among women with benign breast disease seems to be confined entirely to that group of women who have histologic evidence of ductal or lobular cell proliferation on biopsy (about 30 percent of all patients biopsied for benign conditions), and especially those who have atypical hyperplasia (about 3 percent of biopsied patients). The relative risk for developing breast cancer in this group is 4.4 times that of an age-matched population of unselected women. In women with both atypical hyperplasia and a first-degree relative with a history of breast cancer, the risk of subsequent breast cancer is increased about ninefold. Such patients are rare (representing about 1 percent of all biopsies for benign disease), and the *observed* cumulative risk of a patient in this very high risk group developing breast cancer over a 25-year period is about 40 percent; the cumulative risk of a woman in this group dying of breast cancer is less than 10 percent. There is attenuation of this risk with time, since most women who go on to develop breast cancer do so within 10 years of a diagnosis of atypical hyperplasia.

IN SITU BREAST CANCER There are two histologically and clinically distinct variants of carcinoma in situ (CIS): ductal and lobular. Traditionally, both were considered the earliest detectable form of malignant transformation in the breast, but increasingly, lobular CIS (or lobular neoplasia) is viewed as a risk factor akin to atypical hyperplasia. Lobular CIS does not form a palpable tumor and is usually found as an incidental finding in a premenopausal woman biopsied for some other condition. Additional biopsies will usually demonstrate additional foci of lobular CIS in the same or even the contralateral breast, and any attempt to totally excise lobular CIS by any method other than mastectomy is likely to be ineffective. Patients who have no further treatment after a diagnosis of lobular CIS have an increased lifetime risk of subsequently developing an invasive breast cancer with either a ductal or a lobular histology. Without treatment, the cumulative incidence of a subsequent breast cancer of any type (invasive or ductal in situ) is about 25 percent and the cumulative mortality somewhat less than 10 percent. Most of these cancers occur after a latent period of 5 to 20 years and occur as often in the contralateral as in the biopsied breast. For this reason, most physicians now routinely offer these patients one of two treatment options: careful observation or bilateral simple mastectomies and breast reconstruction. A patient's choice between these two disparate options is likely to depend on the anxiety generated by her perception of the risk associated with observation.

Ductal CIS (or intraductal carcinoma) may form palpable tumors. It occurs with almost equal frequency in premenopausal and postmenopausal women and is more often confined to one breast, even to one quadrant of the breast. Thus it is possible to excise this type of cancer totally by more limited surgical procedures than mastectomy. Until recently, ductal CIS was uncommon, accounting for only about 1 percent of all cancers diagnosed in the United States. However, ductal CIS is often the cause of microcalcifications seen in mammograms, and because of the increased use of routine mammography it is estimated that ductal CIS constitutes more than 10 percent of all breast cancers now diagnosed in the United States. Because these changes in incidence and mode of diagnosis are recent, it is not certain that the natural history of the ductal CIS now being diagnosed is the same as that observed in earlier eras. The diagnosis of ductal CIS may be difficult. At one extreme, it may be mistaken for atypical hyperplasia, and at the other, microscopic foci of invasion may be overlooked. Electron microscopy will reveal additional areas of invasion, and this may account for the fact that axillary lymph node metastases are seen in 1 to 2 percent of patients with a diagnosis of ductal CIS.

The natural history of ductal CIS in patients treated with less than a mastectomy has been less extensively studied than that of lobular CIS. These patients, too, are at increased risk of developing a subsequent invasive cancer throughout life, but unlike lobular CIS, this risk is more often expressed in the ipsilateral than in the contralateral breast. Until recently, the standard treatment of ductal CIS was simple mastectomy without node dissection, since only 1 to 2 percent of patients so treated die of breast cancer. Now, wide excision alone or with radiotherapy is used in a substantial percentage of patients. There are seven ongoing randomized trials comparing these two treatments; none utilizes mastectomy alone in a control group, reflecting the desire of women to decide for themselves whether they will undergo a breast-sparing procedure and the increasing acceptance by physicians of lesser surgery for this condition. The first of these randomized trials has been published with 4 years of follow-up. Among women randomized to treatment with wide excision alone, 10 percent subsequently developed a noninvasive and 11 percent an invasive cancer in the ipsilateral breast. In contrast, among women randomized to receive wide excision plus radiotherapy, only 5 percent and 3 percent, respectively, developed a noninvasive or invasive cancer. It is too early to assess the relative cancer mortality associated with these therapies, but it is unlikely that they will be significantly different in light of the long-term follow-up results from similar studies of patients with invasive cancer (see below). In addition, it is too early to determine whether these results apply equally to all the histologic subtypes of ductal CIS. Some, such as the cribriform or micropapillary variants, appear to have much less potential for subsequent recurrence than the comedo type. Until further information is available, either wide excision or wide excision plus radiotherapy may be considered for women diagnosed with ductal CIS, especially for women with small tumors who are fully informed as to the uncertainty surrounding our knowledge regarding the optimal treatment of this type of cancer at this time.

Subsequent risk for invasive cancer in the contralateral breast after mastectomy The women with the highest risk of developing breast cancer are those who have already had one breast cancer. The risk is lifelong and occurs at a rate of 0.5 to 1.0 percent per year of follow-up. Concurrent cancers in both breasts are diagnosed in about 4 percent of patients. However, the prognosis of a patient with two breast cancers, whether concurrent or sequential, is not measurably worse than that of a patient with only one breast cancer. Since the cancer with the worst clinical and pathologic stage determines the patient's overall prognosis, patients with a good prognosis after an initial diagnosis should be monitored carefully to detect a second cancer, should it occur, as early as possible.

PREVENTION Patients who received tamoxifen in the randomized adjuvant therapy trials (see below) were observed to have a significantly decreased incidence of contralateral breast cancer compared with that in the control groups for these studies. In addition, significant decreases in death from heart disease were observed, and data from smaller studies suggest that the incidence of osteoporosis may be decreased in postmenopausal women as well. No similar benefits were seen from the use of cytotoxic therapies. On the basis of these observations, large randomized trials evaluating the potential benefits of tamoxifen in women at high risk of developing breast cancer have begun in the United States and Europe. The primary endpoint in these studies is delay or avoidance of breast cancer onset, but the endpoints of greater importance are reduction in overall mortality, mortality from breast cancer, mortality from heart disease, and fractures from osteoporosis. Since there are not even preliminary data to suggest that overall or cause-specific mortality can be reduced by using tamoxifen in otherwise healthy women, and since there are real and potential toxicities from tamoxifen (see below), it is not recommended that this drug be used for this purpose in women not enrolled in these trials.

SCREENING ASYMPTOMATIC PATIENTS

Seven independent, randomized trials have been performed to evaluate periodic screening mammography in asymptomatic women, and these studies have demonstrated unequivocally that this strategy can reduce breast cancer mortality by 20 to 30 percent, especially in women over the age of 50. Nevertheless, substantial controversies regarding the use of screening mammography persist, including its role in women under age 50, the optimal frequency for examinations, and the amount of the benefit that could be achieved with physical examination alone.

Only one of the studies conducted thus far (the HIP trial) has demonstrated a survival advantage for screening women aged 40 to 49, and the survival benefits for this age group in this study were not seen until the second decade of follow-up. This is in marked contrast to older women, for whom the benefits were apparent within the first 5 years. There are many potential explanations for this seeming difference in efficacy among the two groups. For one, it may be an artifact of study design. Most of these trials were not meant to evaluate screening independently in younger women. Breast cancer is much less common before age 50, and a study would need to be proportionately much larger to reliably detect a benefit of 20 percent in this age group. Canadian investigators have recently published the results of a study specifically designed for women aged 40 to 49. More than 50,000 women were enrolled in the trial, but even then, no survival benefits had emerged by the seventh year of follow-up.

To obtain a definitive answer to this question, the British have recently launched a trial that will eventually enroll 200,000 women under the age of 49. The breasts of younger women are more dense than those of older women, and mammography may be less sensitive in the group aged 40 to 49. This was almost certainly true in the older studies, but in more recent studies the percentage of tumors that can be detected by mammography but not by physical examination is nearly the same in younger and older women. Breast cancers in younger women may grow more rapidly than those in older women, and if so, the lead time during which the cancer can be detected by mammography but has not spread to distant organs may be much shorter in younger women. There is substantial evidence both for and against this proposition. However, if this is the case, it certainly does not make sense to recommend mammograms less frequently in younger women, as is done by many groups now. Finally, it is unlikely that all breast cancer subtypes benefit equally from mammography, and among younger women, there may be a relatively small group with an indolent form of the disease that does benefit. If so, this could explain the delayed benefit after more than 10 years of follow-up in the HIP trial.

Even if mammography results in the same proportional reduction in risk of death among younger and older women, the absolute effects will be smaller. The chance that a woman will die of breast cancer is 0.86 percent between the ages 40 and 49 and 1.23 percent between the ages 55 and 65. With yearly mammography, the chance of dying during these age intervals may be reduced to 0.63 percent and 0.93 percent respectively. Thus the cost/benefit ratio will be less favorable among younger women. These costs include not only the expenditure for mammograms but the human suffering associated with a false-positive examination.

Although the major American trials have evaluated yearly mammography, many of the successful trials in other countries have used intervals of 2 or 3 years. It is likely that most of the benefit is achieved if mammograms are repeated every 2 years, with only a marginal increase in benefit with increased frequency, particularly among older women. No one has yet demonstrated a benefit from the use of a baseline mammogram at age 35 or 40, even though many physicians employ this as a "halfway" measure. The American Cancer Society dropped this from their recommendations in 1992. Most of the benefit from the earliest screening trials derived from the physical examination performed at the same time as the mammogram, but another Canadian study published in 1992 suggests that even with modern mammography techniques, much of the benefit might be achieved with physical examination alone.

Recommendations regarding the women to be screened and the frequency of screening vary widely among professional groups and between countries. However, based on the available evidence, the following guidelines appear reasonable:

1 Women aged 50 and over should undergo an annual or biennial screening examination utilizing both mammography and physical examination.
2 Mammography should generally not be used in women under age 40.
3 Women between the ages of 40 and 49 may elect to undergo periodic screening examinations, but they should be informed about the controversies regarding the use of mammography in this age group.
4 It is widely assumed that the benefits of screening are proportional to the patient's risk of developing breast cancer and that patients with a family history of breast cancer, benign breast disease, or those who are nulliparous should be screened at a younger age or more frequently. These assumptions have not been prospectively or retrospectively evaluated in any study, although in many instances such a policy seems reasonable.

Although real, the risk of radiation-induced cancers is very small and is far outweighed by the benefits in women aged 50 or over and probably in those aged 40 to 49 as well. Ultrasound will not detect microcalcifications, often the only indication of tumor and especially of very small tumors. Thermography results in unacceptably high false-positive and false-negative rates and has not even been shown to be helpful in identifying patients who should undergo mammography. Cancers appearing in patients who perform regular (e.g., monthly) breast self-examination (BSE) are, on average, smaller than those in patients who do not do BSE. The only known toxicity of BSE is the increased anxiety it causes some women. However, all published BSE studies have large length and lead-time biases. These biases occur because apparent survival advantages for patients whose cancers have been found by BSE may be due to a longer clinical observation period from diagnosis to death or to the fact that slower-growing tumors are more often detected by BSE and not due to any improved efficacy of therapy, because the tumor was diagnosed before the onset of metastasis when it is theoretically more curable. It has not yet been shown in properly controlled trials that BSE will actually decrease breast cancer mortality.

DIAGNOSIS AND INITIAL EVALUATION

More than 80 percent of cancers are diagnosed because of a suspicious mass, usually a mass found by the patient. Pain without an immediately apparent mass is a less frequent presenting symptom, and increasingly, breast cancer is being diagnosed on a routine mammogram in a totally asymptomatic patient. Nipple discharge is also an unusual presenting symptom. Most nipple discharges, whether serous or sanguineous, are caused by benign disorders, most commonly an intraductal papilloma. A nipple discharge with a negative test for hemoglobin is almost always benign, but breast cancer is the cause of a hemoglobin-positive discharge in less than 10 percent of such patients.

Physical examination should begin with a visual inspection of the breast while the patient is sitting. An underlying breast cancer may cause a protrusion, asymmetry in breast contour, or a subtle dimpling of the skin due to entrapment of Cooper's ligaments. Recent onset of nipple inversion also may be a sign of breast cancer, but both nipple inversion and asymmetry of breast size are common findings in the normal breast. Palpation of the breast is best performed when the patient is in a supine position. Breast cancers are most often described as irregularly shaped, firm or hard, painless nodules or masses, but in fact they may be of almost any shape or consistency. For this reason, any mass or thickening that is distinctly different from the surrounding tissue (i.e., any "dominant" lesion) should be evaluated more carefully. The most common nonmalignant finding on breast examination is a diffuse, indistinct, and somewhat elastic amalgamation of lumps often mistakenly referred to as "fibrocystic disease" (see above). Well-defined cysts may be quite distinct like a breast cancer, but they have a more elastic character than breast cancer. Benign fibroadenomas are often as firm as breast cancer but can be distinguished by their marble-like smoothness and slippery quality, their appearance in young women, and their recurrent nature. Fat necrosis and sclerosing adenosis, both benign conditions, usually can be distinguished from breast cancer only by biopsy. If there are signs of more locally advanced growth, mastectomy and/or radiotherapy are unlikely to substantially prolong a patient's life. These signs include fixation of the mass to the skin, the pectoralis muscle, or the chest wall; the presence of satellite skin nodules or ulcerations; the finding of matted axillary nodes; or the presence of any supraclavicular lymph nodes. Plugging of the dermal lymphatics will cause skin thickening and exaggeration of the usual skin markings, a process termed *peau d'orange*. When this is extensive and accompanied by inflammation, the patient usually has inflammatory breast cancer, a particularly virulent form of cancer best treated initially with chemotherapy and radiotherapy. Inflammatory breast cancer may be mistakenly diagnosed initially as mastitis, but infections or other inflammatory conditions of the breast are rare except in the first months postpartum or after trauma.

Further evaluation of a suspected cyst might include a repeat examination of the breast immediately following the next menstrual

FIGURE 319-1 Focal compression mammogram shows a clinically occult 1-cm spiculated mass. Biopsy demonstrated infiltrating ductal breast cancer. *(Courtesy of Dr Paul Stomper.)*

period in a premenopausal woman, the use of ultrasound to confirm the impression that the mass is fluid-filled, or removal of the cyst fluid with a fine-gauge needle *and reexamination of the breast immediately and again some weeks later to document that the cyst has disappeared.* The latter is the preferred approach in a symptomatic patient because it will usually relieve the pain and the patient will be reassured that this is not cancer, unless the cyst fluid is grossly bloody or reaccumulates rapidly.

Mammography   If breast examination leads to any suspicion that a mass is malignant, biopsy should be performed. Biopsy should be *preceded* by a mammogram, which may better define the extent of the lesion, demonstrate other suspicious masses, and serve as a baseline obtained before distortion of normal breast architecture by biopsy. Abnormalities on mammogram that suggest a breast cancer include (1) distinct, irregular, often crablike densities (Fig. 319-1), (2) *clusters* of five or more microcalcifications, each less than 1 mm in diameter and all in an area of less than 1 cm (Fig. 319-2), or (3) architectural distortion without a benign explanation such as a scar from a prior biopsy. Although more than 80 percent of suspicious microcalcifications are benign, cancers associated with such microcalcifications are usually the most curable of all breast cancers. Diagnosis can be made by radiologic placement of needles under local anesthesia

FIGURE 319-2 Mammogram shows a clinically occult 1-cm cluster of microcalcifications. Biopsy demonstrated infiltrating ductal breast cancer. *(Courtesy of Dr Paul Stomper.)*

and subsequent biopsy of tissue surrounding the needle ends. The excised tissue should be x-rayed to ensure that the calcifications or other suspicious lesions have been removed, and/or the patient should have a repeat mammogram 4 to 6 weeks after biopsy when the breast is no longer tender.

In almost all instances, incisional or excisional biopsy of the breast may be performed under local anesthesia in a day surgery or an outpatient clinic, thus avoiding the additional risk of general anesthesia and permitting the patient to discuss and adjust to treatment options before undergoing definitive surgical treatment. Fine-needle aspiration and cytologic evaluation also may be diagnostic but are advisable *only* if an experienced cytologist is available and if all suspicious lesions read as negative are followed with a more definitive biopsy procedure. Tissue should be sent routinely for assay of estrogen and progesterone receptors. Additional staging procedures immediately following the diagnosis of breast cancer should include evaluation of those sites to which breast cancer most frequently metastasizes (see below).

NATURAL HISTORY AND PROGNOSTIC FACTORS

The natural history of breast cancer is characterized by long duration and marked heterogeneity. The median survival of patients who refuse all forms of treatment is between 2.5 and 3 years, but the survival of an untreated patient may exceed 20 years. Breast cancer is certainly among the more slowly growing tumors, and it has been estimated that the average tumor doubles about three times per year. If this applies to the preclinical (or prediagnostic) period of tumor growth, then the average breast cancer requires 10 years or more to grow from a single cell to 1 cm, the size at which it can be readily detected by most patients or physicians. Presumably, metastases may occur during much of this preclinical period but likely with greatest frequency during the last 3 to 4 years of preclinical growth, when the tumor mass increases from 10^6 cells to more than 10^9 cells. Microscopic or clinically undetectable micrometastases are well established by the time of diagnosis in a substantial percentage of breast cancer patients. If these patients are treated with local therapy only (i.e., surgery and/or radiotherapy), they will eventually die despite excellent local control of their disease. Because many patients' tumors metastasize late in the preclinical course, early detection with mammography will increase the survival of these patients. Because the growth rate of the disease is so variable, comparisons of treatment effects in even well-defined patient cohorts are often misleading, and large, randomized controlled trials should be used to evaluate all important treatment questions.

Clinical pathologic staging   Clinical staging systems were developed by surgeons to identify *preoperatively* those patients unlikely to benefit from treatment with mastectomy. Although those with large tumor size and palpable axillary adenopathy were found to have a poorer long-term prognosis, the only patients categorically discouraged from undergoing mastectomy were those with signs of locally advanced disease (see above). About 25 to 35 percent of patients with axillary adenopathy will have no histologic evidence of tumor in lymph nodes, and the same percentage of patients without adenopathy *will* have histologic node involvement. Although information on histologic node involvement is of no value in deciding whether a patient should undergo mastectomy, this has proven to be the most accurate and reproducible prognostic factor worldwide. It is convenient to divide patients into three groups: those without node involvement, those with one to three positive nodes, or those with four or more positive nodes (Table 319-2). However, these divisions are arbitrary. A substantial number of node-negative patients will have recurrences and eventually die of breast cancer. Each additional positive node is associated with a worse prognosis, but some patients with more than 10 positive nodes will survive for 10 to 20 years or more. In general, the number of positive lymph nodes correlates with the time of recurrence as well as the probability of recurrence. For the data set

TABLE 319-2   Ten-year survival and survival without recurrence relative to histologic node status at the time of radical mastectomy (no adjuvant systemic therapy given)

Node category	Survival, %	
	Overall	Without recurrence
All patients	60	47
Nodes negative	82	72
Nodes positive	40	25
1–3 nodes positive	54	34
4+ nodes positive	26	16

SOURCE: From Valagussa et al, CA 41:1170, 1978.

shown in Table 319-2, the median time to recurrence was 2.1 years, and the time to death was 4 years for the patients with four or more positive nodes, compared with 4.1 years and more than 10 years, respectively, for those with one to three positive nodes. The hazard of recurrence decreased in all nodal subgroups after the first 3 years but remained fairly constant thereafter. This explains why the effects of therapy on recurrence rate, especially on recurrence in patients with many positive nodes, are apparent after a short follow-up, but the effects of therapy on survival may require much longer follow-up.

Patients with a larger breast mass or a higher clinical stage are more likely to have positive nodes, but within a single-node category the size of the breast cancer has independent prognostic value. This has led to the promulgation of staging systems that combine clinical and pathologic characteristics. However, these systems have changed so frequently and are used so differently by different specialists that the categorization of patients into one of four "stages" has lost all practical meaning. For example, a 3-cm tumor mass and no histologically involved lymph nodes is considered a stage II breast cancer, as is a 1-cm mass with eight positive nodes. Both the prognosis and the likely treatment of these two patients are substantially different. Therefore, a careful description of the patient's cancer, a precise measurement of tumor size, and a simple statement of the number of histologically positive lymph nodes will provide a more accurate description of "stage" than the use of stage numbers I to IV.

Histologic subtypes   More than 80 percent of breast cancers are of the invasive ductal type. The next most common variety , infiltrating lobular, constitutes almost 10 percent of all cancers and has the same prognosis as infiltrating ductal carcinoma. Medullary carcinoma, representing about 5 percent of breast cancers, is less likely to metastasize to regional lymph nodes, but the prognosis of medullary cancers with nodal metastases is the same as that of the other major histologic groups with nodal metastases. The large number of histologic types that make up the remaining 5 percent of breast cancers are generally less malignant.

Tumor grade, defined by the degree of differentiation of cytoplasmic or nuclear features, has been shown repeatedly to correlate with the probability of recurrence or death from breast cancer. Other histologic characteristics that may be important include blood vessel or intramammary lymphatic vessel invasion, mitotic frequency, lymph node sinus histiocytosis, and tumor necrosis. However, the major limitation in the use of tumor histologic features is a lack of reproducibility from one pathologist to another, especially when the pathologist has not been specifically trained and is not very experienced in the use of these grading systems. For this reason, tumor grade is not a very reliable tool for making therapeutic decisions.

Estrogen receptors   Tumors with an estrogen or progesterone receptor (ER or PR) are more likely to respond to endocrine therapy used either as an adjuvant to local therapies soon after diagnosis or as a means of palliating metastatic disease symptoms later in a patient's course. Most studies have demonstrated a significantly better disease-free survival and/or overall survival during the first 10 years of follow-up for patients who have one of these receptors. However,

neither the estrogen nor the progesterone receptor identifies the 20 to 30 percent of node-negative patients likely to have recurrence, and at the end of 5 years, the difference in the recurrence rate among estrogen receptor–positive and –negative patients who are also node-negative is only about 5 percent.

Newer prognostic factors   The percentage of tumor cells undergoing mitosis has been shown in a number of experimental systems to be proportional to the growth fraction (i.e., the percentage of the tumor actually growing at any one point in time) and hence to the growth rate. This growth fraction can be estimated by thymidine labeling and autoradiography to obtain a thymidine labeling index (TLI) or by flow cytometry to estimate the fraction of cells in S phase (SPF). Clinical correlations have shown that a high TLI or high SPF is associated with early relapse and earlier breast cancer death, even after correction for other prognostic factors, such as lymph node and estrogen receptor status. In general, patients with aneuploid tumors or a DNA index greater than unity will have a worse prognosis than patients with predominantly diploid tumors, but early differences in relapse rate are not large, especially among node-negative patients.

Increased levels of growth factors or receptors for growth factors also reflect increased mitotic activity, and several of these have been shown to have prognostic value. The epidermal growth factor receptor (EGFR) has been studied most extensively, and increased levels have been shown to be associated with a shorter time to relapse after initial treatment and a lower likelihood of responding to hormone therapy, even in patients whose tumors are ER-positive. Insulin-like growth factor receptor (IGF-R), somatostatin receptor (SS-R), and tumor growth factor alpha (TGFα) levels are other growth factors or growth factor receptors with prognostic value, although their value relative to other prognostic factors is not yet known.

Cathepsin D, urokinase-plasminogen activator, the products of the gene *nm23,* and adhesion molecules are all thought to be associated with invasion and/or the metastatic process. Angiogenesis is also critical to the continued growth and spread of breast cancer, and there is considerable evidence that angiogenesis factors secreted by the tumor, such as basic fibroblast growth factor (bFGF), are important in this process. Tumor levels of all theses factors have been reported to be increased in patients who relapse early or who have other poor prognostic findings, and in some centers, counts of vessels stained with factor VIII or CD31 are routinely made on newly diagnosed breast cancer.

Multiple genetic alterations have been described in breast cancers, including allelic deletions on chromosome 11 or 13 and amplification of the c-*myc* and *int*-2 genes. As described above, the tumor suppressor gene p53 is mutated in some families at high risk of developing breast cancer, but overexpression of p53 product in breast tumors has been shown to be associated with a worse prognosis as well. However, the most extensively studied is the HER-2/*neu* (or c-*erb*B-2) gene. Both amplification and overexpression of this gene on chromosome 17 are associated with a worse prognosis. This is not too suprising, however, since the HER-2/*neu* ligand and receptor are closely related to EGF and EGFR. Another possible explanation for the poor prognosis of patients with overexpression of HER-2/*neu* may be related to the observation that these patients have tumors relatively resistant to some forms of chemotherapy; ironically, they may have an increased responsiveness to others, especially regimens that include doxorubicin. These studies are the first to identify a specific factor associated with response to chemotherapy.

Before a marker is used routinely in clinical practice, the assay method(s) should be validated in more than one center, the cutoff values defining a poor or good prognostic group should be confirmed using more than one data set, the factor's value relative to other prognostic tests should be established by multivariant analyses, and the size of differences in the disease-free and overall survival of patients in poor and good prognostic categories should be determined in a prospective study with adequate sample size and appropriate patient populations. None of these newer prognostic factors, including TLI, SPF, and ploidy, fulfill all these criteria. Their inappropriate use may, in fact, result in inappropriate treatment or increased patient suffering, since a patient may erroneously conclude that her prognosis is much worse than it really is.

LOCAL THERAPY OF OPERABLE BREAST CANCER

Breast cancers are usually considered "operable" if it is technically possible to remove all cancerous tissue, if the tumor does not involve or has not become fixed to skin or structures deep to the breast, and if the tumor has not metastasized beyond the axillary or internal mammary lymph nodes. It has been demonstrated repeatedly in randomized clinical trials that more extensive surgical procedures will reduce the subsequent likelihood of tumor recurrence on the chest wall, in any remaining breast tissue, or in the nodal areas. However, these trials have failed to demonstrate that the type of surgery used will significantly affect patient survival. The evidence that local therapy has any effect on patient survival comes from the randomized trials of screening mammography (see above), in which it has been demonstrated that early mastectomy results in a lower breast cancer mortality than late mastectomy.

The most extensive surgical procedure is the *radical mastectomy,* in which the breast is removed along with the pectoralis major and minor muscles and some overlying skin (at least 4 cm on each side of the tumor biopsy site), and there is an en bloc resection of all axillary contents, including lymph nodes beyond the subclavian vein. Because of the large cosmetic defect resulting from this procedure, it is not commonly used today, and it is doubtful whether its use is ever indicated, since the same or better local control of disease can be achieved with the use of radiotherapy added to less extensive surgical procedures. Most forms of the modified radical mastectomy leave the pectoralis major muscle intact, require the removal of less skin, and usually involve a less extensive node dissection. A *simple* or *total mastectomy* is the removal of the breast and a small amount of skin. A simple mastectomy with node dissection approximates a modified radical mastectomy. Breast-conserving surgical procedures include wide excision, lumpectomy or tylectomy (Greek *tylos* = "lump"), segmental mastectomy, and quadrantectomy. These all require removal of the mass along with some normal surrounding tissue and differ only in the extent of the tissue excised. A separate incision of either a "sampling" of lymph nodes or a more complete lymph node dissection is possible with all of these procedures.

Radiotherapy When administered after a mastectomy, radiotherapy is usually referred to as *adjuvant,* while radiotherapy given after breast-conserving surgery is often called *primary.* Adjuvant radiotherapy is used less commonly now than it once was because it was not possible to demonstrate in multiple randomized trials that its use prolonged survival. In addition, a small but statistically significant increase in mortality from second tumors and/or cardiovascular disease has been reported in patients who survived more than 10 to 15 years after receiving adjuvant radiotherapy. However, this finding was observed primarily in patients treated with now-outdated radiotherapy techniques.

When breast-conserving therapy is used, the resection margins ideally should be microscopically free of tumor before radiotherapy is given. Usually 4500 to 5000 cGy is administered in divided fractions over about 5 weeks. The same doses of radiotherapy may be administered to the axillary, supraclavicular, and internal mammary nodes, and a boost of 1600 to 1800 cGy may be added to the tumor bed. The treatment of axillary nodal areas and the use of a boost are variable and depend on the tumor characteristics of an individual patient and the treatment philosophy of the radiotherapist. When all areas are treated, primary radiotherapy is as extensive as the radical mastectomy, and local tumor control is as good or better.

The choice between breast-conserving surgery plus radiotherapy and mastectomy will depend on the patient's assessment of the relative benefits and side effects associated with each procedure. The only real advantage of breast-conserving procedures is the greater sense of body integrity and improved cosmesis that may result. This advantage may be lost if the tumor mass is large relative to the size of the breast, thus necessitating almost total removal of the breast to obtain tumor-free margins. Under the best of circumstances, the cosmetic results of limited surgery plus radiotherapy are excellent, and the treated breast may feel entirely normal and appear indistinguishable from the contralateral breast. More often the treated breast will be somewhat smaller with limited induration around the biopsy site; uncommonly (in less than 5 percent of patients) there will be marked induration, breast shrinkage, and distortion of normal breast architecture. Other complications from radiotherapy, including broken bones, brachial plexopathy, and pneumonitis, are uncommon and rarely either cause symptoms or are the source of more than transient symptomatology. There may be a subgroup of patients who have a relatively high recurrence rate (23 percent by the end of 5 years) if treated with breast-conserving surgery and radiotherapy. The histologic appearance of the tumors in these patients is characterized by extensive intraductal carcinoma in *both* the area of invasive carcinoma and adjacent tissues ostensibly free of invasive carcinoma. Although a small intraductal component in an invasive carcinoma is normal, the intraductal component comprises more than 25 percent of all tumor tissue in these patients and appears to be a marker of a tumor likely to be multifocal throughout the breast. Very limited data suggest that patients who have recurrences some years after initial surgery and radiotherapy with tumor confined entirely to the breast or breast and regional lymph nodes may be treated successfully with a secondary mastectomy and that this type of recurrence may not compromise survival.

Breast-conserving surgery *without* radiotherapy is generally not used because of the very high likelihood of local recurrence. In the only randomized trial addressing this issue, patients with tumor-free resection margins who were treated with segmental mastectomy alone had a local recurrence rate of 43 percent by the end of 9 years, compared with 12 percent for patients treated with segmental mastectomy plus radiotherapy. However, the survival of patients in these two groups is not significantly different.

Breast reconstruction Many patients will prefer mastectomy because it requires a shorter period of initial treatment and provides the patient with an added assurance that "all the tumor has been removed." Psychological studies demonstrate that most mastectomy patients have fully recovered from the initial emotional trauma of mastectomy by the end of 1 year. Many patients feel that their lives are simplified and their sense of body integrity restored by surgical reconstruction of the breast. This may be performed at the time of mastectomy or many years later. The procedures used include simple placement of a submuscular (or less commonly, subcutaneous) saline-filled or silicone implant, the use of a tissue expander followed by saline-filled or silicone implant, the transposition of muscle and blood supply from either the back of the abdomen using the latissimus dorsi or the lower rectus abdominis muscle (TRAM flap), or the creation of a free tissue flap using the gluteus maximus muscle anastomosed to the internal mammary vessels. The choice among these procedures will depend on the extent of the patient's prior surgery and radiotherapy, the patient's willingness to undergo additional surgical procedures, and the experience and philosophy of the plastic surgeon. Under the best of circumstances, the reconstructed breast will appear to be exactly the same size and shape as the contralateral breast, but in addition to reconstruction of a nipple, this may require mammoplasty on the contralateral breast and several surgical procedures. There are anecdotal reports of collagen-vascular disease, second cancers, or failure to diagnose a cancer by mammography in an augmented breast, and because of this, the Food and Drug Administration has restricted the use of silicone implants for augmentation mammoplasty but not for reconstruction after a cancer operation. Case-control studies of breast cancer patients with silicone implants have failed to show an increased incidence of second cancers, and it is likely that such a risk, if real, is extremely small.

Node dissection The main purpose of lymph node dissection is diagnostic, not therapeutic (see above). However, the morbidity associated with the treatment of lymph nodes is greater than with any other aspect of local therapy. Even with a limited node sampling, the patient often will complain of lifelong discomfort, hyperesthesia or hypalgesia, and/or a sense of pulling and contraction. When more extensive surgery is used, when the radiotherapy field includes the upper axilla, and especially when both modalities are used, these symptoms increase in frequency and severity. Patients may experience edema of the arm and hand, and on rare occasions the patient may totally lose use of the involved extremity. For this reason, a full node dissection, as employed in the radical mastectomy, followed by radiotherapy, is usually contraindicated, and whenever possible, surgical excision should be limited to lower nodes and radiotherapy to this area avoided altogether.

Summary recommendations for local therapy All patients with invasive operable breast cancer should receive some form of local therapy. In most cases this will be either a modified radical mastectomy (simple mastectomy plus node dissection) or breast-conserving surgery and limited node dissection followed by radiotherapy to the breast. Ideally, the patient will participate in the choice between these treatment alternatives and will see both a surgeon and a radiotherapist in the process of self-education regarding the benefits and limitations of these approaches.

ADJUVANT SYSTEMIC THERAPY

Patients die from breast cancer because of metastases that could not be detected by currently available tests but that occurred months to years prior to the diagnosis and treatment of the local disease. There is no evidence that patients who die of breast cancer live any longer as a result of the local therapy. The patient is either cured or dies at about the same time she would have died without mastectomy or radiotherapy. For this reason, it makes sense that systemic therapies capable of reducing the size of these distant metastatic deposits may prolong the patient's survival. Further, some survival advantage may accrue to the patient even if she is not cured.

This hypothesis has been proven by multiple randomized trials in which thousands of women with operable breast cancer received either local treatment alone or local treatment followed by some form of systemic therapy. These systemic therapies, usually given immediately after or as an "adjuvant" to local treatment, include chemotherapy, tamoxifen, and ovarian ablation. Several meta-analyses or overviews of these trial results have been performed, providing a very accurate estimate of the benefits that might be expected from the use of these therapies in routine clinical practice. Most of the statistics that follow are taken from the overview published in 1992.

Among women aged 50 and older, 90 percent of whom were postmenopausal, the reduction in the odds of recurrence and death as a result of adjuvant tamoxifen use was 20 ± 2 percent and 19 ± 3 percent, respectively, during the first 10 years of follow-up. The benefits of tamoxifen were larger when the analysis was limited to those studies which used at least 2 years of tamoxifen. In an analysis of the chemotherapy trials using the most effective chemotherapy regimens (see below), the reduction in the odds of recurrence and death was 22 ± 3 percent and 14 ± 5 percent, respectively.

Among women less than age 50, most of whom were premenopausal, chemotherapy reduced the odds of recurrence and death by 37 ± 5 percent and 27 ± 6 percent, respectively. Adjuvant ovarian ablation reduced the odds of recurrence by 30 ± 9 percent and of death by 28 ± 9 percent. Among these younger women, adjuvant tamoxifen appeared to be less effective than either of these, with odds reductions of 27 ± 7 percent and 17 ± 10 percent, respectively.

Indirect comparison of these trial results suggests that tamoxifen is more effective than chemotherapy among older women without ovarian function. Chemotherapy suppresses ovarian function in premenopausal women, often inducing a permanent menopause. Taken together, these observations suggest that much of the benefit from adjuvant chemotherapy might be mediated through its effect on the ovary, and it would be reasonable to consider ovarian ablation as an alternative to adjuvant chemotherapy. However, a more appropriate response to these observations would be to perform a randomized trial or direct comparison of these two forms of adjuvant treatment, especially since only about 800 women were included in the ovarian ablation trials, all of which were conducted two to four decades ago. If either chemotherapy or ovarian ablation were 20 to 30 percent better than the other, it would not be possible to detect this difference using the available information.

Using trial results to make decisions about individual patients The effects of treatment may be expressed as either a proportional reduction in the odds of recurrence or death or an absolute difference in the survival of patients randomized to one or the other therapy at a single point in time. In general, the proportional effects will be constant among patients in different risk categories, while the absolute benefits of therapy will be greatest among patients with the highest risk. To better understand this, consider, for example, a trial in which 200 patients are randomized, 100 to each treatment arm of a study. At the end of 5 years of follow-up, 40 patients have died in arm A and 30 patients in arm B. The absolute difference in survival at the end of 5 years is 10 percent (70 percent in arm B minus 60 percent in arm A), but the proportional reduction in mortality is 25 percent (40 deaths expected in arm B if the therapy had no effect minus the 30 deaths actually observed divided by 40). In a second trial with 200 patients, 8 patients have died in arm A and 6 patients in arm B at the end of 5 years. In this case, the absolute difference in survival will be only 2 percent, but the proportional reduction in the odds of death will still be 25 percent.

This example correlates well with the actual results of the adjuvant therapy trials. A 25 percent reduction in the annual odds of death results in an absolute difference in survival of 10 percent at 10 years in patients with histologically positive lymph nodes. This size benefit might be expected from the use of adjuvant chemotherapy or ovarian ablation in premenopausal women or adjuvant tamoxifen in postmenopausal women. However, a 25 percent reduction in the annual odds of death from treating a patient with negative axillary lymph nodes would result in an absolute survival difference of only 6 percent if the patient were in a high-risk node-negative category (i.e., with an untreated risk of dying within 10 years of 24 percent) and 2 percent if the patient had a relatively good prognosis, node-negative breast cancer (i.e., with an untreated risk of dying of 8 percent). A less effective therapy that caused only a 12.5 percent reduction in the annual odds of death would result in a survival difference of only 5 percent at the end of 10 years. This might describe the effect of adjuvant chemotherapy in postmenopausal women.

Despite the large number of prognostic factors studied, it is not possible to identify any patient or group of patients with invasive breast cancer who will definitely not die of breast cancer. The converse is also true: Some patients will beat the odds and will survive many decades to die of causes other than breast cancer despite very bad prognostic features. For this reason, it is impossible to pick out a group of patients for whom adjuvant therapy holds no promise of benefit. Good clinical judgment in the use of adjuvant therapy requires the recognition (1) that the benefits from any therapy vary with the menopausal status of the patient, (2) that some therapies, such as chemotherapy, have substantial acute toxicity, (3) that the vast majority of patients in the good prognostic categories will derive no benefit at all because they have been cured with local therapy alone, and (4) that absolute differences in survival will be relatively small when averaged over all treated patients in the good prognostic groups.

A survival difference of 10 percent between treated and untreated patients does not mean that 10 percent of the patients have been cured and that 90 percent derived no benefit at all. Exactly the same difference might be achieved if every patient had a transient but variable prolongation of life from treatment. For example, one patient

TABLE 319-3 Dose schedules of the drug regimens and endocrine therapies most frequently used to treat early and advanced breast cancer

Drug	Dose schedule
CMF(P) (28-day cycle)	
Cyclophosphamide	100 mg/m^2 PO days 1–14
Methotrexate	60 mg/m^2 IV days 1 and 8
5-Fluorouracil	600 mg/m^2 IV days 1 and 8
Prednisone (optional)	40 mg/m^2 PO days 1–14
CAF (21-day cycle)	
Cyclophosphamide	400–500 mg/m^2 IV day 1
Doxorubicin	40–50 mg/m^2 IV day 1
5-Fluorouracil	400–500 mg/m^2 IV days 1 and 8
Tamoxifen	10 mg PO bid
Megestrol acetate	40 mg PO qid
Aminoglutethimide	250 mg PO bid
+ hydrocortisone	10 mg PO qid

might have lived 3 years from diagnosis without treatment and 4 years if treated with adjuvant systemic therapy, while another would have lived 8 years without and 11 years with treatment. Of course, it is also possible that adjuvant therapy will cure a small minority of patients and prolong the life of most of the rest. If there were a widely acceptable method for estimating the average prolongation of survival, this would be a preferable way of expressing the benefits of adjuvant treatment not only because it would better reflect the true nature of the benefit but also because the patient could then weigh the months of life to be gained against the time spent experiencing the toxicities of treatment. Possibly the closest estimate of the average prolongation of survival from treatment might be obtained by subtracting the median survival of patients randomized to the control arms of the trials included in the overview analysis from that of patients randomized to receive adjuvant therapy. For node-positive patients treated with a therapy that reduces the annual odds of death by 25 percent, this difference in medians is about 2 years. However, there is no method for even approximating the range of survival benefits around this number, and a patient also should know that her benefit could be much shorter than this or as long as several decades.

The selection of an adjuvant therapy regimen (See also Table 319-3) Combinations of drugs, such as the combination of cyclophosphamide, methotrexate, and 5-fluorouracil (CMF), are somewhat more effective than single agents, such as melphalan. While 6 months of chemotherapy is better than 1 month, durations of therapy in the range of 4 to 6 months have been shown to be as effective as more prolonged durations, such as 12 to 24 months. It has now been demonstrated in a large randomized trial that patients given full doses of chemotherapy have a significantly better survival than those treated with much lower doses. Regimens that include doxorubicin (see Table 319-3) or those given at higher doses (so that autologous bone marrow, peripheral blood stem cells, or cytokines such as G-CSF or GM-CSF are required) have not yet been shown to be more effective than CMF, even in patients with many positive lymph nodes. Adjuvant systemic therapy is usually initiated as soon as possible after the completion of local therapy, and it has been argued, largely on theoretical grounds and from uncontrolled clinical observations, that adjuvant chemotherapy should be given before definitive surgery ("neoadjuvant," "protoadjuvant," or "primary chemotherapy"). However, in a large, randomized study, chemotherapy begun 1 month after surgery was as effective as chemotherapy begun within 36 h.

Although there are theoretical reasons why longer durations of tamoxifen therapy may be more effective, there are no published data from randomized trials evaluating different durations of tamoxifen therapy. Among women aged 50 and over, the tamoxifen trials in which the drug was administered for 2 years resulted in a larger benefit than those utilizing 1 year, but no greater benefit was achieved in the trials that used more than 2 years of tamoxifen. The studies among younger women are more difficult to interpret because many

fewer women in the younger age groups were entered into those trials and most trials in younger women evaluated the effect of tamoxifen plus chemotherapy rather than the effect of tamoxifen alone. However, the available evidence suggests that much longer periods (e.g., 5 years) may be needed to demonstrate as much benefit from adjuvant tamoxifen in premenopausal women as can be achieved with 2 years of tamoxifen in postmenopausal women. Randomized trials evaluating different durations of tamoxifen therapy are ongoing. Adjuvant tamoxifen imparts a greater survival benefit to women with estrogen receptor–positive than estrogen receptor–negative tumors, but there is a small benefit in the latter group as well. In fact, the benefits from adjuvant tamoxifen in postmenopausal women with estrogen receptor–negative tumors appear to be as large as the effects of chemotherapy in this age group.

There is probably a small benefit from adding chemotherapy to tamoxifen when treating postmenopausal women and from adding tamoxifen or ovarian ablation to chemotherapy when treating premenopausal women. However, the size of these added benefits may be too small to justify the additional toxicity and cost from using chemohormonal combinations. These questions are also being evaluated in ongoing randomized trials.

Summary recommendations for adjuvant systemic therapy Premenopausal, node-positive patients should routinely receive some form of adjuvant therapy after completion of local therapy. If a formal trial is unacceptable to the patient, 6 months of therapy with CMF or 4 months of therapy with cycloplosphamide and doxorubicin (CA) or CA plus 5-fluorouracil (CAF) might be considered standard. Postmenopausal, node-positive, receptor-positive patients should routinely receive tamoxifen for 2 to 5 years. There is at present no established role for adjuvant systemic therapy in patients with in situ breast cancer or those with very small, node-negative tumors, especially those that are impalpable (e.g., found only by mammography or diagnosed with needle localization) or those that are minimally invasive. The treatment of other groups of patients should be undertaken only after full consideration of the size of the benefits and the nature of the toxicity.

TREATMENT OF DISTANT METASTASES

Breast cancer can and frequently does metastasize to almost every organ in the body but most commonly to skin, lymph nodes, lungs, liver, and bones. More than 10 percent of patients with any metastases will have central nervous system metastases at some point in the course of the disease, and new onset of frequent headaches, personality change, otherwise unexplained vomiting, or localized neurologic dysfunction should lead to a prompt evaluation that includes a head CT scan (or MRI) and cytocentrifuge examination of cerebrospinal fluid. Isolated metastases to the leptomeninges are not uncommon, and visual disturbances may be due to breast cancer metastatic to the choroid. Choroid metastases usually can be seen on funduscopic examination. Breast cancer not infrequently metastasizes to the ovary and adrenal gland, and metastases to the abdomen may mimic ovarian cancer with diffuse peritoneal studding and the development of ascites. Metastases to the skin may occur anywhere and commonly appear on the scalp. A standard evaluation for metastases might include a complete blood count, platelet count, liver function studies, chest x-ray, bone scan, and marker study such as the carcinoembryonic antigen (CEA) and CA15-3 in addition to the investigation of specific signs and symptoms.

CHOOSING AMONG THERAPIES Breast cancer recurrences, even recurrences in the skin or the chest wall or along the mastectomy scar, represent bloodborne metastases and are *never* truly isolated recurrences. Other organs will eventually manifest disease, and the time interval from the first recurrence to the second will be roughly *proportional* to the interval from primary diagnosis to the appearance of the first metastasis, usually referred to as the *disease-free interval* (DFI). Although the treatment of metastases will prolong median survival by some months and may have a profound effect on the survival of a few patients, the major value of treatment for metastatic disease is palliation of symptoms. Surgery and radiotherapy are more certain to shrink disease and palliate symptoms in a given area than systemic therapies. Systemic therapies are more likely to achieve long-term control of the disease throughout the body. Metastases to the brain and the choroid of the eye are almost always treated with radiotherapy. A local recurrence to the chest wall without evidence of distant disease might reasonably be treated with radiotherapy if the DFI is long. Malignant pleural effusions are best treated with complete chest tube drainage followed by sclerosis because the effusion may not clear even in a patient whose disease is otherwise responding to chemotherapy or endocrine therapy. The pain from bone metastases may be relieved by either systemic therapy or radiotherapy, but in a patient with multiple lesions or a short DFI, an initial course of systemic therapy is preferred, since all lesions will be affected by the systemic therapy. If the bone cortex is severely eroded, a surgical approach with placement of stabilizing rods may be preferred, since there is a long period of decreased tensile strength in a bone even after a response to radiotherapy or systemic therapy.

The median survival of all patients with metastatic breast cancer exceeds 2.5 years, and most patients will reach several, and some patients more than a dozen, decision points when treatment should or could be offered. Patients given extensive radiotherapy to bone metastases may not tolerate chemotherapy because of the effect of the radiotherapy on the bone marrow. Patients given chemotherapy may not benefit from endocrine therapy administered secondarily. There is no evidence that the treatment of asymptomatic metastases significantly prolongs survival, and a physician or patient may decide to hold therapy for some period of time both to avoid the toxicity of therapy and to better assess the pace of the disease. An asymptomatic but anxious patient who wishes to "do something" might explore the use of new or more experimental therapies first and hold therapies with known efficacy in reserve.

Endocrine therapy versus chemotherapy The patient most likely to respond to endocrine therapy is one with an estrogen and/or progesterone receptor, a long DFI, disease limited to soft tissues (e.g., lymph nodes, breast, skin) or bone as opposed to viscera, and a prior documented response to endocrine therapy. The ideal patient for chemotherapy is anyone who is symptomatic and who is deemed a poor candidate for endocrine therapy. Although only one-third of unselected patients respond to endocrine therapy, two-thirds of patients with positive receptors and/or others of the characteristics listed above will respond to endocrine therapy. About two-thirds of all patients respond to chemotherapy. There is no evidence that a response to chemotherapy will occur more rapidly. The median duration of response to endocrine therapy, about 12 to 13 months, is somewhat longer than that to chemotherapy, about 9 to 12 months, but this likely reflects differences in the responding patient populations rather than in the efficacy of the therapy. Patients on either therapy may, on occasion, continue to respond for more than a decade. The choice between these two modalities will depend on the relative probability of benefit for an individual patient based on that patient's clinical characteristics.

ENDOCRINE THERAPY Patients who respond to one endocrine therapy frequently respond to a second, often to a third, and on occasion even to a fourth or fifth sequential endocrine manipulation. Patients who fail to respond at all to one form of endocrine therapy are not likely to benefit from a different endocrine therapy. There is little difference in the efficacy of various forms of endocrine therapy, and for this reason, the least toxic therapy is usually used first. For postmenopausal women, this is tamoxifen (see Table 319-3); for premenopausal women, it might be either tamoxifen or ovarian ablation by surgery or radiation. (Studies to determine if leutenizing hormone–releasing hormone agonists are as effective as ovarian ablation are under way.) After response and progression of disease, a postmenopausal woman might be treated with either a progestin,

such as megestrol acetate or medroxyprogesterone acetate, or aminoglutethimide plus hydrocortisone (see Table 319-3).

Side effects of endocrine therapy More than 90 percent of patients treated with tamoxifen have no acute side effects at all. Others experience mild nausea that subsides after several weeks to a month, a flare reaction, menstrual disturbances if premenopausal, or hot flashes. There is an increased frequency of thrombophlebitis and thromboembolic phenomena, and about 30 percent of women on tamoxifen experience vaginal dryness. Like estrogen replacement therapy, tamoxifen treatment is associated with an increased incidence of uterine cancer. The risk appears to increase with the duration of treatment. Tamoxifen has been reported to induce hepatocellular cancer in rats, and two cases have been reported from the million-plus-patient-years of follow-up now available from patients treated with tamoxifen. Thus this seems to be a very rare event, possibly on the order of that seen from the use of oral contraceptives. Preliminary evidence suggests that tamoxifen may decrease heart disease and osteoporosis while increasing the incidence of uterine cancer. Patients usually find weight gain due to increased appetite and fluid retention the most disturbing side effect of progestin therapies.

More than 10 percent of patients with metastatic breast cancer will experience hypercalcemia at some point in the course of their disease. Often this occurs soon after the initiation of endocrine therapy as part of a "flare." In addtion to hypercalcemia, this syndrome is characterized by a sudden increase in bone pain and erythema around skin lesions, an increase in the number and intensity of lesions on bone scan, and an elevation of serum markers such as CEA and CA15-3. These signs and symptoms appear within hours to a few weeks after beginning endocrine therapy and subside by the end of a month. Unless hypercalcemia is life-threatening [calcium $\geq$ 3.5 mmol/L (14 mg/dL)], endocrine therapy should be continued and the underlying symptoms treated with pain medications, fluids, diuretics, and standard regimens for hypercalcemia (see Chap. 357).

CHEMOTHERAPY Although breast cancer responds to a long list of cytotoxic agents, three, and possibly four, appear to be especially effective and non-cross-resistant with each other: cyclophosphamide (C), doxorubicin (A), mitomycin C, and vinblastine. Phase II studies of a new drug, taxol, are also very promising, but the appropriate role for this drug, if any, has not been established. Combinations of these drugs with each other and/or with methotrexate (M) and 5-fluorouracil (F) induce higher response rates and marginally improved survival compared with serial treatment with single agents. The most popular combinations are CMF, CMF plus prednisone, and CAF (see Table 319-3). There is no evidence that survival is substantially improved by prolonged administration of these drugs, but the results of one randomized trial suggest that both response rate and quality of life are improved by some duration in excess of 3 months. A reduction of drug doses below those shown in Table 319-3 is likely to be associated with a lower response rate, but there is as yet no evidence of substantial benefit from exceeding these doses either. The use of very high dose therapy with autologous bone marrow support, peripheral blood stem cells, or cytokines such as G- or GM-CSF has not yet been proven to be beneficial in prolonging survival or improving quality of life.

Side effects of chemotherapy Although the acute side effects of chemotherapy often seem formidable, it has been repeatedly demonstrated in randomized trials that the efficacy of a regimen is a more important determinant of net quality of life than the side effects of treatment for patients with symptomatic, metastatic breast cancer. All these drugs cause dose-related myelosuppression, thrombocytopenia, and, over some months, anemia. Gastrointestinal toxicity may include everything from mild nausea to protracted vomiting, severe mucositis, and diarrhea. Both myelosuppression and gastrointestinal toxicity are mitigated by the addition of prednisone to the regimen. Alopecia may be mild and gradual in onset with the use of CMF or abrupt and total with doxorubicin combinations. Doxorubicin cardiomyopathy occurs with increasing frequency after cumulative doses in excess of 450 mg/m^2 body area have been given. All these agents, and especially the alkylating agents such as cyclophosphamide, are potential carcinogens. CMF and, to a much greater extent, melphalan have been shown to increase the incidence of leukemia and other blood dyscrasias when these drugs are used as adjuvant therapy, but the benefits far outweigh this risk in women with positive lymph nodes or other high-risk features. It is still too early to assess the danger of inducing solid tumors with these drugs, since they usually occur only after a long latent period.

SPECIAL PROBLEMS

Male breast cancer occurs with less than 1 percent of the frequency of female breast cancer. Predisposing risk factors include states of hyperestrogenism, such as Klinefelter's syndrome, schistosomiasis, a family history of breast cancer, and radiation exposure. Gynecomastia, in itself, is not an established risk factor (see Chap. 341). In other respects, male breast cancer is nearly identical to female breast cancer, with a similar prognosis, stage per stage. The primary lesion is usually treated with mastectomy, since most men are not concerned with saving the breast. There are no data from controlled trials regarding the use of adjuvant systemic therapy for men, but the treatment of metastatic disease is nearly identical.

Cystosarcoma phylloides is a rare tumor more closely related to either benign fibroadenoma, from which it apparently arises in most cases, or sarcoma. It metastasizes in less than 5 percent of cases, but the local recurrence rate may exceed 20 percent, especially if it is treated inadequately. Treatment of the benign variety of cystosarcoma phylloides consists of wide excision; for the malignant variety, wide excision or simple mastectomy. Node dissection is rarely indicated.

Paget's disease of the nipple is often mistaken initially for a simple eczema and treated with glucocorticoids. However, a crusting, eroding, or scaling nipple lesion that does not respond promptly to conservative therapy should be biopsied. Histologically, Paget's disease is characterized by noninvasive or minimally invasive tumor cells growing on the undersurface of the nipple. In some cases there will be no other tumor in the breast, and some physicians now treat apparently localized disease with wide excision. However, in over half the cases a mass will be found deep within the breast, in which case the prognosis and treatment of Paget's disease wiil depend on the size of the mass and the presence of involvement. The majority of the patients with Paget's disease will be treated like any other breast cancer patient.

Breast cancer is particularly difficult to diagnose and treat when it occurs *during pregnancy,* but stage per stage the prognosis approximates that of patients diagnosed in a nonpregnant state. There is no evidence that therapeutic abortion improves the prognosis. Mastectomy can be performed in the second and third trimesters, and chemotherapy has been given in the third trimester without observed damage to the fetus. *Pregnancy 2 years or more after diagnosis of breast cancer* is not associated with a higher recurrence rate or shortened survival, and counseling women regarding the advisability of pregnancy depends more on the patient's feelings regarding the possibility of not being able to see her child reach adulthood than about any potential risk to the patient from the pregnancy.

REFERENCES

General, natural history, prognostic factors, epidemiology

HARRIS JR et al: Breast cancer. N Engl J Med 327:319, 1992
HENDERSON IC: What can a woman do about her risk of dying of breast cancer? Curr Probl Cancer 14:165, 1990
———— et al: Breast Cancer, in *Cancer: Principles and Practice of Oncology,* VT De Vita Jr et al (eds). Philadelphia, Lippincott, 1989, pp 1197–1268
MCGUIRE WL, CLARK GM: Prognostic factors and treatment decisions in axillary node-negative breast cancer. N Engl J Med 326:1756, 1992

Familial incidence

GARBER JE: Familial aspects of breast cancer, in *Breast Diseases,* 2d ed, JR Harris et al (eds). Philadelphia, Lippincott, 1991, p 142

Endocrine factors

DUPONT WD, PAGE DL: Menopausal estrogen replacement therapy and breast cancer. Arch Intern Med 151:67, 1991
ROMIEU I et al: Oral contraceptives and breast cancer. Review and meta-analysis. Cancer 66:2253, 1990
STEINBERG KK et al: A meta-analysis of the effect of estrogen replacement therapy on the risk of breast cancer. JAMA 265:1985, 1991

Benign breast disease, in situ carcinoma

DUPONT WD, PAGE DL: Risk factors for breast cancer in women with proliferative breast disease. N Engl J Med 312:146, 1985
FISHER B et al: Lumpectomy compared with lumpectomy and radiation therapy for the treatment of intraductal breast cancer. N Engl J Med 328:1581, 1993
SCHNITT SJ et al: Ductal carcinoma in situ (intraductal carcinoma) of the breast. N Engl J Med 318:898, 1988

Screening

CHU KC et al: Analysis of breast cancer mortality and stage distribution by age for the Health Insurance Plan clinical trial. J Natl Cancer Inst 80:1125, 1988
EDDY DM: Screening for breast cancer. Ann Intern Med 111:389, 1989
———— et al: The value of mammography screening in women under age 50 years. JAMA 259:1512, 1988
MILLER AB et al: Canadian national breast screening study: I. Breast cancer detection and death rates among women aged 40–49 years. Can Med Assoc J 147:1459, 1992

Biology

LIPPMAN ME, DICKSON RB: Mechanisms of growth control in normal and malignant breast epithelium. Rec Prog Hormone Res 45:383, 1989

Local therapy

FISHER B et al: Eight-year results of a randomized clinical trial comparing total mastectomy and lumpectomy with or without irradiation in the treatment of breast cancer. N Engl J Med 320:822, 1989
———— et al: Significance of ipsilateral breast tumor recurrence after lumpectomy. Lancet 338:327, 1991
———— et al: Lumpectomy compared with lumpectomy and radiation therapy for the treatment of intraductal breast cancer. N Eng J Med 328:1581, 1993

Adjuvant therapy

EARLY BREAST CANCER TRIALISTS' COLLABORATIVE GROUP: Systemic treatment of early breast cancer by hormonal, cytotoxic, or immune therapy: 151 randomized trials involving 32,000 recurrences and 25,000 deaths among 77,000 women. Lancet 339:1, 1992
————: *Treatment of Early Breast Cancer.* vol 1: *Worldwide Evidence 1985–1990. A Systematic Overview of All Available Randomized Trials in Early Breast Cancer of Adjuvant Endocrine and Cytotoxic Therapy.* Oxford, Oxford University press, 1990, p 207

Systemic therapy

HENDERSON IC: Endocrine therapy of metastatic breast cancer, in *Breast Diseases,* 2d ed, JR Harris et al (eds). Philadelphia, Lippincott, 1991, p 559
————: Chemotherapy for metastatic disease, in *Breast Diseases,* 2d ed, JR Harris et al (eds). Philadelphia, Lippincott, 1991, p 604
————: Window of opportunity. J Natl Cancer Inst 83:894, 1991
————, HARRIS JR: Principles in the management of metastatic disease: Intergration of local and systemic therapies, in *Breast Diseases,* 2d ed, JR Harris et al (eds). Philadelphia, Lippincott, 1991, p 547

320   MALIGNANT TUMORS OF THE HEAD AND NECK

ROBERT S. LEBOVICS

Primary malignant tumors of the head and neck arise from the multitude of tissues comprising the nasal cavity, paranasal sinuses, pharynx, larynx, salivary glands, and thyroid. Embryologic development and a complex regional anatomy contribute to the various clinical presentations of these malignancies. Tumor size, nodal status, and the presence of metastases define a tumor's classification as well as the stage of disease.

The American Joint Committee on Cancer (AJCC) has developed a standard tumor, node, and metastasis (TNM) staging system. Each anatomic site in the head and neck has its own unique clinical T-stage classification. The head and neck surgeon, for example, will be adept in the subtleties of staging laryngeal cancer involving the supraglottic larynx versus the glottic larynx. Tumors of the salivary glands are staged differently from epithelial tumors of the oropharynx. The AJCC, however, also has developed a uniform staging system for the characterization of regional lymph node (N-stage) disease in the neck (see Table 320-1).

Before definitive therapy, tumors are staged surgically, and malignancy is confirmed pathologically. Adjunctive modalities, such as computed tomography (CT) and magnetic resonance imaging (MRI), do not directly affect what is still a clinical staging system. In practice, however, treatment planning requires the incorporation of data obtained by adjunctive testing. In many institutions, cases of head and neck tumor are routinely presented to a multidisciplinary board of health professionals, including a head and neck surgeon, a radiation oncologist, a medical oncologist, a speech pathologist, and a nutritionist, as well as a diagnostic radiologist and pathologist. A frank exchange of ideas and information among these specialists will result in optimal therapy and allow each cause to be treated as unique.

NOSE AND PARANASAL SINUSES   The nose and the paranasal sinuses consist of a bony framework primarily lined with respiratory epithelium. Malignancies usually arise in either the maxillary or the ethmoid sinuses within this epithelium. Previous exposure to industrial wood products, nickel, and Thorotrast is associated with an increased incidence of malignant sinus tumors. Tumors of either the sphenoid sinus or the frontal sinus are extremely rare.

Symptoms of tumors of the maxillary sinus include facial and dental pain, localized swelling, and epistaxis. Tumors of the ethmoid sinuses may be accompanied by nasal obstruction, epistaxis, and orbital complications (proptosis and epiphora). Noninvasive tests such as CT and MRI may help to image adjacent structures—specifically, the orbit and optic nerves, prevertebral fascia, pterygopalatine fossa, cavernous sinuses, and central nervous system (CNS).

Squamous cell carcinoma is the most common tumor of the sinuses, and adenocystic carcinoma (or cylindroma) is the next most common. Uncommon tumors include adenocarcinomas and malignant melanomas. The 5-year survival rates for tumors of the maxillary and ethmoid sinuses are in the 20 percent range.

Tumors of the nose are similar to malignancies within the paranasal sinuses. Because of the abundance of minor salivary glands, both benign and malignant tumors of salivary gland origin may be manifested by nasal symptoms, including obstruction, epistaxis, foul odor, and secondary infection. Biopsy is critical for diagnosis, and follow-up imaging and staging are essential to the selection of definitive therapy.

NASOPHARYNX   The nasopharynx extends inferiorly from the posterior border of the nose at the choanae down to the junction with the oropharynx. The epithelium is primarily squamous and is richly infiltrated with lymphoid tissue. Esthesioneuroblastomas arise from olfactory epithelium connected to the cribriform plate. These tumors may either grow anteriorly and invade the nose or extend inferiorly and fill the nasopharynx. Superior extension of this tumor results in involvement of the CNS. The nasopharynx also coincides embryologically with the upper pole of the lymphoid tissue of Waldeyer's ring. This abundant tissue helps explain why nasopharyngeal masses may include lymphomas, malignant lymphoepitheliomas, and extramedullary plasmacytomas as well as squamous cell carcinomas in various degrees of differentiation. As in other head and neck tumors, histologic diagnosis of nasopharyngeal malignancies is necessary in addition to TNM staging. Electron microscopy by the surgical pathologist may be needed to confirm a histologic diagnosis. Advanced imaging techniques are usually needed for complete classification of a tumor and for the selection of optimal therapy. Since resectable tumors may invade the CNS, definitive treatment may require craniofacial resection. However, malignancies of lymphoid origins are best managed by irradiation and/or chemotherapy.

Carcinoma of the nasopharynx is infrequent in the United States, where it comprises 4 percent of head and neck malignancies. In China, however, it is more common, particularly in Kwantung Province. The incidence of nasopharyngeal carcinoma among North American–born Chinese is significantly lower than that among native-born Chinese, yet it is still higher than that among North American–born Caucasians. A possible explanation is a focus for genetic susceptibility located on the human leukocyte antigen HLA-A2 histocompatibility locus. Carcinoma of the nasopharynx also has been associated with infection by Epstein-Barr virus. Serum samples can be assayed for IgA antibodies to the viral capsid antigen (VCA) and the early antigen (EA) of this virus; titers can be predictive of prognosis.

Nearly one-half of patients with carcinoma of the nasopharynx present with regional disease in the ipsilateral neck as the only overt clinical finding. If a neck mass is found to contain squamous cell carcinoma cells and there is no known primary tumor site, occult disease within the nasopharynx must be suspected. Surgical endoscopy in addition to random biopsy of high-risk areas in the nasopharynx (including Rosenmüller's fossae) behind the eustachian tubes may help to define the primary tumor site.

Initial treatment for carcinoma of the nasopharynx is generally irradiation to the primary site and to the neck. Surgical treatment of the neck is usually reserved for persistent disease. Because of the proximity of the nasopharynx to the clivus and the base of the skull, locally invasive disease can cause isolated or multiple cranial neuropathies (especially involving cranial nerves I, III, IV, V, VI, IX, X, and XI).

ORAL CAVITY AND OROPHARYNX   The oral cavity extends from the vermilion border of the lips to the junction of the hard and soft palates superiorly and inferiorly to the circumvallate papilla. The area is divided into distinct anatomic regions, including the lips, the buccal mucosa, the alveolar ridge, the hard palate, and the anterior two-thirds of the tongue (i.e., the oral tongue). The oropharynx begins anteriorly with the oral cavity and extends inferiorly to the plane of the hyoid bone and superiorly to the plane of the hard palate. It includes the base of the tongue, the palatine tonsils, and the faucial

---

TABLE 320-1   Diagrammatic representation of TNM staging for head and neck tumors

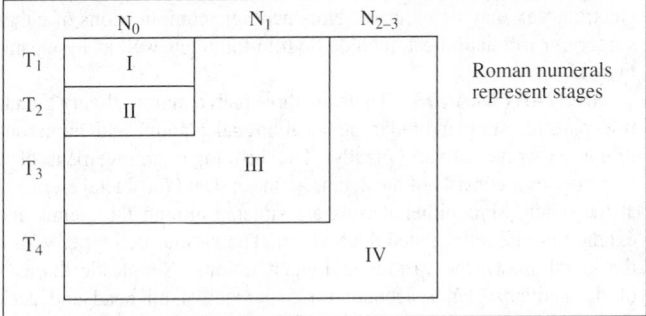

Roman numerals represent stages

Clinical staging of the primary tumor (oral cavity, oropharynx, larynx, thyroid, salivary gland, etc.)

T stages (1–4) are separately defined for each anatomic region.

Clinical staging of neck nodes

N_0 Neck clinically negative for pathologic adenopathy.
N_1 Single ipsilateral node < 3 cm.
N_{2A} Single ipsilateral node 3-6 cm.
N_{2B} Multiple ipsilateral nodes all < 6 cm.
N_{2C} Bilateral or contralateral nodes all < 6 cm.
N_3 Single or multiple nodes, at least one > 6 cm.

Clinical staging of distant sites (brain, lung, bone, liver, etc.)

M_0 No metastatic disease.
M_1 Presence of metastasis (all M_1 tumors are stage IV).

SOURCE: AJCC, 1992.

arch encompassing the soft palate and the anterior pillar. The region inferior to the plane of the hyoid bone begins the hypopharynx, which ends at the cervical opening of the esophagus and is posterior to the true laryngeal framework. The oral cavity, oropharynx, and hypopharynx each has its own T-staging system, and in general, the larger the tumor, the higher the T stage.

Patients with squamous cell carcinoma of the oral cavity and oropharynx usually have associated medical illnesses—specifically, alcohol abuse with possible concurrent hepatic dysfunction. These patients usually also have significant smoking histories, with or without attendant pulmonary disorders. Tobacco chewing and the chewing of betel nut in India are linked to cancer of the oral cavity. Affected patients are frequently cachectic and have significant nutritional deficiencies that are difficult to correct because of odynophagia and/or alcoholism. Some of these patients have impaired cell-mediated immunity, which correlates with increased morbidity. The incidence of second primary squamous cell cancers of the oral cavity is reduced by chemoprevention with cis-retinoic acid. Most patients with squamous cell cancer of the oral cavity, oropharynx, and hypopharynx undergo surgery, radiation therapy, or combined-modality therapy. Chemotherapy is not used as a first-line treatment for carcinoma of the oral cavity and oropharynx. The role of chemotherapy as an adjunct or in nonresectable tumors is subject to debate. As a general rule, for a given T stage, the prognosis is best for tumors of the lips and deteriorates as the site moves toward the hypopharynx. Either stage I or stage II disease usually can be treated effectively by either surgery or irradiation; combined-modality therapy is generally preferred for patients with either stage III or stage IV disease. However, each patient should be evaluated individually by the appropriate specialists, and therapy should be based on multiple considerations, including size of tumor, side effects of planned therapy, and functional status after radical surgery. Regional disease within the neck usually requires neck dissection.

The complications of both irradiation and radical surgery are not trivial. After radiation therapy patients can suffer from xerostomia and be at increased risk for the delayed development of secondary neoplasms. Poor wound healing, fistulas, and major vessel erosion from radiation therapy are significant morbidities. Dry mouth with associated dysphagia should not be trivialized. Radical surgery can often remove a malignancy en bloc; however, both the appearance and the functional and communicative abilities of the patient may be severely compromised.

HYPOPHARYNX The hypopharynx includes the pyriform sinus, the postcricoid region, and the inferoposterior pharyngeal wall. Approximately 5 percent of tumors of the hypopharynx are of minor salivary gland origin; the remaining 95 percent are squamous cell carcinomas. Alcohol abuse and tobacco use are the major etiologic agents for cancer of the hypopharynx. The Plummer-Vinson syndrome, iron-deficiency anemia, and dysphagia secondary to upper esophageal webs are frequently associated with carcinoma of the postcricoid region in nonsmoking women. Hypopharyngeal carcinoma most commonly originates in the pyriform sinus and usually presents in an advanced clinical stage. Symptoms, when present, generally include throat pain, otalgia, and dysphagia. Approximately 80 percent of pyriform sinus lesions are found with cervical node metastases. Because most hypopharyngeal carcinomas present as advanced lesions, therapy usually consists of a total laryngectomy with a partial pharyngectomy and complete neck dissection. Postoperative radiation therapy is usually given. Reconstructive options after radical surgery include myocutaneous flaps, gastric pull-ups, and free jejunal flaps with microvascular reanastomoses. The 5-year survival rate for carcinoma of the hypopharynx in patients undergoing both irradiation and surgery is approximately 40 percent.

LARYNX Cancer of the larynx accounts for fewer than 2 percent of all carcinomas in the United States. The incidence of cancer of the larynx is considerably higher among men than among women (5:1). Tobacco and alcohol abuse are the prime etiologic factors. Lesions of the larynx are frequently detected earlier than those of the hypopharynx because of the associated symptoms.

Hoarseness is the most common symptom of laryngeal cancer and often motivates a patient to seek medical attention. Other associated symptoms include dyspnea, stridor, and severe pain. Dysphagia and odynophagia may be evident, and chronic cough and hemoptysis may indicate large fungating lesions. Late symptoms and signs can include weight loss, halitosis, and regional neck disease.

A clinical diagnosis is frequently made (sometimes in the doctor's office) by either mirror or fiberoptic examination of the pharynx and larynx. Once the diagnosis is suspected, appropriate adjunctive imaging should be undertaken and should be followed by formal staging endoscopy. The supraglottic larynx is embryologically different from the glottic and infraglottic larynx and consequently has a different lymphatic drainage pattern. Tumors of the true vocal cords will therefore behave differently from those originating at superior sites. Surgical endoscopy is critical for staging. Supraglottic, glottic, and infraglottic tumors are staged differently, and precise anatomic definition is a prerequisite to proper treatment. The unique anatomic characteristics of lymphatic drainage in the larynx, along with the existence of local barriers to direct extension of the tumor, theoretically make conservation laryngeal surgery an oncologically sound choice for specialized lesions. Supraglottic (horizontal) laryngectomy may be appropriate for some epiglottic lesions, while hemilaryngectomy (vertical) may be appropriate in carcinoma of the true vocal cords. T_1 and T_2 lesions of the larynx frequently can be treated successfully with irradiation or various vocal cord stripping techniques.

Total laryngectomy with or without neck dissection is reserved for advanced lesions or those which have failed to respond to radiation therapy. The morbidity (both physical and psychologic) associated with a total laryngectomy cannot be overemphasized. Patients undergo a profound change in life-style that few can appreciate preoperatively despite extensive counseling and support. Loss of the upper respiratory airway can result in anosmia and dysgeusia. Because of an open airway in the neck, patients can have a difficult time showering and cannot swim. The most profound effect, however, is loss of speech. Counseling and immediate postoperative training in the use of assistive communication devices are helpful. Some patients develop esophageal speech. Others may undergo procedures such as tracheoesophageal puncture or insertion of various prosthetic devices for the enhancement of their ability to communicate. When these measures fail, an electrolarynx may be required. Nononcologic complications of either surgery or irradiation can include thyroid failure as well as hypoparathyroidism.

SALIVARY GLANDS There are three paired major salivary glands (the parotid, submandibular, and sublingual glands) and numerous minor exocrine salivary glands. The histologic arrangement of a secretory unit consists of the acinus at one end and the ductal elements at the other. Myoepithelial cells are situated around the acinus and extend into the intercalated duct region. The various cell types within the gland spawn the various malignant lesions. Neoplastic diseases of the salivary glands account for 5 percent of all head and neck tumors. Previous radiation therapy has been shown to be associated with the development of pleomorphic adenomas and mucoepidermoid tumors of the major salivary glands, with latencies lasting as long as several years. Persons involved in the manufacture of furniture and woodwork also run an increased risk of minor salivary gland adenocarcinoma, particularly in the sinonasal tract.

Pleomorphic adenoma is the most common tumor of the salivary glands, particularly in the parotid. While this tumor is technically benign and slow-growing, the potential for malignant degeneration exists, and surgical excision is advised in nearly all cases. In fact, nearly all tumors of the major and minor salivary glands require surgical excision because of the significant possibility of malignant degeneration. Table 320-2 lists the histologic classification of salivary tumors. As in all head and neck cancers, AJCC staging according to the TNM system is recommended during the diagnostic evaluation

TABLE 320-2 Salivary gland tumors

Benign
 Pleomorphic adenoma
 Warthin's tumor (papillary cystadenoma lymphomatosum)
 Oncocytoma
 Monomorphic adenoma
Malignant
 Malignant mixed tumor
 Mucoepidermoid carcinoma
 Adenocystic carcinoma
 Adenocarcinoma
 Acinic cell carcinoma
 Squamous cell carcinoma

and before the institution of definitive therapy. As a general rule, the larger the gland, the more likely it is that the tumor is histologically benign. While three-fourths of parotid tumors are histologically benign, the same proportion of minor salivary gland tumors are histologically malignant.

The diagnosis is based on the patient's history and physical examination along with the results of radiographic imaging studies. Paresthesias and pain may be associated with malignant tumors, particularly adenocystic carcinomas. Fine-needle aspiration is a safe method for the preoperative evaluation of salivary neoplasms, although cytologic features can be misleading in establishing a correct tissue diagnosis of malignancy. To date, there is no evidence of tumor tracking by fine-needle cytologic aspiration. The facial nerve is intricately involved with the parotid gland, and weakness in this nerve suggests the presence of a malignant tumor.

Surgical resection is the treatment of choice for salivary gland tumors. Occasionally, malignant tumors invade the facial nerve; if sacrifice of this nerve is required, immediate nerve grafting often using the sural nerve, is the treatment of choice. Reinnervation of the face may take as long as 18 months.

The prognosis of salivary gland tumors is generally a function of the stage of disease as well as tumor histology and grade at the time of initial presentation. This association is especially strong in mucoepidermoid carcinomas and acinic cell carcinomas. In adenocarcinomas and adenocystic carcinomas, the site of origin affects prognosis. Poor outcomes are frequent for tumors originating in the sinonasal tract and the laryngotracheal complex. Facial nerve involvement is especially ominous.

THYROID GLAND (See also Chap. 334) Malignant lesions of the thyroid gland arise from two functionally distinct endocrine cell lines in the thyroid gland. Follicular cells, which secrete thyroid hormone, are the cells of origin for papillary, follicular, and anaplastic carcinoma. The perifollicular cells (C cells) are neural crest derivatives and are the cells of origin for medullary carcinoma of the thyroid gland. Thyroid cancers comprise nearly 10 percent of head and neck tumors. Etiologic factors include previous irradiation to the region and, in some cases, familial syndromes associated with multiple endocrine neoplasia.

Tumors usually present as a neck mass. In some instances, extensive tracheal compression with airway compromise may be the presenting symptom, especially in aggressive neoplasms. Patients frequently complain of hoarseness, particularly in malignant neoplasms. Other risk factors for malignancy include young age, male gender, and a solid, "cold" nodule on a nuclear scan. Except in medullary carcinoma, no clinical or laboratory tests help differentiate benign from malignant thyroid nodules, although aspiration cytology is frequently helpful in defining the malignancy of a lesion.

Papillary carcinoma is the most common cancer of the thyroid; it is frequently multifocal and unencapsulated. A worse prognosis is associated with local tissue invasion and with distant lymphatic spread. Follicular carcinoma is typically solid and encapsulated; it preferentially spreads hematogenously, often involving the lungs and bones. Hürthle cell carcinoma is a variant of follicular cell cancer,

and nuclear aneuploidy is associated with a relatively poor prognosis. Anaplastic carcinoma is highly malignant and has a dismal prognosis. Diagnostic testing for patients suspected of having medullary thyroid carcinoma includes measurement of serum calcitonin. Provocative tests using calcium gluconate and pentagastrin may facilitate early diagnosis.

Surgery is the primary treatment modality for thyroid malignancies. Radioactive iodine administration, hormonal suppression by thyroid hormone supplements, external beam irradiation, and chemotherapy are useful adjuncts in some cases. Tumors whose malignancy is strongly suspected are excised, while benign tumors are generally subjected to a trial of medical management. Effective communication between the endocrinologist and the head and neck surgeon will lead to optimal therapy.

REFERENCES

Advanced techniques for management of head and neck neoplasms. Ontolaryngol Clin North Am 24:1287, 1991
HELLMAN S et al (eds): *Cancer: Principles and Practice of Oncology,* 3d ed, 1989
KOH W et al: Fast neutron radiation for inoperable and recurrent salivary gland cancers. Am J Clin Oncol 12:316, 1989
LEE NK: Molecular biology: the polymerase chain reaction. Head Neck 14:62, 1992
————: Oncogenes. Head Neck 14:235, 1992
MILLION RR: The larynx. Int J Radiat Oncol 23:691, 1992
MOISA II: Neuroendocrine tumors of the larynx. Head Neck 13:498, 1991
PAPARELLA M et al (eds): *Otolaryngology (Head and Neck),* vol 3. Philadelphia, Saunders, 1991
PARSONS JT et al: Twice-a-day irradiation of squamous cell carcinoma. Semin Radiat Oncol 2:29, 1992
PFISTER DC et al: Current status of larynx preservation with multimodality therapy. Oncology 6:33, 1992
SESSIONS RB, DIEHL WL: Thyroid cancer and related nodularity, in *Cancer of the Head and Neck,* 2d ed, E Meyers, JY Suen (eds). New York, Churchill Livingstone, 1989, p 735
WANG CC: *Radiation Therapy for Head and Neck Neoplasms,* 2d ed. New York, Year Book Medical Publishers, 1990

321 OVARIAN CANCER

ROBERT C. BAST, JR. / ANDREW BERCHUCK

Ovarian cancer is neither common nor rare. In incidence, it ranks fifth among all malignancies of women and third among the gynecologic cancers. Ovarian cancer is, however, the most frequent cause of gynecologic cancer death because some two-thirds of cases are detected in advanced stages. Late detection reflects an absence of specific symptoms when disease is localized, as well as the lack of effective strategies for prevention or screening. The prognosis of ovarian cancer depends critically on the histologic type. More than 85 percent of ovarian cancers arise from the epithelium that covers the ovarian surface or that lines inclusion cysts, whereas less than 15 percent develop from ovarian stroma and germ cells. Although relatively rare, germ cell and stromal tumors can be cured in a majority of cases, often with preservation of reproductive function. The more common epithelial ovarian cancers respond to cytoreductive surgery and cytotoxic chemotherapy, but long-term survival is observed in only about a third of all patients with this histotype.

INCIDENCE AND EPIDEMIOLOGY In the United States, a woman's lifetime risk of developing ovarian cancer is 1 in 70. In 1992, some 21,000 cases of ovarian cancer were reported, and about 13,000 women died from the disease. Germ cell tumors generally develop within the first three decades. Stromal tumors can occur at any age. Juvenile granulosa cell and Sertoli-Leydig cell tumors are seen most frequently in younger women, whereas the peak incidence of adult granulosa cell tumors is in the perimenopausal period. The more common epithelial ovarian cancers are seldom encountered in women less than 35 years of age, but the incidence increases sharply with advancing age and peaks at ages 75 to 80. The median age of patients with epithelial ovarian cancer is 60 years. The single most important risk factor for epithelial ovarian cancer is age >40 years.

Most cases of epithelial ovarian cancer are sporadic. Less than 5 percent of ovarian cancer patients belong to families in which ovarian, breast, endometrial, or colon cancer can be tracked as an apparent autosomal dominant trait. In this setting, risk can be as high as 50 percent. Patients with two or more first-degree relatives affected by ovarian cancer are likely to belong to such families, but formal pedigree analysis is required to document risk. A single first-degree relative with ovarian cancer increases a woman's risk by at least threefold, whereas a personal history of breast or colorectal cancer increases the risk of subsequently developing ovarian cancer by twofold.

Among environmental factors, a high-fat diet has been associated with increased risk of epithelial ovarian cancer, as has the intake of lactose in subjects with relatively low tissue levels of galactose-1-phosphate uridyl transferase. Use of talc products has correlated with increased ovarian cancer risk in some studies but not in others. Endocrinologic factors are also important. Early menarche, late menopause, and nulliparity are all associated with increased risk. Conversely, pregnancy, lactation, and oral contraceptive medications decrease the risk of ovarian cancer. Use of oral contraceptives for as long as 5 years can reduce the risk of ovarian cancer by 50 percent. Thus factors that favor prolonged and persistent ovulation increase ovarian cancer risk, whereas factors that suppress ovulation decrease risk. Estrogen replacement does not appear to increase the risk of epithelial ovarian cancer in postmenopausal patients.

HISTOLOGIC CLASSIFICATION Primary ovarian tumors can be divided into three general categories: epithelial, stromal, and germ cell tumors (Table 321-1). In addition, metastases to the ovary can occur from a variety of neoplasms, including fallopian tube, endometrial, breast, colon, gastric, and pancreatic carcinomas, as well as lymphomas and some leukemias. Krukenberg had originally described bilateral metastases to the ovarian stroma from mucin-secreting gastrointestinal cancers.

During embryologic development, the ovarian surface is derived

---

TABLE 321-1   Histologic classification of primary ovarian cancers

EPITHELIAL

Serous
Mucinous
Endometrioid
Clear cell "mesonephroid"
Brenner
Mixed epithelial
Undifferentiated
Unclassified

STROMAL

Granulosa cell
Thecoma, fibroma
Sertoli, Leydig cell tumors
Gynandroblastoma
Lipoid cell tumor
Sarcoma

GERM CELL

Dysgerminoma
Teratoma
Endodermal sinus tumor
Embryonal carcinoma
Polyembryoma
Choriocarcinoma
Mixed germ cell tumors
Gonadoblastoma

---

from the coelomic mesothelium that covers the peritoneal cavity and that also lines the müllerian duct forming the epithelial components of the fallopian tube, endometrium, and endocervix. The flattened epithelium that covers the ovarian surface is thought to retain the potential to differentiate into the cuboidal or columnar epithelia resembling müllerian duct derivatives. Serous, endometrioid, and mucinous ovarian tumors resemble epithelial components of the fallopian tube, endometrium, and endocervix, respectively. Epithelial ovarian cancers can contain a mixture of these different histotypes or can lack differentiation. Within a given histotype, benign, borderline, and frankly malignant ovarian tumors have been described. Borderline ovarian tumors contain histologically transformed cells that lack evidence of invasion. More than 75 percent of borderline lesions are found in early stage and tend to occur in younger women. Recurrence and metastasis of borderline lesions are observed, but the prognosis is dramatically better than that for most ovarian cancers. Benign and borderline ovarian tumors are not necessarily precursors of frankly malignant ovarian cancers, in contrast to cervical dysplastic lesions, which clearly give rise to invasive cervical cancer.

Granulosa, theca, Sertoli, and Leydig cell tumors resemble stromal or "sex-cord" components in the normal ovary. Similar to normal ovarian stroma, these neoplasms can produce estrogens or androgens.

In contrast to testicular lesions, germ cell tumors of the ovary are more often benign than malignant. Dermoid cysts generally contain components of all three germ layers and are most frequently benign. Calcification of bone or teeth can sometimes be detected radiographically. Among the malignant germ cell tumors, dysgerminomas, immature teratomas, endodermal sinus tumors, embryonal carcinomas, and nongestational choriocarcinomas can be differentiated histologically.

EPITHELIAL CANCERS   Biology The ovarian surface epithelium is ordinarily quiescent with a low mitotic index. Following ovulation, surface epithelial cells proliferate to repair the defect produced when a follicle ruptures. Proliferation triggered by repeated ovulation may permit the induction or expression of genetic damage leading to malignant transformation. Invaginations of the surface epithelium can form inclusion cysts. Within the microenvironment of the stroma, proliferation of epithelial cells lining these cysts may be dysregulated.

As in the case of many other neoplasms, epithelial ovarian cancer is a clonal disease that arises from a single cell. Some four to five alterations may be required in growth factors, oncogenes, or tumor suppressor genes to dysregulate growth. Normal ovarian surface epithelial cells express transforming growth factor β that regularly inhibits their growth. A fraction of ovarian cancers appear to have lost this autocrine inhibitory loop. Conversely, a majority of ovarian cancers express both transforming growth factor α and the epidermal growth factor receptor (EGFR) to which it binds, permitting autocrine stimulation of tumor cell proliferation.

Oncogenes associated with ovarian cancers also can encode growth factors or their receptors. The HER-2/*neu* (c-*erb*B-2) gene product, a transmembrane tyrosine kinase growth factor receptor, is overexpressed in one-third of ovarian cancers. Both normal and malignant ovarian epithelia secrete macrophage colony stimulating factor (CSF-1), but only malignant cells appear to express the receptor for this growth factor encoded by the *fms* oncogene. CSF-1 is also a potent chemoattractant for macrophages. Cytokines derived from macrophages, including tumor necrosis factor α, interleukin 1, and interleukin 6, can stimulate ovarian cancer growth. Consequently, tumor-associated macrophages may provide paracrine stimulation rather than inhibition of ovarian tumor growth.

No abnormalities have been detected in the retinoblastoma (Rb) or Wilms' tumor associated suppressor genes, but approximately half of ovarian cancers have lost the normal function of p53, a DNA-binding phosphoprotein that is required for normal growth regulation. Additional suppressor loci are being sought through studies of loss of heterozygosity at different loci within tumor cells. As in many other neoplasms, genetic instability is reflected in aneuploid karyotypes for the majority of advanced ovarian cancers. Using molecular techniques, loss of heterozygosity has been observed at loci on chromosomes 1, 3, 6, 11, and 17, but there is no single karyotypic abnormality that is characteristic of ovarian cancer.

Epithelial ovarian cancer has a distinctive pattern of spread. In addition to lymphatic and hematogenous metastasis, the exfoliation, transperitoneal migration, and implantation of tumor cells can produce multiple metastatic nodules on the visceral and parietal peritoneum. Growth of these nodules and their surrounding stroma produces adhesions leading to mechanical obstruction of the intestine. Invasion of the myenteric plexus also can produce functional ileus. Early implants are found on the hemidiaphragms, particularly on the right, due to the characteristic clockwise circulation of fluid in the peritoneal cavity. Blockade of diaphragmatic lymphatics as well as exudation across tumor capillaries contributes to the intraperitoneal accumulation of ascites fluid. During embryonic development, the ovaries migrate to the pelvis from the level of the renal hilus. Consequently, ovarian lymphatic channels drain to the retroperitoneal lymph nodes at the level of the renal arteries. Retrograde metastases also can occur to femoral and inguinal lymphatics. Hematogenous metastases to the hepatic parenchyma, lung, and brain have been observed, particularly in those individuals whose intraperitoneal disease has been controlled by cytotoxic chemotherapy. Clinically significant metastases to bone are uncommon.

Clinical features and diagnosis Early-stage disease is often asymptomatic and is detected coincidentally by palpating an ovarian mass on pelvic examination. In premenopausal patients, some 95 percent of adnexal masses are benign. Even after menopause, some 70 percent of adnexal masses are benign, but detection of any ovarian enlargement in a postmenopausal patient is an indication for surgical exploration. In premenopausal patients, a mass that enlarges progressively under observation or any mass >8 cm requires exploratory surgery. In addition to primary ovarian cancers, adnexal masses can be produced by functional ovarian cysts, benign ovarian neoplasms, pedunculated uterine fibroids, hydrosalpinx, endometriosis, and inflammatory lesions of the bowel. Transvaginal sonography can aid in confirming the ovarian origin of an adnexal mass and in defining its gross morphology. Bilateral lesions and irregular, complex cysts that contain solid projections are more likely to be malignant.

In postmenopausal patients with a pelvic mass, a markedly elevated serum CA-125 level (>95 U/mL) distinguishes malignant from benign disease with a positive predictive value of 96 percent. CA-125 determinants are expressed on a high-molecular-weight glycoprotein composed of 220-kDa subunits that can be associated with cancers from a number of sites, including the ovary, endometrium, fallopian tube, endocervix, pancreas, breast, lung, and colon. Elevated levels of CA-125 in a patient with a pelvic mass should prompt her referral for initial exploration at an institution capable of proper staging of early ovarian cancer and of cytoreductive surgery for advanced disease.

Progressive enlargement of a localized ovarian cancer can produce urologic or gynecologic symptoms, including urinary frequency, dysuria, obstipation, or constipation. Rarely, torsion of an ovarian mass can produce acute abdominal symptoms. Vaginal bleeding or discharge is not frequently associated with primary ovarian cancer in postmenopausal patients, although premenopausal patients can experience heavy or irregular menstrual periods.

Approximately two-thirds of patients present with stage III or IV disease. Symptoms of more advanced disease include abdominal distention from ascites and ill-defined abdominal pain. Paracentesis usually is not required in a woman with ascites and an adnexal mass, since prompt surgical exploration is already indicated. In addition to a history, physical examination, and complete blood count, the patient's workup should include liver function studies, a serum CA-125 determination, a transvaginal sonogram, a chest film, a mammogram, and, in patients >40 years of age, a barium enema or colonoscopy. Abdominal CT and MRI have a relatively low sensitivity and specificity for diagnosing ovarian cancer and metastatic spread,

precluding their routine use in patients with a unilateral ovarian mass and normal hepatic function.

Prognostic factors Survival is directly related to stage, grade, and the amount of tumor that remains following cytoreductive surgery. Recent studies of cell growth regulation have identified relevant biologic markers. Response to treatment is also an important prognostic factor and can be assessed with serum markers and by "second look" surgical surveillance procedures.

STAGE Stage is assessed at surgical exploration (Table 321-2). In stage I disease, tumor is limited to one or both ovaries. In stage II disease, the pelvic organs are involved without other intraperitoneal spread. In stage III disease, the tumor is limited to the abdominal cavity or retroperitoneum without invasion of the hepatic parenchyma. Stage IV disease involves hepatic parenchymal invasion or tumor spread above the diaphragm.

Careful surgical exploration is required to document early-stage disease. Although a Pfannenstiel incision is sometimes used to remove benign ovarian masses, this approach precludes exploration of the upper abdomen. A midline incision is required for adequate assessment of ovarian cancer. Surgical staging involves examination of both diaphragms, omentectomy, retroperitoneal lymph node sampling, cytologic examination of peritoneal washings, biopsy of any suspicious lesion, as well as random biopsies of apparently normal peritoneal surfaces. Reexploration following simple oophorectomy has resulted in upstaging 30 percent of patients thought to have early-stage disease.

For well-staged patients, 5-year survival in stage I can exceed 90 percent, and that in stage II, approximates 70 to 80 percent. Contemporary management produces a 20 to 30 percent long-term survival in stage III and approximately 5 percent in stage IV.

TUMOR BURDEN With advanced disease, cytoreductive surgery is thought to be of benefit. If the bulk of tumor can be removed, leaving nodules no greater than 1.5 cm, the prognosis of patients is no worse than if only 1.5-cm disease had been present before surgery. Whether this reflects the underlying biology of the disease or the benefit from tumor removal cannot be resolved from studies presently available. Patients whose tumor can be optimally cytoreduced have a median survival of some 39 months compared with 17 months in

---

TABLE 321-2 Staging of primary ovarian cancer

Stage I		Growth limited to the ovaries
	Ia	Growth limited to one ovary with an intact capsule and without ascites or tumor on the external surface
	Ib	Growth limited to both ovaries with intact capsules and without ascites or tumor on the external surfaces
	Ic	Growth limited to one or both ovaries with tumor on the ovarian surface(s) or with rupture of the capsule(s) or ascites present containing malignant cells or with positive peritoneal washings
Stage II		Growth involving one or both ovaries with pelvic extension
	IIa	Extension and/or metastasis to the uterus and/or tubes
	IIb	Extension to other pelvic tissues
	IIc	Growth involving one or both ovaries with metastasis to uterus, tubes, or pelvis with tumor on the ovarian surface or with rupture of the capsule(s) or ascites present containing malignant cells or with positive peritoneal washings
Stage III		Tumor involving one or both ovaries with peritoneal implants outside the pelvis and/or positive retroperitoneal or inguinal nodes. Superficial liver metastasis indicates stage III disease. Tumor is limited to the true pelvis, but with histologically proven malignant extension to small bowel or omentum
	IIIa	Tumor grossly limited to the true pelvis with negative nodes but with histologically confirmed microscopic seeding of abdominal peritoneal surfaces
	IIIb	Tumor of one or both ovaries with histologically confirmed implants of abdominal peritoneal surfaces, none exceeding 2 cm in diameter. Nodes negative.
	IIIc	Abdominal implants >2 cm in diameter and/or positive retroperitoneal or inguinal nodes
Stage IV		Growth involving one or both ovaries with distant metastasis. If pleural effusion is present, there must be positive cytologic test results to allot a case to stage IV. Parenchymal liver metastasis indicates stage IV.

patients with suboptimal cytoreduction in collected series. Patients with bulky disease remaining after surgery rarely experience long-term survival. Only approximately 35 percent of patients with stage III or IV ovarian cancer can be optimally cytoreduced.

HISTOLOGIC GRADE AND CELL TYPE Well-differentiated tumors are associated with a better prognosis than are moderately or poorly differentiated tumors. In some series, clear cell carcinomas are associated with a worse prognosis than are tumors of other histologic types, but among the epithelial ovarian cancers of similar stage, the tumor grade is more important than histologic subtype.

BIOLOGIC MARKERS Expression of EGFR, expression of *fms*, and overexpression of *erb*B-2 are all poor prognostic factors for ovarian cancer. Coexpression of these transmembrane tyrosine kinase growth factor receptors and their ligands may provide autocrine growth stimulation or alter resistance to cytotoxic chemotherapy. An aneuploid karyotype is also associated with a poor prognosis, particularly in borderline lesions.

SERUM MARKERS Tumor burden can be assessed during therapy in more than 80 percent of patients with the serum marker CA-125. When elevated prior to treatment, serum CA-125 levels have correlated with the clinical disease course in 90 percent of instances studied. In addition, elevations of CA-125 have preceded clinical disease recurrence by an average of 3 months, and persistently rising CA-125 values are consistently associated with progressive disease. Elevation of CA-125 (>35 U/mL) at the time of a "second look" surveillance procedure predicts persistence of disease with 96 percent accuracy. When CA-125 levels return to <35 U/mL prior to second look, small-volume residual disease can, however, still be found in 60 percent of cases. Finally, the rate at which CA-125 normalizes correlates with findings at second look procedures and survival. An apparent CA-125 half-life of <20 days is associated with a significantly better prognosis than a half-life of >20 days.

"SECOND LOOK" SURGICAL SURVEILLANCE PROCEDURES At second look laparotomy performed after 3 to 6 months of cytotoxic chemotherapy, 50 to 70 percent of patients with stage III or IV disease will be found to have persistent disease, whereas more than 90 percent of patients with stage I and II disease will be disease-free, suggesting that this procedure may not be required for patients with early-stage ovarian cancer at presentation. If gross disease is found, median survival is only approximately 12 months, whereas persistence of microscopic disease is associated with a median survival of 36 to 48 months. Although a pathologic complete response correlates with a median survival >60 months, 30 to 50 percent of patients who have a negative second look will eventually develop recurrent cancer. Whether or not reresection of disease at second look has therapeutic benefit cannot be resolved from the studies currently available.

Screening strategies Since a majority of patients with stage I and II disease can be cured using conventional therapy, earlier detection of ovarian cancer could improve survival. Pelvic examination is a relatively insensitive technique for the detection of ovarian cancer in its early stages. Cervical cytology is rarely, if ever, positive in primary ovarian cancer. Transvaginal sonography (TVS) has proven more sensitive than transabdominal sonography for detecting ovarian enlargement. Among some 8000 women screened with TVS, 11 cases of ovarian cancer were detected, with 10 in stage I. Despite high sensitivity, however, some 10 to 15 benign lesions are found at laparotomy for each case of ovarian cancer detected. Careful evaluation of morphology and Doppler flow ultrasound may reduce the number of false-positive tests.

CA-125 also may have a role in early detection of ovarian cancer in that values of the serum marker have been elevated 10 to 20 months prior to the diagnosis of the neoplasm. Sensitivity is limited in that only 60 percent of patients with early-stage ovarian cancer will have an elevated antigen level. In a premenopausal population, false-positive values are also a consideration. The first trimester of normal pregnancy, endometriosis, adenomyosis, uterine fibroids, chronic salpingitis, hepatocellular disease, pleuritis, peritonitis, and, rarely, normal menstruation can all elevate serum CA-125. Among postmeno-pausal patients, however, only about 2 percent will have an elevation of CA-125 (>30 U/mL). In studies performed in Sweden and the United Kingdom, an abnormal CA-125 level has triggered the use of transabdominal sonography, permitting the detection of a majority of ovarian cancer cases with some in early stages of disease. Critical studies have not yet been performed to demonstrate the ability of CA-125 and TVS to improve survival of patients with ovarian cancer. At the present time neither CA-125 nor transvaginal sonography should be used routinely for screening, particularly in premenopausal populations.

Therapeutic considerations STAGES I AND II Current management of low-risk ovarian cancers (stage Ia or b and grade 1 or 2) consists of bilateral salpingo-oophorectomy (BSO), total abdominal hysterectomy (TAH), and surgical staging followed by careful observation. In selected premenopausal patients, reproductive function can be preserved by performing unilateral salpingo-oophorectomy. Patients at higher risk with grade 3 cancers or lesions of any grade that have progressed to stages Ic or II generally receive some type of adjuvant therapy following surgery. Intraperitoneal radionuclide (colloidal ^{32}P), total abdominal irradiation, single alkylating agents, or cisplatin-based combinations of cytotoxic drugs have been utilized in this setting. Although many practitioners use cisplatin-based combination chemotherapy to treat high-risk early-stage ovarian cancer, the superiority of any single approach has not been proven.

STAGES III AND IV Treatment of more advanced ovarian cancer involves TAH-BSO, omentectomy, surgical cytoreduction, and platinum-based chemotherapy for 3 to 6 months. Following cytotoxic chemotherapy, a second look laparotomy is usually performed. With current therapy, more than half of patients will have no evidence of disease by noninvasive evaluation at the completion of chemotherapy, but only about 30 to 40 percent will be free from disease when reevaluated with multiple biopsies at second look. Even in the setting of negative surveillance procedures, ovarian cancer recurs in 30 to 50 percent of patients. If residual disease is found at second look operation, investigational therapy has been attempted. This includes intraperitoneal administration of cisplatin and other compounds, use of novel agents such as taxol, and high-dose therapy with hematopoietic stem cell support.

CYTOTOXIC CHEMOTHERAPY Several different cytotoxic drugs have produced at least temporary regression of ovarian cancer (Table 321-3). Alkylating agents have proven most active, and among the alkylators, platinum-based compounds have had the greatest impact. In early studies, it was difficult to show an advantage of multiple cytotoxic drugs over single alkylating agents. With optimal cytoreduction of tumor, however, use of cyclophosphamide and cisplatin in combination has produced greater long-term survival than has cisplatin alone. Addition of doxorubicin or hexamethylmelamine to the alkylators does not appear to improve response rates or survival within individual studies, although metaanalysis suggests an advantage to the addition of doxorubicin. During the last several years, carboplatin, a cisplatin analogue, has proven less nephrotoxic, ototoxic, neuro-

---

TABLE 321-3 Cytotoxic drugs active against ovarian cancer

Alkylating agents
 Cyclophosphamide
 Ifosfamide
 Melphalan
 Chlorambucil
 Thiotepa
 Cisplatin
 Carboplatin
Antimetabolites
 5-Fluorouracil
 Hydroxyurea
Anthracyclines
 Doxorubicin
Other
 Hexamethylmelamine
 Taxol

toxic, and emetogenic but more myelotoxic than the parent compound. In two large studies, a combination of carboplatin and cyclophosphamide was as effective as, but less toxic than, a combination of cisplatin and cyclophosphamide. With carboplatin, dose can be adjusted based on renal function, which correlates effectively with myelosuppression. Current therapy for ovarian cancer includes cisplatin or carboplatin in combination with cyclophosphamide at 3- to 4-week intervals for six to eight cycles. A clinical response rate of 70 percent can be anticipated in patients with advanced epithelial ovarian cancer who have not been previously treated. Approximately 50 percent of responses will be complete judged by noninvasive techniques, and of these patients, 45 percent will have negative surgical surveillance procedures.

PERSISTENT DISEASE If persistent ovarian cancer is found at second look laparotomy or if disease subsequently recurs, options have included retreatment with platinum-based chemotherapy, intravenous administration of other drugs, intraperitoneal chemotherapy, autologous bone marrow transplantation, and immunotherapy. Retreatment with cisplatin or carboplatin has palliated patients who had previously responded to platinum-based chemotherapy and had a disease-free interval of at least 6 months. Among second-line agents, hexamethylmelamine has been used traditionally but has produced a response rate of <20 percent. Ifosfamide with the urothelial protectant mesna induced a 20 percent response rate. Recently, taxol has produced an objective response in 44 percent of patients who could still respond to cisplatin and in 30 percent of patients whose tumors had become resistant to cisplatin. Taxol is derived from the bark of the yew tree and has been in relatively short supply. New sources are being identified, and partial synthesis of the drug has been achieved. The agent has a novel mechanism of action that depends on stabilizing the polymerization of tubulin into microfilaments and mitotic spindles.

INTRAPERITONEAL THERAPY Intraperitoneal therapy produces a substantial pharmacokinetic advantage that depends on the more rapid clearance of compounds such as cisplatin from the peripheral blood than from the abdominal cavity. After intraperitoneal instillation, tumor cells within the peritoneal cavity are exposed to higher concentrations of drug than can be achieved safely by intravenous administration. Patients who have small (<5 mm) tumor nodules and who have previously responded to intravenous cisplatin are most likely to respond to IP cisplatin. As many as 40 percent of such patients have had a complete response following IP administration of cisplatin.

AUTOLOGOUS BONE MARROW TRANSPLANTATION In retrospective studies, response rates to intravenous therapy appeared to depend on the amount of cisplatin that was delivered per unit time. Substantially higher doses of alkylating agents, including platinum-based drugs, can be given with autologous bone marrow and peripheral stem cell support. Using high doses of multiple alkylating agents followed by stem cell and cytokine support, response rates of 54 to 78 percent have been achieved in patients who had failed all conventional therapy.

IMMUNOTHERAPY Different forms of immunotherapy also have been attempted for residual disease. Intraperitoneal instillation of *Corynebacterium parvum*, interferon-α, interferon-γ, or IL-2 can produce responses in approximately one-third of patients. Current trials of IP immunotherapy are evaluating combinations of interferon with standard cytotoxic drugs. Intraperitoneal administration of monoclonal antibodies linked to radionuclides also have shown activity against small volumes of disease.

STROMAL TUMORS Granulosa cell and theca cell tumors are uncommon lesions that occur most frequently in the first three decades of life. Granulosa cell tumors can produce estrogen, leading to premenarchal vaginal bleeding, menstrual irregularities, or postmenopausal bleeding. Endometrial carcinoma is associated with 5 percent of cases, possibly secondary to chronic estrogenic stimulation of the endometrium. Sertoli and Leydig cell tumors most often produce androgens with consequent virilization but can, on occasion, also produce estrogens.

Three-fourths of granulosa cell tumors present in stage I. Growth of tumors is slow, and recurrence is late, with disease-free intervals extending to 10 years. Treatment includes TAH-BSO. Cytotoxic adjuvant chemotherapy is not of proven value. Radiotherapy is of value only in the palliation of unresectable pelvic disease. For recurrent cancer, several different combinations of drugs have been used for palliative treatment, including cyclophosphamide-doxorubicin-cisplatin and actinomycin D–5-fluorouracil–cyclophosphamide.

GERM CELL TUMORS Germ cell tumors account for less than 5 percent of all ovarian cancers but comprise 75 percent of ovarian carcinomas during the first 3 decades of life. With appropriate treatment, >90 percent of patients can be cured. Histologic types include dysgerminomas, immature teratomas, endodermal sinus tumors, embryonal carcinomas, and choriocarcinomas in descending order of incidence. Endodermal sinus tumors secrete alpha fetoprotein (AFP), choriocarcinomas produce human chorionic gonadotropin (hCG), and embryonal carcinomas can express both markers. Pure dysgerminomas and immature teratomas produce neither AFP nor hCG, but elevated levels of either marker can indicate the presence of a mixed germ cell tumor that requires more aggressive treatment.

Dysgerminomas Approximately 5 percent of dysgerminomas are associated with karyotypic abnormalities of the gonads, including pure gonadal dysgenesis (46XY with bilateral streak gonads), mixed gonadal dysgenesis (45X/46XY with unilateral streak gonad and contralateral testis), or testicular feminization (46XY with bilateral testes). Tumors are bilateral in 10 to 15 percent of cases. Dysgerminomas are histologically similar to seminomas and are exquisitely sensitive to radiotherapy or chemotherapy. For disease in stage Ia, unilateral oophorectomy can be performed without additional treatment and with the expectation that radiotherapy or chemotherapy can salvage any subsequent recurrence. The retroperitoneal lymph nodes are the most frequent site of metastasis. For more advanced or recurrent disease, radiotherapy that spares the contralateral ovary or chemotherapy with bleomycin-etoposide and cisplatin (BEP) can cure the tumor and preserve reproductive function.

Nondysgerminomatous tumors Well-differentiated immature teratomas in stage Ia can be managed with surgery alone and careful follow-up. Poorly differentiated lesions or any tumor in a more advanced stage requires adjuvant chemotherapy with BEP or EP alone. In contrast to most other germ cell tumors, 75 percent of patients with endodermal sinus tumors present with pelvic pain. These aggressive tumors are rarely, if ever, bilateral and are treated with unilateral salpingo-oophorectomy, but adjuvant chemotherapy should be given in all cases. Embryonal carcinomas and the rare nongestational choriocarcinomas can be associated with precocious pseudopuberty or irregular menstrual bleeding. Conservative surgery can be undertaken to preserve reproductive function followed by adjuvant chemotherapy with BEP. Primary ovarian choriocarcinoma is less sensitive to cytotoxic chemotherapy than is gestational choriocarcinoma. Taken together, however, virtually all patients with stage I nondysgerminomatous germ cell tumors can be cured, and 50 to 80 percent of patients who present with disseminated disease also can attain long-term survival.

REFERENCES

ALBERTS DS et al: Improved therapeutic index of carboplatin plus cyclophosphamide versus cisplatin plus cyclophosphamide: Final report by the Southwest Oncology Group of a phase III randomized trial in stages III and IV ovarian cancer. J Clin Oncol 10:706, 1992

BAST RC JR et al: A radioimmunoassay using a monoclonal antibody to monitor the course of epithelial ovarian cancer. N Engl J Med 309:883, 1983

——— et al: Malignant transformation of ovarian epithelium. J Natl Cancer Inst 84:556, 1992

BERCHUCK A et al: Oncogenes in ovarian cancer. Hematol Oncol Clin North Am 6:813, 1992

BOOKMAN MA, BAST RC JR: The immunobiology and immunotherapy of ovarian cancer. Semin Oncol 18:270, 1991

CLARKE-PEARSON DL et al: Ovarian cancer, in *Comprehensive Textbook of Oncology*, 2d ed, AR Moossa et al (eds). Baltimore, William & Wilkins, 1991, pp 1006–1019

EINHORN N et al: Specificity of serum CA 125 radioimmunoassay for early detection of ovarian cancer: A prospective study. Obstet Gynecol 80:14, 1992

JACOBS I, BAST RC JR: Tumor markers for ovarian cancer, in *Manual of Clinical Laboratory Immunology*, 4th ed, NR Rose et al (eds). Washington, American Society for Microbiology, 1992, pp 811–816

JOHNSON SW et al: Mechanisms of drug resistance in ovarian cancer. Cancer 71 (2 suppl):594, 1993

LYNCH HT et al: Genetics and gynecologic cancer, in *Principles and Practice of Gynecologic Oncology*, WJ Hoskins et al (eds). Philadelphia, Lippincott, 1992, pp 27–45

MARKMAN M: Intraperitoneal chemotherapy. Semin Oncol 18:248, 1991

MCGUIRE WP, ROWINSKY EK: Old drugs revisited, new drugs, and experimental approaches in ovarian cancer therapy. Semin Oncol 18:255, 1991

OZOLS RF et al: Epithelial ovarian cancer, in *Principles and Practice of Gynecologic Oncology*, WJ Hoskins et al (eds). Philadelphia, Lippincott, 1992, pp 731–781

PIVER MS et al: Epidemiology and etiology of ovarian cancer. Semin Oncol 18:177, 1991

RUNOWICZ CD et al: Taxol in ovarian cancer. Cancer 71 (4 suppl):1591, 1993

SHPALL EJ et al: High-dose alkylating agent chemotherapy with autologous bone marrow support in patients with stage III/IV epithelial ovarian cancer. Gynecol Oncol 38:386, 1990

STANFORD JL: Oral contraceptives and neoplasia of the ovary. Contraception 43:543, 1991

SWENERTON K et al: Cisplatin-cyclophosphamide versus carboplatin-cyclophosphamide in advanced ovarian cancer: A randomized phase III study of the National Cancer Institute of Canada Clinical Trials Group. J Clin Oncol 10:718, 1992

VAN NAGELL JR JR et al: Ovarian cancer screening in asymptomatic postmenopausal women by transvaginal sonography. Cancer 68:458, 1991

WILLIAMS SD et al: Ovarian germ cell and stromal tumors, in *Principles and Practice of Gynecologic Oncology*, WJ Hoskins et al (eds). Philadelphia, Lippincott, 1992, pp 715–730

YOUNG RC et al: Adjuvant therapy in stage I and stage II epithelial ovarian cancer: Results of two prospective randomized trials. N Engl J Med 322:1021, 1990

322 TESTICULAR CANCER AND OTHER TROPHOBLASTIC DISEASES

MARC B. GARNICK

TESTICULAR CANCER

Carcinoma of the testis is a disease that serves as a model of a curable, solid neoplasm. Patients with localized forms of germinal cell cancer have a high cure rate when treated with either surgery or radiation therapy, and the advanced, metastatic forms, which in the past were almost universally fatal, are now also potentially curable. In 1977, testicular cancer was the third leading cause of cancer death in men between the ages of 15 and 34, but by 1981, the disease was no longer among the top five causes of cancer death in the same age group. The multidisciplinary principles and strategies that evolved for the management of patients with advanced testicular cancer are now being applied to other cancers.

Approximately 6600 new cases are diagnosed annually. The incidence in African-Americans is substantially lower than in whites. There is a peak frequency in early childhood and a larger peak incidence between 20 and 35 years. The disease is uncommon after age 40. A lesion suggestive of testicular neoplasm in a patient over the age of 50 should suggest a lymphoma rather than primary germinal cell carcinoma, especially with bilateral involvement of the testes.

Several factors are known to predispose to development of testicular tumor. Men with a history of cryptorchid (undescended) testes have a several-fold increased risk, intraabdominal testes being more at risk than high inguinal testes. Both the cryptorchid testis itself and the contralateral normally descended testis are at risk, suggesting that some underlying testicular defect may predispose both to maldescent and to tumor development. Although the effectiveness of orchiopexy in reducing risk is not established, it is generally agreed that a high inguinal testis should be brought into the scrotum so that it can be followed carefully. Abdominal testes that cannot be treated in this manner should probably be removed. Other predisposing factors include a history of mumps orchitis, inguinal hernia in childhood, and testicular cancer in the contralateral testis. In the majority of cases, no predisposing factor can be identified.

CLINICAL FEATURES AND DIAGNOSIS The manifestations of testicular cancer range from an asymptomatic nodule or swelling detected while performing testicular self-examination to dyspnea secondary to massive pulmonary metastases. Most testicular cancers are diagnosed because of symptoms related to the testes, but significant delay in making a diagnosis is common and is the result of oversight by physicians and by patients. Thus high school health programs that teach testicular self-examination should be encouraged. Such programs have allowed early diagnosis, leading to more successful treatment outcomes. Most testicular cancers occur in men under age 40, and the public should be educated to the need to seek prompt medical advice for any change in previously normal testes, including the presence of a mass, a feeling of heaviness, pain, hardness, and swelling. Other causes of testicular masses include hydrocele, epididymitis, spermatocele, and orchitis, but to reduce delay in reaching a diagnosis, physicians should consider any testicular mass to be malignant until proven otherwise. Patients with testicular tumors may have pain because of associated nonneoplastic lesions, such as epididymitis.

Back or abdominal pain secondary to retroperitoneal adenopathy, weight loss, dyspnea secondary to pulmonary metastases, gynecomastia, supraclavicular lymphadenopathy, and urinary obstruction also may be present at diagnosis.

A testicular sonogram can aid in establishing the presence of a testicular parenchymal abnormality. Magnetic resonance imaging of the testis can sometimes provide useful information when the results of the physical examination and testicular ultrasound are equivocal. Once the diagnosis of a testicular neoplasm is suspected, a blood sample should be set aside, prior to orchiectomy, for subsequent determination of the tumor marker glycoproteins alpha fetoprotein (AFP) and human chorionic gonadotropin (hCG). The correct operative approach is a high radical inguinal orchiectomy. A transscrotal biopsy of the testis or a transscrotal orchiectomy should never be performed if the diagnosis of testicular cancer is likely. Because the lymphatic drainage of the testis (to the retroperitoneal lymphatics between L1 and L3) differs from that of the scrotum (to superficial and deep inguinal groin nodes), a scrotal incision in the presence of a testicular cancer may predispose to the development of local recurrences and metastases to the inguinal lymphatics. This rarely happens if a high radical inguinal orchiectomy is performed.

CLASSIFICATION AND PATHOLOGY The most widely used classification of testicular tumors is that of Mostofi and is based on the cell type from which the tumor is derived, namely germinal or stromal (Leydig and Sertoli) cells (Table 322-1). Germinal cell tumors, the most common of these tumors and the focus of this chapter, can be subdivided into seminomas and nonseminomas. Seminomas are characterized by large cells with clear cytoplasm in a delicate fibrovascular stroma infiltrated with lymphocytes. Indeed, the granulomatous reaction around the tumor can be so intense as to

TABLE 322-1 Classification of testicular tumors

Germinal cell tumors (95%)
  Single cell tumors (60%)
    Seminomas
    Nonseminomas
      Embryonal cell tumors (yolk sac tumors)
      Teratomas
      Choriocarcinomas
  Combination tumors (40%)
Tumors of gonadal stroma (1–2%)
  Leydig cell
  Sertoli cell
  Primitive gonadal structures
Gonadoblastoma (germinal cell + stomal cell)

SOURCE: After FK Mostofi, Cancer 45:1735, 1980.

suggest a graft-versus-host reaction. These tumors account for about half of all testicular neoplasms and can be divided into typical, spermatocytic, and anaplastic varieties. Germinal cell tumors of the nonseminoma type can be divided into embryonal cell tumors (yolk sac tumors), teratomas, and choriocarcinomas. Embryonal carcinomas are common in children and resemble embryonal carcinomas of the ovary. Choriocarcinomas contain syncytiotrophoblastic cells. Teratomas contain at least two types of germinal cell layers and in childhood are second in frequency to embryonal tumor. Mixed tumors that contain combinations of germinal cell types account for 40 percent of germinal cell tumors; the biology of such tumors is usually determined by the least differentiated (most malignant) elements. All four types of germinal cell tumors also can originate in extragonadal sites, most commonly the mediastinum or brain. Such extragonadal tumors are presumed to arise either from aberrant migration of germinal cells during embryogenesis or, alternatively, from some common precursor stem cell line that gives rise to the germinal cells, the thymus, and the pineal.

From the clinical standpoint, the critical distinction is between *seminomas* and *nonseminomas* based on the histopathology of the orchiectomy specimen. The former must be in pure form; the latter may either be a mixed cancer with both seminomatous and nonseminomatous components or a pure form of a nonseminoma, such as embryonal cell carcinoma, teratoma, or choriocarcinoma. The term *teratocarcinoma* generally refers to a mixed nonseminomatous cancer consisting of teratoma and embryonal cell cancer.

The distinction between seminoma and nonseminoma is important because the staging evaluation and subsequent management in the two differ as a consequence of the relative radioresponsiveness of seminomas compared with the radioresistance of nonseminomas. Radiation therapy to the lymphatics of the abdomen and/or chest is the mainstay of therapy in patients with pure seminoma but is rarely utilized in patients with nonseminoma. In addition, seminomas usually spread via the regional lymphatics to the retroperitoneal nodes of the abdomen and/or to the mediastinal and supraclavicular lymph nodes before gaining access to other visceral structures. Pulmonary and other hematogenous metastases (e.g., hepatic, central nervous system, osseous) are more common in patients with nonseminomas than in patients with seminomas.

BIOLOGIC AND MOLECULAR TUMOR MARKERS Germinal cell cancers of the testis often secrete biologic tumor markers that can be detected in the peripheral blood (see Chap. 327). Following orchiectomy, the presence of such markers in blood reflects the presence of metastatic disease. Such assays also can be valuable in monitoring therapy (marker levels fall with disease regression and increase with disease progression), and elevated levels in blood may predate the detection of new clinical or radiologic metastatic disease by weeks to months. The two most common markers are AFP and hCG. AFP is commonly secreted by embryonal cell cancer; its biologic half-life is approximately 6 days. AFP is not produced by pure seminoma, and its detection implies the presence of nonseminomatous elements, either in the primary lesion itself or in the metastatic site, even when the primary orchiectomy specimen is thought to be a pure seminoma. hCG is secreted by syncytiotrophoblastic giant cells, present most commonly in choriocarcinomas; such giant cells may be present in embryonal cell components and occasionally in so-called pure seminomas. The biologic half-life of hCG is approximately 24 h. hCG may be biologically active, and hCG-enhanced secretion of estrogen by the testis is the cause of gynecomastia in such patients (see Chap. 341). Several cytogenetic markers have recently been associated with germ cell cancer of the testis. Isochromosome 12p(i)(12p) is present in the majority of all forms of germ cell neoplasms and when present in multiple copies may be associated with a poorer prognosis.

STAGING EVALUATION The function of staging is to determine whether the cancer is localized to the testis or to regional lymphatics or is widely disseminated. Such information is necessary to determine if disease is amenable to local or regional therapy. If the disease is disseminated at presentation, the initial staging evaluation serves as a baseline in assessing subsequent response. Since the approach to staging and management is dictated by the pathologic diagnosis of the orchiectomy specimen, the appropriate evaluation will be outlined for each.

Pure seminoma The routine workup involves careful physical examination, an abdominal-pelvic computed tomographic (CT) scan to determine the presence of retroperitoneal adenopathy or visceral involvement, a chest x-ray with or without lung tomography, measurement of routine chemistries, and assessment of the biologic markers (AFP and hCG). In most cases, the biologic markers are undetectable. If AFP is elevated, the patient should be treated as having a nonseminoma, even though the pathologic interpretation is pure seminoma.

The portals for radiation therapy for pure seminomas were traditionally determined on the basis of bipedal lymphangiography. However, the necessity of lymphangiography for such purposes is less imperative today because CT scanning may provide similar information.

If plasma hCG is elevated in a patient with a diagnosis of pure seminoma, a search should be made for syncytiotrophoblastic giant cells. Otherwise, there may be some uncertainty as to whether occult foci of nonseminomatous components are responsible for the hCG production. Also, if the physical or radiographic examinations fail to reveal any evidence of metastatic disease and the hCG level is elevated before orchiectomy, it is necessary to follow the level of hCG sequentially. If the marker does not decline as predicted by its biologic half-life, the presence of occult metastatic cancer should be considered.

Nonseminoma The staging evaluation outlined for the seminoma is employed for the patient with a nonseminomatous germinal cell tumor of the testis. On the basis of these noninvasive staging studies, patients can be categorized as having stage I, early stage II, advanced stage II, or stage III disease. Patients with stage I disease have no clinical, radiographic, or marker evidence of tumor presence beyond the confines of the testis. Patients with early stage II have nonpalpable, small, retroperitoneal adenopathy on CT scans, usually measuring <4 to 5 cm. Advanced stage II is defined as retroperitoneal lymphadenopathy measuring >5 cm on CT scan or palpable retroperitoneal adenopathy with disease limited to lymphatics below the diaphragm. Stage III disease includes visceral involvement below the diaphragm (e.g., liver or bowel) or above the diaphragm (e.g., lung or supraclavicular lymphadenopathy). Furthermore, patients with stage III disease can be further subdivided according to anatomic location and extent of disease. Treatment decisions are often based on volume of disease in stage III patients.

Conceptually, patients with testicular cancer can be categorized pathologically as having either *seminoma* or *nonseminoma* and staged as having either "early" or "advanced" disease. Patients with *early* disease would be considered to have stage I and early stage II disease, while patients with *advanced* disease have advanced stage II or any form of stage III disease. This formulation allows rational decision making for nearly all categories of disease.

TREATMENT MODALITIES ACCORDING TO HISTOLOGY AND STAGE (Table 322-2) **Early seminoma** These patients have either a normal abdominal CT scan or retroperitoneal lymphadenopathy measuring less than 5 cm in greatest diameter. Most such patients are treated with abdominal radiotherapy, delivering 30 Gy (3000 rad) to the subdiaphragmatic lymph nodes and ipsilateral groin and a 6-Gy (600-rad) boost in areas of known disease. Although prophylactic mediastinal and supraclavicular radiation therapy was used in the past, this practice is generally not employed today. When treated with radiation following orchiectomy, patients with clinical stage I disease have a 95 to 97 percent cure rate, and patients with early stage II disease have an 85 to 90 percent survival rate.

As with stage I nonseminoma (see below), a policy of surveillance has been recommended for stage I seminoma following orchiectomy. This strategy potentially avoids the use of radiotherapy in patients cured with orchiectomy alone. In those who relapse, radiotherapy or

TABLE 322-2 Testicular cancer: General approach to management and cure rates*

	Seminoma	% Cure	Nonseminoma	% Cure
Stage I	XRT or surveillance[†]	95–97	RPLND or surveillance[†]	97
Early stage II	XRT	85–90	RPLND ± chemo[a] or Chemo[a]	85–90
Advanced stage II Stage III	Chemo[a]	80–85	Chemo[a] ± TRS ± Chemo[b]	80–85

* XRT = radiation therapy, delivered to subdiaphragmatic lymphatics; RPLND = retroperitoneal lymph node dissection; chemo[a] = combination chemotherapy (see Table 322-3); TRS = tumor-reductive surgery; chemo[b] = additional chemotherapy given if surgical specimen reveals viable cancer.
† Must be done in context of clinical protocol, with detailed follow-up and a compliant patient.

TABLE 322-3 Commonly used chemotherapy programs for advanced testicular cancer

BEP	PVB	VAB-6
Etoposide	Vinblastine	Vinblastine
Bleomycin	Bleomycin	Bleomycin
Cisplatin	Cisplatin	Cisplatin
		Cyclophosphamide
		Actinomycin D

chemotherapy is then instituted with excellent results. Such surveillance programs must be performed within the context of a clinical trial and require highly motivated and compliant patients.

Advanced seminoma In the past, patients with large retroperitoneal masses or mediastinal involvement were often treated with radiation therapy to fields including the subdiaphragmatic lymph nodes, whole abdomen, mediastinum, and supraclavicular nodes; however, survival rates were only 40 to 70 percent. If these patients subsequently suffered a relapse in an area outside the radiation therapy field, the ability to administer myelosuppressive combination chemotherapy was diminished and was associated with drug-related morbidity. Today, most patients with advanced forms of seminoma are treated initially with combination chemotherapy that includes cisplatin. Substantial tumor shrinkage occurs in the majority of patients. However, the proper management for partially regressed retroperitoneal masses following chemotherapy is controversial. Patients are restaged following chemotherapy, and depending on the individual treatment protocol, further treatment with chemotherapy, surgery, or radiation therapy is addressed.

Stage I nonseminoma Patients with stage I nonseminoma are routinely treated with a retroperitoneal lymph node dissection (RPLND), using either a transabdominal or a thoracoabdominal approach. The rationale for this operation is based on the inexact data generated from the noninvasive staging evaluation of the retroperitoneal lymphatics. The false-negative rate of abdominal CT scans in patients with clinical stage I disease is 35 to 40 percent. Thus surgical removal of the retroperitoneal lymph nodes not only serves as therapy but also determines the need for possible additional therapy. If microscopic disease is detected and surgically removed, an 85 to 90 percent cure rate can be expected following RPLND.

More recently, a policy of orchiectomy followed by surveillance has been used for selected stage I nonseminoma patients. This strategy avoids a retroperitoneal lymph node dissection in a large percentage of patients. If relapse occurs, chemotherapy can then be instituted, with achievement of greater than 90 percent cure rates.

Stage II nonseminoma The optimal management of patients with retroperitoneal lymphadenopathy measuring between 2 and 5 cm on CT scan is controversial. While RPLND may be curative, a relapse rate of 30 to 45 percent can be expected. If relapse occurs after RPLND, combination chemotherapy can be administered, or chemotherapy may sometimes be given as an adjuvant to RPLND. Alternatively, combination chemotherapy can be given prior to RPLND. If complete resolution of disease is achieved following chemotherapy, RPLND would not be performed, obviating the need for the operation in this subset of patients.

Advanced stage (bulky stage II or stage III) nonseminoma The most common chemotherapy program includes cisplatin, bleomycin, and etoposide (BEP program). Other very active chemotherapeutic agents used in association with cisplatin include vinblastine and bleomycin (PVB program) or actinomycin D, cyclophosphamide,

vinblastine, and bleomycin (VAB program) (Table 322-3). The use of these agents is associated with complete remission in as many as 80 to 85 percent of patients when administered cyclically over a 9- to 12-week period.

Following such therapy, patients are then restaged (with physical, radiographic, and biochemical examinations) to assess the response of areas which previously contained disease and to determine the need for additional therapy. Large abdominal masses may undergo astonishing regression. Pulmonary nodules often resolve completely, and biologic markers frequently return to normal after chemotherapy. If a residual abdominal or pulmonary mass persists despite normal levels of plasma markers, surgical removal of the mass(es) should be undertaken. Table 322-4 outlines current recommendations. Preoperatively, it is difficult to determine the nature of such residual masses. Approximately 20 percent contain residual, viable cancer; 40 percent contain fibrosis, necrosis, or hemorrhage; and an additional 40 percent demonstrate the phenomenon of "teratomatous transformation." The latter is thought to result either from chemotherapy-induced differentiation of the primary mass into a teratoma or from the selective elimination of the more malignant elements of the mass but persistence of residual teratomatous components. If either fibrosis, hemorrhage, or teratoma is found following chemotherapy, additional postoperative chemotherapy is usually not indicated. If, however, residual cancer is demonstrated, additional cisplatin combination chemotherapy is required.

If biologic markers are persistently positive following remission induction chemotherapy, additional chemotherapy is also indicated. "Tumor-reductive" surgery should not be attempted until biologic markers return to normal in most cases. Some patients experience complete resolution of physical, radiographic, and biochemical marker abnormalities after cisplatin-containing chemotherapy and may require no additional chemotherapy or surgery following their program of chemotherapy.

Testicular cancer which is refractory of BEP or other cisplatin-containing programs may sometimes respond to the addition of ifosfamide. Ifosfamide has been approved by the FDA for third-line treatment with other antineoplastics for patients with refractory germ cell tumors. The combination of cisplatin, etoposide, and ifosfamide will result in a second or third remission, which may be durable, in approximately 25 percent of patients. The use of autologous bone marrow transplantation with high-dose chemotherapy remains a

TABLE 322-4 Advanced testicular cancer, nonseminoma: Approach to management after initial chemotherapy

Biologic markers*	Radiographic abnormalities	Therapeutic choice
Positive	Present or absent	Additional chemotherapy[†]
Normal	Present	TRS[‡] ± chemotherapy[§]
Normal	Absent	Observation

* Alpha fetoprotein and human chorionic gonadotropin.
† Chemotherapy with a "second-line" program, with attempts to "normalize" biologic markers.
‡ Tumor-reductive surgery.
§ Additional chemotherapy determined by presence of "viable" cancer in surgical specimen. Chemotherapy withheld if surgical specimen contains only fibrosis or teratoma.

potential therapy for patients with refractory germ cell tumors. Although still investigational, a small percentage of patients can achieve long-term remission and even cure.

FOLLOW-UP OF PATIENTS WITH TESTICULAR CANCER All patients with testicular cancer, regardless of pathology or stage, require meticulous follow-up with monthly physical examinations, chest x-rays, and assessment of markers for 18 to 24 months. Patients with stage I disease who are treated with a surveillance policy following orchiectomy will need frequent abdominal-pelvic CT scanning in addition to the other follow-up evaluations. The frequency of these tests can be decreased in the third or fourth year following diagnosis. The goal is to detect relapse when the tumor burden is minimal. Most relapses from testicular cancer occur within the first 2 years following diagnosis, but late relapses do occur.

SIDE EFFECTS OF THERAPY **Radiation therapy and surgery** Infertility can result both from radiation therapy and RPLND. Because these modalities are generally reserved for the management of early-stage patients, a full discussion with patients about the potential loss of fertility is appropriate. Although of questionable benefit, the possibility of sperm banking should be considered prior to the initiation of either definitive radiation therapy for early-stage seminomas or RPLND for early-stage nonseminomas. Modifications in the surgical technique of RPLND (limited nerve-sparing dissection) may decrease the incidence of fertility loss and ejaculatory disturbances.

Combination chemotherapy When standard BEP programs are employed, the major side effects are myelosuppression, potential for nephrotoxicity, nausea and vomiting, weight loss, anemia, ileus, pulmonary toxicity, ototoxicity, peripheral neuropathy, Raynaud's phenomenon, alopecia, hypomagnesemia, and stomatitis. Neuromuscular and gastrointestinal toxicity were more frequent in vinblastine-containing programs. Infertility is usual during therapy, although fertility may return years after completion of therapy. The use of the chemotherapy programs requires skill on the part of the treating physician and should not be attempted by the occasional user. With proper expertise, these side effects can often be minimized. Hemorrhagic cystitis, which can occur with ifosfamide, can be minimized by concomitant use of the uroprotector mesna.

Bleomycin is known to cause pulmonary toxicity (see Chap. 218), and special precautions must be taken in patients who have received bleomycin and are scheduled for a surgical procedure. The acute respiratory distress syndrome has occurred in some and is thought to be related to excessive fluid overload and high inspired oxygen concentration (FI_{O_2}) during the operative procedure. Current recommendations now call for the FI_{O_2} to be maintained at ≤24 percent and for patients to be kept in a hypovolemic or euvolemic state in the perioperative period. Such measures seem to minimize the postoperative pulmonary complications. Hypercholesterolemia is found in a substantial percentage of cured patients years following completion of cisplatin-containing therapy.

THE EXTRAGONADAL GERMINAL CELL SYNDROME Patients with extragonadal germinal cell tumors may present with a large anterior mediastinal mass, central nervous system abnormalities, or retroperitoneal disease. The response to therapy is generally lower when compared with primary testicular cancer, justifying the need for more intensive therapy. Many patients relapse years after the original diagnosis, leading to a lower cure rate compared with patients with primary testicular cancer. However, a proportion of these patients may be cured when treated with chemotherapy and tumor-reductive surgery. In addition, patients with "undifferentiated" cancer of the mediastinum or retroperitoneum may have an unrecognized form of extragonadal germinal cell cancer. Biologic markers and immunohistochemical staining of the biopsy material for AFP or hCG may provide useful clues. If positive, these patients should be treated as if they have potentially curable advanced testicular cancer. Extragonadal germ cell neoplasms have been associated with a spectrum of non-treatment-related hematologic abnormalities, including idiopathic thrombocytopenia, acute megakaryocytic leukemia, myelodysplasia, and malignant histiocytosis.

OTHER TROPHOBLASTIC DISEASES

Trophoblastic tumors of females encompass all proliferative trophoblastic growths that develop from pregnancy and are hence entitled *gestational trophoblastic neoplasms*. Gestational trophoblastic tumors arise most commonly from antecedent molar pregnancies but also may follow term and ectopic pregnancy and spontaneous abortions. The incidence of choriocarcinoma occurring during a term pregnancy is approximately 1 in 150,000, and approximately 75 percent of these patients demonstrate metastatic disease, the lungs being the most frequent site of metastases. The incidence of choriocarcinoma occurring with an ectopic pregnancy is approximately 1 in 5000; the incidence with spontaneous abortion is approximately 1 in 15,000.

Pathologically, the morphology of gestational trophoblastic neoplasms includes the complete and partial hydatidiform mole, invasive mole, and choriocarcinoma. The distinction between *complete* and *partial* is based on gross and microscopic appearance and karyotype. Complete moles usually demonstrate the absence of fetal or embryonic tissue; such tissue is present in a partial mole. Most complete moles have a 46,XX chromosome pattern; partial moles generally have a triploid karyotype, with the extra set of chromosomes of paternal derivation.

Based on data generated by the New England Trophoblastic Disease Center, presenting signs of patients with complete hydatidiform mole are abnormal vaginal bleeding (>90 percent), anemia (>50 percent), enlargement of the uterus (>50 percent), toxemia of pregnancy (25 percent), hyperemesis gravidarum (25 percent), and infrequently, hyperthyroidism and trophoblastic emboli to the lung. Patients with trophoblastic moles often present with the signs and symptoms of a spontaneous abortion, with vaginal bleeding being the most common feature.

Following evacuation of the molar pregnancy, approximately 15 percent of patients demonstrate localized uterine invasion, and 4 percent demonstrate metastatic disease, most often associated with choriocarcinoma.

Gestational trophoblastic neoplasms can be staged according to the FIGO staging system. Stage I is tumor localized to the uterus; stage II is tumor involving the pelvis and/or vagina; stage III is tumor involving the lung; stage IV is tumor involving other organs. The stage of the patient is generally determined after an extensive diagnostic evaluation, including a history and physical examination, measurement of hCG levels, and routine biochemical and hematologic evaluation. The metastatic workup generally includes a chest x-ray, abdominal-pelvic ultrasonography, evaluation of the liver for hepatic metastases, and, on occasion, angiography of abdominal or pelvic organs. In individuals with choriocarcinoma and documented metastases, hCG values are often measured in the cerebral spinal fluid to detect asymptomatic central nervous system involvement. Likewise, stool guaiac tests are often done to rule out lesions to the gastrointestinal tract.

The most important aspect of gestational trophoblastic neoplasms is the fact that there is a 100 percent cure rate in patients with stages I to III and approximately an 85 percent cure rate in patients with stage IV. Depending on the extent of disease and the level of hCG in the bloodstream, individuals are treated with evacuation of their pregnancy or chemotherapy. For patients having a good prognosis, single-agent methotrexate or actinomycin D are generally employed, while high-risk patients are generally treated with combination chemotherapy, including methotrexate, actinomycin D, and cyclophosphamide. More recently, for patients with evidence of metastatic disease, more intensive programs, including vinblastine, bleomycin, and cisplatin, have been used with excellent success. Treatment is continued until baselines of hCG have returned to normal.

Many patients can expect normal reproductive function following treatment. There is, however, an increased incidence of repeat episodes of moles or gestational trophoblastic neoplasms in subsequent pregnancies. The sequential determination of hCG has been extremely valuable in the monitoring of such patients.

REFERENCES

BERKOWITZ RS, GOLDSTEIN DP: Management of molar pregnancy and gestation trophoblastic disease, in *Gynecologic Oncology*, RC Knapp, RS Berkowitz (eds). New York, Macmillan, 1986

BOYLE P, ZARIDZE DG: Risk factors for prostate and testicular cancer. Eur J Cancer 29A(7):1048, 1993

EINHORN EH, DONOHUE JP: *cis*-Diamminedichloroplatinum, vinblastine, and bleomycin combination chemotherapy in disseminated testicular cancer. Ann Intern Med 87:293, 1977

FUNG CY, GARNICK MB: Clinical stage I carcinoma of the testis: A review. J Clin Oncol 6:734, 1988

GARNICK MB: Advanced testicular cancer: Treatment choices in the "land of plenty" (editorial). J Clin Oncol 3:294, 1985

GIETEMA JA et al: Long-term follow-up of cardiovascular risk factors in patients given chemotherapy for disseminated nonseminomatous testicular cancer. Ann Intern Med 116:709, 1992

NICHOLS CR et al: Hematologic neoplasia associated with primary mediastinal germ cell tumors: An update. N Engl J Med 322:1425, 1990

POTTERN LM et al: Tresticular cancer risk among young men: Role of cryptorchidism and inguinal hernia. J Natl Cancer Inst 74:377, 1985

ROTH BJ, NICHOLS CR (eds): Testicular cancer. Semin Oncol 19:117, 118, 1992

STEPHENS RL, WILLIAMSON SK: Clinical stage I testicular cancer: Orchiectomy without node dissection (editorial). Ann Intern Med 109:179, 1988

WILLIAMS SD et al: Treatment of disseminated germ-cell tumors with cisplatin, bleomycin, and either vinblastine or etoposide. N Engl J Med 316:1435, 1987

――― et al: Immediate adjuvant chemotherapy versus observation with treatment at relapse in pathological stage II testicular cancer. N Engl J Med 317:1433, 1987

323　HYPERPLASIA AND CARCINOMA OF THE PROSTATE

ARTHUR I. SAGALOWSKY / JEAN D. WILSON

PROSTATIC HYPERPLASIA

Development of prostatic hyperplasia is an almost universal phenomenon in aging men. The prostate weighs only a few grams at birth; at puberty it undergoes androgen-mediated growth and reaches the adult size of about 20 g by age 20. It remains stable in size for about 25 years, and during the fifth decade a second growth spurt commences in the majority of men. Consequently, the disorder affects men over the age of 45 and increases in frequency with age so that by the eighth decade more than 90 percent of men have prostatic hyperplasia at autopsy. Because of refinements in prostatic surgery, the disorder is not a major cause of death, but it is a leading cause of morbidity in elderly men. The prostate surrounds the urethra, and prostatic hyperplasia is the most common cause of obstruction to urinary outflow in men. Overall, prostatic surgery is performed in about 10 percent of men at some time. The disorder occurs in all populations but is less common in the Orient. The mean age for development of symptomatic disease is about 65 years for whites and about 60 years for blacks. Prostatic hyperplasia does not predispose to the development of prostatic cancer.

PATHOGENESIS Unlike the pubertal growth spurt which involves the gland diffusely, prostatic hyperplasia begins in the periurethral region as a localized proliferation and progresses to compress the remaining normal gland. Histologically, the hyperplastic tissue is nodular and composed of varying amounts of glandular epithelium, stroma, and smooth muscle. The hyperplasia can compress and obstruct the urethra; rarely, the hyperplastic gland grows posteriorly to obstruct the rectum and cause constipation.

The pathogenesis is not well understood, but two necessary features for the process are aging and the presence of testes; whether the testes play a direct or permissive role is not known, but the active androgen that mediates prostatic growth at all ages is dihydrotestosterone, which is formed within the prostate from plasma testosterone (see Chap. 339). In the castrated dog, hormonal therapy that increases dihydrotestosterone levels in the prostate causes prostatic enlargement comparable with that seen in spontaneous canine prostatic hyperplasia. Estradiol levels in men increase with age (absolutely or relative to testosterone levels), and in dogs estrogen acts synergistically with dihydrotestosterone to induce prostatic growth by enhancing the amount of androgen receptor protein in the tissue. Consequently, the role of aging in the development of prostatic hyperplasia might be explained if estradiol augments dihydrotestosterone action in humans as well.

DIAGNOSIS Urethral obstruction results from the elongation, tortuosity, and compression of the posterior urethra, but there is no straightforward relationship between obstruction and prostate size; indeed, severe obstruction can occur when the hyperplasia does not exceed the size of the normal gland. Early symptoms can be minimal because compensatory hypertrophy of the detrusor musculature of the bladder can compensate for the resistance to urine flow. With increasing obstruction, diminution in the caliber and force of the urinary stream, hesitancy in initiating voiding, postvoiding dribbling, the sensation of incomplete emptying, and on occasion urinary retention supervene. These *obstructive* symptoms must be distinguished from *irritative* symptoms such as dysuria, frequency, and urgency that also can result from inflammatory, infectious, or neoplastic causes. As the amount of residual urine increases, nocturia, overflow urinary incontinence, and a palpable bladder may be present. Eventually, the manifestations of chronic urinary retention and obstruction supervene, or acute urinary retention can be precipitated by infection, tranquilizing drugs, or alcohol. On occasion, profound obstruction can be compensated to the extent that symptoms are minimal or absent, and patients present with obstructive uropathy.

During digital rectal examination, the prostate should be characterized with regard to size, consistency, and shape. Hyperplasia commonly produces a smooth, firm, elastic enlargement, but obstruction can occur in the absence of abnormalities on rectal examination. Ultrasonography with a rectal probe or magnetic resonance imaging allows a quantitative estimate of prostate size but ordinarily provides no information beyond that provided by rectal examination. The presence of upper urinary tract obstruction and the extent of bladder emptying can be documented by an intravenous pyelogram with postvoiding film or renal sonogram with sonographic determination of bladder residual urine. Cystourethroscopy is indicated to evaluate vesicle neck obstruction. Measurement of urine flow rate and/or residual urine volume is recommended to document the degree of obstruction to outflow. More detailed urodynamic evaluation is occasionally required to rule out other causes of voiding dysfunction such as neurogenic bladder.

TREATMENT Because the majority of men above age 60 have some degree of prostatic hyperplasia, the presence of the disorder by itself is not an indication for treatment. In men who lack definite indications for intervention, it is advisable that they be examined periodically to determine the natural history of the process. Many patients who receive no therapy experience no progression in symptoms over many years. Several forms of medical or surgical treatment exist for men with more advanced symptoms. Treatment with luteinizing hormone–releasing hormone (LHRH) analogues or an inhibitor of the steroid 5α-reductase enzyme (finasteride) shrinks prostatic glandular hyperplasia by lowering tissue dihydrotestosterone levels. Therapy with alpha-adrenergic antagonists lowers bladder neck and urethral resistance but is not approved by the U.S. Food and Drug Administration for this purpose. Both finasteride and alpha-adrenergic antagonists produce moderate and durable improvements in symptoms in some patients and may be useful in symptomatic patients who do not wish to undergo surgery, but the long-term effectiveness of medical therapy is not established.

Surgery has been and is still the benchmark treatment. Indications for surgery include decrease in urine flow of sufficient magnitude to cause discomfort, persistent residual urine, acute urinary retention due to obstruction with no reversible precipitating cause, and hydronephrosis. Transurethral prostatectomy is the usual procedure of choice.

Open prostatectomy for massive glands may employ either retropubic, suprapubic, or perineal approaches. Newer surgical alternatives include simple transurethral incision prostatotomy or transurethral laser-induced prostatectomy. Nonsurgical interventional therapies receiving intense study include indwelling urethral stents and balloon dilatation of the prostate.

PROSTATIC CARCINOMA

Cancer of the prostate is the most common malignancy in men in the United States and is the second most common cause of cancer death in men above age 55 (after carcinomas of the lung and colon). In the United States there are approximately 132,000 newly diagnosed cases and more than 33,000 deaths from the disorder each year. Only about a third of cases identified at autopsy are manifest clinically. The disease is rare before age 50, and the incidence increases with age. The frequency varies in different parts of the world. The United States has 14 deaths per 100,000 men per year compared with 22 for Sweden and 2 for Japan. However, Japanese immigrants to the United States develop prostatic cancer at a frequency similar to other men in this country, suggesting that an environmental factor is the principal cause for population differences. The disease is more common among American blacks than whites; the reason for this difference is not known.

CLASSIFICATION   Some carcinomas of the prostate are slow-growing and may persist for long periods without causing significant symptoms, whereas others behave aggressively. It is not known whether tumors can become more malignant with time. Insight into the natural history of a given tumor is provided by careful histopathologic grading, surgical evaluation of the pelvic lymph nodes, and measurement of the primary lesion, a size less than 1.5 mL in volume carrying a good prognosis.

Histologic grading   Over 95 percent of prostatic cancers are adenocarcinomas that arise in the prostatic acini. Adenocarcinoma may begin anywhere in the prostate but has a predilection for the periphery. The tumors are frequently multifocal. Variability in cellular size, nuclear and nucleolar shape, glandular differentiation, and the content of acid phosphatase and mucin may occur within a single specimen, but the most poorly differentiated area of tumor (i.e., the area with the highest histologic grade) appears to determine its biologic behavior. In the Gleason grading scheme, the dominant and any other glandular histologic patterns are independently assigned numbers from 1 to 5 (best to least differentiated), and these numbers are summed to give a total score of 2 to 10 for each tumor. Such grading is reproducible and correlates with the course of the disease and with patient survival.

The remaining prostatic cancers are divided among squamous cell and transitional cell carcinomas that arise in the prostatic ducts, carcinoma of the prostatic utricle (a müllerian duct remnant), carcinosarcomas that arise in the mesenchymal elements of the gland, and occasional metastatic tumors (usually carcinoma of the lung, melanoma, or lymphoma). These tumors will not be considered further.

DIAGNOSIS   Symptoms and signs   Both early and advanced carcinoma of the prostate may be asymptomatic at the time of diagnosis, and more than 80 percent of patients have stage C or D disease at the time of diagnosis (see below). In symptomatic subjects, common presenting complaints (in descending order) include dysuria, difficulty in voiding, increased urinary frequency, complete urinary retention, back or hip pain, and hematuria. A high index of suspicion should be entertained in all men over age 40 with dysuria, frequency, or difficulty in voiding in the absence of mechanical urethral obstruction. Additional complications of advanced disease may include spinal cord compression for dual metastases, deep venous thrombosis and pulmonary emboli, and myelophthisis.

Digital rectal examination   Palpation of the prostate is the most appropriate test for detection of all stages of disease other than stage A. Indeed, the importance of the rectal examination in the routine physical examination of men cannot be stressed too strongly. The posterior surfaces of the lateral lobes, where carcinoma begins most often, are easily palpable on digital rectal examination. Carcinoma characteristically is hard, nodular, and irregular, but induration also may be due to fibrous areas in benign prostatic hyperplasia, to focal infarcts, or to calculi as well as to tumor. The midline furrow between the lateral lobes may be obscured by either benign or malignant enlargement. Local extraprostatic extension of tumor into the seminal vesicles also can be detected by rectal examination. Scrotal and/or lower extremity lymphedema secondary to infiltration of pelvic lymph nodes indicates extensive disease.

Biochemical markers   Elevation of serum prostate-specific antigen (PSA) level is the most sensitive test for the early detection of prostatic cancer. PSA level may be elevated with localized disease, whereas elevation of acid phosphatase level usually indicates extraprostatic disease. Following diagnosis and treatment, serial determinations of PSA are the best available means for assessing response. No technique of assay for either PSA or acid phosphatase (including counterimmune electrophoresis and radioimmunoassay) is sufficiently specific or sensitive for routine screening studies, and serum PSA level can be elevated in benign states, including prostatic hyperplasia, prostatitis, and prostatic infarction.

Imaging   With the use of transrectal prostatic sonography, carcinoma is revealed as hypoechoic densities within the peripheral zone. The procedure is a sensitive means of identifying prostate cancer but is not specific enough for use as a screening test. Ultrasonography is also useful for directing needle biopsy and for documenting the degree of extension of the tumor into bladder and seminal vesicles. Magnetic resonance imaging (MRI) and to a lesser degree computed tomography (CT) of the prostate also may be helpful in defining the extent of tumor and locating nodes for aspiration needle biopsy. Transrectal prostatic sonography is recommended if either the digital rectal examination is positive or the PSA level is elevated. The findings on sonography, the amount of PSA elevation relative to prostate size, and the index of suspicion for carcinoma by history all affect the decision of whether or not to perform a biopsy. The combined use of these modalities allows early detection of large numbers of prostatic cancers and an increased proportion of localized and curable lesions. The biologic significance of individual lesions remains to be defined. Whether early diagnosis leads to improved survival and decreased morbidity from prostatic cancer requires further study.

Biopsy   Biopsy of the prostate is essential for establishing the diagnosis and is indicated when an abnormality is detected by palpation or elevation of serum PSA level and/or by imaging or when lower urinary tract symptoms occur in men who have no known cause of obstruction. Core-needle biopsy may be performed transperineally or transrectally with less risk of bacterial contamination with the former and more precise sampling with the latter. Transrectal prostatic biopsy with a rapid-fire spring-loaded needle under sonography provides the most accurate sampling of the index lesion and the remainder of the gland and is the preferred technique. Fine-needle aspiration cytology offers immediate diagnosis with minimal patient discomfort and morbidity. Open perineal biopsy is performed infrequently because it carries the risk of at least temporary impotence and is a more extensive surgical procedure. Transurethral biopsy is also used infrequently because most early lesions are in the peripheral reigons of the gland.

Staging and assessment of metastatic disease   Adenocarcinoma of the prostate may spread by three routes: direct extension, the lymphatics, and the bloodstream. The prostatic capsule is a natural boundary against growth of tumor into adjacent structures, but direct extension occurs upward into the seminal vesicles and bladder floor. Lymphatic spread can best be assessed by surgical exploration; the frequency with which it occurs correlates with the size and histologic grade of the tumor. Only about one-tenth of tumors with a grade of less than 5 have lymph node involvement, while more than 70 percent of tumors with a Gleason grade of 9 or 10 have coexisting lymphatic

324   SKIN CANCER

CARL V. WASHINGTON, JR.

Nonmelanoma skin cancer is the most common cancer in the United States, with an estimated annual incidence of more than 600,000 cases. Basal cell carcinomas (BCC) account for 70 to 80 percent of nonmelanoma skin cancers. Squamous cell carcinomas (SCC), while representing only about 20 percent of nonmelanoma skin cancers, are more significant because of their ability to metastasize. Incidence rates have risen dramatically over the past decade. While more common in men, this sexual difference has become less pronounced in recent years.

ETIOLOGY   The cause of BCC and SCC is multifactorial, with environmental and host factors being important. Recognized host factors besides age and sex include Celtic descent, fair complexion, tendency to sunburn easily, radiodermatitis, thermal burns, and certain scars and chronic ulcerations. Several heritable conditions have been associated with skin cancer (e.g., xeroderma pigmentosum). Among environmental causes, exposure to sunlight, principally the ultraviolet-B (UV-B) spectrum, appears to be the most significant. Abundant evidence exists to support the role of chronic cutaneous exposure to UV-B in skin cancer pathogenesis. The incidence of these tumors increases with decreasing latitudes. The vast majority develop on sun-exposed areas of the head and neck and are more common on the left side in the United States and the right side in England, presumably related to additional asymmetric exposure during driving. A higher incidence occurs in those with outdoor occupations. As thinning of the earth's protective ozone shield progresses, further increases in the incidence of skin cancer can be anticipated. Among chemical carcinogens, arsenic is the most important. Exposure is usually through medicinals or well water. Skin cancer in affected individuals may be seen with or without other cutaneous markers of chronic arsenism (e.g., arsenical keratoses). Drug- or disease-induced immunosuppression also predisposes to skin cancer. Transplantation patients on chronic immunosuppressive therapy are particularly prone to SCC. The frequency of skin cancer is proportional to the duration of immunosuppression and the extent of sun exposure. Human papillomaviruses (HPV) and UV-B may act as cocarcinogens. Skin cancer is not an uncommon finding in patients infected with the human immunodeficiency virus (HIV) and may be more aggressive in this setting (see Chap. 279). As the life span of HIV-infected persons increases, skin cancer may become a greater problem.

CLINICAL PRESENTATION   Basal cell carcinoma   BCC is a malignancy arising from epidermal basal cells. Several clinical types of BCC occur. The most common is the noduloulcerative BCC, which begins as a small pearly nodule, often showing small telangiectatic vessels on its surface. The nodule increases slowly in size and may undergo central ulceration. Variable amounts of melanin may be present within the tumor. BCC with heavier accumulations of pigment represent the pigmented BCC. While clinically no more aggressive than the noduloulcerative variant, it may be mistaken for malignant melanoma. The morpheaform (fibrosing) BCC manifests as a solitary, flat or slightly depressed, indurated, whitish or yellowish plaque. Borders are typically indistinct. Of BCC variants, this is the most aggressive and likely to recur. Superficial BCC consists of one or several erythematous, scaling plaques that slowly enlarge. Although more commonly found on the trunk and extremities, the head and neck are also affected. The lesions may be confused with benign inflammatory dermatoses, especially nummular eczema and psoriasis.

Squamous cell carcinoma   Primary cutaneous SCC is a malignant neoplasm of keratinizing epidermal cells. Unlike BCC, which has a very low metastatic potential, SCC can metastasize and grow rapidly. The clinical features of SCC vary widely. Commonly SCC appears as an ulcerated nodule or a superficial erosion on the skin or lower lip, but it also may present as a verrucous papule or plaque.

Unlike BCC, overlying telangiectasias are uncommon. Margins of this tumor may be ill-defined, and fixation to underlying structures may occur. Cutaneous SCC may develop anywhere on the body but usually arises on sun-damaged skin.

SCC has several premalignant forms (actinic keratosis, actinic cheilitis, and some cutaneous horns) and in situ forms (e.g., Bowen's disease) that are confined to the epidermis. Actinic keratoses (AK) and cheilitis are hyperkeratotic papules and plaques which occur on sun-exposed areas. While the potential for malignant degeneration is low in any individual lesion, the risk of SCC increases with larger numbers of lesions. Bowen's disease presents as a scaling, erythematous plaque which may occur on sun-exposed or protected sites. Individual lesions may develop into invasive SCC in up to 20 percent of cases. Controversy exists regarding the association of Bowen's disease with internal malignancy; however, recent evidence suggests no significant relationship when other predisposing factors (e.g., arsenic) are absent. Treatment of premalignant and in situ lesions reduces the subsequent risk of invasive disease.

TREATMENT   Basal cell carcinoma   Treatment modalities used with BCC include (1) electrodesiccation and curettage (ED&C), (2) excision, (3) cryosurgery, (4) radiation therapy, (5) Mohs micrographic surgery (MMS), (6) topical chemotherapy, and (7) intralesional interferon. Mode of therapy is directed by location of the tumor, histologic subtype, presence of recurrent disease, and various patient characteristics. ED&C remains the most commonly employed method by dermatologists. This method is selected for less aggressive tumors (e.g., noduloulcerative, superficial). It is best avoided in recurrent lesions, histologically aggressive tumors (e.g., morpheaform), deeply invasive or very large lesions, or in locations with high recurrence rates (e.g., nasolabial folds, medial canthus). Excision, which offers the advantage of histologic control, is usually selected for more aggressive tumors, those in high-risk locations, or in many instances for aesthetic demands. Radiation therapy, while not employed as frequently as surgical modalities, offers an excellent chance for cure in many BCC. It is useful in patients not considered surgical candidates and as a surgical adjunct in high-risk tumors. Cryosurgery utilizing liquid nitrogen may be used in certain low-risk tumors but requires specialized equipment (i.e., cryoprobes) to be used effectively for advanced neoplasms. Mohs micrographic surgery is a specialized type of surgical excision which allows for the ultimate in histologic control and preservation of uninvolved tissue. It is reserved for recurrent lesions, high-risk locations, larger and ill-defined lesions, and where maximal tissue conservation is critical (e.g., eyelids). Topical chemotherapy with 5-fluorouracil (5-FU) has limited usefulness in the management of BCC and should be used only for treating superficial BCC. Recent reports have demonstrated the effectiveness of intralesional interferon in certain primary tumors. The natural history of BCC is that of a slowly enlarging locally invasive neoplasm. The metastatic potential of BCC has been estimated to be 0.0028 to 0.1 percent.

Squamous cell carcinoma   The therapy of cutaneous SCC should be based on an analysis of risk factors influencing biologic behavior. These include size, location, degree of histologic differentiation, and age and physical condition of the patient. Surgical excision, radiation, and MMS are standard methods of treatment. Cryosurgery and ED&C have been used successfully in small primary tumors. The natural history of SCC depends on tumor and host characteristics. Tumors arising on actinically damaged skin have a lower metastatic potential than those on protected surfaces. Metastatic frequency of cutaneous SCC, reported at 0.3 to 3.7 percent, is lower than that of mucosal SCC. Tumors occurring on the lower lip have a metastatic potential approaching 11 percent. Metastases from SCC arising in burn scars, chronic ulcerations, and the genitalia have higher rates.

PREVENTION   Since the vast majority of skin cancers are related to chronic UV-B exposure, potential exists to dramatically reduce the incidence through patient and physician education. Emphasis should be placed on preventive measures beginning early in life. Patients must understand that damage from UV-B begins early, despite the fact that cancers develop years later. Regular use of sunscreens should be encouraged. Avoidance of tanning salons and sun exposure during midday (10 A.M. to 2 P.M.) is recommended. Precancerous and in situ lesions should be treated early. Chemoprophylaxis using synthetic retinoids is useful in controlling new lesions in some patients with multiple tumors.

REFERENCES

AUBRY F et al: Risk factors of squamous cell carcinoma of the skin. Cancer 55:907, 1985

FRIEDMAN RJ et al (eds): *Cancer of the Skin*. Philadelphia, Saunders, 1991, pp 27–94

GALLAGHER RP et al: Trends in basal cell carcinoma, squamous cell carcinoma, and melanoma of the skin from 1973 through 1987. J Am Acad Dermatol 23:413, 1990

KWA RE: Biology of cutaneous squamous cell carcinoma. J Am Acad Dermatol 26:1, 1992

TABLE 325-1 Risk factors for cutaneous melanoma
High risk (>50-fold increased risk)
Persistently changing mole
Atypical moles in patient with two family members with melanoma
Adulthood vs. childhood
>50 nevi ≥ 2 mm
Intermediate risk (~10-fold)
Family history of melanoma
Sporadic atypical moles
Congenital nevi (?)
Caucasians vs. blacks or Asians
Personal history of prior melanoma
Low risk (2- to 4-fold)
Immunosuppression
Sun sensitivity or excess exposure

SOURCE: Adapted from Rhodes et al.

325 MELANOMA AND OTHER PIGMENTED SKIN LESIONS

ARTHUR J. SOBER / HOWARD K. KOH

Pigmented skin lesions are among the most common findings on physical examination. The challenge is to distinguish cutaneous melanoma, which may be lethal, from the remainder, which with rare exception are benign.

Melanoma originates from melanocytes, pigment cells present normally in epidermis and sometimes in dermis. This tumor affects approximately 32,000 individuals per year in the United States, resulting in 6700 deaths. The incidence has increased dramatically (300 percent increase in the past 40 years); it can affect adults of all ages, even young individuals (onset from midteens); it has distinct clinical features which make it detectable at a time when cure by surgical excision is possible; and it is located on the skin surface, where it is visible. If the incidence continues to increase at the present rate, within a decade, lifetime risk of melanoma will approximate 1 percent or higher.

The reason for the increased incidence is uncertain but may stem from increased recreational sun exposure, especially early in life. Individuals of similar ethnic background who emigrate after childhood to areas of high sun exposure (Israel, Australia) have lower melanoma rates than individuals of similar age either born in these countries or who emigrated before age 10. Individuals most susceptible to development of melanoma are those with fair complexions, red or blond hair, blue eyes, and freckles and who are poor tanners and easy sunburners. In one literature survey, 9 of 11 studies linked increased melanoma risk to history of sunburn. Other factors associated with increased risk include family history of melanoma (approximately 1 in 10 melanoma patients have a family member with melanoma), presence of an atypical mole (dysplastic nevus), a giant congenital melanocytic nevus, a small to medium-sized congenital melanocytic nevus (see below), the presence of a higher than average number of ordinary melanocytic nevi, and immunosuppression (Table 325-1). A 64-fold increased risk for individuals with 50 or more moles ≥ 2 mm in size has been reported. Melanoma is relatively infrequent in heavily pigmented peoples. Dark-skinned populations (natives of India, Puerto Rico), blacks, and Orientals have rates one-seventh to one-tenth that noted for lighter-skinned Caucasians.

CLINICAL CHARACTERISTICS There are four types of cutaneous melanoma (Table 325-2). Three of these—superficial spreading melanoma, lentigo maligna melanoma, and acral lentiginous melanoma—have a period of superficial (so-called radial) growth when the lesion increases in size but does not penetrate deeply. It is during the radial growth period that melanoma is most capable of being

cured by surgical excision. The fourth type, nodular melanoma, does not have a recognizable radial growth phase and usually presents as a deeply invasive lesion, fully capable of early metastasis. When tumors begin to penetrate deeply into the skin, they are in the so-called vertical growth phase. Melanomas with radial growth phases are characterized by irregular and sometimes notched borders, variation in pigment pattern, and variation in color. Increase in size or change in color is noted by the patient in 70 percent of early lesions. Bleeding, ulceration, and pain are late signs and are of little help in early recognition. Nodular melanomas are dark brown–black to blue-black nodules. Melanoma may occasionally be amelanotic, where only the biopsy of a new or changing skin nodule histologically establishes the diagnosis. Lentigo maligna melanoma usually confines itself to chronically sun-damaged, sun-exposed sites (face, neck, back of hands) in older individuals. Acral lentiginous melanoma occurs on palms, soles, nail beds, and mucous membranes. While this type occurs in whites, it is most frequent (along with nodular melanoma) in blacks and Asians. Superficial spreading melanoma is most frequent in whites. Melanomas arising in dysplastic nevi (see below) are usually of this type. The back is the most common site for melanoma in men. In women, the back and the lower leg (from knee to ankle) are frequent sites.

PROGNOSTIC FACTORS The most important prognostic factor is stage at time of presentation. (See later discussion of revised staging categories.) Five-year survival for clinical stages I and II (primary tumor; no clinical evidence of disease elsewhere) is about 85 percent. For clinical stage III (clinically palpable regional nodes that contain tumor), a 5-year survival of about 50 percent is noted when only one node is involved and about 15 to 20 percent when four or more nodes are involved. Five-year survival for clinical stage IV (disseminated disease) is less than 5 percent. Fortunately, the majority of melanomas are diagnosed in clinical stages I and II. Within stages I and II, a gradient of prognosis can be delineated based on the thickness of the primary tumor (Table 325-3). This system is based on the rationale that the likelihood of metastasis should correlate with tumor volume, with thickness the best single index of tumor volume. Melanomas less than 0.76 mm thick are usually cured by surgical removal (5-year survival rates range from 96 to 99 percent). Approximately 40 percent of primary melanomas now fall into a low-risk category (thickness < 1 mm). When low-risk patients develop metastases, the primary tumors often exhibit either extensive microscopic features of regression or a vertical growth phase. Approximately 60 percent of individuals with melanomas ≥ 3.65 mm thick will develop metastatic disease and die from their melanoma. These thick tumors are almost always raised substantially above the plane of the skin. Two intermediate categories of thickness exist (Table 325-3). Certain anatomic sites affect prognosis. The favorable sites appear to be forearm and leg (excluding feet), while unfavorable sites include scalp, hands, feet, and mucous membranes. Survival for women in stages I and II is, in general, more favorable than for men, perhaps in part because of earlier diagnosis; women frequently have melanomas large lesions or lesions on anatomic sites where excisional biopsy may not be feasible (such as the face, hands, or feet), an incisional biopsy through the most nodular or darkest area of the lesion is acceptable; this should represent the vertical growth phase of the primary tumor. Data from prospective studies do not support the concern that an incisional biopsy might facilitate the spread of melanoma.

STAGING   Once the diagnosis of malignant melanoma has been confirmed, the tumor must be staged to determine prognosis and treatment. The history should probe for evidence of metastatic disease, such as malaise, weight loss, headaches, visual difficulty, or bone pain. The physical examination should be especially directed to the skin, regional draining lymph nodes, central nervous system, liver, and spleen. In the absence of signs or symptoms of metastasis, few laboratory or radiologic tests are indicated for staging purposes. Aside from a chest x-ray and, possibly, liver function tests, no other tests or scans are routinely indicated unless the history or physical examination suggests metastasis to a specific organ. Specifically, liver-spleen scans and computed tomography have a low yield and are not cost-effective. However, once signs of metastasis exist, favored sites of spread, such as the liver, lungs, bone, and brain, should be scanned.

Traditional staging categories have been stage I (confined to the skin), stage II (spread to regional lymph nodes), and stage III (distant metastases). Approximately 80 percent of patients with melanoma now present with stage I disease. The American Joint Commission on Cancer (AJCC) has promoted a four-stage system to divide patients more easily by risk group. This system splits the former stage I patients into low risk (new stage I: ≤1.5 mm thick) and high risk (new stage II: >1.5 mm thick).

SURGICAL MANAGEMENT   For a newly diagnosed stage I cutaneous melanoma, wide surgical excision of the lesion with a margin of normal skin is necessary to remove all malignant cells and minimize local recurrence. The outdated "5-cm rule," which states that the normal skin within 5 cm of the edge of the primary cutaneous melanoma should be excised, often requires split-thickness skin grafts and is cosmetically disfiguring. Narrower margins allow for primary closure and may obviate the need for grafts or flaps without compromising overall survival rates. The appropriate width of the narrow margin is a source of controversy. A World Health Organization trial prospectively randomized between 1-cm and 3-cm margins in 612 patients with thin malignant melanomas (≤2 mm in thickness) reported that the thinner surgical margin resulted in higher rates of local recurrence but no difference in nodal metastases, distant metastases, disease-free survival, or overall survival after 7½ years of follow-up. For thicker stage I lesions, definitive data are not available, but margins up to 3 cm appear to be reasonable. Once again, for lesions on the face, hands, and feet, strict adherence to margins must give way to individual considerations about the constraints of surgery and minimization of morbidity. In all instances, however, inclusion of subcutaneous fat in the surgical specimen facilitates adequate thickness measurement and assessment of surgical margins by the pathologist.

ELECTIVE REGIONAL NODE DISSECTION   Elective regional node dissection in AJCC stage II disease (without palpable adenopathy) has been advocated, based on the hypothesis that melanoma metastasizes in an orderly fashion from the skin to regional lymph nodes and finally to distant sites. Hence surgical excision of nodal micrometastases could theoretically provide definitive treatment at a time of relatively low tumor burden and, hopefully, improve survival. The efficacy of this procedure remains controversial; while some retrospective series suggest a survival benefit, two randomized studies examining this question in patients with limb melanomas and clinical stage I disease showed no survival advantage for wide local excision followed by immediate elective regional node dissection compared with wide local excision followed by delayed dissection (only if nodes became palpable). Furthermore, the procedure has associated morbidity, and some lesions, especially those on the trunk, have

ambiguous nodal draining sites, making it difficult to decide which area to dissect. In such situations, lymphoscintigraphy can be utilized to define the nodes that serve as the primary drainage area. Certainly not all patients with clinical stage I disease require node dissections. Patients with lesions < 0.75 mm thick have excellent prognoses and need no node dissection; at the other extreme, patients with lesions > 3.50 mm have such a high risk for distant metastases that the possible benefit of an elective node dissection would be negated. A subset of patients with AJCC stage II lesions of intermediate thickness may benefit from elective regional node dissection, but there is no consensus about which patients should undergo this procedure. Ongoing randomized studies may resolve this issue.

ADJUVANT THERAPY   For patients free of disease but at high risk for metastasis, adjuvant therapy that complements surgery is needed to destroy occult micrometastases, prolong disease-free survival, and improve cure rates. Many strategies have been tried, including chemotherapy, nonspecific immunotherapy [such as immunization with bacillus Calmette-Guérin (BCG)], chemoimmunotherapy, and radiation therapy. However, such studies have been hampered by suboptimal stratification, inclusion of those at low risk, lack of randomization, small sample size, or inadequate length of follow-up. Hence no consistent evidence documents adjuvant therapy as effective in prolonging life. Current trials include studies of various melanoma vaccines to heighten the host immune response against micrometastases.

TREATMENT OF METASTATIC DISEASE   Melanoma can metastasize to any organ, the brain being a particularly favored site. Metastatic melanoma is generally incurable, and survival in patients with visceral metastases is generally less than 1 year. Thus the goal of treatment is usually palliative to improve the quality of life. Patients with soft-tissue and node metastases fare better than those with liver and brain metastases. If metastases are limited to regional nodes (AJCC stage III disease), a therapeutic lymph node dissection is indicated. Surgical excision of a single metastasis to the lung or surgically accessible brain site can be associated with prolonged survival. More often, however, patients subsequently have multiple brain metastases that require radiation and glucocorticoids. Radiation therapy can provide local palliation for recurrent tumors or metastatic sites. Chemotherapy has a response rate of only 20 to 25 percent and rarely induces complete remission. The most commonly used single agents are imidazole carboximide (dacarbazine), cisplatin, or the nitrosoureas. Combination chemotherapy does not result in consistent improvement in remission and survival rates compared with those of a single agent. Patients who have advanced regional disease isolated to a limb may benefit from hyperthermic limb perfusion with melphalan, which concentrates the chemotherapeutic agents and minimizes systemic leakage.

The lack of response to traditional treatments has spawned many trials using agents such as retinoids, high-dosage chemotherapy with autologous bone marrow transplantation, interferons, antipigmentary agents, and antibodies conjugated to isotopes, drugs, and toxins. Of all these investigational therapies, adoptive immunotherapy has received the most attention. This treatment involves exposing lymphocytes from melanoma patients to interleukin 2 (IL-2) to generate and expand lymphokine-activated killer cells (LAK cells); these LAK cells are then reinfused in conjunction with IL-2 administration. This therapy may have particular relevance to melanoma because the immune system is suspected of having a critical role in the control of melanoma metastases. However, the early response rate appears to be only about 20 percent; most of these remissions are partial, are seen in patients with skin or lung metastases, and are of short duration. In addition, treatment with IL-2 has considerable toxicity, attributable primarily to a capillary leak syndrome. Research is now focusing on improving remission rates while minimizing the toxicity; trials include high-dose IL-2, either alone or with LAK cells, with even more potent tumor-infiltrating lymphocytes, or with chemotherapeutic agents, biologic response modifiers, or other agents. The continued lack of curative treatment for metastatic disease underscores the importance of early detection and prevention of malignant melanoma to decrease avoidable mortality.

REFERENCES

ALBERT L et al: Dysplastic melanocytic nevi and cutaneous melanoma: Markers of increased melanoma risk for affected individuals and blood relatives. J Am Acad Dermatol 7:69, 1990

ARMSTRONG BK: Epidemiology of malignant melanoma: Intermittent or total accumulated exposure to the sun. J Dermatol Surg Oncol 14:835, 1988

BALCH CM et al (eds): Cutaneous Melanoma: Clinical Management and Treatment Results Worldwide, 2d ed. Philadelphia, Lippincott, 1992

CLARK WH JR et al: The histogenesis and biologic behavior of primary human malignant melanoma of the skin. Cancer Res 29:705, 1969

FRIEDMAN RJ et al: Malignant melanoma in the 1990s: The continued importance of early detection and the role of physician examination and self-examination of the skin. CA 41:201, 1991

HO VC, SOBER AJ: Therapy for cutaneous melanoma: An update. J Am Acad Dermatol 22:159, 1990

KOH HK et al: Adjuvant therapy of cutaneous malignant melanoma: A critical review. Med Ped Oncol 13:244, 1985

————: Cutaneous melanoma. N Engl J Med 325:171, 1991

RHODES AR: Neoplasms: Benign neoplasias, hyperplasias, and dysplasias of melanocytes, in Dermatology in General Medicine, TB Fitzpatrick et al (eds). New York, McGraw-Hill, 1987, pp 877–946

———— et al: Risk factors for cutaneous melanoma. JAMA 258:3146, 1987

RIGEL DS et al: Dysplastic nevi. Markers for increased risk for melanoma. Cancer 63:386, 1989

ROSENBERG SA: The immunotherapy and gene therapy of cancer. J Clin Oncol 10:180, 1992

SOBER AJ et al: Early recognition of cutaneous melanoma. JAMA 242:2795, 1979

VERONESI U et al: Delayed regional lymph node dissection in stage 1 melanoma of the skin of the lower extremities. Cancer 49:2420, 1982

————, CASCINELLI N: Narrow excision (1 cm margin), a safe procedure for thin cutaneous melanoma. Arch Surg 126:438, 1991

326 METASTATIC CANCER OF UNKNOWN PRIMARY SITE

RICHARD M. STONE

The presenting findings in up to 10 percent of cancer patients may not yield definitive identification of the site of origin of the neoplasm. Such patients with cancer of unknown primary site present difficult diagnostic and therapeutic dilemmas. First, since the number of additional studies which could be ordered may be vast, costly, and/or uncomfortable for the patient, the strategy involved in the "search for the primary" must consider what, if any, result the precise identification of the site of origin will have on the patient's treatment and length of survival. Second, while those individuals with cancer of unknown primary site fare poorly (median survival <6 months), there are subgroups of patients who are more likely to benefit from treatment and, in some cases, to enjoy long intervals without evidence of disease. The literature provides a poor guide for the care of such patients due to the largely retrospective nature of the reports, the heterogeneity of the tumors, the selection bias in small individual retrospective studies, and the variability in both the definition of the syndrome and the thoroughness of the evaluation performed to identify a primary site.

The biologic behavior of metastatic cancers of unknown primary site is unique compared with that of other nonhematopoietic neoplasms. Such cancers as breast and prostate are relatively uncommon causes of metastatic malignancy of unknown primary origin. In patients with breast cancer, for example, a breast lesion is almost always identified either prior to or simultaneously with the documentation of metastatic disease. Moreover, cancers presenting with an unknown primary site often display unusual patterns of metastatic spread (e.g., pancreatic cancer presenting with bony metastases). The predominance of tumor bulk located in distant sites rather than in the

tissue of origin suggests that the genetic lesions accounting for the development of such malignancies convey a distinctly aggressive phenotype. Frequently, biopsy of an involved site will reveal a poorly differentiated histology, which represents the morphologic correlate of this biologic behavior. The relative propensity of tumor deposits in patients with metastatic cancer of unknown primary site to grow in distant locations also implies that the malignant cells may proliferate in the absence of the specific host factors (e.g., growth-promoting proteins, vascular supply) important in the development of more typical cancers. Although physiologic and genetic data which might account for the distinctive natural history of neoplasms of unknown origin are scant, cell lines derived from tumors obtained from patients with this syndrome may have abnormalities of chromosome 1, a karyotype generally associated with advanced malignancy.

DEFINITION   While there is no universally accepted definition of the syndrome of metastatic cancer of unknown primary site, a helpful approach has been proposed by Ultmann and Phillip. They suggest that an occult primary neoplasm should fulfill each of the following criteria: (1) biopsy-proven malignancy, (2) history, physical examinations, chest film, complete blood counts, urinalysis, and stool test for occult blood not indicative of a primary site, (3) histologic evaluation not consistent with a primary tumor at the biopsy site, and (4) additional diagnostic studies failing to identify the primary site. Such additional diagnostic tests could include, for example, colonoscopy in a patient whose rectal examination discloses guaiac-positive stool or a meticulous otolaryngologic examination in a patient who presents with squamous cell carcinoma in a cervical node. With increased understanding of the natural history of certain tumors and with the routine use of computed tomographic (CT) scanning as well as detailed pathologic studies, there are many cases which may fulfill the definition of cancer of unknown primary site, yet where there is a reasonable suspicion that a given organ is the probable site of origin.

DIAGNOSTIC EVALUATION   History and physical examination Though usually unrevealing, a thorough history and physical examination should be carried out to elicit easily obtainable clues regarding the primary site. The patient should be questioned concerning epigastric pain, which, if present, would mandate careful exclusion of pancreatic carcinoma as well as other gastrointestinal malignancies. Symptoms referable to a given location (e.g., new cough, hematochezia, hemoptysis, change in bowel habits, unusual vaginal bleeding, nipple discharge) should prompt an aggressive, yet specific, diagnostic approach. Occupational exposure to asbestos, for example, would make the prior probability of mesothelioma much higher. The absence of prior smoking reduces the likelihood of lung cancer but, of course, does not exclude it. A history of fulguration of a skin lesion, colonic polypectomy, dilation and curettage, or prostate biopsy should prompt a review of the original histology. Other than inferences drawn from the location of the involved area (see below), the physical examination will probably be unrevealing unless a thorough pelvic and rectal examination has not been performed previously.

Additional studies   In females with metastatic adenocarcinoma or poorly differentiated carcinoma, mammography should be performed. The use of abdominal/pelvic CT scans may lead to identification of the primary site in as many as 35 percent of patients and will certainly reduce the number of cases of pancreatic cancer in which the primary site is obscure before death. It is reasonable to obtain tumor markers such as an alpha fetoprotein (AFP), beta human chorionic gonadotropin (βhCG), carcinoembryonic antigen (CEA), CA-125 (associated with ovarian cancer), and prostate-specific antigen (PSA). However, since many different adenocarcinomas elaborate either CEA or CA-125, or both, the value of these markers resides in following response to therapy rather than in the identification of a primary site. Moreover, poorly differentiated colonic tumors frequently fail to elaborate CEA, and patients with benign prostate hypertrophy may have modestly elevated PSA levels, reducing the reliability of these markers in defining the primary site in a patient with metastatic cancer. Numerous studies have shown a lack of benefit of contrast studies (upper gastrointestinal series, barium enema, or intravenous pyelogram) in

TABLE 326-1   Suggested clinical evaluation of patients with metastatic cancer of unknown primary site

	Evaluate
History	Smoking history, asbestos exposure, abdominal pain

Physical examination	Lymph nodes, thyroid, skin
	  Men: prostate
	  Women: breasts, pelvic examination

Laboratory evaluation	Stool for occult blood, urinalysis, CBC, liver function tests, serum prostate specific antigen (PSA), βhCG, AFP, CEA, CA-125 (women), CXR, CT abdomen, mammography
Pathologic evaluation	See Table 326-2.

patients with metastatic cancer of unknown primary site who have no specific symptoms or no findings referable to the gastrointestinal or urinary tracts. Moreover, autopsy series reveal that the most likely primary site of origin includes epithelial tissues such as lung, stomach, colon, and kidney which give rise to tumors that respond poorly to chemotherapy, minimizing the impact of such a diagnosis. A summary of a reasonable diagnostic approach is found in Table 326-1.

Pathologic review   The most important aspect in the evaluation of the patient with metastatic cancer of unknown primary site is to derive maximal information from the tissue obtained at biopsy. Vital clues pertaining to the primary site and ultimately to the patient's management can be obtained by careful review of light microscopic, immunohistochemical, ultrastructural, immunologic, and molecular biologic findings. First, if there is any question concerning the adequacy of the original biopsy sample for either confirmation of malignancy or performance of additional specialized studies, rebiopsy is mandated. The clinician must have a close working relationship with a pathologist skilled in the evaluation of tumor specimens, especially when the organ of origin is uncertain. On either the initial or subsequent biopsy, plans may be made to process the tissue for (1) routine fixation for light microscopic, histochemical, and immunohistochemical analysis, (2) freezing for DNA isolation or for additional immunologic evaluation (e.g., certain antibody-based detection methods cannot be applied to fixed, paraffin-embedded tissue), and (3) fixation, usually in glutaraldehyde, for ultrastructural analysis. Fresh tissue may be disaggregated into single-cell suspension for short-term culture for purposes of cytogenetic analysis.

If routine histologic analysis fails to suggest the tissue of origin (e.g., gland formulation in adenocarcinoma, psammoma bodies in ovarian or thyroid cancer, or spindle architecture in sarcomas), special histochemical studies may be helpful. For example, mucin positivity is helpful in recognizing poorly differentiated adenocarcinoma. Based on light microscopic review, including histochemical analysis, approximately half of those with metastatic cancer of unknown primary site are determined to have adenocarcinoma, an additional quarter have squamous cell carcinoma, usually of head and neck or lung origin, and the remainder are poorly differentiated neoplasms. In the latter group, immunohistochemical, cytogenetic, and molecular biologic studies can be extremely useful in detecting sarcoma, germ cell carcinoma, lymphoma, melanoma, or other tumors whose diagnosis would suggest a more specific therapeutic approach.

IMMUNOHISTOCHEMICAL ANALYSIS   Antibodies to specific cell components and the ability to detect binding by sensitive visualization methods such as peroxidase or streptavidin-biotin permit the characterization of tumors that fail to be characterized when standard techniques are employed. Since in most situations no single antibody is of sufficient specificity to identify the primary site with certainty, a battery of such reagents must be employed. Table 326-2 provides a list of antigens that may be assessed by immunohistochemical analysis in an undifferentiated or poorly differentiated specimen. It is particularly important to exclude the diagnosis of lymphoma by employing antibodies reactive to the leukocyte common antigen (LCA, CD45). The presence of LCA suggests that the patient has a

TABLE 326-2   Possible pathologic evaluation of biopsies from patients with metastatic cancer of unknown primary site

Evaluation/findings	Suggested primary site
HISTOLOGY (HEMATOXYLIN AND EOSIN STAINING)	
Psammoma bodies, papillary configuration	Ovarian, thyroid
Signet ring cells	Stomach
IMMUNOHISTOLOGY	
Leukocyte common antigen (LCA, CD45)	Lymphoid neoplasm
Leu-M1	Hodgkin's disease
Epithelial membrane antigen	Carcinoma
Cytokeratin intermediate filaments	Carcinoma
CEA	Carcinoma
HMB 45	Melanoma
Desmin	Sarcoma
Thyroglobulin	Thyroid carcinoma
Calcitonin	Medullary carcinoma of the thyroid
Myoglobin	Rhabdomyosarcoma
PSA/prostatic acid phosphatase	Prostate
AFP	Liver, stomach, germ cell
Placental alkaline phosphatase	Germ cell
B, T cell markers	Lymphoid neoplasm
S-100	Neuroendocrine
Gross cystic fluid protein	Breast, sweat gland
FLOW CYTOMETRY	
B, T cell markers	Lymphoid neoplasm
ULTRASTRUCTURE	
Actin-myosin filaments	Rhabdomyosarcoma
Secretory granules	Neuroendocrine tumors
Desmosomes	Carcinoma
Premelanosomes	Melanoma
CYTOGENETICS	
Isochromosome 12p;12q(−)	Germ cell
t(11;22)	Ewing's sarcoma, primitive neuroectodermal tumor
t(8;14)*	Lymphoid neoplasm
3p(−)	Small cell lung carcinoma; renal cell carcinoma, mesothelioma
t(X;18)	Synovial sarcoma
t(12;16)	Myxoid liposarcoma
t(12;22)	Clear cell sarcoma (melanoma of soft parts)
t(2;13)	Alveolar rhabdomyosarcoma
RECEPTOR ANALYSIS	
Estrogen/progesterone receptor	Breast
MOLECULAR BIOLOGIC STUDIES	
Immunoglobulin, *bcl*-2, T cell receptor gene rearrangement*	Lymphoid neoplasm

* Or any other rearrangement involving an antigen-receptor gene.

lymphoid neoplasm and will respond to therapy with the same likelihood as if there was no diagnostic ambiguity. Compared with the usually poor prognosis in patients with metastatic carcinoma of unknown primary site, such a finding is indeed welcome news; long-term disease-free survival in patients with diffuse large cell lymphoma is approximately 40 percent when a regimen such as CHOP (cyclophosphamide, doxorubicin, vincristine, and prednisone) is employed. The immunohistochemical detection of specific types of filament proteins is helpful in the identification of carcinomas and sarcomas. The presence of keratin suggests carcinoma, since essentially all epithelial tumors contain this protein. However, certain sarcomas, mesotheliomas, and germ cell tumors are also keratin-positive, emphasizing the need for the judicious use of a battery of immunohistochemical markers. Sarcomas may react with antibodies to desmin. Breast, prostate, and thyroid carcinomas can each be suggested if the tissue reacts with antibodies to prostate-specific antigen or prostatic alkaline phosphatase, gross cystic fluid protein, or thyroglobulin, respectively. Sarcoma subgroups including rhabdomyosarcoma (myoglobin) and angiosarcoma or Kaposi's sarcoma (factor VIII) also may be identified immunohistochemically. The finding of AFP, βhCG, or placental alkaline phosphatase staining is very helpful in assigning a germ cell origin. The S-100 protein is present in virtually all primary and metastatic melanomas, including the amelanotic variety, the latter being difficult to classify by routine techniques. However, S-100 positivity is also found in many other tumors of neuroendocrine origin (e.g., small cell lung cancer, carcinoid, neuroepithelioma); a more specific marker for melanomas is the HMB 45 (human melanoma black) antigen.

OTHER DIAGNOSTIC APPROACHES Ultrastructural analysis with electron microscopy can identify cell junctions (i.e., desmosomes, typical of epithelial cancers), neuroendocrine granules, melanosomes, and muscle filaments that can be very helpful in arriving at the tissue of origin. Though not widely utilized, cytogenetic analysis on solid tumors represents a means of classifying neoplasms associated with specific chromosomal translocations or other genetic abnormalities (see Table 326-2). Fresh tissue may be required for detection of estrogen or progesterone receptors where breast cancer is a possibility or for the determination of antigens (such as those found on certain T cells) that are not fixation-resistant. In addition to immunologic analysis, lymphomas can be diagnosed by isolating DNA from tissues and using molecular approaches to detect immunoglobulin, T cell receptor, bcl-2, or other lymphoid-specific gene rearrangement. Since minimal amounts of template DNA are required for amplification by polymerase chain reaction, paraffin-embedded tissue blocks may yield sufficient diagnostic material. As additional tumors are found to have specific acquired chromosomal rearrangements or mutations in genes controlling growth and differentiation, the detection of altered DNA and/or altered gene products will yield additional diagnostic capabilities.

TREATMENT Patients with cancer of unknown primary site have a median age of 62 years. However, regardless of age, the exclusion of treatable and potentially curable neoplasms is important. Patients with squamous cell carcinoma have a median survival somewhat greater (9 months) than do those with adenocarcinoma or unclassifiable neoplasms (4 to 6 months). If laboratory studies lead to a significant probability that the neoplasm is either a lymphoma, germ cell tumor, sarcoma, neuroendocrine tumor, or breast or prostate cancer, then disease-appropriate therapy should be administered. Patients who are found to have either lymphoma or germ cell neoplasm may be cured with combination chemotherapy. In other malignancies, effective palliative chemotherapy (sarcoma, breast, neuroendocrine tumor) or hormonal therapy (breast, prostate) should be strongly considered. Thus, for example, patients with neuroendocrine tumors are expected to respond to cisplatin-based chemotherapy. However, many patients, even after exhaustive pathologic review, will be left with a diagnosis of metastatic cancer (usually carcinoma or poorly differentiated malignancy) of unknown primary site. Despite these discouraging facts, patients often can be categorized as having one of several clinical features or syndromes suggesting a specific form of potentially beneficial therapy (see Table 326-3).

Unrecognized extragonadal germ cell cancer syndrome In the late 1970s, investigators identified a subset of patients with poorly differentiated carcinoma of unknown primary site who were extremely responsive to chemotherapy. These patients displayed one or more of the following features: age less than 50; tumor involving midline structures, lung parenchyma, or lymph nodes; an elevated serum AFP or βhCG level; evidence of rapid tumor growth; or tumor responsiveness to previously administered radiotherapy or chemotherapy. The administration of cisplatin-based chemotherapy has led to long-term survival in a sizable number of patients with these features, suggesting that their tumors behaved in a manner analogous to germ cell neoplasms. If all patients with poorly differentiated carcinoma are treated with a chemotherapy regimen designed for those with

TABLE 326-3 Presentations dictating specific therapy in patients with metastatic cancer of unknown primary site

Clinicopathologic features	Suspected primary site	Suggested therapy
Squamous cell carcinoma, cervical node	Head and neck cancer	Radical neck dissection; XRT
Carcinoma, axillary nodes (female)	Breast cancer	Breast XRT or mastectomy, systemic adjuvant therapy
Peritoneal carcinomatosis (female)	Ovarian cancer	Debulking surgery, cisplatin-based chemotherapy
Poorly differentiated cancer, age <50, lung or retroperitoneal or mediastinal mass or lymph nodes, elevated βhCG or AFP	Germ cell (extragonadal)	Cisplatin/VP-16–based chemotherapy
Adenocarcinoma, liver metastases, elevated CEA	Gastrointestinal malignancy	Colonoscopy, 5-FU/leucovorin

germ cell cancer (e.g., cisplatin plus etoposide or vinblastine, and often with bleomycin), about one-quarter will respond completely and a third will experience partial responses. Approximately one in six is likely to survive more than 5 years without evidence of disease. Furthermore, abnormalities of chromosome 12 similar to those described in patients with proven germ cell cancer have been detected by karyotypic analysis of clinical specimens from patients with this syndrome.

Peritoneal carcinomatosis in women Women presenting with increased abdominal girth and a pelvic mass or pain and who are found to have adenocarcinoma throughout the peritoneal cavity also may benefit from platinum-based chemotherapy. While breast cancer or a gastrointestinal malignancy also could produce these findings, peritoneal carcinomatosis is most commonly ascribed to ovarian cancer, even in those with apparently normal ovaries at the time of laparotomy. Especially if psammoma bodies or a papillary configuration is noted at the time of pathologic examination or if the CA-125 level is elevated, women with adenocarcinoma of the peritoneal cavity without a clear primary site should receive maximum surgical cytoreduction followed by cisplatin-based therapy. The stage-specific response to such therapy appears to be comparable with that observed in patients with proven ovarian cancer.

Carcinoma in an axillary lymph node in a female Women with an axillary mass proven to be adenocarcinoma or poorly differentiated carcinoma should receive treatment appropriate for stage II breast cancer whether or not a careful breast examination or mammography suggests the diagnosis of primary breast cancer and whether or not estrogen or progesterone receptors are detectable in the node. Although no lesion may be found in the breast if an immediate mastectomy is performed, patients with this syndrome who are followed and observed without local therapy have a high rate of developing primary breast tumors. Appropriate therapy would generally include either modified radical mastectomy or breast irradiation for purposes of reducing the risk of local recurrence. In addition, adjuvant systemic therapy (chemotherapy and/or tamoxifen, depending on menopausal status and whether or not estrogen receptor protein was found in the axillary tumor) to reduce the risk of developing evident metastatic breast cancer should be considered. Whether or not such systemic therapy should be administered prior to, rather than after, definitive local treatment is controversial. Women with axillary metastases without an obvious breast primary appear to have the same likelihood of prolonged disease-free survival as patients with typical stage II breast cancer.

Cervical lymph nodes It has long been recognized that patients presenting with a neck mass should be considered to have a primary tumor of the upper aerodigestive tract, usually termed *head and neck cancer,* until proven otherwise. Especially if pathologic analysis suggests squamous histology and the node is located in a high or midcervical area, a careful ear, nose, and throat examination, including direct laryngoscopy, nasopharyngoscopy, and random blind biopsies, should be undertaken. A thyroid examination and scan also must be performed to rule out a primary thyroid tumor, especially if the histology is not definitely squamous. Definitive local therapy (external beam radiation or radical neck dissection) possibly followed by platinum-based chemotherapy may lead to prolonged survival in some patients.

Adenocarcinoma and liver metastases Though not as well characterized as the unrecognized germ cell cancer syndrome and not as responsive to therapy, liver metastases proven to be adenocarcinoma have a significant likelihood of a primary stomach, biliary, or colorectal tumor. An elevated serum CEA level in this setting would provide further evidence suggesting a gastrointestinal malignancy. A flexible sigmoidoscopy or colonoscopy may be reasonable to rule out a potentially obstructive colonic lesion. Even if endoscopy fails to detect a tumor (in which case, depending on its size, resection would offer benefit), treatment with a combination of 5-fluorouracil plus leucovorin may offer palliation to some patients with presumed metastatic gastrointestinal malignancy. Given the severe and even life-threatening diarrhea that may be a consequence of this particular regimen, combined with the relative resistance of gastrointestinal tumors to chemotherapy, patients should be selected carefully prior to embarking on such therapy.

Patients not falling into one of the preceding categories should be treated palliatively. In some patients, observation is appropriate. For example, individuals without evidence of additional metastatic disease who have undergone resection of a solitary pulmonary nodule containing malignant cells may actually have undergone definitive therapy for a small primary lung tumor. Radiation therapy is indicated in patients with local disease causing bony pain or neurologic compromise. Combination chemotherapy is frequently employed in patients with an unknown primary site; however, response rates to "all purpose" regimens [e.g., FAM (5-fluorouracil, doxorubicin, mitomycin C) or FACP (5-fluorouracil, doxorubicin, cyclophosphamide, cisplatin)] are generally under 50 percent, with complete responses occurring in less than 25 percent of patients. Mitomycin C–containing regimens are associated with the risk of hemolytic-uremic syndrome. In some series, patients with a good performance status or whose disease is limited to soft tissue sites have been found more likely to respond to therapy. While patients responding to treatment have been thought to survive longer than those who do not, this seeming benefit of chemotherapy is probably related to the inherent characteristics of the tumor.

Before initiating a trial of combination chemotherapy in a patient with metastatic cancer of unknown primary site, the potential benefits must be weighed carefully against the certainty of toxicity. While some randomized studies have reported a benefit of one form of therapy over another, these reports are generally plagued by small numbers of patients and inadequate control of potential prognostic variables. Depending on motivation, eligibility, and availability, patients with metastatic cancer of unknown primary site may be candidates for evaluation of new (phase I) therapies.

REFERENCES

BELL CW et al: Unknown primary tumors: Establishment of cell lines, identification of chromosomal abnormalities, and implications for a second type of tumor progression. Cancer Res 49:4311, 1989

ELLERBROEK N et al: Treatment of patients with isolated axillary nodal metastases from an occult primary carcinoma consistent with breast origin. Cancer 66:1461, 1990

FLETCHER JA et al: Diagnostic relevance of clonal cytogenetics in malignant soft tissue tumors. N Engl J Med 324:436, 1991

HAINSWORTH JD et al: Cisplatin-based combination chemotherapy in the treatment of poorly differentiated carcinoma and poorly differentiated adenocarcinoma of unknown primary site: Results of a 12-year experience. J Clin Oncol 10:912, 1992

——— et al: Poorly differentiated carcinoma of unknown primary site: Clinical usefulness of immunoperoxidase staining. J Clin Oncol 9:1931, 1991

HORNING SJ et al: Lymphomas presenting as histologically unclassified neoplasms: Characteristics and response to treatment. J Clin Oncol 17:1281, 1989

PASTERZ R et al: Prognostic factors in metastatic carcinoma of unknown primary. J Clin Oncol 4:1652, 1986

RABER MN et al: Unknown primary tumors. Curr Opin Oncol 4:3, 1992

SPORN JR, GREENBERG BR: Empiric chemotherapy in patients with carcinoma of unknown primary site. Am J Med 88:49, 1990

STRNAD CM et al: Peritoneal carcinomatosis of unknown primary site in women. Ann Intern Med 111:213, 1989

ULTMANN JE, PHILLIPS TL: Cancer of unknown primary site, in Principles and Practice of Oncology, 3d ed, VT DeVita et al (eds). Philadelphia, Lippincott, 1990, chap 56

327 ENDOCRINE MANIFESTATIONS OF NEOPLASIA

LAWRENCE A. FROHMAN

Hormone secretion by tumors of nonendocrine tissue has been recognized for more than 60 years. Initially, the majority of reported cases were associated with hypoglycemia and hypercalcemia, but the term *ectopic hormone secretion* was first used in relation to Cushing's syndrome caused by adrenocorticotropin (ACTH) secretion from a variety of tumors. The spectrum of ectopic hormone secretion has expanded as a result of increased clinical awareness and the availability of sensitive assay techniques. However, the use of the term *ectopic* has been questioned with the recognition that hormones once believed to be tissue-specific may have widespread sites of production; i.e., gonadotropins are produced by the normal gonad and intestine, thyrotropin-releasing hormone (TRH) and ACTH by the pancreas, and somatostatin by the kidney and thyroid C cells. Nevertheless, the original term serves to distinguish tumor-associated hormone production from syndromes due to excess secretion of a hormone characteristically associated with a specific endocrine gland.

THEORIES OF ECTOPIC HORMONE SECRETION Several pathogenic mechanisms have been proposed to explain ectopic hormone secretion. The "sponge" theory assumed a selective uptake of the circulating hormone by tumor tissue with subsequent release on tumor cell death. This concept was abandoned, however, after the demonstration of arteriovenous differences of hormones across tumor vascular beds, the presence of hormone mRNA in tumor tissue, and hormone biosynthesis by tumors in vitro. The theory that random mutations resulted in altered DNA sequences and gene products also was discounted when it was established that the production of ectopic hormones by tumors is not random, i.e., that certain tumors are commonly associated with specific endocrinopathies. A third theory, that of gene derepression, proposed that regions of the genome not normally expressed become active and are transcribed in tumors, presumably as a result of loss of normal transcription suppressors during neoplastic transformation. Two other explanations also have been proposed: *cellular dedifferentiation*, a theory that neoplastic cells revert to a more primitive level and again produce peptide hormones that were produced normally at an earlier developmental stage, and *arrested differentiation*, whereby hormone secretion is due to persistence of a function present during development because of a failure (maturational arrest) of the developmental process. Arguments against these theories include an absence of evidence that cells can retrace their pathways of differentiation and that incompletely differentiated cells routinely secrete the hormone in question. Although the pathogenesis of ectopic hormone secretion is still unclear, the mechanism is likely the result of persistent activation of selected gene expression by an oncogene.

CRITERIA FOR DIAGNOSIS Criteria for the diagnosis of ectopic hormone secretion have changed as more precise laboratory methodology made it possible to recognize clinically inapparent cases (Table 327-1). Although many of these criteria cannot be satisfied in

1 Association of a neoplasm with a syndrome attributable to excessive hormone secretion or with inappropriately elevated plasma and/or urine levels of a hormone not normally produced by the tissue from which the tumor is derived
2 Failure of plasma and/or urine hormone levels to respond to normal homeostatic suppression
3 Exclusion of other possible causal mechanisms for hormone hypersecretion
4 Reduction in hormone levels after tumor-specific therapy
5 Arteriovenous step-up gradients of hormone across tumor
6 Demonstration of hormone in tumor tissue
7 Biosynthesis and/or secretion of hormone by tumor tissue in vitro
8 Demonstration in the tumor of hormone-specific messenger RNA by cell-free translation or hybridization with cDNA

individual cases, the majority have been fulfilled in the commonly recognized syndromes.

TUMOR TYPES ASSOCIATED WITH ECTOPIC HORMONE SE-CRETION Ectopic secretion of hormones is associated with a variety of tumors. Although original reports of these syndromes described primarily lung carcinomas, carcinoids, thymomas, and fibrosarcomas, virtually all tumors have the potential of hormone secretion. Nevertheless, the frequency of occurrence of ectopic hormone secretion among various tumor types is not random. The tumors most frequently associated with clinically recognized ectopic hormone production are small cell lung carcinomas, carcinoids, and pancreatic islet tumors. Carcinoid tumors are generally found in the lung or the gastrointestinal tract. Gastrointestinal carcinoids may be present in either the foregut or the hindgut, although it is primarily foregut tumors that are hormonally active. In the lung these tumors are usually endobronchial and may remain undetected for long periods. There are many morphologic similarities between bronchial carcinoid tumors and small cell carcinoma of the lung. Indeed, the two types may have a common cell of origin, namely the Kulchitsky cell, a bronchial mucosal cell that has been called a neuroendocrine cell of the lung because of its peptide-containing granules observed on electron microscopy. A bombesin-like peptide (related to gastrin-releasing peptide) is present in Kulchitsky cells during fetal life and is the most frequent peptide produced by small cell carcinoma of the lung. Ectopic hormone secretion is also associated with other types of lung tumors, most commonly the squamous type of bronchogenic carcinomas.

In the 1960s Pearse proposed the theory that certain hormone-secreting cells are components of a "diffuse neuroendocrine system." Such cells were originally considered to be of neural crest or neuroectodermal origin and were designated APUD (amine precursor uptake and decarboxylation) cells on the basis of their ability to decarboxylate precursors of biogenic amines. Later it was discovered that many of these cells also produce the enzyme neuron-specific enolase and other neurosecretory cell markers. A corollary of the APUD theory was that tumors derived from APUD cells have the capability of hormone secretion. At present, the APUD theory appears invalid for several reasons. First, all APUD cells are not of neuroectodermal origin. Second, the APUD function of these cells is not inherently linked with peptide hormone production, and third, some ectopic hormone-secreting tumors do not possess APUD characteristics. Nevertheless, the fact that particular tumor types secrete certain hormones is useful in evaluating these syndromes.

CHARACTERIZATION OF ECTOPIC HORMONES Type of hormone secreted Of the four classes of hormones—steroids, monoamines, substituted amino acids, and peptides/proteins—only the latter are secreted ectopically. Although the explanation is not known with certainty, the ectopic production of peptide/protein hormones requires less complicated derangements in cell metabolism. For example, an oncogene serving as an inducer or enhancer of gene transcription may increase the expression of a gene coding for a peptide hormone. However, the synthesis of steroids, thyroid hormones, and monoamines requires multiple enzymatic steps and specifically

targeted translocation of the precursor molecules through various cell compartments. It is extremely unlikely that this degree of cell specialization would occur as a consequence of activation of one or several oncogenes.

Ectopic secretion of nearly all peptide hormones has been reported. These hormones may be grouped according to their usual site of origin (Table 327-2). The first group of hormones, common to the central nervous system and gastrointestinal tract, is most frequently secreted by carcinoids, small cell lung carcinomas, and pancreatic islet tumors. The second group, normally produced by the fetoplacental unit and/or the anterior pituitary, tends to be produced by gastrointestinal, hepatic, adrenal, and gonadal tumors. The third group, which includes insulin-like growth factors and parathyroid hormone–related protein, tends to be produced by mesenchymal, hepatic, genitourinary, breast, and squamous cell lung tumors. In addition to the hormones listed, other humoral factors are believed responsible for tumor-associated syndromes such as hypertrophic osteoarthropathy, polyneuropathy, hypophosphatemic osteomalacia, and anorexia.

Relation to naturally secreted hormones The primary amino acid sequences of all ectopically secreted hormones analyzed to date are identical to those of the native hormones. However, differences in structure between ectopically secreted and native hormones can occur as a result of incomplete or abnormal processing of the precursor hormone. Several abnormal forms of ectopic hormones have been defined: (1) large-molecular-weight species due to incomplete enzymatic cleavage of the precursor (proopiomelanocortin), (2) small-molecular-weight fragments due to unregulated intracellular processing (fragments of growth hormone–releasing hormone), and (3) altered glycosylation species (microheterogeneity) due either to failed cleavage of carbohydrate residues during postribosomal hormone processing (glycosylated ACTH) or failure of normal glycosylation (the alpha subunit common to the gonadotropins and TSH). The usual consequence of such altered biosynthetic processing is a hormone variant with diminished biologic activity. If modification of hormone structure is sufficient to cause loss of all biologic activity, ectopic secretion is not accompanied by clinical manifestations. Furthermore, even if a neoplastic cell can synthesize and store a biologically active hormone, a syndrome of hormone excess will not result if an effective secretory mechanism is absent. The frequency with which either an inactive hormone is synthesized or an active hormone is synthesized but not secreted is probably greater than that of classical ectopic hormone secretion, since only a small percentage of tumors that contain ectopic hormones cause clinically recognizable syndromes attributable to hormone hypersecretion.

Other considerations Hormones may be secreted by both benign and malignant tumors. Although hormone secretion normally requires a high level of cellular differentiation, an incompletely differentiated tumor may still retain secretory capability. For example, the process of granule formation and hormone storage is not generally expressed by hormone-secreting tumors; consequently, the concentration of hormone in the tumor is usually low compared with that in endocrine glands. Overall hormone secretion per unit weight is also less, and as a result, considerable tumor mass is usually present before ectopic hormone secretion is clinically apparent. One notable exception is the relatively benign, highly differentiated neoplasm, usually a carcinoid or pancreatic islet tumor, that contains and secretes hormone at a level comparable with that of normal endocrine tissue and is sufficiently small to escape detection for long periods.

Many tumors produce multiple hormones. In some this is due to the existence of a common precursor for multiple hormones; e.g., ACTH, lipotropins, melanocyte-stimulating hormones (MSHs), and endorphins are all derived from a single precursor, proopiomelanocortin (POMC), and both vasoactive intestinal peptide (VIP) and peptide histidyl-methionine (PHM) are encoded in a single precursor. In other instances, multiple hormones are produced in the absence of common precursors, e.g., production of ACTH, calcitonin, and somatostatin by medullary thyroid carcinoma and by small cell carcinoma of the lung. In some tumors separate cells secrete individual hormones,

TABLE 327-2   Spectrum of ectopic hormone production

Group/hormone	Tumor type Common	Tumor type Infrequent	Group/hormone	Tumor type Common	Tumor type Infrequent
NEUROENDOCRINE-GASTROINTESTINAL					
Adrenocorticotropin, β-lipotropin, endorphins, MSHs, enkephalins	Lung carcinoma (small cell), thymoma, pancreatic islet tumors, carcinoid, thyroid medullary carcinoma, pheochromocytoma, parotid tumor, prostatic carcinoma, renal carcinoma	Squamous cell, adenocarcinoma, and large cell carcinoma of the lung; breast carcinoma, colon carcinoma, gallbladder tumors, testicular carcinoma, uterine carcinoma, laryngeal carcinoma, plasmacytoma, bladder small cell carcinoma	Somatostatin	Lung carcinoma (small cell), carcinoid, pheochromocytoma	
			Calcitonin	Lung carcinoma (small cell), carcinoid	Breast carcinoma, pheochromocytoma
			Gastrin	Lung carcinoma (small cell)	Ovarian carcinoma
Vasopressin, oxytocin, neurophysin	Lung carcinoma (small cell, anaplastic, adenocarcinoma), carcinoid	Pancreatic carcinoma, duodenal carcinoma	Vasoactive intestinal peptide	Lung carcinoma (small cell), pancreatic islet tumors	
			Insulin		Gastric carcinoma, lung carcinoma, carcinoid
Corticotropin-releasing hormone	Lung carcinoma (small cell), carcinoid	Pituitary gangliocytoma, medullary carcinoma of thyroid	Glucagon		Lung carcinoma, carcinoid, renal carcinoma
Growth hormone–releasing hormone	Carcinoid, pancreatic islet adenoma, lung carcinoma, (small cell)	Adrenocortical adenoma, neurofibroma, endometrial carcinoma, pheochromocytoma, pituitary gangliocytoma	Gastrin-releasing peptide (bombesin-like)	Lung carcinoma, carcinoid	Medullary carcinoma of thyroid
FETOPLACENTAL AND/OR ANTERIOR PITUITARY					
Chorionic gonadotropin (and subunits)	Lung carcinoma, gastric carcinoma, ovarian carcinoma, adeno- and islet cell carcinoma of the pancreas, hepatoma, genitourinary tract tumors	Testicular carcinoma, ovarian carcinoma, adrenocortical carcinoma, breast carcinoma, melanoma, carcinoid	Growth hormone		Lung carcinoma (large cell), carcinoid, pancreatic islet tumor
			Prolactin		Lung carcinoma, renal carcinoma, gonadoblastoma, ovarian teratoma
Placental lactogen	Lung carcinoma (small cell)	Lymphoma, pheochromocytoma, hepatoma			
OTHERS					
Tissue growth factors (primary insulin-like growth factor II)	Mesenchymal tumors (i.e., fibrosarcoma), hepatoma, adrenocortical carcinoma, pancreatic/bile duct carcinoma	Lung carcinoma, ovarian carcinoma, neuroblastoma, Wilms's tumor	Parathyroid hormone–related protein	Renal carcinoma, lung carcinoma (squamous), hepatoma, pancreatic islet tumors	GI tract tumors, parotid tumors, genitourinary tract tumors, melanoma, breast carcinoma
			1,25-Dihydroxy vitamin D	Lymphoma	
Erythropoietin	Cerebellar hemangioblastoma, uterine fibroma, renal carcinoma	Adrenocortical carcinoma, hepatoma, pheochromocytoma	Parathyroid hormone		Ovarian carcinoma

whereas in others multiple hormones are produced by the same cell. Furthermore, variation may occur in cell lines cloned from such tumors, suggesting that gene expression may be unstable in succeeding generations of tumor cells both in vitro and in vivo.

FREQUENCY   The frequency of ectopic hormone secretion varies with the criteria used for diagnosis. The most frequently encountered syndromes are those of ACTH hypersecretion, hypercalcemia, and organic hypoglycemia. Ectopic ACTH secretion occurs in approximately 15 to 20 percent of patients with Cushing's syndrome. Thus consideration of this diagnosis is of great importance. Similarly, nearly half of patients with hypercalcemia unrelated to volume depletion, excess ingestion of vitamin D, or sarcoidosis have a malignancy rather than hyperparathyroidism, and of these, about 70 percent secrete a hypercalcemic peptide, parathyroid hormone–related protein, that has parathyroid hormone–like biologic activity and whose amino-terminal 13 amino acids are identical to those of parathyroid hormone. In contrast, hypoglycemia due to ectopic production of insulin-like growth factor II is infrequent in patients suspected of having an insulinoma, and ectopic growth hormone–releasing hormone (GRH) secretion is a rare (<1 percent) cause of acromegaly.

CONSEQUENCES OF ECTOPIC HORMONE SECRETION   The consequences of ectopic hormone secretion may be of greater significance than the tumor itself. This is particularly true for patients with benign or slowly growing malignant ACTH- or gastrin-producing tumors in whom fulminant Cushing's syndrome or bleeding peptic ulceration may be life-threatening. In others, the hormone may cause medical problems that shorten the life span beyond that attributable to the tumor itself, i.e., severe hypercalcemia, hyponatremia, or hypoglycemia.

The symptoms of ectopic hormone secretion may be the presenting manifestations of the neoplasm or occur late in the course of the disease. The rapidity of onset of the clinical manifestations of hormone hypersecretion affects the frequency with which the syndrome is recognized. For example, excessive secretion of ACTH or vasopressin is clinically evident within weeks or months; thus a fully developed syndrome can be associated with rapidly growing malignant as well as benign tumors. In contrast, acromegaly due to ectopic GRH secretion typically requires years to become apparent and therefore is observed only when caused by benign or slowly growing malignant neoplasms. Ectopic hormone secretion, once established, does not necessarily persist for as long as the tumor is present. Hormone secretion may cease or decline to clinically insignificant levels either spontaneously or in response to radiation or chemotherapy. Hormone secretion usually, but not invariably, recurs with tumor relapse.

In addition to effects on the host, ectopic hormone secretion has numerous important biologic implications. Since tumor-secreted factors that exhibit biologic effects are not unique substances, their identification and characterization can assist in the search for the naturally occurring (eutopic) peptide. For example, tumor-secreted GRH was the source for the purification, isolation, and structural characterization of hypothalamic GRH. In addition, characterization of tumor-produced parathyroid hormone–related protein has resulted in the identification of a new hormone normally found in skin (keratinocytes), the central nervous system, lactating breast, pancreatic islets, and other tissues.

DIAGNOSIS Occasionally, the clinical manifestations of ectopic hormone secretion are so distinctive that they suggest the diagnosis before any hormones have been measured. The development of gynecomastia in the absence of associated diseases such as cirrhosis or testicular failure may suggest the presence of ectopic gonadotropin secretion, while Cushing's syndrome and increased pigmentation or severe muscle weakness (due to hypokalemia) point to ectopic ACTH secretion.

More commonly, however, clinical manifestations of hormone excess are subtle or absent. In such instances, basal serum levels of hormones, e.g., ACTH, may be elevated out of proportion to the biologic effects observed. This may be the result of the presence of ACTH precursor molecules that have little or no biologic activity. Identification of these abnormal forms can be accomplished by molecular sieve chromatography or by multiple, site-specific radioimmunoassays of serum. Similarly, disproportionate elevations of hCG may reflect the presence of the glycoprotein alpha subunit, which is biologically inactive but exhibits cross-reactivity in some radioimmunoassays. A specific alpha-subunit assay is used to confirm the diagnosis.

In other instances, the diagnosis of ectopic hormone secretion may be suggested by finding suppressed levels of hormones that are subject to feedback inhibition. Low or undetectable levels of insulin or parathyroid hormone in the presence of hypoglycemia or hypercalcemia are suggestive of tumors that secrete insulin-like growth factor II or parathyroid hormone–related protein, respectively.

Alterations in normal feedback regulation also may provide clues that elevated circulating hormone levels are derived from ectopic sources. Patients with ectopic ACTH production do not respond to suppression by glucocorticoids or to stimulation by corticotropin-releasing hormone (presumably because of the absence of appropriate receptors in the tumor tissue), an observation that helps distinguish them from patients with pituitary-dependent Cushing's disease. Apparent suppression of ACTH, which has been noted in several case reports, could be explained by intermittent secretion of ACTH by the tumor (an uncommon and poorly understood phenomenon of ectopic hormone secretion).

If the diagnosis is still in doubt, or if the source of ectopic secretion is unknown, selective venous catheterization may be an effective means of locating the tumor. As long as the tumor is actually secreting hormone at the time of study, a step-up gradient in the concentration of the hormone is of value in tumor localization and/or a search for metastases.

THERAPY Primary treatment of ectopic hormone–secreting tumors should be directed, if possible, toward removal of the tumor. Measurement of circulating hormone levels can serve as a marker for completeness of tumor excision or of the effect of radiation and chemotherapy, e.g., small cell carcinoma of the lung. In addition, recurrence of tumor may be heralded by reappearance of elevated

hormone levels prior to mass effects of the tumor. However, occasional tumors may not secrete hormones at recurrence, so one cannot rely solely on hormone measurements as a marker of tumor activity.

Frequently, the tumor cannot be removed or is metastatic at the time of diagnosis. In such cases, two other approaches are available for eliminating the effects of ectopic hormone secretion. Octreotide, a long-acting somatostatin analogue, may be effective in inhibiting growth hormone–releasing hormone secretion, VIP secretion, and the clinical symptoms of the carcinoid syndrome.

The other approach involves blocking the action of the hormone when its secretion cannot be altered. Pharmacologic agents may interfere with hormone effects on target tissues. Examples include (1) demeclocycline to inhibit vasopressin action on the renal tubule in the syndrome of inappropriate antidiuretic hormone (SIADH) associated with malignancy and (2) ketoconazole and/or mitotane to inhibit adrenal steroidogenesis in the ectopic ACTH syndrome. Alternatively, surgical removal of the target tissue may avoid life-threatening complications and permit relatively symptom-free long-term survival if the tumor is benign or slowly growing. Examples include adrenalectomy for the ectopic ACTH syndrome and gastrectomy for recurrent gastrointestinal bleeding caused by gastrin-producing tumors. This form of therapy is used infrequently as more specific pharmacologic agents have become available.

ECTOPIC HORMONES AS MARKERS FOR NEOPLASIA With the initial recognition of ectopic hormone secretion, it was hoped that measurement of these hormones would provide a generally applicable means of screening for clinically silent tumors. As knowledge of the spectrum of ectopic hormone secretion has increased, however, this hope has faded. The list of ectopically secreted hormones has lengthened to the point that cost considerations preclude this form of screening. Even if the number of hormones were not as extensive, the limited correlation of tumor site and type with secretion of specific hormones necessitates an extensive workup to localize the tumor. Screening programs, when performed, have yielded few positive results. Moreover, evidence is lacking that earlier diagnosis, as a result of such procedures, reduces morbidity or mortality. Consequently, screening for ectopic hormone production is not justified in routine cancer detection programs.

REFERENCES

BURTIS WJ et al: Immunochemical characterization of circulating parathyroid hormone–related protein in patients with humoral hypercalcemia of cancer. N Engl J Med 322:1106, 1990

DOPPMAN JL: The search for occult ectopic ACTH-producing tumors. Endocrinology 2:41, 1992

————et al: Ectopic adrenocorticotropic hormone syndrome: Localization studies in 28 patients. Radiology 172:115, 1989

FROHMAN LA, DOWNS TR: Ectopic GRH syndrome, in Acromegaly, R Robbins et al (eds). New York, Plenum, 1987

KRENNING EP et al: Localisation of endocrine-related tumours with radioiodinated analogue of somatostatin. Lancet 1(8632):242, 1989

LEINUNG MC, et al: Diagnosis of corticotropin-producing bronchial carcinoid tumors causing Cushing's syndrome. Mayo Clin Proc 65:1314, 1990

MARTIN TJ, SUVA LJ: Parathyroid hormone–related protein in hypercalcaemia of malignancy. Clin Endocrinol (Oxf) 31:631, 1989

MUDDLE AH et al: Ectopic production of 1,25-dihydroxyvitamin D by B-cell lymphoma as a cause of hypercalcemia. Cancer 59:1543, 1987

ORTH D: Ectopic hormone production, in Endocrinology and Metabolism, 2d ed, P Felig et al (eds). New York, McGraw-Hill, 1987

PASS HI et al: Management of the ectopic ACTH syndrome due to thoracic carcinoids. Ann Thorac Surg 50:51, 1990

PHILIPPE J et al: Expression of peptide hormone genes in human islet cell tumors. Diabetes 37:1647, 1988

RUSSELL, PJ et al: Ectopic hormone production by small cell undifferentiated carcinomas. Mol Cell Endocrinol 71:1, 1990

SANO T et al: Growth hormone–releasing hormone–producing tumors: Clinical, biochemical, and morphological manifestations. Endocrinol Rev 9:357, 1988

STREWLER GJ, NISSENSON RA: Peptide mediators of hypercalcemia of malignancy. Annu Rev Med 41:35, 1990

TABARIN A et al: Use of ketoconazole in the treatment of Cushing's disease and ectopic ACTH syndrome. Clin Endocrinol 34:63, 1991

WYNICK D et al: Symptomatic secondary hormone syndromes in patients with established malignant pancreatic endocrine tumors. N Engl J Med 319:605, 1988

328   PARANEOPLASTIC NEUROLOGIC SYNDROMES

ROBERT H. BROWN, JR.

Neoplasia can alter neurologic function in numerous ways, as outlined in Table 328-1. Several neurologic syndromes have been delineated which are a consequence of a remotely located neoplasm but do not arise from direct involvement of the nervous system by metastasis or from a known secondary complication of cancer or its therapy (e.g., malnutrition, opportunistic infection, drug-induced neuropathy). These paraneoplastic syndromes, outlined in Table 328-2, share several characteristics. They are clinically dramatic, arising subacutely in weeks or even days to produce neurologic symptoms that may be profoundly disabling. They may precede detection of the neoplasm by months or even years; their recognition should prompt a timely search for a malignant tumor. More than one syndrome may arise with a given neoplasm. In general, as outlined in Table 328-2, certain syndromes are associated with particular types of tumors. The diagnosis of a paraneoplastic neurologic disorder depends primarily on (1) the presence of a recognized clinical syndrome, (2) careful exclusion of other cancer-related disorders (as in Table 328-1), and (3) in some instances, confirmatory laboratory studies, including serum or cerebrospinal fluid (CSF) antibodies with specific patterns of reactivity (see Table 328-3) or electromyographic studies typical of myasthenia gravis or myasthenic syndrome. CSF may show protein elevation and a mild lymphocytic pleocytosis.

INCIDENCE   Studies of the incidence of these syndromes are problematic because the conditions are rare and classifications vary. In one series, these syndromes were detected in about 7 percent of nearly 1500 patients with tumors, although recent studies suggest that the incidence is somewhat lower. The paraneoplastic syndrome is encountered in up to one-sixth of all ovarian tumors, one-seventh of lung tumors, and less frequently in stomach, prostate, and breast cancers. The tumors most frequently associated with paraneoplastic syndromes are small cell lung carcinoma (47 percent), stomach (12 percent), breast (12 percent), ovary (9 percent), and colon (6 percent) tumors.

PATHOLOGIC CHANGES   Pathologic features of these syndromes have been well defined. One group of paraneoplastic syndromes is characterized by *encephalomyelitis,* in which perivascular lymphocytosis, microglial proliferation, and loss of neurons occur. While these changes may be diffuse throughout the neuraxis, they often predominate in a specific anatomic location that dictates the resulting clinical abnormalities. Thus, as outlined below, the manifestations of limbic encephalitis may differ from those of brainstem encephalitis. Inflammation may be evident in dorsal root

TABLE 328-1   Effects of malignancy on the nervous system

Direct invasion
Metastatic invasion
  A Parenchymatous
  B Vascular (neoplastic angioendotheliosis)
  C Meningeal (meningeal carcinomatosis)
Opportunistic infections
  A Bacterial (e.g., listeria)
  B Nonbacterial
    1 Typical and atypical viral (e.g., progressive multifocal
      leukoencephalopathy)
    2 Fungal (e.g., cryptococcus)
Complications of antineoplastic therapy
  A Radiation (e.g., radiation necrosis)
  B Chemotherapy (e.g., vincristine neuropathy)
Metabolic complications
  A Nutritional deficiency
  B Ectopic hormone production
Paraneoplastic syndromes

ganglia or in gray and white matter of the spinal cord, respectively, producing ganglioradiculitis or subacute poliomyelitis. Inflammatory destruction of the sensory neuronal cell bodies (hence the term *neuronopathy*) in the dorsal root ganglia results in wallerian degeneration of axons in both peripheral nerves and corresponding ascending sensory long tracts (posterior columns of the spinal cord).

In a second pathologic form of paraneoplastic disease, severe *focal degeneration* or loss of neurons occurs without inflammation. This is exemplified by the selective but widespread loss of Purkinje neurons in the cerebellum in subacute cortical cerebellar degeneration. This disorder may occur in isolation or concurrently with findings of encephalomyelitis in other areas of the brain or spinal cord. In some cases of paraneoplastic cerebellar degeneration there may be accompanying cerebellar inflammation. In other paraneoplastic syndromes the associated pathologic changes occur in the peripheral nervous system, consisting of multifocal demyelination, myonecrosis, or abnormalities in the neuromuscular junction.

PATHOGENESIS   Several mechanisms have been invoked to explain these disorders, including release by the tumor of neurotoxic substances, common viral or retroviral infections of tumor and neural tissues, and both humoral and cellular autoimmune reactivity to antigens shared between the tumor and the affected neural cells. Some paraneoplastic disorders are characterized by serum and CSF antibodies with highly specific patterns of reactivity with neural tissue or muscle. These are exemplified by the Lambert-Eaton myasthenic syndrome and myasthenia gravis, in which circulating antibodies react with pre- and postsynaptic proteins, respectively. Both syndromes have been reproduced in animals by passive administration of fractionated immunoglobulins (see Chap. 386). In some cases of paraneoplastic cerebellar degeneration, serum and CSF antibodies react specifically with cerebellar cytoplasmic antigens. In other instances, immunoglobulins from patients with a number of different paraneoplastic neurologic syndromes may produce similar patterns of reactivity with neural tissue. Thus antibodies recognizing neuronal nuclear antigens are common in patients with small cell carcinoma of the lung. Similar findings may be present in subacute sensory neuronopathy. In these cases, it appears that one or more pathogenic antibodies, possibly cross-reacting with antigens on the tumor, may provoke autoimmune neural injury in more than one region of the neuraxis. Detection of such antibodies may confirm that an evolving neurologic disorder is of paraneoplastic origin even though the antibodies are not diagnostic of a specific neurologic syndrome. Evidence suggests that some antigens may be specifically targeted by subsets of lymphocytes within affected areas of the brain.

TREATMENT   Treatment of the paraneoplastic disorders is difficult and often unsuccessful. Resection of the underlying malignancy is surprisingly ineffective, although there are isolated reports of symptomatic improvement following tumor removal. Immune suppression is also of little benefit; plasmapheresis or intravenous pooled globulin may ameliorate Lambert-Eaton syndrome.

The salient features of the major paracarcinomatous neurologic syndromes are discussed below (reviewed in detail by Posner) (see Table 328-2).

BRAIN, CEREBELLUM, AND SPINAL CORD   Visual paraneoplastic syndromes   Patients with carcinoma of the lung (and rarely, breast, cervix, or endometrium) may develop progressive, painless loss of vision with photosensitivity due to loss of retinal photoreceptors. The electroretinogram is typically abnormal. This cancer-associated retinopathy (CAR) is commonly associated with high titers of serum antibodies to one or more CAR antigens including a 23-kDa protein.

Paraneoplastic encephalomyelitis   Small cell lung carcinoma may precipitate an encephalomyelitis of variable distribution and, in consequence, variable but often overlapping clinical presentations. In addition, it is often accompanied by an inflammatory paraneoplastic sensory neuronopathy (see below). Serum and CSF from patients with paraneoplastic encephalomyelitis and neuropathy often �onstrate antibodies to neuronal nuclear antigens. This anti-Hu

TABLE 328-2 Paraneoplastic neurologic syndromes

Site	Evolution	Clinical features*	Cancer	Pathology
BRAIN AND CEREBELLUM				
Photoreceptor, retinal degeneration	Weeks to months	Painless visual loss progressing to blindness[1]	SCLC,[†] rarely cervical cancer	Loss of rods and cones, infiltration of retina with mononuclear cells
Subacute cortical cerebellar degeneration	Weeks to months	Cerebellar ataxia, dysarthria[2,3]	SCLC, ovarian and breast cancer, Hodgkin's disease	Loss of Purkinje cells
Opsoclonus-myoclonus	Weeks	Dancing eyes and feet, cerebellar ataxia, and possibly encephalopathy[2,4]	Neuroblastoma, bronchogenic carcinomas	In adults, degeneration of dentate nuclei
Paraneoplastic encephalo-myelitis				
Limbic encephalitis	Weeks to months	Agitated, confusional state, memory loss followed by dementia[2]	SCLC, ovarian and other cancers	Neuronal loss; gliosis in medial temporal lobe, amygdala and elsewhere in limbic system, perivascular and meningeal infiltration
Brainstem encephalitis	Days to weeks	Nystagmus, diplopia, vertigo, ataxia, dysarthria, dysphagia[2]	SCLC, other cancers	Neuronal loss in brainstem, inflammatory changes as above
SPINAL CORD				
Necrotizing myelopathy	Hours, days, or weeks	Para- or quadriplegia with arreflexia, sensory loss and bladder dysfunction	SCLC, lymphoma	Severe necrosis of gray and white matter
Subacute motor neuronopathy	Weeks or months	Flaccid weakness, muscle atrophy, legs affected more than arms[2]	Non-Hodgkin's lymphoma	Inflammation of ventral horns loss of anterior horn cells
PERIPHERAL NERVE				
Subacute sensory neuronopathy	Weeks to months	Severe sensory loss with arreflexia[2] and ataxia, paresthesias, pain	SCLC and other lung tumors	Inflammation and neuronal degeneration in dorsal root ganglia, secondary axon loss
Acute demyelinating neuritis (Guillain-Barré, AIDP)	Hours to days	Ascending paralysis, arreflexia, possibly ascending sensory loss, high spinal fluid protein	Hodgkin's disease	Segmental demyelination inflammation of peripheral nerves
Chronic inflammatory demyelinating polyneuropathy (CIDP)	Weeks to months	Chronic progressive or relapsing weakness with sensory loss, high spinal fluid protein	Rarely lung, breast, and gastric cancer, lymphoma, myeloma	As in AIDP
Neuropathy with paraproteinemia	Weeks to months	Chronic, may be predominantly sensory or motor[‡]	Myeloma, osteosclerotic myeloma	As in AIDP
Sensorimotor neuropathy	Weeks to months	Distal motor and sensory loss[2]	SCLC and other tumors	Axonopathy, some segmental loss of myelin
NEUROMUSCULAR JUNCTION				
Lambert-Eaton myasthenic syndrome	Weeks to months	Proximal weakness, fatiguability, dry mouth, possibly ptosis[6]	SCLC, breast, prostate, stomach tumors	Disruption of active zones on presynaptic terminals
Myasthenia gravis	Weeks to months	Weakness, fatiguability, ptosis, diplopia[7]	Thymoma	Disruption of postsynaptic junctional membrane folds
MUSCLE				
Polymyositis	Months to years	Proximal weakness, myalgias, possibly cardiomyopathy, high serum creatine kinase	Association with malignancy unclear, possibly breast, ovary, lung tumors, lymphoma	Lymphocytic inflammation of muscle interstitium, myofiber necrosis, phagocytosis
Necrotizing myopathy	Days to weeks	Rapidly progressive proximal weakness, possibly dysphagia, dyspnea	Bronchial carcinoma, SCLC	Severe myonecrosis with minimal inflammation or phagocytosis

* Superscript denotes possible association with antibody (listed Table 328-3).
† Small cell lung carcinoma.
‡ May be associated with a serum IgG or IgA M component.

antibody recognizes a 37-kDa protein specific to neuronal nuclei. The major features of paraneoplastic encephalomyelitis include the following.

LIMBIC ENCEPHALITIS   In some cases, the encephalitis is limited to or most extensive within limbic structures such as the hippocampus and amygdala, producing affective changes in personality (anxiety and agitated depression), selective, early memory loss suggestive of Korsakoff psychosis, or confusion and hallucinations. In some cases the initial presentation is an amnesic syndrome. The affective disorder often prompts psychiatric evaluation. Abnormalities of the electroencephalogram or overt seizures may be present early in the syndrome. While cognition may initially be spared, dementia becomes common as the disorder progresses; symptoms referable to encephalitic involvement in other regions are often superimposed.

TABLE 328-3 Defined antibodies associated with paraneoplastic neurologic syndromes*

Antibody	Paraneoplastic syndrome	Tumor	Antigen
[1]CAR ab	Cancer-associated retinopathy	SCLC[†]	Recoverin, 25-kDa calcium-binding cone protein
[2]Anti-Hu	Encephalomyelitis, sensory neuronopathy	Predominantly SCLC[†]	37-kDa CNS nuclear protein
[3]Anti-Yo	Cerebellar degeneration	Gynecologic tumors, breast	Cerebellar leucine-zipper protein
[4]Anti-Ri	Opsoclonus-myoclonus	Breast	55- and 80-kDa CNS nuclear protein
[5]Anti-MAG IgM M protein	Demyelinating neuropathy	Myeloma	Myelin-associated glycoprotein (MAG)
[6]LEMS ab	Lambert-Eaton myasthenic syndrome	SCLC	Presynaptic calcium channel
[7]MG ab	Myasthenia gravis	Thymoma	Postsynaptic acetyl-choline receptor

* Other patterns of antibody reactivity also have been described for some of these syndromes.
† Small cell lung cancer.

BRAINSTEM ENCEPHALITIS Symptoms of brainstem encephalitis relate directly to the distribution of pathologic findings. The predominant symptoms are due to medullary involvement producing nausea, vomiting, nystagmus, vertigo, and ataxia. A syndrome suggestive of progressive bulbar palsy with marked dysarthria and dysphagia may occur with pontine nuclei involvement. Mesencephalic inflammation and neuronal loss result in nuclear or internuclear eye movement abnormalities with disabling diplopia and oscillopsia. Rostral midbrain and nigral involvement may cause rigidity and in some cases stupor and coma.

CEREBELLAR ENCEPHALITIS Inflammatory changes are rare in the cerebellar cortex but may be severe in deep cerebellar nuclei such as the dentate nucleus, causing myoclonus.

MYELITIS In paraneoplastic myelitis, the gray matter of the cord is diffusely infiltrated with leukocytes leading to profound neuronal degeneration. The myelitis may be widespread through the cord or restricted to a few segmental levels. Anterior horn cell destruction typically produces muscle weakness and neurogenic atrophy which is often asymmetric. There may be selective involvement of the neck, upper extremities, or lower extremities. Corticospinal signs (hyperreflexia, weakness, Babinski signs) result from involvement of this tract in the cord or brainstem. The corticospinal tract dysfunction (and in some cases motor neuronopathy) should not be confused with motor neuron disease; typical amyotrophic lateral sclerosis does not appear to arise as a paraneoplastic complication. The appearance of sensory symptoms and signs in a patient with cancer usually denotes either dorsal root ganglioradiculitis or inflammation of the posterior horns (see below).

NECROTIZING MYELOPATHY This is a rare complication of malignancy presenting clinically as a subacute transverse myelitis, often in a thoracic location. It can be distinguished from the less fulminant encephalomyelitis described above by the evolution of an intensely necrotic, central thoracic cord lesion which tails off rostrally and caudally over several segmental levels. In some instances, there are multiple necrotic foci within the cord. Clinical findings include leg (and possibly arm) plegia, sensory loss, and urinary bladder sphincter abnormalities. The lesion is frequently initially asymmetric, mimicking the Brown-Séquard syndrome. In severe cases, the CSF protein and cell count are increased and myelography demonstrates focal cord swelling. Although not all cases are associated with tumor, cancers of the lung, lymphoma, and leukemia are known to occur in such patients.

Opsoclonus-myoclonus A syndrome of opsoclonus, myoclonus, and ataxia ("dancing eyes, dancing feet") occurs in both children and adults. About one-half of affected children have differentiated neuroblastomas, usually located in the thorax. In adults, the syndrome may be associated with solid tumors such as bronchial carcinoma. The onset is subacute, and in some patients the syndrome persists for months, to be followed by permanent encephalopathy or retardation. Pathologic findings in adults include prominent neuronal degeneration in the dentate nucleus of the cerebellum suggesting a relationship to cortical cerebellar degeneration. In some individuals, this syndrome responds to glucocorticoids or treatment of the cancer. A subgroup of women developing opsoclonus with breast cancer has been found to have an antibody (anti-Ri) directed against 55- and 80-kDa antigens on neuronal nuclei and in the tumor.

Subacute cortical cerebellar degeneration (SCCD) This is a subacute progressive cerebellar disorder characterized by profound truncal and appendicular ataxia evolving over a period of weeks in association with gynecologic tumors, oat cell carcinoma, or Hodgkin's disease. Symptoms referable to the brainstem include vertigo, dysarthria, diplopia, nystagmus, and corticospinal signs. In general, any nonfamilial ataxia arising in patients over age 45 should raise the suspicion of this entity. By contrast with paraneoplastic encephalomyelitis described above, the predominant pathologic finding in SCCD is widespread loss of cerebellar Purkinje neurons with astrogliosis and secondary loss of Purkinje cell axons. Many cases are associated with dementia for which an anatomic basis has not been well established. The CSF commonly reveals a mild pleocytosis; cerebellar atrophy may be evident on magnetic resonance imaging (MRI) or computed tomographic (CT) scan.

Several types of anti-Purkinje cell antibodies have been detected in sera of patients with SCCD. Women with cancer of the breast or ovary and SCCD demonstrate anti-antibodies (anti-Yo) recognizing cytoplasmic Purkinje cell proteins of about 34 and 62 kDa. The former is a recently cloned, novel neuronal protein expressed selectively in cerebellar Purkinje cells. A different cytoplasmic antigen is recognized by immunoglobulins from patients with SCCD and adenocarcinoma of the lung. In other patients with small cell lung carcinoma and SCCD, anti-Hu antibodies are present (see Table 328-3).

PERIPHERAL NERVES A number of clinical syndromes affecting the peripheral nerves occur in association with malignancy. *Subacute paraneoplastic sensory neuronopathy,* arguably the most clinically distinctive, is a ganglioradiculitis that may present with paraneoplastic encephalomyelitis. Other paraneoplastic neuropathies are more difficult to distinguish from noncarcinomatous neuropathies. However, their recognition is important because they are relatively common and their manifestations may precede the diagnosis of the underlying neoplasia. Neuropathy may be demonstrated in as many as 50 percent of patients with lung cancer using electrophysiologic criteria. In evaluating a paracarcinomatous neuropathy, it is helpful to ascertain whether the neuropathy (1) affects motor fibers, sensory fibers, or both, (2) predominantly involves axon or myelin, or (3) occurs with an abnormal serum paraprotein.

Subacute sensory neuronopathy This disorder primarily affects the axon, with relative sparing of myelin. The typical pathology is a ganglioradiculitis, as noted earlier. Clinically, the onset is characterized by the subacute development of paresthesias and pain (sometimes severe) in the distal limbs and associated truncal sensory ataxia. The sensory ataxia may be profoundly disabling. Although often initially restricted only to arms or legs, the symptoms eventually affect all four extremities. In a majority of cases, the underlying malignancy is oat cell cancer of the lung; the paraneoplastic neuropathy may precede the diagnosis of the tumor by more than a year. The serum of some patients contains anti-Hu antibodies.

Acute inflammatory demyelinating polyneuritis (AIDP, Guillain-Barré) This syndrome, discussed in detail in Chap. 383, may be associated with Hodgkin's disease. It is characterized by subacutely ascending paralysis, sensory loss which is often mild by comparison with the motor deficits, areflexia, and a characteristic elevation of CSF protein without pleocytosis. Histopathology reveals lymphocytic infiltration of nerves, segmental demyelination, and relative axonal sparing.

Chronic inflammatory demyelinating polyneuropathy (CIDP) Included here are a group of chronic progressive or relapsing inflammatory demyelinative peripheral neuropathies which are distinguished from acute polyneuritis by the time course, more prominent involvement of sensory nerves, lack of involvement of autonomic nerves, and responsiveness to immunotherapy. As in Guillain-Barré syndrome, the demyelinative nature of these neuropathies is defined physiologically by slowed nerve conduction velocities or dispersion of compound muscle action potentials; as in AIDP, the pathologic hallmark is segmental loss of myelin with relative preservation of axons as revealed in teased single fiber preparations. In some cases, physiologic studies may reveal only marginal slowing of conduction, whereas the biopsy demonstrates clearly selective myelin loss. Sural nerve biopsy may fail to reveal any alterations if the demyelination is proximal (and therefore detectable only with electrophysiologic methods). Elevation of CSF protein helps confirm the diagnosis.

CIDP usually occurs without any association with neoplasia. Rarely, however, it can occur in association with solid tumors of lung, breast, and stomach. It also may present in patients with Waldenström's macroglobulinemia, gamma heavy chain disease, and lymphoma. In many instances, paraneoplastic CIDP is characterized by the presence of a serum paraprotein, typically a monoclonal immunoglobulin ("M component"). As many as 20 percent of patients with monoclonal gammopathies of undetermined cause later develop hematologic disease, including malignancies.

Two chronic demyelinating neuropathies are particularly distinctive in this context. The first is associated with a monoclonal IgM that reacts with a myelin-associated glycoprotein (MAG) in peripheral nerve myelin. This pattern of reactivity occurs in about half of patients with an IgM gammopathy and neuropathy. This IgM anti-MAG neuropathy is more sensory than motor; it is slowly progressive. It remains to be established whether the anti-MAG antibody is a cause or consequence of the demyelination. The second distinctive subtype of CIDP occurs with osteosclerotic myeloma and monoclonal IgG or IgA antibodies that do not react with MAG. This polyneuropathy is predominantly motor and often quite indolent, although it may eventually produce severe limb muscle wasting. Sensory and autonomic findings are unusual. A related group of CIDP patients develop polyneuropathy, organomegaly, endocrinopathy, the M protein, and skin changes (POEMS syndrome); one-half have osteosclerotic myeloma and IgG or IgA M proteins with lambda light chains. Some patients with demyelinative neuropathies and IgM M proteins respond well to immunosuppressive therapy. Those with osteosclerotic myeloma may improve after treatment of the underlying plasmacytoma, particularly if it is solitary.

Sensorimotor neuropathy This category of mixed sensory and motor axonopathy is the most common paraneoplastic neuropathy. Symptoms depend on the severity of the neuropathy and may include muscle wasting and weakness, distal limb parasthesia, and sometimes pain. Pathologically, there is noninflammatory degeneration of axons and mild myelin loss, presumably secondary to the axonopathy. Paraneoplastic sensorimotor neuropathy has been reported with several types of tumors (lung oat cell, breast, stomach) and hematologic malignancies (Hodgkin's disease, lymphoma, multiple myeloma). In amyloidosis, itself often associated with myeloma, there may be an axonal neuropathy with intraneural deposition of amyloid fibrils derived from immunoglobulin light chains. Axonal neuropathy has been reported as a manifestation of occult insulinoma, possibly as a consequence of hypoglycemia. Infrequently, these neuropathies remit spontaneously; often they progress even with aggressive treatment of the underlying malignancy.

Subacute motor neuronopathy Another particularly striking paracarcinomatous disorder of peripheral nerves is a subacutely progressive motor neuropathy that causes slowly progressive weakness in the legs heralding an otherwise occult lymphoma. Pathologic

changes include loss of motor neurons in the anterolateral gray matter of spinal cord, gliosis, loss of myelin in ventral roots, and some Schwann cell proliferation. Although there is no clearly effective treatment for this condition, many patients seem to improve following immunosuppressive therapy for the malignancy. In other patients, progression of the weakness may cease independently of the status of the lymphoma.

NEUROMUSCULAR JUNCTION Lambert-Eaton myasthenic syndrome (See also Chap. 386) This syndrome, which occurs either in association with malignancy or autoimmune disease, is characterized by weakness, myalgias, and fatigability. It is typically more severe in the lower extremities and in the proximal muscles. Ptosis may be seen. Dysautonomic features are common and may include dryness of the mouth and eyes, impotence, diminished sweating, and orthostatic symptoms. The disorder afflicts men more often than women. The incidence of associated malignancy is 70 percent in men and 25 percent in women. In most cases of either sex, the tumor is a small cell carcinoma of the lung.

The predominant clinical finding is striking reduction in strength at rest with transient improvement in power on repetitive maximal exertion. Tensilon has no effect or may slightly improve strength. Electromyography demonstrates motor unit potentials whose amplitude is low at rest but which increases with exercise or tetanic stimulation; this contrasts with the electromyographic findings in myasthenia gravis (see Chap. 386). Electron microscopy of the presynaptic motor nerve terminals at the neuromuscular junction reveals a decrease in numbers of structures believed to correspond to voltage-sensitive calcium channels. Lambert-Eaton syndrome is considered to be an autoimmune disorder associated with diminished quantal release of acetylcholine. It is associated with other autoimmune disorders and appears to be HLA-linked (B8 and DRw3 antigens). In paraneoplastic Lambert-Eaton syndrome, physiologic data incriminate antibodies directed against voltage-dependent calcium channels present both on the tumor and at distal motor nerve terminals. Treatment is directed toward the underlying neoplasm or autoimmune disease or toward augmentation of acetylcholine release with drugs that prolong presynaptic depolarization and thereby enhance calcium influx. Guanidine hydrochloride and 3,4-diaminopyridine may be beneficial either in autoimmune or paraneoplastic Lambert-Eaton myasthenic syndrome; plasma exchange and immunosuppression also may be effective.

Myasthenia gravis This disorder, discussed elsewhere in detail (Chap. 386), is characterized by exercise-induced muscle weakness caused by an antibody-mediated reduction in the numbers of acetylcholine receptors at the postsynaptic junction. About 15 percent of cases are associated with thymoma; many arise concurrently with other autoimmune or thyroid disorders.

MUSCLE Polymyositis-dermatomyositis This subject is discussed in Chap. 384. While an increased incidence of malignancy in elderly patients with dermatomyositis has long been suggested, this concept has recently been challenged by a retrospective analysis of experience with polymyositis at the Mayo Clinic.

Necrotizing myopathy Carcinoma of the bronchus may rarely be associated with a fatal subacute widespread necrotizing myopathy that involves all muscles including bulbar and diaphragmatic muscles. Intrafusal muscle fibers are also involved. Deep tendon reflexes are preserved. Muscle undergoes degeneration without phagocytosis or significant inflammatory response. The cause of the necrotizing process is unknown.

OTHER Several other neurologic syndromes have been reported to be paraneoplastic but are less well characterized. *Stiff-man syndrome,* or diffuse hypertonia due to loss of inhibitory spinal interneurons, may arise in association with carcinoma. In the nonneoplastic stiff-man syndrome, autoantibodies have been detected that react with glutamic acid decarboxylase, an enzyme essential for the synthesis of gamma aminobutyric acid, a central nervous system inhibitory neurotransmitter. Nonfamilial, subacute *chorea* and *dystonia* occur with oat cell carcinoma of the lung. *Optic neuritis* may develop as a paraneoplastic disorder, but it is difficult to exclude direct involvement of the optic nerve or chiasm by cancer cells or indirect effects of the underlying malignancy, as outlined in Table 328-1.

REFERENCES

CASCINO TL: Medical complications of systemic cancer. Med Clin North Am 77:265, 1993

DALMAU J et al: Anti-Hu–associated paraneoplastic encephalomyelitis/sensory neuronopathy: A clinical study of 71 patients. Medicine 71:59, 1992

DROPCHO EJ et al: Antineuronal (anti-Ri) antibodies in a patient with steroid-responsive opsoclonus-myoclonus. Neurology 43:207, 1993

FATHALLAH-SHAYKH H et al: Cloning of a leucine zipper protein recognized by the sera of patients with antibody-associated paraneoplastic cerebellar degeneration. Proc Natl Acad Sci USA 88:3451, 1991

FURNEAUX HM et al: Characterization of a cDNA encoding a 34-kDa Purkinje neuron protein recognized by sera from patients with paraneoplastic cerebellar degeneration. Proc Natl Acad Sci USA 86:2873, 1989

HENSON RA, URICH H: *Cancer and the Nervous System.* Oxford, Blackwell, 1982

KINSBOURNE M: Myoclonic encephalopathy of infants. J Neurol Neurosurg Psychiatry 25:271, 1964

LENNON VA, LAMBERT EH: Autoantibodies bind solubilized calcium channel–omega-conotoxin complexes from small cell lung carcinoma: A diagnostic aid for Lambert-Eaton myasthenic syndrome. Mayo Clin Proc 64:1498, 1989

LUQUE FA et al: Anti-Ri: An antibody associated with paraneoplastic opsoclonus and breast cancer. Ann Neurol 29:241, 1991

POLANS AS et al: A photoreceptor calcium-binding protein is recognized by autoantibodies obtained from patients with cancer-associated retinopathy. J Cell Biol 112:981, 1991

POSNER JB: Paraneoplastic syndromes. Neurol Clin 9:919, 1991

SAKAI K et al: Isolation of a complementary DNA clone encoding an autoantigen recognized by an anti-neuronal cell antibody from a patient with paraneoplastic cerebellar degeneration. Ann Neurol 28:692, 1990

SZABO A et al: HuD, a paraneoplastic encephalomyelitis antigen, contains RNA-binding domains and is homologous to Elav and Sex-lethal. Cell 67:325, 1991

THIRKILL CE et al: The cancer-associated retinopathy antigen is a recoverin-like protein. Invest Ophthalmol Vis Sci 33:2768, 1992

section 1 Endocrinology

329 HORMONES AND HORMONE ACTION

JEAN D. WILSON

Communication between cells is largely mediated by the endocrine, nervous, and immune systems. The nervous system was originally considered distinct from the endocrine system—information was thought to be carried either by neural impulses or by chemical mediators in the blood—but it is now clear that they constitute one coordinated network. Not only may neurotransmitters such as norepinephrine circulate in blood as hormones, but neural impulses have major effects on the release of chemical mediators such as testosterone and insulin. This interlocking relationship is most apparent in the hypothalamus, which serves as the highest integrative center for the two systems. Hence, a single neuroendocrine system evolved to integrate and coordinate the metabolic activities of the organism. Endocrinology deals largely with the chemical mediators in this system, but proper understanding of the role of hormones requires knowledge of the autonomic nervous system (Chap. 68) and of the metabolic capacities of cells.

The formulation of endocrinology has been blurred in additional ways. The term *hormone* originally referred to substances that are secreted into the circulation and act as chemical effectors in other tissues. However, the capacity to form such chemical mediators is not limited to so-called endocrine organs. Some hormones, such as angiotensins II and III, are formed in the bloodstream itself. Others, such as testosterone in women and dihydrotestosterone and estradiol in men, are in part secreted and in part formed in extraglandular tissues from circulating precursors, so-called prohormones. Still other chemical mediators circulate only in restricted compartments such as the hypothalamic-pituitary portal system and do not reach the systemic circulation in appreciable quantities. Finally, certain hormones, such as insulin, dihydrotestosterone, and thyrotropin-releasing hormone (TRH), have paracrine actions in the same tissues in which they are formed and exert actions at distal sites, whereas other chemical mediators, such as müllerian-inhibiting substance, exert local actions exclusively.

BIOCHEMISTRY

SYNTHESIS The approximately 100 known mammalian hormones fall into three major categories—peptides or peptide derivatives, steroids, and amines. In the case of peptide hormones, genes code for messenger RNA, which is then translated into protein precursors. These proteins undergo posttranslational cleavage (preproparathyroid hormone → proparathyroid hormone → parathyroid hormone) and/or processing (thyroglobulin → thyroxine → triiodothyronine) to form the active hormone recognized by the target tissues. The distinct feature of peptide hormones is that one or a few structural genes code for the amino acid sequence of the peptide, and other genes are responsible for the alteration of the peptide to its final form. In the case of peptide hormones with subunits, the different subunits may be derived either from a single precursor (insulin) or from separate precursors ([luteinizing hormone (LH)]. Furthermore, the same peptide hormone (somatostatin) can be formed from different prohormones encoded by distinct genes, individual prohormones such as proopiomelanocortin can be metabolized to different hormones in different cells, depending on the complement of processing enzymes in the cell in question, and the primary transcripts of the calcitonin gene can be alternatively spliced in different tissues to form messenger RNA for either calcitonin or calcitonin-related peptide. Peptide hormones may also be formed ectopically in malignancies of nonendocrine origin such as carcinoma of the lung and may be formed in small amounts in normal nonendocrine tissues (see Chap. 327).

In the case of steroid hormones the fundamental precursor—cholesterol (for most steroid hormones) or 7-dehydrocholesterol (for vitamin D metabolites)—undergoes a series of enzymatic transformations to form the final products. At least six enzymes and consequently a minimum of six genes are required to transform cholesterol to estradiol. Because of the number of enzymes required, the synthesis of steroids from cholesterol is unusual in malignancies of nonendocrine tissues. However, many tissues—malignant and nonmalignant—that cannot form steroid hormones de novo from cholesterol contain enzymes that convert circulating steroids to other hormones; examples are the conversion of androgens to estrogens by trophoblastic tumors and by normal adipocytes and the conversion of progesterone to deoxycorticosterone by the kidney.

Amine hormones are synthesized by a series of reactions similar to those involved in steroid hormone synthesis except that the precursors are amino acids. For example, tyrosine is the precursor for epinephrine and norepinephrine (see Chap. 68).

STORAGE Most tissues that synthesize hormones have a limited capacity to store the completed product. For example, the normal adult testes contain only about one-sixth of the quantity of testosterone needed for daily production, and consequently the testicular pool turns over several times to provide the normal daily output of hormone. Even when tissues have special storage organelles for hormone, the amount of hormone stored is usually limited: the insulin granules in the pancreatic beta cell ordinarily contain amounts of insulin sufficient only for short-term, reserve needs. (In contrast, nerve endings may contain a several-day supply of norepinephrine.) The limited capacity to store hormones in tissues is a chemical consequence of their unsuitability for incorporation into any of the three main storage compartments of the body (lipids, glycogen, or protein). For example, most steroid hormones are too polar to be stored in large quantities in lipid compartments, and peptide and amine hormones are unsuitable for incorporation into proteins. As a consequence, the body pools of most hormones tend to be small. The major exceptions to this rule are those instances in which the precursor forms of hormone can be stored either as protein or in neutral lipid compartments; the normal thyroid gland contains the equivalent of a 2-week supply of thyroid hormones in the form of the protein thyroglobulin, and the precursor and intermediate forms of vitamin D can be stored in considerable quantity in hepatic lipid.

RELEASE The biochemical mechanisms involved in the release process are incompletely understood. In some instances they involve conversion of insoluble to soluble derivatives (proteolysis of thyroglobulin to thyroid hormones). In others, release is due to exocytosis of storage granules (insulin, glucagon, prolactin, growth hormone). Finally, release may involve passive diffusion of newly synthesized molecules such as steroid hormones down activity gradients into plasma; under this circumstance the rate of hormone release is a function of the rate of hormone synthesis and the blood flow to the tissue.

Because of the limited capacity for storage, most hormones are released into plasma at a pace reflecting the rates of formation. The pituitary trophic hormones [LH, adrenocorticotropin (ACTH), thyrotropin (TSH)] act in their target tissues to influence rates of both hormone synthesis and release. Even when peptide hormones are stored in granules, initial release of the stored material is followed by an enhanced rate of synthesis (as, for instance, the two-phase release of insulin induced by glucose infusion). For some hormones, major diurnal, sleep-related, developmental, and neural factors influence hormone release; again, it is assumed that in most of these instances synthesis and release are tightly linked.

The rate of hormone release in many instances is periodic or rhythmic, the cycle varying in frequency from minutes to hours (ultradian), to daily (circadian), to months or years (infradian). Hormones such as LH and follicle-stimulating hormone (FSH) are released in a pulsatile fashion with bursts of secretion occurring in a repetitive pattern: ACTH (and cortisol) release varies during a 24-h cycle, and thyroid hormone release can vary on longer cycles. Whether this intermittent release is a function of alterations in synthetic rates, changes in blood flow, or other mechanisms is uncertain, but most such cycles are under neurogenic control. In many instances the physiologic significance of pulsatile release is not fully understood, but in some instances changes in frequency or amplitude of the release pattern have profound effects on hormone function; i.e., the pulsatile administration of luteinizing hormone–releasing hormone (LHRH) stimulates the release of LH by the pituitary, whereas the constant infusion of the same amount of hormone per unit time has the opposite effect. Furthermore, changes in frequency or amplitude of hormone release may characterize specific disease states; loss of the diurnal rhythm of cortisol release is characteristic of the early phase of Cushing's disease, and pulsatile release of LHRH is blunted in anorexia nervosa. Finally, understanding the rhythms by which hormones are released is essential for interpreting plasma hormone levels.

TRANSPORT Hormones are transported via lymph, blood, and extracellular fluids from sites of release to sites of cellular action and ultimately of metabolic inactivation and degradation. The plasma is probably a passive diluent for most peptide and amine hormones, and this feature explains the short half-lives (3 to 7 min) for most nonglycosylated peptide hormones. (Glycoprotein hormones such as human chorionic gonadotropin, or hCG, have longer half-lives.) The more insoluble a hormone in water, the more important the role of transport proteins; for example, thyroid and steroid hormones are largely transported in protein-bound form. No transport protein yet characterized is exclusive; for example, testosterone can be transported both by a specific binding protein [testosterone-binding globulin (TeBG)] and by albumin; thyroxine can be transported both by prealbumin and by thyroxine-binding globulin (TBG). Protein-bound hormone (HP) cannot enter most cellular compartments and serves as a reservoir from which free hormone (H) is liberated for diffusion into intracellular compartments:

$$H + P \rightleftharpoons HP$$

Distribution of bound and free hormone in plasma is determined by the amount of hormone, the amount of binding protein, and the binding affinity of hormone for the protein. However, in the intact organism the effective level of free hormone is influenced by additional factors. When the rate of dissociation of a hormone from a binding protein is rapid, the functional free fraction in vivo is also influenced by capillary transit time and membrane permeability.

The relation between free and bound hormone is complex: First, the free (dialyzable) fraction in vitro generally underestimates the actual free fraction available in vivo because hormone bound to weak binding proteins such as albumin (in contrast to that bound to specific, high-affinity binding proteins) rapidly dissociates from the albumin as the free fraction diffuses from the capillary; consequently the albumin-bound hormone can function in vivo as a free fraction. Under some conditions, measurement of the dialyzable fraction does provide a useful index of the in vivo apparent free fraction. However, in hypoalbuminemic states, the in vitro free (dialyzable) fraction may increase when the in vivo free hormone level is actually diminished. In addition, in those tissue compartments such as liver in which proteins including hormone-transport protein complexes are cleared (in contrast to peripheral tissues in which only the free hormone enters the cell) free hormone levels have lesser effects on hormone uptake by the tissue.

Second, the distribution of hormones between plasma and tissue is a function of the balance between tissue binding proteins and plasma binding proteins. Therefore, levels of true or apparent free hormone may not reflect the amounts of hormone within cells.

Third, only the free hormone interacts with receptors in target cells and participates in the regulatory feedback mechanisms that control the rates of hormone synthesis. As a consequence, changes in the amount of transport protein alone cannot cause endocrine pathology in the steady state, provided the remainder of the endocrine feedback loop is intact. For example, profound elevations or decreases in TBG (either because of genetic or other factors) are both compatible with a euthyroid state. To illustrate, an increase in TBG would lower the level of free (dialyzable) hormone and lower the amount bound to albumin; as a consequence TSH secretion would increase, and the output of thyroxine by the thyroid would increase *until* TBG is again saturated so that the level of free hormone returns to the normal range, at which time TSH levels and thyroid hormone secretion also return to normal. Likewise, a decrease in TBG would temporarily increase the level of free hormone, and TSH secretion and thyroxine output would fall until the free level returns to normal.

To summarize, a change in the amount of a specific, high-affinity binding protein can cause profound alterations in hormone levels but by itself does not cause either a steady state hormone excess or deficiency, provided the regulatory feedback mechanisms that control hormone synthesis are intact. In contrast, alteration of the amount of a binding protein may cause endocrine pathology when hormone formation is not regulated by ordinary feedback control mechanisms or when feedback control mechanisms are deranged. For example, testosterone production in women is not regulated by testosterone levels, and alterations in TeBG levels in women may alter the steady state levels of free testosterone. Likewise, changes in TBG levels in a hypothyroid patient receiving a fixed dose of levothyroxine can cause alterations in free thyroxine levels.

DEGRADATION AND TURNOVER The plasma level (PL) of any hormone is dependent on two factors—the secretion rate (SR) of the hormone and the rates of metabolism and excretion, the so-called metabolic clearance rate (MCR):

$$PL = SR/MCR \quad \text{or} \quad SR = MCR \times PL$$

Metabolic clearance of hormones is accomplished by several mechanisms. Only small fractions of hormones are excreted intact in urine or bile. Degradation and inactivation of the hormone can take place in target tissues, in nontarget tissues such as liver and kidneys, or in both target and nontarget tissues. Peptide hormones are in general inactivated by proteases, largely in target tissues. Hormone metabolism frequently facilitates excretion of steroid and thyroid hormone by rendering them soluble in urine or bile. Thyroid hormones are deiodinated, deaminated, and deconjugated primarily by the liver. Steroid hormones are reduced, hydroxylated, and converted into glucuronide and sulfate conjugates. Biliary conjugates may be hydrolyzed in the gastrointestinal tract and reabsorbed into the circulation. The degradative mechanisms for different hormones have one common feature, namely, that alternative pathways exist for the catabolism of all hormones described to date.

Because of the nature of feedback control of hormone secretion, changes in rates of hormone degradation alone, like changes in plasma protein binding, do not cause endocrine pathology, provided the feedback control mechanisms that regulate synthesis are intact. For example, in severe liver disease and in myxedema, the degradation of glucocorticoids by the liver is impaired; as a consequence the turnover of cortisol slows, but the plasma level does not rise because secretion of ACTH is inhibited. Thus, a normal level of free hormone is maintained by decreasing the rate of cortisol secretion. The opposite is the case when glucocorticoid degradation is enhanced (as in thyrotoxicosis); in this situation cortisol secretion rises to keep the level of the hormone normal.

Although changes in rates of hormone degradation alone do not result in hormone deficit or excess, they may cause profound alterations in endocrine pharmacology. Thus, ordinary doses of glucocorticoids may cause the Cushing syndrome in patients with myxedema or liver disease, and consequently glucocorticoid dosage must be reduced in both conditions. Likewise, doses of glucocorticoids may have to be increased in the presence of hyperthyroidism. In addition, the development of hyperthyroidism in a patient with inadequate adrenal reserve can precipitate adrenal crisis by accelerating the rate of glucocorticoid catabolism. Thus, in circumstances in which the normal control mechanisms that regulate hormone synthesis are either circumvented or inoperative, changes in rates of hormone degradation may aggravate or cause pathology.

REGULATION OF HORMONE PRODUCTION

As stated above, fluctuations of hormone levels in the normal person are determined primarily by changes in rates of production. A unifying feature of all endocrine systems is the fact that the production of most hormones is regulated directly or indirectly by the metabolic activity of the hormone itself. This regulation is accomplished through a series of negative (and positive) feedback loops (Fig. 329-1). In some cases a fairly constant blood level of hormone is required, and some sensing device must exist to monitor either the hormone level itself or some related function such as plasma osmolality, blood glucose, plasma calcium, or body sodium content. For example, hormones produced in response to pituitary trophic hormones (cortisol, thyroxine, gonadal steroids) feed back on the hypothalamic-pituitary system to regulate their own rates of secretion. Similarly, parathyroid hormone and insulin are secreted in response to feedback signals from serum calcium and glucose levels, respectively. Feedback systems are generally more complex than this description indicates, sometimes operating indirectly by several steps; when the hormone itself acts as the direct regulator of feedback (testosterone on the hypothalamic-pituitary axis), the effect is mediated by the same receptor-effector system by which the hormone acts in other target tissues. An example of positive feedback is the stimulation of LH release by estradiol prior to ovulation. Nonhormonal and environmental factors may alter both positive and negative feedback control mechanisms or the response to such control.

A usual feature of the feedback systems is rapidity of action; indeed, most respond within minutes or hours to varying metabolic demands to maintain homeostatic control within a narrow range. The main exceptions relate to gametogenesis in the ovary and testis (see Chaps. 339 and 340). In both instances, a complex differentiative process functions in the steady state so that sperm production tends

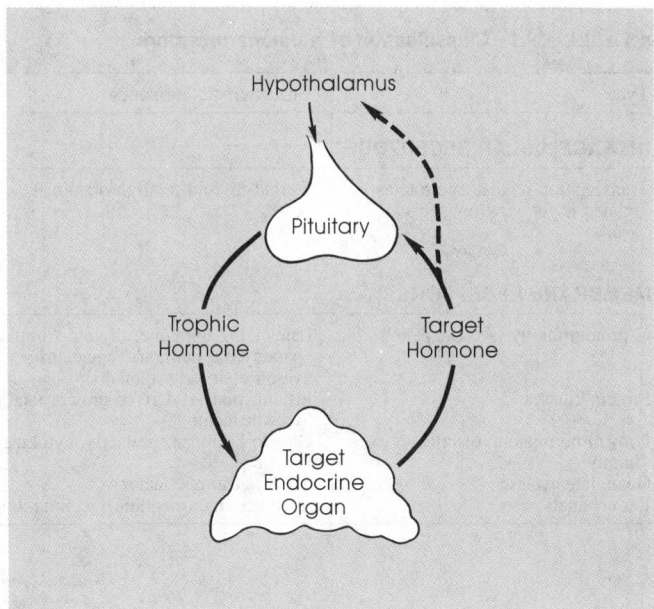

FIGURE 329-1 Feedback control of an endocrine organ such as the adrenal, thyroid, or gonads by the pituitary.

to be relatively constant from day to day whereas ovulation is cyclic. Spermatogenesis and sperm export require approximately 2 months to complete so that changes in FSH levels may not result in altered levels of sperm in the ejaculate for long periods.

The fact that the secretion of hormones is under regulatory control has several important clinical implications. First, the significance of plasma levels of hormones may be interpretable only if the appropriate regulatory factors are taken into account (Fig. 329-2). The meaning of a borderline low plasma thyroxine may become clear only when thyroid-stimulating hormone (TSH) is measured simultaneously; likewise, plasma insulin and parathyroid hormone levels may be interpretable only in conjunction with simultaneous measurements of plasma glucose and calcium, respectively. Second, the finding of simultaneous elevations of hormone pairs (or hormone regulatory factor pairs) in the absence of evidence of hormone excess suggests the presence of a hormone-resistance state. For example, simultaneous elevation of plasma glucose and insulin is characteristic of insulin resistance, and simultaneous elevation of LH and testosterone suggests androgen resistance. In contrast, simultaneous elevation of hormone pairs in the presence of signs of hormone excess suggests a trophic hormone–secreting tumor. Third, insight into the regulatory control of hormone secretion is the basis for the various dynamic tests of hormone reserve and hormone secretion (see Chap. 330).

FIGURE 329-2 Relation between target hormone level and trophic hormone level in normal and disease states (e.g., TSH and thyroid hormones, ACTH and cortisol, LH and testosterone).

TABLE 329-1   Classification of hormone receptors

Type	Characteristic hormones	Disease states due to mutant receptor components
INTRACELLULAR RECEPTORS		
Transcription regulatory proteins related to the viral oncogene *erb*A	Steroid-thyroid family, vitamin A	Testicular feminization and related syndromes; cortisol resistance; vitamin D–dependent rickets, type II; thyroid hormone resistance; pseudohypoaldosteronism
MEMBRANE RECEPTORS		
G protein family (see Chap. 69)	Luteinizing hormone, thyroid-stimulating hormone, parathyroid hormone, epinephrine, somatostatin, vasopressin, glucagon	Pseudohypoparathyroidism, nephrogenic diabetes insipidus
Protein kinases	Insulin, platelet-derived growth factor, epidermal growth factor	Diabetes mellitus with profound insulin resistance
Growth hormone–prolactin family	Growth hormone, prolactin, cytokines, nerve growth factor	Laron dwarfism
Guanylate cyclase	Atrial natriuretic factor	
Ion channels	Acetylcholine (nicotinic), gamma-amino butyric acid	Myasthenia gravis

MECHANISMS OF HORMONE ACTION

The first step in hormone action is the binding of the hormone to specific macromolecules in the cell, so-called hormone receptors. These receptors can either be located intracellularly or in the cell membrane, and membrane-bound receptors in turn fall into several distinct classes (Table 329-1). Insight into the chemical nature of these receptors and into the mechanisms by which they participate in signal transduction has been accelerated by the cloning of the cDNAs and the genes that encode these proteins (see Chap. 61).

INTRACELLULAR RECEPTORS   Most steroid and thyroid hormones are transported in plasma bound to carrier proteins (Fig. 329-3). The protein-bound hormones (HP) are in dynamic equilibrium with small amounts of free hormones (H) that diffuse by a passive mechanism into cells. In most instances the principal form of the hormone secreted into plasma (cortisal, progesterone, aldosterone, estradiol) undergoes no further metabolism within the cell and is responsible for hormone action within the target cell. Other hormones (thyroxine, testosterone) undergo chemical conversion to more active forms (triiodothyronine and dihydrotestosterone).

H binds to specific receptor proteins (R) in the cytoplasm or nucleus to form a hormone-receptor complex (HR). The hormone-receptor complex has the capacity to bind to specific regulatory sequences in DNA (so-called hormone regulatory elements) and thus acts to control the rate of transcription. As the result of this interaction with DNA new messenger RNAs (mRNAs) are formed, and the synthesis of cytoplasmic proteins is enhanced. The cytoplasmic proteins, in turn, mediate the effects of the hormone.

The cloning of the cDNAs for the various receptors revealed that receptors of this class bear a striking homology to the viral oncogene *erb*A and to each other. The fact that members of this family of hormone-dependent transcription factors are similar in structure suggests that these receptors have evolved from a common ancestral transcription factor. Each contains a hormone-binding domain, a DNA-binding domain, and an *N*-terminal variable or immunodominant domain (Fig. 329-4). An interesting feature of this class of receptors is that more than one receptor exists for certain hormones (thyroid hormones) and that candidate receptors have been identified for which no ligand is known. Elucidation of the structures of these receptors made it possible to analyze the mutations that impair hormone action and cause several hormone-resistance syndromes (see below).

MEMBRANE-BOUND RECEPTORS   G protein family   Receptors that bind GTP (G proteins) all work by similar mechanisms but are capable of mediating a complex range of actions. In every case, binding of ligand to the receptor produces a conformational change that causes GTP to bind to the protein at a special site. The active G protein then binds to a target protein and initiates a regulatory cascade involving one (or more) intracellular mediators including adenylate cyclase, phospholipase C, and arachidonic acid. The receptors of this class are monomeric proteins with an extracellular domain that binds ligand, an intracellular G protein–binding domain, and seven transmembrane-spanning regions. Elucidation of the molecular biol-

FIGURE 329-3   Mechanism of action of hormones with intracellular receptors. H = hormone; P = plasma transport protein; R = receptor; R* = activated receptor; mRNA = messenger RNA.

FIGURE 329-4   Intracellular receptors of the thyroid-steroid class. The areas of greatest homology (DNA-binding domain) are shown by the slanted bars, the areas of intermediate homology (hormone-binding domain) are shown by the stippled areas, and the areas with the least homology are shown by the open regions.

FIGURE 329-5 Schematic representation of the insulin receptor. As the result of the binding of insulin to the alpha subunit the protein kinase function of the beta receptor is activated, and both exogenous protein substrates and the beta subunit itself are phosphorylated.

ogy of the G protein has provided insight into the actions of drugs and signaling mechanisms in addition to hormones and into the pathophysiology of pseudohypoparathyroidism (see Chaps. 69 and 357 and below).

Protein kinases Receptors of this class, such as the insulin receptor and the epidermal growth factor (EGF) receptor, are glycoproteins typically composed of two alpha subunits and two beta subunits which are linked by sulfhydryl bonds (Fig. 329-5). The alpha subunits are extracellular and contain the hormone binding site, and the beta subunits are transmembrane proteins. The beta subunit of the receptor is a hormone-regulated protein kinase capable of phosphorylating itself and other substrates on tyrosine residues using ATP as the phosphate source. In the case of insulin the tyrosine activity of the receptor is essential for hormone action. Point mutations in the coding sequence of receptor genes that prevent the protein kinase activity can cause profound resistance to insulin action (see below). Exactly how receptor kinase activity is transmitted into hormone action is not entirely clear. Several endogenous substrates of the enzyme have been identified, and physiologic effects of the hormone may either be indirect or direct consequences of the phosphorylation of the substrates or of the receptor itself. The nerve growth factor receptor has an extracellular domain similar to that of the EGF and insulin receptors.

Receptors of the growth hormone/prolactin class The growth hormone receptor is a protein of approximately 600 amino acids that contains a single, centrally located transmembrane domain. Interestingly, the high-affinity growth hormone–binding protein in plasma corresponds to the extracellular hormone-binding domain of the growth hormone receptor and is believed to be cleaved from the receptor, but the role of the plasma protein in the regulation of growth is undefined. The growth hormone receptor shares approximately a 25 percent homology with the prolactin receptor [which is present in long (~ 600 amino acid) and short (~ 300 amino acid) forms] suggesting that the two receptors have evolved from a common ancestral gene. The mechanism(s) by which these receptors mediate hormone action is unclear. Mutations that impair the function of the growth hormone receptor are responsible for Laron dwarfism (see below).

Other membrane-bound receptors The receptor for atrial natriuretic factor is a guanylate cyclase that spans the plasma membrane; the extracellular portion of the receptor binds the hormone, and the intracellular portion of the protein synthesizes guanosine-3′,5′-monophosphate (cyclic GMP) which serves as the second messenger for the hormone (see Chap. 69). The nicotinic acetylcholine receptor channel is a membrane-spanning complex of proteins that forms a true ion channel containing a central pore that can be opened and closed by ligand-binding-induced conformational change to allow sodium and potassium ions to cross the membrane and hence cause depolarization of cells that contain the receptors. Autoantibodies that block the function of this receptor cause myasthenia gravis (see Chap. 380).

Receptors for gamma-aminobutyric acid and glycine, which mediate inhibitory activity in the central nervous system, show a high degree of homology with the acetylcholine receptor, suggesting that ligand-gated ion channels may be derived from a common ancestral gene.

ENDOCRINE DISORDERS

Endocrinopathy can result from hormone deficiency, hormone excess, or resistance to hormone action, and abnormalities in more than one endocrine system may coexist in the same individual.

DEFICIENCY STATES With few exceptions (calcitonin) hormone deficiency results in pathologic manifestations. The study of clinical disorders that result from hormone deficiency or absence played an important role in the evolution of endocrinology as a discipline. Such studies were followed by attempts to extract the responsible hormone from normal endocrine tissues, characterize the chemical nature (and ultimately synthesize the molecule), and administer the hormone to replace the deficit. The treatment of hypothyroidism by the administration of thyroid hormone is probably as successful as any therapeutic measure in medicine. Because clinical deficiency states can be induced in experimental animals by destruction or removal of the endocrine organ, an enormous amount is known about the pathophysiology of the deficiency states (diabetes mellitus, pituitary and adrenal insufficiency, hypothyroidism, and hypogonadism).

The nature of the destructive processes that cause failure of the endocrine organs is also understood in many instances; these include infections (adrenal insufficiency due to tuberculosis), infarction (postpartum pituitary failure) and tissue death from other causes (diabetes mellitus secondary to pancreatitis), tumors (null cell tumors of the pituitary), autoimmune processes (Hashimoto's thyroiditis), dietary inadequacy (hypothyroidism due to iodine deficiency), and hereditary defects in hormone synthesis (pituitary dwarfism). In certain forms of diabetes mellitus, the cause may be a hereditary predisposition that renders the pancreas subject to destruction by several mechanisms (see Chap. 337). In other endocrine-deficiency diseases the etiology of the defect is unidentified (congenital anorchia).

HORMONE EXCESS With few exceptions (testosterone in men, progesterone in men and women) hormone excess causes pathologic effects. Four general types of hormone excess are recognized. In one, the hormone is overproduced by the gland that is the usual site of its production (hyperthyroidism, acromegaly, Cushing's disease); such excess production results from failure of circumvention of the feedback control mechanisms that regulate production of the hormone in the normal state, but the underlying mechanism is often obscure because animal models for the diseases are rare. The second type of hormone excess results when a hormone is produced by a tissue (usually malignant) that ordinarily is not a major endocrine organ (for example, ACTH production in oat cell carcinoma of the lung, thyroid hormone secretion by struma ovarii). Such hormone-excess states have been described for many hormones (see Chap. 327). A third type of hormone-excess state involves the overproduction of hormones in peripheral tissues from circulating precursors; for example, overproduction of estrogen in liver disease because of diversion of the hormone secreted during the time of study. In the case of hormones formed principally in peripheral tissues (estradiol and dihydrotestosterone in men, triiodothyronine in both sexes) radioactive precursors can be administered, and the rates of conversion to the metabolites in question can be measured for assessment of overall production rates. Alternatively, as described above, clearance rates of hormones can be measured and, together with mean plasma levels, used to estimate secretion rates. Unfortunately, these various techniques are complex and expensive to perform, require use of radioactive isotopes, and can be done in only a few centers.

DYNAMIC TESTS OF HORMONE RESERVE AND REGULATION
When hypo- or hyperfunction is severe, measurement of the level of hormone in blood or urine may be satisfactory for making a diagnosis, particularly when the tests demonstrate appropriate feedback relationships; e.g., low plasma testosterone coupled with high plasma LH indicates primary testicular failure. In less clear-cut instances, however, stimulation tests are useful in establishing the significance of borderline low values. Likewise, suppression tests are used to document the presence of hyperfunction of endocrine systems. All such dynamic tests are designed to take advantage of the known feedback control mechanisms for various hormones (Fig. 329-1).

Two types of stimulation tests are in common use. In one, endogenous hormone production or action is blocked (cortisol production by metyrapone, estradiol action by clomiphene), and the capacity of the pituitary to respond by increasing endogenous production of the trophic hormone and/or the capacity of the target tissue to respond are then assessed; ideally such tests measure the integrity of an entire hypothalamic–pituitary–target tissue loop. In the other type of stimulation test, the trophic hormone itself is administered under some standardized regimen, and the capacity of the target tissue to respond is determined (cortisol levels before and after ACTH administration). Stimulation tests are particularly useful in four situations: (1) assessing hormone status when precise quantification of plasma levels is difficult or imperfect (ACTH), (2) assessing endocrine status when static tests are borderline low, (3) distinguishing primary from secondary (pituitary) causes of endocrine failure, and (4) assessing gonadal reserve in prepubertal subjects in whom plasma gonadotropins and gonadal steroids are difficult to interpret.

Suppression tests are useful for the diagnosis of hyperfunction because the hyperfunctioning gland by definition does not operate under normal control mechanisms. Suppression can either be quantitatively or qualitatively abnormal. For example, the feedback control of the pituitary may be reset to respond to high levels of the suppressing hormone (pituitary ACTH secretion in Cushing's disease), or secretion can be autonomous (ACTH secretion by carcinoma of the lung). In principle, the feedback regulator is administered, and the degree of inhibition of hormone secretion is assessed for the endocrine system in question (change in radioactive iodine uptake after administration of thyroid hormones, change in cortisol secretion after the administration of potent exogenous glucocorticoids, suppressibility of plasma growth hormone by glucose).

The clinical usefulness of dynamic tests of endocrine function is limited by the fact that they are altered by a multitude of secondary factors. Age, coexisting disease states, and concurrent drug regimens all interact to influence responsiveness and hence to limit the specificity of such tests. In particular, psychiatric disorders such as endogenous depression may impair endocrine dynamic tests in the absence of specific endocrine pathology.

HORMONE RECEPTORS AND ANTIBODIES   The measurement of hormone receptors in biopsy material from target tissues or in fibroblasts propagated from biopsy material is useful—for example, in the diagnosis of partial hormone-resistance states such as rickets due to vitamin D resistance, hyperglycemia and hyperinsulinemia associated with insulin resistance, and male pseudohermaphroditism due to androgen resistance (see Chap. 329). In selected laboratories the techniques of molecular biology can be applied to provide specific information about the structure of mutant receptors. Likewise, under selected conditions measurement of antibodies to hormones (such as

antibodies to thyroid hormones that can cause hypothyroidism) or antibodies to target tissues (adrenal gland, gonads, thyroid) may be essential for the assessment of endocrine status. With certain exceptions (antibodies to thyroid tissue) these tests are not widely available.

TISSUE EFFECTS   Perhaps the ideal hormone test is the measurement of the peripheral end result of hormone action in the target tissues for the hormone. For example, demonstration of the capacity to concentrate urine maximally following water restriction indicates that the hypothalamic mechanisms that control the function of the posterior pituitary are intact, that the posterior pituitary has a normal capacity to secrete vasopressin, that the vasopressin receptor is intact, and that the postreceptor effector mechanisms for the hormone are operative. Optimally such a test assesses the function of the entire pathway of hormone secretion and action. In practice, many such tests are imperfect. For example, even though vasopressin secretion is normal, intrinsic renal disease can result in a fixed low urine osmolality and thus distort the interpretation of the functional test of vasopressin action. In other instances the tests are difficult to perform and subject both to artifact and to influences from diverse parameters (for example, the metabolic rate is increased by fever even when thyroid function is normal). For these reasons, the identification of additional specific tissue markers for hormone action would be very useful.

IMAGING PROCEDURES   Developments in imaging have had a profound impact in endocrinology and provide better means of identifying abnormalities in almost every endocrine system, from delineating small lesions of the pituitary and hypothalamus, to measuring bone densitometry to assess metabolic bone disease, to the noninvasive localization of functioning parathyroid tissue in patients with persistent or recurrent hyperparathyroidism. Because the rate of technologic advance in the field is so rapid, the literature evaluating the effectiveness (and limitations) of up-to-date processes inevitably lags.

A major problem in the interpretation of imaging procedures stems from the fact that small nodules of no functional significance are known from autopsy studies to occur in the pituitary, the adrenal, and, less commonly, the testes. The natural history of these nonfunctioning adenomas is not well understood; the vast majority appear to remain limited in size and nonfunctional for life, but in rare instances they may evolve into autonomous and/or hyperfunctioning tumors. In addition, malignancies—both metastatic and primary—can occur in these tissues. Now lesions of this size can be recognized in life, and the incidental discovery of adrenal and pituitary masses is a common result of CT scans or MRI performed for other reasons. Several types of criteria have been proposed for deciding which of these masses are likely to be benign and which should be removed. For example, by one guideline solid, endocrinologically silent lesions of the adrenal smaller than 3.5 cm may be followed safely with serial CT scans whereas larger lesions deserve further workup such as sonographically guided percutaneous needle biopsy or exploratory surgery. Additional experience will be required to establish the validity of these and other criteria for the assessment of such masses.

Another unresolved issue stems from the fact that it is not always clear which imaging procedure is best in a given clinical situation. In some instances evidence will be accrued that will make clear the indications for one or another procedure. In other instances definite guidelines may be harder to develop, as in the choice of MRI versus CT for delineation of the anatomy of the hypothalamic-pituitary system. In some patients small lesions are best seen with MRI whereas in others lesions in the same areas—equally small and with similar histologic features—are better delineated with CT. As a consequence, there is a tendency in the workup of complicated cases to order both procedures routinely. Although this practice is justified in some cases, the costs of diagnostic workups are thereby inflated.

An unexpected dividend of the developments in imaging is that it is now possible to chart the natural history of endocrine disease in a different way, as in the occasional documentation of hemorrhage into a pituitary tumor that eventuates in development of the empty sella syndrome or the uncovering of a functioning adrenal adenoma when biochemical or clinical evidence of Cushing's disease is minimal.

REFERENCES

BELLDEGRUN A et al: Incidentally discovered mass of the adrenal gland. Surg Gynecol Obstet 163:203, 1986

GORDEN P, WEINTRAUB BD: Radioreceptor and other functional hormone assays, in *Williams Textbook of Endocrinology*, 8th ed, JD Wilson, DW Foster (eds). Philadelphia, Saunders, 1992, pp 1647–1661

GRIFFIN JE: Dynamic tests of endocrine function in *Williams Textbook of Endocrinology*, 8th ed, JD Wilson, DW Foster (eds). Philadelphia, Saunders, 1992, pp 1663–1670

HAMPER UM et al: Primary adrenocortical carcinoma: Sonographic evaluation with clinical and pathologic correlation in 26 patients. Am J Roentgenog 148:915, 1987

VAITUKAITIS JL: Hormone assays, in *Endocrinology and Metabolism*, P Felig et al (eds). New York, McGraw-Hill, 1987, p 165

YALOW RS: Radioimmunoassay of hormones, in *Williams Textbook of Endocrinology*, 8th ed, JD Wilson, DW Foster (eds). Philadelphia, Saunders, 8th 1992, p 1635

331 NEUROENDOCRINE REGULATION AND DISEASES OF THE ANTERIOR PITUITARY AND HYPOTHALAMUS

GILBERT H. DANIELS / JOSEPH B. MARTIN

The pituitary, appropriately titled the master gland, produces six major hormones and stores an additional two hormones (Fig. 331-1). Growth hormone (GH) regulates growth and has important influences on intermediary metabolism (see Chap. 332). Prolactin (PRL) is necessary for lactation. Luteinizing hormone (LH) and follicle-stimulating hormone (FSH) control the gonads in men and women. Thyroid-stimulating hormone (TSH, thyrotropin) regulates thyroid

FIGURE 331-1 The relationship between the hypothalamus and pituitary. See text for details.

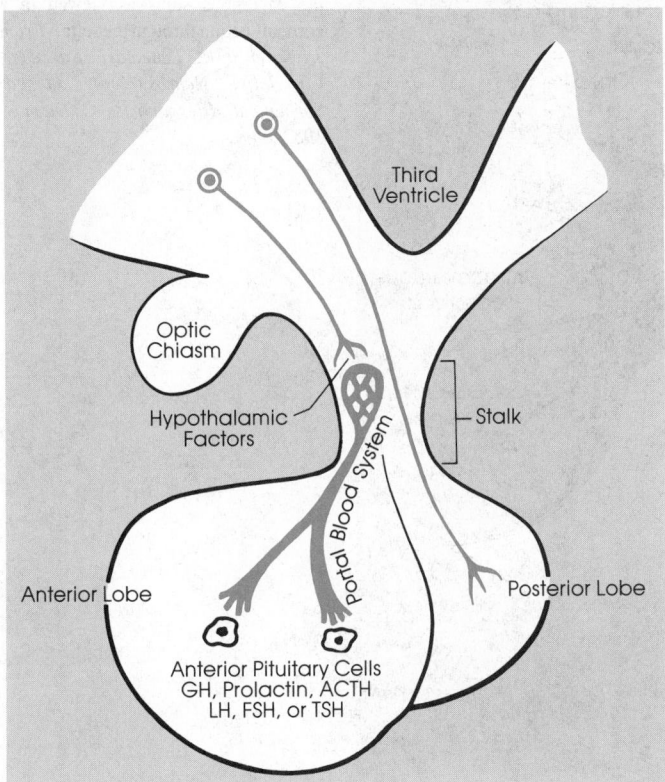

function. Adrenocorticotropin (ACTH) controls glucocorticoid function of the adrenal cortex. These hormones are all synthesized in the anterior pituitary. Vasopressin (AVP; antidiuretic hormone, ADH) and oxytocin are produced in neurons of the hypothalamus and stored in the posterior lobe of the pituitary (see Chap. 333). Vasopressin (AVP) controls water conservation by the kidneys; oxytocin is necessary for milk let-down during lactation and may aid in parturition.

A feedback relationship exists between the anterior pituitary and its three target endocrine glands—the gonads, the adrenal cortex, and the thyroid. When the gonads fail or are removed, the concentrations of LH and FSH rise, a condition known as *primary hypogonadism*. When the adrenal cortex is removed or destroyed, *primary adrenal insufficiency* (or Addison's disease) results, and the serum ACTH concentration increases. Thyroid failure results in the characteristic rise in TSH of *primary hypothyroidism*.

When the pituitary gland is removed or destroyed, loss of the trophic hormones results in secondary hypogonadism, adrenal insufficiency, or hypothyroidism. Growth hormone and prolactin function are also lost. AVP and oxytocin function are not affected by destruction of the pituitary provided their site of origin in the hypothalamus is intact.

The pituitary is, in turn, under the control of the hypothalamus, which produces a number of chemical mediators. These hormones are synthesized in the hypothalamus and enter the portal vascular system, which carries them through the pituitary stalk to the anterior lobe (see Fig. 331-1). Interruption of the pituitary stalk is followed by reduction in the release of GH, LH, FSH, TSH, and ACTH from the anterior pituitary. This implies that stimulatory influences from the hypothalamus are necessary for release of these hormones. In contrast, the level of prolactin rises after interruption of the stalk, implying a normal tonic inhibitory hypothalamic influence on prolactin secretion. The rise in prolactin secretion indicates that stalk section does not lead to pituitary destruction. If the stalk section is not at too high a level, AVP and oxytocin release continue principally from axons that terminate in the median eminence of the hypothalamus. With hypothalamic ablation, the levels of GH, LH, FSH, TSH, ACTH, AVP, and oxytocin fall, whereas prolactin levels increase (see Fig. 331-1).

Most hypothalamic factors that control secretion of the pituitary hormones are peptides (Table 331-1). Growth hormone–releasing hormone (GHRH) is the dominant influence on GH release, and

TABLE 331-1 Anterior pituitary and hypophysiotropic hormones

Pituitary hormone	Hypophysiotropic hormones	
	Name	Structure
Thyrotropin (TSH)	Thyrotropin-releasing hormone (TRH)	Tripeptide
Adrenocorticotropin (ACTH)	Corticotropin-releasing hormone (CRH)	41 Amino acids
	Vasopressin[*]	
Luteinizing hormone (LH)	Luteinizing hormone–releasing hormone (LHRH)	Decapeptide
Follicle-stimulating hormone (FSH)	LHRH	Decapeptide
Growth hormone (GH)	Growth hormone–releasing hormone (GHRH)	44 Amino acids
	Growth hormone release–inhibiting hormone[†] (somatostatin, GIH)	14 Amino acids
Prolactin	Prolactin release–inhibiting factor (PIF)	Dopamine
	Prolactin-releasing factor (PRF)[‡]	Peptide

[*] Other peptides are also important in ACTH release.
[†] Somatostatin also inhibits TRH-stimulated TSH release.
[‡] TRH stimulates prolactin release.

somatostatin acts as an inhibitory hormone for GH release. Although LH and FSH levels vary independently in physiologic states, one releasing hormone [luteinizing hormone–releasing hormone (LHRH), also called gonadotropin-releasing hormone (GnRH)] plays a major role in controlling their release. Thyrotropin-releasing hormone (TRH) controls TSH release and also may influence prolactin release. Corticotropin-releasing hormone (CRH) and other factors control ACTH release. In addition, dopamine acts as a prolactin inhibitory factor (PIF).

Pituitary tumors may lead to hormonal over- or underproduction or may cause mechanical problems by impinging on neighboring structures. The most common syndromes produced by pituitary tumors are due to prolactin and GH excess. Prolactin excess leads to galactorrhea and/or hypogonadism; GH excess leads to gigantism and acromegaly. ACTH-secreting tumors produce Cushing's disease; after bilateral adrenalectomy for Cushing's disease, further enlargement of ACTH-secreting tumors and hyperpigmentation (Nelson's syndrome) may develop. TSH-secreting tumors are rare causes of hyperthyroidism. Gonadotropin-secreting tumors are paradoxically most often associated with hypogonadism. Large pituitary tumors may cause partial or complete hypopituitarism by compression of the adjacent normal gland or pituitary stalk and are associated with visual field disturbances due to compression of the optic chiasm with other neurologic disturbances caused by invasion of cavernous sinuses or cranial fossae.

Hypothalamic disease may cause hypopituitarism, with the exception that secretion of prolactin may be increased. Diabetes insipidus due to AVP deficiency is virtually diagnostic of hypothalamic disease or of high interruption of the pituitary stalk. Disturbances of thirst, temperature regulation, appetite, and blood pressure may occur with hypothalamic disorders as well. Large hypothalamic masses may lead to visual field disturbances, obstruction of the third ventricle, and invasion of surrounding brain tissue.

ANATOMY AND EMBRYOLOGY

The pituitary gland (hypophysis) sits within the sella turcica ("Turkish saddle") of the sphenoid bone at the base of the skull and is composed principally of the anterior (adenohypophysis) and posterior lobes (neurohypophysis). The intermediate lobe is rudimentary in humans. The normal adult pituitary gland weighs between 0.4 and 0.8 g.

The pituitary is separated from the brain by the diaphragma sella, an extension of the dura mater, and from the sphenoid sinus anteriorly and inferiorly by a thin layer of bone. The lateral walls of the sella abut on the cavernous sinuses, which contain the internal carotid arteries and cranial nerves III, IV, V, and VI. The optic chiasm is slightly anterior to the pituitary stalk, just above the diaphragma sella. Thus tumors of the pituitary may lead to visual field defects, to cranial nerve palsies, or to invasion of the sphenoid sinus (Fig. 331-2).

The hypothalamus extends anteriorly to the margin of the optic chiasm and posteriorly to include the mammillary bodies. Superiorly, the hypothalamic sulcus of the third ventricle separates the thalamus from the hypothalamus. The rounded inferior base of the hypothalamus forms the tuber cinereum. The central portion of the base (termed the *infundibulum* or *median eminence*) is formed by the floor of the third ventricle and continues inferiorly to form the pituitary stalk. The releasing factors are synthesized in neurons situated along the margins of the third ventricle. They project fibers that terminate in the median eminence adjacent to the portal capillaries.

The cell bodies of the supraoptic and paraventricular nuclei of the hypothalamus produce vasopressin and oxytocin, which travel down nerve axons in the supraopticohypophyseal and paraventriculohypophyseal nerve tracts to reach the posterior lobe.

The communication between the hypothalamus and the anterior pituitary is chemical rather than physical. Releasing factors produced by hypothalamic neurons reach the anterior pituitary via the portal system to stimulate or inhibit hormone production. Some of the

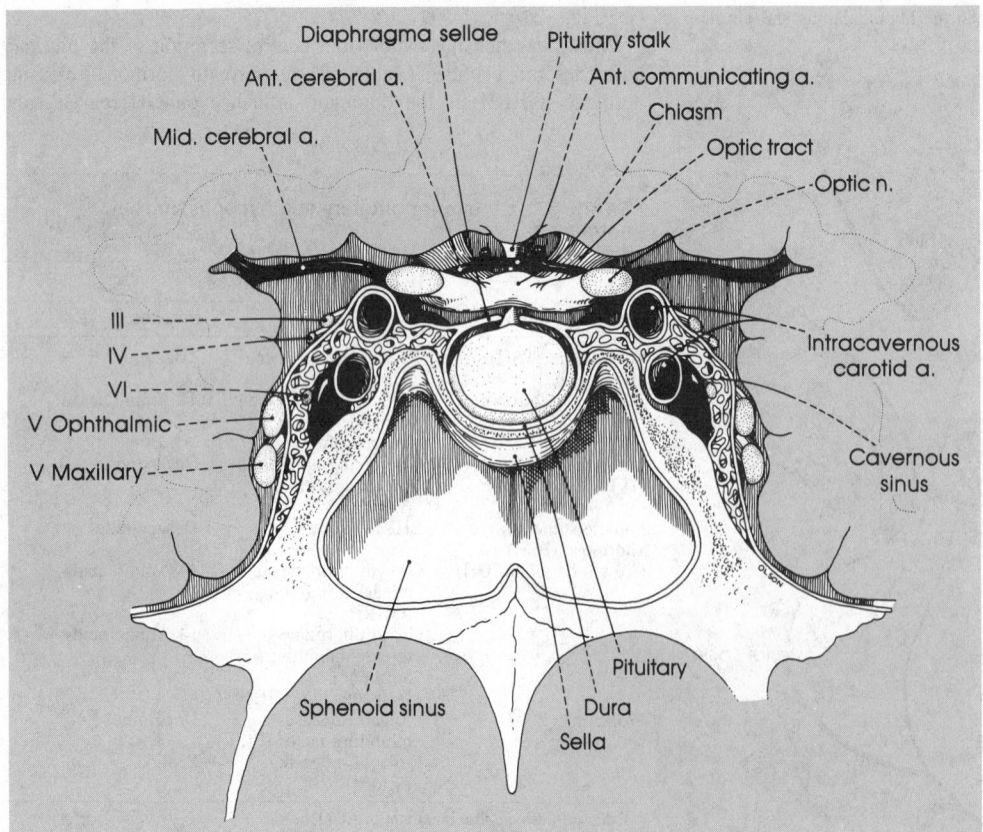

FIGURE 331-2 The relationship between the pituitary, cranial nerves, and the cavernous sinus as viewed in a coronal section through the sella. *(From JA Taren in RC Schneider et al (eds), Correlative Neurosurgery, 3d ed, Springfield, Ill., Charles C Thomas, 1982.)*

vasopressin-containing neurons also terminate in the median eminence, and vasopressin can stimulate release of ACTH and GH.

The anterior pituitary has the highest blood flow of any tissue in the body [0.8 (mL/g)/min]. The blood supply reaches the anterior pituitary by a circuitous route through the hypothalamus. Two derivatives of the internal carotid arteries, the superior hypophyseal arteries (SHA), branch in the subarachnoid space around the pituitary stalk and terminate in the capillary network of the median eminence. These capillaries have a fenestrated endothelium which allows easy access to the hypothalamic releasing hormones. Transport of substances from the capillaries to the median eminence is also facilitated because the median eminence lies outside the blood-brain barrier. The capillaries then coalesce to form 6 to 10 straight veins known as the *hypothalamic-pituitary portal circulation*. These veins constitute the main blood supply to the anterior lobe and supply it with nutrients as well as information from the hypothalamus. A direct arterial blood supply to the anterior lobe is also present, but the magnitude and importance of that circulation are uncertain. The posterior pituitary is supplied entirely by blood from the inferior hypophyseal arteries.

The anterior lobe is formed from the lateral proliferation of Rathke's pouch, an outpouching from the floor of the embryonic oral cavity. Rathke's pouch is met by a diverticulum from the floor of the third ventricle, which forms the posterior lobe.

Rathke's pouch is closed off by proliferation of the anterior and posterior lobe and forms a thin residual cleft in the gland (Rathke's cleft). This cleft may persist as a cyst lined with cuboidal or columnar epithelium. Since the pituitary rotates as it grows, these cysts usually lie in a position superior to the pituitary gland. The further growth and proliferation of these cysts can give rise to craniopharyngiomas, tumors that generally occupy a suprasellar position. Development of the sphenoid bone separates the pituitary from the oral cavity. Remnants of the pituitary, known as *pharyngeal pituitaries*, occasionally persist within or below the sphenoid bone. These remnants may produce pituitary hormones and occasionally develop into pituitary tumors.

Five distinct cell types in the anterior pituitary secrete six different hormones: lactotrophs (prolactin), somatotrophs (GH), gonadotrophs (LH and FSH), thyrotrophs (TSH), and corticotrophs (ACTH). The physiologic role of the other hormones and chemicals produced in the pituitary is uncertain.

PROLACTIN

PHYSIOLOGY The lactotrophs constitute 15 to 20 percent of the normal pituitary and increase to 70 percent during pregnancy. The prolactin gene on chromosome 6 codes for a precursor molecule that is larger than the circulating hormone. The predominant form of the processed hormone contains 198 amino acids (23,000 mol wt) in a single polypeptide chain containing three intrachain disulfide bonds. Higher-molecular-weight forms of prolactin, up to 100,000 mol wt ("big" and "big-big" prolactin), may be present in small amounts in the circulation of normal persons and in larger amounts in patients with pituitary adenomas; these molecules react in prolactin radioimmunoassays but do not have normal biologic potency.

Prolactin is essential for lactation. Receptors for the hormone are present in human breast and gonads, whereas in other animals they are found in additional tissues. Prolactin promotes breast cancer in rodents; a similar connection has not been established in human breast cancer (see Chap. 319).

During pregnancy, increasing estrogen production stimulates the growth and replication of the pituitary lactotrophs and causes increased prolactin secretion. The pituitary doubles in size during pregnancy and returns to normal after delivery. Prolactin during pregnancy prepares the breast for postpartum lactation. High estrogen levels inhibit prolactin action at the breast so that lactation does not commence until estrogen levels decline post partum. Prolactin levels

rise in the fetus beginning at about 25 weeks, probably owing to maternal estrogen transfer and stimulation of the fetal pituitary. The level falls rapidly after delivery, reaching a nadir by 2 to 4 weeks post partum. High concentrations of prolactin are present in amniotic fluid, probably of both uterine and placental origin. The functional significance of this prolactin is unknown.

Under normal circumstances, prolactin secretion by the anterior pituitary is restrained by the hypothalamus. With hypothalamic destruction or pituitary stalk section, prolactin secretion increases, and serum concentrations rise. The release of prolactin from pituitary cells after stalk section in animals requires the autocrine release of vasoactive intestinal peptide (VIP) by pituitary cells. The hypothalamic inhibitory factor for prolactin appears to be dopamine, although peptide inhibitory factors have been described. The arcuate and paraventricular nuclei of the hypothalamus produce dopamine; dopamine travels down axons to nerve terminals in the median eminence, where it is released (tuberoinfundibular dopamine system) into the portal circulation and reaches the anterior pituitary to inhibit prolactin release via interactions with pituitary D_2 receptors (adenylate cyclase–linked dopamine receptors). The intravenous administration of dopamine (2 µg/min per kilogram of body weight) or the oral administration of dopamine precursors (e.g., levodopa) or dopamine agonists (e.g., bromocriptine) inhibits prolactin release. Increased blood prolactin appears to increase hypothalamic dopamine production, which, in turn, partially inhibits prolactin release via a "short" feedback loop.

The prolactin rise during suckling appears to require a prolactin-releasing factor, which has not yet been conclusively identified. VIP may be responsible, since it is a potent stimulator of prolactin release. Suckling-induced prolactin rise is blocked by serotonin antagonists, such as methysergide, which suggests an influence of serotonin on prolactin release. TRH is also a potent stimulator of prolactin release; indeed, the lowest dose of TRH capable of stimulating TSH stimulates prolactin release as well. However, TSH and prolactin release are under independent control in most physiologic states; lactation does not lead to TSH elevation, and primary hypothyroidism is rarely associated with prolactin excess.

Prolactin concentrations rise during sleep, a phenomenon that requires the input of higher centers into the hypothalamus. Stress-related prolactin release can be blocked by opiate antagonists such as naloxone and is probably mediated by endogenous opioids. Morphine can stimulate prolactin release, which may contribute to the amenorrhea of narcotic addiction, but basal prolactin secretion is not influenced by opiate antagonists.

HYPERPROLACTINEMIA Clinical features Prolactin excess (hyperprolactinemia) has many causes, is associated with hypogonadism and/or galactorrhea, and may indicate the presence of a pituitary adenoma or hypothalamic disease. Of women with amenorrhea, 10 to 40 percent have hyperprolactinemia, and about 30 percent of women with amenorrhea and galactorrhea have prolactin-secreting pituitary tumors.

The hypogonadism associated with hyperprolactinemia appears to be due to inhibition of hypothalamic release of LHRH, resulting in a decrease in LH and FSH secretion. This functional hypogonadism can be regarded, in part, as a desirable physiologic mechanism whereby breast feeding causes decreased fertility and delayed resumption of menses. In general, the higher the plasma prolactin, the greater is the likelihood of amenorrhea. Milder degrees of hyperprolactinemia in women cause irregular menses or infertility due to a shortened luteal phase. Prolactin excess in men can cause impotence and infertility. In some series, 8 percent of men with impotence and 5 percent of men with infertility have hyperprolactinemia. With prolactin elevation, FSH and LH levels in men decline, and serum testosterone is often low.

Galactorrhea, defined as milk production in a patient who is not post partum, is present in 30 to 90 percent of hyperprolactinemic women (see Chap. 341). The variation in incidence reflects, in part, variation in the intensity with which clinicians search for this finding.

TABLE 331-2 Causes of hyperprolactinemia

PHYSIOLOGIC STATES

A Pregnancy
B Nursing (early)
C "Stress"
D Sleep
E Nipple stimulation
F Food ingestion

DRUGS

A Dopamine receptor antagonists
　1 Phenothiazines
　2 Butyrophenones
　3 Thioxanthenes
　4 Metoclopramide
　5 Sulpiride
B Dopamine-depleting agents
　1 Methyldopa
　2 Reserpine
C Estrogens
D Opiates

DISEASE STATES

A Pituitary tumors
　1 Prolactinomas
　2 Adenomas secreting GH and prolactin
　3 Adenomas secreting ACTH and prolactin (Nelson's syndrome and Cushing's disease)
　4 Nonfunctioning chromophobe adenomas with pituitary stalk compression
B Hypothalamic and pituitary stalk disease
　1 Granulomatous diseases especially sarcoidosis
　2 Craniopharyngiomas and other tumors
　3 Cranial irradiation
　4 Stalk section
　5 Empty sella
　6 Vascular abnormalities including aneurysm
　7 Lymphocytic hypophysitis
　8 Metastatic carcinoma
C Primary hypothyroidism
D Chronic renal failure
E Cirrhosis
F Chest wall trauma (including surgery, *herpes zoster*)
G Seizures

Galactorrhea may occur without hyperprolactinemia, particularly in parous women. However, galactorrhea is often a clue to prolactin excess; when galactorrhea is coupled with amenorrhea, hyperprolactinemia is present in 75 percent of patients. Hyperprolactinemia in men rarely causes gynecomastia or galactorrhea (see Chap. 341).

Differential diagnosis Prolactin excess has several mechanisms: (1) autonomous production (pituitary adenomas), (2) decreased dopamine or dopamine inhibitory action (e.g., due to hypothalamic disease or drugs that block dopamine synthesis, dopamine release, or dopamine action), (3) stimuli that overcome the normal dopaminergic inhibition (e.g., estrogens, possibly hypothyroidism), and (4) decreased clearance of prolactin (renal failure). No single suppression test can separate physiologic from pharmacologic or pathologic causes of hyperprolactinemia (Table 331-2).

Prolactin concentrations are slightly higher (<20 μg/L) in women than in men (<15 μg/L). During pregnancy, prolactin concentrations begin to increase during the second trimester and peak at term; maximal values are 100 to 300 μg/L, usually less than 200 μg/L. A pregnancy test is mandatory in all patients with hyperprolactinemic amenorrhea, as it is with amenorrhea alone. The mean prolactin level declines post partum but rises with each suckling episode. Over several months basal and suckling-stimulated prolactin concentrations diminish; by 4 to 6 months post partum, basal prolactin levels are normal, and the suckling-induced rise is absent despite continued nursing. Prolactin levels rise within 1 h of feeding and after seizures.

A careful drug history should be obtained in hyperprolactinemic patients. Dopamine-blocking drugs (e.g., phenothiazines, butyrophe-

nones, metoclopramide) and dopamine-depleting drugs (e.g., methyldopa and reserpine) are important causes of hyperprolactinemia. Chronic cocaine use causes modest hyperprolactinemia. Prolactin concentrations are usually less than 100 μg/L with these agents, provided renal failure is not present. However, concentrations as high as 275 μg/L have been reported. Although high-dose estrogens cause hyperprolactinemia, oral contraceptives containing low doses of estrogen do not.

End-stage renal failure is associated with elevated serum prolactin in 70 to 90 percent of women and 25 to 60 percent of men. This contributes to hypogonadism in some patients with renal failure. Both decreased prolactin clearance and increased prolactin secretion may contribute to this elevation. The increased prolactin in cirrhosis of the liver has not been adequately explained.

Severe primary hypothyroidism may cause a mildly elevated serum prolactin, either due to elevated TRH or decreased dopaminergic tone. Since primary hypothyroidism also may cause enlargement of the sella turcica, mimicking a pituitary adenoma, thyroid function tests are essential in all patients with elevated serum prolactin. Rarely, primary adrenal insufficiency causes reversible serum prolactin elevation.

In 10,000 "normal" adults working at a single plant in Japan, the prevalence of hyperprolactinemia greater than 75 μg/L was 0.4 percent. Many different etiologies were found.

If a fasting hyperprolactinemic subject is not pregnant, post partum, cirrhotic, postictal, on medications, hypothyroid, or in renal failure, disease of the pituitary or hypothalamus is likely. Ectopic production of prolactin by nonpituitary tumors occurs rarely if at all. Diseases of the hypothalamus or pituitary stalk cause moderate prolactin elevation (usually less than 150 μg/L). Hyperprolactinemia occurs in 20 to 50 percent of patients with hypothalamic tumors.

Prolactin-secreting pituitary adenomas (prolactinomas) are arbitrarily divided into microadenomas (<10 mm) and macroadenomas (≥10 mm). Large, nonfunctioning pituitary adenomas also may cause modest prolactin elevation, thought to be due to stalk compression and impairment of dopamine delivery to the gland. Acromegalics (25 to 45 percent), some patients with Nelson's syndrome, and rare Cushing's patients have elevated serum prolactin levels.

Laboratory evaluation Serum prolactin levels should be measured in all people with unexplained hypogonadism or galactorrhea. If basal prolactin concentration is elevated, further evaluation is warranted after establishing that minimal prolactin elevations (e.g., less than 30 μg/L) are not due to stress or related to food intake. Blood sampling from an indwelling catheter after a 90-min rest period will exclude "needle stick" hyperprolactinemia. Levels should be assessed after fasting or more than 1 h after eating. Although there is no simple test to distinguish the various causes of hyperprolactinemia, a serum prolactin level of over 300 μg/L is diagnostic of a pituitary adenoma; a serum prolactin of over 150 μg/L in a nonpregnant patient is usually caused by a pituitary adenoma. Administration of dopamine agonists, such as bromocriptine, lowers prolactin regardless of the etiology and, therefore, is not useful as a differential test (Fig. 331-3). The majority of patients with prolactinomas have only a minimal or no rise in prolactin in response to TRH, as compared with the normal rise of 200 percent or more and the intermediate response (usually a doubling of serum prolactin) in patients with hypothalamic disease and those on dopamine-blocking agents. Unfortunately, the response to TRH is too variable to be of diagnostic value in individual patients.

In general, patients with unexplained hyperprolactinemia require magnetic resonance imaging (MRI) or contrast-enhanced computed tomography (CT) scanning of the hypothalamus and pituitary. Pituitary macroadenomas are easily visualized on these scans, but microadenomas (<10 mm) may be more difficult to delineate. Patients with amenorrhea and minimal prolactin elevations also may have hypothalamic lesions (e.g., craniopharyngiomas) or large "nonfunctioning" pituitary adenomas. When no radiologic abnormalities are found, the disorder is designated *idiopathic hyperprolactinemia*, although a

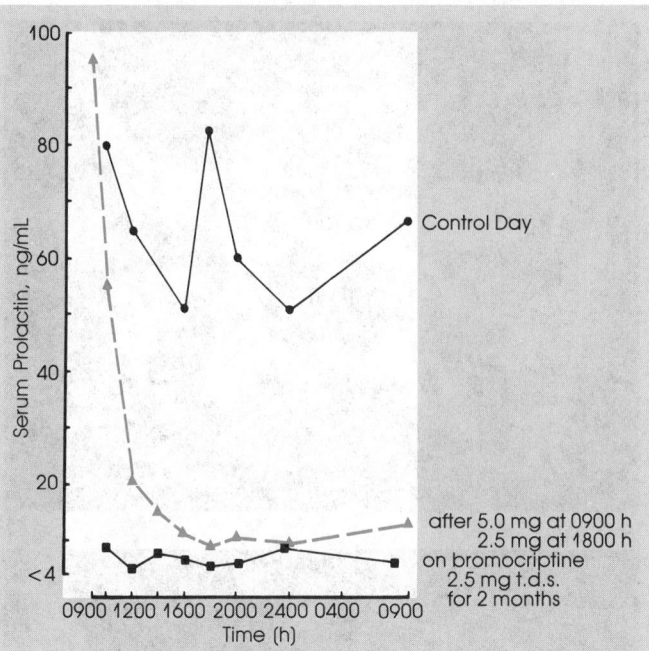

FIGURE 331-3 Changes in serum prolactin concentration in a woman with "idiopathic" hyperprolactinemia after an initial 5-mg dose of bromocriptine and when maintained on 7.5 mg daily. *(From GH Besser and MO Thorner, Postgrad Med J 52:66, 1976.)*

microadenoma may still be present. Sella tomography is not a useful screening test for small pituitary adenomas because of the high frequency of false-positive and false-negative results.

Microprolactinomas do not cause hypopituitarism (except for hypogonadism). If a small pituitary lesion is seen in a patient with hypopituitarism and hyperprolactinemia, sarcoidosis or other lesions involving the pituitary stalk should be suspected rather than a microprolactinoma. In patients with macroprolactinomas or hypothalamic lesions, evaluation of pituitary function and formal visual field examinations are essential.

Prolactinomas PATHOLOGY Prolactinomas are the most common functional pituitary adenomas. Small unsuspected microadenomas are found in 6 to 24 percent of unselected autopsies; 40 percent of these small tumors contain prolactin by immunologic staining techniques, but the fraction that actually secrete prolactin is unknown. About 70 percent of macroadenomas previously thought to be nonfunctioning are, in fact, prolactinomas. Prolactin-secreting pituitary carcinomas are rare.

Prolactinoma size correlates with hormonal output; in general, the larger the tumor, the higher are the prolactin levels. Large pituitary tumors with modest prolactin elevation (50 to 100 μg/L) are not true prolactinomas and differ in their biologic behavior. Microprolactinomas cause only hyperprolactinemia and hypogonadotropism, whereas macroprolactinomas may influence other pituitary hormones and cause headaches, visual field disturbances, and other structural problems.

CLINICAL PRESENTATION Microprolactinomas are more common than macroprolactinomas, and 90 percent of patients with microprolactinomas are women. In contrast, 60 percent of patients with macroprolactinomas are men. Irregular menses, amenorrhea, and galactorrhea are likely to result in early diagnosis, and this may partially explain the preponderance of microadenomas in women. Sexual dysfunction occurs in most men with prolactinomas, but this is the presenting complaint in 15 percent or less. Although delay in seeking medical help probably explains the larger tumors in men, more aggressive tumor behavior in men has not been excluded.

Estrogens promote the growth of lactotrophs, but an etiologic role has not been established for oral contraceptives in the pathogenesis of prolactinomas. Many women with prolactinomas first develop galactorrhea while on oral contraceptives or develop amenorrhea when the drug is discontinued. Some of these women may have been started on oral contraceptives for irregular menses that were the consequence of a prolactinoma. Although amenorrhea after discontinuing oral contraceptives is rare (about 2 percent), about a third of patients with postpill amenorrhea have prolactinomas. Development of galactorrhea in a woman on oral contraceptives mandates a prolactin determination. About 5 to 7 percent of prolactinoma patients have never menstruated (primary amenorrhea), making this an important treatable cause of primary amenorrhea. Prolactinomas may grow during pregnancy, and 15 percent of prolactinoma patients are first diagnosed in the postpartum period.

Women with prolactinomas who desire pregnancy need special consideration. Medical treatment of patients with microprolactinomas results in uneventful pregnancies 95 to 98 percent of the time; the remainder may develop headaches or visual field disturbances due to tumor enlargement that rarely requires therapy. Asymptomatic enlargement of microprolactinomas, as ascertained by radiologic studies, occurs in about 5 percent. With macroprolactinomas, the complications of tumor growth during pregnancy are more common. Symptomatic tumor enlargement occurs in about 15 percent of these patients, although prior therapy with bromocriptine may decrease this risk. The majority of patients who develop symptoms do so during the first trimester.

In prolactinoma patients, the effect of pregnancy on prolactin secretion is variable. A further rise in prolactin during pregnancy may not occur even in patients in whom tumor growth occurs. Prolactin concentrations should be measured periodically throughout pregnancy in women with prolactinomas. An increase in serum prolactin of more than 300 to 400 μg/L during pregnancy usually signals tumor growth; when this occurs, the postpartum prolactin level is usually greater than the prepartum level. Patients with stable or declining prolactin concentrations during pregnancy may have lower prolactin concentrations after pregnancy than before. In such patients, infarction or involution of the adenomas may have occurred during pregnancy. Rarely, macroprolactinomas in men grow during replacement testosterone therapy, presumably as a result of extraglandular conversion of testosterone to estrogen. The safety of oral contraceptives is uncertain, but such therapy is unlikely to cause significant tumor growth.

THERAPY The natural history of untreated hyperprolactinemia is incompletely understood. Although large pituitary adenomas must begin as small tumors, most microadenomas do not progress to macroadenomas. In general, 90 to 95 percent of untreated microprolactinomas remain stable or exhibit decreased serum prolactin concentrations over 7 years of follow-up. Serum prolactin returns to normal in a third of patients with idiopathic hyperprolactinemia (who may harbor microprolactinomas) followed for 5 years without therapy; the number increases to two-thirds if the basal prolactin is less than 40 μg/L. In 30 patients with varying degrees of hyperprolactinemia (30 to 260 μg/L) followed for a mean of 5.2 years, the prolactin level increased by more than 50 percent in a fifth, and another fifth had signs of enlargement on CT scans. The prolactin decreased by more than 50 percent in a third of the patients and returned to normal in a fifth. Abnormal x-rays returned to normal in a sixth of the patients.

Thus not all patients with microprolactinomas need therapy. Women with microprolactinomas require therapy when they desire pregnancy, have decreased libido or troublesome galactorrhea, desire regular menses, or are at risk for osteoporosis. Men with microadenomas should be treated for decreased potency or libido or when infertility is a problem. Most patients with macroprolactinomas require therapy.

Dopamine agonist drugs lower prolactin concentrations in virtually all hyperprolactinemic patients (see Fig. 331-3). Ovulatory menses and fertility are restored in more than 90 percent of premenopausal women, underscoring the direct relationship between hyperprolactinemia and amenorrhea. Bromocriptine, an ergot derivative with dopamine agonist actions, is the only effective prolactin-lowering agent licensed for this purpose in the United States. Bromocriptine should be given twice daily with food or a snack to prevent gastrointestinal irritation; some patients may be treated once a day. Therapy should begin with 1.25 mg at bedtime to minimize the side effects of nausea, vomiting, fatigue, nasal stuffiness, and postural hypotension. Gastrointestinal intolerance to oral bromocriptine may be circumvented when the drug is administered via the vagina; however, the drug is not currently licensed for vaginal administration. The dosage is gradually increased to an average of 2.5 mg twice daily. However, doses up to 15 mg/d may be required to return the prolactin concentration to normal with macroprolactinomas. Although the drug is expensive, it is effective in all forms of hyperprolactinemia and often abolishes nonhyperprolactinemic galactorrhea as well. Long-lasting parenteral and oral dopamine agonists and newer non-ergot-derived oral dopamine agonists are effective and in some cases better tolerated than bromocriptine; they are not yet licensed in the United States.

Bromocriptine is the therapy of choice for patients with microprolactinomas who have one of the indications for treatment discussed above. Prolactin concentrations return to normal in almost all who tolerate the medication, usually within days of achieving full therapeutic dosages (see Fig. 331-3). Menses usually resume within 2 months but may be delayed up to a year. Since pregnancy may occur without resumption of menses, a barrier contraceptive is recommended until menses become regular. In this way, bromocriptine can be stopped with the first missed period when pregnancy has occurred. Bromocriptine use during pregnancy is not, however, associated with an increased risk of congenital anomalies or fetal wastage. The effects of bromocriptine are usually not permanent, but a sixth of microprolactinoma patients maintain normal prolactin concentrations after stopping the drug.

In patients with macroprolactinomas, bromocriptine usually lowers the serum prolactin level and decreases tumor size (Fig. 331-4), but both effects may be incomplete. In men, testosterone concentrations usually begin to increase after 3 months of therapy but may remain subnormal. Normal sperm counts are achieved in some. Almost 90 percent of premenopausal women regain cyclic menses.

Tumor shrinkage is most rapid in the first 3 months of therapy. By 3 months, 40 percent of tumors decrease by more than 50 percent in size. Most tumors demonstrate some shrinkage; more important, abnormal visual fields improve with medical therapy in 90 percent of patients. If the visual field defect does not resolve within a short period of time (1 to 3 months), surgery should be performed. Of patients treated for 12 months without additional therapy 90 percent show tumor shrinkage of more than 50 percent. Prolactin levels fall to 20 percent of baseline in more than 90 percent and return to normal in about a third. After more than 2 years of therapy, the dosage of bromocriptine can often be reduced but rarely discontinued. In patients with persistent symptomatic hyperprolactinemia despite partial response to bromocriptine, radiation therapy or surgical debulking may be appropriate.

Although prolactin concentrations rapidly return to pretreatment levels when long-term bromocriptine is stopped, tumor regrowth may be delayed for months or years. When considering pregnancy in a patient with a macroprolactinoma, this slow regrowth should be kept in mind. Patients who conceive after prolonged bromocriptine therapy may be at less risk of tumor growth during pregnancy. In the United States, bromocriptine is generally stopped when pregnancy is confirmed; if tumor-related symptoms develop during pregnancy, bromocriptine should be reinstituted. However, many physicians outside the United States use bromocriptine throughout pregnancy in patients with macroprolactinomas. There is no evidence that bromocriptine has an adverse effect on the fetus.

Only 10 percent of large nonfunctioning pituitary adenomas with hyperprolactinemia due to stalk compression shrink with bromocriptine therapy, although prolactin concentrations usually return to normal. Alternative therapies are required. There are isolated reports

FIGURE 331-4 Frontal CT scan of a man with a large prolactin-secreting macroadenoma. (*Top*) Pretreatment scan. (*Bottom*) Scan after 1 year of treatment with bromocriptine. The upper border of the tumor is shown by arrows. *(From Molitch et al.)*

of patients with large prolactinomas refractory to bromocriptine whose tumors shrink when tamoxifen, an estrogen antagonist, is added.

Following transsphenoidal resection of microprolactinomas, serum prolactin concentration returns to normal in up to 80 to 90 percent of patients, usually within 24 h. This procedure has low morbidity and mortality. Unfortunately, recurrence rates average 17 percent after "successful" surgery and may be as high as 40 percent after 6 years of follow-up. Surgery is appropriate for women with microprolactinomas who desire pregnancy and who cannot tolerate or do not wish to take dopamine agonist drugs. Surgery may be more difficult in patients with microprolactinoma treated for more than 3 months with bromocriptine; some surgeons report increased fibrosis with a higher complication rate and lower success rate in this situation.

Surgery, whether by transsphenoidal or transcranial approach, is rarely curative for macroprolactinomas. Surgery may be necessary for patients with persistent visual field defects despite bromocriptine and for those intolerant of dopamine agonists. Tumors with large cystic or hemorrhagic components may require surgical decompression for relief of visual symptoms or headaches. Prolactin concentrations return to normal in about 30 percent of patients treated surgically, but recurrence rates may be as high as 80 percent in this subgroup. Long-term bromocriptine therapy is usually required after surgical therapy.

Radiation therapy plays a limited role in the treatment of prolactinomas. Conventional radiation therapy [4500 cGy (4500 rad) over 25 days] causes a slow decline in serum prolactin concentration. Although prolactin concentrations return to normal in about 30 percent of microprolactinomas 2 to 10 years after radiation therapy, we rarely treat microprolactinomas with radiation. The risks of hypopituitarism make this a poor fourth choice after medical, surgical, or no therapy. Radiation therapy may be necessary in macroprolactinomas with rapid or persistent tumor growth despite dopamine agonist therapy and surgery or after surgery alone in patients intolerant of dopamine agonists. The respective roles of conventional radiation, focused gamma radiation (''gamma knife''), and heavy-particle radiation (proton beam) are not established.

PROLACTIN DEFICIENCY Prolactin deficiency is manifested as an inability to lactate. Failure of lactation is often the earliest clue to panhypopituitarism resulting from pituitary infarction during the peripartum period. The lateral wings of the pituitary have a precarious blood supply; most lactotrophs reside in this area. During pregnancy, the hypertrophied and hyperplastic lactotrophs are at risk for necrosis. If systemic hypotension develops, as with postpartum hemorrhage, the hypertrophic and hyperplastic lactotrophs may infarct (Sheehan's syndrome). Patients with diabetes mellitus are susceptible to peripartum pituitary infarction even in the absence of significant hemorrhage. Autoimmune pituitary destruction (lymphocytic hypophysitis) also may occur during late pregnancy but often is associated with elevated prolactin levels.

Many prolactin radioimmunoassays cannot distinguish normal from low concentrations; hence prolactin stimulation tests are needed to diagnose prolactin insufficiency. After administration of TRH or chlorpromazine, a rise in serum prolactin of less than 200 percent suggests prolactin deficiency. If prolactin deficiency is present, evaluation of other pituitary hormones is necessary as well to define other manifestations of hypopituitarism.

GROWTH HORMONE

PHYSIOLOGY Growth hormone (GH, somatotropin) is secreted by somatotrophs, which make up about 50 percent of the anterior pituitary cells. The normal pituitary contains 3 to 5 mg GH and secretes 500 to 875 μg GH per day. GH shares an 85 percent structural identity with human placental lactogen (hPL, chorionic somatomammotropin). GH and hPL genes are on chromosome 17 and appear to have originated by gene duplication. Human growth hormone is a single-polypeptide chain of 191 amino acids (22,000 mol wt) and contains two intrachain disulfide bonds; it is cleaved from a larger precursor molecule (28,000 mol wt). Alternative splicing of this precursor yields a 20-kDa GH molecule of reduced biologic and immunologic activity. GH is stored in cytoplasmic granules in a high-molecular-weight polymeric form. A variant form of GH (GH-V) is found in the placenta, is the dominant form of GH circulating in the third trimester of pregnancy, and is a potent somatogen.

Multiple forms of GH exist in the circulation. The dominant form is monomeric GH (22 kDa), but larger, oligomeric forms (e.g., ''big'' GH, 44,000 mol wt) and smaller forms (e.g., 20 kDa) are present as well. All these variants contribute to the total circulating GH concentration. Several binding proteins for GH contribute to the heterogeneity of circulating GH. The high-affinity GH-binding protein, which is specific for the 22-kDa GH, appears to be a cleavage product of the GH receptor from the liver and possibly other tissues. A lower-affinity binding protein binds both the 22-kDa active and 20-kDa inactive GH.

Pulsatile release of GH is characteristic. Circulating levels are immeasurably low for much of the day, punctuated by four to eight bursts after meals or exercise, during slow-wave sleep, or without obvious cause. The half-life of the hormone in plasma is 20 to 30 min. GH secretion is low in infancy, slightly higher during early childhood, and dramatically increased during puberty. GH secretion is lower in adults than during puberty. After the third decade, a progressive (but individually variable) decline in GH secretion occurs.

GH is necessary for normal linear growth. GH deficiency causes short stature; GH excess (prior to epiphyseal closure) leads to gigantism. GH does not appear to be the principal direct stimulator of growth but acts indirectly by stimulating the formation of other hormones. These factors, known as *somatomedins* (SM, somatotropin-mediating hormones) or *insulin-like growth factors* (IGF), are GH-dependent and are responsible for growth stimulation (also see Chap. 332). Somatomedin C (insulin-like growth factor I, IGF-I/SM-C), the most important somatomedin for postnatal growth, is produced in the liver, chondrocytes, kidney, muscle, pituitary, and gastrointestinal tract. The liver is the main source of circulating IGF-I/SM-C. IGF-I/SM-C is a basic protein (7600 mol wt) that circulates bound to carrier proteins (IGF-binding proteins). Although the role of these carriers is under investigation, their net effect is to increase the half-life of circulating IGF-I/SM-C to 3 to 18 h as compared with the half-life of 20 to 30 min for unbound hormone. As a consequence, the concentration of IGF-I remains relatively constant throughout the day, in contrast to the fluctuating levels of GH itself. How the liver and other tissues integrate the GH pulses into IGF-I/SM-C and IGF-binding protein production is not known. Local tissue generation of IGF-I/SM-C, particularly in bone, may play an important role in growth mediation through its paracrine effects.

IGF-I is structurally similar to proinsulin and exerts some insulin-like actions. Furthermore, GH is a trophic factor for insulin release, facilitating its release in response to various secretagogues, and GH-deficient individuals have impaired insulin release to glucose challenge. Technically, one might consider insulin a somatomedin.

During the prenatal and neonatal period, growth is independent of GH, as shown by the normal birth length of GH-deficient children born to GH-deficient mothers. Nevertheless, IGF-I/SM-C levels are elevated during pregnancy; the concentration correlates with that of hPL, which may regulate IGF-I/SM-C production. IGF-I/SM-C levels at birth are lower than those of adults and rise gradually during childhood to reach the adult range by age 8 to 10 years. IGF-I/SM-C levels are dependent on nutritional status, declining in states of malnourishment. Elevated serum IGF-I/SM-C concentrations are present during the pubertal growth spurt, presumably accounting for the pubertal growth acceleration.

Although IGF-I/SM-C concentrations correlate with linear growth, the correlation is inexact, and therefore, GH may have some direct influence on growth or cause somatomedin generation in target cells.

GH exerts additional metabolic effects, including stimulation of the incorporation of amino acids into protein. Although most of this action is somatomedin-mediated, GH can directly stimulate amino acid uptake in certain systems. Some amino acids, such as arginine, are potent stimuli for GH release.

GH may have a direct effect as an insulin antagonist that inhibits glucose uptake by tissues. Patients with GH deficiency are prone to insulin-induced hypoglycemia; patients with GH excess develop insulin resistance. GH is one of the counterregulatory hormones that help restore a low blood sugar to normal (see Chap. 338). Hypoglycemia is a potent GH stimulus, and an acute rise in blood sugar inhibits GH release. Paradoxically, patients with type I diabetes mellitus have increased GH concentrations. GH increases free fatty acid release from adipocytes. The absence of this effect may be responsible for the pudgy appearance of children with GH deficiency and the higher percent body fat in adults with GH deficiency. Increased serum free fatty acid concentrations tend to blunt GH release. GH opposes the action of insulin on sugar uptake and fatty acid release and complements the anabolic action of insulin on amino acid uptake.

GH is controlled by a dual hypothalamic regulation (Table 331-3). Secretion is stimulated by growth hormone–releasing hormone (GHRH, somatocrinin) and inhibited by growth hormone release–

TABLE 331-3   Growth hormone regulation

Class of agent	Stimulation	Inhibition
Hypothalamic factors	GHRH	Somatostatin
Amines	Alpha-adrenergic stimuli (norepinephrine, clonidine)	Beta-adrenergic stimuli
	Beta-adrenergic blockers (propranolol)	Alpha-adrenergic blockers (phentolamine, dibenzyline)
	Dopaminergic stimuli (levodopa, bromocriptine, apomorphine)	Dopamine blockers (chlorpromazine)
	Serotonergic stimuli (L-tryptophan)	Serotonin blockers (methysergide, cyproheptadine)
Hormones	Decreased IGF-I/SM-C	Increased IGF-I/SM-C (obesity)
	Estrogen	Progestogens
	Vasopressin	Glucocorticoids*
	Glucagon	
Fuels	Hypoglycemia†	Increased blood sugar
	Decreased free fatty acids	Increased free fatty acids
	Amino acids (arginine)†	
Others	Exercise†	
	Stress†	
	Sleep	
	Acetylcholine	

* Acutely, glucocorticoids stimulate GH release.
† Probably mediated through alpha-adrenergic stimulation.

inhibitory hormone (somatostatin, somatotropin release–inhibitory factor, SRIF). GHRH appears to play the more important role, since stalk section leads to failure of GH release. Although GHRH- and somatostatin-containing neurons are separate, they have reciprocal interconnections.

Growth hormone–releasing hormone   GHRH has 44 amino acids, 29 of which are necessary for full potency. GHRH belongs to a family of molecules that includes secretin, glucagon, vasoactive intestinal peptide (VIP), and gastric inhibitory peptide (GIP). The arcuate nucleus of the hypothalamus is the major site of GHRH production, although a few such neurons are in the ventromedial nucleus as well. Axons containing the peptide project to the median eminence and terminate on the portal vessels. GHRH is also present in the mucosa of the small intestine.

GHRH stimulates GH release and synthesis in vitro and in vivo, an effect that is calcium-dependent and appears to be mediated by cyclic adenosine monophosphate (cyclic AMP). GHRH enhances GH gene transcription and stimulates c-*fos*, a growth signal–transducing oncogene. Intravenous injection of GHRH (0.1 to 3.3 μg/kg body weight) produces a peak GH response at 30 to 60 min with a return to baseline by 2 to 3 h postinjection (Fig. 331-5).

Somatostatin   Somatostatin, a cyclic tetradecapeptide, is the most widely distributed of the hypothalamic releasing hormones. The primary hypothalamic sources are the periventricular and medial preoptic areas of the anterior hypothalamus. Somatostatin is found in neurosecretory granules of axons that terminate in the median eminence. In addition to its function as a hormone, somatostatin is synthesized and distributed throughout the brain and serves as a neurotransmitter in many areas, including the spinal cord, brainstem, and cerebral cortex. Somatostatin is also present in the gastrointestinal tract and other organs. Somatostatin-secreting cells (D cells) of the pancreatic islets participate in the regulation of insulin and glucagon secretion, an example of paracrine regulation by this hormone (see Chap. 337).

Somatostatin is produced by processing of a larger precursor molecule and exists in both 28– and 14–amino acid forms. The 28–amino acid somatostatin has a longer half-life and is a more potent inhibitor of GH, TSH, and insulin secretion. Somatostatin 14 has a greater affinity for hypothalamic and cortical receptors and is more potent in inhibition of glucagon release, splanchnic blood flow, intestinal motility, and gastric exocrine secretion. Somatostatin analogues are effective in the therapy of acromegaly, secretory pancreatic tumors, carcinoid syndrome, and other conditions.

Somatostatin inhibits GH secretion and decreases the GH response to secretagogues without altering GH mRNA levels. Somatostatin also lowers serum TSH in normal and hypothyroid individuals and blunts TSH release in response to TRH. Somatostatin probably mediates the secondary hypothyroidism that may develop in GH-deficient children treated with GH. Somatostatin has no significant effect on the release of prolactin, gonadotropins, or ACTH in normal subjects but may lower ACTH concentrations in patients with Nelson's syndrome. Somatostatinomas are rare pancreatic islet cell or duodenal tumors that secrete somatostatin (see Chap. 276).

Growth hormone release is under complex physiologic control (see Table 331-3). The various mediators appear to act through GHRH and somatostatin. IGF-I/SM-C has an important feedback effect on GH secretion. An increased IGF-I/SM-C concentration inhibits GH release both through increased somatostatin production and by a direct

FIGURE 331-5   Response to GHRH-44 (1 μg/kg) in eight men and eight women. The shaded area shows the full range of responses at each time point and the error bars indicate the mean ± 1 SD. (*From MC Gelato et al, J Clin Endocrinol Metab 59:200, 1984.*)

Elapsed Time, minutes

action on the pituitary. A decrease in IGF-I/SM-C, as induced by starvation, leads to a compensatory increase in GH release.

A number of neurotransmitters influence GH release:

1 Hypothalamic dopamine, the important prolactin inhibitory factor, stimulates GH through an effect on GHRH. Dopamine has a direct but weak inhibitory effect on GH release; this effect is overwhelmed by its hypothalamic stimulation of GHRH secretion. Oral administration of dopamine precursors or agonists that cross the blood-brain barrier, such as levodopa, apomorphine, or bromocriptine, causes an increase in serum GH concentration. The effects of these stimuli can be utilized to test the adequacy of GH secretion (GH reserve).
2 Alpha-adrenergic agonists, such as clonidine, stimulate GHRH and GH release, whereas phentolamine, an alpha blocker, prevents the GH rise. A number of GH stimulators, including insulin hypoglycemia, arginine, and exercise, act through alpha-adrenergic mechanisms. Beta-adrenergic blockers potentiate the GH-stimulatory effect of clonidine (and of some other agents, including levodopa), possibly by inhibiting somatostatin secretion.
3 Serotonin agonists stimulate GH release, and the nocturnal surge in GH secretion may be mediated by serotonin, since cyproheptadine (a serotonin antagonist) blocks the sleep-induced GH rise.
4 Acetylcholine increases GH release by inhibiting somatostatin. Acetylcholinesterase inhibitors increase basal GH and the GH response to GHRH.

Obesity blunts GH release in response to many stimuli, including GHRH itself. Weight reduction restores normal GH dynamics. In contrast, malnourished individuals, including women with anorexia nervosa, often have increased GH secretion and plasma concentration, partly the result of a decreased serum IGF-I/SM-C level. Oral glucose administration decreases serum GH and the GH response to GHRH. Arginine also stimulates GH release by inhibiting somatostatin release.

A number of hormones influence GH release. Most factors that stimulate GH release are more potent in women than in men, an effect mediated by estrogen. In testing GH reserve in children, estrogen priming may be necessary before adequate GH release can be demonstrated. Although estrogen increases GH concentration, it decreases its biologic effect by blocking somatomedin production. This is similar to the estrogen effect on prolactin, in which secretion is stimulated but its action in promoting lactation is inhibited. Chronic glucocorticoid administration inhibits GH release and may blunt somatomedin action as well, explaining the potent growth-inhibiting effects of these agents in children. Acute administration of glucocorticoids stimulates GH release, although the response is reduced or absent in obese individuals. ACTH and TH deficiency may be associated with reversible GH deficiency. GH-releasing peptide (GHRP) is a synthetic hexapeptide that stimulates pituitary GH release but does not interact with GHRH or opiate receptors. The therapeutic potential of this peptide is being explored.

GROWTH HORMONE EXCESS: ACROMEGALY AND GIGANTISM   Clinical features
GH excess results in acromegaly, an insidious, chronic debilitating disease associated with bony and soft tissue overgrowth (Table 331-4). Acromegaly occurs most frequently in middle age, with a mean age at diagnosis of 40 years in men and 45 in women. It is uncommon, with an estimated prevalence of 50 to 70 cases per million and an incidence of 3 to 4 cases per million per year. These figures may represent an underestimation due to underdiagnosis of the disorder. When GH excess develops prior to epiphyseal closure in children, increased linear growth and gigantism develop. Tumors may be more aggressive and cause more rapid onset of acromegaly in younger patients.

Most patients have soft tissue and bone enlargement which results in increased hand, foot, and hat size, prognathism, enlargement of the tongue, wide spacing of the teeth, and coarsening of facial features; these are rarely the presenting complaint. Acromegalics are said to look more like each other than like their own family members (Fig. 331-6). Laryngeal hypertrophy and sinus enlargement lead to a

TABLE 331-4   Acromegaly—Manifestations

Location	Symptoms	Signs
General	Fatigue Increased sweating Heat intolerance Weight gain	
Skin and subcutaneous tissue	Enlarging hands, feet Coarsening facial features Oily skin Hypertrichosis	Moist, warm, fleshy, doughy handshake Skin tags Acanthosis nigricans Increased heel pad
Head	Headaches	Parotid enlargement, frontal bossing
Eyes	Decreased vision	Visual field defects
Ears		Otoscope speculum cannot be inserted
Nose-throat–paranasal sinuses	Sinus congestion	Enlarged furrowed tongue
	Increased tongue size	Tooth marks on tongue
	Malocclusion Voice change	Widely spaced teeth Prognathism
Neck		Goiter Obstructive sleep apnea Enlarged sinuses
Cardiorespiratory system	Congestive heart failure	Hypertension Cardiomegaly Left ventricular hypertrophy
Genitourinary system	Decreased libido Impotence Oligomenorrhea Infertility Kidney stones	
Neurologic system	Paresthesias Hypersomnolence	Carpal tunnel syndrome
Muscles	Weakness	Proximal myopathy
Skeletal system	Joint pains (shoulders, back, knees)	Osteoarthritis

hollow-sounding voice. A moist, doughy handshake, increased skin tags, acanthosis nigricans, and oily skin are common.

Acromegaly is more than a cosmetically disfiguring disease. Patients feel weak and tired. The basal metabolic rate increases, which, in turn, causes increased sweating. Obstructive sleep apnea may be an important cause of hypersomnolence. The majority have neurologic and musculoskeletal symptoms, including headaches, paresthesias (often due to carpal tunnel syndrome), muscle weakness, and arthralgias (particularly involving the shoulders, back, and knees). The cartilage hypertrophy and osseous overgrowth often lead to degenerative arthritis, kyphoscoliosis, and on occasion spinal stenosis. Hypertension occurs in about one-third and is characterized by suppressed renin and aldosterone secretion associated with expansion of plasma volume and total-body sodium. Almost all hypertensive acromegalics and about half of nonhypertensive acromegalics have increased left ventricular mass or left ventricular wall thickness. Although it is not established whether a specific cardiomyopathy occurs, acromegalics may develop congestive heart failure in the absence of other known underlying heart disease. Amenorrhea may occur with or without hyperprolactinemia, and hirsutism is often noted. Depression may persist after successful therapy for acromegaly. Many organs, including the liver and kidneys, increase in size with no evidence of functional impairment. Goiter, which probably results from IGF-I stimulation of thyroid cell growth, is common: 3 to 7 percent of patients are hyperthyroid. Some series report abdominal pain and inguinal hernias each in about one-third of patients and nasal polyps in as many as 15 percent. Intracranial aneurysms coexist in 10 percent or less.

Patients with acromegaly probably have a shortened life expectancy with increased deaths from cardiovascular, cerebrovascular, and

FIGURE 331-6 Serial photographs of a patient with acromegaly taken at ages 28, 49, 55, and 65 years, 6 months after removal of a GH-secreting adenoma. Note the gradual increase in the size of the nose, lips, and skin folds, particularly the nasolabial skin fold and forehead. *(From S Reichlin, Med Grand Rounds 1:9, 1982.)*

respiratory disease and, in some studies, from malignancies. In studies in which modern therapy was available, deleterious effects on life expectancy are less striking. Patients with coexisting diabetes mellitus have increased mortality. Skin tags appear to correlate with increased prevalence of colonic polyps and possibly with carcinoma of the colon. Bowel surveillance by colonoscopy has been suggested.

Laboratory investigation Insulin resistance occurs in 80 percent, although abnormal glucose tolerance (20 to 40 percent) and clinical diabetes mellitus (13 to 20 percent) are less common. Hypercalciuria is frequent, apparently due to increased levels of circulating 1,25-dihydroxyvitamin D; renal stones occur in about one-fifth of patients. Hypercalcemia, when it occurs, is not due to acromegaly per se but suggests primary hyperparathyroidism as part of the multiple endocrine neoplasia 1 (MEN 1) syndrome (see Chap. 343). GH causes increased renal tubular reabsorption of phosphate by an undefined mechanism. Elevation of serum phosphate occurs in about one-half of patients. Hyperprolactinemia occurs in up to one-half of patients and is responsible for much of the associated galactorrhea, amenorrhea, and decreased libido.

Pathophysiology Well-defined pituitary adenomas are found in almost all patients with acromegaly and gigantism. The tumors tend to occur in the lateral wings of the sella, where normal somatotrophs are found in abundance. Occasionally, tumors are found in ectopic locations along the lines of migration of Rathke's pouch, such as the sphenoid sinus or parapharyngeal regions.

GH levels correlate, on average, with tumor size. Tumors tend to be larger and may be more aggressive in younger patients. At the time of diagnosis, 75 percent of somatotroph adenomas are macroadenomas; 70 percent, however, are less than 20 mm at diagnosis. Two-thirds or more of prolactinomas are microadenomas at the time of diagnosis. Aggressive screening for acromegaly on the basis of subtle clinical clues might lead to early diagnosis while tumors are still small.

Immunohistochemical staining and electron microscopy of somatotroph tumors help to predict their behavior. Densely granulated tumors have slower growth. GH-secreting carcinomas are rare and should be diagnosed only in the presence of distant metastases. Tumors that cause local invasion are called *invasive adenomas*.

Current evidence suggests a primary pituitary etiology for acromegaly. Most GH-secreting (and other pituitary) tumors are monoclonal in origin. A cellular mutation may lead to GH hypersecretion (and presumably tumor growth as well) in some patients. About 40 percent of somatotroph tumors have a mutation in the alpha subunit of a stimulatory G protein (Gs) (see Chap. 69). These G proteins normally couple surface signals to cyclic AMP production within the cells. Activation of Gs proteins is associated with GTP binding to the alpha subunit, which allows the alpha subunit to stimulate cyclic AMP production. The normal free subunit has intrinsic GTPase activity, which inactivates GTP, preventing continued cyclic AMP stimulation. The mutant alpha subunit in acromegalic patients does not possess GTPase activity; hence continued cyclic AMP stimulation results. Tumors containing these mutations tend to be smaller than those in which the mutation is absent. Further evidence for a primary etiology is the finding that peripheral concentrations of GHRH are low. Although these findings do not exclude hypothalamic GHRH excess or somatostatin deficiency as the cause in some patients, this possibility has no direct support. Abnormal GH pulsations in some surgically "cured" acromegalics could be due to an underlying hypothalamic disorder, residual tumor, or previous GH excess.

GHRH-induced acromegaly is rare (<1 percent in a one series) but is clinically indistinguishable from acromegaly caused by pituitary adenomas; prolactin excess may occur in this syndrome. This diagnosis should be considered when pituitary somatotroph hyperplasia, rather than an adenoma, is diagnosed histologically. Bronchial carcinoids and pancreatic islet cell tumors are the most likely to secrete GHRH ectopically, but small cell carcinoma of the lung, medullary thyroid carcinoma, and carcinoids of the small intestine and thymus contain GHRH as well. Many of the tumors associated with GHRH production also cause ectopic ACTH production. Hypothalamic gangliocytomas, hamartomas, and gliomas can produce GHRH (as well as somatostatin) and cause somatotroph hyperplasia and acromegaly. GHRH is not routinely measured in acromegalics unless somatotroph hyperplasia is present or an appropriate nonpituitary tumor is discovered.

Isolated ectopic production of GH has been described in a patient with a pancreatic islet cell tumor; the tumor size in this instance (420 g) suggests inefficient GH production, since GH-secreting pituitary tumors are usually small.

Diagnosis Patients with acromegaly have symptoms for an average of 9 years and often see several physicians before the diagnosis is made. Newly consulted physicians are more likely to suspect the diagnosis than is one who has watched the insidious progress of the disease. When suggestive facial features are noted, a comparison with old pictures may be helpful (see Fig. 331-6).

Basal or random GH determinations may be elevated in normal persons, particularly in women and people with uncontrolled diabetes mellitus, renal failure, or stress; random GH determinations should not be used to screen for acromegaly. Two screening tests are available, namely, measurements of glucose-suppressed GH concentrations and IGF-I/SM-C concentrations. GH concentrations are measured 60 to 120 min after the oral administration of 100 g glucose. Although a serum GH concentration of <5 μg/L has traditionally been accepted as normal, a postsuppression value of <2 μg/L is a more rigorous criterion and should be applied. Acromegalics usually have a GH concentration after glucose administration of >10 μg/L; some suppress to values below 5 but rarely to below 2 μg/L. IGF-I/SM-C concentrations also provide an excellent screening test for acromegaly. Pitfalls include unreliable commercial assays, failure to use age-adjusted normals (especially during puberty), and possible false-negative tests with starvation. Measurements of serum IGF-I/SM-C concentration correlate with disease activity even in patients with basal GH concentrations below 10 μg/L. As GH values rise to >20 μg/L, IGF-I/SM-C concentrations plateau; this may explain why dramatic falls in GH after therapy do not cause clinical improvement. Although GH concentrations decline, IGF-I/SM-C may remain near maximal until GH falls below 20 μg/L.

GH concentrations in acromegaly may vary during the day, although they are never undetectable as in normal persons. After glucose administration to acromegalics, the GH concentrations usually are unchanged or increase, but some GH lowering may occur. GH levels increase in response to insulin-induced hypoglycemia and arginine infusion, and the response to GHRH is enhanced in most acromegalics. Somatostatin infusion lowers GH concentration but usually not to normal values. In addition, GH-secreting pituitary tumors respond to stimuli that do not affect normal somatotrophs: TRH increases GH in 80 percent, and LHRH increases GH in about 10 to 15 percent. Dopamine agonists stimulate GH release in normal persons but inhibit GH release in most acromegalics.

All patients with large pituitary adenomas should be screened with GH measurements, preferably after glucose ingestion. In rare cases patients with elevated serum GH and IGF-I/SM-C concentrations may have large pituitary tumors without clinical evidence of acromegaly. This syndrome is unexplained.

Radiologic investigation is necessary once the laboratory tests confirm the clinical suspicion of acromegaly. Although conventional skull x-rays or coned-down views of the sella turcica are abnormal in 90 percent of patients with acromegaly, MRI or CT scanning provides better definition of tumor size and is necessary for therapeutic planning. Additional clues to the diagnosis of acromegaly on conventional skull x-rays include thickening of the skull with increased bone density, enlargement of the paranasal sinuses and proliferation of the mastoid air cells, and prognathism if the jaw is included. On bone x-rays one may see enlarged vertebral bodies with anterior lipping, tufting of the distal phalanges of the hands and feet, increased thickness and lengthening of the ribs and clavicles, and bowing of the femur, tibia, and fibula. Soft tissue x-rays demonstrate increased thickness of the heel pad (>18 mm in women and 21 mm in men).

Testing for hypopituitarism and for increased prolactin should be performed. Large somatotroph adenomas commonly cause neurologic abnormalities (visual field defects or oculomotor or abducens nerve lesions). In addition, acromegaly may be associated with hyperparathyroidism and pancreatic islet cell tumors in the MEN I syndrome and rarely with pheochromocytomas or hyperaldosteronism (see Chap. 343). The alpha subunit of the glycoprotein hormones may be oversecreted in acromegaly and may serve as an additional marker of tumor regrowth.

Therapy The objectives of therapy are (1) return of GH and IGF-I/SM-C levels to normal, (2) stabilization or decrease in tumor size, and (3) preservation of normal pituitary function. The available modalities are variably successful in achieving these goals, and none is perfect. Although GH values of <5 μg/L are frequently interpreted as representing cures, a value of <2 μg/L with a normal IGF-I/SM-C level is a better criterion; patients with GH values between 2 and 5 μg/L may have persistent symptoms and increased IGF-I/SM-C concentrations.

Transsphenoidal surgery has the advantage of producing a rapid therapeutic response; it is potentially curative and is the procedure of choice. Anesthesiologists should be alerted to the potential of a difficult intubation due to anatomic changes in the jaw, tongue, epiglottis, and larynx. GH concentrations may fall to normal within hours, and soft tissue (but not bony) enlargement may melt away, even before the patient has been discharged from the hospital. The success of this procedure depends on the completeness of the resection and hence on the size of the tumor. In expert hands, apparent cure rates (GH below 5 μg/L) average 75 percent in patients with preoperative GH levels of <40 μg/L but only 35 percent in those with preoperative GH levels >40 μg/L. More stringent criteria, such as a GH level of <2 μg/L and normal IGF-I/SM-C level, are rarely used; the surgical cure rate is probably closer to 20 to 40 percent when these criteria are applied. This may explain why tumor regrowth and recurrent acromegaly are more common than previously appreciated. Persistent GH response to TRH stimulation may have predictive value in assessing risk of relapse, even in those patients with "normal" postoperative GH concentrations. Hypopituitarism may occur in 10 to 20 percent of patients with larger tumors, but up to 10 percent of patients with pituitary insufficiency prior to surgery regain normal function.

Heavy-particle pituitary radiation is successful in lowering GH concentrations in acromegaly but is slow in accomplishing this goal. Patients with suprasellar extension of the pituitary adenoma are generally excluded from this therapy. The Harvard cyclotron utilizes the Bragg peak with proton irradiation, achieving up to 12,000 cGy (12,000 rad) to the center of the pituitary adenoma. In patients with mean pretherapy GH concentration of 60 μg/L, GH concentrations are <5 μg/L in 29 percent of patients at 2 years, 40 percent at 4 years, 75 percent at 10 years, and 92 percent by 20 years. The risk of hypopituitarism is at least 20 percent.

Conventional pituitary radiation [4500 cGy (4500 rad) over 5 weeks] also has its proponents. GH generally falls 50 percent after 2 ± 1 years. GH concentrations of <5 μg/L occur in 50 percent at 5 years and in 70 percent at 10 years (after a mean pretherapy GH level of 60 μg/L). GH concentrations of <2.5 μg/L occur in 40 percent, and values <1 μg/L are seen in 20 percent at 10 to 15 years. Hypopituitarism is a common sequela, and up to 50 percent of patients require replacement therapy. The hypopituitarism is probably due to hypothalamic damage, which is possibly less common with focused heavy particles or gamma radiation. Higher doses of focused radiation [4000 to 7000 cGy (4000 to 7000 rad)] can be delivered with the cobalt 60 gamma unit ("gamma knife"), which delivers collimated radiation through multiple portals (over 200 in some units) that converge on the target in question. The radiation is delivered in a single session; radiation delivery to the tumor is the equivalent of two to three times the dosage of conventional radiation. Reports to date do not suggest an advantage (apart from convenience) over conventional radiation, either in terms of efficacy or risk of hypopituitarism; however, the data are still preliminary. We employ heavy-particle or conventional radiation in patients who have failed surgery and medical therapy or when surgery is contraindicated or is refused by the patient.

Bromocriptine is a useful adjunct to other modalities of therapy but rarely is successful alone. Clinical improvement is reported in up to 90 percent of patients with dosages of 20 to 60 mg/d. Objective decrease in hand and ring size as well as improvement in diabetes mellitus may occur in the absence of decreasing GH values. However, GH concentrations fall to <10 μg/L in only 35 percent, and values of <5 μg/L are achieved in only 21 percent; IGF-I/SM-C levels return to normal in only 8 percent. Tumor size decreases rarely.

The long-acting somatostatin analogue octreotide lowers GH to <5 μg/L and IGF-I/SM-C to normal in half of acromegalics. Modest tumor regression occurs in 30 to 50 percent of patients. The drug must be administered subcutaneously. Dosages average 100 to 200 μg every 8 h but range from 50 to 250 μg every 6 to 12 h to a maximum of 1500 μg/d. Constant subcutaneous pump therapy also has been employed. Temporary side effects are minimal and include local pain, steatorrhea, and abdominal cramps; the risk of cholelithiasis is substantial and may be due to decreased gallbladder contractility. Octreotide is 2000 times as potent as somatostatin in inhibiting GH secretion but only 1.5 to 2 times as potent an inhibitor of insulin secretion. Although impairment of glucose tolerance or worsening of diabetes mellitus may occur, the GH-lowering effects of the drug may improve glucose tolerance. Inhibition of TSH does not result in hypothyroidism. Headaches disappear quickly, possibly due to an effect on cerebral blood flow. The role of this agent as a primary

PRIMARY HYPOTHYROIDISM Thyroid gland failure (primary hypothyroidism) leads to compensatory hypertrophy of the thyrotrophs. With thyroid failure of long duration, the pituitary gland and the sella turcica may enlarge, occasionally causing visual field defects. Although TSH-secreting tumors may develop in animals after thyroid gland removal, the increased TSH and pituitary size in human hypothyroidism is not autonomous and decreases with thyroid hormone replacement. Since hyperprolactinemia also may occur in patients with primary hypothyroidism, pituitary enlargement (hyperplasia) may be incorrectly diagnosed as a prolactinoma; however, the return to normal of prolactin concentrations with thyroid hormone therapy excludes that diagnosis. Severe primary hypothyroidism occasionally may cause impaired release of GH and ACTH after appropriate stimuli (so-called pituitary myxedema), and hypothyroid children may develop precocious puberty. These abnormalities are all corrected with thyroid hormone therapy.

SECONDARY HYPOTHYROIDISM Hypothyroidism due to pituitary or hypothalamic disease may be difficult to diagnose. With primary hypothyroidism, serum TSH commonly rises before thyroid hormone concentrations decline below the normal range. No similar early laboratory clue exists in secondary hypothyroidism. Patients with central hypothyroidism usually do not have goiter, and many have deficiencies of other pituitary trophic hormones.

Some patients with hypothalamic hypothyroidism have mild TSH elevations, rather than normal or low concentrations, as expected. Although the TSH elevations rarely exceed 10 mU/L, they are above the expected range for hypothyroidism due to TSH deficiency. Biologically inactive but immunologically active thyrotropin is present in such cases. After TRH injection, TSH concentration rises, and the biologic potency of the TSH is increased. This suggests an additional role for TRH in controlling the biologic activity of the TSH molecule by controlling its rate of glycosylation. Although subclinical primary hypothyroidism is also characterized by mild TSH elevations, the two conditions are easily distinguished. Patients with central hypothyroidism and TSH elevations have markedly decreased T_4 concentrations; patients with subclinical hypothyroidism have normal or near-normal T_4 concentrations. TSH concentrations must not be used to guide replacement therapy in central hypothyroidism because TSH concentrations fall before full replacement is achieved; rather, peripheral levels of T_4 and free T_4 should be monitored. Severe illness may cause laboratory changes indistinguishable from central hypothyroidism, part of the so-called sick euthyroid syndrome.

PITUITARY (TSH-INDUCED) HYPERTHYROIDISM Hyperthyroidism is not usually a disease of TSH overproduction. However, two types of TSH-mediated hyperthyroidism are recognized:

1 Pituitary tumors. These are usually macroadenomas with autonomous TSH secretion, unresponsive to thyroid hormone suppression or TRH stimulation. A hallmark of such tumors is overproduction of the glycoprotein hormone alpha subunit (TSH alpha), with a serum molar ratio of alpha to intact TSH of greater than 1:1. The free alpha subunit may be an important tumor marker and differs from the native alpha subunit in that one of its amino acids is carbohydrate-blocked and hence cannot combine with beta subunits. These tumors may produce other pituitary hormones in addition to TSH, most commonly GH. TSH and TSH alpha subunit secretion may decrease with octreotide therapy. Therapy is generally directed to the pituitary tumor, but control of hyperthyroidism may require radioactive iodine or antithyroid drugs.
2 Pituitary resistance to thyroid hormone. In this situation, thyroid hormone fails to inhibit TSH secretion appropriately in the absence of a pituitary adenoma. Since TSH secretion is not inhibited, TSH rises and stimulates thyroid hormone overproduction. The peripheral tissues are not resistant to thyroid hormone, and clinical hyperthyroidism results. The pituitary resistance to thyroid hormone is incomplete, since TSH can be suppressed with supraphysiologic levels of thyroid hormone and stimulated further with TRH; bromocriptine or octreotide may lower TSH as well. Pituitary

resistance is usually diagnosed after thyroid gland ablation, when TSH cannot be lowered to normal values with the usual therapeutic doses of thyroid hormone. However, once the hyperthyroidism has been treated, pituitary resistance is of no clinical consequence, although the TSH measurements cannot be utilized to monitor adequacy of hormone replacement.

ADRENOCORTICOTROPIN

PHYSIOLOGY ACTH is produced by corticotrophs, which comprise about 15 percent of anterior pituitary cells, located principally in the central portion. ACTH is synthesized as part of a large precursor molecule termed *pro-opiomelanocortin* (POMC, 265 amino acids). ACTH contains 39 amino acids, with near complete biologic activity residing in the *N*-terminal 26 amino acids. In the anterior pituitary POMC is cleaved to yield ACTH, β-lipotropin, and an *N*-terminal precursor.

ACTH controls the release of cortisol from the adrenal cortex. Although aldosterone is primarily controlled by the renin-angiotensin system, ACTH also stimulates aldosterone release acutely. Other derivatives of the POMC molecule, such as γ-melanocyte-stimulating hormone (γ-MSH), also influence aldosterone production and are found in increased concentrations in the plasma of patients with idiopathic hyperaldosteronism. Patients with ACTH deficiency have near-normal aldosterone production and do not require mineralocorticoid replacement therapy.

Corticotropin-releasing hormone (CRH) is the major but not exclusive regulator of ACTH release. CRH contains 41 amino acids on a single polypeptide chain. CRH is produced primarily by neurons of the paraventricular nuclei of the hypothalamus but is also present in other areas of the brain, including the limbic system and cortex, as well as in the pancreas, gut, and adrenal medulla. Circulating CRH, which is largely of nonhypothalamic origin, is bound to a high-affinity binding protein. The placenta has the highest concentration outside the nervous system. CRH stimulates cyclic AMP production and regulates intracellular calcium and increases the concentration of POMC mRNA. Vasopressin potentiates the ACTH-releasing properties of CRH through a cyclic AMP–independent mechanism and may play a physiologic role in ACTH release. Naloxone, an opiate antagonist, releases CRH (and hence ACTH) in humans.

ACTH is released in pulses with an overriding circadian rhythm. With a normal sleeping pattern, ACTH concentration is highest in the early morning (around 4 A.M.) and lowest in late evening. The characteristic diurnal rhythm of plasma cortisol occurs in response to these ACTH changes. In primary adrenal insufficiency (Addison's disease), cortisol concentrations fall and ACTH concentrations rise. This results in hyperpigmentation owing to the melanocyte-stimulating properties of ACTH. Cortisol administration inhibits ACTH release, a phenomenon dependent on both the rate of rise of cortisol and its absolute concentration. Increased plasma cortisol inhibits CRH-induced ACTH release and also may inhibit CRH release. When supraphysiologic doses of glucocorticoids are given for prolonged periods, the hypothalamic-pituitary–adrenal cortex axis may remain suppressed for months after the drugs have been stopped, probably as the result of prolonged hypothalamic CRH suppression (see Chap. 335).

Stress, including hypoglycemia, surgery, and psychic distress, stimulates ACTH release, in part via increased CRH release. However, the magnitude of the ACTH release is greater than can be achieved during maximal stimulation with CRH. With severe illness, the requirements for cortisol may increase up to tenfold; failure to achieve these levels of cortisol during such periods may result in clinical adrenal insufficiency when adrenal reserve is impaired.

The immune system is tightly linked to the hypothalamic-pituitary-adrenal (HPA) axis. Glucocorticoids inhibit immune function, and immune mediators such as interleukin 1 are potent stimulators of ACTH secretion. These mediators may explain at least part of the link between "stress" and activation of the HPA axis, the subsequent cortisol response serving to limit the immune response.

In normal persons, ACTH circulates in low concentrations [2 to 18 pmol/L (10 to 80 pg/mL)]. It is difficult to measure ACTH in plasma and often not possible to separate low from normal values using commercial assays. Random ACTH measurements have little clinical significance. Tests for adrenal insufficiency and excess rely primarily on measurements of cortisol and its metabolites rather than on measurement of ACTH.

ACTH EXCESS (CUSHING'S DISEASE AND NELSON'S SYNDROME) Clinical features

Cortisol excess is characterized by a central distribution of adipose tissue, muscle weakness, purplish striae, hypertension, amenorrhea, osteoporosis, fatigue, and psychiatric abnormalities. This syndrome may be caused by pituitary or ectopic ACTH overproduction, adrenal tumors, or exogenous glucocorticoid administration.

The presence of cortisol excess is established by the finding of increased excretion of urine free cortisol and/or 17-hydroxycorticosteroids that fails to decrease appropriately after either overnight (1 mg at midnight) or 2-day low-dose dexamethasone administration (0.5 mg every 6 h for eight doses). Additional suppression (and occasionally stimulation) tests are required to determine whether the Cushing's syndrome is due to a pituitary lesion. In patients with pituitary ACTH hypersecretion, high-dose overnight dexamethasone administration (8 mg at midnight) results in greater than 50 percent reduction in the 8 A.M. plasma cortisol. Two-day dexamethasone administration (2 mg every 6 h for eight doses) generally results in greater than 60 percent suppression of urine 17-hydroxycorticosteroids and greater than 90 percent suppression of urine free cortisol. Urine 17-hydroxycorticosteroids increase after metyrapone administration in Cushing's disease. Plasma ACTH levels are normal or high-normal and show an exaggerated increase after CRH administration. Pituitary ACTH hypersecretion (Cushing's disease) is caused by a corticotroph microadenoma in 90 percent of patients and by a macroadenoma in most of the rest. Corticotroph hyperplasia has been documented in a few cases. The microadenomas are often small (3 to 6 mm or less) and may be difficult to find even with the use of gadolinium-enhanced MRI. Previously, pituitary surgery was often recommended on the basis of dynamic testing alone. However, bilateral inferior petrosal sinus catheterization with or without CRH administration to localize the site of ACTH production can be used to confirm the pituitary source of ACTH production and to localize adenomas. when all imaging studies are negative. Nelson's syndrome (characterized by hyperpigmentation despite adequate glucocorticoid replacement therapy) is caused by growth of the residual pituitary tumor after bilateral adrenalectomy in patients with pituitary Cushing's disease. These tumors are usually easily identified on MRI or CT scanning and may exhibit aggressive growth patterns.

Treatment Transsphenoidal microsurgery is successful in treating microadenomas in about 75 percent of patients. When surgery is successful, plasma cortisol concentrations fall almost to zero and often remain low for many months owing to delayed recovery of CRH and ACTH secretion by the hypothalamus and normal remaining pituitary. However, adrenal function eventually returns to normal in most patients. Cushing's syndrome may recur, however, even after apparently curative surgery. Previously, bilateral adrenalectomy was the therapy of choice for patients with pituitary Cushing's disease. Unfortunately, after this procedure, enlarging pituitary adenomas with increased skin pigmentation (Nelson's syndrome) develop in 10 to 30 percent of patients.

Ectopic ACTH production is a relatively common disorder and can cause great difficulty in diagnosis (see Chaps. 327 and 335). When ACTH production is caused by rapidly growing tumors such as oat cell carcinoma of the lung, symptoms of Cushing's syndrome are blunted. Rather, patients have hypokalemia, muscle weakness, weight loss, and hyperpigmentation. ACTH concentrations often exceed 66 pmol/L (300 pg/mL) and do not change with dexamethasone administration. ACTH concentrations may be lower in IRMA assays

than in radioimmunoassays; the IRMA assays do not measure larger fragments of the POMC molecule. When slow-growing tumors such as thymic carcinoids, bronchial carcinoids, medullary carcinoma of the thyroid, and pancreatic islet cell tumors produce ACTH, the typical features of Cushing's syndrome are common. In the latter group, ACTH measurements and cortisol response to dexamethasone administration may mimic those found in patients with pituitary adenomas. However, with ectopic ACTH production, ACTH concentrations generally do not change after CRH administration. When differentiation between pituitary and ectopic ACTH production is uncertain, bilateral inferior petrosal sinus catheterization is necessary. Cushing's syndrome can rarely be caused by ectopic production of CRH itself.

ACTH DEFICIENCY (SECONDARY ADRENAL INSUFFICIENCY)

ACTH deficiency may be isolated or occur in association with other anterior pituitary hormone deficiencies. Reversible isolated ACTH deficiency is common after long-term glucocorticoid administration. If glucocorticoids are withdrawn suddenly in this situation or continued in physiologic doses when severe illness is present, adrenal insufficiency may occur (see Chap. 335). Symptoms include nausea, vomiting, fatigue, joint discomfort, and dizziness, and there may be fever, hypotension, hyponatremia, and hypoglycemia. Reversible dementia may occur in the elderly. Although cortisol is necessary for free water excretion, it is not needed for potassium excretion. Hence patients with ACTH deficiency are hyponatremic but not hyperkalemic as are patients with primary adrenal insufficiency. Hyperpigmentation does not occur. These factors make diagnosis of secondary adrenal insufficiency more difficult than that of primary adrenal insufficiency. Isolated ACTH deficiency may occur without prior glucocorticoid therapy and may be of hypothalamic or pituitary origin. The diagnosis is often missed.

In general, patients undergoing pituitary surgery need to be treated with "stress" doses of glucocorticoids until normal adrenal function can be demonstrated postoperatively. All patients with pituitary macroadenomas or hypothalamic disease require testing of the pituitary-adrenal axis, but when pituitary surgery is planned, testing can be limited in focus until after surgery is completed.

THE ENDOGENOUS OPIOID PEPTIDES

The endogenous opioid peptides bind to a family of opioid receptors. The endorphins, enkephalins, and dynorphins, although chemically related, arise from different biosynthetic pathways (Fig. 331-7). In the pituitary, β-endorphin, the most abundant endorphin, is synthesized as part of a larger precursor molecule (pro-opiomelanocortin, POMC) that also contains the full sequence of ACTH, α-melanocyte-stimulating hormone (α-MSH), β-MSH, and β-lipotropin (β-LPH) (Fig. 331-8). This biosynthetic pathway represents the only pathway for pituitary ACTH synthesis. Hence ACTH and β-endorphin biosynthesis are inextricably linked in the pituitary. In adrenal insufficiency, plasma levels of both ACTH and β-endorphin are elevated; likewise, glucocorticoid administration decreases the levels of both. CRH stimulates the release of both ACTH and β-endorphin in a parallel manner; in Nelson's syndrome, the plasma levels of both ACTH and β-endorphin are elevated. Ectopic production of ACTH by tumors is also accompanied by β-endorphin excess. Although it was hoped that differential processing of POMC by tumors would allow separation of pituitary from ectopic ACTH production, analysis of metabolites is rarely helpful in individual cases. Production of "big" and "big-big" ACTH by tumors reflects the incomplete processing of the POMC precursor. Alternative processing of POMC occurs within other tissues. Therefore, although different cell types may synthesize the same primary gene product, the final profile of hormone secretion can differ completely. The hypothalamus also produces POMC in neurons and may convert POMC to smaller fragments than the anterior pituitary.

Two other opioid precursors give rise to potent endogenous

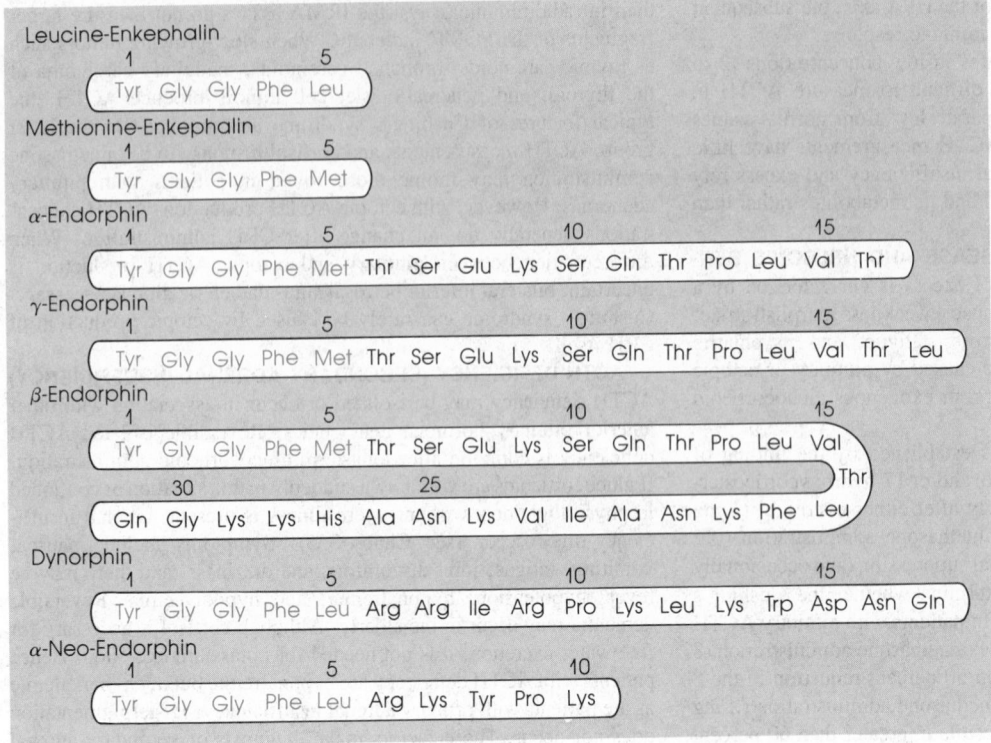

FIGURE 331-7 Structure of several endogenous opiate peptides. The amino-terminal (leftmost) four amino acids are identical in each peptide. At position 5, a methionine or leucine is found.

opioids, including the enkephalins, dynorphins, and neoendorphins. Proenkephalin A gives rise to four copies of met-enkephalin, one copy of leu-enkephalin, and several other opioid compounds; proenkephalin B (also called *prodynorphin*) includes the sequence for the potent opioid dynorphin, several neoendorphins, and other opioids. These opioid precursors are produced in many parts of the brain, including various hypothalamic nuclei. Opioids are also produced in the adrenal medulla, where they are packaged and released with epinephrine both in normal individuals and in patients with pheochromocytomas.

The pituitary is the richest site of endorphin in the body. ACTH- and endorphin-containing cells are found in the anteromedial region of the anterior lobe, at the posterior boundary of the anterior lobe, and in nerve fibers of the posterior lobe. The endorphin- and ACTH-synthesizing neurons of the hypothalamus also project to other regions of the brain. The limbic system contains substantial quantities of immunoreactive β-endorphin, suggesting a role in memory, learning, and emotion.

Neurons containing the enkephalins are even more widely distributed in the central nervous system. Levels are particularly high in the dorsal horn of the spinal cord, a region that contains opiate receptors and is involved in the transmission of pain (see Chap. 11). Enkephalins may act at this location to inhibit pain transmission by sensory nerves. Enkephalin concentrations in the myenteric plexus of the longitudinal muscles of the gastrointestinal tract are higher than in the brain. Enkephalin is released as part of the sympathetic response to stress together with epinephrine and norepinephrine; plasma enkephalin levels are high in patients with pheochromocytoma.

Two approaches have been employed to define the physiologic role of the endogenous opiates: assessment of the effects of administration of morphine or endogeneous opiate peptides and study of the effects of antagonists. Five opiate receptor types have been identified, making it difficult to draw general conclusions from the use of antagonists. Naloxone blocks the effects of endogenously secreted opiates on mu and epsilon receptors, revealing a tonic or physiologic role of opiate peptides. The opiates themselves inhibit gonadotropin release; this may explain the amenorrhea of narcotic addicts. Opiates decrease the function of the pituitary-adrenal axis in humans and stimulate GH and prolactin secretion. Naloxone causes elevations of LH and FSH levels and may prevent the stress-mediated rise in prolactin levels. ACTH and cortisol are elevated only after high doses of naloxone. Naloxone may inhibit vasopressin release in some patients with the syndrome of inappropriate vasopressin secretion (SIADH).

Physiologic actions for these hormones may include (1) morphine-like analgesic properties, (2) euphoria and other behavioral effects, and (3) neurotransmitter and neuromodulator functions. The peptides may play a role in memory, learning, response to stress, reproduction, pain transmission, and regulation of appetite, temperature, and respiration. In addition, the placebo response, acupuncture-mediated analgesia, stress-induced amenorrhea, and the pathogenesis of shock may be mediated in part by enkephalins and the endorphins. Tranquilization, irritability, agitation, violent behavior, catalepsy, narcolepsy, catatonia, the smoking habit, alcoholism, and drug addiction may all be due to biochemical abnormalities of this system.

FIGURE 331-8 Biosynthetic pathway for β-endorphin in the pituitary gland. A single precursor protein, pro-opiomelanocortin (POMC) (molecular weight of approximately 31,000), is initially synthesized from translation of a gene that encodes the structure of adrenocorticotropin (ACTH), β-lipotropin (β-LPH), and β-endorphin. Prohormone-type cleavages can generate other hormones from the same precursor, although this occurs in tissues other than the pituitary. Abbreviations: MSH = melanocyte-stimulating hormone; LPH = lipotropin; CLIP = corticotropin-like intermediate peptide; ACTH = adrenocorticotropin.

DISEASES OF THE HYPOTHALAMUS AND PITUITARY

Diseases that affect the hypothalamus and pituitary can have both endocrine and nonendocrine manifestations.

HYPOTHALAMUS The human hypothalamus weighs only about 4 g; hypothalamic dysfunction occurs only when disease is bilateral. Tumors in this region are often slow-growing and may achieve large size before symptoms appear. Signs of hydrocephalus due to third ventricle obstruction may coexist with hypopituitarism and hypothalamic dysfunction. Neurologic symptoms and signs may be caused by compression of the optic nerve, chiasm, or tract (see Chap. 19). Large tumors may affect frontal or temporal lobe function.

Nonendocrine functions of the hypothalamus include:

1 Food intake and feeding behavior. The basal hypothalamus controls maintenance of a stable weight. Several regions of the hypothalamus are implicated in hunger and satiety. The ventromedial nucleus is known to be involved in satiety, but it now appears that anterior hypothalamic regions are also concerned. Stimulation of appetite and termination of food ingestion are affected by many neuropeptides and neurotransmitters. Appetite is stimulated by γ-aminobutyric acid (GABA), dopamine, β-endorphin, enkephalin, and neuropeptide Y; appetite is inhibited by serotonin, norepinephrine, cholecystokinin, neurotensin, TRH, naloxone, somatostatin, and vasoactive intestinal peptide (VIP). Hypothalamic obesity in humans is usually associated with lesions in the vicinity of the ventromedial nucleus; this obesity appears to involve a resetting of the weight set point. With tumors in this area, aggressive behavior and marked hyperphagia (possibly related to rapid gastric emptying) occur until the new weight set point is reached. Patients often demonstrate decreased activity and finicky eating once the new set point is reached. Other factors including thyroid and adrenal hormones also influence feeding behavior. Acute hypothalamic damage often causes hyperglycemia, whereas chronic damage may rarely be associated with hypoglycemia.

2 Temperature regulation. The anterior hypothalamus contains warm- and cold-sensitive neurons that respond to local and environmental thermal gradients (see Chaps. 16 and 398). The posterior hypothalamus generates the signals necessary for heat dissipation, and serotonin stimulates heat production, which is blocked by norepinephrine and epinephrine. The temperature increase associated with infections is generated by the hypothalamus. Phagocytic cells throughout the body produce interleukin 1 (endogenous pyrogen), which stimulates the anterior hypothalamus to produce prostaglandin E_2. Prostaglandin E_2 raises the thermostat set point, leading to heat conservation (e.g., vasoconstriction) and increased heat production (e.g., muscle shivering) until blood and core temperatures match the new hypothalamic set point.

Abnormalities of temperature regulation may occur with hypothalamic disease. Hypothermia is a rare consequence of diffuse hypothalamic disease. Paroxysmal hypothermia due to sweating and vasodilatation is accompanied by fatigue, decreased alertness, hypoventilation, and arrhythmias; this syndrome is not prevented by anticonvulsants. Acute hyperthermia may accompany acute pathologic processes such as hemorrhage into the third ventricle, hypothalamic surgery, or hypothalamic infarction. Poikilothermia (a change in body temperature of greater than 1°C with change in environmental temperature) is usually a consequence of posterior hypothalamic disease. Paroxysmal hyperthermia with episodic shaking chills, spiking fevers, and autonomic phenomena is uncommon but may respond to anticonvulsants. It is important to remember that adrenal insufficiency can cause fever or hypothermia and that hypothyroidism may cause hypothermia.

3 Sleep-wake cycle. Lesions in the sleep center of the anterior hypothalamus result in insomnia and agitation, as in some patients with encephalitis. The posterior hypothalamus is important for arousal and maintenance of the waking state; posterior hypothalamic destruction due to ischemia, encephalitis, or trauma can result in a hypersomnolent state from which arousal is possible. Larger lesions extending to the reticular formation of the rostral midbrain cause coma (see Chap. 26).

4 Memory and behavior. Lesions of the ventromedial hypothalamus and premammillary region result in loss of short-term memory, often with Korsakoff's syndrome. However, dorsomedial thalamic lesions correlate best with memory loss (see Chap. 377). Longer-term memory is often intact. Large hypothalamic lesions also may cause symptoms and signs of dementia. The role of ACTH, ACTH fragments, vasopressin, and oxytocin in memory integration is under investigation. Rage reactions may result with ventromedial lesions, and lateral hypothalamic destruction may cause an apathetic state.

5 Thirst. The hypothalamus is the center for vasopressin production and for the control of thirst by serum osmolality. Impaired thirst may occur with hypothalamic lesions; rarely, primary polydipsia without diabetes insipidus is a consequence of hypothalamic lesions (see Chap. 333).

6 Autonomic nervous system function. Parasympathetic outputs are organized in the anterior hypothalamus; sympathetic pathways in the posterior hypothalamus. Diencephalic epilepsy is a rare syndrome associated with paroxysms of autonomic hyperactivity. This syndrome is not clearly epileptic in nature and does not usually respond to anticonvulsants. The clinical picture may mimic that of pheochromocytoma.

A diencephalic syndrome in children, characterized by emaciation, hyperkinesis, and inappropriate affect, often with a cheerful disposition, can be caused by invasive tumors of the anterior and basal hypothalamus. Most of these children die by the age of 2 years, but in those who survive the clinical picture changes to one of increased appetite with obesity, irritability, and rage reactions.

In general, slow-growing tumors produce dementia, disturbances of food intake (obesity or emaciation), and endocrine dysfunction. Acute destructive processes are more likely to cause coma or disturbances of the autonomic nervous system.

Diseases of the anterior hypothalamus include craniopharyngiomas, gliomas of the optic nerve, sphenoid ridge meningiomas, granulomatous disease (including sarcoidosis), germinomas, and aneurysms of the internal carotid artery. Suprasellar pituitary adenomas and tuberculum sella meningiomas may grow into the hypothalamus as well. Lesions of the posterior hypothalamus include gliomas, hamartomas, ependymomas, germinomas, and teratomas.

Precocious puberty, particularly in males, can be associated with "pinealomas." However, these pinealomas actually are germinomas, and the precocious puberty appears to result from the ectopic production of hCG by these tumors rather than from an effect on pituitary gonadotropins.

Craniopharyngiomas Craniopharyngiomas arise from remnants of Rathke's pouch and represent 3 to 5 percent of all intracranial neoplasms. Most of these tumors are suprasellar, but about 15 percent are intrasellar. The tumors are usually cystic or partially cystic, often contain calcium, and are lined with stratified squamous epithelium. Although craniopharyngiomas are usually manifested in childhood, 45 percent of patients are over age 20, and 20 percent are over age 40 at the time of diagnosis.

Children usually present with signs of increased intracranial pressure due to hydrocephalus (80 percent), including headache, vomiting, and papilledema. Visual abnormalities such as loss of vision and field cuts are found in 60 percent. Short stature is sometimes found (7 to 40 percent), but retarded bone age is more common. Delayed sexual development occurs in about 20 percent, and diabetes insipidus may be present.

About 80 percent of adults present with visual complaints, and an additional 10 percent have visual abnormalities on careful testing. Papilledema is present in about 15 percent of adults. Headaches (40 percent), mental deterioration or personality change (26 percent), and hypogonadism (35 percent) are relatively common in adults. Hyperprolactinemia is present in one-third to one-half of patients, but prolactin levels rarely exceed 100 to 150 μg/L. Diabetes insipidus (15 percent), weight gain (15 percent), and panhypopituitarism (7 percent) may occur as well. Rarely, the cyst contents spill into the cerebrospinal fluid, causing a picture of aseptic meningitis. Craniopharyngiomas may enlarge and become symptomatic during pregnancy.

Suprasellar calcification (see Fig. 331-15) in a flocculent, granular, or curvilinear pattern is present on skull x-rays in most children and in some adults with craniopharyngioma. Calcification is evident on CT scan in most of these adults, however. Hypothalamic germinomas may calcify as well. Skull x-ray abnormalities include calcification, sellar enlargement, and signs of increased intracranial pressure in 90 percent of children and 60 percent of adults.

Therapy of craniopharyngiomas is often unsatisfactory. Total removal often results in major functional deficits. We generally favor biopsy and partial resection followed by conventional radiation as a more conservative approach. Tumors less than 3 cm in diameter have a better prognosis.

Germ cell tumors   Germinomas originate in the posterior third ventricle, in the anterior third ventricle (supra- or intrasellar), or in both locations (also see Chap. 322). Germinomas (also known as *atypical teratomas*) were previously confused with parenchymal tumors of the pineal (pinealomas); when located in the anterior third ventricle, they were known as "ectopic pinealomas." Germinomas often infiltrate the hypothalamus and occasionally metastasize to the cerebrospinal fluid or distant sites.

The majority of patients have diabetes insipidus in association with variable anterior pituitary insufficiency. Precocious puberty may occur in boys, probably due to hCG production by these tumors. Diplopia, headache, vomiting, lethargy, weight loss, and hydrocephalus are common. The tumors usually begin in childhood but may be diagnosed in young adults. Because germinomas are radiosensitive, early recognition is important. Germinomas of the nonseminoma type may produce hCG and/or alpha fetoprotein, whereas pure seminomas rarely produce tumor markers (see Chap. 369). Elevated cerebrospinal fluid concentrations of hCG or alpha fetoprotein are virtually diagnostic; when elevated, a biopsy is generally unnecessary. When tumor markers are absent, a biopsy should be considered. When the tumor is located in the anterior third ventricle, biopsy by the transsphenoidal route is often possible. Tumors in the pineal region are more difficult to biopsy, leading some authors to recommend empirical radiation therapy or chemotherapy, whereas others prefer surgical biopsy or debulking followed by radiation and chemotherapy (see Chap. 369).

PITUITARY ADENOMAS   Pituitary adenomas account for about 10 to 15 percent of intracranial neoplasms. They can cause anterior pituitary hormonal imbalance, structural problems related to invasion of surrounding structures, or syndromes of hormone excess. Small pituitary tumors are present in 6 to 24 percent of adults at autopsy. Incidental pituitary tumors (pituitary "incidentalomas") are recognized with increasing frequency now that cranial MRI and CT scans are commonly performed.

Pathology   Pituitary tumors were previously classified as basophilic, acidophilic, or chromophobic on the basis of hematoxylin and eosin staining. Corticotroph adenomas are generally basophilic; the more densely granulated prolactin-secreting tumors are acidophilic; the majority of prolactinomas, sparsely granulated GH-secreting tumors, TSH-secreting and gonadotropin-secreting tumors, and nonsecreting tumors are all chromophobic. Because this classification provides little insight into hormone production, it has been abandoned. Many nonfunctioning pituitary tumors, however, are still referred to as "chromophobes." One classification is based on immunohistochemical staining: corticotroph (ACTH and POMC), somatotroph (GH), thyrotroph (TSH), gonadotroph (LH and FSH), and lactotroph (prolactin).

Pituitary tumors can also be classified by size and invasive characteristics. The following classification is used by Kovacs and Horvath. Microadenomas are <10 mm; macroadenomas are ≥10 mm in greatest diameter. Microadenomas may cause hormonal overproduction but do not cause hypopituitarism, structural problems, or sellar enlargement. Intrapituitary adenomas are within the substance of the pituitary gland; intrasellar adenomas are confined to the sella. Diffuse adenomas may fill the sella and cause focal sellar wall erosions. The distinction between intrasellar and diffuse adenomas may be difficult to make. Invasive adenomas erode through the sella into surrounding tissues, including but not limited to the sphenoid bone, cavernous sinuses, optic chiasm, third ventricle, and brain. Pituitary carcinomas are rare but can give rise to distant metastases.

Endocrine manifestations   Anterior pituitary hormone overproduction is suspected on clinical grounds and confirmed by appropriate laboratory evaluation (see Table 331-5). The most common secretory pituitary tumors are prolactinomas. They cause galactorrhea and hypogonadism, including amenorrhea, infertility, and impotence. GH-secreting tumors are the next most common secretory pituitary tumors and cause acromegaly or gigantism. Next in frequency are corticotroph (ACTH-secreting) adenomas, which cause cortisol excess (Cushing's disease). Although glycoprotein hormone–secreting pituitary adenomas are common by histologic criteria, clinical syndromes of excess LH, FSH, or TSH are rare. TSH-secreting adenomas are a rare cause of hyperthyroidism. Paradoxically, most patients with gonadotropin-secreting adenomas have hypogonadism, although testicular enlargement or testosterone excess may occur.

About 15 percent of patients with tumors that come to surgery have adenomas that secrete more than one pituitary hormone. The most common combination is GH and prolactin, and other common patterns are GH-TSH, GH-prolactin-TSH, and ACTH-prolactin. Most of these tumors have one cell secreting two hormones (unimorphous), but some tumors have two or more cell types, each of which produces a single hormone (polymorphous).

Prolactinomas in women and corticotroph adenomas in both sexes are usually diagnosed while still microadenomas. In contrast, the majority of patients with acromegaly and most men with prolactinomas have macroadenomas at the time of diagnosis. Glycoprotein hormone–secreting tumors are also usually quite large at the time of diagnosis.

About 30 to 40 percent of pituitary adenomas that come to surgery are apparently nonsecretory, although most stain immunohistochemically for pituitary hormones. These statistics are influenced by the fact that most prolactinomas do not require surgery. In some cases, particularly in the case of gonadotropin-secreting tumors, hormonal secretion is overlooked. Some of the "nonfunctioning" pituitary tumors, as well as some functional ones, secrete part of the glycoprotein hormone molecule, most commonly the alpha subunit. In general, tumors without endocrine-related symptoms are large at the time of diagnosis and often cause structural problems. Alpha subunit excess is a frequent finding in patients with TSH-secreting adenomas, and LH beta may be hypersecreted in patients with gonadotropin-secreting tumors.

Null cell tumors (no specific hormones identified by immunostaining) also are generally large when diagnosed, since no hormonal overproduction is present to provide early clues to diagnosis. Oncocytomas are nonsecretory pituitary adenomas with abundant mitochondria, commonly found in older men.

Pituitary adenomas are occasionally part of the multiple endocrine neoplasia type 1 (MEN 1) syndrome (see Chap. 343). This dominantly inherited disease causes adenomas of the pituitary gland, secretory tumors of the endocrine pancreas, and hyperparathyroidism involving multiple parathyroid glands. Pituitary adenomas may secrete GH or prolactin or may be nonfunctioning. Insulinomas and gastrinomas are the most common pancreatic tumors in MEN 1. Pancreatic GHRH-secreting tumors can cause acromegaly and pituitary hyperplasia.

Mass effects of pituitary tumors   VISUAL FIELD DEFECTS   The optic chiasm lies anterior and superior to the pituitary gland, usually 8 to 13 mm above the diaphragma sella, and in 80 percent of normal persons overlies the pituitary fossa; in about 15 percent the chiasm is anterior to the tuberculum sella (prefixed), and in 5 percent it

TABLE 331-5 Pituitary hormone evaluation

Hormone	Excess	Deficiency
Growth hormone	*1* Measurement of plasma growth hormone 1 h following glucose PO *2* Measurement of IGF-I/SM-C	*1* Measurement of plasma growth hormone 30, 60, and 120 min after one of the following: 　*a* Regular insulin 0.1 to 0.15 unit/kg IV 　*b* Levodopa 10 mg/kg PO 　*c* L-*Arginine 0.5 mg/kg intravenously over 30 min* *2* Measurement of IGF-I/SM-C
Prolactin	*1* Measurement of basal serum prolactin, preferably fasting	*1* Measurement of serum prolactin 10 to 20 min after one of the following: 　*a* TRH 200 to 500 μg IV 　*b* Chlorpromazine 25 mg IM
TSH	*1* Measurement of T_4, free T_4 index, T_3, TSH, TSH alpha	*1* Measurement of T_4, free T_4, free T_4 index, TSH
Gonadotropins	*1* Measurement of FSH, LH, LH beta, testosterone, FSH beta, FSH response to TRH	*1* Measurement of basal LH, FSH in postmenopausal women; no measurements in menstruating, ovulating women *2* Testosterone, FSH, and LH in men
ACTH	*1* Measurement of urine free cortisol* *2* Dexamethasone suppression by one of the following: 　*a* Measurement of 8 A.M. plasma cortisol after administration of 1 mg dexamethasone at midnight 　*b* Measurement of 8 A.M. plasma cortisol or 24-h urine 17-hydroxysteroids or free cortisol after 0.5 mg dexamethasone PO q 6 h for 8 doses† *3* High-dose dexamethasone suppression by one of the following: 　*a* Measurement of plasma cortisol after 8 mg dexamethasone PO at midnight 　*b* Measurement of 8 A.M. plasma cortisol or 24-h urine 17-hydroxysteroids or free cortisol after 2 mg dexamethasone q 6 h for 8 doses *4* Metyrapone response (same protocol as for deficiency testing) *5* Response of plasma ACTH to ovine corticotropin releasing hormone (1 μg/kg body wt)	*1* Measurement of serum cortisol at 30 and 60 min following regular insulin 0.05 to 0.15 units per kilogram IV *2* Metyrapone response by one of the following: 　*a* Measurement of plasma 11-deoxycortisol at 8 A.M. after 30 mg/kg body wt metyrapone at midnight (maximal dose 2 g) 　*b* Measurement of 24-h urinary 17-hydroxycorticoids or plasma 11-deoxycortisol day of and day after 750 mg metyrapone q 4 h for 6 doses† 　*c* Measurement of 24-h urinary 17-hydroxycorticoids day of and day after 500 mg metyrapone q 2 h for 12 doses† *3* ACTH stimulation test: Measurement of plasma cortisol and aldosterone at 0 and 60 min after IM or IV administration of 0.25 mg cosyntropin *4* ?Response of plasma ACTH to ovine corticotropin-releasing hormone (1 μg/kg body weight)
Arginine vasopressin (AVP)	*1* Measurement of serum sodium and osmolality, urine osmolality in presence of normal renal, adrenal, thyroid function *2* Simultaneous measurement of serum osmolality and ADH levels	*1* Comparison of urine osmolality and serum osmolality under conditions of increased AVP secretion‡ *2* Simultaneous measurement of serum osmolality and AVP levels

* Tests 1 and 2 establish the diagnosis of Cushing's syndrome. Tests 3, 4, and 5 localize the Cushing's disease to the pituitary gland. Often bilateral inferior petrosal sinus catheterization will be necessary.

† Give food with metyrapone, patient hospitalized.

‡ May be achieved by water deprivation or saline administration.

overlaps the dorsum sella posteriorly (postfixed). Since 90 percent of the chiasmal axons originate in the macula, loss of central vision is an early finding. Foggy or dim vision is also described by many patients.

The most common visual field defect in patients with pituitary adenomas is a bitemporal hemianopsia, and about 8 percent of patients develop complete loss of vision in one eye with a temporal defect in the opposite eye. Alternatively, patients may demonstrate bitemporal scotomas rather than hemianopsia, particularly with a rapidly growing lesion in association with a prefixed chiasm (see Chap. 19). For this reason, visual field examinations must assess more than the lateral fields of vision. Of those patients with visual field defects, about 9 percent have a single eye defect, most commonly a superior temporal defect. Occasionally, there is a monocular field loss such as a central scotoma that mimics nonpituitary lesions. Pituitary adenomas causing visual field defects are macroadenomas with suprasellar extension; sellar enlargement is the rule.

OCULOMOTOR PALSIES Pituitary adenomas may extend laterally, invade the cavernous sinuses, and cause oculomotor palsies. When this occurs, visual field defects are usually not present. Involvement of the third cranial nerve is most common and may mimic diabetic third nerve neuropathy in that pupillary reactivity is usually preserved (see Chap. 19). Additional findings associated with lateral extension of the adenoma may include involvement of the fourth and sixth cranial nerves, pain or numbness in the distribution of the fifth cranial nerve, and compression or obstruction of the carotid artery.

Headaches are common in patients with larger tumors and are also present in the majority of patients with acromegaly. Headaches may be exacerbated by coughing. Headaches are thought to be due to stretching of the diaphragma sella but may be vascular in origin and

may be referred to several locations, including the vertex of skull and to retroorbital, frontooccipital, frontotemporal, or occipital-cervical areas.

Very large pituitary tumors may invade the hypothalamus and cause hyperphagia, abnormal temperature regulation, loss of consciousness, and loss of hormonal input from the hypothalamus. Obstructive hydrocephalus involving the third ventricle or causing diabetes insipidus is less common with pituitary adenomas than with craniopharyngiomas. Tumor invasion of the temporal lobe may cause complex partial seizures; invasion of the posterior fossa may be associated with brainstem dysfunction, and invasion into the frontal lobes causes alterations in mental state and frontal release signs.

PITUITARY APOPLEXY Acute hemorrhagic infarction of a pituitary adenoma may cause a dramatic syndrome including severe headache, nausea, vomiting, and depression of consciousness. Ophthalmoplegia, visual and pupillary disturbances, and meningismus may be present. Most of these symptoms are caused by direct pressure from the tumor, whereas meningismus results from blood in the cerebrospinal fluid. The syndrome may either evolve slowly over a period of 24 to 48 h or may lead to sudden death.

Pituitary apoplexy is found most commonly in patients with somatotroph or corticotroph adenomas, but it may be the first clinical manifestation of a pituitary tumor. Both anticoagulation and radiotherapy predispose to hemorrhagic infarction. Rarely, pituitary apoplexy produces "autohypophysectomy" with "cure" of acromegaly, Cushing's disease, or hyperprolactinemia. Hypopituitarism is a common sequela; although hormonal measurements may be normal during the acute phase, cortisol and gonadal steroid concentrations decline over the ensuing days, and thyroxine concentrations decline over weeks. Diabetes insipidus is rare.

It is important to differentiate between pituitary apoplexy and a leaking aneurysm; MRI may allow this distinction to be made, but angiography is often required. Acute pituitary apoplexy is generally considered a neurosurgical emergency and may require acute decompression of the pituitary, generally via the transsphenoidal route. Many pituitary tumors contain small hemorrhagic foci that are clinically silent.

Therapy of pituitary adenomas Ideal therapy for pituitary adenomas would permanently correct hormonal hypersecretion without causing hypopituitarism and would shrink or remove the tumor mass without additional morbidity or mortality. Therapy for microadenomas may achieve both these goals, whereas therapy for macroadenomas is usually less successful. In considering therapy, it is critical to weigh the disability due to the tumor against any disability that may arise from the treatment. Regardless of tumor size, the therapy should not be worse than the disease. Potentially serious diseases such as Cushing's disease or acromegaly may require more aggressive treatment than do prolactinomas. (See also sections on individual pituitary hormones in this chapter.)

MEDICAL THERAPY Bromocriptine, a dopamine agonist, is the therapy of choice in the United States for most patients with microprolactinomas who require therapy. Bromocriptine corrects hyperprolactinemia in almost all patients with microprolactinomas; however, when the drug is stopped, prolactin levels often return to pretreatment levels. More potent dopapime agonists are available outside the United States.

Bromocriptine side effects of nausea, gastric irritation, and postural hypotension can be minimized by initially giving a low dose (1.25 mg) at bedtime with a snack. Other side effects include headache, fatigue, abdominal cramps, nasal congestion, and constipation. The dosage is gradually increased to a twice-daily schedule (most commonly 2.5 mg bid). Vaginal bromocriptine is better tolerated by some patients.

Bromocriptine is also effective in large prolactin-secreting macroadenomas. (Nonfunctioning macroadenomas with minimal prolactin elevation must be excluded.) Prolactin is lowered by at least 80 percent in 90 percent and to normal values in about 37 percent of patients. Abnormal visual fields return to normal in most; the tumor shrinks by 50 percent in about 40 percent of patients within 3 months. Tumor shrinkage may be accompanied by reversal of hypopituitarism. With giant adenomas, bromocriptine-induced tumor shrinkage may rarely cause a devastating intracranial hemorrhage. Prolactin levels quickly rise when bromocriptine is stopped; however, tumor regrowth may be delayed.

Surgery is required when visual field defects do not rapidly return to normal (e.g., after 1 to 3 months of bromocriptine). Symptomatic hyperprolactinemia with inadequate response to bromocriptine requires further therapy with surgery and/or radiation. In the United States, bromocriptine is usually stopped at the onset of pregnancy and reinstituted if tumor regrowth is symptomatic; alternatively, bromocriptine can be continued throughout pregnancy, although it is not licensed for this indication in the United States.

The somatostatin analogue octreotide is the most effective adjunctive therapy in acromegaly; it also may be appropriate as temporary primary therapy or in preparation for surgery. Bromocriptine is an effective adjunct in some patients with acromegaly, particularly those with coexistent hyperprolactinemia. GH concentrations rarely return to normal, but symptomatic improvement and tumor shrinkage may occur. Bromocriptine or octreotide (though not licensed for this purpose) should be considered in acromegalic subjects whose GH or IGF-I/SM-C levels remain elevated following surgery or who are waiting for radiation therapy to be effective. Nonfunctioning and gonadotropin-secreting adenomas usually shrink 10 percent or less in response to bromocriptine, even when high doses are used. Octreotide also may be useful adjunctive therapy in patients with TSH-secreting adenomas.

SURGERY Transsphenoidal surgery of pituitary microadenomas is safe and frequently corrects hormonal oversecretion. Hormonal overproduction is corrected within 24 h in 75 percent of patients with Cushing's disease due to corticotroph microadenomas, acromegaly with GH concentrations of <40 μg/L, and microprolactinomas associated with serum prolactin concentrations of <200 μg/L. The initial success rate for microprolactinomas varies among institutions, with reported figures ranging from 50 to 95 percent. Unfortunately, after initially successful surgery, hyperprolactinemia recurs in about 17 percent of patients followed for 3 to 5 years and possibly in 50 percent after 5 to 10 years. The recurrence rates after initially successful surgery in acromegaly and Cushing's disease are not well established but are substantial.

The mortality rate for transsphenoidal surgery of microadenomas is 0.27 percent, with a morbidity rate of about 1.7 percent, based on 2600 surgical procedures. Major complications include cerebrospinal fluid rhinorrhea, oculomotor palsy, and visual loss.

Pituitary surgery is less successful with larger secretory tumors. In patients with serum prolactin concentrations of >200 μg/L or GH concentrations of >40 μg/L, hormone concentrations return to normal in only 30 percent following surgery. Surgery is successful in about 40 to 60 percent of patients with Cushing's disease due to corticotroph macroadenomas. Recurrence rates with these secretory macroadenomas after a surgery-induced remission are uncertain; in the case of prolactin-secreting tumors, hyperprolactinemia recurs in 10 to 80 percent of patients. Whether pretreatment with octreotide in acromegalic patients with invasive macroadenomas improves the surgical success rate is under investigation.

Although visual field abnormalities are usually reversible with surgery, cure of the tumor is unlikely. The intrasellar portion of tumors invading the cavernous sinus may be debulked, but parasellar extension remains. Early series noted an 85 percent symptomatic recurrence (due to structural problems such as visual field defects) over 10 years in patients treated with surgery alone. When radiation therapy was used in combination with surgery, the 10-year recurrence was 15 percent. These series antedated modern radiologic techniques, hormone measurements, and medical therapy and may not be applicable to current practice.

Surgery for macroadenomas has a mortality rate of around 0.86 percent and a morbidity rate of about 6.3 percent. Hypopituitarism occurs in an additional 10 percent of patients. Transient diabetes insipidus occurs in about 5 percent, and permanent diabetes insipidus occurs in 1 percent. Major complications of surgery for macroadenoma include cerebrospinal fluid rhinorrhea (3.3 percent), permanent visual loss (1.5 percent), permanent oculomotor palsy (0.6 percent), and meningitis (0.5 percent).

We generally treat microprolactinomas with bromocriptine. However, we recommend surgery for those patients with microprolactinoma who require therapy and are intolerant of dopamine agonists. Surgery generally does not result in hypopituitarism in this relatively benign disease. Surgery is usually our treatment of choice in patients with acromegaly or Cushing's disease because in most instances rapid reversal of hormonal hypersecretion is essential and because cure can often be achieved. Since Cushing's disease and acromegaly are serious diseases, more extensive surgery that results in hypopituitarism may be required.

RADIATION THERAPY Conventional radiation therapy is effective in preventing tumor growth (70 to 90 percent) but is unsatisfactory in the acute management of pituitary hyperfunction. Therapy generally consists of 4500 cGy (4500 rad) at 1.8 Gy (180 rad) per day over 5 weeks using rotational techniques. GH values of <5 μg/L are achieved in half of acromegalics after 5 years and in 70 percent after 10 years; values of <2.5 μg/L are achieved in 40 percent and <1 μg/L in only 20 percent by 10 to 15 years. Data on IGF-I/SM-C are not readily available. Conventional radiation alone is rarely successful in treating corticotroph adenomas in adults. The major complications of conventional radiation are hypopituitarism in up to 50 percent and posttherapy lassitude and fatigue lasting many months in the majority. Whether subtle cognitive defects occur is less certain. We generally use radiation as an adjunct to surgery and medical therapy for patients with continued symptomatic hormonal oversecretion (GH and prolactin) and for those with substantial residual tumor after surgery or when tumor regrowth is rapid. Slow tumor regrowth over 5 or 6 years is usually treated with repeat surgery.

The "gamma knife" delivers 4000 to 10,000 cGy (4000 to 10,000 rad) through several hundred portals in a single session, thought to be equivalent to two to three times the total dose given by conventional radiation. Preliminary results using 4000 to 7000 cGy for acromegaly are comparable with those for conventional radiation. Therapy for Cushing's disease with 7000 to 10,000 cGy is apparently successful in up to 75 percent of adults; this is comparable to heavy-particle therapy (see below) and apparently more effective than conventional radiation therapy.

Heavy-particle therapy with proton beam or alpha particles is effective in treating secretory adenomas, but response is slow. Tumors with suprasellar extension or tissue invasion are generally excluded from such series. With proton beam therapy at the Harvard cyclotron, radiation doses of up to 14,000 cGy (14,000 rad) can be given safely without damage to surrounding structures. At 2 years, 28 percent of acromegalics achieve GH values of <5 μg/L; this response increases to 56 percent at 5 years and 75 percent by 10 years. Values of IGF-I/SM-C are not reported. With Cushing's disease proton beam corrects the hypercortisolism in 55 percent at 2 years and in 80 percent by 5 years. Proton beam therapy effectively lowers ACTH and stops growth of most corticotroph adenomas in patients with Nelson's syndrome, with the exception of adenomas that are invasive at the time of therapy. Long-term results for treatment of other tumors with proton beam therapy are not available.

Complications of heavy-particle therapy include hypopituitarism in at least 20 percent of patients, although the exact long-term prevalence of this complication is uncertain. Visual field defects and oculomotor dysfunction, usually temporary, have been reported in about 1.5 percent of patients. The major drawback of all forms of radiotherapy is the length of time that must elapse before hormonal hypersecretion is corrected.

Bromocriptine (or another dopamine agonist, where available) is the therapy of choice for macroprolactinomas. Surgery and/or radiation therapy is not usually necessary but may be required for patients with persistent structural problems, symptomatic hyperprolactinemia, or intolerance to dopamine agonists. Patients with nonfunctioning macroadenomas, including "incidentalomas," require transsphenoidal surgery when the macroadenoma is symptomatic, near the optic chiasm, or growing on serial MRI or CT scans. Indications for conventional and heavy-particle radiation are discussed below. Heavy-particle therapy (or possibly the "gamma knife") is an effective alternative to surgery in patients with acromegaly, Cushing's disease, or large intrasellar nonfunctioning tumors who have contraindications to or refuse surgery. We prefer bilateral adrenalectomy in patients whose pituitary Cushing's disease is not cured by one or two transsphenoidal operations; others employ heavy-particle or "gamma knife" radiation. Persistent acromegaly is treated with medical and/or radiation therapy. Transfrontal surgery is occasionally required, particularly in patients with giant adenomas.

Pituitary adenomas may be discovered during MRI or CT scanning of the brain for other purposes (pituitary "incidentaloma"). With pituitary microadenomas, hormonal overproduction must be identified and treated; hypopituitarism and structural symptoms do not occur. A follow-up scan at 6 months, then yearly for 2 years, and subsequently every 2 to 5 years seems reasonable.

Pituitary macroadenomas, however discovered, need to be evaluated for hormonal over- and underproduction and structural effects, including visual field abnormalities. The approach to the hormonally active tumor has been described above. Should nonfunctioning tumors be treated with bromocriptine? Is prophylactic surgery or radiation therapy indicated? How often should the MRI and endocrine evaluations be repeated? The answers are unknown. We tend to recommend surgery for tumors directly abutting on the optic chiasm. For other tumors, MRI scans should be repeated at 6 and 12 months and yearly

thereafter. If growth occurs, surgery or radiation with conventional radiation, "gamma knife," or protons may be indicated. Ten to fifteen percent of tumors shrink with bromocriptine therapy; how many stabilize without therapy is unknown.

HYPOPITUITARISM *Hypopituitarism* refers to deficiency of one or more pituitary hormones and has many causes (Table 331-6). Pituitary hormone deficiency may be congenital or acquired (see Chap. 332). Isolated GH or gonadotropin deficiency is common. Temporary ACTH deficiency as a consequence of long-term glucocorticoid therapy is also common, but permanent isolated deficiency of ACTH or TSH is rare. Deficiency of any of the anterior pituitary hormones may occur at the level of the pituitary gland or the hypothalamus. When diabetes insipidus is present, the primary defect is almost invariably in the hypothalamus or high pituitary stalk, often in conjunction with mild hyperprolactinemia and anterior pituitary hypofunction.

Manifestations of hypopituitarism depend on the specific pituitary hormones that are lacking. Growth failure due to GH deficiency is a common presenting complaint in children. GH deficiency in adults causes more subtle manifestations such as fine wrinkling around the eyes and mouth and in subjects with diabetes mellitus increased sensitivity to insulin. The cardiovascular mortality of GH-deficient individuals is increased. Complaints related to gonadotropin deficiency include amenorrhea and infertility in women and testosterone deficiency and decreased libido, decreased beard and body hair, and preservation of a youthful scalp hairline in men. TSH deficiency causes hypothyroidism with fatigue, cold intolerance, and puffy skin in the absence of goiter. ACTH deficiency results in cortisol deficiency, manifested by fatigue; decreased appetite; weight loss; decreased skin and nipple pigmentation; abnormal response to stress characterized by fever, hypotension, and hyponatremia; and a high mortality rate. Unlike primary adrenal insufficiency (Addison's disease) ACTH deficiency does not cause hyperpigmentation, hyperkalemia, or salt loss. With combined ACTH and gonadotropin deficiency, axillary and pubic hair may be lost. Children with combined GH and cortisol deficiency often develop hypoglycemia. AVP deficiency causes diabetes insipidus with polyuria and increased thirst. When pituitary adenomas impair anterior pituitary function, GH is often the first hormone to be compromised, followed by deficiencies of gonadotro-

TABLE 331-6 Causes of hypopituitarism

Isolated hormone deficiencies
  1 Congenital or acquired deficiencies
Tumors
  1 Large pituitary adenomas
  2 Pituitary apoplexy
  3 Hypothalamic tumors, e.g., craniopharyngiomas, germinomas, chordomas, meningiomas, gliomas, and others
  4 Metastatic carcinoma
Inflammatory diseases
  1 Granulomatous disease, e.g., sarcoidosis, tuberculosis, syphilis, granulomatous hypophysitis
  2 Eosinophilic granuloma
  3 Lymphocytic hypophysitis (autoimmune)
Vascular diseases
  1 Sheehan's postpartum necrosis
  2 ? Diabetic peripartum necrosis
  3 Carotid aneurysm
Destructive-traumatic events
  1 Surgery
  2 Stalk section
  3 Radiation (conventional—hypothalamus; heavy-particle—pituitary)
  4 Trauma
Developmental anomalies
  1 Pituitary aplasia
  2 Basal encephalocoele
Infiltration
  1 Hemochromatosis
  2 Amyloidosis
"Idiopathic" causes
  1 ?Autoimmune disease

pins, TSH, and ACTH. Panhypopituitarism may be accompanied by inappropriate secretion of vasopressin (see Chap. 333).

Etiology Damage to the anterior pituitary is commonly due to a pituitary adenoma (with or without infarction), pituitary surgery, heavy-particle pituitary irradiation, closed head trauma, or infarction during the postpartum period (Sheehan's syndrome). Postpartum pituitary infarction occurs in the setting of hemorrhage with systemic hypotension; vasospasm is thought to mediate the pituitary destruction that ensues. The enlarged pituitary gland of pregnancy may be more vulnerable to ischemia. Inability to lactate is the most common initial clinical clue, and other symptoms of hypopituitarism may unfold over months or years. The condition is sometimes diagnosed years after the primary event. Although clinical diabetes insipidus is rare in this setting, a decreased vasopressin response to appropriate stimuli is common. Patients with diabetes mellitus are also prone to develop hypopituitarism late in pregnancy.

Lymphocytic hypophysitis that causes hypopituitarism is primarily a disease of women either during pregnancy or in the postpartum period. In this syndrome, a mass lesion is often seen on MRI or CT scanning which, when biopsied, consists of lymphocytic infiltration. Lymphocytic hypophysitis is due to autoimmune pituitary destruction and often occurs with other autoimmune diseases such as Hashimoto's (autoimmune) thyroiditis and gastric atrophy (see Chaps. 334 and 343). Circulating antibodies to prolactin cells have been identified in some patients. It is not clear whether autoimmune hypophysitis is a common cause of "idiopathic" hypopituitarism in adults.

Hypothalamic or pituitary stalk damage has many causes (see Table 331-6). Certain lesions in this region, such as sarcoidosis, metastatic carcinoma, germinomas, histiocytosis, and craniopharyngiomas, commonly cause diabetes insipidus along with hypofunction of the anterior pituitary. Pituitary insufficiency, resulting from conventional radiation to the brain or the pituitary, is thought to be largely hypothalamic in origin, although diabetes insipidus generally does not occur.

"Functional" hypopituitarism is common. Anorexia nervosa, severe stress, and major illness are all associated with reversible LHRH deficiency. Emotional stress in children may cause GH deficiency and cessation of growth (*psychosocial dwarfism*). Severe illness may be associated with TSH and free T_4 deficiency (part of the "sick euthyroid" syndrome). ACTH deficiency occurs after long-term suppression of the hypothalamic-pituitary-adrenal axis; fortunately, ACTH deficiency is not a consequence of severe illness.

Diagnosis (See Table 331-5) To diagnose GH deficiency, the most reliable GH stimulus is insulin-induced hypoglycemia in which the blood sugar declines to less than 2.2 pmol/L (40 mg/dL) (Fig. 331-9). A GH concentration of >10 μg/L after hypoglycemia, levodopa, or arginine effectively excludes GH deficiency. Measuring the basal GH or serum IGF-I/SM-C concentration is less reliable, because GH levels are undetectable in normal persons for much of the day and because IGF-I/SM-C concentrations in patients with GH deficiency may overlap the normal range. Integrated 24-h GH secretion may be low in some short children with normal response to GH provocative stimuli.

Cortisol deficiency is potentially life-threatening. Basal cortisol function may be preserved in the face of extensive pituitary destruction; consequently, the ability of pituitary ACTH secretion to increase in response to "stress" must be assessed. Either the insulin tolerance test or the metyrapone test can be used to determine the adequacy of ACTH reserve; the ACTH stimulation test is a safer but less sensitive alternative. ACTH secretory dysfunction may occur after radiation therapy. Despite normal insulin tolerance tests, these individuals have low 24-h integrated cortisol secretion and excretion; symptomatic improvement occurs with glucocorticoid therapy.

The insulin tolerance test is safely performed on an outpatient basis in younger patients without heart disease or diseases predisposing to seizures (see Fig. 331-9 and Table 331-5). Both cortisol and GH responses are measured. If hypopituitarism is strongly suspected, a lower dose of regular insulin (0.05 to 0.1 units per kilogram of body

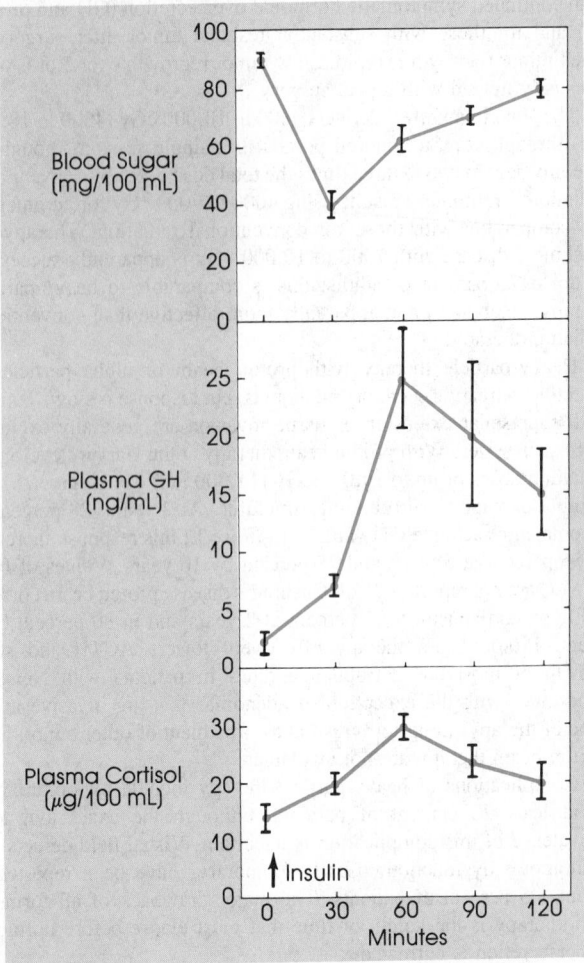

FIGURE 331-9 The insulin tolerance test. After an intravenous injection of regular insulin (0.1 unit per kilogram of body weight) a fall in blood sugar and rise in plasma GH and cortisol is expected. This test permits evaluation of both GH and ACTH in patients with pituitary disease. (*After KJ Catt, Lancet 1:933, 1970.*)

weight) should be employed. After adequate hypoglycemia, the peak plasma cortisol level should be greater than 500 nmol/L (19 μg/dL), although other criteria have been suggested. Since the metyrapone test can precipitate acute adrenal insufficiency in patients with low basal cortisol secretory rates, it should always be performed in the hospital setting when the 8 A.M. basal plasma cortisol level is less than 230 nmol/L (9 μg/dL). A normal response to metyrapone administration (see Table 331-5) has been variably defined, but one criterion is an increase of plasma 11-deoxycortisol to greater than 200 nmol/L (7.5 μg/dL) and of the urinary 17-hydroxysteroids to at least twofold over baseline, usually to a value greater than 60 μmol/d (22 mg/d). The plasma cortisol must concomitantly fall to less than 110 nmol/L (4 μg/dL) to ensure that there has been an adequate stimulus for ACTH release if these criteria have not been met. Although ACTH responses to insulin-hypoglycemia and metyrapone have not been well-standardized, a peak ACTH concentration of >40 pmol/L (200 pg/mL) is considered normal.

The rapid ACTH stimulation test (see Table 331-5) may be the safest and most convenient screening test for determining the adequacy of the pituitary-adrenal axis. Since the response of the adrenal gland to exogenous ACTH is dependent on prior endogenous ACTH exposure, it follows that patients with profound ACTH deficiency will have a deficient adrenal response to exogenous ACTH stimulation. However, the rapid ACTH stimulation test may be normal in some patients with abnormal insulin tolerance tests and therefore may not detect all who are at risk for stress-induced adrenal insufficiency.

Thus, whereas an abnormal ACTH stimulation test is indicative of an abnormal pituitary-adrenal axis, a normal response in the rapid ACTH stimulation test [cortisol >500 nmol/L (19 µg/dL)] does not always establish that the pituitary-adrenal axis is normal.

Gonadotropin function is easier to evaluate. In women with regular menses, gonadotropin secretion is normal, and gonadotropin measurements are superfluous. Likewise, a man with a normal serum testosterone level and normal spermatogenesis need not have gonadotropins measured. In postmenopausal women, gonadotropin levels are elevated (an endogenous stimulation test); "normal" levels suggest gonadotropin deficiency. Estrogen deficiency in women and testosterone deficiency in men in the absence of elevated gonadotropins imply gonadotropin deficiency.

To diagnose central hypothyroidism (thyrotropin deficiency), the serum T_4 and free T_4 (or T_3 resin uptake and free T_4 index) should first be measured. If these are in the midnormal range, TSH function is likely to be normal. If T_4 and free T_4 are low and the serum TSH level is not elevated, central hypothyroidism is present. Minimal TSH elevation (with bioinactive TSH) can occur in hypothalamic hypothyroidism, usually with low free T_4 concentrations. Mild central hypothyroidism, a consideration in patients with known pituitary disease who have low-normal T_4 and free T_4 concentrations, remains a clinical diagnosis. Before considering the diagnosis of isolated TSH deficiency in patients with the biochemical features of central hypothyroidism without evidence of other pituitary hormone deficiency, it is important to exclude the thyroxine-binding globulin (TBG) deficiency syndrome (low T_4, increased T_3 resin uptake, low to low-normal free T_4 index, normal TSH) and the "sick euthyroid" syndrome (low T_4, low free T_4 or free T_4 index, normal or low TSH) (see Chap. 334).

Several diagnostic tests utilize hypothalamic-releasing hormones to assess pituitary reserve. While these tests are *not helpful* in assessing the adequacy of anterior pituitary function, they can be useful in certain situations. In patients with isolated gonadotropin deficiency, the gonadotropin response to gonadorelin (synthetic LHRH) may be useful in predicting which patients will respond to therapy with gonadorelin. CRH testing may be useful in the differential diagnosis of Cushing's syndrome but does not indicate whether the pituitary-adrenal axis will respond appropriately to stress. TRH stimulation testing is useful in some patients in supporting the diagnosis of hyperthyroidism, recurrent acromegaly, or gonadotropin-secreting tumors and in those cases in which documentation of prolactin deficiency is necessary to support a diagnosis of more generalized anterior pituitary hormone deficiency (e.g., mild central hypothyroidism). TRH testing is not necessary in the evaluation for central hypothyroidism and is not reliable in separating pituitary from hypothalamic hypothyroidism. "Mega" tests with multiple releasing hormones have little clinical utility.

Therapy Multiple hormones must be replaced in patients with panhypopituitarism, but cortisol replacement is most important. We prefer prednisone for matters of convenience and cost, but many physicians use cortisone acetate or hydrocortisone (cortisol). Prednisone (5 to 7.5 mg) or cortisone acetate (20 to 37.5 mg) can be given to some patients as a single morning dosage, whereas others require divided doses (two-thirds at 8 A.M., one-third at 3 A.M.). Hypopituitary patients may require lower daily glucocorticoid dosages than do patients with Addison's disease and do not require mineralocorticoid replacement. In stress situations or when preparing these patients for pituitary or other surgery, higher doses of glucocorticoids should be administered (e.g., for major surgery, hydrocortisone hemisuccinate 50 to 75 mg IM/IV every 6 h or methyl prednisolone sodium succinate 15 mg IM/IV every 6 h). Levothyroxine is the therapy of choice in central hypothyroidism (0.05 to 0.15 mg/d). The free T_4 levels should be monitored rather than TSH. Since thyroxine accelerates the degradation of cortisol and can precipitate adrenal crisis in patients with limited pituitary reserve, glucocorticoid replacement should always precede levothyroxine therapy in panhypopituitarism. Hypogonadism in women is treated with estrogen-progestogen combinations

FIGURE 331-10   X-ray of the sella, lateral view. Note (1) planum sphenoidal, (2) limbus sphenoidal, (3) sulcus chiasmaticus, (4) tuberculum sellae, (5) sella floor with distinct lamina dura, (6) dorsum sellae, (7) anterior clinoid, and (8) sphenoid sinus. *(From SM Wolpert, in KD Post et al, eds, The Pituitary Adenoma, New York, Plenum, 1980.)*

and in men with testosterone esters by injection. To achieve fertility, gonadotropins must be administered by injection in patients with pituitary disease, whereas gonadorelin may be successful in those with hypothalamic disease. GH deficiency is not currently treated in adults; in children, GH administration usually is required, but GHRH injections may be effective in those with hypothalamic disease (see Chap. 332). Diabetes insipidus is treated with nasal desmopressin (usually 0.05 to 0.1 mL twice a day) (see Chap. 333).

RADIOLOGY OF THE PITUITARY   Conventional posteroanterior and lateral skull x-rays define the contours of the sella turcica (Fig. 331-10). Abnormalities that may be identified on these films include enlargement, erosions, hyperostosis, and calcification in the region of the sella. However, detailed study of pituitary and hypothalamic lesions requires MRI or CT scanning (Fig. 331-11). Anterior tomograms of the sella may be required to delineate the bony anatomy before transsphenoidal surgery; however, the high radiation doses delivered by tomography and the limited information provided make routine tomography obsolete. Angiography may be required when an aneurysm or vascular malformation is suspected as a cause of an enlarged sella; MRI often obviates the need for this study.

MRI imaging (usually before and after intravenous injection of the contrast agent gadolinium DPTA; see Chap. 365) is the imaging study of choice for pituitary and hypothalamic abnormalities. Details of the optic chiasm, pituitary stalk, pituitary gland itself, intracavernous portion of the carotid artery, and relation to the cavernous sinus can be delineated on MRI scanning (Figs. 331-11 and 331-12). Advantages over CT scanning include lack of radiation, lack of iodinated contrast material, superior tissue contrast, and direct multiplanar capability. MRI is clearly superior to CT scanning in delineating microadenomas, visualizing the optic chiasm, and detecting cavernous sinus invasion. Patients with severe claustrophobia, those with ferrometallic aneurysm clips, and those with pacemakers require CT imaging. The use of sedatives and a prone position may allow patients with mild claustrophobia to tolerate the MRI. MRI is less useful when details of bony erosion or calcification are desired. Specific CT scan problems include radiation to the lens of the eye, artifacts due to bone and dental amalgam, and limited soft tissue density resolution.

The normal pituitary has an appearance similar to brain white matter on most MRI images; it has a height of 3 to 7 mm, although values up to 9 mm can be found, particularly in young women. The upper aspect is flat, concave, or, in younger patients, convex. The stalk is midline and is generally less than 2 mm in diameter. The posterior pituitary usually has a bright signal on T1-weighted images;

FIGURE 331-11 Coronal T1-weighted MRI scan through the posterior portion of the supraoptic hypothalamus (*). Note the anterior pituitary (1), cavernous sinus with internal carotid artery (5), proximal optic tracts (14), pituitary stalk (17), medial temporal lobes (24), and third ventricle (III). *(From Quint.)*

10 percent of normal individuals lack this intense signal. Cerebrospinal fluid appears dark on T1-weighted images and bright on T2-weighted images and is easily visualized within the sella in patients with the empty sella syndrome (Fig. 331-13). The normal pituitary gland, stalk, and cavernous sinus all show enhanced signal after intravenous gadolinium on T1-weighted images. Microadenomas do not enhance or have delayed enhancement, allowing improved resolution of these lesions (see Fig. 331-12). Five minutes after gadolinium administration, this contrast may no longer be evident. Stalk deviation and upward bulging of the pituitary suggest a microadenoma but are not specific. Up to 20 percent of normal persons show pituitary abnormalities on contrast-enhanced CT scan or MRI. In random autopsies, up to one-fourth of individuals have small pituitary abnormalities (e.g., microadenomas, cysts, metastatic tumors, pituitary infarcts), but it is unclear whether such abnormalities correspond to the focal abnormalities on CT and MRI scanning.

Localization of corticotroph adenomas in patients with Cushing's disease may be helpful in directing the surgical approach. MRI in this situation may be negative in 30 percent or more, and incidental nonfunctioning adenomas may be present in some patients with pituitary Cushing's disease. Petrosal catheterization is useful when the MRI is negative and when the question of ectopic versus pituitary Cushing's disease is unresolved. Whether it is necessary in all presumed pituitary Cushing's disease is uncertain. In patients with modest prolactin elevations, the purpose of pituitary and hypothalamic imaging is to exclude larger pathologic entities. Whether a microprolactinoma is actually visualized is less important, since this disorder is generally treated medically.

Pituitary macroadenomas causing sella enlargement with or without bony erosion may be suspected after conventional radiography. However, these findings are not specific. Additional findings on skull x-rays in acromegaly may include prognathism, enlarged paranasal sinuses, hyperostosis of the external occipital protuberance, increased density of the central bone of the sella, and an enlarged square sella

FIGURE 331-12 *A.* Coronal noncontrast T1-weighted MRI scan demonstrates pituitary gland asymmetry *(arrow)* compatible with a pituitary microadenoma. Cavernous internal carotid artery (5), optic chiasm (13), sphenoid sinus (21), and temporal lobe (24). *B.* Coronal contrast (gadolinium) enhanced T1-weighted MRI scan identifies a 4-mm right paramidline microadenoma *(arrows).* *(From Quint.)*

FIGURE 331-13 Empty sella. Coronal contrast-enhanced T1-weighted MRI scan through the pituitary region demonstrates an enlarged sella turcica (*arrows*) with normally enhancing pituitary tissue (16) displaced inferiorly. Note the optic chiasm (13) and intracavernous carotid artery (5). (*From Quint.*)

FIGURE 331-14 Macroadenoma. MRI scan through the pituitary region demonstrates a large sellar mass (*arrows*) elevating the optic chiasm (13) and invading the right cavernous sinus (*arrowheads*). The contrast-enhanced study differentiates the nonenhancing optic chiasm (13) from the enhancing tumor. (*From Quint.*)

with tapered tuberculum. GH-secreting adenomas may calcify and regress to leave a calculus or stone.

Macroadenomas are well delineated on MRI. Coronal views are best (Fig. 331-14) for optic chiasm compromise, invasion of the cavernous sinus, vascular encasement, and invasion of the base of the skull. The medial wall of the cavernous sinus is thin and not directly visualized. The lateral wall of the cavernous sinus is an important landmark; the presence of tissue between the lateral wall of the cavernous sinus and the internal carotid artery is a reliable sign of invasion. Macroadenomas are hyperdense on T2-weighted images in one-third to one-half of patients; the remainder are isointense. Old hemorrhage or cyst formation results in a focally hyperintense signal and may be seen in up to 22 percent of macroadenomas (see below). (With hemorrhage, the signal is bright on T1 and T2; with fluid, the signal is of low intensity on T1 and bright on T2). Approximately one-fifth of patients with macroadenomas have a partially empty sella due to tumor degeneration or necrosis and the presence of cerebrospinal fluid density within the sella. The enlargement of the residual pituitary distinguishes this entity from the primary empty sella (see below), where the residual pituitary is normal in size. Pituitary hyperplasia (e.g., thyrotroph hyperplasia in primary hypothyroidism or lactotroph hyperplasia in pregnancy) appears as a symmetrically enlarged pituitary.

Pituitary apoplexy is caused by a sudden increase in the size of pituitary macroadenoma due to hemorrhage or infarction; enlargement of the sella is almost always evident on plain films. Acute hemorrhage (<7 days) is hypointense or isotense to brain on T1- and T2-weighted images. During the subacute stage (7 to 14 days), signal intensity is increased in the periphery of the hematoma (due to hemoglobin breakdown products such as methemoglobin), with the center remaining hypointense. After 14 days (chronic stage), the entire hematoma appears bright on T1- and T2-weighted images.

Craniopharyngiomas can often be suspected on the basis of nodular or curvilinear calcification in the suprasellar region on x-ray (Fig. 331-15). This calcification is visible in 80 to 90 percent of children and in about half of adults. On CT scanning, cystic components are present with ring or nodular calcification in most children and 80 percent of adults. The findings on MRI are variable; some cysts are cerebrospinal fluid–like in their behavior, some are not as intense as cerebrospinal fluid on T1 but brighter than cerebrospinal fluid on T2, whereas others mimic subacute hemorrhage, being hyperintense on

FIGURE 331-15 Lateral skull x-ray in a patient with a craniopharyngioma. Note dense calcification in suprasellar region (*arrow*).

FIGURE 331-16 The findings in patients with the empty sella syndrome. (*Left panel*) The normal anatomic relationships. With the empty sella syndrome (*right panel*), ballooning of the sella results when an arachnoid diverticulum herniates through an incompetent diaphragma sellae. (*After Jordan et al.*)

T1 and T2. Calcification is usually not seen on MRI unless large amounts are present. Some craniopharyngiomas are primarily solid.

Most meningiomas of the sellar region cause abnormalities on routine skull films that include calcifications of the tumor and hyperostosis of the planum sphenoidale or of the chiasmatic sulcus. Meningiomas also may cause sella enlargement and thereby mimic pituitary adenomas. Meningiomas may be difficult to see on MRI without enhancement because they are isodense to gray matter. Almost all enhance with gadolinium, as they do with iodine contrast–enhanced CT. Delayed scanning (after 45 min) may be necessary with MRI to allow the normal enhancement of the pituitary gland and mucosal surfaces to dissipate. Vascular encasement of the carotid artery is common with meningiomas but rare with other sella region tumors.

Aneurysms in the region of the sella contain concentric calcifications demonstrable on plain skull films in about 30 percent of patients. Aneurysms can cause sella enlargement, usually with lateral depression and erosion of the sella floor. Many aneurysms are visualized on MRI with the dark appearance of a flow void as blood flows through the lumen. Multilamellated thrombi appear as a high signal on T1; adjacent brain may show a low signal on T2 due to hemosiderin deposition. In difficult cases, especially those with complete thrombosis, additional studies may be required such as digital substraction angiography, conventional angiography, and/or magnetic resonance angiography.

Other pathologic entities in the sellar region may be noted with MRI or CT scanning. In hemochromatosis, the pituitary is dark, particularly on T2-weighted images, due to iron deposition. Additional suprasellar masses include optic chiasm or hypothalamic gliomas, metastases to the hypothalamus or pituitary salk, germinomas, sarcoid granulomas, histiocytosis, dermoid tumors, epidermoid tumors, and arachnoid cysts.

THE ENLARGED SELLA–EMPTY SELLA SYNDROME   Enlargement of the sella can be caused by pituitary adenomas, hypothalamic masses and cysts, aneurysms, primary hypothyroidism or hypogonadism, and increased intracranial pressure. It also can occur in patients with the primary empty sella syndrome (Fig. 331-16). In this situation, the sella tends to be symmetrically ballooned without bony erosion. The suprasellar subarachnoid space herniates through an incomplete diaphragma sella (Fig. 331-16) so that the sella is filled with cerebrospinal fluid (CSF) within an arachnoid-lined sac. An incomplete diaphragma sella is thought to be a prerequisite. It is not clear whether transient or persistent increased CSF pressure is necessary to produce sella enlargement in these patients, but CSF pressure is generally normal when measured. The pituitary is flattened and pushed to one side but tends to function normally. The fact that the CSF fills the sella can be demonstrated best with MRI scanning (see Fig. 331-13).

It is important to differentiate the primary empty sella from the enlarged partially empty sella due to a degenerated pituitary adenoma.

In the former the pituitary volume is usually normal, whereas in the latter the pituitary volume is generally increased.

Most patients with the primary empty sella syndrome are obese, multiparous women with headaches; about 30 percent have hypertension. It is of interest that multiparity, obesity, and hypertension are associated with increases in CSF pressure. Selection bias cannot be excluded in case reports, since skull x-rays may be obtained in patients with headaches, which, in turn, uncovers the enlarged sella. Endocrine abnormalities are uncommon. The report that antipituitary antibodies are present in 70 percent of these patients is therefore difficult to understand. Hyperprolactinemia occurs on occasion, possibly due to stalk stretching or coincidental microprolactinomas. GH secretory reserve is often abnormal in these patients, probably the result of obesity. Spontaneous CSF rhinorrhea and pseudotumor cerebri have each been reported in about 10 percent of the cases, but this may represent a bias of ascertainment. CSF rhinorrhea often requires surgical correction. Visual field defects have been reported and are thought to be caused by herniation of the optic chiasm into the sella turcica. Once the diagnosis of the empty sella syndrome is established by MRI or CT scan, further diagnostic studies are superfluous, and the therapy is reassurance.

REFERENCES

General

BLACK PMcL et al: *Secretory Tumors of the Pituitary Gland*. New York, Raven, 1984

BURKE CW: The pituitary megatest: Outdated. Clin Endocrinol 36:133, 1992

BURROW GN et al: Microadenomas of the pituitary and abnormal sellar tomograms in an unselected autopsy series. N Engl J Med 304:156, 1981

CROWLEY WR, ARMSTRONG WE: Neurochemical regulation of oxytocin secretion in lactation. Endocrinol Rev 13:33, 1992

HERMAN V et al: Clonal origin of pituitary adenomas. J Clin Endocrinol Metab 71:1427, 1990

HOLLENHORST RW, YOUNGE BR: Ocular manifestations produced by adenoma of the pituitary gland: Analysis of 1000 cases, in *Diagnosis and Treatment of Pituitary Tumors*, PO Kohler, GT Ross (eds). Amsterdam, Excerpta Medica, 1973, p 53

JENKINS JS, NUSSEY SS: The role of oxytocin: Present concepts. Clin Endocrinol 34:515, 1991

JONES A: Radiation oncogenesis in relation to the treatment of pituitary tumours. Clin Endocrinol 35:379, 1991

JUNEAU P et al: Malignant tumors of the pituitary gland. Arch Neurol 49:555, 1992

KLIBANSKI A: Editorial: Further evidence for a somatic mutation theory in the pathogenesis of human pituitary tumors. J Clin Endocrinol Metab 71:1415, 1990

——, ZERVAS NT: Diagnosis and management of hormone-secreting pituitary adenomas. N Engl J Med 324:822, 1991

LAMBERTS SWJ: The role of somatostatin and its analogues in the diagnosis and treatment of tumors. Endocrinol Rev 12:450, 1991

MARTIN JB, REICHLIN S: *Clinical Neuroendocrinology*, 2d ed. Philadelphia, Davis, 1987

MOLITCH ME (ed): Pituitary tumors: Diagnosis and management. Endocrinol Metab Clin North Am 16:3, 1987

——, RUSSELL EJ: The pituitary "incidentaloma." Ann Intern Med 112:925, 1990

PRYSOR-JONES RA, JENKINS J: Vasoactive intestinal peptide and anterior pituitary function. Clin Endocrinol 29:677, 1988

SCHEITHAUER BW et al: The pituitary gland in pregnancy: A clinicopathologic and immunohistochemical study of 69 cases. Mayo Clin Proc 65:461, 1990

Prolactin

BEVAN JS et al: Dopamine agonists and pituitary tumor shrinkage. Endocrinol Rev 13:220, 1992

CUNNAH D, BESSER M: Management of prolactinomas. Clin Endocrinol (Oxf) 34:231, 1991

FERRARI C et al: Functional characterization of hypothalamic hyperprolactinemia. J Clin Endocrinol Metab 55:897, 1982

KATZ E et al: Increased levels of bromocriptine following vaginal as compared to oral administration. Fertil Steril 55:882, 1991

MOLITCH ME: Pregnancy and the hyperprolactinemic woman. N Engl J Med 321:1364, 1985

———— et al: Bromocriptine as primary therapy for prolactin-secreting macroadenomas: Results of a prospective multicenter study. J Clin Endocrinol Metab 60:698, 1985

MORIONDO P et al: Bromocriptine treatment of microprolactinomas: Evidence of stable prolactin decrease after drug withdrawal. J Clin Endocrinol Metab 60:764, 1985

SCHLECTE J et al: The natural history of untreated hyperprolactinemia: A prospective analysis. J Clin Endocrinol Metab 68:412, 1989

TSAGARAKIS S et al: Megavoltage pituitary irradiation in the management of prolactinomas: Long-term follow up. Clin Endocrinol 34:399, 1991

VANCE ML et al: Bromocriptine. Ann Intern Med 100:78, 1984

———— et al: Treatment of prolactin-secreting pituitary macroadenomas with the long-acting non-ergot dopamine agonist CV 205-502. Ann Intern Med 112:668, 1990

WOOD DF et al: Dopamine, the dopamine D2 receptor and pituitary tumours. Clin Endocrinol 35:455, 1991

Growth hormone

ASA SL et al: A case for hypothalamic acromegaly: A clinicopathological study of six patients with hypothalamic gangliocytomas producing growth hormone-releasing factor. J Clin Endocrinol Metab 58:796, 1984

BARKAN AL: Acromegaly: Diagnosis and treatment. Endocrinol Metab Clin North Am 18:277, 1989

———— et al: Preoperative treatment of acromegaly with long-acting somatostatin analogue SMS 201-995: Shrinkage of invasive pituitary macroadenomas and improved surgical remission rate. J Clin Endocrinol Metab 67:1040, 1988

BAUMANN G: Growth hormone heterogeneity: Genes, isohormones, variants, and binding proteins. Endocrinol Rev 12:424, 1991

EASTMAN RC et al: Conventional supervoltage irradiation is an effective treatment for acromegaly. J Clin Endocrinol Metab 48:931, 1979

EDDY RL et al: Human growth hormone release: Comparison of provocative test procedures. Am J Med 56:179, 1974

EZZAT S, MELMED S: Are patients with acromegaly at increased risk of neoplasia? J Clin Endocrinol Metab 72:245, 1991

FROHMAN LA: Therapeutic options in acromegaly. J Clin Endocrinol Metab 72:1175, 1991

————, JANSSON J-O: Growth hormone–releasing hormone. Endocrinol Rev 7:223, 1986

HO KKY et al: Impact of octreotide, a long-acting somatostatin analogue, on glucose tolerance and insulin sensitivity in acromegaly. Clin Endocrinol 36:271, 1992

LAWRENCE JH et al: Successful treatment of acromegaly: Metabolic and clinical studies in 145 patients. J Clin Endocrinol Metab 31:180, 1970

MARCUS R et al: Effects of short-term administration of recombinant human growth hormone to elderly people. J Clin Endocrinol Metab 70:519, 1990

MELMED S: Acromegaly. N Engl J Med 322:966, 1990

————: Etiology of pituitary acromegaly. Endocrinol Metab Clin North Am 21:539, 1992

———— et al: Pathophysiology of acromegaly. Endocrinol Rev 4:271, 1983

MOSES AC et al: Bromocriptine therapy in acromegaly: Use in patients resistant to conventional therapy and effect on serum levels of somatomedin C. J Clin Endocrinol Metab 53:752, 1981

MURUAIS C et al: Corticosteroid-induced growth hormone secretion in normal and obese subjects. Clin Endocrinol 35:485, 1991

REICHLIN S: Somatostatin. N Engl J Med 309:1495, 1983

ROSS DA, WILSON CB: Results of transsphenoidal microsurgery for growth hormone-secreting pituitary adenomas in a series of 214 patients. J Neurosurg 68:854, 1988

RUDMAN D et al: Effects of human growth hormone in men over 60 years old. N Engl J Med 323:1, 1990

SANO T et al: Growth hormone–releasing hormone–producing tumors: Clinical, biochemical and morphological manifestations. Endocrinol Rev 9:357, 1988

THORNER MO, VANCE ML: Growth hormone 1988. J Clin Invest 82:745, 1988

———— et al: Extrahypothalamic growth-hormone–releasing factor (GRF) secretion is a rare cause of acromegaly: Plasma GRF levels in 177 acromegalic patients. J Clin Endocrinol Metab 59:846, 1984

———— et al: Stereotactic radiosurgery with the cobalt-60 gamma unit in the treatment of growth hormone–producing pituitary tumors. Neurosurgery 29:663, 1991

TSH

BECK-PECCOZ P et al: Decreased receptor binding of biologically inactive thyrotropin in central hypothyroidism: Effect of treatment with thyrotropin-releasing hormone. N Engl J Med 312:1085, 1985

———— et al: Treatment of hyperthyroidism with the somatostatin analogue SMS 201-995. J Clin Endocrinol Metab 68:208, 1989

BIGOS ST et al: Spectrum of pituitary alterations with mild and severe thyroid impairment. J Clin Endocrinol Metab 46:317, 1978

FAGLIA G et al: Inappropriate secretion of thyrotropin by the pituitary. Horm Res 26:79, 1987

MAGNER JA: Thyroid-stimulating hormone: Biosynthesis, cell biology and bioactivity. Endocrinol Rev 11:354, 1990

Gonadotropins and alpha subunits

DANESHDOOST L et al: Recognition of gonadotroph adenomas in women. N Engl J Med 324:589, 1991

HESELTINE DM et al: Testicular enlargement and elevated serum inhibin concentrations occur in patients with pituitary macroadenomas secreting follicle-stimulating hormone. Clin Endocrinol 31:411, 1989

JAMESON JL et al: Glycoprotein hormone genes are expressed in clinically non-functioning pituitary adenomas. J Clin Invest 80:1472, 1987

KATZNELSON L et al: Imbalanced follicle-stimulating hormone β-subunit hormone biosynthesis in human pituitary adenomas. J Clin Endocrinol Metab 74:1343, 1992

MARSHALL JC, KELCH RP: Gonadotropin-releasing hormone: Role of pulsatile secretion in the regulation of reproduction. N Engl J Med 313:1459, 1986

MOGHISSI KS: Clinical applications of gonadotropin-releasing hormones in reproductive disorders. Endocrinol Metab Clin North Am 21:125, 1992

OPPENHEIM DS, KLIBANSKI A: Medical therapy of glycoprotein hormone–secreting pituitary tumors. Endocrinol Metab Clin North Am 18:339, 1989

———— et al: Prevalence of alpha-subunit hypersecretion in patients with pituitary tumors. J Clin Endocrinol Metab 64:1187, 1990

SNYDER PJ: Gonadotroph cell adenomas of the pituitary. Endocrinol Rev 6:552, 1985

———— et al: Secretion of uncombined subunits of luteinizing hormone by gonadotroph cell adenomas. J Clin Endocrinol Metab 59:1169, 1984

TSATSOULIS A et al: Bioactive gonadotrophin secretion in man. Clin Endocrinol 35:193, 1991

WEISS J et al: Hypogonadism caused by a single amino acid substitution in the β-subunit of luteinizing hormone. N Engl J Med 326:179, 1992

WHITCOMB RW, CROWLEY WF JR: Clinical review 4: Diagnosis and treatment of isolated gonadotropin-releasing hormone deficiency in men. J Clin Endocrinol Metab 70:3, 1990

ACTH

BATEMAN A et al: The immune-hypothalamic-pituitary-adrenal axis. Endocrinol Rev 10:92, 1989

BORST GC et al: Discordant cortisol response to exogenous ACTH and insulin-induced hypoglycemia in patients with pituitary disease. N Engl J Med 306:1462, 1982

CHROUSOS GP et al: The corticotropin-releasing factor stimulation test: An aid in the evaluation of patients with Cushing's syndrome. N Engl J Med 310:622, 1984

FLACK MR et al: Urine free cortisol in the high-dose dexamethasone suppression test for the differential diagnosis of the Cushing syndrome. Ann Intern Med 116:211, 1992

IMURA H et al: Cytokines and endocrine function: An interaction between the immune and neuroendocrine systems. Clin Endocrinol (Oxf) 35:107, 1991

LORIAUX DL, NIEMANN L: Corticotropin-releasing hormone testing in pituitary disease. Endocrinol Metab Clin North Am 20:363, 1991

ORME SM, BELCHETZ PE: Isolated ACTH deficiency. Clin Endocrinol (Oxf) 35:213, 1991

ORTH DN: Corticotropin-releasing hormone in humans. Endocrinol Rev 13:164, 1992

SCHLAGHECKE R et al: The effect of long-term glucocorticoid therapy on pituitary response to exogenous corticotropin-releasing hormone. N Engl J Med 326:226, 1992

STREETEN DHP et al: Normal and abnormal function of the hypothalamic-pituitary-adrenal system in man. Endocrinol Rev 5:371, 1984

TAHIR AH, SHEELER LR: Recurrent Cushing's disease after transsphenoidal surgery. Arch Intern Med 152:977, 1992

Endorphins

DELITALA G: Opioid peptides and pituitary function: Basic and clinical aspects, in *Brain Endocrinology*, 2d ed, M Motta (ed). New York, Raven, 1991, p 217

IMURA H et al: Endogenous opioids and related peptides: From molecular biology to clinical medicine. J Endocrinol 107:147, 1985

KROMER W: Endogenous and exogenous opioids in the control of gastrointestinal motility and secretion. Pharmacol Rev 40:121, 1989

LUNDBLAD JR, ROBERTS JL: Regulation of pro-opiomelanocortin gene expression in the pituitary. Endocrinol Rev 9:135, 1988

PFEIFFER A, HERZ A: Endocrine actions of opioids. Horm Metabol Res 16:386, 1984

Hypothalamus

BRAY GA, GALLAGHER TFJ: Manifestations of hypothalamic obesity in man: A comprehensive investigation of eight patients and a review of the literature. Medicine 54:301, 1974

DINARELLO CA: Interleukin 1 and the pathogenesis of the acute phase response. N Engl J Med 54:301, 1984

PLUM F, VAN UITERT R: Nonendocrine disease and disorders of the hypothalamus, in *The Hypothalamus*, S Reichlin et al (eds). New York, Raven, 1978, pp 415–473

Craniopharyngiomas

BANNA M: Craniopharyngiomas in adults. Surg Neurol 1:202, 1973

————: Craniopharyngioma: Based on 160 cases. Br J Radiol 49:206, 1976

FISCHER EG et al: Treatment of craniopharyngiomas in children, 1971–1980. J Neurosurg 62:486, 1985

Hypopituitarism

ABBOUD CF: Laboratory diagnosis of hypopituitarism. Mayo Clin Proc 61:35, 1986

ARAFAH BM: Reversible hypopituitarism in patients with large nonfunctioning pituitary adenomas. J Clin Endocrinol Metab 62:1173, 1986

ASA SL et al: Lymphocytic hypophysitis of pregnancy resulting in hypopituitarism: A distinct clinicopathologic entity. Ann Intern Med 95:166, 1981

EDWARDS OM, CLARK JDA: Post-traumatic hypopituitarism. Medicine 62:281, 1986

MUIR A, MACLAREN NK: Autoimmune diseases of the adrenal glands, parathyroid glands, gonads and hypothalamic-pituitary axis. Endocrinol Metab Clin North Am 20:619, 1991

OELKERS W: Hyponatremia and inappropriate secretion of vasopressin (antidiuretic hormone) in patients with hypopituitarism. N Engl J Med 321:492, 1989

ROSEN T, BENGTSSON BA: Premature mortality due to cardiovascular disease in hypopituitarism. Lancet 336:285, 1990

VELDHUIS JD, HAMMOND JM: Endocrine function after spontaneous infarction of the human pituitary: Report, review, and reappraisal. Endocrinol Rev 1:100, 1980

Radiology

BRUNETON JN et al: Normal variants of the sella turcica. Radiology 131:99, 1979

CHAKERES DW et al: Magnetic resonance imaging of pituitary and parasellar abnormalities. Radiol Clin North Am 27:265, 1989

CONSTINE LS et al: Hypothalamo-pituitary dysfunction after radiation for brain tumors. N Engl J Med 328:87, 1993

GLICK RP, TIESI JA: Subacute pituitary apoplexy: Clinical and magnetic resonance imaging characteristics. Neurosurgery 27:214, 1990

JOHNSON MR et al: The evaluation of patients with a suspected pituitary microadenoma: Computed tomography compared to magnetic resonance imaging. Clin Endocrinol 36:335, 1992

JORDAN RM et al: The primary empty sella syndrome: Analysis of the clinical characteristics, radiographic features, pituitary function, and cerebrospinal fluid adenohypophysial hormone concentrations. Am J Med 62:569, 1977

QUINT DJ: Hypothalamic, pituitary, and pineal imaging, in *Endocrine Imaging*, MP Sandler et al (eds). Norwalk, Conn, Appleton & Lange, 1992

WOLPERT SM: The radiology of pituitary adenomas. Endocrinol Metab Clin North Am 16:553, 1987

332   DISORDERS OF GROWTH

RAYMOND L. HINTZ

NORMAL GROWTH   Children may grow rapidly over relatively short periods of time, and the physician must be aware of normal standards for growth and development as a function of age. A record of these changes can be utilized as a sensitive indicator of general health. Minimal aberrations in health may be reflected first in a deviation from the normal growth rate; conversely, an actively growing child seldom has a serious systemic disease. Thus height and growth rate provide important information.

Both longitudinal and cross-sectional studies indicate that differences exist in growth among different ethnic groups. However, normal, well-nourished children have remarkably similar growth patterns. For example, the average length of children, which at birth is about 50 cm, increases by about 25 cm in the first year of life, 12.5 cm in the second year, and 6.0 cm per year thereafter until puberty. This formula can be used to estimate average height up to about 10 years of age. Nomograms have been constructed to give a more accurate picture of average growth and the range of normal deviations from the mean (Figs. 332-1 and 332-2).

CONTROL OF GROWTH   Growth involves an increase in both the total number of cells and the synthesis of macromolecules by individual cells. The relative importance of these processes varies from organ to organ and with age. The control and integration of growth also vary among tissues and with the stage of development.

Prenatal growth   Prenatal development exemplifies the complexities of the integration and control of growth. During this time, a single cell becomes a complex organism in which billions of cells work in harmonious concert. The growth rate is astounding; the most rapid growth rate occurs during the second trimester. The control of prenatal growth is under different mechanisms from those in the postnatal period. Growth hormone and thyroid hormone have relatively minor effects on growth during prenatal life. Prenatal growth rates are dependent on uterine blood flow and other maternal influences and are less dependent on the factors that determine ultimate stature. At birth, the correlation between body length and adult height is weak ($r = 0.3$); by 2 years of age, the correlation between body length and adult height is stronger ($r = 0.7$), indicating that the factors influencing adult stature begin operating early in postnatal life.

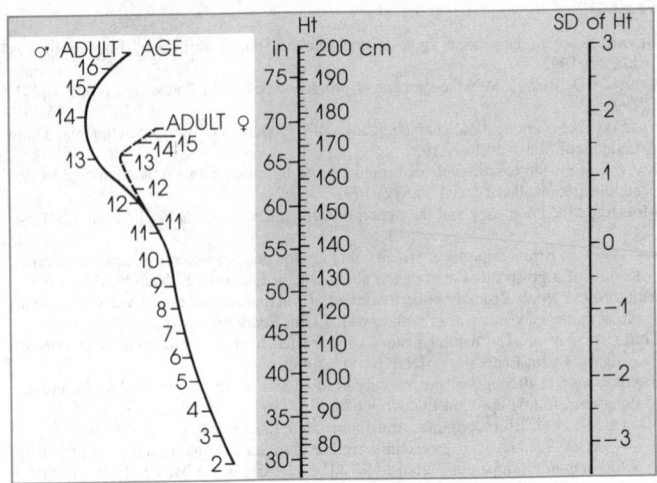

FIGURE 332-1   Nomogram for height of boys and girls.

Genetic factors   Stature is a polygenic trait (see Chap. 60), so there is no simple method of predicting on the basis of genetic factors the adult height of any given child. However, there is a correlation between the mean height of parents and the mean heights attained by their children.

Nutrition   The next most important factor affecting growth is nutrition. Severe nutritional deprivation, as in marasmus or kwashiorkor (see Chap. 72), impairs growth, as may selective deficiencies of vitamins and minerals, such as vitamin D, and subclinical deficiencies of nutrients. The trend toward increased adult stature over the last century may be due to improvement in diet, especially to an increase in protein intake during the period of rapid growth during infancy.

Hormones   GROWTH HORMONE   Growth hormone (GH or somatotropin) plays the central role in the modulation of growth of children from birth until the completion of puberty. In the total absence of GH, linear growth occurs at about half to a third the normal rate. GH also plays a role in the control of body anabolism throughout life.

GH is a member of a family of hormones that includes pituitary prolactin and human placental lactogen (hPL) (see Chap. 331). The most common form of GH in the pituitary and in the circulation is the 22,000-Da ("22K") form. This is the hormone that was purified and sequenced from human pituitary glands. The second most abundant form is a 20,000-Da ("20K") form. This variant is coded by the same gene sequence as the 22K growth hormone, but a segment of a coding exon in the growth hormone gene is not transcribed, thus resulting in a shorter hormone. Whether this variant fulfills some specific metabolic function is not clear; the 20K form seems to have

FIGURE 332-2   Nomogram for growth rate in boys and girls.

equivalent growth-promoting activity but may have less effect on carbohydrate function than the 22K form.

GH secretion is under both positive and negative hypothalamic control (see Chap. 331). The somatotropin release-inhibiting factor (somatostatin, SRIF) is a 14-amino-acid peptide that is widely distributed in tissues outside the hypothalamus and is a potent inhibitor of the secretion of many hormones, including insulin, glucagon, and gastrin.

The biologic action of GH-releasing hormone (GRH, somatocrinin) is contained in the first 29 amino acids of the 44-amino-acid peptide, and the amino-terminal amino acid is crucial for its biologic action. Patients with idiopathic GH deficiency may have a deficiency of GRH rather than an inability to make GH in the pituitary. Indeed, half or more individuals with GH deficiency respond to prolonged pulsatile administration of GRH with an increase in plasma GH and with an accelerated growth rate.

The secretion of somatostatin and GRH, and hence the release of GH, is under the influence of several factors (Fig. 332-3). Higher centers in the central nervous system have synapses that terminate on hypothalamic cells that secrete somatostatin and GRH and exert both positive and negative influences. In addition, both GH and the GH-controlled insulin-like growth factors influence the secretion or action of GRH and somatostatin. The secretion of GH is episodic, with a relatively short (10- to 15-min) half-life in plasma. A significant proportion of GH in serum is bound to a GH-binding protein GHBP that is structurally related to the GH receptor. Although small amounts of GH are secreted during waking periods, most GH secretion occurs during sleep, especially during third- and fourth-stage sleep.

THE INSULIN-LIKE GROWTH FACTORS   Although GH may exert some direct effects on growth, most of its growth-promoting actions are mediated by the insulin-like growth factor (IGF) or somatomedin peptides. Two human IGF peptides, IGF-I and IGF-II, have about 50 percent structural homology with human insulin and 70 percent homology with each other. Somatomedin C (SM-C) and IGF-I are structurally and functionally equivalent. The IGF peptides are bound tightly to six specific plasma proteins (IGFBPs) and have half-lives of hours rather than minutes. Levels of IGF-I and IGFBP-3 are dependent on GH secretion and are consequently high in acromegaly and low in hypopituitarism. Levels are also age-dependent, with low levels in early childhood, a peak during adolescence, and a decline after the age of 50 years. The plasma levels of IGF-II are also dependent on the presence of a minimal amount of GH, but supraphysiologic increases in GH do not result in a further increase in IGF-II. Thus the values of IGF-II are low in hypopituitarism but are not elevated in acromegaly. Plasma levels of IGF-II are constant from 1 year of age to beyond the eighth decade of life.

THYROID HORMONE   Unlike the pattern of growth with GH deficiency, the total absence of thyroid hormone causes an almost complete cessation of linear growth. Thus adequate thyroid hormone appears to be an absolute prerequisite for normal growth. There are several potential mechanisms for this phenomenon. Thyroid hormones exert direct effects on cell metabolism, and thyroid hormone deficiency results in diminished GH secretion in response to stimulation. In addition, the action of IGF-I on cartilage cells may be dependent on thyroid hormone.

GONADAL STEROIDS   Androgens and estrogens exert their major stimulation of growth at puberty. Much of the pubertal growth spurt is due to these hormones. Androgens have a direct stimulatory effect on the growth and maturation of bone, cartilage, and muscle. Estrogens appear to have a biphasic action, stimulating growth at low levels and inhibiting growth at high levels.

INSULIN   Insulin has strong anabolic actions separate from its effects on carbohydrate metabolism. These actions include stimulation of protein synthesis and cell division. The excessive growth of infants of diabetic mothers may be the consequence of high levels of plasma insulin in the fetus. The close structural relationship of insulin to the IGF group of growth factors and the ability of insulin to bind to the IGF-I receptor may explain some of these effects of insulin at high levels. However, insulin also has growth-stimulating actions of its own at low levels in some cell types. The role of insulin in the control of normal growth is still unclear.

OTHER FACTORS   Nerve growth factor, which is structurally related to the insulin-IGF family of peptides, has actions on the development of sympathetic neurons and possibly on the maintenance and repair of other neurons. Epidermal growth factor has potent actions on the maturation of the skin and also acts on other cell types. Platelet-derived growth factor is released from platelets upon clotting and is also a potent mitogen for many cells. The plasma levels, control mechanisms, interactions with other growth-stimulating peptides, and physiologic roles of these growth factors remain to be elucidated.

DIAGNOSIS OF GROWTH DISORDERS   Most individuals with short stature do not have a disease in the usual sense but exhibit some deviation from the normal growth pattern (Table 332-1). Thus the first step in dealing with growth disorders is to identify those individuals with a normal variation in stature who presumably do not require treatment.

Height and growth rate   An important factor in the differential diagnosis of short stature is to determine the height percentile of the patient as compared with others of the same age (see Fig. 332-1). A straightedge is placed on the patient's age and height. The intercept on the right-hand scale estimates the number of standard deviations (SD) from the mean height for age. In general, the further away the patient is from the mean height for age, the more likely that short stature is due to disease. A height above the −2-SD level indicates that the patient is likely normal. The growth rate also should be determined, if possible, either from existing growth data or by observation (see Fig. 332-2). A growth rate consistently below the mean is a cause for concern.

Because short stature is common, clinical judgment plays a large role in the approach to this problem. Individuals with severe short stature (−3 SD or greater for age) should undergo immediate evaluation, while those with less severe short stature may be serially observed so that the growth rate can be assessed. A consistently low

FIGURE 332-3   Feedback control of growth hormone secretion. GH = growth hormone; GHRH = growth hormone–releasing hormone; SM = somatomedins (insulin-like growth factors). Stimulating influences are shown by arrows in color. Inhibitory influences are shown in black.

TABLE 332-1   Causes of short stature

Diagnosis	Usual practice, %	Referral center, %
Constitutional growth delay	98	80
GH deficiency	0.1	10
Hypothyroidism	0.2	4
Systemic disease	0.3	3
Chromosomal disorders	0.1	1
Bone-cartilage dysplasia	0.3	1
Psychosocial disorders	1	1

SOURCE: Modified from Horner et al, 1978.

growth rate should lead to further investigation. The diagnosis of constitutional delay is one of exclusion. In general, if hypothyroidism, GH deficiency, and the more common systemic diseases have been excluded, it is reasonable to observe the patient. However, the boundaries between "normal" and "disease" may be blurred, and the indications for treatment may change. Furthermore, continued failure to maintain a normal growth rate is an indication for reinvestigation.

History   Important features in the history include the weight and gestational age at birth, growth and development in early infancy, and presence of systemic disease. It is also crucial to assess the stature of the parents and first- and second-degree relatives and to review the growth and pubertal development patterns of parents, siblings, and other relatives. A family history of late pubertal development may be helpful diagnostically.

Physical examination   The body proportions must be evaluated. Relatively short limbs compared with the trunk suggest either long-standing hypothyroidism or one of the chondrodystrophies such as achondroplastic dwarfism; but more subtle forms of chondrodystrophy may be difficult to recognize (see also Chap. 351). It is also important to note the height-to-weight ratio. A short child who is underweight for height may have malnutrition or systemic disease. On the other hand, a child who is short but overweight is more likely to have endocrine disease. Patients with Cushing's syndrome, GH deficiency, or hypothyroidism are frequently relatively overweight for their height. Specific physical findings may suggest specific syndromes (Table 332-2).

Laboratory evaluation   Laboratory tests may either confirm the clinical impression or reveal unsuspected pathology. Assessment of bone age is useful to indicate possible pathology and to estimate final adult height. Because the manifestations of hypothyroidism may be minimal, thyroid function should be assessed routinely. IGF-I and IGFGP-3 measurements are also useful screening procedures, since most patients with GH deficiency have low values. Syndromes of GH resistance, such as Laron dwarfism, are characterized by low IGF-I levels and high GH levels. Appropriate tests may be ordered to screen for other disease states (as summarized in Table 332-3). Any girl with unexplained short stature should have a chromosomal karyotype.

TESTING OF GH SECRETION   Because GH secretion is episodic and therefore variable, random measurements of plasma GH are not adequate tests of GH deficiency. Some GH stimulation tests for screening for GH deficiency are summarized in Table 332-4 (also see Chap. 331). Because of the long half-life of IGF-I and IGFBP-3, a random measurement during the day is an accurate reflection of the mean plasma concentration. If care is taken to use age-related standards, measurements and IGF-I and IGFBP-3 provide a reasonable screen for GH deficiency. Low levels of IGF-I or IGFBP-3 should lead to more extensive evaluation. The other tests listed are indirect and largely nonphysiologic ways of provoking the release of GH. In our clinic, a GH level of 10 μg/L (10 ng/mL) after a clonidine test is considered a normal response. If that level is not achieved, more

TABLE 332-3   Screening laboratory investigations in short stature

Test or x-ray	Disorder
Serum thyroxine	Hypothyroidism
IGF-I and IGFBP-3	GH deficiency
Bone age	Constitutional delay, hypothyroidism, GH deficiency
Lateral skull film	Craniopharyngioma or other central nervous system lesion
Serum calcium	Pseudohypoparathyroidism
Serum phosphate	Vitamin D–resistant rickets
Serum bicarbonate	Renal tubular acidosis
Blood urea nitrogen	Renal failure
Complete blood count	Anemia, nutritional disorder
Sedimentation rate	Inflammatory disease of bowel
Chromosomal karyotype	Gonadal dysgenesis or other abnormality

TABLE 332-2   Physical findings in syndromes of short stature

Syndrome	Specific physical findings
GH deficiency	Frontal bossing, central obesity, high-pitched voice
Hypothyroidism	Dry skin, coarse hair, immature facies
Cushing's syndrome	Central obesity, striae, hypertension
Gonadal dysgenesis	Webbed neck, multiple pigmented nevi, shield chest, delayed sexual development
Pseudohypoparathyroidism	Moon facies and obesity, short metacarpals, mental retardation
Bone-cartilage dysplasia	Abnormal proportions, macrocephaly
Russell-Silver dwarfism	Small at birth, "pointed" facies, asymmetry

definitive testing of GH reserve should be carried out as described in Chap. 331.

TREATMENT WITH GH   GH deficiency   The only established use of human GH is in the treatment of children who are GH-deficient. Only between 1 in 4000 and 1 in 20,000 children have a GH deficiency. About half of these cases are due to idiopathic GH deficiency, and the other half are secondary to tumor and/or radiation therapy. In approximately one-third of the latter cases, GH deficiency is isolated, and in the other two-thirds, there are multiple pituitary hormone deficiencies. If short stature is due to a systemic disease

TABLE 332-4   Screening tests for assessing GH secretion

IGF-I RADIOIMMUNOASSAY*

Age (years)	Male Range, μg/L	Female Range, μg/L
1–2	31–160	11–206
3–4	45–230	75–320
5–6	51–288	70–320
7–8	157–385	125–396
9–10	136–308	123–330
11–12	180–440	191–462
13–14	220–616	286–660
15–16	200–836	242–660
17–18	286–627	240–506

IGFBP-3 RADIOIMMUNOASSAY*

Age	Range, mg/L	Mean, mg/L
1–12 months	0.5–1.2	1.3
1–5 years	1.4–3.0	2.1
5–7 years	1.5–3.4	2.4
7–9 years	2.1–4.2	3.0
9–11 years	2.0–4.8	3.3
11–13 years	2.1–6.2	3.8
13–15 years	2.2–5.9	4.2
15–18 years	2.5–4.8	3.8
Adults, 20–30 years	2.0–4.2	3.0

CLONIDINE TEST OF GH RELEASE

NPO after midnight
Administration of clonidine by mouth:

Body weight, kg	Dose, mg
5–15	0.05
15–25	0.10
25–35	0.15
35–50	0.20
>50	0.25

Samples for measurement of GH at 0, 60, and 90 min
Side effects: Postural hypotension and somnolence
Keep patient supine until after postural hypotension is gone
Normal response: Greater than or equal to 10 μg/L (10 ng/mL) on any sample

* Age-related normals (may vary with assay).

such as renal failure, treatment is directed toward the underlying disease state. Similarly, short stature due to hypothyroidism or cortisol excess is managed by treatment of the primary disorder. In general, the earlier the disorder is diagnosed and treated, the more successful is the growth response; if treatment of the underlying disease is delayed until after puberty, little or no improvement in stature can be expected.

Unlike the broad species specificity of peptide hormones such as insulin, GH exhibits limited species specificity. Human GH stimulates linear growth in children with GH deficiency, whereas the bovine hormone is ineffective in humans. The collection of pituitary glands from autopsy material for the preparation of human GH did not supply adequate amounts of hormone for the treatment of all children who had GH deficiency, let alone provide sufficient material for the evaluation of GH for other conditions. Furthermore, the distribution of human pituitary GH in the United States and several other countries was discontinued in 1984 because of the development of Creutzfeldt-Jakob disease in patients who had been treated with human GH. The availability since 1985 of synthetic GH has relieved the supply problem. Hormone is readily available for patients with GH deficiency, and the potentially unlimited supply has allowed exploration of other therapeutic uses of GH, including the treatment of gonadal dysgenesis.

Most children with GH deficiency respond to GH treatment with an acceleration of growth rate to normal or above normal rates. As with other hormones, there is a dose-response curve to GH. The doses that have been tested range from 0.02 to 0.2 units (0.01 to 0.1 mg) per kilogram of body weight administered as a subcutaneous injection daily. There is a wide variation in response, but the higher dosages usually result in higher average growth rates. It is possible that in selected clinical circumstances dosages of GH higher than those currently recommended should be administered. Treatment may be started at a daily dose of 0.05 or 0.1 unit/kg (0.025 or 0.050 mg/kg). The majority of GH-deficient patients have a good growth response to this dosage. If the patient fails to show an adequate growth rate, the dose can be increased until an adequate growth response is obtained or until the upper limit of 1.50 units/kg of body weight per week is achieved. As doses of GH are increased above this level, the risk of glucose intolerance increases, particularly in children who are prediabetic.

An alternative method under study for the treatment of GH deficiency is the use either of GH-releasing hormone (GHRH) or GH-releasing peptide (GHRF). Since at least half of children with GH deficiency are able to secrete GH in response to GHRH, this approach may ultimately be useful for those patients.

Short stature of other causes   IDIOPATHIC SEVERE SHORT STATURE   Growth hormone has been given to some patients with growth failure not due to GH deficiency. Many children with severe short stature (more than 2.5 SD below the mean for age) do not have GH deficiency. Some of these children without GH deficiency are responsive to GH treatment. Many of these patients have low IGF-I, IGFBP-3, and/or GHBP levels and may have a partial defect in the control of GH secretion. Many such children have a short-term increase in growth rate in response to GH therapy; whether the final height of these children after GH treatment is greater than their predicted height is not established. Furthermore, it is not known whether there are serious long-term side effects.

GONADAL DYSGENESIS   GH also may have a role in the treatment of gonadal dysgenesis (see Chap. 62). The majority of women with gonadal dysgenesis have an average adult height between 135 and 142 cm. Androgens can cause a short-term increase in the rate of growth of girls with the disorder but do not result in an increase in final adult stature. The use of GH at modest doses is also associated with an increase in the rate of growth. Results of multicenter group studies utilizing synthetic GH either alone or in combination with androgens are encouraging in terms of both initial growth response and increases in final height.

SKELETAL DISORDERS   Growth hormone also has been used to treat small numbers of subjects with a wide variety of other growth disorders, including bone-cartilage dysplasias and other genetic syndromes associated with short stature. It is not clear whether GH is of use in any of these disorders.

REFERENCES

BAUMANN G: Growth hormone heterogeneity: Genes, isohormone, variants and binding proteins. Endocr Rev 12:424, 1991

BLIZZARD R et al: Idiopathic short stature: Results of a one-year controlled study of human growth hormone treatment. J Pediatr 115:713, 1989

BLUM WF et al: A specific radioimmunoassay for the growth hormone–dependent somatomedin binding protein: Its use for diagnosis of growth hormone deficiency. J Clin Endocrinol Metab 70:1291, 1990

BROWN P: Potential epidemic Creutzfeldt-Jakob disease from human growth hormone therapy. N Engl J Med 313:728, 1985

FRASIER SD: A review of growth hormone stimulation tests in children. Pediatrics 53:929, 1974

GRUMBACH M: Growth hormone therapy and the short end of the stick. N Engl J Med 319:238, 1988

HINDMARSH PC et al: Wider indications for treatment with biosynthetic human growth hormone in children. Clin Endocrinol 34:417, 1991

HINTZ RL: Growth factors. Curr Opin Pediatr 2:786, 1990

———: Untoward events in patients treated with GH in the USA. Horm Res 38(suppl 1):44, 1992

——— et al: Efficacy of growth hormone therapy in patients without classically defined growth hormone deficiency. Growth Genet Horm 8(suppl 1):10, 1992

HORNER JM et al: Growth deceleration patterns in constitutional short stature: An aid to diagnosis. Pediatrics 62:529, 1978

LANTOS J et al: Ethical issues of growth hormone therapy. JAMA 261:1020, 1989

LEE PDK et al: Efficacy of insulin-like growth factor I levels in predicting the response to provocative growth hormone testing. Pediatr Res 27:45, 1990

ROSENFELD RG et al: Six-year results of a randomized, prospective trial of human growth hormone and oxandrolone in Turner's syndrome. J Pediatr 49:121, 1992

TANNER JM, DAVIS PSW: Clinical longitudinal standards for height and height velocity for North American children. J Pediatr 107:317, 1985

———, ISREALSOHN WJ: Parent-child correlations for body measurements of children between the ages of one month and 7 years. Ann Hum Genet 26:245, 1963

——— et al: Effect of human growth hormone treatment for 1 to 7 years on growth of 100 children with growth hormone deficiency, inherited smallness, Turner's syndrome, and other complaints. Arch Dis Child 46:317, 1985

THORNER MO et al: Growth hormone–releasing hormone and growth hormone–releasing peptide as potential therapeutic modalities. Acta Paediatr Scand (Suppl) 376:29, 1990

VIPANI OV et al: Prevalence of severe growth hormone deficiency. Br Med J 2:427, 1977

333 DISORDERS OF THE NEUROHYPOPHYSIS

ARNOLD M. MOSES / DAVID H. P. STREETEN

Axons from two largely independent hypothalamic-neurohypophyseal systems in the supraoptic and paraventricular nuclei extend through the pituitary stalk to the posterior pituitary. Hormones (vasopressin and oxytocin), formed within separate ganglion cells, migrate down the axons as part of precursor proteins. They are stored in secretory granules within the nerve terminals in the neurohypophysis and are released by exocytosis into the bloodstream in response to appropriate stimuli. Vasopressin or antidiuretic hormone (AVP or ADH) controls water conservation, and its release is coordinated with the activity of the thirst center that regulates fluid intake. Oxytocin stimulates uterine contractions and milk ejection.

VASOPRESSIN SYNTHESIS, RELEASE, AND ACTION

SYNTHESIS   Vasopressin (AVP) is synthesized in the magnocellular neurons of the anterior hypothalamus. It is translated as a preprohormone which is altered in the Golgi apparatus to form a prohormone that is packaged into neurosecretory vesicles. While the prohormone is being transported to axonal terminals, enzymes generate

AVP, a 10,000 molecular weight protein called *neurophysin*, and a 39-amino-acid glycopeptide. All three products are released into the peripheral circulation.

ACTIONS AVP conserves water by concentrating the urine. It binds to the V_2 receptor on the contraluminal surface of the distal tubular epithelium, mainly in the collecting ducts. At this site AVP enhances the hydrosmotic flow of water from the lumen to the medullary interstitium and assists in maintaining constancy of the osmolality and volume of body fluids. High concentrations of AVP acting on V_1 receptors can cause vasoconstriction, as in response to severe hypotension or to infusion of vasopressin for treatment of bleeding esophageal varices.

AVP, perhaps from axons that terminate in the cerebrum, may play a role in learning and memory, and AVP from fibers in the median eminence may influence corticotropin secretion.

NORMAL HORMONE LEVELS AVP concentrations in plasma and urine can be measured by radioimmunoassay. The results may be expressed either as units based on pressor activity in the rat or in terms of weight of purified vasopressin. Arginine vasopressin has a biologic activity of approximately 400 units per milligram (1 mU = 2.5 ng = 2.3 pmol). The neurohypophysis under conditions of random fluid intake contains approximately 8 units, or 18 nmol (20 µg), of AVP. Under the same conditions, peripheral plasma AVP concentration ranges from 1.4 to 5.6 pmol/L (1.5 to 6 ng/L). At the latter plasma level and above, urine osmolality is maximal. The AVP concentration in blood fluctuates, with a maximum late at night and in the early morning and a minimum in the early afternoon. Under conditions of normal hydration, healthy subjects release approximately 370 to 1400 pmol (400 to 1500 ng) from the pituitary and excrete 23 to 80 pmol (25 to 90 ng) AVP in urine in 24 h. During 24 to 28 h of dehydration, the amount released increases three to five times with consequent increases in plasma and urinary levels.

METABOLISM Inactivation of AVP occurs largely in liver and kidneys, a major mechanism being the cleavage of the terminal glycinamide to produce a biologically inactive substance. Approximately 7 to 10 percent of secreted AVP is excreted in the urine as active hormone.

CONTROL OF AVP RELEASE The release of AVP is influenced by a number of stimuli.

Osmoregulation Under normal conditions, AVP release is primarily regulated by osmoreceptors in the hypothalamus. Changes in the concentrations of plasma solutes to which the cellular membrane is impermeable cause alterations in the volume of the osmoreceptor cells, which in turn alter the electric activity of the neurons and control AVP release. Osmotic changes that stimulate release also enhance production of AVP. The servomechanism between effective plasma osmolality and AVP release normally maintains plasma osmolality within a very narrow range. The mean plasma osmolality of normal subjects following a water load of 20 mL/kg of body weight is 281.7 mmol/kg plasma water, and the osmolality that initiates AVP release following infusion of hypertonic saline solution into water-loaded subjects is 287.3 mmol/kg. Thus the increase in plasma osmolality from full diuresis to the initiation of antidiuresis by hypertonic saline solution is only 5.6 mmol/kg, or 2 percent.

The infusion of hypertonic saline solution into water-loaded subjects causes a linear rise in plasma osmolality with time. After an interval, there is an abrupt, progressive fall in free water clearance without a significant change in solute or creatinine excretion. We have defined the osmotic threshold for AVP release as the plasma osmolality at the onset of antidiuresis under these conditions. In 73 normal subjects, this occurred at a mean plasma osmolality of 287 mmol/kg. The osmotic threshold for AVP release also may be determined, with very similar results, by constructing a linear regression line between simultaneously obtained plasma osmolality and either plasma or urine AVP concentration during hypertonic saline infusion and extrapolating the regression line to the *x*-axis intercept (plasma osmolality).

Volume regulation Decreases in plasma volume, through effects on stretch receptors in the left atrium and perhaps in the pulmonary veins, stimulate the release of AVP by reducing the tonic inhibitory impulses from the left atrium to the hypothalamus. The neural impulses travel via the vagi to the reticular formation of the midbrain and diencephalon and thence to the supraoptic and paraventricular nuclei, where they are integrated with the other stimuli that affect AVP release. Positive-pressure breathing, quiet standing, and vasodilatation may activate this mechanism, which serves to restore plasma volume, even at times overriding osmotic inhibition of AVP release. Following volume contraction, circulating AVP concentrations may reach 10 times the levels induced by hypertonicity. Increased plasma volume inhibits AVP release by the reverse mechanisms, leading to a diuresis and correction of the hypervolemia. Negative-pressure breathing, recumbency, lack of gravitational force (as in space travel), submersion in water, and exposure to cold may activate this mechanism.

Baroreceptor regulation Activation of carotid and aortic baroreceptors in response to hypotension causes release of AVP. Hypotension due to blood loss is the most potent stimulus and may at times raise plasma levels of AVP to 560 pmol/L (600 ng/L). These concentrations of AVP may cause vasoconstriction, which probably plays a role in the restoration of blood pressure.

Neural regulation Many neurotransmitters and neuropeptides in the hypothalamus play a role in regulating and modulating the release of AVP. Acetylcholine stimulates AVP release by its nicotinic action on supraoptic neurons. Angiotensin II, histamine, bradykinin, and neuropeptide Y probably stimulate AVP release. Norepinephrine, prostaglandins, and dopamine stimulate or inhibit AVP release, depending on the experimental conditions. Gamma aminobutyric acid appears to act as an inhibitory neurotransmitter; serotonin and substance P are also present in the supraoptic nucleus, but their influence on magnocellular neuron activity is not clear. The regulatory action of opioid peptides on AVP release is unclear, with reports indicating stimulation, inhibition, or no effect. Though the roles of these and other transmitters and peptides are still poorly defined, the antidiuretic actions of stress, emesis, and pain and the diuretic actions of hypnosis, psychological conditioning, and inhalation of carbon dioxide indicate that higher centers have an important influence on the release of AVP.

Aging Aging is associated with enhanced AVP release in response to a rising plasma osmolality and a progressive increase in plasma AVP concentration. These changes appear to place the older individual at greater risk of developing water retention and hyponatremia, despite a concomitant decline in maximal renal concentrating capacity in response to AVP, which is usually evident beyond 60 years of age.

Pharmacologic influences Pharmacologic agents that can stimulate AVP release include nicotine, morphine, vincristine, vinblastine, cyclophosphamide, clofibrate, chlorpropamide, and some tricyclic anticonvulsants and antidepressants. Ethanol has diuretic properties by inhibiting neurohypophyseal function under a variety of conditions. Some narcotic antagonists also inhibit AVP release. Experimentally, chlorpromazine, reserpine, and phenytoin all inhibit the loss of AVP from the pituitary and the rise in urinary excretion of AVP that result from water deprivation. In humans, phenytoin and chlorpromazine may inhibit AVP release and produce diuresis.

AVP RESPONSE TO WATER DEPRIVATION AND TO WATER LOAD Water deprivation provides both an osmotic and a volume stimulus to vasopressin release by increasing plasma osmolality and decreasing plasma volume. The maximum urinary osmolality after water deprivation depends on renal medullary osmolality and other intrarenal factors. In response to fluid deprivation for 18 to 24 h in normal individuals, plasma osmolality rarely rises above 292 mmol/kg. The resultant stimulation of AVP release increases plasma AVP concentration to 7.4 to 14 pmol/L (8 to 15 ng/L).

The administration of water lowers plasma osmolality and expands blood volume, inhibiting the release of AVP via both osmoreceptor and atrial volume receptor mechanisms. An oral water load of 20 mL/kg in normal adults results in a fall in plasma osmolality to a mean of 281.7 mmol/kg and causes a maximum diuresis in 1 to 1½ h with free water clearance rising to approximately 12 mL/min and urine osmolality falling to 40 to 60 mmol/kg. The delay in reaching maximal diuresis is accounted for by the time involved in absorption of water from the gut, in metabolizing previously secreted vasopressin, and in renal recovery from the action of vasopressin.

INTERACTION OF OSMOTIC AND VOLUME INFLUENCES

Under conditions of water deprivation and of water loading, volume and osmotic influences act in parallel to influence AVP release. In other circumstances, volume and osmotic influences may be competitive, and changes in plasma volume can modify the effects of hypertonic stimuli on AVP release. Osmotic factors ordinarily predominate to maintain plasma osmolality within a narrow range. Larger changes in blood volume, such as those induced by hemorrhage, may blunt and eventually overcome the osmotic influences, and hypotension can activate arterial baroreceptors to exert a powerful stimulus to the elaboration of AVP and override simultaneous inhibiting influences.

RELATION BETWEEN AVP RELEASE AND THIRST-INDUCED WATER INTAKE

Under normal conditions, there is close coordination between AVP release and thirst, both of which are regulated by small changes in plasma osmolality. The perception of thirst generally becomes apparent when plasma osmolality exceeds 292 mmol/kg. Thus water intake is not stimulated until the urine is maximally concentrated. Angiotensin II increases thirst and AVP release under conditions of extracellular volume depletion. Normally, therefore, water losses lead to slight hypernatremia which increases thirst and fluid intake to restore and maintain normal plasma osmolality. In contrast, when there is loss of thirst perception (adipsia), fluid losses are uncorrected, and hypernatremia occurs even though AVP release is adequate to concentrate the urine maximally.

EFFECTS OF GLUCOCORTICOIDS

Hormones of the adrenal cortex and the posterior pituitary have antagonistic effects on water excretion. Cortisol elevates the osmotic threshold for AVP release elicited by hypertonic saline infusion in water-loaded normal subjects, and glucocorticoids protect against water intoxication and overcome the impaired response to water loading in adrenal insufficiency.

Although the impaired ability to dilute the urine in adrenal insufficiency may be due in part to excessive circulating AVP, glucocorticoids also can act directly on the renal tubules to decrease water permeability and increase excretion of solute-free water in the absence of AVP.

CELLULAR MECHANISM OF AVP ACTIVITY

The mechanism of action of AVP in the renal tubule is shown in Fig. 333-1: (1) AVP binds to contraluminal V_2 receptor sites, (2) the receptor-hormone complex activates adenylate cyclase in the same contraluminal membrane via a guanine nucleotide binding stimulatory protein (see Chap. 69), (3) the production of cyclic AMP is increased, (4) the cyclic AMP is translocated to the luminal cell membrane where it activates a membrane-bound protein kinase, (5) the activated protein kinase causes the phosphorylation of membrane proteins, and (6) permeability of the luminal membrane to water is increased. The AVP-generated cyclic AMP may be inactivated by a phosphodiesterase. AVP also stimulates prostaglandin E_2 production, which, in turn, acts as a feedback inhibitor of adenylate cyclase activation.

The final event in the transtubular movement of water is the appearance of particle aggregates in the luminal membrane of the cell (Fig. 333-2). This aggregation relieves the rate-limiting barrier to water flow. In the presence of the aggregates, water molecules can move passively along an osmotic gradient. The transtubular movement of water depends also on the integrity of the microtubular system.

Various cations and drugs influence the action of AVP. Calcium and lithium inhibit the adenylate cyclase response to vasopressin. Lithium also interferes with a subsequent biochemical action, as does potassium deficiency. Demeclocycline inhibits adenylate cyclase

FIGURE 333-1 Schematic representation of the cellular action of vasopressin. The increased water permeability of responsive cells involves the V_2 receptor for vasopressin. Uninterrupted arrows denote steps that have been defined, interrupted arrows with question marks, postulated steps. ADH = antidiuretic hormone or vasopressin; i and s = inhibitory and stimulatory guanine nucleotide regulatory proteins; cAMP-PDE = phosphodiesterase; IMPs = intramembranous particles. (*From H Valtin, in EE Windhager, ed., Handbook of Physiology, Sect. 8: Renal Physiology, New York, Oxford, 1992.*)

stimulation by AVP and also inhibits the cyclic AMP–dependent protein kinase. In contrast, chlorpropamide increases AVP-induced activation of adenylate cyclase.

DEFICIENCY OF VASOPRESSIN: DIABETES INSIPIDUS

Diabetes insipidus refers to the passage through the body of a large quantity of dilute fluid. This state of excessive water intake and hypotonic polyuria may be due to failure of AVP release in response to normal physiologic stimuli (central or neurogenic diabetes insipidus) or failure of the kidney to respond to AVP (nephrogenic diabetes insipidus).

PATHOPHYSIOLOGY Deficiency of vasopressin release in response to the appropriate stimuli can result from lesions at several functional sites in the physiologic chain of events that regulates hormone release. Four types of central diabetes insipidus can be defined. Patients of the first type show very little rise in urine osmolality, even with a marked increase in plasma osmolality (1, Fig. 333-3) and no evidence of AVP release during hypertonic saline infusion. They are essentially devoid of releasable AVP. In the second type there is an abrupt increase in urine osmolality during dehydration (2, Fig. 333-3), but there is no evidence of an osmotic threshold during saline infusion. These patients have a defective osmoreceptor mechanism but can release AVP in response to the hypovolemia of severe dehydration. The third type of patient has some rise in urine osmolality with increasing plasma osmolality (3, Fig. 333-3) and has an elevated osmotic threshold for AVP release. These patients have a sluggish release mechanism due to a high-set osmoreceptor. In the fourth type of patient, urine and plasma osmolality coordinates are shifted to the right of normal (4, Fig. 333-3). AVP release in these patients is initiated at a normal plasma osmolality but is subnormal in amount.

FIGURE 333-2 Virtual absence of particle clusters in renal collecting duct luminal membrane obtained from untreated Brattleboro (congenital diabetes insipidus) rat (*top*). Appearance of particle clusters (arrows) after treatment with AVP (*bottom*). (*From MC Harmanci et al, Am J Physiol 235:F440, 1978.*)

The second to fourth types of patients may develop a good antidiuresis in response to nausea, nicotine, methacholine, chlorpropamide, or clofibrate, indicating that the synthesis and storage of AVP are sufficient to allow for adequate urinary concentrating ability in the presence of an appropriate stimulus to release. In rare instances, patients of the second to fourth types may present with asymptomatic hypernatremia associated with mild or no polyuria.

ETIOLOGY The causes of central diabetes insipidus in 135 patients who satisfied the criteria described under "Diagnostic Tests" (below) and who had had the disorder for at least 6 months are shown in Table 333-1. Diabetes insipidus frequently starts in childhood or early adult life (median age of onset 24 years) and is more common in males than females. The major causes are as follows: (1) *Neoplastic* or *infiltrative lesions* of the hypothalamus or pituitary, including pituitary adenomas, craniopharyngiomas, germinomas, pinealomas, metastatic tumors, leukemia, histiocytosis X, and sarcoidosis, caused diabetes insipidus in 37 patients. In approximately 60 percent of these patients partial or complete loss of anterior pituitary function was present. (2) *Pituitary* or *hypothalamic surgery* caused diabetes insipidus in 32 patients and was usually associated with anterior hypopituitarism. Surgically induced diabetes insipidus usually develops between 1 and 6 days after surgery and often disappears after a few days. It may recur and become chronic after an "interphase" of 1 to 5 days. Removal of the posterior lobe of the pituitary induces permanent diabetes insipidus only if the pituitary stalk is sectioned high enough to induce retrograde degeneration of most neurons of the supraoptic nucleus. (3) *Severe head injuries*, usually associated with fractures of the skull, caused diabetes insipidus in 24 patients and were associated with anterior hypopituitarism in about one-sixth of patients. Spontaneous remissions of traumatic diabetes insipidus may occur even after 6 months, presumably because of regeneration of disrupted axons within the pituitary stalk. (4) *Idiopathic diabetes insipidus* (in 34 patients) usually starts in childhood and is seldom (<20 percent) associated with anterior pituitary dysfunction. This diagnosis can be made only after a careful search has failed to reveal evidence of a tumor, infiltrative or vascular lesion, or other presumptive cause of AVP deficiency. The presence of anterior hypopituitarism or hyperprolactinemia or radiologic evidence of lesions within or above the sella should stimulate a continuing search for a causative lesion at 3- to 12-month intervals. The diagnosis of idiopathic diabetes insipidus is made with increasing confidence as the duration of negative findings on follow-up increases. The number of neurons in

FIGURE 333-3 Relation of plasma and urinary osmolality during hydration and dehydration in normal adult subjects (shaded area) and in four types of patients with diabetes insipidus.

TABLE 333-1 Characteristics of 135 cases of long-standing* central diabetes insipidus diagnosed by the authors at SUNY Health Science Center, Syracuse. Categories are arranged in order of increasing median age of onset.

| | Age of onset, years | | | | Percent of cases |
Cause	Median[†]	Range	Males	Females	
Histiocytosis	2	1–30	3	2	4
Primary brain tumor —postoperative[‡]	15	6–50	9	11	15
Primary brain tumor —preoperative[§]	18	7–58	17	3	15
Idiopathic	20	<1–66	20	14	25
Head trauma	22	5–48	15	9	18
Nontraumatic encephalomalacia	43	15–73	3	4	5
Ruptured cerebral aneurysm	39		1	0	1
Post-hypophysectomy	42	24–68	4	8	9
Sarcoidosis	42		0	1	1
Metastatic cancer	56	32–72	6	5	8
			(58%)	(42%)	

* Longer than 6 months or until death.
† Median age of entire group = 24 years.
‡ 16 cases were of craniopharyngioma.
§ 5 cases were glioma, 7 germinoma, and 4 craniopharyngioma.

the supraoptic and paraventricular nuclei may be decreased in idiopathic diabetes insipidus, and circulating antibodies to hypothalamic nuclei may be present. In rare instances, diabetes insipidus may be inherited as an isolated defect or as part of an autosomal recessive syndrome (DIDMOAD) consisting of diabetes insipidus (DI), diabetes mellitus (DM), optic atrophy (OA), and deafness (D) (also called the *Wolfram syndrome*; see Chap. 343). (5) Seven patients had nontraumatic encephalomalacia from a variety of causes, including shock, cardiopulmonary arrest, hypertensive encephalopathy, poisoning, and meningitis. All the patients were brain dead and maintained on total life support systems.

Diabetes insipidus may appear during pregnancy and cease a few days after delivery, or it may commence after parturition in women with Sheehan's syndrome, especially when cortisol deficiency is treated. Mild symptoms of diabetes insipidus may either increase or improve during pregnancy. AVP-resistant diabetes insipidus also may develop during pregnancy, perhaps due to increased circulating levels of placental vasopressinase. Fortunately, such patients respond to treatment with desmopressin.

CLINICAL MANIFESTATIONS *Polyuria, excessive thirst,* and *polydipsia* are almost invariably present in diabetes insipidus. Characteristically, these symptoms are sudden in onset, both when the disorder first presents itself and whenever the effects of administered vasopressin disappear during long-term therapy. In severe cases, the urine is pale in color, and the volume may be immense (up to 16 to 24 L/d), requiring micturition every 30 to 60 min throughout the day and night. More frequently, however, urine volume is only moderately increased (2.5 to 6 L/d), and occasionally it may be less than 2 L/d, causing no complaints on the part of the patient. Urinary concentration (less than 290 mmol/kg, specific gravity less than 1.010) is below that of the serum in severe cases but may be higher than that of serum (290 to 600 mmol/kg) in mild diabetes insipidus.

The slight rise in serum osmolality resulting from hypotonic polyuria stimulates thirst. Large volumes of fluid are imbibed, and cold drinks are preferred, patients often going to great trouble to secure cold fluids. Although thirst is probably secondary to loss of water, the administration of vasopressin may relieve or reduce thirst, even in the absence of fluid intake.

Normal function of the thirst center ensures that polydipsia closely matches polyuria, so dehydration is seldom detectable except by a mild elevation of serum sodium. However, when replenishment of excreted water is inadequate, dehydration may become severe, causing weakness, fever, psychic disturbances, prostration, and death. These features are associated with a rising serum osmolality and serum sodium concentration, the latter sometimes exceeding 175 mmol/L. Adipsia does not occur in idiopathic diabetes insipidus, but it may result from impaired function of the hypothalamic thirst center because of extension of the same abnormality that caused the diabetes insipidus. Alternatively, dehydration can occur during unconsciousness produced by surgical anesthesia, head trauma, or other causes.

Hydronephrosis and renal failure may complicate polyuria, especially in patients who fail to empty their bladders adequately because of bladder atony, urethral strictures, or other causes.

DIAGNOSTIC TESTS The cause of hypotonic polyuria can usually be recognized by a pragmatic clinical approach. Even though stimuli such as nausea, nicotine administration, hypoglycemia, and hypotension may release AVP, the results are clinically irrelevant. It is of little consequence to the patient with symptomatic diabetes insipidus that one or more nonosmotic stimuli retains its capacity to release AVP. The following procedures, which utilize plasma and urine osmolality determinations, are readily available, reliable, and safe, and they allow the physician to establish the diagnosis and to initiate therapy rapidly. Measurements of plasma or urine AVP are expensive and time-consuming and are only occasionally needed, when osmolality measurements are inconclusive (Fig. 333-4). Diagnostic tests should not be performed in the presence of untreated thyroid or adrenocortical deficiency or when there is an osmotic diuresis (e.g., uncontrolled diabetes mellitus).

FIGURE 333-4 Relationship between plasma osmolality (Posm) and urinary AVP excretion (U$_{AVP}$) in normal subjects (shaded area on left), patients with central diabetes insipidus (shaded area on right), and patients with nephrogenic diabetes insipidus (individual data points). Correlates in patients with SIADH fall to the left of the normal range. [*From AM Moses, in P Czernichow and AG Robinson (eds), Frontiers of Hormone Research, vol 13: Diabetes Insipidus in Man, Basel, Karger, 1985.*]

Assessment of the relation of plasma to urine osmolality The normal relationship between plasma osmolality (assuming no increase in blood urea or glucose) and urine osmolality is indicated in Fig. 333-3. If several simultaneously determined plasma and urine osmolalities in a patient with polyuria fall substantially to the right of the shaded area, the patient has central or nephrogenic diabetes insipidus. The latter diagnosis can be made if the response to injected vasopressin is subnormal (see "Dehydration Test," below) or if plasma or urinary AVP concentration is increased. The practice of relating plasma to urine osmolality is useful, particularly in postoperative neurosurgical cases or after head trauma, where its use can lead quickly to the differentiation of diabetes insipidus from parenteral fluid excess. If necessary, intravenous hydration can be slowed temporarily, and repeated plasma and urine osmolalities can be plotted as in Fig. 333-3, to determine whether the relationship is normal.

Dehydration test Comparison of the urinary osmolality after dehydration with that after vasopressin administration is a simple and reliable way of diagnosing diabetes insipidus and of differentiating vasopressin deficiency from other causes of polyuria. This test should be combined with the assessment of the relationship between plasma and urine osmolality.

The maximal urinary concentrating capacity varies among individuals, and no absolute lower limits of "normal" can be defined in patients with nonspecific illnesses in whom AVP is produced in adequate amounts. It is impossible to distinguish between deficiency and sufficiency of AVP release solely by the level of the urinary osmolality attained after specified periods of water deprivation. On the other hand, if after prolonged dehydration vasopressin administration induces a further rise in urinary osmolality, there is a strong implication that vasopressin deficiency exists.

PROCEDURE

1 Fluids are withheld long enough to result in stable hourly urinary osmolalities (an hourly increase of < 30 mmol/kg for at least three successive hours). This is usually associated with a loss in body weight of at least 1 kg. In patients whose daily urinary volumes exceed 10 liters, the fluid deprivation should begin between 4 A.M. and 6 A.M. so that the patient can be carefully watched and the test terminated if weight loss exceeds 2 kg or the clinical condition deteriorates. In patients whose urinary volumes are only mildly increased or who are hyponatremic, water deprivation may be started about midnight.

2 Urine specimens are collected hourly for osmolality measurements from 6 A.M. at least until noon and preferably until the osmolality is stable for three consecutive hours.

3 After the third hour of stable urinary osmolality, the patient is given vasopressin as 5 units aqueous arginine vasopressin or 1 μg desmopressin by subcutaneous injection or 10 μg desmopressin by nasal spray.

4 Plasma osmolality is determined immediately before the injection of vasopressin, and urinary osmolality is measured on the specimen collected between 30 and 60 min after the injection.

Vital signs should be monitored during the procedure, but when the test is performed as described, adverse effects are rare.

INTERPRETATION In subjects with normal pituitary function, urinary osmolality does not rise by more than 9 percent after the injection of vasopressin, whatever the maximal urinary osmolality achieved after dehydration alone. In central diabetes insipidus, the rise in urinary osmolality after vasopressin exceeds 9 percent. To ensure adequacy of dehydration, plasma osmolality before the vasopressin injection should be above 288 mmol/kg. Patients who have polyuria from renal diseases, potassium depletion, or nephrogenic diabetes insipidus (see below) usually show little rise in urinary osmolality with dehydration and no further rise after vasopressin injection. Patients with compulsive water drinking (primary polydipsia) often require prolonged water deprivation before plasma osmolality reaches 288 mmol/kg and before a plateau in urinary osmolality is reached; urinary osmolality rises by < 9 percent after the administration of exogenous vasopressin.

Hypertonic saline infusions These tests are sometimes necessary to differentiate between primary polydipsia and partial central diabetes insipidus. In the former the osmotic threshold is low, normal, or slightly increased, while in the latter it is substantially increased or absent. See references for details.

DIFFERENTIAL DIAGNOSIS Diabetes insipidus must be distinguished from other types of hypotonic polyuria (primary polydipsia and nephrogenic diabetes insipidus) and from states of osmotic diuresis (Table 333-2). Several are recognizable by the history

---

TABLE 333-2 Major polyuric syndromes

Primary disorders of water intake or output
A Excessive water intake
   1 Psychogenic polydipsia
   2 Hypothalamic disease: histiocytosis X, sarcoidosis, trauma
   3 Drug-induced polydipsia
     a Thioridazine
     b Chlorpromazine
     c Anticholinergic drugs (dry mouth)
B Inadequate tubular reabsorption of filtered water
   1 Vasopressin deficiency
     a Central diabetes insipidus
     b Drug-induced inhibition of AVP release
       (1) Narcotic antagonists
   2 Renal tubular unresponsiveness to AVP
     a Nephrogenic diabetes insipidus (congenital and familial)
     b Nephrogenic diabetes insipidus (acquired)
       (1) Several chronic renal diseases, after obstructive uropathy, unilateral renal arterial stenosis, after renal transplantation, after acute tubular necrosis
       (2) Potassium deficiencies, including primary aldosteronism
       (3) Chronic hypercalcemias, including hyperparathyroidism
       (4) Drug-induced: lithium, methoxyflurane anesthesia, demeclocycline
       (5) Various systemic disorders: multiple myeloma, amyloidosis, sickle cell anemia, Sjögren's syndrome
Primary disorders of renal absorption of solutes (osmotic diuresis)
A Glucose: diabetes mellitus
B Salts, especially sodium chloride
   1 Various chronic renal diseases, especially chronic pyelonephritis
   2 After various diuretics, including mannitol

(e.g., following lithium or mannitol administration, surgery under methoxyflurane anesthesia, or renal transplantation). In others the physical examination or simple laboratory procedures will indicate the diagnosis (evidence of glycosuria, renal disease, sickle cell anemia, hypercalcemia, or potassium depletion, including primary aldosteronism).

Congenital nephrogenic diabetes insipidus is usually inherited as an X-linked recessive trait. Affected males are totally resistant to vasopressin, while heterozygote females are asymptomatic or have mild polyuria. In several families the abnormal gene is localized to the Xq28 region of the long arm of the X chromosome. Almost all these patients have a V_2 receptor abnormality. Nephrogenic diabetes insipidus also may be inherited as an autosomal recessive trait or may occur sporadically. Females with sporadic disease appear to have a defect in the pathway of AVP action distal the V_2 receptor, and some of them respond to large doses of desmopressin. V_1 receptor–mediated functions are normal in patients with congenital nephrogenic diabetes insipidus.

When patients with nephrogenic and central diabetes insipidus cannot be differentiated by simpler means, documentation of elevated plasma or urinary AVP concentration in relation to plasma osmolality (Fig. 333-4) or of a high AVP concentration in relation to urine osmolality will allow the diagnosis of nephrogenic diabetes insipidus.

Primary polydipsia Primary or psychogenic polydipsia may be difficult to differentiate from diabetes insipidus and occurs in two forms. Chronic overingestion of water results in hypotonic polyuria and is often confused with diabetes insipidus. The intermittent ingestion of large quantities of fluid also may lead to water intoxication and dilutional hyponatremia even though urinary diluting capacity is normal. This phenomenon is rare because normal adults can excrete between 10 and 14 mL/min of solute-free water, and it is unusual to ingest more water than this.

Polydipsia and polyuria may be erratic, even in the chronic form of primary polydipsia. This is in contrast to the sustained polydipsia and polyuria of diabetes insipidus. These patients often have no nocturnal polyuria. Of 17 patients with sustained primary polydipsia, 10 were female and 7 were male, with a median age of onset of 34 years (range 14 to 48). In three patients the onset of primary polydipsia followed head trauma, two had hypothalamic sarcoidosis, one was the sister of a patient with congenital nephrogenic diabetes insipidus, one was mentally retarded, and one had a hypothalamic lesion of unknown cause. The remaining nine patients had moderate to severe psychiatric disturbances, and some were taking psychoactive drugs with anticholinergic properties. The syndrome also has been described in patients with anorexia nervosa who drink huge quantities of water. There is a predisposition toward dilutional hyponatremia in patients who ingest excessive fluids when urinary diluting capacity is impaired by therapeutic agents such as nonsteroidal anti-inflammatory drugs or thiazide diuretics.

The diagnosis is usually evident from the combination of low plasma and urinary osmolalities. The relationship between urine and plasma osmolality during water deprivation is typically normal or supranormal (to left of normal in Fig. 333-3). There is an absent or minimal rise in urine osmolality after injection of vasopressin at the plateau of urine osmolality during dehydration. Because chronic overingestion of water may suppress release of AVP, and because chronic polyuria may cause a wash-out of the medullary osmotic gradient, urine osmolality may be subnormal in relation to plasma osmolality (to right of normal in Fig. 333-3). Therefore, it may be difficult, if not impossible, to differentiate primary polydipsia from partial central diabetes insipidus. Indeed, patients may have both problems. Treatment of these patients with vasopressin, even under close supervision, usually results in water intoxication.

A simple diagnostic approach to patients with hypotonic polyuria is shown in Fig. 333-5.

Determination of the cause of hypotonic polyuria Once the type of the hypotonic polyuria is established, the cause must be determined (see "Etiology"). Even though treatment of the underlying

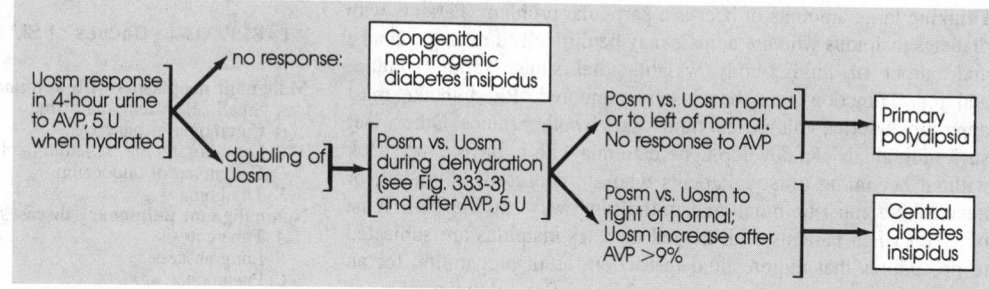

FIGURE 333-5 Approach to hypotonic polyurias.

disease only rarely causes the polyuria to regress, the underlying disease can at times be treated with success (e.g., germinoma). In this sense, the development of the polyuria can be considered a tumor marker.

The patient's history can reveal important clues such as age of onset and duration of disease, presence in other members of the family, constancy of symptoms, preference for cold or lukewarm fluids, head trauma, evidence of anterior pituitary deficiency, symptoms suggesting a space-occupying lesion, etc. Examination may reveal evidence of endocrine deficiency or excess (particularly hyperprolactinemia) or of malignant, granulomatous, or infectious disease. Routine laboratory tests and chests radiographs may provide important information.

Most patients with newly diagnosed central diabetes insipidus and primary polydipsia should have a magnetic resonance imaging study of the pituitary-hypothalamic area. In addition to providing insight into the underlying pathologic abnormality, the presence or absence of the posterior pituitary hyperintense signal with appropriate T_1-weighted imaging may confirm the diagnosis, since the signal is absent in central diabetes insipidus and present in primary polydipsia. Information obtained from lumbar puncture or even, at times, hypothalamic biopsy may diagnose lesions observed by magnetic resonance imaging. If magnetic resonance imaging is negative in patients with central diabetes insipidus, it should be repeated at increasing time intervals.

TREATMENT (See Table 333-3) Diabetes insipidus can be treated by hormone replacement. As is true of most peptides, oral administration of vasopressin is ineffective. Aqueous arginine vasopressin may be administered subcutaneously in doses of 5 to 10 units and usually has a duration of action of 3 to 6 h. The main use of this preparation is in initial management of unconscious patients with acute onset of diabetes insipidus following head trauma or a neurosurgical procedure. Its short duration of action allows recognition of the recovery of neurohypophyseal function and minimizes the development of water intoxication in patients receiving intravenous fluids.

Desmopressin has prolonged antidiuretic activity and is almost completely devoid of pressor effects. When used intranasally in amounts between 10 and 20 μg (0.1 to 0.2 mL) or by subcutaneous injection (1 to 4 μg), it has an antidiuretic action for 12 to 24 h in most patients. This analogue is the drug of choice in the treatment of most patients with diabetes insipidus. Lypressin is a nasal spray; a single application may result in an antidiuresis lasting approximately 4 to 6 h. Nasal absorption of both analogues may be decreased in the presence of an upper respiratory infection or allergic rhinitis. In such circumstances and in unconscious or uncooperative patients with diabetes insipidus, desmopressin should be given by subcutaneous injection.

Patients with diabetes insipidus who have some residual releasable AVP (types 2 to 4) may respond to oral treatment with chlorpropamide, clofibrate, or carbamazepine. Chlorpropamide stimulates AVP release and potentiates the antidiuretic action of submaximal amounts of AVP. Doses of 200 to 500 mg, usually taken once daily, are sufficient for an antidiuretic response. Its action starts within several hours of administration and usually lasts for 24 h. Chlorpropamide also may restore thirst perception and thus be useful in patients with thirst center defects. Oral hypoglycemic agents are rarely used because of hypoglycemia and other undesirable side effects.

The only way to treat most patients with nephrogenic diabetes insipidus is by solute restriction and administering thiazides or other diuretics. The resulting sodium depletion causes a fall in glomerular filtration rate with enhanced reabsorption of fluid in the proximal portion of the nephron and decreased delivery of sodium to the ascending limb of the loop of Henle and consequently reduced capacity to dilute the urine. Some women with congenital nephrogenic diabetes insipidus and some patients with lithium-induced polyuria have been treated effectively by injecting large doses of desmopressin.

When antidiuretic therapy is initiated in patients with longstanding diabetes insipidus care must be taken to avoid excessive drinking, which could result in water intoxication. Education about drinking according to thirst must be reinforced constantly in some patients.

TABLE 333-3 Agents used in treatment of diabetes insipidus

	Dose form	Usual dose	Duration of action, h
CENTRAL DIABETES INSIPIDUS			
Hormone replacement:			
Aqueous arginine vasopressin	10 or 20 units/ampul	5–10 units subcutaneously	3–6
Desmopressin	2.5 and 5.0 mL intranasal preparations, 100 μg/mL; 1- or 10-mL ampul, for injection, 4 μg/mL	10–20 μg intranasally or 1–4 μg subcutaneously	12–24
Lypressin	5-mL bottle, 50 units/mL	2–4 units intranasally	4–6
Nonhormonal agents:			
Chlorpropamide	100- and 250-mg tablets	200–500 mg daily	
Clofibrate	500-mg capsules	500 mg four times daily	
Carbamazepine	200-mg tablets	400–600 mg daily	
NEPHROGENIC DIABETES INSIPIDUS			
Hydrochlorothiazide	50-mg tablets	50–100 mg daily	
Chlorthalidone	50-mg tablets	50 mg daily	

Drinking large amounts of beer is a particular problem. Patients with diabetes insipidus who are adipsic may be difficult to manage. Intake and output of fluids, body weight, vital signs, serum sodium, and renal function must be closely monitored. Fluid intake must approximate urine volume and fluid losses by other routes. Otherwise, such individuals can develop hypernatremia with hypovolemic shock without becoming thirsty. Patients who are confused, obtunded, or unconscious must be monitored in the same way. Special care must be taken when patients with treated diabetes insipidus are subjected to procedures that require fluid restriction, as in preparation for an intravenous pyelogram, or hydration, as after administration of chemotherapy. In the former situation fluid intake must be restricted to conform to urine output. In patients receiving antidiuretic therapy fluids should not be administered beyond the amounts determined by thirst or urine output. If high urine flow rates are necessary, antidiuretic therapy can be discontinued, or furosemide may be administered while antidiuretic therapy is continued.

SYNDROMES ASSOCIATED WITH VASOPRESSIN EXCESS

Excessive blood levels or actions of vasopressin are associated with and probably cause water retention in several circumstances:

1 As a mechanism for *prevention of a rise in plasma osmolality* which would otherwise result from sodium retention in edema associated with congestive heart failure, cirrhosis with ascites, nephrosis, orthostatic edema, myxedema, and treatment with sodium-retaining drugs (fludrocortisone, nonsteroidal anti-inflammatory agents, and others)

2 As a mechanism of *defense against hypovolemia and/or hypotension* in subjects with adrenal insufficiency, excessive fluid loss (from vomiting, diarrhea, drug-induced diuresis, and excessive sweating), fluid deprivation, and probably positive-pressure respiration

3 As a consequence of *drug- or disease-induced release of vasopressin from the neurohypophysis* caused by:

   a Central nervous system disorders: head trauma, subdural hematoma, subarachnoid hemorrhage, cerebral vascular thrombosis, brain tumor, cerebral atrophy, acute encephalitis, acute psychosis, tuberculous and other meningitides

   b Drugs that release or potentiate the action of AVP: chlorpropamide, vincristine, vinblastine, cyclophosphamide, carbamazepine, general anesthetics, tricyclic antidepressants

4 In *ectopic AVP production and release:*

   a From *neoplastic tissue:* small cell carcinoma of lung, pancreatic carcinoma, lymphosarcoma, Hodgkin's disease, reticulum cell sarcoma, thymoma, carcinoma of duodenum or bladder

   b From *inflammatory lung diseases:* tuberculosis, lung abscess, pneumonias, empyema

5 *Other conditions:* Guillain-Barré syndrome, lupus erythematosus, acute intermittent porphyria, severe renovascular hypertension, and old age

SYNDROME OF INAPPROPRIATE AVP SECRETION OR SIADH

SIADH is the term applied to vasopressin excess of types 3 to 5 above, associated with hyponatremia without edema (Table 333-4). In these patients, the AVP excess is considered to be inappropriate because it occurs in the presence of plasma hypoosmolality. SIADH is analogous to abnormalities produced by administration of vasopressin and water to normal subjects. Although it may be conceptually valid to consider the AVP excess to be inappropriate in adrenal insufficiency and the edematous, hypovolemic, and hypotensive disorders listed in 1 and 2 above, their different pathogenic mechanisms and treatments make it clinically advisable not to consider these disorders as variants of the SIADH.

   Pathogenesis of SIADH The ectopic origin of authentic AVP from neoplasms and pulmonary tissue of the types listed above has been documented by tissue analysis. Neoplastic cells obtained from

TABLE 333-4 Causes of SIADH

Malignant neoplasms with autonomous AVP release
  A Small cell carcinoma of lung
  B Carcinoma of pancreas
  C Lymphosarcoma, reticulum cell sarcoma, Hodgkin's disease
  D Carcinoma of duodenum
  E Thymoma
Nonmalignant pulmonary diseases
  A Tuberculosis
  B Lung abscess
  C Pneumonia
  D Viral pneumonitis
  E Empyema
  F Chronic obstructive airways disease
Central nervous system disorders
  A Skull fracture
  B Subdural hematoma
  C Subarachnoid hemorrhage
  D Cerebral vascular thrombosis
  E Cerebral atrophy
  F Acute encephalitis
  G Tuberculous meningitis
  H Purulent meningitis
  I Guillain-Barré syndrome
  J Lupus erythematosus
  K Acute intermittent porphyria
Drugs
  A Chlorpropamide
  B Vincristine
  C Vinblastine
  D Cyclophosphamide
  E Carbamazepine
  F Oxytocin
  G General anesthesia
  H Narcotics
  I Tricyclic antidepressants
Miscellaneous causes
  A Hypothyroidism
  B Positive pressure respiration

the tumors of patients with SIADH can synthesize, store, and release AVP. Both AVP and its associated neurophysin are elevated in the plasma of over 60 percent of patients with small cell carcinoma of the lung. There is excellent correlation between the increases in plasma AVP and neurophysin concentrations on the one hand and the clinical responses to treatment or the recurrences of disease on the other. Vasopressin also has been demonstrated in tuberculous lung tissue. It seems likely, but has not been established, that intracranial lesions (meningitis, encephalitis, trauma, vascular accidents) cause stimulation of AVP release from the neurohypophysis. Some drugs, such as vincristine, chlorpropamide, and carbamazepine, stimulate excessive release of AVP from the neurohypophyseal system, and others (e.g., chlorpropamide and nonsteroidal anti-inflammatory agents) potentiate the antidiuretic action of secreted AVP.

   Excessive release or excessive renal tubular effect of vasopressin results in the excretion of a concentrated urine (with a urinary osmolality usually over 300 mmol/kg) despite a subnormal plasma osmolality and serum sodium concentration. Sodium excretion in the urine is maintained (usually above 20 mmol/L) by hypervolemia, suppression of the renin-angiotensin-aldosterone system, and increased plasma concentration of atrial natriuretic peptide. However, urinary sodium concentration may be below 20 mmol/L if sodium intake is low, but is higher if sodium intake is unrestricted. Blood urea nitrogen and uric acid concentrations tend to fall because of plasma dilution and increased excretion of nitrogenous compounds. Because of the hypervolemia, blood pressure shows no orthostatic fall, but in spite of hypervolemia there is no recumbent hypertension (except when plasma angiotensin II is simultaneously elevated in angiotensinogenic hypertension) and no edema (for an unknown reason). The extracellular hypotonicity leads to intracellular edema, and severe symptoms may result from cerebral edema.

   Clinical manifestations of SIADH In general, the rate of fall in serum sodium concentration is more important in producing the neurologic features of SIADH than the absolute magnitude of the fall.

When SIADH is mild, with serum Na concentrations of 130 to 135 mmol/L, or develops gradually over several weeks, symptoms may be absent or limited to anorexia, nausea, and vomiting, such as occurs in other forms of hyponatremia. When hyponatremia is severe or acute in onset, body weight increases, and the symptoms of cerebral edema become predominant, including restlessness, irritability, confusion, coma, and convulsions associated with nonspecific EEG changes. Edema is almost always absent.

Diagnosis SIADH should be suspected in patients who have hyponatremia and a concentrated urine (osmolality >300 mmol/kg) associated with lethargy and in the absence of edema, orthostatic hypotension, and features of dehydration. The diagnosis of SIADH is made when other causes of enhanced AVP release are excluded. The diagnosis is supported by the finding of blood urea nitrogen, serum uric acid, creatinine, and albumin concentrations in the low-normal or subnormal range. However, it is essential in making the diagnosis to differentiate SIADH from (a) the *dilutional hyponatremias* listed in 2 above, particularly adrenocortical insufficiency, in which orthostatic hypotension with tachycardia and an elevated or high-normal BUN are characteristic, (b) the *edematous states* listed in 1 above, particularly hypothyroidism and congestive heart failure with hyponatremia, (c) *hypertensive states* associated with hyponatremia caused by renovascular stenosis or diuretic therapy, (d) *primary polydipsia* which is always associated with a dilute urine (osmolality < 150 mmol/kg), (e) *pseudohyponatremia* associated with excessive plasma glucose, triglyceride, or protein concentrations [conditions (a) through (e) are easily recognizable by the associated plasma abnormalities], and (f) the *"sick-cell" syndrome*, in which hyponatremia is due to a subnormal setting of the hypothalamic osmoreceptors, associated usually with a chronic, debilitating disease.

When the diagnosis of SIADH is not obvious after excluding other causes of hyponatremia, a positive diagnosis can usually be made with a *water-load test*. The water-load test is particularly useful in differentiating patients with a low-set osmoreceptor (who excrete the water normally) from all other hyponatremic states associated with a concentrated urine. This test should not be performed unless or until the serum sodium concentration has been elevated to a safe level (above 125 mmol/L) by restriction of water intake and/or, if necessary, by saline administration. The patient is asked to drink the water load (20 mL/kg of body weight up to 1500 mL) in 10 to 20 min, and urine is collected in hourly samples, with the patient recumbent between voidings, for 4 to 5 h in the morning. At least 65 percent of the water load should be excreted in 4 h or 80 percent in 5 h, and the lowest urinary osmolality, usually reached in the second hour, should be below 100 mmol/kg. It is essential, to prevent water intoxication in patients who fail to excrete the water load normally, to allow no further water intake for the rest of that day. Failure to excrete the water load may occur in adrenal insufficiency or renal insufficiency, as well as in SIADH. It is important to appreciate, too, that SIADH cannot be diagnosed in the presence of severe pain, nausea, "stress," hypovolemia, hypotension, or other conditions that can stimulate AVP release even in the presence of plasma hypotonicity.

Measurements of plasma or urinary AVP (P_{AVP}, U_{AVP}) are useful adjuvants in establishing the diagnosis of SIADH. Plasma AVP is often immeasurable in hyponatremic states but is detectable, even after a water load, in SIADH. The correlates of plasma osmolality (Posm) versus P_{AVP} or U_{AVP} concentration fall to the left of the normal values in SIADH (Fig. 333-4) and in the other hyponatremic states associated with a concentrated urine. Thus, in most patients with SIADH, P_{AVP} and U_{AVP} concentrations, which may fluctuate widely, are unrelated to concomitant changes in Posm. Occasionally, this lack of correlation between Posm and P_{AVP} or U_{AVP} may be inconsistent. Rarely, for instance, the baseline, unstimulated AVP level may be inappropriately elevated and may fail to change as Posm is raised until the Posm reaches the normal range. Further increases in Posm induced by hypertonic saline infusion or water deprivation may then result in normal or subnormal increases in P_{AVP} or U_{AVP}. This unusual phenomenon may reflect uncontrolled "leakage" of AVP into the circulation.

The diagnostic approach to SIADH is depicted in Fig. 333-6.

Treatment Restriction of fluid intake to 800 to 1000 mL daily is essential. Since this intake is almost always exceeded by urinary output plus insensible fluid loss, a negative water balance ensues that results in gradual, daily reduction in weight, a progressive rise in serum Na concentration and osmolality, and symptomatic improvement. It is useful to verify the effectiveness of fluid restriction by documenting the changes in weight and serum Na concentration daily, until serum Na exceeds 135 mmol/L.

Unless and until the underlying cause of the SIADH can be corrected, fluid intake should be restricted continuously, to maintain normonatremia. In addition to restriction of fluid intake, 5% sodium chloride solution, 200 to 300 mL, should be infused intravenously over 3 to 4 h in patients with severe confusion, convulsions, or coma. It is important to avoid the possibility of inducing pontine myelinosis by not raising the serum Na concentration too rapidly. The possibility of causing congestive heart failure is remote as long as fluid is restricted but may be further reduced by the simultaneous administration of furosemide intravenously.

Attempts should be made to identify and correct the cause of the SIADH as soon as possible. The administration of water-retaining drugs should be stopped. Treatment of hypothyroidism with thyroxine should be initiated. Pulmonary tuberculosis and other pulmonary infections should be treated appropriately, and meningitis or other CNS disorders should be sought and treated, if present. When a malignant tumor is the source of autonomous AVP release and SIADH, surgery, radiation, and/or chemotherapy is often symptomatically beneficial even if the underlying neoplasm cannot be cured.

Antagonism of the release or action of AVP is not often necessary

FIGURE 333-6 Approach to diagnosis of SIADH in patients with hyponatremia.

*Orthostatic hypotension and tachycardia, prerenal azotemia, etc.

**Water excretion test should only be performed when serum Na concentration has risen above 125 mEq/L, after water deprivation for as long as may be necessary.

and seldom successful. Although phenytoin inhibits AVP release, it is seldom effective in SIADH. Drugs that block the effect of AVP on the renal tubule may occasionally be useful. Demeclocycline is the most potent inhibitor of AVP action available for chronic administration, in doses of 900 to 1200 mg/d. Patients receiving demeclocycline should be followed carefully to detect any evidence of renal failure, bacterial superinfection, or excessive drug-induced water loss. Lithium salts interfere with AVP action on tubular water reabsorption and can cause polyuria by this mechanism. Unfortunately, lithium can cause serious side effects in hyponatremic patients and for this reason is not recommended for treatment of SIADH.

Prognosis The prognosis of SIADH depends on the cause. Drug-induced SIADH is rapidly and completely corrected by withdrawal of the causative agent. Similarly, the effective treatment of pulmonary or CNS infections can result in improvement and eventual cure of SIADH. Although SIADH resulting from small cell carcinoma of the lung or other malignancies can often be controlled with vigorous restriction of fluid intake, the underlying malignancy determines the prognosis in these patients.

PARAVENTRICULAR-NEUROHYPOPHYSEAL SYSTEM AND OXYTOCIN

CHEMISTRY AND PHYSIOLOGY Oxytocin, a nonapeptide that differs by two amino acids from vasopressin, is produced in the cell bodies of the paraventricular nuclei and to a lesser extent in those of the supraoptic nuclei. It is synthesized and transported in neurosecretory granules by way of neuronal axons to the neurohypophysis, where it is stored or released, in conjunction with an oxytocin-specific neurophysin. Oxytocin release is stimulated by nerve impulses from the hypothalamus that cause depolarization of the neurosecretory terminals of the posterior pituitary and subsequent release of oxytocin through a calcium-dependent process, similar to the mechanism for vasopressin release. Estrogen stimulates release of oxytocin and its neurophysin. The secretion of oxytocin, as well as of vasopressin, is inhibited by ethanol. Some stimuli such as pain apparently release oxytocin and vasopressin simultaneously, but most stimuli release the two hormones independently. Oxytocin is liberated during suckling, whereas vasopressin is released in much greater quantities than is oxytocin after an osmotic stimulus or hemorrhage. Manipulation or distention of the female genital tract, artificially or during parturition, is a more effective stimulus to oxytocin release than suckling.

Oxytocin acts on the membranes of myometrial and myoepithelial cells to cause an increased force of contraction. Sensitivity of the myometrium to oxytocin increases with the duration of pregnancy, and a role for oxytocin in the initiation and maintenance of labor is probable but not established. Oxytocin may have survival value to the offspring, since it may hasten the final stages of birth and lessen the chances of anoxia. Oxytocin also exerts a contractile action on the myometrium postpartum and contracts the myoepithelial cells of the mammary alveoli, causing them to expel milk from the secretory tissue to the nipple. In the human, oxytocin is 100 times more potent than vasopressin in its milk-ejecting activity. In contrast, the antidiuretic potency of oxytocin relative to vasopressin is about 1:200. Oxytocin probably does not exert any significant physiologic effect other than on the uterus and breast.

One milligram of purified preparation of oxytocin contains 450 IU of hormone, and the amount of oxytocin in the posterior pituitary is similar to that of vasopressin. Even though there is no known role of oxytocin in the male, the male neural lobe stores oxytocin in amounts similar to those in the female. Plasma oxytocin concentration in both men and women exhibits episodic increases, with values ranging from a low of approximately 1 to 4 pmol/L (1.25 to 5 ng/L) but with no diurnal variation. In normal women there is a midcycle increase in plasma oxytocin concentration from a preovulatory value of approximately 2 pmol/L (2.5 ng/L) to a peak value of 4 to 8 pmol/L (5 to 10 ng/L) at the time of ovulation. During labor, plasma oxytocin concentrations may reach high levels, with a rapid fall to prepartum levels after delivery. During suckling, plasma oxytocin levels of the mother vary but are usually about 10 to 20 pmol/L (12 to 25 ng/L). The half-life of oxytocin in plasma is about 3 to 5 min. Removal of oxytocin from the circulation is mainly by the kidneys and liver, although the uterus and mammary gland may remove some.

CLINICAL USE OF OXYTOCIN The clinical use of oxytocin is limited to the induction of labor, control of hemorrhage following incomplete abortion and curettage, and treatment of impaired milk ejection. For discussion of the obstetric uses of oxytocin, the reader is referred to textbooks on obstetrics. Care must be taken because oxytocin may cause uterine rupture and fetal death. The antidiuretic action of oxytocin can be elicited with single intravenous doses of as little as 100 mU. Maximal antidiuresis is reached with 40 to 50 mU/min. Since 10 to 40 units of oxytocin per liter of dextrose is often used in obstetric practice, water intoxication may result. The vasodilatory action of oxytocin may cause sudden death of obstetric patients with heart disease because of hypotension, tachycardia, and arrhythmias. Anesthetics may modify the cardiovascular responses to oxytocin. For instance, in patients under cyclopropane anesthesia, oxytocin produces more hypotension but less tachycardia than in unanesthetized subjects. The vasodilatory effect of oxytocin can be blocked by vasopressin.

REFERENCES

BARTTER FC, SCHWARTZ WB: The syndrome of inappropriate secretion of antidiuretic hormone. Am J Med 42:790, 1967

BICHET DG et al: Hemodynamic and coagulation responses to 1-desamino (8-D-arginine) vasopressin in patients with congenital nephrogenic diabetes insipidus. N Engl J Med 318:881, 1988

CROSS BA, LENG G: *Progress in Brain Research*, vol 60: *The Neurohypophysis: Structure, Function and Control*. Amsterdam, Elsevier, 1983

CZERNICHOW P, ROBINSON AG: *Frontiers of Hormone Research*, vol 13: *Diabetes Insipidus in Man*. Basel, Karger, 1985

DURR JA: Diabetes insipidus in pregnancy. Am J Kidney Dis 9:276, 1987

GASH DM, BOER GJ (EDS): *Vasopressin: Principles and Properties*. New York, Plenum, 1987

MILLER M et al: Recognition of partial defects in antidiuretic hormone secretion. Ann Intern Med 73:721, 1970

MOSES AM: Osmotic thresholds for AVP release using plasma and urine AVP and free water clearance. Am J Physiol 256:R892, 1989

———, STREETEN DHP: Pathophysiologic and pharmacologic alterations in the release and action of ADH. Metabolism 25:697, 1976

——— et al: Marked hypotonic polyuria resulting from nephrogenic diabetes insipidus with partial sensitivity to vasopressin. J Clin Endocrinol Metab 59:1044, 1984

——— et al: Two distinct pathophysiological mechanisms in congenital nephrogenic diabetes insipidus. J Clin Endocrinol Metab 66:1259, 1988

——— et al: The use of T_1-weighted magnetic resonance imaging to differentiate between primary polydipsia and central diabetes insipidus. Am J Neuroradiol 13:1273, 1992

REICHLIN S: *The Neurohypophysis. Physiological and Clinical Aspects*. New York, Plenum, 1984

ROBERTSON GL: The regulation of vasopressin function in health and disease. Rec Progr Hormone Res 33:333, 1977

334   DISEASES OF THE THYROID*

LEONARD WARTOFSKY

Normal function of the thyroid gland is directed to the secretion of L-thyroxine (T_4) and 3,5,3'-triiodo-L-thyronine (T_3), the active thyroid hormones that influence a diversity of metabolic processes (Fig. 334-1). Diseases of the thyroid are manifested by qualitative or quantitative alterations in hormone secretion, enlargement of the thyroid (goiter), or both. Insufficient hormone secretion results in *hypothyroidism* or *myxedema*, in which decreased caloric expenditure (hypometabolism) is a principal feature. Conversely, excessive secre-

* Revision and update of work by the late Sidney Ingbar.

FIGURE 334-1 Structural formulas of thyroxine, its precursors, and certain of its metabolites.

tion of hormone results in hypermetabolism and other features termed *hyperthyroidism* or *thyrotoxicosis*. Enlargement of the thyroid gland (normally 15 to 20 g in adults) may be generalized or focal. Generalized enlargements may not be symmetric, the right lobe tending to enlarge more than the left. Goiters may be associated with increased, normal, or decreased hormone secretion, depending on the underlying disturbance. Focal enlargement usually reflects neoplastic disease, either benign or malignant, the former sometimes responsible for hypersecretion of hormone and hyperthyroidism, the latter rarely so. Any goiter may compress adjacent structures in the neck or mediastinum.

EMBRYOLOGY, ANATOMY, AND HISTOLOGY

The thyroid originates embryologically from an evagination of the pharyngeal epithelium with some contribution from the lateral pharyngeal pouches. Progressive descent of the midline thyroid anlage gives rise to the thyroglossal duct, which extends from the foramen cecum near the base of the tongue to the isthmus of the thyroid. Remnants of tissue may persist along the course of this tract as "lingual thyroid," thyroglossal cysts or nodules, or a structure contiguous with the thyroid isthmus called the *pyramidal lobe*. The latter is usually not discernible, except when the remainder of the gland is enlarged. Rarely, lingual thyroid may be the sole functioning thyroid tissue. In such cases, its secretion may or may not be sufficient to maintain a normal metabolic (euthyroid) state. Thyroid aplasia and functional failure of ectopic thyroid tissue are causes of sporadic neonatal hypothyroidism (1 in every 4000 or 5000 newborns), which responds to early treatment.

The fetal thyroid acquires the capacity to concentrate and organify iodine at about 10 weeks' gestation. Both T_4 and thyroid-stimulating hormone (thyrotropin, TSH) are detectable in the blood soon thereafter and increase in concentration during the second trimester. The increase in serum T_4 is due both to increasing thyroid secretion and to the appearance in plasma of thyroxine-binding globulin (TBG), and the increase in TSH is a reflection of the maturation of the fetal hypothalamus with resulting secretion of thyrotropin-releasing hormone (TRH). Maternal TRH readily crosses the placenta and may play a role in the development of the fetal pituitary-thyroid axis. Maternal TSH, by contrast, does not cross the placenta. T_3 is detectable in the blood later during the second trimester, but its concentration in blood and amniotic fluid remains low until shortly

after parturition. By contrast, the concentration of its analogue, $3,3',5'$-triiodo-L-thyronine (reverse T_3, rT_3), is increased in fetal blood and amniotic fluid relative to that in maternal blood (see Fig. 334-1). These differences are due to qualitative alterations in T_4 metabolism in the fetus. The low T_3 in fetal blood and amniotic fluid in the face of a high maternal concentration indicates that maternal-fetal transfer of T_3 is minimal, and the same is true of T_4. Hence T_4 from the fetal thyroid is the major thyroid hormone available to the fetus. Except for the possible effect of maternal TRH, therefore, the fetal pituitary-thyroid axis is a functional unit distinct from that of the mother.

The normal adult thyroid contains two lobes joined by an isthmus and lies just anterior and caudad to the cartilages of the larynx. Fibrous septa divide the gland into pseudolobules which, in turn, are composed of vesicles, called *follicles* or *acini*, surrounded by a capillary network. Normally, the follicle walls are composed of cuboidal epithelium. The lumen is filled with a proteinaceous *colloid*, which contains a unique protein, *thyroglobulin*, within the peptide sequence of which T_4 and T_3 are synthesized and stored. The thyroid contains a second smaller population of cells, the C cells. They are the source of calcitonin and give rise to medullary thyroid carcinoma when they undergo malignant transformation.

THYROID HORMONE ECONOMY: NORMAL PHYSIOLOGY

The term *thyroid hormone economy* denotes the processes involved in the synthesis of hormones within the thyroid gland, their transport in the circulation, their action and metabolism within the peripheral tissues, and the regulatory mechanisms that maintain a normal supply of thyroid hormones.

HORMONE SYNTHESIS AND SECRETION Thyroid hormone synthesis depends on entry into the thyroid of adequate quantities of iodine, a constituent of T_4 and T_3; normal iodine metabolism within the gland; and synthesis of a receptor protein for iodine, thyroglobulin. The structure of thyroglobulin favors iodination and particularly formation of T_4 and T_3. Secretion of normal quantities of hormone, in turn, requires both a normal rate of hormone synthesis and a process for the hydrolysis of thyroglobulin and liberation of active hormones. Iodine enters the thyroid in the form of inorganic or ionic iodide, whose source is iodide derived either from the deiodination of thyroid hormones or of iodinated agents that the patient may have received or from iodide ingested in food, water, or medication. Formerly, a dietary iodine intake of approximately 0.2 mg/d was considered normal in the United States, and this was sufficient to sustain a plasma iodide concentration of approximately 40 nmol/L (0.5 µg/dL). However, owing to iodine contamination of some foods and to the widespread use of iodine in drugs, vitamin preparations, and antiseptic agents, the average iodine intake has increased to about 0.5 mg/d, and in some areas may be as high as 1 mg/d, with corresponding increases in plasma iodide concentration. Iodide is removed from the plasma by the thyroid, kidneys, and salivary and gastrointestinal glands, but since iodide that enters gastrointestinal secretions is reabsorbed, net clearance is effected by the thyroid and kidneys. In effect, the thyroid and kidneys compete for plasma iodide. Renal clearance is largely a function of glomerular filtration rate and is not influenced by humoral factors or plasma iodide concentration; the kidney is normally a passive participant in this competition. Hence adjustments in the rate of iodide uptake by the thyroid relative to the rate of urinary excretion are mediated by changes in thyroid rather than renal avidity.

The synthesis and secretion of the active thyroid hormones can be divided into four sequential steps (Fig. 334-2). The first involves active transport of iodide into the thyroid cell and follicular lumen. This occurs at a rate that exceeds passive diffusion of iodide out of the gland, with the result that the thyroid maintains concentration gradients for iodide (thyroid/plasma concentration ratios) of substantial magnitude (usually of 25 but up to 500 or more under certain conditions). Energy for iodide transport depends on oxidative metabolism within the gland. The second step in hormone biosynthesis involves oxidation of iodide to a higher valence form that is capable of iodinating tyrosyl residues in thyroglobulin, a glycoprotein of approximately 660,000 mol wt that is synthesized within the follicular cell. Oxidation of iodide is effected by a peroxidase, which utilizes hydrogen peroxide generated during the course of oxidative metabolism within the gland. Organic iodinations occur at the cell-colloid

FIGURE 334-2 Schema depicting pathways in the synthesis and secretion of thyroid hormones and mechanisms for the suprathyroidal and intrathyroidal regulation of thyroid function. Small, solid arrows indicate pathways of iodine metabolism; open arrows indicate stimulation; cross-hatched arrows indicate inhibitory influences. TRH, thyrotropin-releasing hormone; TSH, thyroid-stimulating hormone; IPO, iodide peroxidase; prot., thyroid protease; peptid., thyroid peptidase; MIT, monoiodotyrosine; DIT, diiodotyrosine; T₄, thyroxine; T₃, 3,5,3′-triiodothyronine.

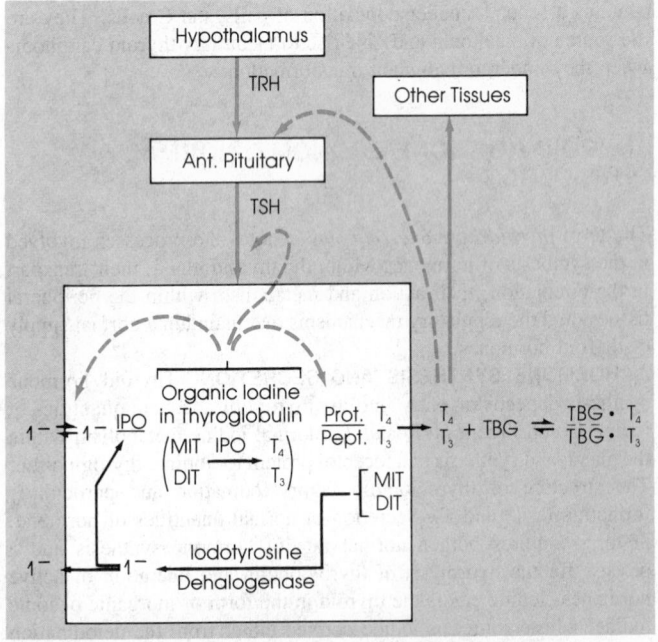

interface, where they take place to a large extent in newly synthesized thyroglobulin undergoing exocytosis into the follicular lumen. The consequence is the formation of the peptide-bound, hormonally inactive precursors monoiodotyrosine (MIT) and diiodotyrosine (DIT). Subsequently, these iodotyrosines undergo oxidative condensation, again through the mediation of peroxidase. This coupling reaction occurs within the thyroglobulin molecule and yields a variety of iodothyronines, including T_4 and T_3. Although minute quantities of thyroglobulin are detectable in the blood, most thyroglobulin is retained for a time within the gland, serving as a storage vehicle for the thyroid hormones. Liberation of the active hormones into the blood involves pinocytosis of follicular colloid at the apical margin of the cells to form colloid droplets. The droplets fuse with thyroid lysosomes to form "phagolysosomes," in which thyroglobulin is hydrolyzed by proteases. The final step is release of the free iodothyronines T_4 and T_3 into the blood. The thyroid is the only source of endogenous T_4; in contrast, thyroid secretion normally accounts for only about 20 percent of the T_3 produced, the remainder being generated in extraglandular tissues by the enzymatic removal of the 5′-iodine from the outer ring of T_4. Inactive iodotyrosines liberated by the hydrolysis of thyroglobulin are stripped of their iodine by an intrathyroid enzyme, iodotyrosine dehalogenase. Normally, iodide so liberated is reutilized in the synthesis of hormone, but a small proportion is lost into the blood (iodide leak); iodine leaks may become large under certain circumstances.

The thyroid also concentrates other monovalent anions such as pertechnetate, which is available as the radioactive isotope sodium [⁹⁹ᵐTc]pertechnetate. Unlike iodide, little pertechnetate is organically bound; hence its duration of stay within the thyroid is short. This property, together with its short physical half-life, makes pertechnetate a valuable radionuclide for imaging the thyroid by scintillation scanning.

The foregoing reactions are subject to inhibition by a variety of agents termed *goitrogens*, since, by virtue of their ability to inhibit hormone synthesis and indirectly stimulate TSH secretion, they induce goiter formation. Inorganic anions such as perchlorate and thiocyanate inhibit iodide transport and thereby reduce substrate for hormone formation. The goiter and hypothyroidism that follow, however, can be prevented or relieved by doses of iodide sufficiently large to enable adequate quantities to enter the gland by passive diffusion. The commonly employed antithyroid agents, such as the derivatives of thiourea and mercaptoimidazole, exert more complex actions on hormone biosynthesis. These agents inhibit the initial oxidation (organic binding) of iodide, decrease the proportion of DIT relative to MIT, and block coupling of iodotyrosines to form the hormonally active iodothyronines. The latter reaction is the most sensitive. Thus the synthesis of hormonally active iodothyronines may be decreased, although the total incorporation of iodine by the thyroid is inhibited but little. In contrast to the effect of the monovalent anions, the goitrogenic action of thioureas is not overcome by large quantities of iodine. Indeed, certain weak goitrogens, such as sulfonamides and antipyrine, are more potent when given with iodide, an effect not understood. Iodine itself, when given acutely in large doses, blocks the organic binding and coupling reactions. This action (Wolff-Chaikoff effect) is normally transient, but prolonged administration of iodide may be associated with continued inhibition of hormone synthesis and development of goiter, with or without hypothyroidism (iodide myxedema). Many patients with Graves' disease, especially after treatment with radioiodine or surgery, or with Hashimoto's disease are sensitive to the blocking effect of iodide and develop hypothyroidism when given iodides chronically. The fetal thyroid is similarly sensitive, and pregnant women should not be given iodide in large amounts because of the danger of inducing goitrous hypothyroidism in the fetus. Iodide in large doses is capable of inhibiting proteolysis of thyroglobulin and hormone release, an effect readily demonstrable in hyperfunctioning thyroids and responsible for the ameliorative action of iodides in hyperthyroidism. Excess iodide also may induce thyrotoxicosis in susceptible individuals, as discussed below. Lithium, which is administered as the carbonate salt in some patients with depression has several effects on intrathyroidal iodine metabolism, one of which is to inhibit hormone release. Glucocorticoids causes a decrease in serum thyroid hormone levels due to inhibition of TSH secretion and decreased T_4 binding to TBG. Serum T_3 is also decreased in part because of inhibition of T_4 to T_3 conversion. A direct inhibitory action of glucocorticoids on the thyroid may occur in Graves' disease, possibly by inhibition of thyroid-stimulating immunoglobulins. Dexamethasone, in conjunction with iodide, can effect a rapid reduction in the degree of thyrotoxicosis.

HORMONE TRANSPORT AND METABOLISM

HORMONE TRANSPORT In the blood, T_4 and T_3 are almost entirely bound to plasma proteins. T_4 is bound, in decreasing order of intensity, to thyroxine-binding globulin (TBG), to a T_4-binding prealbumin (transthyretin, TTR), and to albumin. High-density lipoproteins transport about 3 percent of circulating T_4 and 6 percent of T_3. By virtue of its intense affinity for T_4, TBG is the major determinant of normal binding. T_4 and its binding proteins interact in a reversible binding equilibrium in which the majority of the hormone is bound and a small proportion (normally about 0.03 percent) is free. While TTR transports only about 15 percent of circulating T_4, its contribution to free hormone is comparable to that from TBG owing to its higher dissociation constant. T_3 is not significantly bound by TTR and is bound 10 to 20 times less firmly by TBG than T_4. As a consequence, the normal proportion of free T_3 (approximately 0.3 percent) is 8 to 10 times greater than that of T_4. Only the free or unbound hormone is available to tissues; therefore, the metabolic state correlates more closely with the concentration of free than with the concentration of total hormone in plasma, and homeostatic regulation of thyroid function is directed toward maintenance of a normal concentration of free hormone. Moreover, the relatively weak binding of T_3 accounts for its more rapid onset and offset of action. Disturbances of thyroid hormone–plasma protein interaction are of two general types (see Table 334-1). In the first, the thyroid-pituitary axis is intrinsically normal, and the homeostatic control of thyroid hormone secretion is intact. Under these circumstances, disordered binding interactions result from alterations in thyroid hormone binding. For example, an increase in TBG initially lowers the concentration of free hormone and thus diminishes the quantity of hormone available to tissues. Total hormone concentration in serum then increases until the concentration of free hormone is restored to normal. The increase in total hormone concentration counterbalances the decrease in the free proportion; as a result, the absolute concentration of free hormone is normal, and the metabolic state of the patient is normal. Opposite changes occur when the concentration of TBG declines. Table 334-2 summarizes those states associated with primary alterations in

the concentration of TBG. Primary disturbances in thyroid hormone binding also occur when other binding proteins in blood are increased or when abnormal binding proteins appear. These are discussed below.

The second type of disturbance of thyroid hormone–binding interactions results from a primary alteration in the concentration of thyroid hormones in the blood, as in hypothyroidism or thyrotoxicosis. Here, normal homeostatic control of thyroid hormone secretion is lost, either because of disease within the control mechanism itself or because an intact control mechanism is incapable of overcoming the effects of disease elsewhere. Under these circumstances, the concentration of TBG is changed little, if at all, and the concentration of free hormone varies directly with the total concentration of hormone. Since homeostatic mechanisms cannot restore the concentration of free hormone to normal, primary changes in thyroid function cause persistent changes in the concentration of total and free hormone and, consequently, alterations in the metabolic state.

HORMONE METABOLISM Following penetration into the cell, T_4 and T_3 undergo reactions that lead ultimately to their excretion or inactivation. Thyroid hormones undergo sequential removal of single iodine atoms (monodeiodinations) that ultimately yields the thyronine nucleus stripped of iodine. Deiodinative pathways account for approximately 70 percent of T_4 and T_3 disposal. In the case of T_4, the most important of these is the 5'-monodeiodination that leads to the generation of T_3. Since approximately 30 percent of T_4 is converted to T_3, and since T_3 has approximately three times the metabolic potency of T_4, virtually all the metabolic action of T_4 can be ascribed to the action of the T_3 that it gives rise to. Normally, extraglandular formation accounts for about 80 percent of the T_3 in the blood and of overall T_3 production, the remainder coming from thyroid secretion. As a consequence, abnormal states and pharmacologic agents that impair T_3 formation lower the serum T_3 concentration (Table 334-3). When patients with thyroid hypofunction are treated with synthetic T_4 (levothyroxine) to sustain serum T_4 concentrations within or somewhat above the normal range, normal or nearly normal serum

---

TABLE 334-2 Circumstances associated with altered concentration of TBG

Increased TBG	Decreased TBG
Pregnancy	Androgens
Newborn state	Large doses of glucocorticoid
Oral contraceptives and other sources of estrogen	Chronic liver disease
	Severe systemic illness
Tamoxifen	Active acromegaly
Infectious and chronic active hepatitis	Nephrosis
	Genetically determined
Biliary cirrhosis	Asparaginase
Acute intermittent porphyria	
Perphenazine	
Genetically determined	

TABLE 334-1 Classification of the varieties of disordered thyroid hormone–plasma protein interactions

Type of abnormality	Serum T_4 and T_3	Percent FT_4 and FT_3 or RT_3U	FT_4 and FT_3 or FT_4I and FT_3I
PRIMARY ABNORMALITY IN TBG			
Increased concentration	↑	↓	N
Decreased concentration	↓	↑	N
PRIMARY DISORDER OF THYROID FUNCTION			
Hypothyroidism	↓	↓	↓
Hyperthyroidism	↑	↑	↑

NOTE: FT_4 = free T_4; FT_3 = free T_3; FT_4I = free T_4 index; FT_3I = free T_3 index; RT_3U = resin-T_3 uptake; TBG = thyroid-binding globulin.

TABLE 334-3 States associated with decreased peripheral conversion of T_4 to T_3

PHYSIOLOGIC

Fetal and early neonatal life
? Old age

PATHOLOGIC

Fasting
Malnutrition
Systemic illness
Physical trauma
Postoperative state
Drugs (propylthiouracil, dexamethasone, propranolol, amiodarone)
Radiographic contrast agents (ipodate, ipanoate)

T_3 concentrations are maintained. The generalization that the thyroid secretes relatively little T_3 does not apply to states in which the thyroid is hyperfunctioning or under increased stimulation by TSH. Under these conditions, the T_3/T_4 ratio of the secretory product and the serum concentration of T_3 relative to that of T_4 are increased. In addition, when T_4 production is decreased, as in early thyroid failure or iodine deficiency, the T_3/T_4 concentration ratio in blood is increased still further by an autoregulatory mechanism that leads to an increase in the efficiency of T_3 formation.

Approximately 40 percent of T_4 disposal is accounted for by monodeiodination at the 5 position of its inner ring to yield reverse T_3 (rT_3); this process accounts for nearly all rT_3 produced. rT_3 has little, if any, metabolic potency; therefore, the relative rates of outer- and inner-ring monodeiodination of T_4 determine the quantity of metabolically active hormone available. Factors that impair T_3 formation almost invariably increase serum rT_3 concentrations. This increase is not due to an increase in the production of rT_3 from T_4, but rather to a decrease in the 5'-monodeiodination of rT_3 to yield 3,3'-diiodothyronine ($3,3'T_2$); i.e., both the decreased conversion of T_4 to T_3 and the decreased degradation of rT_3 are due to a selective impairment of 5'-monodeiodination.

A second major pathway of metabolism of T_4 and T_3 and of their metabolites is conjugation in the liver, principally with glucuronate and sulfate. Conjugates either undergo deiodination locally or are secreted into the bile, but the magnitude of the enterohepatic circulation in humans is unknown. Reabsorption is incomplete at best, since the fecal excretion of T_4, T_3, and their iodine-containing metabolites accounts for approximately 20 percent of overall T_4 disposal. About 20 percent of T_4 and T_3 undergoes oxidative deamination and decarboxylation of the alanine side chain to yield tetraiodo- and triiodothyroacetic acid (tetrac and triac, respectively).

Under certain circumstances, changes in hormone synthesis and metabolism are the major determinant of the rates of metabolic clearance of T_4 and T_3. Both phenobarbital and phenytoin increase the metabolic clearance of thyroid hormones without increasing the proportion of free hormone in the blood. Indeed, in the case of phenytoin, both total and free T_4 concentrations are diminished. Nevertheless, a normal metabolic state is maintained, possibly because of an increase in T_3 formation.

HORMONE ACTION   The thyroid hormones influence the growth and maturation of tissues, cell respiration and total energy expenditure, and the turnover of essentially all substrates, vitamins, and hormones, including the thyroid hormones themselves. Some hormone actions on cell metabolism may be mediated at the level of the mitochondrion to influence oxidative metabolism and at the level of the plasma membrane and endoplasmic reticulum to influence the activity of Ca^{2+}-ATPase and transcellular flux of substrates and cations. However, the primary action of the hormone is exerted via binding to one or more intracellular receptor complexes, which, in turn, bind to specific regulatory sites in the chromosomes to influence genomic expression (see Chap. 329). There are two classes of thyroid hormone receptor (TR) which are encoded by two different genes, TRα and TRβ, located on chromosomes 17 and 3, respectively. By alternative splicing, these two genes, in turn, generate additional isoforms (e.g., α_1, α_2, β_1, β_2, etc.). The TR proteins are part of a superfamily of genes encoded by mRNAs of cellular (c-) homologues of the avian retroviral v-erb A proto-oncogene. The TR genes, c-erbA-α (TRα) and c-erb-A-β (TRβ), encode receptor proteins with a T_3-binding domain and a DNA-binding domain. The DNA-binding domain attaches to regulatory sequences in those target genes with T_3-regulated transcription (e.g., TSH, prolactin, growth hormone). In an interaction stabilized by TR auxiliary proteins (TRAPs), the activation and modulation of rates of transcription are mediated by regulatory sequences called *thyroid response elements* (TRE). Thus, in the pituitary, the binding of T_3-TR complexes to TRE serves to inhibit the expression of genes for the synthesis of the α and β subunits of TSH. While pituitary may contain the highest concentrations of TR, all tissues with high-affinity nuclear T_3 binding express TRα and

TRβ receptors. High concentrations of c-erb A-β_1 are found in brain, liver, heart, and kidney. The variable lack of T_3 responsiveness in different tissues ("resistance") is due to point mutations in the T_3-binding domain of the c-erbA-β receptor (see below).

THYROID HORMONE RESISTANCE   Generalized thyroid hormone resistance (GTHR) is a syndrome characterized by reduced responsiveness to elevated levels of thyroid hormone. The resistance to thyroid hormone action is associated with elevated circulating levels of free T_4 and free T_3, inappropriately normal or elevated (i.e., nonsuppressed) serum TSH, and intact TSH responsiveness to TRH. Kindreds have been described whose members express variable patterns of resistance, and responsiveness of target tissues may vary within the same individual. At the molecular levels, the varied phenotypes appear to be due to different gene mutations altering function of the c-erbA-β receptor. Clinical features include short stature, hyperactivity, attention deficits with mental deficiency or learning disability, and goiter. While GTRH patients are either euthyroid or hypothyroid, the differential diagnosis includes isolated pituitary resistance to thyroid hormone and a TSH-secreting pituitary tumor, disorders in which the patients usually present with hyperthyroidism. Indications for treatment of GTHR vary depending on the clinical features, but the presence of increased serum TSH reflects the need for supplemental thyroid hormone, the dosage requirement depending on parameters of tissue responses to thyroid hormone.

REGULATION OF THYROID FUNCTION   Thyroid function is regulated by two general mechanisms, one suprathyroid and one intrathyroid (Fig. 334-2). The proximate mediator of suprathyroid regulation is thyrotropin (thyroid-stimulating hormone, TSH), a glycoprotein secreted by basophilic (thyrotropic) cells in the anterior pituitary. TSH stimulates thyroid hypertrophy and hyperplasia; accelerates most aspects of intermediary metabolism in the thyroid; enhances synthesis of nucleic acid and protein, including thyroglobulin; and stimulates the synthesis and secretion of thyroid hormones. These actions result from binding of TSH to specific receptors in the surface of the follicular cell and subsequent activation of the plasma membrane enzyme adenylate cyclase. The resulting increase in the cellular cyclic 3',5'-adenosine monophosphate (cyclic AMP) concentration initiates most or all TSH responses.

Regulation of TSH secretion, in turn, is effected by two opposing influences at the level of the thyrotropic cell. Thyrotropin-releasing hormone (TRH), a tripeptide of hypothalamic origin, stimulates the secretion and synthesis of TSH, whereas thyroid hormones both inhibit the TSH secretory mechanism directly and antagonize the action of TRH. Thus homeostatic control of TSH secretion is exerted in a negative-feedback manner by thyroid hormones, and the threshold for feedback inhibition is apparently set by TRH. TRH reaches the pituitary via the hypophyseal portal blood system and binds to specific high-affinity receptors on the plasma membrane of the thyrotropic cell. Either activation of the adenylate cyclase system or a concomitant translocation of extracellular calcium into the cell initiates release of TSH. In addition to stimulating release of stored TSH, TRH enhances new synthesis of TSH via transcription and translation of the gene for the β subunit. TRH also plays a role in posttranslational processing of TSH, as indicated by the fact that TSH in patients with hypothalamic hypothyroidism has reduced biologic activity. The negative-feedback effect of the thyroid hormones appears to take place entirely at the level of the thyrotropic cell. Experimentally, thyroid hormones inhibit production of TRH mRNA and TRH prohormone as well as reduce the number of TRH receptors on the thyrotropic cell, thus impairing its responsiveness to TRH. The major negative-feedback action of the thyroid hormones is at the pituitary level, mediated by binding of the hormones to TR in the nucleus of the thyrotropic cell, resulting in reduced expression of the genes for α and β subunits of TSH. The principal arbiter of thyroid hormone action within the pituitary is T_3, both that generated locally from intrapituitary T_4 and that derived from plasma. To what extent T_4 itself is effective within the pituitary is uncertain, but other factors modify the secretion of TSH and its response to TRH. Both somatostatin and dopamine appear to be physiologic inhibitors of TRH secretion. Estrogens enhance responsiveness to TRH, whereas glucocorticoids inhibit this function. Catecholamines also play a role, with α_1-adrenergic pathways being inhibitory and α_2 pathways being stimulatory. Experimentally, tumor necrosis factor and interleukin 1 inhibit TSH secretion, possibly playing a role in the sick euthyroid syndrome.

Intrathyroid regulation of thyroid function is also important. In some manner, changes in glandular organic iodine content cause reciprocal changes in thyroid iodide transport activity and regulate growth, amino acid uptake, glucose metabolism, and nucleic acid synthesis. These influences are evident in the absence of TSH stimulation and hence may be termed *autoregulatory*, but their most important role is to modify (iodine-enrichment inhibiting and iodine-depletion enhancing) the response to TSH, probably by influencing the generation of cyclic AMP consequent to TSH stimulation. Cytokines may exert stimulatory or inhibitory effects on thyroid hormone synthesis or secretion and on interactions with TSH and in vitro, but the physiologic and pathophysiologic significance of these substances (e.g., atrial natriuretic peptide, tumor necrosis factor, transforming growth factor, epidermal growth factor, endothelin, etc.) remains to be clarified.

LABORATORY TESTS

Laboratory tests of thyroid hormone economy can be divided into five general categories: direct tests of thyroid function, tests related to the concentration and binding of thyroid hormones in blood, metabolic indexes, tests of the homeostatic control of thyroid function, and miscellaneous tests that do not fit into other categories.

DIRECT TESTS OF THYROID FUNCTION Among all tests designed to assess thyroid status, only those which involve in vivo administration of radioactive iodine test glandular function per se, and measurement of the *thyroid radioactive iodine uptake* (RAIU) is the most common. ^{131}I has been used for this purpose, but ^{123}I is preferable because of the lower radiation dose that it delivers. The administered radioiodine mixes uniformly with the endogenous iodide in the extracellular fluid and, in the steady state, can be used to assess what percentage of the iodide entering and leaving the extracellular space per unit time is accumulated by the thyroid. The RAIU is measured 24 h after administration of the isotope, since it usually reaches a plateau value at this time, but in severe thyroid hyperfunction it may peak early. The RAIU varies inversely with the plasma iodide concentration and directly with the functional state of the thyroid. At usual levels of iodine intake in the United States (up to 1 mg/d), the normal 24-h RAIU is approximately 10 to 30 percent of the administered dose. Consequently, this test discriminates poorly between normal and hypothyroid states. Values above the normal range, however, usually indicate thyroid hyperfunction and are useful in the diagnosis of hyperthyroidism. The RAIU is also a part of the thyroid suppression test (see below).

One valuable application of the RAIU is in the diagnosis of thyrotoxicosis associated with a low value of the RAIU. These include iodine-induced hyperthyroidism, thyrotoxicosis factitia, inadvertent ingestion of ground meat containing thyroid glands ("hamburger toxicosis"), and the spontaneously resolving thyrotoxicosis associated with painless chronic thyroiditis or subacute thyroiditis.

TESTS RELATED TO HORMONE CONCENTRATION AND BINDING IN BLOOD Until the evolution of highly sensitive assays for TSH, measurement of the concentration of T_4 and/or T_3 in serum, in conjunction with some assessment of hormone binding, was the traditional means of confirming a clinical diagnosis of hyperthyroidism or hypothyroidism. Highly specific and sensitive radioimmunoassays are used to measure *serum T_4* and T_3 concentrations and rarely for the measurement of *serum rT_3* concentration. The approximate normal ranges are 60 to 150 nmol/L (5 to 12 μg/dL) for T_4, 1 to 3 nmol/L (70 to 190 ng/dL) for T_3, and 0.2 to 0.6 nmol/L (10 to 40 ng/dL) for rT_3.

As mentioned above, alterations in the intensity of hormone binding by plasma proteins, as well as alterations in the rate of hormone secretion, influence the concentration of hormone in the blood. However, only alterations in hormone secretion lead to steady state alterations in the concentration of free hormone. Because they most consistently reflect the rate of hormone production, free hormone concentrations usually correlate better with the metabolic state than do total hormone concentrations. The free T_4 concentration (FT_4) can be measured directly by equilibrium dialysis of serum enriched with a tracer quantity of labeled T_4. The percent of T_4 that is dialyzable or free is thereby determined, and the product of this value and the total T_4 is the FT_4. However, since the dialysis technique is cumbersome, it has been replaced by indirect assays (see below). One traditional method, the in vitro uptake test, represents an indirect assessment of hormone binding, is simple to perform, and usually provides the same information as free T_4. Here, the serum is enriched with labeled T_4 or labeled T_3 and is then incubated with an insoluble, particulate matter, such as resin or charcoal, that binds free hormone. The percent of labeled hormone taken up by the particulate material varies inversely with both the concentration of unoccupied sites among the serum proteins and their affinity for the particular hormone being used. Labeled T_3 is usually used in preference to labeled T_4, since it is less strongly bound in the serum and hence yields higher and more accurate uptake values (resin T_3 uptake, RT_3U). In most clinical conditions, values of the RT_3U are proportionate to those of the percent of FT_4 and percent of FT_3. This proportionality reflects the fact that in normal serum, T_4 and T_3 are mainly bound by a common binding site on TBG. Therefore, alterations in binding produced by an excess or deficiency of TBG or by an excessive or insufficient supply of T_4 do not seriously disturb the relationship between the intensity of T_4 binding and that of T_3. Under these conditions, therefore, one may calculate a *free T_4 index* (FT_4I) and a *free T_3 index* (FT_3I) as the product of the RT_3U and the total T_4 and T_3 concentrations, respectively, and these are proportional to the actual FT_4 and FT_3.

Primary alterations in plasma TBG concentration (see Table 334-2) produce changes in the RT_3U that are inverse and approximately proportionate to those in the serum T_4 and serum T_3; as a result, the FT_4I and FT_3I remain normal. By contrast, alterations in T_4 secretion cause changes in the percent FT_4 and RT_3U that are in the same direction as those in serum T_4. As a result, the FT_4 and FT_4I deviate from normal values more markedly than do the percent FT_4 and RT_3U alone. Immunoradiometric (IRMA) and chemiluminescent assay methods for the direct measurement of FT_4 provide reliable results in a wide range of disorders and may replace measurement of total T_4, RT_3U, and FT_4I in the diagnosis of thyrotoxicosis and hypothyroidism.

As noted earlier, several disorders are characterized by increased plasma binding of T_4 in which, because the protein involved is not TBG, the intensity of T_4 binding relative to that of T_3 is abnormal. Most commonly, binding of T_4 is enhanced, while that of T_3 is increased little, if at all. Included among these disorders is *familial dysalbuminemic hyperthyroxinemia (FDH)*, inherited as an autosomal dominant trait, in which the plasma concentration of an albumin variant with an unusually high affinity for T_4 is increased. As a result, the serum T_4 is markedly elevated, but in keeping with the euthyroid state, FT_4 is normal. Because the RT_3U does not reflect the increase in the intensity of T_4 binding, calculated values of the FT_4I are increased, often leading to a mistaken diagnosis of thyrotoxicosis. Similar findings occur when there is *increased T_4 binding by transthyretin* (TTR, TBPA) or when the patient, usually one with autoimmune thyroid disease, develops *circulating antibodies* against T_4 itself.

In the foregoing disorders, serum T_4 is increased owing to an increase in T_4 binding, and the FT_4 and metabolic state are normal. They are therefore classified among the disorders that lead to a state of *euthyroid hyperthyroxinemia*, a term that implies the presence of hyperthyroxinemia not caused by intrinsic thyroid disease (Table 334-4). The mechanism responsible for these findings is variable and in some cases uncertain. The increases in total T_4 do not appear to

TABLE 334-4 States associated with euthyroid hyperthyroxinemia

Disorder	FT$_4$	FT$_4$I	T$_3$	TSH	Comments
Increased T$_4$ binding					See Tables 334-1 and 334-2
A Increased TBG	N	N	↑	N	Autosomal dominant inheritance
B FDH	N	↑	N,Sl ↑	N	Increased concentration (islet-cell tumor) or affinity
C Increased TBPA binding	N	↑	N	N	Anti-T$_3$ antibody may be present
D Anti-T$_4$ antibody	N	↑	N	N	
Pituitary and peripheral thyroid hormone resistance	↑	↑	↑	↑	If only pituitary resistant, patient thyrotoxic
Various disorders					
A Sick euthyroid syndrome	↑, N	↑	↓	N, ↓	Uncommon; poorly understood
B Acute psychiatric illness	↑, N	↑	N, ↑	N, ↑	Remits without treatment in several weeks
C Hyperemesis gravidarum	↑	↑	N	↓	Remits in several weeks
Drugs					
A Inhibitors of T$_3$-formation	↑	↑	↓	↑	Particularly ipodate and iopanoate
1 Radiographic contrast agents					
2 Propranolol	↑	↑	↓	N, ↑	Especially with large doses
3 Amiodarone	↑	↑		↑	Increased TSH during first several months
B Heparin	↑	↑	N	—	Requires only small intravenous doses
C Levothyroxine therapy	↑	↑	N	↓	Hyperthyroxinemia in about 50% of cases

NOTE: FT$_4$ = free T$_4$ concentration; FT$_4$I = free T$_4$ index calculated from an in vitro T$_3$ uptake test; TSH = basal serum TSH concentration and response to TRH; N = normal; Sl = slightly.

have any impact on the metabolic state, but hyperthyroidism may be mistakenly diagnosed.

Some states are associated with an increased thyroid secretion of T$_3$, at least relative to the secretion of T$_4$. As a result, the serum T$_3$ concentration is disproportionately high relative to the serum T$_4$. This is apparently a consequence of hyperfunction of the follicular cell, since it is seen in all varieties of hyperthyroidism and in early thyroid failure, in which the gland is exposed to enhanced stimulation by TSH. Accordingly, the serum T$_3$ concentration and the derived FT$_3$I are generally superior to the corresponding values for T$_4$ in the diagnosis of hyperthyroidism. In *early* hypothyroidism, by contrast, the serum T$_3$ concentration and FT$_3$I are often normal despite subnormal values for the serum T$_4$ and FT$_4$I. Consequently, the serum T$_3$ concentration is not reliable for the diagnosis of hypothyroidism.

Measurement of the serum rT$_3$ concentration is valuable in differentiating the "low T$_3$ syndrome" (see below) from intrinsic hypothyroidism; in the former the serum rT$_3$ concentration is increased, whereas in the latter it is usually subnormal.

METABOLIC INDEXES Tests in this category assess the metabolic impact of thyroid hormone. Though tests of this type have value in the investigative setting, none of sufficient sensitivity, specificity, and ease of performance is available for routine use. Measurements of oxygen consumption in the basal state (basal metabolic rate, BMR) were once a mainstay in the diagnosis of thyroid disease but are now of historic interest. Several blood tests may be abnormal in patients with thyroid disease, but lack of specificity limits their utility. For example, serum concentrations of creatine phosphokinase and, less frequently, lactate dehydrogenase and aspartate aminotransferase are increased in hypothyroidism and may be slightly decreased in

hyperthyroidism. The changes are nonspecific, and appreciation of them is important only in avoiding the inference that other diseases which produce similar changes are present. The concentrations in serum of testosterone-binding globulin (TeBG), the iron storage protein ferritin, and angiotensin-converting enzyme are thyroid hormone–dependent and are, therefore, increased in thyrotoxicosis, but they are of no value in the diagnosis of thyroid disease. Increases in the *serum cholesterol concentration* are common in hypothyroidism of thyroid origin, and decreases in serum cholesterol are common in thyrotoxicosis. *Systolic time indexes*, such as the preejection period and pulse-wave arrival time, are prolonged in hypothyroidism and shortened in hyperthyroidism. They may be of value in monitoring thyroid replacement therapy in elderly patients or in patients with coexisting heart disease.

TESTS OF HOMEOSTATIC CONTROL Measurement of the basal *serum TSH concentration* is useful in the diagnosis of both advanced and subclinical hypothyroidism. The latter state represents a stage in the evolution of hypothyroidism, in which a structural or functional abnormality that impairs hormone synthesis is compensated for by hypersecretion of TSH. In thyrotoxic states, serum TSH concentration is almost always low or undetectable. While the original radioimmunoassays could not distinguish between normal and subnormal values, immunoradiometric or chemiluminescent techniques employing monoclonal antibodies provide exquisite sensitivity. Thyrotoxic patients tend to have undetectable levels (<0.1 mU/L), while values in most normal subjects range between 0.3 and 3.0 mU/L in these assays (Fig. 334-3). Thus these assays offer a significant advantage over conventional radioimmunoassays (RIA) and may be useful in confirming the diagnosis of hyperthyroidism as well as that of hypothyroidism.

FIGURE 334-3 Utility of sensitive TSH assay in evaluation of suspected thyroid dysfunction in ambulatory patients.

Serum TSH concentrations are absolutely or inappropriately elevated relative to serum FT_4 and FT_3 values in patients with TSH-induced hyperthyroidism. This rare syndrome results either from a TSH-secreting pituitary adenoma or resistance of the TSH secretory mechanism to feedback inhibition by T_4 and T_3. Measurement of serum TSH is the best means of distinguishing between untreated hypothyroidism of thyroid origin, in which the values are invariably increased, and pituitary or hypothalamic hypothyroidism, in which the values are usually low or within the normal range. Occasional patients with hypothyroidism of hypothalamic or pituitary origin secrete a form of TSH that is immunoactive but not bioactive. Here, serum TSH concentrations may be elevated rather than depressed.

The *thyrotropin-releasing hormone (TRH) stimulation test* assesses the functional state of the TSH-secretory mechanism and has diagnostic value in diverse circumstances. Following the intravenous injection of TRH in normal subjects, the serum TSH level begins to increase within minutes, reaches a maximum between 20 and 45 min, and then rapidly declines. The nature of the pituitary feedback mechanism is such that when hypothalamic-pituitary function is normal, one would expect an increased response to TRH when the thyrotropic cell senses a deficiency of thyroid hormone, particularly T_3, and a decreased or absent response when there is thyroid hormone excess. Thus, except in the rare instances of pituitary resistance to thyroid hormone, in which responses are usually normal, thyrotoxicosis is invariably accompanied by a blunted or absent TSH response to TRH. Owing to extreme sensitivity of the TSH-secretory mechanism to feedback inhibition, diminished responses to TRH commonly occur in apparently euthyroid patients with serum T_4 or T_3 levels within the normal range but with marginally increased T_4 or T_3 output from autonomously functioning toxic adenomas or toxic multinodular goiters. Blunted TRH responses also may be seen in some patients with euthyroid Graves' disease. In addition, responses to TRH are often decreased in elderly individuals, especially men. Despite these exceptions, a subnormal or absent response to TRH has been employed as a confirmatory test for thyrotoxicosis. With the availability of highly sensitive TSH assays, the TRH test is rarely used for this purpose. TRH tests are of even less value in the diagnosis of hypothyroidism. Responses are increased in patients with primary hypothyroidism, but the magnitude of increase is generally proportional to the extent of increase in basal serum TSH. Some patients with pituitary hypothyroidism have subnormal responses, and some with TRH deficiency due to hypothalamic disease have a near-normal response, but these responses are not seen consistently. Further, in as many as one-fourth of patients with hypothyroidism due to hypothalamic-pituitary disease, basal serum TSH levels are normal or slightly elevated, and the response to TRH is exaggerated, although some of this TSH may not be bioactive.

The *thyroid suppression test* is used to assess whether thyroid function is under normal homeostatic control. Normally, exogenous thyroid hormone suppresses pituitary TSH secretion, resulting in a decrease in the RAIU. Since liothyronine is usually employed for the test (100 μg/d for 7 to 10 days), the resulting decline in serum T_4, as well as in the RAIU, can serve as an index of suppression. A normal suppressive response is a decrease of the RAIU to less than half the control value and a decline of the serum T_4 to low normal or subnormal values. A normal suppression test is incompatible with and excludes a diagnosis of hyperthyroidism. An abnormal suppression test is always present in hyperthyroidism, irrespective of the underlying cause; this indicates either autonomy of thyroid function, the presence of an abnormal (non-TSH) thyroid stimulator, or unremitting hypersecretion of TSH. An abnormal suppression test is not pathognomonic of hyperthyroidism, however, since it may persist after treatment of hyperthyroidism in Graves' disease and is seen in about half the euthyroid patients with the ophthalmopathy of Graves' disease.

Because of the risk of adverse effects of exogenous thyroid hormone, especially liothyronine, in elderly patients and in those with cardiovascular disease, and since the TRH test is almost entirely devoid of undesirable side effects, either the latter test or highly sensitive TSH measurement has almost entirely supplanted the thyroid suppression test in the diagnosis of hyperthyroidism.

MISCELLANEOUS TESTS Various tests that do not assess thyroid function are of value in defining the nature of the thyroid disorder or in planning therapy. For example, high titers of *antithyroid peroxidase* (anti-TPO, antimicrosomal) *antibodies* or *antithyroglobulin antibodies* are found in the serum of most patients with Hashimoto's disease and in many with primary thyroprivic hypothyroidism or Graves' disease. In the latter, the serum also contains antibodies against the TSH receptor on thyroid plasma membranes. In general, these are capable of inhibiting the receptor binding of TSH (TSH-binding inhibitory immunoglobulins, TBII) and of stimulating the production of cyclic AMP therein (thyroid-stimulating antibodies or immunoglobulins, TSAb or TSI). The clinical utility of tests for TBII and TSI stems from the fact that the disappearance of the factors from the serum during a course of antithyroid therapy implies the likelihood of a long-term remission of hyperthyroidism when therapy is withdrawn. In some patients, analogous antibodies have no intrinsic stimulatory effect but block the response to endogenous TSH and produce nongoitrous hypothyroidism. Both stimulatory and blocking anti-TSH receptor antibodies have the ability to cross the placenta and, as a consequence, to produce transient hyperthyroidism (neonatal Graves' disease) or hypothyroidism, respectively, in the newborn. Measurement of these antibodies during the last months of pregnancy makes it possible to assess the likelihood of the disorders developing in the neonate.

Some patients, most commonly those with autoimmune thyroid disease, develop *circulating antibodies against T_3 or T_4*, or both. In RIAs for these hormones, because the endogenous antibody competes with the exogenous antibody for binding of the added labeled ligand, spurious high or low values for the concentration of the hormone are obtained, depending on the technique of RIA used. The true concentration of the hormone, as determined in extracts of the serum, is increased owing to the additional binding sites provided by the antibody, but antibody-bound hormone is unavailable for metabolic action. In the case of anti-T_3 antibodies, which are the more common, values of the RT_3U are low because endogenous antibody competes with the resin for binding of the added labeled T_3. Such antibodies can be detected by adding labeled hormone to serum, separating the immunoglobulins from other serum proteins, and demonstrating that they bind the labeled hormone.

Along with several other thyroid disorders, differentiated carcinomas of the thyroid release thyroglobulin into the bloodstream. As a consequence, measurements of the *serum thyroglobulin* by RIA have value not in the initial diagnosis of thyroid carcinoma but in assessing the adequacy of initial therapy and in monitoring for recurrence or dissemination of the disease. In patients with thyrotoxicosis, subnormal serum thyroglobulin concentrations together with decreased values of the RAIU suggest thyrotoxicosis factitia.

Imaging by *scintiscanning* permits localization of sites of accumulation of radioiodine or sodium [^{99m}Tc]pertechnetate. This technique is useful for defining areas of increased or decreased function within the thyroid and for detecting retrosternal goiter, ectopic thyroid tissue, hemiagenesis of the thyroid, and functioning metastases of thyroid carcinoma. Ultrasonic examination of the thyroid is also useful for differentiating cystic nodules from those which are solid. Since ultrasonic scans provide an accurate indication of size, are noninvasive, and apparently have no injurious effects, sequential scans can be employed to assess changes in the size of the thyroid as a whole or of discrete nodules over time or in response to treatment.

SICK EUTHYROID SYNDROME

Severe illness, physical trauma, or physiologic stress can induce changes in one or more aspects of thyroid hormone economy, leading to findings referred to as the *sick euthyroid syndrome* (SES). Abnormalities in SES include alterations in the peripheral transport and metabolism of the thyroid hormones, the regulation of TSH secretion, and in some cases thyroid function itself. Acting alone or together, these lead to changes in the concentrations of the circulating thyroid hormones, both total and free, that serve to define the several variants of the SES. Because of the frequency and nonspecificity of the disorders that cause it, SES is probably a more common cause of abnormalities in the concentration of thyroid hormones in the blood than intrinsic thyroid disease.

NORMAL-T_4 VARIANT OF SES Decreased production of T_3 owing to inhibition of the peripheral $5'$-monodeiodination of T_4 is a consistent feature of the SES. This is reflected in a decrease in the serum total T_3 concentration that varies in severity with that of the illness. In moderately ill patients, serum total T_4 concentration is within the normal range. A decrease in the intensity of protein binding, greater for T_4 than for T_3, is an additional accompaniment. As a result, values of the RT_3U are moderately increased, and the percent FT_4 is increased to a proportionately greater extent. As a consequence, values of the free T_4 index (FT_4I) and those of the free T_4 concentrations (FT_4) are often increased. Serum rT_3 concentrations are increased, owing to a decrease in the plasma clearance of rT_3 secondary to inhibition of its $5'$-monodeiodination. The plasma clearance rate of T_4 is increased, probably as a result of decreased T_4 binding, and this, in the face of normal T_4 concentrations, indicates that the overall rate of T_4 degradation and production is increased. Production rates for T_3 are decreased, and those for rT_3 are normal. Serum TSH concentration and the response of serum TSH to TRH are generally normal, although they may increase and then return to normal as recovery from the illness takes place. Despite the reduction in the serum T_3 concentration, this variant of the SES can be separated from intrinsic thyroid disease because the serum T_4 and TSH are normal and because the serum T_3 is not useful for diagnosing hypothyroidism.

LOW-T_4 VARIANT OF SES In more seriously ill patients, T_3 production rates and serum total and free T_3 concentrations decrease still further, and abnormalities in hormone binding increase in severity. As a consequence, serum T_4 concentrations decrease into the hypothyroid range. This is partly but not entirely due to decreased T_4 binding, since values of the FT_4 are frequently subnormal. These are probably the result of decreased T_4 production in the most severely ill patients and are secondary to decreased secretion of TSH. Serum TSH concentrations appear normal by conventional assay but are low with sensitive TSH assays, and TRH responses are often blunted. Hence, in this variant of the SES, there is an inappropriate hyposecretion of TSH, considering the low serum total and free T_4 and T_3 concentrations, and a diagnosis of pituitary hypothyroidism may be suggested. While the cause is unknown, low TSH in this setting may be due to effects of cytokines such as interleukin 1 and tumor necrosis factor on the pituitary. With resolution of the underlying illness, TSH levels rise, heralding recovery, and may be transiently elevated until T_4 and T_3 levels are restored to normal. Production rates for rT_3 are diminished, owing to the decreased availability of its precursor T_4; nonetheless, serum rT_3 concentrations are increased, owing to retardation of its degradation, and this provides an important means of differentiating the SES from pituitary hypothyroidism, in which serum rT_3 concentrations are low. In patients with primary hypothyroidism who have associated illness, serum TSH levels remain elevated, although generally lower than they otherwise would be.

HIGH-T_4 VARIANT OF SES An unusual variant of the SES (approximately 1 percent of sick patients) is associated with increased serum total and free T_4 concentrations during acute illness and return to normal thereafter. This variant is most often seen in elderly women, many of whom have received medications that contain iodine. The principal source of diagnostic confusion is with the syndrome of "T_4 toxicosis," i.e., true thyrotoxicosis upon which illness has been superimposed, so that serum T_4 concentrations are increased and serum T_3 concentrations are normal. In the latter, however, serum rT_3 concentrations are higher, values of the serum total T_3 and FT_3I

are higher, TSH is usually undetectable, and TRH responses are blunted to absent.

ABNORMALITIES IN HORMONE BINDING IN SES Multiple factors are responsible for the decreased binding of T_4 and, to a lesser extent, T_3 in the SES. Illness is associated with decreased synthesis of TTR and a decrease in its serum concentration, but the extent to which this contributes to decreased T_4 binding is uncertain. In chronically ill patients, serum TBG concentration is subnormal. Most often, however, the extent of decreased T_4 binding cannot be explained by decreases in serum TTR and TBG, and an inhibitor of hormone binding may be responsible. Its nature is uncertain, but it may be one or more fatty acids, which also may be responsible for diminished conversion of T_4 to T_3.

The importance of the SES is that the changes in circulating thyroid hormone concentrations should not be confused with those due to intrinsic thyroid or pituitary disease. Unresolved questions are whether the metabolic impact of thyroid hormone in peripheral tissues is decreased in the SES and whether the syndrome is a beneficial or adverse response to illness. There is no evidence that patients with low T_4 and T_3 of SES benefit from treatment with thyroid hormones.

SIMPLE (NONTOXIC) GOITER

Endemic goiter implies an etiologic factor or factors common to a particular geographic region. The term has been defined as the presence of generalized or localized thyroid enlargement in more than 10 percent of the population. *Sporadic* goiter arises in nonendemic areas as a result of factors that do not affect the population generally. Since these terms fail to define the causes of such goiters, and since thyroid enlargement of diverse etiology may exist in both endemic and nonendemic regions, it is prudent to employ a general term such as *simple* or *nontoxic goiter*. Simple or nontoxic goiter can be defined as any enlargement of the thyroid gland that does not result from an inflammatory or neoplastic process and that is not initially associated with thyrotoxicosis or myxedema.

ETIOLOGY AND PATHOGENESIS Simple goiter is sometimes due to a definable cause of impaired thyroid hormone synthesis, such as iodine deficiency, ingestion of a goitrogen, or a defect in a hormone biosynthetic pathway, but in most instances its cause is unknown. Whatever the cause, the clinical manifestations reflect the operation of a common pathophysiologic mechanism. Simple goiter occurs when one or more factors impair the capacity of the thyroid to secrete sufficient hormones to meet the needs of the peripheral tissues. Although this has been presumed to lead to increased secretion of TSH, concentrations of TSH in the serum of patients with established simple goiter are usually normal. Hence some other mechanism of goitrogenesis may be operative. A likely possibility is that depletion of glandular organic iodine accompanying impaired hormone synthesis increases the responsiveness of the thyroid to normal levels of TSH. The resulting increases in both functioning thyroid mass and cellular activity overcome mild impairment of hormone synthesis; thus the patient is metabolically normal, though goitrous. When the underlying disorder is severe, compensatory responses, now including hypersecretion of TSH, are inadequate to overcome the impairment, and the patient is both goitrous and hypothyroid. Thus simple goiter cannot be clearly separated in the pathogenic sense from goitrous hypothyroidism. Specific causes of simple goiter may exist with or without hypothyroidism (Table 334-5). Defective iodination of thyroglobulin may be an important cause in many patients. The possibility that goiter can be due to antibodies that stimulate thyroid growth but not function remains to be substantiated.

PATHOLOGY The histopathology of the thyroid in simple goiter varies with the etiology and the stage at which the examination is made. In its initial stages, the gland exhibits a uniform hypertrophy, hyperplasia, and hypervascularity. As the disorder persists or undergoes repeated exacerbations and remissions, uniformity of thyroidal

TABLE 334-5 Classification of the causes of hypothyroidism

THYROID

A Thyroprivic
  1 Congenital development defect
  2 Primary idiopathic
  3 Postablative (radioiodine, surgery)
  4 Postradiation (e.g., for lymphoma)
B Goitrous
  1 Heritable biosynthetic defects
  2 Maternally transmitted (iodides, antithyroid agents)
  3 Iodine deficiency
  4 Drug-elicited (aminosalicylic acid, iodides, phenylbutazone, iodoantipyrine, lithium)
  5 Chronic thyroiditis (Hashimoto's disease)
  6 Interleukin 2 and lymphokine-activated killer cells

SUPRATHYROID (TROPHOPRIVIC)

A Pituitary
  1 Panhypopituitarism
  2 Isolated TSH deficiency
B Hypothalamic
  1 Congenital defects
  2 Infection (encephalitis)
  3 Neoplasm
  4 Infiltrative (sarcoidosis)

SELF-LIMITED

A Following withdrawal of suppressive thyroid therapy
B Subacute thyroiditis and chronic thyroiditis with transient hypothyroidism (usually after a phase of thyrotoxicosis)

---

architecture is lost. Occasionally, the greater part of the gland may display a uniform involution or hyperinvolution with colloid accumulation. More often, areas of involution are interspersed with patchy areas of focal hyperplasia. Fibrosis may demarcate hyperplastic or involuted nodules. These may resemble true neoplasms (adenomas). Areas of hemorrhage and irregular calcification may be present. The evolution of the multinodular stage is almost always accompanied by the development of functional autonomy. Indeed, heterogeneity of structure and function and a degree of functional autonomy are the hallmarks of the mature stage of this disorder.

CLINICAL MANIFESTATIONS In simple goiter, the clinical manifestations arise solely from enlargement of the thyroid, since the metabolic state is normal. In goitrous hypothyroidism, symptoms caused by thyromegaly are accompanied by signs and symptoms of hormonal insufficiency. Mechanical sequelae include compression and displacement of the trachea or esophagus, occasionally with obstructive symptoms if the goiter becomes sufficiently large. Superior mediastinal obstruction may occur with large retrosternal goiters. Signs of compression can be induced in the case of large retrosternal goiters when the patient's arms are raised above the head; suffusion of the face, giddiness, or syncope may result from this maneuver (Pemberton's sign). Hoarseness due to compression of the recurrent laryngeal nerve is rare in simple goiter and suggests neoplasm. Sudden hemorrhage into a nodule may lead to an acute, painful swelling in the neck and may produce or enhance compressive symptoms. Hyperthyroidism may supervene in long-standing multinodular goiter (toxic multinodular goiter). In both endemic and sporadic multinodular goiter, the ingestion of excess iodide may result in the development of thyrotoxicosis (jodbasedow phenomenon).

In regions where iodine deficiency is severe, goitrous enlargement also may be associated with varying degrees of hypothyroidism. Cretinism, both goitrous and nongoitrous, occurs with increased frequency in the children of goitrous parents in many countries where goiter is common. Although iodine deficiency is doubtless a factor in the etiology of endemic goiter, the frequency of goiter differs greatly among persons with equally severe iodine deficiency. In such instances, dietary or waterborne goitrogens appear to be important

conditioning factors. In some areas, these goitrogens may be sufficient to cause goiter in the absence of iodine deficiency.

DIAGNOSIS The diagnosis of simple goiter requires, first, demonstration of a euthyroid state and, second, demonstration of normal serum T_4 and T_3 concentrations. The former may be difficult because manifestations of thyrotoxicosis may be subtle or atypical, especially among the elderly (see the section "Toxic Multinodular Goiter"). The latter may be problematic, since serum T_4 and especially T_3 concentrations may be near the upper limit of the normal range. In addition, the fact that serum T_3 concentrations may decrease in the euthyroid elderly complicates interpretation of this test. The RAIU is usually normal but may be increased in the presence of iodine deficiency or a biosynthetic defect. Thus a measurable TSH by a highly sensitive technique is the best index of euthyroidism. Indeed, subclinical thyrotoxicosis may be secondary to the functional autonomy of the goiter and consequently cause a decrease in both basal TSH and TSH response to TRH. Differentiation of nontoxic goiter from Hashimoto's disease is facilitated by the greater frequency of multinodularity in the former and by the presence of high titers of circulating antimicrosomal or antithyroglobulin antibodies in the latter. In some instances, emergence of a strongly dominant nodule may suggest the presence of a carcinoma. This is especially true if bleeding has caused it to increase in size rapidly and to lose the ability to accumulate iodine or pertechnetate. Appropriate radiographic studies (computed tomography, magnetic resonance imaging) and flow volume measurement should be recorded in the presence of significant substernal extension with potential for upper airway obstruction.

TREATMENT The object of treatment is to reduce the size of the goiter, either by relieving external encumbrances to hormone formation or by providing sufficient quantities of exogenous hormone to inhibit TSH secretion and thereby put the thyroid gland at rest. In disorders characterized by decreased thyroid iodide stores, such as iodine deficiency or impairment of the thyroid iodide-concentrating mechanism, small doses of iodide may prove effective. Occasionally, a known extrinsic goitrogen can be withdrawn. Most commonly, however, no specific etiologic factor can be detected, and thyroid hormone therapy is required. For this purpose, levothyroxine (L-thyroxine) is the agent of choice. In the younger patient with the early diffuse stage of simple goiter, treatment is instituted with 100 µg levothyroxine daily, and the dose is increased over the next month or so to a maximum of 150 or 200 µg/d (average dose of 1.7 µg/kg body weight per day). Complete suppression would imply reduction of serum TSH to levels less than 0.1 mU/L by an ultrasensitive assay. Until uncertainties about the association of long-term excess thyroid hormone therapy and loss of bone mineral (osteopenia) are resolved, patients should be titrated to slightly less than a fully suppressive dose. Adequacy of suppression also may be assessed by measuring the RAIU, which should decrease to less than 5 percent of the administered dose at 24 h. Lesser decreases indicate only partial suppression, which may reflect the presence of autonomous foci demonstrable by scanning techniques. In the elderly or the patient with long-standing multinodular goiter, an ultrasensitive TSH measurement or a TRH stimulation test should be undertaken before initiating treatment with levothyroxine to determine whether significant functional autonomy is present. If such is indicated by an undetectable basal TSH or a diminished or absent TSH responsiveness to TRH, suppressive therapy with levothyroxine is contraindicated, since such patients are or will eventually become thyrotoxic. Rather, consideration should be given to radioiodine ablation of the autonomous foci (see later section "Toxic Multinodular Goiter"). On the other hand, if the basal TSH or the TSH response to TRH is normal, excluding significant functional autonomy, treatment with levothyroxine can be initiated. In the elderly patient, the initial dose should not exceed 50 µg/d, and the dosage should be gradually increased, partial rather than complete suppression of the value for basal TSH and/or the RAIU being the end point. It is the practice to obtain a thyroid scan as part of the initial evaluation of all patients with multinodular goiter. In those patients in whom full suppressive doses of thyroxine are indicated, it is desirable to repeat the RAIU and scan (suppression scan), when practical, to ascertain the efficacy of suppression and/or the presence of autonomous foci.

Results of therapy vary widely. The early diffuse, hyperplastic goiter responds well, with regression or disappearance in 3 to 6 months. In the author's experience, the later, nodular stage responds less favorably, and significant reduction in gland size is achieved only in about one-third of cases; however, in the remainder, suppressive treatment may forestall further glandular growth. Internodular tissue regresses more often than do nodules themselves. The latter may therefore appear to become more prominent during treatment. After maximum regression of the goiter, suppressive medication may be maintained for prolonged periods, reduced to minimal levels, or at times withdrawn. In an unpredictable manner, goiter may remain relieved or recur. In the latter instances, if appropriate studies rule out malignancy, suppressive therapy should be reinstituted and continued indefinitely. In areas of endemic iodine deficiency, the size and prevalence of goiter and the frequency of cretinism can be reduced by the provision of iodized salt or water or the periodic injection of iodized oil.

Surgical therapy of simple goiter is physiologically unsound, but it may occasionally be necessary to relieve obstructive symptoms, especially those that persist after a trial of medical therapy. Large substernal goiters with partial upper airway obstruction also have been treated by radioactive iodine with moderate success. Surgical exploration of nodular goiter also may be indicated in some individuals when evidence suggests carcinoma. However, the concept that subtotal resection of multinodular nontoxic goiter affords effective prophylaxis against the development of thyroid carcinoma is unsound. If for some reason subtotal thyroidectomy has been performed, levothyroxine in a usual dose of about 1.7 μg/kg body weight daily is recommended to inhibit regenerative hyperplasia and further goitrogenesis.

HYPOTHYROIDISM

Hypothyroidism can result from any of a variety of abnormalities that lead to insufficient synthesis of thyroid hormone. Hypothyroidism dating from birth and resulting in developmental abnormalities is termed *cretinism*. The term *myxedema* connotes severe hypothyroidism in which there is accumulation of hydrophilic mucopolysaccharides in the ground substance of the dermis and other tissues, leading to thickening of the facial features and doughy induration of the skin.

ETIOLOGY AND PATHOGENESIS A classification of hypothyroidism is presented in Table 334-5. Overall, the primary thyroid varieties account for approximately 95 percent of cases, only 5 percent or less being suprathyroid in origin. In thyroprivic hypothyroidism, loss of thyroid tissue leads to inadequate synthesis of thyroid hormone, despite maximum stimulation of any thyroid remnant by TSH. The most common cause of thyroprivic hypothyroidism is surgical or radioiodine ablation of the thyroid gland in the treatment of Graves' disease. Thyroprivic hypothyroidism also may occur as a primary idiopathic disorder. The most common cause of primary hypothyroidism is autoimmunity and is associated with circulating antithyroid antibodies and in some cases may result from the action of antibodies that block the TSH receptor. It may coexist with diabetes mellitus and other diseases in which circulating autoantibodies are found, such as pernicious anemia, systemic lupus erythematosus, rheumatoid arthritis, Sjögren's syndrome, and chronic hepatitis. In addition, hypothyroidism can be one manifestation of a polyglandular endocrine deficiency state in which autoantibodies cause variable insufficiency of thyroid, adrenal, parathyroid, and gonadal function (see Chap. 343). All these diseases, including isolated primary hypothyroidism, are associated with an increased frequency of specific HLA haplotypes. Finally, a developmental defect may result in failure of the gland to function adequately, leading to sporadic nongoitrous cretinism or

juvenile hypothyroidism. A self-limited period of hypothyroidism is common in the course of subacute thyroiditis and in the syndrome of "painless thyroiditis," including the postpartum variant and usually after a temporary period of thyrotoxicosis. Owing to a persisting lack of TSH stimulation, intrinsically euthyroid subjects from whom chronic suppressive therapy is abruptly withdrawn experience a several-week period of thyroid hypofunction.

Inability to synthesize adequate quantities of thyroid hormone leads to hypersecretion of TSH and hence goiter. If this compensatory response is inadequate, goitrous hypothyroidism ensues. The most common cause of goitrous hypothyroidism in North America is Hashimoto's disease, in which defective organic binding of iodide and abnormal secretion of iodoproteins are frequent. Iodide-induced goiter with or without hypothyroidism appears to arise from an intrinsic defect in the organic binding mechanism, which permits a persistent Wolff-Chaikoff effect. Euthyroid patients with Graves' disease, especially after surgery or radioiodine treatment, those with Hashimoto's disease, and the normal fetus are particularly susceptible to iodide-induced goiter. In view of the susceptibility of the fetal thyroid to iodide, with resulting goiter and hypothyroidism, iodine in large doses should not be given during pregnancy. Less common causes of goitrous hypothyroidism are hereditary defects in hormone biosynthesis and ingestion of drugs that induce defects in hormone biosynthesis, such as aminosalicylic acid and lithium. Finally, in areas of environmental iodine deficiency, goitrous cretinism and hypothyroidism can occur on an endemic basis. Diminished thyroid reserve occurs as a stage in the evolution of both thyroprivic and goitrous hypothyroidism.

Rarely, long-standing hypothyroidism may lead to diffuse, nodular, or adenomatous thyrotroph hyperplasia. These patients may present with headache, visual field defects, abnormal pubertal development, galactorrhea, and pituitary enlargement, all of which disappear with levothyroxine therapy. Such patients have marked elevations in serum TSH, whereas in hypothyroidism of suprathyroid origin, the thyroid is intrinsically normal but is deprived of stimulation by TSH. Deprivation of TSH, most commonly the result of postpartum pituitary necrosis or a tumor of the pituitary or adjacent regions, results in pituitary hypothyroidism. Hypothalamic hypothyroidism is less common and results from inadequate secretion of TRH.

CLINICAL PICTURE The appearance of children with hypothyroidism depends on the age at which the deficiency began and the promptness with which replacement therapy was instituted. Cretinism may be manifested at birth but usually becomes evident within the first several months, depending on the extent of thyroid failure. Hypothyroidism is present in approximately 1 in every 5000 neonates and manifests itself in persistence of physiologic jaundice, hoarse cry, constipation, somnolence, and feeding problems; since clinical diagnosis is difficult and early treatment is crucial for normal intellectual development, all neonates should be screened for hypothyroidism with measurements of the serum T_4 or TSH. In later months, delay in reaching the normal milestones of development becomes evident, and the physical characteristics of the cretin appear. These include short stature, coarse features with protruding tongue, broad flat nose, widely set eyes, sparse hair, dry skin, protuberant abdomen with an umbilical hernia, impaired mental development, retarded bone age, epiphyseal dysgenesis, and delayed dentition.

In the older child, the clinical manifestations of hypothyroidism are intermediate between those of infantile and adult hypothyroidism. Retardation of linear growth is manifested by shortness of stature, and retardation of sexual maturation results in delayed puberty. Poor performance at school may call attention to the diagnosis. Variable manifestations of adult hypothyroidism are present. X-ray examination reveals delayed union of the epiphyses.

In the adult, early symptoms of hypothyroidism are nonspecific and of insidious onset. In the elderly patient, symptoms may be erroneously attributed to aging or other disorders such as Parkinson's disease, depression, or Alzheimer's disease. They may include fatigue, lethargy, constipation, cold intolerance, stiffness and cramping of the muscles, the carpal tunnel syndrome, and menorrhagia. Over the succeeding months, intellectual and motor activity slows, appetite declines, and weight increases. The hair becomes dry and tends to fall out, and the skin becomes dry. The voice becomes deeper and hoarse, and auditory acuity may deteriorate. Obstructive sleep apnea may occur. Ultimately, the clinical picture of florid myxedema appears, with dull expressionless face, sparse hair, periorbital puffiness, large tongue, and pale, cool skin that feels rough and doughy. Thyroid tissue is not readily palpable, except in the goitrous variety of hypothyroidism. The heart is enlarged owing to both dilation and pericardial effusion; if the heart is small, pituitary hypothyroidism (with secondary adrenal insufficiency) or coincident primary adrenal insufficiency (Schmidt's syndrome) should be considered. Adynamic ileus may cause megacolon or intestinal obstruction. Rarely, psychiatric symptoms or cerebellar ataxia may dominate the clinical picture. The relaxation phase of the deep tendon reflexes is characteristically prolonged, the so-called hung-up reflex. If left untreated, the patient with severe long-standing hypothyroidism may pass into a hypothermic, stuporous state (*myxedema coma*) that may be fatal. Respiratory depression is an important component of this state, and hence arterial P_{CO_2} may be increased. Factors that predispose to myxedema coma include cold exposure, trauma, infection, and administration of central nervous system depressants. Hyponatremia may result from impaired water excretion and from disordered regulation of vasopressin secretion.

LABORATORY TESTS The single most useful measurement is the serum TSH, which is increased in the thyroprivic and goitrous varieties and is usually normal or undetectable in pituitary or hypothalamic hypothyroidism (see Fig. 334-3). In the latter instances, hyposecretion of TSH is usually accompanied by hyposecretion of other pituitary hormones (see Chap. 331). A decrease in serum T_4 and in the FT_4I is common to all varieties of hypothyroidism. In the primary thyroid varieties, the serum T_3 may be decreased to a lesser extent than the serum T_4, presumably because the compensatory hypersecretion of TSH leads to a relative preponderance of T_3 secretion. In thyroprivic hypothyroidism, the decreased RAIU is of limited diagnostic utility because of the low value for the lower limit of the normal range. In goitrous hypothyroidism, the RAIU may be increased or display an abnormal pattern of accumulation or retention.

Manifestations of the hypothyroid state include an increased serum cholesterol level in hypothyroidism of thyroid (but not pituitary) origin and increased concentrations of serum creatine phosphokinase, aspartate transaminase, and lactate dehydrogenase. Systolic time intervals are altered in that the preejection period is prolonged and the ratio of the preejection period to left ventricular ejection time is increased. Electrocardiographic changes include bradycardia, low-amplitude QRS complexes, and flattened or inverted T waves. In primary thyroprivic hypothyroidism, pernicious anemia occurs in about 12 percent of patients; histamine-fast achlorhydria and circulating antigastric parietal cell antibodies are more common.

Some patients who appear clinically euthyroid display laboratory evidence of early thyroid failure (subclinical hypothyroidism). In mild cases, serum TSH and its response to TRH administration are increased, while serum T_4 and T_3 concentrations are normal. When thyroid failure is more advanced, serum T_4 concentration is decreased, but the serum T_3 concentration is normal or nearly so owing to TSH-induced hypersecretion of T_3 relative to T_4 and perhaps to more efficient conversion of T_4 to T_3. Subclinical hypothyroidism is most often seen in patients with Hashimoto's disease or those with Graves' disease who have been treated with ^{131}I or surgery and are usually in the evolution of frank hypothyroidism.

DIFFERENTIAL DIAGNOSIS Little difficulty is experienced in diagnosing the classic picture of cretinism or juvenile and adult hypothyroidism. Occasionally, an infant with Down's syndrome may be confused with a cretin. However, the characteristic eye changes, Brushfield's spots in the iris, hyperextensibility of the joints, and normal skin and hair texture distinguish Down's syndrome from cretinism. Chronic nephritis and the nephrotic syndrome may simulate

TABLE 334-6 Approximate therapeutic equivalence of various thyroid hormone preparations

Preparation	Average daily oral maintenance dose	Serum T_4	Undesirable lability in serum T_3
Levothyroxine	125 μg	Slightly increased	−
Liothyronine	50 μg	Decreased	+ +
Liotrix ($T_4/T_3 = 4:1$)	2 units	Normal	+
Thyroid extract, USP	120–180 mg	Normal	+

myxedema, particularly because of the facial puffiness and pallor. The nephrotic patient may have anemia, hypercholesterolemia, and anasarca, and the serum T_4 may be decreased if TBG is lost into the urine. However, the FT_4I is normal or increased, the serum T_3 concentration is often subnormal, as in any severe systemic illness owing to impaired peripheral generation from T_4, and the serum TSH concentration is normal.

TREATMENT Hormones available for the treatment of hypothyroidism (Table 334-6) include the synthetic hormones levothyroxine (L-thyroxine), liothyronine (L-triiodothyronine), and liotrix (a combination of the two). A preparation of natural origin still occasionally used is thyroid extract, USP. Because of their uniform potency, the author prefers the synthetic preparations and specifically levothyroxine. Unlike liothyronine, liotrix, and even thyroid extract, ingestion of levothyroxine does not lead to abrupt increases in serum T_3 concentration, which can be dangerous in the older patient or in the patient with coexisting heart disease. Rather, a stable T_3 concentration is attained through continuous generation from administered levothyroxine.

In most instances, a normal metabolic state should be restored gradually, especially in the elderly or the patient with heart disease, since sudden increases in metabolic rate may tax cardiac or coronary reserve. In adults, an initial daily dose of 25 μg levothyroxine can be increased by 25- to 50-μg increments at 4-week intervals until a normal metabolic state is attained. The dose necessary to sustain a normal metabolic state is usually about 1.7 μg/kg body weight per day, and this dose usually results in a serum T_4 at or somewhat above the upper limit of the normal range. The serum T_3 is superior to the serum T_4 as an indicator of the metabolic state in the patient receiving levothyroxine. Because of its long half-life, levothyroxine is administered as a single daily dose. The optimal dose is determined by clinical criteria and measurements of serum TSH by an ultrasensitive assay. In the patient with pituitary or hypothalamic disease, serum T_3 is the most useful parameter to follow. Elevations of the former indicate that treatment is insufficient and of the latter that it is excessive.

In neonatal, infantile, and juvenile hypothyroidism, full replacement therapy should be begun as soon as possible; otherwise, the chances of normal intellectual development and growth are poor. Infants and children require doses of levothyroxine that are disproportionately large in relation to body size. *In known or strongly suspected pituitary and hypothalamic hypothyroidism, thyroid replacement should not be instituted until treatment with hydrocortisone has been initiated*, since acute adrenocortical insufficiency may be precipitated by an increase in metabolic rate.

In some adults, hypothyroidism should be treated rapidly. This includes patients with myxedema coma and, because of the extreme sensitivity to central nervous system depressants, hypothyroid patients being prepared for emergency surgery. Here, intravenous administration of levothyroxine, in conjunction with the use of hydrocortisone, is indicated.

THYROTOXICOSIS

The term *thyrotoxicosis* denotes the clinical, physiologic, and biochemical findings that result when the tissues are exposed to, and

TABLE 334-7   **Varieties of thyrotoxicosis**

ASSOCIATED WITH THYROID HYPERFUNCTION*

A   Excess production of TSH (rare)
B   Abnormal thyroid stimulator
   1 Graves' disease
   2 Trophoblastic tumor
C   Intrinsic thyroid autonomy
   1 Hyperfunctioning adenoma
   2 Toxic multinodular goiter

NOT ASSOCIATED WITH THYROID HYPERFUNCTION†

A   Disorders of hormone storage
   1 Subacute thyroiditis
   2 Chronic thyroiditis with transient thyrotoxicosis
B   Extrathyroid source of hormone
   1 Thyrotoxicosis factitia
   2 "Hamburger toxicosis"
   3 Ectopic thyroid tissue
      a Struma ovarii
      b Functioning follicular cacinoma

*   Associated with increased RAIU unless body iodine burden is excessive.
†   Associated with decreased RAIU.

respond to, excess thyroid hormone. Rather than a specific disease, thyrotoxicosis can originate in a variety of ways (Table 334-7). The first, and most important, encompasses those diseases that lead to sustained overproduction of hormone by the thyroid gland itself. Here, hyperfunction of the gland variously results from excessive secretion of TSH, a rare cause associated with pituitary tumor or with resistance to thyroid hormone in the pituitary but not in peripheral tissues; the action of an abnormal, homeostatically unregulated thyroid stimulator of extrapituitary origin, as in Graves' disease or hyperthyroidism in association with Hashimoto's disease or trophoblastic tumors; or the development of one or more areas of autonomous hyperfunction within the gland itself. The second category encompasses the thyrotoxic states associated with subacute thyroiditis and the syndrome termed *chronic thyroiditis with spontaneously resolving thyrotoxicosis;* an excess of preformed hormone leaks from the gland owing to the presence of inflammatory disease. New hormone formation is decreased, however, owing to the suppression of TSH secretion by the hormone excess and in some cases to the inflammatory injury itself. Since the inflammatory disorders are transitory, and since stores of preformed hormone are ultimately depleted, the thyrotoxicosis in these disorders is self-limited and is often followed by a transient period of thyroid hormone insufficiency. The third category of thyrotoxicosis is one in which the source of excess hormone is outside of the thyroid gland itself, as in thyrotoxicosis factitia, the ingestion of meat contaminated with animal thyroids ("hamburger toxicosis"), the rare functioning metastatic thyroid carcinoma, or struma ovarii.

Although the foregoing disorders are associated with thyrotoxicosis, not all are associated with *hyperthyroidism*, a term which should be used to denote only those conditions in which sustained hyperfunction of the thyroid leads to thyrotoxicosis. Thus thyrotoxic states can be classified according to whether or not they are associated with hyperthyroidism. This distinction has implications for diagnosis and for treatment. In hyperthyroidism, hyperfunction of the thyroid is reflected in an increased RAIU, whereas in the nonhyperthyroid thyrotoxic states, thyroid function (as reflected in the RAIU) is subnormal. Further, treatment of thyrotoxicosis by means intended to decrease hormone synthesis (antithyroid agents, surgery, or radioiodine) is appropriate in hyperthyroidism but is inappropriate and ineffective in other forms of thyrotoxicosis.

Though the specific diseases that cause thyrotoxicosis each make their own imprint on the clinical picture, the manifestations of the thyrotoxic state are largely the same. Since the first considered and most common is Graves' disease, the common manifestations of thyrotoxicosis are described in relation to Graves' disease.

GRAVES' DISEASE

Graves' disease, also known as Parry's or Basedow's disease, is a disorder with three major manifestations: hyperthyroidism with diffuse goiter, ophthalmopathy, and dermopathy. The three major manifestations need not appear together. Indeed, one or two need never appear, and moreover, the three may run courses that are largely independent of one another.

PREVALENCE   Graves' disease is a relatively common disorder that occurs at any age but is especially common in the third and fourth decades. The disease is more frequent in women. In nongoitrous areas, the ratio of predominance in women may be as high as 7:1. In areas of endemic goiter, the ratio is lower. Genetic factors play an important role; there is an increased frequency of haplotypes HLA-B8 and -DRw3 in Caucasian, HLA-Bw36 in Japanese, and HLA-Bw46 in Chinese patients with the disease. Not surprisingly, there is a distinct familial predisposition to Graves' disease. In addition, among family members, a clinical and immunologic overlap exists with respect to Hashimoto's disease, primary thyroprivic hypothyroidism, and pernicious anemia and probably with respect to other diseases with prominent autoimmune features. In occasional patients, the picture may change from Graves' disease to Hashimoto's disease, or vice versa, and rarely, patients with primary myxedema later become hyperthyroid. Thus it is proper to consider Graves' disease, Hashimoto's disease, and primary myxedema as closely related autoimmune thyroid diseases.

ETIOLOGY AND PATHOGENESIS   The cause is unknown. In view of the varied manifestations and their differing courses, it is possible that no single factor is responsible for the entire syndrome. With respect to hyperthyroidism, the central disorder is a disruption of homeostatic mechanisms that normally adjust hormone secretion to meet the needs of peripheral tissues. This homeostatic disruption results from the presence in plasma of an abnormal thyroid stimulator, first recognized when it was shown that the serum of patients with Graves' disease releases radioiodine from the prelabeled guinea pig or mouse thyroid. In view of its prolonged duration of action relative to that of TSH in this bioassay system, this material was designated the *long-acting thyroid stimulator* (LATS). LATS activity in the mouse assay is due to thyroid-stimulating immunoglobulins (TSI) of the IgG class elaborated by lymphocytes of patients with Graves' disease. When human thyroid tissue is used as the assay system, the measured end points are stimulation of colloid droplet or cyclic AMP generation in thyroid cells, slices, or membranes (thyroid-stimulating antibodies, TSAb) and inhibition of the binding of TSH to its receptors in human thyroid tissue (TSH-binding inhibitory immunoglobulins, TBII). These factors represent antibodies against the thyroid TSH receptor (TRAb). Activities of this type are also found in serum of some patients with euthyroid ophthalmic Graves' disease, occasional patients with Hashimoto's disease, and some euthyroid relatives of patients with Graves' disease. Presumably, the absence of thyrotoxicosis in such instances reflects predominance of blocking versus stimulatory TRAbs or intrinsic thyroid disease that prevents a hyperthyroid response. Disappearance of stimulatory factors from the serum during antithyroid treatment augurs well for long-term remission after treatment is withdrawn. Thus, while the basic cause of Graves' disease is not understood, an immunoglobulin or family of immunoglobulins directed against the TSH receptor mediates the thyroid stimulation. A heritable abnormality in immune surveillance may permit particular lymphocytes to survive, proliferate, and secrete the stimulatory immunoglobulins in response to precipitating factors.

The pathogenesis of the ophthalmic component is more enigmatic. One proposed mechanism is the development of antibodies against specific antigens in the extraocular muscles. Nothing is known of the pathogenesis of the dermopathy.

PATHOLOGY   In Graves' disease, the *thyroid gland* is diffusely enlarged, soft, and vascular. The pathology is that of parenchymatous hypertrophy and hyperplasia, characterized by increased height of the epithelium and redundancy of the follicular wall, giving the picture of papillary infoldings and cytologic evidence of increased activity. Such hyperplasia is usually accompanied by lymphocytic infiltration that reflects the immune aspect of the disease and correlates with levels of antithyroid antibodies in the blood. Following iodine medication, there is colloid storage, which sometimes causes enlargement and increased firmness of the gland. Graves' disease is associated with generalized lymphoid hyperplasia and infiltration and occasionally with enlargement of the spleen or thymus. Thyrotoxicosis may lead to degeneration of skeletal muscle fibers, enlargement of the heart, fatty infiltration or diffuse fibrosis of the liver, decalcification of the skeleton, and loss of body tissue (including fat deposits, osteoid, and muscle).

The *ophthalmopathy* is characterized by an inflammatory infiltrate of the orbital contents, exclusive of the globe, with lymphocytes, mast cells, and plasma cells. The orbital musculature is often enlarged due to infiltration with lymphocytes, mucopolysaccharides, and edema, which with fat largely accounts for the increased volume of the orbital contents that causes the globe to protrude. Muscle fibers show degeneration and loss of striations, with ultimate fibrosis.

The *dermopathy* of Graves' disease is characterized by thickening of the dermis, which is infiltrated with lymphocytes and with hydrophilic, metachromatically staining mucopolysaccharides.

CLINICAL MANIFESTATIONS The manifestations comprise those that reflect the associated thyrotoxicosis and those specifically related to Graves' disease. The former vary in intensity with the severity of the thyrotoxicosis, the age of the patient, duration of the illness, and the presence of disease in other organs, such as the heart.

Manifestations of thyrotoxicosis Common manifestations include nervousness, emotional lability, inability to sleep, tremors, frequent bowel movements, excessive sweating, and heat intolerance. Weight loss is usual despite a well-maintained or increased appetite. Proximal muscle weakness is present, with loss of strength often manifested by difficulty in climbing stairs. In premenopausal women, oligomenorrhea and amenorrhea tend to occur. Dyspnea, palpitations, and, in older patients, enhancement of angina pectoris or cardiac failure may occur. In general, nervous symptoms dominate the clinical picture in younger individuals, whereas cardiovascular and myopathic symptoms predominate in older subjects.

Usually, the patient appears anxious, restless, and fidgety. The skin is warm and moist with a velvety texture, and palmar erythema is present. Separation of the fingernail from the nailbed (Plummer's nail) is common, especially on the ring finger. The hair is fine and silky. A fine tremor of the fingers and tongue, together with hyperreflexia, is characteristic. *Ocular signs* include a characteristic stare with widened palpebral fissures, infrequent blinking, lid lag, and failure to wrinkle the brow on upward gaze. These signs result from sympathetic overstimulation and usually subside when the thyrotoxicosis is corrected. They are to be distinguished from the *infiltrative ophthalmopathy* characteristic of Graves' disease, discussed below.

Cardiovascular findings include a wide pulse pressure, sinus tachycardia, atrial arrhythmias (especially atrial fibrillation), systolic murmurs, increased intensity of the apical first sound, cardiac enlargement, and, at times, overt heart failure. A to-and-fro, high-pitched sound may be audible in the pulmonic area and may simulate a pericardial friction rub (Means-Lerman scratch).

Manifestations of Graves' disease The distinctive manifestations of Graves' disease, diffuse hyperfunctioning goiter, ophthalmopathy, and dermopathy, appear in varying combinations and in varying frequency, goiter being the most common. Premature graying of the hair and patchy vitiligo are not specific to Graves' disease and are common in other autoimmune disorders.

The *diffuse toxic goiter* may be asymmetric and lobular. The presence of a bruit over the gland usually signifies that the patient is thyrotoxic, but it may rarely be present in other disorders in which the thyroid is hyperplastic. Venous hums and carotid souffles should be distinguished from true thyroid bruits. An enlarged pyramidal lobe of the thyroid may be palpable.

The clinical signs associated with the *ophthalmopathy* of Graves' disease may be divided into two components: the spastic and the mechanical. The former includes the stare, lid lag, and lid retraction that accompany thyrotoxicosis and account for the "frightened" facies and eye signs previously described. These findings need not be associated with proptosis, may be ameliorated by adrenergic antagonists, and usually return to normal after correction of thyrotoxicosis. The mechanical component includes proptosis of varying degrees with ophthalmoplegia and congestive oculopathy characterized by chemosis, conjunctivitis, periorbital swelling, and the potential complications of corneal ulceration, optic neuritis, and optic atrophy. When exophthalmos progresses rapidly and becomes the major concern in Graves' disease, it is termed *progressive* and, if severe, *malignant exophthalmos*. The term *exophthalmic ophthalmoplegia* refers to the ocular muscle weakness that results in impaired upward gaze and convergence and strabismus with varying degrees of diplopia. Exophthalmos may be unilateral early but usually progresses to bilateral involvement.

The *dermopathy* usually occurs over the dorsum of the legs or feet and is termed *localized* or *pretibial myxedema*. It occurs in patients with past or present Graves' disease and is not a manifestation of hypothyroidism. About half of cases occur during the active stage of thyrotoxicosis. The affected area is usually demarcated from normal skin by the fact that it is raised, thickened, has a *peau d'orange* appearance and may be pruritic and hyperpigmented. The lesions are usually discrete, assuming a plaquelike or nodular configuration but in some instances are confluent. Clubbing of the fingers and toes with characteristic bony changes that differ from those of hypertrophic pulmonary osteoarthropathy may accompany the dermal changes (*thyroid acropachy*).

DIAGNOSIS When severe, Graves' disease presents little difficulty in diagnosis. Florid thyrotoxicosis is manifested by weakness, weight loss despite good appetite, nervous instability, tremor, intolerance to heat, sweating, palpitations, and hyperdefecation. When associated with diffuse thyroid enlargement, often accompanied by a bruit, and particularly when associated with ophthalmopathy, the clinical picture is virtually unique. In such instances, laboratory tests documenting undetectable TSH and increased RAIU, serum T_4 and T_3, RT_3U, and FT_4I serve as baselines for evaluation of therapy rather than necessary diagnostic aids. Occasionally, laboratory tests reveal a normal RAIU, normal serum T_4 and RT_3U, and elevated serum T_3 and FT_3I (T_3 toxicosis).

In less severe cases, particularly when ophthalmopathy is lacking, the diagnosis may be more difficult, since the symptoms of mild thyrotoxicosis are similar to those of other disorders (see "Differential Diagnosis" below). Presence of a goiter makes the diagnosis of hyperthyroidism likely, but careful palpation is necessary to determine whether toxic multinodular goiter, toxic adenoma, or subacute thyroiditis is present, since treatment of these disorders may differ from that of diffuse toxic goiter. Absence of thyroid enlargement makes the diagnosis of Graves' disease less likely but does not exclude it. In mild cases, confirmatory laboratory tests assume great importance. Unfortunately, mild thyrotoxicosis is often associated with marginal abnormalities in laboratory tests or values within the upper limit of the normal range. In such instances, an ultrasensitive TSH assay or the TRH stimulation test assumes crucial importance.

In a few (usually older) patients, the clinical picture may be one of apathy rather than hyperactivity, and evidence of hypermetabolism may be slight (*apathetic thyrotoxicosis*). In such patients, myopathic features may be pronounced. More often, cardiovascular manifestations predominate, since mild hyperthyroidism may produce severe disability in patients with underlying heart disease. Hence *all patients with unexplained cardiac failure or atrial arrhythmias should be examined for thyrotoxicosis*.

DIFFERENTIAL DIAGNOSIS Signs and symptoms of several nonthyroid disorders may simulate certain aspects of the thyrotoxic syndrome. Anxiety is a prominent feature of thyrotoxicosis, and there is thus some overlap in the symptomatology of thyrotoxicosis with that of anxiety states. Tachycardia, tremulousness, irritability, weakness, and fatigue are common to both disorders. In anxiety, however, the peripheral manifestations of excessive thyroid hormones are absent; the skin is usually cold and clammy rather than warm and moist. Weight loss, when present in emotional anxiety, is characteristically accompanied by anorexia, whereas in thyrotoxicosis the appetite is generally increased. Thyrotoxicosis can occasionally be confused with such disorders as metastatic carcinoma, cirrhosis of the liver, hyperparathyroidism, sprue, myasthenia gravis, and muscular dystrophy. Hypokalemic periodic paralysis is more common in thyrotoxic patients, especially in Oriental and Latin American men. Signs and symptoms of thyrotoxicosis may overlap with those of pheochromocytoma, which can cause heat intolerance, sweating, tachycardia with palpitations, and a hypermetabolic state. In the preceding disorders and in other conditions considered in the differential diagnosis, laboratory tests usually make it possible to differentiate them from thyrotoxicosis.

When bilateral ophthalmopathy is accompanied by goiter and thyrotoxicosis, the origin of the ophthalmopathy in Graves' disease is virtually certain. The presence of unilateral ophthalmopathy, even when associated with thyrotoxicosis, raises the possibility of some other intraorbital or intracranial disease. In the euthyroid patient with either unilateral or bilateral ophthalmopathy, other causes that must be excluded are cavernous sinus thrombosis, sphenoidal ridge meningioma, retrobulbar tumors, including leukemic deposits, and the rare granulomatous disorder pseudotumor oculi. Exophthalmos also may be seen in certain systemic disorders, such as uremia, accelerated hypertension, chronic alcoholism, chronic obstructive pulmonary disease, superior mediastinal obstruction, and Cushing's syndrome. Ophthalmoplegia in the absence of infiltrative manifestations can be confused with that which occurs in diabetes mellitus, myasthenia gravis, and myopathies. When doubt exists about the cause of ophthalmopathy, the demonstration of significant titers of TSI or TBII or of an abnormal TRH stimulation or thyroid suppression test suggests that the cause is Graves' disease, though not all patients with "euthyroid Graves' disease" demonstrate abnormal responses. In such cases, ultrasonography, magnetic resonance imaging, or computed tomography of the orbits is valuable in demonstrating characteristic thickening of the extraocular muscles.

When a thyrotoxic state occurs in a patient lacking the characteristic ophthalmopathy of Graves' disease, other causes of thyrotoxicosis must be considered. Careful palpation of the thyroid and studies with radioactive iodine are important in this regard. A symmetric, diffuse goiter of moderate or large size suggests the diagnosis of Graves' disease, especially if a bruit is present. However, the uncommon patient whose hyperthyroidism is secondary to an excess of TSH (associated with a *pituitary tumor* or resistance to feedback suppression of TSH secretion) or an abnormal stimulator of trophoblastic origin (*hydatidiform mole* or *choriocarcinoma of uterus* or *testis;* see Chap. 327) may present in this way. A single, prominent thyroid nodule or multiple nodules suggest *toxic adenoma* or *toxic multinodular goiter*, respectively. Tenderness of the thyroid associated with firm nodularity suggests *subacute thyroiditis*, while a small, firm, nontender goiter is consistent with chronic thyroiditis with spontaneously resolving thyrotoxicosis. The foregoing disorders are discussed in later sections. Absence of a palpable thyroid gland suggests an extrathyroid source of hormone, such as ectopic thyroid tissue *(struma ovarii)* or, more commonly, self-administration of hormone *(thyrotoxicosis factitia)*. Studies with radioactive iodine are also helpful. Except when hormone overproduction is secondary to increased iodine intake, values of the RAIU are increased in all disorders producing hyperthyroidism. Conversely, thyrotoxicosis that is not the result of hyperthyroidism is characterized by subnormal values of the RAIU. Subacute thyroiditis and chronic thyroiditis with spontaneously resolving thyrotoxicosis are the most common. Ectopic thyroid tissue producing thyrotoxicosis is rare. Here, the RAIU, as measured over the thyroid, is low, since TSH secretion is suppressed, but urinary excretion of radioactive iodine is slowed, owing to accumulation by the ectopic tissue.

Functioning ectopic tissue can be located by scintillation scanning. Thyrotoxicosis factitia most frequently occurs in medical or paramedical personnel or in those who have easy access to thyroid hormone. The disorder resembles thyrotoxicosis caused by ectopic thyroid tissue in that the patient's thyroid is suppressed. Consequently, the RAIU is very low, and most of administered radioactive iodine is excreted promptly in the urine. When the disorder is caused by ingestion of preparations containing T_4, such as levothyroxine or thyroid extract, the serum T_4 is increased. On the other hand, when caused by liothyronine, the serum T_4 is subnormal. Irrespective of the preparation, the serum T_3 is increased, but more so when liothyronine is the offending agent. Measurement of serum thyroglobulin is useful to confirm thyrotoxicosis factitia. Levels are elevated in Graves' disease and thyroiditis but are subnormal with exogenous thyroid hormone suppression. The demonstration of elevated titers of TRAbs in the blood also provides strong evidence that Graves' disease is the cause of thyrotoxicosis.

TREATMENT Hyperthyroidism Hyperthyroidism is often characterized by cyclic phases of exacerbation and remission, each of unpredictable onset and duration. Moreover, long-standing disease may be associated with progressive thyroid failure, probably consequent to chronic thyroiditis, with the supervention of hypothyroidism or decreased thyroid reserve. These characteristics have important implications in the choice of and response to therapy.

The major treatments are directed to limiting the quantity of thyroid hormones the gland can produce. Antithyroid agents interpose a chemical blockade to hormone synthesis, the effect of which is operative only as long as the drug is administered. Thus the agents can control active thyrotoxicity but probably do not prevent exacerbation at some subsequent period. The second major approach is ablation of thyroid tissue, thereby limiting hormone production. This may be achieved either by surgery or by radioactive iodine. Since these procedures induce permanent anatomic alterations of the thyroid, they can control the active phase and are more likely to prevent later exacerbation or recurrence. On the other hand, surgery or radiation is more likely to lead to hypothyroidism, either shortly after treatment or with the passage of years.

Each therapy has advantages and disadvantages, indications and contraindications. The latter are more often relative than absolute. In general, a trial of long-term antithyroid therapy is desirable in children, adolescents, young adults, and pregnant women but also may be employed in older patients. Indications for ablative procedures include relapse or recurrence following drug therapy, a large goiter, drug toxicity, failure to follow a medical regimen, or failure to return for periodic examinations. Subtotal thyroidectomy may be elected for patients under the age of 30 in whom ablative therapy is required; however, opinions differ, and some authorities employ radioactive iodine in the treatment of patients in the second or third decades. Surgery is also preferable in patients with very large goiters or with a coincident nonfunctioning nodule, especially if there is a history of radiation to the head and neck. Radioactive iodine is the ablative procedure of choice in older patients, in patients who have had previous thyroid surgery, and in those in whom systemic disease contraindicates elective surgery.

In patients selected for *long-term antithyroid therapy*, satisfactory control can almost always be achieved if sufficient drug is administered. Most patients can be managed with propylthiouracil, 100 to 150 mg every 6 or 8 h. Larger doses may be required for initial control. Methimazole is at least as effective as propylthiouracil when administered in one-tenth the dosage. However, propylthiouracil has the advantage of inhibiting the peripheral conversion of T_4 to T_3, thereby bringing about more rapid symptomatic improvement. Once euthyroidism is achieved, the daily dosage may be reduced to the smallest amount that controls the thyrotoxicosis. In some clinics the initial dose is continued and is supplemented with levothyroxine. By this latter regimen, hypothyroidism from overdosage of antithyroid drugs can be prevented. The undesirable consequences of hypothyroidism, such as enhancement of ophthalmopathy and enlargement of the goiter, may thereby be forestalled. In one study, combined therapy was associated with lower titers of TRAbs and a reduced risk of recurrence at the termination of therapy. The duration of antithyroid drug therapy is difficult to predict in the individual patient and may be a function of the natural course of the disease. The longer the course of therapy, the more likely it is that the patient will remain well when the drug is discontinued. In general a 12- to 24-month course is employed, following which one-third to one-half of patients remain well for a prolonged period or indefinitely. The likelihood of a prolonged remission is increased by a decrease in goiter size, reversion of the thyroid suppression test and TRH stimulation test to normal, or disappearance of TRAbs from the serum during treatment.

Leukopenia is the principal undesirable side effect of antithyroid drugs. A complete blood count should be obtained prior to initiating therapy to identify those patients with leukopenia related to Graves' disease. Mild transient leukopenia may occur with antithyroid drugs in approximately an additional 10 percent of patients and is not necessarily an indication for discontinuing therapy. When the absolute number of polymorphonuclear leukocytes reaches 1500 per cubic millimeter or less, antithyroid medication should be discontinued. Allergic rashes and drug sensitivity occur on occasion. These may disappear with antihistamine therapy at the same or reduced dosage of antithyroid agent, but it is probably preferable when sensitivity reactions occur to change to another drug. On rare occasions (in less than 0.2 percent), agranulocytosis occurs. This may be sudden in onset. Hepatitis, drug fever, and arthralgias occur on occasion. In the author's view, severe sensitivity reactions, including agranulocytosis, dictate the abandonment of antithyroid therapy rather than recourse to an alternate drug.

Iodide inhibits the release of hormones from the hyperfunctioning thyroid gland, and its ameliorative effects occur more rapidly than those of agents that inhibit hormone synthesis. Hence its main use is in patients with actual or impending thyrotoxic crisis and in patients with severe cardiac disease. The response to iodide alone is often incomplete and transient. Furthermore, by expanding the thyroid store of hormone, iodide may prolong the latency of response to antithyroid therapy. Therefore, iodide is safely used only in conjunction with the antithyroid agents. If the clinical course is sufficiently severe to require iodide administration, antithyroid drugs are usually the primary therapeutic agents and should be given in large doses prior to iodide. Iodide is also useful in controlling thyrotoxicosis following ^{131}I administration, during the period in which the therapeutic effect of radioiodine has not yet taken place. Large doses of *glucocorticoids* (2 mg dexamethasone every 6 h) reduce the serum T_4 concentration when relief of thyrotoxicosis is urgent. The iodinated x-ray contrast agent sodium ipodate has a similar effect. Iodine liberated from this agent inhibits thyroid secretion of T_4 and T_3, and serum T_3 is further reduced by the inhibition by ipodate of peripheral T_3 formation. Daily doses of 1 g orally are effective, but the same precautions concerning the use of iodine therapy are applicable to ipodate.

Owing to the adrenergic component in thyrotoxicosis, various *adrenergic antagonists* have been employed in its management. Of these, propranolol is the agent of choice because of its relative freedom from side effects. In doses of 40 to 120 mg/d, propranolol alleviates such adrenergic manifestations as sweating, tremor, and tachycardia and may reduce to some extent the conversion of T_4 to T_3. However, propranolol should be used only as adjunctive therapy, since the underlying metabolic abnormalities are not affected. Moreover, although the diminution in heart rate and cardiac work may be beneficial, the blocking of adrenergic support of myocardial contractility requires caution in its use in the patient with coexisting heart failure, unless rate- or rhythm-related. As adjunctive therapy, propranolol is useful during the period when the response to conventional antithyroid agents or to radioiodine therapy is being awaited and in the management of thyrotoxic crisis. It has been employed as the sole agent in preparation for thyroidectomy, but its use in this setting is not recommended, since it does not render the patient euthyroid, with a likely greater risk of surgically induced crisis.

Radioactive iodine (*[131]I*) affords a relatively simple, effective, and economical means of treating thyrotoxicosis. It can produce the ablative effects of surgery without the operative and postoperative complications. The principal disadvantage of ^{131}I therapy, in the dosage usually employed, is its tendency to produce hypothyroidism with a frequency that increases with time. As many as 40 to 70 percent of patients may develop this complication within 10 years after treatment. Although hypothyroidism is treatable, once diagnosed, the insidious onset may obscure the diagnosis until serious complications develop. Hence some recommend that all patients be treated with large doses of ^{131}I to ensure relief of thyrotoxicosis and then placed on permanent physiologic replacement doses of thyroid hormone.

There is no evidence of carcinogenic or leukemogenic effects of radioiodine when given to adults in the doses commonly used in treating hyperthyroidism. However, the susceptibility to carcinogenesis may be increased in the thyroids of children. Mutagenic effects have not been reported and would be difficult to document. For these reasons, many physicians prefer to reserve radioiodine therapy for patients over 30 years of age or those unlikely to have children subsequently. Moreover, the longer the life expectancy after ^{131}I therapy, the greater is the likelihood that hypothyroidism will develop. Among younger patients, therefore, only those with recurrent thyrotoxicosis following surgery, those who refuse surgery, and those with complicating illness that contraindicates surgery are candidates for radioiodine therapy. In elderly patients, treatment with large doses of radioiodine is the general method of choice so that the undesirable effects of incomplete treatment or recurrence can be avoided. In patients with significant ophthalmopathy, it may be prudent to administer glucocorticoids for approximately 2 weeks before and 6 weeks after the ^{131}I dose to reduce the likelihood of exacerbation of eye disease.

The usual therapeutic dose of [131]I [approximately 5.9 MBq (160 μCi) per gram of estimated gland weight] leads to a high frequency of hypothyroidism. As a result, some authorities continuing to use this dose regularly administer prophylactic replacement doses of thyroid hormone. Others have administered smaller doses [approximately 3.0 MBq/g (80 μCi/g)]. However, this does not diminish the frequency of late hypothyroidism but merely delays its onset. Moreover, the smaller dose is less likely to relieve thyrotoxicosis within a relatively short period. Antithyroid agents can be employed, however, to speed the attainment of a eumetabolic state, and propranolol can be given to relieve symptoms while the effect of the ^{131}I is taking hold. There is general agreement that patients with coexisting cardiac disease should receive ^{131}I in large doses in view of the hazard of recurrent thyrotoxicosis.

Radiation thyroiditis is an occasional immediate complication of ^{131}I therapy. It commonly appears within 7 to 10 days and is associated with accelerated release of hormone into the blood. Rarely, radiation thyroiditis may cause thyrotoxic crisis (see below), most commonly in the elderly thyrotoxic patient with other systemic illness. For these reasons, patients with severe hyperthyroidism or underlying heart disease should be rendered eumetabolic with antithyroid agents before ^{131}I is administered. Interruption of antithyroid therapy for 3 to 4 days before and after ^{131}I treatment suffices to permit adequate accumulation and retention of administered [131]I. Propranolol may be used as an adjunct both before and after ^{131}I administration but should not be relied on to provide adequate prophylaxis if given alone. The swelling that accompanies radiation thyroiditis may contraindicate the use of large doses of ^{131}I in patients with large retrosternal goiters.

Before radioactive iodine was introduced, *subtotal thyroidectomy* was the standard form of ablative therapy, and it is still employed in younger patients in whom antithyroid therapy is unsuccessful. Although precise preoperative programs differ, several general principles should be emphasized. Patients should first be rendered euthyroid by means of antithyroid agents. Only then should iodide (five drops of Lugol's solution a day for approximately 10 days) be administered concomitantly to effect an involutional response in the gland. Antithyroid drugs should not be discontinued merely because treatment with iodide is instituted. The response of the patient, and not the calendar, should dictate when surgery is performed.

Hazards of subtotal thyroidectomy include immediate complications, such as anesthetic accidents, hemorrhage sometimes leading to respiratory obstruction, and damage to the recurrent laryngeal nerve leading to vocal cord paralysis. Later complications include wound infection, hemorrhage, hypoparathyroidism, and hypothyroidism. Subtotal thyroidectomy should be performed by a surgeon experienced in this procedure; under this condition, surgery is effective and relatively safe. Postoperative recurrences are uncommon. However, carefully conducted follow-up studies reveal that hypothyroidism follows surgery more frequently than previously suspected, although not as commonly as with conventional doses of ^{131}I.

The *treatment of hyperthyroidism during pregnancy* is a subject of some disagreement. Most physicians believe that antithyroid therapy is preferable to surgery, which should not be performed in any event during the first and third trimesters. Antithyroid agents carry less risk to the patient and the pregnancy. Further, since they traverse the placental barrier, they have the theoretical advantage of preventing fetal and neonatal hyperthyroidism when maternal titers of TRAbs are high. As a clue to the risk of fetal hyperthyroidism, assays of such stimulators should be conducted in pregnant women with a history of Graves' disease, whether treated or not. On the other hand, the major disadvantage of antithyroid therapy is the possibility of inducing hypothyroidism in the fetus. T_4 and T_3 traverse the human placenta from mother to fetus only slowly, and simultaneous administration of thyroid hormone and antithyroid drugs to the mother will not protect the fetus from hypothyroidism. Hence the cardinal rule in using the antithyroid agents in pregnancy is that the dosage should be the smallest necessary to control hyperthyroidism in the mother. From the laboratory standpoint, the physician should aim to keep the serum TSH and the FT_4 concentration within the normal limits, remembering that pregnancy is normally associated with some elevation of the serum total T_4 owing to an increase in serum TBG concentration. Since pregnancy appears to attenuate the severity of hyperthyroidism, control can often be achieved with maintenance doses of 200 mg propylthiouracil daily or less. At this dose, fetal goiter or hypothyroidism has not been a problem. Patients who require doses of 300 mg/d or more during the first trimester should probably be treated by subtotal thyroidectomy during the middle trimester. The author believes that patients carried through pregnancy on antithyroid agents should not be given propranolol as adjunctive treatment, in view of reports that the agent may cause fetal growth retardation and neonatal respiratory depression. Propylthiouracil tends to be favored over methimazole, even though earlier reports of fetal anomalies with the latter agent have not been confirmed. Advantages of propylthiouracil include its effect on inhibiting conversion of T_4 to T_3 and its higher degree of protein binding, which retards its excretion into breast milk. Radioiodine should never be administered to a pregnant woman, and all women of childbearing age who are about to receive ^{131}I should have a pregnancy test performed first.

Ophthalmopathy, dermopathy When severe and progressive, ophthalmopathy is the most difficult component of Graves' disease to treat satisfactorily. Fortunately, in most patients the disorder runs a benign course that is largely independent of the hyperthyroidism. In most instances, the activity of even moderately severe disease declines and disappears with time, although some exophthalmos and ophthalmoplegia may persist. In mild disease, considerable benefit may be obtained from simple measures, such as elevating the head at night, administering diuretics to reduce edema, and providing tinted glasses for protection from sun, wind, and foreign bodies. A 1% solution of methylcellulose or plastic shields may prevent corneal drying in patients unable to oppose the lids during sleep. In more severe cases, as evidenced by progressive exophthalmos, chemosis, ophthalmoplegia, or loss of vision, large doses of prednisone (100 to 120 mg/d) should be administered, since this is usually effective in reducing the edematous and infiltrative components. With improve-

ment, the dosage is reduced to the lowest effective level to minimize the effects of glucocorticoid excess. Orbital radiation may be helpful in some patients with acute, severe infiltrative manifestations, particularly when administered concomitantly with glucocorticoids. In cases that progress despite these measures, orbital decompression, i.e., removal of part of the bony orbit, is required to relieve intraorbital pressure. The management must always be conducted in concert with an ophthalmologist.

In general, treatment of associated hyperthyroidism should be carried out as if ophthalmopathy were not present, since the mode of treatment of the hyperthyroidism does not influence the course of the ocular disease. Whether ^{131}I therapy may aggravate ophthalmopathy remains controversial. It is agreed, however, that hypothyroidism should be avoided.

Severe dermopathy can be alleviated by the topical application of glucocorticoids.

TOXIC MULTINODULAR GOITER

Toxic multinodular goiter is an occasional consequence of long-standing simple goiter, although the proportion of cases in which this complication arises is uncertain. In areas of nonendemicity, the cause of nontoxic multinodular goiter is usually indeterminate. Hence it is unclear whether a specific factor underlies those cases of nontoxic multinodular goiter that progress to thyrotoxic phase. Common to many nontoxic multinodular goiters, even in areas of iodine sufficiency, the iodine content of thyroglobulin is decreased, suggesting either a conditioned deficiency of iodine or an impairment of its normal incorporation into the protein. There is no pathologic feature to distinguish the nontoxic from the toxic multinodular goiter. However, the transition from nontoxic to toxic nodular goiter involves the development of functional autonomy, i.e., independence from TSH stimulation in one or more areas of the gland. Scattered foci of functional autonomy are demonstrable early in the disease process and increase in size and number as time passes so that approximately a fourth of seemingly euthyroid patients with nontoxic nodular goiter display, as evidence of functional autonomy, subnormal or absent responses to TRH administration. As judged from scintillation scanning, functional patterns may be of two types. In the more common, iodine accumulation occurs diffusely in patchy foci throughout the gland. The less common pattern is that of iodine accumulation in one or more discrete nodules within the gland, the remainder appearing to be essentially nonfunctional. Histologic and autoradiographic studies reveal marked heterogeneity of structure and function, the two being poorly correlated. In both endemic and sporadic nontoxic multinodular goiter, administration of iodides may lead to the development of thyrotoxicosis (jodbasedow), a complication consonant with the functional autonomy of this disorder.

Because it arises in long-standing simple goiter, toxic multinodular goiter is a disease of the aging or elderly. For this reason, and because of the nature of the underlying disease, the clinical presentation differs from that in Graves' disease. Ophthalmopathy is rare and would signal the emergence of Graves' disease superimposed on simple goiter. Some patients have typical thyrotoxicosis. Often, however, the degree of thyrotoxicosis is less severe than that in Graves' disease, although its physiologic impact on specific organ systems may be great. Notable among these is the cardiovascular system, in which arrhythmias or congestive failure may be precipitated or accentuated by thyrotoxicosis that may be manifested only by subtle findings in other areas (apathetic hyperthyroidism). Weakness and wasting may predominate, frequently with loss of appetite rather than hyperphagia, suggesting the presence of a carcinoma.

In some patients, a definitive diagnosis of toxic nodular goiter is difficult to establish. On the one hand, enlargement or nodularity of the gland may escape detection because the patient has a short neck or is kyphotic or because the thyroid is substernal. When this is the case, and when the clinical findings suggest thyrotoxicosis, RAIU and scintiscan are particularly helpful. On the other hand, even when a nodular goiter is palpable, the presence of mild but clinically significant thyrotoxicosis may be difficult to confirm, since values of the serum total T_4 and T_3, FT_4, and FT_4I are often only near or slightly above normal. For example, a value for the serum T_3 that would be normal for a young adult may represent an increase in the elderly patient, since serum T_3 usually declines with age. Despite their value in situations such as this, thyroid suppression tests should rarely be undertaken in the elderly patient because of the hazard of adverse cardiovascular responses. Unfortunately, although a normal response to TRH would exclude a diagnosis of thyrotoxicosis in a patient with a nodular goiter, subnormal responses do not establish the diagnosis. Responses to TRH decline in the elderly, especially in men, and seemingly euthyroid patients with nodular goiter may respond subnormally to TRH as a reflection of at least partial functional autonomy of the thyroid gland. An undetectable basal TSH and absent response to TRH by an ultrasensitive assay imply thyrotoxicosis (see Fig. 334-3). When laboratory findings do not permit a clear diagnosis of thyrotoxicosis but suggestive clinical findings are present, a therapeutic trial of antithyroid drugs may be indicated.

Radioactive iodine is the treatment of choice for toxic multinodular goiter. In contrast to Graves' disease, large doses [740 to 1110 MBq (20 to 30 mCi)] are usually required owing to the generally lower RAIU and to the variable degree of function throughout the gland. Moreover, the physiologic instability of the elderly patient makes definitive treatment urgent. For the same reason, it is usually wise to initiate therapy with antithyroid agents, withholding radioiodine until a euthyroid state is achieved, thereby forestalling an exacerbation of thyrotoxicosis should radiation thyroiditis occur. Unless contraindicated, propranolol is often useful in controlling manifestations of thyrotoxicosis both before and after radioiodine therapy, while its therapeutic effect is awaited. Hypothyroidism is an uncommon consequence of radioiodine treatment of toxic multinodular goiter owing to the variable activity of differing portions of the gland, which permits previously quiescent areas to function in place of those destroyed by ^{131}I.

UNUSUAL VARIETIES OF THYROTOXICOSIS

Thyrotoxicosis is also seen in other disorders, including follicular adenoma of the thyroid and various forms of thyroiditis, which are discussed in later sections. This section will consider still other unusual causes of thyrotoxicosis and unusual ways in which thyrotoxicosis may present.

UNUSUAL CAUSES OF THYROTOXICOSIS Rarely, hyperthyroidism and thyrotoxicosis are the result of sustained hypersecretion of TSH from either a *TSH-secreting pituitary adenoma* or a selective *resistance of the TSH-secretory mechanism* to feedback inhibition by thyroid hormones. The resistance syndromes in which both the pituitary and peripheral tissues are relatively resistant to thyroid hormones are discussed above. TSH-secreting pituitary adenomas can be distinguished, in many cases, by radiologic evidence of pituitary tumor, by the fact that the concentration of free α subunits of TSH in serum is elevated, and by the fact that the response of the serum TSH to TRH is negligible. In the variant caused by pituitary resistance, subunit concentrations are not grossly elevated, and the TSH response to TRH is usually normal.

Patients with *trophoblastic tumor*, either choriocarcinoma or hydatidiform mole, frequently display elevations, sometimes marked, of serum total and free T_4 and T_3 concentrations. In addition to signs of pregnancy, the usual manifestations of thyrotoxicosis may be present, but ophthalmopathy is absent. Thyroid hyperfunction is caused by a circulating thyroid stimulator of trophoblastic origin, which is human chorionic gonadotropin (hCG), and the diagnosis may be confirmed by the finding of extremely high blood or urine levels of βhCG. Abnormal thyroid function tests remit promptly after removal of the tumor.

Thyrotoxicosis factitia is a form of thyrotoxicosis without hyperthyroidism that results from purposeful or inadvertent ingestion of large amounts of thyroid hormone. The syndrome is usually a form of malingering and occurs most commonly in women with an underlying psychiatric disorder, usually paramedical personnel, or in patients who have taken thyroid hormones in the past or who have relatives who take thyroid hormones. In such patients, endogenous thyroid function is suppressed, as evidenced by subnormal values of the RAIU and serum thyroglobulin concentration. Serum TSH is suppressed, and both serum T_4 and T_3 concentrations are increased if the patient is taking a preparation that contains T_4, whereas the serum T_3 concentration is elevated and the serum T_4 depressed in patients taking T_3 alone. Factitious hyperthyroidism also has been described in people who ingest large quantities of ground meats contaminated with thyroid tissue.

Very rarely, thyrotoxicosis with a low RAIU is the result of excess hormone secretion by *ectopic thyroid tissue*, either widespread functioning metastases of thyroid carcinoma or struma ovarii.

The *jodbasedow phenomenon* refers to the induction of thyrotoxicosis in a previously euthyroid patient as a result of exposure to iodine. It typically occurs in areas of endemic iodine deficiency when measures to increase iodine intake or body iodine stores are implemented. The presumption is that the supplemental iodine permits functionally autonomous thyroid tissue to produce and secrete excessive hormone. A similar phenomenon can occur in patients with nontoxic multinodular goiter who receive large doses of iodide. Since such patients tend to be elderly with the danger of serious cardiovascular manifestations should thyrotoxicosis ensue, large doses of iodine should not be given to those with multinodular goiter. Similarly, in such patients, pharmaceuticals containing iodine, such as x-ray contrast media, should be used only when indicated and with consideration of the possible hazard of the jodbasedow phenomenon. When a contrast study is indicated under these conditions, it may be judicious to administer large doses of propylthiouracil (450 to 600 mg/d) prior to and for a week after the procedure. Some patients may develop hyperthyroidism following exposure to large quantities of iodine despite the fact that after iodine is withdrawn, they recover, thyroid function appears to be entirely normal, and evidence of functional autonomy is lacking.

UNUSUAL PRESENTATIONS OF THYROTOXICOSIS **T_3 toxicosis** Thyrotoxicosis in which serum T_4 is normal or low in the absence of a deficiency of TBG, while the serum T_3 is increased, is termed *T_3 toxicosis*. Although the production rate of T_3 is disproportionately increased relative to that of T_4 in hyperthyroidism, in some this discrepancy is exaggerated. This may occur in association with Graves' disease, multinodular goiter, or hyperfunctioning adenoma. The diagnosis should be suspected in a patient with clinical manifestations of thyrotoxicosis in whom the serum T_4 and FT_4 are normal or low and the RAIU is normal or increased. These features, together with the frequently palpable goiter, serve to differentiate this disorder from liothyronine-induced thyrotoxicosis factitia. In contrast to nonthyroidal disorders that mimic thyrotoxicosis, patients with this disorder demonstrate nonsuppressibility of thyroid function in response to exogenous T_3, undetectable serum TSH, and absent responses to TRH. In many patients, thyrotoxicosis with increased serum T_3 and normal serum T_4 precedes emergence of typical increases in both, either during an initial episode of hyperthyroidism or more commonly during recurrence after previous treatment. In some patients in whom symptoms of thyrotoxicosis fail to regress completely during antithyroid therapy despite return of the serum T_4 concentration to normal, the serum T_3 concentration is persistently elevated. Such patients are likely to experience a recurrence of thyrotoxicosis when antithyroid therapy is withdrawn.

T_4 toxicosis In most patients with hyperthyroidism, the serum T_3 is increased to a relatively greater extent than is the serum T_4. This reflects the fact that in hyperthyroidism, T_3 generated from T_4 peripherally is supplemented by release of substantial quantities of T_3 from the thyroid. However, thyrotoxicosis may sometimes be associated with a clear elevation of serum T_4 and a seemingly normal serum T_3 concentration. This syndrome of T_3 *toxicosis* occurs most commonly in the setting of prior excess iodine exposure in patients who are elderly, ill, or both and is, therefore, usually seen in a hospital setting. Increased iodine intake favors T_4 biosynthesis. In the absence of a history of excess iodine, the combination of high serum T_4 and normal serum T_3 concentration presumably reflects inhibition of peripheral T_3 generation from T_4, with persistence of T_3 secretion along with T_4 from the thyroid.

MAJOR COMPLICATIONS OF THYROTOXICOSIS

CARDIAC DISEASE   Thyrotoxicosis causes increases in both systolic and diastolic cardiac function, probably secondary to effects on the expression of genes for the contractile protein, myosin. Untreated, the increased work eventually progresses to decompensation. As a consequence of this and peripheral effects of thyroid hormone, a variety of burdens are imposed on the heart. Hypermetabolism of the peripheral tissues increases both the metabolic and nonmetabolic (heat-loss) circulatory load, while direct effects of thyroid hormone on the myocardium cause rapid filling and increase the force, velocity, and rate of ventricular contraction. As a result, cardiac work and cardiac output are increased. Moreover, atrial irritability is enhanced, leading to arrhythmias, most importantly atrial fibrillation. In the patient with a normal heart, these burdens are usually tolerated. In the patient with underlying heart disease, however, cardiac insufficiency may be precipitated or aggravated. As would be expected, this complication is more common in the elderly patient and the patient with toxic multinodular goiter, sometimes as the most prominent manifestation of the thyrotoxic state. In patients with cardiac insufficiency, clues to the presence of thyrotoxicosis include atrial fibrillation, relatively rapid circulation time, increased cardiac output (high-output failure), and resistance to the usual therapeutic doses of digitalis.

Treatment is directed at rapid alleviation of thyrotoxicosis and restoration of cardiac compensation. The former objective is best met by treatment with large doses of an antithyroid agent, followed by iodine if the clinical situation is urgent. In less severe cases, radioiodine treatment is preceded by antithyroid drug treatment alone. The cardiac decompensation is managed in the usual manner, employing larger than usual doses of digitalis but with care to avoid digitalis intoxication as thyrotoxicosis is alleviated. Adrenergic antagonists should be used with caution in the presence of cardiac failure, unless failure is the consequence primarily of disturbance of cardiac rate or rhythm.

THYROTOXIC CRISIS   Thyrotoxic crisis or storm causes a fulminating increase in the signs and symptoms of thyrotoxicosis. In the past, this disturbance usually occurred postoperatively in patients poorly prepared for surgery. However, with the preoperative use of antithyroid drugs and iodide and with appropriate therapy to control metabolic factors, weight, and nutritional status, postoperative thyrotoxic crisis should not occur. At present, so-called medical storm is more common and occurs in untreated or inadequately treated patients. It is precipitated by surgical emergency or complicating illness, usually sepsis. The syndrome is characterized by extreme irritability, delirium or coma, fever to 41°C or more, tachycardia, restlessness, hypotension, vomiting, and diarrhea. Rarely, the picture may be more subtle, with apathy, prostration, and coma, but with only slight elevation of temperature. Such postoperative complications as sepsis, septicemia, hemorrhage, and transfusion or drug reactions may mimic thyrotoxic crisis. The physiologic factor(s) that initiates thyrotoxic crisis is unknown. It does not appear to be an acute increase in the severity of thyroid hyperfunction. Rather, it may represent a shift from protein-bound to free hormone secondary to circulating inhibitors to binding in systemic illness.

Treatment consists of providing supportive therapy while undertaking measures to alleviate thyrotoxicosis as rapidly as possible.

Supportive therapy includes treatment of dehydration and the intravenous administration of glucose and saline, vitamin B complex, and glucocorticoids. The latter are indicated because of the increased glucocorticoid requirements in thyrotoxicosis and because adrenal reserve may be reduced. Patients should be placed in a cooled, humidified oxygen tent, and if hyperpyrexia is present, a cooling blanket should be used. Digitalization is required to control ventricular rate in those with atrial fibrillation. If shock exists, intravenous pressor agents should be employed. Therapy of the hyperthyroidism consists of blockade of hormone synthesis by the immediate and continued administration of large doses of an antithyroid agent (e.g., 100 mg propylthiouracil every 2 h). If the patient is unable to swallow the medication, the tablets should be triturated and given by nasogastric tube or per rectum, since parenteral preparations are unavailable. Following initiation of antithyroid therapy, hormone release is inhibited through the administration of large doses of iodine intravenously or by mouth. The iodinated x-ray contrast agent sodium ipodate can be administered instead of iodine and has the added action of inhibiting the peripheral conversion of T_4 to T_3. Doses of 1 g/d are effective. Adrenergic antagonists are an important, and perhaps critical, part of the therapeutic regimen in the absence of cardiac failure. Propranolol can be administered in doses of 40 to 80 mg every 6 h. If medications cannot be taken orally, 2 mg propranolol may be given intravenously, with careful electrocardiographic monitoring. Large doses of dexamethasone (e.g., 2 mg every 6 h) also should be administered, since they inhibit hormone release, impair the peripheral generation of T_3 from T_4, and provide adrenal support. Indeed, with the combined use of propylthiouracil, iodine, and dexamethasone, the serum T_3 concentration generally returns to normal within 24 to 48 h. Dexamethasone may be tapered thereafter, while antithyroid therapy and iodine must be continued until a normal metabolic state is approached, at which time iodine is progressively withdrawn and plans are made for definitive treatment.

NEOPLASMS

The prevalence of solitary nodules of the thyroid gland increases with age, averaging 6.4 percent of women and 1.5 percent of men. Many palpable thyroid nodules thought to be solitary are actually part of a multinodular thyroid gland. High-resolution ultrasound identifies nodules in a third of patients being evaluated for nonthyroid indications, and autopsy studies reveal thyroid nodules in as many as 50 percent of necropsies. In general, a nodule must reach a size of 1 cm in diameter to be detectable by palpation. In addition to thyroid neoplasms, the differential diagnosis of apparent thyroid nodules includes cysts, adenopathy, cystic hygroma, parathyroid tumors, and laryngocele. True intrathyroidal nodules usually represent colloid adenomas or simple follicular adenomas.

THYROID ADENOMAS   True adenomas, as contrasted with localized adenomatous areas, are encapsulated and compress contiguous tissue. Adenomas vary in size and are classified into three histologic types: papillary, follicular, and Hürthle cell. The follicular adenomas can be subdivided according to the size of the follicles into colloid or macrofollicular, fetal or microfollicular, and embryonal varieties. There is variation in physiologic differentiation, as judged by the ability to concentrate radioiodine. The more highly differentiated adenomas (follicular) are the most common and are the most likely to mimic the function of normal thyroid tissue. Though the function may be responsive to TSH stimulation, it usually differs from that of normal thyroid tissue in being autonomous; i.e., the basal activity is independent of TSH stimulation. Adenomas of this type are usually unifocal, presenting as a single nodule. Often the patient reports that the nodule has grown slowly over many years. Initially, its function is insufficient to disturb hormonal equilibrium, though its capacity to accumulate radioiodine is evident in scintiscans as an area of increased density within the still-functioning extranodular tissue (*"warm" nodule*). At this stage, demonstration of the inherent autonomy requires scintiscanning while the patient is receiving suppressive doses of exogenous thyroid hormone (suppression scan). With time, the nodule grows larger, its function increasing until it is sufficient to suppress TSH secretion. Consequently, the remainder of the gland undergoes relative atrophy and loss of function, and the scintiscan reveals radioiodine accumulation only in the region of the nodule (*"hot"* nodule). At this time, TSH is suppressed ("chemical" thyrotoxicosis), but the patient may or may not be overtly thyrotoxic. Frank thyrotoxicosis usually supervenes eventually (*toxic adenoma*) and may be precipitated by iodine exposure such as from radiographic contrast dyes. Relative to its overall rate of occurrence, hyperfunctioning adenoma is a frequent cause of T_3 toxicosis. Hyperfunctioning adenomas are amenable to ablation by surgery or ^{131}I. Large doses of the latter are usually required to bring about prompt cure. Although it has been thought that radiation damage would be confined solely to the hyperfunctioning nodule being treated with ^{131}I, the remaining tissue being spared, this may not always be the case, since some patients with hyperfunctioning adenoma become euthyroid after treatment with ^{131}I only to become hypothyroid years later.

Hyperfunctioning nodules are rarely the seat of carcinoma. However, hyperfunctioning adenomas may undergo hemorrhagic necrosis. The resulting pain and nodularity may suggest subacute thyroiditis. Subsequently, there is loss of function and the appearance of a *"cold"* nodule on scintiscanning, since the remainder of the thyroid will have resumed function. When this happens, the nodule is likely to be mistaken for a carcinoma. Indeed, hypofunctioning, hemorrhagic adenomas and thyroid cysts account for the majority of cold nodules initially suspected of being carcinomas.

MALIGNANT TUMORS OF THE THYROID Due to its rich vascular supply, the thyroid is a common site of secondary or metastatic cancers from primary tumors elsewhere. Some common sources include malignant melanoma and carcinoma of the lung, breast, and esophagus. The thyroid also may be the site of lymphoproliferative disease, namely *thyroid lymphoma*, which constitutes about 5 percent of all thyroid malignancies. Of the latter, large cell histocytic (or immunoblastic) lymphoma is the most common and typically occurs in women between the ages of 55 and 75 who often have chronic lymphocytic thyroiditis with positive serum antithyroglobulin or anti-TPO antibodies. Indeed, the risk of this tumor is so much higher in elderly patients with Hashimoto's thyroiditis that an enlarging thyroid mass should be considered as thyroid lymphoma until an expedient evaluation rules out the diagnosis. Prognosis depends on cell type and the extent of disease beyond the neck. Variable success rates have followed therapy with combinations of surgery, radiation, and chemotherapy.

Primary thyroid carcinomas may be classified into two varieties depending on whether the lesion arises in thyroid follicular epithelium or from the parafollicular or C cells. The latter disorder, *medullary thyroid carcinoma* (MTC), may occur in four presentations: 80 percent are sporadic and 20 percent are familial, occurring as part of multiple endocrine neoplasia (MEN) types 2A or 2B or in a familial non-MEN setting. In familial forms, the diagnosis of early disease may be made in family members by screening measurements of serum calcitonin. The MEN syndromes are discussed separately below (see Chap. 343). The peak incidence of the sporadic form is in the sixth and seventh decades of life, and patients usually have cervical lymph node metastases at presentation. The tendency of the tumor and involved lymph nodes to calcify may be a clue to the diagnosis when calcification is noted on x-rays of the neck. Serum calcitonin serves as a tumor marker for residual disease after treatment, and the serum levels correlate with tumor burden. The mainstay of therapy is surgical excision; external radiation and chemotherapy have a palliative role for recurrent or residual disease.

Carcinomas of follicular epithelium Of the three general histologic types, *papillary* and *follicular carcinomas* tend to be slow growing and account for 70 and 15 percent, respectively, of all thyroid cancers, while *anaplastic carcinoma* is the least common, comprising approximately 5 percent of thyroid cancers. *Anaplastic*

carcinoma usually occurs in the sixth to seventh decade of life. The tumor is histologically undifferentiated, largely composed of spindle and giant cells, rapidly growing, and highly malignant. Despite radical surgery, the prognosis is dismal, with survival in months rather than years but best in younger patients with early disease. The lesion is rapidly fatal owing to extensive local invasion which is refractory to external radiation and to radioiodine therapy because the tumor does not concentrate iodine. That many patients may have coexistent differentiated carcinoma suggests that anaplastic tumors arise from the former, and metastases of papillary or follicular carcinoma can undergo late malignant dedifferentiation. Anaplastic thyroid carcinoma may be confused with lymphoma and sarcoma, and positive immunocytochemical stains for keratin or the cytoskeletal protein vimentin help to confirm the diagnosis. While thyroglobulin staining may be positive due to entrapped follicular cells or colloid, measurements of serum thyroglobulin are of no diagnostic value as a tumor marker for this tumor in contrast to the situation in well-differentiated thyroid cancer. The lack of calcitonin immunoreactivity will differentiate anaplastic carcinoma from undifferentiated medullary thyroid carcinoma.

Follicular carcinoma tends to occur in older individuals, histologically resembles normal thyroid epithelium, is encapsulated, and differs from benign follicular adenoma only by the presence of capsular and/or vascular invasion. These tumors may be classified as minimally, moderately, or highly invasive, and prognosis varies accordingly. One subtype of follicular carcinoma, the Hürthle cell tumor, tends to be more invasive and have a less favorable clinical course. Follicular carcinoma undergoes early hematogenous spread, and the patient may present with a distant metastasis, usually in lung, bone, or the central nervous system. Lesions in bone are osteolytic. Like papillary carcinoma, large primary lesions are associated with worse prognosis, but even small lesions may metastasize widely. Rarely, the functioning mass of metastatic follicular carcinoma may be so great as to cause increased serum levels of thyroxine and/or triiodothyronine and clinical thyrotoxicosis. Follicular carcinoma or follicular elements in papillary carcinoma are responsible for those instances in which thyroid carcinoma, in situ or in metastases, accumulates significant quantities of ^{131}I. The third and most common type of tumor, *papillary carcinoma*, has a bimodal frequency, i.e., peaks occurring in the second or third decade and again in later life. This lesion is slowly growing, usually nonencapsulated, and typically may spread through the thyroid capsule to structures in the surrounding neck, especially the regional lymph nodes, where it may remain indolent for many years. Prognosis is a function of the size of the original lesion, with tumors of less than 2 cm having an excellent potential outcome. The presence of involved lymph nodes may be associated with greater risk for recurrence but not apparently with increased mortality. Acceleration of the disease may take place at any time. Follicular elements are usually present in both the primary lesion and its metastases. Papillary carcinoma is the most common thyroid malignancy after radiation exposure to the head and neck in childhood. Tumors in this setting are usually multicentric, thereby meriting more extensive thyroidectomy, but they are associated with a good prognosis.

DIAGNOSIS AND MANAGEMENT The diagnosis and management of thyroid carcinoma are interwoven with the management of the nodular goiter. In the past, this subject has evoked a wide disparity of views among authorities, stemming from seemingly contradictory data. On the one hand, surgically excised specimens of thyroid nodules, particularly solitary nodules, revealed a high frequency of carcinoma (as much as 20 percent in some series). On the other hand, despite the frequency of nodular goiter in the general population (approximately 4 percent), the frequency of thyroid carcinoma, either newly diagnosed or as a cause of death, is low. These respective data led either to vigorous or to conservative approaches to the management of nodular goiter. The discordance can be explained by the ability of the physician to select for surgery those patients who are at high risk of harboring thyroid carcinoma, with consequent weighting of statistics from surgical series. With the advent of fine-needle aspiration biopsy this capability has increased, bringing us closer to the as yet unrealized aim of operating only on those patients whose thyroids harbor carcinoma and avoiding surgery in patients whose thyroids do not.

Several features suggest the presence of carcinoma. Recent growth of a thyroid nodule or mass, especially if rapid and unaccompanied by tenderness and hoarseness, is a source of suspicion. Of particular importance is a history of x-ray to the head or neck or upper mediastinum in infancy or childhood, since this is associated with a high incidence of thyroid disease, including carcinoma, later in life. Nodular disease develops in approximately 20 percent of patients so exposed and may not be apparent until 30 years or more after the radiation exposure. Among patients in this group who have palpable nodules, approximately a third have thyroid carcinoma at surgery, often multicentric and sometimes metastatic. Risk for neoplasia correlates directly with younger age at exposure, female sex, and larger radiation dose. Patients who do not undergo surgery should be followed indefinitely and may be candidates for levothyroxine therapy.

Skillful palpation of the thyroid provides important information. A nodule in an otherwise normal gland (solitary nodule) creates more suspicion of thyroid tumor than does one nodule among many, since the latter is more likely to be part of a diffuse process, such as simple goiter. In addition, carcinomas are usually firm or hard in consistency and nontender. Fixation to surrounding structures and lymphadenopathy are late features, although patients may present with a midline mass above the thyroid isthmus (Delphian node) or lateral cervical adenopathy. Since purely cystic lesions, especially those which are less than a few centimeters in diameter, are less likely to reflect malignancy than solid lesions, transillumination is sometimes helpful, and ultrasonograms (see below) are particularly so. Age and sex of the patient also influence the clinical decision. Benign nodular lesions are more common in women than in men, malignant nodular lesions less so. Hence nodular lesions in men create more suspicion of carcinoma than in women.

Laboratory tests are of little assistance in differentiating between malignant and nonmalignant thyroid nodules. Overall thyroid function is usually normal. Except in patients with medullary thyroid carcinoma, in whom serum calcitonin concentrations may be elevated, tumor markers are of little value. Elevations of serum thyroglobulin are present in many patients with differentiated thyroid carcinoma but are not useful in the initial diagnosis, since they may be elevated in patients with benign adenoma, simple goiter, or Graves' disease. Soft-tissue x-rays of the neck may be of assistance, since finely stippled calcification within the thyroid suggests the presence of psammoma bodies within a papillary carcinoma and more dense calcifications may signify medullary carcinoma.

Fine-needle aspiration for cytology is the initial procedure of choice in the evaluation of most patients (Fig. 334-4). The technique is simple to learn, free of complications, and applicable to most nodules. Optimal application of that technique rests on obtaining a satisfactory specimen and the availability of experienced histopathologic interpretation of the specimen obtained. When such is available, aspiration biopsy provides a reliable means of differentiating between benign and malignant nodules in all except highly cellular lesions or follicular lesions, where evidence of vascular invasion may be required to differentiate benign from malignant forms. Needle aspirates of papillary carcinoma may reveal psammoma bodies, lymphocytes suggestive of Hashimoto's disease, and large pink follicular cells with large pale nuclei ("Orphan Annie cells") and numerous nucleoli. Despite the occasional occurrence of false-positive and -negative results, the procedure can reduce the number of operations performed for nodules that prove to be benign. Further, a diagnosis of carcinoma permits planning of the surgery to be undertaken preoperatively.

While fine-needle aspiration for cytology is the keystone in the approach to the management of the patient with nodular goiter, less specific measures such as ultrasonography or scintillation scanning also may be useful. Although only approximately 20 percent of nonfunctioning thyroid nodules prove to be malignant, demonstration that a nodule is "cold" on scintiscan adds substantial weight to the other factors suggesting carcinoma. Nodules that are hyperfunctioning are rarely malignant. Ultrasonograms of the thyroid have value in demonstrating whether nodules are cystic, solid, or a mixture of the two. Cystic nodules can be aspirated, a procedure that is often curative, and their contents should be subjected to cytopathologic examination. Solid or mixed lesions are consistent with tumor but may be either benign or malignant.

When the cytologic results are equivocal, the physician must decide whether to continue to observe the patient; to administer suppressive doses of thyroid hormone in the expectation that the suspect nodule will shrink or disappear—a hope that in the author's experience is usually unrealized; or to proceed to excisional biopsy and thyroidectomy. Patients in whom the author chooses the latter course include those with a history of radiation to the thyroid and one or more clearly palpable nodules, as well as young men and women with solitary cold nodules, particularly if hard, nontender, and changing rapidly in size. In the remainder, thyroid hormone

FIGURE 334-4 Diagnostic approach to the solitary nodule.

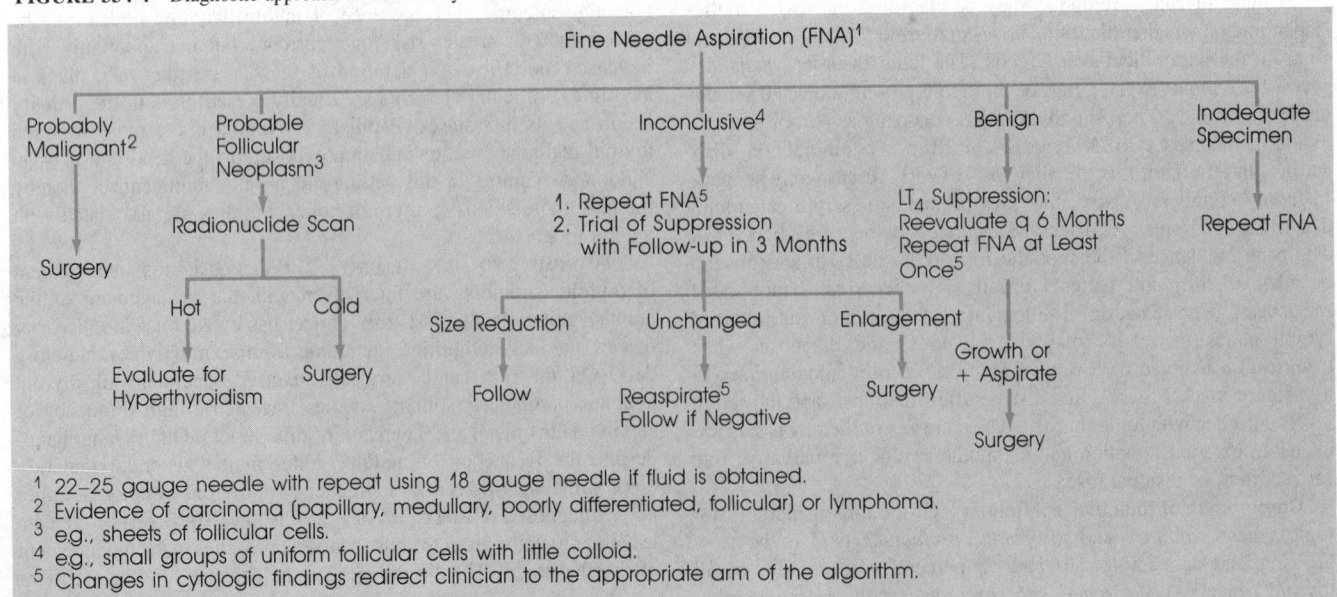

1 22–25 gauge needle with repeat using 18 gauge needle if fluid is obtained.
2 Evidence of carcinoma (papillary, medullary, poorly differentiated, follicular) or lymphoma.
3 e.g., sheets of follicular cells.
4 e.g., small groups of uniform follicular cells with little colloid.
5 Changes in cytologic findings redirect clinician to the appropriate arm of the algorithm.

therapy with repeat aspiration cytology in 3 to 6 months is recommended.

Regardless of the operative procedure planned, surgery for thyroid carcinoma should be performed by a surgeon experienced in the procedure. Should surgery be delayed, suppressive therapy with levothyroxine is often recommended preoperatively to facilitate the operative procedure and perhaps decrease the likelihood of tumor dissemination. In patients in whom a definitive preoperative diagnosis has not been made, the suspected lesion is removed en bloc with a wide margin of surrounding tissue and is examined by frozen section. Opinions vary as to the preferable procedure when carcinoma is found. For lesions of 2 cm or less that are not multicentric and that have not metastasized, some recommend ipsilateral lobectomy, isthmectomy, and possibly contralateral partial lobectomy. Despite its higher rate of morbidity, the author prefers a near-total thyroidectomy, especially for lesions >2 cm, in view of the frequency of seeding of tumor throughout the gland by transglandular lymphatic spread and of evidence that both recurrence rates and subsequent mortality are lower after the more extensive operation. Regional lymph nodes should be explored and removed if there is evidence of involvement, but radical neck dissection is not justified. If permanent sections reveal carcinoma when frozen sections had failed to do so and the initial procedure was limited, secondary surgery should be undertaken to remove residual thyroid tissue, preferably within a few days. A more complete thyroidectomy is warranted for follicular carcinoma in view of its tendency to metastasize to distant sites. This is so because the metastases do not concentrate adequate ^{131}I in the presence of residual normal thyroid tissue, which acts to both compete for the ^{131}I and restrain the increment in serum TSH required to stimulate uptake.

The postoperative necessity for thyroid remnant ablation with radioiodine and subsequent periodic radioisotopic scanning for residual or recurrent disease varies with the histologic type of cancer, size of lesion, presence of metastases, and other indications of invasiveness or aggressiveness. Radioiodine treatment of known residual disease is associated with clinical improvement and reduced recurrence rates, but it is not clear whether mortality rates are benefited by prophylactic postoperative ablation. Papillary cancers of <1.5 cm and unaccompanied by nodal metastases tend to have an excellent prognosis, and it is questionable whether ablation of residual normal thyroid bed and subsequent scanning are necessary. The author favors a more conservative approach in such cases, only administering levothyroxine suppression with periodic follow-up determinations of serum thyroglobulin levels.

Total-body scintiscanning with ^{131}I is the method employed to evaluate for residual normal or malignant thyroid tissue in the neck or distant metastases. Postoperatively, if replacement therapy is initiated with liothyronine (50 to 75 μg/day) rather than levothyroxine, a more rapid increase in TSH secretion is seen when the liothyronine is withdrawn some 3 weeks later. After an additional 2 or 3 weeks without any thyroid hormone replacement, when the serum TSH concentration has risen to the range of 50 mU/L, a large scanning dose of ^{131}I [185 to 370 MBq (5 to 10 mCi)] is administered and whole-body scans are obtained at 72 h. If residual thyroid tissue is found, as is usually the case, a thyroid ablating dose of 1850 MBq (50 mCi) of ^{131}I is administered, and if functioning metastases are present, the dose is doubled. Suppressive therapy with levothyroxine is reinstituted 24 to 48 h later. Approximately 1 week after administration of the second dose of ^{131}I, whole-body scans are repeated, since the larger dose of radioiodine may permit demonstration of functioning metastases not seen after the smaller initial dose. When this proves to be the case, some clinics withdraw suppressive therapy, administer an additional 3700 MBq (100 mCi) of ^{131}I, and then reinstitute suppressive therapy with levothyroxine. Future availability of recombinant human TSH for parenteral injection promises to obviate the discontinuation of thyroid hormone therapy for scanning. In some patients, only measurements of serum thyroglobulin before and after

TSH injection might be performed, with follow-up scanning solely in those in whom a significant rise in thyroglobulin is seen.

Patients are reexamined approximately 6 months after the initial operation and at least every 6 months for several years thereafter. At these examinations, the neck is palpated for evidence of recurrence or metastases, which often can be treated with selective surgical removal. Blood is drawn for a serum thyroglobulin measurement, since elevated values in patients receiving suppressive therapy signal the presence of metastatic disease. At the initial 6-month examination, patients in whom metastases had previously been found are prepared for a whole-body scan as described above. Those in whom no metastases had been demonstrated by earlier scans are not rescanned unless the serum thyroglobulin is elevated but are rescanned approximately 1 year after the initial surgery. Patients in whom whole-body scans are positive are reentered into the therapeutic algorithm, as described above. Those in whom scans are negative continue to be reexamined and have measurements of serum thyroglobulin concentrations at regular intervals. If both serum thyroglobulin concentrations and scans are unrevealing, patients are scanned for the last time after approximately 3 years, unless serum thyroglobulin concentrations rise. In some patients, serum thyroglobulin may be elevated despite the absence of demonstrable functioning metastases. Such patients obviously cannot be treated with ^{131}I but should be studied with x-rays and bone scans to ascertain the site of the thyroglobulin-secreting metastases and to determine whether they may be amenable to external radiation.

A program of this nature, involving near-total thyroidectomy, long-term suppressive therapy, and treatment of functioning metastases with radioiodine reduces the recurrence rate and prolongs survival in patients with papillary carcinoma of the thyroid. Follicular carcinoma should be treated with even greater vigor, since the results are generally less favorable. Because follicular carcinoma metastasizes to lung and bone, appropriate follow-up x-rays and measurements of serum thyroglobulin should be obtained. Mixed differentiated tumors with both follicular and papillary elements tend to behave biologically as papillary tumors and should be so managed. Radioiodine treatment of medullary thyroid carcinoma is usually not successful, those cases showing some reduction in serum calcitonin possibly representing a rare variant of mixed medullary and follicular cancer. Treatment of anaplastic carcinoma is largely palliative; most patients die within 6 months of diagnosis.

THYROIDITIS

Thyroiditis embraces disorders of differing etiology. *Pyogenic thyroiditis* and *chronic fibrosing (Riedel's) thyroiditis* are rare. Pyogenic thyroiditis is usually anteceded by a pyogenic infection elsewhere and is characterized by tenderness and swelling of the thyroid, redness and warmth of the overlying skin, and constitutional signs of infection. Treatment consists of antibiotic therapy and incisional drainage if a fluctuant area within the thyroid should occur. Patients with AIDS may present with thyroiditis due to unusual organisms such as *Pneumocystis carinii*. Riedel's thyroiditis is a disorder in which intense fibrosis of the thyroid and surrounding structures, leading to induration of the tissues of the neck, may be associated with mediastinal and retroperitoneal fibrosis. The principal importance of this disorder is that it requires differentiation from thyroid neoplasia. The other forms of thyroiditis, comprising subacute thyroiditis, chronic thyroiditis with transient thyrotoxicosis, and Hashimoto's thyroiditis, are more common. They are notable for their different clinical courses and for the fact that each can be associated, at one time or another, with a euthyroid, thyrotoxic, or hypothyroid state.

SUBACUTE THYROIDITIS This disorder, also termed *granulomatous, giant cell,* or *de Quervain's thyroiditis,* is viral in origin. Symptoms of thyroiditis usually follow those of an upper respiratory infection and include pronounced asthenia, malaise, and symptoms referable to stretching of the thyroid capsule, principally pain over the thyroid or pain referred to the lower jaw, ear, or occiput. Referred pain may predominate. These symptoms may smolder for weeks before the diagnosis is suspected. Less commonly, the onset is acute, with severe pain over the thyroid, fever, and occasionally symptoms of thyrotoxicosis. Physical findings include exquisite tenderness and nodularity of the thyroid, which may be unilateral but usually involves other areas of the gland. Although local or referred pain is usual, occasional patients have other features typical of the disease but no pain.

Two laboratory findings are characteristic: a high erythrocyte sedimentation rate (ESR) and a depressed RAIU. Values for the remaining tests depend on the stage of the disease in which they are obtained. Early, many patients are mildly thyrotoxic owing to leakage of hormone from the gland. The serum T_4 and T_3 are high, and TSH is undetectable. Later, as glandular hormone is depleted, the patient may pass through a hypothyroid phase, in which serum T_4 and T_3 are low and TSH is increased. Diagnosis of the thyrotoxic phase is especially troublesome in the painless variant because the patient may be thought to have Graves' disease or toxic nodular goiter and therapy inappropriate for subacute thyroiditis may be instituted. Demonstration of a low RAIU usually serves to differentiate subacute thyroiditis from these other causes of hyperthyroidism. Differentiation of painless subacute thyroiditis from chronic thyroiditis with transient thyrotoxicosis is discussed below.

The disorder may smolder for months but eventually subsides with a return of normal thyroid function. In mild cases, aspirin suffices to control the symptoms. In more severe cases, glucocorticoids (prednisone, 20 to 40 mg/d) are generally effective. Propranolol can be used to control associated thyrotoxicosis. When the RAIU and serum T_4 return to normal, therapy can be withdrawn without recurrence of symptoms.

CHRONIC THYROIDITIS WITH TRANSIENT THYROTOXICOSIS

This term denotes a disorder in which a self-limited episode of thyrotoxicosis is associated with a histologic picture of chronic lymphocytic thyroiditis that differs from that of Hashimoto's disease. This syndrome has been variously designated as painless thyroiditis, silent thyroiditis, hyperthyroiditis, chronic thyroiditis with spontaneously resolving hyperthyroidism, or, as the author prefers, chronic thyroiditis with transient thyrotoxicosis (CT/TT). Designations that imply the existence of hyperthyroidism are inappropriate, since ongoing production of thyroid hormone is negligible and the RAIU is decreased.

The syndrome occurs in patients of any age, although it occurs mainly in women. Manifestations of thyrotoxicosis are usually mild but may be severe. The thyroid is nontender, firm, symmetric, and enlarged slightly or moderately. Laboratory features include elevations of the serum T_4 and T_3 concentrations consonant with the thyrotoxicosis and a markedly depressed RAIU. The ESR is normal or slightly elevated, rarely exceeding 50 mm/h, and antithyroid antibodies, when present, are in low titer.

The etiology, pathogenesis, and pathophysiology of this disorder are unclear. Viral antibody titers show no characteristic patterns. It is presumed that thyrotoxicosis results from leakage of hormone from the gland, as in subacute thyroiditis. Low values for the RAIU, in turn, reflect hormonal suppression of TSH secretion and not increased plasma iodine, since urinary iodine excretion is not greatly elevated. Some degree of thyroid malfunction is indicated by failure of the RAIU to respond briskly to exogenous TSH stimulation.

Thyrotoxicosis in CT/TT usually abates within 2 to 5 months. Many patients have recurrent episodes of thyrotoxicosis of similar nature, sometimes following pregnancy (postpartum thyroiditis). The thyrotoxic phase may be followed in several months by a phase of self-limited hypothyroidism. The latter, particularly in the postpartum period, may be the only component of the disease that is diagnosed because the thyrotoxic phase may be very brief. While there appears to be wide geographic variation in incidence, on average, 4 to 8 percent of pregnant women may experience the syndrome post partum.

This disorder, in the thyrotoxic phase, can be differentiated from Graves' disease by demonstration of a depressed RAIU and absence of increased urinary iodine excretion. The latter serves also to exclude the jodbasedow syndrome. When these data are available, the disorder must be differentiated from other causes of thyrotoxicosis with a low RAIU, principally subacute thyroiditis. Lack of tenderness or nodularity of the thyroid and absence of marked elevation of the ESR tend to exclude the latter diagnosis. Patients with either functioning ectopic thyroid tissue or thyrotoxicosis factitia characteristically respond to exogenous TSH stimulation with a brisk increase in RAIU. Definitive diagnosis of CT/TT can be made by thyroid biopsy.

Since the thyroid is not hyperfunctioning in this disorder, measures used in the treatment of hyperthyroidism are useless. Propranolol and mild sedatives are administered until the thyrotoxicosis abates.

HASHIMOTO'S THYROIDITIS   This disorder, also termed *lymphadenoid goiter*, is a common chronic inflammatory disease of the thyroid in which autoimmune factors play a prominent role. It occurs most frequently in women of middle age and is the most common cause of sporadic goiter in children. Evidence of the participation of autoimmune factors includes the lymphocytic infiltration of the gland and the presence in the serum of increased concentrations of immunoglobulins and antibodies against several components of thyroid tissue. Of these, the most important from the clinical standpoint are the antithyroglobulin antibody detected by the tanned red cell agglutination and antithyroid peroxidase (anti-TPO or antimicrosomal) antibody detected by immunofluorescence, complement fixation, or the more sensitive immunosorbent (ELISA) technique. These autoantibodies probably reflect but do not cause the thyroid destruction noted in autoimmune thyroid disease. Hashimoto's thyroiditis also coexists with some frequency with other diseases of an autoimmune nature, including pernicious anemia, Sjögren's syndrome, chronic active hepatitis, systemic lupus erythematosus, rheumatoid arthritis, adrenal insufficiency, diabetes mellitus, and Graves' disease itself (see Chap. 343). These disorders, as well as Hashimoto's disease itself, also occur frequently in family members of patients with Hashimoto's disease. An association of HLA-DR3 and -DR5 with the atrophic and goitrous forms of Hashimoto's disease, respectively, has been noted.

Goiter is the outstanding feature. The enlargement involves the entire gland but not necessarily symmetrically. Typically, the consistency is rubbery, the margins are scalloped, and the general outline of the gland is preserved. The pyramidal lobe may be prominent. Early in the disease the patient is metabolically normal; however, even then decreased thyroid reserve is often manifest in an increase in serum TSH. The RAIU may be elevated early, reflecting the secretion of physiologically inactive iodoproteins, but the serum T_4 and T_3 are normal, and the patient is euthyroid. As the disease progresses, thyroid failure, at first subclinical, may supervene owing to progressive replacement of thyroid parenchyma by lymphocytes or fibrous tissue. The thyroid failure is evident first in a rise in serum TSH concentration. With time, the serum T_4 concentration declines, though the serum T_3 remains normal. Eventually, the serum T_3 concentration falls below normal, and frank hypothyroidism supervenes. Autoimmune thyroiditis including Hashimoto's disease may account for as many as 90 percent of cases of hypothyroidism. High titers of anti-TPO antibody are almost always present. High titers also may occur in other thyroid disorders, particularly primary thyroprivic hypothyroidism and Graves' disease, but with lesser frequency. Although the foregoing findings usually suffice to permit a diagnosis, histologic confirmation may be obtained by needle biopsy. In view of the frequency with which hypothyroidism is either present or eventually develops, treatment with replacement doses of levothyroxine is indicated. In some patients, such therapy is associated with regression of goiter. Pregnant women with high antibody titers may be at higher risk for miscarriage independent of the thyroid status.

Occasional patients present with hyperthyroidism in association with a thyroid gland that is unusually firm and with high titers of circulating antithyroid antibodies, a combination which suggests, probably correctly, the concurrence of Graves' disease and Hashimoto's thyroiditis ("Hashitoxicosis"). In others, hyperthyroidism may supervene in a patient known to have Hashimoto's thyroiditis, presumably due to the emergence of clones of lymphocytes that produce stimulatory anti-TSH receptor antibodies. Hyperthyroidism in association with Hashimoto's thyroiditis is treated in a conventional manner, but ablative therapy is less commonly employed, since the associated chronic thyroiditis tends to limit the duration of thyroid hyperfunction and also predisposes the patient to the development of hypothyroidism after surgical or radioiodine treatment.

REFERENCES

BLACK EG et al: Serial serum thyroglobulin measurements in the management of differentiated thyroid carcinoma. Clin Endocrinol 27:115, 1987

BURCH HB, WARTOFSKY L: Life-threatening thyrotoxicosis: Thyroid storm. Endocrinol Metab Clin North Am (in press)

———: Management of Graves' ophthalmopathy. Endocrinol Rev (in press)

CLARK OH, DUH Q-Y: Thyroid cancer. Med Clin North Am 75:211, 1991

DEGROOT LJ: Diagnostic approach and management of patients exposed to irradiation to the thyroid. J Clin Endocrinol Metab 69:925, 1989

FRADKIN JE, WOLFF J: Iodine-induced thyrotoxicosis. Medicine 62:1, 1983

HAMBURGER JI: The autonomously functioning thyroid nodule: Goetsch's disease. Endocrinol Rev 8:439, 1987

HASHIZUME K et al: Administration of thyroxine in treated Graves' disease: Effects on the level of antibodies to thyroid-stimulating hormone receptors and on the risk of recurrence of hyperthyroidism. N Engl J Med 324:947, 1991

HAY ID et al: American Thyroid Association assessment of current free thyroid hormone and thyrotropin measurements and guidelines for future clinical assays. Clin Chem 37:2002, 1991

HENNESSEY JV et al: L-Thyroxine dosage: A re-evaluation of therapy with contemporary preparations. Ann Intern Med 105:11, 1986

HEUFELDER AE, GORMAN CA: Radioiodine therapy in the treatment of differentiated thyroid cancer: Guidelines and considerations. Endocrinologist 1:273, 1991

MAHONEY KM, WARTOFSKY L: Significance of alterations in thyroid function tests in the critical care setting. J Intensive Care Med (in press)

MAXON HR, SMITH HS: Radioiodine-131 in the diagnosis and treatment of metastatic well differentiated thyroid cancer. Endocrinol Metab Clin North Am 19:685, 1990

MAZZAFERRI EL: Papillary thyroid carcinoma: Factors influencing prognosis and current therapy. Semin Oncol 14:315, 1987

McDOUGAL IR: Graves' disease: Current concepts. Med Clin North Am 75:79, 1991

MOSEKILDE L et al: Effects of thyroid hormones on bone and mineral metabolism. Endocrinol Metab Clin North Am 19:35, 1990

NICOLOFF JT, SPENCER CA: The use and misuse of the sensitive thyrotropin assays. J Clin Endocrinol Metab 71:553, 1990

O'CONNOR G, DAVIES TF: Human autoimmune thyroid disease: A mechanistic update. Trends Endocrinol Metab 1:266, 1990

OPPENHEIMER JH et al: Advances in our understanding of thyroid hormone action at the cellular level. Endocrinol Rev 8:288, 1987

RIDGWAY EC: Clinician's evaluation of a solitary thyroid nodule. J Clin Endocrinol Metab 74:231, 1992

WARTOFSKY L: Use of sensitive TSH assay to determine thyroid hormone therapy and avoid osteoporosis. Annu Rev Med 42:341, 1991

335 DISEASES OF THE ADRENAL CORTEX

GORDON H. WILLIAMS / ROBERT G. DLUHY

BIOCHEMISTRY AND PHYSIOLOGY

STEROID NOMENCLATURE Steroids contain as their basic structure a cyclopentenoperhydrophenanthrane nucleus consisting of three 6-carbon hexane rings and a single 5-carbon pentane ring (Fig. 335-1). The carbon atoms are numbered in a sequence beginning with ring A. Adrenal steroids contain either 19 or 21 carbon atoms. The C_{19} steroids have methyl groups at C-18 and C-19. C_{19} steroids with a ketone group at C-17 are termed *17-ketosteroids*. The C_{19} steroids have predominant androgenic activity. The C_{21} steroids have a 2-carbon side chain (C-20 and C-21) attached at position 17 and methyl groups at C-18 and C-19. C_{21} steroids with a hydroxyl group at

FIGURE 335-1 Basic steroid structure and nomenclature.

position 17 are termed *17-hydroxycorticosteroids*. The C_{21} steroids have either glucocorticoid or mineralocorticoid properties. *Glucocorticoid* signifies a C_{21} steroid with predominant action on intermediary metabolism; *mineralocorticoid* indicates a C_{21} steroid with predominant action on the metabolism of sodium and potassium.

BIOSYNTHESIS OF ADRENAL STEROIDS Cholesterol, derived from the diet and from endogenous synthesis, is the starting compound in steroidogenesis. Uptake of cholesterol by the adrenal cortex is mediated by the low-density lipoprotein (LDL) receptor. With long-term stimulation of the adrenal cortex by ACTH, the number of LDL receptors increases. The three major adrenal biosynthetic pathways lead to the production of glucocorticoids (cortisol), mineralocorticoids (aldosterone), and adrenal androgens (dehydroepiandrosterone). Separate zones of the adrenal cortex synthesize specific hormones; this reflects the enzymatic capacity of each zone to carry out certain transformations and hydroxylations (Fig. 335-2). The outer (glomerulosa) zone is mainly involved in aldosterone biosynthesis, and the inner (fasciculata-reticularis) zone is the site of cortisol and androgen biosynthesis.

STEROID TRANSPORT Some steroid hormones, e.g., testosterone and cortisol, circulate to a considerable extent bound to plasma proteins. Cortisol occurs in the plasma in three forms: free cortisol, protein-bound cortisol, and cortisol metabolites. *Free cortisol* refers to physiologically active hormone that is not protein-bound and, therefore, a form of cortisol acting directly on tissue sites. Normally, less than 5 percent of circulating cortisol is free. Only the unbound cortisol and its metabolites are filterable at the glomerulus. Increased quantities of free steroid are excreted in the urine in states characterized by hypersecretion of cortisol, as the unbound fraction of plasma cortisol rises. *Protein-bound cortisol* is reversibly bound to circulating plasma proteins. There are two cortisol-binding systems of plasma. One is a high-affinity, low-capacity alpha$_2$ globulin termed *transcortin* or *cortisol-binding globulin* (CBG), and the other is a low-affinity, high-capacity protein, *albumin*. The binding affinity of CBG for cortisol is reduced in areas of inflammation, thus increasing the local concentration of free cortisol. CBG in normal humans can bind approximately 700 nmol of cortisol per liter of plasma (25 μg/dL).

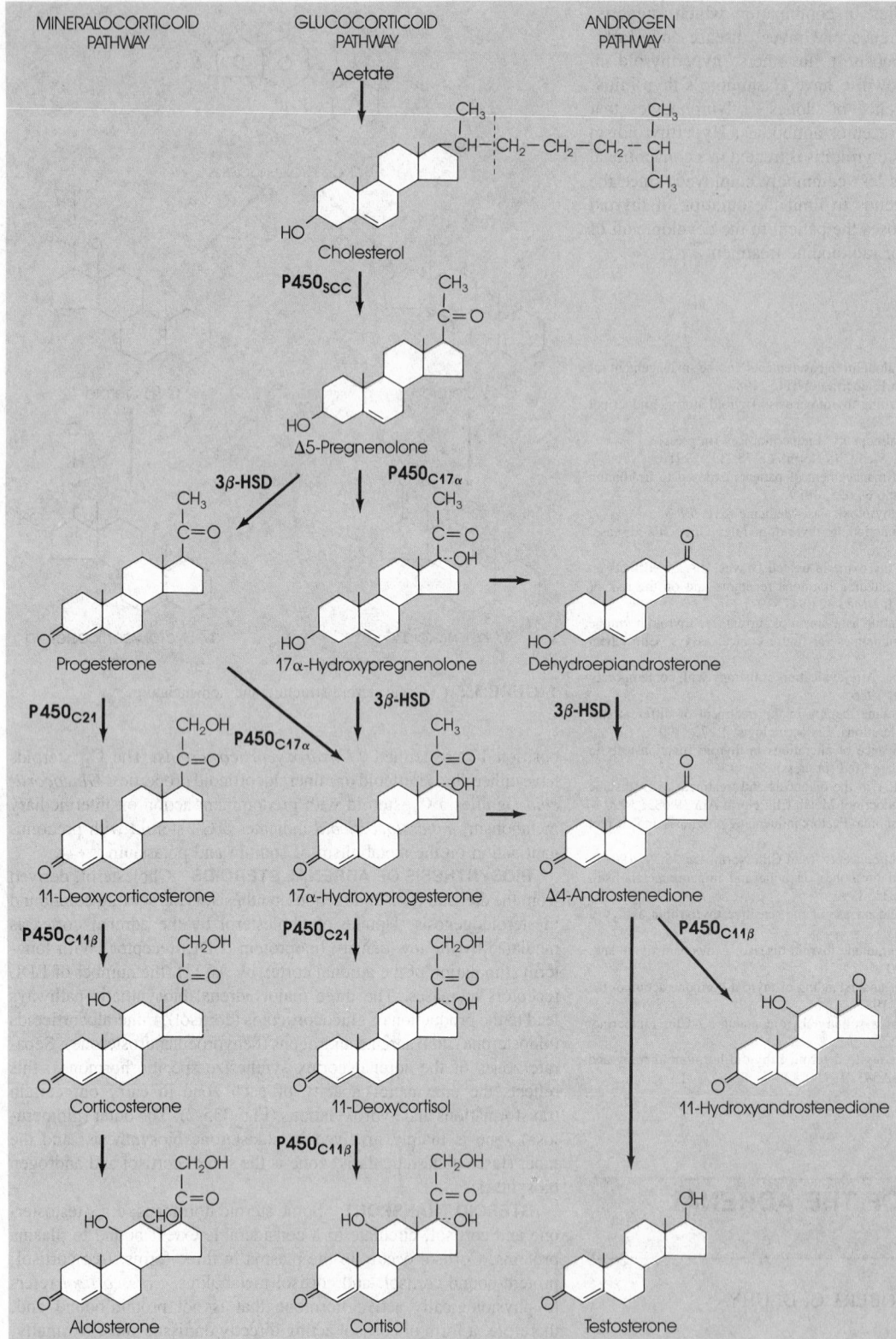

FIGURE 335-2 Biosynthetic pathways for adrenal steroid production; major pathways to mineralocorticoids, glucocorticoids, and androgens. Circled letters and numbers denote specific enzymes: $P450_{SCC}$ = cholesterol side chain cleavage enzyme; 3β-HSD = 3β-hydroxysteroid dehydrogenase; $P450_{C11\beta}$ = C-11 hydroxylase; $P450_{C17\alpha}$ = C-17 hydroxylase; $P450_{C21}$ = C-21 hydroxylase.

When the concentration of cortisol exceeds this level, the excess becomes bound in part to albumin, and a greater proportion circulates unbound. For example, when the total cortisol level is 1400 nmol/L (50 μg/dL) 25 percent will be free. The CBG level is increased in high-estrogen states (e.g., pregnancy, oral contraceptive administration). The rise in CBG is accompanied by a parallel rise in protein-bound cortisol, with the result that the plasma cortisol concentration is elevated. However, the free cortisol levels probably remain normal, and manifestations of glucocorticoid excess are absent. Most synthetic glucocorticoid analogues bind less efficiently to CBG (approximately 70 percent binding). This may explain the propensity of some synthetic analogues to produce cushingoid effects at low dosage. *Cortisol metabolites* are biologically inactive and bind only weakly to circulating plasma proteins.

Aldosterone is bound to proteins to a smaller extent than either testosterone or cortisol, and an ultrafiltrate of plasma contains as much as 50 percent of the circulating aldosterone. The limited binding by plasma protein influences aldosterone metabolism.

STEROID METABOLISM AND EXCRETION Glucocorticoids

The daily secretion of cortisol ranges between 40 and 80 μmol (15 and 30 mg), with a pronounced diurnal cycle. Cortisol is distributed in a volume of body fluids approximating the total extracellular fluid space, with more than 90 percent in the protein-bound fraction. The plasma concentration of cortisol is determined by the rate of secretion, the rate of inactivation, and the rate of excretion of free cortisol. The liver is the major organ responsible for steroid inactivation. The major pathway is reduction of ring A and conjugation of the reduced products with glucuronic acid at position C-3 to form water-soluble compounds. The 11β-hydroxysteroid dehydrogenase converts cortisol to the inactive cortisone in the liver and kidney. The activity of this enzyme is influenced by the level of circulating thyroid hormone, the oxidative reaction being increased in hyperthyroidism.

Mineralocorticoids In normal subjects on a normal salt intake, the average daily secretion of aldosterone ranges between 0.1 and 0.7 μmol (50 and 250 μg). Since aldosterone is only weakly bound to proteins, its volume of distribution is larger than that of cortisol and approximates 35 L. During a single passage through the liver, more than 75 percent of circulating aldosterone is normally inactivated by ring A reduction and conjugation with glucuronic acid. However, under certain conditions, such as congestive failure, this inactivation is reduced.

From 7 to 15 percent of aldosterone is excreted in the urine as a glucuronide conjugate, from which free aldosterone is released on standing at pH 1. This *acid-labile conjugate* is formed in the liver and kidney. For average salt intake, the 24-h urine excretion of the acid-labile conjugate ranges from 15 to 50 nmol (5 to 19 μg), that of the reduced derivative from 70 to 100 nmol (25 to 35 μg), and that of the nonconjugated, nonreduced free aldosterone from 0.5 to 2 nmol (0.2 to 0.6 μg).

Adrenal androgens The major androgen secreted by the adrenal is dehydroepiandrosterone (DHEA) and its C-3 sulfuric acid ester. From 15 to 30 mg of these compounds is secreted daily. Smaller amounts of androstenedione, 11β-hydroxyandrostenedione, and testosterone are secreted. DHEA is the major precursor of the urinary 17-ketosteroids. Two-thirds of the urine 17-ketosteroids in the male are derived from adrenal metabolites, and the remaining one-third comes from testicular androgens. In the female, almost all urine 17-ketosteroids are derived from the adrenal.

Steroids passively diffuse through the cell membrane and bind to intracellular receptors (see Chap. 329). These receptors are part of a superfamily of transcription regulatory factors that include the thyroid hormone receptor. Glucocorticoid receptors are of two types: I and II. The type I receptor is the same as the mineralocorticoid receptor. Mineralocorticoids do not bind to the type II receptor, but most glucocorticoids bind to either receptor, although with different affinities. After the steroid binds to the receptor, the steroid-receptor complex is transported to the nucleus, where it binds to specific sites on steroid-regulated genes, modifying mRNA levels and then protein synthesis. Because cortisol binds to the mineralocorticoid (type I glucocorticoid) receptor with equal affinity to aldosterone, mineralocorticoid specificity is achieved by local metabolism of cortisol to the inactive cortisone, which binds only minimally to the type I receptor. The glucocorticoid effects of other steroids, such as high-dose progesterone, correlate with their relative binding affinities for the type II glucocorticoid receptor. Inherited defects in the glucocorticoid receptor cause glucocorticoid resistance states. These individuals have high levels of cortisol but do not have manifestations of hypercortisolism.

ACTH PHYSIOLOGY ACTH (corticotropin) (see Chap. 331) is an unbranched polypeptide containing 39 amino acids. ACTH and a number of other peptides (lipotropins, endorphins, and melanocyte-stimulating hormones) are processed from a larger precursor molecule of 31,000 mol wt—pro-opiomelanocortin (POMC) (see Chap. 331 and Fig. 335-3). POMC is made in a variety of tissues, including brain, anterior and posterior pituitary, and lymphocytes. The actual peptide secreted varies depending on the tissue. In the anterior pituitary, ACTH is synthesized and stored in basophilic cells. The basophilic staining of the corticotrophs is the result of the glycosylation of ACTH and related peptides. Much of the potential for the corticotropic actions of ACTH is present in smaller polypeptide fragments; the *N*-terminal 18-amino-acid structure retains full biologic potency, and shorter *N*-terminal fragments exhibit partial biologic activity. Release of ACTH and related peptides from the anterior pituitary gland is governed by a "corticotropin-releasing center" in the median eminence of the hypothalamus, which upon stimulation releases a peptide with a chain of 41 amino acids (corticotropin-releasing hormone, CRH) that travels via the pituitary stalk portal bloodstream to the anterior pituitary, where it effects the release of ACTH (Fig. 335-4). Some related peptides such as β-lipotropin (β-LPH) are released in equimolar concentrations with ACTH, suggesting enzymatic cleavage from the parent POMC prior to or concomitant with the secretory process. However, β-endorphin levels may not correlate with circulating levels of ACTH depending on the nature of the stimulus. The functions and regulation of secretion of the related peptides derived from POMC are not understood.

The major factors controlling ACTH release include CRH, free cortisol concentration in plasma, stress, and the sleep-wake cycle (see Fig. 335-4). The plasma level of ACTH varies during the day as a result of its pulsatile secretion but roughly follows a diurnal pattern, with a peak just prior to waking and a nadir before retiring. After several days on a new sleep-wake cycle, the pattern is altered to conform to the new cycle. ACTH and cortisol levels also increase in response to eating. Stress (e.g., pyrogens, surgery, hypoglycemia, exercise, and severe emotional trauma) also can enhance ACTH release. Stress-related secretion of ACTH abolishes circadian periodicity but is, in turn, suppressed by prior high-dose glucocorticoid administration. The secretion of ACTH following stress and the normal pulsatile, diurnal ACTH release are regulated by CRH; this is the so-called open feedback loop. CRH secretion, in turn, is influenced by hypothalamic neurotransmitters. For example, serotoninergic and cholinergic systems stimulate the secretion of CRH and ACTH; there is contradictory evidence regarding the inhibitory effects of alpha-adrenergic agonists and gamma-aminobutyric acid (GABA) on CRH release. In addition, there may be direct pituitary effects

FIGURE 335-3 Schematic representation of the probable structure of the 31,000–mol wt pro-opiomelanocortin molecule. (*From DT Krieger, JB Martin, N Engl J Med 304:880, 1981. By permission of the New England Journal of Medicine.*)

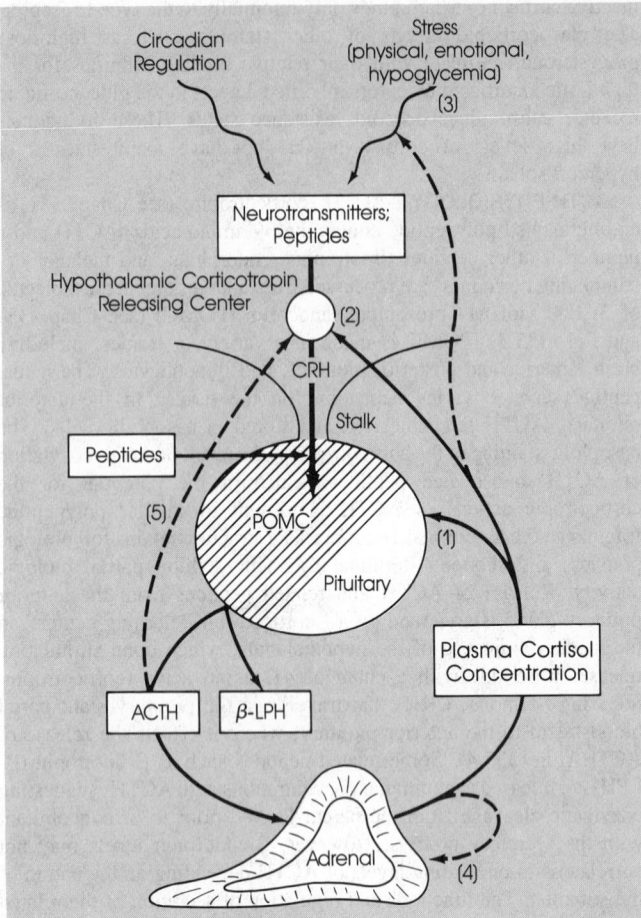

of these neurotransmitters. There is also evidence for peptidergic regulation of ACTH release. For example, β-endorphin and enkephalin inhibit and vasopressin and angiotensin II augment the secretion of ACTH. The immune system also influences the hypothalamic-pituitary-adrenal axis. For example, the cytokine interleukin 1 (IL-1) stimulates CRH secretion. Finally, ACTH release is regulated by the free cortisol level in plasma. Cortisol decreases the responsiveness of adrenal corticotropic cells to CRH; i.e., in the presence of cortisol, more CRH is required to produce a given increment of ACTH. The response of the POMC mRNA to CRH is also inhibited by glucocorticoids. In addition, glucocorticoids inhibit CRH release. This servomechanism establishes the primacy of blood cortisol concentration in the control of ACTH secretion. The inhibition of ACTH occurs in two phases: (1) an early fast feedback, mediated via the type I glucocorticoid receptor, lasting less than 10 min and dependent on both the rate of increase of glucocorticoid levels and the specific glucocorticoid administered, and (2) a time-dependent delayed feedback, likely mediated by the type II glucocorticoid receptor, probably due to inhibition of synthesis of the precursor protein. The suppression of ACTH secretion that results in adrenal atrophy following *prolonged* glucocorticoid therapy may be primarily related to suppression of hypothalamic CRH release, since exogenous CRH administration in this circumstance produces a rise in plasma ACTH. Cortisol also exerts feedback on higher brain centers (hippocampus, reticular system, and septum) and perhaps on the adrenal cortex (see Fig. 335-4).

The biologic half-life of ACTH in the circulation is less than 10 min. The action of ACTH is also rapid; within minutes of its release, the concentration of steroids in the adrenal venous blood increases. ACTH stimulates steroidogenesis via activation of the membrane-bound adenyl cyclase. Adenosine-3',5'-monophosphate (cyclic AMP), in turn, activates protein kinase enzymes, thereby resulting in the phosphorylation of proteins that activate steroid biosynthesis (see Chap. 69).

RENIN-ANGIOTENSIN PHYSIOLOGY (See also Chap. 209)   Renin is a proteolytic enzyme that is produced and stored in the granules of the juxtaglomerular cells surrounding the afferent arterioles of glomeruli in the kidney. Renin exists both in active and inactive forms. Whether the inactive form is a precursor ("prorenin") or is a product formed after release is uncertain. The juxtaglomerular apparatus consists of both the juxtaglomerular cells and the cells of the macula densa. Renin acts on the basic substrate angiotensinogen (a circulating alpha$_2$ globulin made in the liver) to form the decapeptide angiotensin I (Fig. 335-5). Angiotensin I is then enzymatically transformed by converting enzyme, present in many tissues, particularly in the pulmonary vascular endothelium, to the octapeptide

FIGURE 335-4 The hypothalamic-pituitary-adrenal axis. The dominant feedback control of plasma cortisol is on the pituitary gland (1) and on the hypothalamic corticotropin-releasing center (2). Feedback of plasma cortisol also may act on higher nerve centers (3) and/or on the adrenal gland itself (4). There also may be a short feedback inhibition of CRH by ACTH (5). Hypothalamic neurotransmitters influence CRH release; serotoninergic and cholinergic systems stimulate the secretion of CRH and ACTH; alpha-adrenergic agonists and gamma-aminobutyric acid (GABA) probably inhibit CRH release. The opioid peptides β-endorphin and enkephalin inhibit and vasopressin and angiotensin II augment the secretion of CRH and ACTH. CRH = corticotropin-releasing hormone; β-LPH = β-lipotropin; POMC = pro-opiomelanocortin.

FIGURE 335-5 The interrelationship of the volume and potassium feedback loops on aldosterone secretion. Integration of signals from each loop determines the level of aldosterone secretion.

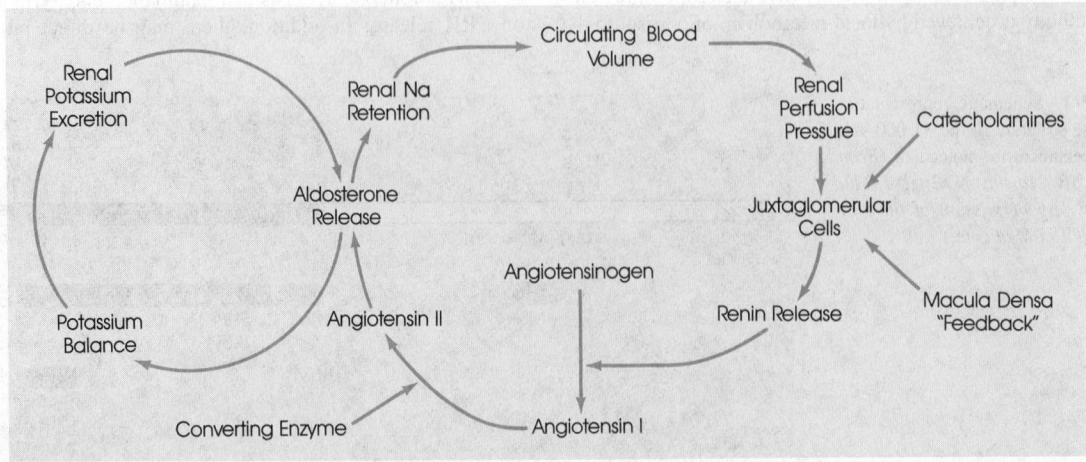

angiotensin II by splitting off the two *C*-terminal amino acids. Angiotensin II is a potent pressor agent and exerts its action by a direct effect on arteriolar smooth muscle. In addition, angiotensin II stimulates production of aldosterone by the zona glomerulosa of the adrenal cortex; the nonapeptide, angiotensin III, also may stimulate aldosterone production. Angiotensinases rapidly destroy angiotensin II (half-life approximately 1 min), while the half-life of renin is more prolonged (10 to 20 min). In addition to circulating renin-angiotensin, many tissues have a local renin-angiotensin system and the ability to produce angiotensin II. These include the uterus, placenta, vascular tissue, heart, brain, and particularly the adrenal cortex. While the role of locally generated angiotensin II is not established, it may be involved in growth and modulation of function of the adrenal cortex and vascular smooth muscle.

Renal renin release is controlled by four interdependent factors, and the amount of renin released is a composite of the effects of all four. The *juxtaglomerular cells*, which are specialized myoepithelial cells cuffing the afferent arterioles, act as miniature pressure transducers, sensing renal perfusion pressure and corresponding changes in afferent arteriolar perfusion pressures. For example, under conditions of a reduction in circulating blood volume, there is a corresponding reduction in renal perfusion pressure and, therefore, in afferent arteriolar pressure (see Fig. 335-5). This is perceived by the juxtaglomerular cells as a decreased stretch exerted on the afferent arteriolar walls. The juxtaglomerular cells then release increasing quantities of renin within the kidney circulation. This results in the formation of angiotensin I, which is converted in the kidney and peripherally to angiotensin II by converting enzyme. Angiotensin II influences sodium homeostasis via two major mechanisms: it changes renal blood flow so as to maintain a constant glomerular filtration rate, thereby changing the filtration fraction of sodium, and it stimulates the adrenal cortex to release aldosterone. Increasing plasma levels of aldosterone lead to increasing renal sodium retention and thus result in expansion of extracellular fluid volume, which, in turn, dampens the initiating signal for renin release. In this context, the renin-angiotensin-aldosterone system subserves volume control by appropriate modifications of renal hemodynamics and tubular sodium transport.

A second control mechanism for renin release centers in the *macula densa* cells, a group of distal convoluted tubular epithelial cells in direct apposition to the juxtaglomerular cells. They may function as chemoreceptors, monitoring the sodium (or chloride) load presented to the distal tubule, and such information may be conveyed to the juxtaglomerular cells, where appropriate modifications in renin release take place. Under conditions of increased delivery of filtered sodium to the macula densa, increasing release of renin is capable of decreasing glomerular filtration rate, thereby reducing the filtered load of sodium.

The *sympathetic nervous system* regulates release of renin in response to assuming the upright posture. The mechanism is either a direct effect on the juxtaglomerular cell to increase adenyl cyclase activity or an indirect effect on either the juxtaglomerular or the macula densa cells by way of a vasoconstrictive action on the afferent arteriole.

Finally, circulating factors influence renin release. Increasing dietary *potassium* directly decreases renin release; decreasing potassium intake increases renin release. The significance of this potassium effect is unclear. *Angiotensin II* itself can exert a negative feedback control on renin release independent of alterations in renal blood flow, pressure, or aldosterone secretion. *Atrial natriuretic peptides* also inhibit renin release. Thus the control of renin release is complex, consisting of both *intrarenal* (pressor receptor and macula densa) and *extrarenal* (sympathetic nervous system, potassium, angiotensin, etc.) mechanisms. A given level of renin secretion probably reflects all these factors, with the intrarenal mechanism predominating.

GLUCOCORTICOID PHYSIOLOGY   The division of adrenal steroids into glucocorticoids and mineralocorticoids is arbitrary in that most glucocorticoids have some mineralocorticoid-like properties.

The descriptive term *glucocorticoid* is applied to those adrenal steroids with a predominant action on intermediary metabolism. The principal glucocorticoid is cortisol (hydrocortisone). This effect on intermediary metabolism is mediated by the type II glucocorticoid receptor. The physiologic actions of the glucocorticoids include the regulation of protein, carbohydrate, lipid, and nucleic acid metabolism. Glucocorticoids raise the blood glucose level by acting as an insulin antagonist and by suppressing the secretion of insulin, thereby inhibiting glucose uptake in peripheral tissues and promoting hepatic synthesis of glucose (gluconeogenesis). The actions on protein metabolism appear to be mainly catabolic in effect, with an increased protein breakdown and nitrogen excretion. Glucocorticoids increase hepatic glycogen content and promote hepatic gluconeogenesis. These actions are in large part explained by the mobilization of glycogenic amino acid precursors from peripheral supporting structures, such as bone, skin, muscle, and connective tissue, due to protein breakdown and inhibition of protein synthesis and amino acid uptake. Glucocorticoid-induced hyperaminoacidemia also facilitates gluconeogenesis by stimulating glucagon secretion. Glucocorticoids act directly on the liver to stimulate the synthesis of certain enzymes, such as tyrosine amino transferase and tryptophan pyrrolase. Glucocorticoids inhibit the synthesis of nucleic acids in most body tissues, but in the liver RNA synthesis is stimulated. Glucocorticoids regulate fatty acid mobilization by enhancing activation of cellular lipase by lipid-mobilizing hormones (e.g., catecholamines and pituitary peptides).

The actions of cortisol on structural protein and on adipose tissue vary in different parts of the body. For example, pharmacologic doses of cortisol can deplete the protein matrix of the vertebral column (trabecular bone), but long bones (primarily compact bone) are affected only minimally; peripheral adipose tissue mass decreases, whereas abdominal and interscapular fat may accumulate.

Glucocorticoids have anti-inflammatory properties, which are probably related to their actions on the microvasculature as well as to cellular effects. Cortisol maintains normal vascular responsiveness to circulating vasoconstrictor factors and opposes the increase in capillary permeability characteristic of acute inflammation. Glucocorticoids cause a polymorphonuclear leukocytosis; the circulating leukocyte mass is increased due to release from the bone marrow of mature cells as well as to inhibition of their egress through the capillary wall. Glucocorticoids produce a depletion of circulating eosinophils and of lymphoid tissue, specifically T cells (thymus-derived lymphocytes). The mechanism is by redistribution from the circulation into other compartments. Thus cortisol impairs cellular-mediated immunity. Glucocorticoids also inhibit the production or action of the local mediators of inflammation such as the lymphokines and prostaglandins. These actions occur via the type II glucocorticoid receptor, and the effects are blocked by inhibitors of RNA and protein synthesis. Glucocorticoids inhibit actions and production of immune interferon by T lymphocytes and the production of lymphocyte-activating factor (interleukin 1) by macrophages. The action of glucocorticoids in suppressing fever may be explained by the latter effect, since IL-1 appears to be identical to endogenous pyrogen, which can activate the hypothalamic fever center. Glucocorticoids also inhibit the production of T cell growth factor (IL-2) by T lymphocytes. Glucocorticoids reverse macrophage activation and antagonize the action of migration-inhibiting factor (MIF), leading to reduced adherence of macrophages to vascular endothelium. Glucocorticoids inhibit prostaglandin and leukotriene production by inhibiting the activity of phospholipase A_2, thus blocking release of arachidonic acid from phospholipids. Finally, glucocorticoids inhibit the inflammatory actions induced by bradykinin and serotonin, such as increased vascular permeability. It is probably only at pharmacologic dosages that antibody production is reduced and lysosomal membranes stabilized, thereby suppressing the release of proteolytic acid hydrolases stored in these cytoplasmic organelles.

Cortisol levels are responsive within minutes to a variety of physical (trauma, surgery, exercise) and psychological stresses (anxiety, depression). Hypoglycemia and fever are also potent stimuli of ACTH and cortisol secretion. The reasons why elevated glucocorticoid levels protect the organism under stress are not understood, but in the absence of glucocorticoids, such stresses may cause hypotension, shock, and death. For these reasons, glucocorticoid administration should always be increased in individuals with hypofunction of the pituitary-adrenal axis during stress.

Cortisol has a major action on the distribution and excretion of body water. It subserves the extracellular fluid volume by retarding the migration of water into cells. It promotes renal water excretion by suppressing the secretion of vasopressin, increasing the rate of glomerular filtration, and acting directly on the renal tubule, the consequence being to guard against water intoxication by increasing solute-free water clearance. Glucocorticoids also have weak mineralocorticoid-like properties, and increasing doses produce renal tubular sodium reabsorption and increased urine potassium excretion. Glucocorticoids also can influence behavior; emotional disorders may occur with either excesses or deficits of cortisol. Lastly, cortisol suppresses the secretion of pituitary POMC and peptides derived from this precursor molecule (ACTH, β-endorphin, and β-lipotropin) as well as the secretion of hypothalamic CRH and vasopressin.

MINERALOCORTICOID PHYSIOLOGY   The major mineralocorticoid, aldosterone, has two important activities: (1) It is a major regulator of extracellular fluid volume, and (2) it is a major determinant of potassium metabolism. These effects are mediated by binding of aldosterone to the type I glucocorticoid (mineralocorticoid) receptor in target tissues (see Chap. 329). Volume is regulated through a direct effect on the renal tubular transport of sodium. Aldosterone acts predominantly at the distal convoluted tubule, where it causes a decrease in the excretion of sodium and an increase in excretion of potassium. The reabsorption of sodium ions causes a fall in the transmembrane potential, thus enhancing the flow of positive ions out of the cell into the lumen. The major intracellular singly charged positive ion is potassium. Since its concentration in the cell is forty- to eightyfold greater than in the lumen, potassium passively follows this relative electric gradient to restore the normal positive charge to the lumen. The reabsorbed sodium ions are then transported out of the tubular epithelial cells into the interstitial fluid of the kidney and from there into the renal capillary circulation. Water passively follows the transported sodium.

Hydrogen ion is also abundant in the tubular epithelial cell. Since its concentration is greater in the lumen than in the cell, it is actively secreted, but the reduced intraluminal positivity allows more hydrogen to be secreted with the same amount of energy. Aldosterone and other mineralocorticoids also act on the epithelium of the salivary ducts, sweat glands, and gastrointestinal tract to cause reabsorption of sodium in "exchange" for potassium ions.

When normal individuals are given aldosterone (or deoxycorticosterone), an initial period of sodium retention is followed by a natriuresis, and sodium balance is reestablished after 3 to 5 days. As a result, edema does not develop. This phenomenon is referred to as the *escape phenomenon*, signifying an "escape" by the renal tubules from the sodium-retaining action of chronically administered aldosterone. While renal hemodynamic factors may play a role in the escape, the level of atrial natriuretic peptide also increases. Importantly, there is no evidence of escape from the potassium-losing effects of mineralocorticoids.

Three primary mechanisms control aldosterone release—the renin-angiotensin system, potassium, and ACTH (Table 335-1). The renin-angiotensin system is the major system for control of extracellular fluid volume, via regulation of aldosterone secretion (see Fig. 335-1). In effect, the renin-angiotensin system maintains the circulating blood volume constant by causing aldosterone-induced sodium retention during periods registered as volume deficiencies and by decreasing aldosterone-dependent sodium retention under conditions in which volume is registered as being ample.

Potassium ions directly regulate aldosterone secretion independently of circulating renin-angiotensin (see Fig. 335-5). However, potassium stimulates the adrenal production of angiotensin II, and

TABLE 335-1   Factors regulating aldosterone biosynthesis

Factors	Effects
Renin-angiotensin system	Stimulate
Sodium ion	Inhibit (?physiologic)
Potassium ion	Stimulate
Neurotransmitters	
Dopamine	Inhibit
Serotonin	Stimulate
Pituitary hormones	
ACTH	Stimulate
Non-ACTH pituitary hormones (e.g., growth hormone)	Permissive (for optimal response to sodium restriction)
Unidentified pituitary factors	Stimulate
β-Endorphin	Stimulate
γ-MSH	Permissive
Natriuretic factors	
Atrial peptide	Inhibit
Ouabain-like factors	Inhibit

administration of converting-enzyme inhibitors blocks the synthesis of locally generated angiotensin II and reduces the aldosterone response to potassium. In normal humans, oral potassium loading increases aldosterone secretion, excretion, and plasma levels. In addition, an increase in serum potassium of as little as 0.1 mmol/L increases plasma aldosterone levels under certain circumstances.

Physiologic amounts of ACTH stimulate aldosterone secretion acutely, but this action is not sustained if ACTH is infused for periods greater than 10 to 12 h. Most studies relegate ACTH to a minor role in the control of aldosterone. For example, subjects on long-term high-dose glucocorticoid therapy and with presumed complete suppression of ACTH have normal aldosterone secretory responses to sodium restriction. Therefore, chronic ACTH deficiency per se does not alter glomerulosa cell responsiveness.

The prior dietary intake of both potassium and sodium can alter the magnitude of the aldosterone response to acute stimulation. Increasing potassium intake or decreasing sodium intake sensitizes the response of the glomerulosa cells to acute stimulation by ACTH, angiotensin II, and/or potassium.

Neurotransmitters (dopamine and serotonin) and some peptides, such as atrial natriuretic peptide, γ-melanocyte-stimulating hormone (γ-MSH), β-endorphin, and an unidentified pituitary aldosterone-stimulating factor, also participate in the regulation of aldosterone secretion (see Table 335-1). Thus the control of aldosterone secretion involves both stimulatory and inhibitory factors.

ANDROGEN PHYSIOLOGY   Androgens regulate male secondary sexual characteristics and can cause virilizing symptoms in women. They produce these actions by binding to high-affinity cytoplasmic receptors.

Steroids with predominant androgenic activity have 19 carbon atoms (see Fig. 335-1). The principal adrenal androgens are dehydroepiandrosterone (DHEA), androstenedione, and 11-hydroxyandrostenedione. DHEA and androstenedione are weak androgens, and they exert their effects via conversion in extraglandular tissues to the potent androgen testosterone. The release of adrenal androgens is stimulated by ACTH, not by gonadotropins. With ACTH stimulation, 17-ketosteroids increase. It follows that adrenal androgens are suppressed by exogenous glucocorticoid administration.

LABORATORY EVALUATION OF ADRENOCORTICAL FUNCTION

The basic assumption in the measurement of plasma or urinary steroids is that they accurately reflect adrenal *secretory* rates of that steroid. A disadvantage of urine *excretion* values is that they may not truly reflect the secretion rate because of improper collection or altered metabolism. Measurement of the actual adrenal secretory rate of a given steroid would be preferable but is more difficult, involving

TABLE 335-2 Range of normal values for tests of adrenal function

Test	Normal value, range
Plasma cortisol, nmol/L (μg/dL):	
8 A.M.	140–690 (5–24)
4 P.M.	80–330 (3–12)
Cortisol secretory rate, nmol/d (mg/d)	14–69 (5–25)
Urinary free cortisol, nmol/d (μg/d)	55–275 (20–100)
17-Hydroxycorticosteroids, μmol/d (mg/d)	5.5–28 (2–10)
Plasma testosterone, nmol/L (ng/mL):	
Men	10–35 (3–10)
Women	<3.5 (<1)
Plasma dehydroepiandrosterone (DHEA), nmol/L (μg/L)	7–31 (2–9)
Plasma DHEA sulfate, μmol/L (μg/L)	1.3–6.7 (500–2500)
Plasma 11-deoxycortisol (S), nmol/L (μg/dL)	<30 (<1)
Plasma 17OH progesterone, nmol/L (μg/L):	
Women	
Follicular phase	0.6–3 (0.2–1)
Luteal phase	1.5–10.6 (0.5–3.5)
Men	0.2–9 (0.06–3)
Plasma aldosterone, pmol/L (ng/dL) (100 mmol Na, 60–100 mmol K, supine, 8 A.M.)	<240 (<8)
Aldosterone secretion, nmol/d (μg/d) (100 mmol Na, 600–100 mmol K)	140–690 (50–250)
Aldosterone excretion, nmol/d (μg/d) (100 mmol Na, 60–100 mmol K)	14–53 (5–19)
Plasma renin activity (μg/L)/h [(ng/mL)/h] (100 mmol Na, 60–100 mmol K, supine, 8 A.M.)	1–2.5 (1–2.5)
Plasma angiotensin II, ng/L (pg/mL) (100 mmol Na, 60–100 mmol K, supine, 8 A.M.)	10–30 (10–30)
Plasma ACTH, pmol/L (pg/mL) (8 A.M.)	<18 (<80)

isotope dilution techniques following administration of a radioactive steroid. Plasma levels reflect the level of secretion only at the time of measurement. The plasma level (PL) is dependent on two factors: the secretion rate (SR) of the hormone and the rate at which it is metabolized, i.e., its metabolic clearance rate (MCR). These three factors can be related mathematically as follows:

$$PL = \frac{SR}{MCR} \quad \text{or} \quad SR = MCR \times PL$$

BLOOD LEVELS (See Table 335-2) **Peptides** ACTH and angiotensin II can be measured by immunologic techniques. However, because of their low concentration and instability in plasma, special precautions are required when specimens are collected. In addition, ACTH levels fluctuate from moment to moment, and a circadian rhythm is superimposed on basal ACTH secretion, with lower levels in the early evening than in the morning. Angiotensin II levels also vary diurnally and are influenced by dietary sodium intake and posture. Both upright posture and sodium restriction elevate angiotensin II levels.

Most clinical determinations of the renin-angiotensin system, however, involve measurements of peripheral *plasma renin activity* (PRA) in which the renin activity is gauged by the generation of angiotensin I during a standardized incubation period. This method depends on the presence of sufficient angiotensinogen in plasma as substrate. The generated angiotensin I is then measured by radioimmunoassay. Plasma renin activity depends on dietary sodium intake and whether the patient is ambulatory. In normal humans, a diurnal rhythm for PRA is characterized by peak values in the morning with decreases in activity in the afternoon.

Steroids Cortisol and aldosterone are both secreted episodically, and levels generally vary during the day, with peak values in the morning and low levels in the evening. In addition, the plasma level of aldosterone, but not of cortisol, is increased by dietary potassium loading, sodium restriction, or assuming the upright posture. Measurement of the sulfate conjugate of DHEA is a useful index of adrenal androgen secretion, since little is formed in the gonads and the half-life is 7 to 9 h.

URINE LEVELS The urine *17-hydroxycorticosteroid* assay measures steroids with a ''dihydroxyacetone'' C-17 side chain, i.e., with hydroxyl groups on C-17 and C-21 and a ketone group on C-20. Therefore, this determination includes cortisol, cortisone, tetrahydrocortisol, tetrahydrocortisone, and 11-deoxycortisol (see Fig. 335-2). Normally, daytime (7 A.M. to 7 P.M.) excretion exceeds night values (7 P.M. to 7 A.M.).

The urine *17-ketosteroids* contain a ketone group at C-17 (see Fig. 335-1). They originate either in the adrenal gland or the gonad. In normal women, 90 percent or more of total urinary 17-ketosteroids is derived from the adrenal gland, while in men only 60 to 70 percent is of adrenal origin. Urine 17-ketosteroid values are highest in young adults and decline with age.

The determination of urinary free cortisol is more useful than 17-hydroxysteroid measurements because elevated values correlate with states of hypercortisolism, reflecting changes in the unbound, physiologically active levels of circulating cortisol.

A carefully timed urine collection is a prerequisite for all excretory determinations. Urinary creatinine should be measured simultaneously to demonstrate the accuracy and adequacy of the collection procedure. Adjustments for body size can be made; e.g., normal subjects excrete 8 to 20 μmol (3 to 7 mg) of 17-hydroxycorticosteroids per gram of creatinine.

STIMULATION TESTS Stimulation tests are useful in documenting the existence of a hormonal deficiency state. A standardized and specific stimulus for the production and release of a given hormone is applied, and the quantity of the released hormone can then be measured.

Tests of glucocorticoid reserve Within minutes after initiation of an infusion of ACTH, cortisol levels increase in adrenal venous blood. This responsiveness of the adrenal gland to ACTH is utilized as an index of the ''functional reserve'' of the gland for production of cortisol. Under maximal ACTH stimulation, the cortisol secretion increases tenfold to 800 μmol/d (300 mg/d). Such maximal stimulation can be obtained only with prolonged ACTH infusions. For clinical purposes, the functional adrenal reserve for cortisol production is standardized with a 24-h ACTH infusion. Synthetic α^{1-24}-ACTH (cosyntropin) is usually given in 500 to 1000 mL normal saline at a rate of 2 units per hour for 24 h. Normal subjects increase 17-hydroxysteroid excretion rates to at least 70 μmol/d (25 mg/d), and plasma cortisol levels exceed 1100 nmol/L (40 μg/dL). In patients with secondary adrenal insufficiency, the maximal 17-hydroxysteroid excretion rate is 8 to 55 μmol/d (3 to 20 mg/d) and the plasma cortisol value at 24 h ranges between 280 and 1100 nmol/L (10 and 40 μg/dL). Patients with primary adrenal insufficiency have smaller responses.

A screening test (the so-called rapid ACTH stimulation test) involves the administration of 25 units (0.25 mg) of cosyntropin intravenously or intramuscularly and measurement of plasma cortisol levels before and 30 and 60 min later; the test can be performed at any time of the day. The most clear-cut criterion for a normal response is a stimulated cortisol level >500 nmol/L (18 μg/dL), and the minimal stimulated normal increment of cortisol is >200 nmol/L (7 mg/dL) above baseline. However, severely ill patients with elevated basal cortisol levels may show no further increases following acute ACTH administration.

Tests of mineralocorticoid reserve and stimulation of the renin-angiotensin system Stimulation tests utilize protocols of programmed volume depletion, such as sodium restriction, diuretic administration, or upright posture. A simple, potent test consists of severe sodium restriction and upright posture. After 3 to 5 days of a 10-mmol sodium intake, aldosterone secretion or excretion rates should increase two- to threefold over control. Supine morning plasma aldosterone levels usually increase three- to sixfold. In addition, plasma levels increase two- to fourfold in response to 2 to 3 h of upright posture.

Stimulation tests on normal dietary sodium intake may be carried out by the administration of a potent diuretic, such as 40 to 80 mg furosemide, followed by 2 to 3 h of upright posture. The normal response is a two- to fourfold rise in plasma aldosterone levels.

FIGURE 335-6   A 20-year-old woman with Cushing's syndrome due to a right adrenal cortical adenoma. *A*. Two years prior to surgery, age 18. *B*. One month prior to surgery, age 20. *C*. One year after surgery, age 21.

Diagnosis   The diagnosis of Cushing's syndrome depends on the demonstration of increased cortisol production and the failure to suppress endogenous cortisol secretion normally when dexamethasone is administered. Once the diagnosis is established, further testing is designed to determine the etiology of the hypercortisolism (Fig. 335-7 and Table 335-5).

TABLE 335-5   Diagnostic tests to determine the type of Cushing's syndrome

Test	Pituitary macro-adenoma	Pituitary-hypothalamic dysfunction or micro-adenoma	Ectopic ACTH or CRH production	Adrenal tumor
Measurement of plasma ACTH	↑ to ↑↑	N to ↑	↑ to ↑↑↑	↓
Percent who respond to high-dose dexamethasone	<10	95	<10	<10
Percent who respond to CRH	>90	>90	<10	<10

NOTE: N, normal; ↑, elevated; ↓, decreased. See text for definition of a response.

For initial screening, the overnight dexamethasone suppression test is recommended (see above). In difficult cases (e.g., in obesity), measurement of a 24-h free cortisol excretion rate also can be used as a screening test. A level greater than 275 nmol/d (100 μg/d) is suggestive of Cushing's syndrome. The definitive diagnosis is then established by failure to suppress urinary cortisol to less than 80 nmol/d (30 μg/d), plasma cortisol to less than 140 nmol/L (5μg/dL), or 17-hydroxysteroid excretion to less than 8 μmol/d (3 mg/d) after a standard low-dose dexamethasone suppression test (0.5 mg every 6 h for 48 h). Owing to diurnal variability, plasma cortisol and, to a certain extent, ACTH determinations are not meaningful when performed in isolation, but demonstration that the normal fall in P.M. levels of plasma corticoid does not occur may be useful.

Determining the etiology of Cushing's syndrome is complicated by the lack of specificity of all tests available and the spontaneous,

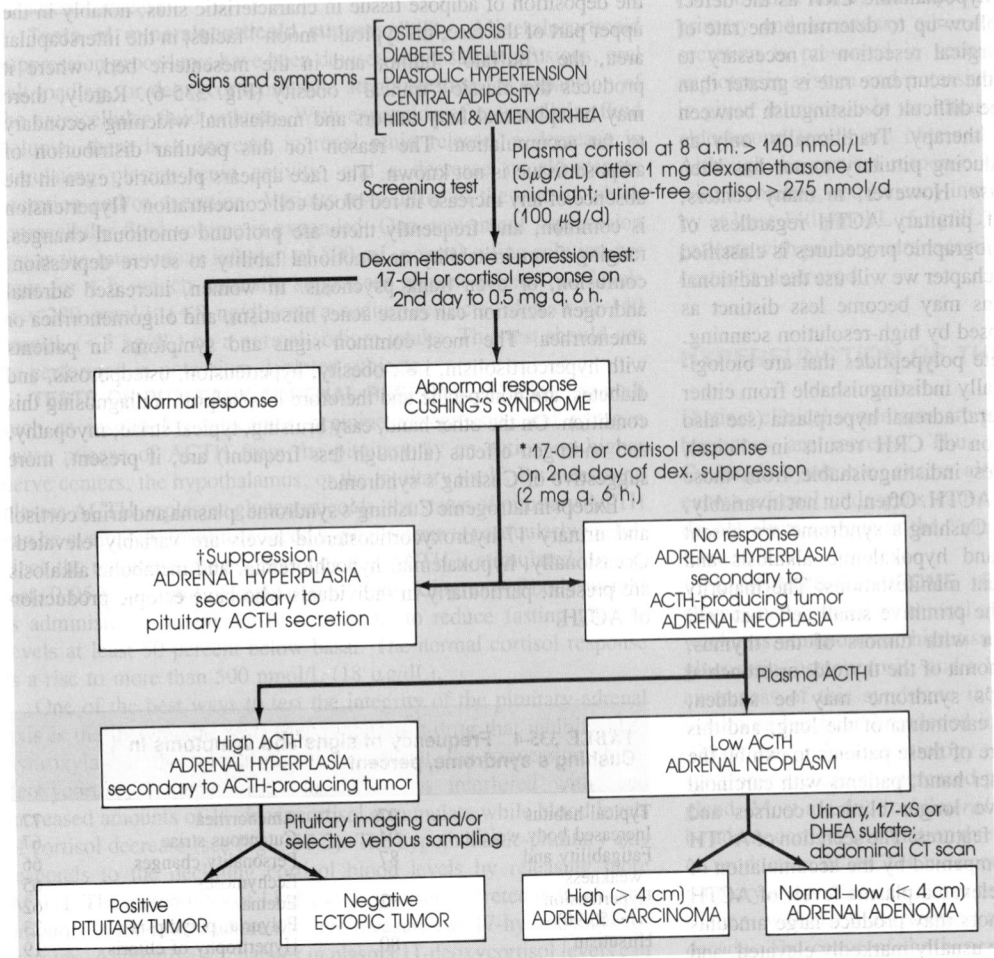

FIGURE 335-7 Diagnostic flowchart for evaluating patients suspected of having Cushing's syndrome.

*The 17-hydroxycorticosteroid response to metyrapone (750 mg given orally every 4 h for six doses) may be used as an alternative test to the high-dose dexamethasone test (2 mg given orally every 6 h). Increased urinary 17-hydroxycorticosteroid excretion following metyrapone occurs in the majority of patients with adrenal hyperplasia secondary to pituitary ACTH secretion; no response suggests an adrenal neoplasm or adrenal hyperplasia secondary to a nonendocrine ACTH-producing tumor.

†This group of patients probably contains subjects with both pituitary-hypothalamic dysfunction and pituitary microadenomas. In some instances, a pituitary microadenoma may be visualized by MRI scanning of the sella turcica.

sometimes clinical, changes in hormonal secretion, often dramatic, that may occur in the tumors producing this syndrome (periodic hormonogenesis). No test has a specificity greater than 95 percent, and it may be necessary to use a combination of tests to arrive at the correct diagnosis. A particularly useful step to distinguish patients with an ACTH-secreting pituitary microadenoma or hypothalamic-pituitary dysfunction from those with other forms of Cushing's syndrome is to determine the response of cortisol output to high-dose dexamethasone administration (2 mg every 6 h for 2 days). Indeed, when the diagnosis of Cushing's syndrome is clear-cut on the basis of baseline urinary and plasma assays, the high-dose dexamethasone suppression test may be utilized without performing the preliminary low-dose suppression test. The high-dose suppression test provides close to 100 percent specificity if the criteria are a suppression of urinary free cortisol by greater than 90 percent and/or 17-hydroxysteroid levels by greater than 65 percent. Occasionally, in individuals with bilateral nodular hyperplasia and/or ectopic CRH production, steroid output is also suppressed. Failure to suppress cortisol production after low- and high-dose dexamethasone administration (see Table 335-5) is usual in patients with adrenal hyperplasia secondary to an ACTH-secreting pituitary macroadenoma or ACTH-producing tumors of nonendocrine origin and in those with adrenal neoplasms.

Theoretically, plasma ACTH levels should be useful in distinguishing the various causes of Cushing's syndrome, particularly in separating the ACTH-dependent from the ACTH-independent causes. In general, this is true for the ACTH-independent etiologies of the syndrome, since most adrenal tumors have low or undetectable ACTH levels. Furthermore, ACTH-secreting pituitary macroadenomas and ACTH-producing nonendocrine tumors usually have elevated ACTH levels. In the ectopic ACTH syndrome, ACTH levels may be elevated above 110 pmol/L (500 pg/mL), with the majority above 40 pmol/L (200 pg/mL). In Cushing's syndrome, as the result of a microadenoma or pituitary-hypothalamic dysfunction, ACTH levels range from 10 to 30 pmol/L (50 to 150 pg/mL) [normal <18 pmol/L (<80 pg/mL)], with half of values within the normal range. However, two problems hinder the utilization of ACTH levels in the differential diagnosis of Cushing's syndrome. First, it is difficult to collect and measure ACTH levels, and second, ACTH levels may be similar in individuals with hypothalamic-pituitary dysfunction, pituitary microadenomas, ectopic CRH production, and ACTH production from some nonendocrine tumors (especially carcinoid tumors) (see Table 335-5).

Because of these difficulties, several additional tests have been advocated, e.g., the metyrapone and the CRH infusion tests. The rationales underlying these tests are similar: Steroid hypersecretion secondary to an adrenal tumor or the ectopic production of ACTH will suppress the hypothalamic-pituitary axis so that inhibition of pituitary ACTH release can be demonstrated by either test. Thus most patients with pituitary-hypothalamic dysfunction and/or a microadenoma have an increase in steroid or ACTH secretion in response to metyrapone and CRH administration, while most ectopic ACTH-producing tumors and adrenal tumors will not. Most pituitary macroadenomas also respond to CRH, while their response to metyrapone is variable. The utility of the CRH infusion test, however, is uncertain, since only a limited number of studies have been performed and since CRH is not clinically available for testing. In addition, false-positive and -negative CRH tests in patients with nonendocrine and pituitary tumors have been reported.

The major diagnostic dilemma in Cushing's syndrome is to distinguish between those individuals with microadenoma of the pituitary and/or pituitary-hypothalamic dysfunction from some paraendocrine tumors (e.g., carcinoids or pheochromocytoma) that ectopically produce CRH and/or ACTH. Clinical manifestations are similar unless the ectopic tumor produces other symptoms, such as diarrhea and flushing from a carcinoid tumor or episodic hypertension from a pheochromocytoma. Sometimes one can distinguish between ectopic and pituitary ACTH production by using metyrapone or CRH tests as noted above. In these situations, computed tomography (CT) scan of the pituitary gland is usually within normal limits. Magnetic

resonance imaging (MRI) with the enhancing agent gadolinium may be superior to CT scanning in demonstrating a pituitary microadenoma in some patients with Cushing's disease. However, finding a structural feature consistent with an adenoma does not prove that the lesion is secreting ACTH. In fact, as the resolution of scanners becomes greater, more variations of the normal pituitary anatomy will be imaged. For this reason, selective venous sampling for ACTH is employed in some centers. Demonstration of a gradient between ACTH level in the petrosal sinus and in peripheral blood localizes the source of ACTH overproduction to the pituitary gland but does not distinguish pituitary-dependent adrenal hyperplasia from pituitary hyperplasia secondary to a tumor producing CRH. CRH levels should be measured in the peripheral blood prior to petrosal sinus sampling. No reliable test is available to make this distinction if the ectopic tumor is not seen or if it produces no other hormones.

The diagnosis of *cortisol-producing adrenal adenoma* is suggested by disproportionate elevations in baseline urine 17-hydroxycorticosteroid or free-cortisol levels with only modest rises or suppression of urinary 17-ketosteroids or plasma DHEA sulfate. Adrenal androgen secretion is usually reduced in these patients owing to the cortisol-induced suppression of ACTH and subsequent involution of the androgen-producing zona reticularis.

The diagnosis of *adrenal carcinoma* is suggested by a palpable abdominal mass and by *markedly* elevated baseline values of *both* urine 17-hydroxysteroids and plasma DHEA sulfate. Plasma and urine cortisol levels are variably elevated. Adrenal carcinoma is usually resistant to both ACTH stimulation and dexamethasone suppression. Markedly elevated adrenal androgen secretion often leads to virilization in the female. Feminizing estrogen-producing adrenocortical carcinoma usually presents with gynecomastia in the male and dysfunctional uterine bleeding in the female. These adrenal tumors secrete increased amounts of androstenedione which is peripherally converted to the estrogens estrone and estradiol (see Chap. 341). Functioning adrenal carcinomas that produce Cushing's syndrome are most often associated with elevated values for the intermediates of steroid biosynthesis (especially 11-deoxycortisol), suggesting inefficient conversion of the intermediates to the final product. Approximately 20 percent of adrenal carcinomas are not associated with endocrine syndromes and are presumed to be nonfunctioning or to produce biologically inactive steroid precursors. In addition, the excessive production of gonadal steroids is not detectable in certain situations (e.g., androgens in adult men).

Differential diagnosis PSEUDOCUSHING'S SYNDROME A variety of groups may present problems in diagnosis; these are patients with obesity, chronic alcoholism, depression, and acute illness of any type. Extreme *obesity* is uncommon in Cushing's syndrome; furthermore, with exogenous obesity, the adiposity is generalized, not truncal. On adrenocortical testing, abnormalities in patients with exogenous obesity are usually modest. Basal urine steroid excretion levels in obese patients are either normal or slightly elevated, a finding similar to their cortisol secretory values. Some patients have elevated conversion of secreted cortisol into excreted metabolites. *Urinary* and *blood cortisol* levels are normal, and the diurnal pattern in blood and urine levels is normal. Patients with *chronic alcoholism* and *depression* share similar abnormalities in steroid output: modestly elevated urine cortisol and 17-hydroxysteroids, absent diurnal rhythm of cortisol levels, and resistance to suppression with dexamethasone (particularly overnight and low dose). In contrast to alcoholic subjects, depressed patients do not have clinical signs and symptoms of Cushing's syndrome. Following discontinuation of alcohol and/or improvement in the emotional status, steroid testing usually returns to normal. A normal cortisol response to insulin-induced hypoglycemia may distinguish these patients from subjects with Cushing's syndrome. *Acutely ill* subjects often have abnormal laboratory tests and fail to suppress with dexamethasone, since major stress (such as pain or fever) interrupts the normal regulation of ACTH secretion. A rare cause of hypercortisolism without cushingoid stigmata is *primary cortisol resistance*; the resistance is incomplete because patients do

FIGURE 335-8   Computed tomography is the preferred method for visualizing the adrenal glands. The adrenal glands are indicated by arrows. *A*. The normal right adrenal gland is adjacent to the inferior vena cava (V) as it emerges from the liver. Approximately 90 percent of the right adrenal glands appear as linear structures extending posteriorly from the inferior vena cava into the space between the right lobe of the liver and the crus of the diaphragm. The normal left adrenal gland is lateral to the left crus of the diaphragm and below the stomach. The majority of left adrenal glands are shaped like an inverted V or Y. *B*. Adrenal CT scan of a patient with ectopic ACTH production. Both adrenal glands (*arrows*) are enlarged (compare with *A*). In contrast, only 50 percent of patients with bilateral adrenal hyperplasia secondary to pituitary ACTH hypersecretion show enlargement of the adrenals when imaged by CT scan. *C*. CT scan of a patient with Cushing's syndrome with biochemical evidence only of cortisol overproduction. The left adrenal has been replaced by a racquet-shaped 2-cm tumor (*arrow*). Attenuation of the tumor is low because of its high lipid content. *D*. CT scan in a patient with Cushing's syndrome and biochemical evidence of an adrenal carcinoma. In contrast to *C*, the right-sided mass has a heterogeneous appearance and is larger in size—usual characteristics of an adrenal carcinoma.

not exhibit signs of adrenal insufficiency. *Iatrogenic Cushing's syndrome*, induced by the administration of glucocorticoids, is indistinguishable by physical findings from endogenous adrenocortical hyperfunction. This situation can be distinguished by measuring blood or urine cortisol levels or urinary 17-hydroxysteroid excretion in a basal state where the levels are low secondary to suppression of the pituitary-adrenal axis. The severity of iatrogenic Cushing's syndrome is related to the total steroid dose, to the biologic half-life of the steroid preparation, and to the duration of therapy. Also, individuals on afternoon and evening doses of steroid develop Cushing's syndrome more readily and on smaller total daily steroid doses than do patients on a steroid program limited to morning doses only. The enzymatic disposition and binding of administered steroids also differ among patients.

Radiologic evaluation for Cushing's syndrome   The preferred radiologic study to visualize the adrenals is CT scan of the abdomen (Fig. 335-8). This procedure has largely replaced previous invasive procedures (such as selective adrenal arteriography and venography) and 19-[^{131}I]iodocholesterol scanning; the CT scan is of value both in localizing adrenal tumors and in differentiating them from bilateral hyperplasia. All patients believed to have hypersecretion of pituitary ACTH should have a pituitary MRI scan with the contrast agent gadolinium. Even with this technique small microadenomas may be undetectable; alternatively, false-positive masses due to nonsecretory variations of the normal pituitary anatomy may be imaged.

Evaluation of asymptomatic adrenal masses   With abdominal CT scanning, many incidental adrenal masses are discovered. This is not surprising, since 10 to 20 percent of subjects at autopsy have adrenocortical adenomas. The first step in evaluating such patients is to determine if the tumor is functioning by appropriate screening tests. However, in 90 percent of the cases, tumors detected incidentally at the time of abdominal CT scanning are nonfunctioning. Fortunately, they also are seldom malignant. Yet nonfunctioning tumors raise difficult therapeutic questions. Since 20 percent of adrenal carcinomas are nonfunctioning, one could argue that all such lesions should be removed. However, the frequency of adrenal carcinomas is low compared with the frequency of benign cortical adenomas (less than 1 percent), and surgery is not indicated in most cases. The size of the tumor sometimes is of value; adrenal carcinomas are rarely smaller than 3 cm in diameter, and adrenal adenomas are usually smaller than 6 cm (see Fig. 335-8). If surgery is not performed, a repeat CT scan in 3 to 6 months is usually required for followup.

Therapy ADRENAL NEOPLASMS When an adenoma or carcinoma is diagnosed, adrenal exploration is performed with excision of the tumor. Because of the possible atrophy of the contralateral adrenal, the patient is treated pre- and postoperatively as if for total adrenalectomy even when a unilateral lesion is suspected, the routine being similar to that for an Addisonian patient undergoing elective surgery (Table 335-11).

Despite operative intervention, most patients with adrenal carcinoma die within 3 years of diagnosis. Metastases occur most often to liver and lung. The principal antitumor drug used to treat metastatic adrenocortical carcinoma is mitotane (*o,p′*-DDD), an isomer of the insecticide DDT. This drug suppresses cortisol production and decreases plasma and urine steroid levels. Although its cytotoxic action is relatively selective for the glucocorticoid-secreting zone of the adrenal cortex, the zona glomerulosa also may be inhibited. Because mitotane also alters the extraadrenal metabolism of cortisol, plasma and urinary cortisol levels must be assessed to titrate the effect. The drug is usually given in divided doses three to four times a day, with the dose increased gradually to 8 to 10 g daily. At higher doses, almost all patients experience gastrointestinal side effects (anorexia, diarrhea, or vomiting) or neuromuscular side effects (lethargy, somnolence, or dizziness). All patients treated with mitotane should be placed on long-term maintenance glucocorticoid therapy, and in some, mineralocorticoid replacement is appropriate. In approximately one-third of patients, regression of both tumor and metastases occurs, but long-term survival is limited. In many patients, mitotane only inhibits steroidogenesis and does not cause regression of tumor metastases. Osseous metastases are usually refractory to the drug and should be treated with radiation therapy. Mitotane also can be given as adjunctive therapy after surgical resection of an adrenal carcinoma, although there is no evidence this improves survival.

BILATERAL HYPERPLASIA Patients with hyperplasia have a relative or absolute increase in ACTH levels. Since therapy would logically be directed at reducing ACTH levels, the ideal primary treatment for ACTH- or CRH-producing tumors, whether in the pituitary or ectopic, is surgical removal. Occasionally, this is not possible because the disease, particularly with ectopic ACTH production, is often far advanced. In this situation, "medical" or surgical adrenalectomy may be indicated to correct the hypercortisolism.

Controversy exists as to the proper treatment for bilateral adrenal hyperplasia when the source of the ACTH overproduction is not apparent. In some centers, these patients (especially patients with a positive high-dose dexamethasone suppression test) have surgical exploration of the pituitary via a transsphenoidal approach in anticipation of a microadenoma being found. These explorations prove fruitful in between 20 and 70 percent of the cases, depending on the skill of the surgeon and the ability of the radiologist to localize the microadenoma preoperatively. In equivocal circumstances, selective petrosal sinus venous sampling may be performed, or the patient may be referred to an appropriate center if the procedure is not locally available. In the event that a microadenoma is not found at the time of exploration, total hypophysectomy may be needed. Complications of transsphenoidal surgery include cerebrospinal fluid rhinorrhea, diabetes insipidus, panhypopituitarism, and optic or cranial nerve injuries. Furthermore, these pituitary neoplasms may recur if the primary abnormality actually resides in the hypothalamus.

In other centers, total adrenalectomy is the treatment of choice. Cure with this procedure is close to 100 percent. The adverse effects include the certain need for lifelong mineralocorticoid and glucocorticoid replacement therapy and a 10 to 20 percent probability of a pituitary tumor developing over the next 10 years, many requiring surgical therapy (Nelson's syndrome). It is uncertain whether in these

individuals (see Chap. 331) the tumor develops de novo or is present prior to bilateral adrenalectomy but is so small that it is not detected by routine procedures. Periodic radiologic evaluation of the pituitary gland by MRI and serial ACTH levels should be obtained in any individual who has undergone bilateral adrenalectomy for Cushing's syndrome. Often, such pituitary tumors become locally invasive and impinge on the optic chiasm or extend into the cavernous or sphenoid sinuses. Thus an aggressive surgical approach is often followed by postoperative irradiation.

In a few centers, pituitary radiation is the primary treatment for pituitary ACTH overproduction, with the use of either conventional external or alpha (proton-beam) radiation. The latter, while more effective, has a greater incidence of ocular motor palsy and hypopituitarism than does conventional radiation therapy. The long lag time between treatment and remission and the fact that the remission rate is less than 50 percent often contraindicate the use of external pituitary radiation in the presence of rapidly progressive or severe Cushing's syndrome.

Finally, in occasional patients in whom a surgical approach is not feasible, medical therapy directed at reducing hypothalamic CRH release either by administering the serotonin antagonist cyproheptadine or the inhibitor of GABA transaminase sodium valproate has been successful in reducing cortisol secretion. Bromocriptine, a dopaminergic agonist, also suppresses ACTH output in occasional patients.

If ACTH levels cannot be lowered successfully by any of the above treatment modalities, then "medical" or surgical adrenalectomy may be indicated (Table 335-6). Inhibition of steroidogenesis also may be indicated in severely cushingoid subjects prior to surgical intervention. Chemical adrenalectomy may be accomplished by the administration of the inhibitor of steroidogenesis, ketoconazole (600 to 1200 mg/d). In addition, mitotane (2 or 3 g/d) and/or the blockers of steroid synthesis aminoglutethimide (1 g/d) and metyrapone (2 or 3 g/d) have been effective either alone or in combination. Mitotane is slow in onset of action (over weeks). Hypoadrenalism is a risk with all these agents, and replacement steroids may be required.

ALDOSTERONISM Aldosteronism is a syndrome associated with hypersecretion of the major adrenal mineralocorticoid aldosterone. *Primary* aldosteronism signifies that the stimulus for the excessive aldosterone production resides within the adrenal gland; in *secondary* aldosteronism, the stimulus is extraadrenal.

Primary aldosteronism In the original case of excessive and inappropriate aldosterone production, the disease was the result of an *aldosterone-producing adrenal adenoma* (Conn's syndrome). The majority of cases involve a unilateral adenoma, usually small and occurring with equal frequency on either side. Rarely, primary aldosteronism occurs in association with adrenal carcinoma. It is twice as common in women as in men, occurs between the ages of 30 and 50, and is present in approximately 1 percent of unselected hypertensive patients. Many cases have clinical and biochemical features characteristic of primary aldosteronism, but a solitary adenoma is not found at surgery. Instead, these patients have *bilateral cortical nodular hyperplasia*. In the literature this disease has been alternatively termed "pseudo" primary aldosteronism, idiopathic hyperaldosteronism, or nodular hyperplasia. The cause is unknown.

TABLE 335-6 Treatment modalities for patients with adrenal hyperplasia secondary to pituitary ACTH hypersecretion

Reduce pituitary ACTH production
 A Transsphenoidal resection of microadenoma
 B Radiation
 C Treatment with hypothalamic serotonin antagonist (cyproheptadine) or GABA-transaminase inhibitor (sodium valproate)*

Reduce or eliminate adrenocortical cortisol secretion
 A Bilateral adrenalectomy
 B Medical adrenalectomy (metyrapone, mitotane, aminoglutethimide, ketoconazole)*

---

* Not curative but effective as long as chronically administered in selected patients.

tion (accelerated phase of hypertensive disease). The secondary aldosteronism is characterized by hypokalemic alkalosis, moderate to severe increases in plasma renin activity, and moderate to marked increases in aldosterone levels (see Chap. 209).

Secondary aldosteronism with hypertension also can be caused by a rare renin-producing tumor in so-called primary reninism. These patients have the biochemical characteristics of renal vascular hypertension; however, the primary defect is renin secretion by a juxtaglomerular cell tumor. The diagnosis can be made by the absence of changes in renal vasculature and/or demonstration of a space-occupying lesion in the kidney by radiographic techniques and documentation of unilateral increases in renal vein renin activity. Rarely, these tumors arise in tissues such as the ovary.

Secondary aldosteronism is present in many forms of *edema*. Increased aldosterone secretion rates are usual in patients with edema as a result of either cirrhosis or the nephrotic syndrome. In congestive heart failure, elevated aldosterone secretion varies depending on the severity of cardiac decompensation. The stimulus for aldosterone release in these conditions appears to be *arterial hypovolemia* and/or hypotension. Diuretic therapy often exaggerates the secondary aldosteronism via volume depletion; when this happens, hypokalemia and, on occasion, alkalosis can become prominent features.

Secondary hyperaldosteronism rarely occurs without edema or hypertension (Bartter's syndrome). This syndrome is characterized by the signs of severe hyperaldosteronism (hypokalemic alkalosis) with moderate to marked increases in renin activity but normal blood pressure and absence of edema. Renal biopsy shows juxtaglomerular hyperplasia. The pathogenesis may be a defect in the renal conservation of sodium or chloride and/or an increased production of prostaglandins. The renal loss of sodium is thought to stimulate renin secretion and subsequent aldosterone production. Hyperaldosteronism produces potassium depletion, with the hypokalemia further elevating plasma renin activity. In some cases, the hypokalemia may be potentiated by a defect in renal conservation of potassium. Increased production of prostaglandins is present but is probably not a primary abnormality, since administration of inhibitors of prostaglandin synthesis only temporarily reverses the features of this syndrome (see Chap. 244).

SYNDROMES OF ADRENAL ANDROGEN EXCESS The syndromes of adrenal androgen excess result from excess production of dehydroepiandrosterone and androstenedione, which are converted to testosterone in extraglandular tissues; the elevated testosterone levels account for most of the androgenic effects. Adrenal androgen excess may be associated with the secretion of greater or smaller amounts of other adrenal hormones and may, therefore, present as "pure" syndromes of virilization or as "mixed" syndromes associated with excessive production of glucocorticoids and some characteristics of Cushing's syndrome.

Clinical signs and symptoms The signs and symptoms of androgen excess can be divided into four areas: hirsutism, oligomenorrhea, acne, and virilization. Clinically, it is important to distinguish between hypertrichosis, simple hirsutism, and hirsutism associated with virilization. Hypertrichosis is an increased hair growth in males or females anywhere on the body. In contrast, hirsutism is limited to females and is hair growth in a male pattern of distribution. In most cases of simple hirsutism, there is no known cause for the increased hair growth. On the other hand, if the patient is virilized as well as hirsute, increased levels of androgens are usually present (see Chap. 49). In general, the degree of virilization reflects both the duration and the degree of excess androgen secretion, although significant virilization can result from minimal changes in testosterone production, and a significant increase in testosterone production may be associated with minimal signs of virilization. The occurrence of oligomenorrhea in a hirsute patient increases the probability that an excess secretion of androgens will be found. Thus the evaluation of the hirsute patient should include a careful history of the onset of menarche, past and present menstrual history, and reproductive capacity and a careful physical examination for signs and symptoms of androgen excess.

Etiology As in other states of adrenocortical hyperfunction, the syndromes associated with androgen excess may result from hyperplasia, adenoma, or carcinoma (the latter two having been discussed above). Adrenal androgen overproduction also may arise from *congenital adrenal hyperplasia*, owing to enzymatic defects. In these patients, increased adrenal androgen production is associated either with excess or decreased secretion of mineralocorticoids or decreased production of glucocorticoids. Since, in humans, cortisol is the principal adrenal steroid regulating ACTH elaboration, and since the ACTH stimulates both cortisol and adrenal androgen production, an enzymatic interference with cortisol synthesis may result in the enhanced secretion of adrenal androgens. In severe congenital virilizing hyperplasia, the adrenal output of cortisol may be so compromised as to cause glucocorticoid deficiency despite anatomic adrenal hyperplasia.

Congenital adrenal hyperplasia is the most common adrenal disorder of infancy and childhood. These children usually have severe enzyme deficiencies (see Chap. 342). The deficiency of enzymes is the result of autosomal recessive mutations. Partial adrenal enzyme deficiencies can be expressed after adolescence, predominantly in women with hirsutism and oligomenorrhea but minimal virilization. Late-onset adrenal hyperplasia may account for 5 to 25 percent of women with hirsutism and oligomenorrhea, depending on the patient population.

Congenital adrenal hyperplasia is secondary to one of several defects in steroid synthesis. To date, defects have been described in the $P450_{C21}$, $P450_{C18}$, $P450_{C17\alpha}$, and $P450_{C11\beta}$ hydroxylases and in 3β-hydroxysteroid dehydrogenase (3β-HSD) (see Fig. 335-2). While the cDNAs for these enzymes have been cloned, the diagnosis of specific enzyme deficiencies with genetic techniques is not practical for routine use. These enzyme deficits usually occur singly. $P450_{C21}$ deficiency is closely linked to the histocompatibility leukocyte antigen (HLA-B) locus of chromosome 6 so that HLA typing and/or DNA polymorphism can be used to detect the heterozygous carriers and to diagnose affected individuals in some families (see Chap. 64). The clinical expression in the different disorders is variable, ranging from virilization of the female ($P450_{C21}$) to feminization of the male (3β-HSD). (See also Chap. 342.)

Adrenal virilization in the female at birth is associated with ambiguous external genitalia (*female pseudohermaphroditism*). The onset of virilization is most probably after the fifth month of embryonic development. At birth there may be enlarged genitalia in the male infant and enlargement of the clitoris, partial or complete fusion of the labia, and sometimes a urogenital sinus in the female. If the labial fusion is nearly complete, the female infant has external genitalia resembling a penis with hypospadias. In the *postnatal* period, congenital adrenal hyperplasia is associated with virilization in the female and isosexual precocity in the male. The excessive androgens result in accelerated growth, with bone age exceeding chronologic age. Since epiphyseal closure is hastened by excessive androgens, growth stops, but truncal development continues, giving the characteristic appearance of a child of short stature with a well-developed trunk.

The most common form of congenital adrenal hyperplasia (95 percent of cases) is a result of impairment of $P450_{C21}$. In addition to cortisol deficiency, there is an associated reduction in aldosterone secretion in approximately one-third of the patients. Thus, with $P450_{C21}$ deficiency, adrenal virilization occurs with or without an associated salt-losing tendency due to aldosterone deficiency (see Fig. 335-2).

$P450_{C11\beta}$ deficiency may cause a "hypertensive" variant of congenital adrenal hyperplasia. Hypertension and hypokalemia can occur because of the impaired conversion of 11-deoxycorticosterone to corticosterone, resulting in the accumulation of 11-deoxycorticosterone, a potent mineralocorticoid. The presence of hypertension is variable. Increased shunting again occurs into the androgen pathway.

$P450_{C17\alpha}$ deficiency is characterized by hypogonadism, hypokalemia, and hypertension. This rare disorder causes decreased production of cortisol and shunting of precursors into the mineralocorticoid pathway with hypokalemic alkalosis, hypertension, and suppressed plasma renin activity. Usually, 11-deoxycorticosterone production is elevated. Because $P450_{C17\alpha}$ hydroxylation is required for biosynthesis of adrenal androgens and for biosynthesis of gonadal testosterone and estrogen, this defect is associated with sexual immaturity, high urinary gonadotropin levels, and low urinary 17-ketosteroid excretion. Female patients have primary amenorrhea and lack of development of secondary sexual characteristics. Because of deficient androgen production, male patients either have ambiguous external genitalia or a female phenotype (male pseudohermaphroditism). Exogenous glucocorticoids can correct the hypertensive syndrome, and treatment with appropriate gonadal steroids results in sexual maturation.

With 3β-HSD deficiency, conversion of pregnenolone to progesterone is impaired, with the result that pathways to both cortisol and aldosterone are "blocked," with shunting then occurring into the adrenal androgen pathway via 17α-hydroxypregnenolone to dehydroepiandrosterone. Since dehydroepiandrosterone is a weak androgen, and because this enzyme deficiency is also present in the gonad, the genitalia of the male fetus may be incompletely virilized or feminized. Conversely, in the female, overproduction of dehydroepiandrosterone may produce partial virilization.

Diagnosis The diagnosis of *congenital adrenal hyperplasia* should be considered in all infants exhibiting "failure to thrive," particularly those having episodes of acute adrenal insufficiency or salt wasting or showing sustained hypertension. The diagnosis is further suggested by the finding of hypertrophy of the clitoris, fused labia, or urogenital sinus in the female and isosexual precocity in the male. In infants and children with a $P450_{C21}$ block, increased urine 17-ketosteroid excretion and increased plasma DHEA sulfate are typically associated with an increase in the blood levels of 17-hydroxyprogesterone and the excretion of its urinary metabolite pregnanetriol. Demonstration of elevated levels of 17-hydroxyprogesterone in amniotic fluid at 14 to 16 weeks of gestation allows prenatal detection of affected female infants.

The diagnosis of a *salt-losing form of congenital adrenal hyperplasia* due to defects in $P450_{C21}$ is suggested by episodes of acute adrenal insufficiency with hyponatremia, hyperkalemia, dehydration, and vomiting. These infants and children often crave salt and exhibit laboratory signs of concomitant deficits in both cortisol and aldosterone secretion.

With the *hypertensive form of congenital adrenal hyperplasia* due to $P450_{C11\beta}$ deficiency, 11-deoxycorticosterone and 11-deoxycortisol accumulate. Both urine 17-ketosteroid and 17-hydroxycorticosteroid excretion may be elevated, since 11-deoxycortisol is included in the analysis. The diagnosis is secured by demonstrating increased levels of 11-deoxycortisol in the blood or increased amounts of tetrahydro-11-deoxycortisol in the urine. Elevation of 17-hydroxyprogesterone levels does not imply a concomitant $P450_{C21}$ deficiency.

The finding of very high levels of urine dehydroepiandrosterone with low levels of pregnanetriol and of cortisol metabolites in urine is characteristic of children with 3β-HSD deficiency. Marked salt wasting may also occur.

Adults with *late-onset adrenal hyperplasia* (partial deficiency of $P450_{C21}$, $P450_{C11\beta}$, or 3β-HSD) are characterized by normal or moderately elevated urinary 17-ketosteroids and plasma DHEA sulfate. A high basal level of a precursor of cortisol biosynthesis (such as 17-hydroxyprogesterone, 17-hydroxypregnenolone, or 11-deoxycortisol) or elevation of the precursor after ACTH stimulation confirms the diagnosis of a partial deficiency. It is uncertain how long ACTH needs to be infused to unmask the enzyme deficiency, but measuring steroid precursors 60 min after the bolus administration of ACTH is usually sufficient. Adrenal androgen output is easily suppressed by the standard low-dose (2 mg) dexamethasone test.

Differential diagnosis The causes of hirsutism can be divided into four broad categories: familial, idiopathic, androgen excess, and drugs. In general, the first two conditions are not associated with other signs of androgen excess, i.e., oligomenorrhea, significant acne,

TABLE 335-7   **Causes of hirsutism in women**
Familial
Idiopathic
Ovarian
A   Polycystic ovaries; hilus cell hyperplasia
B   Tumor: arrhenoblastoma, hilus cell, adrenal rest
Adrenal
A   Congenital adrenal hyperplasia
B   Noncongenital adrenal hyperplasia (Cushing's)
C   Tumor: virilizing carcinoma or adenoma

or virilization. Likewise, drug-induced hirsutism is usually not associated with other signs and symptoms of androgen excess, unless the drug is an androgen. The drugs that produce an increase in body hair include phenothiazines, minoxidil, and phenytoin. Each of these drugs, particularly minoxidil, produces a generalized increase in hair growth, not just an increase in hair growth in androgen target areas. The mechanism may be related to the ability of these drugs to convert vellus into terminal hair follicles.

If drugs are excluded, the only known causes of hirsutism amenable to treatment are those secondary to excess production of androgens by either the adrenal or the ovary.

In the female, the differential diagnosis of hirsutism and virilization is between adrenal and ovarian etiologies (Table 335-7). *Sudden onset of progressive hirsutism and virilization* suggests an adrenal or ovarian neoplasm. *Adrenal adenomas and carcinomas* may cause a pure or mixed virilizing syndrome. Since adrenal androgens are weak compared with gonadal androgens, adrenal virilization is characterized by *large increments in urine 17-ketosteroid excretion.* Virilizing adrenal adenomas are rare. *Virilizing adrenal carcinomas,* the most common adrenal tumors causing virilization, are associated with high plasma DHEA sulfate levels and high urinary 17-ketosteroid excretion rates, and, as a rule, exceed 6 cm in size. Cortisol levels and 17-hydroxycorticosteroid excretion are normal or moderately elevated. Failure to reduce 17-ketosteroid levels and plasma DHEA sulfate levels to normal following dexamethasone suppression (0.5 mg given orally every 6 h for 2 days) further supports a diagnosis of virilizing adrenal tumor and excludes congenital adrenal hyperplasia. The most common virilizing *ovarian tumor* is the arrhenoblastoma, but other ovarian tumors, such as adrenal rest tumor, granulosa cell tumor, hilar cell tumor, and Brenner tumor, have been associated with virilization. Virilization due to ovarian tumors is usually characterized by normal levels of urinary 17-ketosteroids and DHEA sulfate, since the neoplasm usually secretes the potent androgen testosterone. Occasionally, increases in 17-ketosteroid excretion occur in some patients with ovarian neoplasms, but baseline 17-ketosteroid excretion in excess of 100 μmol/d (30 mg/d) is rare with the exception of adrenal rest tumors. Like adrenal neoplasms, ovarian tumors are not suppressed by dexamethasone. With the exception of adrenal rest tumors, these tumors are largely independent of ACTH stimulation. Elevations of plasma testosterone do not localize the neoplasm to the ovary, since testosterone can be elevated subsequent to peripheral conversion of adrenal precursors, such as DHEA (see Chap. 340).

The most common ovarian cause of excess androgen production is ovarian hyperthecosis or polycystic ovaries (see Chap. 340). As opposed to ovarian or adrenal tumors, virilization is less common with polycystic ovaries, whereas hirsutism is quite frequent. Many of these patients are obese and have hyperinsulinemia and glucose intolerance. Acanthosis nigricans may be present. Although the 17-ketosteroid excretion is partially reduced by dexamethasone, the residual level is often greater than in normal subjects. Plasma levels and production rates of androstenedione and, to a lesser extent, testosterone are usually increased. Follicle-stimulating hormone (FSH) levels tend to be lower than normal, and luteinizing hormone (LH) levels may be tonically elevated, leading to the characteristic increased LH/FSH ratio. The laboratory findings in patients with hirsutism-virilizing syndromes are summarized in Table 335-8.

TABLE 335-8 Laboratory evaluation of hirsutism-virilizing syndromes

	Ovarian		Adrenal			
	PCO	Ovarian tumor	CAH	Adrenal neoplasm	Cushing's syndrome	Idiopathic
Urinary 17-ketosteroids, plasma DHEA sulfate	N↑	N	N↑	↑↑↑	N↑	N
Plasma testosterone	N↑	↑↑	N↑	N↑	N↑	N
LH/FSH ratio	N↑	N	N	N	N	N
Precursors of cortisol biosynthesis:						
Basal	N	N	N↑	N↑	N	N
Following ACTH infusion	N	N	↑↑	N↑	N	N
Cortisol following overnight dexamethasone suppresion test	N	N	N	↑	↑	N

NOTE: CAH, congenital adrenal hyperplasia; PCO, polycystic ovary syndrome; N, normal; ↑, elevated.

Treatment Treatment of adrenal virilism is dictated by the type of lesion. Patients with *congenital adrenal hyperplasia* have a fundamental defect of cortisol deficiency with resultant excessive ACTH secretion, producing hyperplasia of the adrenal glands and causing additional "shunting" into the adrenal androgen pathway. Therapy in these patients consists of daily administration of glucocorticoids to suppress pituitary ACTH secretion. Because of its cost and intermediate half-life, prednisone is the drug of choice except in infants, in whom hydrocortisone is usually used. In adults with late-onset adrenal hyperplasia, the smallest single bedtime dose of a long- or intermediate-acting glucocorticoid to suppress pituitary ACTH secretion should be administered. The amount of steroid required by children with congenital adrenal hyperplasia is approximately 1 to 1.5 times the normal cortisol production rate of 33 to 35 μmol (12 to 13 mg) cortisol per square meter of body surface area per day and is given in divided doses two or three times per day. The dosage schedule is governed by repetitive analysis of the urinary 17-ketosteroids, plasma DHEA sulfate, and/or precursors of cortisol biosynthesis. Skeletal growth and maturation also must be closely monitored, since overtreatment with glucocorticoid replacement therapy retards linear growth.

HYPOFUNCTION OF ADRENAL CORTEX

Adrenocortical hypofunction includes all conditions in which adrenal steroid hormone secretion falls below the requirements of the body. Adrenal insufficiency may be divided into two general categories: (1) those associated with primary inability of the adrenal to elaborate sufficient quantities of hormone and (2) those associated with a secondary failure due to a primary failure in the elaboration of ACTH (Table 335-9).

PRIMARY ADRENOCORTICAL DEFICIENCY (ADDISON'S DISEASE) Addison's description of "general languor and debility,

---

TABLE 335-9 Classification of adrenal insufficiency

Primary adrenal insufficiency
  A Anatomic destruction of gland (chronic and acute)
    1 "Idiopathic" atrophy (autoimmune)
    2 Surgical removal
    3 Infection (tuberculous, fungus, viral–especially in AIDS patients)
    4 Hemorrhage
    5 Invasion: metastatic
  B Metabolic failure in hormone production
    1 Congenital adrenal hyperplasia
    2 Enzyme inhibitors (metyrapone, ketoconazole, aminoglutethimide)
    3 Cytotoxic agents (mitotane)
  C ACTH-blocking antibodies
Secondary adrenal insufficiency
  A Hypopituitarism due to hypothalamic-pituitary disease
  B Suppression of hypothalamic-pituitary axis
    1 Exogenous steroid
    2 Endogenous steroid from tumor

---

remarkable feebleness of the heart's action, irritability of the stomach, and a peculiar change of the color of the skin" summarizes the dominant clinical features. Advanced cases are usually easy to diagnose, but recognition of the disease in its early phases may present a real challenge.

Incidence Primary adrenocortical insufficiency is relatively rare, may occur at any age, and affects both sexes equally. Because of increasing therapeutic use of steroids, secondary adrenal insufficiency is relatively common.

Etiology and pathogenesis Addison's disease results from progressive adrenocortical destruction, which must involve more than 90 percent of the glands before signs of adrenal insufficiency appear. The adrenal is a frequent site for chronic granulomatous diseases, predominantly tuberculosis but also histoplasmosis, coccidioidomycosis, and cryptococcosis. In early series, tuberculosis was responsible for 70 to 90 percent of cases; however, the most frequent cause at present is *idiopathic* atrophy, and an autoimmune mechanism is probably responsible. Rarely, other lesions are encountered, such as bilateral hemorrhage, tumor metastases, amyloidosis, or sarcoidosis.

Half of patients have circulating adrenal antibodies. While some antibodies cause adrenal destruction, IgG antibodies can cause Addison's disease by blocking the binding of ACTH to its receptors. Some patients also have antibodies to thyroid, parathyroid, and/or gonadal tissue (see also Chap. 343). There is also an increased incidence of chronic lymphocytic thyroiditis and of premature ovarian failure, type I diabetes mellitus, and hyperthyroidism in patients with idiopathic adrenal insufficiency. The occurrence of two or more of these autoimmune endocrine disorders in the same individual defines the polyglandular autoimmune syndrome type II. Additional disorders include pernicious anemia, vitiligo, alopecia, nontropical sprue, and myasthenia gravis. Within families, multiple generations are affected by one or more of the above diseases. Type II polyglandular syndrome is the result of a mutant gene on chromosome 6 and is associated with the HLA alleles B8 and DR3.

The combination of parathyroid and adrenal insufficiency and chronic mucocutaneous moniliasis constitutes a distinct syndrome (type I polyglandular autoimmune syndrome). Other autoimmune diseases in these patients include pernicious anemia, chronic active hepatitis, alopecia, primary hypothyroidism, and premature gonadal failure. There is no HLA association; this syndrome is an autosomal recessive trait, often with multiple affected siblings. The type I syndrome usually presents during childhood, whereas the type II syndrome is usually expressed in adulthood. The mechanisms by which genetic predisposition and/or autoimmunity interact in the pathogenesis of these disorders are unknown.

Clinical suspicion of adrenal insufficiency should be high in patients with AIDS (see Chap. 279). Cytomegalovirus regularly involves the adrenal glands (so-called CMV necrotizing adrenalitis), and *Mycobacterium avium-intracellulare*, *Cryptococcus*, and Kaposi's sarcoma involvement of the adrenals also have been reported. Adrenal insufficiency in AIDS patients may not be manifest, but tests of adrenal reserve are frequently abnormal. When interpreting tests of

TABLE 335-10 Frequency of symptoms and signs in Addison's disease, percent

Weakness	99	Pigmentation of mucous membranes	82
Pigmentation of skin	98		
Weight loss	97	Abdominal pain	34
Anorexia, nausea, and vomiting	90	Salt craving	22
		Diarrhea	20
Hypotension (<110/70)	87	Constipation	19
		Syncope	16
		Vitiligo	9

adrenocortical function, it is important to consider medications that might potentiate or cause adrenal failure (rifampin, phenytoin, ketoconazole, and opiates).

Clinical signs and symptoms Adrenocortical insufficiency caused by gradual adrenal destruction is characterized by an insidious onset of slowly progressive fatigability, weakness, anorexia, nausea and vomiting, weight loss, cutaneous and mucosal pigmentation, hypotension, and occasionally hypoglycemia (Table 335-10). However, the spectrum may vary, depending on the duration and degree of adrenal hypofunction, from a complaint of mild chronic fatigue to the fulminating shock associated with acute massive destruction of the glands described by Waterhouse and Friderichsen.

Asthenia is the cardinal symptom. Early it may be sporadic, usually most evident at times of stress; as adrenal function becomes more impaired, weakness progresses until the patient is continuously fatigued, necessitating bed rest.

Hyperpigmentation may be striking, but its absence does not exclude this diagnosis. It commonly appears as a diffuse brown, tan, or bronze darkening of both exposed and unexposed parts such as elbows or creases of the hand and of areas normally pigmented such as the areolas about the nipples. Bluish black patches may appear on the mucous membranes. Some patients develop dark freckles, and irregular areas of vitiligo may appear paradoxically. As an early sign, patients may notice persistent tanning following sun exposure.

Arterial hypotension with postural accentuation is frequent, and blood pressures may be in the range of 80/50 or less.

Abnormalities of gastrointestinal function often are the presenting complaint. Symptoms vary from mild anorexia with weight loss to fulminating nausea, vomiting, diarrhea, and ill-defined abdominal pain, which may be so severe as to be confused with an acute abdomen. In addition, patients frequently have personality changes, usually excessive irritability and restlessness. Enhancement of the sensory modalities of taste, olfaction, and hearing is reversible with therapy. Axillary and pubic hair may be decreased in women due to loss of adrenal androgen production.

Laboratory findings In the early phase of gradual adrenal destruction, there may be no demonstrable abnormalities in the routine laboratory parameters, but adrenal reserve is decreased, i.e., basal steroid output may be normal, but a subnormal increase occurs after stress. Adrenal stimulation with ACTH uncovers abnormalities in this stage of the disease with a subnormal response and/or failure of cortisol levels to rise over basal. In more advanced stages of adrenal destruction, serum sodium, chloride, and bicarbonate levels are reduced while the serum potassium level is elevated. The hyponatremia is due to both loss of sodium into the urine (due to aldosterone deficiency) and movement into the intracellular compartment. This extravascular sodium loss depletes extracellular fluid volume and accentuates hypotension. Elevated plasma vasopressin and angiotensin II levels may contribute to the hyponatremia through impairment of free water clearance. The hyperkalemia is due to a combination of aldosterone deficiency, impaired glomerular filtration, and acidosis. Basal levels of cortisol and aldosterone are subnormal and fail to increase following ACTH administration. Mild to moderate hypercalcemia occurs in 10 to 20 percent of patients for unclear reasons. The electrocardiogram may show nonspecific changes, and the electroencephalogram exhibits a generalized reduction and slowing. There may be a normocytic anemia, a relative lymphocytosis, and a moderate eosinophilia.

Diagnosis The diagnosis of adrenal insufficiency should be made only with ACTH stimulation testing to assess adrenal reserve capacity for steroid production (see above for ACTH test protocols). In *severe adrenal insufficiency*, the cortisol secretory rate is markedly decreased, and this may be ascertained indirectly by the finding of low to absent 24-h urine cortisol, 17-hydroxycorticosteroids, and 17-ketosteroids. With *mild adrenal insufficiency* (decreased adrenal reserve), urine and blood steroid values overlap the normal range; thus a diagnosis of adrenal insufficiency should never be excluded solely on the basis of normal basal urine steroid determinations. Plasma cortisol values vary from zero to the lower range of normal. Aldosterone secretion is usually low, resulting in salt wasting and rises in plasma renin levels. In primary adrenal insufficiency, plasma ACTH and associated peptides (β-lipotropin) are elevated because of loss of the usual cortisol-hypothalamic-pituitary feedback relationship, whereas in secondary adrenal insufficiency, plasma ACTH values are low or "inappropriately" normal (Fig. 335-11).

Differential diagnosis Since weakness and fatigue are common complaints, clinical diagnosis of early adrenocortical insufficiency is frequently difficult. However, mild gastrointestinal distress with weight loss, anorexia, and a suggestion of increased pigmentation make mandatory ACTH stimulation testing to rule out adrenal insufficiency, particularly before steroid treatment is begun. Weight loss is useful in evaluating the significance of weakness and malaise. Racial pigmentation may be a problem, but a *recent* and progressive *increase* is usually reported by the patient with gradual adrenal destruction. Hyperpigmentation is usually absent when adrenal destruction is rapid, as in bilateral adrenal hemorrhage. Hyperpigmenta-

FIGURE 335-11 Diagnostic flowchart for evaluating patients with suspected adrenal insufficiency. Plasma ACTH levels are low in secondary adrenal insufficiency. In adrenal insufficiency secondary to pituitary tumors or idiopathic panhypopituitarism, other pituitary hormone deficiencies are present. On the other hand, ACTH deficiency may be isolated, as seen following prolonged use of exogenous glucocorticoids.

Since the isolated blood levels obtained in these screening tests may not be definitive, the diagnosis should always be confirmed by a continuous 24-h ACTH infusion. Normal subjects and patients with secondary adrenal insufficiency may be distinguished by insulin tolerance or metyrapone testing.

tion in other diseases also may present a problem, but the appearance and distribution of pigment in Addison's disease are usually characteristic. When doubt exists, measurement of ACTH levels and testing of adrenal reserve with the infusion of ACTH provide clear-cut differentiation.

Treatment All patients with Addison's disease should receive specific hormone replacement. Like diabetics, these patients require careful education about their disease. Since the adrenal gland elaborates three general classes of hormones, of which two, glucocorticoids and mineralocorticoids, are of primary clinical importance, replacement therapy should correct both deficiencies. Cortisone (or cortisol) is the mainstay of treatment. Cortisone dosage varies from 12.5 to 50 mg/d, with the majority of patients taking 25 to 37.5 mg in divided doses. Cortisol (30 mg/d) or prednisone (7.5 mg/d) in divided doses also may be given for substitution therapy. Patients are advised to take their glucocorticoid replacement medication with meals or, if this is impractical, with milk or an antacid because the drugs may increase gastric acidity. This is particularly important because if the steroid is biologically active, e.g., cortisol, prednisolone, and dexamethasone, it may exert local effects on the gastric mucosa. In addition, the larger proportion of the dose (e.g., 25 mg cortisone) is taken in the morning, and the remainder (12.5 mg cortisone) is taken in the late afternoon to simulate the normal diurnal adrenal rhythm. Some patients exhibit insomnia, irritability, and mental excitement after initiation of therapy; in these, the dosage should be reduced. Other indications for smaller doses are hypertension, diabetes mellitus, or active tuberculosis.

Since this amount of cortisone or cortisol fails to replace the mineralocorticoid component of the adrenal gland, supplementary hormone is usually needed. This is accomplished by the daily oral administration of 0.05 to 0.1 mg fludrocortisone. Patients also should be instructed to ingest an ample intake of sodium (3 to 4 g/d). Adequacy of mineralocorticoid therapy can be assessed by measurement of blood pressure and serum electrolytes. Blood pressure should be normal and without postural change; serum sodium, potassium, creatinine, and urea nitrogen levels also should be normal.

Complications of glucocorticoid therapy, with the exception of gastritis, are *rare* in the dosage used in the treatment of Addison's disease. Complications of mineralocorticoid therapy occur more frequently and include hypokalemia, edema, hypertension, cardiac enlargement, or even congestive failure due to sodium retention. Periodic measurements of body weight, serum potassium level, and blood pressure are useful. All patients with adrenal insufficiency, including bilaterally adrenalectomized patients, should carry medical identification, should be instructed in the parenteral self-administration of steroids, and should be registered with a medical alerting system.

Special therapeutic problems During periods of intercurrent illness, the dose of cortisone or cortisol should be increased to 75 to 150 mg/d. When oral administration is not possible, parenteral routes should be employed. Likewise, before surgery or dental extractions, supplemental glucocorticoids should be administered. Patients also should be advised to increase the dose of fludrocortisone and to add salt to their otherwise normal diet during periods of excessive exercise with sweating, during extremely hot weather, and with gastrointestinal upsets. For a representative program of steroid therapy for the patient with adrenal insufficiency who is undergoing a major operation, see Table 335-11. This schedule is designed to mimic on the day of surgery the output of cortisol in normal individuals undergoing prolonged major stress (10 mg/h, 250 to 300 mg/d). Thereafter, if the patient is progressing well and is afebrile, the dose of cortisol is tapered by 20 to 30 percent daily. Parenteral mineralocorticoid administration is unnecessary at cortisol doses greater than 100 mg/d because of the mineralocorticoid effects of cortisol at such dosages.

SECONDARY ADRENOCORTICAL INSUFFICIENCY Pituitary ACTH deficiency causes *secondary* adrenocortical insufficiency. ACTH deficiency may be selective, as is seen following prolonged administration of excess glucocorticoids, or may occur in association with multiple pituitary tropic hormone deficiencies (panhypopituitar-

TABLE 335-11 Steroid therapy schedule for Addisonian patient undergoing a major operation*

	Cortisol infusion, continuous, mg/h	Cortisol (orally)		Fludro-cortisone (orally), 8 A.M.
		8 A.M.	4 P.M.	
Routine daily medication		20	10	0.1
Day before operation		20	10	0.1
Day of operation	10			
Postoperative:				
Day 1	5–7.5			
Day 2	2.5–5			
Day 3	2.5–5 *or*	40	20	0.1
Day 4	2.5–5 *or*	40	20	0.1
Day 5		40	20	0.1
Day 6		20	20	0.1
Day 7		20	10	0.1

* All steroid doses are given in milligrams. An alternative approach is to give cortisol as an IV bolus every 6 h on the day of operation (see text).

ism) (see Chap. 331). Patients with secondary adrenocortical hypofunction may have many symptoms and signs in common with Addisonian patients but are *characteristically not hyperpigmented*, since ACTH and related peptide levels are low. In fact, plasma ACTH levels distinguish between primary and secondary adrenal insufficiency, since they are elevated in the former and decreased to absent in the latter. Patients with total pituitary insufficiency also have manifestations of multiple hormone deficiencies. An additional feature distinguishing primary from secondary adrenocortical insufficiency is the *near-normal level of aldosterone secretion* seen in the presence of pituitary and/or isolated ACTH deficiencies (see Fig. 335-11). Patients with pituitary insufficiency may present with hyponatremia, which may be dilutional or secondary to subnormal increments in aldosterone secretion in response to severe sodium restriction. However, severe *dehydration, hyponatremia*, and *hyperkalemia* are characteristic of severe mineralocorticoid insufficiency and favor a diagnosis of primary adrenocortical insufficiency.

Patients receiving long-term steroid therapy, despite physical findings of Cushing's syndrome, develop adrenal insufficiency because of prolonged pituitary-hypothalamic suppression and adrenal atrophy secondary to the loss of endogenous ACTH. These patients have two deficits, a loss of adrenal responsiveness to ACTH and a failure of pituitary ACTH release. They are characterized by low blood cortisol and ACTH levels, low baseline steroid excretion, and abnormal ACTH and metyrapone responses. Most patients with steroid-induced adrenal insufficiency eventually recover normal hypothalamic-pituitary-adrenal responsiveness, but response time varies from days to months. The rapid ACTH test is a convenient assessment of recovery of hypothalamic-pituitary-adrenal function. Since the plasma cortisol concentrations after injection of cosyntropin and during insulin-induced hypoglycemia usually correlate closely, the rapid ACTH test assesses the integrated hypothalamic-pituitary-adrenal function (see "Tests of Pituitary-Adrenal Responsiveness," above). Additional testing to assess endogenous pituitary ACTH reserve includes the standard metyrapone and the insulin tolerance tests.

Glucocorticoid therapy in patients with secondary adrenocortical insufficiency does not differ from that for the primary disorder. Mineralocorticoid therapy is usually not necessary, since aldosterone secretion is preserved.

ACUTE ADRENOCORTICAL INSUFFICIENCY Acute adrenocortical insufficiency may result from several processes. Adrenal crisis is a rapid and overwhelming intensification of chronic adrenal insufficiency, usually precipitated by sepsis or surgical stress. Another involves an acute hemorrhagic destruction of both adrenal glands. In children this is usually associated with septicemia with *Pseudomonas* or meningococcemia (Waterhouse-Friderichsen syndrome). In adults, anticoagulant therapy or a coagulation disorder may result in bilateral adrenal hemorrhage. Occasionally, bilateral adrenal hemorrhage in the newborn results from birth trauma. Hemorrhage has been observed during pregnancy, following idiopathic adrenal vein thrombosis, and as a complication of venography (e.g., infarction of an adenoma). A third, and probably the most frequent, cause of acute insufficiency results from the rapid withdrawal of steroids from patients with adrenal atrophy secondary to chronic steroid administration. Acute adrenocortical insufficiency also may occur in patients with congenital adrenal hyperplasia or those with decreased adrenocortical reserve when they are given drugs capable of inhibiting steroid synthesis (mitotane, ketoconazole) or increasing steroid metabolism (phenytoin, rifampin).

Adrenal crisis The long-term survival of patients with adrenocortical insufficiency largely depends on prevention and treatment of adrenal crisis. Consequently, the occurrence of infection, trauma (including surgery), gastrointestinal upsets, or other stress requires an immediate increase in hormone. In untreated patients, preexisting symptoms are intensified. Nausea, vomiting, and abdominal pain may become intractable. Fever may be severe or absent. Lethargy deepens into somnolence, and hypovolemic vascular collapse ensues. In contrast, patients previously maintained on chronic glucocorticoid therapy may not exhibit dehydration or hypotension until preterminally, since mineralocorticoid secretion is usually preserved. In all patients in crisis, a precipitating cause should be sought.

Treatment is primarily directed toward the repletion of circulating glucocorticoids and the replacement of the sodium and water deficits. Hence an intravenous infusion of 5% glucose in normal saline solution should be started with a bolus intravenous infusion of 100 mg cortisol followed by a continuous infusion of cortisol at a rate of 10 mg/h. An alternative approach is to administer a 100-mg bolus of cortisol intravenously every 6 h. However, only the continuous infusion maintains the plasma cortisol constantly at stress levels [>830 nmol/L (30 μg/dL)]. Effective treatment of hypotension consists of glucocorticoid replacement and aggressive repletion of sodium and water deficits. If the crisis was preceded by prolonged nausea, vomiting, and dehydration, several liters of saline solution may be required within the first few hours. Vasoconstrictive agents (such as dopamine) may be indicated in extreme conditions as adjuncts to volume replacement. With large doses of steroid, e.g., 100 to 200 mg cortisol, the patient receives a maximal mineralocorticoid effect, and supplementary mineralocorticoid is superfluous. Following improvement, the steroid dosage is tapered over the next few days to maintenance levels, and mineralocorticoid therapy is reinstituted if needed (see Table 335-11).

HYPOALDOSTERONISM

Isolated aldosterone deficiency accompanied by normal cortisol production occurs in association with hyporeninism, as an inherited biosynthetic defect, postoperatively following removal of aldosterone-secreting adenomas, during protracted heparin or heparinoid administration, in pretectal disease of the nervous system, and in severe postural hypotension.

The feature common to all patients with hypoaldosteronism is the inability to increase aldosterone secretion appropriately during salt restriction. Most patients have unexplained hyperkalemia often exacerbated by restriction of dietary sodium intake. In severe cases, urine sodium wastage occurs on a normal salt intake, whereas in milder forms, excessive losses of urine sodium occur only during salt restriction.

Most cases of isolated hypoaldosteronism occur in patients with a deficiency in renin production (so-called hyporeninemic hypoaldosteronism). This syndrome is seen most commonly in adults with mild renal failure and diabetes mellitus in association with hyperkalemia and metabolic acidosis out of proportion to the state of renal impairment. Plasma renin levels fail to rise normally following sodium restriction and postural changes. The pathogenesis is uncertain. Possibilities include renal disease (most likely), autonomic neuropa

thy, extracellular fluid volume expansion, and a defect in conversion of renin precursors to active renin. Aldosterone levels also fail to rise normally following salt restriction and volume contraction; this is probably related to the hyporeninism, since biosynthetic defects in aldosterone secretion cannot usually be demonstrated. In these patients, aldosterone secretion increases promptly following ACTH stimulation, but it is uncertain whether the magnitude of the response is normal. On the other hand, the level of aldosterone appears to be subnormal in relationship to the hyperkalemia.

Hypoaldosteronism also can be associated with high renin levels. In many of these subjects, there is an inability to transform the C-18 methyl group of corticosterone to the C-18 aldehyde of aldosterone probably due to a defect in corticosterone methyloxidase. These patients have low to absent aldosterone secretion, elevated plasma renin levels, and elevated values for the intermediates of aldosterone biosynthesis (corticosterone and 18-hydroxycorticosterone). Severely ill patients also may have hyperreninemic hypoaldosteronism. Patients with this syndrome have a high mortality rate (80 percent). Hyperkalemia is not part of this syndrome. Possible explanations for the hypoaldosteronism include adrenal necrosis (uncommon) or a shift in steroidogenesis from mineralocorticoids to glucocorticoids, possibly related to prolonged ACTH stimulation.

Before considering the diagnosis of isolated hypoaldosteronism in a patient with hyperkalemia, "pseudohyperkalemia" (e.g., hemolysis, thrombocytosis) should be excluded by measuring the plasma potassium level. The next step is to demonstrate a normal cortisol response to ACTH stimulation. Then stimulated (upright posture, sodium restriction) renin and aldosterone levels should be measured. Low renin–low aldosterone levels establish a diagnosis of hyporeninemic hypoaldosteronism. High renin–low aldosterone levels are consistent with an aldosterone biosynthetic defect or a selective unresponsiveness to angiotensin II. Finally, elevated renin and aldosterone levels suggest primary renal unresponsiveness to aldosterone, so-called pseudohypoaldosteronism.

The treatment of isolated hypoaldosteronism is to replace the mineralocorticoid deficiency. For practical purposes, the oral administration of 0.05 to 0.15 mg fludrocortisone daily should restore electrolyte balance if salt intake is adequate (e.g., 150 to 200 mmol/d). However, patients with hyporeninemic hypoaldosteronism usually require higher doses of mineralocorticoid to correct the hyperkalemia. This poses a risk in patients with hypertension and mild renal insufficiency and/or congestive heart failure. Therefore, an alternative approach is to administer furosemide, which can ameliorate acidosis and hyperkalemia, and reduce the salt intake. Occasionally, a combination of these two approaches is efficacious.

NONSPECIFIC CLINICAL USE OF ADRENAL STEROIDS

The widespread utilization of glucocorticoids emphasizes the need for a thorough understanding of the metabolic effects of these agents. Before instituting adrenal hormone therapy, the expected gains should be weighed against the undesirable actions.

HOW SERIOUS IS THE DISORDER? In a patient with unexplained shock or in whom other measures have failed, the physician need not hesitate to employ large-dosage steroid therapy. In contrast, one should exercise restraint in administering steroids to a patient with early rheumatoid arthritis who has not been tried on physiotherapy, analgesics, and general medical care.

HOW LONG WILL GLUCOCORTICOID THERAPY BE REQUIRED? The use of intravenous steroids for a period of 24 to 48 h for life-threatening situations such as status asthmaticus or pseudotumor cerebri has little or no contraindication, in contrast to the initiation of chronic steroid therapy for asthma, arthritis, or psoriasis. In the latter instances, the almost certain development of Cushing's syndrome of some degree must be weighed against the potential benefit. These side effects should be minimized by a careful

SPEISER PW et al: Disease expression and molecular genotype in congenital adrenal hyperplasia due to 21-hydroxylase deficiency. J Clin Invest 90:584, 1992

STEWART PM et al: Mineralocorticoid activity of liquorice: 11-Beta-hydroxysteroid dehydrogenase deficiency comes of age. Lancet 2:821, 1987

——— et al: Syndrome of apparent mineralocorticoid excess. A defect in the cortisol-cortisone shuttle. J Clin Invest 82:340, 1988

STRAUSS KW: Endocrine complications of the acquired immunodeficiency syndrome. Arch Intern Med 151:1441, 1991

SUDA T et al: Effects of corticotropin-releasing hormone and dexamethasone on proopiomelanocortin messenger RNA level in human corticotroph adenoma cells in vitro. J Clin Invest 82:110, 1988

ULICK S: Two uncommon causes of mineralocorticoid excess: Syndrome of apparent mineralocorticoid excess and glucocorticoid-remediable aldosteronism. Endocrinol Metab Clin North Am 20:269, 1991

——— et al: Defective ring A reduction of cortisol as the major metabolic error in the syndrome of apparent mineralocorticoid excess. J Clin Endocrinol Metab 74:593, 1992

WILLIAMS GH, DLUHY RG: Diagnostic imaging of the adrenal gland, in *Endocrinology*, 2d ed, LG DeGroot et al (eds). Orlando, Grune & Stratton 1989, p 1633

WULFRATT NM et al: Immunoglobulins of patients with Cushing's syndrome due to pigmented adrenocortical micronodular dysplasia stimulate in vitro steroidogenesis. J Clin Endocrinol Metab 66:301, 1988

336 PHEOCHROMOCYTOMA

LEWIS LANDSBERG / JAMES B. YOUNG

Pheochromocytomas produce, store, and secrete catecholamines. They are usually derived from the adrenal medulla but may develop from chromaffin cells in or about sympathetic ganglia (extraadrenal pheochromocytomas or paragangliomas). Related tumors that secrete catecholamines and produce similar clinical syndromes include chemodectomas derived from the carotid body and ganglioneuromas derived from the postganglionic sympathetic neurons.

The clinical features and morbidity of these tumors are due predominantly to the release of catecholamines. Hypertension is the most common manifestation, and hypertensive paroxysms or crises, often spectacular and alarming, occur in over half the cases.

Pheochromocytoma occurs in approximately 0.1 percent of the hypertensive population but is, nevertheless, an important correctable cause of high blood pressure. Indeed, it is usually curable if properly diagnosed and treated but may be fatal if undiagnosed or mistreated. Postmortem series indicate that the majority of pheochromocytomas are unsuspected clinically even when the tumor is related to the fatal outcome.

PATHOLOGY Location and morphology In adults, approximately 80 percent are unilateral and solitary, 10 percent are bilateral, and 10 percent are extraadrenal. In children, a fourth of tumors are bilateral, and an additional fourth are extraadrenal. Solitary lesions inexplicably favor the right side. Although pheochromocytomas may grow to large size (over 3 kg), most weigh less than 100 g and are less than 10 cm in diameter. The tumors are highly vascular.

The tumors are made up of large, polyhedral, pleomorphic chromaffin cells. Less than 10 percent are malignant. As with other endocrine tumors, malignancy cannot be determined by the histologic appearance; local invasion of surrounding tissues or distant metastases indicate malignancy.

FAMILIAL PHEOCHROMOCYTOMA In approximately 5 percent of cases, pheochromocytoma is inherited as an autosomal dominant trait either alone or in combination with other abnormalities such as multiple endocrine neoplasia (MEN) type 2a (Sipple's syndrome) or type 2b (mucosal neuroma syndrome) (see Chap. 343), von Recklinghausen's neurofibromatosis, or von Hippel–Lindau's retinal cerebellar hemangioblastomatosis. Bilateral adrenal pheochromocytomas are common in the familial syndromes; within MEN kindreds, over half of pheochromocytomas are bilateral. A familial syndrome should be suspected in any patient with bilateral pheochromocytomas.

EXTRAADRENAL PHEOCHROMOCYTOMAS Extraadrenal pheochromocytomas usually weigh 20 to 40 g and are less than 5 cm in diameter. Most are located within the abdomen in association with the celiac, superior mesenteric, and inferior mesenteric ganglia. Approximately 1 percent are in the thorax, 1 percent are within the urinary bladder, and less than 1 percent are in the neck, usually in association with the sympathetic ganglia or the extracranial branches of the ninth or tenth cranial nerves.

Catecholamine synthesis, storage, and release Pheochromocytomas synthesize and store catecholamines by processes resembling those of the normal adrenal medulla (Chap. 68). Little is known about the mechanisms of catecholamine release from pheochromocytomas, but changes in blood flow and necrosis within the tumor may be the cause in some instances. These tumors are not innervated, and catecholamine release does not result from neural stimulation. Pheochromocytomas also store and secrete a variety of peptides, including endogenous opioids, neuropeptide Y, and chromagranin A (see Chap. 68). These peptides may contribute to the clinical manifestations in selected cases, as noted below.

EPINEPHRINE, NOREPINEPHRINE, AND DOPAMINE Most pheochromocytomas contain and secrete both norepinephrine and epinephrine, and the percentage of norepinephrine is usually greater than in the normal adrenal. Most extraadrenal pheochromocytomas secrete norepinephrine exclusively. Rarely, pheochromocytomas produce epinephrine alone, particularly in association with MEN. Although epinephrine-producing tumors may cause a preponderance of metabolic and beta-receptor effects, in general the major catecholamine secreted cannot be predicted from the clinical presentation. Increased production of dopamine and homovanillic acid (HVA) is uncommon with benign lesions but may occur with malignant pheochromocytoma.

CLINICAL FEATURES Pheochromocytoma occurs at all ages but is most common in young to midadult life. Some series show a slight female preponderance. Most patients come to medical attention as a result of hypertensive crisis, paroxysmal symptoms suggestive of seizure disorder or anxiety attacks, or hypertension that responds poorly to conventional treatment. Less commonly, unexplained hypotension or shock in association with surgery or trauma will suggest the diagnosis. Most have hypertension in association with headaches, excessive sweating, and/or palpitations.

Hypertension Hypertension is the most common manifestation. In approximately 60 percent of cases the hypertension is sustained, although significant blood pressure lability is usually present, and half of patients with sustained hypertension have distinct crises or paroxysms. The other 40 percent have blood pressure elevations only during an attack. The hypertension is often severe, occasionally malignant, and may be resistant to treatment with standard antihypertensive drugs.

Paroxysms or crises The paroxysm or crisis occurs in over half of patients. In an individual patient the symptoms are often similar with each attack. The paroxysms may be frequent or sporadic, at intervals as long as weeks or months. With time, the paroxysms usually increase in frequency, duration, and severity.

The attack usually has a sudden onset. It may last from a few minutes to several hours or longer. Headache, profuse sweating, palpitations, and apprehension, often with a sense of impending doom, are common. Pain in the chest or abdomen may be associated with nausea and vomiting. Either pallor or flushing may occur during the attack. The blood pressure is elevated, often to alarming levels, and is usually accompanied by tachycardia.

The paroxysm may be precipitated by any activity that displaces the abdominal contents. In some cases a particular stimulus may induce an attack in a characteristic fashion, but in others no clearly defined precipitating event can be found. Although anxiety may accompany the attacks, mental or psychological stress does not usually provoke a crisis.

Other distinctive clinical features Symptoms and signs of an increased metabolic rate, such as profuse sweating and mild to moderate weight loss, are common. Orthostatic hypotension is a consequence of diminished plasma volume and blunted sympathetic reflexes. Both these factors predispose the patient with unsuspected pheochromocytoma to hypotension or shock during surgery or trauma.

CARDIAC MANIFESTATIONS Sinus tachycardia, sinus bradycardia, supraventricular arrhythmias, and ventricular premature contractions all have been noted. Angina and acute myocardial infarction may occur even in the absence of coronary artery disease. Catecholamine-induced increase in myocardial oxygen consumption and, perhaps, coronary spasm may play a role in these ischemic events. Electrocardiographic changes, including nonspecific ST-T wave changes, prominent U waves, left ventricular strain patterns, and right and left bundle branch blocks may be present in the absence of demonstrable ischemia or infarction. Cardiomyopathy, either congestive with myocarditis and myocardial fibrosis or hypertrophic with concentric or asymmetric hypertrophy, may be associated with heart failure and cardiac arrhythmias. Noncardiogenic pulmonary edema may be due to either shifts in extracellular fluid, altered pulmonary capillary permeability, or increased pulmonary venous tone.

CARBOHYDRATE INTOLERANCE Over half of patients have impaired carbohydrate tolerance due to suppression of insulin and stimulation of hepatic glucose output. The impaired glucose tolerance rarely requires treatment with insulin and disappears after removal of the tumor.

HEMATOCRIT The elevated hematocrit is secondary to diminished plasma volume. Rarely, production of erythropoietin by the tumor may cause a true erythrocytosis.

OTHER MANIFESTATIONS Hypercalcemia has been attributed to the ectopic secretion of parathyroid hormone–related protein. Fever and an elevated sedimentation rate have been reported in association with the production of interleukin 6. Elevated temperature more commonly reflects catecholamine-mediated increases in metabolic rate and diminished heat dissipation secondary to vasoconstriction. Polyuria is an occasional finding, and rhabdomyolysis with myoglobinuric renal failure may result from extreme vasoconstriction with muscle ischemia.

PHEOCHROMOCYTOMA OF THE URINARY BLADDER Pheochromocytoma within the wall of the urinary bladder may result in typical paroxysms in relation to micturition. The location within the bladder wall is responsible for symptoms while the tumors are quite small, and consequently, catecholamine excretion may be normal or minimally elevated. Hematuria is present in over half, and the tumor can often be visualized at cystoscopy.

Adverse drug interactions Severe and occasionally fatal paroxysms have been induced by opiates, histamine, adrenocorticotropin, saralasin, and glucagon. These agents appear to release catecholamines directly from the tumor. Indirect-acting sympathomimetic amines, including methyldopa (when administered intravenously), may cause an increase in blood pressure by releasing catecholamines from the augmented stores within nerve endings. Drugs that block neuronal uptake of catecholamines, such as tricyclic antidepressants or guanethidine, may enhance the physiologic effects of circulating catecholamines. Indeed all medications should be carefully considered and cautiously administered in patients with known or suspected pheochromocytoma.

Associated diseases Pheochromocytoma is associated with medullary carcinoma of the thyroid in the MEN syndrome types 2a and 2b and with hyperparathyroidism in MEN 2a (see Chap. 343). Hypercalcemia, resolving after tumor resection, also has been described in the absence of parathyroid disease, as described above. Individuals at risk for MEN 2a and 2b should be screened periodically for pheochromocytoma by assay of a 24-h urine sample for catecholamines, including measurement of epinephrine. Pheochromocytoma should be excluded or removed before thyroid or parathyroid surgery.

The association of pheochromocytoma and neurofibromatosis is not common. Nevertheless, since incomplete forms of neurofibromatosis may be associated with pheochromocytoma, minor manifestations such as café au lait spots, vertebral abnormalities, or kyphoscoliosis should increase the suspicion of pheochromocytoma in a patient with hypertension. The incidence of pheochromocytoma in some

kindreds with von Hippel–Lindau disease may be as high as 10 to 25 percent. Many of these are unsuspected clinically and diagnosed postmortem.

The incidence of cholelithiasis is 15 to 20 percent. Cushing's syndrome is a rare association, usually a consequence of ectopic secretion of ACTH by the pheochromocytoma or, less commonly, by a coexistent medullary carcinoma of the thyroid.

DIAGNOSIS The diagnosis is established by the demonstration of increased excretion of catecholamines or catecholamine metabolites. The diagnosis can usually be made by the analysis of a single 24-h urine sample, provided the patient is hypertensive or symptomatic at the time of collection.

Biochemical tests The assays employed include vanillylmandelic acid (VMA), the metanephrines, and unconjugated or "free" catecholamines (Chap. 68). Although much has been written about the relative specificity and sensitivity of the different assays, they are probably equivalent provided they are properly performed. Accuracy of diagnosis is improved when two of the three determinations are employed, although this is not essential as a screening procedure. The following considerations apply to all the urinary tests: (1) Despite claims for the adequacy of determinations made on random urine samples, analysis of a full 24-h urine sample is preferable. Creatinine should be determined as well to assess the adequacy of collection. (2) Where possible, the collection should be made when the patient is at rest, on no medication, and without recent exposure to radiographic contrast media. Where it is not practical to discontinue all medications, drugs known specifically to interfere in the assays (as noted below) should be avoided. (3) The urine should be acidified and refrigerated during and after collection. (4) With high-quality assays, dietary restrictions are minimal and should be specified by the laboratory performing the analyses. (5) Although most patients with pheochromocytoma excrete increased catecholamines and catecholamine metabolites, the yield is increased in patients with paroxysmal hypertension if a 24-h urine collection is initiated during a crisis.

FREE CATECHOLAMINES The upper limit of normal for total catecholamines is between 590 and 885 nmol (100 and 150 μg) per 24 h. In most patients with pheochromocytoma, values in excess of 1480 nmol (250 μg) per day are obtained. Measurement of epinephrine is often of value, since increased epinephrine excretion [over 275 nmol (50 μg) per 24 h] is usually due to an adrenal lesion and may be the only abnormality in cases associated with MEN. False-positive increases in catecholamine excretion result from exogenous catecholamines and related drugs such as methyldopa, levodopa, labetalol, and sympathomimetic amines, which may elevate catecholamine excretion for up to 2 weeks. Endogenous catecholamines from stimulation of the sympathoadrenal system also may increase urinary catecholamine excretion. Relevant clinical situations include hypoglycemia, strenuous exertion, central nervous system disease with increased intracranial pressure, and clonidine withdrawal.

METANEPHRINES AND VMA In most laboratories, the upper limit of normal is 7 μmol (1.3 mg) of total metanephrine and 35 μmol (7.0 mg) of VMA excretion per 24 h. In most patients with pheochromocytoma, the increase in these urinary metabolites is considerable, often more than three times the normal range. Metanephrine excretion is increased by exogenous and endogenous catecholamines and by treatment with monoamine oxidase inhibitors; propranolol may cause a spurious increase in metanephrine excretion, since a propranolol metabolite interferes in the commonly utilized spectrophotometric assay. VMA is less affected by endogenous and exogenous catecholamines but is spuriously increased by a variety of drugs, including carbidopa. VMA excretion is decreased by monoamine oxidase inhibitors.

PLASMA CATECHOLAMINES Measurement of plasma catecholamines has a limited application. The care required in obtaining basal levels (Chap. 68); the lack of readily available, reliable plasma assays; and the satisfactory results with urinary determinations make measurement of plasma catecholamines unnecessary in most cases. Plasma catecholamine levels are affected by the same drugs and physiologic perturbations that increase urinary catecholamine excretion. In addition, alpha- and beta-adrenergic receptor blocking agents may elevate plasma catecholamines by impairing clearance.

When the clinical features suggest pheochromocytoma and the urinary assays are borderline, measurement of plasma catecholamines may be worthwhile. Markedly elevated basal levels of total catecholamines support the diagnosis, although approximately one-third of patients with pheochromocytoma have normal or slightly elevated basal values. The usefulness of plasma catecholamine determinations may be increased by agents that suppress sympathetic nervous system activity. Clonidine and ganglionic blocking agents (Chap. 68) reduce plasma catecholamine levels in normal subjects and in patients with essential hypertension. These drugs have little effect on catecholamine levels in patients with pheochromocytoma. In patients with elevated or borderline basal catecholamine values, failure to suppress plasma or urinary levels with clonidine supports the diagnosis of pheochromocytoma.

Pharmacologic tests   Reliable methods for the measurement of catecholamines and catecholamine metabolites in urine have rendered obsolete both the provocative and adrenolytic tests, which are nonspecific and entail considerable risk. A modified version of the adrenolytic test may be of some use, however, as a therapeutic trial in a patient in hypertensive crisis with features suggestive of pheochromocytoma. A positive response to phentolamine (5-mg bolus following a 0.5-mg test dose) is a reduction in blood pressure of at least 35/25 mmHg that becomes maximal after 2 min and persists for 10 to 15 min. The pharmacologic response is never diagnostic, and biochemical confirmation is essential. Provocative tests in normotensive patients are potentially dangerous and rarely indicated. However, a glucagon provocative test may be of use in patients with paroxysmal hypertension and nondiagnostic basal catecholamine levels. Glucagon has a negligible effect on blood pressure or plasma catecholamine levels in normal or hypertensive subjects. In patients with pheochromocytoma, on the other hand, glucagon may increase both blood pressure and circulating catecholamine levels. The elevation in plasma catecholamine concentration, moreover, may occur without a blood pressure response. It must be emphasized, however, that life-threatening pressor crises have occurred after administration of glucagon to patients with pheochromocytoma, so the test should never be performed casually. Careful continuous monitoring of the blood pressure is required, intravenous access must be adequate, and phentolamine must be at hand to terminate the test if a significant pressor reaction ensues.

Differential diagnosis   Since the manifestations may be protean, the diagnosis must be considered and excluded in many patients with suggestive clinical features. In patients with essential hypertension and "hyperadrenergic" features such as tachycardia, sweating, and increased cardiac output, and in patients with anxiety attacks associated with blood pressure elevations, analysis of a 24-h urine collection is usually decisive in excluding the diagnosis. Repeated determinations on urine collected during attacks may be necessary, however, before the diagnosis can be excluded with certainty. The clonidine suppression and glucagon stimulation tests may be helpful in excluding the diagnosis in difficult cases. Pressor crises associated with clonidine withdrawal or the use of monoamine oxidase inhibitors (Chap. 68) may mimic the paroxysms of pheochromocytoma. Factitious crises may be produced by self-administration of sympathomimetic amines in psychiatrically disturbed patients.

Intracranial lesions, particularly posterior fossa tumors or subarachnoid hemorrhage, may cause hypertension and increased excretion of catecholamines or catecholamine metabolites. While this is most common in patients with an obvious neurologic catastrophe, the possibility of subarachnoid or intracranial hemorrhage secondary to pheochromocytoma should be considered. Diencephalic or autonomic epilepsy may be associated with paroxysmal spells, hypertension, and increased plasma catecholamine levels. This rare entity may be difficult to distinguish from pheochromocytoma, but an aura, an abnormal electroencephalogram, and a beneficial response to anticonvulsant medications will often suggest the proper diagnosis.

MANAGEMENT   Preoperative management   The induction of stable alpha-adrenergic blockade is the basis of preoperative management and provides the foundation for successful surgical treatment. Once the diagnosis is established, the patient should be placed on phenoxybenzamine to induce a long-lived, noncompetitive alpha-receptor blockade. The usual initial dose is 10 mg every 12 h with increments of 10 to 20 mg added every few days until the blood pressure is controlled and the paroxysms disappear. Because of the long duration of action, the therapeutic effects are cumulative, and the optimal dose must be achieved gradually with careful monitoring of supine and upright blood pressures. Most patients require between 40 and 80 mg phenoxybenzamine per day, although 200 mg or more may be necessary. Phenoxybenzamine should be administered for at least 10 to 14 days prior to surgery. Over this time, the combination of alpha-receptor blockade and a liberal salt intake will restore the contracted plasma volume to normal. Before adequate alpha-adrenergic blockade with phenoxybenzamine is achieved, paroxysms may be treated with intravenous phentolamine. Prazosin, the selective $alpha_1$ antagonist, has been employed in the preoperative management of a small number of patients. Doses in the range of 1.5 to 2.5 mg every 6 h have effectively controlled blood pressure and paroxysms. The role of this and other longer-acting selective $alpha_1$ antagonists in the management of pheochromocytoma has not been established. They may be useful as antihypertensive agents in patients with suspected pheochromocytoma while workup is in progress, since they are usually better tolerated than phenoxybenzamine and will prevent serious pressor crises if pheochromocytoma is present. Nitroprusside, calcium channel blocking agents, and possibly angiotensin-converting enzyme inhibitors reduce blood pressure in patients with pheochromocytoma. Nitroprusside may be useful on occasion in the treatment of pressor crises.

Beta-adrenergic receptor blocking agents should be given only after alpha blockade has been induced, since administration of such agents by themselves may cause a paradoxic increase in blood pressure by antagonizing beta-mediated vasodilatation in skeletal muscle. Beta blockade is usually initiated when tachycardia develops during the induction of alpha-adrenergic blockade. Low doses often suffice, and a reasonable starting dose is 10 mg propranolol 3 to 4 times per day, increased as needed to control the pulse rate. Beta blockade is effective for catecholamine-induced arrhythmias, particularly those potentiated by anesthetic agents.

Preoperative localization of the tumor   Surgical removal of pheochromocytoma is facilitated if the location of the tumor or tumors can be established preoperatively. Once pheochromocytoma is diagnosed, localization should be undertaken while the patient is being prepared for surgery. Computed tomography (CT) or magnetic resonance imaging of the adrenals is usually successful in identifying intraadrenal lesions. Conventional roentgenograms and CT of the chest usually suffice to identify intrathoracic lesions. If these studies are negative, abdominal aortography (once alpha-adrenergic blockade is complete) may identify extraadrenal pheochromocytomas within the abdomen, since these lesions are often supplied by a large aberrant artery. If aortography and CT fail to localize the lesion, venous sampling at different levels of the inferior and superior vena cava may reveal catecholamine gradients in the region drained by the tumor; this area may then be restudied by selective angiography or scanning by CT. An additional localization technique involves a radionuclide scintiscan after administration of an investigational radiopharmaceutical [131I]metaiodobenzylguanidine (MIBG). This agent is concentrated by the amine uptake process and produces an external scintigraphic image at the site of the tumor. This type of scanning may be useful in characterizing lesions discovered by CT when biochemical confirmation is indeterminate, as well as in localizing extraadrenal pheochromocytomas. Percutaneous fine-needle aspiration of chromaffin tumors is contraindicated; indeed, pheochromocytoma should be considered before adrenal lesions are aspirated.

Surgery Surgery is best performed in centers with experience in the preoperative, anesthetic, and intraoperative management of pheochromocytoma. In experienced hands, surgical mortality is 2 or 3 percent.

Monitoring during the surgical procedure should include continuous recording of arterial pressure, central venous pressure, and electrocardiogram; in the presence of cardiac disease or if congestive failure has been present, pulmonary capillary wedge pressure should be monitored. Adequate fluid replacement is crucial. Intraoperative hypotension responds better to volume replacement than to vasoconstrictors. Hypertension and cardiac arrhythmias are most likely during induction of anesthesia, intubation, and manipulation of the tumor. Intravenous phentolamine is usually sufficient to control the blood pressure, but nitroprusside may be required. Propranolol may be given in the treatment of tachycardia or ventricular ectopy.

PHEOCHROMOCYTOMA IN PREGNANCY Spontaneous labor and vaginal delivery in unprepared patients are usually disastrous for mother and fetus. In early pregnancy, the patient should be prepared with phenoxybenzamine, and the tumor should be removed as soon as the diagnosis is confirmed. The pregnancy need not be terminated, but the operative procedure itself may result in spontaneous abortion. In the third trimester, treatment with adrenergic blocking agents should be undertaken; when the fetus is of sufficient size, cesarean section may be followed by extirpation of the tumor. Although the safety of adrenergic blocking drugs in pregnancy is not established, these agents have been administered in several cases without obvious adverse effect.

UNRESECTABLE AND MALIGNANT TUMORS In cases of metastatic or locally invasive tumor or in patients with intercurrent illness that precludes surgery, long-term medical management is required. When the manifestations cannot be adequately controlled by adrenergic blocking agents, the concomitant administration of metyrosine may be required. This agent inhibits tyrosine hydroxylase, diminishes catecholamine production by the tumor, and often simplifies chronic management. Malignant pheochromocytoma frequently recurs in the retroperitoneum and metastasizes most commonly to bone and lung. Although these are resistant to radiotherapy, combination chemotherapy has had limited success in malignant tumors. [131I]metaiodobenzylguanidine (MIBG) has had limited success in the treatment of malignant pheochromocytoma.

PROGNOSIS AND FOLLOW-UP The 5-year survival after surgery is usually over 95 percent, and the recurrence rate is less than 10 percent. After successful surgery, catecholamine excretion returns to normal in about 1 week and should be measured to ensure complete tumor removal. Catecholamine excretion should be assessed at the reappearance of suggestive symptoms or yearly for several years, if the patient remains asymptomatic. In malignant pheochromocytoma, the 5-year survival is less than 50 percent.

Complete removal cures the hypertension in approximately three-fourths. In the remainder, hypertension recurs but is usually well controlled by standard antihypertensive agents. In this group, either underlying essential hypertension or irreversible vascular damage induced by catecholamines may cause the persistence of the hypertension.

REFERENCES

AVERBUCH SD et al: Malignant pheochromocytoma: Effective treatment with a combination of cyclophosphamide, vincristine, and dacarbazine. Ann Intern Med 109:267, 1988

BRAVO EL, GIFFORD RW: Pheochromocytoma: Diagnosis, localization, and management. N Engl J Med 311:1298, 1984

BROWN MJ et al: Increased sensitivity and accuracy of phaeochromocytoma diagnosis achieved by use of plasma-adrenaline estimations and a pentolinium-suppression test. Lancet 1:174, 1981

DALY PA, LANDSBERG L: Pheochromocytoma: Diagnosis and management. Baillieres Clin Endocrinol Metab 6:143, 1992

DUNCAN MW et al: Measurement of norepinephrine and 3,4-dihydroxyphenylglycol in urine and plasma for the diagnosis of pheochromocytoma. N Engl J Med 319:136, 1988

FUDGE TL et al: Current surgical management of pheochromocytoma during pregnancy. Arch Surg 115:1224, 1980

FUKUMOTO S et al: Pheochromocytoma with pyrexia and marked inflammatory signs: A paraneoplastic syndrome with possible relation to interleukin-6 production. J Clin Endocrinol Metab 73:877, 1991

GLUSHIEN AS et al: Pheochromocytoma: Its relationship to the neurocutaneous syndromes. Am J Med 14:318, 1953

HAMILTON BP et al: Measurement of urinary epinephrine in screening for pheochromocytoma in multiple endocrine neoplasia type II. Am J Med 65:1027, 1978

HORTON WA et al: Von Hippel-Lindau disease: Clinical and pathological manifestations in nine families with 50 affected members. Arch Intern Med 136:769, 1976

JONES DH et al: The biochemical diagnosis, localization and followup of phaeochromocytoma: The role of plasma and urinary catecholamine measurements. Q J Med 49:431, 1980

KHAIRI MRA et al: Mucosal neuroma, pheochromocytoma and medullary thyroid carcinoma: Multiple endocrine neoplasia type 3. Medicine 54:89, 1975

KREMPF M et al: Use of m-(131I) iodobenzylguanidine in the treatment of malignant pheochromocytoma. J Clin Endocrinol Metab 72:455, 1991

LAURSEN K, DAMGAARD-PEDERSON K: CT for pheochromocytoma diagnosis. AJR 134:277, 1980

MACDOUGALL IC et al: Overnight clonidine suppression test in the diagnosis and exclusion of pheochromocytoma. Am J Med 84:993, 1988

MANGER WM, GIFFORD RW JR: *Pheochromocytoma*. New York, Springer-Verlag, 1977

MCCORKELL SJ, NILES NL: Fine-needle aspiration of catecholamine-producing adrenal masses: A possibly fatal mistake. Am J Roentgenol 145:113, 1985

PALUBINSKAS AJ et al: Localization of functioning pheochromocytomas by venous sampling and radioenzymatic analysis. Radiology 136:495, 1980

REINIG JW, DOPPMAN JL: Magnetic resonance imaging of the adrenal. Radiologe 26:186, 1986

ROSS EJ et al: Preoperative and operative management of patients with pheochromocytoma. Br Med J 1:191, 1971

ST JOHN WM, GIFFORD RW JR: Prevalence of clinically unsuspected pheochromocytoma. Mayo Clin Proc 56:354, 1981

SHEMIN D et al: Pheochromocytoma presenting as rhabdomyolysis and acute mycoglobinuric renal failure. Arch Intern Med 150:2384, 1990

SISSON JC et al: Scintigraphic localization of pheochromocytoma. N Engl J Med 305:12, 1981

SJOERDSMA A et al: Pheochromocytoma: Current concepts of diagnosis and treatment. Ann Intern Med 65:1302, 1966

STEINER AL et al: Study of a kindred with pheochromocytoma, medullary thyroid carcinoma, hyperparathyroidism and Cushing's disease: Multiple endocrine neoplasia, type 2. Medicine 47:371, 1968

STEWART AF et al: Hypercalcemia in pheochromocytoma. Ann Intern Med 102:776, 1985

337 DIABETES MELLITUS

DANIEL W. FOSTER

Diabetes mellitus is the most common endocrine disease. The true frequency is difficult to ascertain because of differing standards of diagnosis but probably is between 1 and 2 percent if fasting hyperglycemia is the criterion for diagnosis. The disease is characterized by metabolic abnormalities and by long-term complications involving the eyes, kidneys, nerves, and blood vessels. The patient population is not homogeneous, and several distinct diabetic syndromes have been delineated.

DIAGNOSIS The diagnosis of symptomatic diabetes is not difficult. When a patient presents with signs and symptoms attributable to an osmotic diuresis and is found to have hyperglycemia, essentially all physicians agree that diabetes is present. There is likewise little disagreement about an asymptomatic patient with persistently elevated fasting plasma glucose concentrations. The problem arises with the asymptomatic patient who for one reason or another is considered to be a potential diabetic but has a normal fasting glucose concentration in plasma. Such patients are often given an oral glucose tolerance test, and if abnormal values are found, they are diagnosed as having impaired glucose tolerance or diabetes. There seems to be little question that normal glucose tolerance is strong evidence against the presence of diabetes; the predictive value of a positive test is less

FIGURE 337-1 Schematic representation of the HLA D (class II) region. Gene products are determined by constituent α and β chains, each of which is encoded by a separate gene. The α chain at DR is invariant. *(From JM Baisch, JD Capra, Curr Biol 1:385, 1991, by permission.)*

are neutral. For example, HLA DQβ$_1$*0302 (which codes for one allele of the β chain of HLA DQ) is a susceptibility gene, while HLA DQβ$_1$*0301 is associated with a low risk for IDDM. HLA DQβ$_1$*0602 appears to be dominantly protective, overriding the high-risk DQβ$_1$*0302 gene when both are present. Terminology in the HLA field changes rapidly. DQβ$_1$*0301 was formerly known as DQw7 or DQw3.1, DQβ$_1$*0302 was previously known as DQw8 or DQw3.2, and DQβ$_1$*0602 was known as DQw1.2.

How might differing HLA alleles function in predisposition to or protection from IDDM? Probably by exhibiting varying affinity for diabetogenic peptides to be presented to the immune system. Thus HLA DQβ$_1$*0302 might bind a diabetogenic peptide with greater affinity for presentation on the cell surface than DQβ$_1$*0301. Conversely, a dominant protective allele (which presumably would not present antigen in such a way as to activate the immune system) might bind the diabetogenic peptide with such high affinity as to effectively "steal it" from a susceptibility gene even when both are present, thereby preventing the disease. Although the DQβ chain alleles appear to predict risk for diabetes most precisely, they may well be influenced by interaction with α chains. Thus T cell recognition of a DQβ$_1$*0302 is modified by the associated DQα allele. The situation is further complicated by the fact that α and β chains from different HLA molecules may interact to form new dimers, a process called *transcomplementation*. Some authors have found that susceptibility to autoimmune diabetes is linked to decreased expression of class I HLA molecules on splenocytes and lymphocytes in NOD mice (which get autoimmune diabetes) and in humans. The meaning of this finding and its reproducibility are not clear.

While emphasis has been placed on the HLA region as a site for regulatory genes and the development of type 1 diabetes, it is likely that one or more other genes are also involved. It also has been reported that HLA associations found in children may not operate when the disease begins in adults.

Environmental event As noted earlier, the fact that a significant proportion of monozygotic twins remain discordant for diabetes (one twin with, the other without) has suggested that nongenetic factors are required for expression of diabetes in humans. Similar arguments derive from the fact that HLA identity or haploidentity does not ensure concordance.

The environmental factor in many cases is believed to be a virus capable of infecting the beta cell. A viral etiology was originally suggested by seasonal variations in the onset of the disease and what appeared to be more than a chance relationship between appearance of diabetes and preceding episodes of mumps, hepatitis, infectious mononucleosis, congenital rubella, and coxsackievirus infections. The viral hypothesis gained support from studies showing that certain strains of encephalomyocarditis virus cause diabetes in genetically susceptible mice. The isolation of a coxsackievirus B4 from the pancreas of a previously healthy boy who died following an episode of ketoacidosis and the induction of diabetes in experimental animals inoculated with the isolated virus also suggested that viruses can cause diabetes in humans. A rise in titer of neutralizing antibody to coxsackievirus over the weeks prior to death of the patient indicated that the virus was recently acquired. Further support for the viral theory comes from the observation that congenital rubella is associated

with subsequent development of IDDM in about 20 percent of affected individuals in the United States. Cytomegalovirus genes have been found in the genome of a fifth of patients with type 1 diabetes. Retroviral genes are also found consistently in the beta cells of NOD mice. Presumably viral infections of the pancreas could induce diabetes by two mechanisms: direct inflammatory disruption of islets or induction of an immune response.

Despite its attractiveness, considerable caution should be reserved for the viral theory. Serologic studies seeking evidence of recent viral infection in patients with new-onset insulin-dependent diabetes are inconclusive at best.

Great interest has been generated by reports that exposure to cow's milk or milk products early in life predisposes to autoimmune diabetes. The environmental trigger proposed is bovine albumin operating through the mechanism of molecular mimicry. In the initial study, diabetic subjects had antibodies to bovine albumin with a subset specific for a 17-amino acid epitope providing maximal association with the disease. The latter antibodies bind to a 69-kDa protein on the surface of the pancreatic beta cell. The idea would be that exposure to cow's milk induced an immune response to the 17-amino acid fragment in some infants. Cross-reactivity with the p69 antigen would destroy beta cells expressing this peptide. Not universally present on beta cells, p69 can be induced through the action of interferon-γ produced by intermittent viral infections. These results, while intriguing, have not been confirmed at the time of this writing.

Insulitis In animals, macrophages and activated T lymphocytes infiltrate the pancreatic islets prior to or simultaneously with development of diabetes. Lymphocytes are also found in the islets of young persons dying from new-onset diabetes, and radioactively labeled lymphocytes localize in the pancreas in humans with IDDM. These findings are in accord with the observation that immune endocrinopathies in general are associated with lymphocytic infiltration of the affected tissue. It is not clear, however, that insulitis is primary to the destructive sequence in autoimmune diabetes. Some workers believe the cellular infiltration to be an epiphenomenon.

Conversion of the beta cell from "self" to "nonself" and activation of the immune system There seems to be little doubt that the immune system mediates beta cell destruction in type 1 diabetes. The disease is frequently associated with other autoimmune endocrinopathies such as adrenal insufficiency and Hashimoto's thyroiditis; pancreas transplanted from a nondiabetic monozygotic twin into the diabetic twin is rapidly destroyed without evidence of rejection in the absence of immunosuppression, and temporary reversal of clinical symptoms occurs with early use of cyclosporine. Moreover, a majority of patients have antibodies directed against insulin and other beta cell antigens. Since the immune system normally does not attack "self" tissues, it is probably acceptable to define IDDM as an autoimmune disease.

The mechanism by which this occurs is not known. As noted earlier, an environmental trigger appears to be required (frequently, if not always). The putative environmental agent could be a virus, a toxin, or a food. The agent might act in one of several ways. Direct destruction of beta cells by a virus or toxin might expose cryptic antigens to the immune system, invoking an immune response. A relative deficiency of early complement components might impair clearing of islet cell viruses (analogous to persistent hepatitis B infection in some patients with chronic active hepatitis), thereby prolonging cryptic antigen stimulation of the immune system. Alternatively, the agent might form a neoantigen in association with normal membrane structures or newly expressed class II HLA molecules of the susceptibility type (see below). Another popular hypothesis is the aforementioned *molecular mimicry*, a term referring to chance homology between a foreign antigen and a short stretch of amino acids in normal tissue. The best-known example is acute rheumatic fever, where immune response to group A streptococci results in cross-reacting attack on the heart. Once cytotoxic T cells and plasma cells are activated against a particular antigenic epitope (armed), they seek and destroy any cell bearing the epitope. The bovine milk albumin hypothesis mentioned earlier invoked molecular mimicry. It is of interest that homology exists between a coxsackievirus protein and glutamic acid decarboxylase (GAD). Antibodies against GAD are common in subjects with type 1 diabetes.

A third possibility, currently less popular, is that viral infection, via cytokine release, induces HLA D-region molecules in the pancreas (where they are not normally present), converting one or more cell types into antigen-presenting cells.

It is possible that some patients may have a purely genetic form of the disease. In neonatal life, autoreactive T cells are normally destroyed in the thymus ("clonal deletion"). Any cells escaping the thymus are rendered anergic or suppressed in the periphery by regulatory T cells. Failure of either process could leave a repertoire of cells capable of responding to "self" antigens following cell injury. In support of the possibility that a contributing factor in autoimmune disease is suboptimal removal or regulation of autoreactive T cells, intrathymic injection of islets prevents diabetes in the BB rat, a species manifesting an autoimmune form of the disease. Presumably the presence of additional beta cell antigens in the thymus allows the removal of autoreactive lymphocytes capable of responding to islet tissue.

In summary, the precise mechanisms remain a mystery, but activated immune attack is believed to be the fundamental process causing IDDM.

Destruction of beta cells and development of IDDM Because persons developing insulin-dependent diabetes often have a rather abrupt onset of symptomatic hyperglycemia with polyuria and/or ketoacidosis, it was long assumed that beta cell damage occurred rapidly. It is now believed that in most cases there is a slow loss of insulin reserve over a few to many years. This insight came from studies of discordant monozygotic diabetic twins and triplets in whom one twin or triplet developed diabetes long after the index case. In the slow course the earliest sign of abnormality is the development of islet cell antibodies at a time when there is no elevation of the blood sugar and glucose tolerance is normal. Insulin responses to a glucose load are intact. A phase then ensues in which the only metabolic abnormality is decreased glucose tolerance. Fasting blood sugar remains normal. In the third stage fasting hyperglycemia develops, but ketosis does not occur even when the diabetes is poorly controlled. The clinical appearance is that of non-insulin-dependent diabetes mellitus. With time, however, insulin dependence and ketoacidosis may develop, especially with stress. Many nonobese patients with non-insulin-dependent diabetes mellitus may have a slow autoimmune form of the disease, as mentioned earlier.

The immune-directed destruction of beta cells probably involves both humoral and cell-mediated mechanisms, the latter being more important. Islet cell antibodies have different specificities. Originally, they were generically defined as cytoplasmic and surface (complement-fixing), but specific antigens have now been identified. These include insulin, proinsulin, two forms of glutamic acid decarboxylase (GAD 65 and GAD 67), carboxypeptidase H, two ganglioside antigens (GT3 and GM2-1), ICA 69 (an antibody reacting with the 69-kDa bovine albumin peptide), and antibodies directed against the glucose transporter of the beta cell (GLUT 2). The GAD 65 antibody is equivalent to the earlier described 64-kDa antibody. A subset of anti-GAD antibodies appears to react with human and rat but not mouse islets. These "restricted" islet cell antibodies appear to be linked to the protective HLA allele $DQ\beta_1*0602$ and thus may be a mark of resistance to development of diabetes rather than prediction that the disease will occur, as is usually the case.

A variety of cells appear to carry out the beta cell attack with natural killer cells, activated cytotoxic T lymphocytes (CD8), and macrophages each having a part. The final common pathway of cell destruction may be at least partially due to release of cytokines such as interleukin 1 (IL-1) and tumor necrosis factor alpha (TNFα) from activated macrophages. Experimentally, mixtures of cytokines (IL-1, TNFα, interferon-γ, and lymphotoxin) appear to act synergistically and are more potent than single agents. Purified beta cells are reported to be less sensitive to cytokine toxicity than beta cells in intact islets, suggesting that some effects may be indirect.

By the time overt diabetes appears, most insulin-producing cells have disappeared. In one study, pancreatic mass at autopsy averaged 40 g in type 1 diabetes versus 82 g in controls. Endocrine cell mass in subjects with IDDM decreased from 1395 to 413 mg, and beta cells, which averaged 850 mg in normal individuals, were unmeasurable. Since alpha cells remained essentially intact, the ratio of glucagon- to insulin-producing cells approached infinity.

PATHOGENESIS OF NON-INSULIN-DEPENDENT DIABETES Little progress has been made in understanding the pathogenesis of non-insulin-dependent diabetes mellitus.

Genetics Although the disease runs in families, modes of inheritance are not known except for the variant known as *maturity-onset diabetes of the young* (MODY). MODY is usually manifested by mild hyperglycemia in young persons who are resistant to ketosis. Four lines of evidence suggest transmission as an autosomal dominant trait. First, three-generation direct transmission has been demonstrated in over 20 families. Second, a 1:1 ratio of diabetic to nondiabetic children is found when one parent has the disease. Third, about 90 percent of obligate carriers have diabetes. Fourth, direct male-to-male transmission excludes X-linked inheritance.

Genetic studies have shown a clear linkage between MODY and mutations in the glucokinase gene located on the short arm of chromosome 7. The abnormality is not found in ordinary NIDDM. A polymorphism in the glycogen synthase gene has been reported in some patients with typical NIDDM, but its significance is not known. Glycogen synthase is an attractive candidate because glycogen synthesis is impaired in NIDDM. However, the A_2 allele presumed to mark diabetes was present in only 30 percent of the study group of 107 patients (8 percent in controls). No HLA relationships have been identified, and autoimmune mechanisms are not thought to be operative. It is highly likely that more than one gene is involved in NIDDM, but a number of candidate molecules have proved unrewarding in the search for informative mutations. These include the glucose transporter molecules GLUT 2 and GLUT 4 (which transport glucose across the plasma membrane in pancreas/liver and muscle/fat, respectively), the insulin receptor, and the amyloidogenic peptide of islets called *amylin*. Whatever its nature, the genetic influence is powerful, since the concordance rate for diabetes in monozygotic twins with type 2 disease approaches 100 percent. Risk to offspring and siblings of patients with NIDDM is higher than in type 1 diabetes. Nearly four-tenths of siblings and one-third of offspring eventually develop abnormal glucose tolerance or frank diabetes.

Pathophysiology Patients with type 2 NIDDM have two physiologic defects: abnormal insulin secretion and resistance to insulin action in target tissues. Which of the abnormalities is primary is not known. Descriptively, three phases can be recognized in the usual clinical sequence. In the first, the plasma glucose remains normal despite demonstrable insulin resistance because insulin levels are elevated. In the second phase, insulin resistance tends to worsen so that despite elevated insulin concentrations, glucose intolerance becomes manifested by postprandial hyperglycemia. In the third phase, insulin resistance does not change, but insulin secretion declines, resulting in fasting hyperglycemia and overt diabetes.

with a reference standard of defined composition such as bread. Although in principle the approach is attractive because it measures actual glycemic response to foods, its applicability to the general diabetic population is not established. One of the problems is that a glycemic index determined for a food ingested by itself may not apply in a normal mixed meal.

The importance of diet in the management of diabetes varies with type of disease. In insulin-dependent patients, particularly those on intensive insulin regimens, the composition of the diet is not of critical importance, since adjustment of insulin can cover wide variations in food ingestion. In non-insulin-dependent patients not treated with exogenous insulin, more rigorous adherence to a fixed diet is required, since endogenous insulin reserve is limited. Such patients cannot respond to increased demand produced by excess calories or increased intake of rapidly absorbed carbohydrate.

Insulin Insulin is required for treatment of all patients with IDDM and many patients with non-insulin-dependent disease. If the physician does not use oral agents (see below), all diet-unresponsive NIDDM subjects must be given the hormone. It is fairly easy to control the symptoms of diabetes with insulin, but it is difficult to maintain a normal blood sugar throughout 24 h even if one utilizes multiple injections of regular insulin or infusion pumps. In the Diabetes Control and Complications Trial (see below), where teams of health care workers attempted to return the blood glucose level to normal or near normal with much more frequent professional input than is usual in clinical situations, blood glucose levels and hemoglobin A_{1c} concentrations remained above normal in most subjects. It is even more difficult to maintain normal blood sugars utilizing traditional insulin therapy given as one or two injections a day. Nondiabetic subjects maintain the plasma glucose concentration within a narrow range at all times despite episodic food intake. When a meal is eaten, a prompt rise in insulin release occurs such that absorbed carbohydrate is rapidly transported into the liver and other tissues. Even after meals, therefore, the plasma glucose level in normal subjects does not rise into the hyperglycemic or glycosuric range. As the plasma glucose level falls under the influence of insulin, release of the hormone is damped, and counterregulatory hormones enter the circulation to prevent hypoglycemia, ensuring smooth control of plasma glucose throughout the absorptive process. The patient treated with insulin by injection cannot reproduce these physiologic responses. If enough insulin is given to keep the postprandial glucose normal, inevitably too much insulin will be present during the postabsorptive phase, and hypoglycemia will result.

No single standard exists for patterns of administration of insulin, and treatment plans vary from physician to physician and with a given physician in different patients. Three treatment regimes will be described: conventional, multiple subcutaneous injections (MSI), and continuous subcutaneous insulin infusion (CSII). MSI or CSII is required in intensive treatment schedules designed to protect against complications. *Conventional insulin therapy* involves the administration of one or two injections a day of intermediate-acting insulin such as zinc insulin (lente insulin) or isophane insulin (NPH insulin) with or without the addition of small amounts of regular insulin. If the newly diagnosed subject is not in acute distress, therapy can be started as an outpatient, provided instructions in diet, insulin use, and monitoring are adequate and the physician or nurse-clinician can be reached by telephone for consultation. Adults of normal weight may be started on 15 to 20 units a day (the estimated daily insulin production rate in nondiabetic subjects of normal size is about 25 units a day). Obese patients, because of insulin resistance, may be started on 25 to 30 units a day. It is preferable to use the same quantity of insulin for several days before changing, the one exception being the hypoglycemic patient, for whom the dose should be decreased immediately unless a nonrecurrent cause of hypoglycemia (such as excessive exercise) is present. Generally, changes should be no more than 5 or 10 units per step. It is probable that a single injection of insulin provides adequate control only in patients who have some residual capacity for insulin secretion. Poorly controlled

TABLE 337-6 Adjusting insulin dosage in conventional insulin therapy*

Blood glucose		Regular insulin, units	
mmol/L	mg/dL	Breakfast (to be mixed with intermediate dosage)	Supper
2.8–5.5	51–100	8	4
5.6–8.3	101–150	10	5
8.4–11.1	151–200	12	6
11.2–13.9	201–250	14	7
14.0–16.6	251–300	16	8
>16.6	>300	20	10

* Once the patient has most blood sugars in the reasonable range, a prescription can be written for varying the regular insulin dosage as illustrated. The prescription in this case was for a patient in reasonable control on 25 units of NPH plus 10 units of regular before breakfast and 10 units of NPH plus 5 units of regular before supper. Change in metabolic status may require adjustments in both intermediate insulin and the sliding scale of regular insulin.

patients should be placed on split therapy, with about two-thirds of the total insulin given before breakfast and the remainder before supper. Two injections are almost always used when the total dose reaches 50 or 60 units a day but are helpful at smaller doses as well, since the peak action of intermediate insulins appears to be dose-related; i.e., a low dose may exhibit maximal activity earlier and disappear sooner than a large dose. Many physicians routinely add regular insulin to the intermediate dose even at initiation of therapy. Thus, in a single-dose schedule, one might begin with 20 units of intermediate and 5 units of regular insulin rather than 25 units of intermediate alone. This practice is based on the concept that the regular insulin lowers the plasma glucose level rapidly, after which the more slowly absorbed insulin maintains the lowered level. Most patients on twice-daily insulin injections are also treated with a mixture of intermediate and regular insulin; e.g., 25 units NPH plus 10 units of regular before breakfast and 10 units of NPH plus 5 units of regular before supper. Commercial premixed insulin (70/30 intermediate/regular) is acceptable and convenient for many patients. All patients should be taught to decrease insulin when significant extra activity or exercise is anticipated. The proper decrement must be determined by trial and error, although a reduction of 5 to 10 units is a reasonable first step. The blood glucose–lowering effect of exercise is due primarily to increased energy demands in previously noncontracting muscle. Extra regular insulin can be taken before a meal that contains extra calories or food ordinarily not allowed (e.g., when the diabetic must eat out at a banquet or the teenager goes out on a date). For patients willing to self-monitor plasma glucose level, an algorithm for adjusting insulin can be provided. A typical protocol is shown in Table 337-6. Patients with complicated control problems may require hospitalization, where frequent plasma glucose determinations can guide therapy.

The *multiple subcutaneous insulin injection technique* most commonly involves administration of intermediate- or long-acting insulin in the evening as a single dose together with regular insulin prior to each meal. Home glucose monitoring by the patient is necessary if the goal is the return of the plasma glucose level to normal. One approach to initiation of therapy involves administration of 25 percent of the previous daily insulin dose in the patient's conventional regimen at bedtime as intermediate insulin (NPH or lente insulin), with the other 75 percent given as regular insulin divided such that 40, 30, and 30 percent is given 30 min before breakfast, lunch, and supper, respectively. Alternatively, a three-injection schedule can be utilized by omitting the night intermediate insulin and giving a long-acting insulin, such as insulin zinc extended (ultralente insulin) or protamine zinc insulin (PZI insulin), before the evening meal. Adjustments of dosage depend on response of the plasma glucose. A number of different protocols have been utilized, all of which represent sliding scales of insulin based on the plasma glucose level. A typical schedule based on home monitoring of the plasma glucose level is shown in

TABLE 337-7   Adjusting insulin dosage in a multiple-injection schedule*

Initiation of therapy
1 0.6 to 0.7 units insulin per kilogram body weight
2 25% NPH at 9 P.M.; 75% regular in divided doses
   (40% before breakfast, 30% before lunch, 30% before supper)
3 Adjust NPH every 48 h based on fasting blood glucose
   <3.3 mmol/L (<60 mg/dL)   − 2 units
   >5.0 mmol/L (>90 mg/dL)   + 2 units
4 Adjust regular insulin every 48 h based on 1-h postprandial glucose
   <3.3 mmol/L (<60 mg/dL)   − 2 units
   >7.8 mmol/L (>140 mg/dL)   + 2 units
Daily therapy
   Preprandial glucose

mmol/L	mg/dL	Regular insulin, units
<3.3	<60	− 2
3.4–5.0	61–90	No change
5.1–6.7	91–120	+ 1
6.8–8.3	121–150	+ 2
8.4–11.0	151–200	+ 3
11.1–13.9	201–250	+ 4
>13.9	>250	+ 6

* With initiation of therapy insulin dosage is changed until target range is reached (see Table 337-8). After initial stabilization a variable insulin schedule is prescribed to maintain tight control. For example, if the patient after initiation is found to generally require 12 units of regular insulin before breakfast but has a prebreakfast blood sugar of 8.9 mmol/L (160 mg/dL), 15 units of regular insulin instead of the usual 12 would be taken.
SOURCE: Adapted from Schiffrin and Belmonte.

Table 337-7. Individual patients may require different dosages. For specific details, the reader should consult one of the published papers utilizing the technique (e.g., Schriffrin and Belmonte). MSI can be effective in controlling the plasma glucose level and in some studies appears to match goals achieved with CSII.

Continuous subcutaneous insulin infusion involves use of a small battery-driven pump that delivers insulin subcutaneously into the abdominal wall, usually through a 27-gauge butterfly needle. With CSII, insulin is delivered at a basal rate continuously throughout the day, with increased rates programmed prior to meals. Adjustments in dosage are made in response to measured capillary glucose values in a fashion similar to that used in MSI. Ordinarily, about 40 percent of the total daily dose is given at the basal rate, the remainder being administered as preprandial boluses. There is little question that CSII can improve diabetic control relative to conventional therapy. Most patients report positive feelings of well-being as control improves. The danger of hypoglycemia is real, especially during the night in patients who maintain the plasma glucose consistently below 5.5 mmol/L (100 mg/dL). A fall in plasma glucose of 2.7 mmol/L (50 mg/dL) may not be important if the starting value is 8.3 mmol/L (150 mg/dL) but may be fatal if it occurs against a steady-state level of 3.3 mmol/L (60 mg/dL). Several deaths from hypoglycemia have occurred in pump users. There is also an increased frequency of diabetic ketoacidosis in persons utilizing CSII. Pumps should be prescribed only in disciplined and motivated patients who are followed by physicians with extensive experience in their use.

In some centers, catheters for the insulin infusion pumps have been placed intravenously rather than subcutaneously. While few difficulties have been reported, this procedure appears unwise for routine use. Intraabdominal insulin pumps with reservoirs refillable from outside the body have been tried on experimental protocols. At present, no advantage is apparent except that a pump does not have to be worn externally. Administration of insulin by nasal insufflation, although attractive in principle, has not proved practical and is no longer under commercial development.

For surgical procedures in diabetic patients, intermediate insulin is omitted, and treatment is carried out with regular insulin alone. An effective method is to add 10 to 20 units of insulin to a liter of 5% glucose in water with infusion at a rate of 100 to 150 mL/h. Measurement of plasma glucose in capillary blood allows change of rate to avoid significant hypo- or hyperglycemia. It is also possible to administer 10 units of regular insulin subcutaneously and infuse 5% or 10% glucose at rates sufficient to avoid major changes in glucose concentration. Following surgery, a sliding scale can be constructed for use in postoperative management.

Types of Insulin   A variety of insulins are available for use in the treatment of diabetes. Rapidly acting preparations are used in diabetic emergencies and in CSII and MSI programs. Intermediate-acting preparations are used in conventional and MSI regimens. Long-acting formulations are used almost exclusively in three-injection MSI schedules. Peak effects and duration vary from patient to patient and depend not only on route of administration but on dose. Insulin action in patients treated for long periods appears to be delayed, probably because of the presence of anti-insulin antibodies in plasma. In one study in diabetic subjects, regular insulin given subcutaneously had its onset of action at about 1 h, reached a peak at 6 h, and had measurable effects on average for 16 h, whereas in normal persons onset is within minutes, maximal action is around 2 h, and duration is only 6 to 8 h. With NPH insulin, diabetic patients exhibited an onset of action at 2.5 h, a peak at 11 h, and a total period of action of 25 h, more closely approximating values in normal subjects.

Commercial insulins are prepared in concentrations of 100 units per milliliter (U100), although higher concentrations can be obtained (e.g., U500). All animal insulins are purified such that proinsulin contamination is extremely low. Most patients are now treated with synthesized "human" insulin. The amino acid sequence is identical to that of the human hormone, and biologic activity appears to be equivalent. Complications of insulin therapy such as insulin allergy, fat atrophy, and fat hypertrophy are less common than with animal insulins but still occur.

Lente and NPH insulin are used in most conventional therapy and are roughly equivalent in biologic effects, although lente appears to be slightly more immunogenic and to mix less well with regular insulin than does NPH.

Self-monitoring of glucose   For many years, effectiveness of treatment for diabetes was followed by reviewing symptoms (such as frequency of nocturia) and measurement of glucose in the urine by semiquantitative techniques. Since the renal threshold for glucose in normal persons is in the range of 10 to 11 mmol/L (180 to 200 mg/dL) plasma glucose and may increase with the appearance of renal disease, assessment of glycosuria is of little value. Most insulin-requiring patients now monitor control and alter therapy based on self-measurement of the capillary blood sugar. In addition to the fact that such measurements are necessary in all treatment schedules utilizing variable insulin dosage, the ability to assess the blood glucose as needed has other positive benefits. It bestows a sense of confidence and independence in the patient, has a reinforcing effect on therapeutic goals (e.g., the effect of dietary indiscretion can be immediately seen), serves to give early warning of incipient hypoglycemia, and allows documentation of hypoglycemia when suggestive symptoms are present.

Although the blood glucose level can be estimated visually utilizing reagent strips, it is generally preferable to use an instrument for readings. This is so because it is difficult for many patients to extrapolate accurately between the color changes and because subjective wishes may influence the extrapolation. It is harder to ignore a number appearing in a machine. A variety of glucose analyzers are available. Cost of equipment is reasonable, and many insurance carriers reimburse its purchase. The patient needs to have supervised training in the technique, and simultaneous checks of the blood sugar in a laboratory should be done periodically to test the accuracy of the self-analysis. Repeated studies show that patients can measure blood glucose accurately using these techniques.

Although urine testing for glucose is now rarely used to follow diabetes, the measurement of ketones in the urine remains important.

Goals of therapy   Intensive insulin therapy designed to control the blood glucose level as near normal as possible has for many years been considered mandatory during pregnancy and after renal transplantation. Maintenance of a normal blood glucose level during and prolonged. Some patients have required massive glucose infusions for days following the last dose of sulfonylurea. For this reason, hospitalization is mandatory in patients with sulfonylurea-induced hypoglycemia.

The biguanides metformin and phenformin are oral agents used outside the United States. Phenformin was removed from the market by the Food and Drug Administration because of a possible association with lactic acidosis. Metformin has not been introduced in the United States. The drugs are thought to lower blood glucose by inhibiting hepatic gluconeogenesis, although they also may enhance insulin receptor number or activity. Biguanides should not be given to patients with renal disease and should be stopped if nausea, vomiting, diarrhea, or any intercurrent illness appears.

Another class of oral agents, thiazolidine derivatives, is currently under study for treatment of NIDDM. Pioglitazone, prototypical of the class, lowers blood glucose, free fatty acids, and triglycerides and appears to reduce insulin resistance, possibly by increasing insulin receptor kinase activity.

Two naturally occurring peptides are under investigation as adjuncts to treatment in NIDDM. Both insulin-like growth factor 1 (IGF-1, somatomedin C) and glucagon-like peptide 1 (GLP-1), a peptide derived from the proglucagon molecule, lower blood glucose level in normal subjects and in patients with diabetes. The GLP-1 (7-36) and (7-37) amides are the lead insulinotropins under development. Their ultimate usefulness is not established.

Monitoring control of diabetes For those patients who measure blood glucose frequently for adjustment of insulin dosage, an estimate of mean ambient glucose concentrations is readily available. For other patients, and as a check on accuracy of the self measurements, most diabetologists measure hemoglobin A_{1c} to assess long-term control. Hemoglobin A_{1c}, a fast-moving minor hemoglobin component, is present in normal persons but increases in the presence of hyperglycemia. Its enhanced electrophoretic mobility is due to nonenzymatic glycation of the amino acids valine and lysine.

Glucose in the aldehyde (linear) configuration condenses with a free amino group to form a Schiff base (aldimine or pre-A_{1c}). The Schiff base undergoes a rearrangement to form hemoglobin A_{1c}, a ketoamine. Aldimine formation is reversible so that pre-A_{1c} is labile, while ketoamine formation is irreversible and thus stable. Pre-A_{1c} levels change rapidly with alterations in glucose concentrations and do not reflect long-term control, although they are measured in chromatographic methods for determining hemoglobin A_{1c}. Pre-A_{1c} must thus be removed to assess true Hb A_{1c} values accurately. Many laboratories employ high-performance liquid chromatography to make the measurement. A colorimetric method utilizing thiobarbituric acid also does not measure the labile pre-A_{1c} fraction. When properly assayed, the percent of glycated hemoglobin gives an estimate of diabetic control for the preceding 3-month period. Normal values must be obtained for each lab; on average, nondiabetic subjects have Hb A_{1c} values of less than 6 percent, while levels in poorly controlled patients may reach 10 to 12 percent. Measurement of glycated hemoglobin gives an objective assessment of metabolic control. Discrepancies between reported plasma glucose values and hemoglobin A_{1c} concentrations suggest either that measurement or reporting of the former is not accurate. Measurement of glycated albumin, because of its short half-life, can be used to monitor diabetic control over a 1- to 2-week period but clinically is rarely used.

ACUTE METABOLIC COMPLICATIONS In addition to hypoglycemia, patients with diabetes are susceptible to two major acute metabolic complications: diabetic keotacidosis and hyperosmolar, nonketotic coma. The former is a complication of insulin-dependent diabetes, while the latter usually occurs in the setting of non-insulin-dependent disease. Ketoacidosis rarely, if ever, develops in true NIDDM.

Diabetic ketoacidosis Diabetic ketoacidosis appears to require insulin deficiency coupled with a relative or absolute increase in glucagon concentration. It is often caused by cessation of insulin intake but may result from physical (e.g., infection, surgery) or

emotional stress despite continued insulin therapy. In the former case, the concentration of glucagon rises secondary to insulin withdrawal, while in stress the operative stimulus for glucagon release is probably epinephrine. In addition to stimulating glucagon secretion, epinephrine presumably blocks release of the small amount of residual insulin found in some subjects with IDDM and inhibits insulin-induced glucose transport in peripheral tissues. These hormonal changes have multiple effects, but two are critical: (1) They induce maximal gluconeogenesis and impair peripheral utilization of glucose, causing severe hyperglycemia. Glucagon facilitates gluconeogenesis by inducing a fall in fructose-2,6-bisphosphate, an intermediate that stimulates glycolysis through activation of phosphofructokinase and blocks gluconeogenesis by inhibiting fructose bisphosphatase. When fructose-2,6-bisphosphate concentrations fall, glycolysis is inhibited, and gluconeogenesis is enhanced. The resultant hyperglycemia induces an osmotic diuresis that leads to the volume depletion and dehydration that characterize the ketoacidotic state. (2) They activate the ketogenic process and thus initiate development of metabolic acidosis. For ketosis to occur, changes must be produced in both adipose tissue and the liver. Free fatty acids from adipose stores represent the primary substrate for ketone body formation, and plasma levels of free fatty acids must rise if high rates of ketogenesis are to develop. However, fatty acids delivered to the liver are simply reesterified and stored as hepatic triglyceride or converted into very low density lipoproteins and transported back into the circulation unless the hepatic oxidative machinery for fatty acids is activated. While free fatty acid release is enhanced directly by insulin deficiency, accelerated fatty acid oxidation in the liver is primarily induced by glucagon, via action on the carnitine palmitoyltransferase system of enzymes responsible for the transport of fatty acids into the mitochondria. When long-chain fatty acids reach the liver, they are first esterified to coenzyme A (CoA). The fatty acyl CoA cannot traverse the mitochondrial membranes until it is transesterified with carnitine. As shown in Fig. 337-3, carnitine palmitoyltransferase I transesterifies fatty acyl-CoA to fatty acylcarnitine, which then traverses the inner mitochondrial membrane via translocase. Reversal of the reaction occurs internally under the influence of carnitine palmitoyltransferase II. In the fed state, carnitine palmitoyltransferase I is inactive, and as a consequence, long-chain fatty acids cannot reach the β-oxidative enzymes for ketone body production. During starvation or uncontrolled diabetes, the system is activated; under these circumstances, the rate of ketogenesis is a first-order function of the concentration of fatty acids reaching transferase I.

Glucagon (or a change in the glucagon/insulin ratio) activates the transport system in two ways. First, glucagon causes a rapid fall in hepatic malonyl-CoA content. It does so by interrupting the sequence glucose-6-phosphate $\rightarrow$ pyruvate $\rightarrow$ citrate $\rightarrow$ acetyl-CoA $\rightarrow$ malonyl-CoA via the previously mentioned decrease in fructose-2,6-bisphosphate. Glucagon also inhibits acetyl-CoA carboxylase, the enzyme that converts acetyl-CoA to malonyl-CoA. Malonyl-CoA, the first committed intermediate in the synthesis of fatty acids from glucose, is a competitive inhibitor of carnitine palmitoyltransferase I, and a fall in its concentration activates the enzyme. Second, glucagon causes a rise in hepatic carnitine concentration, which then drives the reaction toward fatty acylcarnitine formation by mass action. These events are summarized schematically in Fig. 337-4. At high plasma fatty acid concentrations, hepatic uptake of fatty acids is sufficient to saturate both oxidative and esterifying pathways, resulting in fatty liver, hypertriglyceridemia, and ketoacidosis. Overproduction of ketones by the liver is the primary event in ketotic states, but limitation of peripheral utilization also plays a role at high concentrations of acetoacetate and β-hydroxybutyrate.

Clinically, ketoacidosis begins with anorexia, nausea, and vomiting, coupled with an increased rate of urine formation. Abdominal pain may be present. If untreated, altered consciousness or frank coma may occur. Initial examination usually shows Kussmaul respiration, together with signs of volume depletion. Rarely, the latter is sufficient to cause vascular collapse and renal shutdown. Body temperature is

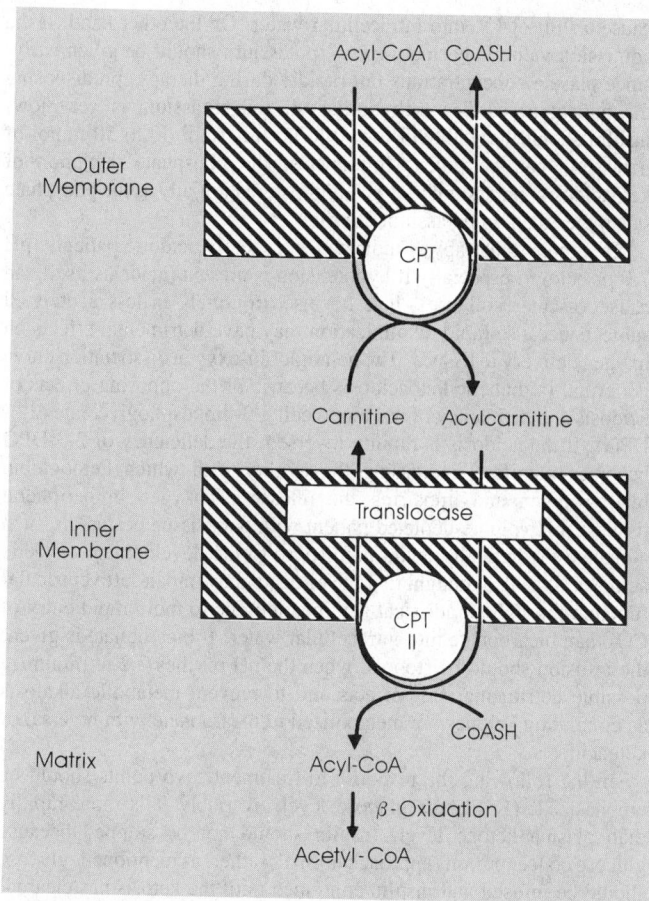

FIGURE 337-3   The carnitine palmitoyltransferase system. Long-chain fatty acyl-CoA molecules require transesterification to carnitine to traverse the inner mitochondrial membrane. Once across, the transesterification is reversed, and the fatty acyl-CoA is oxidized to either ketone bodies (liver) or CO_2 and water with the generation of ATP (nonhepatic tissues). CPT 1 is the rate-limiting step, controlled by malonyl-CoA levels in tissue. CPT 1, carnitine palmitoyltransferase 1; CPT II, carnitine palmitoyltransferase II.

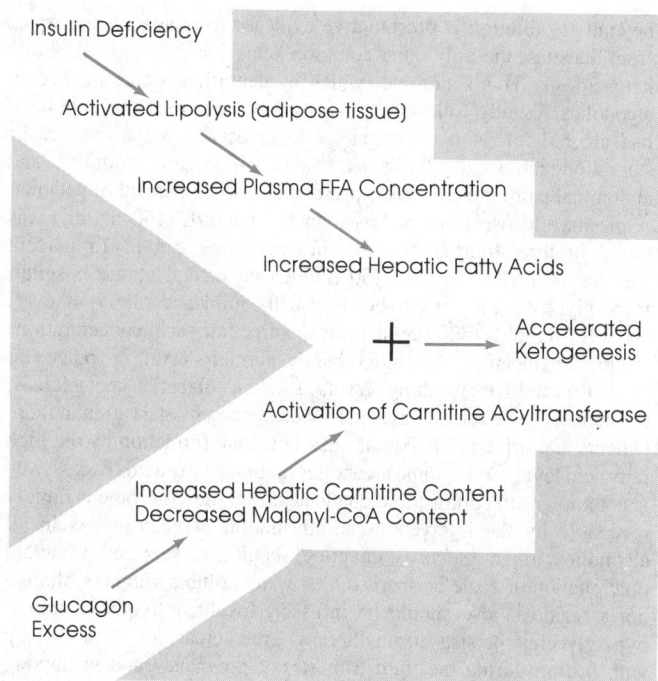

FIGURE 337-4   The regulation of ketogenesis. Significant production of acetoacetate and β-hydroxybutyrate by the liver requires provision of adequate free fatty acid substrate and activation of fatty acid oxidation. Lipolysis is primarily increased by insulin deficiency while the fatty acid oxidative sequence is activated primarily by glucagon. The immediate signal for oxidation is a fall in malonyl CoA content. *(After JD McGarry, DW Foster, Am J Med 61:9, 1976.)*

normal or below normal in uncomplicated keotacidosis: hence fever suggests the presence of infection. Leukocytosis, frequently very marked, is a feature of diabetic acidosis per se and may not indicate infection.

The characteristic metabolic abnormalities of diabetic coma are shown in Table 337-10. Several features deserve comment. The metabolic acidosis and anion gap are almost totally accounted for by the elevated plasma levels of acetoacetate and β-hydroxybutyrate, although other acids (e.g., lactate, free fatty acids, phosphates) contribute. Despite initial potassium concentrations that are normal to high, there is a total-body potassium deficit of several hundred millimoles. Similarly, initial serum phosphorus may be high despite depletion of body stores. Magnesium deficiency also may be present. The serum sodium concentration tends to be low in the face of modest osmolar concentration because of the hyperglycemia that draws intracellular water into the plasma space. A very low serum sodium level (e.g., 110 mmol/L) suggests an artifact due to severe hypertriglyceridemia. Newer autoanalyzers remove triglycerides before assay, eliminating this artifact. Hypertriglyceridemia is common in ketoacidosis and is the consequence of both impaired activity of lipoprotein lipase (a disposal defect) and the hepatic overproduction of very low density lipoproteins. If a fat meal has been ingested prior to the onset of keotacidosis, chylomicrons may make up a major portion of the circulating fat. Lipemia is usually visible if the triglyceride concentration is above 4.5 mmol/L (400 mg/dL). True hyponatremia may occur if the patient has vomited repeatedly and continued to drink water. Prerenal azotemia, reflecting volume depletion, is usually

modest in degree and reversible with treatment. The serum amylase level may be elevated, and frank pancreatitis can occur.

The diagnosis of ketoacidosis in a patient known to have insulin-dependent diabetes is not difficult. Its appearance in a patient not previously diagnosed requires differentiation from the other common causes of metabolic acidosis with an anion gap: lactic acidosis, uremia, alcoholic ketoacidosis, and certain poisonings. The first step is to test the urine for glucose and ketones. If urine ketones are negative, another cause for the acidosis is likely. If positive, plasma examination is required to be certain that something more than starvation ketosis is present. Since quantitative determinations of acetoacetate and β-hydroxybutyrate are not routinely available, semi-quantitative tests must be done using ketone reagent strips. Serial dilutions of plasma can be made and tested. A strong test may occur in undiluted plasma owing to starvation alone; a strong reaction

TABLE 337-10   Initial laboratory findings in diabetic ketoacidosis

Series:	Dallas*	Los Angeles†	Washington‡
Age, y	38	36	43
Glucose, mmol/L (mg/dL)	26(475)	37(675)	41(733)
Sodium, mmol/L	132	131	132
Potassium, mmol/L	4.8	5.3	6.0
Bicarbonate, mmol/L	<10	6	10
BUN, mmol/L (mg/dL)	9(25)	11(32)	15(42)
Acetoacetate, mmol/L	4.8	—	—
β-Hydroxybutyrate, mmol/L	13.7	—	—
Free fatty acids, mmol/L	2.1	—	2.3
Lactate, mmol/L	4.6	—	—
Osmolarity, mosmol/liter	310	323	331

* Eighty-eight consecutive episodes of ketoacidosis at Parkland Memorial Hospital (DW Foster, unpublished observations).
† Mean data from 308 episodes of nonfatal ketoacidosis (PM Beigelman, Diabetes 20:490, 1971).
‡ Mean data from 10 episodes of ketoacidosis (JE Gerich et al, Diabetes 20:228, 1971).

beyond 1:1 dilution is presumptive evidence for ketoacidosis. Apart from diabetes, the only other common ketoacidotic state is alcoholic ketoacidosis. This syndrome, which by definition occurs in chronic alcoholics, usually follows a debauch, but the patient may not have had alcohol for 24 h or longer. It never occurs in the absence of starvation and frequently is associated with severe vomiting and abdominal pain. Pancreatitis is present in up to 75 percent of patients. A plasma glucose level of less than 8.3 mmol/L (150 mg/dL) was found in three-fourths of cases in one series and in 15 percent was less than 2.8 mmol/L (50 mg/dL) on arrival at the hospital. Hyperglycemia may occur but is usually mild and rarely, if ever, above 17 mmol/L (300 mg/dL). Plasma free fatty acid concentrations are higher (mean 2.9 mmol/L) than in normal starvation (range 0.7 to 1.0 mmol/L), reaching levels seen in diabetic keotacidosis. Presumably the liver is activated for ketogenesis by starvation in these patients and driven to maximal rates of ketone formation by the high fatty acid levels. Why some alcoholics mobilize fatty acids excessively is not known. In contrast to diabetic acidosis, the syndrome is rapidly reversible by the intravenous administration of glucose. As in all alcoholics given glucose, thiamine should be supplied to avoid precipitation of acute beriberi. (Other water-soluble vitamins, though not as critical, also should be infused.) Insulin is required only if hyperglycemia persists during therapy. True ketoacidosis can develop with fasting during the third trimester of pregnancy and in nursing mothers who do not eat, but the complication is rare.

Diabetic ketoacidosis cannot be reversed without insulin. For decades, 50 or more units of insulin was given per hour until ketosis was reversed, but now most patients are treated by "low-dose" insulin schedules in which 8 to 10 units of insulin is infused intravenously each hour. Most diabetic acidosis can be reversed adequately with low-dose treatment, but some patients do not respond. Presumably the insulin resistance that is characteristic of diabetic ketoacidosis is more pronounced in these patients than in responsive subjects. The problem is that resistant subjects cannot be identified prospectively. For this reason, it is probably preferable to give 25 to 50 units of insulin as an initial intravenous bolus, followed by an infusion of 15 to 25 units an hour until ketoacidosis is reversed. There are no known toxic effects of larger insulin doses, since maximal physiologic response is obtained once insulin receptors are saturated regardless of how much insulin is given. The advantage of the higher dosage schedule is that it ensures saturation of the receptors in the face of competing antibodies or other resistance factors. High concentrations of insulin probably accelerate the reversal of ketoacidosis by acting via the IGF-1 receptor. Hormonal interaction with this receptor can lower the blood glucose level by a mechanism independent of the insulin receptor. Diabetic ketosis has been reversed by IGF-1 therapy in a patient with severe insulin resistance. If physicians choose to use the low-dose insulin schedule, they should be alert to the possibility of resistance. Should acidosis persist unabated after several hours of treatment, larger amounts of insulin are clearly indicated. Keotacidosis also can be treated adequately with intramuscular (but not subcutaneous) insulin.

Therapy of ketoacidosis also requires intravenous fluids. The usual fluid deficit is 3 to 5 L, and both salt solutions and free water are needed. Between 1 and 2 L of isotonic saline or Ringer's lactate should be given rapidly intravenously on arrival, with additional amounts determined by urine output and clinical assessment of the fluid state. When the plasma glucose level falls to about 17 mmol/L (300 mg/dL), 5% glucose solutions should be added, both as a source of free water and as a prophylactic measure to prevent the late cerebral edema syndrome. The latter is a rare complication of ketoacidosis occurring most often in children. It is suspected when the patient remains comatose or lapses into coma following reversal of acidosis.

Potassium replacement is always necessary, but the time of administration will vary. The initial potassium level is often high despite a total-body deficit because of the severe acidosis. In this case, the cation will ordinarily not be needed until 3 to 4 h after initiation of therapy when reversal of acidosis and the action of insulin

cause a shift of K^+ into intracellular water. On the other hand, if the admission value is normal or low, potassium should be given early, since plasma concentrations fall rapidly during therapy, predisposing the patient to cardiac arrhythmias. If the potassium is very low, insulin should be withheld for 60 to 90 min until 40 to 50 mmol of potassium can be given. In view of the phosphate depletion of ketoacidosis, potassium may be administered initially as the phosphate salt rather than as potassium chloride.

Bicarbonate therapy is indicated in severely acidotic patients (pH 7.0 or below), especially if hypotension is present (acidosis itself can cause vascular collapse). It is not used routinely in less acutely ill subjects because rapid alkalinization may have detrimental effects on oxygen delivery to tissues. The hemoglobin-oxygen dissociation curve is normal in diabetic ketoacidosis because of the opposing effects of acidosis and deficiency of red blood cell 2,3-diphosphoglycerate (2,3-DPG). If the acidosis is rapidly reversed, the deficiency of 2,3-DPG becomes manifest, increasing the avidity with which hemoglobin binds oxygen and impairing the release of oxygen in peripheral tissues. In a volume-depleted patient with poor tissue perfusion, such a change theoretically could predispose to the development of lactic acidosis. It is also thought that bicarbonate may impair left ventricular function through paradoxical acidification due to more rapid entry of CO_2 than bicarbonate into intracellular water. If bicarbonate is given, the infusion should be stopped when the pH reaches 7.2 to minimize possible detrimental side effects and to prevent metabolic alkalosis as circulating ketones are metabolized to bicarbonate with reversal of ketoacidosis.

In the following the response to treatment, two points should be emphasized. (1) Plasma glucose level invariably falls more rapidly than plasma ketone level. Insulin should not be stopped because glucose concentrations approach normal; rather, as mentioned, glucose should be infused and insulin continued until the ketosis has cleared. (2) Plasma ketone values are not very helpful. The testing materials measure acetoacetate and acetone but not β-hydroxybutyrate. Since β-hydroxybutyrate must be oxidized to acetoacetate prior to utilization, it is characteristic for the plasma ketones measured by reagent strip to remain stable or even rise early in therapy at a time when total ketone concentration (acetoacetate plus β-hydroxybutyrate) is falling. Because β-hydroxybutyrate and acetoacetate represent a redox couple in equilibrium with mitochondrial NADH/NAD concentrations, vascular collapse or severe hypoxia may mask the presence of ketoacidosis because acetoacetate is reduced to β-hydroxybutyrate. Under these circumstances, the β-hydroxybutyrate/acetoacetate ratio, normally about 3:1, may reach 7:1 or 8:1. Paradoxically, in such a situation ketosis may seem to worsen as the patient gets better because of conversion of β-hydroxybutyrate to acetoacetate when the circulation is reestablished and tissue oxygenation is restored. The key parameters to follow are the pH and the calculated anion gap, since these give a more accurate assessment of therapeutic progress. The usual picture is for the pH to rise and the anion gap to narrow even though the plasma bicarbonate level remains low. The persistently low bicarbonate is the consequence of hyperchloremia that develops because of rapid infusion of sodium chloride, the loss of potential bicarbonate from the body in urine as ketones, and exchanges with intracellular buffers. Some patients demonstrate a persistent anion gap despite clinical improvement and a rising pH. Presumably, the unmeasured anion derives from tissue buffers. If the anion gap remains elevated and pH is persistently low, this indicates insulin resistance and requires an aggressive increase in the amount of insulin administered. On the other hand, persistence of the anion gap does not indicate resistance when present in the face of clinical improvement, a rising pH, and clearing of urine ketones.

All patients should be followed with a flow sheet outlining amounts and timing of insulin and fluids together with a record of vital signs, urine volume, and blood chemistries. Without such a record, therapy tends to become chaotic.

Most patients with diabetic ketoacidosis recover when properly treated. While mortality in large series is reported to be around 10 percent, the majority of deaths result from late complications rather than from ketoacidosis itself. The major causes are myocardial infarction and infection, particularly pneumonia. Poor prognostic signs on admission include hypotension, azotemia, deep coma, and associated illness. In children, cerebral edema is a common cause of death (less frequent in adults). The cause of the brain swelling is not known. Theories include osmotic disequilibrium between brain and plasma as glucose is rapidly lowered, decreased plasma oncotic pressure due to infusion of large amounts of saline, and insulin-induced ion flux across the blood-brain barrier. Whatever the mechanism, mortality rates are high. Diagnosis is usually made by computed tomographic (CT) scan. Treatment involves the bolus infusion of 1 g mannitol per kilogram of body weight in the form of a 20% solution. Although of questionable benefit, dexamethasone is also usually given: 12 mg initially, then 4 mg every 6 h. If there is no response, hyperventilation to an arterial P_{CO_2} of about 28 mmHg should be carried out by an anesthesiologist or pulmonary specialist.

Other acute complications of ketoacidosis include vascular thrombosis and the adult respiratory distress syndrome. The former is induced by volume depletion, hyperosmolarity, increased viscosity of blood, and changes in clotting factors favoring thrombosis. The cause of the pulmonary lesion is not known; it is probably not related to the metabolic acidosis, since respiratory distress syndrome occurs in hyperosmolar coma as well. Acute gastric dilatation is another rare complication. An unusual infection associated with ketoacidosis is mucormycosis (see below). Table 337-11 summarizes the complications of diabetic ketoacidosis and its treatment.

Hyperosmolar coma Hyperosmolar, nonketotic diabetic coma is usually a complication of non-insulin-dependent diabetes. It is a syndrome of profound dehydration resulting from a sustained hyperglycemic diuresis under circumstances in which the patient is unable to drink sufficient water to keep up with urinary fluid losses. Commonly an elderly diabetic patient—often living alone or in a nursing home—develops a stroke or infection which worsens hyperglycemia and prevents adequate water intake. The full-blown syndrome probably does not occur until volume depletion has become severe enough to decrease urine output. Hyperosmolar coma also has been precipitated by therapeutic procedures such as peritoneal dialysis or hemodialysis, tube feeding of high-protein formulas, high-carbohydrate infusion loads, and the use of osmotic agents such as mannitol

and urea. Phenytoin, steroids, immunosuppressive agents, and diuretics also have been reported to initiate the disorder.

The absence of ketoacidosis is important in the pathophysiology. When ketoacidosis develops, nausea, vomiting, and air hunger bring the patient to the physician before extreme dehydration can occur. Such a protective mechanism is not operative in ketoacidosis-resistant, maturity-onset diabetes. Interestingly, hyperosmolar coma can occur in insulin-dependent diabetic patients given sufficient insulin to prevent ketosis but insufficient to control hyperglycemia. Although unusual, the same person may present on one occasion with ketoacidosis and on the next with hyperosmolar coma.

The reason for the absence of ketoacidosis in maturity-onset diabetes is not known. The hepatic ketogenic machinery is not impaired, since the patients frequently have ketone concentrations in the starvation range (2 to 4 mmol/L). Free fatty acid levels are lower in hyperosmolar coma than in ketoacidosis, and substrate deficiency may limit ketone formation. That this is the sole mechanism seems unlikely, since some patients with hyperosmolar coma have high levels of free fatty acids in plasma. A more likely explanation is that insulin concentrations in the portal vein of persons with NIDDM are higher than those of insulin-dependent subjects and prevent full activation of the hepatic carnitine palmitoyltransferase system. Other possibilities include glucagon resistance, previously mentioned, and maintenance of high malonyl-CoA levels via increased Cori cycle activity. The *Cori cycle* refers to conversion of circulating glucose to lactate in peripheral tissues with return of lactate to the liver for gluconeogenesis. Lactate is an excellent substrate for malonyl-CoA synthesis.

Clinically, patients present with extreme hyperglycemia, hyperosmolality, and volume depletion, coupled with central nervous system signs ranging from clouded sensorium to coma. Seizure activity—sometimes Jacksonian in type—is not unusual, and transient hemiplegia may be seen. Infections, particularly pneumonia and gram-negative sepsis, are common and indicate a grave prognosis. Pneumonia is often due to gram-negative organisms. A high index of suspicion for infection should be maintained, and routine culture of the blood and spinal fluid is indicated. Because of the extreme dehydration, plasma viscosity is high, and widespread in situ thrombosis has been found at post mortem. Bleeding, probably the consequence of disseminated intravascular coagulation, and acute pancreatitis may accompany the illness.

The laboratory findings in two large series are shown in Table 337-12. Plasma glucose is generally around 55 mmol/L (1000 mg/dL), about twice the value seen in ketoacidosis. The serum osmolality is extremely high, but because of the hyperglycemia, the absolute serum sodium concentration is often not elevated.[3] Prerenal azotemia with marked elevation of blood urea nitrogen (BUN) and creatinine is characteristic. A mild metabolic acidosis is present, plasma bicarbonate on average being about 20 mmol/L. The acidosis is due to a combination of starvation ketosis, retention of inorganic acids secondary to renal hypoperfusion, and a modest elevation of plasma lactate, the latter the consequence of volume depletion. If the bicarbonate is less than 10 mmol/L and plasma ketones are not elevated, it can be assumed that lactic acidosis is present.

The mortality rate in hyperosmolar coma is high (>50 percent). As a consequence, immediate treatment is urgent. The most important measure is rapid administration of large amounts of intravenous fluids to reestablish the circulation and urine flow. The average fluid deficit is 10 to 11 L. While free water will ultimately be needed, initial therapy should be with isotonic salt solutions, and 2 to 3 L should be given over the first 1 to 2 h. Subsequently, half-strength saline

TABLE 337-11 Clues to complications in diabetic ketoacidosis

Complication	Clues
Acute gastric dilatation or erosive gastritis	Vomiting of blood or coffee-ground material
Cerebral edema	Obtundation or coma with or without neurologic signs, especially if occurring after initial improvement
Hyperkalemia	Cardiac arrest
Hypoglycemia	Adrenergic or neurologic signs; rebound ketosis
Hypokalemia	Cardiac arrhythmias
Infection	Fever
Insulin resistance	Unremitting acidosis after 4–6 h of adequate therapy
Myocardial infarction	Chest pain, appearance of heart failure; appearance of hypotension despite adequate fluids
Mucormycosis	Facial pain, bloody nasal discharge, blackened nasal turbinates, blurred vision, proptosis
Respiratory distress syndrome	Hypoxemia in the absence of pneumonia, chronic pulmonary disease, or heart failure
Vascular thrombosis	Strokelike picture or signs of ischemia in nonnervous tissue

SOURCE: Adapted from DW Foster, in *Current Therapy in Endocrinology and Metabolism 1985–1986*, DT Krieger, CW Bardin (eds), Toronto/Philadelphia, Decker, 1985.

[3] Serum osmolality can be estimated from the formula Serum osmolality (mosmol/L) = 2 [Na$^+$ + K$^+$] + glucose (mmol/L) + BUN (mmol/L). Glucose and blood urea nitrogen (BUN) can be converted to milliosmoles per liter by dividing concentrations in milligrams per deciliter by 18 and 2.4, respectively. In practice, the contribution of the BUN is often ignored, since it contributes to total osmolality but does not reflect the free-water deficit. There are situations in which an increased osmolality is not equivalent to dehydration. Severe alcohol intoxication is one example, the ethanol itself providing the measured milliosmoles.

TABLE 337-12 Initial laboratory findings in hyperosmolar coma

Series:	Brooklyn*	Washington†
Age, y	60	57
Glucose, mmol/L (mg/dL)	65(1166)	54(976)
Sodium, mmol/L	144	142
Potassium, mmol/L	5	5
Chloride, mmol/L	99	98
Bicarbonate, mmol/L	17	22
BUN, mmol/L (mg/dL)	31(87)	23(65)
Creatinine, mmol/L (mg/dL)	490(5.5)	—
Free fatty acids, mmol/L	0.73	0.96
Osmolarity, mosmol/L	384	374

* Mean data from 33 episodes of hyperosmolar coma (AA Arieff, HJ Carroll, Medicine 51:73, 1972).
† Mean data from 20 episodes of hyperosmolar coma (JE Gerich et al, Diabetes 20:228, 1971).

TABLE 337-13 Lesions of diabetic retinopathy

Background	Proliferative
Increased capillary permeability	New vessels
Capillary closure and dilatation	Scar (retinitis proliferans)
Microaneurysms	Vitreal hemorrhage
Arteriovenous shunts	Retinal detachment
Dilated veins	
Hemorrhages (dot and blot)	
Cotton-wool spots	
Hard exudates	

can be used. As the glucose level approaches normal, 5% dextrose can be given as a vehicle for free water. While hyperosmolar coma may be reversed by fluids alone, insulin should be given to control the hyperglycemia more rapidly. Many authors recommend small doses of insulin, but larger amounts may be necessary, particularly in the obese patient. Potassium salts are usually required earlier in the treatment of hyperosmolar coma than in ketoacidosis because the intracellular shift of plasma K^+ during therapy is accelerated in the absence of acidosis. If lactic acidosis is present, sodium bicarbonate should be given until tissue perfusion can be reestablished. Antibiotics are required if infection complicates the picture.

LATE COMPLICATIONS OF DIABETES The diabetic patient is susceptible to a series of complications that cause morbidity and premature mortality. While some patients may never develop these problems and others note their onset early, on average, symptoms develop 15 to 20 years following the appearance of overt hyperglycemia. A given patient may experience several complications simultaneously, or a single problem may dominate the picture.

Circulatory abnormalities Atherosclerosis occurs more extensively and earlier than in the general population. The cause for this accelerated atherosclerosis is not known, although, as discussed below, nonenzymatic glycation of lipoproteins may be important. The atherosclerotic lesion appears to be initiated by oxidized low-density lipoproteins (LDL) (not native LDL) in a complicated cascade that operates through the acetyl-LDL or scavenger receptor. Both high-density lipoproteins (HDL) and antioxidants have the capacity to impair LDL oxidation, thereby exerting an antiatherogenic action. In experimental animals, diabetes accelerates the oxidative process. Although lipoproteins are often in the normal range, HDL levels tend to be low, while LDL levels are high normal or high. A high LDL/HDL ratio favors atherogenesis, and with lower HDL levels reverse cholesterol transport (from established lesions) would be impaired. Lipoprotein (a) levels are elevated in IDDM but not NIDDM.

Other factors of potential importance are increased platelet adhesiveness, possibly due to enhanced thromboxane A_2 synthesis, and decreased prostacyclin synthesis. Hyperglycemia has been reported to increase secretion of endothelin-1 in vitro, and production of nitric oxide is diminished in aortas of diabetic rats and the coronary microvasculature of humans. These findings have not been confirmed in human diabetes. Endothelin is a powerful vasoconstrictor and is mitogenic for vascular smooth muscle, while nitric oxide is a vasodilator, is antimitogenic in vascular smooth muscle, and inhibits platelet aggregation. Advanced glycation end products may be important, as discussed below.

Atherosclerotic lesions produce symptoms in a variety of sites. Peripheral deposits may cause intermittent claudication, gangrene, and, in men, organic impotence on a vascular basis. Surgical repair of large-vessel lesions may be unsuccessful because of the simultaneous presence of widespread disease of the small vessels.

Coronary artery disease and stroke are common. Silent myocardial infarction is thought to occur with increased frequency in diabetes and should be suspected whenever symptoms of left ventricular failure appear suddenly. Diabetes also may be associated with the clinical picture of cardiomyopathy, in which heart failure occurs in the face of angiographically normal coronary arteries and the absence of other identifiable causes of heart disease. As in nondiabetic subjects, smoking is a major risk factor for both coronary and peripheral vascular disease and should be avoided. Hypertension is also a significant risk factor in many diabetic patients.

Retinopathy Diabetic retinopathy is a leading cause of blindness in the United States. On the other hand, most patients never become blind. Retinopathic lesions are divided into two large categories, *simple* (background) and *proliferative* (Table 337-13). The earliest sign of retinal change is an increased capillary permeability that is evidenced by leakage of dye into the vitreous humor after fluorescein injection. Occlusion of retinal capillaries follows, with subsequent formation of saccular and fusiform aneurysms. Arteriovenous shunts also occur. The vascular lesions are accompanied by proliferation of lining endothelial cells and a loss of the pericytes that surround and support the vessels. Hemorrhages into the inner retinal areas are dot-shaped, while bleeding into the more superficial nerve fiber layer causes flame-shaped, blot, or linear lesions. Preretinal hemorrhages characteristically have a boat-shaped appearance. Exudates are of two types. Cotton-wool spots can be shown by angiography to be microinfarcts—nonperfused areas surrounded by a ring of dilated capillaries. A sudden increase in the number of cotton-wool spots represents an ominous prognostic sign and may herald the appearance of rapidly advancing retinopathy. Hard exudates are more common than cotton-wool spots and probably represent leakage of protein and lipids from damaged capillaries. Retinal edema due to the previously mentioned increase in vascular permeability is most often seen in the posterior pole of the eye, often in association with hard exudates. If the edema is in the macular region, visual acuity may be seriously and permanently impaired. Macular edema should be suspected when loss of visual acuity is not corrected by glasses, especially if posterior pole exudates are seen. Edema is difficult to recognize without slit-lamp examination or stereoscopic fundal photographs. Consultation with a retinal surgeon should be sought early, since vision may be spared by laser therapy of the macular edema.

The fundamental characteristics of proliferative retinopathy are new vessel formation and scarring. The stimulus for neovascularization may be retinal hypoxia secondary to capillary or arteriolar occlusion. Two serious complications of proliferative retinopathy are vitreal hemorrhage and retinal detachment. Either may cause a sudden loss of vision in one eye.

The frequency of diabetic retinopathy appears to vary with the age of onset as well as the duration of the disease. Approximately 85 percent of patients eventually develop the complication, but some never develop lesions even after 30 years of disease. Retinopathy appears to develop earlier in older patients, but proliferative retinopathy is less common. Some 10 to 18 percent of patients with simple retinopathy progress to proliferative disease in a 10-year period. About half of patients with proliferative disease progress to blindness within 5 years. Proliferative retinopathy appears to be more common in insulin-treated patients than in those not treated with insulin.

Treatment for diabetic retinopathy is photocoagulation. Such treatment decreases the incidence of hemorrhage and scarring and is always indicated when new vessel formation occurs. Photocoagulation is also useful in treatment of microaneurysms, hemorrhages, and macular edema even if the proliferative stage has not begun. Panretinal photocoagulation is often used to diminish retinal demands for oxygen in the hope that the stimulus for neovascularization will be decreased. In this technique, several thousand lesions are produced over a 2-week period. Complications of photocoagulation are within the acceptable range. Some loss of peripheral vision is inevitable with extensive burns. Another surgical technique, pars plana vitrectomy, is utilized for treatment of nonresolving vitreal hemorrhage and retinal detachment. Postoperative complications are more frequent than with photocoagulation and include retinal tears, retinal detachment, cataracts, recurrent vitreal hemorrhage, glaucoma, infection, and loss of the eye. Hypophysectomy, once widely performed for diabetic retinopathy, is no longer recommended. There is hope that inhibition of angiogenesis by drugs such as the experimental heparin analogue beta-cyclodextrin tetradecasulfate may prevent proliferative retinopathy. All patients with diabetic retinopathy should be followed by retinal specialists.

Diabetic nephropathy Renal disease is a leading cause of death and disability in diabetes. About half of end-stage renal disease in the United States is now due to diabetic nephropathy. Approximately 35 percent of patients with insulin-dependent diabetes develop this complication. Prevalence in NIDDM varies from 15 to 60 percent depending on ethnic background. Pima Indians have the highest rates, while Europeans have the lowest. It is probable that nephropathy, like other complications, is influenced by the genetic background of the patient. Some families with multiple diabetic members rarely have renal disease, while in others more than 80 percent of persons at risk have nephropathy.

Diabetic nephropathy involves two distinct pathologic patterns that may or may not coexist: diffuse and nodular. The former, which is more common, consists of widening of the glomerular basement membrane together with generalized mesangial thickening. In the nodular form, large accumulations of PAS-positive material are deposited at the periphery of the glomerular tufts, the Kimmelstiel-Wilson lesion. In addition, there may be hyalinization of afferent and efferent arterioles, "drops" in Bowman's capsule, fibrin caps, and occlusion of glomeruli. Deposition of albumin and other proteins occurs in both glomeruli and tubules. The most specific lesions of diabetic glomerulosclerosis are hyalinization of afferent glomerular arterioles and the Kimmelstiel-Wilson nodules. Clinical renal dysfunction in diabetes does not correlate well with the histologic abnormalities.

Diabetic nephropathy may be functionally silent for long periods (10 to 15 years). At onset, the kidneys are usually enlarged with "superfunction" (i.e., glomerular filtration rates may be 40 percent above normal). The next stage is the appearance of *microproteinuria* (microalbuminuria), the excretion of albumin in the range of 30 to 300 mg/d. Normal persons excrete less than 30 mg/d. Microalbuminuria is not detected by reagent sticks for urinary protein, which generally become positive only when proteinuria is greater than 550 mg/d, a degree of leakage termed *macroproteinuria*. Microalbuminuria appears to be due primarily to decreased concentration of anionic heparan sulfate–proteoglycan in the glomerular basement membrane. Since microalbuminuria is initially transient and can be induced by mechanisms other than diabetes, diagnosis requires an excretion rate of albumin greater than 15 μg/h (30 mg/d) in two of three samples collected in a 6-month period. Persistent leakage of protein greater than 50 mg/d is predictive of subsequent macroproteinuria. Interestingly, microalbuminuria also appears to predict cardiovascular mortality in diabetes. Once the macroproteinuric phase begins, there is a steady decline in renal function, with glomerular filtration rate falling, on average, about 1 mL/min per month. A plot of the reciprocal of the serum creatinine against time usually results in a straight line and allows prediction of the rate of deterioration. Ordinarily, azotemia begins about 12 years after diagnosis of diabetes. The nephrotic syndrome may occur prior to azotemia. Progression of renal disease is accelerated by hypertension.

There is no specific treatment for diabetic nephropathy. Meticulous control of diabetes can reverse microalbuminuria in some patients, and diabetic nephropathy may be slowed in its progression, as shown in the intensive treatment group of the DCCT. Hypertension must be treated aggressively whenever present. Angiotensin-converting enzyme inhibitors appear to be useful in slowing progression of diabetic nephropathy. They should be used in hypertensive patients with diabetes and may have a role in normotensive subjects with microalbuminuria. Low-protein diets may be useful, based on experimental studies in animals and humans. Once the azotemic phase is reached, treatment does not differ from that for other forms of renal failure. Chronic dialysis and renal transplantation are routine in patients with renal failure due to diabetes. Hyporeninemic hypoaldosteronism, which is associated with renal tubular acidosis, may require alkalinizing solutions (Shohl's solution) and avoidance of external potassium loads. Potassium tends to rise in parallel with hyperglycemia in the syndrome, since in the absence of aldosterone potassium loads must be disposed of intracellularly under the influence of insulin. Hyperglycemia, reflecting insulin deficiency, indicates impairment of the disposal pathway. Rarely, fludrocortisone may be required to control hyperkalemia.

Diabetic neuropathy Diabetic neuropathy may affect every part of the nervous system, with the possible exception of the brain. While it is rarely a direct cause of death, it is a major cause of morbidity. Distinct syndromes can be recognized, and several different types of neuropathy may be present in the same patient. The most common picture is that of *peripheral polyneuropathy*. Usually bilateral, the symptoms include numbness, paresthesias, severe hyperesthesias, and pain. The pain, which may be deep-seated and severe, is often worse at night. It is occasionally lancinating or lightning in type, resembling tabes dorsalis (pseudotabes). Fortunately, extreme pain syndromes are usually self-limited, lasting from a few months to a few years. Involvement of proprioceptive fibers leads to abnormalities of gait and development of typical Charcot joints, particularly in the feet. Loss of arch with multiple fractures of tarsal bones is a common finding by x-ray. On physical examination, absent stretch reflexes and loss of vibratory sense are early signs. Diabetic neuropathy also may cause delay in return of the ankle reflex identical to that seen in hypothyroidism. *Mononeuropathy*, though less common than polyneuropathy, also may occur. Characteristically, there is a sudden wrist drop, foot drop, or paralysis of the third, fourth, or sixth cranial nerves. Other single nerves, including the recurrent laryngeal, have been reported to be involved. Mononeuropathy is characterized by a high degree of spontaneous reversibility, usually over a several-week period. *Radiculopathy* is a sensory syndrome in which pain occurs over the distribution of one or more spinal nerves, usually in the chest wall or abdomen. The severe pain may mimic herpes zoster or an acute surgical abdomen. Like mononeuropathy, the lesion is usually self-limited. *Autonomic neuropathy* may present in a variety of ways. The gastrointestinal tract is a prime target, and there may be esophageal dysfunction with difficulty in swallowing, delayed gastric emptying, constipation, or diarrhea. The last is often nocturnal. Incompetence of the internal anal sphincter may mimic diabetic diarrhea. Orthostatic hypotension and frank syncope may occur. Cardiorespiratory arrest and sudden death, thought to be due solely to autonomic neuropathy, have been reported. Bladder dysfunction or paralysis is particularly distressing and often leads to the necessity of chronic catheter drainage. Impotence and retrograde ejaculation are additional manifestations in men. Erectile dysfunction is associated with a failure of nitric oxide generation in the penile vasculature. Deficiency of vasoactive intestinal polypeptide (VIP) may also be involved. Clues to autonomic neuropathy can be obtained by clinical tests such as measuring response of the heart rate to the Valsalva maneuver or standing. In both tests the subject has an electrocardiograph running for assessment of heart rate. In the former, the subject blows against an aneroid or mercury manometer to 40 mmHg pressure for 15 s. The test is performed three times with a rest period of 1 min in between. Normally the heart rate speeds during Valsalva such that the ratio of the longest interval between beats after release to the shortest interval during the test is greater than 1.2. In autonomic neuropathy involving the parasympathetic system the ratio is less than 1.1. Similarly, the ratio at the thirtieth beat after standing relative to that at the fifteenth beat should be greater than 1.0. It is less than 1.0 in autonomic neuropathy. Diabetic *amyotrophy* is likely a form of neuropathy, although atrophy and weakness of the large muscles in the upper leg and pelvic girdle resemble primary muscle disease. Anorexia and depression may accompany amyotrophy. Because of the weight loss, such patients are often thought to have a paraneoplastic neuropathy.

Treatment of diabetic neuropathy is unsatisfactory in most respects. When pain is severe, it is easy for the patient to become habituated or addicted to narcotics or powerful nonnarcotic analgesics such as pentazocine. If the pain requires something stronger than aspirin, acetaminophen, or other nonsteroidal anti-inflammatory agents, codeine is the drug of choice. Phenytoin is used by some physicians, but others have not found it helpful. Combination therapy with amitriptyline and fluphenazine causes relief of pain in some patients and is worth trying. The recommended dosage is 75 mg amitriptyline at bedtime and 1 mg fluphenazine three times a day. Mononeuropathies and radiculopathies usually require no specific therapy because they are self-limited. Diabetic diarrhea often responds to treatment with diphenoxylate and atropine or loperamide. Orthostatic hypotension is best treated by having the patient sleep with the head of the bed elevated, avoidance of sudden assumption of the upright position, and the use of full-length elastic stockings. Occasionally, volume expansion with fludrocortisone is required, as in other forms of orthostatic hypotension.

Experimental therapy with aldose reductase inhibitors and myoinositol have failed to provide significant clinical benefit, although enhanced regeneration of nerves has been reported in humans treated with an aldose reductase antagonist. Topical application of capsaicin is occasionally helpful with burning pain syndromes and hyperesthesia.

Diabetic foot ulcers   A special problem in the diabetic patient is the development of ulcers of the feet and lower extremities. The ulcers appear to be due primarily to abnormal pressure distribution secondary to diabetic neuropathy. The problem is accentuated when there is bony distortion in the feet. Callus formation is usually the initial abnormality. Alternatively, the ulcer may be initiated by ill-fitting shoes which cause blister formation in patients whose sensory deficits preclude recognition of pain. Cuts and punctures from foreign bodies such as needles, tacks, and glass are common, and a foreign body of which the patient is unaware may be found in the soft tissue. For this reason, all patients with ulcers should have x-rays made of the feet. Vascular disease with diminished blood supply contributes to development of the lesion, and infection is common, often with multiple organisms. While no specific therapy is available for diabetic ulcers, supportive treatment often can lead to salvation of the leg without amputation. One approach is simply to put the patient to bed using hydrotherapy and debridement to remove nonviable tissue. Others recommend casting the leg with plaster to redistribute weight bearing and protect the lesion. Pending culture, initial antibiotic therapy for infected ulcers without systemic signs might be cefoxitin or ampicillin-sulbactam. If signs of sepsis are present, ampicillin-sulbactam plus gentamicin or aztreonam may be prescribed.

All patients should be instructed about proper foot care in an attempt to prevent ulcers. Feet should be kept clean and dry at all times. Patients with neuropathy should not be allowed to walk barefoot, even in the home. Properly fitted shoes are essential. This is a particular problem with women, since an adequate shoe is not often stylish. The feet should be carefully inspected daily for callus, infection, abrasions, or blisters and the physician consulted for any potentially troublesome lesion. Treatment with growth factors (e.g., fibroblast growth factor) may prove useful in the future.

What causes the complications of diabetes?   The cause of diabetic complications is not known and may be multifactorial. Major emphasis has been placed on the polyol pathway, wherein glucose is reduced to sorbitol by the enzyme aldol reductase. Sorbitol, which appears to function as a tissue toxin, has been implicated in the pathogenesis of retinopathy, neuropathy, cataracts, nephropathy, and aortic disease. The mechanism is perhaps best worked out in experimental diabetic neuropathy, where sorbitol accumulation is associated with a decrease in myoinositol content, abnormal phospho-inositide metabolism, and a decrease in Na^+, K^+-ATPase activity. In experimental models, primacy of the polyol pathway in initiating neuropathy was proven by showing that inhibition of aldol reductase prevented the fall in tissue myoinositol content and the decrease in ATPase activity. Myoinositol deficiency was not found in sural nerve biopsies from humans with diabetic neuropathy, in contrast to animals. Aldol reductase inhibition also has been shown to prevent experimental cataracts and retinopathy. It thus seems possible that neuropathy and retinopathy are primarily due to activation of the polyol pathway. It also may play a role in diabetic nephropathy.

A second mechanism of potential pathogenetic importance is glycation of proteins. (Current terminology uses *glycation* for nonenzymatic addition of hexoses to proteins and *glycosylation* for enzymatic addition.) The effect of such glycation on hemoglobin has been mentioned, but multiple proteins in the body are altered in the same way, often with disturbed function. Examples include plasma albumin, lens protein, fibrin, collagen, lipoproteins, and the glycoprotein recognition system of hepatic endothelial cells. Particularly intriguing is the effect of glycation on lipoproteins. Glycated LDL is not recognized by the normal LDL receptor, and its plasma half-life is increased. Conversely, glycated HDL turns over more rapidly than native HDL. It also has been reported that glycated collagen traps LDL at rates two to three times greater than normal collagen.

Glycated collagen is less soluble and more resistant to degradation by collagenase than native collagen. However, it is not clear that this is related either to the basement membrane thickening or to the tight, waxy skin syndrome with limited joint mobility (scleroderma-like) seen in some patients with insulin-dependent diabetes (see "Miscellaneous Abnormalities," below). Although it is attractive to presume that nonenzymatic glycation of protein plays a role in some degenerative complications, the evidence is less direct than with the polyol pathway. Linkage between the polyol pathway and the glycation sequence occurs as a result of the glycation of collagen and other proteins by fructose generated from sorbitol. The rate of glycation with fructose is seven or eight times faster than with glucose.

Glycated proteins also form *advanced glycation end products* (AGE) through a series of biochemical reactions that are poorly understood. Receptors for AGE are present on macrophages and endothelial cells. Binding of AGE to the receptors may induce the release of cytokines, endothelin-1, and tissue factor. The latter plays a preeminent role in the initiation of coagulation. Experimentally, AGE formation may be impaired or prevented by aminoguanidine, an agent currently in clinical trials in humans. In animals, it has a beneficial effect in prevention of retinopathy, nephropathy, and neuropathy (commonly called *microvascular complications*), but it is projected to have its major effect in atherosclerotic complications (commonly called *macrovascular complications*).

Increased blood flow has been postulated to play an initiating role in diabetic complications, possibly by increasing filtration of macromolecules that function as tissue toxins. There is supportive evidence for a role of hyperperfusion in diabetic nephropathy, but the hemodynamic hypothesis does not appear as attractive as the first two.

Can diabetic complications be prevented by meticulous control of diabetes?   As mentioned earlier, the strongest evidence that the answer is yes comes from the Diabetes Control and Complications Trial (DCCT). Additional clinical evidence supports the view that metabolic environment per se influences or causes complications independent of genetic factors. For example, kidneys from donors who have neither diabetes nor a family history of diabetes develop characteristic lesions of diabetic nephropathy within 3 to 5 years after transplantation into a diabetic recipient. Diabetic nephropathy did not develop when a kidney was transplanted into a diabetic subject whose disease had been reversed by pancreatic transplantation prior to renal transplantation. It also has been reported that kidneys manifesting diabetic nephropathy demonstrated reversal of the lesion when transplanted into normal recipients. All these findings suggest that hyperglycemia or some other aspect of the abnormal metabolism of diabetes causes or influences the development of complications. On the other hand, additional factors, probably genetic, must normally play a role. This follows from the fact that diabetic subjects with decades of poor control may escape the ravages of the late complications and from the fact that typical diabetic complications may be found in patients at the time of diagnosis of diabetes or even in the absence of hyperglycemia.

Meticulous control with insulin infusion pumps has been reported to decrease microalbuminuria, improve motor nerve conduction velocity, lower plasma lipoproteins, and decrease capillary leakage of fluorescein in the retina. Width of the capillary basement membrane in skeletal muscle also has been decreased. The changes are small in general, however, and of questionable biologic significance. Thus firm evidence does not exist to show that late complications can be *reversed* by long-term near-normalization of the plasma glucose level. Progression of retinopathy has been reported despite successful reversal of diabetes by pancreatic transplantation. The progression of diabetic complications after return of the plasma glucose level to normal or near normal has been termed *hyperglycemic memory*. Some investigators suggest that the mechanism is formation of advanced glycation end products during hyperglycemia which, being irreversible, continue their effects long term.

As discussed earlier, the question of intensive therapy for all patients with diabetes remains open at the time of this writing pending evidence that the results achieved in DCCT can be matched in the general population. Care of persons with diabetes is often delivered by nonspecialists who do not have available teams of support personnel, as was the case in the DCCT. There seems little question, however, that the thrust of treatment will be toward tighter control.

Miscellaneous abnormalities of diabetes Diabetes affects almost every system in the body. Space limitations preclude discussion of all associated features, but several deserve comment. *Infections* in persons with diabetes may not occur more frequently than in normal subjects, but they tend to be more severe. This may be due to impaired leukocyte function, a frequent accompaniment of poor control. In addition to common infections of the skin, urinary tract, lungs, and bloodstream, four unusual conditions appear to have specific relationship with diabetes. *Malignant external otitis*, usually due to *Pseudomonas aeruginosa*, tends to occur in older patients and is characterized by severe pain in the ear, drainage, fever, and leukocytosis. Soft tissues around the ear are swollen and tender. A mound of granulation tissue is characteristically present internally at the junction of the osseous and cartilaginous portions of the ear. The facial nerve becomes paralyzed in half the cases, and other cranial nerves also may be involved. Facial nerve paralysis is a poor prognostic sign, and mortality approximates 50 percent in this subset of patients. A 6-week course of ticarcillin or carbenicillin together with tobramycin is the treatment of choice. Ciprofloxacin, imipinem + cilastin, or third-generation parenteral antipseudomonal cephalosporin also may be used. Surgical debridement is often necessary. *Rhinocerebral mucormycosis* is a rare fungal infection which usually develops in patients during or following an episode of diabetic ketoacidosis. Organisms are from the genera *Mucor*, *Rhizopus*, and *Absidia*. Onset is sudden with periorbital and perinasal swelling, pain, bloody nasal discharge and increased lacrimation. The nasal mucosa and underlying tissues become black and necrotic. Cranial nerve palsies are not uncommon. There may be thrombosis of the internal jugular vein or

sinuses of the brain. Proptosis, chemosis, and retinal vein engorgement indicate cavernous sinus thrombosis. Untreated, death usually occurs in a week to 10 days. Amphotericin B and aggressive debridement are the indicated therapies. *Emphysematous cholecystitis* tends to affect diabetic men (in contrast to ordinary cholecystitis, a disease predominantly present in women). Gangrene of the gallbladder is 30 times more frequent than in the usual forms, accounting for high rates of perforation and a mortality rate 3 to 10 times higher than in ordinary cholecystitis. Diagnosis is made when gas is seen in the gallbladder wall on plain films of the abdomen. Clostridial species are frequently cultured from bile, but other organisms may be present. Treatment is cholecystectomy coupled with broad-spectrum antibiotics. Mezlocillin plus metronidazole is adequate initial coverage. *Emphysematous pyelonephritis* is signaled by the presence of gas in the kidney or perirenal space. Antibiotic therapy is usually ineffective, and nephrectomy may be required. Mortality rates of 80 percent have been reported.

Hypertriglyceridemia is common in diabetes and is usually due to insulin deficiency. Both overproduction of very low density lipoproteins in the liver and a disposal defect in the periphery appear to be operative. The latter is a consequence of lipoprotein lipase deficiency, an insulin-dependent enzyme. Some patients exhibit hyperlipemia even when diabetic control is adequate and likely have a primary familial hyperlipoproteinemia that is independent of diabetes. Patients who do not respond to dietary therapy should be treated for hypertriglyceridemia and hypercholesterolemia with drugs, as in nondiabetic subjects (see Chap. 344).

A variety of skin lesions occur in diabetes. *Necrobiosis lipoidica diabeticorum* is a plaquelike lesion with a central yellowish area surrounded by a brownish border. It is usually found over the anterior surfaces of the legs. Ulceration may occur. *Diabetic dermopathy* ("shin spots") is also usually located over the anterior tibial surface. The lesions are small rounded plaques with a raised border which may crust at the edges and ulcerate centrally. Several plaques may be arranged in linear fashion. Pigmentation is not prominent early, but as the lesion heals, a depressed scar occurs with diffuse brown discoloration. A rarer abnormality is *bullosis diabeticorum*. The bullae may be superficial with clear serum or may be mildly hemorrhagic. The cause is unknown. *Infestations of the skin* with *Candida* and dermatophytes are common, and bacterial infections of a variety of types occur. In women, *vaginal moniliasis* may be troublesome during hyperglycemic-glycosuric periods. While the symptoms respond to nystatin or gentian violet, recurrence is inevitable unless glycosuria is reversed. *Atrophy of adipose tissue* may occur at the site of insulin injections even with recombinant human insulin. *Hypertrophy* of fat also may occur, producing a lipoma-like lesion visible on physical examination.

Hyperviscosity occurs in diabetes, and *platelets aggregate abnormally*. The latter may be caused by increased thromboxane synthesis. *Wound healing* is impaired in experimental diabetes but probably is not a major factor clinically. An interesting accompaniment of insulin-dependent diabetes is the presence of *joint contractures* (Dupuytren's contracture) coupled with *tight, waxy skin* over the dorsum of the hands. The hands resemble those in patients with scleroderma. The cause of the tendon contractures is unknown, although alterations of cross-linking in collagen has been proposed. Patients with the joint contracture–waxy skin syndrome appear to have accelerated development of other diabetic complications. *Scleredema* is a common finding in diabetes. The lesion is a thickening of the skin over the shoulders and upper back that resembles scleroderma. The condition is benign.

Patients with diabetes may have additional illnesses. For example, there is a significant prevalence of eating disorders in young women with IDDM.

NONROUTINE THERAPY Transplantation with whole pancreas or segments has cured diabetes in a number of patients but is usually performed only when kidney transplantation is required. However,

KOBAYASHI M et al: Pioglitazone increases insulin sensitivity by activating insulin receptor kinase. Diabetes 41:476, 1992

MARKS JB, SKYLER JS: Immunotherapy of type I diabetes mellitus. J Clin Endocrinol Metab 72:3, 1991

RAVID M et al: Long-term stabilizing effect of angiotensin-converting enzyme inhibition on plasma creatinine and on proteinuria in normotensive type II diabetic patients. Ann Intern Med 118:577, 1993

ROBERTSON RP: Pancreatic and islet transplantation for diabetes—Cures or curiosities? N Engl J Med 327:1861, 1992

SANTIAGO JV: Intensive management of insulin dependent diabetes: Risks, benefits, and unanswered questions. J Clin Endocrinol Metab 75:977, 1992

SCHIFFRIN A, BELMONTE MM: Comparison between subcutaneous insulin infusion and multiple injections of insulin: A one year prospective study. Diabetes 31:255, 1982.

SKYLER JS: Insulin pharmacology. Med Clin North Am 72:1337, 1988

Insulin resistance

FLIER JS: Syndromes of insulin resistance: From patient to gene and back again. Diabetes 41:1207, 1992

TAYLOR SI: Molecular mechanisms of insulin resistance: Lessons from patients with mutations in the insulin receptor gene. Diabetes 41:1473, 1992

338 HYPOGLYCEMIA

DANIEL W. FOSTER / ARTHUR H. RUBENSTEIN

Maintenance of the plasma glucose concentration within narrow bounds is essential for health. Hypoglycemia is dangerous (in the short run more serious than hyperglycemia) because glucose is the primary energy substrate of the brain. Its absence, like that of oxygen, produces deranged function, tissue damage, or even death if the deficit is prolonged. The vulnerability of the brain to hypoglycemia is due to the fact that it cannot utilize circulating free fatty acids as an energy source in contrast to other tissues of the body. Short-chain metabolites of the free fatty acids acetoacetic and β-hydroxybutyric acid (*ketone bodies, ketoacids*) are efficiently oxidized by the brain and can protect the central nervous system from damage by hypoglycemia when present at moderate concentrations in plasma. However, development of ketosis requires a number of hours. Ketogenesis is not, therefore, an effective protective mechanism against acute hypoglycemia. Preservation of central nervous system function in the early phases of fasting or during hypoglycemia thus requires a prompt increase in the production of glucose by the liver. At the same time, glucose utilization in other tissues is diminished by provision of free fatty acids as alternative substrate. These adaptive mechanisms are hormonally controlled and, under ordinary circumstances, are extremely effective. Occasionally, however, the system breaks down or is overwhelmed, resulting in the clinical syndrome of hypoglycemia.

DEFENSE AGAINST HYPOGLYCEMIA The hypoglycemic states can best be understood as derangements of normal fuel metabolism. Under ordinary circumstances, energy needs are met by exogenous substrate derived from food. Oxidation of the constituent molecules of food to carbon dioxide and water is accompanied by the generation of adenosine triphosphate (ATP), the principal high-energy compound of the body. In one sense, life can be defined as the continued ability to generate ATP (and related high-energy nucleotides) for the preservation of cellular integrity in all its manifestations. When caloric intake is greater than immediate oxidative needs, as after the usual meal, excess substrate is stored as fat, structural protein, and glycogen. Substrate flux in this phase of metabolism, called *anabolic*, proceeds from intestine to liver to utilization and storage sites. Insulin is the primary hormone mediating the anabolic phase, and counterregulatory hormone levels are suppressed.

The *catabolic* phase of metabolism begins about 5 to 6 h after a meal. Normally, the only significant catabolic period is during the overnight fast, but under some circumstances, particularly serious illness, it may be prolonged. During fasting/catabolism, a series of metabolic adjustments maintains the plasma glucose in a safe range

for central nervous system metabolism and provides energy for other tissues in the body. First, the liver is activated for glucose production, and second, a lipid economy is established for most other tissues of the body. Initially, glucose from the liver is derived almost exclusively from hepatic glycogen. Because there are only about 70 g of glycogen stored in the human liver, glycogenolysis can only sustain the plasma glucose for a short time, ordinarily 8 to 10 h. Exercise may shorten the protective period, as may the stress of severe illness. To compensate for glycogen depletion, gluconeogenesis begins early, with flux of substrate from muscle and adipose tissue stores to liver and then to utilization sites.

The precursors for hepatic glucose synthesis are lactate/pyruvate and amino acids (primarily alanine) derived from muscle and glycerol released from adipose tissue by lipolysis. Amino acids constitute the primary substrate for gluconeogenesis. Most of the lactate is recycled from preformed glucose (*Cori cycle*), the only net contribution coming from the breakdown of muscle glycogen. Glycerol is initially a minor substrate but increases in importance with time. With prolonged fasting, the kidney also becomes a gluconeogenic organ and contributes to total glucose production. The primary renal substrate for gluconeogenesis is glutamine, not alanine. Proteolysis required to provide amino acids for gluconeogenesis accounts for the negative nitrogen balance of starvation. The same mechanism is operative in the stress of trauma, surgery, and severe infection. In quantitative terms, the liver produces about 11 μmol/kg per minute (2 mg/kg per minute) of glucose in the initial phases of fasting. Higher glucose turnover indicates increased utilization of glucose, an important consideration in the differential diagnosis of hypoglycemia.

The switch to fat metabolism is accomplished by activation of the hormone-sensitive lipase in adipose tissue, which hydrolyzes stored triglycerides to long-chain fatty acids and glycerol. The long-chain fatty acids have two fates. The bulk (normally about 120 g/d) is utilized directly, and the remainder (about 40 g/d) is oxidized in the liver to acetoacetic and β-hydroxybutyric acids. Ketoacids can be utilized efficiently as an energy source by most tissues (liver only minimally), but their primary importance is as backup substrate for the brain, as noted above. The shift of most tissues to lipid metabolism is important because the preferential oxidation of free fatty acids and ketones in place of glucose spares the latter for utilization by the central nervous system.

Catabolic metabolism is initiated by a fall in insulin concentration in plasma and secretion of the four counterregulatory hormones: glucagon, epinephrine, cortisol, and growth hormone. In addition, norepinephrine is released directly from sympathetic neurons. Glucagon is the primary hormone of glucose maintenance, and epinephrine plays a backup or secondary role. The latter is particularly important in the defense against hypoglycemia in diabetes mellitus, where the glucagon response is lost early (see Chap. 337). Cortisol and growth hormone function by antagonizing insulin action, and promoting mobilization of substrate and activation of gluconeogenesis.

The anabolic and catabolic phases of metabolism are summarized in Table 338-1. Breakdown in any of the adaptive mechanisms can lead to hypoglycemia.

SYMPTOMATOLOGY Symptoms of hypoglycemia fall into two main categories: those induced by an *excessive secretion of epinephrine* and those due to *dysfunction of the central nervous system*. Rapid epinephrine release causes sweating, tremor, tachycardia, anxiety, and hunger. Central nervous system (CNS) symptoms include dizziness, headache, clouding of vision, blunted mental acuity, loss of fine motor skill, confusion, abnormal behavior, convulsions, and loss of consciousness. When the onset of hypoglycemia is gradual, CNS symptoms predominate, and the epinephrine phase may not be recognizable. With more rapid drops in plasma glucose (as in insulin reactions), adrenergic symptoms are prominent. In the diabetic subject, adrenergic symptoms may not be manifest if severe neuropathy is present.

The level of plasma glucose required to activate hormonal defenses and to produce symptoms varies. The literature is confusing because

TABLE 338-1 The feeding-fasting cycle

Phase	Primary hormone	Plasma substrates	Substrate flux	Active process

Anabolic*	Insulin	↑ Glucose
		↑ Triglycerides
		↑ Branched-chain amino
		  acids
		↓ Free fatty acids
		↓ Ketones
			Splanchnic bed → storage
			  and utilization sites
				Glycogen storage
				Protein synthesis
				Triglyceride formation

Catabolic†	Glucagon	↓ Glucose ↓ Triglycerides ↑ Alanine and glutamine‡ ↑ Free fatty acids ↑ Ketones	Storage sites → liver and utilization sites	Glycogenolysis Gluconeogenesis Proteolysis Lipolysis Ketogenesis

* Expected findings during the first several hours after ingestion of a mixed meal of fat, carbohydrate, and protein.
† The major catabolic phase occurs during the overnight fast, although partial catabolic cycles occur between meals.
‡ Arrows indicate plasma concentrations except for alanine and glutamine. While arterial concentrations of these amino acids are relatively constant, uptake by the liver and intestine is increased in the catabolic phase.

many experimental studies use "arterialized" venous blood samples (drawn from a hand vein in a heated box), while in clinical practice plain venous blood is ordinarily used. The latter may be as much as 1 mmol/L (18 mg/dL) lower than the arterialized sample. Clinically recognizable symptoms in persons without diabetes are regularly produced when venous plasma glucose concentrations fall below 2.5 mM (45 mg/dL) if the plasma glucose is lowered acutely, as by insulin injection. In the defense against acute hypoglycemia, progressive responses occur as the glucose levels fall. In one study in normal persons (arterialized venous samples), insulin secretion ceased at 4.6 mmol/L glucose (83 mg/dL), glucagon and epinephrine were released at 3.8 mmol/L (68 mg/dL), growth hormone at 3.7 mmol/L (67 mg/dL), and cortisol at 3.2 mmol/L (58 mg/dL). Thus protective mechanisms are activated before the symptomatic threshold is reached. Although overt symptoms are not present, evidence of CNS dysfunction may be demonstrable with minimal decrements of plasma glucose. In a study utilizing auditory evoked potentials as a sensitive indicator of CNS function, abnormalities were seen in normal persons with a drop in glucose in arterialized venous blood from 4.8 to 4.0 mmol/L (87 to 72 mg/dL). When blood glucose is sustained at 4.0 mmol/L (72 mg/dL), counterregulatory release eventually occurs (2 to 3 h) despite the fact that no symptoms are produced. Major symptoms of CNS dysfunction may not occur until plasma glucose concentrations approximate 1 mmol/L (20 mg/dL). This is so because normal persons have the capacity to increase cerebral blood flow sufficiently to deliver adequate glucose to the brain even with low concentrations. Cerebral atherosclerosis, with its nonelastic blood vessels, compromises this protective mechanism and allows symptomatic distress at higher glucose levels. Symptoms (adrenergic or CNS) due to hypoglycemia are unlikely with a plasma glucose above 2.8 mmol/L (50 mg/dL) in nondiabetic persons, recognizing that the physiologic sequence induced by hypoglycemia is subliminal CNS dysfunction, adrenergic symptoms, and then overt CNS dysfunction. Poorly controlled patients with diabetes mellitus appear to develop symptoms at higher glucose concentrations, and meticulously controlled diabetic patients have a lowering of the symptomatic threshold and may exhibit the syndrome of *hypoglycemia unawareness* (see Chap. 337). Some patients with insulinoma also have a lowering of the glucose threshold required to induce counterregulatory hormone release and epinephrine-induced symptoms.

A rare syndrome that mimics the CNS manifestations of hypoglycemia has been described in which blood glucose is normal but cerebrospinal fluid (CSF) glucose is low, presumably due to a defect in the glucose transporter molecule, GLUT 1. Seizures may result.

CLASSIFICATION It is traditional to classify hypoglycemia as either *postprandial* (reactive) or *fasting*. Pathologically low plasma glucose concentrations occur in the former only in response to meals, while they occur in the latter only after fasting for a few to many hours. Patients with fasting hypoglycemia (particularly those with insulinomas) may exhibit a reactive component, but reactive patients

do not have symptoms when food is withdrawn. Fasting hypoglycemia usually means that a disease process is associated with the lowered plasma glucose, but symptoms suggestive of postprandial hypoglycemia are often found in the absence of recognizable disease.

CAUSES OF HYPOGLYCEMIA Postprandial hypoglycemia
The most common cause of postprandial hypoglycemia is alimentary hyperinsulinism (Table 338-2). Patients who have undergone gastrectomy, gastrojejunostomy, pyloroplasty, or vagotomy are subject to hypoglycemia following meals, presumably because of rapid gastric emptying with brisk absorption of glucose and excessive insulin release. Glucose concentrations fall more rapidly than insulin under these circumstances, and the resulting insulin-glucose imbalance leads to hypoglycemia. Ingestion of fructose or galactose induces hypoglycemia in children with fructose intolerance and galactosemia (see Chap. 354), respectively. Leucine intake rarely can cause the syndrome in susceptible infants. Diabetes mellitus in its early phase is usually listed as a cause of reactive hypoglycemia, but in our experience, symptomatic hypoglycemia as a premonitory symptom of diabetes is uncommon. Prediabetics, who by definition are normoglycemic, may have a late fall in plasma glucose after oral glucose tolerance testing, but this pattern is similar to that frequently present in asymptomatic, healthy individuals (see below).

Idiopathic alimentary hypoglycemia consists of two syndromes: *true hypoglycemia* and *pseudohypoglycemia*. In the former, adrenergic symptoms appear postprandially and are accompanied by a low plasma glucose at the time the symptoms appear spontaneously during everyday life. The symptoms are relieved by ingestion of carbohydrate, which raises the plasma glucose. Such patients are rare. The mechanism is unknown, although subtle dysfunction of the gastrointestinal tract might be operative. Some patients with true postprandial hypoglycemia turn out to have insulinomas (see below). *Pseudohypoglycemia* describes the condition of patients who reproducibly develop adrenergic symptoms suggestive of hypoglycemia 2 to 5 h after a meal but who do not have low plasma glucose concentrations when symptoms appear spontaneously in everyday life. The condition is often self-diagnosed, with "confirmation" coming from a 5-h glucose tolerance test that reveals a lower than "normal" plasma glucose between 2 and 5 h.

Two questions have to be asked about pseudohypoglycemia. First, what are the symptoms (which may be incapacitating) due to? Second,

TABLE 338-2 Causes of postprandial (reactive) hypoglycemia

A Alimentary hyperinsulinism
B Hereditary fructose intolerance
C Galactosemia
D Leucine sensitivity
E Idiopathic

can a valid diagnosis of hypoglycemia be made by a glucose tolerance test? The symptoms of nervousness, weakness, tremor, tachycardia, dizziness, and sweating reported by these patients are probably due to epinephrine release. Many otherwise normal persons experience similar symptoms at some time in their lives and may even have gained relief by eating. Patients with pseudohypoglycemia, on the other hand, develop the symptoms regularly and repetitively. In one study, 80 consecutive subjects with reproducible postprandial symptoms were studied by 5-h glucose tolerance testing. Hypoglycemia was considered to be present if (1) the plasma glucose fell below 3.3 mmol/L (60 mg/dL) during the test, (2) symptoms or signs compatible with hypoglycemia were present, and (3) at least a doubling of plasma cortisol occurred 30 to 90 min after the nadir of plasma glucose (suggesting hypoglycemia sufficient to activate the hypothalamic-pituitary-adrenal axis). Only 18 of the 80 (23 percent) who by history were candidates for postprandial hypoglycemia fulfilled these criteria. Twenty-five percent of asymptomatic matched normal controls also met all three criteria. When the patients and controls were tested after a mixed meal, no subject in either group had a plasma glucose below 3.3 mmol/L (60 mg/dL), yet 14 of the 18 patients (78 percent) had symptoms typical of those occurring after glucose tolerance testing. The absence of hypoglycemia after mixed meals despite the presence of typical symptoms has been observed in other studies. *Pseudohypoglycemia* appears to be an accurate descriptive term for the syndrome and is preferable to "idiopathic postprandial syndrome," which also has been used. Many such patients are thought to have stress or anxiety as a predisposing factor. Presumably they have enhanced catecholamine release following a meal, or they might be abnormally sensitive to normal postprandial norepinephrine/epinephrine release. Insulin can stimulate epinephrine release in humans if hypoglycemia is prevented. Whether enhanced insulin release plays a role in the pseudohypoglycemia syndrome is not known.

Fasting hypoglycemia   The causes of fasting hypoglycemia are many, but in all there is an imbalance between the production of glucose by the liver and its utilization in peripheral tissues. In some, hypoglycemia is due primarily to a defect in glucose production, while in others, the problem is excess glucose utilization. Both defects may be present. For example, with insulin excess there is driven glucose utilization coupled with blunted hepatic glucose production. The latter is caused by insulin's capacity to block the glycogenolytic/gluconeogenic effects of the counterregulatory hormones. Dual defects are probably operative in disorders of fat oxidation and non-insulin-producing tumors as well.

Supply-side hypoglycemia (impaired production of glucose) characteristically requires much less glucose during therapy than does *demand-side hypoglycemia* (overutilization of glucose) (Table 338-3). As noted above, glucose production during a fast approximates 11 μmol/kg per minute (2 mg/kg per minute) in normal persons, but with insulin-induced hypoglycemia, glucose utilization increases to about 67 μmol/kg per minute (12 mg/kg per minute). Thus, if more than 56 mmol (10 g) of glucose per hour is required to prevent or reverse hypoglycemia, it can be assumed that overutilization is present.

UNDERPRODUCTION OF GLUCOSE   As discussed earlier, the production of glucose by the liver initially involves the breakdown of stored glycogen and subsequently depends on gluconeogenesis, the synthesis of glucose from precursors delivered to the liver from peripheral tissues. The causes of inadequate production of glucose during fasting can be grouped into five categories: (1) hormone deficiencies, (2) defects in glycogenolytic or gluconeogenic enzymes, (3) inadequate substrate delivery, (4) liver disease, and (5) drugs. Hypopituitarism and adrenal insufficiency are the most common hormone deficiency states causing hypoglycemia. Defects in catecholamine or glucagon release are rare. Enzymic abnormalities causing hypoglycemia are generally seen in children and not adults. Glucose-6-phosphatase deficiency is the classic example of a defect in glycogen breakdown, but hypoglycemia may occur in young children with deficiencies of

TABLE 338-3   Major causes of fasting hypoglycemia

PRIMARILY DUE TO UNDERPRODUCTION OF GLUCOSE

A **Hormone deficiencies**
  1 Hypopituitarism
  2 Adrenal insufficiency
  3 Catecholamine deficiency
  4 Glucagon deficiency
B **Enzyme defects**
  1 Glucose-6-phosphatase
  2 Liver phosphorylase
  3 Pyruvate carboxylase
  4 Phosphoenolpyruvate carboxykinase
  5 Fructose-1,6-diphosphatase
  6 Glycogen synthetase
C **Substrate deficiency**
  1 Ketotic hypoglycemia of infancy
  2 Severe malnutrition, muscle wasting
  3 Late pregnancy
D **Acquired liver disease**
  1 Hepatic congestion
  2 Severe hepatitis
  3 Cirrhosis
  4 Uremia (probably multiple mechanisms)
  5 Hypothermia
E **Drugs**
  1 Alcohol
  2 Propranolol
  3 Salicylates

PRIMARILY DUE TO OVERUTILIZATION OF GLUCOSE

A **Hyperinsulinism**
  1 Insulinoma
  2 Exogenous insulin
  3 Sulfonylureas
  4 Immune disease with insulin or insulin receptor antibodies
  5 Drugs: quinine in falciparum malaria, disopyramide, pentamidine
  6 Endotoxic shock
B **Appropriate insulin levels**
  1 Extrapancreatic tumors
  2 Systemic carnitine deficiency
  3 Deficiency in enzymes of fat oxidation
  4 3-Hydroxy-3-methylglutaryl-CoA lyase deficiency
  5 Cachexia with fat depletion

hepatic glycogen phosphorylase and in other forms of glycogen storage disease (Chap. 350). The inability to make glycogen because of inadequate glycogen synthetase activity also renders the infant susceptible to fasting hypoglycemia. In addition to glucose-6-phosphatase, three other enzymes are necessary for gluconeogenesis: pyruvate carboxylase, phosphoenolpyruvate carboxykinase, and fructose-1,6-bisphosphatase (fructose-1,6-diphosphatase) (Fig. 338-1). Hypoglycemia can occur with decreased activities of any of these enzymes, often in association with lactic acidosis. The cause of lactic acidosis in these disorders is not known, although impaired hepatic lactate uptake due to the gluconeogenic defect probably plays a role. Substrate deficiency appears to be one of the mechanisms operative in ketotic hypoglycemia of infancy, since alanine turnover in such patients is low. Inadequate substrate supply also may contribute to hypoglycemia in malnutrition, muscle-wasting states, chronic renal failure, and late pregnancy. Acquired liver disease can cause serious hypoglycemia. Hepatic congestion due to right-sided heart failure is particularly troublesome, and severe viral hepatitis or cirrhosis also can cause hypoglycemia. Hypothermia, especially in association with alcohol, may cause very low levels of plasma glucose. Slowed enzymatic activity of the liver is the likely mechanism. The hypoglycemia of renal failure has multiple causes. In addition to impairing substrate delivery, uremic toxins may suppress hepatic gluconeogenesis, and decreased renal clearance of insulin and impairment of renal gluconeogenesis may contribute to the problem.

A number of drugs, in addition to insulin and sulfonylureas, cause hypoglycemia. Alcohol induces hypoglycemia only after a period of fasting sufficient to deplete liver glycogen stores. In this circumstance, hepatic glucose production is dependent on gluconeogenesis. The

FIGURE 338-1 Scheme of hepatic carbohydrate metabolism. Only the sequences for gluconeogenesis, glycogen synthesis, and glycogenolysis are shown.

oxidation of ethanol in the liver generates high concentrations of NADH, the reduced form of nicotinamide adenine dinucleotide (NAD). The increased NADH/NAD ratio diverts oxaloacetate into malate formation, diminishing its availability to the gluconeogenic sequence via the action of phosphoenolpyruvate carboxykinase (see Fig. 338-1). The normal pathway of gluconeogenesis from pyruvate is thus blocked, leading to a drop in hepatic glucose output and hypoglycemia. Large amounts of ethanol are not required to produce this syndrome, and plasma alcohol concentrations may be as low as 5.4 mmol/L (25 mg/dL) at the time symptoms occur. Ethanol-induced hypoglycemia usually occurs in adults but can be seen in children who drink alcohol unknowingly. Salicylates (in children) and propranolol are the next most frequently involved drugs. Propranolol presumably causes difficulty in fasting patients or insulin-requiring diabetic subjects by impairing the glycogenolytic response. In diabetes the drug also may prevent recognition of impending hypoglycemia by blunting the symptomatic response to epinephrine release. Other drugs have been reported to cause hypoglycemia in isolated cases, but the relationship is often unproved. Some drugs enhance glucose utilization. Pentamidine and disopyramide cause hyperinsulinism, the former by beta cell cytolysis ("insulin leak") and the latter by an unknown mechanism, perhaps as a direct insulin secretagogue. Quinine given in falciparum malaria has been reported to cause hyperinsulinemic hypoglycemia, but the issue is clouded because hypoglycemia occurs in untreated malaria as well, possibly secondary to malnutrition, liver involvement, or cytokine release.

OVERUTILIZATION OF GLUCOSE Overutilization of glucose occurs in two settings: when hyperinsulinism is present and when plasma insulin concentrations are low. There are basically four causes of hyperinsulinemic hypoglycemia: insulinoma, exogenous insulin administration, sulfonylureas, and a peculiar form of insulin autoimmunity. *Insulinoma* is used generically here to include single solid tumors, microadenomatosis, and islet cell hyperplasia (nesidioblastosis), a rare syndrome in adults. Hypoglycemia in a diabetic taking prescribed insulin or oral agents is not a diagnostic problem. The difficulty comes when a nondiabetic subject induces hypoglycemia

deliberately and surreptitiously because of psychiatric disturbance, raising the possibility of an insulin-producing tumor. The differential diagnosis between insulinoma and factitious hypoglycemia is considered below. Rarely, hypoglycemia with hyperinsulinism occurs in autoimmune disease associated with antibodies to endogenous insulin. Mechanisms are not well understood, although dissociation of free insulin from hormone-antibody complexes at inappropriate times is probably most important. Idiotypic antibodies (antibodies against the anti-insulin antibodies) also might function as insulin agonists with the insulin receptor. By binding insulin, the antibodies also may induce excessive insulin release from the pancreas. Some patients have alternating insulin resistance/hyperglycemia and hypoglycemia. Insulin autoantibodies have been seen most frequently in subjects with hyperthyroidism treated with methimazole, but presumably they might arise in any autoimmune syndrome. Antibodies directed against the insulin receptor, usually a cause of insulin resistance, also may induce hypoglycemia with high plasma insulin levels. Under these circumstances, the configuration of the antibody is thought to allow it to activate the insulin receptor, simultaneously blocking access of native insulin and impairing its clearance.

Sepsis with endotoxinemia causes hyperglycemia followed by hypoglycemia in experiment animals. The excess insulin release is thought to be caused by sepsis-associated cytokine release, probably acting directly on the beta cell.

Hypoglycemia in the context of glucose overutilization and appropriately low plasma insulin concentrations occurs in two situations. The first is in association with solid extrapancreatic tumors, usually of large size. The most common are of mesothelial origin and include fibromas and sarcomas. The syndrome also can be seen with hepatomas, carcinomas of the gastrointestinal tract, renal cell carcinomas, and adrenal cancers. The mechanism of the hypoglycemia is not clear, although high levels of insulin-like growth factor (IGF-2) may play a role. The physiologic role of IGF-2 is not known, and it is not clear whether it produces hypoglycemia through its own receptor or by interacting with the insulin receptor. One patient with tumor-associated hypoglycemia was reported to have an increased number of insulin receptors in liver, muscle, and circulating mononuclear cells, but the significance of the finding is not clear.

Symptomatic hypoglycemia due to overutilization also may occur in situations where free fatty acids and ketones are not available for oxidation in muscle and other tissues. Patients with *systemic carnitine deficiency* can have severe hypoglycemia. In this condition, carnitine, which is necessary to transport fatty acids into mitochondria for oxidation, is low in plasma, muscle, liver, and other tissues. As a consequence, peripheral tissues cannot utilize fatty acids for energy production, and the liver cannot make ketone bodies as alternative substrate. The result is that all tissues become glucose-dependent, exceeding the capacity of the liver to meet the demand. Other features of systemic carnitine deficiency include nausea, vomiting, elevated blood ammonia levels, and hepatic encephalopathy. The illness thus constitutes one form of the Reye syndrome. (In *myopathic carnitine deficiency,* only muscle is involved, and a polymyositis-like syndrome without hypoglycemia is produced.) Nonketotic (or hypoketotic) hypoglycemia with secondary systemic carnitine deficiency and the Reye syndrome also accompany *deficiencies of medium- and long-chain acyl-CoA dehydrogenases and 3-hydroxy-3-methylglutaryl-CoA lyase (HMG-CoA lyase).* The first two enzymes operate in the fatty acid oxidative sequence, while HMG-CoA lyase catalyzes the conversion HMG-CoA to acetoacetate and acetyl-CoA in the ketogenic cycle. Any time there is a block in fatty acid oxidation or ketone formation a secondary carnitine deficiency may develop. Accumulated acyl-CoA is transesterified to form acyl carnitine, which is then lost in the urine. Systemic carnitine deficiency in the absence of enzymic defect probably is due to a primary renal leak. It is not known whether the block in ketone production per se leads to hypoglycemia or whether secondary carnitine deficiency is required. If the former, ketones must become a primary (necessary) substrate during an extended fast. Hypoglycemia is less common with deficiency of *carnitine palmitoyltransferases.* Presumably, the defect is not complete in most patients, allowing some fatty acid oxidation to occur so that the tendency to hypoglycemia is minimized. The clinical picture is that of an exercise-induced myopathy with myoglobinuria. Hypoglycemia also occurs in patients with cachexia due to advanced cancer. At autopsy, no recognizable triglyceride stores are present in adipose tissue, suggesting free fatty acid deficiency as the primary mechanism.

Causes of hypoglycemia in hospitalized patients Frequencies of diagnoses vary in different series. Drugs are the most common cause, the three most frequent being insulin, sulfonylureas, and alcohol. It has been estimated that 60 percent of the time one of these three agents is involved when hypoglycemia is diagnosed. Renal failure is responsible for about 15 percent of cases overall. Liver disease (about 15 percent), malnutrition (about 10 percent), and sepsis (about 5 percent) are also common causes. A high index of suspicion for insulinoma, solid tumors, enzymatic defects, or hormonal deficiencies should be engendered by the finding of hypoglycemia in nondiabetic persons without uremia, liver disease, cachexia, or history of alcohol intake.

DIAGNOSIS Fasting hypoglycemia If a person with diabetes mellitus presents with symptoms of hypoglycemia, it is usually safe to conclude that no special diagnostic tests are needed, since the hypoglycemia is almost always related to therapy. If a nondiabetic develops similar symptoms—particularly if confusion, loss of consciousness, or convulsions are present—it is critical to draw blood for assay before intravenous glucose is administered. *The best time to obtain diagnostic laboratory tests with spontaneous hypoglycemia is at presentation.* The goal is to assess plasma insulin level and counterregulatory hormone response while the plasma glucose is low. Assays should be carried out for glucose, insulin, insulin-connecting peptide (C peptide), cortisol, drugs, and toxins, especially sulfonylureas and alcohol. It is often wise to freeze a separate sample of plasma for subsequent tests (e.g., proinsulin, carnitine, insulin antibodies, lactate) should the diagnosis not be clear from initial evaluation. Demonstration that hypoglycemia is accompanied by inappropriate insulin levels sharply narrows the clinical possibilities. Routine laboratory examinations also may be helpful. For example, the absence of ketones or the presence of a metabolic acidosis may be clues to the primary problem.

Once the patient has become alert (assuming altered mental status is present on arrival), it is important to take a detailed history and carry out a physical examination. Special emphasis should be placed on food intake in the preceding 24 h and the possibility of drug ingestion. Signs of heart failure and hepatic congestion should be sought, and the presence and thickness of the adipose tissue mass should be noted. Pigmentation of the skin may suggest Addison's disease. Workup includes liver function studies and computed tomographic (CT) scanning or abdominal sonography (to look for solid tumors in the retroperitoneal space or abdominal cavity). Patients with enzyme defects and rare hormonal deficiencies (epinephrine, glucagon) usually require evaluation in referral centers, since definitive assays for these hormones and enzymes are not routinely available. For reasons cited above, it is important to quantitate the amount of glucose required to prevent recurrent hypoglycemia during acute phase therapy; i.e., if 8 to 10 g of glucose per hour is sufficient to prevent hypoglycemia, diminished glucose production is probably operative. A requirement for higher infusion rates suggests enhanced glucose utilization.

If the patient has a history compatible with hypoglycemia but does not have symptoms at the time of examination, hospitalization for fasting has traditionally been required. The fast should be carried out for at least 72 h unless symptoms develop. Plasma glucose, insulin, C peptide, and cortisol should be measured every 6 h. Occasionally, quantitation of plasma free fatty acids, glucagon, and total ketones is helpful. (For glucagon, a protease inhibitor such as aprotinin must be added.) Two points are at issue. First, does the patient have fasting hypoglycemia? Second, is the hypoglycemia associated with hyperinsulinism? Neither question is easy to answer. There is no definitive lower limit of plasma glucose that unequivocally defines pathologic hypoglycemia during a 72-h fast. Values of the nadir in one study are shown in Table 338-4. Women usually develop lower levels than men. Another series reported mean minimal levels of 3.4 mmol/L (62 mg/dL) in men and 2.9 mmol/L (52 mg/dL) in women during a 72-h fast. However, values as low as 1.2 mmol/L (22 mg/dL) may occur in normal women without symptoms. On balance, a presumptive diagnosis of hypoglycemia is probably justified if the plasma glucose falls below 2.5 mmol/L (45 mg/dL) in venous blood at any time during the fast, provided typical symptoms are induced. The diagnosis of hypoglycemia is strengthened if symptoms are rapidly relieved by administration of carbohydrate. If symptoms are not produced, the diagnosis of hypoglycemia should be made with caution.

Absolute insulin values are not always helpful in diagnosing hyperinsulinism. In normal subjects when glucose concentrations rise, insulin levels also increase, and when plasma glucose concentrations fall, insulin release is inhibited. This means that plasma insulin concentrations must be interpreted in the light of the simultaneously determined glucose value. Thus a "normal" absolute insulin level may be abnormal in the face of hypoglycemia, while high absolute levels may be appropriate if the glucose concentration is elevated.

Plasma insulin concentration generally reaches background levels for the assay when the plasma glucose falls below about 4.6 mmol/L (83 mg/dL), as noted earlier. While some studies have shown lower cutoff points, it is probable that any measurable insulin concentration should be considered suspicious if the venous plasma glucose is below 2.5 mmol/L (45 mg/dL). If hyperinsulinism is not demonstrated, one of the other causes of fasting hypoglycemia must be sought.

Some investigators screen for insulinoma utilizing outpatient tests. The C-peptide suppression test is based on the fact that suppression of the release of endogenous insulin and C peptide during insulin infusion is impaired in persons with insulinomas. The results are influenced by age and obesity. Less well standardized tests involve intravenous tolbutamide infusion and rigorous exercise in the fasted state. However, the 72-h fast remains the gold standard when the patient cannot be tested during a spontaneous hypoglycemic episode.

Should hypoglycemia not develop during fasting, insulinoma or other hypoglycemia-producing organic disease is unlikely, although insulinomas may rarely (~2 percent) exhibit no depression of the

TABLE 338-4 Mean plasma glucose and insulin during fasting

Assay	Subjects	Hours of fast				
		0*	24	36	48	72
Glucose mmol/L (mg/dL)	Men	4.7 (85)	4.6 (83)	4.3 (78)	4.3 (78)	3.9 (71)
	Women	4.6 (83)	3.5 (63)	2.8 (50)	2.6 (46)	2.7 (48)
Insulin pmol/L (μU/mL)	Men	100 (14)	64 (9)	57 (8)	57 (8)	43 (6)
	Women	86 (12)	43 (6)	29 (4)	21 (3)	29 (4)

* Zero values were obtained after overnight fast. Results are mean values for 20 normal men and 60 normal women.
SOURCE: TJ Merimee, JE Tyson, Diabetes 26:161, 1977.

plasma glucose even during a prolonged fast. Insulinomas rarely present solely as postprandial hypoglycemia. Diagnosis usually is suspected in such cases because inappropriate insulin levels are shown during the postmeal episodes.

Postprandial hypoglycemia In patients presumed to have postprandial hypoglycemia, the most widely used test has been a 5-h oral glucose tolerance examination. Since normal persons may have chemical hypoglycemia without symptoms in the glucose tolerance test while subjects with pseudohypoglycemia have symptoms in the absence of hypoglycemia following meal testing, the 5-h glucose tolerance test should be abandoned as a tool for diagnosis. The only unequivocal diagnostic test for true pseudohypoglycemia is the demonstration of a low plasma glucose concentration (less than 2.5 mmol/L, or 45 mg/dL) during spontaneously developed symptoms. Some physicians utilize a home glucose analyzer in diagnosis. If no hypoglycemia is demonstrated during one week of testing (on arising, 2 h after each meal, at bedtime, and during symptoms), the diagnosis of true postprandial hypoglycemia is rejected. Most authors consider home testing unreliable because of inaccuracies of measurements in the hypoglycemic range. Patients with pseudohypoglycemia usually have slightly elevated glucose concentrations during spontaneous attacks because of the hyperglycemic action of epinephrine, the stress hormone that induces the symptoms.

Insulinoma versus factitious hypoglycemia The self-induction of hypoglycemia by the injection of insulin or the ingestion of sulfonylureas is so common as to equal or exceed the incidence of insulinoma. The demonstration of hyperinsulinism during hypoglycemia cannot, therefore, be taken as definitive evidence of the presence of an islet cell tumor. Factitious disease should always be suspected when hypoglycemic symptoms appear in medical personnel or families of diabetic patients. Several tests are helpful in distinguishing insulinoma from factitious hypoglycemia once hyperinsulinism has been established. Patients with insulinoma tend to have high concentrations of proinsulin in plasma (>20 percent of total insulin). Plasma proinsulin is not elevated by the administration of commercial insulin preparations or sulfonylureas. Measurement of the insulin connecting peptide (C peptide) will indicate whether the insulin circulating in plasma is of endogenous or exogenous origin. When insulin is cleaved from its precursor proinsulin molecule, C peptide is released into the portal vein in a 1:1 ratio with insulin. Thus, in patients with insulinoma, C-peptide concentrations should parallel the plasma insulin values. The characteristic pattern in factitious hypoglycemia due to insulin injection is a high circling level of insulin with relatively suppressed C-peptide values because exogenous insulin, which does not contain C-peptide, suppresses endogenous insulin release in normal persons, as described earlier. Antibodies to insulin are helpful if present because they usually indicate chronic insulin injection. Sulfonylureas elevate both the C-peptide and insulin concentrations in plasma. Therefore, factitious hypoglycemia due to oral agents can only be diagnosed by a high index of suspicion coupled with assay of the drug in plasma or urine. The differential characteristics of insulinoma and the two types of factitious hypoglycemia are shown in Table 338-5.

TREATMENT The initial treatment of serious hypoglycemia (producing confusion or coma) is the intravenous administration of a bolus of 25 or 50 g glucose as a 50% solution followed by constant infusion of glucose until the patient is able to eat a meal. The importance of the meal is due to the fact that hepatic glycogen repletion is not effective with small quantities of intravenous glucose. Patients in the overutilization category may require large amounts of intravenous glucose to maintain consciousness. It is not enough to infuse 5% dextrose at a rate of 1 to 2 mL/min and assume the patient is protected (20% to 30% dextrose solutions may be required in some cases). Frequent measurement of capillary glucose concentrations should be carried out using glucose-sensitive reagent strips to assess effectiveness of glucose infusion rates. Intravenous glucose usually can be stopped once the patient has eaten, but this can only be determined by trial. Adrenergic reactions without central nervous

TABLE 338-5 Differential diagnosis of insulinoma and factitious hyperinsulinism

Test	Insulinoma	Exogenous insulin	Sulfonylurea
Plasma insulin	High	Very high*	High
Insulin/glucose ratio	High	Very high	High
Proinsulin	Increased	Normal or low	Normal
C peptide	Increased	Normal or low[†]	Increased
Insulin antibodies	Absent	± Present[‡]	Absent
Plasma or urine sulfonylurea	Absent	Absent	Present

* Total plasma insulin in patients with insulinoma is rarely above 1435 pmol/L (200 μU/mL) in the basal state and often much lower. Values greater than 7175 pmol/L (1000 μU/mL) are highly suggestive of exogenous insulin injection.
[†] C peptide may be normal in absolute terms, but low in relation to the increased insulin value. See text for C peptide suppression test.
[‡] Insulin antibodies may not be present if only a few injections have been given, especially with purified insulin.

system abnormalities can be treated with oral carbohydrate and do not require parenteral therapy.

Hypoglycemia from sulfonylureas may last for prolonged periods (days) (Fig. 338-2). It is common for patients to lapse back into coma if glucose infusions are stopped too soon. The reason for the prolonged effect is not always clear, though drug interactions, hepatic disease, and renal failure may play a role in some cases.

Surgery is the treatment of choice for insulinoma. Localization of the tumor is best accomplished by ultrasound, and endoscopic ultrasound has the greatest sensitivity. Intraoperative ultrasound is also used if preoperative localization has not been possible. CT, magnetic resonance imaging, and arteriography are not as reliable. If the tumor cannot be found in the pancreas or located in an extrapancreatic site at the time of surgery, stepwise pancreatectomy (from tail to head) should be carried out with frozen sections made of sequential slices. Capillary glucose should be measured at each stage of the resection if the tumor is not obvious. A rise in plasma glucose may indicate removal of a small, nonpalpable lesion. In general, resection is stopped with an 85 percent pancreatectomy, even if the tumor is not found, to avoid malabsorptive complications. While a majority of patients are cured by surgery, as many as 15 percent have persistent hypoglycemia. Postoperative complications include acute pancreatitis, peritonitis, fistulas, pseudocyst formation, and chronic hyperglycemia (acquired diabetes).

Medical treatment is indicated in insulinoma only in preparation for surgery or after failure to find the tumor at operation. Two drugs are available, diazoxide and octreotide, a long-acting octapeptide analogue of somatostatin. Diazoxide can be given intravenously or orally in doses of 300 to 1200 mg/d. Because of its salt-retaining properties, it must be accompanied by a diuretic. Octreotide is given subcutaneously in divided doses of 100 to 600 μg/d. It may cause nausea and diarrhea and predispose to cholelithiasis. Treatment of metastatic insulin-producing carcinomas is unsatisfactory. It has been reported that streptozocin and doxorubicin are superior to streptozocin plus fluorouracil (median survival 2.2 and 1.4 years, respectively). Chlorozotocin, a nitrosourea-containing molecule similar to streptozocin, is currently under study. It appears to have fewer toxic side effects than streptozocin. Despite the generally poor prognosis, occasional patients with insulin-producing islet cell carcinomas survive for long periods.

Therapy of other forms of recurrent hypoglycemia, apart from hormone replacement in pituitary or adrenal insufficiency, is dietary. In most cases, avoidance of fasting is all that is required. This is critical in diseases of fat oxidation or ketone synthesis. If intercurrent illness prevents eating, hospitalization for intravenous glucose is absolutely required. A high-protein, low-carbohydrate diet often relieves symptoms in patients with pseudohypoglycemia. With true alimentary hypoglycemia, it is probably important to keep the size of the individual meals small. The practice of giving massive amounts

FIGURE 338-2 Prolonged and refractory hypoglycemia in factitious hypoglycemia due to chlorpropamide in an alcoholic. Note continued hypoglycemia despite the infusion of glucose at rates up to 50 g/h. (*From RM Jordan et al, Arch Intern Med 137:390, 1977. Copyright 1977, American Medical Association. Used by permission.*)

of vitamin E, crude adrenocortical extract, and trace metals to patients with pseudohypoglycemia is useless even if harmless (which has not been established).

REFERENCES

CHARLES MA et al: Comparison of oral glucose tolerance tests and mixed meals in patients with apparent idiopathic postabsorptive hypoglycemia: Absence of hypoglycemia after meals. Diabetes 30:465, 1981

CRYER PE: Glucose counterregulation: Prevention and correction of hypoglycemia in humans. Am J Physiol 264:E149, 1993

DAVIS SN, CHERRINGTON AD: The hormonal and metabolic responses to prolonged hypoglycemia. J Lab Clin Med 121:21, 1993

DE FEO P et al: Modest decrements in plasma glucose concentration cause early impairment in cognitive function and later activation of glucose counterregulation in the absence of hypoglycemic symptoms in normal man. J Clin Invest 82:436, 1988

FERNER RE, NEIL HAW: Sulphonylureas and hypoglycaemia. Br Med J 296:949,1988

GRUNBERGER G et al: Factitious hypoglycemia due to surreptitious administration of insulin: Diagnosis, treatment, and long-term follow-up. Ann Intern Med 108:252, 1988

MARKS V: Recognition and differential diagnosis of spontaneous hypoglycemia. Clin Endocrinol 37:309, 1992

MERIMEE TJ: Insulin-like growth factors in patients with nonislet cell tumors and hypoglycemia. Metabolism 35:360, 1986

MOERTEL CG et al: Streptozocin-doxorubicin, streptozocin-fluorouracil, or chlorozotocin in the treatment of advanced islet-cell carcinoma. N Engl J Med 326:519, 1992

PANDIT MK et al: Drug-induced disorders of glucose tolerance. Ann Intern Med 118:529, 1993

SERVICE FJ: Hypoglycemias. J Clin Endocrinol Metab 76:269, 1993

——— et al: Insulinoma: Clinical and diagnostic features of 60 consecutive cases. Mayo Clin Proc 51:417, 1976

——— et al: C-peptide suppression test: Effects of gender, age, and body mass index; implications for the diagnosis of insulinoma. J Clin Endocrinol Metab 74:204, 1992

339   DISORDERS OF THE TESTES

JAMES E. GRIFFIN / JEAN D. WILSON

The testes produce sperm and the steroid hormones that regulate male sexual life. Both functions are under complex feedback control by the hypothalamic-pituitary system so that the testes have biosynthetic and regulatory features similar to those of the ovary and the adrenal. Testicular hormones are also responsible for the formation of the

basic male phenotype during embryogenesis. The function of the embryonic testis and the disorders of sexual differentiation are described in Chap. 342.

PHYSIOLOGY AND REGULATION OF TESTICULAR FUNCTION

The testis consists of two components—clusters of interstitial or Leydig cells that produce androgenic steroids and a system of spermatogenic tubules for the production and transport of sperm.

THE LEYDIG CELL   Testosterone synthesis   The biochemical pathway by which the 27-carbon sterol cholesterol is converted to androgens and estrogens is depicted in Fig. 339-1. Cholesterol can either be synthesized de novo in the Leydig cell or derived from plasma lipoproteins. Five enzymatic transformations are required for the conversion of cholesterol to testosterone. In this process, the side chain of cholesterol is cleaved in two steps to reduce the size from 27 to 19 carbons, and the A ring of the steroid is converted to the Δ^4-3-keto configuration. The five enzyme reactions are cholesterol side chain cleavage (P450$_{SCC}$), 3β-hydroxysteroid dehydrogenase/isomerase (3β-HSD), 17α-hydroxylase (P450$_{17\alpha}$), 17,20-lyase (P450$_{17\alpha}$), and 17β-hydroxysteroid oxidoreductase (17β-HSOR). Both 17α-hydroxylase and 17,20-lyase activities are present in a single cytochrome P450$_{17\alpha}$. The first four reactions take place in the adrenal as well as the testis.

The rate-limiting process in testosterone synthesis is the conversion of cholesterol to pregnenolone by the P450$_{SCC}$; luteinizing hormone (LH) from the pituitary regulates the activity of this enzyme and of other enzymes in the pathway. Additional steroids including estradiol are synthesized in small amounts in the Leydig cell.

Testosterone secretion and transport   Only about 70 nmol (20 µg) of testosterone is stored in the normal testes, so the total hormone content turns over about 200 times each day to provide the average of 17 to 20 µmol (5 to 6 mg) that is secreted into plasma in normal young men (Fig. 339-2). Testosterone is transported in plasma bound to protein, largely to albumin and to a specific transport protein, testosterone-binding globulin (TeBG, also called *sex hormone–binding globulin*, SHBG). The bound and unbound fractions in plasma are in dynamic equilibrium, only about 1 to 3 percent being unbound. The fraction of circulating testosterone available for entry into tissues approximates the sum of the free and albumin-bound fractions or about half the total plasma testosterone.

FIGURE 339-2 Androgen and estrogen production in normal young men. Average production of androstenedione and testosterone is shown in the top boxes, and mean daily production of estrone and estradiol is shown in the lower boxes. Estrogen is formed by extraglandular aromatization (*braces*) or by direct secretion from the testes. Vertical arrows indicate the rates of extraglandular aromatization of androgens, and the horizontal arrows indicate the interconversion of androgen and estrogens by 17β-hydroxysteroid dehydrogenase. Thus estradiol arises from plasma testosterone, from estrone, and from direct secretion by the testes. (*Adapted from PC MacDonald et al.*)

FIGURE 339-1 Pathways of androgen formation in the testis and the conversion of androgens to other active hormones in peripheral tissues.

Peripheral metabolism of androgens Testosterone serves as a circulating precursor (or prohormone) for the formation of two other types of active metabolites that mediate many of the physiologic processes involved in androgen action (see Fig. 339-1). Testosterone can be 5α-reduced to dihydrotestosterone, which performs many of the differentiative, growth-promoting, and functional actions involved in male sexual differentiation and virilization. Circulating androgens in both sexes also can be converted to estrogens in extraglandular tissues. In men, estrogens act in some instances in concert with androgens but also can have effects independent of or opposite to those of androgens. Thus the physiologic effects of testosterone are the result of the combined effects of testosterone itself plus those of the active androgen and estrogen metabolites of the parent molecule. (In normal men, small amounts of estradiol and dihydrotestosterone are also derived by direct secretion from the testes and indirectly from the weak adrenal androgen androstenedione.)

The quantitative relation between circulating androgens and the formation of estrogen in normal young men is illustrated diagrammatically in Fig. 339-2. The production rates of testosterone and androstenedione average about 20 and 10 μmol (6 and 3 mg), respectively, per day. All estrone production [averaging about 240 nmol (66 μg) per day] can be accounted for by formation from circulating precursors. The mean estradiol production is approximately 170 nmol (45 μg)

per day; about 35 percent is derived from circulating testosterone, 50 percent is derived from the weak estrogen estrone, and 15 percent is secreted directly into the circulation by the testes. When gonadotropin levels are elevated, the amount of estradiol secretion by the testes is increased.

The 5α-reduced and estrogenic metabolites can exert local (paracrine) actions in the tissues in which they are formed or enter the circulation and act as hormones at other sites. Circulating dihydrotestosterone is formed principally in the androgen target tissues; estrogen formation takes place in many tissues, the most significant being adipose tissue. The overall rate of extraglandular estrogen formation increases with increasing amounts of adipose tissue and with age.

Plasma testosterone and its active metabolites are converted to inactive metabolites in the liver and excreted predominantly in the urine; approximately half the daily turnover is excreted in the form of urinary 17-ketosteroids (primarily androsterone and etiocholanolone), and the remainder is excreted as polar metabolites (diols, triols, and conjugates).

Gonadotropin regulation and testosterone secretion Testosterone secretion is regulated by pituitary LH (Fig. 339-3). (For the details of pituitary function, see Chap. 331.) Follicle-stimulating hormone (FSH) may augment testosterone secretion, possibly by inducing maturation of the Leydig cell. Testosterone also regulates the sensitivity of the pituitary to the hypothalamic-releasing factor luteinizing hormone–releasing hormone (LHRH, also called *gonadotropin-releasing hormone*, GnRH). Although the pituitary can convert testosterone to dihydrotestosterone and to estrogens, testosterone itself is the primary regulator of gonadotropin secretion. Testosterone also acts in the central nervous system to slow the rate of LHRH formation or secretion and consequently to decrease the frequency of pulsatile LH release. Under ordinary circumstances, LH secretion is exquisitely sensitive to the feedback effects of testosterone, with complete suppression following the administration of amounts of exogenous androgen that approximate the normal daily secretory rate of testosterone (about 20 μmol or 6 mg). However, prolonged elevation of plasma LH (as in testicular deficiency) renders the pituitary less sensitive to negative feedback control by exogenous androgen.

Neither the plasma concentration of testosterone nor that of LH is constant, each fluctuating in a pulsatile manner that reflects changes in secretory rates (Fig. 339-4). Major sleep-related surges in the pulsatile secretion of both LH and testosterone signal the initiation of male puberty. In young adults, diurnal variation in the magnitude of

FIGURE 339-3 Regulation of testosterone and sperm production by LH and FSH. (C, cholesterol; T, testosterone.)

FIGURE 339-4 Twenty-four-hour pattern of plasma LH and testosterone in a normal man sampled every 20 min. (*Reprinted from Griffin and Wilson.*)

this episodic secretion of LH and testosterone occurs with peak morning levels of testosterone about 25 to 30 percent higher than late afternoon values.

Androgen action The major functions of androgen are regulation of LH secretion, formation of the male phenotype during sexual differentiation, and induction of sexual maturation and function at puberty. The cellular mechanisms by which androgens perform these functions are summarized schematically in Fig. 339-5. Testosterone (T) enters the cell by passive diffusion. Inside the cell T can be converted to dihydrotestosterone (D) by the 5α-reductase enzymes 1 and 2; 5α-reductase 2 is responsible for dihydrotestosterone formation in most androgen target tissues. T or D is then bound to the androgen-receptor protein in the nucleus (R). The hormone-receptor complex (TR or DR) attaches to specific chromosomal sites; as a result, new messenger RNA is transcribed, and new protein appears within the cytoplasm of the cell. The androgen receptor protein is coded by a gene on the long arm of the X chromosome; it contains 917 amino acids and has a molecular mass of about 110 kDa. It is similar in structure to other steroid hormone receptors and has distinct hormone-binding, DNA-binding, and functional domains (see Chap. 329). Estradiol acts by a mechanism similar to that of androgens but involving its own receptor (see Chap. 340).

Although testosterone and dihydrotestosterone bind to the same receptor, their physiologic roles differ. The testosterone-receptor complex regulates gonadotropin secretion and is responsible for the wolffian stimulation phase of sexual differentiation (see Chap. 342), whereas the dihydrotestosterone-receptor complex is responsible for external virilization during embryogenesis and the major portion of androgen action during sexual maturation and adult sexual life. The question of which hormone controls spermatogenesis is unresolved. The mechanism by which two hormones can interact with the same receptor but have different physiologic effects is also not well understood. Dihydrotestosterone binds to the receptor much more tightly than does testosterone, and hence its formation serves to amplify the hormonal signal.

THE SEMINIFEROUS TUBULE AND SPERMATOGENESIS Normal function of the seminiferous tubule is dependent on the pituitary and on the adjacent Leydig cells, both FSH and androgen being essential for normal spermatogenesis (see Fig. 339-3). The major site of FSH action is the Sertoli cell in the seminiferous tubules. The seminiferous tubule also contains androgen receptors. Androgen appears to be essential for spermatogenesis, whereas FSH is required for spermatid maturation. The normal adult testes produce more than 200 million sperm per day.

The Sertoli cell cannot synthesize steroid hormones de novo and is dependent on testosterone that diffuses in from adjacent Leydig cells. Sertoli cells can convert testosterone to estradiol and to dihydrotestosterone. The seminiferous tubules also produce the peptide hormones inhibin, which exerts a negative feedback control, and activin, which feeds back positively on FSH secretion by the pituitary (see Fig. 339-3). Testosterone and estradiol also can inhibit FSH secretion.

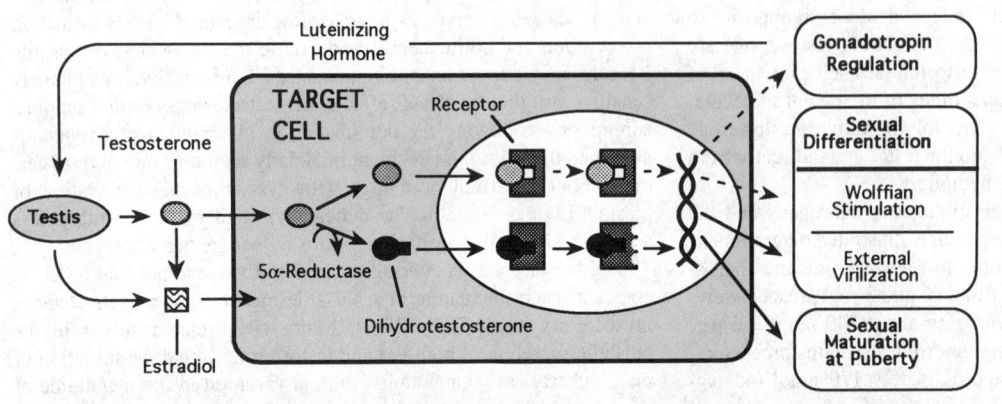

FIGURE 339-5 Current concepts of androgen action.

The interlocking system in which two pituitary hormones regulate testicular function provides a precise dual-control mechanism by hormonal signals from Leydig cells and the spermatogenic tubules that feed back on the hypothalamic-pituitary system to regulate their own function (see Fig. 339-3).

ASSESSMENT OF TESTICULAR FUNCTION

LEYDIG CELL FUNCTION **History and physical examination** The assessment of Leydig cell function and androgen status should include inquiry about the presence at birth of developmental abnormalities of the urogenital tract, the timing and extent of sexual maturation at puberty, the rate of beard growth, and the current libido, sexual function, strength, and energy. Inadequate Leydig cell function or androgen action during embryogenesis may manifest by the presence of hypospadias, cryptorchidism, or microphallus. If Leydig cell failure occurs prior to puberty, sexual maturation will not occur, and the individual will develop the features termed *eunuchoidism*, including an infantile amount and distribution of body hair, poor development of skeletal muscles, and failure of closure of the epiphyses so that the arm span is more than 5 cm greater than the height and the lower body segment (heel to pubic) more than 5 cm longer than the upper body segment (pubic to crown). Detection of postpubertal Leydig cell failure requires a high index of suspicion and appropriate laboratory assessment. One reason is that decreased sexual function in adult men may be caused by nonendocrine as well as endocrine factors. The second is that certain functions that require androgens for initiation continue unabated when Leydig cell failure occurs, and functions that eventually regress may do so very slowly. For example, the frequency of shaving may not decrease for months or years because of slow decline in the rate of beard growth once established.

Plasma testosterone and dihydrotestosterone levels Plasma testosterone is measured by radioimmunoassay. Testosterone is secreted into plasma in a pulsatile fashion every 60 to 90 min (see Fig. 339-4); a single random sample provides a result within ±20 percent of the true mean value only two-thirds of the time, while three equally spaced samples 15 to 20 min apart provide a more accurate assessment. The samples do not need to be assayed separately, and aliquots of the three samples should be pooled for a single determination. The range of plasma testosterone in normal adult men is 10 to 35 nmol/L (3 to 10 ng/mL). In adult men, the plasma values vary somewhat throughout the day and at different times of the year, but these variations are not as great as those for plasma cortisol and are not significant in routine clinical assessment. Plasma levels of testosterone correlate in general with testosterone secretory rates as measured by isotope infusion. Estimation of TeBG concentration by radioimmunoassay is sometimes useful in the interpretation of total plasma testosterone levels. Bioavailable testosterone in plasma can be estimated by measuring the non-TeBG-bound fraction of testosterone.

The plasma testosterone value in prepubertal children is statistically higher in boys than in girls, the range in both being 0.2 to 0.7 nmol/L (0.05 to 0.2 ng/mL). The rise in plasma testosterone at the start of male puberty begins as a result of sleep-related nocturnal gonadotropin surges, so during the initial phases, plasma testosterone and LH are higher at night than during the day. Random daytime levels of plasma testosterone increase gradually as puberty progresses and reach adult levels at about age 17.

Dihydrotestosterone is also measured by radioimmunoassay. In young men, the plasma dihydrotestosterone level is about one-tenth the testosterone value and averages around 2 nmol/L (0.6 ng/mL). In older men with benign prostatic hyperplasia, plasma dihydrotestosterone levels average about 3 nmol/L (0.9 ng/mL).

Urinary 17-ketosteroids The measurement of urinary 17-ketosteroids is not a valid way to assess testicular function because testosterone contributes only about 40 percent of daily urinary 17-ketosteroids in men. The bulk of urinary 17-ketosteroids is derived from adrenal androgens.

Plasma LH Plasma LH is also measured by radioimmunoassay. LH is also secreted in a pulsatile fashion and fluctuates more widely than does plasma testosterone so that in adult men an isolated random plasma LH is likely to be within ±20 percent of true mean value only a third of the time. Again, assay of a pool of plasma composed of equal portions of three samples drawn 15 to 20 min apart as described above provides a value approaching the true mean. In early puberty, plasma LH secretion increases only during sleep, but the pulsatile secretion in the adult is of similar magnitude during sleep and waking periods. The normal plasma LH values should be established for a given laboratory. The usual normal range in adult men is 5 to 20 IU/L. Bioactive LH can be assessed in some laboratories by the rat interstitial cell assay and may be detectable at times when the immunoreactive LH is undetectable. A low plasma testosterone concentration can be interpreted correctly only if plasma LH is also measured simultaneously, and likewise, the "appropriateness" of a given plasma testosterone value must be interpreted in relation to the plasma testosterone value. For example, a low plasma testosterone coupled with a low LH implies hypothalamic or pituitary disease, whereas the finding of a low plasma testosterone and a high LH suggests primary testicular insufficiency (see Chap. 330).

Response to gonadotropin stimulation Leydig cell function is difficult to assess prior to puberty when both LH and testosterone levels are low, and it is common to measure response of plasma testosterone to gonadotropin stimulation as an index of Leydig cell capacity. Normal prepubertal boys respond to 3 to 5 days of injection of 1000 to 2000 IU human chorionic gonadotropin (hCG) with an increase in plasma testosterone to about 7 nmol/L (2 ng/mL); the magnitude of the response increases with the initiation of puberty and peaks in early puberty.

Response to luteinizing hormone–releasing hormone The responsiveness of the pituitary gland to luteinizing hormone–releasing hormone (LHRH) changes at the time of puberty. Prior to puberty, quantitative responses of LH and FSH are similar. With pubertal development, the LH response to acute administration of LHRH increases, while the FSH response remains the same. The amount of LH released following acute administration of LHRH probably reflects the amount of stored hormone in the pituitary. When 100 μg LHRH is given subcutaneously or intravenously to normal men, LH levels usually increase four- to fivefold, with the peak level at 30 min. However, the range of response is broad, some normal men having less than a doubling of LH levels. In general, the peak LH following a single LHRH injection correlates with the basal levels. In primary testicular failure, measurement of basal LH is usually sufficient, and measurement of LHRH response adds little to aid the diagnosis. Men with either pituitary disease or hypothalamic disease may have a normal or an abnormal LH response to acute administration of LHRH. Therefore, a normal response is of no diagnostic value either in determining the presence of disease or in distinguishing hypothalamic from pituitary disease. A subnormal response is of value in establishing that an abnormality exists, even though the site is not determined. The LHRH test is most useful in the evaluation of men with secondary hypogonadism and subnormal LH response to acute administration of LHRH. If daily infusions of LHRH for a week lead to the development of a normal acute LH response, a hypothalamic etiology is likely.

SEMINIFEROUS TUBULE FUNCTION **Examination of the testes** Evaluation of the testes is an essential portion of the physical examination. The seminiferous tubules account for about 60 percent of testicular volume. The prepubertal testis measures about 2 cm in length and 2 mL in volume and grows during puberty to reach the adult proportions by age 16. When damage to the seminiferous tubules occurs prior to puberty, the testes are small and firm, whereas the testes are usually small and soft following postpubertal damage (the capsule, once enlarged, does not contract to its previous size). Testes in adults average 4.6 cm in length (range 3.5 to 5.5 cm), corresponding to a volume of 12 to 25 mL. Advanced age does not influence testicular size, so the significance of small testes is the same at all ages in the adult. Testis size varies among ethnic groups. Asian men have smaller testes than western Europeans, independent of differences in body size. Because of the possible causal role in infertility, the presence of varicocele should be sought by palpation with the patient standing.

Semen analysis   Seminal fluid analysis is performed on samples obtained by masturbation into a glass container after 24 to 36 h abstinence. Analysis should be performed within an hour. The normal ejaculate volume is 2 to 6 mL. Immediately after ejaculation, the seminal fluid coagulates, followed within 15 to 30 min by liquefaction. Estimation of motility should be made on undiluted seminal fluid; more than 60 percent of the sperm should be motile and of normal morphology. The normal range for sperm density is generally considered to be greater than 20 million per milliliter, with a total count of more than 60 million per ejaculate, but the definition of a minimally adequate ejaculate is not clear. Some men with low sperm counts are nevertheless fertile. This uncertainty as to the lower level of sperm density, percent motility, and percent normal forms in fertile semen stems from two issues. First, many factors produce temporary aberrations in sperm count, and in men who present with semen of equivocal quality it is necessary to examine three or more ejaculates to determine whether abnormal findings are permanent or temporary. Second, the seminal fluid is routinely evaluated by tests that do not assess the functional capacity of sperm. Methods to measure sperm penetration of bovine cervical mucus and zona-free hamster ova are not sufficiently standardized to permit general use.

Plasma FSH   Plasma FSH, as measured by specific radioimmunoassay, usually correlates inversely with spermatogenesis. In normal adult men, the range of plasma FSH is 5 to 20 IU/L. Men with intact hypothalamic-pituitary axes have elevations of FSH when damage to the germinal epithelium is severe.

Testicular biopsy   Testicular biospy is useful in some patients with oligospermia and azoospermia both as an aid in diagnosis and as an indication of feasibility of treatment. For example, a normal testicular biopsy and a normal FSH in an azoospermic man suggest obstruction of the vas deferens, which may be surgically correctable.

ESTROGENIC FUNCTION   Examination of the breasts   Breast enlargement (gynecomastia) is the most consistent feature of feminizing states in men (see Chap. 341). Gynecomastia is due to the proliferation of both glandular and adipose tissue. The presence of gynecomastia should be sought by examining the sitting patient using the fingers to grasp glandular tissue. Palpation with the flat of the hand while the patient is supine may result in failure to detect early or minimal breast enlargement. In obese men it is important to try to define the edge of the rim of glandular tissue that separates it from adipose tissue of the chest wall.

Plasma estrogen   As discussed above, most of the estradiol and all the estrone produced in normal men is formed by extraglandular aromatization of circulating androgens. Plasma estradiol is usually less than 180 pmol/L (50 pg/mL) in normal men; plasma estrone is somewhat higher but usually less than 300 pmol/L (80 pg/mL). Elevated estrogen production and elevated plasma levels can be due to elevations in plasma precursors (liver or adrenal disease), to increases in extraglandular aromatization (obesity), or to increased production by the testes (testicular tumors or androgen resistance).

PHASES OF NORMAL TESTICULAR FUNCTION

The phases of male sexual life can be defined in terms of the plasma testosterone value (Fig. 339-6). In the male embryo, the production of testosterone by the testes commences at about 7 weeks of gestation. Shortly thereafter plasma testosterone attains a high value that is maintained until it falls late in gestation so that at the time of birth plasma testosterone is only slightly higher in males than in females. Shortly after birth, plasma testosterone in the male infant again begins to rise and remains elevated for approximately 3 months, falling to low levels by age 6 months to 1 year. The concentration then remains

FIGURE 339-6   Phases of male sexual life. *(Reprinted from Griffin and Wilson.)*

low (but slightly higher in boys than in girls) until the onset of puberty, when it begins to rise in boys, reaching adult levels by about age 17. The mean plasma level remains more or less constant in the adult until late middle age and then declines slowly during the later decades of life. During the third, or adult, phase of male sexual life, sperm production becomes sufficient to allow reproduction to take place. The physiologic events that take place during these various phases differ, as do the pathologic consequences of derangements in testicular function at different stages of life. Male sexual differentiation during embryogenesis is considered in Chap. 342. The role of the surge of testosterone formation during the first year of life is not certain. However, in primates, neonatal activation of the hypothalamic-pituitary-testicular axis is important for subsequent normal pubertal development. The focus of this chapter is on testicular pathophysiology during puberty, adulthood, and old age.

ABNORMALITIES OF TESTICULAR FUNCTION

PUBERTY   The factors that control the onset of puberty are poorly understood and may reside in the hypothalamic-pituitary system, the testes, or the adrenal. Prior to the onset of puberty, gonadotropin secretion by the pituitary is low but appears to be under regulatory control by the testes, since prepubertal castration results in a rise in plasma gonadotropin levels. This suggests that prior to puberty the negative feedback control of gonadotropin secretion is exquisitely sensitive to the small amount of circulating testosterone. The onset of puberty is heralded by sleep-associated surges in gonadotropin secretion. Later in puberty the rises in LH and FSH persist throughout the day. Thus, with maturation, the hypothalamic-pituitary system becomes less sensitive to negative feedback control, and the consequences are a higher mean plasma testosterone, maturation of the testes, and the onset of spermatogenesis. The rise in gonadotropin secretion is the consequence of both an increase in LHRH secretion and an increased sensitivity of the pituitary to LHRH. Plasma levels of bioactive LH increase even more than those of the immunoreactive hormone. The somatic changes at the time of puberty are secondary to the rise in plasma testosterone. Growth of the accessory organs of male reproduction (the penis, the prostate, the seminal vesicles, and the epididymides) accounts for about one-fourth of androgen-mediated nitrogen retention during puberty. Accelerated linear growth is accompanied by growth of muscle and connective tissue, accounting for the major portion of nitrogen retention at puberty. The principal androgen-sensitive muscles are those of the pectoral region and the shoulder. The characteristic hair growth of male puberty involves development of mustache and beard; regression of the scalp line; appearance of body, extremity, and perianal hair; and extension of the pubic hair upward into a diamond-shaped pattern. Growth of axillary and pubic hair is initiated under the control of adrenal androgens and is promoted by testicular androgens. The larynx enlarges, and the vocal cords become thickened, resulting in a lowering of the pitch of the voice. Hemoglobin levels increase about 10 g/L. These various androgen-mediated growth and maturation processes reach some limiting value so that once puberty is completed the administration of pharmacologic doses of androgen has no further effect. The entire process is heralded by testicular enlargement beginning at age 11 to 12 and is usually completed within 5 years, although some aspects of virilization, such as growth of the chest hair, may continue over a decade or more.

The events of normal male puberty are variable in onset, duration, and sequence. The central issue in dealing with disorders of puberty is separating instances of true absence or precocity from subjects at the extremes of normal variation. The use of staging criteria that correlate developmental and anatomic landmarks with chronologic age is useful in making this distinction. (See Marshall and Tanner.)

Sexual precocity Development of premature sexual characteristics appropriate for the phenotype, i.e., virilization in boys, is termed *isosexual precocity. Heterosexual precocity* refers to feminizing syndromes in boys.

ISOSEXUAL PRECOCITY Sexual development prior to age 9 in boys is generally considered abnormal. *True precocious puberty* or *complete isosexual precocity* occurs when both premature virilization and spermatogenesis take place, and *precocious pseudopuberty* or *incomplete isosexual precocity* refers to virilization unaccompanied by spermatogenesis, indicating that androgen formation is not the result of premature activation of the hypothalamic-pituitary system. This distinction is blurred in practice because pure virilizing syndromes may cause activation of gonadotropin secretion secondarily and thus be followed by development of spermatogenesis. Furthermore, local androgen production in the testis, as in Leydig cell tumors, can cause local areas of spermatogenesis around the tumor and limited sperm production. We therefore prefer a simple two-part classification: virilizing syndromes (in which hypothalamic-pituitary activity is appropriate for age) and premature activation of the hypothalamic-pituitary system.

Virilizing syndromes can result from Leydig cell tumors, human chorionic gonadotropin (hCG)–secreting tumors, adrenal tumors, congenital adrenal hyperplasia (most commonly 21-hydroxylase deficiency), androgen administration, or Leydig cell hyperplasia. In all these situations, plasma testosterone is inappropriately elevated for the age. Leydig cell tumors are rare in children but should be suspected when the testes are asymmetric in size (see Chap. 322). Virilizing adrenal tumors secrete large amounts of adrenal androgen (mainly androstenedione and dehydroepiandrosterone, some of which is converted to testosterone) and consequently cause elevated 17-ketosteroid secretion. Glucocorticoid administration does not suppress 17-ketosteroid excretion to normal in patients with testicular or adrenal tumors, in contrast to the prompt decrease that occurs following such treatment in congenital adrenal hyperplasia. Congenital adrenal hyperplasia leads to elevated 17-hydroxyprogesterone levels and as a consequence elevated androgen levels (see Chaps. 335 and 342). When this disorder is treated with glucocorticoids, true precocious puberty can then result if sufficient hypothalamic maturation has been produced by the increased androgen levels.

Gonadotropin-independent sexual precocity in boys may occur as a result of autonomous Leydig cell hyperplasia in the absence of Leydig cell tumor formation. The disorder is inherited as a male-limited autosomal disorder either from affected fathers to sons or from mothers who are unaffected carriers. Virilization begins usually by age 2. Testosterone levels are elevated, often to the adult male range; however, immunoreactive and bioactive LH levels and the LH response to LHRH are prepubertal. Many of these boys were mistakenly thought to have true precocious puberty in the past because of the presence of spermatogenesis.

Premature activation of the hypothalamic-pituitary system may be ''idiopathic'' or due to central nervous system (CNS) tumors, infections, or injuries. Such early hypothalamic-pituitary activation typically is associated with characteristics of normal puberty, i.e., sleep-related gonadotropin secretion, elevated plasma bioactive LH, and enhanced gonadotropin response to LHRH. Since the diagnosis of idiopathic true precocious puberty is one of exclusion, rare patients later prove to have been misclassified and to have an identifiable CNS abnormality. With improved means of diagnosis, such as computed tomographic scans and magnetic resonance imaging, delays in diagnosis will probably be less frequent.

Management of sexual precocity due to steroid- or gonadotropin-producing tumors, congenital adrenal hyperplasia, or CNS abnormality is directed toward the primary disease. In boys with Leydig cell hyperplasia, attempts have been made to lower plasma testosterone with medroxyprogesterone acetate or ketoconazole, but the long-term effectiveness of these agents is unknown. Idiopathic true precocious puberty and true precocious puberty due to inoperable CNS lesions are treated with LHRH analogue therapy, resulting in reversal of the pubertal maturation including decreased rate of skeletal development.

HETEROSEXUAL PRECOCITY Feminization in prepubertal boys can result from absolute or relative increases in estrogen due to a variety of causes (see Chap. 341).

Delayed or incomplete puberty The separation of failure of puberty from variants of normal is one of the most difficult problems in endocrinology. Some patients fail to show the normal spurt of growth and sexual development at the usual time but eventually commence puberty by age 16 or older. Adolescence may then either progress rapidly, or there may be a slow development and growth that continues until ages 20 to 22. Many men with delayed onset of puberty attain heights within the normal adult range. At times the history reveals that a parent or sibling has shown a similar pattern of development. The major problem is to separate this group of patients with delayed puberty from patients with organic disorders that impair puberty. Panhypopituitarism and hypothyroidism can cause pubertal failure in males (see Chaps. 331 and 334). Absent puberty also can result from primary disease of the testis, including defects in testicular development; this diagnosis is suspected on the basis of low plasma testosterone and elevated FSH and LH levels. Hereditary androgen resistance (in which plasma testosterone and LH levels are both high) usually results in hereditary male pseudohermaphroditism but in milder cases may be manifested by absent or incomplete puberty (see Chap. 342).

The most frequent finding in boys with absent puberty is both low plasma testosterone and low gonadotropin levels; in these patients it is necessary to distinguish boys with delayed puberty from those with isolated gonadotropin deficiency or idiopathic *hypogonadotropic hypogonadism (Kallman syndrome)*. The manifestations of isolated gonadotropin deficiency vary from boys with eunuchoidal features and testes of prepubertal size to those with partial manifestations of LH and/or FSH deficiency and partial degrees of testicular enlargement and pubertal development. Anosmia or hyposmia and cryptorchidism are common. The disorder is inherited as an X-linked recessive trait or an autosomal dominant trait with variable expressivity. Serum FSH and LH levels are usually below the normal male range, and plasma testosterone levels are low for age. The secretion of other pituitary hormones is usually normal. The defect appears to be in the synthesis or release of LHRH with the resultant gonadotropin pattern ranging from absence of pulsatile LH secretion to defects in amplitude and frequency of LH secretion; the administration of synthetic LHRH for a sufficient period corrects the endocrine abnormalities and initiates spermatogenesis. If untreated, these patients usually remain in the prepubertal state indefinitely. A prepubertal manifestation is microphallus, in which the size of the penis is below the fifth percentile for the age. Indeed, a fourth or more of isolated prepubertal microphallus is due to hypogonadotropic hypogonadism. Distinction between this disorder and delayed puberty is particularly difficult in patients of early or midpubertal age; the presence of microphallus, anosmia, or a family history of hypogonadotropic hypogonadism may help to establish the diagnosis. In the absence of such evidence, differentiation of the two states may become clear only after several years of observation. In some cases the response of plasma LH to LHRH stimulation may be helpful in suggesting that puberty is imminent.

ADULT ABNORMALITIES OF TESTICULAR FUNCTION At the completion of puberty, plasma testosterone levels reach the adult level of 10 to 35 nmol/L (3 to 10 ng/mL) throughout the day, plasma gonadotropins are 5 to 20 IU/L each for LH and FSH, and sperm production is sufficient to allow reproduction. The adult set of the complex regulatory system (see Fig. 339-3) is sustained in the normal man for more than 40 years. However, the system is subject to a variety of influences, at the level of both the testes and the hypothalamic-pituitary system. Spermatogenesis is exquisitely sensitive to alterations in temperature, and brief increases either in systemic or local temperature (as in a hot bath) can be followed by temporary decreases in sperm production. The system is likewise subject to influence by diet, drugs, alcohol, environmental agents, and psychological stress, all of which may cause temporary decreases in sperm count.

Persistent abnormalities of testicular function in adults can be due to hypothalamic-pituitary disorders (see Chap. 331), testicular defects, or abnormalities of sperm transport. Certain of these conditions tend to affect Leydig cell function or spermatogenesis selectively, but most cause both underandrogenization and infertility (Table 339-1). The interlocking of defective Leydig cell function and infertility is a consequence of the dependence of spermatogenesis on androgen formation. Even partial decreases in testosterone production can cause infertility. Certain disorders (hyperprolactinemia, radiation, cyclophosphamide therapy, autoimmunity, paraplegia, androgen re-

sistance) can cause either isolated infertility or a combined defect in testicular function in different subjects.

Hypothalamic-pituitary disorders Disorders of the hypothalamus and pituitary can impair secretion of gonadotropins (and cause decreased androgen production and decreased spermatogenesis) either as a portion of generalized disease of the anterior pituitary (see Chap. 331) or as an isolated defect, usually hypogonadotropic hypogonadism, in which secretion of both LH and FSH are impaired; hypogonadotropic hypogonadism can be either congenital or, rarely, an acquired idiopathic defect. Alternatively, gonadotropin secretion can be altered by factors other than hypothalamic-pituitary pathology. For example, elevation of plasma cortisol in the *Cushing syndrome* can depress LH secretion independent of a space-occupying lesion of the pituitary. Some patients with *congenital adrenal hyperplasia* have suppressed gonadotropin secretion and consequent infertility. *Hyperprolactinemia* (as the consequence either of pituitary adenomas or of drugs such as phenothiazines) has been associated with combined Leydig cell and seminiferous tubule dysfunction, presumably the consequence of inhibition of LH and FSH secretion by prolactin. Occasionally, impaired fertility in hyperprolactinemia is associated with normal gonadotropin and androgen levels and is presumed to result from direct inhibition of spermatogenesis by prolactin. *Hemochromatosis* impairs testicular function most commonly as the result of effects on the pituitary; less often it affects the testis directly (see Chap. 345). The use of *androgens* for purposes other than replacement therapy is often associated with impaired sperm production (see below). In several other conditions, testosterone levels may be decreased in association with normal LH levels, and the mechanism is less clear. Men with massive obesity have decreased TeBG and decreased levels of total and bioavailable testosterone that return toward normal with weight loss. Obesity may be part of the mechanism for decreased testosterone levels in the subset of such men with Pickwickian syndrome (see Chap. 229). Some men with seizures of temporal lobe origin also have a hormonal pattern consistent with hypogonadotropic hypogonadism.

Testicular defects Abnormalities of testicular function in the adult can be grouped into several categories: developmental and structural defects of the testes, acquired testicular defects, and disorders secondary to systemic and/or neurologic disease.

DEVELOPMENTAL ABNORMALITIES The *Klinefelter syndrome* (both the classic and mosaic forms) and the *XX male syndrome* are usually not recognized until after the time of expected puberty (see Chap. 342). Some developmental defects cause infertility in the presence of normal androgen production. These include varicocele, germinal cell aplasia, and cryptorchidism. *Varicocele* may be of etiologic importance in as much as one-third of all male infertility. It is caused by retrograde flow of blood into the internal spermatic vein that eventuates in progressive, often palpable dilatation of the peritesticular pampiniform plexus of veins. Varicocele occurs in about 10 to 15 percent of men in the general population and in 20 to 40 percent of men with infertility and is thought to result from incompetence of the valve between the internal spermatic vein and the renal vein. It is more common on the left (85 percent). Unilateral varicocele increases the blood flow and the temperature of both testes as a result of the extensive anastomoses of the venous systems. The increased scrotal (and testicular) temperature is believed to be the cause of the poor-quality semen and infertility (the testes do not have the usual 2°C lower temperature than that of the abdominal cavity). The findings on semen analysis are usually nonspecific, with all parameters showing some abnormality. In some studies, surgical resection results in improved fertility, with the best results (70 percent pregnancy rate) obtained in men whose preoperative sperm counts are over 10 million per milliliter.

Some patients with *germinal cell aplasia* (the Sertoli cell–only syndrome) have a positive family history and may constitute a specific group in whom the germinal epithelium is missing with resulting azoospermia; plasma testosterone and LH values are normal, and plasma FSH levels are elevated. Other patients with identical histologic

---

TABLE 339-1 Abnormalities of adult testicular function

Infertility with underandrogenization	Infertility with normal virilization
Hypothalamic-pituitary:	
Panhypopituitarism	
Isolated gonadotropin deficiency	Isolated FSH deficiency
Cushing's syndrome	Congenital adrenal hyperplasia
Hyperprolactinemia	Hyperprolactinemia
Hemochromatosis	Androgen use
Testicular:	
Developmental and structural defects	
Klinefelter's syndrome*	Germinal cell aplasia
XX male	Cryptorchidism
	Varicocele
	Immotile cilia syndrome
Acquired defects	
Viral orchitis*	*Mycoplasma* infection
Trauma	
Radiation	Radiation
Drugs	Drugs
(spironolactone, alcohol,	(cyclophosphamide)
ketoconazole,	
cyclophosphamide)	
Environmental toxins	Environmental toxins
Autoimmunity	Autoimmunity
Granulomatous disease	
Associated with systemic diseases	
Liver disease	Febrile illness
Renal failure	Celiac disease
Sickle cell disease	
Neurologic disease (myotonic	Neurologic disease (paraplegia)
dystrophy and paraplegia)	
Androgen resistance	Androgen resistance
Sperm Transport:	
	Obstruction of the epididymis or vas deferens (cystic fibrosis, diethylstilbesterol exposure, congenital absence)

* The common testicular causes of underandrogenization and infertility in adults—Klinefelter's syndrome and viral orchitis—are associated with small testes.

and clinical findings have androgen resistance or a history of viral orchitis or cryptorchidism. Consequently, a variety of conditions are commonly lumped under this term. The syndrome accounts for less than 10 percent of patients with azoospermia.

Unilateral *cryptorchidism*, even when corrected prior to puberty, is associated with abnormal semen in many individuals. This suggests that even in unilateral cryptorchidism the testicular abnormality is usually bilateral.

The *immotile cilia syndrome* is an autosomal recessive defect characterized by immotility or poor motility of the cilia of the airways and of the sperm. Kartagener's syndrome is a subgroup of the immotile cilia syndrome associated with situs inversus, chronic sinusitis, and bronchiectasis (see Chap. 221). The immotile sperm cannot fertilize. The structural abnormality leading to impaired motility of cilia can usually be defined by the electron-microscopic appearance. The specific defects that are known to cause the syndrome include defects in the dynein arms, spokes, or microtubule doublets. Cilia from epithelia and sperm tails from the same individual exhibit the same defects, but the pulmonary manifestations may be minor. *Other structural defects of sperm* that are less well understood can apparently lead to immotile sperm without involvement of cilia in the lung.

ACQUIRED TESTICULAR DEFECTS The most common cause of acquired testicular failure in the adult is *viral orchitis*. The responsible viruses include mumps virus, echovirus, lymphocytic choriomeningitis virus, and group B arboviruses. The orchitis is due to actual infection of the tissue by virus rather than to indirect effects of the infection. Orchitis is the most common complication of mumps, occurring in as many as one-fourth of adult men with the disease. In about two-thirds the orchitis is unilateral, and in the remainder it is bilateral. Orchitis usually develops within a few days after the onset of parotitis but may precede it. The testis may return to normal size and function or undergo atrophy. Atrophy is believed to be due both to direct effects of the virus on the seminiferous tubules and to ischemia secondary to pressure and edema within the taut tunica albuginea. Semen analysis returns to normal in three-fourths of men with unilateral involvement and in only one-third of men with bilateral orchitis. Atrophy is usually perceptible within 1 to 6 months after the orchitis subsides, and the degree of atrophy is not necessarily proportional to the severity of the acute orchitis or the development of infertility. Unilateral atrophy occurs in approximately one-third of cases of mumps orchitis, and bilateral atrophy occurs in about one-tenth.

Trauma is the second most common cause of secondary atrophy of the testes. The exposed position of the testis in the scrotum renders it susceptible to both thermal and physical trauma—particularly in individuals with hazardous occupations.

The testes are sensitive to *radiation damage;* decreased secretion of testosterone appears to be a consequence of diminished testicular blood flow. Doses higher than 200 mGy (20 rad) cause increases in plasma FSH and LH levels and damage to the spermatogonia. After doses of about 800 mGy (80 rad), oligospermia or azoospermia develops. Higher doses may obliterate the germinal epithelium, except for occasional stem and Sertoli cells. Fractionated radiation may have a more profound effect than single-dose radiation. Recovery of sperm density occurs in a dose-related fashion, and complete recovery of sperm density to preradiation levels may require as long as 5 years. Permanent infertility can occur after radiation therapy of malignant lymphoma despite shielding of the testes. Permanent androgen deficiency in adult men is uncommon after doses of radiation in the therapeutic range; however, most boys receiving direct testicular radiation for acute lymphoblastic leukemia have permanently low plasma testosterone levels.

In general, *drugs* interfere with testicular function in one of four ways—inhibition of testosterone synthesis, blockade of the peripheral action of androgen, enhancement of estrogen levels, or direct inhibition of spermatogenesis. Certain drugs have multiple effects, and agents such as guanethidine that block the sympathetic nervous system can impair sexual function in men whose pituitary-testicular axis is normal.

Spironolactone and ketoconazole block the synthesis of androgen by interfering with the late reactions in androgen biosynthesis. Spironolactone and cimetidine compete with androgen for the cytoplasmic receptor protein and thus interfere with androgen action in the target cell. Testosterone levels may be low and estradiol levels may be elevated in patients taking large amounts of marijuana, heroin, or methadone, although the exact reasons are unclear. Alcohol, when consumed in excess for prolonged periods, causes decreased plasma testosterone, independent of liver disease or malnutrition. Elevated plasma estradiol and decreased plasma testosterone levels have been reported in men taking digitalis.

Antineoplastic and chemotherapeutic agents commonly interfere with spermatogenesis. Cyclophosphamide causes azoospermia or extreme oligospermia within a few weeks after the initiation of therapy. Cessation of therapy is followed by a return of spermatogenesis within 3 years in about half of patients. Combination chemotherapy for acute leukemia, Hodgkin's disease, and other malignancies also may impair Leydig cell function. In pubertal boys this is manifested by decreased serum testosterone and elevated LH levels; in adult men testosterone levels do not decline, and the impaired Leydig cell function may only be detected as an enhanced LH response to LHRH. The alkylating agents in the chemotherapeutic regimens seem to be responsible for Leydig cell toxicity.

Because of the potentially toxic effects of many physical and chemical agents on spermatogenesis, the occupational and recreational history should be carefully evaluated in all men with infertility. Known environmental hazards include chemicals, such as the nematocide dibromochloropropane, cadmium, and lead, microwaves, and ultrasound.

Testicular failure also occurs as a part of a generalized disorder of *autoimmunity* in which multiple primary endocrine deficiencies coexist (Schmidt's syndrome) and in which circulating antibodies to the basement membrane of the testes are present (see Chap. 343). Sperm antibodies are also a cause of isolated male infertility. In some instances, such antibodies may be secondary phenomena resulting from duct obstruction or vasectomy. *Granulomatous diseases* also can destroy the testes, the most common such disorder being leprosy. Testicular atrophy occurs in 10 to 20 percent of men with lepromatous leprosy, the result of direct invasion of the tissue by the mycobacteria. The tubules are involved initially, followed by endarteritis and destruction of Leydig cells.

TESTICULAR ABNORMALITIES ASSOCIATED WITH SYSTEMIC DISEASE The common systemic diseases that cause underandrogenization and infertility are liver disease and renal failure. In *cirrhosis of the liver*, a combined testicular and pituitary abnormality leads to decreased testosterone production independent of the direct toxic effects of ethanol. Although plasma LH is elevated, the level may be below the expected range given the degree of androgen deficiency. This is most likely the result of inhibition of LH secretion by estrogen in patients with chronic liver disease. Increased estrogen production results from impaired hepatic extraction of adrenal androstenedione and subsequent increased extraglandular conversion to estrone and estradiol. In effect, estrogen precursors are shunted to sites of extraglandular aromatization. Testicular atrophy and gynecomastia are present in about half of men with cirrhosis, and many such men are impotent.

In chronic *renal failure*, decreased androgen synthesis and diminution of sperm production develop in the setting of elevated plasma gonadotropins. The elevated LH is due to increased production as well as reduced clearance but is incapable of effecting normal testosterone production. In addition, about one-fourth of men with chronic renal failure have hyperprolactinemia. Low testosterone coupled with normal or increased plasma estrogen levels probably account for the presence of gynecomastia in about half of men on chronic hemodialysis. The role of the hyperprolactinemia in decreasing testosterone production is unclear. About half of men with renal failure on dialysis experience decreased libido and impotence. The etiology of the testicular abnormalities in renal failure is not well understood. Improvement in testosterone production with hemodialysis is incomplete, but successful transplantation may lead to return of testicular function to normal.

Men with *sickle cell anemia* usually have impaired secondary sexual development, and testicular atrophy is present in one-third. The defect may be either at the testicular or hypothalamic-pituitary level. Abnormalities in Leydig cell function, frequently accompanied by decreased sperm density, have been noted in a variety of chronic systemic diseases, including protein-energy *malnutrition*, advanced *Hodgkin's disease* and *cancer* prior to chemotherapy, and *amyloidosis*. Most of these disorders cause a lowered plasma testosterone level coupled with a normal to increased plasma LH level, suggesting combined hypothalamic-pituitary and testicular defects. The low plasma testosterone is not the result of inhibitors that interfere with the binding to TeBG and hence is not analogous to the sick euthyroid syndrome. Similar hormone changes occur following *surgery, myocardial infarction*, and severe *burns* and thus may be a nonspecific effect of illness.

The temporary decrease in sperm density after *acute febrile illness* usually occurs in the absence of any changes in testosterone production. Infertility in men with *celiac disease* is associated with a hormonal pattern typical of androgen resistance, namely elevated testosterone and LH levels. *Neurologic diseases* associated with altered testicular function include myotonic dystrophy and paraplegia. In myotonic dystrophy, small testes may be associated with abnormalities of both spermatogenesis and Leydig cell function. Spinal cord lesions resulting in paraplegia lead to a temporary decrease in testosterone levels and persistent defects in spermatogenesis; some patients retain the capacity to obtain erection and to ejaculate.

ANDROGEN RESISTANCE   Defects of the androgen receptor cause resistance to the action of androgen usually associated with defective male phenotypic development, infertility, and underandrogenization (see Chap. 342). A less severe form of androgen resistance, associated with infertility due to oligo- or azoospermia in otherwise phenotypically normal men, may cause a significant fraction of infertility previously classified as idiopathic azoospermia.

Impairment of sperm transport   Disorders of sperm transport may cause infertility in as many as 6 percent of infertile men with normal virilization. The obstruction may be unilateral or bilateral, congenital or acquired. In men with unilateral obstruction of sperm transport, the infertility may result from antisperm antibodies. Obstructive azoospermia at the level of the epididymis also occurs in association with chronic infections of the paranasal sinuses and lungs. Tuberculosis, leprosy, and gonorrhea are rare causes of acquired obstruction of ejaculatory structures. Congenital defects of the vas deferens can occur as an isolated abnormality associated with absence of the seminal vesicles (and consequently absence of fructose in the ejaculate), in patients with *cystic fibrosis* (on occasion the principal manifestation of the disease), or in men whose mothers received *diethylstilbestrol* during pregnancy.

At least 40 percent of infertile men have infertility of unknown etiology; none of the preceding conditions is found on careful search. The therapy in all forms of male infertility, except surgically correctable varicocele, vas deferens obstruction, or treatable endocrinopathy, is unsatisfactory. Empirical therapy with androgens or gonadotropins has no significant effect on fertility. Although the semen quality may improve with such treatment, the pregnancy rate is usually no greater than in infertile men given no therapy (25 percent fertility in patients followed for a year). This latter fact should be kept in mind, namely, that spontaneous resolution may occur in up to one-fourth of patients with idiopathic infertility followed with no treatment. Many forms of male infertility associated with some motile sperm in the semen can be treated by in vitro fertilization.

Fertility control in the male   A variety of approaches to fertility control in men have been tried, including use of the condom as a safe barrier method that also prevents sexually transmitted disease. Another widely used technique is ligation of the vas deferens, a procedure that has been successful in large numbers of men and can be performed on an outpatient basis. The time required for azoospermia to occur following the operation depends on the number of sperm in the terminal vas deferens and ejaculatory ducts at the time of surgery but is usually less than 40 days. Azoospermia should be documented in each case to prove effectiveness. No deleterious effects on either testosterone production or the hypothalamic-pituitary axis have been documented. Despite reports of immune-complex–associated accelerated atherosclerosis in vasectomized nonhuman primates, there does not appear to be any association between vasectomy and atherosclerosis in men. Vasectomy should only be recommended for men requesting permanent sterilization. Only about 30 to 40 percent of men subjected to vasovasostomy for reanastomosis of the vas subsequently achieve fertility.

OLD AGE   Beginning at about age 60, mean plasma total and bioavailable testosterone concentrations decline. Nevertheless, though statistically lower than levels in young men, the concentrations of testosterone in elderly men usually remain within the normal range. The cause of the decreased testosterone level is likely decreased Leydig cell numbers in the testes. There is also a decline in seminiferous tubule function and decreased sperm production in older men. Plasma LH and FSH levels are usually increased in elderly men, and an increase in the rate of conversion of androgen to estrogen in peripheral tissues results in a decrease in the effective ratio of androgen to estrogen. These latter endocrine changes may play a role in the development of prostatic hyperplasia and possibly in development of gynecomastia in aging men (see Chap. 341). Male sexual function gradually declines after early adulthood, but there is no convincing evidence that hormonal changes have any direct bearing on changes in sexual function with age.

Prostatic hyperplasia   See Chap. 323.

Cancer of the prostate   See Chap. 323.

DISORDERS OF ALL AGES   Testicular tumors (See Chap. 322) Chorionic gonadotropin is present in normal testes, and it is not surprising that plasma gonadotropins may be elevated in testicular tumors. Indeed, an elevated plasma level of the beta subunit of human chorionic gonadotropins (hCG-β) serves as a sensitive and specific marker of tumor activity in some men with germ cell tumors. Plasma levels of the beta subunit are elevated in all patients with choriocarcinoma, in one-third of embryonal carcinomas and teratocarcinomas, and rarely in seminomas. There is a good correlation between change in hCG-β levels and response to therapy.

Elevated estradiol and testosterone production in patients with testicular tumors can arise by at least two mechanisms. In trophoblastic tumors and in tumors of Leydig and Sertoli cells, production of both hormones occurs autonomously in the tumor tissue itself; in these instances, plasma gonadotropin levels and hormone production by the uninvolved portions of the testes are depressed, and azoospermia is common. However, when gonadotropins are secreted by the tumor, the gonadotropin acts to increase estradiol and testosterone production in the unaffected areas of the testes, and azoospermia is uncommon. When estrogens and androgens are formed (directly or indirectly) by the tumors, feminization, virilization, or no obvious change may result, depending on the pattern of hormones produced and the age of the patients. Other cellular markers of testicular tumor activity have been described in individual cases, including alpha fetoprotein.

Gynecomastia   See Chap. 341.

HORMONAL THERAPY

ANDROGENS   Pharmacologic preparations   Effective androgen therapy requires the use of chemically modified analogues of testosterone. When testosterone itself is administered by mouth, it is absorbed into the portal blood and degraded promptly by the liver so that insignificant amounts reach the systemic circulation; when injected parenterally, testosterone is rapidly absorbed from the injection vehicle and rapidly degraded. As a consequence, effective androgen therapy requires either the administration in a slowly absorbed form of testosterone (dermal patches or micronized oral preparation) or the administration of modified analogues. Such chemical modifications either retard the rate of absorption or catabolism, so as to sustain effective blood levels, or enhance the androgenic potency of each molecule, so that full androgenic effects can be achieved at a lower blood level of the drug. Three types of modification of the molecule have received widespread clinical application (Fig. 339-7), namely, esterification of the 17β-hydroxyl group, alkylation at the 17α position, and modification of the ring structure, particularly substitutions at the 2, 9, and 11 positions. Most agents actually contain combinations of ring structure alterations and either 17α-alkylation or esterification of the 17ß-hydroxyl. Esterification serves to decrease the polarity of the molecule. Consequently, the steroid is more soluble in the fat vehicles used for injection, and release of the steroid into the circulation is slowed. Most esters must be injected parenterally. The more carbon molecules in the acid esterified, the more prolonged is the action. Esters such as testosterone cypionate and testosterone enanthate can be injected every 1 to 3 weeks. Because the esters are hydrolyzed before the hormones act, the effectiveness of therapy can be monitored by assaying plasma testosterone level with time following administration.

The oral effectiveness of 17α-alkylated androgens (such as methyltestosterone and methandrostenolone) is due to slower hepatic catabolism than occurs with testosterone itself so that the alkylated derivatives escape degradation by the liver and reach the systemic circulation. For this reason, 17α-methyl or -ethyl substitution is a common feature of most orally active androgens. Unfortunately, all 17α-alkylated steroids may cause abnormalities of liver function, and for this reason they have a limited role in medicine.

Other alterations of the ring structure of the androgen molecule

FIGURE 339-7 Some of the androgen preparations available for pharmacologic use.

have been adopted empirically. In some instances the modification slows the rate of inactivation, in others it enhances the potency of a given molecule, and in still others it alters the conversion to other active metabolites. For example, the potency of fluoxymesterone may be due to the fact that, unlike most androgens, it is a poor precursor for conversion to estrogens in peripheral tissues. Transdermal preparations of testosterone in which a testosterone-loaded patch is applied each day are under evaluation. This therapy avoids the wide swings in serum testosterone values that occur between injections of testosterone esters.

Side effects of androgens All androgens carry the risk of inducing virilization in women. Early manifestations include acne, coarsening of the voice, hirsutism, and menstrual irregularities. If treatment is discontinued as soon as these effects develop, the manifestations may slowly subside. Long-term side effects such as male-pattern baldness, worsening of the hirsutism and voice changes, and hypertrophy of the clitoris are largely irreversible. There is considerable variation in the frequency and degree to which these signs develop in women, probably because of individual differences in susceptibility, in steady state blood levels of hormone, and in duration of therapy. In general, the younger the patient, the more striking are the virilizing signs; nevertheless, florid virilization also can occur in adult women. At physiologic replacement doses, testosterone esters have no known side effects in mature men. At supraphysiologic doses, however, gonadotropin secretion is inhibited, the testes decrease in volume, and the sperm count falls (indeed, low sperm counts may persist for as long as 9 months after cessation of androgen abuse). The so-called toxic side effects differ among the different agents and depending on the clinical setting in which they are used.

Retention of a limited amount of sodium is an inevitable consequence of androgen therapy, but in patients with underlying heart disease or renal failure or when androgens are administered in enormous amounts, the degree of sodium retention may lead to edema. Although androgens do not cause malignancy, they may promote growth of and intensify pain from carcinoma of the prostate and from breast carcinoma in men.

Feminizing side effects of androgen therapy in men are poorly understood. Testosterone itself can be converted (aromatized) in extraglandular tissues to estradiol. In contrast, 5α-reduction of the molecule precludes estrogen formation. The most common manifestation of feminization is the development of gynecomastia. Such breast enlargement is common in children given androgens and correlates with an increase in urinary estrogens, possibly because of a greater capacity to convert androgens to estrogens in childhood. The administration of testosterone esters to men results in an increase in plasma estrogen levels. In men with normal liver function, gynecomastia usually develops only after high doses of androgens.

All 17α-alkylated androgens can produce liver function abnormalities such as elevation of plasma alkaline phosphatase and conjugated bilirubin. The incidence of clinical liver disease probably depends on the previous integrity of the liver, but jaundice may occur in the absence of preexisting liver disease. 17α-Alkylated drugs also cause an increase in a variety of plasma proteins that are synthesized in the liver. The most serious complications of 17α-alkylated androgen therapy are the development of peliosis hepatis (blood-filled cysts in the liver) and hepatoma. These disorders were initially described in patients with aplastic anemia, many of whom had Fanconi anemia, itself a predisposing factor for the development of malignancy. However, both lesions also have been reported in patients who received substituted androgens for a variety of other causes, including use by athletes. There may be a similar increased incidence of hepatocellular neoplasms in women taking oral contraceptives. In some individuals these tumors regress and follow a benign course after discontinuation of the drugs; and in others the course is rapidly fatal.

One indication for the use of 17α-alkylated androgens is in hereditary angioedema; in this disorder the desired therapeutic benefit (increase in the level of the inhibitor of the first component of complement) may actually be a side effect of the 17-alkylated steroid rather than an effect of the parent androgen itself. As a consequence, weak androgens such as danazol are effective in this disorder (see Fig. 339-7). Danazol is also used in the management of endometriosis (see Chap. 48).

Replacement therapy The aim of androgen therapy in hypogonadal men is to restore or bring to normal male secondary sexual characteristics (beard, body hair, external genitalia) and male sexual behavior and to mimic the hormonal effects on somatic development (hemoglobin, muscle mass, nitrogen balance, and epiphyseal closure). Since an assay for plasma testosterone is available for monitoring therapy, the treatment of androgen deficiency is almost universally successful. The parenteral administration of a long-acting testosterone ester such as 100 to 200 mg testosterone enanthate at 1- to 2-week intervals results in a sustained increase in plasma testosterone to the normal male range. Such esters act only through the release of testosterone itself into the circulation. If the hypogonadism is primary and of long duration (as in the Klinefelter syndrome), suppression of plasma LH to the normal range may not occur for many weeks, if at all. Considerable variability exists in the relation between plasma testosterone and male sexual behavior, but in postpubertal testicular failure (even of many years duration) resumption of normal sexual activity is usual following adequate replacement. Androgen does not restore spermatogenesis in hypogonadal states, but the volume of the ejaculate (derived largely from the prostate and seminal vesicles) and other male secondary sex characteristics return to normal. The effects of endogenous androgen on hemoglobin, nitrogen retention, and skeletal development are also reproduced.

In patients of all ages in whom hypogonadism developed prior to expected puberty (such as patients with hypogonadotropic hypogonadism), it is appropriate to bring plasma testosterone slowly into the adult range. When therapy is commenced at the time of expected puberty in such patients, the normal events of puberty proceed in the usual fashion. If therapy is delayed until after the time of usual puberty, the degree to which normal virilization will occur is variable, but many patients undergo a relatively complete anatomic and functional maturation. Intermittent low-dose androgen therapy is indicated in prepubertal hypogonadal boys with microphallus to bring the external genitalia into the normal range. If such patients are monitored closely and given androgens only for short periods, such therapy usually has no adverse effects on somatic growth.

In boys of pubertal age with either isolated hypogonadotropic hypogonadism or primary testicular deficiency, the usual practice is to institute androgen therapy between the ages of 12 and 14 years, depending on the subjective need for sexual development. The initial administration of small doses of testosterone esters followed by a gradual increase to 100 to 150 mg/m^2 of body surface area every 1 to 3 weeks should result in a normal pubertal growth spurt. The time from the start of treatment to the appearance of secondary sex characteristics is variable. Penile development, deepening of the voice, and other secondary sexual characteristics usually commence during the first year of treatment. In normal boys, puberty extends over several years, and treatment designed to replicate normal development does not shorten the process greatly.

Testosterone exerts its full action only in the presence of a balanced hormonal environment and, particularly, in the presence of adequate levels of growth hormone. Consequently, prepubertal boys with coexisting growth hormone and androgen deficiency exhibit a diminished response to androgens unless growth hormone is given simultaneously.

Pharmacologic uses Androgens have been used for a variety of disorders unassociated with hypogonadism, in the hope that potential benefits from the nonvirilizing actions of the agents (such as increase in nitrogen retention and muscle mass, increased hemoglobin, etc.) would outweigh any deleterious actions of the drugs. The most common nonreplacement uses of androgen have been attempts to improve nitrogen balance in catabolic states, self-administration by

athletes in the belief that muscle mass and/or athletic performance will be improved, attempts to enhance erythropoiesis in refractory anemias including the anemia of renal failure, treatment of hereditary angioedema and endometriosis, and management of growth retardation of various etiologies. Most expectations of beneficial effects in these disorders have been illusory for two reasons. First, pharmacologic doses of androgens do little, if anything, in men beyond the normal testicular androgen, and in women the virilizing side effects of androgens are formidable. Second, no androgen has been devised that exhibits only the nonvirilizing effects of the hormone. This is not surprising in view of the fact that all actions of androgens are mediated by a single high-affinity receptor protein in the cytoplasm (see Fig. 339-5).

The most pervasive form of androgen abuse is by male athletes in the expectation that muscle development and athletic performance will be improved. In fact, however, in adequately controlled studies such therapy does not improve performance consistently. However, published trials of efficacy involve the administration of drugs at smaller doses than are usually taken by athletes; since the drugs at high dosage have multiple side effects, some of which preclude studies of efficacy in a double-blind fashion, it is not clear whether the question of efficacy can ever be resolved scientifically. Under no circumstances do putative benefits outweigh the risks associated with androgen abuse, a practice that cannot be condemned too harshly. The only established indications for androgen therapy outside of male hypogonadism are in selected patients with anemia due to bone marrow failure, hereditary angioedema, or endometriosis and as an adjunct to growth hormone therapy.

Parenteral administration of testosterone esters to normal men results in little effects of any kind, except for the suppression of gonadotropin secretion by the hypothalamic-pituitary system and a consequent decrease in the production of sperm. There is no established contraindication to their administration to men with those disorders (such as short stature) where their use has been advocated, but the efficacy is not yet established. However, in women, the virilizing side effects preclude androgen use in all except life-threatening situations. Even in potentially fatal diseases in women, such as bone marrow failure, great care must be exercised in androgen use.

GONADOTROPINS Treatment with gonadotropins is utilized to establish or restore fertility in patients with gonadotropin deficiency of all causes. Two gonadotropin preparations are available: human menopausal gonadotropins (hMG) (purified from the urine of postmenopausal women) and human chorionic gonadotropin (hCG) (purified from the urine of pregnant women). hMG contains 75 IU FSH and 75 IU LH per vial. hCG has little FSH activity and resembles LH in its ability to stimulate testosterone production by Leydig cells. Because of the expense of hMG, treatment is usually begun with hCG alone, and hMG is added later to stimulate the FSH-dependent stages of spermatid development. A high ratio of LH to FSH activity and a long duration of treatment (3 to 6 months) are necessary to bring about maturation of the prepubertal testes. Once spermatogenesis is restored in hypophysectomized patients or initiated in hypogonadotropic hypogonadal men by combined therapy, it can usually be maintained with hCG alone.

Men with oligospermia of unknown etiology also have been treated with gonadotropins; the incidence of fertility in such patients is probably no greater than in untreated controls.

The dosage of hCG required to maintain a normal testosterone level varies from 1000 to 5000 IU weekly. A number of regimens have been utilized to induce maturation of spermatogenesis. Most involve starting with 2000 IU hCG three or more times a week until most of the clinical parameters, including plasma testosterone levels, are normal. hMG (usually one ampul) is then added three times a week to complete the development of spermatogenesis. After spermatogenesis has regressed, the length of therapy required to restore spermatogenesis may be as long as 12 months.

LUTEINIZING HORMONE–RELEASING HORMONE AND LHRH ANALOGUES LHRH (gonadorelin) is available for endocrine testing. LHRH therapy is used by some physicians for chronic therapy of the infertility of hypogonadotropic hypogonadism. It is necessary to administer LHRH in frequent boluses (25 to 200 ng/kg of body weight every 2 h), requiring the use of portable infusion pumps or periodic nasal application. In general, LHRH does not appear to be more efficacious than gonadotropin in returning sperm counts to normal. LHRH analogues (leuprolide and nafarelin) are available for the suppression of gonadotropin secretion and induction of hypogonadism. In prostatic cancer, testicular androgen production can be blocked by monthly injection of 7.5 mg leuprolide in depot form.

REFERENCES

CARR BR, GRIFFIN JE: Fertility control and its complications, in *Williams' Textbook of Endocrinology*, 8th ed, JD Wilson, DW Foster (eds). Philadelphia, Saunders, 1992, pp 1007–1031

DAVIS JE: Male sterilization. Clin Obstet Gynaecol 6:97, 1979

DE KRETSER DM: The effects of systemic disease on the function of the testis. Clin Endocrinol Metabol 8:487, 1979

———, ROBERTSON DM: The isolation and physiology of inhibin and related proteins. Biol Reprod 40:33, 1989

GOLDZIEHER JW et al: Improving the diagnostic reliability of rapidly fluctuating plasma hormone levels by optimized multiple-sampling techniques. J Clin Endocrinol Metab 43:824, 1976

GRIFFIN JE, WILSON JD: Disorders of the testes and male reproductive tract, in *Williams' Textbook of Endocrinology*, 8th ed, JD Wilson, DW Foster (eds). Philadelphia, Saunders, 1992, pp 799–852

GRUMBACH MM, STYNE DM: Puberty: Ontogeny, neuroendocrinology, physiology, and disorders, in *Williams' Textbook of Endocrinology*, 8th ed, JD Wilson, DW Foster (eds). Philadelphia, Saunders, 1992, pp 1139–1221

LAUE L et al: Treatment of familial male precocious puberty with spironolactone and testolactone. N Engl J Med 320:496, 1989

MACDONALD PC et al: Origin of estrogen in normal men and in women with testicular feminization. J Clin Endocrinol Metab 49:905, 1979

MARSHALL WA, TANNER JM: Variation in the pattern of pubertal changes in boys. Arch Dis Child 45:13, 1970

MASSEY FJ et al: Vasectomy and health: Results from a large cohort study. JAMA 252:1023, 1984

NIESCHLAG E: Care for the infertile male. Clin Endocrinol (Oxf) 38:123, 1993

SANTORO N et al: Hypogonadotropic disorders in men and women: Diagnosis and therapy with pulsatile gonadotropin-releasing hormone. Endocr Rev 7:11, 1986

SIGMAN M, HOWARDS SS: Male infertility, in *Campbell's Urology*, 6th ed, PC Walsh et al (eds). Philadelphia, Saunders, 1992, pp 661–705

SNYDER PF, LAWRENCE DA: Treatment of male hypogonadism with testosterone enanthate. J Clin Endocrinol Metab 51:1335, 1980

WHITCOMB RN, CROWLEY WF: Hypogonadotropic hypogonadism: GnRH therapy, in *Current Therapy in Endocrinology and Metabolism*, 4th ed, CW Bardin (ed). Toronto, Decker, 1991, pp 273–275

WILSON JD: Androgen abuse by athletes. Endocr Rev 9:181, 1988

———, GRIFFIN JE: The use and misuse of androgens. Metabolism 29:1278, 1980

YING S-Y: Inhibins, activins, and follistatin: Gonadal proteins modulating the secretion of hormone. Endocr Rev 9:267, 1988

340 DISORDERS OF THE OVARY AND FEMALE REPRODUCTIVE TRACT

BRUCE R. CARR / JEAN D. WILSON

The ovary is the source of ova for reproduction and of the hormones that regulate female sexual life. The anatomic structure, response to hormonal stimuli, and secretory capacity of the ovary are different at different periods of life. This chapter will review normal ovarian physiology as a background for understanding abnormalities of the ovary and other tissues of the female reproductive tract.

DEVELOPMENT, STRUCTURE, AND FUNCTION OF THE OVARY

EMBRYOLOGY During the third week of gestation, the primordial germ cells arise from the endoderm lining the yolk sac at the caudal end of the embryo. The germ cells migrate to the genital ridge adjacent to the mesonephric kidney by the fifth week of gestation and undergo mitotic divisions. The gonads exist in an undifferentiated state until the seventh week of fetal life, at which time the primitive ovary can be differentiated from the testis (see Chap. 342). Estrogen formation in the ovary commences between weeks 8 and 10, and by 10 to 11 weeks of gestation, some oogonia in the developing ovarian cortex begin developing into primary oocytes. The ovary contains a finite number of germ cells, the maximal number of about 7 million oogonia being reached by the fifth to sixth month of gestation. Afterward, the germ cells decrease in number through a process of atresia such that only 1 million remain at birth, 400,000 are present at the time of menarche, and only a few remain at menopause. Two X chromosomes are required for normal development of the ovary; in individuals with a 45,X karyotype, ovarian development occurs, but the rate of atresia is accelerated so that only a fibrous streak remains at the time of birth (see Chap. 342).

After the oogonia cease to proliferate, meiosis commences, proceeds until the diplotene stage of the first meiotic division is completed, and remains stationary until the time of onset of ovulation at puberty. From the fifth month of fetal life, the primordial follicle consists of the primary oocyte arrested in meiosis, a single surrounding layer of granulosa cells, and a basement membrane that separates the primordial follicle from surrounding stromal (interstitial) tissues.

PUBERTAL MATURATION Final maturation of ovarian follicles commences during puberty. The two major hormones that regulate follicular development are the pituitary gonadotropins—follicle-stimulating hormone (FSH) and luteinizing hormone (LH) (Fig. 340-1). During the second trimester of fetal development, the plasma gonadotropins rise to levels equivalent to those at menopause. This peak in gonadotropin levels may be causally related to the simultaneous peak in replication of oocytes. The hypothalamic-pituitary axis (the so-called gonadostat) undergoes maturation and becomes sensitive after the second trimester to negative feedback by steroid hormones, particularly estrogen and progesterone produced in the placenta. The circulating gonadotropins decrease thereafter and are almost undetectable at the time of birth. In the neonate, concomitant with the decrease in estrogen and progesterone levels due to separation from the placenta at birth, there is a rebound increase in gonadotropin secretion that persists for the first few months of life. With continued maturation of the hypothalamic-pituitary system, the gonadostat becomes sensitive to negative feedback by the low levels of circulating steroid hormones, and plasma gonadotropins again decrease.

As the time of puberty nears, a decrease in the sensitivity of the gonadostat allows for increased secretion of FSH and LH, possibly secondary to increased episodic or pulsatile secretion of luteinizing hormone–releasing hormone (LHRH) by the hypothalamus (see Chap. 331). A sleep-induced, pulsatile pattern of LH secretion then ensues, the first step in the development of a cyclic pattern of gonadotropin secretion (see Fig. 340-1). The increase in estrogen secretion subsequently exerts a positive feedback which leads to an exaggeration of the pulsatile release of LH and eventually to ovulation and the menarche, after which mean plasma gonadotropin concentrations reach adult values in which day and night levels are similar. After the menopause, plasma gonadotropin levels rise, plateau 5 to 10 years later, and remain fairly constant until the eighth to ninth decade of life when the levels may fall. Although ovarian function is regulated primarily by LH and FSH, the ovary is a source of several peptide and protein hormones and growth factors that may play a role in ovarian function.

With the development at puberty of decreased sensitivity of the hypothalamic-pituitary centers to circulating steroid hormones, LHRH release by the hypothalamus increases, gonadotropin secretion by the pituitary is enhanced, ovarian estrogen secretion increases, and the anatomic changes of puberty ensue. At age 10 to 11, the first secondary sexual characteristics begin to appear in girls, namely, development of the breast buds (thelarche), followed by the development of pubic hair (pubarche), and later by the development of

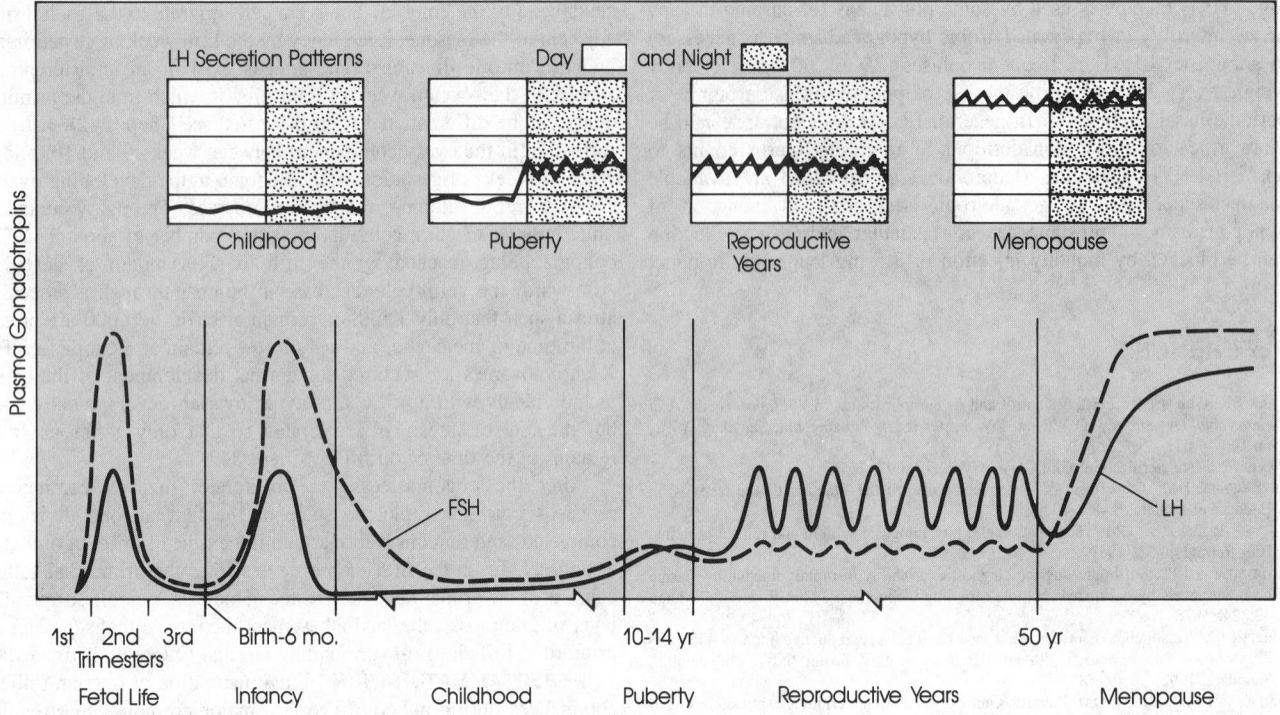

FIGURE 340-1 Pattern of gonadotropin secretion during different stages of life in women. FSH (follicle-stimulating hormone), LH (luteinizing hormone). The secretory patterns of LH during the waking hours (clear area) and night (stippled area) for each stage are indicated in the upper insets. (*After C Faiman et al.*)

axillary hair (adrenarche). The appearance of pubic and axillary hair is believed to be the result of an increase in adrenal androgens, commencing at approximately 6 to 8 years of age. A growth spurt ensues, and peak growth rate is attained at a mean age of 12 years.

The culmination of puberty is the onset of predictable, cyclic menses. The average time between the beginning of breast development and the onset of menses (menarche) is 2 years. During the first few years after menarche, menstrual cycles are often irregular and unpredictable due to anovulation. The age of menarche is variable and is determined in part by socioeconomic and genetic factors as well as general health. In the United States, the mean age of menarche is believed to have decreased at a rate of 3 to 4 months per decade over the last 100 years and is now around 13 years, a decrease believed to be due to an improvement in nutrition. A critical body weight of around 48 kg or a critical combination of weight, body water, and body fat is associated with development of hypothalamic insensitivity to circulating steroids that leads to increased secretion of gonadotropins and finally to menarche. Obese girls with a body weight 20 to 30 percent above ideal have earlier menarche than girls with normal weights. In contrast, participation in certain sports or ballet, malnutrition, and chronic debilitating disease can delay menarche.

MATURE OVARY **Morphology** The anatomic components and function of the adult ovary are illustrated schematically in Fig. 340-2. Under the influence of gonadotropins, a group of primary follicles is recruited, and by day 6 to 8 of the menstrual cycle, one follicle becomes mature or "dominant," a process characterized by accelerated growth of granulosa cells and enlargement of the fluid-filled antrum. The recruited follicles not destined to ovulate begin to undergo degeneration, similar to the atresia observed in other follicles during embryogenesis. Just prior to ovulation, meiosis resumes in the ova of the dominant follicle, and the first meiotic division is completed with formation of the first polar body. Rapid enlargement of the antrum (up to 10 to 25 mm in size) occurs with an associated increase in follicular fluid, followed by a thinning of the follicular surface and formation of a conical stigma. Ovulation from the dominant follicle occurs some 16 to 23 h after the LH peak or 24 to 38 h after the

onset of the LH surge as the result of rupture of the follicular wall at the area of the stigma, followed by expulsion of the ovum together with a mass of surrounding granulosa cells called *cumulus cells*. The rupture is believed to result from the action of hydrolyzing enzymes on the surface of the follicle, possibly under the control of prostaglandins. The second meiotic division begins after the egg is fertilized by a sperm, and the second polar body is then extruded. Following ovulation, the formation of the corpus luteum begins in the retained remnant of the ovulated follicle; the remaining granulosa and theca cells increase in size and accumulate lipids and a yellow pigment, lutein, to become "luteinized." The basement membrane that separated the granulosa cells from the stroma and blood vessels breaks, and capillaries, fibroblasts, and lymphatics from the theca invade the granulosa cells and reach the central cavity, thereby filling it with blood. After a period of 14 ± 2 days (the functional life of the corpus luteum), regression of vessels and atrophy of the corpus luteum commence and eventuate in replacement of the corpus luteum by a fibrous scar, the corpus albicans. The factors that limit the life span of the human corpus luteum are not known. However, if pregnancy occurs, the corpus luteum persists under the influence of placental or chorionic gonadotropins, and progesterone is produced by the corpus luteum for the support of early pregnancy.

Hormone formation STEROID HORMONES Like other steroid hormones, ovarian steroids are derived from cholesterol (Fig. 340-3). The ovary can synthesize cholesterol de novo from 2-carbon precursors and also can utilize cholesterol from circulating low-density lipoproteins (LDL) as substrate for steroid hormone formation (Fig. 340-4). Virtually all ovarian cells are believed to possess the complete enzymatic complement required for the conversion of cholesterol to estradiol (see Fig. 340-3); however, different cell types within the ovary contain different amounts of these enzymes so that the principal steroids produced differ in the various compartments. For example, the corpus luteum forms progesterone and 17-hydroxy-progesterone predominantly, whereas theca and stromal cells convert cholesterol to the androgens androstenedione and testosterone. Granulosa cells are particularly rich in the aromatase responsible for conversion of androgens to estrogen and utilize as substrates for this

FIGURE 340-2 Developmental changes in the adult ovary during a complete 28-day cycle.

process androgens synthesized in the granulosa cells and the adjacent theca cells.

The principal sites of action of LH and FSH are also illustrated in Figs. 340-3 and 340-4. LH acts primarily to regulate the first step in steroid hormone biosynthesis, namely, the conversion of cholesterol to pregnenolone, and also induces subsequent enzymes in the pathway. FSH acts to regulate the final process by which androgens are aromatized to estrogens. As a consequence, in the absence of FSH, LH enhances substrate flow and the formation of androgens and/or progesterone, whereas FSH action is impeded in the absence of LH because of diminished substrate for aromatization.

Estrogens Naturally occurring estrogens are 18-carbon steroids characterized by an aromatic A ring, a phenolic hydroxyl group at C-3, and either a hydroxyl group (estradiol) or a ketone (estrone) at C-17 (see Fig. 340-3). (For the numbering of the steroid ring, see Fig. 339-1.) The principal estrogen secreted by the ovary and the most potent naturally occurring estrogen is estradiol. Estrone is also secreted by the ovary, but the principal source of estrone is from extraglandular conversion of androstenedione in peripheral tissues. Estriol (16-hydroxyestradiol), the most abundant estrogen in urine, arises from the 16-hydroxylation of estrone and estradiol. Catechol estrogens are formed by hydroxylation of estrogens at the C-2 or C-4 position and may act as the intracellular mediators of some estrogen action. Estrogens promote development of the secondary sexual characteristics in women and cause uterine growth, thickening of the vaginal mucosa, thinning of the cervical mucus, and development of the ductular system of the breasts. The mechanism of estrogen action in target tissues is similar to that for other steroid hormones and involves the binding to a nuclear steroid receptor and enhancement of the transcription of messenger RNA, which in turn causes increased protein synthesis in the cell cytoplasm (see Chap. 329).

Progesterone Progesterone, a 21-carbon steroid (see Fig. 340-3), is the principal hormone secreted by the corpus luteum and is responsible for progestational effects, namely, induction of secretory activity in the endometrium of the estrogen-primed uterus in preparation for implantation of the fertilized egg. Progesterone also induces a decidual reaction in endometrium. Other effects include inhibition of uterine contractions, increased viscosity of cervical mucus, glandular

development of the breasts, and increase in basal body temperature (thermogenic effect).

Androgens The ovary synthesizes a variety of 19-carbon steroids, including dehydroepiandrosterone, androstenedione, testosterone, and dihydrotestosterone, principally in stromal and thecal cells. The major ovarian 19-carbon steroid is androstenedione (see Fig. 340-3), part of which is secreted into plasma and the remainder of which is converted to estrogen in granulosa cells or to testosterone in the interstitium. In peripheral tissues, androstenedione also can be converted to testosterone and to estrogens. Only testosterone and dihydrotestosterone are true androgens that interact with the androgen receptor and induce virilizing signs in women (see Chaps. 49 and 339).

OTHER HORMONES Other ovarian hormones play an uncertain role in human physiology. *Relaxin*, a polypeptide hormone produced by the human corpus luteum as well as by the decidua, causes softening of the cervix and loosening of the symphysis pubis in preparation for parturition in animals. *Oxytocin, vasopressin*, and other hypothalamic and pituitary hormones are also present in granulosa and/or luteal cells, but their function in these cells is unknown. *Follicular inhibin* or *folliculostatin* (the equivalent of testicular inhibin) is secreted by the follicle and is believed to inhibit the release of FSH by the hypothalamic-pituitary unit. *Activin* is also secreted by the follicle and may enhance FSH secretion. *Follicle regulatory protein* (FRP) of human follicular fluid inhibits granulosa secretion and growth. *Gonadocrinins*, peptides purified from rat follicular fluid, stimulate the release of both FSH and LH from the pituitary in vitro and in vivo. Granulosa cells secrete *oocyte maturation inhibitor* (OMI), a factor that prevents premature ovulation. In addition, in the gonads of both sexes a *meiosis-inducing substance* (MIS) triggers the onset of meiosis, an event that occurs earlier in ovarian than in testicular development. A variety of growth factors produced locally (including IGF1, IGF2, TGFα, and TGFβ) influence steroid secretion by the ovary.

The normal menstrual cycle The menstrual cycle is usually divided into a follicular or proliferative phase and a luteal or secretory phase (Fig. 340-5). The secretion of FSH and LH is fundamentally under negative feedback control by ovarian steroids (particularly estradiol) and probably by inhibin, but the response of gonadotropins

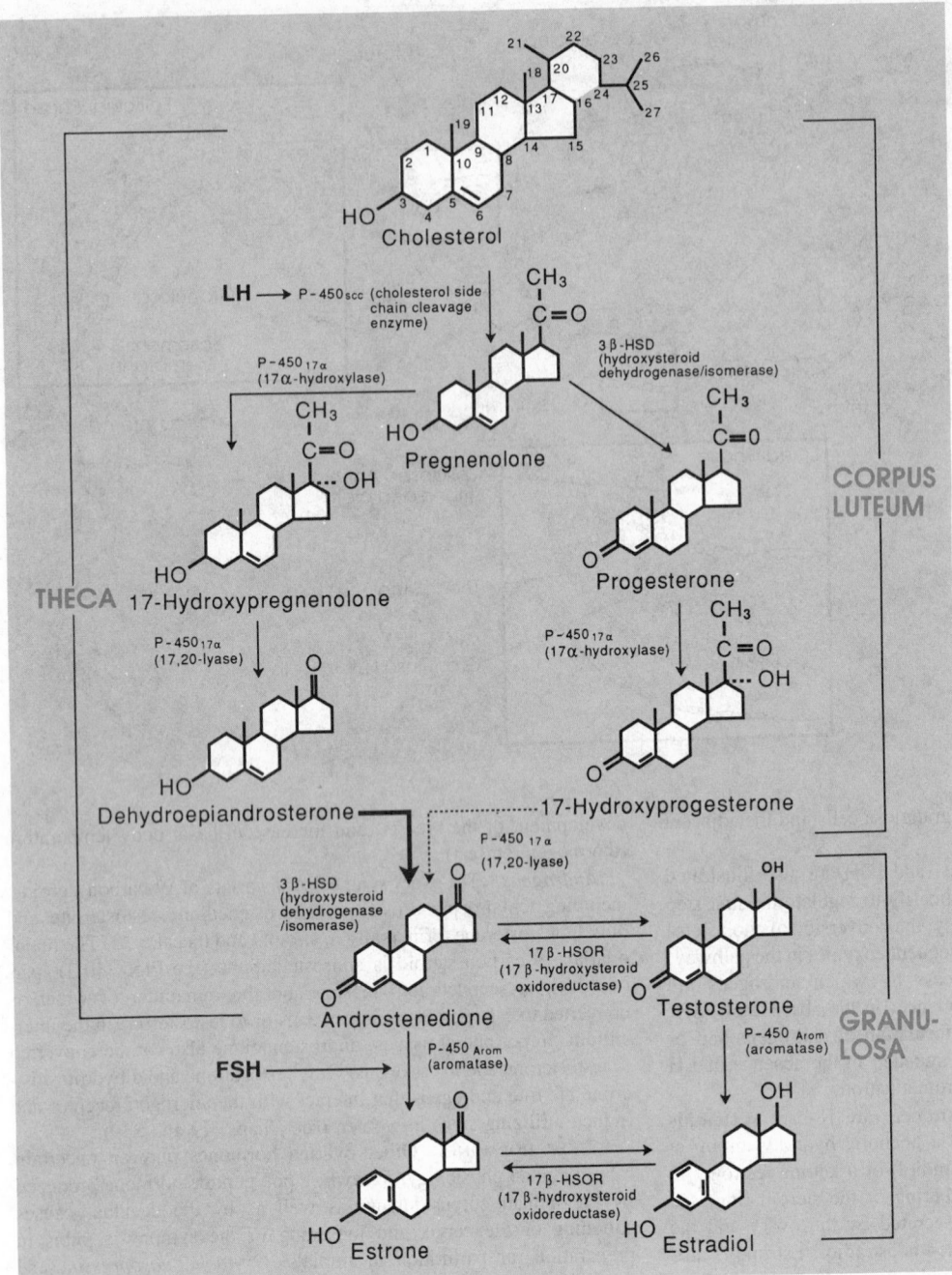

FIGURE 340-3 The principal pathway of steroid hormone biosynthesis in the ovary. Although every ovarian cell probably contains the complete enzyme complement required for the formation of estradiol from cholesterol, the amounts of the various enzymes and consequently the predominant hormones formed differ among the various cell types. The major enzyme complements for the corpus luteum, stroma, and granulosa cells are shown by the brackets; as a consequence these cells produce predominantly progesterone and 17-OH progesterone, androgen, and estrogen, respectively. The major sites of action of LH and FSH in mediating this pathway are shown in the horizontal arrows. The dotted line emphasizes that the metabolism of 17-hydroxyprogesterone is limited in the human ovary. (*From BR Carr, in JD Wilson and DW Foster, eds,* Williams' Textbook of Endocrinology, *8th ed, Philadelphia, Saunders, 1992.*)

to different levels of estradiol varies. FSH secretion is inhibited progressively as estrogen levels increase—typical negative feedback. In contrast, LH secretion is suppressed maximally by estrogen in low amounts and is enhanced in response to a rising and sustained elevation of estradiol—so-called positive feedback control. Negative feedback of estrogen involves both the hypothalamus and pituitary, whereas positive feedback operates primarily at the level of the pituitary.

The length of the normal menstrual cycle is defined as the time from the onset of one menstrual bleeding episode to onset of the next. In women of reproductive age, the menstrual cycle averages 28 ± 3 days, and the mean duration of flow is 4 ± 2 days. Longer menstrual cycles (usually characterized by anovulation) occur at menarche and prior to menopause. At the end of one menstrual cycle and in the face of a waning corpus luteum, plasma levels of estrogen and progesterone fall, and circulating levels of FSH increase concomitantly. Under the influence of increasing levels of FSH, follicular

recruitment is initiated to effect development of the follicle that will be dominant during the next cycle.

After the onset of menses, follicular development continues, but FSH levels decrease. Approximately 8 to 10 days prior to the midcycle LH surge, plasma estradiol levels begin to rise as the result of secretion of estradiol by the granulosa cells of the enlarging dominant follicle. During the second half of the follicular phase, LH levels also begin to rise (positive feedback). Just prior to ovulation, estradiol secretion reaches a peak and then falls. Immediately thereafter, a further rise in the plasma level of LH mediates the final maturation of the follicle, followed by follicular rupture and ovulation 16 to 23 h after the LH peak. Concomitant with the rise in LH is a smaller increase in the level of plasma FSH, the physiologic significance of which is unclear. Plasma progesterone also begins to rise just prior to midcycle and facilitates the positive feedback action of estradiol on LH secretion.

At the onset of the luteal phase, plasma gonadotropins decrease

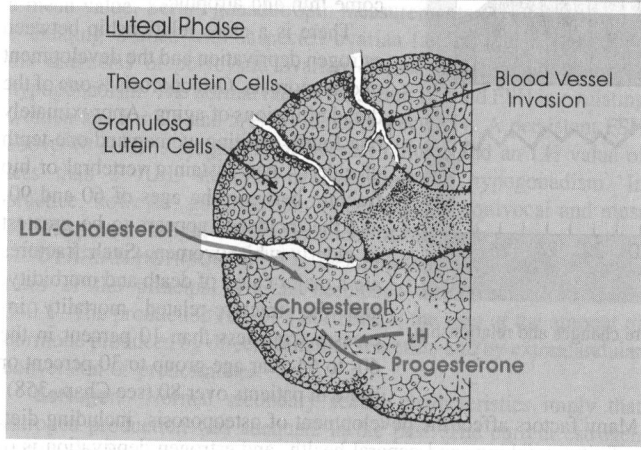

FIGURE 340-4 Cellular interactions in the ovary during the follicular phase (top) and luteal phase (bottom); LDL (low-density lipoprotein), FSH (follicle-stimulating hormone), and LH (luteinizing hormone). (*From BR Carr et al, 1982.*)

and plasma progesterone increases. A secondary rise in estrogens causes further gonadotropin suppression. Near the end of the luteal phase, progesterone and estrogen levels fall, and FSH levels begin to rise to initiate the development of the next follicle (usually in the contralateral ovary) and the next menstrual cycle.

The endometrium lining the uterine cavity undergoes marked alterations in response to the changing plasma levels of ovarian hormones (see Fig. 340-5). Concomitant with the decrease in plasma estrogen and progesterone and the decline of corpus luteum function in the late luteal phase, intense vasospasm occurs in the spiral arterioles supplying blood to the endometrium, followed by an ischemic necrosis, endometrial desquamation, and bleeding. This vasospasm is caused by locally synthesized prostaglandins. The onset of bleeding marks the first day of the menstrual cycle. By the fourth to fifth day of the cycle, the endometrium is thin. During the proliferative phase glandular growth of the endometrium is mediated by estrogen. After ovulation, increased progesterone leads to further thickening of the endometrium, but the rapid growth slows. The endometrium then enters the secretory phase characterized by tortuosity of the glands, curling of the spiral arterioles, and glandular secretion. As corpus luteum function begins to wane in the absence of conception, the sequence of events leading to menstruation is again set into action.

Biphasic changes in basal body temperature are characteristic of the ovulatory cycle and are mediated by alterations in progesterone

levels (see Fig. 340-5). An increase in basal body temperature of 0.3 to 0.5°C begins after ovulation, persists during the luteal phase, and returns to the normal baseline (36.2 to 36.4°C) after the onset of the subsequent menses (see Chap. 16).

Cellular interactions in the ovary during the normal cycle LH stimulates thecal cells surrounding the follicle to form androgens, and androstenedione diffuses across the basement membrane of the follicle into granulosa cells, where it is aromatized to estrogen (see Figs. 340-3 and 340-4).

The increase of FSH late in the preceding menstrual cycle stimulates growth and recruitment of the primary follicles by enhancing granulosa cell proliferation, resulting ultimately in the formation of the dominant follicle. In the granulosa cells, FSH also stimulates activity and the amount of aromatase that converts androstenedione to estrogen. Enhanced secretion of estradiol causes an increase in the number of estradiol receptors and further proliferation of granulosa cells. In the late follicular phase, FSH, in concert with estradiol, causes induction of LH receptors on the granulosa cells. LH acts via these receptors to increase progesterone secretion at midcycle. The amount of progesterone formed by the follicle is believed to be limited by the availability of LDL-cholesterol to serve as substrate for steroidogenesis and by the fact that most of the progesterone formed is converted to androstenedione by thecal cells. Prior to ovulation, the granulosa cells of the follicle are bathed in follicular fluid but have limited access to circulating blood and consequently to plasma LDL. As depicted in Fig. 340-4, the granulosa cells become vascularized after ovulation, and plasma LDL-cholesterol is made available to serve as the major substrate for progesterone synthesis by the corpus luteum. Thus increased progesterone synthesis by the corpus luteum is the consequence of increased substrate availability. The peak in progesterone secretion by the corpus luteum is attained 8 days after ovulation at the time of maximal vascularization of the granulosa cells.

MENOPAUSE The *menopause* is defined as the final episode of menstrual bleeding in women. However, the term is used commonly to refer to the period of the female climacteric that encompasses the transitional period between the reproductive years up to and beyond the last episode of menstrual bleeding. During this period, there is a gradual but progressive loss of ovarian function and a variety of endocrine, somatic, and psychological changes.

The median age of women at the time of cessation of menstrual bleeding is 50 to 51 years. Since the life expectancy in women is close to 80 years, approximately one-third of life occurs after cessation of reproductive function. Preceding the menopause, the pattern of menstrual cycles is variable, but the interval between menses usually becomes longer. In addition, there is an increase in the mean levels of plasma FSH and LH, despite the continuation of ovulatory cycles. Thus, the ovary appears to become less responsive to gonadotropins prior to the menopause.

The menopause is the consequence of the exhaustion of ovarian follicles. The decrease in the number of ova begins in intrauterine life; by the time of the menopause, few ova remain, and these appear to be nonfunctional. Only a small number of ova are lost as the result of ovulation during reproductive life, the majority of follicles and associated ova being lost by atresia. The cessation of follicular development results in a drop in the production of estradiol and other hormones, which, in turn, causes a loss of negative feedback on the hypothalamic-pituitary centers. In turn, the levels of plasma gonadotropins increase, with FSH levels rising earlier and to a greater extent than those of LH (Figs. 340-1 and 340-6). The higher concentration of FSH than LH in postmenopausal women may result from the decrease in inhibin secretion by the ovary, from the fact that FSH is cleared from plasma less rapidly than LH, and possibly from the loss of positive feedback on LH production by estradiol. Intravenous administration of LHRH to menopausal women results in a pronounced increase in the secretion of both FSH and LH, consistent with the enhanced hypothalamic-pituitary secretory activity in other forms of primary ovarian failure.

Isosexual precocious puberty Isosexual precocious puberty in girls can be divided into three major categories (Table 340-2).

TRUE PRECOCIOUS PUBERTY True precocious puberty is characterized by an early but otherwise normal sequence of pubertal development, including increased secretion of gonadotropins and ovulatory menstrual cycles. Constitutional or idiopathic precocious puberty comprises 90 percent of cases. In these individuals, no cause for the premature maturation of the central nervous system–hypothalamic-pituitary axis can be identified, and the diagnosis is one of exclusion. As many as half these individuals have abnormal electroencephalograms. Premature appearance of secondary sexual characteristics and of ovulatory cycles with the accompanying risk of fertility may result in significant emotional disturbances. Therefore, prompt initiation of therapy is imperative. LHRH analogues inhibit estrogen synthesis and thus inhibit precocious puberty, and they may prevent premature closure of the epiphyses and the resultant short stature.

About 10 percent of cases are due to organic brain diseases, including brain tumors (hypothalamic gliomas, astrocytomas, ependymomas, germinomas, and hamartomas), encephalitis, meningitis, hydrocephalus, head injury, tuberous sclerosis, and neurofibromatosis. It is essential to separate this group of patients from those with the idiopathic disorder, and patients designated as idiopathic occasionally prove to have such tumors. Fortunately, most patients with organic lesions serious enough to cause precocious puberty have obvious neurologic signs and symptoms. Evaluation of all patients with precocious puberty should include, at a minimum, skull films and computed tomographic (CT) scans or magnetic resonance imaging (MRI) of the brain. The success of treatment depends on the nature of the lesion, but surgical and radiation treatment of well-localized tumors is occasionally successful.

A rare cause of isosexual precocity is virilizing congenital adrenal hyperplasia due to 21-hydroxylase deficiency in girls in whom treatment is delayed until 4 to 8 years of age. After initiation of glucocorticoid replacement, such individuals may undergo true isosexual precocious puberty (see Chap. 335).

PRECOCIOUS PSEUDOPUBERTY Precocious pseudopuberty occurs when girls feminize as a consequence of enhanced estrogen formation but do not ovulate or develop cyclic menses. Ovarian cysts or tumors that secrete estrogen (granulosa-theca cell tumors) are the most frequent cause of precocious pseudopuberty. Granulosa-theca cell tumors associated with intestinal polyps and pigmentation of the mucous membranes occur in the Peutz-Jeghers syndrome. Other ovarian tumors that secrete estrogens (or androgens that can be converted to estrogens at extraglandular sites) include dysgerminomas, teratomas, cystadenomas, and ovarian carcinomas (also see Chap. 321). Ovarian tumors usually can be detected by rectoabdominal examination, and sonography, CT scans, MRI, and/or laparoscopy also may be of help. Ovarian teratomas and choriocarcinomas and other carcinomas that secrete hCG do not cause precocious puberty in girls unless there is concomitant secretion of estrogen by the tumor (hCG or LH in the absence of FSH does not induce ovarian estrogen production). Rarely, feminizing tumors of the adrenal cause isosexual precocious puberty, either by formation of estrogens directly or by secretion of weak androgens to serve as estrogenic precursors in extraglandular tissues.

Other causes of precocious pseudopuberty include the following: (1) The McCune-Albright syndrome (polyostotic fibrous dysplasia), characterized by café au lait spots, cystic fibrous dysplasia of bones, and sexual precocity. Some of these individuals have increased gonadotropin secretion, whereas others have functional ovarian cysts in the presence of low gonadotropins, which represents a form of gonadotropin-independent sexual precocity. Occasionally, this disorder leads to true precocious puberty (see Chap. 343). (2) Primary hypothyroidism in which secretion of thyrotropin-releasing hormone (TRH) as well as secretion of other hypothalamic hormones is enhanced, leading to increased FSH levels and ovarian estrogen secretion, frequently with galactorrhea. (3) The Russell-Silver syndrome, or congenital asymmetry associated with short stature and precocious feminization. (4) Estrogen-containing medications, including use of estrogen-containing creams for diaper rash or the ingestion of meat from estrogen-treated animals or poultry or any estrogen by mouth.

INCOMPLETE ISOSEXUAL PRECOCITY This term is used to describe the premature development of a single pubertal event and encompasses several entities. The appearance of breast budding prior to the age of 8 (premature thelarche) without other evidence of estrogen secretion and without premature bone maturation is believed to be due to a transient increase in estrogen secretion or a temporary increase in sensitivity to the small amounts of circulating estrogens formed prior to puberty. Usually, the disorder is self-limited and resolves spontaneously. Occasionally, axillary hair and/or pubic hair (so-called *premature adrenarche* and *pubarche*) appear without any other secondary sexual development. The phenomenon is associated with adrenal androgen secretion in the range of normal puberty and can be distinguished from syndromes of virilization by the absence of clitoromegaly. It requires no treatment, and patients enter puberty at about the average time.

Heterosexual precocity Virilization in a prepubertal female is usually due to congenital adrenal hyperplasia or to androgen secretion by an ovarian or adrenal tumor. The manifestations of virilization are described in Chap. 49. Virilization in girls with congenital adrenal hyperplasia usually takes place in a background of variable sexual ambiguity (see Chap. 342).

Evaluation of sexual precocity The evaluation of sexual precocity involves a careful history and physical examination, including rectoabdominal examination, abdominal sonography, determination of bone age, and measurement of thyroid hormones, TSH, and gonadotropins (and androgen or estrogen levels when appropriate). Skull films and further diagnostic tests are indicated if a neurologic disorder is suspected and no evidence of ovarian or adrenal tumor is found.

REPRODUCTIVE YEARS Disorders of the menstrual cycle
ABNORMAL UTERINE BLEEDING Between menarche and the menopause, almost every woman experiences one or more episodes of abnormal uterine bleeding, here defined as any bleeding pattern that differs in frequency, duration, or amount from the pattern observed during a normal menstrual cycle. A variety of descriptive terms (such as *menorrhagia*, *metrorrhagia*, and *menometrorrhagia*) have been used to characterize patterns of abnormal uterine bleeding. A more logical approach is to divide abnormal uterine bleeding into those patterns associated with ovulatory cycles and those associated with anovulatory cycles.

OVULATORY CYCLES Normal menstrual bleeding with ovulatory cycles is spontaneous, regular, cyclic, and predictable and frequently associated with discomfort (dysmenorrhea). Deviations from this pattern associated with cycles that are still regular and predictable are most often due to organic disease of the outflow tract. For example, regular but prolonged and excessive bleeding episodes unassociated with bleeding dyscrasias (hypermenorrhea or menorrhagia) can result from abnormalities of the uterus such as submucous leiomyomas, adenomyosis, or endometrial polyps. Regular, cyclic, predictable menstruation characterized by spotting or light bleeding is termed *hypomenorrhea* and is due to obstruction of the outflow tract as from intrauterine synechiae or scarring of the cervix. Intermenstrual bleeding between episodes of regular, ovulatory menstruation is also often due to cervical or endometrial lesions. An exception to the association between organic disease of the uterus and abnormal uterine bleeding is the occurrence of episodes of regular bleeding more frequently than 21 days apart (polymenorrhea). These cycles may be a normal variant.

ANOVULATORY CYCLES Uterine bleeding that is unpredictable with respect to amount, onset, and duration and is usually painless is described as *dysfunctional uterine bleeding*. This disorder is not due to abnormalities of the uterus but rather to chronic anovulation and occurs when there is interruption of the normal progressive sequence of follicular and luteal phases under the influence of a dominant follicle and its resulting corpus luteum. As discussed above, normal uterine bleeding in ovulatory cycles is due to progesterone withdrawal and requires that the endometrium first be primed with estrogen (when castrates or postmenopausal women are given progesterone, withdrawal bleeding usually does not occur).

Dysfunctional uterine bleeding can occur in women who have a transient disruption of the synchronous hypothalamic-pituitary-ovarian patterns necessary for regular ovulatory cycles, most often at the extremes of the reproductive life, namely, in the early menarche and in the perimenopausal period, but also as the secondary consequence of temporary stresses or intercurrent illnesses.

On the other hand, primary *dysfunctional uterine bleeding* can result from at least three pathophysiologic mechanisms.

1 *Estrogen withdrawal bleeding* occurs when estrogen is given to a castrate or postmenopausal woman and then withdrawn. As in other types of dysfunctional uterine bleeding, this form of menstrual bleeding is usually painless.

2 *Estrogen breakthrough bleeding* occurs when there is prolonged continuous estrogen stimulation of the endometrium not interrupted by cyclic progesterone secretion and withdrawal. This is the most common type of dysfunctional uterine bleeding and is usually due to anovulation associated with chronic acyclic estrogen production as in women with polycystic ovarian disease. Such women may have histories of irregular, unpredictable menses, oligomenorrhea, or amenorrhea (see below). Alternatively, estrogen breakthrough bleeding can occur in hypogonadal women given estrogens chronically rather than intermittently or in women with estrogen-secreting tumors of the ovary. Estrogen breakthrough bleeding may be profuse and is unpredictable with respect to duration, amount of flow, and time of occurrence. The endometrium is typically thin because its repair between episodes of bleeding is incomplete.

3 *Progesterone breakthrough bleeding* occurs in the presence of abnormally high ratios of progesterone to estrogen, e.g., in women on continuous low-dose oral contraceptives.

The approach to a patient with dysfunctional uterine bleeding begins with a careful history of menstrual patterns and prior hormonal therapy. Since not all bleeding from the urogenital tract is from the uterus, rectal, bladder, and vaginal or cervical sources must be excluded by physical examination. If the bleeding is from the uterus, a pregnancy-related disorder such as abortion or ectopic pregnancy also must be excluded. Once the diagnosis of dysfunctional uterine bleeding is established, a rational approach to management is as follows: During a first episode of dysfunctional bleeding the patient can simply be observed, provided the bleeding is not copious and no evidence of bleeding dyscrasia is present. If bleeding is moderately severe, control can be achieved with relatively high dose estrogen oral contraceptives for 3 weeks. Alternatively, a regimen of three or

four low-dose oral contraceptive pills per day for 1 week followed by tapering to the usual dosage for up to 3 weeks is also effective. If uterine bleeding is more severe, hospitalization, bed rest, and intramuscular injections of estradiol valerate (10 mg) and hydroxy-progesterone caproate (500 mg) or intravenous or intramuscular conjugated estrogens (25 mg) usually control the bleeding. After initial treatment, iron replacement should be instituted, and recurrence can be prevented by cyclic oral contraceptives for 2 to 3 months (or more if pregnancy is not desired). Alternatively, menses should be induced every 2 to 3 months with medroxyprogesterone acetate, 10 mg by mouth once or twice a day for 10 days. If hormone therapy fails to control uterine bleeding, an endometrial biopsy, hysteroscopy, or dilatation and curettage may be required for diagnosis and therapy. Indeed, uterine sampling may be indicated prior to hormone therapy in women at risk for endometrial cancer (i.e., in women approaching the age of menopause or in the massively obese); endometrial cancer is rare in ovulatory women of reproductive age.

AMENORRHEA An acceptable definition of amenorrhea is failure of menarche by age 16, irrespective of the presence or absence of secondary sexual characteristics, or the absence of menstruation for 6 months in a woman with previous periodic menses. However, women who do not fulfill these criteria should be evaluated if (1) the subject and/or her family are greatly concerned, (2) no breast development has occurred by age 14, or (3) any sexual ambiguity or virilization is present (Chap. 342). Amenorrhea is usually categorized as either primary (in a woman who has never menstruated) or secondary (in a woman in whom menstruation is present for a variable time and then ceases); some disorders can cause either primary or secondary amenorrhea. For example, most women with gonadal dysgenesis have primary amenorrhea, but some have some follicles and ovulate for short periods so that pregnancies may rarely occur. Furthermore, patients with chronic anovulation (polycystic ovarian disease) most often have secondary amenorrhea but may present with primary amenorrhea. For these reasons, categorization of amenorrhea into primary and secondary types is less helpful in the differential diagnosis than a classification based on the major underlying physiologic derangements: (1) anatomic defects, (2) ovarian failure, and (3) chronic anovulation with or without estrogen present.

Anatomic defects A variety of anatomic or structural defects of the female genital tract can preclude menstrual bleeding. Starting from the caudal end of the female genital tract, labial agglutination or fusion is often associated with disorders of sexual development, particularly female pseudohermaphroditism (congenital adrenal hyperplasia or exposure to maternal androgens in utero) (see Chap. 342). Congenital defects of the vagina, imperforate hymen, and transverse vaginal septae also can cause amenorrhea. These women frequently have accumulation of menstrual blood behind the obstruction and may have cyclic, predictable episodes of abdominal pain.

More severe müllerian anomalies include müllerian agenesis (the Mayer-Rokitansky-Küster-Hauser syndrome; see Chap. 342), second in frequency only to gonadal dysgenesis as a cause of primary amenorrhea. Women with this syndrome have a 46,XX karyotype, female secondary sex characteristics, and normal ovarian function, including cyclic ovulation, but have absence or severe hypoplasia of the vagina. The uterus usually consists of only rudimentary bicornuate cords, but if the uterus contains endometrium, cyclic abdominal pain and accumulation of blood may occur as in other forms of outlet obstruction. One-third of patients have abnormalities of the urogenital tract, and one-tenth have skeletal anomalies, usually involving the spine. The major diagnostic problem is separating müllerian agenesis from complete testicular feminization, in which 46,XY genetic males with testes differentiate as phenotypic women with a blind vaginal pouch and an absent uterus. Women with testicular feminization have feminized breasts but a paucity of pubic and axillary hair. The disorder is due to a defect in the androgen-receptor protein that causes profound resistance to the action of testosterone (see Chap. 342). Testicular feminization can be diagnosed by demonstrating a male level of serum testosterone or a 46,XY karyotype, whereas demonstration of a 46,XX karyotype, biphasic basal body temperatures characteristic of ovulating women, and elevated levels of progesterone during the luteal phase establish the diagnosis of müllerian agenesis.

A rare cause of absence of the uterus in 46,XY phenotypic women who are sexually infantile is the so-called testicular regression syndrome or testicular agenesis (see Chap. 342).

Other abnormalities of the uterus that cause amenorrhea include obstruction due to scarring or stenosis of the cervix, often resulting from surgery, electrocautery, laser therapy, or cryosurgery. Destruction of the endometrium (Asherman's syndrome) may follow vigorous curettage, usually in association with postpartum hemorrhage or therapeutic abortion complicated by infection. This diagnosis is confirmed by hysterosalpingography or by direct vision of the endometrial scarring or synechiae using a hysteroscope.

Treatment of disorders of the outflow tract is surgical. Repair of vaginal agenesis results in normal menstruation and potential fertility only if an intact uterus is present.

Ovarian failure   Primary ovarian failure is associated with elevated plasma gonadotropins and can result from several causes. The most frequent cause is *gonadal dysgenesis*, in which the germ cells are lacking and the ovary is replaced by a fibrous streak (also see Chaps. 62 and 342). Women with gonadal dysgenesis can be divided into two broad groups on the basis of chromosomal karyotype. The most common is due to deletion of genetic material in the X chromosomes and accounts for about two-thirds of gonadal dysgenesis. A 45,X karyotype is found in about half, and most have somatic defects, including short stature, webbed neck, shield chest, and cardiovascular defects, collectively termed the *Turner phenotype*. The remainder with identifiable abnormalities of the X chromosome have chromosomal mosaicism with or without associated structural abnormalities of the X chromosome. The most common form of mosaicism is 45,X/46,XX. Gonadal tumors are rare in 45,X patients, but gonadal malignancies may occur in women with chromosomal mosaicism involving the Y chromosome. Therefore, a chromosomal analysis should be obtained in all cases of amenorrhea associated with ovarian failure, and the streak gonad should be removed if a Y chromosome is present. Another means of identifying the presence of a Y chromosome is to amplify the sex-determining regions of the Y chromosome (SRY) by means of the polymerase chain reaction (see Chap. 342). Approximately 90 percent of individuals with gonadal dysgenesis associated with partial or complete deletion of the X chromosome never have menstrual bleeding, and the remaining 10 percent have sufficient follicles to experience menses and, rarely, fertility; the menstrual and reproductive lives of such individuals are invariably brief.

A tenth of subjects with bilateral streak gonads have a normal 46,XX or 46,XY karyotype and are said to have *pure gonadal dysgenesis*. These individuals have either normal or above-average stature due to failure of estrogen-mediated epiphyseal closure in the presence of a normal chromosomal constitution. Pure gonadal dysgenesis does not constitute a phenotypic or chromosomally homogeneous disorder (see Chap. 342). Approximately one-tenth of such individuals with a 46,XY karyotype develop signs of virilization, including clitoromegaly, and have an increased incidence of tumors in the gonadal streaks; as a consequence, gonadal streaks should be removed prophylactically as discussed above when a Y chromosome is present. Approximately two-thirds of women with 46,XX gonadal dysgenesis experience no menses, while the remainder have one or more menstrual episodes and are occasionally fertile.

Other causes of ovarian failure and amenorrhea include deficiency of the P450$_{17\alpha}$ enzyme that encodes 17α-hydroxylase and 17,20-lyase activities, premature ovarian failure, the resistant-ovary syndrome, and ovarian failure secondary to chemotherapy or radiation therapy for malignancy. *17α-Hydroxylase deficiency* is characterized by primary amenorrhea, sexual infantilism, and hypertension that is due to increased production of desoxycorticosterone (DOC), whereas women with *17,20-lyase deficiency* have primary amenorrhea and sexual infantilism with normal blood pressure (see Chaps. 335 and

342). The diagnosis of *premature ovarian failure* or *premature menopause* is applied to women who cease menstruating prior to age 40. The ovaries are similar to the ovaries of postmenopausal women, namely, paucity or absence of follicles as the result of accelerated follicular atresia. Premature ovarian failure due to ovarian antibodies may be one component of polyglandular failure together with adrenal insufficiency, hypothyroidism, and other autoimmune disorders (see Chap. 343). A rare form of ovarian failure is the *resistant-ovary syndrome*, in which the ovaries contain many follicles arrested in development prior to the antral stage, possibly because of resistance to the action of FSH in the ovary. To differentiate this disorder from the 46,XX variety of pure gonadal dysgenesis, both of which are associated with sexual immaturity, it is necessary to perform ovarian biopsy. However, such a distinction is not clinically useful, since the conventional treatment of infertility in both conditions is usually unsuccessful. Women with ovarian failure who desire pregnancy have been treated with hormone replacement and transfer of donor embryos to the uterine cavity or fallopian tubes.

CHRONIC ANOVULATION   At least 80 percent or more of gynecologic endocrine problems result from chronic anovulation. Women with chronic anovulation fail to ovulate spontaneously but may ovulate with appropriate therapy. The ovaries of such women do not secrete estrogen in a normal cyclic pattern; it is clinically useful to differentiate those women who produce sufficient estrogen to have withdrawal bleeding after progestogen therapy from those who fail to produce enough estrogen to have progesterone withdrawal bleeding and who often have hypothalamic-pituitary dysfunction.

Chronic anovulation with estrogen present   Women with chronic anovulation who experience withdrawal bleeding after progestogen administration are said to be in a state of "estrus" due to the acyclic production of estrogen, largely estrone, by extraglandular aromatization of circulating androstenedione. The most common term for this disorder is *polycystic ovarian disease* (PCOD), a syndrome characterized by infertility, hirsutism, obesity, and amenorrhea or oligomenorrhea. When spontaneous uterine bleeding occurs in subjects with PCOD, it is unpredictable with respect to time of onset, duration, and amount, and on occasion the bleeding can be severe. The dysfunctional uterine bleeding is usually due to estrogen breakthrough (see above).

The disorder, which may be transmitted as an autosomal dominant or X-linked trait, was originally described by Stein and Leventhal as characterized by enlarged, polycystic ovaries, but the syndrome and its accompanying endocrine abnormalities are now known to be associated with a variety of pathologic findings in the ovaries, only some of which result in enlargement of the ovaries and none of which are pathognomonic. The most common finding is a white, smooth, sclerotic ovary with a thickened capsule, multiple follicular cysts in various stages of atresia, a hyperplastic theca and stroma, and rare or absent corpora albicans. Other ovaries have hyperthecosis in which the ovarian stroma is hyperplastic and may contain lipid-laden luteal cells. Thus the diagnosis of PCOD is a clinical one, based on the coexistence of chronic anovulation and varying degrees of androgen excess.

In most women with PCOD, menarche occurs at the expected time, but uterine bleeding is unpredictable in onset, duration, and amount. Amenorrhea ensues after a variable time, although primary amenorrhea occurs in some women. Signs of androgen excess (hirsutism) usually become evident around the time of menarche. One formulation suggests that this disorder originates as an exaggerated adrenarche in obese girls (Fig. 340-7). The combination of elevated adrenal androgens and obesity would result in increased formation of extraglandular estrogen and lead to an acyclic positive feedback on LH secretion and negative feedback on FSH secretion so that the characteristic LH/FSH ratios in plasma would be greater than 2. The increased LH levels could then lead to hyperplasia of the ovarian stroma and theca cells and increased androgen production, which in turn would provide more substrate for peripheral aromatization and perpetuate the chronic anovulation. In the advanced state the ovary

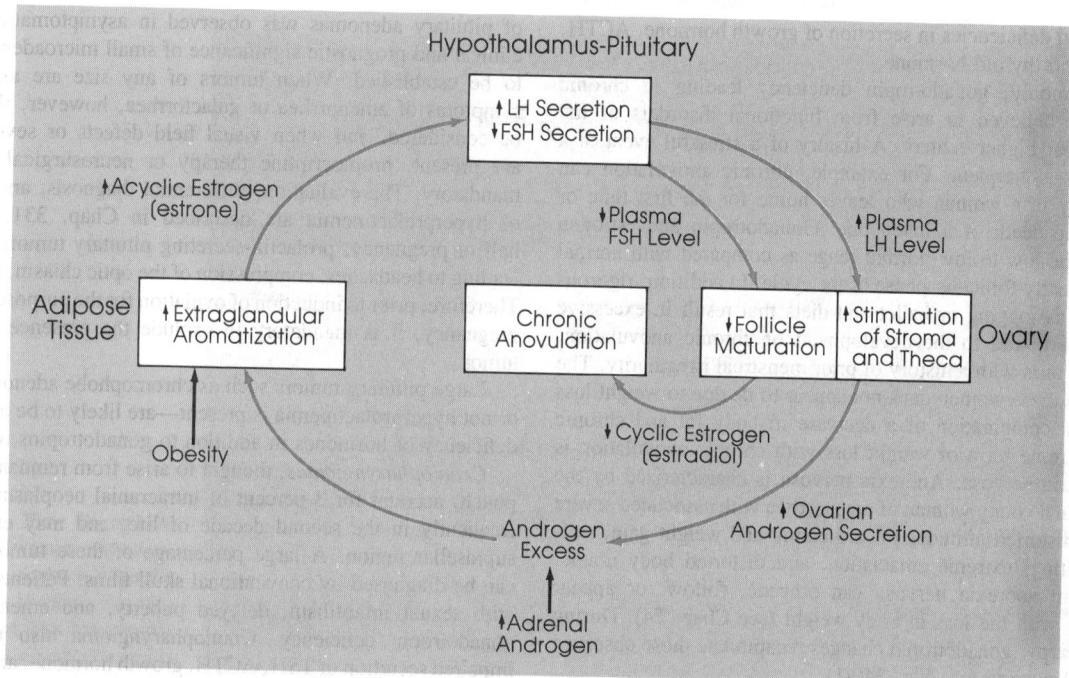

FIGURE 340-7 Proposed mechanism for the initiation and perpetuation of chronic anovulation in polycystic ovarian disease (PCOD). This cycle may be entered or initiated via adrenal androgen excess or obesity, both of which result in enhanced extraglandular formation of estrogens. The therapy of PCOD involves interruption of the cycle at various sites. (*From SSC Yen and RB Jaffe, 1986, and from U Goebelsmann in DR Mishell, Jr, and V Davajan.*)

is the major site of androgen production, but the adrenal may continue to secrete excess androgen as well. The greater the obesity, the more this sequence would be perpetuated because adipose tissue stromal cells aromatize androgens to estrogens, which in turn exaggerates inappropriate LH release by positive feedback.

Thus the fundamental defect in PCOD is viewed as one of inappropriate signals to the hypothalamus and pituitary. In fact, the hypothalamic-pituitary axis responds appropriately to high levels of estrogen, and ovulation can be induced with antiestrogens such as clomiphene citrate. Increased levels of plasma endorphins and inhibin may contribute to the perpetuation of the defect. The concept that the fundamental defect is one of inappropriate signals is supported by the findings in the ovary itself. Ovarian follicles from women with PCOD have low aromatase activity, but normal aromatase can be induced when the follicles are treated with FSH. In short, the anovulation is not due to an intrinsic abnormality in the ovary itself but rather the result of FSH deficiency and LH excess. An association exists between PCOD or hyperthecosis, virilization, acanthosis nigricans, and insulin resistance; in the ovary, insulin may interact via the insulin-like growth factor receptors to enhance androgen synthesis in insulin-resistant states.

Treatment of PCOD is directed toward interrupting this self-perpetuating cycle and can be accomplished in several ways, including decreasing ovarian androgen secretion (wedge resection or oral contraceptive agents), decreasing peripheral estrogen formation (weight reduction), and enhancing FSH secretion [administration of clomiphene, human menopausal gonadotropin (hMG), LHRH (gonadorelin) by portable infusion pump, or purified FSH (urofollitropin)]. The choice of therapy depends on the clinical findings and the needs of the patient. Attempt at weight reduction is appropriate in all who are obese. If the woman is not hirsute and does not desire pregnancy, periodic withdrawal menses can be induced with medroxyprogesterone acetate 10 days per month; such treatment prevents development of endometrial hyperplasia. If the woman is hirsute but does not desire pregnancy, the ovarian (and possibly the adrenal) component of androgen production can be suppressed with combined estrogen-progestogen oral contraceptive agents. Combined oral contraceptives are also indicated if prolonged or excessive menstrual bleeding is present. Once androgen excess is controlled,

treatment of previously existing hair growth by shaving, depilatories, or electrolysis may be indicated (see Chap. 49). If the woman wants to become pregnant, induction of ovulation is necessary. The drug of choice for this purpose is clomiphene, which promotes ovulation in three-fourths of cases, or treatment with hMG, urofollitropin, or gonadorelin. Pretreatment with LHRH analogues prior to hMG, urofollitropin, or gonadorelin has been utilized to improve ovulation and pregnancy rates. Wedge resection of the ovaries is rarely indicated today because of the development of adhesions but may be successful on occasion.

Chronic anovulation with estrogen present also may occur with tumors of the ovary. These include granulosa-theca cell tumors, Brenner tumors, cystic teratomas, mucous cystadenomas, and Krukenberg tumors (also see Chap. 321). These tumors can either secrete excess estrogen themselves or produce androgens that can then be aromatized in extraglandular sites. As a result, chronic anovulation and the clinical features of PCOD are produced. Occasionally, areas of the ovary not involved with tumors show the characteristic histologic changes of PCOD. Other causes of chronic anovulation with estrogen present include adrenal production of excess androgen (usually adult-onset adrenal hyperplasia due to partial $P450_{C21}$ deficiency) and various thyroid disorders.

Chronic anovulation with estrogen absent Women with chronic anovulation who have low or absent estrogen production and do not experience withdrawal bleeding after progestogen treatment usually have hypogonadotropic hypogonadism due either to pituitary disease or to any of several organic or functional disorders of the central nervous system.

Isolated hypogonadotropic hypogonadism associated with defects of smell (olfactory bulb defects) is known as the *Kallman syndrome* (see Chaps. 331 and 339). Affected women are sexually infantile with a eunuchoid habitus and appear to have a defect in either the synthesis or release of LHRH. A variety of rare hypothalamic lesions also can impair LHRH production and cause hypogonadotropic hypogonadism; these include craniopharyngioma, germinoma (pinealoma), glioma, Hand-Schüller-Christian disease, teratomas, endodermal-sinus tumors, tuberculosis, sarcoidosis, and metastatic tumors that cause suppression or destruction of the hypothalamus. Central nervous system trauma and radiation also can cause hypothalamic tion and embryo transfer (IVF-ET) may be tried. Indications for the use of IVF-ET in infertile couples include tubal obstructive disease, cervical factors, endometriosis, oligospermia, and unexplained infertility. Multiple follicles are induced with clomiphene and/or gonadotropins, and follicles are obtained by laparoscopy or transabdominal or transvaginal aspiration with ultrasound monitoring. After fertilization and cleavage, embryos are transferred to the uterine cavity. Although pregnancy rates vary, successful pregnancy has been reported in as many as 30 percent of cases after IVF-ET. Other techniques include a modification of IVF-ET known as *gamete-intrafallopian transfer* (GIFT), in which a mixture of sperm and ova are introduced into the end of the fallopian tube at laparoscopy, and intrauterine insemination after gonadotropin stimulation.

Medical aspects of pregnancy The possibility of pregnancy should be considered in all women of reproductive age who are evaluated for medical illness or considered for surgery. Procedures such as x-ray exposure, drugs, and anesthetics may be harmful to the developing fetus, and a variety of medical problems may worsen during pregnancy, including hypertension; diseases of the heart, lungs, kidney, and liver; and metabolic and endocrine disorders. Indeed, all women who present with abnormal vaginal bleeding or amenorrhea during the reproductive years should be assumed to have a complication of pregnancy, such as incomplete abortion, ectopic pregnancy, or trophoblastic disease (hydatidiform mole or choriocarcinoma). Women who present with these complications of pregnancy often have histories of abdominal pain and vaginal bleeding and may have evidence of intraabdominal hemorrhage.

Choriocarcinoma is a particular problem because of its protean manifestations. Half these malignancies follow pregnancies complicated by hydatidiform mole, and the remainder occur after spontaneous abortion, ectopic pregnancy, or normal deliveries. Patients may present with intraabdominal bleeding due to rupture of the uterus, liver, or ovary, with pulmonary manifestations (cough, hemoptysis, pleuritic pain, dyspnea, and respiratory failure) or gastrointestinal symptoms, usually chronic blood loss or melena. In addition, patients can present with cerebral metastases or renal involvement. The diagnosis can be established by demonstrating an elevated level of the β subunit of hCG in plasma. Treatment and cure are possible with chemotherapeutic agents (dactinomycin and/or methotrexate). (For manifestations of choriocarcinoma in men, see Chap. 322.)

Ovarian tumors See Chap. 321.

TREATMENT

PROGESTOGENS The major use of progestogen is in conjunction with estrogen to ensure the full maturation of the endometrium, both in combination birth control pills and in the therapy of hypogonadal states. In certain circumstances, however, progestogen therapy is appropriate by itself—to induce a progestational effect on the estrogen-primed endometrium (diagnostic tests for the evaluation of amenorrhea), to inhibit pituitary gonadotropins (the progestogen-only birth control pill or progestogen-containing implants) for contraception, for prophylaxis to prevent hyperplasia in PCOD, and for palliation in endometrial and breast carcinoma or treatment of endometriosis. Even when a direct progestational effect is desired, the available oral drugs substitute a synthetic derivative for the naturally occurring hormone. Oral progestogens include medroxyprogesterone acetate, megestrol acetate, norethindrone, norgestrel, and micronized progesterone. Parenteral agents include progesterone in oil, medroxyprogesterone acetate suspension, and 17-hydroxyprogesterone caproate. Vaginal progesterone suppositories are used for treatment of luteal phase defects, and progestogen implants are available for long-term contraception.

The most common undesirable side effect is breakthrough bleeding, which occurs when progestogens are used continuously. Other complications include nausea, vomiting, and hirsutism. Abnormal liver function is a side effect of those derivatives with alkyl substitution

FIGURE 340-9 The circulating forms of administered estrogenic drugs.

in the 17α position. Progestogens are contraindicated if pregnancy is known or suspected because of the risk of birth defects.

ESTROGENS Estrogens are used for four purposes—the treatment of gonadal failure, control of fertility, management of dysfunctional uterine bleeding, and management of carcinoma of the breast. (The management of carcinoma of the breast is discussed in Chap. 319.) However, none of the presently available orally active or parenteral hormones replaces the pattern of concentration of estradiol characteristic of the normally cycling, premenopausal woman (see Fig. 340-5). Estrogens that can be given by mouth are either nonsteroidal agents (such as diethylstilbestrol) that mimic the action of estradiol, estrogen conjugates that must be hydrolyzed before they become active (estrogen sulfates, predominantly estrone sulfate from pregnant mare's urine), or estrogen analogues that cannot be metabolized to estradiol (mestranol, quinestrol) (Fig. 340-9). Even when micronized estradiol is given orally, it is rapidly converted in the body to estrone. Because oral therapy neither replaces nor mimics the daily secretory pattern of the lost hormone, such therapy must be viewed as a pharmacologic substitution rather than a physiologic replacement. Likewise, the use of parenteral estrogens rarely mimics the physiologic situation. Parenteral preparations of conjugated estrogens, like the oral derivatives, are poor precursors of estradiol, and estradiol esters (estradiol benzoate and valerate) rarely cause plasma estradiol levels that mimic the normal monthly secretory pattern of the hormone. Transdermal estrogen results in constant levels of blood estrogen and is effective in the treatment of menopausal symptoms. The side effects of estrogen substitution differ at various times of life.

Hypoestrogenism In women with decreased estrogen production, whether due to disease of the ovaries (gonadal dysgenesis) or to hypogonadotropic hypogonadism, treatment with cyclic estrogens should be instituted at the time of expected puberty for development and maintenance of female secondary sexual characteristics and prevention of osteoporosis. The most commonly used medications are conjugated estrogens (0.625 to 1.25 mg/d by mouth) or ethinyl estradiol or its precursors (0.02 to 0.05 mg/d by mouth). The addition of medroxyprogesterone acetate (5 to 10 mg/d) is recommended by most physicians during the last several days of monthly estrogen treatment to prevent development of endometrial hyperplasia during long-term estrogen treatment. Abnormal bleeding in women receiving estrogen replacement requires histologic evaluation of the endometrium. Such substitution therapy or the use of oral contraceptives (see below) also may be used for the purpose of suppressing pituitary gonadotropins, as in women with PCOD, in whom the major therapeutic aim is suppression of ovarian androgen production prior to the time when fertility is desired.

Temporary administration of estrogens in larger quantities (up to two times the usual adult maintenance dose) may be necessary to induce full development of secondary sexual characteristics in girls and for the control of menopausal symptoms. Even larger doses of parenteral estrogens (10 mg estradiol valerate or 25 mg conjugated estrogen) in conjunction with progestogen may be required in some instances of dysfunctional uterine bleeding. In addition to the potential long-term side effects of all estrogens (see below), high doses may cause specific problems, including nausea, vomiting, and edema.

Fertility control Since the use of all contraceptive methods is associated with diverse side effects, an understanding of the use, methods of actions, and consequences of these agents is important to all physicians. Furthermore, since pregnancy may aggravate a variety of chronic illnesses, fertility control should be recommended in many patients.

To be effective, fertility control requires patient acceptance and compliance. The most widely utilized methods include (1) rhythm and withdrawal techniques, (2) barrier methods, including the condom, jellies, foam, suppositories, and diaphragms, (3) intrauterine devices (IUD), (4) hormonal contraceptives, (5) sterilization, and (6) abortion.

The rhythm and withdrawal technique and the barrier methods are effective if used correctly and consistently but in actual practice result in high failure rates because of imperfect compliance. Nevertheless, these methods carry the lowest incidence of side effects, and the side effects, when produced, are minor except for local allergic reactions. When the rhythm method is combined with self-evaluation of the preovulatory part of the menstrual cycle (i.e., evaluation of cervical mucus) plus home LH testing, it is an effective method of contraception. Use of these methods should be recommended when there is a relative or absolute contraindication to other therapy.

The most widely utilized nonsurgical methods of contraception, the IUD and birth control pills, are effective but may be associated with significant side effects.

IUD The success rates of most IUDs are 95 to 98 percent. Only two devices are marketed in the United States. Both are T-shaped, cause minimal pain at insertion, and are associated with low expulsion rates. One of these IUDs contains copper, which enhances effectiveness, and is replaced at 8-year intervals. The other contains slow-release progesterone, which makes annual replacement necessary. The IUD is believed to prevent pregnancy by the induction of a chronic inflammatory reaction in the endometrium, resulting in an unfavorable environment for the implantation of the blastocyst, although some evidence suggests that IUDs prevent fertilization.

Once the IUD is inserted, it is necessary to check periodically to be certain that the device is in place. Both minor and serious side effects can occur. Intermenstrual spotting and increased bleeding and pain or cramps at the time of menses are frequent causes of discontinuation of the IUD. In addition, the device may be expelled spontaneously during a menstrual period without the subject being aware of its loss. The most serious side effect is pelvic infection, occasionally leading to the development of tuboovarian abscess and subsequent infertility. Pelvic infection is more frequent than in users of oral or barrier contraceptives but no more common than in women using no contraception. Women with multiple sex partners are at greatest risk for pelvic infection. For this reason, use in nulligravida women is not advocated by many gynecologists. In addition, pregnancy with an IUD in place is more likely to be ectopic because intrauterine but not extrauterine pregnancies are inhibited. Because of the increased incidence of spontaneous and septic abortions when IUDs are in place, the device should be removed if pregnancy is detected. Any user who develops persistent, severe bleeding, lower abdominal pain, fever, or discharge should have the IUD removed.

ORAL CONTRACEPTIVES Oral contraceptive agents have been used by over 200 million women worldwide and by 1 of 4 women in the United States under age 45. These agents are popular because of ease of administration, low pregnancy rate (less than 1 percent), and a relatively low incidence of side effects.

The most widely utilized oral contraceptive pills are either combination tablets or triphasic formulations. A list of oral contraceptives marketed in the United States is given in Table 340-3. Combination oral contraceptive tablets contain one of two synthetic estrogens (mestranol or ethinyl estradiol) and one of five synthetic progestogens (norethindrone, norethindrone acetate, norethynodrel, norgestrel, ethynodiol diacetate desogestrel and norgestimate). The agents now available all contain no more than 50 μg ethinyl estradiol or its equivalent. The combination or triphasic tablets are taken for 21 consecutive days followed by 7 days' rest. Progestogen-only tablets are taken continuously on a daily basis. Presumably, the ideal contraceptive contains the lowest amount of steroid to minimize side effects but an amount that is at the same time sufficient to prevent pregnancy or breakthrough bleeding. The triphasic tablets, containing 35 μg or less of estrogen and less than 1 mg progestogen, come closest to this goal.

Oral contraceptives inhibit ovulation by suppressing FSH and LH secretion. As a consequence, the secretion of all ovarian steroids is also suppressed, including estrogen, progesterone, and androgen (Fig. 340-10). These agents also exert minor direct inhibitory effects on the reproductive tract, altering the cervical mucus and thereby decreasing sperm penetration and decreasing the motility and secretions of the fallopian tubes and uterus.

The death rates associated with oral contraceptives and other forms of birth control are summarized in Table 340-4. Up to age 40, the mortality rates in women using oral contraceptives and IUDs are lower than in women using no form of contraception (this difference results from the increased risk of death associated with pregnancy). The decrease in death rate below age 40 is even more striking in nonsmokers than in smokers using contraceptives. In fact, the death rates in nonsmoking women aged 15 to 24 who use oral agents are lower than those with other forms of fertility control. The increased death rates in women using rhythm or barrier techniques probably results from the higher failure rate and the consequent risk of pregnancy in such women. Oral contraceptive agents are not recommended for smoking women after age 35 and for women of all ages who are at increased risk for myocardial infarction.

Despite the overall safety of these agents, users are at risk for several serious side effects. In most retrospective and prospective studies, an increased incidence has been found for *deep vein thrombosis* and *pulmonary embolism*. The relative increased risk varies from two- to twelvefold and is greater for women taking tablets containing more than 50 μg estrogen. The use of oral contraceptives is also associated with an increased risk of thromboembolism after surgery, and for this reason, these agents should be discontinued at least 1 month prior to elective surgery. In retrospective studies there is a 3- to 9-times increased risk for *thromboembolic stroke* and a twofold greater risk for *hemorrhagic stroke* in users of oral contraceptives. However, three large prospective studies have demonstrated only a slight increase in hemorrhagic stroke in oral contraceptive users. Therefore, the drugs should be discontinued in women who experience visual complaints or severe headaches. Smoking and age increase the risk for stroke as well as the frequency of death from complications of deep venous thrombosis, pulmonary emboli, and myocardial infarction.

A small rise in blood pressure while taking oral contraceptives is common, and 5 percent of women develop significant *hypertension* (blood pressure greater than 140/90) after 5 years of continuous use. Estrogens induce the synthesis of a variety of proteins by the liver, including the renin substrate angiotensinogen. The resulting increased formation of angiotensin is believed to be involved in the development

TABLE 340-3 Composition of currently marketed oral contraceptives

Name	Estrogen	μg	Progestogen	mg
COMBINATION-TYPE				
Fixed type				
Estrogen content = 50 μg:				
Ortho-Novum 1/50	Mestranol	50	Norethindrone	1.0
Norinyl 1/50	Mestranol	50	Norethindrone	1.0
Ovcon 50	Ethinyl estradiol	50	Norethindrone	1.0
Ovral	Ethinyl estradiol	50	Norgestrel	0.5
Demulen	Ethinyl estradiol	50	Ethynodiol diacetate	1.0
Norlestrin 2.5/50	Ethinyl estradiol	50	Norethindrone acetate	2.5
Norlestrin 1/50	Ethinyl estradiol	50	Norethindrone acetate	1.0
Estrogen content <50 μg:				
Ortho-Novum 1/35	Ethinyl estradiol	35	Norethindrone	1.0
Norinyl 1 + 35	Ethinyl estradiol	35	Norethindrone	1.0
Modicon	Ethinyl estradiol	35	Norethindrone	0.5
Brevicon	Ethinyl estradiol	35	Norethindrone	0.5
Ovcon 35	Ethinyl estradiol	35	Norethindrone	0.4
Demulen 1/35	Ethinyl estradiol	35	Ethynodiol diacetate	1.0
Loestrin 1.5/30	Ethinyl estradiol	30	Norethindrone acetate	1.5
Loestrin 1/20	Ethinyl estradiol	20	Norethindrone acetate	1.0
Nordette	Ethinyl estradiol	30	Levonorgestrel	0.15
Lo-Ovral	Ethinyl estradiol	30	Norgestrel	0.3
Biphasic type				
Ortho-Novum 10/11				
First 10 days	Ethinyl estradiol	35	Norethindrone	0.5
Next 11 days	Ethinyl estradiol	35	Norethindrone	1.0
Triphasic type				
Ortho-Novum 7/7/7				
First 7 days	Ethinyl estradiol	35	Norethindrone	0.5
Second 7 days	Ethinyl estradiol	35	Norethindrone	0.75
Third 7 days	Ethinyl estradiol	35	Norethindrone	1.0
Tri-Norinyl				
First 7 days	Ethinyl estradiol	35	Norethindrone	0.5
Next 9 days	Ethinyl estradiol	35	Norethindrone	1.0
Next 5 days	Ethinyl estradiol	35	Norethindrone	0.5
Triphasil				
First 6 days	Ethinyl estradiol	30	Levonorgestrel	0.05
Second 5 days	Ethinyl estradiol	40	Levonorgestrel	0.075
Third 10 days	Ethinyl estradiol	30	Levonorgestrel	0.125
Tri-Levein				
First 6 days	Ethinyl estradiol	30	Levonorgestrel	0.05
Second 5 days	Ethinyl estradiol	40	Levonorgestrel	0.075
Third 10 days	Ethinyl estradiol	30	Levonorgestrel	0.125
PROGESTOGEN ONLY				
Micronor	None		Norethindrone	0.35
Nor Q.D.	None		Norethindrone	0.35
Ovrette	None		Norgestrel	0.075

of hypertension. Alternatively, the progestogen component of oral contraceptives may be associated with increased risk of hypertension. In most cases, blood pressure returns to normal when oral contraceptives are discontinued.

Serum lipids and lipoproteins are altered in women on oral contraceptives, the nature of the change depending on the specific components of the oral contraceptives. In general, estrogens increase serum high-density (HDL) and very low density lipoproteins (VLDL). Progestogens depress the concentration of HDL. However, with oral contraceptives containing less than 35 μg estrogen, lipoproteins change little if at all.

A few women taking oral contraceptives develop *impairment of glucose tolerance* as manifested by abnormal glucose levels and elevated plasma insulin after an oral glucose load, both of which usually return to normal after discontinuing the agents. Because juvenile-onset and adult-onset diabetes may be associated with increased incidence of cardiovascular disease, it is preferable to utilize other forms of contraception in these individuals.

Oral contraceptives should not be used by women with abnormal liver function tests or in women with acute or chronic liver disease. A rare complication linked to the long-term use of oral contraceptives is the development of peliosis hepatis, which can cause death due to sudden rupture and hemorrhage of the liver. Cholestatic jaundice may

occur in those women predisposed to the development of the syndrome of recurrent jaundice of pregnancy.

Oral contraceptives cause an increased concentration of cholesterol in the bile, which is probably the cause for the twofold increase in *cholelithiasis* and cholecystitis in women on oral contraceptives.

Estrogens induce elevation of a variety of proteins secreted by the liver, including cortisol-binding globulin (CBG), testosterone-binding globulin (TeBG), and thyroxine-binding globulin (TBG). Consequently, various laboratory tests of adrenal and thyroid function may be altered and must be interpreted with caution (see Chaps. 330 and 334). Oral contraceptives also slightly lower plasma ACTH levels, possibly due to an inhibitory effect on ACTH secretion or cortisol catabolism. Finally, serum prolactin levels are slightly elevated in women on oral contraceptives, but such treatment is not believed to play a role in the development of pituitary prolactinomas.

Other effects of oral contraceptive pills include minor dyspepsia, breast discomfort, weight gain, development of pigmentation of the face (chloasma), which is augmented by exposure to the sun, and a variety of psychological effects, such as depression and changes in libido. There is no convincing evidence that oral contraceptive use is associated with significant increase in the incidence of cancer of the uterus, cervix, or breast. In fact, oral contraceptives have many beneficial effects including control of dysmenorrhea and anovulatory

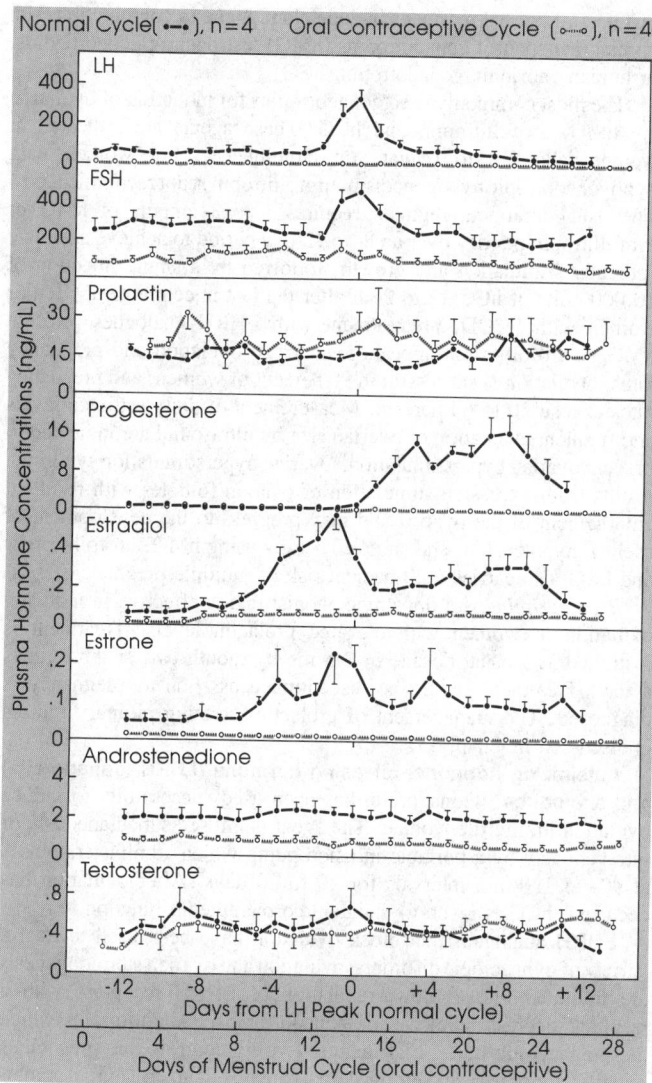

Normal Cycle(•--•), n = 4   Oral Contraceptive Cycle (○----○), n = 4

FIGURE 340-10   The mechanism of action of the birth control tablet. Mean daily plasma hormone concentrations during the ovarian cycle are shown for four ovulating women and four women treated with combination-type oral contraceptives. Data for the normal ovarian cycle are presented in relationship to the day of the LH peak; day 1 of the contraceptive cycle corresponds to the first day of uterine bleeding. The values are the mean ± SE obtained from four women. (*From BR Carr et al, 1979.*)

bleeding, prevention of sexually transmitted diseases, and decreased incidence of endometrial and ovarian cancer.

The absolute contraindications to the use of oral contraceptives include previous thromboembolic disorders, cerebral vascular or coronary artery disease, known or suspected carcinoma of the breast or estrogen-dependent neoplasia, undiagnosed abnormal genital bleeding, or known or suspected pregnancy. Relative contraindications must be weighed against the risk-versus-benefit ratio of the oral contraceptive pills and include hypertension, migraine headaches, diabetes mellitus, uterine leiomyomas, sickle cell anemia, hyperlipemia, and elective surgery.

OTHER STEROID CONTRACEPTIVES   Types of steroid contraception other than the conventional oral contraceptives include (1) postcoital contraception and (2) injectable steroids, including progestogen-containing implants. Use of high-dose estrogen for 5 days during the fertile part of the cycle (the morning-after pill) is an effective method of contraception but is associated with significant side effects, particularly nausea. Administration of progestogens by injection or vaginal rings is used infrequently in the United States.

Estrogen treatment of the menopause   The rationale for use of estrogens in postmenopausal women is based on the belief that such therapy may relieve many of the disorders of the menopause, including osteoporosis, and indeed of aging itself. In some parts of the United States, by the mid-1970s as many as half of women in the menopausal age group used one or more forms of estrogen replacement for a median period of 5 years, accounting for more than 30 million prescriptions per year.

The menopause is not associated with a simple state of estrogen deprivation, since some estrogens continue to be produced, but is instead a state of altered estrogen metabolism; the predominant estrogen becomes estrone formed by extraglandular conversion of prehormone rather than estradiol secretion by the ovary. As is true for all estrogen therapy, the estrogen treatment of the menopause is actually a pharmacologic substitution of one or another estrogen analogue for the physiologic estradiol rather than a physiologic replacement of the missing steroid. Estrogens available for replacement therapy include conjugated estrogens, estrogen substitutes (diethylstilbestrol), synthetic estrogen (ethinyl estradiol or derivatives), micronized estradiol, estrogen-containing vaginal creams, and estrogen-containing dermal patches. Regimens associated with low risk of complications include (1) cyclic estrogen therapy in the lowest effective dose for 25 days per month or continuous estrogens given each day of the month and (2) estrogens plus the addition of progestogen during the last 10 to 13 days of estrogen therapy, or low-dose continuous progestogen plus estrogen given daily.

The most clear-cut early benefit of estrogen therapy in the menopause is the relief of vasomotor instability (hot flashes) and of atrophy of the urogenital epithelium and skin. Estrogen therapy ameliorates these symptoms in the majority of cases. When estrogen therapy is designed to treat hot flashes alone, such therapy should be continued for only a few years, since hot flashes tend to diminish after 3 to 4 years in untreated women.

Several lines of evidence indicate that routine estrogen therapy is beneficial in preventing the complications of menopausal osteoporosis, especially in high-risk women (i.e., thin white women). First, in women undergoing premature menopause, the incidence and complication rates of osteoporosis are increased, and long-term estrogen replacement appears to be beneficial. Second, estrogen

TABLE 340-4   Annual death rates associated with fertility control per 100,000 women

Contraceptive techniques	Age group					
	15–19	20–24	25–29	30–34	35–39	40–44
None (birth-related)	7.0	7.4	9.1	14.8	25.7	28.2
Oral contraceptives						
Smokers	2.4	3.6	6.8	13.7	51.4	117.6
Nonsmokers	0.5	0.7	1.1	2.1	14.1	32.0
IUD	1.3	1.1	1.3	1.3	1.9	2.1
Abortion	0.5	1.1	1.3	1.9	1.8	1.1
Barrier methods (birth-related)	1.5	1.4	1.0	0.8	1.3	7.6

SOURCE: Adapted from Ory.

therapy has short-term positive effects on calcium balance and long-term beneficial effects on bone density. Third, in women given estrogen therapy, the incidence of fractures is decreased.

Of the potential side effects, the possibility of an increased risk of endometrial carcinoma is perhaps most worrisome. The relative risk of developing endometrial adenocarcinoma in estrogen users is between 6 and 8. The risk is increased with duration and dosage of estrogen but is less in women given combination estrogen-progestogen therapy.

Despite the large body of evidence linking endometrial carcinoma and estrogen use, two types of doubt have been raised about the clinical significance of the association. First, some epidemiologists have argued that the increased risk associated with estrogens has been exaggerated because of problems inherent in obtaining adequate controls in retrospective analyses. Second, despite an increased incidence of endometrial carcinoma in the United States, there was no concomitant increased mortality from this disease. Indeed, the increased incidence apparently involves low-grade malignancies which may be difficult to distinguish histologically from various forms of hyperplasia. These forms of malignancy have little effect on life expectancy.

Apprehension concerning worsening of hypertension and thromboembolic disease appears to be due to reports of the effects of estrogen-progestogen oral contraceptives during the reproductive years and not to estrogen use in menopausal women. There is no documented evidence that low-dose estrogen therapy in the menopause increases the incidence or the severity of thromboembolic disease, breast cancer, or hypertension. Low-dose estrogen treatment in the menopause does not appear to influence the development of atherosclerosis, myocardial infarction, or stroke. Strong evidence suggests that, in fact, estrogens may decrease the incidence of death from myocardial infarction. There is a slightly increased risk for the development of gallbladder disease with estrogen use in the menopause.

A reasonable approach to the use of estrogens in the menopause is as follows: (1) For long-term use, estrogens should be given in the minimal effective doses (0.625 mg conjugated estrogen orally or 0.01 to 0.02 mg ethinyl estradiol orally per day or transdermal estradiol 0.05 mg every 3 to 4 days). Except when hot flashes preclude intermittent use, the agents are often prescribed for 25 days each month followed by a rest period. (For women with an intact uterus, it is the practice in some clinics to give estrogens alone for 15 days, estrogen plus a daily progestogen for an additional 10 to 13 days, and nothing for a week. Other regimens include continuous estrogen treatment plus cyclic progestogens or low-dose continuous progestogens.) (2) Such replacement therapy is indicated routinely in women undergoing premature menopause (surgically induced or spontaneous) at least until the age of normal menopause. (3) Estrogen therapy is also indicated routinely in women of all ages who have severe hot flashes or symptomatic atrophy of the urogenital epithelium. Hot flashes rarely persist for longer than 4 years, so if given for this purpose, the duration of therapy can be limited. (4) In women who have had prior hysterectomy, potential benefits of treatment appear to outweigh the dangers. In women who do not have a uterus, cyclic or continuous estrogen without progestogen is recommended. Whether estrogens should be given routinely to all women with intact uteri is unsettled, but the authors prescribe it routinely in the absence of contraindications in hopes of ameliorating osteoporosis (in combination with calcium). (5) Each woman receiving estrogens must be monitored indefinitely at yearly intervals.

DRUGS TO INDUCE OVULATION   The most common treatment for ovulation induction in women with PCOD is *clomiphene*. This antiestrogen is believed to act as an antiestrogen in the hypothalamus and allow FSH to rise to stimulate follicular development and ultimately result in ovulation. Clomiphene therapy is usually begun in a dose of 50 mg by mouth daily for 5 days commencing on the fifth day of progestogen-induced uterine bleeding. If ovulation does not occur, the dose may be increased to 100 or 150 mg/d. Such treatment results in ovulatory cycles in 60 percent of women with PCOD. Additional regimens include clomiphene in combination with human menopausal gonadotropins (hMG), estrogen, glucocorticoids, or human chorionic gonadotropin (hCG).

The most commonly used gonadotropins for induction of ovulation are hMG, urofollitropin, and hCG. These agents are indicated in women who fail to ovulate on clomiphene. (For women with hypogonadotropic hypogonadism, urofollitropin is not recommended.) The usual treatment regimen requires 1 to 3 ampuls of hMG or urofollitropin per day over an 8- to 12-day period to achieve adequate follicular stimulation and growth, followed by a single injection of 10,000 units of hCG 12 to 24 h after the last injection of hMG. For women with PCOD, pretreatment with LHRH analogues prior to hMG or urofollitropin appears to improve ovulation and pregnancy rates. Ovulation is successful in 90 percent of women, and pregnancy rates exceed 50 to 60 percent. Measurement of daily estrogen levels and frequent evaluation of ovarian size by ultrasound are indicated to prevent ovarian hyperstimulation. Ovarian hyperstimulation syndrome results from excessive stimulation of ovarian follicles with resultant enlargement of the ovaries and may progress to the development of ascites, hypotension, and shock. Therapy using hMG, urofollitropin, and hCG also carries a 20 percent risk of multiple pregnancies.

Bromocriptine is a dopamine agonist that is effective in inducing ovulation in women with elevated prolactin levels. Treatment is instituted at a usual dosage of 2.5 mg by mouth two or three times a day. Treatment should be discontinued as soon as pregnancy is diagnosed. The management of prolactin-secreting pituitary tumors is discussed in Chap. 331.

Luteinizing hormone–releasing hormone (LHRH, gonadorelin) and analogues   Gonadorelin has been used successfully to induce ovulation in infertile women. The agent is infused subcutaneously or intravenously by a portable infusion pump which administers pulses at 90- to 120-min intervals for 10 to 20 days. After ovulation has occurred, hCG is given to maintain corpus luteum function.

LHRH analogues that block ovulation have been used to treat a variety of gynecologic disorders; ovulation and ovarian steroidogenesis are inhibited due to down-regulation of LHRH receptors with a resultant decreased release of gonadotropins. Conditions in which these agents are under trial include fertility control, true precocious puberty, endometriosis, uterine leiomyomas, hirsutism, and, in combination with gonadotropins, ovulation induction and in vitro fertilization.

OTHER DISORDERS OF THE FEMALE REPRODUCTIVE TRACT

VULVA   Most disorders of the vulva are due to venereal disease, most commonly syphilis (painless chancre), condylomata acuminata (venereal warts), and herpes vulvitis (painful ulcers) (see Chap. 88). All other lesions of the vulva, particularly in older women, must be biopsied. Early biopsy of cancer of the vulva is mandatory, because when it becomes symptomatic (pruritus and bleeding), it has often progressed to an advanced stage.

VAGINA   Infections of the vagina usually present as vaginal discharge and pruritus. The most frequent organisms are *Trichomonas, Candida albicans*, and *Gardnerella vaginalis* (also see Chap. 88). The diagnosis is made by microscopic examination of the discharge, and appropriate therapy can be instituted utilizing vaginal or oral antibiotics.

Abnormalities of the vagina and cervix in female offspring of women given diethylstilbestrol during pregnancy include adenosis of the vagina as well as structural abnormalities of the vagina, cervix, and uterus; the risk of developing a rare form of vaginal cancer (adenocarcinoma, clear cell type) is increased (2 per 10,000 exposed women). Periodic examination of women at risk should commence at ages 12 to 14, and reevaluation should be undertaken after any episode of abnormal bleeding.

CERVIX Preinvasive lesions of the cervix (also known as *cervical intraepithelial neoplasia*) as well as invasive carcinoma of the cervix can be detected reliably by obtaining a Papanicolaou smear (Pap smear). Current recommendations by the American Cancer Society are that a Pap smear be obtained every 3 years after 2 negative Pap smears were obtained at yearly intervals. However, many gynecologists recommend yearly Pap smears, especially in patients with more than one sexual partner.

UTERUS Only 40 percent of endometrial adenocarcinoma is detected by Pap smear. In women at high risk for endometrial carcinoma (obesity, history of chronic anovulatory cycles, diabetes, hypertension, estrogen treatment), yearly endometrial sampling should be performed. Low-dose oral estrogen therapy rarely causes breakthrough or withdrawal bleeding in menopausal women. Therefore, irrespective of whether the patient is on estrogen therapy, occurrence of postmenopausal bleeding makes it mandatory to obtain a tissue diagnosis to exclude endometrial cancer either by endometrial sampling or by curettage.

One of the most common disorders of the uterus and the most frequent tumor of women (1 of 4 women affected) is the uterine leiomyoma, or fibroid tumor. Three-fourths of women with leiomyoma are asymptomatic, and the diagnosis is made on routine pelvic examination. When associated with excessive menstrual blood loss, excessive size or rapid growth, or significant pelvic pain (see Chap. 48), the preferred treatment is surgical removal by hysterectomy if there is no desire for further childbearing. In young women, myomectomy may on occasion be indicated when infertility or repeated fetal wastage is a manifestation or where future childbearing is desired.

FALLOPIAN TUBES AND OVARIES Infectious pelvic inflammatory disease is a common disorder of the fallopian tubes and usually becomes symptomatic after a menstrual period; the symptoms include fever, chills, abdominal pain, and vaginal discharge, and pelvic tenderness on physical examination is common. The initiating organism most often is *Chlamydia trachomatis* or *Neisseria gonorrhoeae*, but tuboovarian abscess and sterility are probably caused by mixed aerobic and anaerobic superinfections and require wide-spectrum antibiotic treatment (see Chap. 89).

Endometriosis is a benign disorder characterized by the presence and proliferation of endometrial tissue (stroma and glands) outside the endometrial cavity. The clinical manifestations are variable. Endometriosis occurs most commonly between the ages of 30 and 40 and is found incidentally at the time of surgery in approximately one-fifth of all gynecologic operations. The fertility rate is significantly reduced in affected women. The disorder usually involves the posterior cul-de-sac or the ovaries and can give rise to ovarian enlargement (endometriomas), although it also may involve sites distant to the pelvis (lung, umbilicus). The most significant symptom is pelvic pain, characteristically dysmenorrhea (see Chap. 48). However, the frequency and degree of pelvic symptomatology correlate poorly with the extent of disease. Other symptoms include dyspareunia, pain with defecation, and infertility. The characteristic physical findings are multiple tender nodules palpable along the uterosacral ligament at the time of rectal-vaginal examination, a posteriorly fixed uterus, or enlarged cystic ovaries. The diagnosis can only be confirmed by direct visualization, usually at diagnostic laparoscopy. Treatment depends on the degree of involvement and the desires of the patient and includes observation for mild disease with no associated infertility or pain, hormonal suppressive therapy (see infertility), conservative surgery if fertility is desired, or removal of the uterus, tubes, and ovaries in severe disease. Endometriosis is rarely found after the menopause.

Any adnexal mass that persists for more than 6 weeks or is larger than 6 cm must be evaluated. Although ovarian cysts and neoplasms compose the largest group of pelvic adnexal masses (see above), tumors of the fallopian tubes, uterus, gastrointestinal tract, or urinary tract also should be considered. Sonography or radiographic evaluation is often helpful in identifying the nature of the adnexal mass prior to surgical exploration.

REFERENCES

ADASHI E: Putative intraovarian regulators. Semin Reprod Endocrinol 7:1, 1989

CARR BR: Disorders of the ovary and reproductive tract, in *Williams' Textbook of Endocrinology*, 8th ed, JD Wilson, DW Foster (eds). Philadelphia, Saunders, 1992, pp 733–798

———, BLACKWELL RE (eds): *Textbook of Reproductive Medicine*. Norwalk, Appleton & Lange, 1992

———, GRIFFIN JE: Fertility control and its complications, in *Williams' Textbook of Endocrinology*, 8th ed, JD Wilson, DW Foster (eds). Philadelphia, Saunders, 1992, pp 1007–1031

——— et al: Plasma levels of adrenocorticotropin and cortisol in women receiving oral contraceptive steroid treatment. J Clin Endocrinol Metab 49:346, 1979

——— et al: Plasma lipoprotein regulation or progesterone biosynthesis by human corpus luteum tissue in organ culture. J Clin Endocrinol Metab 52:875, 1981

——— et al: The role of lipoproteins in the regulation of progesterone secretion by human corpus luteum. Fertil Steril 38:303, 1982

CUNNINGHAM FG et al: *Williams' Obstetrics*, 18th ed. Norwalk, Appleton-Lange, 1989

D'ARMIENTO M et al: McCune-Albright syndrome: Evidence for autonomous multiendocrine hyperfunction. J Pediatr 102:584, 1983

DIZEREGA GS, HODGEN GD: Folliculogenesis in the primate ovarian cycle. Endocrinol Rev 2:27, 1981

DMOWSKI WP: Endocrine properties and clinical applications of danazol. Fertil Steril 31:237, 1979

ERICKSON GF et al: Functional studies of aromatase activity in human granulosa cells from normal and polycystic ovaries. J Clin Endocrinol Metab 49:514, 1979

——— et al: The ovarian androgen producing cells: A review of structure/function relationships. Endocr Rev 6:371, 1985

FAIMAN C et al: Patterns of gonadotropins and gonadal steroids throughout life. Clin Obstet Gynecol 3:467, 1976

FILSHIE M, GUILLEBAND J (eds): *Contraception: Science and Practice*. London, Butterworths, 1989

FUTTERWEIT W: *Polycystic Ovarian Disease*. New York, Springer-Verlag, 1984

GEMZELL C, WANG CF: Outcome of pregnancy in women with pituitary adenoma. Fertil Steril 31:363, 1979

GLUCKMAN PD et al: The human fetal hypothalamus and pituitary gland, in *Maternal-Fetal Endocrinology*, D Tulchinksy, KJ Ryan (eds). Philadelphia, Saunders, 1980

GOLDZIEHER JW: Polycystic ovarian disease. Fertil Steril 35:371, 1981

GRUMBACH MM, CONTE FA: Disorders of sex differentiation, in *Williams' Textbook of Endocrinology*, 8th ed, JD Wilson, DW Foster (eds). Philadelphia, Saunders, 1992, pp 853–952

———, STYNE DM: Puberty: Ontogeny, neuroendocrinology, physiology and disorders, in *Williams' Textbook of Endocrinology*, 8th ed, JD Wilson, DW Foster (eds). Philadelphia, Saunders, 1992, pp 1139–1222

HATCHER RA et al: *Contraceptive Technology 1990–1992*. New York, Irvington, 1992

HERBST AL et al: *Comprehensive Gynecology*. 2d ed. St. Louis, Mosby, 1992

HSUEH AJW et al: Hormonal regulation of the differentiation of cultured ovarian granulosa cells. Endocr Rev 5:76, 1984

JONES HW JR et al (eds): *In Vitro Fertilization*. Baltimore, Williams & Wilkins, 1986

JUDD HL et al: Estrogen replacement therapy: Indications and complications. Ann Intern Med 98:195, 1983

KAPLAN SA (ed): *Clinical Pediatric Endocrinology*. Philadelphia, Saunders, 1990

KASE N, WEINGOLD A: *Principles and Practice of Clinical Gynecology*. New York, Wiley, 1983

KELCH RP: Management of precocious puberty. N Engl J Med 312:1057, 1985

KNOBIL E, NEILL JD (eds): *The Physiology of Reproduction*. New York, Raven, 1988

MISHELL DR JR, DAVAJAN V (eds): *Reproductive Endocrinology, Infertility, and Contraception*, 2d ed. Philadelphia, Davis, 1986

PIEPER DR et al: Ovarian gonadatropin-releasing hormone (GnRH) receptors: Characterization, distribution, and induction by GnRH. Endocrinology 108:1148, 1981

RIGGS BL et al: Effect of the fluoride/calcium regimen on vertebral fracture occurrence in postmenopausal osteoporosis. N Engl J Med 306:446, 1982

ROSS JL et al: A preliminary study of the effect of estrogen dose on growth in Turner's syndrome. N Engl J Med 309:1104, 1983

SCULLY RE: Ovarian tumors: A review. Am J Pathol 87:686, 1977

SEIBEL MM: A new era in reproductive technology. N Engl J Med 318:828, 1988

SHEARMAN RP (ed): *Clinical Reproductive Endocrinology*, Edinburgh, Churchill Livingston, 1985

SITTERI PK, MACDONALD PC: Role of extraglandular estrogen in human endocrinology, in *Handbook of Physiology*, sec 7, Endocrinology, SR Geiger et al (eds). Washington, American Physiological Society, 1973, p 615

SPEROFF L: Menopause. Semin Reprod Endocrinol 1:1, 1983

——— et al: *Clinical Gynecologic Endocrinology and Infertility*, 4th ed. Baltimore, Williams & Wilkins, 1989

STEINGOLD KA et al: Treatment of hot flashes with transdermal estradiol administration. J Clin Endocrinol Metab 61:627, 1985

STUDD JWW, WHITEHEAD MI (eds): *The Menopause*. Oxford, Blackwell, 1988

STYNE DM, GRUMBACH MM: Disorders of puberty in the male and female, in *Reproductive Endocrinology*, SSC Yen, RB Jaffe (eds). Philadelphia, Saunders, 1991, pp 11–54

THOMPSON JD, ROCK JA: *Te Lindes Operative Gynecology*. Philadelphia, Lippincott, 1992

WALLACH EE, KEMPERS RD: *Modern Trends in Infertility and Contraception Control*, vol 3. Baltimore, Williams & Wilkins, 1985

WENTZ AC et al: *Gynecologic Endocrinology and Infertility*, Baltimore, Williams & Wilkins, 1988

YEN SSC: Neuroendocrine regulation of the menstrual cycle. Hosp Prac 14:84, 1979

————: Clinical application of gonadotropin-releasing hormone and gonadotropin-releasing hormone analogs. Fertil Steril 39:257, 1983

————, JAFFE RB (eds): *Reproductive Endocrinology*, 3d ed. Philadelphia, Saunders, 1991

YING SY et al: Gonadocrinins: Peptides in ovarian follicular fluid stimulating the secretion of pituitary gonadotropins. Endocrinology 108:1206, 1981

341 ENDOCRINE DISORDERS OF THE BREAST

JEAN D. WILSON

Examination of the breasts is an important part of the physical examination. The breasts are the site of fatal and preventable disease in women and provide clues to underlying systemic illness in both men and women. The internist frequently does not examine the male breast and is apt to refer the evaluation of the female breast to a gynecologist. It is the duty of every physician to distinguish the abnormal from the normal at the earliest possible stage and to call for assistance if there is any doubt. (For cancer of the breast see Chap. 319.)

ENDOCRINE CONTROL OF THE BREAST There is no histologic or functional difference in the breasts of boys and girls prior to the onset of puberty, but a profound sexual dimorphism in breast development ensues at the time of puberty. The endocrine control of female breast development is illustrated in Fig. 341-1. The pubertal growth of the female breast is dependent primarily on the action of estradiol, which induces the growth, division, and elongation of the tubular duct system and maturation of the nipples. In men the administration of estrogen is equally effective in this regard. To produce true alveolar development at the ends of the ducts, however, the synergistic action of progesterone is required, a ratio of estrogen to progesterone of 1:20 to 1:100 being optimal. Once the anatomic development of the ducts and alveoli is complete, the continued action of estrogen and progesterone does not appear to be required for lactation itself.

The endocrine control of milk formation is complex, requiring, in addition to appropriate priming by estrogen and progesterone, specific lactogenic hormone and the permissive action of glucocorticoid, insulin, thyroxine, and, in some species, growth hormone. There are

FIGURE 341-1 Endocrine control of female breast development and function at various stages of life.

Stage	Duct System	Major Hormones	Permissive Hormones
Prepubertal		None	Unknown
Adult		Estrogen (progesterone)	
Pregnancy		Estrogen Progesterone Prolactin Human Placental Lactogen	Insulin Thyroxine Glucocorticoids Growth Hormone
Lactation		Prolactin Oxytocin	

two lactogenic hormones. Human placental lactogen (hPL or chorionic somatomammotropin) is secreted in large amounts by the placenta during the latter part of gestation and prepares the breast for milk production. hPL disappears from the fetal (and maternal) circulation shortly after termination of pregnancy. Pituitary prolactin (see Chap. 331) plays the critical role in the initiation and maintenance of lactation during the puerperium. The plasma level of prolactin rises during pregnancy; during late pregnancy and lactation, 60 to 80 percent of the anterior pituitary may consist of prolactin-secreting cells.

Unlike most pituitary hormones, the predominant regulation of prolactin secretion is negative, i.e., under ordinary basal conditions one or more inhibitory hypothalamic hormones, the most important being dopamine, is delivered to the pituitary via the hypothalamic portal system and inhibits the release of prolactin into the blood (see Chap. 331). Most factors that influence prolactin secretion do so by affecting the synthesis or release of the inhibiting factor(s). Basal prolactin levels fall following delivery, but prolactin secretion is enhanced by stimulation of the breasts, such as the act of nursing (the so-called sucking reflex), a phenomenon that is probably mediated by the reflex release of oxytocin. In the postgestational state, the normal woman is capable of forming about a liter of milk per day containing 38 g fat, 70 g lactose, and 12 g protein. Normal lactation can be suppressed by the administration of estrogens or diethylstilbestrol, which inhibit milk production by direct effects on the breast, or bromocriptine, which inhibits prolactin secretion by the pituitary. Alternatively, if a woman does not nurse or empty her breasts postpartum, lactation usually ceases of its own accord in 1 to 2 weeks.

GALACTORRHEA Exactly what constitutes nonpuerperal or inappropriate lactation is not always clearly defined in the literature. According to the studies of Friedman and Goldfein, no breast secretion whatsoever can be demonstrated in normal, regularly menstruating nulligravid women, but breast secretions can be demonstrated in a fourth of normal women who have been pregnant in the past; thus breast secretions may be of no clinical significance in these instances. Spontaneous leakage of milk from the breasts is usually of more importance than milk that must be expressed. A second problem is related to the composition of the breast secretions. When the secretion is milky or white, it is safe to assume that it contains fat, casein, and lactose and is in fact milk; however, when the secretion is brown or greenish, it rarely contains normal milk constituents and consequently may not result from an underlying endocrinopathy. Milk also must be distinguished from blood or bloody discharges that may be due to neoplasms of the breast. It also should be kept in mind that the composition of milk constituents may increase upon repeated sampling from low, colostrum-like values to those typical of milk (see Chap. 319). With these problems in mind, galactorrhea can be defined as inappropriate production of milk that is persistent or worrisome to the patient, recognizing that in some instances no underlying pathology may be demonstrated.

Since the action of a lactogenic hormone is necessary for the initiation of milk production, it is logical to consider galactorrhea as a consequence of deranged prolactin physiology. However, as indicated above, a complex endocrinologic milieu is necessary for lactation, and in many instances in which prolactin is elevated, both in women who have not been appropriately primed and in men, no production of milk takes place. As a consequence, hyperprolactinemia is more common than galactorrhea. Furthermore, while enhanced prolactin secretion is necessary for the initiation of lactation, continued production can be maintained in the presence of minimally or intermittently elevated prolactin levels so that basal plasma prolactin levels are not always elevated in patients with galactorrhea. For example, repeated stimulation of the nipples of women who have previously been pregnant can cause galactorrhea with minimal elevations of basal prolactin (the wet nurse phenomenon). Perhaps the strongest evidence for a critical role for prolactin in galactorrhea is the fact that administration of bromocriptine, which suppresses plasma prolactin levels, causes a disappearance of galactorrhea even when the basal plasma prolactin levels are normal.

Differential diagnosis Galactorrhea is due either to a failure of the normal hypothalamic inhibition of prolactin release, to enhanced prolactin-releasing factor(s), or to autonomous prolactin secretion by tumors (Table 341-1). Pituitary stalk section results in a striking increase in prolactin secretion, as the result of the interruption of the delivery of prolactin inhibitory factors to the pituitary. Likewise, many drugs that influence the central nervous system (including virtually all psychotropic agents, methyldopa, reserpine, and antiemetics) cause enhanced prolactin release, presumably by inhibiting synthesis or release of dopamine or prolactin inhibitory factors such as dopamine. Estrogens enhance prolactin levels by an uncertain mechanism. Extrapituitary central nervous system diseases presumably cause galactorrhea by interfering with delivery of the inhibitory factors to the pituitary (central nervous system sarcoidosis, craniopharyngioma, pinealoma, encephalitis, meningitis, hydrocephalus, hypothalamic tumors).

In primary hypothyroidism, galactorrhea results from enhanced prolactin-releasing activity. Thyrotropin-releasing hormone (TRH) stimulates prolactin release, and thyroid hormone replacement cures the galactorrhea. A similar mechanism, as the result of enhanced secretion of oxytocin, may cause the galactorrhea of breast trauma.

Enhanced prolactin release also can occur from pituitary or nonpituitary tumors. Three types of pituitary tumors (see Chap. 331) may be associated with galactorrhea: pure prolactin-secreting tumors (micro- or macroadenomas), mixed tumors that secrete both growth hormone and prolactin and result in acromegaly with galactorrhea, and some null cell adenomas. The latter may interfere with the delivery of inhibitory factors to the pituitary. Prolactin also can be secreted by other malignancies such as bronchogenic carcinoma, and hydatidiform moles and choriocarcinomas may secrete placental lactogen.

In four published series totaling more than 500 carefully studied patients, a pituitary tumor was identified in about one-fourth of the patients, other known causes could be identified in another fourth or fifth, and the remaining half fall into the idiopathic category. Many patients prove ultimately to have prolactin-secreting pituitary tumors, some probably have subtle disorders of hypothalamic function, and in others a drug-related cause may have been missed, but the fact remains that no satisfactory diagnosis is reached in many patients. When normal menses and galactorrhea coexist, the likelihood of establishing a diagnosis is poor.

Galactorrhea is unusual in men, even in the presence of profound elevations of plasma prolactin; when it does occur, it is usually upon the background of a feminizing state (see below).

Diagnostic evaluation If hyperprolactinemia is present, the workup is fundamentally that of a pituitary tumor once drug causes and hypothyroidism are excluded (see Chap. 331). Even when a specific cause cannot be identified and the diagnosis of idiopathic galactorrhea is made by exclusion, it is necessary to remember that pituitary tumors may subsequently become manifest. The higher the prolactin values and the more persistent the galactorrhea, the greater is the likelihood of such a development.

Treatment Breast binders can be effective in patients with mild galactorrhea of unknown etiology, presumably by preventing stimulation of the nipple and the consequent perpetuation of lactation. The aim of treatment in other instances is to correct the elevated prolactin, and resection of pituitary tumor, cessation of causative drugs, or correction of hypothyroidism is often followed by the disappearance of galactorrhea. Bromocriptine, which suppresses plasma prolactin, has been used to treat idiopathic hyperprolactinemia, prolactin-secreting tumors of the pituitary (see Chap. 331), and even in women with normoprolactinemic galactorrhea. This drug not only suppresses lactation but also may cause resumption of menstrual cycles (and even fertility) in patients with amenorrhea and galactorrhea.

GYNECOMASTIA A central issue in the evaluation of breast tissue in adult men is the separation of the normal from the abnormal. The incidence of active gynecomastia in autopsy data is between 5 and 9 percent, but Nuttall and colleagues have reported that approximately 40 percent of normal men and up to 70 percent of hospitalized men have palpable breast tissue. The reason for this discrepancy is not clear. On the one hand, it may be difficult to distinguish true breast tissue from masses of adipose tissue without true breast enlargement (lipomastia); in such cases, true gynecomastia can be separated from lipomastia by mammography or by sonography. Alternatively, the incidence of gynecomastia may have increased, or the autopsy data may underestimate the frequency of palpable breast tissue. Regardless, we are left with major uncertainties; the finding of gynecomastia (distinct from lipomastia) could indicate underlying pathology or a normal variant. For the purposes of this discussion, we shall assume that any palpable breast tissue in men (except for the three so-called physiologic states) can be due to an underlying endocrinopathy and deserves a limited evaluation.

Early gynecomastia is characterized by proliferation of both the fibroblastic stroma and the duct system, which elongates, buds, and duplicates. As gynecomastia persists, progressive fibrosis and hyalinization are associated with regression of epithelial proliferation. Eventually, the number of ducts decreases. Resolution occurs by reduction in size and epithelial content with gradual disappearance of the ducts, leaving hyaline bands that eventually disappear.

Growth of the breast in men, as in women, is mediated by estrogen and results from disturbances of the normal ratio of active androgen to estrogen in plasma or within the breast itself. As described in Chap. 339 estradiol formation in the normal man occurs principally by the conversion of circulating androgens to estrogens in extraglandular tissues; the normal ratio of production of testosterone to estradiol in adult men is approximately 100:1 (6 mg versus 45 μg), and the normal ratio of the two hormones in plasma is about 300:1. Growth of the breast ensues in men when this effective ratio decreases significantly as the result of diminished testosterone production or action, enhanced estrogen formation, or both processes occurring simultaneously.

Enlargement of the male breast can be a normal physiologic phenomenon at certain stages of life or the result of several pathologic states (Table 341-2).

Physiologic gynecomastia In the *newborn*, transient enlargement of the breast is due to the action of maternal and/or placental estrogens. The enlargement usually disappears in a few weeks but may persist longer. *Adolescent* gynecomastia is common at some time during puberty. The median age of onset is 14; it is often asymmetric, occasionally unilateral for a portion of its course, and frequently tender, and it regresses so that by age 20 only a small number of men have palpable vestiges of gynecomastia in one or both breasts. Although the origin of the excess estrogen has not been identified, the onset of gynecomastia correlates with transient elevations of plasma estradiol prior to the completion of puberty so that the

---

TABLE 341-1   Classification of galactorrhea

Failure of normal hypothalamic inhibition of prolactin release
- A Pituitary stalk section
- B Drugs (phenothiazines, butyrophenones, methyldopa, tricyclic antidepressants, opiates, reserpine, verapamil)
- C Central nervous system disease, including extrapituitary tumors and null cell adenomas of the pituitary

Enhanced prolactin-releasing factor
- Hypothyroidism
- Sucking reflex and breast trauma

Autonomous prolactin release
- A Pituitary tumors
    - *1* Prolactin-secreting tumors
    - *2* Mixed growth hormone and prolactin-secreting tumors
    - *3* Chromophobe adenomas
- B Ectopic production of human placental lactogen and/or prolactin
    - *1* Hydatidiform moles and choriocarcinomas
    - *2* Bronchogenic carcinoma and hypernephroma

Idiopathic

TABLE 341-2   Differential diagnosis of gynecomastia

PHYSIOLOGIC GYNECOMASTIA

Newborn
Adolescence
Aging

PATHOLOGIC GYNECOMASTIA

Deficient production or action of testosterone:
　Congenital defects:
　　Congenital anorchia
　　Klinefelter syndrome
　　Androgen resistance (testicular feminization and Reifenstein syndrome)
　　Defects of testosterone synthesis
　Secondary testicular failure:
　　Viral orchitis
　　Trauma
　　Castration
　　Neurologic and granulomatous diseases
　　Renal failure
Increased estrogen production:
　Estrogen secretion:
　　Testicular tumors
　　True hermaphroditism
　　Carcinoma of the lung and other tumors producing hCG
　Increased substrate for extraglandular aromatase:
　　Adrenal disease
　　Liver disease
　　Malnutrition
　　Hyperthyroidism
　　Increase in extraglandular aromatase
Drugs:
　Estrogens (diethylstilbestrol, birth control pills, digitalis, estrogen-containing cosmetics, estrogen-contaminated foods, phytoestrogens)
　Drugs that enhance endogenous estrogen secretion (gonadotropins, clomiphene)
　Inhibitors of testosterone synthesis and/or action (ketoconazole, metronidazole, alkylating agents, cisplatin, spironolactone, cimetidine, flutamide, etomidate)
　Unknown mechanisms (busulfan, isoniazid, methyldopa, tricyclic antidepressants, penicillamine, diazepam, omeprazole, calcium-channel blockers, angiotensin-converting enzyme inhibitors, marijuana, heroin)
Idiopathic

androgen/estrogen ratio is low. *Gynecomastia of aging* also occurs in otherwise healthy men. Forty percent or more of aged men have gynecomastia. A likely explanation is the increase with age in the conversion of androgens to estrogens in extraglandular tissues. Abnormal liver function or drug therapy may be contributing causes in such men.

Pathologic gynecomastia Pathologic gynecomastia can result from one of three basic mechanisms: deficiency in testosterone production or action (with or without a secondary increase in estrogen production), increase in estrogen production, or drugs (Table 341-2). Most of the individual disorders that cause primary and secondary testicular failure have been discussed in Chap. 339. The fact that a deficiency in testosterone production by itself can cause gynecomastia is illustrated by the syndrome of congenital anorchia in which normal (or slightly low) estradiol production in the presence of profoundly decreased testosterone production results in florid gynecomastia. This mechanism is also responsible in some patients with Klinefelter syndrome and in men with testicular failure from other causes. In the inherited syndromes of androgen resistance, such as testicular feminization, deficient androgen action and increased testicular estrogen production are both present.

A primary increase in estrogen production can result from a variety of causes. Increased testicular estrogen secretion may result from elevations in plasma gonadotropins, for example, in cases of aberrant production of chorionic gonadotropin by testicular tumors or by bronchogenic carcinoma, from the ovarian elements in the gonads of men with true hermaphroditism, or as the result of direct secretion by testicular tumors (particularly Leydig cell and Sertoli cell tumors). Increased conversion of androgen to estrogens in extraglandular tissues can be due either to increased availability of substrate for extraglandular estrogen formation or to increased amount of the enzymes of estrogen formation in peripheral tissues. Increased substrate availability for extraglandular conversion can result from increased production of androgens such as androstenedione (congenital adrenal hyperplasia, hyperthyroidism, and most feminizing adrenal tumors) or because of diminished catabolism of androstenedione by the usual pathways (liver disease). Increased amount of extraglandular aromatase can be caused by a rare hereditary abnormality or by tumors of the liver or adrenal gland.

Drugs can cause gynecomastia by several mechanisms. Many drugs either act directly as estrogens or cause an increase in plasma estrogen activity, for example, in men receiving diethylstilbestrol for prostatic carcinoma and in transsexuals in preparation for sex-change operations. Boys and young men are particularly sensitive to estrogen and can develop gynecomastia after the use of dermal ointments containing estrogen or after the ingestion of milk or meat from estrogen-treated animals. The gynecomastia of digitalis ingestion is usually attributed to an estrogen-like side effect of the drug, but in the experience of the author it usually occurs in men with abnormal liver function. A second mechanism of drug-induced gynecomastia is illustrated by gonadotropin, such as human chorionic gonadotropin, which causes enhanced testicular secretion of estrogen. Other drugs cause gynecomastia by interfering with testosterone synthesis (ketoconazole and alkylating agents) and/or testosterone action, for instance, by blocking the binding of androgen to its cytosol receptor protein in target tissues (spironolactone and cimetidine). Finally, drugs that cause gynecomastia by mechanisms which have not been defined include busulfan, ethionamide, isoniazid, methyldopa, tricyclic antidepressants, penicillamine, omeprazole, angiotensin-converting enzyme inhibitors, diazepam, marijuana, and heroin. In some instances, the feminization is due to effects of drugs on liver function.

Diagnostic evaluation The evaluation of patients with gynecomastia should include (1) a careful drug history, (2) measurement and examination of the testes (if both are small, a chromosomal karyotype should be obtained; if they are asymmetric, a workup for testicular tumor should be instituted), (3) evaluation of liver function, and (4) endocrine evaluation to include measurement of serum androstenedione or 24-h urinary 17-ketosteroids (usually elevated in feminizing adrenal states), measurement of plasma estradiol and hCG (helpful if elevated but usually normal), and measurement of plasma luteinizing hormone (LH) and testosterone. If LH is high and testosterone is low, the diagnosis is usually testicular failure; if LH and testosterone are both low, the diagnosis is most likely increased primary estrogen production (e.g., a Sertoli cell tumor of the testis); and if both LH and testosterone are elevated, the diagnosis is either an androgen-resistance state or a gonadotropin-secreting tumor.

A satisfactory diagnosis can be made in only half or less of patients referred for gynecomastia. This implies either that the diagnostic techniques are not sufficiently refined to recognize mild disturbances, that many causes of gynecomastia are as yet undefined, that the causes may be transient and difficult to diagnose, or, as suggested by Nuttall, that gynecomastia may in some instances be normal rather than due to a pathologic state. Because of the problem of separating the normal from the pathologic, gynecomastia should probably be routinely worked up only if the drug history is negative, if the breast is tender (indicating rapid growth), or if the breast mass is larger than 4 cm in diameter. In other instances, a decision to perform an endocrine evaluation depends on the clinical context. For example, gynecomastia associated with signs of underandrogenization should be evaluated.

Treatment When the primary cause can be identified and corrected, the breast enlargement usually subsides promptly and eventually disappears. For example, androgen replacement therapy may produce dramatic improvement in men with testicular insufficiency. However, if the gynecomastia is of long duration (and fibrosis has replaced the original ductal hyperplasia), correction of the primary defect may not be followed by resolution. In such instances and when the primary cause cannot be corrected, surgery is the only effective therapy. Indications for surgery include several psychologic and/or cosmetic problems, continued growth, or a suspected malignancy. Although the relative risk of carcinoma of the breast is increased in men with gynecomastia, it is rare nevertheless. Prophylactic radiation of the breasts prior to the institution of diethylstilbestrol therapy is effective in preventing gynecomastia and has a low complication rate in elderly men. In rare patients who have painful gynecomastia and who are not candidates for other therapy, treatment with antiestrogens such as tamoxifen may be indicated.

REFERENCES

Galactorrhea

CAVANAUGH J et al: Gynecomastia and cirrhosis of the liver. Arch Intern Med 150:563, 1990

CHOTINER HC et al: Lactose and casein content of nonpuerperal breast secretion. J Reprod Med 22:267, 1979

FRANTZ AG, WILSON JD: Endocrine disorders of the breast, in *Williams' Textbook of Endocrinology*, 8th ed, JD Wilson, DW Foster (eds). Philadelphia, Saunders, 1992, p 593

FRIEDMAN S, GOLDFEIN A: Breast secretions in normal women. Am J Obstet Gynecol 104:846, 1969

JOHNSON DG et al: Prolactin secretion and biological activity in females with galactorrhoea and normal circulating prolactin concentrations at rest. Clin Endocrinol 22:661, 1985

KLEINBERG DL et al: Galactorrhea: A study of 235 cases, including 48 with pituitary tumors. N Engl J Med 296:589, 1977

KOPPELMAN MCS et al: Hyperprolactinemia, amenorrhea, and galactorrhea. A retrospective assessment of twenty-five cases. Ann Intern Med 100:115, 1984

KULSKI JK et al: Changes in the milk composition of nonpuerperal women. Am J Obstet Gynecol 139:597, 1981

PADILLA SL et al: The efficacy of bromocriptine in patients with ovulatory dysfunction and normoprolactinemic galactorrhea. Fertil Steril 44:695, 1985

RUIZ-VELASCO V: Hyperprolactinemia and mammary prostheses. A report of eight cases. J Reprod Med 31:267, 1986

SAUER HJ: Physiology of lactation and factors affecting lactation. Obstet Gynecol Clin North Am 14:615, 1987

TURKSOY RN et al: Diagnostic and therapeutic modalities in women with galactorrhea. Obstet Gynecol 56:323, 1980

YAMAGUCHI M et al: Effects of nocturnal hyperprolactinemia on ovarian luteal function and galactorrhea. Eur J Obstet Gynecol 34:187, 1991

Gynecomastia

ANDERSON JA, GROOM JB: Male breast at autopsy. Acta Pathol Microbiol Immunol Scand 90:191, 1982

CIMORA GA et al: Percutaneous oestrogen-induced gynecomastia: A case report. Br J Plast Surg 35:209, 1982

DE GASPARO M et al: Antialdosterones: Incidence and prevention of sexual side effects. J Steroid Biochem 32:223, 1989

FASS D et al: Radiotherapeutic prophylaxis of estrogen-induced gynecomastia: A study of late sequela. Int J Radiation Oncology Bio Phys 12:407, 1986

FELDMAN D: Ketoconazole and other imidazole derivatives as inhibitors of steroidogenesis. Endocr Rev 7:409, 1986

FRANTZ AG, WILSON JD: Endocrine disorders of the breast, in *Williams' Textbook of Endocrinology*, 8th ed, JD Wilson, DW Foster (eds). Philadelphia, Saunders, 1992, p 953

KORENMAN SG: The endocrinology of the abnormal male breast. Ann NY Acad Sci 464:400, 1986

MABUCHI K et al: Risk factors for male breast cancer. J Natl Cancer Inst 74:371, 1985

MAHONEY CP: Adolescent gynecomastia: Differential diagnosis and management. Pediatr Clin North Am 37:1389, 1990

MCDERMOTT MT et al: Tamoxifen therapy for painful idiopathic gynecomastia. South Med J 83:1283, 1990

NIEWOEHNER CV, NUTTALL FQ: Gynecomastia in a hospitalized male population. Am J Med 77:633, 1984

NUTTALL FQ: Gynecomastia as a physical finding in normal men. J Clin Endocrinol Metab 48:338, 1979

ROSE DP: Endocrine epidemiology of male breast cancer (review). Anticancer Res 8:845, 1988

342 DISORDERS OF SEXUAL DIFFERENTIATION

JEAN D. WILSON / JAMES E. GRIFFIN

Sexual differentiation is a sequential and ordered process. *Chromosomal sex*, established at the moment of fertilization, determines *gonadal sex*, and *gonadal sex*, in turn, causes the development of *phenotypic sex*, in which the male or female urogenital tract is formed (Table 342-1). A disturbance of any step in this process during embryogenesis may result in a disorder of sexual differentiation. Known causes of such disorders include environmental insults as in the ingestion of a virilizing drug during pregnancy, nonfamilial aberrations of the sex chromosomes as in 45,X gonadal dysgenesis, developmental birth defects of multifactorial etiology as in most cases of hypospadias, and hereditary disorders resulting from single gene mutations as in the testicular feminization syndrome.

Limitations of knowledge make it necessary to make empirical assignments as to the nature of the derangement in certain disorders. Nevertheless, a specific diagnosis usually can be made as the result of genetic, endocrine, phenotypic, and chromosomal assessment. As a consequence, appropriate gender assignment can be made, even in extreme instances of ambiguous genitalia, and tailoring of the phenotype can be undertaken when appropriate.

NORMAL SEXUAL DIFFERENTIATION

The first process in sexual differentiation is the establishment of chromosomal sex, the heterogametic sex (XY) being male and the homogametic sex (XX) female. The embryos of both sexes then develop in an identical fashion until approximately 40 days of gestation. The second phase of sexual differentiation is the conversion of the indifferent gonad into a testis or an ovary. The differentiation of the indifferent gonad into a testis is mediated by one or more sex-determining genes on the short arm of the Y chromosome (SRY); indeed, no matter how many X chromosomes are present (as in 47,XXY, 48,XXXY, etc.), a testis will develop as long as a Y chromosome is present. The final process, the translation of gonadal sex into phenotypic sex, is the consequence of the type of gonad formed and the endocrine secretions of the fetal gonads. The development of phenotypic sex results in the formation of the male and female urogenital tracts.

The internal urogenital tract is derived from the wolffian and müllerian ducts that exist side by side in early embryos of both sexes

---

TABLE 342-1 Classification of disorders of sexual development

Disorders of chromosomal sex
  Klinefelter syndrome
  XX male
  Gonadal dysgenesis
  Mixed gonadal dysgenesis
  True hermaphroditism
Disorders of gonadal sex
  Pure gonadal dysgenesis
  Absent testis syndrome
Disorders of phenotypic sex
  Female pseudohermaphroditism
    Congenital adrenal hyperplasia
    Nonadrenal female pseudohermaphroditism
    Developmental disorders of müllerian ducts
  Male pseudohermaphroditism
    Abnormalities in androgen synthesis
    Abnormalities in androgen action
    Persistent müllerian duct syndrome
    Development defects of male genitalia

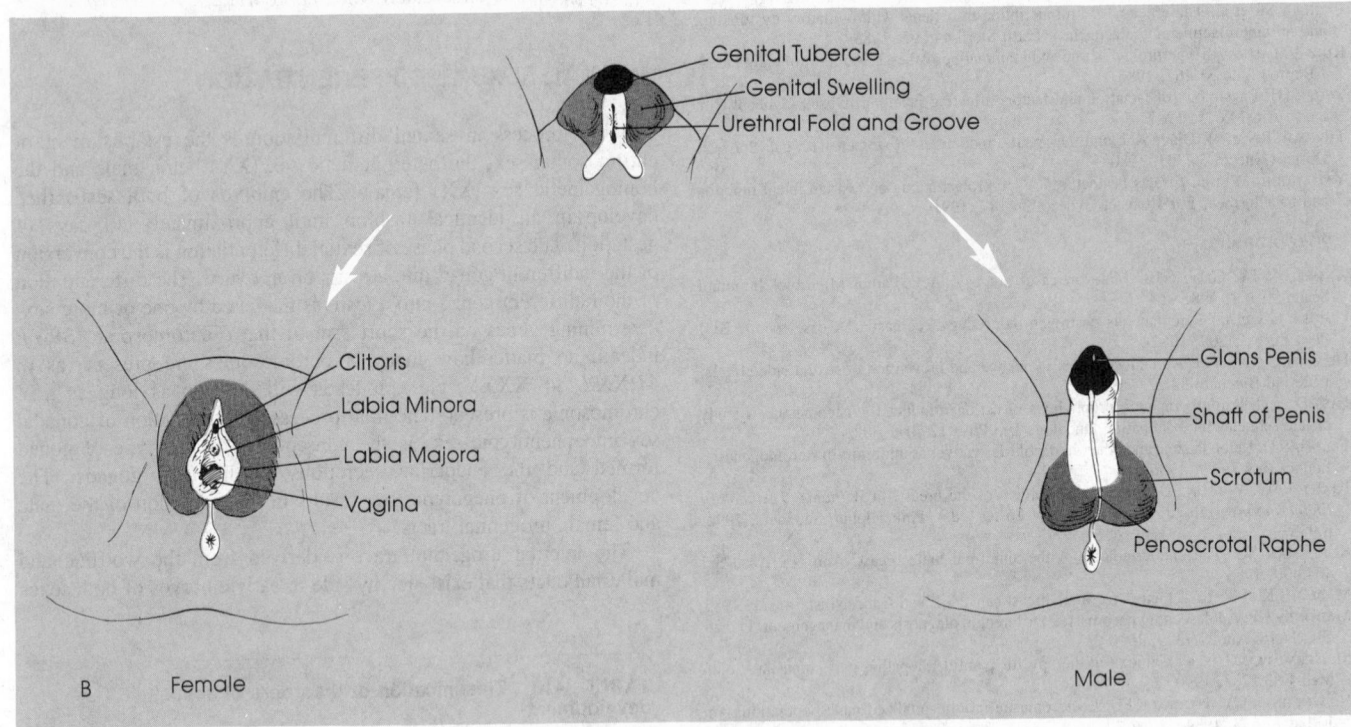

FIGURE 342-1   Normal sexual differentiation. *A*. Internal urogenital tract. *B*. External genitalia.

(Fig. 342-1*A*). In the male the wolffian ducts give rise to the epididymides, vasa deferentia, and seminal vesicles, and the müllerian ducts disappear. In the female the fallopian tubes, uterus, and upper vagina are derived from the müllerian ducts, and the wolffian ducts regress. The external genitalia and urethra in the two sexes develop from common anlage—the urogenital sinus and the genital tubercle, folds, and swellings (Fig. 342-1*B*). The urogenital sinus gives rise to the prostate and prostatic urethra in the male and to the urethra and lower portion of the vagina in the female. The genital tubercle is the origin of the glans penis in the male and the clitoris in the female. The urogenital swellings become the scrotum or the labia majora, and the urethral folds develop into the labia minora or fuse to form the shaft of the penis and the male urethra.

In the absence of the testis, as in the normal female or in the male embryo castrated prior to the onset of gonadal differentiation, phenotypic sex develops along female lines. Thus masculinization of the fetus is the positive result of action of hormones from the fetal testis, whereas female development does not require the presence of the ovary. Phenotypic sex normally conforms to chromosomal sex. That is, chromosomal sex determines gonadal sex, and gonadal sex, in turn, controls phenotypic sex.

The formation of the male phenotype is vested in the action of three hormones. Two—müllerian-inhibiting substance and testosterone—are secretory products of the fetal testis. Müllerian-inhibiting substance (MIS, also termed *antimüllerian hormone*, AMH) is a protein hormone that acts to suppress the müllerian ducts and prevent

TABLE 342-2 Clinical features of the disorders of chromosomal sex

Disorder	Common chromosomal complement	Gonadal development	External genitalia	Internal genitalia	Breast development	Comment
Klinefelter syndrome	47,XXY *or* 46,XY/47,XXY	Hyalinized testes	Normal male	Normal male	Gynecomastia	Most common disorder of sexual differentiation; tall stature.
XX male	46,XX	Hyalinized testes	Normal male	Normal male	Gynecomastia	Shorter than normal men; increased incidence of hypospadias. Similar to Klinefelter syndrome. May be familial.
Gonadal dysgenesis (Turner syndrome)	45,X *or* 46,XX/45,X	Streak gonads	Immature female	Hypoplastic female	Immature female	Short stature and multiple somatic abnormalities. May be 46,XX with structurally abnormal X chromosome.
Mixed gonadal dysgenesis	46,XY/45,X *or* 46,XY	Testis and streak gonad	Variable but almost always ambiguous; 60% reared as female	Uterus, vagina, and one fallopian tube	Usually male	Second most common cause of ambiguous genitalia in the newborn; tumors common.
True hermaphroditism	46,XX *or* 46,XY *or* mosaics	Testis and ovary or ovotestis	Variable but usually ambiguous; 60% reared as males	Usually a uterus and urogenital sinus; ducts correspond to gonad	Gynecomastia in 75%	May be familial.

development of the uterus and fallopian tubes in the male. Testosterone acts directly to stimulate virilization of the wolffian duct and is the precursor for the third embryonic male hormone, dihydrotestosterone (see Chap. 339). Dihydrotestosterone, which is formed from circulating testosterone, promotes development of the male urethra and prostate and formation of the penis and scrotum. Thus testosterone and dihydrotestosterone function during fetal life to induce formation of the male urogenital tract by the same intracellular machinery by which they act in postembryonic life (Chap. 339).

The secretion of testosterone by the fetal testis approaches a maximum by the eighth to tenth week of gestation, and formation of the sexual phenotypes is largely completed by the end of the first trimester. During the latter phases of gestation, the ovarian follicles develop and the vagina matures in the female and descent of the testes and growth of the external genitalia take place in the male.

DISORDERS OF CHROMOSOMAL SEX

Disorders of chromosomal sex (Table 342-2) occur when the number or structure of the X or Y chromosomes is abnormal (see Chap. 62).

KLINEFELTER SYNDROME Clinical features Klinefelter syndrome is characterized by small, firm testes, azoospermia, gynecomastia, and elevated levels of plasma gonadotropins in men with two or more X chromosomes. The common karyotype is either a 47,XXY chromosomal pattern (the classic form) or 46,XY/47,XXY mosaicism. The disorder is the most frequent major abnormality of sexual differentiation, the incidence being around 1 in 500 men.

Prepubertally, the testes are small but otherwise appear normal. After puberty, the disorder is manifest as infertility, gynecomastia, or occasionally underandrogenization (Table 342-3). Hyalinization of the seminiferous tubules and azoospermia are consistent features of the 47,XXY variety. The small, firm testes are characteristically less than 2 cm and always less than 3.5 cm in length (corresponding to 2- and 12-mL volume, respectively). The increased mean body height is the result of an increased lower body segment. Gynecomastia ordinarily develops during adolescence, is generally bilateral and painless, and may become disfiguring (see Chap. 341). Obesity and varicose veins occur in one-third to one-half, and mild mental deficiency, social maladjustment, abnormalities of thyroid function, diabetes mellitus, and pulmonary disease may be present. The risk of breast cancer is 20 times that of normal men (but only about a

fifth that in women). Most have a male psychosexual orientation and function sexually as normal men.

The mosaic variant comprises about 10 percent of the patients, as estimated by chromosomal karyotypes on peripheral blood leukocytes. The frequency of this variant may be underestimated, since chromosomal mosaicism may be present in the testes in subjects whose peripheral leukocyte karyotype is normal. The mosaic form is usually not as severe as the 47,XXY variety, and the testes may be normal in size (see Table 342-3). The endocrine abnormalities are less severe, and gynecomastia and azoospermia are less common. Indeed, occasional mosaic subjects may be fertile. In some the diagnosis may not even be suspected because of the minor manifestations.

Approximately 30 additional variants of Klinefelter syndrome have been described, including those with uniform cell lines (such as 48,XXYY, 48,XXXY, and 49,XXXXY) and a variety of mosaicisms of the X chromosome with or without associated structural abnormalities of the X. In general, the greater the degree of chromosomal abnormality (and in mosaic forms the more cell lines that are abnormal), the more severe are the manifestations.

Pathophysiology The classic form is due to meiotic nondisjunction of the chromosomes during gametogenesis (Fig. 342-2). About 40 percent of the responsible meiotic nondisjunctions occur during spermatogenesis, and 60 percent occur during oogenesis. Advanced maternal age is a predisposing factor. The mosaic form is thought to

TABLE 342-3 Characteristics of patients with classic versus mosaic Klinefelter syndrome*

	47,XXY, %	46,XY/47,XXY, %
Abnormal testicular histology	100	94[†]
Decreased length of testis	99	73[†]
Azoospermia	93	50[†]
Decreased testosterone	79	33
Decreased facial hair	77	64
Increased gonadotropins	75	33[†]
Decreased sexual function	68	56
Gynecomastia	55	33[†]
Decreased axillary hair	49	46
Decreased length of penis	41	21

* Table based on 519 XXY patients and 51 XY/XXY patients.
[†] Significantly different at $p < .05$ or better.
SOURCE: After Gordon et al.

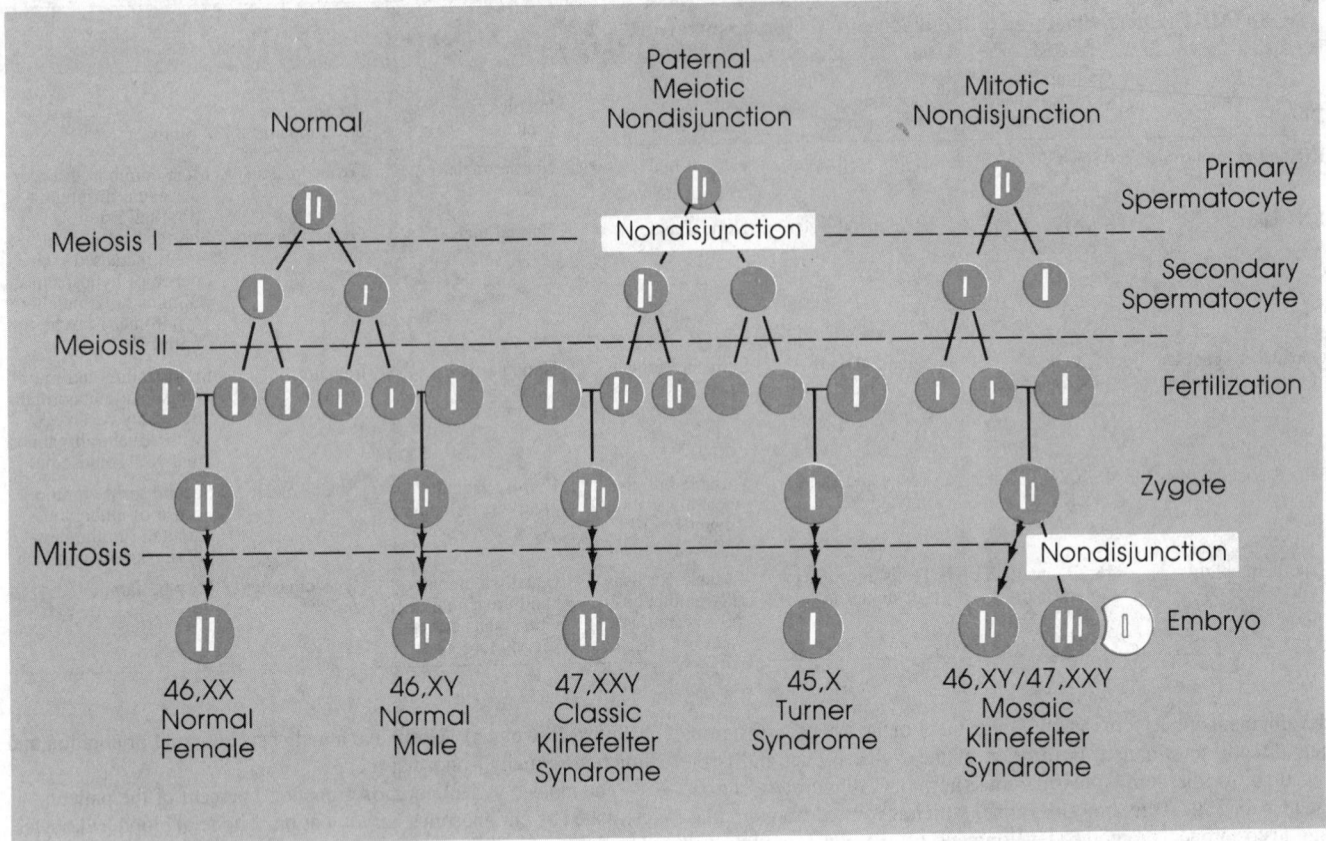

FIGURE 342-2 Schema for normal spermatogenesis and fertilization showing effects of meiotic and mitotic nondisjunction leading to classic Klinefelter syndrome, Turner syndrome, and mosaic Klinefelter. The schema would be similar if the abnormal events took place during oogenesis.

result from chromosomal mitotic nondisjunction after fertilization of the zygote and can take place either in a 46,XY zygote (see Fig. 342-2) or a 47,XXY zygote. The latter defect, or double nondisjunction (meiotic and mitotic), may be the usual cause and thus explain why the mosaic form is less frequent than the classic disorder.

Plasma follicle-stimulating hormone (FSH) and luteinizing hormone (LH) levels are usually high; FSH shows the best discrimination, and little overlap occurs with normal individuals, a consequence of the consistent damage to the seminiferous tubules. The plasma testosterone level averages half normal, but the range of values overlaps the normal range. Mean plasma estradiol levels are elevated, the cause of which is not entirely clear. Early, the testes may secrete increased amounts of estradiol in response to the elevated plasma LH level, but the testicular secretion of estradiol (and testosterone) eventually declines. Elevated plasma estradiol late in the course is probably due to a combination of a decreased metabolic clearance rate and an increased rate of conversion of testosterone to estradiol in extragonadal tissues. The net result both early and late is a variable degree of insufficient androgenization and enhanced feminization. The feminization, including gynecomastia, depends on the ratio of circulating estrogen to androgen (relative or absolute), and subjects with lower plasma testosterone and higher plasma estradiol levels are more likely to develop gynecomastia (see Chap. 341). The normal feedback inhibition of testosterone on pituitary LH secretion is diminished. Subjects with untreated Klinefelter syndrome may have enlarged or abnormal sella turcicas, presumably secondary to the persistent inadequate testosterone feedback and hyperplasia of the gonadotrophs. It is not known whether true adenoma formation occurs.

Management No method is available for reversing the infertility, and surgical removal is the treatment for the gynecomastia. Some underandrogenized patients benefit from supplemental androgen, but such treatment may worsen the gynecomastia, presumably by providing increased androgen substrate for the conversion to estrogens in the peripheral tissues. Androgen should be administered in the form of testosterone cypionate or testosterone enanthate (see Chap. 339). Following the administration of testosterone, the plasma LH level returns to normal only after several months, if at all.

XX MALE SYNDROME The incidence of a 46,XX karyotype in phenotypic males is approximately 1 in 20,000 to 24,000 male births. Affected individuals have absence of all female internal genitalia and male psychosexual identification. Indeed, the findings resemble those in Klinefelter syndrome: the testes are small and firm (generally less than 2 cm), gynecomastia is frequent, the penis is normal to small in size, azoospermia and hyalinization of the seminiferous tubules are usual, mean plasma testosterone level is low, plasma estradiol level is elevated, and plasma gonadotropin levels are high. Affected individuals differ from typical Klinefelter patients only in that average height is less than in normal men, the incidence of mental deficiency is not increased, and the incidence of hypospadias is increased.

The majority of XX males whose DNA is probed with Y-chromosome DNA fragments containing the SRY gene are positive for Y-related DNA; thus an X-Y interchange appears to be the common cause of the disorder. Other 46,XX males are negative for all Y-specific DNA, suggesting that these cases are the consequence of mutation in a downstream, autosomal or X-linked gene involved in development of the testes. The management is similar to that of Klinefelter syndrome.

GONADAL DYSGENESIS (TURNER SYNDROME) **Clinical features** Gonadal dysgenesis is characterized by primary amenorrhea, sexual infantilism, short stature, multiple congenital anomalies, and bilateral streak gonads in phenotypic women with any of several defects of the X chromosome. This condition should be distinguished from (1) mixed gonadal dysgenesis in which a unilateral testis and a contralateral streak gonad may be present, (2) pure gonadal dysgenesis in which bilateral streak gonads are associated with a normal 46,XX or 46,XY karyotype, normal stature, and primary amenorrhea, and (3) the Noonan syndrome, an autosomal dominant disorder of males and females characterized by webbed neck, short stature, congenital heart disease, cubitus valgus, and other congenital defects despite normal karyotypes and normal gonads.

The incidence is estimated at 1 in 2500 newborn females. The diagnosis is made either at birth because of the associated anomalies or more frequently at puberty when amenorrhea and failure of sexual development are noted in conjunction with the associated anomalies. Gonadal dysgenesis is the most common cause of primary amenorrhea, accounting for a third of such patients. The external genitalia are unambiguously female but remain immature, and there is no breast development unless the patient is treated with exogenous estrogen. The internal genitalia consist of infantile fallopian tubes and uterus and bilateral streak gonads located in the broad ligaments. Primordial germ cells are present transiently during embryogenesis but disappear as the result of an accelerated rate of atresia (see Chap. 340). After the age of expected puberty, these streaks lack identifiable follicles and ova but contain fibrous tissue that is indistinguishable from normal ovarian stroma.

The associated somatic anomalies primarily involve the skeleton and connective tissue. Lymphedema of the hands and feet, webbing of the neck, low hairline, redundant skin folds on the back of the neck, a shieldlike chest with widely spaced nipples, and a low birth weight are features that suggest the diagnosis in infancy. In addition, the facies may be characterized by micrognathia, epicanthal folds, prominent low-set or deformed ears, a fishlike mouth, and ptosis. Short fourth metacarpals are present in half, and 10 to 20 percent have coarctation of the aorta. In adults, the average height rarely exceeds 150 cm. Associated conditions include renal malformations, pigmented nevi, hypoplastic nails, tendency to keloid formation, perceptive hearing loss, unexplained hypertension, and autoimmune disorders. Hypothyroidism is present in 20 percent.

Pathophysiology About half have a 45,X karyotype, approximately one-fourth have mosaicism with no structural abnormality (46,XX/45,X), and the remainder have a structurally abnormal X chromosome with or without mosaicism (see Chap. 62). The 45,X variety may result from chromosome loss during gametogenesis in either parent or a mitotic error during one of the early cleavage divisions of the fertilized zygote (see Fig. 342-2). Short stature and other somatic features result from loss of genetic material on the short arm of the X chromosome. Streak gonads result when genetic material is missing from either the long or short arm of the X. In individuals with mosaicism or structural abnormalities of the X, phenotypes on average are intermediate in severity between that seen in the 45,X variety and the normal. In some patients with hypertrophy of the clitoris, there is an unidentified fragment of a chromosome present in addition to the X chromosome, assumed to be an abnormal Y; malignancy may develop in the streak gonads in this subset of patients. Rarely, familial transmission of gonadal dysgenesis can be the result of a balanced X-autosome translocation (see Chap. 62). Analysis of chromosomal karyotype is necessary to establish the diagnosis and to identify the fraction with Y chromosomal elements and a high chance of developing malignancy in the streak gonads.

Sparse pubic and axillary hair develop at the time of expected puberty, the breasts remain infantile, and no menses occur. Serum FSH is elevated in infancy, falls during midchildhood to the normal range, and increases to castrate levels at the age of 9 or 10. At this time, the serum LH level is also elevated, and plasma estradiol levels are low [<40 pmol/L (<10 pg/mL)]. Approximately 2 percent of 45,X subjects and 12 percent of mosaic subjects have sufficient residual follicles to allow some menstruation. Indeed, occasional pregnancy has been reported in minimally affected individuals; the reproductive life in such individuals is brief.

Management At the anticipated time of puberty, replacement therapy with estrogen should be instituted to induce maturation of the breasts, labia, vagina, uterus, and fallopian tubes (see Chap. 340). Linear growth and bone maturation rates are approximately doubled

during the first year of treatment with estradiol, but the eventual height of patients rarely approaches the predicted height. Combination therapy with oxandrolone and/or growth hormone accelerates growth, but it is not established whether such therapy has an effect on final height (see Chap. 332).

Gonadal tumors are rare in 45,X patients but have occurred in several patients with mosaicism involving the Y chromosome; consequently, streak gonads should be removed in any patient with evidence of virilization or a Y-containing cell line.

MIXED GONADAL DYSGENESIS **Clinical features** Mixed gonadal dysgenesis is an entity in which phenotypic males or females usually have ambiguous genitalia and a testis on one side and a streak gonad on the other. Most have 45,X/46,XY mosaicism, but the clinical entity is not confined to that chromosomal pattern. The incidence is unknown, but in most hospitals the disorder is the second most common cause of ambiguous genitalia in the neonate after congenital adrenal hyperplasia.

About two-thirds of such children are reared as females. Many have ambiguous genitalia, including some degree of phallic enlargement, a urogenital sinus, and varying degrees of labioscrotal fusion. In most the testis is located intraabdominally; individuals with a testis in the inguinal or scrotal position are usually reared as males. A uterus, vagina, and at least one fallopian tube are almost invariably present.

The prepubertal testis appears relatively normal. The postpubertal testis contains abundant mature Leydig cells, but the seminiferous tubules lack germinal elements and contain only Sertoli cells. The streak gonad, a thin, pale, elongated structure located either in the broad ligament or along the pelvic wall, is composed of ovarian stroma. At puberty the testis secretes androgen, and virilization and phallic enlargement both occur. Feminization is rare; when it occurs, estrogen secretion from a gonadal tumor should be suspected.

Approximately a third of such patients exhibit the somatic features of 45,X gonadal dysgenesis, i.e., low posterior hairline, shield chest, multiple pigmented nevi, cubitus valgus, webbing of the neck, and short stature (height less than 150 cm).

Approximately two-thirds have the 45,X/46,XY karyotype, and the remainder have a 46,XY karyotype or a variant mosaicism. The 45,X/46,XY karyotype is not necessarily associated with abnormal sexual development, and it may be discovered incidentally in phenotypically normal men and women. In addition, females with bilateral streak gonads and males with bilateral dysgenetic testes may have this karyotype. The origin of 45,X/46,XY mosaicism is best explained by the loss of a Y chromosome during an early mitotic division of an XY zygote similar to the postulated loss of the X chromosome in the 46,XY/47,XXY mosaicism shown in Fig. 342-2.

Pathophysiology It has been assumed that the 46,XY cell line stimulates testicular differentiation, whereas the 45,X stem leads to the development of the contralateral streak gonad, but actual comparisons between karyotype and phenotypic expression have failed to substantiate such a relationship. Furthermore, there is no clear correlation between the percentage of cells cultured from blood or skin containing 45,X or 46,XY and the degree of gonadal development or of somatic anomalies.

Both masculinization and müllerian duct regression in utero are incomplete. Since Leydig cell function is normal at puberty, inadequate virilization in utero may be the result of delayed development of a testis that is ultimately capable of normal Leydig cell function. Alternatively, the fetal testis may simply be incapable of synthesizing adequate amounts of müllerian-inhibiting substance and androgen.

Management For the older child or adult in whom gender is fixed prior to diagnosis, the central issue in management is the possibility of tumor development in the gonads. The overall incidence of gonadal tumors is about 25 percent. Seminomas occur more frequently than gonadoblastomas, and the tumors may occur prior to puberty. The tumors occur most frequently in patients with a female phenotype who lack the somatic features typical of 45,X gonadal dysgenesis and are more common in intraabdominal testes than in the streak gonad. When the diagnosis is established in phenotypic females, early exploratory laparotomy and prophylactic gonadectomy should be undertaken both because gonadal tumors may occur in childhood and because the testis secretes androgen at puberty and thus causes virilization. Such subjects, like those with gonadal dysgenesis, are then given estrogen to induce and maintain feminization.

When the diagnosis is established in phenotypic males during late childhood or in adults, the management is more complicated. Phenotypic males with mixed gonadal dysgenesis are infertile (no germinal elements are present in the testes) and have a high risk of developing gonadal tumors. Which testes can be safely conserved? In general, the following observations apply: (1) tumors develop in scrotal streak gonads but not in scrotal testes, (2) tumors that develop in intraabdominal testes are always associated with ipsilateral müllerian duct structures, and (3) tumors in streak gonads are always associated with tumors in the contralateral abdominal testis. Based on these observations, it is recommended that (1) all streak gonads should be removed, (2) scrotal testes should be preserved, and (3) intraabdominal testes should be excised unless they can be relocated in the scrotum and are not associated with ipsilateral müllerian duct structures. Decisions as to reconstructive surgery of the phallus depend on the nature of the defect.

When the diagnosis is established in early infancy and the genitalia are ambiguous, gender assignment is usually female. Resection of the enlarged phallus and gonadectomy can then be accomplished in infancy, sometimes in one procedure. If the decision is for male gender assignment, the same criteria apply as to which testes should be removed in infants as in older males.

TRUE HERMAPHRODITISM   Clinical features   True hermaphroditism is a condition in which both an ovary and a testis or a gonad with histologic features of both (ovotestis) is present. To justify the diagnosis, there must be histologic documentation of both types of gonadal epithelium, the presence of ovarian stroma without oocytes not being sufficient. The incidence is unknown, but more than 400 cases have been reported. Three categories are recognized: (1) one-fifth are bilateral—testicular and ovarian tissue (ovotestes) on each side, (2) two-fifths are unilateral—an ovotestis on one side and an ovary or a testis on the other, and (3) the remainder are lateral—a testis on one side and an ovary on the other.

The external genitalia display all gradations of the male-to-female spectrum. Two-thirds are sufficiently masculinized to be reared as males. However, less than one-tenth have normal male external genitalia; most have hypospadias, and more than half have incomplete labioscrotal fusion. Two-thirds of phenotypic females have an enlarged clitoris, and most have a urogenital sinus. Differentiation of the internal ducts usually corresponds to the adjacent gonad. Although an epididymis usually develops adjacent to a testis, development of the vas deferens is complete in only one-third. Of the patients with an ovotestis, three-fourths have an epididymis, two-thirds have a fallopian tube, one-tenth have a vas deferens, and one-tenth have both a vas deferens and a fallopian tube. A uterus is usually present, although it may be hypoplastic or unicornuate. The ovary usually occupies the normal position, but the testis or ovotestis may be found at any level along the route of embryonic testicular descent, frequently associated with an inguinal hernia. Testicular tissue is present in the scrotum or the labioscrotal fold in one-third, in the inguinal canal in one-third, and in the abdominal area in one-third.

Variable feminization and virilization ensue at puberty, three-fourths develop gynecomastia, and about half menstruate. In phenotypic men, menstruation presents as cyclic hematuria. Ovulation occurs in approximately one-fourth and is more common than spermatogenesis. In men, ovulation may present as testicular pain. Fertility has been reported in women following removal of an ovotestis and in a man who fathered two children. Congenital malformations of other systems are rare.

Pathophysiology   About two-thirds of subjects have a 46,XX karyotype, a tenth have a 46,XY karyotype, and the remainder are chimeras or mosaics in which a Y cell line is present. The mechanism responsible for the gonadal development is unknown. Even though

not demonstrable with conventional karyotyping methods, it was assumed that sufficient genetic material from the Y chromosome was present (as the result of translocation, nondisjunction, or mutation) to induce the development of testicular tissue. Indeed, approximately a fourth of 46,XX true hermaphrodites have genetic sequences indicative of Y to X translocation. In rare instances, multiple sibs with a 46,XX karyotype are affected, possibly the result of an autosomal or X-linked mutation. The cause of the remaining instances of the 46,XX disorder is unknown.

Because corpora lutea are present in the ovaries of more than one-fourth of subjects, it can be deduced that a female neuroendocrine axis is present and functions normally in such individuals. Feminization (gynecomastia and menstruation) is the result of secretion of estradiol by the ovarian tissue present. In masculinized patients, secretion of androgen predominates over secretion of estrogen, and some produce sperm.

Management   When the diagnosis is made in a newborn or early infant, gender assignment depends on the anatomic features. In older children and adults, gonads and internal duct structures that are contradictory to the predominant phenotype (and the gender of rearing) should be removed, and when necessary, the external genitalia should be modified appropriately. Although gonadal tumors are rare in true hermaphroditism, a gonadoblastoma has been reported in an individual with an XY cell line. Consequently, the possibility of future tumor development must be taken into account when the decision regarding conservation of gonadal tissue is made.

DISORDERS OF GONADAL SEX

Disorders of gonadal sex result when chromosomal sex is normal, but for one of several reasons differentiation of the gonads is abnormal. Thus gonadal sex does not correspond to chromosomal sex.

PURE GONADAL DYSGENESIS   Clinical features   Pure gonadal dysgenesis is a disorder in which phenotypic females with gonads and genitalia characteristic of gonadal dysgenesis (bilateral streaks, infantile uterus and fallopian tubes, and sexual infantilism) have normal height, few if any somatic anomalies, and either a normal 46,XX or 46,XY karyotype. This disorder is only about one-tenth as common as gonadal dysgenesis. It is genetically distinct from gonadal dysgenesis, but it cannot be distinguished clinically from instances of gonadal dysgenesis associated with minimal somatic abnormalities. The height is normal or greater than normal, some subjects being over 170 cm. Estrogen levels vary from profound deficiency typical of 45,X gonadal dysgenesis to some breast development and appearance of menses that terminate in an early menopause. About 40 percent have some feminization. Axillary and pubic hair are scanty, and the internal genitalia consist of müllerian derivatives only.

Tumors may develop in the streak gonads, particularly dysgerminoma or gonadoblastoma in the 46,XY disorder. Such tumors may be heralded by the development of virilizing signs or a pelvic mass.

Pathophysiology   Although chromosomal mosaicisms have been described under this nosology, the designation here is restricted to subjects with uniform 46,XX or 46,XY karyotypes. (Those with mosaicism are variants of gonadal dysgenesis or mixed gonadal dysgenesis, as described above.) The rationale for this restricted definition is based on the fact that both the XX and XY varieties can result from single gene mutations that are presumed to involve gene(s) essential for gonadal development. Several sibships have been reported in which more than one individual is affected with the 46,XX type of the disorder, frequently the result of consanguineous matings, suggesting an autosomal recessive pattern of inheritance. Familial occurrence of the 46,XY variety also has been described; in some the mutation appears to be inherited in an X-linked recessive pattern, while in other families the occurrence is compatible with a male-limited autosomal recessive inheritance. In some sporadic patients with the 46,XY form of the disorder, the SRY region of the short arm of the Y chromosome is deleted, and in two 46,XY subjects, mutations in the SRY gene have been described. In both the 46,XX and the 46,XY forms the disorder prevents differentiation of ovary or testis, respectively; the development of the female phenotype is the consequence of the failure of gonadal development. As in all individuals with nonfunctional gonads, gonadotropin secretion is elevated and estrogen secretion is low.

Management The management of the estrogen deficiency is identical to that in gonadal dysgenesis; namely, appropriate estrogen replacement therapy is initiated at the time of expected puberty and maintained in adult life (see Chap. 340). Because of the high frequency of gonadal tumors in the 46,XY variety, the streak gonads should be removed once the diagnosis is made. The development of virilizing signs is indication for immediate surgery. The natural history of the gonadal tumors in this disorder is uncertain, but the prognosis after surgical removal is usually good.

THE ABSENT TESTES SYNDROME (ANORCHIA, TESTICULAR REGRESSION, GONADAL AGENESIS, AGONADISM) Clinical features

A spectrum of phenotypes has been described in 46,XY males with absent or rudimentary testes but in whom unequivocal evidence exists that endocrine function of the testis (e.g., invariable müllerian duct regression and variable testosterone synthesis) was present at some time during embryonic life. This rare disorder can be distinguished from pure gonadal dysgenesis in which no evidence can be inferred for gonadal function during embryonic development. The disorder varies in its manifestations from complete failure of virilization through varying degrees of incomplete virilization of the external genitalia to otherwise normal males with bilateral anorchia.

The purest form is represented by 46,XY females with absent testes, sexual infantilism, and absence of both müllerian duct derivatives and accessory organs of male reproduction. Such individuals differ from 46,XY pure gonadal dysgenesis in that no gonadal remnant can be identified, including no streak gonad, and in the absence of müllerian derivatives. Testicular failure must have occurred between the onset of formation of müllerian-inhibiting substance and the secretion of testosterone, i.e., after development of the seminiferous tubules but before the onset of Leydig cell function.

In others, the testicular failure must have occurred later in gestation, and these individuals may constitute problems in gender assignment. In some, failure of müllerian regression is more pronounced than failure of testosterone secretion, but none exhibit normal müllerian development. In those with more extensive virilization, the external genitalia are phenotypically male, but rudimentary oviducts and vasa deferentia may coexist internally.

At the final extreme is the syndrome of bilateral anorchia in which phenotypic men have absence of müllerian structures and gonads but male development of the wolffian system and external genitalia. Microphallus implies that failure of androgen-mediated growth occurred late in embryogenesis after anatomic development of the male urethra was complete. Persistent gynecomastia may or may not develop.

Pathophysiology The pathogenesis is not understood. Sibships with multiple affected individuals have been described. The testicular regression could be the result of mutant genes, teratogen, or trauma. Multiple instances of agonadism in the same family have been reported, some of which are unilateral and others bilateral. Some subjects in whom no testes can be identified at laparotomy have blood testosterone values clearly above the castrate range, presumably derived from remnant testes.

Management The management of the two extremes is clear-cut. Sexually infantile, phenotypic females should be treated like gonadal dysgenesis; namely, they should be given adequate estrogen to ensure appropriate breast and female somatic development, and any coexisting vaginal agenesis should be treated by surgical or medical means. Likewise, phenotypic males with anorchia should be given androgen replacement to allow normal male secondary sexual development. The cases with incomplete virilization or ambiguous development of the external genitalia are more complex and require hormonal therapy at the time of expected puberty and individual assessment as to whether surgical therapy is appropriate.

DISORDERS OF PHENOTYPIC SEX

FEMALE PSEUDOHERMAPHRODITISM Congenital adrenal hyperplasia CLINICAL FEATURES The pathways by which glucocorticoids are synthesized in the adrenal gland and androgens are formed in the testis and adrenal are summarized in Fig. 342-3. Three

FIGURE 342-3 Pathways of glucocorticoid and androgen synthesis. Note abnormal conditions corresponding to impaired enzyme reactions.

reactions are common to the formation of glucocorticoids and androgens (cholesterol side chain cleavage, 3β-hydroxysteroid dehydrogenase/isomerase, and 17α-hydroxylase); impairment of any of these reactions results in deficiency of glucocorticoid and androgen synthesis and consequently in both congenital adrenal hyperplasia (due to enhanced ACTH levels) and defective virilization of the male embryo (male pseudohermaphroditism). Two enzyme reactions are involved exclusively in androgen synthesis (17,20-lyase and 17β-hydroxysteroid oxidoreductase); deficiency in either results in pure male pseudohermaphroditism with normal glucocorticoid synthesis. Deficiency of either of the terminal two enzymes of glucocorticoid synthesis (21-hydroxylase and 11β-hydroxylase) results in defective formation of hydrocortisone; the compensatory increase in ACTH secretion causes adrenal hyperplasia and a secondary increase in androgen formation that results in virilization in the female or precocious masculinization in the male.

The *adrenal insufficiency* in these disorders may produce equally severe and life-threatening problems in both sexes and is described in detail in Chap. 335. The major features of congenital adrenal hyperplasia are listed in Table 342-4. From the standpoint of *abnormal sexual development*, some defects in steroidogenesis result in female pseudohermaphroditism, and some cause male pseudohermaphroditism. (3β-Hydroxysteroid dehydrogenase/isomerase deficiency can cause either male or female pseudohermaphroditism, but since incomplete virilization of the male is more common, it will be discussed as a form of male pseudohermaphroditism.)

Congenital adrenal hyperplasia due to classic 21-hydroxylase deficiency is the most common cause of ambiguous genitalia in the newborn, with an incidence of between 1 in 5000 and 1 in 15,000 lives births in Europe and the United States; it may or may not be associated with mineralocorticoid deficiency (salt loss) (see Table 342-4). Virilization is usually apparent at birth in the female and within the first 2 to 3 years of life in the male. Manifestations in females include hypertrophy of the clitoris with ventral binding (chordee), partial fusion of the labioscrotal folds, and variable virilization of the urethra. The internal female structures and ovaries remain unaltered, and the wolffian ducts regress normally, probably because adrenal function begins relatively late in embryogenesis. The external appearance of affected females is similar to that of a male with bilateral cryptorchidism and hypospadias. The labioscrotal folds are bulbous and rugated and resemble a scrotum. Rarely, the virilization is so severe that development of a complete male penile urethra and prostate results in errors in sex assignment at birth.

Radiography following the injection of radiopaque dye into the external genital orifice is helpful in demonstrating the presence of a vagina, uterus, and sometimes even fallopian tubes. In a few cases, virilization of the female is slight or absent at birth and becomes evident in later infancy, adolescence, or adulthood, presumably as the result of allelic variation of the mutant genes (the so-called nonclassic or late-onset form of the disorder). The untreated female with the classic disorder grows rapidly during the first year of life and has progressive virilization. At the time of expected puberty there is a failure of normal female sexual development and absence of menstruation. In both sexes, rapid somatic maturation results in premature epiphyseal closure and a short adult height.

Since male phenotypic differentiation is normal, the condition is usually not recognized in the male at birth in the absence of overt adrenal insufficiency. However, early growth and maturation of the external genitalia, appearance of secondary sex characteristics, coarsening of the voice, frequent erections, and excessive muscular development are noticeable in the first few years of life. Virilization in the male can follow either of two patterns. Excessive adrenal androgens can inhibit gonadotropin production so that the testes remain infantile in size despite the acceleration of masculinization. Such untreated adult men are capable of erection and ejaculation but have no spermatogenesis. Alternatively, adrenal androgen secretion can activate a premature maturation of the hypothalamic-pituitary axis and initiate a true precocious puberty including early maturation of spermatogenesis (see Chap. 339). The untreated male is also subject to the development of ACTH-dependent "tumors" of the testis composed of adrenal rest cells.

In classic 21-hydroxylase deficiency, which accounts for about 95 percent of congenital adrenal hyperplasia, decreased production of hydrocortisone leads to increased release of ACTH, enlargement of the adrenal glands, and partial or complete compensation of the defect in the secretion of hydrocortisone. In about half, the enzyme defect appears to be partial, and cortisol secretion is normal. This form is termed "simple virilizing." In the remainder, deficiency of the enzyme is more complete; the enlarged adrenal fails to produce adequate amounts of cortisol and aldosterone leading to severe salt wastage with anorexia, vomiting, volume depletion, and collapse within the first few weeks of life, the so-called salt-losing form of 21-hydroxylase deficiency. In all untreated patients, overproduction of the cortisol precursors prior to the 21-hydroxylase step occurs, leading to increase in plasma progesterone and 17-hydroxyprogesterone. These act as weak aldosterone antagonists at the receptor level and in the compen-

TABLE 342-4 Forms of congenital adrenal hyperplasia

Deficiency	Cortisol	Aldosterone	Degree of virilization of females	Failure of virilization in males	Dominant steroid secreted	Comment
Classic 21-hydroxylase, partial (simple virilizing or compensated)	Normal	↑	+ + + +	0	17-Hydroxy-progesterone	Most common type (95% of total); from one- to two-thirds salt losers
Severe (salt-losing)	↓	↓	+ + + +	0	17-Hydroxy-progesterone	
11β-Hydroxylase (hypertension)	↓	↓	+ + + +	0	11-Deoxycortisol and 11-deoxy-corticosterone	Hypertension
3β-Hydroxysteroid dehydrogenase/isomerase	0	0	+	+ + + +	Δ⁵-3β-OH compounds (dehydroepiandrosterone)	Probably second most common, usually salt loss
17α-Hydroxylase	↓	↓	0	+ + + +	Corticosterone and 11-deoxy-corticosterone	No feminization of female, hypertension
Cholesterol side chain cleavage enzyme	0	0	0	+ + + +	Cholesterol(?)	Rare, usually salt loss

sated form result in greater than normal aldosterone production to maintain normal sodium balance. Increased substrate availability is also responsible for the increase in androgen synthesis in the disorder.

Female pseudohermaphroditism also may occur in 11β-hydroxylase deficiency. In this disorder, a block in hydroxylation at the 11 carbon results in the accumulation of 11-deoxycortisol and deoxycorticosterone (DOC), a potent salt-retaining hormone that causes hypertension rather than salt loss. The clinical features that stem from glucocorticoid deficiency and androgen excess are similar to those in 21-hydroxylase deficiency.

PATHOPHYSIOLOGY Both disorders are due to autosomal recessive mutations. The carrier frequency for P450$_{C21}$ deficiency is about 1 in 50. Because the gene is located on the sixth chromosome close to the HLA-B locus, carriers of the disorder (as well as homozygotes) within a given family can be identified on the basis of the HLA haplotype. At the molecular level the mutations that give rise to 21-hydroxylase deficiency are even more polymorphic; indeed, deletions of portions of the gene (10 to 30 percent), conversion of the gene from a functional state to a form that is not transcribed normally (10 percent), and point mutations (60 to 75 percent) have been characterized in different families with the disorder. The classic disorder is due to mutations that severely reduce enzyme activity, and less severe mutations cause the nonclassic or late-onset variety. 11β-Hydroxylase activity is encoded by two genes on chromosome 8; the molecular biology of P450$_{11β}$ deficiency has not been characterized in extensive detail, but there are at least two variants, namely, the classic and late-onset types.

For discussion of the endocrine pathology see Chap. 335. In brief, urinary excretion of ketosteroids is elevated, as is the excretion of the major metabolites that accumulate proximal to the enzymatic blocks. Plasma ACTH is elevated. In P450$_{C21}$ deficiency, 17-hydroxyprogesterone accumulates in blood and is excreted predominantly as pregnanetriol. In P450$_{11β}$ deficiency, 11-deoxycortisol accumulates in blood and is excreted predominantly as tetrahydrocortexolone.

MANAGEMENT Gender assignment should correspond to the chromosomal and gonadal sex, and appropriate surgical correction of the external genitalia should be undertaken as early as possible. This is of importance because appropriately treated men and women are capable of fertility. However, if the correct diagnosis is made late (after 3 years of age), gender assignment should be changed only after careful consideration of the psychosexual background.

Treatment with appropriate glucocorticoids prevents the consequences of hydrocortisone deficiency, arrests the rapid virilization, and prevents premature somatic and epiphyseal maturation. The suppression of the abnormal steroid secretion results in cure of the hypertension in patients with 11β-hydroxylase deficiency and allows normal onset of menses and development of female secondary sex characteristics in both disorders. In males, glucocorticoid therapy suppresses adrenal androgens and results in normal gonadotropin secretion, testicular development, and spermatogenesis. Measurements of plasma 17-hydroxyprogesterone, androstenedione, ACTH, and renin levels have all been used to assess adequacy of replacement therapy. In severe 21-hydroxylase deficiency associated with salt loss or elevated plasma renin activity, treatment with mineralocorticoids is also indicated. In such patients, the monitoring of plasma renin is useful for determining the adequacy of mineralocorticoid replacement.

Other causes of female pseudohermaphroditism Female pseudohermaphroditism also may occur in babies born to mothers with virilizing tumors of the ovary (e.g., arrhenoblastomas or luteomas of pregnancy) and, rarely, to mothers with virilizing adrenal tumors. In the past, the administration to pregnant women of progestational agents with androgenic side effects (such as 17α-ethinyl-19-nortestosterone) to prevent abortion resulted in masculinization of female fetuses.

Developmental disorders of müllerian ducts (congenital absence of the vagina, müllerian agenesis) CLINICAL FEATURES Congenital hypoplasia or absence of the vagina in combination with abnormal or absent uterus (the Mayer-Rokitansky-Kuster-Hauser syndrome) is second to gonadal dysgenesis as a cause of primary amenorrhea. Most patients are ascertained after the time of expected puberty because of failure to menstruate. The height is normal, and the breasts, axillary and public hair, and habitus are feminine in character. The uterus can vary from almost normal, lacking only a conduit to the introitus, to the characteristic rudimentary bicornuate cords with or without a lumen. In some patients, cyclic abdominal pain indicates that sufficient functional endometrium is present to result in retrograde menstruation and/or hematometra.

About one-third have abnormal kidneys, most commonly agenesis, ectopy, fused kidneys of the horseshoe type, or solitary ectopic kidneys located in the pelvis. Skeletal abnormalities are present in one-tenth; two-thirds involve the spine, and limb and rib abnormalities account for the remainder. Specific bone abnormalities include wedge vertebrae, fused rudimentary or asymmetric vertebral bodies, and supernumerary vertebrae. The Klippel-Feil syndrome (congenital fusion of the cervical spine, short neck, low posterior hairline, and painless limitation of cervical movement) is a frequent association.

PATHOPHYSIOLOGY The karyotype is 46,XX. Familial occurrence has been described. The pattern of inheritance in most familial cases is consistent with a sex-limited autosomal dominant mutation. Sporadic cases may represent new mutations of the type responsible for the familial disorder or be multifactorial in etiology. In the familial cases, expressivity is variable; some affected family members have skeletal or renal abnormalities only, and some have other abnormalities of müllerian derivatives such as a double uterus. Bilateral renal aplasia in stillborn infants is commonly associated with absence of the uterus and vagina. Thus the family history should be probed for isolated skeletal and renal abnormalities and for stillbirths that might result from congenital absence of both kidneys. Ovarian function is normal, and successful pregnancies have occurred after corrective vaginal surgery in patients with normal uteri.

MANAGEMENT Vaginal agenesis can be treated by surgical or nonsurgical means. Surgical repair generally utilizes a split-thickness skin graft around a solid rubber mold for the creation of an artificial vagina. Medical treatment consists of the repeated application of pressure against the vaginal dimple with a simple dilator to cause development of adequate vaginal depth. In view of complication rates of 5 to 10 percent in surgical series, medical treatment should be tried in most, and surgery should be reserved for patients in whom a well-formed uterus is present and the possibility of fertility exists. Frequent coitus or instrumental dilatation is essential for maintaining the neovagina formed by either technique.

MALE PSEUDOHERMAPHRODITISM Defective virilization of the male embryo (male pseudohermaphroditism) can result from defects in androgen synthesis, defects in androgen action, defects in müllerian duct regression, and uncertain causes. Four-fifths of male pseudohermaphrodites have normal androgen synthesis.

Abnormalities in androgen synthesis CLINICAL FEATURES Enzymatic defects that result in defective testosterone synthesis (see Fig. 342-3) can cause incomplete virilization of the male embryo during embryogenesis (Tables 342-4 and 342-5). Each of the defects blocks a step in the conversion of cholesterol to testosterone. Three are common to the synthesis of other adrenal hormones as well: cholesterol side chain cleavage, 3β-hydroxysteroid dehydrogenase/isomerase, and 17α-hydroxylase or P450$_{17α}$. Consequently, their deficiency results in congenital adrenal hyperplasia (see Table 342-4) as well as male pseudohermaphroditism. Two others (17,20-lyase and 17β-hydroxysteroid oxidoreductase) are unique to the pathway of androgen synthesis, and their deficiency results only in male pseudohermaphroditism. Since androgens are obligatory precursors of estrogens, synthesis of estrogen is also low in affected men and women in all but the terminal defect (17β-hydroxysteroid oxidoreductase deficiency).

The adrenal dysfunction is described in Chap. 335, and the present discussion concerns the abnormal sexual development. In 46,XY

TABLE 342-5   Anatomic, genetic, and endocrine profile of hereditary male pseudohermaphroditism

Disorder	Inheritance	Phenotype Müllerian ducts	Wolffian ducts	Spermatogenesis	Urogenital sinus	External genitalia
DEFECTS IN TESTOSTERONE SYNTHESIS						
Five enzyme deficiencies	Autosomal or X-linked recessive	Absent	Variable development	Normal or decreased	Variable from male to female	Generally female
DEFECTS IN ANDROGEN ACTION						
Steroid 5α-reductase 2 deficiency	Autosomal recessive	Absent	Male	Normal or decreased	Female	Clitoromegaly
Receptor disorders: Complete testicular feminization	X-linked recessive	Absent	Absent	Absent	Female	Female
Incomplete testicular feminization	X-linked recessive	Absent	Male	Absent	Female	Clitoromegaly and posterior fusion
Reifenstein syndrome	X-linked recessive	Absent	Variable development	Absent	Variable from male to female	Incomplete male development
Infertile male syndrome	X-linked recessive	Absent	Male	Absent or decreased	Male	Male
Undervirilized fertile male	X-linked recessive	Absent	Male	Normal or decreased	Male	Male
DEFECTS IN MÜLLERIAN REGRESSION						
Persistent müllerian duct syndrome	Autosomal or X-linked recessive	Rudimentary uterus and fallopian tubes	Male	Normal	Male	Male

subjects there is usually no trace of uterus or fallopian tubes, indicating that the müllerian-inhibiting function of the testis during embryogenesis was normal. The masculinization of the urogenital tract and external genitalia and the degree of virilization at puberty vary from almost normal to absent, and therefore, the clinical picture spans the range from men with mild hypospadias to phenotypic women who prior to puberty resemble patients with complete testicular feminization. This variability is the consequence of varying severity of the enzymatic defects in different patients and of varying effects of the steroids that accumulate proximal to the metabolic blocks in the different disorders. In patients with partial defects and in whom the plasma testosterone level is normal, the diagnosis can only be made by measuring the steroids that accumulate proximal to the metabolic block.

Cholesterol side chain cleavage enzyme (P450$_{SCC}$) *deficiency (lipoid adrenal hyperplasia)* is an autosomal recessive disorder in which virtually no urinary steroids (either 17-ketosteroids or 17-hydroxycorticoids) can be detected. The defect is prior to the formation of pregnenolone and is assumed to involve the side-chain cleavage enzyme that is encoded on chromosome 15 and is responsible for the conversion of cholesterol to pregnenolone. The syndrome is associated with salt wasting and profound adrenal insufficiency, and most affected individuals die during infancy. At autopsy, the adrenals and testes are enlarged and infiltrated with lipid. Affected males are incompletely masculinized, whereas affected female infants have normal genital development. The gene for the human enzyme is located on chromosome 15.

3β-Hydroxysteroid dehydrogenase/isomerase deficiency is due to an autosomal recessive mutation of the 3β-HSD gene on chromosome 1 that causes varying failure of masculinization and development of a vagina in male infants. Female infants may be modestly virilized at birth due to the weak androgenic potency of dehydroepiandrosterone, the major steroid secreted. If the enzyme is absent in both the adrenal and testis, no urinary steroids contain a Δ^4-3-keto configura-

tion, whereas in patients in whom the defect is partial or affects only the testis, the urine may contain normal or elevated levels of Δ^4-3-ketosteroids. Most patients have marked salt wasting and profound adrenal insufficiency, and long-term survival in untreated cases occurs only in states of partial deficiency. Affected males may experience an otherwise normal male puberty except for profound gynecomastia. In these individuals, a low-normal blood testosterone level is accompanied by elevated Δ^5 precursors. The enzyme in different tissues must be under complex control, since deficiency of the enzyme in the testis may be less severe than in the adrenal and the enzyme activity in the liver appears to be encoded by a different gene.

17α-Hydroxylase-17,20-lyase (P450$_{17α}$) *deficiency* impairs the introduction of the 17-hydroxyl and the scission of the C-17,20 carbon bond that convert pregnenolone and progesterone to dehydroepiandrosterone and androstenedione, respectively. These reactions are mediated by a single cytochrome, P450$_{17α}$, encoded on chromosome 10, and it is unclear why both reactions occur in the ovary and testis, whereas in the adrenal 17-hydroxyprogesterone is largely converted to glucocorticoids and mineralocorticoids rather than the 19-carbon steroids. Likewise, it is unclear why some patients have selective impairment of either 17α-hydroxylase or 17,20-lyase activity; the distinction between these activities must be functional and may involve the relative concentration of steroid substrates and competing enzymes. Whatever the explanation, the clinical consequences of 17α-hydroxylase and 17,20-lyase deficiencies are different.

17α-Hydroxylase deficiency characteristically results in hypogonadism, absence of secondary sex characteristics, hypokalemic alkalosis, hypertension, and virtually undetectable hydrocortisone secretion in phenotypic women. The secretion of both corticosterone and desoxycorticosterone (DOC) by the adrenal is elevated, and urinary 17-ketosteroids are low. Aldosterone secretion is low due to high plasma DOC and depressed angiotensin levels and returns to normal after suppressive doses of hydrocortisone are administered. In 46,XX subjects, amenorrhea, absent sexual hair, and hypertension are

| Breast | Endocrine profile relative to normal male | | |
	Testosterone production	Estrogen production	LH
Usually male	Normal to decreased	Variable	High
Male	Normal	Normal	Normal or increased
Female	High	High	High
Female	High	High	High
Female	High	High	High
Usually male	Normal or high	Normal or high	Normal or high
Usually male	Normal or high	Normal or high	Normal or high
Male	Normal	Normal	Normal

common, but since gonadal steroids are not required for female development during embryogenesis, the phenotype is that of a normal prepubertal woman. In males, the deficiency results in defective virilization that varies from complete male pseudohermaphroditism to ambiguous genitalia with perineoscrotal hypospadias and, in some, gynecomastia. Adrenal insufficiency does not develop, since the secretion of both corticosterone (a weak glucocorticoid) and DOC (a mineralocorticoid) is elevated. Hypertension and hypokalemia are prominent features of the disorder (even in the neonatal period) and remit after suppression of the DOC secretion by adequate glucocorticoid replacement.

17,20-lyase deficiency in males is associated with normal function of the adrenal cortex and a variable pattern of male pseudohermaphroditism. In the majority there is genital ambiguity at birth, with some virilization at the time of expected puberty. Rare 46,XY patients have had a female phenotype and no virilization at the time of expected puberty. The disorder has been recognized in one 46,XX woman with sexual infantilism. A number of mutations in the P450$_{17\alpha}$ gene on chromosome 10 have been described.

17β-Hydroxysteroid oxidoreductase (17β-HSOR) *deficiency* involves the final step in testosterone biosynthesis, reduction of the 17-keto group of androstenedione. This is the most common of the enzymatic defects in testosterone synthesis. Affected 46,XY males usually have a female phenotype with a blind-ending vagina and absence of müllerian derivatives, but inguinal or abdominal testes and virilized wolffian duct structures are present. At the time of expected puberty, both virilization (with phallic enlargement and development of facial and body hair) and a variable degree of female breast development take place. In some untreated patients, reversal of gender behavior from female to male occurs at puberty. Androgen and estrogen dynamics have not been elucidated in detail, but the 17-keto reduction of estrone to estradiol by the gonads is also low. 17β-Hydroxysteroid oxidoreductase is normally present in many tissues besides the gonads, and only the gonadal enzyme appears to be

defective in this disorder. Plasma testosterone level may be in the low-normal range, making it essential to document elevation in plasma androstenedione to make the diagnosis. It is not clear how many genes encode this activity.

PATHOPHYSIOLOGY These various disorders are inherited as autosomal recessive traits. The pattern of steroid secretion and excretion depends on the site of the various metabolic blocks (see Fig. 342-3). In general, gonadotropin secretion is high, and as a consequence, many individuals with incomplete defects are able to compensate so that the steady state levels of end products such as testosterone may be normal or almost normal.

In some cases of male pseudohermaphroditism, testosterone formation is deficient for reasons other than a single enzyme defect in androgen synthesis. These include disorders in which Leydig cell agenesis (possibly due to absence of the LH receptor) or the secretion of a biologically inactive LH molecule is thought to be the primary defect. In addition, as described above, in several disorders including familial 46,XY pure gonadal dysgenesis, sporadic dysgenetic testes, and the absent testis syndrome, deficient testosterone production is secondary to abnormal gonadal development.

MANAGEMENT Therapy with glucocorticoids and in some instances mineralocorticoids is indicated in those disorders causing adrenal hyperplasia. The decision as to the management of the genital abnormalities depends on the individual case. Fertility has not been reported, and its consideration does not enter into sex assignment. In genetic females there is no problem (except in diagnosis), in that affected individuals are raised appropriately as females and suitable estrogen replacement is administered at the time of expected puberty to promote development of normal secondary sex characteristics. The decision as to whether newborn males with ambiguous genitalia should be raised as males or females depends on the anatomic defect; in general, the more severely affected should be raised as females, and corrective surgery of the genitalia and removal of the testes should be undertaken as early as possible. In such subjects estrogen therapy is also indicated at the appropriate age to allow development of normal female secondary sex characteristics. In individuals raised as males, corrective surgery is indicated for any coexisting hypospadias, and monitoring of plasma androgens and estrogens should be undertaken at the time of expected puberty to determine whether supplemental testosterone therapy is appropriate.

Abnormalities in androgen action Several disorders of male phenotypic development result from abnormalities of androgen action. The spectrum of phenotypes is described in Tables 342-4 and 342-5. In these disorders, testosterone formation and müllerian regression are normal, but male development is impaired to a variable degree as a result of resistance to androgen action in the target cells.

STEROID 5α-REDUCTASE 2 DEFICIENCY This autosomal recessive disorder is characterized by (1) severe perineoscrotal hypospadias, (2) a blind vaginal pouch of variable size opening either into the urogenital sinus or into the urethra, (3) testes with normal epididymides, vasa deferentia, and seminal vesicles, and termination of the ejaculatory ducts into the blind-ending vagina, (4) a female habitus without female breast development but with normal axillary and pubic hair, (5) the absence of female internal genitalia, (6) normal male plasma testosterone, and (7) masculinization to a variable degree at the time of puberty.

The fact that virilization during embryogenesis is defective only in the urogenital sinus and the external genitalia provided insight into the fundamental abnormality. Testosterone, the androgen secreted by the fetal testis, is responsible for differentiation of the wolffian duct into the epididymis, vas deferens, and seminal vesicle, whereas dihydrotestosterone mediates virilization of the urogenital sinus and the external genitalia. Consequently, a failure of dihydrotestosterone formation in a male embryo would be expected to cause the phenotype observed in this disorder, normal male wolffian duct derivatives with defective masculinization of the external genitalia and urogenital sinus. Since testosterone itself regulates LH secretion (see Chap. 339), plasma LH level is normal or minimally elevated. As a result, testosterone and estrogen production rates are those of normal men, and gynecomastia does not develop.

The fact that 5α-reductase 2 enzyme is deficient in this disorder was established by assay of biopsied tissues and cultured fibroblasts from affected individuals. Deletions or point mutations in the gene encoding steroid 5α-reductase 2 have been identified in most families studied. Approximately 40 percent are compound heterozygotes.

RECEPTOR DISORDERS   The androgen receptor is a typical member of the steroid/thyroid family of receptors with steroid-binding, DNA-binding, and functional domains and is encoded by a gene on the long arm of the X chromosome. A variety of mutations of this gene impair receptor function and hence impair male phenotypic differentiation and/or virilization.

Clinical features   Complete testicular feminization is a common form of male pseudohermaphroditism; estimates of frequency vary from 1 in 20,000 to 1 in 64,000 male births. It is the third most common cause of primary amenorrhea in phenotypic women after gonadal dysgenesis and congenital absence of the vagina. The features are characteristic. Namely, a woman is ascertained either because of inguinal hernia (prepubertal) or primary amenorrhea (postpubertal). The development of the breasts after puberty, the general habitus, and the distribution of body fat are female in character so that most patients have a truly feminine appearance. Axillary and pubic hair is absent or scanty, but some vulval hair is usually present. Scalp hair is that of a normal woman, and facial hair is absent. The external genitalia are unambiguously female, and the clitoris is normal. The vagina is short and blind-ending and may be absent or rudimentary. All internal genitalia are absent except for testes that contain normal Leydig cells and seminiferous tubules without spermatogenesis. The testes may be located in the abdomen, along the course of the inguinal canal, or in the labia majora. Occasionally, remnants of müllerian or wolffian duct origin are present in the paratesticular fascia or in fibrous bands extending from the testis. Patients tend to be rather tall, and bone age is normal. Psychosexual development is unmistakably female with regard to behavior, outlook, and maternal instincts.

The major complication of undescended testes in this disorder, as in all forms of cryptorchidism, is the development of tumors (Chap. 322). Since affected individuals undergo a normal pubertal growth spurt and feminize successfully at the time of expected puberty, and since testicular tumors rarely develop until after puberty, it is usual to delay castration until after the time of expected puberty. Prepubertal castration is indicated if the testes are present in the inguinal region or the labia majora and result in discomfort or hernia formation. (If hernia repair is indicated prepubertally, most physicians prefer to remove the testes at the same time to limit the number of operative procedures.) If the testes are removed prepubertally, estrogen therapy is required at the appropriate age to ensure normal growth and breast development. When castration is performed postpubertally, menopausal symptoms and other evidence of estrogen withdrawal supervene, and suitable estrogen replacement is indicated (see Chap. 340).

Incomplete testicular feminization is about one-tenth as frequent as the complete form. In the incomplete disorder there is minor virilization of the external genitalia (partial fusion of the labioscrotal folds and/or some degree of clitoromegaly), normal pubic hair, and some virilization as well as feminization at the time of expected puberty. The vagina is short and blind-ending, but in contrast to the complete form, the wolffian duct derivatives are often partially developed. The management of patients with the complete and incomplete forms of testicular feminization differs. Since patients with the incomplete disorder virilize at the time of expected puberty, gonadectomy should be performed before the expected time of puberty in all prepubertal patients with clitoromegaly or posterior labial fusion.

Reifenstein syndrome is the term applied to forms of incomplete male pseudohermaphroditism initially described by a number of eponyms (Reifenstein syndrome, Gilbert-Dreyfus syndrome, Lubs syndrome). Each of these phenotypes was originally assumed to be a distinct entity, but these syndromes are now known to constitute variable manifestations of mutations of the androgen receptor. The most common phenotype is a man with perineoscrotal hypospadias and gynecomastia, but the spectrum of defective virilization in affected families ranges from men with azoospermia to phenotypic women with pseudovaginas. Axillary and pubic hair is normal, but chest and facial hair is minimal. Cryptorchidism is common, the testes are small, and azoospermia is present. Some have defects in wolffian duct derivatives such as absence or hypoplasia of the vas deferens. Since the psychological development in most in unequivocally male, the hypospadias and cryptorchidism should be corrected surgically. The only successful form of treatment of the gynecomastia is surgical removal.

The *infertile male syndrome* may be the most common disorder of the androgen receptor and is not actually a form of male pseudohermaphroditism. Some such individuals are minimally affected subjects in families with Reifenstein syndrome with azoospermia as the only manifestation of the receptor abnormality. More commonly, subjects present with male infertility and have negative family histories; indeed, a disorder of the androgen receptor may be present in a fifth or more of men with idiopathic azoospermia. The *undervirilized fertile male* is another manifestation of an androgen receptor defect. In these families, affected men have gynecomastia and undervirilization, and some are fertile.

Pathophysiology   The karyotype is 46,XY, and the mutant gene is X-linked. The frequency of a positive family history varies from about two-thirds of patients with testicular feminization and Reifenstein syndrome to only occasional patients with the infertile male syndrome. The patients with a negative family history are believed to be the result of new mutations.

Hormone dynamics are similar in all disorders of the androgen receptor. Plasma testosterone levels and rates of testosterone production by the testes are normal or higher than normal. The elevated testosterone production is caused by the high mean plasma level of LH, which, in turn, is due to defective feedback regulation caused by resistance to the action of androgen at the hypothalamic-pituitary level. Elevated LH concentration is responsible also for the increased estrogen production by the testes (see Chap. 339). (In normal men, most estrogen is derived from peripheral formation from circulating androgens, but when the plasma LH level is elevated, the testes secrete increased amounts of estrogen into the circulation.) Thus resistance to the feedback regulation of LH secretion by circulating androgens results in elevated plasma LH levels, and this, in turn, results in the enhanced secretion of both testosterone and estradiol by the testes. Gonadotropin levels rise even higher (and menopausal symptoms may develop) when the testes are removed, indicating that gonadotropin secretion is under partial regulatory control. Presumably, in the steady state and in the absence of an androgen effect, estrogen alone regulates LH secretion, a control purchased at the expense of an elevated plasma estrogen concentration for a male. The hormonal changes in the infertile male syndrome are similar to those in the other receptor disorders but less marked. Some men with this syndrome do not have an elevation of plasma LH or plasma testosterone level.

Feminization in these disorders is the result of two interlocking phenomena. First, androgens and estrogens have antagonistic effects, and virilization occurs in normal men when the ratio of androgen to estrogen is 100:1 or greater; in the absence of androgen action, the cellular effect of estrogen is unopposed. Second, the testicular production of estradiol is greater than that of the normal male (although less than that of the normal female). Variable degrees of androgen resistance coupled with variably enhanced estradiol production result in different degrees of defective virilization and enhanced feminization in the four clinical syndromes.

Each of these syndromes is the result of an abnormality of the androgen receptor. In some families, the fundamental defect is due to the deletion of a portion of the gene; more commonly, the disorder is due to point mutations in the coding sequence leading to premature termination codons or amino acid substitutions in the hormone-binding domain. Some families with clinical syndromes typical of an androgen receptor disorder have normal androgen binding in fibroblasts. In many of these families, point mutations in the DNA-binding domain are responsible for the androgen resistance.

Persistent müllerian duct syndrome Men with this uncommon disorder have testes and normal phenotypic development and in addition have fallopian tubes, a uterus, an upper vagina, and variable development of the vas deferens. The disorder is heterogeneous. In one type, one or both testes are descended, and the uterus and ipsilateral fallopian tube are in the inguinal canal or scrotum; both testes and fallopian tubes may be present in the hernia sac or can be drawn into it. The other type is associated with high bilateral cryptorchidism and no hernias. In both types, the vasa deferentia are embedded in the wall of the uterus, a feature that complicates surgical procedures designed to preserve potential fertility. Most patients have uninformative family histories, but in some the condition is inherited as an autosomal recessive trait. Because the external genitalia are well developed and the patients masculinize normally at puberty, it is assumed that during the critical stage of embryonic differentiation the fetal testes produce a normal amount of androgen. However, müllerian regression does not occur. Utilizing immunoassays, subjects can be divided into two groups. In the MIS-positive group, levels of müllerian-inhibiting substance (MIS) in serum and testes are normal, and it is postulated that the MIS receptor is defective. In the MIS-negative group, serum MIS is absent or decreased, and one such patient has been shown to have single-nucleotide substitution that inserts a premature stop codon that results in a truncated hormone. To minimize the chance of tumor development and to maintain virilization, orchiopexy should be performed. Malignancy in the uterus or vagina has not been described, and because the vasa deferentia are closely associated with the broad ligaments, the uterus and vagina should be left in place to avoid disruption of the vasa deferentia during removal and consequently to preserve possible fertility.

Developmental defects of the male genitalia HYPOSPADIAS Hypospadias is a congenital anomaly in which the urethra terminates in an abnormal position along the midline of the ventral surface of the penis at some site between the normal urethral meatus and the perineum. This malformation is often associated with ventral contraction and bowing of the penis (chordee) and occurs in 0.5 to 0.8 percent of male births in the United States. It is common to categorize hypospadias as glandular (involving the glans penis), penile, or perineoscrotal. Since androgens control penile development, hypospadias is believed to result form some defect in androgen formation or androgen action during embryogenesis. Indeed, hypospadias occurs in most disorders of male sexual differentiation. A rare cause of hypospadias is maternal ingestion of progestational agents early in pregnancy. However, the known causes (single-gene defects, chromosomal abnormalities, and maternal drug ingestion) at best can account for only about one-fourth of cases, and the etiology of most remains unknown. The management is surgical.

CRYPTORCHIDISM The normal descent of the testis is perhaps the most poorly understood portion of male sexual differentiation, with regard both to the nature of the forces that result in the movement and to the hormonal factors that regulate the process. In anatomic terms, testicular descent can be divided into three phases: (1) transabdominal movement of the testis from its site of origin above the kidney to the inguinal ring, (2) formation of the opening in the inguinal canal (processus vaginalis) through which the testis exits the abdominal cavity, and (3) actual movement of the testis through the inguinal canal to its permanent site in the scrotum. This entire process occurs over a 6- to 7-month period during gestation, beginning at about the sixth week and not completed in some until after birth. Impairment of any of the above anatomic events can be responsible for the failure of descent of one or both testes. About 3 percent of full-term and 30 percent of premature male infants have at least one cryptorchid testis at birth, but completion of descent can occur within the first few weeks of life, so the incidence of failure of descent by

6 to 9 months of age is only 0.6 to 0.7 percent. It is this latter category of maldescent that requires intervention.

Permanent cryptorchidism can be classified as intraabdominal (10 percent), canalicular (in the inguinal canal) (20 percent), high scrotal (40 percent), or obstructed (30 percent), in which maldescent is due to a physical barrier between the inguinal pouch and the inlet of the scrotum. These disorders must be distinguished from the temporarily retracted normal testis.

The cryptorchid testis functions poorly after puberty, but the extent to which maldescent is the result of an abnormality of the testis or the cause of abnormal function is unknown. Two general theories have been advanced as to the etiology—inadequate intraabdominal pressure and deficient endocrine function of the testis either because of deficient testosterone synthesis or inadequate formation of müllerian-inhibiting substance. Indeed, defects that result in inadequate development of intraabdominal pressure of inadequate development of the testes can cause cryptorchidism. As is true for hypospadias, however, the known causes of cryptorchidism constitute only a small fraction of the cases, and the etiology in most remains to be identified. Two complications of cryptorchidism are important; spermatogenesis cannot occur at the temperature of the abdominal cavity, and it is therefore necessary to correct the process as early as possible to allow possible fertility. The fact that infertility is common in men who have been treated for unilateral as well as bilateral cryptorchidism suggests that maldescent is usually the consequence rather than the cause of the testicular malfunction. There is also a greater frequency of malignancy in undescended testes, and all should be surgically corrected for this reason (see Chap. 322).

REFERENCES

DE LA CHAPELLE A: The etiology of maleness in XX men. Hum Genet 58:105, 1981

DONAHOE PK et al: Mixed gonadal dysgenesis, pathogenesis and management. J Pediatr Surg 14:287, 1979

EDMAN CD et al: Embryonic testicular regression: A clinical spectrum of XY agonadal individuals. Obstet Gynecol 49:208, 1977

GEORGE FW, WILSON JD: Sex determination and differentiation, in *The Physiology of Reproduction*, E Knobil, JD Neill (eds). New York, Raven, 1988, vol 1, pp 3–26

GORDON DL et al: Pathologic testicular findings in Klinefelter's syndrome. 47,XXY vs 46,XY/47,XXY. Arch Intern Med 130:726, 1972

GRIFFIN JE: Androgen resistances: The clinical and molecular spectrum. N Engl J Med 336:611, 1992

———, WILSON JD: Disorder of sexual differentiation, in *Campbell's Textbook of Urology*, 6th ed, PC Walsh et al (eds). Philadelphia, Saunders, 1992, pp 1509–1542

——— et al: The androgen resistance syndromes: 5α-Reductase deficiency, and related disorders, in *The Molecular and Metabolic Basis of Inherited Disease*, 7th ed, CR Scriver et al (eds). New York, McGraw-Hill, in press

——— et al: Congenital absence of the vagina. The Mayer-Rokitansky-Kuster-Hauser syndrome. Ann Intern Med 85:224, 1976

GRUMBACH MM, CONTE FA: Disorders of sexual differentiation, in *Williams' Textbook of Endocrinology*, 8th ed, JD Wilson, DW Foster (eds). Philadelphia, Saunders, 1992, pp 853–951

GUERRIER D et al: The persistent müllerian duct syndrome: A molecular approach. J Clin Endocrinol Metab 68:46, 1989

JOSSO N et al: Anti-müllerian hormone and intersex states. Trends Endocrinol Metab 2:227, 1991

LEONARD JM et al: The classification of Klinefelter's syndrome, in *Genetic Mechanism of Sexual Development*, HL Vallet, IH Porter (eds). New York, Academic, 1979

McPHAUL MJ et al: The spectrum of mutations in the androgen receptor that causes androgen resistance. J Clin Endocrinol Metab 76:17, 1993

MILLER, WL: Molecular biology of steroid hormone synthesis. Endocrinol Rev 9:295, 1988

NEW M et al: Congenital adrenal hyperplasia and related conditions, in *The Metabolic Basis of Inherited Disease*, 6th ed, CR Scriver et al (eds). New York, McGraw-Hill, 1989, pp. 1881–1917

RAMSAY M et al: XX True hermaphroditism in Southern African blacks: An enigma of primary sexual differentiation. Am J Hum Genet Vol 43:4, 1988

SIMPSON JL: Gonadal dysgenesis and sex chromosome abnormalities: Phenotypic-karyotypic correlations, in *Genetic Mechanisms of Sexual Development*, HL Vallet, IH Porter (eds). New York, Academic, 1976

——— et al: XY gonadal dysgenesis: Genetic heterogeneity based upon clinical observations, H-Y antigen status and segregation analysis. Hum Genet 58:91, 1981

SINCLAIR AH et al: A gene from the human sex-determining region encodes a protein with homology to a conserved DNA-binding motif. Nature 364:240, 1990

WILSON JD et al: Steroid 5α-reductase 2 deficiency. Endocr Rev 14:577, 1993

YANASE T et al: 17α-Hydroxylase/17,20-lyase deficiency: From clinical investigation to molecular definition. Endocr Rev 12:91, 1991

ZAH W et al: Mixed gonadal dysgenesis. A case report and review of the world literature. Acta Endocrinol Suppl 197:3, 1975 undergo parathyroid exploration. In MEN 1 there is, in addition, an additional criterion for operative intervention; hypercalcemia may stimulate gastrin overproduction and development of ZES in MEN 1, a feature that may be reversed by restoration of normocalcemia. There is less agreement regarding the necessity for parathyroid exploration in individuals who do not meet these criteria, and observation over a several-year period may be appropriate in a MEN 1 patient with asymptomatic hyperparathyroidism.

When surgery is indicated for hyperparathyroidism in MEN 1, the preferred procedure is to identify and remove all parathyroid tissue at the time of primary operation and to implant parathyroid tissue in multiple packets in the nondominant forearm. Consequently, if reoperation is necessary, surgical removal of single or multiple packets of tissue can be performed under local anesthesia with titration of tissue removal to return the serum calcium concentration to normal. A second approach is to remove $3\frac{1}{2}$ parathyroid glands from the neck, carefully marking the location of residual tissue so that the remaining tissue can be located easily during subsequent surgery.

PANCREATIC ISLET TUMORS   (See Chap. 276 for discussion of the treatment of pancreatic islet tumors not associated with MEN 1.) Two contradictory lines of thought exist as to the management of pancreatic islet cell tumors in MEN 1. First, the pancreatic islet cell tumors are multicentric, malignant about a third of the time, and result in the death of 10 to 20 percent of patients. Second, pancreatic islet tissue is required for insulin production and glucose homeostasis; removal of all pancreatic islets to prevent malignancy will result in diabetes mellitus, a disease with long-term complications equivalent to those of the potential malignancy. These contradictions make it difficult to formulate clear-cut guidelines, but several general concepts appear to be valid. First, surgical removal of islet cell tumors producing insulin, glucagon, VIP, GHRH, or CRH is appropriate, because medical therapy for these disorders is generally ineffective. Second, gastrin-producing islet cell tumors causing ZES can be managed by either surgical or medical approaches. The latter tumors are frequently multicentric, and the surgical cure rate is low. The availability of H-2 receptor antagonists (cimetidine or ranitidine) and an H^+,K^+-ATPase inhibitor (omeprazole) provides effective long-term alternatives to surgery for control of the ulcer diathesis, although high doses are required and the long-term safety of the drugs for this use has not been established. If a single tumor can be identified, a surgical approach seems reasonable in most cases. In patients with multicentric tumors or in those with hepatic metastasis, medical therapy is appropriate. Third, in families in which there is a high incidence of malignant islet cell tumors causing death, total pancreatectomy at an early age may be justified to prevent development of metastatic disease.

Long-term management of metastatic islet cell carcinoma is unsatisfactory. Hormonal abnormalities and their clinical sequelae can sometimes be controlled medically. For example, ZES can be effectively managed with H-2 receptor antagonists or omeprazole. The somatostatin analogue octreotide is useful in the management of carcinoid and the watery diarrhea syndrome but less effective for tumors that secrete gastrin, insulin, or glucagon. Bilateral adrenalectomy may be required for ectopic ACTH syndrome if medical therapy is ineffective (see Chap. 335). The islet cell carcinomas frequently metastasize to the liver but may grow slowly. Hepatic artery embolization may reduce tumor mass in patients with extensive hepatic metastasis, and chemotherapy, although not curative, may reduce tumor mass.

PITUITARY TUMORS   Treatment of prolactin-secreting pituitary tumors with bromocriptine usually returns the serum prolactin level to normal and prevents further tumor growth (see Chap. 331). Surgical removal of a prolactinoma is rarely curative, although surgical debulking may be indicated for large tumors that cause mass effects. Transsphenoidal resection of ACTH- or GH-producing neoplasms may be successful, although serum GH and insulin-like growth factor 1 concentrations may be returned to normal by octreotide therapy. Nonfunctioning tumors or those that produce the alpha subunit of the pituitary glycoprotein hormones are best managed surgically. Radiation therapy may be useful for large or recurrent tumors.

MULTIPLE ENDOCRINE NEOPLASIA TYPE 2   Clinical manifestations   The association of thyroid carcinoma and pheochromocytoma can be subcategorized into two major syndromes (see Table 343-1). Multiple endocrine neoplasia type 2A (MEN 2A) is the combination of medullary thyroid carcinoma, hyperparathyroidism, and pheochromocytoma. Two subvariants of MEN 2A are familial medullary thyroid carcinoma only (FMTC) and MEN 2A in association with cutaneous lichen amyloidosis. Multiple endocrine neoplasia type 2B is the combination of medullary thyroid carcinoma, pheochromocytoma, mucosal neuromas, intestinal ganglioneuromatosis, and marfanoid-like features.

MULTIPLE ENDOCRINE NEOPLASIA TYPE 2A   Medullary thyroid carcinoma is the most common manifestation. The fully developed neoplasm is located characteristically at the junction of the upper one-third and lower two-thirds of each lobe of the thyroid gland and appears grossly as chalky white to yellow lesions; tumors greater than 1 cm in size are frequently associated with local or distant metastasis. This tumor usually develops in childhood, beginning as hyperplasia of the C-cells, or calcitonin-producing cells, of the thyroid. Measurement of the serum calcitonin level after injection of a stimulator of release such as calcium or pentagastrin makes it possible to diagnose this disorder when the likelihood of metastasis is low.

Pheochromocytoma occurs in approximately 50 percent of MEN 2A patients and causes typical symptoms, including palpitations, nervousness, headaches, and sometimes sweating. About half the tumors are bilateral, and in the remainder, the contralateral adrenal normal. More than 50 percent of patients who have had unilateral adrenalectomy develop a pheochromocytoma in the contralateral gland over an 8- to 10-year period. A second characteristic of these pheochromocytomas is the disproportionate increase in epinephrine secretion relative to that of norepinephrine. Patients with minimal abnormalities of epinephrine secretion may be asymptomatic. Finally, capsular invasion is common in pheochromocytoma associated with MEN 2, but malignant behavior is rare.

Primary hyperparathyroidism occurs in 15 to 20 percent of MEN 2A gene carriers, with a peak incidence in the third or fourth decade. In a few families, hyperparathyroidism occurs early and may be significant. The clinical presentation of hyperparathyroidism does not differ from that in other forms of primary hyperparathyroidism (see Chap. 353), with renal nephrolithiasis being common. Diagnosis is established by the finding of hypercalcemia, hypophosphatemia, hypercalciuria, and an inappropriately high serum intact parathyroid hormone concentration. Multiglandular parathyroid hyperplasia is the most common histologic finding, although with long-standing disease adenomatous changes may be superimposed on hyperplasia.

MULTIPLE ENDOCRINE NEOPLASIA TYPE 2B   The association of medullary thyroid carcinoma, pheochromocytoma, mucosal neuromas, a marfanoid habitus, and the absence of hyperparathyroidism is designated MEN 2B. Medullary thyroid carcinoma in MEN 2B is similar to that in MEN 2A except that development of C-cell hyperplasia and microscopic carcinoma occurs early and metastatic disease may be present prior to 1 year of age. Indeed, medullary thyroid carcinoma with MEN 2B commonly causes death in the second or third decade of life. However, the prognosis is not invariably bad even in patients with metastatic disease; a number of multigenerational families with this disorder exist.

Pheochromocytoma occurs in more than half of MEN 2B patients and does not differ significantly from that in MEN 2A. Hypercalcemia is rare in MEN 2B, and most examples of hypercalcemia are thought to be caused by bone metastases.

The mucosal neuromas constitute the most distinctive feature. They are present on the tip of the tongue, under the eyelids, and throughout the gastrointestinal tract and are true neuromas and should be differentiated from the neurofibromas associated with neurofibromatosis. The presence of the neuromas and a marfanoid body habitus form a distinct clinical picture recognizable even in childhood. Children also may present with gastrointestinal symptoms, including increased gas, intermittent obstruction, and diarrhea caused by neuromas.

Genetics and pathophysiology The genetic locus for all four variants of the MEN 2 syndrome has been mapped to the pericentromeric region of chromosome 10, most likely on the proximal long arm (see Fig. 343-1). The nature of the genetic defect is unclear, but the mechanism of tumorigenesis differs from MEN 1 in that there is no evidence for involvement of a "tumor suppressor gene" in the pathogenesis. The hypothesis that best fits the experimental evidence is that a mutation in a single allele of the MEN 2 gene stimulates hyperplasia of the several cell types involved in this syndrome. Subsequent mutational events at other genetic loci on chromosome 1p, 22q, 3p, or 9 may be involved in the progression of the disease.

Treatment SCREENING FOR MULTIPLE ENDOCRINE NEOPLASIA TYPE 2 Death from medullary thyroid carcinoma can be prevented by early thyroidectomy. The currently accepted form of screening utilizes annual pentagastrin or combined pentagastrin-calcium stimulation of calcitonin release from the thyroidal C-cell to identify medullary thyroid carcinoma or its precursor lesion, C-cell hyperplasia, in children before development of metastatic disease. Screening of individuals at risk should begin in early childhood, preferably before age 5. The pentagastrin test involves measurement of serum calcitonin basally and 2, 5, 10, and 15 min after bolus injection of 5 μg pentagastrin per kilogram of body weight. Patients should be warned before injection of epigastric tightness, nausea, warmth, and tingling of extremities and reassured that the symptoms will last approximately 2 min. It is sometimes difficult to differentiate between a mildly abnormal test result in a normal child and the first evidence of abnormality in an affected child. This issue can be resolved either by repetitive pentagastrin testing or by genetic approaches to testing.

The identification of polymorphic DNA sequences closely linked to the MEN 2 locus has made it possible to identify gene carriers with 90 to 99 percent certainty. Genetic testing is not perfect because of the potential for recombination between the disease gene and closely linked polymorphic DNA sequences. For this reason, many investigators utilize both genetic and calcitonin testing to determine which children should undergo thyroidectomy.

Screening studies for pheochromocytoma in subjects at risk should be performed on a regular (usually annual) basis. The goal is to identify a pheochromocytoma before it causes significant symptoms or is likely to cause sudden death, an event most commonly associated with large tumors. The measurement of basal plasma or 12-h urine catecholamines can be performed easily in conjunction with pentagastrin testing. Radiographic studies, such as MRI or CT scans, are generally reserved for individuals with abnormal screening tests or with symptoms suggestive of pheochromocytoma (see Chap. 336).

Measurement of serum calcium and parathyroid hormone levels every 2 to 3 years provides an adequate screen for hyperparathyroidism, except in those families in which hyperparathyroidism is a prominent component, in whom measurements should be made annually.

TREATMENT OF MEDULLARY THYROID CARCINOMA Hereditary medullary thyroid carcinoma is a multicentric disorder. Total thyroidectomy with a central lymph node dissection should be performed in children with abnormal calcitonin responses. More than 90 percent of children in whom thyroidectomy was performed on the basis of calcitonin screening remain without evidence of disease more than 15 years after surgery, whereas 15 to 25 percent of patients in whom the diagnosis is made on the basis of clinical findings die from metastatic disease within 15 years.

In adults with medullary thyroid cancer greater than 1 cm in size, metastases to regional lymph nodes are common. Total thyroidectomy with central lymph node dissection and selective dissection of other regional chains provide the best chance for cure. In patients with significant local metastatic disease, external radiotherapy may prevent local recurrence or reduce tumor mass but does not alter the course. Chemotherapy is also not curative but may reduce tumor mass.

TREATMENT OF PHEOCHROMOCYTOMA The long-term goal for management of pheochromocytoma is to prevent death and cardiovascular complications. Pheochromocytomas detected by screening studies should be removed surgically through an anterior abdominal approach. The major question is whether to remove both adrenal glands at the time of primary surgery or to remove only the affected adrenal. Issues to be considered in making this decision include the possibility of malignancy (fewer than 10 reported cases), the likelihood of development of pheochromocytoma in the apparently unaffected gland (may occur over an 8- to 10-year period), and the risks of adrenal insufficiency caused by removal of both glands. Most but not all clinicians recommend removal only of the affected gland and leave the contralateral gland in place unless inspection during surgery reveals an abnormality. If both adrenals are removed, glucocorticoid and mineralocorticoid replacement is mandatory.

TREATMENT OF HYPERPARATHYROIDISM Hyperparathyroidism has been managed by one of two approaches. Removal of $3\frac{1}{2}$ glands with maintenance of the remaining half gland in the neck is the usual procedure. In families in whom hyperparathyroidism is a prominent manifestation and recurrence is common, total parathyroidectomy with transplantation of parathyroid tissue into the nondominant forearm is the preferred approach. The advantage of the latter approach is the ease of subsequent removal of parathyroid tissue if hypercalcemia recurs.

OTHER GENETIC TUMOR SYNDROMES A number of mixed syndromes exist in which the neoplastic associations differ from those usually found in MEN 1 or 2 (see Table 343-1).

IMMUNOLOGIC SYNDROMES AFFECTING MULTIPLE ENDOCRINE ORGANS

The polyglandular autoimmune syndromes (PGA) are designated type I, type II, and type III (Table 343-2). The type I syndrome starts in childhood and is characterized by mucocutaneous candidiasis, hypoparathyroidism, and adrenal insufficiency. Hypoparathyroidism is unusual in the type II or III syndromes, which are seen in adults. All the syndromes may cause adrenal insufficiency.

POLYGLANDULAR AUTOIMMUNE SYNDROME TYPE I PGA type I usually is recognized in the first decade of life. Although the manifestations vary, ultimately, the triad of mucocutaneous candidiasis, hypoparathyroidism, and adrenal insufficiency is seen. This disorder is also called *autoimmune polyendocrinopathy-candidiasis-ectodermal dystrophy* (APECED). Other features include dystrophy of the dental enamel with hypoplasia of the teeth and nails, vitiligo and keratopathy, gonadal failure, and thyroid or gastric parietal cell dysfunction resulting in primary hypothyroidism or pernicious anemia. Destruction of the β cells of the pancreatic islets and development of insulin-dependent (type I) diabetes are less common than in the type II syndrome. Some patients develop autoimmune hepatitis or malabsorption. At the outset, only one organ

---

TABLE 343-2 Disease associations in polyglandular autoimmune syndromes (PGA)

PGA I	PGA II	PGA III
Mucocutaneous candidiasis	Adrenal insufficiency	Type I diabetes mellitus and autoimmune thyroid disease or adrenal insufficiency and autoimmune thyroid disease (Hashimoto's)
Hypoparathyroidism	Autoimmune thyroid disease	
Addison's	Type I diabetes mellitus	
Hypogonadism	Hypogonadism	
Alopecia	Myasthenia gravis	
Hypothyroidism	Vitiligo	
Malabsorption	Alopecia	
Chronic active hepatitis	Pernicious anemia	
Vitiligo	Celiac disease	
Pernicious anemia		

may be involved, but the number of systems involved increases with time so that patients eventually manifest two to five components of the syndrome.

In a Finnish series, 78 percent of patients had a nonendocrine presentation, with oral candidiasis the most common initial finding. Although candidiasis occurs in most patients, the symptoms are often mild and can easily be missed. Involvement of the parathyroid glands usually occurs before adrenal insufficiency develops. More than 60 percent of postpubertal women become hypogonadal, whereas only about 15 percent of men develop testicular failure. APECED is not a disease of childhood exclusively, since the endocrine components, including adrenal insufficiency or hypoparathyroidism, may not develop until the fourth decade. Thus patients and their families should be followed long term for early detection and treatment of new manifestations of this syndrome.

POLYGLANDULAR AUTOIMMUNE SYNDROME TYPE II   Type I diabetes mellitus is the most common manifestation of PGA type II and occurs in approximately half of affected families. Mucocutaneous candidiasis does not occur. This disorder, which tends to develop later in life than PGA type I, was first described by Schmidt in patients who had lymphocytic infiltration of the adrenal and thyroid glands at autopsy and who had family members with type I diabetes and hypogonadism. The autoimmune thyroid disease causes either Hashimoto's thyroiditis or hyperthyroidism; however, many patients with antimicrosomal and antithyroglobulin antibodies never develop abnormalities of thyroid function. Thus these antibodies alone are poor predictors of future disease. Dermatologic manifestations, including vitiligo, alopecia totalis, and alopecia areata (alopecia occurring in scattered areas), are common. Antibodies against the melanocyte may explain the localized areas of depigmentation. A few patients develop transient hypoparathyroidism with hypocalcemia as the result of antibodies that block the action of parathyroid hormone. Up to 25 percent of patients with myasthenia gravis and an even higher percentage who have myasthenia and a thymoma have polyglandular autoimmune syndrome type II (see Chap. 386).

POLYGLANDULAR AUTOIMMUNE SYNDROME TYPE III   In certain families, abnormalities of only two endocrine glands, either diabetes mellitus and autoimmune thyroid disease or adrenal insufficiency in association with Hashimoto's thyroiditis, occur in a heritable manner. In these families, the syndrome never extends to the full spectrum of organ involvement of the PGA type II syndrome.

GENETICS AND PATHOGENESIS   Type I PGA syndrome shows no HLA associations and is inherited as an autosomal recessive trait. In contrast, the type II and III syndromes are usually associated with the DR3 or DR4 haplotypes, or both, and are inherited as autosomal dominant traits. Epidemiologic studies of twins with either type I diabetes mellitus or Graves' disease revealed that only about 50 percent of the noninvolved identical twins develop these diseases. Thus additional environmental factors must activate the immune disregulation, even in individuals who inherit the tendency to develop the disease. In type I diabetes mellitus and other autoimmune diseases, the concept of molecular mimicry has been advanced to explain how environmental factors may trigger the disease in a genetically susceptible individual. Certain foreign antigens such as rubella viral capsid proteins or cow's milk proteins may share an epitope with a common antigen expressed on the surface of the human β cell. Activation of the immune system by the foreign antigen would initiate an immune attack on both the antigens and result in destruction of the β cell. Anti-insulin and anti-islet cell antibodies have been used in research studies as markers to predict the later development of type I diabetes mellitus. Studies of monozygotic twins or relatives of patients with known type I diabetes have shown that the process of β cell failure may develop slowly, with up to 8 years from the time of antibody detection to the development of hyperglycemia. Patients with the PGA syndromes may have a variety of organ-specific autoantibodies directed against many different target antigens. Some of the antibodies are only markers of autoimmunity and recognize cytoplasmic components of various endocrine cells (antithyroglobulin and antimicrosomal antibodies). However, other antibodies may be disease-specific, like those that fix complement and destroy a particular target or those directed against the acetylcholine, TSH, or parathyroid hormone receptors that interfere with the function of the hormone and thus may cause the various disorders seen in these patients.

Diagnosis and treatment   The clinical manifestations of adrenal insufficiency often develop slowly and may be difficult to detect. The disease can be fatal if not diagnosed and treated appropriately. Thus all patients and family members with the suspected PGA syndromes should be screened prospectively to diagnose and treat the various components of the syndrome in a timely manner. The most effective screening test for adrenal disease is a cosyntropin stimulation test (see Chap. 335). A fasting blood glucose level can be obtained to screen for hyperglycemia. Additional screening tests should include studies of thyroid function, including measurements of thyroid-stimulating hormone and serum thyroxine, measurements of luteinizing hormone (LH), follicle-stimulating hormone (FSH), and testosterone levels in men, and assessment of LH and FSH levels in women. In families with suspected type I PGA syndrome, calcium and phosphorus levels are also measured. These screening studies should be performed every 1 to 2 years up to about age 50 in families with PGA type II and III syndrome and until about age 40 in patients with type I syndrome.

With the exception of Graves' disease, the management of each of the endocrine components of the disease involves hormone replacement and is covered in detail in the chapters on adrenal, thyroid, gonadal, and parathyroid disease (Chaps. 334, 335, 339, 340, and 357). Because primary hypothyroidism can mask adrenal insufficiency by prolonging the half-life of cortisol, administration of thyroid hormone to a patient with unsuspected adrenal insufficiency can precipitate adrenal crisis. Thus one needs to screen for adrenal disease and, if present, to initiate treatment with glucocorticoids prior to or concurrently with the thyroid hormone replacement.

OTHER AUTOIMMUNE ENDOCRINE SYNDROMES   **Insulin receptor antibodies**   Insulin resistance, defined as a decrease in the biologic response to a given amount of insulin, occurs commonly in patients with obesity, severe infections, trauma, or surgery, as well as in individuals with acromegaly or Cushing's syndrome, in whom growth hormone or cortisol excess can antagonize the action of insulin. In contrast, rare insulin-resistance syndromes occur in patients who develop spontaneous antibodies directed against insulin receptor. These antibodies block the normal insulin signal transduction pathway. Conversely, other classes of anti-insulin receptor antibodies can activate the receptor and can cause hypoglycemia and must be considered in the differential diagnosis of fasting hypoglycemia (see Chap. 337).

Anti-insulin receptor antibodies with insulin resistance and acanthosis nigricans, type B insulin resistance   These patients are typically middle-aged women who acquire insulin resistance in association with other autoimmune disorders such as systemic lupus erythematosus or Sjögren's syndrome. Vitiligo, alopecia, Raynaud's phenomenon, and arthritis also may be seen. Other autoimmune endocrine disorders, including hyper- or hypothyroidism and hypogonadism, occur rarely. A mossy, hyperpigmented, thickened skin lesion, typical of acanthosis nigricans, is prominent on the dorsum of the neck and other skin fold areas in the axillae or groin. However, acanthosis nigricans also may occur in patients with obesity or polycystic ovarian syndrome, also associated with insulin resistance, and thus is not diagnostic of this form of insulin resistance. This syndrome is called the *type B insulin resistance syndrome* and must be differentiated from type A insulin resistance syndromes, which are secondary to a variety of molecular defects in the insulin receptor gene that result in mutations which alter insulin receptor signaling.

The anti-insulin receptor antibodies block the interaction of the hormone with its receptor and impair its action to varying degrees. Activation of the receptor by the antibodies also may result in receptor down-regulation and impair insulin action. The degree of insulin resistance can be quite variable. Some patients with acanthosis nigricans show normal to mild glucose intolerance with a compensatory increase in insulin secretion that is only detected when insulin levels are measured. Others have severe diabetes mellitus requiring massive doses of insulin (several thousand units per day) to lower the blood glucose levels. The nature of the antibodies determines the manifestations. Although insulin resistance is more common, fasting hypoglycemia can be present from the first or develop during the course of the disease. The hypoglycemia results from interactions of insulinomimetic classes of antibodies with insulin receptor.

Anti-insulin antibodies and ataxia telangiectasia Ataxia telangiectasia is an autosomal recessive disorder with insulin-resistant diabetes mellitus, ataxia, telangiectasia, immune abnormalities, and an increased incidence of malignancies. This disorder is also associated with anti-insulin antibodies.

Autoimmune insulin syndrome with hypoglycemia Spontaneous polyclonal insulin-binding autoantibodies, typically found in patients with other autoimmune disorders, can bind the insulin released in response to meals and release it later to cause hypoglycemia, often several hours or more after a meal. Fasting hypoglycemia may be caused by release of insulin from these antibodies during a fast. Most cases of the syndrome have been described from Japan, and there may be a genetic component. The anti-insulin antibodies may interfere in the insulin assay and falsely elevate the insulin levels. A finding of normal C-peptide levels in this situation suggests a false-positive insulin measurement. In plasma cell dyscrasias such as multiple myeloma, the plasma cells may produce monoclonal antibodies against insulin and cause hypoglycemia by a similar mechanism.

Antithyroxine antibodies and hypothyroidism Circulating autoantibodies against thyroid hormones in patients with both immune thyroid disease and plasma cell dyscrasias such as Waldenström's macroglobulinemia can bind thyroid hormones, decrease their biologic activity, and result in primary hypothyroidism.

Plasma cell dyscrasia with polyneuropathy, organomegaly, endocrinopathy, M proteins, and skin changes (POEMS syndrome The features of this syndrome are highlighted by an acronyn that emphasizes its important features: *p*olyneuropathy, *o*rganomegaly, *e*ndocrinopathy, *M* proteins, and *s*kin changes (POEMS). The most important feature is a severe, progressive sensorimotor polyneuropathy associated with a plasma cell dyscrasia. Localized collections of plasma cells (plasmacytomas) can cause sclerotic bone lesions and produce monoclonal IgG or IgA proteins. Endocrine manifestations include amenorrhea in women and impotence and gynecomastia in men. Hyperprolactinemia, due to loss of normal inhibitory control of the lactotroph by the hypothalamus, may be associated with other central nervous system manifestations, including papilledema, and increased cerebrospinal fluid pressure and protein. Type II diabetes mellitus occurs commonly, whereas primary hypothyroidism and adrenal insufficiency are less frequent. Skin changes include hyperpigmentation, thickening of the dermis, hirsutism, and hyperhidrosis. Hepatomegaly and lymphadenopathy occur in about two-thirds of the cases, and splenomegaly is seen in about one-third. Other manifestations include peripheral edema, ascites, pleural effusions, and fever.

The systemic nature of the disorder may cause confusion with other connective tissue diseases. The endocrine manifestations suggest an autoimmune basis of the disorder, but circulating antibodies against endocrine cells have not been demonstrated. Thus the pathophysiologic basis for the POEMS syndrome is uncertain. Therapy directed against the plasma cell dyscrasia such as local radiation of bony lesions or chemotherapy may result in improvement.

TABLE 343-3 Other disorders with common polyglandular manifestations

Condition	Clinical features	Hypothalamic-pituitary	Thyroid	Parathyroid	Pancreas	Adrenal	Gonads	Inheritance/molecular defect
Ataxia-telangiectasia	Early ataxia, Oculocutaneous telangiectasia, Immunologic deficiency	Occasional diminished pituitary reserve			Diabetes mellitus	Cortical hypoplasia	Dysgenic gonads: gonadoblastomas in females	Autosomal recessive
Pseudohypoparathyroidism	Short stature, Short metacarpals and metatarsals, Round facies, Ectopic calcification	Variable deficiency of all pituitary hormones including prolactin	Hypo- or hyperthyroidism	Elevated parathyroid hormone levels with normo- or hypocalcemia	Diabetes mellitus		Ovarian failure	Mutation of the GS$_{s\alpha}$ subunit
Myotonic dystrophy	Muscular dystrophy, Premature baldness, Mental retardation	Gonadotropin and growth hormone abnormalities	Hypothyroidism		Diabetes mellitus		Primary gonadal failure	Insertion of unstable CTG repeat in myotonic dystrophy gene on chromosome 19
Noonan syndrome	Short stature, Ptosis, Webbed neck, Pulmonary stenosis	Gonadotropin deficiency	Thyroiditis				Primary gonadal failure	Autosomal dominant
Fanconi syndrome	Short statuure, Bone marrow hypoplasia, Abnormal skin pigmentation, Radial malformations	Panhypopituitarism			Diabetes mellitus	Adrenal atrophy	Gonadal atrophy	Autosomal recessive
Werner syndrome	Premature aging, Atrophic skin, Cataracts, Early osteopenia		Papillary thyroid carcinoma		Diabetes mellitus		Gonadal atrophy	Autosomal recessive

Type of endocrine involvement

Immune nodular adrenal hyperplasia A rare form of Cushing's syndrome, nodular adrenal hyperplasia can occur due to several causes. Some patients have antibodies against the adrenal gland that stimulate adrenal cortical cell growth and result in hyperplasia and excess glucocorticoid production.

MISCELLANEOUS DISORDERS WITH ENDOCRINE MANIFESTATIONS

A variety of other clinical and genetic disorders are associated with multiple endocrine manifestations (Table 343-3).

REFERENCES

AHONEN P et al: Clinical variation of autoimmune polyendocrinopathy-candidiasis-ectodermal dystrophy (APECED) in a series of 68 patients. N Engl J Med 322:1829, 1990

BARDWICK PA et al: Plasma cell dyscrasia with polyneuropathy, organomegaly, endocrinopathy, M protein, and skin changes: The POEMS syndrome. Medicine 59:311, 1980

FRIEDMAN E et al: Clonality of parathyroid tumors in familial multiple endocrine neoplasia type 1. N Engl J Med 321:213, 1989

GAGEL RF: Multiple endocrine neoplasia, in William's Textbook of Endocrinology, 8th ed, JD Wilson, DW Foster (eds). Philadelphia, Saunders, 1992, pp 1537–1553

—— et al: The clinical outcome of prospective screening for multiple endocrine neoplasia type 2a: An 18-year experience. N Engl J Med 318:478, 1988

KAHN CR et al: The syndromes of insulin resistance and acanthosis nigricans: Insulin-receptor disorders in man. N Engl J Med 294:739, 1976

LARSSON C et al: Multiple endocrine neoplasia type 1 gene maps to chromosome 11 and is lost in insulinoma. Nature 322:85, 1988

NEUFELD M et al: Two types of autoimmune Addison's disease associated with different polyglandular autoimmune (PGA) syndromes. Medicine 60:355, 1981

RIZZOLI R et al: Primary hyperparathyroidism in familial multiple endocrine neoplasia type I: Long-term follow-up of serum calcium levels after parathyroidectomy. Am J Med 78:467, 1985

SIMPSON NE: The exploration of the locus or loci for the syndromes associated with medullary thyroid cancer (MTC) on chromosome 10, in Hereditary Tumors, ML Brandi, R White (eds). New York, Raven, 1991, pp 55–67

SKOGSEID B et al: Multiple endocrine neoplasia type 1: A 10-year prospective screening study in four kindreds. J Clin Endocrinol Metab 73:281, 1991

section 2   Disorders of intermediary metabolism

344   THE HYPERLIPOPROTEINEMIAS AND OTHER DISORDERS OF LIPID METABOLISM

MICHAEL S. BROWN / JOSEPH L. GOLDSTEIN

The *hyperlipoproteinemias* are disturbances of lipid transport that result from accelerated synthesis or retarded degradation of lipoproteins that transport cholesterol and triglycerides through plasma. Elevated plasma lipoprotein levels are important clinically because they can cause two life-threatening diseases: atherosclerosis and pancreatitis. A reduction in cholesterol-carrying lipoproteins, achieved by diet and drugs, reduces the risk of myocardial infarction in subjects with hyperlipoproteinemia. Some hyperlipoproteinemias are the direct result of *primary* defects in the synthesis or degradation of lipoprotein

particles. Other hyperlipoproteinemias are *secondary*; that is, the elevated plasma lipoprotein level occurs as part of a constellation of abnormalities caused by an underlying disorder in a related metabolic system, such as thyroid hormone deficiency or insulin deficiency. The primary hyperlipoproteinemias can be divided into two broad categories: (1) *single-gene disorders* that are transmitted by simple dominant or recessive mechanisms and (2) *multifactorial disorders* with complex inheritance patterns in which multiple variant genes, each having a subtle effect, interact with environmental factors to produce varying degrees of hyperlipoproteinemia in members of a family.

ROLE OF LIPOPROTEINS IN LIPID TRANSPORT The lipoproteins are globular particles of high molecular weight that transport nonpolar lipids (primarily *triglycerides* and *cholesteryl esters*) through the plasma. A general model for the structure of a lipoprotein particle is shown in Fig. 344-1. Each lipoprotein particle contains a nonpolar *core*, in which many molecules of hydrophobic lipid are packed to form an oil droplet. This hydrophobic core, which accounts for most

FIGURE 344-1 *A.* Diagrammatic representation of the structure of a typical plasma lipoprotein particle. The *core* of the spherical lipoprotein particle is composed of two nonpolar lipids, triglyceride and cholesteryl ester, which are present in different lipoproteins in varying amounts. The nonpolar core is surrounded by a *surface coat* composed primarily of phospholipids. Apoproteins are exposed at the surface and extend into the core. Variable amounts of unesterified cholesterol are interdigitated with the phospholipids of the surface coat. The composition of the five major classes of lipoproteins in human plasma is summarized in Table 344-1. *B.* Two nonpolar lipids, triglyceride and cholesteryl ester. For them to be assimilated into tissues, the ester bonds between the fatty acids and either glycerol (triglycerides) or cholesterol (cholesteryl esters) must be broken by lipoprotein lipase and the lysosomal cholesterol esterase, respectively.

TABLE 344-1   Characteristics of the major classes of lipoproteins in human plasma

Lipoprotein class	Major lipids	Major apoproteins	Density, g/mL	Diameter, nm	Electrophoretic mobility
Chylomicrons and remnants	Dietary triglycerides	AI, AII, B48, CI, CII, CIII, E	<1.006	800–5000	Remains at origin
VLDL	Endogenous triglyc-erides	B100, CI, CII, CIII, E	<1.006	300–800	Pre-β
IDL	Cholesteryl esters, tri-glycerides	B100, CIII, E	<1.019	250–350	Slow pre-β
LDL	Cholesteryl esters	B100	1.019–1.063	180–280	β
HDL	Cholesteryl esters	AI, AII	1.063–1.210	50–120	α

of the mass of the particle, consists of triglycerides and cholesteryl esters in varying proportions. Surrounding the core is a polar *surface coat* of phospholipids that stabilize the lipoprotein particle so that it can remain in solution in the plasma. In addition to phospholipids, the polar coat contains small amounts of unesterified cholesterol. Each lipoprotein particle also contains specific proteins (termed *apoproteins*) that are exposed at the surface. The apoproteins bind to specific enzymes or transport proteins on cell membranes, thus directing the lipoprotein to its sites of metabolism.

Table 344-1 describes the characteristics of the five major classes of lipoproteins that normally circulate in human plasma. These lipoprotein classes differ in the composition of the nonpolar lipids in the core, in the composition of the apoproteins, and in density, size, and electrophoretic mobility.

Lipid transport: The exogenous pathway   Figure 344-2 shows the pathways by which lipoproteins transport lipids in plasma. The largest amounts of lipoproteins are involved in the transport of dietary fat, which amounts to more than 100 g triglyceride and about 1 g cholesterol per day. Within intestinal epithelial cells, dietary triglycerides and cholesterol are incorporated into large lipoprotein particles called *chylomicrons*. The chylomicrons are secreted into the intestinal lymph and pass into the general circulation for transport to the capillaries of adipose tissue and skeletal muscle, where they adhere to binding sites on the capillary walls. While bound to these endothelial surfaces, the chylomicrons are exposed to the enzyme *lipoprotein lipase*. The chylomicrons contain an apoprotein, apoprot-

ein CII, that activates the lipase, liberating free fatty acids and monoglycerides (Fig. 344-3). The fatty acids pass through the endothelial cells and enter the underlying adipocytes or muscle cells, where they are either reesterified to triglycerides or oxidized.

After the core triglycerides have been removed, the remainder of the chylomicron dissociates from the capillary endothelium and reenters the circulation. It has now been transformed into a particle that is relatively poor in triglyceride and enriched in cholesteryl esters. It also has undergone an exchange of apoproteins with other plasma lipoproteins. The net result is the conversion of the chylomicron to a *chylomicron remnant particle*, enriched in cholesteryl esters and apoproteins B48 and E. This remnant travels to the liver, where it is taken up with great efficiency. This uptake is mediated by the binding of apoprotein E to specific receptors, called *chylomicron remnant receptors*, on the surface of the hepatocytes. The surface-bound remnants are taken into the cell and degraded within lysosomes by a process called receptor-mediated endocytosis (see Fig. 344-3). The overall result of the chylomicron transport process is to deliver dietary triglyceride to adipose tissue and cholesterol to the liver.

Some of the cholesterol that reaches the liver is converted to bile acids, which are excreted into the intestine to act as detergents and facilitate the absorption of dietary fat. In addition, some cholesterol is excreted into the bile without metabolism to bile acids. The liver also distributes cholesterol to other tissues by the endogenous pathway, which is discussed below.

Lipid transport: The endogenous pathway   Triglyceride synthesis in the liver is enhanced when the diet contains excess carbohydrates. The liver converts the carbohydrate to fatty acids, esterifies the fatty acids with glycerol to form triglycerides, and secretes the triglyceride into the bloodstream in the core of *very low density lipoprotein (VLDL)*. The VLDL particles are relatively large, carry 5 to 10 times more triglycerides than cholesteryl esters, and contain a form of apoprotein B, designated B100, that differs from the apoprotein B48 of chylomicrons (see Table 344-1).

The VLDL particles are transported to tissue capillaries, where they interact with the same lipoprotein lipase enzyme that catabolizes chylomicrons. The core triglycerides of the VLDL particles are hydrolyzed, and the fatty acids are used for triglyceride synthesis within adipose tissue. The remnants generated from the action of lipoprotein-lipase on VLDLs are designated *intermediate-density lipoprotein (IDL)*. A portion of the IDL particles is catabolized by the liver through binding to receptors called *low-density lipoprotein (LDL) receptors*, which are distinct from the chylomicron remnant receptors. The remaining IDLs remain in plasma, where they undergo a further transformation in which nearly all the residual triglycerides are removed. During this conversion, all the apoproteins are removed from the particle with the exception of apoprotein B100. The result is the transformation of the IDL particle into cholesterol-rich LDL. The core of LDL is composed almost entirely of cholesteryl esters, and the surface coat contains only one apoprotein, apoprotein B100. In humans, a relatively high fraction of IDL escapes hepatic uptake, and consequently, humans have relatively high circulating levels of LDL. Indeed, about three-fourths of the total cholesterol in normal human plasma is contained within LDL particles.

FIGURE 344-2   Model for plasma triglyceride and cholesterol transport in humans. The details of this model are described in the text. VLDL, very low density lipoprotein; IDL, intermediate-density lipoprotein; LDL, low-density lipoprotein; HDL, high-density lipoprotein; LCAT, lecithin:cholesterol acyltransferase; LP lipase, lipoprotein lipase; FFA, free fatty acids. The major apoprotein for each class of lipoproteins is shown. Other apoproteins are also present, and these are listed in Table 344-1.

A. Extracellular Digestion of Triglyceride-rich Lipoproteins

B. Receptor-mediated Endocytosis of Cholesterol-rich Lipoproteins

FIGURE 344-3 Comparison of the mechanisms by which triglyceride-rich lipoproteins and cholesterol-rich lipoproteins deliver their core lipids to target tissues. Triglycerides are hydrolyzed by an extracellular enzyme (LPL) that is attached to endothelial cells and operates at the endothelial surface. Cholesteryl esters are hydrolyzed by an intracellular enzyme, acid lipase, that is located in lysosomes and cleaves the esters that enter cells via receptor-mediated endocytosis. TG, triglycerides; LPL, lipoprotein lipase; VLDL, very low density lipoproteins; CE, cholesteryl esters; IDL, intermediate-density lipoproteins; LDL, low-density lipoproteins; FFA, free fatty acid. The apoproteins responsible for the interactions (CII, B, and E) are indicated.

One function of LDL is to supply cholesterol to a variety of extrahepatic parenchymal cells, such as adrenal cortical cells, lymphocytes, and renal cells. These cells have *LDL receptors* localized on the cell surface. LDL that binds to this receptor is taken up by receptor-mediated endocytosis and digested by lysosomes within the cells (see Fig. 344-3). The cholesteryl esters of LDL are hydrolyzed by a lysosomal cholesteryl esterase (acid lipase), and the liberated cholesterol is used for membrane synthesis, as a precursor for steroid hormone synthesis, and as a regulatory molecule that suppresses the synthesis of new LDL receptors. Like extrahepatic tissues, the liver also has abundant LDL receptors; it uses the LDL-cholesterol for synthesis of bile acids and for generation of free cholesterol, which is secreted into the bile. In humans, 70 to 80 percent of LDL is removed from plasma by the LDL receptor pathway. Much of the remainder is degraded by a scavenger cell system in phagocytic cells in the reticuloendothelial system. In contrast to the receptor-mediated pathway for LDL degradation, the scavenger cell pathway is thought to function solely to degrade LDL when the lipoprotein reaches high concentrations in plasma rather than to supply cholesterol to cells.

As the membranes of parenchymal and scavenger cells undergo turnover and as cells die and are renewed, unesterified cholesterol is released into plasma, where it binds initially to *high-density lipoprotein (HDL)*. This unesterified cholesterol is then coupled to a fatty acid in an esterification reaction catalyzed by the plasma enzyme *lecithin:cholesterol acyltransferase (LCAT)*. The cholesteryl esters that are formed on the surface of HDL are transferred to VLDL and eventually appear in LDL. This establishes a cycle by which LDL delivers cholesterol to extrahepatic cells and by which cholesterol is returned to LDL from extrahepatic cells via HDL. Most of the cholesterol released from extrahepatic tissues is transported to the liver for excretion in the bile.

DIAGNOSIS OF HYPERLIPOPROTEINEMIA A number of diseases cause elevations in the concentrations of one or more lipoprotein classes in plasma. In general, these abnormalities are detected by the finding of an elevated concentration of triglycerides or cholesterol in fasting plasma, a condition called *hyperlipidemia*. The value for plasma cholesterol represents the total cholesterol, which includes both cholesteryl esters and unesterified cholesterol. The plasma cholesterol and triglyceride levels provide information regarding the nature of the lipoprotein particle that is increased. An isolated elevation in plasma triglycerides indicates that the concentrations of chylomicrons or VLDL are increased. On the other hand, an isolated elevation of plasma cholesterol nearly always indicates that the concentration of LDL is increased. Frequently, both triglycerides and

cholesterol are elevated. Such a combined abnormality may be produced by a marked elevation in chylomicrons or VLDL, in which case the ratio of triglyceride to cholesterol in plasma will be greater than 5:1. Alternatively, there may be an elevation of both VLDL and LDL, in which case the triglyceride/cholesterol ratio in plasma is usually less than 5:1.

The definition of hyperlipoproteinemia is arbitrary because plasma lipid and lipoprotein levels exhibit a bell-shaped distribution in the population, without clear separation between normal and abnormal values. Since lipoprotein concentrations are influenced by diet and other environmental factors, standards must be established for the population under consideration. Usually, arbitrary statistical limits of normal concentrations are selected, based on the examination of a large number of healthy-appearing subjects of different ages. The usual cut-off limit is the upper 5 to 10 percent of values (i.e., the 90th to 95th percentile values). However, analysis of blood lipid levels in individuals from industrialized and more agrarian cultures indicates that lipid and lipoprotein concentrations that are "normal" in a statistical sense are not necessarily healthy. As a working rule, hyperlipoproteinemia is considered to be present whenever the plasma cholesterol level exceeds 5.2 mmol/L (200 mg/dL) or the triglyceride level exceeds 2.2 mmol/L (200 mg/dL).

The various combinations of elevated lipoproteins that occur in disease states have been divided into six lipoprotein types or patterns (Table 344-2). Most of the lipoprotein types can be caused by several different genetic diseases (Table 344-3); conversely, some genetic diseases can produce more than one lipoprotein type. In addition, each of the abnormal lipoprotein types can occur as a secondary

TABLE 344-2 Patterns of lipoprotein elevation in plasma (lipoprotein types)

Lipoprotein pattern	Major elevation in plasma	
	Lipoprotein	Lipid
Type 1	Chylomicrons	Triglycerides
Type 2a	LDL	Cholesterol
Type 2b	LDL and VLDL	Cholesterol and triglycerides
Type 3	Chylomicron remnants and IDL	Triglycerides and cholesterol
Type 4	VLDL	Triglycerides
Type 5	VLDL and chylomicrons	Triglycerides and cholesterol

TABLE 344-3   Characteristics of the primary hyperlipoproteinemias resulting from single-gene mutations

Genetic disorder	Primary biochemical defect	Plasma lipoprotein elevation (pattern)	Typical clinical findings	Lipoprotein pattern in affected relatives	Drug therapy First choice	Other
Familial lipoprotein lipase deficiency	Deficiency of lipoprotein lipase	Chylomicrons (1)	Eruptive xanthomas, pancreatitis	1	None	None
Familial apoprotein CII deficiency	Deficiency of apoprotein CII	Chylomicrons and VLDL (1 or 5)	Pancreatitis	1 or 5	None	None
Familial type 3 hyperlipoproteinemia	Abnormal apoprotein E of VLDL	Chylomicron remnants and IDL (3)	Palmar and tuberous xanthomas; premature atherosclerosis	3, 2a, 2b, or 4	Gemfibrozil	Nicotinic acid; HMG CoA reductase inhibitor
Familial hypercholesterolemia	Deficiency of LDL receptor	LDL (2a, rarely 2b)	Tendon xanthomas; premature atherosclerosis	2a (rarely 2b)	Bile acid–binding resin plus HMG CoA reductase inhibitor	Nicotinic acid; probucol
Familial hypertriglyceridemia	Unknown	VLDL (rarely chylomicrons) (4, rarely 5)	Premature atherosclerosis (eruptive xanthomas, rarely)	4 (rarely 5)	Gemfibrozil; nicotinic acid	
Multiple lipoprotein–type hyperlipidemia (familial combined hyperlipidemia)	Unknown	LDL and VLDL (2a, 2b, or 4, rarely 5)		2a, 2b, or 4 (rarely 5)	Gemfibrozil; nicotinic acid	HMG CoA reductase inhibitor

consequence of another metabolic disease (Table 344-4). Hence the lipoprotein type must be considered a shorthand notation to describe an abnormal lipoprotein pattern in plasma and not a designation of a specific disease.

Ordinarily, the simple measurement of plasma lipid levels, coupled with a clinical assessment, is sufficient to classify the type of lipoprotein abnormality present (see Table 344-2). Occasionally, electrophoresis of the plasma on agarose gels is useful either when an elevation in remnant particles is suspected (type 3 lipoprotein pattern giving a "broad beta" band on electrophoresis) or when chylomicronemia is a possibility (type 1 pattern). When the total cholesterol level exceeds 6.2 mmol/L (240 mg/dL), HDL levels should be measured, since low levels of this lipoprotein class are statistically associated with an increased risk of myocardial infarction (see Chap. 208). The level of HDL can be estimated in clinical laboratories using standardized lipoprotein separation techniques.

THERAPEUTIC APPROACHES   The first approach for treatment of all hyperlipoproteinemias is dietary. Individuals who are overweight should be placed on a weight-reducing regimen. Virtually all patients with hyperlipoproteinemia, either primary or secondary, can be treated with a single diet that is low in cholesterol and saturated animal fats and relatively (but not absolutely) high in polyunsaturated vegetable oils, which reduce concentrations of plasma LDL.

The second therapeutic aim is to eliminate aggravating factors, such as diabetes mellitus, alcoholism, or hypothyroidism. Patients with hyperlipoproteinemia also should be encouraged to reduce all other risk factors that predispose to atherosclerosis. These include cessation of smoking, treatment of hypertension, maintenance of a good exercise and physical fitness program, and control of blood glucose in subjects with diabetes mellitus (see Chap. 208).

The final aspect of therapy involves the use of drugs that lower plasma concentrations of lipoproteins, either by decreasing their production or by increasing their removal from plasma. The drugs available for this purpose are discussed below.

PRIMARY HYPERLIPOPROTEINEMIAS RESULTING FROM SINGLE-GENE MUTATIONS

FAMILIAL LIPOPROTEIN LIPASE DEFICIENCY   This rare autosomal recessive disorder is attributable to the absence or marked reduction in the activity of the enzyme lipoprotein lipase. This deficiency leads to a metabolic block in the metabolism of chylomi-

crons, causing these lipoproteins to accumulate to massive levels in plasma.

Clinical features   The disease usually presents in infancy or childhood with recurrent attacks of abdominal pain. The pain is caused by pancreatitis occurring as a consequence of the massive elevation of chylomicrons in plasma. Affected individuals intermittently develop eruptive xanthomas, small yellowish papules, frequently surrounded by an erythematous base, that appear predominantly on the buttocks and other pressure-sensitive surfaces. The xanthomas are caused by the deposition of large amounts of chylomicron triglycerides in cutaneous histiocytes. Triglycerides are also deposited in phagocytes of the reticuloendothelial system, producing hepatomegaly, splenomegaly, and foam cell infiltration of the bone marrow. When the level of chylomicrons in the blood is massively elevated [i.e., plasma triglyceride level greater than 22 mmol/L (2000 mg/dL)], the blood appears pale and creamy and is said to be *lipemic*. When viewed with the ophthalmoscope, the retina is pale, and the retinal vessels are white, producing the appearance of lipemia retinalis. Despite the massive elevation of plasma triglycerides, accelerated atherosclerosis does not occur.

Pathogenesis   Affected individuals have two copies of a mutant lipoprotein lipase gene. The activator of lipoprotein lipase, apoprotein CII, is present in normal amounts. The parents are obligate heterozygotes for the lipoprotein lipase defect, but they are usually normal clinically. As a result of the deficiency of lipoprotein lipase in homozygotes, chylomicrons cannot be metabolized normally, and the level of chylomicrons in the blood rises to high levels after a fat meal. In normal individuals, chylomicrons disappear from the blood after a 12-h fast. However, in affected patients, high levels of chylomicrons are found in the plasma even after several days of fasting or ingestion of a fat-free diet.

The circulating chylomicrons inflame the pancreas when they pass through its capillaries. Within the capillary lumen in the pancreas, chylomicrons are exposed to small amounts of pancreatic lipase that leaks from the tissue. Partial hydrolysis of the triglycerides and phospholipids of the chylomicron produces toxic products, including fatty acids and lysolecithin, that break down tissue membranes, produce further leakage of lipase from the pancreatic acinar cells, and eventually cause fulminant pancreatitis.

Diagnosis   The diagnosis of familial lipoprotein lipase deficiency is suggested by the finding of lipemic plasma in a young individual who has been fasting for at least 12 h. This lipemic plasma, when collected in the presence of EDTA, has a characteristic appearance

TABLE 344-4   Clinical disorders associated with secondary hyperlipoproteinemia

Underlying disorder	Plasma lipoprotein elevation				Lipoprotein type	Proposed mechanism for hyperlipoproteinemia	Associated abnormality of carbohydrate metabolism
	Chylomicrons	IDL	VLDL	LDL			
ENDOCRINE AND METABOLIC							
Diabetes mellitus	+		+ + +		4 (rarely 5)	Increased secretion of VLDL Decreased catabolism of VLDL and chylomicrons due to reduced lipoprotein lipase activity	Insulin deficiency or resistance
von Gierke's disease (glycogen storage disease, type I)	+		+ + +		4 (rarely 5)	Increased secretion of VLDL Decreased catabolism of VLDL and chylomicrons due to reduced lipoprotein lipase activity	Hypoglycemia with decreased insulin secretion
Lipodystrophies (congenital and acquired forms)			+ +		4	Increased secretion of VLDL	Insulin resistance
Cushing's syndrome			+	+ +	2a or 2b	Increased secretion of VLDL with conversion to LDL	Insulin resistance
Sexual ateliotic dwarfism (isolated growth hormone deficiency)			+ +	+ +	2b	Increased secretion of VLDL with conversion to LDL	Insulin deficiency or resistance
Acromegaly			+		4	Increased secretion of VLDL	Insulin resistance
Hypothyroidism		+		+ + +	2a (rarely 3)	Decreased catabolism of VLDL and IDL	
Anorexia nervosa				+ +	2a	Reduced biliary excretion of cholesterol and bile acids	
Werner's syndrome				+ +	2a	Unknown	Insulin resistance
Acute intermittent porphyria				+ +	2a	Unknown	
DRUG-INDUCED							
Alcohol	+		+ + +		4 (rarely 5)	Increased secretion of VLDL in individuals genetically predisposed to hypertriglyceridemia	
Oral contraceptives	+		+ + +		4 (rarely 5)	Increased secretion of VLDL in individuals genetically predisposed to hypertriglyceridemia	Insulin resistance
Glucocorticoids			+	+ +	2a or 2b	Increased secretion of VLDL with conversion to LDL	Insulin resistance
RENAL							
Uremia			+ + +		4	Decreased catabolism of VLDL due to reduced lipoprotein lipase activity	Insulin resistance
Nephrotic syndrome			+ +	+ + +	2a or 2b	Increased secretion of VLDL Direct secretion of LDL from liver Decreased catabolism of VLDL and LDL	
HEPATIC							
Primary biliary cirrhosis and extrahepatic biliary obstruction					↑ Cholesterol ↑ Phospholipids ↑ Lipoprotein X	Diversion of biliary cholesterol and phospholipids into bloodstream	
Acute hepatitis (nonfulminant)			+ + +		4	Decreased hepatic secretion of lecithin: cholesterol acyltransferase (LCAT)	

TABLE 344-4 Clinical disorders associated with secondary hyperlipoproteinemia (continued)

Underlying disorder	Plasma lipoprotein elevation				Lipoprotein type	Proposed mechanism for hyperlipoproteinemia	Associated abnormality of carbohydrate metabolism
	Chylomicrons	IDL	VLDL	LDL			
HEPATIC (continued)							
Hepatoma				+ +	2a	Lack of feedback inhibition of hepatic cholesterol synthesis by dietary cholesterol	
IMMUNOLOGIC							
Systemic lupus erythematosus	+ +				1	Presence of IgG or IgM that binds heparin, thereby decreasing activity of lipoprotein lipase	
Monoclonal gammopathies (myeloma, macroglobulinemia, lymphoma)	+ +	+ +	+ +		3 or 4	Presence of IgG or IgM that forms immune complex with chylomicron remnants and/or VLDL, thereby decreasing their catabolism	
STRESS-INDUCED							
Emotional stress, acute myocardial infarction, extensive burns, acute gram-negative sepsis			+ +		4	Increased secretion and decreased catabolism of VLDL	

after it has incubated overnight in a refrigerator at 4°C. A white layer of cream (which consists of chylomicrons) appears at the top of the tube. The layer beneath the cream is clear. The diagnosis of familial lipoprotein lipase deficiency is supported by the finding of a type 1 pattern on lipoprotein electrophoresis. It is confirmed by the demonstration that lipoprotein lipase levels in plasma fail to increase following the infusion of heparin. In normal individuals, intravenous heparin releases lipoprotein lipase from its binding sites within the capillary endothelium, and increased amounts of enzyme can then be assayed in the plasma. Gel electrophoresis of VLDL apoproteins in patients with lipoprotein lipase deficiency shows a normal amount of activator apoprotein CII, thus distinguishing these patients from those with the related disorder, familial apoprotein CII deficiency (see below).

Treatment The symptoms and signs of the disease recede when the patient is placed on a fat-free diet. Every attempt should be made to maintain the fasting plasma triglyceride level below 11 mmol/L (1000 mg/dL) to prevent pancreatitis. It has been found empirically that the chronic fat intake in affected adults must be less than 20 g/d to prevent symptomatic hyperlipemia. Since medium-chain triglycerides are not incorporated into chylomicrons, they have been employed to help achieve normal caloric intake. The diet should be supplemented with fat-soluble vitamins.

FAMILIAL APOPROTEIN CII DEFICIENCY This rare autosomal recessive disorder is due to the absence of apoprotein CII, an essential cofactor for lipoprotein lipase. Deficiency of this peptide creates a functional lipoprotein lipase deficiency, thus producing a syndrome that is similar but not identical to familial lipoprotein lipase deficiency (see above). Because of the apoprotein CII deficiency, lipoprotein lipase is not activated, and its two substrate lipoproteins, chylomicrons and VLDL, accumulate in the blood, thus causing hypertriglyceridemia (type 1 or type 5 lipoprotein pattern). The disorder is diagnosed in children or adults on the basis of recurrent attacks of pancreatitis or by milky plasma detected by chance. The diagnosis is made by showing an absence of apoprotein CII on gel electrophoresis of VLDL apoproteins. Transfusion of normal plasma (which contains abundant

apoprotein CII) into the patient is followed by a dramatic fall in plasma triglyceride levels. Heterozygotes, who have 50 percent reduction in apoprotein CII levels, may exhibit slightly elevated triglyceride concentrations but do not have pancreatitis. Treatment involves use of a fat-restricted diet throughout life. In case of severe pancreatitis, transfusion of 1 or 2 units of normal plasma is helpful. As compared with patients with familial lipoprotein lipase deficiency, subjects with homozygous apoprotein CII deficiency are generally detected at a later age, accumulate more VLDL in their plasma, and rarely show cutaneous eruptive xanthomas. The reason for these clinical differences is not known.

FAMILIAL TYPE 3 HYPERLIPOPROTEINEMIA This is an inherited disorder in which the plasma concentrations of both cholesterol and triglycerides are elevated owing to the accumulation in plasma of remnant-like particles derived from the partial catabolism of VLDL. Also called *familial dysbetalipoproteinemia*, the disorder is transmitted by a single-gene mechanism, but its expression appears to require the presence of contributory environmental and/or genetic factors (discussed below).

Clinical features Affected individuals characteristically do not manifest hyperlipidemia or any clinical feature of the disease until after age 20. A unique clinical feature is the occurrence of two types of cutaneous xanthomas: xanthoma striata palmaris, which appear as orange or yellow discolorations of the palmar and digital creases, and tuberous or tuberoeruptive xanthomas, which are bulbous cutaneous xanthomas that may vary from pea to lemon size. The tuberous xanthomas are characteristically located over the elbows and knees. Xanthelasmas of the eyelids also occur but are not unique to this disorder (see "Familial Hypercholesterolemia," below).

Severe and fulminant atherosclerosis involves the coronary arteries, the internal carotids, and the abdominal aorta and its branches. The sequelae include premature myocardial infarctions, strokes, intermittent claudication, and gangrene of the lower extremities. Patients who develop clinical manifestations of this disorder often have hypothyroidism, obesity, or diabetes mellitus as aggravating factors.

Pathogenesis The hyperlipidemia is caused by the accumulation of large lipoprotein particles that contain both triglycerides and cholesteryl esters. These particles consist of chylomicron remnants produced from the catabolism of chylomicrons and IDL produced from the catabolism of VLDL through the action of lipoprotein lipase. In normal subjects, chylomicron remnant particles are rapidly taken up by the liver, and hence they are barely detectable in plasma. A portion of the IDL is also taken up by the liver, while the rest is converted to LDL. In patients with type 3 hyperlipoproteinemia, the uptake of IDL and chylomicron remnants by the liver is blocked, and these lipoproteins accumulate to high levels in plasma and tissues, producing xanthomas and atherosclerosis.

The mutation responsible for this disease involves the gene that encodes the structure of apoprotein E, a protein normally found in IDL and chylomicron remnants. This protein binds with very high affinity to both the chylomicron remnant receptor and the LDL receptor. Apoprotein E thus mediates the rapid uptake of chylomicron remnants and IDL by the liver. The gene for apoprotein E is polymorphic in the population. There are three common alleles, designated E^2, E^3, and E^4, with approximate frequencies of 0.12, 0.75, and 0.13 in the population. Each allele specifies a distinctive form of apoprotein E that differs from the others by a single amino acid substitution. This structural alteration allows each protein to be detected by isoelectric focusing. The three alleles create six genotypes: E^2/E^2, E^3/E^3, E^4/E^4, E^2/E^3, E^2/E^4, and E^3/E^4. Type 3 hyperlipoproteinemia occurs only in individuals who are homozygous for the E^2 allele (genotype E^2/E^2). The protein produced by the E^2 allele is defective in its ability to bind to the liver receptors that mediate uptake of chylomicron remnants and IDL, as a result of which these particles accumulate in plasma.

The frequency of the E^2/E^2 genotype in the population is about 1 in 100. Yet the frequency of type 3 hyperlipoproteinemia is only about 1 in 10,000. Thus only 1 percent of the individuals having genotype E^2/E^2 have symptomatic disease. Familial type 3 hyperlipoproteinemia occurs only in those individuals who are homozygous for the E^2 allele and who are also unable to compensate for the abnormal function of the E protein. The inability to compensate may be caused by the independent inheritance of another defect in lipoprotein metabolism, such as familial hypercholesterolemia or multiple lipoprotein–type hyperlipoproteinemia (see below). When an individual is a heterozygote for one of these dominant diseases and is also homozygous for the E^2 allele, he or she expresses the syndrome of type 3 hyperlipoproteinemia. The expression of hyperlipoproteinemia is also brought out when an individual of genotype E^2/E^2 develops hypothyroidism, diabetes mellitus, or obesity. It should be emphasized that heterozygotes for the E^2 allele never show the clinical syndrome of familial type 3 hyperlipoproteinemia.

In addition to the relatively common E^2 allele, rare mutant alleles also occur at the apo E locus. Some of these produce autosomal dominant as well as recessive forms of type 3 hyperlipoproteinemia.

Diagnosis The diagnosis is suggested by the finding of palmar or tuberous xanthomas in a patient with elevated plasma levels of both cholesterol and triglyceride. Approximately 80 percent of symptomatic patients exhibit these xanthomas. The diagnosis is also suggested when a moderate elevation in the plasma concentration of both cholesterol and triglyceride occurs in such a way that the absolute concentrations of cholesterol and triglyceride are similar [e.g., the plasma cholesterol is about 7.8 mmol/L (300 mg/dL) and the triglyceride level is about 3.4 mmol/L (300 mg/dL)]. However, this finding does not always hold true and becomes especially unreliable when the disease is in severe exacerbation, in which case the plasma triglyceride level tends to rise higher than the cholesterol level.

The diagnosis is supported by the finding of a so-called broad beta band on lipoprotein electrophoresis (type 3 pattern). This appearance results from the presence of chylomicron remnants and IDL. The diagnosis can be established in specialized laboratories by two procedures. First, the plasma can be subjected to ultracentrifugation, and the chemical composition of the VLDL fraction can be measured. In affected patients, the VLDL fraction contains IDL and chylomicron remnants that have a relatively high ratio of cholesterol to triglyceride. Second, the diagnosis can be confirmed by the finding of homozygosity for the E^2 allele on isoelectric focusing of the proteins extracted from the remnant particles.

Treatment A vigorous search for occult hypothyroidism should be made, including measurement of plasma thyroid-stimulating hormone (TSH) levels. If hypothyroidism exists, levothyroxine should be instituted. Patients who have hypothyroidism show a dramatic lowering of lipid levels with treatment. In addition, attempts should be made to control obesity and diabetes mellitus through diet and insulin treatment. If these measures are not successful, patients with type 3 hyperlipoproteinemia should be treated with a fibric acid, such as gemfibrozil or clofibrate. Affected patients usually show a dramatic and sustained reduction in plasma lipid levels when treated with these drugs. Nicotinic acid may be effective in the severely hyperlipidemic patient who does not respond to gemfibrozil or clofibrate.

FAMILIAL HYPERCHOLESTEROLEMIA This common autosomal dominant disorder affects approximately 1 in every 500 persons. It is caused by a mutation in the gene for the LDL receptor. Heterozygotes manifest a two- to threefold elevation in the concentration of total plasma cholesterol which is attributable to an elevation in the level of LDL. Patients with two mutant LDL receptor genes (called *familial hypercholesterolemia homozygotes*) have six- to eightfold elevations in plasma LDL-cholesterol levels.

Clinical features Heterozygotes with familial hypercholesterolemia can be diagnosed at birth because their umbilical cord blood contains a two- to threefold increase in the concentration of LDL and hence a similar increase in total cholesterol. The elevated levels of plasma LDL persist throughout life, but symptoms typically do not develop until the third or fourth decade. The most important feature is the occurrence of premature and accelerated coronary atherosclerosis. Myocardial infarctions begin to occur in affected men in the third decade and peak in the fourth and fifth decades. By age 60, approximately 85 percent have experienced a myocardial infarction. In women, the incidence of myocardial infarction is also increased, but the mean age of onset is delayed 10 years as compared with men. Heterozygotes for this disorder constitute about 5 percent of all patients who have a myocardial infarction.

Xanthomas of the tendons constitute the second major clinical manifestation of the heterozygous state. These xanthomas are nodular swellings that typically involve the Achilles and other tendons about the knee, elbow, and dorsum of the hand. They are formed by the deposition of LDL-derived cholesteryl esters in tissue macrophages. The macrophages are swollen with lipid droplets and form foam cells. Cholesterol is also deposited in the soft tissue of the eyelid, producing xanthelasma, and within the cornea, producing arcus corneae. Whereas tendon xanthomas are essentially diagnostic of familial hypercholesterolemia, xanthelasma and arcus corneae also occur in many adults with normal plasma lipid levels. The incidence of tendon xanthomas in familial hypercholesterolemia increases with age, and up to 75 percent of heterozygotes display this sign. The absence of tendon xanthomas does not rule out familial hypercholesterolemia.

Approximately 1 in 1 million persons in the general population inherits two copies of the familial hypercholesterolemia gene and is a homozygote for the disorder. These individuals have marked elevations in the plasma level of LDL from birth. A unique type of planar cutaneous xanthoma is often present at birth and always develops within the first 6 years of life. These xanthomas are raised, yellow, plaquelike lesions at points of cutaneous trauma, such as the knees, elbows, and buttocks. Xanthomas are almost always present in the interdigital webs of the hands, particularly between the thumb and index finger. Tendon xanthomas, arcus corneae, and xanthelasma are also characteristic. Coronary artery atherosclerosis frequently has its clinical onset before age 10, and myocardial infarction has been reported as early as 18 months of age. In addition, cholesterol deposition in the aortic valve may produce symptomatic aortic stenosis. Homozygotes usually succumb to the complications of myocardial infarction before age 20.

Obesity and diabetes mellitus do not occur with increased frequency in familial hypercholesterolemia. A slender body habitus is the rule.

Pathogenesis The primary defect resides in the gene for the LDL receptor. Studies of DNA from affected individuals indicate that at least 150 mutant alleles occur at this locus. These mutant alleles can be grouped into three classes. The most common, designated *receptor-negative,* specifies a gene product that is nonfunctional. The second most frequent mutant, designated *receptor-defective,* produces a receptor that has 1 to 10 percent of normal LDL binding activity. The third type, designated *internalization-defective,* produces a receptor that binds LDL normally but is unable to transport the receptor-bound lipoprotein into the cell. This rare allele produces the so-called internalization defect.

Phenotypic homozygotes possess two mutant alleles at the LDL receptor locus, and hence their cells show a total or near-total inability to bind or take up LDL. Heterozygotes have one normal allele and one mutant allele at the LDL receptor locus, and hence their cells are able to bind and take up LDL at approximately half the normal rate.

Because of the reduction in LDL receptor activity, LDL catabolism is blocked, and the level of LDL in plasma rises in a manner that is inversely proportional to the reduction in LDL receptors. In addition to the impaired catabolism of LDL, LDL production is increased. Enhanced production of LDL has been attributed to the lack of an LDL receptor on liver cells. The liver fails to remove IDL from the plasma normally, with the result that an increased amount of IDL is converted to LDL. This overproduction of LDL, together with its inefficient catabolism, accounts for the high concentrations in affected patients. The elevated LDL levels causes an increase in the uptake of LDL by scavenger cells, which accumulate at various sites in the body, producing xanthomas.

The accelerated coronary atherosclerosis in familial hypercholesterolemia results from the high LDL levels, which lead to an enhanced infiltration of LDL into the artery wall following episodes of endothelial damage. The large amounts of LDL that penetrate the artery wall cannot be cleared from the interstitial space by the scavenger cells, and atherosclerosis ultimately results. Some of the lipids in LDL may undergo oxidation when the lipoprotein enters the artery wall, and the resultant products may be toxic to endothelial cells, thereby accelerating the damage. High LDL levels also may act to accelerate platelet aggregation at sites of endothelial injury, thereby enhancing the growth of the atherosclerotic plaque (see Chap. 208).

Diagnosis The diagnosis of heterozygous familial hypercholesterolemia is suggested by the finding of an isolated elevation of plasma cholesterol, with a normal concentration of plasma triglycerides. Such an isolated elevation in plasma cholesterol is usually due to an elevation in the plasma concentration of LDL alone (type 2a pattern). However, most individuals in the general population with type 2a hyperlipoproteinemia do not have familial hypercholesterolemia. Rather, they have a form of polygenic hypercholesterolemia that puts them on the upper end of the bell-shaped curve for the general population (see "Polygenic Hypercholesterolemia," below). Type 2a hyperlipoproteinemia is also caused by multiple lipoprotein–type hyperlipidemia and familial defective apo B100 (discussed below). In addition, a variety of metabolic disorders, including hypothyroidism and nephrotic syndrome, can cause type 2a hyperlipoproteinemia (see Table 344-4).

Among individuals who have a type 2a lipoprotein pattern, those with heterozygous familial hypercholesterolemia can be distinguished from those with polygenic hypercholesterolemia and multiple lipoprotein–type hyperlipidemia on several grounds. (1) In familial hypercholesterolemia the plasma cholesterol level tends to be higher. A plasma cholesterol level in the range of 9 to 10 mmol/L (350 to 400 mg/dL) is highly suggestive of heterozygous familial hypercholesterolemia.

However, many patients with heterozygous familial hypercholesterolemia have cholesterol levels of 7 to 9 mmol/L (285 to 350 mg/dL), a range in which the other disorders cannot be excluded. (2) The occurrence of tendon xanthomas virtually establishes the diagnosis of familial hypercholesterolemia, since such xanthomas usually do not occur in patients with other forms of hyperlipidemia. (3) In cases in which the diagnosis is in doubt, other family members should be surveyed. In familial hypercholesterolemia, half the first-degree relatives show an elevated plasma cholesterol level. Hypercholesterolemia in relatives is particularly informative when it occurs in children, since elevated levels of cholesterol in childhood are characteristic of familial hypercholesterolemia but not of the other disorders.

Approximately 10 percent of heterozygotes with familial hypercholesterolemia have a concomitant elevation in plasma triglyceride levels (type 2b pattern). In these cases, the disease is difficult to differentiate from multiple lipoprotein–type hyperlipidemia. The finding of a tendon xanthoma or a hypercholesterolemic child in the family establishes the diagnosis of familial hypercholesterolemia.

Differentiating heterozygous familial hypercholesterolemia from familial defective apo B100 is more difficult. The latter is caused by a missense mutation at amino acid 3500 in apo B100. This mutation interferes with the ability of apo B to bind to LDL receptors and thus results in hypercholesterolemia. Affected heterozygotes often have a positive family history of hypercholesterolemia, coronary atherosclerosis, and tendon xanthomas. The easiest way to distinguish this disorder from heterozygous familial hypercholesterolemia is by direct detection of the apo B100 mutation using polymerase chain reaction (PCR)–based molecular techniques (see Chap. 61).

The diagnosis of homozygous familial hypercholesterolemia ordinarily affords no problem, providing the physician is familiar with the clinical picture. Most patients are first seen by dermatologists in childhood because of the cutaneous xanthomas. Occasionally, the presentation is delayed until the onset of angina pectoris or until the child suffers a syncopal episode owing to the xanthomatous aortic stenosis. The finding of a cholesterol level greater than 16 mmol/L (600 mg/dL) with normal triglyceride values in a nonjaundiced child is highly suggestive of the diagnosis. Both parents should have elevated cholesterol levels and other features of heterozygous familial hypercholesterolemia.

In specialized laboratories, the diagnosis of both heterozygous and homozygous familial hypercholesterolemia can be made by direct measurement of the number of LDL receptors on cultured skin fibroblasts or freshly isolated blood lymphocytes. Homozygous familial hypercholesterolemia has been diagnosed in utero by the absence of LDL receptors on cultured amniotic fluid cells. The mutant genes for the LDL receptor also can be visualized directly in genomic DNA from affected individuals by using restriction enzyme digests, Southern blots, or the polymerase chain reaction (PCR) (see Chap. 61).

Treatment Inasmuch as the atherosclerosis in this disorder is a consequence of the long-standing elevation in plasma LDL levels, every effort should be made to lower the plasma LDL level into the normal range. Patients should be placed on a diet that is low in cholesterol, low in saturated fats, and high in polyunsaturated fats. This generally means the avoidance of milk, butter, cheese, chocolate, shellfish, and fatty meats and the addition of polyunsaturated cooking oils such as corn oil and safflower oil. With such a diet, heterozygotes usually show a 10 to 15 percent drop in plasma cholesterol level.

Bile acid–binding resins, such as cholestyramine, should be added to the regimen when dietary therapy fails to lower the cholesterol levels to the normal range. These resins trap the bile acids excreted by the liver into the intestine and prevent their reabsorption. The liver responds to bile acid depletion by converting additional cholesterol into bile acids. This leads to an enhanced production of LDL receptors by the liver, which, in turn, lowers the plasma level of LDL. Unfortunately, affected subjects also respond to bile acid depletion by enhancing cholesterol synthesis in the liver, and this compensatory response ultimately limits the long-term success of bile acid sequestrant therapy. With the combination of diet and bile acid–binding resins, the extent of reduction in plasma cholesterol level usually is in the range of 15 to 20 percent in heterozygotes. The addition of nicotinic acid may help to block the compensatory increase in hepatic cholesterol synthesis, thus allowing a further lowering of the cholesterol. Major side effects of bile acid–binding resins include gastrointestinal bloating, cramps, and constipation. The major side effect of nicotinic acid is hepatotoxicity; it also produces flushing and headaches in most patients. Probucol also has been used for the treatment of familial hypercholesterolemia. It is an antioxidant that retards the progression of atherosclerosis in animal models. Its effectiveness in humans is not established.

A new class of drugs shows great promise for treatment of hypercholesterolemia. These drugs inhibit 3-hydroxy-3-methylglutaryl coenzyme A (HMG CoA) reductase, an enzyme in the cholesterol biosynthetic pathway. This class includes lovastatin, pravastatin, and simvastatin. When cholesterol synthesis is inhibited, the production of LDL is diminished and the clearance of LDL by the liver is enhanced as a result of an increased production of LDL receptors. These two effects combine to lower plasma LDL levels by 30 to 50 percent. The HMG CoA reductase inhibitors are even more effective when given together with a bile acid–binding resin such as cholestyramine. The major side effects of this class of drugs are myopathy (0.5 percent) and asymptomatic but persistent increases in plasma transaminases (1.9 percent). A more severe myopathy with rhabdomyolysis is seen rarely in patients who are treated with reductase inhibitors plus immunosuppressive drugs, gemfibrozil, nicotinic acid, or erythromycin.

Heterozygotes often show a moderate to marked lowering of plasma cholesterol level in response to the creation of an intestinal anastomosis that bypasses the ileum. This operation has the same functional effect as bile acid–binding resins; i.e., it accelerates the loss of bile acids in the stool. In certain patients in whom drug therapy is not tolerated, the creation of an ileal bypass may be indicated.

Homozygotes tend to be more resistant to treatment, probably because they are unable to increase production of LDL receptors. In general, combination therapy consisting of diet, a bile acid–binding resin, nicotinic acid, and HMG CoA reductase inhibitors has little effect. Ileal bypass is uniformly ineffective. Several homozygous children have responded to surgical creation of a portacaval anastomosis. At least four homozygous children have been treated with liver transplantation, which provided LDL receptors and lowered LDL levels by 70 to 80 percent. The use of a continuous-flow blood cell centrifuge to perform plasma exchanges at monthly intervals lowers the cholesterol in all homozygotes. After each plasma exchange, the plasma cholesterol level drops to about 8 mmol/L (300 mg/dL) and then gradually rises over the ensuing 4 weeks to the pretreatment level. In one version of this procedure, plasma is exchanged with normal plasma or albumin. In another version, called *LDL apheresis*, plasma is passed extracorporeally over columns that remove apo B100–containing lipoproteins (VLDL, IDL, and LDL) but do not absorb HDL or other plasma proteins. The effluent is then returned to the patient. If facilities are available, plasma exchange is the treatment of choice for homozygotes.

Several studies have shown that cholesterol-lowering therapy retards the progression, and in some instances induces actual regression, of atherosclerotic plaques in the coronary arteries of patients with heterozygous familial hypercholesterolemia. The studies used serial coronary angiography to document these changes, which took place over periods of 2 to 3 years. Several different drug regimens and ileal bypass operations were employed to lower blood cholesterol, and the antiatherosclerotic effect seems to be independent of the regimen employed. These and other studies also documented a reduction in myocardial infarctions and other symptoms of coronary artery disease following such treatment. None of these studies has had sufficient statistical power to document a prolongation of life in treated patients.

FAMILIAL HYPERTRIGLYCERIDEMIA   This is a common autosomal dominant disorder in which the concentration of VLDL is elevated in the plasma, causing hypertriglyceridemia.

Clinical features   Affected individuals do not usually express hypertriglyceridemia until puberty or early adulthood. Thereafter, the fasting plasma triglyceride level tends to be moderately elevated in the range of 2 to 6 mmol/L (200 to 500 mg/dL) (type 4 lipoprotein pattern). The typical patient exhibits the clinical triad of obesity, hyperglycemia, and hyperinsulinemia. Hypertension and hyperuricemia are also frequent.

The incidence of atherosclerosis is increased. In one study, affected patients constituted 6 percent of all individuals with myocardial infarction. However, it has not been established that the hypertriglyceridemia per se causes the increased atherosclerosis. As discussed above, many patients with this disease have diabetes, obesity, and hypertension. Each of these disorders by itself may predispose to atherosclerosis. Hypertriglyceridemic subjects also tend to have reduced levels of HDL, which predisposes to atherosclerosis and which may account for the observed association of hypertriglyceridemia and myocardial infarction. Xanthomas are not a characteristic feature of familial hypertriglyceridemia.

Affected patients ordinarily have mild to moderate hypertriglyceridemia but may develop a severe exacerbation when exposed to a variety of precipitating factors. These include poorly controlled diabetes mellitus, excessive consumption of alcohol, ingestion of birth control pills containing estrogen, and the development of hypothyroidism. In response to any of these stimuli, the plasma triglyceride level can rise to more than 11 mmol/L (1000 mg/dL). During exacerbations, such patients develop *mixed hyperlipidemia;* that is, they show an elevation in the concentration of both VLDL and chylomicrons (type 5 lipoprotein pattern). Whenever the concentration of chylomicrons rises to high levels, patients are predisposed to the formation of eruptive xanthomas and the development of pancreatitis. With treatment of the exacerbating condition, the chylomicron-like particles disappear from plasma, and the concentration of triglycerides returns to the moderately elevated basal condition.

In certain families, some patients exhibit a severe mixed hyperlipidemia, even in the absence of known exacerbating factors. This is the so-called familial type 5 hyperlipidemia. Other individuals in the same family may have only the mild form of the disease with moderate hypertriglyceridemia and no hyperchylomicronemia (type 4 pattern).

Pathogenesis   Familial hypertriglyceridemia is transmitted as an autosomal dominant trait, implying a mutation in a single gene. However, the nature of the mutant gene and the mechanism by which it produces hypertriglyceridemia have not been identified. It is likely that the disorder is genetically heterogeneous; that is, the hypertriglyceridemia phenotype in different families may result from different mutations.

Some patients with familial hypertriglyceridemia seem to have an underlying defect in the ability to catabolize the triglycerides of VLDL. When VLDL production rates become elevated due to obesity or diabetes, they are unable to increase the catabolism of VLDL proportionately, and hypertriglyceridemia results. The reason for this defect in catabolism is not apparent. Lipoprotein lipase activity increases normally in plasma after the administration of heparin, and no abnormalities of lipoprotein structure have been identified.

The increased prevalence of diabetes mellitus and obesity in this syndrome is believed to be fortuitous, owing to the fact that both conditions tend to increase VLDL production and hence to exacerbate hypertriglyceridemia. In family studies, one can find relatives who have diabetes without hypertriglyceridemia and relatives who have hypertriglyceridemia without diabetes, indicating that the two are inherited by independent mechanisms. When an individual inherits the gene(s) for diabetes as well as the gene for hypertriglyceridemia, the hypertriglyceridemia is more severe, and such a person is more apt to come to medical attention. Similarly, an individual with familial hypertriglyceridemia who has a normal weight usually has mild hypertriglyceridemia and is less likely to come to medical attention. However, if obesity develops, the hypertriglyceridemia worsens, and a diagnosis is more likely to be made.

Diagnosis A moderate elevation in the plasma triglyceride level, together with a normal cholesterol level, raises the possibility of familial hypertriglyceridemia. In most patients, the plasma is clear to somewhat cloudy on inspection. Chylomicrons typically are not found at the top of the plasma after overnight refrigeration. Electrophoresis of the plasma reveals an increase in the pre-β fraction (type 4 lipoprotein pattern). As mentioned above, an occasional patient exhibits severe hypertriglyceridemia with an elevation in both chylomicrons and VLDL. In this case, a cream layer develops on top (chylomicrons) and a cloudy infranatant (VLDL) is present after overnight storage of plasma in the refrigerator (type 5 lipoprotein pattern).

Given an individual who has an elevation in VLDL levels with or without an elevation in chylomicrons, there is no simple test to determine whether this subject has familial hypertriglyceridemia or hypertriglyceridemia due to some other genetic or acquired cause, such as multiple lipoprotein–type hyperlipidemia or sporadic hypertriglyceridemia. In a typical case of familial hypertriglyceridemia, half the first-degree relatives have hypertriglyceridemia and no relatives have isolated hypercholesterolemia. Measurement of plasma lipid levels in children is not helpful inasmuch as the disease is typically not manifest until the time of puberty.

Treatment Attempts should be made to control all the exacerbating conditions. Caloric restriction is required in the obese subject. The dietary content of saturated fat also should be limited. Alcohol and oral contraceptives should be avoided. Diabetes mellitus, if present, should be treated vigorously. Thyroid function should be checked, and hypothyroidism should be treated if found. If the preceding measures fail, some patients respond to the administration of gemfibrozil or nicotinic acid. The mechanism of action of neither drug is well defined. Patients with severe hypertriglyceridemia frequently show a dramatic response to a fish oil diet. If a patient with hypertriglyceridemia has an especially low level of HDL-cholesterol, the prognosis for coronary artery disease is relatively poor, and therapeutic efforts must be especially vigorous.

MULTIPLE LIPOPROTEIN–TYPE HYPERLIPIDEMIA This common disorder, which is also called *familial combined hyperlipidemia*, is inherited as an autosomal dominant trait. Affected individuals in a single family characteristically show one of three different lipoprotein patterns: hypercholesterolemia (type 2a), hypertriglyceridemia (type 4), or both hypercholesterolemia and hypertriglyceridemia (type 2b). The level of HDL tends to be below normal

Clinical features Hyperlipidemia is not present in childhood. Elevations in the plasma cholesterol and/or triglyceride level appear at puberty and continue throughout life. The lipid elevations tend to be mild and vary from time to time so that affected individuals may have a mildly elevated cholesterol level at one examination and/or a mildly elevated triglyceride level at another time. Xanthomas are not a feature. However, premature atherosclerosis occurs, and the incidence of myocardial infarction in middle age is elevated in affected women as well as men.

Patients usually have a strong family history of premature coronary artery disease. This disorder is found in about 10 percent of all patients who have a myocardial infarction. The frequency of obesity, hyperuricemia, and glucose intolerance is increased in affected individuals, especially those with hypertriglyceridemia. However, this association is not as striking as in familial hypertriglyceridemia.

Pathogenesis The disease is transmitted within families as an autosomal dominant trait, implying a mutation in a single gene. Family studies show that about half the first-degree relatives of an affected individual have hyperlipidemia. However, blood lipid levels are variable among affected individuals in the same family as well as in the same individual at different times. About one-third of hyperlipidemic relatives have hypercholesterolemia (type 2a lipopro-

tein pattern), one-third hypertriglyceridemia (type 4), and one-third both hypercholesterolemia and hypertriglyceridemia (type 2b). In most affected relatives, the plasma lipid levels tend to be just above the 95th percentile for the population and to dip into the normal range intermittently.

While the extent (if any) of the genetic heterogeneity and the nature of the underlying biochemical mechanisms are not known, some affected individuals may have an elevated rate of secretion of VLDL by the liver. Others may be heterozygous for a mutation in the gene for lipoprotein lipase. Depending on the interplay of factors governing the efficiency of conversion of VLDL to LDL and the efficiency of catabolism of LDL, this overproduction of VLDL may manifest itself alternatively as an elevation in plasma VLDL levels (hypertriglyceridemia), an elevation in LDL levels (hypercholesterolemia), or both. The hyperlipidemia is worsened by diabetes, alcoholism, and hypothyroidism.

Diagnosis No clinical or laboratory methods exist by which to determine whether an individual with hyperlipidemia has the multiple lipoprotein–type disorder. The 2a, 2b, and 4 lipoprotein patterns can each occur in patients with several other diseases (see Tables 344-3 and 344-4). However, this disorder should be suspected in any individual whose hyperlipoproteinemia is mild and whose lipoprotein type changes with time. The diagnosis is supported by the finding of multiple abnormal lipoprotein types in relatives. The diagnosis can be ruled out by the finding of tendon xanthomas in the patient or the patient's relatives or by the finding of hypercholesterolemia in a relative under the age of 10 years.

Treatment Therapy should be directed at the predominant lipid elevated at the time of examination. General measures such as weight reduction, restriction of dietary saturated fat and cholesterol, and avoidance of alcohol and oral contraceptives are useful. Triglyceride elevations may respond to nicotinic acid or gemfibrozil. When only the cholesterol level is elevated, an HMG CoA reductase inhibitor should be given. Bile acid–binding resins should be avoided since lowering of cholesterol levels with such a drug is sometimes accompanied by an increase in triglyceride levels.

PRIMARY HYPERLIPOPROTEINEMIAS OF UNKNOWN ETIOLOGY

POLYGENIC HYPERCHOLESTEROLEMIA By definition, 5 percent of individuals in the general population have LDL-cholesterol levels that exceed the 95th percentile and therefore have hypercholesterolemia (type 2a or type 2b lipoprotein patterns). On average, among every 20 such hypercholesterolemic persons, 1 person has the heterozygous form of familial hypercholesterolemia, and 2 have multiple lipoprotein–type hyperlipidemia. The remaining 17 have a form of hypercholesterolemia, designated *polygenic hypercholesterolemia*, that owes its origin not to a single mutant gene but rather to a complex interaction of multiple genetic and environmental factors.

Most of the factors that place an individual in the upper part of the bell-shaped curve for cholesterol levels are not known. It is likely that subtle genetic differences exist among people with regard to many processes governing cholesterol metabolism. For example, among normal people there may be genetic polymorphisms in the proteins that govern the rates of intestinal cholesterol absorption, bile acid synthesis, cholesterol synthesis, and LDL synthesis or catabolism. Certain unfavorable combinations of these mildly altered proteins, coupled with an environmental challenge, such as a diet high in cholesterol or saturated fat, may raise the plasma cholesterol level.

Clinically, polygenic hypercholesterolemia can be distinguished from familial hypercholesterolemia and multiple lipoprotein–type hyperlipidemia in two ways: (1) family studies (hyperlipidemia is present in no more than 10 percent of first-degree relatives in polygenic hypercholesterolemia in contrast to 50 percent in the other two disorders) and (2) examination for tendon xanthomas (absent in both polygenic hypercholesterolemia and multiple lipoprotein–type hyperlipidemia but present in about 75 percent of adult heterozygotes with familial hypercholesterolemia).

Certain patients with polygenic hypercholesterolemia respond to dietary restriction of saturated fat and cholesterol. Other patients require drug therapy. An HMG CoA reductase inhibitor and a bile acid–binding resin with or without nicotinic acid also may be used.

FAMILIAL HYPERALPHALIPOPROTEINEMIA This entity is characterized by elevated plasma levels of HDL, also called *alpha lipoprotein*. The plasma levels of LDL, VLDL, and triglycerides are normal. The elevated HDL causes a slight elevation in the total plasma cholesterol level. Although a selective elevation in plasma HDL-cholesterol can be observed in individuals after exposure to chlorinated hydrocarbon pesticides, in alcoholism, and after administration of estrogen, most cases of hyperalphalipoproteinemia have a genetic basis. In some families, hyperalphalipoproteinemia is inherited as an autosomal dominant trait, while in others a multifactorial or polygenic basis is suspected. Individual subjects with familial hyperalphalipoproteinemia show no distinctive clinical features.

Hyperalphalipoproteinemia is associated with a slightly increased longevity and an apparent protection against myocardial infarction. The mechanism for the increase in plasma HDL levels in this disorder has not been determined.

SECONDARY HYPERLIPOPROTEINEMIAS

A number of clinical disorders produce secondary hyperlipoproteinemias. These are summarized in Table 344-4. The most frequently encountered forms of secondary hyperlipoproteinemia occur in association with diabetes mellitus, consumption of alcohol, and ingestion of oral contraceptives.

DIABETES MELLITUS Three distinct patterns of hypertriglyceridemia occur in patients with diabetes mellitus. Classic *diabetic hyperlipidemia* consists of a massive elevation in the plasma triglyceride level that occurs in patients who have suffered from insulin deficiency or insulin resistance for many weeks or months. Such insulin-deprived patients develop a progressive increase in concentration of plasma VLDL and eventually of chylomicrons as well. Triglyceride levels as high as 280 mmol/L (25,000 mg/dL) are seen. Eruptive xanthomas, lipemia retinalis, and hepatomegaly can occur. Ketosis is frequently present, but severe acidosis is not characteristic. This form of massive hyperlipoproteinemia is seen only in partial insulin deficiency. Patients with this form of diabetic hyperlipidemia usually respond to a fat-free diet and to the administration of insulin, although triglyceride levels may not return entirely to normal.

The second type of hypertriglyceridemia in diabetics is associated with acute ketoacidosis. Such patients usually exhibit a mild hyperlipidemia with elevations of VLDL but not chylomicrons. On occasion, however, marked elevations of triglyceride are seen with lipemia retinalis. In this case, both VLDL and chylomicrons are present.

The third type of hypertriglyceridemia is a mild to moderate elevation in plasma VLDL that persists even when patients appear to be adequately treated for their diabetes. This chronic triglyceride elevation generally occurs in patients who are obese. Inasmuch as most patients with well-controlled diabetes have normal plasma triglyceride levels, the occasional patient with persistent hypertriglyceridemia is likely to have an underlying familial hyperlipoproteinemic disorder. Indeed, family studies indicate that many of these patients have inherited the trait for familial hypertriglyceridemia in a pattern independent of the inheritance of diabetes mellitus.

The insulin deficiency or insulin resistance of diabetes produces a high VLDL level by two mechanisms. With acute insulin deprivation there is an increase in VLDL secretion from the liver as a secondary response to the increased mobilization of free fatty acids from adipose tissue. As the state of insulin deprivation becomes prolonged, the rate of removal of VLDL and chylomicrons from the circulation declines because lipoprotein lipase activity becomes diminished.

ALCOHOL CONSUMPTION In any individual, the daily consumption of large amounts of ethanol can produce a mild, asymptomatic elevation in the plasma triglyceride level due to an elevation of VLDL. However, in a subgroup ethanol ingestion regularly produces massive and clinically significant hyperlipidemia with elevations in both VLDL and chylomicrons (type 5 lipoprotein pattern). In most of this group, the VLDL level remains mildly elevated (type 4 lipoprotein pattern), even in the basal state after recovery from the severe alcoholic hyperlipidemia. This suggests that these individuals have a form of familial hypertriglyceridemia or multiple lipoprotein–type hyperlipidemia that is exacerbated and converted to a type 5 pattern by the ethanol ingestion.

Ethanol elevates the plasma triglyceride level primarily because it inhibits fatty acid oxidation and enhances fatty acid synthesis in the liver. The excess fatty acids are esterified to triglyceride. Some of this excess triglyceride accumulates in the liver, producing the characteristic enlarged fatty liver of alcoholics. The remainder of the newly formed triglyceride is secreted into plasma, resulting in an increased secretion of VLDL. In those who develop massive alcoholic hyperlipidemia, there appears to be a partial defect in the catabolism of these VLDL particles. As the concentration of VLDL increases, the lipoprotein begins to compete with chylomicrons for hydrolysis by lipoprotein lipase, and the plasma concentration of chylomicrons also rises.

In severe alcoholic hyperlipidemia, eruptive xanthomas and lipemia retinalis are frequent. The most serious complication, pancreatitis, may be difficult to diagnose, since elevated triglyceride levels can interfere with the estimation of serum amylase. There is no evidence to indicate that pancreatitis can cause hyperlipidemia; rather, the hyperlipidemia is the cause of the pancreatitis.

Plasma from patients with alcoholic hyperlipidemia is creamy in appearance. If a blood sample is drawn in calcium edetate and the plasma placed in the refrigerator at 4°C overnight, the chylomicrons float to the top, and the infranatant layer is turbid, owing to the combined elevation of VLDL and chylomicrons (type 5 pattern).

ORAL CONTRACEPTIVES The ingestion of estrogen-containing birth control pills causes an increase in the VLDL secretion rate from the liver. In most women the catabolism of VLDL also increases so that the overall increase in plasma triglyceride level is modest. However, in women who have an underlying genetic disorder (such as familial hypertriglyceridemia or multiple lipoprotein–type hyperlipidemia), the plasma VLDL-triglyceride level can increase markedly, and hyperchylomicronemia can develop when estrogen-containing medications are taken. These women generally have mild hypertriglyceridemia prior to the institution of oral contraceptive therapy, and they presumably are unable to increase VLDL catabolism in response to the stimulation of VLDL production. The elevated VLDL prevents the normal catabolism of chylomicrons by lipoprotein lipase, and secondary hyperchylomicronemia ensues. When the latter develops, severe pancreatitis can occur.

Ingestion of oral contraceptives may be a risk factor in promoting thromboembolic disease in young women, especially those with preexisting hypercholesterolemia. Thus it is important to measure the plasma cholesterol and triglyceride levels prior to the institution of birth control therapy. The finding of hyperlipidemia is a contraindication to the use of these drugs.

RARE DISORDERS OF LIPID METABOLISM

Table 344-5 summarizes the clinical and pathophysiologic features of five rare autosomal recessive disorders of lipid metabolism. In two—abetalipoproteinemia and Tangier disease—the major effect of the abnormality is to cause a decrease in lipid levels in plasma. In two—cerebrotendinous xanthomatosis and sitosterolemia—the major effect of the inborn error is to cause an accumulation of unusual sterols in tissues. In LCAT deficiency, the underlying mutation produces both an abnormal pattern of lipoproteins in plasma and an accumulation of unesterified cholesterol in tissues.

TABLE 344-5 Rare autosomal recessive disorders of lipid metabolism

Disorder	Typical age of onset	Plasma lipid abnormality	Major clinical manifestations	Pathogenesis	Treatment
Abetalipoproteinemia	Early childhood	Very low cholesterol and triglyceride levels	Malabsorption of fat, ataxia, neuropathy, retinitis pigmentosa, acanthocytosis	Defective synthesis of apoprotein B leads to absence of chylomicrons, VLDL, and LDL in plasma	Vitamin E
Tangier disease	Childhood	Low cholesterol; triglycerides, normal to slightly elevated	Large orange tonsils, corneal opacities, relapsing polyneuropathy. No premature atherosclerosis	Absence of HDL from plasma leads to generation of abnormal chylomicron remnants, which are taken up and stored as cholesteryl esters in phagocytic cells	None
Lecithin:cholesterol acyltransferase (LCAT) deficiency	Young adult	Total plasma cholesterol level variable with marked decrease in esterified cholesterol and increase in unesterified cholesterol; elevated VLDL level; structure of all lipoproteins is abnormal	Corneal opacities, hemolytic anemia, renal insufficiency, premature atherosclerosis	Decreased LCAT activity in plasma leads to accumulation of excess unesterified cholesterol in plasma and body tissues	Fat-restricted diet, kidney transplantation
Cerebrotendinous xanthomatosis	Young adult	None	Progressive cerebellar ataxia, dementia and spinal cord paresis, subnormal intelligence, tendon xanthomas, cataracts	Defective synthesis of primary bile acids in liver leads to increased hepatic synthesis of cholesterol and cholestanol, which accumulate in brain, tendons, and other tissues	None
Sitosterolemia	Childhood	Elevated levels of plant sterols in plasma, elevated or normal levels of cholesterol, normal triglyceride levels	Tendon xanthomas	Increased intestinal absorption of dietary cholesterol, sitosterol, and other plant sterols with accumulation in plasma and tendons	Diet low in plant sterols and cholesterol

REFERENCES

BROWN MS, GOLDSTEIN JL: A receptor-mediated pathway for cholesterol homeostasis. Science 232:34, 1986

————, ————: Drugs used in the treatment of hyperlipoproteinemias, in *Goodman and Gilman's The Pharmacological Basis of Therapeutics,* 8th ed, AG Gilman et al (eds). New York, Pergamon, 1990, chap 36

BRUNZELL JD: Familial lipoprotein lipase deficiency and other causes of the chylomicronemia syndrome, in *The Molecular and Metabolic Basis of Inherited Disease,* 7th ed, CR Scriver et al (eds). New York, McGraw-Hill, in press, chap 59

CONNOR WE et al: Reduction of plasma lipids, lipoproteins and apoproteins by dietary fish oils in patients with hypertriglyceridemia. N Engl J Med 312:1210, 1985

GOLDSTEIN JL et al: Familial hypercholesterolemia, in *The Molecular and Metabolic Basis of Inherited Disease,* 7th ed, CR Scriver et al (eds). New York, McGraw-Hill, in press, chap 62

HAVEL RJ: Lowering cholesterol, 1988: Rationale, mechanisms and means. J Clin Invest 81:1653, 1988

HOBBS HH et al: The LDL receptor locus and familial hypercholesterolemia: Mutational analysis of a membrane protein. Annu Rev Genet 24:133, 1990

KRAMSCH DM, BLANKENHORN DH: Regression of atherosclerosis: Which components regress and what influences their reversal? Wien Klin Wochenschr 104:2, 1992

MAHLEY RW, RALL SC: Type III hyperlipoproteinemia (dysbetalipoproteinemia): The role of apolipoprotein E in normal and abnormal lipoprotein metabolism, in *The Molecular and Metabolic Basis of Inherited Disease,* 7th ed, CR Scriver et al (eds). New York, McGraw-Hill, in press, chap 61

SCRIVER CR et al: *The Molecular and Metabolic Basis of Inherited Disease,* 7th ed. New York, McGraw-Hill, in press, chaps 56, 57, 63–65.

345 HEMOCHROMATOSIS

LAWRIE W. POWELL / KURT J. ISSELBACHER

DEFINITION Hemochromatosis is a disorder of iron storage in which an inappropriate increase in intestinal iron absorption results in deposition of excessive quantities of iron in parenchymal cells with eventual tissue damage and functional impairment of the organs involved, especially the liver, pancreas, heart, and pituitary. In 1889, von Recklinghausen named the disease *hemochromatosis* and the iron-storage pigment *hemosiderin* because he believed that the pigment was derived from the blood. The terms *hemosiderosis* and *siderosis* are often used to describe the presence of stainable iron in tissues, but quantitative measurement of tissue iron is necessary for accurate assessment of body iron status (see below and Chap. 303). *Hemochromatosis* implies present or potentially severe progressive iron overload leading to fibrosis and organ failure. Cirrhosis, diabetes mellitus, arthritis, cardiomyopathy, and hypogonadotrophic hypogonadism are the usual manifestations. Although there is debate about definitions, it seems logical to use the following terminology: (1) *genetic or hereditary hemochromatosis*—the disease now known to be due to the inheritance of a mutant gene that is tightly linked to the HLA-A6 locus on the short arm of chromosome 6, and (2) *acquired hemochromatosis*—iron overload and tissue injury secondary to other disease, usually an iron-loading anemia such as thalassemia or sideroblastic anemia, in which increased erythropoiesis is ineffective. In these acquired iron-loading disorders, massive iron deposits in parenchymal tissues can lead to the same clinical and pathologic features as in hereditary hemochromatosis.

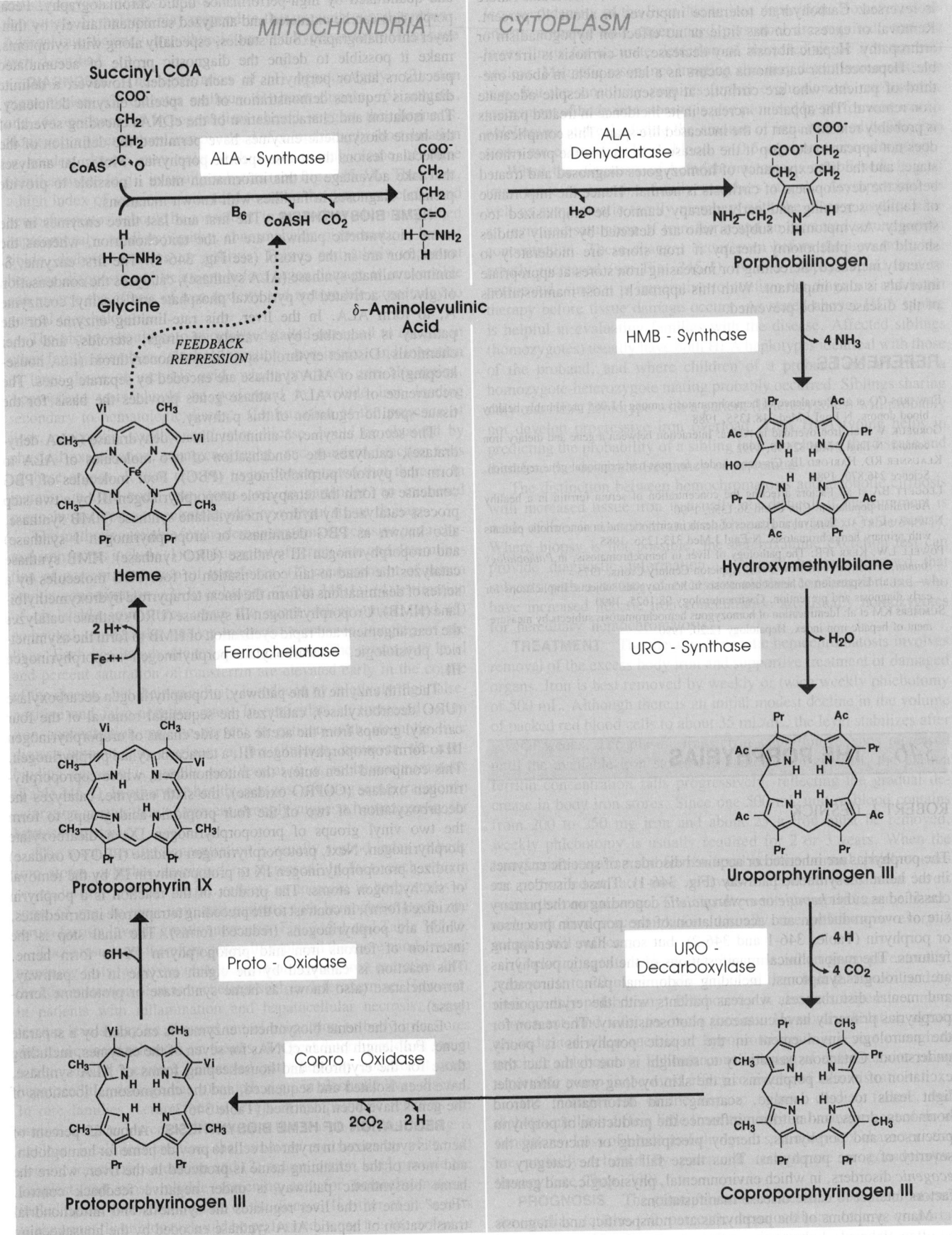

FIGURE 346-1 The human heme biosynthetic pathway.

TABLE 346-1 Classification of the human porphyrias

Type/porphyria	Deficient enzyme	Inheri-tance*	Photosensi-tivity	Neurovisceral symptoms
HEPATIC PORPHYRIAS				
ALA dehydratase deficiency	ALA dehy-dratase	AR	−	+
Acute intermittent porphyria (AIP)	HMB synthase	AD	−	+
Hereditary copro-porphyria (HCP)	COPRO ox-idase	AD	+	+
Variegate por-phyria (VP)	PROTO ox-idase	AD	+	+
Porphyria cutanea tarda (PCT)	URO decar-boxylase	AD	+	−
ERYTHROPOIETIC PORPHYRIAS				
X-linked sider-oblastic anemia (XLSA)	ALA synthase	XLR	−	−
Congenital eryth-ropoietic por-phyria (CEP)	URO synthase	AR	+ + +	−
Erythropoietic protoporphyria (EPP)	Ferrochelatase	AD	+	−

* AR = autosomal recessive; AD = autosomal dominant; XLR = X-linked recessive.

the liver is used for the synthesis of the cytochrome P450 enzymes, hepatic ALA synthase and the cytochrome P450s are induced in a coordinated fashion.

In erythroid cells, different regulatory mechanisms control production of heme for hemoglobin. The erythroid-specific ALA synthase encoded on the X chromosome is expressed at higher levels than the hepatic gene encoded on chromosome 3. In addition, an erythroid-specific control mechanism regulates iron transport into erythroid

TABLE 346-2 The major metabolites accumulated in the human porphyrias

Type/porphyria	Increased erythrocyte porphyrins	Porphyrin excretion*	
		Urine	Stool
HEPATIC PORPHYRIAS			
ALA dehydratase deficiency	—	ALA, COPRO III	
Acute intermittent porphyria (AIP)	—	ALA, PBG	—
Hereditary copro-porphyria (HCP)	—	ALA, PBG, COPRO III	COPRO III
Variegate por-phyria (VP)	—	ALA, PBG COPRO III	COPRO III, PROTO IX
Porphyria cutanea tarda (PCT)	—	URO I, 7-car-boxylate, porphyrin	Isocopro
ERYTHROPOIETIC PORPHYRIAS			
X-linked sider-oblastic anemia (XLSA)	—	—	—
Congenital eryth-ropoietic por-phyria (CEP)	URO I	URO I	COPRO I
Erythropoietic protoporphyria (EPP)	PROTO IX	—	PROTO IX

* ALA = δ-aminolevulinic acid; PBG = porphobilinogen; COPRO I = coproporphyrin I; COPRO III = coproporphyrin III; ISOCOPRO = isocoproporphyrin; URO I = uroporphyrin I; URO III = uroporphyrin III; PROTO = protoporphyrin IX

TABLE 346-3 The heme biosynthetic genes and their chromosomal locations

Structural gene	cDNA and genomic sequences characterized	Chromosomal assignment
ALA synthase		
Housekeeping	+	3p21
Erythroid	+	Xp11.21
ALA dehydratase	+	9q34
HMB synthase	+	11q23 → qter
URO synthase	+	10q25.3 → 26.3
URO decarboxylase	+	1p34
COPRO oxidase	−	9
PROTO oxidase	−	14q31 → q32
Ferrochelatase	+	18q21.3

cells. During erythroid differentiation, the activities of the heme biosynthetic enzymes increase in a coordinated fashion.

THE HEPATIC PORPHYRIAS

The rapid onset of neurologic symptoms is characteristic of the acute hepatic porphyrias. During an acute attack, individuals have markedly elevated plasma and urinary concentrations of the porphyrin precursors ALA and PBG, which originate from the liver.

ALA DEHYDRATASE–DEFICIENT PORPHYRIA This disease is a rare autosomal recessive trait that has been described in four unrelated males in Europe. Onset and severity of the disease are variable, presumably depending on the amount of residual ALA dehydratase activity. Treatment and prevention of the neurologic complications are the same as for other acute porphyrias (see below).

Clinical features The clinical presentation is variable. The first reported cases were two unrelated German men who had the onset during adolescence of abdominal pain and neuropathy, resembling acute intermittent porphyria (AIP; see below). The third patient, a Swedish infant, presented with failure to thrive and required transfusions and parenteral nutrition. Presumably, the earlier age of onset and more severe manifestations reflect a more complete enzyme deficiency. The fourth patient, a Belgian male, developed an acute motor polyneuropathy and polycythemia at age 63.

Diagnosis All four had increased urinary ALA and coproporphyrin levels. ALA dehydratase activity was reduced in erythrocytes (<5 percent of normal). It should be noted that both succinylacetone (which accumulates in hereditary tyrosinemia and is structurally similar to ALA) and lead inhibit ALA dehydratase and cause increased urinary excretion of ALA and manifestations that resemble those of the acute porphyrias. Therefore, lead intoxication and hereditary tyrosinemia (fumarylacetoacetase deficiency) should be considered in the differential diagnosis of the ALA dehydratase–deficient porphyria. Immunologic studies in the four reported cases demonstrated the presence of nonfunctional enzyme proteins that cross-reacted with anti-ALA dehydratase antibodies. DNA analysis revealed different missense mutations that resulted in the amino acid substitutions G133R and V275M in the infantile-onset case and R240W and A274T in one of the juvenile-onset cases.

Heterozygotes are clinically asymptomatic and do not excrete increased levels of ALA but can be detected by demonstration of intermediate levels of erythrocyte ALA dehydratase activity or by the presence of a specific mutation in the ALA dehydratase gene. The prenatal diagnosis of this disorder has not been made but should be possible by determination of the ALA dehydratase activity in cultured chorionic villi or amniocytes.

Treatment Treatment is similar to that in AIP (see below). The severely affected infant was supported by hyperalimentation and periodic blood transfusions. Continued failure to thrive led to a liver transplant, which did not improve the hematologic manifestations.

ACUTE INTERMITTENT PORPHYRIA This hepatic porphyria is an autosomal dominant condition resulting from the half-normal level

Clinical features HCP is influenced by the same factors that cause attacks in AIP. The disease is latent before puberty, and symptoms are more common in women. Neurovisceral symptoms and other clinical features are virtually identical to those of AIP. Photosensitivity may resemble that in PCT and VP. Cutaneous lesions may begin in childhood in homozygous cases.

Diagnosis Coproporphyrin is markedly increased in the urine and feces when this disease is symptomatic and sometimes when there are no symptoms. Urinary ALA and PBG are increased during acute attacks but may return to normal when symptoms resolve. Although the diagnosis can be confirmed by measuring COPRO oxidase activity, assays are not widely available and require cells other than erythrocytes.

Treatment Attacks of neurologic symptoms are treated as in AIP (see above). Phlebotomy and chloroquine are not effective in patients with cutaneous lesions.

VARIEGATE PORPHYRIA (VP) This hepatic porphyria results from the deficient activity of PROTO oxidase, is inherited as an autosomal dominant trait, and can present with neurologic symptoms, photosensitivity, or both.

Clinical features Neurovisceral signs and symptoms develop after puberty and are indistinguishable from those of AIP or HCP (see above). Attacks are provoked by the same drugs, steroid hormones, and nutritional factors that are detrimental in AIP. Skin manifestations are more common than in HCP but usually occur apart from the neurovisceral symptoms. Since the skin lesions in VP, HCP, and PCT are not distinguishable by clinical examination or biopsy, these conditions must be diagnosed by measurements of porphyrins and porphyrin precursors in blood, urine, and feces.

VP is particularly common in South Africa, where 3 of every 1000 whites have the disorder. Most are descendants of a couple who emigrated from Holland to South Africa in 1688. Homozygous VP has been described; photosensitivity, neurologic symptoms, and developmental disturbances, including growth retardation, were noted in infancy or childhood. All cases had increased erythrocyte zinc protoporphyrin levels, a characteristic finding in all homozygous porphyrias so far described.

Dual porphyria, the simultaneous occurrence of VP and familial PCT, has been documented in several kindreds. *Chester porphyria* was described in a large family from Great Britain in which individuals had acute porphyric attacks and evidence of both PROTO oxidase and HMB synthase deficiencies. Photosensitivity was not observed. It is unclear whether Chester porphyria is a variant of VP or AIP.

Diagnosis When VP is symptomatic, fecal protoporphyrin and coproporphyrin and urinary coproporphyrin are increased. Urinary ALA and PBG are increased during acute attacks. Plasma porphyrins are increased, particularly when there are cutaneous lesions. VP can be distinguished rapidly from all other porphyrias by examining the fluorescence emission spectrum of porphyrins in plasma at neutral pH. This is particularly useful for differentiating VP from PCT.

Assays of PROTO oxidase activity in cultured fibroblasts or lymphocytes are not widely available. Some latent cases of VP can be diagnosed by measurement of fecal porphyrins in relatives of VP patients.

Treatment Acute attacks are treated with hematin as in AIP. Other than avoiding sun exposure, there are few effective measures for the skin lesions. β-Carotene, phlebotomy, and chloroquine are not helpful.

THE ERYTHROPOIETIC PORPHYRIAS

In the erythropoietic porphyrias, elevated bone marrow erythrocyte and plasma porphyrins become deposited in the skin and lead to cutaneous photosensitivity.

X-LINKED SIDEROBLASTIC ANEMIA (XLSA) This anemia results from the deficient activity of the erythroid form of ALA synthase and is associated with ineffective erythropoiesis, weakness, and pallor.

Clinical features Males with XLSA develop refractory hemolytic anemia, pallor, and weakness during infancy. They have secondary hypersplenism, become iron overloaded, and can develop hemosiderosis. The severity of these symptoms depends on the level of residual erythroid ALA synthase activity and on the responsiveness of the specific mutation to pyridoxal 5'-phosphate supplementation (see below). Peripheral blood smears reveal a hypochromic, microcytic anemia with striking anisocytosis, poikilocytosis, and polychromasia; the leukocytes and platelets appear normal. Hemoglobin content is reduced, and the mean corpuscular volume and mean corpuscular hemoglobin concentration are decreased.

Diagnosis Bone marrow examination reveals a hypercellular marrow with a left shift and megaloblastic erythropoiesis with an abnormal maturation. A variety of Prussian blue–staining sideroblastic forms are observed. Urinary porphyrin precursors and both urinary and fecal porphyrins are normal. The level of erythroid ALA synthase is decreased in bone marrow, but this enzyme is difficult to measure in the presence of the normal housekeeping enzyme. Definitive diagnosis requires the demonstration of specific mutations in the erythroid ALA synthase gene.

Treatment The severe anemia may respond to pyridoxine supplementation. This cofactor is essential for ALA synthase activity, and mutations in the pyridoxine binding site of the enzyme have been found in several responsive patients. Cofactor supplementation may obviate the need for periodic transfusions or reduce their frequency. Unresponsive patients may be transfusion-dependent and require chelation therapy.

CONGENITAL ERYTHROPOIETIC PORPHYRIA (CEP) This autosomal recessive porphyria, also known as *Gunther's disease,* is due to deficiency of URO synthase and is associated with hemolytic anemia and cutaneous lesions. CEP is characterized by accumulation of the type I isomers of uroporphyrin and coproporphyrin.

Clinical features Cutaneous photosensitivity is usually severe and begins in early infancy. The skin over sun-exposed areas is friable. Bullae and vesicles are prone to rupture and infection. Skin thickening, focal hypo- and hyperpigmentation, and hypertrichosis of the face and extremities are characteristic. Secondary infection can lead to disfiguring of the face and hands. Porphyrins are deposited in teeth and in bones. As a result, the teeth are reddish brown and fluoresce on exposure to long-wave ultraviolet light. Hemolysis is probably due to the marked increase in erythrocyte porphyrins and leads to splenomegaly. A milder form of the disease occurs with onset of symptoms in adulthood.

Diagnosis Uroporphyrin and coproporphyrin (mostly isomer I) accumulate in the bone marrow, erythrocytes, plasma, urine, and feces. The diagnosis should be confirmed by demonstration of markedly deficient URO synthase activity. The disease can be detected in utero by measuring porphyrins in amniotic fluid and URO synthase activity in cultured amniotic cells or chorionic villi. Molecular analyses of the mutant alleles from over 20 unrelated patients have revealed the presence of gene rearrangements, an mRNA processing defect, and several point mutations that cause amino acid substitutions.

Treatment Blood transfusions sufficient to suppress erythropoiesis appear to be the most effective form of treatment, but this strategy is complicated by iron overload. Splenectomy may reduce hemolysis and reduce transfusion requirements. Protection from sunlight and from minor skin trauma is important. β-Carotene may be of some value. Complicating bacterial infections should be treated promptly. Bone marrow transplantation has been reported in only one patient, who subsequently died from transplant complications.

ERYTHROPOIETIC PROTOPORPHYRIA (EPP) This condition is due to the partial deficiency of ferrochelatase and is inherited as an autosomal dominant trait. Protoporphyrin accumulates in erythroid cells and plasma and is excreted in bile and feces. EPP is the most common erythropoietic porphyria and, after PCT, the second most common porphyria.

Clinical features Skin photosensitivity usually begins in childhood. The skin manifestations of EPP differ from those of other porphyrias. Vesicular lesions are uncommon. Redness, swelling, burning, and itching can develop within minutes of sun exposure and resemble angioedema. Symptoms may seem out of proportion to visible skin lesions. Vesicles and bullae are absent or sparse and may occur in only 10 percent of cases. Chronic skin changes may include lichenification, leathery pseudovesicles, labial grooving, and nail changes. Severe scarring is rare, as are pigment changes, friability, and hirsutism.

The primary source of excess protoporphyrin is the bone marrow reticulocyte. Erythrocyte protoporphyrin is free (not complexed with zinc) and is mostly bound to hemoglobin. In plasma protoporphyrin is bound to albumin. Hemolysis and anemia are usually absent or very mild.

Liver function is usually normal. However, in some patients, accumulation of protoporphyrin causes chronic liver disease that can progress to liver failure and death. The hepatic complications are often preceded by increasing levels of erythrocyte and plasma protoporphyrin and probably result, in part, from protoporphyrin accumulation in the liver. Protoporphyrin is insoluble, forms crystalline structures in liver cells, and can decrease hepatic bile flow. Gallstones composed at least in part of protoporphyrin occur in some patients.

Some obligate heterozygotes are asymptomatic and have little or no increase in erythrocyte protoporphyrin. Thus there is phenotypic variation in this disease.

Diagnosis Protoporphyrin concentrations are increased in bone marrow, circulating erythrocytes, plasma, bile, and feces. Urinary porphyrin and porphyrin precursors are normal. Decreased ferrochelatase activity can be demonstrated in cultured lymphocytes or fibroblasts.

Treatment Oral β-carotene (Hoffman-LaRoche) (120 to 180 mg/d) improves tolerance to sunlight in many patients. Adjustment in dosage may be needed to maintain serum carotene levels in the recommended range of 10 to 15 μmol/L (600 to 800 μg/dL). Mild skin discoloration due to carotenemia is the only significant side effect. The beneficial effects of β-carotene may involve quenching of singlet oxygen or free radicals. Unfortunately, this drug appears less effective in other forms of porphyria associated with photosensitivity.

Treatment of hepatic complications is difficult. However, cholestyramine and other porphyrin absorbents such as activated charcoal may interrupt the enterohepatic circulation of protoporphyrin and promote its fecal excretion, leading to some improvement. Splenectomy may be helpful when the disease is accompanied by hemolysis and significant splenomegaly. Caloric restriction and drugs or hormone preparations that may induce the heme pathway in liver or impair hepatic excretory function should be avoided. Iron deficiency should be prevented or treated. Transfusions or intravenous heme therapy may suppress erythroid and hepatic protoporphyrin production and are sometimes clinically beneficial. Liver transplantation has been carried out in some patients with severe liver complications.

REFERENCES

ANDERSON KE et al: A GnRH analogue prevents cyclical attacks of porphyria. Arch Intern Med 150:1469, 1990

COTTER PD et al: Enzymatic defect in "X-linked" sideroblastic anemia: Molecular evidence for erythroid δ-aminolevulinate synthase deficiency. Proc Natl Acad Sci USA 89:4028, 1992

DESNICK RJ, ANDERSON KE: Disorders of heme biosynthesis: The porphyrias, in *Hematology: Basic Principles and Practices*, R Hoffman et al (eds). New York, Churchill Livingstone, 1991, pp 350–367

KAPPAS A et al: The porphyrias, in *The Metabolic Basis of Inherited Disease*, CR Scriver et al (eds). New York, McGraw-Hill, 1990, pp 1305–1366

MOORE MR et al: *Disorders of Porphyrin Metabolism*. New York, Plenum, 1987

MUSTAJOKI P, NORDMANN Y: Early administration of heme arginate for acute porphyric attacks. Ann Intern Med (in press)

PLEWINSKA M et al: δ-Aminolevulinate dehydratase deficient porphyria: Identification of the molecular lesions in a severely affected homozygote. Am J Hum Genet 49:167, 1991

WARNER CA et al: Congenital erythropoietic porphyria: Identification and expression of exonic mutations in the uroporphyrinogen III synthase gene. J Clin Invest 89:693, 1992

347 GOUT AND OTHER DISORDERS OF PURINE METABOLISM

ROBERT L. WORTMANN

Gout encompasses a heterogeneous group of disorders that occur alone or in combination and include (1) hyperuricemia, (2) attacks of acute, typically monarticular, inflammatory arthritis, (3) tophaceous deposition of urate crystals in and around joints, (4) interstitial deposition of urate crystals in renal parenchyma, and (5) urolithiasis. *Hyperuricemia,* the cardinal biochemical feature and prerequisite for gout, is defined as a plasma urate concentration greater than 420 μmol/L (7.0 mg/dL) and is an indication of increased total-body urate. Hyperuricemia can result from increased production of urate, decreased excretion of uric acid, or a combination of the two processes. When hyperuricemia exists, plasma and extracellular fluids are supersaturated with respect to urate and conditions exist that favor crystal formation and tissue deposition. These conditions may result in the clinical manifestations included in the term *gout.*

URIC ACID METABOLISM Uric acid is the final breakdown product of purine degradation in humans. It is a weak acid with pK_a's of 5.75 and 10.3. Urates, the ionized forms of uric acid, predominate in plasma, extracellular fluid, and synovial fluid, with approximately 98 percent existing as monosodium urate at pH 7.4. Monosodium urate is easily ultrafiltered and dialyzed from plasma. Binding of urate to plasma proteins has little physiologic significance.

Plasma is saturated with monosodium urate at a concentration of 415 μmol/L (6.8 mg/dL) at 37°C. At higher concentrations, plasma is therefore supersaturated with urate, and potential exists for urate crystal precipitation. However, precipitation does not occur even at plasma urate concentrations as high as 4800 μmol/L (80 mg/dL). Why urate forms stable supersaturated solutions in plasma is unclear but may relate to the presence of solubilizing substances.

Uric acid is more soluble in urine than in water, possibly because of the presence of urea, proteins, and mucopolysaccharides. The pH of urine greatly influences its solubility. At pH 5.0, urine is saturated with uric acid at concentrations ranging from 360 to 900 μmol/L (6 to 15 mg/dL). At pH 7.0, saturation is reached at concentrations between 9480 and 12,000 μmol/L (158 and 200 mg/dL). Ionized forms of uric acid in urine include mono- and disodium, potassium, ammonium, and calcium urates.

Although purine nucleotide synthesis and breakdown occur in all tissues, urate is produced only in tissues that contain xanthine oxidase, primarily liver and small intestine. The amount of urate in the body is the net result of the amount produced and the amount excreted (Fig. 347-1). Urate production varies with the purine content of the diet and the respective rates of purine biosynthesis, degradation, and salvage. Normally, two-thirds to three-fourths of urate produced is excreted by the kidneys, and most of the remainder is eliminated through the intestines. A three-component model that includes glomerular filtration and both tubular secretion and reabsorption is proposed for the renal handling of uric acid in humans (Fig. 347-2). Approximately 8 to 12 percent of urate filtered by the glomeruli is excreted in the urine as uric acid. After filtration, 98 to 100 percent of the urate is reabsorbed. Approximately half the reabsorbed urate is secreted back into the proximal tubule, and 40 to 44 percent of that is again reabsorbed.

Serum urate concentrations vary with age and sex. Most children have serum urate concentrations of 180 to 240 μmol/L (3.0 to 4.0 mg/dL). Levels begin to rise during puberty in males but remain low in females until menopause. Although the cause of this sex variation is not completely understood, it is in part due to higher functional excretion of urate in females and is attributable to hormonal influences. Mean serum urate values for adult men and premenopausal women are 415 and 360 μmol/L (6.8 and 6.0 mg/dL), respectively. After

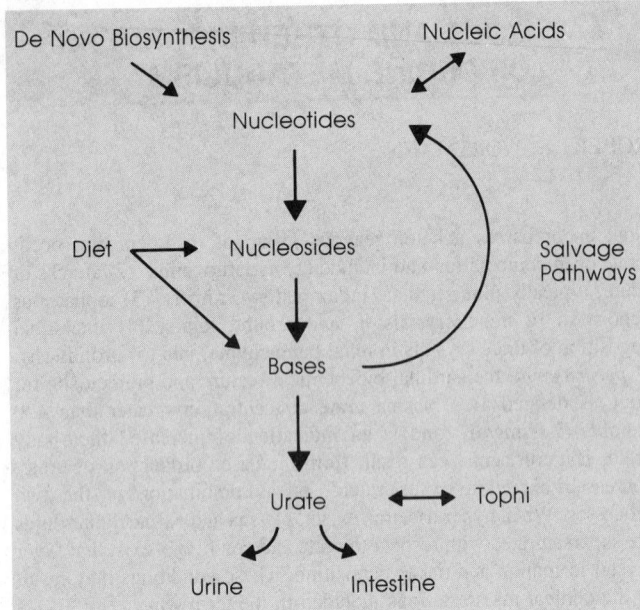

FIGURE 347-1 The total-body urate pool is the net result between urate production and excretion. Urate production is influenced by dietary intake of purines and the rates of de novo biosynthesis of purines from nonpurine precursors, nucleic acid turnover, and salvage by phosphoribosyltransferase activities. The formed urate is normally excreted by urinary and intestinal routes. Hyperuricemia can result from increased production, decreased excretion, or a combination of both mechanisms. When hyperuricemia exists, urate can precipitate and deposit in tissues as tophi.

menopause, values for women increase to approximate those of men. Adult concentrations rise steadily over time and vary with height, body weight, blood pressure, renal function, and alcohol intake.

HYPERURICEMIA

Hyperuricemia may be defined as a plasma (or serum) urate concentration greater than 420 μmol/L (7.0 mg/dL). This definition is based on physicochemical, epidemiologic, and disease-related criteria. Physicochemically, hyperuricemia is the concentration of urate in the blood that exceeds the solubility limits of monosodium urate in plasma, 415 μmol/L (6.8 mg/dL). In epidemiologic studies, hyperuricemia is defined by the mean plus 2 standard deviations of values determined from a randomly selected healthy population. In a major study, 95 percent of unselected individuals had serum urate concentrations below 420 μmol/L (7.0 mg/dL). Finally, hyperuricemia can be defined in relation to the risk of developing disease. The risk of developing gout or urolithiasis increases with urate concentrations greater than 420 μmol/L (7.0 mg/dL) and escalates in proportion to the degree of elevation. Hyperuricemia has a prevalence of between 2.0 and 13.2 percent in ambulatory adults and somewhat higher in hospitalized individuals.

CAUSES OF HYPERURICEMIA It is useful to classify hyperuricemia in relation to the underlying physiology, i.e., whether the hyperuricemia results from increased production, decreased excretion, or a combination of the two (Fig. 347-1, Table 347-1).

Increased urate production Diet provides an exogenous source of purines and, accordingly, contributes to the serum urate concentration in proportion to its purine content. Strict restriction of purine intake reduces the mean serum urate concentration by as little as 60 μmol/L (1.0 mg/dL) and urinary uric acid excretion by approximately 1.2 mmol/d (200 mg/d). Because about 50 percent of ingested RNA purine and 25 percent of ingested DNA purine appear in the urine as uric acid, foods high in nucleic acid content have a significant effect

FIGURE 347-2 Schematic for handling of uric acid by the kidney. Components are illustrated with the percentage of filtered urate.

on the serum urate level. Such foods include liver, "sweetbreads" (i.e., thymus and pancreas), kidney, and anchovy.

Endogenous sources of purine production also influence the serum urate concentration (Fig. 347-3). De novo purine biosynthesis, the formation of a purine ring from nonring structures, is an 11-step process that results in formation of inosinate (IMP). The first step combines phosphoribosylpyrophosphate (PRPP) and glutamine and is catalyzed by amidophosphoribosyltransferase (amidoPRT) activity. The rate of purine biosynthesis and consequent urate production is determined, for the most part, by this enzyme. AmidoPRT is regulated by the substrate PRPP, which drives the reaction forward, and by the end products of biosynthesis (IMP and other ribonucleotides), which provide feedback inhibition. A second regulatory pathway is the salvage of purine bases by hypoxanthine phosphoribosyltransferase (HPRT). HPRT catalyzes the combination of the purine bases hypoxanthine and guanine with PRPP to form the respective ribonucleotides IMP and GMP. Increased salvage activity thus retards de novo synthesis by reducing PRPP levels and increasing concentrations of inhibitory ribonucleotides.

Serum urate concentrations are closely coupled to the rates of de novo purine biosynthesis. An X-linked disorder that causes an increase in activity of the enzyme PRPP synthetase causes increased PRPP production and accelerated de novo biosynthesis. PRPP is a substrate and allosteric activator of amidoPRT, the first enzyme in the de novo pathway. Individuals with this inborn error of metabolism have

TABLE 347-1 Classification of hyperuricemia

Urate overproduction	Decreased uric acid excretion	Combined mechanism
Primary idiopathic	Primary idiopathic	Glucose-6-phosphatase deficiency
HPRT deficiency	Renal insufficiency	Fructose-1-phosphate aldolase deficiency
PRPP synthetase overactivity	Polycystic kidney disease	Alcohol
Hemolytic processes	Diabetes insipidus	Shock
Lymphoproliferative diseases	Hypertension	
Myeloproliferative diseases	Acidosis	
Polycythemia vera	Lactic acidosis	
Psoriasis	Diabetic ketoacidosis	
Paget's disease	Starvation ketosis	
Glycogenosis III, V, and VII	Berylliosis	
Rhabdomyolysis	Sarcoidosis	
Exercise	Lead intoxication	
Alcohol	Hyperparathyroidism	
Obesity	Hypothyroidism	
Purine-rich diet	Toxemia of pregnancy	
	Bartter's syndrome	
	Down syndrome	
	Drug ingestion	
	Salicylates (>2 g/d)	
	Diuretics	
	Alcohol	
	Levodopa	
	Ethambutol	
	Pyrazinamide	
	Nicotinic acid	
	Cyclosporine	

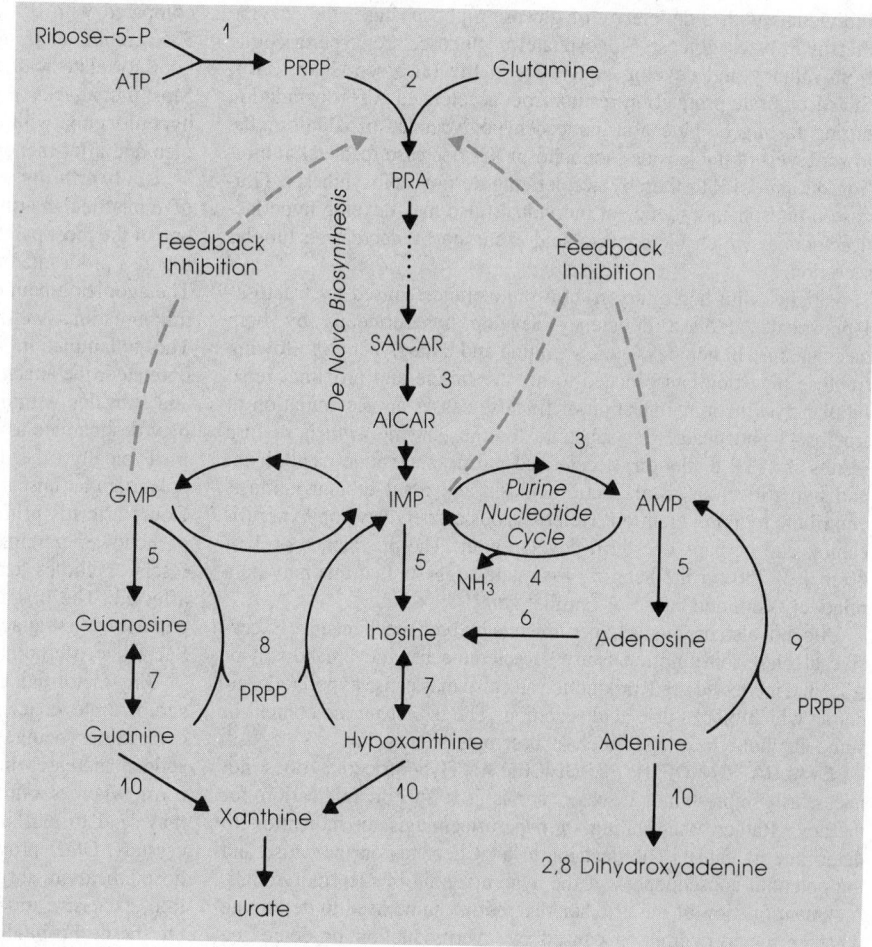

FIGURE 347-3 Abbreviated scheme of purine metabolism. (1) Phosphoribosylpyrophosphate (PRPP) synthetase, (2) amidophosphoribosyltransferase (amidoPRT), (3) adenylosuccinate lyase, (4) adenylate (AMP) deaminase, (5) 5'-nucleotidase, (6) adenosine deaminase, (7) purine nucleoside phosphorylase, (8) hypoxanthine phosphoribosyltransferase (HPRT), (9) adenine phosphoribosyltransferase (APRT), and (10) xanthine oxidase. PRPP, phosphoribosylpyrophosphate; PRA, phosphoribosylamine; SAICAR, succinylaminoimidazole carboxamide ribotide; AICAR, aminoimidazole carboxamide ribotide; GMP, guanylate; IMP, inosinate; AMP, adenylate.

overproduction of purines, hyperuricemia, and hyperuricaciduria and develop uric acid calculi and gout before age 20.

Similarly, individuals deficient in HPRT have hyperuricemia, hyperuricaciduria, uric acid calculi, and gout because of urate overproduction. HPRT deficiency is also X-linked. A complete deficiency of HPRT, the Lesch-Nyhan syndrome, is also associated with self-mutilation, choreoathetosis, and other neurologic problems. Individuals with partial HPRT deficiency, the Kelley-Seegmiller syndrome, only experience gout and renal calculi. HPRT deficiency enhances urate biosynthesis in two ways. PRPP is accumulated as a result of decreased utilization in the salvage pathway and, in turn, provides increased substrate for amidoPRT and de novo biosynthesis. In addition, decreased formation of the nucleoside monophosphates IMP and GMP via the salvage pathway decreases feedback inhibition on amidoPRT, further enhancing de novo biosynthesis.

Accelerated purine nucleotide degradation also can cause hyperuricemia, e.g., with conditions of rapid cell turnover, proliferation, or cell death, as in leukemic blast crises, cytotoxic therapy for malignancy, hemolysis, or rhabdomyolysis. Nucleic acids released from cells are hydrolyzed by the sequential activities of nucleases and phosphodiesterases, forming nucleoside monophosphates, and then are degraded to nucleosides, bases, and urate. Hyperuricemia can result from excessive degradation of skeletal muscle ATP after strenuous physical exercise or status epilepticus and in glycogen storage diseases types III, V, and VII. The hyperuricemia of myocardial infarction, smoke inhalation, and acute respiratory failure also may be related to accelerated breakdown of ATP.

Decreased uric acid excretion As many as 98 percent of individuals with primary hyperuricemia and gout have a defect in the renal handling of uric acid. This is evidenced as a lower than normal ratio of urate clearance to glomerular filtration rate (or urate to inulin clearance rate) over a wide range of filtered loads. As a result, gouty

individuals excrete approximately 40 percent less uric acid than nongouty individuals for any given plasma urate concentration. Uric acid excretion increases in gouty and nongouty individuals when plasma urate levels are raised by purine ingestion or infusion, but in subjects with gout, plasma urate concentrations must be 60 to 120 μmol/L (1 to 2 mg/dL) higher than normal to achieve equivalent uric acid excretion rates.

Altered uric acid excretion could theoretically result from decreased glomerular filtration, decreased tubular secretion, or enhanced tubular reabsorption. Decreased urate filtration does not appear to cause primary hyperuricemia but does contribute to the hyperuricemia of renal insufficiency. Although hyperuricemia is invariable in chronic renal disease, the correlation between serum creatinine, urea nitrogen, and urate concentration is poor because although uric acid excretion per unit of glomerular filtration rate increases progressively with chronic renal insufficiency, tubular secretory capacity tends to be preserved, tubular reabsorptive capacity is reduced, and extrarenal clearance of uric acid increases as renal damage becomes more severe.

Decreased proximal tubular secretion of urate may cause the hyperuricemia in individuals with gout and no evidence of urate overproduction. Decreased tubular secretion of urate also causes the secondary hyperuricemia of acidosis. Diabetic ketoacidosis, starvation, ethanol intoxication, lactic acidosis, and salicylate intoxication are accompanied by accumulations of organic acids (β-hydroxybutyrate, acetoacetate, lactate, or salicylates) that compete with urate for tubular secretion. In some subjects with gout, hyperuricemia may be due to enhanced reabsorption of uric acid distal to the site of secretion, a mechanism known to be responsible for the hyperuricemia of extracellular volume depletion such as with diabetes insipidus or diuretic therapy.

Combined mechanisms Both increased urate production and decreased uric acid excretion may contribute to hyperuricemia.

Individuals with a deficiency of glucose-6-phosphatase, the enzyme that hydrolyzes glucose-6-phosphate to glucose, are hyperuricemic from infancy and develop gout early in life (also see Chap. 350). Increased urate production results from accelerated ATP degradation during fasting or glucagon-induced hypoglycemia. In addition, the lower levels of nucleoside monophosphates decrease feedback inhibition on amidoPRT, thereby accelerating de novo biosynthesis. Glucose-6-phosphatase–deficient individuals also may develop hyperlacticacidemia, which blocks uric acid excretion by decreasing tubular secretion.

Patients with hereditary fructose intolerance caused by fructose-1-phosphate aldolase deficiency develop hyperuricemia by both mechanisms. In hemozygotes, vomiting and hypoglycemia following fructose ingestion can proceed to hepatic failure and proximal renal tubular dysfunction. Ingestion of fructose causes an accumulation of fructose-1-phosphate, the substrate for the enzyme, which in turn results in ATP depletion, accelerated purine nucleotide catabolism, and hyperuricemia. Both lactic acidosis and renal tubular acidosis contribute to urate retention. Heterozygous carriers develop hyperuricemia, and perhaps one-third develop gout. The prevalence of 1 of 80 to 1 of 250 for the heterozygous state suggests that this may be a relatively common cause of familial gout.

Alcohol also promotes hyperuricemia by both mechanisms. Excessive alcohol consumption causes accelerated hepatic breakdown of ATP and increased urate production and also may cause hyperlacticacidemia which blocks uric acid secretion. The higher purine content in some alcoholic beverages such as beer may be a factor.

EVALUATION OF HYPERURICEMIA Hyperuricemia does not necessarily represent a disease, nor is it a specific indication for therapy. Rather, the finding of hyperuricemia is an indication to determine its cause. The decision to treat depends on the cause and the potential consequences of the hyperuricemia in each individual.

Quantification of the uric acid excretion can be used to determine whether hyperuricemia is caused by overproduction or decreased excretion. On a purine-free diet, men with normal renal function excrete less than 3.6 mmol/d (600 mg/d). Thus the hyperuricemia of individuals who excrete more uric acid per day while on a purine-free diet is due to purine overproduction, and that in those excreting less is due to decreased excretion. If the assessment is performed while the patient is on a regular diet, the level of 4.2 mmol/d (800 mg/d) can be used as the discriminating value. With renal insufficiency, less urate is filtered in the glomeruli and less uric acid appears in the urine. Consequently, in the presence of renal insufficiency, a lower 24-h urinary uric acid value does not necessarily rule out urate overproduction, but an elevated value provides strong evidence of urate overproduction. Spuriously high values can occur if the patient is taking a uricosuric agent at the time of urine collection. Glucocorticoids, ascorbic acid, salicylates in doses greater than 2 g/d, and other agents that promote urate excretion interfere with the interpretation of results.

Assessment of the ratio of uric acid to creatinine (or the ratio of uric acid clearance to creatinine clearance) in spot or random urine samples is not a reliable method to screen for urate overproduction. However, this is a useful tool for evaluating individuals with acute renal failure suspected of having acute uric acid nephropathy (see below).

COMPLICATIONS OF HYPERURICEMIA Although the manifestations of gout can occur in almost any combination, the typical sequence involves progression through asymptomatic hyperuricemia, acute gouty arthritis, interval or intercritical gout, and chronic or tophaceous gout. Nephrolithiasis can occur before or after the first attack of gouty arthritis.

The prevalence of hyperuricemia is estimated to range between 2.0 and 13.2 percent and the prevalence of gout varies between 1.3 and 3.7 percent in the general population. The higher the serum urate concentration, the more likely an individual is to develop gout. In one large study, the incidence of gout was 4.9 percent for individuals with serum urate concentrations of 540 μmol/L (9.0 mg/dL) or more compared with 0.5 percent for those with values between 415 and 535 μmol/L (7.0 and 8.9 mg/dL). Similarly, the complications of gout correlate with the duration and severity of the hyperuricemia. Most first attacks of gouty arthritis follow 20 to 40 years of sustained hyperuricemia with a peak age of onset between 40 and 60 years for men and after menopause for women.

Gouty arthritis The benchmark feature of gout is the acute attack of monarticular arthritis. The first attack begins explosively and is one of the most painful events experienced. Occasionally, individuals report a prodrome or previous episodes of milder pain lasting hours. The agonizing pain of acute gout is accompanied by signs of intense inflammation: swelling, erythema, warmth, and exquisite tenderness. The inflammation may be accompanied by low-grade fever. If untreated, the attack usually peaks 24 to 48 h after the first symptoms and subsides within 7 to 10 days. The skin over the involved part may desquamate as the episode resolves.

Typically, the initial attack affects only one joint, although polyarticular onsets occur and may be more common in women. Gouty arthritis primarily affects peripheral joints, particularly those of the lower extremities. In addition, periarticular sites such as plantar fascia, Achilles tendon insertions, or other tenosynovia can be affected. The first metatarsophalangeal joint is involved in over 50 percent of first attacks and in 90 percent of individuals at some time. Sacroiliac, sternomanubrial, and spinal involvement occurs rarely.

Any factor that causes either an abrupt increase or decrease in the serum urate concentration may provoke an acute attack, the best correlations being with factors that cause a rapid fall. In theory, sudden increases in urate concentration may cause new crystals to form, whereas a drop in serum and extracellular urate concentrations may lead to partial dissolution and shedding of previously formed crystals. Other provocative factors include stress, trauma, infection, hospitalization, surgery, starvation, weight reduction, hyperalimentation, excessive food intake, alcohol, and medications (Table 347-2). Of these, hospitalization and medications are probably the most significant. Acute gouty attacks occur in 20 to 86 percent of individuals with a history of gout when they are hospitalized for medical or surgical reasons. The stress of a severe illness, changes in medication, shifts in fluid status or electrolytes, and general anesthesia probably contribute to the exacerbations. Attacks can follow the use of thiazide diuretics that cause hyperuricemia or after initiation of allopurinol or other therapies to lower serum urate.

Occasional attacks of acute gouty arthritis occur in the absence of hyperuricemia. Presumably most such attacks can be explained by factors that lower serum concentrations, temporarily altering the usual hyperuricemic state (and that perhaps triggered the attack). Occasionally, hyperuricemia cannot be documented despite repeated attempts. Gout could theoretically develop anytime synovial fluid is supersaturated with urate. Free water is cleared from the joint space more rapidly than urate, and if the amount of synovial fluid containing a normal concentration of urate increases because of trauma or edema, then the urate concentration within the joint would temporarily increase as the problem resolved and the water was more rapidly cleared. Supersaturated concentrations of urate could cause the formation of crystals and precipitate an attack.

TABLE 347-2 Medications with uricosuric activity

Acetohexamide	Glyceryl guaiacolate
ACTH	Glycopyrrolate
Ascorbic acid	Halofenate
Azauridine	Meclofenamate
Benzbromarone	Phenolsulfonphthalein
Calcitonin	Phenylbutazone
Chlorprothixene	Probenecid
Citrate	Radiographic contrast agents
Dicumarol	Salicylates (>2 g/2d)
Diflunisal	Sulfinpyrazone
Estrogens	Tetracycline that is outdated
Glucocorticoids	Zoxazolamine

FIGURE 347-4 Chronic tophaceous gout. The left panel shows deformities of the foot in a 65-year-old man with a long history of gouty arthritis. On the right are tophi in an olecranon bursa and in the fingers of a 25-year-old man with Kelley-Seegmiller syndrome (partial HPRT deficiency).

Some individuals experience only a single gouty attack in their lifetime; others experience recurrence. Although the interval between first and second attacks may be over 40 years, three-fourths of individuals have a second attack within 2 years. The terms *interval gout* or *intercritical gout* describe the periods between attacks of acute arthritis when the individual has no joint complaints. In severe cases, unless therapeutic intervention occurs, chronic gouty arthritis develops with time. The pain-free intercritical periods shorten, and acute attacks occur with increased frequency, last longer, and involve more joints. The intensity of attacks may lessen somewhat, and involvement becomes polyarticular. Chronic gout is characterized by persistent polyarticular low-grade pain with superimposed acute or subacute inflammation. During this stage, tophi become apparent on physical examination (Fig. 347-4). Although there is individual variability, the rate of urate deposition in joint tissues and of articular destruction correlates with duration and severity of hyperuricemia. In general, approximately 10 years elapse between the first attack of the gouty arthritis and appearance of tophi. During the interim, however, destruction of cartilage and bone occurs, as evidenced by the radiographic changes (Fig. 347-5).

Pathogenesis Acute gout results from the interaction between urate crystals and polymorphonuclear leukocytes (Fig. 347-6) and involves activation of humoral and cellular inflammatory mechanisms. Urate crystals activate complement through both the classic and alternate pathways. Hageman factor and the contact system of coagulation are also activated and result in generation of bradykinin, kallikrein, and plasmin. The interaction of urate crystals with neutrophils results in the release of lysosomal enzymes, oxygen-derived free radicals, leukotriene and prostaglandin metabolites, collagenase, and protease. Phagocytosis of crystals by neutrophils causes release of crystal-induced chemotactic factor (CCF). CCF, leukotriene B_4 (LTB_4), and the activated complement component C5a are all chemotactic and contribute to the marked polymorphonuclear leukocyte response in the initial phase of acute arthritis. With time, phagocytic mononuclear cells replace the polymorphonuclear cells. Urate crystals cause these cells to release prostaglandins (PGE_2), lysosomal enzymes, tumor necrosis factor alpha, and interleukins 1 and 6 (IL-1 and IL-6). Synovial lining cells also participate in the inflammatory response by releasing inflammatory mediators.

The inflammatory potential of urate crystals is greatly affected by the presence of absorbed proteins. Absorbed purified IgG causes enhanced crystal-induced platelet secretion, increased superoxide generation, and increased lysosomal enzyme release from polymorphonuclear leukocytes. On the other hand, apoprotein B, a component

FIGURE 347-5 Radiographic changes in gout are the result of urate deposition. At first deposits are microscopic and are undetectable by x-ray. With persistent hyperuricemia, tophi enlarges to involve juxtaarticular bone and are apparent radiographically but not on physical examination. If unaltered by therapy, tophi continue to enlarge and become obvious in physical examination. The classic radiographic change of gout is a bony erosion. The location can be intraarticular, paraarticular, or at a distance from the joint. The erosions tend to be round and surrounded by a sclerotic border, giving a "punched out" appearance. There may be an "overhanging margin or lip." Nodular soft tissue prominence develops as the tophi enlarge. Joint spaces are typically preserved until late in the disease when secondary degenerative changes may occur. The left panel shows classic advanced changes of tophaceous gout including soft tissue distortion and erosion with sclerotic margins and overhanging edges. The right panel shows an erosive lesion in the interphalangeal joint in a patient with no tophi found on physical examination.

FIGURE 347-6 Crystals of monosodium urate in polymorphonuclear leukocytes and synovial fluid.

of very low density, low-density, and intermediate-density lipoproteins, inhibits urate crystal–induced stimulation of neutrophils. Apoprotein B is not normally present in synovial fluid and, because of its size, probably does not have access to that compartment under normal conditions. When synovitis develops, larger molecules, including lipoproteins, enter the joint space, bind to urate crystals, and, perhaps, play a role in terminating the attack.

Tophi are aggregates of monosodium urate monohydrate crystals that are generally surrounded by a giant cell, foreign body–type mononuclear cell inflammatory reaction. They can form in extraarticular and articular structures and cause deformity and destruction of hard and soft tissues. In joints, they lead to destruction of cartilage and bone, triggering secondary degeneration changes.

Renal disease Despite the invariable hyperuricemia in renal failure, gouty arthritis occurs in less than 1 percent of patients with chronic renal failure. Since most gouty arthritis follows 20 to 40 years of sustained hyperuricemia, most patients with renal failure are probably not hyperuricemic long enough to accumulate the necessary urate load. In addition, individuals with chronic renal insufficiency show diminished inflammatory responses to urate crystals injected subcutaneously. Polycystic disease of the kidneys is an exception, with a prevalence between 24 and 36 percent. The mechanism for this association is unknown.

Chronic renal failure patients on long-term hemodialysis can experience recurrent acute arthritis or periarthritis. Some of these attacks are gout due to urate crystal deposition, and others are caused by crystals of calcium phosphate (apatite) or calcium oxalate.

Gout is an important cause of morbidity in some recipients of renal allografts. From 7 to 12 percent of individuals who receive cyclosporine and glucocorticoids for maintenance immunosuppression develop acute gouty arthritis with a mean duration of about 24 months between transplantation and first attack. In contrast, gouty attacks are very rare in transplant recipients maintained with azathioprine and glucocorticoids. In cyclosporine-treated transplant recipients, urate synthesis is normal and urate clearances are decreased compared with azathioprine-treated controls. Concomitant diuretic therapy may enhance the hyperuricemic effects of cyclosporine.

In addition to the association with renal insufficiency, hyperuricemia causes several renal problems: (1) nephrolithiasis, (2) urate nephropathy, a rare cause of renal insufficiency attributed to monoso-dium urate crystal deposition in the renal interstitium, and (3) uric acid nephropathy, a reversible cause of acute renal failure resulting from deposition of large amounts of uric acid crystals in the renal collecting ducts, pelvis, and ureters.

NEPHROLITHIASIS Individuals with gout commonly develop nephrolithiasis. Nephrolithiasis may precede the onset of gouty arthritis in 40 percent of individuals with both conditions. In gout, the prevalence of nephrolithiasis correlates with the serum and urinary uric acid concentrations, reaching approximately 50 percent with serum urate levels of 770 μmol/L (13 mg/dL) or urinary uric acid excretion over 6.5 mmol/d (1100 mg/d).

Not all kidney stones that occur in individuals with gout are composed of uric acid. Stones composed of calcium oxalate, calcium phosphate, or those salts combined with uric acid occur in approximately 15 percent of cases. Uric acid may act as a nidus on which calcium oxalate can precipitate and grow. Furthermore, uric acid stones can develop in individuals with no other manifestations of gout, only 20 percent of whom are hyperuricemic. Some nongouty individuals with calcium oxalate stones have hyperuricemia or hyperuricaciduria.

URATE NEPHROPATHY Urate nephropathy, sometimes referred to as *urate nephrosis,* is a late manifestation of severe gout and is characterized histologically by deposits of monosodium urate crystals surrounded by a giant cell inflammatory reaction in the medullary interstitium and pyramids and can cause chronic renal insufficiency. The disorder is rare and cannot be diagnosed in the absence of gouty arthritis. Clinically, the lesions may be silent or associated with proteinuria, hypertension, and renal insufficiency.

Prior to the advent of antihyperuricemic agents and aggressive treatment for asymptomatic hypertension, renal failure was the cause of death in up to 25 percent of individuals with gout. Postmortem evaluations of kidneys from patients with gout frequently revealed urate crystals, pyelonephritis, and vascular changes. At present, aging or coexisting diseases that cause nephropathy, such as cardiovascular disease, hypertension, or independently occurring intrinsic renal disease, are usually responsible for the decreased renal function that may develop in gout.

URIC ACID NEPHROPATHY This reversible cause of acute renal failure is due to precipitation of uric acid in renal tubules and collecting ducts that causes obstruction to urine flow and is not a component of gout. Uric acid nephropathy develops following sudden urate overproduction and marked hyperuricaciduria. Factors that favor uric acid crystal formation include dehydration and acidosis. This form of acute renal failure occurs most often during an aggressive "blastic" phase of leukemia or lymphoma prior to or coincident with cytolytic therapy but also has been observed in individuals with other neoplasms, following epileptic seizures, and after vigorous exercise with heat stress. Autopsy studies have demonstrated intraluminal precipitates of uric acid, dilated proximal tubules, and normal glomeruli. Animal studies suggest that the initial pathogenic events include obstruction of collecting ducts with uric acid and obstruction of distal renal vasculature.

If recognized, uric acid nephropathy is potentially reversible. Appropriate therapy has reduced the mortality from 47 percent to practically nil. Serum levels cannot be relied on for diagnosis because this condition has developed in the presence of urate concentrations ranging from 720 to 4800 μmol/L (12 to 80 mg/dL). The distinctive clinical finding is the urinary uric acid concentration. In most forms of acute renal failure with decreased urine output, urinary uric acid content is either normal or reduced, and the ratio of uric acid to creatinine is less than 1. Because the decreased urine output in acute uric acid nephropathy is due to massive uricaciduria, the ratio of uric acid to creatinine in a random urine sample or 24-h specimen is greater than 1 and therefore is essentially diagnostic.

MANAGEMENT Asymptomatic hyperuricemia For many years, fear of adverse outcomes caused physicians to prescribe urate-lowering agents for asymptomatic hyperuricemia. Today, with perhaps one exception, no data indicate that treatment of asymptomatic hyperuricemia is cost-effective or beneficial. That exception is in individuals with neoplastic disease who are about to receive cytolytic therapy and are at risk for acute uric acid nephropathy.

Although hyperuricemic individuals are at risk for developing gouty arthritis, especially those with higher serum urate levels, treatment of asymptomatic hyperuricemia to prevent the first attack of gouty arthritis is not indicated because most people who are hyperuricemic never develop gout. Furthermore, organ damage does not appear to occur prior to a first gouty attack. Neither structural kidney damage nor tophi are identifiable before that event. Reduced renal function cannot be attributed to asymptomatic hyperuricemia, and treatment of asymptomatic hyperuricemia does not alter the progression of renal dysfunction in patients with renal disease. Although nephrolithiasis is common in gouty patients, and although a number of individuals with nephrolithiasis are hyperuricemic, the risk of stone formation in people with asymptomatic hyperuricemia is not established. Nor is hyperuricemia an independent risk factor for atherosclerotic cardiovascular disease.

Thus, other than for prevention of acute uric acid nephropathy, the routine treatment of asymptomatic hyperuricemia cannot be justified. In fact, routine screening for asymptomatic hyperuricemia is not recommended. If hyperuricemia is diagnosed, however, the cause should be determined. Causal factors should be corrected if the condition is secondary, and associated problems such as hypertension, hypercholesterolemia, diabetes mellitus, and obesity should be controlled. Treatment of asymptomatic hyperuricemia with antihyperuricemia agents entails inconvenience, cost, and potential toxicity and should not be prescribed.

Symptomatic hyperuricemia Initially, therapy should be directed toward relieving symptoms. Both gouty arthritis and nephrolithiasis are excruciatingly painful. Once the presenting symptoms are controlled, a decision must be made whether to initiate antihyperuricemic therapy.

Acute gouty arthritis As with any disease, appropriate and effective treatment requires accurate diagnosis. Few conditions can be diagnosed with more certainty or treated more successfully than gout. Thus a specific diagnosis provides insight into prognosis and treatment. A definitive diagnosis requires aspiration of the involved joint or tissue and demonstration of intracellular monosodium urate crystals in synovial fluid polymorphonuclear leukocytes or in tophaceous aggregates. Using polarized light microscopy with a first-order red compensator, the strong negative birefringence of the needle-shaped crystals can be appreciated easily. The triad of acute monarticular arthritis, hyperuricemia, and a dramatic response to colchicine provides presumptive evidence for gouty arthritis. These criteria, however, are a poor substitute for crystal identification, because some patients with gout are not hyperuricemic at the time of the attack. In addition, colchicine may be effective for other disorders, especially pseudogout (calcium pyrophosphate dehydrate crystal deposition disease) and calcific (basic calcium phosphate or apatite) tendinitis. These diseases that can mimic acute gout may occur in individuals who happen to be hyperuricemic. Finally, acute gouty arthritis can coexist with septic arthritis, psoriatic arthritis, systemic lupus erythematosus, rheumatoid arthritis, osteoarthritis, and pseudogout.

Once the diagnosis of gouty arthritis is secure, the choice of therapeutic agents includes colchicine, a nonsteroidal anti-inflammatory drug (NSAID), or intraarticular glucocorticoids. Regardless of the choice, the effectiveness of the agent is dependent on when it is used. Each will work if started early; none works quickly if initiated late in the course of the attack.

Colchicine, the traditional agent used, inhibits the release of leukocyte-derived crystal-induced chemotactic factor (CCF). Oral doses of 0.6 mg are given every hour until improvement is noted, gastrointestinal side effects develop, or 10 doses have been taken without relief (in which case the diagnosis may be questioned). Although highly effective, oral colchicine cannot be tolerated by up to 80 percent of people because of abdominal pain, diarrhea, and nausea. Colchicine also can be given intravenously, but administration

by this route is potentially dangerous and should be used with extreme caution despite the fact that intravenous use can eliminate the gastrointestinal side effects (provided the drug is not also being taken orally). A single dose of 1 mg diluted in 20 mL normal saline is usually adequate. A second dose can be repeated 6 to 12 h later, but doses greater than 2 mg and repeated injections beyond 24 h are not recommended. Absolute contraindications for intravenous colchicine therapy include depressed bone marrow function, renal disease (creatinine clearance less than 10 mL/min, oliguria, or anuria), liver disease (liver function tests over twice the upper limit of normal), and sepsis.

Because of its relative specificity for acute gouty arthritis, oral colchicine is the agent of choice for the ambulatory patient in whom the diagnosis is not certain. If the diagnosis is certain, NSAID may be more appropriate because of better tolerance. Indomethacin is the usual agent, but ibuprofen, naproxen, tolmetin, sulindac, piroxicam, ketoprofen, and flurbiprofen have all been used effectively. The action of these agents is less specific for gout than that of colchicine, but they are effective, especially if used early in the attack. Treatment is begun with the highest approved dose of the selected agent and is continued until 3 to 4 days after all signs of inflammation have completely resolved. These agents are contraindicated in patients with active peptic ulcer disease; should be used in caution in patients with heart failure, other edematous states, or hypertension because of potential problems from sodium retention; and may precipitate hyperkalemia and renal insufficiency.

Intraarticular injection of glucocorticoids also may be used for acute gout. This is most useful when the patient cannot take oral medications, when colchicine and NSAIDs are contraindicated, or in refractory cases. ACTH injection and oral glucocorticoids have been employed for acute gouty arthritis but are not recommended for routine use.

Intercritical and chronic gout The term *intercritical* (or *interval*) *gout* applies to the period after the acute gouty attack has resolved and the patient is asymptomatic. It is at that time that the decision must be made whether to initiate antihyperuricemic therapy. All authors agree that hyperuricemia should be treated in patients with recurrent attacks, those with chronic gout or evidence of tophi, and individuals with gouty arthritis and nephrolithiasis. Some maintain that the first attack of acute gouty arthritis alone is sufficient indication. Others argue that first attacks are easily, inexpensively, and effectively treated and postpone urate-lowering therapy until one or more additional attacks occur.

Sustained hyperuricemia provides a definite risk to bone and cartilage for those with gouty arthritis. If hyperuricemia is not controlled, urate deposits enlarge and become radiographically evident before subcutaneous tophi develop. In a study of patients with intercritical gout, 42 percent had radiographic changes characteristic of bony tophi despite no evidence of tophi on physical examination (see Fig. 347-5). One cannot predict from the frequency of acute attacks, the history of therapy, or the serum urate levels at the time of evaluation which patients will show bony changes.

Before starting treatment with urate-lowering agents, the patient should be free of all signs of inflammation and have begun colchicine for prophylaxis. The sudden drop in serum urate with the initiation of allopurinol or uricosuric therapy may prolong or precipitate an acute attack. Colchicine, at a dose of 0.6 mg orally one to three times a day, is about 90 percent effective in preventing subsequent gout attacks. Rarely, a reversible colchicine-induced neuromuscular toxicity may be manifested by subacute myopathy and axonal neuropathy with elevated serum creatinine kinase levels. This toxicity is most common in individuals with renal insufficiency and is reversible when colchicine is discontinued.

Once antihyperuricemic therapy is initiated, the dosage used should maintain the serum urate at or below 300 μmol/L (5.0 mg/dL). Extracellular fluid is saturated with urate at a concentration of approximately 415 μmol/L (6.8 mg/dL). If the serum urate remains above this level, tissue deposition of urate crystals will continue. A

TABLE 349-1 Summary of lysosomal storage diseases

Disorder*	Heterogeneity (onset)	Enzyme deficiency	Stored material	Neurologic
G_{M1} gangliosidosis (90)	Infantile (birth) Juvenile (6–20 mo) Adult	β-Galactosidase	G_{M1} ganglioside Glycoproteins Keratan sulfate	Mental retardation, seizures, blindness; later in juvenile form, variable in adults
Tay-Sachs and variants, G_{M2} gangliosidosis (92)	Infantile (3–6 mo) Juvenile Adult forms	Hexosaminidase A	G_{M2} ganglioside	Mental retardation, seizures, blindness; later in juvenile form
Sandhoff, G_{M2} gangliosidosis (92)	Infantile (3–6 mo)	Hexosaminidase A and B	G_{M2} ganglioside Globoside	Mental retardation, seizures, blindness
G_{M2} gangliosidosis, AB variant (92)	Findings similar to Tay-Sachs except primary defect is a ganglioside activator protein.			
Krabbe, galactosylceramide lipidosis (87)	Infantile (2–6 mo) Late onset	Galactosylceramide β-Galactosidase	↑ Galactoscerebroside/ sulfatide ratio	Mental retardation, leukodystrophy; variable in late onset
Metachromatic leukodystrophy, sulfatide lipidosis (88)	Late infantile (1–4 yr) Juvenile (4–20 yr) Adult	Arylsulfatase A (cerebroside sulfatase)	Galactosyl sulfatides	Mental retardation, leukodystrophy, psychosis and dementia in adults
Sphingolipid activator protein 1 deficiency (77)	Findings similar to metachromatic leukodystrophy except primary defect is activator protein.			
Niemann-Pick, sphingomyelin lipidosis (84,85)	Infantile neuropathic (1–4 mo) Late onset neuropathic Visceral	Sphingomyelinase in types A and B but not type C	Sphingomyelin Cholesterol	Mental retardation, ataxia, and seizures in neuropathic forms
Gaucher, glucosylceramide lipidosis (86)	Infantile (1–12 mo) Juvenile (2–6 yr) Adult	β-Glucocerebrosidase	Glucosylceramide	Mental retardation; spastic, later flaccid, ataxia in juvenile; no neurologic symptoms in adult form
Fabry, trihexosyl ceramidosis (89)	Hemizygous males Heterozygous females	α-Galactosidase A	Trihexosylceramide	Painful neuropathy
Acid lipase deficiency (82)	Infantile Wolman's disease (0–3 mo) Late onset cholesteryl ester storage disease (CESD)	Acid lipase	Cholesteryl ester Triglyceride	Mental retardation but mild related to growth failure in Wolman; none in CESD
Farber, ceramide deficiency (83)	Infantile (0–4 mo) Rare juvenile	Ceramidase	Ceramide	Occasional mental retardation, but may be secondary to somatic features
Pompe, glycogen storage type II (78)	Infantile (0–6 mo) Juvenile Adult	Acid maltase (α-1,4- and α-1,6-glucosidase)	Glycogen	Probably normal mentally
Fucosidosis (81)	Infantile (3–12 mo) Juvenile	α-Fucosidase	Glycopeptides Glycolipids Oligosaccharides	Mental retardation
Mannosidosis (81)	Infantile (6–18 mo) Milder form	α-Mannosidase	Oligosaccharides	Mental retardation
Aspartylglucosaminuria (81)	Young adult onset	Aspartylglucosamine amidase	Aspartylglucosamine Glycopeptides	Mental retardation
Mucopolysaccharidosis IH and IS (79)	Infantile Hurler (6–12 mo) Intermediate Adult Scheie	α-Iduronidase	Dermatan sulfate Heparan sulfate	Mental retardation, absent in Scheie
Hunter, mucopolysaccharidosis II (79)	Severe infantile (6–12 mo) Mild juvenile	Iduronosulfate sulfatase	Dermatan sulfate Heparan sulfate	Mental retardation, less in mild form

* Numbers in parentheses refer to the chapters in Scriver et al., 7th ed., in which the disorder is discussed in detail.

TABLE 349-1 Summary of lysosomal storage diseases *(continued)*

Liver and/or spleen enlargement	Skeletal dysplasia	Ophthalmic	Hematologic	Genetics	Unique manifestations
+ + + + Less in juvenile, variable in adult	+ + + + Variable in juvenile and adult forms	Cherry red spot in 50% of infantile; corneal clouding variable but more in adults	Foam cells Vacuolated lymphocytes	AR[†]	Coarse facies, edema, macroglossia, mucopolysacchariduria; early blindness in infantile, milder in juvenile; in adults often spondyloepiphyseal dysplasia ± mucopolysacchariduria
0	0	Cherry red spot in infantile form, rare in juvenile	0	AR	Macrocephaly, hyperacusis in infantile; increased in Ashkenazic Jews
0	0	Cherry-red spot	0	AR	Macrocephaly, hyperacusis, visceral histiocytosis
0	0	Optic atrophy	0	AR	Extreme irritability, ↑ CSF protein, fever, globoid cell neuropathology
0	0	Optic atrophy, less in juvenile and adult forms	0	AR	↑ CSF protein and early gait abnormalities in late infantile; peripheral neuropathy
+ + + + Less prominent in late onset forms	0	Macular degeneration and cherry red spot in neuronopathic forms	Distinctive foam cell Vacuolated lymphocytes	AR	Pulmonary infiltrates, brownish skin, infantile neuronopathic form increased in Ashkenazic Jews, sea-blue histiocytes
+ + + + Hypersplenism common	+ +	Usually normal	Distinctive foam cell	AR	Adult form includes ↑ acid phosphatase, pathologic fractures; Ashkenazic Jewish predilection
0	0	Corneal dystrophy, vascular lesions, cataracts	0	X-linked Fabry's Disease	Cutaneous angiokeratoma, vascular thromboses, hypohidrosis
+ + +	0	0	Foam cells Vacuolated lymphocytes	AR	Adrenal calcification, anemia, vomiting and poor growth in Wolman; hepatic fibrosis and ↑ blood cholesterol in CESD
+/−	?	Mild macular degeneration	0	AR	Arthropathy—subcutaneous, periarticular and visceral nodules (lipogranulomatosis); ↑ CSF protein
Mild hepatomegaly	0	0	0	AR	Lethal skeletal and cardiac myopathy in infantile; primarily skeletal myopathy in adults
+ +	+ +	0	Vacuolated lymphocytes Foam cells	AR	Coarse facies, increased sweat electrolytes, angiokeratoma in juvenile
+ + +	+ +	Cataracts, corneal clouding	Vacuolated lymphocytes Granulated neutrophils	AR	Coarse facies, enlarged tongue
0	+ +	Lens opacities	Vacuolated lymphocytes	AR	Coarse facies, detectable by urine amino acid analysis
+ + +	+ + + +	Corneal clouding	Granulated lymphocytes	AR	Coarse facies, cardiovascular involvement, joint stiffness
+ + +	+ + + +	Retinal degeneration, no significant corneal clouding	Granulated lymphocytes	X-linked	Coarse facies, cardiovascular involvement, joint stiffness

[†] AR = autosomal recessive.

(Table continues next page)

TABLE 349-1 Summary of lysosomal storage diseases (continued)

Disorder*	Heterogeneity (onset)	Enzyme deficiency	Stored material	Neurologic
Sanfilippo A, muco-polysaccharidosis III A (79)		Heparan N-sulfatase (sulfamidase)		
Sanfilippo B, muco-polysaccharidosis III B (79)	Late infantile (1–4 yr)	N-Acetyl-α-glucosaminidase	Heparan sulfate	Severe mental retardation
Sanfilippo C, muco-polysaccharidosis III C (79)		Acetyl-CoA:α-glucosaminide N-acetyl-transferase		
Sanfilippo D, mucopolysac-charidosis III D (79)		N-Acetylglucosamine-6-sulfate sulfatase		
Morquio, mucopolysacchar-idosis IV (79)	Some variation	N-Acetylgalactosamine-6-sulfate sulfatase	Keratan sulfate	0
Maroteaux-Lamy, muco-polysaccharidosis VI (79)	Variation in severity and cardiovascular involvement	N-Acetylhexosamine-4-sulfate sulfatase (arylsulfatase B)	Dermatan sulfate	0
β-Glucuronidase deficiency, mucopolysaccharidosis VII (79)	Few patients; infantile to adult forms	β-Glucuronidase	Dermatan sulfate ? Heparan sulfate	Mental retardation ? Absent in some adults
Multiple sulfatase deficiency (88)	Late infantile (1–4 yr)	Arylsulfatases A, B, and C Other sulfatases	Sulfatides Mucopolysaccharides	Mental retardation
Sialidosis (81)	Congenital, infantile, juvenile, cherry-red spot myoclonus	Glycoprotein neuramini-dase (sialidase)	Sialyloligosaccharides	Mental retardation, myoclonus
Galactosialidosis (91)	Infantile Juvenile	Protective glycoprotein	Sialyloligosaccharides	Mental retardation
Mucolipidosis II, I cell disease (80)	Infantile (0–3 mo)	UDP-N-acetylglucosamine (GlcNAc):glycoprotein GlcNAc-1-phosphotransferase	Glycoproteins Glycolipids	Mental retardation
Mucolipidosis III, pseudo-Hurler polydystrophy (80)	Late infantile (>2 yr)		Glycoproteins Glycolipids	Mild mental retardation
Mucolipidosis IV	Infantile	? Ganglioside neuramin-idase	? Multiple	Mental retardation
Neuronal ceroid lipofus-cinoses	Late infantile Juvenile Adult	Unknown	"Ceroid" "Lipofuscin"	Mental retardation, dementia variable in adults, seizures

* Numbers in parentheses refer to the chapters in Scriver et al., 7th ed., in which the disorder is discussed in detail.
‡ AR = autosomal recessive.

and recurrent infection. The family history may reveal similarly affected siblings or consanguinity in autosomal recessive disease or other affected male family members in X-linked disorders. Ethnic background may be helpful because several lipid storage diseases are more frequent in Ashkenazic Jews, and mannosidosis and aspartylglucosaminuria may occur with increased frequency in Scandinavian populations. The juvenile form of sialidosis is frequent in the Japanese.

On physical examination, the head circumference may be enlarged. Increased somatic growth may occur early in the course of some mucopolysaccharidoses and glycoprotein storage diseases, while short stature is a later finding in many disorders. Ophthalmologic examination should include slit-lamp and careful funduscopic examination. Enlargement of the tongue, coarsening of the facies, and hepatosplenomegaly may occur. Skeletal findings may include gibbus deformity, broadening of the long bones, and joint stiffness. Cutaneous findings are rare except in fucosidosis, sialidosis, Fabry disease, and Hunter disease. Careful neurologic examination should attempt to

distinguish the extent of involvement of gray matter, white matter, and peripheral nerves. Preliminary diagnostic studies should include examination of the peripheral blood smear for vacuolated or granulated leukocytes, urinary screening for mucopolysaccharide, and radiologic bone survey. The preferred method of diagnosis is to use the preceding information to select specific enzyme assays in serum, leukocytes, or cultured skin fibroblasts. If a mucopolysaccharide screening test is positive, or if clinical findings are suggestive, quantitative mucopolysaccharide analysis can be carried out. If a specific diagnosis is not readily established, biopsy of skin, bone marrow, rectal mucosa, liver, peripheral nerve, conjunctiva, or other tissue for light and electron microscopy can be helpful. Electron-microscopic findings can direct one toward or away from the general category of lysosomal storage diseases based on the presence or absence of engorged lysosomes. Again, enzyme assay is the proper method for diagnosis of the standard disorders. When significant evidence favors a lysosomal storage disease but no enzyme deficiency is demonstrable, chemical

TABLE 349-1 Summary of lysosomal storage diseases *(continued)*

Liver and/or spleen enlargement	Skeletal dysplasia	Ophthalmic	Hematologic	Genetics	Unique manifestations
+	+	0	Granulated lymphocytes	AR	Mild coarsening of facies
+	Severe, distinctive	Corneal clouding	Granulated neutrophils	AR	Severe deformity, odontoid hypoplasia, aortic regurgitation
++	++++	Corneal clouding	Granulated neutrophils and lymphocytes	AR	Mild coarsening of facies, joint stiffness, valvular heart disease
+++	+++	Corneal clouding	Granulated neutrophils	AR	Coarse facies, ↑ vascular involvement
+	MPS features	Retinal degeneration	Vacuolated and granulated cells	AR	Icthyosis, combined MPS and metachromatic leukodystrophy phenotype
++ Less in late form	++ Less or absent in late form	Cherry red spot	Vacuolated lymphocytes	AR	MPS phenotype in all but cherry red spot myoclonus
++ Less in juvenile	++	Cherry red spot, corneal clouding	Vacuolated lymphocytes	AR	Angiokeratoma in juvenile; dysotosis multiplex
0/+	++++	Corneal clouding	Vacuolated and granulated neutrophils	AR	Coarse facies, inclusions in cultured fibroblasts, normal mucopolysacchariduria
0	+++	Corneal clouding	Vacuolated plasma cells	AR	Coarse facies, inclusions in cultured fibroblasts, joint contractures, valvular heart disease, normal mucopolysacchariduria
0	0	Corneal clouding, retinal degeneration	0	AR	Diagnosis based on electron microscopy; ? Ashkenazic Jewish predilection
0	0	Optic atrophy, macular degeneration, retinitis pigmentosa	Vacuolated lymphocytes Granulated neutrophils	AR	Electron microscopy helpful, degree of genetic heterogeneity unknown

analysis of biopsy tissue from liver or brain may be an appropriate research starting point.

The diagnosis of lysosomal storage diseases in adults is often difficult, although studies such as bone marrow aspiration in Gaucher disease and renal biopsy in Fabry disease may be pathognomonic. The diagnosis is difficult in the face of insidious, slowly progressive neurologic and psychiatric symptoms as described below for deficiencies of aryl sulfatase A, hexosaminidase A, or β-galactosidase. Erroneous diagnoses are common in these disorders, and a high index of suspicion is required. Lysosomal α-glucosidase deficiency mimics muscular dystrophy (see Chap. 385).

HETEROGENEITY There is extensive clinical, biochemical, and molecular heterogeneity within the lysosomal storage diseases. The biochemical genetic principles underlying this heterogeneity are reviewed in Chaps. 60 and 61. In general, structural genes for lysosomal enzymes produce propeptides that undergo posttranslational modification to become glycoproteins, often resulting in a series of electrophoretic variants, or isozymes. These isozymes may hydrolyze one or a variety of substrates, and the substrate specificity of particular isozymes may vary. Differences in substrate specificity also arise from the occurrence of similar but genetically distinct enzymes, e.g., the β-galactosidases. Mutations within a gene may totally eliminate or reduce enzyme activity, alter posttranslational modification, or alter the activity of the enzyme for specific substrates.

In most instances, different mutations within the structural genes for lysosomal enzymes account for varying degrees of severity from individual to individual and for the diverse combinations of visceral, skeletal, neurologic, ocular, and other manifestations. The heterogeneity is increased further by the recessive nature of most of the conditions, and many affected individuals are compound heterozygotes. In this instance, either one or both genes may encode some form of residual enzyme activity for one or more substrates. Patients with intermediate clinical phenotypes for mucopolysaccharidosis type I (MPS I) are likely examples of compound heterozygotes. At a molecular level, the majority of lysosomal storage disease patients might prove to be compound heterozygotes. Although it is useful to characterize clinical phenotypes as infantile, juvenile, adult, neuropathic, or nonneuropathic, the existence of different mutant alleles and of compound heterozygotes provides an explanation for those occasional patients who appear aberrant or intermediate as compared with the usual phenotype. Another type of heterogeneity is illustrated by MPS III A, B, C, and D, which are very similar disorders caused by different gene defects. Thus biochemical heterogeneity can underlie apparent clinical homogeneity.

Further complexity results from the fact that certain enzyme activities are derived from complexes of nonidentical subunits. As a consequence, different mutations can cause deficiency of the same enzyme, e.g., hexosaminidase A deficiency in Tay-Sachs and Sandhoff diseases, and can explain multiple enzyme deficiencies due to a single-gene defect as in Sandhoff disease. Genetic disorders that affect the posttranslational modification of lysosomal enzymes and defects in the lysosome itself also may cause lysosomal storage diseases. The mucolipidoses II and III are situations in which a single-gene defect alters the ability of a number of lysosomal enzymes to enter the lysosome. Thus mutations outside the structural genes for the enzymes can account for further heterogeneity. Better understanding of the identity, subunit structure, posttranslational processing, and substrate specificities of lysosomal enzymes should provide further insight into phenotypic and genotypic heterogeneity.

Clinical diagnosis is facilitated but also somewhat complicated by the widespread use of synthetic substrates for measuring lysosomal enzyme activities. These substrates often measure a group of related activities attributable to different enzymes. Thus the activity of β-galactosidase using an artificial substrate may represent the sum of various β-galactosidases encoded by different structural genes and having different substrate specificities. Clinical reliability generally is achieved by manipulating in vitro conditions to reflect that enzyme activity whose deficiency is characteristic of a clinical disorder. Genetic heterogeneity has, however, resulted in individuals with a mutant enzyme that either hydrolyzes the natural substrate and not the artificial substrate or vice versa. This is exemplified by the normal individuals who have hexosaminidase A deficiency using artificial substrate and by patients with Tay-Sachs disease who have substantial levels of hexosaminidase A activity with artificial substrates. The presence or absence of disease correlates with ability to hydrolyze the natural G_{M2} ganglioside substrate. These phenomena have considerable significance for identification of affected patients, for heterozygote screening, and for prenatal diagnosis. They indicate the need to go beyond artificial substrate enzyme assays if normal results occur in the face of overwhelming clinical, electron-microscopic, or chemical evidence of a storage disease.

MANAGEMENT AND PREVENTION   Specific therapy is rarely effective in lysosomal storage diseases at present (see "Gaucher Disease," below, for some exceptions), and care is largely symptomatic. The relentless, progressive course in many instances represents a tragic burden. Splenectomy has been useful in type I Gaucher disease in the past, and transplantation is effective in reversing the renal failure in Fabry disease. Attempts at more specific therapy have focused on enzyme replacement, fibroblast transplantation, and bone marrow transplantation. The greatest success with enzyme replacement is in Gaucher disease, and the availability of recombinant enzymes offers somewhat more favorable prospects for additional enzyme replacement in the future. Bone marrow transplantation is primarily a research modality. Patients with life-threatening or severely disabling somatic manifestations who have an HLA-identical, unaffected sibling are the best candidates for bone marrow transplantation. The most distressing manifestations of the majority of lysosomal storage diseases involve the central nervous system and are less amenable to enzyme replacement or bone marrow transplantation.

Genetic counseling is important in the management of these disorders. All the lysosomal storage diseases in which the specific enzyme deficiency is known either have been or presumably could

be diagnosed in utero, since lysosomal enzyme activities are expressed in cultured amniotic fluid cells as well as in cultured skin fibroblasts. Prenatal diagnosis also can be made using chorionic villus biopsy, and the possibility of earlier diagnosis is attractive to families at high risk. Heterozygote detection in close relatives is sometimes possible, although it can be difficult to achieve adequate statistical confidence using biochemical methods. Molecular methods using mutation detection or linkage analysis are more reliable where applicable. Heterozygote detection is further complicated by random inactivation of X chromosomes in female carriers of X-linked diseases, and women at risk in such families should be counseled using molecular data where possible. More widespread approaches to prevention require identification of heterozygous couples prior to the birth of an affected offspring. The feasibility of this approach has been demonstrated by heterozygote testing programs for Tay-Sachs disease. Such programs could result in a decreased frequency of these disorders through extensive testing and appropriate reproductive decisions by the rare couples at risk for affected offspring; the high frequency of the heterozygous state in Ashkenazic Jews and reliable methods for carrier detection for Tay-Sachs disease have facilitated this program. Molecular analysis of mutations complements biochemical methods for Tay-Sachs testing and makes possible carrier detection for Gaucher disease in the Ashkenazic population. Efficient, accurate heterozygote detection methods would be needed to apply this approach to other diseases and to populations with lower heterozygote frequencies. Even under optimal conditions, genetic variants may cause false-positive or false-negative results in any screening process. Population-based carrier screening is not feasible for most lysosomal storage diseases.

MOLECULAR ANALYSIS   Most of the genes encoding lysosomal enzymes have been cloned and sequenced. Many specific mutations are identified, and sometimes it is possible to correlate the genotype with the severity of the phenotype, as discussed for Tay-Sachs and Gaucher diseases below. There is extensive molecular heterogeneity, and many patients are compound heterozygotes. Molecular diagnosis generally can supplement but not replace enzymatic diagnosis. When a small number of mutations accounts for the majority of the defective gene copies, as in the case of Tay-Sachs and Gaucher diseases in the Ashkenazic population, mutation analysis is extremely valuable. Mutation detection and linkage analysis are also helpful in cases of prenatal diagnosis, where pseudodeficiency or biochemical difficulties can lead to diagnostic errors. The availability of the cloned cDNAs also improves the prospects for enzyme replacement using recombinant protein and for somatic gene therapy.

SPECIFIC DISORDERS

SPHINGOLIPIDOSES G_{M1} **gangliosidosis** G_{M1} gangliosidosis is due to deficiency of β-galactosidase. The features of the infantile form are summarized in Table 349-1. The juvenile form is characterized by a later onset, survival to the latter half of the first decade of life, neurologic impairment and seizures, and milder skeletal and ocular findings. In adults, one phenotype (sometimes called *Morquio B*) includes corneal clouding, normal intelligence, and spondyloepiphyseal dysplasia similar to that seen in MPS IV. Other adults have minimal bony abnormalities but exhibit spasticity, ataxia, or myoclonus. Patients with slowly progressive extrapyramidal signs with prominent dystonia, cerebral and caudate atrophy, and absence of visceral findings have been misdiagnosed as juvenile parkinsonism. A high index of suspicion is necessary to recognize the diverse phenotypes caused by β-galactosidase deficiency in juvenile and adult patients, since a wide range of skeletal, ocular, neurologic, and visceral findings can occur. Isozymes of β-galactosidase occur, but the diversity of phenotypes is believed to be due to different mutations in the same structural gene. All forms of G_{M1} gangliosidosis have an autosomal recessive inheritance. The frequency of the disease is low, with fewer than 50 patients reported for any given phenotype. Patients with isolated β-galactosidase deficiency must be distinguished from those with galactosialidosis, the combined deficiency of neuraminidase and β-galactosidase.

G$_{M2}$ gangliosidosis Tay-Sachs disease is a relatively common inborn error of metabolism. Although it is clinically similar to Sandhoff disease, the two are genetically distinct, with deficiency of hexosaminidase A in the former and hexosaminidase A and B in the latter. An additional disorder, called the *AB variant* of G$_{M2}$ gangliosidosis, is due to a deficiency of a protein factor (activator) necessary for activity of the enzyme against natural substrate. The presenting features are similar in all the infantile disorders and include a developmental delay beginning in the third to sixth month with subsequent, rapidly progressive neurologic deterioration. Macrocephaly, seizures, retinal cherry red spots, and an augmented startle response to sound suggest the diagnosis. The diagnosis is confirmed by enzyme assay. Most juvenile-onset patients with hexosaminidase deficiency present with dementia, seizures, and ocular findings, and some have an atypical spinocerebellar degeneration.

The neurologic manifestations of hexosaminidase A deficiency in adults are variable. Ataxia, dysarthria, lower motor neuron disease, pyramidal signs, and recurrent psychosis are common. Misdiagnoses have included Kugelberg-Welander spinal muscular atrophy, amyotropic lateral sclerosis, cerebellar or spinocerebellar ataxia, atypical Friedreich ataxia, muscular dystrophy, dementia, schizophrenia, and others. The manifestations are slowly progressive, and if considered, the diagnosis is easily established by serum enzyme assay.

Sandhoff disease is nonallelic with Tay-Sachs disease, whereas the juvenile forms of hexosaminidase deficiency are usually allelic with Tay-Sachs disease. Tay-Sachs disease is the most frequent form of hexosaminidase deficiency, the risk being about 100 times higher in Ashkenazic Jews than in other ethnic groups. All forms of G$_{M2}$ gangliosidosis are autosomal recessive. Hexosaminidase B is composed of β subunits whose structural locus is on chromosome 5, while hexosaminidase A is composed of α and β subunits with the structural locus for the α subunit on chromosome 15. Thus there is a defect in the α subunit in Tay-Sachs disease and in the β subunit in Sandhoff disease.

Although no specific therapy is available, extensive programs for heterozygote detection have been carried out in which more than half a million people have been tested and hundreds of couples at risk have been identified. Almost 2000 prenatal diagnoses have been performed, and the frequency of affected births has been reduced by 80 to 90 percent in the Jewish population in the United States and Canada.

Molecular studies have identified four mutations that account for over 95 percent of the mutant genes in the Ashkenazic population; a large deletion mutation is common in the French Canadian population. Presently, mutational and enzyme analyses are both accurate for carrier detection in the Ashkenazic population, but the two together are slightly better than either alone; enzyme assays are preferable outside the Ashkenazic and French Canadian populations because of molecular heterogeneity. Most patients with adult G$_{M2}$ gangliosidosis have the milder G269S mutation [substitution of glycine (G) for serine (S) at position 269] in a compound heterozygote state with a severe infantile allele.

LEUKODYSTROPHIES Krabbe galactosylceramide lipidosis or globoid cell leukodystrophy is an infantile disease due to deficiency of galactosylceramide β-galactosidase (see Table 349-1). Rapid neurologic deterioration and death occur within 1 to 2 years of onset. Premortem diagnosis is accomplished by enzyme assay. The presence of globoid cells in the brain is a characteristic postmortem finding. Galactosylceramide β-galactosidase is distinct from the β-galactosidase that is deficient in G$_{M1}$ gangliosidosis. Krabbe disease is an autosomal recessive disorder, and diagnosis can be made prenatally. Juvenile or adult forms are rare.

Deficiency of arylsulfatase A (cerebroside sulfatase) is the basis of metachromatic leukodystrophy, a lipid storage disease with a frequency of 1 in 40,000. The age of onset is later than that in Tay-Sachs disease or Krabbe disease. Patients usually attain the ability to walk and frequently present with gait abnormalities in the second to fourth year of life. Initially the patients may be hypotonic with decreased deep tendon reflexes, the latter reflecting peripheral nerve involvement. The disease progresses over the first decade to include ataxia, increased muscle tone, decorticate or decerebrate posturing, and eventual loss of all contact with surroundings. Rare patients with a juvenile form of metachromatic leukodystrophy have the clinical onset between 4 and 20 years of age and progress more slowly.

The adult form deserves special mention as an example of the difficulties presented by subtle, slowly progressive forms of lysosomal storage disease. The onset is in the second to fifth decade with a slowly progressive dementia. Emotional difficulties, motor dysfunction, and indistinct speech are often present. Even though conduction velocity in peripheral nerves is usually diminished, the deep tendon reflexes are often increased. Typical misdiagnoses include organic dementia, multiple sclerosis, and schizophrenia; psychiatric hospitalization is common. Premortem diagnosis was rare in the past, but the presence of periventricular hypodensities of white matter on computed tomographic scan or abnormalities of periventricular white matter on magnetic resonance imaging of the brain may suggest the diagnosis, which should be confirmed by enzyme assay.

Although some diagnostic studies have been performed on urine, leukocytes or fibroblasts are preferable for diagnostic enzyme assay. Arylsulfatase A is measured using artificial substrate, but the assay is complicated by low levels of activity in normal individuals (psuedodeficiency) and moderate levels of residual activity in some patients. Analysis of mutations in the various forms of metachromatic leukodystrophy and delineation of a pseudodeficiency allele may be helpful in resolving diagnostic problems. A few patients with a phenotype similar to metachromatic leukodystrophy have deficiency of a sphingolipid activator protein. Arylsulfastase A deficiency also occurs in multiple sulfatase deficiency.

NIEMANN-PICK DISEASE Niemann-Pick disease is a sphingomyelin lipidosis. In disease types A and B, there is deficiency of sphingomyelinase, an enzyme that hydrolyzes sphingomyelin to yield ceramide and phosphorylcholine. The most common disorder, Niemann-Pick type A, begins shortly after birth with hepatosplenomegaly, failure to thrive, and neurologic impairment. Retinal cherry red spots occur, but seizures and hypersplenism are rare. The diagnosis is made by recognition of the distinctive Niemann-Pick cell in the bone marrow and is confirmed by enzyme assay. Niemann-Pick type B disease is a relatively benign disorder with hepatosplenomegaly, sphingomyelinase deficiency, and sometimes pulmonary infiltrates, but there is no neurologic involvement. Niemann-Pick type C disease is characterized by sphingomyelin lipidosis and progressive neurologic deterioration in childhood. Type C disease is not due to sphingomyelinase deficiency but is associated with a massive lysosomal accumulation of cholesterol due to an incompletely characterized defect in intracellular utilization of cholesterol.

GAUCHER DISEASE Gaucher disease is a glucosylceramide lipidosis caused by deficiency of β-glucocerebrosidase, commonly known as β-glucosidase. An infantile form is characterized by early onset, marked hepatosplenomegaly, and severe neurologic progression to early death. A juvenile form with milder neurologic involvement exists. The type 1, or nonneuronopathic, form (commonly called adult Gaucher) is the most common lysosomal storage disease. The diagnosis of Gaucher disease should be established by enzyme analysis, and mutational analysis also should be performed. All forms of Gaucher disease have an autosomal recessive genetic basis and are allelic disorders. Type 1 is about 30 times more frequent in Ashkenazic Jews, with an incidence in this group of at least 1 in 1000 births. Absence of neurologic involvement is the criterion for inclusion in the type 1 or adult category.

Clinical manifestations include incidental discovery of painless splenomegaly; thrombocytopenia, anemia, or leukopenia secondary to hypersplenism; and bone pain. The course is variable, ranging from confinement to a wheelchair early in life to asymptomatic diagnosis in the ninth decade. Most patients have a mild course with relatively normal life expectancy. Partial or total splenectomy may be required. Pneumococcal vaccine should be administered prior to splenectomy. Careful management of postsplenectomy infection risks is important, and prophylactic antibiotics are recommended. The extent of bone disease is variable and includes bone pain, pathologic fractures, vertebral collapse, and aseptic necrosis of the femoral head. Bone pain with fever is termed *psuedoosteomyelitis*. MRI is particularly effective in defining the bony abnormalities. Moderate hepatic dysfunction is common, and rarely, severe hepatic failure, portal hypertension, pulmonary infiltrates, and pulmonary hypertension may develop. Serum acid phosphatase is characteristically elevated. A distinctive storage cell is present in the bone marrow in all forms of Gaucher disease, but enzyme assay should be performed because the Gaucher cell also may be found in patients with granulocytic leukemia and myeloma.

Four mutations account for 96 percent of the mutations in the Ashkenazic population. These findings opened the way for genotype/phenotype correlations and carrier screening in that population. One mutation, designated N370S [substitution of serine (S) for asparagine (N) at position 370], is mild; a single copy of this mutation in a compound heterozygote does not cause neurologic involvement, and homozygosity for this mutation is associated with a particularly mild phenotype. In fact, homozygosity for the N370S phenotype was found in 2 of 453 "normal" Ashkenazic individuals.

A major change in the treatment for Gaucher disease is the availability of aglucerase for enzyme replacement therapy. Aglucerase is a modified form of β-glucosidase prepared from human placenta. Treatment improves anemia and thrombocytopenia, decreases organomegaly, and decreases bone pain. Although this treatment may reduce or eliminate the need for splenectomy, the cost is about $300,000 per year. Recombinant enzyme is undergoing clinical trials; however, cost is likely to remain a major obstacle, and the dosage and indications for treatment are subjects of current investigation.

FABRY DISEASE Fabry disease involves the accumulation of a trihexoside, galactosylgalactosylglucosylceramide, due to deficiency of α-galactosidase A. The disorder is X-linked. The most severe symptoms occur in hemizygous males, with an incidence of about 1 in 40,000; milder symptoms occur in heterozygous females. Painful neuropathy is the most prominent symptom in younger men. The pain may be constant or cause intermittent crises of burning pain particularly in the palms and soles. Painful crises may mimic appendicitis or renal colic, and associated low-grade fever may lead to misdiagnoses of inflammatory processes.

The diagnosis can be suggested by the astute dermatologist or ophthalmologist. Cutaneous manifestations include angiokeratoma and decreased sweating. The angiokeratoma occur as clusters of red angiectases in the superficial skin. They do not blanch with pressure and are located on the trunk, perineal area, penis, and scrotum. The anhidrosis or hypohidrosis can predispose to heat stroke with vigorous exercise, as in military training. A characteristic corneal opacity occurs in males and in most heterozygous females. Lenticular opacities and tortuosity of the conjunctival and retinal vessels also occur.

Cardiovascular manifestations include direct involvement of the myocardium with lipid deposition, arrhythmias, valvular dysfunction, and myocardial infarction. Cerebral vascular manifestations secondary to involvement of small vessels are not rare, and frank cerebral hemorrhage can occur. Deposition of lipid in the kidney results in progressive renal impairment with renal failure in middle age (see also Chap. 241). The mean age at death of males not treated for renal failure was 41 years in one study. The diagnosis is often recognized at renal biopsy on the basis of lipid vacuoles in glomerular and tubular epithelial cells.

Heterozygous females are affected more mildly, but corneal dystrophy and cutaneous manifestations may be present. Life expectancy is near normal in women, although the more serious complications occur rarely.

Therapeutic intervention of several types may be helpful. Counsel-ing regarding the risks of hypohidrosis is important. Painful neuropathy frequently responds to administration of phenytoin. Renal failure can be treated by chronic dialysis, and the patients are acceptable candidates for transplantation because the donor kidney will not be impaired by the disease. Since the central nervous system is spared, the disease is a candidate for enzyme replacement therapy.

ACID LIPASE DEFICIENCY The infantile form of acid lipase deficiency, Wolman disease, is listed in Table 349-1. Cholesteryl ester storage disease in adulthood and adolescence is a rare disorder with mild phenotypic features by comparison. The usual features are hepatosplenomegaly, lipid deposition in the liver, and increased plasma cholesterol. Hepatic fibrosis, esophageal varices, and poor growth may occur.

GLYCOPROTEIN STORAGE DISORDERS Fucosidosis, mannosidosis, and aspartylglucosaminuria are rare, autosomal recessive disorders involving hydrolases that degrade polysaccharide linkages. Glycolipids as well as glycoproteins are accumulated in fucosidosis. All are characterized by neurologic impairment and varying somatic involvements (see Table 349-1). Fucosidosis and mannosidosis are most often lethal disorders in childhood, while aspartylglucosaminuria is a late-onset lysosomal storage disease with prominent mental retardation and a prolonged course. Abnormal sweat electrolytes and cutaneous angiokeratomas are distinctive in fucosidosis, and an unusual cartwheel-type cataract occurs in mannosidosis. Aspartylglu-cosaminuria is remarkable in that urinary amino acid analysis is diagnostic with an increase of aspartylglucosamine. The disorder is more frequent in the Finnish population. Sialidosis encompasses a group of phenotypes associated with glycoprotein neuraminidase (sialidase) deficiency. The phenotypes include an adult cherry red spot myoclonus syndrome, infantile and juvenile presentations with mucopolysaccharidosis-like phenotypes, and a congenital presentation with hydrops fetalis. Many patients previously classified as having mucolipidosis I have been proven to have mannosidosis or sialidosis. Some patients with sialidosis have β-galactosidase deficiency as well as neuraminidase deficiency. The combined β-galactosidase and neuraminidase deficiency is due to a defect in a "protective protein." Each of the glycoprotein storage diseases can be diagnosed by appropriate enzyme assay.

MUCOPOLYSACCHARIDOSIS (MPS) The mucopolysaccharidoses represent a broad spectrum of disorders due to deficiencies of one of a group of enzymes that degrade three classes of mucopolysaccharides: heparan sulfate, dermatan sulfate, and keratan sulfate. The MPS phenotype includes coarse facies, corneal clouding, hepatosplenomegaly, joint stiffness, hernias, dysostosis multiplex, mucopolysaccharide excretion in the urine, and metachromatic staining in peripheral leukocytes and bone marrow. Various components of the MPS phenotype are also found in the mucolipidoses, glycoprotein storage disorders, and other lysosomal storage diseases. Detailed clinical and radiologic evaluation and identification of the type of MPS excreted in the urine help to narrow the diagnostic possibilities. Diagnosis requires assay of specific enzymes in various tissues such as cultured skin fibroblasts.

Hurler or MPS IH disorder is the prototype MPS. Virtually all the components of the phenotype mentioned above are expressed in a severe degree. Nasal congestion and grossly visible corneal clouding are early features. Excessive growth during the first year of life is followed by poor growth late in the course. Radiologic features include enlargement of the sella turcica with a distinctive "shoe-shaped" fossa, broadening and shortening of the long bones, and hypoplasia and beaking of the vertebrae in the lumbar area. The vertebral beaking gives rise to an accentuated kyphosis or gibbus deformity. Death occurs within the first decade; postmortem findings include hydrocephalus and cardiovascular disease with occlusion of the coronary arteries. The biochemical defect is α-iduronidase deficiency with accumulation of heparan sulfate and dermatan sulfate.

MPS IS or Scheie syndrome, a clinically distinct disorder with childhood onset but adult survival, is characterized by joint stiffness, corneal clouding, aortic regurgitation, and usually normal intelligence.

Surprisingly, this much milder disorder is also the result of α-iduronidase deficiency; it is allelic with Hurler syndrome, as shown by lack of cross-correction of enzyme activity in cocultures of skin fibroblasts. Phenotypes occur that are clearly intermediate between Hurler and Scheie syndromes. It is believed that patients with an intermediate phenotype represent genetic compounds with one Hurler allele and one Scheie allele. Although genetic compounds must occur, in any one case their existence is difficult to distinguish from mutations of intermediate severity unless molecular analysis is performed.

Hunter or MPS II syndrome is distinguishable from the Hurler phenotype by the absence of gross corneal clouding and the X-linked recessive inheritance. The infantile form resembles the Hurler disease phenotype, and a milder form allows survival into adulthood. The severe and mild forms are allelic, and both are X-linked and share the same enzyme deficiency (iduronosulfate sulfatase).

Sanfilippo mucopolysaccharidoses (MPS III A, B, C, and D) are distinguished by the accumulation of heparan sulfate without dermatan or keratan sulfate and by the marked central nervous system involvement with milder somatic involvement. Sanfilippo mucopolysaccharidosis usually is diagnosed in the evaluation of mental retardation in childhood. Because the somatic features of this MPS are mild, the condition can be overlooked in the evaluation of an apparently isolated central nervous system problem. Death usually occurs during the second or third decade. The MPS III disorders are approximate genocopies. That is, four different enzyme deficiencies give rise to relatively indistinguishable clinical phenotypes with the same storage product. The four MPS III disorders can be diagnosed and distinguished by enzyme assay (see Table 349-1).

Morquio or MPS IV syndrome is distinguished by the absence of mental retardation and the presence of a distinctive bony dystrophy which can be classified as a spondyloepiphyseal dysplasia. Marked hypoplasia of the odontoid process can cause cervical dislocation and usually leads to some degree of spinal cord compression. Aortic regurgitation is frequent. The deficiency of N-acetylgalactosamine-6-sulfate sulfatase is the basis for this condition. Bone changes similar to those in Morquio syndrome also occur in one form of β-galactosidase deficiency. Maroteaux-Lamy or MPS VI disorder is characterized by prominent osseous involvement, corneal clouding, and normal intellect. Allelic forms with variable severity but the same deficiency of arylsulfatase B(N-acetylhexosamine-4-sulfate sulfatase) have been described. MPS VII, or β-glucuronidase deficiency, has been described in only a few patients with a rather complete MPS phenotype. Extreme variability from a lethal infantile form to a mild adult disease occurs.

MUCOLIPIDOSES *Mucolipidosis* is a general term for lysosomal storage diseases involving some combination of MPS, glycoprotein, oligosaccharide, and glycolipids. The category of mucolipidosis I probably can be abandoned, since most or all of these patients actually have a specific glycoprotein storage disease.

Mucolipidosis II, or I cell disease, is an early-onset disorder with mental retardation and an MPS phenotype. The distinctive features are striking inclusions in cultured skin fibroblasts and markedly elevated serum levels of lysosomal enzymes. The disorder has an autosomal recessive basis and is now known to represent a defect in the posttranslational processing of lysosomal enzymes. Mucolipidosis III, or pseudo-Hurler polydystrophy, is a milder disorder with many aspects of the MPS phenotype, particularly dysostosis multiplex. The disorder presents in the first decade with joint stiffness, the diagnosis of rheumatoid arthritis often being considered. The major handicaps are progressive physical disabilities, particularly claw hand deformity and hip dysplasia. Mild mental retardation is common. Aortic and/or mitral valvular disease is routinely present, although often not functionally significant. Survival into adult life with possible stabilization of the condition is characteristic, with greater disability in males than in females. Inclusions in cultured skin fibroblasts and elevation of serum lysosomal enzymes are essentially identical with the findings in mucolipidosis II, suggesting that these are allelic disorders. The primary defect in mucolipidosis II and III is deficiency of UDP-N-acetylglucosamine (GLcNAc):glycoprotein GLcNAc-1-phosphotransferase, an enzyme involved in posttranslational synthesis of the oligosaccharide portion of the lysosomal enzymes.

NEURONAL CEROID LIPOFUSCINOSES The neuronal ceroid lipofuscinosis disorders include a wide clinical spectrum with onset in childhood, juvenile, or adult periods. It is uncertain if these disorders are true lysosomal storage diseases, indeed whether single or multiple biochemical genetic disorders are present. The clinical features include central nervous system deterioration with cerebral atrophy, usually commensurate with the degree of impairment. Seizures, particularly myoclonic jerks, are prominent. Ocular involvement with optic atrophy, retinitis pigmentosa, and macular degeneration is present in the infantile and juvenile disorders but often absent in adult forms. Autosomal recessive inheritance is likely in most instances. The neuropathologic findings form the basis of the descriptive term for the disease. Electron microscopy demonstrates abnormal inclusions within lysosomes throughout a wide variety of tissues, despite the rather isolated clinical neurologic involvement. The presence of curvilinear bodies, electron-dense material, and fingerprint profiles on electron microscopy of white blood cells, liver biopsy, or muscle biopsy can be helpful diagnostically.

OTHER LYSOSOMAL STORAGE DISEASES Glycogen storage disease type II (Pompe disease) is the prototype lysosomal storage disease. The predominant clinical features of skeletal and cardiac myopathy are described in Chap. 350. Some rarer disorders are included in Table 349-1. Multiple sulfatase deficiency is an autosomal recessive disorder characterized by a deficiency of five or more cellular sulfatases: aryl sulfatase A, aryl sulfatase B, other mucopolysaccharide sulfatases, and a nonlysosomal steroid sulfatase. The clinical picture combines features of metachromatic leukodystrophy, an MPS phenotype, and ichthyosis. Other neurodegenerative diseases may eventually be classifiable as lysosomal storage diseases. Disorders such as juvenile dystonic lipidosis, neuroaxonal dystrophy, Hallervorden-Spatz disease, and other candidates exist. In addition, it is not unusual to identify patients with distinctive clinical features suggestive of lipidosis, mucolipidosis, or mucopolysaccharidosis, in which none of the present biochemically identifiable disorders can be identified. For these reasons, the number of distinct lysosomal storage diseases is likely to continue to increase.

REFERENCES

BEUTLER E: Gaucher's disease. N Engl J Med 325:1354, 1991

———: Gaucher disease: New molecular approaches to diagnosis and treatment. Science 256:794, 1992

DURAND P, O'BRIEN JS (eds): *Genetic Errors of Glycoprotein Metabolism.* Berlin, Springer-Verlag, 1982

NAVON R et al: Hexosaminidase A deficiency in adults. Am J Med Genet 24:179, 1986

NEUFELD EF: Lysosomal storage diseases. Annu Rev Biochem 60:257, 1991

SCRIVER CR et al (eds): *The Molecular and Metabolic Basis of Inherited Disease,* 7th ed. New York, McGraw-Hill, in press

WALTZ G et al: Adult metachromatic leukodystrophy. Arch Neurol 44:225, 1987

350 THE GLYCOGEN STORAGE DISEASES

ARTHUR L. BEAUDET

The glycogen storage diseases are a group of genetic disorders involving the pathways for storage of carbohydrate as glycogen and for its utilization to maintain blood sugar and to provide energy. Some forms are not associated with actual increases in glycogen content in tissues.

Glycogen is a highly branched polymer of glucose with the majority of residues in 1,4 linkage and with 7 to 10 percent of residues in 1,6 linkage. The treelike structure undergoes addition and removal of residues at its periphery. Glycogen synthesis begins by covalent attachment of glucose to a tyrosine residue on a protein, glycogenin. Through addition of glucose, individual particles can grow to include up to 60,000 glucose residues. Various forms of glycogen particles are distinguishable by electron microscopy. Liver generally contains less than 70 mg glycogen per gram of tissue, and muscle usually contains less than 15 mg/g, but these levels fluctuate as a consequence of feeding and hormonal stimuli. Abnormalities of glycogen structure can result either from decreased or increased branching.

The metabolic pathways involved in glycogen synthesis and breakdown are outlined in Fig. 350-1. These pathways differ among tissues; for example, certain reactions are active in liver but trivial or absent in muscle, and some enzyme functions are encoded by different genes in muscle and liver. Plasma glucose enters the cell and is phosphorylated by glucokinase or hexokinase. The former enzyme is found in liver where it accomplishes the majority of phosphorylation of glucose, while multiple hexokinases are distributed more widely in tissues. Glucose-6-phosphate (Glc-6-P) is converted to glucose-1-phosphate (Glc-1-P) in a reversible reaction catalyzed by phosphoglucomutase. Uridine diphosphate glucose (UDP-Glc) is synthesized from Glc-1-P and UTP by UDP-Glc pyrophosphorylase. Genetic deficiency has not been documented for any of these hepatic enzymes except that heterozygous glucokinase deficiency is a rare cause of type 2 diabetes mellitus (see Chap. 337). Glycogen is then elongated by the addition from UDP-Glc of individual glucose residues to an existing polymer. This reaction is catalyzed by glycogen synthase, which is encoded by separate genes in liver and muscle and is highly regulated, being stimulated by insulin and inhibited by epinephrine or glucagon. The regulation involves both phosphorylation of multiple sites to inhibit the enzyme and relief of the inhibition by the allosteric effect of Glc-6-P. Synthesis of a normally branched glycogen structure also requires the action of a branching enzyme (1,4-α-glucan:1,4-α-glucan-6-glucosyltransferase) which transfers a 1,4-linked oligosaccharide to a 1,6-linkage position.

Glucose is mobilized from glycogen by a complex group of enzyme reactions. Glycogen is acted on directly by the active form of phosphorylase, phosphorylase a, to remove individual glucose units and yield Glc-1-P. Phosphorylase is encoded by different gene products in muscle and in liver. In both tissues, the enzyme can exist in an active phosphorylated form and in an inactive dephosphorylated form. Phosphorylase is a dimer of identical subunits, and both forms of the enzyme are subject to complex allosteric regulation. The inactive phosphorylase b is converted to the active form by phosphorylase b kinase. Phosphorylase b kinase also exists in an active phosphorylated form and in an inactive dephosphorylated form. Phosphorylase b kinase is a multimer of four nonidentical subunits $(\alpha,\beta,\gamma,\delta)_4$, and the δ chain is identical with the calcium-binding protein calmodulin. The rate of glucose mobilization by this system is regulated by a cascade of kinase reactions, including cyclic AMP-dependent protein kinase. Epinephrine and glucagon act to increase blood sugar via this cascade system by activation of phosphorylase and simultaneous inactivation of glycogen synthase. Glycogen also is acted on directly by a debranching enzyme which carries out the debranching process by first transferring an oligosaccharide from a branch point to leave a single 1,6-linked glucose residue and then hydrolyzing the 1,6 linkage. Thus the debrancher enzyme has both glucan transferase activity (oligo-1,4 → 1,4-transferase) and a glucosidase (amylo-1,6-glucosidase) activity and yields a single residue to glucose for each branch point removed. The Glc-1-P generated by phosphorylase, as mentioned above, must be further metabolized to Glc-6-P by phosphoglucomutase. In the liver, Glc-6-P is transported by a specific translocase to the inner surface of the endoplasmic reticulum for hydrolysis by Glc-6-P. The Glc-6-P system may require as many as six distinct proteins for proper function, including the catalytic protein, a Glc-6-P transport protein, and a phosphate transport protein. Free glucose derived from this system is able to exit the hepatic cell to maintain blood levels. Many genetic deficiencies occur in the enzymes required for the conversion of glycogen to free glucose in the liver, and these cause the hepatic-hypoglycemic forms of glycogen storage disease.

If glycogen is used as a direct energy source, as in muscle, Glc-6-P and Glc-1-P must enter the pathways for glycolysis. Again, numerous enzymes are required in muscle for proper breakdown of glycogen and entry into the glycolytic pathway and tricarboxylic acid cycle. The enzymatic steps associated with genetic deficiency states in muscle include muscle phosphorylase, debranching enzyme, muscle phosphofructokinase (PFK), and probably muscle phosphoglycerate mutase (PGAM) and lactate dehydrogenase (LDH) M subunit.

The lysosomal enzyme α-glucosidase, which is structurally and metabolically separate from the above-described pathways, is capable of degrading both 1,4 and 1,6 linkages in glycogen to give free glucose. This enzyme has widespread distribution in tissues, but its deficiency affects primarily skeletal and cardiac muscle.

CLASSIFICATION   The clinical manifestations, diagnostic criteria, and therapy for glycogen storage diseases can be formulated in terms of the metabolic pathway outlined above (Table 350-1). According to this schema, two broad categories of disease can be delineated—those with a *hepatic-hypoglycemic* pathophysiology and those with a *muscle-energy* pathophysiology. Diseases with individualized pathophysiology also occur. It is suggested that disorders be designated by the specific protein deficiency, i.e., glucose-6-phosphatase deficiency. Although the roman numeral designations for types I through VII are in widespread use, numbering for higher types is confused and is to be avoided. Eponyms are of historical interest.

The hepatic-hypoglycemic disorders include glucose-6-phosphatase deficiency (type Ia), Glc-6-P microsomal translocase deficiency (type Ib), rarer type I subtypes, debrancher enzyme deficiency (type III), hepatic phosphorylase deficiency (type VI), and X-linked and autosomal forms of phosphorylase b kinase deficiency. Within this group, a distinction can be made between those disorders in which Glc-6-P and its metabolites are likely to be elevated (various forms of type I) and those disorders where Glc-6-P and related metabolites are likely to be decreased. This explains why increased glycolysis and lactic acidosis occur in type I disease but not in other forms of hepatic-hypoglycemic disease. Likewise, various forms of type I disease are distinct because gluconeogenesis, galactose, and fructose cannot contribute effectively to maintenance of blood sugar, in contrast to the other forms of hepatic-hypoglycemic disease. The glycemic response to epinephrine or glucagon tends to be blunted in the hepatic-hypoglycemic disorders. Dietary therapy with frequent feeding is a rational approach to the hepatic-hypoglycemic disorders and is tailored to reduce protein and to eliminate sources of galactose and fructose in type I disease.

The muscle-energy disorders include muscle phosphorylase deficiency (type V), phosphofructokinase deficiency (type VII), phosphoglycerate mutase deficiency, and LDH M-subunit deficiency. The clinical picture is one of muscle pain, myoglobinuria, and elevation of muscle enzymes in serum following vigorous exercise. The interruption of the pathway from glycogen to lactate with the accompanying failure to oxidize NADH is the unifying theme in these disorders. The failure of blood lactate to increase in response to exercise is a useful diagnostic test for the muscle-energy deficiency disorders. Debrancher enzyme deficiency constitutes an overlap syndrome; it presents primarily as a hepatic-hypoglycemic disorder in childhood, but serious muscle weakness occurs in some adults.

Two other disorders are best considered individually. Deficiency of lysosomal α-glucosidase is a lysosomal storage disease without major impact on either carbohydrate metabolism or maintenance of blood sugar (see Chap. 349). The major pathologic process in branching enzyme deficiency is a severe hepatic cirrhosis, possibly due to the harmful effects of the abnormal glycogen that accumulates. Glycogen content is generally normal, and the ability to maintain a normal blood sugar is not impaired.

HEPATIC-HYPOGLYCEMIC DISEASES   Glucose-6-phosphatase deficiency, type Ia   CLINICAL FEATURES   Glucose-6-phosphatase deficiency, or von Gierke disease, is an autosomal recessive

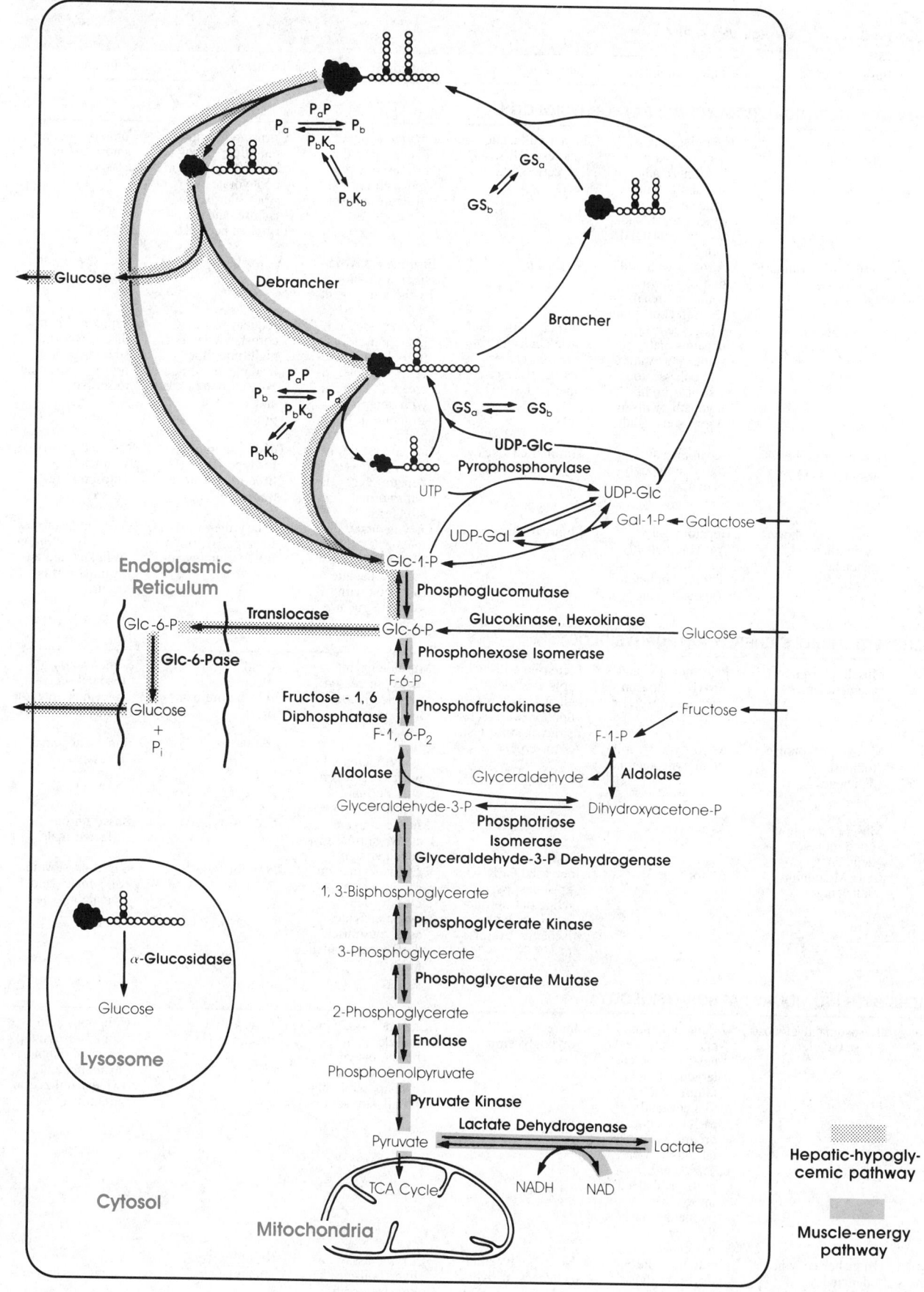

FIGURE 350-1   Metabolic pathways related to glycogen storage disease. A hypothetical composite cell is shown depicting both hepatic and muscle pathways. The shaded areas depict pathways that are blocked in the hepatic-hypoglycemic diseases or in the muscle-energy diseases. Nonstandard abbrevia-tions are as follows: GS_a, active glycogen synthase; GS_b, inactive glycogen synthase; P_a, active phosphorylase; P_b, inactive phosphorylase; P_aP, phosphor-ylase *a* phosphatase; P_bK_a, active phosphorylase *b* kinase; P_bK_b, inactive phosphorylase *b* kinase.

TABLE 350-1 Glycogen storage diseases

Type	Basic defect*	Clinical findings	Laboratory	Diagnosis	Treatment	Comments
DISORDERS WITH HEPATIC-HYPOGLYCEMIC PATHOPHYSIOLOGY						
Ia von Gierke	Glucose-6-phosphatase deficiency	Hypoglycemia, hepatomegaly, bleeding diathesis, short stature, delayed adolescence, hepatic adenomas, enlarged kidneys	Increased lactate, cholesterol, triglyceride, and uric acid	Enzyme assay on liver or intestine, increased glycogen with normal structure in liver	Cornstarch, and/or nighttime, feeding, 60–70% carbohydrate, restrict sucrose and lactose, and allopurinol as needed	Common, severe, autosomal recessive
Ib	Glc-6-P microsomal translocase deficiency	As for Ia with addition of neutropenia and recurrent infection	As for Ia	Enzyme assay on liver with and without detergent	As for Ia	Rare, severe, autosomal recessive
III Cori	Debrancher enzyme deficiency	Hypoglycemia, hepatomegaly, some short stature and delayed adolescence, mild myopathy worsening in some adults	Normal lactate and uric acid; increased cholesterol, triglyceride, and SGOT	Enzyme assay on liver, muscle, or fibroblasts; leukocytes variable; increased glycogen with abnormal structure in liver and muscle	Frequent feeding, cornstarch, and/or nighttime tube feeding for some, 50% carbohydrate and 15–20% protein	Common, intermediate severity, some hepatic fibrosis, autosomal recessive
VI Hers	Hepatic phosphorylase deficiency	Hepatomegaly, variable hypoglycemia	Minimal changes, ? hyperlipidemia	Enzyme assay on liver, increased hepatic glycogen with normal structure	Dietary therapy as for type III, often little treatment required	Rare and poorly characterized; ? autosomal recessive
Formerly VIb, VIII, or IX	Hepatic phosphorylase b kinase deficiency	Hepatomegaly, variable hypoglycemia, occasional findings in heterozygous females	Minimal changes	Enzyme assay on leukocytes, fibroblasts, or liver; increased hepatic glycogen with normal structure	Dietary therapy as for type III, often little treatment required	Very mild but may be fairly common; X-linked and autosomal forms occur.
DISORDERS WITH MUSCLE-ENERGY PATHOPHYSIOLOGY						
V McArdle	Muscle phosphorylase deficiency	Pain, cramps, and mylgobinuria on strenuous exercise	Increased CPK with episodes, deficient lactate production with ischemic exercise test	Muscle enzyme assay, increased muscle glycogen with normal structure	Avoid exercise, glucose or fructose before exercise	Some clearly autosomal recessive, male preponderance
VII	Muscle phosphofructokinase deficiency	As for type V, mild hemolytic anemia	As for type V	Muscle enzyme assay, increased muscle glycogen with normal structure	As for type V	Rare, autosomal recessive
	Muscle phosphoglycerate mutase deficiency	As for type V	As for type V	Muscle enzyme assay, normal glycogen content	? As for type V	Based on one affected male
	LDH M-subunit deficiency	As for type V	Increased CPK with episodes; pyruvate but not lactate rises with ischemic exercise test	LDH isozymes on serum, erythroctyes or leukocytes; enzyme assay on muscle; ? glycogen content normal	? As for type V	Based on sibship of 3 males and 1 female affected
DISORDERS WITH INDIVIDUAL PATHOPHYSIOLOGY						
II Pompe	Lysosomal α-glucosidase deficiency	*Infantile:* hypotonia, muscle weakness, cardiac enlargement and failure, enlarged tongue, fatal early; *juvenile:* progressive skeletal muscle weakness; *adult:* progressive skeletal muscle weakness, pulmonary insufficiency presentation	Increased CPK, no hypoglycemia	Enzymes assay on muscle or fibroblasts, enzyme assay on leukocytes possible but pitfalls are serious	No effective treatment	Common, autosomal recessive, prenatal diagnosis available and widely utilized in infantile
VI Andersen	Brancher enzyme deficiency	Infantile failure to thrive, cirrhosis and liver failure, extreme hypotonia and weakness in some, fatal early	No hypoglycemia, changes of liver disease	Enzyme assay on liver, muscle, leukocytes or fibroblasts; glycogen content not remarkable but structure abnormal	No effective treatment	Very rare, autosomal recessive

* These defects provide the preferred nomenclature for the diseases.

genetic disorder with an incidence of 1 in 100,000 to 400,000. The disorder is usually manifested during the first 12 months of life by symptomatic hypoglycemia or by the recognition of hepatomegaly. Occasional patients experience hypoglycemia in the immediate neonatal period, and rare patients never have hypoglycemia. Characteristic findings include a full-cheeked, rounded facial appearance, a protuberant abdomen due to marked hepatomegaly, and thin extremities. Hyperlipidemia may cause eruptive xanthomas and lipemia retinalis. Splenomegaly is usually mild or absent, although massive enlargement of the left lobe of the liver may be mistaken for enlargement of the spleen. Growth is usually normal for the first few months of life; growth retardation then supervenes, and adolescence is delayed. Mental development is usually normal except for injury from hypoglycemia.

The characteristic profound symptomatic hypoglycemia may be associated with blood glucose levels below 0.8 mmol/L (15 mg/dL). Liver enzymes are mildly elevated if at all. The presence of lactic acidosis is helpful in diagnosing this disorder, although blood lactate may be normal in the fed state in young infants. However, these patients are relatively resistant to development of ketosis. Hyperlipidemia is frequent and involves elevation of both cholesterol and triglycerides. Hypertriglyceridemia can be extreme, with levels as high as 60 mmol/L (5000 mg/dL) or higher. Hyperuricemia due both to decreased renal excretion and increased production is frequent and often becomes more severe after adolescence. The rise in plasma glucose following administration of epinephrine or glucagon is impaired, as is the rise in blood glucose following administration of galactose by mouth. The pathogenesis of most of the metabolic abnormalities is not well understood; lactic acidosis may be due to increased glycolysis, and other abnormalities, including poor growth, may be the result of chronically altered levels of insulin and glucagon. Renal enlargement can be demonstrated by radiologic or sonographic techniques. Mild renal tubular dysfunction or the Fanconi syndrome may occur. Moderate anemia is usually due to recurrent nosebleeds and chronic acidosis but may become severe after prolonged acidosis. A bleeding diathesis is due to a platelet dysfunction.

Once type Ia disease is suspected clinically, the diagnosis is established by liver biopsy. Type Ia disease is suggested by lactic acidosis, an abnormal galactose tolerance test, or renal enlargement. Proper handling of biopsy material should be arranged to distinguish the various subtypes Ia, Ib, etc. Sufficient material for enzyme assay may be obtained by needle biopsy provided the bleeding time is normal, or alternatively, open liver biopsy provides more tissue for analysis. Microscopic examination of liver reveals increased glycogen in cytoplasm and nuclei; lipid vacuoles in hepatocytes are prominent, and fibrosis is usually absent.

The hypoglycemia and lactic acid acidosis may be life-threatening. Other troublesome features include short stature, delayed adolescence, and hyperuricemia. During adult years, uric acid nephropathy and glomerulosclerosis may lead to renal failure. Hepatic adenomata are common after adolescence. There is a significant risk of hepatic malignant degeneration, often during the third decade, and subjects who live long enough may be at increased risk for atherosclerosis.

TREATMENT The mainstay of management is frequent feeding. The most widely used approach in children has been the combination of frequent daytime feeding by mouth and continuous nighttime feeding by nasogastric tube (see Chap. 75). The regimen should include approximately 60 percent carbohydrate, and no significant portion of carbohydrate should come from sources containing galactose or fructose, which cannot be utilized effectively to maintain blood sugar. Uncooked cornstarch feeding provides a convenient, economical, and palatable source of slowly digested glucose polymer, and cornstarch therapy has become an important form of dietary treatment for this disease. The ability of a family to carry out such a program is a significant variable, but in some instances the metabolic abnormalities and the rate of growth have improved substantially. Optimal management requires a team attentive to the dietary and psychosocial needs of patient and family. Control of elevated plasma

urate may require the addition of allopurinol. This regimen provides a reasonably optimistic short-term prognosis, and limited long-term follow-up data indicate that the risk of malignancy may be reduced. Portacaval anastomosis is no longer used in the management of glycogen storage disease. Prenatal diagnosis is not possible at present except by fetal liver biopsy.

Glc-6-P microsomal translocase deficiency, type Ib Glc-6-P microsomal translocase deficiency, historically referred to as *pseudo type I*, has an incidence of one-fifth to one-tenth that of type Ia. The term *microsomal translocase* describes the capacity to transport Glc-6-P into the endoplasmic reticulum. The clinical features are similar to those in type Ia, but unique features include neutropenia, impaired neutrophil migration, and recurrent pyogenic infections; in general, type Ib is more severe than Ia. Laboratory findings, responses to tolerance tests, and management are similar in the two disorders.

Type Ib disease was initially distinguished from type Ia by the presence of normal glucose-6-phosphatase activity on assay of biopsy tissue in the presence of detergent. However, glucose-6-phosphatase activity is low in type Ib disease when fresh tissue is homogenized and assayed in the absence of detergent. These results have been interpreted to imply a genetic deficiency of a microsomal Glc-6-P transport system as a primary defect in type Ib glycogen storage disease. The cause for the neutropenia and abnormal neutrophil migration is unknown, although the disease suggests a role for Glc-6-P transport in these cells.

Debrancher deficiency, type III CLINICAL FEATURES Debrancher enzyme deficiency, also known historically as *Cori disease*, is an autosomal recessive disorder and is one of the more frequent forms of glycogen storage diseases, occurring with a particularly high frequency in North African Jews. Symptomatic disease in the newborn period is unusual, and patients usually present with hypoglycemia or hepatomegaly during the first year of life. The physical findings are similar to those in type Ia, except that splenomegaly is more prominent, but the clinical course tends to be less severe. The skeletal or cardiac myopathy is usually mild or insignificant in childhood but may be disabling and progressive in adults. Some patients with myopathy are first diagnosed as adults because the features in childhood were mild and overlooked. Patients with enzyme deficiency in both liver and muscle are sometimes classified as type IIIa and those free of muscle involvement as type IIIb, but the molecular basis for the tissue specificity is unknown, since there is evidence for a single gene.

Fasting hypoglycemia occurs in about 80 percent of patients. The glucose response after glucagon or epinephrine is abnormal in the fasting state but may be normal shortly after eating because the terminal glucose residues in glycogen can be mobilized. The galactose tolerance test is usually normal. Ketosis is prominent, and blood lactate is normal. Serum transaminase is elevated, and further increases may occur with minor illnesses. Blood cholesterol and triglyceride are elevated in about two-thirds. Hyperuricemia is rare.

Two diagnostic modalities are used to establish the diagnosis—analysis of glycogen and measurement of debranching enzyme in tissue samples. The glycogen content of red blood cells and liver is increased in almost all, whereas glycogen content of muscle is increased only in some. Documentation of abnormal structure of glycogen with the use of spectrophotometric techniques is a more consistent finding than the increase in glycogen content. The establishment of the diagnosis by enzymatic assay is complicated by both methodologic problems and genetic heterogeneity. Both debrancher functions—the glucan transferase activity and glucosidase activity—are believed to reside in a single polypeptide, but various subtypes of the disease have been described. While the diagnosis can be made in some patients using red cells, leukocytes, or fibroblasts, it is generally preferable to document the abnormal glycogen structure and the enzyme deficiency directly in biopsy material from liver or muscle. The pathologic findings in liver are similar to those in type Ia except for less lipid deposition and more prominent fibrous septae.

With regard to growth retardation and abdominal protuberance,

EDS, and a subset of patients with primary generalized osteoarthritis have mutations in the gene for procollagen II similar to the mutations in the same gene that cause lethal CDs. At the moment, there is still disagreement as to the best diagnosis for such patients in that some clinical investigators feel that after a mutation similar to those seen in the early-onset diseases is identified, the patients should be reclassified as having mild forms of OI, EDS, or CD even though they did not have definitive evidence of the early-onset diseases or seek medical attention until they were adults. The debate is fueled by the fact that many of the clinical classifications are based on variable clusters of signs and symptoms for which there are few objective criteria. However, some patients with late-onset diseases of connective tissue such as osteoporosis, osteoarthritis, and aneurysms inherit the disorders in a manner consistent with single-gene defects. Therefore, it may be necessary to expand greatly the category of diseases currently referred to as heritable disorders of connective tissues.

DEFINITION AND COMPOSITION OF CONNECTIVE TISSUES

The connective tissues are composed of distinctive macromolecules, many of which are also major constituents of the lung, the kidney, the walls of blood vessels, the vitreous gel of the eye, and the synovial fluid. Also, essentially all organs and tissues contain small amounts of the same macromolecules assembled into membranes and septa. Therefore, most of these structures are now regarded as connective tissues.

The distinguishing feature of connective tissues, however, is that they contain specific macromolecules that are assembled into an insoluble extracellular matrix (Table 351-1). The macromolecules include at least 18 different types of collagens, the related fiber-associated proteins known as *elastin* and *fibrillin*, a series of proteoglycans, and components whose structure and function have been only partially defined.

Differences in the connective tissues of bone, skin, and cartilage are in part explained by differences in their content of specific components (see Table 351-1). For example, tendons and ligaments consist primarily of type I collagen fibrils associated with small amounts of other components that probably help organize the type I collagen fibrils into larger fibers and fiber bundles. Cartilage consists primarily of fibrils of type II collagen in the form of arcade-like structures that are distended by the presence of highly charged proteoglycans. The extracellular matrix of large blood vessels such as the aorta contains collagens that provide tensile strength and elastin that provides elasticity. Differences among the connective tissues also depend on the three-dimensional organization of the molecular components. The type I collagen fibrils in tendon are packed into thick, parallel bundles of fibers. In skin, fibrils of the same type I collagen are randomly oriented in the plane of the skin. In cortical bone, type I collagen fibrils are deposited in intricate helical arrays around haversian canals.

BIOSYNTHESIS OF CONNECTIVE TISSUE Assembly of the connective tissues is largely governed by the principle of self-assembly, whereby a molecular subunit of the correct size, shape, and surface properties binds to other molecules with the same structure, or with similar structures, in a spontaneous but ordered manner. The molecular mechanisms and driving forces are similar to those involved in the formation of large crystals from supersaturated solutions.

The principle of self-assembly in connective tissue is best illustrated by the assembly of collagen into fibrils. The molecule of a fibril-forming collagen is a long, thin rod consisting of three polypeptide α chains that are wrapped into a rigid, ropelike triple helix (Fig. 351-1). The molecule has a triple-helical conformation, because each of the three α chains has a simple, repetitive amino acid sequence of about 1000 amino acids in which glycine (Gly) appears as every third amino acid. Therefore, the sequence of each α chain can be designated as $(-Gly-X-Y-)_{333}$, where X and Y represent amino acids other than glycine. To fold into a triple helix, it is essential that every third amino acid in an α chain is glycine, the smallest amino acid, since this residue must fit in a sterically restricted space where the three chains of the triple helix come together. Many of the X- and Y-position amino acids are the ring amino acids proline and hydroxyproline that give rigidity to the triple-helical structure. The remaining X- and Y-position amino acids form clusters of hydrophobic and charged regions on the surface of the molecule that direct how one molecule

TABLE 351-1 Constituents of various connective tissues

Connective tissue	Known constituents	Approximate amounts (% dry wt)	Characteristics or functions
Skin, ligaments, tendons	Type I collagen	80	Bundles of fibrils
	Type III collagen	5–15	Thin fibrils
	Type IV collagen, laminin, nidogen	<5	In basal laminae under epithelium and in blood vessels
	Types V, VI, and VII collagens	<5	Functions unclear
	Elastin, fibrillin	<5	Provide elasticity
	Fibronectin	<5	Associated with collagen fibers and cell surfaces
	Proteoglycans* and hyaluronate	0.5	Provide resiliency
Bone (demineralized)	Type I collagen	90	Complex fibril network
	Type VI collagen	1–2	Function unclear
	Proteoglycans	1	Function unclear
	Osteonectin, osteocalcin, osteopontin, α2-glycoprotein, sialoproteins	1–5	Probably initial or regulate mineralization
Aorta	Type I collagen	20–40	Fibril network
	Type III collagen	20–40	Thin fibrils
	Elastin, fibrillin	20–40	Provide elasticity
	Type IV collagen, laminin, nidogen	<5	Form basal lamina
	Types V and VI collagens	<2	Functions unclear
	Proteoglycans	<3	Provide resiliency
Cartilage	Type II collagen	40–50	Arcades of thin fibrils
	Type IX collagen	5–10	Links type II fibrils
	Type X collagen	5–10	Surrounds hypertrophic cells
	Type XI collagen	<10	Function unclear
	Proteoglycans and hyaluronate	15–50	Provide resiliency

* As discussed in text, at least five proteoglycans have now been identified. They differ in the structures of their core proteins and their contents of mucopolysaccharide side chains of chondroitin-4-sulfate, chondroitin-6-sulfate, dermatan sulfate, and keratin sulfate. Basil lamina contain a proteoglycan with a side chain of heparan sulfate that resembles heparin.

FIGURE 351-1 Schematic representation of synthesis of a type I collagen fibril by a fibroblast. *A.* Intracellular steps in the assembly of the procollagen molecule. Hydroxylations and glycosylations of the proα chains begin soon after the amino termini pass into the cisternae of the rough endoplasmic reticulum and continue after the three chains associate through their carboxy-terminal propeptides and become disulfide linked. *B.* Cleavage of procollagen to collagen, self-assembly of the collagen molecule into quarter-staggered fibrils, and cross-linking of the molecules in the fibrils. Cleavage of the propeptides may occur within crypts of the fibroblast, as shown here, or some distance from the cell. *(From DJ Prockop and KI Kivirikko. Used with permission.)*

spontaneously binds to other collagen molecules and thereby self-assembles into the large collagen fibrils found in tissues (see Fig. 351-1).

More than 18 different collagens have been identified. Most are minor constituents that probably have highly specialized functions. About one-third of fibrillar collagens are found in tissues as long, highly ordered fibrils with a characteristic banding pattern by electron microscopy. Type I collagen is the most abundant and is found as cross-striated fibrils in a large number of tissues (see Table 351-1). It is composed of two identical α chains called α1(I) and one α2(I) chain. Type II collagen, a similar fibrillar collagen in cartilage, is composed of three identical´ chains called α1(II). Type III collagen, the third most abundant fibrillar collagen, is found in smaller amounts in many tissues that contain type I collagen and in large amounts in large blood vessels and is composed of three identical chains called α1(III). The nonfibrillar collagens are similar to the fibrillar collagens in that they contain -Gly-X-Y- sequences of amino acids that form triple-helical domains, but they also contain large globular domains. Self-assembly of most of the nonfibrillar collagens usually involves binding together of the globular domains to form network-like structures. For example, the type IV collagen in basement membranes self-assembles into a complex three-dimensional network that provides a diffusion barrier in the renal glomerulus and pulmonary alveolus and provides support for epithelial and endothelial cells in these tissues and in skin, the gastrointestinal tract, and blood vessels.

Because fibrillar collagens spontaneously self-assemble into fibrils, they are first synthesized as larger and more soluble precursors called *procollagens*. The procollagen forms of type I, II, and III collagens are 1.5 times the mass of the corresponding collagens due to the presence of amino acid sequences that are called *propeptides* and are located at both the *N* terminus and the *C* terminus of the proα chains of the procollagens.

The biosynthesis of procollagens involves a large number of intracellular processing steps (see Fig. 351-1) and an unusual self-assembly whereby the three chains fold into a triple-helical conforma-

tion. As the proα chains of procollagen are translated from mRNAs on ribosomes, they pass into the cisternae of the rough endoplasmic reticulum. Hydrophobic signal peptides at the *N* terminus are cleaved, and a series of additional posttranslational reactions begin. Proline residues in the Y position of the repeating -Gly-X-Y- sequences are converted to hydroxyproline by prolyl hydroxylase, requiring oxygen, iron, and ascorbic acid. Lysine residues in the Y position are similarly hydroxylated to hydroxylysine by a specific lysyl hydroxylase. Many of the hydroxylysine residues are further modified by glycosylation with galactose or with galactose and glucose. A large mannose-rich oligosaccharide is assembled on the *C*-terminal propeptide of each chain. As the last amino acids are incorporated into the proα chains, they are released into the cisternae of the rough endoplasmic reticulum. At this stage two proα1(I) and one proα2(I) chains associated through their *C*-propeptides. The association of the proα chains is directed by the structure and the surface properties of the globular *C*-propeptides. After the *C*-propeptides assemble correctly, the structure is locked in place by the formation of interchain disulfide bonds. Posttranslational modifications of the proα chains continue until each chain acquires a critical level of about 100 hydroxyproline residues. Then a few of the -Gly-X-Y- sequences at the *C* terminus of the protein that are very rich in hydroxyproline fold into a triple-helical conformation. The short region of triple helix becomes a nucleus for self-assembly of the triple helix of the whole protein, much like a nucleus for crystallization, in that the triple-helical conformation in one -Gly-X-Y- sequence induces the next -Gly-X-Y- sequence to fold into the same conformation. As a result, the conformation is propagated in a zipper-like fashion from the *C* terminus to the *N* terminus of the molecule and the entire α-chain domain becomes a continuous triple helix. Once the protein is folded, it passes from the rough endoplasmic reticulum to other membranous compartments and is secreted. The requirement for ascorbic acid in the hydroxylation of prolyl residues by prolyl hydroxylase explains why wounds fail to heal in scurvy (see Chap. 72). If a sufficient number of proline residues are not converted to hydroxyproline, the protein cannot fold into a triple helix that is stable at body temperature. The abnormal protein accumulates in the cisternae of the rough endoplasmic reticulum and is slowly degraded.

After secretion, procollagen is processed to collagen by cleavage of the N-propeptides by procollagen N-proteinase and of the C-propeptides by procollagen C-proteinase. In the case of type I procollagen, the processing by the two proteinases converts the soluble precursor to type I collagen, whose solubility is less than 1 µg/mL under the same conditions. The 1000-fold decrease in solubility as procollagen is converted to collagen provides the entropic energy that drives the spontaneous self-assembly of the collagen into fibrils. The assembly of collagen into fibrils is, again, similar to the process of crystallization of a small molecule from a supersaturated solution. Collagen monomers first assemble into a nucleus that grows by addition of monomers in a manner that is determined by the structure of the nucleus. The initial nucleus for fibril assembly probably involves few molecules and has been difficult to define. However, structures intermediate between the initial nucleus and the final fibrils are readily detected in in vitro systems. The intermediate structures have pointed and highly symmetrical tips and grow by addition of monomers to the pointed tips. The nucleus, the intermediate structures, and the final fibril can all be assembled spontaneously from a single kind of collagen such as type I or type II, but other fibrils are assembled as copolymers in which two or more collagens are incorporated into the same fibril simultaneously. Alternatively, a second collagen or a proteoglycan can bind to the surface of a growing fibril or to a fully formed fibril and thereby influence the final structure and the functional properties of the fibrils. The final structure of the fibrils in tissues is also influenced by the pressure and tensions on the fibrils, particularly after their tips are inserted into muscle and bone. The tension on tendons, for example, probably makes the thin fibrils that are initially assembled to coalesce into large fiber bundles. The initial self-assembly of collagen into fibrils, however, involves a large number of specific interactions along the surface of each rodlike molecule and therefore can only be altered by molecules that bind either to the surface of the large, rodlike monomer or to the surfaces of the growing fibrils. For this reason, assembly of collagen fibrils is less subject to influence of other components than the crystallization of small molecules.

Self-assembled collagen fibers have considerable tensile strength, and the strength is increased by cross-linking reactions that form covalent bonds between α chains in one molecule and α chains in adjacent molecules. The first step in cross-linking is oxidation by lysyl oxidase of amino groups on a few lysine or hydroxylysine residues to form aldehydes. The aldehydes then interact to form a complex series of stable covalent bonds that may or may not involve enzymatic reactions.

Collagen fibers in most tissues of normal adults undergo very little metabolic turnover. One exception to this is the collagen fibrils that undergo repeated degradation and synthesis as part of the continual remodeling of bone. During growth and development, however, the collagen fibrils in all tissues undergo repeated synthesis, degradation, and resynthesis. The degradation of collagen fibers in tissues is initiated by collagenase in leukocytes, fibroblasts, synovial cells, or related cell types. The collagenases cleave the collagen molecule at a point about three-quarters of the distance from its N terminus. The cleavage apparently triggers unfolding of the molecules on the surface of a fibril and further degradation by other proteinases.

Although the collagen in many adult tissues is metabolically stable, the turnover changes under some circumstances. In starvation, a large fraction of the collagen in skin and other connective tissues is degraded, thus providing amino acids for gluconeogenesis. Large losses of collagen also occur in most connective tissues during immobilization or prolonged periods of low-gravitational stress. In rheumatoid arthritis, pannus invasion of articular cartilage causes a rapid degradation of the collagen in the tissue, and prolonged or excessive treatment with glucocorticoids decreases the collagen content of most connective tissues, including bone, by decreasing the rate of collagen synthesis. The decreases in collagen content weaken the tissues. In many pathologic states, however, collagen is deposited in excess. With injury to any tissue, the inflammatory response is usually followed by increased deposition of collagen fibrils in the form of fibrotic tissue and scars that primarily consist of type I collagen. The increased deposition of collagen fibrils during the repair process is largely irreversible and therefore is a major feature of the pathologic changes in hepatic cirrhosis, pulmonary fibrosis, atherosclerosis, and nephrosclerosis and in the scarring in tissues such as skin and ligaments following surgery or trauma.

The biosynthesis of all collagens involves essentially the same steps of assembly and processing. Assembly of nonfibrillar collagens such as the type IV of basement membranes does not, however, involve cleavage of the globular domains at the ends of the protein, since the globular domains are required for the self-assembly of the proteins. Elastin assembly appears to be closely related to the collagen biosynthetic pathway, since a few of the prolyl residues in the protein are hydroxylated to hydroxyproline by prolyl hydroxylase. The elastin monomer, however, is a single polypeptide that does not fold into a defined three-dimensional structure and is not synthesized as a larger precursor molecule. Instead, it is slowly secreted from cells into extracellular compartments, where it forms amorphous deposits around previously deposited microfibrils. The elastin deposits then become covalently cross-linked through oxidation of lysine residues to aldehydes by the same lysyl oxidase that initiates the cross-linking of collagen. The microfibrils in elastin deposits are largely composed of fibrillin, a large protein that forms beadlike strands. The amorphous deposits of elastin and fibrillin also may contain additional components that have not yet been identified.

The synthesis of proteoglycans begins with assembly of a core protein in the cisternae of the rough endoplasmic reticulum. The core protein then undergoes modifications by a series of sugar and sulfate transferases that generate large side chains of glycosaminoglycans. At least five proteoglycans have been identified by differences in the structures of their core proteins. The major proteoglycan of cartilage, called *aggrecan*, has a core protein of about 2000 amino acids to which are bound multiple side chains of chondroitin sulfate and keratin sulfate, distinctive mucopolysaccharides consisting of highly charged and repetitive disaccharide sequences. After secretion from cells, the aggrecan monomer binds to a smaller protein called a *link protein*. The complex of core protein and link protein then spontaneously binds to a long chain of hyaluronic acid to form a huge copolymer called a *proteoglycan aggregate*. The large and highly charged proteoglycan aggregate binds water and small ions and thereby provides a large swelling pressure and resiliency to cartilage. Smaller proteoglycans such as decorin, biglycan, and fibromodulin have smaller core proteins with somewhat different mucopolysaccharide side chains. They do not form large aggregates with hyaluronate but bind to fibrils of collagens or fibronectin and may thereby help regulate the assembly of fibrils or their spatial orientation. One group of small proteoglycans known as *syndecans* are bound to the plasma membranes of cells and may have a role in migration of cells along fibrils or in signal transduction.

The assembly of bone follows much the same principles as the assembly of other connective tissues (see also Chap. 356). The first step is deposition of osteoid tissue that consists largely of type I collagen fibrils (see Fig. 351-1). Mineralization of osteoid occurs by steps that are still incompletely defined; proteins such as osteopontin and osteocalcin probably bind to the collagen fibrils and chelate calcium to initiate mineralization. Small proteoglycans such as decorin or fibromodulin also may have a role in mineralization.

MUTATIONS THAT PRODUCE DISEASES OF CONNECTIVE TISSUES Because of the large number of tissue-specific macromolecules present in connective tissues, a large number of gene-protein systems are candidates for mutations that might cause pathologic changes in the tissues. However, the situation appears to be simpler than originally assumed in that most forms of the diseases are caused by mutations in the genes for the structural proteins of connective tissues, and many are in the genes for collagens. Because most of the diseases involve defects in structural proteins, most are inherited as autosomal dominant traits. Also, many involve synthesis of structurally abnormal proteins instead of simply a decrease in the amount of the protein synthesized. The deleterious effects of the structurally abnormal proteins are largely explained by the consequences they have for the assembly of macromolecules into the insoluble extracellular matrix.

The most complete data on mutations causing heritable disorders of connective tissue are available on OI. Over 90 percent of patients with OI have mutations in either the gene for the proα1(I) chain or the gene for the proα2(I) chain of type I procollagen (the COL1A1 and COL1A2 genes). In patients with mild disease, some of the mutations decrease expression of protein from one allele of the genes. Most of the mutations in patients with severe OI cause synthesis of a structurally abnormal but partially functional proα chain (Figs. 351-2 and 351-3). The mutations that cause synthesis of structurally abnormal proα chains include partial gene deletions, partial gene duplications, and RNA splicing mutations. The most common mutations, however, are single-base mutations that substitute amino acids with bulkier side chains for the obligate glycine residues that appear as every third amino acid in the triple-helical domain of a proα chain (Fig. 351-4). The structurally abnormal proα chains exert their effects primarily through one of three molecular mechanisms (see Fig. 351-2). First, the presence of an abnormal proα chain in a procollagen molecule containing two normal proα chains can prevent folding of the protein into a triple-helical conformation and lead to degradation of the whole molecule in a process called *procollagen suicide*. Similar dominant negative mutations are seen with other multisubunit proteins. The net result of procollagen suicide is a marked reduction in the amount of collagen available for fibril assembly. Second, the presence of one abnormal proα chain in a procollagen molecule can interfere with cleavage of the N-propeptide from the protein by procollagen N-proteinase. The persistence of the N-propeptide on a fraction of the molecules produced by fibroblasts interferes with the self-assembly of normal collagen synthesized by the same cell so that thin and irregular collagen fibrils are formed. Third, the substitution of a bulkier amino acid for glycine can produce a change in the conformation of the molecule. Because the abnormal collagen can copolymerize with normal collagen, a small amount of collagen with an abnormal conformation can cause assembly of collagen fibrils that are abnormally branched (see Fig. 351-3) or abnormally thick and short. Also, copolymerization of the mutated collagen with normal collagen can

FIGURE 351-2 Schematic summary of three mechanisms (see text) whereby mutations that cause biosynthesis of structurally abnormal proα1(I) or proα2(I) chains of type I procollagen interfere with either the assembly of the protein (*A*) or its processing to normal collagen fibrils (*B*). (*From DJ Prockop et al, Am J Med Genet 34:60, 1989. Used with permission.*)

slow fibril assembly and decrease the total amount of collagen incorporated into fibrils.

There are several reasons why the type I procollagen genes harbor most of the mutations that cause OI. One, because collagen fibrils are a principal source of the strength of bone, the structure is weakened by any mutation that reduces the amount or distorts the normal geometry of collagen. The self-assembly of collagen fibrils is easily disrupted by a defective subunit that can participate in the assembly process but has the wrong structure. For example, the substitution of a bulky amino acid for a single glycine in one proα chain can interfere

FIGURE 351-3 Space-filling model showing a cysteine substitution of glycine α1-748 of type I procollagen (*on the left*) and darkfield light micrographs (*on the right*) of fibrils formed from control type I collagen at 32°C (*A*) and from the mixture of normal and mutated type I collagen containing the same cysteine substitution (*B*). (*From A Vogel et al, J Biol Chem 263:19249, 1988; and KE Kadler et al, Biochemistry 30:5081, 1991. Used with permission.*)

(accordina femora) may be present. For unclear reasons, the long bones may be either unusually thick or unusually thin. In types III and IV, multiple fractures from minor physical stress can produce progressive and severe deformities. Kyphoscoliosis may cause respiratory impairment, cor pulmonale, and predisposition to pulmonary infections. The appearance on radiographs of "popcorn-like" deposits of mineral on the ends of long bones is usually an ominous sign. Some patients develop progressive and severe neurologic symptoms because of basilar compression and communicating hydrocephalus.

In all forms of OI, bone mineral density in unfractured bone is decreased compared with that of age-matched controls. However, the degree of intrinsic osteopenia may be difficult to evaluate because recurrent fractures limit exercise and thereby exacerbate the decrease in bone mass. Surprisingly, the healing of fractures appears to be normal.

Ocular changes   The sclerae can be normal, slightly bluish, or bright blue. The blueness is probably caused by a thinness of the collagen layers of the sclerae that allows the choroid layers to be seen. Blue sclerae, however, are an inherited trait in some families without evidence of increased bone fragility.

Dentinogenesis imperfecta   The teeth may be normal, moderately discolored, or grossly abnormal. The enamel generally appears normal, but the teeth may have a characteristic amber, yellowish brown, or translucent bluish gray color because of improper deposition or deficiency of dentin. The deciduous teeth are usually smaller than normal, whereas permanent teeth are frequently bell-shaped and restricted at the base. In some patients, the teeth readily fracture and need to be extracted. The defect in dentin is directly attributable to the fact that normal dentin is rich in type I collagen. Similar tooth defects, however, occur in some families without any evidence of OI.

Hearing loss   Hearing loss is common. It usually begins during the second decade of life and can be detected in 90 percent of subjects over age 30. The loss can be conductive, sensorineural, or mixed and ranges widely in severity. The middle ear usually exhibits maldevelopment, deficient ossification, persistence of cartilage in areas that are normally ossified, and abnormal calcium deposits.

Associated features   Many patients and families show involvement of other connective tissues. Some have thin skin that scars extensively. Others have extreme joint laxity with permanent dislocations indistinguishable from those of EDS. A few have cardiovascular manifestations such as aortic regurgitation, floppy mitral valves, mitral incompetence, and fragility of large blood vessels. For unknown reasons, some patients develop a hypermetabolic state with elevated serum thyroxine levels, hyperthermia, and excessive sweating.

Molecular defects   Most patients with OI have mutations in one of the two genes for type I procollagen. A third or more of the patients with type I OI have as yet undefined mutations in the proα1(I) gene that decrease the steady state levels of the mRNA for proα1(I) chains and decrease the rates of synthesis of proα1(I) chains relative to those for proα2(I) chains. In more severe forms (types II, III, and IV), most of the mutations cause synthesis of structurally abnormal proα chains whose effects are amplified by the three molecular mechanisms discussed above (see Fig. 351-2). The mutations that change the structure of the protein near the N-proteinase cleavage site cause accumulation of a partially processed procollagen and produce lax joints more characteristic of type VII EDS rather than OI. Mutations that change the structure in the middle or near the C terminus tend to produce severe or lethal variants of OI. It is difficult, however, to deduce a more precise correlation between the site or nature of the mutation and the clinical phenotype (see Fig. 351-4). Rare patients are homozygous with two mutated alleles for proα1(I) or proα2(I) chains.

Mosaicism in germ line cells and in somatic cells   Most of the lethal variants of OI are the result of new autosomal dominant mutations. The frequency of a second child with lethal OI in the same family, however, is about 7 percent because of germ line mosaicism in one of the parents. The presence of germ line mosaicism was demonstrated directly in several fathers of patients with type II OI in that the mutated gene was found in a fraction of their sperm. Apparently normal parents of children with severe OI also may have somatic cell mosaicism in that the mutated allele is present in a fraction of somatic cells such as fibroblasts, leukocytes, and hair root cells. Because of the possibility of germ line mosaicism, asymptomatic parents of a child with severe OI should be counseled that the chance of a recurrence is not negligible.

Diagnosis   The diagnosis is usually made on the basis of clinical criteria alone. The presence of fractures together with either blue sclerae, dentinogenesis imperfecta, or family history of the disease is usually sufficient to make the diagnosis. Other possible causes of pathologic fractures must be excluded, including battered child syndrome, nutritional deficiencies, malignancies, and other heritable disorders such as CDs and hypophosphatasia (Table 351-3). X-rays usually reveal a decrease in bone density that can be verified by photon or x-ray absorptiometry. There is no consensus, however, as to whether the diagnosis can be made by microscopy of bone specimens. With research procedures, a molecular defect in type I procollagen can be demonstrated in half or more of patients by incubating skin fibroblasts with radioactive amino acids and then analyzing the proα chains by polyacrylamide gel electrophoresis. The analysis detects decreases in the rate of synthesis of proα1(I) chains relative to proα2(I) chains, abnormally long pro-α chains, abnormally short proα chains, and proα chains that are posttranslationally overmodified because of an amino acid substitution that delays folding of the triple helix. The mutations themselves can be defined in most patients by DNA sequencing of mRNA-derived cDNAs or sequencing of genomic DNAs. Because each proband and family usually has a "private" mutation, extensive analysis of 5000 or more bases in each of the two genes is required to identify the exact mutation. After a mutation in a type I procollagen gene is identified, a test based on the polymerase chain reaction can be used to screen family members at risk and for prenatal diagnosis.

Treatment   Treatment is ineffective. Many patients have successful careers despite severe deformities. Patients with mild disorder may need little treatment when fractures decrease after puberty, but women require special attention during pregnancy and after menopause, when fractures again increase. More severely affected children require a comprehensive program of physical therapy, surgical management of fractures and skeletal deformities, and vocational education.

Many of the fractures are only slightly displaced and have little soft tissue swelling. Therefore, they can be treated with minimal support or traction for a week or two followed by a light cast. If fractures are relatively painless, physical therapy can be initiated early. A judicious amount of exercise is obviously important to

TABLE 351-3   Differential diagnosis of OI

Age	Diagnosis	Distinguishing features
At birth	Hypophosphatasia	Unmineralized skull
	Achondrogenesis	Unmineralized vertebrae
	Thanatophoric dwarfism	H-shaped vertebrae
	Asphyxiating thoracic dystrophy	Cylindrical thorax
	Achondroplasia	Large head, short, tubular bones
Infancy	Battered child syndrome	Skull and rib fractures more common
	Immobilization osteogenesis	
	Scurvy	
	Congenital syphilis	
Childhood	Homocystinuria	Marfanoid appearance and mental deficiency
	Celiac disease	Steatorrhea, anemia
	Adrenal cortical tumor	
	Glucocorticoid therapy	

SOURCE: After R Smith et al, *The Brittle Bone Syndrome: Osteogenesis Imperfecta*, London, Butterworths, 1983, p 128.

prevent loss of bone mass secondary to physical inactivity. Some physicians advocate insertion of steel rods into long bones to correct limb deformities; the risk/benefits and cost/benefits of such procedures are difficult to evaluate. Aggressive conventional intervention is usually warranted for pneumonia and cor pulmonale. For severe hearing loss, excellent results have been reported with stapedectomy or replacement of the stapes with a prosthesis. Moderately to severely affected patients probably should be evaluated periodically to anticipate possible neurologic problems. About half of patients have a substantial increase in growth if treated during childhood with growth hormone. Treatment with bisphosphorates and related agents to decrease bone loss has been discussed, but no controlled studies have been reported.

A program for careful orthotic management developed by Bleck and a program for compressive management developed by Marini are useful guides. Counseling and emotional support for patients and parents is important, and lay organizations to provide help in these areas have now been formed in most countries. Prenatal ultrasonography will detect severely affected fetuses at about 16 weeks of pregnancy. Diagnosis by analysis for synthesis of abnormally migrating proα chains or by DNA sequencing can be carried out in chorionic villa biopsies at 8 to 12 weeks of pregnancy.

EHLERS-DANLOS SYNDROME The Ehlers-Danlos syndrome (EDS) is a group of heritable disorders characterized by hyperelasticity of the skin and hypermobile joints (Fig. 351-8).

Classification into types Beighton initially identified five types of EDS based primarily on the extent to which the skin, joints, and other tissues are involved (Table 351-4). Type I is the classical, severe form of the disease, with both severe joint hypermobility and skin changes that make it velvety in texture, hyperextensible, and easily scarred. Type II is similar to type I but milder. In type III, joint hypermobility is more prominent than the skin changes, and in type IV, the skin changes are far more prominent than the joint changes. A striking feature of type IV, however, is that the patients have a strong predisposition to sudden death from rupture of large blood vessels or the large bowel. Type V is similar to type II but characterized by X-linked inheritance. Type VI usually can be distinguished by the presence of scoliosis, ocular fragility, and a cone-shaped deformity of the cornea (keratoconus). Type VII is characterized by marked joint hypermobility that is difficult to distinguish from type III except by the specific molecular defects in the processing of type I procollagen to collagen. Type VIII is distinguished by periodontal changes. The remaining types IX, X, and XI were defined on the basis of preliminary biochemical and clinical data, but these classifications have not proven useful. Because of overlapping signs and symptoms, many patients and families cannot be assigned to any of the nine defined types of EDS.

Incidence Figures on the incidence of EDS have been difficult to develop, largely because patients with mild skin or joint symptoms rarely seek medical attention. Also, it is difficult to define the normal range of variation for features such as joint mobility or skin elasticity. An incidence of about 1 in 5000 births is gaining acceptance, although a higher value has been reported for a predominantly black population. Types I, II, and III account for most of the diagnosed patients.

Skin The changes vary from unusually thin and velvety skin to skin that is either dramatically hyperextensible ("rubber man" syndrome) or easily torn or scarred. Patients with type I develop characteristic "cigarette-paper" scars. In type IV, extensive scars and hyperpigmentation develop over bony prominences, and the skin may be so thin that subcutaneous blood vessels become visible. In type VIII, the skin is more fragile than hyperextensible, and it heals with atrophic, pigmented scars. Easy bruisability is a feature of several types of EDS.

Ligament and joint changes Laxity and hypermobility of joints vary from mild to unreducible dislocations of hips and other large joints. In milder forms, patients learn to reduce dislocations themselves and to avoid them by limiting physical activity. In more severe forms, surgical repair is required. Some patients have progressive difficulty

FIGURE 351-8 Schematic representation of the skin and joint changes in EDS. Girl in upper right has type VII EDS with dislocations of both hips that were not correctable by surgery. *(From DJ Prockop and NA Guzman, Hosp Pract 12(12):61, 1977. Used with permission.)*

with age, but severe joint laxity is compatible with a normal life span.

Associated changes Mitral valve prolapse occurs, particularly in type I. Pes planus and mild to moderate scoliosis are common. Extreme joint laxity and repeated dislocations may lead to degenerative arthritis. Hernias are frequent in patients with type I. In type VI, the eye may rupture with minimal trauma, and kyphoscoliosis can produce respiratory impairment. Sclerae are frequently blue in type VI.

Molecular defects The molecular defects in the type I, type II, and type III variants of EDS are unknown. Electron microscopy of the skin from some patients has shown an unusual morphology of collagen fibers, but similar features are seen occasionally in normal skin.

TABLE 351-4 Clinical features, mode of inheritance, and biochemical defects in EDS

Type	Clinical features	Inheritance*	Biochemical defect
I, gravis	Soft, velvety, hyperextensible skin; easy bruising; "cigarette paper" scars; hypermobile joints; varicose veins; prematurity	AD	Not known
II, mitis	Similar to EDS type I but less severe	AD	Not known
III, familial hypermobility	Soft skin, no scarring, marked hypermobility	AD	Not known
IV, acrogeric, ecchymotic, vascular	Thin, translucent skin with visible veins; increased bruisability, skin and joints have normal extensibility; arterial, bowel, and uterine rupture	AD	Mutations in type III procollagen (see Fig. 351-6)
V, X-linked	Similar to EDS type II	XLR	Not known
VI, ocular-scoliotic	Soft, velvety, hyperextensible skin; hypermobile joints; scoliosis; ocular fragility and keratoconus	AR	Lysyl hydroxylase deficiency
VII, arthrochalasis multiplex congenita	Marked joint hypermobility, soft skin with normal scarring	AD	A. Structural defect in the proα1(I) chain
		AD	B. Structural defect in the proα2(I) chain
		AR	C. Procollagen *N*-proteinase deficiency
VIII, periodontal	Generalized periodontitis, skin similar to EDS type II	AD	Not known
IX, cutis laxa occipital horn syndrome	Vacant, now recategorized as a disorder of copper transport		
X	Similar to EDS type II	AR	Possible defect in fibronectin
XI, familial joint instability	Vacant, now recategorized with familial articular hypermobility syndromes		

* AD, autosomal dominant; AR, autosomal recessive; XLR, X-linked recessive.
SOURCE: After PH Byers, in *Clinical Medicine*, Philadelphia, Harper & Row, 1983, p. 1; and P Beighton et al, Am J Med Genet 29:581, 1988.

Most patients with type IV have a defect either in the synthesis or structure of type III procollagen, a finding consistent with the fact that these patients are prone to spontaneous rupture of the aorta and intestines, tissues rich in type III collagen. The thinness and scarring of skin are more difficult to explain, since type III constitutes a small fraction of the collagen in skin (see Table 351-1). The mutations identified in the type III procollagen gene include partial gene deletions, RNA splicing mutations, and single-base mutations that cause substitution of amino acids with bulkier side chains for glycine (see Fig. 351-6). In brief, most of the mutations lead to synthesis of abnormal but partially functional proα1(III) chains that produce procollagen suicide or alter fibril formation by the same mechanisms that amplify the effects of mutations in the genes for type I procollagen. Similar mutations in type III procollagen also can cause aortic aneurysms in individuals without other evidence of EDS type IV, MS, or other defined heritable disorders of connective tissue.

Type VI is caused by a deficiency of lysyl hydroxylase. Mutations in the gene for this enzyme have been defined in two families. In one family, the mutation produced a premature stop codon, and in the other the mutation produced a large duplication of the gene. Deficiency of lysyl hydroxylase causes synthesis of a collagen that is deficient in its content of hydroxylysine and as a result does not form stable cross-links.

Type VII is a defect in the conversion of procollagen to collagen in patients with marked joint hypermobility. The defect can be caused either by mutations that make type I procollagen resistant to cleavage by procollagen *N*-proteinase or by mutations that decrease the activity of the enzyme. In type VIIA, the mutations alter the cleavage site in the proα1(I) chain. In type VIIB, the mutations alter the cleavage site in the proα2(I) chain. Both types are dominantly inherited. Type VIIC is caused by mutations that decrease the activity of procollagen *N*-proteinase. It is inherited as an autosomal recessive trait. In all three forms of type VII EDS, the persistence of the *N*-propeptide on the molecule causes the formation of fibrils that are thin and irregular in cross section. Since most patients do not have clinical osteopenia, the thin and irregular fibrils apparently suffice for the mineralization of bone but do not provide the necessary tensile strength for ligaments and joint capsules.

The cause of type VIII is unknown. Type IX is a disorder of copper transport. The syndrome, also referred to as *Menkes' syndrome*, is due to an X-linked defect and is associated with cutis laxa, hypopigmentation, unusual hair ("kinky"), vascular aneurysms, neurologic degeneration, and mental retardation. Mutations in a gene coding for a copper-transporting ATPase cause the disease. Type X EDS may be caused by defects in fibronectin, but no specific mutations have been defined. (See also Chaps. 78 and 353.)

Diagnosis The diagnosis of EDS is based primarily on clinical criteria. Biochemical assays and gene analyses for known molecular defects in EDS are difficult and time-consuming, but specific diagnostic tests should be available in the future for families in which the mutations have been defined.

Treatment There is no specific therapy. Surgical repair and tightening of joint ligaments require careful evaluation of individual patients, since the ligaments frequently will not hold sutures. Patients with easy bruisability should be evaluated for other bleeding disorders. Patients with type IV EDS and members of their families probably should be evaluated at regular intervals by sonography and related techniques for early detection of aneurysms. Surgical repair of aneurysms may be difficult because of increased friability of tissues, and there is limited experience with elective surgery in such patients. Also, women with type IV EDS should be counseled about the increased risk of uterine rupture, bleeding, and other complications of pregnancy.

CHONDRODYSPLASIAS The chondrodysplasias (CDs) are heritable disorders of skeletal growth that produce dwarfism with abnormal body proportions. The category also includes some individuals with normal stature and body proportions who have features such as characteristic ocular changes or cleft palate that are common in more severe CDs. Also, many patients with CD develop degenerative joint changes that are difficult to distinguish from osteoarthritis. Therefore, mild CDs in adults may be difficult to differentiate from primary generalized osteoarthritis. Some authors refer to the disorders as "skeletal dysplasias," but CD is a more widely used term because most of the diseases produce changes in cartilage and because the effects on the bony skeleton appear to be secondary to effects on cartilage.

Classifications of the diseases Over 150 distinct types of CDs with 8 major subtypes have been defined in the literature (Table 351-5). The classifications have been based on a variety of criteria such as "bringing death" (thanatophoric), causing "twisted" bones (diastrophic), primarily affecting metaphyses (metaphyseal), primarily affecting epiphyses (epiphyseal), and producing characteristic histologic changes such as an apparent increase in the fibrous material seen in the epiphyses (fibrochondrogenesis). Also, a number of eponyms have been introduced based on the first or most comprehensive case reports. Severe forms of the diseases produce gross distortions of most cartilaginous structures and of the eye (see Table 351-1). Mild forms are more difficult to classify. Among the features are cataracts, degeneration of the vitreous and retinal detachment, high forehead, hypoplastic facies, cleft palate, short and thin extremities, and gross distortions of the epiphyses, metaphyses, and joint surfaces.

Incidence Data on the frequency of most CDs are not available, but the incidence of the Stickler syndrome has been estimated as high as 1 in 10,000. Therefore, the diseases are probably among the more common heritable disorders of connective tissue.

Molecular defects Because most CDs produce dramatic changes in the appearance of cartilage, most are probably caused by a mutation in a gene for one of the structural proteins in the matrix of cartilage (see Table 351-1). To date, however, the only gene explored extensively for such mutations is the gene for type II procollagen (COL2A1) (see Fig. 351-7).

DNA linkage studies with the COL2A1 gene demonstrated that specific alleles of the gene were frequently coinherited with the Stickler syndrome and with arthroophthalmopathy, a condition characterized by myopia and lattice degeneration of the vitreous and frequently associated with cleft palate, hypoplastic facies, variable skeletal changes, and early-onset degenerative arthritis. In one series,

half of families demonstrated linkage to the COL2A1 gene. Subsequently, direct analysis of the COL2A1 gene demonstrated that four unrelated families had different mutations that produced premature termination codons for translation of the mRNA. The consequences of premature termination codons were not explicitly defined, but they probably caused synthesis of shortened proα1(II) chains that lack C-terminal propeptides and therefore are not incorporated into type II procollagen and do not contribute to the assembly of type II collagen fibrils. A decrease in the amount of type II collagen in the eye is consistent with the lattice degeneration of the vitreous and retinal detachment. A decrease in type II collagen fibers also explains the cleft palate, the skeletal changes, and the degenerative arthritis of joints. As with OI, however, it is less clear why other mutations in the same COL2A1 gene cause other phenotypes (see Fig. 351-7). For example, a mutation that substituted an aspartate for a glycine codon was seen in a family defined as having the Wagner syndrome because they had the ocular changes characteristic of the Stickler syndrome but no evidence of extraocular tissue involvement.

Defects of the COL2A1 gene in more severe CDs include one exon deletion, one partial gene duplication, one RNA splicing mutation, and five glycine substitutions (see Fig. 351-7). The clinical phenotypes range from lethal at birth (hypochondrogenesis and achondrogenesis II/hypochondrogenesis) to severe spondyloepiphyseal dysplasia. Again, there is no apparent relationship between the site or nature of the mutation and the phenotype. Although the data are incomplete, about half of patients with severe CDs have mutations in the gene for type II procollagen, and the remainder are likely to have mutations in genes for other molecules.

Of special interest, two different mutations in the COL2A1 gene replace arginine codons in the triple-helical domain with codons for cysteine. Cysteine is not found in the triple-helical domain of type II collagen from any species, and the presence of cysteine in the type II collagen introduces an abnormal disulfide cross-link in collagen. One of the cysteine-for-arginine substitutions was found in affected members of a large family with primary generalized osteoarthritis and minimal evidence of a CD. The other was found in a family with a mild spondyloepiphyseal dysplasia. In brief, mutations in the COL2A1 gene, like mutations in the genes for type I and type III procollagen, can cause a spectrum of diseases from lethal conditions to common disorders such as osteoarthritis.

Diagnosis The diagnosis of severe forms of CD is made on the basis of analysis of the physical appearance, x-ray findings, histologic changes, and clinical course (Table 351-5).

Treatment No definitive therapy is available. Symptomatic treatment is directed toward secondary features such as degenerative arthritis. Many patients require joint replacement surgery and corrective surgery for cleft palates. Ocular changes should be monitored carefully for the development of cataracts and for the need for laser therapy to prevent retinal detachment. Patients probably should be advised to avoid obesity and contact sports. Counseling for the serious psychological problems of short stature is critical, and support groups have formed in many countries. Ultrasonography is sometimes successful for prenatal diagnosis but less frequently than with OI. Specific tests should be available in the future for the CDs caused by mutations in the COL2A1 gene.

MARFAN SYNDROME Severe Marfan syndrome (MS) is characterized by a triad of features: (1) long, thin extremities frequently associated with other skeletal changes, (2) reduced vision as the result of dislocations of the lenses (ectopia lentis), and (3) aortic aneurysms that typically begin at the base of the aorta. Milder forms of the disorder, particularly those with only the skeletal changes, are difficult to classify.

Classification The severe form is usually due to a mutation in a single allele of the fibrillin gene (FBN1). At the same time, MS must be distinguished from related syndromes: (1) homocystinuria that frequently causes ectopia lentis and some of the same skeletal changes as the MS, (2) congenital contractural arachnodactyly that causes similar skeletal changes but none of the other features of MS,

---

TABLE 351-5 Classifications of chondrodysplasias

Achondrodysplasia family
  Achondroplasia
  Hypochondroplasia
  Thanatophoric dysplasia
Spondyloepiphyseal dysplasia (SED) family
  Achondrogenesis type IA
  Achonodrogenesis type IB
  Achondrogenesis type II
  Hypochondrogenesis
  SED congenita
  Strudwick syndrome
  Stickler syndrome
  Kniest dysplasia
Chondrodysplasia punctata family
  Rhizomelic chondrodysplasia punctata
  Conradi-Hünermann disease
  X-linked dominant chondrodysplasia punctata
  Chondrodysplasia punctata associated with Xp
Short rib (-polydactyly) family
  Ellis-van Creveld syndrome
  Asphyxiating thoracic dysplasia
  Short rib–polydactyly syndrome type I
  Short rib–polydactyly syndrome type II
Metatropic dysplasia family
  Metatropic dysplasia
  Metatropic-like dysplasia
Metaphyseal chondrodysplasia family
  Metaphyseal chondrodysplasia, Jansen type
  Metaphyseal chondrodysplasia, Schmid type
  Metaphyseal chondrodysplasia, McKusick type
Brachyolmia family
  Brachyolmia, Hobaek type
  Brachyolmia, Maroteaux type
  Brachyolmia, autosomal dominant type
Acromelic dysplasia family
  Peripheral dysostosis
  Achodysplasia
  Trichorhinophalangeal syndrome type I
  Trichorhinophalangeal syndrome type II

SOURCE: After Spranger J. Eur J Pediatr 151:407, 1992; WA Horton and JT Hecht.

(3) familial ectopia lentis not associated with other features of MS, and (4) familial aortic aneurysms that result from a more common autosomal dominant disorder not associated with other features of MS, type IV EDS, or other known disorders of connective tissue.

Incidence and inheritance   MS has an incidence of about 1 in 10,000 in most racial and ethnic groups. The disorder is inherited as an autosomal dominant trait, but at least one-quarter of patients do not have an affected parent and therefore their disorders probably are due to new mutations.

Skeletal changes   Patients are usually tall compared with other members of the same family and have long limbs. The ratio of the upper segment (top of the head to top of the pubic ramus) to the lower segment (top of the pubic ramus to the floor) is usually 2 standard deviations below mean for age, race, and sex. The fingers and hands are long and slender and have a spider-like appearance (arachnodactyly). Many patients have severe chest deformities, including depression (pectus excavatum), protrusion (pectus carinatum), or asymmetry. Scoliosis is usually accompanied by kyphosis. High-arched palate and high pedal arches or pes planus are common. A few patients have joint hypermobility similar to that in mild EDS, but joint mobility is usually normal.

Cardiovascular changes   Cardiovascular abnormalities are the major source of morbidity and mortality. Mitral valve prolapse develops early in life and in about one-quarter progresses to mitral valve regurgitation of increasing severity because of redundancy of the leaflets, stretching of the chordae tendinae, and dilatation of the valvulae annulus. Dilatation of the root of the aorta and the sinuses of Valsalva may be detected by echocardiography in utero. The rate of dilatation is unpredictable, but the dilatation can cause aortic regurgitation, dissection of the aorta, and rupture. Dilatation is probably accelerated by physical and emotional stress, as well as by pregnancy.

Ocular changes   The dislocation of the lens may be readily apparent, but diagnosis usually requires pupillary dilatation and slit-lamp examination. The displacement is usually not progressive but may contribute to the formation of cataracts. The ocular globe is frequently elongated, most patients are myopic, and some develop retinal detachment. A few patients have lattice degeneration and retinal tears; most have adequate vision.

Associated changes   Striae may occur over the shoulders and buttocks. Otherwise the skin is normal. A number of patients develop spontaneous pneumothorax. Inguinal and incisional hernias are common. Marked dilatation of the dural sac is seen frequently in CT scans, but the condition is usually asymptomatic. Characteristically, patients are thin with little subcutaneous fat, but adults may develop centripetal fat accumulation.

Molecular defects   Most patients with the classical features of MS have mutations in a gene for fibrillin, a glycoprotein of 350 kDa that is a major component of elastin-associated microfibrils. These microfibrils are abundant in large blood vessels and the suspensory ligaments of the lens. Patients are heterozygous for the mutations, and many of the mutations appear to change amino acid codons at various sites along the protein. The function of fibrillin has not been defined, but the data suggest that fibrillin self-assembles into a fibrillar structure and that the conformation and surface properties of the entire molecule are critical for normal assembly. Therefore, the functional consequences of mutations that change the amino acid sequence of fibrillin may be similar to the effects of mutations that change the conformation of a fibrillar collagen (see Figs. 351-2, 351-4, 351-6, and 351-7). Although only a few mutations have been specifically identified, most patients with the classical syndrome are thought to have mutations in the same gene located on the long arm of chromosome 15 (FBN1), since extensive studies demonstrated linkage of the mutated genes to the same site. In addition, DNA linkage studies indicate that the gene causing familial ectopia lentis without any other signs of MS is also located on chromosome 15, but it is unclear whether the gene is identical with FBN1. Two families with a Marfan-related syndrome characterized by congenital contractural

arachnodactyly demonstrate linkage to a second fibrillin gene located on chromosome 5 (FBN2). A third fibrillin gene (FBN3) is presented on chromosome 17, but no defect has yet been linked to the gene. Also, two patients with atypical forms of the syndrome apparently have defects in the proα2(I) chain of type I procollagen. Therefore, patents with classical MS have mutations in genes other than the FBN gene on chromosome 15.

Diagnosis   The diagnosis is easily established if the patient and other members of the family have dislocated lenses, aortic dilatation, and long and thin extremities together with kyphoscoliosis or other chest deformities. The diagnosis is frequently made if ectopia lentis and an aneurysm of the ascending aorta occur in the absence of a Marfan habitus or a positive family history. All patients in whom the diagnosis is suspected should have a slit-lamp examination and an echocardiogram. Also, homocystinuria (see Table 351-3) should be ruled out by a negative cyanide-nitroprusside test for disulfides in the urine. A few patients with types I, II, and III EDS have ectopia lentis but lack the Marfan habitus and instead have characteristic skin changes not present in MS. Patients with familial aortic aneurysms tend to develop aneurysms at the base of the abdominal aorta. The location of the aneurysms, however is, variable, and the high incidence of aortic aneurysms (1 in 100) makes the differential diagnosis difficult unless other features of MS are clearly present. A few families with familial aortic aneurysms have mutations in the gene for type III procollagen (see Fig. 351-6).

Treatment   There is no established treatment, but several investigators have recommended use of propranolol or other beta-adrenergic blocking agents to delay or prevent aortic dilatation. Surgical replacement of the aorta, aortic valve, and mitral valve has been successful in some patients, and all patients should be followed carefully with echocardiography and other techniques for evaluation of cardiovascular changes. Patients probably should be advised of the risks of severe physical and emotional stress and of pregnancy.

The scoliosis tends to be progressive and should be treated by mechanical bracing and physical therapy if greater than 20 degrees or by surgery if it progresses to greater than 45 degrees. Estrogen has been tried in girls with scoliosis, but the results are inconclusive. Dislocated lenses rarely require surgical removal, but patients should be followed closely for retinal detachment. Pyeritz has summarized current protocols for the management of patients.

Diagnostic tests based on detection of fibrillin defects in cultured skin fibroblasts or DNA analysis of the gene may be available in the near future.

EPIDERMOLYSIS BULLOSA   Epidermolysis bullosa (EB) is a group of disorders in which the skin and related epithelial tissues break and blister as the result of minor trauma. As with most heritable disorders of connective tissues, the clinical manifestations range from lethal to mild disorders.

Classifications   Three major categories are defined on the basis of the level at which blistering occurs: EB simplex for blistering in the epidermis, EB junctional for blistering in the dermal-epidermal junction, and EB dystrophica for blistering in the dermis. More than 20 subtypes have been separated on the basis of the clinical findings together with ultrastructural and immunohistologic changes in skin.

Incidence   The incidence of EB in the United States is estimated to be 1 in 50,000.

Molecular defects   The molecular basis of several specific variants of EB has been defined. Some of the first information came from experiments with transgenic mice in which mice expressing a gene for a truncated keratin (keratin 14) developed intraepidermal blistering similar to that seen in patients with EB simplex. Subsequently, point mutations in the same gene were found in two patients with the herpetiformis variant of EB simplex. In addition, point mutations in another keratin gene (keratin 5) were identified in several other patients with EB simplex. The structure-function relationships of the multiple keratins found in the epithelium have not been defined. The findings in transgenic mice and in patients suggest that the proteins are similar to collagens in that a large part of the conformation and surface properties of the monomers must be preserved for normal function.

In EB dystrophica, DNA linkage studies established that both dominantly and recessively inherited forms of the disease are coinherited with specific alleles of the genes for type VII collagen (COL7A1). Type VII collagen is seen in electron micrographs of skin as strandlike fibrils that anchor the basal lamina to the collagen fibrils of the dermis. Anchoring fibrils are decreased in number or absent in skin from patients with EB dystrophica. Therefore, mutations in the gene for type VII collagen can account for the clinical syndrome.

The gene or genes at fault in EB junctional are still unknown.

Diagnosis   The diagnosis is based on skin that readily breaks and forms blisters. EB simplex, which affects only the epidermis, is generally milder than either EB junctional or EB dystrophica. EB dystrophica variants are generally associated with large and prominent scars. Classification within specific subtypes usually requires ultrastructural microscopy.

Treatment   The treatment is symptomatic. Bruckner-Tuderman has reviewed the diagnostic criteria and management.

ALPORT SYNDROME   (See also Chaps. 234 and 241)   The Alport syndrome (AS) is a heritable disorder characterized by hematuria. Two forms of the disease are now recognized: (1) classic AS, which is inherited as an X-linked disorder with hematuria, sensorineural deafness, and conical deformation of the anterior surface of the lens (lenticonus), and (2) nonclassical AS, which is inherited as an autosomal trait that causes hematuria but not deafness or lenticonus.

Incidence   The incidence of AS is about 1 in 10,000 in the general population and as high as 1 in 5000 in some ethnic groups.

Molecular defects   Electron microscopy of kidneys from patients with classic AS demonstrated that the glomerular basement membrane was up to five times thicker than normal and that the lamina densa was distorted and split. DNA linkage studies demonstrated that the gene at fault is located on the long arm of the X chromosome (Xq22). The subsequent discovery that the $\alpha5(IV)$ chain of type IV collagen is also encoded on the long arm of the X chromosome spurred extensive analysis of the gene in the disease, and several mutations were identified. Most of the mutations are large deletions or gene rearrangements that probably cause decreased synthesis of $\alpha5(IV)$ chains. In the hemizygous male who inherits only the mutated gene, therefore, none of these chains is likely to be synthesized. The absence of the $\alpha5(IV)$ chains probably explains the manifestations. The most abundant type IV collagen in most basement membranes consists of two $\alpha1(IV)$ chains and one $\alpha2(IV)$ chain in the form of a large, rodlike molecule with globular ends and a long triple-helical domain that is interrupted by short sequences that do not form triple helices. The molecules self-assemble through both the globular ends and the triple-helical domains to form a complex, three-dimensional network. Since $\alpha5(IV)$ chains are similar in structure to $\alpha1(IV)$ or $\alpha2(IV)$ chains, they probably are assembled into monomers of a similar type IV collagen, either as homotrimers of $\alpha5(IV)$ chains or together with the $\alpha3(IV)$ and $\alpha4(IV)$ chains found in some basement membranes. No disease-causing mutations in the genes for $\alpha1(IV)$, $\alpha2(IV)$, $\alpha3(IV)$, or $\alpha4(IV)$ chains have been identified.

The cause of nonclassic AS with hematuria but without deafness is unknown.

Diagnosis   The diagnosis of classic AS is based on X-linked inheritance of hematuria, sensorineural deafness, and lenticonus. Because of the X-linked transmission, women are usually less severely affected than men and are generally underdiagnosed. The hematuria progresses to nephritis and may cause renal failure in late adolescence in affected males and at older ages in some women. The sensorineural deafness is primarily in the high-tone range. It frequently can be detected only by an audiogram and usually is not progressive. The lenticonus rarely occurs without nephritis and is considered to be pathognomonic of classic AS.

Treatment   There is no known treatment. DNA tests should soon be available for prenatal diagnosis.

REFERENCES

BARKER DF et al: Identification of mutations in the COL4A5 collagen gene in the Alport syndrome. Science 248:1224, 1990

BLECK EE: Non-operative treatment of osteogenesis imperfecta: Orthotic and mobility management. Clin Orthop 159:115, 1981

BOYE E et al: Major rearrangements in the $\alpha5(IV)$ collagen gene in three patients with Alport syndrome. Genomics 11:1125, 1991

BRUCKNER-TUDERMAN L: Epidermolysis bullosa, in *Connective Tissue and Its Heritable Disorders*, PM Royce, B Steinmann (eds). New York, Wiley-Liss, 1993, p. 507

BYERS PH: Osteogenesis imperfecta, in *Connective Tissue and Its Heritable Disorders*, PM Royce, B Steinmann (eds). New York, Wiley-Liss, 1993, p 317

FLINTER FA et al: Genetics of classic Alport's syndrome. Lancet 2:1005, 1988

HORTON WA, HECHT JT: The chondrodysplasias, in *Connective Tissue and Its Heritable Disorders*, PM Royce, B Steinmann (eds). New York, Wiley-Liss, 1993 p 641

KUIVANIEMI H et al: Mutations in collagen genes: Causes of rare and some common diseases in humans. FASEB J 5:2052, 1991

MARINI JC: Osteogenesis imperfecta: Comprehensive management. Adv Pediatr 35:391, 1988

———— et al: Evaluation of growth hormone axis and responsiveness to growth stimulation of short children with osteogenesis imperfecta. Am J Med Genet 45:21, 1993

McKUSICK VA: *Heritable Disorders of Connective Tissue*, 4th ed. St Louis, Mosby, 1972

PROCKOP DJ: Mutations in collagen genes as a cause of connective-tissue diseases. N Engl J Med 326:540, 1992

————, KIVIRIKKO KI: Heritable diseases of collagen. N Engl J Med 311:376, 1984

PYERITZ RE: The Marfan syndrome, in *Connective Tissue and Its Heritable Disorders*, PM Royce, B Steinmann (eds). New York, Wiley-Liss, 1993, p 437

SILLENCE DO: Osteogenesis imperfecta: An expanding panorama of variance. Clin Orthop 191:11, 1981

STEINMANN B et al: The Ehlers-Danlos syndrome, in *Connective Tissue and Its Heritable Disorders*, PM Royce, B Steinmann (eds). New York, Wiley-Liss, 1993, p 351

UITTO J, CHRISTIANO AM: Molecular genetics of the cutaneous basement membrane zone: Perspectives on epidermolysis bullosa and other blistering skin disorders. J Clin Invest 90:687, 1992

---

352   INHERITED DISORDERS OF AMINO ACID METABOLISM AND STORAGE

LEON E. ROSENBERG

All polypeptides and proteins are polymers of 20 different amino acids. Eight of these, referred to as *essential*, cannot be synthesized by humans and must be obtained from dietary sources. The others are formed endogenously. Although most of the body's amino acids are "tied up" in proteins, small intracellular pools of *free* amino acids are in equilibrium with extracellular reservoirs in plasma, cerebrospinal fluid, and the lumina of the gut and kidney. Physiologically, amino acids are more than mere "building blocks." Some (glycine, glutamate, γ-aminobutyric acid) are neurotransmitters. Others (phenylalanine, tyrosine, tryptophan, glycine) are precursors of hormones, coenzymes, pigments, purines, or pyrimidines. Each has a unique degradative pathway by which its nitrogen and carbon components are used for the synthesis of other amino acids, carbohydrates, and lipids.

Current concepts of inherited metabolic diseases are based to a considerable degree on investigations of amino acid disorders. More than 70 such disorders are now known, the catabolic defects (approximately 60) discussed in this chapter far outnumbering the transport abnormalities (approximately 10) considered in Chap. 353. Each of these disorders is rare—the incidences range from 1 in 10,000 for cystinuria or phenylketonuria to 1 in 200,000 for homocystinuria or alkaptonuria. Collectively, however, they occur in perhaps 1 in 500 to 1 in 1000 live births.

The salient features of inherited disorders of amino acid catabolism are summarized in Table 352-1. In general, these disorders are named for the compound that accumulates to highest concentration in blood (-*emias*) or urine (-*urias*). For many conditions (often called *aminoacidopathies*), the parent amino acid is found in excess; for

TABLE 352-1 Inherited disorders of amino acid catabolism *(continued)*

Amino acid(s) affected	Disorder or condition	Enzyme defect	Clinical manifestations*			
			Mental retardation	Neuropsychiatric dysfunction	Protein intolerance	Metabolic ketoacidosis
CATIONIC *(continued)*						
Ornithine	Hyperornithinemia-hyperammonemia-homocitrullinuria	Mitochondrial ornithine translocator (?)	+	+	+	−
	Hyperornithinemia	Ornithine-D-aminotransferase	−	−	−	−
UREA CYCLE						
Carbamylphosphate	Hyperammonemia (type I)	Carbamylphosphate synthetase I	+	+	+	−
N-acetylglutamate	Hyperammonemia (type IA)	N-acetylglutamate synthetase	?	+	+	−
Ornithine	Hyperammonemia (type II)	Ornithine transcarbamylase	±	+	+	−
Citrulline	Citrullinemia	Argininosuccinate synthetase	+	+	+	−
Argininosuccinic acid	Argininosuccinic aciduria	Argininosuccinase	+	+	+	−
Arginine	Argininemia	Arginase	+	+	+	−
BRANCHED-CHAIN						
Valine	Hypervalinemia	Valine aminotransferase	+	+	+	−
Leucine, isoleucine	Hyperleucine-isoleucinemia	Leucine-isoleucine aminotransferase	+	+	+	−
Valine, leucine, isoleucine	Classic branched-chain ketoaciduria	Branched-chain ketoacid dehydrogenase	+	+	+	
	Intermittent branched-chain ketoaciduria	Branched-chain ketoacid dehydrogenase	±	−	+	+
Leucine	Isovaleric acidemia	Isovaleryl CoA dehydrogenase	±	±	+	+
	β-Methylcrotonyl glycinuria	β-Methylcrotonyl CoA carboxylase	+	+		+
	β-Hydroxy-β-methylglutaric aciduria	β-Hydroxy-β-methylglutaryl CoA lyase	−	+	+	+
Isoleucine, valine	α-Methylacetoacetic aciduria	β-Ketothiolase	±	±	+	+
	Propionic acidemia (pcc A, B, C)‡	Propionyl CoA carboxylase	±	±	+	+
	Propionic acidemia (bio)‡	Holocarboxylase synthetase; biotinidase	+	±	+	+
	Methylmalonic acidemia (mut)‡	Methylmalonyl CoA mutase	±	±	+	+
	Methylmalonic acidemia (cbl A)‡	Cobalamin (vitamin B_{12}) reductase (mitochondrial) (?)	±	±	+	+
	Methylmalonic acidemia (cbl B)‡	Cobalamin (vitamin B_{12}): ATP adenosyltransferase	±	±	+	+

* +, Regularly present; ±, sometimes present; −, absent; ?, uncertain; all designations refer to manifestations in untreated disorder.
† AR, autosomal recessive; XL, X-linked; (AR), probably autosomal recessive.
‡ Designations in parentheses refer to complementation groups.

pteridine, tetrahydrobiopterin, is cofactor (Fig. 352-1). Tyrosine and dihydrobiopterin are the products of this catalytic system, the latter being reconverted to tetrahydrobiopterin by a second enzyme, dihydropteridine reductase. In classic phenylketonuria, activity of the hydroxylase apoenzyme, encoded by a gene in the q22–q24.1 region of chromosome 12, is almost totally deficient. Six different mutations leading to such complete deficiency are recognized. These include missense changes, splicing defects, and partial deletions. Benign hyperphenylalaninemia results from a less complete deficiency, and transient hyperphenylalaninemia (sometimes called *transient phenylketonuria*) is caused by a delayed maturation of the hydroxylase apoenzyme. In "malignant" hyperphenylalaninemia, however, persistent impairment of hydroxylating activity results not from abnormality in the apohydroxylase but from tetrahydrobiopterin deficiency due to blocks in the pathway by which tetrahydrobiopterin is synthesized from GTP or deficiency of dihydropteridine reductase, the enzyme that regenerates tetrahydrobiopterin from dihydrobiopterin (see Fig. 352-1). This reductase system is also utilized by tyrosine hydroxylase and tryptophan hydroxylase.

The hyperphenylalaninemias are autosomal recessive traits that occur in about 1 in 10,000 births. Classic phenylketonuria, which accounts for nearly two-thirds of these, is widely distributed among whites and Orientals. It is rare in blacks. Phenylalanine hydroxylase activity in obligate heterozygotes is low but higher than in affected homozygotes. Heterozygous carriers are clinically well but may have slightly increased phenylalanine concentrations in plasma.

Phenylalanine accumulation in blood and urine and reduced tyrosine formation are direct consequences of the impaired hydroxylation. In untreated phenylketonuria and in its tetrahydrobiopterin-deficient variants, plasma concentrations of phenylalanine become sufficiently high [greater than 1200 μmol/L (20 mg/dL)] to activate alternative pathways of metabolism and lead to formation of phenylpyruvate, phenylacetate, phenyllactate, and other derivatives that are rapidly cleared by the kidney and excreted in urine. Plasma concentrations of several other amino acids are moderately reduced, probably secondary to inhibition of gastrointestinal absorption or impairment of renal tubular reabsorption by excess phenylalanine. The severe brain damage is due to several consequences of phenylalanine

Ammonia intoxication	Other	Inheritance pattern[†]
+		AR
−	Gyrate atrophy of choroid and retina	AR
+		AR
+		?
+		XL
+		AR
+		AR
+		AR
−		?
−		?
−	"Maple syrup" odor	AR
−		AR
±	"Sweaty feet" odor	AR
−	"Cat's urine" odor	AR
		?
+		AR
+		AR
−		AR
+		AR
+		AR
+		AR

FIGURE 352-1 Pathways, enzymes, and coenzymes involved in the hyperphenylalaninemias. Blocked-in symbols highlight points of etiologic or therapeutic significance to the various genetic defects underlying these disorders. Abbreviations: GTP, guanosine triphosphate; GTP-CH, guanosine triphosphate cyclohydrolase; DNT, dihydroneopterin triphosphate; 6-PTS, 6-pyruvoyltetrahydropterin synthase; BH₄, tetrahydrobiopterin; BH₂, dihydrobiopterin; DHPR, dihydropteridine reductase; PAH, phenylalanine hydroxylase.

classic phenylketonuria. Children with tetrahydrobiopterin deficiency, however, are the most unfortunate. Seizures appear early, followed by progressive cerebral and basal ganglia dysfunction (rigidity, chorea, spasms, hypotonia). Most succumb to secondary infection within a few years despite early diagnosis and vigorous treatment.

A number of women with phenylketonuria who have been treated since infancy have reached adulthood and become pregnant. More than 90 percent of their offspring are markedly retarded, and many have additional congenital anomalies such as microcephaly, growth retardation, and congenital heart defects. Since these children are heterozygous, not homozygous for a phenylketonuria mutation, the clinical manifestations must be attributed to damage produced by the elevated maternal concentrations of phenylalanine to which they have been exposed in utero. This alarming syndrome is called *maternal phenylketonuria*.

DIAGNOSIS Plasma phenylalanine concentrations are usually normal at birth in the hyperphenylalaninemias but rise rapidly after institution of protein feedings and are usually abnormal by day 4. Since diagnosis and initiation of dietary treatment of classic phenylketonuria must occur before the child is 30 days of age if developmental retardation is to be prevented, most newborns in North America and Europe are screened by determinations of blood phenylalanine concentration using the Guthrie bacterial inhibition assay. Infants with abnormal values are followed up with more quantitative fluorometric or chromatographic assays. In classic phenylketonuria and in tetrahydrobiopterin deficiency, values greater than 1200 μmol/L (20 mg/dL) are regularly observed. In transient or benign hyperphenylalaninemia, concentrations are usually lower but above control values of less than 60 μmol/L (1 mg/dL). Separation of classic phenylketonuria from its benign variants depends on following serial plasma phenylalanine concentrations as a function of age and dietary restriction. In transient hyperphenylalaninemia, plasma values return to normal within 3 to 4 months. In benign hyperphenylalaninemia, dietary restriction produces a more profound fall in plasma phenylalanine than in classic phenylketonuria. Deficiency of tetrahydrobiopterin must be considered in any child with hyperphenylalaninemia who develops progressive neurologic impairment despite prompt diagnosis and dietary treatment. These variants, which account for 1 to 5 percent of phenylketonuric children, can be diagnosed by enzyme assay on cultured fibroblasts. Administration of oral tetrahydrobiopterin loads also can distinguish children with classic phenylketonuria (who show no chemical response) from those with tetrahydrobiopterin deficiency (who exhibit a sharp fall in plasma phenylalanine). Prenatal diagnosis of classic phenylketonuria is now

accumulation: competitive inhibition of transport of other amino acids required for protein synthesis, impaired polyribosome formation or stabilization, reduced myelin synthesis, and inadequate formation of norepinephrine and serotonin. Phenylalanine is a competitive inhibitor of tyrosinase, a key enzyme in the pathway of melanin synthesis. This block, plus reduced availability of the melanin precursor tyrosine, accounts for the hypopigmentation of hair and skin.

CLINICAL MANIFESTATIONS No abnormalities are apparent at birth, but untreated children with classic phenylketonuria fail to attain early developmental milestones and demonstrate progressive impairment of cerebral function. Most require chronic institutionalization within a few years of birth because of the hyperactivity, seizures, and severe mental retardation. Electroencephalographic abnormalities, "mousy" odor of skin, hair, and urine (due to phenylacetate accumulation), and a tendency to hypopigmentation and eczema complete the devastating clinical picture. In contrast, affected children who are detected at birth and treated promptly show none of these abnormalities. Children with transient hyperphenylalaninemia or with the benign variant are not at risk for the clinical consequences of untreated feasible using DNA-based tests capable of detecting specific mutations or linked restriction fragment length polymorphisms (RFLPs). Dihydropteridine reductase deficiency and the blocks in tetrahydrobiopterin synthesis also can be detected in utero using assays on cultured amniocytes.

TREATMENT Classic phenylketonuria is the first inherited metabolic disease in which prevention of the accumulation of the offending metabolite prevented the dire clinical consequences. This is accomplished by a special diet in which the bulk of protein is replaced by an artificial amino acid mixture low in phenylalanine. By supplementing this formula with a small amount of natural foods, sufficient dietary phenylalanine is provided for normal growth but does not produce markedly increased quantities of phenylalanine in blood. Ordinarily, plasma phenylalanine concentrations are maintained between 180 and 700 μmol/L (3 and 12 mg/dL).

Such diet therapy must be instituted during the first month of life. Even then, modest nervous system dysfunction is often seen. Because uncontrolled hyperphenylalaninemia results in brain damage throughout childhood (and perhaps in adults), dietary restriction should be continued indefinitely in classic phenylketonuria. The transient and benign forms of hyperphenylalaninemia do not require long-term dietary restriction. As mentioned earlier, children with tetrahydrobiopterin deficiency deteriorate despite dietary phenylalanine restriction; efficacy of pteridine cofactor replacement is under study. Such patients may be helped, however, by a regimen in which dietary phenylalanine restriction is combined with supplements of levodopa and 5-hydroxytryptophan. Finally, the deleterious consequences of maternal phenylketonuria can be minimized by instituting dietary phenylalanine restriction prior to conception and continuing such treatment throughout gestation. This means that women with phenylketonuria should stay on a phenylalanine-restricted diet from birth through the childbearing years.

THE HOMOCYSTINURIAS

The homocystinurias are seven biochemically and clinically distinct disorders (see Table 352-1), each characterized by increased concentration of the sulfur-containing amino acid homocystine in blood and urine. The most common form results from reduced activity of cystathionine β-synthase, an enzyme in the transsulfuration pathway by which methionine is converted to cysteine. The other forms are the result of impaired conversion of homocysteine to methionine, a reaction catalyzed by homocysteine:methyltetrahydrofolate methyltransferase and two essential cofactors, methyltetrahydrofolate and methylcobalamin (methyl–vitamin B_{12}). Depending on the underlying disorder, some patients show chemical and, in some instances, clinical improvement following administration of specific vitamin supplements (pyridoxine, folate, or cobalamin).

CYSTATHIONINE β-SYNTHASE DEFICIENCY Definition Deficiency of this enzyme leads to increased concentrations of methionine and homocystine in body fluids and to decreased concentrations of cysteine and cystine. The clinical hallmark is dislocated optic lenses. Mental retardation, osteoporosis, and thrombotic vascular disease are frequent.

Etiology and pathogenesis The sulfur atom of the essential amino acid methionine is transferred ultimately to cysteine by the transsulfuration pathway (Fig. 352-2). In one of these steps, homocysteine condenses with serine to form cystathionine. This reaction is catalyzed by the pyridoxal phosphate–dependent enzyme cystathionine β-synthase. The gene for this homodimeric enzyme has been mapped to the q21 region of chromosome 21. The condition is common in Ireland (1 in 40,000 births) but rare elsewhere (less than 1 in 200,000 births).

Homocysteine and methionine accumulate in cells and body fluids; cysteine synthesis is impaired, resulting in reduced concentrations of this amino acid and its disulfide form cystine. In approximately half of patients, synthase activity in liver, brain, leukocytes, and cultured

fibroblasts is undetectable. In the remaining patients, tissues retain 1 to 5 percent of normal activity, and this residual activity often can be stimulated by pyridoxine supplementation. Heterozygous carriers of this autosomal recessive trait show no reproducible chemical abnormalities in body fluids but have reduced tissue synthase activity.

Homocysteine interferes with the normal cross-linking of collagen, an effect that likely plays an important role in the ocular, skeletal, and vascular complications. Altered collagen in the suspensory ligament of the optic lens and in bone matrix may account for the dislocated lenses and osteoporosis. Similarly, interference with normal ground substance metabolism in vascular walls may predispose to the arterial and venous thrombotic diathesis. Increased platelet adhesiveness may result from homocysteine accumulation, thereby contributing to the thrombotic occlusive disease so often observed. Recurrent cerebrovascular accidents secondary to thrombotic disease may account for the mental retardation, but direct chemical effects on cerebral cell metabolism have not been excluded.

Clinical manifestations More than 80 percent of homozygotes for complete synthase deficiency have dislocated optic lenses. This abnormality usually appears by 3 to 4 years of age and often results in glaucoma and impaired visual acuity. Mental retardation occurs in about half of such patients, often accompanied by ill-defined behavioral disturbances. Osteoporosis is a common radiologic finding (seen in two-thirds of patients by age 15) but rarely causes clinical disease. Life-threatening vascular complications, probably initiated by damage to vascular endothelium, are the major cause of morbidity and mortality. Occlusion of coronary, renal, and cerebral arteries with attendant tissue infarction can occur during the first decade of life. Nearly one-quarter of patients die of vascular disease before age 30. These vascular complications seem to be exacerbated by angiographic procedures. Importantly, pyridoxine-responsive patients have milder clinical manifestations in all regards. Heterozygous carriers for synthase deficiency (about 1 in 70 in the population) and others with high concentrations of plasma homocysteine may be at increased risk for premature coronary, peripheral, and cerebral occlusive vascular disease.

Diagnosis The cyanide-nitroprusside test is a simple way of demonstrating increased excretion of sulfhydryl-containing compounds in urine. Since cystine and S-sulfocysteine also give a positive test, other disorders of sulfur metabolism must be excluded, but this is usually possible on clinical grounds. Distinction of cystathionine β-synthase deficiency from other causes of homocystinuria usually can be accomplished by measurements of plasma methionine, which tend to be increased in synthase-deficient patients and normal or low in those with impaired methionine formation (see below). Diagnostic confirmation depends on measurements of synthase activity in tissue extracts. Heterozygotes can be identified by measurement of peak serum homocystine after an oral methionine load and by measurement of tissue synthase activity.

Treatment As with classic phenylketonuria, effective treatment depends on early diagnosis. A number of infants diagnosed in the newborn period have been treated successfully with methionine-restricted, cystine-supplemented diets. Their clinical course is benign compared with that of untreated affected siblings. In approximately half of patients, oral pyridoxine (25 to 500 mg/d) produces a fall in plasma and urinary methionine and homocystine and an increase in cystine concentration in body fluids. This effect probably reflects a modest increase in synthase activity in cells of patients in whom the defect is characterized either by reduced affinity for cofactor or by accelerated degradation of mutant enzyme. Since such vitamin supplementation is apparently harmless, it should be tried in all patients. There are no reports of the effect of the initiation of pyridoxine supplementation soon after birth. Similarly, there are no data regarding pyridoxine supplements in heterozygous carriers.

5,10-METHYLENETETRAHYDROFOLATE REDUCTASE DEFICIENCY Definition In this form of homocystinuria, methionine concentrations in body fluids are normal or decreased because deficiency of 5,10-methylenetetrahydrofolate reductase leads to im-

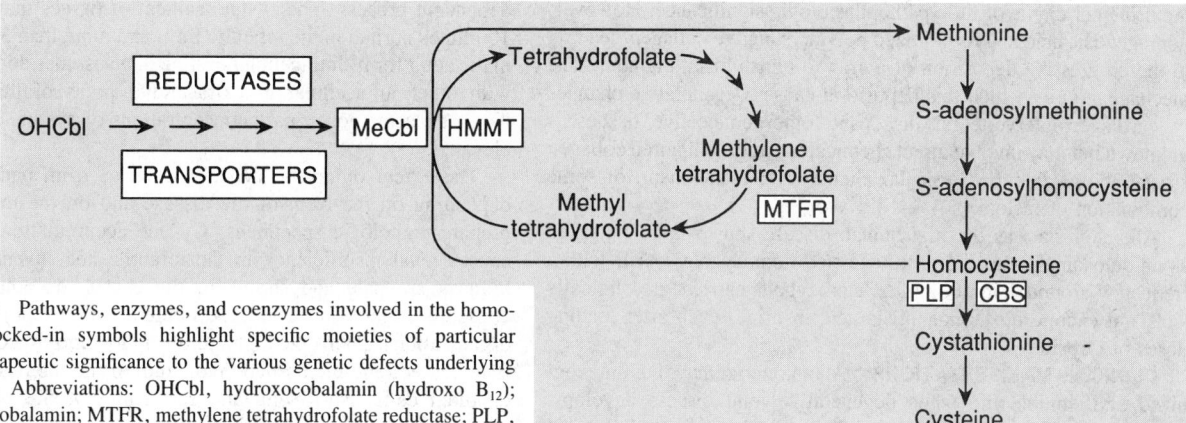

FIGURE 352-2 Pathways, enzymes, and coenzymes involved in the homocystinurias. Blocked-in symbols highlight specific moieties of particular etiologic or therapeutic significance to the various genetic defects underlying these disorders. Abbreviations: OHCbl, hydroxocobalamin (hydroxo B_{12}); MeCbl, methylcobalamin; MTFR, methylene tetrahydrofolate reductase; PLP, pyridoxal phosphate; CBS, cystathionine β-synthase.

paired synthesis of 5-methyltetrahydrofolate, a cofactor in the enzymatic formation of methionine from homocysteine (see Fig. 352-2). Central nervous system dysfunction occurs in most patients.

Etiology and pathogenesis 5-Methyltetrahydrofolate:homocysteine methyltransferase catalyzes the conversion of homocysteine to methionine. The methyl group transferred in this reaction comes from 5-methyltetrahydrofolate, which is converted to tetrahydrofolate in the process. 5-Methyltetrahydrofolate, in turn, is synthesized enzymatically from 5,10-methylenetetrahydrofolate by 5,10-methylenetetrahydrofolate reductase. Thus reductase activity controls both methionine synthesis and tetrahydrofolate generation. This series of reactions is critical to normal DNA and RNA synthesis. A primary defect in the reductase activity results, secondarily, in deficient methyltransferase activity and impaired conversion of homocysteine to methionine. Methionine deficiency and impaired nucleic acid synthesis may contribute to the central nervous system dysfunction. The disorder appears to be inherited as an autosomal recessive trait.

Clinical manifestations More than 25 children with homocystinuria due to reductase deficiency have been reported. The most severely affected have developmental retardation and cerebral atrophy early in life. Others have behavioral disturbances (catatonia) during the second decade or mild retardation. Presumably the severity of the clinical manifestations reflects the severity of the reductase deficiency.

Diagnosis and treatment The combination of increased concentrations of homocystine in body fluids with normal or decreased concentrations of methionine should suggest this entity. Serum folate concentrations are low in some patients. Confirmation requires direct reductase assays in tissue extracts (brain, liver, cultured fibroblasts). Although therapeutic experience is limited, one teenage girl with a catatonic psychosis responded dramatically, both chemically and clinically, to folate supplements (5 to 10 mg/d). When the folate was withdrawn, behavior worsened. This observation suggests that early diagnosis followed by folate supplementation may forestall neurologic or psychiatric disturbances.

DEFICIENCY OF COBALAMIN (VITAMIN B_{12}) COENZYME SYNTHESIS Definition Five other forms of homocystinuria also reflect impaired conversion of homocysteine to methionine. The primary defects in these entities, however, are in the synthesis of methylcobalamin, a cobalamin (vitamin B_{12}) coenzyme required by methyltetrahydrofolate:homocysteine methyltransferase (see Fig. 352-2). In some, methylmalonic acid accumulates in body fluids because of impaired synthesis of a second coenzyme, adenosylcobalamin, required for isomerization of methylmalonyl coenzyme A (CoA) to succinyl CoA. These disorders are designated cblC, D, E, F, and G.

Etiology and pathogenesis As with 5,10-methylenetetrahydrofolate reductase deficiency, each disorder impairs remethylation of homocysteine. Since methylcobalamin is required for methyl-group transfer from methyltetrahydrofolate to homocysteine, impaired cobalamin metabolism leads to deficient methyltransferase activity. The

defects responsible for impaired synthesis of methylcobalamin involve one of several steps in lysosomal or cytosolic activation of the vitamin precursor (see Fig. 352-2). In the cblF disorder, the transport of cobalamins out of lysosomes is impaired. In cblC and D, a reductase needed for formation of both methylcobalamin and adenosylcobalamin is deficient. In cblE and G, some component required to maintain a reduced form of cobalamin on the methyltransferase apoenzyme is impaired. Somatic cell genetic studies indicate that each of these abnormalities is distinct and imply that all are inherited as autosomal recessive traits.

Clinical manifestations More than 25 patients—mostly children—with these defects in cobalamin metabolism have been described. Although clinical manifestations vary, abnormalities include developmental delay, dementia, spasticity, megaloblastic anemia, and pancytopenia. It is not possible to define a specific clinical syndrome for each of the defects in cobalamin metabolism.

Diagnosis and treatment Homocystinuria, homocystinemia, and hypomethioninemia are the chemical hallmarks. Methylmalonic acidemia, too, has been noted in those defects resulting from defective synthesis of both cobalamin coenzymes. These findings also may be present in juvenile- or adult-onset pernicious anemia in which intestinal cobalamin absorption is impaired. Measurement of serum cobalamin concentrations, low in pernicious anemia and normal in patients with defective conversion of cobalamin vitamin to coenzymes, helps in the differential diagnosis. Definitive diagnosis depends on demonstrating impaired coenzyme synthesis in cultured cells. Treatment of affected children with cobalamin supplements (1 to 2 mg/d) causes homocystine and methylmalonate excretion to fall to near normal values; the hematologic and neurologic deficits also have lessened to a variable degree in several patients. Intervention early in life seems to offer the best long-term prognosis.

ALKAPTONURIA

DEFINITION Alkaptonuria is a rare disorder of tyrosine catabolism in which deficiency of homogentisic acid oxidase leads to excretion of large amounts of homogentisic acid in urine and accumulation of oxidized homogentisic acid pigment in connective tissues (ochronosis). After many years, ochronosis produces a distinctive form of degenerative arthritis.

ETIOLOGY AND PATHOGENESIS Homogentisic acid is an intermediate in the catabolism of tyrosine. Activity of homogentisic acid oxidase, the enzyme that catalyzes the opening of the phenolic ring yielding maleylacetoacetic acid, is deficient in liver and kidney of patients with alkaptonuria, and homogentisic acid accumulates in cells and body fluids. Patients have minimally increased concentrations of homogentisic acid in blood because it is rapidly cleared by the kidney. The excretion of as much as 3 to 7 g homogentisic acid in the urine per day is of little pathophysiologic significance. However, homogentisic acid and its oxidized polymers bind to collagen, leading to the progressive deposition of a gray to bluish black pigment. The mechanism(s) by which this deposition causes degenerative changes in cartilage, intervertebral disk, and other connective tissues is unknown but may involve direct chemical irritation, impaired collagen cross-linking, disturbed articular chondrocyte metabolism, or some combination of factors.

Alkaptonuria was the first human disease shown to be inherited as an autosomal recessive trait. Affected homozygotes occur with a frequency around 1 in 200,000. Heterozygous carriers are clinically well and excrete no homogentisic acid in urine, even after loading doses of tyrosine.

CLINICAL MANIFESTATIONS   Alkaptonuria may go unrecognized until middle life when degenerative joint disease develops. Prior to this time, the tendency of the patient's urine to darken on standing may go unnoticed, as may slight discoloration of the sclerae and ears. The latter manifestations are generally the earliest external evidence of the disorder and develop after age 20 to 30. Foci of gray-brown scleral pigment and generalized darkening of the concha, anthelix, and finally, helix of the ear are typical. Ear cartilages may be irregular and thickened. *Ochronotic arthritis* is heralded by pain, stiffness, and some limitation of motion of the hips, knees, and shoulders. Acute arthritis may resemble rheumatoid arthritis, but small joints are usually spared. Limitation of motion and ankylosis of the lumbosacral spine are common late manifestations. Pigmentation of heart valves, larynx, tympanic membranes, and skin occurs, and occasional patients develop pigmented renal or prostatic calculi. Degenerative cardiovascular disease may be increased in older patients.

DIAGNOSIS   A patient whose urine darkens to blackness on standing must be suspected of having alkaptonuria but, because of modern plumbing conditions, is not often observed. The diagnosis is usually made from the triad of degenerative arthritis, ochronotic pigmentation, and urine that turns black upon alkalinization. Homogentisic acid in urine may be identified presumptively by other tests: upon addition of ferric chloride, a purple-black color is observed; treatment with Benedict's reagent yields a brown color; addition of a saturated silver nitrate solution produces an immediate black color. These screening tests can be confirmed by chromatographic, enzymatic, or spectrophotometric determinations of homogentisic acid. X-rays of the lumbar spine are virtually pathognomonic. They show degeneration and dense calcification of the intervertebral disks and narrowing of the intervertebral spaces.

TREATMENT   There is no specific treatment for ochronotic arthritis. Joint manifestations might be mitigated if homogentisic acid accumulation and deposition could be curbed by dietary restriction of phenylalanine and tyrosine, but the long course of the disease has discouraged such therapeutic attempts. Ascorbic acid impedes oxidation and polymerization of homogentisic acid in vitro, but the efficacy of this form of treatment has not been established. Symptomatic treatment is similar to that for osteoarthritis (Chap. 296).

CYSTINOSIS

DEFINITION   Cystinosis is a rare disorder characterized by the intralysosomal accumulation of free cystine in body tissues. This results in the appearance of cystine crystals in the cornea, conjunctiva, bone marrow, lymph nodes, leukocytes, and internal organs. Three variants have been identified: an infantile (nephropathic) form leading to the Fanconi syndrome and renal insufficiency in the first decade, a juvenile (intermediate) form in which renal disease is manifest during the second decade, and an adult (benign) form characterized by deposition of cystine in the cornea but not in the kidney.

ETIOLOGY AND PATHOGENESIS   The basic defect involves impaired efflux of cystine from lysosomes rather than an abnormality in cystine catabolism. Lysosomal cystine efflux is an active, ATP-

dependent process. The cystine content of tissues may be more than 100 times normal in the infantile form and more than 30 times normal in the adult form. Intracellular cystine in lysosomes does not exchange with other intracellular or extracellular pools of this amino acid. Neither plasma nor urinary concentrations of cystine are particularly elevated.

The extent of crystal deposition varies from patient to patient, depending on the form of the disease and on the methods used to prepare pathologic specimens. Cystine accumulation in the kidney causes renal insufficiency in the infantile and juvenile forms. The kidneys are pale and shrunken, the capsule is adherent, and the corticomedullary junction is obscured. Microscopically, nephron organization is interrupted, glomeruli are hyalinized, connective tissue is increased, and the normal epithelium of the tubules is replaced by cuboidal cells. Narrowing and shortening of the proximal tubule produce the swan neck deformity that is characteristic of but not specific for cystinosis. Patchy depigmentation and degeneration of the peripheral retina occurs in the infantile and juvenile forms. Cystine crystals also may be deposited in the cornea, ocular conjunctiva, or uvea.

Each form appears to be inherited as an autosomal recessive trait. Obligate heterozygotes have intracellular cystine concentrations intermediate between those of normal persons and affected patients but are free of clinical abnormalities.

CLINICAL MANIFESTATIONS   In the infantile form, abnormalities are usually apparent by 4 to 6 months of age. Growth retardation, vomiting, fever, vitamin D–resistant rickets, polyuria, dehydration, and metabolic acidosis are prominent. Generalized proximal tubular dysfunction (the Fanconi syndrome) leads to hyperphosphaturia and hypophosphatemia, renal glycosuria, generalized aminoaciduria, hypouricemia, and often hypokalemia. Pyelonephritis may contribute, along with interstitial fibrosis, to progressive glomerular insufficiency. Death due to uremia or intercurrent infection usually occurs before age 10. Ocular manifestations are prominent. Photophobia is usually demonstrable within the first few years of life due to cystine deposits in the cornea, and retinal degeneration may appear even earlier.

In contrast, patients with the adult form have only ocular abnormalities. Photophobia, headache, and burning or itching of the eyes are major complaints. Glomerular and tubular function and the integrity of the retina are preserved. The findings in the juvenile variant fall between these extremes. Ocular and renal manifestations do not become significant until the second decade. The renal lesion, albeit milder than that in the infantile form, eventually leads to renal insufficiency.

DIAGNOSIS   Cystinosis must be considered in any child with vitamin D–resistant rickets, the Fanconi syndrome, or glomerular insufficiency. Hexagonal or rectangular cystine crystals can be detected in the cornea (by slit-lamp examination), in leukocytes from peripheral blood or bone marrow, or in biopsies of rectal mucosa. Diagnosis can be confirmed by quantification of cystine in peripheral blood leukocytes or cultured fibroblasts. The infantile form has been diagnosed prenatally by the demonstration of increased cystine content in cultured amniotic fluid cells.

TREATMENT   The adult form is benign and requires no treatment. Symptomatic treatment of renal disease in the infantile or juvenile form does not differ from that of other forms of chronic renal insufficiency: maintenance of adequate fluid intake to prevent dehydration; correction of the metabolic acidosis; and ingestion of supplementary calcium, phosphate, and vitamin D to heal the rickets. Such measures are effective in maintaining growth, development, and well-being in affected children for a time. Two specific therapies have been attempted. Cystine-restricted diets do not prevent progression of renal disease. This is not surprising given the nature of the primary defect and the large amount of cystine produced endogenously by cellular protein turnover. Whereas the early use of thiol reagents such as penicillamine and dimercaprol yielded no long-term benefits, administration of the free thiol cysteamine slows the progression of renal dysfunction, improves growth, and dissolves corneal cystine crystals. This compound acts in lysosomes by forming a mixed disulfide with cysteine that can be transported out of the organelle by a different transporter from that deficient in the disease.

The most successful form of therapy for nephropathic cystinosis is renal transplantation. Hundreds of affected children with end-stage renal disease have been so treated. Those patients who tolerated the procedure and did not develop immunologic problems have had return of kidney function toward normal. The transplanted kidneys have not developed the functional abnormalities typical of cystinosis (i.e., the Fanconi syndrome or glomerular insufficiency). Patients may, however, continue to accumulate cystine in the cornea and other ocular tissues. Because the usual life span of a transplanted kidney is generally 15 to 20 years, some patients with the infantile form of cystinosis have received two or more transplanted kidneys.

PRIMARY HYPEROXALURIA

DEFINITION Primary hyperoxaluria is the designation for two rare disorders characterized by chronic excessive urinary excretion of oxalic acid and by calcium oxalate nephrolithiasis and nephrocalcinosis. Typically, patients with both forms develop renal insufficiency early in life and die of uremia. At postmortem examination, calcium oxalate deposits are widespread in renal and extrarenal tissues, a condition referred to as *oxalosis*.

ETIOLOGY AND PATHOGENESIS The metabolic basis for the primary hyperoxalurias involves pathways of glyoxylate metabolism. In type I hyperoxaluria, urinary excretion of oxalate and of the oxidized and reduced forms of glyoxylate is increased. The excessive synthesis of these substances results from a block in glyoxylate metabolism. The primary defect in most patients is deficiency of the hepatic peroxisomal enzyme alanine:glyoxylate amino transferase. In the remainder the transferase is misdirected to mitochondria and is, thereby, nonfunctional. The resulting expansion of the glyoxylate pool leads to enhanced oxidation of glyoxylate to oxalate and to enhanced reduction of glyoxylate to glycolate. Each of these 2-carbon acids is then excreted in excess in the urine. In type II hyperoxaluria, L-glyceric acid is excreted in excess along with oxalate. In this condition, activity of D-glyceric acid dehydrogenase, which catalyzes the reduction of hydroxypyruvate to D-glyceric acid in the catabolic pathway of serine metabolism, is absent in leukocytes (and presumably other tissues). The accumulated hydroxypyruvate is instead reduced by lactic dehydrogenase to the L-isomer of glycerate, which is excreted in the urine. The reduction of hydroxypyruvate is coupled in some way to the oxidation of glyoxylate to oxalate, thus causing the formation of increased oxalate. Both disorders appear to be inherited as autosomal recessive traits. Heterozygotes are asymptomatic.

Stone formation, nephrocalcinosis, and oxalosis are due to insolubility of calcium oxalate. Extrarenal deposits of oxalate are prominent in the heart, walls of arteries and veins, male urogenital tract, and bone.

CLINICAL MANIFESTATIONS Nephrolithiasis and oxalosis may be manifest during the first year of life. Most patients experience renal colic or hematuria between ages 2 and 10 and succumb to uremia before age 20. With the onset of uremia, patients may develop severe peripheral arterial spasm and necrosis with resulting vascular insufficiency. Oxalate excretion falls as renal failure worsens. In patients with delayed onset of symptoms, survival to age 50 or 60 has been reported, despite recurrent nephrolithiasis.

DIAGNOSIS Oxalate excretion in normal children or adults is less than 0.5 mmol (60 mg) per 1.73 m^2 surface area per day. Patients with type I or type II hyperoxaluria generally excrete two to four times this amount. Distinction between the two types depends on measurements of the other organic acids that identify them: glycolic acid in type I and L-glyceric acid in type II. Since patients with pyridoxine deficiency or chronic ileal disease may excrete excessive amounts of oxalate, these conditions must be excluded.

TREATMENT There is no satisfactory treatment. Urinary oxalate concentration can be transiently reduced by increasing the urinary flow rate. Large doses of pyridoxine (100 mg/d) may reduce urinary oxalate, but long-term effects are not dramatic. A diet high in phosphate content seems to reduce the frequency of attacks of renal colic, but oxalate excretion is unaffected. Finally, after renal transplantation renal function is lost because of calcium oxalate deposition in the transplanted kidney. The beneficial effects of combined liver-kidney transplantation observed in a single patient warrant additional study.

REFERENCES

BOERS GHJ et al: Heterozygosity for homocystinuria in premature peripheral and cerebral occlusive arterial disease. N Engl J Med 313:709, 1985

EISENSMITH RC, WOO SLC: Molecular basis of phenylketonuria and related hyperphenylalaninemias: Mutations and polymorphisms in the human phenylalanine hydroxylase gene. Hum Mutat 1:13, 1992

FENTON WA, ROSENBERG LE: Inherited disorders of cobalamin transport and metabolism, in *The Molecular and Metabolic Basis of Inherited Disease*, 7th ed, CR Scriver et al (eds). New York, McGraw-Hill, in press

GAHL WA et al: Lysosomal transport disorders, in *The Molecular and Metabolic Basis of Inherited Disease*, 7th ed, CR Scriver et al (eds). New York, McGraw-Hill, in press

HILLMAN RE: Primary hyperoxalurias, in *The Molecular and Metabolic Basis of Inherited Disease*, 7th ed, CR Scriver et al (eds). New York, McGraw-Hill, in press

LADU BN: Alcaptonuria, in *The Molecular and Metabolic Basis of Inherited Disease*, 7th ed, CR Scriver et al (eds). New York, McGraw-Hill, in press

MUDD SH et al: Natural history of homocystinuria due to cystathionine β-synthase deficiency. Am J Hum Genet 37:709, 1985

—— et al: Disorders of transsulfuration, in *The Molecular and Metabolic Basis of Inherited Disease*, 7th ed, CR Scriver et al (eds). New York, McGraw-Hill, in press

PLATT LE et al: Maternal phenylketonuria collaborative study, obstetric aspects and outcome: The first 6 years. Am J Obstet Gynecol 166:1150, 1992

PURDUE PE et al: Mistargeting of peroxisomal L-alanine:glyoxylate aminotransferase to mitochondria in primary hyperoxaluria patients depends upon activation of a cryptic mitochondrial targeting sequence by a point mutation. Proc Natl Acad Sci USA 88:10900, 1991

ROSENBERG LE, SCRIVER CR: Disorders of amino acid metabolism, in *Metabolic Control and Disease*, 8th ed, PK Bondy, LE Rosenberg (eds). Philadelphia, Saunders, 1980, pp 583–776

SCRIVER CR et al: The hyperphenylalaninemias, in *The Molecular and Metabolic Basis of Inherited Disease*, 7th ed, CR Scriver et al (eds). New York, McGraw-Hill, in press

353 INHERITED DEFECTS OF MEMBRANE TRANSPORT

LEON E. ROSENBERG / ELIZABETH M. SHORT

The passage of many molecules across plasma cell membranes depends on transport systems that owe their specificity to membrane receptor and "carrier" proteins. These membrane constituents recognize individual molecules or structurally related substances and catalyze their transmembrane movement by mechanisms poorly understood. The disorders considered in this chapter have three features in common: each is characterized by a specific defect in the transport of one or more compounds; each is inherited as a dominant or recessive trait, implying that a single genetic locus is involved; and each is presumed to reflect a primary alteration in a specific membrane protein. Many of these defects have been well characterized physiologically. The mutation in one of these disorders has been identified, namely, the intestinal glucose transporter gene in a family with glucose-galactose malabsorption syndrome.

More than 20 inherited disorders of membrane transport have been described (Table 353-1). Most affect the gut and/or kidney only. Classes of substrates represented include amino acids, sugars, cations, anions, vitamins, and water. Some are discussed elsewhere in this text. Those impairing the transport of amino acids, hexoses, urate, and chloride are discussed here as examples of the abnormalities encountered.

TABLE 353-1 Genetic disorders of membrane transport

Class of substance and disorder	Individual substrates	Tissues manifesting transport defect	Proposed molecular basis of defect	Major clinical manifestations	Mode of inheritance	Location of discussion
AMINO ACIDS						
Classic cystinuria	Cystine, lysine, arginine, ornithine	Proximal renal tubule, jejunal mucosa	Mutation of shared dibasic-cystine transport protein	Cystine nephrolithiasis	Autosomal recessive	Chap. 353
Dibasicaminoaciduria	Lysine, arginine, ornithine	Proximal renal tubule, jejunal mucosa	Mutation of dibasic transport protein	Type I: Benign Type II: Protein intolerance, hyperammonemia, retardation	Autosomal recessive	Chap. 353
Hypercystinuria	Cystine	Proximal renal tubule	Mutation of cystine transport protein	Some risk of cystine nephrolithiasis	Autosomal recessive	Chap. 353
Lysinuria	Lysine	Proximal renal tubule, jejunal mucosa	Mutation of lysine transport protein	Seizures, physical and mental retardation	Possible autosomal recessive	Chap. 353
Hartnup disease	Neutral amino acids	Proximal renal tubule, jejunal mucosa	Mutation of shared neutral amino acid transport protein	Constant neutral aminoaciduria, intermittent symptoms of pellagra	Autosomal recessive	Chap. 353
Tryptophan malabsorption	Tryptophan	Jejunal mucosa	Mutation of tryptophan transport protein	Indoluria, ?hypercalcemia, ?nephrocalcinosis	Probable autosomal recessive	Chap. 353
Methionine malabsorption	Methionine	Jejunal mucosa	Mutation of methionine transport protein	α-Hydroxybutyricaciduria, white hair, mental retardation, convulsions, hyperpneic attacks, edema	Probable autosomal recessive	Chap. 353
Histidinuria	Histidine	Proximal renal tubule, jejunal mucosa	Mutation of histidine transport protein	Mental retardation	Autosomal recessive	Chap. 353
Iminoglycinuria	Glycine, proline, hydroxyproline	Proximal renal tubule, jejunal mucosa	Mutation of shared glycine–imino acid transport protein	None	Autosomal recessive	Chap. 353
Dicarboxylicaminoaciduria	Glutamic acid, aspartic acid	Proximal renal tubule, jejunal mucosa	Mutation of shared dicarboxylic amino acid transport protein	None	Probable autosomal recessive	Chap. 353
Cystinosis	Cystine	Lysosomal membranes	Mutation of cystine transport protein	Renal failure, hypothyroidism, blindness	Autosomal recessive	Chap. 352
HEXOSES						
Renal glycosuria	D-Glucose	Proximal renal tubule	Mutation of D-glucose transport protein	Glycosuria with normal blood glucose	Autosomal recessive	Chap. 353
Glucose-galactose malabsorption	D-Glucose D-Galactose	Jejunal mucosa, proximal renal tubule	Mutation of shared Na^+-dependent glucose-galactose transport protein	Watery diarrhea on feeding glucose, lactose, sucrose, or galactose	Autosomal recessive	Chaps. 254, 353
LIPIDS						
Familial hypercholesterolemia	Cholesterol	Fibroblasts, lymphoid lines, leukocytes	Mutation of membrane LDL–cholesterol receptor protein	Hypercholesterolemia, tendon xanthomas, arcus corneae, coronary artery atherosclerosis	Autosomal dominant	Chap. 344
URATE						
Hypouricemia	Uric acid	Proximal renal tubule	Mutation of urate transport protein	Hypouricemia, hyperuricosuria, ?hypercalcinuria	Autosomal recessive	Chap. 353
ANIONS						
Familial hypophosphatemic rickets	Inorganic phosphate	Proximal renal tubule, jejunal mucosa	Mutation of inorganic phosphate transport protein	Hypophosphatemia, phosphaturia, phosphatopenic rickets/ osteomalacia	X-linked dominant	Chap. 358

TABLE 353-1   Genetic disorders of membrane transport *(continued)*

Class of substance and disorder	Individual substrates	Tissues manifesting transport defect	Proposed molecular basis of defect	Major clinical manifestations	Mode of inheritance	Location of discussion
ANIONS *(continued)*						
Congenital chloridorrhea	Chloride	Ileal and colonic mucosa	Mutation of Cl^-/H^+ uptake pump of Cl^-/HCO_3^- exchange pump carrier protein	Hydramnios, watery diarrhea, elevated fecal chloride, achloriduria, metabolic alkalosis with volume depletion, hyperaldosteronism	Autosomal recessive	Chaps. 254, 353
Cystic fibrosis	Chloride	Lung, pancreas, sweat gland	Mutation of ion channel protein	Pulmonary, pancreatic destruction	Autosomal recessive	Chap. 222
Familial goiter	Inorganic iodide	Thyroid gland, salivary gland, gastric mucosa	Mutation of iodide transport protein	Congenital hypothyroidism (cretinism), goiter	Probable autosomal recessive	Chap. 334
CATIONS						
Distal renal tubular acidosis (type I—gradient)	Hydrogen ion	Distal renal tubule	Mutation of distal tubule H^+ pump carrier protein	Hyperchloremic acidosis, hypokalemia, acquired nephrocalcinosis, and hypercalcinuria	Autosomal dominant	Chap. 244
Proximal renal tubular acidosis (type II—HCO_3^- wasting)	Hydrogen ion	Proximal renal tubule	Mutation of proximal tubule H^+ pump carrier protein	Hyperchloremic acidosis, bicarbonate wasting	Probable autosomal recessive	Chap. 244
Menkes' disease	Copper	Duodenal and jejunal intestinal cells	Possible serosal transport protein or intracellular transport defect	Severe mental retardation, pili torti (kinky hair), typical facies, arterial tortuosity, excess Wormian bones, thermal instability	X-linked recessive	Chaps. 78
Lethal diarrhea	Sodium ion	Jejunal intestinal cells	Mutation of Na^+/H^+ proton exchange pump	Watery diarrhea, severe sodium depletion, and acidosis	Recessive?	Chap. 254
WATER						
Nephrogenic diabetes insipidus (AVP-resistant)	Water	Distal renal tubule	Lack of activation of AVP-responsive luminal membrane adenylate cyclase, possible defect in receptor or enzyme protein	Polyuria, polydipsia, hyposthenuria	X-linked recessive	Chap. 244
VITAMINS						
Juvenile pernicious anemia	Cobalamin (vitamin B_{12})	Ileal mucosa	Mutation of receptor for intrinsic factor–cobalamin complex	Megaloblastic anemia	Autosomal recessive	Chap. 304
Folate malabsorption	Folic acid	Small bowel	Mutation of folate transport protein	Megaloblastic anemia	Autosomal recessive	Chap. 304
OTHER						
Sialic acid storage	Sialic acid (monosaccharide)	Lysosomes	Mutation of sialic acid transport protein	Retardation	Autosomal recessive	Chap. 349

DISORDERS OF AMINO ACID TRANSPORT

As noted in Table 353-1, 10 disorders of amino acid transport have been described. Five (cystinuria, dibasicaminoaciduria, Hartnup disease, iminoglycinuria, and dicarboxylicaminoaciduria) show transport abnormalities for structurally related amino acids, thereby implying the existence of group-specific membrane receptors or carriers. With the exception of iminoglycinuria and dicarboxylicaminoaciduria, the defects have important clinical consequences. The remaining five disorders affect the transport of only one amino acid, implying the existence of substrate-specific transport systems. Each of these conditions affects transport in the kidney, gut, or both; none has been shown to alter transport in other tissues.

CYSTINURIA   Definition   Cystinuria, the most common inborn error of amino acid transport, is characterized by impaired tubular reabsorption and excessive urinary excretion of the dibasic amino acids lysine, arginine, ornithine, and cystine. A similar transport defect exists in the intestinal mucosa. Because cystine is the least soluble of the naturally occurring amino acids, its overexcretion predisposes to the formation of renal, ureteral, and bladder stones. Such stones are responsible for the signs and symptoms of the disorder.

Etiology and pathogenesis Massive excretion of cystine and the other dibasic amino acids occurs only in classic cystinuria. The disorder, inherited as an autosomal recessive trait, is believed to result from alterations in a membrane carrier protein essential for transport of this group of amino acids in the apical brush border of proximal renal tubule and small intestinal cells. The protein has a greater affinity for ornithine and arginine than for lysine and cystine. Although the renal clearance of all four amino acids is increased in homozygotes, the presence of some residual transport capacity for these compounds plus the existence of three other disorders marked by selective excretion of members of this group (dibasicaminoaciduria, hypercystinuria, lysinuria) argues for the existence of at least three discrete renal transport systems for these amino acids: one for each amino acid alone; one shared by lysine, arginine, and ornithine; and one for all four amino acids.

Whereas urinary excretion patterns and renal clearance abnormalities in all homozygotes are similar, evidence for three variants has come from studies of intestinal transport in homozygotes and of urinary excretion in heterozygotes. Type I homozygotes lack mediated intestinal transport of cystine, lysine, arginine, and ornithine; heterozygotes have normal urinary amino acid excretion patterns. Type II homozygotes lack mediated lysine transport in the gut but retain some capacity for cystine transport; heterozygotes have moderately increased urinary excretion of each of the four amino acids. Type III homozygotes retain some capacity for mediated intestinal transport of the four involved substrates; heterozygotes have modestly increased urinary lysine and cystine.

Clinical manifestations Cystinuria is among the most common inborn errors, with a frequency of 1 in 10,000 to 1 in 15,000 in many ethnic groups. Two-thirds of adults with cystinuria are type I homozygotes. Cystine stones account for 1 to 2 percent of all urinary tract calculi. The maximum solubility of cystine in the physiologic urinary pH range of 4.5 to 7.0 is about 1200 μmol/L (300 mg/L). Since affected homozygotes regularly excrete 2400 to 7200 μmol (600 to 1800 mg) daily, crystalluria and stone formation are a constant threat. Stone formation usually becomes manifest in the second or third decade but may occur in the first year of life. Symptoms and signs are those typical of urolithiasis: hematuria, flank pain, renal colic, obstructive uropathy, and infection (see Chap. 245). Recurrent urolithiasis may lead to progressive renal insufficiency.

Diagnosis The presence of cystine in a urinary tract stone is pathognomonic of cystinuria. However, since half the stones in cystinuric subjects are of mixed composition, and since as many as 10 percent may contain no detectable cystine, a urinary nitroprusside test should be done on all patients with urolithiasis to exclude this diagnosis. The nitroprusside test is also positive (appearance of a cherry red color) in some heterozygotes for cystinuria; in patients with hypercystinuria, homocystinuria, and cysteine β-mercaptolactate disulfiduria; and in the presence of acetone in the urine. When cystine content exceeds 1000 μmol/L (250 mg/L), cystine crystals may be seen in the sediment of acidified, concentrated, chilled urine. These hexagonal crystals are pathognomonic of cystine overexcretion in patients not taking sulfonamides.

Diagnostic confirmation of cystinuria depends on demonstration of the characteristic amino acid excretion pattern in the urine. Selective excretion of cystine, lysine, arginine, and ornithine can be demonstrated by paper chromatography or electrophoresis, and quantitative determinations can be made by column chromatography. Quantitation is important for differentiating some heterozygotes from homozygotes and for documenting the reduction of free cystine excretion during therapy.

Treatment Management is aimed at reducing the concentration of cystine in urine. The most important treatment is maintenance of a large urine volume. Fluid ingestion in excess of 4 L/d is essential, and 5 to 7 L/d is optimal. Urinary cystine excretion should measure less than 1000 to 1200 μmol/L (250 to 300 mg/L). The daily fluid ingestion necessary to maintain this dilution of excreted cystine should be spaced over the waking hours, with one-quarter to one-third of the total volume ingested at bedtime. Stones can be prevented and even dissolved by such hydration. It must be made clear to the cystinuric subject that water is a drug. Solubility of cystine rises sharply in urine above pH 7.5, and urinary alkalinization can be therapeutic in some situations. Vigorous administration of sodium bicarbonate, acetazolamide, and polycitrates is required to maintain a persistently alkaline pH, but this measure introduces the danger of inducing formation of calcium oxalate, calcium phosphate, and magnesium ammonium phosphate stones and of producing nephrocalcinosis.

Another treatment involves administration of penicillamine, which undergoes sulfhydryl-disulfide exchange with cystine to form the mixed disulfide of penicillamine and cysteine. Since this disulfide is more than 50 times as soluble as cystine, penicillamine (in doses of 1 to 3 g/d) reduces free cystine excretion markedly, thereby preventing new stone formation and promoting dissolution of existing calculi. Unfortunately, side effects include acute serum sickness, agranulocytosis, pancytopenia, immune glomerulitis, and the Goodpasture syndrome. Thus its use should be reserved for patients who fail to respond to hydration alone or who are in a high-risk category (one remaining kidney, renal insufficiency). Those patients unable to tolerate penicillamine may benefit from α-mercaptopropionylglycine, an experimental drug whose mechanism of action is similar to that of penicillamine but whose structure, and hence toxicity, is different. As many as two-thirds of patients unable to tolerate penicillamine may take α-mercaptopropionylglycine without ill effects. Captopril, a sulfhydryl-containing antihypertensive agent, is ineffective in reducing cystine excretion. When medical management fails, urologic surgery is required. An occasional patient may require renal transplantation because of renal failure.

DIBASICAMINOACIDURIA This disorder is characterized by a defect in renal tubular reabsorption of lysine, arginine, and ornithine but not of cysteine. The disorder almost surely reflects mutations in the gene(s) coding for a widely distributed transport protein used solely by the three dibasic amino acids. Two variants are each apparently inherited as an autosomal recessive trait. Manifestations are related to the losses of ornithine, arginine, and perhaps lysine.

In the common form of dibasicaminoaciduria (type II), also known as *lysinuric protein intolerance* and more common in Finland (1 in 60,000) than elsewhere, homozygotes show defective intestinal transport of dibasic amino acids as well as exaggerated renal losses. The transport defect affects basolateral rather than luminal membrane transport. Uptake of these substances is also defective in cultured fibroblasts and hepatocytes. Affected patients present in childhood with hepatosplenomegaly, protein intolerance, and episodic ammonia intoxication. Plasma concentrations of lysine, arginine, and ornithine are reduced. The clinical findings have been attributed to hyperammonemia resulting from insufficient amounts of arginine and ornithine to maintain proper function of the urea cycle. Treatment includes dietary protein restriction and supplementation with citrulline, a neutral amino acid whose intestinal and hepatic transport are unimpaired, and which, when metabolized to arginine and ornithine, fuels the urea cycle. With 2.0 to 8.0 g of oral citrulline daily, dietary protein intake can be increased and growth improved in children. Obligate heterozygotes are healthy and show no excess urinary loss of dibasic amino acids.

Type I dibasicaminoaciduria has been described in a large French-Canadian kindred. The proband was moderately mentally retarded. Her urinary losses of dibasic amino acids were not as great as those seen in type II homozygotes. The condition differed from type II by the presence of modest excesses of dibasic amino acids in urine of both asymptomatic parents. Several chemically affected members of the family also were symptom-free. Other families containing asymptomatic heterozygotes have been identified by urinary screening programs. Type I disease may involve the same transport system as that impaired in the more common type II disorder.

HARTNUP DISEASE Pellagra-like skin lesions, variable neurologic manifestations, and aminoaciduria for the monoaminomonocarboxylic amino acids with neutral or aromatic side chains characterize this disease. Alanine, serine, threonine, valine, leucine, isoleucine, phenylalanine, tyrosine, tryptophan, glutamine, asparagine, and histidine are excreted in urine in quantities 5 to 10 times normal, and intestinal transport for these same amino acids is defective. The clinical manifestations result from nutritional deficiency of the essential amino acid tryptophan, caused by the combination of intestinal malabsorption and renal loss. Manifestations are episodic, related, at least in part, to metabolic demands for tryptophan. Only a small fraction of patients with the chemical findings of this disorder develop a pellagra-like syndrome, implying that manifestations depend on factors over and above the transport defect.

The major pathway of tryptophan metabolism leads to the synthesis of niacin and nicotinamide-adenine dinucleotide (NAD). This pathway supplies about half the daily niacin needs. In patients with Hartnup disease, the renal and intestinal transport defect for tryptophan leads to niacin deficiency. The transport defect likely reflects abnormalities of a group-specific system for neutral amino acids. Some residual reabsorptive capacity persists for each involved amino acid. This suggests that they are transported by other carrier systems as well, a conclusion supported by the identification of patients with substrate-specific transport errors for tryptophan, methionine, and histidine.

Hartnup disease is inherited as an autosomal recessive trait. Homozygotes occur with a frequency of about 1 in 24,000 births. Heterozygotes exhibit no clinical or chemical abnormalities.

Pellagra is the clinical syndrome produced by dietary niacin deficiency, and its features are those of Hartnup disease (see Chap. 77). The diagnosis of Hartnup disease should be suspected in any patient with pellagra without a history of dietary niacin deficiency. The neurologic and psychiatric manifestations range from attacks of cerebellar ataxia to mild emotional lability to frank delirium and usually accompany exacerbations of the erythematous, eczematoid skin rash. Fever, sunlight, stress, and sulfonamide therapy provoke clinical relapses. Diagnosis is made by detection of the neutral aminoaciduria that does not occur in dietary niacin deficiency. Treatment is directed at niacin repletion and includes a high-protein diet and daily nicotinamide supplementation (50 to 250 mg). Tryptophan ethyl esters also can bypass the absorption defect.

IMINOGLYCINURIA This benign autosomal recessive trait is characterized by excessive urinary excretion of glycine and the imino acids proline and hydroxyproline. Homozygotes occur with a frequency of about 1 in 16,000. The enhanced excretion of glycine, proline, and hydroxyproline reflects a defect in the tubular transport system shared by these three compounds. An intestinal transport defect also may be present. This suggests that more than one mutation may lead to iminoglycinuria, a thesis corroborated by the demonstration that obligate heterozygotes from some but not all families have glycinuria. No consistent clinical abnormalities have been reported in homozygotes, who are usually detected by urinary amino acid screening programs. Individuals with iminoglycinuria should be reassured as to the benign nature of the disturbance.

DICARBOXYLICAMINOACIDURIA Selective urinary loss and exaggerated endogenous renal clearance of glutamic and aspartic acids have been described in two unrelated children. Intestinal absorption of these dicarboxylic amino acids was impaired in one. This patient suffered from recurrent hypoglycemia; the other was asymptomatic.

SUBSTRATE-SPECIFIC DEFECTS IN AMINO ACID TRANSPORT Rare pedigrees exist in which individuals have defective renal tubular reabsorption and/or impaired intestinal absorption of a single free amino acid. These disorders, each apparently inherited as an autosomal recessive trait, suggest that transport of amino acids is catalyzed by substrate-specific as well as group-specific transport mechanisms.

Hypercystinuria Two siblings exhibited modest cystinuria without excessive urinary excretion of lysine, arginine, or ornithine. Fractional tubular reabsorption of cystine was reduced to about 80 percent of the filtered load, and up to 250 mg/d was excreted in the urine. Intestinal absorption of cystine was normal. Both were clinically well, although the cystine excretion places them at risk for cystine urolithiasis. Cystine excretion by the parents was normal.

Lysinuria A child with selective impairment of renal tubular reabsorption of lysine has been described. Endogenous lysine clearance was increased; intestinal transport was impaired; plasma lysine was reduced. Mental and growth retardation and seizures were present. A lysine-supplemented diet stimulated growth. Urinary lysine excretion was normal in the parents.

Histidinuria Two siblings, each with mental retardation, exhibited a selective renal transport defect for histidine. Urinary loss of histidine approached 40 to 50 percent of the filtered load, and intestinal transport of histidine also was defective. The clinically normal parents had normal urinary excretion but a modest defect in intestinal absorption of histidine. In two additional cases of isolated histidinuria myoclonic seizures occurred.

Methionine malabsorption Children from two pedigrees have shown an intestinal transport defect for methionine. One may have had a renal transport defect as well. This disorder was detected because of urinary excretion of α-hydroxybutyric acid, a by-product of the intestinal bacterial breakdown of the unabsorbed methionine. This compound, which gives an odor resembling malt or dried celery to the urine, appears to be responsible for the white hair, attacks of hyperpnea, convulsions, edema, and mental retardation. Treatment of one of these children with a methionine-restricted diet caused improvement in all clinical manifestations.

Tryptophan malabsorption An isolated defect in intestinal absorption of tryptophan has been described in two siblings. The renal tubular reabsorption of tryptophan was normal. A number of indoles were excreted in stool and urine. These compounds result from chemical degradation of unabsorbed tryptophan by intestinal bacteria and may be present in patients with Hartnup disease as well. Because of concomitant renal disease, hydrolytic enzymes were released into the urine, acted on the indoles found there, and led to the formation of a blue pigment, indigotin. This sequence of events earned this condition the sobriquet "blue-diaper syndrome." No pellagra-like symptoms were described. The mother also excreted indole compounds, suggesting that she is a carrier of this trait.

DISORDERS OF HEXOSE TRANSPORT

Nondiabetic melituria occurs in a number of conditions. Pentoses, hexoses, heptoses, and disaccharides have been identified in the urine; all except sucrose yield a positive test for reducing substances. Some meliturias result from diffuse renal injury, others from ingestion of nonmetabolizable sugars. In still others the sugars accumulate in blood owing to deficient activity of catabolizing enzyme systems and "spill" into the urine. Only among the hexoses have specific inherited disorders of sugar transport been identified. The existence of renal glycosuria and intestinal glucose-galactose malabsorption as heritable, autosomal recessive disorders points to the existence of at least two specific carrier proteins for hexoses in human jejunal and renal brush border membranes: one for glucose and one shared by glucose and galactose.

RENAL GLYCOSURIA To avoid confusion with diabetes mellitus, Marble's criteria for the diagnosis of renal glycosuria should be followed: (1) glycosuria in the absence of hyperglycemia, (2) constant glycosuria with little fluctuation related to diet, (3) normal (or slightly flat) oral glucose tolerance test, (4) identification of urinary reducing substance as glucose, and (5) normal storage and utilization of carbohydrates. The Fanconi syndrome, in which renal glycosuria occurs as part of generalized proximal tubular dysfunction, also should be excluded. The condition is benign, but occasionally glycosuria may be great enough to cause polyuria and polydipsia. Even more rarely, dehydration or ketosis may develop under conditions of stress such as pregnancy or starvation.

In normal persons, glucose is present in the glomerular filtrate at a concentration equal to that in plasma water and is reabsorbed throughout the proximal renal tubule by a sodium-dependent, phloriz-in-inhibitable transport process. Reabsorptive capacity exceeds normal plasma glucose concentration. Thus glucose does not appear in the urine until the threshold for reabsorption is reached. The plasma concentration at which filtered glucose begins to escape proximal tubular reabsorption is usually around 10 mmol/L (200 mg/dL). Maximal renal reabsorptive capacity is exceeded at a filtered load of around 2 mmol (325 mg)/min per 1.73 m^2 body surface area, and this value is defined as the tubular maximum for glucose (TmG).

Two patterns of glycosuria are recognized: type A, characterized by a reduced tubular maximum reabsorptive capacity, and type B, showing a reduced threshold for glycosuria, an increased "splay" in the titration curve, and a normal TmG. Renal glycosuria occurs in homozygotes for either of these recessively inherited mutations and in compound heterozygotes for these presumably allelic mutations. Modest reduction in renal threshold or TmG is present in heterozygotes in some families; modest glycosuria occurs in such family members when plasma glucose is elevated. The gene responsible for renal glycosuria segregates with the HLA haplotype, suggesting that it is located on chromosome 6. No linkage disequilibrium was observed, and no specific HLA antigens have been associated with renal glycosuria.

GLUCOSE-GALACTOSE MALABSORPTION   In this condition, infants develop a profuse, watery diarrhea when fed milk or foods containing lactose, sucrose, glucose, or galactose. Fructose or carbo-hydrate-free formulas are well tolerated. A specific defect in intestinal absorption of glucose and galactose can be demonstrated by oral tolerance tests that produce little or no increase in plasma glucose or galactose. The primary defect involves the sodium/hexose cotrans-porter in the intestinal and renal brush border. Active D-glucose and D-galactose transport is absent in affected children, and intermediate transport capacity is present in their parents. These findings confirm the specificity and the autosomal recessive inheritance of the disorder. Treatment with a glucose- and galactose-free diet leads to resolution of symptoms in childhood. Although the basic transport defect is present throughout life, most patients show an improved tolerance for glucose and galactose with age.

A number of these patients have renal glycosuria at normal plasma glucose concentrations. Renal titration studies generally demonstrate a reduced threshold for glucose reabsorption (type B renal glycosuria) and a normal TmG. Urinary glucose loss is not as severe as in isolated renal glycosuria. This finding suggests the presence of multiple glucose transport proteins in the kidney. One, responsible for the bulk of glucose reabsorption and specific for glucose only, is affected in renal glycosuria; another, shared by glucose and galactose and responsible for transporting less of the filtered load of glucose, is affected in glucose-galactose malabsorption. Either the former is not present in intestinal mucosa, or the shared system is more important in that tissue. In both disorders, transport of sugars in all other tissues is normal, reflecting the multiplicity and tissue specificity of membrane transport proteins.

DEFECTIVE URATE TRANSPORT: HYPOURICEMIA

Individuals with a selective defect in renal tubular reabsorption of sodium urate have marked hypouricemia. Since little serum urate is bound to plasma proteins, failure to reabsorb filtered urate results in a serum urate ranging from 12 to 110 μmol/L (0.2 to 1.8 mg/dL). Moderate uricosuria is present, and 25 percent of patients have renal calculi.

Renal urate clearance normally averages 15 percent of glomerular filtration rate, and the excreted urate is composed both of filtered urate that has escaped reabsorption and of secreted urate. Subjects with isolated hypouricemia have urate clearances averaging from 33 to 85 percent of the filtration rate; in some, urate clearance exceeds the glomerular filtration rate. Studies with probenecid, which blocks tubular reabsorption of urate, and pyrazinamide, which blocks tubular secretion, reveal that 11 of the 16 families described have a presecretory urate reabsorptive defect, and 5 have defective transport affecting the entire tubule. In 4 families hypercalciuria due to enhanced intestinal calcium absorption is also present, but in others only uricosuria has been demonstrated. The defect is inherited as an autosomal recessive trait. Urate transport appears to be normal in nonrenal tissue. Obligate heterozygotes have moderately increased urate clearance. The defect is presumed to reflect mutation of one or both of the proximal renal tubular membrane proteins that transport sodium urate. The findings in these families support the hypothesis that renal urate reabsorption is controlled by more than one transport protein.

DEFECTIVE ANION TRANSPORT: CHLORIDORRHEA

This rare, autosomal recessive disease results from impairment of active transport of chloride in the ileum and colon. Absence of chloride-bicarbonate ion exchange causes profound symptoms even before birth (polyhydramnios and absence of meconium). Massive watery diarrhea is apparent from the first days of life. This fluid loss, with its attendant impairment of electrolyte homeostasis, is life-threatening. A hypokalemic, hypochloremic, hyponatremic metabolic alkalosis develops with dehydration and secondary hyperaldosteron-ism. Fecal fluid contains an excess of chloride ion over the sum of the accompanying cations sodium and potassium. Fecal chloride concentration always exceeds 90 mmol/L when volume and serum electrolyte disturbances are corrected, and this chloridorrhea is diagnostic. Renal chloride transport is normal. Decreased urine chloride results from the kidney's attempts to conserve salt and water.

Treatment requires adequate, lifelong repletion of electrolyte and fluid losses. Exact replacement of water, sodium chloride, and potassium chloride can prevent the growth and psychomotor retardation and the development of progressive renal damage. The renal lesion, with hyalinized glomeruli, juxtaglomerular hyperplasia, calcifications, and arteriolar changes, is probably a result of chronic volume depletion. Treatment of hyperreninemia and hypokalemia with prostaglandin inhibitors may reduce renal damage but does not alter intestinal symptoms or the need for chronic sodium chloride repletion.

REFERENCES

DESJEUX JF: Congenital selective Na$^+$ D-glucose cotransport defects leading to renal glycosuria and congenital selective intestinal malabsorption of glucose and galactose, in *The Molecular and Metabolic Basis of Inherited Disease*, 7th ed, CR Scriver et al (eds). New York, McGraw-Hill, in press

ELSAS LJ, ROSENBERG LE: Renal glycosuria, in *Strauss and Welt's Diseases of the Kidney*, 3d ed, LE Earley, CW Gottschalk (eds). Boston, Little, Brown, 1979, pp 1021–1028

HOLMBERG C, PERHEENTUPA J: Congenital chloride diarrhoea (CCD), in *Population Structure and Genetic Disorders*, AW Erikson et al (eds). New York, Academic, 1980, pp 596–599

KAMOUN PP et al: Renal histidinuria. J Inherited Metab Dis 4:217, 1981

LEVY HL: Hartnup disorder, in *The Molecular and Metabolic Basis of Inherited Disease*, 7th ed, CR Scriver et al (eds). New York, McGraw-Hill, in press

MILLINER DS: Cystinuria. Endocrinol Metab Clin North Am 19:889, 1990

ROSENBERG LE: Intestinal hexose transport in familial glucose-galactose malabsorption, in *Membranes and Disease*, L Bolis et al (eds). New York, Raven, 1976, pp 253–262

———, SCRIVER CR: Disorders of amino acid metabolism, in *Metabolic Control and Disease*, 8th ed, PK Bondy, LE Rosenberg (eds). Philadelphia, Saunders, 1980, pp 616–645

Segal S, Thier SO: Cystinurias, in *The Molecular and Metabolic Basis of Inherited Disease*, 7th ed, CR Scriver et al (eds). New York, McGraw-Hill, in press

Short EM, Rosenberg LE: Renal aminoaciduria, in *Strauss and Welt's Diseases of the Kidney*, 3d ed, LE Earley, CW Gottschalk (eds). Boston, Little, Brown, 1979, pp 975–1020

Simell O: Lysinuric protein intolerance and other cationic aminoacidurias, in *The Molecular and Metabolic Basis of Inherited Disease*, 7th ed, CR Scriver et al (eds). New York, McGraw-Hill, in press

Sperling O: Hereditary renal hypouricemia, in *The Molecular and Metabolic Basis of Inherited Disease*, 7th ed, CR Scriver et al (eds). New York, McGraw-Hill, in press

Weitz R, Sperling O: Hereditary renal hypouricemia: Isolated tubular defect of urate reabsorption. J Pediatr 96:850, 1980

354 GALACTOSEMIA, GALACTOKINASE DEFICIENCY, AND OTHER RARE DISORDERS OF CARBOHYDRATE METABOLISM

KURT J. ISSELBACHER

DEFINITION *Galactosemia* refers to any of three inborn errors of galactose metabolism. *Classic galactosemia* is due to the deficiency of galactose-1-phosphate uridyl transferase (GALT) and is typically associated with cataract formation, mental retardation, and cirrhosis. The second disorder, *galactokinase deficiency*, leads primarily to cataract formation. The third, *UDP-galactose-4-epimerase deficiency*, is the rarest of the group; few cases have been described, and the eventual outcome is uncertain.

PATHOGENESIS Lactose, the main carbohydrate in milk, is a disaccharide containing galactose and glucose; when ingested, it is hydrolyzed by intestinal lactase. Normally, the absorbed galactose is converted to glucose in the liver. The first reaction in this pathway is the phosphorylation of galactose to galactose-1-phosphate by galactokinase (specified by a gene on chromosome 17):

$$\text{Galactose} + \text{ATP} \xrightarrow{\text{galactokinase}} \text{galactose-1-phosphate}$$

The next step involves the conversion of galactose-1-phosphate to glucose-1-phosphate by GALT (the gene for which is on chromosome 9):

$$\text{Galactose-1-phosphate} + \text{UDP-glucose} \xrightarrow{\text{GALT}}$$

$$\text{UDP-galactose} + \text{glucose-1-phosphate}$$

The uridine diphosphate (UDP) sugars can be reversibly interconverted by an epimerase reaction (UDP-galactose-4-epimerase):

$$\text{UDP-galactose} \rightleftharpoons \text{UDP-glucose}$$

Galactose also can be metabolized by alternative pathways. It can be converted (reduced) in the presence of NADPH (or NADH) to galactitol (dulcitol) by aldose reductase. It also can be oxidized to a limited extent by galactose dehydrogenase, leading to the formation of galactonic acid, xyulose, and CO_2. These pathways account for limited galactose metabolism in patients with galactosemia.

In galactokinase deficiency, galactose accumulates in the blood and tissues. In the lens, galactose is converted by aldose reductase to galactitol, a sugar to which the lens is impermeable. As a consequence, excessive hydration occurs which, together with a decrease in glutathione in the lens, leads to cataract formation.

In classic galactosemia, GALT deficiency results in tissue accumulation of galactose-1-phosphate and galactose. As in galactokinase deficiency, cataracts develop secondary to galactitol accumulation in the lens. It is assumed that the cirrhosis and mental retardation of

classic galactosemia are related to increased amounts of galactose-1-phosphate in these tissues. Elevated blood galactose levels may lead to a decreased hepatic output of glucose and hence to hypoglycemia. In the kidney and intestine, accumulation of galactose and galactose-1-phosphate appears to lead to an inhibition of amino acid transport. In female homozygotes there is an increased incidence of hypergonadotrophic hypogonadism in which ovarian failure develops at an early age, and this complication may persist despite dietary therapy.

Both galactokinase and GALT deficiencies are transmitted as autosomal recessive traits. Heterozygotes for these disorders have half-normal enzyme levels but are asymptomatic. Maternal deficiency of galactokinase, together with lactose intake during pregnancy, may contribute to cataract formation during fetal development. However, not all persons with decreased GALT enzyme activity in their cells are carriers of classic galactosemia. Some individuals homozygous for another gene, called the *Duarte variant*, normally have half-normal GALT levels and are asymptomatic. This group can be differentiated from classic galactosemia heterozygotes on the basis of the electrophoretic properties of the mutant enzyme. In both galactokinase deficiency and classic galactosemia there is a functional deficiency or absence of the involved enzyme. Classic galactosemia is due to a variety of mutations in regions of the gene that are highly conserved throughout evolution. This molecular heterogeneity may help to explain diverse clinical outcomes in patients. Mutations in the variable (less conserved) regions of the gene contribute to polymorphisms accounting for normal function of GALT but with altered electrophoretic mobility.

The incidence of classic galactosemia is about 1 per 50,000 births in the white population. Approximately 0.8 to 1.3 percent of the population are heterozygotes for the GALT gene, and about 10 percent carry the Duarte variant. During screening of newborns for galactosemia, the most frequent cause of an abnormal result is compound heterozygosity for the Duarte variant and for classic galactosemia in which GALT levels are about 17 percent of normal. Such individuals are clinically asymptomatic.

CLINICAL FEATURES Symptoms of classic galactosemia usually begin within days to weeks after birth. The infant usually is reluctant to ingest breast milk or milk formulas, develops vomiting, shows poor nutrition, and fails to thrive. Jaundice, hepatomegaly, and evidence of liver disease may develop. Cataracts are usually not present at birth but develop gradually over weeks to months. Mental retardation becomes evident after 6 to 12 months and is usually not reversible. Infants with classic galactosemia are subject to bacterial sepsis (especially with *Escherichia coli*), and this may be the leading cause of death in the neonatal period. The only consistent feature of galactokinase deficiency is cataract formation.

DIAGNOSIS Galactokinase deficiency should be suspected in infants or children with cataract formation who have non-glucose-reducing substances in the urine. The diagnosis is made by demonstrating the deficiency of galactokinase in red blood cells.

Classic galactosemia must be considered when one or more of the clinical features described above are found. If the patient is ingesting milk, reducing sugar is present in the urine but gives a negative glucose oxidase reaction (i.e., is not glucose) and is identified as galactose by other techniques, such as chromatography. If the child is vomiting, has a poor food intake, or is on intravenous glucose feedings, galactose may not be present in the urine. The definitive diagnosis is made by demonstrating a lack or deficiency of red cell GALT by one of several techniques. The disease also can be diagnosed prenatally by enzyme studies on culture amniocentesis cells or by demonstrating increased galactitol in amniotic fluid. A nonenzymatic glycosylation of hemoglobin, analogous to that in diabetes mellitus, can be detected in patients with galactosemia as manifested by increased concentrations in the blood of Hb A_{lab} rather than Hb A_{lc}.

In the neonatal period galactosemia needs to be differentiated from primary liver disease. With liver damage, galactose removal from the blood is impaired, and elevated blood galactose levels and galactosuria insulin receptors, diminished affinity of the receptor for insulin, and postreceptor defects have all been reported. Mutations in the insulin receptor have been identified in some patients. Insulin in the plasma of affected subjects is biologically active. Although glucagon levels are high (indicating insulin resistance in the alpha cell of the islets of Langerhans) and free fatty acid concentrations are elevated, ketoacidosis is unusual. One patient had recurrent episodes of metabolic acidosis considered to be ketoacidosis, but concentrations of acetoacetate and β-hydroxybutyrate were characteristic of fasting ketosis, not diabetic ketoacidosis; presumably lactate or other organic acids were involved.

True ketoacidosis may be infrequent because insulin resistance is less severe in liver and skeletal muscle than in adipose tissue. Glycogen levels in the liver are high (insulin stimulates glycogen synthesis), and branched-chain amino acids fall normally or near normally in response to injected insulin. Elevated insulin levels in portal vein plasma would counteract the actions of glucagon in the insulin-responsive hepatocyte (see Chap. 338). This would prevent activation of ketone body synthesis in liver and ensure utilization of incoming fatty acids for triglyceride/VLDL synthesis. The elevated long-chain fatty acids in the plasma are of dietary origin and fall toward normal with restriction of dietary fat. Diabetes mellitus accompanying lipodystrophy appears to be typical apart from insulin resistance, including the propensity to develop late degenerative complications. High levels of insulin in plasma and resistance to ketoacidosis distinguish this condition from type I (autoimmune) insulin-dependent diabetes mellitus, although both conditions begin in childhood or early adult life.

2 *Hypertriglyceridemia with accumulation of both chylomicrons and very low density lipoproteins in the blood.* Eruptive xanthomas, lipemia retinalis, and recurrent pancreatitis may be seen. Although lipoprotein lipase is low, as noted, and there is a defect in disposal of triglycerides in the atrophied fat tissue, the major cause for the hypertriglyceridemia is overproduction of VLDL in the liver. This overproduction is probably driven by the elevated free fatty acids in blood, since dietary fat restriction results in a fall of VLDL production rates toward normal. Hyperinsulinemia may contribute by enhancing hepatic fat synthesis.

3 *A hypermetabolic state with normal thyroid function.* Basal metabolic rates are usually elevated, although thyroid hormone values (thyroxine, triiodothyronine, reverse triiodothyronine) are normal. Patients do not gain weight with excessive caloric intake, indicating a facile capacity to waste calories as heat. Food intakes as high as 21,000 kJ (5000 kcal)/d are not unusual. One 16-month-old child ate 10,000 kJ (2400 kcal) daily. Following thyroidectomy in one patient, the basal metabolic rate decreased but did not return to normal; symptoms and signs of hypothyroidism supervened, requiring treatment with thyroid hormone despite continued high metabolic rates. It thus seems clear that hypermetabolism is not due to hyperthyroidism. There is also no evidence of mitochondrial disease. The most likely explanation for the increased metabolic rate is enhanced "futile" cycles with wastage of ATP. Increased sympathetic nervous system activity may play a role. There is no evidence for adrenal medullary dysfunction.

Course and treatment Patients with generalized lipodystrophy may die at an early age. Hepatic failure, hemorrhage from esophageal varices, and renal failure are common causes of death. Despite the almost constant hypertriglyceridemia, symptomatic coronary artery disease is rare. Recurrent pancreatitis may be life-threatening. There is no specific treatment for lipodystrophy, although dietary fat restriction is generally recommended. Medium-chain triglyceride supplementation has been reported to be of benefit. Because of insulin resistance, large amounts of insulin are often required to control the plasma glucose. Gemfibrozil is usually prescribed to lower triglycerides but is often ineffective. In patients with recurrent pancreatitis, nicotinic acid may be prescribed to lower triglycerides.

ACQUIRED PARTIAL LIPODYSTROPHY This is the most common of the lipodystrophies and usually affects women. Fat atrophy occurs in the upper half of the body, including the face, but spares the lower extremities. Rarely, the lower half of the body is affected, leaving the upper torso intact. Occasionally, the lesion affects only one side. The other anatomic features of generalized lipodystrophy are usually absent, and liver disease is unusual. Proteinuria, with or without the nephrotic syndrome, occurs more frequently than in other forms. The complement system is abnormal, and C3 levels tend to be low. C3 nephritic factor, a polyclonal IgG immunoglobulin that interacts with alternative pathway convertase (C3b Bb) to augment C3 activation, is present in serum. C3 levels may be low in unaffected first-degree relatives, but C3 nephritic factor is absent. Complement abnormalities disappeared after renal transplantation in one subject. Dermatomyositis and Sjögren's syndrome may occur. Rarely, partial lipodystrophy progresses to the generalized form of the disease.

An unusual form of partial lipodystrophy is mandibuloacral dysplasia, a syndrome with typical features of lipodystrophy, including insulin resistance, hypermetabolism, and increased glucose production. Other features include hypoplasia of the mandibles and clavicles with lytic bone lesions, wrinkled skin, and joint contractures. Some patients have hypogonadism, short stature, and alopecia.

LIPODYSTROPHY WITH DOMINANT TRANSMISSION This variant is characterized by fat atrophy of the limbs and trunk with sparing of the face, which may actually be rounded. The neck also may be exempt. The disease usually begins at puberty but may not appear until middle age. Males are rarely affected. In families with the Rieger anomaly, onset tends to be in infancy. Insulin resistance and hyperglycemia are usual, and severe hypertriglyceridemia with eruptive xanthomas may occur. The labia majora are hypertrophied, and polycystic ovaries may be seen. Acanthosis nigricans is usually present. Liver and renal disease do not occur.

LOCALIZED LIPODYSTROPHY Localized lipodystrophy takes several patterns. Centrifugal lipodystrophy (*lipodystrophia centrifugalis abdominalis infantilis*) has been mentioned already. Annular lipoatrophy is a bandlike ring of fat atrophy encircling a limb or the ankles. Occasionally, only half the limb is involved, in which case the term often used is *lipoatrophia semicircularis*. On biopsy, inflammatory infiltrates are usually present in the areas of fat atrophy. Localized lipodystrophy also may occur secondary to injection of insulin, iron dextrans, triamcinolone, and diphtheria/pertussis/tetanus vaccine.

MULTIPLE SYMMETRIC LIPOMATOSIS

Multiple symmetric lipomatosis, a disease found predominantly in men, is characterized by formation of nonencapsulated lipomas in various areas. Two patterns of distribution are noted. In the *type I* variant, lipomas are primarily in the nape of the neck and in the supraclavicular and deltoid regions, resulting in an extraordinary bull-necked appearance (*Madelung collar*). Extension into the mediastinum may produce obstruction of the trachea or vena cava. Fat over the remainder of the body appears normal. In the *type II* pattern, lipomas are not localized to the neck but extend down over the body, giving the appearance of simple obesity. Correct diagnosis requires recognition that the fat masses are symmetric and that the distal arms and legs are spared. Deep lipomatosis is absent in type II disease, and vena caval and tracheal compression do not occur.

Multiple symmetric lipomatosis may occur sporadically or in families. Autosomal dominant transmission has been postulated in the latter. Alcoholism is common. Coexisting folate deficiency, macrocytic anemia, and abnormal liver function may be due to alcohol and not lipomatosis. Neuropathy, which may be sensory, motor, or autonomic, is prominent, and neuropathic foot ulcers may be present. Histologic evidence from sural nerve biopsies suggests that the neuropathy is integral to the disease and not due to alcohol. The lesion is a chronic distal atrophy without the axonal degeneration and demyelination characteristic of alcohol injury.

Metabolic abnormalities include hyperuricemia, hypertriglyceridemia (VLDL, chylomicrons), and paradoxically, an elevation of high-density lipoproteins (HDL) as well. Diabetes mellitus has not been reported, although hyperinsulinism may be present. A few patients have had renal tubular acidosis.

The cause of multiple symmetric lipomatosis is not known. The fat cells are slightly smaller than normal, suggesting hyperplasia. Isolated adipocytes appear to have a marked increase in lipoprotein lipase activity and a defect in adrenergic lipolysis. Lipolytic response to cyclic AMP is intact, suggesting an abnormality at the hormone receptor/adenylate cyclase unit. The biochemical abnormalities are not present in all cases.

There is no treatment except for surgical removal of lipomas that cause compression. They also may be removed for cosmetic reasons.

OTHER LIPOMATOSES

MEDIASTINOABDOMINAL This lipomatosis may be a variant of multiple symmetric lipomatosis. The syndrome comprises (1) exertional dyspnea due to compression of airways by lipomas of the mediastinum, (2) massive enlargement of the abdomen (pseudoascites) due to intraperitoneal and retroperitoneal fat, and (3) abnormal glucose tolerance or diabetes mellitus. The metabolic abnormalities and enzymic changes in adipocytes are identical with those in multiple symmetric lipomatosis except that HDL levels are not elevated.

PELVIC Pelvic lipomatosis is characterized by nonmalignant overgrowth of dense, unencapsulated fat in pelvic spaces enveloping the pelvic viscera. The disease is almost always present in men, the male-to-female ratio being 18:1. Symptoms are of bladder dysfunction (frequency, dysuria, hematuria), constipation, and vague abdominal pain. The constricting pelvic fat may cause bilateral ureteral obstruction with hydronephrosis and renal failure. Hypertension is common. Radiographic studies show a deformed bladder, deviation of the ureters, displacement of rectosigmoid junction, and hydronephrosis in advanced cases. MRI examination or CT scan reveals the compressing fat. The cause is not known. There is no treatment except surgery to remove the fat and relieve upper urinary tract obstruction.

EPIDURAL Epidural lipomatosis is a syndrome of spinal cord compression due to adipose tissue. It causes back pain, radicular pain, or compression of the cord. The syndrome is most often seen with chronic glucocorticoid therapy and may occur in Cushing's syndrome. Cord compression requires laminectomy, but otherwise a trial of decreased steroid dosage should be undertaken.

ACUTE PANNICULITIS (NODULAR FAT NECROSIS)

The appearance of single or multiple crops of tender nodules in subcutaneous fat with a histologic picture of fat cell necrosis, infiltration of inflammatory cells, and development of fat-filled macrophages (foam cells) is the hallmark of acute panniculitis. The nodules range in size from 0.5 to 10 cm and may be firm or fluctuant. They are usually, but not always, tender. On occasion they drain an oily solution, and suppuration may occur. Individual lesions last from 1 to 8 weeks before disappearing, and a pigmented depressed area may be left at the involved site. While some patients have only nodular panniculitis, which may or may not be relapsing, others develop fever, abnormal liver function, involvement of the bone marrow with leukemoid response, bleeding tendencies, nodular pulmonary lesions, and evidence of pancreatic disease with elevated plasma amylase and lipase levels. In the past this constellation of findings was called *Weber-Christian disease*. However, since painful or nonpainful panniculitis may result from a variety of conditions,

Weber-Christian disease is not a specific entity, and the term should probably be abandoned.

It is not possible to develop a firm classification of acute panniculitis since the lesions may appear in sporadic fashion with many conditions. One classification system is given in Table 355-4.

Panniculitis without systemic disease is usually due to trauma (sometimes factitiously induced) or cold. For example, in equestrian cold panniculitis the lesions appear in the outer thighs of persons riding horseback for several hours in icy weather. One variant, subcutaneous fat necrosis of the newborn, may be due to a combination of obstetric trauma and hypothermia.

Panniculitis with systemic disease can be divided into several large categories. Collagen vascular disease is a frequent cause, although few patients with connective tissue disorders develop this complication. Lupus is probably most common, and scleroderma is second. Nodular fat necrosis occurs in about 2 to 3 percent of patients with lupus and is more common in discoid than in systemic lupus. Lymphomas and histiocytosis represent a second category. Histiocytic cytophagic panniculitis (HCP) is characterized by fever, serositis (pleural effusions), hepatosplenomegaly, panniculitis, anemia, leukopenia, thrombocytopenia, and coagulation defects. The characteristic lesion is the "beanbag" histiocyte containing ingested lymphocytes, red cells, and platelets. While some patients have a benign course, the majority have a fatal outcome due to hemorrhagic complications. Malignant T cell lymphoma occasionally involves subcutaneous tissue directly and may mimic HCP. Infiltrating T lymphocytes in HCP are of clonal origin, suggesting that subcutaneous T cell lymphomas are a malignant counterpart or late transformation phase of HCP. Deficiencies of α_1-antitrypsin have been found in a number of patients with acute panniculitis. It is postulated that the α_1-antitrypsin deficiency predisposes to panniculitis secondary to trauma and induces a hyperactive immune response. Panniculitis with systemic symptoms, including fever and hepatitis, also has been seen with light chain paraproteinemia and acquired deficiency of C_1 inhibitor in the classic complement-generating sequence. Severe pancreatic disease also may cause acute panniculitis. One distinct syndrome has been called *disseminated fat necrosis* and is described below. Panniculitis rarely may be associated with generalized lipodystrophy, especially the acquired type. Rare causes of panniculitis include gout, familial Mediterranean fever, Nasu disease (see above), drugs (glucocorticoids, aspartame), renal failure, atheromatous emboli, and infection. Eosinophilic panniculitis may be seen with vasculitis, parasitic infestation, lymphomas, and atopic dermatitis.

Acute panniculitis can only be diagnosed histologically. Once the lesion is identified, a search for the cause must be made. If systemic symptoms are present and the course is rapidly downhill, the primary differential diagnosis is between collagen vascular disease, lymphoproliferative disorder, and pancreatitis or pancreatic cancer. Milder cases raise the possibility of α_1-antitrypsin deficiency.

Treatment is often unsatisfactory. Some patients with histiocytic cytophagic panniculitis respond to combined chemotherapy with cyclophosphamide, bleomycin, and prednisone. Patients with α_1-antitrypsin deficiency may respond to dapsone but should be given

---

TABLE 355-4 Causes of panniculitis

Panniculitis without systemic disease
  Trauma
  Cold
  Subcutaneous fat necrosis of the newborn
Panniculitis with systemic disease
  Connective tissue disorders (lupus erythematosus, scleroderma)
  Lymphoproliferative disease (lymphoma, histiocytosis)
  α_1-Antitrypsin deficiency
  Pancreatic disease (cancer, pancreatitis)
  Generalized lipodystrophy
  Paraproteinemia with C1 inhibitor deficiency
  Miscellaneous (see text)

α_1-antiprotease concentrate (60 mg/kg body weight weekly) if this fails.

DISSEMINATED FAT NECROSIS

Disseminated fat necrosis (also called *metastatic fat necrosis*) is a syndrome in which patients with pancreatitis (two-thirds) or carcinoma of the pancreas (one-third) develop lesions that appear to be similar to or identical with nodular panniculitis. The fat necrosis has a predilection for periarticular sites. Fever is almost invariably present. Arthritis occurs in about 60 percent of cases and may be severe, resulting in destruction of the joint. Often there are sinus tracts running from the site of subcutaneous fat necrosis into the joint space, leading to deposition of necrotic material. Lytic bone lesions may underlie the site of fat necrosis. Polyserositis and vasculitis may be present. Since complement levels are low and immunofluorescent staining shows deposition of complement and IgG, the syndrome resembles, in some respects, lupus-associated panniculitis. Serologic studies for lupus have not been systematically carried out. However, antinuclear antibody (ANA) and rheumatoid factor are undetectable in some patients.

Disseminated fat necrosis may be due to release of pancreatic enzymes into blood or lymph, and these enzymes may initiate fat necrosis at distal sites. Presumably, free fatty acids released by pancreatic lipase and phospholipase A_2, both of which may be elevated in serum, induce tissue necrosis, with trypsin playing an ancillary role. Experimentally, necrosis can be induced in pericardial, subpleural, and subcutaneous fat by ligation of pancreatic ducts. Amylase and lipase levels may be elevated in pleural, pericardial, and ascitic fluid. These enzymes also have been found in fluid aspirated from subcutaneous nodules. The possibility that release of aberrant pancreatic enzyme into the blood is the cause is supported by the occurrence of disseminated fat necrosis in patients with pancreatic–portal vein fistulas. On the other hand, an immune mechanism cannot be ruled out, given that polyserositis is common and that low complement levels and vasculitis may be present. The meaning of the eosinophilia that frequently accompanies disseminated fat necrosis is not known.

Mortality rates are high (even in the absence of pancreatic carcinoma), and death may occur in weeks to months. No treatment is known. Infusion of the protease inhibitor aprotinin appeared to have beneficial effects in one patient.

ADIPOSIS DOLOROSA

Adiposis dolorosa (Dercum's disease) is characterized by painful circumscribed adipose tissue deposits in subcutaneous tissues of the extremities and of other parts of the body. Juxtaarticular areas, particularly the knees, are the most common sites. Lesions vary from 0.5 to 5.0 cm. Pain and paresthesias may occur spontaneously or result from pressure. Affected subjects are frequently women (30:1). They are usually obese. The syndrome is associated with weakness, fatigue, emotional instability, and occasional dementia. The condition rarely begins until after menopause. Most cases are sporadic, but familial occurrence has been noted with a presumed dominant inheritance. Multiple associations have been reported, but they are probably chance phenomena. Autopsy reports from early in the century suggested abnormalities of the pituitary and other endocrine glands, but modern endocrinologic evaluations have not been undertaken.

Biopsy of affected sites may show no abnormalities, but granulomas with giant cell formations are usually seen. Fat necrosis is rare, thus separating the condition from acute panniculitis.

Treatment is unsatisfactory, although intravenous lidocaine has apparently provided relief in two cases.

REFERENCES

Lipodystrophy

BILLINGS JK et al: Lipoatrophic panniculitis: A possible autoimmune inflammatory disease of fat. Report of three cases. Arch Dermatol 123:1662, 1987

CHUN SI et al: Membranous lipodystrophy: Primary idiopathic type. J Am Acad Dermatol 24:844, 1991

CUTLER DL et al: Insulin-resistant diabetes mellitus and hypermetabolism in mandibulo-acral dysplasia: A newly recognized form of partial lipodystrophy. J Clin Endocrinol Metab 73:1056, 1991

DUNNIGAN MG et al: Familial lipoatrophic diabetes with dominant transmission: A new syndrome. Q J Med 43:33, 1974

FRANKLIN B et al: Very low-density lipoprotein metabolism in an unusual case of lipoatrophic diabetes. Metabolism 33:814, 1984

GARG A et al: Peculiar distribution of adipose tissue in patients with congenital generalized lipodystrophy. J Clin Endocrinol Metab 75:358, 1991

KLEIN S et al: Generalized lipodystrophy: In vivo evidence for hypermetabolism and insulin-resistant lipid, glucose, and amino acid kinetics. Metabolism 41:893, 1992

LILLYSTONE D, WEST RJ: Lipodystrophy of limbs associated with insulin resistance Arch Dis Child 50:737, 1975

SEIP M: Generalized lipodystrophy, in *Ergebnisse der Inneren Medizin und Kinderheil-kunde*, P Frick et al (eds). Berlin, Springer-Verlag, 1971, pp 59–95

WACHSLICHT-RODBARD H et al: Heterogeneity of the insulin-receptor interaction in lipoatrophic diabetes. J Clin Endocrinol Metab 52:416, 1981

WILSON DE et al: Eucaloric substitution of medium chain triglycerides for dietary long chain fatty acids in acquired total lipodystrophy: Effects on hyperlipoproteinemia and endogenous insulin resistance. J Clin Endocrinol Metab 57:517, 1983

Multiple symmetric lipomatosis

ENZI G: Multiple symmetric lipomatosis: An updated clinical report. Medicine 63:56, 1984

LEUNG NWY et al: Multiple symmetric lipomatosis (Launois-Bensaude syndrome): Effect of oral salbutamol. Clin Endocrinol 7:601, 1987

POLLOCK M et al: Neuropathy in multiple symmetric lipomatosis. Madelung's disease. Brain 111:1157, 1988

RUZICKA T et al: Benign symmetric lipomatosis Launois-Bensaude. Report of ten cases and review of the literature. J Am Acad Dermatol 17:663, 1987

Mediastinoabdominal lipomatosis, pelvic lipomatosis, and epidural lipomatosis

ENZI G et al: Mediastino-abdominal lipomatosis: Deep accumulation of fat mimicking a respiratory disease and ascites. Clinical aspects and metabolic studies *in vitro*. Q J Med 53:453, 1984

FESSLER RG et al: Epidural lipomatosis in steroid-treated patients. Spine 17:183, 1992

HEYNS CF: Pelvic lipomatosis: A review of its diagnosis and management. J Urol 146:267, 1991

Acute panniculitis

ALEGRE VA, WINKELMANN RK: Histiocytic cytophagic panniculitis. J Am Acad Dem…atol 20:177, 1989

ARONSON IK et al: Panniculitis associated with cutaneous T-cell lymphoma and cytophagocytic histiocytosis. Br J Dermatol 112:87, 1985

HYTIROGLOU P et al: Histiocytic cytophagic panniculitis: Molecular evidence for a clonal T-cell disorder. J Am Acad Dermatol 27:333, 1992

PASCUAL M et al: Recurrent febrile panniculitis and hepatitis in two patients with acquired complement deficiency and paraproteinemia. Am J Med 83:959, 1987

PATTERSON JW: Differential diagnosis of panniculitis, in *Advances in Dermatology*, 6th ed, JP Callen et al (eds). St Louis, Mosby–Year Book, 1991, pp 309–330

PETERS MS, SU WPD: Panniculitis. Dermatol Clin 10:37, 1992

SMITH KC et al: Panniculitis associated with severe α_1-antitrypsin deficiency: Treatment and review of the literature. Arch Dermatol 123:1655, 1987

WINKELMANN RK: Panniculitis in connective tissue disease. Arch Dermatol 119:336, 1983

Disseminated fat necrosis

PHILLIPS MR JR et al: Inflammatory arthritis and subcutaneous fat necrosis associated with acute and chronic pancreatitis. Arthritis Rheum 23:355, 1980

POTTS JR: Pancreatic–portal vein fistula with disseminated fat necrosis treated by pancreaticoduodenectomy. South Med J 84:632, 1991

WILSON HA et al: Pancreatitis with arthropathy and subcutaneous fat necrosis. Evidence for the pathogenicity of lipolytic enzymes. Arthritis Rheum 26:121, 1983

Adiposis dolorosa

ATKINSON RL: Intravenous lidocaine for the treatment of intractable pain of adiposis dolorosa. Int J Obes 6:351, 1982

section 3 Disorders of bone and mineral metabolism

356 CALCIUM, PHOSPHORUS, AND BONE METABOLISM: CALCIUM-REGULATING HORMONES

MICHAEL F. HOLICK / STEPHEN M. KRANE /
JOHN T. POTTS, JR.

BONE STRUCTURE AND METABOLISM (See also Chap. 358) Bone is a dynamic tissue that is constantly remodeled throughout life. The arrangement of compact and cancellous bone provides a combination of strength and density suitable for mobility. In addition, bone provides a reservoir for calcium, magnesium, phosphorus, sodium, and other ions necessary for the support of homeostatic functions. The skeleton is highly vascular and receives about 10 percent of the cardiac output.

The properties of bone are a function of its extracellular components. The structure consists of a solid mineral phase in close association with an organic matrix, of which 90 to 95 percent is type I collagen (see Chap. 351). The noncollagenous portion of the organic matrix contains proteins derived from serum (albumin and α_2-HS glycoproteins), α-carboxyglutamic acid (GLA)-containing proteins (*bone GLA protein*, or *BGP*, or *osteocalcin* and a matrix GLA protein), the glycoprotein *osteonectin*, the phosphoprotein *osteopontin*, sialoproteins, *thrombospondin*, and other less well characterized proteins. Some of these proteins may function in initiating mineralization and in binding of the mineral phase to the matrix. The mineral phase is made up of calcium and phosphate, best characterized as a poorly crystalline hydroxyapatite, although the calcium/phosphate molar ratio is less than the 1.67 molar ratio of hydroxyapatite [empirical formula $Ca_{10}(PO_4)_6(OH)_2$]. In addition, other ions are present, predominantly in the surface layers. The mineral phase of bone is deposited initially in intimate relation to the collagen fibrils and is found in specific locations within the "holes" between the collagen fibrils. This architectural arrangement of mineral and matrix results in a two-phase material uniquely suited to withstand mechanical stresses. The formation and the localization of the inorganic phase are determined in part by the organic matrix.

Cells of mesenchymal origin, *osteoblasts*, synthesize and secrete the organic matrix. Mineralization of the matrix, largely in *osteons* (haversian systems), begins soon after the matrix is secreted (primary mineralization) but is not completed until after several weeks (secondary mineralization). Osteoblasts are characterized by their location and morphology, the presence of a specific skeletal form of alkaline phosphatase, the presence of receptors for parathyroid hormone (PTH) and 1,25-dihydroxyvitamin D [$1,25(OH)_2D$], and the ability to synthesize specific matrix proteins such as type I collagen, osteocalcin, and osteopontin. As an osteoblast secretes matrix, which is then mineralized, the cell becomes surrounded by matrix and becomes an *osteocyte*, still connected with its blood supply through a series of canaliculi. Resorption of bone is carried out mainly by *osteoclasts*. Osteoclasts are multinucleated cells formed by fusion of precursor hematopoietic stem cells related to the mononuclear phagocyte series. Resorption of bone takes place in scalloped spaces (Howship's lacunae) where the osteoclasts are attached through a specific $\alpha v\beta 3$ integrin to components of the bone matrix such as osteopontin. This

zone (clear zone) contains contractile proteins. The resorbing end of the cell forms a specialized ruffled border. Mineral and matrix are removed in this space where the ruffled border is folded and is in contact with the bone. Proteins, including a specialized proton pump ATPase, are found in the ruffled border membrane, which contributes to the production of a unique acid environment in the enclosed extracellular compartment and results in solubilization of the mineral phase. This area is also rich in protein encoded by the oncogene c-*src* and in the src phosphorylation substrate p80/85. In addition to the proton pump, carbonic anhydrase (type II isoenzyme) is required to maintain the acid pH. Other features of osteoclasts include the presence of tartrate-resistant acid phosphatase, cell surface receptors for calcitonin, sodium pumps of the kidney type, bicarbonate/chloride exchanger of the band 3 family, and an ability to resorb mineralized bone. The bone matrix is resorbed in the acid environment adjacent to the ruffled border by acid hydrolyases following solubilization of the mineral phase. Several soluble ligands modulate the differentiation of osteoblasts or osteoclasts from precursor cells and modulate the function of the differentiated cells, particularly the colony stimulating factors and interleukins 6 and 11 (IL-6 and IL-11). Bone is a storehouse for growth regulatory factors. Some that affect osteoblast function include transforming growth factors (TGFβ I and II), acidic and basic fibroblast growth factors (FGF), platelet-derived growth factors (PDGF), and insulin-like growth factors (IGF-1 and -2). In addition, several proteins have the capacity to induce ectopic bone formation and may have a role in bone remodeling, e.g., osteoinductive factor, osteogenin, and bone morphogenic proteins. Other cytokines modulate resorption through effects on osteoclasts, e.g., interleukin 1 (IL-1), tumor necrosis factor (TNF), interferon-γ, and colony stimulating factors (CSFs). Some of these effects on osteoclasts are mediated by osteoblasts and adjacent stromal fibroblasts in the marrow. For example, PTH receptors are not found on mature osteoclasts, and PTH increases osteoclastic bone resorption by first acting on osteoblasts or stromal fibroblasts. $1,25(OH)_2D$ receptors are found in precursor cells, which can differentiate into monocytes or osteoclasts, and $1,25(OH)_2D$ promotes differentiation along the osteoclast pathway. Some cytokines such as IL-1 and TGFα may induce local production of prostaglandins and other cytokines such as IL-6 and CSFs. What had initially been termed *osteoclast-activating factor* is currently thought to reflect the presence of cytokines such as IL-1, TNFα, TNFβ (lymphotoxin), and probably others as well.

In the embryo and in the growing child, bone develops by remodeling and replacing previously calcified cartilage (endochondral bone formation), or it is formed without a cartilage matrix (intramembranous bone formation). New bone, whether in infants or in adults during repair, has a relatively high ratio of cells to matrix and is characterized by coarse fiber bundles of collagen that are interlaced and randomly dispersed (woven bone). In adults, the more mature bone is organized with fiber bundles regularly arranged in parallel or concentric sheets (lamellar bone). In long bones, deposition of lamellar bone in a concentric arrangement around blood vessels forms the haversian systems. Growth in length of bones is dependent on proliferation of cartilage cells and on the endochondral sequence at the growth plate. Growth in width and thickness is accomplished by formation of bone at the periosteal surface and by resorption at the endosteal surface with the rate of formation exceeding that of resorption. In adults, after the epiphyses close, growth in length and endochondral bone formation cease, except for some activity in the cartilage cells beneath the articular surface. Even in adults, however, remodeling of bone (remodeling of haversian systems as well as trabecular bone) continues through life. Newly forming surfaces are characterized by smooth character, by uptake of tetracycline, and by relatively low mineral density and are covered by active osteoblasts. The osteoid seam that results from the lag in mineralization of the newly formed organic matrix is about 12 μm in width. An index of the rate of bone formation can be obtained by examination of undemineralized sections of bone biopsies from individuals who have received tetracycline for two periods separated by a drug-free interval. The distance between the fluorescent bands on the sections reflects the new bone formed. Resorption areas are characterized by irregular configurations and the presence of osteoclasts (Fig. 356-1). Resorption precedes formation and is more intense, but it does not persist as long as formation. In adults, approximately 4 percent of the surface of trabecular bone (such as iliac crest) is involved in active resorption, whereas 10 to 15 percent of trabecular surfaces is covered with osteoid. Radioisotope studies indicate that as much as 18 percent of the total skeletal calcium is deposited and removed each year. Thus bone is an active metabolizing tissue that requires an intact blood supply. The remodeling of bone is somehow related to the mechanical stresses to which it is subjected. Bone also serves as an important reservoir of mineral ions such as calcium, which are critical for a variety of processes.

The response of bone to fractures, infection, and interruption of blood supply and to expanding lesions is relatively limited. Dead bone must be resorbed, and new bone must be formed, a process carried out in association with growth of new blood vessels into the involved area. In injuries that disrupt the organization of the tissue, such as a fracture in which apposition of fragments is poor and motion exists at the fracture site, the progenitor stromal cells differentiate into cells with functional capacities different from those of osteoblasts, and varying amounts of fibrous tissue and cartilage are formed. When

FIGURE 356-1 Schematic representation of bone remodeling surfaces in trabecular bone. Most bone surfaces in adults are involved in neither formation nor resorption. Such surfaces are usually smooth, have no osteoid seam, and are covered either by no visible cells or by flattened cells. Active formation surfaces are smooth and covered by osteoblasts which have an osteoid seam (*clear*), normally no thicker than 12 μm. The calcification front is located at the junction of the osteoid seam and mineralized bone (*stippled*). Inactive formation surfaces are not covered by osteoblasts but by only a few flattened cells. Active resorption surfaces are irregular or scalloped and contain multinucleated osteoclasts. The latter are not seen on inactive resorption surfaces.

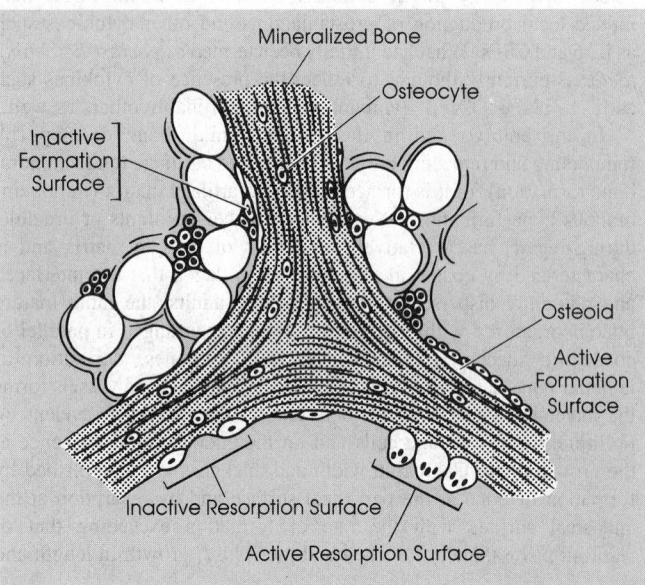

Inactive Formation Surface
Mineralized Bone
Osteocyte
Osteoid
Active Formation Surface
Inactive Resorption Surface
Active Resorption Surface

there is good apposition with fixation and little motion at the fracture site, repair occurs predominantly by formation of new bone without other scar tissue. Remodeling of this bone occurs along lines of force determined by mechanical stresses that are somehow translated into biologic response.

Expanding lesions in bone, such as tumors, induce resorption at the surface in contact with the tumor. A bowing deformity causes increased new bone formation at the concave surface and resorption at the convex surface, all seemingly designed to produce the strongest mechanical structure. Even in a disorder as architecturally disruptive as Paget's disease, remodeling is dictated by mechanical forces. Thus the plasticity of bone is due to cells interacting with each other and with the environment.

Mechanisms of bone formation and resorption   Bone formation is an orderly process in which inorganic mineral is deposited in relation to an organic matrix. The mineral phase is composed of calcium and phosphorus, and the concentration of these ions in the plasma and extracellular fluid (ECF) influences the rate at which mineral is formed. In vitro, mineralization can proceed, and crystals of hydroxyapatite can grow at concentrations of calcium and phosphorus similar to those in an ultrafiltrate of plasma. However, the concentration of these ions at the sites of mineralization is unknown, and the cells involved (osteoblasts, osteocytes) may determine the local concentration of calcium, phosphorus, and other ions. Collagens from a variety of sources can catalyze the nucleation of a mineral phase of calcium and phosphorus from solutions of these ions, and the initial mineral phase is deposited in specific locations in the holes produced by the particular packing arrangement of the collagen molecules. The organization of collagen probably influences the amount and type of mineral phase formed in bone. The primary structures of type I collagen in skin and bone tissues are similar. There are differences, however, in posttranslational modifications of type I collagen such as hydroxylation, glycosylation, and the type, number, and distribution of intermolecular cross-links. In addition, the "holes" in the packing structure of the collagen are larger in mineralized collagen of bone and dentin than in unmineralized collagens such as tendon. The fact that single amino acid substitutions in the helical portion of either the α1 or α2 chains of type I collagen due to mutations in the *COL1A1* or *COL1A2* genes in osteogenesis imperfecta disrupt the organization of bone indicates the importance of the fibrillar matrix in the structure of bone (see also Chap. 351). The noncollagenous organic components such as osteocalcin, osteonectin, or osteopontin also may play a role in the formation of the mineral phase of bone. Alkaline phosphatase is a marker for osteoblasts, and cellular levels of this enzyme correlate with mineralization potential of osteoblasts. Although mineralization defects occur in individuals with mutations in the alkaline phosphate gene that cause decreased alkaline phosphatase activity (hypophosphatasia), the function of alkaline phosphatase in mineralization is not completely understood. Inorganic pyrophosphate is a potent inhibitor of mineralization at concentrations below those necessary to bind calcium ions. Since alkaline phosphatase in osteoblasts and other cells can catalyze the hydrolysis of inorganic pyrophosphate a neutral pH, this enzyme could regulate mineralization by controlling the concentrations of pyrophosphate. In addition, macromolecular inhibitors such as proteoglycan aggregates also may influence mineralization. In cartilage undergoing calcification, mineralization may be initiated in membrane-bound vesicles outside the cells.

In bone, the calcium phosphate solid phase at the inception of mineralization is brushite ($CaHPO_4·2H_2O$). As mineralization progresses, the solid phase is a poorly crystalline hydroxyapatite with a relatively low (~1.2) calcium/phosphate molar ratio. With age and maturation, the perfection of the crystal and the calcium/phosphate ratio increase. Fluoride ions, when incorporated into the mineral phase, decrease the proportion of amorphous calcium phosphate and enhance the crystal structure.

There is a limit for the concentration of calcium and phosphorus ions in the ECF below which mineralization will not occur. A "solubility product" for bone mineral is difficult to calculate because the mineral phase itself is of variable composition and the various components in ECF that regulate this solubility product are not known. Nevertheless, when the concentrations of calcium and phosphorus in ECF are excessive, a mineral phase may form in areas that are not normally mineralized.

When bone is resorbed, calcium and phosphorus ions are released into the ECF, and the organic matrix is then resorbed. The fact that bone resorption takes place in the region of the osteoclast adjacent to the bone surface, where the extracellular pH is low, suggests that an acid environment is required for solubilization of bone mineral. The alkaline phosphatase of bone cells is an ectoenzyme that is released into the ECF. Increased circulating levels of the bone-derived enzyme are correlated with rates of bone formation. Other circulating markers of bone formation include osteocalcin and type I procollagen carboxy-terminal peptides. Urinary markers for bone resorption are hydroxy-proline, hydroxylysine and its glycosides, and the bone-specific hydroxypyridinium collagen cross-links.

CALCIUM METABOLISM There are about 1 to 2 kg calcium in the average adult body, over 98 percent of which is in the skeleton. The calcium of the mineral phase at the surface of the crystals is in equilibrium with the ECF, but only a minor proportion of the total calcium (about 0.5 percent) is exchangeable. The calcium in ECF is critical for a variety of functions, and it is remarkably constant. In normal adults, the range of plasma concentration is 2.2 to 2.6 mmol/L (8.8 to 10.4 mg/dL). The calcium in plasma is in three forms: as free ions, bound to plasma proteins, and, to a small extent, as diffusible complexes. The concentration of free calcium ions, mean 1.2 mmol/L (4.8 mg/dL), influences many cellular functions and is subjected to tight hormonal control, especially through parathyroid hormone (PTH), as described below. The concentration of serum proteins is an important determinant of calcium ion concentration; most is bound to albumin. Ionized calcium can be measured directly with the use of calcium-specific electrodes. If ionized calcium cannot be measured, certain approximations can be utilized to distinguish the protein bound from the ionized fraction. One formula that approximates the amount of calcium bound to protein is

$$\% \text{ protein-bound Ca} = 0.8 \times \text{albumin (g/L)}$$
$$+ 0.2 \times \text{globulin (g/L)} + 3$$

A simplified correction is sometimes used to indicate whether a stated total serum calcium concentration is abnormal when serum proteins are low. The correction is to add 1 mg/dL to serum calcium for every g/dL that serum albumin is below 4.0 g/dL. If the serum calcium, for example, is 7.8 mg/dL (a subnormal value) and the serum albumin is only 3.0 mg/dL, then the stated serum calcium is corrected by adding 1 mg/dL; the corrected value of 8.8 mg/dL is within the normal range. These rough approximations generally agree with measurements of ionized calcium in patients with subnormal serum proteins.

Calcium ions inside the cell mediate a variety of cellular functions (see also Chap. 69). Most of the cellular calcium is in the form of insoluble complexes. The concentration of free calcium within the cell, which is critical for functional regulation, is low, approximately 0.1 μmol/L; thus the gradient between plasma and intracellular free calcium is about 10,000 to 1. This gradient is tightly regulated. The concentration of calcium ions in the ECF is kept constant by processes that constantly feed calcium into and withdraw calcium from the extracellular fluid. Calcium enters the plasma via absorption from the intestinal tract and by resorption of ions from the bone mineral. Calcium leaves the ECF via secretion into the gastrointestinal tract (~100 to 200 mg/d), urinary excretion (~50 to 300 mg/d), deposition in bone mineral, and losses in sweat (up to 100 mg/d). Bone resorption and formation are tightly coupled, approximately 12 mmol (500 mg) calcium entering and leaving the skeleton daily (Fig. 356-2).

The average dietary calcium intake for most adults in the United States is approximately 15 to 20 mmol/d (0.6 to 0.8 g/d). However, with the heightened awareness of the role of adequate calcium intake for the prevention of osteoporosis, many adults on supplements have

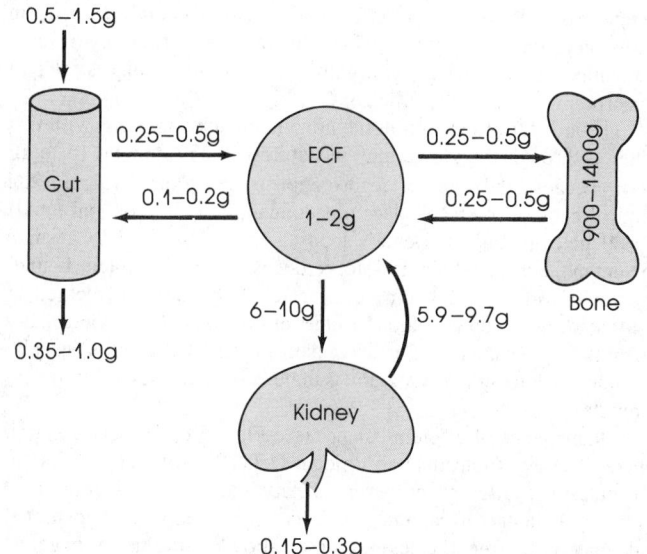

FIGURE 356-2 Calcium homeostasis. Schematic illustration of calcium content of extracellular fluid (ECF) and bone as well as of diet and feces; magnitude of calcium flux per day as calculated by various methods is shown at sites of transport in intestine, kidney, and bone. Ranges of values shown are approximate and chosen to illustrate certain points discussed in text. In intestine, absorption efficiency varies inversely with dietary calcium (chronic adaptation). This is reflected in typical quantities absorbed and excreted in feces; with 0.5-g intake, 50 percent absorption is depicted to occur (0.25 g), but at 1.5 g only 30 percent (0.5 g). Endogenous fecal calcium, the 0.1 to 0.2 g secreted into the intestinal lumen daily, is constant and does not vary with calcium intake or absorption. Quantities of calcium depicted as filtered, reabsorbed, and excreted at the kidney are chosen arbitrarily to indicate that at lower rates of filtration of calcium (expected at lower glomerular filtration rates), most is reabsorbed (e.g., 5.85 of 6 g), leading to urinary excretion of 150 mg; at higher rates of filtration (at high dietary calcium intake), slightly less is reabsorbed (e.g., 9.7 of 10 g), leading to a higher urinary excretion, 300 mg. In all situations, renal calcium reabsorption exceeds 95 percent of filtered load. Urinary calcium excretion is seen, therefore, to increase by only 150 mg despite a 1-g increase in dietary intake. In conditions of calcium balance, rates of calcium release from and uptake into bone are equal.

an intake of 20 to 37 mmol/d (0.8 to 1.5 g/d). In adults, less than half of dietary calcium is absorbed. Calcium absorption increases during periods of rapid growth in children, in pregnancy, and in lactation and decreases with advancing age. Most of the calcium is absorbed in the proximal small intestine, and the efficiency of absorption decreases in the more distal intestinal segments. Both active transport and diffusion-limited absorption are involved; the former is more important in the upper and the latter is more important in the lower intestine. Both processes are influenced by vitamin D through the action of its metabolites. All forms of calcium in the diet may not be equally absorbed; calcium as the chloride is probably absorbed more efficiently than that in other preparations.

Calcium is also secreted into the lumen of the gastrointestinal tract. When radioactive calcium is administered intravenously, it appears in the feces, making possible calculations of *endogenous fecal calcium* (see Fig. 356-2). Higher estimates of calcium losses in intestinal juices have been made by other techniques. Secretion of calcium into the intestinal lumen is constant and independent of absorption. If calcium availability in the diet is low [<12 mmol/d (500 mg/d)], positive calcium balance requires an efficiency of absorption greater than 30 to 40 percent.

The urinary calcium excretion of normal adults on average calcium intakes ranges between 2.5 and 10 mmol/d (100 and 400 mg/d). When the dietary calcium is below 5 mmol/d (200 mg/d), urinary calcium excretion is usually less than 5 mmol/d (200 mg/d). However, in most normal individuals, the level of dietary intake over a wide range has relatively little effect on urinary calcium. Hence, in individuals on diets low in calcium, this relative inefficiency of renal calcium conservation leads to negative calcium balance unless calcium absorption is maximally efficient (see Fig. 356-2).

The amount of calcium in the urine is minute compared with that filtered through the glomerulus [about 150 to 250 mmol/d (6 to 10 g/d)] because the rates of reabsorption of the filtered calcium are high. Reabsorption takes place predominantly in the proximal tubule (~60 percent) and in Henle's loop (~25 percent) and to a small extent in the distal tubule. It is not certain whether non-protein-bound, nonionic forms of calcium (e.g., calcium citrate) are cleared at different rates. The excretion of other electrolytes affects the urinary excretion of calcium. For example, urinary calcium is usually proportional to urinary sodium; sulfate also increases calcium excretion.

Maintenance of calcium balance (see Fig. 356-2) is dependent on the efficiency of intestinal absorption. Deficiency of PTH or vitamin D, intestinal disease, or severe dietary calcium deprivation may provide challenges to calcium homeostasis that cannot be compensated adequately by renal calcium conservation, resulting in negative calcium balance. Increased bone resorption may protect against ECF calcium depletion even in states of chronic negative calcium balance but only at the expense of progressive bone loss.

Pathophysiology Decrease in the concentration of free calcium ions in plasma results in increased neuromuscular irritability and tetany. This syndrome is characterized by peripheral and perioral paresthesias, carpal spasm, pedal spasm, anxiety, seizures, bronchospasm, laryngospasm, Chvostek's, Trousseau's, and Erb's signs, and lengthening of the QT interval of the electrocardiogram. In infants, tetany may be manifested only by irritability and lethargy. The level of calcium ions that determines which features of tetany will be manifested varies among individuals. Tetany is also influenced by the concentration of other components of the ECF. For example, hypomagnesemia and alkalosis lower whereas hypokalemia and acidosis raise the threshold for tetany.

Increases in total serum calcium are usually accompanied by increases in calcium ions and may be associated with anorexia, nausea, vomiting, constipation, hypotonia, depression, and occasionally lethargy and coma. Persistent hypercalcemia, especially when accompanied by normal or elevated levels of serum phosphate, may cause ectopic deposition of a solid phase of calcium and phosphate in walls of blood vessels, connective tissue about the joints, gastric mucosa, cornea, and renal parenchyma. Hypercalcemia per se alters renal function in addition to the pathologic effects of calcium phosphate deposition.

PHOSPHORUS METABOLISM Phosphorus is a major component of bone and of all other tissues and in some form is involved in almost all metabolic processes. The total amount of phosphorus in the normal adult is about 32 mol (1 kg), of which about 85 percent is in the skeleton.

In fasting plasma, most of the phosphorus is present as inorganic orthophosphate in concentrations of approximately 0.9 to 1.3 mmol/L (2.8 to 4 mg/dL). In contrast to calcium, where about 50 percent is bound, only about 12 percent of the phosphorus in plasma is bound to proteins. Free HPO_4^{2-} and $NaHPO_4^-$ normally are about 75 percent of the total phosphorus, and free $H_2PO_4^-$ is 10 percent. Since so many species are present, depending on pH and other factors, it is the convention to express concentrations in terms of mass of elemental phosphorus, i.e., millimoles per liter or milligrams per deciliter. Total phosphorus levels are higher in children and in women after the menopause. There is a circadian variation in phosphorus concentration even during a 24-h fast, mediated in part by the adrenal cortex. The nadir occurs between 9 A.M. and 12 noon, followed by an increase to a plateau in the afternoon and another small peak after midnight. The magnitudes of the peaks and troughs vary with phosphorus intake but occur regardless of whether the intake is high or low. Dietary restriction of phosphorus that only modestly decreases the morning fasting levels may abolish the afternoon rise. Despite changes in

serum phosphorus levels of nearly twofold, serum ionized calcium levels do not change significantly.

During phosphate depletion, phosphaturia decreases before serum phosphorus declines. This adaptive response of increasing tubular transport when luminal concentrations are decreasing is an intrinsic property of these cells. There is also heterogeneity of phosphorus transport among different segments of proximal renal tubules. Tubular fluxes of phosphorus rather than hypophosphatemia per se may be critical in modulating effects of hypophosphatemia such as the stimulation of 25(OH)D-1α-hydroxylase. Conversely, increased phosphorus loads and increased renal tubular phosphorus fluxes result in decreased renal tubular reabsorption and increased clearance of phosphorus and suppress the activity of 25(OH)D-1α-hydroxylase (see below). Ingestion of carbohydrate depresses serum phosphorus acutely by 0.3 to 0.5 mmol/L (1 to 1.5 mg/dL), presumably as the result of cellular uptake and formation of phosphate esters. Ingestion of phosphorus per se increases serum levels. Therefore, for the interpretation of serum levels and urinary clearances, samples should be obtained in the fasting state. Decreases in plasma phosphorus also occur during induction of alkalosis.

Whereas dietary calcium is inefficiently absorbed from the intestine, phosphorus absorption is remarkably efficient. At low levels of intake (less than 2 mg/kg of body weight per day), 80 to 90 percent of ingested phosphorus is absorbed. Even with levels of intake greater than 10 mg/kg of body weight per day in the form of dairy products, cereals, eggs, and meat, absorption is about 70 percent. Hypophosphatemia due to deficient intestinal absorption is unusual except when nonabsorbable antacids are consumed; the antacids bind phosphorus and prevent absorption from the intestinal lumen.

The major control of phosphorus economy is exerted at the level of the kidney. Phosphorus filtered through the glomerulus is largely reabsorbed in the proximal tubule (there is homeostatically important distal reabsorption as well) so that only about 10 to 15 percent of the filtered load is normally excreted. When filtered loads of phosphorus decrease, proximal tubular reabsorption increases. Conversely, when phosphorus loads are increased, tubular reabsorption decreases and clearance rises. Thus the urinary excretion of phosphorus normally reflects dietary intake, and conservation or elimination of excessive amounts depends on adequate renal handling (Fig. 356-3). There is no good evidence for renal tubular phosphate secretion. Proximal reabsorption of phosphorus is dependent on parallel sodium reabsorption, but whereas the sodium rejected by the proximal tubule may be reabsorbed distally, the rejected phosphorus is not. Therefore, volume expansion and decreased sodium reabsorption increase phosphorus clearance; similarly, diuretics that act proximally, such as acetazolamide, are phosphaturic parallel to the degree to which they are natriuretic.

Pathophysiology No direct symptoms result from hyperphosphatemia. When high levels are maintained for long periods, however, the driving force for mineralization is increased, and calcium phosphate may be deposited in abnormal sites. Ectopic calcification of this type is encountered in untreated chronic renal failure, with severe hypercalcemia, and in vitamin D intoxication. *Tumoral calcinosis* is a rare heritable disorder in which ectopic calcification is associated with hyperphosphatemia and normal glomerular filtration rates (GFR). The disorder is characterized by high ratio of phosphorus tubule maximum (TmP) to GFR and increased serum levels of 1,25(OH)$_2$D. The latter is a paradoxical finding and presumably is related to the abnormal renal tubular phosphate fluxes. In contrast, severe acute hypophosphatemia may cause anorexia, dizziness, bone pain, proximal muscular weakness, and waddling gait. Significant hypophosphatemia is encountered in severe alcoholics and may be aggravated after repletion of nutrients, in the course of therapy of diabetic ketoacidosis, and for various reasons in severely ill, hospitalized elderly patients (see also Chap. 359). Myopathy in severe hypophosphatemia may be accompanied by elevations in serum creatinine kinase levels and by rhabdomyolysis. Severe congestive cardiomyopathy may occur with chronic hypophosphatemia, and restoration of phosphorus

FIGURE 356-3 Phosphate homeostasis. Schematic illustration of inorganic phosphorus content (termed here *phosphate*) in extracellular fluid (ECF) and bone as well as diet and feces; magnitude of phosphorus flux per day as estimated by various methods is shown at transport sites in intestine, kidney, and bone. Range of values shown illustrates special features of phosphorus metabolism discussed in text. Intestinal phosphorus absorption is highly efficient, 85 percent at a lower intake (0.5 g of a 0.6-g intake) and 70 percent at a higher intake (1.4 g of a 2.0-g intake). Estimates of magnitude of endogenous fecal phosphate are less well established than for calcium. Contribution of at least 0.15 g is estimated to be added to the nonabsorbed phosphorus to provide a total of 0.2 g fecal phosphorus at the low intake level. At high phosphorus dietary intakes, no correction for endogenous fecal phosphate is calculated. Higher quantities of phosphorus are excreted in urine at all levels of dietary intake than for corresponding intakes of calcium; quantities excreted match closely the quantities absorbed, thereby maintaining phosphorus balance (no correction in this illustration is made for endogenous fecal phosphorus). Note that renal phosphorus reabsorption, in contrast to high and relatively invariant renal calcium reabsorption, varies from a low of 75 percent of filtered load to greater than 85 percent. The compartment labeled ICF refers to intracellular phosphorus, both organic and inorganic; rapid shifts of phosphorus into cells (and corresponding, possibly slower, efflux of phosphorus from cells) contribute to changes in ECF phosphorus. These shifts between ECF and ICF and phosphorus release from and uptake by bone are equal in conditions of phosphorus balance.

deficits leads to prompt reversal. Respiratory muscle weakness in severe hypophosphatemia also may improve with phosphate repletion. The bone pain and waddling gait are attributed to the osteomalacia that develops as a result of phosphate depletion. The muscular weakness may be due either to direct effects of hypophosphatemia on nerves and muscle or, in some instances, to the effects of hyperparathyroidism (either primary or secondary) which may have a role in the etiology of the hypophosphatemia. Phosphorus depletion in children may cause defective growth. Hypophosphatemia results in decreased levels of 2,3-diphosphoglyceric acid and adenosine triphosphate (ATP) in erythrocytes, which in turn alter the dissociation of oxyhemoglobin so that less oxygen is delivered to tissues. Hemolytic anemia may result from impairment of the ability of erythrocytes to deform in small vessels.

VITAMIN D

Vitamin D is a hormone, not a vitamin. With adequate exposure to sunlight, no dietary supplements are needed. The active principle of

vitamin D is synthesized under metabolic control via successive hydroxylations in the liver and kidney and is transported through the blood to its target tissues (the small intestine and bone), where it regulates calcium homeostasis. Calcium and phosphate ions, parathyroid hormone, and possibly other peptide and steroid hormones regulate the renal metabolism of vitamin D. Analysis of hereditary and acquired defects in these processes has provided new insights into the pathophysiology of several disorders involving calcium, phosphorus, and bone metabolism. These discoveries culminated in the chemical synthesis of active vitamin D metabolites and analogues, the clinical use of $1\alpha,25$-dihydroxyvitamin D_3 [1,25(OH)$_2D_3$] (calcitriol) in many vitamin D–resistant disorders, and the development of assays for measuring vitamin D metabolites in blood to define suspected abnormalities in vitamin D metabolism.

PHOTOBIOGENESIS OF VITAMIN D Vitamin D_3 is a derivative of 7-dehydrocholesterol (provitamin D_3), the immediate precursor of cholesterol. When skin is exposed to sunlight or certain artificial light sources, the ultraviolet radiation enters the epidermis and causes transformation of 7-dehydrocholesterol to vitamin D_3. Wavelengths between 290 and 315 nm are absorbed by the conjugated double bonds at C_5 and C_7 of 7-dehydrocholesterol and fragment the B ring between C_9 and C_{10} to yield a 9,10-secosterol (*seco* means "split"), previtamin D_3 (Fig. 356-4). Previtamin D_3 is biologically inert but spontaneously undergoes a temperature-dependent molecular rearrangement of its conjugated triene system (three double bonds) to form the thermally stable 9,10-secosterol, vitamin D_3 (see Fig. 356-4). At body temperature it takes approximately 24 h for previtamin D_3 to convert completely into vitamin D_3. Wide changes in skin surface do not affect the rate of this conversion because the process occurs in the actively growing layers of the epidermis, where the temperature is relatively constant; changes in the core body temperature also have little effect on this reaction. Once vitamin D_3 is synthesized, it is translocated from the epidermis into the circulation by the vitamin D–binding protein. Thus vitamin D_3 is made in the skin from previtamin for many hours after a single sun exposure (see Fig. 356-4). Although melanin in the skin competes with 7-dehydrocholesterol for ultraviolet photons and thus can limit the synthesis of previtamin D_3, the photochemical isomerization of previtamin D_3 and vitamin D_3 to biologically inert products appears to be more important in preventing excessive production of previtamin D_3 and vitamin D_3 during prolonged exposure to the sun.

Aging decreases the capacity of the skin to produce vitamin D_3; greater than fourfold reduction occurs after the age of 70 years. Topical sunscreens can reduce or prevent the cutaneous vitamin D_3 production by absorbing the solar radiation responsible for previtamin D_3 synthesis in the skin. Other factors that affect the cutaneous synthesis of vitamin D_3 include altitude, geographic location, time of day, and area of exposure. Latitude has profound effects on the cutaneous synthesis of vitamin D_3. As the zenith angle of the sun increases with approaching winter, more of the high-energy ultraviolet photons responsible for previtamin D_3 synthesis are absorbed by the ozone layer. In Boston (42°N) and in Edmonton (52°N), the absorption of these photons is so complete that essentially no vitamin D_3 is made in the skin between the months of November through February and October through March, respectively. When the entire body is exposed to sufficient sunlight to cause mild erythema, the increase in the blood vitamin D is about equivalent to consuming an oral dose of 10,000 to 25,000 international units (1 IU = 0.025 μg) of vitamin D. Only when skin irradiation is insufficient to produce the required quantities of vitamin D_3 is dietary supplementation needed to prevent skeletal mineralization defects. Fish liver oils, a natural source of vitamin D, were used widely for the treatment of rickets early in this century. The fortification of milk and some cereals with either crystalline vitamin D_2 (see Fig. 356-4) or vitamin D_3 prevents rickets and osteomalacia. However, a survey of the vitamin D content in milk from five Eastern states revealed that 71 percent did not contain 80 to 120 percent of the amount of vitamin D on the label and 20 percent of samples of skim milk did not contain detectable vitamin D. Although type II who are unable to respond to physiologic concentrations of 1,25(OH)₂D (because of mutations that impair receptors for this hormone) appear to have no demonstrable in vivo defects in the cellular immune response and in the growth of skin (with the exception of the associated alopecia) and other tissues. When these patients receive infusions of calcium, the metabolic bone disease is reversed. Although the use of $1,25(OH)_2D$ (calcitriol) for the treatment of leukemia is not efficacious, the antiproliferative activity of calcitriol and its analogue calcipotriene provides the rationale for the use of these compounds in the treatment of psoriasis.

Most measurements of circulating $1,25(OH)_2D$ in various physiologic or pathologic states utilize a receptor/competitive binding assay (Table 356-2). Serum concentrations of vitamin D and 25(OH)D vary with the season and with vitamin D intake. Serum concentrations of $1,25(OH)_2D$, however, appear to be unaltered by seasonal variation, by increases in dietary vitamin D, or by exposure to sunlight; as long as vitamin D supplies and circulating concentrations of 25(OH)D are sufficient, metabolic influences control the renal 25(OH)D-1α-hydroxylase to ensure a closely regulated circulating concentration of $1,25(OH)_2D$. The serum concentration of $1,25(OH)_2D$ ranges from 40 to 160 pmol/L (16 to 65 pg/mL). The serum half-life of $1,25(OH)_2D$ is from 3 to 6 h.

When concentrations of calcium in plasma fall below normal, secretion of PTH is enhanced, resulting in increased production of $1,25(OH)_2D$. The principal physiologic regulation of the production of $1,25(OH)_2D$ appears to involve changes in serum extracellular calcium concentrations that result in reciprocal changes in secretion of PTH, the latter controlling, possibly through actions on serum or tissue phosphorus concentrations, the rate of $1,25(OH)_2D$ production. Other factors that enhance $1,25(OH)_2D$ production include estrogen, prolactin, and growth hormone. Humans adapt to increased calcium requirements during growth, pregnancy, and lactation by increasing the efficiency of intestinal calcium absorption, possibly by enhancing 25(OH)D-1α-hydroxylase activity. During the first two trimesters of pregnancy, the concentrations of $1,25(OH)_2D$ increase in proportion to the concentrations of the vitamin D–binding protein; concentrations of free $1,25(OH)_2D$ do not change. During the last trimester, the need for calcium for mineralization of the fetal skeleton is met by an increase in the free concentrations of $1,25(OH)_2D$, which in turn enhance maternal intestinal calcium absorption.

PATHOPHYSIOLOGY OF DISORDERS OF VITAMIN D NUTRITION AND METABOLISM *Hypovitaminosis D* results from inadequate endogenous production of vitamin D_3 in the skin, insufficient dietary supplementation, and/or the inability of the small intestine to absorb adequate amounts of vitamin D from the diet. Resistance to the effects of vitamin D can result from (1) use of drugs that antagonize vitamin D action, (2) alterations in the metabolism of vitamin D, or (3) deficient or defective receptors for $1,25(OH)_2D$. The consequences of hypovitaminosis D include (1) disturbances of mineral ion metabolism and secretion of PTH and (2) mineralization defects in the skeleton (e.g., rickets in children, osteomalacia in adults). The changes in the skeleton are described in Chap. 358. With regard to calcium metabolism, lack of vitamin D action leads to insufficient intestinal calcium absorption and hypocalcemia. The latter stimulates the secretion of PTH (secondary hyperparathyroidism), which enhances calcium release from bone and decreases calcium clearance by the kidney and tends to blunt the hypocalcemia. (Late in the course of untreated hypovitaminosis D, severe hypocalcemia develops.) Hypophosphatemia is more marked than hypocalcemia, especially in early stages of vitamin D deficiency. The efficiency of intestinal phosphate absorption is also decreased. The increased secretin of PTH, although partially effective in minimizing hypocalcemia, leads to urinary phosphate wasting through decreases in renal tubular reabsorption. This latter effect is the most significant factor in causing hypophosphatemia. With an adequate GFR, the predominant changes are hypophosphatemia, moderate or slight hypocalcemia, increased levels of PTH, and low levels of 25(OH)D (see Table 356-1). As discussed in Chap. 358 defects in skeletal mineralization may accompany these disturbances in mineral ion metabolism.

Although the conversion of vitamin D to 25(OH)D is impaired in severe chronic liver disease, there is no strong correlation between low serum 25(OH)D levels and osteopenia. Patients with nephrotic syndrome with more than 4 g/d of proteinuria may have low 25(OH)D levels due to the loss in the urine of the vitamin D-binding protein with its associated tightly bound 25(OH)D. Circulating levels of 25(OH)D also may be decreased when the catabolism of 25(OH)D is increased, as in sarcoidosis and hyperparathyroidism. Chronic anticonvulsant therapy also can cause the development of osteomalacia or rickets; mineralization defects are worse in patients on multiple drug therapy and when vitamin D intake or exposure to sunlight is inadequate. Anticonvulsant drugs have multiple effects on calcium metabolism. Phenobarbital induces hepatic microsomal enzymes, alters the kinetics of the vitamin D-25-hydroxylase, and stimulates bile secretion, which result in decreased serum concentrations of vitamin D and 25(OH)D. Phenytoin and phenobarbital inhibit intestinal calcium transport and bone mineral mobilization, independent of effects of vitamin D metabolism.

Glucocorticoids in high doses cause disturbances in calcium metabolism and osteoporosis but do not induce osteomalacia and rickets. Glucocorticoids directly inhibit vitamin D–mediated intestinal calcium absorption and bone mineral mobilization and enhance the sensitivity of bone cells to $1,25(OH)_2D$ by stabilizing the $1,25(OH)_2D$ receptor or by increasing the affinity or number of receptors. Patients receiving glucocorticoids chronically may have depressed circulating levels of $1,25(OH)_2D$; the mechanism(s) is unknown.

A genetic defect in the hepatic 25-hydroxylation of vitamin D has not been described, but in one inherited disorder of calcium and bone metabolism renal production of $1,25(OH)_2D$ is defective. In the syndrome of pseudovitamin D–deficient rickets (also known as vitamin D–dependent rickets type I; see Chap. 358), circulating levels of $1,25(OH)_2D$ are low, but the therapeutic response to physiologic doses of calcitriol (0.25 to 1.0 μg/d) is normal. These findings are accounted for by a deficiency in renal 25(OH)D-1α-hydroxylase activity. In patients with a similar phenotype, pseudovitamin D–resistant rickets (vitamin D–dependent rickets type II), mutations that impair the $1,25(OH)_2D$ receptors alter hormone binding or DNA

TABLE 356-2 Serum concentrations of 1,25(OH)₂D in disorders of calcium, phosphorus, and bone metabolism

Disease states	Serum 1,25(OH)₂D
Vitamin D deficiency	↓ *
Renal failure:	
GFR > (30 mL/min)/1.7 m²	↓ or N
GFR < (30 mL/min)/1.7 m²	↓
Hypoparathyroidism	↓ or N
Pseudohypoparathyroidism	↓ or N
Vitamin D–dependent rickets:	
Type I	↓
Type II	↑
X-linked vitamin D–resistant rickets	↓ or N
Tumor-induced osteomalacia	↓
Oncogenic hypercalcemia	↓
Some lymphomas	↑
Hyperparathyroidism	↑
Sarcoidosis, tuberculosis, silicosis	↑
Idiopathic hypercalciuria	N or ↑
Williams' syndrome	↑
Vitamin D intoxication	N or ↑

* Serum 1,25(OH)₂D concentrations are normal or elevated in occasional patients with biopsy-proven osteomalacia and undetectable or low circulating concentrations of 25(OH)D. These patients also have secondary hyperparathyroidism, and they may represent a partially treated state; if a small amount of vitamin D is obtained from the diet or generated in the skin in these patients, the vitamin is efficiently converted to 1,25(OH)₂D. The net effect is low or undetectable circulating concentrations of 25(OH)D along with normal or elevated concentrations of 1,25(OH)₂D. However, in extreme vitamin D deficiency, circulating concentrations of 1,25(OH)₂D are low or undetectable.

NOTE: ↓ = decreased; N = normal; ↑ = increased; GFR = glomerular filtration rate.

binding of the receptor-hormone complex. Individuals with this disorder have high circulating levels of $1,25(OH)_2D$; administration of high doses of vitamin D produce further increases in the levels of $1,25(OH)_2D$.

In patients with X-linked hypophosphatemic rickets, serum concentrations of $1,25(OH)_2D$ are normal or low. Since hypophosphatemia is a potent stimulator of the renal $25(OH)D-1\alpha$-hydroxylase, levels of $1,25(OH)_2D$ should be high. In this syndrome there is a functional defect in the $25(OH)D-1\alpha$-hydrolase even in the presence of normal circulating levels of $1,25(OH)_2D$. Therefore, the combination of calcitriol and phosphate supplements is superior to therapy with phosphate supplements alone (Chap. 358). In patients with mild to moderate chronic renal failure [GFR > 0.5 mL/s (> 30 mL/min)] and decreased phosphate clearance, hyperphosphatemia and acidosis play important roles in suppressing the renal production of $1,25(OH)_2D$ despite high circulating concentrations of PTH. With progressive destruction of the renal cortex, the reserves of the $25(OH)D-1\alpha$-hydroxylase are depleted to a point at which the kidney is unable to produce sufficient $1,25(OH)_2D$ to maintain calcium homeostasis, even when serum phosphorus concentrations are normal. Under these circumstances, replacement therapy with calcitriol is most beneficial (Chap. 358). Aging decreases the responsiveness of the renal $25(OH)D-1\alpha$-hydroxylase to PTH, results in small decreases in circulating levels of $1,25(OH)_2D$, and may contribute to decreased calcium absorption in the elderly.

Patients with hypocalcemia due to hypoparathyroidism or pseudo-hypoparathyroidism have lower than normal mean serum concentrations of $1,25(OH)_2D$, although individual values may be in the normal range. In these patients, small replacement doses of calcitriol (0.25 to 1.0 μg/d; see Chap. 357) are effective even when the serum $25(OH)D$ concentrations are elevated. These observations suggest that absent or ineffective action of PTH decreases the activity of renal $25(OH)D-1\alpha$-hydroxylase. It is not known to what extent serum $1,25(OH)_2D$ concentrations would be restored if the hyperphosphatemia were adequately controlled.

Patients with tumor-induced (oncogenic) osteomalacia have low levels of serum phosphorus and $1,25(OH)_2D$. These tumors presumably secrete a substance(s) that causes renal phosphorus wasting and inhibits the synthesis of $1,25(OH)_2D$; after removal of the tumor, the serum phosphorus and $1,25(OH)_2D$ levels return to normal.

In disorders such as sarcoidosis (and other chronic granulomatous disorders), lymphomas, idiopathic hypercalciuria, and Williams' syndrome there is enhanced synthesis of $1,25(OH)_2D$ from $25(OH)D$ (see Table 356-2). Hypercalcemia and hypercalciuria in sarcoidosis are associated with elevated circulating concentrations of $1,25(OH)_2D$; granulomas and pulmonary alveolar macrophages from patients with sarcoidosis synthesize $1,25(OH)_2D$. Normal pulmonary macrophages also can be induced to metabolize $25(OH)D$ to $1,25(OH)_2D$ in vitro when exposed to lipopolysaccharides from the cell wall of gram-negative bacteria or to interferon-γ. Most patients with tumor-induced hypercalcemia have low circulating concentrations of $1,25(OH)_2D$ (see Table 356-2). The exceptions are patients with several types of lymphoma (including T cell, mixed histiocytic-lymphocytic, and B cell immunoblastic lymphomas) where hypercalcemia is associated with elevated concentrations of $1,25(OH)_2D$. In one report, surgical excision of a solitary splenic lymphoma resulted in rapid return of elevated serum $1,25(OH)_2D$ and calcium levels to normal, suggesting that the lymphoma metabolized $25(OH)D$ to $1,25(OH)_2D$ in an unregulated manner. Patients with hypercalcemia and elevated blood levels of $1,25(OH)_2$ due to unregulated extrarenal production of the hormone respond to glucocorticoids with a decrease in the circulating concentrations of $1,25(OH)_2D$ and calcium. Patients with primary hyperparathyrodisim, hypercalciuria, and renal stones, on average, have elevated circulating levels of $1,25(OH)_2D$. Similarly, in some instances of idiopathic hypercalciuria, intestinal calcium absorption is inappropriately increased. Approximately one-third of these patients have elevated circulating $1,25(OH)_2D$. These findings are consistent with the hypothesis that excessive $1,25(OH)_2D$ production is responsi-

ble for the hyperabsorption of calcium by the small intestine. Infants with hypercalcemia associated with supravalvular aortic stenosis, mental retardation, and elfin facies (*Williams' syndrome*) also have elevated serum concentrations of $1,25(OH)_2D$. It is not clear whether the increased levels result from abnormal synthesis or degradation of $1,25(OH)_2D$.

PHARMACOLOGY AND SOURCES OF VITAMIN D AND ITS METABOLITES Casual exposure to sunlight provides most humans with their vitamin D requirement. For the elderly who wish to take advantage of this natural source of vitamin D, exposure of hands, face, and arms to a suberythemal dose of sunlight two to three times a week is usually adequate. If the patient plans to remain outdoors in sunlight after the initial exposure, a sunscreen with a protection factor of at least 15 (SPF-15) should be applied to help prevent the damaging effects caused by excessive chronic overexposure to sunlight. A variety of over-the-counter vitamin preparations contain 400 IU of either vitamin D_2 or vitamin D_3. More potent preparations of vitamin D (calciferol) are available in capsule and tablet form (50,000 IU), as oil (500,000 IU/mL), and in oral solution (8000 IU/mL). A single oral dose of 50,000 IU of vitamin D_2 increases the circulating concentrations of vitamin D from less than 25 nmol/L (10 ng/mL) to 130 to 260 nmol/L (50 to 100 ng/mL) within 12 to 24 h; the plasma half-life is about 2 days. Serum concentrations of $25(OH)D$ and $1,25(OH)_2D$ are not changed by these doses of vitamin D. For treatment of vitamin D deficiency, 50,000 IU of vitamin D twice a week for several weeks raises the circulating concentration of $25(OH)D$ into the normal range; in the presence of secondary hyperparathyroidism, the circulating concentrations of $1,25(OH)_2D$ can increase to supranormal levels [up to 600 pmol/L (250 pg/mL)]. $25(OH)D_3$ (calcifediol) is available in capsules containing either 20 or 50 μg. This drug may be useful in treating vitamin D deficiency [low $25(OH)D$ concentrations] in patients with severe liver dysfunction. Pharmacologic doses are used to treat disorders of $25(OH)D$ metabolism; in pharmacologic doses, $25(OH)D_3$ is believed to act via interaction with the receptor for $1,25(OH)_2D$. $1,25(OH)_2D$ (calcitriol) is available in capsules containing 0.25 or 0.5 μg and as a solution for intravenous use (1.0 and 2.0 μg/mL). Calcitriol is efficacious in a variety of disorders (see Chap. 357). 1α-Hydroxyvitamin D_3 $[1(OH)D_3]$ is a potent $1,25(OH)_2D_3$ agonist that is used in Europe and Japan. The structure of this analogue is identical to that of the natural renal hormone with the exception that it lacks a C_{25} OH (Fig. 356-6). In humans, this analogue is rapidly metabolized by the liver to $1,25(OH)_2D_3$. Topical preparations of calcitriol (3 μg/g) and calcipotriene (50 μg/g) are available in Europe for the treatment of psoriasis. When used over a large surface area, both can cause hypercalcemia.

When vitamin D is chemically manipulated to rotate the A ring through 180 degrees, the C_3 β-OH assumes a geometric position that mimics the C_1 α-OH (see Fig. 356-6). These compounds, called *pseudo-1α-hydroxyvitamin D analogues*, include the clinically useful dihydrotachysterol (DHT). This analogue is less effective in stimulating intestinal calcium transport on a weight basis than either vitamin D or $1,25(OH)_2D$, but because it does not require 1α-hydroxylation to be active on intestinal calcium transport, it is 3 to 10 times more potent than vitamin D in disease states that impair renal $25(OH)D-1\alpha$-hydroxylase, such as hypoparathyroidism and chronic renal failure. Dihydrotachysterol is efficiently metabolized in the liver to 25-hydroxy-DHT, which is the biologically active form.

PARATHYROID HORMONE **Physiology** The function of PTH is to maintain ECF calcium concentration. The hormone acts directly on bone and kidney and indirectly on intestine through its effects on synthesis of $1,25(OH)_2D$ to increase serum calcium concentrations; in turn, PTH production is closely regulated by the concentration of serum ionized calcium. This feedback system is the critical homeostatic mechanism for maintenance of ECF calcium. Any tendency toward hypocalcemia, as might be induced by calcium-deficient diets, is counteracted by an increased secretion of PTH. This in turn (1) acts to increase the rate of dissolution of bone mineral, thereby

FIGURE 356-6 Structure of 1,25-dihydroxyvitamin D_3, i.e. $1\alpha,25(OH)_2D_3$, and some of its clinically important analogues. When vitamin D_3, is hydrogenated, its A ring is rotated 180°, placing the 3β-OH in a pseudo 1α spatial orientation. This analogue, dihydrotachysterol (DHT_3) is metabolized by a liver 25-hydroxylase (step 25) to 25-hydroxydihydrotachysterol, i.e., $25(OH)DHT_3$. It is believed that $25(OH)DHT_3$ is the biologically active form that mimics $1,25(OH)_2D_3$ in its activity. Two clinically important analogues of $1\alpha,25(OH)_2D_3$ include its 25-deoxy derivative 1α-hydroxyvitamin D_3, i.e., $1\alpha(OH)D_3$, and calcipotriene. $1\alpha(OH)D_3$ is metabolized in the liver by 25-hydroxylase to $1\alpha,25(OH)D_3$. Calcipotriene is an analogue that is currently being used in Europe for the topical treatment of psoriasis.

increasing the flow of calcium from bone into blood, (2) reduces the renal clearance of calcium, returning more of the calcium filtered at the glomerulus into ECF, and (3) increases the efficiency of calcium absorption in the intestine. The relative physiologic importance in minute-to-minute calcium homeostasis of stimulation of calcium transport in bone, kidney, and intestine is not established, but immediate control of blood calcium is probably due to effects of the hormone on bone and, to a lesser extent, on renal calcium clearance. Maintenance of steady state calcium balance, on the other hand, probably results from the effects of the hormone on $1,25(OH)_2D$ levels and hence on the efficiency of intestinal calcium absorption. As much as 12 mmol (500 mg) calcium is transferred between ECF and bone each day (a large amount in relation to the total ECF calcium pool), and PTH has a major effect on this transfer. The homeostatic role of the hormone serves to preserve calcium concentration in blood acutely at the cost of bone destruction. The action of PTH on kidney to increase the reabsorption of filtered calcium also may contribute to rapid regulation of blood calcium concentration.

PTH has a dual action on bone, the *calcium replacement* and the *bone remodeling* effects. There is an increased rate of release of calcium from bone into blood after administration of PTH, the time needed to observe the change varying with the dose of hormone and the overall metabolic status (influenced by age, diet, etc.). Usually

30 min to 1 h is required to detect a significant increase in blood calcium, but with the use of radioisotopes, changes in bone calcium release can be seen within minutes. When studied carefully in animals, a rapid efflux of calcium out of blood into bone, presumably into bone cells, precedes the release of calcium from bone. On the other hand, the chronic effects of PTH, mainly an increase in the number of osteoclasts and a general increase in the remodeling of bone, are apparent only hours after the hormone is given. These latter actions, which involve increased protein synthesis, persist for hours after PTH has been given. The administration of PTH intermittently over days in animals leads to a net stimulation of bone formation rather than bone breakdown. Human studies in vitro and in vivo confirm that chronic intermittent hormone administration can lead to anabolic actions in skeleton rather than merely increased turnover. This skeletal anabolic action of PTH is being studied in clinical trials, but the extent and mechanism of the effect are still poorly understood. Osteoblasts mediate principally the bone-forming response of PTH and indirectly stimulate osteoclasts. Osteoclasts are the principal bone-resorbing cells.

Osteoblastic cells but not osteoclasts have receptors for PTH. The action of PTH on osteoclasts is indirect, through cytokines released from osteoblasts to activate osteoclasts; e.g., osteoblasts must be present along with osteoclasts for PTH to activate osteoclasts to resorb bone. The nature of the cytokines that stimulate osteoclasts is a subject of major interest. IGF-1, interleukin-6, GM-CSF, and possibly other agents are candidates, but the definitive messenger(s) has not been determined.

Chemistry The complete amino acid sequences of PTH from cow, pig, rat, and human have been defined. The peptides consist of a single-chain structure composed of 84 amino acids. The molecules lack cysteine or cystine; the sequences of the four forms of the hormone are similar. The sequence of chicken PTH has been deduced from the nucleotide sequence of the cloned cDNA. This molecule differs from the mammalian hormones. One large sequence deletion in the middle of the molecule, and a larger addition near the carboxyl terminus result in a molecule of 88 rather than 84 amino acids. There is, however, marked conservation in the amino-terminal portion needed for biologic actions of the molecule.

Some structural requirements for the binding of the hormone to receptors and hence for its biologic activity have been defined. Synthetic fragments containing the amino-terminal sequence residues 1–34 (or even shorter sequences, 2–26 being minimally active) exert the known biologic actions of the hormone on mineral ion transport in kidney and bone and, by stimulating the renal 25-hydroxyvitamin D-1α-hydroxylase, stimulate intestinal calcium absorption.

Fragments shortened at the amino terminus lose binding affinity more slowly than capacity to stimulate biologic response. The peptide composed of sequences 7–34 is a competitive inhibitor of the binding of active hormone to receptors in vitro but is a weak inhibitor in vivo.

Biosynthesis, secretion, and metabolism and mode of action Several larger molecular forms have been identified in the biosynthetic sequence leading from gene transcription and translation to final packaging of the 84-amino acid peptide in secretory granules prior to secretion. The earliest detected precursor, *preproparathyroid hormone*, consists of 115 amino acids; this molecular form is converted to an intermediate form of 90 amino acids termed *proparathyroid hormone*, and then to the secreted product of 84 amino acids, PTH. PTH shares with other polypeptides and proteins destined for secretion from cells this complex pattern of initial synthesis as a larger molecule which is then reduced in size by several cleavages prior to secretion. The regulation of these sequential steps in PTH biosynthesis is poorly understood except by analogy with regulatory steps in biosynthesis, transport, and packaging of other proteins destined for secretion. The hydrophobic regions of the preproparathyroid hormone are similar to preprotein-specific regions of other cell-secreted proteins and serve a role in guiding transport of the polypeptide from sites of synthesis on polyribosomes through the endoplasmic reticulum to secretory granules. In one kindred with hypoparathyroidism, a mutation disrupts the critical hydrophobic sequence and interferes with hormone secretion.

The genes for bovine, rat, and human PTH have been cloned, and the gene structures from these three species are highly homologous. Studies with cloned and expressed PTH genes in vitro have demonstrated regions for control of gene expression at the transcriptional level, including sites for interaction and regulation by $1,25(OH)_2D$ and its receptor and "upstream" silencer elements as well as sites in which ambient calcium concentration regulates transcription. These in vitro observations are not well understood in terms of physiologic regulation of PTH biosynthesis and secretion; the rate of processing of hormone precursors and the proteolytic destruction and turnover of the hormone itself (posttranslational regulation of hormone production) may be more central to hormone availability than changes in rates of transcription. It does not appear that changes in transcriptional activity of the PTH gene in the normal physiologic range of levels of blood calcium and $1,25(OH)_2D$ nor in short-term environmental stresses (e.g., fasting for 24 h) are important in control of blood levels of the hormone. Control is exerted by precise and rapid variation of rates of processing of preformed hormone under the control of ECF calcium.

Blood calcium concentration over wide ranges controls the secretion of PTH; the ionized fraction of blood calcium is the important determinant of hormone secretion. Hormone secretion increases steeply to a maximum value of fivefold above basal rates of secretion as calcium concentration falls from normal to the range of 1.9 to 2.0 mmol/L (7.5 to 8.0 mg/dL) (measured as total calcium). Beta-adrenergic agonists such as epinephrine and H-2 agonists also may increase hormone secretion, but the physiologic significance of these secretagogues is not established. Furthermore, drugs such as propranolol or cimetidine do not reproducibly decrease circulating PTH levels.

Magnesium may influence hormone secretion in the same direction as calcium but is a less potent secretagogue. It is unlikely that physiologic variations in magnesium concentration affect PTH secretion, but severe intracellular magnesium deficiency impairs PTH secretion.

The hormone secreted in vivo by normal bovine and human parathyroid glands and from parathyroid adenomas is indistinguishable by immunologic criteria and by molecular size from the 84-amino acid peptide (molecular weight 9500) extracted from glands. However, much of the immunoreactive material found in the circulation of humans and animals (cow, dog) is smaller than the extracted or secreted hormone. The principal circulating fragments of immunoreactive hormone (approximate molecular weight 7000) lack a portion of the critical amino-terminal sequence required for biologic activity and, hence, are biologically inactive fragments (so-called middle- and carboxyl-terminal fragments). Study of these fragments suggests that an endopeptidase cleaves the molecule into at least two types of

pieces. Much of the proteolysis of hormone occurs in the liver and kidney.

The proteolytic process should result in formation of a second fragment (molecular weight 2000 to 3000) representing the amino-terminal, biologically active portion of the hormone. Hormone fragments as well as intact hormone are also released from the gland. However, fragments corresponding only to the middle- and carboxyl-terminal portions have been detected so far in effluent blood. If biologically active fragments do actually survive hormone proteolysis within the gland or in peripheral sites, such amino-terminal fragments could be alternative active hormonal species. After much study, certain conclusions can be drawn. There is no convincing evidence for circulating amino-terminal fragments. Circulating biologically active fragments are also not detected after analysis of products produced by peripheral metabolism. Peripheral metabolism of PTH does not appear to be regulated by physiologic states (high versus low calcium, etc.); hence peripheral metabolism of hormone, although responsible for rapid clearance of secreted hormone, appears to be a high-capacity, metabolically invariant catabolic process.

The rate of clearance of the secreted 84-amino acid peptide from blood is more rapid than the rate of clearance of the biologically inactive fragment(s) corresponding to the middle- and carboxyl-terminal regions of the molecules that result from peripheral metabolism or glandular secretion. Hence measurements of PTH in blood by most earlier immunoassays provided only an overall index of parathyroid gland activity rather than a direct measure of biologically active hormone. Changes in the rate of production or clearance of fragments can change the concentration of immunoreactive hormone without influencing the rate of hormone secretion. Such discordance between concentrations of immunoreactive hormone and biologically active peptide occurs, for example, in renal failure, since the kidney seems to be the principal route of excretion of inactive hormone fragments. The problems inherent in accurate measurements of PTH in blood due to the heterogeneity of circulating forms of the molecule are now circumvented by use of double-antibody assays that detect only the intact molecule (as discussed in Chap. 357).

Parathyroid hormone–related protein The application of the techniques of molecular biology together with careful physiologic and clinical studies led to the cloning and subsequent physiologic evaluation of the parathyroid hormone–related protein (PTHrP) responsible for hypercalcemia in cancer patients, a syndrome that resembles hyperparathyroidism. This protein, now appreciated to be a paracrine or autocrine factor, plays a role both in fetal development and in adult physiology. Many different cell types produce PTHrP, including brain, pancreas, heart, lung, mammary tissue, placenta, endothelial cells, and smooth muscle.

PTH and PTHrP, although distinctive proteins and products of different genes, share considerable functional and structural homology (Fig. 356-7) and may have evolved from an ancestral gene. The

FIGURE 356-7 Schematic diagram to illustrate similarities and differences in structure of human PTH and human PTHrP. Close structural (and functional) homology exists between the first 30 amino acids of hPTH and hPTHrP. The PTHrP sequence may be 144 amino acid residues in length or longer. PTH is only 84 residues long; after residue 30, there is little structural homology

between the two. Dashed lines in the PTHrP sequence indicate homology; underlined residues, although different from those of PTH, still represent conservative changes (charge or polarity preserved). Eleven amino acids are identical, and a total of 21 of 30 are homologues.

structure of the gene for human PTHrP, however, is more complex than that of PTH, containing multiple exons and multiple sites for alternate splicing patterns during formation of the messenger RNA. Protein products of 141, 139, and 173 amino acids are produced. The varying molecular forms have multiple potential internal cleavage sites, and the biologic roles of these various molecular species and the nature of the circulating forms of PTHrP are unclear. The assays currently available are based on a variety of immunologic methods. Furthermore, multiple PTHrP products are synthesized, and other molecular forms may result from tissue-specific degradation at accessible internal cleavage sites. In fact, it is uncertain whether PTHrP circulates at all in normal human adults; as a paracrine factor, PTHrP may be produced, act within, and be destroyed locally within tissues.

PTHrP may have little to do with calcium homeostasis, except in disease states (Chap. 357), when large tumors, especially of the squamous cell type, lead to massive overproduction of PTHrP, which then circulates. PTHrP (see Fig. 356-7) shares a significant homology with PTH in the critical amino terminus that allows it to bind to the PTH receptor; synthetic molecules corresponding to the first 34 amino acids of PTHrP bind to and activate the PTH receptor indistinguishably from effects seen with PTH. This finding explains much of the confusion in earlier clinical studies of the humoral hypercalcemia of malignancy (Chap. 357).

PTHrP exerts important developmental influences in calcium and bone biology. Gene knockout studies in mice reveal a lethal deformity in the fetuses made homozygous for deletion of the PTHrP gene in which animals are born with a severe skeletal deformity of the chondrodysplastic type. In fetal animals, PTHrP directs transplacental calcium transfer, and high concentrations of PTHrP are produced in mammary tissue and secreted into milk. Human and bovine milk, for example, contains very high concentrations of the hormone. The

biologic significance of the latter is unknown. PTHrP also may play a role in uterine contraction.

HORMONE ACTION   The action of PTH at the biochemical level involves receptor-mediated effects on second messengers in target cells (see also Chap. 69). Stimulation of enzyme activity (adenyl cyclase, phospholipase C) during hormone–target cell membrane interaction leads to an increase in second messengers, including intracellular cAMP, products of polyphosphoinositol metabolism, and transmembrane and intracellular fluxes of calcium. PTH interacts with a specific receptor/adenylate cyclase complex on plasma membranes of target cells consisting of hormone receptor, enzyme catalytic unit (adenylate cyclase), and a guanyl nucleotide (GTP or GDP)–binding regulatory protein (G protein). The latter protein consists of α subunits that bind GTP and dissociate from the remainder of the G protein complex. The α subunit with bound GTP complexes with adenylate cyclase, thereby activating the enzyme to increase the rate of cAMP production from ATP. Hydrolysis of the GTP to GDP on the α subunit leads to reassociation of the G units and reduction in adenylate cyclase activity. The receptor, when activated by hormone binding, drives the G protein cycle by binding the α subunit portion and catalyzing the GDP/GTP exchange. Other G proteins link hormone action to phospholipase C; rapid changes in intracellular calcium concentrations within cells may be independent of phospholipase C stimulation.

The multiplicity of PTH actions on target cells in kidney and bone and the variety of second messengers—cAMP, IP$_3$, DAG, and Ca^{2+}—raise obvious questions as to the mechanism whereby specific responses are mediated. With many other hormonal systems, several different, although related, receptor subtypes direct hormone responses to individual second-messenger pathways by favoring coupling to one versus another G protein species; the concept is illustrated for PTH in Fig. 356-8A.

FIGURE 356-8   Schematic models of possible mechanisms of PTH action. Depicted in *A* is the hormone response systems seen with numerous hormones and predicted for PTH before cloning of the receptor; namely, several distinctive but closely related receptor types each mediate PTH–binding effects on distal cellular biological responses by coupling preferentially to different G proteins—G$_s$, G$_q$, etc.—which, in turn, activate a particular cellular second messenger such as cyclic AMP (cAMP), diacylglycerol (DAG), inositol triphosphate (IP$_3$), calcium Ca^{++}), or other specific receptor pathways indicated by ? Certain cells preferentially express one receptor type and, hence, one biological response is predominant.

Depicted in *B* is the actual result found so far with the cloning of the PTH receptor from several species. Only one receptor is present, which couples to multiple G proteins and effector pathways; in this model, cellular specificity or other factors (hormone levels, receptor expression levels) determine which pathway is activated predominantly in one cell type versus another. Although one form of receptor so far has been identified with PTH and PTHrP, multiple receptors of the type shown in *A* may yet be identified, and both mechanisms of control of PTH action may be used in vivo, varying from one target organ or cell to another.

However, only one molecular species has been detected in kidney and bone in human, rat, and other animal species, suggesting that a single PTH receptor (Fig. 356-8*B*) can be coupled to more than one G protein second-messenger kinase pathway. The receptors for PTH and calcitonin (the two receptors share close homology) are polypeptides of 500 to 600 amino acids. The primary amino acid sequence predicts the structures illustrated in Fig. 356-9: an extracellular domain, seven hydrophobic membrane-spanning domains connected by three extracellular and three intracellular loops, and a carboxyl-terminal intracellular domain. The extracellular regions are involved in hormone binding, and the intracellular domains, after hormone activation, bind G protein subunits to transduce hormone signaling into cellular responses through stimulation of second messengers by activated G protein subunits.

The details of the biochemical steps by which an increased intracellular concentration of cAMP, IP$_3$, or DAG lead to changes in calcium and phosphate ion translocation are unknown. Stimulation of protein kinases (protein kinase A, cAMP; protein kinase C, DAG) and calcium transport channels is associated with a variety of hormone-specific tissue responses, some of which are cAMP-dependent and others cAMP-independent. These responses include inhibition of phosphate and bicarbonate transport and stimulation of calcium transport and renal 1α-hydroxylase in the kidney. The responses in bone include effects on collagen synthesis; alkaline phosphatase activity; ornithine decarboxylase, citrate decarboxylase, and glucose-6-phosphate dehydrogenase activity; DNA, protein, and phospholipid synthesis; and calcium and phosphate transport. Ultimately, these cellular biochemical events lead to an integrated hormonal response in bone turnover and calcium homeostasis.

Pathophysiology   In hyperparathyroidism, PTH is overproduced by tumors of the parathyroid or hyperplasia involving all glands. The excess hormone results in hypercalcemia secondary to increased intestinal calcium absorption [increased synthesis of 1,25(OH)$_2$D], reduced renal calcium clearance, and increased bone calcium release. Bone turnover increases in all patients, and resorption exceeds formation in many. Individual patients respond to the excess hormone variably at intestinal, renal, and bone target sites; the factors influencing the response from patient to patient are not known.

Hypophosphatemia results from the actions of the excessive PTH on renal tubular phosphate reabsorption. Hypophosphatemia in turn aggravates the hypercalcemia by increasing the synthesis of 1,25(OH)$_2$D and by increasing the sensitivity of the bone to PTH. Hypophosphatemia also may interfere with the normal mineralization of bone, leading to a mixed picture of increased resorption and deficient mineralization in adjacent skeletal sites.

Hypoparathyroidism causes hypocalcemia and hyperphosphatemia, a reversal of the response seen with hormone excess. See Chap. 357 for details of the clinical syndromes.

CALCITONIN (See also Chap. 343)   Calcitonin is a hypocalcemic peptide hormone that, in many ways, acts as the physiologic antagonist to parathyroid hormone. The hypocalcemic activity of calcitonin is accounted for primarily by inhibition of osteoclast-mediated bone resorption and secondarily by stimulation of renal calcium clearance. These effects are mediated by receptors on osteoclasts and renal tubular cells. Calcitonin exerts additional effects presumably through binding to receptors present in brain, gastrointestinal tract, and the immune system (Fig. 356-9). The hormone, for example, has analgesic effects exerted directly on cells in the hypothalamus and related structures, possibly by interacting with receptors for related peptide hormones, such as calcitonin gene–related peptide (CGRP) or amylin. The latter ligands have specific high-affinity receptors and also can bind to and trigger calcitonin receptors. The calcitonin receptors as deduced from the nucleotide sequences of the cDNA, contain seven transmembrane α-helical domains similar to the G protein–coupled receptors. The calcitonin, PTH, and PTHrP receptors are sufficiently different from other G protein–coupled receptors as to constitute a distinct subfamily. Other members of this subfamily include receptors for secretin, vasoactive intestinal peptide, growth hormone–releasing hormone, and gastric inhibitory peptide. Interaction of calcitonin with its receptors activates signal transduction pathways that, like those for PTH, involve distinct G proteins. Thus calcitonin can stimulate adenylyl cyclase and protein kinase A as well as protein kinase C and induce calcium transients as well. These specific G protein interactions probably involve distinct amino acid sequences in a single receptor protein.

The thyroid is the major source of the hormone, and the cells involved in calcitonin synthesis arise from neural crest tissue. During embryogenesis, these cells migrate into the ultimobranchial body, derived from the last branchial pouch. In submammalian vertebrates, the ultimobranchial body constitutes a discrete organ, anatomically separate from the thyroid gland, but in mammals, the ultimobranchial gland fuses with and is incorporated into the thyroid gland.

The naturally occurring calcitonins consist of a peptide chain of 32 amino acids. There is a considerable variability in sequence among species. The entire chain of 32 amino acids appears to be required for biologic activity in the intact animal, although fragments function

FIGURE 356-9   Schematic illustration of predicted structure of PTH and calcitonin receptors contains one large extracellular domain, seven membrane-spanning domains, three extracellular loops connecting the membrane-spanning domains on the cell surface, one large intracellular domain, and three intracellular loops. Backbone structure is of the PTH receptor; shaded residues are common between PTH and the CT receptor.

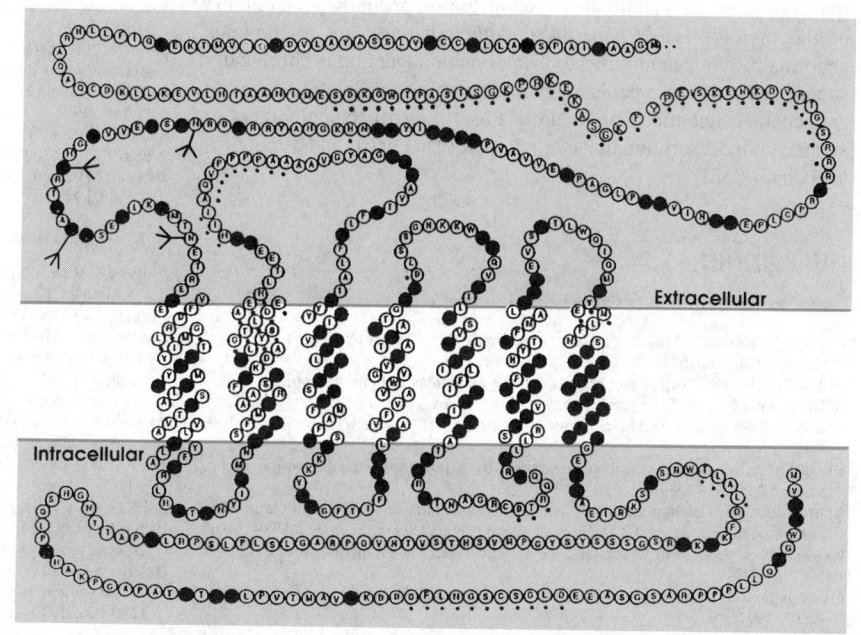

in in vitro systems. Calcitonin from salmon is 10 to 100 times more potent than mammalian forms in lowering serum calcium in animals; eel calcitonin is also potent. Slow turnover may in part explain the greater potency of salmon calcitonin, but the hormone binds more tightly to receptor sites as well. Calcitonin is synthesized as a precursor molecule that is four times larger than calcitonin itself. Analysis of the sequence of the coding portions of the gene for rat calcitonin indicates that at least two peptides flank calcitonin, from which they are separated by basic residues. It is likely (in analogy with the common precursor for ACTH and endorphin) that these peptides are released along with calcitonin. There is no known biologic function for these noncalcitonin peptides.

There are two calcitonin genes, α and β, located on chromosome 11 in the general region of the beta globulin and parathyroid hormone genes. The two genes are sometimes called calcitonin/CGRP-1 and / CGRP-2. The transcription of these genes is complex. Two different messenger RNA molecules are transcribed from the α gene; one is translated into the precursor for calcitonin, and the other message is transcribed into an alternate product, calcitonin gene–related peptide (CGRP). CGRP is synthesized wherever the calcitonin message is expressed, e.g., in medullary carcinoma of the thyroid. The β, or CGRP-2, gene is transcribed into the messenger RNA for CGRP in the central nervous system (CNS) in animals; this gene is silent for calcitonin production. CGRP has cardiovascular actions and may serve a neurotransmitter or developmental role in CNS.

The secretin of calcitonin is under the direct control of blood calcium: An increase in calcium causes an increase and a decrease in calcium causes a decrease in calcitonin levels. Once secreted, calcitonin disappears from the circulation with a half-life of 2 to 15 min.

The concentration of calcitonin in the peripheral blood of normal humans is lower than that in many other species. Basal and stimulated immunoreactive calcitonin levels are lower in women than in men and tend to decrease with age to a greater extent in women.

In animals, calcitonin acts to lower both blood calcium and blood phosphate by inhibiting bone resorption and by increasing urinary calcium and phosphate clearance. The actions of calcitonin on kidney and bone are in turn modulated by the regulation of calcitonin production by serum calcium. The view that calcitonin serves to protect against hypercalcemia is thus explained by the hypocalcemic effects of calcitonin triggered in response to hypercalcemia.

In humans, changes in calcium and phosphate metabolism are not seen despite extreme variations in hormone production; no definite effects are attributable to calcitonin deficiency (totally thyroidecto-mized patients receiving only replacement thyroxine) or excess (patients with the calcitonin-secreting tumor, medullary carcinoma of the thyroid) (see Chap. 343). Although there are no obvious abnormalities in calcium metabolism, bone remodeling is chronically suppressed, and these patients are refractory to the skeletal actions of exogenous calcitonin. Calcitonin is a useful pharmacologic agent to suppress bone resorption in Paget's disease (Chap. 361) and osteoporosis (Chap. 358).

REFERENCES

Calcium, phosphorous, and bone metabolism

AVIOLI LV, KRANE SM (eds): *Metabolic Bone Disease and Clinically Related Disorders.* Philadelphia, Saunders, 1990
AZRIA M: The value of biomarkers in detecting alterations in bone metabolism. Calcif Tissue Int 45:7, 1989
BARON R: Polarity and membrane transport in osteoclasts. Connect Tissue Res 20:109, 1988
BLAIR HC et al: Osteoclastic bone resorption by a polarized vacuolar proton pump. Science 245:855, 1989
BRINGHURST FR: Calcium and phosphate distribution, turnover, and metabolic actions, in *Endocrinology,* 2d ed, LJ DeGroot et al (eds). Philadelphia, Saunders, 1989, p 805
CANALIS E et al: Growth factors and the skeletal system. J Endocrinol Invest 12:577, 1989
CANALIS E et al: Growth factors and cytokines in bone cell metabolism. Annu Rev Med 42:17, 1991

COHN DV et al (eds): *Calcium Regulating Hormones and Bone Metabolism: Bone and Clinical Aspects.* Amsterdam, Excerpta Medica, 1992
DELMAS PD: Clinical use of biochemical markers of bone remodeling in osteoporosis. Bone 13:S17, 1992
EPSTEIN S: Serum and urinary markers of bone remodeling: Assessment of bone turnover. Endocrine Rev 9:437,1988
ERICKSEN EF: Normal and pathological remodeling of human trabecular bone: Three dimensional reconstruction of the remodeling sequence in normals and in metabolic bone disease. Endocrine Rev 7:379, 1986
EVERED D, HARNETT S (eds): *Cell and Molecular Biology of Vertebrate Hard Tissues.* Chichester, Wiley, 1988
HOROWITZ MC: Cytokines and estrogen in bone: Anti-osteoporotic effects. Science 260:626, 1993
KANDERS B et al: Interaction of calcium nutrition and physical activity on bone mass in young women. J Bone Min Res 3:145, 1988
KATZ EP et al: The structure of mineralized collagen fibrils. Connect Tissue Res 21:149, 1989
KLEEREKOPER M, KRANE SM (eds): *Clinical Disorders of Bone and Mineral Metabolism.* New York, Mary Ann Liebert, 1989
MARCUS R: Biochemical markers of bone remodeling, in *Clinical Disorders of Bone and Mineral Metabolism,* M Kleerekopper, SM Krane (eds). New York, Mary Ann Liebert, 1989, p 49
MUNDY GR: Identifying mechanisms for increasing bone mass. J Natl Inst Health Res 1:65, 1989
PARFITT AM: The coupling of bone formation: A critical analysis of the concept and of its relevance to the pathogenesis of osteoporosis. Metab Bone Dis Relat Res 4:1, 1982
————: The cellular basis of bone remodeling: The quantum concept reexamined in light of recent advances in the cell biology of bone. Calcif Tissue Int 36:S37, 1984
PORTALE AA et al: Physiologic regulation of the serum concentration of 1,25-dihydroxyvitamin D by phosphorus in normal men. J Clin Invest 83:1494, 1989
POUILLES JM et al: Sensitivity of dual-photon absorptiometry in spinal osteoporosis. Calcif Tissue Int 43:329, 1988
RAISZ LG, KREAM BE: Regulation of bone formation. N Engl J Med 309:29, 1983
ROBEY PG: The biochemistry of bone. Endocrinol Metab Clin North Am 18:859, 1989
ROODMAN GD: Interleukin-6: An osteotropic factor? J Bone Miner Res 7:474, 1992
SAGE EH, BORNSTEIN P: Extracellular proteins that modulate cell-matrix interactions. SPARC, tenascin, and thrombospondin. J Biol Chem 266:14831, 1991
SLAVKIN H, PRICE P (eds): *Chemistry and Biology of Mineralized Tissues.* Amsterdam, Excerpta Medica, 1992
SORIANO P et al: Targeted disruption of the c-*src* proto-oncogene leads to osteopetrosis in mice. Cell 64:693, 1991
SUDA T et al: Modulation of osteoclast differentiation. Endocr Rev 13:66, 1992
UEBELHART D et al: Urinary excretion of pyridinium crosslinks: A new marker of bone resorption in metabolic bone disease. Bone Miner 8:87, 1990
———— et al: Effect of menopause and hormone replacement therapy on the urinary excretion of pyridinium cross-links. J Clin Endocrinol Metab 7:367, 1991
URIST MR et al: Bone cell differentiation and growth factors. Science 220:680, 1983
WOZNEY JM et al: Novel regulators of bone formation: molecular clones and activities. Science 242:1528, 1988

Vitamin D

ADAMS JS et al: A role for endogenous arachidonate metabolites in the regulated expression of the 25-hydroxyvitamin D 1-hydroxylation reaction in cultured alveolar macrophages from patients with sarcoidosis. J Clin Endocrinol Metab 70:595, 1990
BARAN D et al: 1α,25-Dihydroxyvitamin D₃–induced increments in hepatocyte cytosolic calcium and lysophosphatidylinositol: Inhibition by pertussis toxin and 1β,25-dihydroxyvitamin D₃. J Bone Miner Res 5:517, 1990
HOLICK MF: Vitamin D: biosynthesis, metabolism, and mode of action, in *Endocrinology,* LJ DeGroot et al (eds). New York, Grune & Stratton, 1989, vol 2, pp 902–926
———— et al: The vitamin D content of fortified milk and infant formula. N Engl J Med 326:1178, 1992
KRALL E et al: Effect of vitamin D intake on seasonal variation in parathyroid hormone secretion in postmenopausal women. N Engl J Med 321:1777, 1989
PIKE JW: Vitamin D₃ receptors: Structure and function in transcription. Annu Rev Nutr 11:189, 1991
REICHEL H et al: The role of the vitamin D endocrine system in health and disease. N Engl J Med 320:981, 1989
TILYARD MW et al: Treatment of postmenopausal osteoporosis with calcitriol or calcium. N Engl J Med 326:356, 1992

Parathyroid hormone and calcitonin

ABBAS SK et al: Stimulation of ovine placental calcium transport by purified natural and recombinant parathyroid hormone–related protein (PTHrP) preparations. Q J Exp Physiol 74:549, 1989
ABOU-SAMRA AB et al: Expression cloning of a common receptor for parathyroid hormone and parathyroid hormone–related peptide from rat osteoblast-like cells: A single receptor stimulates intracellular accumulation of both cAMP and inositol triphosphates and increases intracellular free calcium. Proc Natl Acad Sci USA 89:2732, 1992
ARNOLD A et al: Mutation of the signal peptide-encoding region of the preproparathyroid hormone gene in familial isolated hypoparathyroidism. J Clin Invest 86:1094, 1990
BRINGHURST FR et al: Cloned, stably expressed parathyroid hormone (PTH)/PTH–related peptide receptors activate multiple messenger signals and biological responses in LLC-PK₁ kidney cells. Endocrinology 132:2090, 1993
BUDAYR AR et al: Increased serum levels of PTH-like protein in malignancy-associated hypercalcemia. Ann Intern Med 111:807, 1989
BURTIS WJ et al: Immunochemical characterization of circulating parathyroid hormone–related protein in patients with humoral hypercalcemia of malignancy. N Engl J Med 322:1106, 1990

DEMAY MB et al: Sequences in the human parathyroid hormone gene that bind the 1,25-dihydroxyvitamin D₂ receptor and mediate transcriptional repression in response to 1,25-dihydroxyvitamin D₃. Proc Natl Acad Sci USA 89:8097, 1992

FORCE T et al: A cloned porcine renal calcitonin receptor couples to adenyl cyclase and phospholipase C. Am J Physiol 262:F1110, 1992

GARDELLA TJ et al: Mutational analysis of the receptor activating region of human parathyroid hormone. J Biol Chem 266:13141, 1991

GORN AH et al: The cloning characterization and expression of a human calcitonin receptor from an ovarian carcinoma cell line. J Clin Invest 90:1726, 1992

GRILL V et al: PTH-related protein: Elevated levels in both humoral hypercalcemia of malignancy and hypercalcemia complicating breast cancer. J Clin Endocrinol 73:1309, 1991

HAYMAN JA et al: Expression of parathyroid hormone–related protein in normal skin and in tumors of skin and skin appendages. J Pathol 158:293, 1989

HENDERSON JR et al: Circulating concentrations of PTH-like peptide in malignancy and in hyperparathyroidism. J Bone Miner Res 5:105, 1990

JUPPNER H et al: A G-protein–linked receptor for parathyroid hormone and parathyroid hormone–related protein. Science 254:1024, 1991

KAO PC et al: PTH-related peptide in plasma of patients with hypercalcemia and malignancy lesions. Mayo Clin Proc 65:1399, 1990

KARAPLIS AC et al: Gene-encoding parathyroid hormone–like peptide: Nucleotide sequence of the rat gene and comparison with the human homolog. Mol Endocrinol 4:441, 1990

——— et al: Disruption of parathyroid hormone–related peptide gene leads to a multitude of skeletal abnormalities and preinatal mortality. J Bone Miner Res 7(suppl 1):abst 1, 1992

LIM SK et al: Full-length chicken parathyroid hormone: Biosynthesis in *Escherichia coli* and analysis of biological activity. J Biol Chem 266:3709, 1991

LIN HY et al: Expression cloning of an adenylate cyclase–coupled calcitonin receptor. Science 254:1022, 1991

MARTIN TJ et al: Parathyroid hormone–related protein: Biochemistry and molecular biology. CRC Crit Rev Biochem Mol Biol 26:377, 1991

NIKOLS GA et al: Hypotension and cardiac stimulation due to the parathyroid hormone–related protein, humoral hypercalcemia of malignancy factor. Endocrinology 125:834, 1989

——— et al: Hypercalcemia and ectopic secretion of PTH by an ovarian carcinoma with rearrangement of the gene for PTH. N Engl J Med 323:1324, 1990

NUSSBAUM SR, POTTS JT JR: Immunoassays for parathyroid hormone 1–84 in the diagnosis of hyperparathyroidism. J Bone Miner Res 6:543, 1991

POTTS JT JR: Chemistry of the calcitonins. Bone Miner 16:169, 1992

RATCLIFFE WA et al: Immunoreactivity of plasma parathyrin-related peptide. Clin Chem 37:1781, 1991

SCHIPANI E et al: Identical complementary deoxyribonucleic acids encode a human renal and bone parathyroid hormone (PTH)/PTH–related peptide receptor. Endocrinology 132:2157, 1993

SUVA LJ et al: A parathyroid hormone–related protein implicated in malignant hypercalcemia: Cloning and expression. Science 237:893, 1987

THIEDE M et al: Human renal carcinoma expresses two messages encoding a parathyroid hormone–like peptide: Evidence for the alternative splicing of a single copy gene. Proc Natl Acad Sci USA 85:4605, 1988

WIMALAWANSA SJ: Calcitonin: Molecular biology, physiology, pathophysiology and its therapeutic uses, in *Advances in Bone Regulatory Factors: Morphology, Biochemistry, Physiology and Pharmacology*, AB Pecile (ed). London, Plenum Press, 1990, p 121

YAMAMOTO M et al: Suckling-mediated increases in urinary phosphate and 3′,5′-cyclic adenosine monophosphate excretion in lactating rats: Possible systemic effects of parathyroid hormone–related protein. Endocrinology 129:2614, 1991

ZAIDI M et al: Evidence that the action of calcitonin on rat osteoclasts is mediated by two G proteins acting via separate post-receptor pathways. J Endocrinol 126:473, 1990

ZAJAC JD et al: Regulation of gene transcription and proliferation by parathyroid hormone is blocked in mutant osteoblastic cells resistant to cyclic AMP. Mol Cell Endocrinol 87:69, 1992

evaluation? What are the most probable causes of hypercalcemia, and how can they be diagnosed?

Whenever hypercalcemia is confirmed, a definitive diagnosis must be established. Although hyperparathyroidism, a frequent cause of asymptomatic hypercalcemia, is a chronic disorder in which manifestations, if any, may be expressed only over months or years, hypercalcemia also can be the earliest clue to the presence of malignancy, the second most common cause of hypercalcemia in the adult. The causes of hypercalcemia are numerous (Table 357-1), but hyperparathyroidism and cancer account for 90 percent of cases. Diagnosis can usually be established. However, the optimal management of asymptomatic hyperparathyroidism is still unsettled, and treatment of the hypercalcemia of cancer is difficult.

Before undertaking an evaluation of hypercalcemia, it is essential to be sure that true hypercalcemia, not a false-positive laboratory test, is present. Hypercalcemia is a chronic problem, and it is cost-effective to obtain several serum calcium measurements; these tests need not be in the fasting state. False-positive calcium tests are usually the result of inadvertent hemoconcentration during blood collection or elevation in serum proteins, particularly albumin. Measurement of ionized calcium is technically feasible, but there is no advantage, except in research applications, to measurement of ionized rather than total calcium.

Clinical features alone are helpful in differential diagnosis. Hypercalcemia in an adult who is asymptomatic is usually due to primary hyperparathyroidism. In most cases of malignancy-associated hypercalcemia the disease is not occult; rather, symptoms of the underlying malignancy bring the patient to the physician, and hypercalcemia is discovered during the workup. In patients with malignancy, the interval between detection of hypercalcemia and death is often less than 6 months. Accordingly, if an asymptomatic individual has had hypercalcemia or some manifestation of hypercalcemia, such as kidney stones, for more than 1 or 2 years, it is unlikely that malignancy is the cause. As discussed below, however, differentiating primary hyperparathyroidism from *occult* malignancy can occasionally be a problem, and careful evaluation of patients is required, particularly when the duration of the hypercalcemia is unknown.

Hypercalcemia not due to hyperparathyroidism or malignancy can result from excessive vitamin D action, high bone turnover from any of several causes, or from renal failure (Table 357-1). The sensitivity and specificity of various diagnostic tests for the differential diagnosis were previously not optimal, but newer parathyroid hormone (PTH) immunoassays based on double-antibody methods are reliable. Dietary history and a history of ingestion of vitamins and drugs are often helpful in recognizing some of the less frequent causes. Except in malignancy-associated hypercalcemia, acute management of the hypercalcemia is usually successful prior to the institution of definitive

357 DISEASES OF THE PARATHYROID GLAND AND OTHER HYPER- AND HYPOCALCEMIC DISORDERS

JOHN T. POTTS, JR.

HYPERCALCEMIA

Hypercalcemia can be a manifestation of a serious illness such as malignancy or can be detected coincidentally by laboratory testing in a patient with no obvious illness. Management is a particular problem when the patient is asymptomatic. The number of patients recognized with asymptomatic hypercalcemia has increased severalfold in the last two decades. Does the hypercalcemia always require further

TABLE 357-1 Classification of causes of hypercalcemia

Parathyroid-related:	Vitamin D–related:
1 Primary hyperparathyroidism	*1* Vitamin D intoxication
a Solitary adenomas	*2* ↑ 1,25(OH)₂D; sarcoidosis and other granulomatous diseases
b Multiple endocrine neoplasia	*3* Idiopathic hypercalcemia of infancy
2 Lithium therapy	
3 Familial hypocalciuric hypercalcemia	**Associated with high bone turnover:**
	1 Hyperthyroidism
Malignancy-related:	*2* Immobilization
1 Solid tumor with metastases (breast)	*3* Thiazides
2 Solid tumor with humoral mediation of hypercalcemia (lung, kidney)	*4* Vitamin A intoxication
3 Hematologic malignancies (multiple myeloma, lymphoma, leukemia)	**Associated with renal failure:**
	1 Severe secondary hyperparathyroidism
	2 Aluminum intoxication
	3 Milk-alkali syndrome

are reversed by parathyroidectomy; in these patients there appears to be a cause-and-effect relationship. Generally, however, the fact that hyperparathyroidism is common in elderly patients, in whom there are often other problems, suggests the possibility that such problems as hypertension, renal deterioration, and depression may not be parathyroid-related and suggests caution in recommending surgery as a cure for these conditions in hyperparathyroid patients. It is not apparent why some patients with hyperparathyroidism have no symptoms, while others with similar biochemical abnormalities develop symptomatic disease.

Neuromuscular manifestations include proximal muscle weakness, easy fatigability, and atrophy of muscles. The clinical signs in these patients may be so striking as to suggest a primary neuromuscular disorder. The distinguishing feature is the complete regression of neuromuscular disease after surgical correction of the hyperparathyroidism.

Gastrointestinal manifestations of hyperparathyroidism are sometimes subtle and include vague abdominal complaints and disorders of the stomach and pancreas. Again, cause and effect are unclear, except in certain situations, such as the multiple endocrine syndromes. In MEN 1 patients with hyperparathyroidism, duodenal ulcer is a result of the associated pancreatic tumors that secrete excessive quantities of gastrin (the Zollinger-Ellison syndrome). Pancreatitis has been reported in association with hyperparathyroidism, but the incidence and the mechanism are not established.

Chondrocalcinosis and pseudogout are said to be sufficiently frequent in hyperparathyroidism that screening of such patients is warranted. Occasionally, pseudogout is the initial manifestation.

DIAGNOSIS   The diagnosis is made primarily on clinical grounds. The newer immunoassays for PTH are reliable and cost-effective. Since hypercalcemia can be the presenting evidence for malignancy or other serious disease, a thorough evaluation of possible etiologies, including hyperparathyroidism, is indicated even in asymptomatic subjects. If the diagnosis of hyperparathyroidism is suspected after such an evaluation, a decision may be made to follow the patient rather than to recommend surgery.

Hypercalcemia is the most common manifestation—either sustained or intermittent hypercalcemia. Careful consideration must be given to the justification for surgical exploration in the absence of hypercalcemia. So-called normocalcemic hyperparathyroidism, i.e., surgically proven hyperparathyroidism accompanied by a normal calcium level but elevated values of immunoreactive PTH (iPTH), is rare in the absence of renal failure or gastrointestinal disease. If such patients have coexisting conditions that interfere with the calcium-elevating actions of PTH, such as chronic renal failure, severe malabsorption, or vitamin D deficiency, then the lack of calcium elevation need not argue against the presence of true hyperparathyroidism. Confusing situations can arise, however, in patients with recurrent kidney stones who are suspected of having hyperparathyroidism because of elevated iPTH levels but who have normal serum calcium. These patients may have true normocalcemic hyperparathyroidism. In situations in which the symptoms call for an early definitive diagnosis, it may be useful to search for postabsorptive hypercalcemia (detectable in certain patients when fasting hypercalcemia is absent) or to use a provocative test with benzothiadiazides (see below).

Hypercalciuria is common in hyperparathyroidism. However, PTH actually reduces calcium clearance, and the daily excretion of calcium in urine is lower than in patients with equivalent degrees of hypercalcemia from nonparathyroid causes.

Serum phosphate is usually low but may be normal, especially if renal failure has developed. Hypophosphatemia is a less useful diagnostic finding than hypercalcemia for two reasons. First, phosphate levels are influenced by dietary intake, diurnal variations, and other factors; to be useful, samples must be obtained in the morning under fasting conditions. Second, patients with severe hypercalcemia of all causes may have a low serum phosphate.

Many tests based on renal responses to excess parathyroid hormone (renal calcium and phosphate clearance; blood phosphate, chloride, magnesium; urinary or nephrogenous cyclic AMP) have been proposed and used in the past. These tests have low specificity for hyperparathyroidism, are not cost-effective, and have been replaced by the improved PTH immunoassays.

TREATMENT   *Medical treatment*   Medical treatment involves two separate issues. If hypercalcemia is severe and symptomatic, then the calcium must be lowered (the measures are described below). Hypercalcemia is not symptomatic in most patients with hyperparathyroidism, and it is usually not difficult to control the hypercalcemia. Simple hydration will often suffice to lower the calcium concentration to values below 2.9 mmol/L (11.5 mg/dL). There have been discussions in the past about whether chronic management of the hypercalcemia of hyperparathyroidism should be undertaken with oral phosphate therapy. Lowering the calcium concentration by phosphate is accompanied by an increase in iPTH levels in blood; it is unclear whether the increased PTH levels would cause more or less organ deterioration. There have been no systemic trials to evaluate the effects of medical therapy for hypercalcemia.

Rather, the usual issue is to decide whether surgical intervention is required. If not, medical management consists of following the patient without specific therapy but monitoring bone and renal function periodically to ensure that silent osseous and renal deterioration does not occur. In postmenopausal women with hyperparathyroidism who are either unwilling or unable to undergo parathyroid surgery, estrogen therapy may retard demineralization of the skeleton and reduce blood and urinary calcium levels.

The natural history of the disease has been studied in several centers. Several hundred patients have been followed in attempts to afford a rational explanation for the benefits of surgery versus the risks of medical observation. Large-scale randomized, prospective clinical trials have not been undertaken, however. Rather, the long-term effects of hyperparathyroidism have been assessed in patients who do not have kidney stones, osteitis fibrosa cystica, or other clear-cut symptoms. Of principal concern is the possibility of progressive loss of bone density, a worrying problem in women who face the problem of age-dependent and estrogen-deficient bone loss in the absence of hyperparathyroidism. The concern is that such patients, even though asymptomatic, will suffer a degree of bone loss due to PTH excess that will leave them more vulnerable later in life to developing symptomatic osteoporosis.

The importance of the topic of asymptomatic hyperparathyroidism led the National Institutes of Health to hold a Consensus Conference on Management of Asymptomatic Hyperparathyroidism in 1991. *Asymptomatic hyperparathyroidism* was defined as the clinical profile of patients with documented (presumptive) hyperparathyroidism without signs or symptoms attributable to the disease. It was emphasized that surgery to correct the hyperparathyroidism is always an acceptable approach, if feasible medically, but surveillance may be justified in patients over the age of 50 with minimal calcium elevation when renal function and bone mass are close to normal and remain so during careful monitoring.

Three of the important questions addressed were: (1) *What is the most accurate, cost-effective method of diagnosing hyperparathyroidism? (2) Are there patients with asymptomatic hyperparathyroidism who can safely be followed, and should they be? (3) If not operated on, how should asymptomatic patients be monitored and managed?*

The recommendation was that the diagnosis of primary hyperparathyroidism can best be established by demonstrating persistent hypercalcemia (artifactual elevation in serum calcium concentration should be eliminated) and an elevated serum PTH concentration. The panel agreed that the improved PTH assay is sensitive, specific, and reliable and that other tests are usually unnecessary.

As to which asymptomatic patients should be followed medically, the consensus was that a subgroup of patients over age 50 is appropriate for medical monitoring if certain criteria are met and the patients wish to avoid surgery.

Patients under age 50 should be routinely operated on, given the long surveillance that would be required. Other guidelines for recommending surgery in patients with asymptomatic hyperparathyroidism include the following:

1 Elevation of serum calcium, more than 0.25 to 0.40 mmol/L (1 to 1.6 mg/dL) above the upper limit of normal for the laboratory.

2 History of an episode of life-threatening hypercalcemia, such as an episode induced by dehydration and recurring illness.

3 Reduction of creatinine clearance by greater than 30 percent compared with age-matched controls (the author finds it difficult to use this criterion as an absolute, given the multiplicity of factors that affect creatinine clearance with age).

4 Presence of kidney stones detected by abdominal radiograph.

5 Elevation of 24-h urinary calcium excretion above 400 mg.

6 Reduction of bone mass more than 2 standard deviations below normal by one of several noninvasive methods of measuring bone mass.

Practical considerations that favor surgery include concern that consistent follow-up would be unlikely or that coexistent illness would complicate management. Asymptomatic patients should be monitored regularly. Surgical correction of hyperparathyroidism can always be undertaken when indicated, since the success rate is high (greater than 90 percent), mortality is low, morbidity is minimal, and cure is common. The goals of monitoring are early detection of worsening hypercalcemia, deteriorating bone or renal status, or other complications of hyperparathyroidism. Cortical bone mass is principally at risk in untreated primary hyperparathyroidism. Some data indicate that there is also an increased risk of vertebral bone fracture in patients with untreated hyperparathyroidism, suggesting that cancellous bone is also at risk. Cancellous bone loss may be a particular problem when vitamin D and calcium intakes are low.

Although patients have reduced bone mass at the time of initial detection, there may be little further loss over years of subsequent follow-up. It is not clear which technique of bone mass monitoring should be used routinely and how much reduction from normal or change should be considered an indication for surgery. The use of single-photon absorptiometry to follow cortical bone is relatively easy and inexpensive; in the United States at least, increased loss of cancellous bone and increased risk of vertebral fractures are unusual. Consequently, the monitoring of spinal bone mass by dual-energy x-ray absorptiometry need not be undertaken. The consensus panel did not make a recommendation as to estrogen use in patients for whom surgery was not elected because there was too little cumulative experience with such therapy.

Surgical treatment   Parathyroid exploration is best undertaken by an experienced surgeon with the help of an experienced pathologist. Certain features help in predicting the pathology; for example, in familial cases multiple abnormal glands are likely. However, some critical decisions regarding management can be made only during the operation. The examination by frozen section of tissue removed at surgery helps direct the subsequent course of the operation.

As discussed under etiology, there are many unresolved issues to consider in surgery for hyperparathyroidism. At the extreme of conservatism, the surgical approach is based on the view that typically only one gland (the adenoma) is abnormal. If an enlarged gland is found, a normal gland should be sought. If a biopsy of a normal-sized second gland confirms its histologic and therefore presumed functional normality, no further exploration, biopsy, or excision is needed. At the other extreme is the minority viewpoint that not only should all four glands be sought but also most of the total parathyroid tissue mass should be removed.

The concern with the former approach is that the rate of recurrence of hyperparathyroidism may be high because a second abnormal gland will sometimes be missed; the latter approach could involve unnecessary surgery and an unacceptable rate of hypoparathyroidism.

The majority viewpoint, judged by surgical reviews, is in favor of conservative surgery, i.e., removal of what is usually only one enlarged gland but only after four-gland exploration to eliminate the possibility that more than one gland is abnormal. When normal glands are found in association with one enlarged gland, excision of the single adenoma leads to cure or symptom-free disease in most such patients.

Known hyperplasia, as predicted in familial cases, poses more difficult questions of surgical management. Once a diagnosis of hyperplasia is established, it is necessary to identify all the glands. Two different schemes for surgical management have been proposed. One is that three glands be totally removed and the fourth gland be partially excised; care is taken to leave a good blood supply for the remaining gland. Other surgeons advocate total parathyroidectomy with immediate transplantation of a portion of a removed, minced parathyroid gland into the muscles of the forearm with the view that even if recurrence of residual gland enlargement and hyperfunction is seen, surgical excision is easier from the ectopic site in the arm. Cryopreservation is also being explored, but functional survival of the glands is unclear. When parathyroid carcinoma is encountered, the tissue should be widely excised; care must be taken to avoid rupture of the capsule to prevent local seeding of the tumor.

If no glandular abnormalities are found in the neck, the issue of further exploration must be decided. There are documented cases of five or six parathyroid glands and, therefore, of unusual locations for adenomas. A variety of techniques have been developed to aid in the preoperative localization of the abnormal parathyroid tissue; usually these techniques are used only in patients with unsuccessful neck explorations before further surgery is undertaken. The early techniques featured either selective intraarterial angiography or selective venous catheterization of the thyroid venous plexus and adjacent areas coupled with radioimmunoassay for PTH. The techniques were often successful but not better than the rate of success of an experienced parathyroid surgeon in finding the abnormal tissue at the first operation, so such procedures are not warranted. Less invasive techniques also have been utilized for preoperative localization, including ultrasound, computed tomography of the neck and mediastinum, differential scanning after simultaneous radiothallium and technetium administration, and intraarterial digital angiography; the yield for these procedures in preoperative localization is also insufficiently high to warrant their use except when the initial surgery is unsuccessful.

Ultrasound is reported to detect abnormal parathyroid tissue in 60 to 70 percent of cases and has been advocated for lesions in the vicinity of the thyroid; it is less successful for lesions in the anterior mediastinum. The technique may assist the surgeon even in the initial operation by directing the surgery to the side of the neck where the abnormal gland is located. Computed tomography has a similar success rate and is more helpful with mediastinal glands, although false-positive results are noted. The subtraction of the technetium image, which targets the thyroid, from the radiothallium image, which targets both thyroid and parathyroid, has led to successful preoperative localization in approximately half of patients undergoing a second exploration.

Several generalizations seem warranted. Localization and removal of a single abnormal parathyroid gland at the first operation are usually successful depending on the experience of the surgeon (greater than 90 percent success for experienced surgeons). Preoperative localization techniques, therefore, which are less than 90 percent successful, should be reserved for patients in whom initial exploration is unsuccessful. When a second parathyroid exploration is indicated, ultrasound, computed tomography, and thallium-technetium scanning should probably be combined with selective digital arteriography in one of the centers specializing in these techniques. At one center, long-term cures have been achieved with selective embolization or injection of large amounts of contrast material into the end-arterial circulation feeding the parathyroid tumor.

A decline in serum calcium occurs within 24 h after successful surgery; usually blood calcium falls to low-normal values for 3 to 5 days until the remaining parathyroid tissue resumes hormone secretion. Intraoperative monitoring of PTH levels by rapid PTH immunoassays may be useful in guiding the surgery, especially in patients who are reexplored after an initial unsuccessful operation. Severe postoperative hypocalcemia is likely only if osteitis cystica is present or if injury to all the normal parathyroid glands has occurred during surgery.

In general, patients with good renal and gastrointestinal function, who do not have symptomatic bone disease and a large deficit in bone mineral, have few problems with postoperative hypocalcemia. The extent of postoperative hypocalcemia varies with the surgical approach. If all glands are biopsied, hypocalcemia may be more prolonged and may be transiently symptomatic. Symptomatic hypocalcemia is more likely to occur after second parathyroid explorations, when normal parathyroid tissue may have been removed at the unsuccessful initial operation and when the manipulation and/or biopsy of the remaining normal gland has been more extensive in the search for the missing adenoma. Patients with hyperparathyroidism have efficient intestinal calcium absorption due to the increased levels of 1,25(OH)$_2$D stimulated by parathyroid excess. Once hypocalcemia signifies successful surgery, patients can be put on a high calcium intake or be given oral calcium supplements. Despite manifestations of mild hypocalcemia, most patients do not require parenteral therapy and do not experience severe symptoms. If the serum calcium falls below 2 mmol/L (8 mg/dL), *in particular if the phosphate level simultaneously rises*, the possibility of hypoparathyroidism must be considered. Coexistent hypomagnesemia should be checked for, since it interferes with PTH secretion and causes a relative hypoparathyroidism. Parenteral calcium replacement at a low level should be instituted if symptomatic hypocalcemia supervenes. Such symptoms include a general sense of anxiety and positive Chvostek and Trousseau signs coupled with serum calcium consistently below 2 mmol/L (8 mg/dL). For parenteral therapy, calcium (gluconate or chloride) solutions are prepared at a concentration of 1 mg/mL in 5% dextrose in water. The rate and duration of intravenous therapy are determined by the severity of the symptoms and the response of the serum calcium. A rate of infusion of 0.5 to 2 (mg/kg)/h or 30 to 100 mL/h of a 1 mg/mL solution usually suffices to relieve symptoms. Generally, parenteral therapy is required for only a few days. If symptoms become severe or if the need for parenteral calcium continues for more than 2 to 3 days, replacement therapy with a vitamin D analogue and/or oral calcium (2 to 4 g/d) should be started (see below). It is cost-effective to use calcitriol (doses of 0.5 to 1.0 μg/d) because of the rapidity of onset and rapidity of cessation of action, in contrast to vitamin D per se (see below). A sudden rise in blood calcium after several months of vitamin D replacement may indicate restoration of parathyroid function to normal. It is also appropriate to monitor serum PTH serially to estimate gland function in such patients.

Magnesium deficiency also may complicate the postoperative course. Magnesium deficiency impairs the secretion of PTH, and therefore, hypomagnesemia should be corrected whenever detected. Magnesium chloride is effective by mouth, but this compound is not widely available. Accordingly, repletion is usually parenteral. Since the depressant effect of magnesium on central and peripheral nerve functions does not occur below 2 mmol/L (normal range 0.8 to 1.2 mmol/L), parenteral replacement can be given rapidly. A cumulative dose as great as 0.5 to 1 mmol/kg of body weight can be administered if severe hypomagnesemia is present; often, however, total doses of 12 to 12 mmol are sufficient. The magnesium is given either as an intravenous infusion over 8 to 12 h or in divided doses intramuscularly (magnesium sulfate, USP).

LITHIUM THERAPY Lithium, used in the management of bipolar depression and other psychiatric disorders, causes hypercalcemia in approximately 10 percent of patients. The parathyroids are involved in mediation of the hypercalcemia, and PTH levels may be elevated. The hypercalcemia is dependent on continued lithium treatment, remitting and recurring when lithium is stopped and restarted. In a few patients, parathyroid adenomas were present. Histologic findings in the remaining parathyroid glands in these patients have not been described, but the implication is that there is a single abnormal gland.

The presence of hypercalcemia does not correlate with plasma lithium level, but the frequency with which hypercalcemia occurs is sufficiently high to support a causal relationship between lithium and the hypercalcemia, particularly the dependence of the hypercalcemia on the continuation of the lithium. It is presumed that in most cases an adenoma is not present, merely hyperfunctioning glands. Lithium, at the levels achieved in blood in treated patients, can be shown in vitro to shift the curve describing PTH secretion as a function of calcium level to the right; i.e., higher calcium levels are required to lower PTH secretion. It is logical to assume that this effect can cause elevated PTH and consequent hypercalcemia in otherwise normal individuals. If careful studies were done, elevated PTH levels might be found in more patients treated with lithium than the 10 percent in whom frank hypercalcemia is detected. The adenomas reported in some hypercalcemic patients with lithium therapy may reflect the presence of an independently occurring parathyroid tumor; a permanent effect of lithium on parathyroid gland growth need not be implicated, since the majority of patients have complete reversal of hypercalcemia when lithium is stopped. On the other hand, evidence suggesting monoclonality in large parathyroid glands in some patients with renal failure and secondary hyperparathyroidism implies that long-standing stimulation of parathyroid cell replication may predispose to development of adenomas such as those seen in primary hyperparathyroidism; hence chronic lithium stimulation of the parathyroids may be risk factor for adenoma formation. Long-term follow-ups have not been reported; many patients are continued on lithium to treat psychiatric problems. These patients are presumably best managed according to the principles used in asymptomatic hypercalcemia independent of lithium administration. If troubling symptoms or signs, such as rising blood calcium levels, progressive bone demineralization, or kidney stones, develop, it may be necessary to try alternate psychotropic medication. It does not seem wise to recommend parathyroid surgery unless hypercalcemia and elevated PTH persist after lithium is discontinued.

Familial hypocalciuric hypercalcemia Familial hypocalciuric hypercalcemia (familial benign hypercalcemia; FHH) is inherited as an autosomal dominant trait. Affected individuals are frequently discovered because of asymptomatic hypercalcemia; surgical exploration of the parathyroids is not indicated because parathyroidectomy does not cure the disorder. It is therefore important to separate such patients from those with primary hyperparathyroidism.

The pathophysiology is not understood, and there is no single biochemical marker to distinguish these patients from patients with primary hyperparathyroidism. The genetic defect maps to a locus on chromosome 3. A defect in a calcium channel or a calcium signaling mechanism is suspected. The aggregate evidence serves to separate FHH clinically from primary hyperparathyroidism. The majority of patients with primary hyperparathyroidism have less than 99 percent renal calcium reabsorption, and most patients with FHH exceed 99 percent reabsorption. The hypercalcemia may be detectable in affected members of the kindreds in the first decade of life, whereas hypercalcemia rarely occurs in primary hyperparathyroidism and the MEN syndromes under the age of 10 years. The iPTH values may be elevated in FHH, but the values are usually normal or lower for the same degree of calcium elevation than in patients with primary hyperparathyroidism. Recurrent surgery in a few patients led to permanent hypoparathyroidism, but hypocalciuria persisted nevertheless; the hypocalciuria, therefore, is not PTH-dependent. Serum magnesium levels are, on average, higher in FHH than in primary hyperparathyroidism.

Few clinical signs or symptoms are present in patients with FHH. Unlike the MEN syndromes, other endocrine abnormalities are not present. Most patients are detected as a result of family screening after the diagnosis has been made in one member of the kindred. All too commonly, the initial patient is operated on without reversal of the hypercalcemia. At operation, the glands appear normal, or a moderate degree of hyperplasia of all parathyroid glands is seen. No patient has had reversal of hypercalcemia by surgery unless all the parathyroid tissue has been inadvertently removed, rendering the patient hypoparathyroid, a most undesirable result. The high renal calcium reabsorption (parathyroid independent) and the prompt recurrence of hypercalcemia as long as any parathyroid tissue remains establish that there is some abnormality in the regulation of the ratio of extracellular to intracellular calcium concentration or some abnormal mechanisms of calcium sensing in cell membranes in the kidney and parathyroid gland. The exact nature of this disorder and its natural history are not clear yet, but since the parathyroid glands are permissive rather than responsible for the syndrome, parathyroid surgery is not appropriate, nor, in view of the lack of symptoms, is medical treatment needed to lower the calcium.

MALIGNANCY-RELATED HYPERCALCEMIA Clinical syndromes and mechanisms of hypercalcemia Hypercalcemia due to malignancy is common (occurring with 10 to 15 percent of certain types of tumor, such as lung carcinoma), often severe and difficult to manage, confusing as to etiology, and sometimes difficult to distinguish from primary hyperparathyroidism. Traditionally, hypercalcemia in malignancy was thought to be due to a local invasion and destruction of bone by tumor cells; many cases are now known to result from the elaboration by the malignant cells of humoral mediators of hypercalcemia.

Although the presence of malignancy is often clinically obvious, hypercalcemia can occasionally be due to an occult tumor. With occult malignancy, diagnosis and definitive treatment must be accomplished quickly if the patient is to be protected from the complications of the underlying malignancy.

Humoral hypercalcemia of malignancy occurs in patients with cancers of the lung and kidney in which bone metastases are absent, minimal, or not detectable clinically. The clinical picture resembles primary hyperparathyroidism (hypophosphatemia accompanies hypercalcemia), and elimination or regression of the primary tumor leads to disappearance of the hypercalcemia. Ectopic production of PTH by the tumor was initially felt to be responsible, but the disorder is in fact due to humoral mechanisms unrelated to ectopic PTH production.

Many patients with the humoral hypercalcemia of malignancy have elevated urinary nephrogenous cyclic AMP excretion, hypophosphatemia, and increased urinary phosphate clearance, findings compatible with the actions of a humoral agent that emulates PTH action. On the other hand, these patients generally have lower iPTH levels than patients with hyperparathyroidism. Using double-antibody assays of greater specificity, in fact, patients with the hypercalcemia of malignancy have either undetectable or suppressed immunoreactive PTH levels, consistent with non-PTH mechanisms. Other features of the syndrome differ from true hyperparathyroidism. Patients may have high, rather than low, renal calcium clearance (relative to serum calcium when compared to true hyperparathyroidism) and low to normal levels of 1,25-dihydroxyvitamin D [$1,25(OH)_2D$], all consistent with mediation by humoral factors distinct from PTH.

The histologic character of the tumor is more important than the extent of skeletal metastases in predicting hypercalcemia. Small cell carcinoma (oat cell) and adenocarcinoma of lung, although the most common lung tumors associated with skeletal metastases, rarely cause hypercalcemia. By contrast, as many as 10 percent of patients with squamous cell carcinoma of the lung develop hypercalcemia. Histologic studies of bone in patients with squamous cell or epidermoid carcinoma of the lung, in sites invaded by tumor as well as areas remote from tumor invasion, reveal bone remodeling, including osteoclastic and osteoblastic activity. In contrast, minimal evidence of skeletal metabolic activation is seen despite extensive skeletal metastases of small cell (oat cell) carcinoma.

Agents other than PTH are responsible for hypercalcemia, and only certain tumor types produce these factors. At least two general mechanisms of hypercalcemia are suspected. Most solid tumors associated with hypercalcemia, particularly squamous cell and renal tumors, produce and secrete cellular factors that are believed to cause increased bone resorption and to mediate the hypercalcemia through systemic actions on the skeleton as a whole by stimulation of bone resorption. On the other hand, direct bone marrow invasion occurs with other tumors, both hematologic malignancies such as leukemia, lymphoma, and multiple myeloma and solid tumors such as breast carcinoma. Substances produced by cells involved in the marrow response to the tumors promote resorption of bone through local destruction and may be identical or analogous to some of the known lymphokines and cytokines.

A classification of the hypercalcemia of malignancy is given in Table 357-2. Multiple myeloma and other hematologic malignancies involving the bone marrow have been typically considered as one group; bone destruction and hypercalcemia are believed to be caused through local mechanisms of malignant cells spread widely throughout the marrow spaces. Breast carcinoma is typical of solid tumors that cause hypercalcemia through *localized osteolytic destruction*, probably mediated by locally secreted tumor products that may differ from those involved in multiple myeloma or lymphoma. Finally, solid tumors not involving bone may cause hypercalcemia by secretion of a humoral mediator. In other instances, etiologic mechanisms may overlap.

In addition to the bone-resorbing factors elaborated by malignant cells in patients with hypercalcemia of malignancy, there may be variable synergism and antagonism between various bone-active agents secreted by the tumors. In some patients with the humoral hypercalcemia of malignancy, osteoclastic resorption may be generalized, and there is an absence of an osteoblastic or bone-forming response to the surge of bone resorption, implying some inhibition of the normal coupling of formation and resorption. Cooperativity and antagonism in the skeletal actions of locally released cytokines may include blockade of cytokine-induced bone resorption by interferon or related cytokines, both the bone-resorbing and bone-resorbing-blocking cytokines being secreted in response to interactions among tumor cells and host inflammatory cells. Thus the interaction of more than one substance may determine whether hypercalcemia develops in a particular patient.

Several hormones, hormone analogues, cytokines, and growth factors have been implicated as the result of clinical assays, in vitro tests, or chemical isolation. In some lymphomas, typically B cell lymphomas, there is an increased blood level of $1,25(OH)_2D$. It is not clear whether the increased $1,25(OH)_2D$ is produced by stimulation of the renal 1α-hydroxylase or by lymphocytes; the latter seems likely, based on studies with the malignant cells. The search for etiologic mechanisms in hematologic malignancies has focused on the production of distinctive bone-resorbing factors by activated normal lymphocytes and by myeloma and lymphoma cells. This factor(s), termed *osteoclast activation factor* (OAF), now appears to represent the biologic action of several different cytokines, probably interleukin 1 and lymphotoxin or tumor necrosis factor, two closely related cytokines.

More than one factor may be responsible for humorally mediated hypercalcemia in patients with solid tumors, but as discussed in the

---

TABLE 357-2 Classification of tumor hypercalcemia

HEMATOLOGIC MALIGNANCIES

A Local bone destruction (OAF, interleukin 1, tumor necrosis factor, lymphotoxin)
  Multiple myeloma
  Lymphomas
B Humoral mediation [$1,25(OH)_2D$, PTH-rP]
  Lymphomas

SOLID TUMORS

A Local bone destruction (prostaglandin, E series)
  Some breast cancers
B Humoral mediation (PTH-rP, ?other agents)
  Lung (squamous cell)
  Kidney
  Urogenital tract
  Other breast cancers

preceding chapter, a specific factor termed *parathyroid hormone–related protein* (PTH-rP) that resembles but is distinct from PTH fulfills criteria of a humoral agent for the hypercalcemia syndrome. This factor binds equivalently to the PTH receptor and activates the receptor in a manner indistinguishable from PTH itself. As discussed in Chap. 356, immunoassays for PTH-rP are complicated by the heterogeneity of the circulating forms of the peptide. Nonetheless, elevated levels of PTH-rP are present in patients with the typical syndrome of humoral hypercalcemia of malignancy. The complexity of the etiologic mechanisms, however, are illustrated by several findings. For example, some breast carcinoma cells produce high levels of PTH-rP, and a distinctive type of T cell lymphoma/leukemia syndrome due to HTLV-I infection is also associated with severe hypercalcemia and high levels of circulating PTH-rP. In most instances, in contrast, breast carcinoma is believed to cause hypercalcemia by local stimulation of osteoclasts directly by products secreted by the metastatic breast carcinoma cells and associated inflammatory cells. Breast carcinoma cells produce and secrete prostaglandins of the E series, which are potent local stimulators of bone-resorbing cells.

Several aspects of the hypercalcemia of malignancy remain unclear. Levels of urinary cyclic AMP rise in test animals treated with synthetic PTH-rP, but $1,25(OH)_2D$ levels also rise, which is at variance with the fact that many patients with the humoral hypercalcemic syndrome have normal or depressed levels of $1,25(OH)_2D$. Tumor-derived growth factors, believed to act as autocrine regulators to maintain the transformation and growth of tumor cells, and cellular growth factors produced by nonmalignant cells are also potent bone-resorbing agents in vitro. Still other factors potentially involved in tumor hypercalcemia are known only by their bone-resorbing properties and lack of stimulation of renal or bone cell cyclic AMP production. Several of these factors stimulate production of prostaglandins of the E_2 type.

Assays to detect PTH-rP using different approaches (single-antibody, double-antibody, different epitopes) give similar results, but there are discrepancies perhaps relating to the methodologic difficulties listed above. Most data indicate undetectable (or low) levels in normal subjects, elevated levels in many cancer patients with the humoral syndrome, and high levels in human milk. Thus, although identification of PTH-rP represents a singular advance, it is not established to what extent the substance constitutes the sole pathophysiologic mechanism in the humoral hypercalcemia of malignancy.

Diagnostic issues and treatment Ordinarily, the diagnosis of hypercalcemia secondary to tumor is not difficult to make because the tumor symptoms are prominent at the time the hypercalcemia is detected. Indeed, the hypercalcemia may be noted incidentally during the workup of a patient with known or suspected malignancy. Patients with malignancy and hypercalcemia may have a coexistent parathyroid adenoma, some reports suggesting an incidence as high as 10 percent.

Laboratory testing becomes critical when occult carcinoma is a possibility. Levels of iPTH by the newer double-antibody technique are undetectable or extremely low in tumor hypercalcemia, as would be expected with the mediation of the hypercalcemia by a nonparathyroid agent (the hypercalcemia suppressing the normal parathyroid glands). This improvement in the usefulness of the PTH assay is a significant advance in laboratory diagnosis. (Earlier assays gave equivocal results.) Assays for PTH-rP should be helpful; low or undetectable PTH and elevated PTH-rP would focus attention on the presence of an occult malignancy.

Clinical suspicion that malignancy is the cause of the hypercalcemia is heightened when symptoms associated with the paraneoplastic syndromes, such as weight loss, fatigue, muscle weakness, and unexplained skin rash, or symptoms specific for a particular tumor are present. Squamous cell tumors are most frequently associated with hypercalcemia, and the tumors most frequently arise in the lung, kidney, and urogenital tract. X-ray examinations can focus on these areas when clinical evidence is unclear. Bone scans with technetium-

labeled diphosphonate are useful for detection of osteolytic metastases; the sensitivity is high, but specificity is low; results must be confirmed by conventional x-rays to be certain that areas of increased uptake are due to osteolytic metastases per se. Bone marrow biopsies are helpful in patients with anemia or abnormal peripheral blood smears.

Treatment of the hypercalcemia of malignancy must be considered in the perspective of the individual patient. Control of the tumor is the principal objective, and reduction of tumor mass is usually also the key to satisfactory control of hypercalcemia. If a patient has severe hypercalcemia yet has an excellent chance for effective tumor therapy, treatment of the hypercalcemia should be vigorous. If hypercalcemia, on the other hand, is an accompaniment of the late stages of a tumor that is resistant to therapy, the treatment of the hypercalcemia should not be vigorous, since hypercalcemia can have a mild sedating effect. Standard therapies for hypercalcemia (discussed below) are applicable to patients with malignancy.

VITAMIN D–RELATED HYPERCALCEMIA Hypercalcemia related to abnormal vitamin D action can be due to *excessive ingestion* of vitamin D or *abnormal metabolism* of the vitamin. Abnormal metabolism of the vitamin is usually acquired in association with some widespread granulomatous disorder, but one rare hereditary form of vitamin D sensitivity in infants is associated with other developmental anomalies. As discussed in Chap. 356, vitamin D metabolism is carefully regulated, particularly the activity of the renal 1α-hydroxylase responsible for the production of $1,25(OH)_2D$. Many details of the regulation of 1α-hydroxylase remain unclarified, but the normal feedback suppression by $1,25(OH)_2D$ on the enzyme seems to work less well in infants than in adults and operates poorly, if at all, in ectopic sites, as distinct from the renal tubule; these facts explain the occurrence of hypercalcemia secondary to excessive $1,25(OH)_2D_3$ production in certain infants (Williams' syndrome) and in adults with granulomatous disease (sarcoidosis) or certain lymphomas.

Vitamin D Intoxication The chronic ingestion of large doses of vitamin D, usually at least 50 to 100 times the normal physiologic requirement (doses in excess of 50,000 to 100,000 units per day), is required to produce hypercalcemia in normal individuals. In animals, vitamin D intoxication causes increased bone resorption as well as increased intestinal calcium absorption. In humans, excessive vitamin D action leads to an increase in intestinal calcium absorption, but it is not known whether increased bone resorption contributes to the hypercalcemia.

The immediate mechanism for the hypercalcemia is presumed to be an excessive production of $1,25(OH)_2D$ as a consequence of an increase in the substrate for the renal 1α-hydroxylase; namely, $25(OH)D$ production is less tightly regulated than is the production of $1,25(OH)_2D$. Hence concentrations of $25(OH)D$ average 5 to 10 times above normal in patients on high-dose vitamin D, whether therapeutically, as in hypoparathyroidism, or accidentally, as in vitamin D intoxication. $25(OH)D$ has a definite, if low, biologic activity in intestine and bone. Hence part of vitamin D intoxication may be attributable to the high levels of $25(OH)D$ itself, as well as supernormal levels of $1,25(OH)_2D$.

The diagnosis is substantiated by documenting elevated levels of $25(OH)D$. Hypercalcemia is usually controlled by restriction of dietary calcium intake and appropriate attention to hydration. These measures, plus discontinuation of vitamin D, usually lead to satisfactory management, but vitamin D stores in fat may be substantial, and vitamin D intoxication may persist for weeks after vitamin D ingestion is terminated. Such patients are responsive to glucocorticoids, which in doses of 100 mg of hydrocortisone per day, or its equivalent, usually return calcium levels to normal over several days; severe intoxication may require intensive therapy.

Sarcoidosis and other granulomatous diseases Normal relations between $25(OH)D$ and the product, the active metabolite $1,25(OH)_2D$, are not maintained in patients with sarcoidosis and other granulomatous diseases. There is a positive correlation between $25(OH)D$ levels (reflecting vitamin D intake) and the circulating concentrations of 1,25(OH)$_2$D; normally there is no increase in 1,25(OH)$_2$D with increasing 25(OH)D levels due to multiple feedback controls on the activity of the renal 1α-hydroxylase (see Chap. 356). In patients with sarcoidosis, the site of synthesis of 1,25(OH)$_2$D is believed to be in macrophages or other cells associated with granulomatous deposits. Hypercalcemia has been reported in an anephric sarcoidosis patient in association with increased 1,25(OH)$_2$D levels. Macrophages obtained from granulomatous tissue form 1,25(OH)$_2$D at an increased rate when 25(OH)D is provided as substrate. The usual regulation of active metabolite production by calcium or PTH does not operate in these patients; hypercalcemia does not lead to a reduction in the blood levels of 1,25(OH)$_2$D in patients with sarcoidosis. PTH-independent production of 1,25(OH)$_2$D is indicated by reports of normal 1,25(OH)$_2$D production in a patient with sarcoidosis and hypoparathyroidism. Clearance of 1,25(OH)$_2$D from blood may be decreased in sarcoidosis as well.

Even normocalcemic patients with sarcoidosis have unregulated production of 1,25(OH)$_2$D in response to vitamin D loading. Exposure to sunlight or administration of as little as 9000 units of vitamin D daily is followed by increased levels of the active metabolite. Treatment with moderate doses of glucocorticoids leads to a reversal of the hypercalcemia, as in other cases of excessive vitamin D action such as vitamin D intoxication, and reversal of the abnormal responsiveness of 1,25(OH)$_2$D levels to vitamin D challenge. Presumably, glucocorticoid administration causes multiple effects in the disease, and both excessive production of the metabolite and the responsiveness to it in target organs are blocked.

Variation in reported frequency of hypercalcemia in sarcoidosis (10 percent or less in recent reports, 60 percent or more in older reports) is probably explained in part by the common use of glucocorticoids to control pulmonary complications and other manifestations of the granulomatous disease. Lytic lesions also occur in bone so that increased bone resorption could play a role in some cases. In most, however, hypercalcemia is directly related to an increased intestinal calcium absorption. Clinically, hypercalcemia is usually a manifestation of disseminated disease. Hence pulmonary involvement is usual; chest x-ray may reveal a diffuse fibronodular infiltrate and/or prominent hilar adenopathy. Levels of angiotensin converting enzyme are elevated; blood gamma globulin also may be elevated. The most useful diagnostic procedure is demonstration of noncaseating granulomas in liver or lymph node biopsy. Hypercalcemia due to sarcoidosis can be elusive when many of the typical features of the disease are lacking (see section on differential diagnosis).

Management of the hypercalcemia in these patients can be accomplished by avoiding excessive sunlight exposure and by limiting vitamin D and calcium intake; glucocorticoids in the equivalent of 100 mg hydrocortisone per day or less usually are sufficient to control hypercalcemia when it occurs. Presumably, however, the abnormal sensitivity to vitamin D and abnormal regulation of 1,25(OH)$_2$D synthesis will persist as long as the disease is active. PTH levels are usually suppressed and 1,25(OH)$_2$D levels are elevated, but primary hyperparathyroidism and sarcoidosis may occur in some patients.

Idiopathic hypercalcemia of infancy This unusual disorder, sometimes referred to as *Williams' syndrome*, consists of multiple congenital development defects, including supravalvular aortic stenosis, mental retardation, and an elfin facies, in association with hypercalcemia due to abnormal sensitivity to vitamin D. The syndrome was first recognized in England after the commencement of fortification of milk with vitamin D. Hypercalcemia develops with vitamin D intakes as small as 2000 to 4000 units per day. Levels of 1,25(OH)$_2$D are elevated, ranging from 46 to 120 nmol/L (150 to 500 pg/mL). The mechanism of the abnormal sensitivity to vitamin D and of the increased circulating levels of 1,25(OH)$_2$D is unclear. The children become hypercalcemic because of excessive intestinal calcium absorption. The abnormality in vitamin D metabolism and the increased sensitivity to vitamin D intake do not occur after the first year of life. Treatment is restriction of calcium intake. Occasionally, the hypercalcemia can be severe, and calcium values

above 4 mmol/L (16 mg/dL) are recorded. Treatment with glucocorticoids in the doses used for vitamin D intoxication or sarcoidosis, adjusted for body weight, rapidly reverses the hypercalcemia.

HYPERCALCEMIA ASSOCIATED WITH HIGH BONE TURNOVER

Hyperthyroidism As many as 20 percent of hyperthyroid patients have high-normal or mildly elevated serum calcium concentrations; hypercalciuria is even more common. The hypercalcemia seems due to increased bone turnover, with bone resorption exceeding bone formation. Severe calcium elevations are not typical, however, and the presence of such suggests a concomitant disease such as hyperparathyroidism. Indeed, patients with thyrotoxicosis are more sensitive to the hypercalcemic effects of PTH. Usually, the diagnosis is obvious, but signs of hyperthyroidism may occasionally be occult, particularly in the elderly. Hypercalcemia is managed by specific therapy of the hyperthyroidism.

Immobilization Immobilization in adults is rarely associated with hypercalcemia in the absence of an associated disease but may cause hypercalcemia in children and adolescents, particularly after spinal cord injury and paraplegia or quadriplegia. With resumption of some ambulation, the hypercalcemia in children usually returns to normal spontaneously.

The mechanism appears to involve a disproportion between rates of bone formation and bone resorption. Hypercalciuria and increased mobilization of skeletal calcium can be seen in normal volunteers subjected to extensive bed rest, although hypercalcemia does not usually occur. Immobilization in an adult with an underlying disease associated with high bone turnover, such as Paget's disease, may cause hypercalcemia.

Thiazides Administration of benzothiadiazines (thiazides) can cause hypercalcemia in patients with high rates of bone turnover, such as patients with hypoparathyroidism treated with high doses of vitamin D. Traditionally, thiazides are associated with aggravation of hypercalcemia in primary hyperparathyroidism but this effect can be seen in other high-bone-turnover states as well. The mechanism of action of the drugs is complex, but the overall result seems to be to impose a challenge to calcium homeostasis by actions on renal calcium excretion, on bone-calcium turnover, and on parathyroid action. Thiazide administration in normal individuals causes a transient increase in blood calcium (but usually within the high normal range) which reverts to preexisting levels after a week or more of continued administration. If hormonal function and calcium and bone metabolism are normal, homeostatic controls are reset to counteract the calcium-elevating effect of the thiazides. In the presence of hyperparathyroidism or increased bone turnover from another cause, homeostatic mechanisms are ineffective. The abnormal effects of the thiazide on calcium metabolism disappear within days of cessation of the drug.

Many aspects of the action of the thiazides on calcium metabolism remain unclear. The drug clearly augments PTH responsiveness of target cells of bone and renal tubule. Chronic thiazide administration leads to reduction in urinary calcium excretion; the hypocalciuric effect of the drug appears to reflect the enhancement of proximal tubular resorption of sodium and calcium in response to sodium depletion. Some of this renal action reflects augmentation of PTH actions and is more pronounced in subjects with intact parathyroid secretion. However, a substantial hypocalciuric effect can be achieved in hypoparathyroid patients on high-dose vitamin D and oral calcium replacement if sodium intake is restricted. This finding is the rational for the use of thiazides as an adjunct to therapy in hypoparathyroid patients as discussed below.

Vitamin A intoxication Vitamin A intoxication is a rare cause of hypercalcemia. Most vitamin A intoxication is a side effect of excessive intake of the vitamin. Calcium levels can be elevated into the 3 to 3.5 mmol/L (12 to 14 mg/dL) range after the ingestion of 50,000 to 100,000 units of vitamin A daily (10 to 20 times the minimum daily requirement). The patients have typical features of severe hypercalcemia, which include fatigue and anorexia. They may have severe muscle and bone pain. The excess vitamin A intake is presumed to increase bone resorption.

Diagnosis can be established by history and by measurements of vitamin A levels in serum, which may be increased severalfold above normal. Occasionally, skeletal x-rays reveal periosteal calcifications, particularly in the hands. Withdrawal of the vitamin is usually associated with the prompt disappearance of the hypercalcemia and reversal of the skeletal changes. As in vitamin D intoxication, administration of 100 mg/d hydrocortisone or its equivalent leads to a rapid return of the serum calcium to normal.

HYPERCALCEMIA ASSOCIATED WITH RENAL FAILURE Severe secondary hyperparathyroidism Secondary hyperparathyroidism occurs when partial resistance to the metabolic actions of the hormone leads to excessive PTH production. Parathyroid gland hyperplasia occurs because resistance to the normal level of the hormone leads to hypocalcemia, which, in turn, is a stimulus to enlargement of the parathyroid glands with resultant increased secretion of PTH. This concept is based on studies in experimental animals with renal failure and phosphate retention and studies of the treatment of patients with diphosphonates that block skeletal resorptive response. In Fig. 357-2 is illustrated the pathophysiology of hormone production in secondary hyperparathyroidism. When the parathyroid secretory reserve is tested by deliberately lowering blood calcium, the extent of rise in PTH for each decrement of plasma calcium is greater with parathyroid hyperplasia than with normal glands. There is, therefore,

FIGURE 357-2 The relation between blood calcium and iPTH in normal subjects and subjects with secondary (2°) hyperparathyroidism. This model of secondary hyperparathyroidism assumes that there is an increased mass of parathyroid tissue. The lower line represents normal secretory patterns, and the upper line describes the exaggerated secretion (steeper slope) typical of secondary hyperparathyroidism. When calcium level in blood is raised by calcium infusion and multiple measurements of PTH and calcium are made, some portion of hormone secretion in normals is constant despite high calcium levels in blood (nonsuppressible secretion), and this secretion is higher in hyperparathyroidism. An elevation of blood calcium from low normal levels [(2 mmol/L (8 mg/dL)] to high normal levels [(2.2 mmol/L (9 mg/dL)] results in a reduction in PTH in both normal and hyperparathyroid individuals, but true involution of secondary hyperparathyroidism with treatment can be confirmed only by showing a return of the exaggerated response curve to normal.

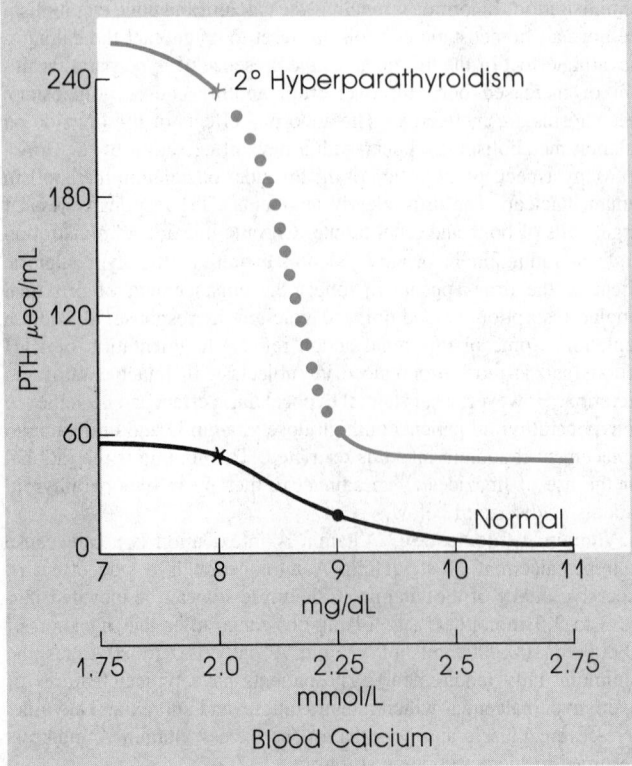

a higher concentration of hormone at any given level of calcium concentration. Since a portion of PTH secretion by each individual parathyroid cell is not suppressible by any degree of elevation of blood calcium concentration, larger glands (more cells) have a higher hormone output at the hypercalcemic end of the dose-response curve.

Secondary hyperparathyroidism occurs in patients with renal failure, osteomalacia (vitamin D deficiency), and pseudohypoparathyroidism (deficient response to PTH at the level of the receptor). The clinical manifestations of secondary hyperparathyroidism vary in these states. Hypocalcemia seems to be the common denominator in secondary hyperparathyroidism. Primary and secondary hyperparathyroidism can be distinguished conceptually by the autonomous nature of the growth of the parathyroid glands in primary hyperparathyroidism (presumably irreversible) and the adaptive increase in parathyroid gland size in secondary hyperparathyroidism (presumably reversible). In fact, reversal over weeks from an abnormal pattern of secretion, presumably accompanied by an involution of parathyroid gland mass to a normal pattern of function, can be monitored in patients treated with bisphosphonate after the drug is withdrawn (see Fig. 357-2). In some patients with secondary hyperparathyroidism, enlarged glands are monoclonal in origin. This phenomenon must mark conversion of the parathyroid glands from a state of reversible hyperplasia (polyclonal) to an irreversible growth defect (monoclonal); presumably, a more serious state of glandular hyperfunction occurs after the monoclonal transformation. Clinically, this concept has been referred to as *tertiary hyperparathyroidism.*

In progressive kidney disease, the initial tendency to hypocalcemia seems attributable to two causes: phosphate retention that develops because of the reduced excretion of phosphate and reduced concentrations of 1,25(OH)$_2$D associated with progressive renal damage. The two disturbances reduce skeletal responsiveness to PTH. The deficiency of 1,25(OH)$_2$D also interferes with the absorption of calcium from the intestine, already impaired in uremia. The ultimate pathophysiologic consequences in any given patients with chronic renal failure represent the outcome of competing physiologic adaptations, stimuli that cause parathyroid gland hyperplasia (tendency toward hypercalcemia and excessive bone resorption) versus those which modify the hormonal responsiveness of the end organs—bone, gut, and residual renal tubules (tendency toward hypocalcemia, hyperphosphatemia, and reduced bone resorption). Typically patients with renal failure exhibit hyperphosphatemia (renal retention and increased bone breakdown) and a low normal or moderately low blood calcium (calcium-lowering action of the phosphate level and reduced availability of calcium from bone and gut). In patients with severe secondary hyperparathyroidism, hypercalcemia and hyperphosphatemia both develop due to an increase in bone resorption; parathyroid hypersecretion "overshoots" the degree of resistance to hormone action; the monoclonal expansion of parathyroid gland mass may play a role in the "overshoot" and hypercalcemia.

In addition to hypercalcemia and hyperphosphatemia, patients with secondary hyperparathyroidism may develop bone pain, ectopic calcification, and pruritus. The bone disease in patients with secondary hyperparathyroidism and renal failure is usually termed *renal osteodystrophy.* Concomitant osteomalacia (vitamin D and calcium deficiency) and osteitis fibrosa cystica (excessive PTH action on bone) may occur. In fact, osteitis fibrosa cystica is now more common in untreated renal failure than in primary hyperparathyroidism.

Judicious medical therapy, which includes reduction of excessive blood phosphate by dietary phosphate restriction plus the use of nonabsorbable antacids (or, to avoid excess aluminum ingestion, calcium-containing antacids, either of which tie up phosphate in the gut) and careful, selective addition of calcitriol (0.25 to 2.0 μg/d), may reverse severe secondary hyperparathyroidism. Intravenous administration of calcitriol has been reported to cause long-term involution of secondary hyperparathyroidism (this experimental approach is designed, in part, to suppress PTH synthesis). As illustrated in Fig. 357-2, involution of the parathyroids then occurs; reduction of increased cellular mass causes the exaggerated secretory response to return to normal. The level of PTH at any given level of blood calcium is now more appropriate, and excessive parathyroid action is reversed. Somewhat paradoxically, during successful medical reversal of secondary hyperparathyroidism, elevated serum calcium (and phosphate) levels return to normal despite the administration of increased amounts of calcium and vitamin D metabolites that might have been expected to aggravate the hypercalcemia.

Aluminum intoxication Aluminum intoxication occurs in patients on chronic dialysis; manifestations include acute dementia and unresponsive and severe osteomalacia. Bone pain, multiple nonhealing fractures, particularly of the ribs and pelvis, and a proximal myopathy may occur. Hypercalcemia develops when attempts are made to treat these patients as one treats those with severe secondary hyperparathyroidism and renal osteodystrophy due to renal failure, as discussed above, namely, by administration of vitamin D or calcitriol. Acute hypercalcemia occurs after administration of vitamin D because of impaired skeletal responsiveness. Aluminum is present at the site of osteoid mineralization, and osteoblastic activity is minimal. Presumably, these patients are unable to incorporate the increased blood calcium into the skeleton. Prevention is accomplished by avoidance of aluminum excess in the dialysis regimen; treatment involves mobilizing aluminum through the use of the chelating agent deferoxamine. Aluminum is mobilized from bone and, being tightly bound to the chelating agent, can be removed via dialysis. After aluminum toxicity is reversed, patients may show typical features of renal osteodystrophy and secondary hyperparathyroidism. They can then be managed like other patients with secondary hyperparathyroidism with renal disease. A failure to recognize the syndrome is associated with persistence of the disabling bone disease and a fatal course due to progressive features or to hypercalcemia inadvertently induced by treatment with vitamin D.

Milk-alkali syndrome The milk-alkali syndrome can cause several clinical presentations—acute, subacute, and chronic—all of which feature hypercalcemia, alkalosis, and renal failure. The disorder is due to an excessive ingestion of calcium and absorbable antacids such as milk or calcium carbonate and is less frequent since nonabsorbable antacids and H-2 receptor antagonists such as cimetidine and ranitidine became available for the treatment of peptic ulcer disease.

Individual susceptibility must be important in pathogenesis, since many patients are treated with calcium carbonate without developing the syndrome. One variable is the fractional calcium absorption as a function of calcium intake. Some individuals absorb a high fraction of calcium, even with intakes as high as 2 g and more of elemental calcium per day, instead of reducing calcium absorption with high intake, as occurs in most normal subjects. Resultant mild hypercalcemia after meals in such patients is postulated to be the critical factor in the generation of alkalosis. With the development of hypercalcemia, increased sodium excretion and some depletion of total-body water occur. These phenomena and perhaps, additionally, some suppression of endogenous PTH secretion due to mild hypercalcemia would lead to increased bicarbonate resorption. This bicarbonate retention then would lead to alkalosis in the face of continued calcium carbonate ingestion. Alkalosis per se causes selective enhancement of calcium resorption in the distal nephron, thus aggravating the hypercalcemia. The cycle of mild hypercalcemia → bicarbonate retention → alkalosis → renal calcium retention → severe hypercalcemia perpetuates and aggravates hypercalcemia and alkalosis as long as calcium and absorbable alkali are ingested.

Acute hypercalcemia and alkalosis occurring within days of beginning calcium and alkali ingestion, *acute milk-alkali syndrome*, is manifested by weakness, myalgia, irritability, and apathy. The impairment of renal function, including reduced renal concentrating ability and tubular dysfunction as well as hypercalcemia and alkalosis, reverses rapidly upon stopping the intake of calcium and alkali.

The far-advanced milk-alkali syndrome, sometimes referred to as *Burnett's syndrome*, is due to long-standing calcium and alkali ingestion. Severe hypercalcemia, irreversible renal failure, and phos-

phate retention may be accompanied by ectopic calcification. Some improvement may result when the ingestion of calcium and alkali is reduced, but prior to the availability of renal dialysis, renal failure led to death. There is an intermediate or subacute form in which the renal failure is reversible over a period of weeks after withdrawal of excessive calcium and alkali intake.

DIFFERENTIAL DIAGNOSIS: SPECIAL TESTS Differential diagnosis of hypercalcemia is best achieved by using clinical criteria, but the radioimmunoassay for PTH, as now modified, is useful in distinguishing among major causes. The clinical features that deserve major emphasis are the presence or absence of symptoms or signs of disease and evidence of chronicity. If one discounts fatigue or depression, patients with *asymptomatic hypercalcemia* have primary hyperparathyroidism in well over 90 percent of instances; symptoms of malignancy are usually present when hypercalcemia is due to cancer. Disorders other than hyperparathyroidism and malignancy cause no more than 10 percent of cases of hypercalcemia, and some of the nonparathyroid causes are associated with clear-cut manifestations such as renal failure.

Chronicity is the second most important clinical criterion. If hypercalcemia has been manifest for more than 1 year, malignancy can usually be excluded as the cause of hypercalcemia. A striking feature of malignancy-associated hypercalcemia is the rapidity of the course, whereby signs and symptoms of the underlying malignancy are evident within months of the detection of hypercalcemia. Hyperparathyroidism is the likely diagnosis in patients with *chronic hypercalcemia*. Diseases such as sarcoidosis are rare causes of chronic hypercalcemia. A careful *history* of dietary supplements and drug use will often readily reveal intoxication with vitamins D or A or the use of thiazides.

Although clinical considerations are helpful in arriving at the correct diagnosis of the cause of hypercalcemia, appropriate laboratory testing is essential for definitive diagnosis (Table 357-3). Theoretically, the radioimmunoassay for PTH should separate hyperparathyroidism from all other causes of hypercalcemia, those with hyperparathyroidism having elevated levels of iPTH despite hypercalcemia and patients with malignancy and the other causes of hypercalcemia (except for other disorders mediated by PTH such as lithium-induced hypercalcemia) having levels of hormone below normal or undetectable. Early assays sometimes gave equivocal results, but assays based on the double-antibody method separate from those with primary hyperparathyroidism hypercalcemic patients with malignancy (Fig. 357-3), thus establishing the method as possessing the relevant specificity and sensitivity to serve the central test in the differential diagnosis (see Table 357-3). $1,25(OH)_2D$ levels are elevated in many (but not all) patients with primary hyperparathyroidism and are also increased in states of vitamin D intoxication, particularly sarcoidosis. In other disorders associated with hypercalcemia, concentrations of $1,25(OH)_2D$ are low or, at the most, normal. Since not all patients with hyperparathyroidism, however, have elevated $1,25(OH)_2D$ levels, and since not all nonparathyroid hypercalcemic patients have suppressed $1,25(OH)_2D$, the test is of low specificity and not cost-effective in

TABLE 357-3 Differential diagnosis of hypercalcemia

Clinical issues alone	
>90% due to hyperparathyroidism or cancer	
If asymptomatic or chronic	Hyperparathyroidism most likely
Use of PTH assay	
If PTH level increased (or rarely normal)	Hyperparathyroidism confirmed
If PTH level decreased (or undetectable)	*Acute presentation*—with or without symptoms—screen carefully for malignancy
	Chronic—malignancy unlikely, sarcoidosis or other rarer cause

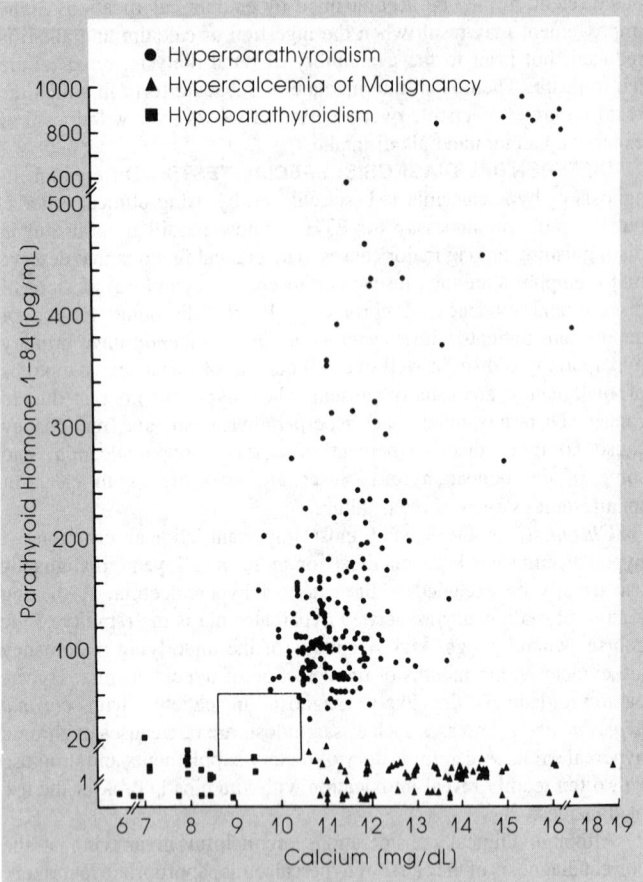

FIGURE 357-3 Levels of iPTH detected in patients with primary hyperpara-thyroidism, hypercalcemia of malignancy, and hypoparathyroidism. *(From Nussbaum and Potts.)*

differential diagnosis per se; measurement of 1,25(OH)$_2$D is of critical value in establishing the cause of hypercalcemia in sarcoidosis and certain B cell lymphomas.

PTH levels are elevated in chronic renal failure; the elevation seen in early assays reflects, in part, accumulation of fragments secondary to renal failure rather than true parathyroid oversecretion. Results with the double-antibody assay correlate well with independent evidence for parathyroid gland overactivity. Patients with sarcoidosis have low or undetectable levels of iPTH. No systematic surveys have been reported of the results of double-antibody PTH radioimmunoassays in many of the other non-parathyroid-related causes of hypercalcemia shown in Table 357-1 largely because of the infrequency with which the disorders are encountered, but it is predicted that they will be low or undetectable.

In summary, iPTH values are elevated in greater than 90 percent of parathyroid-related causes of hypercalcemia, undetectable or low in malignancy-related hypercalcemia, and undetectable or normal in vitamin D-related and high-bone-turnover–related causes of hypercalcemia (although there is a paucity of data for these latter categories).

Measurements of nephrogenous cyclic AMP are of limited value in distinguishing primary hyperparathyroidism and malignancy. Elevation of nephrogenous cyclic AMP occurs in some patients with malignancy and in essentially all patients with primary hyperparathyroidism. Specific laboratory tests are of utility in diagnosing particular disorders (such as thyrotoxicosis), and the newer immunoassays for PTH-rP are helpful in diagnosing certain types of malignancy-associated hypercalcemia.

Some general recommendations can be made as to the differential diagnosis of hypercalcemia. Two independent causes of hypercalcemia in the same person, although reported, are rare. If a specific disease traditionally associated with hypercalcemia (see Table 357-1) is

clinically evident, it is reasonable to assume that the disease is responsible for the hypercalcemia. It is cost-effective, in view of the specificity and speed of the PTH radioimmunoassay and the high frequency of hyperparathyroidism in hypercalcemic patients, to measure the iPTH level in all hypercalcemic patients unless malignancy is clinically evident or a specific diagnosis of a nonparathyroid disease is obvious. If hypercalcemia disappears in response to control of hyperthyroidism or after reduction of excessive intake of fat-soluble vitamins or alkali and calcium, in the cases of vitamin D intoxication and milk-alkali syndrome, respectively, there is no need to search for a second cause of hypercalcemia. If specific treatment does not lead to a reversal of the hypercalcemia, a search for an additional cause, by detailed laboratory testing, must be undertaken. It also follows that the management of the patient with the hypercalcemia of malignancy focuses on management of the malignancy.

When the diagnosis is unclear, either because the patient is asymptomatic or because chronic illness obscures manifestations that might indicate the presence of malignancy, the following general approach can be used: If the patient is *asymptomatic* and there is evidence by history of *chronicity* to the hypercalcemia, hyperparathyroidism is almost certainly the cause. If iPTH levels (usually measured at least twice) are elevated, little additional evaluation is necessary. Hyperparathyroidism is never confirmed until abnormal parathyroid tissue is removed surgically and hypercalcemia is corrected, but patients with asymptomatic hypercalcemia can be presumed to have the diagnosis on the basis of elevated concentration of iPTH. If there is a family history suggestive of other endocrine abnormalities, screening for multiple endocrine neoplasia should be undertaken in the patient and family.

If the patient does not have clear-cut symptoms and there is only a short history or no clue as to the duration of the hypercalcemia, *occult malignancy* must be considered. If the iPTH levels with the double-antibody technique are increased, the diagnosis of asymptomatic hyperparathyroidism is established.

If patients with recent-onset hypercalcemia have clear-cut systemic symptoms and/or the iPTH levels are not elevated, then a thorough workup must be undertaken for malignancy, including chest x-ray, computed tomography of chest and abdomen, and bone scan. Attention also should be paid to clues for underlying hematologic disorders such as anemia, increased plasma globulin, and abnormal serum immunoelectrophoresis; bone scans can be negative in patients with multiple myeloma.

Finally, if a patient with *chronic hypercalcemia* is *asymptomatic* but iPTH values are not elevated, and if malignancy seems unlikely on clinical grounds (*chronicity*), it is useful to search for other chronic causes of hypercalcemia, such as occult sarcoidosis. Table 357-3 summarizes the approach.

MEDICAL TREATMENT OF HYPERCALCEMIA The acute treatment of hypercalcemia is usually successful. The serum calcium concentration can be decreased by 0.7 to 2.2 mmol/L (3 to 9 mg/dL) within 24 to 48 h in most patients, enough to relieve acute symptoms, prevent death from hypercalcemic crisis, and permit diagnostic evaluation. However, the chronic medical management of hypercalcemia is less satisfactory unless the underlying cause can be corrected because available therapies are inconvenient and may be toxic.

Hypercalcemia develops because of excessive skeletal calcium release, increased intestinal calcium absorption, or inadequate renal calcium excretion. Understanding the particular pathogenesis helps guide therapy. For example, hypercalcemia in patients with osteolytic metastases or acute immobilization is primarily due to excessive skeletal calcium release and is, therefore, minimally improved by restriction of dietary calcium. On the other hand, patients with vitamin D hypersensitivity or vitamin D intoxication have excessive intestinal calcium absorption, and restriction of dietary calcium is beneficial. Decreased renal function or extracellular fluid depletion decreases urinary calcium excretion. If additional abnormalities, such as increased bone breakdown, are present, hypercalcemia will develop. This may happen, for example, when patients with resorptive bone disease become dehydrated. In such situations, rehydration may rapidly reduce or reverse the hypercalcemia, even though bone resorption and urinary calcium excretion are increased.

Hydration, increased salt intake, mild and forced diuresis The first principle of treatment is to restore *normal hydration*. Many hypercalcemic patients are dehydrated because of vomiting, inanition, and/or hypercalcemia-induced defects in urinary concentrating ability. The resultant drop in glomerular filtration rate is accompanied by an additional decrease in renal tubular sodium and calcium clearance. Restoring a normal extracellular fluid volume corrects these abnormalities and increases urine calcium excretion by 2.5 to 7.5 mmol/d (100 to 300 mg/d). Increased urinary sodium excretion to 400 to 500 mmol/d increases urinary calcium excretion even further than simple rehydration. After rehydration has been achieved, saline can be administered or furosemide or ethacrynic acid can be given twice daily to depress the tubular reabsorptive mechanism for calcium (care must be taken to prevent dehydration). The combined use of these therapies can increase urinary calcium excretion to 12.5 mmol/d (500 mg/d) or higher in most hypercalcemic patients. Since this is a substantial percentage of the exchangeable calcium pool, the serum calcium concentration usually falls 0.25 to 0.75 mmol/L (1 to 3 mg/dL) within 24 h. Precautions should be taken to prevent potassium and magnesium depletion; calcium-containing renal calculi are a potential complication.

Under life-threatening circumstances, the preceding approach can be pursued more aggressively, giving as much as 6 L isotonic saline (900 mmol sodium) daily plus furosemide or equivalent in doses up to 100 mg every 1 to 2 h or ethacrynic acid in doses to 40 mg every 1 to 2 h. Urinary calcium excretion may exceed 25 mmol/d (1000 mg/d), and the serum calcium may decrease by 1 mmol/L (4 mg/dL) or more within 24 h. Depletion of potassium and magnesium is inevitable unless replacements are given; pulmonary edema can be precipitated. The potential complications can be reduced by careful monitoring of central venous pressure and plasma or urine electrolytes; a bladder catheter may be necessary. This treatment approach should be immediately supplemented with agents to block bone resorption

that become effective within a few days, since forced diuresis is difficult to sustain even in patients with good cardiopulmonary and renal function.

Bisphosphonates The bisphosphonates are analogues of pryophosphate, with high affinity for bone, especially in areas of increased bone turnover. These bone-seeking compounds are stable in vivo because phosphatase enzymes cannot hydrolyze the central carbon-phosphorus-carbon bond. The bisphosphonates are concentrated in areas of high bone turnover and are taken up by and inhibit osteoclast action; the detailed mechanism of action is not well understood. Bisphosphonates may alter proton pump function or impair the release of acid hydrolases into the excellular lysosomes contiguous with mineralized bone. They also may inhibit the differentiation of monocyte-macrophage precursors into osteoclasts.

Etidronate, a first-generation bisphosphonate, is poorly absorbed and, like most bisphosphonates, generally must be given intravenously to be effective. At times, the continuation of oral etidronate after intravenous therapy may be useful to control hypercalcemia.

A newer class of bisphosphonates has more favorable efficacy and longer duration of action (Table 357-4). Pamidronate is a potent inhibitor of osteoclast-mediated skeletal resorption yet does not cause mineralization defects as ordinary doses. (Pamidronate is approved by the FDA for intravenous use for hypercalcemia of malignancy.) Several additional bisphosphonates (alendronate, toludronate, and risidronate) that are highly potent and have a favorable ratio of blocking resorption over inhibiting bone formation are undergoing clinical trials in the United States. Between 60 and 90 mg pamidronate, given as a single intravenous dose, returns serum calcium to normal in 80 to 100 percent of patients for weeks or months.

While the bisphosphonates have similar structures, efficacy, toxicity, and side effects vary. Etidronate therapy results in hyperphosphatemia, through a direct renal mechanism, whereas hypophosphatemia is seen following therapy with other bisphosphonates. Toxicities of the aminobisphosphonates include low-grade fever in as many as 20 percent of patients, likely related to release of cytokines from osteoclasts, monocytes, and macrophages, and possibility,

---

TABLE 357-4 Therapies for severe hypercalcemia

Treatment	Onset of action	Duration of action	Advantages	Disadvantages
MOST USEFUL THERAPIES				
Hydration with saline	Hours	During infusion	Rehydration invariably needed	
Forced diuresis; saline + loop diuretic	Hours	During treatment	Rapid action	Cardiac decompensation, intensive monitoring electrolyte disturbance hypokalemia, hypomagnesemia
Bisphosphonates				
1st generation: etidronate	1–2 days	5–7 days in doses used	First available bisphosphonate; intermediate onset of action	Hyperphosphatemia; 3-day infusion
2d generation: pamidronate	1–2 days	10–14 days after high dose	High potency; intermediate onset; prolonged duration of action	Fever in 20%; hypophosphatemia hypocalcemia, hypomagnesemia
Calcitonin	Hours	2–3 days	Rapid onset of action; useful as adjunct in severe hypercalcemia	Often limited calcium lowering, rapid tachyphylaxis
OTHER THERAPIES				
Gallium nitrate	Day after 5-day administration	7–10 days	High potency	Length of IV administration; cannot be used with renal failure
Plicamycin	3–4 days	Days	Potent antiresorptive	Liver, kidney, and marrow toxicity; bleeding
Phosphate				
Oral	24 h	During use	Low toxicity if P < 4 mg/dL	Limited use except as adjuvant or chronic therapy
Intravenous	Hours	During use and 24–48 h afterward	Rapid action, highly potent	Ectopic calcification; severe hypocalcemia
Glucocorticoids	Days	Days, weeks	Oral therapy, antitumor agent	Active only in certain malignancies; glucocorticoid side effects
Dialysis	Hours	During use and 24–48 h afterward	Useful in renal failure; onset of effect in hours; can immediately reverse life-threatening hypercalcemia	Complex procedure, reserved for extreme or special circumstances

reversible hepatocellular injury (Table 357-4). Overall, second-generation bisphosphonates are now the agents of choice in several hypercalcemia, particularly that associated with malignancy.

Calcitonin Calcitonin acts within minutes of its administration, through receptors on osteoclasts, to decrease the release of skeletal calcium, phosphorus, and hydroxyproline. In addition, inhibition of renal tubular calcium reabsorption may, in part, contribute to its rapid onset of action. In various reports, however, the administration of 2 to 8 U/kg of body weight intravenously, subcutaneously, or intramuscularly every 6 to 12 h caused variable and minimal lowering of calcium in some patients. Tachyphylaxis, a well-known phenomenon with this drug, may explain the variable results. This escape from the hypocalcemic effects of calcitonin is seen in vitro, where it can be prevented by glucocorticoids. In vivo in humans, administration of glucocorticoids in combination with calcitonin may augment or prolong the action of calcitonin; in some patients, particularly those with lymphoproliferative malignancies, continued lowering of calcium may last for as long as 10 days. In other studies, however, the prevention of tachyphylaxis by glucocorticoids was not impressive. Calcitonin therapy with the salmon, porcine, and human sequences, as currently used, rarely returns serum calcium to normal and can best be viewed as a nontoxic therapy with a very rapid onset of action and definite, although limited, efficacy. However, in life-threatening hypercalcemia, calcitonin can be used while waiting for a more sustained effects from plicamycin, gallium, or bisphosphonate. Calcitonin therapy may be associated with transient nausea, cramping, abdominal pain, and flushing.

Plicamycin For the acute management of hypercalcemia, plicamycin (mithramycin), which inhibits bone resorption, has been a useful therapeutic agent. Plicamycin must be given intravenously, either as a bolus injection or by slow infusion. The usual dose is 25 μg/kg of body weight. In some patients, 10 μg/kg of body weight can be given twice a week for chronic therapy. Treatment should not be repeated until hypercalcemia recurs, because the toxicity of the drug is dependent on the frequency of treatment and the total dosage. Careful monitoring is needed if repeated doses are used. The major side effects are thrombocytopenia, hepatocellular necrosis with increased lactic acid dehydrogenase (LDH) and aspartate aminotransferase (AST) levels, and decreased levels of clotting factors with resultant epistaxis, bruising, hemorrhage, and bleeding gums. Azotemia, proteinuria, and hypocalcemia may occur. Hypophosphatemia, hypokalemia, nausea, vomiting, stomatitis, and facial swelling may occur. Toxicity is rare when only one or two doses are used and can be minimized by repeating single doses only when hypercalcemia recurs. Toxic effects other than hemorrhage can usually be reversed by stopping the drug. Use of plicamycin has been largely replaced by the less toxic second-generation bisphosphonates.

Gallium nitrate Gallium nitrate exerts a hypocalcemic action by inhibiting bone resorption and altering the structure of bone crystals. The major disadvantages appear to be the 5-day duration of infusion and the potential for nephrotoxicity. Alternative, shorter-dosage regimens have not been reported. (Gallium nitrate is approved by the FDA for the treatment of hypercalcemia; further clinical experience should help define its ultimate role.)

Other therapies Glucocorticoids increase urinary calcium excretion and decrease intestinal calcium absorption when given in pharmacologic doses (e.g., 40 to 200 mg prednisone daily in divided doses), but they also cause negative skeletal calcium balance. In normal subjects and in patients with primary hyperparathyroidism, glucocorticoids neither increase nor decrease the serum calcium concentration. In patients with hypercalcemia due to certain osteolytic malignancies, however, glucocorticoids may be effective as a result of antitumor effects. The malignancies in which hypercalcemia responds to glucocorticoids include hematologic malignancies such as multiple myeloma, leukemia, Hodgkin's disease, other lymphomas, and carcinoma of the breast, at least early in the course. Glucocorticoids are also effective in treating hypercalcemia due to vitamin D intoxication and sarcoidosis. In all the preceding situations, the hypocalcemic effect develops over several days, and the usual glucocorticoid dosage is 40 to 100 mg prednisone (or its equivalent) daily in four divided doses. The side effects of chronic glucocorticoid therapy may be acceptable in some circumstances.

Hypercalcemia complicated by renal failure is difficult to manage; dialysis is often the treatment of choice. Peritoneal dialysis with calcium-free dialysis fluid can remove 5 to 12.5 mmol (200 to 500 mg) of calcium in 24 to 48 h and lower the serum calcium concentration by 0.7 to 3 mmol/L (3 to 12 mg/dL). Large quantities of phosphate are lost during dialysis, and serum inorganic phosphate concentrations usually fall, thus aggravating hypercalcemia. Therefore, the serum inorganic phosphate concentration should be measured after dialysis, and phosphate supplements should be added to the diet or to dialysis fluids if necessary.

Phosphate therapy, oral or intravenous, has a role in certain circumstances. Patients with primary hyperparathyroidism are frequently hypophosphatemic, and hypercalcemia of other causes also may be complicated by hypophosphatemia. Hypophosphatemia decreases the rate of calcium uptake into bone, increases intestinal calcium absorption, and directly and indirectly stimulates bone breakdown. These effects aggravate hypercalcemia, and correcting hypophosphatemia lowers the serum calcium concentration. The usual treatment is 1 to 1.5 g phosphorus per day for several days, given in four divided doses to minimize the chances of developing hyperphosphatemia. Such therapy has been administered for prolonged periods in selected patients. It is generally believed but not established that toxicity will not occur if the phosphate therapy is limited to restoring serum inorganic phosphate concentrations to normal rather than making them supranormal.

Raising the serum inorganic phosphate concentration above normal does decrease serum calcium levels, sometimes strikingly. Intravenous phosphate is one of the most dramatically effective treatments available for severe hypercalcemia but is toxic and even dangerous so that it is used rarely and *only* in severely hypercalcemic patients with cardiac or renal failure. A dose of 1500 mg phosphate phosphorus or more intravenously over 6 to 8 h leads to a prompt decrease in serum calcium of as much as 1.2 to 2.5 mmol/L (5 to 10 mg/dL) in patients with initially normal serum inorganic phosphate concentrations. This therapy should be employed only in extreme emergencies for two reasons. First, fatal hypocalcemia can be produced by excessive dosage; serum calcium should be measured frequently if intravenous phosphate is administered. Second, unlike sodium chloride, sodium phosphate does not remove calcium from the body. In fact, urine calcium generally declines, and fecal calcium declines or remains the same. The decline in serum calcium reflects a redistribution of calcium within the body. There is a rapid efflux of calcium with no change in calcium influx to the circulation, findings indicative of precipitation of calcium phosphate salt. The calcium precipitates in bone, and metastatic calcification also may occur in patients receiving oral or intravenous phosphate therapy for hypercalcemia. Indeed, hyperphosphatemia can cause metastatic calcification in normocalcemic animals. Thus administration of intravenous phosphate in patients with compromised renal function who cannot have diuretic therapy is justifiable only as an emergency treatment.

Inorganic phosphate is commercially available for oral use in liquid, powder, and capsule form and as a liquid for intravenous use. It is important to calculate doses in terms of phosphate phosphorus (see Table 357-5).

Summary The various therapies for hypercalcemia are listed in Table 357-4. The choice depends on the underlying disease, the severity of the hypercalcemia, the serum inorganic phosphate level, and the renal, hepatic, and bone marrow function. Mild hypercalcemia [3 mmol/L (12 mg/dL) or less] can usually be managed by the sequence of hydration followed by intravenous sodium chloride and, if needed, small doses of furosemide or ethacrynic acid. Severe hypercalcemia [3.7 mmol/L (15 mg/dL)] requires rapid correction. Calcitonin should be given for its rapid, albeit short-lived, blockade of bone resorption, and intravenous pamidronate should be administered,

TABLE 357-5 Commercially available phosphate preparations

	1000 mg P	mmol Na	mmol K
ORAL PREPARATIONS			
Neutraphos (1250-mg capsule)	4 caps	28.5	28.5
Neutraphos-K (1450-mg capsule)	4 caps	—	57
Phos-Tabs (860-mg tablet)	6 tabs	—	51
Fleets Phospho-Soda (liquid)	6.7 mL	40	—
INTRAVENOUS PREPARATIONS			
In-Phos	40 mL	65	8
Hyper-Phos-K	15 mL	—	50

SOURCE: After RM Neer and JT Potts Jr, in *Endocrinology*, LJ DeGroot et al (eds), 2d ed, Philadelphia, Saunders, 1989, with permission.

although its onset of action is delayed for 1 to 2 days. Hence aggressive sodium-calcium diuresis with intravenous saline and large doses of furosemide and ethacrynic acid works but should be initiated only if appropriate monitoring is available and cardiac function is adequate.

There is a role for oral phosphate therapy in chronic management of hypercalcemia, but its utility may be superseded by the bisphosphonates. Phosphate supplements should only be administered if hyperphosphatemia is not present.

Severe dietary calcium restriction should be employed and glucocorticoids should be administered judiciously if intestinal absorption is enhanced (in sarcoidosis, vitamin D intoxication). Dialysis is appropriate for hypercalcemia complicating acute or chronic renal failure.

Chronic therapy of hypercalcemia poses greater problems of toxicity. One satisfactory regimen for chronic use is a combination of dietary calcium restriction, administration of sodium chloride with or without furosemide or ethacrynic acid to maintain high urinary calcium, and moderate-dose oral phosphate (the patient is kept normophosphatemic). Some of the effective remedies (plicamycin, glucocorticoids, high-dose oral phosphate) may have significant toxicity when used chronically. Oral bisphosphonates, if proven nontoxic, may become the chronic treatment of choice in cases of hypercalcemia where increased bone resorption is responsible for the disturbance in calcium metabolism.

HYPOCALCEMIA

PATHOPHYSIOLOGY OF HYPOCALCEMIA: CLASSIFICATION BASED ON MECHANISM
Chronic hypocalcemia is less common than hypercalcemia; causes include chronic renal failure, hereditary and acquired hypoparathyroidism, vitamin D deficiency, pseudohypoparathyroidism, and hypomagnesemia.

Critically ill patients may have *transient hypocalcemia* in association with severe sepsis, burns, acute renal failure, and extensive transfusions with citrated blood. Acute hypocalcemia in association with certain medications is also usually transient and may have no symptoms. Although as many as half of patients in intensive care setting are reported to have calcium concentrations below 2.1 mmol/L (8.5 mg/dL), less than 10 percent have a reduction in ionized calcium. Patients with severe sepsis may have a decrease in ionized calcium (true hypocalcemia), but in other severely ill subjects, hypoalbuminemia is the cause of the reduced total calcium concentration. Alkalosis, however, increases calcium binding to proteins, and in this setting, direct measurements of ionized calcium should be made.

Medications such as protamine, heparin, and glucagon may cause transient hypocalcemia. These forms of hypocalcemia, apparent or real, are usually not associated with tetany and resolve with improvement in the overall medical condition. The hypocalcemia after repeated transfusions of citrated blood also usually resolves quickly.

Patients with acute *pancreatitis* have hypocalcemia that persists during the acute inflammation and varies in degree with the severity of the pancreatitis. The cause of hypocalcemia in pancreatitis remains unclear. PTH values are variously reported to be low, normal, or elevated, and both resistance to PTH and impaired PTH secretion have been postulated. Occasionally, a chronic low total-blood calcium and low ionized calcium concentration are detected in an elderly patient without obvious cause and with a paucity of symptoms of hypocalcemia; the pathogenesis is unclear.

Chronic hypocalcemia, however, is usually symptomatic and requires treatment. Neuromuscular and neurologic manifestations of chronic hypocalcemia include muscle spasms, carpopedal spasm, facial grimacing, and in extreme cases, laryngeal spasm and convulsions. Respiratory arrest may occur. Increased intracranial pressure occurs in some patients with long-standing hypocalcemia, often in association with papilledema. Mental changes include irritability, depression, and psychosis. The QT interval on the electrocardiogram is prolonged, in contrast to its shortening with hypercalcemia. Arrhythmias occur, and digitalis effectiveness may be reduced. Intestinal cramps and chronic malabsorption may occur. Chvostek's or Trousseau's sign can be used to confirm latent tetany.

The classification of hypocalcemia shown in Table 357-6 is based on the premise that PTH is responsible for minute-to-minute regulation of plasma calcium concentration within narrow limits and, therefore, that the occurrence of hypocalcemia must mean a failure of the homeostatic action of PTH. Failure of the PTH response can occur if PTH is absent due to hereditary or acquired gland failure, if the hormone is ineffective at target organs, or if the action of the hormone is overwhelmed by the loss of calcium from the extracellular fluid at a rate faster than it can be replaced.

PTH ABSENT Hypoparathyroidism, whether hereditary or acquired, has a number of common components. Acute and chronic symptoms of untreated hypocalcemia are shared by both types of hypoparathyroidism, although typically the onset of hereditary hypoparathyroidism is more gradual and hereditary hypoparathyroidism is associated with developmental defects. In earlier decades, acquired hypoparathyroidism secondary to surgery in the neck was

TABLE 357-6 Functional classification of hypocalcemia (excluding neonatal conditions)

PTH ABSENT

A Hereditary hypoparathyroidism
B Acquired hypoparathyroidism
C Hypomagnesemia

PTH INEFFECTIVE

A Chronic renal failure
B Active vitamin D lacking
  1 ↓ dietary intake or sunlight
  2 Defective metabolism:
    Anticonvulsant therapy
    Vitamin D–dependent rickets type I
C Active vitamin D ineffective
  1 Intestinal malabsorption
  2 Vitamin D–dependent rickets type II
D Pseudohypoparathyroidism

PTH OVERWHELMED

A Severe, acute hyperphosphatemia
  1 Tumor lysis
  2 Acute renal failure
  3 Rhabdomyolysis
B Osteitis fibrosa after parathyroidectomy

more common than hereditary hypoparathyroidism, but the frequency of surgically induced parathyroid failure has diminished as a result of parathyroid gland preservation and the use of nonsurgical treatment of hyperthyroidism. Basal ganglia calcification and extrapyramidal syndromes are more common and earlier in onset in hereditary hypoparathyroidism. Pseudohypoparathyroidism, an example of ineffective PTH action rather than a failure of parathyroid gland production, shares several features with hypoparathyroidism, including extraosseous calcification and extrapyramidal manifestations such as choreoathetotic movements and dystonia. Papilledema and raised intracranial pressure occur in both states, as do chronic changes in fingernails and hair and lenticular cataracts, the latter usually reversible with treatment of hypocalcemia. Certain skin manifestations, including alopecia and candidiasis, occur exclusively in hereditary hypoparathyroidism.

Hypocalcemia associated with hypomagnesemia is associated with both deficient PTH release and impaired responsiveness to the hormone (see also Chap. 360). Patients with hypocalcemia secondary to hypomagnesemia have absent or low levels of circulating PTH, indicative of diminished hormone release despite maximum physiologic stimulus by hypocalcemia. Plasma PTH levels return to normal with correction of the hypomagnesemia. Thus hypoparathyroidism associated with low levels of PTH in blood can be due to hereditary gland failure, acquired gland failure, or acute but reversible gland dysfunction (hypomagnesemia). Patients with acquired or hereditary hypoparathyroidism also have hyperphosphatemia and absent or low levels of $1,25(OH)_2D$.

Hereditary hypoparathyroidism Hypoparathyroidism can occur as an isolated entity without other endocrine or dermatologic manifestations (idiopathic hypoparathyroidism) or, more typically, in association with other abnormalities such as defective development of the thymus or failure of function of other endocrine organs such as the adrenal thyroid or ovary (see also Chap. 343). Idiopathic and hereditary hypoparathyroidisms are often manifest within the first decade but may appear later.

One rare form of hypoparathyroidism due to congenital aplasia of the parathyroid glands is manifested shortly after birth; there is a linkage between defective development of the thymus and the parathyroid glands. The disorder is termed the *DiGeorge syndrome*, or the *third and fourth branchial pouch syndrome*, is associated with congenital cardiovascular and other developmental defects. Most patients die in early childhood with severe infections, hypocalcemia and seizures, or cardiovascular complications. Some patients survive into adulthood. Milder, incomplete forms are recognized. Most cases are sporadic. Cytogenetic abnormalities involving chromosome 22 are reported.

Hypoparathyroidism can occur in association with other diverse developmental defects or as part of a complex hereditary autoimmune syndrome involving failure of the adrenals, the ovaries, and the parathyroids in association with recurrent mucocutaneous candidiasis, alopecia, vitiligo, and pernicious anemia (see Chap. 343). In many cases, antibodies to endocrine organs are present; there is, in addition, a failure of cell-mediated immunity. The inheritance of the autoimmune syndrome appears to be autosomal recessive, and some unaffected family members show antibodies to endocrine tissue without evidence of endocrine failure. The disorder is usually referred to as autoimmune polyglandular deficiency.

Hereditary hypoparathyroidism occurs also as an isolated entity without any other defects. The mechanism of inheritance varies from one kindred to another. Autosomal dominant, autosomal recessive, and X-linked inheritance patterns have all been identified. In one family in which the disorder was transmitted as an autosomal dominant trait, a structural abnormality in the PTH gene has been identified. The defect in the signal sequence needed for processing of the hormone before secretion rather than in the structural portion interferes with PTH secretion. In one kindred with autosomal recessive inheritance, the homozygous mutant allele has a mutation in the first gene intron which causes a splicing defect in mRNA production. Most

kindreds, however, have no clue as to the genetic origin of the hypoparathyroidism.

Treatment of hypoparathyroidism is similar to that for acquired hypoparathyroidism and pseudohypoparathyroidism, although specific features of each disease require additional treatments. Replacement therapy with vitamin D or calcitriol combined with a high oral calcium intake usually suffices to regulate blood calcium and phosphate levels satisfactorily. Oral calcium and vitamin D restore the overall calcium-phosphate balance but do not reverse the lowered urinary calcium reabsorption typical of hypoparathyroidism. Therefore, care must be taken to avoid excessive urinary calcium excretion after vitamin D and calcium replacement therapy; otherwise, kidney stones can develop. Thiazide diuretics lower urine calcium by as much as 100 mg/d in hypoparathyroid patients on vitamin D, provided patients are maintained on a low-sodium diet. Use of thiazides seems to be of benefit in mitigating hypercalciuria.

Acquired hypoparathyroidism *Acquired chronic hypoparathyroidism* is usually the result of inadvertent surgical removal of all the parathyroid glands; in some instances, not all the tissue is removed, but the remainder undergoes compromise of vascular supply secondary to fibrotic changes in the neck after surgery. In the past, the most frequent cause of acquired hypoparathyroidism was surgery for hyperthyroidism. Hypoparathyroidism now usually occurs after surgery for hyperparathyroidism when the surgeon, facing the dilemma of removing too little tissue and thus not curing the hyperparathyroidism, removes too much.

Parathyroid function is not totally absent in all patients with postoperative hypoparathyroidism, but suitable therapy varies greatly from patient to patient irrespective of the type of hypoparathyroidism or the question of residual parathyroid activity.

Even rarer causes of acquired chronic hypoparathyroidism include radiation-induced damage subsequent to radioiodine therapy of hyperthyroidism or glandular damage in patients with hemochromatosis or hemosiderosis after repeated blood transfusions. Chronic infections may involve one or more of the parathyroids but usually do not cause permanent hypoparathyroidism because all four glands are not usually involved.

Transient hypoparathyroidism is frequent following surgical exploration for hyperparathyroidism. Often, after a variable period of hypoparathyroidism, normal parathyroid function returns due to hyperplasia or recovery of remaining tissue. Occasionally, recovery occurs months after surgery. The management of transient postoperative hypoparathyroidism is discussed under the surgical treatment of hyperparathyroidism. The treatment of chronic acquired hypoparathyroidism is similar to that used with idiopathic hypoparathyroidism: replacement with calcitriol and oral calcium.

Hypomagnesemia Hypomagnesemia of a severe degree is associated with severe hypocalcemia (see also Chap. 360). Restoration of the total-body magnesium deficits leads to rapid reversal of hypocalcemia. There are least two causes of the hypocalcemia—impaired secretion and reduced responsiveness to PTH.

Hypomagnesemia is generally classified as primary or secondary; primary hypomagnesemia is due to hereditary defects in intestinal absorption or renal reabsorption of magnesium. Secondary hypomagnesemia, a more common condition, occurs on a nutritional basis or as a result of acquired intestinal or renal disorders. The most common causes of the secondary disorder are chronic alcoholism with poor nutritional intake, intestinal malabsorption syndromes, and parenteral nutrition in which magnesium replacement is omitted.

Magnesium in extracellular fluid has effects similar to those of calcium on secretion of PTH; hypermagnesemia suppresses and hypomagnesemia stimulates PTH secretion. Effects of magnesium on hormone secretion are normally of little physiologic significance, however, because the effects of calcium dominate. Greater change in magnesium than in calcium is needed to influence hormone secretion. Nonetheless, hypomagnesemia, if it influences hormone secretion at all, might be expected to increase hormone secretion. It is therefore surprising to find that severe hypomagnesemia is associated with blunted secretion of PTH. The explanation for the paradox is that severe, chronic hypomagnesemia reflects intracellular magnesium deficiency; severe intracellular magnesium deficiency interferes with secretion and peripheral responses to PTH. The mechanism of the cellular defects due to hypomagnesemia is unknown, although a defective adenylate cyclase response (for which magnesium may serve as a cofactor) has been proposed.

Severe hypocalcemia is often seen when serum magnesium is substantially below the normal range of 0.8 to 1.2 mmol/L (2 to 3 mg/dL). In most cases in which hypomagnesemia is associated with hypocalcemia, serum magnesium is below 0.4 mmol/L (1.0 mg/dL).

PTH levels are usually undetectable or inappropriately low despite the extreme stimulus of severe hypocalcemia, and acute repletion of magnesium leads to a rapid increase in PTH concentration. The overall data indicate that PTH secretion is blunted in virtually all patients with severe hypomagnesemia; thus absolute or relative hypoparathyroidism seems to be the rule in patients with hypocalcemia secondary to hypomagnesemia.

In addition, diminished peripheral responsiveness to administered PTH occurs in some patients, as manifested by subnormal response in urinary phosphorus and urinary cyclic AMP excretion after administration of exogenous PTH to hypomagnesemic patients who are hypocalcemic. Both blunted PTH secretion and lack of renal response to administered PTH can occur in the same patient. When acute magnesium repletion is undertaken, the restoration of PTH concentrations to normal or supranormal levels may precede by several days the restoration of normal serum calcium.

Overall, blunted PTH secretory response in hypomagnesemia seems the real cause of hypocalcemia. The fact that impaired peripheral responsiveness, particularly renal response, is more variable from patient to patient suggests that an even greater degree of magnesium deficiency is required to induce end-organ resistance than to impair hormone secretion.

Several other features have been noted. The brisk response in hormone secretion following magnesium repletion, sometimes demonstrable within minutes of giving a large parenteral dose of magnesium, indicates that hormone biosynthesis is not impaired, only secretion. Serum phosphate levels are often not elevated, as they usually are in patients with acquired or idiopathic hypoparathyroidism, probably because phosphate deficiency is a frequent accompaniment of hypomagnesemia. Magnesium wasting may occur in chronic renal disease; magnesium is usually elevated in acute renal failure but is usually normal in chronic renal failure.

Repletion of magnesium is the cure of the condition, and attention must be given to restoring the intracellular deficiency, which may be considerable. After intravenous magnesium administration, serum magnesium may return transiently to the normal range, but unless replacement therapy is adequate, serum magnesium will rapidly fall to subnormal levels again. If renal function is normal, a useful indicator of restoration of magnesium deficiency is the urinary magnesium excretion; magnesium is retained by the kidney until magnesium deficiencies are repleted. Intracellular deficits can be as great as 50 mmol or more. Parenteral administration of 10 to 14 mmol magnesium usually reverses the signs of magnesium deficiency. If the cause of the hypomagnesemia is renal magnesium wasting, treatment may have to be administered chronically to prevent recurrence.

PTH INEFFECTIVE   PTH can be considered ineffective when the hormone receptor–guanyl nucleotide-biding protein complex is defective or when PTH action to promote calcium absorption from the diet is interfered with because of a primary deficiency of vitamin D or because of conditions in which vitamin D is ineffective (receptor or synthesis defects) or in chronic renal failure in which the calcium-elevating action of PTH is opposed by several different processes associated with uremia.

Despite diverse pathophysiologic mechanisms, these latter conditions involving ineffectiveness of PTH (excluding the rare condition of defective PTH-receptor response) often involve, but are not limited

to, the unavailability of vitamin D as a cofactor for PTH. Hypocalcemia is usually mild and is accompanied by hypophosphatemia. Typically, hypophosphatemia is more severe than hypocalcemia due to the increased secretion of PTH. Increased PTH is only partly effective in elevating blood calcium, but its ability to promote renal phosphate excretion is only slightly impaired in vitamin D deficiency. Varying degrees of bone disease with impaired mineralization and/or frank osteomalacia are the more frequent and harmful consequences of chronic renal failure or inadequate or ineffective vitamin D action due to the hypophosphatemia.

Pseudohypoparathyroidism, on the other hand, has a distinct pathophysiology from the other disorders of ineffective PTH action. Pseudohypoparathyroidism most closely resembles conditions in which there is an absence of PTH synthesis and secretion and is manifested, in the untreated state, by hypocalcemia and hyperphosphatemia. The cause of the disease, however, is defective hormone binding to the receptor or deficient activation of guanyl nucleotide-binding proteins, resulting in failure to increase intracellular cyclic AMP (see below).

Chronic renal failure   Severe abnormalities in mineral and bone metabolism occur in chronic renal failure, and improved medical management of chronic renal failure and/or a more indolent course of the renal disease allow many patients to survive long enough for renal osteodystrophy, the mixed bone disease associated with renal failure, to became an important feature. The roles of phosphate retention and impaired production of $1,25(OH)_2D$ are recognized as the principal factors responsible for inducing calcium deficiency, secondary hyperparathyroidism, and frequently a picture of severe bone disease. The uremic state appears to be associated also with impairment of intestinal absorption by factors other than defects in vitamin D metabolism. Nonetheless, treatment with supraphysiologic amounts of vitamin D or calcitriol leads to satisfactory calcium absorption.

Hyperphosphatemia per se in renal failure tends to lower blood calcium concentration by several actions; these include extraosseous deposition of calcium and phosphate, impaired sensitivity of the skeleton to the bone-resorbing action of PTH, reduced $1,25(OH)_2D$ production by surviving renal tissue, and reduction in calcium absorption due to trapping of calcium in insoluble form as calcium phosphate complexes. In animals, prevention of hyperphosphatemia by dietary means can block the development of secondary hyperparathyroidism, emphasizing the importance of phosphate retention in the pathogenesis of secondary hyperparathyroidism and the associated disorders of mineral and bone metabolism in renal failure. Low levels of $1,25(OH)_2D$ are due to hyperphosphatemia and to destruction of renal tissue and are critical in the hypocalcemia.

Therapy of chronic renal failure (see Chaps. 237 and 238) involves careful management of patients prior to dialysis as well as adjustment of dialysis regimens once this becomes necessary. Attention should be paid to restriction of phosphate in the diet, use of phosphate-binding antacids such as those based on aluminum hydroxide or calcium-containing salts which serve as phosphate binders and as a source of needed calcium supplementation and which avoid the problem of aluminum intoxication, provision of an adequate calcium intake by mouth, usually 1 to 2 g/d, and supplementation with 0.25 to 1.0 μg/d calcitriol. Each patient must be monitored closely. The aims of therapy are to restore normal calcium balance to prevent osteomalacia and secondary hyperparathyroidism. Renal osteodystrophy, as discussed earlier, is the principal disabling feature of chronic renal failure related to calcium metabolism. Reduction of hyperphosphatemia and restoration of normal intestinal calcium absorption by calcitriol can improve blood calcium concentration and reduce the manifestations of secondary hyperparathyroidism.

Vitamin D deficiency due to inadequate diet and/or sunlight Vitamin D deficiency is more common in the United States than previously recognized. Biopsies of bone in elderly patients with hip fracture (documenting osteomalacia) and abnormal concentrations of vitamin D metabolites, PTH, calcium, and phosphate have established that vitamin D deficiency may occur in as many as 25 percent of elderly patients, particularly in areas where there is little ambient sunlight. Concentrations of 25(OH)D are at the lower limits of normal or below normal in these patients. Quantitative histomorphometry of bone biopsy specimens reveals widened osteoid seams consistent with osteomalacia. PTH hypersecretion compensates for a tendency of the blood calcium level to fall, but with the consequence of inducing renal phosphate wasting and a combined mineral ion abnormality that results in osteomalacia.

The genesis of vitamin D deficiency is impaired intake of dairy products that are enriched with vitamin D, lack of vitamin supplementation, and reduced sunlight exposure in the elderly, particularly in winter in northern latitudes.

Treatment involves the administration of vitamin D and provision of 1 to 1.5 g calcium in the diet. Vitamin D supplementation should aim to provide several times the recommended daily requirement in younger people, which is probably a safe recommendation; a dosage of 1000 to 2000 units of vitamin D per day is satisfactory. Vitamin D is usually not available in small-dose forms. Hence the administration of a capsule containing 50,000 units of vitamin D once monthly is safe in elderly patients who have osteomalacia. The increased awareness of the importance of calcium supplementation, particularly in women, even without supplementation of vitamin D, may lessen the frequency of this problem. Severe hypocalcemia is rarely seen in the moderately severe vitamin D deficiency of the elderly, but vitamin D deficiency needs to be considered in the differential diagnosis of mild hypocalcemia.

Defective vitamin D metabolism ANTICONVULSANT THERAPY Anticonvulsant therapy with any of several agents induces a state of acquired vitamin D deficiency by increasing the conversion of vitamin D into inactive compounds. The more marginal the degree of vitamin D intake in the diet, the more likely that anticonvulsant therapy will lead to abnormalities in mineral and bone metabolism. The syndrome at its extreme involves severe rickets with bone fractures, hypocalcemia, hypophosphatemia, and on occasion severe proximal myopathy. More often, frank hypocalcemia is not detected, and mild osteomalacia is the only clinical symptom. In other patients on long-term anticonvulsant therapy, no symptoms or signs are present, but bone density is lower than normal and responds favorably to vitamin D supplementation.

Anticonvulsants stimulate the hepatic microsomal mixed-oxidase enzymes and hence increase the rate of clearance of vitamin D and its metabolites. Phenytoin also impairs intestinal calcium absorption independent of effects on vitamin D; the drug also has deleterious effects on bone cell function in vitro, including inhibition of collagen synthesis. All manifestations of the syndrome can nevertheless be reversed with adequate vitamin D supplementation.

Although 1,25(OH)$_2$D levels are lower for the degree of vitamin D intake in patients treated with chronic anticonvulsants than in the normal population, there is a great deal of variation. The greater prevalence of the disorder in some European populations and in children in homes for the mentally retarded probably reflects the lower vitamin D intake of those groups. Restoration of bone mineral mass and reversal of hypocalcemia, when seen, can be accomplished with vitamin D replacement plus added oral calcium. Adjustments in dose are indicated depending on the age and body size of the patient, but approximately 50,000 units of vitamin D weekly plus 1 g elemental calcium per day for several months is usually sufficient. Alternatively, administration of one 50,000-unit capsule of vitamin D monthly may be preventive if anticonvulsant therapy must be given chronically.

VITAMIN D–DEPENDENT RICKETS TYPE I   Rickets can be due to *resistance* to the *action* of vitamin D as well as to vitamin D deficiency. Vitamin D–dependent rickets type I, previously termed *pseudo-vitamin D–dependent rickets*, differs from vitamin D–resistant rickets in that it is less severe and the biochemical and radiographic abnormalities can be reversed with large doses of the vitamin.

Clinical features include hypocalcemia, often with tetany or convulsions, hypophosphatemia, secondary hyperparathyroidism, and osteomalacia, often associated with skeletal deformities and increased alkaline phosphatase. Doses of vitamin D or calcifediol, 100 to 1000 times above the usual amounts, are required to heal the bone disease, whereas physiologic amounts of calcitriol cure the disease. This finding fits with the pathophysiology. The disorder, an autosomal recessive trait, is due to a defect in conversion of 25(OH)D to 1,25(OH)$_2$D. Plasma levels of 1,25(OH)$_2$D are low or undetectable even after administration of large doses of vitamin D or calcifediol. Response to high doses of vitamin D or calcifediol is probably due to direct actions of high levels of 25(OH)D. Treatment requires careful adjustment of calcitriol dose, particularly during growth periods.

Active vitamin D ineffective INTESTINAL MALABSORPTION   Mild hypocalcemia, secondary hyperparathyroidism, severe hypophosphatemia, and a variety of nutritional deficiencies occur with gastrointestinal diseases. Hepatocellular dysfunction can lead to reduction in 25(OH)D levels, as in portal or biliary cirrhosis of the liver. Malabsorption of vitamin D and its metabolites, including 1,25(OH)$_2$D, may occur in a variety of intestinal diseases, hereditary or acquired. Hypocalcemia itself can lead to steatorrhea, due to deficient production of pancreatic enzymes and bile salts. Depending on the disorder, vitamin D or its metabolites can be administered parenterally, thereby guaranteeing adequate blood levels of active metabolites.

VITAMIN D–DEPENDENT RICKETS TYPE II   Pseudo-vitamin D–dependent rickets can be due to defective response as well as to defective production of 1,25(OH)$_2$D. This disorder, vitamin D–dependent rickets type II, results from any of several types of end-organ resistance to the active metabolite, including absence or qualitative defects of the intracellular receptor protein for the hormone and postreceptor blocks in hormone action (see Chap. 329). The clinical features are similar to those with the type I disorder and include hypocalcemia, hypophosphatemia, secondary hyperparathyroidism, and rickets. Plasma levels of 1,25(OH)$_2$D are elevated at least three times above normal, in keeping with the refractoriness of the end organs. Severe alopecia totalis may commence early in life. Patients with this disorder usually require much higher doses of vitamin D or vitamin D metabolites than with the type I disorder.

Pseudohypoparathyroidism   Pseudohypoparathyroidism (PHP) is a hereditary disorder characterized by symptoms and signs of hypoparathyroidism, typically in association with distinctive skeletal and developmental defects. The hypoparathyroidism is due to a deficient end-organ response to PTH. Excessive secretion of PTH is the consequence of hyperplasia of the parathyroids, a response to the resistance to hormone action. The entity is actually a syndrome in which various individuals and kindreds exhibit different aberrancies in hormone receptor complex response. Studies, both clinical and basic, have clarified some aspects of this still confusing syndrome, including the variable spectrum of the clinical features, the pathophysiology, the genetic defects, and the hereditary patterns.

Most patients show a characteristic phenotype usually referred to as *Albright's hereditary osteodystrophy* (AHO). Short stature, round face, skeletal anomalies (brachydactyly), and heterotopic calcification constitute the AHO phenotype. The patients have low calcium and high phosphate, as do patients with true hypoparathyroidism. PTH levels, however, are elevated, and resistance to hormone action can be demonstrated as, for example, by defective urinary cyclic AMP response to PTH administration. The cases are commonly familial; not all kindreds show the AHO phenotype but only the abnormal mineral metabolism. A few patients are resistant to PTH but exhibit normal urinary cyclic AMP response (responses in calcium and phosphate seemingly blocked after the adenyl cyclase step).

At least part of the defect is attributable in the majority of patients (those with the AHO phenotype) to inheritance of one defective allele that must encode the α subunit of the guanyl nucleotide–binding protein ($G_{s\alpha}$). This defect seems to account for a diminished response to PTH (approximately 50 percent of normal, consistent with one defective allele). However, in some kindreds there are individuals with a distinctive AHO phenotype who, while unaffected with symptoms or signs of defective mineral metabolism, still have a demonstrable 50 percent reduction in assays of $G_{s\alpha}$ subunits (so-called pseudopseudohypoparathyroidism). Hence the defective guanyl nucleotide subunit concentration is not itself sufficient to explain the pathophysiology. Perhaps another independently inherited allelic defect so far undetected is needed to provide full expression of the disordered mineral metabolism.

Since the defective $G_{s\alpha}$ subunit function was recognized, attention has focused on the molecular mechanism of the defective guanyl nucleotide–binding protein function. The gene encoding this subunit has been cloned (chromosome 20); multiple defects have now been identified, including abnormalities in splice junctions associated with deficient mRNA production and point mutations that would result in a protein unit with defective function. The commonly held view that the disease is an X-linked disorder has given way, with a combination of careful family and molecular genetic studies, to the view that the subset with hereditary osteodystrophy is due to an autosomal dominant mode of inheritance (chromosome 20). The inheritance of the variant disorder in which individuals have no abnormalities in mineral metabolism despite an abnormal gene for $G_{s\alpha}$ is not understood.

A working classification of the various forms of pseudohypoparathyroidism is given in Table 357-7. The classification scheme is based on the signs of ineffective parathyroid hormone action (low calcium and high phosphate), urinary cyclic AMP response to exogenous PTH, the presence or absence of Albright's hereditary osteodystrophy (AHO), and assays of the concentration of the $G_{s\alpha}$ subunit of the adenylate cyclase enzyme (see Chap. 69). Using these criteria, there are four types: pseudohypoparathyroidism (PHP) type I, subdivided into a and b categories; PHP-II; and pseudopseudohypoparathyroidism (PPHP). Individuals with PHP-I, the most common of the disorders, show a deficient response in urinary cyclic AMP following administration of exogenous parathyroid hormone. Pseudohypoparathyroidism type II refers to patients with hypocalcemia and hyperphosphatemia who have a normal urinary cyclic AMP response to PTH. These patients are assumed to have a defect in the response to PTH at a locus beyond that of cyclic AMP production, although at least some patients reported to have PHP-II may instead have occult vitamin D deficiency. It is disputed whether PHP-II is a discrete phenotypic and genotypic entity because vitamin D deficiency and an associated hypocalcemia can result in a clinical picture of enhanced cyclic AMP response to administered PTH yet a blunted phosphatemic response (the hallmark of the PHP-II syndrome). Patients with the PHP-I syndrome are divided into type a, with reduced activity of the stimulatory G-protein subunit ($G_{s\alpha}$) in in vitro assays, and type b, with normal amounts of $G_{s\alpha}$ in erythrocytes. Subjects with PHP-Ia have shortened metacarpals and metatarsals and the other features of Albright's hereditary osteodystrophy syndrome and commonly show resistance to hormones in addition to PTH. Patients with PHP-Ib have a normal phenotype without the AHO syndrome. Fibroblasts cultured from the skin of some patients with PHP-Ib show a much reduced response of cyclic AMP accumulation to PTH, consistent with the presence of a defective receptor. A subset of these patients, however, have a normal response to cyclic AMP production in fibroblasts in vitro.

Patients with PPHP have typical features of the hereditary osteodystrophy syndrome despite normal serum calciums and normal response of urinary cyclic AMP to exogenous PTH. These individuals are usually first-degree relatives of patients with PHP-Ia, and patients initially classified as having PPHP have subsequently developed mild hypocalcemia. Patients with PPHP on average have levels of $G_{s\alpha}$ subunits that are half normal. These various features suggest that PPHP is a mild variant of PHP-Ia and illustrate the heterogeneity of the defect in PTH responsiveness. Further studies will be necessary to clarify the pathogenesis of these disorders.

The mineral deposits in ectopic sites may include true bone, whereas bone formation in ectopic sites never occurs in idiopathic hypoparathyroidism. Amorphous deposits of calcium and phosphate are found in the basal ganglia in about half of patients. The defects in metacarpal and metatarsal bones are sometimes accompanied by abnormal phalanges as well, possibly reflecting premature closing of the epiphyses. The typical findings are abnormally short fourth and fifth metacarpals and metatarsals. The defects are usually bilateral. Exostoses and radius curvus are frequent. Impairments in olfaction and taste and unusual dermatoglyphic abnormalities have been reported. There is little improvement in mental status even after adequate therapy with calcium and vitamin D.

The diagnosis can usually be made without difficulty. Positive family history for developmental defects and/or the presence of developmental defects characteristic of PHP-Ia, including brachydactyly, in association with the signs of hypoparathyroidism, low calcium, and high phosphate, make the diagnosis likely on clinical grounds. On the other hand, patients with PHP-Ib or PHP-II do not have phenotypic abnormalities. Here the clue is hypocalcemia with high PTH levels. In PHP-Ib, administration of exogenous parathyroid hormone can lead to detection of the blunted cyclic AMP response; such tests are usually used to confirm the diagnosis even in PHP-Ia. Low levels of $G_{s\alpha}$ subunits in erythrocyte membranes can also distinguish patients with PHP-Ia from those with PHP-Ib. Patients in both categories have elevated serum PTH, particularly if they are hypocalcemic. The diagnosis of PHP-II is more complex, in that cyclic AMP responses in urine are, by definition, normal. Since vitamin D deficiency itself can result in dissociation between phosphaturic and urinary cyclic AMP responses to exogenous PTH, vitamin D deficiency must be excluded before diagnosis of PHP-II can be made.

Treatment of PHP is similar to that of hypoparathyroidism, except that the dose of vitamin D and calcium is usually lower than that required in true hypoparathyroidism, presumably because the defect in PHP is only partial (a 50 percent reduction in $G_{s\alpha}$). Variations in individual responses make it necessary to establish the optimal therapeutic program for each patient, based on maintaining the appropriate blood calcium concentration and urinary calcium excretion.

PTH overwhelmed Occasionally, loss of calcium from the extracellular fluid is so severe that PTH cannot compensate. Such situations include severe, acute hyperphosphatemia, often in association with renal failure, or acute pancreatitis, conditions in which there is rapid efflux of calcium from extracellular fluid. Severe hypocalcemia can occur quickly; PTH rises in response to hypocalcemia but does not

---

TABLE 357-7 Classification of pseudohypoparathyroidism (PHP) and pseudopseudohypoparathyroidism (PPHP)

Type	Hypocalcemia, hyperphosphatemia	Response of Urinary cAMP to PTH	Serum PTH	G_s subunit deficiency	AHO	Resistance to hormones in addition to PTH
PHP-Ia	Yes	↓	↑	Yes	Yes	Yes
PHP-Ib	Yes	↓	↑	No	No	No
PHP-II	Yes	Normal	↑	No	No	No
PPHP	No	Normal	Normal	Yes	Yes	±

NOTE: ↓ = decreased; ↑ = increased; AHO = Albright's hereditary osteodystrophy.

return blood calcium to normal. The chance of hypocalcemia is enhanced when renal failure is present.

Severe, acute hyperphosphatemia Severe hyperphosphatemia occurs in situations associated with extensive tissue damage or cell destruction (see also Chap. 359). The combination of an increased release of phosphate from muscle and an impaired ability to excrete phosphorus secondary to the renal failure causes moderate to severe hyperphosphatemia, the latter causing calcium loss from the blood and hypocalcemia of mild to moderate severity. Hypocalcemia is usually reversed with tissue repair and restoration of renal function as phosphorus and creatinine values return to normal. There may even be a mild hypercalcemic period in the oliguric phase of recovery of renal function. This sequence, severe hypocalcemia followed by mild hypercalcemia, reflects widespread deposition of calcium in muscle with subsequent redistribution of some of the calcium to the extracellular fluid after restoration of phosphate levels to normal.

Other causes of hyperphosphatemia that lead to hypocalcemia include hypothermia, massive hepatic failure, and hematologic malignancies, either because of high cell turnover as part of the malignancy or because of cell destruction when chemotherapy is instituted.

Treatment is directed toward lowering of blood phosphate by the administration of phosphate-binding antacids or dialysis, often needed for the management of renal failure. Although calcium replacement may be necessary if hypocalcemia is severe and symptomatic, calcium administration during the hyperphosphatemic period may increase extraosseous cellular calcium deposition, thereby aggravating ultimate tissue damage. Although the levels of $1,25(OH)_2D$ may be low during the hyperphosphatemic phase and may return to normal during the oliguric phase of recovery, mineral ion imbalance per se seems to be the principal pathophysiologic mechanism.

Osteitis fibrosis after parathyroidectomy Severe hypocalcemia after parathyroid surgery is less common now that osteitis fibrosa cystica is an infrequent manifestation of hyperparathyroidism. When osteitis fibrosa cystica is severe, however, bone mineral deficits can be large, and after parathyroidectomy, blood calcium levels can fall to the hypocalcemic range and remain depressed for days if calcium replacement is inadequate. The mechanism of the hypocalcemia is complex. Increased cellularity of bone in severe osteitis fibrosa cystica involves both osteoblastic and osteoclastic cells. High levels of PTH enhance bone-blood exchange, with resorption favored over formation; an abrupt decrease in PTH levels with surgery leaves bone formation favored over resorption. Calcium loss from blood is increased, and temporary hyporesponsiveness of bone to the bone-resorbing actions of PTH (lowered hormone levels after parathyroid surgery in the presence of receptor down-regulation) may add to the imbalance between bone resorption and bone formation. Treatment may require parenteral administration of calcium; addition of calcitriol and oral calcium supplementation may hasten the ability to withdraw parenteral calcium supplementation and/or reduce the amount needed.

DIFFERENTIAL DIAGNOSIS Care must be taken to ensure that true hypocalcemia is present; in addition, acute transient hypocalcemia can be a manifestation of a variety of severe, acute illnesses, as discussed above. *Chronic hypocalcemia*, however, can usually be ascribed to a few disorders associated with an absence of PTH or its ineffectiveness. Important clinical criteria include the duration of the illness, signs or symptoms of associated disorders, and the detection of features that suggest a hereditary abnormality in calcium and bone metabolism. A nutritional history can be helpful in detecting a low intake of vitamin D and calcium in the elderly, and a history of excessive alcohol intake can be the clue to magnesium deficiency.

Hypoparathyroidism and pseudohypoparathyroidism are typically lifelong illnesses; hence a recent onset of hypocalcemia in an adult is usually due to nutritional deficiencies, renal failure, or intestinal disorders that result in vitamin D deficiency or ineffective vitamin D action. A history of seizure disorder raises the issue of anticonvulsive medication. Neck surgery, even long past, can be associated with a delayed onset of postoperative hypoparathyroidism. Developmental defects, particularly in childhood and adolescence, may point to the

diagnosis of pseudohypoparathyroidism. Rickets and a variety of neuromuscular syndromes and deformities may indicate ineffective vitamin D action, either due to hereditary defects in vitamin D metabolism or, rarely, to vitamin D deficiency.

A pattern of *low calcium* with *high phosphorus* in the absence of renal failure or massive tissue destruction almost invariably means hypoparathyroidism or pseudohypoparathyroidism. A *low calcium* and a *low phosphorus* points to absent or ineffective vitamin D, thereby rendering the action of PTH on calcium metabolism ineffective. The relative ineffectiveness of PTH in vitamin D deficiency, anticonvulsant therapy, gastrointestinal disorders, and hereditary defects in vitamin D metabolism leads to secondary hyperparathyroidism as a compensation. The relatively unopposed action of the excess PTH on renal tubule phosphate transport, less dependent on vitamin D sufficiency than calcium transport, accounts for renal phosphate wasting and hypophosphatemia.

Exceptions to these patterns may occur. Most forms of hypomagnesemia are due to long-standing nutritional deficiency, and despite the fact that the hypocalcemia is due principally to an acute absence of PTH, phosphate levels are usually low rather than elevated as in hypoparathyroidism. Chronic renal failure is often associated with hypocalcemia and hyperphosphatemia, despite secondary hyperparathyroidism.

Diagnosis is usually established by application of the PTH radioimmunoassay, tests for vitamin D metabolites, and measurements of the urinary cyclic AMP response to exogenous PTH. In hereditary and acquired hypoparathyroidism and severe hypomagnesemia, PTH is either undetectable or in the normal range, especially with double-antibody assays; this result in a hypocalcemic patient is supportive of hypoparathyroidism, as distinct from ineffective PTH action, in which even mild hypocalcemia is associated with elevated PTH levels. Hence a failure to detect elevated PTH levels establishes the diagnosis of hypoparathyroidism; elevated levels suggest the presence of secondary hyperparathyroidism, as found in many of the situations in which the hormone is ineffective due to associated abnormalities in vitamin D action. Assays for $25(OH)D$ and $1,25(OH)_2D$ can be quite helpful. Low or low normal $25(OH)D$ indicates vitamin D deficiency due to lack of sunlight, inadequate vitamin D intake, or intestinal malabsorption. A low level of $1,25(OH)_2D$ in the presence of elevated concentrations of PTH suggests ineffective PTH action, including chronic renal failure, severe vitamin D deficiency, vitamin D–dependent rickets type I, and pseudohypoparathyroidism. Recognition that mild hypocalcemia, rickets, and hypophosphatemia are due to chronic anticonvulsant therapy is made by history.

TREATMENT OF HYPOCALCEMIA The chronic management of hypoparathyroidism or pseudohypoparathyroidism, chronic renal failure, and hereditary defects in vitamin D metabolism features the use of vitamin D or vitamin D metabolites and calcium supplementation. Vitamin D itself is the least expensive form of vitamin D replacement and is frequently used in the management of uncomplicated hypoparathyroidism and disorders associated with ineffective vitamin D action. When vitamin D is used prophylactically, as in the elderly or in those with chronic anticonvulsant therapy, there is a wider margin of safety than with the more potent metabolites. On the other hand, most of the conditions in which vitamin D is administered for chronic management of hypocalcemia require the use of 50 to 100 times the daily replacement doses because the formation of $1,25(OH)_2D$ is deficient. In such situations, vitamin D is no safer than the active metabolite because intoxication does occur with high-dose vitamin D therapy. Calcitriol is more rapid in onset of action and also has a short biologic half-life; in high doses, vitamin D is stored in body tissues and is cleared slowly.

One to five micrograms per day of vitamin D or calcifediol and slightly lower doses of calcitriol (0.25 to 1.0 μg/d) are required to prevent rickets in normal subjects. In contrast, 500 to 3000 μg of vitamin D_2 or D_3 is typically required in hypoparathyroidism; doses of calcifediol are also high (several hundred micrograms per day) compared with doses required in euparathyroid individuals. The dose of calcitriol is unchanged in hypoparathyroidism, since the defect is in hydroxylation by the 1α-hydroxylase.

The slightly greater therapeutic efficacy of calcifediol than vitamin D₃ when the metabolism of the vitamin is impaired may be due to superior metabolic availability for the renal 1α-hydroxylase or to direct action directly by 25(OH)D at receptors in target tissues. Vitamin D is metabolized to a variety of compounds other than the principal product, 25(OH)D. Calcifediol bypasses these alternate pathways and is directly available for metabolism to 1,25(OH)₂D. In hypoparathyroidism and in hereditary defects in renal 1α-hydroxylase, the efficiency of formation of 1,25(OH)₂D from 25(OH)D is low, but some formation does occur with high substrate levels. Calcifediol has about 1 percent of the potency of calcitriol in vivo and in vitro tests of vitamin D responsiveness.

Unless a loading dose is given, 2 to 4 weeks or even longer are required to achieve the maximum calcium replacement action of vitamin D or calcifediol; again, the onset of action of calcifediol is slightly more rapid. Calcitriol can be given for hypoparathyroidism at the same dose required for the prevention of rickets in euparathyroid individuals, 0.2 to 1.0 μg/d. Its onset of action is days rather than weeks. When vitamin D or calcifediol is withdrawn, weeks are required for the disappearance of the biologic effects, compared with a few days for calcitriol.

Patients with hypoparathyroidism should be given 2 to 3 g elemental calcium by mouth each day. The two agents, vitamin D (or vitamin D metabolites) and oral calcium, can be varied independently. Higher doses of vitamin D or its metabolites increase the efficiency of intestinal calcium absorption; higher intakes of oral calcium permit adequate calcium assimilation despite a lower efficiency of intestinal calcium absorption. When hypercalcemia occurs during the treatment of chronic hypocalcemia, the withdrawal of the supplemental oral calcium is effective in lowering calcium within 24 h, even more rapidly than withdrawal of calcitriol. Most patients with hypoparathyroidism can be managed with high-dose vitamin D therapy combined with 2 to 3 g oral calcium per day. If hypocalcemia alternates with episodes of hypercalcemia, then administration of calcitriol will often make management easier.

The administration of thiazide diuretics in the usual antihypertensive doses and sodium restriction in patients with hypoparathyroidism lowers urinary calcium excretion. This hypocalciuric effect allows the calcium and vitamin D supplementation to be reduced. Patients will have a lower urinary calcium excretion at any given level of blood calcium on thiazides. The treatment also may protect against the development of kidney stones, a potential complication of the long-term management of hypoparathyroidism. If on dialysis, patients with chronic renal failure and hypocalcemia can have adjustments in dialysate calcium concentrations as an alternative to vitamin D and calcium supplementation. The doses of vitamin D and calcium required for the management of pseudohypoparathyroidism are usually lower than those required for hypoparathyroidism, reflecting incomplete resistance to the action of PTH in pseudohypoparathyroidism. The acute treatment of hypomagnesemia is discussed above.

REFERENCES

AHN TG et al: Familial isolated hypoparathyroidism: A molecular genetic analysis of 8 families with 23 affected persons. Medicine 65:73, 1986

ARNOLD A et al: Mutation of the signal peptide-encoding region of the preproparathyroid hormone gene in familial isolated hypoparathyroidism. J Clin Invest 86:1084, 1990

BENSON L et al: Hyperparathyroidism presenting as the first lesion in multiple endocrine neoplasia type 1. Am J Med 82:731, 1987

BILEZIKIAN JP: Etiologies and therapy of hypercalcemia. Endocrinol Metab Clin North Am 18:389, 1989

BUDAYR AR et al: Increased serum levels of PTH-like protein in malignancy-associated hypercalcemia. Ann Intern Med 111:807, 1989

BURTIS WJ et al: Immunochemical characterization of circulating parathyroid hormone–related protein in patients with humoral hypercalcemia of malignancy. N Engl J Med 322:1106, 1990

CHOU YH et al: The gene responsible for familial hypocalciuric hypercalcemia maps to chromosome 3 in four unrelated families. Nature Genet 1:295, 1992

FIBISON WJ et al: Molecular studies of DiGeorge syndrome. Am J Hum Genet 46:888, 1990

FITCH N: The identification and inheritance of Albright's hereditary osteodystrophy. Am J Med Genet 11:11, 1982

FLEISCH H: Bisphosphonates: Pharmacology and use in the treatment of tumor-induced hypercalcemia and metastatic bone disease. Drugs 42:919, 1991

FRIEDMAN E et al: Clonality of parathyroid tumors in familial multiple endocrine neoplasia type 1. N Engl J Med 321:213, 1989

FUKAGAWA M et al: Suppression of parathyroid gland hyperplasia by 1,25(OH)₂D₃ pulse therapy. N Engl J Med 315:421, 1990

GEJMAN PV et al: Genetic mapping of the Gs-alpha subunit gene (GNAS1) to the distal long arm of chromosome 20 using a polymorphism detected by denaturing gradient gel electrophoresis. Genomics 9:782, 1991

GIDDING SS et al: Unmasking of hypoparathyroidism in familial partial DiGeorge syndrome by challenge with disodium edentate. N Engl J Med 319:1589, 1988

GRILL V et al: PTH-related protein: Elevated levels in both humoral hypercalcemia of malignancy and hypercalcemia complicating metastatic breast cancer. J Clin Endocrinol 73:1309, 1991

HENDERSON JR et al: Circulating concentrations of PTH-like peptide in malignancy and in hyperparathyroidism. J Bone Miner Res 5:105–112, 1990

JAMESON JL, ARNOLD A: Recombinant DNA strategies for determining the molecular basis of endocrine disorders. J Endocrinol Metab 70:301, 1990

KAO PC et al: PTH-related peptide in plasma of patients with hypercalcemia and malignancy lesions. Mayo Clin Proc 65:1399, 1990

LEVINE MA, DEILY JR: Identification of multiple mutations in the gene encoding the alpha subunit of Gs in patients with pseudohypoparathyroidism Ia. Abstracts of the Annual Meeting of the American Society for Bone and Mineral Research, Atlanta, GA, 1990

MALLETTE LE, EICHORN E: Effects of lithium carbonate on human calcium metabolism. Arch Intern Med 146:770, 1986

MARX SJ: Familial hypocalciuric hypercalcemia, in *Primer on the Metabolic Bone Diseases and Disorders of Mineral Metabolism*, MJ Favus (ed). Richmond, VA, William Byrd Press, 1990, p 113

MAYNARD FM: Immobilization hypercalcemia following spinal cord injury. Arch Phys Med Rehabil 67:41, 1986

MOTOKURA T et al: Cloning and characterization of human cyclin D3, a cDNA closely related in sequence to the PRAD1/cyclin D1 proto-oncogene. J Biol Chem 267:20412, 1992.

MUDDE AH et al: Ectopic product of 1,25-dihydroxyvitamin D by B-cell lymphoma as a cause of hypercalcemia. Cancer 59:1543, 1987

NEUFELD M et al: Autoimmune polyglandular syndromes. Pediatr Ann 9:43, 1980

NUSSBAUM SR, POTTS JT JR: Immunoassays for parathyroid hormone 1-84 in the diagnosis of hyperparathyroidism. J Bone Miner Res 6(suppl 2):S43, 1991

ORWOLL ES: The milk-alkali syndrome: Current concepts. Ann Intern Med 97:242, 1982

PARFITT AM et al: Asymptomatic primary hyperparathyroidism discovered by multichannel biochemical screening: Clinical course and considerations bearing on the need for surgical intervention. J Bone Miner Res 6(suppl 2):S97, 1991

PARKINSON DB, THAKKER RV: A donor splice site mutation in the parathyroid hormone gene is associated with autosomal recessive hypoparathyroidism. Nature Genet 1:149, 1992

PATTEN JL et al: Mutation in the gene encoding the stimulatory G protein of adenylyl cyclase in Albright's hereditary osteodystrophy. N Engl J Med 322:1412, 1990

POTTS JT JR et al (eds): Proceedings of the NIH Consensus Development Conference on Diagnosis and Management of Asymptomatic Primary Hyperparathyroidism. J Bone Miner Res 6(suppl 2):S1–S166, 1991

RALSTON SH et al: Comparison of aminohydroxypropylidene diphosphonate, mithramycin and corticosteroids/calcitonin in treatment of cancer-associated hypercalcemia. Lancet 2:907, 1985

——— et al: Cancer-associated hypercalcemia: Morbidity and mortality. Ann Intern Med 12:499, 1990

RATCLIFFE WA et al: Immunoreactivity of plasma parathyrin-related peptide. Clin Chem 37:1781, 1991

ROSENBERG CL et al: Coding sequence of the overexpressed transcript of the putative oncogene PRAD1/cyclin D1 in two primary human tumors. Oncogene 8:519, 1993

SCHWINDINGER WF et al: Identification of a novel missense mutation in the gene encoding the alpha subunit of the stimulatory G protein of adenylyl cyclase in a subject with Albright hereditary osteodystrophy. Abstracts of the 74th Annual Meeting of the Endocrine Society, San Antonio, TX, 1992

STUCKEY BGA et al: Fasting calcium excretion and parathyroid hormone together distinguish familial hypocalciuric hypercalcaemia from primary hyperparathyroidism. Clin Endocrinol 27:525, 1987

THAKKER RV et al: Association of parathyroid tumors in multiple endocrine neoplasia type 1 with loss of alleles on chromosome 11. N Engl J Med 321:218, 1988

——— et al: Mapping the gene causing X-linked recessive idiopathic hypoparathyroidism to Xq26–Xq27 by linkage studies. J Clin Invest 86:40, 1990

WARRELL RP et al: A randomized double-blind study of gallium nitrate compared with etidronate for acute control of cancer related hypercalcemia. J Clin Oncol 9:1467, 1991

WEINSTEIN LS et al: Mutations of the Gs alpha-subunit gene in Albright hereditary osteodystrophy detected by denaturing gradient gel electrophoresis. Proc Natl Acad Sci USA 87:8287, 1990

WILSON DI et al: A prospective cytogenetic study of 36 cases of DiGeorge syndrome. Am J Hum Genet 51:957, 1992

WINTER WE et al: Autosomal dominant hypoparathyroidism with variable, age-dependent severity. J Pediatr 103:387, 1983

358   METABOLIC BONE DISEASE

STEPHEN M. KRANE / MICHAEL F. HOLICK

OSTEOPOROSIS

GENERAL CONSIDERATIONS *Osteoporosis* is the term used for diseases of diverse etiology that cause a reduction in the mass of bone per unit volume. The reduction in mass is not accompanied by a significant decrease in the ratio of the mineral to the organic phase, nor by any known abnormality in bone mineral or organic matrix. Histologically, the disorder is characterized by a decrease in cortical thickness and in the number and size of the trabeculae of cancellous bone. Individual trabecular plates are abnormally perforated and may be fractured, and trabecular connectivity is reduced. The osteoid seams, however, are of normal width. Osteoporosis is the most common of the metabolic bone diseases (disorders in which all the skeleton is involved) and is an important cause of morbidity in the elderly.

The remodeling of bone (its formation and resorption) is a continuous process. In osteoporosis, the bone mass *is* decreased, indicating that the rate of bone resorption must exceed that of bone formation. Bone formation is higher in cortical than in cancellous bone. This difference is exaggerated by the normal menopause and exaggerated further in patients with osteoporosis because rates of formation of cancellous bone tend to be lower in patients with osteoporosis, particularly in women after the menopause. The fact that about a third of postmenopausal women have high skeletal turnover, assessed by whole-body retention of ^{99m}Tc-methylene diphosphonate and by other biochemical markers, could reflect the greater relative contribution of cortical remodeling in this group. After closure of epiphyses and cessation of longitudinal growth, there is a period of consolidation with a decrease in cortical porosity. When peak adult bone mass is reached at about age 30 to 35 for cortical bone and probably earlier for trabecular bone, rates of bone formation and resorption are relatively low (compared with the period of growth spurt) and approximately equal. The normal balance between bone formation and resorption results in maintenance of skeletal mass. The rates of remodeling differ, however, not only in cortical compared with trabecular bone but also in individual bones or portions of bones. Most of the bone surfaces are "inactive" and not involved at any given time either in formation or resorption. Active surfaces may be distributed randomly, but formation and resorption are locally coupled as units. Resorption areas are covered by osteoclasts if active; bone formation surfaces are characterized by the presence of osteoid seams and are covered by active osteoblasts. Resorption precedes formation and is probably more intense, but it does not last as long as formation. As a consequence, there are normally more sites of active formation than of resorption. Bone turnover is high when there are many units active and low when there are few. Unless formation compensates for resorption, bone mass decreases. In both sexes after age 40 to 50 there is a slow rate of loss of cortical bone of about 0.3 to 0.5 percent per year. In women around the menopause, an accelerated loss of cortical bone is superimposed on the age-related loss. Loss of trabecular bone begins at an earlier age in both sexes but is probably greater in degree in women. The rate of bone loss in women also may be accelerated around the time of menopause. The cumulative losses of bone mass range from 20 to 30 percent in men and 40 to 50 percent for some women. In general, the bone loss involves predominantly trabecular bone in the spine and distal radius in women and the spine and hip in both women and men. The fact that loss is not uniform has been documented with techniques such as single- and dual-photon absorptiometry, quantitative computed tomography, x-ray–based dual-energy densitometry, and neutron activation analysis of total-body calcium. For example, the rate of loss is greater in the metacarpals, the femoral neck, and the vertebral bodies than in the midshaft of the femur, the tibia, and the skull.

Although, as noted, skeletal turnover may be increased, turnover is usually normal or low. Bone formation is low in the majority, but the degree of reduction varies with the different bone surfaces. The major remodeling abnormalities in patients with vertebral crush fractures are a reduced frequency of activation of remodeling units and a decrease in the function of osteoblasts. Even in those individuals with increased bone resorption, however, bone formation does not compensate. At some critical point if the difference between rates of formation and resorption is maintained, loss of bone substance may become so marked that the bone can no longer resist the normal mechanical forces to which it is subjected, and fracture results. This problem is most evident following perforation of bony trabecular plates. The template for formation of new bone is lost, and loss of bone is rapid as bone resorption continues and is even more uncoupled from resorption. Osteoporosis usually becomes a clinical problem following fracture. Although the level of reduction in bone mass sufficient to result in fractures after minimal trauma is variable, the bone mineral density as measured by x-ray–based dual-energy absorptiometry (DEXA) is an excellent predictor of fracture risk. The strength of bones such as vertebrae depends on "quality" (e.g., trabecular connectivity and arrangement) as well as mineral density. For example, horizontal trabeculae of the cancellous bone of vertebrae are preferentially lost in osteoporosis. Additional factors such as the adequacy of ligamentous support and the age-related changes in the intervertebral disks influence the susceptibility to fracture. Microfractures are frequent. In elderly individuals with osteoporosis, age- or drug-related impairments of vision, hearing, and other neurologic and intellectual functions are additional contributions to the occurrence of fractures.

In the process of remodeling lamellar bone in adults, most of the net resorption occurs at the corticoendosteal surface. The abnormal remodeling in osteoporosis follows the same pattern; the bone loss includes cancellous bone, cortical bone at the endosteal surface, and intracortical bone, resulting in enlargement of the medullary cavity and thinning of the cortex. Since bone formation at the periosteum continues at a slow rate, the diameter of the bone does not decrease, and the periosteal surface retains its smooth configuration. In addition, the cancellous bone also undergoes progressive resorption, with some trabeculae being resorbed at rates faster than others, particularly those vertebral trabeculae with horizontal orientation.

The age-related loss of bone begins earlier and proceeds more rapidly in women, and there is a trend toward acceleration of bone loss before the menopause. All the reasons for this age-associated bone loss are not known, although several risk factors have been identified. In general, white women have a greater risk than black women, and white men have a greater risk than black men. One explanation for these population differences is that the bone mass at skeletal maturity is one determinant of the bone mass at subsequent ages. The lower incidence of osteoporosis and hip fracture in black men and women has been attributed to a higher bone mineral content in blacks than in whites despite the fact that bone formation is lower in blacks. Since formation and resorption are usually coupled, and since bone mass is increased, bone resorption (and turnover) also must be reduced. Osteoporotic subjects are frequently less muscular and have lower average body weight. Patients who are kept at complete bed rest and astronauts in microgravity can lose approximately 1 percent of their bone mass each month. Exercise may have a beneficial effect in maintaining bone mass. The facts that accelerated bone loss accompanies the menopause in some women and that premature osteoporosis occurs after premature surgical menopause suggest that estrogens play a major role in preventing bone loss. Furthermore, osteoporotic women as a group may have an earlier menopause than age-matched nonosteoporotic women. Osteoporotic women also have a higher incidence of smoking; cigarette smoking might directly affect bone remodeling or have secondary effects on ovarian function. Excessive alcohol consumption, which can result in decreased bone formation, also is a risk factor for osteoporosis. Dietary calcium intake during the first three decades of life influences the ultimate peak bone mass. Calcium intake during adult life also has a small effect on bone mass and risk of fracture. Inability to synthesize adequate amounts of 1α,25-dihydroxyvitamin D [1,25(OH)$_2$D] may play a role in the decreased calcium absorption, possibly because of decreased sensitivity of the 25(OH)D-1α-hydroxylase to parathyroid hormone or impaired activity of the renal 25(OH)D-1α-hydroxylase.

Local production of selected cytokines appears to mediate the effects of estrogen deficiency in enhancing osteoclast-mediated bone resorption. Peripheral blood monocytes from patients with osteoporosis secrete more interleukin 1 (IL-1), and in women with postmenopausal osteoporosis the increased production of IL-1 is suppressed by estrogen treatment. IL-1 and other cytokines such as tumor necrosis factor α (TNF-α) stimulate production of IL-6 by osteoblasts and other mesenchymal cells. IL-6 is probably the most important cytokine in the excessive recruitment of osteoclasts that is a common feature of the abnormal bone remodeling in postmenopausal osteoporosis. Although osteoporosis occurs with Cushing's syndrome, there is no established role for adrenal steroids in the osteoporosis associated with the menopause or advancing age.

Excessive acid intake, particularly in the form of high-protein diets, may contribute to "dissolution" of bone in an attempt to buffer the extra acid. Acidosis also may increase osteoclast function directly. Prolonged use of heparin as an anticoagulant is also associated with osteoporosis, and heparin potentiates bone resorption in vitro. Subjects with osteoporosis have increased numbers of mast cells, presumably capable of producing heparin and other substances that modulate bone cell function, in the bone marrow. Circumscribed and diffuse areas of osteoporosis occur in patients with systemic mastocytosis.

As mentioned earlier, the remodeling of bone is responsive to mechanical forces. The early response to immobilization in the normal skeleton is an increase in bone resorption while bone formation remains normal or is decreased; later there is a compensatory increase in bone formation. In osteoporosis, immobilization tends to aggravate the defect by increasing the gap between formation and resorption. A sedentary life may reduce mechanical forces exerted on the skeleton and increase the tendency to bone loss.

CLASSIFICATION (See Table 358-1) In some instances, osteoporosis is a feature of another disease such as Cushing's syndrome. Osteoporosis is also characteristic of certain heritable diseases of connective tissue such as osteogenesis imperfecta (see Chap. 351). In most cases of osteoporosis, however, no other disease is apparent. One form occurs in children or young adults of both sexes and with normal gonadal function and is frequently termed *idiopathic osteoporosis*, although most of the other forms are also of unknown pathogenesis. So-called *type I osteoporosis* occurs in a subset of postmenopausal women who are between 51 and 75 years of age and is characterized by an accelerated and disproportionate loss of trabecular bone. Fractures of vertebral bodies and the distal forearm are common complications. Decreased parathyroid gland function may be compensatory to increased bone resorption. So-called *type II osteoporosis* is found in a large proportion of women and men over the age of 70 and is associated with fractures of the femoral neck, proximal humerus, proximal tibia, and pelvis. These skeletal sites contain both cortical and trabecular bone. Circulating levels of parathyroid hormone (PTH) tend to be high. Both groups have decreased mean circulating levels of 1,25(OH)$_2$D.

GENERAL CLINICAL FEATURES Although osteoporosis is a generalized disorder of the skeleton, its major clinical sequelae result from fractures of the vertebrae, wrist, hip, humerus, and tibia. The most frequent symptoms from vertebral body fractures are pain in the back and deformity of the spine. Pain usually results from collapse of the vertebrae especially in the dorsal and lumbar regions, is typically acute in onset, and often radiates around the flank into the abdomen. Such episodes may occur after sudden bending, lifting, or jumping movements that may seem to have been trivial; on some occasions they cannot be related to trauma. The pain may be increased

TABLE 358-1 Classification of osteoporosis

Common forms, unassociated with other disease
  A Idiopathic osteoporosis (juvenile and adult)
  B Type I osteoporosis
  C Type II osteoporosis
Osteoporosis as a common feature
  A Hypogonadism
  B Hyperadrenocorticism
  C Chronic glucocorticoid administration
  D Hyperparathyroidism
  E Thyrotoxicosis
  F Malabsorption
  G Scurvy
  H Calcium deficiency
  I Immobilization
  J Chronic heparin administration
  K Systemic mastocytosis
  L Adult hypophosphatasia
  M Associated with other metabolic bone diseases
Osteoporosis as a feature of heritable disorders of connective tissue
  A Osteogenesis imperfecta
  B Homocystinuria due to cystathionine synthase deficiency
  C Ehlers-Danlos syndrome
  D Marfan's syndrome
Osteoporosis is associated but pathogenesis is not understood
  A Rheumatoid arthritis
  B Malnutrition
  C Alcoholism
  D Epilepsy
  E Primary biliary cirrhosis
  F Diabetes mellitus
  G Chronic obstructive pulmonary disease
  H Menkes' syndrome

even with slight movements such as turning in bed or the Valsalva maneuver. Bed rest may relieve the pain temporarily, only for it to recur in spasms of variable duration. Radiation of pain down one leg is uncommon, and symptoms or signs of spinal cord compression are rare. The acute episodes of pain also may be accompanied by abdominal distention and ileus, thought to be due to retroperitoneal hemorrhage, but the use of narcotics also contributes to the ileus. Loss of appetite and muscular weakness also may be present. Episodes of pain usually subside after several days to a week, and by 4 to 6 weeks patients may be fully ambulatory and able to resume normal activities. Although acute pain may be minimal, nagging, deep, dull, uncomfortable sensations may be localized to the area of fracture and brought about by straining or sudden changes in position. Patients may be unable to sit up in bed and have to arise by rolling over on the side and then propping themselves up. Most patients have disappearance or diminution of pain between episodes of vertebral body collapse. Others do not have acute episodes but complain of backache made worse by standing or sudden movement. Tenderness is common over involved areas of the spinous processes or rib cage. Some patients have an associated disease such as osteoarthritis of facet joints to account for chronic back pain. When collapse fractures of vertebral bodies do occur, they are usually anterior, producing a wedge-shaped deformity and contributing to loss in height. This is particularly common in the middorsal region, where collapse may be unassociated with pain but may result in a dorsal kyphosis and exaggerated cervical lordosis described as a "dowager's" or "widow's" hump. Postural slumping with increase in existing curves also contributes to the loss of height. Scoliosis is also common. Generalized skeletal pain is uncommon, and between fractures most patients are free of pain. Although recurrent episodes of vertebral collapse, increasing spine deformity, and loss of height are common, the course in any one subject is not predictable, and there may be intervals of several years between fractures.

RADIOLOGIC FEATURES Prior to fracture and collapse, the osteoporotic vertebral body shows a decrease in mineral density, increase in prominence of vertical striations due to a relatively greater loss of the horizontally oriented trabeculae, and prominence of the end plates. The bodies may become increasingly biconcave because of weakening of the subchondral plates, microfractures, and expansion of the intervertebral disks, resulting in the so-called codfish vertebrae. When collapse occurs, it usually produces a decrease in the anterior height of the vertebral body and irregularity in the anterior cortex (Fig. 358-1). Older compression fractures may show reactive changes and osteophytes about the anterior margins. Most osteoporotic fractures occur in the middle and lower thoracic and upper lumbar vertebral bodies. Fractures of isolated vertebral bodies of T4 or higher should suggest malignancy. Although the cortices of long bones may be thin because of excessive endosteal resorption, the outer margins are sharp in contrast to the typical effects of the subperiosteal resorption of hyperparathyroidism. Pseudofractures or Looser's zones do not occur in the absence of osteomalacia, but it may be impossible to distinguish osteoporosis from osteomalacia on radiologic grounds alone. In the absence of fractures, standard roentgenograms are insensitive indicators of bone loss, since as much as 30 percent decrease in bone mass may not be appreciated. Other procedures are required to establish whether a given individual has a sufficient decrease in bone mass to be at risk for fracture. Dual-energy x-ray absorptiometry is an excellent technique because of its sensitivity, ability to scan the entire skeleton, low radiation exposure, and short scanning time. Single- and dual-photon absorptiometry and quantitative computed tomography (CT) also can detect small (1 to 2 percent) changes in the bone mineral density of the hip and lumbar spine.

LABORATORY FINDINGS The concentrations of calcium and inorganic phosphorus in the blood are usually normal. Slight hyperphosphatemia occurs in women who are past the menopause. The alkaline phosphatase in uncomplicated instances is normal but may increase after fractures. About 20 percent of postmenopausal women with osteoporosis have hypercalciuria. Urinary excretion of peptides containing hydroxyproline, an index of bone resorption, is usually

FIGURE 358-1 Lateral views of the lumbar spine of a 54-year-old man with idiopathic osteoporosis. A typical anterior compression fracture is indicated by the arrow.

normal or slightly increased in those with high-turnover osteoporosis. Serum levels of osteocalcin (bone GLA protein), urinary excretion of hydroxypyridinium cross-link compounds, and uptake of ^{99m}Tc-methylene diphosphonate also correlate with the rate of bone turnover.

DIFFERENTIAL DIAGNOSIS Since decrease in skeletal mass is a universal feature of aging, it is difficult to evaluate asymptomatic decreased bone density, determined radiographically, in older women, especially when unaccompanied by marked increase in biconcavity of vertebral bodies or fractures. Quantitative measurement of bone mass is, however, a predictor of future fractures. In the presence of bone pain with or without fracture or deformity, it is important to establish the presence or absence of known causes of osteoporosis as listed in Table 358-1 and to be certain that osteoporosis is the correct diagnosis. Malignancies of various types, particularly *multiple myeloma, lymphoma, leukemia,* and *metastatic carcinoma,* may result in diffuse loss of bone, especially the trabecular bone of the vertebral column, even in the absence of hypercalcemia. The absence of anemia, elevated erythrocyte sedimentation rate, abnormal electrophoretic patterns of serum proteins, and Bence Jones proteinuria is helpful in eliminating the possibility of multiple myeloma. However, needle bone biopsy or marrow aspiration may be appropriate in instances of severe osteoporosis with fractures. Quantitative histomorphometry on standard biopsy samples from the iliac crest is a research tool but is available in some referral laboratories. Bone biopsy samples must be properly fixed, not demineralized, and embedded in plastic to rule out osteomalacia, however.

Radiologic evidence of osteoporosis is common in patients with primary *hyperparathyroidism,* who may not have osteitis fibrosa (discrete lytic lesions of varying size and subperiosteal resorption) or elevation of serum alkaline phosphatase. Although mild asymptomatic primary hyperparathyroidism is not a major risk factor in osteoporosis, it does contribute to accelerated bone loss. An element of secondary hyperparathyroidism may be present in some elderly patients with type II osteoporosis and in others with impairment of renal function, inadequate oral calcium intake, or decrease of intestinal calcium absorption. Increased numbers of osteoclasts may be present in bone biopsy specimens from such patients.

Osteomalacia may mimic osteoporosis or coexist with it, yet specific radiologic signs of osteomalacia may not always be present. Although the presence of abnormalities such as low or undetectable circulating levels of 25-hydroxyvitamin D [25(OH)D] and/or hypophosphatemia suggests the possibility of osteomalacia, bone biopsy may be essential for diagnosis, as discussed below. Since osteomalacia is more responsive to therapy (e.g., vitamin D in hypovitaminosis D or phosphate supplements in phosphate depletion) than the usual case of osteoporosis, such diagnostic procedures are often warranted. Subclinical vitamin D deficiency with associated secondary hyperparathyroidism may be more common in elderly women than previously recognized, and treatment of postmenopausal women with small doses of vitamin D$_3$ (20 µg or 800 IU daily) may reduce the risk of hip fractures and other nonvertebral fractures.

In an occasional patient with *Paget's disease,* the radiologic features may be almost purely lytic and be confused with osteoporosis. However, high alkaline phosphatase levels and moderately or markedly increased urinary excretion of hydroxyproline-containing peptides are clues to the presence of Paget's disease. Scanning procedures with bone-seeking isotopes are not helpful in differential diagnosis if fractures are present because fractures cause preferential uptake of isotope. However, in the absence of fractures, "hot spots" suggest tumor or early Paget's disease, particularly if present in the appendicular skeleton.

IDIOPATHIC OSTEOPOROSIS *Idiopathic osteoporosis* occurs in younger men and in premenopausal women in whom no other etiologic factor is detected. These patients probably have a number of different disorders with superficial resemblances. In some women, the onset of the disease appears to be related to pregnancy and may represent a transient failure in homeostatic mechanisms, such as failure to increase circulating levels of 1,25(OH)$_2$D and hence to protect the maternal skeleton from the stresses of childbirth (see Chap. 356). Some patients have low levels of serum alkaline phosphatase, though not low enough to fulfill diagnostic criteria for *hypophosphatasia*. Estrogens are ineffective in therapy. Losses of calcium and phosphorus are probably excessive, and it is unwise to permit women with osteoporosis to breast-feed because calcium losses via lactation are appreciable. Some patients have a disorder similar to mild forms of osteogenesis imperfecta and may thus have defects in type I collagen genes, although such features as family history, blue sclerae, and deafness are lacking. The course is variable; although recurrent episodes of fractures are characteristic, progressive deterioration does not occur in all patients, and in some the clinical problem is benign. Juvenile osteoporosis is a rare disorder with onset usually between the ages of 8 and 14 years and is characterized by the abrupt appearance of bone pain and fractures after minimal trauma. In many cases the disorder is self-limited, and recovery takes place spontaneously within 4 or 5 years.

GLUCOCORTICOID EXCESS Glucocorticoid excess does not appear to be involved in osteoporosis of the idiopathic variety or in the type I or II disorder. Osteoporosis, however, commonly accompanies Cushing's syndrome, both endogenous and exogenous, and in some instances is rapidly progressive, especially in children and in women over age 50. Bone loss of glucocorticoid excess is accounted for by a combination of low rates of bone formation (depressed osteoblastic oppositional rate) and high rates of bone resorption reflected in the hypercalciuria that accompanies increased activation frequency of bone remodeling units. A part of the latter may be the result of glucocorticoid-induced secondary hyperparathyroidism, although increases in circulating PTH are not found consistently. Glucocorticoids, however, potentiate the effects of PTH and $1,25(OH)_2D$ on bone cells in vitro. Glucocorticoids depress collagen synthesis in many tissues, as evidenced by delayed wound healing, thinning of the dermis, striae, and tendency to blue sclerae. In some disorders in which glucocorticoids are administered in pharmacologic doses, such as rheumatoid arthritis, a tendency to thin skin and osteoporosis is initially present, and the skeletal effects of the glucocorticoids may become particularly apparent. Even low dosages of glucocorticoids may accelerate bone loss in postmenopausal women and men with rheumatoid arthritis. Blood levels of $25(OH)D$ are normal or slightly decreased, and blood levels of $1,25(OH_2)D$ are usually normal. Glucocorticoids inhibit intestinal calcium absorption by a direct, vitamin D-independent action on the intestine. Osteomalacia is not observed histologically. Once osteoporosis develops in adults with Cushing's syndrome, the abnormality may persist indefinitely following alleviation of the glucocorticoid excess. In children, however, cure of the Cushing's syndrome may result in striking improvement in the appearance of the spine due to new endochondral bone formation around the less dense, older osteoporotic bone. Likewise, increase in bone mass, increase in serum osteocalcin levels (indicative of increased osteoblastic function), and decrease in urinary hydroxyproline excretion may occur in young adults following therapy of Cushing's syndrome. Withdrawal of glucocorticoids or decrease of the dose by alternate-day schedule is important to halt progression of the osteoporosis. Anabolic steroids are not effective in this regard. The defect in intestinal calcium absorption may be overcome by administering calcitriol $[1,25(OH)_2D_3]$ in oral doses of 0.5 to 1.0 μg/d plus 1 g supplemental oral calcium daily. Such regimens with or without calcitonin (e.g., 400 IU/d intranasally) are effective in preventing glucocorticoid-induced bone loss. Vitamin D metabolites such as calcifediol $[25(OH)D]$ also may be effective. It is important to monitor serum and urinary calcium levels at intervals of 2 to 4 months. In Cushing's syndrome, spontaneous, symptomless fractures may occur in ribs and pubic and ischial rami even in the absence of marked osteoporosis of the spine. These fractures often heal partially with an exuberant calcified callus surrounding a radiolucent zone of nonunion, superficially resembling the pseudofractures of osteomalacia. If they appear in the thorax superimposed on the lungs, they may be confused with nodules suggesting primary or metastatic tumor.

GONADAL DEFICIENCY Receptors for estrogens are in osteoblasts, and estrogens may function in these cells by stimulating production of substances that are anabolic for bone such as somatomedin C (insulin-like growth factor 1) or by reducing the production of catabolic cytokines by osteoblasts and mononuclear phagocytes. Estrogen is deficient in the postmenopausal woman, and the administration of estrogen to such an individual reduces the negative calcium balance and decreases urinary hydroxyproline excretion. Estrogens are particularly useful in retarding the bone loss in women who have oophorectomy at an early age and in preventing the development of osteoporosis following the menopause. Bone mass is also decreased in women athletes who are amenorrheic, such as marathon runners. Such women are particularly prone to tibial stress fractures. In patients of either sex castrated at an early age, the adult skeleton is smaller to begin with, and therefore, age-related losses are more significant. Bone density is also decreased in women with hyperprolactinemia and in men with hypogonadism of all types.

THYROTOXICOSIS In many patients with hyperthyroidism, excessive bone resorption, occasionally marked in degree and far exceeding that in the usual patient with osteoporosis, can be associated with increased excretion of calcium and phosphorus in urine and feces. The excessive bone resorption is usually accompanied by a compensatory increase in bone formation. PTH secretion is decreased, and levels of $1,25(OH)_2D$ are normal or low. If the hyperthyroidism is of short duration, skeletal losses are inconsequential. In patients with chronic hyperthyroidism, however, especially in women after the menopause, this accelerated bone loss becomes significant, and it is important to eliminate hyperthyroidism as a contributing cause of osteoporosis. Hypothyroid patients treated with excessive doses of levothyroxine also may have accelerated loss of bone mass. Although typical osteitis fibrosa (resorption lacunae containing osteoclasts and a fibrous stroma) may be seen on biopsy, the skeletal lesions have the radiologic appearance of osteoporosis.

ACROMEGALY Hypercalciuria and overall net negative calcium balance occur in acromegaly, and occasionally, osteoporosis is an associated finding. The secondary panhypopituitarism and the associated gonadal insufficiency may be factors in production of the osteoporosis. In adult animals, growth hormone decreases endosteal resorption and stimulates bone formation, and it is therefore unlikely that excessive secretion of growth hormone in itself produces osteoporosis.

DIABETES MELLITUS Individuals with juvenile or adult-onset diabetes mellitus have a decreased bone mass. In some series, the incidence of hip fractures is increased, but studies of large groups of diabetic subjects have not revealed abnormal calcium metabolism or significant bone disease specifically attributable to the diabetes.

CALCIUM DEFICIENCY AND MALABSORPTION Although calcium deficiency may be a factor, it cannot be the sole or major cause in idiopathic, senile, or postmenopausal osteoporosis. Osteoporosis is an associated finding in a significant number of cases of steatorrhea, prolonged obstructive jaundice, and lactose intolerance and in patients following gastrectomy. Other patients may have a specific defect in calcium absorption or a failure to adapt adequately to a low-calcium diet either by increasing the percentage of dietary calcium absorbed or by decreasing urinary calcium excretion. Presumably, vitamin D is adequate in these instances to prevent osteomalacia.

HERITABLE DISORDERS OF CONNECTIVE TISSUE In the strict sense, the bone disease of osteogenesis imperfecta is osteoporosis (see Chap. 351). *Osteogenesis imperfecta* is clinically, genetically, and biochemically heterogeneous. Type I osteogenesis imperfecta is the autosomal dominant form, characterized by mild to moderate bone fragility, blue sclerae, and premature deafness. The frequency of fractures tends to decrease around puberty, and another period of increased incidence occurs in women after the menopause. Type II is the lethal perinatal disorder. Type III is characterized by severe bone fragility, progressive bone deformity, and white sclerae. In type IV, sclerae are white, but other features are similar to those of type I disease. Many instances of osteogenesis imperfecta of all types have

FIGURE 358-2 Photomicrograph of an undemineralized section stained with Goldner method of an iliac crest bone biopsy from a 45-year-old man with chronic renal failure maintained on hemodialysis. Almost the entire surface is covered by osteoid (O) readily distinguished from mineralized bone (MB). The thickness of the osteoid seams exceeds 100 μm in several areas.

is also characterized by inadequate mineralization of the matrix of cartilage in the growing epiphyseal plate. Calcification in the interstitial regions of the hypertrophic zone is defective, the growth plate increases in thickness, the columns of cartilage cells (usually highly ordered) are disorganized, and there is a variable cupping of the epiphyses. The rachitic bones are often incapable of withstanding usual mechanical stresses and tend to undergo bowing deformities. If rickets is untreated, growth at the epiphyseal plates is slowed, and the eventual length of the long bones is diminished.

It has not been established whether vitamin D, through one of its metabolites, has a major direct effect on mineralization as long as the supply of mineral ions is adequate. Its primary roles after metabolic conversion to 25(OH)D and 1,25(OH)$_2$D are to regulate and enhance absorption of calcium ions from the intestinal lumen and, possibly, to enhance differentiation of stem cells to form osteoclasts. Insufficiency of the active metabolites of vitamin D leads to decreased intestinal absorption of calcium and decreased mobilization of calcium from bone, resulting in hypocalcemia. This stimulates increased synthesis and secretion of PTH and hyperplasia of the parathyroid glands. The increased circulating concentration of PTH tends to increase plasma calcium and enhances renal phosphate clearance, which, in turn, produces hypophosphatemia. When the concentration of phosphorus in the extracellular fluid falls below a critical level, mineralization cannot proceed normally. In severe vitamin D deficiency, normal levels of serum calcium cannot be maintained, and the driving force for mineralization is further decreased. The absence of some critical metabolite of vitamin D that acts directly on the skeleton also may play a role in the defective mineralization of rickets and osteomalacia.

Phosphate depletion alone can produce osteomalacia, as in patients consuming large amounts of nonabsorbable antacids and in persons with excessive renal loss of phosphate due to decreased tubular reabsorption. Secondary hyperparathyroidism is usually not present in these patients. Hypophosphatemia per se produces mineralization defects despite its effect on increasing the activity of the renal 25(OH)D-1α-hydroxylase, but it cannot account for the osteomalacia in all the disorders listed in Table 358-3. In chronic renal failure, for example, plasma phosphate levels are not decreased and usually are

increased. Similarly, plasma phosphorus levels are not depressed in infants and children with osteomalacia secondary to hypophosphatasia, a hereditary deficiency in alkaline phosphatase. Osteomalacia in some patients with chronic renal failure is associated with accumulation of aluminum in bone, and the aluminum probably plays a role in production of the mineralization defect.

CLINICAL FINDINGS The clinical manifestations of rickets are the result of skeletal deformities, susceptibility to fractures, weakness and hypotonia, and disturbances in growth. In extreme instances of vitamin D-deficiency rickets, hypocalcemia may cause tetany which, when severe, may be accompanied by laryngeal spasm and seizures. In infants and young children, features include listlessness, irritability, and often profound hypotonia and muscular weakness. As the disorder progresses, children become unable to walk without support. Abnormal parietal flattening and frontal bossing develop in the skull. The calvaria are softened (craniotabes), and sutures may be widened. Prominence of the costochondral junctions is called the "rachitic rosary," and the indentation of the lower ribs at the site of attachment of the diaphragm is known as *Harrison's groove*. If untreated, deformities of the pelvis and extremities progress, with bowing particularly common in the tibia, femur, radius, and ulna. Fractures are frequent, dental eruption is often delayed, and enamel defects are common.

The presentation of osteomalacia in adults is usually more insidious. The skeletal deformities may be overlooked, and the features of the underlying disorder may dominate, as, for example, in the vitamin D deficiency of adult celiac disease. Symptoms, when they occur, include diffuse skeletal pain and bony tenderness. Pain about the hips may result in an antalgic gait. Muscular weakness may be difficult to distinguish from hesitancy to move because of skeletal pain. Proximal weakness may mimic that of primary muscle disorders and contribute to the waddling gait. Pain and weakness may cause patients to be confined to bed and chair. Many factors, including secondary hyperparathyroidism, contribute to the myopathy. Clinical improvement in the myopathy usually results from specific therapy such as vitamin D repletion in nutritional osteomalacia, phosphate replacement in renal hypophosphatemia, or correction of acidosis. Fractures of the involved bones may occur with minimal trauma. When the ribs are involved, severe deformities may develop in the thoracic cage, and the collapse of vertebral bodies may produce loss of height.

RADIOLOGIC FEATURES In rickets, radiologic alterations are most evident at the epiphyseal growth plate, which is increased in thickness, cupped, and hazy at the metaphyseal border due to decreased calcification of the hypertrophic zone and inadequate mineralization of the primary spongiosa. The trabecular pattern of the metaphyses is abnormal, the cortices of the diaphyses may be thinned, and the shafts may be bowed.

In osteomalacia, decrease in bone density is usually associated with loss of trabeculae and thinning of the cortices. The radiologic changes may be indistinguishable from those in osteoporosis. Trabecular patterns may be blurred, producing a homogeneous ground glass appearance. The specific finding that suggests osteomalacia is the presence of radiolucent bands ranging from a few millimeters to several centimeters in length, usually perpendicular to the surface of the bones. They are particularly common at the inner aspects of the femur, especially near the femoral neck, in the pelvis, in the outer edge of the scapula, in the upper fibula, and in the metatarsals (Figs. 358-3 and 358-4). These radiolucent bands, called *pseudofractures* or *Looser's zones*, occur most often at sites where major arteries cross the bones and are thought to be due to the mechanical stress of the pulsation of these vessels. On radionuclide bone scans the pseudofractures appear as hot spots. Subperiosteal erosions along the diaphyseal cortices are sometimes seen in secondary hyperparathyroidism.

Increased rather than decreased density of bones may be observed in patients with renal tubular disorders rather than with vitamin D deficiency and may produce a striking thickening of the cortices and trabeculae of spongy bone. Despite the increase in mass of bone per

FIGURE 358-3 Radiographs of the scapula of a 58-year-old woman with phosphate diabetes. The presence of a pseudofracture or Looser's zone is indicated by the arrow.

unit volume, the trabeculae are covered with thickened osteoid seams typical of osteomalacia. Similar findings may occur in patients with chronic renal failure. The reason for the hyperostosis is unknown; the bone is architecturally abnormal and subject to fracture with minimal trauma.

LABORATORY FINDINGS Changes in serum concentrations of calcium, inorganic phosphorus, 25(OH)D, and 1,25(OH)₂D vary with the different disorders (see Chap. 356). In vitamin D deficiency, whether due to dietary lack, inadequate sunlight exposure, or intestinal malabsorption, serum calcium levels are normal or low, whereas phosphorus and 25(OH)D levels are consistently low, the latter usually <20 nmol/L (<8 ng/mL) depending on the assay. In contrast, levels of 1,25(OH)₂D may be normal or elevated due to secondary hyperparathyroidism. Eventually, when levels of 25(OH)D become so low that there is inadequate substrate for the renal 25(OH)D-1α-hydroxylase, then the serum level of 1,25(OH)₂D also declines. In adults, the lower limit of serum phosphorus concentration is around 0.9 mmol/L (2.8 mg/dL); in children, the lower limit of normal is closer to 1.3 to 1.5 mmol/L (4.0 to 4.5 mg/dL). In *severe* vitamin D depletion, hypocalcemia may be sufficient to produce tetany. Mild acidosis and generalized aminoaciduria result from secondary hyperparathyroidism. As a rule, patients with renal tubular disorders have normal serum calcium levels and hypophosphatemia. Other laboratory findings, such as glucosuria, aminoaciduria, acidosis, and hypouricemia, reflect variable degrees of disturbance of proximal tubular function or features of the underlying disease (e.g., low plasma ceruloplasmin in Wilson's disease or abnormalities of immunoglobulins in multiple myeloma). In chronic renal failure, hyperphosphatemia and hypocalcemia are usually accompanied by normal 25 (OH)D and low 1,25(OH)₂D levels. In nephrotic syndrome, serum 25(OH)D levels can be low due primarily to urinary losses of protein-bound 25(OH)D. Serum phosphorus levels are also normal or elevated in hypophosphatasia. Increased excretion of hydroxyproline-containing peptides occurs when secondary hyperparathyroidism and excessive bone resorption are associated with the defect in mineralization. Alkaline phosphatase levels in plasma are usually elevated in rickets or osteomalacia, but typical and even severe osteomalacia, especially that due to renal tubular disorders, may be accompanied by normal levels or borderline elevations. Levels may increase during the early phases of therapy.

DIETARY VITAMIN D DEFICIENCY AND INADEQUATE ENDOGENOUS SYNTHESIS Most foods unfortified with vitamin D contain insufficient amounts of the vitamin to prevent rickets in growing children or osteomalacia in adults living in temperate-zone cities. As discussed in Chap. 356, in the absence of supplements, vitamin D must be formed endogenously through the ultraviolet irradiation of precursor 7-dehydrocholesterol in the skin. Many factors decrease the formation of vitamin D₃ from its precursor: increased melanin pigmentation, hyperkeratosis, sunscreens, limited exposure of the body, short days of sunlight, oblique angle of ultraviolet irradiation, and factors in the atmosphere, such as smog, which prevent adequate penetration of solar ultraviolet radiation. Since fortification of milk and routine use of vitamin D supplements for infants have been in

FIGURE 358-4 Radiograph of the femurs of a 47-year-old woman with Fanconi's syndrome of adult onset. The presence of multiple pseudofractures is indicated by the arrows.

effect, deficiency is unusual in the United States. Poor, dark-skinned infants living in crowded northern cities are most susceptible. Furthermore, elderly individuals with insufficient sun exposure, particularly those who are housebound or in nursing homes, drink no milk, and receive no vitamin D supplements, may have low serum levels of 25(OH)D, secondary hyperparathyroidism, and increased frequency of hip fractures. Intestinal absorption of vitamin D is normal in the elderly.

VITAMIN D LOSS AND INTESTINAL MALABSORPTION Osteomalacia may occur with intestinal malabsorption such as in adult celiac disease and regional enteritis. Prior to the discovery of gluten sensitivity in some of these cases, celiac disease was among the more common disorders underlying osteomalacia. Vitamin D absorption, which normally occurs via chylomicrons, is impaired in diseases causing steatorrhea, such as chronic biliary obstruction. Patients with cholestatic liver disease or extrahepatic biliary obstruction may have low serum levels of 25(OH)D and osteomalacia due not only to poor vitamin D absorption but also to decreased hepatic production of 25(OH)D. Osteomalacia is less frequent in chronic pancreatic insufficiency. Patients who have had gastric surgery for peptic ulcer disease or gastric bypass for obesity also may develop osteomalacia, possibly due to malfunction of the proximal small bowel. Additional factors may contribute to the osteomalacia in patients with small-bowel disease, such as inadequate absorbing surface and failure of intestinal cells to respond to the active metabolites of vitamin D. Secondary hyperparathyroidism is usually present in intestinal malabsorption, as in dietary lack of vitamin D, and may be particularly severe in patients who develop osteomalacia following intestinal bypass surgery. Some patients who lack vitamin D, usually associated with intestinal malabsorption, have normal circulating levels of 1,25(OH)$_2$D despite low or undetectable levels of 25(OH)D. In these individuals, the normal levels of 1,25(OH)$_2$D may be accounted for by ingestion of sufficient vitamin D in hospital diets to produce substrate 25(OH)D for 1α-hydroxylation by the renal enzyme that is increased in activity due to secondary hyperparathyroidism. In other patients, circulating 1,25(OH)$_2$D levels may not reflect levels at critical target cells.

ABNORMAL METABOLISM OF VITAMIN D Serum 25(OH)D levels are reduced in some instances of parenchymal and obstructive liver disease, but these findings have not been correlated with quantitative histologic studies of bone. Patients consuming anticonvulsant drugs such as phenobarbital, phenytoin, or carbamazepine may develop rickets or osteomalacia. For a given intake of vitamin D, patients on chronic anticonvulsant therapy have lower serum levels of calcium and 25(OH)D. Consumption of anticonvulsants may be especially important in individuals whose intake of vitamin D is marginal, who are nonambulatory and confined indoors, who have chronic recurrent infections, or in whom mild intestinal malfunction exists as in the postgastrectomy state. As discussed in Chap. 356, the anticonvulsant drugs have multiple actions on calcium homeostasis.

Two autosomal recessive syndromes associated with rickets have been termed *vitamin D–dependent rickets* (also see Chap. 329). Features of *type I vitamin D–dependent rickets* include hypocalcemia, hypophosphatemia, short stature, skeletal deformities of rickets, dental enamel hypoplasia, frequently marked elevations of serum alkaline phosphatase activity, generalized aminoaciduria, and secondary hyperparathyroidism. Circulating levels of 1,25(OH)$_2$D are low or undetectable. Treatment with massive doses of vitamin D or small doses of calcitriol reverses the abnormal biochemical findings, induces healing of the rickets, and restores the rate of skeletal growth. The abnormalities are due to mutations that impair the renal 25(OH)D-1α-hydroxylase. By linkage analysis, the disorder has been mapped to chromosome 12q14. Lifelong replacement therapy with calcitriol is required. *Type II vitamin D–dependent rickets*, also termed *hereditary resistance to 1,25(OH)$_2$D*, has many clinical features of the type I syndrome. Rickets is usually of early onset but varies in severity in different kindreds. Distinguishing features include alopecia, which may develop during the first few months of age, and multiple

milia and epidermal cysts. The type II disorder is due to mutations that impair structure and function of the 1,25(OH)$_2$D receptor. Different molecular abnormalities in different kindreds include mutations that impair binding of the receptor to DNA, mutations that cause the formation of incomplete receptor molecules, and mutations that cause single amino acid substitutions in the protein. This disorder also maps by linkage analysis to chromosome 12 in a locus close to but distinct from that for type I vitamin D–dependent rickets.

Abnormalities in vitamin D metabolism, not on a genetic basis, and osteomalacia may occur in patients on long-term total parenteral nutrition. Some of these individuals have hypoparathyroidism, but this cannot account for the osteomalacia. Serum levels of 25(OH)D are normal, although levels of 1,25(OH)$_2$D may be low. Aluminum has been detected in increased amounts in plasma, urine, and bone and may play a role in genesis of the osteomalacia similar to that postulated in patients with renal failure on chronic hemodialysis.

RENAL TUBULAR DISORDERS Rickets and osteomalacia occur in association with a variety of disorders of proximal renal tubular function. These disorders have in common increased renal clearance of inorganic phosphorus and hypophosphatemia with normal or near-normal glomerular filtration rate. Increased phosphate clearance with resultant hypophosphatemia is usually an isolated defect with no other abnormalities except for increased urinary glycine excretion (hyperglycinuria). X-linked hypophosphatemia (also called *phosphate diabetes* or *vitamin D–resistant rickets*) is an X-linked dominant disorder characterized by rickets in an otherwise well-nourished, healthy-appearing child. When the child begins to walk and bear weight, lower limb deformities appear and become progressively worse. The rate of linear growth is at first normal and then slowed. Many of these individuals develop a unique disorder of tendons, ligaments, and joint capsules characterized by calcification or, more probably, ossification of insertions of tendons and ligaments and joint capsules (enthesopathy). In some patients, spontaneous remissions may be followed by recurrences in adult life, e.g., with pregnancy and lactation. Hypophosphatemia is due to defective renal conservation of phosphate, which in turn is due to defective phosphate transport across the luminal membrane of proximal renal tubular cells. [A model of the human disease occurs in a strain of hypophosphatemic (Hyp) mice.] On the basis of analysis of restriction fragment polymorphism studies in several kindreds of X-linked hypophosphatemia, the gene has been mapped to the short arm of the X chromosome (Xp22.31-p21.3). The responsible gene has not been identified. In affected individuals, the serum levels of 25(OH)D are normal, and the levels of 1,25(OH)$_2$D are in the low-normal range. Whereas the induction of hypophosphatemia in normal individuals results in stimulation of 25(OH)D-1α-hydroxylase and an increase in the levels of 1,25(OH)$_2$D, altered renal tubular cellular phosphate fluxes in X-linked hypophosphatemia fail to stimulate the hydroxylase. Thus levels of 1,25(OH)$_2$D, although in the normal range, are inappropriately low relative to the phosphate depletion. The skeletal mineralization defect is due both to the low ambient phosphate levels and to an intrinsic defect in osteoblast function possibly related to that in the renal tubular cells. Effective therapy therefore requires both phosphate repletion with large amounts of oral phosphate and treatment with calcitriol (see below). Such combined therapy reverses the osteomalacia of trabecular bone surfaces, corrects the microscopic periosteocytic mineralization defects, and results in improvement in longitudinal growth. After the rickets is healed, however, defects in phosphate clearance and hypophosphatemia persist, and medical therapy is still required. The effects of excessive calcitriol administration, such as nephrocalcinosis and nephrolithiasis, must be avoided. Adults with X-linked hypophosphatemia frequently have pseudofractures; osteoarthritis in the sacroiliac joints, wrists, knees, hips, and feet; and marked enthesopathy. Another variant of hereditary rickets has been termed *hereditary hypophosphatemic rickets with hypercalciuria*. Muscular weakness, not a feature of X-linked hypophosphatemia, may be present. These individuals, whose disorder is probably inherited as an autosomal recessive trait, have normocalcemia, hypophosphatemia, and striking absorptive hypercalciuria; the latter disappears after fasting and returns after oral calcium loading. Levels of $1,25(OH)_2D$ in serum are elevated, in contrast to low-normal levels in X-linked hypophosphatemia. These elevations of serum $1,25(OH)_2D$ are an appropriate response of the $25(OH)D\text{-}1\alpha$-hydroxylase to phosphate depletion. Phosphate replacement induces healing of the rachitic lesions.

Sporadic cases of hypophosphatemia also have been described in adults in whom family histories are negative and proximal muscle weakness is a prominent feature (see also Chap. 359). These patients also are best treated with a combination of calcitriol and inorganic phosphorus. As mentioned above, secondary hyperparathyroidism is not present in most untreated patients with renal tubular disorders associated with rickets and osteomalacia.

In other patients, the disorder in tubular function may be more widespread, involving (besides phosphorus) glucose, potassium, amino acids, and uric acid; the various combinations are termed the *de Toni-Debré-Fanconi syndrome*. The more complete renal tubular defects may occur sporadically or in families. In some instances, the lesion is part of a more widespread disorder, as in Wilson's disease and cystinosis. Fanconi syndrome also may be a feature of plasma cell myeloma, where it is attributed to toxic effects of deposited Bence Jones protein. Similarly, osteomalacia and renal tubular acidosis have been observed in Sjögren syndrome with increased urinary excretion of beta_2 microglobulin and retinol-binding protein. The acidosis of proximal tubular defects also plays a role in development of osteomalacia, possibly by altering metabolism of vitamin D or the renal handling of calcium and phosphorus. In this regard, osteomalacia has accompanied the hyperchloremic acidosis or ureterocolic anastomosis.

TUMOR-ASSOCIATED (ONCOGENOUS) OSTEOMALACIA Osteomalacia and hypophosphatemia with high renal phosphate clearance occur with a variety of mesenchymal tumors, including giant cell tumors (benign or malignant), reparative granulomas, hemangiomas, fibromas, and other mesenchymal neoplasms. A similar syndrome occurs in patients with prostatic carcinoma. In some instances, removal of the tumor resulted in return of renal phosphorus clearance to normal, rise in serum phosphorus levels, and healing of the osteomalacia (or rickets in children). Serum $1,25(OH)_2D$ levels are low or undetectable, although chronic administration of sufficient calcitriol to raise circulating levels of this metabolite to normal does not alter renal phosphorus clearance or serum phosphorus concentrations. Humoral factors released by these tumors may impair proximal tubular functions such as 1α-hydroxylation of $25(OH)D$ *and* phosphate transport.

CHRONIC RENAL FAILURE Osteomalacia is common in patients with chronic renal failure; it tends to be the predominant type of renal osteodystrophy in younger patients and is more frequent in those with the lower plasma levels of calcium and phosphorus. A component of secondary hyperparathyroidism and osteitis fibrosa is almost always present. The defect itself probably involves a decreased conversion of $25(OH)D$ to $1,25,(OH)_2D$ either because of insufficient viable renal cortical tissue or the inhibitory effect of hyperphosphatemia on renal $25(OH)D\text{-}1\alpha$-hydroxylase activity. In addition, there may be a primary defect in intestinal calcium absorption. Part of the secondary hyperparathyroidism also may be due to decreased phosphate clearance and subsequent hyperphosphatemia. Under circumstances of hyperphosphatemia and near-normal plasma concentration of calcium, the presence of inhibitors probably causes the defective mineralization. In some patients, the osteomalacia responds to large doses of vitamin D or dihydrotachysterol or to small doses of calcitriol or calcifediol. However, some patients with renal osteodystrophy do not respond to pharmacologic doses of vitamin D or to calcitriol. In some, accumulation of aluminum in the bone accounts for the vitamin D–refractory osteomalacia. Aluminum deposits can be identified at the mineralization fronts, and bone apposition rates are low. These individuals have high levels of aluminum and uncoupling of matrix deposition and mineralization. Individuals with lower amounts of aluminum develop

a form of "aplastic" bone disease where matrix deposition and mineralization are more closely coupled. Deferoxamine can mobilize aluminum from bone and other tissues and is effective therapy. In some patients with renal osteodystrophy, the total bone mass may be increased (osteosclerosis), resulting in increased density of bone. This is particularly evident in the spine, where a characteristic appearance is that of dense bone at the superior and inferior margins of the vertebral bodies with more radiolucent central portions ("rugger jersey sign"). Histologically, although there is more bone per unit area, each trabecula is covered by a wide osteoid seam.

HYPOPHOSPHATASIA Rickets is a feature of a deficiency of alkaline phosphatase in infants and children termed *hypophosphatasia*. There are four forms of hypophosphatasia, i.e., lethal perinatal, infantile, childhood, and adult. Rickets occurs in the infantile and childhood forms. In adults, the disorder may not be recognized until middle age, but there is frequently a history of early loss of deciduous or permanent teeth. Osteomalacia and calcium pyrophosphate deposition disease occur in the adult form. The severe perinatal and infantile forms are inherited as autosomal recessive traits; the pattern of inheritance in the other forms is uncertain. The low levels of circulating alkaline phosphatase activity are explained by a deficiency of the tissue-nonspecific enzyme (bone-liver-kidney). Missense mutations have been demonstrated in the alkaline phosphatase gene.

Although alkaline phosphatase is abundant in osteoclasts, its function in mineralization is not established. In hypophosphatasia, there is increased urinary excretion of phosphoethanolamine and increased circulating levels of pyridoxal-5'-phosphate. The metabolic origin of the phosphoethanolamine is not established. Concentrations of pyridoxal-5'-phosphate are not elevated intracellularly, and the extracellular increases are consistent with the function of alkaline phosphatase as an ectoenzyme; whether alterations of pyridoxal-5'-phosphate metabolism contribute to the clinical abnormalities is not known. Inorganic pyrophosphate (PPi) is a substrate for alkaline phosphatase, which accounts for increased levels of PPi in urine and plasma and for the increased incidence of calcium pyrophosphate deposition disease in hypophosphatasia. Since PPi also can function to inhibit growth of the calcium-phosphate mineral phase, excessive concentrations of PPi may cause the rickets and osteomalacia. There is no effective therapy.

OTHER DISORDERS ASSOCIATED WITH DEFECTIVE MINERALIZATION Disturbances in mineralization may be seen in patients consuming high doses of fluoride ion and in patients with Paget's disease treated with diphosphonates such as etidronate. Some decrease in mineralization of newly forming matrix, increase in surface covered by osteoid, and increase in the width of the osteoid seams may occur in conditions that are not usually considered as osteomalacia except by these criteria. Examples include patients with the osteitis fibrosa of hyperparathyroidism following surgical cure. In these circumstances, there is a temporary imbalance between the rate at which mineral is supplied to bone and the rate at which bone matrix is formed. Biopsies in some of these conditions show a normal calcification front. Wide osteoid seams and hypophosphatemia are also seen in children with osteopetrosis, in whom there is inadequate resorption of bone and calcified cartilage but active bone formation.

A condition that resembles osteomalacia and is associated with a coarsened, mottled bony trabecular pattern, pseudofractures, and bone pain but normal plasma levels of calcium and phosphorus is *fibrogenesis imperfecta ossium*. The bone has a distinctive histologic appearance, with wide osteoid seams, distortion of the birefringent pattern of normal bone, and abnormal collagen fibers by electron microscopy. The nature of the abnormality is not known.

TREATMENT OF RICKETS AND OSTEOMALACIA In rickets and osteomalacia due to dietary absence of vitamin D or inadequate exposure to sunlight, vitamin D_2 (ergocalciferol) or vitamin D_3 (cholecalciferol) is given orally in doses of 800 to 4000 IU (0.02 to 0.1 mg) daily for 6 to 12 weeks, followed by daily supplements of 200 to 400 IU, which are adequate to prevent the development of the disorder in otherwise normal subjects. In infants and children, such treatment causes improvement in muscle tone and strength, increase in serum calcium and phosphorus levels, and decrease in alkaline phosphatase levels after several weeks. Radiologic evidence of healing is evident within weeks and may be complete by a few months. Calcium supplements and larger initial doses of vitamin D may be necessary in infants and children with tetany. In adults with nutritional osteomalacia, healing of pseudofractures may be evident within 3 to 4 weeks after therapy with as little as 2000 IU (0.5 mg) vitamin D daily. Healing is complete usually by 6 months.

Patients with osteomalacia due to intestinal malabsorption do not respond to small doses of vitamin D. In the presence of active steatorrhea, daily oral doses of vitamin D of 50,000 to 100,000 IU (1.25 to 2.5 mg) and large doses of calcium (e.g., 15 g calcium lactate or 4 g calcium carbonate orally per day) may be required. In some instances, oral vitamin D is ineffective, and the parenteral route is required (e.g., 10,000 IU/d intramuscularly). Another approach is the use of artificial ultraviolet B radiation or exposure to sunlight in addition to supplemental calcium. Small doses of calcitriol (0.5 to 1.0 μg daily) are usually effective in this form of osteomalacia. Inorganic phosphate therapy is not indicated either in deficiency or in intestinal malabsorption of the vitamin, since hypocalcemia will develop and intestinal calcium absorption will remain inadequate. In all patients in whom large doses of vitamin D are used, serum calcium and 25(OH)D levels should be monitored periodically. Semiquantitative urinary calcium measurements are inadequate.

In patients on anticonvulsants, it is usually necessary to continue the drugs while adding 4000 to 40,000 IU/d of vitamin D and to monitor levels of serum calcium and serum 25(OH)D until a therapeutic response (evidence of radiologic healing, improvement in symptoms) is obtained.

Treatment of rickets and osteomalacia in the presence of renal tubular disorders is more difficult. In the past, the X-linked form of hypophosphatemic osteomalacia was treated with large doses of vitamin D (from 50,000 to several hundred thousand IU/d), but skeletal responses were rarely complete. The use of dihydrotachysterol, a pseudo-1α(OH)D analogue, 0.2 to 0.6 mg orally per day, in place of vitamin D had the advantage of shorter onset and duration of action and more consistent skeletal healing. With such therapy, radiologic evidence of healing in many patients is incomplete; some hypophosphatemia persists, linear skeletal growth remains abnormally slow, and bony deformities continue to develop. In addition, hypercalcemia and its consequences are potential hazards. Currently, oral supplements of inorganic phosphate in divided doses of phosphorus, 1.0 to 3.6 g/d, and calcitriol, 0.5 to 2.0 μg/d, constitute the best regimen to restore skeletal growth and heal the bone disease. In some adults therapy with inorganic phosphate alone abolishes muscle weakness and bone pain and produces radiologic and histologic healing. The addition of calcitriol improves calcium balance and helps decrease secondary hyperparathyroidism and maintain a sufficient level of serum phosphorus to permit complete healing. In some patients there may be temporary increase in bone pain and rise in serum alkaline phosphatase during the early phases of treatment. In the osteomalacia associated with the chronic acidosis of renal tubular disorders, the use of alkali may be of value in supplementing therapy with phosphate and calcitriol. In patients with ureterosigmoidostomy, oral sodium bicarbonate can reverse acidosis, improve serum phosphate level, and heal the bone disease; with maintenance doses of alkali, recurrence of symptoms can be prevented.

Patients with nephrotic syndrome and low serum 25(OH)D levels benefit from modest vitamin D supplementation. In chronic renal failure, high doses of vitamin D, similar to those needed to treat osteomalacia of renal tubular disorders, are used. Dihydrotachysterol at doses of 0.2 to 1.0 mg daily and small doses of calcitriol are equally effective in treating hypocalcemia and osteodystrophy resulting from chronic renal failure. The recommended initial dose of calcitriol is 0.25 μg/d. If after 2 to 4 weeks on this dose the biochemical parameters are unaltered, the dose is increased by 0.25 μg/d every 2 to 4 weeks until a satisfactory clinical biochemical

response (including elevation of serum calcium levels and decrease in PTH levels) is obtained. The usual dose is 0.5 to 1.0 μg/d. Calcitriol also may be administered intravenously (1.0 to 2.5 μg three times weekly) in patients on dialysis, particularly to treat refractory osteitis fibrosa. Because there are no regulatory mechanisms to control the biological responses to calcitriol, there is a high incidence of transient hypercalciuria and hypercalcemia, especially initially. Thus serum calcium should be monitored frequently during the first 1 to 2 months of therapy and less frequently once a stable dose has been established. Since calcitriol has a short duration of action and is not stored in fat depots, hypercalcemia usually resolves in 2 to 7 days after the dose is discontinued or decreased. Phosphate supplements are, of course, contraindicated in the usual patient with chronic renal failure. Occasionally, however, hypophosphatemia may result from the excessive use of nonabsorbable antacids or from excessive removal of phosphate through hemodialysis.

In patients who have had rickets in childhood, the abnormal mechanical stress of severe deformities may contribute to the development of degenerative joint disease, particularly in hips and knees. Osteotomies at the proper time after healing may prevent this complication and the requirement for more extensive arthroplasties later in life.

REFERENCES

Osteoporosis

AVIOLI LV, KRANE SM (eds): *Metabolic Bone Disease and Clinically Related Disorders*. Philadelphia, Saunders, 1990

BERGKVIST L et al: The risk of breast cancer after estrogen and estrogen-progestin replacement. N Engl J Med 321:293, 1989

BILLER BMK et al: Mechanisms of osteoporosis in adult and adolescent women with anorexia nervosa. J Clin Endocrinol Metab 68:548, 1989

BOIVIN G et al: Fluoride content in human iliac bone: Results in controls, patients with fluorosis, and osteoporotic patients treated with fluoride. J Bone Miner Res 3:497, 1988

BUCHANAN JR et al: Effect of excess endogenous androgens on bone density in young women. J Clin Endocrinol Metab 67:937, 1988

CHEEMA C et al: Effects of estrogen on circulating "free" and total 1,25-dihydroxyvitamin D and on the parathyroid–vitamin D axis in postmenopausal women. J Clin Invest 83:537, 1989

CIVITELLI R et al: Bone turnover in postmenopausal osteoporosis: Effect on calcitonin treatment. J Clin Invest 82: 1268, 1988

COLE WG et al: New insights into the molecular pathology of osteogenesis imperfecta. Q J Med 70, 1, 1989

DEMPSTER DW: Bone histomorphology in glucocorticoid-induced osteoporosis. J Bone Miner Res 4:137, 1989

———, LINDSAY R: Pathogenesis of osteoporosis. Lancet 341:797, 1993

DIAMOND T et al: Ethanol reduces bone formation and may cause osteoporosis. Am J Med 86:282, 1989

DRINKWATER BL et al: Bone mineral content of amenorrheic and eumenorrheic athletes. N Engl J Med 311:277, 1984

EASTELL R et al: Colles' fracture and bone density of the ultradistal radius. J Bone Miner Res 4:607, 1989

ETTINGER B et al: Postmenopausal bone loss is prevented by treatment with low-dosage estrogen with calcium. Ann Intern Med 106:40, 1987

FINKELSTEIN JS et al: Osteoporosis in men with idiopathic hypogonadotropic hyogonadism. Ann Intern Med 106:354, 1987

GALLAGHER JC et al: Epidemiology of fractures of the proximal femur in Rochester, Minnesota. Clin Orthop 150:163, 1980

HEANEY RP et al: Thinking straight about calcium. N Engl J Med 328:503, 1993

HEDLUND LR, GALLAGHER JC: Increased incidence of hip fracture in osteoporotic women treated with sodium fluoride. J Bone Miner Res 4:223, 1989

HODSMAN AB, DROST DJ: The response of vertebral bone mineral density during the treatment of osteoporosis with sodium fluoride. J Clin Endocrinol Metab 69:932, 1989

HOLBROOK TL et al: Dietary calcium and risk of hip fracture: 14-year prospective population study. Lancet 2:1046, 1988

HOROWITZ MC: Cytokines and estrogen in bone: Anti-osteoporotic effects. Science 260:626, 1993

HUPPERT LC: Hormonal replacement therapy: Benefits, risks, doses. Med Clin North Am 71:23, 1987

JENSEN J et al: Cigarette smoking, serum estrogens, and bone loss during hormone-replacement therapy early after menopause. N Engl J Med 313:973, 1985

KRANE SM, SCHILLER AL: Metabolic disease, in *Endocrinology*, 2d ed, LJ DeGroot et al (eds). Philadelphia, Saunders, 1989, vol 2, p 1151

LINDSAY R: Prevention and treatment of osteoporosis. Lancet 341:801, 1993

——— et al: Prevention of spinal osteoporosis in oophorectomised women. Lancet 2:1151, 1980

MAMELLE N et al: Risk-benefit ratio of sodium fluoride treatment in primary vertebral osteoporosis. Lancet 2:361, 1988

MARIE PJ et al: Osteocalcin and deoxyribonucleic acid synthesis in vitro and histomorphometric indices of bone formation in postmenopausal osteoporosis. J Clin Endocrinol Metab 69:272, 1989

NABULSI AA et al: Association of hormone-replacement therapy with various cardiovascular risk factors in postmenopausal women. N Engl J Med 328:1069, 1993

NAGANT DE DEUXCHAISNES C: Therapy for skeletal disorders. Curr Opin Rheumatol 1:98, 1989

PAK CYC et al: Safe and effective treatment of osteoporosis with intermittent slow release sodium fluoride: Augmentation of vertebral bone mass and inhibition of fractures. J Clin Endocrinol Metab 68:150, 1989

PARFITT AM: Dietary risk factors for age-related bone loss and fractures. Lancet 2:1181, 1983

——— et al: Relationship between surface, volume, and thickness of iliac trabecular bone in aging and in osteoporosis: Implications for the microanatomic and cellular mechanisms of bone loss. J Clin Invest 72:783, 1985

POCOCK NA et al: Recovery from steroid-induced osteoporosis. Ann Intern Med 107:319, 1987

PRIOR JC et al: Spinal bone loss and ovulatory disturbances. N Engl J Med 323:1221, 1990

PROCKOP DJ: Mutations that alter the primary structure of type I collagen. J Biol Chem 265:15349, 1990

REGINSTER JY et al: Relationship between whole plasma calcitonin levels, calcitonin secretory capacity, and plasma levels of estrone in healthy women and postmenopausal osteoporotics. J Clin Invest 83:1073, 1989

REID IR et al: Effect of calcium supplementation on bone loss in postmenopausal women. N Engl J Med 328:460, 1993

RIGGS BL, MELTON LJ III: Evidence for two distinct syndromes of involutional osteoporosis. Am J Med 75:899, 1983

———, ———: Involutional osteoporosis. N Engl J Med 314:1676, 1986

——— et al: Incidence of hip fractures in osteoporotic women treated with sodium fluoride. J Bone Miner Res 2:123, 1987

——— et al: Effect of fluoride treatment on the fracture rate in postmenopausal women with osteoporosis. N Engl J Med 322:802, 1990

———, ———: The prevention and treatment of osteoporosis. N Engl J Med 327:620, 1992

RIIS B et al: Does calcium supplementation prevent postmenopausal bone loss? N Engl J Med 316:173, 1987

RYAN PJ et al: Osteoporosis and chronic back pain: A study with single-photon emission computed tomography bone scintigraphy. J Bone Miner Res 7:1455, 1992

SAMBROOK P et al: Prevention of corticosteroid osteoporosis: A comparison of calcium, calcitriol, and calcitonin. N Engl J Med 328:1747, 1993

SEEMAN E et al: Risk factors for spinal osteoporosis in men. Am J Med 75:977, 1983

——— et al: Effect of early menopause on bone mass in normal women and patients with osteoporosis. Am J Med 85:213, 1988

SILVERBERG SJ et al: Abnormalities in parathyroid hormone secretion and 1,25-dihydroxyvitamin D_3 formation in women with osteoporosis. N Engl J Med 320:277, 1989

SMITH R et al: Osteoporosis of pregnancy. Lancet 1:1178, 1985

SPENCER H et al: Chronic alcoholism: Frequently overlooked cause of osteoporosis in men. Am J Med 80:393, 1986

STEINBERG KK et al: Sex steroids and bone density in premenopausal and perimenopausal women. J Clin Endocrinol Metab 69:533, 1989

STEPAN JJ et al: Castrated men exhibit bone loss: Effect of calcitonin treatment on biochemical indices of bone remodeling. J Clin Endocrinol Metab 69:523, 1989

STEWART AF et al: Calcium homeostasis in immobilization: An example of resorptive hypercalciuria. N Engl J Med 306:1136, 1982

STORM T et al: Effect of intermittent cyclical etidronate therapy on bone mass and fracture rate in women with postmenopausal osteoporosis. N Engl J Med 322:1265, 1990

TILYARD MW et al: Treatment of postmenopausal osteoporosis with calcitriol or calcium. N Engl J Med 326:357, 1992

WATTS et al: Intermittent cyclical etidronate treatment of postmenopausal osteoporosis. N Engl J Med 323:73, 1990

WEINSTEIN RS, BELL NH: Diminished rates of bone formation in normal black adults. N Engl J Med 319:1698, 1988

WHITEHEAD MI, FRASER D: Controversies concerning the safety of estrogen replacement therapy. Am J Obstet Gynecol 156:1313, 1987

WILSON RJ et al: Mild asymptomatic primary hyperparathyroidism is not a risk factor for vertebral fractures. Ann Intern Med 109:959, 1988

Osteomalacia

ANDRESS DL et al: Osteomalacia and aplastic bone disease in aluminum-related osteodystrophy. J Clin Endocrinol Metab 65:11, 1987

ANDRESS DL et al: Intravenous calcitriol in the treatment of refractory osteitis fibrosa of chronic renal failure. N Engl J Med 321:274, 1989

BONKOVSKY HL et al: Prevalence and prediction of osteopenia in chronic liver disease. Hepatology 12:273, 1990

BURNSTEIN MI et al: The enthesopathic changes of hypophosphatemic osteomalacia in adults: Radiologic findings. AJR 153:785, 1989

CHARHON SA et al: Effects of parathyroidectomy on bone formation and mineralization in hemodialyzed patients. Kidney Int 27:426, 1984

CHINES A, PACIFICI R: Antacid and sucralfate-induced hypophosphatemic osteomalacia: A case report and review of the literature. Calcif Tissue Int 47:291, 1990

COLLINS N et al: A prospective study to evaluate the dose of vitamin D required to correct low 25-hydroxyvitamin D levels, calcium, and alkaline phosphatase in patients at risk of developing antiepileptic drug-induced osteomalacia. Q J Med 78:113, 1991

DAWSON-HUGHES B et al: Effect of vitamin D supplementation on wintertime and overall bone loss in healthy postmenopausal women. Ann Intern Med 115:505, 1991

DELVIN EE et al: Vitamin D nutritional status and related biochemical indices in an autonomous elderly population. Am J Clin Nutr 48:373, 1988

DIAMOND TH: Metabolic bone disease in primary biliary cirrhosis. J Gastroenterol Hepatol 5:66, 1990

FRASER D, SCRIVER CR: Hereditary rickets and osteomalacia associated with abnormalities in vitamin D metabolism (calcipenic rickets) or phosphate homeostasis (phosphopenic rickets), in Endocrinology, 2d ed, LJ DeGroot et al (eds). Philadelphia, Saunders, 1989, vol 2, p 1080

GALLAGHER JC: Vitamin D metabolism and therapy in elderly subjects. South Med J 85:2S43, 1992

GLORIEUX FH: Disturbances of phosphate metabolism—Effects on bone, in Metabolic Bone Disease: Cellular and Tissue Mechanism, CS Tam et al (eds). Boca Raton, Fla, CRC Press, 1988, p 215

———: Rickets, the continuing challenge. N Engl J Med 325:1875, 1991

GODSALL JW et al: Vitamin D metabolism and bone histomorphometry in patients with antacid-induced osteomalacia. Am J Med 77:747, 1984

HARDY DC et al: X-linked hypophosphatemia in adults: Prevalence of skeletal radiographic and scintigraphic features. Radiology 171:403, 1989

HARRELL RM et al: Healing of bone disease in X-linked hypophosphatemic rickets/osteomalacia: Induction and maintenance with phosphorus and calcitriol. J Clin Invest 75:1858, 1985

HARVEY JA et al: Lack of effect of 24,25-dihydroxyvitamin D_3 administration on parameters of calcium metabolism. J Clin Endocrinol Metab 69:467, 1989

HENDERSON JB et al: Blunted seasonal variation in serum 25-hydroxy vitamin D and increased risk of osteomalacia in vegetarian London Asians. Eur J Clin Nutr 46:509, 1992

HENTHORN PS et al: Different missense mutations at the tissue-nonspecific alkaline phosphatase gene locus in autosomal recessively inherited forms of mild and severe hypophosphatasia. Proc Natl Acad Sci USA 89:9924, 1992

HOCKBERG Z et al: 1,25-dihydroxyvitamin D resistance, rickets, and alopecia. Am J Med 77:805, 1984

HODSMAN AB et al: Vitamin D-resistant osteomalacia in hemodialysis patients lacking secondary hyperparathyroidism. Ann Intern Med 94:629, 1981

——— et al: Bone aluminum and histomorphometric features of renal osteodystrophy. J Clin Endocrinol Metab 54:439, 1982

HUTCHISON FN, BELL NH: Osteomalacia and rickets. Semin Nephrol 12:127, 1992

KLEEREKOPER M, KRANE SM (eds): Clinical Disorders of Bone and Mineral Metabolism. New York, Mary Ann Liebert, 1989

KLEIN GL, COLVURN JW: Metabolic bone disease associated with total parenteral nutrition. Adv Nutr Res 6:67, 1984

——— et al: Bone disease in burn patients. J Bone Miner Res 8:337, 1993

KONISHI K et al: Hypophosphatemic osteomalacia in von Recklinghausen neurofibromatosis. J Med Sci 301:322, 1991

KUMAR R: Hepatic and intestinal osteodystrophy and the hepatobiliary metabolism of vitamin D. Ann Intern Med 98:662, 1983

LABUDA M et al: Two hereditary defects related to vitamin D metabolism map to the same region of human chromosome 12q13–14. J Bone Miner Res 7:1447, 1992

LEICHT E et al: Tumor-induced osteomalacia: Pre- and postoperative biochemical findings. Horm Metab Res 22:640, 1990

LIPS P et al: The effect of vitamin D supplementation on vitamin status and parathyroid function in elderly subjects. J Clin Endocrinol Metab 67:644, 1988

MALLOY PJ et al: Abnormal binding of vitamin D receptors of deoxyribonucleic acids in a kindred with vitamin D–dependent rickets, type II. J Clin Endocrinol Metab 68:263, 1989

MCELDUFF A, POSEN S: Parathyroid hormone sensitivity in familial X-linked hypophosphatemic rickets. J Clin Endocrinol Metab 69:386, 1989

MIYAUCHI A et al: Hemangiopericytoma-induced osteomalacia: Tumor transplantation in nude mice causes hypophosphatemia and tumor extracts inhibit renal 25-hydroxyvitamin-1-hydroxylase activity. J Clin Endocrinol Metab 67:46, 1988

MONTE NESTO JT et al: Osteomalacia secondary to renal tubular acidosis in a patient with primary Sjögren's syndrome. Clin Exp Rheumatol 9:625, 1991

NORDAL KP, DAHL E: Low dose calcitriol versus placebo in patients with predialysis chronic renal failure. J Clin Endocrinol Metab 67:929, 1988

PARFITT AM et al: Metabolic bone disease with and without osteomalacia after intestinal bypass surgery: A bone histomorphometric study. Bone 6:211, 1985

PETERSON DJ et al: X-linked hypophosphatemic rickets: A study (with literature review) of linear growth response to calcitrol and phosphate therapy. J Bone Miner Res 7:583, 1992

POLISSON RP et al: Calcification of entheses associated with X-linked hypophosphatemic osteomalacia. N Engl J Med 313:1, 1985

PORTALE AA et al: Physiologic regulation of the serum concentration of 1,25-dihydroxyvitamin D by phosphorus in normal men. J Clin Invest 83:1494, 1989

RALPHS JR et al: Ultrastructural features of the osteoid of patients with fibrogenesis imperfecta ossium. Bone 10:243, 1989

SCRIVER CR et al: X-linked hypophosphatemia: An appreciation of a classic paper and a survey of progress since 1958. Medicine 70:218, 1991

STONE MD et al: A neuroendocrine cause of oncogenic osteomalacia. J Pathol 167:181, 1992

SULLIVAN W et al: A prospective trial of phosphate and 1,25-dihydroxyvitamin D_3 therapy in symptomatic adults with x-linked hypophosphatemic rickets. J Clin Endocrin Metab 75:879, 1992

VILLAREAL DT et al: Subclinical vitamin D deficiency in postmenopausal women with low vertebral bone mass. J Clin Endocrinol Metab 72:6281, 1991

WEBB AR et al: An evaluation of the relative contributions of exposure of sunlight and of diet on the circulating concentrations of 25-hydroxyvitamin D in an elderly nursing home population in Boston. Am J Clin Nutr 51:1075, 1990

WEIDNER N: Review and update: oncogenic osteomalacia-rickets. Ultrastruct Pathol 15:317, 1991

WHYTE MP: Hypophosphatasia, in The Molecular and Metabolic Basis of Inherited Disease, 7th ed, CR Scriver et al (eds). New York, McGraw-Hill, in press, chap 136

359 DISORDERS OF PHOSPHORUS METABOLISM

JAMES P. KNOCHEL

Phosphorus is the most abundant intracellular anion and is critical for membrane structure, transport, and energy storage. The role of phosphate ions in tissues explains the systemic nature of cellular injury consequent to phosphorus deficiency.

At a plasma pH of 7.4, inorganic phosphate in plasma is a 4:1 mixture of HPO_4^{2-} and $H_2PO_4^{2-}$. The sum of the products of the valences of these ions $(4 \times 2^- + 1 \times 1^-)$ divided by the sum of the ions $(4 + 1)$ is equal to 9/5 or an average valence of 1.8. Of the average 700 g of phosphorus in the body, 85 percent is in the skeleton, about 15 percent is in soft tissues, and 0.1 percent is in extracellular fluid. The phosphorus in extracellular fluid is in a freely diffusible form that (1) permits excretion of hydrogen ions as phosphate buffer into the urine and (2) is in diffusion equilibrium with cytosolic inorganic phosphate in cells.

A normal adult consumes approximately 1 g phosphorus each day. Soluble phosphates in dairy products and meat are almost completely absorbed, predominantly in the midjejunum. Insoluble phosphates, in vegetables and seeds, are absorbable provided the phosphate can be digested from its ligand. For example, phosphorus in corn and oats is partly in the form of phytic acid; these foods contain little phytase, which splits phytic acid (inositol hexaphosphate) into phosphate and inositol, and hence phosphorus from this source may be poorly absorbed. Thus corn and oats may be rachitogenic in man if they are the major components of the diet. Addition of rye bran to the diet, which contains phytase, increases the bioavailability of phosphorus from these sources.

Phosphorus absorption is under the influence of vitamin D, and phosphorus excretion is under the control of parathyroid hormone. Parathyroid hormone decreases tubular phosphate reabsorption and increases excretion into the urine. The effect of vitamin D on phosphate reabsorption by the kidney is relatively minor. The quantity of soluble phosphorus available for absorption from the diet varies, and excretion of phosphorus in the urine on a given day depends directly on absorption. Accordingly, the range for phosphorus excretion in health is very broad.

HYPOPHOSPHATEMIA

CAUSES Hypophosphatemia has many causes (Table 359-1). The finding of hypophosphatemia is not always a reliable indicator of deficiency, since a total-body deficit of phosphorus may exist in the face of hyperphosphatemia, such as, for example, in diabetic ketoacidosis.

Hypophosphatemia can be moderate or severe. Decreased dietary intake is an unusual cause of hypophosphatemia because of the ubiquitous and abundant distribution of the mineral in foods. Decreased absorption of phosphorus from the small intestine occurs in a variety of malabsorptive states, but simple diarrhea is usually not a cause. One of the most common causes of hypophosphatemia is respiratory alkalosis. Indeed, discovery of hypophosphatemia should lead to a search for potentially serious causes of hyperventilation such as sepsis or otherwise unsuspected alcohol withdrawal. Reduction of intracellular P_{CO_2} and elevation of pH increase the activity of phosphofructokinase, the rate-limiting enzyme of glycolysis. Phosphorylation of glucose intermediates causes cellular uptake of phosphorus and hypophosphatemia. Administration of insulin and consumption of nutrients that stimulate insulin release are also common causes of hypophosphatemia. Insulin stimulates phosphorus uptake by cells. Cellular phosphorus uptake also occurs in patients recovering from hypothermia as a result of reactivation of metabolism. Certain rapidly

TABLE 359-1   Causes of hypophosphatemia

Decreased dietary intake
Decreased intestinal absorption
  A Vitamin D deficiency
  B Malabsorption
  C Steatorrhea
  D Secretory diarrhea
  E Vomiting
  F PO_4-binding antacids
Shifts from serum into cells
  A Respiratory alkalosis
    1 Sepsis
    2 Alcohol withdrawal
    3 Heat stroke
    4 Neuroleptic malignant syndrome
    5 Hepatic coma
    6 Salicylate poisoning
    7 Gout
    8 Panic attacks
    9 Psychiatric depression
  B Hormonal effects
    1 Insulin
    2 Glucagon
    3 Epinephrine
    4 Androgens
    5 Glucocorticoids
    6 Anovulatory hormones
  C Nutrient effects
    1 Glucose
    2 Fructose
    3 Glycerol
    4 Lactate
    5 Amino acids
    6 Xylitol
  D Cellular uptake syndromes
    1 Recovery from hypothermia
    2 Burkitt's lymphoma
    3 Histiocytic lymphoma
    4 Acute myelomonocytic leukemia
    5 Acute myelogenous leukemia
    6 Treatment of pernicious anemia
    7 Hungry bone syndrome
      a Following parathyroidectomy
      b Acute leukemia
Increased excretion into the urine
  A Hyperparathyroidism
  B Renal tubular defects
    1 Renal rickets
    2 Polyostotic fibrous dysplasia
    3 Postrenal transplantation
    4 Oncogenic osteomalacia
  C Aldosteronism
  D Licorice ingestion
  E Volume expansion
  F Inappropriate secretion of vasopressin
  G Mineralocorticoid administration
  H Glucocorticoid therapy
  I Diuretics

growing malignancies may take up enough phosphate to cause hypophosphatemia. Deposition of bone mineral following parathyroidectomy also may be a cause. Hypocalcemia consequent to saline infusion causes release of parathyroid hormone. Thus volume expansion and parathyroid hormone both reduce tubular reabsorption of phosphorus. A number of other conditions associated with chronic volume expansion may cause hypophosphatemia.

Severe hypophosphatemia is defined as phosphorus levels in serum below 0.3 mmol/L (1.0 mg/dL). Many of the conditions that result in such low levels are associated with prolonged hyperventilation with respiratory alkalosis or reflect rapid cellular uptake (Table 359-2). Respiratory alkalosis does not cause phosphorus deficiency but may reduce serum phosphorus values to 0.1 mmol/L (0.3 mg/dL) and urinary phosphorus excretion to virtually undetectable levels. Severe hypophosphatemia and severe total-body deficiency of phosphorus occur in patients with poor dietary intake who consume phosphate-binding antacids. Similarly, treatment of diabetic ketoacidosis results in hypophosphatemia. Reduction of serum phosphorus below 0.3 mmol/L (1.0 mg/dL) suggests, but does not prove, the existence of

TABLE 359-2 Causes of severe hypophosphatemia

Chronic alcoholism and alcohol withdrawal
Dietary deficiency and phosphate-binding antacids
Severe thermal burns
Recovery from diabetic ketoacidosis
Hyperalimentation
Nutritional recovery syndrome
Respiratory alkalosis
Therapeutic hyperthermia
Neuroleptic malignant syndrome
Recovery from exhaustive exercise
Renal transplantation
Acute renal failure

serious phosphorus depletion. In chronic alcoholics, reduction of phosphorus content of skeletal muscle may occur because of a renal phosphate leak. The resulting phosphorus deficiency may cause a reduction of muscle magnesium and potassium and accumulations of calcium, sodium, chloride, and water. These findings are not necessarily associated with elevations of creatine phosphokinase activity that would reflect acute muscle damage. However, during withdrawal from alcohol, phosphorus is often taken up rapidly into skeletal muscle or liver, resulting in severe hypophosphatemia, and in this instance hypophosphatemia may precipitate acute rhabdomyolysis.

Most patients with diabetic ketoacidosis are not severely depleted of phosphorus. Although, on the one hand, metabolic acidosis and insulin deficiency mobilize intracellular phosphate stores and lead to their excretion into the urine, most patients have not been sick long enough for severe phosphorus deficiency to occur. On the other hand, patients with hypophosphatemia and hypokalemia, in the presence of severe diabetic ketoacidosis, are likely severely depleted of phosphorus and potassium and require treatment. The history usually shows that this type of patient with diabetic ketoacidosis has been sick for many days, has not had significant vomiting, has maintained a good intake of fluids, and has excreted phosphorus briskly for a period of many days, thus establishing severe deficiency. Such patients probably represent no more than 5 percent of cases of diabetic ketoacidosis.

MANIFESTATIONS The manifestations of phosphorus deficiency are listed in Table 359-3; many of these can occur simultaneously.

Phosphate trapping is an acute disorder resulting from reduction of intracellular inorganic phosphate concentration. The most common cause is administration of intravenous fructose. Fructose is metabolized by only three tissues in the body—the liver, the small bowel epithelium, and the proximal tubule of the kidney. When glucose is taken up into liver cells and phosphorylated by hexokinase, the resulting glucose-6-phosphate inhibits hexokinase, producing a smoothly regulated uptake of glucose that does not deplete or trap stores of inorganic phosphate. When fructose is administered intravenously, it is taken up into liver cells, where it is converted to fructose-1-phosphate by the enzyme fructokinase. Fructose-1-phosphate does not inhibit fructokinase, thus permitting rapid uptake of fructose into liver cells and consumption or trapping of available stores of inorganic phosphate. Reduced intracellular phosphate concentration activates AMP deaminase and nucleotidase. The consequent reduction of adenylate compounds is reflected by increased uric acid production and hyperuricemia. Acute reduction of ATP, which is bound to magnesium, is heralded by a modest rise of magnesium in serum. Acute liver cell damage may occur. Disturbances of renal function also may occur after intravenous fructose. Hepatic and renal metabolic disturbances that follow fructose administration are preventable by infusing inorganic phosphate. Whether oral fructose affects intestinal epithelium in a similar manner is not known.

Rhabdomyolysis predictably occurs in chronic alcoholics who become acutely hypophosphatemic during the course of alcohol withdrawal. Hypophosphatemic rhabdomyolysis also occurs rarely during treatment for diabetic ketoacidosis, during the course of hyperalimentation, or while refeeding patients with malnutrition. In alcoholics, evidence of muscle cell injury precedes the occurrence of

hypophosphatemia. Presumably, severe hypophosphatemia triggers induction of acute rhabdomyolysis. This syndrome can be reproduced experimentally. It does not occur if hypophosphatemia is prevented during hyperalimentation.

Cardiomyopathy occurs in severe phosphorus depletion. The manifestations include reduction in cardiac output, hypotension, impaired pressor responsiveness to cathecholamines, and a reduced threshold to ventricular arrhythmias.

Respiratory insufficiency occurs in malnourished patients receiving intravenous nutrients with inadequate phosphorus who become progressively hypophosphatemic over 8 or 10 days. Profound weakness causes failure of diaphragm function, hypoxia, and respiratory acidosis. Despite severe hypophosphatemia, these patients rarely develop rhabdomyolysis, presumably because they had no preexistent muscle damage. The initial clue may be an inability to extubate a patient from a ventilator at the anticipated time. This syndrome is seldom seen in chronic alcoholics because rhabdomyolysis in such patients may correct hypophosphatemia spontaneously. Rapid correction of chronic respiratory acidosis also may cause hypophosphatemia and diaphragm weakness. In these patients, administration of phosphorus rapidly corrects muscle weakness and respiratory insufficiency.

Erythrocyte dysfunction is due to a decrease in 2,3-diphosphoglycerate (2,3-DPG) content. The red cell is the only tissue in the body that produces this substance. Both 2,3-DPG and ATP facilitate dissociation of oxyhemoglobin and promote oxygen delivery to tissue. Reduced 2,3-DPG and ATP both enhance affinity of oxygen for hemoglobin and reduce tissue oxygenation. This mechanism may explain central nervous system dysfunction in hypophosphatemia. Hemolysis due to phosphorus deficiency probably does not occur.

Leukocyte dysfunction due to phosphorus deficiency results in impaired phagocytosis and opsonization. As a result, chronic hypophosphatemia increases susceptibility to bacterial and fungal infections.

Skeletal demineralization is an important effect of phosphorus deficiency, especially in patients with a poor dietary intake who simultaneously ingest phosphate-binding antacids. Under conditions of increased bone turnover, in normal children or in adults with Paget's disease, hyperparathyroidism, or bony metastases, demineralization may occur at such a rate as to cause hypercalcemia. Osteopenia, bone pain, and a syndrome resembling osteomalacia occur in chronic phosphorus deficiency.

Metabolic acidosis may occur in children or adults with phosphorus deficiency due to vitamin D deficiency. Reduced phosphorus intake results in mobilization of hydroxyapatite from bone that serves to maintain normal levels of serum phosphorus. Hypercalciuria occurs normally as a result of phosphorus deprivation. Severe hypophosphatemia has two important metabolic effects on the kidney. First, inorganic phosphate excretion into the urine falls so that hydrogen excretion as NaH_2PO_4 into the urine is eliminated. Second, phosphorus deficiency also elevates renal intracellular pH, which results in a profound decrease in ammonia production. The reduction in ammonia production eliminates hydrogen excretion as ammonium ions (NH_4^+). Since excretion of hydrogen as phosphate buffer or ammonium accounts for nearly all the kidney's capacity to secrete acid, it is surprising that phosphorus deficiency is only rarely associated with metabolic acidosis. The explanation lies in the fact that mobilization

TABLE 359-3 Hypophosphatemic syndromes

Phosphate trapping
Rhabdomyolysis
Cardiomyopathy
Respiratory insufficiency
Erythrocyte dysfunction
Leukocyte dysfunction
Skeletal demineralization
Metabolic acidosis
Nervous system dysfunction

of hydroxyapatite from bone provides carbonate ions, which, in turn, buffer the retained hydrogen ions that otherwise would be excreted in the urine. Under conditions in which hydroxyapatite cannot be mobilized during phosphorus deprivation (e.g., vitamin D deficiency, severe magnesium deficiency, and perhaps aluminum poisoning), buffer cannot be mobilized adequately, and metabolic acidosis ensues.

Nervous system dysfunction is a distinctive and predictable feature of severe hypophosphatemia and phosphorus deficiency. This syndrome usually occurs in the setting of refeeding or hyperalimentation-induced hypophosphatemia that develops over the course of 8 to 10 days. Such patients become irritable and apprehensive and hyperventilate sufficiently to cause paresthesias and numbness. Profound muscular weakness is followed by dysarthria, confusion, obtundation, convulsive seizures, coma, and death. Alternatively, ascending motor paralysis with or without sensory disturbances may resemble the Guillain-Barré syndrome. In such cases, the cerebrospinal fluid is normal. Ophthalmoplegia, diplopia, and dysphagia suggest botulism, and poorly defined defects in color perception (metachromatopsia) suggests cerebral cortical dysfunction. In these patients, as in those with respiratory failure, spontaneous rhabdomyolysis does not occur despite severe hypophosphatemia.

TREATMENT   Before initiating treatment for hypophosphatemia, the cause should be ascertained. Measurement of arterial pH and blood gases and of phosphorus concentration in the urine is helpful.

Milk is an excellent source of phosphorus, containing 33 mmol/L (100 mg/dL). Phosphate salts are also available for oral use. They are less likely to cause diarrhea in phosphorus-deficient patient than in a normal person. Phosphorus salts cannot be given by intramuscular or subcutaneous injection, but sodium phosphate and potassium phosphate are available for intravenous use. The potassium salt should be given when hypokalemia and hypophosphatemia coexist. A safe dosage regimen for treatment of alcoholics who are hypophosphatemic, hypokalemic, and hypomagnesemic is the infusion each 8 to 12 h of 1 L of 0.5 normal NaCl in 5% glucose containing 9 mmol of potassium phosphate and 4.2 mmol $MgSO_4$ (2.0 mL of 50% $MgSO_4$ solution). Serum concentrations of potassium, magnesium, and phosphate should be monitored closely. Such infusions should be stopped when oral intake becomes possible.

Hyperphosphatemia should be avoided because it can cause severe hypocalcemia and crystal deposition in important structures, including blood vessels, the eye, lung, heart, and kidney. Fatal alveolar diffusion block has occurred, especially if the patient is alkalotic.

HYPERPHOSPHATEMIA

Defined in adults as an elevation of serum phosphorus above 1.67 mmol/L (5 mg/dL), hyperphosphatemia is a common finding with many causes (Table 359-4). Abnormal positively charged serum proteins, as in plasma cell dyscrasias, may cause marked elevations of phosphorus. In one instance, the serum concentration was 4.5 mmol/L (13.5 mg/dL), and each millimole of myeloma protein bound 15 molecules of phosphate.

Decreased renal excretion of phosphorus is the most common cause of hyperphosphatemia. Since parathyroid hormone (PTH) is phosphaturic, hyperphosphatemia is a cardinal feature of hypoparathyroidism, either as a primary disorder or in patients whose renal cAMP response to PTH is abnormal (pseudohypoparathyroidism type I) or those whose phosphaturic response to PTH is suppressed (pseudohypoparathyroidism type II).

Of interest, severe hypomagnesemia causes marked suppression of PTH in plasma despite hypocalcemia but does not cause hyperphosphatemia. Hyperphosphatemia occurs in tumoral calcinosis, pseudoxanthoma elasticum, infantile hypophosphatasia, and hyperostosis because of decreased renal excretion. Untreated severe hyperthyroidism apparently increases cellular catabolism sufficiently to elevate serum phosphorus despite increased phosphorus loss in the urine. Acromegaly or administration of growth hormone causes modest hyperphosphatemia. Presumably, the higher phosphorus levels in

TABLE 359-4   Causes of hyperphosphatemia

BINDING TO SERUM PROTEINS

Plasma cell dyscrasias

DECREASED RENAL EXCRETION

Renal insufficiency
Hypoparathyroidism
Pseudohypoparathyroidism, types I and II
Tumoral calcinosis
Pseudoxanthoma elasticum
Infantile hypophosphatasia
Hyperostosis
Hyperthyroidism
Growth hormone activity
Adrenal insufficiency
Bisphosphonate therapy

INCREASED INTESTINAL ABSORPTION

Phosphorus-containing cathartics
Medication with vitamin D compounds
Granulomatous diseases producing vitamin D
 Sarcoidosis
 Tuberculosis

INTERNAL REDISTRIBUTION

Acute metabolic acidosis
Acute respiratory acidosis
Reduced insulin level
Clonidine administration

CELLULAR RELEASE

Rhabdomyolysis
Organ infarction
Tumor lysis
 Burkitt's lymphoma
 Lymphoblastic lymphoma
 Metastatic small cell carcinoma
Thyrotoxicosis
Acute hemolysis

PARENTERAL ADMINISTRATION

Intravenous phosphate salts
Lipid (phospholipid) infusion

children partly reflect growth hormone activity. Hyperphosphatemia occurs in untreated adrenal insufficiency because of volume contraction, metabolic acidosis, and possibly reduced glomerular permeability. Mild hyperphosphatemia may occur with biphosphonate therapy because of increased tubular reabsorption of phosphorus.

Hyperphosphatemia secondary to increased absorption from the gut occurs during administration of excess phosphate salts by mouth or from the colon as a result of enemas that contain phosphorus. Overmedication with vitamin D and production of vitamin D by granulomatous tissue such as sarcoidosis and tuberculosis can cause hyperphosphatemia. Both acute metabolic and acute respiratory acidosis may decompose cellular organic phosphates, reduce phosphorylation, and result in diffusion of phosphorus from the cell and hyperphosphatemia. Reduced insulin levels or clonidine administration also can cause hyperphosphatemia. Cellular release of phosphorus may cause hyperphosphatemia, particularly in rhabdomyolysis, infarction of other tissues, tumor lysis, or hemolysis. Severe hyperphosphatemia after intravenous infusion of phosphate salts is a particular danger in patients who are acidotic or oliguric. Finally, infusion of compounds containing phospholipids for parenteral nutrition has caused hyperphosphatemia.

REFERENCES

ANGELI P et al: Hypophosphatemia and renal tubular dysfunction in alcoholics. Gastroenterology 100:502, 1991

BLACHLEY J et al: Fluid and electrolyte disorders associated with alcoholism and liver disease, in *Fluid and Electrolytes*, JP Kokko, RL Tannen (eds). Philadelphia, Saunders, 1990, chap 11, pp 649–688

DAVIS SV et al: Reversible depression of myocardial performance in hypophosphatemia. Am J Med Sci 295:183, 1988

FULLER TJ et al: Reversible depression in myocardial performance in dogs with experimental phosphorus deficiency. J Clin Invest 62:1194, 1978

JOHNSON MA et al: Adenosine triphosphate turnover in humans. J Clin Invest 84:990, 1989

KNOCHEL JP: Hypophosphatemia and phosphorus deficiency, in *The Kidney*, 4th ed, B Brenner, F Rector (eds). Philadelphia, Saunders, 1991

———: Central nervous system manifestations of hypophosphatemia and phosphorus depletion, in *Metabolic Brain Dysfunction in Systemic Disorders*, AC Arief, RC Griggs (eds). Boston, Little, Brown, 1992, chap 10, pp 183–204

———: Hypophosphatemia and rhabdomyolysis. Am J Med 92:455, 1992

KOTANKO P: Hyperphosphatemia in multiple myeloma. N Engl J Med 326:1781, 1992

LEVI M et al: Disorders of phosphate and magnesium metabolism, in *Disorders of Bone and Mineral Metabolism*, FC Coe, MJ Favus (eds). New York, Raven, 1992, chap 28, pp 587–610

VEECH RL et al: Cytosolic phosphorylation potential. J Biol Chem 254:6538, 1979

360   DISORDERS OF MAGNESIUM METABOLISM

JAMES P. KNOCHEL

Magnesium is the most abundant intracellular divalent cation. The total magnesium content of a normal man is 12.4 mmol (0.3 g) per kilogram of body weight. Of this, 1 percent is extracellular, 31 percent is in cells, and 67 percent is in bone. Serum magnesium ranges between 0.8 and 1.2 mmol/L (2 and 3 mg/dL). Of this, the unbound diffusible concentration is about 0.6 mmol/L (1.4 mg/dL). It exists in two forms in cells, one in solution which is in equilibrium with the diffusible form in plasma and a larger quantity bound to organic components. Since most magnesium inside cells is bound to ATP, in accordance with the principle of mass action, MgATP is in equilibrium with free magnesium ions. Thus shifts in free magnesium concentration may help regulate stores of ATP. From the opposite viewpoint, if ATP is acutely reduced, e.g., by infusion of fructose intravenously, freed magnesium ions diffuse from the cell, and serum magnesium rises. Since ATP is critical to nearly all metabolic transformations, a normal concentration of serum magnesium is essential to maintain adequate stores of this important nucleotide.

The ideal intake of magnesium for an adult is 15 to 20 mmol/d (36 to 48 mg/d). Foods rich in magnesium include seed grains, nuts, peas, and beans. Fresh meat, fish, and most fresh fruits contain relatively small amounts of magnesium. Magnesium is absorbed primarily in the jejunum and ileum, and healthy persons absorb about 30 to 40 percent of ingested magnesium. This may increase to 70 percent when intake is low or magnesium deficiency exists. Vitamin D deficiency reduces magnesium absorption. When magnesium intake is restricted, fecal excretion becomes negligible, and urinary excretion decreases to 0.5 to 1 mmol/d (12 to 24 mg/d). Thus magnesium retention by the kidney is very efficient. Magnesium excretion depends on glomerular filtration of the unbound fraction, of which 25 percent is reabsorbed in the proximal tubule and 50 to 60 percent is reabsorbed in the loop of Henle. Loop diuretics, such as ethacrynic acid, bumetanide, or furosemide, cause greater excretion of magnesium than do diuretics such as thiazides that act on the distal tubule. Magnesium excretion is increased by expanding extracellular fluid volume by ingestion of water and salt, and aldosterone decreases reabsorption of magnesium by the renal tubule. Magnesium excretion increases sharply when the concentration in serum exceeds 0.8 mmol/L (2 mg/dL).

Slight hypomagnesemia occurs in athletically trained individuals, hypermetabolic states such as pregnancy and cold acclimatization, or after experimental administration of thyroid hormone.

MAGNESIUM DEFICIENCY

When any of the three major intracellular elements is deprived or lost, whether magnesium, potassium, or phosphorus, losses of the others usually follow. For this reason, deficiency of a single intracellular component almost never occurs. A diet devoid of magnesium causes depletion of phosphorus and potassium in skeletal muscle. Selective potassium deficiency may cause reductions in magnesium and phosphorus. Phosphorus deficiency may cause reductions in potassium and magnesium contents of tissue. The usual somatic responses to selective deprivation of one major intracellular element are anorexia, cellular atrophy, a negative nitrogen balance, and net loss of the other two major intracellular elements. Shrinkage of the cell and expulsion of the elements not deprived help to maintain a normal intracellular composition.

During hyperalimentation, a different situation prevails. Provision of a diet that is otherwise replete but deficient in one major intracellular element promotes an anabolic state, and the protoplasm that is synthesized has a major deficit of the ion being deprived. In these situations, serious derangements of cellular composition include accumulations of sodium, chloride, calcium, and water, suggesting a major interference with cellular ion transport. Indeed, elevation of cellular calcium, by activating proteases and phospholipases, may be an important cause of cellular injury under these conditions.

As in deficiencies of other major intracellular elements, deficiency of body magnesium can exist even when serum values are normal. In addition, certain tissues become deficient before others. The definition of a true deficit of an intracellular element is reduction of its ratio to nitrogen in tissue. In muscle, this ratio is about 0.3 mmol (7 mg) magnesium per gram of nitrogen. Red cell magnesium content decreases in all species during magnesium deficiency, whereas muscle magnesium content remains normal in some species. Because of the inconsistency of tissue levels, and because measurement of tissue magnesium is difficult, the clinician must rely on serum magnesium levels to detect magnesium deficiency or excess.

THE CLINICAL PHYSIOLOGY OF MAGNESIUM DEFICIENCY
Volunteers fed a diet deficient in magnesium eventually develop characteristic symptoms and findings. Within 3 to 7 days after reducing dietary magnesium intake to less than 0.5 mmol (12 mg) per day, renal excretion of magnesium declines to below 0.5 mmol (12 mg) per day. Anorexia, nausea, vomiting, lethargy, and weakness develop within weeks. Characteristic symptoms of magnesium deficiency consist of paresthesias, muscular cramps, irritability, decreased attention span, and mental confusion. These complaints may require months to appear.

The physical findings are manifestations of the associated hypocalcemia. These are positive Trousseau and Chvostek signs, peculiar movements of the fingers best described as athetoid tetany, and, on occasion, convulsions. Muscle fasciculations may be precipitated by a blow with a neurologic hammer to muscle. About half of patients with selective magnesium depletion become hypokalemic. In animals, rhabdomyolysis may occur. Cardiac arrhythmias, disturbances of conduction, and even ventricular fibrillation and cardiac arrest can occur in patients with coexisting hypokalemia and hypomagnesemia. In such instances, hypokalemia may be the cause of the associated ECG abnormalities. Digitalis potentiates the severity and potential danger of arrhythmias. In the presence of QT prolongation, polymorphic ventricular tachycardia (torsades des pointes) may occur that responds to magnesium salts. The causes of magnesium deficiency are shown in Table 360-1.

Hypocalcemia usually does not develop until serum magnesium falls below 0.5 mmol/L (1.2 mg/dL). Although mild magnesium deficiency may increase release of parathyroid hormone, severe hypomagnesemia [levels below 0.4 mmol/L (1 mg/dL)] blocks release of parathyroid hormone. The resulting hypocalcemia may be severe. In addition, magnesium deficiency impairs the normal calcemic response to parathyroid hormone at the level of the skeleton. Hypocalcemia can become sufficiently severe to cause tetany. Al-

TABLE 360-1 Causes of hypomagnesemia

Primary nutritional disturbances
  A Inadequate intake
  B Total parenteral nutrition
  C Refeeding syndrome
Gastrointestinal disorders
  A Specific absorptive defects
  B Malabsorption syndromes
    1 Enteric fistulas
    2 Nontropical sprue
    3 Whipple's disease
    4 Intestinal lymphoma
    5 Chronic pancreatic insufficiency
    6 Biliary diversion
    7 Giardiasis
    8 Short bowel syndrome
  C Prolonged diarrhea
  D Prolonged nasogastric suction
  E Pancreatitis
Endocrine disorders
  A Hyperparathyroidism
  B Hypoparathyroidism
  C Hyperthyroidism
  D Primary hyperaldosteronism
  E Bartter's syndrome
  F Diabetic ketoacidosis
  G Alcoholic ketoacidosis
  H Administration of epinephrine
  I Syndrome of inappropriate secretion of antidiuretic hormone
  J "Hungry bone" syndrome after parathyroidectomy
Chronic alcoholism, alcoholic withdrawal
Increased renal excretion
  A Ethanol ingestion
  B Idiopathic
  C Following renal transplantation
  D Cisplatin therapy
  E Aminoglycoside therapy
  F Amphotericin B therapy
  G Capreomycin therapy
  H Viomycin therapy
  I Diuretic administration
    1 Furosemide
    2 Ethacrynic acid
    3 Acetazolamide
    4 Thiazides
    5 Chlorthalidone
    6 Osmotic agents
  J Recovery phase of acute tubular necrosis
  K Pentamidine therapy
  L Theophylline toxicity
  M Colony stimulating factor therapy

though tetany has been reported in patients with hypomagnesemia independently of hypocalcemia, both conditions usually exist in patients with this finding. In most cases the tetany with hypomagnesemia does not respond to infusions of calcium and requires correction of magnesium levels. The hypocalcemia also responds only to magnesium replacement therapy, usually requiring 2 to 7 days for correction. In patients whose hypomagnesemia is caused by steatorrhea, administration of magnesium salts intravenously can cause prompt and sometimes explosive release of parathyroid hormone. In rare instances, acute hypercalcemia can occur.

Hypokalemia in patients with magnesium deficiency is less well understood. Aldosterone production may be enhanced, thus permitting loss of potassium into the urine. It is difficult to correct the potassium deficiency with supplemental potassium salts. However, administration of magnesium salts sufficient to correct the hypomagnesemia promptly reduces potassium excretion and corrects the hypokalemia. For this reason, it should be kept in mind that hypokalemia refractory to potassium supplements may be due to magnesium deficiency.

GASTROINTESTINAL CAUSES OF MAGNESIUM DEFICIENCY
Familial hypomagnesemia is manifested during childhood and is caused by reduced absorption of dietary magnesium. The most common cause of magnesium deficiency in adults is intestinal malabsorption and steatorrhea, as in nontropical sprue, the short

bowel syndrome, chronic pancreatic insufficiency, or biliary diversion. Because of unabsorbed fat, complexes of nonabsorbable magnesium–fatty acid soaps form in the intestinal lumen. When long-standing, hypomagnesemia in such cases is often associated with hypocalcemia, hypokalemia, and hypophosphatemia. Because of steatorrhea, disorders related to malabsorption of fat-soluble vitamins, especially vitamins K, A, and D, may coexist. It is important to recognize that vitamin D deficiency associated with hypomagnesemia can cause weakness due to proximal myopathy in association with pain in the lower back and hips resulting from osteomalacia.

Magnesium deficiency also occurs after prolonged nasogastric suction in patients who have not received adequate magnesium salts. Acute hypomagnesemia, along with acute hypocalcemia, can occur in acute hemorrhagic pancreatitis when magnesium– and calcium–fatty acid soaps form in situ as a result of tissue necrosis.

ENDOCRINE CAUSES OF HYPOMAGNESEMIA
Mild hypomagnesemia occurs in poorly controlled diabetes mellitus. Moderate hypomagnesemia may occur in hyperparathyroidism, hypoparathyroidism, hyperthyroidism, and primary hyperaldosteronism, as well as during recovery from diabetic ketoacidosis. In primary hyperaldosteronism, aldosterone enhances magnesium excretion directly and acts via volume expansion to cause net losses of magnesium. These effects can be reversed by spironolactone. Hypomagnesemia may occur in hypokalemic and hyponatremic patients with the syndrome of inappropriate secretion of vasopressin (antidiuretic hormone). Presumably, this is the result of increased aldosterone production and overexpansion of extracellular volume. Epinephrine and other potent beta agonists may cause transient hypomagnesemia, presumably because of uptake of magnesium ions into adipose tissue as fatty acids are released. Furthermore, as catecholamines cause release of fatty acids into the blood, insoluble fatty acid–magnesium and fatty acid–calcium complexes form in serum. If serum is centrifuged, the precipitates settle to the bottom of the tube, and spurious hypomagnesemia and hypocalcemia can be diagnosed.

HYPOMAGNESEMIA ASSOCIATED WITH ALCOHOLISM
Ethanol causes a transient loss of magnesium into the urine. Alcoholics with a reasonably normal nutrient intake and normal intestinal function usually have normal or only slightly depressed magnesium levels in blood. The total-body deficit of magnesium in chronic alcoholics is modest, amounting to 100 to 150 mmol (2.4 to 3.6 g). However, during alcoholic withdrawal, hypomagnesemia may occur in association with acute hypophosphatemia and acute hypokalemia. Simultaneously, urinary excretion of magnesium, PO_4, and potassium falls. Thus hypomagnesemia occurs both because of net deficit and because of a shift into cells during withdrawal. In animals, sustained ethanol administration in intoxicating doses causes severe depletion of phosphorus, moderate depletion of magnesium and potassium, and increases in intracellular sodium, chloride, water, and calcium. Selective depletion of phosphorus also causes magnesium wasting and muscle magnesium deficiency. The same findings occur in muscle of severely alcoholic patients. In acute alcohol withdrawal, respiratory alkalosis and insulin release stimulated by administration of nutrients act in concert to incorporate phosphate into cells. Increased ATP synthesis as a result of phosphate movement into cells may cause increased magnesium binding and worsen hypomagnesemia.

In alcoholics with intestinal malabsorption and steatorrhea, hypomagnesemia can be severe in association with hypocalcemia, hypophosphatemia, and hypokalemia. Although a relationship between hypomagnesemia and alcoholic withdrawal seizures has been suggested, alcoholics in a withdrawal state display prominent respiratory alkalosis, which lowers the threshold for seizure activity. Thus the relationship of hypomagnesemia to seizures in this setting is not clear. Furthermore, correction of hypomagnesemia in a withdrawing alcoholic appears to have no favorable effect on the withdrawal syndrome.

Magnesium deficiency may play a role in the temporary hypertension that occurs during alcohol withdrawal. Independently of alcohol, magnesium deficiency causes accumulation of calcium in smooth muscle and increases vascular tone. Magnesium salts reduce arteriolar tone by reducing cytosolic calcium. Accumulation of calcium potentiates the pressor response to circulating catecholamines. Withdrawing alcoholics nearly always have elevations of circulating catecholamines. Thus the combined effects of magnesium depletion, calcium accumulation in cells, and elevated levels of catecholamines may explain the occurrence of hypertension and the favorable effect of calcium channel blocking drugs under such circumstances.

MAGNESIUM DEFICIENCY DUE TO INCREASED RENAL EXCRETION Hypomagnesemia also can result from impaired renal tubular reabsorption. Most of these states are associated with renal potassium wasting and hypokalemia, and some patients are hypercalciuric. Transient hypomagnesemia due to reduced renal tubular reabsorption may follow renal transplantation.

Aminoglycosides, cisplatin, diuretics, and cyclosporine can cause magnesium wasting in the urine. Aminoglycosides cause hypomagnesemia and hypokalemia as a result of impaired tubular reabsorption. Hypomagnesemia develops after prolonged treatment and usually in patients who have received more than 8.0 g of aminoglycosides. Total recovery is the rule after the drug is stopped. Most patients treated with cisplatin develop hypomagnesemia that can be severe; hypokalemia is less common. Renal tubular mitochondrial injury may be responsible for these events. Even after cisplatin is withdrawn, the nephron defect may persist for months, years, or for life. Of interest, calcitriol may enhance magnesium wasting in patients with cisplatin nephrotoxicity who are also hypomagnesemic and hypocalcemic. About a fourth of patients treated with cyclosporine and prednisone after renal transplantation develop serum magnesium levels below 0.5 mmol/L (1.2 mg/dL). Loop diuretics are potent magnesuric agents, but hypomagnesemia is frequent in patients medicated with diuretics. Patients who receive large doses of diuretics or who receive two or more diuretics that act at different sites in the nephron are more likely to develop hypomagnesemia. Treatment with pentamidine, theophylline, and granulocyte-macrophage colony stimulating factor has each caused hypermagnesuria and hypomagnesemia.

TREATMENT OF HYPOMAGNESEMIA AND MAGNESIUM DEFICIENCY Treatment of hypomagnesemia and its associated disorders should be aimed at correcting the cause. Patients with inadequate dietary intake or with disorders that reduce intestinal absorption or cause excessive losses into the urine can often be corrected by oral administration of magnesium salts. Patients with potentially serious cardiac arrhythmias or with nausea and vomiting should be given intravenous magnesium sulfate. Magnesium sulfate heptahydrate ($MgSO_4 \cdot 7H_2O$) has a molecular weight of 234; thus 1 mL of a 50% solution contains 2.1 mmol (50 mg) of magnesium. The usual adult dose of 50% magnesium sulfate is 2 mL every 6 h on the first day and half this quantity on each of the following 3 to 4 days. Magnesium sulfate may be given intramuscularly, but this is painful and may cause elevation of creatine phosphokinase levels, reflecting muscle damage and thus blunting the value of measurements of the enzyme to detect rhabdomyolysis. It is preferable to infuse magnesium in a dose of 4.1 mmol (1 g) magnesium sulfate every 6 h. Patients who require intravenous magnesium sulfate are often hypokalemic and hypophosphatemic. Potassium phosphate and potassium chloride may be included with magnesium sulfate in 0.5% saline containing 5% glucose. The total potassium content in each infusion bottle should represent one-fourth the amount determined to be necessary each day. In patients with adequate urine flow, such solutions can be given in a quantity of 750 mL every 6 h until nausea and vomiting disappear and oral intake becomes possible. In patients with tetany due to magnesium deficiency, although hypocalcemia coexists, calcium is generally ineffective, and infusions of magnesium salts usually require 2 h or more to relieve the tetany. Up to a full day may be required for all signs of latent tetany, such as the Chvostek and Trousseau signs, to disappear completely. Several oral preparations of magnesium salts are available. Thus 5 mL of magnesium hydroxide–containing antacids (Maalox, Gelusil, Mylanta) each contains 14 mmol (340 mg) of

magnesium. However, there are two theoretical objections to the use of these preparations: they contain aluminum salts that may be hazardous if renal impairment is present, and they bind phosphate in the gut, which by itself promotes loss of magnesium. Other preparations include magnesium chloride tablets, magnesium gluconate tablets, and commercially available magnesium oxide powder. Since both spironolactone and triamterene cause retention of magnesium and potassium, these drugs may be useful adjuncts to maintain normal serum magnesium balance in patients taking diuretics.

Considerable attention has been focused on the role of hypomagnesemia or magnesium deficiency in cardiac arrhythmias under a variety of circumstances, including alcoholic withdrawal, open-heart surgery, coronary angioplasty, myocardial infarction, congestive heart failure, and the multiple organ failure syndrome. In some of these situations, there appears to be an inverse relationship between serum magnesium levels and potentially dangerous ventricular arrhythmias. Although therapeutic and prophylactic treatment with $MgSO_4$ appears to be efficacious, it is controversial whether these patients are actually magnesium deficient. The favorable effect of magnesium under these conditions is probably the result of nonspecific antiarrhythmic properties and electrical stabilization of membranes.

HYPERMAGNESEMIA

Patients with end-stage renal disease frequently have modest hypermagnesemia that can be aggravated by ingesting magnesium-containing compounds such as antacids or cathartics. Surreptitious ingestion of magnesium salts as a cathartic may be identified by demonstration of hypermagnesemia in serum and fecal magnesium concentration above 25 mmol/L (60 mg/dL). Rhabdomyolysis causes hypermagnesemia because of release from injured muscle. Adrenal insufficiency also may cause modest hypermagnesemia. Half of patients with familial benign hypocalciuric hypercalcemia have modest hypermagnesemia. Pronounced hypermagnesemia (6.5 mmol/L) has been described in patients with near-drowning in the Dead Sea in Jordan or Basque Lake in British Columbia. Magnesium concentrations in water from these sources average 164 and 174 mmol/L, respectively. In the Dead Sea, survivals in near-drowning cases have been attributed to pronounced hypercalcemia because of the extreme calcium levels in this water.

Symptomatic hypermagnesemia is uncommon and is usually precipitated by inadvertent overdosage with magnesium salts or is deliberately induced to treat patients with eclampsia. Infants born of eclamptic mothers treated with magnesium may be hypermagnesemic. Magnesium can reduce neuromuscular transmission and act as a central nervous system depressant. Symptoms of hypermagnesemia usually correspond to serum levels. Nausea usually appears at between 2 and 4 mmol/L (5 and 10 mg/dL). Sedation, hypoventilation with respiratory acidosis, decreased deep tendon reflexes, and muscle weakness appear at levels between 8 and 14 mmol/L (20 and 34 mg/dL). Hypotension, bradycardia, and diffuse vasodilatation appear at 10 to 20 mmol/L (24 to 48 mg/dL). Areflexia, coma, and respiratory paralysis occur at 20 to 30 mmol/L (48 to 72 mg/dL). Patients treated for eclampsia must be observed very carefully for signs of magnesium intoxication. If this occurs, symptoms and findings can generally be reversed promptly by infusion of calcium salts, since these ions electrically oppose one another at their sites of action. Administration of saline and furosemide may help promote excretion of magnesium. Hemodialysis is also effective.

REFERENCES

ALFREY AC et al: Evaluation of body magnesium stores. J Lab Clin Med 84:153, 1974

ANDERSON R et al: Skeletal muscle phosphorus and magnesium deficiency in alcoholic myopathy. Miner Electrolyte Metab 4:106, 1980

BRADY HR et al: Mitochondrial injury: An early event in cisplatin toxicity to renal proximal tubules. Am J Physiol 258:F1181, 1990

CRONIN RE et al: Skeletal muscle injury after magnesium depletion in the dog. Am J Physiol 243:F113, 1982

———, et al: Magnesium deficiency, in *Advances in Internal Medicine*, GH Stollerman (ed). Chicago, Year Book Medical Publishers, 1983, chap 28, pp 509–533

D'ANGELO EKG et al: Magnesium relaxes arterial smooth muscle by decreasing intracellular Ca^{2+} without changing intracellular Mg^{2+}. J Clin Invest 89:1988, 1992

FINE KD et al: Diagnosis of magnesium-induced diarrhea. N Engl J Med 324:1012, 1991

KNOCHEL JP: Hypophosphatemia in the alcoholic. Arch Intern Med 140:613, 1980

KROENKE K et al: The value of serum magnesium determination in hypertensive patients receiving diuretics. Arch Intern Med 147:1553, 1987

MOSSERI M et al: Electrocardiographic manifestations of combined hypercalcemia and hypermagnesemia. J Electrocardiol 23:235, 1990

PORATH A et al: Dead Sea water poisoning. Ann Emerg Med 18:121, 1989

RALSTON MA et al: Serum and tissue magnesium concentrations in patients with heart failure and serious ventricular arrhythmias. Ann Intern Med 113:841, 1990

SHILES ME: Magnesium in health and disease. Annu Rev Nutr 8:429, 1988

TZIVONI D et al: Treatment of torsade de pointes with magnesium sulfate. Circulation 77:392, 1988

VELOSO D et al: The concentrations of free and bound magnesium in rat tissues. J Biol Chem 248:4811, 1973

VICTOR M: The role of hypomagnesemia and respiratory alkalosis in the genesis of alcohol withdrawal symptoms. Ann NY Acad Sci 215:235, 1973

WHANG R et al: Frequency of hypomagnesemia in hospitalized patients receiving digitalis. Arch Intern Med 145:655, 1985

361 PAGET'S DISEASE OF BONE

STEPHEN M. KRANE

Paget's disease of bone (osteitis deformans) is usually focal but may be widespread. The initial event is excessive resorption of bone by cells such as osteoclasts, followed by the replacement of normal marrow by vascular, fibrous connective tissue. At some stage and to a variable degree, the resorbed bone is replaced by coarse-fibered, dense trabecular bone organized in haphazard fashion. The irregular and often rapid deposition of this new bone, to a great extent still lamellar, causes an increase in the number of prominent, irregular cement lines that give the bone its characteristic "mosaic" pattern. Most lesions show both excessive resorption and chaotic new bone formation.

INCIDENCE The prevalence is difficult to determine because the disease is often asymptomatic and is frequently detected when roentgenograms are obtained for other reasons or because of a high level of alkaline phosphatase on routine blood screening. On the basis of autopsy examination, the incidence is estimated to be about 3 percent in individuals over age 40; there is increased likelihood of occurrence with increasing age. The incidence varies in different parts of the world. Figures based on radiologic surveys indicate less than a 1 percent frequency in the adult populations in the United States, Great Britain, and Australia. In India, Japan, the Middle East, and Scandinavia, the disease is rare.

ETIOLOGY The cause is unknown. No convincing evidence of endocrine abnormality has been produced. Likewise, although pagetic bone can be exceedingly vascular, it has not been established that the vascular abnormality is primary. Some of the manifestations can be suppressed with glucocorticoids, salicylates, and cytotoxic drugs, but there is no convincing evidence that the fundamental lesion is inflammatory. Intranuclear inclusions have been found by electron microscopy in osteoclasts in pagetic bone but not in osteoclasts or other bone cells in normal persons or patients with other bone diseases with the exception of pyknodysostosis. Some of the inclusions resemble nucleocapsids of viruses belonging to the measles group. Indirect immunofluorescence and immunoperoxidase studies using antibodies to measles virus support the suggestion that the inclusions are indeed measles virus nucleocapsids. Measles virus nucleocapsid mRNA also has been detected by in situ hybridization in bone cells from patients with Paget's disease. Other evidence suggests that the inclusions are due to respiratory syncytial virus. In one area of England, ownership of dogs is more common in pagetic subjects than

in controls, suggesting that a canine virus (e.g., canine distemper) might be the infective agent. Thus different viral agents might be responsible for Paget's disease in different patients.

PATHOPHYSIOLOGY The characteristic feature is increased resorption of bone accompanied by an increase in bone formation, which is usually adequate to compensate. In the early phase bone resorption predominates (e.g., in the variant *osteoporosis circumscripta*), and the bones are exceedingly vascular. This has been termed the *osteoporotic, osteolytic,* or *destructive phase* of disease in which the external calcium balance may be negative. Commonly, the excessive resorption is followed closely by formation of new pagetic bone. In this so-called mixed phase of the disease, the rate of bone formation is so geared to that of bone resorption that the magnitude of the increase in bone turnover is not reflected in the overall calcium balance.

As the activity decreases, a progressive decrease in resorptive rate relative to formation rate may occur, eventually leading to the occurrence of hard, dense, less vascular bone (the so-called *osteoplastic* or *sclerotic phase*) and a positive external calcium balance. The rates of bone turnover may be increased enormously in patients with active Paget's disease, occasionally more than 20 times normal. Quantitative histomorphometry of bone biopsies confirms the extent of remodeling with marked increase in resorption surfaces and deep scalloped lacunae containing osteoclasts and increased numbers of osteoblasts lining the edges. Increased generation and overactivity of osteoclasts are considered the major abnormality. The osteoclasts are larger than normal and contain multiple pleomorphic nuclei and nuclear and cytoplasmic inclusions that resemble viral nucleocapsids. Increased numbers of osteoclast-like multinucleated cells are generated from hematopoietic precursors in long-term marrow cultures from individuals with Paget's disease compared with normal individuals. Production of the cytokine interleukin 6 (IL-6) by the pagetic marrow cells is increased. Thus IL-6 could act as a local factor that contributes to the increased osteoclast formation and activity in this disease. The calcification rate is also increased. The normal hematopoietic marrow is replaced by a loose stroma which may be highly vascular. The magnitude of the increase in turnover varies with the extent as well as the activity of the disease. The increase correlates with the increased plasma levels of bone alkaline phosphatase, which are higher in Paget's disease than in any other condition with the exception of hereditary hyperphosphatasia. Although increased bone resorption enhances release of calcium and phosphate ions from bone, utilization of these ions for new bone formation and, presumably, feedback control of parathyroid hormone secretion usually maintain the concentration of calcium ions in the plasma at normal levels. The concentration of phosphate in the plasma is normal or slightly elevated. When marked imbalance between bone formation and resorption occurs in favor of resorption, as after prolonged immobilization or fractures, urinary calcium excretion may be increased, and rarely, hypercalcemia may occur. If, on the other hand, bone formation exceeds resorption (relatively uncommon), circulating levels of parathyroid hormone may be increased. Significant increases in trabecular bone resorption and osteoid surfaces in normal bone from patients with Paget's disease may be due to compensatory, secondary hyperparathyroidism. Resorption involves the organic phase of bone as well as the mineral phase. While the inorganic ions of the mineral phase are reutilized for bone formation, amino acids such as hydroxyproline and hydroxylysine and the hydroxypyridinium cross-link compounds are released during resorption of the collagen matrix of bone and are not reutilized for collagen biosynthesis. The urinary excretion of small peptides containing hydroxyproline is increased, reflecting the increased bone resorption. Peptides of about 1500 to 5000 mol wt containing hydroxyproline and other amino acids in proportions characteristic of collagen are also excreted in increased amounts in the urine and are correlated with increased bone formation. Other markers for increased matrix synthesis include elevated levels of osteocalcin (bone-GLA protein) (see Chap. 356) and procollagen extension fragments in plasma.

RADIOLOGIC CHANGES The radiologic findings reflect the underlying pathology and the phase of the disease that predominates at the time of the examination. The pelvic bones are most commonly involved, followed by the femur, skull, tibia, lumbrosacral spine, dorsal spine, clavicles, and ribs; small bones are not as frequently diseased. The lytic phase of the disease may be overlooked except when it occurs in the skull as *osteoporosis circumscripta*, with areas of sharply demarcated radiolucency in the frontal, parietal, and occipital bones. In the long bones, the lytic areas are usually first seen at one end, from which they progress toward the other end with a V-shaped advancing edge. The lesion may produce expansion of the cortex and exhibit features suggesting malignancy. Usually the lytic area is followed by a zone of increased density, representing the new bone formation of the mixed phase of the disease. In general, the bone shows enlargement with irregularly widened cortex in a coarse, striated pattern and increased density, occasionally focal in distribution. Perpendicular lines of radiolucency (cortical infractions) are frequent and occur on the convex side of bowed long bones, particularly the femur and tibia. Transverse fractures also may occur, some initiated at the sites of these cortical infractions. The remodeling of the pagetic bone usually follows the lines of stress produced by muscle pull or gravity, accounting for the characteristic lateral bowing of the femur or anterior bowing of the tibia and the tendency for most of the dense bone to be deposited on the concave side of the bowed bone. In the skull, in the mixed stage, there is enlargement and thickening, especially of the outer table, with irregular areas of increased density, often spotty (Fig. 361-1). Basilar invagination is common with involvement of the base of the skull. The changes in the pelvis also consist of bone resorption and new bone formation and are frequently accompanied by a characteristic thickening of the pelvic brim. In the sclerotic phase of the disease, the bone may show uniform increase in density, often in the absence of striations. This is common in the facial bones but is occasionally seen as well in the vertebrae, where a homogeneous, dense pattern gives an "ivory" appearance similar to that typical of Hodgkin's disease, although the involved vertebrae are not enlarged in Hodgkin's disease. Computed tomography is useful in defining atypical lesions, particularly where neoplastic involvement is suspected. Technetium 99m diphosphonate bone scans are indicated to document the extent of disease when therapy is contemplated or to confirm the diagnosis when radiologic findings are inconclusive. Gallium 67 scans also have been used to define the extent of bone involvement.

FIGURE 361-1 Lateral roentgenogram of the skull from a 58-year-old woman with Paget's disease of bone.

CLINICAL PICTURE The clinical presentation is a function of the extent of the disease, the particular bones involved, and the presence of complications. Many patients are asymptomatic. In these individuals, the disorder is discovered during radiologic examination of the pelvis or spine for an unrelated disease or complaint or because of the finding of an elevated level of plasma alkaline phosphatase. Other individuals may gradually become aware of a swelling or deformity of a long bone or develop a disturbance in gait due to unequal length of and change in the distribution of mechanical forces in the lower extremities. Enlargement of the skull is often not noticed by the patients, or they may be aware of increasing hat size. Pain in the face and headache are initial complaints in some; backache and pain in the lower extremities are common. The pain is usually dull but may be shooting or knifelike. Back pain is most common in the lumbar region and may radiate into the buttocks or lower extremities. This pain is probably due to the pagetic process itself, to distortion of articular facets, and to secondary osteoarthritis. Pain in the lower extremities may be associated with the transverse cortical infractions along the convex lateral surface of the femur or the anterior surface of the tibia. Often the new lytic lesions detected on bone scan are the most painful. Pain also may be due to involvement of the hip joint resembling degenerative joint disease and characterized by narrowing of the joint space, bony lipping at the margin of the acetabulum, and deepening of the acetabulum. Angioid streaks may be present in the retina. Hearing loss is due to direct involvement of the ossicles of the inner ear or of bone in the region of the cochlea or to impingement by bone on the eighth cranial nerve in the auditory foramen. More serious neurologic complications can result from overgrowth of bone at the base of the skull (platybasia) and compression of the brainstem. Compression of the spinal cord with paraplegia has been observed, particularly with involvement of the middorsal spine. Pathologic fractures of vertebrae also may produce spinal cord lesions.

COMPLICATIONS Blood flow may be markedly increased in extremities involved with Paget's disease. There is proliferation of blood vessels in pagetic bone, but anatomic and functional studies have not confirmed the presence of arteriovenous fistulas. Although blood flow is increased in bone, cutaneous vasodilatation in the pagetic extremities accounts for the increased warmth noted clinically. When the disease is widespread, involving one-third or more of the skeleton, the increased blood flow may be associated with *high cardiac output* and rarely with so-called high-output heart failure. However, heart disease in individuals with Paget's disease is usually due to the same conditions that occur in other patients of similar age. *Pathologic fracture* may occur in the destructive phase of the disease. In the weight-bearing bones fractures are often incomplete, multiple, and on the convex side of the bone. They may occur spontaneously or follow slight trauma; the lesions are painful but heal spontaneously with no major disability. More serious fractures also may occur. Complete fractures are often transverse as if the bone were snapped like a piece of chalk. Under these circumstances the fracture may upset the delicate balance between bone formation and resorption in favor of resorption. At this stage the imbalance may be reflected by increased urinary calcium excretion, and in rare instances the serum calcium level may rise to dangerous levels.

There is no characteristic level of urinary calcium excretion, although calcium excretion tends to be higher when the resorptive phase predominates. This may be a factor which accounts for the somewhat higher incidence of *urinary stone* in these patients. Secondary changes in the cartilage of the hip joints and knees may result in articular symptoms. Hyperuricemia and gout commonly occur in men with Paget's disease, and calcific periarthritis may occur.

Sarcoma is the dread complication. The incidence is probably no greater than 1 percent, although higher incidence has been noted in some series that include many patients with polyostotic involvement. The sarcomas most frequently arise in the femur, humerus, skull, facial bones, and pelvis and rarely in the vertebrae. In about 20 percent the tumors are multicentric. Histologically, they are usually osteosarcomas, although fibrosarcomas and chondrosarcomas also have been found. Increase in pain and swelling are the common complaints that lead to recognition of the sarcomas. The extent and character of the neoplastic involvement are established by computed tomography and/or magnetic resonance imaging. The level of alkaline phosphatase in the serum of patients with sarcomas usually reflects the activity and extent of the Paget's disease. In occasional patients, an "explosive rise" of the phosphatase level may accompany the growth of the sarcoma, whereas in patients with limited Paget's disease, phosphatase levels may be only slightly elevated and give no clue to the development of the malignant lesion. The prognosis is poor following the development of sarcomas, and ablative surgery is rarely successful. Although chemotherapy is successful for treatment of some osteosarcomas in children, such regimens have little effect on survival of patients in whom osteosarcomas develop on the background of Paget's disease. Reparative granulomas resembling giant cell tumors may be locally destructive, but they do not metastasize.

THERAPY Most patients require no treatment, since the disease is localized and does not cause symptoms. Indications for therapy include persistent pain in involved bones, neural compression, rapidly progressive deformity resulting in disabling disturbance of posture and/or gait, high-output congestive heart failure, hypercalcemia, severe hypercalciuria with or without formation of renal stones, repeated fractures or nonunion, and preparation for major orthopedic surgery. Nonsteroidal anti-inflammatory drugs such as *indomethacin,* 25 mg three or four times daily, may relieve pain, especially in the presence of hip involvement. *Glucocorticoids* suppress the disease but only in large doses (greater than 60 mg prednisone per day), which are usually not tolerated and, therefore, are not recommended. It is of interest that the high cardiac output of some patients may be reduced significantly after only a few days of glucocorticoid treatment. Orthopedic procedures also have a role in the management of selected cases. Total hip replacement may be indicated, and osteotomy may correct marked bowing deformities, particularly of the tibia. In patients with fractures or orthopedic procedures or in patients immobilized for any reason, urinary and serum calcium levels should be measured at intervals to anticipate the development of hypercalciuria and hypercalcemia. Early ambulation and adequate fluid intake are essential. If hypercalcemia does occur under these circumstances, intravenous infusion of the bisphosphonate pamidronate disodium (see below) is recommended in dosage of 20 mg over 2 to 6 h repeated each day for 3 to 4 days.

Several agents reduce the excessive bone resorption of Paget's disease and are of possible therapeutic value. The administration of porcine, salmon, and human *calcitonins* for prolonged periods to pagetic patients causes a decrease in plasma alkaline phosphatase and in urinary hydroxyproline excretion. Treatment with calcitonin causes variable decrease in bone pain due to suppression of the pagetic lesion and an independent, centrally mediated analgesic effect. Calcitonin also induces improvement in neurologic symptoms and decrease in elevated cardiac output. Some patients have not continued to respond to porcine and salmon calcitonins, possibly because of the development of neutralizing antibodies. These individuals usually continue to exhibit a satisfactory response to human calcitonin. In others, the development of secondary hyperparathyroidism has been postulated as the cause for a diminished response, although this cannot account for resistance in all cases. The calcitonins are probably most useful in patients with pain in areas of pagetic involvement not due to associated joint disease. The dose of salmon calcitonin (the form available in the United States) is 50 to 100 MRC units daily given subcutaneously. In most cases, it is possible to reduce the dose to three times weekly. In severe cases, alkaline phosphatase levels decrease, but not to the normal range. The disorder relapses after weeks or months when the calcitonin is discontinued. Some patients develop a sensation of warmth and/or nausea 30 min to several hours after injection. This may occur after initiating treatment or after months or years of therapy. The etiology is unknown, but the

symptoms may be severe enough to discontinue the medication. The use of nasal spray formulations of calcitonin is under investigation.

Although cytotoxic drugs such as plicamycin and dactinomycin have been used in the past to treat Paget's disease, they no longer have a place in therapy, since other agents are safer and more effective. *Etidronate,* a bisphosphonate compound, given orally in doses up to 20 mg/kg body weight per day, is effective in reducing bone resorption in almost all affected individuals and in producing clinical improvement in some. Biochemical indices may be brought to normal, but in most the responses are incomplete. Serum alkaline phosphatase and urinary hydroxyproline excretion remain decreased for several months after withdrawal of the drug and only gradually return to pretreatment levels. In doses of 20 mg/kg of body weight per day for periods of 6 months or longer and even with lower doses, mineralization of new bone may be inhibited (osteomalacia), predisposing to fracture. Some patients develop disabling pain over pagetic lesions within weeks or months of starting treatment that may be severe enough to warrant discontinuing the drug. Radiographs in some instances show an increase in bone lysis that heals when the drug is stopped. It is therefore recommended that doses of 5 mg or occasionally 10 mg/kg of body weight per day be used for 6-month periods. Treatment should be reinstituted within 3 to 12 months if biochemical relapse occurs.

Newer bisphosphonates that result from substitutions at R_1 and R_2 of the

$$
\begin{array}{c}
R_1 \\
| \\
-P-C-P- \\
| \\
R_2
\end{array}
$$

bond are now used in therapy in Europe, and several should soon be available in the United States. These compounds (alendronate, clodronate, pamidronate, risendronate, and tiludronate) are more potent than etidronate and in doses that are effective in completely suppressing the pagetic lesions do not inhibit mineralization. Pamidronate, as already discussed, is approved for treatment of hypercalcemia. These drugs should replace etidronate in the therapy of Paget's disease. Several dosage schedules have been used, such as 15 to 20 mg pamidronate intravenously over 2 to 6 h daily or several times per week for 4 to 10 treatments. Higher intravenous doses may produce fever and flulike symptoms. With such a program, urinary hydroxyproline excretion returns to normal within weeks, and serum alkaline phosphatase becomes normal within months. Remission usually lasts for more than 12 months and for up to 5 years in some patients.

The oral bioavailability of all the bisphosphonates is poor (~ 1 percent), but oral treatment with each of the preceding agents is effective. The major problems with oral treatment are gastrointestinal (nausea, vomiting, mucosal erosions). Although the bisphosphonates and calcitonins act primarily to decrease bone resorption, the rate of new bone formation subsequently falls. As a result, the state of high bone turnover is shifted to a state of lower turnover, where rates of formation and resorption are still apparently geared to each other. In this lower turnover state, collagen fibers of the bone matrix are deposited in a more orderly fashion similar to normal bone.

REFERENCES

Bone HG, Kleerekoper M: Clinical review 39: Paget's disease of bone. J Clin Endocrinol Metab 75:1179, 1992

Harinck HIJ et al: Relation between signs and symptoms in Paget's disease of bone. Q J Med 226:133, 1986

Huvos AG: Osteogenic sarcoma of bones and soft tissues in older persons. Cancer 57:1442, 1986

——— et al: Osteogenic sarcoma associated with Paget's disease of bone: A clinicopathologic study of 65 patients. Cancer 52:1489, 1983

Krane SM: Paget's disease of bone, in *Current Therapy of Endocrinology and Metabolism,* CW Bardin (ed). Philadelphia, BC Decker, 1991, pp 456–460

McDONALD DJ, SIM FH: Total hip arthroplasty in Paget's disease. J Bone Joint Surg 69A:766, 1987

NAGANT DE DEUXCHAISNES C, KRANE SM: Paget's disease of bone: Clinical and metabolic observations. Medicine 43:233, 1964

REBEL A (ed): Symposium on Paget's disease. Clin Orthop 217:1, 1987

ROODMAN GR et al: Interleukin 6: A potential autocrine/paracrine factor in Paget's disease of bone. J Clin Invest 89:46, 1992

SERET P et al: Sarcomatous degeneration of Paget's bone disease. J Cancer Res Clin Oncol 113:392, 1987

SINGER FR, KRANE SM: Paget's disease of bone, in Metabolic Bone Disease, LV Avioli, SM Krane (eds). Philadelphia, Saunders, 1990, pp 546–615

———, WALLACH S (eds): Paget's Disease of Bone. New York, Elsevier 1991, pp 1–313

STRICKBERGER SA et al: Association of Paget's disease of bone with calcific aortic valve disease. Am J Med 82:953, 1987

TABLE 362-1 Causes of hyperostosis

1 Endocrine disorders
  a Primary hyperparathyroidism
  b Hypothyroidism
  c Acromegaly
2 Radiation osteitis
3 Chemical poisoning
  a Fluoride
  b Elemental phosphorus
  c Beryllium
  d Arsenic
  e Vitamin A intoxication
  f Lead
  g Bismuth
4 Osteomalacic disorders
  a Renal tubular osteomalacia (vitamin D resistance or phosphate diabetes)
  b Chronic renal glomerular failure
5 Osteosclerosis (localized) associated with chronic infection
6 Osteosclerotic phase of Paget's disease
7 Osteoscleorsis associated with carcinomatous metastases, malignant lymphoma, and hematologic disorders (myeloproliferative disorders, sickle cell disease, leukemia, multiple myeloma, systemic mastocytosis)
8 Osteosclerosis of erythroblastosis fetalis
9 Osteopetrosis
  a Infantile (malignant, autosomal recessive form)
  b Adult (benign, dominant form)
  c Intermediate form with carbonic anhydrase II deficiency and renal tubular acidosis
10 Unclassified diseases
  a Pyknodysostosis
  b Osteomyelosclerosis
  c Hyperostosis corticalis generalisata
  d Hyperostosis generalisata with pachydermia
  e Hereditary hyperphosphatasia
  f Progressive diaphyseal dysplasia (osteopathia hyperostotica multiplex infantilis; Camurati-Engelmann disease)
  g Melorheostosis
  h Osteopoikilosis
  i Hyperostosis frontalis interna

362 HYPEROSTOSIS, NEOPLASMS, AND OTHER DISORDERS OF BONE AND CARTILAGE

STEPHEN M. KRANE / ALAN L. SCHILLER

HYPEROSTOSIS

A number of disease states have in common an increase in the mass of bone per unit volume (hyperostosis) (Table 362-1). Such increase in bone mass is detected radiologically as increased density of the bone, often associated with a variable disturbance in the architecture of the tissue. In the absence of quantitative histomorphometric data, it is usually not possible to distinguish between an increase in bone mass due to excessive formation of new bone or to decreased resorption of bone already formed. When bone deposition is rapid, the new bone may be of the woven type, but if the process is more chronic, true lamellar bone is formed. The additional bone may be located at the periosteum, within the compact bone of the cortex, or in the trabeculae of the cancellous regions. In the medullary area, the new bone is deposited on and between the trabeculae and encroaches on the medullary spaces. Typical examples of such responses are seen in areas adjacent to tumors or in association with infection. In some diseases, the increase in bone mass may be spotty, as in osteopoikilosis, whereas in others, most of the skeleton may be involved, as in the malignant form of osteopetrosis in children. The increase in mass is usually not due to an excessive amount of mineral relative to matrix, except in disorders such as osteopetrosis, where islands of calcified cartilage may persist. (The mineral density of calcified cartilage is greater than that of bone.) In some diseases, such as the osteosclerosis of renal insufficiency, the bone mass and radiodensity may be increased, even though the new bone formed is poorly mineralized and contains widened osteoid seams. Hyperostosis could be due to dysfunction of osteoblasts or osteoclasts. It is of interest, therefore, that infection of newborn mice produces an osteopetrosis-like phenotype in which osteoblast progenitors appear to induce increased bone formation. In human osteopetrosis of the relatively benign and sporadic type, however, viral nucleocapsid particles have been found in osteoclasts, and it is possible that viral infection causes disordered function in these cells to account for the excessive bone mass.

Several of these conditions are discussed in more detail in other chapters, although some generalizations are pertinent. Bone that is denser than normal may be seen occasionally in the osteitis fibrosa associated with hyperparathyroidism. When the hyperparathyroidism is successfully treated, the rate of bone resorption decreases abruptly out of proportion to the rate of bone formation; this imbalance may lead to the production of areas of bone density greater than in the surrounding skeleton, especially in the healing of brown tumors. In addition, intermittent low levels of parathyroid hormone act directly on osteoblasts, to increase bone formation. In hypothyroidism, the rates of both bone formation and resorption may be decreased, but when the balance is in favor of formation, bones are of increased density but normal architecture. Increased bone density also occurs in some instances of osteomalacia associated with disturbances in renal tubular function. The increased mass of bone occurs together with widened osteoid seams, as in chronic renal glomerular insufficiency. In the vertebral bodies, the bone appears denser in transverse bands at the upper and lower margins, with a relatively radiolucent center. This "sandwich" appearance is similar to that seen in some patients with osteopetrosis and has been termed by the British the *rugger jersey sign*. Skeletal hyperostosis, including cortical hyperostoses, periostitis, and tendon and ligament ossification, is also a complication of long-term therapy with synthetic retinoids such as isotretinoin.

OSTEOPETROSIS Osteopetrosis (Albers-Schönberg or marble bone disease) is clinically, biochemically, and genetically heterogeneous. Although osteopetrosis has multiple causes, a defect in bone resorption is always the underlying mechanism. Several genetically determined forms of osteopetrosis in rodents may serve as models for the human diseases. Some can be cured by bone marrow transplantation from a normal littermate and probably represent stem cell defects. Two other forms of osteopetrosis, in *op/op* mice and *tl/tl* toothless rats, are not cured by bone marrow transplantation, however. These animals have few osteoclasts, and those which are present express osteoclast enzymes weakly. The *op/op* mice have a defect in the coding region of the gene for colony stimulating factor 1 (CSF-1, also known as M-CSF, the M standing for macrophage), and the skeletal defects in these animals and in *tl/tl* rats can be reversed by treatment with CSF-1. Another form of osteopetrosis has been produced in transgenic mice by "knockout" of the c-*src* gene by homologous recombination; c-*src* and its phosphorylation substrate, P80/85 are expressed at high levels in osteoclasts. Human homologues of these rodent diseases have not yet been demonstrated. The most severe form in human infants is also due to defects in differentiation and/or function of osteoclasts. Infantile osteopetrosis is manifested in utero and progresses after birth with anemia, hepatosplenomegaly, hydrocephalus, cranial nerve involvement, and death, often due to infections. The disorder is usually inherited as an autosomal recessive trait. Several attempts to transplant bone marrow from normal donors to provide normal osteoclast precursor cells have been successful, and osteopetrotic bone has been repopulated with functioning osteoclasts of donor origin that produce radiologic and/or bone biopsy evidence of bone resorption. One infant received a bone marrow transplant from a brother with successful response lasting more than 4 years, although vision was not restored. In other individuals with osteopetrosis, peripheral blood monocyte function is defective. In still other cases of osteopetrosis, clinical improvement has been obtained using high doses of calcitriol.

Less fulminant forms of osteopetrosis occur in older children and adults. In some of the latter, the disorder appears to be sporadic. In others, the osteopetrosis is inherited as an autosomal dominant trait and is progressive with increasing age; anemia is not as severe, neurologic abnormalities are not as frequent, and recurrent pathologic fractures are the main feature. Although most cases are in infants and children, many are discovered first in adult life when roentgenograms are obtained because of fractures or unrelated diseases. There is no predilection for either sex. Even the inherited adult disorder is heterogeneous. Type I is characterized by increased thickness of the cranial vault, whereas rugger jersey sign and "endo bones" in the pelvis are features of type II. A defect in modeling of endosteal bone is present in both types, and there is an additional defect in the remodeling of trabecular bone in type II osteopetrosis.

An "intermediate" form of osteopetrosis has been described in several kindreds in which the skeletal abnormality is associated with renal tubular acidosis and cerebral calcification. This form, which is inherited as an autosomal recessive defect, is compatible with long survival and is associated with a virtual absence of one of the isoenzymes of carbonic anhydrase (carbonic anhydrase II). Carbonic anhydrase II is a major component of the enzyme system required for generation of the unique acid environment adjacent to the ruffled border of the osteoclast, and deficiency of carbonic anhydrase results in disordered bone resorption. Bone resorption is depressed. In some instances, islands of unresorbed calcified cartilage are encased in bone. The defect in remodeling results in disorganization of bone structure with thickened cortices and lack of funnelization of metaphyses. Despite increased density, the bone is abnormal mechanically and fractures readily. Osteomalacia or rickets is sometimes a component of the osteopetrosis in children (Fig. 362-1).

The histologic changes are reflected in the roentgenograms (Fig. 362-2), which reveal uniformly dense, sclerotic bone often without distinction between the cortical and cancellous regions. In the severe infantile form, there is persistence of the primary spongiosa with central calcified cartilage cores surrounded by woven bone. Osteoclasts are often increased in number but apparently do not function properly. Osteoclasts may be morphologically normal or have loss of the ruffled borders, suggesting that a spectrum of changes may occur. The variability may reflect heterogeneity in this syndrome, as in the osteopetrosis in rodents. The long bones are usually involved, with increased density along the entire shaft. Foci of increased density may be seen in the epiphyses corresponding to regions of unresorbed calcified cartilage. The metaphyses have a characteristic clubbed or splayed appearance. Horizontal bandings of increased density alternating with zones of decreased density in the long bones and vertebrae suggest that the defect is intermittent during periods of growth. The skull, pelvis, ribs, and other bones may be involved. The phalanges and the distal humerus may appear normal.

Encroachment of bone on the marrow cavity, particularly in the malignant infantile disorder, is associated with anemia of the myelophthisic type with foci of extramedullary hematopoiesis in liver, spleen, and lymph nodes and enlargement of these organs. Neurologic abnormalities are associated with encroachment on cranial nerves and include optic atrophy, nystagmus, papilledema, exophthalmos, and impairment of extraocular motility. Facial paralysis and deafness are frequent; trigeminal lesions and anosmia are less common. In infants, macrocephaly, hydrocephalus, and convulsions may occur, and

FIGURE 362-2 Roentgenogram of the spine and pelvis of a 55-year-old man with the more benign, dominant form of osteopetrosis.

FIGURE 362-1 Lateral roentgenogram of the thorax of a 9-month-old boy with the "malignant" form of osteopetrosis. Note the uniform increase in mineral density of the vertebral bodies and the marked flaring of the ends of the ribs (arrows), indicative of rickets.

infections such as osteomyelitis are frequent. Renal tubular acidosis is a feature of the osteopetrosis associated with a deficiency in carbonic anhydrase II.

In the milder dominant osteopetrosis, about half the patients have no symptoms, and the disorder is discovered incidentally on roentgenograms. Other patients present because of fractures, bone pain, osteomyelitis, and cranial nerve palsies.

Fractures are a complication even with trivial trauma. Healing of such fractures is usually satisfactory, although delayed union may occur. When the disease is manifested first in adult life, fractures may be the only clinical problem. Levels of calcium and alkaline phosphatase in the plasma are usually normal in adults, although in children hypophosphatemia and moderate hypocalcemia have been noted. Serum acid phosphatase levels are usually increased.

The skeletal defect is not the same in all forms of osteopetrosis, and within a clinical subtype, genetic and biochemical heterogeneity is common. As mentioned, in several children with severe osteopetrosis, bone marrow transplants from HLA-identical siblings have resulted in histologic and radiologic increases in bone resorption and variable improvement in anemia, vision, hearing, and growth and development.

Unfortunately, it is not always possible to find appropriate donors, or patients may not be good candidates for bone marrow transplantation. In patients with the lethal forms, calcitriol therapy is associated with the appearance of osteoclasts with normal ruffled borders and other evidence for increased bone resorption.

PYKNODYSOSTOSIS *Pyknodysostosis* is a form of osteosclerosis that superficially resembles osteopetrosis. It is one of the types of short-limbed dwarfism associated with bone fragility and a tendency to fracture with minimal trauma. Nevertheless, life span is usually normal. In addition to a generalized increase in bone density, features include short stature, separated cranial sutures, hypoplasia of the mandible, kyphoscoliosis and deformities of the trunk, persistence of deciduous teeth, progressive acroosteolysis of the terminal phalanges, high, arched palate, proptosis, blue sclerae, and a pointed, beaked nose. Life span is usually unaffected, and the patient usually presents because of frequent fractures. Pyknodysostosis is inherited as an autosomal recessive trait. In one case, levels of plasma calcitonin were intermittently elevated, and the response of the plasma calcitonin to infusions of calcium and glucagon was exaggerated. The gene that causes this disorder may be located on the short arm of a small acrocentric chromosome.

OSTEOMYELOSCLEROSIS *Osteomyelosclerosis* is a disorder in which the marrow cells are replaced by diffuse fibroplasia, occasionally accompanied by osseous metaplasia. When the latter is prominent, increased skeletal density is seen on roentgenograms. In early stages woven bone may be found in intratrabecular locations, whereas in more advanced stages woven bone is observed in the medulla. The disorder is probably a phase in the course of the myeloproliferative disorders and is characteristically accompanied by extramedullary hematopoiesis.

Hyperostosis corticalis generalisata (van Buchem's disease) is characterized by osteosclerosis of the skull (base and calvaria), lower jaw, clavicles, and ribs and thickening of the diaphyseal cortices of the long and short bones. Alkaline phosphatase levels in the serum are elevated, and the disorder may be due to increased formation of bone of normal structure. The major manifestations are due to neural compression and consist of optic atrophy, facial paralysis, and perception deafness. In *hyperostosis generalisata with pachydermia* (Uehlinger), the sclerosis is due to increased formation of subperiosteal spongy bone and involves the epiphyses, metaphyses, and diaphyses. Pain, swelling of joints, and thickening of the skin of the lower arms are common.

HEREDITARY HYPERPHOSPHATASIA This disorder is characterized by severe structural deformities of the skeleton with increase in thickness of the calvaria, large homogeneous areas of increased density at the base of the skull, and widening and loss of normal architecture of the shafts and the epiphyses of the long and short bones. There is a failure to deposit normal bone, with haphazard

orientation of lamellae suggesting active remodeling that resembles Paget's disease of bone. Osteoclasts with multiple nuclei characteristic of Paget's disease and the typical "mosaic" pattern of faceted units of lamellar bone are not found, however. Levels of plasma alkaline phosphatase and urinary excretion of hydroxyproline peptides and other collagen degradation products are markedly increased. The disorder is apparently inherited as an autosomal recessive trait. Calcitonin therapy may be of value in some of these patients.

PROGRESSIVE DIAPHYSEAL DYSPLASIA A disorder in which a symmetric thickening and increased diameter of the diaphyses of long bones occurs, particularly in femurs, tibias, fibulas, radii, and ulnas, has been termed *progressive diaphyseal dysplasia* (Camurati-Engelmann disease). Pain over affected areas, fatigue, abnormal gait, and muscle wasting are the major manifestations. Serum alkaline phosphatase levels may be elevated, and on occasion, hypocalcemia and hyperphosphatemia may be found. Other abnormalities include anemia, leukopenia, and elevated erythrocyte sedimentation rate. Clinical and biochemical improvement may result from the use of glucocorticoids.

MELORHEOSTOSIS This rare condition usually begins in childhood and is characterized by a slowly progressive linear hyperostosis in one or more bones of one limb, usually in a lower extremity. All segments of the bone may be involved, with sclerotic areas that have a "flowing" distribution. The involved limb is often extremely painful. Soft tissue masses, not connected to bone, are often mineralized and are composed of osseous or cartilaginous tissue. Other types of soft tissue masses are associated with joint contractures or consist of fibrofatty, lymphatic, or vascular tissue.

OSTEOPOIKILOSIS This benign autosomal dominant trait is usually discovered by chance. It is characterized by dense spots of trabecular bone less than a centimeter in diameter, usually of uniform density, that are located in the epiphyses and adjacent parts of the metaphyses. All bones may be involved except the skull, ribs, and vertebrae.

HYPEROSTOSIS FRONTALIS INTERNA *Hyperostosis frontalis interna* is an abnormality of the inner table of the frontal bones of the skull consisting of smooth, rounded enostoses covered by dura and projecting into the cranial cavity. These enostoses are usually less than 1 cm at their greatest diameter and usually do not extend posteriorly beyond the coronal suture. The abnormality is found almost exclusively in women, who are frequently obese, hirsute, and have a variety of neuropsychiatric complaints (Morgagni-Stewart-Morel syndrome). However, hyperostosis frontalis interna also occurs in women with no obvious illness or particular associated disease. The finding in the skull may be a manifestation of a generalized metabolic disorder.

NEOPLASMS OF BONE

Primary neoplasms of the skeletal system reflect in their histology the cellular and extracellular components of the skeleton. However, it is not always possible to prove that a tumor arises from the same type of tissue that it produces. The precursor cells of bone tissue are derived from distinct cell lines in which the osteoclasts arise from hematopoietic stem cells and the osteoblasts arise from stromal stem cells. The primitive stromal stem cells can differentiate into chondroblasts and fibroblasts as well as osteoblasts. Neoplasms can arise from all these cell types. Each of these cells can produce its characteristic extracellular matrix, and neoplasms arising from them may thus be recognized. Primary neoplasms of bone can arise also from other hematopoietic, vascular, and neural elements.

PATHOPHYSIOLOGY Neoplasms in bone induce resorption of skeletal tissue. This bone resorption results from production by the tumor cells of factors that stimulate osteoclast function and/or recruitment and differentiation of the osteoclast hematopoietic precursor cells. One of the factors produced by the tumor cells is the parathyroid hormone-related protein (PTHrP) that interacts with the

PTH receptor (see also Chap. 357). Other factors that induce bone resorption by modulating recruitment, differentiation, and/or activation of osteoclasts include cytokines such as transforming growth factor alpha; interleukins 1, 6, and 11; tumor necrosis factor alpha; lymphotoxin; and tumor necrosis factor beta derived from the tumor, resident bone cells, or infiltrating mononuclear inflammatory cells. What was initially termed "osteoclast activating factor" is now known to include cytokines such as interleukin 1 and lymphotoxin produced by monocytes and lymphocytes. Prostaglandin or other eicosanoid production by some tumors also may mediate bone resorption. T lymphocytes infected with some viruses can metabolize circulating 25(OH)D to 1,25(OH)$_2$D, which also may stimulate bone resorption. Tumors also may alter blood supply to bone by obstructing vessels or inducing angiogenesis. Tumors also may produce reaction in surrounding bone and alter the normal contour. The epiphyseal plate, articular cartilage, cortex, and periosteum of bone often offer a barrier to the spread of neoplastic tissue. Alteration of the contour of the cortex is not due to "expansion" but to remodeling of the bone in the area and formation of new bone with the new contour. Some tumors induce primarily an osteoblastic or sclerotic reaction in surrounding bone, which results in increased radiodensity. Primary neoplasms may be less radiopaque than surrounding bone or more radiopaque depending on the degree of calcification or ossification of the matrix and the density of the tissue. Bone tumors may be recognized because of (1) the presence of a mass in the soft tissues, (2) deformity of a bone, (3) pain and tenderness, or (4) pathologic fractures. Tumors of bone also may be detected incidentally on roentgenograms obtained for other reasons. Although it is usually possible to classify bone tumors as benign or malignant, prediction of the clinical outcome on histologic and radiologic criteria is not always possible.

The extent of the lesions should be defined by standard and computed tomographic techniques and magnetic resonance imaging, if available. Lesions also can be assessed by bone scans utilizing ^{99m}Tc polyphosphonate. There are numerous pitfalls in the clinical diagnosis and interpretation of histologic features of tumors of bone. However, proper evaluation and selection of therapy require evaluation of both radiographic and histologic features. Management, therefore, requires cooperation of the orthopedist, oncologist, radiologist, radiotherapist, and pathologist.

BENIGN TUMORS   The most common benign tumors are *osteochondromas* (exostoses) and *endochondromas* (which may be multiple in Ollier's disease), *giant cell tumors, unicameral bone cysts, osteoid osteomas, and nonossifying fibromas* (fibrous cortical defects). As a rule, benign tumors are not painful except for osteoid osteomas, chondroblastomas, and chondromyxoidfibroma. The usual clinical problem is that of slowly progressing mass, pathologic fracture, or deformity. Treatment is usually accomplished by resection or curettage and bone grafting. When wide resection of tissue is necessary, insertion of metal and plastic prostheses or allograft transplantation may preserve limb function.

MALIGNANT TUMORS   The most common malignant tumor of bone is multiple myeloma (see Chap. 280). Primary lymphoma also may arise locally in bone. Malignant tumors of nonhematopoietic origin include osteosarcomas, chondrosarcomas, fibrosarcomas, and Ewing's tumor. Giant cell tumors may be included here because they may metastasize, especially after incomplete curettage, and are locally destructive. *Osteogenic sarcomas* are presumed to arise from osteoprogenitor cells and have a wide variation in histopathology, with at least 12 histologic types. These tumors always contain woven bone, at least in small foci, and may contain in addition cartilaginous and fibrous elements. They are most common in the second and third decades and are less common under age 10 and over age 40. Genetic factors are important in the genesis of osteosarcomas particularly in children. Between 30 and 40 percent of patients with retinoblastoma have a hereditary predisposition to the tumor as well as to other cancers, particularly osteosarcomas. This predisposition has been mapped to chromosome 13q14, the locus of the retinoblastoma (*Rb*)

gene. The *Rb* gene, which functions normally as a tumor suppressor by forming complexes with several viral-encoded oncoproteins, is inactivated on one allele in these patients as well as in others with sporadic neoplasms, where the gene inactivation is derived from somatic events. Thus homozygosity for the mutant *Rb* allele in the osteoblast precursor could lead to osteosarcoma in the same way that homozygosity at the same allele in a retinoblast could lead to retinoblastoma. Other tumor suppressor genes also may predispose to osteosarcoma. For example, in patients with the multifocal osteosarcoma subtype, mutations have been identified in a highly conserved region of the p53 gene. When osteosarcomas occur in older individuals, e.g., in those with Paget's disease of bone or prior exposure to ionizing radiation, it is probable that mutations in the *Rb*, p53, or other genes are responsible for the abnormal growth and other features of the malignant osteoblasts. In primary osteogenic sarcomas, the lesions usually arise in the metaphyseal region of long bones, especially in the distal femur, proximal tibia, and proximal humerus. The most common symptoms are pain and swelling which may be present for weeks or months. The roentgenographic features of osteosarcomas depend on the degree of bone destruction, the extent to which mineralized bone is formed by and within the tumor, and the type of reaction in the surrounding bone. Thus the lesions may vary from purely lytic lesions to dense areas containing radiopaque lumps, clouds, or spicules of tumor bone in varying patterns of organization. Discontinuities may occur in the cortex surrounding the lesion. In other cases, hyperostotic periosteal reactions may involve grossly layered bone. If the tumor grows rapidly, it may destroy the cortex and penetrate the soft tissue surrounding the bone; it leaves only a cuff of periosteal new bone at the peripheral margin of the tumor, just at the point of penetration (Codman's triangle). High plasma alkaline phosphatase levels in those sarcomas which are predominantly osteogenic parallel the course of the tumor. In general, high levels of serum alkaline phosphatase activity correlate with a poor prognosis. When lesions are adequately treated by amputation or wide resection, chemotherapy, or radiation, the level of alkaline phosphatase falls, and when metastases appear, the level rises again, often reaching values higher than those present initially. When values are initially high, the course is often rapidly fatal. Metastases occur primarily by the hematogenous route, especially to the lung.

The prognosis of osteosarcoma was very poor prior to development of effective chemotherapy, with radiologic evidence of pulmonary metastases usually occurring within a year following surgical excision that was potentially curative. The course varies with the type of tumor; for example, a high-grade histologic variant has a very poor prognosis unless treated with aggressive chemotherapy, whereas the less common low-grade intramedullary type has a better prognosis. In the typical intramedullary type of osteosarcoma, death occurs within 6 months from the onset of detectable pulmonary metastases, suggesting that the lesions in the lungs were present at the time of surgery or that cells were shed from the tumor during the operation.

The management of bone tumors in general has been improved by the introduction of a reliable staging system. The staging is based on the histologic grade of the lesion, flow cytometric analysis of tumor DNA content, and assessment as to whether the lesion is confined to a skeletal compartment or has metastasized. Several chemotherapeutic programs are efficacious. The disease-free and overall survival rates after 4 to 5 years in patients with no demonstrable metastases have increased from about 20 percent with ablative surgery alone to 80 percent or higher with current treatment programs. Since microscopic metastatic foci must be present when the bone tumors are first recognized, aggressive adjuvant chemotherapy is now routine. Chemotherapeutic programs include high-dose methotrexate with leucovorin rescue and various combinations of doxorubicin, cisplatin, bleomycin, cyclophosphamide, and dactinomycin. Amputation or surgical resection of the sarcoma leaving a wide margin of normal tissue is generally carried out. More frequently, a limb-sparing procedure is attempted, particularly in distal femoral osteosarcomas, with allograft bone and cartilage transplants and/or prosthetic devices used to preserve the joint. Resection of isolated pulmonary metastases combined with chemotherapy also may improve survival in younger individuals with primary osteosarcomas. The prognosis of osteosarcoma occurring on the background of Paget's disease in adults is still poor despite chemotherapy.

Chondrosarcomas are distinguishable from osteogenic sarcomas. In contrast to the latter, chondrosarcomas usually arise in adulthood and old age, with the peak incidence in the fourth, fifth, and sixth decades. Most are located in the pelvic girdle, ribs, and diaphyseal portions of the femur and humerus; distal portions of the extremities are involved rarely. Chondrosarcomas probably arise by malignant transformation in enchondromas and more rarely in the cartilaginous cap of osteochondromas. As a rule, chondrosarcomas are slow growing and slow to recur. Radiographically, the lesions appear destructive, with mottled increases in radiodensity which reflect the variable degree of calcification of cartilaginous matrix and ossification. Radical excision is the treatment of choice. Histologic grading of the tumor can be valuable for predicting prognosis and determining appropriate surgical therapy.

Ewing's tumor This is a malignant sarcoma composed of small, round cells that occurs most frequently in the first three decades of life. Most are located in the long bones, although any bone may be involved. No specific tumor marker is available for Ewing's sarcoma, and light and electron microscopy are most useful tools in diagnosis. A characteristic cytogenetic feature in Ewing's sarcoma is a reciprocal translocation of the long arms of chromosomes 11 and 22. Although Ewing's sarcoma is highly malignant, it responds to chemotherapy and radiation with overall survival rates approaching 60 to 70 percent. Limb-sparing surgery with resection of the involved bone is coupled with chemotherapy, and radiation is used for metastatic disease or if the surgical margins contain tumor cells. Chemotherapy with doxorubicin, cyclophosphamide, vincristine, and dactinomycin improves survival of patients with Ewing's sarcoma, including some with metastatic disease.

TUMORS METASTATIC TO BONE The skeleton is a common site for metastases from carcinomas and occasionally even from sarcomas. Skeletal metastases may be silent or produce symptoms by the same mechanisms as primary tumors, i.e., pain, swelling, deformity, encroachment on hematopoietic tissue in the marrow, compression of spinal cord or nerve roots, and pathologic fractures. In addition, rapidly lytic skeletal metastases can result in hypercalcemia. The bones involved most commonly are the vertebrae, proximal femur, pelvis, ribs, sternum, and proximal humerus, in that order of frequency. The carcinomas that most frequently metastasize to bone arise in prostate, breast, lung, thyroid, kidney, and bladder. Malignant cells reach the skeleton via the bloodstream. Those which survive may proliferate and distort the normal architecture, probably by production of substances that cause dissolution of both mineral phase and organic matrix.

Osteolysis most often results from modulation of osteoprogenitor cells to osteoclasts in the surrounding bone. Some mediators involved in induction of osteoclasts were described earlier in this section. Some carcinoma cells also may act directly to resorb bone. Carcinomatous metastases (which are usually predominantly osteolytic) arise from thyroid, kidney, and lower bowel. Other tumors induce an *osteoblastic* response in which the new bone does not arise from the tumor itself but is induced from normal skeletal cells by some product(s) of the tumor cells. The resulting lesion may be more dense than the surrounding tissue. Occasionally, the increase in radiodensity is uniform, simulating osteosclerosis. Carcinoma of the prostate characteristically produces osteoblastic metastases. Carcinoma of the breast can cause both osteolytic and osteoblastic metastases. Malignant carcinoid tumors arising from the embryonic foregut and hindgut metastasize to bone with high frequency, producing an osteoblastic reaction. Hodgkin's disease in bone also produces an osteoblastic response both focal and diffuse. More malignant lymphomas in bone produce predominantly destructive lesions. As a rule, osteolytic metastases are the ones associated with hypercalcemia, hypercalciuria,

and increased excretion of hydroxyproline-containing peptides (reflecting matrix destruction); they are usually associated with normal or only slightly increased levels of serum alkaline phosphatase. Osteoblastic metastases, on the other hand, may cause more marked elevations of serum alkaline phosphatase and may be associated with hypocalcemia. With some metastases (as in carcinoma of the breast), there may be phases in which osteolysis predominates (with hypercalciuria, hypercalcemia, and normal alkaline phosphatase levels) alternating with phases in which alkaline phosphatase levels rise and the skeletal lesions become more sclerotic.

Treatment of skeletal metastases is usually palliative. In slowly growing localized lesions (as in some instances of carcinoma of the thyroid or occasionally in carcinoma of the kidney), local radiation is useful to relieve pain or reduce compression of surrounding structures. Many patients with carcinomas of breast or prostate survive for years even after extensive skeletal metastases are recognized. Castration and estrogen therapy or receptor antagonists may slow the progress of the lesions in patients with metastatic prostatic carcinoma (see Chap. 323). When patients with mammary cancer are treated with estrogens or androgens, the character of the reaction to the metastases may temporarily shift from a predominantly osteoblastic to a lytic phase with resultant hypercalcemia (see Chap. 319).

Intravenous administration of bisphosphonates such as pamidronate diminishes bone pain and reduces the incidence of fracture and indices of excessive bone resorption in patients with osteolytic metastases, e.g., from breast cancer. Pamidronate also alleviates bone pain in patients with metastatic prostate carcinoma. The bone pain in patients with metastatic carcinoma also may be relieved by the use of levodopa. Hypercalcemia in patients with malignant tumors is not due solely to skeletal metastases, although this is the most common cause. Production of circulating stimulators of osteoclast differentiation, such as PTHrP, is another cause of the humoral hypercalcemia of malignancy. Hypercalcemia per se, whether spontaneous or induced by therapy, may produce anorexia, polyuria, polydipsia, depression, and eventually coma. In addition, nephrocalcinosis can result from hypercalcemia, and death may result from renal insufficiency. Intravenous pamidronate is effective in treatment of the hypercalcemia of malignancy due either to humoral factors such as PTHrP or to local factors produced by metastases in bone.

OTHER DISORDERS OF BONE AND CARTILAGE

FIBROUS DYSPLASIA (McCUNE-ALBRIGHT SYNDROME) This syndrome is characterized by osteitis fibrosa disseminata, areas of pigmentation, and endocrine dysfunction, with precocious puberty in females. The bony lesions, called *fibrous dysplasia*, may occur in the absence of the other features. The fundamental nature of the disorder is unknown; the disease does not appear to be heritable, although it has been reported to affect monozygotic twins. The disease occurs with equal frequency in both sexes.

Incidence The disease may be divided into three main categories: (1) monostotic, (2) polyostotic, and (3) McCune-Albright syndrome and its variants. The monostotic form is the most common. The lesions can be asymptomatic, associated with local pain, or predispose to pathologic fracture. The majority of the lesions are in the ribs or in the craniofacial bones, especially the maxillas. Many other bones may be affected, however, such as metaphyseal or diaphyseal portions of the proximal femurs or tibias. Monostotic fibrous dysplasia is most often diagnosed between 20 and 30 years of age. There are usually no associated skin lesions. Approximately a quarter of the individuals with the polyostotic form have more than half the skeleton involved by disease. One side of the body may be affected, and the lesions may be distributed segmentally in a limb, particularly in the lower extremities. Craniofacial lesions are present in approximately half of patients with the polyostotic form. Whereas the monostotic form is usually detected in young adults, fractures and skeletal deformities occur in childhood in the polyostotic form; the disease is generally more severe and deforming with early clinical onset. Lesions, especially monostotic lesions, may become quiescent around the time of puberty and may worsen during pregnancy. McCune-Albright syndrome (polyostotic fibrous dysplasia, multiple café au lait spots, and sexual precosity) is more common (10:1) in females. Short stature is ascribed to premature closure of the epiphyses. The most frequent extraskeletal manifestations are the skin lesions.

Pathology   All forms of fibrous dysplasia have a similar histologic appearance, although cartilage is more commonly involved in the polyostotic form. The marrow cavity is filled by gritty, gray-pink, rubbery tissue that replaces the normal cancellous bone. Often, the endosteal cortical surface is scalloped. Histologically, the lesions contain benign-appearing fibroblastic tissue arranged in a loose whorled pattern (Fig. 362-3). The grittiness is due to irregularly arranged woven bone spicules, most of which lack osteoblastic palisading or rimming, which are embedded in the fibrous tissue. These bone spicules also may have prominent cement lines. In approximately 10 percent of cases, islands of hyaline cartilage are present, and more rarely, myxoid tissue may predominate in young patients. Examination by polarized light and with the use of special stains indicates a contiguity of collagen fibers of the osseous and marrow tissue. In the polyostotic form, cystic degeneration may be characterized by the presence of hemorrhage with hemosiderin-containing macrophages and osteoclast-type giant cells in the periphery of the cyst. Malignant transformation of either monostotic or polyostotic fibrous dysplasia occurs but with a frequency of less than 1 percent. The malignant change is usually detected in the third or fourth decades in individuals who have had lesions first identified in childhood. In about a third of the cases the neoplasms arise in previously radiated lesions. Ossifying fibroma of long bones is a peculiar fibroosseous cortical lesion which may be a variant of fibrous dysplasia. It is most common in the tibial shaft of teenagers. Although benign, the lesion has a tendency to recur if not adequately excised.

Radiologic changes   The roentgenographic appearance of the lesions is that of a radiolucent area with a well-delineated, smooth or scalloped border, typically associated with focal thinning of the cortex of the bone (Fig. 362-4). Fibrous dysplasia and Paget's disease of bone are two disorders that can cause a bone to become larger than normal. The lesions of fibrous dysplasia are not usually cysts in the strict sense, since they are not fluid-filled cavities. They occasionally appear multiloculate. The so-called ground glass appearance reflects the content of the thin spicules of calcified, woven bone. Frequently, deformities are present such as coxa vara, shepherd's-crook deformity of the femur, bowing of the tibia, Harrison's grooves, and protrusio acetabuli. Involvement of facial bones, usually with lesions of increased radiodensity, may create a leonine appearance (leontiasis ossea). Fibrous dysplasia of the temporal bones can cause progressive

FIGURE 362-4 Roentgenogram of the upper extremity from a 33-year-old woman with fibrous dysplasia of bone. Typical lesions involve the entire humerus as well as the scapula and proximal ulna.

loss of hearing and obliteration of the external ear canal. Advanced skeletal age in females is correlated with sexual precocity but also may be seen in males without sexual precocity. The lesions tend to spare the epiphyseal regions before puberty, but in older individuals fibrous dysplasia may develop in the epiphyses. Occasionally, a focus of fibrous dysplasia may undergo cystic degeneration with an enormous distortion of the shape of the bone and mimic the so-called aneurysmal bone cyst.

Clinical picture   The clinical course is variable. Skeletal lesions are usually detected because of localized pain, deformities, or fractures. Other symptoms ascribable to bone involvement are headache, seizures, cranial nerve abnormalities, hearing loss, narrowing of the external ear canal, or even spontaneous scalp hemorrhages if there is craniofacial bone disease. In some females and even less commonly in males, sexual precocity is the presenting complaint, occasionally before the appearance of skeletal symptoms. Serum calcium and phosphorus values are usually normal. In approximately one-third of patients, levels of serum alkaline phosphatase may be elevated to high values, and urinary hydroxyproline excretion is often increased. In some subjects, high cardiac output similar to that in extensive Paget's disease may be found. In general, patients with extensive involvement have widespread disease when symptoms first appear, whereas when disease is mild at the onset, extensive disease does not usually develop.

The cutaneous pigmentation in most patients with McCune-Albright syndrome consists of isolated dark-brown to light-brown macules which tend to remain on one side of the midline (Fig. 362-5). The border is usually, although not always, irregular or jagged ("coast of Maine") in contrast to the smooth borders of the pigmented macules of neurofibromatosis ("coast of California"). As a rule, there are fewer than six of the lesions, which range in size from 1 cm to those covering very large areas, particularly the back, buttocks, or

FIGURE 362-3 Photomicrograph of the lesion of fibrous dysplasia. Note spicules of dark-staining woven bone (WB) surrounded by loose fibroblastic tissue.

FIGURE 362-5 Typical pigmented café au lait lesion of the skin in an 11-year-old boy with polyostotic fibrous dysplasia. The border has the jagged "coast of Maine" appearance that is characteristic of McCune-Albright's syndrome. Note that the lesion is limited to one side (left) of the body.

sacral regions. When the lesions are present in the scalp, the overlying hair may be more deeply pigmented than that over the remainder of the scalp. Localized alopecia is associated with osteomas of the skin, and such lesions tend to have concordance with the skeletal lesions. The pigmentation tends to be on the same side as the skeletal lesions and actually overlie them. Occasionally, neurofibromatosis and fibrous dysplasia coexist.

The sexual precocity occurs more commonly in females than in males (see also Chaps. 339 and 340). Premature vaginal bleeding and development of axillary and pubic hair and of breasts are the main features. In the few ovaries that have been examined, no corpora lutea have been seen. In the few cases where measurements have been reported, the girls have high estrogen levels and low or undetectable gonadotropins. Estrogen receptors have been measured in the bone lesions. It is therefore not surprising that precocious sexuality is not limited to patients with cranial involvement. The characteristic pigmented macules are usual but not invariable. Another endocrine abnormality that occurs with increased frequency is hyperthyroidism. Rarer associations include Cushing's syndrome, acromegaly, possibly hypogonadotropic hypogonadism, and soft tissue myxomas. Hypophosphatemic osteomalacia also may accompany fibrous dysplasia and resembles the disorder associated with other skeletal and nonskeletal tumors. Sexual precocity and adrenal and thyroid hyperfunction in association with fibrous dysplasia are due to autonomous end-organ activity, not to pituitary or hypothalamic dysfunction. Thus luteinizing hormone (LH) or follicle-stimulating hormone (FSH) levels are low and do not show the expected early pubertal nocturnal rise and are not responsive to luteinizing hormone–releasing hormone (LHRH). Furthermore, treatment with LHRH analogues does not suppress gonadal steroid secretion or reverse sexual precocity. The multiple endocrine hyperfunction and possibly the fibrous dysplasia lesions in the disorder may be due to defects in the G protein–cyclic AMP–protein kinase A–dependent pathway. Activating mutations have been identified in the G protein that stimulates adenylyl cyclase ($G_{s\alpha}$) by nucleotide sequence analysis of $G_{s\alpha}$ cDNA in tissues from affected patients. The mutations presumably result in constitutive activation of signal transduction pathways and induce end-organ hyperfunction. Since germ line mutations might be lethal, somatic mutations may occur early in embryogenesis in patients with McCune-Albright syndrome so that affected individuals are mosaics. It is of interest that the error in Albright's hereditary osteodystrophy (pseudohypoparathyroidism) is the converse of that found in the

McCune-Albright syndrome (fibrous dysplasia). In the former, mutations in $G_{s\alpha}$ proteins result in *deficient* activity and decreased responsiveness to hormones that function through cAMP-mediated signal transduction pathways.

Although the lytic lesions of fibrous dysplasia resemble the brown tumors of hyperparathyroidism, the age of the patient, normal calcium levels, increased density of bone in the skull, and areas of cutaneous pigmentation identify the former condition. Fibrous dysplasia and hyperparathyroidism may coexist, however. Neurofibromas may involve bone and produce cutaneous pigmentation as well as nodules in the skin. The pigmented macules of neurofibromatosis are more numerous and more widely distributed than in fibrous dysplasia, usually have smooth borders, and tend to involve areas such as the axillary folds. Other lesions that have roentgenographic features similar to those of isolated fibrous dysplasia are unicameral bone cysts, aneurysmal bone cysts, and nonossifying fibromas. Leontiasis ossea is most often due to fibrous dysplasia, although other disorders also may produce this appearance, such as craniometaphyseal dysplasia, hyperphosphatasia, and, in adults, Paget's disease.

Treatment Fibrous dysplasia is not curable. The symptoms, however, can be managed using a variety of orthopedic procedures such as casting, osteotomy with internal fixation, curettage, and bone grafting depending on the lesion and the age of the patient. Indications for such procedures include progressive deformity, nonunion of fractures, and pain unresponsive to conservative treatment. Calcitonin may be effective in treatment of widespread disease associated with bone pain and high serum alkaline phosphatase levels (see Chap. 361).

DYSPLASIAS AND CHONDRODYSTROPHIES A variety of diseases of bone and cartilage have been called *dystrophies* or *dysplasias*. The *osteochondrodysplasias* are heritable disorders of connective tissue that are characterized by primary abnormalities of cartilage that lead to disturbances in cartilage and bone growth and development. They comprise more than 100 distinct entities, which can be distinguished based on clinical, genetic, and radiologic features. The biochemical (and genetic) defects have been identified in few of these conditions. Genetic errors have been demonstrated at various steps in the metabolism of glycosaminoglycans (mucopolysaccharides) to account for the abnormal phenotypes in the Hunter and Hurler syndromes (also see Chap. 349), and mutations in collagen genes have been identified in several forms of the skeletal dysplasias. For example, mutations in the type II collagen gene have been found in Stricker syndrome, Kniest dysplasia, other chondrodysplasias associated with osteoarthritis, and in a related syndrome, spondyloepiphyseal dysplasia, and deletion in one type X collagen allele has been found in a form of metaphyseal chondrodysplasia. Mutations in several genes, e.g., types II, IX, and X collagen genes, in transgenic mice result in phenotypes that resemble several of the human disorders (also see Chap. 351). Eventually, it should be possible to classify many of these disorders based on the genetic and biochemical defects. At present, however, a useful scheme is that proposed by Rubin based on the consideration of errors in modeling of bone and cartilage (Table 362-2). Other clinical and genetic features form the basis of a classification by Rimoin. Pathologic processes in the skeletal dysplasias may be expressed as a deficiency (hypoplasia) or excess (hyperplasia) in relation to normal development.

Spondyloepiphyseal dysplasia The *spondyloepiphyseal dysplasias* are disorders in which abnormalities of growth occur in various bones, including the vertebrae, pelvis, carpal and tarsal bones, and the epiphyses of tabular bones. On the basis of roentgenographic findings, this group can be divided into (1) those with generalized platyspondyly, (2) those with multiple epiphyseal dysplasias, and (3) those with epiphysometaphyseal dysplasias. *Morquio's syndrome*, in which there is a defect in degradation of glycosaminoglycans (therefore a "mucopolysaccharidosis"), is inherited as an autosomal recessive trait and is associated with corneal opacities, dental defects, variable disturbances in intellect, and increased urinary excretion of keratosulfate, and it belongs in the first group. Other forms of spondyloepiphy-

TABLE 362-2 Working classification of bone dysplasias

Epiphyseal dysplasias
A Epiphyseal hypoplasias
  1 Failure of articular cartilage: spondyloepiphyseal dysplasia, congenita and tarda
  2 Failure of ossification of center: multiple epiphyseal dysplasia, congenita and tarda
B Epiphyseal hyperplasia
  1 Excess of articular cartilage: dysplasia epiphysialis hemimelica

Physeal (growth plate) dysplasias
A Cartilage hypoplasias
  1 Failure of proliferating cartilage: achondroplasia, congenita and tarda
  2 Failure of hypertrophic cartilage: metaphyseal dysostosis, congenita and tarda
B Cartilage hyperplasias
  1 Excess of proliferating cartilage: hyperchondroplasia
  2 Excess of hypertrophic cartilage: enchondromatosis

Metaphyseal dysplasias
A Metaphyseal hypoplasias
  1 Failure to form primary spongiosa: hypophosphatasia, congenita and tarda
  2 Failure to absorb primary spongiosa: osteopetrosis, congenita and tarda
  3 Failure to absorb secondary spongiosa: craniometaphyseal dysplasia, congenita and tarda
B Metaphyseal hyperplasia
  1 Excessive spongiosa: familial exostosis

Diaphyseal dysplasias
A Diaphyseal hypoplasias
  1 Failure of periosteal bone formation: osteogenesis imperfecta, congenita and tarda
  2 Failure of endosteal bone formation: idiopathic osteoporosis
B Diaphyseal hyperplasias
  1 Excessive periosteal bone formation: Engelmann's disease
  2 Excessive periosteal bone formation: hyperphosphatasia

seal dysplasia, some of which are accounted for by defects in type II collagen, may not be recognized until late in childhood or young adult life. Flat vertebral bodies are associated with other abnormalities in shape and alignment. The disordered development of the capital femoral epiphyses leads to irregularities in shape and flattening of the femoral heads and early onset of osteoarthritis of the hips.

Achondroplasia *Achondroplasia* is a physeal dysplasia in which dwarfism results from decrease in the proliferation of cartilage in the growth plate. This disorder is among the more common types of dwarfism and is inherited as an autosomal dominant trait. Histologic sections through the growth plate show a thin zone of cartilage cells with absence or abbreviation of the normal columnar arrangement and zone of provisional calcification, although endochondral ossification may not be completely disorganized. Formation of the primary spongiosa is reduced, since there is often a transverse bar of bone sealing off the plate from further endochondral ossification. Formation and maturation of the secondary ossification centers and articular cartilage are not disturbed, however. Appositional growth at the metaphysis continues, with resulting flare in this region of the bone; intramembranous bone formation at the periosteum is normal. The abnormal proliferation at the growth plate, leaving other areas relatively unaffected in the tubular bones, causes production of short bones that are proportionately thick. The length of the spine is almost always normal. The appearance of short limbs with a normal trunk is characteristically accompanied by a large head, saddlenose, and an exaggerated lumbar lordosis. The disease is usually recognized at birth. Those who survive the period of infancy usually have normal mental and sexual development, and life span may be normal. Spinal deformity nevertheless may lead to a cord compression and nerve root encroachment, especially in those with kyphoscoliosis. Homozygous achondroplasia is a more serious disorder and a cause of neonatal death. In view of the observations in spondyloepiphyseal dysplasia, several of the achondroplasias also may eventually be explained on the basis of defects in genes encoding extracellular matrix components of cartilage such as proteoglycan core protein, types II, IX, or X collagens, or link protein.

Enchondromatosis (dyschondroplasia, Ollier's disease) This is also a disorder affecting the growth plate in which the hypertrophic cartilage is not resorbed and ossified in a normal fashion. It results in masses of cartilage with disorderly arrangement of the chondrocytes showing variable proliferative and hypertrophic changes. These masses are located in the metaphyses in close association with the growth plate in very young patients but often are diaphyseal in teenagers and young adults. The disorder is usually recognized in childhood by the appearance of deformities or retardation in growth. The most common sites of involvement are the ends of long bones, usually in the region where rate of growth is most marked. The pelvis is often involved, but ribs, sternum, and skull are seldom affected. There is also a tendency toward unilateral involvement. Chondrosarcoma develops occasionally in the enchondromata. The association of enchondromatosis and cavernous hemangiomata in the soft tissues including the skin is known as *Maffucci's syndrome*.

Multiple exostoses (diaphyseal aclasis or osteochondromatosis) This is a disorder of the metaphysis, inherited as an autosomal dominant character, in which areas of the growth plate become displaced, presumably by growing through a defect in the perichondrium or so-called ring of Ranvier. The spongiosa forms within the mass as vessels invade the cartilage. Therefore, the diagnostic radiographic finding is the direct continuity of the mass to the marrow cavity of the parent bone with absence of underlying cortex. Usually the growth of these exostoses ceases when growth of the adjacent plate ceases. The lesions may be solitary or multiple and are usually located in the metaphyseal areas of long bones with the apex of the exostosis directed toward the diaphysis. Often the lesions produce no symptoms, but occasionally, interference with the function of a joint or tendon or compression of nerves may result. Dwarfism may occur. The metacarpals may be shortened, resembling those seen in Albright's hereditary osteodystrophy. Multiple exostoses are sometimes seen in patients with pseudohypoparathyroidism.

An exostosis may suddenly begin to enlarge long after growth should have ceased, and rarely, chondrosarcomas may develop from the cartilage cap of an exostosis. Although pregnancy may stimulate growth of an exostosis that clinically may mimic malignancy, the lesion merely undergoes exuberant endochondral ossification and cartilage hyperplasia without malignant changes.

RELAPSING POLYCHONDRITIS See Chap. 299.

TIETZE'S SYNDROME (COSTOCHONDRAL SYNDROME) See Chap. 299.

REFERENCES

Hyperostosis

BENLI IT et al: Epidemiological, clinical and radiological aspects of osteopoikilosis. J Bone Joint Surg 74B:504, 1992

BOLLERSLEY J et al: Structural and histomorphometric studies of iliac crest trabecular and cortical bone in autosomal dominant osteopetrosis: A study of two radiological types. Bone 10:19, 1989

BOSTMAN OM et al: Osteosarcoma arising in a melorheostoric femur. J Bone Joint Surg 69A:1232, 1987

BYERS PH et al: Research perspectives in heritable disorders of connective tissue. Matrix 12:333, 1992

CAUDLE RJ et al: Melorheostosis of the hand: A case report with long-term follow-up. J Bone Joint Surg 69A:1229, 1987

CHAN Y-L et al: Dialysis osteodystrophy: A study involving 94 patients. Medicine 64:296, 1985

COCCIA PF et al: Successful bone-marrow transplantation for infantile malignant osteopetrosis. N Engl J Med 302:701, 1980

―――― et al: Cells that resorb bone. N Engl J Med 310:456, 1984

COINDRE JM et al: Histomorphometric analysis of sclerotic bone from idiopathic myeloid metaplasia (nine cases). J Pathol 144:163, 1984

CRISP AJ, BRENTON DP: Engelmann's disease of bone - a systemic disorder? Ann Rheum Dis 41:183,1982

DIGIOVANNA JJ et al: Extraspinal tendon and ligament calcification associated with long-term therapy with etretinate. N Engl J Med 315:1177, 1986

EDELSON JG et al: Pycnodysostosis: Orthopedic aspects with a description of 14 new cases. Clin Orthop 280:263, 1992

EINHORN TA et al: Hyperphosphatasemia in an adult: Clinical, roentgenographic, and histomorphometric findings and comparison to classical Paget's disease. Clin Orthop 204:253, 1986

GEBHARDT MC, MANKIN HJ: The diagnosis and management of bone tumors, in *Metabolic Bone Disease*, LV Avioli, SM Krane (eds). Philadelphia, Saunders, 1990, pp 753–792

GENANT HK et al: Osteosclerosis in primary hyperparathyroidism. Am J Med 59:104, 1975

GOLDMAN AB et al: Case report 778. Skeletal Radiol 22:206, 1993

IAVARONE A et al: Germ-line and somatic p53 gene mutations in multifocal osteogenic sarcoma. Proc Natl Acad Sci USA 89:4207, 1992

JACCOBSON HG: Dense bone—too much bone: Radiological considerations and differential diagnosis, part II. Skeletal Radiol 13:97, 1985

JOHNSON CC et al: Osteopetrosis: A clinical, genetic, metabolic and morphologic study of the dominantly inherited benign form. Medicine 47:149, 1968

KAPLAN FS et al: Successful treatment of infantile malignant osteopetrosis by bone-marrow transplantation. J Bone Joint Surg 70A:617, 1988

KEY L et al: Treatment of congenital osteopetrosis with high-dose calcitriol. N Engl J Med 310:409, 1984

KRAEMER KH et al: Prevention of skin cancer in xeroderma pigmentosum with the use of oral isotretinoin. N Eng J Med 318:1633, 1988

KUIVANIEMI H et al: Mutations in collagen genes; causes of rare and some common diseases in humans. FASEB J 5:2052, 1991

MARKS SC et al: Administration of colony stimulating factor-1 corrects some macrophage, dental, and skeletal defects in an osteopetrotic mutation (toothless, *tl*) in the rat. Bone 13:89, 1992

MAJZOUB JA, SCULLY RE: A six-year-old boy with multiple bone lesions, repeated fractures, and sexual precocity. N Engl J Med 328:496, 1993

SCHOTLAND HM et al: Neurofibromatosis 1 and osseous fibrous dysplasia in a family. Am J Med Gen 43:815, 1992

SHAPIRO F et al: Variable osteoclast appearance in human infantile osteopetrosis. Calcif Tissue Int 43:67, 1988

SHELDON J et al: Englemann's disease (progressive diaphyseal dysplasia): A review and presentation of two cases with abnormal phosphate retention. Metab Bone Dis Rel Res 2:307, 1981

SINGER FR: Osteopetrosis. Semin Nephrol 12:191, 1992

SLAVKIN H, PRICE P (eds): Chemistry and Biology of Mineralized Tissues. Amsterdam, Excerpta Medica, 1992, pp 1–550

SLY WS et al: Carbonic anhydrase II deficiency in 12 families with the autosomal recessive syndrome of osteopetrosis with renal tubular acidosis and cerebral calcification. N Engl J Med 313:139, 1985

THOMPSON RC Jr et al: Hereditary hyperphosphatasia. Am J Med 47:209, 1969

TRICHE T, CAVAZZANA A: Round cell tumors of bone, in *Bone Tumors*, KK Unni (ed). New York, Churchhill Livingstone, 1988, pp 199–223

ULLRICH SJ et al: the p53 tumor suppressor protein, a modulator of cell proliferation. J Biol Chem 267:15259, 1992

VAN BUCHEM FSP et al: Hyperostosis corticalis generalisata. Am J Med 33:387, 1962

WEINBERG RA: Tumor suppressor genes. Science 254:1138, 1991

WEINSTEIN LS et al: Activating mutations of the stimulatory G protein in the McCune-Albright syndrome. N Engl J Med 325:1688, 1991

WHYTE MP, MURPHY WA: Osteopetrosis and other sclerosing bone disorders, in *Metabolic Bone Disease*, LV Avioli, SM Krane (eds). Philadelphia, Saunders, 1990, pp 616–658

WULFSBERG EA et al: Chondrodysplasia punctata: A boy with X-linked recessive chondrodysplasia punctata due to an inherited X-Y translocation with a current classification of these disorders. Am J Med Genet 43:823, 1992

Neoplasms of bone

BACCI G et al: Therapy for primary non-Hodgkin's lymphoma of bone and comparison of results with Ewing's sarcoma: Ten years' experience at the Istituto Ortopedico Rizzoli. Cancer 57:1468, 1986

——— et al: Neoadjuvant chemotherapy for osteosarcoma of the extremity. Clin Orthop 224:268, 1987

ETTINGER LJ et al: Adjuvant adriamycin and cisplatin in newly diagnosed, nonmetastatic osteosarcoma of the extremity. J Clin Oncol 4:353, 1986

GEBHARDT MC, MANKIN HJ: The diagnosis and management of bone tumors, in *Metabolic Bone Disease*, LV Avioli, SM Krane (eds). Philadelphia, W.B. Saunders Co., pp 753–792, 1990

GOORIN AM et al: Osteosarcoma: Fifteen years later. N Engl J Med 313:165, 1985

HAN M-T et al: Aggressive thoractomy for pulmonary metastatic osteogenic sarcoma in children and young adolescents. J Pediatr Surg 16:928, 1981

HAYES FA et al: Metastatic Ewing's sarcoma: Remission induction and survival. J Clin Oncol 5:1199, 1987

VAN HOLTEN-VERZANTVOORT AT et al: Reduced morbidity from skeletal metastases in breast cancer patients during long-term bisphosphonate (APD) treatment. Lancet 2:983, 1987

HUVOS AG: Osteogenic sarcoma of bones and soft tissues in older persons. A clinicopathologic analysis of 117 patients older than 60 years. Cancer 57:1442, 1986

——— et al: Osteogenic sarcoma associated with Paget's disease of bone. A clinicopathologic study of 65 patients. Cancer 52:1489, 1983

IAVARONE A et al: Germ-line and somatic p53 gene mutations in multifocal osteogenic sarcoma. Proc Natl Acad Sci USA 89:4207, 1992

KLEEREKOPER M, KRANE SM (EDS): *Clinical Disorders of Bone and Mineral Metabolism.* New York, Mary Ann Liebert, pp 1–-649, 1989

MANKIN HJ et al: The use of frozen cadaveric allografts in the management of patients with bone tumors of the extremities. Orthop Clin North Am 18:275, 1987

MISER JS et al: Preliminary results of treatment of Ewing's sarcoma of bone in children and young adults: Six months of intensive combined modality therapy without maintenance. J Clin Oncol 6:484, 1988

SCHILLER AL: Diagnosis of borderline cartilage lesions of bone. Semin Diag Pathol 2:42, 1985

SIMON MA, NACHMAN J: The clinical utility of preoperative therapy for sarcomas. J Bone Joint Surg 68A:1458, 1986

——— et al: Limb-salvage treatment versus amputation for osteosarcoma of the distal end of the femur. J Bone Joint Surg 68A:1331, 1986

SUIT HD et al: Treatment of the patient with stage M_0 soft tissue sarcoma. J Clin Oncol 6:854, 1988

SUTOW WW et al: Survival after metastasis in osteosarcoma. Natl Cancer Inst Monogr 56:227, 1981

UNNI KK et al: Conditions that stimulate primary neoplasms of bone. Pathol Ann 15(Part 1):91, 1980

WINKLER K et al: Neoadjuvant chemotherapy of osteosarcoma: Results of a randomized cooperative trial (COSS-82) with salvage chemotherapy based on histological tumor response. J Clin Oncol 6:329, 1988

YUNIS EJ, BARNES L: The histologic diversity of osteosarcoma. Pathol Ann 21(Part 1):121, 1986

Other disorders of bone and cartilage

AKESON WH et al: *Symposium on Heritable Disorders of Connective Tissue.* St. Louis, Mosby, 1982

ALBRIGHT FA et al: Syndrome characterized by osteitis fibrosa disseminata, areas of pigmentation and endocrine dysfunction, with precocious puberty in females. Report of five cases. N Engl J Med 216:727, 1937

BENEDICT PH et al: Melanotic macules in Albright's syndrome and in neurofibromatosis. JAMA 205:618, 1968

GRABIAS SL, CAMPBELL CJ: Fibrous dysplasia. Orthop Clin North Am 8:771, 1977

HARRIS RI: Polyostotic fibrous dysplasia with acromegaly. Am J Med 78:539, 1985

HARRIS WH et al: The natural history of fibrous dysplasia: An orthopaedic, pathological and roentgenographic study. J Bone Joint Surg (BR) 44A:207, 1962

KAPLAN FS et al: Estrogen receptors in bone in a patient with polyostotic fibrous dysplasia (McCune-Albright syndrome). N Engl J Med 319:421, 1988

LEE B et al: Identification of the molecular defect in a family with spondyloepiphyseal dysplasia. Science 244:978, 1989

NAGER GT et al: Fibrous dysplasia: A review of the disease and its manifestations in the temporal bone. Ann Otol Rhinol Laryngol 91(suppl 92):1, 1982

PALOTIE A et al: Predisposition to familial osteoarthrosis linked to type II collagen gene. Lancet 1:924, 1989

RIMOIN DL: The chondrodystrophies. Adv Hum Genet 5:1, 1975

RUBIN P: Dynamic Classification of Bone Dysplasias. Chicago, Year Book, 1964

SAMBROOK PN et al: Synovial complications of spondylepiphyseal dysplasia of late onset. Arthritis Rheum 31:282, 1988

SILLENCE DO et al: Neonatal dwarfism. Pediatr Clin North Am 25:431, 1978

STEPHENSON RB et al: Fibrous dysplasia. An analysis of options for treatment. J Bone Joint Surg 69A:409, 1987

TRICHE T, CAVAZZANA A: Round cell tumors of bone, in *Bone Tumors*, KK Unni (ed). New York, Churchhill Livingstone, 1988, pp 199–223

WEINBERG RA: Tumor suppressor genes. Science 254:1138, 1991

YABUL SM et al: Malignant transformation of fibrous dysplasia. A case report and review of the literature. Clin Orthop 281, 1988

PART FOURTEEN NEUROLOGIC DISORDERS

363 APPROACH TO THE PATIENT WITH NEUROLOGIC DISEASE

JOSEPH B. MARTIN*

Symptoms and signs of disordered nervous system function are among the most frequent in clinical medicine. Because neurologic disorders may affect cognitive function with disturbances in language, perception, and memory, as well as produce specific symptoms referable to subcortical structures, spinal cord, peripheral nerve, or muscle, the symptoms and signs presented to the physician are numerous and diverse. A careful assessment of the character and pattern of the symptoms, their temporal profile, and associated complaints, together with a focused neurologic examination, permit a conclusion to be reached among various alternatives.

These considerations are made more complicated by the difficulties that often arise in distinguishing so-called neurologic from psychiatric diseases. In general, the neurologist has defined disease of the nervous system as any condition that produces a visible anatomic or definable biochemical lesion. However, it is now recognized that many primary neurologic disorders, some of which present with severe clinical manifestations, fail to show any demonstrable neuropathologic or neurochemical abnormality, even when scrutinized by the most modern techniques of neurobiology. Torsion dystonia, tardive dyskinesia, and Gilles de la Tourette's syndrome, for example, are considered to be neurologic disorders, some with a clear-cut genetic basis, yet no defined structural abnormality has been reported. The possibility that such disorders are caused by abnormalities of neurotransmitter release or of receptor function is currently viewed as likely because they occur after drug treatment or show partial response to various neuropharmacologic agents. In other disorders traditionally treated by the psychiatrist, in particular the major psychoses of schizophrenia and of manic-depressive disease, accumulated evidence based on genetic analysis, responses to neuroactive agents, and documented neuroendocrine-biochemical abnormalities suggest that these, too, are primary disorders of nervous system function (see Chap. 389). This conclusion is supported further by observations that similar psychotic symptoms can be observed in patients with readily identifiable lesions of the nervous system (chronic complex partial seizures, brain tumor) or after the administration of certain drugs, such as lysergic acid or amphetamines.

Despite the importance of these areas of overlap between neurology and psychiatry, most neurologic conditions for which a patient seeks general medical care are due to readily demonstrated disease processes. It is the task of the clinician to develop a neurologic method of analysis that will result in accurate diagnosis of the site of the disorder and of its likely cause. Only then can effective approaches to management and treatment be developed.

In this and the subsequent sections, neurology and psychiatry are considered separately because many of the approaches to diagnosis and treatment remain distinct even today. In the chapters that follow, neurologic disorders and diseases are described as they present to the neurologist or general internist. Currently accepted explanations in terms of anatomy, physiology, pharmacology, and chemistry are offered. The section on psychiatric disorders is found in Chap. 389. Dependency syndromes are described in Chaps. 390 to 393.

THE NEUROLOGIC METHOD OF CLINICAL EVALUATION The strategy used in evaluating a patient with neurologic illness is to begin with the question, What portion of the neural axis is likely to be involved in causing the neurologic symptoms? The first clues to defining the anatomic area of involvement appear in the history, and the examination is then directed to confirm or rule out these impressions and to clarify uncertainties suggested by the history. A more detailed examination of a particular region of the central nervous system (CNS) or peripheral nervous system is often indicated. For example, optokinetic nystagmus may be an important part of the examination in a patient with a left hemiparesis and dressing apraxia but irrelevant to the examination of a patient complaining of burning feet. In a patient who presents with a history of ascending paresthesia and weakness, the examination should be *directed* toward deciding, among other things, if the location of the lesion is the spinal cord or peripheral nerves. Notations regarding muscle stamina or endurance might be crucial to the examination of a patient with myasthenia gravis, as opposed to the usual tests of peak muscle power. What one does in the neurologic examination depends on what the questions are; the questions are formulated by a properly taken history.

Deciding "where the lesion is" accomplishes the task of delimiting the number of possible etiologies to a manageable, finite size. In addition, this strategy safeguards against making really tragic errors. Symptoms of recurrent vertigo, diplopia, and nystagmus should not trigger "multiple sclerosis" as an answer (etiology) but "brainstem" or "pons" (location); then a diagnosis of brainstem arteriovenous malformation will not be missed because it is not considered. Similarly, the combination of optic neuritis and spastic ataxic paraparesis should not suggest only multiple sclerosis; CNS syphilis and vitamin B_{12} deficiency (both treatable) also can cause these findings. When the question, "Where is the lesion?" is answered, then the question, "What is the lesion?" can be addressed.

The neurologic history A bewildering array of clinical abnormalities requires documentation and interpretation during the neurologic evaluation of a patient. The analysis becomes difficult because similar symptoms and signs may present in a patient with any of several disorders. A number of general principles relevant to obtaining a complete neurologic history are important for the physician, whether a generalist or a specialist. Careful attention to the description of the symptoms as experienced by the patient and substantiated by family members or friends permits, in many instances, an accurate localization and determination of the probable cause of the complaints even before an examination of the patient has been undertaken. Two principles should be followed. First, each complaint ought to be pursued as far as possible in an effort to delineate (before the examination) where the lesion might be or, more important, *to formulate a set of questions to be answered by the examination.* A patient complains of weakness of the right upper limb. What are the associated features? Is this weakness for brushing the hair or opening a twist-top can? Second, in neurology—where many of the diseases are due to *anatomically restricted* lesions—*negative* associations may be crucial. A patient with a right hemiparesis without a language

* The author acknowledges the prior contributions of Raymond D. Adams to this chapter.

deficit likely has a different lesion (and likely etiology) than a patient with a right hemiparesis and aphasia. Additional important factors that aid in defining the nature of the neurologic disorder include:

1 *Temporal course of the illness.* It is particularly important to ascertain the precise rate of appearance and progression of the symptoms experienced by the patient. A paroxysmal onset of a neurologic complaint, occurring within seconds or minutes, usually indicates a cerebrovascular lesion or a seizure. Attention to the temporal march of symptoms may help define a focal seizure, a transient cerebral ischemic attack (TIA), or the onset of a migraine. For example, the onset of sensory symptoms located in one extremity that spread over a few seconds to adjacent portions of that extremity and then to the other limb or to the face suggests a seizure. A more gradual onset involving less discrete regions of the extremities points to the possibility of a TIA. A similar but slower progression of sensory change occurring in a young person together with other symptoms of headache, nausea, or visual disturbance suggests migraine. In general, the march of a migraine is slower than that of seizure, and a TIA tends to be more generalized in location on the side of the body or extremities. The presence of positive sensory symptoms or motor movements suggests a seizure; in contrast, transient loss of a function (negative symptom) suggests a TIA. A stuttering onset where symptoms appear, stabilize, regress, and then progress over hours or days also suggests the presence of impending vascular ischemia. In some cases, a demyelinating process may produce new symptoms over the course of a few hours. Progressing symptoms associated with the systemic manifestation of fever, stiff neck, and altered level of consciousness or awareness suggest the possibility of an infectious process. The course of the illness over years in terms of remissions and exacerbations offers additional clues to the nature of the process. Recurrent neurologic symptoms involving any level of the neuraxis with partial or complete recovery suggest the possibility of multiple sclerosis. Slowly progressive disorders without remissions tend to be characteristic of a neurodegenerative disorder.

2 *Subjective descriptions of the complaint.* Patient vocabularies are often limited, and symptoms are interpreted within the experience of the patient. Descriptions are highly introspective and subject to the patient's degree of intelligence and general familiarity with medical terminology. The same words often mean very different things to individual patients. For example, ''dizziness'' may be a description applied by the patient to impending syncope, to a sense of giddiness, or to true vertigo. ''Numbness'' may mean a complete loss of feeling, a positive sensation of tingling, or paralysis. ''Blurring of vision'' may be used to describe unilateral visual loss, as in amaurosis fugax, or diplopia. It is important to determine the level of understanding that the patient exhibits with respect to the complaint in order to assess accurately the precise significance of the symptom.

3 *Corroboration of the history by other close associates.* It is often useful to obtain additional information from family, friends, or observers to corroborate or expand the patient's description. Memory loss, personality change, drug abuse, excess alcohol intake, and other factors may severely impair the ability of patients to describe accurately their subjective experiences or prevent them from being completely open and forthright about the factors that have contributed to the illness. Complaints of loss of consciousness that may be due to syncope or seizures necessitate seeking details from patients and family to ascertain the exact circumstances. Major manifestations of depression and anxiety may mask or color the presentation given by the patient. Failure to note these underlying factors that interfere with the patient's performance may result in the incorrect interpretation that the complaints are actually due to structural disease of the brain.

4 *Family history.* Many neurologic disorders, particularly those presenting in childhood or early adulthood, are familial or inherited conditions. It is important to ascertain the familial frequency of

occurrence of systemic diseases such as hypertension, heart disease, or stroke, which may affect the nervous system. It is essential to inquire about the possibility of consanguinity of the parents or of the existence of similar symptoms in other members of the family. These may provide clues to a propensity toward a hereditary neurologic condition. It is critical to distinguish between a *negative* family history and an *incomplete* family history. It is insufficient to simply ask, Is there any similar illness in any member of your family? A negative response to such an inquiry may mean that there is, in fact, no such illness in the patient's family, but it also may mean that the patient is unfamiliar with relatives or their medical histories. It is wise to elicit specific positive or negative data about relatives as follows: Are your parents living? If so, are they well? If not, what illness did they have, and how did they die? It should always be remembered that maternity is a fact, but paternity is only an assumption.

It is also important to elicit family history data regarding all illnesses rather than just neurologic and psychiatric disorders. Many familial neurologic illnesses are associated with signs and symptoms in other systems (e.g., the phakomatoses, hepatocerebral disorders, neuroophthalmic syndromes, etc.).

5 *Medical illnesses.* Many neurologic illnesses occur in the context of systemic disorders. A history of allergy and asthma may suggest the onset of polyarteritis, with mononeuritis multiplex. Previous or current medical illnesses such as diabetes mellitus, hypertension, and abnormalities of blood lipids may be relevant to evolving symptoms that affect the nervous system. Similarly, the presence of systemic diseases that have an increased association with peripheral neuropathy should be explored. Most patients with coma in a hospital setting can be shown to have a metabolic, toxic, or infectious process.

6 *The patient's perception of the disease.* It is frequently helpful to ask patients what they perceive to be wrong. Patients who complain of failing memory are often concerned that they have early symptoms of Alzheimer's disease. Patients with headaches may fear that a tumor or an impending stroke is a possibility. Patients with sensory symptoms frequently are concerned about the possibility of multiple sclerosis. The patient may seek medical attention because a relative or friend has been diagnosed with a serious neurologic illness.

7 *Drug use and abuse and toxin exposure.* It is essential to inquire about the history of drug use, both prescribed and illicit. Complaints of yellow vision may occur with digitalis administration. Excessive vitamin administration may lead to peripheral neuropathy, as has been demonstrated in the case of pyridoxine. Aminoglycoside antibiotics may exacerbate symptoms of weakness in patients with disorders of neuromuscular transmission, such as myasthenia gravis. Dizziness may be secondary to ototoxicity caused by the aminoglycosides. In eliciting a history of drug use it is often necessary to be quite specific and to use lay terminology. Most patients are, for example, unaware that over-the-counter sleeping pills, cold preparations, and diet pills are actually drugs. Alcohol, the most prevalent neurotoxin, is often not recognized as such by patients. History of environmental or industrial exposure to neurotoxins may provide the essential clue; consultation with the patient's family or employer may be required.

8 *History of malignancy.* Patients with prior malignancy can present with unexpected and unusual neurologic complications. Malignant tumors may present with nervous system metastases or occasionally with a paraneoplastic syndrome. In a patient with history of malignancy, it is important to ask whether chemotherapy or radiotherapy was given.

9 *Formulating an impression of the patient.* Use the opportunity while taking the history to form an impression of the patient. Is there evidence of anxiety, depression, hypochondriasis? Are there any clues to defects of language, memory, inappropriate behavior, or secondary gain? The neurologic assessment begins as soon as the patient walks into the room and the first introduction is made.

The neurologic examination After obtaining a complete medical and neurologic history, the physician should have reliable clues to the portions of the nervous system to be examined. By the elicitation of specific signs it is then determined whether the nervous system is affected and, if so, to what degree and which part. The anatomic localization of the lesion assumes special significance in neurology, since certain diseases are known to affect certain regions of the nervous system and not to involve others. Recognition of a constellation of symptoms and signs (a syndrome) points to the possible existence of certain diseases and to the exclusion of others.

A systematic neurologic examination should encompass a survey of all functions from the cerebrum to peripheral nerve and muscle, i.e., from the mental status examination to the simplest reflexes. Such a detailed examination requires the performance of a series of physical tests aimed at eliciting the functional capacities of each part of the nervous system. The examiner must acquire skills that come only from the repeated use of the same techniques and instruments on a large number of normal and abnormal individuals. Errors and serious omissions are avoided if the examination procedure is orderly and systemic, beginning with mental (cerebral) functions and continuing with cranial nerves, then with motor, reflex, and sensory functions of the arms, trunk, and legs, and finishing with an analysis of posture and gait.

The mental status is already appreciated while the history is being taken. But rather profound disorders of recent memory or of spatial organization may be missed unless specifically tested for. Faults of memory, incoherence of thought, dominating ideas, peculiarities of mood and outlook, aphasic errors, problems of articulation, and loss of insight and judgment should be sought. If abnormalities are noted, a more formal analysis of these functions is undertaken along the lines suggested in Chaps. 25, 27, and 28. The function of each cranial nerve is then examined in order, beginning with olfaction (see Chaps. 18, 19, 20, and 380). Examination of the motor system should include estimates of power of each of the major muscle groups, evidence of atrophy or fasciculation, and assessment of the tone of the musculature during passive manipulations, looking for signs of spasticity, rigidity, or hypotonia (as outlined in Chaps. 21 and 382). Speed and coordination of the limbs are assessed. Next, prevailing postures and the stance and gait are evaluated (Chap. 22). The tendon reflexes are examined for evidence of increased or decreased (or absent) response or of asymmetry between right and left sides or between arms and legs. The superficial cutaneous reflexes, abdominal and plantar, are then evaluated. Touch, pain, vibration, and joint-position sense are tested as the final part of the examination (see Chap. 24).

This detailed neurologic examination is undertaken only if there are symptoms of disturbed nervous system functioning. If none are present, it suffices to do an abbreviated examination which includes evaluation only of pupils, ocular movements, optic fundi, facial movements, speech, strength of arm and leg muscles, tendon and plantar reflexes, pain and vibratory sensation in hands and feet, and gait. All this can be completed in 3 to 5 min. The findings, even in the short examination, should be recorded in the patient's record for future reference.

Two additional points about the examination are worth noting. First, in recording observations, it is important for the physician to describe what is found rather than to apply a poorly defined medical term (i.e., "patient groans to sternal rub" rather than "obtunded"). Second, if the patient's complaint is brought out by some activity, reproduce the activity in the office. If the complaint is of dizziness when raising the right arm and turning the head to the left, have the patient do it. If pain occurs after walking two blocks, have the patient demonstrate it, and repeat the examination.

Experience teaches that the neurologic examination may be normal even in patients with a serious neurologic disease, such as one which causes seizures or syncope. Or the patient may arrive in a coma with no available history, and the examination proceeds along the lines described in Chap. 26. An inadequate history may to some extent be replaced by a succession of examinations from which the course of the illness may be plotted.

The formulation of the problem and establishment of an etiologic diagnosis The clinical data obtained from the history and the examination are assembled into one of the known syndromes and are interpreted and translated in terms of neuroanatomy and neurophysiology. From the syndrome the physician should be able to determine the anatomic localization(s) that best explains the clinical findings. The anatomic localization, mode of onset and course of illness, other medical data, and laboratory findings are then integrated. Finally, the etiologic diagnosis is reached, and therapy appropriate for the disorder is proposed.

Laboratory tests The proper selection of tests is important to arrive at an anatomic, but more particularly an etiologic, diagnosis. The laboratory assessment of a patient with positive neurologic findings may include (1) serum electrolytes, complete blood count, and renal, liver, and endocrine studies, (2) cerebrospinal fluid (CSF) examination, (3) imaging studies of the CNS (see Chap. 365), or (4) electrophysiologic studies (see Chap. 366).

Lumbar puncture Lumbar puncture should be considered (1) to measure CSF pressure and to obtain a sample for cellular, chemical, and bacteriologic examination, (2) to administer spinal anesthetics, antibiotics, or antineoplastic agents, and (3) to inject contrast substances for myelography or a radioactive substance [e.g., indium or radioactive iodinated serum albumin (RISA)] for the study of CSF dynamics and to aid in the diagnosis of hydrocephalus or CSF leak.

Lumbar puncture carries a risk if the CSF pressure is high (evidenced by headache and papilledema), for it increases the possibility of fatal cerebellar or tentorial herniation. In patients in whom this possibility exists, it is wise first to obtain a CT or MRI scan to exclude a mass lesion before proceeding to a lumbar puncture. However, if it seems important in a given case of suspected increased intracranial pressure to have the information yielded by CSF examination, the lumbar puncture may be performed with a fine-bore (22- or 24-gauge needle). If the pressure is over 400 mmHg, one should obtain the necessary sample of fluid, remove the needle, and then, according to the suspected clinical disease and the patient's condition, administer mannitol in a dose of 0.75 to 1.0 mg/kg. Unless contraindicated, dexamethasone should be started in a dose of 4 to 6 mg every 6 h in cases of tumor, cerebral trauma, hemorrhage, and certain types of encephalitis (acute hemorrhagic leukoencephalitis, herpes simplex encephalitis).

Cisternal puncture and lateral cervical puncture (C1–C2) are safe procedures in the hands of the expert but should not be performed by those without experience. Cisternal puncture is sometimes necessary in instances of spinal block to perform myelography above a lesion.

Lumbar puncture should always be done under sterile conditions. If local anesthetic is injected into and beneath the skin, the procedure should be painless. Failure to enter the lumbar subarachnoid space after two or three trials can usually be corrected by doing the puncture with patients in the sitting position and then assisting them to lie on their side for pressure measurements and fluid removal. The "dry tap" is more often due to an improperly placed needle than to a pathologic obliteration of subarachnoid space by a compressive lesion of the spinal cord or by chronic adhesive arachnoiditis. A bloody tap due to penetration of a meningeal vessel may result in confusion of the diagnosis if it is wrongly interpreted as indicating hemorrhage into the subarachnoid space. Lumbar puncture should be undertaken with particular care in patients with thrombocytopenia or disorders of blood coagulation because serious hemorrhage into the extradural or intradural space may occur.

CSF should be studied for (1) pressure and "dynamics," (2) color, including centrifugation, if blood is present, to examine the supernatant for xanthochromia, (3) number and type of cells and presence of microorganisms, (4) protein, sugar, and other chemical measurements, (5) exfoliative cytology using Millipore filters, (6) VDRL determination and appropriate serologic precipitation reactions (including cryptococcal antigen in patients with immunologic suppression, e.g., AIDS), (7) protein immunoelectrophoresis for determination of gamma globulin levels and other special biochemical tests (for NH_3, pH, CO_2, enzymes, etc.), and (8) bacteriologic cultures and virus isolation. Normal values of CSF constituents are shown in the Appendix.

The principal complication of lumbar puncture is a headache caused by a drop in CSF pressure. Such headaches are worsened by an upright posture and usually disappear in a few hours. Severe cases may require nonsteroidal anti-inflammatory drugs or epidural injection of an autologous "blood patch."

REFERENCES

ADAMS RD, VICTOR M: *Principles of Neurology*, 5th ed. New York, McGraw-Hill, 1993
DEJONG RN: *The Neurologic Examination*. New York, Harper & Row, 1979
FISHMAN RA: *Cerebrospinal Fluid in Diseases of the Nervous System*, 2d ed. Philadelphia, Saunders, 1992
SWANSON PD: *Symptoms and Signs in Neurology*. Philadelphia, Lippincott, 1984

364 IMPACT OF NEUROBIOLOGY AND MOLECULAR GENETICS ON NEUROLOGY

JOSEPH B. MARTIN

Advances in molecular genetics, neurobiology, and brain imaging are having a major impact on neurology and psychiatry. These advances are changing our understanding of how the brain is constructed and of the way it functions. They are also expanding the repertoire of experimental approaches, some of which may be successful in solving clinical problems and offering new therapeutic approaches. Molecular genetic discoveries have made possible a more rational taxonomy for many of the inherited diseases that affect the central and peripheral nervous systems, enable new approaches for understanding the molecular basis of development (and degeneration) of the nervous system, and permit presymptomatic or prenatal diagnosis.

The advances have occurred on several fronts, which are now beginning to coalesce. The identification of genes responsible for several of the inherited neurologic diseases has provided insight into their pathogenesis (Table 364-1). Research in molecular structure has disclosed several proteins that subserve receptor and membrane channel functions. Elucidation of the genes that encode for neurotransmitters and their receptors has led to new understanding of neurotransmitter signal transduction and of intercellular and intracellular communication. These discoveries have major implications for drug development by permitting identification of more selective receptor agonists and antagonists. There is also new insight into the mechanisms of cellular injury and neuronal death. The ability to analyze neuronal structure and function extends also to the intact brain. Positron emission tomography (PET), magnetoencephalography, and in vivo magnetic resonance spectroscopy now provide powerful techniques for analysis of the functional organization of the brain (see also Chap. 365).

MOLECULAR GENETICS Applications of molecular biology have already had a major effect on the clinical neurosciences. In the case of inherited neurologic diseases, the use of DNA probes that demonstrate restriction fragment length polymorphisms (RFLPs), combined with linkage analysis in affected pedigrees, have made possible the chromosomal localization of the mutant gene in Huntington's disease (see Chap. 370), familial Alzheimer's disease (see Chap. 370), neurofibromatosis types I and II (see Chap. 370), Friedreich's ataxia (see Chap. 370), spinal muscular atrophy, torsion dystonia, Wilson's disease, and several types of familial CNS tumors including retinoblastoma and von Hippel-Lindau disease (see Table 364-1). The use of linkage analysis with chromosome-specific RFLPs is the first step toward localization and eventual characterization of the abnormal

gene product, a process referred to as *reverse genetics*, i.e., analysis of gene structure to study the abnormal cellular protein, an approach more correctly referred to as *positional cloning*.

In several conditions this approach has already affected clinical practice. In Duchenne's dystrophy, and Becker's X-linked disorders, the muscle abnormality results from failure to encode for a membrane-attached protein, *dystrophin*, which is absent from skeletal muscle in virtually all patients with the Duchenne variant of the disorder (see Chap. 385). In Becker's dystrophy dystrophin is present but is abnormal in amount or in size. Dystrophin is also present in smooth muscle, cardiac muscle, and brain. Its presence in the brain presumably accounts in some way yet to be defined for the frequent occurrence of mental retardation in individuals with Duchenne's dystrophy. The discovery of dystrophin demonstrates elegantly the power of molecular genetics. Decades of effort attempting to define the protein abnormality in Duchenne's dystrophy had been unsuccessful. The quantities of dystrophin present in muscle are so minute that it could not have been characterized by current biochemical approaches.

In retinoblastoma, identification of the protein encoded by the normal allele of the gene (a growth suppressor gene) that is absent from the tumor has provided insight into cellular growth. It is postulated that an inherited mutation affects one allele of the normal gene. If this is followed by a "second hit" mutation that eliminates the function of the second allele in one of the cells in the developing retina, the cell growth suppressor cannot be synthesized. The consequence is the abnormal division of cells in the retina and tumor formation (see also Chap. 63). Another tumor associated with hereditary retinoblastoma is osteosarcoma. A similar mechanism for tumor formation may be involved in Wilms' tumor (on chromosome 11) and in the von Hippel-Lindau syndrome, which leads to hemangioblastoma, pheochromocytoma, and renal cell carcinoma (see Table 364-1).

The application of DNA diagnostics has provided new approaches to presymptomatic and prenatal diagnosis of Huntington's disease, Duchenne's dystrophy, retinoblastoma, and von Hippel-Lindau disease (Table 364-1).

CHARACTERIZATION OF NEW NEUROTRANSMITTER CANDIDATES More than 60 neurotransmitter candidates have been identified in the brain based upon localization within synaptic vesicles, release with depolarization, and interactions with postsynaptic receptors. The functions of these agents, many of which are small-molecular-weight peptides (neuropeptides), remain obscure in many cases. But some are known to modulate functions such as pain transmission (opioid peptides), satiety (cholecystokinin), and thirst (angiotensin).

The discovery of these molecules has made possible new approaches to defining neuronal populations in the human brain by immunohistochemical staining, autoradiography, and in situ messenger RNA hybridization. This information has made it possible to delineate the subclasses of cells affected in neurodegenerative diseases, such as Alzheimer's, Parkinson's, and Huntington's disease. Realiza-

TABLE 364-1 Molecular genetics of neurologic disorders

Chromosome location	Disorder	Principal clinical findings/phenotype	Mode of inheritance	Genotype/gene product	Genetic testing?	Ref. (or Chap.)
1p36.2-p36.1	Neuroblastoma	Related to tumor location and metastases, opsoclonus, myoclonus.	Usually sporadic.	Tumors commonly show hemizygous (one copy) of regions of chromosome 1p. Genomic amplification of N-*myc* occurs.	Tumor analysis for hemizygous state possible.	369
1q21.2-q23	Charcot-Marie-Tooth peripheral neuropathy, Type IB	Onset 2d-3d decade. Distal weakness in legs, less affected in arms. Decreased reflexes, minimal sensory changes. Demyelinating disorder with hypertrophic neuropathy.	AD	Unknown.	Not available.	383
1q21	Gaucher's disease	Infantile, juvenile, and adult forms. Mental retardation, spasticity or ataxia.	AR	Mutations in gene encoding ß-glucocerebrosidase.	Available.	349
2p24	Hypobetalipoproteinemia	Fat malabsorption, neuropathy, sensory loss, ataxia, retinitis pigmentosa, acanthocytosis.	AR	Defect in apolipoprotein B-100. Genetic basis unknown.	Not available.	383
2q33-qter	Cerebrotendinous xanthomatosis	Progressive cerebellar ataxia, dementia, weakness, mental retardation, tendon xanthomas.	AR	Defective synthesis in bile acids in liver.	Not available.	344
2q35	Waardenburg's syndrome, type I	Deafness, white forelock, abnormal pigmentation due to developmental defect caused by defective neural crest migration.	AD	Mutant gene is a member of the paired box-containing (PAX-3) gene family; DNA binding proteins.	Possible in selected families.	54, Tassabehji et al (1992)
3p25	von Hippel-Lindau disease	Retinal vascular malformations, hemangioblastomas,	AD	Tumor suppressor gene identified.	Possible in selected families.	378, Latif et al
3p14.2	G$_{M1}$-gangliosidosis	Mental retardation, seizures, blindness.	AR	Mutations in gene for ß-galactosidase.	Widely available.	349
3q	Retinitis pigmentosa 1	Night blindness, peripheral field loss, blindness, abnormal EEG.	AD	Mutations in gene that encodes rhodopsin.	Possible in families with identified mutations.	19
4p16.3	Huntington's disease	Chorea, dementia.	AD	CAG triplet repeats 5' end of gene that encodes a novel protein huntingtin.	Yes.	370, MacDonald et al (1993)
4p16.1	Wolf-Hirschhorn syndrome	Mental retardation, peculiar facies.	Sporadic	Deletion 4p16.	No.	
4q35	Facioscapulohumeral muscular dystrophy	Typical weakness atrophy. Face and shoulder muscles.	AD	Unknown.	Possible by linkage testing in large families.	385
5q12.2-q13.3	Spinal muscular atrophy (SMA) type 1,2,3	Weakness, muscle atrophy, diminished or absent reflexes.	AR	Unknown.	Linkage testing possible.	372
5q1.13	G$_{M2}$-gangliosidosis (Sandhoff disease)	Mental retardation, seizures, blindness.	AR	Mutations in A-B hexosaminidase.	Widely applied.	349
6p21.3	Epilepsy, juvenile myoclonic	Tonic-clonic seizures, myoclonus, onset 8–20 years, EEG abnormal.	AD	Unknown.	Linkage testing possible in some pedigrees.	367
6p24-23	Spinocerebellar ataxia 1 (SCA1)	Ataxia, progressive dementia, spasticity.	AD	Expansion of CAG repeats in gene.	Possible.	372/381
6p21.1-cen	Retinitis pigmentosa, peripherin-related	Night blindness, peripheral visual loss leading to blindness.	AD	Mutations in RDS/peripherin gene, a rod photoreceptor membrane protein.	Possible in families with identified mutations.	Kajiwara et al (1993)
7q35	Myotonia congenita (Thomsen disease)	Myotonia, symptoms variable in severity	AD	Mutation in muscle chloride channel gene.	Possible.	385
9p.13	Galactosemia	Cataracts, mental retardation, cirrhosis.	AR	Deficiency of galactose-1-phosphate uridyl transferase.	Prenatal diagnosis by measuring enzyme.	354
9q12-13	Friedreich's ataxia	Onset in puberty; ataxia; dysarthria; absent DTRs; decreased vibration, joint position sense; 1/50,000 incidence.	AR	Unknown.	97% reliable.	370
9q31-33	Familial dysautonomia Riley-Day syndrome	Sensory and autonomic dysfunction, occurs in Ashkenzi-Jewish population.	AR	Unknown.	Possible.	163

(continued)

TABLE 364-1 Molecular genetics of neurologic disorders (*continued*)

Chromosome location	Disorder	Principal clinical findings/Phenotype	Mode of inheritance	Genotype/gene product	Genetic testing?	Ref. (or Chap.)
9q34	Tuberous sclerosis 1	1/10,000 births, mental retardation, seizures, adenoma sebaceum.	AD	Unknown.	Not reliable.	378
9q34	Torsion dystonia	Dystonia, torticollis, occurs in both Ashkenazi-Jewish and non-Jewish pedigrees.	AD	Unknown.	97% reliable.	370
11q22.3-q23.1	Ataxia telangiectasia	Cerebellar degeneration, oculocutaneous telangiectasia, immunodeficiency, endocrinopathy.	AR	Unknown.	Not available.	278
11q24.1-q24.2	Acute intermittent porphyria	Confusion, coma, peripheral neuropathy with proximal weakness.	AD	Defect in porphobilinogen deaminase. Gene defect not defined.	Not available.	346
12q23-24.1	Spinocerebellar ataxia 2 (SCA2)	Ataxia, clinically indistinguishable from SCA1.	AD	Unknown.	Possible by linkage.	372
13q14.1-q14.2	Retinoblastoma	40% hereditary, 60% nonhereditary, multiple tumors in inherited form.	AR	*Rb* gene mutations or deletions cause disease. Rb protein is 105-kDa tumor suppressor.	Detection of carriers and presymptomatic diagnosis.	19, 60
13q14-q21	Wilson's disease	Kayser-Fleischer ring in cornea, movement disorder, progressive neurologic deficit if untreated.	AR	Unknown.	Not available.	348
14q21-q31	Krabbe's disease	Mental retardation, leukodystrophy.	AR	Enzyme defect, galactosylceramide, ß-galactoside.	Possible.	349
14q24.3	Alzheimer's disease, early onset	Dementia, memory loss, typical AD.	AD	Unknown.	Not available.	370
15q11	Prader-Willi/Angelman syndrome	Prader-Willi: hypotonia, hypogonadism, hyperphagia, hypopigmentation. Angelman: movement disorder, ataxia, reverse mental retardation.	Sporadic	Deletion mutation defect due to unequal expression of maternal or paternal alleles. Prader-Willi due to active paternal allele, Angelman to active maternal allele.	Cytogenetics in individual patients.	Wagstaff et al
15q23-q24	Tay-Sachs disease, G_{M2}-gangliosidosis	Mental retardation, delayed development, seizures, blindness.	AR	Mutations in hexosaminidase A.	Widely available.	349
16p12.1	Batten disease—Juvenile neuronal lipofuscinosis	Dementia, paralysis, white matter disease.	AD	Unknown.	Possible.	Mitchison et al
16p3	Tuberous sclerosis 2	Hamartomas, epilepsy, mental retardation.	AD	Unknown.	Not available.	378
17p13.3	Miller-Dieker lissencephaly syndrome	Microcephaly, micrognathia, epilepsy, pathology shows smooth brain (agyria) due to failure of cortical neuronal migration.	AD	17p13 deletion, gene of homologue of ß-transducin.	Cytogenetics possible.	Reiner et al
17p11.2	Charcot-Marie-Tooth Type 1A	Motor and sensory neuropathy, distal muscle atrophy, areflexia, pes cavus, decreased nerve conduction velocities.	AD	Mutation or duplication in peripheral myelin protein gene, PMP-22.	Possible in families with demonstrated mutations.	383, Pentao et al (1992)
17q11.2	Von Recklinghausen neurofibromatosis, NF1	Multiple neurofibromas, 1/3500 individuals, café au lait spots, malignant gliomas, Lisch nodules.	AD	Encodes neurofibromin, a member of the GTPase activating protein (GAP) family.	Possible in families with demonstrated mutations.	378
17q23.1-q25.3	Hyperkalemic periodic paralysis	Myotonia, periodic areflexic paralysis.	AD	Point mutation sodium channel.	Possible.	387
18q11.2-q12.1	Familial amyloid neuropathy due to mutations in transthyretin	Sensorimotor cardiac neuropathy.	AD	Over 40 different point mutations in gene for transthyretin.	Yes.	383
18q22.1	Tourette's syndrome	Familial, but not all cases linked to this chromosomal site.	AD?	Unknown.	No.	370
19q13.3	Myotonic dystrophy	Multisystem disorder, cataracts, myotonia, weakness, frontal baldness, mental retardation.	AD, anticipation	CTG repeats 3' end of myotonin protein kinase.	Yes.	385
19q13.1	Malignant hyperthermia	Sensitivity to volatile anesthetics, muscle contraction.	AD	Mutation in ryanodine receptor.	Yes.	398

(continued)

TABLE 364-1 Molecular genetics of neurologic disorders (*continued*)

Chromosome location	Disorder	Principal clinical findings/Phenotype	Mode of inheritance	Genotype/gene product	Genetic testing?	Ref. (or Chap.)
19q12-q13.2	Central core disease of muscle	Hypotonia, weakness.	AD	Mutation in ryanodine receptor.	Yes.	385
19q13.2	Alzheimer's disease, late-onset	Memory loss, dementia.	AD	Apolipoprotein E4 association.	Not available.	370
20pter-p12	Gerstmann-Straussler disease	Spongioform encephalopathy with dementia, myoclonus.	AD	Prion protein mutation.	Yes.	375
20pter-p12	Familial Creutzfeldt-Jakob disease	Spongioform encephalopathy with dementia, myoclonus.	AD	Prion protein mutation.	Yes.	375
20q	Benign neonatal familial epilepsy	Onset early in life, remits by 1 year, small percentage have mental retardation.	AD	Unknown.	Not available.	367
21q21.3-q22.05	Familial Alzheimer's disease with amyloid precursor protein mutation	Rare cause of early onset Alzheimer's disease.	AD	Mutation in amyloid precursor protein.	Possible.	370
21q22.1-q22.2	Familial amyotrophic lateral sclerosis	Weakness, muscle atrophy, spasticity, increased DTRs. About 5% of cases are familial.	AD	Point mutations in Cu, Zn-superoxide dismutase (SOD1). In 40 percent of families.	Possible.	370, Rosen et al (1993)
21q21.3-q22.05	Familial cerebral amyloid angiopathy (Dutch type)	Cerebral hemorrhage.	AD	Point mutation in amyloid precursor protein (APP).	Possible.	370
21q22.3	Epilepsy, progressive myoclonic	Rare, dementia and other neurologic findings.	AD (probably)	Unknown.	Not available.	367
22q1.11	Neurofibromatosis type II (NFII)	Acoustic neuromas, bilateral.	AD	Deletions in the gene that encodes for merlin, a 587 amino acid cytoskeletal protein.	Yes.	378, Trofatter et al (1993)
22q11.21-q13.1	Acoustic neuroma, meningioma	Acoustic neuromas, bilateral. Meningiomas.	AD	Deletions in merlin gene	Yes.	369
22q13-13qter	Metachromatic leukodystrophy	Mental retardation, leukodystrophy, dementia.	AR	Several mutations in gene encoding for arylsulfatase A have been identified.	Enzyme measurement available, DNA diagnosis possible.	383
Xp22.3	Kallmann syndrome	Anosmia with hypogonadism (GnRH deficiency), syndrome due to failure of neuronal migration.	X-LR	Mutations in gene (*KALIG-1*) which encodes protein with homology to neural cell adhesion (N-CAM) molecules.	Possible.	339/340
Xp21.2	Duchenne's muscular dystrophy and Becker's muscular dystrophy	Onset of muscular weakness in early life, progressive. Becker's is more benign.	X-LR	Mutations in the dystrophin-encoding gene.	Widely available.	385, Ahn and Kunhal (1993)
Xp11.4	Norrie disease	Failure of normal brain development.	X-LR	Gene encodes small protein with homology to glycosylated mucins.	Possible.	Meindl et al
Xq12-q13	Menkes disease	Progressive neurologic deterioration, kinky or steely hair, pallor, death in childhood.	X-LR	Mutations in a gene (*MCI*) that encodes a protein that regulates cation transport (probably including copper).	Possible.	Vulpe et al (1993)
Xq21.3-q22	Spinal muscular atrophy; Kennedy disease	Muscular weakness.	X-LR	Trinucleotide repeats in androgen receptor gene.	Possible.	372
Xq22	Pelizaeus-Merzbacher disease	Progressive neurologic deterioration.	X-LR	One-quarter of patients have mutation in proteolipid protein gene.	Not available.	Strautnieks et al
Xq22	Fabry disease	Painful neuropathy.	X-LR	Enzyme defect in α-galactosidase A	Possible.	241/349
Xq13	Charcot-Marie-Tooth, X-linked-1 dominant	Neuropathy, with weakness and sensory loss.	X-LR	Unknown.	Not available.	383
Xq21.2	Choroideremia	Retinitis pigmentosa, visual loss due to degeneration of pigment epithelium and choroid.	X-LR	Gene isolated encodes geranylgeranyl transferase that prenylates several proteins.	Possible.	Cremers et al
Xq21-q22	Spastic paraplegia, X-linked	Midlife onset, spasticity, weakness, urinary frequency.	X-LR	Unknown.	Not available.	370
Xq26-q27.2	Lesch-Nyhan syndrome	Mental retardation.	X-LR	HPRT deficiency.	90% have point mutation in exon 9 of HPRT gene.	347

(*continued*)

TABLE 364-1   Molecular genetics of neurologic disorders (*continued*)

Chromosome location	Disorder	Principal clinical findings/Phenotype	Mode of inheritance	Genotype/gene product	Genetic testing?	Ref. (or Chap.)
Xq27.3	Fragile-X syndrome	Decreased head size, prominent forehead, large ears, macro-orchidism, mental retardation.	X-LR	Gene characterized by trinucleotide 5′ repeats of CGG. Gene identified as *FMR*-1.	Yes.	62 and 378
Xq28	Adrenoleukodystrophy	Mild neuropathy, spastic paraparesis, baldness, hypogonadism, hypoadrenalism.	X-LR	Gene characterized.	Possible.	377
Xq28	Emery-Dreifuss muscular dystrophy	Onset before age 10, benign course characterized by slowly progressive proximal weakness, cardiac arrhythmias may occur.	X-LR	Unknown.	Not available.	385

Abbreviations: AD, autosomal dominant; AR, autosomal recessive; X-LR, X-linked recessive; HPRT, hypoxanthine-guanine phosphoribosyltransferase.
SOURCE: Martin JB, Ann Neurol, vol. 34, 1993.

tion that dopamine cells are affected in Parkinson's disease led to therapy with levodopa. In Huntington's disease, it has been possible to define the subsets of neurons affected by the degenerative process in the striatum and to show selective sparing of other cell types (see Chap. 370). Although this has not led yet to specific theories about the mechanisms of cell death, it has resulted in speculations about potentially beneficial therapeutic strategies.

Many of these newly discovered neuropeptides appear to share nerve terminals and often even secretory vesicles with conventional neurotransmitters. It appears likely that neuropeptides exert profound modulatory effects on the actions of the primary neurotransmitter. In other cases the peptide may influence neuronal plasticity, growth, or differentiation. A most surprising discovery was the recognition that nitric oxide (NO), synthesized in neurons by the enzyme nitric oxide synthase, acts after cellular release to exert a variety of effects on neural tissues. First recognized as an endothelial cell–derived muscle cell relaxant (nitrates dilate blood vessels, as in the treatment for angina), NO can be both beneficial and toxic to brain cells. Subclasses of neurons contain NO synthase, as for example do NADPH diaphorase-positive neurons of the striatum, and NO release in normal quantities can activate other neurons. Excessive release can prove toxic. Other gases, such as carbon monoxide, may also serve modulatory roles in nervous tissue.

BIOCHEMICAL CLASSIFICATION OF RECEPTOR SUBTYPES
Some of the most important insights from neurobiology have resulted from the cloning of the genes of several neurotransmitter and hormone receptors that are critical to brain function. Based on pharmacologic analysis alone it was difficult to account for the diverse effects mediated by molecules of low molecular weight. For example, pharmacologic analysis of acetylcholine disclosed muscarinic and nicotinic effects. With the biochemical elucidation of acetylcholine receptor subtypes and by means of molecular cloning techniques and molecular probes, it is now established that multiple forms of muscarinic (M1, M2, M3, M4, and M5) and nicotinic (N1 and N2) receptors exist in the brain and that their distribution varies from region to region. Thus, differences in receptor subtypes expressed in different regions of the brain can account for the complex multiple effects of the medications acting on cholinergic receptors. The molecular specificities of the various receptor subtypes provide sensitive systems with which to search for selective agonists and antagonists. For example, M1 agonists may facilitate memory. Regional differences in the distribution of the subtypes of the nicotinic cholinergic receptor in the central nervous system make it possible to explore the neurologic basis of nicotine addiction.

Identification of the subclasses of the alpha- and beta-adrenergic, serotoninergic, gamma-aminobutyric acid (GABA), and glutamatergic receptors makes it possible to correlate structure and function and

provide a rational basis for molecular classification of drug actions. In the case of the GABA receptor, structural features that account for the interaction of barbiturates and benzodiazepines can now be recognized.

Subclasses of glutamate receptors mediate excitatory amino acid neurotransmitter effects. Glutamate, one of the most abundant of all neurotransmitters in the brain, functions to promote rapid neurotransmitter depolarization by opening membrane channels that permit diffusion of sodium and potassium ions. These rapid effects are mediated by two receptor subtypes, identified by ligand binding with kainate and AMPA. The identification of an additional subtype of glutamate receptor which binds *N*-methyl-D-aspartate (the *NMDA receptor*) made possible identification of additional glutamate functions. The NMDA receptor appears to mediate other functions that heretofore were classed in the category of plasticity, a process considered important, for example, in memory and learning. The NMDA subtype of glutamate receptor is linked to a voltage-sensitive channel that responds to repetitive activation by the opening of an ion channel. The actions of calcium permit transduction of electrical events into molecular changes that can alter neuronal function permanently, i.e., change cellular function to subserve a memory or learning response.

Based on definitive experimental results, it is now clear that activation of the NMDA receptor can also have deleterious effects on the cell, whereby calcium entry induces *neurotoxicity* that, if sufficiently severe, can lead to neuronal cell death. This mechanism may explain some of the extensive neuronal cell damage that occurs in ischemia, hypoxia, epilepsy, and, perhaps, neurodegenerative diseases (see Choi).

These findings have resulted in great interest in the development of new drugs that might selectively block the NMDA receptor, thereby minimizing the effects of ischemia or hypoxia that occur in stroke or after cardiorespiratory arrest. The profound potential of this work is illustrated by the demonstration that NMDA receptor blockade induced even several hours after the neuronal insult may be "neuroprotective."

Cloning of cellular membrane channels (sodium, potassium, calcium) also has had a profound effect on defining mechanisms of neuronal excitability. It is anticipated that these findings will lead to the discovery of more effective drugs for epilepsy, neuroprotection, and migraine.

BRAIN IMAGING   The development of computed tomography and proton imaging by magnetic resonance has revolutionized our ability to define lesions in the brain and spinal cord (see Chap. 365). Other techniques have been developed to make it possible to study brain function as well as structure by the application of positron emission tomography (PET), single photon emission computed tomography (SPECT), magnetoencephalography, and nuclear magnetic resonance spectroscopy (NMRS).

PET scanning involves the use of positron-emitting radionuclides with short half-lives in which particle disintegration is captured in a three-dimensional array by multiple sensors positioned about the head. With the use of radioisotopes for carbon (^{13}C), oxygen (^{15}O), and fluorine (^{18}F), it is possible to measure cerebral blood flow, cerebral oxygen metabolism, and cerebral glucose uptake (with ^{18}F-labeled deoxyglucose). The last technique employs the principles developed by Sokoloff and colleagues, who first used the technique of labeled deoxyglucose combined with tissue section autoradiography. PET scanning also can define regional changes in cerebral function associated with stroke, Alzheimer's disease, Huntington's disease, and schizophrenia, and it identifies foci of hyperactivity associated with epilepsy.

Perhaps the most creative use of PET techniques has been analysis of cognitive function. Two theories of language had emerged from studies in neurology and linguistics. The first proposed that language function occurs serially, i.e., an object is first seen in the occipital lobes, its name is recalled by the temporal lobes, and the information is then sent to the frontal lobes, which direct formation of speech. PET studies have now confirmed the second of these hypotheses, which suggested from linguistic analysis that language occurs in a parallel array. Posner and colleagues, using subtraction techniques to isolate activity associated with a particular language task, have shown clearly that brain processing occurs simultaneously in several of the regions underlying a set of neurologic functions. These kinds of analyses now permit regionalized functional study of the brain in a manner not hitherto expected by the physical limits set by three-dimensional imaging using positron emitters. Regional studies of this kind have also shown that brain blood flow changes that occur in panic disorder and anticipatory anxiety correlate with anatomic loci in the temporal lobes.

There have also been important advances in the use of radioligands for neurotransmitter receptors. The imaging of dopamine and of dopamine receptors in the basal ganglia has been achieved in both normals and in patients with Parkinson's disease and with 1-methyl-4-phenyl-1,2,3,6-tetrahydropyridine (MPTP) poisoning. In the latter case deficits in basal ganglion function in asymptomatic subjects exposed to MPTP raise the possibility of identifying subclinical deficits and of following subjects over time to determine eventual outcome and prognosis. MRI techniques can also be applied to functional studies in the brain. Blood flow changes, measured in real time, have been detected by MRI in the visual cortex in subjects exposed to visual stimulation. Mapping of the brain by MRI, PET, and magnetoencephalography is now being actively pursued in many laboratories.

SPECT imaging has been made possible by refinements in detection systems for single photon emitters. The resolution of SPECT does not yet reach the capacity of PET, but the longer half-lives of the isotopes and the simplicity of the detection systems make it less expensive and potentially more widely available. Its potential includes measurement of radioligand binding to receptors and determination of cerebral blood flow. Thus far, studies with SPECT have delineated regional changes in brain metabolism and blood flow in the neurodegenerative diseases.

NMR spectroscopy offers an opportunity to assess brain function at the subcellular molecular level. The technique uses natural emissions from atomic nuclei activated by magnetic fields to measure endogenous molecules. Potential nuclei include ^{31}P, ^{13}C, ^{23}Na, ^{7}Li, in addition to ^{1}H. The promise of analysis of ^{31}P is the closest to realization. It is possible to quantitate several phosphate-containing compounds (phosphocreatine, ATP, ADP, and inorganic phosphorus). The combination of spectral analysis with topical NMR permits localization within superficial regions of the brain. It can be anticipated that further refinements of this technique will make possible measurement of brain metabolism with spatial resolution that may exceed that of PET.

REFERENCES

AHN AH, KUNKEL LM: The structural and functional diversity of dystrophin. Nature Genet 3:283, 1993

BLUMENFELD A et al: Localization of the gene for familial dysautonomia on chromosome 9 and definition of DNA markers for genetic diagnosis. Nature Genet 4:160, 1993

BREAKEFIELD XO, CAMBI F: Molecular genetic insights into neurologic diseases, in Annual Review of Neuroscience, vol 10, WM Cowan et al (eds). Palo Alto, Annual Reviews, 1987, pp 535–594

BROWN GG et al: In vivo ^{13}P NMR profiles of Alzheimer's disease and multiple subcortical infarct dementia. Neurology 39:1423, 1989

BUCKLEY NJ et al: Antagonist binding properties of five cloned muscarinic receptors expressed in CHO-K1 cells. Molec Pharmacol 35(4):469, 1989

CHOI D: Glutamate neurotoxicity and diseases of the nervous system. Neuron 1:623, 1989

COOPER JR et al: The Biochemical Basis of Neuropharmacology. New York, Oxford University Press, 1986

CREMERS FPM et al: An autosomal homologue of the choroideremia gene colocalizes with the Usher syndrome type II locus on the distal part of chromosome 1q. Hum Mol Gen 1:71, 1992

GUSELLA JF et al: DNA markers for nervous system diseases. Science 225:1320, 1984

KAJIWARA K et al: A null mutation in the human peripherin RDS gene in a family with autosomal dominant retinitis punctata albescens. Nature Genet 3:208, 1993

KATIF F et al: Identification of the von Hippel-Lindau disease tumor suppressor gene. Science 260:1317, 1993

KAUPPINEN RA et al: Applications of magnetic resonance spectroscopy and diffusion-weighted imaging to the study of brain biochemistry and pathology. Trends Neurosci 16:88, 1993

MACDONALD M et al: A novel gene containing a trinucleotide repeat that is expanded and unstable on Huntington's disease chromosomes. Cell 72:971, 1993

MARTIN JB: Molecular genetics: Applications to the clinical neurosciences. Science 238:765, 1987

——: Molecular genetic studies in the neuropsychiatric disorders. Trends Neurosci 12:130, 1989

MARTIN JB: Molecular genetics in neurology. Ann Neurol vol. 34, 1993

MEINDL A et al: Norrie disease is caused by mutations in an extracellular protein resembling C-terminal globular domain of mucins. Nature Genet 2:139, 1992

MEISSEN GJ et al: Predictive testing for Huntington's disease with use of a linked DNA marker. N Engl J Med 318:535, 1988

MITCHISON HM et al: Fine genetic mapping of the Batten disease locus (CLN3) by haplotype analysis and demonstration of allelic association with chromosome 16p microsatellite loci. Genomics 16:455, 1993

PENTAO L et al: Charcot-Marie-Tooth type-1A duplication appears to arise from recombination at repeat sequences flanking the 1.5 Mb monomer unit. Nature Genet 2:292, 1992

PETTEGREW JW et al: ^{31}P nuclear magnetic resonance studies of phosphoglyceride metabolism in developing and degenerating brain: Preliminary observations. J Neuropathol Exp Neurol 46:419, 1987

POSNER EM et al: Localization of cognitive operations in the human brain. Science 240:1627, 1988

REINER O et al: Isolation of a Miller-Dieker lissencephaly gene containing G-protein β-subunit-like repeats. Nature 364:717, 1993

ROSEN DR et al: Mutations in Cu/Zn superoxide dismutase gene are associated with familial amyotrophic lateral sclerosis. Nature 362:59, 1993

REIMAN EM et al: Neuroanatomical correlates of anticipatory anxiety. Science 243:1071, 1989

ROWE CC et al: Localization of epileptic foci with postictal single photon emission computed tomography. Ann Neurol 26:660, 1989

SHULMAN RG et al: Nuclear magnetic resonance imaging and spectroscopy of human brain function. Proc Natl Acad Sci USA 90:3127, 1993

SNYDER SH: Drug and neurotransmitter receptors: New perspectives with clinical relevance. JAMA 261:3126, 1989

——, BREDT DS: Biological roles of nitric oxide. Sci Amer May 1992:68

STRAUTNIEKS S et al: Pelizaeus-Merzbacher disease: Detection of mutations Thr 181-Pro and Leu 223-Pro in the proteolipid protein gene, and prenatal diagnosis. Am J Hum Genet 51:871, 1992

TASSABEHJI M et al: Waardenburg's syndrome patients have mutations in the human homologue of the Pax-3 paired box gene. Nature 355:635, 1992

TROFATTER JA et al: A novel Moesin-like, Ezrin-like, Radixin-like gene is a candidate for the neurofibromatosis-2 tumor suppressor. Cell 72:791, 1993

VULPE C et al: Isolation of a candidate gene for Menkes disease and evidence that it encodes a copper-transporting ATPase. Nature Genet 3:273, 1993

WAGSTAFF J et al: Maternal but not paternal transmission of 15q11-13-linked nondeletion syndrome leads to phenotypic expression. Nature Genet 1:291, 1992

section 1 The central nervous system

365 IMAGING OF THE NERVOUS SYSTEM

KENNETH R. DAVIS / JOSEPH B. MARTIN

Advances in imaging have revolutionized the ability to visualize brain and spinal cord lesions that cause neurologic dysfunction. These developments have followed the application to clinical problems of computed tomography (CT) in the 1970s, magnetic resonance imaging (MRI) in the 1980s, and positron emission tomography (PET) and single-photon emission computed tomography (SPECT) in the past decade. Magnetic resonance spectroscopy (MRS), as well as MR perfusion and diffusion studies, have promise for the study of function in the central nervous system (CNS) like that currently possible with PET and SPECT.

COMPUTED TOMOGRAPHY CT scanning provides a sensitive and reproducible method for evaluating suspected lesions in the CNS. It has been replaced by MRI as the procedure of choice for imaging of the brain and spinal cord, although it remains more widely available than MRI. Its principal utility is when rapid information about the state of the CNS is desired, and it is particularly important for decisions related to emergent surgical versus medical management of patients with the sudden onset of a neurologic deficit. Such conditions include acute head or spinal trauma, stroke where a differentiation between hemorrhage and infarction is important, and other circumstances where a decision as to immediate operative intervention is important. CT continues to have an advantage over MRI in emergency settings in patients with acute neurologic deterioration. It has high specificity, particularly for the demonstration of acute hemorrhage, where its imaging capacity exceeds that of MRI.

CT is also widely used for the evaluation of lesions that involve bone, such as metastatic disease at the base of the skull. However, the radionuclide bone scan provides a more sensitive generalized evaluation for bone metastases than CT or MRI. Calcification within lesions of the brain is demonstrated best by CT rather than MRI. CT is also the better imaging method for fractures of the face, temporal bone, and base of the skull. It is also an important imaging technique for evaluating fractures of the spine, although soft tissue encroachment upon the spinal cord is better visualized by MRI.

MAGNETIC RESONANCE IMAGING MRI is useful in the following circumstances:

1 Screening for metastatic disease. With the administration of intravenous MRI contrast material containing gadolinium, metastatic tumors can be visualized within the brain parenchyma, as well as primary tumors that cause a breakdown of the blood-brain barrier (Fig. 365-1). Imaging with gadolinium-DTPA is more sensitive for these conditions than noncontrast MR or CT with contrast. It is also preferred for visualization of pituitary tumors, acoustic neurinomas (Fig. 365-2), and other posterior fossa tumors, where CT artifacts from dental fillings on coronal scans of the sellar region and from nearby bony structures in the posterior fossa may prevent clear delineation of the lesion.

2 Imaging of demyelinating diseases such as multiple sclerosis (MS) and other white matter disorders of the brain and spinal cord (Fig. 365-3). It is possible to visualize small (2 to 5 mm) white matter lesions and to watch their progress over time. Contrast enhancement may make it possible to determine the acute perivascular involvement of new active lesions in MS. It is also the method of choice for evaluation of the leukodystrophies and for other white matter diseases such as senescent white matter ischemia (leukoariosis or Binswanger's disease) (see Chap. 368).

3 Screening for the presence of arteriovenous malformation (AVM) and aneurysms, particularly when family members at risk require evaluation (Fig. 365-4). MRI is followed by angiography if more detailed visualization is necessary in preparation for surgical intervention, or if the findings are equivocal. Development of MRI methods for evaluation of blood flow (MR angiography) promises to improve the ability to delineate blood flow and vascular lesions, including encroachment upon the lumen by atheromatous plaques in the carotid and vertebral basilar systems (Fig. 365-5).

A   B

FIGURE 365-1 Cerebral metastases. Magnetic resonance scan of the brain showing many more obvious enhancing lung metastases on the T1-weighted image (*arrows*) with intravenous contrast material (A) than on the T2-weighted image prior to contrast injection (B).

A   B

FIGURE 365-2 Acoustic neurinoma. MRI with intravenous contrast material clearly depicts the intracanalicular (*arrow*) and cerebellopontine angle cistern (*double arrows*) components of an acoustic neurinoma on axial (*A*) and coronal (*B*) views. (*Courtesy of R.G. Gonzalez, M.D.*)

A   B   C

FIGURE 365-3 Multiple sclerosis. *A*. Proton-density MRI reveals multiple periventricular hyperintense multiple sclerosis plaques. T2-weighted MRI of the spine shows a hyperintense plaque within the conus medullaris (*B*) and the upper cervical cord (*C*), respectively (*arrows*), in different patients. (*Courtesy of S. Sweriduk, M.D.*)

4 Evaluation of congenital and developmental abnormalities of the CNS. These include the Chiari malformation, porencephalic cysts, mesial temporal sclerosis (as a cause of epilepsy), as well as a variety of inherited abnormalities affecting the CNS (e.g., tuberous sclerosis).

5 Detection of posterior fossa vascular lesions. Small lacunes can be visualized within the brainstem that are not visible on CT scan (see Chap. 368). It is also the procedure of choice for the demonstration of small hemorrhages more than several days old in the posterior fossa. MR angiography is capable of visualizing basilar and vertebral artery flow (Fig. 365-5).

6 Lesions intrinsic to the spinal cord. Particularly advantageous is the ability to examine the entire spinal cord and canal, a technique that has led to improved management, particularly of thoracic disc syndromes. Myelopathy should be evaluated first with an MRI to differentiate intramedullary from extramedullary lesions. Metastatic disease affecting the spinal cord from an epidural location is easily visualized by MRI. It is also the best method for the demonstration of intrinsic spinal cord lesions including tumors (Fig. 365-6), syringomyelia, and areas of demyelination (Fig. 365-3). Use of intravenous contrast material may provide increased sensitivity or improved characterization of a lesion (Fig. 365-7). As compared to the myelo-

gram, MRI allows visualization within and around the entire cord. The postmyelography CT scan is limited in the full evaluation of the spine because a large number of slices, and hence excessive time, are required. MRI is the choice for acute spinal cord syndromes caused by extramedullary lesions, including epidural abscess and metastases. Leptomeningeal metastases are also best evaluated by gadolinium-enhanced MR scans. Osteomyelitis of the spine and secondary abscess are readily visualized by MRI (Fig. 365-8).

7 Although MRI is useful in the evaluation of all vertebral disc and spondylosis problems, it is particularly valuable for patients who have had previous back surgery. Following the administration of intravenous contrast material, it is possible to visualize extradural granulation tissue and to determine whether fibrosis (scarring) or recurrent disc protrusion is contributing to root symptoms. Fibrous granulation tissue usually shows early enhancement following intravenous contrast material, whereas a disc fragment may show delayed slight enhancement 15 to 20 min after injection.

8 Developmental lesions of the spinal cord such as syringomyelia, tethered cord, lipomas, and cavernous hemangiomas. MRI can demonstrate vascular lesions that subsequently may require angiography for definition, but may also demonstrate small intramedullary lesions that are not visible on the angiogram.

FIGURE 365-4   Cerebral aneurysm. MR angiography indicates the presence of a large aneurysm originating from the left internal carotid artery. A, aneurysm. Single arrow: left carotid artery. Double arrows: right carotid artery. Angle arrowhead: basilar artery. Double arrowheads: vertebral arteries. (*Courtesy of D. Mikulis, M.D.*)

However, the problems of taking care of patients in the MRI scanner, particularly those who are unconscious on life-support systems, who have gunshot wounds, or who are in MRI-incompatible tongs or halos for spinal traction or immobilization, limit the use of MRI. In these circumstances, it may be necessary to obtain a myelogram performed with a water-soluble, nonionic contrast material that permits a subsequent CT-myelogram.

MYELOGRAPHY   If the MRI is insufficient to account for the clinical presentation, it may be necessary to perform a myelogram or CT-myelogram in which a water-soluble, nonionic contrast material is instilled into the subarachnoid space. Films are usually taken at the time of contrast injection and followed by a CT scan of the appropriate regions. The procedure is particularly useful in cervical spondylosis where an MRI may not demonstrate detail of a herniated

FIGURE 365-5   Basilar artery stenosis. MR angiogram of the vertebral basilar circulation showing stenosis of the midbasilar artery (*arrow*) with turbulent flow artifact above the stenosis. Double arrows: vertebral arteries. Arrowhead: normal lower basilar artery. (*Courtesy of Gilbert Vezina, M.D.*)

A   B

FIGURE 365-6   Ependymoma. *A.* T1-weighted sagittal MRI of the cervical spine made without intravenous contrast shows expansion of the cervical cord by an ependymoma (*arrow*) with mixed hypointense signal intensities. *B.* Following intravenous injection of gadolinium-DTPA contrast, the T1 image shows enhancement of a portion of the tumor (*double arrows*) that would be most likely to yield a positive biopsy.

disc or osteophyte. The safety of new nonionic, water-soluble contrast materials has made myelography a more feasible procedure associated with less risk. Iophendylate myelography, no longer performed, did not permit subsequent CT evaluation. Furthermore, residual iophendylate after myelography produced artifacts on subsequent MR scans. A CT-myelogram may be particularly useful in cervical disc disease and spondylosis to demonstrate narrowing of the neural foramen and to differentiate an osteophyte (hard disc) from soft disc material, if this is not optimally visualized on MRI. For tumors of the vertebral foramen, such as neurofibromas, a myelogram and CT-myelogram are not often necessary, given the availability of MRI and use of intravenous contrast material (see Fig. 365-7). Seeding of tumors along roots in the cauda equina is often visualized on MRI, but such tumors may be too small to be identified or not enhance with intravenous contrast material. In this circumstance, a myelogram followed by a CT-myelogram may be the best choice. Herniated lumbar disc is usually detected by MRI (Fig. 365-9), but some physicians still prefer to have the anatomic details confirmed by CT and myelography prior to surgery. If the MRI is normal or equivocal, a myelogram or CT-myelogram may demonstrate enlarged veins in cases of suspected spinal AVM prior to deciding on spinal angiography. MRI may detect flow voids of the AVM and an abnormal signal within the cord. Where AVM is suspected a CT-myelogram followed by a spinal angiogram is the next step after an unremarkable MRI. Finally, a CT-myelogram may be the examination of choice in spinal cord injury where ferromagnetic metal stabilization has been used and MRI-incompatible life-support systems are required. In these circumstances, it is difficult to perform an adequate MRI.

INTERVENTIONAL RADIOLOGY   It is now possible to navigate into small vessels using maneuverable microcatheters and to visualize the vasculature and tip of the microcatheter by high-resolution, digital fluoroscopic equipment with real-time roadmapping capabilities. The decrease in the time required for microcatheter entry and visualization of target vessels results in faster studies at lower risk. The studies are usually performed by transfemoral retrograde catheterization using specialized coaxial microcatheters that can enter small vessels in the distribution of the anterior, middle, and posterior cerebral, vertebral, basilar, external carotid, or spinal circulations. This technique, along

FIGURE 365-7 Neurofibroma. T1-weighted axial MRI of the spine through the D2-3 neural foramen reveals a hypointense foraminal and extraforaminal neurofibroma (*arrow*) extending into the left paraspinal region (*A*) that enhances (*double arrows*) with intravenous contrast (*B*).

FIGURE 365-8 Osteomyelitis of the spine. T2-weighted sagittal MRI indicates hyperintense signal of the remaining D11-12 disc space (*arrow*) between the collapsed, slightly hyperintense surrounding vertebral bodies. These findings are caused by disc space infection and surrounding osteomyelitis. Posterior extension of the epidural mass represents epidural granulation tissue and abscess (*arrowhead*).

with availability of polymerizing glues such as *n*-butyl-cyanoacrylate, microcoils, and various particulate agents, such as polyvinyl alcohol (PVA) and gelfoam, makes endovascular embolization treatment of AVMs possible. Treatment is usually partial, to facilitate surgical resection, but occasionally is primary and definitive. The development of detachable balloons that are attached to microcatheters has made possible the endovascular treatment of fistulas, such as carotid-cavernous or vertebral-venous fistulas. Detachable balloons and platinum coils, such as the thermoelectric detachable type, can be used to occlude intracranial and cavernous aneurysms or the parent feeding vessel. Temporary inflation of nondetachable balloons is used to predict deficiencies of neurologic function that may follow permanent surgical or balloon occlusion of vessels. Selective micro-catheterization of a vessel supplying an AVM followed by injection of amobarbital also can be used to test for adverse neurologic effect prior to embolization. Nondetachable balloons may be used to dilate and treat certain cases of vasospasm secondary to subarachnoid hemorrhage from an aneurysm. Finally, preoperative embolization is often used to reduce vascularity in tumors such as meningiomas, glomus jugulare, and angiofibromas prior to surgical removal.

POSITRON EMISSION TOMOGRAPHY PET is based upon three-dimensional reconstruction of brain sections using positron-emitting radionuclides. By utilization of a number of individual radionuclides and radiolabeled moieties, it provides an opportunity to measure quantitatively: regional cerebral blood flow, blood volume, oxygen metabolism, glucose transport and metabolism, and neurotransmitter metabolism; and it permits neurotransmitter receptor localization. PET can provide spatial resolution approaching 3 to 5 mm definition in sequential slices.

Cerebrovascular disease In acute ischemic injury to the brain, PET studies demonstrate functional alterations in blood flow and oxygen metabolism when the CT scan may be normal; however, the difficulty in obtaining emergency PET studies limits its usefulness in this setting. MRI scans do show acute changes in stroke more readily than CT and are now widely used. In the assessment of long-term neurologic dysfunction after a stroke, PET scanning with deoxyglucose may show focal abnormalities that extend well beyond the lesions seen on CT or MRI. Analysis in such circumstances may provide insight into neural connections important for cognition.

Epilepsy The PET application most useful in epilepsy is assessment of glucose metabolism by measurement of brain uptake and phosphorylation of [18F]fluorodeoxyglucose (FDG). The methods are based on those developed by Sokoloff and colleagues for 2-deoxyglucose autoradiography in tissue sections. The PET scan summates approximately 40 min of local cerebral glucose metabolism and allows assessment of regional variations. PET studies have been most useful in patients with focal seizures. About 70 percent of patients with partial (focal) seizures that are refractory to medical treatment show zones of decreased glucose metabolism in the interictal state. The site of hypometabolism correlates with the epileptic focus in many patients. The same region often shows enhanced glucose metabolism if it is measured during a seizure discharge. In patients with temporal lobe seizures, it is common to find hypometabolism in one lobe.

The application of FDG-PET to evaluation of epilepsy patients undergoing consideration for surgical treatment is useful for confirming the unilaterality of sites producing electrical discharges and, in

A   B

FIGURE 365-9 Herniated and extruded disc at L5-S1. *A.* The sagittal proton density MRI shows the abnormal hypointense disc (*arrow*) producing a large extradural defect. *B.* Using a 110-degree flip angle, the axial multiplanar gradient echo image shows the disc lateralized to the left (*double arrows*) compressing the S1 root sleeve and thecal sac as well as extruding caudally into the lateral recess of S1.

some cases, rendering intracerebral recordings unnecessary (Fig. 365-10).

Neurodegenerative diseases Parkinson's nigrostriatal disease, caused by degeneration of the dopaminergic nigrostriatal pathway, can be demonstrated by [^{18}F]6-fluoro-L-dopa (^{18}F-FD) and PET. Decreased accumulation of ^{18}F-FD occurs in the striatum in Parkinson's disease and during normal aging. 6-Fluoro-L-dopa is decarboxylated to 6-fluoro-L-dopamine by the enzyme aromatic L-amino acid

FIGURE 365-10 Preoperative CT, MRI, and FDG-PET images of a patient with infantile spasms (epilepsy). Right side of the brain is to the viewer's left. CT and MRI failed to show abnormalities. Interictal PET studies revealed right occipitotemporal hypometabolism, matching the surface EEG localization of interictal discharges. (*Used with permission of Harry Chugani and Annals of Neurology.*)

decarboxylase, and the product then enters nerve terminals. PET allows visualization of the entrapped labeled dopamine. Decreased dopamine levels have been demonstrated in patients with Parkinson's disease induced by 1-methyl-4-phenyl-1,2,3,6-tetrahydropyridine and in asymptomatic drug addicts exposed to the drug, who presumably have subclinical degeneration of the nigrostriatal pathway.

Abnormalities also can be detected by FDG-PET in the basal ganglia in Huntington's disease (decreased metabolism) and in the brainstem and cerebellum in degenerative diseases such as olivopontocerebellar degeneration and Friedreich's ataxia (decreased metabolism). Decreased oxygen extraction and metabolism in the cerebral cortex may be demonstrated in Alzheimer's disease and in schizophrenia. Abnormalities in dopamine receptors have also been documented in schizophrenia. PET studies are also valuable in neuropsychological studies.

Although PET is at present primarily a research tool, its increasing availability in medical centers for cardiac imaging (see Chap. 191) makes likely more widespread application to other neurologic and psychiatric disease.

SINGLE-PHOTON EMISSION COMPUTED TOMOGRAPHY

SPECT depends on gamma-emitting radionuclides attached to molecules that can readily cross the blood-brain barrier. SPECT allows for concurrent blood flow determination and visualization of neurotransmitter receptors. For example, [^{123}I]isopropyl amphetamine (IMP) and [^{99m}Tc]d, 1-hexamethyl-propylene-amine-oxime–labeled iodoamphetamine have been used to demonstrate abnormalities in epilepsy, Alzheimer's disease, and Parkinson's disease. However, present SPECT technology is relatively nonquantitative and insensitive in demonstrating changes, and its spatial resolution is considerably less than that of PET. On the other hand, SPECT is less expensive and more widely available. It is now widely acknowledged as a potentially important diagnostic tool for differentiation of dementia caused by Alzheimer's disease from that caused by vascular disease (multi-infarct dementia) (see Chap. 25).

MAGNETIC RESONANCE SPECTROSCOPY

MRS offers the potential of assessing brain function at metabolic and molecular levels. MRS uses naturally occurring nonradioactive measurements of ^{31}P, ^{13}C, ^{23}Na, ^{7}Li, and ^{1}H. The ^{31}P MR spectrum can detect tissue concentrations of the phosphomonoesters phosphocholine and inorganic orthophosphate, the phosphodiesters glycerol-3-phosphoethanolamine and glycerol-3-phosphocholine, the triphosphate ATP, and other phosphorus-containing molecules including phosphocreatinine. The ^{31}P MR spectrum gives quantitative analysis of these compounds in vivo with the potential of three-dimensional resolution within the brain. ^{1}H spectroscopy offers the ability to measure lactate concentrations and neuronal markers such as *N*-acetyl aspartate. At present, much of the work in this area is experimental.

MAGNETIC SOURCE IMAGING

Magnetic source imaging (MSI) is based on electromagnetic field shifts created by brain electrical activity. MSI provides a new, still largely experimental method to map activity in the brain.

REFERENCES

ATLAS SW (ed): *Magnetic Resonance Imaging of the Brain and Spine.* New York, Raven, 1991

CHUGANI HT et al: Infantile spasms: I. PET identifies focal cortical dysgenesis in cryptogenic cases for surgical treatment. Ann Neurol 27:406, 1990

DUARA R et al: Positron emission tomography in Alzheimer's disease. Neurology 36:879, 1986

EDELMAN R, HESSELINK, J (eds): *Clinical Magnetic Resonance Imaging.* Philadelphia, Saunders, 1990

———, WARACH S: Magnetic resonance imaging. N Engl J Med 328:708, 1993

FELIX R et al: Brain tumors: MR imaging with gadolinium-DTPA. Radiology 156:681, 1985

JOHNSON KA et al: Single photon emission computed tomography in Alzheimer's disease: Abnormal iofetamine I 123 uptake reflects dementia severity. Arch Neurol 45:392, 1988

JUNCK L et al: PET imaging of human gliomas with ligands for the peripheral benzodiazepine binding site. Ann Neurol 26:752, 1989

LATCHAW RE (ed): *MR and CT Imaging of the Head, Neck and Spine.* 2d ed. Chicago. Mosby Year Book, 1991

LEE SH et al (eds): *Cranial MRI and CT,* 3d ed. New York, McGraw-Hill, 1992

McCARTHY G et al: Echo-planar magnetic resonance imaging studies of frontal cortex activation during word generation in humans. Proc Natl Acad Sci USA 90:4952, 1993

McGEER PL et al: Positron emission tomography in patients with clinically diagnosed Alzheimer's disease. Can Med Assoc J 134:597, 1986

MODIC MT et al (eds): *Magnetic Resonance Imaging of the Spine.* Chicago, Year Book, 1989

PETTEGREW JW et al: ^{31}P nuclear magnetic resonance study of the brain in Alzheimer's disease. J Neuropath Exp Neurol 47:235, 1988

PHELPS ME, MAZZIOTTA JC: Positron emission tomography: Human brain function and biochemistry. Science 228:799, 1985

PRICHARD JW, BRASS LM: New anatomical and functional imaging methods. Ann Neurol 32:395, 1992

QUAST MJ et al: The evolution of acute stroke recorded by multimodal magnetic resonance imaging. Magn Reson Imaging 11:465, 1993

ROSS JS et al: Magnetic resonance angiography of the extracranial carotid arteries and intracranial vessels: A review. Neurology 39:1369, 1989

SMITH ME et al: Clinical worsening in multiple sclerosis is associated with increased frequency and area of gadopentetate dimeglumine enhancing magnetic resonance imaging lesions. Ann Neurol 33:480, 1993

WILLIAMS AL, HAUGHTON VM (eds): *Cranial Computed Tomography. A Comprehensive Text.* St. Louis, Mosby, 1985

WONG DF et al: Positron emission tomography reveals elevated D$_2$ dopamine receptors in drug-naive schizophrenics. Science 234:1558, 1986

ZAWADZKI MB, NORMAN D: *Magnetic Resonance Imaging of the Central Nervous System.* New York, Raven, 1987

---

366   ELECTROPHYSIOLOGIC STUDIES OF THE CENTRAL AND PERIPHERAL NERVOUS SYSTEMS

MICHAEL J. AMINOFF

ELECTROENCEPHALOGRAPHY

The electrical activity of the brain (the electroencephalogram or EEG) is easily recorded from electrodes placed on the scalp. The potential difference between pairs of electrodes on the scalp (bipolar derivation) or between individual scalp electrodes and a relatively inactive common reference point (referential derivation) is amplified and displayed on paper or the screen of an oscilloscope. The findings depend on the patient's age and level of arousal. The rhythmic activity normally recorded represents the postsynaptic potentials of vertically oriented pyramidal cells of the cerebral cortex, and is characterized by its frequency. In normal awake adults lying quietly with the eyes closed, an 8-13 Hz alpha rhythm is seen posteriorly in the EEG, intermixed with a variable amount of generalized faster (beta) activity, and it is attenuated when the eyes are opened (Fig. 366-1). During drowsiness, the alpha rhythm is also attenuated; with light sleep, slower activity in the theta (4–7 Hz) and delta (<4 Hz) ranges becomes more conspicuous.

The EEG is best recorded from several different electrode arrangements (montages) in turn, and activating procedures are generally undertaken in an attempt to provoke abnormalities. Such procedures commonly include hyperventilation (for 3 or 4 min), photic stimulation, sleep, and the deprivation of sleep on the night prior to the recording.

Electroencephalography is relatively inexpensive and may aid clinical management in several different contexts.

THE EEG AND EPILEPSY   The EEG is most useful in evaluating patients with suspected epilepsy. The presence of *electrographic seizure activity,* i.e., of abnormal, repetitive, rhythmic activity having an abrupt onset and termination, clearly establishes the diagnosis. The absence of such electrocerebral accompaniment does not exclude a seizure disorder, however, because there may be no change in the scalp-recorded EEG during simple or complex partial seizures. It is often not possible to obtain an EEG during clinical events that may represent seizures, especially when such events occur unpredictably or infrequently. The development of portable equipment to record the EEG continuously on cassettes for 24 h or longer in ambulatory patients

FIGURE 366-1 *A*. Normal EEG showing a posteriorly situated 9-Hz alpha rhythm that attenuates with eye opening. *B*. Abnormal EEG showing irregular diffuse slow activity in an obtunded patient with encephalitis. *C*. Irregular slow activity in the right central region, on a diffusely slowed background, in a patient with a right parietal glioma. *D*. Periodic complexes occurring once every second in a patient with Creutzfeldt-Jakob disease. Horizontal calibration: 1 s; vertical calibration: 200 μV in A, 300 μV in other panels. (*From Aminoff, 1992.*) In this and the following figure, electrode placements are indicated at the left of each panel and accord with the international 10:20 system. A, earlobe; C, central; F, frontal; Fp, frontal polar; P, parietal; T, temporal; O, occipital. Right-sided placements are indicated by even numbers, left-sided placements by odd numbers, and midline placements by Z.

has made it easier to capture the electrocerebral accompaniments of such clinical episodes, and monitoring by this means is sometimes helpful in confirming that seizures are occurring, characterizing the nature of clinically equivocal episodes, and determining the frequency of epileptic events.

The EEG findings may also be helpful in the interictal period by showing certain abnormalities that are strongly supportive of a diagnosis of epilepsy. Such *epileptiform activity* consists of bursts of abnormal discharges containing spikes or sharp waves. The presence of epileptiform activity is not specific for epilepsy, but it has a much greater prevalence in epileptics than normal subjects. When epileptiform activity is found in the EEG of a patient with episodic behavioral disturbances that clinically might be epileptic in nature, the likelihood that epilepsy is the correct diagnosis is markedly increased.

The EEG findings also have been used in classifying seizure disorders and selecting appropriate anticonvulsant medication for individual patients (Fig. 366-2). The episodic generalized spike-wave activity that occurs both during and between seizures in patients with typical absences (petit mal epilepsy) contrasts with the normal findings, focal interictal epileptiform discharges, or ictal patterns found in patients with complex partial seizures. These latter seizures may have no correlates in the scalp-recorded EEG or may be associated with abnormal rhythmic activity of variable frequency, a localized or generalized distribution, and a stereotyped pattern that varies with the patient. Focal or lateralized epileptogenic lesions are important to recognize, especially if surgical treatment is contemplated. Intensive long-term monitoring of clinical behavior and the EEG is required for operative candidates, however, and this generally also involves recording from intracranially placed electrodes (which may be subdural, extradural, or intracerebral in location).

The findings in the routine scalp-recorded EEG may indicate the prognosis of seizure disorders: in general, a normal EEG implies a better prognosis than otherwise, whereas an abnormal background or profuse epileptiform activity suggests a poor outlook. The EEG findings are not helpful in determining which patients with head injuries, stroke, or brain tumors will go on to develop seizures, because in such circumstances epileptiform activity is commonly encountered regardless of whether seizures occur. The EEG findings

are sometimes used to determine whether anticonvulsant medication can be discontinued in epileptic patients who have been seizure-free for several years, but the findings provide only a general guide to prognosis: further seizures may occur after withdrawal of anticonvulsant medication despite a normal EEG or, conversely, may not occur despite a continuing EEG abnormality. The decision to discontinue anticonvulsant medication is made on clinical grounds, and the EEG does not have a useful role in this context except for providing guidance when there is clinical ambiguity or the patient requires reassurance about a particular course of action.

The EEG has no role in the management of tonic-clonic status epilepticus except when there is clinical uncertainty whether seizures are continuing in a comatose patient. In patients treated by pentobarbital-induced coma for refractory status epilepticus, the EEG findings are useful in indicating the level of anesthesia and whether seizures are occurring. During status epilepticus, the EEG shows repeated electrographic seizures or continuous spike-wave discharges. In nonconvulsive status epilepticus, a disorder which may not be recognized unless an EEG is performed, the EEG may also show continuous spike-wave activity (''spike-wave stupor'') or, less commonly, repetitive electrographic seizures (complex partial status epilepticus).

THE EEG AND COMA The EEG tends to become slower as consciousness is depressed, regardless of the underlying cause (Fig. 366-1). Other findings may also be present and may suggest diagnostic possibilities, as when electrographic seizures are found or there is a focal abnormality indicating a structural lesion. The response of the EEG to external stimulation is helpful prognostically because electrocerebral responsiveness implies a lighter level of coma than a nonreactive EEG. Serial records provide a better guide to prognosis than a single record and supplement the clinical examination in following the course of events. As the depth of coma increases, the EEG becomes nonreactive and may show a burst-suppression pattern, with bursts of mixed-frequency activity separated by intervals of relative cerebral inactivity. In other instances there is a reduction in amplitude of the EEG until eventually electrocerebral activity cannot be detected. Such electrocerebral silence does not necessarily reflect irreversible brain damage, because it may occur in hypothermic patients or with drug overdose. The prognosis of electrocerebral

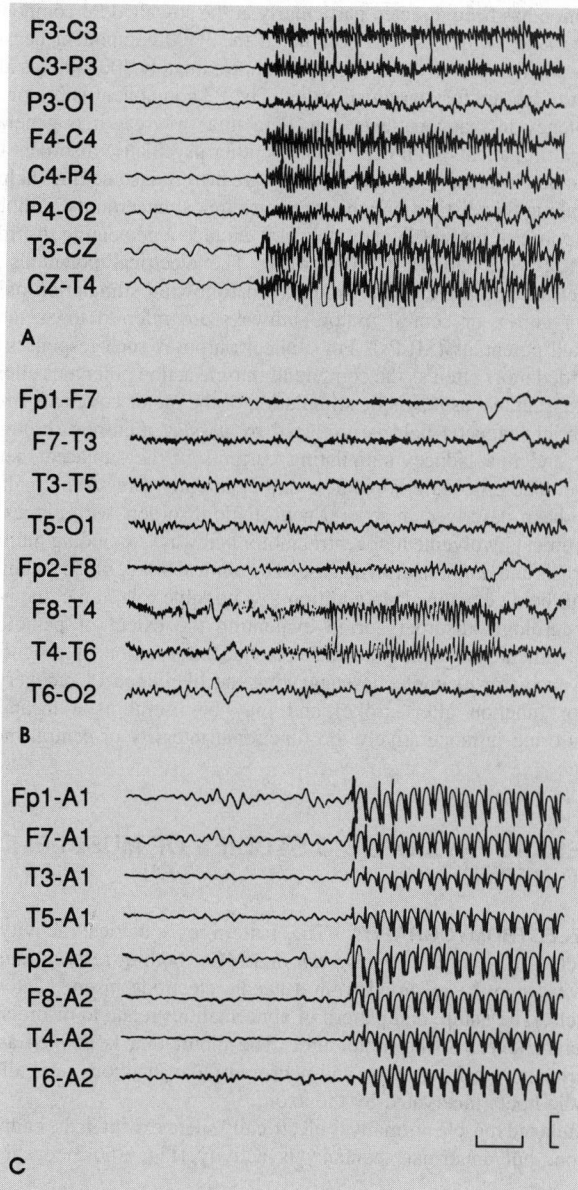

FIGURE 366-2 Electrographic seizures. *A.* Onset of a tonic seizure showing generalized repetitive sharp activity with synchronous onset over both hemispheres. *B.* Burst of repetitive spikes occurring with sudden onset in the right temporal region during a clinical spell characterized by transient impairment of external awareness. *C.* Generalized 3-Hz spike-wave activity occurring synchronously over both hemispheres during an absence (petit mal) attack. Horizontal calibration: 1 s; vertical calibration: 400 μV in A, 200 μV in B, and 750 μV in C. (*From Aminoff, 1992.*)

silence, when recorded using an adequate technique, depends upon the clinical context in which it is found. In patients with severe cerebral anoxia, for example, electrocerebral silence in a technically satisfactory record implies that useful cognitive recovery will not occur.

The EEG is usually normal in patients with locked-in syndrome and helps in distinguishing this disorder from the comatose state with which it is sometimes confused clinically.

THE EEG IN OTHER NEUROLOGIC DISORDERS In the developed countries, CT scanning and MRI have taken the place of EEG as a noninvasive means of screening for focal structural abnormalities of the brain, such as tumors, infarcts, or hematomas (Fig. 366-1). Nonetheless, the EEG is still used for this purpose in many parts of the world, although infratentorial or slowly expanding lesions may fail to cause any abnormalities. Focal slow-wave disturbances,

a localized loss of electrocerebral activity, or more generalized electrocerebral disturbances are common findings, but provide no reliable indication about the nature of the underlying pathology.

The EEG is also helpful for diagnostic purposes when it reveals the characteristic but nonspecific abnormalities found in certain neurologic disorders. The presence of complexes occurring with a regular repetition rate (so-called periodic complexes) in dementing disorders, for example, supports a diagnosis of Creutzfeldt-Jakob disease (Fig. 366-1) or subacute sclerosing panencephalitis, depending upon the appearance and frequency of the complexes and the clinical context. Focal or lateralized periodic slow-wave complexes, sometimes with a sharpened outline, in patients with an acute encephalopathy suggest a diagnosis of herpes simplex encephalitis, and periodic lateralized epileptiform discharges are commonly found with acute hemispheric pathology such as a hematoma, abscess, or rapidly expanding tumor.

The EEG generally slows in metabolic encephalopathies, and triphasic waves may be present. The findings do not permit differentiation of the underlying metabolic disturbance but help to exclude other encephalopathic processes by indicating the diffuse extent of cerebral dysfunction.

The EEG findings in dementia are nonspecific and usually do not distinguish between the different causes of cognitive decline except in rare instances when Creutzfeldt-Jakob disease or subacute sclerosing panencephalitis is responsible. The EEG may be normal or diffusely slowed, and the EEG findings alone cannot indicate whether a patient is demented or distinguish between dementia and pseudodementia.

EVOKED POTENTIALS

SENSORY EVOKED POTENTIALS The noninvasive recording of spinal or cerebral potentials elicited by stimulation of specific afferent pathways is an important means of monitoring the functional integrity of these pathways, but does not indicate the pathologic basis of lesions involving them. Such evoked potentials (EPs) are so small compared to the background EEG activity that responses to a number of stimuli have to be recorded and averaged with a computer in order to permit their recognition and definition. The background EEG activity, which has no fixed temporal relationship to the stimulus, is averaged out by this procedure.

Visual evoked potentials (VEPs) are elicited by monocular stimulation with a reversing checkerboard pattern, and are recorded from the occipital region in the midline and on either side of the scalp. The component of major clinical importance is the so-called P100 response, a positive peak having a latency of approximately 100 ms. Its presence, latency, and symmetry over the two sides of the scalp are noted. Amplitude may also be measured, but changes in size are much less helpful for the recognition of pathology. VEPs are most useful in detecting dysfunction of the visual pathways anterior to the optic chiasm. In patients with acute severe optic neuritis the P100 is frequently lost or grossly attenuated; as clinical recovery occurs and visual acuity improves, the P100 is restored but with an increased latency that generally remains abnormally prolonged indefinitely. The VEP findings are therefore helpful in indicating previous or subclinical optic neuritis. They may also be abnormal with ocular abnormalities and with other causes of optic nerve disease, such as ischemia or compression by a tumor. Normal VEPs may be elicited by flash stimuli in patients with cortical blindness.

Brainstem auditory evoked potentials (BAEPs) are elicited by monaural stimulation with repetitive clicks, and are recorded between the vertex of the scalp and the mastoid process or ear-lobe. A series of potentials, designated by roman numerals, occur in the first 10 ms after the stimulus, and represent in part the sequential activation of different structures in the pathway between the auditory nerve (wave I) and the inferior colliculus (wave V) in the midbrain. The presence, latency, and interpeak latency of the first five positive potentials recorded at the vertex are evaluated. The findings are helpful in screening for acoustic neuromas, detecting brainstem pathology, and evaluating comatose patients. The BAEPs are normal in coma due to metabolic/toxic disorders or bihemispheric disease, but abnormal in the presence of brainstem pathology.

Somatosensory evoked potentials (SEPs) are recorded over the scalp and spine in response to electrical stimulation of a peripheral (mixed or cutaneous) nerve. The configuration, polarity, and latency of the responses depend on the nerve that is stimulated and on the recording arrangements. SEPs are used to evaluate proximal (otherwise inaccessible) portions of the peripheral nervous system and the integrity of the central somatosensory pathways.

Clinical utility of sensory evoked potentials   EP studies may detect and localize lesions in afferent pathways in the CNS. They have been used particularly to investigate patients with suspected multiple sclerosis, the diagnosis of which requires the recognition of lesions involving several different regions of the central white matter. In patients with clinical evidence of only one lesion, the electrophysiologic recognition of abnormalities in other sites helps to suggest or support the diagnosis, but does not establish it unequivocally. In patients with suspected multiple sclerosis (or other neurologic disorders) who have vague, ill-defined complaints, the organic basis of symptoms may be supported by the presence of EP abnormalities in the appropriate afferent pathway. MRI is also helpful in detecting lesions in patients with possible multiple sclerosis, but electrophysiologic studies are cheaper and monitor the functional rather than anatomic status of the afferent pathways under study. Moreover, the electrophysiologic studies occasionally reveal abnormalities missed by MRI or vice versa. The two techniques therefore complement each other. Normal electrophysiologic (or imaging) findings do not exclude multiple sclerosis when this is a clinical possibility. In established multiple sclerosis, the use of EP studies to follow the disorder or its response to treatment is of uncertain value and unjustified at the present time.

EP abnormalities occur in disorders other than multiple sclerosis that involve the afferent pathways under test. Even multimodality EP abnormalities are not specific for MS; they may occur in AIDS, Lyme disease, systemic lupus erythematosus, neurosyphilis, spinocerebellar degenerations, familial spastic paraplegia, and deficiency of vitamin E or B$_{12}$. The diagnostic utility of the electrophysiologic findings therefore depends upon the circumstances in which they are found. Abnormalities may aid in the localization of lesions to broad areas of the CNS, but attempts at precise localization on electrophysiologic grounds are misleading because the generators of many components of the EP are unknown.

The EP findings are sometimes of prognostic relevance. Bilateral loss of those SEP components that are generated in the cerebral cortex implies that cognition may not be regained in posttraumatic or postanoxic coma, and EP studies may also be useful in evaluating patients with suspected brain death. In patients with spinal cord injuries, SEPs have been used to indicate the completeness of the lesion—the presence or early return of a cortically generated response to stimulation of a nerve below the injured segment of the cord indicates an incomplete lesion and thus a better prognosis for functional recovery than otherwise. Intraoperative monitoring of function in neural structures placed at risk by the surgical procedure may permit the early recognition of dysfunction, but whether this enables any permanent deficit to be averted or minimized by alteration of the responsible operative manipulation has not been established.

Visual and auditory acuity have been determined by ophthalmologists and audiologists using EP techniques in patients whose age or mental state precludes their cooperation for behavioral testing.

COGNITIVE EVOKED POTENTIALS   Certain EP components depend upon the mental attention of the subject and the setting in which the stimulus occurs, rather than simply on the physical characteristics of the stimulus. Such "event-related" or "endogenous" potentials (ERPs) are related in some manner to the cognitive aspects of distinguishing an infrequently occurring target stimulus from other stimuli occurring more frequently. For clinical purposes,

attention has been directed particularly at the so-called P3 component of the ERP, which is also designated the P300 component because of its positive polarity and latency of approximately 300–400 ms after onset of an auditory target stimulus. The P3 component is prolonged in latency in many patients with dementia, whereas it is generally normal in patients with depression or other psychiatric disorders that might be mistaken for dementia. ERPs are therefore sometimes helpful in making this distinction when there is clinical uncertainty, although a response of normal latency does not exclude a dementing disorder.

MOTOR EVOKED POTENTIALS   The electrical potentials recorded from muscle or the spinal cord following stimulation of the motor cortex or central motor pathways are referred to as motor evoked potentials (MEPs). For clinical purposes such responses are recorded most often as the compound muscle action potentials elicited by transcutaneous magnetic stimulation of the motor cortex. A strong but brief magnetic field is produced by passing a current through a coil, and this induces stimulating currents in the subjacent neural tissue. The procedure is painless and apparently safe. Abnormalities have been described in several neurologic disorders with clinical or subclinical involvement of central motor pathways, including multiple sclerosis and motor neuron disease. The clinical utility of the technique is still being examined. In addition to a possible role in the diagnosis of neurologic disorders or in evaluating the extent of pathologic involvement, the technique may provide information of prognostic relevance (for example, in suggesting the likelihood of recovery of motor function after stroke) and may be useful as a means of monitoring intraoperatively the functional integrity of central motor tracts.

ELECTROPHYSIOLOGIC STUDIES OF MUSCLE AND NERVE

ELECTROMYOGRAPHY   The pattern of electrical activity in muscle (i.e., the *electromyogram* or EMG), both at rest and during activity, may be recorded from a needle electrode inserted into the muscle. The nature and pattern of abnormalities relate to disorders at different levels of the motor unit. The motor unit is defined as an anterior horn cell, its axon and neuromuscular junctions, and all the muscle fibers innervated by the axon.

Relaxed muscle normally is electrically silent except in the endplate region, but abnormal spontaneous activity (Fig. 366-3) occurs in

FIGURE 366-3   Activity recorded during EMG. *A.* Spontaneous fibrillation potentials and positive sharp waves. *B.* Complex repetitive discharges recorded in partially denervated muscle at rest. *C.* Normal triphasic motor unit action potential. *D.* Small, short-duration, polyphasic motor unit action potential such as is commonly encountered in myopathic disorders. *E.* Long-duration polyphasic motor unit action potential such as may be seen in neuropathic disorders.

various neuromuscular disorders. Fibrillation potentials and positive sharp waves (which reflect muscle fiber irritability) and complex repetitive discharges are most often—but not always—found in denervated muscle and may also occur after muscle injury and in certain myopathic disorders, especially inflammatory disorders such as polymyositis. Fasciculation potentials (which reflect the spontaneous activity of individual motor units) are characteristic of neuropathic disorders, especially those with degeneration of anterior horn cells (such as amyotrophic lateral sclerosis). Myotonic discharges—high-frequency discharges of potentials derived from single muscle fibers that wax and wane in amplitude and frequency—are the signature of myotonic disorders such as myotonic dystrophy or myotonia congenita, but occur occasionally in polymyositis or other, rarer, disorders.

Slight voluntary contraction of a muscle leads to activation of a small number of motor units. The potentials generated by any muscle fibers of these units that are within the pick-up range of the needle electrode will be recorded (Fig. 366-3). The parameters of normal motor unit action potentials depend on the muscle under study and age of the patient, but their duration is normally between 5 and 15 ms, amplitude is between 200 µV and 2 mV, and most are bi- or triphasic; the number of units activated depends on the degree of voluntary activity. The incidence of small, short-duration, polyphasic motor unit action potentials (i.e., having more than four phases) is usually increased in myopathic muscle, and an excessive number of units is activated for a specified degree of voluntary activity. By contrast the loss of motor units that occurs in neuropathic disorders leads to a reduction in number of units activated during a maximal contraction and an increase in their firing rate; the configuration and dimensions of the potentials may also be abnormal depending on the duration of the neuropathic process and on whether reinnervation has occurred.

Electromyography (EMG) enables disorders of the motor units to be detected and characterized as either neurogenic or myopathic. In neurogenic disorders, the pattern of affected muscles may localize the lesion to the anterior horn cells or to a specific site as the axons traverse a nerve root, limb plexus, and peripheral nerve to their terminal arborizations. The findings do not enable a specific etiologic diagnosis to be made, however, except in conjunction with the clinical findings and results of other laboratory studies.

The findings may provide a guide to the severity of an acute disorder of a peripheral or cranial nerve (by indicating whether denervation has occurred and the completeness of the lesion), and whether the pathologic process is active or progressive in chronic or degenerative disorders such as amyotrophic lateral sclerosis. Such information is important for prognostic purposes.

Various quantitative EMG approaches have been developed. The most common is to determine the mean duration and amplitude of 20 motor unit action potentials using a standardized technique. The technique of macro-EMG provides information about the number and size of muscle fibers in a larger volume of the motor unit territory, and has also been used to estimate the number of motor units in a muscle. Scanning EMG is a computer-based technique that has been used to study the topography of motor unit action potentials and, in particular, the spatial and temporal distribution of activity in individual units. Both of these latter approaches are of limited interest except to specialists and merit no further discussion. The technique of single-fiber EMG is of immediate clinical relevance, however, and is discussed separately below.

NERVE CONDUCTION STUDIES Recording of the electrical response of a muscle to stimulation of its motor nerve at two or more points along its course (Fig. 366-4) permits conduction velocity to be determined in the fastest-conducting motor fibers between the points of stimulation. Similarly, sensory nerve conduction studies are performed by determining the conduction velocity and amplitude of action potentials in sensory fibers when these fibers are stimulated at one point and the responses are recorded at another point along the course of the nerve. In adults, conduction velocity in the arms is

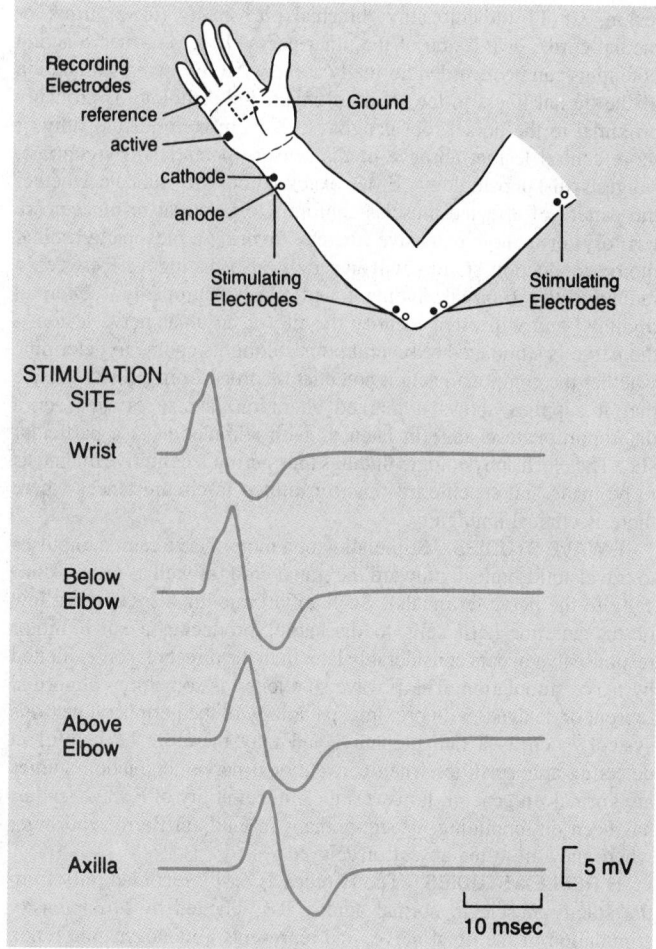

FIGURE 366-4 Arrangement for motor conduction studies of the ulnar nerve. Responses are recorded with a surface electrode from the abductor digiti minimi muscle to supramaximal stimulation of the nerve at different sites, and are shown in the lower panel. (*From Aminoff, 1987.*)

normally between 50 and 70 m/s, and in the legs is between 40 and 60 m/s.

Nerve conduction studies complement the EMG examination, enabling the presence and extent of peripheral nerve pathology to be determined. They are particularly helpful in determining whether sensory symptoms are arising from pathology proximal or distal to the dorsal root ganglia (in the former instance, peripheral sensory conduction studies will be normal) and whether neuromuscular dysfunction relates to peripheral nerve disease. In patients with a mononeuropathy, they are invaluable as a means of localizing a focal lesion, determining the extent and severity of the underlying pathology, providing a guide to prognosis, and detecting subclinical involvement of other peripheral nerves. They enable a polyneuropathy to be distinguished from a mononeuropathy multiplex when this is not possible clinically, an important distinction because of the etiological implications. Nerve conduction studies provide a means of following the progression and therapeutic response of peripheral nerve disorders, and may suggest the underlying pathologic basis in individual cases. Conduction velocity is often markedly slowed and conduction block may occur in the acquired demyelinating neuropathies, whereas conduction velocity is normal or slowed only mildly, sensory nerve action potentials are small or absent, and there is EMG evidence of denervation in axonal neuropathies.

The utility and complementary role of EMG and nerve conduction studies are best illustrated by reference to a common clinical problem. Numbness and paresthesias of the little finger and associated wasting of the intrinsic muscles of the hand may result from a spinal cord lesion, C8/T1 radiculopathy, brachial plexopathy (lower trunk or medial cord), or a lesion of the ulnar nerve. If sensory nerve action potentials can be recorded normally at the wrist following stimulation of the digital fibers in the affected finger, the pathology is probably proximal to the dorsal root ganglia, i.e., there is a radiculopathy or more central lesion; absence of the sensory potentials, by contrast, suggests distal pathology. EMG examination will indicate whether the pattern of affected muscles conforms to radicular or ulnar nerve territory, or is more extensive (thereby favoring a plexopathy); ulnar motor conduction studies will generally also distinguish between a radiculopathy (normal findings) and ulnar neuropathy (abnormal findings) and will often identify the site of an ulnar nerve lesion—the nerve is stimulated at several points along its course to determine whether the compound action potential recorded from a distal muscle that it supplies shows a marked alteration in size or area, or a disproportionate change in latency, with stimulation at a particular site. The electrophysiologic findings thus permit a definitive diagnosis to be made and specific treatment instituted in circumstances where there is clinical ambiguity.

F WAVE STUDIES   Stimulation of a motor nerve causes impulses to travel antidromically toward the spinal cord (as well as orthodromically to the nerve terminals). Such antidromic impulses cause a few of the anterior horn cells to discharge, producing a small motor response that occurs considerably later than the direct response elicited by nerve stimulation. The F wave so elicited is sometimes abnormal (absent or delayed) with proximal pathology of the peripheral nervous system, such as a radiculopathy, and may therefore be helpful in detecting abnormalities when conventional nerve conduction studies are normal. In general, however, the clinical utility of F wave studies has been disappointing, except perhaps in Guillain-Barré syndrome, where they are often absent or delayed.

H REFLEX STUDIES   The H reflex is easily recorded only from the soleus muscle in normal adults. It is elicited by low-intensity stimulation of the tibial nerve, and represents a monosynaptic reflex in which spindle (Ia) afferent fibers constitute the afferent arc and alpha motor axons the efferent pathway. The H reflexes are often absent bilaterally in elderly patients or with polyneuropathies, and may be lost unilaterally in S1 radiculopathies.

MUSCLE RESPONSE TO REPETITIVE NERVE STIMULATION The size of the electrical response of a muscle to supramaximal electrical stimulation of its motor nerve relates to the number of muscle fibers that are activated. Neuromuscular transmission can be tested by several different protocols, but the most helpful is to record with surface electrodes the electrical response of a muscle to supramaximal stimulation of its motor nerve by repetitive (2 to 3 Hz) shocks delivered before and at selected intervals after a maximal voluntary contraction.

There is normally little or no change in size of the compound muscle action potential following repetitive stimulation of a motor nerve at 2 to 3 Hz with stimuli delivered at intervals after voluntary contraction of the muscle for about 20 to 30 s, even though preceding activity in the junctional region influences the release of acetylcholine and thus the size of the endplate potentials elicited by a test stimulus. This is because more acetylcholine is normally released than is required to bring the motor endplate potentials to the threshold for generating muscle fiber action potentials. In disorders of neuromuscular transmission this safety factor is reduced. Thus, in myasthenia gravis repetitive stimulation, particularly at a rate of between 2 and 5 Hz, may lead to a depression of neuromuscular transmission, with a decrement in size of the response recorded from affected muscles. Similarly, immediately after a period of maximal voluntary activity, single or repetitive stimuli of the motor nerve may elicit larger muscle responses than before, indicating that more muscle fibers are responding. This postactivation facilitation of neuromuscular transmission is followed by a longer-lasting period of depression, maximal between 2 and 4 min after the conditioning period and lasting for as long as 10 min or so, during which responses are reduced in size.

Decrementing responses to repetitive stimulation at 2 to 5 Hz are common in myasthenia gravis but may also occur in the congenital myasthenic syndromes. In Lambert-Eaton myasthenic syndrome, in which there is defective release of acetylcholine at the neuromuscular junction, the compound muscle action potential elicited by a single stimulus is generally very small. With repetitive stimulation at rates of up to 10 Hz, the first few responses may decline in size, but subsequent responses increase. If faster rates of stimulation are used (20 to 50 Hz), the increment may be dramatic so that the amplitude of compound muscle action potentials eventually reaches a size that is several times larger than the initial response. In patients with botulism, the response to repetitive stimulation is similar to that in Lambert-Eaton syndrome, although the findings are somewhat more variable and not all muscles are affected.

SINGLE-FIBER ELECTROMYOGRAPHY   The technique of single-fiber EMG is particularly helpful in detecting disorders of neuromuscular transmission. A special needle electrode is placed within a muscle and positioned to record action potentials from two muscle fibers belonging to the same motor unit. The time interval between the two potentials will vary in consecutive discharges, and this is called the *neuromuscular jitter*. The jitter can be quantified as the mean difference between consecutive interpotential intervals, and is normally between 10 and 50 μs. This value is increased when neuromuscular transmission is disturbed for any reason, and in some instances impulses in individual muscle fibers may fail to occur because of impulse blocking at the neuromuscular junction. Single-fiber EMG is more sensitive than repetitive nerve stimulation or determination of acetylcholine receptor antibody levels in diagnosing myasthenia gravis.

Single-fiber EMG can also be used to determine mean fiber density of motor units (i.e., mean number of muscle fibers per motor unit within the recording area) and to estimate the number of motor units in a muscle, but this is of less immediate clinical relevance.

BLINK REFLEXES   Electrical or mechanical stimulation of the supraorbital nerve on one side leads to two separate reflex responses of the orbicularis oculi—an ipsilateral R1 response having a latency of approximately 10 ms and a bilateral R2 response with a latency in the order of 30 ms. The trigeminal and facial nerves constitute the afferent and efferent arcs of the reflex, respectively. Abnormalities of either nerve or intrinsic lesions of the medulla or pons may lead to uni- or bilateral loss of the response, and the findings may therefore be helpful in identifying or localizing such pathology.

TESTS OF AUTONOMIC FUNCTION

Noninvasive tests of autonomic function are becoming increasingly important for the recognition of small-fiber peripheral neuropathies and in defining central dysautonomias, such as the Shy-Drager syndrome. Invasive tests, such as microneurography, provide information of considerable academic importance, but because of their specialized nature and limited clinical utility they are not discussed further.

Tests of *heart-rate responses* to various maneuvers are easy to perform, safe, reproducible, and provide clinically relevant information. One such test is to record the heart-rate response to deep breathing for 1 min at a rate of approximately six breaths per minute. In normal persons a tachycardia occurs during inspiration and a bradycardia during expiration. The difference in heart rate between inspiration and expiration is age-dependent, but is usually more than about 15 beats per minute. Heart-rate variation of less than 10 is clearly abnormal, and suggests vagal dysfunction. The Valsalva ratio, which depends on both vagal and sympathetic function, is also a sensitive indicator of autonomic dysfunction. It is determined from the maximum heart rate generated during a forced expiratory maneuver and the slowest heart rate following the maneuver. It is conveniently recorded with an electrocardiograph—the longest interbeat interval after the maneuver is divided by the shortest interbeat interval during it. Another approach is to record the heart-rate changes that occur with change from a supine to erect posture; the heart rate increases in the first 15 s or so and then slows. The ratio of the heart rates or the R-R intervals at the 30th and 15th beats after standing, which is age-dependent, has therefore been used as an index of vagal function.

Sudomotor function has been evaluated in various ways. Perhaps the easiest is the thermoregulatory sweat test, in which the patient's body temperature is increased by 1°C by radiant heat from a heat cradle, and the presence and distribution of sweat is noted by a change in color of an indicator powder placed on the skin. This provides information about the integrity of pre- and postganglionic sympathetic fibers, and the distribution of abnormalities may suggest the underlying pathology. Because it is so time consuming, however, alternative approaches have been favored. One simple approach is to measure the skin potential in response to electrical stimulation. This depends upon activation of sweat glands, but is of limited utility because only an absent response, and not the latency or size of the response, indicates an abnormality. The test is therefore nonquantitative, and the response habituates rapidly, further complicating interpretation. The quantitative sudomotor axon reflex test (QSART) is more complicated, but is sensitive, specific, and reproducible. The function of postganglionic sudomotor fibers is evaluated in selected sites in the limbs by accurate determination of sweat output in response to iontophoresed acetylcholine.

Adrenergic function can be tested most easily by recording the blood pressure with the patient supine and then tilted into a 60° head-up position. Other approaches include recording the rise in systolic and diastolic blood pressure, and in heart rate, to sustained hand grip. Sympathetic efferent activity can also be evaluated qualitatively by determining whether peripheral blood flow is reduced, or arterial blood pressure is increased, by emotional stress (such as from a sudden loud noise or attempted mental arithmetic despite being distracted).

REFERENCES

AMINOFF MJ: *Electromyography in Clinical Practice: Electrodiagnostic Aspects of Neuromuscular Disease,* 2d ed. New York, Churchill Livingstone, 1987

AMINOFF MJ (ed): *Electrodiagnosis in Clinical Neurology,* 3d ed. New York, Churchill Livingstone, 1992

DALY DD, PEDLEY TA (eds): *Current Practice of Clinical Electroencephalography,* 2d ed. New York, Raven Press, 1990

EBERSOLE JS (ed): *Ambulatory EEG Monitoring.* New York, Raven Press, 1988

KIMURA J: *Electrodiagnosis in Diseases of Nerve and Muscle,* 2d ed. Philadelphia, Davis, 1989

NIEDERMEYER E, LOPES DA SILVA F (eds): *Electroencephalography,* 3d ed. Baltimore, Urban & Schwarzenberg, 1993

367 THE EPILEPSIES AND CONVULSIVE DISORDERS

MARC A. DICHTER

The *epilepsies* are a group of disorders characterized by chronic, recurrent, paroxysmal changes in neurologic function caused by abnormalities in the electrical activity of the brain. They are estimated to affect between 0.5 and 2 percent of the population and can occur at any age. Each episode of neurologic dysfunction is called a *seizure.* Seizures may be *convulsive* when they are accompanied by motor manifestations or may be manifest by other changes in neurologic function (i.e., sensory, cognitive, emotional events). Epilepsy can be acquired as a result of neurologic injury or a structural brain lesion and also can occur as a part of many systemic medical diseases.

Epilepsy also occurs in an *idiopathic* form in an individual with neither a history of neurologic insult nor other apparent neurologic dysfunction and may have a genetic cause. Isolated, nonrecurrent seizures may occur in otherwise healthy individuals for a variety of reasons, and under these circumstances, the individual is *not* said to have epilepsy.

CLASSIFICATION OF SEIZURES AND EPILEPSY SYNDROMES

The neurologic manifestations of epileptic seizures are varied, ranging from a brief lapse of attention to a prolonged loss of consciousness with abnormal motor activity. The proper classification of the kinds of seizures which an individual is experiencing is important for an appropriate diagnostic workup, prognostic evaluation, and selection of therapy. The classification of epileptic seizures provided in this chapter is based on the International League Against Epilepsy (ILAE) classification of epileptic seizures. It emphasizes the clinical seizure type and ictal (seizure-associated) and interictal (between-seizure) electroencephalographic pattern (Table 367-1), whereas etiology, anatomic substrate, and pathways of spread are not major considerations. The older terminology of grand mal, petit mal, and psychomotor or temporal lobe epilepsy has been integrated into the current scheme. In addition to identifying the seizure types which an individual is experiencing, it is also useful to categorize the clinical context within which the seizures occur. Epilepsy syndromes which take into account the age of the patient, types of seizures, presence of underlying neurologic lesion, etc. help define groups of patients with relatively predictable prognoses and for whom specific therapies are indicated. A detailed description of these syndromes is beyond the scope of this chapter. However, Table 367-2 summarizes the ILAE classification of the epilepsies and epilepsy syndromes.

The major underlying premise of the seizure classification is that some seizures (partial or focal seizures) start in one area of brain (cortex) and either remain localized or secondarily generalize (i.e., spread throughout the brain), whereas other seizures appear to be generalized from their earliest manifestation.

PARTIAL OR FOCAL SEIZURES Partial or focal seizures begin with the activation of neurons in one area of cortex. The specific clinical symptoms depend on the area of cortex involved and imply

---

TABLE 367-1 Classification of epileptic seizures

PARTIAL OR FOCAL SEIZURES

Simple partial seizures (with motor, sensory, autonomic, or psychic signs)
Complex partial seizures (psychomotor or temporal lobe seizures)
Secondary generalized partial seizures

PRIMARY GENERALIZED SEIZURES

Tonic-clonic (grand mal)
Tonic
Absence (petit mal)
Atypical absence
Myoclonic
Atonic
Infantile spasms

STATUS EPILEPTICUS

Tonic-clonic status
Absence status
Epilepsia partialis continua

RECURRENCE PATTERNS

Sporadic
Cyclic
Reflex (photomyoclonic, somatosensory, musicogenic, reading epilepsy)

specific musical compositions (musicogenic epilepsy), tactile stimulation (somatosensory-induced epilepsy), or reading (reading or language epilepsy). The latter usually consists of brief myoclonic jerks of the jaw, cheek, and tongue which occur during silent or oral reading and may progress to generalized tonic-clonic seizures.

PATHOPHYSIOLOGY OF EPILEPSY

Epileptic seizures can be induced in any normal human (or vertebrate) brain with a variety of different electrical or chemical stimuli. The ease and rapidity with which these seizures can occur and the stereotyped nature of the seizures produced suggest that the normal brain, particularly the cerebral cortex, contains within its fine anatomic and physiologic structure a mechanism which is inherently unstable and which can be influenced in many different ways to produce a seizure. Thus many different kinds of metabolic abnormalities and anatomic lesions of brain can produce seizures, and conversely, there is no pathognomonic lesion of the epileptic brain.

The hallmark of the altered physiologic state of epilepsy is a rhythmic and repetitive hypersynchronous discharge of many neurons in a localized area of the brain. A reflection of this hypersynchronous discharge can be observed in the EEG. The EEG records the integrated electrical activity generated by synaptic potentials in neurons in the superficial layers of a localized area of cortex. Normally, the EEG records unsynchronized activity during periods when the mind is actively working or mildly synchronized activity when the mind is in a restful state (i.e., alpha waves during relaxation with closed eyes) or during various stages of sleep. In the epileptic focus, neurons in a small area of the cortex are activated for a brief period (50 to 100 ms) in an unusually synchronized manner and are then inhibited. This produces a larger, sharper waveform in the EEG—the spike discharge—followed by a slow wave. If the synchronous neuronal discharge occurs repetitively over several seconds, a focal seizure follows; if it spreads through the brain and lasts for many seconds or minutes, a complex partial or generalized seizure (the ictus) will occur, and the EEG can have a variety or appearances depending on which areas of brain are involved and how the primary discharging areas project to the superficial cortex. During the seizure, the EEG may display low-voltage fast activity or high-voltage spikes or spike and wave discharges throughout both hemispheres.

During the interictal spike discharge, the neurons in the epileptic focus undergo a large membrane depolarization (the depolarizing shift, or DS) accompanied by action potential generation. After the DS, the neurons hyperpolarize and stop firing for several seconds. In areas around the discharging focus, the neurons are inhibited throughout the spike discharge. Thus it appears as if the epileptic discharge is limited to a localized area of cortex by a ring of inhibition around the focus and slightly delayed inhibition within the focus. When the epileptic focus undergoes a transition from the isolated discharges to a seizure, the post-DS inhibition disappears and is replaced by a depolarizing potential. Neurons in contiguous areas and in synaptically connected distant areas are then recruited into the seizure and become activated. Local cortical circuits, long association pathways (including callosal), and subcortical pathways are all utilized for the spread of the discharges. Thus a focal seizure can spread locally or generalize throughout the brain. Widely ramifying thalamocortical pathways are likely to be responsible for the rapid generalization of some forms of focal epilepsy and primary generalized epilepsy as well.

A number of metabolic events occur within the brain during the epileptic discharges which may contribute to the development of the focus, to the transition to seizures, or to postictal dysfunction. During the discharges, extracellular potassium concentration increases and extracellular calcium concentration decreases. Both these changes have profound effects on neuronal excitability and neurotransmitter release and on neuronal metabolism. Neurotransmitters and neuropeptides are also released in unusually large amounts during seizure discharges. Some of these substances can have prolonged actions on

central neurons and may be responsible for prolonged postictal phenomena such as Todd's paralysis. In addition to the ionic effects, seizures produce increases in cerebral blood flow to the primary involved areas, increases in glucose utilization, and alterations in oxidative metabolism and local pH. It is possible that these events are not just consequences of the seizures but actually contribute to the development of the seizure activity and that manipulation of such factors could become an effective means for controlling seizures.

There are many mechanisms by which seizures can develop in either normal or pathologic brains. Three common mechanisms include (1) diminution of inhibitory mechanisms [especially synaptic inhibition due to gamma-aminobutyric acid (GABA)], (2) enhancement of excitatory synaptic mechanisms [especially those mediated by the N-methyl-D-aspartate (NMDA) component of glutamate responses], and (3) enhancement of endogenous neuronal burst firing (usually by enhancing voltage-dependent calcium currents). Different forms of human epilepsy may be caused by any one or combination of these mechanisms. For example, in some forms of chronic focal epilepsy, inhibitory interneurons appear to be preferentially lost or inhibitory efficacy is reduced; in other models, and possibly in cases of human hippocampal sclerosis, aberrant recurrent excitatory connections may form among surviving neurons; under other circumstances, neurons may develop enhanced burst firing either because of injury or secondary to genetic factors. In primary generalized absence epilepsy, thalamic neurons with large, low-threshold, transient, voltage-dependent calcium currents may be responsible for generating the diffusely synchronous cortical spike and wave activity.

Currently available antiepileptic drugs appear to operate on several of these mechanisms. Phenytoin, carbamazepine, barbiturates, and valproic acid all appear able to block voltage-dependent sodium channels in a use- and/or voltage-dependent manner such that individual action potentials are relatively unaffected but high-frequency repetitive firing is reduced. The barbiturates and benzodiazepines can enhance GABA-mediated inhibition. Ethosuximide appears to block a low-threshold, transient calcium current in neurons. At present, no drugs are available for clinical use which specifically block excitatory synaptic systems, but much effort is being expended in this direction.

There are a number of animal models in which epilepsy is caused by genetic factors. The best characterized of these is a group of mice in which single-gene mutations cause either absence or tonic-clonic seizures. It is clear from studies of these mice that alterations in a single gene can cause an entire epilepsy syndrome, including multiple seizure types, that different genotypes can produce very similar epilepsy phenotypes, and that interactions between genes can produce intermediate phenotypes. In no case, however, is the genetic basis of the epileptic activity yet understood. Given how many ways seizures can be induced in normal animals, it is likely that a great variety of genetic lesions will produce epilepsy as part of their phenotypic expressions. At the level of human epilepsy, several genetic syndromes have been localized to specific chromosomes (JME possibly to chromosome 6, benign familial neonatal convulsions to chromosome 20, myoclonic epilepsy of the Unverricht-Lundborg type to chromosome 21), and one complex syndrome (myoclonic epilepsy with ragged red fibers) has been localized to a single mutation in mitochondrial DNA.

Electrical stimulation is another mechanism by which seizures can easily be produced in a normal brain. At certain current strengths and stimulus frequencies, seizure discharges are produced and become self-sustaining beyond the original stimulus. Generalized tonic seizures result. At lower stimulus parameters, only brief afterdischarges may occur. However, if afterdischarge-eliciting stimuli are repeated at regular intervals (which may even be as infrequent as one stimulation per day), the afterdischarge duration and spread throughout the brain will increase until generalized seizures occur to the same stimulus which was originally subthreshold. Eventually, spontaneous seizures may occur without any further electrical stimulation. This phenomenon has been called *kindling*. Its relationship to the development of epilepsy, after either an early lesion or trauma, or to the issue of whether the occurrence of seizures themselves tends to foster the continued development of a seizure focus in man has not been resolved.

THE CAUSES OF EPILEPSY

The likely cause of a given seizure depends on the age of the patient and the type of seizure (Table 367-3). In young infants, anoxia or ischemia before or during birth; intracranial birth injury; metabolic disturbances such as hypoglycemia, hypocalcemia, and hypomagnesemia; congenital malformations of the brain; and infections are the most common causes of seizures. In the young child, trauma and infections are common causes of epilepsy, although idiopathic seizures (possibly caused by genetic factors) account for the majority of patients.

Genetic factors can influence the development of epilepsy and also have been shown to affect EEG patterns in general. Patients with primary generalized seizures, especially absence and myoclonic seizures, have a higher familial incidence of epilepsy than is found in the normal population, and relatives of such patients have higher incidences of dysrhythmic EEGs, even when they do not have seizures. The mode of inheritance of epilepsy susceptibility appears complicated for many syndromes and probably represents multiple genes with variable penetrance.

Young children also frequently (approximately 2 to 5 percent of the population) develop seizures with febrile illnesses. These febrile convulsions are short, generalized tonic-clonic convulsions which occur during the early phases of a febrile illness in children between the ages of 3 months and 5 years. Febrile seizures must be distinguished from seizures which are triggered by central nervous system infections which coincidentally produce fever (meningitis or encephalitis). There is minimal likelihood that the child will develop epilepsy or any neurologic impairment from the febrile convulsion if the seizure lasts less than 5 min, is generalized rather than focal, and is not associated with any interictal EEG abnormalities or abnormalities on neurologic examination. There may be a family history of this kind of febrile seizure. Febrile seizures of this kind are probably best treated with quick and relatively vigorous attempts to keep children from developing excessive fevers during various childhood illnesses but without specific antiepileptic medication. Some pediatricians prefer to maintain children susceptible to febrile convulsions on phenobarbital medication; others advocate administration of benzodiazepines at the first sign of illness. On the other hand, if the febrile convulsion is prolonged or focal or is associated with an abnormal EEG, or if the child has a neurologic abnormality, there is a significant risk of subsequent epilepsy. These children should be treated with chronic antiepileptic therapy.

In adolescents and young adults, head trauma is a major cause of focal epilepsy. Epilepsy can be caused by any kind of serious head injury, with the likelihood of developing recurrent seizures being proportional to the extent of the damage. Injuries which either cause dural penetration or produce posttraumatic amnesia of more than 24 h duration may result in a 40 to 50 percent incidence of later epilepsy, while the incidence with closed head injuries with cerebral contusion varies from 5 to 25 percent. Brief concussions or nonpenetrating head injuries without loss of consciousness are not usually epileptogenic. Seizures which occur immediately or within the first 24 h of injury are not associated with a poor prognosis, whereas seizures occurring after the first day and within the first 2 weeks indicate a high likelihood of posttraumatic epilepsy. Most recurring seizures develop by 2 years after the injury. Approximately 50 percent of patients with posttraumatic seizures spontaneously recover, 25 percent have medically controllable seizures, and 25 percent have seizures that are much more intractable to antiepileptic medication. The effectiveness of prophylactic anticonvulsant medication after head trauma still requires adequate documentation.

In the adolescent or young adult age group, generalized tonic-clonic seizures tend to be idiopathic or are associated with drug abuse (especially cocaine) or alcohol use or withdrawal. Arteriovenous malformations may present as focal seizures in this age group. Between the ages of 30 and 50 years, brain tumors become more common causes of seizures and may be present in 30 percent of patients with new focal seizures. In general, the incidence of seizures is higher with slowly growing brain tumors involving the cerebrum, such as meningiomas or low-grade gliomas, than with the more malignant types. However, seizures can occur in individuals with any kind of central nervous system mass lesion.

Above age 50, cerebrovascular disease is the most common cause of focal or generalized seizures. Seizures can occur acutely in patients with an embolus, hemorrhage, or, more rarely, a thrombosis but more often as a late sequel to these lesions. Seizures also can result from "silent" cerebral infarctions in patients with no known cerebrovascular disease. Brain tumors, either primary or metastatic, also present with seizures in the older age group.

At any age, a variety of medical diseases can produce metabolic disturbances which may present as seizures. Uremia, hepatic failure, hypo- or hypercalcemia, hypo- or hyperglycemia, and hypo- or hypernatremia may be associated with myoclonic seizures or generalized tonic-clonic seizures.

EVALUATION OF THE PATIENT WITH A SEIZURE

Individuals with seizures present to physicians either in an emergency room setting during the acute attack or in an office setting days after the epileptic event. In the former case, the seizure may be the presenting symptom of serious central nervous system disorder which requires immediate diagnosis and therapy. In the latter case, the seizure may be a symptom of a more chronic neurologic dysfunction, and a different approach is warranted.

Initial emergency evaluation is directed toward ensuring adequate ventilation and perfusion and stopping the seizure (see "Treatment"). Once the patient is medically stable, the investigation is directed at determining the cause of the seizure. Often a careful history (either from the patient, if recovered, or from a friend or relative), a physical examination, and a few blood studies can provide the diagnosis.

A history indicating a focal component to the seizure [e.g., an aura, a focal motor or sensory symptom at onset, a postictal focal deficit (Todd's paralysis)] indicates a high likelihood of an underlying

TABLE 367-3 The causes of seizures

Infant (0–2)	Perinatal hypoxia and ischemia Intracranial birth injury Acute infection Metabolic disturbances (hypoglycemia, hypocalcemia, hypomagnesemia, pyridoxine deficiency) Congenital malformation Genetic disorders
Child (2–12)	Idiopathic Acute infection Trauma Febrile convulsion
Adolescent (12–18)	Idiopathic Trauma Drug, alcohol withdrawal Arteriovenous malformations
Young adult (18–35)	Trauma Alcoholism Brain tumor
Older adult (>35)	Brain tumor Cerebrovascular disease Metabolic disorders (uremia, hepatic failure, electrolyte abnormality, hypoglycemia) Alcoholism

structural/pathologic etiology of the seizure and directs the evaluation accordingly. A recent febrile illness accompanied by headaches, change in mental status, or confusion suggests an acute central nervous system infection (either meningitis or encephalitis) and indicates the need for urgent examination of the cerebrospinal fluid. In this context, a complex partial seizure may be the presenting symptom of herpes simplex encephalitis. A history of headache and/ or change in mental functioning preceding the seizure, coupled with signs of either increased intracranial pressure or a focal neurologic deficit, suggests an underlying mass lesion (tumor, abscess, arteriovenous malformation) or a chronic subdural hematoma. A magnetic resonance imaging (MRI) or computed tomographic (CT) scan (both without and with contrast) should be performed for a more definitive diagnosis.

The general physical examination may provide important etiologic information. Gum hyperplasia is usually the result of chronic phenytoin therapy. Exacerbation of a chronic seizure disorder due to intercurrent infection, alcohol, or cessation of therapy is a common cause of patients presenting to an emergency room. Skin examination may reveal the port wine facial stain of Sturge-Weber disease (with accompanying cerebral calcifications) or the stigmata of tuberous sclerosis (adenoma sebaceum and shagreen patches) or neurofibromatosis (subcutaneous nodules, café au lait spots). Body or limb asymmetries may indicate hypotrophic somatic development contralateral to a congenital or infantile cerebral lesion.

The history or physical examination also may reveal evidence of chronic alcoholism. Heavy alcohol users commonly have seizures for any of several reasons—old cerebral contusion (secondary to trauma), chronic subdural hematoma, metabolic derangements of undernutrition and liver disease, central nervous system infection, or alcohol withdrawal ("rum fits"). Seizures occurring during alcohol use or withdrawal, in the absence of other causes, are usually brief, generalized tonic-clonic seizures which occur singly or in a flurry of two or three. Once the flurry is over, chronic antiepileptic treatment is unnecessary, since they are usually self-limiting. Seizures in alcoholics which occur at other times should be treated, but this group of patients presents a particular challenge because of lack of compliance and metabolic problems which complicate drug therapy.

Routine blood studies will indicate if the seizure was caused by hypoglycemia, hypo- or hypernatremia, or hypo- or hypercalcemia. These biochemical abnormalities should be corrected and the cause determined. In addition, other less common causes of seizures can be sought with appropriate tests: thyrotoxicosis, acute intermittent porphyria, and lead or arsenic intoxication.

In the older patient, a seizure may indicate an acute cerebrovascular accident or may be a delayed effect of an old cerebral infarct (even a silent one). The manner in which further evaluation proceeds is dictated by the patient's age, cardiovascular status, and accompanying symptoms.

Generalized tonic-clonic seizures can occur in neurologically normal individuals after moderate sleep deprivation. Such seizures can be seen in individuals working double shifts, in college students around examination time, and in soldiers returning from short leaves of absence. Similarly, brief myoclonic jerks or a generalized tonic-clonic seizure can occur after a vasovagal syncopal episode. In these situations, if all investigations are normal, such individuals do not require further treatment.

If the patient's history, physical examination, and blood chemistries are all normal after a seizure, it is likely that the seizure was "idiopathic" and was not caused by a serious underlying CNS lesion. However, tumors or other mass lesions may be entirely asymptomatic, and every older child and adult with an unexplained seizure should have an EEG and an MRI or CT scan (both without and with contrast) and should be reevaluated at regular intervals (3 to 6 months).

The EEG is important in relation to the differential diagnosis of the seizure, the determination of the cause of the seizure, and the proper classification of the seizure. When the diagnosis of a seizure is in doubt, such as, for example, when trying to distinguish seizures from syncope, the presence of a paroxysmal EEG abnormality supports the diagnosis of epilepsy. For this purpose, special activation procedures (sleep recording, photic stimulation, or hyperventilation), special EEG leads (sphenoidal, nasopharyngeal, nasoethmoidal) for recording from deep structures, or prolonged monitoring, even on an ambulatory basis, can be employed. The EEG also can reveal focal abnormalities (spikes, sharp waves, or focal slow waves) which would indicate the possibility of a focal neurologic lesion even if the seizure symptomatology appeared generalized from the outset.

The EEG is also used to help classify seizures. It can distinguish focal seizures with secondary generalization from primary generalized seizures and is especially useful in the differential diagnosis of brief lapses of consciousness. Absence seizures are always accompanied by bilateral spike and wave discharges, whereas complex partial seizures are accompanied by either focal paroxysmal spikes or slow waves or by a normal surface EEG. In cases of absence seizures, the EEG may reveal that the patient is having many more small seizures than was clinically apparent and may help in monitoring antiepileptic drug therapy.

Lumbar puncture is performed in those situations where acute or chronic CNS infections or subarachnoid hemorrhage is suspected. MRI and CT scans provide definitive information about anatomic lesions. MRI is capable of demonstrating hippocampal sclerosis and/ or atrophy in a subset of patients with complex partial seizures. Positron emission tomography (see Chap. 365) can identify seizure foci, but the technique remains primarily experimental. Similarly, magnetoencephalography is undergoing experimental assessment for its efficacy to localize seizure discharges.

DIFFERENTIAL DIAGNOSIS OF SEIZURES

SYNCOPE VERSUS SEIZURE Sudden loss of consciousness, usually without convulsive movements, presents a common diagnostic problem in both children and adults (see Chap. 17). Faints are often preceded by a feeling of light-headedness, of the room spinning, of a flush and are often, but not always, precipitated by an environmental stimulus such as prolonged standing in a hot, crowded area, the sight of blood, a fright, etc. In older people, pure syncope is most often secondary to cardiovascular problems, such as Stokes-Adams attacks, tachyarrhythmias, or orthostatic hypotension, and these may occur with or without a warning. A clear focal onset of the event (i.e., abnormal smell, head turning, staring, etc.) favors seizure as the cause. In addition, convulsive muscular contractions, tongue biting, or incontinence commonly accompany seizures but are much less common with fainting spells. Occasionally, vasovagal or other types of fainting episodes can be accompanied by either clonic movements or brief generalized tonic-clonic seizures. If the original loss of consciousness can be ascribed to a clear nonepileptic cause (e.g., the patient was having blood drawn or a dental procedure at the time), it is not necessary to regard the episode as a manifestation of epilepsy, and antiepileptic drug therapy is not indicated.

When the origin of a syncopal episode is in doubt, the patient should undergo a complete cardiovascular evaluation, an EEG with sleep recording, and, if available, prolonged ambulatory EEG monitoring. If the EEG shows paroxysmal activity (which is often brought out by drowsiness and sleep onset) and the patient has no signs of cardiac arrhythmia with electrocardiographic monitoring or of valvular disease on echocardiogram, it is likely that the syncopal episode represented a seizure, and the patient should be evaluated and treated accordingly.

TRANSIENT ISCHEMIC ATTACKS AND MIGRAINE Transient ischemic attacks (TIAs) and migraine episodes can present as a transient alteration in neurologic function (usually without loss of consciousness) which may be confused diagnostically with focal seizures. Neurologic dysfunction due to ischemia (TIA or migraine) is often a negative symptom (i.e., loss of feeling, numbness, visual field deficit, paralysis), whereas deficits due to focal seizure activity are often positive (twitching, paresthesias, visual distortion, or hallucination), although this distinction is not absolute. Brief stereotyped episodes which conform to dysfunction in a single vascular territory in an individual with either known vascular disease, heart disease, or risk factors for vascular disease (diabetes, hypertension) are more likely TIAs. However, since cerebral infarcts are a common cause of subsequent seizures in older patients, a paroxysmal EEG focus should be sought.

Classic migraine headaches with a visual aura, unilateral headache, and gastrointestinal upset are usually easy to distinguish from seizures. However, some migraine patients have only "migraine equivalents" such as a hemiparesis, numbness, or aphasia and may not have subsequent headache. These episodes, especially when they occur in older individuals, are hard to distinguish from TIAs but also may represent focal seizures. The presence of loss of consciousness after some forms of vertebrobasilar migraine and the common occurrence of headaches after seizures make this differential diagnosis more difficult. The slower development of neurologic dysfunction in migraine (often occurring over minutes) is the most helpful point. Nevertheless, occasionally such patients need to be investigated for all three problems with an MRI or CT scan, carotid studies, and specialized EEG procedures before a diagnosis can be made. In some cases, a therapeutic trial with antiepileptic drugs (which, interestingly, can prevent migraines as well as seizures in some patients) will be necessary for the final diagnosis.

PSEUDOSEIZURES AND "HYSTERICAL" SEIZURES Some patients with complex partial seizures may have bizarre behavioral manifestations of their seizures. These may consist of abrupt changes in personality, feelings of impending doom or of undirected fear, abnormal bodily sensations, episodic forgetfulness, or brief repetitive motor activities such as picking at one's clothes or stamping a foot. Some of these patients also have personality disorders, and a significant proportion have had psychiatric treatment. It is common, especially if these patients do not have tonic-clonic seizures or loss of consciousness and when these patients appear emotionally disturbed, for these episodes of complex partial seizures to be called *pseudoseizures, psychopathic fugues*, or *"hysterical" seizures*. This incorrect diagnosis is often reinforced by a "normal" EEG interictally or even during one of these episodes. It must be emphasized that seizures (as well as interictal discharges) can arise from foci deep in temporal lobe structures with *no* surface EEG manifestations. This has been demonstrated repeatedly with depth electrode recordings. Moreover, deep temporal seizures can be manifest only by the kinds of phenomena described above and may be free of the usual seizure phenomena of motor convulsions and loss of consciousness.

In a small number of cases, individuals present with seizure-like events which upon investigation turn out to be pseudoseizures or, rarely, frank malingering. Often these individuals have had true seizures in the past or are acquainted with an individual with epilepsy. Such pseudoseizures can be quite difficult to distinguish from true seizures. They are characterized by nonphysiologic events such as a progression of twitching from one hand to the other without spread to subjacent ipsilateral face or leg areas, twitching of all four extremities without loss of consciousness (or with surreptitious loss of consciousness), or careful attention to avoiding injury by moving away from a wall or bed edge while having motor convulsions. In addition, pseudoseizures, especially in adolescent girls, may have frankly sexual overtones, with pelvic thrusting or genital manipulation. While many forms of complex partial seizures can occur with normal surface EEGs, generalized tonic-clonic seizures always produce abnormal EEGs both during and after the seizure. In addition, most generalized tonic-clonic seizures and many complex partial seizures of moderate duration are accompanied by rises in serum prolactin (during a 30-min postictal period), whereas pseudoseizures are not. Although not an absolute distinguishing point, such measurements, especially if positive, can be very helpful in characterizing the origin of a given "spell." After careful observation, especially with video-EEG monitoring, and after establishing a relationship with the patient,

pseudoseizures can sometimes be elicited by suggestion. Frequently, when patients are appropriately confronted with this diagnosis, they respond well, and the pseudoseizures are eliminated or greatly reduced in frequency.

TREATMENT OF SEIZURES

Treatment of the patient with a seizure disorder is directed at eliminating the cause of the seizures, suppressing the expression of the seizures, and dealing with the psychosocial consequences which may occur as a result of the neurologic dysfunction underlying the seizure disorder or from the presence of a chronic disability.

If the seizure disorder is a result of a metabolic disturbance, such as hypoglycemia or hypocalcemia, restoration of normal metabolic function is usually accompanied by cessation of the seizures. If the seizures are caused by a structural brain lesion, such as a brain tumor, arteriovenous malformation, or cerebral cyst, removal of the offending lesion may eliminate the seizures. However, long-standing lesions, even nonprogressive ones, can result in gliosis and chronic denervation. These changes may lead to chronic epileptic foci which will not be eliminated by the subsequent removal of the original lesion. In such cases, surgical extirpation of the epileptic brain regions may be necessary for control of the epilepsy (see "Neurosurgical Approaches to Epilepsy," below).

There is complex interrelationship between the limbic system and neuroendocrine function which may have significant implications for patients with epilepsy. Normal hormonal fluctuations may influence the frequency of seizures. Some women have a marked change in the pattern of their seizures during particular parts of the menstrual cycle (catamenial epilepsy), while others may have changes in seizure frequency in response to oral contraceptives or pregnancy. In general, estrogens tend to exacerbate seizures, while progesterones tend to be more protective.

In addition, epilepsy can cause changes in neuroendocrine function. Some patients with epilepsy, especially those with complex partial seizures, also may have an associated reproductive endocrine dysfunction. Disorders in sexual interest, especially hyposexuality, are frequently observed. In addition, women may have polycystic ovary disease, and men may have disturbances in potency. Interestingly, some patients with these endocrine disorders have not had clinical seizures but have significantly abnormal EEGs (often with temporal discharges). Whether the epilepsy causes the endocrine and/or behavioral dysfunction or whether the two conditions are separate manifestations of a common underlying neuropathologic process is not known. However, endocrine manipulation can sometimes be useful in controlling some forms of seizures, and antiepileptic medication may be a useful adjunct for treating some forms of endocrine dysfunction.

PHARMACOLOGIC CONTROL OF EPILEPSY The fundamental modality for the treatment of epilepsy is pharmacologic therapy. The goal is to protect the patient from having seizures without interfering with normal cognitive function (or, in the child, with development of normal intellectual function) and without producing harmful systemic side effects. If possible, the individual should be treated with the lowest possible dose of a single antiepileptic medication. Precise knowledge of the kind of seizure the patient is having, the spectrum of action of the available antiepileptic medications, and a few basic pharmacokinetic principles can result in the complete control of seizures in approximately 60 percent of patients with epilepsy. Many patients appear to be resistant to medications or develop unnecessary side effects because the medications chosen are not appropriate for the kind(s) of seizure or are not administered in the optimal doses.

The availability of serum levels of antiepileptic drugs makes it possible to optimize dosage regimens for individual patients and to monitor drug compliance. Thus patients can be placed on a medication, and after a suitable equilibration period (usually several weeks, but at least five "half-lives"), the amount of medication in the serum can be determined and compared with standard "therapeutic ranges" established for each drug. Utilizing blood levels to adjust doses can compensate for individual patient variability in absorption or metabolism of drugs.

Many antiepileptic drugs are bound by serum proteins, and it is the unbound, or "free," drug which is in equilibrium with extracellular spaces within the brain; this level correlates best with seizure control. However, "total" drug is measured in the serum by conventional

TABLE 367-4 Commonly used antiepileptic drugs

Generic name	Trade name	Principal uses	Dosage	Half-life	Therapeutic range	% Protein bound	Toxic effects Neurologic	Toxic effects Systemic	Drug interactions
Phenytoin (PTN) (diphenyl-hydantoin)	Dilantin	Tonic-clonic (grand mal) Partial	300–400 mg/d (3–5 mg/kg, adult) (4–7 mg/kg, child)	24 h (with wide variation)	10–20 µg/mL	90	Ataxia Incoordination Confusion Cerebellar Skin rash	Gum hyperplasia Lymphadenopathy Hirsutism Osteomalacia	Level increased by INH, dicoumarol, sulfonamides Level decreased by CBZ, phenobarbital Altered folate metabolism Folate interferes with effects
Carbamazepine CBZ	Tegretol	Tonic-clonic Partial	600–1200 mg/d (20–30 mg/kg, child)	13–17 h	4–12 µg/mL	80	Ataxia Dizziness Diplopia Vertigo	Bone marrow suppression Gastrointestinal irritation Hepatotoxicity	Level decreased by phenobarbital, PTN Level increased by erythromycin
Phenobarbital	Luminol	Tonic-clonic Partial	60–120 mg/d (1–5 mg/kg, adult) (3–6 mg/kg, child)	90 h (shorter in children)	10–50 µg/mL	40–60	Sedation Ataxia Confusion Dizziness Decreased libido Depression	Skin rash	Level increased by VPA, PTN Enhances metabolism of other drugs via liver enzyme induction
Primidone	Mysoline	Tonic-clonic Partial	750–1000 mg/d (10–25 mg/kg)	Primidone, 8 h PEMA, 24–48 h Phenobarbital, 90 h	Primidone, 2–10 µg/mL Phenobarbital, 10–50 µg/mL	Small for primidone or PEMA	Same as phenobarbital		
Sodium val-proate (valproic acid, VPA)	Depakene Depakote	Absence Atypical absence Myoclonic Tonic-clonic (Partial)	750–1250 mg/d (30–60 mg/kg)	15 h	50–100 µg/mL	80–94	Ataxia Sedation Tremor	Hepatotoxicity Bone marrow suppression Gastrointestinal irritation Weight gain Transient alopecia Hyperammonemia	May precipitate absence status if given with clonazepam Increases free PTN Decreases phenobarbital Increases active CBZ metabolites
Ethosuximide	Zarontin	Absence (petit mal)	750–1250 mg/d (20–40 mg/kg)	60 h, adult 30 h, child	40–100 µg/mL	Small	Ataxia Lethargy	Gastrointestinal irritation Skin rash Bone marrow suppression	
Methsuximide	Celontin	Absence (complex partial)	600–1200 mg/d	38–50 h	10–30 µg/mL (N-desmethyl methsux-imide)	Small	Ataxia Lethargy	Same as ethosuximide	Increases PTN level Increases phenobarbital from primidone
Clonazepam	Klo-nopin	Absence Atypical absence Myoclonic	1–12 mg/d (0.1–0.2 mg/kg)	24–48 h	5–70 ng/mL	50	Ataxia Sedation Lethargy	Anorexia	May precipitate ab-sence status if given with VPA
Trimethadione	Tridione	Absence Atypical absence (use only with in-tractable seizures)	900–2100 mg/d (20–60 mg/kg)	6–13 days (for dimetha-dione)	700 µg/mL (for dimetha-dione)	Small	Sedation Blurred vision	Skin rash Bone marrow suppression Nephrosis Hepatitis	
Lamotrigine	Lamictal	Partial	300–500 mg/d (depends on concomitant AEDs)	25 h 13 h (with PTN, CBZ, PHB, PRIM) 60–70 h (with VPA)	Unknown	55%	Headache Dizziness Ataxia Diplopia	Skin rash Nausea	PTN, CBZ, Barbitu-rates shorten half life VPA prolongs half life Decrease VPA level
Gabapentin	Neu-rontin	Partial	900–1200 mg/d (up to 2400 mg/d if necessary and tol-erated)	5–7 h	Unknown	None	Dizziness Somnolence Ataxia	Gastrointestinal irritation	None

assays. Under most circumstances, this is adequate for determining if the antiepileptic drug is in the therapeutic range. Occasionally, serum antiepileptic drug levels will be high, yet the patient continues to have seizures without any "physiologic" side effects of the drug. In these cases, it is possible that serum protein binding is higher than expected and that the patient is "undermedicated" in relation to the "free" drug available. Increase in dose may produce control without any untoward side effects (despite a blood level above "therapeutic range"). Similarly, individuals with impaired liver or renal function may have low serum proteins or circulating "toxins" which reduce drug binding. In these cases, toxicity may appear at unusually low serum levels because of a relatively higher "free" level of drug.

Intensive long-term EEG and video monitoring has demonstrated that careful characterization of seizures and selection of antiepileptic drugs can significantly increase seizure control in many patients whose seizures had previously been considered intractable to conventional antiepileptic drugs. In fact, often these patients can have one or more of their multiple drugs removed while still achieving better control.

INDICATIONS FOR USE OF SPECIFIC DRUGS   Generalized tonic-clonic seizures (grand mal)   There are four medications which are of proven value in this very common form of seizure—phenytoin (or diphenylhydantoin), carbamazepine, phenobarbital (and other long-acting barbiturates), and valproic acid (Table 367-4). Most patients will be controlled by adequate doses of any one of these, although individual patients may respond better to one or another. The choice among them often relates to minimizing undesirable side effects.

Phenytoin often can produce effective control with no sedation and very little, if any, intellectual impairment. However, phenytoin produces gum hyperplasia in some individuals, coarsening of facial features, and mild hirsutism, all of which can lead to long-term changes in appearance, which is especially unpleasant for young women. Phenytoin may produce lymphadenopathy and, in very high doses, may be toxic to the cerebellum.

Carbamazepine is equally effective and does not have many of the side effects seen with phenytoin. Cognitive function is well preserved. However, carbamazepine may exacerbate generalized spike-wave discharges in the EEG and absence seizures, even in patients who had only previously experienced generalized tonic-clonic seizures. Carbamazepine can cause gastrointestinal upset and may cause bone marrow suppression with mild to moderate falls in peripheral white count (3.5 to 4×10^3 per microliter) which can occasionally become severe and which must be watched carefully. In addition, carbamazepine can produce hepatotoxicity. For these reasons, a complete blood count and liver function tests should be performed before starting carbamazepine and at 2-week intervals for a period after initiating therapy.

Phenobarbital is also effective against tonic-clonic seizures and has none of the systemic side effects mentioned above. It commonly causes sedation and a dulling of intellect, however, especially early in its use, and this may lead to poor compliance. The sedation is dose-dependent and may limit the amount of drug which can be given to achieve complete control. However, if control can be achieved with nonsedative doses of phenobarbital, it can be a safe regimen. Primidone is a barbiturate which is metabolized to phenobarbital and phenylethylmalonamide (PEMA). In children, the barbiturates can produce a state of hyperactivity and hyperirritability which will limit their usefulness. Barbiturates also may exacerbate depression.

Valproic acid (sodium valproate) is also effective for tonic-clonic seizures and does not produce sedation or interfere with cognitive function. It can cause gastrointestinal irritation, patchy hair loss, excessive weight gain, bone marrow suppression (especially thrombocytopenia), hyperammonemia, and hepatic dysfunction (including rare instances of fatal progressive hepatic failure which appear to be idiosyncratic rather than dose-related and more common in children under 2 years of age). A complete blood count with platelet count and liver function tests should be performed before beginning therapy and at biweekly intervals after initiating therapy for a suitable period until the safety of the drug is established in the individual patient.

In addition to their systemic side effects, all four of these drugs have neurologic toxicities at higher doses. Nystagmus is common at therapeutic blood levels, but ataxia, dizziness, tremor, intellectual dulling, forgetfulness, confusion, and even stupor may occur with increasing blood concentrations. These are reversible when blood levels fall back to therapeutic levels.

Partial seizures, including complex partial seizures (temporal lobe epilepsy)   Three of the four groups of drugs which are useful for tonic-clonic seizures are also effective for partial seizures. Carbamazepine and phenytoin are the drugs of choice, while the barbiturates also may be effective. Valproic acid has more variable effects. Felbamate is a new drug recently approved by the FDA for use in partial seizures with or without secondary generalization and in children with multiple seizure types associated with the Lennox Gastaut syndrome. Its side effects include gastrointestinal upset, anorexia, and insomnia, but in general it is well tolerated. Felbamate has important interactions with some other antiepileptic drugs (see Table 367-4). At present, two other anti-epileptic drugs (lamotrigine and gabapentin) have also been approved by the FDA Advisory Panel for use in partial seizures. The relevant pharmacologic data for both are included in Table 367-4.

In general, complex partial seizures are difficult to control, and such patients may require more than one medication (i.e., carbamazepine and phenobarbital, or phenytoin and phenobarbital, or any one of the primary drugs and high doses of methsuximide) and may become candidates for neurosurgical intervention. These are the kinds of seizures for which many epilepsy centers are conducting trials of new antiepileptic drugs.

Other primary generalized seizures [absence (petit mal), atypical absence, myoclonic]   These seizures respond to different classes of medications than either tonic-clonic or focal seizures. For simple absence, ethosuximide and valproic acid are the drugs of choice. Side effects of ethosuximide include gastrointestinal upset, behavior changes, dizziness, and lethargy, but these are not often troublesome. For more difficult to control atypical absence seizures and for myoclonic seizures, valproic acid is the drug of choice. Clonazepam (a benzodiazepine) also can be used for atypical absence and myoclonic seizures, but its effectiveness is often limited by the development of tolerance. It can cause drowsiness and irritability but usually does not cause other systemic side effects. Trimethadione was one of the first antiabsence drugs, but it is now rarely used because of its potential toxicity.

Approximately one-third of children who present with "pure" absence seizures also have tonic-clonic seizures at some later time. The question of whether these children should be treated prophylactically with an anti–tonic-clonic seizure medication has not been resolved. Since valproic acid is effective against both classes of seizures, its use has been increasing in children with absence. The concurrent use of phenobarbital with antiabsence drugs for this purpose should be avoided because it may interfere with therapy for the absence. Clinical trials are underway with several new antiepileptic drugs, including lamotrigine, felbamate, and vigabatrin. None is approved for clinical use in the United States.

Status epilepticus   Generalized tonic-clonic status epilepticus is a life-threatening medical emergency, but overzealous and incautious treatment can produce more harm than good. Patients are in danger from hyperpyrexia and acidosis (from prolonged muscle activity) and, less commonly, hypoxia or compromise of respiratory function. Immediate treatment for status is protection of the airway, protection of the tongue (with a soft object, large enough not to be swallowed, between the clenched teeth), protection of the head, and then establishment of a secure parenteral (IV) access. A bolus of 50% glucose in water (after blood is drawn for analysis), even if hypoglycemia is not expected, may stop the seizures. All further intravenous medication should be given after respiratory and circulatory support are available.

Phenytoin, 1000 to 1500 mg (18 to 20 mg/kg) in a slow IV "push" (not in 5% dextrose in water—phenytoin precipitates in this low-pH solution), no faster than 50 mg/min, is one of the drugs of choice. It does not depress respiration but may produce mild atrioventricular block and, if given too rapidly, can cause a serious fall in blood pressure. Blood pressure and ECG should be monitored.

The benzodiazepines, diazepam (10 mg) or lorazepam (4 mg, followed by another 4 mg if necessary), are also effective in stopping status epilepticus when administered intravenously. These drugs may depress respiratory function (or even cause respiratory arrest), and measures for respiratory support should be available before they are administered. The use of a benzodiazepine after phenobarbital administration carries a particular risk. The benzodiazepines are short-acting drugs in these circumstances, and after they are administered, a second, longer-acting antiepileptic such as phenytoin is usually required to prevent recurrence of seizures.

Phenobarbital, in a dose of 10 to 20 mg/kg (up to 1 g), divided into two to four doses at 30- to 60-min intervals, also can be administered for status epilepticus. Phenobarbital causes respiratory depression and should not be used immediately after treatment with IV diazepam.

If tonic-clonic seizures cannot be controlled within 30 to 60 min with the above sequence, the likelihood of serious neurologic sequelae or death becomes very high. These patients often have a serious underlying cause for the status epilepticus, such as cerebral hypoxia, sepsis, or some metabolic derangement. Serious consideration needs to be given to anesthetizing the patient with barbiturates or inhalation anesthetics, with EEG monitoring, to ensure that cessation of electrical seizure activity accompanies cessation of motor convulsions.

After stopping the seizures, it is imperative to determine the cause of the status epilepticus in order to prevent its recurrence. In most adults, the cause can be determined and is usually tumor, vascular disease, infection, cerebral damage, or precipitous withdrawal from alcohol or antiepileptic medication. In children, the incidence of idiopathic status is higher (approximately 50 percent), and the remaining cases are divided between acute brain illnesses such as purulent meningitis, encephalitis, and dehydration with electrolyte disturbances and chronic encephalopathies. Tonic-clonic status epilepticus is a dangerous condition; the mortality may be over 10 percent, with another 10 to 30 percent of patients being left with permanent neurologic sequelae.

NEUROSURGICAL TREATMENT OF EPILEPSY   If a structural lesion (i.e., tumor, cyst, abscess, etc.) is causing recurrent seizures, the removal of that lesion and nearby diseased brain will often eliminate the seizures or make them easier to control. Some patients, however, have uncontrollable seizures without a demonstrable structural lesion. These are often complex partial seizures with ictal and interictal EEG abnormalities emanating from one or both temporal lobes. Some patients have demonstrable lesions in the hippocampus (sclerosis or atrophy) visible by high-resolution MRI. Many surgical series have shown that if the epileptogenic lesion can be clearly localized to the depths of one temporal lobe, neurosurgical removal of that temporal lobe can result in complete elimination of the seizures or significant improvement in 60 to 95 percent of the patients. Individuals with epileptic foci in temporal neocortex or other neocortical areas often have a somewhat lower chance of such success but may still be helped significantly. Localization often depends on intensive EEG monitoring and may require intracranial recordings from the temporal or frontal lobes. In a high percentage of cases, the removed temporal lobe can be shown to have microscopic pathology, such as hippocampal (or "Ammon's horn") sclerosis (loss of pyramidal cells in the hippocampus), a hamartoma, or cortical ectopia.

Some individuals with complex partial seizures also develop a psychiatric illness characterized most often as a borderline personality disorder with certain specific behavioral manifestations, including hypergraphia, hyperreligiosity, lack of sense of humor, and disordered sexuality. The psychiatric aspects of this illness may result from the epilepsy or may be produced independently by the same underlying brain lesion which produces the epilepsy. The personality disorder may not significantly change after epilepsy surgery, even if the seizures are controlled.

TREATMENT OF A SINGLE SEIZURE   Some individuals present with a single, brief, generalized tonic-clonic seizure and, after complete evaluation, are found to have a normal EEG and no underlying cause for the seizure. Some of these individuals (between 40 and 70 percent, depending on the series) go on to have recurrent seizures. The decision to treat such a patient with several years (at least) of antiepileptic medication must be made on an individual basis, considering the patient's life style, risks from a sudden loss of consciousness, and feelings about medications.

CESSATION OF ANTIEPILEPTIC DRUG THERAPY   Many patients with epilepsy require antiepileptic drug therapy for life. However, a large proportion of epileptic patients become seizure-free on appropriate medication, and approximately half of such patients can eventually stop their medications and remain seizure-free. Individuals with the best chance of remaining seizure-free after medication discontinuation meet the following criteria: no seizures for 2 to 4 years, relatively few seizures before control was attained, only required a single medication for control, normal neurologic examination, no structural lesion causing the seizures, normal EEG at the end of the therapeutic period. (An abnormal EEG is not, however, a contraindication to discontinuing medication.) When considering the discontinuance of antiepileptic therapy, the consequences of the recurrence of seizures must be considered carefully. One inopportune seizure in a previously well-controlled patient who is not used to taking precautions may be a life-threatening event or lead to loss of a driver's license or loss of employment. Nevertheless, since all medications carry some risk of toxicity, and since medication compliance in a healthy individual is often variable, it is worth a careful trial of medication tapering in individuals who meet the above criteria and are willing to accept the risk.

EPILEPSY AND PREGNANCY   Most women with epilepsy can undergo uneventful pregnancies and deliver healthy babies—even those taking antiepileptic medications. During the pregnant state, however, body metabolism changes, and close attention must be given to antiepileptic drug levels. Sometimes relatively high doses have to be given to ensure therapeutic levels. Most women who are well controlled before pregnancy will remain so during pregnancy and delivery. Women whose seizures are not under good control before becoming pregnant are at higher risk for having increased difficulties during the pregnancy.

One of the most serious complications of pregnancy, toxemia, often presents as a generalized tonic-clonic convulsion in the third trimester. This seizure is a symptom of a severe neurologic disturbance and is not a manifestation of epilepsy, nor is it more common in epileptic women. The toxemic state must be treated in order to control the seizures.

There is a two- to fivefold higher incidence of significant fetal malformations in offspring of epileptic women, and this is likely due to a combination of a genetic predisposition in this population as well as a low, but real, incidence of medication-induced malformations. Among those malformations which do occur, a syndrome consisting of cleft lip and palate, heart defects, digital hypoplasia, and nail dysplasia has been identified which was initially ascribed to phenytoin ("fetal-hydantoin syndrome") but also has been associated with other antiepileptic drugs.

Although it would be ideal for women contemplating pregnancy to have their antiepileptic drugs discontinued, it is likely that for a large number of women this would result in recurrence of seizures, which would, in the long run, be more harmful for both mother and baby. If patients meet the criteria for discontinuance of medication, this should be done with a suitable interval before pregnancy is to occur. Other patients should be tapered to a minimal effective dosage and, if possible, be maintained on only one medication. There are no clear data indicating differences in safety for phenobarbital, phenytoin, or carbamazepine when used alone. Less experience is available for valproate. Phenobarbital, primidone, and phenytoin can cause transient and reversible deficiency in vitamin K–dependent clotting factors in the neonate, and this should be treated promptly. Babies exposed to chronic barbiturates in utero are often transiently sluggish, hypotonic, jittery, and may show signs of barbiturate withdrawal. These babies should be considered at risk for neonatal problems and should be withdrawn slowly from barbiturates and closely observed in the nursery during the neonatal period.

DRIVING AND EPILEPSY Each state has its own regulations for determining when an individual with epilepsy can obtain a driver's license, and several states have laws about the physician's obligations in either reporting epileptic patients to the registry or informing the patients of their responsibilities to do so. In general, patients can drive after a seizure-free interval (on or off medications) which ranges from 6 months to 2 years. In some states there is no fixed interval, but the individual is required to have a physician's letter attesting to seizure control. It is the physician's responsibility to warn the patient with epilepsy of the risks of driving when seizures are not under control.

SOCIAL AND EDUCATIONAL REHABILITATION Many people with epilepsy attain adequate control of their seizures and are able to attend school, obtain employment, become involved in relationships, and live relatively normal lives. Some individuals are more disabled by the fact that they have epilepsy than by the seizures themselves and unduly restrict their activities or withdraw from social interactions. These individuals need to have their psychosocial concerns professionally treated. Children with epilepsy tend to have more problems in school than their peers, but every effort should be made to keep these children integrated into the mainstream of the educational process while supplying additional help in the form of academic tutoring or psychological counseling.

REFERENCES

BERKOVIC SF et al: Hippocampal sclerosis in temporal lobe epilepsy demonstrated by magnetic resonance imaging. Ann Neurol 29:175, 1991

CALLAGHAN N et al: Withdrawal of anticonvulsant drugs in patients free of seizures for two years. N Engl J Med 318:942, 1988

CENDES F et al: MRI volumetric measurement of amygdala and hippocampus in temporal lobe epilepsy. Neurology 43:719, 1993

COMMISSION ON CLASSIFICATION AND TERMINOLOGY OF THE ILAE: Proposal for revised clinical classification of epileptic seizures. Epilepsia 22:489, 1981

———: Proposal for revised clinical classification of epilepsies and epileptic syndromes. Epilepsia 30:3898, 1989

DELGADO-ESCUETA A, JANZ D: Consensus guidelines: Preconception counseling, management, and care of the pregnant woman with epilepsy. Neurology 42(suppl 5):149, 1992

DICHTER M, AYALA GF: Cellular mechanisms of epilepsy: A status report. Science 237:157, 1987

———, BUCHHALTER J: The genetic epilepsies, in The Molecular and Genetic Basis of Neurological Diseases, R Rosenberg et al (eds). Boston, Butterworth, 1993, pp 925–950

EMERSON R et al: Stopping medication in children with epilepsy. N Engl J Med 304:1125, 1981

ENGEL J: Clinical neurophysiology, neuroimaging, and the surgical treatment of epilepsy. Curr Opin Neurol Neurosurg 6:240, 1993

ENGEL J JR: Seizures and Epilepsy. Philadelphia, Davis, 1989

——— (ed): Surgical Treatment of the Epilepsies. New York, Raven, 1987

HAJEK M et al: Mesiobasal versus lateral temporal lobe epilepsy—Metabolic differences in the temporal lobe shown by interictal F-18-FDG positron emission tomography. Neurology 43:79, 1993

LAIDLAW J, RICHENS A (eds): A Textbook of Epilepsy, 3d ed. London, Churchill Livingstone, 1988

LEHESJOKI AE et al: Localization of a gene for progressive myoclonus epilepsy to chromosome 21q22. Proc Natl Acad Sci (USA) 88:3696, 1991

LEPPERT M et al: Benign familial neonatal convulsions linked to genetic markers on chromosome 20. Nature 337:647, 1989

LEPPIK IF et al: Felbamate for partial seizures: Results of a controlled clinical trial. Neurology 41:1785, 1991

LEVY R et al (eds): Antiepileptic Drugs, 3d ed. New York, Raven, 1989

MATTSON R, CRAMER J: Epilepsy, sex hormones and antiepileptic drugs. Epilepsia 26(S):S40, 1985

——— et al: Comparison of carbamazepine, phenobarbital, phenytoin, and primidone in partial and secondarily generalized tonic-clonic seizures. N Engl J Med 313:145, 1985

NOBELS JL: Molecular genetics and epilepsy, in Recent Advances in Epilepsy, T Pedley, B Meldrum (eds). Edinburgh, Churchill Livingstone, 1992, pp 1–13

SO EL: Update on epilepsy. Med Clin North Am 77:203, 1993

TEMKIN N et al: A randomized, double-blind study of phenytoin for the prevention of post-traumatic seizures. N Engl J Med 323:497, 1990

368 CEREBROVASCULAR DISEASES

J. PHILIP KISTLER / ALLAN H. ROPPER / JOSEPH B. MARTIN

Cerebrovascular disease, the third leading cause of death after heart disease and cancer in developed countries, has an overall prevalence of 794 per 100,000. In the United States, it is estimated that more than 400,000 patients are discharged each year from hospitals after a stroke. The loss of these patients from the work force and the extended hospitalization they require during recovery make the economic impact of the disease one of the most devastating in medicine.

PATHOGENESIS AND PATHOLOGY OF STROKE Cerebrovascular disease is caused by one of several pathologic processes involving the blood vessels of the brain. The process may (1) be intrinsic to the vessel, as in atherosclerosis, lipohyalinosis, inflammation, amyloid deposition, arterial dissection, developmental malformation, aneurysmal dilation, or venous thrombosis; (2) originate remotely, as occurs when an embolus from the heart or extracranial circulation lodges in an intracranial vessel; (3) result from decreased perfusion pressure or increased blood viscosity with inadequate cerebral blood flow; or (4) result from rupture of a vessel in the subarachnoid space or intracerebral tissue.

A *stroke* is the acute neurologic injury occurring as a result of one of these pathologic processes and is manifested either as brain infarction or hemorrhage. Approximately 80 percent of strokes are due to ischemic cerebral infarction and 20 percent to brain hemorrhage. An infarcted brain is pale initially. Within hours to days, the gray matter becomes congested with engorged, dilated blood vessels and minute petechial hemorrhages. When an embolus blocking a major vessel migrates, lyses, or disperses within hours, recirculation into the ischemic area causes hemorrhagic infarction that may aggravate edema formation from blood-brain barrier disruption. A primary intracerebral hemorrhage damages the brain directly at the site of the hemorrhage by compressing the surrounding tissue.

The brain is unable to repair itself and only forms fibrogliotic scar tissue at the site of infarction or hemorrhage; therefore, the most effective therapy for stroke is prevention. After a stroke, therapy is directed toward minimizing subsequent worsening of the infarction or hemorrhage, preventing a second stroke, or decreasing edema. Therapy in ischemic stroke is aided by a precise diagnosis that determines the primary vascular pathology, the extent and location of the stroke, and the collateral circulation. The clinical presentation and temporal profile of a stroke often suggests the cause. Diagnosis includes imaging studies (CT and MRI) and noninvasive laboratory tests (carotid and transcranial Doppler ultrasonography and magnetic resonance angiography).

Primary risk factors for stroke include hypertension, hypercholesterolemia, and smoking as the most important for arteriosclerotic cerebrovascular disease, atrial fibrillation or recent myocardial infarction for cardiogenic embolism, and hypertension for primary intracerebral hemorrhage. Hypertension also causes lipohyalinosis, the primary pathologic lesion of lacunar stroke. Virtually every type of cardiac disease is associated with increased risk for stroke.

ISCHEMIC CEREBROVASCULAR DISEASE: GENERAL REMARKS

Ischemic cerebrovascular disease is divided into two broad categories, thrombotic and embolic (Table 368-1). Cerebral embolic strokes usually occur abruptly but may present with stuttering, fluctuating symptoms. Thrombotic strokes are heralded in 50 to 75 percent of patients by transient symptoms, transient ischemic attacks (TIAs), or a minor stroke leading to a more devastating event.

TABLE 368-1   Causes of ischemic stroke

THROMBOSIS

A   Atherosclerosis
B*   Arteritis: Temporal arteritis, granulomatous arteritis, polyarteritis, Wegener's granulomatosis, granulomatous arteritis of the great vessels (Takayasu's arteritis, syphilis)
C*   Dissections: Carotid, vertebral, or intracranial arteries at the base of the brain (spontaneous or traumatic)
D*   Hematologic disorders: Polycythemia first-degree or second-degree, sickle cell disease, thrombotic thrombocytopenic purpura, etc.
E*   Cerebral mass effect compressing intracranial arteries: Tentorial herniation—post-cerebral artery; giant aneurysm—middle cerebral artery compression
F*   Miscellaneous: Moyamoya disease, fibromuscular dysplasia, Binswanger's disease

VASOCONSTRICTION

A*   Cerebral vasospasm following subarachnoid hemorrhage
B*   Reversible cerebral vasoconstriction: Etiology unknown, following migraine, trauma, eclampsia of pregnancy

EMBOLISM

A   Atherothrombotic arterial source: Bifurcation common carotid artery, carotid siphon, distal vertebral artery, aortic arch
B*   Cardiac source
　　1   Structural heart disease
　　　a   Congenital: mitral valve prolapse, patent foramen ovale, etc.
　　　b   Acquired: following myocardial infarction, marantic vegetation, etc.
　　2   Dysrhythmia, atrial fibrillation, sick sinus syndrome, etc.
　　3   Infection: acute bacterial endocarditis
C*   Unknown source
　　1   Healthy child or adult
　　2   Associations: hypercoagulable state secondary to systemic disease, carcinoma (especially pancreatic), eclampsia of pregnancy, oral contraceptives, lupus, anticoagulants, factor C deficiency, factor S deficiency, etc.

* May occur in patients under 30.

TIA SYNDROME   TIAs can be conveniently divided into three types: (1) large vessel low-flow TIA, (2) embolic TIA, and (3) lacunar or small penetrating vessel TIA. *Low-flow TIAs* are brief (usually minutes to a few hours), recurrent, and stereotyped. They are often associated with a tightly stenotic atherosclerotic lesion at the internal carotid artery origin or in the intracranial portion of the internal carotid artery (siphon) when collateral flow from the circle of Willis to the ipsilateral middle or anterior cerebral artery is impaired (Figs. 368-1 and 368-2). Other important causes include atherosclerotic stenotic lesions in the middle cerebral artery stem or at the junction of the vertebral and basilar artery (see Fig. 368-2). Any obstructive vascular process listed in Table 368-1 in the extra- or intracranial arteries can cause a low-flow TIA syndrome if collateral flow to the potentially ischemic brain is also impaired (see Figs. 368-1A–C and 368-2).

Embolic TIAs are characterized by discrete, usually single, more prolonged (hours) episodes of focal neurologic symptoms. The embolus may arise from a pathologic process in an artery, usually extracranial, or from the heart. If symptoms or signs persist beyond 24 h, an ischemic stroke with infarction has occurred. However, symptoms that last less than 24 h also may be associated with ischemic infarction. If the primary pathologic process is thought to be embolic, a diligent search for its source is necessary before therapy to prevent future stroke is initiated. *Lacunar or penetrating vessel TIAs* occasionally occur due to transient cerebral ischemia from stenosis of one of the intracerebral penetrating vessels arising from the middle cerebral artery stem, the basilar or vertebral artery, or the circle of Willis (see Fig. 368-2). Occlusion of these small intracerebral penetrating vessels is usually due to lipohyalinosis from hypertension but also may arise from atheromatous disease at their origin. Occasionally, recurrent stereotyped TIAs occur. In this case, the term *lacunar* or *small-vessel TIAs* seems appropriate.

FIGURE 368-1   Arrangement of the major arteries of the right side carrying blood from the heart to the brain. Also shown are vessels of collateral circulation that may modify the effects of cerebral ischemia (*A,B,C*). Not shown is the circle of Willis, which also provides a source for collateral circulation. *A.* The anastomotic channels between the distal branches of the anterior and middle cerebral artery, termed borderzone or watershed anastomotic channels. Note that they also occur between the posterior and middle cerebral arteries and the anterior and posterior cerebral arteries. *B.* Anastomotic channels occurring through the orbit between branches of the external carotid artery and ophthalmic branch of the internal carotid artery. *C.* Wholly extracranial anastomotic channels between the muscular branches of the ascending cervical arteries and muscular branches of the occipital artery that anastomose with the distal vertebral artery. Note that the occipital artery arises from the external carotid artery, thereby allowing reconstitution of flow in the vertebral from the carotid circulation. *(Courtesy of C.M. Fisher, M.D.)*

STROKE SYNDROME   The clinical characteristics and temporal course of ischemic stroke are produced by the same pathophysiologic mechanism responsible for TIAs: (1) large vessel thrombosis with low flow, (2) artery-to-artery, cardiogenic, or unknown-source embolism, or (3) small intracerebral penetrating vessel occlusion producing a lacuna. Of the many causes of primary thrombotic and embolic stroke listed in Table 368-1, thrombosis complicating atherosclerosis accounts for most cases of thrombotic stroke, and embolus of an unknown or cardiac source accounts for most cases of embolic stroke. The symptoms and signs resulting from an ischemic stroke differ depending on the precise location of the occlusion and the extent of the spared collateral flow. The following descriptions apply to

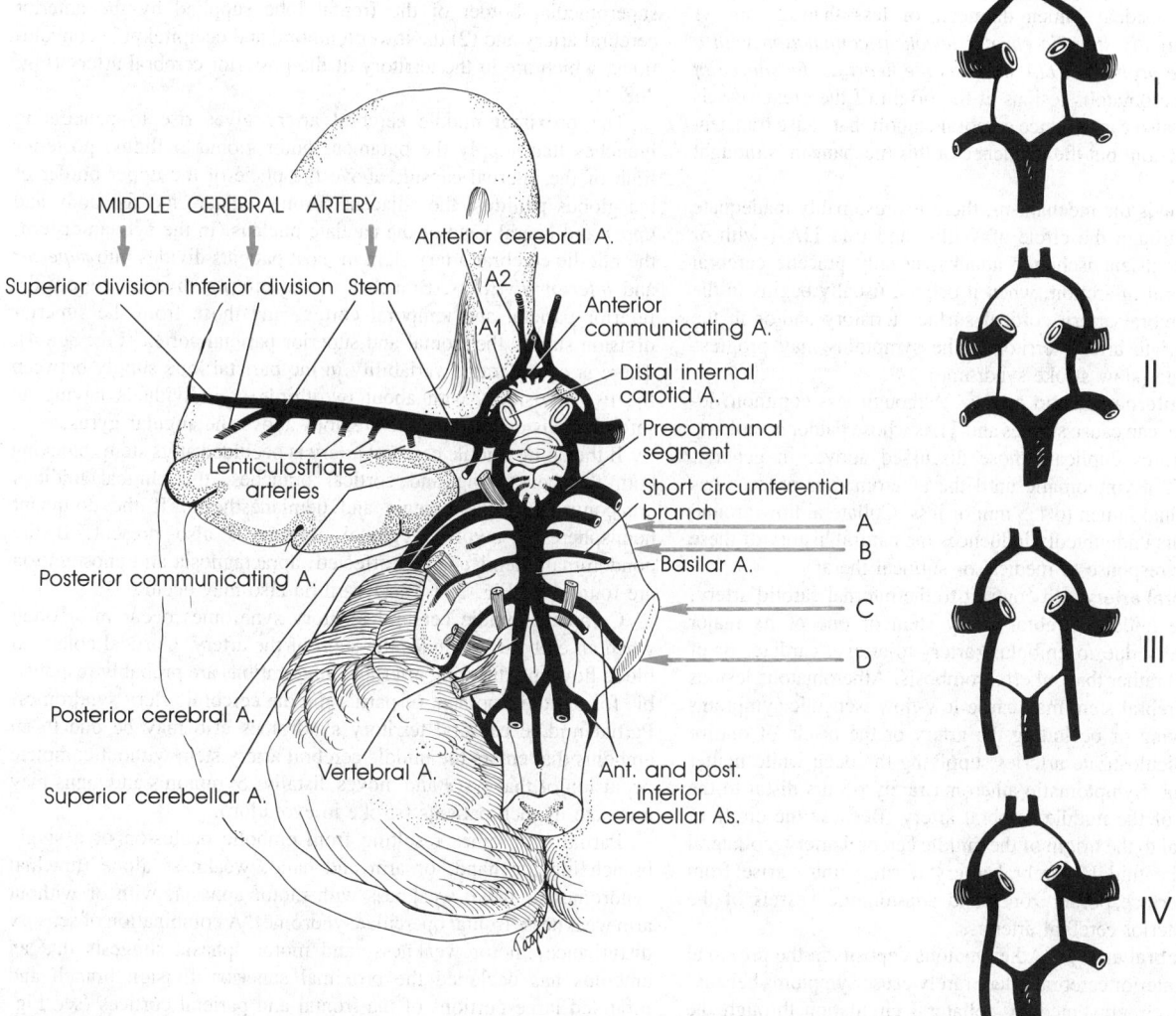

MIDDLE CEREBRAL ARTERY

Superior division Inferior division Stem

Anterior cerebral A.

A2

A1

Anterior communicating A.

Distal internal carotid A.

Precommunal segment

Short circumferential branch

Basilar A.

A
B
C
D

Lenticulostriate arteries

Posterior communicating A.

Posterior cerebral A.

Superior cerebellar A.

Vertebral A.

Ant. and post. inferior cerebellar As.

I

II

III

IV

FIGURE 368-2 Diagram of the brainstem, cerebellum, inferior right frontal lobe, and temporal lobe transected. Principal branches of the vertebral basilar arterial system are pictured. Small branches of the vertebral and basilar artery that penetrate the medulla and pons are not pictured. The stem of the middle cerebral artery with its small, deep penetrating lenticulostriate arteries and the circle of Willis with its small, deep penetrating branches are shown. Roman numerals I, II, III, and IV represent some of the possible variations of the circle of Willis due to atresia of one or more of its arterial components. *A, B, C,* and *D* arrows point to the four cross sections of the brainstem diagrammed below (*D* = Fig. 368-7, *A* = Fig. 368-8, *B* = Fig. 368-9, *C* = Fig. 368-10). Although typical vascular syndromes of the pons and medulla have been designated by the shaded areas in Figs. 368-7 to 368-10, the shading is arbitrary. Great variability in infarct size and location occurs when the basilar or vertebral arteries or one of their penetrating branches becomes occluded. This variability is because of variation in arterial anatomic location and available collateral circulation. Thus the stroke syndromes produced are often atypical, incomplete, or merge with one another. (*Courtesy of C.M. Fisher, M.D.*)

infarction and ischemia in specific arteries due to atherothrombosis, although similar syndromes may occur with other types of arterial pathology, after primary embolic stroke, and occasionally after primary intracerebral hemorrhage.

ATHEROTHROMBOTIC DISEASE OF THE INTERNAL CAROTID ARTERY AND ITS BRANCHES

PATHOPHYSIOLOGY The origin of the internal carotid artery is the most common site of atherosclerosis and superimposed atherothrombosis that leads to TIA or stroke. Less often, disease at the siphon (S-shaped portion of the internal carotid artery in the cavernous sinus) or in the proximal segment (stem) of the middle or anterior cerebral arteries may be responsible. Rarely, the origin of the common carotid artery may be the site.

Internal carotid artery Atherosclerosis in the proximal internal carotid artery is usually most severe in the first 2 cm and arises from the posterior wall, often extending downward into the common carotid artery. Atherosclerosis at this site is often heralded by a minor stoke or TIA caused by embolism or, less frequently, low flow.

Emboli arising from a stenotic or ulcerated atherosclerotic lesion at the origin of the internal carotid artery may cause occlusion of the ophthalmic artery, the middle cerebral artery stem or one of its branches, or, less often, the anterior cerebral artery. Small platelet emboli that occlude the ophthalmic artery branches cause transient monocular blindness (*amaurosis fugax*). Larger emboli composed of platelet-fibrin clot may occlude the primary and secondary branches of the middle cerebral artery leading to discrete and easily recognizable neurologic syndromes. Large emboli may occlude the proximal "stem" of the middle cerebral artery, leading to devastating ischemia of the entire middle cerebral territory (deep white matter, lenticular nuclei, and cortical surface). In some instances, only deep infarction occurs because collateral flow through the cortical surface is sufficient (see Fig. 368-1A). Large emboli may partially occlude a major vessel or may migrate or lyse and disperse, causing a neurologic deficit that fluctuates (stroke in evolution) or resolves.

In some patients, an ulcerated plaque may be the only lesion in the carotid bifurcation, but more often there is an accompanying stenosis with a residual lumen diameter of less than 2 mm. *A nonstenotic or slightly stenotic carotid lesion in conjunction with a stroke or a single prolonged TIA suggests the heart as the source of the embolus.* Atheromatous lesions at the origin of the great vessels in the aortic arch also can produce cerebral emboli that cause transient ischemia or infarction, but the incidence of this mechanism is thought to be low.

When *low flow* is the mechanism, there is presumably inadequate collateral flow through the circle of Willis, and true TIAs, with or without retinal transient ischemic attacks, usually precede cerebral infarction. Cerebral infarction, when it occurs, usually begins in the distal middle cerebral artery cortical surface territory and/or in the distal lenticulostriate artery territory. The symptoms may progress slowly or fluctuate (slow stroke syndrome).

Intracranial internal carotid artery   Although less common, lesions in the siphon can cause strokes and TIAs whose pathophysiologic and clinical features duplicate those discussed above. In general, siphon stenosis is asymptomatic until the atheromatous process has reduced the residual lumen to 1.5 mm or less. Collateral flow around the circle of Willis undoubtedly influences the natural history of these lesions and their response to medical or surgical therapy.

Middle cerebral artery   In contrast to the internal carotid artery, occlusion of the middle cerebral artery stem or one of its major branches is usually due to embolus (artery-to-artery, cardiac, or of unknown source) rather than atherothrombosis. Atheromatous lesions in the middle cerebral stem may cause low-flow ischemic symptoms either by narrowing or occluding the artery or the origin of one or more of the lenticulostriate arteries supplying the deep white matter and basal ganglia. Symptomatic atheroma rarely occurs distal to the first bifurcation of the middle cerebral artery. Because the circle of Willis is proximal to the origin of the middle cerebral artery, collateral blood flow to the middle cerebral artery territory must arise from small cortical surface border zones and anastomotic vessels of the anterior and posterior cerebral arteries.

Anterior cerebral artery   Atheromatous deposits in the proximal segment of the anterior cerebral artery rarely cause symptoms because the occlusion is circumvented by collateral circulation through the anterior communicating artery. However, if the anterior communicating artery is congenitally atretic or if the atheromatous lesion occurs distal in the anterior cerebral artery, TIAs and stroke may occur.

CLINICAL SYNDROMES   Middle cerebral artery   The cortical branches of the middle cerebral artery supply the lateral surface of the hemisphere except for (1) the frontal pole and a strip along the superomedial border of the frontal lobe supplied by the anterior cerebral artery and (2) the lower temporal and occipital pole convolutions, which are in the territory of the posterior cerebral artery (Fig. 368-3).

The proximal middle cerebral artery gives rise to penetrating branches that supply the putamen, outer globus pallidus, posterior limb of the internal capsule above the plane of the upper border of the globus pallidus, the adjacent corona radiata, and the body and upper and lateral head of the caudate nucleus. In the sylvian cistern, the middle cerebral artery stem in most patients divides into *superior* and *inferior divisions*. Branches of the inferior division supply the inferior parietal and temporal cortex, and those from the superior division supply the frontal and superior parietal cortex (Fig. 368-4). There is considerable variability in the parietal lobe supply between the two divisions, with about two-thirds of individuals having an inferior division that supplies regions above the angular gyrus.

If the entire middle cerebral artery is occluded at its stem, blocking both the penetrating and cortical branches, the clinical findings are contralateral hemiplegia and hemianesthesia. If the dominant hemisphere is involved, global aphasia is also present. If the nondominant hemisphere is affected, apractagnosia and anosognosia are found (see Fig. 368-4). Dysarthria also may occur.

Complete middle cerebral territory syndromes occur most often when an embolus occludes the stem of the artery. Cortical collateral blood flow and differing arterial configurations are probably responsible for the development of partial middle cerebral artery syndromes. Partial middle cerebral territory syndromes also may be due to an embolus that enters the middle cerebral artery stem without complete occlusion or that lyses and moves distally. Symptoms and signs may fluctuate in such patients (stroke in evolution).

Partial syndromes resulting from embolic occlusion of a single branch include hand, or arm and hand, weakness alone (brachial syndrome) or facial weakness with motor aphasia, with or without arm weakness (frontal opercular syndrome). A combination of sensory disturbance, motor weakness, and motor aphasia suggests that an embolus has occluded the proximal superior division branch and infarcted large portions of the frontal and parietal cortices (see Fig. 368-4). If Wernicke's aphasia occurs without weakness, the inferior division of the middle cerebral artery supplying the posterior part (temporal cortex) of the dominant hemisphere is probably involved (see Fig. 368-4). Jargon speech and an inability to comprehend written and oral language are prominent features, often accompanied by a

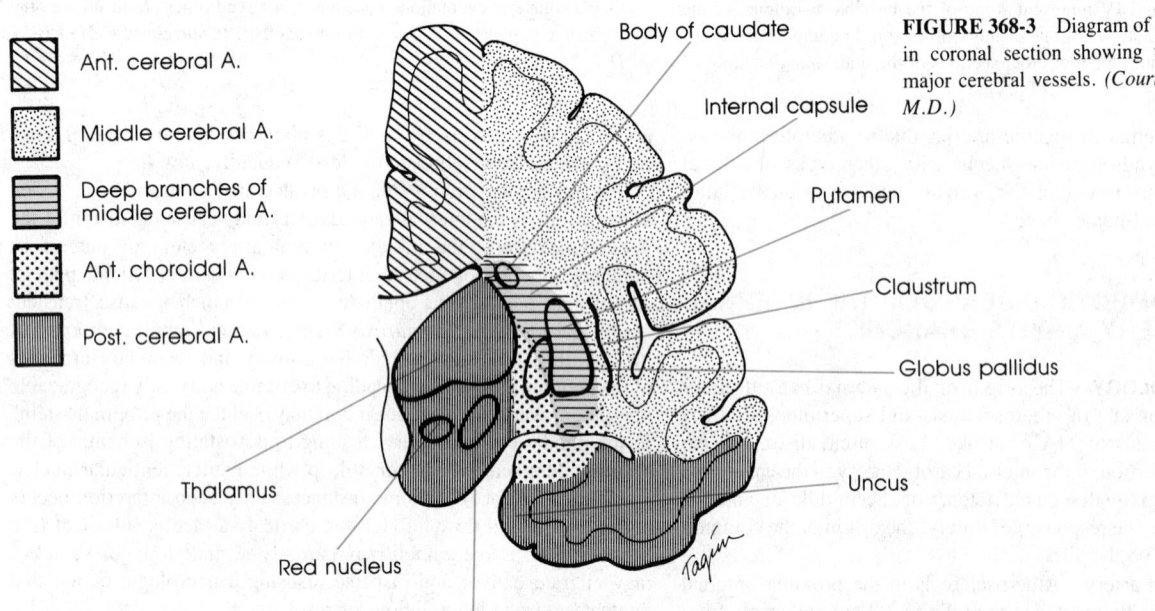

Ant. cerebral A.

Middle cerebral A.

Deep branches of middle cerebral A.

Ant. choroidal A.

Post. cerebral A.

Body of caudate

Internal capsule

Putamen

Claustrum

Globus pallidus

Uncus

Thalamus

Red nucleus

Subthalamic body

FIGURE 368-3   Diagram of a cerebral hemisphere in coronal section showing the territories of the major cerebral vessels. (*Courtesy of C. M. Fisher, M.D.*)

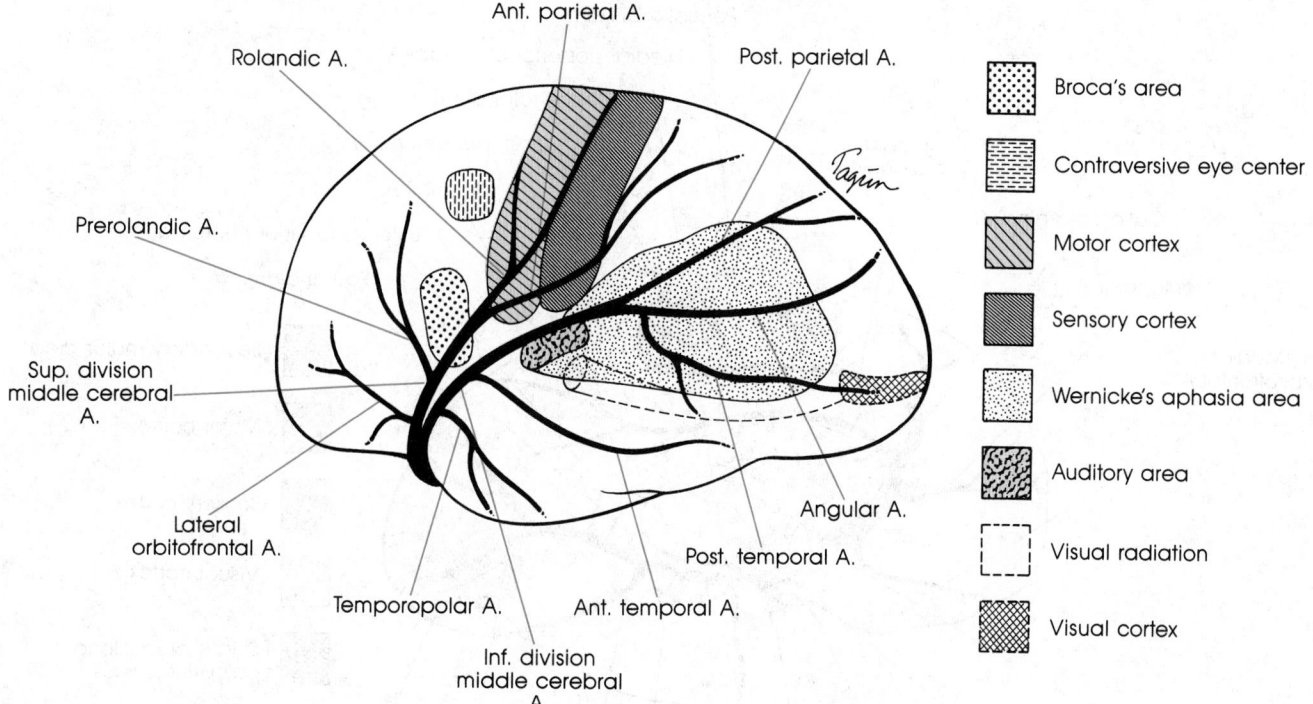

FIGURE 368-4 Diagram of a cerebral hemisphere, lateral aspect, showing the branches and distribution of the middle cerebral artery and the principal regions of cerebral localization. Note the bifurcation of the middle cerebral artery into a superior and inferior division (*Courtesy of C. M. Fisher, M.D.*)

Signs and symptoms	Structures involved
Paralysis of the contralateral face, arm, and leg; sensory impairment over the same area (pinprick, cotton touch, vibration, position, two-point discrimination, stereognosis, tactile localization, barognosis, cutaneographia)	Somatic motor area for face and arm and the fibers descending from the leg area to enter the corona radiata and corresponding somatic sensory system
Motor aphasia	Motor speech area of the dominant hemisphere
Central aphasia, word deafness, anomia, jargon speech, sensory agraphia, acalculia, alexia, finger agnosia, right-left confusion (the last four comprise the Gerstmann syndrome)	Central, suprasylvian speech area and parietooccipital cortex of the dominant hemisphere
Conduction aphasia	Central speech area (parietal operculum)
Apractognosia of the minor hemisphere (amorphosynthesis), anosognosia, hemiasomatognosia, unilateral neglect, agnosia for the left half of external space, dressing "apraxia," constructional "apraxia," distortion of visual coordinates, inaccurate localization in the half field, impaired ability to judge distance, upside-down reading, visual illusions (e.g., it may appear that another person walks through a table)	Nondominant parietal lobe (area corresponding to speech area in dominant hemisphere); loss of topographic memory is usually due to a nondominant lesion, occasionally to a dominant one
Homonymous hemianopsia (often homonymous inferior quadrantanopsia)	Optic radiation deep to second temporal convolution
Paralysis of conjugate gaze to the opposite side	Frontal contraversive field or fibers projecting therefrom

contralateral superior quadrantanopsia. Hemineglect or spatial agnosia without weakness indicates that the inferior division of the middle cerebral artery in the nondominant hemisphere is involved.

Anterior cerebral artery The anterior cerebral artery is divided into two segments: the precommunal (A1) circle of Willis, or stem, which connects the internal carotid artery to the anterior communicating artery, and the postcommunal (A2) segment distal to the anterior communicating artery (see Fig. 368-2). The A1 segment of the anterior cerebral artery gives rise to several deep penetrating branches that supply the anterior limb of the internal capsule, the anterior perforate substance, amygdala, anterior hypothalamus, and the inferior part of the head of the caudate nucleus (see Fig. 368-3).

Infarction in the territory of the anterior cerebral artery is uncommon and most often due to embolism rather than atherothrombosis. Occlusion of the A1 segment of the anterior cerebral artery is usually well tolerated because of collateral flow. If both A2 segments arise from a single anterior cerebral stem (contralateral A1 segment atresia), then the occlusion affects both hemispheres. Profound abulia (a delay in verbal and motor response) and bilateral pyramidal signs with paraplegia result. Occlusion of a single A2 segment of the anterior

cerebral artery results in the contralateral symptoms noted in the legend of Fig. 368-5.

Anterior choroidal artery This artery arises from the internal carotid artery and supplies the posterior limb of the internal capsule and the white matter posterolateral to it, through which pass some of the geniculocalcarine fibers (Figs. 368-3 and 368-6). The complete clinical syndrome of anterior choroidal artery occlusion consists of contralateral hemiplegia, hemianesthesia (hypesthesia), and homonymous hemianopsia. However, because this territory is also supplied by penetrating vessels of the middle cerebral stem and the posterior communicating and posterior choroidal arteries, syndromes with minimal deficits may occur, and patients frequently recover partially or completely.

Internal carotid artery The clinical picture of internal carotid occlusion varies depending on whether the cause of ischemia is propagated thrombus, embolism, or low flow. The cortex supplied by the middle cerebral territory is most often affected. With a competent circle of Willis, however, occlusion can be entirely asymptomatic. Less often, there is massive infarction of the deep white matter and cortical surface from propagation of a thrombus up

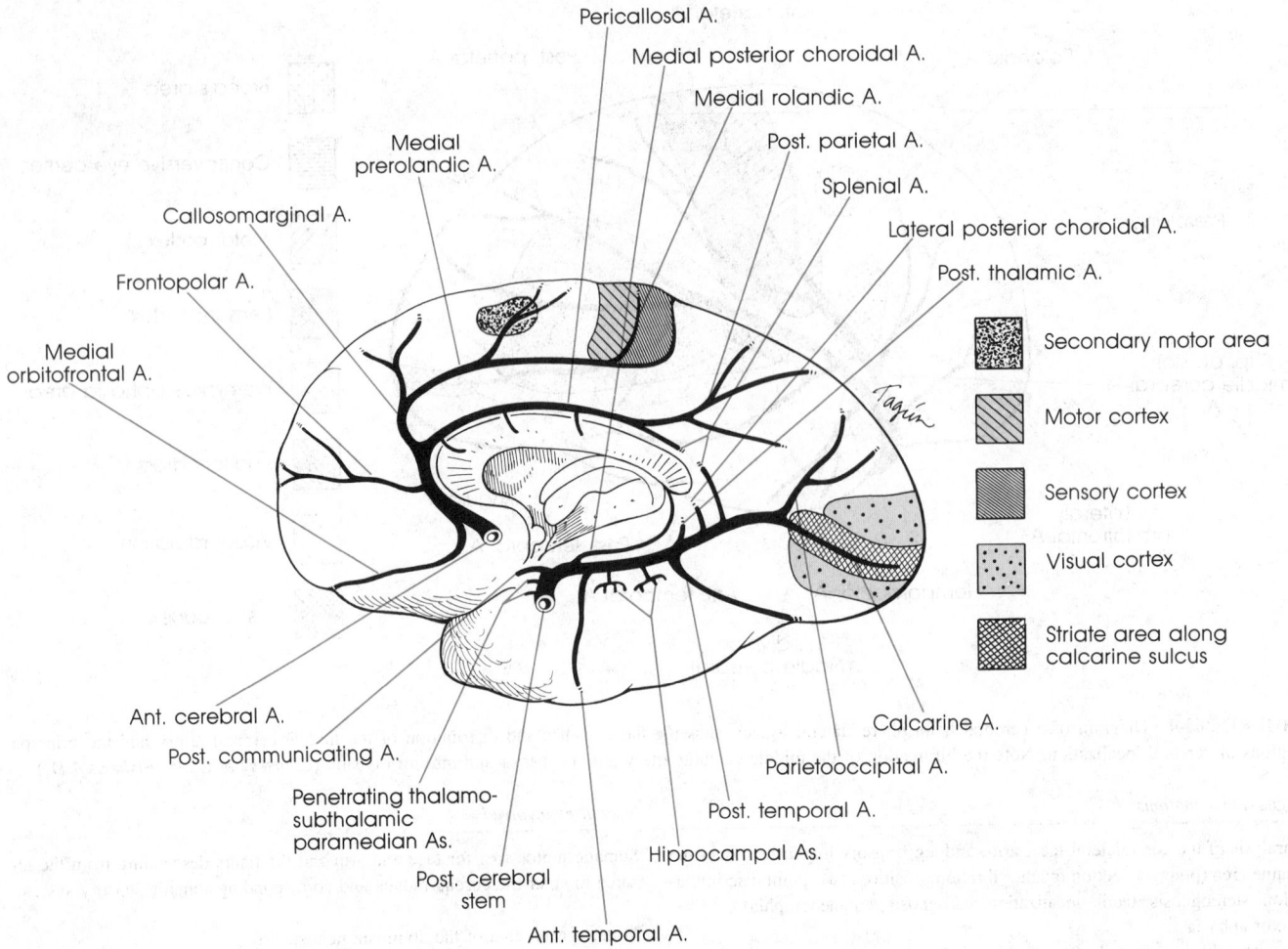

FIGURE 368-5 Diagram of a cerebral hemisphere, medial aspect, showing the branches and distribution of the anterior cerebral artery and the principal regions of cerebral localization. (*Courtesy of C. M. Fisher, M.D.*)

Signs and symptoms	Structures involved
Paralysis of opposite foot and leg	Motor leg area
A lesser degree of paresis of opposite arm	Involvement of arm area of cortex or fibers descending to corona radiata therefrom
Cortical sensory loss over toes, foot, and leg	Sensory area for foot and leg
Urinary incontinence	Sensorimotor area in paracentral lobule
Contralateral grasp reflex, sucking reflex, gegenhalten (paratonic rigidity)	Medial surface of the posterior frontal lobe (?) supplemental motor area
Abulia (akinetic mutism), slowness, delay, intermittent interruption, lack of spontaneity, whispering, reflex distraction to sights and sounds	Uncertain localization—probably cingulate gyrus and medial inferior portion of frontal, parietal, and temporal lobes
Impairment of gait and stance (gait apraxia)	Frontal cortex near leg motor area
Dyspraxia of left limbs, tactile aphasia in left limbs	Corpus callosum

the internal carotid artery, into the middle cerebral stem, or from embolization to the stem of the middle cerebral artery. Symptoms are identical to middle cerebral stem occlusion (see above). When the origins of both the anterior and middle cerebral arteries are occluded by embolus to the top of the carotid artery, abulia and/or stupor occurs with hemiplegia, hemianesthesia, and aphasia or anosognosia. When the posterior cerebral artery arises from the internal carotid artery (an unusual configuration called a *fetal posterior cerebral artery*), it also may become occluded and give rise to symptoms referable to its peripheral territory (see Figs. 368-5 and 368-6).

Carotid occlusion may cause low-flow infarction if the circle of Willis is incomplete. The territory of the distal cortical branches of the middle cerebral artery tends to be involved, giving rise to transient or stepwise, progressive hip, shoulder, or arm weakness. Other TIAs suggestive of carotid insufficiency include recurrent unilateral tongue, lip, cheek, or hand numbness, with or without motor weakness.

In addition to supplying the ipsilateral brain, the internal carotid artery perfuses the optic nerve and retina via the ophthalmic artery (see Fig. 368-1). In about 25 percent of symptomatic internal carotid disease, transient recurrent monocular blindness (TMB or amaurosis fugax) warns of the lesion. Patients may describe a shade that seems to sweep up, down, or across the field of vision or may say that the periphery of vision fades away. They also may complain that their vision was blurred in that eye or that the upper or lower half of vision disappeared. In most cases, these symptoms last only a few minutes. Rarely, ophthalmic or central retinal artery occlusion develops at the time of stroke.

Common carotid artery All the neurologic symptoms and signs of internal carotid occlusion also may be present with occlusion of the common carotid artery. Bilateral common carotid arterial occlusion at their origin may occur in "pulseless disease," or the aortic arch syndrome (see Chap. 210). Clues to this condition are absence of

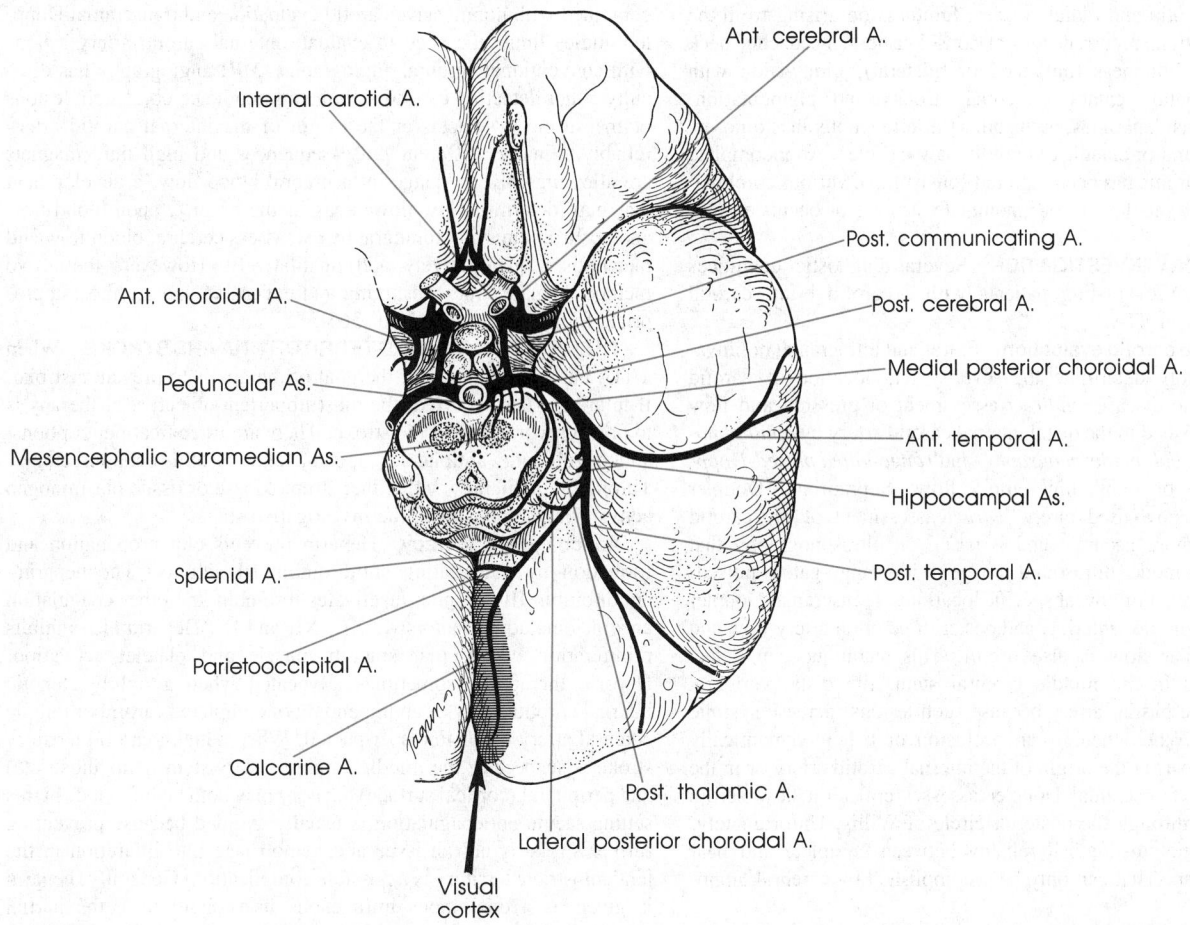

FIGURE 368-6 Inferior aspect of the brain with the branches and distribution of the posterior cerebral artery and the principal anatomic structures shown. (*Courtesy of C. M. Fisher, M.D.*)

Signs and symptoms	*Structures involved*
Peripheral territory (see also Fig. 368-5)	
Homonymous hemianopsia (often upper quadrantic)	Calcarine cortex or optic radiation nearby
Bilateral homonymous hemianopsia, cortical blindness, awareness or denial of blindness; tactile naming, achromatopsia (color blindness), failure to see to-and-fro movements, inability to perceive objects not centrally located, apraxia of ocular movements, inability to count or enumerate objects, tendency to run into things which the patient sees and tries to avoid	Bilateral occipital lobe with possibly the parietal lobe involved.
Verbal dyslexia without agraphia, color anomia	Dominant calcarine lesion and posterior part of corpus callosum
Memory defect	Hippocampal lesion bilaterally or on the dominant side only
Topographic disorientation and prosopagnosia	Usually with lesions of nondominant, calcarine, and lingual gyrus
Simultagnosia, hemivisual neglect	Dominant visual cortex, contralateral hemisphere
Unformed visual hallucinations, peduncular hallucinosis, metamorphopsia, teleopsia, illusory visual spread, irreminiscence, paliopsia, distortion of outlines, central photophobia	Calcarine cortex
Complex hallucinations	Usually nondominant hemisphere
Central territory	
Thalamic syndrome: sensory loss (all modalities), spontaneous pain and dysesthesias, choreoathetosis, intention tremor, spasms of hand, mild hemiparesis	Posteroventral nucleus of thalamus; involvement of the adjacent subthalamus body or its afferent tracts
Thalamoperforate syndrome: crossed cerebellar ataxia with ipsilateral third nerve palsy (Claude's syndrome)	Dentatothalamic tract and issuing third nerve
Weber's syndrome: third nerve palsy and contralateral hemiplegia	Third nerve and cerebral peduncle
Contralateral hemiplegia	Cerebral peduncle
Paralysis or paresis of vertical eye movement, skew deviation, sluggish pupillary responses to light, slight miosis and ptosis (retraction nystagmus and "tucking" of the eyelids may be associated)	Supranuclear fibers to third nerve, interstitial nucleus of Cajal, nucleus of Darkschewitsch, and posterior commissure
Contralateral rhythmic, ataxic action tremor; rhythmic postural or "holding" tremor (rubral tremor)	Dentatothalamic tract (?)

pulsation in carotid and radial arteries, faintness on arising from the horizontal position, recurrent loss of consciousness, headache, neck pain, transient blindness (unilateral or bilateral), dim vision with exercise, premature cataracts, retinal atrophy and pigmentation, atrophy of the iris, leukomas, peripapillary arteriovenous anastomoses, optic atrophy, and/or claudication of the jaw muscles. An incomplete aortic arch syndrome has been reported consisting of various combinations of carotid, subclavian, or innominate stenosis or occlusion (see below).

LABORATORY INVESTIGATION   Several diagnostic techniques are available for evaluating patients with a carotid bruit, carotid territory stroke, or TIA.

Noninvasive carotid evaluation   Extra- and intracranial noninvasive tests reliably determine the severity and location of carotid atherothrombotic disease. *Indirect* assessment of pressure and flow can be accomplished in the distal internal carotid artery by *ophthalmodynamometry, oculoplethysmography,* and *range-gated pulsed-Doppler assessment* of ophthalmic artery flow. Supraorbital Doppler examination is now used rarely. *Direct* assessment of the carotid bifurcation is more accurate and is based on ultrasonography that combines a B-mode ultrasound image with range-gated pulsed-Doppler assessment of flow at specific locations. Transcranial Doppler assessment of middle, anterior, and posterior cerebral artery flow and of vertebrobasilar flow is also useful. This technique can detect stenotic lesions in the middle cerebral stem, the distal vertebral arteries, and the basilar artery because such lesions increase systolic flow velocity. When there is an occlusion or a hemodynamically significant stenosis at the origin of the internal carotid artery or in the carotid siphon, transcranial Doppler assesses collateral flow across the anterior or through the posterior circle of Willis. Unfortunately, these tests cannot distinguish reliably between complete and near carotid occlusion. That can only be accomplished by cerebral angiography.

Cerebral angiography   Cerebral angiography performed by selective extracranial dye injection after transfemoral catheterization remains the most reliable method of assessing the cerebrovascular system. It can (1) detect ulcerative lesions, severe stenosis, and formation of mural thrombus at the bifurcation of the common carotid artery, (2) visualize atherothrombotic disease or dissection in the carotid siphon or intracranial vessels, (3) demonstrate collateral circulation around the circle of Willis and on the cortical surface, and (4) show embolic occlusion of cerebral branch vessels. Although angiography cannot measure blood flow directly, the timing of dye arrival reflects relative pressures in major vessels and may demonstrate compromised flow in the internal carotid artery system.

The advantages of selective cerebral angiography must be balanced in each patient against complications that occur in 2 to 12 percent. The principal risks are aortic or carotid artery dissection and embolic stroke. Cholesterol emboli from aortic arch atheroma rarely can cause watershed cerebral infarction and renal failure. A skilled angiographer and careful attention to hydration reduce these risks. Because of the risks, attention is now being directed to the development of magnetic resonance angiographic imaging (see Chap. 365).

Brain imaging   Brain imaging remains the most important acute test once a stroke has occurred. *Computed tomographic* (CT) *scans* immediately exclude hemorrhage as the cause of stroke, but they may fail to show small ischemic strokes in the posterior fossa or be imprecise because of bone artifact. CT scans also may miss infarction on the cortical surface. Furthermore, they cannot detect cerebral infarction reliably for the first 24 to 48 h (see Chap. 365).

Magnetic resonance imaging (MRI) reliably documents the extent and location of infarction not only in the cortical surface, but also in the deep white matter and in the posterior fossa within 1 h of its onset. It also documents primary intracranial hemorrhage. The higher the field strength, the more reliable and precise the image will be. Using high field strengths (1.5 Tesla) and different pulse sequencing, blood flow may be imaged in the extracranial arteries and in the large intracranial extracerebral vessels. In many cases, *MRI angiography*

combined with noninvasive carotid evaluation and transcranial Doppler studies limits the need to evaluate internal carotid artery lesions with conventional cerebral angiography. MRI angiography has difficulty either detecting carotid siphon and middle cerebral stem lesions or measuring a stenosis at the origin of the internal carotid artery reliably. Finally, different pulse sequences and high field magnets are allowing MRI to image intracerebral blood flow, a development that may determine low-flow areas in the brain. Xenon-blood-flow and positron-emission tomography can assess cerebral blood flow and metabolism quantitatively and qualitatively. However, these two methods remain time-consuming and expensive and are most appropriate for research (see Chap. 365).

THERAPY FOR CAROTID TERRITORY TIA AND STROKE   When a TIA has been diagnosed, the goal of therapy is to prevent a stroke. If infarction has occurred, the most important objective of therapy is to prevent worsening of the stroke. There are three treatment options: anticoagulation, antiplatelet agents, and carotid endarterectomy. Thrombolytic therapy with either streptokinase or tissue plasminogen activator agents is still in the investigative stage.

Anticoagulant therapy   Heparin prevents clot propagation and formation by potentiating antithrombin III activity. The heparin–antithrombin III complex inactivates thrombin and other coagulation enzymes including factors X, XII, XI, and IX. Heparin also inhibits proliferation of vascular smooth muscle and platelet activation. Heparin therapy is sometimes advocated when a tightly stenotic internal carotid artery or an impending or completed carotid or middle cerebral artery occlusion is suspected. When a major carotid territory stroke is suspected, the middle cerebral artery stem (lenticulostriate) and peripheral (cortical surface) territory may both be infarcted. In this setting, acute anticoagulation is usually avoided because preventing further stroke is not an issue and hemorrhage into infarction in the lenticulostriate territory is a possible complication. Generally, heparin is given as a continuous intravenous infusion to raise the partial thromboplastin time to 1.5 to 2.5 times control. A 1000- to 10,000-unit bolus may be given prior to initiating the continuous infusion.

Sodium warfarin (Coumadin) inhibits the activation of vitamin K, the essential cofactor in the activation of the vitamin K–dependent coagulation proteins. Chronic oral anticoagulation with sodium warfarin is considered in patients when an embolic or low-flow TIA or stroke is related to carotid siphon or middle cerebral stem stenosis. It is also considered for 6-month trial to prevent subsequent embolism when the internal carotid artery is known to have been occluded recently. Although several studies have suggested that sodium warfarin is effective in these clinical settings, a randomized study is required to document conclusively the effectiveness of either oral anticoagulation or antiplatelet agents. It is well established that the risk of hemorrhage is directly related to the intensity of anticoagulation. Therefore, low-intensity warfarin anticoagulation (prothrombin time ratio 1.2 to 1.5 times control or international normalized ratio 1.5 to 2.7 or 2 to 3) is usually used (see "Embolism," below). When the standard medical contraindications are present, antiplatelet therapy becomes the only option.

Antiplatelet therapy   Studies of the effect of antiplatelet agents on the natural history of TIAs and minor stroke all suffer from a lack of precise understanding of the pathophysiologic condition underlying the ischemic event. Aspirin has been the most widely studied antiplatelet agent. Paradoxically, aspirin has dual effects: It inhibits platelet formation of thromboxane A_2, a platelet-aggregating, vasoconstricting prostaglandin, but it also inhibits the formation of prostacyclin, an antiaggregating, vasodilating prostaglandin derived from endothelial cells. Aspirin in low doses predominantly inhibits the production of thromboxane A_2; therefore, many physicians recommend aspirin in doses of 300 mg or less per day.

Dipyridamole acts by inhibiting platelet phosphodiesterase, which is responsible for the breakdown of cyclic adenosine monophosphate (AMP). The resulting elevation in cyclic AMP inhibits the aggregation of platelets. There is no reliable evidence to suggest that dipyridamole alone prevents ischemic stroke. In one study in patients with prosthetic valves, there was a nonstatistically significant suggestion that warfarin in combination with dipyridamole helped prevent embolism. Ticlopidine is thought to inhibit platelet binding to fibrinogen, and recent studies have shown it to be comparable to aspirin in preventing stroke in patients with TIAs or stroke. Unfortunately, these studies also suffer from failure to define precisely the pathophysiologic cause of the cerebral symptoms. Ticlopidine has the disadvantage of incurring a small risk of leukopenia, diarrhea, and rash. It is recommended for use as an antiplatelet agent only if aspirin is contraindicated or fails.

Carotid endarterectomy Carotid endarterectomy is the treatment of choice for patients who have had a low-flow or embolic TIA or minor stroke resulting from a tightly stenotic (>70 percent stenosis) arteriosclerotic lesion at the origin of the internal carotid artery. Its efficacy has been documented by three randomized trials. However, none of them found a statistically significant improvement in subsequent ipsilateral stroke when endarterectomy is performed on lesions that are not tightly stenotic. One of the trials is continuing to randomize patients with a 30 to 70 percent stenotic internal carotid artery origin lesion and ipsilateral carotid territory symptoms. Each trial has had a combined surgery and angiography complication rate of less than 4 percent. It is clear that the morbidity is lowest when patients are properly selected from a cardiac/medical risk point of view and an experienced team of surgeons, physicians, and nurses manages the patients. Reliable guidelines have now been developed to exclude patients with an unacceptable cardiac risk. Unless the combined anesthesia and surgical morbidity and mortality are less than 5 percent, medical therapy is probably the best choice. Because in one study endarterectomy carried a 26 percent benefit for stroke reduction compared with aspirin, the latter might not be the best medical therapy. Low-intensity warfarin anticoagulation may be better. It is often considered in patients with symptomatic tightly stenotic carotid stenosis who carry too high a risk for surgery.

Antiedema and general medical therapy Cerebral edema occurs in most ischemic infarctions but is rarely a problem unless large middle cerebral stem territory infarction occurs. When edema with mass effect is evident on CT or MRI and the patient becomes drowsy, it is best to keep the patient slightly dehydrated with a normal or elevated serum sodium level. If symptoms worsen, therapy with mannitol to keep the serum osmolarity above 300 mosmol/L is helpful. Serious cerebral edema usually begins 48 to 72 h after the stroke and begins to resolve by the second week. In all patients with acute carotid territory ischemic stroke and hypertension, it is best not to lower the blood pressure rapidly. The expanded use of anticoagulant therapy to prevent subsequent stroke has the added advantage of helping to prevent phlebitis in patients with a hemiparesis.

Experimental therapies Therapies designed to protect the brain under conditions of extreme ischemia are being actively studied. Therapies designed to reduce blood viscosity have been effective in the laboratory setting but have not been clearly effective in the clinical setting of prolonged ischemia. Nonetheless, they carry little risk and may be of benefit. It is probably best to keep the hematocrit slightly low, at 35 percent, if there is prolonged cerebral ischemia in the stroke process. Calcium channel antagonists have not convincingly limited infarct size. Experimental studies with glutamate receptor antagonists (specifically the NMDA subtype; see Chap. 364), show promise of reducing stroke size.

ASYMPTOMATIC CAROTID BIFURCATION STENOSIS WITH A BRUIT The natural history of asymptomatic atherosclerotic lesions of the carotid bifurcation that produce a bruit is uncertain. There is evidence that the tighter the stenotic lesion, the more likely symptoms are to occur over time. Patients with tightly stenotic lesions that are hemodynamically significant (residual lumen diameter 1.5 mm or less, 75 percent stenosis) may be at higher risk of embolic stroke. Although such patients have reduced flow in the distal internal carotid artery, they remain asymptomatic because of adequate collateral flow in circle of Willis. Clot may form in the low-flow carotid and may be associated with artery-to-artery embolism.

A high-pitched prolonged carotid bruit fading into diastole is often associated with such tightly stenotic lesions. As the stenosis grows tighter and flow distal to the stenosis becomes reduced, the bruit becomes fainter and finally disappears when occlusion is imminent. Noninvasive carotid testing combined with transcranial Doppler assessment of collateral flow across the anterior circle of Willis helps identify such lesions and document progression.

Medical therapy (aspirin 325 mg/d) generally has been recommended for patients with asymptomatic carotid stenosis. However, patients with hemodynamically significant lesions, particularly if they have progression in severity, may benefit from low-morbidity carotid endarterectomy. However, surgery should be considered only in the absence of significant cardiac disease and when the physiologic age of the patient will allow the benefits of endarterectomy over time. Randomized trials comparing medical and surgical therapy may reliably identify patients with tightly stenotic hemodynamically significant lesions and establish criteria for choosing one treatment over the other.

ATHEROTHROMBOTIC DISEASE OF THE VERTEBROBASILAR–POSTERIOR CEREBRAL ARTERY SYSTEM

The two vertebral arteries join to form the basilar artery at the pontomedullary junction. The basilar artery divides into two posterior cerebral arteries in the interpeduncular fossa (see Fig. 368-2). Each of these major arteries gives rise to long and short circumferential branches and to smaller deep penetrating branches that supply the cerebellum, medulla, pons, midbrain, subthalamus, thalamus, hippocampus, and medial temporal and occipital lobes. Atherosclerosis has a predilection for the origin and the distal segments of the vertebral arteries, the proximal basilar artery, and the origin of the major and minor branches of the vertebral, basilar, and posterior cerebral arteries. Predictably, atheromatous disease at each site carries its own unique natural history, produces its own clinical syndromes, and has its own specific therapeutic implications.

POSTERIOR CEREBRAL ARTERY **Pathophysiology** In 70 percent of cases, both posterior cerebral arteries arise from the bifurcation of the basilar artery; in 22 percent, one or the other comes from the ipsilateral internal carotid artery; in 8 percent, both come from the ipsilateral internal carotid artery (see Fig. 368-2) via the posterior communicating arteries. The precommunal segment (mesencephalic portion) of the true posterior cerebral artery is atretic in such cases (see Fig. 368-2).

Atheroma formation at the top of the basilar artery or along the precommunal segment of the posterior cerebral artery may cause symptoms by narrowing one or more of the small brainstem-penetrating branches (see Figs. 368-2 and 368-6) that supply the middle cerebral peduncles, the substantia nigra, red nucleus, oculomotor nuclei, midbrain reticular formation, subthalamic nucleus of Luys, decussation of superior cerebellar peduncles, the medial longitudinal fasciculus, and the medial lemniscus. The artery of Percheron (the posterior thalamosubthalamoparamedian artery) is a single artery that arises from either the right or the left precommunal segment of the posterior cerebral artery. It divides in the subthalamus to supply the inferomedial and anterior portions of the thalamus and subthalamus bilaterally. The thalamogeniculate branches, which also originate from the precommunal portion of the posterior cerebral artery, supply the dorsal, dorsomedial, anterior, and inferior thalamus and the medial geniculate body. The medial posterior choroidal artery supplies the superior dorsomedial and dorsoanterior thalamus and the medial geniculate body in addition to the tela choroidea of the third ventricle. The lateral posterior choroidal artery supplies the choroid plexus of the lateral ventricle.

Atheroma in the posterior cerebral artery distal to the junction with the posterior communicating artery (see Fig. 368-6) may occlude small circumferential branches that course around the midbrain to supply the lateral part of the cerebral peduncles, medial lemniscus, tegmentum of the midbrain, superior colliculi, lateral geniculate body, and posterolateral nucleus of the thalamus, choroid plexus, and hippocampus. On the rare occasions when atheroma occur more distally in the posterior cerebral artery (see Fig. 368-6), occlusion may produce ischemia and infarction in the inferomedial temporal lobe, parahippocampal and hippocampal gyri, and occipital lobe—including the calcarine cortex and the visual association areas 18 and 19.

Clinical manifestations   The site of atheromas and the degree of narrowing determine the clinical syndrome. Although factors of collateral circulation or serum viscosity may play a role in some cases, embolic occlusion is the usual cause of stroke in this vascular territory. Two syndromes are commonly observed: (1) midbrain, subthalamic, and thalamic signs, which are due to disease of the precommunal segment of the posterior cerebral artery or of its penetrating branches and (2) cortical temporal and occipital lobe syndromes, due to occlusion of the postcommunal segment.

PROXIMAL PRECOMMUNAL SYNDROMES (CENTRAL TERRITORY)   If the proximal posterior cerebral artery is occluded, infarction usually occurs in the ipsilateral or bilateral subthalamus and medial thalamus and in the ipsilateral cerebral peduncle and midbrain, producing concomitant signs (see Fig. 368-6). If the posterior communicating artery is atretic, the peripheral territory supplied by posterior cerebral artery is also affected (see Fig. 368-6). If the posterior cerebral artery is completely occluded at its origin, hemiplegia secondary to infarction of the cerebral peduncle occurs. Involvement of the red nucleus and/or dentatorubrothalamic tract can produce contralateral ataxia. A third nerve palsy with contralateral ataxia (Claude's syndrome) or with contralateral hemiplegia (Weber's syndrome) may result. If the subthalamic nucleus of Luys is involved, contralateral hemiballismus may occur. Occlusion of the artery of Percheron produces paresis of upward gaze and drowsiness and is often associated with abulia. Extensive infarction in the midbrain of the subthalamus occurring with bilateral posterior cerebral stem occlusion is usually secondary to embolism. Coma, bilateral pyramidal signs, and "decerebrate rigidity" occur in this setting.

Atheromatous occlusion of the penetrating branches of the thalamic and thalamogeniculate arteries produces less extensive thalamic and thalamocapsular lacunar syndromes. The *thalamic syndrome of Déjerine and Roussy* is the best known. Its main feature is contralateral hemisensory loss of both superficial sensation (pain and temperature) and deep sensation (touch and proprioception). Occasionally, it may affect only pain and temperature or vibration and joint position sense. After a few weeks or months, an agonizing, searing pain may develop in the affected areas. Patients describe the pain as tight, drawing, icy, and knifelike. It is devastatingly persistent and responds poorly to analgesics. Occasionally, anticonvulsants are beneficial. If the posterior limb of the internal capsule is involved, hemiparesis or hemiplegia may accompany the hemisensory syndrome. Other associated motor signs include hemiballismus, choreoathetosis, intention tremor, incoordination, and posturing of the hand and arm, particularly while walking.

POSTCOMMUNAL SYNDROMES (PERIPHERAL OR CORTICAL TERRITORY) (See also Fig. 368-6)   Occlusion of the posterior cerebral artery causes infarction of the cortical surface of the medial temporal and occipital lobes. Contralateral homonymous hemianopsia is the usual manifestation. Occasionally, only the upper quadrant of the visual field is involved. If the visual association areas are spared and only the calcarine cortex is involved, the patient is aware of visual defects. Central vision may be spared if middle cerebral artery branches supply the macular region of the occipital pole. Medial temporal lobe and hippocampal involvement may cause an acute disturbance in memory, particularly if it occurs in the dominant hemisphere, but the defect usually clears because memory has bilateral representation. If the dominant hemisphere is affected and the infarct extends to involve the splenium of the corpus callosum, the patient may demonstrate alexia without agraphia. Visual agnosia for faces, objects, mathematical symbols, and colors and anomia with paraphasic errors (amnestic aphasia) also may occur in this setting even without callosal involvement. Occlusion of the posterior cerebral artery can produce peduncular hallucinosis (visual hallucinations of brightly colored scenes and objects).

Bilateral infarction in the distal posterior cerebral arteries produces cortical blindness. The patient is often unaware of the blindness. The clinical clue to the site is a finding of normal pupillary reaction to light. Tiny islands of vision may persist, and the patient then reports that vision fluctuates as images are captured in the preserved portions. Rarely, only peripheral vision is lost and central vision is spared, resulting in "gun-barrel" vision. A constellation of symptoms termed *Balint's syndrome* can occur with unilateral or bilateral visual association area lesions. It includes optic ataxia (inability to visually guide limb movements), ocular ataxia (inability to direct eyes to a precise point in the visual field), inability to enumerate objects in a picture or extract meaning from a picture, and inability to avoid objects seen in one's path. Balint's syndrome is seen most often with bilateral infarctions, secondary to low flow in the distal posterior and/or middle cerebral "watershed" territories as occurs after arrest. Embolic occlusion of the top of the basilar artery can produce a clinical picture that includes any or all of the central or peripheral territory symptoms. Its hallmark is suddenness of onset and bilaterality of symptoms, including ptosis and somnolence (see above in the discussion of the artery of Percheron).

Laboratory evaluation   Infarction in the peripheral territory of the posterior cerebral artery can be documented easily by CT or MRI. Infarction in the central territory of the posterior cerebral artery, particularly in territories supplied by the penetrating branches of the posterior cerebral artery, is not reliably detected by CT scanning. MRI can detect infarctions greater than 0.5 cm in this area. MRI angiography and intracranial Doppler may identify atherosclerotic stenotic lesions in the proximal posterior cerebral artery.

Therapy   Because infarction in the territory of the posterior cerebral artery is usually secondary to embolism from the vertebrobasilar system or from the heart, treatment with anticoagulants to prevent further embolic events is appropriate. Transient ischemic symptoms in the territory of the posterior cerebral artery may result from atherothrombotic stenosis of its proximal portion or one of its penetrating branches (lacunar TIA). The natural history of such atheromatous disease is unknown. Thus the efficacy of anticoagulants versus antiplatelet therapy is still uncertain.

VERTEBRAL AND POSTERIOR INFERIOR CEREBELLAR ARTERIES   The *vertebral artery*, which arises from the innominate artery on the right and the subclavian artery on the left, divides into four anatomic segments. The first segment extends from its origin to its entrance into the sixth or fifth transverse vertebral foramen. The second segment traverses the vertebral foramina from C6 to C2. The third segment passes through the transverse foramen and circles around the arch of the atlas to pierce the dura at the foramen magnum. The fourth segment courses upward to join the other vertebral artery to form the basilar artery; only the fourth segment gives rise to branches that supply the brainstem and cerebellum. The *posterior inferior cerebellar artery* in its proximal segments supplies the lateral medulla and, in its distal branches, the inferior surface of the cerebellum. Anastomotic channels exist among the ascending cervical arteries, the thyrocervical arteries, the occipital artery (branch of the external carotid artery), and the second segment of the vertebral artery (see Fig. 368-1). In 10 percent of patients, one vertebral artery is too small to contribute significant blood to the brainstem.

Atherothrombotic lesions have a predilection for the first and fourth segments of the vertebral artery. Although the atheromatous narrowing in the first segment (the origin) may be significant, it seldom produces brainstem ischemic strokes. Collateral flow from the contralateral vertebral artery or the ascending cervical and ascending thyrocervical or occipital arteries is usually sufficient to prevent ischemia (see Fig. 368-1D). When one vertebral artery is atretic and an atherothrombotic lesion threatens the origin of the other, the only avenues for collateral circulation are through the ascending cervical artery, the thyrocervical artery, and the occipital artery or by retrograde flow down the basilar artery via the posterior communicating artery (see Fig. 368-2 and 368-6). In this setting, low flow in the vertebrobasilar system exists and TIAs may occur. In addition, incipient thrombosis in the proximal basilar or distal vertebral system may occur. If the subclavian is blocked proximal to the origin of the vertebral artery, exercise of the left arm may draw blood from the vertebrobasilar insufficiency (*subclavian steal*). It rarely leads to significant vertebrobasilar ischemia.

Atheroma in the fourth segment of the vertebral artery can occur proximal to or distal to the origin of the posterior inferior cerebellar artery, as well as at the junction with the other vertebral artery to form the basilar artery. When it is proximal to the origin of the posterior inferior cerebellar artery, a critical narrowing can threaten the lateral medulla and posteroinferior surface of the cerebellum.

Although atheromatous disease rarely narrows the second and third segments of the vertebral artery, this region is subject to dissection, fibromuscular dysplasia, and, rarely, encroachment by osteophytic spurs within the vertebral foramina.

Clinical manifestations *True transient cerebral ischemic attacks* resulting from vertebral artery insufficiency cause dizziness or vertigo, numbness of the ipsilateral face and contralateral limbs, diplopia, hoarseness, dysarthria, and dysphagia. Hemiparesis is rare. Such TIAs are usually short (up to 10 to 15 min) and repetitive.

When *infarction* ensues, it most often affects the lateral medulla with or without the posteroinferior cerebellum (Wallenberg's syndrome). Its features are listed in Fig. 368-7. In 70 to 80 percent of the cases, the syndrome occurs after ipsilateral vertebral artery occlusion; in the remainder, it results from posterior inferior cerebellar artery occlusion. Atherothrombotic occlusion of the medullary penetrating branches of the vertebral or posterior inferior cerebellar artery results in partial syndromes of the ipsilateral, lateral, or medial medulla.

Rarely, a medial medullary syndrome occurs in which the pyramid becomes infarcted, causing a contralateral hemiparesis of the arm and leg, sparing the face. If the medial lemniscus and emerging hypoglossal nerve fibers are involved, contralateral loss of joint position sense and ipsilateral tongue weakness occur.

Cerebellar infarction with edema formation can lead to *sudden respiratory arrest* due to raised intracranial pressure in the posterior fossa. Drowsiness, Babinski signs, dysarthria, and bifacial weakness may be absent or present only briefly before respiratory arrest ensues. Gait unsteadiness, dizziness, nausea, and vomiting may be the only early symptoms and signs and should arouse suspicion of this impending complication.

Laboratory evaluation When true TIAs occur in the territory of the lateral medulla, it becomes important to determine the adequacy of blood flow in the distal vertebral artery and the posterior inferior cerebellar artery. CT scanning may detect a large cerebellar infarction in the territory of the posterior inferior cerebellar artery. MRI can detect cerebellar infarction earlier and, with high-resolution scanning, can detect lateral medullary infarction. MRI angiography can determine the patency of the vertebral artery and occasionally the posterior inferior cerebellar artery. Cerebral angiography is rarely necessary if MRI angiography is available in evaluating stroke in this territory. Transcranial Doppler analysis of flow in the vertebral artery determines its patency, but its sensitivity in detecting distal vertebral artery stenotic lesions is limited.

Therapy Four important therapeutic issues arise in managing patients with ischemia or infarction in the territory of the vertebral or posterior inferior cerebellar artery. First, the ensuing edema may be life-threatening. It should be treated with osmotic agents (mannitol); surgical decompression may be necessary. Second, thrombosis of the fourth segment of the vertebral artery may send clots into the basilar artery or emboli into the basilar or posterior cerebral arteries. Symptoms or signs of basilar insufficiency may ensue. Acute anticoagulation with heparin is advocated in such cases in an effort to prevent

clot propagation. Third, some physicians argue for the prophylactic use of heparin in acute vertebral artery occlusion whether or not basilar artery symptoms have occurred. Chronic anticoagulation has not been recommended after the acute phase of the stroke has passed. Fourth, when one vertebral artery is symptomatic with atheromatous disease and the contralateral vertebral is congenitally atretic or already occluded, basilar ischemia may ensue and proximal basilar thrombosis may develop. Despite its potential hazards, acute anticoagulation with heparin, followed by chronic warfarin anticoagulation, is recommended in such patients. When the same circumstance occurs but the symptomatic vertebral atherothrombotic lesion lies immediately proximal to the posterior inferior cerebellar artery, occipital to posterior inferior bypass grafting has been recommended. The efficacy of this surgery is unproven, and it should be considered only after anticoagulation therapy has failed.

BASILAR ARTERY **Pathophysiology** Branches of the basilar artery supply the base of the pontis and superior cerebellum and fall into three groups: (1) paramedian, 7 to 10 in number, which supply a wedge of pons on either side of the midline, (2) short circumferential branches, 5 to 7 in number, which supply the lateral two-thirds of the pons and middle and superior cerebellar peduncles, and (3) 2 bilateral long circumferential arteries (superior cerebellar and anterior inferior cerebellar arteries) which course around the pons to supply the cerebellar hemispheres.

Atheromatous lesions can occur anywhere along the basilar trunk but are most often in the proximal basilar and distal vertebral segments. Typically, lesions occlude either the proximal basilar and one or both vertebral arteries. The clinical picture varies depending on the availability of retrograde collateral flow from the posterior communicating arteries.

Although atherothrombosis occasionally occludes the top of the basilar artery, emboli from the heart or proximal vertebral or basilar segments are more common.

Clinical manifestations Because the brainstem contains many structures in close approximation, a diversity of clinical syndromes may emerge with ischemia. Involvement of the corticospinal tracts, corticobulbar tracts, medial and superior cerebellar peduncles, spinothalamic tracts, and cranial nerve nuclei causes the common symptoms and signs (Figs. 368-8 to 368-10).

Unfortunately, the symptoms of transient ischemia or infarction in the territory of the basilar artery often do not indicate whether the basilar artery itself or one of its branches is diseased, yet the distinction has important implications for therapy. The picture of complete basilar insufficiency, however, is easy to recognize. A combination of bilateral long tract signs (sensory and motor) with signs of cranial nerve and cerebellar dysfunction suggests this diagnosis. A "locked-in" state of quadriplegia occurs with bilateral basis pontis infarction. Coma due to dysfunction of the reticular activating system and quadriplegia with cranial nerve signs suggest complete and devastating pontine and upper midbrain infarction. The therapeutic goal, however, is to recognize impending basilar occlusion before such a devastating infarction occurs. A series of TIAs and a slowly progressive, fluctuating stroke become extremely significant when they herald an atherothrombotic occlusion of the distal vertebral or proximal basilar artery.

TRANSIENT ISCHEMIC ATTACKS Transient ischemic attacks in the proximal basilar distribution may produce dizziness (often described by patients as "swimming," "swaying," "moving," "unsteadiness," or "light-headedness"). Patients may complain that the room is upside down or that the floor seems to move toward them. Other symptoms that warn of basilar thrombosis include diplopia, dysarthria, facial or circumoral numbness, and hemisensory symptoms. In general, symptoms of basilar branch TIAs affect one side of the brainstem, whereas symptoms of basilar artery TIAs usually affect both sides, though a "herald" hemiparesis has been emphasized as an initial symptom of basilar occlusion. Most often TIAs, whether due to impending occlusion of the basilar artery or of a basilar branch, are short-lived (5 to 30 min) and repetitive, occurring several times a

Medial longitudinal fasciculus
12th N. nucleus
Tractus solitarius with nucleus
Vestibular nucleus
Restiform body
Nucleus ambiguus—motor 9 + 10
Cerebellum
Olivocerebellar fibers
Descending nucleus and tract–5th N.
Medial lemniscus
Descending sympathetic tract
Dorsal spinocerebellar tract
10th N.
Ventral spinocerebellar tract
MEDULLARY SYNDROME:
Spinothalamic tract
Lateral
Medial
Pyramid   Inferior olive
12th nerve

FIGURE 368-7 (*Courtesy of C. M. Fisher, M.D.*)

Signs and symptoms	Structures involved
1 Medial medullary syndrome (occlusion of vertebral artery or of branch of vertebral or lower basilar artery)	
On side of lesion:	
Paralysis with atrophy of half the tongue	Ipsilateral twelfth nerve
On side opposite lesion:	
Paralysis of arm and leg sparing face; impaired tactile and proprioceptive sense over half the body	Contralateral pyramidal tract and medial lemniscus
2 Lateral medullary syndrome (occlusion of any of five vessels may be responsible—vertebral, posterior inferior cerebellar, superior, middle, or inferior lateral medullary arteries)	
On side of lesion:	
Pain, numbness, impaired sensation over half the face	Descending tract and nucleus fifth nerve
Ataxia of limbs, falling to side of lesion	Uncertain—restiform body, cerebellar hemisphere, cerebellar fibers, spinocerebellar tract (?)
Nystagmus, diplopia, oscillopsia, vertigo, nausea, vomiting	Vestibular nucleus
Horner's syndrome (miosis, ptosis, decreased sweating)	Descending sympathetic tract
Dysphagia, hoarseness, paralysis of palate, paralysis of vocal cord, diminished gag reflex	Issuing fibers ninth and tenth nerves
Loss of taste	Nucleus and tractus solitarius
Numbness of ipsilateral arm, trunk, or leg	Cuneate and gracile nuclei
On side opposite lesion:	
Impaired pain and thermal sense over half the body, sometimes face	Spinothalamic tract
3 Total unilateral medullary syndrome (occlusion of vertebral artery): Combination of medial and lateral syndromes	
4 Lateral pontomedullary syndrome (occlusion of vertebral artery): Combination of lateral medullary and lateral inferior pontine syndromes	
5 Basilar artery syndrome (the syndrome of the lone vertebral artery is equivalent): A combination of the various brainstem syndromes plus those arising in the posterior cerebral artery distribution	
Bilateral long tract signs (sensory and motor; cerebellar and peripheral cranial nerve abnormalities)	Bilateral long tract; cerebellar and peripheral cranial nerves
Paralysis or weakness of all extremities, plus all bulbar musculature	Corticobulbar and corticospinal tracts bilaterally

day. The pattern suggests intermittent reduction of flow rather than recurrent embolism.

INFARCTION   Atherothrombotic occlusion of the basilar artery with brainstem infarction usually causes *bilateral* brainstem signs. Sometimes only gaze paresis or internuclear ophthalmoplegia associated with ipsilateral hemiparesis, i.e., a particular combination of cranial nerve and long tract (sensory and/or motor) deficits, signifies

bilateral brainstem ischemia. More often, bilateral basis pontis signs coexist with unilateral or bilateral pontine tegmental signs.

Symptomatic atherothrombotic occlusion of a branch of the basilar artery usually causes *unilateral* symptoms and signs involving motor, sensory, and cranial nerves. Occlusion of the long circumferential branches of the basilar artery produces specific clinical syndromes depending on the artery involved.

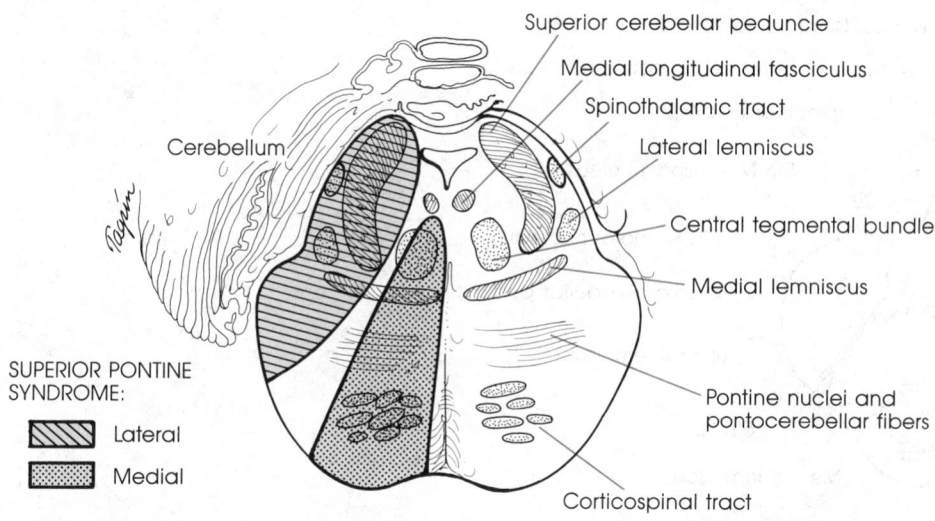

Superior cerebellar peduncle
Medial longitudinal fasciculus
Spinothalamic tract
Lateral lemniscus
Central tegmental bundle
Medial lemniscus
Pontine nuclei and pontocerebellar fibers
Corticospinal tract
Cerebellum

SUPERIOR PONTINE SYNDROME:

Lateral

Medial

FIGURE 368-8 (*Courtesy of C. M. Fisher, M.D.*)

Signs and symptoms	Structures involved
1 Medial superior pontine syndrome (paramedian branches of upper basilar artery)	
On side of lesion:	
Cerebellar ataxia (probably)	Superior and/or middle cerebellar peduncle
Internuclear ophthalmoplegia	Medial longitudinal fasciculus
Myoclonic syndrome, palate, pharnyx, vocal cords, respiratory apparatus, face, oculomotor apparatus, etc.	Localization uncertain—central tegmental bundle (?), dentate projection (?), inferior olivary nucleus (?)
On side opposite lesion:	
Paralysis of face, arm, and leg	Corticobulbar and corticospinal tract
Rarely touch, vibration, and position are affected	Medial lemniscus
2 Lateral superior pontine syndrome (syndrome of superior cerebellar artery)	
On side of lesion:	
Ataxia of limbs and gait, falling to side of lesion	Middle and superior cerebellar peduncles, superior surface of cerebellum, dentate nucleus
Dizziness, nausea, vomiting; horizontal nystagmus	Vestibular nucleus
Paresis of conjugate gaze (ipsilateral)	Pontine contralateral gaze
Skew deviation	Uncertain
Miosis, ptosis, decreased sweating over face (Horner's syndrome)	Descending sympathetic fibers
Static tremor reported in one case	Dentate nucleus (?), superior cerebellar peduncle (?)
On side opposite lesion:	
Impaired pain and thermal sense on face, limbs, and trunk	Spinothalamic tract
Impaired touch, vibration, and position sense, more in leg than arm (there is a tendency to incongruity of pain and touch deficits)	Medial lemniscus (lateral portion)

SUPERIOR CEREBELLAR ARTERY Occlusion of the superior cerebellar artery results in severe ipsilateral cerebellar ataxia (middle and/or superior cerebellar peduncles), nausea and vomiting, dysarthria, and contralateral loss of pain and temperature sensation over the extremities, body, and face (spino- and trigeminothalamic tract). Partial deafness, ataxic tremor of the ipsilateral upper extremity, Horner's syndrome, and palatal myoclonus may occur rarely. Partial syndromes occur frequently (see Fig. 368-8).

ANTERIOR INFERIOR CEREBELLAR ARTERY Occlusion of the anterior inferior cerebellar artery produces variable degrees of infarction because the size of this artery and the territory it supplies vary inversely with those of the posterior inferior cerebellar artery. The principal symptoms include ipsilateral deafness, facial weakness, true vertigo (whirling dizziness), nausea and vomiting, nystagmus, tinnitus and cerebellar ataxia, Horner's syndrome, and paresis of conjugate lateral gaze. The opposite side of the body loses pain and temperature sensation. An occlusion close to the origin of the artery may cause corticospinal tract signs (see Fig. 368-10).

Occlusion of one of the five to seven short circumferential branches of the basilar artery affects the lateral two-thirds of the pons and/or middle or superior cerebellar peduncle, whereas occlusion of one of the 7 to 10 paramedian branches of the basilar artery affects a wedge-shaped area on either side of the medial pons (see Figs. 368-8 to 368-10). Many brainstem syndromes with cranial nerve abnormalities and crossed hemiplegia have been given eponyms, e.g., Weber, Claude, Benedict, Foville, Raymond-Cestan, Millard-Gubler.

Laboratory evaluation MRI scanning can detect brainstem infarction due to either basilar artery or basilar branch occlusion. MRI angiography combined with transcranial Doppler analysis may eventually replace conventional angiography in documenting basilar artery potency. CT scanning is not reliable in detecting brainstem infarcts but can show hemorrhages and assess mass effect after large cerebellar infarctions.

Selective cerebral arteriography remains the best method to define atherothrombotic disease of the basilar artery. Arteriography entails potential morbidity and may precipitate the very stroke one is seeking

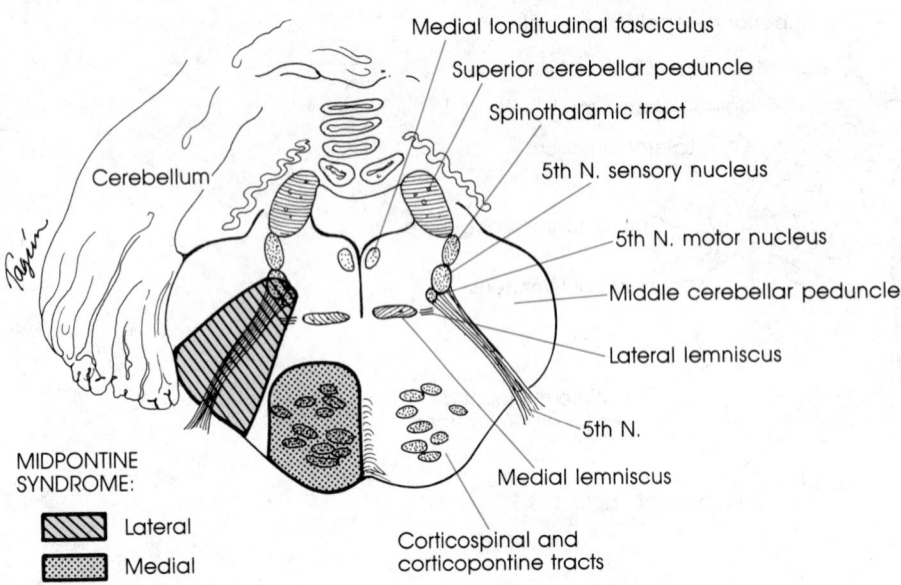

Medial longitudinal fasciculus
Superior cerebellar peduncle
Spinothalamic tract
5th N. sensory nucleus
5th N. motor nucleus
Middle cerebellar peduncle
Lateral lemniscus
5th N.
Medial lemniscus
Corticospinal and corticopontine tracts
Cerebellum
MIDPONTINE SYNDROME:
Lateral
Medial

FIGURE 368-9 *(Courtesy of C. M. Fisher, M.D.)*

Signs and symptoms	*Structures involved*
1 Medial midpontine syndrome (paramedian branch of midbasilar artery)	
On side of lesion:	
Ataxia of limbs and gait (more prominent in bilateral involvement)	Pontine nuclei
On side opposite lesion:	
Paralysis of face, arm, and leg	Corticobulbar and corticospinal tract
Variable impaired touch and proprioception when lesion extends posteriorly	Medial lemniscus
2 Lateral midpontine syndrome (short circumferential artery)	
On side of lesion:	
Ataxia of limbs	Middle cerebellar peduncle
Paralysis of muscles of mastication	Motor fibers or nucleus of fifth nerve
Impaired sensation over side of face	Sensory fibers or nucleus of fifth nerve
On side opposite lesion:	
Impaired pain and thermal sense on limbs and trunk	Spinothalamic tract

to prevent. It is recommended only when MRI angiography fails to detect the clinically suspected basilar arterial lesion that, if known, would influence patient management. Occasionally, injection of angiographic dye in the posterior circulation precipitates a delirious state sometimes associated with cortical blindness. This reversible state can last for 24 to 38 h or, rarely, several days.

Therapy Impending basilar occlusion causing transient or fluctuating symptoms should be treated with short-term anticoagulation with intravenous heparin, after MRI or CT scanning has excluded hemorrhage. When basilar artery stenosis or occlusion is associated with minor or improving stroke, long-term anticoagulation with warfarin is recommended. If, on the other hand, basilar branch disease is the cause, then the rationale for using warfarin is uncertain. While embolism from the heart or from atheroma in the distal vertebral system may occlude a penetrating basilar branch, this is unlikely. Therefore, long-term control of blood pressure and antiplatelet therapy are recommended as preventive measures in the management of small-vessel basilar branch disease. Because of the long-term accumulative risk of anticoagulation therapy, it is generally reserved for symptomatic large-vessel atherothrombotic disease.

LACUNAR DISEASE

The term *lacunar infarction* refers to infarction following atherothrombotic or lipohyalinotic occlusion of *one* of the penetrating branches

of the circle of Willis, middle cerebral artery stem, or vertebral and basilar arteries.

PATHOPHYSIOLOGY The middle cerebral artery stem, the arteries comprising the circle of Willis (A1 segment of the anterior cerebral artery, anterior and posterior communicating arteries, and precommunal segment of the posterior cerebral arteries), and the basilar and vertebral arteries all give rise to 100- to 300-µm-diameter branches that penetrate the deep gray and white matter of the cerebrum or brainstem (see Fig. 368-2). Each of these small branches can be thrombosed either by atherothrombotic disease at its origin or by the development of lipohyalinotic thickening. Thrombosis of these vessels causes small infarcts that are referred to as *lacunes*. They range in size from as small as 3 to 4 mm to 1 to 2 cm. Hypertension is the principal risk factor for such small-vessel disease. Lacunar infarcts represent approximately 20 percent of all strokes.

CLINICAL MANIFESTATIONS Lacunar infarcts cause recognizable stroke syndromes that usually evolve over hours or longer. Transient symptoms (lacunar TIAs) may herald a lacunar infarct; they may occur several times a day and last only a few minutes. When infarction occurs, it usually causes a sudden deficit, but it may evolve in a progressive fashion over a few days. Recovery often begins within hours or days after the infarct and over weeks or months may be complete or result in minimal residual deficit. In some cases, significant disability persists.

The most common lacunar syndromes are the following:

1 Pure motor hemiparesis from an infarct in the posterior limb of

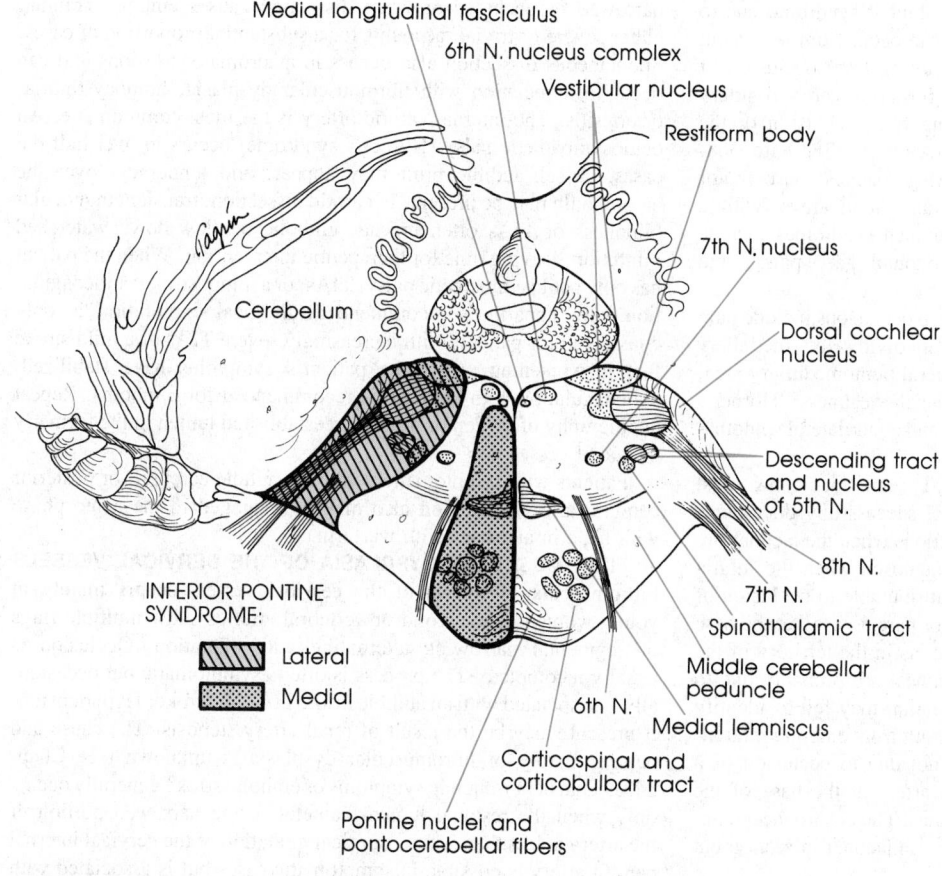

Medial longitudinal fasciculus
6th N. nucleus complex
Vestibular nucleus
Restiform body
7th N. nucleus
Dorsal cochlear nucleus
Descending tract and nucleus of 5th N.
8th N.
7th N.
Spinothalamic tract
Middle cerebellar peduncle
Medial lemniscus
6th N.
Corticospinal and corticobulbar tract
Pontine nuclei and pontocerebellar fibers
Cerebellum

INFERIOR PONTINE SYNDROME:
Lateral
Medial

FIGURE 368-10 *(Courtesy of C. M. Fisher, M.D.)*

Signs and symptoms	Structures involved
1 Medial inferior pontine syndrome (occlusion of paramedian branch of basilar artery)	
On side of lesion:	
Paralysis of conjugate gaze to side of lesion (preservation of convergence)	"Center" for conjugate lateral gaze
Nystagmus	Vestibular nucleus
Ataxia of limbs and gait	Middle cerebellar peduncle (?)
Diplopia on lateral gaze	Abducens nerve
On side opposite lesion:	
Paralysis of face, arm, and leg	Corticobulbar and corticospinal tract in lower pons
Impaired tactile and proprioceptive sense over half of the body	Medial lemniscus
2 Lateral inferior pontine syndrome (occlusion of anterior inferior cerebellar artery)	
On side of lesion:	
Horizontal and vertical nystagmus, vertigo, nausea, vomiting, oscillopsia	Vestibular nerve on nucleus
Facial paralysis	Seventh nerve
Paralysis of conjugate gaze to side of lesion	"Center" for conjugate lateral gaze
Deafness, tinnitus	Auditory nerve or cochlear nucleus
Ataxia	Middle cerebellar peduncle and cerebellar hemisphere
Impaired sensation over face	Descending tract and nucleus fifth nerve
On side opposite lesion:	
Impaired pain and thermal sense over half the body (may include face)	Spinothalamic tract

the internal capsule or basis pontis. Here, the face, arm, leg, foot, and toes are almost always involved. The weakness may be intermittent (TIA), progress in a stepwise manner, or appear abruptly and may progress to complete paralysis, but improvement occurs in many cases.

2 *Pure sensory stroke* from an infarct in the ventrolateral thalamus.

3 *Ataxic hemiparesis* from an infarct in the base of the pons or *dysarthria and a clumsy hand or arm* due to infarction in the base of the pons or in the genu of the internal capsule.

4 *Pure motor hemiparesis* with "motor aphasia" due to thrombotic occlusion of a lenticulostriate branch supplying the genu and anterior limb of the internal capsule and adjacent white matter of the corona radiata.

Before the advent of hypertensive therapy, multiple lacunes often caused *pseudobulbar palsy* with emotional instability, a slowed abulic state, and bilateral pyramidal signs. This syndrome is now uncommon. Other lacunar syndromes have been described, some not correlated with arterial occlusion. An anarthric pseudobulbar syndrome due to bilateral infarctions in the internal capsule can occur from disease in the lenticulostriate arteries. Syndromes resulting from occlusion of the penetrating arteries of the proximal posterior cerebral artery were discussed above. Syndromes resulting from occlusion of the penetrating arteries of the basilar artery (see Figs. 368-8 to 368-10) include ipsilateral ataxia and crural (leg) paresis, pure motor hemiparesis with horizontal gaze palsy, and hemiparesis with a crossed sixth nerve palsy. Lower basilar branch syndromes include sudden internuclear ophthalmoplegia, horizontal gaze palsy, and appendicular cerebellar ataxia.

Syndromes resulting from vertebral branch occlusions include pure motor hemiparesis sparing the face by involving the medullary pyramid and syndromes that involve the lateral pontomedullary area, which may include vertigo, vomiting, facial weakness, Horner's syndrome, ipsilateral trigeminal numbness, and contralateral spinothalamic sensory loss.

LABORATORY EVALUATION The CT scan documents most supratentorial lacunar infarctions, and MRI successfully documents both supratentorial and infratentorial infarctions when the lacunes are 5 mm or greater. Lacunar infarction is diagnosed when the infarct size is less than 2 cm, and its location is attributable to occlusion of a small penetrating arterial branch of a major parent vessel at the base of the brain. Larger deep white matter infarcts in the territory of the middle cerebral artery (so-called giant lacunes) are probably due to embolism. The CT scan and clinical evaluation may fail to identify cortical surface infarction. *Giant lacunes* result from embolic infarctions in a large-vessel territory. They are not due to occlusion of a single penetrating vessel arising from an artery at the base of the brain. Hence they should not be called lacunes. The electroencephalogram (EEG) is usually normal, or nearly so, in lacunar infarction but abnormal in cortical surface infarction.

THERAPY Lacunar strokes may present with a fluctuating progressive course, and acute reduction in blood pressure may worsen symptoms. Antihypertensive therapy is begun after the patient's symptoms become stable. Whether anticoagulant or antiplatelet agents benefit patients with lacunar TIAs and fluctuating stroke is unknown. Some studies suggest that thalamic lacunes may be associated with minor hemorrhage, since hemosiderin-laden macrophages are sometimes seen at autopsy. This circumstance increases the risk of using heparin. On the other hand, some patients with fluctuating hemiparesis from atherothrombotic disease of a basilar branch or of the middle cerebral stem lenticulostriate arteries may improve coincident with heparin administration. Most physicians, however, do not use anticoagulation in patients with typical lacunar strokes. Long-term therapy after lacunar stroke requires careful control of hypertension to prevent progression of vascular disease.

OTHER CAUSES OF CEREBRAL INFARCTION

VENOUS THROMBOSIS (See also Table 368-1) Lateral or sagittal sinus thrombosis or thrombosis of small cortical veins occurs as a complication of sepsis, intracranial infections (meningitis), conditions associated with hypercoagulable states such as polycythemia and sickle cell anemia, or during pregnancy or administration of oral contraceptives. Venous thromboses may cause an increase in intracranial pressure, headaches, focal seizures, and focal neurologic signs affecting the legs more than the arms. Massive venous infarction with secondary edema may be fatal. The CT scan shows hemorrhagic infarction underlying the occluded veins and may show clot in the posterior sagittal sinus, but the definitive diagnosis is made with angiography.

DISSECTION OF THE CERVICOCEREBRAL ARTERIES Dissection of the large extracranial arteries may cause cerebral infarction and is a frequent cause of stroke in children and young adults. The dissection divides the media of the vessel or separates the intima from the media. TIAs and infarction occur when the vessel is critically

narrowed or occluded or when dissection causes emboli. Trauma, either severe or trivial, accounts for a substantial proportion of cases. Spontaneous dissection also occurs in atheromatous lesions and can occur in association with fibromuscular dysplasia, homocystinuria, or arteritis. The internal carotid artery is the most common site. An oculosympathetic palsy (Horner's syndrome) occurs in over half the cases. A self-audible bruit may appear, and tenderness over the carotid bulb may be present. In carotid dissection, transient monocular blindness or TIAs often precede embolic or "low-flow" watershed infarction, leaving time for therapeutic intervention. When the patient has only oculosympathetic palsy, TIAs, or a minor stroke, anticoagulation with heparin is recommended. Surgical exploration is only considered for patients with increasingly severe TIAs or a mild stroke that is worsening. After the patient's symptoms have stabilized, anticoagulation with warfarin is recommended for 6 months. Repeat angiography often demonstrates a reestablished lumen in the formerly occluded vessel.

Patients with symptomatic vertebral, middle cerebral, or posterior cerebral artery dissection also may be managed in the acute phase with heparin and later with warfarin.

FIBROMUSCULAR DYSPLASIA OF THE CERVICAL VESSELS Fibromuscular dysplasia of the cervical vessels occurs mainly in young women. The carotid or vertebral arteries show multiple rings of segmental narrowing alternating with dilatation. Occlusion is usually incomplete. The process is often asymptomatic but occasionally is associated with an audible bruit, TIAs, or stroke. Hypertension, if present, may be the result of renal artery stenosis. The cause and natural history of fibromuscular dysplasia is unknown (see Chap. 243). Transient ischemic symptoms or embolic stroke generally occurs only when the residual lumen diameter of the narrowed portion of the artery is less than 2 mm. Surgical dilatation of the cervical internal carotid artery is possible in symptomatic cases but is associated with considerable morbidity. Anticoagulation may be more successful than surgery in patients with TIAs of increasing severity.

ARTERITIS Arteritis due to bacterial or syphilitic infection is no longer a common cause of cerebral thrombosis. Other arteritides are rare but can cause cerebral thrombosis (see below and Chaps. 284 and 291). Necrotizing or granulomatous arteritis, occurring alone or in association with generalized polyarteritis nodosa or Wegener's granulomatosis, involves the distal small branches (<2 mm diameter) of the main intracranial arteries and produces small ischemic infarcts in the brain, optic nerve, or spinal cord. The disease, although rare, is relentlessly progressive. The cerebrospinal fluid often has cells. In some cases, glucocorticoid therapy (prednisone, 40 to 60 mg/d) has been helpful, and recently, immunosuppressive drugs have been used with some success (see Chap. 291). Idiopathic giant cell arteritis involving the great vessels arising from the aortic arch (Takayasu's syndrome) may, on rare occasions, cause carotid or vertebral thrombosis. It is an infrequent cause of the aortic arch syndrome in the western hemisphere (see Chap. 210).

TEMPORAL ARTERITIS (CRANIAL ARTERITIS) (See also Chap. 291) This is a relatively common affliction of elderly persons in which the external carotid system, particularly the temporal arteries, is the site of a subacute granulomatous inflammation with an exudate of lymphocytes, monocytes, neutrophilic leukocytes, and giant cells. Usually the most severely affected parts of the artery become thrombosed. Headache or head pain is the chief complaint. Systemic manifestations include anorexia, loss of weight, malaise, and polymyalgia rheumatica. The inflammatory nature of the illness is indicated by one of the following: fever, slight leukocytosis, increased erythrocyte sedimentation rate, and anemia. Occlusion of branches of the ophthalmic artery results in blindness in one or both eyes in over 25 percent of patients. Occasionally, an ophthalmoplegia due to involvement of ocular nerves occurs. An arteritis of the aorta and its major branches, including the carotid, subclavian, coronary, and femoral arteries, has been found at postmortem examination in some cases. Significant inflammatory involvement of intracranial arteries is rare, but strokes occur occasionally on the basis of occlusion of the internal carotid, middle cerebral, or vertebral arteries. The diagnosis depends on the finding of a tender thrombosed or thickened cranial artery and demonstration of the lesion in a biopsy specimen. Glucocorticoids bring striking subjective relief and often prevent blindness. Prednisone is most often used, beginning with large daily doses of 80 to 120 mg and then tapering after 2 to 4 weeks using the erythrocyte sedimentation rate as a guide.

MOYAMOYA DISEASE Moyamoya disease is a poorly understood occlusive disease involving large intracranial arteries, especially the internal carotid artery and the stem of the middle and anterior cerebral arteries. The lenticulostriate arteries develop a rich collateral flow circulation around the middle cerebral occlusive lesion that on cerebral angiography gives the impression of a puff of smoke (*moyamoya*). Other collaterals include transdural anastomoses between the cortical surface branches of the middle cerebral artery and the scalp arteries. The disease mainly occurs in the oriental population but should be suspected when TIAs or stroke occur in children or young adults. Its etiology is unknown. Few pathologic studies have been made; they suggest that hyalinotic fibrous-type material is associated with the arterial narrowing. Because of the occurrence of subarachnoid hemorrhage from rupture of the transdural anastomotic channels, anticoagulation is not recommended in all symptomatic cases. Extracranial-intracranial (EC/IC) bypass grafting has been recommended in some cases, but its efficacy is not established.

ISCHEMIC DISEASES ASSOCIATED WITH HYPERCOAGU-LATION STATE Certain diseases have been associated with ischemic infarction in special clinical circumstances through a mechanism of a hypercoagulable state (see Chaps. 314 and 315). They include polycythemia vera, thrombotic thrombocytopenic purpura, idiopathic thrombocytosis, hyperproteinemia, sickle cell anemia, and familial clotting abnormalities, e.g., protein C deficiency. Furthermore, circulation of anticardiolipin antibodies ("lupus anticoagulant") has been associated with stroke in young adults, although its relative frequency is controversial. Some cases may be due to cerebral embolism (see below), but others seem to be caused by local arterial thrombosis.

REVERSIBLE CEREBRAL SEGMENTAL VASOCONSTRICTION Reversible, widespread cerebral segmental vasoconstriction has been noted in patients with severe headache and fluctuating neurologic symptoms and signs. Sometimes cerebral infarction has ensued. The cause is unknown. Eclampsia, the postpartum period, head injury, migraine, and sympathomimetic intoxication have all been associated with this entity. Angiography is the only means of establishing the diagnosis. The cerebrospinal fluid is normal in most cases, but an elevated protein and slight lymphocytic pleocytosis has been found in some cases. No effective therapy is known. Maintenance of normal systemic arterial pressure or even increasing it modestly with adequate hydration seems important on empirical grounds. Glucocorticoids and vasodilators such as calcium channel blocking agents or intravenous nitroglycerin may be considered.

BINSWANGER'S DISEASE Binswanger's disease (chronic progressive subcortical encephalopathy) is a rare condition in which the subcortical white matter becomes subacutely infarcted. The CT or MRI scan detects periventricular areas of white matter disruption and gliosis. There is lipohyalinosis in the small arteries of the deep white matter, as in hypertension. There are usually associated lacunar or embolic strokes. Binswanger's disease may represent a type of border zone ischemic infarction in the deep white matter between the penetrating arteries of the circle of Willis and of the cortex. Unfortunately, the pathophysiologic basis of the disease remains unknown, and the underlying microvascular pathology may be different in younger patients without hypertension and typical cases in older patients with severe long-standing hypertension. Binswanger's disease is one of the causes of gait disability and abulia in the elderly.

ORAL CONTRACEPTIVE AGENTS Oral contraceptive agents have been associated with an increased incidence of stroke in young women (13.2:100,000 among women who take oral contraceptives compared with 2.8:100,000 among those who do not). In most cases,

there is no vascular occlusion on angiography, or if there is occlusion, it is found to have opened later, suggesting embolism as the cause of the stroke. The source of the embolus, however, is uncertain. Pathologic examination has shown that the affected arteries and the heart are normal. Migraine and cigarette smoking have been associated with increased frequency of strokes in young women on oral contraceptives and suggest that hypercoagulability may predispose to thrombosis formation and/or embolization.

CEREBRAL EMBOLISM

PATHOPHYSIOLOGY Cerebral embolism is the most common cause of ischemic stroke. The heart is the most common source of embolic material, with artery-to-artery embolism, usually arising from an atherothrombotic lesion in the carotid or vertebrobasilar system or ascending aorta, a somewhat less frequent source (see above). Other causes, such as thrombus in the pulmonary vein, fat emboli, tumor emboli, marantic endocarditis, air emboli, paradoxical emboli, and complications of neck or thoracic surgery (see Table 368-1), may occasionally be responsible. Frequently, however, embolic cerebral infarction occurs without an obvious source.

The term *cerebral embolism of unknown source* is used when a sudden stroke occurs and cardiac monitoring, echocardiography, and carotid, vertebral, and transcranial Doppler studies fail to disclose an obvious source. About 40 percent of ischemic strokes fall into this category. The etiology of these presumed emboli poses one of the most perplexing problems in cerebrovascular disease. Sophisticated analyses of activity of the hemostatic system, blood coagulation factors, and autoantibodies show that patients with hypercoagulable states are prone to cerebral embolism. Hypercoagulability may be induced by anticardiolipid antibodies, protein C deficiency, protein S deficiency, antithrombin III deficiency, metastatic tumor, and even surgery. The association of cerebral embolism with these pathophysiologic conditions is suspected, but its incidence is uncertain. Transesophageal echocardiography has identified atheromatous plaques in the ascending aorta as a possible source of central embolism. The incidence and natural history of this lesion are uncertain.

Cardiogenic cerebral embolism is presumed to have occurred when cardiac arrhythmias or structural abnormalities are found or known to be present. Of the cardiac arrhythmias, atrial fibrillation is commonly associated with cerebral embolism. Prospective evidence suggests that independent of other cardiac disease, including mitral stenosis, persistent or paroxysmal atrial fibrillation is the most important cause of cerebral embolism from the heart. The presumed mechanism is thrombus formation in the fibrillating atrial appendage with subsequent embolization. Recent therapeutic trials and natural history studies suggest that age over 60 years is an important risk factor for such embolization. Mitral annulus calcification, left ventricular aneurysm, and left atrial size also may be risk factors.

The most common cause of cerebral embolism from structural heart disease occurs with atherothrombotic cardiovascular disease. *Left ventricular myocardial infarction*, either subendocardial or transmural, represents an important risk for embolus, especially in the first few weeks when mural thrombus formation and maturation usually occur in younger patients (see Chaps. 202 and 203). *Congenital septal defects* have long been associated with cerebral embolism. The deep peripheral venous system is usually the source of *paradoxical emboli*. Transesophageal and bubble echocardiographic techniques can demonstrate a patent foramen ovale as a conduit for cerebral embolism. Mitral valve prolapse is considered a potential source of emboli, but the incidence and natural history require further assessment. Mitral annulus calcification independent of atrial fibrillation has been shown to be a risk factor for ischemic stroke. Cardiogenic embolization during or following coronary artery surgery or intracardiac surgery is a well-recognized complication.

Vegetations of acute and subacute bacterial endocarditis give rise to septic emboli (see Chaps. 200 and 201) that cause large areas of infarction. Small septic infarcts of microscopic size may appear in the brain. Large brain abscesses, however, are not commonly associated with embolism from subacute bacterial endocarditis. Large septic emboli pose a greater risk of hemorrhage into the infarction than nonseptic embolism. Mycotic aneurysms caused by septic emboli may give rise to subarachnoid or intracerebral hemorrhage. Therefore, endocarditis should always be considered when cerebral embolism is suspected. Vegetations on the aortic and mitral valves from rheumatic or marantic endocarditis are also associated with systemic or cerebral emboli. Typically, flat vegetations under the mitral and, to a lesser extent, aortic valve leaflets have been noted in patients with systemic lupus erythematosus (Libman-Sacks vegetations). These may give rise to cerebral embolism and may be a nidus for bacterial endocarditis.

Atrial myxoma may give rise to tumor emboli from the endocardial surface. Signs of pulmonary hypertension or a high erythrocyte sedimentation rate, together with signs of systemic illness (fever, malaise), may help in the differential diagnosis. Thoracic surgery (pulmonary vein embolism) and head and neck surgery (aortic or carotid artery-to-artery emboli) have an uncommon, but definite, association with cerebral embolism.

Embolic infarction depends on the size of the embolic fragment and where it lodges, resulting from the size, location, and clinical findings. Emboli from the heart lodge in the middle cerebral artery or one of its branches 80 percent of the time, in the posterior cerebral artery or its branches 10 percent of the time, and in the vertebral artery or its branches in the remainder. Cardiac emboli rarely reach the anterior cerebral artery. Emboli large enough to occlude the stem of the middle cerebral artery (3 to 4 mm) lead to a large stroke, one that involves both deep gray and white matter and some portion of the cortical surface and its underlying white matter. A smaller embolus may occlude a small cortical or penetrating arterial branch. Characteristically, embolic platelet fibrin clot has a tendency to migrate, lyse, and disperse, accounting for fluctuation in symptoms and, in some cases, complete recovery of the ischemic deficit. The location and size of an infarct also depend on the extent of the spared collateral circulation.

Because emboli migrate and lyse, recirculation into the infarcted brain may cause petechial hemorrhages (*hemorrhagic infarction*). On rare occasions, petechial hemorrhages coalesce to form a significant hemorrhage mass (*hemorrhage into infarction*). This is more likely to occur when the stem of the middle cerebral artery is occluded and large areas of infarction develop in the territory of the lenticulostriate arteries before recirculation occurs.

CLINICAL MANIFESTATIONS   The onset of the neurologic deficit from embolism is sudden and usually maximal. This temporal profile with a neurologic syndrome corresponding to the distribution of a major branch vessel points to cerebral embolism. Sometimes, however, the neurologic deficit may not be complete and, after its sudden onset, may fluctuate. The neurologic signs may wax and wane, lasting only a few minutes or hours, and then partially or completely disappear, suggesting an embolic TIA, or a mild deficit may progress to complete major infarction over hours. The neurologic deficit corresponds to the cerebral cortex supplied by the affected artery. The resulting deficits resemble those caused by occlusive atheromatous lesions (see sections on atherothrombosis and lacunar stroke). Certain neurologic syndromes strongly suggest embolism as their cause. In the middle cerebral artery territory these include (1) the frontal opercular syndrome, in which there is facial weakness and severe aphasia or dysarthria, (2) the brachial or hand plegia syndrome, in which the arm and hand or the hand is paralyzed with or without cortical sensory abnormalities, (3) the syndromes of Broca's or Wernicke's aphasia alone, when the dominant hemisphere is involved, or (4) the syndrome of left visual neglect, when the nondominant parietal lobe is involved. Sudden hemianopic field defect suggests a posterior cerebral artery embolus; sudden foot incoordination or weakness suggests an anterior cerebral territory embolus. Sudden gait unsteadiness may suggest a cerebellar embolus. Sudden sleepiness

and an inability to look up associated with bilateral ptosis suggest an embolus to the top of the basilar artery, specifically to the artery of Percheron (the small vessel supplying both sides of the medial subthalamus and thalamus arising from the top of the basilar artery).

Seizures following cerebral infarction occur most often after embolic infarction and are not associated with deep white matter lacunar infarction. They are associated with supratentorial cortical surface infarction but are infrequent at the onset and are more often the result of gliotic scar that matures months or more after stroke. Seizures after infarction are rare before 6 months and peak in incidence at 12 to 18 months. Many cases of idiopathic epilepsy in the elderly are probably the result of silent cortical infarction.

LABORATORY EVALUATION   Although early CT scanning is usually negative in embolic stroke, it serves to exclude hemorrhage. MRI scanning is better to document the extent and location of the embolic infarction, both supratentorially and infratentorially. Although endocarditis is rarely the cause of cerebral embolism, laboratory evaluation should include a sedimentation rate and blood cultures. Noninvasive carotid studies combined with transcranial Doppler analysis can exclude hemodynamically significant carotid stenosis as the source of emboli if there is any clinical reason to consider this source. Cerebral angiography is considered only when endarterectomy is considered and/or noninvasive tests for significant carotid stenosis have produced equivocal results. An ECG may show an arrhythmia or myocardial infarction that may have been the source of embolism. Echocardiography (conventional or transesophageal) is used to determine whether a cardiac thrombus or ascending aorta lesion was the source of embolism. These techniques are generally insensitive to small clots and are positive in less than 20 percent of patients who have had cerebral emboli.

THERAPY   Therapy of patients with embolic cerebral infarction consists of managing the stroke itself, in both the acute and chronic phases, and of preventing further embolic strokes. When cerebral embolism is suspected, the immediate goal is to keep cerebral perfusion in the ischemic area as adequate as possible. The blood pressure should not be lowered even if hypertension is found unless it is malignant hypertension (see Chap. 209). If the blood pressure is low, raising it is probably advisable in the hours after stroke. An excessive rise above normal may, however, aggravate edema formation. Approximately 5 percent or less of patients with embolic strokes have enough *secondary cerebral edema* to cause clinical problems. Edema seldom becomes problematic until the second or third day but can then cause mass effect for up to 10 days. Two observations governing the severity of the edema associated with cerebral embolism seem to apply. First, in instances of supratentorial embolic infarction, the larger the area of infarct, the more likely it is that edema formation will become a problem. Emboli that lodge in the middle cerebral artery stem are much more likely to cause symptomatic edema formation that leads, in a few patients, to coma and death than are emboli in a distal branch of the middle cerebral artery. Second, small amounts of edema formation in the cerebellum following embolic infarction, usually in the territory of the posterior inferior cerebellar artery (inferior cerebellum), can lead to an acute increase in intracranial pressure in the posterior fossa. The resulting compression of the brainstem may result in sudden coma and respiratory arrest requiring emergency surgical decompression. Water restriction and agents that raise the serum osmolality should be considered early in both instances. Intravenous mannitol is most frequently used to raise the serum osmolarity to approximately 300 mosmol/L; it is given as often as every 2 to 4 h. The acute management of artery-to-artery embolus, in either the carotid or vertebral territory, is discussed above (see "Ischemic Cerebrovascular Disease").

When the deficit is large enough to suggest that the embolus has lodged in the middle cerebral artery stem with corresponding infarction of the basal ganglion, deep white matter, and cortical surface, acute anticoagulation with heparin is generally avoided. On rare occasions, symptomatic basal ganglion hemorrhage into infarcted tissue occurs. But when the stroke is smaller and involves the cortical surface, or when the deficit fluctuates, suggesting partial arterial occlusion, then acute anticoagulation should be considered. For future stroke prevention, chronic anticoagulation with warfarin is general recommended beginning 2 to 5 days after the stroke. A second embolism is rare in the first 3 days. Anticoagulation is usually continued for 6 months. Chronic ventricular failure or a ventricular aneurysm, if present, may indicate a need for longer treatment. Antiplatelet as opposed to anticoagulation therapy has not been assessed adequately in this setting. Lifelong anticoagulation with warfarin may be legitimately considered in patients who have evidence of recurrent embolism or embolism associated with chronic intermittent or sustained atrial fibrillation. Low-intensity anticoagulation (PT 1.2 to 1.5 times control or international normalized ratio, INR, 1.5 to 2.7 or 2 to 3) for patients with chronic, intermittent, or sustained atrial fibrillation has been proven conclusively to be safe and to prevent cerebral embolism. The rate of significant hemorrhage under careful anticoagulation control is the same for warfarin-treated and untreated groups. Aspirin, by contrast, did not demonstrate consistent efficacy for preventing cerebral embolism in this setting. Thus low-intensity warfarin anticoagulation is generally recommended for patients with atrial fibrillation who are over age 60. Higher intensities of anticoagulation (INR > 3) have been used for prosthetic heart valve patients, but they are associated with higher incidence of hemorrhagic complications. It is possible, though as yet unproven, that in nonvalvular atrial fibrillation patients, a lower intensity of anticoagulation (INR 1.4 to 1.9), may be as effective and require less monitoring.

INTRACRANIAL HEMORRHAGE: GENERAL REMARKS

Of the many causes of nontraumatic intracranial hemorrhage, four are particularly common: deep hypertensive and spontaneous lobar intracerebral hemorrhages, ruptured saccular aneurysm, and bleeding from an arteriovenous malformation. Hemorrhage associated with a bleeding disorder and rupture of a mycotic aneurysm are less common. Rare causes include idiopathic brain purpura, brainstem (Duret) hemorrhages associated with brainstem compression during herniation, and small multifocal hemorrhages associated with hypertensive encephalopathy.

HYPERTENSIVE INTRACEREBRAL HEMORRHAGE

PATHOPHYSIOLOGY Hypertensive hemorrhages typically occur in one of four sites: (1) the putamen and adjacent internal capsule, (2) the thalamus, (3) the pons, and (4) the cerebellum. They rarely originate in the central white matter of the hemispheres. A penetrating artery arising from the middle cerebral artery stem, basilar artery, or circle of Willis is generally the source of hemorrhage, the same vessels that are known to be damaged by hypertension.

The hemorrhage begins as a small oval mass and then spreads by dissection, growing in volume and displacing and compressing adjacent brain tissue. Rupture or seepage into the ventricular system may occur. Primary intraventricular hemorrhage is rare.

Most hypertensive intracerebral hemorrhages develop over a few minutes, but some evolve over 30 to 60 min, and others, particularly those associated with anticoagulant therapy, may evolve for as long as 24 to 38 h. Once bleeding stops, it has generally been thought not to start again. Edema in the compressed tissue around the hemorrhage often leads to increasing mass effect and, in some cases, worsening of the clinical state. Within 48 h, macrophages begin to phagocytize the hemorrhage at its outer surface. After 1 to 6 months, the hemorrhage mass is generally resolved to a slitlike orange cavity lined with glial scar tissue and hemosiderin-laden macrophages.

CLINICAL MANIFESTATIONS Hypertensive intracerebral hemorrhages are most common in patients with prolonged, sustained hypertension. Although not particularly associated with exertion,

intracerebral hemorrhages almost always occur while the patient is awake and sometimes when under stress. Unlike the sudden onset of embolism, these strokes usually evolve over a few minutes, with the neurologic signs and symptoms dependent on the site and size of the extravasation. Vomiting and headache are hallmarks of acute hemorrhages that distinguish them from other strokes. Seizures are uncommon but occur in a few instances.

Putamenal hemorrhage, the most common hypertensive hemorrhage, invariably disrupts the internal capsule adjacent to the basal ganglia. Contralateral hemiplegia is therefore the sentinel sign, but when these hemorrhages are large, the patient may become comatose within a few minutes. In milder cases, over 5 to 30 min, the face sags on one side, speech becomes slurred, the arm and leg gradually weaken, and *the eyes deviate away from the side of the hemiparesis*. The paralysis may worsen until the affected limbs become flaccid or extend rigidly with a Babinski sign on the same side. In the worst case, drowsiness gives way to stupor as signs of upper brainstem compression appear. Coma ensues, accompanied by deep, irregular, or intermittent respiration, a dilated and fixed ipsilateral pupil, bilateral Babinski signs, and decerebrate rigidity. Edema formation in the adjacent brain may cause progressive deterioration over 12 to 72 h.

Thalamic hemorrhages also produce a hemiplegia or hemiparesis from pressure on or dissection through the internal capsule adjacent to the thalamus. A prominent sensory deficit involving all modalities is usually present. Aphasia, often with preserved verbal repetition, may occur after hemorrhage into the dominant (left) thalamus, and apractagnosia or mutism occurs in some cases of nondominant hemorrhage. There also may be a transient homonymous visual field defect. Thalamic hemorrhages cause several typical ocular disturbances by virtue of extension medially into the upper midbrain. These include, most characteristically, deviation of the eyes downward and inward so that they appear to be looking at the patient's nose, unequal pupils with absence of light reaction, skew deviation with the eye opposite the hemorrhage displaced downward and medially, ipsilateral ptosis and miosis (Horner's syndrome), absence of convergence, paralysis of vertical gaze, an assortment of lateral gaze abnormalities (paresis or pseudoparesis of the sixth nerve), and retraction nystagmus.

In *pontine hemorrhages*, deep coma with quadriplegia usually occurs over a few minutes. There is often prominent decerebrate rigidity and small (1-mm) pupils that react to light. There is impairment of reflex horizontal eye movements evoked by head turning (doll's-head or oculocephalic maneuver) or by irrigation of the ears with cold water (see Chap. 26). Hyperpnea, severe acute hypertension, and hyperhidrosis are common. Death usually occurs within a few hours, but there are exceptions where consciousness is retained because the hemorrhage is limited to the tegmentum.

Cerebellar hemorrhages usually develop over several hours with repeated vomiting and inability to walk or stand. In mild cases there may be no other neurologic signs; therefore, it is imperative to test gait. Occipital headache and dizziness or vertigo may be prominent symptoms. There is often paresis of conjugate lateral gaze toward the side of the hemorrhage, forced deviation of the eyes to the opposite side, or an ipsilateral sixth nerve palsy. Other less frequent ocular signs include blepharospasm, involuntary closure of one eye, ocular bobbing, and skew deviation. There may be little or no evidence of the usual signs of cerebellar disease, and only a minority of cases show nystagmus or ataxia of the limbs. A mild ipsilateral facial weakness and a diminished corneal reflex are common. Dysarthria and dysphagia may occur. There are no Babinski signs until late in the evolution of the hemorrhage as it expands to the brainstem. As the hours pass, and occasionally with unanticipated suddenness, the patient becomes stuporous, then comatose as a result of brainstem compression, at which point reversal of the syndrome by surgical removal of the clot is seldom successful.

In summary, ocular signs have been highlighted as a method of rapidly localizing hemorrhages. In putamenal hemorrhage, the eyes are deviated to the side opposite the paralysis; in thalamic hemorrhage, the eyes are deviated downward and the pupils may be 3 to 4 mm and unreactive; in pontine hemorrhage, the reflex lateral eye movements are impaired and the pupils are less than 1 mm yet reactive; and in cerebellar hemorrhage, the eyes may be deviated laterally (to the side opposite the lesion) in the absence of paralysis.

LABORATORY EVALUATION The CT scan reliably detects all acute hemorrhages of 1 cm or more in diameter in the cerebral or cerebellar hemispheres. After the first 2 weeks, x-ray attenuation values of clotted blood diminish until they become isodense with surrounding brain. Mass effect and edema may remain. In some cases, a surrounding rim of contrast enhancement appears after 2 to 4 weeks and may persist for months. Small pontine hemorrhages may not be identified because of motion and bone artifact that obscure structures in the posterior fossa. MRI, though more sensitive for delineating posterior fossa lesions, is not necessary in most instances. Images of flowing blood on MRI scan may identify arteriovenous malformations as the cause of the hemorrhage. Angiography is used when the cause of intracranial hemorrhage is uncertain, particularly if the hematoma is not in one of the four usual sites for hypertensive hemorrhage. For example, hemorrhage into the temporal lobe suggests rupture of a middle cerebral artery berry aneurysm. Lumbar puncture carries considerable risk after intracerebral hemorrhage and should generally be avoided unless CT scanning is not available.

THERAPY The size and location of the hematoma determine the treatment and prognosis. Supratentorial hematomas greater than 5 cm in largest diameter generally have a poor prognosis, and infratentorial pontine hematomas greater than 3 cm in size are usually fatal. The occurrence of edema in the week after the intracerebral hemorrhage often worsens the prognosis. The tissue surrounding the hematoma is displaced and compressed but not necessarily infarcted. Hence, in survivors, improvement can result as the hematoma is reabsorbed and the tissue regains its function. Careful management of the patient during the critical acute phase of the cerebral hematoma can lead to considerable recovery.

Surgical removal of an acute supratentorial clot is controversial, but most surgeons have found it necessary on rare occasions. In stuporous patients who still have reflex eye movements and some pupillary reaction, surgery may prevent temporal lobe herniation and irreversible brainstem compression. One important randomized trial has shown a benefit of surgery, though marginal, only in patients in this state. Lifesaving surgery may nonetheless leave major neurologic residua. In contrast, surgical treatment of acute cerebellar hemorrhage is nearly always recommended because it prevents secondary brainstem compression that is the mechanism of death and it offers an excellent prognosis for recovery. If patients are alert without focal brainstem signs and if the cerebellar hematoma is small, acute surgical removal may not be necessary.

Mannitol and other osmotic agents reduce intracranial pressure that has been raised by the volume of the hematoma and edema (see Chap. 376). Glucocorticoids are of uncertain value in curtailing edema from intracerebral hematoma. Monitoring of the intracranial pressure may help to assess medical therapy. Both excessive hypo- and hypertension should be avoided. Toxemia of pregnancy and malignant hypertension associated with acute hemorrhage should be treated cautiously to avoid excessive or precipitous lowering of the blood pressure.

LOBAR INTRACEREBRAL HEMORRHAGE

As control of hypertension in the general population has improved, the relative proportion of hemorrhages outside the basal ganglia and thalamus has increased. These "lobar hemorrhages" appear on CT scan as oval or circular clots in the subcortical white matter. The role of chronic hypertension in their genesis is controversial, but many occur without a history of increased blood pressure. A number of other underlying conditions are found in almost half the cases, the most common being arteriovenous malformation. Others are due to

bleeding diathesis, often associated with warfarin administration; hemorrhages into tumor, usually a melanoma or glioma; and aneurysms of the circle of Willis that bleed into brain substance; and there are a large number whose causes remain undetermined even after extensive study including arteriography. Many of these are presumed to be from arteriovenous malformations or venous angiomas that have become obliterated or are angiographically occult.

Amyloid angiopathy, a cause of both single and recurrent lobar hemorrhages in the elderly, can only be diagnosed by postmortem demonstration that cerebral vessels stain strongly with Congo red. Amyloid is deposited in the walls of the cerebral arteries but not elsewhere in the body. Patients may have multiple hemorrhages, with months between occurrences.

CLINICAL MANIFESTATIONS The neurologic symptoms and signs of lobar hemorrhage appear suddenly, over one to several minutes. Most lobar hemorrhages are small enough to cause a restricted clinical syndrome that simulates an embolus to a vessel supplying one lobe. For example, the major neurologic deficit of occipital hemorrhage is hemianopsia; of left temporal hemorrhage, aphasia and delirium; of parietal hemorrhage, thalamic-like hemisensory loss; and of frontal hemorrhage, arm weakness. Large hemorrhages may be associated with stupor or coma if they secondarily compress the lower thalamus and midbrain, but the greater distance of lobar clots from these vital structures makes coma result less frequently than from putamenal or thalamic hemorrhages.

Most patients with lobar hemorrhages have focal headaches that are attributable to the innervation of adjacent dural vessels; occipital hemorrhage causes pain over the ipsilateral eye; temporal hemorrhage, over the area around or anterior to the ipsilateral ear; frontal hemorrhage, over the forehead or diffusely in the frontal quadrant; and parietal hemorrhage, over the temple region. Stiff neck or seizures are uncommon, but more than half the patients vomit or are initially drowsy.

TREATMENT In awake or drowsy patients, surgical evacuation offers little benefit over medical management with fluid restriction and osmotic agents. Stuporous or comatose patients who do not respond rapidly to medical therapy for raised intracranial pressure should generally have the clot evacuated.

SUBARACHNOID HEMORRHAGE—SACCULAR ANEURYSM

Rupture of an intracranial saccular aneurysm is the most common cause of subarachnoid hemorrhage, followed by arteriovenous malformation. Although autopsy studies have estimated that 5 percent of the population harbor aneurysms, the incidence of bleeding is about 4:100,000 per year. This devastating disease causes a greater than 10 percent mortality during the first day, and another 25 percent succumb in the first 3 months. Of those who survive, more than half are left with major neurologic deficits as a result of the initial hemorrhage or of a delayed complication, such as rehemorrhage, infarction from cerebral vasospasm, or hydrocephalus. Given these alarming figures, the major therapeutic emphasis should be on preventing the initial rupture and, if rupture occurs, preventing the predictable early complications.

PATHOPHYSIOLOGY Saccular aneurysms occur at the bifurcations of the large arteries at the base of the brain and rupture into the subarachnoid space of the basal cisterns. The common sites of saccular aneurysms include the junction of the anterior communicating artery with the anterior cerebral artery, the junction of the posterior communicating artery and the internal carotid artery, the bifurcation of the middle cerebral artery, the top of the basilar artery, the junction of the basilar artery and the superior cerebellar artery or the anterior inferior cerebellar artery, or the junction of the vertebral artery and the posterior inferior cerebellar artery. Approximately 85 percent of cases occur in the anterior circle of Willis; 10 to 30 percent of patients have multiple aneurysms; 10 to 20 percent occur in bilateral identical locations.

As an aneurysm develops, it often forms a neck with a dome. The length of the neck and the size of the dome, factors that are important in planning microsurgical obliteration, vary greatly. The arterial internal elastic lamina disappears at the base of the neck. The media thins, and connective tissue replaces smooth-muscle cells. At the site of rupture (most often the dome), the wall thins to less than 0.3 mm, and the tear that allows bleeding is often no more than 0.5 mm long.

It is not possible to determine which aneurysms are likely to rupture, but limited data suggest that those larger than 7 mm may warrant prophylactic surgical obliteration.

CLINICAL SYMPTOMS, EVOLUTION, AND MANAGEMENT Prodromal symptoms
Prodromal symptoms may suggest the location of an unruptured aneurysm and suggest that it is progressively enlarging. A third nerve palsy, particularly when associated with pupillary dilatation, loss of light reflex, and focal pain above and behind the eye, indicates an expanding aneurysm at the junction of the posterior communicating artery and the internal carotid artery. Prompt surgery is indicated. A sixth nerve palsy may indicate an aneurysm in the cavernous sinus, and visual field defects can occur with an expanding supraclinoid carotid aneurysm. Occipital and posterior cervical pain may signal a posterior inferior cerebellar artery (PICA) or anterior inferior cerebellar artery (AICA) aneurysm. Pain in or behind the eye and in the low temple can occur with an expanding middle cerebral aneurysm.

It is not known for certain if an aneurysm can cause small intermittent bleeding into the subarachnoid space—so-called warning leaks. However, the importance of recognizing the smallest aneurysmal rupture or leak is undeniable. Sudden unexplained headache at any location should raise suspicion of subarachnoid hemorrhage and be investigated by a CT scan to look for blood in the basal cisterns. Often a small subarachnoid hemorrhage will not be seen by CT scan, necessitating a lumbar puncture to detect subarachnoid blood.

Initial clinical presentation: Acute major subarachnoid hemorrhage
At the moment of aneurysmal rupture with major subarachnoid hemorrhage, the intracranial pressure approaches the mean arterial pressure, and cerebral perfusion pressure falls. This may account for the sudden transient loss of consciousness that occurs in up to 45 percent of cases. Sudden loss of consciousness may be preceded by a brief moment of excruciating headache, but most patients first complain of headache upon regaining consciousness. In 10 percent of cases, aneurysmal bleeding may be severe enough to cause loss of consciousness for several days. In about 45 percent of cases, severe headache, usually associated with exertion, is the presenting complaint. The headache is often called by the patient "the worst headache of my life." Words like *explode* and *burst* may be used. It may be "all over" or "in the back of the head and neck." Vomiting is a prominent symptom and when coupled with sudden headache should always raise the question of acute subarachnoid hemorrhage.

Although sudden headache in the absence of focal neurologic symptoms is the hallmark of aneurysmal rupture, focal neurologic deficits may occur (in addition to direct cranial nerve compression by the enlarging aneurysm as noted above). Anterior communicating artery aneurysms or middle cerebral bifurcation aneurysms may rupture into the subdural space, into the basal cisterns of the subarachnoid space, or directly into the underlying brain and form a clot large enough to produce a localized mass effect. The common deficits that result include hemiparesis, aphasia, anosognosia (hemineglect), memory loss, and abulia. An unusual acute unilateral hemispheric swelling with associated focal neurologic signs and stupor occurs rarely, immediately following aneurysmal rupture. Transient interruption of the cerebral circulation, possibly from acute vascular spasm, may underlie this complication.

Initial evaluation
Over 75 percent of cases have evidence of a subarachnoid clot on a noncontrast CT scan obtained within 72 h of aneurysmal rupture. The extent and location of subarachnoid blood may help locate the underlying aneurysm and identify the cause of the initial neurologic deficit. The clot in the subarachnoid space also may help predict the delayed neurologic deficits due to cerebral vasospasm. *A noncontrast CT scan should be done first because arterial enhancement in the basal cisterns may be mistaken for clotted blood.* If the CT scan neither establishes the diagnosis of subarachnoid hemorrhage nor demonstrates a mass lesion or obstructive hydrocephalus, a lumbar puncture should be performed to establish the presence of subarachnoid blood. Lumbar puncture prior to scanning is indicated only if the CT scan is not available at the time of the suspected subarachnoid hemorrhage. Once the diagnosis of subarachnoid hemorrhage from ruptured saccular aneurysm has been established, four-vessel angiography is generally performed to localize and define the anatomic details of the aneurysm and to determine if other unruptured aneurysms exist.

The ECG frequently shows ST-segment and T-wave changes similar to those associated with ischemic coronary heart disease. Prolonged QRS complex, increased QT interval, and prominent "peaked" or deeply inverted symmetric T waves, although suggesting primary cardiac disease, are usually secondary to the intracranial hemorrhage. The cause of these changes is debated, but there is evidence that structural myocardial lesions may occur after acute hemorrhage.

Serum electrolytes are obtained because hyponatremia may develop from urinary sodium loss, possibly due to natriuretic peptides released by the brain or heart.

Initial management
Following subarachnoid hemorrhage, a stuporous or comatose patient may have increased intracranial pressure. Care is required to maintain adequate cerebral perfusion pressure while avoiding excessive elevation of mean arterial pressure. Frequent arterial blood gas determinations are helpful to assess alveolar ventilation. If hypercapnia exists, mechanically assisted ventilation is necessary. If a subdural or intracerebral hematoma mass is causing neurologic deterioration, its surgical removal and, if feasible, obliteration of the aneurysm are undertaken.

Because rebleeding is possible, all patients are put on bed rest in a quiet, preferably darkened room and are given adequate stool softeners to prevent constipation. If headache or neck pain is severe, mild sedation and analgesics are prescribed. Aspirin, an antiplatelet agent, is inappropriate, but acetaminophen, meperidine, and phenobarbitol or other sedatives may be used. Extreme sedation is generally avoided because it can obscure the assessment of initial or delayed neurologic deficits.

Seizures are uncommon at the onset of aneurysmal rupture. The quivering, jerking, and extensor posturing that usually accompany loss of consciousness are probably related to the sharp rise in intracranial pressure. However, phenytoin or phenobarbitol is sometimes given as prophylactic therapy, since a seizure may cause rebleeding.

Glucocorticoids may help reduce the head-and-neck ache caused by the irritative effect of blood in the subarachnoid space, but there is no evidence to suggest they help in treatment of the cerebral edema that is sometimes seen in patients immediately after a subarachnoid hemorrhage, and they are generally omitted.

DELAYED NEUROLOGIC DEFICITS
There are three major causes of delayed neurologic deficits: *rerupture, hydrocephalus,* and *cerebral vasospasm.* Recognizing each of these depends on knowing precisely the cause and character of the initial neurologic findings.

Rerupture
The incidence of rerupture in the first 3 weeks following subarachnoid hemorrhage is 10 to 30 percent. Because rerupture is associated with a 60 percent mortality and poor outcome, early surgery is now generally recommended for stable patients. In the event surgery cannot be accomplished, antifibrinolytic agents may be considered. They have been associated with a reduced incidence of aneurysm rerupture but are also associated with an increased incidence of secondary cerebral infarction, presumably due to vasospasm. Hence antifibrinolytic agents are an option only when the early CT scan suggests that cerebral vasospasm is not likely to follow (see below).

Hydrocephalus   Acute hydrocephalus can cause stupor and coma and requires emergency ventricular drainage. More often, subacute hydrocephalus over a few days or a few weeks causes progressive drowsiness or abulia with incontinence. Differentiating hydrocephalus from symptomatic cerebral vasospasm in the anterior communicating arteries is often difficult. It may clear spontaneously or require temporary ventricular drainage. Permanent ventricular drainage, if necessary, is usually done at the time of aneurysmal surgery. Chronic hydrocephalus similar to normal-pressure hydrocephalus may appear a few weeks to months after subarachnoid hemorrhage. It may present with gait difficulty, incontinence, or slowed mentation (abulia). The clue to the diagnosis may be a lack of initiative in conversation or a failure to recover independence after the aneurysm has been surgically clipped. Ventricular shunting is the treatment of choice.

Cerebral vasospasm   Narrowing of the arteries at the base of the brain following subarachnoid hemorrhage from ruptured saccular aneurysm (*cerebral vasospasm*) can lead to delayed cerebral ischemia and infarction. This *symptomatic cerebral vasospasm* after subarachnoid hemorrhage occurs in approximately 30 percent of patients and is the major cause of delayed morbidity or death. Signs of ischemia usually appear 4 to 14 days after the initial subarachnoid hemorrhage, most frequently at about 7 days. The new deficits may fluctuate and correspond to ischemia in specific arterial territories. The severity and distribution of vasospasm determine whether cerebral infarction will develop. Although the precise mechanism of cerebral vasospasm is uncertain, it seems related to the presence of clotted blood surrounding an artery. Because there are no vasa vasorum around the arteries at the base of the brain, clotted blood prevents cerebrospinal fluid from nourishing the vessels. The current hypothesis suggests that spasmogenic hemoglobin breakdown products from the clot induce vasospasm in the underlying vessel, and reduction in local ATP may then prevent the artery from relaxing.

Clinical evidence suggests that the extent and location of clotted blood on CT scans can be used to predict the incidence, location, and severity of cerebral vasospasm in patients after subarachnoid hemorrhage. A high incidence of symptomatic cerebral vasospasm in the middle and anterior cerebral artery territories has been found in patients with early CT scans showing globular subarachnoid clots larger than 5×3 mm in the basal cisterns or layers of blood 1 mm thick or greater in the cerebral fissures. CT scans less reliably predict vasospasm in the vertebral, basilar, or posterior cerebral arteries. For this purpose, the CT scan should be obtained between 24 and 96 h following subarachnoid hemorrhage, since blood present initially can disappear or "wash out" on a scan obtained after 24 h. With the further passage of time, x-ray attenuation values of clotted blood diminish so that its full extent and location may not be reliably detected after 96 h.

CLINICAL SYNDROMES   Symptomatic severe cerebral vasospasm presents with symptoms referable to the specific arterial territories involved. For example, spasm of the middle cerebral stem or its main branches causes contralateral hemiparesis, dysphasia (dominant hemisphere), anosognosia, or apractagnosia (nondominant hemisphere). Even severe vasospasm may not produce ischemic symptoms if sufficient collateral blood flow develops through border zone anastomotic channels (see Fig. 368-1*A*). Proximal anterior cerebral artery vasospasm is associated with abulia and incontinence, while severe vasospasm of the posterior cerebral artery is associated with hemianopic visual field defects. Severe spasm of the basilar or vertebral arteries occasionally produces focal brainstem ischemia. All these focal neurologic symptoms may develop over a few days, fluctuate, or present abruptly. Transcranial Doppler assessment of proximal middle, anterior, and posterior cerebral and basilar artery flow can now reliably detect the onset of vasospasm prior to symptoms and follow its course and response to therapy.

TREATMENT   Therapeutic efforts to prevent or treat symptomatic cerebral vasospasm have been universally disappointing. The failure to find a satisfactory therapy for cerebral vasospasm has prompted a search for prophylactic measures to prevent or minimize its occurrence.

Treatment with the calcium channel blocking agent nimodipine has been reported in several studies to have beneficial effects, but patients in both the treated and untreated groups developed symptomatic vasospasm.

The most commonly accepted form of therapy for symptomatic cerebral vasospasm is to increase the cerebral perfusion pressure by raising mean arterial pressure through plasma volume expansion and the judicious use of pressor agents, ordinarily phenylephrine or dopamine. Raised perfusion pressure has been associated with symptomatic improvement in some patients, but high arterial pressure may risk rebleeding. The therapies generally require monitoring the central venous pressure, arterial pressure, and, in severe cases, the intracranial and pulmonary artery wedge pressure. If symptomatic vasospasm persists despite optimal medical therapy, then percutaneous intraarterial angioplasty, if available, is considered. It can effectively relieve focal severe symptomatic vasospasm in the arteries at the base of the brain, but it carries the risk of precipitating further ischemic stroke or arterial rupture and requires a highly skilled, experienced team.

Severe cerebral edema in patients with infarction from vasospasm may increase the intracranial pressure enough to reduce cerebral perfusion pressure. Treatment, as outlined in Chap. 376, is with mannitol and hyperventilation. Plasma osmolality is usually raised to approximately 300 mosmol/L. As a last resort, barbiturate-induced coma has been used to reduce intracranial pressure in some patients; it has not been proven to improve outcome.

Surgical interventional neuroradiologic treatment of saccular aneurysm   The advent of the operating microscope has made surgical obliteration of a ruptured saccular aneurysm the safest and most effective means of preventing disastrous rerupture. Recently, acute (day 1 to day 3) surgical management has been advocated, eliminating the problem of rerupture and allowing more aggressive medical treatment of symptomatic cerebral vasospasm. Interventional neuroradiologic techniques, including balloon occlusion of the aneurysm or of the internal carotid artery in a patient with inoperable aneurysm and angioplasty for cerebral vasospasm, are now possible. These new therapeutic strategies hold promise for improving management of patients with subarachnoid hemorrhage.

Giant aneurysms   Giant aneurysms larger than 2 cm in diameter occur at the same sites as small aneurysms. The three most common locations are the intracranial internal carotid, middle cerebral bifurcation, and top of the basilar arteries. Although they can bleed, they usually cause symptoms by compressing the adjacent brain or cranial nerves. Edema formation in the compressed brain can be relentless, compounding the mass effect. It is resistant to treatment and may be fatal. This progression is particularly likely if a giant aneurysm occurs at the bifurcation of the middle cerebral artery. Surgical decompression, until recently, was the only adequate therapy. It is extremely difficult technically and carries a high morbidity in the presence of edema. Newer interventional neuroradiologic procedures may prove helpful (see Chap. 365).

Mycotic aneurysms   Mycotic aneurysms are located distal to the first bifurcation of major arteries of the circle of Willis. Emboli from bacterial endocarditis should be suspected and appropriate blood cultures taken. Because of their distal location in the arterial tree, they rarely leave significant amounts of clotted blood in the basal cisterns, and severe cerebral vasospasm is infrequent. Mycotic aneurysms, however, are subject to rerupture. Although antibiotic therapy may reduce this risk, surgical obliteration may be required.

OTHER CAUSES OF INTRACRANIAL HEMORRHAGE

ARTERIOVENOUS MALFORMATION   An angioma, or hemangioma, consists of a tangle of abnormal vessels forming an abnormal communication between the arterial and venous systems. Most are developmental arteriovenous fistulas in which the constituent vessels enlarge and grow with the passage of time. Angiomas vary in size from a small blemish a few millimeters in diameter to a huge mass of tortuous channels composing an arteriovenous shunt of sufficient magnitude to raise the cardiac output. Hypertrophic dilated arterial "feeders" approach the main lesion, disappear below the cortex, and break up into a network of thin-walled blood vessels which connect directly with draining veins. These often form huge, dilated, pulsating channels carrying away arterial blood. The blood vessels forming the tangle interposed between arteries and veins are usually abnormally thin and do not have a normal structure. Angiomas occur in all parts of the brain, brainstem, and spinal cord, but the larger ones are most frequently in the posterior half of the hemispheres, commonly forming a wedge-shaped lesion extending from the cortex to the ventricular lining.

Angiomas are more frequent in men and may occur in more than one member of a family in the same or successive generations. Although the lesion is present from birth, bleeding or other complaints are most common between the ages of 10 and 30, occasionally as late as the fifties.

The chief clinical symptoms and signs are headache, seizures, and those associated with rupture. When headache occurs (without bleeding), it may be hemicranial and throbbing, like migraine, or diffuse. There may be hemiplegia with headache, resembling hemiplegic migraines. Focal seizures that become generalized occur in about 30 percent of cases and are usually well managed with anticonvulsants. In half of cases, arteriovenous malformations become evident as intracerebral hemorrhages. In most of these cases, the hemorrhage is mainly intraparenchymal with a small amount of spillage into the subarachnoid space. Blood is usually not deposited in the basal cistern, and symptomatic cerebral vasospasm is therefore rare. The threat of rerupture in the first 3 weeks is low, so there is no need to consider the use of antifibrinolytic agents. The hemorrhage may be massive, leading to death acutely, or may be as small as 1 cm in diameter, leading to minor focal symptoms or no deficit. In either case, the hemorrhagic mass may compress the arteriovenous malformation so completely that angiography cannot detect the malformation. Hence, when arteriovenous malformation (AVM) is suspected, angiography is best postponed until the hematoma has completely resolved, i.e., after 6 to 8 weeks. Rarely the angioma is large enough to steal blood away from adjacent normal brain tissue, rendering the surrounding brain ischemic. This deprivation is most often seen when large AVMs in the middle cerebral–posterior cerebral system or middle cerebral–anterior cerebral system extend from the cortical surface to the ventricular system. Hydrocephalus may result when the vein of Galen enlarges as a channel for drainage from the AVM.

Large AVMs of the carotid–middle cerebral system may be associated with a systolic and diastolic bruit (sometimes self-audible) over the eye, forehead, or neck where a bounding, forceful carotid pulse may be perceived. Headache at the onset of AVM rupture is not as prominent or as common as it is with a ruptured saccular aneurysm. Contrast CT scan can often detect the channels of an AVM prior to rupture; newer MRI techniques may prove more sensitive.

Small AVMs, 0.5 cm or less, are usually low-pressure venous angiomas that can bleed slowly. If they have bled, surgical obliteration or resection should be considered.

The management of patients with arterial AVMs is best accomplished by a team approach. Many cases are first assessed and may be treated by interventional neuroradiology. Each case requires a unique approach that takes into account the extent and location of the lesion, the feasibility and safety of the various therapeutic options, and the assumption of a risk of 3 percent per year rate of hemorrhage.

TRAUMA Head injury can result in intracerebral (especially temporal lobe and inferior frontal) hematoma and infratentorial hematomas, subarachnoid bleeding, acute and chronic subdural hematoma formation, and acute epidural hematoma formation. Trauma must be considered in any patient with an unexplained acute neurologic deficit (hemiparesis, stupor, or confusion), particularly if the deficit occurred in the context of a fall. These entities and their distinction from spontaneous hemorrhage are discussed more fully in Chap. 376.

HEMATOLOGIC DISORDERS Intracerebral hemorrhage associated with hematologic disorders (leukemia, aplastic anemia, thrombocytopenic purpura) can occur at any intracranial site and may present as multiple intracerebral hemorrhages. Skin and mucous membrane bleeding is usually evident and offers a diagnostic clue. Intracerebral hemorrhage associated with anticoagulant therapy can occur at any location, often lobar, and may evolve slowly over 24 to 48 h. Fresh frozen plasma and vitamin K are usually given immediately. When intracerebral hemorrhage is associated with aspirin, fresh platelet transfusions may be required.

BRAIN TUMORS Hemorrhage into a brain tumor may be the first manifestation of neoplasm. Choriocarcinoma, malignant melanoma, renal cell carcinoma, and bronchogenic carcinoma are among the most common metastatic tumors associated with intracerebral hemorrhage. Glioblastoma multiforme in adults and medulloblastoma in children also may have areas of intracerebral hemorrhage.

OTHER CAUSES Primary intraventricular hemorrhage is rare. It usually begins intraparenchymally and dissects into the ventricular system without leaving signs of intraparenchymal hemorrhage. Sepsis can cause small petechial hemorrhages through the cerebral white matter. There is no blood in the spinal fluid, and this condition should not be confused with a stroke. Inflammatory disease of the arteries and veins, especially polyarteritis nodosa and lupus erythematosus, can produce hemorrhage into the central nervous system. Most of the time it is associated with hypertension. An intensely inflammatory and hemorrhagic white matter process termed *Hurst's hemorrhagic leukoencephalitis* is probably a type of hyperacute multiple sclerosis. Moyamoya, mainly an obliterative disease that causes ischemic symptoms, also may have multiple small aneurysms that rupture in a small percentage of patients. Hemorrhages into the spinal cord are usually the result of an AVM or metastatic tumor. Epidural spinal hemorrhage usually compresses the cord rapidly and produces a transverse myelopathy (see Chap. 381).

HYPERTENSIVE ENCEPHALOPATHY (See Chap. 209)

In this acute syndrome, severe hypertension is associated with headache, nausea, vomiting, convulsions, confusion, stupor, and coma. Focal or lateralizing neurologic signs, either transitory or lasting, may occur but are infrequent and always suggest some other form of vascular disease (hemorrhage, embolism, or atherosclerotic thrombosis). By the time neurologic manifestations appear, the hypertension has usually reached the malignant state, with retinal hemorrhages, exudates, papilledema (hypertensive retinopathy grade IV), and evidence of renal and cardiac disease. In many, but not all, cases the cerebrospinal fluid pressure and the protein values are both elevated. The hypertension may be essential or due to chronic renal disease, acute glomerulonephritis, acute toxemia of pregnancy, pheochromocytoma, Cushing's syndrome, or ACTH toxicity. Lowering of the blood pressure with hypotensive drugs may reverse the process in several days if permanent damage is not severe. Neuropathologic examination may reveal a cerebral swelling or hemorrhages of various sizes from massive to petechial. A cerebellar pressure cone reflects increased pressure in the posterior fossa, and in some instances lumbar puncture has been fatal. Microscopically, there are small hemorrhages, clusters of microglial cells, minute cerebral infarcts, and necrosis of arterioles.

The term *hypertensive encephalopathy* should be reserved for this syndrome and not for chronic recurrent headaches, dizziness, epileptic seizures, recurrent TIAs, or small strokes which often occur in association with high blood pressure.

REFERENCES

AMARENCO P et al: The prevalence of ulcerated plaques in the aortic arch in patients with stroke. N Engl J Med 326:221, 1992

BAUER KA, ROSENBERG RD: The pathophysiology of the prethrombotic state in humans: Insights gained from studies using markers of hemostatic system activation. Blood 70:343, 1987

BOSTON AREA ANTICOAGULATION TRIAL FOR ATRIAL FIBRILLATION INVESTIGATORS: The effect of low-dose warfarin on the risk of stroke in patients with nonrheumatic atrial fibrillation. N Engl J Med 323:1505, 1990

BOUSSER MG et al: "AICLA" controlled trial of aspirin and dipyridamole in the secondary prevention of athero-thrombotic cerebral ischemia. Stroke 14:5, 1983

CALL GK et al: Reversible cerebral segmental vasoconstriction. Stroke 19:1159, 1988

CANADIAN COOPERATIVE STUDY GROUP: A randomized trial of aspirin and sulfinpyrazone in threatened stroke. N Engl J Med 299:53, 1978

CEREBRAL EMBOLISM STUDY GROUP: Immediate anticoagulation of embolic stroke: Brain hemorrhage and management options. Stroke 15:779, 1984

CHAMBERS BR et al: Outcome in patients with asymptomatic neck bruits. N Engl J Med 315:860, 1986

EAGLE KA, BOUCHER CA: Cardiac risk of noncardiac surgery. N Engl J Med 321:1330, 1989

EC/IC BYPASS STUDY GROUP: Failure of extracranial-intracranial arterial bypass to reduce the risk of ischemic stroke: Results of an international randomized trial. N Engl J Med 313:1191, 1985

EUROPEAN CAROTID SURGERY TRIALISTS' COLLABORATIVE GROUP: MRC European Carotid Surgery Trial: Interim results for symptomatic patients with severe (70–99%) or with mild (0–29%) carotid stenosis. Lancet 337:1235, 1991

EZEKOWITZ MD et al: Warfarin in the prevention of stroke associated with nonrheumatic atrial fibrillation. N Engl J Med 327:1406, 1992

FALKEBORN M et al: Hormone replacement therapy and the risk of stroke—follow-up of a population-based cohort in Sweden. Arch Intern Med 153:1201, 1993

FISHER CM: Clinical syndromes in cerebral thrombosis, hypertensive hemorrhage, and ruptured saccular aneurysm. Clin Neurosurg 22:117, 1975

——: Concerning transient ischemic attacks. Cleve Clin J Med 54:3, 1987

——: Lacunar strokes and infarcts: A review. Neurology 32:871, 1982

——: Late-life migraine accompaniments as a cause of unexplained transient ischemic attacks. Can J Neurol Sci 7:9, 1980

——: Occlusion of the internal carotid artery. Arch Neurol Psychiatry 65:346, 1951

—— et al: The arterial lesions underlying lacunes. Acta Neuropathol (Berl) 12:1, 1969

—— et al: Atherosclerosis of the carotid and vertebral arteries: Extracranial and intracranial. J Neuropathol Exp Neurol 24:455, 1965

—— et al: Cerebral vasospasm with ruptured saccular aneurysm: The clinical manifestations. Neurosurgery 1:245, 1977

—— et al: Lateral medullary infarction: The pattern of vascular occlusion. J Neuropathol Exp Neurol 20:323, 1961

—— et al: Spontaneous dissection of cervico-cerebral arteries. Can J Neurol Sci 5:9, 1978

HINTON RC et al: Symptomatic middle artery stenosis. Ann Neurol 5:152, 1979

HIRSH J et al: Optimal therapeutic range for oral anticoagulants. Chest (Suppl) 95:5S, 1989

KISTLER JP et al: Carotid endarterectomy: Specific therapy based on pathophysiology. N Engl J Med 325:505, 1991

—— et al: The relation of cerebral vasospasm to the extent and location of subarachnoid blood visualized by CT scan: A prospective study. Neurology 33:424, 1983

—— et al: Therapy of ischemic cerebral vascular disease due to atherothrombosis. N Engl J Med 311:27, 100, 1984

KOUDSTAAL PJ et al: Predictors of major vascular events in patients with a transient ischemic attack or nondisabling stroke. Stroke 24:527, 1993

MAYBERG MR et al: For the Veterans Affairs Cooperative Studies Program 309 Trialist Group: Carotid endarterectomy and prevention of cerebral ischemia in symptomatic carotid stenosis. JAMA 266:3289, 1991

NORTH AMERICAN SYMPTOMATIC CAROTID ENDARTERECTOMY TRIAL COLLABORATORS: Beneficial effect of carotid endarterectomy in symptomatic patients with high-grade carotid stenosis. N Engl J Med 325:445, 1991

PETERSEN P et al: Placebo-controlled, randomized trial of warfarin and aspirin for prevention of thromboembolic complications in chronic atrial fibrillation: The Copenhagen AFASAK study. Lancet 1:175, 1989

ROPPER AH, DAVIS KR: Lobar cerebral hemorrhages: Acute clinical syndromes in 26 patients. Ann Neurol 8:141, 1980

WELIN L et al: Analysis of risk factors for stroke in a cohort of men born in 1913. N Engl J Med 317:521, 1987

WOLF PA et al: Atrial fibrillation as an independent risk factor for stroke: The Framingham study. Stroke 22:983, 1991

369 NEOPLASTIC DISEASES OF THE CENTRAL NERVOUS SYSTEM

FRED HOCHBERG / AMY PRUITT

Tumors of the brain, of its meningeal coverings, and of the spinal cord are estimated to cause 90,000 deaths in the United States each year. *Primary* tumors arising within the meninges or the parenchyma of the brain or spinal cord are common at all ages of life. Yet, more than three-quarters of central nervous system (CNS) tumors are *secondary* metastases arising in patients undergoing treatment for systemic cancer. CNS neoplasms claim a disproportionate share of hospital beds, diagnostic tests, and other medical resources. One-fourth of the annual $4 billion cost for the care of cancer patients in the United States is allocated to patients with neoplasms of the CNS.

Although the specialized care of such patients is usually delegated to the neurosurgeon, radiotherapist, or neurooncologist, with the advent of new imaging techniques, the internist is increasingly involved in the initial diagnosis. Late in the course of the disease, such patients again may come under the care of a general physician. The proper care of patients with primary or metastatic tumors of the CNS requires a systematic approach that enables the physician to (1) distinguish tumor from other causes of neurologic dysfunction such as infection, immunosuppression, metabolic derangement, pseudotumor cerebri, or subdural hematoma; (2) make proper use of sophisticated diagnostic techniques, such as magnetic resonance imaging (MRI) and computed tomography (CT), and of more invasive tests, such as spinal fluid evaluation and arteriography; (3) provide early therapy to control cerebral edema and avoid seizure activity; (4) exclude systemic malignancy prior to referring the patient for a brain biopsy; and (5) recognize the medical complications of the tumor and of its therapy.

APPROACH TO THE PATIENT WITH CNS TUMORS

CLASSIFICATION OF TUMORS Both benign and malignant primary CNS tumors are capable of producing neurologic impairment. Primary tumors arise from glial cells (astrocytoma, oligodendroglioma, glioblastoma), ependymal cells (ependymoma), or supporting tissue (meningioma, schwannoma, papilloma of the choroid plexus). In childhood, tumors arise from more primitive cells (medulloblastoma, neuroblastoma, chordoma). Malignant astrocytoma or glioblastoma is the most common type of primary tumor in adults over age 20. A classification of intracranial tumors is given in Table 369-1.

CLINICAL MANIFESTATIONS OF INTRACRANIAL TUMOR Intracranial tumors may be located within the brain substance (intraaxial) or in close proximity to the brain (extraaxial). The latter produce symptoms by compression of the brain. Many of the symptoms caused by intracranial masses reflect tumor expansion within a fixed bony vault into space normally occupied by brain, blood, and cerebrospinal fluid (CSF). The nature and severity of these symptoms depend on the location of the tumor and the rate of its growth. Although brain tissue can accommodate the presence of slowly growing tumors, masses larger than 3 cm in diameter compress the brain, its blood supply, and CSF pathways. This compression is increased by peritumoral edema (vasogenic cerebral edema). Neurologic deterioration occurs as the tumor infiltrates or displaces normal brain structures; as the tumor develops areas of hemorrhage, necrosis, or cyst formation; or as the tumor obstructs the normal flow of CSF, producing hydrocephalus.

TABLE 369-1 Classification of intracranial tumors

Type of tumor	Percent of total
Glioma:	40
Glioblastoma	20
Astrocytoma grades I and II	10
Ependymoma	6
Medulloblastoma	2
Oligodendroglioma	1
Papilloma of choroid plexus	1
Metastases	23
Meningioma	17
Pituitary adenoma	5
Schwannoma	5
Lymphoma	3
Miscellaneous (congenital tumors, PNETs*)	7

*Primitive neuroectodermal tumors.

Symptoms of intracranial tumor may develop in patients with previously diagnosed systemic cancer or in those not known to harbor a malignancy. Patients with intracranial tumor usually present with one or more of the following groups of symptoms: (1) headache with or without evidence of increased intracranial pressure, (2) progressive generalized decline in cognitive abilities or impairment of specific neurologic functions affecting speech and language, gait, or memory, (3) adult-onset seizures or increased frequency or severity of previously documented seizure activity, or (4) focal neurologic symptoms reflecting the particular anatomic site of the tumor, such as those caused by acoustic schwannoma (neuroma) in the cerebellopontine angle, by meningioma of the olfactory groove, sella, or parasellar areas, or by pineal area masses which abut the diencephalon.

Headache is the initial symptom in half of patients with brain tumors. Traction on the dura, blood vessels, or cranial nerves results from local compression, elevation of intracranial pressure, edema, or hydrocephalus. In most patients with supratentorial tumor, pain radiates to the side of the tumor mass, whereas patients with posterior fossa masses describe retroorbital, retroauricular, or occipital pain. Emesis and hiccups, often without nausea, signal development of increased intracranial pressure and are especially common in patients with masses located beneath the tentorium.

Tumors of the frontal lobes may attain considerable size before symptoms develop, and then symptoms often are nonspecific. Subtle, progressive disturbances of mentation, slowness of comprehension, loss of acuity in business affairs, memory disorders, or apathy, lethargy, and drowsiness may be reported. Spontaneity of thought and activity is lost. Incontinence of urine and disordered gait may be seen by family members. The development of a true dysphasia and/or motor weakness signal progression of the tumor or its associated edema into motor cortex and speech areas of the frontoparietal region. Papilledema, choking of the optic nerve head, or loss of retinal venous pulsations follows.

Masses in the temporal lobes are associated with personality changes that may resemble affective or psychotic thought disorders. Various combinations of auditory hallucinations, abrupt shifts in mood, and altered sleep, appetite, and sexual functions are soon interspersed with complex partial seizures, possibly accompanied by visual field defects in the superior quadrants contralateral to the tumor. Temporal tumors force the medial temporal lobe (uncus) through the tentorial notch (uncal herniation). The third cranial nerve is compressed against the diencephalon. The pupil dilates, followed shortly by hemiparesis on the opposite side.

Disorders of communication and vision characterize parietooccipital masses. Receptive aphasia with contralateral hemianopsia characterizes left parietal tumors, while a combination of spatial disorientation, constructional apraxia, and left homonymous hemianopsia bespeaks right parietal tumors.

Seizures occur as the initial symptom in 20 percent of patients with brain tumors. Patients with new onset of epilepsy after the age of 35 must be evaluated for brain tumor. Similar high-risk groups of new seizure patients include those with previously diagnosed systemic cancer, longstanding neurologic diseases (including such neuroectodermal disorders as von Recklinghausen's disease and tuberous sclerosis), or acute or atypical psychiatric disorders. A carefully obtained history may uncover disordered time perceptions (déjà vu or déjà jamais), paroxysms of fear, and clinging "viscous" personality changes in addition to obvious features such as "complex partial" (temporal lobe) seizures or personality changes that antedate the diagnosis by years. Occasionally, the first symptom simulates a transient ischemic attack with no residual deficit or discernible seizure, but more commonly the pattern of clinical seizures provides localizing information. Thus, the "Jacksonian march" of tonic-clonic seizure points to frontal tumors and a sensory march characterizes tumors of the sensory parietal cortex. Metastatic tumors, occupying the junction of gray and white matter, are more likely than are primary tumors to produce acute symptoms evolving in days to weeks. Even more rapid onset of symptoms reflects hemorrhage in tumors of lung, melanoma,

renal cell, choriocarcinoma, or thyroid origins. In contrast, with the exception of oligodendroglioma and malignant astrocytoma, primary brain tumors are unlikely to hemorrhage.

PHYSICAL EXAMINATION OF THE PATIENT WITH SUSPECTED CNS TUMORS When the physician examines a brain tumor suspect who is not previously known to have a systemic cancer, the general examination should include (1) survey of the skin for stigmata of neurocutaneous syndromes or melanoma, (2) a search for enlarged lymph nodes, (3) an examination of the abdomen for hepatic or splenic enlargement, (4) a rectal examination with stool guaiac test, (5) a breast and pelvic examination in female patients, and (6) a cardiopulmonary examination.

The neurologic examination of the patient with suspected brain tumor should focus first on an evaluation of the mental status. The examiner should look for evidence of specific localizing cognitive deficits, such as dysphasia, dyspraxia, or memory loss, in addition to gleaning a sense of any personality change which has occurred. The patient is examined for increased intracranial pressure (papilledema or sixth cranial nerve paresis) and for other cranial nerve abnormalities. Asymmetries of strength, sensation, visual fields, and reflex activity should be sought. Combinations of cranial nerve abnormalities and corticospinal or lumbosacral radicular signs raise suspicion of leptomeningeal metastases (see below).

INVESTIGATION OF THE PATIENT WITH INTRACRANIAL TUMOR Advances in neuroradiology have contributed greatly to the diagnosis and management of patients with suspected neoplastic disease of the CNS. A plan for appropriate diagnostic studies based on the initial MRI or CT scan results is outlined in Table 369-2. The language of neurooncology differs from that of medical oncology, familiar terms such as "benign," "malignant," and "metastasizing" taking on different connotations when the tumor involves the CNS. Benign and malignant tumors are not differentiated in the scheme of Table 369-2 because the initial clinical approach is identical. Although many primary CNS tumors exhibit microscopic characteristics classifiable as "benign" because they are well-differentiated histologically and grow slowly, they are, nevertheless, often incurable. Tumors of identical histology may have very different prognoses, depending on their location and amenability to resection and on the patient's age. Secondary CNS tumors are malignant in the conventional sense, since they represent metastases and invade normal tissue. Both benign and malignant tumors may produce profound, irreversible neurologic impairment. Primary brain tumors, with rare exceptions, do not metastasize outside the CNS; however, virtually all primary brain tumors are capable of diffuse seeding to the leptomeninges. Thus, the approach to *all* intracranial tumors, summarized in Table 369-2, relies on the clinical history and physical examination and on information provided by MRI and CT.

The laboratory evaluation of intracranial tumors Contrast-enhanced and unenhanced MRI and CT have now largely replaced the combination of skull x-ray, electroencephalogram, radionuclide brain scan, and arteriography as the principal tests for the evaluation of patients with suspected brain tumor.

MAGNETIC RESONANCE IMAGING (MRI) MRI is the procedure of choice for the evaluation of neurologic dysfunction in a patient suspected of having cancer. MRI delineates most metastatic and primary tumors of the nervous system (see also Chap. 365). Lesions of the skull base and those in the brainstem, cerebellum, and spinal cord are visualized with greater detail with MRI than with CT, myelographic, or radionuclide images (Fig. 369-1). In addition to great sensitivity and delineation of anatomic detail, MRI offers the advantages of requiring no radiation exposure. The "flow-void" characteristic of MRI images provides a measure of tumor vascularity and may be reconstructed to create an MRI angiogram that may obviate preoperative arteriography (Fig. 369-2). Hemorrhage, seen in metastatic melanoma and glioblastoma, is easily identified as hemoglobin products or as ferritin. Tumors which contain fat (epidermoid, lipoma, craniopharyngioma) are recognized by their "bright" T2 signals as are those growths with cysts containing high concentra-

TABLE 369-2 Evaluation following MRI or CT scan of the patient with suspected neoplastic disease of the brain and spinal cord

CT/MRI result	Possible diagnosis	Pretreatment evaluation	Primary treatment	Secondary treatment
KNOWN SYSTEMIC CANCER: BRAIN				
Normal				
No focal deficits on examination	Infection, metabolic abnormality	Lumbar puncture, exclude infection	See text	——
Focal deficits on examination	Vascular disease, carcinomatous meningitis, seizure, paraneoplastic syndrome, complications of therapy	Lumbar puncture, follow-up MRI 4–6 weeks, gadolinium MRI	See text	Glucocorticoids as needed
Solitary mass	Radioresistant or radiosensitive tumor, unrelated tumor	MRI (Gd-DTPA), metastatic evaluation, surgical opinion	Glucocorticoids, radiation if radiosensitive tumor or active systemic disease found	Glucocorticoids as needed
Multiple masses	Metastases	None	Glucocorticoids, radiation	Glucocorticoids as needed, radiation, chemotherapy as indicated
NO KNOWN SYSTEMIC CANCER: BRAIN				
Normal	No disease	Repeat MRI (Gd-DTPA) in 8–12 weeks if symptoms persist	——	——
Solitary mass	Neoplastic disease, primary or secondary tumor, benign or malignant tumor	Metastatic evaluation, surgical opinion, MRI (Gd-DTPA)	Glucocorticoids, biopsy, radiation	Glucocorticoids as needed
Multiple masses	Neoplastic disease, primary or secondary tumor	Metastatic evaluation	Glucocorticoids and radiation if systemic tumor identified Glucocorticoids, biopsy, and radiation if no systemic tumor is found	See text
KNOWN SYSTEMIC CANCER: SPINAL CORD				
Normal	Nonneoplastic disease Carcinomatous meningitis Paraneoplastic	CSF analysis CSF cytology CT/myelogram	See text	See text
Abnormal	Metastases vs. tumor vs. nonneoplastic	CSF cytology, CT/myelogram, metastatic evaluation, surgical opinion	Glucocorticoids, chemotherapy (meningeal disease), Radiation	See text
NO KNOWN SYSTEMIC CANCER: SPINAL CORD				
Normal	No disease	Further evaluation in 8–12 weeks if symptoms persist (EMG)	See text	——
Abnormal	Metastases vs. primary tumor vs. nonneoplastic	Metastatic evaluation, CSF analysis and cytology, angiography, CT/myelogram, MRI (Gd-DTPA)	See text	——

tions of protein. The interpretation of MRI abnormalities can be very vexing, however. Many patients harbor unexplained white matter abnormalities ("unidentified bright objects," of UBOs) in close proximity to the ventricular system. Extensive areas of T2 signal abnormality on MRI are not clearly correlated with the extent of tumor on CT nor with the histologic tumor margin. These areas reflect cerebral edema, infarction, tumor necrosis, and the effects of prior irradiation and surgery.

Paramagnetic contrast with intravenous gadolinium diethylenetriamine pentaacetic acid (gadolinium DTPA) produces contrast changes in MRI similar to those observed following the use of organic iodides in CT. The combination of paramagnetic agents and higher energy MRI units provides better separation of tumor from nontumor tissue and better resolution of the spinal cord, nerve roots, and brachial plexus. Contrast MRI provides definition of an altered blood-brain barrier. It is useful for targeting stereotactic surgical procedures, delineating the extent of the tumor mass, and measuring tumor volume for longitudinal assessment of the response to therapy. Reconstruction in the coronal and sagittal planes allows detection of masses larger

than 5 mm. Contrast-enhanced tumor margins are defined to within 1 cm of the tumor's histologic border. Echoplanar MRI (fast MRI) provides assessment of blood volume within tumors (see Chap. 365). Gadolinium DTPA administration occasionally produces hypotension and nausea or emesis. The agent is cleared through the kidneys and must be used with caution in hepatic failure because of altered iron metabolism. Because red cell morphology may be altered, gadolinium DTPA should be used with caution in hemolytic anemia.

CT SCAN The virtues of CT remain those of speed, cost, and the delineation of bony density. Contrast-enhanced CT imaging delineates intracranial masses as small as 0.5 cm in diameter. Certain tumors whose density exceeds that of normal brain parenchyma, including meningioma, melanoma, and primary lymphoma, and tumors with spontaneous hemorrhage can be visualized without contrast enhancement. CT scanning may be better than MRI for definition of calcium-containing meningiomas, oligodendrogliomas and pineal region tumors. Tumors commonly appear as homogeneous or ring-enhancing masses surrounded by variable amounts of edema.

Initial unenhanced CT or MRI studies may show no abnormality

A

B

FIGURE 369-1 CT and MRI scans in a 57-year-old woman with a long history of temporal lobe epilepsy. *A*. Contrast-enhanced CT scan showed decreased absorption in the medial left temporal lobe (arrows) with no sign of contrast enhancement. Lesion was present on a CT scan taken 5 years earlier. *B*. Recent T2-weighted image shows a hyperintense circumscribed mass in the same lobe. Biopsy revealed a low-grade astrocytoma.

in meningeal carcinomatosis, small metastases, primary brain lymphoma, or some glial tumors that emerge in the setting of chronic seizure activity. Repeat CT scanning, using single or double doses of contrast, or enhanced MRI, 4 to 5 weeks later, usually provides tumor detection. Enhanced MRI should be performed if the initial CT scan is negative or uncertain and a CNS cancer is suspected. The clinician should be wary of attributing all CT or MRI scan masses to tumor, as ringlike abnormalities may occur in abscesses, in recent cerebral infarction, in the plaques of multiple sclerosis, as a consequence of encephalitis, and in certain vascular malformations with or without hemorrhage. Asymptomatic meningioma and aneurysm are sometimes detected incidentally during evaluation for brain tumors.

Before MRI, brainstem, cerebellar, and spinal cord masses could be further defined by a combination of CT and subarachnoid administration of water-soluble contrast agents. MRI has largely supplanted this procedure except for the preoperative delineation of intradural lesions of the spinal cord.

ANGIOGRAPHY Transfemoral arteriography provides selective visualization of internal carotid and vertebral arteries and their branches. Vessels of malignant tumors are characterized by an angiographic "blush" with enlarged early draining veins, features not seen in association with an intracerebral hemorrhage, infarction, or abscess. The identification on MRI of "flow-voids" has diminished the requirement for arteriograms. Preoperative neurosurgical planning is often aided by knowledge of the vascular anatomy or by embolization of excessively vascularized tumors such as meningioma (see Chap. 365).

MANAGEMENT OF INTRACRANIAL TUMORS   Surgery: biopsy and resection Surgical exploration allows tumor identification in patients with either solitary or multiple intracranial masses. Surgical exploration may be necessary to obtain a diagnosis in patients with

FIGURE 369-2 Meningioma. Gadolinium-enhanced T1 magnetic resonance scan reveals a homogeneous mass attached to the midline falx and superior sagittal sinus. A magnetic resonance angiogram (not shown) revealed patency of the sinus circulation.

multiple CT masses in whom a thorough systemic evaluation, including hemogram, liver function studies, carcinoembryonic antigen, chest x-ray, sputum cytology, radionuclide bone and liver scans, and perhaps intravenous pyelography is unrewarding. Of patients with multiple CNS metastatic lesions, 20 percent have no evidence of systemic cancer.

Tumor biopsy is performed through an open craniotomy or with MRI or CT-guided stereotaxic techniques. The establishment of a diagnosis is important to determine prognosis and treatment. *Resection* is undertaken and may be curative for some primary tumors such as meningioma, ependymoma, oligodendroglioma, and low-grade astrocytoma (see below) in nondominant, frontal, anterior temporal, or occipital locations or in the ventricular system. *Partial resection* improves patient symptoms, often including better seizure control; by diminishing cerebral edema, it reduces dependence on glucocorticoids. Although resection offers little to patients with multiple intracranial lesions, such as those with brain lymphoma, it may be of value for solitary metastases. Resection of a *solitary tumor* in patients with known systemic cancer may be considered if (1) there is a greater than 2-year interval without known residual systemic malignancy, (2) relief of specific symptoms such as hydrocephalus is required, (3) the tumor is known to be radioresistant as in the case of melanoma, sarcoma, and renal or colonic carcinomas, (4) symptomatic tumor recurs after radiation, and (5) the patient's systemic disease is under good control and the cerebral tumor is the limiting factor in quality of survival. For selected patients, this approach offers survival free of neurologic disease of more than 1 year and is superior to radiation therapy alone.

Acute treatment of intracranial tumors Clinical evidence of acute or subacute deterioration, such as stupor, focal neurologic signs, or evidence of transtentorial herniation, requires aggressive management. Treatment is directed to reducing cerebral edema, lowering intracranial pressure, and reducing the risk of seizures. Treatment with daily doses of dexamethasone 30 to 60 mg or methylprednisolone 120 to 200 mg in four to six divided doses reduces cerebral edema and associated surgical morbidity. Glucocorticoids may not control symptoms caused by obstruction of the ventricular system, and emergency ventricular drainage may be required. Anticonvulsant medications, such as phenytoin (to achieve an early morning blood level between 15 to 20 µg/dL) or carbamazepine (to achieve an early morning blood level between 9.5 to 11 µg/dL), are usually prescribed for patients with seizures, though many physicians administer them prophylactically when intracranial tumor has been diagnosed.

PSEUDOTUMOR—BENIGN INTRACRANIAL HYPERTENSION Symptoms of increased intracranial pressure may occur in the absence of demonstrable parenchymal or leptomeningeal tumor or hydrocephalus. However, little distinguishes the symptomatic presentation of true tumor from that of pseudotumor, which includes headache, neck stiffness, visual blurring and obscurations, diplopia, nausea, and vomiting. Papilledema, which may be unilateral or asymmetric, is accompanied by enlargement of the blind spot and altered visual acuity. Pseudotumor usually afflicts young, often obese women; it occurs most often in the absence of systemic cancer and focal neurologic difficulties. The marked increases in intracranial pressure may reflect impaired venous drainage within the brain or skull or may accompany the hormonal alterations of pregnancy, oral contraceptive use, or obesity. Less-common predisposing endocrinologic illnesses include both hypo- and hyperthyroidism, hypoparathyroidism, adrenal insufficiency, and both endogenous and exogenous excess of adrenocorticoids. Rare associations occur with sarcoidosis and lupus erythematosus. A variety of drugs have been implicated, including supplemental vitamin A, tetracycline, nalidixic acid, nitrofurantoin, sulfa preparations, lithium, indomethacin, and phenytoin. The diagnosis is confirmed by the exclusion of an intracranial mass lesion or meningeal cancer. In the presence of a normal or small ventricular system on CT or MRI scan, lumbar puncture carries no risk for brain herniation. Cerebrospinal fluid is invariably under

increased pressure but is otherwise unremarkable. Treatment is aimed at prevention of visual deficits and lasting symptoms of reducing the CSF volume by repetitive lumbar punctures. The removal of an offending drug or metabolic cause will reverse symptoms within 1 week's time. Patients refractory to this may benefit from acetazolamide, furosemide, or short-term glucocorticoid therapy. Lumboperitoneal shunting and surgical subtemporal decompression or optic nerve sheath fenestration are reserved for patients with progressive visual impairment who have failed medical therapy. The outlook for most patients is excellent—fully 80 percent respond to conservative therapy, but as many as 10 percent experience permanent or recurrent visual deficits.

SYSTEMIC CANCER AND THE CNS

CEREBRAL METASTASES The most common CNS tumors are metastatic. The following section discusses the approach to patients who present with a CNS tumor where systemic cancer must be considered.

Pathogenesis and pathology Cerebral metastases occur in one-quarter of patients with systemic cancer. Spread to the calvarium, brain parenchyma, and subarachnoid space occurs through several mechanisms. *Hematogenous tumor embolism* from intermediate sites such as lung and liver is the most common mechanism in solid tumors of the breast and lung and in melanoma. Spread into the spinal canal via the *perivertebral venous system* occurs with uterine, colonic, and prostatic tumors. *Direct extension* of tumors originating in the head and neck may occur through the base of the skull. *Paraspinal direct* infiltration may occur with lymphoma and with prostate and breast carcinomas. *Tumor passage from the eye* or through the choroid plexus to the brain and subarachnoid space occurs in lymphoma and leukemia.

Clinical manifestations Sixty percent of cerebral metastases occur in the setting of diagnosed systemic cancer. Cancers of lung in men and of breast in women account for the largest percentage, although melanoma is the tumor with highest likelihood of spread to the CNS. Of patients with a cerebral metastasis (most often arising in the lung) 20 percent develop neurologic symptoms before discovery of the primary malignancy. At some point after diagnosis of systemic cancer, 25 percent of patients with lung carcinoma, 6 to 20 percent of patients with breast carcinoma, and about 50 percent of those with melanoma (when this last tumor has already metastasized to a site outside the CNS) develop tumors in brain or spinal cord. Patients with recurrent sarcoma or ovarian or colorectal cancer who survive beyond 3 years after the original diagnosis face a heightened risk of neurologic involvement. These tumors rarely accounted for cerebral metastases in the past. In the majority of patients, cerebral metastases occur with systemic relapse (Table 369-3). An exception occurs in patients with lung cancer, where the CNS is frequently either the initial site of presentation or of first demonstrated recurrence in otherwise apparently well-controlled disease. As systemic treatment continues to improve survival, the incidence of CNS involvement can be expected to rise for virtually all tumors.

Diagnosis of cerebral metastases More often than is the case with primary brain tumors, those of metastatic origin occur in a setting of seizure activity, increasingly severe head pain, and motor weakness. These difficulties often evolve in days to weeks. MRI or contrast-enhanced CT scan is the procedure of choice for evaluating patients with known systemic cancer and new neurologic symptoms (Table 369-2). Tumors appear with equal frequency as multiple ring-shaped lesions or solitary masses. Three categories of patients without neurologic symptoms or signs are initially evaluated by MRI or CT. First, patients with lung carcinoma for whom attempted cure with pulmonary lobectomy is planned should have a scan preoperatively, since 5 percent of such patients will have clinically unsuspected cerebral metastases. Second, prophylactic brain radiation for small cell carcinoma of the lung should be preceded by a scan. Third,

TABLE 369-3 Interval between diagnosis of cancer and occurrence of brain metastases

| Tumor | Patients with brain metastases, percent | | | Interval from diagnosis of primary tumor to diagnosis of brain metastasis, percent |
	At diagnosis of primary	Sometime during course of tumor growth	At autopsy	
Lung tumor	10–15	20–30	15–30	90 after 3 months
Breast tumor	1	6–20	15–30	90 after 1 year
Melanoma	6	50	40–80	80 after 1 year
Renal tumor	4	11–13	8–20	90 after 1 year
Colorectal tumor	1	—	1	75 after 2 years
Sarcoma	1	36	—	90 after 1 year

SOURCE: L Weiss et al, *Brain Metastases*, Boston, Hall, 1980; M Deutsch et al, Cancer 34:1607, 1974.

patients with widely disseminated cancer due to breast or testicular tumors, sarcoma, or melanoma who are about to receive systemic chemotherapy often with bone marrow transplantation or as part of experimental treatment should have a scan to stage the disease.

Ten percent of patients with cancer develop neurologic difficulties in the absence of an intracranial mass on CT scan. Most of these will be found to have an abnormality on MRI scan. Focal motor or cranial nerve symptoms, headache, or impaired intellectual performance may reflect cerebrovascular lesions known to be associated with systemic cancer, unwitnessed seizures, meningeal carcinomatosis, paraneoplastic syndromes, or complications of tumor therapy.

Patients with systemic neoplasms can develop several types of cerebrovascular disease. Multiple cerebral infarctions are the most frequent in patients with solid tumors. Patients with lymphoma or leukemia may develop diffuse encephalopathic difficulties from infarcts due to disseminated intravascular coagulation; or may develop focal findings from emboli of nonbacterial thrombotic endocarditis, hemorrhage in the setting of clotting abnormalities, or thrombocytopenia. If the cause is unknown, laboratory studies should be done to exclude a circulating anticoagulant.

Focal deficits in patients with negative MRI or CT scans may result from seizures due to undetectable metastatic disease or may be manifestations of meningeal carcinomatosis or paraneoplastic syndromes (see Chap. 328). Gadolinium-enhanced MRI or repeat CT scan in 4 to 6 weeks often discloses the tumor if present. A lumbar puncture with cytologic examination is mandatory in such patients both to exclude infection and to search for leptomeningeal tumor (see below). CSF pleocytosis with mild elevation of protein may be found with paraneoplastic disorders.

Treatment The common assumption that brain metastases represent a uniform disease has proven invalid. Therapeutic decisions must be based on the type, extent, and radiosensitivity of the primary tumor, the morbidity produced, and the number and location of metastases.

Patients with solitary lesions and little or no active systemic disease should be considered for surgical resection or stereotactic radiosurgical therapy, whereas for those with advanced, widespread systemic cancer, comfort is the prime consideration. Glucocorticoids may be used in such patients to maximize neurologic function and to reduce headache (see "Acute Treatment of Intracranial Tumors").

RADIATION THERAPY After acute symptoms are treated, most patients with multiple cerebral metastases or unresectable solitary lesions receive radiation therapy. Patients with small (<3 cm) metastases are increasingly provided focused *stereotactic radiosurgery* using linear accelerators, "gamma knife," or cyclotron sources. Eighty percent of lesions so treated are rendered necrotic but still appear as enhanced abnormalities on contrast scans. For multiple or larger metastases a common approach is palliative whole-brain radiation totaling about 30 Gy (3000 rad) given in 10 to 15 equal fractions. Three-quarters of patients improve clinically and by CT; over one-half are able to discontinue their glucocorticoid medication for a time. However, only 30 percent of patients who complete radiation therapy survive 6 months and fewer than 20 percent are alive at 1 year. Two-thirds of the latter patients die from recurrent

systemic tumor and not from cerebral disease. Treatment is less effective in the elderly, in those with advanced systemic cancer, and in patients with radiation-resistant tumors such as melanoma and gastrointestinal and lung tumors. Reinstitution of glucocorticoids may be useful when progressive neurologic deterioration recurs.

CHEMOTHERAPY Systemic (intravenous or intraarterial) chemotherapy has been used with some success to treat cerebral metastases of lung (small cell), breast, and testicular origin. Anecdotal reports of brain metastases of breast origin responding to tamoxifen or other systemic chemotherapy have appeared.

LEPTOMENINGEAL METASTASES Pathogenesis and pathology Eight percent of patients with cancer develop diffuse infiltration of the meninges. The cranial and spinal nerve roots are usually affected. Tumors that commonly invade the meninges include non-Hodgkin's lymphoma, leukemia, melanoma, and adenocarcinoma of breast, lung, or gastrointestinal origin.

Clinical manifestations The common symptoms are headache, alteration in mentation, cranial nerve abnormalities, and lumbosacral radiculopathies. Patients may also present with seizures. The MRI or CT scan usually is normal, but may reveal enlarged ventricles. With contrast injections, scans may reveal diffuse enhancement of the meninges over the cerebral hemispheres and at the base of the brain.

A lumbar puncture is required for diagnosis. Three-quarters of patients show a modest CSF mononuclear pleocytosis of 5 to 100 cells. Elevation of protein and lowered glucose content may occur, but demonstration of malignant cells is required to confirm the diagnosis. Repeat lumbar or cervical subarachnoid punctures may be necessary to obtain positive cytology. In the past, myelography was often done in such patients because of back pain and radicular symptoms; it often disclosed multiple small nodules on the nerve roots. MRI studies using surface coils provide equal sensitivity providing that arachnoiditis is not present. Larger lesions can be detected and treated with radiation.

Treatment Treatment of meningeal carcinomatosis usually requires a combination of cranial radiation and intrathecal administration of chemotherapeutic agents. Chemotherapy is given either into the lumbar subarachnoid space or (more effectively) into a reservoir connected to the lateral ventricle. Agents commonly used include methotrexate, triethylenethiophosphoramide (thio-TEPA), cytosine arabinoside, and methylprednisolone either alone or in combination.

About one-half of patients with breast carcinoma respond initially to these treatments, but the median survival is only 7 months. The prognosis is particularly grave for meningeal carcinomatosis of melanoma or lung tumor origin; few responses are seen. A much better prognosis is expected in patients with lymphoma or leukemia with control for 2 or more years being common. Treatment failures reflect tumor drug resistance, poor circulation of drug within the subarachnoid space, and complications arising from chemotherapy and radiation.

TOXIC EFFECTS OF CANCER TREATMENT Chemotherapy Chronic glucocorticoid therapy may induce insulin-dependent diabetes mellitus, myopathy, and aseptic necrosis of the hip and may predispose to thrombophlebitis. In the early stages, the muscle changes reverse with steroid taper and intensive physical therapy. Administration of anticonvulsants is associated with cutaneous allergies. Anticonvulsant doses may need to be adjusted in patients receiving glucocorticoids. Allergy to an anticonvulsant may be masked while the patient receives glucocorticoids and revealed later when the steroid medication is tapered. Confusion and altered mentation may accompany glucocorticoid, L-asparaginase, nitrosourea, and methotrexate treatment. Ataxic syndromes may follow the use of 5-fluorouracil and cytosine arabinoside. Neuropathies of the cranial nerves may occur after nitrosourea and cisplatin administration. Vinca alkaloids may produce cranial and peripheral neuropathies.

Radiation therapy   Radiation therapy may cause toxic effects on the CNS. Acute changes include lethargy, loss of appetite, alterations in mental status, or exacerbation of previous symptoms and signs. These develop within 1 to 2 weeks of its initiation. These effects are usually attributable to worsening cerebral edema and are best treated with increased doses of glucocorticoids. Subacute changes that develop between 3 and 18 months after treatment are ascribed to radiation-induced demyelination and are unresponsive to glucocorticoids. Reappearance of previous neurologic impairment and the appearance of a mass which is indistinguishable from recurrent tumor on MRI or CT scan may occur. These areas of radiation necrosis may be visualized by hypometabolism following the injection of positron-emitting ^{18}F-deoxyglucose (PET scan). Patients who have received spinal radiation may develop Lhermitte's phenomenon with tingling in the back and legs following flexion of the neck.

Between 18 and 60 months after radiation, still other less reversible changes occur. These include retarded growth rate and impaired intellectual development in children who have received more than 30 Gy (3000 rad) of whole-brain radiation. At doses above 50 Gy (5000 rad), adults may exhibit cortical atrophy, communicating hydrocephalus, and hypothalamic dysfunction with elevated prolactin levels and amenorrhea or impotence. Dementia resulting from these changes is irreversible and in the case of hydrocephalus is usually unimproved by ventricular shunting.

The peripheral nervous system also can be affected by radiation therapy. Localized dysfunction of the brachial or lumbosacral plexus may follow radiation in excess of 40 Gy (4000 rad), usually appearing more than 1 year after treatment (see Chap. 383). Unlike peripheral nerve problems due to tumor invasion, radiation plexopathy is commonly painless. Additional tests, including CT scan, may be necessary to distinguish tumor invasion from radiation toxicity. Glucocorticoids may afford some benefit.

PRIMARY BRAIN TUMORS

In the following section, the most common primary brain tumors in adults are discussed by histologic type. Other tumors which occur in characteristic locations and whose presenting symptoms therefore reflect site rather than specific histology are then discussed by location. These include tumors located in the diencephalon-third ventricle, the posterior fossa, and the skull base.

MALIGNANT   ASTROCYTOMA   (GLIOBLASTOMA)   Definition   Malignant astrocytoma or glioblastoma (also known as malignant glioma or grade 3 or 4 astrocytoma) and the less malignant anaplastic astrocytoma account for about one-quarter of the 5000 intracranial gliomas diagnosed yearly in the United States; 75 percent of gliomas in adults are of this category. Because of its profound and uniform morbidity, it contributes more to the cost of cancer on a per capita basis than does any other tumor. The patient, commonly stricken in the fifth decade of life, enters a cycle of repetitive hospitalizations and operations while experiencing the progressive complications associated with relatively ineffective treatments of radiation and chemotherapy.

Pathogenesis and pathology   Epidemiology studies offer few clues to the etiology of malignant astrocytoma. Some tumors arise in patients with long-standing seizure disorders or personality disorders resulting from temporal lobe dysfunction and in scars incurred from

head trauma, suggesting that in certain instances the malignant cells emerge from a more benign glial proliferation. There are rare instances of malignant tumors occurring in families, suggesting a genetic propensity. At least four human oncogenes (*sis, myc, src,* n-*myc*) have been identified in cell lines derived from primary brain tumors, and there is overexpression for the receptors of both platelet-derived (PDGF) and epidermal (EGF) growth factors. Small clusters of tumors have appeared in certain occupational settings, notably in the petroleum processing industry. The tumor has an appearance similar to that produced by a variety of viral agents inoculated into animals. On gross examination, the surrounding normal brain is distorted and infiltrated by yellow tumor tissue containing areas of necrosis, cysts, and hemorrhage. Microscopic examination reveals a highly cellular composite of heterogeneous glial cells with elongated or rounded astrocytes whose processes stain for glial fibrillary acidic protein. Giant cells may be seen along with mitotic figures and the proliferation of small capillaries.

Clinical manifestations   Patients commonly present with a subacute progressive neurologic deficit exhibiting either focal signs or personality changes. Prior mental changes or seizures may antedate tumor diagnosis by months to years. Clinical symptoms may occur abruptly with seizures or with sudden deficits secondary to tumor hemorrhage. CT or MRI reveals a heterogeneous pattern of tumor enhancement interspersed with hypodense foci presumably corresponding to tumor necrosis and edema. Multiple tumors can occur but are uncommon. MRI scans often define more extensive tumor involvement than is indicated on the CT scan.

Malignant astrocytoma can arise in the brainstem, cerebellum, or spinal cord in addition to the more common locations within the white matter of the cerebral hemispheres. The prognosis for any site, unfortunately, has not changed greatly in the last 20 years. Following treatment, less than 6 months of useful function can be expected for most patients before progression of symptoms signals recurrent tumor. Death results in 80 percent of patients from tumor recurrence within 6 to 12 months. Progressive neurologic deterioration is followed by stupor and coma. In patients who survive over 1 year, often young adults, CNS dissemination can occur to the meninges or the ventricular ependyma. Metastasis outside the CNS is extremely rare.

Treatment   Confirmation of histology by biopsy should be performed in most patients; debulking of tumor is recommended if the tumor is located in an area that permits an extensive operation. Large tumor resections are more likely than biopsies to disclose small glioblastoma tumor foci within anaplastic astrocytoma.

Therapeutic modalities are not highly effective. The average life expectancy of 17 weeks for untreated patients is improved by postoperative external beam radiation alone to 47 weeks and by radiation combined with chemotherapy to 62 weeks. A subgroup of young patients under age 50 obtains significant improvement in quality and duration of life. Such patients have a 20 percent 2-year survival after cranial radiation of 55 to 60 Gy (5500 to 6000 rad) combined with adjunctive chemotherapy with the nitrosoureas carmustine (BCNU) or lomustine (CCNU).

Efforts to improve prognosis for this malignancy include trials of implanted radiation sources of isotopic iodine (^{125}I brachytherapy) and twice daily (hyperfraction) radiation. Current chemotherapeutic trials are often based on the localized nature of the tumor and of its recurrence. No superiority over intravenous BCNU has been seen as a result of experimental approaches including the modification of the blood-brain barrier, the administration of oxygen carriers, or the local or arterial instillation of chemotherapeutic agents.

ASTROCYTOMA   Definition   Low-grade astrocytomas occur throughout the brain and spinal cord. The subcortical white matter is the most common site in adults. In children and young adults astrocytomas arise in the optic nerves, cerebellum (cystic, juvenile, pilocytic astrocytoma), and brainstem (pontine glioma). These tumors are also associated with neurofibromatosis (type II) and tuberous sclerosis and are found in 20 percent of patients undergoing temporal lobectomy for control of chronic seizure disorders.

A

B

FIGURE 369-3 *A.* Gadolinium-DTPA-enhanced T1-weighted axial image demonstrating a decreased signal in the right temporoparietal region with no evidence of contrast enhancement. Mild effacement of the body of the left lateral ventricle without midline shift is present. Biopsy showed low-grade glioma. *B.* T2-weighted axial MRI of same tumor showed area of hyperintense signal corresponding to low signal area seen on T1 study.

Pathogenesis and pathology The tumors are avascular without necrosis and contain homogeneous populations of well-differentiated astrocytes. Progress to malignancy is associated with the appearance of mitotic figures and necrotic zones. The astrocytomas are divided into those with good prognosis (80 percent survivorship at 5 years) (cystic cerebellar, "juvenile" pilocytic, giant cell subependymoma) and those with likely recurrence after surgery (infiltrating, gemisto-cytic, and anaplastic).

Clinical manifestations The tumors evolve slowly over several years, producing symptoms by displacement of normal brain or by invasion of white matter tracts. Optic nerve gliomas cause progressive, monocular or bitemporal visual field defects leading eventually to blindness and sometimes proptosis. Hypothalamic compression may cause endocrine dysfunction. Hydrocephalus is rare. In the brainstem, such tumors typically involve several cranial nerves (often the abducens, facial, and trigeminal) and later impinge on corticospinal fibers and medial lemniscal and spinothalamic tracts. These symptoms must be distinguished from those caused by multiple sclerosis, arteriovenous malformations, cysts of cysticercosis and echinococcal origin, and extramedullary tumors such as schwannomas or meningiomas. Cerebellar astrocytomas cause progressive incoordination and gait ataxia combined with abnormalities of eye movements. In supratentorial locations, these tumors may produce seizures before any focal abnormality appears on clinical examination. In *gliomatosis cerebri,* slow infiltration of white matter occurs with atypical individual astrocytes without evidence of localized tumor.

Early use of MRI may allow for earlier diagnosis and intervention (see Figs. 369-1, 369-3, 369-4). MRI often demonstrates white matter abnormalities in patients with normal CT scans and is the preferred procedure for early diagnosis and follow-up. A stable clinical course is common with astrocytoma and repeat radiologic studies may show

FIGURE 369-4 Brainstem glioma in a 9-year-old boy. The medulla and cervical spinal cord are twice as wide as normal. Focal areas of cystic degeneration are seen as hypodense T1 signals. Biopsy revealed an astrocytoma.

little change. The characteristic CT appearance is an indistinct mass that is hypodense with respect to surrounding brain and exhibits little or no contrast enhancement, calcification, or evidence of edema. Malignant degeneration of astrocytomas is heralded by rapid progression of symptoms and signs, evidence of expanded size or altered MRI T2 or CT signal, or the presence of new enhancement on MRI with gadolinium DTPA or CT with iodine contrast. Echoplanar MRI reveals areas of increased "blood flow" in malignant zones while PET studies identify foci of increased glucose uptake.

Treatment As astrocytomas may contain areas of aggressive gliomas, many surgeons argue for early biopsy. This is especially true in the setting of seizure progression or increase in the size of the lesion. Surgical excision can be curative for some cerebellar, optic nerve, and lobar astrocytomas. Cyst drainage and partial resection are feasible for many. Biopsy should be obtained for supratentorial tumors but is less frequently considered for brainstem or spinal cord gliomas. Exceptions to the latter are tumors that have a cystic or extraaxial component. Postoperative radiation is recommended for incompletely resected tumors and for those involving the brainstem (for which multiple daily doses are often provided). Its role in the treatment of excised supratentorial tumors is less clear. The possible benefits of radiation therapy are weighed against the known long natural course of the astrocytoma and the complications of irradiation. Radiation is recommended when symptoms and signs progress or areas of enhancement or enlargement on CT or MRI are observed. Radiation may be safely delayed for several years in apparently totally resected tumors because of the accuracy of MRI and CT scans. The judicious use of glucocorticoids during radiation or when symptoms recur improves function. The median life expectancy is 67 months for supratentorial tumors and 89 months for cerebellar tumors. Average survivals of 15 months after radiation are reported for patients with brainstem tumors. However, the 5-year survival is only 30 percent. Chemotherapy, currently under investigation for brainstem tumors, may offer some improvement in survival.

OLIGODENDROGLIOMA Definition This tumor may develop in isolation or may be mixed with other glial cells. An uncommon tumor, it represents less then 10 percent of all gliomas.

Pathology Microscopic examination discloses rounded cells containing darkly staining nuclei with poorly staining cytoplasm, the "fried egg" appearance. The tumor is prone to spontaneous hemorrhage. Both "benign" and "malignant" forms are seen.

Clinical manifestations Presentation is most commonly in the third or fourth decade and tumors are most frequently in the frontal lobes or within the ventricles. CT reveals a well-defined, low-attenuation mass with fine speckled calcium deposits and small cysts.

Treatment Although the oligodendroglioma is histologically benign, resection is curative in only one-third of patients. Formerly postoperative radiation was recommended for incompletely resected tumors or those with mixed glial or malignant features or with evidence of progression after operation. The malignant transformation of "pure" oligodendroglial or mixed oligodendroglial tumors is more readily diagnosed if contrast-enhanced CT or MRI is used. Fully three-quarters of patients with "pure" or mixed oligodendrogliomas respond to the administration of chemotherapy with PCV (procarbazine, CCNU, vincristine) prior to irradiation. This approach is currently the subject of study.

MENINGIOMA Definition Meningiomas account for 20 percent of brain tumors. They can arise in either the cranium or the spinal canal. They occur more frequently at all sites in women. They are commonly found as asymptomatic tumors at postmortem. When symptomatic they usually present in the fifth or sixth decades.

Pathogenesis and pathology Meningiomas arise from cells of the pia-arachnoid. Common sites include the midline along the falx cerebri and the lateral cerebral convexity, the olfactory groove and along the sphenoid ridge, the tuberculum sellae, foramen magnum, and tentorium of the cerebellum. They also arise on occasion within the ventricles, where on radiographic examination they are indistinguishable from a papilloma of the choroid plexus. Meningio-

mas may coexist with schwannomas in patients with the central form of neurofibromatosis. Both tumor types are related to the loss of a "tumor suppressor" gene on chromosome 22. They occur more frequently in women with breast cancer; some meningiomas contain estrogen and progesterone receptors.

On the basis of microscopic characteristics, meningiomas are divided into seven categories: syncytial, transitional, fibroblastic, microcystic, psammomatous, angioblastic, and malignant. Malignant tumors display mitoses, invade normal brain, and occasionally develop CNS and extraneural metastases. Angioblastic and malignant forms are prone to recur.

Clinical manifestations The clinical presentation reflects the slow expansion of tumor within the skull and spine, with neurologic deficits evolving over many years. Tumors of the parasellar region produce a combination of second, third, fourth, fifth, and sixth cranial nerve deficits. Cerebellopontine tumors may produce a syndrome similar to that of acoustic schwannomas (see "Tumors of the Posterior Fossa," below). Early hearing loss is not a typical finding in meningioma. Parasagittal and frontal tumors may produce seizures or may be entirely asymptomatic, often growing to enormous size before they are discovered. Parasagittal lesions that attain sufficient size may cause spastic paraparesis and incontinence. Falx meningioma should be considered in the differential diagnosis of gait disorders in the middle-aged and elderly. In all locations, meningiomas must be distinguished from similar-appearing dural metastases from breast, prostate, and lung. CT often discloses calcium within a tumor and delineates the close relation between the mass and the dura, falx, or tentorium, as well as the altered bony calvarium. MRI often shows isodense masses that enhance with gadolinium-DTPA. Magnetic resonance angiography identifies tumor vessels supplied by meningeal vessels of the external carotid circulation.

Treatment Tumor site, rather than histology, is the major determinant of outcome. Intraventricular or parasagittal tumors are usually resectable and recurrence is rare. Those in the olfactory groove, sphenoid ridge, and parasellar locations are more difficult to resect completely and are prone to recur. Tumors of the foramen magnum may be totally removed with microneurosurgical techniques (see "Spinal Tumors," below). Radiation, often using beams of small focus, is advocated for malignant meningiomas and for incompletely excised symptomatic tumors of other histologic subtypes. Chemotherapy is without apparent efficacy; but antiprogestational agents are under evaluation.

PAPILLOMA OF THE CHOROID PLEXUS Definition Neoplasms derived from choroid plexus epithelium are rare, representing only 0.5 percent of all intracranial tumors.

Pathogenesis and pathology In children most such tumors occur as aggressive tumors in the lateral ventricles, whereas in adults the fourth ventricle is the most common site. The histologic structure resembles normal choroid plexus, with a connective tissue core covered by a single layer of cuboidal epithelium.

Clinical manifestations Very rare examples of malignant transformation have been described. Metastases to the leptomeninges may occur. The tumor may secrete excessive CSF leading to communicating hydrocephalus.

Treatment Surgery is the treatment of choice and is usually highly successful.

LIPOMA Lipoma can develop anywhere within the brain or spinal cord, though the corpus callosum is the most common location. The association of lipomas with partial or complete agenesis of this structure and with other dysplastic or hamartomatous anomalies such as ectopias, colloid cysts, and epidermoids supports the theory that they are the result of disorders of development. Intraspinal lipomas are most common in the thoracic region and are associated with spina bifida in one-third of cases. All lipomas can be easily demonstrated by MRI. The treatment of symptomatic cranial and spinal lipomas is excision.

DERMOID AND EPIDERMOID TUMOR Definition The distinction between dermoid tumors and epidermoids (true cholesteatomas) is often difficult. Both result from inclusion of ectodermal tissue at the time of closure of the neural groove and soon thereafter.

Pathology and pathogenesis Cholesteatomas are slowly growing tumors that most often afflict young adults, occurring commonly in lateral or midline locations within the skull, i.e., the cerebellopontine angle, the suprasellar region, the fourth ventricle, the pineal region, and over the hemispheres. No clear relationship has been established between cholesteatoma of the cerebellopontine angle and middle ear infection. Dermoid tumors, which are frequently cystic, occur largely in the posterior fossa or in the lumbosacral region. Rarely they are found in suprasellar or pineal regions.

Clinical manifestations Symptoms vary according to the location of these tumors, the general pattern being slow evolution of defects attributable to the specific area with seizures interspersed when the tumor occupies cortical regions. MRI provides excellent delineation.

Treatment Treatment of the cholesteatoma is total surgical removal of the tumor together with its capsule. Dermoid tumors similarly are curable if total surgical excision is possible.

PRIMARY LYMPHOMA OF THE CNS **Definition** Primary lymphomas are now recognized to be relatively common in the CNS. Before 1972, fewer than 25 cases had been identified at the Massachusetts General Hospital over a 50-year period. Since 1980 the tumor has tripled in frequency. Primary lymphoma is distinguished from the more frequent secondary involvement of the meninges that occurs in patients with poorly differentiated non-Hodgkin's lymphomas.

Pathogenesis and pathology The tumor is uncommon in patients without immunologic compromise. It is usually seen in patients with mixed humoral and cellular immune deficits. Three such disorders are recognized: inherited disorders of immunity such as combined immunodeficiency disease, selective IgM deficiency, or selective IgA abnormalities seen with combined immunodeficiency and Wiskott-Aldrich syndrome; AIDS; and therapeutic immunosuppression following organ transplantation or treatment of autoimmune disorders. Epstein-Barr virus (EBV) DNA has been demonstrated within primary lymphoma in 80 percent of immunosuppressed patients, raising the possibility that this agent may play a role in the pathogenesis of this disease.

The tumor may be focal or multicentric in the subcortical white matter, the walls of the ventricles, or the subarachnoid space. Tumor cells are always found in a perivascular distribution. At biopsy, tumor cells are often indistinguishable from normal lymphocytes, leading to an erroneous early diagnosis of "encephalitis" or "nonspecific perivascular inflammation." The B cell populations may be characterized as malignant by the immunohistochemical demonstration of monoclonal immunoglobulin surface proteins. The tumors contain cells defined histologically as immunoblastic or large cell (see Chap. 311). Burkitt-type lymphomas are rarely reported.

Clinical manifestations A history of personality change, focal deficits, or seizures evolving over several weeks in an immunosuppressed patient should raise the suspicion of cerebral lymphoma. Obviously, in these circumstances infection must be excluded. Patients with HIV infection are often treated presumptively for toxoplasmosis and brain lymphoma. In immunosuppressed and nonsuppressed populations, MRI and CT typically reveal multiple periventricular masses which enhance with contrast. T2-weighted MRI abnormalities have disappeared. A characteristic feature, rarely observed with other types of intracranial tumor, is the marked reduction or disappearance of lesions after a few weeks of high-dose glucocorticoid therapy (dexamethasone 5 to 10 mg four times daily). When both symptoms and CT abnormalities resolve after glucocorticoid therapy, remissions lasting several months are common, and steroids can be tapered. Spontaneous remissions without glucocorticoid therapy have been described. The usual clinical course is recurrence after 4 to 6 months, with resistance to steroid administration. Staging of patients should include HIV serologic testing, enhanced MRI or CT, slit lamp eye examination, and immunohistologic examination of CSF cell populations. The tumor may seed the meninges in one-quarter of patients. Systemic lymphoma is found in less than 10 percent of

patients and occurs late in the course of the disease. However, uveitis or vitreitis may occur at the time of presentation or early in the evolution of the disease; when present, it is helpful in the initial diagnosis.

Treatment After biopsy or diagnosis by CSF cytology, the recommended treatment is chemotherapy consisting of high-dose methotrexate and glucocorticoids, alone or in combination with cyclophosphamide, doxorubicin, and vincristine, followed by radiation. Chemotherapy provides therapeutic drug levels in brain parenchyma and most importantly, in the CSF. Partial or complete remission occurs in over three-quarters of patients. When methotrexate is administered prior to radiation, there is a reduced risk of radiation or drug-induced white matter damage. The median survival following chemotherapy and irradiation is in excess of 2 years. Radiation treatment is recommended for immunosuppressed patients with brain lymphoma.

TUMORS OF THE THIRD VENTRICLE AND PINEAL REGION Tumors of the diencephalon often present with a combination of failure of pupillary constriction to light, failure of upward gaze, and neuroendocrine abnormalities. Hydrocephalus due to obstruction to CSF flow at the level of the third ventricle leads to headache. Masses which push down on the diencephalon create the picture of *central herniation:* altered consciousness, Cheyne-Stokes respiration with reserved pupillary reaction. Masses below the diencephalon affect eye movement and pupillary responses. Several categories of tumors occur in close proximity to the diencephalon, hypothalamus, and third ventricle; these are pituitary adenoma, craniopharyngioma, germ-cell neoplasms, pineal tumors, and glial, meningeal, or metastatic tumors.

Uncommon tumors of the pineal region include astrocytomas, glioblastomas, meningiomas, and metastases. Nonneoplastic masses occurring in this region include colloid cysts of the third ventricle (see "Colloid Cysts," below) and parasitic cysts (cysticercosis).

Pituitary adenomas These tumors are described in Chap. 331.

Craniopharyngiomas These tumors arise from remnants of Rathke's pouch, derived from the primitive stomatodeum. They are usually suprasellar in location and cause symptoms by compressing hypothalamus or the optic chiasm (see also Chap. 331). They are easily identified by a "bright" T2 signal on MRI (Fig. 369-5).

Germ-cell tumors DEFINITION Germ-cell tumors, which account for half of all pineal region neoplasms, arise primarily during childhood or early adolescence and include germinoma, teratoma, embryonal carcinoma, endodermal sinus tumor, and choriocarcinoma.

CLINICAL MANIFESTATIONS The most common of these germ-cell tumors is the germinoma. It may occur in the pineal region or at the base of the hypothalamus. It occurs more frequently in males, who present with findings of diabetes insipidus and other neuroendocrine deficiencies, bitemporal visual field defects, paralysis of upward gaze (see Chap. 19), and sometimes hydrocephalus. The typical features of pineal masses occur more commonly with nongerminomatous germ cell tumors. Findings include Parinaud's syndrome—a failure of upward gaze and pupillary dilatation with deficiencies in response to light. Rarely, other signs such as nystagmus retractorius or brainstem signs due to compression may occur. Diagnosis may be assisted by the finding of elevated serum and CSF levels of alpha-fetoprotein (AFP) and of human chorionic gonadotropin (hCG) in germinomas. MRI and CT scans identify tumors of the pineal region *but offer no histologic differentiation.*

TREATMENT Following CT stereotactic biopsy by transcallosal or suboccipital route, radiation is given. Germinomas are radiosensitive; up to 80 percent are cured by doses of cranial radiation sufficient to produce disappearance of the MRI mass while avoiding damage to surrounding hypothalamic tissue. Craniospinal irradiation is provided when the tumor invades the ventricles or subarachnoid space, or is found outside the pineal region. Other histologic subtypes have poorer prognoses and recurrence is common, often with seeding of the cranial nerves and meninges. Recurrences sometimes respond to drug treatment with bleomycin, cisplatin, and vinblastine, which are beneficial in testicular tumors of similar histology.

FIGURE 369-5 This 39-year-old woman presented with headaches and gait disturbance (caused by a craniopharyngioma). On a T1-weighted coronal MRI, a large, lobulated hyperdense mass is visualized in the suprasellar cistern compressing the inferior third ventricle. There is enlargement of the frontal and temporal ventricles.

Pineoblastoma and pineocytoma These tumors account for 20 percent of growths in the pineal region.

PATHOGENESIS AND PATHOLOGY Pineoblastoma and pineocytoma arise from pineal organ cells. The pineoblastoma is a primitive malignant tumor of childhood and early adult life and is indistinguishable both in appearance and natural history from primitive neuroectodermal tumors that arise elsewhere in the CNS. The tumor may contain astrocytic or neuronal elements. Recurrence is invariable and dissemination through the ventricular system and subarachnoid space is frequent.

TREATMENT Brain and neuraxis radiation are recommended, and chemotherapy as outlined above for germ cell tumors has been successful in producing remissions in a few patients. Chemotherapy prior to irradiation is reserved for pineoblastoma. The pineocytoma is a more slowly growing tumor which is often well-demarcated and resembles the normal structure of the pineal. Although histologically benign, it tends to recur, probably because of incomplete removal. It is resistant to radiation.

Colloid cysts PATHOGENESIS AND PATHOLOGY Colloid cysts arise within the anterior third ventricle and are considered to develop from the anlage of the paraphysis, a component of the third ventricle, or possibly from the ependyma itself. The cysts are well-encapsulated and consist of a layer of connective tissue covered with columnar ciliated cells. The cyst is filled with glycoproteinaceous material which stains with periodic acid Schiff (PAS).

CLINICAL MANIFESTATIONS Symptoms occur usually in adults and may be dramatic, with episodes of headache, weakness of the limbs, and loss of consciousness. These symptoms are attributed to intermittent acute hydrocephalus due to blockage of the foramen of

Monro by the mobile cyst. Diagnosis follows MRI identification of the cyst and the visualization of either intact or obstructed CSF flow. Treatment is removal of the cyst.

TUMORS OF THE POSTERIOR FOSSA Tumors of the posterior fossa pose special problems in diagnosis and treatment. Rapidly growing tumors hindering CSF flow in the fourth ventricle or aqueduct of Sylvius may cause obstructive hydrocephalus, and even small mass lesions in the posterior fossa may result in vomiting, lethargy, headache, and papilledema. Slowly growing tumors give rise to progressive signs which are recognized by rather specific syndromes. These include progressive unilateral hearing loss, facial weakness, pain or numbness, and a unilateral sixth nerve deficit occurring with tumors in the cerebellopontine angle. (See Chap. 380 for discussion of cranial nerve symptoms and signs.) Gait ataxia and unilateral cerebellar signs occur with hemangioblastoma, medulloblastoma, or cystic astrocytoma of the cerebellum. Progressive diplopia, cranial nerve abnormalities, and crossed corticospinal tract and reflex abnormalities occur in brainstem glioma. Nuchal and occipital pain are common with all tumors of the posterior fossa. Corticospinal signs develop with further tumor enlargement and encroachment on the brainstem. Cerebellar tumors force the cerebellar tonsils into the foramen magnum. This *tonsil herniation* is accompanied by bradycardia, hypertension and respiratory irregularities when medullary compression occurs.

Acoustic schwannoma DEFINITION The acoustic schwannoma (synonymous with acoustic neuroma) is composed of myelin-forming Schwann cells that cover the acoustic nerve fibers. Schwann cells normally replace oligodendroglia as the nerve leaves the brainstem to enter the internal auditory meatus.

PATHOGENESIS AND PATHOLOGY Schwannomas are slow-growing masses that compress rather than invade normal tissue. When bilateral, they represent an inherited form of schwannoma which is diagnostic of "central" neurofibromatosis (NFII). Other CNS tumors associated with neurofibromatosis or von Recklinghausen's disease are schwannomas of spinal and other cranial nerves, intracranial and spinal meningiomas, gliomas, and ependymomas (see Chap. 378).

CLINICAL MANIFESTATIONS AND TREATMENT Early detection of acoustic schwannomas at a time of minimal hearing deficit and minimal facial motor difficulty is essential, as hearing may be spared by microneurosurgical intervention while the tumor is still restricted to the canal. Brainstem auditory evoked responses, CT and MRI studies, especially with contrast injection, have replaced metrizamide cisternography by enhancing the physician's ability to detect these tumors in their early stages. Recurrent masses are increasingly treated with small field radiation approaches (radiosurgery or gamma knife).

Hemangioblastoma DEFINITION The cerebellar hemangioblastoma is an uncommon tumor that may be solitary but is frequently multiple. When the tumors are multiple, they are considered part of von Hippel-Lindau disease. This autosomal dominant disorder, linked to chromosome 3, typically consists of retinal, cerebellar, and spinal hemangioblastomas and visceral lesions, usually renal and/or pancreatic tumors or cysts. Polycythemia may be present.

PATHOGENESIS AND PATHOLOGY Hemangioblastomas are well-circumscribed and often cystic. The tumor may consist solely of a small nodule attached to the wall of a large cyst. The lesion is usually highly vascular and may be mistaken for an arteriovenous malformation. The microscopic appearance is one of numerous capillary vessels separated by sheets of clear cells with an abundance of intracytoplasmic vacuoles. The tumors are probably derived from capillary endothelial cells.

CLINICAL MANIFESTATIONS Dizziness, ataxia of gait or of the limbs, and symptoms of raised intracranial pressure are characteristic features of the cerebellar hemangioblastoma. The tumors may bleed spontaneously, resulting in a paroxysmal onset of headache and neurologic deficit. The MRI may show vascular "flow voids" or ferritin suggesting old hemorrhage in the wall of a cyst.

TREATMENT Craniotomy with opening of the cerebellar cyst and excision of the mural tumor may be curative. Though the tumor is histologically benign, postoperative recurrences and the appearance of less operable spinal lesions worsen the prognosis. Patients with the von Hippel-Lindau syndrome should have periodic ophthalmologic evaluation for the appearance of retinal angiomas and general medical follow-up for early detection of renal tumors.

Ependymoma PATHOGENESIS AND PATHOLOGY These are glial tumors that occur chiefly in childhood and young adulthood, with a typical cranial location in the fourth ventricle. The tumor is composed of uniform ependymal cells surrounding a central lumen. Spinal ependymomas, which are more common, arise within the dura of the lumbar spine and represent more than half of spinal intramedullary gliomas. In this location, the prognosis is excellent. Supratentorial tumors are often more aggressive in rate of growth.

TREATMENT Resection and radiation to the tumor site results in 5-year survival in excess of 80 percent for spinal cord lesions and between 30 and 50 percent for posterior fossa tumors. The role of chemotherapy in the treatment of local recurrences and of seeding within the subarachnoid space is not established.

PRIMITIVE NEUROECTODERMAL TUMORS (PNET) Several histologic varieties of tumor arise from primitive neuroectodermal tumors (PNET) which contain dense aggregates of small cells with a capacity to differentiate into medulloblasts, astrocytes, oligodendrocytes, ependyma, ganglion cells, or skeletal muscle. Some tumors have several cell types, but all PNETs of the posterior fossa share a propensity for local invasion, subarachnoid dissemination, and extraneural metastases. The initial evaluation should include enhanced MRI scan of the brain and lumbosacral nerve roots as well as cytologic evaluation of CSF.

Medulloblastoma DEFINITION The *medulloblastoma* is the most common variety of PNET. It accounts for 25 percent of childhood brain tumors. However, one-fourth of medulloblastomas occur in patients over age 20.

PATHOGENESIS AND PATHOLOGY In children the tumor is usually located in the midline, in the inferior portion of the vermis of the cerebellum. In adults the cerebellar hemisphere is most often the site of occurrence. It is composed of small, densely staining cells which elicit a brisk glial response. Invasion of the meninges, ventricles, and subarachnoid space is common.

CLINICAL MANIFESTATIONS The common presentation is occipital headache, vomiting and truncal ataxia. Hydrocephalus is frequent. With enlargement of the tumor other signs of brainstem compression emerge. As spinal axis dissemination occurs in one-third of patients, initial evaluation should include CSF cytologic examination and either MRI of the cauda equina or myelography.

TREATMENT Resection of the tumor is usually attempted, followed by radiation in doses of 45 to 50 Gy (4500 to 5000 rad) to the posterior fossa, together with 40 Gy (4000 rad) to the whole brain and 35 to 40 Gy (3500 to 4000 rad) to the spinal cord. Chemotherapy prior to irradiation is under investigation for children and those whose tumors invade the ventricle or have disseminated. Drugs have been used with some success in recurrent tumors. Nitrosourea, procarbazine, and vincristine combined with prednisone and intrathecal methotrexate are advocated. Five-year survival is nearly 75 percent. The posterior fossa remains the major site for recurrence. A pessimistic outlook exists for children under 3 years, those with large tumors, and those with subarachnoid spread. Metastases to lung, liver, vertebrae, and pelvis are reported. Some medulloblastomas may take on features reminiscent of neuroblastoma.

Neuroblastoma DEFINITION The neuroblastoma, a relatively common adrenal tumor, can rarely occur as a primary CNS tumor. Eighty percent of cases present during the first decade of life.

CLINICAL MANIFESTATIONS The most important clue to the presence of neuroblastoma is opsoclonus (see Chap. 328), the presence of which confers a better prognosis.

PATHOGENESIS AND PATHOLOGY Microscopically, neuroblastoma resembles medulloblastoma because of its small dense cells. Variations in pathology occur. Some tumors show differentiation to ganglion cells but do not have a better prognosis. These tumors appear to form

a spectrum of tumors of embryonal origin, ranging from the aggressive, poorly differentiated PNETs to the very well differentiated and quite slow growing neurocytomas. The intraparenchymal tumors found in children resemble in clinical behavior the PNETs, with neuraxis spread and occasional extraneural metastases. CT reveals a hypodense mass with dense uniform enhancement after contrast administration as well as variable hemorrhage and calcification. These tumors may present as slowly growing intraventricular masses in adults and may grow to large size before discovery.

TREATMENT The rarity of these tumors has prevented any randomized therapeutic trials. Optimal treatment may consist of radical excision with postoperative radiation, though definitive evidence that radiation increases survival is lacking. Because of the frequency of local recurrence and CSF metastases, prophylactic spinal irradiation may be justified. A trial of chemotherapy, either pre- or postirradiation may be worthwhile, especially in younger patients with more aggressive-appearing tumors. Long-term follow-up is complete but appears to have a greater than 30 percent 5-year survival. The survival of adults with intraventricular tumors may be better than that of other primitive CNS tumors.

TUMORS OF THE SKULL BASE Tumors in this region produce characteristic clinical presentations that pose unique diagnostic difficulties even with advanced neuroradiologic procedures. Meningiomas, tumors of bone (including epidermoid and dermoid tumors and osteomas), chordomas, schwannomas (neurofibromas) of the cranial nerves, nasopharyngeal carcinoma, and metastases may all present with pain localized to the lower face, ear, or occiput and with involvement of one or more cranial nerves making exit from the skull. Metastases arise commonly from the lung, breast, nasopharynx, testicle, and prostate. Multiple myeloma and occasionally lymphoma may appear at this site. The mass may be palpable or may be visualized on enhanced CT scan, or MRI. These studies usually differentiate successfully other erosive processes of the skull base, including fibrous dysplasia, Paget's disease, xanthomatosis, and osteitis fibrosa cystica. Enlargement of specific cranial nerve foramens may be the first evidence of schwannomas or of *glomus* tumors of the chromaffin cells in the jugular bulb. These last tumors invade temporal and occipital bone and produce hearing abnormalities and lower cranial nerve deficits.

Chordomas arise from remnants of the notochord. Of these, 60 percent are localized in the clivus, 30 percent in the sacral region, and the remaining 10 percent along the extent of the spine and skull base. The chordoma is not easily distinguished in appearance from radiation-sensitive chondrosarcomas and chondroid chordoma. They are highly invasive, expanding along the skull base and causing serial cranial nerve compression, sometimes with invasion of the nasopharynx. Up to one-third may metastasize via the subarachnoid space. A cauda equina syndrome (see ''Spinal Tumors'') results from sacral tumors. Clivus tumors may be difficult to visualize adequately on CT scan but are clearly delineated by MRI. Complete removal is rarely feasible and postoperative radiation therapy is recommended. Radiation with cyclotron-derived protons is followed by 80 percent survival at 5 years and 63 percent at 10 years with minimal complications.

Metastases to the skull base are treated with radiation therapy. In the presence of characteristic patterns of pain and cranial nerve deficit, radiation may be considered to treat presumptive metastases in patients with known systemic malignancy even when radiographic examinations are inconclusive.

SPINAL TUMORS **Pathogenesis and pathology** Tumors of the spinal canal and of the cord are only one-quarter as common as are intracranial tumors. Spinal neoplasms arise from the same types of cells as their counterparts in the cerebrum. They are classified according to location as intramedullary (within the substance of the spinal cord), extramedullary (or intradural), and extradural. Some tumors, such as schwannomas, may be both extradural and intradural. The most frequent location for all types of spinal neoplasms is in the thoracic cord, presumably reflecting its greater total length. These tumors arise from cells of the spinal cord, nerve roots, meninges, vascular structures, or the vertebral column. Tumors of the spinal cord parenchyma are relatively infrequent compared to lesions arising outside the substance of the cord. In one large series, nerve sheath tumors (schwannomas) accounted for 29 percent of all spinal tumors, meningiomas for 25.5 percent, gliomas for 22 percent, and sarcomas for 12 percent. Metastatic lesions represent about 13 percent of all spinal tumors, but as with intracranial tumors, these figures reflect neurosurgical service statistics and metastases are likely to be underrepresented.

Clinical manifestations   Any lesion that narrows the spinal canal sufficiently to encroach on neural structures can give rise to neurologic symptoms. Dysfunction may arise from direct compression of the spinal cord and its nerve roots or from interference with blood supply. The rapid growth of metastatic lesions leads to motor and sensory symptoms over a period of days to weeks, whereas slowly growing astrocytomas and ependymomas produce symptoms over a period of months to years.

Extramedullary tumors (both intradural and epidural) cause symptoms by compressing the spinal cord or nerve roots. The initial symptoms are usually focal back pain and paresthesias followed by sensory loss below the level of the pain, weakness, and bladder and bowel dysfunction. Intramedullary lesions usually extend over several spinal cord segments, and their symptoms and signs are more varied than those of extramedullary tumors. A common pattern is dissociated sensory loss, with pain and temperature sensation impairment in the segments of tumor origin and with sparing of posterior column sensory function. Later, as the tumor grows peripherally, spinothalamic tracts may be involved. Since, in the thoracic and cervical regions, the sacral pain and temperature fibers lie superficial to those fibers representing more rostral regions, the sacral segments may be spared. Atrophy in the appropriate segments due to anterior horn cell involvement may combine with corticospinal tract signs.

These clinical presentations are not diagnostic of spinal cord neoplasm. Transverse myelitis from multiple sclerosis or other causes can lead to rapid onset of spinal cord dysfunction associated with pain, paresthesias, and weakness (see Chap. 381). A similar syndrome can occur as a paraneoplastic process, resulting from a necrotic myelopathy (see Chap. 328). Syringomyelia can produce a chronic syndrome indistinguishable from that produced by intramedullary neoplasms. Other diseases that can lead to a progressive spinal cord syndrome include combined system degeneration due to vitamin B_{12} deficiency, amyotrophic lateral sclerosis, cervical spondylosis, arachnoiditis, vascular anomalies, meningeal carcinomatosis, and spinal stenosis due to a combination of degenerative disk disease and hypertrophy of the ligamentum flavum (see Chap. 381).

Additional specific clinical syndromes occur in two other locations within the spinal canal. *Foramen magnum tumors* may extend into the cervical region or rostrally into the posterior fossa. A combination of signs and symptoms referrable to lower cranial nerves, sensory loss in the distribution of the second cervical segment, posterior headache, and asymmetric sensory and motor involvement of the limbs leads to the suspicion of such a tumor, most commonly a meningioma. *Tumors of the conus medullaris or cauda equina produce* pain in the back, rectum, and/or both legs and may mimic lumbosacral disk disease. With tumor growth, muscle atrophy in the legs associated with sphincter dysfunction and reflex changes usually point to the correct site of involvement.

Diagnosis of spinal cord tumors   MRI has replaced all other modalities in the evaluation of patients suspected to have cancer outside or within the dura of the spinal canal (Fig. 369-6 and 369-7) In most centers MRI can be performed as an emergency procedure. With or without gadolinium, these studies delineate the site, number, and extent of *extradural* deposits, while providing definitive information concerning the enlargement of neural foramens (which occurs with schwannomas), distortion of paraspinal tissues with masses that have grown into the spinal canal from extraneural sites (as with lymphomatous spread), and the intricate anatomy of the cervicomedul-

FIGURE 369-6   Sagittal T1-weighted MRI image of the conus medullaris (arrow) in a 26-year-old male with malignant primitive neuroectodermal tumor.

lary junction (as with meningioma or skull-base chordoma or nasopharyngeal metastases). MRI pictures have supplanted confusing arguments regarding ''complete'' or ''incomplete'' myelographic block. By identifying multiple extradural lesions needless surgery can be avoided and irradiation fields appropriately applied. Intradural, leptomeningeal metastases or tumors within the spinal cord or its roots are equally amenable to MRI visualization, especially when used following injection of gadolinium.

Myelography following the subarachnoid injection of nonionic contrast materials is often used to complement MRI studies or when MRI is unavailable. A small amount of contrast injected prior to CT

FIGURE 369-7   Sagittal MRI of the thoracic spinal cord in a patient with metastatic breast cancer reveals destruction of a vertebral body with epidural tumor mass compressing the spinal cord.

evaluation of the spine is used to elucidate the coexistence of extradural tumor *and* calcified disk fragment, compression fracture of the bony vertebrae, osteomyelitis, or defects from prior surgery or irradiation. Similarly these CT studies identify intradural processes including arachnoiditis, lipomatous masses, and syrinx for which MRI experience remains scanty.

Cerebrospinal fluid removed at the time of myelography should be analyzed for cell count, protein content, and cytology. A specimen stained with Wright's stain should be analyzed and cells examined further after cytocentrifugation. The cell count is usually normal in spinal tumors unless there is meningeal tumor, but protein content is increased in virtually all cases of high-grade spinal cord block. The CSF glucose is usually normal unless there is meningeal tumor invasion.

Treatment   Once the diagnosis of spinal cord tumor is established, rapid treatment is mandatory to maximize neurologic recovery. Extramedullary primary neoplasms are treated with microneurosurgery, and complete resection is usually possible. The most common intramedullary tumors, ependymomas and astrocytomas, usually can only be partially resected and are likely to recur. The role of radiation therapy for slowly growing tumors of this class is not well established; for high-grade astrocytomas a course of postoperative radiation is recommended. Glucocorticoids may improve function temporarily. There is no established role for chemotherapy of spinal neoplasms.

EPIDURAL CANCER: THE PATIENT WITH CANCER AND BACK PAIN   Spinal epidural cancer should be suspected in patients with back pain and known systemic malignancy even in the absence of neurologic signs. Progressive paraparesis with bladder dysfunction and development of a sensory deficit may be avoided by timely MRI imaging of the spine followed by surgical or radiation therapy. The MRI identification of tumor anterior to the spinal cord may pave the way for surgical anterior decompression (Fig. 369-7). High doses of glucocorticoids (up to 100 mg dexamethasone per day) are administered immediately and radiation therapy is usually recommended. The results of treatment in the large series of patients with epidural cancer reported by Gilbert has led to the conclusion that radiation therapy is as effective as surgery in the relief of symptoms. The clinical condition of the patient at the time of diagnosis is the most important factor in prognosis; only 3 percent of patients paraplegic at the time of treatment, regardless of type of therapy, regain ambulation. Reconsideration is being given to surgical decompression as a primary mode of treatment in patients with radioresistant malignancies such as melanoma and lung, prostatic, and colonic cancers and in the setting of paraparesis of recent onset.

REFERENCES

BLACK P McL: Brain tumors. N Engl J Med 324:1471, 1555, 1991

BULLARD DE et al: Oligodendroglioma. An analysis of the value of radiation therapy. Cancer 60:2179, 1987

BYRNE TN, WAXSMAN SG: *Spinal Cord Compression; Diagnosis and Principles of Management.* Philadelphia, FA Davis, 1990

CONSTINE LS et al: Hypothalamic pituitary dysfunction after radiation for brain tumors. N Engl J Med 328:87, 1993

CORBETT JJ et al: Visual loss in pseudotumor cerebri. Arch Neurol 39:461, 1982

GLANTZ MJ et al: Influence of the type of surgery on the histologic diagnosis in patients with anaplastic gliomas. Neurology 41:1741, 1991

GOWLAND P et al: Dynamic studies of gadolinium uptake in brain tumors using inversion-recovery echo-planar imaging. Magn Reson Med 26:241, 1992

GUTIN PH: Recurrent malignant gliomas: Survival following interstitial brachytherapy with high activity iodine 125 sources. J Neurosurg 67:864, 1987

HELWEG-LARSEN S: Recovery of gait following radiation therapy in paralyzed patients with metastatic epidural spinal cord compression. Neurology 40:1234, 1990

HOCHBERG FH et al: The therapy of primary brain lymphoma. J Neuro-Oncol 10:191, 1991

HOCHBERG FJ, MILLER DC: Primary central nervous system lymphoma. J Neurosurg 68:835, 1988

HUGHES EN et al: Medulloblastoma at the Joint Center for Radiation Therapy between 1968 and 1984. The influence of radiation dose on the patterns of failure and survival. Cancer 61:1992, 1988

JANUS TJ et al: Use of [F-18] fluorodeoxyglucose positron emission tomography in patients with primary malignant brain tumors. Ann Neurol 33:540, 1993

JENNINGS MT et al: Intracranial germ cell tumors: Natural history and pathogenesis. J Neurosurg 63:155, 1985

KORNBLITH PL, WALKER M: Chemotherapy for malignant gliomas. J Neurosurg 68:1, 1988

LEVINE AJ, SCHMIDEK HH (eds): *Molecular Genetics of Nervous System Tumors.* New York, Wiley-Liss, 1993

MAHALEY MS: Neuro-oncology index and review—adult primary brain tumors. J Neuro-Oncol 11:85, 1991

PATCHELL R: A randomized trial of surgery in the treatment of single metastases to the brain. N Engl J Med 322:494, 1990

SIDRANSKY D et al: Clonal expansion of P53 mutant cells associated with brain tumor progression. Nature 355:846, 1992

SMOKER WR et al: The role of MR imaging in evaluating metastatic spinal disease. Am J Radiol 149:1241, 1987

WASSERSTROM WR: Diagnosis and treatment of leptomeningeal metastases from solid tumors. Cancer 49:759, 1982

YOUNG DP: Neurology complications of chemotherapy, in *Neurological Complications of Therapy,* A Silverstein (ed). Mount Kisco, NY, Futura Publishing, 1982, p 57

370   ALZHEIMER'S DISEASE AND OTHER DEMENTIAS

M. FLINT BEAL / EDWARD P. RICHARDSON, JR. / JOSEPH B. MARTIN

In classifying diseases of the nervous system, it is customary to designate a group of them as *degenerative*, indicating that they are characterized by gradually evolving, relentlessly progressive neuronal death occurring for reasons that are still largely unknown. The identification of these diseases depends on exclusion of such possible causative factors as infections, metabolic derangements, and intoxications. A considerable proportion of the disorders classed as degenerative are genetic, with either dominant or recessive inheritance. Others, however, occur only sporadically—as isolated instances in a given family.

Classification of the degenerative diseases cannot be based on any exact knowledge of cause or pathogenesis; their subdivision into individual syndromes rests on descriptive criteria based largely on neuropathologic and clinical aspects. This group of diseases presents as several distinct clinical syndromes, the recognition of which can assist the clinician in arriving at a diagnosis.

GENERAL CONSIDERATIONS   The degenerative disorders usually begin insidiously and run a gradually progressive course over many years. Their course is generally more protracted than that of the hereditary metabolic diseases of the nervous system (see Chap. 377). The earliest changes may be so subtle that it often is impossible to assign any precise time of onset. At times the history suggests an abrupt onset of disability—particularly when an injury or some other event in the patient's life has occurred to which illness might conceivably be related. By careful questioning, it is frequently evident that the patient or family has suddenly become aware of a condition that had, in fact, already been present but had passed unnoticed.

The family history is of great importance, and denial of familial occurrence cannot always be taken at face value. Some patients or their relatives are hesitant to disclose that a neurologic disease afflicts the family. In other cases, the extent of the disease affecting other family members may be so slight as to go unnoticed by the family—as may occur, for instance, in the group of the hereditary ataxias. Moreover, small sibships in a family may prevent well-established hereditary diseases from being recognized. Familial occurrence, of course, does not always mean that a disease is hereditary; it may indicate instead that there has been a common exposure to an infective or toxic agent.

Many of the degenerative nervous system diseases progress uninfluenced by therapeutic measures. Caring for such patients is often an anguishing experience for all concerned. In others, such as persons with Parkinson's disease, symptoms can often be alleviated by wise and skillful management. The physician's caring attention may be of great help even when curative measures cannot be offered.

The symptoms and signs of this group of diseases tend to have a bilaterally symmetric distribution. This aspect alone may help to distinguish the disorder from other varieties of neurologic disease. In some patients, in the early stages, one side of the body or one limb may become involved in the presence of normal findings elsewhere. Eventually, despite the asymmetric beginning, the inherently bilateral nature of the process generally asserts itself.

A striking characteristic of the degenerative disorders is that particular anatomic or physiologic systems of neurons may be selectively affected, leaving others entirely intact. This is exemplified in amyotrophic lateral sclerosis, in which the disease process is limited to cerebral and spinal motor neurons, and in some forms of progressive ataxia, in which only the Purkinje cells of the cerebellum are affected. In Friedreich's ataxia and some other syndromes, the disease process affects multiple neuronal systems.

In this respect, certain degenerative neuronal diseases resemble others of known cause, particularly intoxications, where similarly circumscribed effects occur. Diphtheria toxin, for example, produces selective breakdown of peripheral nerve myelin, triorthocresyl phosphate affects the corticospinal tracts in the spinal cord together with the peripheral nerves, and the neurotoxin 1-methyl-4-phenyl-1,2,3,6-tetrahydropyridine (MPTP) brings about death of dopamine-containing neurons in the substantia nigra. Selective involvement of particular neuronal systems is not, however, characteristic of all the degenerative diseases; some are characterized by pathologic changes that are diffuse and unselective.

Typically, the pathologic process in the nervous system is one of slow involution of nerve cell bodies or their axonal extensions, unaccompanied by any intense tissue reaction or cellular response, although the loss of neurons and fibers is often accompanied by hyperplasia of fibrillary astrocytes (gliosis). The cerebrospinal fluid (CSF) shows little, if any, change—at most a slight elevation of protein, without abnormalities in specific proteins, cell count, or other constituents. Moreover, since these diseases invariably result in tissue loss, rather than in new tissue formation, radiologic visualization of the brain, the ventricular system, or subarachnoid space shows either no change or an enlargement of the CSF compartments. These negative laboratory findings thus help to distinguish the degenerative disorders from the other large classes of progressive diseases of the nervous system—tumors and infections.

CLASSIFICATION   Since etiologic classification is impossible, subdivision of the degenerative diseases into individual syndromes rests on descriptive criteria based largely on their clinical aspects and pathologic anatomy. Many of these syndromes are named after distinguished neurologists and neuropathologists. A useful classification is outlined in Table 370-1.

SYNDROMES IN WHICH PROGRESSIVE DEMENTIA PREDOMINATES

In the disease entities that follow, the clinical picture is dominated by gradual loss of intellectual capacities, i.e., by dementia. Other neurologic abnormalities, except in the terminal stages, are absent or relatively insignificant. (For further discussion of dementia, including its clinical evaluation, Chaps. 25 and 27 should be consulted.)

ALZHEIMER'S DISEASE   Alzheimer's disease is perhaps the most important of all the degenerative diseases because of its frequent occurrence and devastating nature. It is the most common cause of dementia in the elderly, with all that this implies in the way of distress for patients and families and economic loss in the form of the costs entailed in the long-term care of patients totally disabled by the disease. Historically, the term *Alzheimer's disease* was applied to progressive dementia coming on in late middle life but preceding the senile period, following the original description by Alois Alzheimer in 1907, in which the illness of a woman dying at the age of 55 was depicted clinically and pathologically. It became usual to classify cases of this kind under the heading of *presenile dementia*. Meanwhile, it became increasingly apparent that very old people dying with progressive mental deterioration, generally referred to as *senile dementia*, showed cerebral lesions that were identical to those found in cases of presenile dementia. Such cases are now designated as *senile dementia of the Alzheimer type*. Current evidence indicates that the disease process is the same, regardless of the age of onset. At the same time, Alzheimer's disease is clearly age-related. It is extremely uncommon in young people and rare in middle age; as age advances, however, it is increasingly frequent, such that its prevalence in persons over 85 years old is estimated to be as high as 47 percent. Advancing age is unmistakably a predisposing factor, but it is incorrect to consider Alzheimer's disease as the inevitable accompaniment of aging. Many elderly people remain mentally unimpaired into the ninth and tenth decades. Genetic predisposition to Alzheimer's disease emerges as a clear-cut pattern in some families; however, these cases comprise less than 20 percent of all cases. There are well-documented familial cases, some following an autosomal dominant pattern of inheritance with linkage to either chromosome 21 or 19. An exception to the statement that Alzheimer's disease is rare in young people occurs in the instance of Down's syndrome (trisomy 21), which leads to the development of the characteristic lesions of Alzheimer's disease in the majority of the patients after 40 years of age.

Pathology   The outstanding pathologic feature is death and disappearance of nerve cells in the cerebral cortex. This leads

---

TABLE 370-1   Clinical classification of the degenerative diseases of the nervous system

Progressive dementia in the absence of other prominent neurologic signs
  A Alzheimer's disease
  B Senile dementia of the Alzheimer type
  C Pick's disease (lobar atrophy)
Syndromes combining progressive dementia with other prominent neurologic abnormalities
  A Mainly in adults
    1 Huntington's disease
    2 Multiple system atrophy combining dementia with ataxia and/or manifestations of Parkinson's disease
    3 Progressive supranuclear palsy (Steele-Richardson-Olszewski)
    4 Diffuse Lewy body disease
    5 Corticodentatonigral degeneration
  B Mainly in children or young adults
    1 Hallervorden-Spatz disease
    2 Progressive familial myoclonic epilepsy
Syndromes of gradually developing abnormalities of posture and movement (see Chap. 371)
  A Paralysis agitans (Parkinson's disease)
  B Striatonigral degeneration
  C Progressive supranuclear palsy (see *II, A, 3* above)
  D Torsion dystonia (torsion spasm; dystonia musculorum deformans)
  E Spasmodic torticollis and other restricted dyskinesias
  F Familial tremor
  G Gilles de la Tourette syndrome
Syndromes of progressive ataxia (see Chap. 372)
  A Cerebellar degenerations
    1 Cerebellar cortical degeneration
    2 Olivopontocerebellar atrophy (OPCA)
  B Spinocerebellar degenerations (Friedreich's ataxia and related disorders)
Central autonomic nervous system failure (Shy-Drager syndrome) (see Chap. 379)
Syndromes of muscular weakness and wasting without sensory changes (motor neuron disease) (see Chap. 372)
  A Amyotrophic lateral sclerosis
  B Spinal muscular atrophy
    1 Infantile spinal muscular atrophy (Werdnig-Hoffmann)
    2 Juvenile spinal muscular atrophy (Wohlfart-Kugelberg-Welander)
    3 Other forms of familial spinal muscular atrophy
  C Primary lateral sclerosis
  D Hereditary spastic paraplegia
Syndromes combining muscular weakness and wasting with sensory changes (progressive neural muscular atrophy; chronic familial polyneuropathies) (see Chap. 383)
  A Peroneal muscular atrophy (Charcot-Marie-Tooth)
  B Hypertrophic interstitial polyneuropathy (Dejerine-Sottas)
  C Miscellaneous forms of chronic progressive neuropathy
Syndromes of progressive visual loss
  A Pigmentary degeneration of the retina (retinitis pigmentosa)
  B Hereditary optic atrophy (Leber's disease)

ultimately to extensive convolutional atrophy, especially in the frontal, parietal, and medial temporal regions. There is a corresponding enlargement of the ventricular system, but this is usually not extreme.

Two kinds of microscopic lesions are distinctive for the disease. The first, originally described by Alzheimer, consists of intraneuronal accumulations of filamentous material in the form of loops, coils, or tangled masses—referred to as *Alzheimer neurofibrillary tangles*. The neuropathologic evidence strongly suggests that these fibrillar masses are of major importance in bringing about the death of neurons. Neurofibrillary tangles and loss of synapses are the neuropathologic features most closely linked to dementia. Electron microscopy reveals accumulations of paired helical filaments that differ from normal neurofilaments and microtubules. Recent studies have shown that a major component is an abnormally phosphorylated form of the microtubule protein tau. Alzheimer neurofibrillary tangles also contain ubiquitin, a protein that marks cells for proteolysis.

Neurofibrillary tangles tend to be most abundant, together with the most extreme degrees of neuronal loss, in the hippocampus and adjacent parts of the temporal lobe—structures that have been found to be of greatest importance in memory function.

The other histopathologic change that characterizes Alzheimer's disease is the presence of intracortical clusters of thickened neuronal processes, both axons and dendrites (collectively referred to as *neurites*), generally in the form of an irregular ring surrounding a spherical deposit of amyloid fibrils. These lesions, which had been recognized before Alzheimer's description of the neurofibrillary change, were termed *senile plaques*. Recent elucidation of their structure has led to their current designation as *neuritic plaques*. They have been shown to contain paired helical filaments identical to those found in the perinuclear cytoplasm of the diseased neurons. One form of plaque, the *diffuse plaque*, consists of amorphous amyloid without neurites.

In many, but not all, cases, identical amyloid deposits may be found in the walls of small meningeal and intracortical arteries, and the question has arisen as to whether this cerebrovascular amyloidosis (often called *cerebral amyloid angiopathy* or *congophilic angiopathy* because of the characteristic staining of amyloid with the dye Congo red) has a close relationship, perhaps even causative, to plaque amyloidosis. Antibodies against the cerebrovascular amyloid cross-react with the amyloid in neuritic plaques. It is as yet unclear where the amyloid in plaques originates—whether from neurons or blood vessels; most investigators favor the former. The amyloid in the blood vessels in Alzheimer's disease, as well as that in the core of neuritic plaques, has been isolated and sequenced. It consists of a 42 to 43 amino acid peptide. Some recent evidence suggests that it may exert neurotoxic effects. The amyloid peptide (β- or A_4-peptide) gene is on chromosome 21, on which the familial Alzheimer's disease gene also has been localized in some families. A recent advance has been the finding that in a handful of families with familial Alzheimer's disease there are point mutations in the amyloid precursor protein. This observation suggests that Alzheimer's disease can be linked to a primary defect in amyloid production or processing, but most cases of familial and sporadic Alzheimer's disease do not have a clear cause (see Chap. 364).

Biochemical studies show that choline acetyltransferase, the key enzyme required for the synthesis of acetylcholine, is decreased in the cerebral cortex in Alzheimer's disease. The major source of neocortical cholinergic innervation is a group of neurons situated in the basal part of the forebrain just beneath the corpus striatum—the nucleus basalis of Meynert. Careful neuropathologic investigations have shown that in Alzheimer's disease this nucleus is a site of major neuronal loss and of frequent Alzheimer neurofibrillary tangles. These studies suggest that impairment of cholinergic transmission may play a part in the clinical expression of the disease. However, attempted therapy with cholinomimetic agents has been largely unsuccessful. Less consistent reductions in cortical norepinephrine and serotonin appear to be caused by neuronal loss in the locus coeruleus and raphé nucleus, respectively. Loss of peptidergic neurons in the cerebral cortex is associated with reduced cortical concentrations of somatostatin and corticotropin releasing factor.

It is anticipated that investigations of the biochemistry of the cerebral lesions in Alzheimer's disease will lead ultimately to an understanding of their pathogenesis. The remarkable discovery that one form of progressive dementia, Creutzfeldt-Jakob disease, is the result of infection with a transmissible virus-like agent has led to the question as to whether Alzheimer's disease and other neuronal degenerations might be due to a similar form of infectious agent (see Chap. 375). All attempts to transmit Alzheimer's disease have failed, however, so that currently an infective basis is thought unlikely.

Clinical manifestations The onset is insidious and subtle, with changes most noticeable first in memory for recent happenings and in other aspects of mental activity. Psychiatric disturbances such as depression, anxiety, or odd, unpredictable quirks of behavior, delusions, and hallucinations may be salient features in the early stages. Progression is usually slow and gradual, and unless other medical conditions supervene, it may smolder on for 10 or more years.

In the milder cases, including those of the senile period, the noteworthy features are those of simple dementia, as described in Chap. 25. More unusual disorders of thought and intellect, including aphasia, apraxic disturbances, and abnormalities of space perception, may be seen, especially in the presenile group. Exceptionally, and only in the advanced stages of the disease, extrapyramidal signs appear; the patient walks in a shuffling manner with short steps, and there is a generalized stiffness of the musculature with slowness and awkwardness of all movements. In some patients, sudden jerklike contractions of various muscles (myoclonus) may occur in the presence of otherwise typical Alzheimer's disease, but this is unusual and should immediately raise the suspicion of Creutzfeldt-Jakob disease (Chap. 375). Terminally, the patient may become nearly decorticate, losing all ability to perceive, think, speak, or move.

Laboratory investigations, including blood and CSF determinations, do not yield any conclusive or pertinent data. There is a diffuse slowing in the electroencephalogram in the more advanced stages of the disease. Enlargement of the ventricular system and subarachnoid space resulting from brain atrophy can be demonstrated by computed tomography (CT) and by magnetic resonance imaging (MRI). These imaging procedures, however, are not decisive for making the diagnosis, especially in the earlier stages, because the degree of cerebral atrophy demonstrated may be no more than that seen in patients of a similar age group who are functioning normally. Recent studies with positron-emission tomography have shown decreased glucose metabolism in the temporal and parietal lobes. During the course of the illness, occasional convulsive seizures may occur, but they are relatively rare and should raise suspicion of other diseases. Terminally, the patient dies from intercurrent disease, in a state of total helplessness. Institutional care is usually necessary long before the end.

Differential diagnosis The physician should recognize that treatable conditions may at first appear to be dementia of the Alzheimer type. Space-occupying lesions, such as chronic subdural hematoma or slowly growing frontal neoplasms (meningioma or glioma), should be excluded. CT and MRI usually demonstrate mass lesions of these kinds, as well as an unsuspected hydrocephalus, which, when treated by a shunt procedure for ventricular decompression, may lead to dramatic improvement in the patient's state. Other treatable conditions producing a dementia-like state include metabolic derangements (liver disease), vitamin B_{12} deficiency, and hypothyroidism. Elderly people may be unusually susceptible to the sedative effects of medications, so chronic drug intoxication may need to be considered. Cerebrovascular disease is not ordinarily a cause of uncomplicated dementia, but finding multiple small infarcts by CT or MRI raises the possibility of multi-infarct dementia. Depression can mimic dementia, particularly in the elderly, in whom it may be all too easy to attribute deficits in thinking, motivation, and memory to cerebral disease (see Chap. 25). Depression may show a most gratifying response to appropriate treatment (see Chap. 389).

The evidence that cholinergic innervation may be impaired in Alzheimer's disease has led to attempts to correct the deficiency pharmacologically. The most recent of these is the acetylcholinesterase inhibitor tetrahydroaminoacridine, which produces limited improvement in some mental status tests but which is compromised by liver toxicity.

Practical measures that may help in the management of cases of Alzheimer's disease are suggested in Chap. 25.

PICK'S DISEASE (LOBAR ATROPHY) This remarkable form of cerebral disease, characterized by circumscribed cerebral atrophy (lobar sclerosis), enters in the differential diagnosis of dementia in the presenile period. It is, however, an extremely rare condition as compared with diffuse cerebral atrophy of the Alzheimer type. Hereditary transmission (as a dominant trait) is frequent in Pick's disease, and women are more frequently affected than men. The age distribution is similar in both these varieties of progressive dementia.

Pathology So striking are the gross pathologic changes in the brain that in typical cases the diagnosis can be made at a glance. Severe atrophy of the anterior portions of the frontal and temporal lobes occurs, and there is a curiously sharp line of demarcation between the atrophied portions and the remainder of the brain, which appears normal or nearly so. In some cases, the frontal atrophy is more prominent; in others, the temporal lobes are more severely involved; in general, both regions are affected. Rarely, the disorder has a predominantly unilateral localization—as in cases described originally by Pick. Atrophic changes also occur in subcortical structures, i.e., the caudate nucleus, putamen, thalamus, and substantia nigra, and in the descending frontopontine fiber system. There are striking changes in nerve cells in the affected regions in most cases. These consist of fibrillary deposits within the cytoplasm—masses of straight fibrils, differing from the paired helical filaments of Alzheimer's disease. In some neurons, densely packed spherical aggregates (Pick bodies) can be seen with silver-impregnation methods. In other affected neurons, the fibrils are more widely dispersed, and the neuronal cytoplasm takes on a rounded, distended appearance, forming "ballooned" cells. Recent evidence suggests that despite the morphologic differences, these neuronal changes are biochemically related to those in Alzheimer's disease, as indicated by common antigenic properties. In rare instances of Alzheimer's disease, disproportionate atrophy of the frontal and temporal lobes may suggest Pick's disease, but in such cases the distinguishing feature is the presence of the characteristic plaques and neurofibrillary tangles, which are not found in Pick's disease.

Clinical manifestations If Pick's disease has any distinctive clinical features, they consist of unusually severe signs of frontal lobe or temporal lobe dysfunction (see Chap. 27). Typical early manifestations are a general impoverishment of mental function, changes in behavior patterns, and a striking lack of insight. Some patients have an early impairment of language with difficulty naming objects or people. The later phases of the disease are characterized by loss of retentive memory (with temporal lobe involvement), loss of all language functions, and, when the frontal lobes are mainly affected, prominent grasp and sucking reflexes. In CT and MRI scans the shrinkage of the cortex and the low density of the white matter in the affected lobes may be diagnostic. Progression, as in Alzheimer's disease, is slow and relentless, the average duration being about 7 years. In the late stages, rigidity, dystonic postures, and perhaps tremor may be prominent features; these can be ascribed to extension of the disease process into the basal ganglia.

Differential diagnosis The considerations already noted with regard to Alzheimer's disease apply to Pick's disease as well.

SYNDROMES COMBINING DEMENTIA WITH OTHER NEUROLOGIC SIGNS

HUNTINGTON'S DISEASE This disorder, characterized by a combination of choreoathetotic movements and progressive dementia usually beginning in midadult life, is transmitted as an autosomal dominant disease. The determining gene is located on the terminal segment of the short arm of chromosome 4. The classic description is that of George Huntington, who, together with his father and grandfather, all physicians, made clinical observations on familial cases living near their home on Long Island, New York. Huntington, writing in 1872, entitled his paper "On Chorea"; subsequently, the disorder described by him came to be known as *Huntington's chorea*. The more general term used in this chapter—Huntington's disease—is preferable, since the disease state comprises more than abnormal movements, and the motor abnormalities often are more complex than would be implied by the unqualified term *chorea*.

Because of its distressing and incapacitating nature and its implications for members of any family in which it appears (50 percent risk in each child of an affected parent), the disease has attracted attention in recent years and has been found to be considerably more frequent and widely distributed than once was thought. It is estimated that there are approximately 25,000 cases in the United States alone. In virtually all cases that come to the notice of a physician, there is a family history of the disease, although occasionally patients present with typical symptoms and no documentable family history; no proven case of a new mutation has occurred. Some of these cases are classified as senile chorea, where family members have died of other causes before the disease became manifest. Genetic testing of at-risk patients with a known family history is now available in many clinical settings.

Pathology Distinctive for Huntington's disease is atrophy of the caudate nucleus and, to a lesser extent, other structures of the basal ganglia (putamen and globus pallidus), out of proportion to any other changes in the brain. The degree of atrophy is directly related to the severity and duration of the disease. In the late stages, the caudate nucleus, which normally forms a convexly rounded eminence in the lateral wall of the lateral ventricle, takes on instead a flattened or concave appearance. As the result of the tissue loss, the ventricular system becomes correspondingly widened, especially the frontal horns. Along with these changes in the basal ganglia, there characteristically is diffuse gyral atrophy, most severe over the convex aspect of the brain.

The atrophy of the caudate nucleus and putamen is seen microscopically to be due to extensive loss of neurons, which stands out in contrast to the intactness of adjacent structures such as the nucleus accumbens septi, the nucleus basalis of Meynert (so strikingly involved in Alzheimer's disease), and the thalamus. Recent studies also show loss of neurons in the cerebral cortex.

There are no morphologically distinctive or characteristic cytopathologic alterations in the neurons in Huntington's disease such as occur in Alzheimer's and some other diseases. Neurochemical studies have shown a striking decrease of γ-aminobutyric acid (GABA) and of its synthesizing enzyme, glutamic acid decarboxylase, in the caudate nucleus, putamen, globus pallidus, and pars reticulata of the substantia nigra, as well as some decrease in choline acetyltransferase in the caudate nucleus. The loss of GABA can be attributed to depletion of the abundant medium-sized *spiny* neurons within the striatum. Spiny neurons are characterized in Golgi studies by a large number of dendritic spines and have been shown to constitute the projection neurons of the striatum. They provide efferents to both the globus pallidus and substantia nigra. In contrast, *aspiny* neurons, with few dendritic spines, are striatal interneurons with locally arborizing axons. In addition to GABA, other neurotransmitters contained within striatal spiny neurons, including substance P, enkephalins, and dynorphin, are similarly depleted in the striatum and its sites of projection.

Recent observations indicate that the peptide neurotransmitters somatostatin and neuropeptide y are relatively increased in the caudate nucleus and putamen in Huntington's disease, and cells identifiable as somatostatin–neuropeptide y neurons (*aspiny* neurons) are selectively preserved—in striking contrast to the loss of other neurons in the same regions. The large aspiny neurons containing acetylcholine are also preserved. The pathophysiologic meaning of this sparing is not clear as yet; its occurrence emphasizes the fact that in Huntington's disease, as in other neuronal system degenerations, selective vulnerability of neurons occurs in a particular region with preservation of others. The pattern of resistance of certain neuronal groups has provided clues to a possible underlying pathogenesis of the disease. The susceptible spiny neurons have dense glutamate inputs from the cerebral cortex. The pattern of cell death can be reproduced experimentally by glutamate receptor agonists that act on the *N*-methyl-D-aspartate subclass of glutamate receptors (see Chap. 364). Recent work shows that the spared aspiny neurons produce nitric oxide, a new neurotransmitter candidate (see Chap. 364). These observations have led to the hypothesis that striatal neurons die as a result of glutamate-induced neurotoxicity.

Clinical aspects The disorder has a prevalence in Europe and North America of 7 to 10 per 100,000 population. The movement disorder generally makes its appearance in early to middle adult years (average age of onset about 35 to 40 years). It is characteristic of the disease that younger patients, with onset of symptoms in the age group of 15 to 40 years, suffer a more severe form of the disorder than older patients, with onset in the 50s and 60s, and the neuropathologic changes in the brain are correspondingly more extensive and severe in the younger as compared with the older patients. Huntington's disease is occasionally manifest in childhood (even before the age of 4); in such cases, transmission usually occurs through the father. Such cases are rare and tend to be characterized more by rigidity than by chorea and by other atypical features such as convulsive seizures and cerebellar ataxia (Westphal variant).

The involuntary movements (bizarre grimacing, respiratory irregularity, faulty articulation of speech, and irregular, arrhythmic, unpatterned movements of the limbs, imparting to the gait a peculiar dancing quality) tend to be less quick and more athetoid than in Sydenham's chorea (see Chap. 21). Some reported cases that on genealogic and pathologic grounds must be classified with Huntington's chorea have shown progressive rigidity rather than choreiform movements, even in the adult. As a general rule, dementia runs parallel with the motor disorder. Occasionally it may appear before or after chorea; very rarely it may be slight or lacking altogether. Neuropsychiatric manifestations of depression, erratic behavior, and emotional outbursts often seriously handicap the patient before dementia or the movement disorder is severe. The advance of the disease is slow, with death occurring, on average, 15 to 20 years after onset of symptoms. Increasing disability from involuntary movements and mental changes result in death from intercurrent infection or, not rarely, suicide.

Differential diagnosis There is no difficulty in the recognition of typical cases. Midlife onset of chorea in a patient with a positive family history together with the slowly progressive course and prominent dementia make the diagnosis straightforward. In patients with a negative family history, the diagnosis is more difficult. Genetic testing is of no benefit in isolated cases because it remains dependent on linkage analysis in affected families. Lack of association with rheumatic fever helps to exclude Sydenham's chorea. Patients with Parkinson's disease, when overdosed with levodopa, may develop a widespread chorea or choreoathetosis, and this, combined with the early dementia that occurs in some patients, can reproduce the picture of Huntington's disease. Phenothiazine drugs may induce generalized chorea, unassociated with dementia, and the movement disorder may persist for months or years after the medication is discontinued (tardive dyskinesia). Typically, tardive dyskinesia spares the forehead and does not impair gait, in contrast to the findings in Huntington's disease. Finally, there is a form of self-limited chorea, which, like other localized dyskinesias, may appear in older persons without identifiable cause. Hepatolenticular degeneration (Wilson's disease) and nonfamilial forms of hepatocerebral degeneration may display clinical abnormalities resembling those of Huntington's disease, but the specific changes characteristic of these disorders, including liver disease, corneal Kayser-Fleischer rings (in Wilson's disease), and the

typical biochemical abnormalities, are absent in Huntington's disease (see Chap. 348). Choreoathetosis appearing during the second postnatal year and lasting throughout life is due to hypoxic birth injury or kernicterus. Sporadic cases of choreiform movements beginning in middle or late life may present a difficult problem in exact diagnosis. The occasional cases of violent choreiform movements produced by vascular lesions, classically in the subthalamic region, are characterized by sudden onset, unilateral distribution (hemiballismus), and a tendency to improve after a period of initial severity. A few cases of acute choreoathetosis have accompanied hyperthyroidism. Virus encephalitis may occasionally be associated with choreiform movements; acute development, fever, and pleocytosis in the CSF help in recognition of such cases. Hereditary acanthocytosis is a rare condition which can mimic Huntington's disease.

Treatment No form of treatment has as yet been devised that halts the relentless progression of this disease, and therapeutic attempts to alleviate the abnormal movements have generally been unsatisfactory. Dopamine receptor antagonists (butyrophenones or phenothiazines) may partially ameliorate the chorea, but the side effects characteristic of this class of drugs limit their use. The depression, which is so common in many patients, usually responds to tricyclic antidepressants. The application of molecular genetic probes for presymptomatic and prenatal testing is available in several centers. However, until the gene itself is discovered, testing can only be performed in families by linkage analysis (see Chaps. 61 and 364).

MULTIPLE-SYSTEM ATROPHY General experience has indicated that cases of multiple affection of neuronal systems may occur in which progressive dementia is combined with varying degrees of ataxia, dysarthria, parkinsonian dyskinesia, and autonomic dysfunction depending on the pattern of anatomic distribution of the pathologic changes (see Chap. 379). For cases of this kind, the general term *multiple-system atrophy* or *degeneration* has been applied. In some, loss of neurons in the cerebellar cortex and in the pontine nuclei and inferior olivary nuclei results in the predominating picture of *olivopontocerebellar degeneration*, to be discussed as one of the syndromes of progressive ataxia. These changes may be combined with similar neuronal loss in the substantia nigra (and in the striatum in striatonigral degeneration), resulting in parkinsonian features (discussed under "Parkinson's Disease"). Cases with loss of neurons in the intermediolateral columns are termed *Shy-Drager syndrome* (see Chap. 379). Pathologically, the disease process is characterized by death and disappearance of the affected cells and an accompanying reactive gliosis, without intracellular inclusions or other distinctive features. The cerebral cortex generally shows little discernible change, so it may be difficult to ascribe a definite pathoanatomic basis for the dementia, which, for this reason, is sometimes designated as *subcortical*. Typically, multiple-system atrophy is a disorder of late adult life, occurring sporadically in some instances and genetically transmitted in others. Further details of individual syndromes are given in later sections.

PROGRESSIVE SUPRANUCLEAR PALSY (STEELE-RICHARDSON-OLSZEWSKI SYNDROME) This disorder is discussed in Chap. 371 among the syndromes characterized by gradually developing abnormalities of posture and movement. It is mentioned here because progressive dementia may accompany the other neurologic abnormalities, although it appears late in the course and generally is not severe.

DIFFUSE LEWY BODY DISEASE Diffuse lewy body disease is a rare illness that presents with progressive dementia or psychosis. Confusional episodes with pronounced impairment of attention occur early. Agitation, hallucinations, and delusions may be prominent features. Parkinsonian signs, which may be absent or mild at the onset, eventually become common, and rigidity is usually severe. Tremor is often absent. Other features include involuntary movements, myoclonus, quadriparesis in flexion, orthostatic hypotension, and dysphagia in some cases. Lewy bodies are found profusely in the brainstem, basal forebrain, hypothalamic nuclei, and neocortex. The course of the illness is relentlessly progressive over several years.

CORTICODENTATONIGRAL DEGENERATION Corticodentato-nigral degeneration with neuronal achromasia is a rare illness which also has been termed *cortical-basal ganglionic degeneration*. Watts and colleagues have studied seven cases. The illness begins between the ages of 55 and 75, and the initial symptoms are loss of dexterity in one limb (usually an arm) combined with rigidity and often a tremor in the limb. The illness then progresses steadily over several months to involve the other limbs, with rigidity, postural imbalance, and masked facies. Dyspraxia is a prominent clinical feature, but dementia is usually mild or absent until late in the clinical course. The findings at autopsy are severe neuronal loss and gliosis in the cerebral cortex, which is greatest in the perirolandic regions, and mild neuronal loss and gliosis in the substantia nigra. In cortical areas, many of the pyramidal neurons are swollen with indistinct nuclei and poorly stained pale cytoplasm ("achromasia").

HALLERVORDEN-SPATZ DISEASE This unusual disorder, often affecting several siblings in a family in a manner suggesting an autosomal recessive trait, is associated with a rather variable clinical picture in which abnormalities of posture and muscle tone, involuntary movements, and progressive dementia predominate. Pathologically, there are characteristic abnormalities in the basal ganglia, suggesting a localized disorder of metabolism. The features of the condition were classically described in an affected family by Hallervorden and Spatz (1922).

Pathology Distinctive for this condition is the accumulation of large amounts of pigmented material in the globus pallidus and pars reticulata of the substantia nigra, resulting in grossly visible brownish discoloration of these regions. Microscopically, there are irregular pigmented, ferruginous concretions and granules of varying brownish or greenish hues depending on the stains used. Although much of this pigment contains iron, serum iron and ferritin are normal, and there is no systemic disorder of iron metabolism. There also is loss of nerve cells. Another feature of the disease is the presence of focal swelling of axons, most probably in their terminal portions; this is especially pronounced in the regions affected by the pigmentary disorder but typically can be found at all levels of the central nervous system, including the cerebral cortex. This neuroaxonal change may link the disease with childhood neuroaxonal dystrophy.

Clinical aspects The disorder typically makes its appearance in childhood or adolescence, with abnormalities in muscle tone and movements, such as rigidity and choreoathetosis. Abnormal postures of the trunk characteristic of torsion spasm (dystonia) may be seen, or the clinical picture may be reminiscent of parkinsonism. Cerebellar ataxia is also present in some instances. Speech becomes indistinct, and there is progressive intellectual impairment. Eventually, the involuntary movements give way to increasing generalized rigidity, and death comes as a rule about 10 years after onset. A few cases of late onset have shown a parkinsonian syndrome.

Differential diagnosis No feature of the clinical picture serves to distinguish this particular disorder from other conditions showing dementia with extrapyramidal motor abnormalities. Wilson's disease must be excluded by appropriate laboratory tests. The clearly progressive course sets this condition apart from clinically similar abnormalities resulting from accidents or illnesses at birth or in the neonatal period. It has lately been demonstrated that following intravenous injection of labeled ferrous citrate, there is a selective uptake of radioactive iron in the region of the basal ganglia; possibly a study of this kind would be helpful in diagnosis. In an advanced case, CT scanning may show extreme atrophy of the brain, especially including the structures of the basal ganglia, but the pigmented deposits do not show any increased radiographic density. In some cases there is lucency in the putamen and globus pallidus. MRI scans show a characteristic pattern of increased density in the globus pallidus surrounded by low density on T2-weighted images. This sign has been termed "eye of the tiger." At present, no effective treatment is known. Treatment with a chelating agent, deferoxamine mesylate, has not shown definite benefit, and levodopa and other antiparkinsonian medications, tryptophan, and megavitamin therapy have been of only temporary and questionable help.

PROGRESSIVE FAMILIAL MYOCLONIC EPILEPSY There are several neurologic disorders that can result in a syndrome of convulsive seizures, myoclonic jerklike contractions of the musculature, and progressive dementia. Those most frequently encountered in practice are subacute sclerosing panencephalitis in children, adolescents, and young adults (Chap. 375) and subacute spongiform encephalopathy (Creutzfeldt-Jakob disease) in older adults (Chap. 375). The syndrome also can occur in some of the rare forms of metabolic familial disorders: neuraminidase deficiency associated with macular cherry red spots (Chap. 349) and ceroid-lipofuscinosis (Chap. 355). When these and other disorders of known cause can be excluded from consideration, there remain some clinicopathologic entities which can appropriately be considered under the heading of the hereditary degenerative diseases. Several families presenting this syndrome have been carefully studied in northern Europe (Sweden and Finland), but there is no specific geographic distribution.

Lafora's disease This variety of recessively inherited progressive myoclonic epilepsy is characterized by distinctive intracytoplasmic inclusions in cerebral neurons, called *Lafora bodies* following their original description by Gonzalo Lafora (1911). These have been found to be composed of polymers of glucose (polyglucosans) and thus indicate a disorder of carbohydrate metabolism, but the biochemical defect that leads to their accumulation is unknown. The Lafora bodies are widely distributed, but they are most numerous in the thalamus, substantia nigra, and dentate nucleus of the cerebellum. Subsequent to Lafora's reports, similar polysaccharide deposits have been found in myocardial and skeletal muscle fibers, skin, and the liver, and it is now possible to establish the diagnosis in the presymptomatic phase by skin or liver biopsy.

The disorder characteristically makes its appearance during childhood or adolescence in the form of recurrent seizures (generalized or restricted), uncontrollable myoclonic jerks, or combinations of the two. With the passage of time, the myoclonic phenomena become increasingly severe, and there is deterioration of all intellectual functions. Death from intercurrent infection generally occurs before age 25. Anticonvulsive treatment may help in controlling the seizures, but there currently is no effective treatment for the underlying disease.

Unverricht-Lundborg disease This is a rare autosomal recessive illness with onset in adolescence of myoclonic and tonic-clonic seizures. Dementia is mild or absent at the outset, but eventually there is a gradual intellectual decline as well as dysarthria, ataxia, and intention tremor. Survival into adulthood is usual. Pathologic studies show widespread degenerative changes without evidence of storage material.

Other varieties of myoclonic epilepsy When Lafora's disease and the metabolic and infective disorders mentioned above have been excluded, there remains a rather heterogeneous group of progressive neurologic illnesses having in common autosomal recessive inheritance, myoclonic phenomena, convulsive seizures, and mild dementia. Ataxia of stance, gait, and limb movements is a prominent feature in most cases—so much so that the term introduced by Ramsay Hunt, *dyssynergia cerebellaris myoclonica*, is often applied. In a few cases, including some of those originally described by Hunt, there is an overlap with Friedreich's ataxia, or with chronic sensorimotor neuropathies (see Chaps. 381 and 383). The neuropathologic changes in the few cases that have come to postmortem examination have varied from case to case. In some, atrophy of the dentate nucleus and its fiber projections has been prominent; in others, there has been loss of neurons, especially Purkinje cells, in the cerebellar cortex; in still others, changes have been confined to long-tract degeneration (posterior columns and spinocerebellar tracts) in the spinal cord; a few patients have had cortical, basal-ganglionic, or retinal lesions. Variations also occur in the age of onset and the rate of progression. Until more is known about the biochemistry and genetics of this group of disorders, no satisfactory classification is possible. For further details of these syndromes, general reference works on neurology, such as that of Adams and Victor, should be consulted.

Treatment with appropriate anticonvulsant medications has been helpful in some mild cases, but phenytoin is contraindicated. l-Tryptophan and carbidopa or valproic acid have ameliorated myoclonus in a few cases.

NORMAL-PRESSURE HYDROCEPHALUS Normal-pressure hydrocephalus (NPH) is a syndrome of communicating hydrocephalus in which intracranial hypertension is either absent or not recognized.

Pathology and pathophysiology Although it is recognized that delayed hydrocephalus can occur after meningitis, head injury, or subarachnoid hemorrhage, the majority of patients presenting with NPH give no history of such an illness. Studies of isotope cisternography indicate that NPH is a communicating hydrocephalus presumed to be due to partial obliteration of the subarachnoid space with defective CSF reabsorption through the arachnoid villi. Whether episodes of increased intracranial pressure occur during the course of the illness is debated. Some patients monitored continuously show fluctuations in CSF pressure including so-called plateau waves.

Clinical manifestations Typically, the patient or family describes a subacute onset, over weeks, months, or sometimes years, of progressive intellectual deterioration accompanied by slowness and restriction of movements, particularly of gait. No single diagnostic gait disorder occurs (see description, Chap. 22). A broad-based stance with hesitant initiation of walking is common. In some patients, ataxic features are present. Hyperreflexia in the legs and extensor plantar responses may be found. Urinary incontinence is noted in less than one-half of patients.

Differential diagnosis Parkinson's disease can be differentiated by its clinical features and the response to carbidopa-levodopa (Sinemet). Bifrontal disease due to tumor (butterfly glioma), metastases, or cerebral infarction can be identifed by CT or MRI. Multi-infarct dementia with gait disorder can be recognized by focal, often asymmetric, neurologic signs and by CT changes. Aqueductal stenosis may present occasionally in late adulthood with hydrocephalus, headaches, dementia, and incontinence. The CT or MRI usually will demonstrate an enlarged third ventricle with normal fourth ventricle.

Treatment The diagnosis can be difficult because of the common association of ventricular enlargement in patients with degenerative brain conditions, particularly Alzheimer's disease. The characteristic gait disorder is the most reliable clinical feature of NPH. CSF pressure in NPH is usually in the normal range of 80 to 150 mmH$_2$O. Isotope cisternography demonstrating reflux into the ventricular system has not proved to determine reliably which patients are likely to improve following a surgical shunt. Temporary benefit in the gait disorder after removal of 25 to 30 mL of CSF has been noted in some patients. When the history of dementia and gait disorder is subacute in onset and accompanied by considerable ventricular dilatation, surgical shunting is warranted. Ventricular-peritoneal shunting is the procedure most commonly performed. Between 40 and 70 percent of patients show benefit after surgery. The gait disorder tends to show a better response to shunting than the dementia (see Black et al. for review).

REFERENCES

General

ADAMS JH et al (eds): *Greenfield's Neuropathology*, 5th ed. New York, Wiley, 1992
ADAMS RD, VICTOR M: *Principles of Neurology*, 5th ed. New York, McGraw-Hill, 1993
ASBURY AK et al: *Diseases of the Nervous System*, vols I and II, 2d ed. Philadelphia, Ardmore Medical Books, Saunders, 1992

Alzheimer's disease

ARRIAGADA PV et al: Neurofibrillary tangles but not senile plaques parallel duration and severity of Alzheimer's disease. Neurology 42:631, 1992
BRAAK H, BRAAK E: Neuropathological staging of Alzheimer-related changes. Acta Neuropathol 82:239, 1991
EVANS DA et al: Prevalence of Alzheimer's disease in a community population of older persons: Higher than previously reported. JAMA 262:2551, 1989

FARRER LA et al: Segregation analysis reveals evidence of a major gene for Alzheimer disease. Am J Hum Genet 48:1026, 1991
GOATE A et al: Segregation of a missense mutation in the amyloid precursor protein with familial Alzheimer's disease. Nature 349:704, 1991
HANSEN L et al: The Lewy body variant of Alzheimer's disease: A clinical and pathologic entity. Neurology 40:1, 1990
KATZMAN R, SAITOH T: Advances in Alzheimer's disease. FASEB J 5:278, 1991
KOSIK KS: Alzheimer's disease: A cell biological perspective. Science 256:780, 1992
McKEE AC et al: Neuritic pathology and dementia in Alzheimer's disease. Ann Neurol 30:156, 1991
PERICAK-VANCE MA et al: Linkage studies in familial Alzheimer disease: Evidence for chromosome 19 linkage. Am J Hum Genet 48:1034, 1991
SELKOE DJ: Amyloid protein and Alzheimer's disease. Sci Am 265:68, 1991
SKOOG I et al: A population-based study of dementia in 85-year-olds. N Engl J Med 328:153, 1993
ST. GEORGE-HYSLOP PH et al: Genetic linkage studies suggest that Alzheimer's disease is not a single homogeneous disorder. Nature 347:194, 1990
YANKNER BA, MESULAM M-M: β-Amyloid and the pathogenesis of Alzheimer's disease. N Engl J Med 325:1849, 1991

Huntington's disease

BEAL MF: Does impairment of energy metabolism result in excitotoxic neuronal death in neurodegenerative illness? Ann Neurol 31:119, 1992
CHAPMAN MA: Canadian experience with predictive testing for Huntington disease: Lessons for genetic testing centers and policy makers. Am J Med Genet 42:491, 1992
DAWSON T et al: A novel neuronal messenger molecule in brain: The free radical, nitric oxide. Ann Neurol 32:297, 1992
HARPER P (ed): *Huntington's disease*. Philadelphia, Saunders, 1992
HUGGINS M et al: Ethical and legal dilemmas arising during predictive testing for adult-onset disease: The experience of Huntington's disease. Am J Hum Genet 47:4, 1990
KOROSHETZ W ET AL: The neurology of Huntington's disease, in *Movement Disorders in Neurology and Neuropsychiatry*, AB Joseph and RR Young (eds). Cambridge, 1992. pp 167–177
MARTIN JB, GUSELLA JF: Huntington's disease: Pathogenesis and management. N Engl J Med 315:1267, 1986
MEISSEN GJ et al: Predictive testing for Huntington's disease with use of a linked DNA marker. N Engl J Med 318:535, 1988
VONSATTEL JP et al: Neuropathological classification of Huntington's disease. J Neuropathol Exp Neurol 44:559, 1985

Miscellaneous

BLACK PM et al: CSF shunts for dementia, incontinence and gait disturbance. Clin Neurosurg 32:632, 1985
BRION S et al: Maladie de pick point de vue anatomo-clinique. Rev Neurol 147:693, 1991
BRYNE EJ et al: Diffuse Lewy disease: Clinical features in 15 cases. J Neurol Neurosurg Psychiatry 52:709, 1989
CRYSTAL HA et al: Antemortem diagnosis of diffuse Lewy body disease. Neurology 40:1523, 1990
GIBB WRG: Cortical Lewy body dementia. Behav Neurol 3:189, 1990
SNOWDEN JS et al: Progressive language disorder due to lobar atrophy. Ann Neurol 31:174, 1992
TISSOT R et al: *La Maladie de Pick*. Paris, Masson, 1975
VANNESTE J et al: Shunting normal-pressure hydrocephalus: Do the benefits outweigh the risks? A multicenter study and literature review. Neurology 42:54, 1992

371 PARKINSON'S DISEASE AND OTHER EXTRAPYRAMIDAL DISORDERS

M. FLINT BEAL / J. STEPHEN FINK / JOSEPH B. MARTIN*

PARKINSON'S DISEASE This is a common condition first named and described by James Parkinson in 1817. His remarkably complete account gives this definition:

Involuntary tremulous motion, with lessened muscular power, in parts not in action and even when supported; with a propensity to bend the trunk forward, and to pass from a walking to a running pace, the senses and intellects being uninjured.

Typically, Parkinson's disease is a disorder of middle or late life, with very gradual progression and a prolonged course. Although it

* The authors acknowledge the contribution of E.P. Richardson and R.D. Adams in previous editions.

has been seen to occur in families (the estimated familial incidence is 1 to 2 percent), it usually is sporadic. It is well recognized, however, that the epidemic encephalitis of von Economo, which occurred in a worldwide distribution in the years following World War I, was followed by a syndrome clinically almost indistinguishable from paralysis agitans. It is usual in such instances to speak of postencephalitic parkinsonism, whereas the term *Parkinson's disease* should be reserved for true paralysis agitans of unknown cause. Parkinson's disease bears no consistent relation to any known disease process such as arteriosclerosis, trauma, or intoxication (except for MPTP, see below), although such conditions have often been invoked as etiologically significant and may at times produce somewhat similar clinical manifestations.

Pathology The most regularly observed changes have been in the aggregates of melanin-containing nerve cells in the brainstem (substantia nigra, locus coeruleus), where there are varying degrees of nerve cell loss with reactive gliosis (most pronounced in the substantia nigra) along with distinctive eosinophilic intracytoplasmic inclusions (Lewy bodies). Similar changes are seen in the nucleus basalis of Meynert. Lesions in pigmented nuclei, but without Lewy bodies, characterize the pathologic findings in postencephalitic parkinsonism, in striatonigral degeneration, and in the Shy-Drager syndrome (discussed below).

Biochemical studies show a decrease of dopamine in the caudate nucleus and putamen, emphasizing the point that Parkinson's disease can be considered an example of neuronal system disease, involving mainly the nigrostriatal dopaminergic system. Confirmation of the importance of the nigrostriatal dopaminergic system arose from observations of the effects of accidental intoxication of drug users by self-injection with 1-methyl-4-phenyl-1,2,3,6-tetrahydropyridine (MPTP), which selectively destroys dopaminergic neurons of the substantia nigra. The typical clinical manifestations of this disease resemble closely those of Parkinson's disease. The pathologic features of MPTP-induced Parkinson's disease, however, differ from those of idiopathic cases in the absence of Lewy bodies and the lack of neuronal loss in the locus coeruleus. The mechanism by which the drug kills substantia nigra neurons may provide new insights about the pathogenesis of the idiopathic illness. Recent studies show that a metabolite of MPTP blocks mitochondrial function. The possibilities of either mitochondrial impairment or excess free-radical formation are leading theories of causation in Parkinson's disease.

Clinical aspects In its fully developed form, Parkinson's disease is easily recognized. The stooped posture, the stiffness and slowness of movement, the fixity of facial expression, and the rhythmic tremor of the limbs, which subsides on active willed movement or complete relaxation, are familiar to every clinician. Although symmetric in the later stages, the disorder typically begins asymmetrically, e.g., as a slight tremor of the fingers of one hand or in one leg. Also typical are more or less general hypokinesia and stiffness of the musculature so that even where tremor is inapparent, the disease may betray itself by a somewhat staring and immobile facial expression, a monotonous voice, a general slowness and diminution of all motor activity, and a curious lack of the little spontaneous movements of postural adjustment that are so characteristic of the normal individual. When tremor is minimal, patients often are able to alleviate it by relaxation or by movement or to hide it by keeping their hands in their pockets. The tremor is generally most pronounced in the hands but may involve the legs (and thus secondarily the trunk), lips, tongue, and neck muscles and is easily seen in the eyelids when they are lightly closed. Its frequency is 4 to 5 per second, but another faster (action) tremor (7 to 8 per second) predominates in some patients (see Chap. 21). There is never total paralysis, although this is implied by the name of the disease; nevertheless, general enfeeblement of voluntary movement is characteristic of the fully developed disorder. Generally accompanying the stopped attitude is the typical festinating gait, whereby the patient, prevented by the abnormality of postural tone from making the appropriate reflex adjustments required for effective walking, progresses with quick shuffling steps at an accelerating pace

as if to catch up with the body's center of gravity. Clinical examination of the tendon and plantar reflexes discloses no abnormalities. There are no sensory changes, although deep aching in joints and muscles may occur. Eventually, even with maximal drug therapy, patients may become so incapacitated by rigidity and tremor as to be helpless in caring for themselves. It has often been observed, however, that even severely disabled patients may, when excited or under great emotional stress, perform complex motor acts quickly and efficiently. Although the temporary alleviation under extreme provocation can never be long maintained, it is nevertheless true that the severity of the symptoms is considerably influenced by emotional factors. Despite the inherently progressive nature of the condition, much can be achieved with good medical management, and patients may continue for years to live effective, happy lives.

Although intellectual deterioration is not a consistent feature of early Parkinson's disease, dementia has been increasingly recognized to be a feature of advanced Parkinson's disease. It eventually afflicts up to one-quarter of all cases.

Differential diagnosis In typical cases, this is not difficult. The extrapyramidal syndromes associated with most diseases of known cause or established nature, such as cerebrovascular disease, cerebral hypoxia (including carbon monoxide asphyxia), or metallic poisoning, differ from Parkinson's disease in a number of respects, such as atypical behavior or tremor, presence of signs of corticospinal tract deficit, or early onset of dementia. These clinical conditions which resemble idiopathic Parkinson's disease are collectively termed *Parkinson syndromes* or *parkinsonism*. The differentiation from postencephalitic parkinsonism may be difficult; a clear history of an attack of epidemic encephalitis (prolonged somnolence, disturbance of consciousness, diplopia) and relatively early age of onset of the disorder, little or no progression of symptoms, relative sensitivity to levodopa, and oculogyric crises may be the only clues to this diagnosis. A neurologic disorder similar to some degree to Parkinson's disease occurs with the prolonged administration of large amounts of reserpine and neuroleptic drugs as the result of their blocking action on dopaminergic transmission. This drug-induced syndrome usually subsides on discontinuation or decrease in the dosage of the drug. MPTP-induced parkinsonism persists because of the destructive effects of the drug on the nigral dopaminergic neurons. Chronic manganese poisoning and other toxins (carbon monoxide, cyanide) also may produce parkinsonism. Parkinsonism very rarely is produced by cerebral neoplasms or other focal lesions, but then only when the nigrostriatal system has been largely destroyed, with relative sparing of the corticospinal projections.

Some Parkinson-like postural and motor abnormalities may be seen following the repeated blows to the head sustained by boxers—in the "punch drunk" syndrome, in which lesions of the substantia nigra are one of the neuropathologic components. In this condition, dementia, ataxia, dysarthria, and inappropriate behavior are prominent, and neuronal cell loss with neurofibrillary tangles is evident in the cerebral cortex.

Multiple bilateral infarcts in the corticospinal pathways and central structures of the brain may produce parkinsonism (so-called arteriosclerotic parkinsonism), but careful clinical assessment of the history and findings, particularly the deep tendon reflexes, serves to distinguish this disorder from true Parkinson's disease. In their fully developed form and with adequate history, other akinetic-rigid syndromes are usually differentiated from idiopathic Parkinson's disease (see below). However, in early stages, idiopathic Parkinson's disease may be indistinguishable from other Parkinson syndromes in up to one-quarter of cases.

Treatment An important part of any therapeutic program is the maintenance of optimal general health and neuromuscular efficiency by planned programs of exercise, activity, and rest; expert physical therapy may be of great help in achieving these ends. In addition, the patient often needs much emotional support in meeting the stress of the illness, in comprehending its nature, and in carrying on courageously in spite of it. Along with these general supportive measures, which are applicable to many chronic illnesses, patients generally require a carefully thought-out program of treatment specifically aimed at counteracting the pathophysiologic disorder that produces their disabilities.

Drug therapy should be adapted to the patient's needs, which vary with the stage of the disease and the predominant manifestation(s). Usually, anticholinergic drugs are most effective in suppressing tremor at rest, and propranolol or primidone is best for action tremor. Levodopa improves akinesia and postural imbalance; anticholinergic drugs have little effect on these two abnormalities.

The decision about whether to treat with a drug and the choice of drug(s) are influenced by the stage of the disease. The scale of Hoehn and Yahr is recommended:

Stage I: Unilateral involvement.
Stage II: Bilateral involvement but no postural abnormalities.
Stage III: Bilateral involvement with mild postural imbalance; the patient leads an independent life.
Stage IV: Bilateral involvement with postural instability; the patient requires substantial help.
Stage V: Severe, fully developed disease; the patient is restricted to bed and chair.

A recent advance in the therapy of Parkinson's disease has been the observation that treatment with deprenyl, a monoamine oxidase B inhibitor, may slow the progression of the illness. Because the drug has some symptomatic benefits, it is not possible to unequivocally conclude that it exerts a neuroprotective effect. Most clinicians now treat patients with mild disease (stages I and II) with deprenyl at a dose of 5 mg bid. The mechanism by which deprenyl is effective is uncertain; a leading theory is that it reduces free-radical formation generated from the oxidation of catecholamines.

Once a patient develops significant disability (stages III, IV, and V), the initiation of therapy with levodopa is required. Levodopa is the most effective drug available for treatment of Parkinson's disease and remains the mainstay of treatment. Levodopa is the precursor of dopamine. Treatment increases dopamine levels in the striatum and restores neurotransmitter balance between dopamine and acetylcholine. It is particularly effective in improving akinesia and rigidity; often, concurrent administration of anticholinergic medications is required to optimally control rest tremor. Postural instability frequently does not respond to levodopa. The initiation of levodopa is predictably accompanied by a rapid and dramatic reduction of symptoms and signs. A lack of response to levodopa (at doses greater than 1,000 mg/d) suggests a clinical condition other than Parkinson's disease. Levodopa is given in combination with a dopa-carboxylase inhibitor (carbidopa) which prevents destruction of levodopa in the bloodstream and peripheral tissues but does not pass the blood-brain barrier. This combination therefore makes it possible to achieve optimal effects with a smaller dosage of levodopa than would otherwise need to be used. In this way, some of the side effects of levodopa, particularly nausea and vomiting, can be greatly reduced. The combination (Sinemet) is available in ratios of 1:4 carbidopa to levodopa (25 mg/ 100 mg) or 1:10 (10 mg/100 mg, 25 mg/250 mg). At all stages of disability it is desirable to use the lowest dose of levodopa that gives satisfactory benefit; this decreases the chances of unwanted side effects such as dyskinesias and hallucinations. A controlled-release formulation (Sinemet CR) is now available consisting of 50 mg carbidopa and 200 mg levodopa. This formulation has a slower onset of effect but lasts for 4 to 6 h, resulting in more sustained clinical benefit. Initial therapy is started with one-half tablet bid (at least 6 h apart) and titrated upward as needed. Some patients are dissatisfied with the delayed onset of response, particularly in the morning. In this instance, the addition of a small amount of standard Sinemet, such as half a 25 mg/100 mg tablet, may be useful. A total daily dosage of levodopa from 200 to 2000 mg can be used. Although levodopa is the cornerstone of therapy, it can be combined with dopamine receptor agonists or anticholinergic drugs.

Direct-acting dopamine receptor agonists are the next most effica-cious agents. Bromocriptine and pergolide are available in the United States, while lisuride is available in some other countries. When used alone in patients with mild disease, a dose of bromocriptine of 15 to 30 mg daily is often effective. Pergolide mesylate was found to be efficacious at a mean dose of 2.6 mg daily as sole therapy. Uncontrolled trials of dopamine agonists indicate that the use of low doses of these agents in the early phase of symptomatic therapy, in combination with lower doses of levodopa, results in fewer clinical fluctuations, particularly end-of-dose loss of efficacy, and dyskinesias than with levodopa alone. The major disadvantage of the early use of agonists is the high cost of dopamine receptor agonists. The side effects of dopamine agonists are much the same as those with levodopa.

Anticholinergics and amantadine are weaker antiparkinsonian agents, but they are useful in the early stages of the illness or as adjuvant drugs later in the disease. Anticholinergics appear to be particularly useful in patients whose tremor is not completely relieved by levodopa and the dopaminergic agonists. Anticholinergic drugs reduce cholinergic transmission by blocking muscarinic receptors. Amantadine releases dopamine from presynaptic terminals and may prove useful in enhancing the effects of levodopa in patients with mild symptoms. The usual dosage is 100 mg bid; larger doses may produce side effects such as skin changes (livedo reticularis), ankle edema, and mental confusion.

Currently available anticholinergic drugs are trihexyphenidyl, benztropine, biperiden, and procyclidine. The usual dose of trihexy-phenidyl is 1 to 2 mg qid. Benztropine has both anticholinergic and antihistaminic properties; the usual dose is 0.5 to 1.0 mg tid. The optimal dose of all these medications varies for each patient and often needs to be adjusted. Low doses of these drugs cause dry mouth but few, if any, other side effects. Larger doses should be given with caution, for in the elderly they may cause confusion, visual and tactile hallucinations, narrow-angle glaucoma, and urinary retention. Anticholinergic drugs may exacerbate dementia and should be withdrawn when dementia becomes clinically evident.

It must be said that although the modern treatment of Parkinson's disease is more successful than any that was available before the introduction of levodopa, including stereotactic surgery, there are still many problems. Underlying much of the difficulty undoubtedly is the fact that none of these therapeutic measures has an effect on the underlying disease process, which consists of neuronal degeneration. Ultimately, a point seems to be reached where pharmacotherapy can no longer compensate for the loss of basal ganglia dopamine. The major difficulties consist of fluctuations or sudden variations in the response to the drugs used (the on-off response), the development of weakness or immobility (akinesia), and dyskinesias. Hallucinations, particularly in the elderly, become more frequent in some patients with moderate to advanced disease. Initial treatment is dosage reduction; however, if this is unsuccessful, the atypical neuroleptic clozapine has been used successfully. Clozapine has little or no extrapyramidal effects, but neutropenia can occur. As time passes, the therapeutic window between an effective dose of levodopa and a dose producing dyskinesias lessens. The dyskinesias consist of choreiform or choreoathetotic movements, which in the advanced stages of the disease alternate with paralyzing akinesia depending on a very narrow dosage variation (50 to 100 mg) of levodopa. Interference with absorption of levodopa may be partially responsible, since continuous intravenous infusions of levodopa result in a stable clinical state. Loss of therapeutic efficacy also occurs: a single dose which at one time was effective for 5 to 6 h may last only an hour or so. Giving smaller amounts of medication more frequently is sometimes efficacious or using a sustained-release preparation of levodopa (Sinemet CR). In addition, agents acting directly on the postsynaptic receptor, such as bromocriptine or pergolide, are sometimes more effective. It has been shown recently that temporary levodopa withdrawal, advocated as a method of dealing with the long-term complications of Parkinson's disease, carries some risk and does not result in sustained improvement in efficacy of levodopa.

As many as one-half of patients with Parkinson's disease have depressive symptoms. They should be treated along the lines suggested in Chap. 389.

The introduction of stereotactic surgery, with the placement of precisely localized focal lesions in central structures in the brain—mainly the ventrolateral thalamus or globus pallidus contralateral to the side of the major symptoms—was an important advance in the attempt to relieve the symptoms of Parkinson's disease. The success that has been achieved with levodopa has largely supplanted these procedures, which, although very beneficial in well-chosen cases, were not without risk and at times were followed by severe disability. Neurosurgical treatment of this kind can still be recommended for patients who are relatively young and who have a severe unilateral disabling or disfiguring tremor unresponsive to medication. Recent interest has focused on adrenal medullary transplants to the striatum. Although initial reports indicated favorable responses, subsequent experience in many centers has failed to confirm the earlier report. Fetal tissue transplants containing substantia nigra neurons may be more effective, but remain experimental.

OTHER AKINETIC-RIGID SYNDROMES In addition to parkinsonism resulting from encephalitis, drugs or toxins, head trauma, or structural causes, akinetic-rigid syndromes may occur in other uncommon degenerative diseases. Often, these akinetic-rigid syndromes are accompanied by other extrapyramidal signs such as chorea, dystonia, ballism, dyskinesias, or myoclonus. The most common of these akinetic-rigid syndromes are *progressive supranuclear palsy (PSP)* and a group of disorders collectively referred to as *multiple-system degenerations*. The latter group of disorders includes the clinically heterogeneous *olivopontocerebellar atrophy (OPCA), striatonigral degeneration*, and the *Shy-Drager syndrome*; the exact clinical designation depends on the predominant clinical features. The multiple-system degenerations have in common lesions within the cerebellum, inferior olives, basal ganglia, pigmented nuclei, pontine nuclei, and spinal cord. In patients with these akinetic-rigid syndromes there is little or no clinical improvement with levodopa. Parkinsonism accompanied by ataxia, corticobulbar signs, and corticospinal deficits would be considered a type of OPCA (see Chap. 372). Signs of autonomic failure (such as orthostatic hypotension, urinary incontinence, and sexual dysfunction) are prominent in the Shy-Drager syndrome (see Chap. 379). In patients in whom parkinsonism progresses more rapidly than idiopathic Parkinson's disease, akinesia/rigidity and postural disturbances but not tremor are prominent, and in those in whom there is little or no clinical improvement with levodopa, the diagnosis of striatonigral degeneration should be considered. Usually it is not possible to clinically distinguish with certainty striatonigral degeneration from idiopathic Parkinson's disease or other akinetic-rigid syndromes. Confirmation of clinical diagnosis of striatonigral degeneration can only be made by postmortem examination of brain. Progressive supranuclear palsy is considered in more detail below. The Shy-Drager syndrome is considered in more detail in Chapter 379.

Parkinsonism may be present in other less common degenerative diseases. Hepatolenticular degeneration (Wilson's disease, Chap. 348) and acquired hepatocerebral degeneration (Chap. 377) are often accompanied by rigidity and bradykinesia. Parkinsonism accompanied by prominent apraxia, asymmetric severe rigidity, action tremor, and preserved intellect suggests the diagnosis of corticobasal ganglionic degeneration (Chap. 370). Parkinsonism also may be present in other degenerative diseases in which dementia is a prominent feature. These disorders include Alzheimer's disease, Pick's disease, Parkinson-dementia-amyotrophic lateral sclerosis (ALS) complex of Guam, Creutzfeldt-Jakob disease, normal-pressure hydrocephalus, a rigid form of Huntington's disease, progressive supranuclear palsy, Hallervorden-Spatz disease, Wilson's disease, and some metabolic diseases (Lafora body disease, ceroid lipofuscinosis) (see Chaps. 370 and 372).

PROGRESSIVE SUPRANUCLEAR PALSY (STEELE-RICHARD-SON-OLSZEWSKI SYNDROME) This disorder, first clearly described in 1963 by Richardson, Steele, and Olszewski, occurs in elderly individuals in approximately the same age period as Parkinson's disease. Moreover, it is among the group of parkinsonian patients that most of the examples of this disease are to be found.

Pathology A loss of neurons and gliosis are found on postmortem examination in the tectum and tegmentum of the midbrain, the subthalamic nuclei of Luys, the vestibular nuclei, and to some extent the ocular nuclei. A characteristic finding is the presence of neurofibrillary tangles similar to those of Alzheimer's disease on light-microscopic examination but differing from them on electron microscopy in that they are composed of straight rather than paired helical filaments. The cause of the disease is unknown. A slow virus has been suspected, but attempts to transfer it to monkeys by the intracerebral inoculation of brain tissue have failed.

Clinical manifestations The clinical features are quite distinctive: disturbances of balance and gait with unexpected falls; rigidity of the neck and other trunk muscles, resembling Parkinson's disease; "masking" of the face; reduction in the volume of the voice; extreme flexion or extension dystonia of the neck; and difficulty in looking down—all these are early symptoms, and any one of them may first bring the patient to a physician. In contrast to idiopathic Parkinson's disease, rest tremor is usually absent in progressive supranuclear palsy. Ophthalmoplegia has been regarded as the cardinal clinical sign of the disease. Typically there is initial impairment of vertical saccadic movements and a loss of the fast component of optokinetic nystagmus usually affecting downward more than upward gaze. With progression of the disease, horizontal eye movements are affected, with oculovestibular reflexes preserved. Symptoms progress over months and years, until the patient becomes virtually anarthric with total loss of voluntary control of eye movements and severe cervical and truncal rigidity. Dementia is usually mild, with forgetfulness, slowing of thought processes, apathy, and impaired ability to manipulate acquired knowledge. There are no impairments of vision, hearing, somatic sensation, or voluntary power, and signs of corticospinal involvement are minimal or absent. The diagnosis should be considered whenever an elderly patient begins to fall repeatedly and inexplicably and has extrapyramidal symptoms with a rigid neck and paralysis of conjugate or vertical gaze.

Treatment Treatment has been largely unsuccessful. Relatively little benefit comes from the administration of the antiparkinsonian group of drugs, although they should be tried. Occasionally, levodopa, or a combination of levodopa with an anticholinergic drug, has helped to diminish some of the symptoms. Idazoxan, which increases norepinephrine neurotransmission, improves motor function in some patients, but it is not available for clinical usage.

TORSION DYSTONIA (TORSION SPASM; DYSTONIA MUSCU-LORUM DEFORMANS) This is a syndrome of sustained muscular contraction frequently causing twisting and repetitive movements that result in abnormal, at times bizarre, postures of the limbs and trunk. Eventually these postures become more or less fixed. Recent studies using segregation analysis have shown that in Jewish and non-Jewish families, idiopathic early-onset generalized dystonia is transmitted as an autosomal dominant disorder with variable penetrance. Genetic studies have shown linkage to a region on chromosome 9. It is to these cases, both hereditary and sporadic, that the term *torsion dystonia* (torsion spasm, dystonia musculorum deformans) is correctly applied. When this disorder occurs in late-adult life, it tends to be focal in onset. In cases of early onset, dystonia tends to generalize. The cause and pathogenesis remain unknown.

Dystonias in which the etiology is known are called *secondary dystonias*. Underlying the secondary dystonias may be any of several pathologic conditions, including lesions of neonatal hypoxia, strokes, Wilson's disease, the pigmented lesions of Hallevorden-Spatz, GM_1 gangliosidosis, ataxia-telangiectasia, or kernicterus.

Pathology Few cases of torsion dystonia not due to one of the definable disease processes indicated above have been adequately studied neuropathologically. Reported results from these cases have led to uncertainty as to what the pathologic-anatomic basis of the clinical state might be, although it was generally assumed that the basal ganglia were diseased. A careful study by Zeman and Dyken, which included comparison of the findings in patients with the disease with control material, failed to demonstrate any neuropathologic abnormality to which the clinical changes could reasonably be attributed. These negative findings, which are perhaps surprising, must not be interpreted as indicating that there is "no disease" in the brain, but rather that the pathologic state is not one that can be disclosed by the usual histopathologic techniques. It may well be that more careful quantitative assessments of certain populations of neurons and studies of the pathophysiology of neurotransmitters will result in further elucidation of this disease.

Clinical manifestations A descriptive classification of the motor abnormalities of dystonia is given in Chap. 21. In the early stages, the involuntary muscular contractions are intermittent and variable in location and severity, but they typically interfere with motor performance by superimposing an unwanted posture on parts in use. One leg may briefly be pulled into a flexed or extended position or one shoulder elevated. Later the lingual, pharyngeal, neck, and thoracic muscles participate, and grimacing may occur. These latter also may be the first and only signs of disease for several years. Progression may be relatively rapid in cases with onset during early childhood but is slow in those beginning in late childhood or adult life. The end result is extreme disability, with grossly distorted postures of the trunk and contractures of the limbs. Affection of face and tongue muscles results in faulty articulation of speech, which eventually becomes incomprehensible. The tendon and plantar reflexes are normal.

Early-onset dystonia characteristically makes its appearance in childhood after a preceding period of normalcy. Typically it becomes evident first in the lower limbs and then evolves, sometimes relatively rapidly, into the generalized state of severe incapacity described above. When onset is in adulthood, it tends to appear first in the upper limbs and to remain more restricted in its extent than the early-onset variety, and progression is less relentless. The late-life sporadic cases are generally similar in character.

A rare form is *dopa-responsive dystonia*. This syndrome appears to be inherited in an autosomal dominant manner with reduced penetrance. Onset is in childhood, with dystonia usually affecting gait. There is diurnal fluctuation with worsening as the day progresses. Most individuals later develop parkinsonism. There is a dramatic response to levodopa therapy.

FOCAL DYSTONIAS In addition to the generalized dystonias noted above, there is a group of focal or segmental dystonias which appear sporadically in adult life. Their clearly involuntary nature and lack of susceptibility to willed control by the patient distinguish them from common tics, habit spasms, and mannerisms. They have often been erroneously interpreted as manifestations of hysteria. If the muscle contraction is frequent and prolonged, aching pain accompanies it—for which the spasm may mistakenly be blamed.

The most frequent and familiar type of focal dystonia is *spasmodic torticollis*. This is a disorder of adults that afflicts women somewhat more frequently than men. It consists of an involuntary turning of the head to one side—intermittent at first, then gradually worsening to the point of being more or less continuous. In some cases, torticollis is the first manifestation of a generalized dystonia, but more usually it remains focal and segmental.

Another frequent focal dystonia of adults is exemplified by *writer's cramp*, in which the dystonic postures and movements occur only during the performance of specific acts, to the extent that carrying out the act in the usual way, such as writing with a pen or pencil, becomes impossible, while other motor activities using the same musculature are unimpaired. An analogous disorder sometimes afflicts musicians.

The combination of blepharospasm and oromandibular dystonia—*cranial dystonia*—is sometimes referred to as Meige's syndrome. When the throat and respiratory muscles are involved, this interferes with speech production, resulting in spasmodic dysphonia. The

muscles of the neck are variably affected. It should be recalled that similar dystonic states (facial-cervical and more extreme dyskinesias) can result from the use of phenothiazine and similar drugs. This sometimes persists after discontinuation of the medication as *tardive dystonia*—a troublesome condition that may resist all forms of treatment.

Differential diagnosis The treatable condition of hepatolenticular degeneration (Wilson's disease) should be seriously considered in any case presenting these motor symptoms, and appropriate measures should be undertaken for its investigation (see Chap. 348). The progressive course and possibly, the family history differentiate the degenerative group of dystonias from the "secondary" dystonias resulting from infections or metabolic disorders occurring at birth or later and structural lesions of the brain such as occur following trauma, strokes, or neoplasms. Hallervorden-Spatz disease, however, cannot be distinguished on clinical grounds alone (see Chap. 370). Rare instances of GM_1 gangliosidosis or other lipid storage diseases may begin in adult life with a dystonic syndrome, and drug-induced (tardive) dystonia must be considered in all cases of focal or generalized dystonia in adults, especially if they have or have had a psychiatric illness.

Treatment This is extremely difficult and often unsatisfactory. In the generalized dystonias, pharmacotherapy should certainly be attempted and, in most patients, needs to be individualized. Marsden and Fahn, whose experience with this disorder is extensive, suggest beginning with an anticholinergic agent such as trihexyphenidyl or ethopropazine and very gradually increasing the dosage until either benefit ensues or intolerable side effects appear. They found that the response in children (who may be able to take as much as 80 mg/d of trihexyphenidyl) was better than in adults, who tolerated the high doses less well, generally because of mental disturbances. In their experience, the next best group of drugs for ameliorating dystonic spasms are the benzodiazepines (such as diazepam or clonazepam), which likewise are used in high dosage after a very gradual introduction and increase (up to 80 mg diazepam daily). Again, children are more tolerant of the side effects (mainly drowsiness). A combination of anticholinergics and benzodiazepines may work out best. Other drugs—both dopaminergic agonists and antagonists, as well as carbamazepine—have been used, occasionally with success. Neuroleptics (dopaminergic antagonists) such as haloperidol, perhaps together with dopamine-depleting drugs (reserpine, tetrabenazine) and anticholinergics, may be useful in the treatment of some refractory dystonias. Dopa-responsive dystonia shows a dramatic response to levodopa, which may warrant a therapeutic trial if this diagnosis is suspected.

The symptoms of the focal dystonias, if not severe, may be more acceptable to the patient than prolonged trials with various drugs or surgical intervention. The most promising therapy for focal dystonia has been injections of botulinum toxin, which blocks acetylcholine release at the neuromuscular junction. Beneficial effects last on average 2 to 6 months. The most responsive of the focal dystonias to botulinum toxin treatments is blepharospasm. Denervative surgical procedures may in some cases be beneficial if only a restricted group of muscles is involved (as in torticollis). Medical management must be adapted to the individual patient's needs. The medications used for the treatment of generalized dystonias also may be useful for some focal dystonias; however, some focal dystonias (e.g., writer's cramp) are uniformly unresponsive to medications.

FAMILIAL TREMOR One of the most common hereditary disorders of the human nervous system is that which gives rise to a fast-frequency (6 to 8 per second) action tremor. This may appear at any age but more often during adolescence and adult years; once started, it lasts throughout life. The heredity is dominant. Probably all cases are not the same, for some patients have tremors of slower frequency, looking more like those of Parkinson's disease, but lacking the slowness of movement, rigidity, and flexed postures of that disorder. In patients of advanced age it is called *senile tremor*. Consumption of alcohol suppresses the fast-frequency forms, as does a beta-adrenergic blocking agent (propranolol) in doses of 20 to 40 mg three times daily. The slightly slower rhythmic action tremors with frequencies of approximately 6 per second do not consistently respond to propranolol or alcohol. Primidone 50 mg at bedtime has recently been found to be effective and has been advocated for use as initial therapy. If there is no response after 1 week, the dose should be increased gradually up to 250 mg at bedtime.

GILLES DE LA TOURETTE SYNDROME This condition, of unknown cause and uncertain pathology, presents with multiple tics, associated with snorting, sniffing, and involuntary vocalizations. It begins in childhood, usually as isolated tics, which are at first difficult to distinguish from habit spasms. Progression occurs over years, and other behavioral findings appear; compulsive touching of others, repeating of words or phrases, and explosive utterance of obscenities (coprolalia). Careful attention to other members of the family has given evidence that the disease is hereditary, with an autosomal dominant pattern of transmission. Obsessive compulsive disorder appears to be an alternate phenotypic expression of the gene in these families.

The course of the illness is unpredictable. In some cases associated mild neurologic abnormalities are found with hyperactivity, disorders of attention, and abnormal psychologic tests. Dementia does not occur. In some patients the condition abates, in others it progresses, leading to serious disability. Treatment is only partially satisfactory. Haloperidol has received the most clinical attention, but side effects are often unacceptable and it should be used only in severe cases and in the smallest effective dosage: 0.25 to 0.5 mg daily. Pimozide has recently been approved for treatment of Gilles de la Tourette. It causes fewer side effects than haloperidol but can cause widening of the QT interval and sudden death at high doses. Therefore, the electrocardiogram should be followed and the dose limited to 0.3 mg/kg per day. Clonidine has proved effective in some cases.

REFERENCES

General

ADAMS JH et al (eds): *Greenfield's Neuropathology*, 5th ed. New York, Wiley, 1992
ADAMS RD, VICTOR M: *Principles of Neurology*, 5th ed. New York, McGraw-Hill, 1993
ASBURY AK et al: *Diseases of the Nervous System*, vols 1 and 2, 2d ed. Philadelphia, Ardmore Medical Books, Saunders, 1992
MARSDEN CD, FAHN S (eds): *Movement Disorders*. London, Butterworth, 1987
WEINER WJ, LANG AE: *Movement Disorders: A Comprehensive Survey*. Mt. Kisco, N.Y., Futura, 1988

Parkinson's disease

BEAL MF: Does impairment of energy metabolism result in excitotoxic neuronal death in neurodegenerative illnesses? Ann Neurol 31:119, 1992
BLOEM BR et al: The MPTP model: Versatile contributions to the treatment of idiopathic Parkinson's disease. J Neurol Sci 97:273, 1990
FAHN S et al (eds): *Recent Advances in Parkinson's Disease*. New York, Raven Press, 1986
FRIEDMAN JH, LANNON MC: Clozapine in the treatment of psychosis in Parkinson's disease. Neurology 39:1219, 1989
HOEHN MN, YAHR MD: Parkinsonism: Onset, progression and mortality. Neurology 17:427, 1967
HUGHES AJ et al: Accuracy of clinical diagnosis of idiopathic Parkinson's disease: A clinico-pathological study of 100 cases. J Neurol Neurosurg Psychiatry 55:181, 1992
LINDVALL O et al: Transplantation of fetal dopamine neurons in Parkinson's disease: One-year clinical and neurophysiological observations in two patients with putaminal implants. Ann Neurol 31:155, 1992
MARSDEN CD: Parkinson's disease. Lancet 1:948, 1990
MOURADIAN MM et al: Modification of central dopaminergic mechanisms by continuous levodopa therapy for advanced Parkinson's disease. Ann Neurol 27:18, 1990
PARKINSON STUDY GROUP: Effect of deprenyl on the progression of disability in early Parkinson's disease. N Engl J Med 321:1364, 1989
RIEDERER P et al: Recent advances in pharmacological therapy of Parkinson's disease. Adv Neurol 60:626, 1993
STANDAERT DG, STERN MB: Update on the management of Parkinson's disease. Med Clin North Am 77:169, 1993

Miscellaneous

ADAMS RD et al: Striatonigral degeneration. J Neuropathol Exp Neurol 23:584, 1964
BERKOVIC SF et al: Progressive myoclonic epilepsies: Specific causes and diagnosis. N Engl J Med 315:296, 1986
CHAN J et al: Idiopathic cervical dystonia: Clinical characteristics. Movement Dis 6:119, 1991

GHIKA J et al: Idazoxan treatment in progressive supranuclear palsy. Neurology 41:986, 1991
GILMAN S: Medical progress: Advances in neurology. N Engl J Med 326:1608, 1992
GOETZ CG et al: Adult tics in Gilles de la Tourette's syndrome: Description and risk factors. Neurology 42:784, 1992
GREENE P et al: Double-blind, placebo-controlled trial of botulinum toxin injections for the treatment of spasmodic torticollis. Neurology 40:1213, 1990
IIVANAINEN M, HIMBERG J-J: Valproate and clonazepam in the treatment of severe progressive myoclonus epilepsy. Arch Neurol 39:236, 1982
JANKOVIC J et al: Cervical dystonia: Clinical findings and associated movement disorders. Neurology 41:1088, 1991
————, SCHWARTZ K: Botulinum toxin injections for cervical dystonia. Neurology 40:277, 1990
KRAMER PL et al: Dystonia gene in Ashkenazi Jewish population is located on chromosome 9q32-34. Ann Neurol 27:114, 1990
LOGIGIAN EL et al: Myoclonus epilepsy in two brothers: Clinical features and neuropathology of a unique syndrome. Brain 190:411, 1986
McGEER EG, McGEER PL: The dystonias. Can J Neurol Sci 15:447, 1988
MESULAM MM, PETERSEN RC: Treatment of Gilles de la Tourette syndrome: Eight-year, practice-based experience in predominantly adult population. Neurology 37:1828, 1987
NYGAARD TG et al: Dopa-responsive dystonia: Long-term treatment response and prognosis. Neurology 41:174, 1991
SETHI KD et al: Hallervorden-Spatz syndrome: Clinical and magnetic resonance imaging correlations. Ann Neurol 24:692, 1988
SINGER HS, WALKUP JT: Tourette syndrome and other tic disorders: Diagnosis, pathophysiology, and treatment. Medicine 70:15, 1991
STEELE JC: Progressive supranuclear palsy. Brain 95:693, 1972
WATTS RL et al: Corticobasal ganglionic degeneration. Neurology 35:178, 1985
ZEMAN W, DYKEN P: Dystonia musculorum deformans: Clinical, genetic and pathoanatomical studies. Psychiatr Neurol Neurochir 70:77, 1967

372 MOTOR NEURON DISEASE AND THE PROGRESSIVE ATAXIAS

ROBERT H. BROWN, JR.

MOTOR NEURON DISEASE (MUSCULAR WEAKNESS AND WASTING WITHOUT SENSORY CHANGES)

AMYOTROPHIC LATERAL SCLEROSIS Amyotrophic lateral sclerosis (ALS) is the most common form of progressive motor neuron disease (Table 372-1). It is a prototypic example of a neuronal system disease and is arguably the most devastating of the neurodegenerative disorders.

Pathology The pathology of the motor neuron degenerative disorders affects two classes of neurons: lower motor neurons (consisting of anterior horn cells in the spinal cord and their brainstem homologues innervating bulbar muscles) and upper motor neurons (emanating from layer five of the motor cortex to descend via the corticospinal and corticobulbar tracts to synapse directly with lower motor neurons or indirectly via interneurons) (see Chap. 21). Typical ALS is characterized by progressive loss of both categories of motor neurons, although variants may involve specific subsets of motor neurons, particularly early in the course of the illness. Thus, in *bulbar palsy* and *spinal muscular atrophy* (or progressive muscular atrophy), the lower motor neurons of brainstem and spinal cord, respectively, are most severely involved, whereas *pseudobulbar palsy* and *primary lateral sclerosis* affect predominantly upper motor neurons innervating the brainstem and spinal cord. The loss of motor neurons is not accompanied by any distinctive or unique cytopathologic features. The affected cells undergo shrinkage, often with some excessive accumulation of the pigmented lipid (lipofuscin) that normally develops in these cells with advancing age, and they eventually disappear. Focal enlargement of proximal motor axons is frequently seen; ultrastructurally, these "spheroids" are composed of accumulations of neurofilaments. Beyond some astroglial proliferation, which is the inevitable accompaniment of all degenerative processes in the central nervous system (CNS), the interstitial and supportive tissues and the macrophage system remain inactive, and there is no inflammation.

TABLE 372-1   Classification of motor neuron disorders

SPORADIC

Upper and lower motor neurons
   Amyotrophic lateral sclerosis
Predominantly upper motor neurons
   Primary lateral sclerosis
Predominantly lower motor neurons
   Multifocal motor neuropathy with conduction block
   Motor neuropathy with paraproteinemia
   Motor-predominant peripheral neuropathies
Other
   Associated with other degenerative disorders
      Olivopontocerebellar atrophy
      Azorean (Machado-Joseph) disease
   Secondary motor neuron disorders (see Table 372-2)

FAMILIAL

Familial amyotrophic lateral sclerosis
   Autosomal dominant
   Autosomal recessive (juvenile)
Spinal muscular atrophies
   SMA I: Infantile: Werdnig-Hoffman disease
   SMA II: Childhood onset
   SMA III: Adolescent onset: Wohlfart-Kugelberg-Welander disease
Familial spastic paraparesis (FSP)
   Familial HTLV-I myelopathy
   Isolated FSP
   Complicated FSP
Hereditary biochemical disorders
   Superoxide dismutase deficiency
   Hexosaminidase A and B deficiency
   Androgen receptor mutation (Kennedy's syndrome)
Miscellaneous
   Arthrogryposis multiplex congenita
   Progressive juvenile bulbar palsy (Fazio-Londe)

The death of the peripheral motor neurons in the brainstem and spinal cord leads to denervation and consequent atrophy of the corresponding muscle fibers. Histochemical and electrophysiologic evidence indicates that in the early phases of the illness denervated muscle may be reinnervated by sprouting of preserved nearby distal motor axon terminals, although reinnervation in this disease is less extensive than in other disorders affecting motor neurons (e.g., poliomyelitis, peripheral neuropathy). As denervation progresses, there is shrinkage of the musculature and muscle fiber atrophy. This muscular atrophy is designated *amyotrophy* in the name for the disease. The loss of upper motor neurons in the cortex results in disappearance of their long axons and myelin sheaths in the corticospinal and corticobulbar tracts (see Chap. 21). The loss of fibers in the corticospinal tracts of the spinal cord, together with the accompanying astrogliosis, imparts a firmness (sclerosis) to the spinal cord (lateral sclerosis). Nerve fiber loss is more extensive in the distal parts of the affected tracts in the lower spinal cord than in the more proximal parts, such as the internal capsule, suggesting that affected neurons undergo a process of "dying back." The disease clearly affects both large pyramidal neurons (Betz cells) of the motor cortex in the precentral gyrus and other long projection neurons involved in voluntary movement and located in the cerebral cortex and selected subcortical nuclei.

The remarkable selectivity of neuronal cell death entirely spares the sensory systems, the neural systems that control coordination of movement, and the components of the brain that are needed for cognition. However, immunostaining indicates that neurons bearing ubiquitin, a marker for degeneration, are also detected in nonmotor systems. Selectivity within the motor system is also seen; motor neurons required for ocular motility (oculomotor, trochlear, and abducens) remain unaffected, as do the parasympathetic neurons in the sacral spinal cord (the nucleus of Onufrowicz or Onuf) which innervate the sphincters of the bowel and bladder.

Clinical manifestations   The manifestations of motor neuron disease are variable depending on whether upper or lower motor neurons are more prominently involved. With lower motor neuron cell death and early denervation, the first evidence of the disease typically is insidiously developing asymmetric weakness, usually first evident distally in one of the limbs. A careful history will often disclose the recent development of cramping with volitional movements, typically in the early hours of the morning (e.g., while stretching in bed). Weakness caused by denervation is associated with progressive wasting and atrophy of muscles and, particularly early in the illness, spontaneous twitching of motor units, or *fasciculations*. In the hands, a preponderance of extensor over flexor weakness is very common. When the initial denervation involves bulbar rather than limb muscles, the first symptoms are difficulty with chewing, swallowing, and movements of the face and tongue. Early involvement of the muscles of respiration may lead to respiratory compromise before the disease is far advanced elsewhere.

With prominent corticospinal involvement, there is hyperactivity of the muscle stretch reflexes (tendon jerks) and, often, spastic resistance to passive movements of the affected limbs. The patient complains of muscle stiffness. Involvement of corticobulbar projections innervating the brainstem results in dysarthria and exaggeration of the motor expressions of emotion leading to involuntary weeping or laughing (*pseudobulbar affect*).

Virtually any muscle group may be the first to show signs of the disease, but as time passes, more and more muscles become involved, until ultimately the disorder takes on a symmetric distribution in all regions. It is characteristic of ALS that, regardless of whether the initial disease involves upper or lower motor neurons, both categories are eventually implicated. Indeed, in the absence of clear involvement of both types of motor neurons, the diagnosis of ALS is questionable. Even in the late stages of the illness, sensory, bowel and bladder, and cognitive functions are preserved. Dementia is not usually a component of ALS, although it may occur in a small subset of patients. Similarly, even when there is severe brainstem disease, ocular motility is spared until the very late stages of the illness.

The illness is relentlessly progressive, leading ultimately to death (usually from respiratory paralysis). In most large series, median survival is from 3 to 5 years. There are rare reports of stabilization or even regression of ALS.

Epidemiology   There are approximately 1 to 3 per 100,000 new cases and about 3 to 5 per 100,000 total cases per year in populations worldwide. Several endemic foci of higher prevalence are described in the western Pacific (e.g., in specific regions of Guam and Papua New Guinea). In the United States and Europe, it is agreed that males are somewhat more frequently affected than females. Although ALS is overwhelmingly a sporadic disorder, approximately 5 to 10 percent of cases are inherited as an autosomal dominant trait.

Differential diagnosis   Because ALS is currently untreatable, it is imperative that potentially remediable causes of motor neuron dysfunction be excluded (Table 372-2). Atypical features that should alert the physician include (1) restriction of disease to either upper or lower motor neurons, (2) involvement of neurons other than motor neurons, and (3) evidence of motor neuronal conduction block on electrophysiologic testing (see Chap. 366). *Compression of the cervical spinal cord* or *cervicomedullary junction* from tumors in the cervical spinal canal or at the foramen magnum or from cervical spondylosis with osteophytes can give rise to weakness, wasting, and fasciculations in the upper limbs and spasticity in the legs, thus closely resembling ALS. The absence of cranial nerve involvement may be helpful in differentiation, although some compressive lesions in the foramen magnum may implicate the twelfth cranial (hypoglossal) nerve as well, with weakness and atrophy of the tongue. Absence of pain or of sensory changes, normal function of bowel and bladder, normal imaging studies of the spine, and absence of changes in cerebrospinal fluid (CSF) all favor ALS rather than spinal cord compression. If doubt exists, magnetic resonance imaging (MRI) and contrast myelography should be performed to visualize the cervical spinal cord and the cervicomedullary junction.

Another entity in the differential diagnosis of ALS is multifocal *motor neuropathy with conduction block* (MMCB). In this disorder, lower motor neuron function is regionally and chronically disrupted

TABLE 372-2 Etiology and investigation of secondary motor neuron disorders

Diagnostic categories	Investigations
Structural lesions	MRI scan head (including
Parasagittal or foramen magnum	foramen magnum), cervical
tumors	spine
Cervical spondylosis	
Chiari malformation or syrinx	
Spinal cord arteriovenous	
malformation	
Infections	CSF examination, culture
Bacterial–tetanus, Lyme	Serum Lyme titers
Viral–poliomyelitis, herpes zoster	Antiviral antibody titers
Retroviral myelopathy	HTLV-I
Intoxications, physical agents	24-h urine for heavy metals;
Toxins–lead, aluminum, other	serum, urine for lead or
metals	aluminum
Drugs–strychnine, phenytoin	
Electric shock	
X-irradiation	
Immunologic mechanisms	Complete blood count,
Plasma cell dyscrasias	sedimentation rate,
Autoimmune	immunoprotein electrophoresis,
polyradiculoneuropathy	anti-G_{M1} antibodies
Paraneoplastic	Anti-Hu antibody, bone marrow
Paracarcinomatous	biopsy
Paralymphomatous	
Metabolic	Fasting blood sugar (FBS),
Hypoglycemia	routine chemistries, including
Hyperparathyroidism	calcium
Hyperthyroidism	Thyroid functions
Deficiency of folate, vitamins	Vitamin B_{12}, folate levels
B_{12}, E	
Malabsorption	24-h stool fat, carotene,
	prothrombin time
Hereditary biochemical disorders	
Superoxide dismutase	Red cell SOD1 deficiency
Androgen receptor defect	Abnormal –CAG– repeat insert
(Kennedy's disease)	
Hexosaminidase deficiency	Lysosomal enzyme screen
Infantile α-glucosidase deficiency	
(Pompe's disease)	
Hyperlipidemia	Lipid electrophoresis
Hyperglycinuria	Urine and serum amino acids

by remarkably focal blocks in nerve conduction. Many cases have associated elevations in serum titers of mono- and polyclonal antibodies to ganglioside G_{M1}; it is hypothesized that the antibodies may selectively produce focal, paranodal demyelination of motor neurons. MMCB is not typically associated with corticospinal signs. In contrast to ALS, MMCB may respond dramatically to intravenous gamma globulin or chemotherapy; it is thus imperative that MMCB be excluded when considering the diagnosis of ALS.

A diffuse *lower motor axonal neuropathy* mimicking ALS sometimes evolves as a component of hematopoietic disorders such as lymphoma. The underlying marrow pathology is often signaled by the presence of an M-component in serum, which, in this clinical setting, should prompt consideration of a bone marrow biopsy. Lyme disease also may cause an axonal lower motor neuropathy.

Other treatable disorders that occasionally can mimic ALS are *chronic lead poisoning* and *thyrotoxicosis*. These disorders may be suggested by the patient's social or occupational history or by unusual clinical features. When the family history is positive, *inherited enzyme disorders* such as hexosaminidase A or α-glucosidase deficiency must be excluded (see Chap. 349). These are readily identified by appropriate laboratory tests. *Benign fasciculations* are commonly a source of concern to the patient. On inspection, they may resemble the fascicular twitchings that accompany motor neuron degeneration. Absence of weakness, atrophy, or denervation on clinical and electrophysiologic examination excludes ALS or other serious neurologic disease. *Poliomyelitis* may lead to a delayed, progressive deterioration of motor neurons which presents clinically with progressive weakness, atrophy, and fasciculations. Its cause is unknown but is thought to reflect sublethal prior injury to motor neurons by poliovirus (see Chap. 375).

Rarely, ALS develops concurrently with features indicative of more widespread neurodegeneration. Thus otherwise typical ALS patients may present with a parkinsonian movement disorder or dementia. It remains unclear whether this reflects the unlikely simultaneous occurrence of two disorders or a primary defect triggering two forms of neurodegeneration. The latter is suggested by the observation that multisystem neurodegenerative diseases may be inherited; rare families are reported with ALS and parkinsonism or ALS and dementia with features of Pick's disease (see Chap. 371).

Familial ALS Several forms of motor neuron disease are inherited (see Table 372-1). Two disorders selectively involve corticospinal and lower motor neurons. The most common is familial ALS. Inherited as an autosomal dominant trait, it is clinically indistinguishable from sporadic ALS. Family linkage studies with DNA probes suggest that there is more than one gene for autosomal dominant ALS; one gene, superoxide dismutase, is on chromosome 21 (see also Chap. 364). There is also a recessive form of hereditary ALS. Unlike sporadic ALS, this begins in childhood and entails very prolonged survival; a locus for this disease has been genetically mapped to the long arm of chromosome 2. *Kennedy's syndrome* is another familial, adult-onset disorder that may mimic ALS (see below).

Treatment There is no treatment for ALS. However, several of the disorders listed in Table 372-2 which resemble ALS are treatable; for this reason, a careful search for such forms of secondary motor neuron disease is warranted. Recently, several motor neuron trophic factors have been cloned and biologically characterized; at least two, ciliary neurotrophic factor (CNTF) and insulin-like growth factor 1 (IGF-1), are in clinical trials in ALS. A variety of rehabilitative aids may substantially assist ALS patients. Foot-drop splints facilitate ambulation by avoiding tripping and by obviating excessive hip flexion. Finger-extension splints can potentiate grip. Respiratory support may be life-sustaining. For patients electing against long-term ventilation by tracheostomy, positive-pressure ventilation by mouth or nose may provide transient (several weeks) relief from hypercarbia and hypoxia.

OTHER LOWER MOTOR NEURON DISORDERS In the varieties of motor neuron disease grouped under this heading, the peripheral motor neurons are affected without evidence of involvement of the corticospinal motor system (Table 372-1).

X-linked spinobulbar muscular atrophy (Kennedy's disease) Kennedy's disease is an X-linked lower motor neuron disorder in which progressive weakness and wasting of limb and bulbar muscles begins in midadult life and is conjoined with androgen insensitivity manifested by gynecomastia and reduced fertility (see Chap. 339). A critical finding distinguishing this disorder from ALS is the absence of signs of hyperreflexia and spasticity. The molecular defect is an expanded trinucleotide repeat (–CAG–) in the first exon of the androgen receptor gene on the X chromosome; this abnormality is readily demonstrated on a small sample of DNA obtained from peripheral blood leukocytes. An inverse correlation appears to exist between the number of –CAG– repeats and the age of onset of the disease.

Adult Tay Sach's disease Hexosaminidase enzyme mutations may cause adult-onset, predominantly lower motor neuronopathies that closely mimic ALS. The condition is slowly progressive. Dysarthria and cerebellar atrophy may occur. The latter may be accompanied by signs of cerebellar incoordination. Rarely, spasticity also may be present (Chap. 349).

Spinal muscular atrophy The spinal muscular atrophies (SMA) are a group of familial disorders all associated with selective lower motor neuron diseases with early age of onset. Despite some phenotypic variability (largely in age of onset), the defect in the majority of families with SMA is genetically linked to a locus on the proximal long arm of chromosome 5 (see also Chap. 364). Each disorder is transmitted as an autosomal recessive trait. Neuropathologically, SMA is characterized by extensive loss of large motor neurons; biopsied muscle reveals evidence of denervation atrophy. *Infantile SMA (SMA I, Werdnig-Hoffmann disease)* has an early onset and is rapidly fatal. In some instances it is apparent even before birth, as indicated by decreased fetal movements late in the third trimester. Although alert, afflicted infants are weak and floppy (hypotonic) and lack muscle stretch reflexes. Death generally ensues within the first year of life. When the family history is unclear, it is difficult in the early weeks and months to distinguish SMA I from benign congenital hypotonia. An electromyogram is helpful by showing denervation, which does not occur in the congenital hypotonias. *Chronic childhood SMA (SMA II)* begins in childhood and progresses slowly. *Juvenile SMA (SMA III, Wohlfart-Kugelberg-Welander disease)* manifests during late childhood or early adolescence and runs a slow, indolent course. Unlike most denervating diseases, in this chronic disorder weakness is greatest in the proximal muscles; indeed, the pattern of weakness may suggest a primary myopathy such as limb girdle dystrophy (see Chap. 385). Electrophysiologic and muscle biopsy evidence of denervation distinguish SMA III from the myopathies.

Miscellaneous forms of lower motor neuron disease In individual families, other syndromes characterized by selective lower motor neuron dysfunction in an SMA-like pattern have been described. There are rare X-linked and autosomal dominant forms of SMA. There is also an ALS variant of juvenile onset, the Fazio-Londe syndrome, which involves mainly the musculature innervated by the brainstem. A component of lower motor neuron dysfunction is also found in some patients with multisystem degenerative disorders such as Machado-Joseph's disease and the related olivopontocerebellar degenerations (see below).

UPPER MOTOR NEURON DISORDERS   Primary lateral sclerosis (PLS) This exceedingly rare disorder arises sporadically in adults in middle to late life. It is characterized by progressive spastic weakness of the limbs, preceded or followed by spastic dysarthria and dysphagia, indicating combined involvement of the corticospinal and corticobulbar tracts. Fasciculations, amyotrophy, and sensory changes are absent; neither electromyography nor muscle biopsy show denervation. On neuropathologic examination there is selective loss of the large pyramidal cells in the precentral gyrus and degeneration of the corticospinal and corticobulbar projections. The lower motor neurons and other neuronal systems are spared. The course of PLS is variable; while long-term survival is documented, the course may be as aggressive as in ALS with approximately 3-year survival from onset to death. Early in its course, PLS raises the question of a diagnosis of multiple sclerosis or other demyelinating diseases such as adrenoleukodystrophy. A myelopathy suggestive of PLS occurs rarely with CNS infection with the retrovirus HTLV-I (see Chap. 375). The clinical course and laboratory testing will distinguish these possibilities. The myelopathy associated with HIV infection occasionally may cause spasticity without sensory changes.

Familial spastic paraplegia (FSP) This disorder is transmitted in most families as an autosomal dominant trait. It is characterized by progressive spastic weakness beginning in the distal lower extremities. It first causes symptoms in the third or fourth decades and typically has long survival with slow progression and with minimal involvement of the arms or of the respiratory musculature. Late in the illness there is commonly urinary urgency and incontinence, sometimes as well as fecal incontinence, but with preservation in males of sexual function. In pure forms of autosomal dominant FSP, ataxia, posterior column sensory loss, and amyotrophy are absent or minimal; however, in some patients, minor sensory changes (impaired vibration and position sense) may be observed in late stages. Mild involvement in some family members may be manifest only as spasticity without noticeable symptoms. Neuropathologically, FSP is associated with degeneration of the corticospinal tracts, which appear nearly normal in the brainstem but show increasing atrophy at more caudal levels in the spinal cord.

Rarely, patients with FSP have involvement of other regions of the nervous system, including lower motor neuron involvement (amyotrophy), mental retardation or mental retardation with skin thickening, optic atrophy, and sensory neuropathy (see review by Harding). In some cases, there is loss of fibers in the ascending posterior columns and the spinocerebellar tracts, features reminiscent of Friedreich's ataxia. These complicated forms of FSP emphasize the challenge inherent in classifying the neurodegenerative disorders until the precise genetic abnormalities are identified; there may be considerable overlap of the clinical phenotypes in diseases otherwise classified as distinct.

MUSCULAR WEAKNESS AND WASTING ASSOCIATED WITH SENSORY CHANGES

PROGRESSIVE NEURAL MUSCULAR ATROPHY Degenerative disorders characterized by progressive weakness and wasting of skeletal muscles combined with sensory changes are usually due to chronic diseases of peripheral nerves; many are hereditary. The most frequent form of hereditary peripheral neuropathy is Charcot-Marie-Tooth (CMT) disease. In its usual form, it occurs as a dominantly inherited demyelinating neuropathy with striking motor and sensory findings on physical examination and slowing of conduction on electrophysiologic studies (see Chap. 383). Many families with dominant CMT show linkage to a duplicated locus on chromosome 17p11.2 containing a gene for a peripheral myelin protein. Some variants of CMT are recessively inherited and predominantly axonal with corresponding motor neuron manifestations. Such cases can be impossible to distinguish from true lower motor neuronopathies on clinical grounds; genetic studies linking affected individuals to known SMA (chromosome 5q) or CMT (e.g., chromosome 17p, chromosome 1, or X) loci may distinguish these entities. Similarly, some forms of Friedreich's ataxia and adrenomyeloneuropathy may have prominent lower motor neuron signs; usually either genetic, radiographic, or biochemical studies will distinguish these from isolated lower motor neuropathy syndromes.

SYNDROMES OF PROGRESSIVE VISUAL LOSS Some neurodegenerative disorders are accompanied by concomitant impairment of the visual system. Thus, in Friedreich's ataxia, there may be slowing of conduction in the optic nerves. Two broad categories of visual pathology have been described: selective degeneration of retinal ganglion cells with secondary optic atrophy and a more diffuse degeneration involving all retinal components. The latter entails subsequent migration of melanin-containing cells of the pigment epithelium into the superficial retinal layers, resulting in pigmentary degeneration of the retina. Historically, this has been described as "retinitis pigmentosa," a misnomer because there is no inflammation within the retina. Some disorders causing retinitis pigmentosa are now documented to arise from genetic defects in mitochondrial DNA or in autosomal genes encoding mitochondrial proteins (see Chap. 385). An important implication of these findings, as yet not firmly established, is that mitochondrial lesions may be implicated in the associated neurodegenerative sensory and motor syndromes. Other inherited forms of retinitis pigmentosa are due to mutations in the photoreceptor rhodopsin (see Chaps. 19 and 364).

THE HEREDITARY ATAXIAS

These conditions present with progressive unsteadiness in standing and walking, along with impaired coordination of the limbs. In the pediatric age group, such conditions are often associated with metabolic disturbances that may give rise to either remitting or chronic progressive imbalance. A detailed review of these metabolic disorders is beyond the scope of this chapter, but an outline of the major entities is included in Table 372-3. In adults, the major diseases of progressive unsteadiness are characterized pathologically by degeneration of the cerebellum and/or its related fiber systems and thus constitute classic examples of the system degenerations. Although sporadic instances occur, hereditary transmission is the outstanding feature in most cases. Accordingly, this group of disorders is often referred to as the *hereditary ataxias*. As with other neurodegenerative disorders, it has

TABLE 372-3 Selected major syndromes of progressive ataxia in adults

INHERITED DEGENERATIVE DISORDERS

Disease	Chromosome
Friedreich's ataxia	9q13-21
Spinocerebellar atrophy 1	6p22-23
Spinocerebellar atrophy 2	12q23-24
Spinocerebellar atrophy 3	Unknown
Machado-Joseph disease	14q24.3-31
Ataxia with vitamin E deficiency	8q

SYSTEMIC DISORDERS

Metabolic disorders
  Mitochondrial disorders
  Abnormal amino and organic acid metabolism
  Urea cycle defects
  Vitamin and cofactor deficiencies
  Enzyme defects
    Hexosaminidase deficiency
    Gamma-glutamyl cysteine synthetase deficiency
    Glutamate dehydrogenase deficiency
  Lipid metabolism disorders
    A- and hypobetalipoproteinemia
    Refsum's disease
    Cerebrotendinous xanthomatosis
DNA repair defects
  Ataxia telangiectasia
  Xeroderma pigmentosum
Inflammatory autoimmune disorders
  Paraneoplastic cerebellar degeneration
  Multiple sclerosis and related disorders
Infections
  Prion or "slow-viral" infection
  Postinfectious cerebellar inflammation

OTHER

Post-hyperthermia
Post-anoxia
Drug-induced disorders
  Phenytoin
  Chronic ethanol abuse
Structural lesions
  Posterior fossa tumors
  Hydrocephalus

proved difficult to devise an absolute classification scheme for these diseases based either on their clinical presentation or on neuropathologic findings. Nonetheless, the following clinicopathologic subdivision of the adult ataxic diseases is useful: (1) cerebellar cortical degeneration, (2) olivopontocerebellar atrophy, and (3) spinocerebellar degenerations, including Friedreich's ataxia.

CEREBELLAR CORTICAL DEGENERATION The principal neuropathologic finding in this disorder is loss of neurons (mainly Purkinje cells) in the cerebellar cortex. The onset of symptoms usually occurs in late adult life. In the majority of patients it is inherited as an autosomal dominant trait, although apparently sporadic cases have been described.

Pathology The loss of Purkinje cells is usually most severe in the superior vermis and adjacent parts of the cerebellar cortex but can be more widely distributed. The granule layer neurons are less affected. In long-standing cases, there is an associated atrophy of neurons in the olivary nuclei of the medulla, apparently representing a transsynaptic retrograde degeneration resulting from the loss of Purkinje cells, to which the olivocerebellar fibers project. In advanced cases, atrophy of the cerebellar cortex can be readily demonstrated by computed tomographic (CT) or MRI scanning. In the purest forms of this disorder, as exemplified by the cases of late onset, slow progression, and dominant inheritance, other neuronal systems remain relatively intact.

Clinical manifestations Incoordination first appears in the legs, resulting in abnormal stance and an unsteady, wavering, lurching gait typical of cerebellar ataxia (see Chap. 22). This gait disturbance is a consequence of degenerative changes in the superior vermis of the cerebellum and adjacent parts of the cerebellar cortex. With more extensive cerebellar involvement, a disturbance in articulation and rhythm of speech occurs, and the arms also become ataxic. There may be nystagmus. The illness progresses gradually, often extending over two or three decades, without appreciably curtailing the life span. Dementia may occur, but it tends to be mild or is a late feature. Cerebellar cortical degeneration with similar features may occur as a component of other ataxic disorders.

In addition to this slowly evolving cerebellar cortical degeneration, there is a subacute diffuse cerebellar cortical degeneration that affects all parts of the cerebellar cortex indiscriminately, often in association with inflammatory changes. This disorder occurs in the presence of malignant neoplastic diseases of various kinds and is referred to as *subacute cortical cerebellar degeneration* (see Chap. 328). This is one of several paraneoplastic neurologic degenerative syndromes that result from an indirect effect of the neoplasm on the CNS.

OLIVOPONTOCEREBELLAR ATROPHY (OPCA) Grouped under this category are a number of similar disorders characterized by a combination of cerebellar cortical degeneration, atrophy of the inferior olivary nuclei secondary to this, and degeneration and disappearance of neurons of the pontine nuclei and their fiber projections in the basis pontis and middle cerebellar peduncles. Five subtypes have been described on the basis of differences in hereditary transmission and in the extent of other abnormalities both within and outside the nervous system. Most instances of OPCA can now be considered to represent a form of multiple system degeneration in which admixtures of parkinsonism, dementia, spasticity, choreoathetosis, retinal degeneration, myelopathy, and peripheral neuropathy may be encountered, these associated findings sometimes obscuring the ataxic component.

Pathology The variants of OPCA provide yet another example of selective premature neuronal death, affecting vulnerable neuronal systems while sparing others. It is not certain what pathologic change results in the dementia that so often accompanies them. It has been generally assumed that abnormalities occur in the cerebral cortex, but examination in typical cases fails to disclose sufficient abnormalities to account for the cognitive and behavioral alterations. The lesions in the basal ganglia and substantia nigra (equivalent to striatonigral degeneration) underlie the features of parkinsonism and of other postural movement disorders that are so frequently seen as manifestations of OPCA. Involvement of the peripheral motor neurons, similar to that encountered in motor neuron diseases, produces the muscular weakness and atrophy that may be encountered. The site of degeneration that leads to the disturbances of ocular motility that typify some cases has not been elucidated.

Clinical manifestations There is considerable variation in the clinical findings of OPCA. Some patients present with a picture of a relatively pure cerebellar ataxia indistinguishable from that seen in patients with atrophy of the cerebellar cortex. Others are characterized by parkinsonian features. Superimposed is an evolving dementia. Accounts of the varied forms of clinical expression can be found in the monographs by Duvoisin and Plaitakis and by Harding.

Genetics and pathogenesis Autosomal dominant inheritance is characteristic in many families. Genetic linkage analysis has localized the mutant gene to the short arm of chromosome 6 in several large families [spinocerebellar atrophy type 1 (SCA1)]. In a large Cuban family, the disease was linked to chromosome 12q23-24 (SCA2). The defect in SCA1 is an expanded -CAG- repeat in a gene expressed in muscle, brain, and other tissues. The function of the protein encoded by this gene has not been fully defined. Data indicate that in some forms of OPCA there may be a reduction in levels of glutamic acid dehydrogenase (GDH) as assayed in fibroblasts and leukocytes. This occurs either as a sporadic disorder or on a familial basis with either dominant or recessive inheritance. The dominant GDH deficiency cases are often of childhood onset with clinical features resembling other types of OPCA. Peripheral neuropathy and slowed saccadic eye movements may be prominent. The observation of GDH deficiency in OPCA has led to the hypothesis that the loss of Purkinje cells and other neurons may be a consequence of elevated levels of glutamate. The possibility that mitochondrial function is deranged in OPCA is supported by reports of individuals with mitochondrial complex I deficiency or myoclonic epilepsy with ragged red fibers (MERRF) who develop degeneration of selected populations of olivary, pontine, dentate, and other neurons with associated long tract (spinocerebellar, posterior column, corticospinal) degeneration. While these features are reminiscent of pathologic findings in OPCA (see below), a specific biochemical defect has yet to be delineated for any form of OPCA or indeed any of the progressive ataxias.

SPINOCEREBELLAR DEGENERATION (FRIEDREICH'S ATAXIA)

This group of ataxic disorders is characterized by degeneration of long ascending and descending fiber systems in the spinal cord, including the spinocerebellar tracts, and concomitant degeneration of peripheral axons and myelin sheaths in the form of chronic peripheral neuronopathy. There is considerable overlap in the clinical and neuropathologic findings of the spinocerebellar and OPCA disorders. The principal clinical feature justifying separation of these groups is the relative sparing of brainstem function in the spinocerebellar disorders. The classic form of hereditary spinocerebellar ataxia is Friedreich's disease, usually inherited as an autosomal recessive trait. First depicted by Nikolaus Friedreich in 1863, it constitutes a relatively distinct symptom complex that generally is inherited in a phenotypically recognized form. In some families, the disorder occurs with dominant inheritance. Recent studies have linked the recessive form of the disease to the long arm of chromosome 9; a specific gene has not been identified (see Chap. 364).

Pathology The principal changes are cell loss in the dorsal root ganglia and secondary degeneration in the posterior columns and spinocerebellar tracts of the cord and in peripheral nerves. Degeneration is also evident in the corticospinal tracts in most cases. The cerebellum is variably affected. In addition to these neuropathologic changes, there occurs in some cases a peculiar form of cardiomyopathy resulting in muscle fiber loss and fibrosis. There are no other associated visceral lesions.

Clinical manifestations As with other progressive ataxias, the disorder first appears in the legs, affecting the individual during late childhood. The patient begins to stagger and lurch in walking and is unsteady on standing. Clumsiness and cerebellar tremor of the hands and arms appear later along with dysarthria and an abnormal rhythm (scanning) of speech. These symptoms result from changes in the dorsal root ganglia, the spinocerebellar tracts, and the cerebellum. The limbs, in addition to being ataxic, generally show considerable weakness. Examination usually discloses nystagmus and skeletal deformities such as kyphoscoliosis, the basis of which is not certain, and a peculiar foreshortening of the feet (pes cavus) with cocking of the toes, best ascribed to atrophy and contractures of the musculature of the feet at a time when the bones of the feet are malleable. Typically, there is an unusual combination of total absence of tendon reflexes with extensor plantar reflexes (Babinski sign). This results from the degeneration of the corticospinal tracts together with the involvement of peripheral sensory neurons that relay afferent signals from muscle spindles. Impairment of position and vibration sense in the extremities is prominent, and in some patients, sensation of pain, temperature, and light touch is diminished in a distal and roughly symmetric distribution consistent with an axonal neuropathy affecting small nerve fibers. Mentation is usually preserved, though a few patients have been of low intelligence or have become demented late in the course of the disease. Survival beyond early adult life is rare, with death frequently the result of associated cardiomyopathy. Survival is somewhat better in families with the dominantly inherited forms of the illness.

Occasionally, mild or fragmentary forms of the disorder (such as pes cavus and absent or hyperactive tendon reflexes) may be encountered with little, if any, disability or progression. Such abnormalities are most likely to be seen in other members of the family of a patient afflicted with the fully developed form of the disease. A related

syndrome, the Roussy-Levy syndrome, shows similarities to Friedreich's ataxia and to peroneal muscular atrophy. Mild ataxia, pes cavus, absent ankle and knee tendon jerks, and atrophy of lower leg muscles occur. In some well-documented cases, the peripheral nerves show hypertrophy due to proliferation of Schwann cells (see Chap. 383). Chronic familial polyneuropathies are particularly difficult to distinguish because they also give rise to sensory ataxia (see Chap. 383). Hereditary forms of ataxia with corticospinal signs (hyperactive tendon reflexes) and sensory disturbances are also known to occur in the adolescent or adult. Familial spastic paraplegia with or without optic atrophy (Behr's syndrome) is another closely related disease. In the absence of a family history and with atypical clinical findings, further diagnostic studies are necessary to exclude congenital malformation, spinal cord compression, foramen magnum tumor, and multiple sclerosis.

Treatment No treatment is of proven value. Because the myocardium may be involved, regular evaluation of cardiac function is prudent.

DIFFERENTIAL DIAGNOSIS OF THE ATAXIAS The slow but relentless progression in the absence of abnormalities in other parts of the nervous system and in the CSF distinguishes the hereditary group from other diseases and other forms of cerebellar ataxia such as may occur with hereditary metabolic diseases, with neoplastic, infectious, or demyelinative disease, or with drug intoxication (e.g., phenytoin) or hyperpyrexia. The degenerative disorders under discussion tend to develop slowly over many years in a setting of otherwise good general health and in the absence of other neurologic symptoms and signs; this, together with the other clinical differences, distinguishes them from such hereditary metabolic diseases as juvenile Gaucher's disease, juvenile Niemann-Pick disease, juvenile hexosaminidase deficiency, and alcoholic cerebellar ataxia or nutritional deficiency disease with or without Wernicke-Korsakoff syndrome. Alcoholic cerebellar degeneration usually develops over a few days to weeks and then may remain more or less unchanged (see Chap. 377). A prolonged deficiency of vitamin E, sometimes arising as an inherited defect, can result in progressive ataxia, incoordination of the limbs, areflexia, and distal loss of proprioception and vibratory sense, mimicking the spinocerebellar degeneration of Friedreich's ataxia (see Chap. 377). Most cases are associated with fat malabsorption.

In the cases associated with carcinoma, the tempo of evolution of the process is relatively rapid, with severe disability coming on within a period of months. Vertigo, diplopia, and nausea may be prominent. In an occasional patient, the neurologic symptoms appear before any evidence of carcinoma. Opsoclonus (rapid side-to-side jerking of the eyes) and oscillopsia (rhythmic movement back and forth of perceived objects) may be conjoined (see Chap. 328). In contrast to the consistently normal CSF findings in the forms of cerebellar degeneration noted above, the CSF in paraneoplastic degeneration may show increased lymphocytes and elevated protein. Finally, the serum and CSF in patients with paracarcinomatous cerebellar degeneration may have high titers of antibodies seen specifically in the paraneoplastic syndromes (e.g., anti-Hu and anti-Yo) (see Chap. 328).

A dominantly inherited, progressive ataxia termed *Machado-Joseph* or *Azorean disease* occurs in Portuguese families of Azorean descent and is linked to a marker on chromosome 14q. This adult-onset disorder shows considerable clinical variability. Its central characteristic is progressive ataxia with eye movement weakness, nystagmus, and eyelid retraction resulting in a prominent stare. Additionally, early-onset patients have a more rapid course with superimposed pyramidal (spasticity) and extrapyramidal (dystonia and rigidity) manifestations. Late-onset patients may show distal amyotrophy and neuropathic sensory loss in addition to the ataxia and eye movement abnormalities. In all ages, memory and cognition are usually spared. Pathologic studies document that this is a multisystem degenerative disorder with features overlapping both the olivopontocerebellar and the spinocerebellar degenerations. There is degeneration of the spinocerebellar tracts and Clarke's columns and loss of brainstem (vestibular nuclei, pontine, dentate nucleus) and spinal motor neurons. Cerebellar Purkinje neurons are spared. The genetic basis for Machado-Joseph disease remains unclear; it is linked to chromosome 14q24 and thus is distinct from SCA1, ataxia with vitamin E deficiency, Friedreich's ataxia, and SCA2, respectively, at loci on chromosomes 6, 8, 9, and 12. It also has been established that Machado-Joseph disease is not an allelic form of Huntington's disease.

NEURODEGENERATIVE DISORDERS ASSOCIATED WITH AUTONOMIC FAILURE (SHY-DRAGER SYNDROME)

Abnormalities of central autonomic nervous system functions, manifest principally by failure to maintain blood pressure and by urinary incontinence, are now recognized to be caused in some cases by a progressive degenerative disorder of the CNS that affects several systems (see Chap. 379). In some patients, the peripheral nervous system is also involved (postganglionic sympathetic neurons). Bradbury and Eggleston in 1925 called attention to the combination of postural hypotension, incontinence, impotence, and abnormality of sweating (anhidrosis). Symptoms of central neurologic origin develop later in many of these patients, consisting predominantly of extrapyramidal or cerebellar dysfunction.

Pathogenesis and pathology The cause of the disorder is unknown. In 1960, Shy and Drager described neuropathologic changes in the brainstem and basal ganglia, and subsequently, others showed a prominent loss of neurons in central regions of the autonomic nervous system, affecting in particular the cells of the intermediolateral column of the thoracic spinal cord. Abnormalities also have been found in peripheral autonomic ganglia (cell loss). In the brainstem and basal ganglia there is widespread symmetric neuronal degeneration affecting the caudate nucleus, substantia nigra, locus coeruleus, olivary nuclei, dorsal vagal nuclei, and, in some cases, the cerebellum. Cell loss is accompanied by gliosis; Lewy bodies typical of Parkinson's disease are present in some cases. For these reasons, many neurologists consider the Shy-Drager syndrome to be a unique form of multisystem degeneration resembling but distinct from either Parkinson's disease or OPCA.

Clinical manifestations The onset is insidious, usually in the sixth or seventh decade. Men are more frequently affected than women. Disturbances of urinary bladder function, including hesitancy and incontinence, postural dizziness and syncope, impotence, and decreased sweating are the presenting manifestations. Symptoms of extrapyramidal dysfunction resembling parkinsonian or cerebellar findings may emerge. The condition becomes severely disabling over the course of 5 to 7 years in most patients. The hallmark of the condition is postural hypotension, defined as a fall in blood pressure greater than 30/20 mmHg on standing upright from a supine position (see Chap. 379). Despite this fall in blood pressure, there is usually a total failure of compensatory tachycardia; the pulse rate fails to change. Autonomic signs of pupillary asymmetry, partial Horner's syndrome, or partial parasympathetic denervation occur in some patients. Anhidrosis is common and can be demonstrated by placing the individual in a warm room after application of a starch-iodine mixture to the skin. The parkinsonian manifestations may be identical to those of idiopathic parkinsonism, although in many patients rigidity and bradykinesia are more prominent than tremor. Cerebellar gait ataxia may be evident. Other findings include laryngeal paralysis and sleep apnea, which may herald the onset of the disease. MRI may demonstrate T2-weighted signal hypointensity in the putamen, globus pallidum, and substantia nigra. Positron emission tomography shows decreased uptake of dopamine derivatives in the putamen and caudate, probably reflecting a loss of nigrostriatal dopaminergic neurons.

Treatment The treatment is symptomatic. The postural hypotension is usually the most disabling initial symptom. Antigravity stockings to minimize pooling of venous blood in the legs are recommended. A leotard that covers the lower abdomen may provide additional benefit. Pharmacologic agents are given to expand blood volume and enhance vascular responsivity. Increased NaCl intake combined with fludrohydrocortisone, 0.05 to 0.2 mg twice daily, is usually beneficial (see Chap 379). In severe cases, adrenergic drugs such as ephedrine, levodopa, or amphetamine may improve the disability. The parkinsonian symptoms often respond initially to Sinemet or bromocriptine, but later in the course most patients become refractory to these agents. Centrally acting alpha agonists (e.g., yohimbine or clonidine or the investigational drug xamoterol) also may be beneficial.

REFERENCES

Motor neuron diseases

BRZUSTOWICZ LM et al: Genetic mapping of chronic childhood-onset spinal muscular atrophy to chromosome 5q11.2–13.3. Nature 344:540, 1990

DALAKAS M, ILLA I: Post-polio syndrome: Concepts in clinical diagnosis, pathogenesis, and etiology. Adv Neurol 56:495, 1991

LA SPADA AR et al: Androgen receptor gene mutations in X-linked spinal muscular atrophy. Nature 352:77, 1991

MUNSAT TL: Poliomyelitis—New problems with an old disease. N Engl J Med 324:1206, 1991

PRADAS J et al: The natural history of amyotrophic lateral sclerosis and the use of natural history controls in therapeutic trials. Neurology 43:751, 1993

ROSEN DR et al: Association of mutations in Cu/Zn cytosolic superoxide dismutase with familial amyotrophic lateral sclerosis. Nature 362:59, 1993

ROWLAND LP (ed): *Advances in Neurology*, vol. 56: *Amyotrophic Lateral Sclerosis and Other Motor Neuron Diseases*. New York, Raven, 1991

SIDDIQUE TS et al: Linkage of a gene causing familial amyotrophic lateral sclerosis to chromosome 21 and evidence of genetic locus heterogeneity. N Engl J Med 324:1381, 1991

SMITH RA (ed): *Handbook of Amyotrophic Lateral Sclerosis*. New York, Marcel Dekker, 1992

Progressive ataxias

CARSON WJ et al: The Machado-Joseph disease locus is different from the spinocerebellar ataxia locus (SCA1). Genomics 13:852, 1992

DUVOISIN RC, PLAITAKIS A (eds): *Advances in Neurology*, vol. 41: *The Olivopontocerebellar Atrophies*. New York, Raven Press, 1984

GILMAN S et al: *Disorders of the Cerebellum*. Philadelphia, Davis, 1981

GISPERT S et al: Chromosomal assignment of the second locus for autosomal dominant cerebellar ataxia (SCA2) to human chromosome 12q23-24.1. Nature Genet 4:295, 1993

HARDING AE: *The Hereditary Ataxias and Related Diseases*. London, Churchill Livingstone, 1984

KAGEYAMA Y et al: An autopsy case of mitochondrial encephalomyopathy with prominent degeneration in olivo-ponto-cerebellar system. Acta Neuropathol 83:99, 1991

KEATS BJ et al: "Acadian" and "classical" forms of Friedreich ataxia are most probably caused by mutations at the same locus. Am J Med Genet 33:266, 1989

KONIGSMARK BW, WEINER LP: The olivopontocerebellar atrophies: A review. Medicine 49:227, 1970

PLAITAKIS A: Olivopontocerebellar atrophy with glutamate dehydrogenase deficiency, in *Handbook of Clinical Neurology*, vol 16: *Hereditary Neuropathies and Spinal Ataxias*, JMBV de Jong (ed). New York, Elsevier Science Publishers, 1991, p 551

RANUM LP et al: Autosomal dominant spinocerebellar ataxia: Locus heterogeneity in a Nebraska kindred. Neurology 42:344, 1992

SUDARSKY L et al: Machado-Joseph disease in New England: Clinical description and distinction from the olivopontocerebellar atrophies. Mov Disord 7:204, 1992.

TAKIYAMA Y et al: The gene for Machado-Joseph disease maps to human chromosome 14q. Nature Genet 4:300, 1993

Miscellaneous

BROOKS DJ et al: The relationship between locomotor disability, autonomic dysfunction, and the integrity of the striatal dopaminergic system in patients with multiple system atrophy, pure autonomic failure, and Parkinson's disease, studied with PET. Brain 113:1539, 1990

LUPSKI JR et al: DNA duplication associated with Charcot-Marie-Tooth disease type IA. Cell 66:219, 1991

MCLEOD JG, TUCK RR: Disorders of the autonomic nervous system: 2. Investigation and treatment. Ann Neurol 21:519, 1987

OBARA A et al: Effect of xamoterol on Shy-Drager syndrome. Circulation 85:606, 1992

SANDRONI P et al: Autonomic involvement in extrapyramidal and cerebellar disorders. Clin Auton Res 1:147, 1991

373 MULTIPLE SCLEROSIS AND OTHER DEMYELINATING DISEASES

STEPHEN L. HAUSER

The demyelinating diseases occupy a unique place in neurology, arising from their frequency and tendency to strike young adults, the diversity of manifestations that challenge the most skilled clinician, and the range of fundamental questions in neurobiology, immunology, virology, and genetics that arise regarding their pathogenesis. These disorders share the common feature of inflammation and selective destruction of central nervous system (CNS) myelin. Their course may be chronic (multiple sclerosis) or acute (acute disseminated encephalomyelitis and acute hemorrhagic leukoencephalitis). The peripheral nervous system (PNS) is generally spared. No specific tests for the demyelinating diseases exist, and diagnosis is based on recognition of the distinctive clinical patterns of CNS injury they produce.

MULTIPLE SCLEROSIS

Multiple sclerosis (MS) is characterized by chronic inflammation, demyelination, and gliosis (scarring). Lesions of MS are classically said to be disseminated in time and space. MS affects 350,000 Americans and is, with the exception of trauma, the most frequent cause of neurologic disability in early to middle adulthood. Indirect evidence supports an autoimmune etiology for MS, perhaps triggered by a viral infection in a genetically susceptible host. As in other chronic inflammatory disorders, the manifestations of MS are variable and range from a benign illness to a rapidly evolving and incapacitating disease. Complications from MS may affect multiple body systems and may require profound adjustments in life-style and goals for patients and their families; hence a multidisciplinary approach is necessary to optimize clinical care.

PATHOLOGIC FEATURES MS derives its name from the multiple scarred areas visible on macroscopic examination of the brain. These lesions, termed *plaques*, are well-demarcated gray or pink areas easily distinguished from surrounding white matter. Occasionally, plaques are also present in gray matter. Plaques vary in size from 1 or 2 mm to several centimeters. The acute MS lesion, rarely found at autopsy, is characterized by perivenular cuffing and tissue infiltration by mononuclear cells, predominantly T lymphocytes and macrophages, and by demyelination. B cells and plasma cells are rarely found. The inflammatory infiltrates appear to mediate the loss of myelin sheaths that surround axis cylinders. As the lesion progresses, large numbers of macrophages and microglial cells (specialized CNS phagocytes of bone marrow origin) scavenge the myelin debris, and proliferation of astrocytes (gliosis) occurs. Proliferation of oligodendrocytes, the myelin-producing cells, is also present initially, but these cells appear to be destroyed as the infiltration and gliosis progress. Gliosis is more severe in MS lesions than in most other neuropathologic conditions. In chronic MS lesions, complete or nearly complete demyelination, dense gliosis, and loss of oligodendroglia are present. In some plaques (chronic active lesions), gradations in histologic findings from the center to the lesion edge suggest that lesions expand by concentric outward growth.

Lesions of MS are typically more numerous than anticipated on the basis of clinical criteria. Selective demyelination with sparing of axon cylinders is the hallmark of the disease, yet partial or total axonal destruction, and in extreme cases cavitation, may occur. Although partial remyelination (shadow plaques) is occasionally present, in most lesions significant remyelination does not occur. The correlation of plaque number and size with clinical symptoms is poor.

Hence an extensive plaque burden may be associated with only mild symptoms, or conversely, minor pathologic findings may be present in some individuals severely disabled during life. Approximately 35 percent of cases are clinically silent with evidence of MS only at autopsy.

PATHOPHYSIOLOGY AND PATHOGENESIS Pathophysiology Experimental studies indicate that demyelination may result in either negative or positive effects on axonal conduction. *Negative conduction abnormalities* consist of slowed axonal conduction, variable conduction block that occurs in the presence of high- but not low-frequency trains of impulses, or complete conduction block. Conduction block in demyelinated fibers also may occur in response to raised temperature or with metabolic changes in the extracellular milieu of axons. *Positive conduction abnormalities* include ectopic impulse generation, spontaneously or following mechanical stress, and abnormal "crosstalk" between demyelinated axons. While the degree to which these negative and positive changes occur in MS is unknown, their presence may explain several characteristics of the disease. For example, conduction block may account for the fluctuations in function that vary from hour to hour and from day to day in MS and for the worsening that follows elevation in core body temperature. Ectopic impulse generation or "crosstalk" might give rise to Lhermitte's symptom, paroxysmal symptoms, or parasthesias (see below). Experimental therapies based on postulated conduction abnormalities in MS have included the use of calcium blockers to reduce the threshold for impulse generation and pharmacologic blockage of voltage-dependent potassium channels (4-aminopyridine) that are exposed in the internodal axon membrane following myelin loss.

Epidemiology MS is approximately twofold more common in females than in males. MS is unusual before adolescence, then rises steadily in incidence from the teens to age 35, and declines gradually thereafter. There is a slightly later age of onset in men than in women. MS beginning as early as age 2 or as late as age 74 is rare but well documented.

Marked differences in the prevalence of MS exist between different populations and ethnic groups. The highest known prevalence (250 per 100,000) occurs in the Orkney islands, located north of the mainland of Scotland, and MS is also common in Scandinavia and throughout northern Europe. In the United States, the prevalence of MS is higher in Caucasians than in other racial groups, consistent with observations in other parts of the world. MS is extremely rare in Japan (2 per 100,000) and is essentially unknown in black Africa, yet Japanese-Americans and black Americans are at significant risk for MS, with respective prevalence rates estimated at one-quarter and one-third that of Caucasian Americans.

MS is in general a disease of temperate climates. In both hemispheres, its prevalence decreases with decreasing latitude. Comparison of North American and European populations indicates that similar prevalence rates and north-south gradients are observed. Migration data in well-defined ethnic populations also support an effect of environment on risk. Children born to parents who have migrated from a high-risk to a low-risk area for MS have a lower lifetime risk than their parents. Conversely, migration from a low-risk to a high-risk area confers an increased risk for MS in the children. Some migration studies, notably those from South Africa and Israel, suggest that a critical environmental exposure in MS occurs prior to the age of 15 years, but these data are based on small numbers of individuals who have migrated at different ages. Other evidence for an environmental effect on MS is derived from apparent point epidemics that have occurred, e.g., the cluster of MS that appeared in the Faroe Islands off the coast of Denmark following the British occupation during World War II.

Genetics Compelling data indicate that susceptibility to MS is inherited. Familial aggregation is known to occur, and first-, second-, and third-degree relatives of patients are at increased risk for the disease. Siblings of MS patients have a 2 to 5 percent lifetime risk for MS, whereas the risk to parents or children of patients is somewhat lower. Concordance of MS is also increased in monozygotic compared with dizygotic twins. The risk of MS to a monozygotic twin of an MS patient is approximately 30 percent, whereas the risk to a dizygotic twin approximates the risk to a nontwin sibling.

Pedigree study of multiple-affected-member families is consistent with the hypothesis that multiple unlinked genes confer susceptibility. Genetic heterogeneity, i.e., independent major genes, also may be present in MS. The major histocompatibility complex (MHC) on chromosome 6 has been identified as one genetic determinant for MS. This complex encodes genes for the histocompatibility antigens (the HLA system) that serve in the context of antigen presentation to T cells. Linkage disequilibrium studies suggest that MS susceptibility is linked to the class II (DR, DQ, and DP) region of the MHC. The DR2(15) DQw1 haplotype is common in Caucasian populations at risk for MS, and some family studies support a genetic effect of the DR2-bearing haplotype on susceptibility. Other HLA haplotypes may be associated with MS in other ethnic populations, but family studies supporting their role have been negative or are lacking. The MHC locus contributes only a small fraction to the genetic effect on MS. Other studies have implicated a role for other genes in MS, including T cell receptor, immunoglobulin heavy chain, and MBP genes.

Immunology Attention has focused on the role of thymus-derived or T lymphocytes in the pathogenesis of MS. T cells reactive against myelin proteins, either myelin basic protein (MBP) or myelin proteolipid protein (PLP), mediate CNS inflammation in experimental allergic encephalomyelitis (EAE), a laboratory model for demyelinating diseases. This has been proven by adoptive transfer experiments in which sensitized T cells from an animal with EAE can transfer disease to a healthy syngeneic recipient. EAE is induced in genetically susceptible animals by immunization with CNS tissue homogenized in an adjuvent. Chronic relapsing/remitting forms of EAE have been described that pathologically resemble human MS. Occasional laboratory accidents have resulted in human inoculation with an EAE homogenate that was followed by development of an acute EAE-like illness, indicating that humans are also susceptible.

Evidence that myelin-reactive T cells play a role in MS is only indirect. The frequency of MBP-reactive T cells appears to be increased in peripheral blood of patients, and such cells carry a high frequency of mutations, indicating that they may have undergone chronic stimulation in vivo. Perhaps more significant, T cells reactive against MBP and PLP are concentrated in CSF in MS compared with their frequency in peripheral blood.

One remarkable feature of the T cell response to MBP in EAE concerns the repertoire of antigen receptor molecules that are present on disease-inducing (encephalitogenic) cells. In rodents, a restricted number of different families of T cell receptor (TCR) genes are expressed by encephalitogenic T cells, and if these cells are removed or rendered inactive, the animal is protected from EAE. This has been accomplished both by passive and active immunization against these families of TCR genes. The majority of T cells do not express TCR genes that are targeted by therapy; hence cellular immunity is preserved and selective immunotherapy achieved. In MS patients, analysis of the T cell response to MBP has revealed that similar restrictions of the T cell repertoire occur in some individuals, although the identity of the TCR genes appears to differ between different patients. Thus specific therapy against MBP-reactive T cells may require that it be tailored to the individual immune response that is present.

Elevated levels of CNS immunoglobulin (Ig) are also characteristic of MS. Some of this antibody can be shown to be oligoclonal, indicating that it is comprised of a small number of different molecules. Oligoclonal Ig is also detected in other chronic inflammatory responses, including infections, and thus is not specific to MS. It is synthesized locally by plasma cells that are present within the CNS. The specific pattern or fingerprint is unique to each patient. Numerous attempts to identify an antigen against which the majority of oligoclonal Ig is directed have been unsuccessful. The appearance of oligoclonal Ig may thus represent a secondary event resulting from chronic inflammation or tissue injury.

It is possible that tissue damage in MS is mediated by cytokine products of activated T cells, macrophages, or astrocytes. For example, the cytokine tumor necrosis factor (TNF) has been found to be selectively toxic to myelin and to oligodendrocytes in vitro. TNF is present in lesions of MS, CSF levels are reported to parallel MS disease activity, and antibodies to TNF have been found to block acute EAE.

Virology Epidemiologic evidence supports the role of an environmental exposure in MS. MS risk also correlates with high socioeconomic status, which may reflect improved sanitation and delayed initial exposures to infectious agents. Some viruses, e.g., poliomyelitis and measles, produce neurologic sequelae that are more common when the age of initial infection is delayed. Despite many claims, no specific virus has been identified in MS. Reports of infection with a human retrovirus related to HTLV-I have not been confirmed. Elevated antibody titers to measles virus are found in different populations of MS patients, but proof of persistent infection has not followed, and MS may occur in individuals with no evidence of prior measles exposure. In animals, the most widely studied model of virus-induced demyelinating disease has been Theiler virus, a murine coronavirus similar to measles and canine distemper virus. Infection with some Theiler strains results in a chronic infection of oligodendrocytes with multifocal perivascular lymphocytic infiltration and demyelination. As is the case for EAE, genetic factors—both MHC-linked and other loci—influence susceptibility to demyelinating disease due to Theiler virus, in part by determining the magnitude of the immune response against viral determinants that occurs.

CLINICAL MANIFESTATIONS (See also Table 373-1) The onset of MS may be dramatic or so mild as to not cause a patient to seek medical attention. In most published series, the most common initial symptoms include weakness in one or more limbs, visual blurring due to optic neuritis, sensory disturbances, diplopia, and ataxia.

Weakness of the limbs may present insidiously as fatigue with exertion, difficulty in climbing stairs, or loss of dexterity associated with increased muscle tone. Patients may report injury and stubbing of the great toe due to a subtle foot drop. At an early stage of the disease, weakness may not be detectable on testing. Increased motor tone (spasticity), hyperreflexia, an extensor plantar response, Hoffmann reflex, and absent superficial abdominal reflex, all indicative of pyramidal tract disease, may be present. Occasionally, a tendon reflex, e.g., a triceps jerk, may be lost due to a focal lesion in the dorsal root entry zone through which the afferent fibers of the motor reflex arc traverse, simulating a peripheral nerve lesion.

Sensory symptoms include paresthesia (tingling, "pins and needles," or, less commonly, pain) or hypesthesia (numbness or a "dead" feeling). The sensory attack may begin in one foot, typically in a great toe, and ascend over hours or several days; at a variable time into the attack, ascending numbness in the other leg appears, and involvement of the perineum and lower trunk may be noted. Involvement of the trunk with a "cord level" is diagnostically helpful because it distinguishes the sensory attack from peripheral neuropathies due to Guillain-Barré syndrome, mononeuropathy multiplex, or toxins. In patients with established sensory deficits, unpleasant

TABLE 373-1 Initial symptoms of MS

Symptom	Percent cases	Symptom	Percent Cases
Weakness	35	Lhermitte	3
Sensory loss	37	Pain	3
Paresthesias	24	Dementia	2
Optic neuritis	36	Visual loss	2
Diplopia	15	Facial palsy	1
Ataxia	11	Impotence	1
Vertigo	6	Myokymia	1
Paroxysmal	4	Epilepsy	1
Bladder	4	Falling	1

SOURCE: After Matthews et al.

complaints of "swollen," "wet," or "tightly wrapped" body parts are common.

Cerebellar involvement results in ataxia of gait and limbs. In advanced MS, dysarthria of cerebellar origin (scanning speech) is common. In individual patients, the contribution of cerebellar involvement to specific symptoms may be difficult to define when motor and sensory deficits are also present.

Optic neuritis, a core symptom of demyelinating disease, produces variable visual loss. It usually begins as visual blurring that may remain mild or progress to severe visual loss, or, rarely, to complete loss of light perception. Symptoms are generally monocular, but attacks may be bilateral. Pain, localized to the orbit or supraorbital area, is typically present and may precede visual symptoms. The pain may worsen with eye movement. Examination may reveal an enlarged pupil, diminished visual acuity, and a paracentral blind spot (scotoma). The optic disc may be visually swollen (papillitis), and a Gunn phenomenon—pupillodilatation on exposure to direct light following constriction by indirect light—may be detected by a swinging flashlight test (see Chap. 19). Funduscopic examination also may detect venous sheathing of retinal vessels. Residual pallor of the optic disc (optic atrophy) commonly follows bouts of optic neuritis. Rarely, uveitis also has been present in patients with otherwise typical MS.

Visual blurring in MS may result from optic neuritis or diplopia. These two causes are distinguished by asking the patient to sequentially cover each eye and observing whether the visual difficulty clears. Diplopia in MS is often due to the development of an internuclear ophthalmoplegia (INO) or to a sixth nerve palsy; ocular muscle palsies due to involvement of the third or fourth cranial nerves are rare. An INO consists of a delay or complete loss of adduction on attempted horizontal gaze to one side accompanied by nystagmus in the abducting eye. Convergence is preserved, distinguishing INO from medial rectus palsy. An INO results from involvement of the crossed medial longitudinal fasciculus that connects contralateral third and sixth cranial nerve nuclei; involvement is usually on the side of the adducting eye. The presence of bilateral INO in an awake patient is virtually diagnostic of MS. Other gaze deficits include horizontal gaze palsy due to ipsilateral lesions of the lateral pontine tegmentum and the "one and a half" syndrome, consisting of a horizontal gaze palsy to one direction and an INO to the other (see Chap. 19).

Trigeminal neuralgia, a lancinating shocklike facial pain, may occur. Typically, trigeminal neuralgia occurs in patients over 50 years of age and is only rarely due to MS (see Chap. 380). Clinical features that raise a question of underlying MS include onset at a young age; bilaterality, if present; objective signs of sensory loss on the affected side; and prolonged pain lasting minutes or hours.

Interruption of motor innervation to the face may result in several clinical syndromes. Facial palsy due to MS may be difficult to distinguish from idiopathic Bell's palsy. In MS, facial palsy is usually not associated with ipsilateral loss of taste sensation or retroaural pain, two characteristics of Bell's palsy. Chronic flickering contractions of the facial musculature, termed *facial myokymia*, are thought to arise from involvement of corticobulbar tracts and, if chronic, are characteristic of MS. Facial hemispasm, while less common than other motor syndromes, also may occur.

Vertigo may appear suddenly and in dramatic fashion with gait unsteadiness and vomiting, and an incorrect diagnosis of labyrinthitis may be made. A brainstem rather than end-organ origin of vertigo may result in associated "neighborhood" signs, including ipsilateral trigeminal or facial nerve involvement, vertical nystagmus, or the presence of type 3 nystagmus on Barany testing (i.e., no latency, no direction reversal, and no fatigue) (see Chap. 18). Hearing loss also may occur in MS but is unusual.

Urinary bladder, and less frequently bowel, urgency or incontinence occurs in most MS patients at some time and may be present at disease onset.

Cognitive dysfunction is common in advanced MS but also may occur in early or mild disease. Rarely, cognitive symptoms are the initial manifestation of the disease. Memory loss is the most common

cognitive change in MS, and impaired judgment or inappropriate jocularity may be noted. Uncontrollable episodes of laughter or crying, occurring either spontaneously or triggered by emotional stimuli (pseudobulbar palsy), may occur. Depression is also common and is generally secondary to the clinical devastation of MS.

Ancillary symptoms Other clinical accompaniments, when present, support consideration of MS in a patient with neurologic complaints of uncertain cause. *Lhermitte's symptom* is a momentary electric-like sensation evoked by neck flexion, other neck movement, or cough. The symptom typically is experienced as a shooting phenomenon that travels down the spine and into the legs. Variants of Lhermitte's symptom include other tingling or painful sensations induced by neck movements, spread to the arms, or induction by movements of the lumbar spine.

Heat sensitivity, i.e., the appearance or worsening of symptoms upon exposure to heat (typically a hot shower), occurs in most patients with MS. One characteristic form of heat sensitivity is Uhthoff's symptom, in which transient visual blurring, generally monocular, occurs with exercise or upon exposure to heat.

Fatigue is present in the majority (up to 88 percent) of MS patients. Fatigue is typically present in midafternoon and may take the form of increased motor weakness with effort, mental fatigue, or lassitude and sleepiness.

Paroxysmal attacks consist of brief, stereotyped, recurrent phenomena. These underrecognized symptoms frequently occur at the onset of MS or early in its course. Typical are "tonic seizures," in which an unpleasant tingling or other sensory sensation is associated with tonic contraction of a limb, face, or trunk. Others consist of paroxysmal dysarthria and ataxia, diplopia, or transient unilateral paralysis, paresthesias, or pain. Attacks may be momentary or persist for 30 s or longer. They generally begin in clusters, occurring many times daily, and the patient may identify precipitating factors, such as particular movements, that trigger attacks.

DISEASE COURSE McAlpine's illustration of the clinical course characteristics of MS are shown in Fig. 373-1. The course may be stratified into three general categories. The first, *relapsing MS,* is characterized by recurrent attacks of neurologic dysfunction. MS attacks generally evolve over days to weeks and may be followed by complete, partial, or no recovery. Recovery from attacks generally occurs within weeks to several months from the peak of symptoms, although rarely some recovery may continue for 2 or more years. The second form of the disease, *chronic progressive MS,* results in gradually progressive worsening without periods of stabilization or remission. This form develops most often in individuals with a prior history of relapsing MS, although in 20 percent of patients no relapses can be recalled. Acute relapses also may occur during the progressive course. A third form, *inactive MS,* is characterized by fixed neurologic deficits of variable magnitude. Most patients with inactive MS have an earlier history of relapsing MS.

While the clinical course of MS is highly variable, some general prognostic indicators can be defined. In one study that assessed function 25 years after the initial diagnosis of MS, 25 percent of patients remained capable of work, and 50 percent were still ambulatory. Other studies have reported a less favorable long-term prognosis, and in general, the longer that a population is followed, the smaller is the proportion of patients with mild disease. Despite these discouraging data, MS may be present for many decades and produce little or no disability in 5 to 10 percent of patients. Favorable prognostic factors include early onset (excluding childhood), a relapsing course, and little residual disability 5 years after onset. By contrast, poor prognosis is associated with a late age of onset (age 40 or older) and a progressive course; these variables are interdependent, since chronic progressive MS tends to begin at a later age than relapsing MS. Disability from chronic progressive MS is usually due to progressive paraplegia or quadriplegia, and in individual patients, the tempo of worsening, once established, tends to persist throughout the disease course. In relapsing MS, disability results from poor or incomplete recovery from attacks in approximately half

FIGURE 373-1 The clinical course of MS. *A.* Severe relapses, increasing disability and early death. *B.* Many short attacks, tending to increase in duration and severity. *C.* Slow progress from onset, superimposed relapses, and increasing disability. *D.* Slow progression from onset without relapses. *E.* Abrupt onset with good remission followed by long latent phase. *F.* Relapses of diminishing frequency and severity; slight residual disability only. *G.* Abrupt onset; few if any relapses after first year; no residual disability. *(From McAlpine, with permission.)*

of patients and from an evolution to chronic progressive MS in the other half.

DIAGNOSIS The diagnosis of MS is usually easily made in young adults with relapsing and remitting symptoms referable to different areas of CNS white matter. Diagnosis is more difficult in a patient with recent onset of neurologic complaints or in a patient with a primary progressive course. In such situations, the patient should be questioned carefully for history of prior attacks that may not be recalled initially. Other presentations that may cause diagnostic uncertainty include symptoms with a rapid or even explosive onset, suggesting a cerebrovascular accident; progressive brainstem syndromes, raising a question of brainstem glioma; cervical myelopathy in the setting of degenerative disk disease; or mild symptoms unaccompanied by objective signs on examination. Rarely, a mass lesion resulting from intense inflammation and swelling may occur in MS and falsely suggest a primary or metastatic tumor.

Examination reveals objective evidence of neurologic disease in the great majority of patients. Abnormal signs on examination are often more widespread than expected from the interview. For example, the MS patient may present with symptoms in one leg and signs in both. This is helpful when it permits exclusion of a single focal lesion as the source of a symptom complex. Other MS patients may experience symptoms unaccompanied by objective neurologic findings on examination. They are frequently misdiagnosed as suffering from a conversion reaction, a label that should be avoided unless rigid diagnostic criteria for that condition are met.

The differential diagnosis of MS will vary depending on the specific clinical situation. Numerous diagnostic formulas have been proposed (see Table 373-2) that, while useful, should not be used in place of sound clinical judgment. No clinical sign or diagnostic test is unique to MS. The appearance of symptoms that are uncommon or rare in MS should call the diagnosis into question; these include

TABLE 373-2 Diagnostic criteria for MS

1 Examination must reveal *objective* abnormalities of the CNS.
2 Involvement must reflect predominantly disease of white matter long tracts, usually including (a) pyramidal pathways, (b) cerebellar pathways, (c) medial longitudinal fasciculus, (d) optic nerve, and (e) posterior columns.
3 Examination or history must implicate involvement of two or more areas of the CNS.
   a MRI may be used in patients below the age of 40 to document a *second* lesion when only one site of abnormality has been demonstrable on examination. A confirmatory MRI must have either four lesions involving the white matter or three lesions if one is periventricular in location. Acceptable lesions must be greater than 3 mm in diameter.
   b Evoked response testing may be used to document a *second* lesion.
4 The clinical pattern must consist of (a) two or more separate *episodes* of worsening involving different sites of the CNS, each lasting at least 24 h and occurring at least 1 month apart or (b) gradual or step-wise *progression* over at least 6 months if accompanied by increased CSF IgG synthesis or two or more oligoclonal bands.
5 Age of onset between 15 and 60 years of age.
6 The patient's neurologic condition could not be better attributed to another disease. Laboratory testing that may be advisable in specific cases includes (a) CSF analysis, (b) MRI of the head or spine, (c) serum B_{12} level, (d) human T cell lymphotropic virus type I (HTLV-I) titer, (e) sedimentation rate, (f) rheumatoid factor, antinuclear, anti-DNA antibodies (SLE), (g) serum VDRL, (h) angiotensin-converting enzyme (sarcoidosis), (i) *Borrelia* serology (Lyme disease), (j) very long chain fatty acids (adrenoleukodystrophy), and (k) serum or CSF lactate, muscle biopsy, or mitochondrial DNA analysis (mitochondrial disorders).

DIAGNOSTIC CATEGORIES

1 Definite MS: All six criteria fulfilled.
2 Probable MS: All six criteria fulfilled except (a) only one objective abnormality despite two symptomatic episodes or (b) one symptomatic episode and unrelated signs detected on examination.
3 At risk for MS: All six criteria fulfilled except one symptomatic episode and corresponding signs detected on examination.

aphasia, extrapyramidal syndromes suggesting Parkinson's disease, chorea, isolated dementia, amyotrophy with fasciculations, peripheral neuropathy, seizures, or coma. In patients with mild symptoms, there is often little to be gained by making a diagnosis of "definite MS," and a wise course of action may be to exclude other, potentially treatable causes of the presenting symptoms.

Systemic lupus erythematosus (SLE) may on rare occasions result in a relapsing or progressive CNS disorder that mimics MS. Other signs of SLE are usually present, including an elevated erythrocyte sedimentation rate (ESR), autoantibodies, and evidence of systemic disease. Neurologic involvement in SLE may simulate optic neuritis or transverse myelitis; the two may occur in succession (neuromyelitis optica; see below). Myelopathy in SLE may be acute or progressive and is due to vasculitis or infarction rather than to primary demyelination. Behçet's disease (see Chap. 290) also may result in a chronic CNS illness with optic neuropathy and myelopathy but more often resembles acute disseminated encephalomyelitis (see below) in its presentation; the characteristic oral and genital lesions, associated uveitis, and predilection for men are distinguishing features. Relapsing/remitting CNS disease also has been described in Sjögren's syndrome (see Chap. 288). Sarcoidosis may produce relapsing/remitting cranial nerve palsies (particularly of the seventh nerve), progressive optic atrophy, or myelopathy that raises a question of MS; associated lymphadenopathy, pulmonary or hepatic involvement, an elevated angiotensin-converting enzyme, and hypercalcemia may be present. Lyme disease (see Chap. 137) may involve the optic nerve, brainstem, or spinal cord in the absence of characteristic rash, fever, or meningoradiculitis. Other chronic infections, notably meningovascular syphilis, may need to be considered. CSF examination may aid in distinguishing these disorders from MS when marked lymphocytosis, polymorphonuclear leukocytes, or a raised protein level is present. MS is a common disorder, and in individual patients it may be difficult to exclude the coexistence of two different diseases.

The acute onset of a focal CNS disturbance in a previously healthy individual may suggest a vascular etiology, either cerebrovascular disease or migraine. Progressive focal deficits should always prompt consideration of a compressive lesion. Primary CNS lymphoma may produce solitary or multiple lesions that enhance by MRI and may resemble acute lesions of MS. The development of a progressive or relapsing brainstem disturbance may be due to a vascular malformation in the posterior fossa. Pontine glioma is distinguished from MS by its tendency to produce progressive deficits that involve contiguous structures. Arnold-Chiari malformation presenting in adulthood may cause cerebellar ataxia, nystagmus, and spastic weakness of the limbs. Headache, a short neck, lower cranial nerve palsies, and a syringomyelic syndrome are useful distinguishing features.

Patients who present with primary progressive myelopathies unaccompanied by relapses may present a diagnostic uncertainty. Focal lesions of the spinal cord may result from cervical spondylosis, extradural tumor, or arteriovenous malformation. Subacute necrotic myelopathy (Foix-Alajouanine) is a rare disorder that presents as a spinal cord syndrome that progresses over weeks to months, may appear to ascend, and generally results in complete loss of function below the level of the lesion; pathology reveals necrosis, venous thrombosis, and in some cases vascular malformation within the substance of the cord.

HTLV-I–associated myelopathy (HAM; tropical spastic paraparesis) is a chronic illness that evolves over years and is characterized by back pain, progressive spasticity affecting predominantly the lower limbs, and bladder symptoms (see Chap. 279). It is caused by a human retrovirus that is endemic to certain parts of the world, including southern Japan and the Caribbean, but cases also have been identified from nonendemic regions, including the United States. Clinical examination invariably confirms evidence of pyramidal tract disease, and signs of posterior column, cerebellar, or cranial nerve involvement also may be present. Peripheral neuropathy, when present, is a useful distinguishing feature. CSF pleocytosis is present in up to 20 percent of cases. Diagnosis is based on identification of specific antibody to HTLV-I in serum and CSF and by direct virus isolation.

Inherited and other degenerative disorders also may be questioned, particularly where familial occurrence or a progressive course is present. Asymmetric clinical signs, a sharply demarcated spinal cord level, an intact peripheral nervous system, and CSF inflammatory changes may point to a correct diagnosis of MS. Subacute combined degeneration may on occasion develop in the absence of characteristic megaloblastic anemia and can be excluded by a normal serum B_{12} level and a Schilling test. Two related inherited defects, cobalamin G mutation and plasma R binder deficiency, are reported to result in MS-like syndromes (see Chap. 77). Mitochondrial disorders, including subacute necrotic encephalopathy (Leigh's disease), mitochondrial encephalopathy with acidosis and stroke (MELAS), and Leber's hereditary optic neuropathy, may be excluded by blood and CSF lactate levels, by muscle biopsy, and by biochemical or DNA identification of the specific deficit (see Chap. 385). Heredity ataxias produce symmetric involvement of posterior columns and corticospinal and spinocerebellar tracts, with or without involvement of the peripheral nervous system. Other single-gene disorders that may present in adulthood and resemble MS include the autosomal recessive disorders metachromatic leukodystrophy and Krabbe disease and the X-linked disorders Fabry disease and adrenoleukodystrophy (ALD). ALD is of particular interest because it is associated with an intense CSF inflammatory response.

Neuromyelitis optica (Devic's syndrome) is an unusual condition characterized by the development of acute bilateral optic neuritis, followed within days to weeks by transverse myelitis, in a previously healthy individual. On occasion, optic neuritis may be unilateral or occur after an initial bout of myelitis. CNS lesions may be necrotizing and severe. CSF findings are variable but in some cases consist of polymorphonuclear pleocytosis and an increase in the protein content. Neuromyelitis optica may present as an initial manifestation of MS but also may occur in ADEM, SLE, or Behçet's disease.

LABORATORY DIAGNOSIS Laboratory support for MS may be derived from CSF analysis, evoked response testing, and neuroimaging. CSF abnormalities consist of mononuclear cell pleocytosis, an elevation in the level of total Ig, and the presence of oligoclonal Ig. In one large series, CSF pleocytosis (>5 cells per microliter) was present in 25 percent of MS patients. CSF cell counts are generally less than 20 cells per microliter in MS, and counts above 50 cells per microliter are unusual but may occur at the onset of disease. Pleocytosis of >75 cells per microliter or a finding of polymorphonuclear leukocytes in CSF makes the diagnosis of MS unlikely. Pleocytosis is present more commonly in young patients with relapsing MS than in older patients with chronic progressive MS or inactive MS. In relapsing MS, CSF cell counts correlate poorly with clinical disease activity, indicating that an inflammatory response may be ongoing even at times of clinical remission.

In approximately 80 percent of patients, the CSF content of IgG is increased in the presence of a normal concentration of total protein. This results from the selective production of IgG within the CNS. Occasional MS patients exhibit mild elevations in the total CSF protein content. Various formulas are employed in different laboratories to quantitate the selective increase of IgG that is present and to distinguish local synthesized IgG from serum IgG that may have passively entered the CNS across an abnormal blood-brain barrier. This is important because, under normal conditions, the proportion of total protein that is IgG is lower in CSF than in serum. One useful formula expresses CSF IgG as a ratio to that of CSF albumin.

Oligoclonal banding of CSF IgG is detected by agarose gel electrophoresis techniques (Fig. 373-2A). Two or more oligoclonal bands are found in 75 to 90 percent of MS patients. The presence of oligoclonal banding correlates with an elevated total IgG level in MS. Oligoclonal banding may be absent at the onset of MS, and in individual patients the number of bands present may increase with time. Other Ig abnormalities in MS CSF include free kappa or lambda light chains and elevated levels of other Ig isotypes including IgA. It is important that paired serum samples be studied in order to exclude a systemic origin to the abnormal CSF protein that is detected.

Metabolites derived from myelin breakdown also may be detected in CSF. Elevated levels of MBP or its fragments may be detected by radioimmunoassay both in MS and in some patients with other neurologic diseases. The sensitivity of different assays employed to detect CSF MBP varies.

Evoked response testing may detect slowed or abnormal conduction in visual, auditory, somatosensory, or motor pathways. These tests employ computer averaging techniques to record the electrical response evoked in the nervous system following repetitive sensory or motor stimuli (see Fig. 373-2B). One or several evoked responses are abnormal in 80 to 90 percent of patients with MS. Testing is of greatest value when it provides evidence of a second lesion in a patient with a single clinically apparent lesion or when it demonstrates an objective abnormality in a patient with subjective complaints and a normal examination. Slowing of evoked response latencies in MS is thought to result from loss of saltatory conduction along the course of demyelinated axons. Nonetheless, these changes, when present, are etiologically nonspecific and are also present in other conditions, including vascular disease, in which selective demyelination does not occur.

Neuroimaging has assumed an important role in the diagnosis and longitudinal assessment of MS and has modified basic concepts of the disease. Computed tomographic (CT) scanning is abnormal in a proportion of patients and may reveal ventricular enlargement, low-density periventricular abnormalities, or focal regions of enhancement following injection of a contrast agent. Magnetic resonance imaging (MRI) is the most useful imaging method available, and abnormal scans are present in greater than 90 percent of patients with definite MS. On inversion-recovery (T1-weighted) imaging, the CNS may appear normal or show darkened punctate foci corresponding to white matter structures. Characteristic changes of MS are best appreciated

A

B

FIGURE 373-2 *A*. Agarose gel electrophoresis of CSF in MS reveals multiple bands in the "slow" IgG region. No banding is present in control (CON) CSF. *B*. Pattern stimulation visual evoked responses recorded from an MS patient reveals a mononuclear latency abnormality. Left eye (OS) response was normal at 115 ms; right eye (OD) response was abnormal with P100 peak delayed in latency at 135 ms. *(Courtesy of Keith Chiappa, MD.)*

with spin-echo (T2-weighted) MRI sequences, in which abnormal areas stand out brightly from the surrounding brain substance (Fig. 373-3*A*). Some T2-weighted bright foci may appear to arise from the ventricular surface and extend in a linear fashion corresponding to a pattern of perivenous demyelination that is observed pathologically (Dawson's fingers). Abnormal foci also may be detected in the spinal cord (Fig. 373-3*B*). Following administration of the contrast agent gadolinium DPTA, enhancement of "active" lesions may be visualized as a result of extravasation of the injected substance across a disrupted blood-brain barrier; these are best appreciated on T1-weighted sequences. Serial MRI studies in relapsing MS indicate that new T2-weighted bright foci appear and may disappear far more frequently than anticipated on the basis of clinical criteria alone. More surprising, similar changes are also present in chronic progressive MS, although abnormal foci in these patients tend to be more confluent than in relapsing MS. These data indicate that in both forms of MS frequent flares of disease activity may be ongoing in the absence of clinical symptoms or signs.

MANAGEMENT Management may be divided into two categories consisting of (1) treatment designed to arrest the disease process and (2) symptomatic management. The importance of longitudinal staging of the status of MS cannot be overemphasized as an aid to decisions

regarding therapy. Many disease scoring systems have been proposed. For gait assessment, one simple and reliable measure is the ambulation index (Table 373-3), which can be rapidly performed in an office or bedside setting.

Treatment designed to arrest the disease process Immunosuppressive drugs remain the cornerstone of therapy, although their efficacy is limited and their chronic use entails considerable risk. It is thus not surprising that differences in opinion exist as to their specific indications. One practical approach to therapy is summarized in Fig. 373-4.

Long the mainstay of MS therapy, ACTH and glucocorticoids are used for their anti-edema and anti-inflammatory effects. Pulse therapy with these agents speeds the tempo of recovery from acute attacks and may modestly improve the degree of recovery that occurs. They are useful as short-term therapy for relapsing MS. There is no evidence that their use alters the long-term course of the disease.

When neurologic symptoms arise in relapsing MS, it is useful to consider whether they result from new inflammatory lesions in the CNS or whether old MS symptoms have reappeared as a nonspecific consequence of infection or other intercurrent illness. The decision whether or not to treat acute attacks with new neurologic symptoms depends on their severity. Mild deficits, which do not impede functioning, can go untreated, while moderate attacks may benefit from a course of intravenous methylprednisolone followed by oral prednisone. In the past, moderate attacks were most frequently treated with oral prednisone alone on an outpatient basis, but a recent trial of acute optic neuritis indicated that the relapse rate was increased

FIGURE 373-3 *A*. Spin-echo MRI sequence in MS demonstrates extensive bright signal abnormalities in periventricular and other white matter areas. *B*. In a different patient, two discrete abnormal areas are present in the cervical cord.

A

B

TABLE 373-3 Ambulation index

0 Asymptomatic; fully active
1 Walks normally but reports fatigue that interferes with athletic or other demanding activities
2 Abnormal gait or episodic imbalance; gait disorder is noticed by family and friends; able to walk 25 ft (8 m) in 10 s or less
3 Walks independently; able to walk 25 ft in 20 s or less
4 Requires unilateral support (cane or single crutch) to walk; walks 25 ft in 20 s or less
5 Requires bilateral support (canes, crutches, or walker) and walks 25 ft in 20 s or less, or requires unilateral support but needs more than 20 s to walk 25 ft
6 Requires bilateral support and more than 20 s to walk 25 ft; may use wheelchair on occasion
7 Walking limited to several steps with bilateral support; unable to walk 25 ft; may use wheelchair for most activities
8 Restricted to wheelchair; able to transfer self independently
9 Restricted to wheelchair; unable to transfer self independently

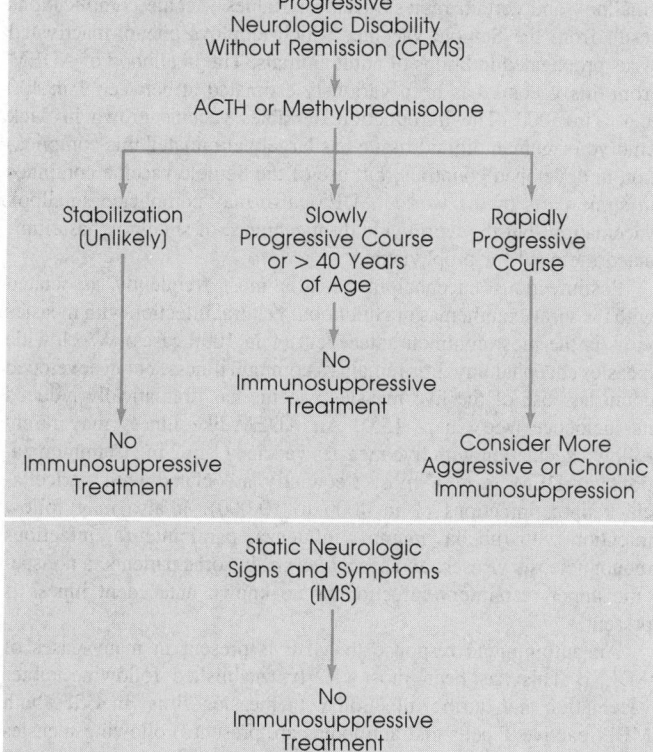

FIGURE 373-4 Therapeutic strategies for MS.

TABLE 373-4 Therapeutic regimens for MS

ACTH

1. Aqueous ACTH (20 U/mL), 80 U is given IV in 500 mL of 5% dextrose and water over 6–8 h for 3 days
2. ACTH gel (40 U/mL) is then given IM in a dose of 40 U every 12 h for 7 days. The dose is then reduced every 3 days as follows:
   35 U bid for 3 days
   30 U bid for 3 days
   50 U qd for 3 days
   40 U pd for 3 days
   30 U qd for 3 days
   20 U qd for 3 days
   20 U every other day for 3 doses

METHYLPREDNISOLONE

Methylprednisolone is mixed in 500 mL D$_5$W and administered slowly, over 4 to 6 h, preferably in the morning:
1000 mg daily for 3 days
500 mg daily for 3 days
250 mg daily for 3 days

METHYLPREDNISOLONE-PREDNISONE

Methylprednisolone, 1000 mg IV daily for 3 days, followed by oral prednisone (1 mg/kg per day) for 14 days

---

by prednisone but not by methylprednisolone-prednisone therapy. Whether these data are generally applicable to the relapsing MS population is unknown, but caution in the use of oral prednisone alone is warranted. Severe MS attacks, which are functionally disabling, may require hospitalization for intravenous treatment with methylprednisolone or ACTH. The effect of ACTH on MS is likely due to stimulation of endogenous cortisol production rather than to direct effects of ACTH itself. One clinical trial found a similar response to intravenous methylprednisolone or ACTH in acute MS attacks. Specific treatment regimens are outlined in Table 373-4, but varied recommendations with respect to dosage and duration of treatment have been proposed. Because of the high incidence of hypomanic reactions to corticosteroids or ACTH in MS, coadministration of lithium carbonate (300 mg two or three times daily) is routinely employed in all the above regimens.

More aggressive therapies have been employed in attempts to limit the number or severity of relapses in relapsing MS or halt chronic progressive MS in patients with rapid neurologic deterioration. The chronic use of glucocorticoids has not proved useful in the treatment of MS, although clinical trials have employed only low dosages. The antimetabolite azathioprine given orally on an outpatient basis is a relatively safe and well-tolerated form of chronic immunosuppression. Its beneficial effect is modest in controlled trials and must be weighed against potential risks that include hepatitis, susceptibility to infection, and a possible increased cancer risk. Pulse therapy with the alkylating agent cyclophosphamide is of benefit to young (<40 years) ambulatory patients with rapidly progressive MS. The side effects associated with treatment are considerable and include nausea, hair loss, a risk of hemorrhagic cystitis, and temporary profound immunosuppression. A modest effect of cyclosporine on the course of chronic progressive MS is also present, but side effects, notably hypertension and reversible renal dysfunction, have limited its widespread use.

More than 100 other therapies have been proposed for treatment of MS. Most represent variants of nonspecific immunosuppression strategies. Conversely, others have attempted to stimulate immunity on the assumption that MS may be caused by a chronic viral infection. One such trial employed interferon-γ (immune), which appeared to trigger attacks of MS in a chronic progressive MS population. One effect of interferon-γ is to increase expression of MHC molecules on the surface of antigen-presenting cells, thus facilitating antigen presentation to T cells. This might have resulted in amplification of an autoimmune response in MS. MHC expression induced by interferon-γ can be abrogated by interferon-β. A recently completed 3-year trial of interferon-β therapy in relapsing-remitting MS indicated that this treatment lessened the frequency of MS attacks by one-third, and reduced by 80 percent disease activity as assessed by MRI. Patients enrolled in this trial were ambulatory without support and had experienced at least two MS attacks in the previous 2 years. This subgroup of MS patients should thus be considered as candidates for chronic treatment with subcutaneously administered interferon-β, which was approved for use in 1993. Whether the beneficial effect of interferon-β on MS is due to its antiviral or immunosuppressive properties is not known.

Patients should be discouraged from seeking out costly studies or potentially hazardous therapies carried out by well-meaning but naive practitioners. The National Multiple Sclerosis Society remains the best source for information on therapeutic options for MS.

Symptomatic therapy Spasticity with stiffness, flexor spasms, and clonus can be functionally disabling and painful. Acute worsening of spasticity may occur with underlying infection (frequently of the urinary tract), obstipation, bedsores, other painful lesions, or injuries.

These precipitants should be sought out and treated specifically. All medications for spasticity have limited efficacy and may produce symptomatic worsening in patients who require stiffness in order to ambulate. Baclofen (15 to 80 mg/d in divided dosages) is the most useful drug available. In refractory cases, oral baclofen in higher dosages (up to 240 mg/d) or intrathecal administration via an indwelling catheter may be effective. Diazepam (2 mg bid or tid) is useful in patients who tolerate its sedative effect, and a single bedtime dose may be especially effective for nocturnal spasms. Dantrolene may produce unacceptable weakness, and its use is reserved for nonambulatory patients. A course of glucocorticoids may be given in exceptional cases where other agents have failed; a beneficial effect may last for several months.

Pain, including trigeminal neuralgia and painful dysesthesias, may respond to carbamazepine (100 to 1200 mg/d in divided, escalating dosages), phenytoin (300 mg/d), or amitriptyline (50 to 200 mg/d). The distinction between dysesthesias due to MS and radiculopathy due to lumbar disk disease may be difficult in patients with unilateral leg pain. Conservative (e.g., *nonsurgical*) therapy is often justified in the absence of convincing signs of nerve root compression.

Paroxysmal symptoms respond to acetazolamide (125 to 250 mg tid) or carbamazepine (up to 1200 mg in divided doses). No treatment for tremor is satisfactory. Isoniazid (up to 1200 mg in divided doses) is reported to benefit postural tremor but is of little practical value for most patients; pyridoxine should be administered concomitantly to prevent peripheral neuropathy. Stereotaxic thalamotomy may be considered in rare cases of disabling tremor in which a unilateral reduction in symptoms is required.

Because specific symptoms of bladder dysfuntion correlate poorly with physiologic findings, urodynamic evaluation is often required. The pathophysiology of abnormal micturition also may change over time in MS. Bladder hyperreflexia is treated with anticholinergics (oxybutynin, 5 mg bid or tid, or propantheline, 7.5 to 15 mg qid). Urinary retention due to bladder hyporeflexia may respond to the cholinergic drug bethanecol (10-50 mg tid or qid). Dyssynergia between detrusor and external sphincter muscles is common in MS, is difficult to treat, and may require a combination of anticholinergic medication to decrease bladder contractions, as well as intermittent catheterization. Supravesical urinary diversion or a chronic indwelling catheter may be required in cases of severe bladder disturbance. Ascorbic acid may reduce the risk of urinary tract infections.

Bowel dysfunction, including constipation and urge incontinence, can be ameliorated by regimentation of bowel function with laxatives and enemas. A low-fiber diet to decrease bulk may be advised for incontinence. Sexual dysfunction may be treated in males by penile implantation, or erections may be achieved pharmacologically using papaverine and phentolamine injections in the corpora cavernosa. Women may experience vaginismus, which may respond to antispasticity medications, or decreased vaginal lubrication leading to dyspareunia, which may be simply treated with lubricants.

Afternoon fatigue may benefit from a shift to an early work schedule or by a regular afternoon nap. Amantadine (100 mg bid) may transiently benefit a small proportion of patients. Emotional lability responds to amitriptyline (25 to 75 mg/d) or to other tricyclic antidepressant medications. It is essential that signs of reactive depression be sought out and specifically treated. Suicide is an important cause of death in MS. Occupational counseling and other support services may assist patients and their families in coping with the effects of the disease. Health maintenance should be emphasized, including stress reduction, a balanced diet, avoidance of rapid weight loss, and adequate rest. There is little evidence linking vaccination with relapses of MS, yet it would be prudent to avoid unnecessary immunizations. Swimming is an ideal form of exercise for many patients because of the buoyant support and hypothermia that is achieved.

Pregnancy may affect the course of MS. Compared with nonpregnant MS patients, pregnant patients experience fewer attacks during gestation but more attacks in the first 3 months postpartum. Both effects appear to be roughly similar in magnitude; thus no effect of pregnancy on disability or on the overall disease course has been identified. It is possible that high levels of prolactin induced in the postpartum period and maintained by breast feeding result in immune stimulation that predisposes to relapses of MS, but in one retrospective study, no effect of breast feeding on attack frequency was found. The advisability of childbearing should be determined primarily by the patient's physical state and available family support.

ACUTE DISSEMINATED ENCEPHALOMYELITIS

DEFINITION AND PATHOGENESIS In contrast to the chronic disorder MS, acute disseminated encephalomyelitis (ADEM) is distinguished by a monophasic course and a frequent association with antecedent immunization (postvaccinial encephalomyelitis) or infection (postinfectious encephalomyelitis). The pathologic hallmark of ADEM consists of widely scattered small foci of perivenular inflammation and demyelination. The illness is sudden in onset and may be neurologically devastating or self-limited.

Postvaccinial encephalomyelitis may follow administration of smallpox and certain rabies vaccines. Rabies vaccine complications result from the Semple vaccine, which employs phenol-inactivated virus propagated in brains of adult animals. The likelihood of ADEM from this vaccine has been variously estimated at between 1 in 400 and 1 in 5000. The introduction of rabies vaccine grown in duck embryo or human diploid tissue has largely eliminated this complication in developed countries, but use of the Semple vaccine continues in some parts of the world. ADEM also may complicate smallpox vaccination, but the worldwide disappearance of smallpox has eliminated the need for prophylaxis.

Postinfectious encephalomyelitis is most frequently associated with the viral exanthemas of childhood. Natural infection with measles virus is the most common antecedent (1 in 1000 cases). Worldwide measles encephalomyelitis remains a common illness, but in developed countries, use of the live measles vaccine has dramatically reduced its incidence (see Chap. 155). An ADEM-like illness may rarely follow vaccination with live measles vaccine (1 to 2 in 10^6 immunizations). ADEM is now most frequently associated with varicella-chickenpox infections (1 in 4000 to 10,000). It also may follow infection with rubella, mumps, influenza, parainfluenza, infectious mononucleosis viruses, and *Mycoplasma*. In some patients, a nonspecific upper respiratory infection or no known antecedent illness is present.

An autoimmune response to MBP is present in many cases of ADEM. This has been most clearly established following rabies vaccination and during infection with measles virus. In CSF, both MBP-reactive T cells and antibodies are present. Following measles infection, induction of immune responses to a variety of CNS constituents may occur, but only the response to MBP correlates with development of ADEM. As noted earlier, many cases of postvaccinial encephalomyelitis almost certainly result from sensitization with brain material that contaminates the viral vaccines. Postinfectious ADEM generally begins late in the course of the viral illness as the exanthem is fading. Many attempts to demonstrate direct viral invasion of the CNS have been unsuccessful. The molecular mechanism responsible for virus-induced triggering of an autoimmune response to MBP is not known but may include molecular mimicry due to common antigens shared between the virus and host protein, CNS injury with secondary sensitization to MBP, or nonspecific effects of virus infection on immune regulation.

CLINICAL MANIFESTATIONS The severity of ADEM is variable. In severe cases, the onset is abrupt, and progression is rapid, over the course of hours to days. In postinfectious ADEM, fever that may have faded reappears, and headache, meningismus, and lethargy progressing to coma may develop. Seizures are common. Signs of disseminated neurologic disease are consistently present. Motor findings may include hemiparesis or quadriparesis and extensor plantar responses. Tendon reflexes may be lost initially, later to become hyperactive. Variable degrees of sensory loss and of brainstem involvement may occur. In ADEM due to complications from chickenpox, cerebellar involvement is often prominent and may dominate the clinical picture. CSF protein is modestly elevated (50 to 150 mg/dL). Lymphocytic pleocytosis, generally 200 cells per microliter or less, occurs in 80 percent of cases. Occasional patients may have higher counts or a mixed polymorphonuclear-lymphocytic pattern during the initial days of the illness. Transient CSF oligoclonal banding has been reported in some patients. MRI scanning may reveal extensive gadolinium enhancement of white matter in brain and spinal cord. Electrophysiologic studies indicate involvement of the peripheral nervous system in a proportion of patients.

Prognosis reflects the severity of the underlying acute illness. Measles encephalomyelitis is associated with an estimated mortality of 5 to 20 percent, and permanent neurologic residua occur in the majority of survivors. Children with encephalopathy may have persistent seizures and behavioral and learning disorders. On rare occasions, recovery from apparent ADEM has been followed by development of a chronic or relapsing/remitting CNS disorder.

DIAGNOSIS Correct diagnosis is easily established in settings of recent vaccination or exanthemous illness. In severe cases with predominantly cerebral involvement, acute encephalitis due to infection with herpes simplex or other viruses may be difficult to exclude. In the absence of a specific viral prodrome or immunization, it may not be possible to distinguish ADEM from acute MS. The simultaneous onset of disseminated symptoms and signs indicating optic nerve, brain, and spinal cord involvement is common in ADEM and rare in MS. Similarly, meningismus, drowsiness or coma, or seizures suggest ADEM. Optic nerve involvement is generally bilateral in ADEM and unilateral in MS, and transverse myelopathy is usually complete in the former and partial in the latter. CSF protein is normal in the great majority of MS patients, lymphocyte counts are rarely above 50 cells per microliter, and polymorphonuclear leukocytes are not present. MRI findings that may support a diagnosis of ADEM include extensive and relatively symmetric white matter abnormalities that also involve the posterior fossa and diffuse gadolinium enhancement of all abnormal areas, indicating active disease and a monophasic course. It is worth emphasizing that MS may on occasion present in an explosive fashion, particularly in children. The clinician is often best advised to classify such cases as "acute demyelinating disease," reflecting this uncertainty.

TREATMENT Treatment consists of intravenous methylprednisolone or methylprednisolone-prednisone in an analogous fashion as employed for MS (see Table 373-4). ACTH also has been reported in uncontrolled studies to be of benefit. Occasional patients may show evidence of relapse shortly following termination of therapy, and in such cases, reinstitution of therapy may be useful.

ACUTE HEMORRHAGIC LEUKOENCEPHALITIS

Acute hemorrhagic leukoencephalitis (AHL) of Weston Hurst is a rare, devastating, and hyperacute demyelinating disorder of unknown etiology. CNS lesions of AHL are characterized by perivenous demyelination and intense infiltration by mononuclear and especially polymorphonuclear inflammatory cells. Vasculitis results in necrosis of the walls of venules, fibrin deposition, and innumerable small hemorrhages scattered throughout the white matter of the hemisphere, brainstem, and spinal cord. Large necrotic foci may form by coalescence of smaller lesions.

The clinical course resembles that of severe forms of ADEM but may be even more explosive in onset and progression. The CSF profile consists of marked pleocytosis (up to 3000 cells per microliter), variable numbers of red blood cells, and elevated protein content. Peripheral blood may show an elevated ESR and leukocytosis. Occasional cases may display mixed features of both ADEM and AHL or evolve from one form to the other during the course of the

acute illness. As in ADEM, immune sensitization to MBP also has been described in AHL. Thus AHL may represent a form of ADEM in which a hyperacute inflammatory response is superimposed on lymphocyte-mediated perivenular demyelination. In animal models of EAE, demyelinating lesions also may be either lymphocytic or polymorphonuclear/hemorrhagic depending on the genetic background of the animal, the immunization regimen, and the adjuvent employed.

The differential diagnosis of AHL includes viral encephalitis, acute bacterial cerebritis, venous thrombosis, or multiple embolic infarctions. Prognosis is generally poor. Death may occur within 2 to 4 days of onset. In some patients, complete neurologic recovery has been observed, and as for ADEM, occasional reports describe the subsequent development of a chronic disease similar to MS. These observations further highlight the diagnostic uncertainties and possible overlap between the clinically defined demyelinating diseases. Therapy for AHL consists of methylprednisolone or methylprednisolone-prednisone regimens (see Table 373-4).

REFERENCES

ADAMS CWM et al: Pathology, histochemistry and immunocytochemistry of lesions in acute multiple sclerosis. J Neurol Sci 92:291, 1989

BECK RW et al: A randomized, controlled trial of corticosteroids in the treatment of acute optic neuritis. N Engl J Med 326:581, 1992

GOODKIN DE et al: Diagnostic criteria for multiple sclerosis research involving multiply affected families. Arch Neurol 48:805, 1991

HARDING AE et al: Occurrence of a multiple sclerosis-like illness in women who have a Leber's hereditary optic neuropathy mitochondrial DNA mutation. Brain 115:979, 1992

HARTUNG HP: Immune-mediated demyelination. Ann Neurol 33:563, 1993

HEMACHUDHA T et al: Myelin basic protein as an encephalitogen in encephalomyelitis and polyneuritis following rabies vaccination. N Engl J Med 316:369, 1987

IFNB MULTIPLE SCLEROSIS STUDY GROUP: Interferon beta-1b is effective in relapsing-remitting multiple sclerosis. I. Clinical results of a multicenter, randomized, double-blind, placebo-controlled trial. Neurology 43:655, 1993

JOHNSON RT et al: Measles encephalomyelitis: Clinical and immunologic studies. N Engl J Med 310:137, 1984

KESSELRING J et al: Acute disseminated encephalomyelitis: MRI findings and the distinction from multiple sclerosis. Brain 113:291, 1990

KURTZKE JF, HYLLESTED K: Multiple sclerosis in the Faroe Islands: II. Clinical update, transmission, and the nature of MS. Neurology 36:307, 1986

MATTHEWS WB et al: McAlpine's Multiple Sclerosis. New York, Churchill Livingston, 1991

MCALPINE D et al: Multiple Sclerosis: A Reappraisal. Edinburgh, Livingstone, 1965

MYRIANTHOPOULOS NC: Genetic aspects of multiple sclerosis, in Handbook of Clinical Neurology, vol. 3: Demyelinating Diseases, JC Koetsier (ed). New York, Elsevier Science Publishers, 1985

PATY DW et al: Interferon beta-1b is effective in relapsing-remitting multiple sclerosis. II. MRI analysis results of a multicenter, randomized, double-blind, placebo-controlled trial. Neurology 43:662, 1993

—— et al: MRI in the diagnosis of MS: A prospective study with comparison of clinical evaluation, evoked potentials, oligoclonal banding, and CT. Neurology 38:180, 1988

SADOVNICK AD et al: Parent-child concordance in multiple sclerosis. Ann Neurol 29:252, 1991

WAKSMAN SG: Clinical course and electrophysiology of multiple sclerosis, in Advances in Neurology, vol 47: Functional Recovery in Neurological Disease, SG Waksman (ed). New York, Raven, 1988.

WEINER HL et al: Intermittent cyclophosphamide pulse therapy in progressive multiple sclerosis: Final report of the Northeast Cooperative Multiple Sclerosis Treatment Group. Neurology 43:910, 1993

YUDKIN PL et al: Overview of azathioprine treatment in multiple sclerosis. Lancet 338:1051, 1991

ZAMVIL SS and STEINMAN L: The T lymphocyte in experimental allergic encephalomyelitis. Annu Rev Immunol 8:579, 1990

374   BACTERIAL MENINGITIS AND BRAIN ABSCESS

W. MICHAEL SCHELD

ACUTE BACTERIAL MENINGITIS

DEFINITION   Bacterial meningitis may be defined as an inflammatory response to bacterial infection of the pia-arachnoid and the cerebrospinal fluid (CSF) of the subarachnoid space. Since the subarachnoid space is continuous through the brain, spinal cord, and optic nerves, infection in this space extends throughout the cerebrospinal axis unless there is obstruction of the subarachnoid space. Ventriculitis is nearly uniformly present in patients with bacterial meningitis.

EPIDEMIOLOGY   Bacterial meningitis remains a common disease worldwide. Although precise figures are unavailable, the incidence of bacterial meningitis is between 4.6 and 10 per 100,000 people per year in the United States. More than 2000 deaths due to bacterial meningitis are reported annually in the United States. Approximately 25,000 cases of bacterial meningitis occur annually, of which about 70 percent occur in children under 5 years of age. The disease is even more common in developing countries. The relative frequency of isolation of various bacterial species as a cause of meningitis is age related (Table 374-1). Gram-negative bacilli (principally *Escherichia coli*, of the K1 capsular type), other enteric bacilli, *Pseudomonas* sp., *Listeria monocytogenes*, and group B streptococci are the major causative agents during the neonatal period. *Haemophilus influenzae* and *Neisseria meningitidis* are the major causes in children beyond 1 month of age. Meningitis in adults is due primarily to meningococci and pneumococci, although disease due to aerobic gram-negative bacilli is observed with increasing frequency, especially in the elderly. *N. meningitidis* is the only major cause of epidemics of bacterial meningitis. Recent trends indicate an increase in the proportion of cases due to gram-negative bacilli and *L. monocytogenes*.

In 1981, it was estimated that *H. influenzae* meningitis developed in approximately 1 in every 500 children during the first 4 years of life. The Centers for Disease Control and Prevention estimate that 29,000 cases due to *H. influenzae*, 4800 cases of pneumococcal meningitis, and 4600 cases of meningococcal disease occurred in the United States during 1973. Similar figures for the 1978–1981 period were reported recently, and the incidence may be increasing, particularly in adults. The overall incidence per 10^5 population per year in the United States during 1986 was 2.9, 1.35, and 1.0 for meningitis due to *H. influenzae* (with significant variability by geographic region), *N. meningitidis*, and *Streptococcus pneumoniae*, respectively (Table 374-2). These most recent figures are derived from a prospective laboratory-based surveillance project in an area with a population of 34 million, 14 percent of the U.S. population. A similar overall incidence for neonatal meningitis of 2.8 cases per 100,000 population

per year was observed in western Sweden during a comparative time period. It is hoped that widespread usage of *H. influenzae* polysaccharide-conjugate vaccines will lead to a marked decline in the incidence of invasive disease due to this pathogen, as observed in the greater Helsinki area since extensive trials with conjunctive vaccines began in 1986.

Meningitis is a major international health problem, as is evident by the recent experience in Africa and South America; explosive and highly fatal outbreaks may occur. At least 30 countries worldwide, including the United States, have reported serious outbreaks of meningococcal meningitis in recent years. During one decade (1973–1982), 4100 cases of meningitis were admitted to a single hospital in Salvador, Brazil, and this disease accounted for 27 percent of all admissions in this interval. The differences in etiology among various studies performed on four different continents are shown in Table 374-3. Worldwide, the three major meningeal pathogens (*H. influenzae*, *N. meningitidis*, and *S. pneumoniae*) account for approximately 75 to 80 percent of cases, but the proportion due to each organism is somewhat variable by geographic region.

ETIOLOGY   At the present time, *H. influenzae* is the most common isolate from cases of bacterial meningitis in the United States. Nearly all cases occur in children under 6 years of age, and more than 90 percent are due to capsular type b strains (see Chap. 112). Meningitis usually follows nasopharyngeal acquisition of a virulent organism with subsequent systemic invasion. *H. influenzae* accounts for only about 0.5 percent of total CSF isolates after 6 years of age, and isolation of this organism from older age groups should suggest the presence of certain predisposing factors, including sinusitis, epiglottitis, pneumonia, otitis media, head trauma with a CSF leak, diabetes mellitus, alcoholism, splenectomy or other asplenic states, and immune deficiency (including hypogammaglobulinemia and AIDS).

Meningitis due to *N. meningitidis* is most often encountered in children and young adults and may occur in epidemics (Chap. 109). Epidemic meningococcal meningitis is usually due to serogroups A or C, although the potential for epidemic spread of any serogroup exists. Type B strains are isolated most frequently in sporadic cases, accounting for approximately 50 percent of all isolates in the United States. Type Y strains are associated with pneumonia. The meningococcus is isolated from approximately 20 percent of all cases of bacterial meningitis in the United States. Nasopharyngeal carriage of virulent organisms also accounts for the initiation of infection. Infection is more likely in patients who have deficiencies in the terminal complement components (C5 to C8, and perhaps C9), the so-called membrane attack complex. Persons with these deficiencies have an 8000-fold increased risk of *Neisseria* infections, although the mortality rates appear to be lower than in patients with an intact complement system. Meningococcal meningitis also may occur in properdin-deficient individuals.

Pneumococcal meningitis is the most frequently observed agent in adults over the age of 30 years and accounts for approximately 15 percent of the total cases of meningitis in the United States (see Chap. 101). Mortality rates remain high, in the 19 to 30 percent range.

TABLE 374-1   Bacterial etiology of meningitis, by age

Organism	Neonates (≤1 month), %	Children (1 month to 15 years), %	Adults (>15 years), %
H. influenzae	0–3	40–60	1–3
S. pneumoniae	0–5	10–20	30–50
N. meningitidis	0–1	25–40	10–35
Gram-negative bacilli	50–60	1–2	1–10
Streptococci	20–40*	2–4	5
Staphylococci	5	1–2	5–15
Listeria species	2–10	1–2	5

* Nearly all isolates are group B streptococci.
SOURCE: After Roos et al.

TABLE 374-2   Bacterial meningitis in five states and Los Angeles County, 1986

Organism	Percent of total cases	Case fatality rate (%)
H. influenzae	45	3
S. pneumoniae	18	19
N. meningitidis	14	13
Group B streptococci	5.7	12
L. monocytogenes	3.2	22
Others	15	18

SOURCE: After Wenger et al.

TABLE 374-3 Etiology of bacterial meningitis in four geographic areas (% of total cases)

Organism	United States, 1978–1981	United Kingdom, 1980–1984	Dakar, Senegal, 1970–1979	Salvador, Brazil, 1973–1982
H. influenzae	48	29	20	23
S. pneumoniae	13	20	29	17
N. meningitidis	20	25	11	32
Group B streptococcus	3	7	4	2
L. monocytogenes	2	2	<0.5	—
Other	8	16	9	8
Unknown	6	—	26	19

SOURCE: After Roos et al.

Pneumococcal infection of the meninges is often associated with distant foci such as pneumonia, otitis media, mastoiditis, sinusitis, or endocarditis. Serious pneumococcal infections may be observed in patients with predisposing conditions, including splenectomy or asplenic states, multiple myeloma, hypogammaglobulinemia, alcoholism, cirrhosis, and the Wiskott-Aldrich syndrome. *S. pneumoniae* is the most common meningeal isolate in head trauma patients who have suffered a basilar skull fracture with subsequent CSF leak.

Although *L. monocytogenes* represents only a small minority of cases of bacterial meningitis in the United States, mortality remains high (see Table 374-2). *Listeria* infection is more likely in neonates, the elderly, alcoholics, cancer patients, and immunosuppressed adults (e.g., renal transplant patients). The incidence of *Listeria* meningoencephalitis may be declining in renal transplant populations due to the frequent use of trimethoprim-sulfamethoxazole prophylaxis. However, up to 30 percent of adults and 50 percent of children with listeriosis have no apparent underlying condition. Serious *Listeria* infections have been associated with several foodborne outbreaks involving contaminated cole slaw, milk, and cheese.

Meningitis due to aerobic gram-negative bacilli is unusual except at the extremes of life. *E. coli* is isolated from 30 to 50 percent of neonates with bacterial meningitis. *Klebsiella* sp., *E. coli,* and *Pseudomonas aeruginosa* also may be isolated following head trauma, neurosurgical procedures, in the elderly, in immunosuppressed patients, and in patients with gram-negative bacteremia. Despite the relative low frequency of meningitis due to this group of microorganisms, the mortality rates remain high. Many of these infections are nosocomial in origin, although community-acquired gram-negative bacillary meningitis appears to be increasing in frequency, particularly among the elderly and in debilitated, alcoholic, or diabetic adults. Staphylococcal meningitis is rare except in patients with indwelling CSF shunts, in whom *Staphylococcus epidermidis* is the most common organism. Meningitis due to *S. aureus* is unusual and accounts for about 1 to 8 percent of cases in various surveys. *S. aureus* is the second most common cause of CSF shunt infections and is also a nosocomial pathogen. Although secondary meningitis in the setting of infective endocarditis is relatively uncommon, most of these infections are due to *S. aureus*. Other important associated conditions include head trauma, abscesses in other organs, neurosurgical procedures, sinusitis, osteomyelitis, pneumonia, cellulitis, decubitus ulcers, and infected intravascular grafts or shunts. Many patients have concomitant conditions, including diabetes mellitus, malignancy, renal failure, and immunosuppression. The mortality of staphylococcal meningitis remains high (about 50 percent in adults), although the prognosis for CSF shunt infections is more favorable.

Group B streptococci are an important cause of neonatal meningitis. These infections may occur as early-onset septicemia associated with premature rupture of the membranes and low-birth-weight or late-onset meningitis more than 7 days after birth. The early-onset form is acquired from the maternal genital tract, whereas the source of the group B streptococci in late-onset disease is more controversial; at least 40 percent of infected infants are born to culture-negative mothers. Rare cases of group B streptococcal meningitis have been reported in adults, including postpartum females following vaginal delivery. Bacteremic infections, usually in older adults, unrelated to

pregnancy occur in the setting of underlying risk factors in the following approximate order of decreasing frequency: diabetes mellitus, malignancy, liver failure or history of alcoholism, neurologic impairment, renal failure, congestive heart failure, use of intravenous catheters, glucocorticoid administration, asplenia, and AIDS. Nevertheless, this is a rare disease in the adult.

Meningitis due to anaerobic bacteria is rare, accounting for less than 1 percent of pyogenic cases. Recovery of anaerobic bacteria from CSF should suggest intraventricular rupture of a brain abscess. Most other cases arise from spread of infection secondary to a contiguous focus of disease and are seen in patients predisposed to focal suppurative intracranial processes.

A plethora of microorganisms have been documented as the cause of meningitis in isolated case reports or in small numbers of patients. Meningitis due to *Flavobacterium meningosepticum* may be a problem in certain neonatal intensive care units, and nosocomial meningitis due to other gram-negative bacilli or *Acinetobacter* sp. appears to be increasing in frequency. Polymicrobial bacterial meningitis with simultaneous recovery of two or more bacterial species from CSF is unusual and accounts for less than 1 percent of cases. The majority of cases occur in adults with a wide spectrum of etiologic agents. Many patients have had tumors in close proximity to the neuraxis, rectal carcinoma, or a fistulous communication with the CNS. Simultaneous isolation of viruses and bacteria from the CSF is rare; only seven well-documented cases have been reported since 1988. Nevertheless, CSF samples are infrequently cultured for both groups of microorganisms, and this occurrence may be a gross underestimate of the actual problem.

PATHOGENESIS AND PATHOPHYSIOLOGY Since most cases of bacterial meningitis are hematogenous in origin, pathogenesis involves sequential steps related to the expression of several different bacterial virulence factors that overcome host defense mechanisms and allow the pathogen to reach, invade, and replicate in the CSF. These pathogenic steps include the following: (1) nasopharyngeal colonization, (2) nasopharyngeal epithelial cell invasion, (3) bloodstream invasion, (4) bacteremia with intravascular survival, (5) traversal across the blood-brain barrier and entry into CSF, and (6) survival and replication within the subarachnoid space.

Nasopharyngeal mucosal colonization and invasion by meningeal pathogens require evasion of secretory IgA, avoidance of ciliary clearance mechanisms, adhesion to the apical epithelial cell membrane, and passage to the basolateral side of the cell. Virtually all clinical isolates of the three major meningeal pathogens secrete IgA proteases that cleave the hinge region of IgA and render it nonfunctional, thereby facilitating bacterial adhesion to the epithelium. Studies using a human nasopharyngeal organ culture model have elucidated the distinct mechanisms of adhesion and invasion by the human pathogens *H. influenzae* and *N. meningitidis*. Infection of human nasopharyngeal organ cultures with either organism results in injury to ciliated epithelial cells with ciliostasis and selective adherence to nonciliated epithelial cells. Meningococcal binding is dependent on expression of cell surface pili, and the organism interacts with epithelial cell microvilli. Meningococci enter nonciliated epithelial cells by an endocytotic process and proceed to the abluminal side by a transcellular route within membrane-bound vacuoles. *H. influenzae,* in contrast, creates separations between apical tight junctions of columnar epithelial cells and invades primarily via an intercellular route. After adhesion to and invasion of the nasopharyngeal epithelium, pathogenic bacteria must enter and survive within the intravascular space prior to penetration of the CNS. Evasion of the host's alternative complement pathway is an important strategy of meningeal pathogens to sustain intravascular survival; this virulence property is largely dependent on expression of capsular polysaccharide. The actual molecular basis for this complement evasion strategy differs among the major meningeal pathogens and has been attributed to meningococcal capsular sialic acid and the *H. influenzae* type b polysaccharide capsule (polyribosoyl-ribose-phosphate). *H. influenzae* is capable of replication within the intravascular space.

Once bacteremia occurs, the bacterial pathogens must invade the CNS. The site and mechanism of meningeal invasion by bacteria, however, are poorly understood. Early studies in an experimental infant rat model of *H. influenzae* meningitis suggested that the dural venous sinuses were the major route of CNS invasion. More recent studies, however, suggest that a nonspecific sterile focal inflammation above the cribriform plate facilitates CNS invasion at this site. Experimental studies also have demonstrated that bacteria may enter the CSF via the choroid plexus related to its exceptional high rate of blood flow and fenestrated capillaries. Three hypotheses are proposed to account for the observed neurotropism of meningeal pathogens and for their entry into the CNS: (1) meningitis is secondary to a sustained bacteremia that must be of sufficient duration and magnitude, (2) adhesion to critical blood-brain barrier components may mediate CNS invasion, supported by the potential role of adhesion of *E. coli* strains to the luminal surface of microvascular cerebral endothelium and the epithelial lining of the choroid plexus and ventricles, and (3) microorganisms are transferred within macrophages or other phagocytic cells entering the CNS by normal cellular trafficking pathways.

Once bacteria cross the blood-brain barrier and enter the CNS, host humoral defense mechanisms, particularly dependent on immunoglobulin and complement activity, are virtually absent, resulting in a significant advantage for the pathogen. Since opsonic activity is often undetectable even in infected CSF, phagocytosis of the encapsulated bacterial pathogens in the fluid medium of the CSF is inefficient. Thus bacterial meningitis represents an infection in an area of impaired host resistance commonly leading to very large bacterial densities in the CSF and mandating the use of bactericidal agents for optimal response to therapy.

Once bacteria enter and replicate within the CSF, subarachnoid space inflammation ensues. This inflammation is largely responsible for the pathophysiologic consequences that contribute to the clinical syndrome of bacterial meningitis, including the following: increased permeability of the blood-brain barrier, cerebral edema (vasogenic, interstitial, and cytotoxic in origin), increased outflow resistance to CSF, cerebral vasculitis, increased intracranial pressure, decreased cerebral blood flow and/or loss of autoregulation of cerebral blood flow, cortical hypoxia, and CSF acidosis.

CSF neutrophilic pleocytosis is a hallmark of subarachnoid space inflammation. Nevertheless, the pathway of neutrophil traversal into the CSF is largely unknown. Adhesion of neutrophils to vascular endothelial cells is a necessary prerequisite for this traversal; pretreatment of endothelial cells in tissue culture with various inflammatory cytokines induces formation of specific adhesion molecules [e.g., endothelial leukocyte adhesion molecule 1 (ELAM-1)], although some of these adhesion molecules have yet to be demonstrated in cerebral endothelium. Leukocyte endothelial cell adhesion is mediated by specific transmembrane glycoproteins expressed on the endothelial cells that interact with specific counterparts on neutrophils. Three families of adhesion molecules may mediate these important interactions, including the immunoglobulin superfamily (e.g., ICAM-1 and ICAM-2), the integrin family (e.g., the CD11/CD18 subfamily), and the selectin family (ELAM-1). The complex interrelationships among these three families, including the inducibility of neutrophil adhesion, and the participation of multiple glycoproteins in diapedesis and the

induction of inflammation are considered in greater detail in Chap. 79. Important for consideration is evidence that blockage of neutrophil adhesion to endothelium by the systemic administration of a monoclonal antibody (IB4) against the CD11/CD18 family of receptors leads to absence of CSF pleocytosis in experimental animal models of meningitis. The CSF pleocytosis following challenge with live microorganisms and cell wall components is prevented. Combination treatment with dexamethasone and monoclonal antibody IB4 is more effective than either agent alone in the prevention of CSF pleocytosis.

Subarachnoid space inflammation is induced by constituents of bacteria. Capsular polysaccharides are remarkably noninflammatory, although bacterial capsule is crucial for intravascular and subarachnoid space survival of meningeal pathogens. Experimental animal studies have documented that the cell wall of gram-positive microorganisms and the endotoxin (lipopolysaccharide, or LPS, or lipooligosaccharide) of gram-negative organisms induce subarachnoid space inflammation. In the case of pneumococcus, intracisternal injection of the major components of the cell wall, teichoic acid and peptidoglycan, induces inflammation. In gram-negative meningitis, the lipid A region of LPS is responsible for the induction of inflammation. CSF inflammatory changes are also invoked following the intracisternal inoculation of *H. influenzae* type b outer membrane vesicles, which may serve as a relevant nonreplicating vehicle for the delivery of the toxic moieties of LPS to host cells in vivo. Pneumococcal cell wall and *H. influenzae* type b LPS elicit subarachnoid space inflammation through the release of various inflammatory mediators within the CNS. Both interleukin 1 (IL-1) and tumor necrosis factor (TNF) appear within CSF rapidly following the intracisternal inoculation of pneumococcal cell wall or LPS from gram-negative bacteria. These proinflammatory cytokines induce subarachnoid space inflammation independently and appear to act synergistically in this effect. In addition, increased CSF concentrations of TNF may be specific for bacterial meningitis, since elevated levels are found in bacterial but not viral meningitis in both experimental animals and humans. The role of other inflammatory cytokines in the induction of subarachnoid space inflammation is less clear. Although interleukin 6 (IL-6) and platelet-activating factor (PAF) are present at increased concentrations in the CSF during the disease, the precise contribution of these inflammatory cytokines within the CNS is unknown. Nevertheless, higher CSF concentrations of TNF and PAF are associated with increased severity of the disease in children.

One of the major pathophysiologic consequences of bacterial meningitis is increased permeability of the blood-brain barrier, which leads to vasogenic cerebral edema. After the intracisternal inoculation of bacterial pathogens in experimental animals, a uniform host response to experimental meningitis at the level of the cerebral capillary endothelium is observed, characterized morphologically by an early and sustained increase in pinocytotic vesicle formation and a progressive increase in separation of intercellular tight junctions. These morphologic alterations correlate with a functional penetration of a marker protein (albumin) across the blood-brain barrier. CSF leukocytes augment changes in permeability late in the disease course. Intracisternal inoculations of pneumococcal cell walls, *H. influenzae* type b LPS, outer membrane vesicles prepared from *H. influenzae*, and various proinflammatory cytokines all induce increased blood-brain permeability in vivo. Encapsulation of *H. influenzae* is not essential for blood-brain barrier injury but facilitates its progression by allowing the organism to escape host clearance mechanisms within the CSF in vivo. Studies that utilize an in situ perfusion protocol of albumin–colloidal gold as tracer as well as complementary immunogold detection of perfused monomeric albumin have localized the site of albumin traversal to the postcapillary venule in the subarachnoid space during bacterial meningitis. Albumin traversal occurs primarily via a paracellular pathway through open intercellular junctions in venular segments, since transcytosis to the abluminal side of the endothelium is minimal. Although gram-negative cell wall components in addition to LPS (e.g., peptidoglycan) may induce subarachnoid space inflammation, the effect is minimal when compared with

LPS alone. The precise primary and secondary messengers governing alterations in blood-brain barrier permeability and the paracellular leak of albumin remain unknown, but ongoing development of in vitro systems of isolated cerebral microvascular endothelial cells may assist in delineating this event at the cellular level. Furthermore, the recent demonstration of elevated concentrations of excitatory amino acids within CSF suggests a role for these substances in the altered blood brain-barrier permeability as well as altered CNS homeostasis.

Another important pathophysiologic consequence of subarachnoid space inflammation is the development of increased intracranial pressure (ICP) caused primarily (but not exclusively) by the development of cerebral edema that may be vasogenic, cytotoxic, and/or interstitial in origin. Vasogenic cerebral edema is primarily a result of increased blood-brain barrier permeability. Cytotoxic cerebral edema results from swelling of the cellular elements of the brain, most likely due to the release of toxic factors from neutrophils and/or bacteria. Interstitial cerebral edema occurring during meningitis is largely due to obstruction of normal CSF pathways with resultant increased CSF outflow resistance. Cerebral edema is always found in experimental animal models of meningitis, as measured by increased brain water content. The attenuation of the observed cerebral edema, raised ICP, and increased CSF outflow resistance with glucocorticoid administration in experimental animal models of meningitis led directly to a reexamination of the potential adjunctive roles for these agents in the treatment of this disease (see below). Cerebral blood flow alterations also have been documented in animal models and in patients with bacterial meningitis. In an infant rhesus monkey model of *H. influenzae* meningitis, certain areas of the cortex (postcentral, temporal, and occipital) were hypoperfused relative to the hypothalamus and midbrain, while the brainstem was hyperperfused, suggesting cerebral cortical hypoperfusion with resultant relative cerebral anoxia as an early physiologic change during *H. influenzae* meningitis. Loss of cerebral autoregulation has been documented in an experimental rabbit model of pneumococcal meningitis. It has been suggested that even minor fluctuations of mean arterial blood pressure may have adverse consequences for patients with meningitis, since autoregulation may be lost, resulting in an increased risk of brain injury from either transient hypotension or hypertension. The blood flow alterations may lead to regional hypoxia, increased brain lactate concentrations secondary to utilization of glucose by anaerobic pathways, and CSF acidosis, which may be a precursor to encephalopathy. It is possible that generation of reactive oxygen intermediates in the microvasculature potentiates these changes in regional cerebral blood flow. Infusion of superoxide dismutase modifies the early alterations in cerebral blood flow in experimental models of pneumococcal meningitis.

PATHOLOGY The pathologic hallmark of bacterial meningitis is a subarachnoid space exudate. On gross examination, the exudate has a typical grayish yellow or yellowish green appearance. It is most abundant in the cisterns at the base of the brain and over the convexities of the cerebral hemispheres in the rolandic and sylvian fissures. Purulent exudate accumulates in the basal cisterns and also, in the absence of obstruction, extends along the spinal cord and nerve sheaths and into the ventricular system. Microscopic examination of the subarachnoid exudate in the early stages demonstrates large numbers of neutrophils and bacteria. Within 2 to 3 days of infection, evidence of inflammation in the wall of the small and medium-sized subarachnoid blood vessels appears. Subintimal arterial infiltration by lymphocytes and neutrophils is relatively unique to infection of the meninges. The meningeal veins become distended and develop mural infection, which may be complicated by focal necrosis of the vessel wall, mural thrombus formation in the lumen, or involvement of the dural sinuses. Hemorrhagic cortical infarction may be the result of cortical venous and dural sinus thrombosis. By the end of the first week of meningeal inflammation, a change in the cellular composition of the subarachnoid exudate occurs. Neutrophils begin to degenerate and are removed by macrophages, derived from meningeal histiocytes. The nuclei of affected neurons and glia cells become shrunken,

pyknotic, and darkly staining. Further infiltration of subependymal tissues and perivascular spaces by neutrophils and lymphocytes occurs. Blockage of normal CSF pathways, particularly in the fourth ventricle through the midline foramen of Magendie and the lateral foramina of Luschka may result in noncommunicating or obstructive hydrocephalus. Interference of CSF absorption via the arachnoid villi may result from accumulation of the fibrinopurulent exudate. Diffuse cerebral edema and/or increased intracranial pressure may lead to life-threatening herniation. Cranial and spinal nerve deficits, focal neurologic deficits, seizure disorders, encephalopathy, and subdural effusions are all recognized complications of meningitis.

CLINICAL MANIFESTATIONS The classic clinical presentation of adults with bacterial meningitis includes headache, fever, and meningismus, often with signs of cerebral dysfunction; these are found in more than 85 percent of patients. Nausea, vomiting, rigors, profuse sweats, weakness, myalgias, and photophobia are also common. The meningismus may be subtle or marked, accompanied by Kernig's and/or Brudzinski's signs. These signs are elicited in only about 50 percent of adults with bacterial meningitis, and their absence does not rule out this possibility. Cerebral dysfunction is manifested primarily by confusion, delirium, or a declining level of consciousness ranging from lethargy to coma. Cranial nerve palsies, especially involving cranial nerves IV, VI, and VII, are found in 10 to 20 percent of cases, occasionally in concert with focal neurologic deficits such as visual field defects, dysphasia, and hemiparesis in a small minority of patients. Seizures occur in about 40 percent of cases. The presence of bilateral sixth nerve palsies, manifested as weakness of the lateral rectus muscles, suggests raised ICP. Papilledema is rare (<1 percent of patients) and should suggest an alternative diagnosis, such as an intracranial mass lesion. Later in the disease course patients may develop signs of increased ICP, including coma, hypertension, bradycardia, and third nerve palsy; these findings are ominous prognostic signs. Focal neurologic deficits, seizure activity, and encephalopathy may arise from cortical and/or subcortical ischemia and/or infarction, raised ICP, or the development of a subdural effusion.

Certain symptoms and/or signs may suggest a specific etiologic diagnosis in patients with meningitis. Meningococcemia with or without meningitis presents with a prominent rash, principally of the extremities, in about 50 percent of patients. Early in the disease process, the rash is often erythematous and macular but typically evolves quickly into a petechial phase with further coalescence into a purpuric form with gun metal gray necrosis in the center of the purpuric regions. This rash often matures rapidly, sometimes with the appearance of new petechial lesions during the performance of the physical examination. A similar rash also may be seen in other forms of meningitis (e.g., due to echovirus type 9, *S. aureus*, *Acinetobacter* sp., and, rarely, *S. pneumoniae* or *H. influenzae*), Rocky Mountain spotted fever or other rickettsioses, *S. aureus* endocarditis, rapidly overwhelming sepsis due to encapsulated bacteria in splenectomized patients, or noninfectious disorders such as vasculitis or thrombotic thrombocytopenic purpura. An additional suppurative focus of infection, typically otitis media, sinusitis, or pneumonia, may be seen in approximately 30 percent of patients with pneumococcal or *H. influenzae* meningitis. Patients with meningitis following a CSF leak may demonstrate rhinorrhea or otorrhea due to a persistent defect.

Conversely, certain subgroups of patients may not manifest many of the classic signs and/or symptoms of bacterial meningitis. Meningismus and/or fever are commonly absent in neonates, and the only clinical clues may be listlessness, high-pitched crying, refusal to feed, irritability, or other nonspecific manifestations. Elderly patients often present insidiously with lethargy or obtundation and with variable signs of meningeal inflammation and no fever. In this subgroup of patients, an altered mental status should not be ascribed to other causes until bacterial meningitis has been excluded by CSF examination. Many of the signs of bacterial meningitis, including alteration in consciousness, are present in patients following neurosurgery and/or head trauma. The diagnosis of meningitis is difficult in this situation, and the physician should have a low threshold for CSF examination if any clinical deterioration occurs.

DIAGNOSIS The diagnosis of bacterial meningitis rests on examination of the CSF, usually following lumbar puncture. When papilledema and/or focal neurologic findings suggestive of an intracranial mass lesion are present, lumbar puncture should be deferred until a computed tomographic (CT) scan or magnetic resonance imaging (MRI) study is performed. Nevertheless, if meningitis remains an important consideration, empirical antimicrobial therapy should be started during the performance of the neuroimaging study. Although CSF cultures may be rendered sterile, the CSF profile will still be suggestive of bacterial meningitis despite empirical antimicrobial therapy during the performance of the procedure.

The typical CSF findings in acute bacterial meningitis consist of an elevated opening pressure, neutrophilic pleocytosis, elevated protein concentration, and hypoglycorrhachia. The opening pressure is elevated in virtually all cases. Values exceeding 600 mL of water suggest cerebral edema, communicating hydrocephalus, or the presence of intracranial suppurative foci. The gross appearance of the fluid may be cloudy or turbid if the white cell count is elevated. Occasionally, the fluid may appear turbid due to the presence of microorganisms in the absence of significant CSF pleocytosis; this is an ominous prognostic sign. Traumatic lumbar puncture may produce a bloody CSF initially but should clear as flow continues. Xanthochromia may occur during meningitis but should suggest the possibility of subarachnoid hemorrhage and in patients with heart valve disease raises the possibility of ruptured mycotic aneurysm. The CSF leukocyte concentration is usually elevated in untreated bacterial meningitis, ranging from 10 to $> 1000 \times 10^3$ per liter with a neutrophilic predominance. Approximately 10 percent of patients present initially with a predominance of lymphocytes in CSF. A very low CSF white cell concentration in bacterial meningitis often has been associated with poor prognosis. Therefore, Gram's stain and culture should be performed on all CSF specimens even in the absence of a CSF pleocytosis. The CSF protein concentration is elevated in virtually all cases of bacterial meningitis, sometimes to an extreme degree when spinal block is present, presumably due to disruption of the blood-brain barrier and/or generation of protein from leukocytes or microorganisms in the subarachnoid space. The CSF glucose concentration is less than 40 mg/dL (<2.2 mmol/L) in approximately 60 percent of patients with bacterial meningitis, and the CSF to serum glucose ratio is less than 0.31 in about 70 percent of patients. The CSF glucose concentration must be compared with simultaneous serum glucose concentration for proper evaluation. A recent analysis found that a CSF glucose level less than 34 mg/dL (1.9 mmol/L), a CSF/blood glucose ratio of less than 0.23, a CSF protein level of greater than 2.2 g/L (220 mg/dL), and more than 2000×10^6 CSF leukocytes per liter or more than 1180×10^6 CSF neutrophils per liter were individual predictors of bacterial as opposed to viral meningitis with 99 percent certainty or better.

CSF examination by Gram's stain should always be performed and permits a rapid and accurate identification of the etiologic agent in approximately 60 to 90 percent of cases of bacterial meningitis (overall sensitivity is approximately 75 percent). The probability of organism detection correlates with bacterial concentrations in CSF. False-positive findings may occur as a result of contamination of collection tubes or the staining reagents. Negative CSF Gram's stains are usually related to prior antimicrobial therapy and low CSF concentrations of microorganisms. The CSF culture is positive in approximately 70 to 85 percent of patients with bacterial meningitis. The probability of identifying an organism may decrease in patients who have received prior antimicrobial therapy. Blood cultures also should be obtained because they are positive in a variable proportion of patients with bacterial meningitis depending on the pathogen.

Many other rapid diagnostic tests have been developed to aid in the diagnosis of bacterial meningitis when the Gram's stain is negative. Countercurrent immunoelectrophoresis (CIE) may be helpful in the detection of specific microbial antigens in CSF with a sensitivity of approximately 62 to 95 percent with high specificity. Nevertheless, newer techniques employing staphylococcal coagglutination or latex agglutination are more rapid and sensitive than CIE (ability to detect bacterial antigen concentrations of approximately 1 ng/mL of CSF). It must be emphasized that a negative test does not rule out infection due to a particular meningeal pathogen. The limulus lysate test is highly sensitive in the detection of LPS within CSF, although it does not distinguish between gram-negative organisms that may be present and the results often do not alter decisions on therapeutic regimen.

Neuroimaging techniques such as CT and MRI have little role in the diagnosis of acute bacterial meningitis but may detect complications and/or a parameningeal source of infection. CT or MRI may be useful in patients with prolonged fever several days after initiation of antimicrobial therapy, with prolonged obtundation or coma in the presence of new or recurrent seizure activity, with signs of increased ICP, or with focal neurologic deficits. MRI is more sensitive than CT for the evaluation of subdural effusions, cortical infarction, and cerebritis but is more difficult to obtain in a critically ill patient. The vast majority of patients with suspected or proven bacterial meningitis do not require a neuroimaging study.

Most patients with suspected bacterial meningitis deserve initial evaluation in an intensive care setting. Multiple complications may ensue, including shock, disseminated intravascular coagulation, the syndrome of inappropriate secretion of vasopressin (antidiuretic hormone), and others. In addition to frequent monitoring, blood cultures and tests for coagulation factors and electrolytes, including renal function, are essential. A chest x-ray may reveal a coexistent pneumonia. Stains of petechiae or purpuric lesions may reveal intracellular cocci in approximately 70 percent of meningococcemia cases. In the presence of frank arthritis, arthrocentesis with culture and stains may yield the etiologic agent.

DIFFERENTIAL DIAGNOSIS Multiple infectious and noninfectious processes may be responsible for an acute meningitis syndrome and can be confused with acute bacterial meningitis, including parameningeal foci of infection (e.g., brain abscess, subdural empyema, and epidural abscess; see below), viral meningitis or encephalitis, CSF syphilis, the neurologic manifestations of Lyme disease, tuberculous meningitis, fungal meningitis, bacterial endocarditis, rickettsial infections such as Rocky Mountain spotted fever, CNS neoplasms, cerebral vasculitis, granulomatous angiitis, sarcoidosis, cyst-related meningitis, subarachnoid hemorrhage, neuroleptic malignant syndrome, chemical meningitis due to drugs, radiocontrast agents, or anesthetics, and various poorly understood chronic or recurrent meningeal syndromes.

TREATMENT Antimicrobial therapy The initial procedure in a patient with suspected bacterial meningitis is performance of a lumbar puncture to obtain CSF for analysis. Patients should receive emergent empirical antimicrobial therapy based on age and underlying disease status if no etiologic agent is identified by Gram's stain or rapid diagnostic tests and the diagnosis of bacterial meningitis is likely. In those few patients who present with focal signs on neurologic examination, a CT scan should be obtained prior to a lumbar puncture. However, if meningitis is a strong possibility, empirical antimicrobial therapy should be instituted immediately. The empirical regimens for presumed bacterial meningitis are based primarily on the age of the host and the likely infecting pathogens. For neonates under 1 month of age, the most likely pathogens are *E. coli*, *S. agalactiae*, and *L. monocytogenes*. Empirical therapy commonly consists of ampicillin plus a third-generation cephalosporin, usually cefotaxime due to the concerns of albumin binding by ceftriaxone and bilirubin metabolism in this age group. An alternative treatment regimen is ampicillin plus an aminoglycoside. In older infants (ages 4 to 12 weeks), infections with either *H. influenzae* or *S. pneumoniae* join the typical neonatal pathogens, and the regimen of choice is ampicillin plus a third-generation cephalosporin. From ages 3 months to 6 years, *H. influenzae* is by far the most common etiologic agent, and empirical therapy with a third-generation cephalosporin may be used. Some authorities still recommend ampicillin plus chloramphenicol or chloramphenicol alone in this age group, but cefuroxime should be avoided. In younger adults, most cases of meningitis are due to *N. meningitidis* or *S. pneumoniae*, and penicillin G or ampicillin are often used. Because of the prevalence of gram-negative aerobic bacilli in older adults (over 50 years of age) and the possibility of *L. monocytogenes* infection, the empirical regimen should consist of ampicillin in combination with a third-generation cephalosporin. In postneurosurgical patients or in those with CSF shunts or foreign bodies in place, the likely infecting organisms include staphylococci, diphtheroids, or gram-negative bacilli, including *P. aeruginosa*. Empirical antimicrobial therapy in these situations should consist of vancomycin plus ceftazidime until culture results are available.

Once the infecting microorganism has been isolated in culture (or identified by other means), antimicrobial therapy can be modified for optimal treatment based on susceptibility results. For bacterial meningitis due to *S. pneumoniae* or *N. meningitidis*, penicillin G or ampicillin remain the drugs of choice, but recent developments may modify these recommendations. "Relatively" penicillin-resistant pneumococci have increased in frequency in recent years. Thus susceptibility testing of pneumococcal isolates from sterile body fluids is mandatory. For relatively resistant strains, a third-generation cephalosporin should be used, and for meningitis due to "highly" penicillin-resistant pneumococci (MIC ≥ 2 μg/mL), vancomycin is commonly recommended, although failures may occur. Meningococcal strains that are relatively resistant to penicillin also have been reported from several areas, particularly Spain. Although most patients harboring these strains have recovered with standard penicillin therapy, a third-generation cephalosporin may be indicated for empirical treatment for adults with meningitis where these strains are prevalent. Approximately 33 percent of *H. influenzae* isolates in the United States produce β-lactamase and are resistant to ampicillin. Fortunately, chloramphenicol resistance is rare in the United States, but it may be found in more than 50 percent of CSF isolates in some countries. Recently, the American Academy of Pediatrics has endorsed the use of the third-generation cephalosporins as empirical therapy in children with bacterial meningitis. Ceftriaxone is clearly superior to cefuroxime in this age group. The third-generation cephalosporins have revolutionized the treatment of gram-negative enteric bacillary meningitis. Cure rates of 78 to 94 percent have been obtained with these agents, and one, ceftazidime, may be used in monotherapy or as part of combination regimens for the care of patients with *Pseudomonas* meningitis. Intrathecal or intraventricular aminoglycoside therapy should be considered for patients with gram-negative aerobic bacillary meningitis if there is no response to systemic therapy alone. The quinolone agents (e.g., ciprofloxacin, pefloxacin, and ofloxacin) have been used in some patients with gram-negative meningitis but should only be considered for adult patients with meningitis due to multi-drug-resistant gram-negative bacilli or in patients failing conventional therapy. The third-generation cephalosporins are, however, inactive against *L. monocytogenes;* therefore, ampicillin is often added empirically for treatment of this organism. In documented *Listeria* meningitis, consideration should be given to a combination of an aminoglycoside and ampicillin to achieve synergy in vivo. In the penicillin-allergic patient, systemic trimethoprim-sulfamethazole, which is bactericidal against *Listeria* in vitro, can be used. Patients with *S. aureus* meningitis should be treated with nafcillin, oxacillin, or vancomycin. Since *S. epidermidis* is the most likely isolate in patients with CSF shunt infection, vancomycin is the drug of choice; rifampin may be added if the patient fails to improve. Shunt removal is often required to optimize therapy.

The duration of therapy for bacterial meningitis is based largely on tradition in the absence of rigorous scientific data. In general, the following treatment durations are recommended: *N. meningitidis:* 7 days; *H. influenzae:* 7 to 10 days; *S. pneumoniae:* 10 to 14 days; and gram-negative aerobic bacilli: 3 weeks. Therapy should be individualized and based on the clinical response; some patients may require longer courses of treatment.

Adjunctive therapy Despite the availability of bactericidal antimicrobial therapy, the morbidity and mortality from bacterial meningitis remain at unacceptably high levels. Recent studies have focused on the pathogenesis and pathophysiology of bacterial meningitis, since the introduction of newer antimicrobial agents may not improve this situation. However, rapidly bactericidal therapy, the desired result of the initiation of antimicrobial agents, may result in accentuated release of proinflammatory bacterial cell wall components into the CSF. Initiation of treatment with bacteriolytic agents in experimental meningitis results in an increase in CSF leukocyte concentration. Antibiotic therapy also results in higher concentrations of free LPS in the CSF of children with *H. influenzae* meningitis during the first day of treatment. Hence anti-inflammatory agents, particularly glucocorticoids or nonsteroidal anti-inflammatory agents, have been shown to decrease the inflammatory response in the subarachnoid space in experimental models of infection (as assessed by CSF pleocytosis) with resultant improvement in many of the pathophysiologic consequences, including blood-brain barrier permeability, cerebral edema, and ICP. Based on these studies and the known effects of glucocorticoids on cytokine generation, these agents have been reevaluated in patients with bacterial meningitis. Several prospective, double-blind, randomized clinical trials have now evaluated dexamethasone as an adjunctive therapy for children with meningitis. Although mortality was not affected, CSF inflammatory indices normalized faster, fever disappeared more rapidly, and the incidence of moderate to severe bilateral sensorineural hearing loss and/or overall neurologic sequelae was reduced. Dexamethasone also reduced mortality in adults and children with pneumococcal meningitis treated in one Egyptian trial. Although concerns have been raised about the routine use of dexamethasone in all patients with bacterial meningitis and virtually no information exists in neonates or older adults, this adjunctive therapy is potentially beneficial in children, particularly those with proven or suspected *H. influenzae* disease. Close monitoring of the hematocrit and stool guaiac for blood loss is essential during therapy. The mechanism of the beneficial effect of dexamethasone is incompletely defined, but CSF concentrations of IL-1β fall more rapidly in children receiving dexamethasone when compared with a placebo control. If dexamethasone is used, it should be administered shortly before or simultaneously with the first dose of antimicrobial agents to maximally attenuate the CSF inflammatory response. The recommended dose of dexamethasone is 0.15 mg/kg per dose, administered four times daily (total of 0.6 mg/kg per day) for 4 days. Studies on the potential role of adjunctive dexamethasone in neonates and adults are in progress.

Other adjunctive therapies may be useful in critically ill patients with bacterial meningitis. Patients with signs of increased ICP may benefit from the insertion of an intracranial pressure monitoring device and vigorous treatment of raised ICP. Elevation of the head of the bed to 30°, hyperventilation to a Pa_{CO_2} of 27 to 30 mmHg, hyperosmolar agents such as mannitol, intravenous lidocaine to reduce transient increases in ICP during endotracheal suctioning, and glucocorticoids may be tried alone or in combination (see Chap. 376). Seizures should be treated promptly to avoid status epilepticus with appropriate agents such as lorazepam or diazepam and/or phenytoin. Occasionally, barbiturates are necessary for control of seizure activity. Another important adjunctive therapy in children with bacterial meningitis is fluid restriction to combat excess secretion of antidiuretic hormone if the patient is not hypotensive. Treatment of shock and/or disseminated intravascular coagulation may be necessary (see Chap. 83). Plasma exchange or plasmapheresis has proven lifesaving in some patients with fulminant meningococcemia, but this treatment modality must be considered experimental at the present time.

PROGNOSIS The overall case fatality rates of the major meningeal pathogens in cases of meningitis encountered in the United States in 1986 are shown in Table 374-2. The mortality rate for *H. influenzae* meningitis is less than 5 percent but may exceed 20 to 25 percent in some developing countries. Meningococcemia without meningitis is associated with a worse prognosis than meningitis alone due to this organism. Pneumococcal meningitis, among the three major pathogens, is associated with the highest mortality rate. Gram-negative aerobic bacillary meningitis is often refractory to therapy, and relapses may occur. In addition, permanent neurologic sequelae are encountered in approximately one-third to one-half of survivors of bacterial meningitis. The major sequelae include hearing loss or language delay, mental retardation, cerebral palsy, seizures, and behavioral problems. Prospective studies have documented persistent sensorineural hearing loss in approximately 10 percent of survivors of bacterial meningitis (approximately 31 percent following pneumococcal meningitis), a finding with critical implications for growth and educational development. Despite an apparent recent decline in the incidence of severe neurologic sequelae among children surviving bacterial meningitis, as measured by learning patterns upon school entry, the public health problems as a result of this disease are significant worldwide.

BRAIN ABSCESS

DEFINITION   Brain abscess is a focal suppurative process within the brain parenchyma of diverse pathogenesis and etiology.

EPIDEMIOLOGY   The incidence of brain abscess has remained relatively stable in the antibiotic era; nevertheless, it is generally regarded as a rare disease, with large autopsy series reporting an occurrence rate of 0.18 to 1.3 percent. It has been estimated that brain abscess accounts for approximately 1 out of every 10,000 general hospital admissions, and about 4 to 10 cases are seen yearly on active neurosurgical services in hospitals of developed countries. Although some series have noted a slightly increased incidence in recent years, this may represent a bias derived through more sensitive diagnostic techniques. In addition, brain abscess remains a significant problem in the developing world, particularly in children in lower socioeconomic regions. Focal suppurative processes of the brain have emerged as an important type of intracranial infection in patients with AIDS. For example, estimates of the prevalence of toxoplasma encephalitis alone have ranged from 2.6 to 30.8 percent in patients with AIDS.

In most series, the male/female ratio has been approximately 2:1, with the median age at presentation of 30 to 40 years. Approximately 25 percent of brain abscesses occur in children less than 15 years of age. Brain abscess in a child less than 2 years of age is distinctly unusual and suggests an associated gram-negative bacillary (especially *Citrobacter diversus*) meningitis. In some series, brain abscess secondary to otitis media displays a bipolar age distribution, with peaks in the pediatric age group and after age 40. In contrast, brain abscess secondary to paranasal sinusitis occurs more commonly between 10 and 30 years of age.

ETIOLOGY   In the preantibiotic era, the most common etiologic agents isolated from brain abscesses were *S. aureus*, streptococci, and coliform bacteria, although no growth was recorded in up to 50 percent of patients. With proper attention to anaerobic culture techniques, the role of anaerobic bacteria in brain abscess has become apparent, and sterile abscesses are less frequently encountered. Microbial isolates from brain abscesses are dependent to a significant degree on the immune status of the host. The etiology of focal CNS infections in patients with AIDS is addressed in Chaps. 279 and 375.

Currently, pyogenic brain abscesses are often (30 to 60 percent) mixed infections. In a summary of 12 separate series of patients with brain abscess, excluding AIDS patients, 61 percent of the isolates were aerobic bacteria, while 32 percent were anaerobic bacteria. Aerobic or microaerophilic streptococci accounted for about one-half of the aerobic isolates and have been noted to be present in approximately 70 percent of all brain abscess patients. The most frequently isolated streptococci include organisms belonging to the *S. milleri* group (*S. anginosus*, *S. constellatus*, *S. intermedius*, etc.). *S. aureus* is isolated from about 15 percent of patients with brain abscess, especially following head trauma or neurosurgery. Aerobic

gram-negative bacilli (e.g., *Proteus* sp., *E. coli*, *Klebsiella* sp., *Enterobacter* sp., and *P. aeruginosa*) have been observed with increased frequency in recent studies, often in mixed culture, and are isolated from 16 to 30 percent of patients. Anaerobes most recently encountered include *Bacteroides* sp. (including *B. fragilis*), *Fusobacterium* sp., anaerobic streptococci, and *Clostridium* sp. Anaerobic bacteria are particularly prevalent pathogens in the setting of underlying chronic otitis or pulmonary disease.

The location of a given brain abscess and its underlying predisposing cause often suggest the most likely etiologic agent(s). Frontal lobe abscesses resulting from a preexisting sinusitis often yield an organism of the *S. milleri* group in pure culture. Furthermore, brain abscess in association with chronic sinusitis is often a mixed infection with an aerobic/anaerobic ratio of approximately 1 to 1.5 in most series. Posttraumatic or postoperative brain abscesses are usually caused by staphylococci. Temporal lobe abscesses are often a complication of otitis media and almost always yield multiple agents upon culture, including streptococci, *Bacteroides* sp., and gram-negative aerobic bacilli. Approximately 33 percent of chronically infected ears yields anaerobes on culture. In contrast to the role of *S. pneumoniae*, *H. influenzae*, and *M. catarrhalis* in acute otitis media, other streptococci, gram-negative aerobes including *P. aeruginosa*, anaerobic cocci, and *Bacteroides* sp. are the most common isolates from chronic otitis media and its intracranial complications. Pneumococci, meningococci, and *H. influenzae* very rarely cause brain abscess, even in association with a purulent meningitis.

In addition, the microbiology of a brain abscess is fundamentally influenced by the immune status of the host. Immunocompromised patients may develop brain abscess due to fungi, and *Toxoplasma gondii* is a major cause of focal CNS lesions in patients with AIDS. Brain abscess in neutropenic patients is usually due to aerobic gram-negative bacteria, *Candida* sp., *Aspergillus* sp., or zygomycosis. Conversely, focal brain abscess in patients with abnormal cell-mediated immunity is commonly due to *T. gondii*, *Nocardia asteroides*, *L. monocytogenes*, *Mycobacterium* sp., or *Cryptococcus neoformans*. *Pseudallescheria boydii* abscess may follow a near-drowning episode. Multiple other fungi, protozoa, and helminths may cause brain abscess.

PATHOGENESIS AND PATHOPHYSIOLOGY   Brain abscesses occur most commonly in association with three distinct clinical settings: (1) a contiguous focus of infection, particularly otitis, sinusitis, or dental infection, (2) hematogenous spread from a distant focus of infection, especially chronic pyogenic lung disease, and (3) following cranial trauma or surgery. The predisposing factor remains undefined in approximately 15 to 20 percent of cases.

A review of multiple series encompassing more than 3500 cases of brain abscess in the past half century reveals that about 45 percent of cases were associated with a contiguous focus of infection (predominantly otitis or sinusitis). Recent data suggest that otogenic brain abscesses are decreasing in frequency, perhaps related to the availability and common use of antimicrobial agents for upper respiratory tract infections. Frequent but inadequate courses of antimicrobial agents for ear or sinus infections have, however, altered the natural history of brain abscess, resulting in puzzling or more subtle clinical presentations. Otogenic brain abscesses are most commonly located in the temporal lobe or cerebellum; conversely 85 to 95 percent of cerebellar abscesses are associated with ear or mastoid infections. Sinusitis as a cause of brain abscess also appears to be decreasing in overall incidence. Rhinogenic abscesses are rare in children and in adults over the age of 60 years. Most brain abscesses in the setting of sinusitis are localized in the frontal lobe. Sphenoid sinusitis is notable for both the frequency and severity of its potential intracranial complications. The diagnosis of this form of sinusitis is often difficult and may lead to therapeutic delay. Cocaine inhalation is an additional risk factor for sphenoid sinusitis and subsequent brain abscess development. Dental infections, often overlooked as a cause of brain abscess, have been implicated in about 10 percent of patients with brain abscess. Periapical abscesses surrounding the teeth are often detected in patients with "cryptogenic brain abscess." Brain abscesses rarely complicate the course of bacterial meningitis in adolescents or adults. Nevertheless, the presence of a brain abscess should be strongly considered in neonates with gram-negative meningitis, particularly due to *Citrobacter* or *Proteus* sp.

Brain abscess is a rare complication of neurosurgical procedures or cranial trauma. CNS infections occur in only 0.6 to 1.7 percent of clean neurosurgical procedures, and brain abscess accounts for only 10 percent of these infections. Brain abscess may, however, complicate penetrating cranial injuries, with an increased risk noted in the setting of gunshot wound complications. Retained bone fragments have been consistently noted as an important risk factor.

Hematogenous brain abscess arising from distant foci of infections account for about 25 percent of cases. These lesions are associated most commonly with pulmonary infections and share the following characteristics: (1) location in the distribution of the middle cerebral artery, (2) initial location at the gray matter–white matter junction, (3) poor encapsulation, and (4) higher mortality. Hematogenous brain abscesses are most likely to present as multiple lesions. Multiple brain abscesses was reported in only 1 to 15 percent in older series; however, with the advent of CT scanning, multiple lesions are now detected in 10 to 50 percent of patients. Important preceding processes have included chronic lung infections (lung abscess, bronchiectasis, and empyema), osteomyelitis, cholecystitis, intraabdominal infection, and/or pelvic sources. Brain abscess has been observed following endoscopic sclerosis of esophageal varices or dilatation of esophageal strictures. Although a transient bacteremia may follow these procedures and is instrumental in the development of a brain abscess, macroscopic CNS lesions are rare complications of bacterial endocarditis. *S. aureus* is the most common cause of endocarditis complicated by intracranial involvement. Hereditary hemorrhagic telangiectasia is an important risk factor for brain abscess, especially in affected patients with clubbing, cyanosis, and/or polycythemia. This condition (Osler-Rendu-Weber syndrome) may be underrecognized in patients with brain abscess. Cyanotic heart disease is recognized in 3 to 14 percent of brain abscess cases and may be the most common underlying process found within brain abscess in children. Tetralogy of Fallot is the most commonly cited anomaly; however, brain abscess may complicate patent foramen ovale, ventricular septal defect, and transposition of the great vessels. The presence of a right-to-left shunt appears to be critical for the development of brain abscess in these patients.

Brain abscess development in any of the above-described clinical settings appears to require a compromised area of brain as the final common pathway. Experimental data suggest that brain is remarkably resistant to infection. Brain abscess development from an area of contiguous infection usually follows two major mechanisms: (1) direct extension through areas of associated osteitis or osteomyelitis and (2) retrograde thrombophlebitic spread via diploic or emissary veins into the intracranial compartment. The polycythemia and systemic hypoxia observed in cyanotic congenital heart disease and hereditary hemorrhagic telangiectasia increase blood viscosity, which may, in concert with a reduction in brain capillary blood flow, result in microinfarction or reduced tissue oxygenation in brain as a nidus for ensuing infection.

PATHOLOGY A solitary brain abscess involves the following brain regions in approximate decreasing order of frequency: frontal $\geq$ frontoparietal > parietal > cerebellar > occipital. This distribution reflects the associated, often contiguous foci of infection. Brainstem, intrasellar, basal ganglia, and thalamic abscesses are rare.

The pathologic evolution of brain abscess has been documented most convincingly in experimental models of infection and appears to involve four histopathologic stages. Importantly, the histopathologic features may correlate with specific findings on CT, which has direct implications for subsequent therapy. The four stages include (1) early cerebritis (days 1 to 3 following intracerebral inoculation of animals), characterized by a perivascular inflammatory response surrounding a developing necrotic center, with profound edema, (2) late cerebritis, with maximal extent of the well-formed necrotic center and the

appearance of fibroblasts and neovascularity in the periphery of the necrotic zone, (3) early capsule formation (days 10 to 13 following intracerebral inoculation of experimental animals), characterized by a well-developed layer of fibroblasts with persistent cerebritis and neovascularity, and (4) late capsule formation, with thickening of the capsule and an abundance of reactive collagen. It should be noted, however, that these stages are somewhat stereotyped, are best described for abscess following infection with alpha-hemolytic streptococci, and may not reflect the sequence in abscesses caused by other microorganisms. Nevertheless, encapsulation is frequently more complete on the cortical side of the abscess when compared with the ventricular side and is often less extensive in abscesses resulting from hematogenous spread than in those arising from a contiguous focus of infection. These observations may explain the propensity for abscesses to rupture medially into the ventricular system rather than into the subarachnoid space. Brain abscess formation is a continuum from cerebritis to a well-encapsulated necrotic focus. Maturity of the lesion(s) is dependent on multiple factors, including local oxygen concentration, the offending microorganism, and the host immune response.

CLINICAL MANIFESTATIONS (See also Table 374-4) The clinical course of a patient with a brain abscess may range from indolent to fulminant; however, the duration of symptoms is 2 weeks or less in about 75 percent of patients. In most cases, the prominent clinical manifestations of brain abscess reflect the expanding intracerebral mass rather than systemic signs of infection. Furthermore, the clinical manifestations are often nonspecific and depend on several variables (e.g., the virulence of the infecting organisms, the patient's immune status, and the location of the abscess or abscesses). Only a minority of patients display the classic triad of fever, headache, and focal neurologic deficits. Headache is most consistently observed (70 percent of patients), but fever is documented in only one-half of patients. Focal neurologic deficits are encountered in about half the cases, and the specific features are dependent on the number and location of the brain abscesses. Focal deficits may include hemiplegia, hemianopsia, cranial nerve abnormalities, and others depending on location. Cerebellar abscess often results in nystagmus, ataxia, vomiting, and dysmetria, whereas frontal lobe abscess is often dominated by headache, drowsiness, inattention, and a generalized deterioration in mental function. Hemiparesis with unilateral motor signs and/or a speech disorder are frequent findings. Seizures are observed in 25 to 45 percent of patients and, when present, are usually generalized. The presence of nausea and vomiting correlates to some degree with the ICP. A change in mental status (lethargy to coma) occurs in most patients, but frank coma on presentation is now infrequently noted and may reflect the availability of improved diagnostic modalities such as CT. Papilledema is observed with varying frequency, does not correlate with the size of the abscess, but appears to be associated closely with the presence of headache and vomiting. Nuchal rigidity (about 25 percent of patients) is observed more commonly with a shorter duration of illness and may lead to confusion with bacterial meningitis. Intrasellar abscess often simulates a pituitary tumor, presenting with headache, visual field defects, and endocrine disturbances.

TABLE 374-4 Clinical manifestations of brain abscess

Symptom/sign	Percent
Headache	70
Triad of fever, headache, focal deficit	<50
Fever	40–50
Focal neurologic deficit	~50
Seizures	25–40
Nausea/vomiting	22–50
Nuchal rigidity	~25
Papilledema	~25

NOTE: Other symptoms/signs are dependent on location.
SOURCE: After Wispelwey et al, 1991.

Since the clinical presentation may be nonspecific and fever is often absent, brain abscess may be confused with several other processes, and the following should be considered in the differential diagnosis: pyogenic meningitis, subdural empyema, epidural abscess, encephalitis, mycotic aneurysm, complicated migraine headache, intracerebral or subarachnoid hemorrhage, cerebral infarction, cerebral venous sinus thrombosis, and primary or metastatic malignancies of the CNS.

DIAGNOSIS   Routine studies of the blood and urine are rarely helpful in the diagnosis of a brain abscess. A moderate peripheral blood leukocytosis may be present, but 40 percent of patients display a completely normal peripheral leukocyte count. The erythrocyte sedimentation rate is often elevated but may be normal in the setting of cyanotic congenital heart disease. Serum C-reactive protein concentrations have been used to differentiate brain abscess from intracranial neoplasms but are inadequate for this purpose. Blood cultures are only occasionally (≤10 percent) positive in patients with a brain abscess.

Although the CSF is often abnormal in patients with brain abscess, the findings are nonspecific, and lumbar puncture is usually contraindicated in a patient with a suspected parenchymal abscess. The diagnostic yield is poor, and the risk of subsequent herniation after the procedure has been reported to be as high as 20 percent. The poor diagnostic yield and significant morbidity of lumbar puncture in the presence of a brain abscess necessitate that this procedure be delayed in patients with a febrile CNS disorder with focal neurologic signs. However, if pyogenic meningitis is also a strong consideration in the individual patient, blood cultures should be obtained and appropriate antimicrobial agents started parenterally before obtaining a neuroradiologic study. Although abnormalities may be noted, skull roentgenograms, electroencephalograms, arteriography, ventriculography, and/or technetium 99m brain scans are rarely necessary in the evaluation of a patient with a suspected brain abscess. Radionuclide brain scans are, however, useful in facilities lacking CT scan or MRI technology.

The introduction of CT and MRI has revolutionized the diagnostic and therapeutic approach to brain abscess. CT is superior to other, older radiologic techniques in the evaluation of paranasal sinuses, mastoids, and the middle ear and should be obtained, along with a chest roentgenogram, in all patients with suspected brain abscess. CT is sensitive (over 95 percent) in the detection of a brain abscess but can give additional crucial information such as the extent of the surrounding edema, the presence of hydrocephalus and/or a midline shift, and the precise localization of the lesion. The typical CT appearance of a brain abscess is a hypodense lesion surrounded by a uniformly enhancing ring upon contrast administration. A variable hypodense area of edema extends beyond the ring. Unfortunately, this CT appearance is not specific for a brain abscess, and other processes, including neoplasm, granuloma, cerebral infarction, or resolving hematoma, may give a similar finding on CT. Furthermore, glucocorticoid use may alter the typical appearance on CT; only about 40 to 60 percent of brain abscesses in patients on glucocorticoid therapy reveal ring enhancement on CT scan. Indium 111–labeled leukocyte scintigraphy may prove complementary to CT in the diagnosis of abscesses in the CNS. However, necrotic tumors may be confused with brain abscess by this methodology, and the concomitant use of glucocorticoids also may produce a false-negative scan.

The data regarding the utility of MRI in the diagnosis and evaluation of a patient with a brain abscess continue to accumulate. MRI permits multiplanar imaging, accentuates the contrast between gray and white matter, and affords a variety of imaging techniques to elucidate pathologic changes. In addition, bony artifact, which may hinder CT interpretation, is not a problem with MRI techniques. MRI appears to be more sensitive than CT in the cerebritis phase of brain abscess development, as well as in the detection of associated cerebral edema. Therefore, MRI may detect early satellite lesions not demonstrated by CT and is often more useful for demonstration of

FIGURE 374-1   MRI of brain abscess. Coronal T_1-weighted spin-echo image following gadolinium-DTPA enhancement demonstrating large necrotic right frontal lobe mass with intense peripheral enhancement and surrounding edema. Multiple complications are also evident: ependymal enhancement in lateral and third ventricles and enhancement of subarachnoid space reflecting ventricular rupture, ventriculitis, and meningitis, and mass effect with midline shift. Aspiration revealed pus and *S. milleri* in pure culture.

extraparenchymal extension of an abscess (i.e., ventricular rupture) than CT (Fig. 374-1). The lack of ionizing radiation, greater tissue characterization, lack of bone artifact, increased sensitivity in follow-up evaluations, and less toxic contrast agents make MRI the procedure of choice in the evaluation of a patient with suspected brain abscess.

THERAPY   The optimal management of most patients with a bacterial brain abscess requires both administration of antimicrobial agents and surgical intervention. CT scanning or MRI should be performed without delay in the patient with neurologic complaints and a predisposing condition suggesting brain abscess, as described above. Results in animal models and humans suggest that focal bacterial infections of the brain parenchyma may be "staged" by a sequential CT scan. Cerebritis is characterized by an area of low density surrounded by ring enhancement (often thick and diffuse) that does not decay on delayed contrast scans obtained 1 h later. In contrast, an encapsulated abscess is characterized by a faint ring on the unenhanced scan and ring enhancement that decays in the delayed CT scan. These parameters may prove useful in planning a combined medical-surgical approach. Since 1971, it has been recognized that early antimicrobial therapy alone, in the absence of surgical intervention, could cure cerebritis without the later development of encapsulated abscess. Subsequent cases claiming "cure" of an encapsulated abscess share many of the following features: (1) the initial diagnosis and resolution of brain abscess(es) were documented by sequential CT scans, usually without aspiration or histopathology; (2) prolonged courses (e.g., ≥8 weeks) of high-dose antibiotic therapy were administered, and (3) evidence of encapsulation often was lacking. Based on experimental animal models of brain abscess and the well-defined CT appearance of the cerebritis stage, medical "cures" of established brain abscess may represent successful resolution of bacterial cerebritis. In general, close cooperation between medical and surgical disciplines is essential for the optimal management of a given patient with suspected brain abscess.

The antimicrobial regimens recommended for the empirical (and specific) therapy of a brain abscess reflect considerations of the microbiology as well as evidence from both animal and human studies evaluating the penetration of a given antimicrobial agent into brain parenchyma and/or brain abscess pus. Unfortunately, no prospective, randomized clinical trials exist to guide the clinician in the choice of an optimal antimicrobial regimen. If CT scanning suggests cerebritis and the patient is neurologically stable, antibiotics can be started and the patient observed. Since the early 1960s, a combination of penicillin G (20 to 24 million units per day IV) plus chloramphenicol (1.0 to 1.5 g IV every 6 h) has been advocated in adults. Penicillin remains a mainstay of therapy because of (1) excellent activity against streptococci, including the *S. milleri* group, complicating contiguous foci of infection, and pyogenic lung disease, (2) activity against most anaerobes encountered in brain abscess patients, (3) favorable results obtained in experimental animal models of brain abscess, and (4) a marked reduction in brain abscess mortality observed after the introduction of penicillin in the 1940s. Chloramphenicol often has been administered concurrently with penicillin in the past because of its high lipid solubility, resulting in brain tissue concentrations often exceeding those present in plasma, and good activity against anaerobic bacteria, including *B. fragilis*. The use of metronidazole for the therapy of brain abscess has increased greatly in recent years and has generally supplanted chloramphenicol because (1) metronidazole is bactericidal against *B. fragilis*, whereas chloramphenicol may be bacteriostatic, (2) metronidazole attains reproducibly excellent concentrations in brain abscess pus, (3) entry of metronidazole into brain abscess pus is not affected by concomitant steroid treatment in contrast to several other antibiotics, (4) chloramphenicol may be degraded by deacylation in pus, as shown in experimental intraabdominal abscess, and (5) metronidazole may have had a salutary affect on mortality, as suggested by several recent retrospective studies. Metronidazole, when substituted for chloramphenicol, may lead to more rapid healing and a lower mortality rate; however, these two agents have never been compared in a prospective, randomized clinical trial. Nevertheless, an antianaerobic agent such as metronidazole is indicated for the treatment of brain abscess complicating otitis media, mastoiditis, or pyogenic lung abscess because anaerobes are often present. Metronidazole should never be used alone to treat a patient with suspected brain abscess. Antianaerobic therapy may not be necessary in addition to penicillin for patients with frontal or ethmoidal sinusitis and brain abscess because *B. fragilis* is an uncommon isolate; however, empirical therapy with at least two agents is mandatory prior to culture confirmation. When staphylococci are proven or suspected, as in posttraumatic or postneurosurgical brain abscess, nafcillin or oxacillin (1.5 to 2 g IV every 4 h) is indicated. Vancomycin may be substituted if either the patient is allergic to penicillin or a methicillin-resistant strain is isolated. The frequent isolation of aerobic gram-negative bacilli in brain abscesses of otitic origin prompts many to add a third-generation cephalosporin or trimethoprim-sulfamethoxazole to the antimicrobial regimen pending culture results. Since *P. aeruginosa* is encountered in this setting of chronic middle ear infection, ceftazidime is a logical empirical choice. Recent data suggest that cefotaxime may be adequate for the majority of streptococcal isolates as well, thereby replacing penicillin as the standard regimen (i.e., cefotaxime plus metronidazole as empirical therapy). Installation of antibiotics into the abscess cavity during aspiration, although frequently employed, has never been studied systematically and has no proven additional benefit.

The relative role of aspiration alone or total excision of a brain abscess in the individual patient remains problematic. Given the current availability of stereotactic CT-guided aspiration and its attendant low morbidity while obtaining an accurate microbiologic and pathologic diagnosis, operative therapy should remain the definitive approach for most patients with brain abscess. If the CT scan or MRI suggests the presence of cerebritis and the patient is neurologically stable, antibiotic therapy as previously outlined should be initiated and the patient observed. If the patient remains stable and the abscess is accessible, CT-guided aspiration is then desirable to facilitate a specific pathologic and microbiologic diagnosis. Although this delay may render subsequent cultures negative, aspiration during the cerebritis stage may be associated with an unacceptable risk of hemorrhage, especially in children. If the lesion appears encapsulated by CT scan criteria, antibiotic therapy should be started and aspiration for diagnosis and drainage performed immediately. Subsequent management will depend on both clinical and radiologic assessments. Multiple aspirations may be required to drain the abscess successfully, and this is a potential disadvantage relative to total excision. Neurologic deterioration or failure of the lesion to resolve on follow-up imaging studies is an indication for further surgery, often excision if feasible. The duration of antimicrobial therapy is empirical and also may relate to the initial surgical procedure. Lesions treated by total excision may require a shorter duration of antimicrobial therapy than those treated with aspiration only. In general, most authorities recommend that patients be treated with at least 4 to 6 weeks of parenteral therapy. Metronidazole may be an exception to this rule because of the high oral bioavailability facilitating oral regimens. Prolonged therapy with oral regimens, if a suitable agent(s) is available against the isolated pathogen(s), is often continued for 2 to 6 months following parenteral therapy but is of no proven benefit when compared with shorter treatment regimens. A cured brain abscess may continue to exhibit contrast enhancement on CT scans for 4 to 10 weeks to up to 6 to 9 months after completion of successful therapy. The management of a focal CNS process in an HIV-infected patient requires a different approach and is discussed in Chap. 375. Empirical therapy for toxoplasmosis is often started if the CT appearance is characteristic in a seropositive patient. Brain biopsy for diagnosis may be considered in patients with a negative toxoplasmosis serology, atypical findings on the CT, or evidence of a disseminated process due to another pathogen.

Adjunctive glucocorticoids are often employed during management of patients with brain abscess, but their role remains controversial. Glucocorticoids may reduce antibiotic entry into the CNS, decrease collagen formation and glial response, and therefore lessen the degree of encapsulation of the brain abscess, or they may alter the CT scan appearance of ring enhancement as inflammation subsides, which may obscure information from sequential CT studies from the assessment of cure. Experimental animal models do not suggest that glucocorticoids alter mortality. Glucocorticoids should be employed in patients with proven or suspected raised ICP. In this circumstance, ICP monitoring may be advisable, and elevation may be controlled with steroids, hyperventilation, mannitol, or a combination of these methods. Anticonvulsants are frequently administered empirically to patients with suspected brain abscess.

PROGNOSIS The mortality rate of brain abscess was about 40 to 60 percent in the preantibiotic era and has remained high until relatively recently. The major reduction of the mortality rate (to about 10 percent) coincides with the advent of CT. The incidence of neurologic sequelae, however, ranges between 30 and 55 percent, and late seizures have been documented in as many as 90 percent of survivors. The relative contributions of medical and surgical approaches to the individual patients continue to be refined. Earlier diagnosis through improved technology and an aggressive medical-surgical approach remain essential for the successful management of this unforgiving CNS infection.

SUBDURAL EMPYEMA

DEFINITION Subdural empyema is a collection of pus in the space between the dura mater and the arachnoid membrane. Subdural empyema accounts for about 20 percent of all localized intracranial infections. Prior to the advent of antimicrobial therapy, the disease was almost always fatal, but with current methods of diagnosis and treatment, mortality rates range from 10 to 30 percent.

EPIDEMIOLOGY Although precise incidence figures are unavailable, subdural empyemas are most often a complication of otorhinologic infection. Males predominate by a ratio of approximately 3:1, and about 70 percent of patients are in the second or third decade of life.

ETIOLOGY In the majority of cases, a single microorganism is responsible for subdural empyema, but many cultures obtained at surgery are sterile because patients are often receiving antimicrobial therapy. In addition, the precise role of anaerobic bacteria in this infection has not been studied carefully because anaerobic techniques are often inadequate or not performed at surgery. Nevertheless, the major pathogens include aerobic and anaerobic streptococci (about 50 percent), staphylococci (about 16 percent), aerobic gram-negative bacilli (3 to 8 percent), and other anaerobic bacteria (about 5 percent). As with brain abscess, the causative organism is somewhat predictable based on the anatomic focus of contiguous infection. Otorhinogenic subdural empyemas are usually caused by streptococci (including members of the *S. milleri* group), whereas staphylococci and anaerobes are unusual. Infections arising from head trauma, surgery, or indwelling foreign devices commonly involve staphylococci and/or aerobic gram-negative bacilli. Subdural empyema rarely complicates meningitis but cases due to *S. pneumoniae* or *H. influenzae* have been described. Rare etiologic agents including *Salmonella* sp., *Campylobacter fetus*, *N. meningitidis*, *Pasteurella* sp., and *Actinomyces* sp.

PATHOGENESIS AND PATHOPHYSIOLOGY The subdural space, normally a potential space rather than an actual space, is divided anatomically into several large compartments by the foramen magnum, tentorium cerebelli, base of the brain, and falx cerebri. Since these spaces are confined anatomically, a developing empyema can quickly evolve into a fatal expanding mass lesion. The pathogenesis usually involves spread of infection to the subdural space via valveless emissary veins in association with thrombophlebitis or by extension of an osteomyelitis of the skull with accompanying epidural abscess. Paranasal sinusitis overwhelmingly predominates as the major precipitating factor in patients with subdural empyema. The frontal sinuses are almost always involved, often with other sinuses as well. The frontal and sphenoid sinuses are intimately associated with the dura mater and are often separated by only a thin bony layer. Only about 10 percent of subdural empyemas are found infratentorially. The lesion may communicate with the contralateral side via the inferior free margin of the falx cerebri. The mastoid or middle ear is the source of subdural empyema in 10 to 20 percent of patients, especially in geographic areas (e.g., Sri Lanka) where delay in therapy of otitis media may be complicated by this event. Otitis or mastoiditis may extend directly into the subdural space via erosion of the tegmen tympani or bone adjacent to the dura mater and air cells or may spread indirectly by way of a progressive thrombophlebitis of the perforating veins. Otitis-induced subdural empyema is localized initially on or around the tentorium. Bacterial meningitis in adults is a very unusual cause of subdural empyema. Nevertheless, this lesion complicates about 2 percent of bacterial meningitis cases in infants and may follow an initially sterile subdural effusion. Other predisposing conditions include cranial trauma, neurosurgical procedures, or infection of a preexisting subdural hematoma. Subdural empyema is metastatic in origin in a small minority of cases (about 5 percent), principally from chronic infection in the chest. Once infection develops in the subdural space, spread along the falx and over the convexities may occur. Septic thrombophlebitis of the cortical veins may evolve and lead to hemorrhage, cerebral infarction, brain edema, and fatal transtentorial herniation.

CLINICAL MANIFESTATIONS Subdural empyema may present as a rapidly progressive life-threatening condition. The symptoms and signs relate to the presence of increased ICP, meningeal irritation, or focal cortical inflammation. In addition, the majority of patients (60 to 90 percent) have evidence of their antecedent infection (e.g., sinusitis or otitis). In general, patients often have a nonspecific illness for days to weeks prior to an acutely ill presentation. The most common symptoms and signs include headache, fever, stiff neck, and focal neurologic deficits. Headache, initially localized to the infected sinus or ear, is a prominent complaint and can become generalized

as the infection progresses. Vomiting is common as ICP rises. Early during the course, about one-half of patients have altered mental status, which can progress to obtundation and/or coma in the absence of treatment. Fever above 39°C is present in most cases. Focal neurologic findings appear after 24 to 48 h of illness and progress rapidly to involvement of the entire cerebral hemisphere. Hemiparesis or hemiplegia are the most common focal findings; although ocular palsy is common, dysphasia, homonymous hemianopsia, cerebellar signs, dilated pupils, and other focal presentations also have been observed. Seizures, either focal or generalized, are found in more than 50 percent of cases. Meningeal irritation (particularly meningismus) is found in 70 to 80 percent of patients, although Kernig's and/or Babinski's signs are less frequently noted. In the absence of treatment, neurologic deterioration occurs rapidly with signs of increased ICP and cerebral herniation. Papilledema develops in less than 50 percent of patients. This fulminant picture may not be seen in several clinical settings, including patients with subdural empyema following cranial surgery and/or trauma, where the presentation may be subacute and subtle, in patients receiving prior antimicrobial therapy, after infection of a subdural hematoma, and/or following a metastatic infection to the subdural space from a chronic focus elsewhere. The clinical manifestations of subdural empyema in infants are similar to those found in adults, except that a bulging anterior fontanelle is a common finding.

DIAGNOSIS As with brain abscess, routine studies of blood, urine, and CSF are of limited value in the evaluation of patients with suspected subdural empyema. Most patients have a peripheral blood leukocytosis, and plain films of the skull may be useful in the demonstration of sinusitis or mastoiditis. Since a high clinical suspicion and rapid diagnosis of this condition are critical for a successful outcome, subdural empyema should be suspected in any patient with a CNS syndrome with fever and focal neurologic findings. Lumbar puncture is contraindicated in this setting because of the risk of cerebral herniation. When performed, CSF findings are nonspecific and include an elevated opening pressure, a moderate neutrophilic pleocytosis, and an increased protein concentration. Unless the course is complicated by coexistent bacterial meningitis, CSF Gram's stain and cultures are negative. Cerebral arteriography was the diagnostic procedure of choice prior to the development of CT scans.

At the present time, CT scan with contrast enhancement and MRI are the diagnostic procedures of choice in patients with suspected subdural empyema. The typical CT appearance is of a crescentic or elliptically shaped area of hypodensity below the cranial vault or adjacent to the falx cerebri. Loculations may be seen, and associated mass effect with displacement of midline structures is common. After the administration of contrast material, a fine intense line of enhancement is seen between the subdural collection and the cerebral cortex. However, false-negative CT scans have been reported; MRI provides greater clarity for morphologic detail and may detect empyema not seen clearly on CT. MRI is of particular value in identifying subdural empyema located at the base of the brain, along the falx cerebri, or in the posterior fossa. On the basis of signal intensity, extraaxial empyemas can be differentiated from sterile effusions and/or chronic hematomas. Both CT and MRI can be useful for the demonstration of sinusitis and otitis, although CT is superior to MRI in bone imaging and should be used in cases of penetrating injury or when osteomyelitis is a consideration. Cerebral arteriography should be employed on an emergent basis when MRI is unavailable and subdural empyema is strongly suspected despite a normal CT scan. Arteriography may establish the presence of a subdural avascular mass and detect spread of the lesion to the contralateral or parafalcine subdural space. As stated above, subdural empyema shows a striking sex and age predilection and should be strongly considered in young males in the second and third decades with appropriate clinical findings.

TREATMENT Subdural empyema is a surgical emergency. While awaiting operative intervention, antibiotics should be chosen based on the suspected source of infection, the known organisms associated with that focus of infection, and the host immune status. A combined medical-surgical approach is optimal for the management of these patients. As with brain abscess, no controlled clinical trials have evaluated different antimicrobial regimens for the treatment of subdural empyema. Empirical therapy often includes penicillin G and/or chloramphenicol in the doses as for brain abscess described above. If staphylococci are suspected, a β-lactamase–stable penicillin (e.g., nafcillin, 1.5 g IV every 4 h) should be used, with vancomycin (about 1 g IV every 12 h in adults) reserved for patients allergic to penicillin or when methicillin resistant *S. aureus* (MRSA) are suspected. Metronidazole is often substituted for chloramphenicol at a loading dosage of 15 mg/kg, followed by 7.5 mg/kg IV every 6 h. Many authorities add a third-generation cephalosporin (often cefotaxime or ceftriaxone) in combination until culture results are available. Ceftazidime is useful in patients in whom *P. aeruginosa* is a consideration (after neurosurgery or trauma, etc.). The duration of therapy is empirical; however, parenteral antibiotics should be continued for 3 to 4 weeks after drainage, depending on the patient's clinical response. Longer periods of intravenous therapy and/or continuation as an oral regimen may be required if an associated osteomyelitis is present.

Although case reports have suggested that subdural empyema may respond to antimicrobial agents alone, the optimal approach requires surgical drainage. The comparative efficacy of multiple burr holes versus an open craniotomy has not been subjected to rigorous clinical trial. All cases should involve close cooperation with a neurosurgical service. Previous studies documenting a lower mortality rate in patients undergoing craniotomy may merely reflect a larger percentage of gravely ill patients treated with burr hole drainage alone because of the greater surgical risk associated with an open craniotomy. Unfortunately, burr holes may be inadequate due to the thickened pus during the course of the infection. Craniotomy is often essential for posterior fossa subdural empyemas and is also needed in the 10 to 20 percent of patients who are initially treated with trephination. When craniotomy is performed, wide exposure should be afforded to allow adequate exploration of all areas where subdural pus is suspected. Although antibiotic irrigation at the time of surgery has become common, there are no data on the potential benefits of this practice. Drains or catheters are often left in the subdural space after the initial drainage, but this practice may increase the risk of nosocomial superinfection. Finally, surgical correction of the antecedent otorhinologic infection also may be necessary on an emergent basis. Adjunctive measures to control raised ICP are also essential. Preoperative use of mannitol, dexamethasone, and/or hyperventilation may be effective in controlling ICP. Glucocorticoids should, however, be tapered rapidly after surgical therapy because of the risk of secondary infection. Anticonvulsants are indicated in patients with seizures.

PROGNOSIS The overall mortality of subdural empyema averages 15 to 25 percent, with severe neurologic sequelae (chiefly disabling hemiparesis or aphasia) found in 5 to 25 percent of survivors. Seizures are documented on follow-up in 8 to 46 percent of patients.

SPINAL SUBDURAL EMPYEMA This rare condition, with approximately 20 to 30 cases reported in the literature, is far less common than spinal epidural abscess. The signs and symptoms include fever, back pain, and subsequent manifestations of spinal cord compression, but tenderness to palpation or percussion along the spine is often absent, in contrast to spinal epidural abscess. Most cases occur following hematogenous dissemination from a distant site of infection, and *S. aureus* is the most common etiologic agent. The presentation may resemble transverse myelitis. MRI is the diagnostic procedure of choice for the detection of suspected spinal subdural empyema, since the extent of the lesion is defined more favorably by MRI when compared with CT. Metrizimide spinal CT is also useful in the diagnosis of this condition. Myelography should be performed when MRI and CT are not available. Myelography may not detect the entire length of the empyema if complete blocks are present within

the spinal canal at multiple levels. Treatment should consist of empirical antibiotics initially directed at *S. aureus*, streptococci, and gram-negative enteric bacilli in association with prompt laminectomy for drainage of the empyema. The antimicrobial regimen is commonly administered for 2 to 4 weeks following surgical drainage.

EPIDURAL ABSCESS

SPINAL EPIDURAL ABSCESS This type of abscess possesses unique clinical features and constitutes an important neurologic and neurosurgical emergency. It is discussed in Chap. 381.

INTRACRANIAL EPIDURAL ABSCESS An *epidural abscess* is defined as a suppurative infection in the epidural space. This space is located between the dura mater and the overlying bone. Cranial epidural abscess often crosses the cranial dura along the emissary veins, so subdural empyema is also often present. Therefore, the etiology, pathogenesis, and bacteriology of intracranial abscess are usually similar to those described for subdural empyema, with an initial focus on infection in the paranasal sinuses, middle ear, or mastoids. The overall incidence of cranial epidural abscess is unknown. In general, it is the third most common localized intracranial infection following brain abscess and subdural empyema in frequency. Only about 10 percent of all epidural abscesses arise in the intracranial epidural space. Unlike the striking sex and age distribution of subdural empyema, intracranial abscesses are rare in young children and have been reported over a wide age range. Above the foramen magnum, the epidural space represents only a potential space, since the dura is essentially adherent to the inner lining of the skull. Infections of the intracranial epidural space result primarily from an extension of a contiguous focus of infection, including sinusitis, mastoiditis, scalp or orbital cellulitis, and rhinocerebral mucormycosis, or as a result of an intracranial defect caused by a skull fracture, neurosurgical procedure, or as a complication of fetal monitoring. In general, epidural abscess is a slowly growing mass, which accounts for its insidious clinical presentation. Intracranial abscesses rarely dissect beyond the base of the skull. Similar to subdural empyema, the organisms responsible for intracranial epidural abscesses are dependent on the underlying mechanism. Aerobic and microaerophilic streptococci predominant in infections of the paranasal sinuses, whereas *S. aureus* or *S. epidermidis* and aerobic gram-negative bacilli are associated with cranial trauma. Many other organisms have been isolated from localized intracranial abscesses, including *Salmonella* sp., *Eikenella corrodens*, *Aspergillus* sp. and the agents of mucormycosis. The onset of symptoms is often insidious and may be overshadowed by the primary focus of infection (e.g., sinusitis or otitis). Headache is a usual complaint, but the patient may otherwise be asymptomatic unless the clinical course is complicated by the development of subdural empyema or involvement of deeper intracranial structures because the epidural abscess usually enlarges slowly and does not produce sudden major neurologic deficits unless complicated by deep extension. However, focal neurologic signs and/or focal generalized seizures may develop ultimately. Without treatment, papilledema or other signs of increased ICP develop as the abscess enlarges. An epidural abscess localized near the petrous bone may present as Gradenigo's syndrome, characterized by involvement of cranial nerves V and VI with unilateral facial pain and weakness of the lateral rectus muscle. If cranial osteomyelitis is present, edema and cellulitis of the face and/or scalp may be present. Attention may be focused on the primary process, such as sinusitis, cellulitis, or skull fracture, allowing a developing intracranial abscess to remain undetected. Thus the striking manifestations of the complications, including an alteration in mental status and a declining level of consciousness (including coma and/or meningismus), may be the first indication of an intracranial process. As with patients with suspected subdural empyema, CT scanning and MRI are the diagnostic procedures of choice for the detection of intracranial epidural abscess. Both studies usually demonstrate a superficial circumscribed area of diminished density, often with contrast enhancement. This rim enhancement is usually thicker and more irregular with an epidural abscess than with subdural empyema. Subgaleal or subperiosteal abscesses, calvarial osteomyelitis, and frontal sinusitis are often associated with intracranial abscesses. MRI offers several advantages over CT scanning in the evaluation of patients with suspected intracranial epidural abscess. Small collections are often identified more accurately with MRI, and streak artifacts from bone are absent. In addition, MRI readily differentiates postoperative and posttraumatic abscesses from sterile effusions and/or chronic extraaxial hematomas with far greater accuracy than CT scanning.

As is the case with other focal suppurative infections of the CNS, a combined medical-surgical therapeutic approach is optimal for management of intracranial epidural abscess. In adults, where 60 to 90 percent of intracranial abscesses are a direct result of extension from paranasal sinusitis or mastoiditis, empirical antimicrobial therapy should be directed against aerobic streptococci, staphylococci, and anaerobic bacteria and commonly involves a combination of agents. When cranial defects are suspected or proven, an antistaphylococcal agent such as a penicillinase-resistant penicillin or vancomycin should be added in the dosages discussed above. All intracranial epidural collections should be drained surgically. Furthermore, appropriate stains and cultures should be obtained at the time of surgery, including investigation for acid-fast bacteria and/or fungi if clinically warranted. The actual procedure employed, e.g., burr holes versus craniotomy or craniectomy, depends on the extent of the lesion and involvement of overlying bone. Dural grafting may be necessary if the dura has been breached by infection, and communications between sinus cavities and the epidural space may require surgical closure later. Perhaps due to its insidious clinical presentation, improved diagnostic accuracy of the CT scan and MRI, and the availability of potent antimicrobial agents, the morbidity and mortality of intracranial epidural abscess are low.

SUPPURATIVE INTRACRANIAL THROMBOPHLEBITIS

EPIDEMIOLOGY AND ETIOLOGY Suppurative intracranial thrombophlebitis is defined by the simultaneous presence of venous thrombosis and suppuration in the intracranial compartment. The process may begin within veins and/or venous sinuses following infection of the paranasal sinuses, middle ear, mastoid, facial skin, or oropharynx and may involve additional vessels by propagation of clot or discontinuous spread. Septic intracranial thrombophlebitis also may complicate the presence of epidural abscess, subdural empyema, or bacterial meningitis. Occasionally, but rarely, metastatic spread of infection from a distant site may lead directly to suppurative intracranial thrombophlebitis. Conditions that increase blood viscosity or coagulability, including dehydration, pregnancy, oral contraceptive use, sickle cell disease, polycythemia, malignancy, or trauma, all increase the likelihood of intracranial thrombosis and suppurative complications. Intracranial venous sinus thrombosis depends, to a large extent, on the close proximity of the dural venous sinuses to other structures involved by antecedent conditions. The usual predisposing conditions for the development of cavernous sinus thrombosis are paranasal sinusitis (especially frontal, ethmoidal, or sphenoidal) or infections of the face or mouth. The most common bacterial pathogens depend on the initial source of infection as follows: (1) staphylococci, aerobic and/or microaerophilic streptococci, gram-negative bacilli, and/or anaerobes with sinusitis, and (2) *S. aureus* secondary to facial infections. Otitis media or mastoiditis may be complicated by the development of lateral sinus thrombosis and/or infection of the superior and inferior petrosal sinuses. Infections of the face, scalp, subdural space, epidural space, or meningitis are associated with suppurative thrombophlebitis of the superior sagittal sinus. Again, the most likely infecting microorganisms depend on the associated primary condition. *S. aureus* is the most important

associated pathogen in patients with cavernous sinus thrombosis and is isolated in more than two-thirds of cases. This predominance reflects the importance of this organism in the associated infections of the face and scalp and in acute sphenoid sinusitis. Less common isolates in patients with cavernous sinus thrombosis include streptococci, pneumococci, gram-negative bacilli, and *Bacteroides* sp.

CLINICAL MANIFESTATIONS Not unexpectedly, the clinical presentation of suppurative cortical thrombophlebitis depends on the location of involvement. In addition, if the cortical venous system is involved, the appearance of neurologic deficits is dependent on the adequacy of collateral venous drainage. Patients with inadequate collateral flow present with impairment of consciousness, focal or generalized seizures (often alternating in character), symptoms of increased ICP, and various focal neurologic findings (e.g., hemiparesis). Aphasia is common when the dominant cerebral hemisphere is involved. The most common complaints in patients with cavernous sinus thrombosis include periorbital swelling (73 percent) and headache (52 percent). Headache is more common when the antecedent condition is sinusitis rather than a facial cellulitis. Other prominent symptoms include diplopia, tearing, photophobia, drowsiness, and ptosis. Fever is present in over 90 percent of patients with cavernous sinus thrombosis. Upon examination, proptosis, chemosis, periorbital edema, and weakness of the extraocular muscles due to involvement of the cranial nerves III, IV, or VI are common. Since the abducens nerve is the only cranial nerve traversing the inferior portion of the cavernous sinus, a lateral gaze palsy may be an early neurologic finding. Papilledema or venous engorgement and a change in mental status are observed in approximately 65 and 55 percent of patients, respectively. Meningitis, often confusing the diagnostic issues, is present in about 40 percent of cases, usually secondary to retrograde spread of thrombophlebitis. About 25 percent of patients also have dilated or sluggishly reactive pupils, decreased visual acuity (frequently progressing to blindness), and dysfunction of cranial nerve V. With spread of the infection to the opposite cavernous sinus, these findings may be duplicated in the opposite eye. In addition, septic cavernous sinus thrombosis may present in two ways. In the acute presentation, the onset between the primary infection (usually a facial cellulitis) and cavernous sinus thrombosis is less than 1 week. The patient appears seriously ill, with a rapid development of symptoms and signs described above and progression to bilateral eye signs. In contrast, some patients present with a more indolent form of cavernous sinus thrombosis, usually secondary to dental infections, otitis media, or paranasal sinusitis. The orbital manifestations are less impressive, and involvement of the contralateral eye is a late and inconsistent finding. Headache is the most prominent finding (> 80 percent) in patients with septic lateral sinus thrombosis, but earache, vomiting, nausea, and vertigo are often present, since otitis media is a common predisposing condition. Fever and abnormal ear findings are observed in the majority of patients (about 80 and 98 percent, respectively); facial pain, altered facial sensation, papilledema, mild nuchal rigidity, and/or a sixth nerve palsy also may be present. Thrombosis of the superior sagittal sinus produces an abnormal mental status progressing to coma, motor deficits, nuchal rigidity, and papilledema. Seizures occur in more than 50 percent of patients. The onset may be subacute, particularly in patients with sinusitis. Involvement of the inferior petrosal sinus may produce ipsilateral facial pain and lateral rectus muscle weakness (Gradenigo's syndrome).

DIAGNOSIS MRI is the diagnostic procedure of choice for the evaluation of patients with suspected suppurative intracranial thrombophlebitis. MRI is far superior to CT in differentiating thrombosis from normal flowing blood. MRI also can reveal the evolution and resolution of the entire venoocclusive process. CT scanning, with and without intravenous contrast enhancement, also permits diagnosis of venous sinus thrombosis, but it is considerably less sensitive and reliable than MRI. The CT appearance usually reveals unilateral or bilateral multiple irregular filling defects in the enhancement of the cavernous sinus with or without orbital inflammatory change. Both MRI and CT can reliably evaluate the paranasal sinuses and provide information concerning subdural and epidural infection, cerebral infarction, cerebritis, hemorrhage, and/or cerebral edema. In the unusual case in which MRI and CT are negative but suspicion of thrombophlebitis is high, carotid arteriography with venous phase studies should be performed. Arteriography reveals narrowing of the intracavernous segment of the carotid sinus in cavernous sinus thrombosis. Orbital venography also may be useful and is the most definitive method of demonstrating cavernous sinus thrombosis. As with other focal suppurative intracranial processes, the lumbar puncture usually demonstrates a mild pleocytosis and an elevated protein concentration. In septic thrombosis of the superior sagittal sinus, however, the CSF finding may be consistent with a frank meningitis, and the causative organism is often isolated on CSF culture. Blood cultures may be positive, especially in patients with a rapidly progressing course. Chest radiographs may reveal evidence of septic pulmonary emboli following propagation of thrombus into the inferior petrosal sinus and the jugular vein.

TREATMENT Analogous to subdural empyema and epidural abscess, empirical therapy should be directed toward gram-positive organisms, including staphylococci, aerobic gram-negative bacilli, and anaerobes. In cavernous sinus thrombosis, a potent antistaphylococcal agent should always be included in the antimicrobial regimen. Nafcillin should be used, with vancomycin reserved for the penicillin-allergic patient and when methicillin-resistant organisms are suspected or proven. Combination regimens including nafcillin or vancomycin plus metronidazole plus a third-generation cephalosporin are often used. Surgical intervention may be required for optimal therapy. Surgical drainage of infected sinuses is necessary when antimicrobial therapy alone is ineffective. Operative intervention for patients with cavernous sinus thrombosis is often employed, especially in the setting of sphenoid sinusitis. Internal jugular vein ligation and thrombectomy have been utilized in patients with lateral sinus vein thrombosis, but the efficacy of these procedures is poorly defined. Surgical therapy also may be necessary for other contiguous foci of infection, e.g., dental abscess. Anticoagulation is controversial. Although anticoagulation may prevent the spread of the thrombus, the benefit is most apparent when initiated early during the course. However, the hazards of intracranial hemorrhage, including bleeding from sites of cortical venous infarction, must be recognized. In the absence of definitive data and specific contraindications, anticoagulation is most likely to be useful early in the course of cavernous sinus thrombosis. Anticoagulation is not recommended for septic lateral sinus thrombophlebitis because the cortical veins overlying the infected mastoid may become occluded, resulting in small venous hemorrhagic infarcts and leading to the consequences of intracerebral hemorrhage.

REFERENCES

CAMPBELL S: Amebic brain abscess and meningoencephalitis. Semin Neurol 13:153, 1993

DINUBILE MJ et al: Septic cortical thrombophlebitis. J Infect Dis 161:1216, 1990

FEIGIN RD et al: Diagnosis and management of meningitis. Pediatr Infect Dis J 11:785, 1992

HELFGOTT DC et al: Subdural empyema, in *Infections of the Central Nervous System,* WM Scheld et al (eds). New York, Raven, 1991, pp 487–498

KILPI T et al: Severity of childhood bacterial meningitis and duration of illness before diagnosis. Lancet 2:406, 1991

KUMAR P, VERMA IC: Antibiotic therapy for bacterial meningitis in children in developing countries. Bull World Health Organ 71:183, 1993

LEBELL MH et al: Dexamethasone therapy for bacterial meningitis: Results of two double-blind, placebo-controlled trials. N Engl J Med 319:964, 1988

ODIO CM et al: The beneficial effects of early dexamethasone administration in infants and children with bacterial meningitis. N Engl J Med 324:1525, 1991

PELTOLA H et al: Rapid disappearance of *Haemophilus influenzae* type b meningitis after routine childhood immunization with conjugate vaccines. Lancet 340:592, 1992

PFISTER HW et al: Spectrum of complications during bacterial meningitis in adults—Results of a prospective clinical study. Arch Neurol 50:575, 1993

PINNER RW et al: Meningococcal disease in the United States–1986. J Infect Dis 164:368, 1991

POMEROY LS et al: Seizures and other neurologic sequelae of bacterial meningitis in children. N Engl J Med 323:1651, 1990

QUAGLIARELLO V, SCHELD WM: Bacterial meningitis: Pathogenesis, pathophysiology, and progress. N Engl J Med 327:864, 1992

ROOS KL et al: Acute bacterial meningitis in children and adults, in *Infections of the Central Nervous System,* WM Scheld et al (eds). New York, Raven, 1991, pp 335–409

SAEZ-LLORENS X et al: Molecular pathophysiology of bacterial meningitis: Current concepts and therapeutic implications. J Pediatr 116:671, 1990

SCHELD WM: Recent advances in the pathophysiology and management of bacterial meningitis. J Infect Dis (in press)

SEYDOUX CH, FRANCIOLI P: Bacterial brain abscesses: Factors influencing mortality and sequelae. Clin Infect Dis 15:394, 1992

SOUTHWICK FS et al: Septic thrombosis of the dural venous sinuses. Medicine 65:82, 1985

SPANOS A et al: Differential diagnosis of acute meningitis. JAMA 262:2700, 1989

STEPHENS DS, FARLEY MM: Pathogenetic events during infection of the human nasal pharynx with *Neisseria meningitidis* and *Haemophilus influenzae*. Rev Infect Dis 13:22, 1991

TUNKEL AR et al: Bacterial meningitis: Recent advances in pathophysiology and treatment. Ann Intern Med 112:610, 1990

TUNKEL AR, SCHELD WM: Pathogenesis and pathophysiology of bacterial meningitis. Ann Rev Med 44:103, 1993

TUREEN JH et al: Effect of hydration status on cerebral blood flow and cerebrospinal fluid lactate acidosis in rabbits with experimental meningitis. J Clin Invest 89:947, 1992

TYLER K, MARTIN JB: *Infectious Diseases of the Central Nevous System*. Philadelphia, FA Davis, 1993

WENGER JD et al: Bacterial meningitis in the United States, 1986: Report of a multistate surveillance study. J Infect Dis 162:1316, 1990

WISPELWEY B, SCHELD WM: Brain abscess, in *Principles and Practices of Infectious Diseases,* 4th ed. GL Mandell et al (eds). New York: Churchill Livingstone, in press

——— et al: Brain abscess, in *Infections of the Central Nervous System,* WM Scheld et al (eds). New York, Raven, 1991, pp 457–486

ZIMMERMAN RD, WEINGARTEN K: Evaluation of intracranial inflammatory disease by CT and MRI, in *Clinical Neuroimaging,* WH Theodore (ed). New York, Liss, 1988, pp 75–100

375 VIRAL AND PRION DISEASES OF THE NERVOUS SYSTEM

KENNETH L. TYLER

Hundreds of viruses have been reported to produce acute infection and injury to the central or peripheral nervous systems. Many aspects of the clinical characteristics of these diseases are determined by whether the infection is limited primarily to the meninges (*meningitis*) or extends to involve the parenchyma of the brain (*encephalitis*) and/ or spinal cord (*myelitis*). Although there are a number of similarities in the basic epidemiology and diagnostic approaches to these disorders, they are discussed separately. Viruses also can produce chronic or persistent infections of the central nervous system (CNS). These disorders are sufficiently different from acute viral infections and from each other as to merit separate consideration. Special emphasis is given to HIV infection of the nervous system, both because of its obvious epidemiologic importance and because of its capacity to produce myriad neurologic syndromes as it attacks virtually every part of the nervous system. An additional group of neurologic disorders, commonly discussed in the context of viral infections, shares the characteristics of being transmissible neurodegenerative diseases (TNDs), although the brunt of recent evidence indicates that they are caused by a novel class of agents, commonly referred to as *prions* ("proteinaceous infectious particles").

ACUTE VIRAL INFECTIONS

VIRAL MENINGITIS   Clinical picture The syndrome of viral meningitis consists of fever, headache, and signs of meningeal irritation coupled with an inflammatory cerebrospinal fluid (CSF) profile typically consisting of a lymphocytic pleocytosis, a slightly elevated protein level, and a normal glucose level. Fever may be accompanied by malaise, myalgia, anorexia, nausea and vomiting, abdominal pain, or diarrhea. It is not uncommon to see a mild degree

TABLE 375-1 Viruses causing aseptic meningitis*

Common	Less common	Rare
Enteroviruses	HSV-1	Adenoviruses
Arboviruses	LCMV	CMV
HIV	Mumps	EBV
HSV-2		Influenza A, B; measles; parainfluenza; rubella; VZV

* CMV = cytomegalovirus; EBV = Epstein-Barr virus; HIV = human immunodeficiency virus; HSV = herpes simplex virus; LCMV = lymphocytic choriomeningitis virus; VZV = varicella-zoster virus.

of lethargy or drowsiness. The presence of more profound alterations in consciousness such as stupor, coma, or marked confusion should prompt consideration of alternative diagnoses. Similarly, the presence of seizures, cranial nerve palsies, or other focal neurologic signs or symptoms suggests parenchymal involvement and is not typical of uncomplicated viral meningitis. The headache associated with viral meningitis is typically frontal or retro-orbital in location and often associated with photophobia and pain on moving the eyes. Nuchal rigidity is present in the majority of cases but may be mild in nature and present only in the terminal portion of neck anteflexion. Evidence of severe meningeal irritation, such as Kernig's and Brudzinski's signs, are generally absent.

Etiology Comprehensive attempts to identify the etiology of individual cases of viral meningitis are rarely made in general practice. In large series, using routine serologic and culture techniques, a specific viral cause can be found in 30 to 70 percent of cases (Table 375-1).

Epidemiology It is impossible to determine the exact incidence of viral meningitis in the United States, since the majority of cases go unreported to public health authorities. There is a striking increase in cases during the summer months, reflecting the seasonal predominance of enterovirus and arbovirus infections, with a peak monthly incidence of about 1 reported case per 100,000 population. The striking seasonal predilections of some of the viruses causing meningitis can provide a valuable clue to diagnosis (Table 375-2), although it is important to recognize that seasonal distributions are relative rather than absolute indicators of frequency.

Laboratory diagnosis CSF EXAMINATION The most important laboratory test in the diagnosis of meningitis is examination of the CSF. The typical profile in cases of viral meningitis is a lymphocytic pleocytosis, slightly elevated protein level, and normal glucose level. Organisms *cannot* be seen on Gram's or acid-fast stained smears or india ink wet mounts of CSF. Polymorphonuclear neutrophils (PMNs) may predominate in the first 48 h of illness, especially in some enteroviral infections, and may last longer when infection is due to echovirus 9 or Eastern equine virus (EEV). Patients with suspected viral meningitis and a PMN pleocytosis should have a follow-up CSF examination after 8 to 12 h to look for the presence of a shift toward mononuclear cells. The presence of a PMN pleocytosis always should prompt consideration of bacterial meningitis or parameningeal infections. The total CSF cell count per microliter in viral meningitis rarely exceeds 1000. The CSF glucose level is typically normal in viral infections, although it may be decreased in cases due to mumps (10 to 30 percent), lymphocytic choriomeningitis virus (LCMV) and, less frequently, echovirus and other enteroviruses, herpes simplex

virus type 2 (HSV-2), or varicella-zoster virus (VZV). As a general rule, a lymphocytic pleocytosis with a low glucose level (≤25 mg/dL) should suggest the presence of fungal, listerial, or tuberculous meningitis or of noninfectious disorders (e.g., sarcoid, neoplastic meningitis).

A number of tests measuring levels of various CSF proteins, enzymes, and mediators, including C-reactive protein, lactic acid, lactate dehydrogenase, neopterin, interleukin 1β (IL-1β), IL-6, soluble IL-2 receptor, beta₂ microglobulin, and tumor necrosis factor (TNF), have been proposed as potential discriminators between viral and bacterial meningitis or as markers of specific types of viral infection (e.g., human immunodeficiency virus, HIV), but most appear to lack sufficient sensitivity and specificity to be truly useful. It has been suggested recently that the presence of detectable TNF-α in the CSF is indicative of bacterial infection and is not found in cases of viral meningitis, although this observation requires further confirmation. Patients with HIV CNS infection often have elevated CSF levels of p24 antigen, and this may be useful in diagnosis.

CSF CULTURE The overall results of CSF culture for the diagnosis of viral infection are disappointing (Table 375-3), presumably reflecting the generally low concentration of infectious virus present and the need to customize isolation procedures for individual viruses. For viral isolation, 2 mL of CSF should be obtained and brought promptly to the microbiology laboratory, where it should be refrigerated and processed as speedily as possible. As a general rule, CSF specimens for viral isolation should never be stored in a freezer (−20°C), since viruses are often unstable at this temperature, and most modern freezers have "frostfree" warmup cycles that are detrimental to viral stability. Storage for more than 24 h is probably best done in a −70°C freezer.

OTHER SOURCES FOR VIRAL ISOLATION It is important to remember that viruses also may be isolated from sites and body fluids other than CSF. Enteroviruses and adenoviruses may be found in feces; arboviruses, some enteroviruses, and LCMV, in blood; mumps and cytomegalovirus (CMV), in urine; and enteroviruses, mumps, and adenoviruses, in throat washings. During enteroviral infections, viral shedding in stool may persist for several weeks. The presence of enterovirus in stool is not diagnostic and may result from residual shedding from a previous enteroviral infection and also can occur in some asymptomatic individuals during enteroviral epidemics.

NUCLEIC ACID AMPLIFICATION Amplification of viral-specific DNA or RNA from CSF using polymerase chain reaction (PCR) amplification or related techniques appears to have great promise as a diagnostic tool. HSV-1 DNA has been amplified from the CSF of patients with herpes simplex encephalitis and recurrent (Mollaret) meningitis even when standard culture techniques have been negative. Successful genomic amplification and detection of picornaviruses (coxsackie, polio) in the CSF of patients with meningitis also have been reported. These techniques will undoubtedly become more widely available in the future.

SEROLOGIC STUDIES In most cases, definitive diagnosis of viral infection depends on documentation of seroconversion between acute phase and convalescent sera (typically obtained after 2 to 4 weeks). Antiviral antibodies also may be measured in CSF (see below). The timing of the antibody response often means that the utility of serologic data is primarily in retrospective establishment of a specific diagnosis, and their value in initial diagnosis and management is limited. Most viral infections of the CNS are associated with

TABLE 375-2 Seasonal prevalence of viruses commonly causing meningitis

Summer–early fall	Fall and winter	Winter and spring	Nonseasonal
Arboviruses Enteroviruses	LCMV	Mumps	HIV HSV

NOTE: Abbreviations as in Table 375-1.

TABLE 375-3 Possibility of culturing specific viruses from CSF

Excellent	Fair	Poor or none
Coxsackie, echo, LCMV, mumps	HIV, adeno, arboviruses (most), HSV-2, VZV, rabies	Polio, HSV-1, EBV, CMV

NOTE: Abbreviations as in Table 375-1.

intrathecal synthesis of antiviral antibody. This results in an elevation in the CSF/serum antibody ratio. Similar elevations also may occur as a result of breakdown in the blood-brain barrier (BBB), but this is typically associated with elevation in the CSF/serum albumin ratio. Obtaining paired CSF and sera for serologic testing may provide additional evidence that an antibody response is the result of CNS infection. The sensitivity of CSF/serum antibody ratio studies may be enhanced by correcting for breakdown of the BBB using the CSF/serum albumin ratio or using CSF/serum antibody ratios of other viruses as controls. Although use of CSF/serum antibody ratio determinations may enhance the sensitivity of diagnosis, the technique still suffers from the delay between onset of infection and appearance of the host's antibody response.

Agarose electrophoresis or isoelectric focusing of CSF gamma globulins may reveal the presence of oligoclonal bands. These have been found in association with a number of viral infections, including HIV, HTLV-I, mumps, subacute sclerosing panencephalitis (SSPE), and progressive rubella panencephalitis. The associated antibodies are often directed against viral proteins. The finding of oligoclonal bands may be of some diagnostic utility, since they are not seen with arbovirus, enterovirus, or HSV infections. It is important to recognize that oligoclonal bands are commonly encountered in certain noninfectious neurologic diseases (e.g., multiple sclerosis) and may be found in nonviral infections (e.g., syphilis, Lyme borreliosis).

OTHER LABORATORY STUDIES   All patients with suspected viral meningitis should have a complete blood count and differential, platelet count, hematocrit, erythrocyte sedimentation rate (ESR), electrolytes, glucose, liver function tests, BUN, creatinine, creatine kinase, aldolase, amylase, and lipase. Abnormalities in specific tests may provide a clue suggesting particular etiologic diagnoses. Magnetic resonance imaging (MRI), computed tomography (CT), electroencephalography (EEG), evoked response studies, electromyography (EMG), and nerve conduction studies are not necessary in the majority of cases and should not be ordered routinely. Their use is best tailored to individual circumstances when atypical presentations or unusual features of particular cases present diagnostic problems.

Differential diagnosis   Perhaps the most important issue in the differential diagnosis is the exclusion of nonviral causes that can mimic viral encephalitis. The major categories of disease that should always be specifically considered and excluded are (1) parameningeal infections or partially treated bacterial meningitis, (2) nonviral infectious meningitides where cultures may be negative (e.g., fungal, tuberculous, or syphilitic disease), (3) neoplastic meningitis, and (4) meningitis secondary to noninfectious inflammatory diseases such as sarcoid, Behçet disease, and the uveomeningitic syndromes. Although the diagnosis of a specific viral etiology in a particular case of viral meningitis can rarely be made on clinical grounds alone, proper attention to epidemiologic, clinical, and laboratory features may substantially narrow the diagnostic possibilities. Statistically, *enteroviruses* (see Chap. 154) are the most common cause of viral meningitis (>80 percent of cases with etiology identified) and should be considered the leading candidates when a typical case occurs in the summer months, especially in a child (<15 years of age) (Table 375-4). However, despite their summer prevalence, it is important to recognize that sporadic cases of enteroviral CNS infection are seen year-round. The physical examination should include a careful search for exanthemata, hand-foot-mouth disease, herpangina, pleurodynia, myopericarditis, and hemorrhagic conjunctivitis, which may be stigmata of enterovirus infections.

Mumps (see Chap. 157) should be considered when meningitis occurs in the late winter or early spring, especially in males (male/female ratio 3:1). With the widespread use of the live attenuated mumps vaccine in the United States, the incidence of mumps meningitis has fallen dramatically. Rare cases of mumps vaccine–associated meningitis have been reported, but they are not usually seen after vaccination with the Jeryl-Lynn strain of virus used in the United States. The presence of orchitis, oophoritis, parotitis, or pancreatitis or elevations in serum lipase and amylase are suggestive

TABLE 375-4   Enteroviruses causing aseptic meningitis

	Polio	Coxsackie	Echo	Entero
Common		A7,9 B2–5	4,6,9,11,16 30	
Less common	1–3	A1–6,8,10, 11,14,16– 18,22,24 B1,6	1–3,5,7,8 12–15,17–23 25,27,28,30 31,33	70,71

but can be found with other viruses. Mumps infection confers lifelong immunity, so a previous history of documented infection excludes this diagnosis. The presence of hypoglycorrhachia (10 to 30 percent) may be an additional diagnostic clue, once other causes have been excluded (see above).

Development of meningitis in the late fall or winter associated with a history of exposure to house mice (*Mus musculus*), pet or laboratory rodents (e.g., hamsters), or their excreta should suggest the possibility of *LCMV infection* (see Chap. 160). Some patients have an associated rash, pulmonary infiltrates, alopecia, parotitis, orchitis, or myopericarditis. Laboratory clues to the diagnosis may include the presence of leukopenia, thrombocytopenia, abnormal liver function tests, or pulmonary infiltrates. Some cases present with a marked CSF pleocytosis (>1000 cells per microliter) and hypoglycorrhachia (<30 percent).

HSV-2 (see Chap. 143) *meningitis* should be suspected in any patient with concomitant primary genital infection, but it also occurs less commonly with recurrent (secondary) episodes of genital disease. Both *HSV-1* and *HSV-2* should be considered in patients with recurrent episodes of aseptic meningitis (Mollaret meningitis), although special techniques, such as PCR amplification of viral genomic material from the CSF, may be required to establish the diagnosis in these cases. *Epstein-Barr virus (EBV) infections* also may produce aseptic meningitis, with or without accompanying evidence of the infectious mononucleosis syndrome. The diagnosis may be suggested by the presence of atypical lymphocytes in the CSF or an atypical lymphocytosis in peripheral blood. *VZV meningitis* should be suspected in the presence of concurrent chickenpox or shingles. Some patients develop a distinctive syndrome of acute cerebellar ataxia. This typically occurs in children and presents with the abrupt onset of limb and truncal ataxia. A similar syndrome occurs less commonly in association with EBV and enteroviral infection.

Arbovirus infections typically occur in the summer months, have clear geographic localization, and occur in epidemics, all factors reflecting the ecology of their transmission through infected insect vectors (see Fig. 375-1 and Table 375-6; see also Chap. 159). Arboviral meningitis should be considered when clusters of meningitis cases occur in a restricted geographic region during the summer or early fall. A history of tick exposure or travel or residence in the appropriate geographic area should suggest the possibility of Colorado tick fever virus (CTFV) or Powassan virus infection, although nonviral diseases producing meningitis (e.g., Lyme disease) or headache with meningismus (e.g., Rocky mountain spotted fever) also may present this way.

HIV infection is discussed more fully below and in Chap. 279. HIV meningitis should be suspected in any patient with known or identified risk factors for HIV infection. Aseptic meningitis appears to be a common manifestation of primary exposure to HIV and may be associated with HIV seroconversion (see Chap. 279). In some patients, seroconversion may be delayed for several months, and in seronegative patients, serology should be repeated after 3- and 6-month intervals. Cranial nerve palsies are more common in HIV meningitis than in other viral infections, most commonly involving cranial nerves V, VII, or VIII.

Treatment   In the usual case of viral meningitis, treatment is symptomatic, and hospitalization is not required. Exceptions to this rule include patients with deficient humoral immunity, neonates with

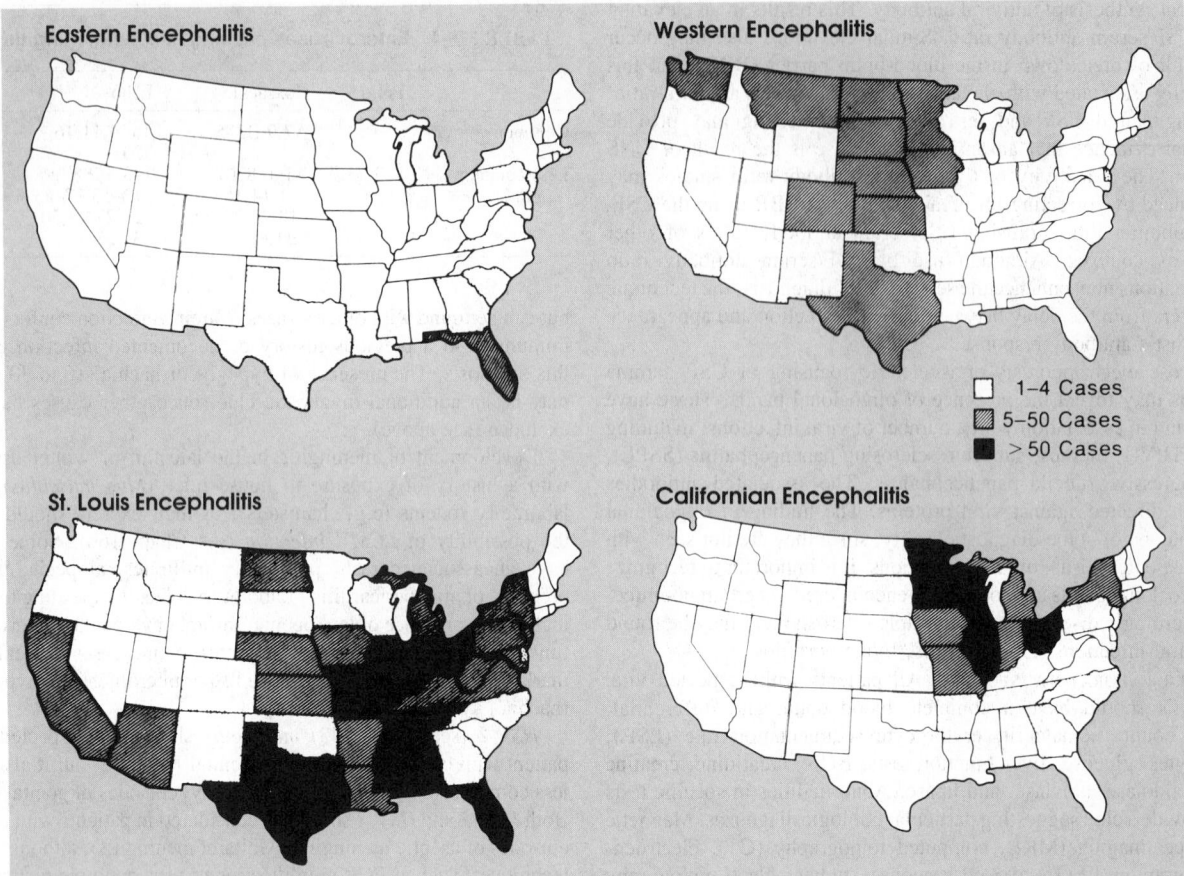

FIGURE 375-1 Geographic distributions of the most commonly encountered arbovirus encephalitides in the United States. (*From RT Johnson, with permission.*)

overwhelming infection, and patients in whom the clinical or CSF profile suggests the possibility of bacterial or other nonviral causes of infection. Patients with suspected bacterial meningitis should receive appropriate empirical therapy pending culture results (see Chap. 374). Patients with deficient humoral immunity may benefit from a trial of intravenous gamma globulin. Oral or intravenous acyclovir may be beneficial to patients with meningitis caused by HSV-1 or HSV-2 and, although rarely indicated, would theoretically be of value in cases of severe EBV or VZV infection. Zidovudine (AZT) or didanosine (formerly dideoxyinosine; ddI) presumably would be of value in the treatment of HIV meningitis, although no clinical trials have been performed. Patients usually prefer to rest undisturbed in a quiet, darkened room. Analgesics can be used to relieve headache, which is often reduced by the initial diagnostic lumbar puncture. Antipyretics may help to reduce fever, which rarely exceeds 40°C. Hyponatremia may develop as a result of the syndrome of inappropriate vasopressin secretion (SIADH), so fluid and electrolyte status should be monitored. Repeat lumbar puncture is only indicated in patients whose fever and symptoms fail to be resolving after a few days or if there is doubt about the initial diagnosis. Vaccination is an effective method of preventing the subsequent development of meningitis and other neurologic complications associated with poliovirus, mumps, and measles infection.

Prognosis In adults, the prognosis for full recovery from viral meningitis is excellent. Rare patients continue to complain of persisting headache, mild mental impairment, incoordination, or generalized asthenia for weeks to months. The outcome in infants and neonates (<1 year of age) is less certain. Intellectual impairment, learning disabilities, hearing loss, and other lasting neurologic sequelae have been reported in some but not all studies; however, their frequency is uncertain.

VIRAL ENCEPHALITIS Definition In distinction to meningitis, where the brunt of the infectious process and associated inflammatory

response is limited to the meninges, in encephalitis there is, in addition, involvement of the brain parenchyma.

Clinical picture In addition to the acute febrile illness with evidence of meningeal involvement characteristic of meningitis, the patient with encephalitis commonly has an altered level of consciousness, an abnormal mental state, and evidence of either focal or diffuse neurologic signs and symptoms. All degrees of altered consciousness may occur, ranging from mild lethargy to deep coma. A patient with encephalitis is not mentally alert and is frequently confused, delirious, and disoriented. Mental aberrations may include hallucinations, agitation, personality change, behavioral disorders, and at times, a frankly psychotic state. Focal or generalized seizures occur in more than 50 percent of patients with severe encephalitis. Virtually every possible type of focal neurologic disturbance has been reported in viral encephalitis, the signs and symptoms reflecting the sites of infection and inflammation. The most commonly encountered focal findings are aphasia, ataxia, hemiparesis (with hyperactive tendon reflexes and extensor plantar responses), involuntary movements (e.g., myoclonic jerks), and cranial nerve deficits (e.g., ocular palsies, facial weakness). Involvement of the hypothalamic-pituitary axis may result in temperature dysregulation, diabetes insipidus, or the development of SIADH. Despite the clear neuropathologic evidence that viruses differ in the regions of the CNS they injure, it is often impossible to reliably distinguish on clinical grounds alone one type of viral encephalitis (e.g., that caused by HSV) from others (see "Differential Diagnosis").

Etiology The number of viruses reported to cause encephalitis is legion. In the United States, there are approximately 20,000 reported cases per year. The same organisms responsible for aseptic meningitis are also responsible for encephalitis, although their relative frequencies differ (Table 375-5).

Laboratory diagnosis CSF EXAMINATION CSF examination should be performed in all patients with suspected viral encephalitis unless contraindicated by the presence of severely increased intracranial pressure (ICP). The characteristic CSF profile is indistinguishable from that of viral meningitis and consists of a lymphocytic pleocytosis, a mildly elevated protein level, and a normal glucose level. A CSF pleocytosis (>5 cells per microliter) occurs in more than 95 percent of patients with documented viral encephalitis, and its absence should prompt a careful search for other causes of an encephalopathy. In rare cases, a pleocytosis may be absent on the initial lumbar puncture, but present subsequently. Patients who are severely immunocompromised by radiation, chemotherapy, or certain lymphoreticular malignancies may fail to mount a CSF inflammatory response. The cell count exceeds 500 cells per microliter in only about 10 percent of patients. Infections with certain arboviruses (Eastern equine encephalitis or California encephalitis), mumps, and LCMV occasionally may result in more than 1000 cells per microliter, but this degree of pleocytosis should suggest the possibility of nonviral infections or other inflammatory processes. Atypical lymphocytes in the CSF may be seen in EBV infection and less commonly with other viruses, including CMV and HSV. The presence of substantial numbers of PMNs after the first 48 h should prompt consideration of bacterial infection, leptospirosis, amebic infection, and noninfectious processes such as acute hemorrhagic leukoencephalitis; however, large numbers of PMNs in the CSF are occasionally present with Eastern encephalitis, echovirus 9, and other enteroviral infections. About 20 percent of patients with encephalitis will have a significant (>500 cells per microliter) number of red blood cells in the CSF in a nontraumatic tap. The pathologic correlate of this may be the presence of a hemorrhagic encephalitis of the type seen with HSV, Colorado tick fever virus (CTFV), and occasionally California encephalitis virus (CEV). A decreased CSF glucose level is distinctly unusual in viral encephalitis and should suggest the possibility of fungal, tuberculous, parasitic, leptospiral, syphilitic, sarcoid, or neoplastic meningitis. Rare patients with mumps, LCMV, or late in the stage of HSV encephalitis may have hypoglycorrhachia.

CSF CULTURE   Attempts to culture viruses from the CSF in cases of encephalitis are often disappointing (see Table 375-3). In particular, it should be noted that cultures are invariably negative in cases of HSV-1 encephalitis.

NUCLEIC ACID AMPLIFICATION   Early reports indicated that this may be an extremely promising approach to the diagnosis of certain types of viral encephalitis. Most studies have focused on PCR amplification of HSV DNA from the CSF of patients with suspected HSV encephalitis, although successful amplification of enteroviral RNA also has been reported (see "Viral Meningitis").

SEROLOGIC STUDIES AND ANTIGEN DETECTION   The basic approach to the serodiagnosis of viral encephalitis is identical to that discussed earlier for viral meningitis. In the case of HSV encephalitis, attention has focused on the detection of HSV antibodies in the CSF. In one large series, antibodies to HSV-1 glycoprotein B were found in 97 percent of biopsy-proven cases of HSV encephalitis. The specificity was 100 percent if the assay was corrected for leakage across the blood-brain barrier using adenovirus antibodies as a marker. In another study, virus glycoprotein antigens (gB, gC, gD, and gE) were found in the CSF of 92 percent of patients with biopsy-proven cases of HSV encephalitis and had a specificity of 82 percent. Unfortunately, the best results with these types of assays occur after the first week of illness. This limits their utility to retrospective diagnostic confirmation rather than acute diagnosis.

CT, MRI, EEG   Patients with suspected encephalitis almost invariably undergo structural imaging studies and often EEG. The utility of these tests is to identify or help exclude alternative diagnoses and to help establish the existence of a focal, as opposed to a diffuse, encephalitic process. The presence of focal findings should always raise the possibility of HSV encephalitis. These are (1) periodic focal spikes on a background of slow or low-amplitude ("flattened") activity with a temporal predominance of EEG, (2) temporoparietal areas of low absorption, mass effect, and contrast enhancement on CT, or (3) areas of increased signal intensity in the frontotemporal,

TABLE 375-5 Viruses causing encephalitis

Common	Less common	Rare
Arboviruses, enteroviruses, HSV-1, mumps	CMV, EBV, HIV, measles, VZV	Adenoviruses, CTFV, influenza A, LCMV, parainfluenza, rabies, rubella

NOTE: Abbreviations as in Table 375-1. Also CTFV = Colorado tick fever virus

cingulate, or insular regions of the brain on T_2-weighted spin-echo MRI images.

BRAIN BIOPSY   The isolation of HSV from brain tissue obtained at biopsy has been considered the gold standard for the diagnosis of HSV encephalitis and has been employed in the major trials of HSV encephalitis therapy conducted by the National Institutes of Allergy and Infectious Diseases Collaborative Antiviral Study Group (NIAID-CASG). Biopsy tissue is cultured for virus and examined histopathologically and ultrastructurally. Biopsy is typically carried out under general anesthesia through a craniectomy. Tissue should be taken from a site that appears to be significantly involved based on clinical and laboratory criteria. The most common practice is to obtain tissue (1 cm^3) from the anterior portion of the inferior temporal gyrus through a subtemporal craniectomy. The sensitivity of brain biopsy exceeds 95 percent, and its specificity is probably greater than 99 percent. Although brain biopsy is not an innocuous procedure, the mortality rate is low (<0.2 percent). Potential morbidity, in addition to that related to general anesthesia, includes local bleeding and edema, the development of a seizure focus, and wound dehiscence or infection. From a practical viewpoint, the incidence of serious morbidity appears to be between 0.5 and 2 percent.

Although brain biopsy was widely employed when vidarabine was the primary therapeutic agent for the treatment of HSV encephalitis, its use has declined substantially with the recognition that empirical acyclovir treatment is safe and associated with minimal complications (see below). The decision about whether to biopsy patients suspected of HSV encephalitis prior to instituting therapy with acyclovir remains controversial. Advocates of the biopsy approach stress the fact that biopsy can lead to identification of potentially treatable non-HSV-related diseases, although the frequency with which this occurs remains controversial. One recent decision-analysis model based on data from the NIAID-CASG trials suggested that as many as 40 percent of biopsy-negative patients may have alternative non-HSV diseases identifiable by brain biopsy, of which 40 percent represent treatable illnesses. These estimates appear excessively high and are not consistent with more recent data or the personal experiences of many neurologists. These data were compiled prior to the widespread use of MRI. It is difficult to believe that these numbers, which included diseases such as tumors, subdural hematomas, adrenoleukodystrophy, subdural empyema, and brain abscess, would be nearly as high if all patients had MRI and CT scans with new-generation scanners. As a general principle, the higher the likelihood that a patient has HSV encephalitis, the easier it is to justify empirical acyclovir therapy without biopsy. Conversely, the lower the probability of HSV encephalitis, the greater is the potential rationale for biopsy. The work of the NIAID-CASG clearly indicates that the capacity of physicians to distinguish between HSV and non-HSV encephalitis on the basis of clinical criteria alone is little better than chance. Among the laboratory tests widely employed to help this differentiation are imaging studies (MRI, CT, brain scan) and EEG. The presence of focally abnormal imaging studies in a patient over age 30 with a CSF lymphocytic pleocytosis (>5 cells per microliter) would seem sufficient to justify empirical therapy. Conversely, a young patient with no evidence of focal process on CT or MRI and a nonfocal EEG may be a candidate for biopsy, because of the diminished prior probability of having HSV encephalitis and the possibility that biopsy may lead to a treatable diagnosis.

Differential diagnosis The initial step in diagnosis is to exclude nonviral causes of the encephalitis syndrome. These can include both infections and noninfectious diseases. Although the list of possibilities is extensive, insight into some of the most common illnesses masquerading as viral encephalitis comes from a list of alternative diagnoses made in patients referred for entry into the NIAID-CASG trials as cases of suspected HSV encephalitis. Among the nonviral diagnoses that mimicked HSV encephalitis were vascular diseases; abscess and empyema; fungal, parasitic, rickettsial, and tuberculous infections; tumors; Reye's syndrome; toxic encephalopathy; subdural hematoma; and systemic lupus erythematosus. Of the nonviral infections, particular attention should be paid to *Listeria, Mycoplasma, Cryptococcus,* and *Mucor* infections, as well as toxoplasmosis and tuberculosis.

Once nonviral causes of encephalitis have been excluded, the major diagnostic impetus is to distinguish HSV from other causes of encephalitis. This distinction is particularly important because in virtually every other instance the therapy is supportive, whereas specific and effective antiviral therapy is available for HSV, and its efficacy is enhanced when therapy is instituted early in the course of infection. HSV encephalitis should be considered when clinical features suggesting involvement of the inferomedial frontotemporal regions of the brain, including prominent olfactory or gustatory hallucinations, anosmia, unusual or bizarre behavior or personality alterations, or memory disturbance, are present. Unfortunately, the results from the NIAID-CASG studies suggest that clinical criteria alone are not reliable in differentiating HSV and non-HSV encephalitis.

Epidemiologic factors may provide important clues that help to limit or focus the diagnostic possibilities. Particular attention should be paid to the season of the year (see Table 375-2), the age of the patient (Table 375-6), the geographic location and travel history (see Fig. 375-1 and Table 375-6), and possible exposure to animal bites, rodents, ticks. *Morbidity and Mortality Weekly Reports* provides regular information about the prevalence of particular viruses causing encephalitis by season and region of the country. State public health authorities provide another valuable resource concerning isolation of particular agents in individual regions.

Treatment Specific antiviral therapy should be initiated when appropriate (see below). Vital functions, including respiration and blood pressure, should be monitored continuously and supported as required. In the initial stages of encephalitis, many patients will require ICU care. Basic management and supportive therapy should include careful monitoring of ICP, fluid restriction and avoidance of hypotonic intravenous solutions, and suppression of fever. Seizures should be treated with standard anticonvulsant regimens, and prophylactic therapy is probably indicated in view of the high frequency of seizures in severe cases of encephalitis (>50 percent). Like all seriously ill, immobilized patients with altered consciousness, encephalitis patients are at risk for aspiration pneumonia, stasis ulcers and decubiti, contractures, deep venous thrombosis and its complications, and infections of indwelling lines and catheters.

Acyclovir (ACV) is of benefit in the treatment of HSV encephalitis and is also useful in selected cases of severe encephalitis due to infection with EBV or VZV. These viruses encode an enzyme, deoxypyrimidine (thymidine) kinase, that phosphorylates ACV to produce ACV-5'-monophosphate (AMP). Host cell enzymes then phosphorylate AMP to form a triphosphate derivative. It is the triphosphate that acts as an antiviral agent by inhibiting viral DNA polymerase and by causing premature termination of nascent viral DNA chains. The specificity of action of ACV depends on the fact that uninfected cells do not phosphorylate significant amounts of ACV to AMP. A second level of specificity is provided by the fact that the ACV triphosphate is a more potent inhibitor of viral DNA polymerase than of the analogous host cell enzymes.

Patients should receive a dose of 10 mg/kg of acyclovir IV every 8 h for a 10-day course. The drug should be diluted to a concentration not exceeding 7 mg/mL. (A 70-kg person would receive a dose of 700 mg, which would be diluted in a volume ≥100 mL.) Each dose should be infused slowly over 60 min rather than by rapid or bolus infusion to minimize the risk of renal dysfunction. Care should be taken to avoid extravasation or intramuscular or subcutaneous administration. The alkaline pH of ACV can cause local inflammation and phlebitis (9 percent). Dose adjustment is required in patients with impaired renal glomerular filtration. CSF penetration is excellent, with average drug levels approximately 50 percent of serum levels. Complications of therapy include elevations in BUN and creatinine levels (5 percent), thrombocytopenia (6 percent), gastrointestinal toxicity (nausea, vomiting, diarrhea) (7 percent), and neurotoxicity, (lethargy or obtundation, disorientation, confusion, agitation, hallucinations, tremors, seizures) (1 percent). ACV resistance may be mediated by changes in either the viral deoxypyrimidine kinase or DNA polymerase. To date, ACV-resistant isolates have not been a significant clinical problem in immunocompetent individuals. However, there has been an increasing number of reports of clinically virulent ACV-resistant HSV isolates from immunocompromised individuals, including those with AIDS.

Sequelae There is considerable variation in the incidence and severity of sequelae in patients surviving viral encephalitis. In the case of Eastern equine encephalitis virus infection, nearly 80 percent of survivors have severe neurologic sequelae. At the other extreme are infections due to EBV, California encephalitis virus, and Venezuelan equine encephalitis virus, where sequelae are extremely rare. Detailed information about sequelae in patients with HSV encephalitis treated with ACV are available from the NIAID-CASG trials. Twenty-six of 32 ACV-treated patients survived (81 percent). Of the 26 survivors, 12 (46 percent) had no or only minor sequelae, 3 (12 percent) were moderately impaired (gainfully employed but not functioning at their previous level), and 11 (42 percent) were severely impaired (requiring continuous supportive care). The incidence and severity of sequelae were directly related to the age of the patient and the level of consciousness at the time of initiation of therapy. Patients with severe neurologic impairment (Glasgow coma score ≤ 6) at initiation of therapy either died or survived with severe sequelae. Young (≤30 years old) patients with good neurologic function at initiation of therapy did substantially better (100 percent survival, 62 percent

---

TABLE 375-6 Features of selected arbovirus encephalitides

	Virus*				
	WEE	EEE	VEE	SLE	CE
Region	West, midwest	Atlantic and Gulf	South	All	East, and North Central
Age	Infants, adults > 50	Children	Adults	Adults > 50	Children
Deaths	5–15 percent	50–75 percent	1 percent	2–20 percent	<1 percent
Sequelae	Low–moderate	80 percent	Rare	20 percent	Rare
Vector	Mosquito	Mosquito	Mosquito	Mosquito	Mosquito
Animal host	Birds	Birds	Horses, small mammals	Birds	Rodents

* CE = California encephalitis virus; EEE = Eastern equine encephalitis virus; SLE = St. Louis encephalitis virus; VEE = Venezuelan equine encephalitis virus; WEE = Western equine encephalitis virus.
SOURCE: After Whitley, 1990 with permission.

normal or mild sequelae) compared with their older (≥30 years) counterparts (64 percent survival, 57 percent normal or mild sequelae).

MYELITIS AND RADICULITIS

The prototypical viral myelitis is the syndrome of acute anterior poliomyelitis caused by polioviruses and rarely by other enteroviruses and possibly EBV and mumps virus. A distinctive syndrome is produced by enterovirus 70. Patients develop acute hemorrhagic conjunctivitis, followed days to weeks later by a poliomyelitis-like syndrome (see below). Some cases of rabies present with an acute ascending paralysis with areflexia which can resemble poliomyelitis or the Guillain-Barré syndrome. Paralytic polio is a rarity in the United States (<20 cases per year), although it remains a major problem in some other regions of the world. Most cases of paralytic polio in the United States occur as a result of the exceedingly rare reversion of vaccine strains to virulence. The cases are divided among those recently vaccinated and unvaccinated nonimmune adults exposed to recently vaccinated children. Occasional outbreaks have occurred in nonimmunized populations such as the Amish in Pennsylvania. Illness typically begins with prodromal symptoms, including fever, headache, myalgia, pharyngitis, nausea and vomiting, and meningeal signs. These are associated with the typical CSF profile of aseptic meningitis. In some patients these symptoms are followed by the development of muscle weakness. The incidence, severity, and pattern of weakness are age-dependent, with more severe disease being seen with increasing age. Young children often develop weakness of one leg, older children weaknesss of both legs, and adults asymmetric quadriparesis often with associated urinary retention. Weakness is associated with fasciculations, loss of deep and superficial reflexes, and the development of atrophy. Involvement of the brainstem (bulbar polio) can result in dysphagia, dysarthria, respiratory impairment, and vasomotor disturbances. Although some patients complain of paresthesias, objective sensory loss is not present.

Viruses also may affect both the anterior and posterior portions of the spinal cord over a considerable longitudinal extent, producing the syndrome of ''transverse'' myelitis. The clinical syndrome is one of acutely developed muscle weakness, which may be of the flaccid hyporeflexic type initially but usually develops into spastic paralysis with hyperreflexia and extensor plantar responses. Sensory loss is almost invariably present and typically involves both pain-temperature and position-vibration, producing a sensory level. Urinary symptoms (retention, overflow incontinence, or in milder cases, hesitancy or decreased voiding sensation) and constipation or even fecal incontinence are present in virtually all patients. Although this syndrome can be caused by a variety of viruses, most cases are due to HSV-2, CMV, VZV, or EBV. Pathologic evidence of myelitis is commonly encountered in severe cases of St. Louis, Eastern, and Western encephalitis. A milder form of the syndrome may be encountered in patients with episodes of herpes genitalia. Especially during the primary outbreak, patients may develop an aseptic meningitis syndrome associated with urinary retention or other symptoms; dysesthesia, paresthesias, or neuralgia in the legs, buttocks, or genital area; and weakness in one or both legs. A chronic viral myelitis is associated with infection by HIV (vacuolar myelopathy) and by HTLV-I (tropical spastic paraparesis, or TSP, and HTLV-I–associated myelopathy, or HAM) (see Chaps. 151 and 279).

HERPES ZOSTER A distinctive clinical syndrome consisting of paresthesias or dysesthesias in a dermatomal distribution followed by a localized cutaneous eruption (''shingles,'' ''zoster'') is commonly associated with VZV infection and rarely may be produced by HSV. Zoster occurs in patients previously infected with chickenpox (varicella). During the initial varicella infection, virus in the skin travels up the sensory nerves to become latent in the sensory ganglia. The mechanisms that account for maintenance of latency and subsequent reactivation remain unknown. Reactivation results in active viral replication in sensory ganglia followed by spread of virus

through nerves to the skin, where a dermatomal vesicular eruption occurs. The incidence of zoster increases with age and is higher in patients with compromised cellular immunity. The typical history is one of several days of itching, tingling, burning, or pain in a dermatomal distribution that is followed after several days by a vesicular eruption consisting of clear vesicles on an erythematous base. The vesicles become cloudy, dry, and crust over after 1 to 2 weeks. The lesions are most commonly found in the thoracic dermatomes, with T5–T10 accounting for approximately two-thirds of cases. Most patients will have hypalgesia and hypesthesia in the affected dermatome. About 5 percent of patients develop motor weakness and atrophy (zoster paresis) in the associated myotome. Forty-five percent of patients over age 50 who develop shingles will experience pain persisting for more than 6 weeks after disappearance of the rash, i.e., *postherpetic neuralgia* (PHN). PHN is almost never seen in children who develop zoster and is rare (6 percent) in adults younger than 50. PHN may benefit from topical therapy with capsaicin ointment, as well as systemic therapy with amitriptyline and carbamazepine. Characteristic syndromes result from zoster eruptions involving the trigeminal and geniculate distribution. In 10 to 15 percent of cases, reactivation of virus in the trigeminal ganglia results in rash in the distribution of the ophthalmic division of the trigeminal nerve (ophthalmic zoster). Vesicular eruption may be conjoined with conjunctivitis, keratitis, ocular muscle palsies, ptosis, and mydriasis. Rare cases are followed by the development of cerebral angiitis involving the ipsilateral carotid and/or middle cerebral arteries. Vascular compromise may lead to hemiplegia, aphasia, or other focal deficits contralateral to the side of the facial eruption. Reactivation of virus in the geniculate ganglion is reported to produce the Ramsay Hunt syndrome, consisting of facial palsy often associated with loss of taste in the anterior tongue, tinnitus, hearing loss, and vertigo. Zoster eruptions are found in the external auditory meatus.

HIV AND OTHER VIRAL NEUROPATHIES Isolated virus-induced peripheral or cranial neuropathies or plexopathies are unusual, with the exception of those associated with HIV infection (see below). CMV has been reported to produce both peripheral neuropathy and brachial plexus neuropathy. A similar syndrome may be seen with EBV. The incidence of CMV neuropathy is clearly increased in patients with AIDS. In some cases there has been evidence for direct viral infection, whereas in others the mechanism appears to be one of virus-induced segmental demyelination. CMV, HSV, EBV, VZV, mumps, and hepatitis B virus (HBV) also have been associated with Guillain-Barré syndrome. An almost identical syndrome can be seen in association with HIV infection, although these patients typically have a CSF pleocytosis rather than the classic albuminocytologic dissociation (elevated protein, no or few cells). Isolated cranial nerve palsies, especially of the facial (VII) nerve (Bell's palsy), have been attributed to VZV (Ramsay Hunt syndrome), HIV, EBV, enteroviruses, mumps, and HSV, although in many cases the etiologic relationship appears rather tenuous. Mumps, measles, and VZV may produce unilateral or bilateral nerve deafness. Seroepidemiologic studies also suggest a possible role for parainfluenza, adenoviruses, and HSV in acute hearing loss.

CHRONIC AND PERSISTENT VIRAL CNS DISEASE

GENERAL CONSIDERATIONS From a practical point of view, chronic and persistent CNS viral diseases can be divided into those caused by conventional viruses and those caused by unconventional agents such as prions (Table 375-7).

HIV A complete discussion of the virologic aspects of HIV infection, of specific complications of HIV infection such as associated opportunistic infections, and of HIV therapy can be found in Chap. 279. We will focus here on the consequences of direct HIV infection on the central and peripheral nervous system.

Neurologic manifestations of HIV infection differ at different stages of illness (Fig. 375-2). Primary HIV infection can be associated

TABLE 375-7 Chronic and persistent CNS diseases caused by viruses and prions

Disease	Agent	Disease	Agent
Progressive multifocal leukoencephalopathy	JC virus	Creutzfeldt-Jakob	Prion
Subacute sclerosing panencephalitis	Measles virus	Gerstmann-Straussler-Scheinker	Prion
Progressive rubella panencephalitis	Rubella virus	Kuru	Prion
Tropical spastic paraparesis	HTLV-I	Fatal familial insomnia	Prion
AIDS	HIV	Alper's	Prion?

with aseptic meningitis and more rarely with an acute encephalopathy. No clinical features clearly differentiate HIV aseptic meningitis from other viral meningitides, although the diagnosis should be strongly considered in patients with known risk factors for HIV infection. The syndrome is characterized by fever, headache, meningeal signs, and in some patients cranial nerve palsies (V, VII, VIII). The CSF shows a mononuclear pleocytosis, elevated protein level, and normal glucose level. HIV can be isolated from CSF, and p24 core protein may be present, which establishes the diagnosis. More commonly, the diagnosis is established by documenting HIV antibody seroconversion and intrathecal HIV antibody synthesis. In suspected cases, follow-up HIV serology should be obtained at 1, 2, and 3 months because seroconversion may be delayed.

Persisting CSF pleocytosis also has been found in otherwise asymptomatic HIV-seropositive individuals. Seropositive individuals also may develop Guillain-Barré syndrome (GBS), chronic inflammatory demyelinating polyneuropathy (CIDP), or myopathy. HIV-associated GBS appears clinically indistinguishable from the syndrome that occurs in non-HIV-infected individuals. Patients present with acute onset of progressive extremity weakness, which may progress to respiratory failure. Bifacial weakness is common. Sensory symptoms may occur, but sensory signs are far less conspicuous than motor findings. All patients are areflexic or severely hyporeflexic. Findings in CIDP are similar but generally progress chronically rather than acutely and are not typically as severe. A diagnostic clue to HIV-associated GBS or CIDP may be the presence of a CSF

FIGURE 375-2 The relative frequency and timing of major neurologic complications of direct HIV infection. Diseases that affect the CNS are shaded with diagonal lines; those which affect the peripheral nervous system are cross-hatched. The height of the boxes is a relative indicator of the frequency of each type of disease. (*From RT Johnson et al, FASEB J 2:2970, 1988, with permission.*)

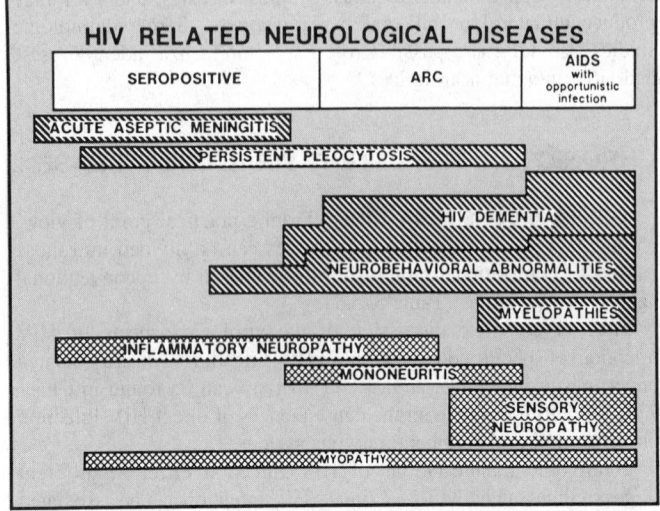

pleocytosis in place of the typical albuminocytologic dissociation (no or few cells, elevated protein) seen in non-HIV cases. Electrophysiologic studies are consistent with demyelination (slowed conduction velocities, prolonged or absent F responses and distal motor latencies, etc.). Extensive controlled trials of therapy in HIV-associated GBS and CIDP are not available. Plasmapheresis is the standard therapy for non-HIV-associated CIDP and GBS. Recent studies suggest that intravenous high-dose immunoglobulin may also be effective and associated with few side effects, although some patients relapse following treatment. Both these treatments should be considered in HIV-positive individuals.

Progression of HIV infection from the asymptomatic state to more clinically advanced disease is associated with an increased incidence of neuropsychological abnormalities, including the development of HIV encephalopathy and dementia, also referred to as *AIDS-dementia complex*. Common early symptoms of cognitive impairment include difficulty concentrating, memory loss, slowness of thought, apathy, depression, social withdrawal, and personality changes. In distinction to "cortical" dementias such as Alzheimer disease, aphasia, apraxia, and agnosia are uncommon, leading some investigators to classify HIV encephalopathy as a "subcortical dementia." At least 50 percent of patients will have associated signs or symptoms of motor dysfunction, including leg weakness, balance difficulty, ataxia, tremor, or pyramidal tract signs (hyperreflexia, extensor plantars). The illness progresses slowly over months, although mean survival time from the onset of severe dementia rarely exceeds 6 months. Laboratory studies are helpful in excluding or diminishing the possibility of other treatable processes. Twenty percent of patients will have CSF lymphocytic pleocytosis (<50 cells per microliter), and 60 percent will have an elevated protein level. Hypoglycorrhachia is rare. CSF beta$_2$ microglobulin concentrations appear to correlate with the severity of HIV encephalopathy and may serve as a useful marker of disease progression or response to antiviral therapy. CT and MRI typically show evidence of diffuse cerebral atrophy with widened sulci and ex vacuo ventricular enlargement. T2-weighted MRI spin-echo images show either patchy or diffuse white matter lesions. EEG findings are nonspecific, although some degree of generalized slowing is almost invariably present.

The neuropathologic hallmarks of AIDS encephalopathy are the presence of multinucleated giant cells (MGC) seen throughout the cortex and white matter, microglial nodules, white matter pallor, and reactive gliosis. The MGCs have been shown to contain HIV particles by electron microscopy and copious amounts of viral antigen and genome by immunocytochemistry and in situ hybridization. They appear to arise by syncytial fusion of infected monocyte-macrophage-microglial cells. These cells contain the bulk of HIV antigen and genome found in brain material. Endothelial cells and oligodendroglia may be found to contain HIV antigen or genome; neurons are rarely, if ever, positive. Neuronal dysfunction is not the result of productive infection with subsequent cell destruction. The mechanism by which HIV infection indirectly produces neuronal injury has not yet been established. Neurons may be injured as a result of cytokines, excitatory neurotoxins, or other soluble factors released by infected immune cells, macrophages, or glia. Alternatively, binding of gp120 or other viral proteins to neurons may result in alterations in ion channel conductance (e.g., Ca^{2+}) or neurotransmitter levels leading to cell injury (see also Chap. 279).

No definitive therapy is available. Both AZT and didanosine have been reported to lead to improvement in some patients, although didanosine's limited CSF penetration may limit its usefulness.

Symptomatic HIV-infected patients also may develop CIDP or mononeuropathy multiplex (MM). MM typically presents with asymmetric multifocal peripheral and/or cranial nerve lesions. These may appear acutely as isolated regions of sensory loss or weakness in a peripheral nerve distribution. The pathogenesis appears to be ischemic injury to nerves resulting from arteritis of the vasa nervorum. In distinction to CIDP, the electrophysiologic studies suggest an axonal rather than a demyelinating lesion.

A distal symmetric painful sensory neuropathy is the most common form of neuropathy encountered in patients with clinically advanced AIDS and is present in at least one-third of patients. Most patients complain of painful distal paresthesias in the feet (''burning feet''), which are often induced in causalgia-like fashion by pressure or contact. Walking may be difficult or impossible, and even minimal contact with blankets or sheets can produce severe discomfort. Findings on examination include a stocking-type sensory loss to pin, temperature, and touch and loss of ankle reflexes. The knee jerks are usually intact. Motor changes (weakness, atrophy) are mild compared with the prominence of sensory signs and symptoms and are usually limited to weakness of the intrinsic foot muscles. Trophic changes, including atrophy of the skin, loss of hair, nail abnormalities, edema, and vasomotor disturbances, may be found. Patients with advanced HIV infection also may develop an autonomic neuropathy characterized by diarrhea, postural hypotension, and cardiac arrhythmias.

Electrophysiologic studies are indicative of a distal sensorimotor axonopathy, which is consistent with findings on nerve biopsy. Conduction velocities and distal latencies are normal, but compound muscle action potentials in the legs and the sural sensory action potential are diminished in amplitude. HIV has been isolated from nerve biopsy specimens, although the source of virus (Schwann cells, axons, inflammatory cells) has not been established definitively. A similar neuropathy has been associated with CMV infection, and CMV antigen and genome can be detected in some biopsy specimens by immunocytochemistry, in situ hybridization, or PCR. The relative importance of HIV and CMV infection in the production of this syndrome remains to be established. Patients receiving either didanosine or dideoxycytidine also may develop neuropathic symptoms, and this should be considered in the differential diagnosis. No adequate therapy exists. Patients with evidence to suggest CMV infection should be treated with ganciclovir. Analgesics, tricyclic antidepressants, anticonvulsants (including phenytoin and carbamazepine), and topical capsaicin ointment may be useful in the control of pain. Mineralocorticoids such as fludrocortisone may help control postural hypotension in patients with autonomic neuropathy.

A chronic progressive myelopathy affecting the posterior and lateral columns of the spinal cord may be seen in 10 to 25 percent of AIDS patients. Patients develop a spastic ataxic paraparesis with diminished position and vibratory sense and urinary incontinence. Tibial somatosensory evoked responses are abnormal in virtually all patients. The clinical features resemble those seen in subacute combined degeneration secondary to vitamin B_{12} deficiency and those of nitrous oxide–induced myelopathy. Most patients (>90 percent) have associated HIV encephalopathy or dementia. Pathologic changes consist of vacuolar degeneration of the white matter of the lateral and posterior columns, typically maximal in the thoracic cord. The vacuolar areas result from severe edema within the myelin sheaths of nerve fibers and contain axonal spheroids and lipid-laden macrophages. HIV has been isolated from the spinal cord of affected individuals, and HIV genome has been found by in situ hybridization, although the role of direct viral infection versus indirect mechanism(s) of injury has not been established. No definitive therapy is available, and treatment with either AZT or didanosine is generally of little benefit.

In addition to vacuolar myelopathy, a variety of other myelopathic syndromes may occur in HIV-infected individuals. Ganglionitis of the lumbar and sacral dorsal root ganglia can result in secondary degeneration of the fasciculus gracilis within the posterior column of the spinal cord. The resulting clinical syndrome includes paresthesias and sensory loss (vibration, position sense) in the legs. Transverse myelitis also may result from infection with HSV, CMV, or both viruses simultaneously. Concurrent HIV and HTLV-I infection can occur, with the latter producing a spastic myelopathy (see next section).

Patients at any stage of HIV infection may develop myopathy. This is typically characterized by slowly progressive polymyositis-like proximal muscle weakness, myalgia, elevated muscle enzymes

(creatine kinase, aldolase, lactate dehydrogenase, SGOT), and a myopathic pattern (brief low-amplitude motor unit potentials) on EMG testing. Muscle biopsy may show inflammation and/or myofiber degeneration and necrosis. Some patients have additional histologic changes, including nemaline rod and cytoplasmic bodies, mitochondrial abnormalities, and ragged red fibers. The pathogenesis of the syndrome has not been established. Direct HIV infection of muscle has not been detected, although HIV-infected monocytes, macrophages, and multinucleated giant cells may surround muscle fibers.

HIV-associated myopathy should be distinguished from myopathy as a complication of AZT therapy. Most patients with AZT myopathy have been on therapy for 6 months or more and often have higher enzyme levels and more pain than non-AZT cases. Biopsy may help with the differential diagnosis, since AZT-related cases show more muscle fiber necrosis and less inflammation than patients with HIV myopathy. Discontinuation of AZT results in resolution of symptoms. Concurrent glucocorticoid therapy may allow continuation of AZT treatment.

TROPICAL SPASTIC PARAPARESIS (TSP), HTLV-I–ASSOCIATED MYELOPATHY (HAM) TSP and HAM are characterized by the development of slowly progressive spastic paraparesis, often associated with a neurogenic bladder (see Chap. 151). Symptoms of these diseases typically appear during the third or fourth decades, and women are affected far more frequently than men. The majority of reported cases have been from Japan (HAM), the Caribbean basin, parts of South America (Panama, Colombia, Peru, Brazil), the Seychelles Islands, and western Africa. Isolated cases have occurred in the southeastern United States and in many other locations. Neurologic examination shows a spastic paraparesis or paraplegia with hyperactive tendon reflexes, clonus, and extensor plantar responses. Although some patients have paresthesias, dyesthesias, or pain in the legs, sensory findings are usually mild (e.g., mild diminution in vibratory sense), and a true sensory level is only rarely found. Additional findings are seen in 5 to 20 percent of cases and can include brisk reflexes in the upper extremities, frontal release responses, cranial nerve abnormalities (optic neuropathy, deafness, nystagmus, diplopia, facial paresis), and cerebellar signs (tremor, dysmetria).

Tropical spastic myelopathies are multifactorial in nature and may be caused by a wide variety of toxic and nutritional factors. Several epidemiologic studies have unequivocally shown that infection with HTLV-I is the cause of an important subset of this disorder. Infection appears to be acquired through blood transfusion, sexual contact, intravenous drug use, and vertical transmission from mother to fetus. HTLV-I–associated cases are characterized by the presence of serum and CSF anti-HTLV-I antibodies. The CSF/serum antibody ratio is elevated, indicative of intrathecal antibody synthesis. HTLV-I–specific CSF oligoclonal bands are often present. Between 25 and 60 percent of patients will have a mild lymphocytic pleocytosis (<50 cells per microliter), and a higher percentage will have a mild elevation in protein. HTLV-I genome can be found in CSF and peripheral blood lymphocytes using Southern blot hybridization or PCR amplification. Virus also can be isolated from CSF and blood of affected individuals.

A number of abnormalities may be found on laboratory tests, although specific diagnosis requires viral isolation or positive serology. MRI of the spinal cord may show evidence of demyelination, and similar findings are occasionally found in the periventricular white matter in the cerebrum. Somatosensory evoked response studies may show evidence of posterior column dysfunction, even when clinical findings are mild or absent. Some patients have evidence of a demyelinating peripheral neuropathy with slowed conduction velocities, increased distal latencies, and slow or absent F waves. Pathologic examination of the spinal cord typically shows symmetrical degeneration of the lateral columns encompassing the corticospinal tracts. Degenerative changes also may involve the posterior columns and spinocerebellar and spinothalamic tracts. There is an associated inflammatory infiltrate in the spinal leptomeninges, cord parenchyma, and surrounding vessels. Myelin destruction may at times resemble the vacuolar myelopathy seen in association with AIDS.

The pathogenesis of the spinal cord disease has not been completely established. Both direct viral injury and immune-mediated processes may play a role in the spinal cord pathology. Recent evidence suggests that HTLV-I–specific cytotoxic T lymphocytes (CTLs) may be important in the production of immune-mediated spinal cord injury.

Definitive therapy is not currently available. Many patients benefit from oral prednisolone or equivalent glucocorticoid therapy. AZT would be expected to be beneficial in limiting viral replication and associated direct cell injury.

PROGRESSIVE MULTIFOCAL LEUKOENCEPHALOPATHY (PML)   As the name implies, PML is a progressive disorder characterized pathologically by multifocal areas of demyelination varying greatly in size and scattered throughout the CNS. In addition to demyelination, there are characteristic cytologic alterations in both astrocytes and oligodendrocytes. Astrocytes are tremendously enlarged and contain hyperchromatic, deformed and bizarre nuclei, and frequent mitotic figures. Oligodendrocytes have enlarged, densely staining nuclei that contain viral inclusions formed by crystalline arrays of JC virus (JCV) particles. Patients often present with visual deficits (45 percent), typically a homonymous hemianopia, and mental impairment (38 percent) (dementia, confusion, personality change). Motor weakness may not be present early but eventually occurs in 75 percent of cases.

CT and MRI remain the most valuable diagnostic studies in suggesting the diagnosis of PML. CT shows hypodense nonenhancing white matter lesions without associated edema or mass effect. Lesions are typically located periventricularly, in the centrum semiovale, in the parietal-occipital region, and in the cerebellum. MRI is more sensitive than CT and reveals hyperintense signal in the white matter on T2-weighted spin-echo images. EEG almost always shows focal or diffuse slowing, and abnormalities may occasionally precede those seen by CT. The CSF is typically normal, although mild elevation in protein and/or IgG may be found. Pleocytosis occurs in less than 25 percent of cases, is predominantly mononuclear, and rarely exceeds 25 cells per microliter. The presence of oligoclonal bands, a substantial pleocytosis, or PMNs or red cells in the CSF should suggest such possibilities as acute multiple sclerosis, acute hemorrhagic leukoencephalitis, HIV-associated leukoencephalomyelopathy, multifocal VZV leukoencephalitis, or postinfectious or vaccinal immune-mediated encephalomyelitis.

Almost all patients (>95 percent) have an underlying immunosuppressive disorder. Prior to the HIV epidemic, common associated diseases included lymphoproliferative disorders, immune deficiency states, myeloproliferative disease, and chronic infectious or granulomatous diseases. Since 1984, the importance of these associated disorders has been dwarfed by that of AIDS. According to some recent estimates, more than 60 percent of currently diagnosed PML cases occur in patients with AIDS. Conversely, it has been estimated that nearly 1 percent of AIDS patients will develop PML. Early indications suggest that the basic clinicopathologic features of AIDS-associated PML do not differ significantly from those of non-AIDS-associated PML. Some patients with AIDS-associated PML have shown significant spontaneous improvement in the absence of therapy. Unfortunately, this appears to be the exception rather than the rule, and most cases pursue the same relentless downhill course to a fatal termination that characterizes almost all reported cases of non-AIDS-associated PML.

Definitive diagnosis depends on identification of the characteristic neuropathologic abnormalities at biopsy or necropsy. The presence of JCV antigen and genomic DNA can be confirmed by immunocytochemistry, in situ hybridization, and PCR amplification on brain tissue. However, detection of JCV antigen or genomic material is not diagnostic of PML unless accompanied by characteristic pathologic changes, since both antigen and genomic material can be found in the brains of normal patients. Between 80 and 90 percent of the population is seropositive for JCV by middle adult life. Virus may remain latent in brain or other tissues and become reactivated during immunosuppression. PML also may result from primary exposure to JCV in an immunocompromised host, since 10 to 20 percent of individuals are seronegative at the time of disease diagnosis. JCV DNA has been amplified from the CSF of patients using PCR, but initial results suggest that this test is relatively insensitive as a diagnostic tool.

SUBACUTE SCLEROSING PANENCEPHALITIS (SSPE)   This is a rare disease, with less than 10 cases per year reported in the United States. The incidence has declined substantially since the introduction of a measles vaccine. Most patients give a history of primary measles infection at an early age (≤2 years), which is followed after a latent interval of 6 to 8 years by the development of a progressive neurologic disorder. Eighty-five percent of cases are between 5 and 15 years of age at diagnosis. Initial manifestations include poor school performance and mood and personality changes. As the disease develops, these nonspecific symptoms give way to progressive intellectual deterioration, focal and/or generalized seizures, myoclonus, ataxia, and visual disturbances. In the late stage of the illness, patients are unresponsive, quadriparetic, and spastic, with hyperactive tendon reflexes and extensor plantar responses. The EEG shows a characteristic periodic pattern with bursts every 3 to 8 s of high-voltage sharp slow waves, followed by periods of attenuated (''flat'') background. The CSF pattern may be diagnostic. The fluid is acellular with a normal or mildly elevated protein level and a markedly elevated gamma globulin level (>20 percent of total CSF protein). CSF antimeasles antibody levels are invariably elevated, and oligoclonal antimeasles antibodies are often present. CT and MRI show evidence of multifocal white matter lesions, cortical atrophy, and ex vacuo ventricular enlargement. Measles virus can be cultivated from brain tissue using special cocultivation techniques. Viral antigen can be identified immunocytochemically, and viral genome can be detected by in situ hybridization or PCR amplification. No definitive therapy is currently available. Treatment with Inosiplex (isoprinosine) (100 mg/kg per day) remains controversial but has been reported to prolong survival and produce clinical improvement in some patients.

The pathogenesis of SSPE remains unclear. Almost all patients with SSPE fail to make an antibody response to the measles virus M (matrix) protein despite an adequate antibody response to other viral proteins. The failure to make antibody apparently results from a lack of viable M protein in infected cells. The M protein is essential for complete virion assembly and release of virus by budding from infected cells. Electron microscopy of virus-infected cells from SSPE patients reveals nucleocapsids but no complete or budding viral particles. Genomic sequencing suggests that viral isolates from SSPE patients contain the gene encoding the M protein. Absence of M protein could theoretically result from transcriptional or translational errors or the production of an unstable protein, although none of these abnormalities has been documented consistently in SSPE. It has been hypothesized that lack of M protein results in intracellular accumulation of incomplete measles virions in brain cells. The host immune response is unable to clear the intracellular infection, and the persisting accumulation leads to neuronal dysfunction.

PROGRESSIVE RUBELLA PANENCEPHALITIS   This is an extremely rare disorder that predominantly affects children with congenital rubella syndrome, although isolated cases have been reported following childhood rubella. All the approximately 20 cases reported to date have been in male children. After a latent period of 8 to 19 years, patients develop progressive neurologic deterioration. The initial manifestations are similar to those seen in SSPE and include decline in school performance, behavioral alterations, and seizures. These are followed by severe progressive dementia, prominent ataxia, pyramidal signs (spasticity, hyperreflexia, extensor plantar responses), and visual deterioration. Myoclonus may be present but is less prominent than in SSPE, whereas cerebellar signs are a great deal more prominent. In the terminal stages of the illness, patients are globally demented, mute, and quadriparetic, often with associated ophthalmoplegia. CSF shows a mild lymphocytic pleocytosis (<40 cells per microliter), slightly elevated protein level (<150 mg/dL), markedly increased gamma globulin level (35 to 50 percent of total protein), and oligoclonal bands. The oligoclonal antibodies are specific for rubella virus antigens. The CSF/serum antirubella antibody ratio is markedly elevated, indicating high levels of intrathecal antirubella antibody synthesis. CT scans show ex vacuo ventricular enlargement with associated cortical atrophy. There may be hypodensity in the white matter, especially in the centrum semiovale. Cerebellar atrophy and associated fourth ventricle enlargement may be especially prominent. The EEG is nondiagnostic but is almost invariably abnormal with diffuse slowing. A few patients have a burst-suppression pattern similar to that encountered in SSPE. Biopsy or autopsy material shows perivascular lymphocytic and plasma cell cuffing in the white matter, leukomalacia of the centrum semiovale, and the atrophic and ex vacuo ventricular changes described above. Virus particles are not seen by electron microscopy, although rubella virus has been isolated from explant and cocultivation cultures of brain biopsy material in one reported case. The pathogenesis of the disease remains unclear. No therapy is currently available. Isoprinosine and amantadine are of no benefit. Universal prevention of both congenital and childhood rubella through the use of the available live attenuated rubella vaccine would be expected to eliminate the disease.

PRION DISEASES

Although traditionally included in discussions of viral diseases of the CNS, a substantial and rapidly accumulating body of research suggests that the transmissible neurodegenerative diseases (TNDs), e.g., kuru, Creutzfeldt-Jakob disease, Gerstmann-Straussler-Scheinker (GSS) syndrome, are not viral diseases at all. The leading hypothesis for the etiology of these diseases suggests that they are caused by a proteinaceous infectious particle (*prion*) devoid of nucleic acid that is encoded by a single-copy host gene (designated *PRNP*) present on the short arm of chromosome 20. The function of the normal cellular isoform of the PRNP gene (*PrP^c*) is unknown, although both membrane-associated and secreted forms exist. Neurons contain high concentrations of PrP^c, which is developmentally regulated. Substantial amino acid homology exists between PrP^c and a chicken protein (*ARIA*) produced by motor neurons that induces acetylcholine receptor activity.

A modified form, *PrP^Sc*, which is resistant to proteolytic digestion and spontaneously aggregates to produce rodlike or fibrillary particles (scrapie-associated fibrils, prion rods) can be isolated from the brains of animals and humans with TNDs. The exact mechanism by which the normal cellular protein (PrP^c) is modified to its pathologic isoform (PrP^Sc), the method by which PrP^Sc replicates itself, and the way PrP^Sc accumulation leads to neuronal degeneration remain unknown.

Epidemiologic and clinical studies indicate that human TNDs can be sporadic (Creutzfeldt-Jakob disease), infectious (kuru, rare cases of Creutzfeldt-Jakob), or genetic (GSS syndrome, familial Creutzfeldt-Jakob disease) in origin. The basic clinical features of each of these diseases are discussed below.

KURU This disease was previously endemic among members of the Fore linguistic tribal group of the Eastern Highlands area of Papua New Guinea. At its peak, the disease affected close to 1 percent of the population, although currently less than 10 cases per year are reported. The cardinal features of the illness were severe cerebellar ataxia with associated involuntary movements, including choreoathetosis, myoclonus, and tremor. These were associated with the subsequent development of mental impairment and frontal release signs. Brain material from affected individuals transmits the disease to primates. No new cases of the disease have been reported among individuals born since the cessation of ritual cannibalism in the affected areas. It has been suggested that ingestion of infected brain material during these rituals was responsible for disease transmission.

CREUTZFELDT-JAKOB DISEASE Most cases are sporadic in nature, although 5 to 15 percent are familial with an autosomal dominant pattern of inheritance. Regions of high incidence and prevalence are scattered throughout the world, most prominently in parts of Libya and North Africa and in Slovakia. Creutzfeldt-Jakob disease is not contagious, but person-to-person spread of the disease has occurred following transplantation of corneas or dural grafts obtained from infected individuals. Isolated cases also have been attributed to improperly decontaminated neurosurgical instruments and stereotactic intracerebral depth electrodes. Approximately 25 cases have been reported in patients with panhypopituitarism who received supplemental cadaveric human growth hormone therapy and in patients who received cadaveric human gonadotropins for treatment of infertility.

Creutzfeldt-Jakob disease typically presents as a rapidly progressive dementia with prominent associated myoclonus. Clinical manifestations are protean and often include combinations of severe and progressive dementia, pyramidal and extrapyramidal motor disturbances, and signs and symptoms of cerebellar dysfunction. Clinical and pathologic subtypes with predominant involvement of specific regions of the brain have been described (e.g., occipital, thalamic, and cerebellar types). Early signs of mental impairment may be manifested as slowness in thinking, difficulty concentrating, impaired judgment, and memory loss. Mood changes and emotional lability may be combined with visual or other types of hallucinations. About a third of patients present initially with prominent cerebellar or visual disturbances, which may initially overshadow the mental impairment. Myoclonus occurs in more than 90 percent of patients and may be provoked or aggravated by startle. Additional motor signs and symptoms can include tremor, clumsiness, and choreoathetosis. As the disease progresses, about two-thirds of patients will develop a parkinsonian extrapyramidal syndrome with hypokinesia and rigidity. Hyperreflexia, spasticity, and extensor plantar responses occur in about half of patients. The clinical presentation of Creutzfeldt-Jakob disease associated with use of cadaveric human pituitary hormone therapy may differ from that of classic Creutzfeldt-Jakob disease. Patients are typically younger and often present with a kuru-like illness in which cerebellar features may be more prominent initially than dementia.

Laboratory tests are helpful in excluding other causes of rapidly progressing dementia. The CSF is typically unremarkable, although the protein level may be mildly elevated. A pleocytosis is unusual and should prompt a thorough search for other processes. It has been suggested recently that two-dimensional isoelectric focusing of CSF proteins may show abnormal protein species, two of which (proteins designated 130 and 131) may be typical of Creutzfeldt-Jakob disease. This test has recently become commercially available; however, additional studies of sensitivity and specificity will be required to establish its diagnostic utility. CT and MRI may show evidence of generalized cortical atrophy, but more typically the degree of clinical dementia appears disproportionate to the amount of tissue loss seen on CT and MRI. In some patients, sequential studies performed at biweekly or monthly intervals may show rapidly progressive loss of brain tissue and ex vacuo ventricular enlargement. The EEG may be quite useful in suggesting the diagnosis. The typical pattern of periodic sharp wave complexes consists of a generalized slow background interrupted by bilaterally synchronous sharp wave complexes occurring at intervals of 0.5 to 2.5 s and lasting for 200 to 600 ms. The classic EEG pattern is found in 75 to 95 percent of cases, although it may not be present very early or in the terminal stages of the disease. Sequential EEG studies may be useful if the initial recording fails to reveal the typical pattern.

The gold standard for diagnosis remains the histologic study of brain material obtained at biopsy or necropsy and the subsequent demonstration of transmissibility to susceptible rodents. The pathologic hallmarks of Creutzfeldt-Jakob disease are spongiform changes (small round vacuoles) within the neuropil, neuronal loss, hypertrophy and proliferation of glial cells, and absence of significant inflammation or white matter involvement. Pathologic changes are maximal in the cortex but are often prominent in the basal ganglia, cerebellum, and thalamus. The brainstem and spinal cord are usually spared. Recent studies suggest that the demonstration of prion proteins in immunoblots of brain material is a sensitive and apparently specific marker for the presence of Creutzfeldt-Jakob disease or related TNDs. The finding of prion rods or scrapie-associated fibrils which may be seen in electron micrographs of prepared brain material also appears to be pathognomonic for TNDs.

Creutzfeldt-Jakob disease is invariably fatal, and no specific therapy is available. A number of drugs, including amantadine, have been reported to slow disease progression in isolated anecdotal case reports; however, the results have not been consistently reproducible.

Recent molecular genetic studies have established an unequivocal linkage between mutations in the PRNP gene and familial cases of Creutzfeldt-Jakob disease. Several mutations have been described, which may correlate with variations in the clinical phenotype of the disease in individual familial clusters. Among the commonly reported mutations are a Lys for Glu substitution in codon 200 and an Asn for Asp substitution in codon 178. Inserts in the PRNP gene also occur in several families with Creutzfeldt-Jakob disease. No consistent PRNP gene mutation has been identified in cases of sporadic Creutzfeldt-Jakob disease. Some recent reports suggest that homozygosity at a polymorphic amino acid residue at codon 129 of the PRNP gene occurs with greater than expected frequency in cases of sporadic and iatrogenic Creutzfeldt-Jakob disease and kuru, although this requires further confirmation.

GERSTMANN-STRAUSSLER-SCHEINKER SYNDROME This is a rare hereditary spinocerebellar degeneration. Patients develop signs and symptoms of progressive cerebellar dysfunction in midlife, evidenced by unsteadiness, clumsiness, incoordination, and progressive gait difficulty. As the illness progresses, the cerebellar findings become increasingly severe and include ataxia, dysarthria, and nystagmus. Some patients have additional findings, which can include parkinsonian, pyramidal and extrapyramidal findings, deafness, blindness, and gaze palsies. In distinction to their prominence in Creutzfeldt-Jakob disease, dementia and myoclonus are either absent or minor features and are overshadowed by the cerebellar dysfunction.

Molecular genetic studies of GSS syndrome families have consistently demonstrated mutations in the PRNP gene. The most common abnormality is a Leu for Pro substitution at codon 102. Additional mutations have included a Val for Ala substitution at codon 117, as well as a point mutation in codon 198. Although the clinical material is limited because of the rarity of the disease, it appears that ataxia is the dominant feature of the disease in families with the codon 102 mutation, whereas ataxia plus dementia is seen in those with the codons 117 and 198 mutations.

PUTATIVE TNDs Fatal familial insomnia (FFI) is a rapidly progressive autosomal dominant disease of middle or later life characterized by intractable insomnia, sympathetic hyperactivity and other autonomic and endocrine disturbances, dysarthria, and motor system abnormalities, including myoclonus, tremor, ataxia, hyperreflexia, and spasticity. Dementia is not prominent, although mild memory and attention deficits are common. Patients often experience complex hallucinations with the characteristics of "enacted dreams." A variety of endocrine abnormalities also may occur, including loss of the normal circadian fluctuations in melatonin, prolactin, and growth hormone secretion, decreased ACTH secretion, and elevated cortisol secretion. Pathologic changes include atrophy and gliosis of specific thalamic nuclei, cerebellar cortex, and inferior olives. One patient has been described who had spongiform changes in the involved areas and periodic sharp wave complexes on EEG, but this appears exceptional rather than typical. Sequencing of the PRNP gene from patients in two families with FFI has shown an Asn for Asp mutation in codon 178, similar to that reported in some cases of familial Creutzfeldt-Jakob disease. Brain material from patients in these two families was found to contain the protease-resistant PrP^{Sc} isoform. There have been no reports to date of successful transmission of the disease from brain material of infected cases.

There is one reported case of transmission of a scrapie-like disease to rodents using brain material from a 2½-year-old child diagnosed as having Alper's disease (progressive infantile poliodystrophy). This has not been confirmed, and no molecular genetic studies on the PRNP gene have been reported from patients with Alper's disease.

REFERENCES

BALE JF: Viral encephalitis. Med Clin North Am 77:25, 1993

BERGER JR et al: Progressive multifocal leukoencephalopathy associated with human immunodeficiency virus infection. Ann Intern Med 107:78, 1987

BOOSS J, ESIRI MM: *Viral Encephalitis.* Oxford, Blackwell Scientific, 1986

BUCHER B et al: Tropical neuromyelopathies and retroviruses: A review. Rev Infect Dis 12:890, 1990

CONNOLLY KJ, HAMMER SM: The acute aseptic meningitis syndrome. Infect Dis Clin North Am 4:599, 1990

GABUZDA DH, HIRSCH MS: Neurologic manifestations of infection with the human immunodeficiency virus. Ann Intern Med 107:383, 1987

GILLESPIE SM et al: Progressive multifocal leukoencephalopathy in persons infected with human immunodeficiency virus, San Francisco 1981–1989. Ann Neurol 30:597, 1991

JEFFERY DR et al: Transverse myelitis—Retrospective analysis of 33 cases, with differentiation of cases associated with multiple sclerosis and parainfectious events. Arch Neurol 50:532, 1993

JOHNSON RT: *Viral Infections of the Nervous System.* New York, Raven, 1982

MANETTO V et al: Fatal familial insomnia: Clinical and pathologic study of five new cases. Neurology 42:312, 1992

McARTHUR JC: Neurological manifestations of AIDS. Medicine 66:407, 1987

McKENDALL RR (ed): *Viral Disease, (Handbook of Clinical Neurology),* vol 56/12. Amsterdam, Elsevier, 1989

MEDORI R et al: Fatal familial insomnia, a prion disease with a mutation at codon 178 of the prion protein gene. N Engl J Med 326:444, 1992

PRUSINER SB: Molecular biology of prion diseases. Science 252:1515, 1991

————: Molecular biology and genetics of neurodegenerative diseases caused by prions. Adv Virus Res 41:241, 1992

ROOS KL (ed): Central nervous system infections. Semin Neurol 12:155, 1992

ROSENBLUM ML et al (eds): *AIDS and the Nervous System.* New York, Raven, 1988

SCHELD WM et al: *Infections of the Central Nervous System.* New York, Raven, 1991

TSAI TF: Arboviral infections in the United States. Infect Dis Clin North Am 5:73, 1991

TYLER KL: Diagnosis and management of acute viral encephalitis. Semin Neurol 4:480, 1984

————, Martin JB: *Infectious Diseases of the Central Nervous System.* Philadelphia, F.A. Davis, 1993

VINKEN PJ et al (eds): *Infections of the Nervous System (Handbook of Clinical Neurology)* vol 34. Amsterdam, North-Holland, 1978

WHITEMAN MLH et al: Progressive multifocal leukoencephalopathy in 47 HIV-seropositive patients—Neuroimaging with clinical and pathologic correlation. Radiology 187:233, 1993

WHITLEY RJ: Viral encephalitis. N Engl J Med 323:242, 1990

————— et al: Vidarabine versus acyclovir therapy in herpes simplex encephalitis. N Engl J Med 314:144, 1986

WOOD M, ANDERSON M: *Neurological Infections (Major Problems in Neurology),* vol 16. Philadelphia, Saunders, 1988

376 TRAUMA OF THE HEAD AND SPINE

ALLAN H. ROPPER

Head injuries are frequent in industrialized countries, affecting many patients in the prime of life. To appreciate the medical and social magnitude of this problem, it needs only to be recognized that almost 10 million Americans have head injuries yearly, about 20 percent serious enough to cause brain damage. Among men under 35 years old, accidents, usually motor vehicle collisions, are the chief cause of death, and over 70 percent of these involve head injury. Minor head injuries are so common that almost all physicians encounter patients requiring immediate care or suffering from various sequelae. Traumatic spinal cord injuries often occur in conjunction with head injury. The two are best considered together in the context of trauma to the nervous system.

Declining mortality from head and spinal cord injuries can be attributed mainly to public health measures, such as use of seat belts and motorcycle helmets, and the development of ambulance systems with trained personnel. A systematic approach to the evaluation of patients with head and spine trauma, beginning at the scene of the accident, has improved outcome. Understanding the pathologic lesions produced by trauma, essential for diagnosis and management, has been revolutionized by the wide availability of computed tomography (CT) scanning.

TYPES OF HEAD INJURIES

SKULL FRACTURES A blow to the skull causes fractures if the elastic tolerance of the bone is exceeded. Significant intracranial lesions accompany two-thirds of skull fractures, and the presence of a skull fracture increases manyfold the chances of an underlying subdural or epidural hematoma. Consequently, fractures assume importance primarily as markers of the site and severity of injury. They also cause cranial nerve injuries and produce entry pathways to the cerebrospinal fluid (CSF) for bacteria (meningitis) and air (pneumocephalus) or for leakage of CSF. Fractures are classified as linear, basilar, compound, or depressed; linear fractures account for 80 percent of all skull fractures and are most often associated with subdural or epidural hematomas. Linear fractures usually extend from the point of impact toward the base of the skull.

Basilar skull fractures are often extensions of adjacent fractures over the convexity of the skull but may occur independently due to stresses on the floor of the middle cranial fossa or occiput. They are usually located parallel to the petrous bone or along the sphenoid bone toward the sella turcica and ethmoidal groove. Most are uncomplicated, but they may cause CSF leak, pneumocephalus, or cavernous-carotid fistula. Fractures of the basal skull bones are often accompanied by signs of hemotympanum (blood behind the tympanic membrane), delayed ecchymosis over the mastoid process (Battle's sign), or periorbital ecchymosis ("racoon sign"). Because routine x-ray examination can fail to disclose basilar fractures, they should be suspected in the presence of these clinical signs. Cerebrospinal fluid also may leak through the cribriform plate or the adjacent sinus and present as a watery discharge from the nose (CSF rhinorrhea). Persistence of rhinorrhea or recurrent meningitis is an indication for a surgical repair of torn dura underlying the fracture. The site of the leak is often difficult to determine, but useful diagnostic tests include metrizamide instillation into the CSF with subsequent CT scans and radionuclide or fluorescein injection into the CSF followed by assessment of uptake by absorptive nasal pledgets. The site of intermittent leaks is rarely delineated; most resolve spontaneously. Sellar fractures also can be radiologically occult, although they are sometimes associated with serious neuroendocrine dysfunction. Occasionally, fractures of the dorsum sella cause sixth or seventh nerve palsies or optic nerve damage. An air-fluid level in the sphenoid sinus suggests a fracture of the sellar floor.

About 20 percent of petrous bone fractures, usually along the long axis of the bone, are associated with facial palsy. Disruption of ear ossicles and CSF otorrhea are other complications. Transverse petrous fractures are less common, almost always damaging the cochlea or labyrinths and often the facial nerve. External bleeding from the ear can result from petrous bone fractures, although local laceration of the external canal from abrasions is more common. Frontal bone fractures are often depressed, involving the frontal and paranasal sinuses and the orbits; anosmia frequently follows if the olfactory filaments in the cribriform plate are disrupted.

Depressed skull fractures are often compound but are commonly neurologically asymptomatic because the impact energy is dissipated in breaking the bone; however, some cause brain contusions and focal signs from the underlying cortical area. Surgical repair and bone elevation with exploration of the dura are required in most cases. Delayed or incomplete debridement of the wound leads to a high incidence of infection. If the skin is lacerated over a skull fracture and the underlying meninges are torn, or if the fracture passes through the posterior wall of a nasal sinus, bacteria or air may enter the cranial cavity resulting in meningitis, abscess formation, or pneumocephalus.

CRANIAL NERVE INJURIES Cranial nerves liable to injury with basilar skull fractures are the olfactory, optic, oculomotor, trochlear, first and second branches of the trigeminal, facial, and auditory. Anosmia and an apparent loss of taste (actually a loss of perception of aromatic flavors, with elementary tastes retained) occurs in approximately 10 percent of serious head injuries, particularly with falls on the back of the head. This results from displacement of the brain and shearing of the olfactory nerve filaments. Recovery usually occurs with residual hyposmia, but if bilateral anosmia persists for several months, the prognosis is poor. Fractures of the sphenoid bone may bruise or transect the optic nerve, resulting in unilateral partial or complete blindness and an unreactive pupil, usually equal in size to the other side, with a preserved consensual light response. Partial optic nerve injuries from closed trauma result in blurring of vision, central or paracentral scotomas, or sector defects. Direct orbital injury may cause short-lived blurred vision for close objects because of reversible iridoplegia. Oculomotor nerve injury causes the globe to turn outward with loss of adduction and vertical movement and a fixed dilated pupil; vision is preserved. Diplopia only on looking down, which suggests trochlear nerve damage from fracture of the lesser sphenoid wing, occurs as an isolated problem from minor injury and may be delayed in appearance for several days. Patients report correction of the diplopia by tilting the head away from the affected eye. Direct facial nerve injury by a basal fracture is present immediately in 3 percent of severe injuries or also may be delayed 5 to 7 days. Petrous fractures, particularly the less common transverse type, are liable to produce this injury. Delayed facial palsy has a good prognosis; its mechanism is not known. Injury to the eighth cranial nerve with fractures of the petrous bone causes loss of hearing, vertigo, and nystagmus immediately after injury; the nystagmus is frequently positional. Deafness due to nerve injury must be distinguished from rupture of the eardrum, blood in the middle ear, or disruption of the ossicles from fracture through the middle ear. A high-tone hearing loss occurs with direct cochlear concussion.

CONCUSSION Concussion refers to an immediate but transient loss of consciousness often described as dazed or "star struck" and associated with a short period of amnesia. It typically occurs after blunt impact or deceleration of the frontal or occipital areas that creates sudden movement of the brain within the skull. In severe cases, a brief convulsion or autonomic symptoms and signs such as facial pallor, bradycardia, faintness with mild hypotension, or sluggish pupillary reaction may occur, but most patients are neurologically normal. Higher primates are particularly susceptible to concussion; in contrast, billy goats, rams, and woodpeckers can tolerate impact velocity and deceleration a hundred times greater than that experienced by humans. The mechanism of loss of consciousness in concussion is believed to be transient electrophysiologic dysfunction of the reticular activating system in the upper midbrain caused by rotation of the cerebral hemispheres on the relatively fixed brainstem. The mechanism of the associated amnesia is not known. Gross and light microscopic changes in the brain are usually absent after concussion, but biochemical and ultrastructural changes such as mitochondrial ATP depletion and local disruption of the blood-brain barrier suggest that complex abnormalities occur. The CT and magnetic resonance (MRI) scans are usually normal, and there are usually no red blood cells in the CSF, as occurs with more severe injuries. Approximately 3 percent of patients who have had concussions will have an intracranial hemorrhage (subdural, epidural, or parenchymal), but the presence of a skull fracture increases the risk.

Amnesia after concussion typically follows a few moments of unresponsiveness after impact. Rarely there is no loss of consciousness. The memory loss spans the time of, and moments before, mild impact injuries but may encompass previous weeks (rarely months) in more severe trauma. Any anterograde amnesia is usually brief and disappears rapidly in alert patients. The extent of retrograde amnesia has been suggested as a rough measure of the severity of injury.

Improvement usually occurs in an orderly progression from most distant to recent memories, with islands of amnesia occasionally remaining in severe cases. Hysterical posttraumatic amnesia is not uncommon and should be suspected when abnormalities of behavior occur, such as a tendency to recount events that cannot be recalled on later testing, bizarre affect, forgetting one's own name, or exaggerated anterograde deficit in comparison with the degree of injury.

A single uncomplicated head injury has not been shown to produce permanent neurobehavioral changes in most patients who are free of preexisting psychiatric problems and substance abuse. In some patients, however, there has been increasing attention to minor problems in memory and concentration that may have an anatomic correlate in small shearing or other microscopic lesions (see below).

CONTUSION, BRAIN HEMORRHAGES, AND SHEARING LESIONS **Hemispheral lesions** Contusions on the surface of the brain and deeper hemorrhages result from mechanical forces that move the hemispheres relative to the skull. Deceleration of the brain against the inner skull causes contusions, either under a point of impact (coup lesion) or in the antipolar area (contrecoup lesion). Trauma sufficient to cause prolonged unconsciousness usually produces contusions varying from small superficial cortical petechiae to hemorrhagic and necrotic destruction of large portions of a hemisphere. Because the motion of the hemispheres brings them into contact with the prominences of the sphenoid and other frontal basal bones, blunt impact, as from an automobile dashboard, typically causes contusions on the orbital surfaces of the frontal lobes and the anterior and basal portions of the temporal lobes. The anterior corpus callosum also may be bruised from striking the falx. With lateral forces, as from the doorframe of a car, contusions occur on the convexity of the hemispheres.

Contusions are visible on CT scan, appearing early as inhomogeneous hyperlucencies from scattered cortical and subcortical blood with mass effect that distorts the lateral ventricles. After several hours, the surrounding edematous tissue appears as a ring of lower density. Confluent, roughly spherical contusions can be distinguished from cerebral hemorrhages because contusions extend to the cortical surface. After a week, some contusions have a surrounding ringlike contrast-enhancing density that may be mistaken for tumor or abscess. Glial and macrophage reactions begin within 2 days, years later resulting in scarred hemosiderin-stained depressions on the surface (*plaques jaune*) that are one source of posttraumatic epilepsy. Large single hemorrhages after minor trauma may occur in patients with a bleeding diathesis or in the elderly, sometimes related to cerebrovascular amyloidosis.

The clinical signs produced by contusions vary with their location and size; most often a hemiparesis or gaze preference is seen, similar to a middle cerebral artery stroke. Bilateral large contusions produce coma with extensor posturing; when contusions are limited to the frontal lobes, an abulic-taciturn state or inappropriate jocularity and indifference occur. Contusions of the temporal lobes cause an aggressive combative syndrome, described below. With large contusions, the secondary effect of progressive edema is the most threatening aspect of the injury. Coma and signs of secondary brainstem compression (pupillary enlargement) then dominate. Seizures soon after trauma are rare with contusions, as indeed they are for several weeks after most acute head injuries.

Deep hemorrhages in the central white matter may result from confluent contusions in the depths of a sulcus. However, ganglionic, diencephalic, and other deep hematomas due to torsion or shearing forces in the brain infrequently occur independently of surface damage. The areas around these hematomas can become edematous, resulting in enlargement of the affected region and progressively raised intracranial pressure.

Another type of white matter, or "shearing," lesion consists of widespread acute disruption of axons at the time of impact. The affected areas of white matter are replaced with glial proliferation over a period of several months. There are characteristically small areas of tissue disruption in the corpus callosum and dorsolateral pons. Widespread axonal shearing lesions in the deep white matter of both hemispheres may explain persistent coma or vegetative state, but small hemorrhages in the midbrain and low diencephalon are as often the cause. Only severe shearing lesions are visualized by CT scanning, as small hemorrhages of the corpus callosum and centrum semiovale; MRI is able to show them throughout the white matter.

On occasion, head trauma causes diffuse brain swelling within a few hours after injury, although CT scanning fails to reveal focal lesions or hemorrhage, particularly in children. The swelling creates a mass effect with disastrous consequences. This problem is probably due to microvascular disruption and greatly increased cerebral blood flow.

Deep cerebral hemorrhages may be delayed several days after severe injury. Sudden neurologic deterioration, often in already comatose patients, or a sustained and unexplained rise in intracranial pressure should therefore prompt a CT scan.

Brainstem hemorrhages A syndrome with coma, midposition or larger pupils unreactive to light, and impaired or absent oculocephalic reflex eye movements results from small linear or oval-shaped hemorrhages in the high midbrain, visible on CT scan, although often delayed in appearance. Although extensor posturing occurs with stimulation, the limbs are otherwise flaccid. This clinical syndrome should be suspected even in the initial absence of a hemorrhage on CT scan. These acute midbrain hemorrhages may be the result of primary injury from rotational forces in the upper midbrain. They also occur from secondary compression of the brainstem by supratentorial hematomas and lateral tissue shifts or pressure from the adjacent temporal lobes. MRI shows many other small brainstem and hemispheric white matter lesions that are related to mechanical disruption of tissue, similar to shearing. In pathologic material from severe, acutely fatal injuries, small linear and oval hemorrhages are found in the low thalamic and subthalamic regions and throughout the midline of the brainstem (*Duret hemorrhages*).

Residual symptoms and signs of primary or secondary brainstem hemorrhages or ischemic lesions include tremor, pupillary enlargement, eye movement abnormalities, or the "locked-in" syndrome (see Chap. 26). Midbrain or diencephalic hemorrhages are the only well-defined direct traumatic brainstem lesions responsible for coma. Most other lesions causing coma and subsequent persistent vegetative state that are unexplained by CT scan are probably due to diffuse axonal shearing injuries in the cerebral hemispheres or severe anoxia-ischemia at the time of trauma.

SUBDURAL AND EPIDURAL HEMATOMAS In severe head injury, hemorrhages beneath the dura (subdural) or between the dura and skull (epidural) may be combined with contusions and other injuries, making it difficult to determine their relative contribution to the clinical state. However, subdural and epidural hematomas often occur as the primary lesion, each with a characteristic clinical and radiologic appearance. Because the mass effect of the hemorrhage and rise in intracranial pressure may be life-threatening, it is important to make an immediate diagnosis by CT scan and carry out surgical evacuation.

Acute subdural hematoma Acute subdural hematomas become symptomatic within minutes to hours after injury. Up to one-third of patients have a lucid interval before coma supervenes, but the majority are drowsy or comatose from the moment of injury. Arousable patients complain of unilateral headache and frequently have a slightly enlarged pupil on that side. Stupor or coma and unilateral pupillary enlargement are the major signs in larger hematomas. Pupillary dilation is usually ipsilateral, but 5 to 10 percent are contralateral to the hematoma. Lateralizing signs such as a hemiparesis are helpful but may be ipsilateral to the clot. The CT scan shows the clot, allowing early evacuation. The degree of midline shift is often disproportionately greater than the size of the clot in one CT scan axial section, but in general, rules relating shift to the level of consciousness, outlined in Chap. 26, remain useful. MRI may fail to demonstrate an acute clot. In an acutely deteriorating patient with diminished alertness and pupillary enlargement, burr holes or an emergency craniotomy are appropriate at times without prior radiographic confirmation of subdural hematoma. A subacute syndrome with drowsiness, headache, confusion, or mild hemiparesis occurring days to 2 weeks after injury is seen in alcoholics and in the elderly.

Direct trauma or surface contusions are not required for acute subdural hemorrhage; acceleration forces alone, as from whiplash, are adequate, especially in the elderly. Most subdural hematomas are small crescentic collections over the hemispheral convexity, adjacent to variable degrees of surface hemorrhagic contusions. Larger clots are thought to be primarily venous in origin, although additional arterial bleeding sites are often found, and some, when explored surgically, appear to be exclusively arterial. Most are located over the frontotemporal region, less often in the inferior middle fossa or over the occipital poles. Less common instances of interhemispheric, posterior fossa, or bilateral convexity clots are difficult to diagnose clinically, although drowsiness and the signs expected for each region can be detected. Small subdural hematomas may be asymptomatic and usually do not require therapy.

Acute epidural hematoma Epidural hematomas evolve more rapidly than subdural hematomas and therefore can be more treacherous. They occur in 1 to 3 percent of all head injuries, in up to 10 percent of severe cases, and are less often associated with underlying cortical damage than subdural hematomas. The majority of patients are unconscious when first seen. A "lucid interval" of several minutes to hours before coma supervenes is said to be most characteristic of epidural hemorrhage, although it is not common and by no means the only cause of this temporal profile.

The location of an epidural hematoma overlying the lateral temporal convexity is explained by its origin from torn dural vessels, most commonly the middle meningeal artery. The majority of patients have fractures of the squamous portion of the temporal bone, through the path of the torn vessel. Frontal, inferior temporal, or occipitoparietal epidural hematomas are less frequent, occurring when fractures disrupt branches of the middle meningeal artery. Dural laceration over the sagittal or lateral sinuses and rupture of small diploic veins are rarer causes. Epidural hematomas strip the tightly attached dura from the inner table of the skull, producing a characteristic lenticular-shaped clot on CT scan. They may be relatively less frequent in the elderly because of the tighter attachment of dura to skull that occurs with aging. Posterior fossa epidural hematomas are rare and difficult to detect clinically (most result from surgery such as resection of an acoustic neuroma).

Chronic subdural hematoma In chronic subdural hematoma, a preceding traumatic cause is less often clear; 20 to 30 percent of patients fail to give a history of injury, particularly elderly patients or those with a bleeding diathesis. The causative injury may be trivial (striking the head against the branch of a tree, a sudden stop in a car with lurching forward, or minor head contact during a fall or faint) and is often forgotten because it was remote in time. A period of weeks, or even months, follows when headaches (common but not invariable), slowed thinking, confusion, changes in personality, seizures, and/or a mild hemiparesis emerges. Fluctuation in the severity of the headache is typical, often with positional changes. Many chronic subdural hematomas are bilateral and give particularly misleading clinical syndromes. The initial clinical impression is often a stroke, brain tumor, drug intoxication, or a depressive, senile, or other type of dementia, the latter because drowsiness, inattentiveness, or incoherence of thought is more prominent than focal signs such as hemiparesis. Hemianesthesia or hemianopsia is seldom observed, probably because the anatomic structures subserving these functions are deep and not easily compressed. The diagnosis should be considered in dementias of rapid onset, particularly if headache is present. The condition does not usually progress unless acute bleeding is superimposed on the chronic hematoma, making the patient comatose with fluctuations of alertness and pupillary dilation. Occasionally patients present with "spells" of hemiparesis or aphasia typically lasting more than 10 min and indistinguishable from transient ischemic attacks. Patients with undetected small bilateral subdural hematomas seem to tolerate surgery, anesthesia, and nervous system depressive drugs poorly, often remaining drowsy or confused for long periods postoperatively.

Skull x-rays are usually normal except for a shift of a calcified pineal body to one side or an occasional unexpected fracture. The CT scan without contrast infusion typically shows a low-density mass over the convexity of the hemisphere, but between 2 to 6 weeks after the initial bleeding may show only a shift of the midline structures and compression of the lateral ventricles because the clot is isodense to adjacent brain. Bilateral chronic hematomas are often missed because of the absence of lateral tissue shifts. A "hypernormal" CT scan with full cortical sulci and small ventricles in an older patient should suggest the diagnosis of bilateral isodense hematomas. Contrast infusion demonstrates a chronic fibrous capsule surrounding the clot. MRI is reliable in identifying a subacute clot. Lumbar puncture is not recommended for diagnosis because of risk of worsening tissue shifts but, if performed, shows xanthochromia and a variable number of red blood cells. Chronic subdural hematomas can gradually expand and then behave clinically like a tumor. Treatment with glucocorticoids alone is sufficient in some cases, but surgical evacuation is most often successful. Fibrous membranes (pseudomembranes) that grow from the dura and encapsulate the region require surgical resection to prevent recurrent fluid accumulation. Small hematomas are largely resorbed, and only the organizing membranes remain, becoming calcified after many years.

PENETRATING INJURIES, COMPRESSIONS, AND LACERATIONS Tangential scalp wounds from bullets can produce neurologic signs or delayed seizures due to small hemorrhages or contusions, even in the absence of missile penetration. Bullets entering the brain cause considerable damage because of tremendous kinetic energy. A cylindrical area of necrosis surrounds the bullet track. Injuries differ with varying projectiles; soft civilian bullets typically shatter on impact and leave a track of metallic fragments with moderate parenchymal damage. Military bullets, because of high velocity and energy, disrupt tissue at great distances from the track and produce massive brain destruction.

Penetrating bullet injuries cause a rapid increase in intracranial pressure for several minutes followed by a drop depending on the volume of secondary hemorrhage and the degree of developing edema. Infection is a risk mainly from shell fragments, shrapnel, grenades, and mines, because such small projectiles carry surface bacteria and dirt into the brain. Most neurosurgeons administer systemic antibiotics prophylactically and perform local debridement in all types of penetrating injuries. Traumatic aneurysms can form as a result of disruption of vessel walls from the shock wave of the projectile; facial-orbital entrance wounds have the highest incidence. The aneurysms have an unpredictable course, but most that rupture do so in the first month. The prognosis for survival after missile injuries is good if consciousness is preserved and poor if coma is present from the outset.

Other intracranial foreign bodies from knives, picks, studguns, or high-speed tool bits may be missed unless skull x-rays are taken after minor penetrating injuries. Surgical removal, debridement, and extensive exploration for hemorrhage and necrotic tissue are required.

TRAUMATIC VASCULAR OCCLUSION AND DISSECTION Minor, sometimes unnoticed, neck trauma can produce dissection (stripping of the intima or the media) of the internal carotid or vertebral arteries. Chiropractic neck manipulation accounts for some cases. Severe blunt trauma to the neck can initiate a dissection several centimeters above the origins of the internal carotid or vertebral arteries. In awake patients there is usually local neck pain over the internal carotid artery, a Horner's syndrome, and headache over the ipsilateral anterior cranium. Some patients with carotid dissection subsequently have large middle cerebral artery strokes with hemiplegia. In drowsy or comatose patients, evidence of dissection or subsequent stroke is difficult to discern but is suggested by unexplained hemiplegia, unilateral miosis, or appearance of cerebral infarction on

CT scan. Angiography demonstrates either the typical "string sign" characterized by an elongated, narrowed lumen extending over 5 to 10 cm or complete occlusion of the carotid artery beginning several centimeters distal to the bifurcation. On rare occasions, basilar skull fractures cause carotid dissection beginning at the point of entry of the artery into the skull. Traumatic "false" aneurysms of the cervical carotid artery result from deep penetrating, and occasionally from nonpenetrating, blunt trauma of the neck. A pulsatile mass and bruit over the artery establish the diagnosis. Traumatic vertebral artery dissection can produce vertigo, vomiting, suboccipital or supraorbital headache, and other signs of lateral medullary ischemia. These symptoms are frequently attributed to vestibular concussion. In comatose patients, the only indication of vertebral artery occlusion may be inferior cerebellar infarction on CT scan.

Preexisting saccular aneurysms may rupture after basilar skull fractures, and this diagnosis should be considered if subarachnoid hemorrhage is profuse and inadequately explained by accompanying subdural blood on CT scan. Vasospasm from traumatic subarachnoid blood may be involved in the development of infarction after head injury.

Cavernous sinus arteriovenous fistulas are serious complications in patients surviving severe head injury. They are first evident as a self-audible bruit (many are also audible to the examiner), proptosis, conjunctival injection, or visual impairment. Angiography shows early filling of the cavernous sinus and its draining tributaries. The fistula generally enlarges, causing increasingly severe local changes around the eye and orbit and decreased chances of visual recovery. About 10 percent, mostly small fistulas, resolve spontaneously. Many surgical approaches have been tried, including ligation of the carotid artery, direct obliteration of the fistula or cavernous sinus, and angiographic-guided balloon embolization. A detachable balloon technique has proved successful in many cases (see Chap. 365).

INTRACRANIAL PRESSURE AND CEREBRAL BLOOD FLOW

Intracranial pressure (ICP) regulation and its relationship to cerebral blood flow (CBF), which is applicable to many pathologic processes including cerebral hemorrhage, encephalitis, and brain edema after stroke, is best understood in the context of head trauma. The components of the intracranial compartment are brain, CSF, and blood. Because the skull limits total intracranial content, the volume of these compartments is compromised by expanding lesions within the cranial cavity. The brain is virtually incompressible; therefore, CSF and blood serve as the main buffers of increasing intracranial volume. The relationship between increments in intracranial volume and the associated rises in ICP, termed *compliance*, approximates an exponential function. ICP is normally between 2 and 12 mmHg. Raised ICP in the range 15 to 40 mmHg, while not harmful by itself, can rapidly result in secondary damage, either by precipitously decreasing cerebral perfusion when ICP approaches blood pressure in the cranium or by associated shifts of brain tissue that damage the upper brainstem. The global damage from increased ICP is therefore ischemic in nature and related to the difference between ICP and blood pressure in the major cerebral arteries. When this pressure difference, termed *cerebral perfusion pressure* or *CPP*, is below 40 to 60 mmHg, raised ICP becomes detrimental to nerve cells; therapy is therefore directed toward maintaining perfusion above this range. The rationale for keeping CPP even higher (i.e., bringing ICP below 15 to 20 mmHg) is to afford a margin of safety should transient increases in ICP occur. Physiologic changes or medications that increase blood pressure do not necessarily improve CPP because increased vascular pressures can exacerbate brain edema in damaged areas, resulting in further increases in ICP that ultimately lower perfusion.

The most important secondary nervous system complication of head injury is raised intracranial pressure arising from the added volume of contusions, hematomas, and the progressive edema surrounding them. A close relationship exists between clinical outcome and ICP in patients with closed head injury. At least 50 percent of patients who die as a result of head injury do so because of uncontrolled rises in ICP, and outcome is inversely related to the level of ICP after acute injury. Aggressive treatment of raised ICP in modern intensive care units is believed to improve survival after severe head injury. The role of direct monitoring of ICP to guide therapy is more controversial.

Resting ICP, CPP, and compliance are spontaneously interrupted by rises in ICP termed *plateau waves* that may be precipitated by iatrogenic maneuvers such as suctioning, physical therapy, excess fluid administration, or pain. Plateau waves are due to a loss of cerebrovascular tone with a resultant increase in cerebral blood volume. Some apparently spontaneous plateau waves are due to mild, often unnoticed hypotension that causes cerebrovascular dilation. Such plateau waves (lasting 1 to 10 min and ranging from 25 to 60 mmHg) are most pronounced in patients with diminished intracranial compliance. They are best appreciated with continuous trend recordings of ICP. Signs of apparent transtentorial herniation such as pupillary enlargement may occur after plateau waves (they more often do not), and occasionally, brain death ensues.

There is little consensus about the importance of alterations in cerebral blood flow caused by head injury. For several minutes to an hour after acute head injury, cerebral blood flow may increase in some patients, although metabolic demands and oxygen consumption are diminished. Autoregulation, the ability of the cerebral vasculature to keep blood flow constant in response to decreased or increased perfusion pressure, is also impaired in damaged regions. Vascular factors have been found to account for approximately two-thirds of the rise in ICP after severe head injury. The blood-brain barrier also becomes more permeable after head injury in badly damaged regions, making edema formation more likely.

There is a complex relationship between raised ICP and clinical signs such as coma and pupillary enlargement that accompany supratentorial masses. ICP represents the accommodation of intracranial contents to additional mass; clinical signs are a parallel barometer of tissue shifts, particularly affecting structures around the tentorial opening. Raised ICP per se does not cause signs until it reaches levels that preclude cerebral perfusion; it then causes global ischemia in a fashion similar to acute hypotension. Coma and other secondary signs resulting from tissue shifts in the region of the tentorial opening are described in Chap. 26. Horizontal midline shift at the level of the pineal body is closely related to the level of consciousness with acute unilateral mass lesions.

Other secondary phenomena after severe head injury cause brain damage and alter outcome. Hypoxia or coagulopathy, for example, are common from a number of causes and, when severe, are associated with a poorer outcome.

CLINICAL SYNDROMES AND TREATMENT OF HEAD INJURY

MINOR INJURY A fully alert and attentive patient presenting after head injury with one or more symptoms of headache, faintness, nausea, a single episode of emesis, difficulty with concentration, or slight blurring of vision has a good prognosis with little risk of subsequent deterioration. Such patients have sustained a concussion or have been dazed and have a brief amnestic epoch surrounding the moment of impact. Occasionally, vasovagal syncope occurs several minutes to an hour after the injury and causes concern. Constant generalized or frontal headache is common in the days following trauma; it is often throbbing or hemicranial in nature, like migraine. The majority of patients with a minor syndrome do not have a skull fracture on skull x-ray or hemorrhage on CT scan. The decision to obtain these tests depends largely on the availability of CT or MRI scanning and clinical signs suggesting that the impact was severe (e.g., prolonged concussion, periorbital or mastoid hematoma, repeated vomiting, etc). Children and young adults are particularly prone to drowsiness, vomiting, and irritability, sometimes delayed for several hours after apparently minor injuries. After a period of observation for several hours, arrangements may be made for the patient to be accompanied home to be observed by family or friends.

Persistent severe headache and repeated vomiting in the context of normal alertness and no focal neurologic signs are usually benign, but CT or MRI scanning and/or skull x-rays should be obtained. Skull fractures increase the likelihood of a subdural or epidural hematoma. Skull x-ray is an acceptable screening method in areas without access to CT scanning. Patients with these exaggerated signs, even if they follow minor injury, deserve observation in the hospital for 24 h. Clinical judgment, the presence of associated noncranial injuries, the availability of others at home, and the examiner's certainty of a normal neurologic examination should guide the need for further surveillance.

INJURY OF INTERMEDIATE SEVERITY Patients who are not comatose but who have persistent confusion, behavioral changes, less than normal alertness, extreme dizziness, or focal neurologic signs such as hemiparesis should be admitted to the hospital and have a CT scan. The clinical syndromes most common in this group, in addition to postconcussive headache and dizziness, unsteadiness, photophobia, and vomiting of minor injury, include (1) delirium with a disinclination to be examined or moved, expletive speech, and resistance if disturbed, often associated with anterior temporal lobe contusions; (2) a quiet, disinterested, slowed mental state (abulia) with dull facial appearance and slight irascibility if bothered, the patient lying quietly with eyes closed when undisturbed, seen with inferior and frontopolar frontal contusions; (3) severe memory loss with poor retrograde and anterograde performance, headache, and photophobia, with medial temporal lobe contusions or diffuse injury; (4) a focal deficit such as aphasia or mild hemiparesis (hemianopsia is rare as an isolated posttraumatic finding), suggesting subdural hematoma or convexity contusion, or rarely, carotid artery dissection and stroke; (5) global confusion with inattention, poor performance on simple mental tasks, fluctuating or slightly erroneous orientation, associated with several types of injuries including the first two described above as well as medial frontal contusions and interhemispheric subdural hematoma; (6) repetitive vomiting, nystagmus, drowsiness, and unsteadiness, usually from a labyrinthine concussion, but occasionally due to a posterior fossa subdural hematoma or vertebral artery dissection; (7) drowsiness alone or with muteness, often unassociated with significant CT scan abnormalities; and (8) diabetes insipidus with or without a frontal-temporal lobe syndrome, from damage to the median eminence or pituitary stalk and adjacent medial cortex.

The syndromes of intermediate severity are usually preceded by brief loss of consciousness, and many are associated with skull fractures. A CT scan is required to exclude surgically remediable subdural or epidural hematomas and to define areas of contusion that later enlarge with edema or coalesce to form intraparenchymal hemorrhages. Paroxysmal or rhythmic EEG abnormalities, in contrast to acute convulsions, are common over the region of a large contusion. Many intermediate injuries are complicated by drug or alcohol intoxication, making toxic screening important.

Close clinical observation in a well-staffed setting is advisable in order to detect increasing drowsiness and change in respiratory pattern or pupillary enlargement and to ensure fluid restriction. Fully awake or slightly drowsy patients with small subdural hematomas may be treated with glucocorticoids and fluid restriction; larger clots, especially with fluctuating or worsening alertness, require surgery. Follow-up CT scanning is advisable. Epidural hematomas causing compression of adjacent brain should be evacuated in patients who have a reasonable chance of recovery from other injuries. Free water intake should be limited, allowing serum osmolarity to rise spontaneously toward 290 mosmol/L. Fever must be treated assiduously with antipyretics or a cooling blanket, and its source must be identified

(usually aspiration). So-called central fever is rare. The routine, acute administration of phenytoin is controversial. About half of neurosurgeons advocate its use, particularly in children and young adults, in the belief that it may reduce the incidence of posttraumatic epilepsy, but the best randomized trial has shown no benefit beyond the first week of drug administration. Glucocorticoids may be useful if there is a contusion, hemorrhage, or edema on the CT scan; otherwise, they complicate management and should be omitted. The possibility of associated cervical spine injuries should be considered in all patients with syndromes of intermediate severity. The neck should be immobilized, and adequate x-rays of the spine should be obtained.

The majority of patients with intermediate injury improve over 1 to 6 weeks. During the first week, alertness, irascibility, memory, and mental performance fluctuate. Behavioral changes such as agitation are most evident at night and sometimes seem to be worsened by large doses of glucocorticoids or CNS-depressant drugs. Haloperidol is useful when used sparingly. Subtle abnormalities of intellectual function, particularly attention, spontaneity, and memory, tend to return toward normal later, and sometimes do so abruptly. Persistent intellectual difficulties are discussed below.

SEVERE HEAD INJURY AND COMA Patients who are stuporous or comatose from the outset require immediate neurologic attention and, often, resuscitation. There is often pupillary enlargement or asymmetry. Persistent unresponsiveness is a grave sign. After the patient is intubated and the blood pressure is stabilized, attention is given to life-threatening noncranial injuries, followed by a survey neurologic examination. The possibility of cervical injuries should not be overlooked, and the cervical spine must be immobilized during the initial assessment. The depth of coma and the size of the pupils are most important. Extensor limb posturing and bilateral Babinski signs, combined with apparently purposeful movements, are common. Asymmetry in limb posture, limb movement, or gaze preference suggests a subdural or epidural hematoma or a large contusion.

As soon as vital functions permit and cervical spine x-rays and a CT scan have been obtained, the patient should be taken to a critical care unit. The finding of an epidural or subdural hematoma or large intracerebral hemorrhage is usually an indication for surgery and intracranial decompression. In one large series, the time between injury and evacuation of acute subdural hematomas was the major determinant of outcome. If such lesions are not present and the patient is still comatose and critically ill, attention is directed toward treating raised ICP. Patients with abnormal CT scans showing contusions, hemorrhages, or tissue shifts are the best candidates for ICP monitoring. The lumbar CSF pressure does not accurately reflect the intracranial pressure and lumbar puncture may increase the risk of brain herniation; therefore, the practice in most head injury treatment centers is to use one of several devices inserted intracranially to measure ICP. The pressure can be monitored continuously, disturbances in compliance and falling CPP can be identified, and appearance of plateau waves can be noted.

The treatment of raised ICP is best guided by direct measurement but may proceed on a presumptive basis using clinical status and CT scan as guides. All potentially exacerbating factors must be eliminated. Hypoxia, hyperthermia, hypercarbia, awkward head positions, and high mean airway pressures from mechanical ventilation all increase cerebral blood volume and ICP. Many, but not all, patients will have lower ICPs when the head and trunk are elevated. If raising the patient's head lowers blood pressure, then cerebral perfusion pressure may be optimal in the supine position. Active management of raised ICP includes induced hypocarbia to an initial level of 28 to 33 mmHg P_{CO_2} and hyperosmolar dehydration with 20% mannitol (0.25 to 1 g/kg every 3 to 6 h), preferably using directly measured ICP as a guide. Otherwise, a serum osmolality of 305 to 315 mosmol/L is desirable, as is ventricular or subarachnoid fluid drainage when possible.

Persistently raised ICP after inception of this conservative therapy generally indicates a poor outcome, but the addition of high-dose barbiturates may further lower ICP. In many instances, barbiturates cause a parallel reduction in ICP and blood pressure without resulting in net improvement in cerebral perfusion. The beneficial effects of barbiturates, aside from their sedative and anticonvulsant activities, are not established, and they can cause disastrous hypotension, so their routine use in severe head injury is not recommended. Further details of treatment of raised ICP are given in Chap. 26. Systolic blood pressure should be maintained above 100 mmHg by vasopressor agents, if necessary, but when pressors are required to support barbiturate use, there is usually little improvement in CPP. Mean blood pressure levels above 110 to 120 mmHg may exaggerate brain edema and are associated with plateau waves; hypertension may be treated with diuretics and beta-adrenergic blocking agents, angiotensin-converting enzyme inhibitors, or intermittent doses of barbiturates. A number of other antihypertensive drugs, including some calcium-channel blockers, are relatively contraindicated because they may raise ICP. Fluid and electrolytes must be administered cautiously, and free water administration should be limited. Administration of phenytoin to prevent seizures is recommended by many neurosurgeons. Antacids by nasogastric tube or directly acting drugs should be administered to keep gastric pH above 3.5 and prevent gastrointestinal bleeding. The use of large doses of glucocorticoids in severe head injury does not improve outcome. Several recent studies suggest that early nutritional support results in earlier neurologic recovery from head injury. If the patient remains comatose, it is worthwhile to repeat the CT scan to exclude a delayed surface or intracerebral hemorrhage. Intensive care salvages some critically ill head-injured patients by concentrating efforts on simple treatments that avoid medical complications, particularly pneumonia and sepsis and preventable increases in ICP. Whether more assiduous control of ICP and CPP will produce better results remains to be proved.

ASSOCIATED DERANGEMENTS OCCURRING WITH SEVERE HEAD TRAUMA   Injuries outside the cranium should be searched for at the outset, because they are likely to be forgotten if not initially noted. In particular, associated spinal, long bone, and abdominal injuries may cause delayed difficulties in management. However, secondary medical complications dominate the intermediate-term intensive care of head trauma patients.

Fluids and electrolytes   Over half of patients who persist in coma for 24 h after head injury develop abnormalities of electrolytes or fluid balance. Frequently these are a consequence of therapy, but the metabolic responses to head trauma are similar to those produced by trauma elsewhere and are important in planning treatment. Daily input-output records and body weights, when possible, are useful. Water restriction and osmotic agents render most patients hyperosmolar and hypovolemic, requiring monitoring of serum osmolality and sodium concentrations. Diabetes insipidus should be suspected if urine output increases and urine specific gravity is low. Replacement of water losses suffices for mild cases, but vasopressin may be required in persistent cases. Serum osmolality above approximately 325 mosmol/L should be avoided because of the associated decrease in cardiac output.

Aldosterone and antidiuretic hormone (vasopressin, AVP) secretion in response to stress favor sodium and free water retention, respectively. The latter usually predominates, leading to mild hypervolemic hyponatremia in untreated patients, but is obscured by concomitant administration of osmotic agents. Severe hyponatremia results from excessive AVP secretion, which may occur with raised ICP, basilar skull fractures, and after prolonged mechanical ventilation. Potassium is lost in head injury because of trauma-induced aldosterone hypersecretion, therapeutic osmotic diuresis, and glucocorticoids. Because potassium is predominantly an intracellular ion, hypokalemia is frequently manifested as a hypochloremic alkalosis with normal or minimally depressed serum potassium and requires adequate replacement therapy with KCl.

Respiratory complications   Some patients with head injuries have hypoxia acutely after injury without obvious pulmonary infiltrates. Aspiration pneumonia presents a great risk; acid burn injury from aspirated gastric contents, infection, and atelectasis may combine to produce the adult respiratory distress syndrome (ARDS) and severe arteriovenous shunting. Some evidence suggests that agents that coat the gastric lining without reducing pH, such as sucralfate, are associated with less aspiration pneumonia than are conventional prophylactic agents for gastric bleeding. ARDS also can occur due to disseminated intravascular coagulopathy, fat embolism, or, rarely, "neurogenic" pulmonary edema. Treatment is similar to other cases of ARDS with positive end-expiratory pressure (PEEP) to allow lowered inspired oxygen concentrations and to prevent further atelectasis. The effect of PEEP on ICP is complex, but PEEP should not be withheld if necessary for oxygenation.

Atelectasis is common in all poorly responsive patients and is treated with chest physical therapy and adequate ventilator tidal volumes. Pulmonary embolism is also a major threat to bedridden patients, and intermittent pneumatic calf compression or modest doses of subcutaneous heparin may be useful prophylaxis. The latter has not predisposed to intracerebral or gastrointestinal bleeding. Early recognition of deep leg vein thrombosis and aggressive treatment by occlusion of the inferior vena cava may prevent later emboli.

Gastrointestinal hemorrhage   The majority of patients with severe head injuries develop gastric erosions, but only a few have clinically significant hemorrhages. Gastrointestinal bleeding usually occurs in the first days to 1 week. Unlike most patients in shock or with stress ulceration, head-trauma patients often have elevated gastric acidity. The synergistic effect of glucocorticoids in causing upper tract hemorrhage has been questioned, but the incidence of viscus perforation, particularly of the cecum, is elevated. Prophylactic treatment with gastric coating agents, as discussed above, with H-2 blockers or with frequent antacid administration to keep gastric pH high, probably reduces gastric hemorrhage in other stress states and is commonly used in head trauma.

Fat embolism   Patients with severe long bone injuries are subject to widespread cerebral fat embolism. This complication is seen less often than previously, perhaps due to better fluid replacement. In the typical case, head injury is a minor part of the overall trauma; in a few, severe cranial injury masks the syndrome. Several days after the bone fractures, restlessness, delirium, or drowsiness progressing to coma in severe cases, seizures, generalized brain edema, and/or hypoxia develops. About half the patients have retinal and conjunctival punctate hemorrhages or visible fat in retinal vessels. A petechial rash, prominent in the anterior axillary folds and supraclavicular fossae, diffuse interstitial infiltrates on the chest x-ray, fat in the urine, and/or renal failure occurs in some patients. Severe reduction in arterial oxygen content is common from widespread lung injury (ARDS). Cerebral fat embolism causes cerebral purpura, mainly in the white matter, due to capillary occlusion by fat globules. There is evidence that cases recognized and treated early have a better prognosis. Massive doses of glucocorticoids, reduction of ICP, and administration of positive-pressure ventilation with high end-expiratory pressures have been claimed to be useful. Heparin or intravenous alcohol are no longer recommended.

Cardiovascular changes   Acute head trauma may cause transient apnea and cardiac arrest. In the absence of overwhelming brain damage, recovery from the arrest is the rule. Subsequently, a sympathoadrenal discharge or raised ICP may cause systemic hypertension, either with the classically associated bradycardia (Cushing response) or, almost as frequently, with tachycardia. Cardiac arrhythmias are common, most notably sinus bradycardia, supraventricular tachycardias, nodal rhythm, and heart block. T-wave inversion and alterations in the ST segment may simulate subendocardial ischemia.

Neurogenic pulmonary edema is a form of ARDS in which the alveoli fill with fluid as they would in congestive heart failure but left ventricular end-diastolic pressure (measured by pulmonary capillary wedge pressure) is normal. A pulmonary vascular leak may be produced when a sudden shift of intravascular volume occurs from the systemic to pulmonary circulation, as occurs transiently with suddenly raised ICP, or there may be a direct neurogenic influence of hypothalamic function on the pulmonary microvasculature. Once

TABLE 376-1 Glasgow Coma Scale for head injury

Eye opening (E):

Spontaneous	4
To loud voice	3
To pain	2
Nil	1

Best motor response (M):

Obeys	6
Localizes	5
Withdraws (flexion)	4
Abnormal flexion posturing	3
Extension posturing	2
Nil	1

Verbal response (V):

Oriented	5
Confused, disoriented	4
Inappropriate words	3
Incomprehensible sounds	2
Nil	1

NOTE: Coma score = E + M + V. Patients scoring 3 or 4 have an 85 percent chance of dying or remaining vegetative, while scores above 11 indicate 5 to 10 percent likelihood of death or vegetative state and 85 percent chance of moderate disability or good recovery. Intermediate scores correlate with proportional chances of patients recovering.

the pulmonary vasculature has been damaged, an alveolar capillary leak may continue despite return of pulmonary vascular pressure to normal. The result is pulmonary edema with normal central venous and wedge pressures after the initial injury.

Hematologic complications A large number of patients demonstrate a mild coagulopathy, and 5 to 10 percent have various degrees of disseminated intravascular coagulation, a harbinger of poor outcome. A correlation may exist between the severity of injury and the level of increased fibrin degradation products in blood. One cause of the coagulopathy is thought to be the release of highly thromboplastic material into the systemic circulation from the damaged brain.

PROGNOSIS Extensive work by Jennet's group in Glasgow and from the Traumatic Coma Data Bank has provided data on the outcome in severe head injury (Table 376-1). Verbal output, eye opening, and the best motor response are important predictors of ultimate outcome. Eighty-five percent of patients with aggregate Glasgow Coma Scale scores of 3 or 4 die 24 h after injury. Yet a number of patients with a poor initial prognosis, including absent pupillary light responses, survive, suggesting that aggressive management is justified in virtually all patients. Patients below approximately 20 years of age, particularly children, may make remarkable recoveries after grave early neurologic signs. In one large study of severe head injury, 55 percent of children had a good outcome at 1 year, compared with 21 percent of adults. Increased intracranial pressure, older age, and signs of cisternal compression and midline shift on CT scan all have poor prognostic significance.

Evoked potentials also have prognostic value in head injury, and their accuracy probably exceeds clinical observations. Somatosensory evoked potentials are the most useful, with bilaterally absent cortical potentials (with more caudal potentials present) being predictive of death or a vegetative state in 85 to 95 percent of patients. Prediction of a good functional outcome in the presence of normal or mildly abnormal tests is less certain.

NEUROPSYCHOLOGICAL OUTCOME AFTER HEAD INJURY

Traumatic damage and cognitive sequelae of head injury both occur in a continuum, but most patients recover to normal after mild injury. There is probably a high rate of temporary inattention and memory and other subtle deficits after all but the mildest injuries. Attention has recently been directed toward a structural basis for the fatigue, dizziness, headache, and difficulty in concentration after mild injury,

termed the *postconcussion syndrome*. Based on experimental models, some investigators believe that subtle axonal shearing lesions or biochemical alterations account for these symptoms despite normal brain imaging, evoked potentials, and EEG. In moderate and severe trauma, neuropsychological changes are found routinely; however, formal testing often shows deficits that are not important in daily functioning. This is partly due to the type of testing and the nature of the control groups. Test scores tend to improve rapidly during the first 6 months after injury, then more slowly for years.

SPINAL CORD TRAUMA

Approximately 10,000 patients a year in the United States, mostly young and otherwise healthy, become paraplegic or quadriplegic because of spinal cord injuries. There are an estimated 200,000 quadriplegics in the country. The majority of cord injuries in civilian life result from damage to the surrounding vertebral column from fracture, dislocation, or both. Vertical compression with flexion is the main mechanism of injury in the thoracic cord, and hyperextension or flexion is the main cause of injury in the cervical cord. Preexisting spondylosis, a congenitally narrowed spinal canal, hypertrophied ligamentum flavum (see Chap. 381), and instability of the apophyseal joints of adjacent vertebrae from diseases such as rheumatoid arthritis predispose to severe spinal cord damage after minor degrees of injury.

PATHOPHYSIOLOGY AND PATHOLOGY OF CORD INJURY Much damage to the spinal cord is due to secondary phenomena in the minutes and hours following injury. Even when a complete transverse myelopathy is evident immediately after impact, some secondary changes are avoidable, and the resultant damage may be reversible. The immediate injury causes pericapillary hemorrhages that coalesce and enlarge, particularly in the gray matter. Infarction of gray matter and early white matter edema are evident within 4 h of experimental blunt injury. Eight hours after injury there is global infarction at the injured level, and only at this point does necrosis of white matter and paralysis below the level of the lesion become irreversible. The necrosis and central hemorrhages enlarge to occupy one or two levels above and below the point of primary impact. Gliosis in these regions results in necrotic areas over several months and may cavitate causing a progressive syringomyelic syndrome.

The early phases of injury are associated with reduced regional blood flow from direct capillary damage and a more prolonged secondary ischemia. A number of interventions, including opiate antagonists, thyrotropin-releasing hormone, local cord cooling, dextran infusion, adrenergic blockade, and hyperbaric oxygen, have been of uncertain clinical usefulness. A large randomized trial has shown the benefit of high doses of methylprednisolone administered within 8 h of injury. This effect may result from inhibition of lipid peroxidation rather than a direct anti-inflammatory action. The critical factor for recoverable function is the time from injury to institution of any therapy. Complete axonal disruption from the immediate trauma or secondary phenomena precludes recovery.

TYPES OF SPINAL CORD INJURY AND THEIR MANAGEMENT Any patient with severe head injury potentially has an associated instability of the spinal column. The care of such patients begins at the scene of the accident. The neck should be immobilized to prevent cord damage, and care should be taken during transport and during the physical and radiologic examinations to avoid neck extension or rotation and to prevent torsion-rotation of the thoracic spine. Blood pressure, respiratory status, and systemic injuries are attended to rapidly. Most patients can be intubated, if necessary, by blind nasotracheal technique without neck extension. High thoracic or cervical cord trauma regularly cause mild hypotension and bradycardia because of functional sympathectomy that responds to infusion of crystalloid or colloid (often corroborated by bilateral ptosis and miosis—Horner's syndrome).

The neurologic examination in the awake patient focuses on neck or back pain, diminished limb power, a sensory level on the trunk, and deep tendon reflexes, usually absent below the level of an acute cord injury. Injuries above C5 cause quadriplegia and respiratory failure. At C5 and C6 the biceps are also weak, and at C4 and C5 the deltoid and supra- and infraspinatus are weak. C7 injuries cause weakness of the triceps, wrist extensors, and forearm pronators. Injuries at T1 and below cause paraplegia; the precise level can be determined from the level of sensory loss. Compression in the low thoracic and lumbar region causes a conus medullaris or cauda equina syndrome (see Chap. 381). Cauda equina injuries are usually incomplete, involving peripheral nerves rather than spinal cord, and therefore are surgically remediable for longer periods after injury than spinal cord compression. In a comatose patient, absent reflexes, especially with small pupils or paradoxical breathing, signify a high cervical cord injury.

The next priority is to exclude a surgically remediable and potentially reversible cord compression due to dislocation of a vertebral body. Many traumatic myelopathies have no clearly associated fracture or dislocation. If x-rays suggest any aberration in the position of vertebrae, then reduction should be undertaken quickly. The role of myelography is controversial, but many neurosurgeons instill a few drops of water-soluble contrast media into the spinal subarachnoid space to demonstrate a block to the flow of CSF by CT scan or conventional myelography. Examination by MRI, when available, can be more useful. Decompression within 2 h of severe injury may lead to some recovery of cord function. With incomplete myelopathies, especially if the limbs are becoming progressively weaker, early decompression is strongly recommended, even many hours after injury. Surgical approaches to decompressing the spinal column depend on the specific nature of the injury. In complete transverse myelopathies beyond 6 to 12 h in duration, decompressive laminectomies are usually unsuccessful in restoring function.

The concerns with spinal column fractures, with or without myelopathy, are threefold: (1) detection of vertebral dislocations causing cord compression, (2) instability caused by fractures that will lead to misalignment and cord compression in the future, and (3) the proper treatment of fractures through the pedicles, facets, or vertebral bodies. Some fractures heal with immobilizaton and time, usually 2 to 3 months; others require surgical fusion to ensure stability.

Atlantoaxial dislocations can cause immediate death from respiratory failure, an event that may occur with no neurologic signs. Rheumatoid arthritis predisposes to this injury. Atlantooccipital dislocations occur predominantly in children and are almost always fatal. "Jefferson's fractures" are burst fractures of the ring of the atlas resulting from a force descending on the vertex of the skull as in diving accidents; they are usually asymptomatic. "Hangman's fractures" are produced by hyperextension and longitudinal distraction of the upper cervical spine, as occurs with penal hanging or striking the chin on a steering wheel in head-on collisions. These are usually fractures through the pedicles of C2 with subluxation anteriorly of C2 on C3. Traction reduction and immobilization allow proper healing.

Hyperflexion dislocation of the cervical vertebrae commonly causes traumatic quadriplegia. Occasionally, a markedly displaced injury is unassociated with neurologic dysfunction, presenting only with neck pain. In most cases, however, minor subluxation is associated with a severe neurologic deficit. Ligamentous disruption presumably allows compression of the cord at the moment of impact, but the vertebral bodies return closer to their original stations afterward. Therefore, any degree of subluxation must be treated as potentially unstable.

Compression fractures of the cervical spine can cause neurologic damage if a bone fragment is driven backward (burst fracture) into the spinal cord. "Teardrop fractures" with crushing of a vertebral body, leaving a fragment of bone anteriorly, are usually associated with ligamentous disruption and spinal instability. Single compression fractures of the thoracic spine are usually stable because the thoracic cage provides support, but they may be associated with anterior cord

compression and require decompression and stabilization with the insertion of metal rods.

Mild hyperextension injuries may cause only disruption of supporting ligamentous structures and be well tolerated. More severe injuries cause vertebral displacement and cord compression. The "central cord syndrome" is produced by brief compression of the cervical cord and disruption of the central gray matter, usually occurring in patients with an already narrow spinal canal, either congenitally or from cervical spondylosis. There is weakness of the arms, often with pinprick loss over the arms and shoulders, and relative sparing of leg power and sensation on the trunk and legs. Abnormality of bladder function is variable. The prognosis for recovery is good.

Thoracolumbar fractures are produced by impact in the high or midback, usually while the patient is bent over. Impingement on the spinal canal results in a complex combination of cauda equina and conus medullaris dysfunction. Pure lumbar fractures produce cauda equina compression. Myelography, MRI, or CT scan allows precise localization, and surgical decompression is usually recommended, even with complete deficits, because the potential for recovery of peripheral nerves is great.

The subsequent care of patients with spinal cord injury is best undertaken in specialized centers. General principles of medical and urologic management are discussed in Chap. 381.

REFERENCES

ADAMS JH et al: Diffuse brain damage of the immediate impact type. Brain 100:489, 1977

BAKAY L, GLASSAUER FE: *Head Injury.* Boston, Little, Brown, 1980

DACEY RG et al: Neurosurgical complications after apparently minor head injury. J Neurosurg 65:203, 1986

EISENBERG HM et al: Report of the Traumatic Coma Data Bank. J Neurosurg 75 (suppl) S1, 1991

GOLDSTEIN M: Traumatic brain injury: A silent epidemic. Ann Neurol 27:327, 1990

LANGFITT TW, GENARELLI TA: Can the outcome from head injury be improved? J Neurosurg 56:19, 1982

LEVIN HS et al: Neurobehavioral outcome following minor head injury: A three center study. J Neurosurg 66:234, 1987

REINUS WR et al: Practical selection criteria for noncontrast cranial computed tomography in patients with head trauma. Ann Emerg Med 22:1148, 1993

ROPPER AH et al (eds): *Neurological and Neurosurgical Intensive Care,* 2d ed. Baltimore, Aspen, 1988

RUFF RM et al: Predictors of outcome following severe head trauma: Follow-up data from the Traumatic Coma Data Bank. Brain Inj 7:101, 1993

STEIN SC et al: Delayed and progressive brain injury in closed-head trauma: Radiological demonstration. Neurosurgery 32:25, 1993

377   NUTRITIONAL AND METABOLIC DISEASES OF THE NERVOUS SYSTEM

MAURICE VICTOR / JOSEPH B. MARTIN

Included under this title are a large and diverse number of disorders of the nervous system. They fall readily into two groups—acquired and inherited. Here the emphasis will be on the *acquired* diseases, since they are essentially disorders of adult life and a major concern to both internists and neurologists. The *inherited* metabolic and nutritional diseases, on the other hand, are predominantly disorders of infancy and childhood and are more appropriately considered in a textbook of pediatrics (see also Chaps. 349 to 352). However, a small number of the inherited diseases permit survival to adolescence or early adult life or may even have their onset during these periods. These latter instances, which need to be differentiated from certain degenerative and acquired metabolic diseases, will be discussed briefly in this chapter and in others, to which the reader will be referred.

DISEASES DUE TO NUTRITIONAL DEFICIENCY

The general aspects of deficiency disease have been presented in Chap. 77, which should be reviewed as an introduction to the deficiency diseases of the nervous system. The term *deficiency*, used here in its strictest sense, designates those diseases or syndromes resulting from the *lack of an essential nutrient in the diet or from a conditioning factor that increases the need for that nutrient*. This category comprises the following neurologic diseases:

1 Wernicke's disease and Korsakoff's psychosis
2 "Alcoholic" cerebellar degeneration
3 Nutritional polyneuropathy
4 Pellagra
5 Deficiency amblyopia (nutritional optic neuropathy)
6 The syndrome of amblyopia, painful neuropathy, and orogenital dermatitis (Strachan's syndrome)
7 Subacute combined degeneration of the spinal cord (vitamin B_{12} deficiency)
8 Folic acid deficiency
9 Vitamin E deficiency

A number of general principles are applicable to all the above diseases. Of the known vitamin deficiencies, the B deficiencies (rarely, vitamin E deficiency) are most important in neurologic disease. Thiamine chloride, nicotinic acid, pyridoxine, pantothenic acid, and possibly folic acid and riboflavin each plays a role in carbohydrate metabolism, upon which the CNS depends for its principal source of energy. These vitamins function as coenzymes in the Krebs tricarboxylic acid cycle; in addition, thiamine is involved in the hexosemonophosphate shunt. Vitamin B_{12} is required for the conversion of methylmalonyl to succinyl coenzyme A and for the conversion of homocysteine to methionine.

Except for subacute combined degeneration of the spinal cord secondary to vitamin B_{12} deficiency and the ocular signs of Wernicke's disease resulting from thiamine deficiency, it is rarely possible to relate the deficiency diseases in humans to the lack of one particular vitamin. For example, polyneuropathy may result from any one of several vitamin deficiencies [thiamine chloride (vitamin B_1), pyridoxine (vitamin B_6), pantothenic acid, and probably B_{12}]. Pellagra, beriberi, and Strachan's syndrome are probably related to a deficiency of several vitamins. It is noteworthy that chronic pyridoxine (vitamin B_6) intoxication also causes a sensory polyneuropathy similar to that caused by its deficiency.

In the western world, deficiency diseases of the nervous system occur most often in the alcoholic population of large urban centers. Alcohol acts mainly by displacing food in the diet, but it also increases the demand for B vitamins, which are necessary to metabolize the carbohydrate furnished by alcohol itself, and it may impair the gastrointestinal absorption of vitamins. Dietary faddism, impaired absorption of dietary nutrients (as occurs in sprue or after gastric plication for the treatment of obesity or resection of the stomach and small bowel), and the use of certain drugs (e.g., isoniazid and hydralazine, which interfere with the enzymatic function of pyridoxine) account for a small number of cases of deficiency disease.

Each of the deficiency diseases may occur in pure form and will be so described. More often they occur in various combinations. Stated in another way, deficiency diseases usually involve both the central and peripheral nervous systems, an attribute that they share with few other categories of disease. Also, the examination of patients with deficiency disease frequently discloses nonneurologic signs of malnutrition such as general wasting, lesions of the skin and mucous membranes, and circulatory abnormalities.

WERNICKE'S DISEASE OR ENCEPHALOPATHY Wernicke originally described an illness of acute onset characterized by mental

disturbance, paralysis of eye movements, and ataxia of gait. Swelling of the optic discs and retinal hemorrhages also were present, and there was a progressive depression of the state of consciousness, leading to death, so that a fatal outcome was at one time considered a universal feature of this disease. Wernicke observed focal vascular lesions in the gray matter around the third and fourth ventricles and aqueduct of Sylvius; he regarded them as inflammatory in nature and named the disease *acute superior hemorrhagic polioencephalitis*. Since Wernicke's time, views regarding this disease have undergone considerable modification.

Symptoms and signs   The most readily recognized abnormalities are the ocular motor signs, and it is difficult to make the clinical diagnosis without them. The usual abnormality is a weakness or paralysis of abduction (abducens palsy) which is invariably bilateral (though rarely symmetric) and accompanied by horizontal diplopia, strabismus, and nystagmus. Three types of nystagmus may occur, horizontal or vertical gaze–evoked nystagmus being the most frequent. A horizontal gaze–evoked nystagmus limited to the abducting eye is characteristic of internuclear ophthalmoplegia. Rarely, one sees an upbeat or downbeat nystagmus in the primary position, accompanied by oscillopsia. Each of these abnormalities may be present alone, but far more often a constellation of signs of disordered motility is present, including supranuclear paralysis of gaze. Horizontal gaze palsy is more frequent than vertical gaze palsy. Rarely an isolated paralysis of downgaze or an isolated paralysis of convergence or divergence occurs. In advanced disease there may be complete loss of ocular movement, and the pupils, which ordinarily are spared, may become miotic and nonreacting. Ptosis is rare. The parenteral administration of thiamine in the early stages results in dramatic improvement of ocular motility although horizontal nystagmus may persist indefinitely.

The *ataxia* affects stance and gait predominantly and may be so severe that the patient cannot stand or walk without support. With specific treatment the disorder of equilibrium improves, and the patient is left with a wide-based, uncertain gait. The mildest degree of ataxia is brought out only by heel-to-toe walking. In contrast to the gross disorder of locomotion, an intention (cerebellar) tremor of the limbs is relatively infrequent. The latter abnormality, when present, affects the legs more than the arms. Scanning speech is present only in isolated cases.

A derangement of mental function is found in about 90 percent of patients and takes one of several forms: (1) The most common is a *global confusional-apathetic state*, characterized by profound listlessness, inattentiveness, indifference to the surroundings, and disorientation. Unconsciousness or deep stupor as the initial abnormality is distinctly rare, but drowsiness is common. Spontaneous speech is minimal. Many questions directed to the patient go unanswered, or the patient may fall asleep while being questioned, a state from which he or she can be readily roused, however. Whatever questions the patient answers betray disorientation in time and place, misidentification of those nearby and an inability to grasp the meaning of the illness or immediate situation. Many of the patient's remarks are irrational and show no consistency from one moment to another. Under these circumstances, a more extensive evaluation of intellectual function is seldom possible. (2) Some patients show a disproportionate disorder of retentive memory, i.e., the Korsakoff amnesic state (see Chap. 25 and further on in this chapter). (3) A relatively small number of patients (less than 20 percent in our series) show the symptoms of alcohol withdrawal, either delirium tremens or a variant thereof.

The symptoms of Wernicke's disease may appear simultaneously and rather acutely, but more often ophthalmoplegia and/or ataxia precede the mental signs by days or weeks.

Wernicke's disease is usually associated with other manifestations of nutritional disease, both neurologic and nonneurologic. In more than 80 percent of patients, a *polyneuropathy* of varying degrees of severity is evident. Rarely, *amblyopia* or *spinal spastic ataxia* may be present. Many patients in the chronic stage demonstrate impaired olfactory discrimination, a defect that is most likely related to the diencephalic lesions (see below). Hypothermia may complicate acute Wernicke's disease.

Full-blown beriberi heart disease occurs only rarely in patients with Wernicke's disease, although indications of *disordered cardiovascular function* such as tachycardia, exertional dyspnea, postural hypotension, and minor electrocardiographic abnormalities are common. Occasionally, the patient dies suddenly, the mode of death suggesting "cardiovascular collapse." Wernicke's disease is characterized by a state of high cardiac output, which is out of proportion to the oxygen consumption. This is probably due to peripheral vasodilatation, which, in turn, may be related to thiamine deficiency. Postural hypotension and syncope are related to impaired function of the automatic nervous system, more specifically to a defect in sympathetic regulation.

Ancillary findings Vestibular function, as measured by the response to standard caloric testing, is always impaired bilaterally and more or less symmetrically in the acute stages of Wernicke's disease (*vestibular paresis*). The cerebrospinal fluid (CSF) is normal or shows only a modest elevation of protein content; protein values above 1.0 g/L (100 mg/dL) or a pleocytosis should always suggest the presence of a complicating illness. In untreated cases of Wernicke's disease, there is invariably an elevation of the *blood pyruvate* and a marked reduction in the *blood transketolase* (a thiamine-dependent enzyme of the hexose monophosphate shunt). Diffuse slowing of the EEG, mild to moderate in degree, occurs in about one-half of patients. On the other hand, total cerebral blood flow and cerebral oxygen and glucose consumption may be greatly reduced in the acute stages and persist for several weeks after the institution of treatment.

Course of the illness Death occurs in 15 to 20 percent of hospitalized patients and is usually due to hepatic failure or to a complicating infection (pneumonia, pulmonary tuberculosis, and septicemia being the most common).

Patients who recover do so in a characteristic manner. Ocular palsies may *begin to improve* within hours after the administration of thiamine and practically always within several days. Failure to respond in this manner raises doubts about the diagnosis of Wernicke's disease. Sixth nerve palsies, ptosis, and vertical gaze palsies recover completely, within a week or two in most cases, but vertical gaze–evoked nystagmus may persist for months. Horizontal gaze palsies recover completely as a rule, but a fine horizontal gaze–evoked nystagmus often remains as a permanent sequela of the disease.

Ataxia improves somewhat more slowly than the ocular motor abnormalities. Approximately half the patients recover incompletely and are left with a slow, shuffling, wide-based gait and an inability to walk tandem. The residual gait disturbance and horizontal nystagmus provide a means of identifying obscure and chronic cases of dementia as alcoholic-nutritional in origin. Vestibular function, as measured by caloric testing, improves at about the same rate as the ataxia of stance and gait, i.e., over a period of weeks or months, and recovery is usually but not always complete.

The symptoms of apathy, drowsiness, and confusion recede gradually, and as they do, the *defect in retentive memory and learning* stands out more clearly (*Korsakoff's psychosis*; see Chap. 25). It needs to be emphasized that Wernicke's disease and Korsakoff's psychosis are not separate diseases, but that the changing ocular and ataxic signs and the transformation of the global confusion state into an amnesic syndrome are successive stages in the recovery of a single disease process. Stated in another way, Korsakoff's psychosis is the psychic component of Wernicke's disease. Hence the symptom complex should be called *Wernicke's disease* when the amnesic state is not evident and the *Wernicke-Korsakoff syndrome* when both the ocular-ataxic and amnesic symptoms are present.

The outcome of the Korsakoff amnesic state varies. Complete or almost complete recovery occurs in less than 20 percent of patients. In the remainder, recovery is slow and incomplete. Depending on the severity of the residual symptoms, the patient may or may not be able to lead a supervised existence out of a hospital. The residual mental state is characterized by large gaps in memory, usually without

confabulation, and an inability of the patient to sort out events in their proper temporal sequence. This late stage of the disease, when the ocular and ataxic signs have receded or are not recognized, is often loosely referred to as "alcoholic deteriorated state" or "alcoholic dementia."

Pathologic findings In patients who die in the acute stages of Wernicke-Korsakoff disease there are symmetrically placed lesions in the paraventricular regions of the thalamus and hypothalamus, the mammillary bodies, periaqueductal region of the midbrain, floor of the fourth ventricle, and anterosuperior folia of the cerebellum, particularly of the vermis. Lesions are invariably found in the mammillary bodies and less consistently in the other areas. Microscopically, the principal change consists of varying degrees of necrosis of parenchymal structures. Many nerve cells and fibers are destroyed; others remain intact and are seen against a background of reactive glial elements, both astrocytes and microgliocytes. The blood vessels are prominent, owing to adventitial and endothelial proliferation. Hemorrhagic lesions are present in a small proportion of cases and are usually of recent origin. The oculomotor and vestibular nuclei are regularly involved, but to a lesser degree.

Clinical-pathologic correlations The ocular motor signs are attributable to lesions in the brainstem affecting the abducens nuclei and eye movement centers in the pons and rostral midbrain (see Chap. 19). The lesions of the vestibular nuclei are probably responsible for the loss of caloric responses and the gross abnormality of equilibrium that characterize the initial stage of the disease. The lack of significant destruction of nerve cells in these lesions accounts for the rapid improvement in oculomotor and vestibular function.

The persistent ataxia of stance and gait is related to the loss of neurons in the superior vermis of the cerebellum; extension of the lesion into the anterior parts of the anterior lobes accounts for the ataxia of individual movements of the legs. These cerebellar lesions are indistinguishable from those of so-called *alcoholic cerebellar degeneration* (see below).

The amnesic defect is related to lesions in the diencephalon, more specifically to those in the medial dorsal nuclei of the thalami. Lesions in the mammillary bodies are probably not critical in respect to memory function since they are found in patients with Wernicke's disease who had shown no disorder of memory during life.

Etiology and pathogenesis The specific factor responsible for most, if not all, of the symptoms of the Wernicke-Korsakoff syndrome is a deficiency of thiamine. The marked sensitivity of the ocular abnormalities to the administration of thiamine accounts for their rapid abatement after the ingestion of a meal or two. The quality of prompt reversibility indicates that the ocular signs are due to a biochemical abnormality and not to irreversible structural changes. On the other hand, the slow and incomplete recovery of the memory defect suggests that this symptom is due to irreversible structural changes, presumably in the medial dorsal nuclei.

The mechanism whereby thiamine deficiency causes brain lesions is not fully understood. Thiamine is a cofactor for several enzymes, including transketolase, pyruvate dehydrogenase, and α-ketoglutarate dehydrogenase. Thiamine deficiency produces a diffuse decrease in cerebral glucose utilization, and lesions in thiamine-deficient experimental animals are diminished by antagonists that block N-methyl-D-aspartate–preferring glutamic acid receptors. This latter finding suggests that the neurotoxicity of thiamine deficiency may be mediated by excitotoxicity evoked by glutamic acid release (see also Chaps. 364 and 370).

The selective vulnerability of certain periventricular regions to a deficiency of thiamine also remains to be explained. McEntee and Mair have pointed out that the lesions lie in the monoamine-containing pathways and have presented evidence that 3-methoxy-4-hydroxyphenylglycol (MHPG), the primary brain metabolite of norepinephrine, is decreased in the CSF of alcoholic patients with Korsakoff's psychosis; moreover, the administration of clonidine, an alpha$_2$-adrenergic agonist, seemed to improve the memory disorder in these patients. These authors have theorized that damage to the ascending norepinephrine-containing neurons in the brainstem and diencephalon is the basis for the amnesia.

The topography of the lesions caused by thiamine deficiency has been studied in rhesus monkeys. Witt and Goldman-Rakic found that the severity and number of brain nuclei affected are related to the duration and number of bouts of thiamine deficiency.

Treatment of the Wernicke-Korsakoff syndrome Wernicke's disease represents a medical emergency, and its recognition demands the immediate administration of thiamine. A delay of a few hours may be crucial in determining whether the patient with ocular and ataxic signs will be prevented from developing an amnesic state and whether the patient with early Korsakoff changes will be restored to a state of mental competency. Although 2 to 3 mg of thiamine may modify the ocular signs, much larger doses are needed to replenish the thiamine stores—50 mg intravenously and 50 mg intramuscularly, the latter dose being repeated each day until the patient resumes a normal diet. The other B vitamins may be given by mouth in the dosages outlined in Chap. 77. If the patient cannot or will not eat, parenteral feeding and administration of B vitamins become necessary.

A particular danger attends the treatment of the severely depleted alcoholic patient with intravenous glucose solutions. Such infusions may exhaust the patient's reserve of B vitamins and either precipitate Wernicke's disease in a previously unaffected patient or cause a rapid worsening of an early form of the disease. For this reason, B vitamins must be administered to all alcoholic patients requiring parenteral glucose. The cardiovascular status of each patient should be monitored carefully. Since these patients are confused and forgetful, they must be supervised continually.

A special problem arises when the patient recovers from the acute phase of the illness and the amnesic psychosis becomes prominent. The disposition of the patient to family, nursing home, or mental institution should be made on the basis of the severity of the mental illness as well as the capacity of the family unit and social circumstances.

NUTRITIONAL POLYNEUROPATHY (See also Chaps. 77 and 383) In the United States, nutritional polyneuropathy is usually a disease of alcoholics. As mentioned above, it is present in most patients with the Wernicke-Korsakoff syndrome, but it often occurs as the sole manifestation of deficiency disease. The peripheral neuropathy of alcoholics ("alcoholic polyneuropathy") does not differ in any fundamental way from neuropathic beriberi. The clinical features of nutritional polyneuropathy and its identity with beriberi are discussed in Chaps. 77 and 383. A deficiency of thiamine chloride, pyridoxine, pantothenic acid, vitamin B_{12}, and perhaps folic acid has been demonstrated in individual cases to cause nutritional polyneuropathy. In the alcoholic patient it is usually not possible to incriminate a particular vitamin.

"ALCOHOLIC" CEREBELLAR DEGENERATION This is the term applied to a common, stereotyped, nonfamilial form of cerebellar ataxia that occurs on a background of prolonged ingestion of alcohol. Usually the symptoms evolve in subacute fashion, i.e., over several weeks or months, sometimes more rapidly. In some patients the symptoms are present in mild but stable form and worsen after an attack of pneumonia or delirium tremens.

The signs are those of cerebellar dysfunction, affecting stance and gait predominantly. The legs are involved more severely than the arms, and nystagmus and speech disturbances occur infrequently. Once established, the signs change very little, although some improvement of gait may follow the cessation of drinking, due probably to improvement in general nutrition and recovery from an associated polyneuropathy.

The pathologic changes consist of degeneration of varying severity of all the neurocellular elements of the cerebellar cortex, particularly of the Purkinje cells, with a striking topographic restriction to the anterior and superior aspects of the vermis and adjacent parts of the anterior lobes of the cerebellum. The disorder of stance and gait is related to the lesion in the vermis, and the ataxia of the limbs to the involvement of the anterior lobes. A similar clinical-pathologic

syndrome is observed occasionally in nutritionally depleted nonalcoholic patients.

CNS disorders in alcoholics not associated with vitamin deficiency Alcoholics are vulnerable to a number of CNS disorders that are attributable neither to nutritional deficiency nor to trauma. There appears to be an increased incidence of hypertension in alcoholics and probably of strokes, both ischemic infarction and spontaneous subarachnoid hemorrhage. Alcoholics as a group also show dilatation of the lateral ventricles and widening of sulci on CT scans or MRI. The nature of these changes is obscure. They do not correlate with mental abnormality, nor do they represent cerebral atrophy insofar as partial and sometimes complete reversal occur with sustained abstinence. Some believe that alcohol can cause intellectual deterioration separate from effects due to nutritional deficiency, but an entity of "alcoholic dementia" has never been established on the basis of clinical and neuropathologic studies. A syndrome of progressive myelopathy occurring in alcoholics also has been described. Such patients are said to show no evidence of nutritional deficiency (B_{12} or folic acid) or of liver disease. The nature of the spinal cord disease is unknown, and a causal relationship to the toxic effects of alcohol remains to be established.

PELLAGRA This disease is described in Chap. 77. Neurologic manifestations are quite diverse. Pellagra is essentially an encephalopathy, although involvement of the spinal cord and peripheral nerves may occur. The early mental symptoms—insomnia, fatigue, anxiety, nervousness, irritability, and depression—may be mistaken for a psychiatric disorder. However, as the disease advances, slowing and inefficiency of mental processes and impairment of memory become apparent. Pellagra may not only cause psychiatric manifestations but occasionally also may result from them because certain mental illnesses, including alcoholism, cause anorexia and dietary deficiency.

The spinal cord involvement in pellagra has not been clearly delineated, perhaps because the mental state of the patients has precluded accurate testing. In general, there is both posterior and lateral column involvement, predominantly the former. Neuropathic signs are difficult to distinguish from other types of nutritional polyneuropathy. Other manifestations such as tremor, extrapyramidal rigidity, suck and grasp reflexes, and coma (referred to in the past as "nicotinic acid–deficiency encephalopathy") have been included in the pellagra syndrome on uncertain grounds, as have various disorders of the special senses.

A *spastic spinal syndrome*, apart from the other symptoms and signs of pellagra, may be a rare manifestation of nutritional deficiency. The chief signs are spastic weakness of the legs with absent abdominal and increased tendon reflexes, clonus, and extensor plantar responses. These signs are usually accompanied by other manifestations of nutritional deficiency, such as Wernicke's disease, amblyopia, and peripheral neuropathy.

Pathologic features The distinctive neuropathologic changes in pellagra are most readily discerned in the large Betz cells of the motor cortex, although the same changes are seen to a lesser extent in the smaller pyramidal cells of the cerebral cortex and cells of the basal ganglia, cranial motor and dentate nuclei, and anterior horns of the spinal cord. The affected cells appear swollen and rounded with eccentric nuclei and loss of Nissl staining. This *central neuritis of pellagra*, as it is called, probably represents a primary affection of the motor cell and not a reaction to interruption of the corticospinal tracts. The spinal cord lesions take the form of a symmetric degeneration of the dorsal columns, especially the fasciculus gracilis, and to a lesser extent of the corticospinal tracts. The posterior column degeneration is probably secondary to degeneration of specific dorsal root ganglion cells.

DEFICIENCY AMBLYOPIA (NUTRITIONAL OPTIC NEUROPATHY, "TOBACCO-ALCOHOL AMBLYOPIA") These terms refer to a characteristic form of visual impairment that complicates nutritional deficiency. The lesion responsible for the visual loss lies in the optic nerve, more or less confined to the zone of the papillomacular bundle; the cornea and other parts of the refractive mechanism are uninvolved.

The main symptoms are dimness or blurring of vision for near and distant objects and impairment of color vision, which worsens progressively and insidiously for several days or weeks. In addition to a reduction in visual acuity, examination discloses the presence of bilateral and roughly symmetric central or centrocecal scotomas, which are larger for colored than for white test objects. Pallor of the temporal portion of the optic disc is observed in some cases. Untreated, this condition progresses to irreversible optic atrophy.

Deficiency amblyopia was common among prisoners of war in the Far East. Although this form of amblyopia had previously been described in association with beriberi (due to thiamine deficiency) and pellagra (due to niacin deficiency), the peak incidence among prisoners coincided with neither of these syndromes but with the syndrome of orogenital dermatitis and "burning feet" (Strachan's syndrome, see below).

In the United States, most, if not all, of the cases of retrobulbar neuropathy attributed to the toxic effects of alcohol or tobacco— so-called tobacco-alcohol amblyopia—are of nutritional origin. Optic neuropathy may occur as the only manifestation of vitamin deficiency, but often it is combined with other evidence of nutritional deficiency, such as peripheral neuropathy and the Wernicke-Korsakoff syndrome.

Although the nutritional origin of this type of amblyopia has been established, a specific vitamin deficiency can rarely be identified. Observations in both humans and experimental animals indicate that a deficiency of thiamine (vitamin B_1), vitamin B_{12}, or perhaps riboflavin may cause lesions in the optic nerves. The notion that cyanide or other substances in tobacco smoke have a toxic effect on the optic nerves is not supported by experimental data.

Treatment consists of the administration of a balanced diet, supplemented with B vitamins, and the interdiction of alcohol where this is the cause of nutritional deficiency.

SYNDROME OF AMBLYOPIA, PAINFUL NEUROPATHY, AND OROGENITAL DERMATITIS (STRACHAN'S SYNDROME)

This is a neurologic syndrome that is probably nutritional in origin but which does not fit readily within the boundaries of beriberi or pellagra. Strachan attributed the disorder to malaria. Originally known as "Jamaican neuritis," the syndrome occurs among the undernourished populations of many tropical countries. Large numbers of patients with this syndrome also were observed in the besieged population of Madrid during the Spanish Civil War and among prisoners of war during World War II in the Middle and Far East. In the United States, this syndrome is observed occasionally in alcoholic patients.

Strachan's syndrome is essentially a disorder of the peripheral and optic nerves. The peripheral nerve disorder results in sensory symptoms and signs (painful paresthesias of the feet, loss of superficial and deep sensation, and ataxia); foot drop and muscle weakness occur rarely. Failing vision, which may go on to complete blindness and pallor of the optic discs, may also occur. Deafness and vertigo are rare; in these respects the syndrome differs from beriberi. Along with the neurologic signs there may be an *orogenital syndrome* consisting of stomatoglossitis, corneal degeneration, and genital dermatitis.

The few pathologic studies of this syndrome show damage to the papillomacular bundle in the optic nerve, and a loss of myelinated fibers in the posterior columns (fasciculus gracilis) of the spinal cord, the latter indicating degeneration of the central processes of the large bipolar sensory neurons of the lumbosacral spinal ganglia. Degeneration of the peripheral processes of small sensory neurons probably accounts for the loss of pain and temperature sensation.

SUBACUTE COMBINED DEGENERATION (SCD) OF THE SPINAL CORD

(See also Chap. 77) This term designates the spinal cord disease that is due to vitamin B_{12} deficiency. The white matter of the brain, optic nerves, and peripheral nerves also may be affected but far less often than the spinal cord. The neurologic and hematologic manifestations (pernicious anemia) of vitamin B_{12} deficiency are distinctive insofar as they are caused not by a lack of this vitamin in the food but by an inability to transfer minute amounts of this nutrient across the intestinal mucosa. Such a nutritional disorder is referred to as a *conditioned deficiency*, since it depends on the lack of an intrinsic factor in the gastric secretions (see Chap. 304). Rarely, neurologic symptoms due to vitamin B_{12} deficiency occur in patients with disease of the distal small intestine (Crohn's disease, lymphoma) or after surgical resection.

Clinical manifestations   Neurologic symptoms are present in the majority of patients with vitamin B_{12} deficiency. The patient first notices general weakness and paresthesias, consisting of tingling, "pins-and-needles" feelings, or other vaguely described sensations in the distal parts of the limbs; either the lower or the upper extremities may be involved first. The paresthesias tend to be persistent, to progress steadily, and to be the source of much distress. As the illness progresses, the gait becomes unsteady, and movements of the limbs, especially the legs, become stiff and awkward.

Early in the course of the illness, when only paresthesias are present, there may be no objective signs. Later, the neurologic examination discloses a disorder of the posterior and lateral columns of the spinal cord, predominantly the former. Loss of vibration sense, the most consistent sign, is more pronounced in the legs than in the arms, and frequently it extends over the trunk. Position sense is involved to a somewhat lesser extent. The motor defects are usually limited to the legs and include weakness, spasticity, changes in the tendon reflexes, clonus, and extensor plantar responses. At first the patellar and Achilles reflexes may be diminished, increased, or absent. With treatment, the reflexes may return to normal or become hyperactive. The gait at first is predominantly ataxic, later ataxic and spastic. If the disease remains untreated, an ataxic paraplegia with variable degrees of spasticity and contracture develops.

A loss of superficial sensation below a segmental level on the trunk, implicating the spinothalamic tracts, occurs rarely, but such a finding should always suggest the possibility of some other disease of the spinal cord. More often the sensory defect takes the form of a blunting of tactile, painful, and thermal sensation over the distal segments of the lower limbs, implicating the peripheral nerves, but such findings are uncommon.

The nervous system involvement in vitamin B_{12} deficiency is characteristically, though not perfectly, symmetric. A definite asymmetry of motor or sensory findings, maintained over a period of weeks or months, should always cast doubt on the diagnosis.

Mental signs are frequent, ranging from irritability, apathy, somnolence, suspiciousness, and emotional instability to a marked confusional or depressive psychosis, or even to intellectual deterioration. Optic neuropathy with impaired acuity and cecocentral scotomas has been reported with all forms of vitamin B_{12} deficiency; variable improvement in acuity occurs once systemic vitamin B_{12} is administered. Dementia and amblyopia are relatively uncommon manifestations of vitamin B_{12} deficiency, but each may occasionally be the initial manifestation of the disease.

Pathology and pathogenesis   The pathologic process takes the form of a diffuse, though uneven, degeneration of the white matter of the spinal cord and sometimes of the brain. At first there is swelling of myelin sheaths, characterized by separation of the myelin lamellae and formation of intramyelinic vacuoles. This is followed by a coalescence of small foci of tissue destruction into larger ones, giving the tissue a vacuolated appearance. The myelin sheaths and the axis cylinders are both affected, the former perhaps earlier and to a greater extent than the latter. Astrocytic gliosis is minimal in the early lesions, but in the more chronic ones gliosis is pronounced. The changes begin in the posterior columns of the lower cervical and upper thoracic cord and spread from this region up and down the cord, as well as forward into the lateral columns. The lesions are not limited to specific systems of fibers within the posterior and lateral funiculi but are scattered irregularly through the white matter. The changes in the optic nerves are similar to those in other types of nutritional neuropathy, i.e., a bilateral degeneration of myelinated fibers in the territory of the papillomacular bundles.

The *pathogenesis* of the nervous system lesions in vitamin B_{12} deficiency is not fully known. Impairment of DNA synthesis probably accounts for the hematologic abnormalities and the production of megaloblasts; however, since neurons do not divide, this mechanism cannot be invoked to explain the central nervous system changes. One of the better-understood functions of vitamin B_{12} is its role as a coenzyme in the methylmalonyl CoA mutase reaction. Impairment of this metabolic step may lead to the production of abnormal fatty acids, which are important building blocks of cell membranes and of myelin. However, Carmel and his colleagues have described a hereditary form of cobalamin deficiency, in which methylmalonyl CoA mutase activity was normal despite the presence of typical neurologic abnormalities. These authors attributed the neurologic abnormalities to an impairment of methionine synthase activity. These and other hypotheses have been reviewed by Beck.

Diagnosis and treatment The chief obstacle to early diagnosis is the lack of parallelism between the hematologic and neurologic signs. This is particularly true of patients who have received folic acid, which serves to maintain a hematologic remission for an indefinite period while the neurologic signs worsen, often to an irreversible stage. Under these circumstances the most reliable diagnostic procedures are the measurement of the serum B_{12} concentration and the two-stage Schilling test (see Chap. 304). In rare instances, even these tests may be inconclusive, in which case the finding of high serum concentrations of cobalamin metabolites—methylmalonic acid and homocysteine—may be diagnostically useful.

The treatment of the neurologic manifestations of vitamin B_{12} deficiency differs in no way from the treatment of the hematologic ones. Patients whose vitamin B_{12} stores have been depleted require large doses of cobalamin—1000 μg intramuscularly each day during hospitalization, then weekly for a month, and then monthly for the remainder of the patient's life.

The most important factor influencing the *response to treatment* is the duration of the neurologic symptoms. Recovery may be complete if therapy is instituted within a few weeks of their onset. For this reason, SCD and the other neurologic complications of vitamin B_{12} deficiency represent medical emergencies. If symptoms have been present for longer than a month or two, only partial recovery can be expected, and in long-standing cases the best that can be expected is the arrest of progression of the disease.

FOLIC ACID DEFICIENCY Despite the frequent occurrence of folic acid deficiency, its role in the pathogenesis of nervous system disease has not been established beyond doubt. The polyneuropathies that occasionally complicate sprue and other malabsorption syndromes and the chronic administration of phenytoin have been attributed, on uncertain grounds, to folate deficiency. With respect to folate deficiency and spinal cord disease, the data are equally limited. Cases have been described in which the neurologic signs of subacute combined degeneration were attributed to folic acid deficiency (see Pincus). In these cases there was no evidence of vitamin B_{12} deficiency, but there was a resolution of both the hematologic and neurologic abnormalities after the institution of folate therapy.

VITAMIN E DEFICIENCY A rare neurologic disorder of childhood, consisting essentially of a spinocerebellar degeneration in association with a polyneuropathy and pigmentary retinopathy, has been related to vitamin E deficiency developing after prolonged intestinal malabsorption (Satya-Murti et al.; Sokol et al.). The same mechanism has been proposed to explain the neurologic disorders that sometimes complicate abetalipoproteinemia, fibrocystic disease, and extensive intestinal resections (Harding et al.). Vitamin E deficiency also occurs in young children with chronic cholestatic hepatobiliary disease. Ataxia, loss of tendon reflexes, ophthalmoparesis, proximal muscle weakness with elevated serum creatine phosphokinase, and decreased sensation are the usual manifestations. These symptoms are referable to parts of the nervous system and musculature known to be involved in animals deprived of vitamin E—degeneration of Clarke's columns, spinocerebellar tracts, posterior columns, nuclei of Goll and Burdach, and sensory roots (Nelson et al.). In affected children, neurologic function improves after the long-term correction of vitamin E deficiency.

NEUROLOGIC SYNDROMES CAUSED BY HYPERVITAMINOSIS Acute toxicity with vitamin A causes symptoms of headache, dizziness, irritability, and drowsiness. Chronic hypervitaminosis A can give rise to chronic increased intracranial pressure or pseudotumor cerebri (see Chap. 77).

The ingestion of pyridoxine in excessive amounts (2 g or more daily) can cause a sensory neuropathy characterized clinically by progressive ataxia, impairment of position and vibration sense, and loss of deep tendon reflexes. Motor function is preserved. The syndrome is reversible with discontinuation of pyridoxine.

ACQUIRED (SECONDARY) METABOLIC DISEASES OF THE NERVOUS SYSTEM

In this important category of neurologic disease, disturbance of cerebral function is due to disease in some other organ system—heart (and circulation), lungs (and respiration), kidneys, liver, endocrine glands, and possibly pancreas. Each of these diseases affects the nervous system in somewhat different ways.

ANOXIC-ISCHEMIC ENCEPHALOPATHY This common and often disastrous condition is caused by a lack of oxygen to the brain, resulting from hypotension or respiratory failure. Sometimes both are responsible, and one cannot say which predominates—hence the ambiguous reference, in clinical records, to "cardiorespiratory failure." The conditions that most often lead to anoxic-ischemic encephalopathy are (1) myocardial infarction; (2) cardiac arrest; (3) hemorrhage, with shock and circulatory collapse; in these situations vascular supply to the brain is compromised before respiration; (4) shock; (5) suffocation (from drowning, strangulation, aspiration of vomitus or blood, compression of the trachea by hemorrhage or a surgical pack, or a foreign body in the trachea); (6) diseases that paralyze the muscles of respiration or compromise the CNS respiratory drive (trauma, vascular disease of the brain, epilepsy), causing respiratory failure followed by cardiac failure; and (7) carbon monoxide (CO) poisoning. In circumstances (4) through (7) respiration fails first and then cardiovascular functions. Hypoxia alone may induce different clinicopathologic consequences than a combination of hypoxia and hypoperfusion (ischemia).

Clinical manifestations Mild degrees of hypoxia cause inattentiveness, impaired judgment, and motor incoordination but have no lasting effects. With severe hypoxia or anoxia, as occurs with cardiac arrest, consciousness is lost within seconds, but recovery will be complete if breathing, oxygenation of blood, and cardiac action are restored within 3 to 5 min. If anoxia persists beyond this time, there is serious and permanent injury to the brain, particularly to those parts in which the efficiency of circulation is marginal (globus pallidus, cerebellum, hippocampus, and the "borderzone regions" of the parietooccipital lobes). Clinically, it is difficult to judge the precise degree of hypoxia-ischemia, since slight heart action or an imperceptible blood pressure may serve to maintain the circulation to some extent. Hence some individuals have made an excellent recovery after cerebral anoxia that allegedly lasted 8 to 10 min or longer. *An important clinical rule is that degrees of hypoxia that at no time abolish consciousness rarely if ever cause permanent damage to the nervous system.* P_{O_2} as low as 2.7 kPa (20 mmHg) is well tolerated if it develops gradually and blood pressure is normal. Also, subjects who demonstrate intact brainstem function (as indicated by normal ciliospinal, oculovestibular, and pupillary light responses and intact doll's-head eye movements) usually have a better outlook for recovery of consciousness and perhaps all their faculties. Conversely, absence of these reflexes and the presence of pupils that are persistently fixed to light indicate a grave prognosis.

Extreme or sustained global ischemia causes brain death (see Chap. 26). Immediately after resuscitation from cardiorespiratory arrest, the physical findings may suggest brain death (dilated, unresponsive pupils, absent brainstem reflexes and respiration, and isoelectric EEG), yet full recovery may occur. However, persistence of the unresponsive state for more than an hour or two invariably carries a poor prognosis. The diagnosis of brain death must be made with caution because anesthesia, drug intoxication, and hypothermia also may cause deep coma, absent brainstem reflexes, and an isoelectric EEG but permit recovery. The problem of brain death is being constantly brought to public attention because of ethical and moral issues that surround the question of discontinuing supportive medical therapy.

Issues of management are most difficult in the patient who has suffered severe anoxic encephalopathy, but one that falls short of causing "brain death." Often breathing and heart action have stabilized by the time the patient is seen by a physician. Neurologic evaluation shows the patient to be profoundly comatose, with eyes slightly divergent and motionless but with reactive pupils, flaccid or intensely rigid limbs, and diminished tendon reflexes. Within a few minutes after cardiac action and breathing have been restored, generalized convulsions and isolated or grouped twitches of muscles (myoclonus) may supervene. Decerebrate or decorticate postures may be present or can be brought out by pinching the limbs, and bilateral Babinski signs can be evoked. Death may occur in the first 24 to 48 h, in a setting of rising temperature, deepening coma, and circulatory collapse. Or, with somewhat lesser degrees of injury, in which the cerebral and cerebellar cortices are partly or completely destroyed but brainstem-spinal structures remain intact, the individual may survive in a state referred to as "irreversible coma" or "persistent vegetative state" (see Chap. 26). The latter patients remain mute, unresponsive, and unaware of their environment for weeks, months, or even years. Criteria that accurately predict the outcome of anoxic encephalopathy early in the comatose period have been developed (see Chap. 26). If intoxication can be excluded, the presence of fixed dilated pupils and paralysis of eye movement for 24 to 48 h, along with marked slowing of the EEG, usually signifies irreversible cerebral damage. Deep coma of this type, lasting more than a few days, is rarely attended by full recovery.

Patients with lesser degrees of injury improve after a period of coma. Consciousness is regained, and then varying degrees of confusion, visual agnosia, extrapyramidal rigidity, or movement disorder (action or intention myoclonus, choreoathetosis, cerebellar ataxia) become manifest. Some of these patients pass quickly through this posthypoxic phase and proceed to make full recovery; others are left with permanent neurologic sequelae. The *posthypoxic syndromes* observed most frequently are (1) *persistent coma or stupor*, and, with lesser degrees of cerebral injury, (2) *dementia*, with or without extrapyramidal signs, (3) *visual agnosia*, (4) *parkinsonism*, (5) *choreoathetosis*, (6) *cerebellar ataxia*, (7) *intention or action myoclonus*, and (8) the *Korsakoff amnesic state*. *Seizures* may continue to be a problem but are uncommon.

A relatively uncommon and unexplained phenomenon is *delayed postanoxic encephalopathy*. Initial improvement, which appears to be complete, is followed after a variable period of time (several days to a week or longer) by a relapse, characterized by apathy, confusion, irritability, and occasionally agitation or mania. A few patients have recovered from this second episode, but in most the neurologic syndrome is a progressive one, with shuffling gait, diffuse rigidity and spasticity, coma, and death after 1 to 2 weeks. Postmortem examination of these patients has shown the major abnormality to be widespread cerebral demyelination. Even more rare is a syndrome in which a period of hypoxia is followed by a slow, deteriorating state, affecting basal ganglia more than cerebral cortex and white matter and progressing for weeks to months until the patient is mute, rigid, and helpless.

The essential *mechanism* in hypoxic encephalopathy is a neuronal lack of oxygen and an arrest of all aerobic metabolic processes necessary to sustain the Krebs tricarboxylic cycle and the electron transport system. Lactic acid accumulates in the tissues. The pathophysiology of delayed progression is not understood. Recent experimental observations suggest that excitatory neurotransmitters, and particularly glutamate, released from hypoxic-ischemic brain tissue

are instrumental in the rapid destruction of neurons (see Choi and Rothman). The restoration of oxygen to the ischemic brain, e.g., following cardiac arrest, may result in reperfusion injury probably related to the effects of oxygen-derived free radicals upon membrane phospholipids.

Diagnosis The diagnosis depends on the history of a hypoxic-ischemic event and evidence of (1) reduced oxygenation of arterial blood [$P_{O_2} < 5.3$ kPa (40 mmHg)], (2) CO intoxication (indicated by its spectroscopic band or cherry red color of the skin for a few minutes to hours after the episode), (3) blood pressures below 9.3 kPa (70 mmHg) systolic, or (4) cardiac arrest. The typical clinical sequence of events after a possible hypoxic-ischemic episode has terminated as outlined above, confirm the diagnosis. Renal damage (anuria) and myocardial infarction also may have occurred and provide corroborative evidence of the hypoxic-ischemic event.

Treatment The treatment of anoxic encephalopathy is directed mainly at the prevention of a critical degree of hypoxic injury. After a clear airway is secured, artificial respiration, external thoracic cardiac massage, the use of a cardiac defibrillator or pacemaker, and open chest surgery all have their place, and every second counts in their prompt utilization. Once cardiac and pulmonary function are restored, there is no evidence that any pharmacologic measure enhances recovery. Barbiturates, glucocorticoids, dimethyl sulfoxide, and benzodiazepines have been given without clear proof of benefit. A small proportion of patients develop diffuse brain swelling after cardiac arrest; this condition is more common in children. This is evidenced by compression of the lateral ventricles and cisterns on CT scan or by very high lumbar CSF pressure. Seizures should be controlled by anticonvulsants. Posthypoxic myoclonus may respond to oral administration of clonazepam 1.5 to 10 mg/d. Other details of treatment are considered in Chap. 26.

HYPERCAPNIC ENCEPHALOPATHY Chronic emphysema and fibrosing lung disease and, in rare instances, an inadequacy of central respiratory drive lead to chronic respiratory acidosis, with an elevation of P_{CO_2} and a reduction in arterial P_{O_2}. Secondary polycythemia and cor pulmonale are common sequelae of these pulmonary diseases.

Clinical manifestations The clinical syndrome consequent on hypercapnia (and hypoxia) consists of generalized or bilateral frontal or occipital headache, often intense and persistent for hours; papilledema; mental dullness, drowsiness, confusion, stupor, and coma; a fast-frequency action tremor and coarse twitching of all the muscles, which are in a state of sustained contraction; and an inability to maintain a fixed posture or interruption of a voluntary movement because of brief lapses of sustained muscle contraction (asterixis). Intermittent drowsiness, indifference and inattention to the environment, reduction of psychomotor activity, imperception of the sequence of events, and forgetfulness constitute the more subtle manifestations of this syndrome.

In fully developed cases, the CSF is under increased pressure, P_{CO_2} may exceed 10 kPa (75 mmHg), and oxygen saturation of the arterial blood ranges from 85 to 40 percent. The EEG reveals slow activity in the delta and theta range, sometimes bilaterally synchronous. The cerebral disorder is said to be due to CO_2 narcosis, but the biochemical mechanism is not known. The danger of administering morphine or sedatives, which blunt the respiratory drive (already depressed by the CO_2 retention), or inhaled O_2, which removes the sole stimulus (low P_{O_2}) to the respiratory center, is now widely recognized.

Treatment Forced ventilation with an intermittent positive-pressure respirator, treatment of heart failure with digitalis and diuretics, venesection to reduce the viscosity of the blood, and antibiotics to combat pulmonary infection are the most effective therapeutic measures. If stupor or coma persists, the arterial O_2 level should be rechecked; it may be critically reduced, and it needs to be raised by controlled O_2 administration to a point [6.7 to 7.3 kPa (50 to 55 mmHg)] where consciousness is improved but the stimulus to respiratory drive is not removed. Also, the pH of the CSF may be very low, in the range of 7.15 to 7.25. In CO_2 narcosis, correction of the acidosis of blood is easier than that of CSF, which tends to lag. The management of respiratory failure is discussed in detail in Chap. 223.

Differential diagnosis   Unlike pure hypoxic encephalopathy, hypercapnia rarely causes prolonged coma and is not a cause of irreversible brain damage. Papilledema and asterixis are important diagnostic features. (Asterixis is also characteristic of liver failure and uremia, and occasionally it is observed in other metabolic disorders.) The syndrome of hypercapnia is apt to be mistaken for brain tumor, a confusional psychosis of nondescript type, or a chronic extrapyramidal syndrome causing myoclonus or chorea.

HYPOGLYCEMIC ENCEPHALOPATHY (See also Chaps. 337 and 338)   This condition is an important cause of episodic confusion, convulsions, coma, and sometimes of hemiparesis and other focal neurologic signs. The essential biochemical abnormality is a critical lowering of the blood glucose concentration to usually less than 1.4 mmol/L (25 mg/dL) (lower in infants), which, if it lasts for many minutes, leads to exhaustion of the cerebral glucose reserve. As cerebral oxidation proceeds without exogenous glucose, the lipid and protein components of neurons are metabolized, and irreversible damage occurs. The severely hypoglycemic patient becomes deeply comatose before permanent damage occurs; consequently, prompt treatment is important.

Etiology   The most common causes of hypoglycemic encephalopathy are (1) accidental or deliberate overdose of insulin or an oral antidiabetic agent, (2) insulin-secreting islet cell tumor or retroperitoneal sarcoma, (3) rare cases of protracted ethanol intoxication, (4) acute, nonicteric hepatic encephalopathy of childhood (Reye's syndrome), and (5) an idiopathic syndrome occurring in the neonatal period. Hypoglycemic encephalopathy was a frequent complication of "insulin shock" therapy of schizophrenia, a form of treatment fortunately no longer used.

Clinical manifestations   As the concentration of blood glucose decreases to about 1.7 mmol/L (30 mg/dL), the initial symptoms (reflecting norepinephrine release) appear—nervousness, hunger, flushed facies, headache, palpitation, anxiety, sweating, and trembling—and these gradually or rapidly give way to signs of cerebral glucopenia, i.e., confusion, drowsiness, focal neurologic signs, and occasionally excitement or overactivity. In the next stage, forced sucking, grasping, motor restlessness, muscular spasms, and finally decerebrate rigidity occur, in that sequence; myoclonic twitching and convulsions frequently develop in this stage. Blood levels of approximately 0.6 mmol/L (10 mg/dL) are associated with deep coma, dilatation of the pupils, pallor, shallow respirations, bradycardia, and hypotonicity of limb musculature—the so-called medullary phase of hypoglycemia. If glucose is administered before the medullary phase is reached, the patient is restored to normal within a few minutes, retracing the aforementioned steps in reverse order. Once the medullary phase appears, and particularly if it persists for a time before the hypoglycemia is corrected, neurologic recovery is delayed for a period of days or weeks and may be incomplete.

A huge dose of insulin that produces severe hypoglycemia, even of relatively brief duration (30 to 60 min), is more dangerous than a series of less severe hypoglycemic episodes from smaller doses of insulin, presumably because the counterregulation mechanisms are likely to be less effective in the former situation. Massive amounts of glucose may have to be infused in order to maintain plasma glucose levels in the normal range (see Chap. 338).

Pathology   The major *neuropathologic effect* is on the cerebral cortex; nerve cells degenerate and are replaced by microgliocytes and astrocytes. The distribution of lesions is similar though not identical to that in hypoxic encephalopathy (the cerebellar cortex is relatively spared in hypoglycemic encephalopathy). The neurologic sequelae of the two disorders are also much alike.

Episodes of chronic hypoglycemia may give rise to two other syndromes, both relatively uncommon. One, termed *subacute hypoglycemia*, is characterized by drowsiness and lethargy, diminution in psychomotor activity, deterioration of social behavior, and confusion.

Oral or intravenous glucose immediately alleviates the symptoms. In the other, *more chronic syndrome*, there is gradual deterioration of intellectual function, raising the question of a presenile dementia, and in some reported instances there have been tremor, chorea, rigidity, cerebellar ataxia, and rarely signs of lower motor neuron involvement ("hypoglycemic amyotrophy"). These subacute and chronic forms of hypoglycemia have been observed with islet cell hyperplasia or tumor, as well as with carcinoma of the stomach, fibrous mesothelioma, carcinoma of the cecum, and hepatoma.

Differential diagnosis   The major clinical differences between hypoglycemia and hypoxia reflect the clinical setting and mode of evolution of the neurologic disorder. With hypoglycemia, the disturbance of cerebral function evolves more slowly than with hypoxia, over a period of 30 to 60 min rather than in a few seconds or minutes. The recovery phase and sequelae of the two conditions are much the same. *Recurrent hypoglycemia*, as occurs with an islet cell tumor, may masquerade for some time as an episodic confusional psychosis or seizure disorder, and diagnosis awaits a period of demonstrably low blood glucose or hyperinsulinism (see Chap. 338).

Correction of the hypoglycemia at the earliest moment is the obvious therapy. It is not known whether hypothermia or other measures will increase the safety period of hypoglycemia or alter the outcome.

HYPERGLYCEMIC COMA   Two coma-producing hyperglycemic syndromes occur, mainly in the diabetic: (1) hyperglycemia with ketoacidosis and (2) hyperosmolar nonketotic hyperglycemia. These are described in Chap. 337.

HEPATIC ENCEPHALOPATHY   Chronic hepatic insufficiency with portacaval shunting of blood is often punctuated by episodes of stupor, coma, and other neurologic symptoms, a state referred to as *hepatic coma* or *portal-systemic encephalopathy*. Also, hereditary hyperammonemic syndromes of infancy may lead to episodic coma with or without seizures. A special type of nonicteric hepatic encephalopathy (Reye's syndrome) occurs in children, presenting as acute brain swelling, in conjunction with rapid enlargement of the liver, fine droplets of fat in hepatocytes, high serum aspartate aminotransferase (AST, SGOT) and other liver enzymes, and very high levels of serum ammonia (see Chap. 270).

Clinical features   The central feature of hepatic encephalopathy in the adult is a derangement of consciousness, presenting first as mental confusion with increased or decreased psychomotor activity, followed by progressive drowsiness, stupor, and coma. Severe brain edema, which can be visualized by MRI, occurs commonly. The confusional state before coma intervenes is frequently combined with characteristic lapses of sustained muscle contraction (asterixis). The EEG becomes abnormal during the earliest stages of the confusional state. Paroxysms of bilaterally synchronous delta waves, characteristically triphasic and prominent in the frontal regions, are at first interspersed with alpha activity and later, as the coma deepens, displace all normal activity. A variable, fluctuating rigidity of the trunk and limbs, grimacing, suck and grasp reflexes, exaggeration or asymmetry of tendon reflexes, Babinski signs, and focal or generalized seizures round out the clinical picture. An elevated CSF glutamine level is found in most patients with severe hepatic encephalopathy, reflecting its synthesis by astrocytes in response to elevated plasma ammonia levels.

The syndrome usually evolves subacutely, over a period of days to weeks, and often terminates fatally. At times it does not advance beyond the stage of drowsiness and confusion with asterixis and EEG changes. This relatively mild form needs to be differentiated from other forms of acute confusional psychosis and delirium. If the metabolic disorder persists for months and years, a mild dementia and a persistent disorder of posture and movement may gradually appear (grimacing, tremor, dysarthria, ataxia of gait, choreoathetosis), and the condition must then be distinguished from other dementing and extrapyramidal syndromes (see later). Hepatic coma is rapidly reversed following successful hepatic transplantation.

Pathology and pathogenesis The striking *neuropathologic finding* in patients who die in a state of hepatic coma is a diffuse increase in the number and size of the protoplasmic astrocytes (Alzheimer type II astrocytes) in the deep layers of the cerebral cortex and in the lenticular nuclei, with little or no alteration in the nerve cells or other parenchymal elements. Brain edema is seen as well, often sufficient to cause cerebellar herniation.

The *pathogenesis* of hepatic encephalopathy is not fully understood. The most plausible theory relates it to an abnormality of nitrogen metabolism, wherein ammonia and/or other amines, which are formed in the bowel by the action of urease-containing organisms on dietary protein and are carried in the portal circulation to the liver, fail to be converted into urea, either because of hepatocellular disease or portal-systemic shunting of blood, or both. As a result, these substances reach the systemic circulation, where they interfere with cerebral metabolism in some obscure way. Other theories of causation have been discussed in Chap. 268 and have been reviewed in detail by Zieve, by Cooper and Plum, and by Butterworth and his colleagues.

Treatment Despite an incomplete understanding of the genesis of hepatic coma, the most effective means of treating this disorder consists of restriction of dietary protein, mechanical cleansing of the colon, oral administration of antibiotics that suppress or eliminate urease-producing organisms in the bowel, and the use of lactulose, an inert sugar that acidifies the colonic contents. Liver transplantation has proved highly efficacious in some patients. Additional methods of treatment, the practicality of which remain to be established, are discussed in Chap. 268.

In *acute fulminant hepatitis*, delirious, confusional, and comatose states also occur, but their mechanisms are not understood. Blood ammonia levels are usually elevated but of unclear significance because of other associated metabolic abnormalities.

CHRONIC HEPATIC ENCEPHALOPATHY (ACQUIRED HEPATO-CEREBRAL DEGENERATION) Clinical manifestations Patients who survive one or more episodes of hepatic coma are occasionally left with residual neurologic abnormalities, such as tremor of the head or arms, asterixis, grimacing, choreatic twitching of the limbs, dysarthria, ataxia of gait, or impairment of intellectual function, and these symptoms may worsen with repeated attacks of stupor and coma. In other patients with hepatic failure, these neurologic abnormalities become manifest in the absence of discrete episodes of hepatic coma. In either event, patients thus afflicted deteriorate neurologically over a period of months or years. As the condition evolves, a characteristic dysarthria, mild ataxia, wide-based, unsteady gait, and choreoathetosis, mainly of the face, neck, and shoulders, are joined in a common chronic syndrome. Mental function is slowly altered—a simple dementia evolves, with indifference to the illness. A coarse rhythmic tremor of the arms, appearing with certain sustained postures, mild corticospinal tract signs, and diffuse EEG abnormalities complete the clinical picture. Other less frequent signs are muscular rigidity, grasp reflexes, tremor in repose, nystagmus, asterixis, and action or intention myoclonus. Many of the neurologic abnormalities that occur as part of acute or subacute hepatic encephalopathy also may be observed in patients with chronic hepatocerebral degeneration, the only difference being that the abnormalities are transient in the former and irreversible in the latter.

The chronic cerebral symptoms, like the transient ones, may occur with all varieties of chronic liver disease. Portacaval or intrahepatic shunts are always present; jaundice, ascites, and esophageal varices are manifest in most of the cases.

Pathology Chronic hepatocerebral degeneration, like acute and subacute hepatic encephalopathy, is characterized by a widespread hyperplasia of protoplasmic astrocytes in the deep layers of the cerebral and cerebellar cortices as well as in the thalamic and lenticular nuclei and many other nuclear structures of the brainstem. In addition, in the chronic disease, medullated fibers and nerve cells are destroyed in the affected areas, and polymicrocavitation is prominent at the corticomedullary junction, in the striatum (particularly in the superior pole of the putamen), and in the cerebellar white matter. Protoplasmic

astrocytic nuclei contain periodic acid Schiff (PAS)–positive glycogen granules. Nerve cells may appear swollen and chromatolyzed, accounting for the so-called Opalski cells. The similarity of these lesions to those observed in the familial form of hepatocerebral disease (Wilson's disease) suggests a common hepatogenesis.

UREMIC ENCEPHALOPATHY Episodic confusion and stupor and other neurologic symptoms may accompany any form of severe renal disease. In addition, a number of neurologic syndromes complicate chronic hemodialysis and kidney transplantation. Chronic polyneuropathy, the most common neurologic complication of renal failure, is discussed in Chap. 383.

Acute uremic encephalopathy The initial cerebral symptoms attributable to uremia consist of apathy, fatigue, inattentiveness, and irritability; later, confusion, disturbances of sensory perception, hallucinations, and stupor supervene. The later symptoms are practically always associated with twitching of the muscles, myoclonic jerks, and asterixis, and the patient may convulse.

Uremic encephalopathy, if associated with irreversible and progressive renal disease, can only be managed with dialysis or renal transplantation (see Chap. 238). Convulsive seizures, which occur in about one-third of cases, often preterminally, respond to relatively low plasma concentrations of phenytoin and phenobarbital.

The brains of patients with uremic encephalopathy and the twitch-convulsive syndrome show hyperplasia of protoplasmic astrocytes in some cases but never to the degree observed in hepatic encephalopathy. Cerebral edema is notably absent. Restoration of renal function corrects the neurologic syndrome, attesting to a biochemical rather than a structural abnormality. Whether this is caused by the retention of organic acids, elevation of phosphate in the CSF, or the action of other toxins has never been settled.

"Disequilibrium syndrome" and dialysis encephalopathy These terms refer to syndromes that commonly complicate hemodialysis or peritoneal dialysis. These treatments induce an acute intracellular shift of water. Intracellular osmolality becomes transiently greater than that of the serum. This gradient induces a syndrome akin to water intoxication. The *disequilibrium syndrome* is characterized by headaches, nausea, muscular cramps, nervous irritability, agitation, drowsiness, convulsions, and intracranial hypertension. The headache develops in approximately 70 percent of patients, while the other symptoms are observed in 5 to 10 percent, usually in those undergoing rapid dialysis or in the early stages of a dialysis program. The symptoms tend to occur in the third or fourth hour of dialysis and last for several hours. Sometimes the symptoms appear 8 to 48 h after completing dialysis (see Chap. 238).

Dialysis encephalopathy or *dialysis dementia* is a now uncommon complication of chronic hemodialysis. It begins with stuttering and dysarthria, coupled with a predominantly motor aphasia, to which are added facial and generalized myoclonus, focal and generalized seizures, personality changes and psychotic episodes, intellectual decline, progressive aphasic disorder, and EEG abnormalities. The last consist of bisynchronous, predominantly frontal or multifocal bursts of slow wave discharges, associated with spikes and sharp waves. The CSF is usually normal. At first these symptoms are intermittent, occurring during or immediately after dialysis and lasting for only a few hours, but gradually they become more persistent and eventually permanent. Once established, the syndrome is usually steadily progressive over a 1- to 15-month period (average survival of 6 months in 42 cases analyzed by Lederman and Henry). A few patients have a waxing and waning course and survive for several years. In some patients the myoclonus and seizures subside for several months under the influence of clonazepam or diazepam.

The neuropathologic changes are subtle and consist of a mild microcavitation of the upper layers of the cerebral cortex. Although the changes are diffuse, some neuropathologic studies indicate that the left (dominant) hemisphere is affected more than the right, and the left frontotemporal operculum more than other parts of the cortex (Winkelman). These findings may explain the striking disturbance of speech and language. Alfrey and his associates found that the cerebral gray matter of patients who died with dialysis encephalopathy contained a much greater amount of aluminum than analogous tissue from dialysis patients without encephalopathy. The aluminum was derived from both the dialysate and orally administered aluminum gels. The concept that dialysis encephalopathy represented a form of aluminum intoxication was supported by the observations that (1) the frequency of dialysis dementia was related to the concentrations of aluminum in the dialysate and (2) deionization of the water used in the dialysate prevented the occurrence of new cases. The possibility that other trace elements contribute to the syndrome has not been excluded.

Kidney transplantation is associated with an increased risk of developing primary cerebral lymphoma, Wernicke's encephalopathy (if not given thiamine), and central pontine myelinolysis. Systemic fungal infections are common at autopsy in patients who have had renal transplants and long periods of immunosuppressive treatment, and in some of these patients there is involvement of the CNS. *Cryptococcus, Aspergillus, Candida, Nocardia,* and *Histoplasma* are the usual organisms. Other CNS infections that complicate transplantation are toxoplasmosis and cytomegalic inclusion disease.

ENCEPHALOPATHIES DUE TO ELECTROLYTE AND ENDO-CRINE DISTURBANCES Only brief reference to these important groups of metabolic encephalopathies can be made here. Detailed accounts are found in the cross-referenced chapters.

Metabolic acidosis (arterial pH <7.30, P_{CO_2} <35 mmHg, HCO_3^- <10 mmol/L) due to diabetes mellitus, renal failure, lactic acidosis, or poisoning with an acid substance produces a syndrome characterized by drowsiness, stupor, and coma with dry skin and Kussmaul breathing, described in Chap. 46. Extreme degrees of *hyperosmolality* of the blood may develop in the course of diabetes mellitus [blood glucose > 22 mmol/L (>400 mg/dL)] and in extreme hypernatremia, resulting in either case in tremulousness, seizures, and coma. The patient may present with focal motor seizures (epilepsia partialis continua). In some instances the movement disorder resembles chorea or the myoclonic twitching of uremia. *Hypokalemia* is characterized by extreme muscular weakness (see Chap. 387) without any abnormality in cerebral function.

Hyponatremia, usually with water intoxication, is another cause of episodic coma, especially in infants. Among the many causes, the syndrome of inappropriate secretion of antidiuretic hormone (SIADH) is of special importance, since it commonly complicates neurologic diseases of many types—head trauma, bacterial meningitis and encephalitis, cerebral infarction and subarachnoid hemorrhage, neoplasm, and sometimes Guillain-Barré disease (see Chap. 333). The diagnosis of SIADH should be suspected in any critically ill neurologic or neurosurgical patient who excretes urine that is hypertonic relative to the plasma. As the hyponatremia develops, there is a decrease in alertness, which progresses through stages of confusion to coma, often with convulsive seizures. Lack of recognition of this state may allow the serum Na^+ to fall to dangerously low levels, 100 mmol/L or lower. Treatment is described in Chap. 333. Replacement with intravenous NaCl in severe cases must be done cautiously because vigorous and rapid correction of severe hyponatremia has been incriminated in the pathogenesis of central pontine myelinolysis (CPM) and related brainstem, cerebellar, and cerebral lesions. Firm therapeutic guidelines for the restoration of severe hyponatremia have yet to be established, but the most careful studies to date indicate that the serum sodium should be raised by no more than 12 mmol/L in the first 24 h and by no more than 20 mmol/L in the first 48 h (Laureno and Karp).

In children more than adults, cholera being an exception, extremely *severe diarrhea* may be attended by an encephalopathy. Irritability, weakness, headache, seizures, stupor, and coma may develop over a period of 2 to 3 days. Presumably this is a metabolic encephalopathy due to loss of fluids and electrolytes and can be corrected by their replacement. This metabolic disturbance carries a grave prognosis unless promptly relieved.

In the *endocrine encephalopathies* the clinical phenomena are even more abstruse. Confusional states may be combined with agitation, hallucinations, delusions, anxiety, and depression. And the duration of the illness may be measured in weeks and months rather than days. Derangement of higher cerebral function may follow the *administration of ACTH or glucocorticoids,* and the same symptoms have been reported in *Cushing's disease* (see Chap. 335). The neurologic manifestations of *thyrotoxicosis* are particularly elusive. Allusions to thyrotoxic psychosis are widely recorded in the medical literature; mental confusion, seizures, manic or depressive attacks, delusions, and chorea occur in various combinations with muscular weakness and atrophy, periodic paralysis, and myasthenia (see Chap. 334). Treatment of the hyperthyroidism gradually restores the patient to a normal mental state. *Myxedematous patients* may show slow mentation and depression, and in a small proportion there is a major change in cerebral function, taking the form of inattentiveness, apathy, and drowsiness or extreme somnolence. These symptoms can usually be reversed within weeks to months by thyroid medication. The association of myxedema and cerebellar ataxia is well documented, but the neuropathologic basis of this disorder remains unclear. In *hyperparathyroidism,* when the serum calcium levels reach 3.7 mmol/L (15 mg/dL) or higher, the patient sinks into a quiet state of inattentiveness, lethargy, and confusion. Stupor, coma, and death may be caused by extreme degrees of *hypercalcemia* such as occur occasionally in cases of hypervitaminosis D and metastatic tumors of the bones. Chronic *hypoparathyroidism,* either idiopathic or following thyroid or parathyroid resection, may rarely give rise to intracranial calcifications and an extrapyramidal motor syndrome. *Adrenal insufficiency* may be attended by episodic confusion, stupor, or coma, without special identifying features (see Chap. 335).

The term *pancreatic encephalopathy* describes a syndrome of agitation and confusion, sometimes with hallucinations and clouding of consciousness, dysarthria, and changing rigidity of the limbs, in association with acute pancreatic disease. The status of this entity is uncertain, and a uniform neuropathologic change has not been discerned. We agree with Pallis and Lewis, who suggest that before such a diagnosis can be entertained in a patient with acute pancreatitis, one needs to exclude delirium tremens, the cerebral effects of shock, renal or hepatic failure, hypoglycemia, diabetic acidosis, hyperosmolality, hypokalemia, hypo- or hypercalcemia, any one of which may complicate the underlying disease(s).

Lactic acidosis may be the cause of an encephalopathy in patients who undergo jejunoileostomy for treatment of morbid obesity. Such patients report episodes of confusion, ataxia, and slurred speech. D-Lactate, an isomer not normally found in the blood and a product of intestinal bacteria, is present in the serum, urine, and stool of these patients. D-Lactate causes encephalopathy by interfering with pyruvate metabolism. Diagnosis is dependent on recognition of metabolic acidosis associated with hyperchloremia and measurement of elevated D-lactate (see Dahlquist; Cross). A more common cause of encephalopathy in patients with jejunoileal shunting is hepatic failure (see Chap. 73).

HEREDITARY METABOLIC DISEASES OF LATE ONSET

Inherited metabolic disorders affecting amino acid metabolism (Chap. 352), lysosomal enzyme functions (Chap. 349), and cerebral lipids (Chap. 349) are generally rare and usually become manifest during infancy or childhood. In this chapter are described a small number of hereditary metabolic disorders that may have their onset in late adolescence and adulthood and may present diagnostic problems because of the similarity of clinical presentation to other more common acquired and degenerative diseases of the nervous system. Noteworthy attributes of these diseases are their chronicity and progressive nature.

METACHROMATIC LEUKODYSTROPHY (See Chap. 349)   Probably the most common member of this category is *adult metachromatic leukodystrophy (MLD).* While the majority of cases appear in early childhood, approximately 25 percent manifest their first symptoms after age 21. Men outnumber women 2:1. The mode of inheritance is autosomal recessive in almost all instances. The onset is insidious, and the course is protracted, over 20 or more years.

Mental symptoms tend to dominate the clinical picture. Failing scholastic performance, forgetfulness, and irrationality occur early in the illness but may be obscured by peculiarities of personality, such as suspiciousness, delusional thinking, and bizarre actions. These latter qualities may raise the question of schizophrenia or immature ("borderline") personality development. Sooner or later a mild cerebellar ataxia presenting as awkwardness and falling, mild pyramidal signs, masked facies, and bizarre postures stamp the illness as neurologic. Eventually, mental processes deteriorate to the point where the patient is helpless, demented, mute, incontinent, and bedfast.

Specific diagnostic tests include (1) the demonstration of a diminished arylsulfatase A activity in white blood cells, serum, and urine, (2) increased excretion of sulfatides in the urine, (3) slowed conduction velocity in nerves, and (4) deposits of metachromatic material in nerve biopsies. No treatment is available.

ADRENOLEUKODYSTROPHY In this X-linked metabolic disorder, either adrenal insufficiency or cerebral symptoms may be the initial manifestation. The cerebral lesions may present as a homonymous hemianopia, cortical blindness, hemiparesis, aphasia, or dementia. The signs are usually asymmetric at first and progress intermittently. Relatively pure polyneuropathic and myelopathic forms also have been described. The diagnosis is usually made by finding a low blood cortisol level in a male with cerebrospinal demyelinating disease, although a purely spinal type, taking the form of a progressive spastic paraparesis, has been described in the heterozygote (female carrier). Increased urinary concentration of C22–C26 fatty acids is diagnostic. Glucocorticoid replacement therapy helps the symptoms of adrenal insufficiency but has no effect on the neurologic disorders. The latter progress intermittently over a few years, and the outcome is usually fatal.

ADULT LIPID STORAGE DISEASES G_{M2} *gangliosidosis* (hexosaminidase A deficiency) has been observed in young adults. Many are from non-Jewish families, and males and females in the same generation are equally affected. Generalized seizures may mark the beginning of a cerebral disorder that later is evidenced by alterations of behavior and intellectual decline. A progressive ataxia and mild signs of corticospinal disease, the combination of which interferes with independent locomotion, clarifies the diagnosis. The fundi and visual function are normal in most cases, but typical cherry red macular spots are seen occasionally. The liver and spleen are normal or slightly enlarged. The CSF protein is normal. CT scans of the brain reveal a modest ventricular enlargement. A slowly developing dementia, cerebellar ataxia, polymyoclonus, and failing vision may characterize the clinical picture in some cases. In yet others, the presenting syndrome has consisted of prominent motor neuron involvement accompanied by muscle cramps, suggesting a diagnosis of spinal muscular atrophy or amyotrophic lateral sclerosis (see Chap. 372). G_{M2} ganglioside is increased in tissue obtained by cerebral biopsy. Membranous cytoplasmic bodies are visualized by electron microscopy of rectal, appendicular, and cortical neurons. *Gaucher's* and *Niemann-Pick* diseases are yet other storage diseases that may present in adult life (see Chap. 349).

Ceroid lipofuscinosis The Kufs type of *ceroid lipofuscinosis* is a lipid storage disease that only becomes evident in adolescence or early adult life. Usually the disease begins with mental deterioration, followed by seizures, ataxia, increasing rigidity, athetotic posturing, and corticospinal signs. Skin and conjunctival biopsies, examined by electron microscopy, show lipofuscin storage material in fibroblasts and endothelial cells.

SUBACUTE NECROTIZING ENCEPHALOMYELOPATHY (LEIGH'S DISEASE) This disease, now classified as a disorder of mitochondrial metabolism, sometimes begins in adolescence and takes the form of a progressive polymyoclonus with seizures and cerebellar ataxia and relatively mild impairment of intellectual function.

SUMMARY These rare forms of hereditary metabolic disease should be considered whenever an adolescent or young adult becomes demented, shows a psychiatric syndrome with decline in cognitive functions, or has seizures (especially with polymyoclonus), failing vision, and cerebellar ataxia in combination with corticospinal signs or a progressive polyneuropathy.

REFERENCES

ADAMS RD, VICTOR M: *Principles of Neurology*, 5th ed. New York, McGraw-Hill, 1993, chaps 38 and 39

ALFREY AC et al: The dialysis encephalopathy syndrome: Possible aluminum intoxication. N Engl J Med 294:184, 1976

ALLEN RH et al: Diagnosis of cobalamin deficiencies: I. Usefulness of serum methylmalonic acid and total homocysteine concentrations. Am J Hematol 34:90, 1990

BECK WS: Neuropsychiatric consequences of cobalamin deficiency. Adv Intern Med 36:33, 1991

BUTTERWORTH RF: Pathophysiology of cerebellar dysfunction in the Wernicke-Korsakoff syndrome. Can J Neurol Sci 20(Supplement 3):123, 1993

—— et al: Ammonia: Key factor in the pathogenesis of hepatic encephalopathy. Neurochem Pathol 6:1, 1987

CARMEL R: Subtle and atypical cobalamin deficiency states. Am J Hematol 34:108, 1990

—— et al: Hereditary defect of cobalamin metabolism (*cblG* mutation) presenting as a neurologic disorder in adulthood. N Engl J Med 318:1738, 1988

CHOI DW, ROTHMAN SM: The role of glutamate neurotoxicity in hypoxic-ischemic neuronal death. Annu Rev Neurosci 13:171, 1990

COOPER AJL, PLUM F: Biochemistry and physiology of brain ammonia. Physiol Rev 67:440, 1987

FLEMING JL et al: Whipple's disease: Clinical, biochemical, and histopathologic features and assessment of treatment in 29 patients. Mayo Clin Proc 63:539, 1988

FRANCIS GS et al: Metachromatic leukodystrophy: Multiple nonfunctional and pseudodeficiency alleles in a pedigree: Problems with diagnosis and counseling. Ann Neurol 34:212, 1993

HARDING AE et al: Spinocerebellar degeneration associated with a selective defect of vitamin E absorption. N Engl J Med 313:32, 1985

HORNBEIN TF et al: The cost to the central nervous system of climbing to extremely high altitude. N Engl J Med 321:1714, 1989

KERTESZ A et al: The structural determinants of recovery in Wernicke's aphasia. Brain Lang 44:153, 1993

KOLODNY EH, BOUSTANY RM: Storage diseases of the reticuloendothelial system, in Nathan D, Oski F (eds): *Hematology of Infancy and Childhood*, 3d ed. Philadelphia, Saunders, 1986

LAURENO R: Central pontine myelinolysis following rapid correction of hyponatremia. Ann Neurol 13:232, 1983

——, KARP BI: Pontine and extrapontine myelinolysis following rapid correction of hyponatremia. Lancet 1:1439, 1988

LEDERMAN RS, HENRY CE: Progressive dialysis encephalopathy. Ann Neurol 4:199, 1978

LINDENBAUM J et al: Neuropsychiatric disorders caused by cobalamin deficiency in the absence of anemia or macrocytosis. N Engl J Med 318:1720, 1988

MULLEN KD: Benzodiazepine compounds and hepatic encephalopathy. N Engl J Med 325:509, 1991

NELSON JS et al: Progressive neuropathologic lesions in vitamin E–deficient rhesus monkeys. J Neuropathol Exp Neurol 40:166, 1981

NORENBERG MD: The role of astrocytes in hepatic encephalopathy. Neurochem Pathol 6:13, 1987

PALLIS CA, LEWIS PD: *The Neurology of Gastrointestinal Disease*. Philadelphia, Saunders, 1974

PINCUS JH: Folic acid deficiency: A cause of subacute combined system degeneration, in Botez MI, Reynolds EH (eds): *Folic Acid in Neurology, Psychiatry, and Internal Medicine*. New York, Raven Press, 1979, pp 427–433

PLUM F, POSNER JB: *Diagnosis of Stupor and Coma*, 3d ed. Philadelphia, Davis, 1980

RAO RVL et al: Glutamatergic synaptic dysfunction in hyperammonemic syndromes. Metab Brain Dis 7:1, 1992

RASKIN NH, FISHMAN RA: Neurologic disorders in renal failure. N Engl J Med 294:143, 1976

RIZZO JF, LESSELL S: Tobacco amblyopia. Am J Ophthalmol 116:84, 1993

SATYA-MURTI S et al: The spectrum of neurologic disorders from vitamin E deficiency. Neurology 36:917, 1986

SCHAUMBURG HH et al: Sensory neuropathy from pyridoxine abuse: A new megavitamin syndrome. N Engl J Med 309:445, 1983

SERDARU M et al: The clinical spectrum of alcoholic pellagra encephalopathy. Brain 111:829, 1988

SOKOL RJ et al: Vitamin E deficiency neuropathy in children with fat malabsorption: Studies in cystic fibrosis and chronic cholestasis. Ann NY Acad Sci 570:156, 1989

VICTOR M: Polyneuropathy due to nutritional deficiency and alcoholism, in Dyck PJ et al (eds): *Peripheral Neuropathy*, 2d ed. Philadelphia, Saunders, 1984, pp 1899–1940

——, ROTHSTEIN J: Neurologic manifestations of hepatic and gastrointestinal diseases, in Asbury AK et al (eds): *Diseases of the Nervous System*, 2d ed. Philadelphia, Saunders, 1992, pp 1442–1455

—— et al: The acquired (nonwilsonian) type of chronic hepatocerebral degeneration. Medicine 44:345, 1965

—————— et al: *The Wernicke-Korsakoff Syndrome and Related Disorders Due to Alcoholism and Malnutrition*. Philadelphia, Davis, 1989

WILKINSON DS, PROCKOP LD: Hypoglycemia: Effects on the nervous system, in Vinken PJ, Bruyn BW (eds): *Handbook of Clinical Neurology*, vol 27. Amsterdam, North-Holland, 1976, pp 53–78

WINKELMAN MD, RICANATI ES: Dialysis encephalopathy: Neuropathologic aspects. Hum Pathol 17:823, 1986

WITT ED, GOLDMAN-RAKIC PS: Intermittent thiamine deficiency in the rhesus monkey: I. Progression of neurological signs and neuroanatomical lesions. Ann Neurol 13:376, 1983

ZIEVE L: Pathogenesis of hepatic encephalopathy. Metab Brain Dis 2:147, 1987

378 NEUROCUTANEOUS SYNDROMES AND OTHER DEVELOPMENTAL DISORDERS OF THE CENTRAL NERVOUS SYSTEM

VERNE S. CAVINESS, JR.*

Developmental disorders that involve the nervous system and are encountered in adult life are the emphasis of this chapter. The discussion is arranged according to broad phenotypic groupings, namely *neurocutaneous* syndromes in which abnormalities of the nervous system are associated with abnormalities of osseous structures and the skin, *developmental* disorders principally affecting the nervous system, and *neuroskeletal* disorders.

NEUROCUTANEOUS SYNDROMES

A large number of neurocutaneous disorders (also known as *phakomatoses*, from phakos, "lentil," "mole," or "freckle") are expressed in a patchy fashion in affected tissues. The most commonly encountered of these, reviewed below, are transmitted by autosomal dominant inheritance. In each of these disorders the severity of expression is highly variable. Where mild, the disorder will be overlooked; telltale features must be sought diligently among family members of affected patients. The chromosomal linkage group has been (provisionally) identified for four of these dominantly transmitted forms (Table 378-1).

NEUROFIBROMATOSIS (VON RECKLINGHAUSEN'S DISEASE)
The dominating feature of this disorder is the neurofibroma, a tumor that arises from the Schwann cells and fibroblasts of the neurilemmal sheath of the peripheral nerve. Two nonallelic heritable forms are now recognized. *Neurofibromatosis type 1* (NF1), carried on chromosome 17, is the classic autosomal dominant neurocutaneous disorder in which tumors involving the sheaths or peripheral nerves are associated with characteristic cream-brown cutaneous lesions (café au lait spots). The neurofibromas themselves are only occasionally symptomatic, as when they result in entrapment of a nerve root at intervertebral foramina or in the unusual instances when they are sarcomatous. The disorder may be associated with other tumors of the central nervous system (CNS) including optic glioma, glioblastoma, and meningioma and rarely with pheochromocytoma (see also Chap. 336). Other associated aberrations include hamartomas of the iris (Lisch nodules), freckling concentrated around the nipples and in the axillae, macrocephaly unassociated with hydrocephalus, stenosis of the aqueduct of Sylvius, leading to obstructive hydrocephalus, and mild degrees of mental retardation, which has been ascribed to dysplasia of the cerebral cortex.

The structure of the NF1 gene is now known. The deduced structure of the encoded protein, *neurofibromin*, suggests that it

* This chapter is in part a revision of one for the 11th edition by G.R. DeLong and R.D. Adams.

TABLE 378-1 Chromosomal locations of dominant mutant genes in the phakomatoses*

Disorder	Chromosome	Phenotypic signature	Mental retardation	Tumors
NF1	17	Café au lait spots, neurofibromas	Occasionally	Multiple types: CNS, PNS, viscera
NF2	22	Bilateral acoustic neuromas	No	Acoustic neuromas; other CNS
TS	9, 16	White spots, adenoma sebacea	Frequent	CNS: tubers, gliomas; viscera
VH-L	3	Cerebral hemangioblastomas, retinal angiomas	No	Angiomas of viscera; renal cell carcinomas

* NF1 and NF2 are neurofibromatosis types 1 and 2; TS, tuberosclerosis; VH-L, von Hippel-Lindau. See also Chap. 364.

should have GTPase activating properties. Neurofibromin under normal circumstances appears to have tumor suppressor properties which are impaired or lost with mutation. The tumor suppressor function is currently thought to be exercised through modulation of the state of phosphorylation of *ras*, a proto-oncogene involved in regulation of cell division and differentiation.

Neurofibromatosis type 2, carried on chromosome 22, is also an autosomal dominant disorder in which neurofibromas involve the acoustic nerves exclusively and usually bilaterally. The acoustic neurinomas may produce deafness and other symptoms and signs of a cerebellopontine angle lesion. They may also be associated with meningiomas and astrocytomas.

TUBEROUS SCLEROSIS (BOURNEVILLE'S DISEASE)
In this condition, cutaneous lesions of multiple types are associated with malformation and tumors of the CNS. Mental deficiency, though not invariable, may be profound and associated with a remarkably intractable seizure disorder. The earliest lesions to emerge are leaf-shaped hypopigmented spots ("white spots") scattered over the trunk and limbs. These are seen most clearly under ultraviolet light (Wood's lamp). The adenoma sebaceum, a hallmark of the disorder, is an angiofibroma, distributed in a butterfly pattern over the cheeks, chin, and forehead. The individual adenomas vary in size from 0.1 to 1.0 cm and are elevated and pinkish or pinkish yellow in color. The skin over the lumbosacral region of the back may be marked by a rough thickening which is yellowish in color like sharkskin or pigskin (shagreen patch). The cutaneous lesions may provide the earliest clue to the causation of mental retardation or infantile epilepsy. Rhabdomyoma of the heart and tumorous malformations (angioleiomyomas) of the kidney, liver, adrenal glands, and pancreas are also characteristic of this disorder. The cardiac rhabdomyoma may be imaged by ultrasound in utero. The disorder is inherited as an autosomal dominant trait: linkage studies with RFLPs in some pedigrees have located the mutant gene to chromosome 9 but in other pedigrees to chromosome 16.

In the brain multiple nodular tumors, composed of abnormal neurons and glial cells, often lie in the plane of the cerebral cortex itself. These can be diagnosed accurately in T2 weighted magnetic resonance scans. If calcified, they may also be visualized by CT scans or skull x-rays. Calcified nodules occur in brain subependymal regions adjacent to the ventricles. If large, they may obstruct the foramen of Monro, causing a unilateral or bilateral hydrocephalus. Masses of subependymal glial tissue forming nodules are likened to "candle gutterings" on the walls of the ventricles. The electroencephalogram is usually abnormal but without specific pattern. The only treatment is symptomatic. When severe epilepsy and mental retardation are present, prognosis for life beyond the third decade is poor. Death is usually due to seizures, associated tumors, or intercurrent diseases.

CEREBELLORETINAL HEMANGIOBLASTOMATOSIS (VON HIPPEL-LINDAU SYNDROME)   This syndrome of retinal and cerebellar hemangioblastoma is inherited as an autosomal dominant disorder (encoded on chromosome 3). (See Table 378-1) The retinal lesions are capillary angiomas, usually multiple, causing progressive loss of vision. The cerebellar hemangioblastomas, which may occur multiply, are slowly growing cystic tumors. These may also occur in the medulla or in the spinal cord where they may be associated with a syrinx. Enlargement of cerebellar tumor may lead to obstructive hydrocephalus with headache, papilledema, and cerebellar ataxia. Only rarely do tumors become symptomatic before adolescence but the diagnosis must be considered in all adults with a cerebellar tumor. Tumors of the CNS are a part of a constellation including angiomas and cysts of the liver, pancreas, and kidneys, and tumors of the epididymis and kidney. The latter may be lethal. Pheochromocytomas may occur in this as in other of the phakomatoses (see Chap. 336). An association with renal cell carcinoma led to localization of the mutant gene on chromosome 3. The mutant gene has recently been identified (see Chap. 364). Polycythemia, presumably the consequence of ectopic production of erythropoietin by the hemangioblastoma, may disappear after excision of the tumor.

ENCEPHALOTRIGEMINAL SYNDROME (STURGE-WEBER DISEASE)   Capillary or cavernous hemangiomas, within but not always limited to the cutaneous distribution of the trigeminal nerve, occur along with a predominantly venous hemangioma that can spread through subjacent leptomeninges. The adjacent cerebral cortex is progressively destroyed, perhaps as a consequence of interruption of local blood flow. The first neurologic symptom is usually a focal seizure on the side opposite the skin lesion. Sensorimotor paralysis or permanent visual field defect, the most common sequelae, may be either of sudden or insidious onset with progression. In time calcium is deposited within the area of involved cortex and may be visualized as a characteristic "railroad track" in conventional x-ray or CT scans. If the skin lesion is within the area of supply of the ophthalmic division of the trigeminal nerve, the occipital lobes are more commonly involved. A facial nevus is more often associated with involvement of the parietal and frontal lobes. The intracranial and cutaneous lesions may also occur separately. The disease is usually sporadic; a familial occurrence consistent with autosomal dominant inheritance is exceptional. Deeply situated arteriovenous malformations rarely coexist. Blindness in the eye on the side of the nevus is nearly always due to glaucoma. Most patients with this malformation survive for many years, often with mental defects and hemiparesis. Intractable seizures and cognitive functions may in some instances be substantially improved by resection of large blocks of involved cerebrum.

Hemangioma of the trunk or upper or lower extremity may be associated with a spinal cord vascular malformation (Klippel-Trenaunay syndrome) and with hypertrophy of the involved extremity. The cord lesion may cause infarction in nervous tissue, producing a spinal sensorimotor paralysis. Surgical exploration and decompression are seldom beneficial.

DEVELOPMENTAL DISORDERS OF THE CNS

Developmental disorders expressed largely or even exclusively as disturbance of neurologic functions afflict a substantial portion of the population. Certain of these, particularly when neurologic disability is severe, are complicated secondarily by restricted general somatic growth, articulatory contractures, and general medical disorders resulting from limited mobility and poor personal care. The discussion will be focussed upon developmental disorders expressed predominantly as malfunction of the forebrain, in particular, of the cerebral hemispheres. Three general syndromes are emphasized: mental retardation where the disability is predominantly in the domains of cognition, language, and memory; autism where socialization is prominently defective; and "cerebral palsy" where disability largely relates to motor function.

MENTAL RETARDATION   Mental retardation specifies an IQ less than 70 resulting from pathophysiologic processes affecting the cerebrum during the developmental period. If IQ is normal, the diagnosis is not applied to more restricted learning disabilities including dyslexia, incompetence with mathematics, and a variety of developmental language disorders. Mental retardation, even if the predominant disability, is conjoined with a complex of other disabilities which include disordered motor function, abnormalities of special senses, such as hearing and sight, and a variety of medical problems.

Etiology and pathogenesis   The specific cause of abnormal cerebral development cannot be defined for as many as half of all mentally retarded persons. For many, the disorder is familial and may be due either to single-gene defects or polygenic inheritance. Among the remaining half in whom the cause can be identified, the recognized causes include the 21 trisomy and fragile X syndromes and intrauterine exposure to alcohol (see Chap. 62). Collectively these few disorders are responsible for a third of mental retardation in this country. Prevalence for each approximates 1:1000 live births. Other identifiable causes include encephaloclastic processes, such as infection, hypoxia/ischemia, trauma, and hydrocephalus, occurring either before or after birth. Intrauterine exposures to infectious and pharmacologic teratogenic agents are also common, e.g., herpes simplex and human immunodeficiency virus (HIV), other viral and protozoal infectious agents, or cocaine and other "recreational" drugs. Malnutrition, hypothyroidism, and other metabolic disorders also may cause mental retardation during intrauterine and postnatal life. Among the general medical conditions is a substantial list of heritable disorders of metabolism. The list is long and includes enzymopathies relating to amino acid, carbohydrate, organic acid, and lipid processing such as phenylketonuria (see Chap. 349), galactosemia (see Chap. 354), propionic aciduria, and disorders of lysosomal enzyme function such as neuronal ceroid lipofuscinosis, the gangliosidoses, and the mucopolysaccharidoses (see also Chaps. 349 and 351).

Many chromosomal and single-gene disorders of metabolism may be diagnosed prenatally. Where diagnosis is made postnatally, it may be critical to do so expeditiously in the case of treatable CNS infections and correctable or manageable metabolic disorders, i.e., cretinism or phenylketonuria. During the first 2 years of life diagnosis and intervention are also critical for malnutrition, a state usually coupled to other socioeconomic deprivations. These deprivations may result in retarded brain growth and mental development that persist into adult life. If, however, such children are "rescued" by refeeding and placement in a stimulating and supportive environment, the effects of early malnutrition are largely reversible, and normal mental development can result.

Clinical manifestations   The defining characteristic of this domain of cerebral disturbance, subnormal IQ, is an inexact but a meaningful predictor of behavioral capabilities. Severely retarded children, those with IQs of less than 20, are virtually unable to look after themselves. Often they never sit up, walk, or stand. Language is rudimentary; at most a few words are understood and uttered. They exhibit only primitive emotional reactions and sphincteric control may never be achieved. Motor mannerisms such as rhythmic rocking, rolling, head banging, and bouncing movements are typical and often are accompanied by bleating sounds and squeals. Music may encourage rhythmic movements. Their physical appearance may be unremarkable. However, if the insult to the brain occurs in utero or early in postnatal life, a variety of physical deformities, particularly microcephaly and variable degrees of joint contracture, are common in this group.

If the mental defect is less pronounced (IQ of 20 to 50), and if specific motor defects do not coexist, then sitting, walking, and speech are acquired, often after a delay. The existence of a cerebral defect may be noted for the first time when the child fails to speak normally during the second and third year of life and seems not to be able to learn the usual household tasks and play activities as well as other children. However, delay in speech development by itself is not a mark of mental retardation, for some children who are intelligent and show remarkable talent in communicating by gesture are slow in talking. Also the deaf child may be singled out by indifference to noise and reduced vocalization but otherwise normal development. Toilet training also may be difficult to accomplish in the retarded child, but again it may be delayed in an otherwise normal child.

The least severely retarded of these individuals (IQ of 50 to 70) grows and develops in many ways not different from the normal child during the early years of life. Their abilities and adaptations merge imperceptibly with those of the general population. Often there is neither somatic nor other specific neurologic abnormality. That the child is handicapped may not be evident until it is apparent that scholastic pursuits are relatively unsuccessful. There may be manifest inability to learn, with poor school progress, and the child with an IQ of 60 to 70 is generally unable to pass the sixth grade. Vocational training is of more value than other types of education. The mildly retarded child may be able to acquire useful occupational skills and to work under careful supervision.

Whereas IQ is a useful index of competence, the clinical and behavioral characteristics of individuals with retarded development cannot be adequately described by this single attribute. In particular, the social competence, which may vary in ways that are not predicted by IQ, may largely determine the life expectations of retarded children. This aspect of behavior should be an organizing theme for education and training. Some mentally retarded persons are pleasant and amiable and achieve a satisfactory social adjustment. At the opposite extreme is the poorly understood syndrome of autism, associated with varying degrees of retardation, in which the child or older person fails to manifest any kind of interpersonal, social contact (see ''Autism,'' below). Many retarded individuals are dull, apathetic, and underactive. Others display an incessant hyperactivity, characterized by a very short attention span, a restless inquisitive searching of the environment, and low frustration tolerance; they may be destructive or recklessly fearless and may seem strangely impervious to injury. As with the mentally normal but hyperactive, inattentive child, improvement in these children can often be achieved by using stimulants and desipramine.

Three specific disorders associated with mental retardation deserve separate description.

Fetal alcohol syndrome The *fetal alcohol* syndrome may be the most prevalent cause of defective cerebral development in industrialized nations. Its estimated frequency in the United States, 1:700 live births, is probably less than the actual occurrence and is even greater than the occurrences of trisomy 21 (Down's syndrome) and the fragile X syndrome. The fully developed disorder includes marked growth retardation, microcephaly, and cardiac valvular lesions. Characteristic facial features include hypotelorism, small palpebral fissures, small nasal bridge, and reduction of the vermilion border of the upper lip. Mental retardation may be profound. However, the less severely affected may have IQs in the normal range but be significantly disabled by attention deficit disorder with hyperactivity and learning disabilities. The severity of the disorder is related to alcohol dose, and the threshold for clinical expression appears to lie in mother's ingestion of 30 to 60 mL of absolute alcohol equivalent per day. Additional risk factors including exposure to multiple drugs or venereally transmitted infectious agents may interact with alcohol abuse. The potential risk to successive offspring is obvious.

Fragile X syndrome The *fragile X chromosome anomaly* is a phenotype that combines dysmorphic somatic characteristics with mental retardation. Cytogenetic analysis shows constriction of the terminal segment of the long arm of the affected X chromosome, and the fragile link is subject to breakage. Expression of the anomaly in standard tissue culture conditions is enhanced by folate deficiency and other modifications. The characteristic phenotype, which generally becomes evident only after puberty, is expressed in approximately 80 percent of males and in 35 percent of females carrying a single affected X chromosome. The mother of an affected male is always a carrier; paradoxically, within a lineage carrying the genetic disorder, there is increasing risk of expression with successive generations.

Stigmata include macro-orchidism in males, possibly large ovaries in females, prognathism, and large everted ears. The skull is narrow and elongate. Mental retardation is usually mild to moderate and associated with dysphonic, sometimes echolalic speech. The association of the fragile X chromosome anomaly and autism in males (see below) has been estimated to be as high as 10 to 15 percent. The fragile X phenotype reflects disruption in the function of the FMR-I gene which is located at the fragile site; the gene becomes disabled through a succession of modifications, rather than just a single modification. These include both the methylation and acquisition of multiple repetitions of a CpG sequence located approximately 150 base pairs 5' to the gene. Susceptibility to this sequence of modifications is acquired during meiosis as a germline ''premutation.'' The repetitions accumulate in successive generations, a phenomenon which explains the increasing expression through successive generations within a lineage. Approximately 60 to 79 repeats correspond to the threshold for clinical expression; 100 percent expression is associated with 90 to 200 repeats. A therapeutic response to treatment with folate has not been substantiated.

Down's syndrome (See Chap. 62) *Down's syndrome* accounts for about 1 percent of all retardation. Trisomy of chromosome 21 or translocation of parts of this chromosome is responsible for the disorder. Older mothers are more apt to have babies with Down's syndrome than are young mothers. The mean age of the mother is 37.

The degree of mental retardation in Down's syndrome varies from mild to severe and is associated with a characteristic facial appearance and small stature. Many stigmata can be recognized in the neonatal period. The head tends to be small and round, with sloping forehead. The ears are set low and are oval, with small lobules. The eyes slant slightly upward and outward owing to the presence of a medial epicanthal fold, which partly covers the angle of the palpebral fissure. The bridge of the nose is poorly developed. The mouth tends to hang open, and the tongue is usually enlarged, heavily fissured, and protruding. Gray-white specks of depigmentation are seen in the iris (Brushfield's spots). The little fingers are often short and curved inward (clinodactyly), owing to a hypoplastic middle phalanx. The hands are broad with a single transverse palmar crease. Lenticular opacities and congenital heart lesions (septal defects) are found in some cases. At birth these children are of average size, but at later periods of life they are characteristically small. The brain is of reduced weight with a relatively simple convolutional pattern. Of the patients who survive to puberty, many live to middle adult life and may develop a premature Alzheimer's type cerebral degeneration (onset in the majority by the age of 40) (see Chap. 370).

CRETINISM (See also Chap. 334) Cretinism and childhood hypothyroidism occur endemically in parts of the world where there is iodine deficiency and in infants everywhere with congenital disorders of thyroid function. The frequency is greater than that of phenylketonuria. For iodine deficiency to produce cretinism the mother must be lacking in iodine during the pregnancy, especially in the first trimester. Diagnosis rests with the clinical picture, for in the iodine-deficient state routine measures of thyroid function may be normal. Jaundice, umbilical hernia, noisy respirations, hypotonia, depression of reflexes, and lethargy are present at birth. Coarse facial features, large tongue, and constipation become manifest later. Among those with endemic cretinism, the neurologic abnormality consists of mental deficiency, deaf-mutism (or lesser degrees of hearing loss), and a combination of flexed posture with spasticity and rigidity of proximal limb musculature. These deficits persist throughout adult life.

AUTISM Autism is a mysterious and provocative condition. Long considered primarily psychiatric or a childhood form of schizophrenia, it is now generally thought to represent an organic defect in brain development characterized by failure to develop communicative language or other form of social communication. The incidence is at least 2 to 5 per 10,000 births; the disorder is approximately 1.5 times as prevalent in males as in females. The essence of the cognitive disorder has been formulated as a defect in "the theory of mind," that is, an impairment in the ability to appreciate what is going on in the minds of other people. In normal children this ability is well developed by age 4. Some autistic persons often show motor and other skills far beyond that expected of a mentally retarded person. Often they are obsessively preoccupied with inanimate objects, such as lights, running water, or spinning objects. Most children with autism prove later to be retarded, and the ultimate level of disability depends largely on the IQ. Some gradually acquire language and may then exhibit certain exceptional talents, such as in mathematics (idiot savant). Up to 30 percent of autistic children eventually manifest temporal lobe epilepsy. Upon reaching adult life they retain all the above characteristics. Not more than 1 in 20 improves significantly. Anecdotal pathologic reports draw attention to structural abnormalities of the limbic part of the forebrain. A blighting of the neocerebellar vermis, although visualized in the sagittal plane by MRI in a limited series of autistic subjects, is now recognized from more extensive study not to be characteristic of the disorder. The cause of autism is unknown and is likely to be multiple. There is no specific therapy.

ABNORMALITIES OF MOTOR FUNCTION (CEREBRAL PALSY)

Cerebral palsy carries the connotation of a developmental disorder of motor function that is present from infancy or early childhood and that is due to a nonprogressive cerebral disorder. The more commonly encountered conditions are spastic diplegia (affecting the legs), hemiplegia (affecting the arm and leg on the same side), and heterogeneous extrapyramidal syndromes. Cerebral infarction resulting from hypoxia and/or ischemia is one determinant of these disorders. For most the abnormal state has its origins before birth in events that go unrecognized. The insult may occur perinatally as a result of obstetrical mishap in 20 percent or less of cases. For some few an encephaloclastic event occurs in early childhood.

Spastic diplegia resulting from a prenatal or perinatal insult to the brain may not attract attention until several weeks or months after birth. There may be a delay in all normal developmental sequences, especially those that depend on the motor system. Once walking is attempted, usually much later than in the normal child, the characteristic stance and gait become manifest. The legs are advanced stiffly in short steps, each describing part of the arc of a circle: adduction is often so strong as to lead to actual crossing (scissors gait), with lower legs slightly splayed out and the feet flexed and turned in, the heels not touching the ground. Crural paraparesis is the rule, though in general associated with at least a mild affection of the arms as well. In the adolescent and adult, the legs tend to be short and small, but the muscles are not markedly atrophic, as in infantile muscular atrophy and dystrophy. Less commonly there may also be pseudobulbar dysarthria and athetosis.

Hemiplegia is a not uncommon condition of infancy and childhood, and a difference in function of the right and left extremities may be noticed soon after birth or during the first 6 to 12 months of life. The parents may be the first to notice that movements of prehension and exploration are carried out with only one arm. The affection of the leg is usually recognized later, i.e., during the first attempt to stand and walk. Mental defect is even less common than with cerebral diplegia and less common than in bilateral hemiplegia. Convulsions occur in 35 to 50 percent of children with congenital hemiplegia and may persist throughout life. If the hemiplegia is acquired during childhood, seizures often accompany the onset. They may be generalized but are frequently unilateral and limited to the hemiplegic side. Often, after a series of seizures, the affected side will be weak for several hours or longer (Todd's paralysis).

In *double hemiplegia*, a less frequent condition, the bilateral weakness of face, arms, and legs arises at any age under conditions of more severe acquired cerebral disease. The arms are severely affected, in contrast to their minimal involvement in cerebral diplegia. A quadriplegic state may occur without bulbar involvement. The condition is relatively rare and may result from a bilateral cerebral lesion or a high cervical cord lesion. Although this may occasionally result from cysts, tumors, and other malformations, it is usually

produced in the infant by fracture-dislocation of the cervical spine, induced during a difficult breech delivery. Similarly, in paraplegia, with weakness or paralysis limited to the legs, the lesion may be either a cerebral form of diplegia or a spinal one. Sphincteric disturbances and a loss of sensation below a certain level on the trunk favor a spinal localization.

The spastic and rigid cerebral diplegias discussed above shade almost imperceptibly into the congenital extrapyramidal syndromes. Many such patients are found in every cerebral palsy clinic and ultimately reach adult medical clinics. Pyramidal tract signs may be absent. The nonprogressive extrapyramidal cases considered here are generally attributable to severe perinatal hypoxia; others represent separate diseases such as erythroblastosis fetalis with kernicterus. These are to be distinguished from the progressive acquired or hereditary postnatal syndromes such as familial athetosis, dystonia musclorum deformans, and cerebellar ataxia.

Congenital choreoathetosis (double athetosis) is probably the most frequent representative of this group. Like the spastic states, it may be recognized only after several months or a year have elapsed. Syndromes may be mixed, however. All combinations of chorea, athetosis, ballismus, myoclonus, and dystonia may be found in a single case, or one or another type of movement disorder may predominate. However, in all instances there is, in addition, a primary defect in voluntary movement. Choreoathetosis varies in severity. In some the disorder is so mild that the abnormal movements are misinterpreted as restlessness or "the fidgets"; in others, every voluntary act is marred by intense involuntary movements, leaving the patient nearly helpless. The severely handicapped patients, even with the help of rehabilitation clinics and corrective orthopedic operations, rarely achieve a degree of motor control that permits them to lead an independent life, and they need supportive treatment and help as adults. In selected patients dorsal rhizotomy may diminish spasticity without augmenting the motor disability and, thus, facilitates a rehabilitative program. Intelligence may be preserved.

Kernicterus was a more common cause of abnormal cerebral development prior to the contemporary practice of restraining early postnatal serum bilirubin concentrations to levels below 250 μmol/L (15 mg/dL). The majority of infants with this disorder die within the first week or two of life, and those who survive are often mentally retarded, deaf, and totally unable to sit, stand, or walk. However, exceptional patients, obviously less damaged, are mentally normal or at most only slightly backward. Either athetosis or ataxia may be present. A few have rigid limbs and a picture not too different from that of cerebral spastic diplegia with involuntary movements. Kernicterus should always be suspected if an extrapyramidal syndrome is accompanied by bilateral deafness and palsy of upward gaze.

NEUROSKELETAL DISORDERS

The skull and vertebral column normally enlarge coordinately with growth of the central nervous system. Abnormalities in the size of the skull can occur secondary to underlying abnormalities of brain development. Abnormalities resulting primarily from derangements of osseous development may lead to aberrations in skull shape and to entrapment of the enclosed nervous system, as in the Chiari and related malformations. Abnormalities of nervous and skeletal systems are characteristically associated with disorders of body configuration and size and with the viscera. The majority of disorders with the neuroskeletal spectrum appear to arise as a consequence of pathologic processes set in motion from the earliest phases of organ formation and CNS development. These pathologic processes, though not well understood, are recognized to have both genetic and nongenetic causes. Among those which have their origins in gene mutation are those which appear to be segmental or multisegmental in their developmental affects; mutation or overexpression of homeotic genes in experimental animals provides models for certain of these complex and mysterious disorders.

SECONDARY MACROCRANIA AND MICROCRANIA Alterations in the circumference of the head greater than (macrocrania) or less than (microcrania) the 98th percentile are considered abnormal. Macrocrania may result from potentially correctable hydrocephalus and is associated with headache, mental dullness, depression, visual blurring, difficulty walking and urinary incontinence. Limited ability to elevate the eyes, ataxia of gait, hyperreflexia in the legs, and Babinski responses are common signs.

Developmental causes of *noncommunicating hydrocephalus* include aqueductal stenosis, the Dandy-Walker malformation in which the CSF escape from the 4th ventricle is obstructed, and the Chiari malformations (see below). Neoplasms or cysts, particularly when located within the ventricular system or impinging upon structures of the posterior fossa, must be excluded. *Communicating hydrocephalus* may develop after recovery from disorders that cause scarring of the leptomeninges, such as intraventricular hemorrhage in the perinatal period, especially in premature infants, and meningitis. Localized head enlargement, associated with mental slowing and contralateral long tract signs, may complicate porencephalic cerebral defects resulting from a focal cerebral injury in the perinatal period of early childhood.

Macrocrania may also be the result of an abnormally large brain (macrocephaly). Benign, or asymptomatic, macrocephaly may be familial. Macrocephaly associated with a characteristic triangular face, moderate impairment of cognitive functions and macrosomia constitute the syndrome of cerebral gigantism (Soto), which in some families appears to be transmitted by autosomal dominant inheritance. Symmetric or asymmetric macrocephaly, seizures, and cognitive impairment may occur with neurofibromatosis. Macrocephaly can also occur in certain lysosomal storage disorders that affect the brain, but such individuals rarely reach adulthood.

Microcrania is most commonly secondary to microcephaly. Typically this is a consequence of lack of brain growth and may result from virtually any heritable or acquired disorder that affects the developing brain. *Microcephaly vera* is a rare but distinctive disorder transmitted by autosomal recessive inheritance and associated mental retardation and brain weight less than 500 g. The face and facial features are distinctively prominent in relation to the small cranium.

PRIMARY DISORDER OF SKELETAL DEVELOPMENT The Chiari malformations are among the most prevalent and complex neuroskeletal malformations. The characteristic feature is entrapment and compression of the rhombencephalon within an underdeveloped posterior cranial fossa (see Marin-Padilla). In the severest forms, typically apparent at birth, the cerebellar vermis, medulla, and 4th ventricle are herniated or extruded into the upper cervical canal (Chiari Type II) or protrude exteriorly as an occipital encephalocele at the base of the skull (Chiari type III). Hydrocephalus and hydromyelia may be associated with meningomyelocele arising from the lumbosacral spinal cord. Milder degrees of herniation of the posteroinferior region of the cerebellum ("tonsils") into the cervical canal with little or no downward displacement of the 4th ventricle (Chiari Type I) or milder degrees of the Chiari II deformity may become symptomatic only in adolescence or adult life. Symptoms typical of adult expression of the Chiari malformation include pain that is localized to the cranial-cervical junction, which is aggravated by head movement or Valsalva maneuver. There may be unsteadiness of gait, dysarthria and dysphagia, corresponding to compromise of cerebellar related connections and lower cranial nerve paresis. Downbeat nystagmus is characteristic.

Syringomyelia or *syringobulbia* occur in association with the Chiari malformations. Syringomyelia, a disorder of the cervical region of the spinal cord, can be viewed as a progressive destructive expansion of a central cavitation of the spinal cord. A variable number of segments of the upper cervical and thoracic cord, or of the medulla and pons in the case of syringobulbia, may be involved. Typically, the commissure and the posterior horns of the central gray and the axonal fascicles of the posterior and lateral columns of the cord are damaged. The neurologic manifestations include impairment of pain and temperature perception in a cape-like distribution and impairment of perception of vibration and joint displacement and spasticity in the lower extremities. To the extent that anterior horn cells are destroyed at cervical segmental levels, muscle atrophy and weakness appear in the upper extremities (see Chap. 381). Extension of the cystic cavity upward into the brainstem can cause facial pain, nystagmus, and lower cranial nerve deficits.

Other disorders of the axial skeleton and the lower spinal cord and cauda equina are also characteristically associated with the Chiari malformation but may occur independently. The osseous anomalies include aberrations of the primary pattern of formation (absence or fusion) or the size of vertebrae, hemivertebra, or fusion of vertebra and scapula (Sprengel deformity). The Klippel-Feil deformity is a complex of osseous and visceral anomalies that include low hair line, platybasia, fusion of cervical vertebra with short neck, and deafness. These malformations may entrap and damage the brain and spinal cord. The disorders of the lower vertebral region may become symptomatic with rapid growth in adolescence or in adult life. Diastematomyelia, the protrusion of a bony spur into the vertebral canal, is of particular importance in adults because it represents a treatable form of deficit. Intermittent, generally progressive disturbances of somatic and visceral motor function, typically associated with pain, may be subtle clues to the diagnosis.

A cauda equina syndrome, that is, impairment of both somatic and visceral sensory and motor functions referable to the lower lumbar and sacral roots, may result from lipomas or dermoid cysts within the lower vertebral canal. A dimple or tuft of hair near the midline in the lumbar region or within the gluteal crease may suggest the persistence of a sinus tract or a deeper lying anomaly affecting vertebral canal and spinal roots. Tethering of the cord to the lower end of the vertebral canal by fibrous bands may result in traction that becomes symptomatic with growth in adolescence. Stenosis of the lumbar vertebral elements may be associated with claudication, that is, symptoms of a cauda equina syndrome that develop with walking.

Computed tomography and magnetic resonance imaging, particularly when utilized in conjunction with myelography for syrinx and other spinal disorders, are sensitive and efficient diagnostic procedures. Images obtained in the midsagittal plane are particularly appropriate for diagnosis of the Chiari malformation and syrinx and for abnormalities of the lumbosacral region. In principle, treatment is surgical. Decompression is appropriate for entrapment and compression, shunting is required for hydrocephalic (or syringomyelic) states. Mass lesions and bony spurs are excised.

SYNOSTOSES AND CRANIOFACIAL DEFORMITIES Cranial synostosis and some other craniofacial anomalies affect principally the rostral region and the vault of the skull. Premature closure of the sagittal suture results in an elongate (scaphocephalic) skull, and premature closure of the coronal sutures causes a broad and foreshortened (brachycephalic) skull. If all major sutures close prematurely, a tower (turricephalic) skull manifests itself by shallow orbits with bulging eyes. Other combinations may affect one or more sutures. Synostosis, particularly when generalized, may result in cerebral compression and hydrocephalus. Less extensive disorders are cosmetically disfiguring. Early surgical correction of the disorders is appropriate.

REFERENCES

ADAMS RD: Neurocutaneous disease, in *Dermatology in General Medicine*, 3d ed, TB Fitzpatrick et al (eds). New York, McGraw-Hill, 1986

———, LYON G: *Neurology of Hereditary Metabolic Diseases of Children*. New York, McGraw-Hill, 1982

BALLING R et al: Undulated, a mutation affecting the development of the mouse. Cell 55:531, 1988

BENSON PF, FENSOM AH: *Genetic Biochemical Disorders*. New York, Oxford Medical Publications, 1986

BERG BO: Current concepts of neurocutaneous disorders. Brain Dev 13:9, 1991

CASKEY CT et al: Triplet repeat mutations in human disease. Science 256:784, 1992

CHASNOFF IJ et al: Cocaine use in pregnancy. N Engl J Med 313:666, 1985

COPP AJ et al: The embryonic development of mammalian neural tube defects. Prog Neurobiol 35:363, 1990

DENCKLA MB, JAMES LS (eds). *An Update on Autism: A Developmental Disorder.* Pediatrics, vol 87, 1991

FRITH U et al: The cognitive basis of a biological disorder: Autism. Trends Neurosci 14:433, 1991

GOMEZ MR: Phenotypes of the tuberous sclerosis complex with revision of diagnostic criteria, in *Tuberous Sclerosis and Allied Disorders*, WG Johnson, MR Gomez (eds). Ann NY Acad Sci, Vol 615, 1991

HARRIS RM et al: Physical mapping within the tuberous sclerosis linkage group in region 9q32-q34. Genomics 15:265, 1993

HUGHES I, NEWTON R: Genetic aspects of cerebral palsy. Dev Med Child Neurol 34:80, 1992

LATIF F et al: Identification of the von Hippel-Lindau disease tumor suppressor gene. Science 260:1317, 1993

LUFKIN T et al: Disruption of the Hox-1.6 homeobox gene results in defects in a region corresponding to its rostral domain of expression. Cell 66:1105, 1991

MARIN-PADILLA M: Clinical and experimental rachischisis, in *Handbook of Clinical Neurology*, PJ Vinken, GW Bruyn (eds). Amsterdam, North Holland Publishing, 1978, pp 159–191

MARTUZA RL, ELDRIDGE R: Neurofibromatosis 2 (bilateral acoustic neurofibromatosis). N Engl J Med 318:684, 1988

ROWLAND LP et al (eds). *Molecular Genetics in Diseases of Brain, Nerve, and Muscles.* New York, Oxford University Press, 1989

SMITH DW: *Recognizable Patterns of Human Malformation*, 3d ed. Philadelphia, Saunders, 1982

SWAIMAN KF: *Pediatric Neurology: Principles and Practice.* St. Louis, Mosby, 1989

VISKOCHIL D et al: The neurofibromatosis type-1 gene. Annu Rev Neurosci 16:183, 1993

VOLPE JJ: *Neurology of the Newborn.* Philadelphia, Saunders, 1987

WALLACE MR, COLLINS FS: Molecular genetics of von Recklinghausen neurofibromatosis, in *Advances in Human Genetics* vol. 20, J Harris, K Hirschhorn (eds). New York, Plenum, 1991, pp 267–307

379   DISORDERS OF THE AUTONOMIC NERVOUS SYSTEM

RONALD J. POLINSKY / JOSEPH B. MARTIN

The regulation of homeostatic functions throughout the body is accomplished by the autonomic nervous system (ANS). An extensive peripheral innervation network combined with central vigilance provides rapid adjustments in vital physiologic mechanisms that are critical to survival. The importance of this regulation is emphasized by the extent and severity of disability resulting from compromised ANS function. The functional anatomy and relevant pharmacology of the sympathetic and parasympathetic components of the ANS are discussed in Chap. 68. This chapter describes the clinical manifestations, diagnosis, and treatment of ANS disorders. Hypothalamic disorders that cause disturbances in homeostasis are discussed in Chaps. 16 and 331.

CLINICAL MANIFESTATIONS   Classification   Disorders of the ANS may result from central or peripheral causes; they may be generalized, segmental, or focal. In many instances, the clinical signs and symptoms are due to interruption of reflex control of autonomic responses. For example, a lesion of the medulla oblongata in the brainstem may paralyze blood pressure responses to postural changes (orthostatic hypotension). Lesions of afferent connections (as in tabes dorsalis or diabetes mellitus) or of the efferent portion of the reflex arc (spinal cord disease, postganglionic autonomic insufficiency) may produce similar effects. Segmental disorders or focal deficits occur in spinal cord disease, in reflex sympathetic dystrophy (causalgia), and in Horner's syndrome (Table 379-1). Diagnosis of the site of reflex interruption is dependent on associated clinical findings, autonomic nervous system tests, and neural imaging.

Another approach to the classification of ANS disorders is based on the presence (or absence) of central nervous system (CNS) signs. The primary value of this approach is that pathophysiology and prognosis differ between these two groups. Subdivision of the two groups is based on special characteristics, e.g., the presence of a positive family history, pathologic characteristics, and the association with sensory/motor neuropathy. Unfortunately, some syndromes do

TABLE 379-1   Classification of ANS Disorders

GENERALIZED ANS DISORDERS

A With CNS signs
1 Multiple system atrophy (Chap. 372)
2 Shy-Drager syndrome (Chap. 372)
3 Olivopontocerebellar degeneration (Chap. 372)
4 Striatonigral degeneration (Chap. 371)
5 Parkinson's disease (Chap. 337)
6 Huntington's disease (Chap. 370)
7 Hypothalamic disorders (Chap. 331)

B Without CNS signs
1 Pure autonomic failure (Bradbury and Eggleston)
2 Guillain-Barré syndrome (occasionally accompanied by CNS signs) (Chap. 383)
3 Chronic idiopathic anhidrosis
4 Postural orthostatic tachycardia syndrome (POTS)
5 Raynaud's syndrome (Chap. 211)
6 Familial dysautonomia—Riley-Day syndrome

SEGMENTAL ANS DISORDERS

A Afferent loop disorders
1 Tabes dorsalis (Chap. 381)
2 Diabetes mellitus (Chap. 337)
3 Spinal cord and root disorders (Chap. 381)
4 Guillain-Barré syndrome (Chap. 383)

B Efferent loop disorders
1 Diabetes mellitus (Chap. 337)
2 Peripheral neuropathy (Chap. 383) (amyloidosis, porphyria, alcoholism)
3 Lambert-Eaton syndrome (Chap. 386)

FOCAL ANS DISORDERS

A Reflex sympathetic dystrophy (Chap. 299)
1 Shoulder-hand syndrome
2 Causalgia

B Horner's syndrome (Chap. 19)

C Reinnervation anomalies
1 "Crocodile" tears (Chap. 380)

not fit easily into any classification scheme. Included in this category are chronic idiopathic anhidrosis, postural orthostatic tachycardia syndrome, and reflex sympathetic dystrophy of which little is known about their causes, pathology, or treatment (see Table 379–1).

Symptoms of autonomic dysfunction   The clinical manifestations of autonomic lesions depend on a number of factors including the organ involved and its normal balance of sympathetic-parasympathetic innervation, the nature of the underlying illness, and the severity and stage of progression (see Table 379–2). However, some generalizations can be made about evolution of autonomic symptoms. *Impotence* often heralds autonomic failure in men and may precede the appearance of other symptoms by more than a decade, making its relevance apparent only in retrospect (see Chap. 47). A decrease in the frequency of spontaneous erections may occur months before loss of nocturnal penile tumescence and development of total impotence. *Bladder dysfunction* also appears early in men and women, particularly in those with CNS involvement. As with other autonomic symptoms, there can be overactivity or loss of function; however, neurogenic bladder with frequency and incontinence is more common than retention. *Gastrointestinal dysfunction* is typically manifested as severe constipation, although diarrhea can occur in some disorders such as diabetes mellitus. Impairment of glandular secretory function may cause difficulty with food intake (decreased salivation) and eye irritation (decreased lacrimation). Occasionally, temperature elevation and vasodilation can result from *anhidrosis* since sweating is an important form of heat dissipation (see Chap. 16).

Orthostatic hypotension is the most disabling feature of autonomic dysfunction. Generally accepted criteria for diagnosis are a postural decrease of 20 mmHg in systolic or 10 mmHg in diastolic blood pressure sustained for at least 3 minutes in the standing position to differentiate autonomic failure from sluggish baroreflex responses that are common in the elderly. Postural hypotension can cause a variety of symptoms including headache, neck/shoulder pain, dimming or

TABLE 379-2   Major clinical manifestations in some generalized autonomic failure syndromes

Disorder	Postural hypotension	Genitourinary dysfunction	Gastrointestinal involvement	Sweating deficit	Other manifestations
Aging	+ +	+	+	+ / −	Postprandial hypotension
Alcoholism	+	+			Tachycardia
Amyloidosis	+ + +	+	+ +	+ +	Dissociated sensory loss
Diabetes mellitus	+ + +	+ +	+ + + +	+	Distal neuropathy
Familial dysautonomia	+ +	+	+ + +	+	Abdominal crises, fevers, ↓ sensitivity to pain
Holmes-Adie syndrome	+ +		+ +	+	Tonic pupils, areflexia, supine hypertension
Multiple system atrophy	+ + + +	+ + +	+ + +	+ + +	Parkinsonian and/or cerebellar dysfunction
Parkinson's disease	+ +	+	+ +	+ / −	Sweating may be increased
Progressive supranuclear palsy	+	+ +	+ + +	+	Rigidity, gaze palsies
Pure autonomic failure	+ + + +	+	+ + +	+ + +	

Abbreviations: ± = Inconsistent or minimal; + = mild; + + = moderate; + + + = severe; + + + + = disabling lack of adrenergic output. Also, insulin can cause profound hypotensive effects.

loss of vision, and weakness. Syncope results when the drop in systemic pressure impairs cerebral perfusion (see Chap. 17). Other manifestations of impaired cardiovascular control from baroreflex dysfunction include supine hypertension, fixed heart rate, and postprandial hypotension.

Autonomic testing   The organizational and functional characteristics of the ANS can be assessed by physiologic and pharmacologic tests. Physiologic methods offer the advantage of ease but are useful primarily for demonstrating the presence of an autonomic lesion, whereas pharmacologic tests can elucidate pathophysiologic abnormalities and guide the development of rational therapy.

VALSALVA RESPONSE   Investigation of blood pressure (BP) control is particularly valuable in eliciting evidence of ANS disorders. The Valsalva response assesses the afferent limb, central integrity, and efferent limb of the baroreceptor reflex. An abnormal Valsalva response indicates a lesion in the pathways responsible for BP control, and analysis of the type of abnormal response can help define the site of the defect. With the use of continuous noninvasive BP recordings using plethysmographic techniques, the integrity of the efferent limb of the baroreflex arc can be evaluated by measuring the BP response to immersion of the hand in ice water (cold pressor test). This test may be invalid if spinothalamic function (pain and temperature) is abnormal. *The presence of an afferent or central lesion can be inferred when a normal cold pressor efferent response is evoked in the presence of an abnormal Valsalva response.* Central vasomotor function can be assessed by examining the BP response to hyperventilation. Sinus arrhythmia and the heart rate response to deep breathing provide physiologic indices of parasympathetic function. These are assessed by measuring the changes in RR interval on the electrocardiogram during phases of respiration.

QUANTITATIVE SUDOMOTOR AXON REFLEX TEST (QSART)   Sweating is induced by release of acetylcholine (ACh) from sympathetic postganglionic fibers. The *sudomotor axon reflex* can be activated by a constant current generator, and ACh-induced sweat release can be quantified (see Low). A reduced or absent response indicates a lesion of the postganglionic sudomotor axon. Abnormalities may be identifiable in patients with autonomic dysfunction (diabetes mellitus, amyloidosis) before clinical symptoms emerge.

ORTHOSTATIC BLOOD PRESSURE RECORDINGS   Beat-to-beat BP measurements determined in supine, 80° tilt, and tilt-back are useful to quantitate orthostatic failure in BP control. It is important to allow a 20-min period of supine rest before assessing changes in BP during tilting.

PHARMACOLOGIC TESTS   Pharmacologic assessments are based on responses to the administration of selectively active drugs. Neurochemical investigations typically provide the rationale for selecting various drugs as probes. For example, low plasma norepinephrine (NE) levels reflect postganglionic involvement in peripheral autonomic disorders. Further definition of specific abnormalities in noradrenergic neuronal function can be achieved by using drugs with

pressor activity. Tyramine, an indirect sympathomimetic, increases blood pressure if neuronal NE stores are adequate and the uptake mechanisms are intact. Up-regulation of postsynaptic noradrenergic receptors, a manifestation of denervating lesions, can be demonstrated by measuring the BP response to NE. Supersensitivity is reflected by a leftward shift of the dose-response curve in contrast to the increased slope that results from decentralization. The chronotropic response to BP elevation using a pure alpha-adrenergic agonist (e.g., phenylephrine) serves as an index of afferent baroreflex function. Measurement of BP and heart rate responses to isoproterenol provide measures of beta$_2$- and beta$_1$-adrenergic cardiovascular functions, respectively.

SPECIFIC SYNDROMES OF ANS DYSFUNCTION   Two neurodegenerative disorders (pure autonomic failure and multiple system atrophy) have been intensively studied in an effort to clarify the distinction between central and peripheral ANS lesions (see Table 379–1).

Pure autonomic failure   This syndrome of isolated, generalized autonomic dysfunction was described by Bradbury and Eggleston in 1925. The etiology is unknown. It occurs in the absence of peripheral neuropathy and is not inherited. The disorder generally begins in the middle decades with insidious onset and affects women more than men. The symptoms, particularly postural hypotension, can be disabling, but the disease does not appear to shorten the life-span. Although the pathologic changes have not been characterized in detail, the clinical and neuropharmacologic characteristics are consistent with primary involvement of postganglionic sympathetic neurons. Low plasma NE, reduced NE response to tyramine, decreased neuronal uptake of NE, and noradrenergic supersensitivity reflect peripheral sympathetic noradrenergic dysfunction.

Multiple system atrophy   The clinicopathologic and neurochemical features of multiple system atrophy differ from those in pure autonomic failure. *The term refers to several overlapping clinical disorders including striatonigral degeneration and olivopontocerebellar atrophy* (see Chap. 372). *Shy-Drager syndrome* is a well-characterized form of multiple system atrophy that is accompanied by autonomic failure. Most patients present with autonomic dysfunction, and somatic neurologic manifestations usually develop within 5 years. Patients with the striatonigral variant exhibit a form of parkinsonism in which bradykinesia and rigidity are more prominent than tremor. Patients with either a pure cerebellar syndrome or striatonigral degeneration may also develop pyramidal tract involvement. Some patients, particularly those with Shy-Drager syndrome, have features of both subtypes (see Chap. 372).

These disorders progress relentlessly to death 7 to 10 years after onset. Normal or elevated plasma NE, defective baroreflex modulation of BP, and low CSF monoamine metabolite levels (MHPG, 5HIAA) are consistent with CNS involvement in this syndrome. From a neuropathologic standpoint, these disorders are classified as primary neuronal degenerations with loss of neurons and gliosis in many

CNS regions including the brainstem, cerebellum, striatum, and intermediolateral zone of the spinal cord.

Pure autonomic failure and multiple system atrophy are relatively uncommon. ANS disorders occurring in Parkinson's disease, Huntington's disease, and progressive supranuclear palsy are more common (see Chap. 371).

Peripheral nerve disorders Peripheral neuropathies are the most common cause of chronic autonomic insufficiency (see Chap. 383). Neuropathies that affect small myelinated and unmyelinated fibers of the sympathetic and parasympathetic nerves occur in diabetes mellitus, amyloidosis, chronic alcoholism, porphyria, and Guillain-Barré syndrome.

DIABETES MELLITUS Autonomic involvement in diabetes may begin at any stage in the disease and often presents with altered vagal function (see Chap. 337). Loss of myelinated fibers in the splanchnic innervation, carotid sinus, and vagus nerves characterize the disorder. Widespread enteric neuropathy can cause profound disturbances in gut motility, achlorhydria, and rectal incontinence and may result in failure of the typical signs of hypoglycemia to appear when sympathetic efferents to the adrenal gland are impaired. Insulin excess may also cause profound hypotension in patients with abnormal blood pressure regulation. Autonomic dysfunction may lengthen the QT interval and enhance the risk of sudden death. The cause of the neuropathy in diabetes is unknown. Hyperglycemia appears to be one risk factor for autonomic involvement. Biochemical and pharmacologic studies in diabetic neuropathy reveal low plasma NE, decreased responses to tyramine and edrophonium, and enhanced pressor responsivity to phenylephrine.

AMYLOID POLYNEUROPATHY Autonomic neuropathy occurs in both sporadic and familial forms of amyloidosis (see Chap. 383). Although patients usually present with a painful neuropathy accompanied by a dissociated sensory loss, autonomic insufficiency can precede the development of the sensorimotor neuropathy. Cardiac and renal impairment are the usual causes of death. Postmortem studies reveal amyloid deposition in many organs including two sites that contribute to autonomic failure: intraneural blood vessels and neurons in autonomic ganglia.

ALCOHOLIC NEUROPATHY Abnormal parasympathetic vagal and efferent sympathetic function occur in chronic alcoholics, and pathologic changes can be demonstrated in the vagus nerves, sympathetic fibers, and ganglia. Impotence is a major problem, but concurrent abnormalities in gonadal hormones may obscure the parasympathetic contribution to this symptom. Autonomic failure generally appears after the onset of peripheral neuropathy, although orthostatic hypotension may be prominent in Wernicke's encephalopathy. Alcoholics with liver disease are more likely to develop autonomic neuropathy. Autonomic involvement may contribute to the high mortality rates in alcoholism.

PORPHYRIA Although each of the porphyrias can cause autonomic dysfunction, the condition is most extensively documented in the acute intermittent type (see Chap. 346). Prominent symptoms include abdominal pain, nausea, vomiting, tachycardia, sweating abnormalities, urinary retention, and hypertension. Abnormal autonomic function can occur both during acute attacks and during remissions. Elevated catecholamine levels during acute attacks correlate with the degree of tachycardia and hypertension. Interestingly, several heme precursors inhibit NE uptake in platelets from patients with acute porphyria.

GULLAIN-BARRÉ SYNDROME Blood pressure fluctuations and arrhythmias can be severe in acute demyelinating polyradiculoneuropathy. Abnormal sweating, sphincter disturbance, and pupillary dysfunction also occur. Fortunately, autonomic dysfunction is minimal in most patients and is rare in the chronic form of the disorder. Pathologic changes have been described in the vagus and glossopharyngeal nerves, the sympathetic chain, and the white rami communicans.

Segmental involvement of the ANS REFLEX SYMPATHETIC DYSTROPHY Reflex sympathetic dystrophy, also referred to as the *shoulder-hand syndrome* or *causalgia*, is characterized by pain,

loss of function, and localized autonomic impairment. Myocardial infarction, limb paralysis, and shoulder trauma can be precipitating events. The pain has a neuropathic character, and the autonomic dysfunction causes localized sweating and changes in blood flow. Abnormal hair and nail growth may accompany edema or atrophy of the skin. Although the pathophysiology is not completely understood, the changes in blood flow and sweating appear to result from localized noradrenergic and cholinergic supersensitivity. An analogous defect, perhaps involving endogenous opioids, could underlie the pain. Treatment of reflex sympathetic dystrophy is a difficult therapeutic challenge (see Chap. 11).

SPINAL CORD LESIONS Spinal cord transection may be attended by autonomic hyperreflexia. The increased autonomic discharge can be elicited by bladder pressure or by other stimuli. This phenomenon affects 85 percent of patients with a spinal cord lesion above the C6 level. Sudden, dramatic increases in blood pressure can lead to intracranial hemorrhage and death.

MULTIPLE SCLEROSIS A variety of abnormalities in autonomic function occur in multiple sclerosis. Abnormal sweating occurs in approximately 40 percent of cases. Impairment of cardiovascular control is less common and usually minor. There does not appear to be any relationship between the severity of the disease and degree of autonomic involvement. However, the sympathetic nervous system can modulate immune mechanisms that could contribute to disease progression.

Inherited disorders Riley-Day syndrome (familial dysautonomia) is an autosomal recessive disorder occurring in Ashkenazic Jews which is associated with decreased tearing, reduced sensitivity to pain, and absent fungiform papillae on the tongue. Episodic abdominal crises and fever are common. Increased sensitivity to intraocular methacholine and absent axon flare response to intradermal histamine injection are useful diagnostic markers. Normal resting plasma NE levels that do not increase upon standing are consistent with an afferent lesion. The mechanism of the increased urinary excretion of homovanillic acid is unclear (see Chap. 364).

A syndrome of dopamine-β-hydroxylase deficiency has been described in siblings and may be hereditary. This rare syndrome is an important model for the development of rational pharmacotherapy. Patients with this condition have a variety of sympathetic failure. Plasma levels of NE and epinephrine are virtually absent while dopamine levels are extremely high. Administration of an unnatural NE precursor, L-dihydroxyphenylserine (L-DOPS), increases plasma NE and greatly improves the symptoms. This compound bypasses the enzymatic block in NE synthesis resulting from the deficiency of dopamine-β-hydroxylase.

Miscellaneous Other conditions associated with autonomic failure include autoimmune disease, infections, toxins, malignancy, and aging. Disorders of the hypothalamus can affect autonomic function and produce, in addition to the symptoms already discussed, abnormalities in temperature control, satiety, sexual function, and circadian rhythms (see Chap. 331).

TREATMENT In most conditions, management of autonomic failure is limited to alleviating the disability caused by the symptoms. If possible, the primary disorder, e.g., diabetes mellitus, should be treated, but this will not generally improve autonomic function. Orthostatic hypotension is the main focus of treatment because it can drastically impair function. Other aspects of autonomic failure may also affect blood pressure control. For example, severe constipation leads to excessive straining that can precipitously lower blood pressure.

Orthostatic hypotension only requires treatment if it causes symptoms. Supine hypertension presents a therapeutic dilemma in some patients. In the early stages patients can maintain normal function by using good judgment and a few precautions. For example, small meals are better tolerated because they mitigate the shunting of blood towards the splanchnic circulation during digestion. Alcohol intake and excessive environmental temperatures should be avoided because vasodilation can precipitously lower blood pressure in patients with deficient baroreflex activity. Drugs that affect blood pressure should be used with caution; many nonprescription medicines contain sympathomimetic agents.

Salt intake should be increased to the maximum tolerated. Sleeping in a reverse Trendelenburg position (head-up tilt) reduces nocturnal diuresis in these patients and helps to minimize supine hypertension. Compressive garments are of questionable value but may be tried; they present a number of practical problems, particularly for individuals with neurogenic bladder and/or neurologic impairment.

Eventually, most patients require drug therapy for management of hypotension. Fludrocortisone, which enhances renal sodium conservation, is the initial drug of choice; potassium supplements are necessary with chronic administration. Inhibitors of prostaglandin synthesis (e.g., ibuprofen) have potent pressor effects in patients with autonomic dysfunction. Other pharmacologic agents have been used with variable success to elevate blood pressure. These include beta-blockers (propranolol, pindolol, xamoterol), sympathomimetics (ephedrine, midodrine), dopamine antagonists (metoclopramide), and venoconstrictors (dihydroergotamine). Other approaches include the vasopressin analogue desmopressin and the somatostatin analogue octreotide. Desmopressin minimizes fluid loss which may play an important role in exacerbating the hypotension in patients with autonomic failure. Octreotide inhibits release of gut peptides, some of which have profound vasodilator and hypotensive effects. Since these substances are typically released after a meal, octreotide is most effective in alleviating postprandial hypotension.

Many patients with ANS failure exhibit exaggerated sensitivity to various drugs. Compounds with hypotensive actions should generally be avoided. Hence, anticholinergic agents are a better initial choice than dopaminergic compounds for parkinsonism. Anesthetic management poses unique problems since these patients have atypical physiologic and pharmacologic responses, abnormal fluid balance, and adrenal medullary insufficiency. More important than the choice of anesthetic is awareness by the physician of the implications autonomic failure may have for peri- and postoperative monitoring and management.

REFERENCES

Arnold JMO et al: Increased venous alpha-adrenoceptor responsiveness in patients with reflex sympathetic dystrophy. Ann Intern Med 118:619, 1993

Bannister R (ed): *Autonomic Failure*, 3d ed. London, Oxford University Press, 1992

————, Oppenheimer DR: Degenerative diseases of the nervous system associated with autonomic failure. Brain 95:457, 1972

Bradbury S, Eggleston C: Postural hypotension: A report of three cases. Am Heart J 1:73, 1925

Dagogojack SE et al: Hypoglycemia-associated autonomic failure in insulin-dependent diabetes-mellitus—Recent antecedent hypoglycemia reduces autonomic responses to, symptoms of, and defense against subsequent hypoglycemia. J Clin Invest 91:819, 1993

Hirayama M et al: Postprandial hypotension—Hemodynamic differences between multiple system atrophy and peripheral autonomic neuropathy. J Auton Nerv Syst 43:1, 1993

Johnson RG: Autonomic involvement in systemic diseases. Curr Opinion Neurol Neurosurg 5:468, 1992

Low PA, Pfeifer MA: Standardization of autonomic function, in PA Low (ed): *Clinical Autonomic Disorders: Evaluation and Management*. Boston, Little Brown, 1992

Man in't Veld AJ et al: Congenital dopamine-β-hydroxylase deficiency: A novel orthostatic syndrome. Lancet 1:183, 1987

McLeod JG: Autonomic dysfunction in peripheral nerve disease. Muscle Nerve 15:3, 1992

————, Tuck RR: Disorders of the autonomic nervous system. Ann Neurol 21:419(1), 519(2), 1987

Polinsky RJ: Clinical autonomic neuropharmacology. Neurol Clin 8:77, 1990

————: Autonomic dysfunction in neurological illness, in *Textbook of Clinical Neuropharmacology*, HL Klawans et al (eds). New York, Raven Press, 1992, pp 537–557

Proceedings of a consensus development conference on standardized measures in diabetic neuropathy: Autonomic nervous system testing. Neurology 42:1823, 1992

Robertson D et al: Isolated failure of autonomic noradrenergic neurotransmission. Evidence for impaired β-hydroxylation of dopamine. N Engl J Med 314:1494, 1986

Shy GM, Drager GA: A neurologic syndrome associated with orthostatic hypotension. Arch Neurol 2:511, 1960

380 DISORDERS OF THE CRANIAL NERVES

MAURICE VICTOR / JOSEPH B. MARTIN

The cranial nerves are susceptible to disorders that rarely affect the spinal peripheral nerves and, for this reason, deserve to be considered separately. This chapter describes the principal syndromes of disordered cranial nerve function and the diseases that cause them. Disorders of taste and smell, vision and ocular movement, and vertigo and deafness are discussed in Chaps. 18 to 20.

OLFACTORY NERVE (See Chap. 20)

OPTIC NERVE

TRANSIENT MONOCULAR BLINDNESS (AMAUROSIS FUGAX) (See also Chap. 368) **Definition** These terms are used interchangeably to designate an attack of transient painless loss of vision in one eye. Frequently it is recurrent.

Clinical manifestations Amaurosis fugax is a common clinical symptom indicative of transient retinal ischemia, usually associated with ipsilateral internal carotid artery stenosis or embolism of the retinal arteries. In some cases the basis for the symptom cannot be discerned.

Typically, the episode of blindness evolves swiftly, in a matter of 10 to 15 s, and is described as a shade that falls smoothly and painlessly over the field of vision until the eye is completely blind. Or a similar obliteration of the visual field may occur from below. The blindness lasts for a few seconds or minutes, sometimes longer, then clears slowly and uniformly, the patient's vision returning in the reverse direction from that in which it was lost. Sometimes there is only a generalized dimness of vision, rather than a complete loss, or only a segment of the visual field may be involved. Many patients who experience amaurosis fugax on the basis of carotid stenosis also have transient attacks of contralateral hemiparesis, but it is uncommon for the two types of attack to occur simultaneously.

Diagnosis The transient visual loss that accompanies classic migraine is of a different type. Often it begins with unformed flashes of light (photopsia) or dazzling zigzag lines (fortification spectra or teichopsia) which move across the visual field for several minutes, leaving scotomatous or hemianopic defects. The patient with migraine may complain of blindness in one eye, but examination usually shows the visual loss to be bilateral and homonymous, i.e., to occupy corresponding halves of both visual fields. The latter abnormality points to an origin in the visual cortex of one occipital lobe. In so-called basilar migraine, in which the neurologic symptoms are referable to the territory of the basilar artery, the transient visual disturbances may occupy the whole of both visual fields.

Investigation and treatment Amaurosis fugax is most commonly a manifestation of ipsilateral internal carotid artery disease. Carotid bruits should be sought, and noninvasive tests for carotid blood flow and lumen diameter should be carried out in every case. The decision of when to proceed to angiography is discussed in Chap. 368. Definitive treatment is dependent on the results of these investigations. In the absence of carotid disease, possible sources of emboli (cardiac or aortic) should be sought. Amaurosis fugax may sometimes herald occlusion of the central retinal artery or anterior ischemic optic neuropathy due to giant cell arteritis or to nonarteritic (atherosclerotic) disease. The sedimentation rate is usually elevated in giant cell arteritis (Chap. 291).

RETROBULBAR OPTIC NEUROPATHY OR NEURITIS Definition This syndrome is characterized by the rapid development (hours or days) of impaired vision in one or both eyes. In the latter case the eyes may be affected either simultaneously or sequentially. The visual loss in such cases is usually the result of acute demyelinative disease of optic nerves, although several other causes of unilateral or bilateral optic nerve disease need also to be considered (see below).

Clinical manifestations The most frequent setting is one in which a child, adolescent, or young adult notes a rapid diminution of vision in one eye (as though a veil or haze covered every object seen). Within a few days the condition may progress to severe loss of vision, but complete blindness is rare. The optic disc and retina may appear normal, but in some patients the disc is hyperemic and elevated with blurring of the disc margins (papillitis). Peripapillary hemorrhages are seen infrequently, and the veins are not engorged. *Papillitis* is distinguished from *papilledema* due to increased intracranial pressure by the acute and often marked reduction of visual acuity that accompanies the former. Also, in retrobulbar neuropathy, movement of the eye or pressure on the globe is often painful. After a few days or weeks the other eye may become similarly involved, with loss, typically, of central vision but with some preservation of peripheral vision. The pupillary light reflex is impaired. With complete or nearly complete interruption of one optic nerve, the pupil fails to react to direct light stimulation but does constrict when light is shone in the healthy eye (consensual reflex). With lesser degrees of optic nerve damage, there may be a failure to sustain pupillary constriction in response to a steady light stimulus ("pupillary escape" or Gunn pupil sign) (see Chap. 19, Fig. 19-3).

In a high percentage of patients, no cause can be found, and after a few days or weeks there is spontaneous recovery of vision. Sometimes a small central scotoma persists. The optic disc later becomes slightly pale due to demyelination, most prominent in the temporal region. The CSF may be normal or may contain from 10 to 20 lymphocytes, and the protein content, particularly the gamma globulin portion, may be increased. Oligoclonal bands are found in some patients.

More than half of such patients will develop the symptoms and signs of multiple sclerosis within 10 to 15 years, and an even higher percentage will do so if the patients are observed for longer periods (see Chap. 373). The prognosis for children with retrobulbar neuropathy is considerably better than that for adults. Multiple sclerosis is the most common cause of a *unilateral retrobulbar neuritis*. Bilateral optic neuritis may occur in association with or slightly in advance of an attack of transverse myelitis, a combination referred to as neuromyelitis optica or Devic disease (Chap. 373).

Diagnosis Other causes of unilateral optic neuropathy include postinfectious or disseminated encephalomyelitis, posterior uveitis, and, much more commonly (particularly in persons > 50 years of age), vascular lesions of the optic nerve. *Anterior ischemic optic neuropathy* (AION) is a condition caused by interruption of blood supply to the optic nerve secondary to atherosclerotic or inflammatory disease of the ophthalmic artery or its posterior ciliary branches (see Chap. 19). It presents clinically as acute, painless, visual loss in one eye, often accompanied by an altitudinal visual field defect. In severe cases, visual loss is complete and permanent. The fundus shows a markedly swollen optic disc surrounded by splinter-shaped peripapillary hemorrhages. Investigations are directed toward excluding temporal arteritis (see Chap. 291). Rarely, microemboli can cause occlusion of the posterior ciliary arteries and AION, following open heart or coronary artery bypass surgery, for example.

Central retinal artery occlusion (CRAO) also presents with sudden blindness. In this entity the optic disc initially appears normal. The retina is infarcted and appears pale with accentuation of the macular cherry red spot. In all cases of unilateral involvement of the optic nerve, tumor (glioma, von Recklinghausen neurofibromatosis, meningioma) needs to be ruled out.

Treatment Acute optic neuropathy due to demyelinative disease usually resolves without specific treatment. Severe visual loss is commonly treated with intravenous methylprednisolone or ACTH as outlined in the section on multiple sclerosis (see Chap. 373), but it should not be treated with oral prednisone alone (see Lessell).

Treatment may hasten recovery from an individual attack but does not prevent further attacks or modify their severity.

TOXIC-NUTRITIONAL OPTIC NEUROPATHY Simultaneous impairment of vision in the two eyes, with central or centrocecal scotomas, occurring over a period of days or weeks, is usually due to a toxic or nutritional disorder rather than to a demyelinative process (see Chap. 377). Impairment of vision due to *methyl alcohol intoxication* is abrupt in onset and is characterized by large symmetric central scotomas, as well as by symptoms of systemic disease and acidosis (see Chap. 395). The lesion is in the retinal ganglion cells and their axons, which constitute the optic nerve. The most important therapeutic measure is the immediate intravenous administration of sodium bicarbonate. Hemodialysis is a useful adjunct because of the slow rate of oxidation of methyl alcohol. Other drugs with proven but less devastating toxic effects on the optic nerve include chloramphenicol, ethambutol, isoniazid, streptomycin, sulfonamides, digitalis, ergot, disulfiram, and heavy metals (see also Chap. 19).

Degenerative diseases may affect the retina or the optic nerves, taking the form of optic atrophy. There are several types of hereditary optic atrophy, a common one being the Leber type, which has been shown to be due to a point mutation in mitochondrial DNA and is therefore maternally inherited (see Chap. 385). An autosomal dominant form of congenital or early infantile optic atrophy and optic atrophy with diabetes mellitus and deafness are equally common. Senile macular degeneration and various forms of retinitis pigmentosa are important causes of visual loss (see Chap. 19).

BITEMPORAL HEMIANOPIA This type of visual disorder is usually related to suprasellar extension of a pituitary adenoma (often with an enlarged sella), but it also may be due to a craniopharyngioma, saccular aneurysm of the circle of Willis, meningioma of the tuberculum sellae (normal sella or thickened tuberculum by radiography), and rarely sarcoidosis, metastatic carcinoma, and Hand-Schüller-Christian disease (see Chap. 331). The lesion involves the decussating nasal fibers from each retina.

OCULOMOTOR, TROCHLEAR, AND ABDUCENS NERVES (See Chap. 19)

TRIGEMINAL NERVE

The trigeminal nerve supplies sensation to the skin of the face and anterior half of the head. Its motor part innervates the masseter and pterygoid masticatory muscles.

PAROXYSMAL FACIAL PAIN (TRIGEMINAL NEURALGIA, TIC DOULOUREUX) Definition The most striking disorder of trigeminal nerve function is tic douloureux, a condition characterized by excruciating paroxysms of pain in the lips, gums, cheek, or chin and, very rarely, in the distribution of the ophthalmic division of the fifth nerve. The disorder occurs almost exclusively in middle-aged and elderly persons. The pain seldom lasts more than a few seconds or a minute or two but may be so intense that the patient winces, hence the term *tic*. The paroxysms recur frequently, both day and night, for several weeks at a time. Another characteristic feature is the initiation of pain by stimuli applied to certain areas on the face, lips, or tongue ("trigger zones") or by movement of these parts. Sensory loss cannot be demonstrated. In studying the relations between stimuli applied to a trigger zone and the paroxysm of pain, it is found that the adequate stimulus for precipitating an attack is a tactile one and possibly tickle, rather than a noxious or thermal stimulus. Usually a spatial and temporal summation of impulses is necessary to trigger an attack, which is followed by a refractory period of up to 2 or 3 min.

The *diagnosis* of this disorder rests on these strict clinical criteria, and the condition must be distinguished from other forms of facial and cephalic neuralgia and pain arising from diseases of the jaw, teeth, or sinuses (see Chap. 14). Tic douloureux is usually without assignable cause; occasionally, when it appears in younger adults, it may be due to a demyelinative plaque at the root entry zone of the fifth nerve. Very rarely it may occur with herpes zoster or a tumor. To a degree that remains uncertain, pain of tic douloureux may be caused by a redundant or tortuous blood vessel in the posterior fossa, causing an irritative lesion of the nerve or its root. Usually, however, lesions such as aneurysms, neurofibromas, or meningiomas affecting the nerve produce a loss of sensation (trigeminal neuropathy, see below).

Treatment The initial treatment of tic douloureux is pharmacologic. Carbamazepine is the drug of choice and is effective initially in 75 percent of patients. Carbamazepine should be started gradually, 100 mg with food, as a single dose, and increased to 200 mg qid. Doses greater than 1200 mg daily provide no additional benefit. Unfortunately, not all patients can tolerate the drug in the doses required to alleviate pain, in which case phenytoin, 300 to 400 mg daily, can be substituted.

If drug treatment fails, surgical therapy should be offered. The most widely applied procedure is percutaneous retrogasserian rhizotomy accomplished by radiofrequency lesions. Injection of glycerol in Meckel's cave is a method preferred by some surgeons. Relief is obtained by either of these procedures in more than 95 percent of patients. The pain recurs in 7 to 31 percent of patients. Complications and morbidity are infrequent in experienced hands. These procedures result in partial numbness of the face and carry a risk of corneal denervation with secondary keratitis when used for rare instances of first-division trigeminal neuralgia.

A third treatment, microvascular decompression, requires a suboccipital craniectomy, a major procedure requiring several days of hospitalization. It has an 80 percent efficacy rate, but the pain may recur, and in a small number of cases, there may be damage to the eighth or seventh nerve. A rare but most troublesome complication of all surgical treatments is the development of anesthesia dolorosa or denervation hypersensitivity. This condition responds poorly to treatment. Tricyclic antidepressants or phenothiazines are usually given with only partial success in alleviating the discomfort.

TRIGEMINAL NEUROPATHY A variety of diseases may affect the trigeminal nerve in addition to those mentioned above. Most present with sensory loss on the face or with weakness of the jaw muscles. Deviation of the jaw on opening indicates weakness of the pterygoids of the side to which the jaw deviates. Tumors of the middle cranial fossa (meningiomas), of the trigeminal nerve (schwannomas), or of the base of the skull (metastatic) may cause a combination of motor and sensory signs. Lesions in the cavernous sinus can affect the first and second divisions of the trigeminal nerve, and lesions of the superior orbital fissure can affect the first (ophthalmic) division. The accompanying corneal anesthesia increases the risk of ulceration (neurokeratitis).

Anesthesia and analgesia of the face have been reported after treatment with stilbamidine (formerly used in the treatment of kala azar and multiple myeloma). Pain and itching may occur during recovery. Rarely, an idiopathic form of trigeminal neuropathy is observed. It is characterized by feelings of numbness and paresthesias, sometimes bilaterally, with loss of sensation in the territory of the trigeminal nerve but without weakness of the jaw. Recovery is the rule, but the symptoms may be troublesome for many months, or even years. Leprosy may involve the trigeminal nerves.

Tonic spasm of the masticatory muscles, known as *trismus*, is symptomatic of tetanus (see Chap. 106). It also may occur as an idiosyncratic reaction in patients treated with phenothiazine drugs; lesser degrees may be associated with disease of the pharynx, temporomandibular joint, teeth, and gums.

FACIAL NERVE

FACIAL PALSY AND FACIAL SPASM The seventh cranial nerve supplies all the muscles concerned with facial expression. The sensory component is small (the nervus intermedius of Wrisberg); it conveys

taste sensation from the anterior two-thirds of the tongue and probably cutaneous impulses from the anterior wall of the external auditory canal. The motor nucleus of the seventh nerve lies anterior and lateral to the abducens nucleus. After leaving the pons, the seventh nerve enters the internal auditory meatus with the acoustic nerve. The nerve continues its course in its own bony channel, the facial canal, and exits from the skull via the stylomastoid foramen. It then passes through the parotid gland and subdivides to supply the facial muscles.

A complete interruption of the facial nerve at the stylomastoid foramen paralyzes all muscles of facial expression. The corner of the mouth droops, the creases and skin folds are effaced, the forehead is unfurrowed, and the eyelids will not close. Upon attempted closure of the lids, the eye on the paralyzed side is seen to roll upward (Bell's phenomenon). The lower lid sags also, and the punctum falls away from the conjunctiva, permitting tears to spill over the cheek. Food collects between the teeth and lips, and saliva may dribble from the corner of the mouth. The patient complains of a heaviness or numbness in the face, but sensory loss is rarely demonstrable and taste is intact.

If the lesion is in the middle ear portion, taste is lost over the anterior two-thirds of the tongue on the same side. If the nerve to the stapedius is interrupted, there is hyperacusis (painful sensitivity to loud sounds). Lesions in the internal auditory meatus also may affect the adjacent auditory and vestibular nerves, causing deafness, tinnitus, or dizziness. Intrapontine lesions that paralyze the face usually affect the abducens nucleus as well, and often the corticospinal and sensory tracts.

If the peripheral facial paralysis has existed for some time and recovery of motor function has begun but is incomplete, a kind of contracture (actually a continuous diffuse contraction) of facial muscles may appear. The palpebral fissure becomes narrowed, and the nasolabial fold deepens. With the passage of time, the face and even the tip of the nose become pulled to the unaffected side. Attempts to move one group of facial muscles may result in contraction of all of them (associated movements, or *synkinesis*). Facial spasms may develop and persist indefinitely, being initiated by every facial movement (*hemifacial spasm*). This condition may represent a transient or permanent sequela to a Bell's palsy but also may be due to an irritative lesion of the facial nerve (e.g., an acoustic neuroma, an aberrant artery that compresses the nerve and is relieved by surgery, or a basilar artery aneurysm). However, in the most common form of hemifacial spasm, the cause and pathology are unknown. Anomalous regeneration of the seventh nerve fibers may result in other troublesome phenomena. If fibers originally connected with the orbicularis oculi come to innervate the orbicularis oris, closure of the lids may cause a retraction of the mouth, or if fibers originally connected with muscles of the face later innervate the lacrimal gland, anomalous tearing (crocodile tears) may occur with any activity of the facial muscles, such as eating. Yet another unusual facial synkinesia is one in which jaw opening causes a closure of the eyelids on the side of the facial palsy (jaw-winking).

BELL'S PALSY Definition The most common form of facial paralysis is idiopathic, i.e., *Bell's palsy*. The incidence rate of this disorder is about 23 per 100,000 annually, or about 1 in 60 or 70 persons in a lifetime. The pathogenesis of the paralysis is unknown. The few autopsied cases of this disease have shown only nondescript changes in the facial nerve and not inflammatory changes, as is commonly presumed.

Clinical manifestations The onset of Bell's palsy is fairly abrupt, maximal weakness being attained by 48 h as a general rule. Pain behind the ear may precede the paralysis for a day or two. Taste sensation may be lost unilaterally, and hyperacusis may be present. In some cases there is mild CSF lymphocytosis. Fully 80 percent of patients recover within a few weeks or months. Electromyography may be of value in distinguishing a temporary conduction defect from a pathologic interruption in the continuity of nerve fibers. Evidence of denervation after 10 days indicates that there has been axonal degeneration and that there will be a long delay (3 months, as a rule) before regeneration occurs and that it may be incomplete. The presence of incomplete paralysis in the first week is the most favorable prognostic sign.

Treatment Protection of the eye during sleep, massage of the weakened muscles, and a splint to prevent drooping of the lower part of the face are the measures generally employed in the management of such cases. A course of prednisone beginning with 60 to 80 mg daily during the first 5 days and then tapered over the next 5 days may be beneficial. Unroofing of the nerve in the facial canal has been practiced, but there is no evidence that this measure is helpful, and it may be harmful.

Differential diagnosis There are many other causes of facial palsy. Tumors that invade the temporal bone (carotid body, cholesteatoma, dermoid) may produce a facial palsy, but the onset is insidious and the course progressive. The *Ramsay Hunt syndrome*, presumably due to herpes zoster of the geniculate ganglion, consists of a severe facial palsy associated with a vesicular eruption in the pharynx, external auditory canal, and other parts of the cranial integument; often the eighth cranial nerve is affected as well. *Acoustic neuromas* frequently involve the facial nerve by local compression (see Chap. 369). Infarcts and tumors are the common pontine lesions that interrupt the facial nerve fibers. Bilateral facial paralysis (facial diplegia) occurs in acute inflammatory polyradiculoneuritis (*Guillain-Barré syndrome*) and in a variety of sarcoidosis known as *uveoparotid fever* (*Heerfordt syndrome*). The *Melkersson-Rosenthal syndrome* consists of a rarely encountered triad of recurrent facial paralysis, recurrent—and eventually permanent—facial (particularly labial) edema, and less constantly, plication of the tongue; many causes of this rare syndrome have been suggested, but none has been established. Leprosy frequently involves the facial nerve.

A puzzling disorder is the *facial hemiatrophy of Romberg*. It occurs mainly in females and is characterized by a disappearance of fat in the dermal and subcutaneous tissues on one side of the face. It usually begins in adolescence or early adult years and is slowly progressive. In its advanced form, the affected side of the face is gaunt, and the skin is thin, wrinkled, and rather brown. The facial hair may turn white and fall out, and the sebaceous glands become atrophic. The muscles and bones are not involved as a rule. Sometimes the atrophy becomes bilateral. The condition is a form of lipodystrophy, and the localization within a dermatome suggests a disorder of some neural trophic factor of unknown nature. There is no treatment other than transplantation of skin and subcutaneous fat by a plastic surgeon.

Facial myokymia refers to a fine rippling activity of the facial muscles; it may be caused by a plaque of multiple sclerosis. *Blepharospasm* is an involuntary recurrent spasm of both eyelids that occurs in elderly persons as an isolated phenomenon or with varying degrees of spasm of other facial muscles (see Chap. 21). Relaxant and sedative drugs are of little help, although in many patients this disorder subsides spontaneously. Severe persistent cases of blepharospasm or hemifacial spasm are now successfully treated by local injection of botulinus toxin into the orbicularis oculi; the spasms are relieved for 3 to 4 months, and the injections can be repeated without morbidity.

All these forms of nuclear or peripheral facial palsy must be distinguished from the supranuclear type. In the latter, the frontalis and orbicularis oculi muscles are involved less than those of the lower part of the face, since the upper facial muscles are innervated by corticobulbar pathways from both motor cortices, whereas the lower facial muscles are innervated only by the opposite hemisphere. In supranuclear lesions there may be a dissociation of emotional and voluntary facial movements, and often some degree of paralysis of the arm and leg or an aphasia (in dominant hemisphere lesions) is conjoined.

VESTIBULAR NERVE

The eighth cranial nerve has two components, vestibular and auditory. Symptoms and signs of involvement of the vestibular portion are

discussed in Chap. 18 and in this section. The auditory nerve and its disorders are discussed in Chap. 20.

MÉNIÈRE'S SYNDROME Definition and clinical manifestations Ménière's disease, or Ménière's syndrome, is the name applied to recurrent vertigo associated with tinnitus and progressive deafness. Tinnitus and/or deafness may be absent during the initial attack(s) of vertigo, but they invariably appear as the disease progresses and are increased in severity during an acute attack. With milder forms of the syndrome the patient may complain more of head discomfort, slight instability, and difficulty in concentration than of vertigo and may be considered to be anxious or depressed. Provided that deafness is not complete, the recruitment phenomenon can be demonstrated (see Chap. 20).

Ménière's disease has its onset most frequently in the fifth decade of life, although younger adults and the elderly are not spared. The pathologic changes are said to consist of a dilatation of the endolymphatic system which leads to a degeneration of the delicate vestibular and cochlear hair cells. The relation of these pathologic changes to the paroxysmal disorder of labyrinthine function is unknown.

Treatment During an acute attack, rest in bed is the most effective treatment, since the patient can usually find a position in which vertigo is minimal. Dimenhydrate, cyclizine, or meclizine in doses of 25 to 50 mg tid is useful in treating more protracted attacks. A low-salt diet is still used in treatment, but its value is difficult to judge. Mild sedative drugs may help the anxious patient between attacks. Usually the deafness is unilateral and progressive, and when it is complete, the vertiginous attacks cease. However, the course is variable, and if the attacks persist in a severe manner, permanent relief can be obtained by surgical destruction of the labyrinth or section of the vestibular portion of the eighth nerve intracranially.

BENIGN POSITIONAL VERTIGO Another disorder of labyrinthine function is characterized by the occurrence of paroxysmal vertigo and nystagmus with the assumption of certain critical positions of the head. This is the positional vertigo of Bárány, of the so-called benign paroxysmal type (see Chap. 18). In refractory cases, in which attacks continue, vestibular exercises may be beneficial.

DIFFERENTIAL DIAGNOSIS OF VERTIGO There are many other causes of acute vertigo, such as purulent labyrinthitis complicating meningitis, serous labyrinthitis due to infection of the middle ear, "toxic labyrinthitis" due to drug intoxication (e.g., with alcohol, quinine, streptomycin, gentamicin, and other antibiotics), motion sickness, trauma, and hemorrhage into the internal ear. In these instances, the attacks of vertigo tend to last longer than in the recurrent form, but in other respects the symptoms are similar. Aminoglycoside antibiotics may damage the fine hair cells of the vestibular end organs and cause a permanent disorder of equilibrium (as well as hearing), especially in older patients (see also Chap. 18).

There has been described a dramatic clinical syndrome, characterized by the abrupt onset of severe vertigo, nausea, and vomiting without tinnitus or hearing loss. The vertigo persists for several days or weeks, and labyrinthine function is permanently ablated on one side. Occlusion of the labyrinthine division of the internal auditory artery would logically explain this syndrome, but pathologic or angiographic confirmation of this hypothesis has so far not been obtained.

Vertigo of vestibular nerve origin may occur with diseases that involve the nerve in the petrous bone or the cerebellopontine angle. Except that it is less severe and is less frequently paroxysmal, it has many of the characteristics of labyrinthine vertigo. The adjacent auditory division of the eighth cranial nerve also may be affected, which explains the frequent association of vertigo with tinnitus and deafness. The function of the eighth cranial nerve may be disturbed by tumors of the lateral recess (especially acoustic neuroma), less frequently by meningeal inflammation in this region and, rarely, by an abnormal vessel that compresses the nerve.

Vestibular neuronitis and *benign recurrent vertigo* are the names applied to a clinical syndrome that occurs mainly in middle-aged and young adults (sometimes in children) and is characterized by the abrupt onset of vertigo, nausea, and vomiting without impairment of hearing. The attacks are brief and leave the patient for some days with a mild positional vertigo. They may occur only once or recur in varying degrees of severity. The cause is unknown. The medical treatment is the same as for Ménière's disease.

A particular variety of paroxysmal vertigo affects children. The attacks occur in a setting of good health and are of sudden onset and brief duration. Pallor, sweating, and immobility are prominent manifestations, and occasionally vomiting and nystagmus occur. No relation to posture or movement of the head has been observed. The attacks are recurrent but tend to cease spontaneously after a period of several months or years. The outstanding abnormality is demonstrated by caloric testing, which shows impairment or loss of vestibular function, bilateral or unilateral, frequently persisting after the attacks have ceased; cochlear function is unimpaired, however. The pathologic basis of this disorder has not been determined.

GLOSSOPHARYNGEAL NERVE

GLOSSOPHARYNGEAL NEURALGIA This form of neuralgia resembles trigeminal neuralgia in many respects but is much less common. The pain is intense and paroxysmal; it originates in the throat, approximately in the tonsillar fossa. In some cases the pain is localized in the ear or may radiate from the throat to the ear because of implication of the tympanic branch of the glossopharyngeal nerve. Spasms of pain may be initiated by swallowing. There is no demonstrable sensory or motor deficit. Cardiac symptoms—bradycardia, hypotension, and fainting—have been reported. A trial of

carbamazepine or phenytoin is the recommended therapy, but if this is unsuccessful, division of the glossopharyngeal nerve near the medulla is the definitive treatment. Percutaneous rhizotomy of glossopharyngeal and vagal fibers in the jugular foramen alleviates pain in some patients.

Very rarely, herpes zoster may involve the glossopharyngeal nerve. Glossopharyngeal neuropathy in conjunction with vagus and accessory nerve palsies may occur with a tumor or aneurysm in the posterior fossa or in the jugular foramen. Hoarseness due to vocal cord paralysis, some difficulty in swallowing, deviation of the soft palate to the intact side, anesthesia of the posterior wall of the pharynx, and weakness of the upper part of the trapezius and sternocleidomastoid muscles make up the syndrome (see Table 380-1, jugular foramen syndrome).

VAGUS NERVE

DYSPHAGIA AND DYSPHONIA Complete interruption of the intracranial portion of one vagus nerve results in a characteristic paralysis. The soft palate droops ipsilaterally and does not rise in phonation. There is loss of the gag reflex on the affected side, as well as the "curtain movement" of the lateral wall of the pharynx, whereby the faucial pillars move medially as the palate rises in saying "ah." The voice is hoarse, slightly nasal, and the vocal cord lies immobile in the cadaveric position, i.e., midway between abduction and adduction. There also may be a loss of sensibility at the external auditory meatus and back of the pinna. Usually no change in visceral function can be demonstrated.

Complete interruption of both vagi is said to be incompatible with life, and this is probably true if the nuclei are involved in the medulla by poliomyelitis or some other disease. However, in the cervical region, both vagi have been blocked with procaine (Novocain), for the treatment of intractable asthma, without mishap. The pharyngeal branches of both vagi may be affected in diphtheria; the voice has a nasal quality, and regurgitation of liquids through the nose occurs during the act of swallowing.

The vagus nerve may be implicated at the meningeal level by neoplastic and infectious processes and within the medulla by tumors, vascular lesions (e.g., the lateral medullary syndrome of Wallenberg), and by motor neuron disease. This nerve may be involved by the inflammatory lesion of herpes zoster. Polymyositis and dermatomyositis, which cause hoarseness and dysphagia by direct involvement of laryngeal and pharyngeal muscles, may be confused with diseases of the vagus nerves. Also, dysphagia is a symptom in some patients with myotonic dystrophy (see Chap. 37 for discussion of nonneurologic forms of dysphagia).

The recurrent laryngeal nerves, especially the left, are most often damaged as a result of intrathoracic disease. Aneurysm of the aortic arch, an enlarged left atrium, and tumors of the mediastinum and bronchi are much more frequent causes of an isolated vocal cord palsy than are intracranial disorders.

When confronted with a case of laryngeal palsy, the physician must attempt to determine the site of the lesion. If it is intramedullary, there are usually other signs, such as ipsilateral cerebellar dysfunction; loss of pain and temperature sensation over the ipsilateral face and contralateral arm and leg, and an ipsilateral Horner syndrome. If the lesion is extramedullary, the glossopharyngeal and spinal accessory nerves are frequently involved (see jugular foramen syndrome, Table 380-1). If it is extracranial in the posterior laterocondylar or retroparotid space, there may be a combination of ninth, tenth, eleventh, and twelfth cranial nerve palsies and a Horner syndrome. Combinations of these lower cranial nerve palsies have a variety of eponymic designations, listed in Table 380-1. If there is no sensory loss over the palate and pharynx and no palatal weakness or dysphagia, the lesion is below the origin of the pharyngeal branches, which leave the vagus nerve high in the cervical region; the usual site of disease is then the mediastinum.

TABLE 380-1 Cranial nerve syndromes

Site	Cranial nerves involved	Eponymic syndrome	Usual cause
Sphenoid fissure (superior orbital)	III, IV, first division V, VI	Foix	Invasive tumors of sphenoid bone; aneurysms
Lateral wall of cavernous sinus	III, IV, first division V, VI, often with proptosis	Foix Tolosa-Hunt	Aneurysms or thrombosis of cavernous sinus; invasive tumors from sinuses and sella turcica; benign granuloma responsive to steroids
Retrosphenoid space	II, III, IV, V, VI	Jacod	Large tumors of middle cranial fossa
Apex of petrous bone	V, VI	Gradenigo	Petrositis; tumors of petrous bone
Internal auditory meatus	VII, VIII		Tumors of petrous bone (dermoids, etc.); infectious processes; acoustic neuroma
Pontocerebellar angle	V, VII, VIII, and sometimes IX		Acoustic neuroma; meningioma
Jugular foramen	IX, X, XI	Vernet	Tumors and aneurysms
Posterior laterocondylar space	IX, X, XI, XII	Collet-Sicard	Tumors of parotid gland, carotid body, and metastatic tumor
Posterior retroparotid space	IX, X, XI, XII and Horner syndrome	Villaret Mackenzie Tapia	Tumors of parotid gland, carotid body, lymph nodes; metastatic tumor; tuberculous adenitis

ACCESSORY NERVE

Isolated involvement of the accessory, or eleventh cranial, nerve can occur anywhere along its route, resulting in partial or complete paralysis of the sternocleidomastoid and trapezius muscles. More commonly, involvement occurs in combination with deficits of the ninth and tenth cranial nerves in the jugular foramen or after exit from the skull (see Table 380-1). An idiopathic form of accessory neuropathy, akin to Bell's palsy, has been described, and it may be recurrent in some cases. Most but not all patients recover.

HYPOGLOSSAL NERVE

The twelfth cranial nerve supplies the ipsilateral muscles of the tongue. The nucleus of the nerve or its fibers of exit may be involved by intramedullary lesions such as tumor, poliomyelitis, or most often motor neuron disease. Lesions of the basal meninges and the occipital bones (platybasia, invagination of occipital condyles, Paget's disease) may compress the nerve in its extramedullary course or in the hypoglossal canal. Isolated lesions of unknown cause can occur. Atrophy and fasciculation of the tongue develop weeks to months after interruption of the nerve.

MULTIPLE CRANIAL NERVE PALSIES

Several cranial nerves may be affected by the same disease process. In this situation, the main clinical problem is to determine whether the lesion lies within the brainstem or outside it. Lesions that lie on the surface of the brainstem are characterized by involvement of adjacent cranial nerves (often occurring in succession) and late and rather slight involvement of the long sensory and motor pathways and segmental structures lying within the brainstem. The opposite is true of intramedullary, intrapontine, and intramesencephalic lesions. The extramedullary lesion is more likely to cause bone erosion or enlargement of the foramens of exit of cranial nerves. The intramedullary lesion involving cranial nerves often produces a crossed sensory or motor paralysis (cranial nerve signs on one side of the body and tract signs on the opposite side).

Involvement of multiple cranial nerves outside the brainstem is frequently the result of trauma (sudden onset), localized infections such as herpes zoster (acute onset), granulomatous disease such as Wegener's granulomatosis (subacute onset), Behçet's disease, or tumors and enlarging saccular aneurysms (chronic development). Of the tumors, neurofibromas, meningiomas, chordomas, cholesteatomas, carcinomas, and sarcomas have all been observed to implicate a succession of lower cranial nerves. Owing to their anatomic relationships, the multiple cranial nerve palsies form a number of distinctive syndromes, listed in Table 380-1. Sarcoidosis has been found to be the cause of some cases of multiple cranial neuropathy, and chronic glandular tuberculosis (scrofula) the cause of a few others. Malignant granuloma of the nasopharynx also may affect multiple cranial nerves, as do nasopharyngeal tumors, platybasia, basilar invagination of the skull, and the Chiari malformation that becomes evident in adult life. A purely motor disorder without atrophy always raises the question of myasthenia gravis (see Chap. 386). Guillain-Barré syndrome commonly affects the facial nerves bilaterally (facial diplegia). In the Fisher variant of the Guillain-Barré syndrome, oculomotor paresis occurs with ataxia and areflexia in the limbs. Wernicke encephalopathy can cause a severe ophthalmoplegia combined with other brainstem signs (see Chap. 377).

An idiopathic form of multiple cranial nerve involvement on one or both sides of the face is occasionally seen. The disease may recur over a period of years with variable degrees of recovery between attacks. The clinical features overlap those of the Tolosa-Hunt orbitocavernous sinus syndrome (Juncos and Beal).

REFERENCES

ADAMS RD, VICTOR M: *Principles of Neurology*, 5th ed. New York, McGraw-Hill, 1993, chap 47

BRODAL A: The cranial nerves, in *Neurological Anatomy in Relation to Clinical Medicine*, 3d ed. New York, Oxford, 1980, chap 7, pp 448–577

BROWNSTONE PK et al: Bilateral superior laryngeal neuralgia. Arch Neurol 37:525, 1980

CHALK C, ISAACS H: Recurrent spontaneous accessory neuropathy. J Neurol Neurosurg Psychiatry 53:621, 1990

DEVINSKY O, FELDMANN E: *Examination of the Cranial and Peripheral Nerves*. New York, Churchill Livingstone, 1988

DURELLI L et al: The Melkersson-Rosenthal syndrome: A case with increased CNS IgG synthesis. Ann Neurol 18:623, 1985

EISEN A, BERTRAND G: Isolated accessory nerve palsy of spontaneous origin: A clinical and electromyographic study. Arch Neurol 27:496, 1972

GROVES J: Bell's (idiopathic) facial palsy, in *Scientific Foundations of Otolaryngology*, R Hinchcliffe, D Harrison (eds). London, Heinemann, 1976, pp 446–459

HAUSER WA et al: Incidence and prognosis of Bell's palsy in the population of Rochester, Minnesota. Mayo Clin Proc 46:258, 1971

JANKOVIC J, BRIN MF: Therapeutic uses of botulinum toxin. N Engl J Med 324:1186, 1991

JANNETTA PJ: Posterior fossa neurovascular compression syndrome other than neuralgias, in *Neurosurgery*, Wilkins RH, Rengachary SS (eds). New York, McGraw-Hill, 1985, pp 1901–1906

JUNCOS JL, BEAL MF: Idiopathic cranial polyneuropathy. Brain 110:197, 1987

KARNES WE: Diseases of the seventh cranial nerve, in *Peripheral Neuropathy*, 3d ed, PJ Dyck et al (eds). Philadelphia, Saunders, 1993, chap 43, pp 818–836

LECKY BRF et al: Trigeminal sensory neuropathy. Brain 110:1463, 1987

LESSELL S: Corticosteroid treatment of acute optic neuritis. N Engl J Med 326:634, 1992

MAYO CLINIC AND MAYO FOUNDATION: *Clinical Examinations in Neurology*, 6th ed., St. Louis, Mosby Yearbook, 1991

SAWLE GV et al: The natural history of non-arteritic anterior ischemic optic neuropathy. J Neurol Neurosurg Psychiatry 53:830, 1990

SELBY G: Diseases of the fifth cranial nerve, in *Peripheral Neuropathy*, 3d ed, PJ Dyck et al (eds). Philadelphia, Saunders, 1993, chap 42, pp 801–817

SWEET WH: The treatment of trigeminal neuralgia (tic douloureux). N Engl J Med 315:174, 1986

————: Percutaneous methods for the treatment of trigeminal neuralgia and other faciocephalic pain; comparison with microvascular decompression. Semin Neurol 8:272, 1988

381 DISEASES OF THE SPINAL CORD

ALLAN H. ROPPER / JOSEPH B. MARTIN

Diseases of the spinal cord are frequently devastating, causing permanent and severe neurologic disability. Small lesions can produce quadriplegia, paraplegia, and sensory deficits far beyond the damage they would inflict elsewhere in the nervous system because the spinal cord contains, in a small cross-sectional area, almost the entire motor output and sensory input systems. Many spinal diseases are reversible, particularly extrinsic cord compression, making acute spinal cord lesions among the most critical of neurologic emergencies.

The stereotypic organization of the spinal cord, innervating the limbs and trunk segmentally through 31 pairs of spinal nerves, makes anatomic diagnosis relatively straightforward. A sensory level, paraplegia, or other typical syndromes usually permit recognition of a spinal cord process. Full assessment of cord disease requires a careful examination supplemented by laboratory tests, including magnetic resonance imaging (MRI), computed tomographic (CT) scanning, myelography, analysis of cerebrospinal fluid (CSF), electromyography, and somatosensory evoked responses. Most deficiencies in evaluating patients with signs of spinal cord disease result from cursory physical examination or inadequate x-rays. Computed tomography and MRI have replaced conventional myelography because of their ease of performance and better resolution; MRI gives particularly valuable information about intrinsic cord structure.

SPINAL COLUMN AND SPINAL CORD ANATOMY RELEVANT TO CLINICAL SIGNS The spinal cord is organized in a uniform somatotopic fashion throughout its length, giving rise to easily identifiable syndromes (see Chaps. 11, 21, and 24). The longitudinal location of lesions is established by the uppermost level of sensory and motor dysfunction. However, the relationship between the vertebral bodies of the spinal column (or their surface markers, the vertebral spines) and the cord segments that underlie them complicates the anatomic interpretation of signs of spinal cord diseases. The level of a spinal cord syndrome is described according to the cord segment affected rather than by the surrounding vertebrae. During embryologic development, growth of the cord lags behind that of the spinal column so that the cord ends behind the first lumbar vertebral body and the lower nerves must take an increasingly downward course to exit in the appropriate vertebral foramen. The upper cervical cord segments lie behind the same numbered vertebral body, whereas the lower cervical segments are located one above each corresponding vertebral body, the upper thoracic cord two segments higher, and the lower thoracic cord, three segments higher. The lumbar and sacral cord segments, which form the conus medullaris, are located behind the ninth thoracic to first lumbar vertebrae. The cervical roots (except C8) exit from neural foramina above their respective vertebral bodies, while thoracic and lumbar roots exit below each body.

CLINICAL SYNDROMES OF SPINAL CORD DISEASE The principal clinical signs of spinal cord damage are a "sensory level," i.e., loss of sensation below a circumferential horizontal line on the trunk, and weakness in the extremities innervated by the descending corticospinal fibers. Sensory symptoms, particularly paresthesias, may begin in the feet (or in one foot) and ascend, giving the impression early on of a polyneuropathy before a fixed sensory level is apparent. Lesions that disrupt descending corticospinal and bulbospinal tracts at a single cord level cause paraplegia or quadriplegia, with increased muscle tone, enhanced deep tendon reflexes, and Babinski signs. A careful examination often also elicits segmental signs that are approximate indicators of the location of a transverse lesion, such as a band of altered sensation at the upper extent of the sensory level (hyperalgesia or hyperpathia), and isolated flaccidity, atrophy, or a single diminished deep tendon reflex. The sensory level to pinprick and temperature sensation is generally one or two segments below the level of an asymmetric lesion but is at the level of the lesion when bilateral. This is a result of the course of sensory fibers that synapse in the dorsal horn and then ascend and cross to the opposite spinothalamic tract. Midline back pain is also an accurate localizing sign, particularly in the thoracic region, where aching interscapular pain may be the first sign of cord compression. Radicular pain marks the primary site of a more laterally placed spinal lesion. Pain from lower cord (conus medullaris) lesions is often referred to the low back.

Early in the course of a severe and acute transverse lesion there may be flaccidity of the limbs rather than spasticity, due to so-called spinal shock. This state may last for several days, rarely for weeks, and may be mistaken for extensive segmental damage or a polyneuropathy, but the reflexes later become increased. Brief clonic or myoclonic limb movements often precede paralysis in acute transverse lesions, particularly those due to infarction. Autonomic dysfunction, mainly urinary retention, is another prominent sign in transverse spinal lesions and should call attention to cord disease.

Much is made of the clinical distinction between intramedullary (within the cord) and extramedullary compressive lesions, but most rules are approximations that do not distinguish one from the other dependably. Features that favor extramedullary lesions include radicular pain, a Brown-Séquard hemicord syndrome (see below), asymmetric lower motor neuron signs in one or two segments, early corticospinal signs, marked sacral sensory loss, and early, prominent CSF abnormalities. On the other hand, poorly localized burning pain, dissociated loss of pain sensation with sparing of joint position sensation, sparing of sensation in the perineal and sacral areas, late corticospinal signs, and normal or minimally altered CSF generally favor an intramedullary lesion. *Sacral sparing* refers to the preservation of pinprick and temperature sensation in the sacral dermatomes, usually S3 to S5, with more rostral areas affected up to the sensory

level. This is usually a dependable sign of intrinsic cord disease damaging the innermost fibers of the spinothalamic tracts while sparing those placed more laterally which subserve sacral sensation.

The *Brown-Séquard syndrome* is an eponym given to an idealized hemicord syndrome consisting of ipsilateral mono- or hemiplegia and loss of joint position and vibration sense, with contralateral loss of pain and temperature (spinothalamic) sensation. The segmental level for pain and temperature loss is sometimes one or two levels below the anatomic lesion. Segmental signs, such as radicular pain, muscle atrophy, or decreased tendon reflexes when they occur, are unilateral.

Lesions limited to or primarily within the central portion of the cord preferentially damage gray matter neurons and segmental tracts crossing at that level. Traumatic contusion, developmental syringomyelia, tumors, and vascular lesions in the territory of the anterior spinal artery are the most common lesions localized to the central cord. Inflammatory diseases occur in this distribution less frequently. In the cervical cord, the central cord syndrome gives arm weakness out of proportion to leg weakness and a "dissociated" sensory loss signifying analgesia (loss of pin sensation) in a cape distribution over the shoulders, lower neck, and upper trunk without anesthesia (loss of touch sensation) or pallanesthesia (loss of vibration sense).

Lesions located in the region of the first lumbar vertebral body or below compress the spinal nerves of the cauda equina and cause a flaccid, areflexic, asymmetric paraparesis usually accompanied by bladder and bowel dysfunction. A sensory level is found in a saddle distribution up to L1, corresponding to the roots carried in the cauda equina. The Achilles and patellar reflexes are diminished or absent. Pain is common and projected to the perineum or thighs. With conus medullaris lesions, pain is less prominent than in cauda equina lesions, and bladder and prominent bowel symptoms occur earlier. Compressive lesions may involve both the cauda equina and conus medullaris, causing a combined syndrome of lower motor neuron signs and hyperflexia or a Babinski sign.

The classic syndrome of the foramen magnum is weakness of the shoulder and arm followed by weakness of the ipsilateral leg, then contralateral leg, and finally, contralateral arm. Masses in this region sometimes produce suboccipital pain spreading to the neck and shoulders. A Horner's syndrome is another clue to a high cervical cord lesion; it does not occur with lesions below T2.

A few nontraumatic diseases are capable of producing sudden "strokelike" myelopathy without preceding symptoms. They include epidural hemorrhage, hematomyelia, cord infarction, nucleus pulposus embolism, and compression by spinal subluxation.

SPINAL CORD COMPRESSION Tumors of the cord Tumors in the spinal canal may be primary or metastatic and are classified as extradural ("epidural") or intradural, and the latter as intra- or extramedullary (inside or outside the cord) (see Chap. 369). The majority of neoplastic lesions are epidural, arising from metastases to the adjacent spinal column. Neoplasms originating in the prostate, breast, and lung, and lymphoma and plasma cell dyscrasias are particularly common, although virtually every malignant tumor has been reported to cause metastatic epidural cord compression. The initial symptom in epidural compression is usually local back pain, often worse in the recumbent position and causing the patient to awaken at night. Radiating radicular pain exacerbated by coughing, sneezing, or straining may accompany the back pain. Pain and local tenderness may precede other symptoms by many weeks. Neurologic signs commonly evolve over several days to a few weeks. The cord syndrome begins with progressive weakness, eventually acquiring all the hallmarks of a transverse myelopathy with paraparesis and a sensory level. A plain radiograph may show lytic or blastic changes or a compression fracture at the level appropriate to the cord syndrome; radionuclide bone scans are frequently positive. CT scan, myelography, and particularly MRI provide the optimal way of demonstrating cord compression. A horizontally widened and flattened cord from extrinsic compression is seen at the margins of the subarachnoid block, and the adjacent vertebral body is usually abnormal (Fig. 381-1).

In the past, emergency laminectomies were considered necessary to treat epidural cord compression by tumor, but treatment with high-dose glucocorticoids and rapid, fractionated radiation therapy has been as successful. Outcome is most closely related to the tumor type and its radiosensitivity. Paraparesis frequently improves within 48 h of the administration of glucocorticoids. Some incomplete or early transverse cord syndromes may still be better treated surgically, but each case must be analyzed individually, taking into account the radiosensitivity of the tumor, distribution of other metastases, and the patient's general medical condition. Whichever therapy is chosen, it is wise to proceed quickly and use glucocorticoids as soon as the diagnosis of cord compression is suspected.

Intradural, extramedullary tumors are a less frequent cause of spinal cord compression and evolve more slowly than extradural lesions. Meningiomas and neurofibromas are the most common causes. Symptoms usually begin with radicular sensory changes and an asymmetric spinal cord syndrome. Radiologic studies show dislocation of the cord to one side and an outline of the tumor within the subarachnoid space. Primary intramedullary tumors of the spinal cord are discussed in Chap. 369.

Compressive myelopathies of all types initially cause moderate elevation of CSF protein concentration, but with complete block of the subarachnoid space, CSF protein concentration rises to the 1 to 10 g/L (100 to 1000 mg/dL) range due to impaired CSF circulation from the caudal sac to the intracranial subarachnoid space. There are usually few or no cells, cytology for malignant cells is usually negative, and CSF glucose concentration remains normal unless there is accompanying widespread carcinomatous meningitis (see Chap. 369).

Epidural abscess This is a treacherous lesion, often misdiagnosed at first (see Chap. 374). The predisposing clinical settings are furunculosis of the back or scalp, bacteremia, or minor back injury. The condition can occur as a complication of local operation or very rarely after lumbar puncture. Spinal osteomyelitis acts as the nidus for the formation of an abscess that subsequently enlarges to compress the cord. The osteomyelitis is usually small and may not be evident on plain radiographs. For several days to 2 weeks there may be only unexplained fever and mild spinal ache with local tenderness; later, radicular pain occurs. As the abscess expands, it rapidly causes cord compression with a transverse syndrome. The proper treatment is rapid decompression by laminectomy and drainage, followed by appropriate antibiotics determined from culture of the purulent material. Incomplete drainage is not uncommon, resulting in a chronic granulomatous and fibrous reaction that may be sterilized with antibiotics but continues to act as a compressing mass. Tuberculous pyogenic abscess formation is still a common cause of epidural abscess in developing countries.

Epidural hemorrhage and hematomyelia Hemorrhage into the spinal cord (hematomyelia) or epidural space produces an acute transverse myelopathy evolving over minutes or hours, accompanied by severe pain. Although these hemorrhages may originate from an arteriovenous malformation, hemorrhage into a tumor, or from anticoagulation with warfarin or another coagulopathy, they are commonly spontaneous. Epidural hematoma may occur in the setting of minor trauma or lumbar puncture. Back and radicular pain precedes weakness by several minutes to hours. Patients may appear to be exaggerating their difficulties if back pain is severe but there are minimal or no neurologic signs. Lumbar epidural hematoma results in loss of both knee and ankle reflexes, whereas retroperitoneal hematomas usually cause only absence of the knee reflexes. A myelogram or MRI defines the mass; CT scan is sometimes normal because the clot cannot be distinguished from adjacent bone. Subdural and subarachnoid clots occur spontaneously or under circumstances similar to those causing epidural hemorrhages. The CSF with epidural hemorrhage is usually clear or contains a few red blood cells; in subarachnoid or subdural hemorrhage the CSF is grossly bloody at first and later becomes discolored to a deep yellow-brown characteristic of blood pigments present in the CSF. There may be, in addition, a pleocytosis and lowered CSF glucose, giving the impression of bacterial meningitis.

Acute disk protrusion Lumbar disk herniation, a common disorder, is discussed in Chap. 15. Thoracic or cervical disk protrusion is less often a cause of spinal cord compression, usually occurring after direct trauma to the spinal column. Degeneration of cervical disk spaces with adjacent osteoarthritic hypertrophy causes a subacute spondylytic compressive myelopathy in the cervical and, less often, the thoracic region (discussed below). Embolism from nucleus pulposus material causing acute spinal cord infarction is also described below.

Other unusual compressive lesions Patients with iatrogenic or primary Cushing's syndrome have a tendency to form foci of epidural fat tissue that rarely can reach a size sufficient to compress the thoracic cord. Extramedullary hematopoiesis also has caused cord compression in hematologic diseases. Eroding aortic aneurysms, echinococcal or other parasitic cysts, gummas, lymphomatoid-granulomatosis, mucopolysaccharidoses, and other rare lesions also can compress the cord.

Arthritic diseases of the spine occur in two clinical forms: a lumbar or cauda equina compression from *ankylosing spondylitis* or cervical cord compression from destruction of the cervical apophyseal or atlantoaxial joints in *rheumatoid arthritis*. Spinal complications arising as one component of severe generalized joint disease in rheumatoid arthritis are often overlooked. Forward subluxation of cervical vertebral bodies or of the atlas on the axis can cause a devastating, even fatal, acute cord compression after minor trauma such as whiplash, or it may present as a chronic compressive myelopathy similar to cervical spondylosis. Separation of the odontoid process from the axis may narrow the upper spinal canal compressing the cervicomedullary junction, particularly during flexion movements.

FIGURE 381-1 Sagittal section MRI showing compression deformity of the T12 vertebral body from metastatic adenocarcinoma (*below arrows*) and compression and displacement of the spinal cord. (*Courtesy of Greg Shoukimas, M.D., Department of Radiology, Massachusetts General Hospital.*)

NONCOMPRESSIVE NEOPLASTIC MYELOPATHIES   Intramedullary metastasis, paracarcinomatous myelopathy, and radiation myelopathy   In the context of known cancer, most myelopathies are compressive. However, when radiologic studies fail to show compression, there is often difficulty distinguishing between several less common entities: intramedullary metastasis, paraneoplastic myelopathy, and radiation myelopathy. In a patient with metastatic cancer and a noncompressive myelopathy, intramedullary metastasis is the most likely diagnosis (see Chap. 328). Back pain is the most common initial symptom, although it is not invariable, followed by progressive spastic paraparesis and, less often, paresthesias. Dissociated sensory loss or sacral sparing, which is characteristic of intrinsic compression, is uncommon, and asymmetric paraparesis with incomplete sensory loss is typical. Myelography, CT scan, or MRI may show a swollen cord without extrinsic compression; in almost half of patients CT or myelography are normal; MRI is more successful in outlining a metastatic mass or primary intramedullary tumor (Fig. 381-2). Intramedullary metastases usually arise from bronchogenic carcinoma and less often from breast cancer and other solid tumors. Metastatic melanoma, an uncommon cause of extrinsic cord compression, more often presents as an intramedullary mass. The pathology of the metastasis is usually a single eccentrically placed nodule that presumably arises from hematogenous dissemination. Radiation therapy may be helpful in appropriate circumstances.

Carcinomatous meningitis, a common form of CNS invasion in malignancy, does not cause a myelopathy unless there is extensive subpial infiltration from adjacent roots causing nodules with secondary compression or infiltration of the cord. An incomplete, painless cauda equina syndrome can result from carcinomatous root infiltration (see Chap. 369). Headache is common, and repeated CSF examinations eventually reveal malignant cells, an elevated protein, and, in some cases, reduced CSF glucose concentration.

A progressive necrotic myelopathy associated with a paucity of inflammation can occur as a remote effect of cancer, usually with solid tumors (paraneoplastic myelopathy). The radiologic studies and CSF are normal, or there may be slightly elevated protein. A subacute progressive spastic paraparesis evolves over days or weeks, usually asymmetrically, with distal paresthesias ascending to establish a sensory level, and late bladder dysfunction. Several adjacent segments of cord are involved (see Chap. 328).

Radiation may produce a delayed subacute progressive myelopathy due to microvascular hyalinization and vascular occlusion (see Chap. 369). It frequently presents a differential diagnostic problem when the cord lies within radiation portals used to treat other structures such as the mediastinal lymph nodes. Differentiation from paraneoplastic myelopathy or intramedullary metastasis is difficult except by circumstantial history of prior radiation.

INFLAMMATORY MYELOPATHIES   Acute myelitis, transverse myelitis, and necrotic myelopathy   These related diseases are characterized by intrinsic inflammation of the cord and a clinical syndrome evolving over several days to 2 or 3 weeks. There may be a virtually complete spinal syndrome (transverse myelitis) or incomplete variants such as a posterior column myelopathy with ascending paresthesias and a sensory level for vibration; ascending, predominantly spinothalamic findings; or a Brown-Séquard syndrome with leg paresis and contralateral spinothalamic-type sensory changes. Many cases follow a viral illness. The most common presenting findings in transverse myelitis are back pain, progressive paraparesis, and asymmetric ascending paresthesias in the legs, later affecting the hands if the disease progresses, creating confusion with Guillain-Barré syndrome. Radiologic studies are necessary to exclude a compressive lesion. The CSF contains 5 to 50 lymphocytes per microliter in most patients, and rarely, polymorphonuclear cells predominate. The inflammatory process is most common in the middle and low thoracic regions, but any level of the cord may be affected. A chronic progressive cervical myelitis has been described, predominantly in older women, and is believed to be a form of multiple sclerosis (see Chap. 373).

In some cases necrosis is profound and may progress intermittently for several months to involve contiguous portions of the cord, reducing much of it to a thin gliotic ribbon. The term *progressive necrotic myelopathy* has been given to this condition. Severe cases of necrotic myelopathy progress to involve virtually the entire cord (necrotic panmyelopathy). When a transverse necrotic lesion occurs before or shortly after optic neuritis, it has been termed *Devic's disease* or *neuromyelitis optica*. All these processes appear to be variants of multiple sclerosis. It is not clear what proportion of patients will ultimately be found to have multiple sclerosis after a single episode of acute transverse myelitis. Estimates have been 15 to 80 percent, a range similar to multiple sclerosis after optic neuritis. The postinfectious demyelinating disorders are usually monophasic and only rarely recur, although fluctuation of symptoms related to a single level of the cord is common (see Chap. 375). Systemic lupus erythematosus and other autoimmune disorders also have been associated with myelitis.

Infectious myelopathy   Several neurotropic viruses can cause myelitis. In the past, the most common form was poliomyelitis. Herpes zoster, preceded by radicular symptoms and rash, is presently the most common cause of viral myelitis. The pathologic process is not restricted to the gray matter and causes a transverse myelopathy. Lymphocytes are always found in the CSF.

The human retroviruses HTLV-I and HIV may be associated with myelopathies (see Chaps. 151 and 375). HTLV-I causes a chronic progressive, noninflammatory cord syndrome with symmetric spastic paraparesis and mild sensory and bladder disturbances. The disease is endemic in several areas, including areas of the Caribbean, South America, and southern Japan. It was identified as *tropical spastic paraparesis* before the virus was known. A myelopathy with vacuolar pathologic changes occurs with HIV infections. There is generally no clear sensory level in the retroviral myelopathies. An inflammatory cauda equina neuritis caused by cytomegalovirus is described in AIDS patients.

Intramedullary cord abscesses caused by bacteria or mycobacteria

FIGURE 381-2   Sagittal MRI showing intrinsic fusiform enlargement of the cervical spinal cord from an intramedullary tumor. The tumor displays a low-density signal (*arrows*). (*Courtesy of Greg Shoukimas, M.D., Department of Radiology, Massachusetts General Hospital.*)

may occur after systemic infections. Chronic meningitic lesions due to syphilis may produce a secondary subpial myelitis and radiculitis that evolve slowly (see below). An intense granulomatous, necrotic, and inflammatory myelitis is peculiar to infestation by *Schistosoma mansoni*, caused by a local response to tissue-digesting enzymes produced by ova from the parasite. Toxoplasmosis also may rarely cause a focal myelopathy.

Toxic myelopathy   A toxic noninflammatory myelopathy, sometimes with optic atrophy, has been reported mainly in Japan and has been linked to ingestion of iodochlorhydroxyquinoline. Most patients have recovered, but many have persistent paresthesias.

Arachnoiditis   This is a nonspecific term referring to inflammation, scarring, and fibrous thickening of the arachnoid membrane that is capable of compressing nerve roots or, rarely, the spinal cord. It is usually a postoperative complication or results from instillation of radiographic dye, antibiotics, or noxious chemicals into the subarachnoid space. The CSF contains cells and an elevated protein concentration soon after the inciting event, but the inflammation then subsides. Bilateral asymmetric radicular limb pain is the most prominent feature, with additional signs of root compression, such as reflex loss. There may be slight fever in acute cases. Back pain and radicular symptoms are attributed to lumbar arachnoiditis more often than justified. Congenital meningeal cul-de-sacs or arachnoid cysts along nerve roots may produce severe radicular pain in midadulthood when the cysts enlarge and distort or exert traction on spinal nerve roots or ganglia. An unexplained delayed paraplegia has been reported after the use of chymopapain for the treatment of disk herniation.

SPINAL CORD INFARCTION   Because the anterior or posterior spinal arteries are not usually involved by atherosclerosis, and only occasionally are affected by angiitis or emboli, most infarctions of the spinal cord are due to distant vascular occlusions or severe hypotension. Aortic thrombosis or dissection causes cord infarction by interrupting the entire radicular and direct arterial supply to the anterior and posterior spinal arteries. The infarction typically occurs in a vascular watershed region of the thoracic cord between the large tributary to the spinal cord arising from the lower aorta, the artery of Adamkiewicz, and the anterior spinal artery arising from the vertebral arteries. The anterior spinal artery syndrome usually appears abruptly, like a stroke, or emerges postoperatively if the proximal aorta has been clamped. In some cases, however, symptoms progress over 24 to 72 h, making diagnosis difficult. Spinal infarction has been reported rarely with systemic arteritis, immune reactions of serum sickness, and after intravascular contrast injection, in the latter heralded by severe back pain at the time of injection.

Cord infarction caused by microscopic fragments of herniated nucleus pulposus may occur after minor trauma, frequently during athletic activities. There is sharp local pain followed by a rapid paraplegia and a transverse cord syndrome evolving over several minutes to an hour. Pulposus tissue is found in small intramedullary vessels and often within the marrow of the adjacent vertebral body. The route from the disk space to marrow and thence to the cord is uncertain. This entity should be suspected in young adults with catastrophic transverse cord syndromes after back injury or exercise.

VASCULAR MALFORMATION OF THE SPINAL CORD   Arteriovenous malformations (AVM) of the spinal cord are rare but may simulate multiple sclerosis, transverse myelitis, spinal cord stroke, or neoplastic compression. They are difficult lesions to detect because of their great clinical variability. AVMs are most often found in the low thoracic or lumbar cord in middle-aged men. The majority begin with an incomplete progressive cord syndrome that may advance subacutely or episodically, like multiple sclerosis, producing bilateral corticospinal, spinothalamic, and posterior column symptoms and signs in any combination. About a third of patients have an abrupt syndrome with a single acute transverse myelopathy from bleeding, which simulates acute myelitis; others present with several acute exacerbations. About half have back or radicular pain, a few have a claudication syndrome similar to lumbar canal stenosis, and rare

patients describe an acute onset with severe, localized back pain. Fluctuation of pain or neurologic signs with exercise, posture, or menses is helpful in suspecting the diagnosis. Bruits over the lesion are rare but should be sought at rest and after exercise. Most patients have mild elevation of CSF protein and a few show CSF pleocytosis. Myelography, CT, or MRI shows a lesion in 75 to 90 percent of cases. The anatomic details of most AVMs can be demonstrated with selective spinal angiography, and simultaneous interventional neuroradiologic embolization has been a major advance in the treatment of the disorder.

The myelopathy caused by AVMs appears to be a noninflammatory gliotic and sometimes necrotic process consistent with ischemia. A special type of dorsal AVM with a prominent progressive intramedullary syndrome (Foix-Alajouanine disease) has been reported with an adjacent necrotic myelopathy. The abnormal vessels have a characteristic thickened, hyalinized wall. Since any necrotic process within the cord may give rise to neovascularization and thick-walled vessels, the pathologic interpretation of this vascular malformation remains controversial. Arteriovenous fistulas outside the spinal cord, including in visceral organs such as the kidney, have been associated with a vascular myelopathy due to large draining veins that traverse the spinal canal.

CHRONIC MYELOPATHIES   Spondylosis   This is a general term for several related degenerative changes of the spine giving rise to compression of the cervical cord and adjacent roots. Cervical spondylosis is primarily a disease of older patients, affecting men more often than women, and consisting of a combination of (1) narrowing of intervertebral disk spaces with nucleus pulposus herniation or annulus bulging, (2) osteophytic spur formation on the dorsal (posterior) aspect of the vertebral bodies, (3) partial subluxation of vertebrae, and (4) hypertrophy of the dorsal spinal ligament and dorsolateral facet articulations (see Chap. 15). The bony changes are reactive in nature, but there is no true arthritis. The most important feature causing spinal cord symptoms and signs is usually a ''spondylitic bar'' formed by osteophytes arising from the dorsal surfaces of adjacent vertebral bodies resulting in a horizontal compression of the ventral cord (Fig. 381-3*A* and *B*). The sagittal diameter of the spinal canal may be narrowed further during neck extension. Extension of the bar laterally and articulatory hypertrophic changes that encroach on the neural foramina cause additional radicular symptoms. Although the radiographic findings of spondylosis are common in the elderly, only a few patients develop myelopathy or radiculopathy, often dependent on a congenitally narrow canal.

Neck and shoulder pain with stiffness are early symptoms; pressure on nerve roots is associated with radicular arm pain, most often in a C5 or C6 distribution. Compression of the cervical cord produces a slowly progressive spastic paraparesis, at times asymmetric, and often accompanied by paresthesias in the feet and hands. Vibratory sense is substantially diminished in the legs in most patients, and occasionally there is a sensory level for vibration on the upper thorax. Coughing or straining often produces leg weakness or radiating arm or shoulder pain. Dermatomal sensory loss in the arms, atrophy of intrinsic hand muscles, increased deep tendon reflexes in the legs, and asymmetric Babinski signs are common. Urinary urgency or incontinence do not occur unless the process is well-advanced. The reflexes in the arms are often diminished at some level, notably the biceps, corresponding to C5–C6 root compression. Either radicular, myelopathic, or combined signs may predominate. The diagnosis should be considered in cases of progressive cervical myelopathy, paresthesias of feet or hands, or wasting of the hands. Spondylosis is also one of the most common causes of gait difficulty in the elderly, often causing increased leg reflexes or Babinski signs.

Plain radiographs demonstrate spondylitic bars, intervertebral narrowing and subluxations, reversal of the normal cervical spine curvature, and reduction of the sagittal diameter of the canal to less than 11 mm, or to 7 mm with neck extension (see Fig. 381-3*A*). CT or MRI are the preferred methods of demonstrating cord compression. The CSF is usually normal or shows a slightly elevated protein

A

B

FIGURE 381-3 *A*. Lateral x-ray of the cervical spine showing spondylitic "bar" formation from the junction of adjacent osteophytes at C6–C7 (*arrow*). *B*. Horizontal CT section at C6 from patient shown in *A* after instillation of water-soluble dye into the subarachnoid space. A spur of the bony osteophyte compresses and distorts the spinal cord (*arrows*).

concentration. Electromyography also may be useful in demonstrating radicular compression.

Cervical spondylosis is both an under- and overdiagnosed disease. Many patients with intrinsic cord processes, particularly amyotrophic lateral sclerosis, multiple sclerosis, and subacute combined degeneration, have had cervical laminectomies in the belief that spondylosis was responsible. There may be temporary improvement, suggesting that there was an element of spondylytic compression, but the underlying intrinsic myelopathy soon progresses. A mild progressive gait disorder with sensory symptoms in the feet and hands caused by cervical spondylosis also may be incorrectly attributed to peripheral neuropathy.

Rest and cervical immobilization with a soft collar are helpful in minor cases, traction may be helpful in others, but an operation is advisable if there are advanced symptoms of gait difficulty, severe hand weakness, or bladder difficulty.

Lumbar stenosis (also discussed in Chap. 15) is an intermittent and chronic compression of the cauda equina usually based on congenital narrowing of the lumbar spinal canal, which is further compromised by disk protrusion or spondylitic changes. Exercise brings about an aching pain in the buttocks, thighs, and calves, frequently sciatic in distribution, ceasing with rest and thereby simulating vascular-induced claudication. During the peak of pain, deep tendon reflexes and sensation may be reduced as compared with the resting state; peripheral vascular studies are normal. Lumbar stenosis and cervical spondylosis commonly occur together, the former probably explaining occasional lower extremity fasciculations in cervical spondylosis.

Degenerative and inherited myelopathies The prototype of the inherited disorders causing spinal cord syndromes is Friedreich's ataxia, a progressive, recessively inherited leg and truncal ataxia of late childhood onset. Intention tremor, clumsiness of the arms, and, later, dysarthria occur. Kyphoscoliosis and pes cavus are common. Areflexia, Babinski signs, and severely impaired vibratory and joint position sense loss are found on examination. Fragmentary or milder forms of the illness occur and overlap with other syndromes, including spastic paraparesis (Strümpell-Lorrain), cerebellar cortical degeneration with ataxia, and olivopontocerebellar atrophy (see also Chap. 372).

Amyotrophic lateral sclerosis (motor neuron disease) must be considered in patients with symmetric spastic paraparesis without sensory findings. It causes a pure motor syndrome with combined corticospinal, corticobulbar, and anterior horn cell involvement. Clinical or electromyographic evidence of widespread muscle fasciculations and denervation, in contrast to the limited segmental denervation of spondylosis, confirms the diagnosis (see Chaps. 372 and 382).

Subacute combined degeneration due to vitamin B$_{12}$ deficiency This treatable myelopathy causes a progressive spastic and ataxic paraparesis and neuropathy, usually with prominent distal paresthesias of the feet and hands. It should be considered in cases simulating cervical spondylosis, late-onset degenerative myelopathies, and symmetric late-onset spinal multiple sclerosis. The disease also can involve the peripheral and optic nerves and the brain. The diagnosis is confirmed by low B$_{12}$ serum concentration and a positive Schilling test. This entity and related nutritional degenerations are discussed in Chap. 377. Whether folate or vitamin E deficiencies can produce a similar syndrome is controversial.

Syringomyelia *Syringomyelia* is a progressive myelopathy characterized pathologically by cavitation of the central spinal cord. It is often idiopathic or developmental (see Chap. 378) but may result from trauma, primary intramedullary tumors, extrinsic compression with central cord necrosis, arachnoiditis, hematomyelia, or necrotic myelitis. The developmental type usually begins in the midcervical cord and extends upward to the medulla or downward as low as the lumbar cord. It commonly takes an eccentric position, often causing unilateral long tract signs or reflex asymmetries. Many cases occur in association with craniovertebral abnormalities, most commonly the Arnold-Chiari malformation, but also including myelomeningocele, basilar skull impression (platybasia), atresia of the foramen of Magendie, or Dandy-Walker cysts (see Chap. 378).

The cardinal signs of syringomyelia correspond to a central high cervical cord syndrome and depend on the extent of the syrinx and associated abnormalities such as the Arnold-Chiari malformation. The classic presentation is (1) sensory loss, usually of a dissociated type (loss of pain and temperature and preservation of touch and vibration senses), which is "suspended" over the nape of the neck, shoulders, and upper arms (cape distribution), and eventually extends to the hands, (2) wasting of muscles in the lower neck, shoulders, arms, and hands, with asymmetric or absent reflexes, and (3) high thoracic kyphoscoliosis. The majority begin asymmetrically with unilateral sensory loss. A number of patients develop loss of pin sensation on the face from damage to the descending tract of the trigeminal nerve in the upper cervical cord. Cough-induced headache and neck pain are common with associated Arnold-Chiari malformations.

A

B

FIGURE 381-4 *A.* Horizontal CT section 1 h after subarachnoid instillation of water-soluble contrast medium showing the cervical spinal cord surrounded by contrast and dye in a large intramedullary syrinx cavity (*arrow*). *B.* Sagittal MRI of same patient as in *A* showing the syrinx cavity and enlargement of the spinal cord (*arrows*). *(Courtesy of Greg Shoukimas, M.D., Department of Radiology, Massachusetts General Hospital.)*

Symptoms in idiopathic cases begin in adolescence or early adulthood, progress irregularly, and frequently arrest for several years. A few patients escape major disability, but over half become wheelchair-bound. Analgesia leads to injuries, burns, and trophic ulcers in the fingertips. Charcot joints in the shoulders, elbows, or knees are common in advanced cases. Prominent lower extremity weakness or hyperreflexia suggests an associated abnormality at the craniovertebral junction. Syringobulbia results from extension of the cavity into the medulla, or rarely the pons, usually occupying the lateral medullary tegmentum. Palatal and vocal cord paralysis, dysarthria, nystagmus, episodic dizziness, tongue weakness, and Horner's syndrome may occur.

The diagnosis can be made dependably from the clinical features, confirmed by finding an enlarged cervical cord on delayed CT images several hours after subarachnoid instillation of metrizamide or another water-soluble contrast material (Fig. 381-4A), but syrinx cavities are shown to greatest advantage by MRI (Fig. 381-4B). The cervicomedullary junction should be examined for associated developmental abnormalities. Therapy is directed at decompressing the cavity to prevent progression of damage and decompressing the spinal canal if the cord is distended. Laminectomies and suboccipital decompression are sometimes recommended when an Arnold-Chiari malformation accompanies an enlarged cervical cord.

Tabes dorsalis   *Tabes* and *meningovascular syphilis* of the spinal cord are presently rare but at one time had to be considered in the differential diagnosis of most spinal cord syndromes. The most common symptoms of tabes are characteristic fleeting and repetitive, lancinating pains occurring mostly in the legs, less commonly in the back, thorax, abdomen, arms, and face. Severe gait and leg ataxia due to loss of position sense occurs in half of patients. Paresthesias, bladder disturbances, and acute abdominal pain with vomiting (visceral crisis) occur in 15 to 30 percent. The cardinal signs of tabes are loss of reflexes in the legs, impaired position and vibratory sense, Romberg's sign, and bilateral Argyll Robertson pupils, which fail to constrict to light but react with accommodation.

Traumatic spinal cord lesions are discussed in Chap. 376.

GENERAL CARE OF THE PATIENT WITH ACUTE PARAPLEGIA OR QUADRIPLEGIA   Protection from secondary damage to the urinary tract is a high priority in the acute stages of paraplegia. The bladder is areflexic, retains urine, and the patient is unaware of bladder distention, making damage to the detrusor muscle from overdistention possible. Urologic rehabilitation requires bladder drainage and avoidance of urinary infection. This is best accomplished by intermittent catheterization by trained personnel. Continuous closed system urinary drainage, which is associated with a higher infection rate than intermittent catheterization, and suprapubic drainage are less desirable alternatives. Patients with acute lesions, especially those causing spinal shock, frequently need special cardiovascular care because of paroxysmal hypertension or hypotension. Ileus and gastric stress ulcers are other potential acute medical problems in patients with complete transverse cord lesions. Cimetidine, ranitidine, or sucralfate may be useful in these circumstances. Pulmonary embolism due to immobilization is a grave early risk occurring in up to one-third of patients after acute cord trauma. Subcutaneous heparin may reduce the risk of early embolic complications. Rarely, spinal injury patients have become hypercalcemic from immobilization.

High cervical cord lesions cause varying degrees of mechanical respiratory failure requiring artificial ventilation. In cases of incomplete respiratory failure with forced vital capacities of 10 to 20 mL/kg, chest physical therapy is useful, and a negative-pressure cuirass may be used to alleviate atelectasis, particularly if the major lesion is below C4. With severe respiratory failure, tracheal intubation (performed over an endoscope if the spine is unstable), followed by tracheostomy, provides tracheal access for ventilation and suctioning. Phrenic nerve pacing may be useful in some patients with lesions at C5 or above.

As clinical signs stabilize, attention should be directed to the psychological state of the patient and the development of a rehabilitation plan framed by realistic expectations. An aggressive program is often remarkably successful with younger and middle-aged patients, allowing return to home and a productive lifestyle.

Chronic nursing care problems can be handled by patients with varying degrees of assistance. The major issues are related to immobilization: skin breakdown over pressure points, urinary sepsis, autonomic instability, and the potential for pulmonary embolism. Early care includes frequent repositioning, application of skin emollients, and soft bed coverings. Specialized beds turn the patient or distribute body weight evenly rather than predominantly on bony prominences. If the sacral cord segments are undamaged, then a large degree of automatic voiding can be entrained. Patients initially void reflexly between catheterizations and later learn to induce voiding with various maneuvers. If residual urinary volumes lead to infection, surgical procedures or an indwelling catheter may be necessary. Bowel regimens and disimpaction are necessary in most patients to ensure at least biweekly evacuation and avoid colonic distention or obstruction.

Severe hypertension and bradycardia occur in response to noxious superficial stimuli, bladder or bowel distention, or surgery, particularly in patients with cervical and high thoracic cord lesions. Flushing and diaphoresis above the level of the lesion may accompany the hypertension. The mechanism of this dysautonomia is not well understood. A potent antihypertensive agent may be necessary, particularly during surgery, but beta-blocking drugs should probably be avoided. Some patients become severely bradycardic with tracheal suctioning; this can be prevented with small doses of atropine.

Detailed aspects of the physical therapy, rehabilitation, and orthotics related to severe spinal cord diseases may be found in specialized texts.

REFERENCES

AMINOFF MJ, LOGUE V: Clinical features of spinal vascular malformations. Brain 97:197, 1974

BAKER AS et al: Spinal epidural abcess. N Engl J Med 293:463, 1975

BERNS DH et al: Magnetic resonance imaging of the spine. Clin Orthop 244:78, 1989

BYRNE TN, WAXMAN SG: Spinal cord compression. Contemporary Neurology Series, vol 33. Philadelphia, Davis, 1990

CHOUCAIR AK: Myelopathies in cancer patients: Incidence, presentation, diagnosis and management, part 1. Oncology 5:71, 1991

GILBERT RW et al: Epidural cord compression from metastatic tumor: Diagnosis and treatment. Ann Neurol 3:40, 1978

GREENBERG HS et al: Epidural spinal cord compression from metastatic tumor: Results with a new treatment protocol. Ann Neurol 8:361, 1980

HACKING HG et al: Factors related to the outcome of inpatient rehabilitation in patients with neoplastic epidural spinal cord compression. Paraplegia 31:367, 1993

JACOBSON S et al: Isolation of HTLV-II from a patient with chronic, progressive neurological disease clinically indistinguishable from HTLV-I-associated myelopathy/tropical spastic paraparesis. Ann Neurol 33:392, 1993

JEFFERY DR et al: Transverse myelitis. Retrospective analysis of 33 cases, with differentiation of cases associated with multiple sclerosis and parainfectious events. Arch Neurol 50:532, 1993

JOHNSON RT, MCARTHUR JC: Myelopathies and retroviral infections. Ann Neurol 21:113, 1987

LOGUE V, EDWARDS MR: Syringomyelia and its surgical treatment. J Neurol Neurosurg Psychiatr 44:273, 1981

MCILROY WJ, RICHARDSON JC: Syringomyelia: A clinical review of 75 cases. J Can Med Assoc 93:731, 1965

ROPPER AH, POSKANZER DC: Prognosis of acute and subacute transverse myelopathy based on early signs and symptoms. Ann Neurol 4:51, 1978

SNOW RB, WEINER H: Cervical laminectomy and foraminotomy as surgical treatment of cervical spondylosis: A follow-up study with analysis of failures. J Spinal Disord 6:245, 1993

UMBACH I, HEILPORN A: Review article: Post-spinal cord injury syringomyelia. Paraplegia 29:219, 1991

section 2 Disorders of nerve and muscle

382 APPROACH TO THE PATIENT WITH NEUROMUSCULAR DISEASE

ROBERT C. GRIGGS / WALTER G. BRADLEY*

The neuromuscular diseases are disorders of the *motor unit* and of the sensory and autonomic peripheral nerves. Each motor unit consists of (1) the *motor neuron cell body*, located in either the spinal cord anterior horn (for muscles innervated by the spinal cord) or a cranial nerve nucleus (for ocular, facial, bulbar musculature), (2) the *axon* of the motor neuron in the peripheral (or cranial) nerve, (3) the *neuromuscular junction*, and, (4) the *muscle fibers* innervated by the motor neuron. The sensory peripheral nerves comprise (1) the *sensory neuron* cell body in the posterior root ganglion, (2) the *central axon* passing to the spinal cord in the posterior root, (3) the *distal axon* in the peripheral nerve, and (4) the *sensory nerve terminal* in skin, muscle, joint capsule, etc. The autonomic nerves are divided into *sympathetic* and *parasympathetic* fiber systems. The sympathetic preganglionic fibers arise from cell bodies in the intermediolateral column of the spinal cord and enter the sympathetic ganglia, where postganglionic fibers arise to innervate blood vessels or viscera. The parasympathetic preganglionic neurons lie in the brainstem and sacral spinal cord, and axons terminate in the viscera, special sensory organs, or skin, which contain the postganglionic neurons and their nerve terminals. Neuromuscular diseases are classified into four groups depending on which portion of the motor unit is involved (see Table 382-1).

The major symptoms of diseases of the motor unit are muscle weakness, wasting, fatigue, cramps, pain, or stiffness. Symptoms of peripheral nerve disease include, in addition, decreased sensation (hypesthesia or hypalgesia), abnormal sensations (paresthesias), or painful sensations (dysesthesias) (see Chap. 24). Symptoms of autonomic nervous system disease include postural dizziness; abnormal cardiac, visceral, and ocular function; and changes in sweating (see also Chap. 379). The symptoms of neuromuscular disease, particularly those of weakness or sensory disturbance, do not necessarily distinguish disorders of the peripheral nervous system from those of the central nervous system. Most neuromuscular diseases are relatively symmetric in contrast to the asymmetry of many central nervous system diseases.

CLINICAL ASSESSMENT

History and physical examination will lead to a diagnosis in a majority of patients with neuromuscular disease. Failure to arrive at a diagnostic impression before routine and sophisticated laboratory studies often leads to diagnostic inaccuracy and confusion. Few of the biochemical, histologic, and electrodiagnostic studies used to evaluate patients with neuromuscular disease are pathognomonic, since nerve and muscle can respond to disease processes in only a limited number of ways.

CLINICAL HISTORY Weakness and fatigue (See Chap. 21) The patient with weakness, particularly when of gradual onset, may not recognize it, emphasizing the useful axiom that "signs of muscle weakness precede symptoms of weakness." Words such as "numbness," "deadness," "tiredness," or "fatigue" may be used by a patient with weakness who is unfamiliar with what is taking place. On the other hand, some complaints of "weakness" result from systemic rather than neuromuscular disease. In such patients,

* The authors acknowledge the contributions of Robert Young and Bhagwan Shahani to this chapter in previous editions.

TABLE 382-1   Classification of neuromuscular disease

Site of involvement	Typical example
Anterior horn cell	
Without upper motor neuron involvement	Spinal muscular atrophy
With upper motor neuron involvement	Amyotrophic lateral sclerosis
Peripheral nerve	
Unifocal	Carpal tunnel syndrome
Multifocal	Mononeuritis multiplex (e.g., polyarteritis nodosa)
Diffuse	Diabetic neuropathy
Neuromuscular junction	Myasthenia gravis
Muscle	Duchenne's muscular dystrophy

strength is often normal or only mildly reduced, since the complaint is usually loss of stamina and endurance. The patient with fatigue should be asked to distinguish between true weakness and the less specific symptoms of lassitude and asthenia. If the patient is unable to perform a normal activity, true weakness is suggested. Objective evidence of weakness is established if symptoms exceed the bounds of normal variation (e.g., double vision, drooping eyelids, difficulty in swallowing, aspiration of food or liquids into the airway) as opposed to the more subjective complaints of inability to lift, carry, or push an object.

The time-course and severity of weakness must be quantitated by questions concerning alterations in functional abilities: for the legs, difficulty in rising from a chair or commode, rising from a squatting position, or climbing up and down stairs and a history of frequent tripping, stumbling, or falling; for the trunk, difficulty in sitting up from supine in bed; or for the arms, difficulty in washing the hair, opening jars, fastening buttons, or raising objects onto a shelf.

Abnormalities of sensation (See Chaps. 24 and 383) Sensory symptoms suggest peripheral nerve disease, although, as with weakness, sensory abnormalities can occur with disease at any level of the nervous system. The characteristics and localization of sensory symptoms in the various peripheral nerve syndromes and diseases are discussed in Chap. 24. In contradistinction to weakness, it is axiomatic that "sensory symptoms precede objective sensory signs."

Muscle pain (See Chap. 23) Muscle aches and pains may suggest inflammatory or metabolic muscle disease but are far more common in bone, joint, and nerve disease. Persistent muscle pain in a patient with normal strength usually results from a cause other than myopathy. Intermittent muscle pain, however, particularly when precipitated by exercise, should raise a consideration of a substrate utilization defect such as a glycogen or lipid storage myopathy. It is important to determine if other factors, such as fasting, precipitate pain and then to inquire about associated findings such as dark urine which may be indicative of myoglobinuria.

Autonomic dysfunction The most common complaint is "dizziness" or "blackouts," which prove to be precipitated by the patient standing up from sitting or lying (see Chap. 17). Loss of potency in the male is frequent in autonomic neuropathies. Explosive diarrhea or cyclical diarrhea-constipation are sometimes present, as is partial urinary retention.

PHYSICAL EXAMINATION   Strength testing Reliable testing of strength requires that the examiner have an adequate frame of reference for normal strength and that the patient be motivated and able to cooperate with testing. As with history taking, it is helpful to quantitate the ability to perform tasks required in daily living. The legs are particularly easy to test by observing walking on heels and toes; rising from a chair, noting whether there is a need to use the arms; rising from a squat; and stepping up onto a chair. It is also important to examine the legs for a *knee-extension lag*, the inability to fully extend the leg against gravity. The number of degrees of extension lag can be measured with a goniometer. Patients with even a minor extension lag almost invariably report frequent tripping and falling. The converse is also true: Patients with muscle weakness

who report frequent falls usually have quadriceps muscle weakness producing a knee-extension lag. Trunk and neck muscles can be tested by having the patient sit up from supine; extending the head over the edge of an examining table is a sensitive method of detecting neck weakness. The arms are not as easily evaluated with function testing: inspection of shoulders for scapular winging as the arms are elevated and watching the patient lift the arms above the head test shoulder girdle function. Hand strength can be judged by determining the degree of difficulty in extracting two fingers from the grip of the patient and by noting the ability of the patient to blanch the knuckles when making a tight fist. When the lesion affects a specific region, e.g., the brachial plexus or the ulnar nerve, it is essential to test each individual muscle of the arm or hand.

Formal muscle testing, assigning a numerical grade to muscle strength, is usually based on the MRC (Medical Research Council of Great Britain) 0 to 5 scale:

5—normal
4—able to oppose gravity plus resistance
3—able to move fully against gravity but not resistance
2—able to move with gravity eliminated
1—trace movement
0—no movement

An important assessment is whether a muscle is indeed *weaker than one would expect*, after making allowances for age, male-female differences, inactivity, or generalized illness. If one has a limited time for the testing of muscle strength, the assessment of function is likely to be of more value than formal muscle testing.

Muscle bulk Muscle atrophy and hypertrophy are often difficult to recognize because of wide variation among normal individuals. The problem is accentuated in young children and in obese patients because of overlying adipose tissue. Atrophy is easier to appreciate when asymmetric. Muscle enlargement or hypertrophy is a normal accompaniment of physical activity. It is occasionally a sign of disease in patients with long-standing spasticity or myotonic disorders. So-called pseudohypertrophy, in which the muscles become enlarged by replacement with connective tissue and fat, may be prominent in certain of the muscular dystrophies but is also seen with spinal muscular atrophy and other denervating conditions. Actual hypertrophy of muscle fibers also may be present in these patients. Muscle enlargement also may be caused by infiltration with substances such as amyloid or by parasitic infestation (e.g., cysticercosis).

Focal muscle swelling may be due to inflammatory infiltrates, calcium deposits, localized myositis, sarcoidosis, ectopic calcification, neoplasms, or tendon rupture. Preservation of some parts of a muscle, while other parts atrophy, may occur in spinal muscular atrophy and some forms of muscular dystrophy, giving an appearance of a focal swelling during muscle contraction ("belly hypertrophy"). Single or multiple muscle masses in a patient without weakness may indicate a neoplastic process.

Pathologic fatigue Patients with disorders of neuromuscular transmission such as myasthenia gravis usually can be shown to fatigue on examination. Sustained upward gaze produces gradual ptosis of the eyelids (curtain sign); eye movements become disconjugate on sustained horizontal gaze; the voice may become hoarse, slurred, or nasal with prolonged speech; or a smile may rapidly become a sneer when the patient cannot maintain facial muscle activity. Inability to sustain limb activity is less easily quantitated, since patients who are weak from any cause may have decreased endurance.

Sensory testing Patients with peripheral neuropathy usually have sensory loss. The distribution of sensory disturbance and the modalities affected are often of diagnostic importance (see Chaps. 24 and 383).

Autonomic testing A fall of systolic blood pressure of more than 20 mmHg from lying to standing indicates impaired autonomic control of peripheral blood vessels. A greater fall often occurs with exercise in the erect position. The pulse rate does not increase

TABLE 382-2 Presenting clinical features of the neuromuscular diseases

	Anterior horn cell	Peripheral nerve	Neuromuscular junction	Muscle
Distribution of weakness	Asymmetric limb or bulbar	Symmetric distal	Extraocular, bulbar, proximal limb	Symmetric limb (bulbar in some)
Atrophy	Marked and early	Moderate	None	Slight early; marked later
Sensory involvement	None	Paresthesias, hypesthesia	None	None
Characteristic features	Fasciculations, cramps	Combined sensory and motor abnormality	Diurnal fluctuation	
Reflexes	Variable (depending on degree of upper motor neuronal involvement)	Decreased out of proportion to weakness	Normal	Decreased in proportion to weakness

normally in response to this hypotension if there is an autonomic neuropathy. Similarly, there is no slowing of the heart rate following a sustained Valsalva maneuver (see Chap. 379).

Other findings Myotonia, fasciculations, myokymia, and other spontaneous activity (Chap. 23) should be sought. Certain disorders such as myotonic dystrophy and facioscapulohumeral dystrophy have distinctive and virtually pathognomonic facial features. Less diagnostic but significant facial weakness is found in other myopathies and in myasthenia gravis. Contractures, particularly of the Achilles tendons, limitation of hip joint movement, and scoliosis may indicate that weakness is of long duration.

DIFFERENTIAL DIAGNOSIS Weaknesses produced by diseases of the motor unit are distinguishable from each other by their distribution, by the time-course of the illness, and by accompanying clinical findings such as muscle bulk and tone, reflexes, and sensory findings. The portion of the motor unit involved by a disease process is usually evident from clinical findings (Table 382-2). Motor neuron diseases (Chap. 372) are suggested in the patient whose weakness is accompanied by prominent atrophy, fasciculations, and lack of sensory involvement. The reflexes may be disproportionately depressed if anterior horn cell disease alone is present or pathologically increased if there is coexistent upper motor neuron disease, such as amyotrophic lateral sclerosis. Peripheral neuropathy (Chap. 383) is suggested by the presence of distal weakness associated with sensory involvement. In general, patients with peripheral neuropathy have depressed reflexes; preservation of reflexes in the presence of significant weakness suggests a cause other than neuropathy. Neuromuscular junction disorders (Chap. 386) are suggested if ocular and bulbar weakness is prominent, particularly if there is *diurnal variation*, with the patient becoming weaker as the day progresses. Pathologic fatigue usually can be demonstrated. Reflexes are preserved in most neuromuscular junction disorders, particularly myasthenia gravis.

Myopathy versus other neuromuscular disease Clinical features which suggest myopathy in contrast to other motor unit diseases include a proximal distribution of weakness, relative preservation or increase of muscle bulk, and the preservation of reflexes. Table 382-3 presents a classification of primary muscle diseases. Many patients with muscle symptoms, however, do not have a primary myopathy, and clinical evaluation discloses disease in another portion of the motor unit or in another system (see Chap. 21). For example, a patient with a denervation produced by nerve root damage from a lumbar disk protrusion may have muscle cramps, pain, and weakness in muscles innervated by those nerve roots. Furthermore, fatigue, weakness, and pain are common accompaniments of derangements of cardiac, hematologic, gastrointestinal, pulmonary, renal, or hepatic function. Despite complaints of weakness and fatigue and the finding of atrophy, it is relatively infrequent for patients with pulmonary or cardiac disease to be mistaken for those with primary muscle disease.

Proximal weakness is so characteristic of myopathies that, by a somewhat circular argument, proximal weakness is usually attributed to "myopathy." In fact, neuropathies such as acute or chronic inflammatory polyneuropathy, the neuromuscular junction disorders, and many anterior horn cell diseases have predominantly proximal weakness. Proximal weakness, occurring in disorders such as hyperthyroidism and hyperparathyroidism and as a result of glucocorticoid

administration, is often termed "myopathic," despite the fact that the underlying pathophysiology of the muscle disorders in these conditions has not been defined.

Acute generalized weakness Weakness developing over the course of less than an hour is usually caused by a metabolic or toxic disorder affecting either the neuromuscular junction or muscle. A sudden alteration in circulating levels of potassium, calcium, sodium, magnesium, or phosphate may result in partial or complete paralysis of muscle. Acute failure of neuromuscular junction transmission may occur with botulism and other toxins, hypermagnesemia, aminoglycoside antibiotics, and other medications. Weakness developing over the course of 24 h may occur in electrolyte, metabolic, and toxic disorders; in periodic paralysis (Chap. 387); and in acute inflammatory myopathies, particularly those related to viral and parasitic infection (Chap. 384) and certain acute polyneuropathies (Chap. 383). Occasionally, patients with more chronic disorders first realize that they are weak when the insidious progression of their weakness produces an abrupt change in function.

Subacute weakness Weakness developing over days is more common in peripheral nerve or neuromuscular junction diseases than in muscle or anterior horn cell disease. Acute inflammatory polyneuropathy (Guillain-Barré syndrome) and porphyric, diphtheritic, and toxic neuropathies are of subacute onset. Myasthenia gravis and other neuromuscular junction diseases also must be considered in the differential diagnosis. Subacute weakness can occur in severe polymyositis and dermatomyositis (see Chap. 384). Weakness from endocrine disorders and certain muscle toxins (see Table 382-3) also

TABLE 382-3 Classification of primary muscle diseases

Hereditary
  A Muscular dystrophy (Chap. 385): Duchenne's, myotonic, facioscapulohumeral, limb-girdle, oculopharyngeal, scapuloperoneal, congenital, distal, and ocular
  B Congenital myopathies (Chap. 385): Central core, nemaline, centronuclear, fiber-type disproportion
  C Metabolic myopathies (Chap. 385):
    1 Glycogen: Deficiencies of phosphorylase, phosphofructokinase, phosphoglyceromutase, acid maltase, others
    2 Lipid: Defective synthesis or transport of carnitine; deficiency of carnitine palmitoyl transferase
    3 Purine nucleotide cycle: Deficiency of myoadenylate deaminase
  D Myotonia (Chap. 385 and 387): Congenita, paramyotonia
  E Periodic paralysis (Chap. 23 and 387): Hypokalemic, hyperkalemic, normokalemic
Inflammatory (Chap. 384)
  A Collagen disease: Systemic lupus erythematosus, rheumatoid arthritis, scleroderma, mixed-connective tissue
  B Sarcoidosis, carcinoid
  C Infections: Numerous, especially viral (influenza B), protozoal (toxoplasmosis), parasitic (trichinosis)
  D Idiopathic: Polymyositis, dermatomyositis, inclusion body myositis
Endocrine and metabolic (Chap. 385)
  A Electrolyte abnormalities: Calcium, phosphate, magnesium, sodium, potassium
  B Endocrine: Hypo- and hyperfunction of thyroid, adrenal, parathyroid, pituitary
Toxic (Chap. 385): Alcohol, opiates, pentazocine, clofibrate, others
Tumors and masses: Primary and metastatic neoplasms, infection, sarcoidosis, myositis ossificans, calcinosis, muscle rupture and hemorrhage

may develop subacutely (Chap. 385). Of the anterior horn cell disorders, only infections with poliomyelitis and other viruses commonly evolve subacutely. Amyotrophic lateral sclerosis occasionally pursues a subacute, severe course.

Slowly progressive weakness *Slowly progressive proximal weakness* evolving over weeks to months may be caused by polymyositis or dermatomyositis or an unsuspected endocrinopathy. When the course has extended for a year or more, however, one of the muscular dystrophies, spinal muscular atrophy, or a neuromuscular junction defect such as myasthenia gravis may be present. Neuropathies are seldom proximal, the major exceptions being acute and chronic inflammatory polyneuropathy, porphyric neuropathy, and diabetic proximal mononeuropathy. *Slowly progressive distal weakness* is more characteristic of peripheral nerve or anterior horn cell disorders than of disorders of muscle or the neuromuscular junction. The only commonly encountered distal myopathy is myotonic dystrophy. Less common disorders such as distal muscular dystrophy, nemaline and centronuclear myopathies, and a variant of polymyositis known as *inclusion body myositis* may present with distal weakness. Prominent distal lower limb weakness is also present in the facioscapulohumeral and scapuloperoneal muscular dystrophies, but proximal involvement is invariably also present in such patients. *Slowly progressive bulbar weakness* is more typical of anterior horn cell or neuromuscular junction disorders than of myopathies. Bulbar weakness (difficulty in speaking, coughing, and swallowing) occurs commonly in motor neuron disease (especially amyotrophic lateral sclerosis) and neuromuscular junction disorders. It is also seen in oculopharyngeal dystrophy, myotonic dystrophy, and polymyositis or dermatomyositis. *Ocular muscle weakness and ptosis* do not occur in motor neuron disease and are uncommon in peripheral neuropathy. Ophthalmoparesis is typical of myasthenia gravis and may occur in myotonic and oculopharyngeal dystrophies. Weakness limited to or predominantly ocular in location (*progressive external ophthalmoplegia*) occurs in disorders such as the Kearns-Sayre syndrome (Chap. 385).

LABORATORY ASSESSMENT

Patients with significantly impaired strength and sensation merit thorough diagnostic study. The sequence of investigations should be based on the test's diagnostic specificity and sensitivity, level of patient discomfort, and cost. Hematologic, renal, and hepatic function and serum electrolytes should be evaluated. In many instances, thyroid, adrenal, and other endocrine studies may be indicated. Other useful diagnostic tests are the serum creatine kinase (CK) level, nerve conduction studies, electromyography, and in many instances muscle biopsy. Nerve biopsy is a more specialized technique with a relatively small number of specific indications (see Chap. 383). Repetitive stimulation of nerve with recording from muscle should be obtained when a neuromuscular junction defect is suspected. Since many diagnostic tests are uncomfortable and expensive, it is important to consider what information is being sought in requesting each test. Confounding features in the investigations also must be understood. For instance, muscle necrosis and inflammation and an elevated serum CK level may occur after minor muscle trauma such as is caused by electromyography and intramuscular injection. Electromyography and muscle biopsy obtained from a muscle affected by past nerve root disease (e.g., from a herniated disk) may show neuropathic abnormalities unrelated to a new disease process. A patient complaining of weakness and fatigue who is found on examination to have no weakness should be examined during exercise. Some of these patients have a metabolic myopathy. Others may have a neuromuscular junction, central nervous system, or psychological problem requiring appropriate investigations.

BIOCHEMICAL EVALUATION OF NEUROMUSCULAR DISEASE Certain enzymes, especially CK, occur in high concentrations in the sarcoplasm of muscle and may leak into blood to serve as an indicator of muscle damage. The serum CK, lactic dehydrogenase (LDH), aspartate aminotransferase (AST, SGOT), and alanine aminotransferase (ALT, SGPT) levels may be elevated in patients with active muscle destruction. Since several of these enzymes are used for screening for abnormalities of organs other than muscle, it is not uncommon for a patient with muscle disease to be first identified by an unexpected elevation in one of these enzymes. The clue to the muscle origin of the increased enzyme levels is that the degree of abnormality decreases in the order CK > LDH > SGOT > SGPT. The serum CK level is the most sensitive test and may be very high (raised more than tenfold) in diseases with muscle fiber necrosis, such as the muscular dystrophies, polymyositis, and rhabdomyolysis. It is frequently slightly elevated in spinal muscular atrophy, amyotrophic lateral sclerosis, and other motor neuron disorders and is usually normal in peripheral neuropathies and neuromuscular junction disorders. Strenuous exercise in normal individuals can elevate the level of serum CK for 6 h or more. Three isoenzymes of CK occur: MM, MB, and BB. MM predominates in skeletal muscle, MB occurs mainly in cardiac muscle, and BB is mainly in brain. Elevations of CK-MB levels are used to indicate the presence of myocardial damage. CK elevation caused by acute muscle injury is usually due to the MM isoenzyme. However, in many patients with long-standing necrotizing muscular diseases and in athletes, the proportion of MB in skeletal muscle rises, and in consequence, the proportion of CK-MB in blood is elevated.

MUSCLE COMPOSITION AND MASS Computed tomography and magnetic resonance imaging can differentiate between muscle fibers, fat, and connective tissue and may show distinctive differences between muscular dystrophy and the other forms of muscle disease. The high cost and the nonspecificity of the findings limit the role of these techniques. Estimations of total muscle mass are of some importance in metabolic studies. A simple decline in muscle mass without weakness is indicative of a process other than a neuromuscular disease, e.g., aging, neoplasm, impaired nutrition, renal or hepatic disease. The 24-h urinary creatinine excretion is the most widely available technique used to estimate muscle mass; it is decreased in patients with wasting from any cause.

METABOLIC, ENDOCRINE, AND OTHER STUDIES Hypo- and hyperkalemia, hypernatremia, hypo- and hypercalcemia, hypophosphatemia, and hypermagnesemia can all cause severe, usually acute, weakness. Serum potassium levels are labile and subject to rapid shifts induced by acidosis or alkalosis. The intracellular concentration of potassium is high, so hemolysis during blood collection may spuriously elevate the potassium level. The extensive muscle damage in rhabdomyolysis may produce a true hyperkalemia. Such elevations in serum potassium level are generally not greater than 0.1 mmol/L, however, unless the serum is stained with hemoglobin, as occurs with hemolysis, or the urine is stained with myoglobin, as occurs with rhabdomyolysis.

Chronic endocrine disorders, either hypo- or hyperfunction of thyroid, adrenal, or parathyroid glands, may cause weakness in the absence of other clinical evidence of endocrinopathy. Rheumatoid arthritis, systemic lupus erythematosus, scleroderma, and the polymyalgia rheumatica syndrome may be complicated by muscle weakness. Tests for these diseases are usually indicated in the evaluation of unexplained muscle pain and weakness. The weakness in most of these disorders is related to disuse atrophy and joint pain; muscle inflammation and evidence of muscle destruction are uncommon. Disorders of muscle mitochondrial function may cause a high plasma lactate level. Other laboratory investigations that may be indicated in patients with peripheral neuropathy include tests for diabetes mellitus; levels of serum vitamin B_{12}, folate, and lipids; serum protein electrophoresis; urinary and serum immunoelectrophoresis; lipoprotein electrophoresis; and urinary porphyrins and heavy metal levels. Diagnostic enzyme determinations are available in white blood cells in certain neuromuscular disorders, such as aryl sulfatase and acid maltase deficiencies.

MYOGLOBINURIA Acute muscle destruction, *rhabdomyolysis* associated with myoglobinuria, occurs with acute toxic, metabolic, inflammatory, infectious, and traumatic muscle damage (see Chap. 384). The molecular weight of myoglobin is lower than that of hemoglobin, so the urine rather than the serum changes color in extensive rhabdomyolysis. Myoglobinuria causes a positive urine test for blood in the absence of urinary erythrocytes. Confirmatory testing for myoglobin uses a specific immunoassay.

EXERCISE TESTING (See Chap. 385) Patients with substrate utilization defects characteristically have decreased exercise tolerance and muscle pain and weakness during or following exercise. Most defects in the enzymatic pathways of glycolysis result in the failure of muscle to generate adenosine triphosphate (ATP) from glycogen and a diminished or absent production of lactic acid. Patients with these disorders can be evaluated with forearm exercise determining the level of venous lactic acid. Patients with disturbance of fatty acid metabolism (such as carnitine palmitoyl transferase deficiency, in which long-chain fatty acids cannot be transferred into mitochondria for beta oxidation) generate lactic acid normally. Patients with myoadenylate deaminase deficiency generate lactate in normal or increased amounts but fail to produce ammonia in the exercise test (Chap. 385). Measurement of specific muscle enzymes can define the cause of the disorder.

ELECTROPHYSIOLOGIC STUDIES OF NEUROMUSCULAR DISEASE

NORMAL MOTOR UNIT PHYSIOLOGY The motor unit is the final common pathway for motor activity of the nervous system, and muscle is the final effector of the motor unit. All movement, posture, and reflex activity results from integrated discharge of large numbers of motor units by spinal and supraspinal mechanisms. The strength of a muscle contraction depends on the number of motor units recruited, the frequency of motor unit discharge, the speed of contraction of muscle fibers in the motor unit, and the nature of the motor unit (whether fatigue-resistant or fatigue-prone). The number of motor units varies greatly among muscles, ranging from as few as 10 in the extraocular muscles, to approximately 100 in the intrinsic muscles of the hands, to several thousand in leg muscles such as the gastrocnemius. The number of muscle fibers per muscle varies up to a thousandfold, from 1000 in extraocular muscles to over 1 million in large leg muscles. The muscle fibers of the motor unit are dispersed randomly within an area of muscle, and fibers innervated by the same anterior horn cell are generally not contiguous. An understanding of the organization of motor units and their patterns of firing is important in the interpretation of clinical and laboratory findings in normal and diseased muscle.

The physiologic characterization of the muscle fibers relates importantly to the exercise capacity of muscle. Motor units that consist of type 1 slow-twitch muscle fibers are designed for continuous and prolonged activity, since their energy supply is derived from the oxidative metabolism of mitochondria. These motor units are smaller and are activated (*recruited*) by low-intensity efforts. High-intensity effort or rapid muscle contraction, such as lifting of a heavy weight or sprinting, recruits larger motor units that consist of rapid-twitch type 2 muscle fibers, which derive their energy supply from anaerobic glycolysis.

As muscles relax, the cessation of firing of individual motor units occurs in a groupwise fashion so that a patient exerting an inadequate effort owing to functional weakness (e.g., malingering), lack of motivation, or pain will frequently have a ratchet-like or "give-way" quality on muscle testing. This may permit the distinction between true and feigned weakness.

ELECTROMYOGRAPHY The normal electromyogram The measurement of electrical activity arising from muscle fibers is usually performed by inserting a needle electrode percutaneously into a muscle. The electrical activity from this electrode is then displayed on a cathode-ray oscilloscope and can be made audible through a loudspeaker. Such studies provide only an average picture of the local

electrical activity of muscle, and normal electrical activity in one area does not exclude the possibility of pathologic phenomena close by.

In a single muscle fiber, as the action potential travels from the neuromuscular junction toward the ends of the muscle fiber, current flows outward through the normally polarized region of the muscle membrane (*sarcolemma*) toward the depolarized zone (zone A, Fig. 382-1). The recording electrode initially becomes slightly positive relative to the reference electrode (wave A). When the depolarized region moves under the recording electrode (zone B), a negative deflection (wave B) occurs. As the active region moves away from the electrode (zone C), the membrane under the electrode become repolarized (wave C). The net result is a triphasic action potential (see Fig. 382-1). The motor unit comprises many such fibers, and hence firing of many fibers of the motor unit produces a more complex waveform (*the motor unit action potential*) resulting from summation of individual single-fiber action potentials. Normal muscle is electrically silent when at rest, once *insertional activity*, produced by the trauma of placing the needle, has died down. When a muscle is voluntarily contracted, motor unit action potentials appear. With increasing strength of contraction, the number and size of the motor unit action potentials increase, until with full contraction individual motor unit potentials can no longer be distinguished, and a *complete recruitment (interference) pattern* is produced.

The abnormal electromyogram SPONTANEOUS ACTIVITY DURING COMPLETE RELAXATION Persistent insertional activity occurs in myotonic disorders, in polymyositis, and in denervated muscles. Spontaneous activity of a single muscle fiber is called *fibrillation*, and of part of or an entire motor unit, *fasciculation*. Triphasic fibrillation potentials and biphasic positive sharp waves can be seen 7 to 25 days after denervation of muscle fibers (depending on the distance of denervated muscle fibers from the site of the nerve lesion) and may persist for several years unless reinnervation occurs. Fibrillation appears with destruction of the motor neuron or its axon and in muscle diseases where a portion of a muscle fiber is separated from its innervated portions by segmental necrosis.

FIGURE 382-1 The single muscle fiber action potential. The shaded area represents the zone of the action potential at each of three positions, A, B, and C, as it sweeps along the muscle fiber from left to right. When the action potential reaches zone A, wave A is seen in the cathode-ray oscilloscope (*CRO*), reflecting the positive potential difference between the active (*vertical arrow*) and the reference (*Ref.*) electrodes. When the action potential reaches zone B, wave B occurs, and when it reaches zone C, wave C is recorded at the active electrode.

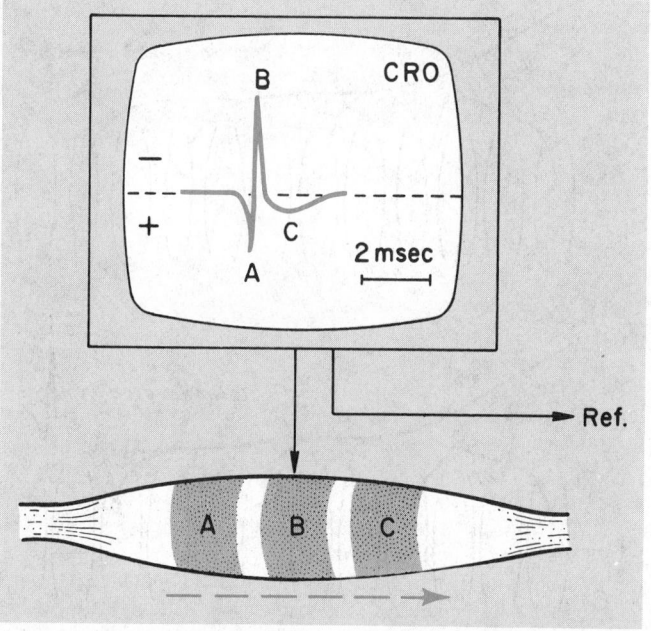

Fasciculations are seen with slowly progressive disease of the anterior horn cells such as amyotrophic lateral sclerosis and progressive spinal muscular atrophy, with compressive nerve root lesions, and in some motor neuropathies. In the syndrome of *benign fasciculations*, the same motor unit tends to fire at a regular rate that is usually faster than that of fasciculations indicative of disease.

In *myotonia*, the sarcolemma is irritable, and repeated muscle depolarization and contraction occur despite voluntary relaxation (see Chap. 385). Such patterns occur in myotonia congenita, myotonic dystrophy, and the periodic paralyses. On electromyography (EMG), myotonia causes high-frequency repetitive discharges that wax and wane in amplitude and frequency, producing a "dive bomber" or "motorcycle" sound on the loudspeaker. *Bizarre, repetitive high-frequency discharges* without waxing and waning are seen in many disorders affecting the motor neurons or muscle. *Coupling of action potentials* into doublets, triplets, or higher multiples of single units occurs in tetany, hemifacial spasm, and myokymia and indicates

FIGURE 382-2 Motor unit potentials. The shaded muscle fibers are functional members of one motor unit; the axon, which enters from the upper left, branches terminally to innervate the appropriate muscle fibers. The motor unit action potential produced by each motor unit is seen in the upper right; its duration is measured between the two small vertical lines. The normal-appearing but unshaded fibers belong to other motor units. *A.* The normal situation, with five muscle fibers in the active unit. *B.* In this myopathic unit, only two fibers remain active; the other three (shrunken and unshaded) have been destroyed by a muscle disease. *C.* Four fibers which belonged to other motor units and had been denervated have now been reinnervated by terminal axon sprouting from the healthy motor unit. Both the motor unit and its action potential are now larger than normal. Note that only under these abnormal circumstances do fibers in the same unit lie next to one another.

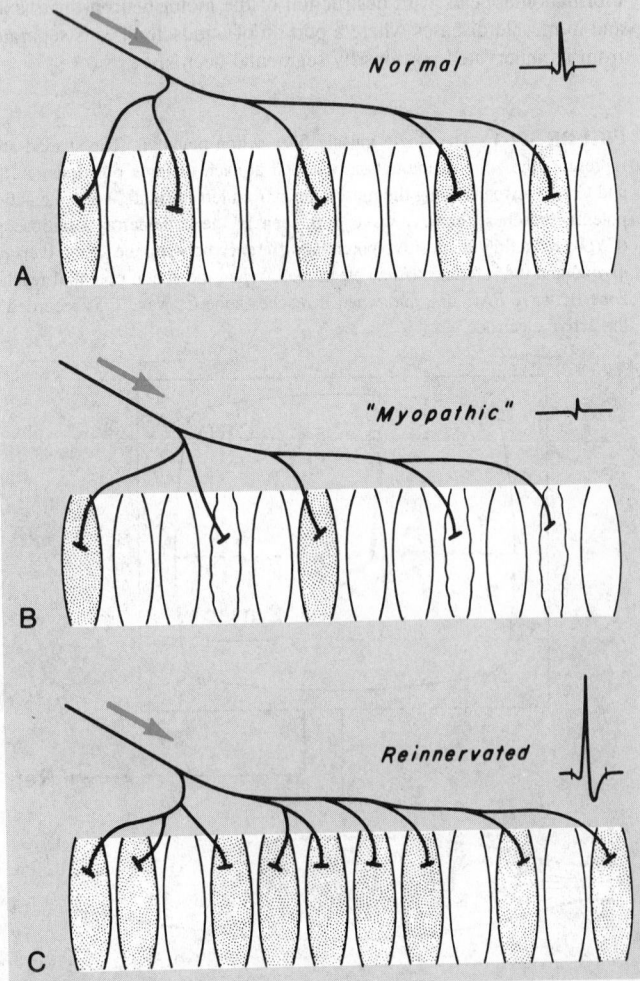

instability in repolarization of the nerve fiber. Electrical silence characterizes *contracture*, as in McArdle's disease and malignant hyperthermia.

ABNORMALITIES IN MOTOR UNIT POTENTIALS   Early in the course of denervation, the remaining motor units are normal, but with the development of reinnervation, the remaining motor units increase in amplitude and become longer in duration and polyphasic (see Fig. 382-2). Conversely, in diseases such as polymyositis, the muscular dystrophies, and other myopathies that destroy scattered fibers within a motor unit (Fig. 382-2), the motor unit action potentials are of lower amplitude and shorter duration and are polyphasic.

In diseases of the central or peripheral nervous system, a *reduced recruitment (interference) pattern* results from maximum voluntary effort because fewer motor units are activated. Conversely, in patients with primary muscle disease, submaximal voluntary effort produces a *full recruitment pattern* despite marked weakness. Because fewer muscle fibers are active, however, the amplitude of the pattern is reduced from normal.

A number of advanced electromyographic techniques, such as single-fiber EMG and macro EMG (see Chap. 366), have been developed to investigate the stability of neuromuscular junction and motor unit reinnervation; their description is beyond the scope of this presentation.

Nerve conduction studies   Stimulation of the larger peripheral motor and sensory nerves permits the recording of their action potentials and provides objective quantitative data of *latency* and *conduction velocity*. The technique is performed by stimulating the nerve with surface electrodes placed over the nerve. The resulting *compound action potential* is recorded by electrodes placed over the nerve proximally in the case of large sensory nerve fibers or over the muscle distally in the case of motor nerve fibers in a mixed motor sensory nerve (see Fig. 382-3). The normal maximum motor and sensory nerve conduction velocities vary from 40 to 80 m/s in different peripheral nerves. Values are approximately half in newborn infants and reach the adult range by 3 to 4 years of age. Normal values have been defined for *distal* or *peripheral latencies* that represent conduction time from the most distal stimulating electrodes, measured in milliseconds from the stimulus artifact to the onset of the response. It is important that the limb be kept warm during nerve conduction studies because subnormal temperatures cause slower conduction velocity. The *compound muscle action potential* obtained by stimulating a mixed motor nerve is of relatively high amplitude (5 to 10 mV) because of the amplification produced by the large number of muscle fibers in each motor unit. Sensory nerve action potentials, lacking this amplification, are of low amplitude (10 to 50 μV) and hence are more difficult to record. In abnormal nerves, sensory nerve action potentials may be small or absent, and sensory conduction measurements may be impossible to record. In contrast, reliable measurement of motor conduction velocities are usually possible even though only a few functional motor nerve fibers remain intact.

Maximum nerve conduction velocity measurements reflect the status of the best surviving of the largest myelinated nerve fibers and may be normal despite extensive loss of nerve fibers. Hence nerve conduction velocity is normal or only slightly below normal in many neuropathies, although the amplitude of the evoked action potential is often reduced. In diseases of peripheral nerves causing severe segmental demyelination, such as chronic inflammatory polyneuropathy, diphtheria, metachromatic leukodystrophy, and the hereditary demyelinating hypertrophic neuropathies, the maximum nerve conduction velocities may be reduced to below half normal. Focal compressions of nerve, as in entrapment syndromes, produce localized slowing of conduction because of demyelination and narrowing of axons at the site of compression. The conduction of proximal segments of the nerves and nerve roots can be studied by F waves and H reflexes (see Chap. 366), or by stimulation of nerve roots by a needle electrode or magnetic stimulator.

Repetitive stimulation tests   In myasthenia gravis, a disorder of the neuromuscular junction, the size of the initial compound muscle

FIGURE 382-3 Measurement of nerve conduction velocity. The median nerve is stimulated through the skin at the wrist (1) or in the antecubital fossa (2), and the resultant compound muscle action potential is recorded as the potential difference between a surface electrode over the thenar eminence (*vertical arrow*) and a reference electrode (*Ref.*) more distally. Sweep 1′ on the cathode-ray oscilloscope (*CRO*) depicts the stimulus artifact (moment of stimulation at 1) followed by the muscle potential. The distal latency is the time *A′* on the CRO sweep (3.0 ms, for example) which corresponds to conduction over distance *A* in the hand. The same is true for sweep 2′ where stimulation is at point 2, and the time from artifact to response is *A′* + *B′*. The maximal motor conduction velocity from points 2 to 1 is obtained by dividing distance *B* by time *B′*.

action potential produced by a supramaximal electrical stimulus to the nerve may be normal. However, after a few stimuli at rates of 2 to 3 Hz, the amplitude of compound muscle action potential declines. It then increases again after the fourth or fifth stimulus. This pattern of decrement followed by increment is characteristic of myasthenia gravis. This defect resembles the partial blockade produced by curare and reflects a postjunctional disorder of synaptic function. The defect is reversed by administration of anticholinesterase medications such as intravenous edrophonium hydrochloride (5 to 10 mg). A progressive decline in the compound muscle action potential with repetitive stimulation also may occur in poliomyelitis, amyotrophic lateral sclerosis, myotonia, and other diseases of the motor unit. Usually, the typical pattern of decrement-increment seen in myasthenia gravis is not present in other disorders.

In the Lambert-Eaton (myasthenic) syndrome, repetitive stimulation causes a facilitation of transmission. Rapid stimulation of nerve (20 to 30 Hz) results in a progressive increase in the amplitude of the muscle action potential, which is small at the first stimulus, to a nearly normal amplitude. This facilitation response is not affected by anticholinesterase drugs.

HISTOPATHOLOGY OF MUSCLE AND NERVE

MUSCLE BIOPSY Biopsy is useful in (1) distinguishing between neurogenic and myopathic processes, (2) recognizing specific disorders of muscle such as muscular dystrophy or the congenital myopa-

thies, (3) identifying specific metabolic defects of muscle by histochemical or biochemical techniques, and (4) diagnosing diseases of connective tissue and blood vessels, such as polyarteritis nodosa, and infections such as trichinosis.

Muscle biopsy is performed under local anesthesia. In children and in adults with diffuse conditions, an adequate specimen often can be obtained by needle biopsy. Open biopsy may be necessary to obtain sufficient tissue to diagnose focal, patchy processes such as myositis or vasculitis. In all instances, the muscle chosen for sampling must be appropriate for the condition suspected, and the specimen must be handled by a laboratory skilled in the evaluation of muscle biopsies. Muscles to be biopsied should generally be only slightly weak. If the biopsy is taken from a muscle that has recently been traumatized by an EMG needle or that has been affected by a preexisting disease (e.g., coincidental nerve root compression), misleading information will be obtained.

Muscle fibers are subdivided into two types which have different staining characteristics with the myosin ATPase reaction at pH 9.4. Type 1 fibers (fatigue-resistant and rich in oxidative enzymes) stain lightly with this reaction, and type 2 fibers (fast-contracting, fatigue-prone, and rich in glycolytic enzymes) stain darkly. Normal muscle has a random distribution of fibers of the two histochemical types.

Denervation, reinnervation A denervated muscle fiber undergoes atrophy, and in the initial stages myofibrils are lost to a greater degree than is sarcoplasm containing the mitochondria, so the muscle fibers appear "super dark" with stains for oxidative enzymes (Fig. 382-4). Such denervated fibers are squeezed by adjacent innervated fibers and therefore become angulated and atrophic. In the initial stages of denervation, because of motor unit overlap, denervated atrophic fibers are distributed randomly throughout the muscle. Remaining motor axons sprout to reinnervate such fibers, eventually producing fiber type grouping. With subsequent death of such enlarged motor units, grouped fiber atrophy occurs. The typical appearance of a denervated and reinnervated muscle is shown in Fig. 382-4*B* and *C*. The fiber diameter distribution in chronically denervated and reinnervated muscle is bimodal, with the atrophic denervated fibers making up one population and the normal-sized (or hypertrophied) innervated fibers making up the other population.

Muscle fiber necrosis and regeneration Damage of the sarcolemma of the muscle fiber allows entry of calcium at high extracellular concentration into the low-calcium environment of the sarcoplasm. Calcium entry activates a neutral protease, initiating proteolysis. Calcium also poisons mitochondrial function and can cause cell death. Invading macrophages phagocytize the muscle fibers. Satellite cells, which provide the basis for regeneration of muscle fibers, are spared in most of the processes that damage muscle. They proliferate and fuse to produce multinuclear myotubes leading to regeneration of the muscle fiber. Characteristically, regenerating fibers are small, are basophilic owing to an increased concentration of RNA, and have large vesicular internalized nuclei. The distribution of muscle fiber diameters in a typical chronic myopathy is broad and unimodal, very different from the bimodal diameter distribution of denervated and reinnervated muscle.

Muscle fiber necrosis and regeneration are common in trauma, Duchenne's muscular dystrophy, polymyositis, and dermatomyositis. Eventually, if the necrosis is sufficiently chronic, regeneration may fail, causing progressive loss of muscle fibers and replacement with fat and fibrous tissue. A chronic myopathy, Duchenne's muscular dystrophy, is illustrated in Fig. 382-5. Differences in the extent and tempo of these processes allow histologic distinction among the muscular dystrophies, inflammatory myopathies, and acute rhabdomyolysis.

Structural changes in muscle fibers Degeneration of muscle fibers without frank necrosis produces structural alteration of individual muscle fibers; disorganization of myofibrils and sarcoplasm produces target fibers (Fig. 382-4*C*), ringbinden (appearance of a portion of the myofibrils wrapped circumferentially around the remaining longitudinal myofibrils), central cores, cytoid bodies, and

FIGURE 382-4 *A.* Normal skeletal muscle biopsy stained for myosin ATPase, pH 9.4. Type 1 fibers are light and type 2 dark. *B.* Chronic denervation-reinnervation showing fiber type grouping. Myosin ATPase, pH 9.4. *C.* Chronic denervation-reinnervation in amyotrophic lateral sclerosis, preparation stained for mitochondrial enzyme, NADH-TR. There are groups of reinnervated type 2 fibers (*light*), and of denervated angulated atrophic fibers, many of them "superdark" and showing target-fiber changes. *D.* Type 2 fiber atrophy. Myosin ATPase, pH 9.4.

nemaline bodies. In one congenital myopathy, the fibers resemble myotubes (centronuclear myopathy). In others, abnormal mitochondria suggest an abnormality of mitochondrial biochemistry, while the presence of vacuoles suggests a disturbance of glycogen or lipid metabolism. Rimmed vacuoles (accumulations of degenerating phospholipid material between myofibrils) occur particularly in oculopharyngeal muscular dystrophy and inclusion-body myositis.

Inflammatory changes Perivascular and interstitial inflammatory cell infiltration with lymphocytes and macrophages is characteristic of polymyositis and dermatomyositis. Necrosis and regeneration of muscle fibers are also present. In some instances, atrophy of the fibers located on the periphery of muscle fasciculi (*perifascicular atrophy*) is prominent and can be an indicator of inflammatory myopathy, even though a focus of inflammation is not present in the muscle taken at biopsy. Muscle biopsy may show vasculitis in patients with collagen diseases or granulomas in patients with sarcoidosis.

Changes specific to fiber type Pathologic changes may be restricted to one fiber type in the muscle. The most common such condition is type 2 fiber atrophy (Fig. 382-4*D*), which occurs in a wide range of disorders that limit activity such as disuse, muscle pain, joint pain, and upper motor neuronal dysfunction. Atrophy of type 1 fibers is less frequent and occurs in myotonic dystrophy, rheumatoid arthritis, and some congenital myopathies.

NERVE BIOPSY Nerve biopsy is more difficult and more traumatic than muscle biopsy and is useful in only a limited number of specific circumstances (see Chap. 383). The sural nerve in the leg or

FIGURE 382-5 *A.* Normal muscle (hematoxylin-eosin). *B.* Duchenne's muscular dystrophy, showing hyalin fibers, fiber degeneration, loss of fibers and fibrosis (hematoxylin-eosin).

the superficial radial nerve at the wrist are the usual biopsy sites. Both are sensory nerves and may show no changes in pure motor neuropathies. The biopsy procedure is performed under local anesthesia, and specimens are obtained for light and electron microscopy and for teasing of individual nerve fibers. Nerve biopsy aids in (1) distinguishing between segmental demyelination and axonal degeneration, (2) identifying inflammatory neuropathies, and (3) establishing specific diagnoses such as amyloidosis, sarcoidosis, leprosy, vasculitis, and several metabolic neuropathies. Full evaluation of the nerve biopsy requires the facilities of a laboratory with special interest and experience in peripheral nerve pathology. Light microscopic examination of biopsied nerves is of limited value, showing only gross changes such as vasculitis, inflammation, infiltration by granuloma or amyloid, loss of axons, and axonal degeneration. More information is obtained by electron microscopy and studies of single teased nerve fibers. Some diseases affect specific nerve fiber types. For instance, large myelinated fibers are affected in Friedreich's ataxia and unmyelinated fibers in familial amyloidosis. Quantitative morphometry (measurement of the number of nerve fibers and the distribution of their diameters) can therefore be of additional help. Two basic pathologic processes may be seen in nerve biopsies.

Segmental demyelination Diseases may attack either myelin or the Schwann cell, causing the myelin sheath to undergo degeneration but leaving the axon essentially unchanged. Healing of this segmental demyelination proceeds through a phase of abnormally thin myelin sheaths, which may eventually return to normal thickness. However, even after apparent recovery of segmental demyelination, single teased nerve fiber studies demonstrate short and variable lengths of the internodes (distance between the nodes of Ranvier). If this process is progressive, *onion-bulb formation* occurs, with thinly remyelinated fibers lying at the center of concentric lamellae of redundant Schwann cell cytoplasm.

Axonal degeneration Death of the nerve cell body or section of the axon at any level will lead to degeneration of the distal parts of the axon with secondary degeneration of the myelin sheath. If the nerve cell body remains intact proximally, there is attempted axonal regeneration with sprouting. Such nerve sprouts (*clusters*) are characteristic of degenerating and regenerating axonal neuropathy.

Pathologic changes in neuropathies Axonal degeneration is most common in toxic, inherited, traumatic, and ischemic diseases. Segmental demyelination may occur in the inherited and autoimmune inflammatory disorders; in the latter condition, inflammatory cell infiltration may be seen. A mixed picture of axonal degeneration and segmental demyelination, together with a vasculopathy, is characteristic of diabetes mellitus. Some specific pathologic changes may indicate the probable etiology of a neuropathy. The deposition of IgM on the myelin-associated glycoprotein of the myelin sheaths in IgM gammopathies can be detected by immunofluorescence techniques. The deposition leads to an increase in myelin periodicity. Amyloid fibrils are present in amyloid neuropathy. Specific inclusions may be seen in the Schwann cells in metachromatic leukodystrophy and adrenomyeloleukodystrophy.

GENERAL THERAPEUTIC CONSIDERATIONS

Cardiac Most disorders of skeletal muscle also involve cardiac muscle. Symptomatic cardiac dysfunction is relatively uncommon, however, perhaps because the limited exercise capacity of the patient with weakness decreases demands on cardiac performance. Relatively specific electrocardiographic abnormalities occur in Duchenne's dystrophy and infantile acid maltase deficiency. Cardiac conduction disorders including complete heart block occur in patients with myotonic dystrophy. An electrocardiogram should be obtained in all patients with neuromuscular disease, particularly in patients with myopathies.

Respiratory Diminished pulmonary function in patients with acute or chronic neuromuscular disease may progress to ventilatory failure. The earliest manifestation of respiratory muscle weakness

is a decrease in maximum expiratory and inspiratory pressures. Diaphragmatic weakness in particular may be substantial in patients with neuromuscular disease and should be evaluated by examining pulmonary function while the patient is both supine and sitting. Diaphragmatic weakness causes a decrease in pulmonary function when measured in the supine compared with the erect position. Paradoxical abdominal movements may be evident. Patients with chronic respiratory failure may be maintained with home respiratory support. The possible occurrence of cor pulmonale from insidious respiratory failure should be considered in any patient with neuromuscular disease who develops ankle edema or other signs of heart failure.

Physical therapy Physical therapy is of greatest value in patients with muscle weakness when joint contractures are developing and when enforced immobility, such as an injury, results in decreased activity. Exercises may increase strength in muscles weakened by disease just as in normal persons, but there is little evidence that exercise improves functional abilities. However, therapeutic standing in patients with marginal leg and trunk function has considerable psychological benefit and may help to preserve bone mineralization and cardiovascular reflexes.

Dietary modification Dietary restriction is often necessary in patients with muscle weakness, since caloric expenditure is decreased because of immobility and loss of muscle mass. Development of obesity further compromises already reduced mobility, worsens pulmonary function, and may depress ventilatory drive. Unless there is specific evidence for malabsorption of vitamin B_{12} or vitamin E, neither these nor any other vitamin has a specific role in the treatment of neuromuscular disease. Certain vitamins are hazardous in excessive dosages, including vitamins B_6, A, and D (see Chaps. 77 and 357).

Bracing In patients with distal leg weakness, particularly of foot dorsiflexion, ankle-foot orthoses can restore gait to nearly normal. With more proximal weakness, however, leg braces diminish mobility and are of value only in enabling patients who are unable to walk to perform therapeutic standing. In most adults, even this use of braces is impractical because such standing in braces usually requires assistance.

Scoliosis Spinal deformity complicates many neuromuscular diseases, particularly those which occur before puberty. Duchenne's dystrophy, spinal muscular atrophy, and congenital myopathies are particularly liable to this complication. Once full long-bone growth has been achieved, many of these patients should have surgical correction of the scoliosis. Severely impaired pulmonary function is a contraindication to such therapy; therefore, patients with progressive scoliosis need careful sequential follow-up to determine the appropriate timing for surgery.

GENETIC EVALUATION AND COUNSELING (See also Chap. 385) Management of the patient with hereditary muscle disease should include careful family pedigree analysis and genetic counseling. The family history may initially be negative in many patients with autosomal dominant diseases such as Charcot-Marie-Tooth disease, myotonic dystrophy, and facioscapulohumeral dystrophy because of the variable expressivity of the disorders. The availability of chromosomal markers for linkage analysis and of specific tests for gene abnormalities has made carrier detection, antenatal diagnosis, and early diagnosis of disease feasible in most hereditary neuromuscular diseases (e.g., in Duchenne's and myotonic dystrophy). The availability of therapy for disorders such as periodic paralysis, myotonia, and certain metabolic myopathies and of preventive measures in disorders such as malignant hyperthermia provides a strong impetus for early diagnosis. History alone is often inadequate for family evaluation. Physical examination or inspection of photographs of family members will often identify mildly afflicted individuals, providing clues to the characteristic facial or other features of the disorder. Molecular biologic techniques now permit specific diagnosis of certain neuromuscular diseases by identification of an abnormal or missing gene product. Thus the protein dystrophin is lacking in muscle of patients with Duchenne's dystrophy (see Chap. 385), and the sodium channel is abnormal in hyperkalemic periodic paralysis (see Chap. 387).

REFERENCES

BROOKE MH: *A Clinician's View of Neuromuscular Disease*, 2d ed. Baltimore, Williams and Wilkins, 1986

CARPENTER S, KARPATI G: *Pathology of Skeletal Muscle*. New York, Churchill Livingstone, 1984

DYCK PJ et al (eds): *Peripheral Neuropathy*, 3d ed. Philadelphia, Saunders, 1993

ENGEL AG, FRANZINI-ARMSTRONG C (eds): *Myology*, 2d ed. New York, McGraw-Hill, 1994

KIMURA J: *Electrodiagnosis in Diseases of Nerve and Muscle*, 2d ed. Philadelphia, Davis, 1989

OH SJ: *Electromyography; Neuromuscular Transmission Studies*. Baltimore, Williams and Wilkins, 1988

383 DISEASES OF THE PERIPHERAL NERVOUS SYSTEM

ARTHUR K. ASBURY

The basic processes affecting nerve and muscle and the approach to diseases of nerve and muscle are set forth in Chap. 382. The first purpose here is to build upon that base by providing an overview of the wide array of peripheral neuropathies that afflict humans. Peripheral neuropathy is a general term indicating disorder of peripheral nerve of any cause; the manifestations may be so bewildering and complex that it is difficult for the physician to know where to begin and how to proceed. Therefore the second purpose here is to develop a logical approach and assessment scheme (summarized in Fig. 383-1) which will guide the examiner to correct diagnoses and management decisions.

GENERAL DESCRIPTION OF NEUROPATHIC SYNDROMES

The prototypical picture of polyneuropathy occurs with acquired toxic or metabolic neuropathic states. From a symptom standpoint, the first noticeable features tend to be sensory and consist of tingling, prickling, burning, or bandlike dysesthesias in the balls of the feet or tips of the toes, or in a general distribution over the soles. Symmetry of symptoms and findings in a distal graded fashion is the rule, but occasionally dysesthesias appear in one foot a brief time before the other or may be more pronounced in one foot. Some care and judgment is needed to avoid confusion with mononeuropathy multiplex. If the polyneuropathy remains mild, no objective motor or sensory signs may be detectable.

With progression, pansensory loss is usually found over both feet, ankle jerks are lost, and weakness of dorsiflexion of the toes, best demonstrated in the great toe, may be present. In some instances, the process begins with weakness in the feet, usually dorsiflexion of the toes and feet without subjective sensory symptoms. As worsening occurs, sensory loss moves centripetally in a graded "stocking" fashion, and the patient may complain that the feet have a numb or "wooden" feeling or may say "I feel as though I'm walking on stumps." Patients experience difficulty walking on their heels during examination and their feet may slap while walking. Later, the knee jerk reflex disappears and foot drop becomes more apparent. By the time sensory disturbance has reached the upper shin, dysesthesias are usually noticed in the tips of the fingers. The degree of spontaneous pain varies, but is often considerable. Light stimuli to hypesthetic areas, once perceived, may be experienced as extremely uncomfortable (hyperpathia). Unsteadiness of gait may be out of proportion to muscle weakness because of proprioceptive loss.

FIGURE 383-1 Flowchart approach to the evaluation of peripheral neuropathies. (*After Asbury, 1983.*)

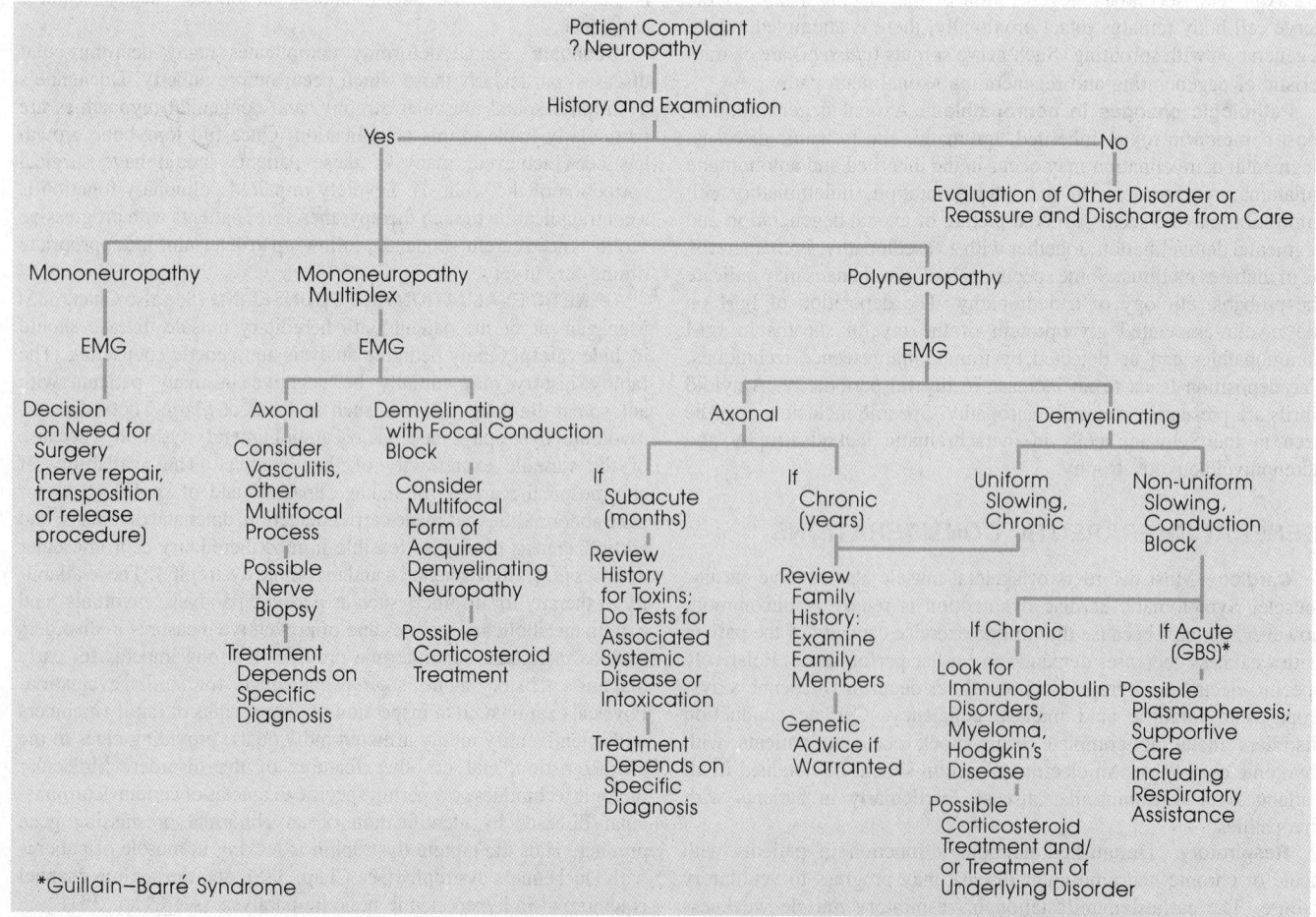

*Guillain–Barré Syndrome

Worsening proceeds in a centripetal, symmetrically graded manner with muscle atrophy, pansensory loss, and areflexia and with motor weakness that is usually greater in the extensor muscles than in corresponding flexor groups. When the sensory disturbance reaches mid thigh, generally a tent-shaped area of hypesthesia on the lower abdomen may be demonstrated. This will grow broader, and the apex will extend rostrally toward the sternum as the neuropathy worsens. By this time, patients generally cannot stand or walk or hold objects in their hands.

In the most extreme cases, ventilatory capacity may be impaired along with sphincteric function. Hypesthesia at the crown of the scalp may be present and spread radially into both the trigeminal and C2 distribution. Considering the entire sequence, nerve fibers are affected according to length of axon without regard to root or nerve trunk distribution—hence, the aptness of the term "stocking-glove" to describe the pattern of sensory deficit. In general, the motor deficit is also graded, distal, and symmetric.

Variations on the general sequence outlined above are manifold and explain the diversity of clinical syndromes encountered. Variations include the rate of evolution; fluctuations in the course; the eventual degree of severity; the presence or absence of positive motor and sensory symptoms; the symmetry of features and their distribution in terms of proximal versus distal, arms versus legs, and motor versus sensory; the relative proportion of dysfunction attributable to large fiber deficit and to small fiber deficit; and the determination, mainly by electrodiagnostic examination, of axonal versus demyelinating processes.

ASSESSMENT AND DIAGNOSIS OF NEUROPATHY **Taking the first step** Clues to the diagnosis of specific peripheral neuropathies often lie in unnoted or readily forgotten events occurring weeks or months prior to the onset of symptoms. Inquiry should be made about recent viral illnesses; other systemic symptoms; institution of new medications; potentially toxic exposures to solvents, pesticides, or heavy metals; the occurrence of similar symptoms in family members or coworkers; habits concerning alcohol; and the presence of known preexisting medical disorders. It is also useful to ask patients if they would otherwise feel well if free of their neuropathic symptoms, to obtain an idea of the presence or absence of an underlying systemic illness.

It is important to learn how symptoms first appeared. Even with distal polyneuropathies, symptoms may appear in the sole of one foot a few days or a week before the other, but usually the patient will describe a distal graded disturbance that moves evenly and symmetrically in centripetal fashion. Tingling dysesthesias will appear in the fingertips only when similar symptoms have reached the level of the knees. It is important to determine whether symptoms first appeared in the distribution of individual digital nerves involving only one-half of a digit at a time and then gradually spread to become coalescent. This pattern of onset raises strong suspicions of a multifocal process (mononeuropathy multiplex) such as might be encountered with a systemic vasculitis or cryoglobulinemia.

The evolution of neuropathy ranges from rapid worsening over a few days to an indolent process extending many years. Polyneuropathies with a slowly progressive course lasting more than 5 years are most likely to be genetically determined, particularly if the major manifestations are distal atrophy and weakness with few or no positive sensory symptoms. Exceptions are diabetic polyneuropathy and paraproteinemic neuropathies in which the progression may be insidious over 5 to 10 years. Axonal degenerations of toxic or metabolic origin tend to evolve over several weeks to a year or more, and the rate of progression of demyelinating neuropathies is highly variable, ranging from a few days in Guillain-Barré syndrome to many years in others.

Major fluctuations in the course of neuropathy raise two possibilities: (1) relapsing forms of neuropathy; or (2) repeated toxic exposures. A slow fluctuation in symptoms taking place over weeks or months (reflecting changes in the activity of neuropathy) should not be confused with day-to-day variation or diurnal undulation of symptoms.

The latter are common to all neuropathic disorders. An example is carpal tunnel syndrome in which dysesthesias may be prominent at night but absent during the day.

In polyneuropathies, the findings are symmetric on both sides of the body. If only one foot slaps when the patient walks, the process is not symmetric and the possibility of a multifocal process is raised. In addition, in acquired symmetric polyneuropathies, the muscles of extension and abduction tend to be weakened to a greater extent than the muscles of flexion and adduction. Hence, weakness in lower legs often affects the peronei and anterior tibial muscles, with attendant foot drop and weakness of eversion, more than the gastrocnemius group or foot inverters. In most polyneuropathies the legs are more severely affected than the arms and the distal muscles more than the proximal ones. There are exceptions to this rule, as in lead neuropathy, in which manifestation of bilateral wrist drop may predominate, and occasionally in porphyric neuropathy, in which arms may be more affected than legs and proximal muscles more than distal.

Palpation of the nerve trunk to detect enlargement is a frequently forgotten part of the neurologic examination. In mononeuropathies, the entire course of the nerve trunk in question should be explored manually for focal thickening; the presence of neurofibroma, point tenderness, or Tinel's phenomenon (generation of a tingling sensation in the sensory territory of the nerve by tapping along the course of the nerve trunk); and elicitation of pain by putting the nerve trunk on stretch. In leprous neuritis, fusiform thickening of nerve trunks is frequent, and beading of nerve trunks may be encountered in amyloid polyneuropathy. In genetically determined hypertrophic neuropathies uniform thickening of all nerve trunks may occur, often to the caliber of a clothesline or larger.

Most neuropathies involve nerve fibers of all sizes, but on occasion selective damage may be restricted either to large or to small fibers. In a polyneuropathy affecting mainly small fibers, diminished pinprick and temperature sensation, often with burning painful dysesthesias, may predominate along with autonomic dysfunction but with relative sparing of motor power, balance, and tendon jerks. Selected cases of amyloid and distal diabetic polyneuropathies fall into this category. In contrast, large-fiber polyneuropathy is characterized by areflexia, imbalance, relatively minor cutaneous sensory deficit, and variable but often severe motor dysfunction.

In addition to a history and a physical examination, other measures need to be undertaken routinely in the evaluation of a patient with neuropathy. Electrodiagnostic examination is a key procedure in all patients. For patients with polyneuropathy or mononeuropathy multiplex, standard tests should include a complete blood count and erythrocyte sedimentation rate, urinalysis, chest x-ray, postprandial blood glucose, and serum protein electrophoresis. Further tests should be dictated by the formulation arrived at via the combined history and physical and electrodiagnostic examination (see Fig. 383-1).

Taking the next step The next step is electrodiagnostic examination. It is not generally possible to make the distinction between axonal versus demyelinating disorders on clinical examination alone; here electrodiagnostic analysis is particularly useful. Electrodiagnostic features of demyelination are slowing of nerve conduction velocity (NCV), dispersion of evoked compound action potentials (CAPs), conduction block (major decrease in amplitude of muscle CAP upon proximal stimulation of its nerve as compared to distal stimulation), and marked prolongation of distal latencies. In contrast, axonal neuropathies are characterized by a reduction in amplitude of evoked CAPs with relative preservation of NCV. The distinction between a primarily demyelinating neuropathy from one that is primarily axonal is crucial because of the differing approaches to diagnosis and management.

If in a particular instance of progressive polyneuropathy of subacute or chronic evolution the electrodiagnostic findings are those of an axonopathy, a long list of metabolic states and exogenous toxins comes into consideration (see Tables 383-1 and 383-2). If the course is protracted over several years, it raises the likelihood of the neuronal (axonal) form of peroneal muscular atrophy (HMSN-II); family

TABLE 383-1 Polyneuropathy associated with systemic diseases

Systemic disease/Occurrence	Axonal*			Demyelinating*			Sensory vs. motor†	Autonomic*	Comment
	Acute	Subacute	Chronic	Acute	Subacute	Chronic			
Diabetes mellitus/Common	−	±	+	−	±	+	S, SM, rarely M	± to +	See Table 383-4
Uremia/Sometimes	±	+	+	−	−	−	SM	±	Controllable with proper dialysis; curable with successful renal transplant
Porphyria (3 types)/Rare	+	±	−	−	−	−	M or SM	± to +	May be proximal > distal and may have atypical proximal sensory deficits
Hypoglycemia/Rare	±	+	±	−	−	−	M	−	Usually with insulinoma; arms often > legs
Vitamin deficiency, exclude B$_{12}$/Sometimes	−	+	+	−	−	−	SM	±	Involves thiamine, pyridoxine, folate, pantothenic acid; probably others
Vitamin B$_{12}$ deficiency/Sometimes	−	±	+	−	−	−	S	−	Neuropathy overshadowed by myelopathy
Critical illness (sepsis)/Common	−	+	±	−	−	−	M > S	−	Severely ill, sepsis patients, often on ventilator
Chronic liver disease/Sometimes	−	−	−	−	−	+	S or SM	−	Usually mild or subclinical
Primary biliary cirrhosis/Rare	−	±	+	−	−	−	S	−	Intraneural xanthomas
Primary systemic amyloidosis/Rare	−	±	+	−	−	−	SM	+	Also in amyloidosis with myeloma or macroglobulinemia
Hypothyroidism/Rare	−	−	−	−	±	+	S	−	May respond to thyroid replacement
Chronic obstructive lung disease/Rare	−	±	+	−	−	−	S or SM	−	Severe pulmonary insufficiency
Acromegaly/Rare	−	−	+	−	−	−	S	−	Carpal tunnel syndrome also frequent
Malabsorption (sprue, celiac disease)/Sometimes	−	±	+	−	−	−	S or SM	±	Basis for neuropathy unclear; deficiency?
Carcinoma (sensory)/Rare	−	+	+	−	−	−	Pure S	−	Due to gangliitic neuronopathy; mostly small cell lung or breast carcinoma; paraneoplastic
Carcinoma (sensorimotor)/Sometimes	−	+	+	−	−	−	SM	±	Sensorimotor axonal neuropathy; mostly with lung carcinoma
Carcinoma (late)/Common	−	+	+	−	−	−	S > M	±	Mild, probably related to weight loss and wasting
Carcinoma (demyelinating)/Sometimes	−	−	−	+	+	±	SM		Acute or relapsing demyelinating neuropathy
HIV infection/Sometimes	−	±	+	−	−	−	S ≫ M		Late stages of AIDS; other neuropathies occur; see text
Lyme disease/Sometimes	−	±	+	−	−	−	S > M		Variable picture; see text
Lymphoma including Hodgkin's/Sometimes	−	+	+	+	+	±	See above	±	Same as with carcinomatous types
Polycythemia vera/Rare	−	±	+	−	−	−	S	−	Also many CNS manifestations; often shooting pains in limbs
Multiple myeloma lytic type/Sometimes	−	±	+	−	−	−	S, M, or SM	±	Symptomatic neuropathy uncommon, subclinical neuropathy frequent
Multiple myeloma‡: osteosclerotic or solitary plasmacytoma/Sometimes	−	−	±	−	±	+	SM	−	May show severe slowing of nerve conduction velocity
Benign monoclonal gammopathy:									
IgA	−	±	+	−	−	−	SM	−	IgM$_\kappa$ (or occasionally
IgG	−	±	+	−	−	−	SM	−	IgM$_\lambda$) may bind to my-
IgM /Sometimes	−	−	−	−	±	+	SM or S	−	elin-associated glyco-protein or glycolipids
Cryoglobulinemia/Sometimes	−	±	+	−	−	−	SM	−	May be mononeuropathy multiplex in presentation

*± = sometimes; + = usual.
†S = sensory; M = motor; SM = sensorimotor.
‡Some cases associated with POEMS syndrome (see text).

members must be examined and additional attention given to the family history. Alternatively, if the electrodiagnostic findings indicate primary demyelination of nerve, the approach is entirely different. The possibilities then include acquired demyelinating neuropathy, thought to be immunologically mediated, and genetically determined neuropathies, some of which are marked by uniform and drastic slowing of nerve conduction velocities.

The flowchart in Fig. 383-1 summarizes the clinical and electrodiagnostic approach to evaluation and management of a neuropathic disorder. Using this scheme, the clinician determines for each patient the tempo, distribution, severity, and functional impairment, and other features previously discussed, making a clinical judgment as to whether the problem represents a mononeuropathy, a mononeuropathy multiplex, or a polyneuropathy. Often this distinction is obvious.

TABLE 383-2 Polyneuropathy associated with drugs or environmental toxins

	Axonal*			Demyelinating*			Sensory vs. motor[†]	Autonomic*	CNS*	Comment
	Acute	Subacute	Chronic	Acute	Subacute	Chronic				
DRUGS										
Amiodarone (anti-arrhythmic)	−	−	+	−	−	+	SM	−	−	Dose-dependent neuropathy, reversible by decreasing dose
Aurothioglucose (antirheumatic)	±	±	−	+	+	−	SM	−	−	Idiosyncratic reaction, ? immune-mediated
cis-Platinum (antineoplastic)	−	+	−	−	−	−	S	−	−	Severe sensory neuropathy, also ototoxicity; dose-related
Dapsone (dermatologic including leprosy)	−	±	+	−	−	−	M	−	−	Dose-related pure motor neuropathy
Disulfiram (antialcohol)	±	+	+	−	−	−	SM	−	±	Usually occurs after months of treatment
Hydralazine (antihypertensive)	−	±	+	−	−	−	S > M	−	−	A pyridoxine antagonist
Isoniazid	−	±	+	−	−	−	SM	±	−	A pyridoxine antagonist; neurotoxic in slow acetylators
Metronidazole (antiprotozoal)	−	−	±	−	−	−	S or SM	−	+	Dose-related central-peripheral distal axonopathy
Misonidazole (radiosensitizer)	−	±	+	−	−	−	S or SM	−	+	Neurotoxicity is the limiting factor
Nitrofurantoin (urinary antiseptic)	−	±	+	−	−	−	SM	−	−	Generally total dose-related; renal failure enhances toxicity
Nucleoside neuropathies (ddC, ddI, d4T) (antiretrovirus)	±	+	+	−	−	−	S ≫ M	−	?	Dose-related; painful
Phenytoin (anticonvulsant)	−	−	+	−	−	−	S > M	−	−	After 20-30 years of phenytoin use
Pyridoxine (vitamin)	−	±	+	−	−	−	S	−	−	Occurs with large intake: >500 mg/d
Vincristine (antineoplastic)	−	+	+	−	−	−	S > M	−	−	Sensory symptoms common, hands > feet; motor signs ominous; should stop treatment
TOXINS										
Acrylamide (flocculant; grouting agent)	−	±	+	−	−	−	S > M	±	+	Large-fiber neuropathy; sensory ataxia
Arsenic (herbicide; insecticide)	±	+	+	−	−	−	SM	±	±	Skin changes, Mees' lines in nails; painful; systemic effects
Diphtheria	−	−	−	+	+	−	SM	−	−	Clinically very rare; can be confused with GBS
γ-Diketone hexacarbons (solvents)	−	±	+	−	−	+	SM	±	+	Neurofilamentous swelling of axons; these solvents now in restricted use
Inorganic lead	−	−	+	−	−	−	M > S or M	−	±	Selective motor neuropathy with prominent wrist drop
Organophosphates	−	±	+	−	−	−	SM	−	+	Brain and spinal cord also affected, the latter irreversibly
Thallium (rat poison)	−	+	+	−	−	−	SM	−	+	Also alopecia, Mees' lines in nails; painful

*± = sometimes, + = usual.
[†]S = sensory; M = motor; SM = sensorimotor.
The following drugs and environmental toxins are also neurotoxic, mainly to the peripheral nervous system.

Drugs	Environmental toxins
Amitriptyline, chloramphenicol, colchicine, ethambutol, glutethimide, nitrous oxide, perhexiline maleate, sodium cyanate, suramin, thalidomide, L-tryptophan, vinarabine	Allyl chloride, buckthorn berry, carbon disulfide, dimethylaminoproprionitrile, (DMAPN), ethylene oxide, methyl bromide, polychlorinated biphenyls, styrene, trichlorethylene, vacor

With the sum of clinical and electrodiagnostic information in hand, the differential diagnostic possibilities and management options will have been narrowed to only a few. The remainder of this chapter deals with the details of this formulation.

Electrodiagnosis As seen in Fig. 383-1, electrodiagnosis is a key part of the evaluation of any neuropathy. See Chap. 382 for details of technique and interpretation. For example, electrodiagnosis helps one to be certain about the presence or absence of a sensory involvement when this is not clear by clinical examination alone. It provides information about the distribution of subclinical findings, thus sharpening the diagnostic focus. The general questions that may be posed by the clinician to the electrodiagnostician include

1 The distinction between disorders primary to nerve or to muscle (neuropathy versus myopathy).

2 The distinction between root or plexus involvement and more distal nerve trunk involvement.

3 The distinction between generalized polyneuropathic processes and widespread multifocal nerve trunk affection.

4 The distinction between upper and lower motor neuron weakness.

5 The distinction, in a given generalized polyneuropathic process, between primary demyelinating neuropathy and axonal degeneration.

6 The assessment, in both primary axonal and demyelinating neuropathies, of many factors bearing on the nature, activity, and likely prognosis of the neuropathy.

7 The assessment, in mononeuropathies, of the site of the lesion and its major effect on nerve fibers, especially the distinction between demyelinating conduction block and wallerian degeneration.

8 The characterization of disorders of the neuromuscular junction.

9 The identification, often in muscle of normal bulk and strength, of important features such as chronic partial denervation, fasciculations, and myotonia.

10 The analysis of cramp, and its distinction from physiologic contracture.

Nerve biopsy The sural nerve at the ankle is the preferred site for cutaneous nerve biopsy. There are few indications to employ this invasive technique. The main one is in asymmetric and multifocal neuropathic disorders producing a clinical picture of mononeuropathy multiplex, the basis of which is still unclear after other laboratory investigations are complete. Diagnostic considerations include vasculitis, amyloidosis, leprosy, and occasionally sarcoidosis. Nerve biopsy is also helpful when one or more cutaneous nerves are palpably enlarged. Another clinical application is in establishing the diagnosis in some genetically determined childhood disorders such as metachromatic leukodystrophy, Krabbe's disease, giant axonal neuropathy, and infantile neuroaxonal dystrophy. In all of these recessively inherited diseases, both the central nervous system (CNS) and the peripheral nervous system (PNS) are affected.

There is a tendency to carry out sural nerve biopsy in distal symmetric polyneuropathies of subacute or chronic evolution. This practice is discouraged because it is a low-yield measure. Nerve biopsy in this situation is only useful as part of an approved research protocol when the biopsy will provide crucial information not otherwise obtainable.

POLYNEUROPATHY Although this term connotes a widespread symmetric process, usually distal and graded, polyneuropathies present a high degree of diversity because of the extreme variability of tempo, severity, mix of sensory and motor features, and presence or absence of positive symptoms. The patient with a fulminant, severely dysesthetic sensory neuropathy and alopecia who is in the early phases of thallium intoxication bears little similarity to the patient with a 40-year history of insidiously progressive clumsiness of gait whose findings are foot drop, lower leg atrophy, pes cavus, and minimal asymptomatic distal sensory deficit (i.e., peroneal muscular atrophy, either type I or II; see Table 383-3). These two patients fall near opposite ends of the spectrum of polyneuropathy.

The classification of peripheral neuropathies has become increasingly complex as the capacity to discriminate new subgroups and identify new associations with toxins and systemic disorders improves. Further, our grasp of the pathophysiologic basis for the clinical phenomena observed in neuropathy has increased rapidly (see Chap. 382). But these advances are primarily descriptive; little or no progress has been made in understanding the fundamental pathogenic events in nervous tissue that eventuate in any one of the polyneuropathies.

The important features of each major grouping of polyneuropathies are summarized below and key aspects of specific polyneuropathies may be found in Tables 383-1 to 383-5.

Acute axonal polyneuropathy In this setting the term acute means evolution over days, making these neuropathies relatively uncommon. Included are porphyric neuropathy and massive intoxications, often suicidal or homicidal in intent. For example, an individual receiving a large dose of arsenic (e.g., 100 mg of arsenous oxide) will become violently ill in a few hours with vomiting, diarrhea, and circulatory collapse. In 1 to 3 days serious renal and liver failure will ensue, and between 14 and 21 days painful polyneuropathy will appear, often as the systemic disorder abates. Progression occurs for 2 or 3 weeks, but following a plateau, recovery requires months.

Subacute axonal polyneuropathy Subacute, meaning to evolve in weeks, characterizes many instances of toxic and metabolic polyneuropathy, but perhaps even more of these are chronic in evolution (months to years). Scanning the appropriate columns in Tables 383-1 and 383-2 provides many possibilities. Management in almost all instances involves removing from contact the offending agent or treating the associated systemic order.

Chronic axonal polyneuropathy This category includes many more types of polyneuropathy, in part because the term chronic subsumes neuropathies that have progressed over a period as short as 6 months to as long as 60 years. As a rough approximation, slow worsening for more than 5 years, absence of positive symptoms, mainly motor deficit, and absence of systemic disorder all favor a genetically determined neuropathy. Although these are mostly autosomal dominant in inheritance pattern, recessively inherited and X-linked varieties also occur, including a form phenotypically resembling dominantly inherited peroneal muscular atrophy (HMSN-II) and also adrenomyeloneuropathy (Table 383-3). To complete the picture, an array of rare autosomal recessive neuropathies occur in childhood (Table 383-3).

Acute demyelinating polyneuropathy For all practical purposes, this category is synonymous with Guillain-Barré syndrome (GBS). This acute, frequently severe and fulminant polyneuropathy occurs at a rate of one case per million population per month, or approximately 3500 cases per year in the United States and Canada. Incidence patterns are similar worldwide. In over two-thirds, an infection, usually viral, either clinically overt or evidenced by serum titer rise, precedes the onset of neuropathy by 1 to 3 weeks. Herpes infections [cytomegalovirus, Epstein-Barr virus (EBV)] account for a large proportion of virus-triggered cases. Some cases appear to be triggered by *Campylobacter jejuni* gastroenteritis. A small proportion, less than 5 percent, occur within 1 to 4 weeks of a surgical procedure. GBS occurs on a background of lymphoma, including Hodgkin's disease, and in lupus erythematosus more frequently than can be attributed to chance alone. Although the weight of evidence suggests that GBS is immune-mediated, the immunopathogenesis remains obscure. In 1976 to 1977, a flurry of some 500 cases followed in the wake of the national swine flu vaccination program in the United States. This exceeded by severalfold the baseline incidence expected in this period in those vaccinated. The epidemiologic features of this outbreak resembled a point-source epidemic with an ''incubation'' period of 1 to 6 weeks. The reason why swine flu vaccine appears to have triggered GBS in 1976 to 1977 has never been discovered. In subsequent annual flu vaccine programs in the United States, no excess cases of GBS have been identified.

The clinical features of GBS typically include areflexic motor paralysis with mild sensory disturbance coupled with an acellular rise of total protein in the cerebrospinal fluid by the end of the first week of symptoms. Most patients with GBS require hospitalization, and about 30 percent will need ventilatory assistance at some point during the illness. The prognosis is good; approximately 85 percent of patients will make a complete or nearly complete recovery. The mortality rate is 3 to 4 percent. Management is generally supportive care, but plasmapheresis also has a role. Large, multicenter, controlled trials in North America and Europe have demonstrated a beneficial effect of plasmapheresis, if initiated in the first 2 weeks of illness. Intravenous administration of high-dose immunoglobulin (2 g/kg body weight given over 5 days) is probably as effective as plasmapheresis. In contrast, glucocorticoid treatment has not been shown to be effective.

TABLE 383-3 Genetically determined neuropathies

Genetic disorder	Inheritance pattern	Age of onset	Basic process	Other features*	Other systems involved	Metabolic defect	Comment
Peroneal muscular atrophy (HMSN-I)†	Dominant; large duplication on chr. 17 in most families	Decades 2–3	Demyelinating	Hypertropic change with onion bulbs; marked ↓ NCV	Rare; bony defects	Defective myelin protein?	Pes cavus, motor deficit predominates
Peroneal muscular atrophy (HMSN-II)†	Dominant	Decades 3–5	Axonal	Marked ↓ NAP; NCV sl. decreased	–	Unknown	Same as HSMN-I
Hereditary amyloid neuropathies	Dominant	Decades 3–6	Axonal	Small fiber involvement; endoneurial amyloid deposition	Some families—cornea; kidneys	Point mutations in transthyretin (prealbumin) in most families	Dysautonomia often prominent. Genetic defect on chromosome 18.
Hereditary sensory neuropathy (HSN-I)	Dominant	Decades 1–3	Neuronopathic	DRG neurons selectively involved	Sensorineural deafness, some families	Unknown	Frequent distal mutilation—hands and feet
Porphyric neuropathy	Dominant	Adult life	Axonal	Neuropathy part of attacks; may be recurrent	Widespread cellular abnormality	Enzyme defects in porphyrin pathway	Acute intermittent porphyria, variegate porphyria, and erythropoietic porphyria
Hereditary liability to pressure palsy	Dominant	Decades 2–3	? Demyelinating	Tomaculous changes in myelin	–	Unknown	Mostly ulnar, peroneal, and brachial plexus
Fabry's disease	X-linked	Young males	Neuronopathic	Sensory neuronopathy, small DRG neurons	Kidney, skin, lung	Accumulation of ceramide-trihexoside	Neuropathy painful; often die of renal failure
Peroneal muscular atrophy	X-linked	Infancy to 2d decade	Axonal or demyelinating	Heterozygote females may have symptoms	–	Unknown	Localizes to long arm of X chromosome
Adreno-myeloneuropathy	X-linked	Young males	? Axonal	Mild neuropathy, spastic paraparesis, baldness, hypogonadism	Adrenal cortex, cerebral white matter, spinal cord	Accumulation of very long chain fatty acids	Phenotypic variant of adrenoleukodystrophy: dietary therapy possible
Hereditary sensory neuropathy (HSN-II)	Recessive	Decades 1–3	Neuronopathic	DRG neurons selectively involved	–	Unknown	May be less severe than HSN-I
Déjerine-Sottas neuropathy (HMSN-III)	Recessive	1st decade	Demyelinating	Hypertrophic change with onion bulb formation	May be mentally retarded	Unknown	Marked nerve trunk enlargement
Refsum's disease	Recessive	1st or 2d decade	Demyelinating	Hypertropic change with onion bulb formation	Retinitis pigmentosa, ichthyosis, sensorineural deafness	Defect in α-oxidation of β-methylated fatty acids	Low phytanate diet, plasmapheresis therapy
Ataxia-telangiectasia	Recessive	Decade 1 or 2	Axonal	Neuropathy moderate	Cell nuclear aneuploidy, skin and scleral telangiectasia, cerebellar atrophy, immunopathy	Basic defect unknown	High incidence of early neoplasia
Abetalipo-proteinemia	Recessive	Decade 1 or 2	Neuronopathic	Large DRG neurons	Retinitis pigmentosa, acanthocytosis of red blood cells	Absence of all lipoprotein-containing apo B	Proprioceptive disturbance marked, minimal small fiber deficit
Giant axonal neuropathy	Recessive	1st decade	Axonal	Massive segmented accumulation of neurofilaments in axons	Slowly progressive encephalopathy with Rosenthal fibers	Generalized disorder of 10-nm filaments	Intermediate filament masses in other cell types
Metachromatic leukodystrophy	Recessive	1st decade	Demyelinating	Schwannopathy with cerebroside accumulation	Cerebral white matter disease predominates	Defect of arylsulfatase A	Infantile, juvenile, and adult onset forms
Globoid cell leukodystrophy	Recessive	1st decade	Demyelinating	Schwannopathy with galactocerebroside accumulation	Cerebral white matter disease predominates	Defect of β-galactosidase	Characteristic clefts in Schwann cell cytoplasm
Friedreich's ataxia	Recessive linked to chr. 9	1st decade	Axonal	Spinocerebellar and corticospinal tracts involved; also 1° sensory neuron	Cardiomyopathy; usual cause of death	Controversial	Ataxia is both sensory and cerebellar

* chr. = chromosome; DRG = dorsal root ganglia; NAP = nerve action potential; NCV = nerve conduction velocity; sl = slightly; HMSN = hereditary motor-sensory neuropathy; HSN = hereditary sensory neuropathy.
† Both forms are also collectively referred to as Charcot-Marie-Tooth neuropathy.

Other acute demyelinating polyneuropathies are rare and include buckthorn berry intoxication and diphtheritic polyneuritis (see Table 383-2).

Subacute demyelinating polyneuropathy Neuropathies in this category are heterogeneous in origin, although all are acquired. Most common is a relapsing and remitting neuropathy which has many clinical features in common with GBS, but differs from GBS in tempo, course, and absence of discernible triggering events (see "Acquired Demyelinating Neuropathies," below). Previously mentioned toxins (buckthorn berry, diphtheria toxin, aurothioglucose) may also induce a picture of widespread subacute demyelination of peripheral nerves (see Table 383-2).

TABLE 383-4   Classification of diabetic neuropathies

Symmetric
1 Distal, primarily sensory polyneuropathy
  a Mainly large fibers affected
  b Mixed*
  c Mainly small fibers affected*
2 Autonomic neuropathy
3 Chronically evolving proximal motor neuropathy*†

Asymmetric
1 Acute or subacute proximal motor neuropathy*†
2 Cranial mononeuropathy†
3 Truncal neuropathy*†
4 Entrapment neuropathy in the limbs

*Often painful.
†Recovery, partial or complete, is likely.

Chronic demyelinating polyneuropathy   Although more common than the subacute neuropathies, chronic polyneuropathy with demyelinating features encompasses a wide diversity of disorders, including hereditary neuropathies, inflammatory neuropathies, and other acquired neuropathies associated with diabetes mellitus, dysproteinemias, other metabolic states, and some chronic intoxications. To complicate matters, many of these disorders present an electrodiagnostic picture of mixed axonal-demyelinative findings. Frequently it is difficult to determine which process, axonal degeneration or demyelination, is the primary event. Aspects of many of these neuropathies are included in Table 383-1 to 383-5 and in the sections below.

SPECIAL CATEGORIES OF NEUROPATHY   Hereditary neuropathies   The major characteristics of this highly variegated group of disorders are summarized in Table 383-3. With the exception of the porphyric neuropathies, the onset of neuropathic dysfunction is insidious and progression is indolent over years or decades. Most of these diseases are quite rare with the striking exception of the dominantly inherited peroneal muscular atrophies (HMSN-I and HMSN-II; see Table 383-3). In peroneal muscular atrophy, phenotypic expression is often variable, so that affected family members of a propositus may have no symptoms and minimal neurologic findings but (in HMSN-I) may still show severe reduction of nerve conduction velocity.

Acquired demyelinating neuropathies   These fall into two major groups, the acute form called Guillain-Barré syndrome and more chronic forms, usually referred to as chronic inflammatory demyelinat-ing polyradiculoneuropathy (CIDP). The entire group of acquired demyelinating neuropathies constitutes a significant proportion of all cases of polyneuropathy and shares a distinctive clinical, electrophysiologic, and pathologic pattern. The diagnosis rests upon recognition of the clinical pattern and of other features, including elevated cerebrospinal fluid protein level, electrophysiologic changes (marked slowing of conduction velocities, delayed late responses, prolonged distal latencies, dispersion of evoked responses, and evidence of conduction block), and pathologic changes of low-grade inflammation, endoneurial edema, and demyelination-remyelination of peripheral nerves. The course of GBS is acute and monophasic, whereas the more chronic forms pursue either a slowly progressive or a relapsing course. Cases with an intermediate course occur frequently enough to blur the diagnostic delimitation of GBS from the more chronic type of acquired demyelinating neuropathy (CIDP).

Pathogenically, this group of neuropathies is generally agreed to be immune-mediated, but the specific antigens involved and the crucial events of the immune response and why it is activated are uncertain. Also unknown is whether GBS and CIDP share a common immunopathogenesis.

Management of CIDP involves a judicious mix of glucocorticoid therapy; plasmapheresis; immunosuppressants such as azathioprine, cyclophosphamide or cyclosporine; and high-dose intravenous immunoglobulin. These powerful agents are used only if the disorder is severe enough to threaten walking.

Diabetic neuropathies   Classifications of the neuropathies of diabetes mellitus are found in Table 383-4. Although this provides a satisfactory frame of reference, the limitations inherent in classifying diabetic neuropathies should be understood. The most serious limitation is that most patients will not fit neatly into any single category, but rather will have overlapping clinical features of several. For instance, many diabetics with distal, primarily sensory polyneuropathy also can be shown to have autonomic dysfunction, usually in the form of vasomotor disturbance in the limbs and abnormalities of sweating. Similarly, patients who develop a proximal motor syndrome may have dysautonomic features (including sexual impotence in males) and some degree of distal sensory polyneuropathy. To compound matters, such patients appear at risk to develop a cranial mononeuropathy.

Classifying the diabetic neuropathies tells us nothing of the pathogenesis of the neuropathic lesion. Rather, attempts at classification represent an educated guess at identifying the apparent anatomic sites of disorder and the critical clinical features. Pain is a frequent

TABLE 383-5   Sensory neuropathies

Cause or association	Course	Fiber size affected		Neuronopathy	Comment
		Small	Large		
TOXINS/DRUGS					
cis-Platinum (antineoplastic)	Sub/Chr	+	+ +	+	Dose-related
Pyridoxine (megadose)	Sub/Chr	+	+ +	+/−	Dose-related
Taxol (antineoplastic)	Acu/Sub	+ +	+	−	NGF may be protective
SYSTEMIC DISEASES					
Paraneoplastic	Sub	+	+ +	+ +	Most SCLC and breast
Sjögren syndrome	Sub/Chr	+/−	+	+ +	Variable presentation
Dysproteinemia (mainly IgMk)	Chr	+	+ +	−	Demyelinating; may bind to MAG
IDIOPATHIC					
Sporadic	Acu	+/−	+ +	+ +	Poor recovery
Sporadic	Chr	+/−	+ +	?	Sensory ataxia
HEREDITARY					
Many varieties (see Table 383-3)	Chr	Variable		Some	Progressive

Abbreviations: + + = most; + = some; ± = occasionally; Acu = acute; Sub = subacute; Chr = chronic; NGF = nerve growth factor; MAG = myelin-associated glycoprotein; SCLC = small cell lung carcinoma.

feature of diabetic neuropathies (see Table 383-4) but is variable in incidence and degree and is subjective in nature. The term diabetic amyotrophy should be avoided because of its ambiguity.

Diabetic neuropathies tend to occur in the setting of long-standing hyperglycemia (decades) whether insulin-dependent or not. By far the most common neuropathies related to diabetes mellitus are the diffuse sensory and autonomic types (categories 1 and 2 under "Symmetric" in Table 383-4). Sensory and autonomic polyneuropathy, chronic and indolent in evolution, may first be noticed in the third or fourth decade in patients with juvenile-onset diabetes but tends to occur after age 50 in patients with adult-onset diabetes. Focal and multifocal types of neuropathy are less common but quite dramatic (categories 1, 2, and 3 under "Asymmetric" in Table 383-4). They rarely occur before the age of 45 and are usually subacute or acute in onset. Cranial mononeuropathies refer to isolated sixth or third nerve palsies. The latter spares the pupil in three-fourths of cases, and some local pain or headache occurs in one-half. Truncal, or thoracoabdominal, neuropathy is painful, involves one or more intercostal or lumbar nerves unilaterally, and frequently coexists with the asymmetric proximal motor neuropathy. Femoral and obturator nerve–innervated muscles (quadriceps femoris, iliopsoas, adductor magnus) and loss of knee jerk on that side are the most evident features of asymmetric proximal motor neuropathy. Sensory deficit is minor, but pain in the hip and anterior thigh may predominate. Common to all of these multifocal and focal neuropathies is the strong likelihood of subsidence of pain within weeks to a year and partial or complete recovery of function. The same is true of symmetric proximal motor neuropathy (category 3 under "Symmetric" in Table 383-4).

Focal and multifocal diabetic neuropathies are considered to be ischemic in origin, and the basis for symmetric polyneuropathies, thought by some to involve abnormality of nerve metabolism, includes the possibility of ischemia.

Management of diabetic neuropathies is directed toward optimal control of hyperglycemia and symptomatic pain suppression. The role of aldose reductase inhibitors in preventing or reversing diabetic complications, including neuropathy, remains unclear. Entrapment neuropathies are frequently amenable to surgical decompression procedures.

Neuropathies with dysproteinemia An association between polyneuropathy and both multiple myeloma and macroglobulinemia has been recognized for many years. With commonly encountered multiple myeloma (MM) having either lytic or diffuse osteoporotic bone lesions, clinically overt polyneuropathy is relatively infrequent, occurring in approximately 5 percent of patients. These neuropathies are sensorimotor, may be severe, and generally do not reverse with successful suppression of the myeloma. In most cases, electrodiagnostic and pathologic features are consistent with a process of axonal degeneration.

In contrast, myeloma with osteosclerotic features, although representing only 3 percent of all myelomas, is associated with polyneuropathy in almost one-half of cases. These neuropathies, which may also occur with solitary plasmacytoma, seem to be different from those linked to MM in that they (1) often respond to radiation or removal of the primary lesion, (2) are more frequently demyelinating in character, (3) are associated with different monoclonal proteins and light chains (almost all lambda as opposed to mostly kappa in MM), and (4) frequently occur in association with other systemic findings. These include skin thickening, hyperpigmentation, hypertrichosis, organomegaly, endocrinopathy, anasarca, papilledema, and clubbing of fingers (POEMS syndrome: *p*olyneuropathy, *o*rganomegaly, *e*ndocrinopathy, *m* protein, and *s*kin changes). A great deal of attention has been paid to this curious syndrome in Japan, where it is more prevalent, but the underlying mechanism remains unknown, other than abnormality of lambda light chains.

Benign monoclonal gammopathy with an IgM serum spike, and usually with kappa light chains, is described in association with demyelinating polyneuropathy that often follows a protracted course

and indolent progression. In about one-quarter of cases, the monoclonal serum protein binds to normal human peripheral myelin, specifically to myelin-associated glycoprotein. Immunocytochemical studies show binding of IgM to nerve obtained at biopsy or autopsy of these patients, but in a pattern different from that seen following incubation of sections of nerve with the IgM serum. Incubated nerves show uniform staining of the entire expanse of compact myelin sheath, but in vivo deposited IgM can be demonstrated to localize more selectively, probably at sites of myelin splitting, the latter a phenomenon characteristic of most dysglobulinemic neuropathies. Whether the IgM bound to nerve in vivo plays a role in damaging nerve is unresolved.

Neuropathies with HIV infection Neuropathies are common in HIV infection, but different types of neuropathy are seen according to the stage of the disease. GBS or CIDP are the neuropathies likely to occur following conversion to seropositivity and during the asymptomatic phase of HIV infection. Treatment is the same as for HIV-negative patients. In later, symptomatic stages, subacute to chronic mononeuritis multiplex, axonal in nature, can occur. In some cases, vasculitis of the vasa nervorum has been demonstrated.

The most common neuropathy is a distal symmetrical mainly sensory polyneuropathy that evolves slowly in the late symptomatic stages of HIV infection, and frequently coexists with symptomatic encephalopathy and myelopathy (see Table 383-1 and Chap. 279). Improvement of this polyneuropathy with zidovudine treatment has been claimed. Also in the late stages, a severe, destructive subacute polyradiculopathy involving the cauda equina may be seen; it is caused by an opportunistic infection of roots with cytomegalovirus. Ganciclovir, started early, can arrest the disorder.

Neuropathies with Lyme disease In the aftermath of primary infection by the tick-borne spirochete *Borrelia burgdorferi*, a focal or multifocal radiculoneuropathy may occur weeks, months, or even years later. Although usually sensory and either dysesthetic or painful, the distribution is variable, affecting cranial nerves and spinal roots or nerves in a patchy asymmetrical fashion. Neuropathy is often chronic and persistent; CSF pleocytosis is the rule. In many, improvement occurs spontaneously, but the course is shortened by treatment with antibiotics, usually intravenous ceftriaxone (see Chap. 137).

Autonomic neuropathy The autonomic nervous system regulates the visceral organs and vegetative functions. Many pharmacologic agents modify specific autonomic functions, but autonomic neuropathy (dysautonomia) with structural changes in pre- and postganglionic neurons can also occur. Usually autonomic neuropathy is a manifestation of a more generalized polyneuropathy also affecting somatic peripheral nervous function, as in diabetic neuropathy, GBS, and alcoholic polyneuropathy, but occasionally syndromes of pure pandysautonomia are encountered. Symptoms of dysautonomia are mainly negative (i.e., loss of function) and include postural hypotension with faintness or syncope, anhidrosis, hypothermia, bladder atony, obstipation, dry mouth and dry eyes from failure of salivary and lacrimal glands to secrete, blurring of vision from lack of pupillary and ciliary regulation, and sexual impotence in males. Positive phenomena (hyperfunction) may also occur and include episodic hypertension, diarrhea, hyperhidrosis, and either tachycardia or bradycardia.

Pure motor neuropathy Disorder affecting any level of the motor unit—anterior horn cell (can be called *motor neuronopathy*), motor axon, or neuromuscular junction—can result in a purely lower motor syndrome without sensory disturbance. Distinguishing anterior horn cell disorders from motor axonopathies may be difficult clinically because they share manifestations (weakness, muscle denervation atrophy, hypo- or areflexia, fasciculations). Electrodiagnostic examination may also fail to localize the primary site of the lesion (neuropathic versus neuronopathic) unless the lesion is demyelinative in nature, in which case it is by definition neuropathic.

Examples of motor neuronopathies include the lower motor form of amyotrophic lateral sclerosis, poliomyelitis, hereditary spinal muscular atrophies, and adult variant of hexosaminidase A deficiency. Motor neuropathies may be seen with lead or dapsone intoxication, occasionally with porphyria, and also with multifocal motor neuropathy. The latter is a chronic asymmetrical disorder of midlife that may be associated with high titers of antiganglioside antibodies (particularly anti-G_{M1}), persistent conduction block electrodiagnostically, or both. Neuromuscular junction disorders (e.g., Lambert-Eaton myasthenic syndrome, tick bite paralysis, other toxic neuromuscular blockade) can be recognized and localized electrodiagnostically. Some motor-sensory polyneuropathies have predominant motor symptoms and signs, such as hereditary motor-sensory neuropathies, GBS, and CIDP, but the subclinical sensory component is readily demonstrated electrodiagnostically or by quantitative sensory testing.

Pure sensory neuropathy Clinical presentations involving primary sensation only (see Chap. 24) are not uncommon. Manifestations may: (1) be pansensory; (2) reflect mainly large afferent fiber involvement with deficits of vibratory and proprioceptive sense, areflexia, and sensory ataxia with or without tingling dysesthesias; or (3) reflect mainly small afferent fiber involvement with numbness and cutaneous hypesthesia to pin-prick and temperature stimuli, often with painful burning dysesthesias. The pattern of distribution, although variable, is often distal and symmetrical, particularly for large-fiber neuropathies.

The most severe and widespread of these pure sensory syndromes exhibit poor or no recovery, suggesting irreversible lesions of nerve cell bodies or dorsal root and trigeminal ganglion cells. These are frequently referred to as *sensory neuronopathies*. With sensory neurotoxins, moderate doses lead to potentially reversible neuropathy, but high doses appear to cause neuronopathy (see Table 383-5).

Plexopathy This term refers to disorders of either the brachial or lumbosacral plexus. Lesions of the brachial plexus are characterized by motor and sensory signs different from those expected either in mononeuropathies of the upper limb or in polyneuropathies. The usual causes are direct trauma to the plexus, idiopathic brachial neuritis (also called neuralgic amyotrophy), cervical rib or band, infiltration by malignant tumor, or prior radiation therapy. When the upper parts of the brachial plexus, arising from cervical roots 5 through 7, are affected, weakness and atrophy of shoulder girdle and upper arm muscles occur. Injuries to the lower brachial plexus, arising from the eighth cervical and first thoracic roots, produce distal arm weakness, atrophy, and focal sensory deficit in the forearm and hand. In general, idiopathic brachial neuritis, radiation damage greater than 60 Gy (6000 rad), and particular types of trauma (arm jerked downward) result in damage to the upper portions of the brachial plexus. In contrast, infiltration by malignant tumor, cervical rib or band, and certain other types of trauma (arm jerked upward) cause damage to the lower brachial plexus. Lumbosacral plexopathies are less common; they may be due to idiopathic lumbosacral plexitis, retroperitoneal hemorrhage, malignant tumor infiltration, or occur in association with long-standing diabetes mellitus.

Miscellaneous causes of neuropathy Ischemia of nerve severe enough to produce clinical symptoms has as its basis the widespread compromise of blood flow in the vasa nervorum. Typically, this is the result of small-vessel disease involving the vasa nervorum directly, as occurs with vasculitis, rather than large-vessel disease, such as atherosclerosis. Clinically, widespread disease of the vasa nervorum produces mononeuropathy multiplex, which electrodiagnostically has the features of a patchy axonal process.

Cold exerts deleterious effects on peripheral nerve directly without an intermediate step of ischemia being necessary. Cold injury to nerve occurs after prolonged exposure, usually of a limb, to moderately low temperatures, as with immersion of the feet in seawater; actual freezing of tissue is not required. Axonal degeneration of myelinated fibers is the pathologic expression of cold injury. Frequently limbs affected by cold injury to nerve show sensory deficit and dysesthesias, cutaneous vasomotor instability, pain, and marked sensitivity to minimal cold exposure, which persist for many years. The pathophysiology of these phenomena is uncertain.

TROPHIC CHANGES IN SEVERE NEUROPATHY   The array of observable changes in completely denervated muscle, bone, and skin, including hair and nails, is well known, if incompletely understood. It is unclear what portion of the changes is due purely to denervation versus that caused by disuse, immobility, lack of weight bearing, and particularly recurrent, unnoticed, painless trauma. Considerable evidence favors the view that ulceration of skin, poor healing, tissue resorption, neurogenic arthropathy, and mutilation are the result of repeated heedless injury to insensitive parts. This sequence of events is avoidable with proper attention to and care of the insensitive parts by both patient and physician.

RECOVERY FROM NEUROPATHY In contrast to axons in the CNS, peripheral nerve fibers have an excellent capability to regenerate under proper circumstances. The process of regeneration following axonal degeneration may take from 2 months to more than a year, depending on the severity of the neuropathy and the length of regeneration required. Whether regeneration takes place depends upon the subsidence of the initial basis for neuropathy. This could be removal from contact with a neurotoxic substance or correction of an abnormal metabolic state. A deficit secondary to demyelination may recover rapidly since intact axons may remyelinate in just a few weeks. For example, a patient with GBS, in whom demyelination but no secondary axonal degeneration has occurred, may recover to normal strength from bedfastness and paralysis of arms and legs in as little as 3 to 4 weeks.

MONONEUROPATHY MULTIPLEX (MULTIFOCAL NEUROPATHY) This term means simultaneous or sequential involvement of individual noncontiguous nerve trunks, either partially or completely, evolving over days to years. Since the disease process underlying mononeuropathy multiplex involves peripheral nerves in a multifocal and random fashion, there is a tendency, as worsening occurs, for the neurologic deficit to become less patchy and multifocal and more confluent and symmetric. Some patients present initially with a distal symmetric neuropathy. Attention to the pattern of early symptoms is therefore important in making the judgment that a particular neuropathy is indeed a mononeuropathy multiplex.

Once that issue is settled, the next question is whether the process is primarily axonal or demyelinating. Almost one-third of all adults with the clinical syndrome of mononeuropathy multiplex have a clear-cut picture of a demyelinating disorder usually with multiple foci of persistent conduction block by electrodiagnostic examination. More intensive study of this subgroup suggests that the multifocal demyelinating neuropathy represents part of the spectrum of chronic acquired demyelinating neuropathy, that is, CIDP. Management of this multifocal subgroup is the same as for CIDP. (See "Acquired Demyelinating Neuropathies," above.)

The remaining two-thirds of patients with mononeuropathy multiplex have a picture by electrodiagnostic examination of axonal involvement that is heterogeneously distributed. Although ischemia would be suspected as the basis of neuropathy in these patients, only about one-half can be shown to have a process, usually vasculitis, affecting the vasa nervorum. Management of those with proven vasculitis of vasa nervorum is the same as treatment for systemic vasculitis (see Chap. 291). The others remain undiagnosed even on follow-up, and the basis for their mononeuropathy multiplex is uncertain. Management in this group is conservative and many patients will stabilize or recover, at least partially.

In individuals in whom vasculitic change in vasa nervorum can be demonstrated, any one of a large number of underlying disorders may be responsible. The primary vasculitides of the polyarteritis nodosa group constitute the most frequent basis, followed closely by the vasculitis syndrome occurring in the course of other connective tissue disorders. In descending order of frequency, the latter are rheumatoid arthritis, systemic lupus erythematosus, and mixed connective tissue disease. Other rarer causes of mononeuropathy multiplex due to nerve ischemia from occlusion of vasa nervorum include mixed cryoglobulinemia, Sjögren's syndrome, Wegener's granulomatosis, progressive systemic sclerosis, Churg-Strauss allergic granulomatosis, and hypersensitivity angiitides. Management of the neuropathy in each instance is predicated upon the appropriate treatment of the responsible disease.

Mononeuropathy multiplex syndrome may also be seen as a manifestation of leprosy, sarcoidosis, certain types of amyloidosis, hypereosinophilia syndrome, cryoglobulinemia, and multifocal types of diabetic neuropathy.

MONONEUROPATHY Mononeuropathy means focal involvement of a single nerve trunk and therefore implies a local causation. Direct trauma, compression, and entrapment are the usual causes. Ulnar neuropathies, due to lesions either at the ulnar groove or in the cubital tunnel, and median neuropathy due to compression in the carpal tunnel constitute the great majority of mononeuropathies encountered in clinical practice. These are described below, and other common mononeuropathies are listed in Table 383-6.

In the absence of a history of trauma to the nerve trunk, factors favoring conservative management include sudden onset, no motor deficit, few or no sensory findings even though pain and sensory symptoms might be present, and no evidence of axonal degeneration by electrodiagnostic criteria. Factors favoring surgical intervention include chronicity and worsening neurologic deficit on examination, particularly if motor, and electrodiagnostic evidence that the lesion has produced a degree of wallerian degeneration.

Ulnar nerve Complete ulnar paralysis results in a characteristic claw-hand deformity owing to wasting and weakness of many of the small hand muscles and hyperextension of the fingers at the metacarpophalangeal joints and flexion at the interphalangeal joints. The flexion deformity is most pronounced in the fourth and fifth fingers. Sensory loss occurs over the fifth finger, the ulnar aspect of the fourth finger, and the ulnar border of the palm. The superficial

TABLE 383-6 Some common mononeuropathies

Nerve	Origin (spinal segments)	Muscles innervated	Usual site of lesion	Clinical features	Comments
UPPER EXTREMITY					
Suprascapular	C5, C6	Supraspinatus Infraspinatus	Suprascapular notch of scapula	Weakness of lateral rotation of the humerus	No sensory deficit
Long thoracic	C5–C7	Serratus anterior	Variable	Winging of scapula	No sensory deficit
Axillary	C5, C6	Deltoid, teres minor	Near shoulder joint	Weakness of shoulder abduction; atrophy of shoulder	Sensory deficit similar to C5 dorsal root lesion (see Figs. 24-2 and 24-3)
Radial	C5–T1	Triceps, brachioradialis, wrist, finger, and thumb extensors	Spiral groove of humerus	Wrist drop most obvious, also finger and thumb extensors paralyzed	Saturday night palsy (acute compression) is frequent cause
Posterior interosseous branch	C7, C8	Finger and thumb extensors	Edge of supinator muscle below elbow	Finger drop; wrist relatively spared	No sensory deficit
Ulnar	C8, T1	Ulnar flexor of the wrist, long flexors of 4th and 5th digits, and most intrinsic hand muscles	Ulnar groove at the elbow	Weakness of finger adduction and abduction and thumb adduction (see text); interosseous atrophy, claw-hand	May be acute or insidious; sensory symptoms/signs are distinctive (Figs. 24-2 and 24-3); see also text
			Cubital tunnel	Same as above	Often pain over medial proximal forearm (cubital tunnel)
			Medial base of palm	Intrinsic hand muscles only, interosseous atrophy	No sensory deficit
Median	C6–T1	Abductor pollicis brevis; more proximal muscles include forearm pronator, long finger and thumb flexors	Carpal tunnel	Characteristic sensory symptoms and deficit and inability to make a circle with thumb and index finger	Sensory deficit as per Figs. 24-2 and 24-3 (see text); known as carpal tunnel syndrome
Anterior interosseous branch	C7–T1	Long flexors of thumb and index and middle fingers	Anterior interosseus branch below the elbow	Weakness of pinch; pain in volar forearm	No sensory deficit
LOWER EXTREMITY					
Femoral	L2–L4	Iliopsoas (hip flexor) and quadriceps femoris (knee extensor)	Proximal to inguinal ligament	Knee buckling; absent knee jerk; weak anterior thigh muscles with atrophy	Association with diabetes mellitus; sensory disturbance as per Fig. 24-2
Lateral femoral cutaneous branch	L2, L3	None	Inguinal ligament	Dysesthetic hyperpathia of lateral thigh	Known as meralgia paresthetica
Obturator	L3, L4	Thigh adductors	Intrapelvic or at pubis	Weakness of hip adduction	Sensory deficit on medial thigh
Sciatic	L4–S3	Hamstring muscles, hip abductor and all muscles below the knee	Near sciatic notch	Severe lower leg and hamstring weakness; flail foot; severe disability	Uncommon except from war wounds
Posterior tibial	L5–S2	Calf muscles (proximally), toe flexors and other intrinsic foot muscles	Tarsal tunnel, near medial malleolus	Pain and numbness of sole, weak toe flexors	Known as tarsal tunnel syndrome
Peroneal	L4–S1	Dorsiflexors of toes and foot, evertors of foot	At neck of fibula	Foot drop and weakness of foot eversion	Sensory deficit is similar in distribution to L5, S1 sensory roots

location of the nerve at the elbow makes it a common site of pressure palsy. The ulnar nerve may also become entrapped just distal to the elbow in the cubital tunnel formed by the aponeurotic arch linking the two heads of the flexor carpi ulnaris. Also, prolonged pressure on the base of the palm, as occurs with use of hand tools or bicycle riding, may result in damage to the deep palmar branch of the ulnar nerve, causing weakness of the small hand muscles but no sensory loss.

Median nerve The median nerve in the carpal tunnel lies in close quarters with nine tendons. Entrapment of the nerve at the wrist (carpal tunnel syndrome) may be secondary to excessive use of the wrist, tenosynovitis with arthritis, or local infiltration, for example, by a thickening of connective tissue as in acromegaly or by deposit of amyloid or by one of the mucopolysaccharidoses. Other systemic diseases associated with an increased incidence of carpal tunnel syndrome are hypothyroidism, rheumatoid arthritis, and diabetes mellitus, but underlying diseases account for only a small fraction of all cases. The main symptoms of carpal tunnel syndrome are nocturnal paresthesias of thumb, index, and middle fingers. With worsening, numbness demonstrable by pin examination occurs in that distribution, and eventually weakness and atrophy of the abductor pollicis brevis (thenar eminence) becomes evident. Treatment of carpal tunnel syndrome is surgical section of the carpal ligament to relieve entrapment. Incomplete lesions of the median nerve between the axilla and wrist may result in causalgia (a particularly severe type of burning pain; see Chap. 11).

OTHER FOCAL NEUROPATHIES Peripheral nerve tumors These are mostly benign and can arise on any nerve trunk or twig. Although peripheral nerve tumors occur anywhere in the body including the spinal roots and cauda equina, many are subcutaneous in location and present as a soft swelling, sometimes with a purplish discoloration of the skin. Two major categories of peripheral nerve tumors are recognized: neurilemmoma (schwannoma) and neurofibroma. Neurilemmomas are usually solitary and grow within the nerve sheath, rendering the tumor relatively easy to dissect free. In contrast, neurofibromas tend to be multiple, grow within the endoneurial substance, rendering them difficult to dissect, may undergo malignant changes, and are the hallmark of von Recklinghausen's neurofibromatosis (NF1). This disease is characterized by an autosomal dominant inheritance pattern, any number of neurofibromas from one to thousands, five or more café au lait–pigmented skin lesions greater than 1.5 cm (80 percent of patients), axillary freckles (93 percent of patients), an increased incidence of seizure disorder and mental retardation and an exceptionally high rate of spontaneous mutation (see Chap. 378). The gene for NF1 is on chromosome 17, and its protein product, neurofibromin, is a large, widely expressed protein that appears to regulate the proto-oncogene *ras.*

Herpes zoster This is a sensory neuritis due to varicella-zoster infection and is characterized by acute inflammation of one or more dorsal root ganglia. Lancinating pain and hyperalgesia over the skin surface supplied by affected roots occur for 3 to 4 days, followed by the appearance of herpetic eruption in the same segment characterized by painful raised blisters on reddened bases. If the inflammatory process spreads to involve adjacent motor roots of anterior horns of the cord, segmental motor weakness and wasting appear. Paralysis of the oculomotor nerves may occur in conjunction with ophthalmic division involvement of the trigeminal ganglion (ophthalmoplegic zoster). Facial paralysis may occur with involvement of the geniculate ganglion and herpetic eruption on the ipsilateral tympanic membrane or external ear canal (Ramsay Hunt syndrome).

In less than 5 percent, neuropathic pain persists in the dermatomal distribution of the affected ganglia. The pain, known as *postherpetic neuralgia,* is intense, burning, hyperpathic, unrelenting, and often dominates the lives of those affected. Advancing age is a risk factor for this outcome. In some patients blunting of the pain to tolerable levels is achieved by use of carbamazepine or a tricyclic antidepressant such as desipramine (see also Chap. 11).

Leprous neuritis This is a major worldwide cause of neuropathy. *Mycobacterium leprae* organisms readily invade Schwann cells in cutaneous nerve twigs, particularly those associated with unmyelinated nerve fibers. Two major forms of leprous neuritis are recognized, tuberculoid and lepromatous, which actually represent the far ends of a spectrum of disease, the middle of which is called dimorphous leprosy (patchy and multifocal involvement of skin and nerve). Treatment depends upon where in the spectrum a given case is classified (see Chap. 131). Tuberculoid (high-resistance) leprosy is restricted to a single patch of hypesthetic or anesthetic skin in any location. The skin patch is frequently thickened, reddened, or hypopigmented. If a superficially placed nerve trunk, typically a cutaneous nerve, courses just beneath the area of affected skin, it may be engulfed in the inflammatory reaction, resulting in an associated mononeuropathy. Such a nerve may be palpably enlarged and beaded. Lepromatous (low-resistance) leprosy is marked by immunologic tolerance and widespread skin thickening, cutaneous anesthesia, and anhidrosis, sparing only the warmest parts of the body, notably the axilla, groin, and beneath the scalp hair. Motor signs (focal weakness and atrophy) result from damage to mixed nerves lying close to the skin, particularly the median, ulnar, peroneal, and facial nerves.

Bell's palsy This seventh nerve palsy is due to inflammation of the facial nerve in the facial canal, the basis for which remains obscure. Edema may play a part leading to compression of nerve fibers, with resulting acute unilateral paralysis of facial muscles (see Chap. 380).

Sarcoidosis This may involve single or multiple peripheral nerves, producing asymmetric mononeuritis or polyneuritis. Unilateral or bilateral facial paralysis is described in association with parotitis and uveitis (Heerfordt's syndrome).

Polyneuritis cranialis This is a relapsing and remitting mononeuropathy multiplex restricted to cranial nerves. It is usually associated with indolent tuberculous cervical adenitis (scrofula) or sarcoidosis. Treatment of the underlying condition will halt the cranial nerve palsies.

Acknowledgment

By arrangement with the publishers, portions of this section also appear in substantially the same form in Asbury AK: Diseases of peripheral nerve, in *Diseases of the Nervous System,* 2d ed, AK Asbury, GM McKhann, WI McDonald (eds). Philadelphia, Saunders, 1992.

REFERENCES

ASBURY AK: New aspects of disease of the peripheral nervous system, in *Harrison's Textbook of Internal Medicine, Update IV.* McGraw-Hill, New York, 1983, pp 211–229

———, GILLIATT RW: *Peripheral Nerve Disorders: A Practical Approach.* London, Butterworth, 1984

BAROHN RJ et al: Peripheral nervous system involvement in a large cohort of human immunodeficiency virus infected individuals. Arch Neurol 50:167, 1993

CHANCE PF et al: DNA deletion associated with hereditary neuropathy with liability to pressure palsies. Cell 72:143, 1993

DAWSON DM et al: *Entrapment Neuropathies,* 2d ed. Boston, Little, Brown, 1991

DYCK PJ et al (eds): *Peripheral Neuropathy,* 3d ed. Philadelphia, Saunders, 1992

HELLER S, WARD JD: Neurologic consequences of hypoglycemia and pathogenic mechanisms involved in diabetic neuropathy. Curr Opin Neurol Neurosurg 6:423, 1993

———: *Diabetic Neuropathy.* Philadelphia, Saunders, 1987

LAYZER RB: *Neuromuscular Manifestations of Systemic Disease,* vol 25: *Contemporary Neurology Series.* Philadelphia, Davis, 1984

RAIVICH G, KREUTZBERG GW: Nerve growth factor and regeneration of peripheral nervous system. Clin Neurol Neurosurg 95:S84, 1993

ROPPER AH et al: *Guillain Barré Syndrome.* Philadelphia, FA Davis, 1991

STEWART JD: *Focal Peripheral Neuropathies.* New York, Elsevier, 1987

SUTER U et al: Progress in the molecular understanding of hereditary peripheral neuropathies reveals new insights into the biology of the peripheral nervous system. Trends Neurosci 16:50, 1993

384 DERMATOMYOSITIS AND POLYMYOSITIS

RUP TANDAN / WALTER G. BRADLEY

Dermatomyositis and polymyositis are conditions of presumed autoimmune etiology in which the skeletal muscle is damaged by a nonsuppurative inflammatory process dominated by lymphocytic infiltration. The term *polymyositis* is applied when the condition spares the skin and the term *dermatomyositis* when polymyositis is associated with a characteristic skin rash. One-third of cases are associated with various connective tissue disorders, such as rheumatoid arthritis, lupus erythematosus, mixed connective tissue disorder, and progressive systemic sclerosis, and one-tenth with a malignancy.

ETIOLOGY The precise cause of these diseases is unknown, but interplay between host genetic factors, viral infection of muscle, and autoimmune mechanisms is probably contributory. Familial occurrence of these diseases, and the increased frequency of HLA-DR3 and -DRw52 antigens in patients, suggest an underlying genetic and immunologic predisposition. Experimental viral myositis can be induced in animals by coxsackie virus. A mild inflammatory myopathy can occur with influenza and coxsackie viruses in humans. However, the several electron-microscopic observations of virus-like particles in muscle fibers in dermatomyositis or polymyositis have not been confirmed by virus isolation or demonstration of rising viral antibody titers, and the disease has not been passed into animals by injection of extracts of skeletal muscles. Nevertheless, the presence of serum antibodies to several cytoplasmic ribonucleoproteins involved in translation (especially histidyl tRNA synthetase or Jo-1 and signal recognition particle, SRP) may result from an immune response to an altered virus that serves as an immunogen in polymyositis. These antibodies probably represent a cross-reactive phenomenon.

A lymphocyte-mediated disease resembling polymyositis has been reported in laboratory animals injected with muscle antigens together with Freund's adjuvant (experimental allergic myositis). Recent immunohistochemical and muscle co-culture studies indicate that muscle fiber necrosis in polymyositis and inclusion body myositis probably derive from activation of T cells of the cytotoxic-suppressor types, accompanied by T helper-inducer cells and macrophages present in the inflammatory infiltrates. In dermatomyositis, deposition of immunoglobulins and the C_{5b-9} complement membrane attack complex (MAC) has been demonstrated on intramuscular blood vessels even in unaffected or minimally involved regions of muscle, suggesting that humorally mediated blood vessel damage initiates the angiopathy that precedes muscle destruction. The final pathway for muscle fiber damage in dermatomyositis may be T helper cell-dependent stimulation of B cells, with resultant antibody-mediated cytotoxicity.

CLASSIFICATION The classification of the dermatomyositis-polymyositis group that is most widely used and which was proposed before the recent advances in the understanding of the immunology of these diseases, is given in Table 384-1. This classification is based partly on known differences in etiology and has a number of drawbacks, as noted below. Other uncommon associations of polymyositis are sarcoidosis, giant cell myositis with thymoma, and myositis

TABLE 384-1 Classification of polymyositis-dermatomyositis

Group I:	Primary idiopathic polymyositis
Group II:	Primary idiopathic dermatomyositis
Group III:	Dermatomyositis (or polymyositis) associated with neoplasia
Group IV:	Childhood dermatomyositis (or polymyositis) associated with vasculitis
Group V:	Polymyositis (or dermatomyositis) with associated collagen vascular disease

SOURCE: Classification suggested by Bohan et al.

in systemic infections due to viruses, toxoplasma, or parasites. A focal infective myositis due to streptococcal or staphylococcal infection is mostly seen in the tropics. Focal nodular myositis is a variant of polymyositis where focal areas of myositis cause hot, often painful, multifocal muscle masses. Inclusion body myositis is an inflammatory myopathy with characteristic clinical and pathologic features (see below).

INCIDENCE Current estimates that the annual incidence of the inflammatory myopathies is about five per million of the population are probably too low; we estimate that the incidence may be as high as two to three per hundred thousand population.

CLINICAL MANIFESTATIONS Group 1: Primary idiopathic polymyositis This group comprises about one-third of all cases of inflammatory myopathy. It is usually insidiously progressive over weeks, months, or even years. Rarely the disease is acute, producing severe muscle weakness in a matter of days or even rhabdomyolysis. The disease may develop at any age and in either sex. Females outnumber males 2:1.

The patients first become aware of weakness of the proximal limb muscles, especially the hips and thighs, and find difficulty in arising from the squatting or kneeling position and in climbing or descending stairs. When shoulder girdle muscles are involved, placing an object on a high shelf or combing the hair becomes difficult. Occasionally the disease is more restricted, affecting only the neck, the shoulder, or the quadriceps muscles. Pain of an aching type in the buttocks, thighs, and calves is experienced in about 10 percent of the cases, and tenderness on palpation in another 20 percent. Early symptoms of dysphagia and weakness of flexor muscles of the neck in a patient with a chronic myopathy suggest the diagnosis of polymyositis.

When the patient is first seen, there may be weakness of the muscles of the trunk, the pectoral and pelvic girdles, the upper arms and thighs, the anterior neck, more so than the posterior, and the pharynx. Ocular muscles are almost never affected except in a rare association with myasthenia gravis. The distal muscles are spared in about 75 percent of cases. Muscle atrophy, contractures, and diminished tendon reflexes are rare in early myositis and never as pronounced as in muscular dystrophies and denervating conditions. When the reflexes are disproportionately reduced, carcinoma with polymyositis and polyneuropathy or the Lambert-Eaton syndrome should be considered. Occasionally, the reflexes may be paradoxically brisk in dermatomyositis-polymyositis, perhaps due to irritation of muscle spindle receptors by the inflammation.

At presentation about 25 percent of patients have dysphagia, about 5 percent have significant respiratory impairment, and 5 percent are unable to walk. Dysphagia is due to involvement of striated muscles of the pharynx and upper esophagus. At some time in the course of the disease cardiac abnormalities are observed in about 30 percent of cases; these include ECG changes, arrhythmias, and heart failure secondary to myocarditis. About half of the fatal cases have pathologic evidence of cardiac disease with necrosis of myocardial fibers, usually with only modest inflammatory reaction. The frequency of myocardial infarction may be increased in those treated for long periods with glucocorticoids. In a few cases there is dyspnea due to lymphocytic pneumonitis, obliterating bronchiolitis, pulmonary edema, or pulmonary fibrosis. Arthralgia, Raynaud's phenomenon, and rarely, low-grade fever may also be present.

Group II: Primary idiopathic dermatomyositis This group comprises just over one-third of all cases of myositis. The skin changes may precede or follow the muscle syndrome and include a localized or diffuse erythema, maculopapular eruption, scaling eczematoid dermatitis, or, rarely, an exfoliative dermatitis. The classic lilac-colored (heliotrope) rash is on the eyelids, bridge of the nose, cheeks (butterfly distribution), forehead, chest, elbows, knees and knuckles, and around the nail beds. Itching may be troublesome in some cases. The skin lesions may be subtle and easily overlooked. Periorbital edema is frequent, particularly in acute cases. The skin lesions may occasionally ulcerate. Subcutaneous calcification may occur, especially in children.

The typical rash and myositis allow a diagnosis of dermatomyositis, and such cases may be placed in this category (group II, Table 384-1) if idiopathic and into groups III, IV, and V if there are other features, namely malignancy, vasculitis in children, and an established collagen vascular disease. There should be concern about an underlying malignancy in patients with dermatomyositis over the age of 60.

Group III: Polymyositis or dermatomyositis with neoplasia This syndrome, which comprises about 8 percent of all cases of myositis, is categorized separately, although muscle and skin changes are indistinguishable from those in the other groups. Malignancy, however, is uncommon in myositis seen in children and in association with a connective tissue disorder. The malignancy may antedate or postdate the onset of the myositis by up to 2 years. The incidence of this paraneoplastic syndrome is higher in patients with dermatomyositis over the age of 60; therefore, in such patients a thorough history and clinical examination (including breast and rectal) must be supplemented by hemogram, biochemical profile, serum protein electrophoresis and immunofixation, screening for carcino-embryonic antigen, urine analysis for blood and cytology, stool samples for occult blood, chest x-ray, sputum for cytology, and bone scan seeking clues for an underlying malignancy. This relatively inexpensive search often uncovers most malignancies; undirected radiologic screening procedures are costly and unhelpful in improving the yield. The most common malignancies are lung, ovary, breast, gastrointestinal tract, and myeloproliferative disorders. The myositis is a paraneoplastic syndrome, the cause of which may lie in an altered immune status or an occult viral infection of the muscle.

Group IV: Childhood polymyositis and dermatomyositis associated with vasculitis This group comprises about 8 to 20 percent of all cases of myositis in various series. Inflammatory myopathy in childhood is frequently associated with skin involvement and clinical or pathologic evidence of vasculitis in skin, muscles, gastrointestinal tract, and other organs. Degeneration and loss of capillaries in a perifascicular distribution occur in the skeletal muscles; often necrotizing lesions of the skin, and ischemic infarction of kidneys, gastrointestinal tract, and rarely brain may be seen. Consequently, some authors have reported mortality rates of up to one-third in childhood dermatomyositis, though most have found that the prognosis is better than in adult dermatomyositis-polymyositis. One limitation of the classification of Bohan et al. is that it is not clear whether or not all cases of childhood myositis should be included in group IV. Subcutaneous calcification is frequently present in childhood dermatomyositis.

Group V: Polymyositis or dermatomyositis with an associated connective tissue disorder This "overlap group" of myositis comprises about one-fifth of all cases that occur in association with several connective tissue diseases. Progressive systemic sclerosis, rheumatoid arthritis, mixed connective tissue disease (the rheumatologic overlap disorder), and lupus erythematosus are the most common associated conditions; polyarteritis nodosa and rheumatic fever are more rarely associated. Criteria for placement in the "overlap group" combine the demonstration of the appropriate clinical and laboratory abnormalities required for the diagnosis of the connective tissue disorder together with clinical and laboratory evidence of myositis. The diagnosis of myositis is often difficult in patients with a connective tissue disorder producing arthritis, since this may often produce muscle weakness with type II fiber atrophy. Moreover, perivascular inflammatory foci are common in muscle in connective tissue disorders. Demonstration of increased serum creatine kinase (CK), electromyography (EMG), and muscle biopsy are often required to make this diagnosis. Though patients in this overlap group usually respond to glucocorticoid therapy, the prognosis for recovery of function is poorer than in pure dermatomyositis-polymyositis. Dysphagia in group V patients with progressive systemic sclerosis is often due to involvement of the smooth muscle of the distal third of the esophagus.

Other disorders associated with myositis SARCOIDOSIS AND POLYMYOSITIS The skeletal muscle contains noncaseating granulomas with Langhans-type multinuclear giant cells in at least one-quarter of patients with sarcoidosis. Symptomatic polymyositis is, however, uncommon. Regenerating multinuclear myoblasts resemble Langhans' giant cells, which has led to misdiagnosis in many of the cases reported in the literature to have "sarcoid myositis." Giant cell or granulomatous polymyositis and myocarditis, sometimes associated with myasthenia gravis, have been recorded in patients with thymomas.

FOCAL NODULAR MYOSITIS A syndrome of acutely developing and painful focal inflammatory nodules, sometimes occurring sequentially in different muscles, has been termed *focal nodular myositis*. The pathologic appearance and response to therapy are similar to those in generalized polymyositis. The differential diagnosis includes, when single, a muscle tumor (sarcoma or rhabdomyosarcoma) or proliferative fasciitis and myositis and, when multiple, muscle infarcts such as can occur in polyarteritis nodosa.

INFECTIOUS POLYMYOSITIS Rare cases of polymyositis have clear-cut evidence of being due to known pathogens such as toxoplasma (Chap. 177), viruses (Chap. 154), and spirochetes (Lyme disease). Antibody screening will suggest the diagnosis in such cases. Trichinosis may be confused with idiopathic polymyositis, particularly if the history of raw pork ingestion is not obtained. The symptoms of trichinosis are variable and depend upon the parasitic load. Low-grade fever, muscle pain of variable degree, conjunctival and periorbital edema, and fatigue are frequent. Weakness is generally mild. Heavy infestation is often associated with central nervous system symptoms of delirium, coma, or focal neurologic deficit. The frequent myocardial involvement is manifested by tachycardia and ECG changes. The diagnosis is made by the history of ingestion of undercooked pork, marked eosinophilia, sensitivity to intradermal *Trichina* antigen, and the appearance of serum antibodies to *Trichina* during the course of the disease. Occasionally the diagnosis is not recognized until a muscle is biopsied. Pyomyositis, a suppurative inflammation of muscle due to staphylococci or streptococci, is mainly seen in the tropics but has recently been reported in patients with AIDS. The presentation is that of a diffuse abscess of the muscle.

MYOPATHY IN HIV INFECTION Polymyositis occurs in AIDS, which is caused by infection with the human immunodeficiency virus (HIV) (see Chap. 279). It may be the presenting manifestation of the disorder or, rarely, be due to therapy with zidovudine (AZT). Profound weight loss greater than 10 percent of baseline body weight with associated chronic diarrhea or weakness characterizes the HIV wasting syndrome; a myopathy, among other causes, may underlie this entity. Raised serum CK, EMG evidence of myopathy, and muscle fiber necrosis with or without inflammatory infiltrates occur in AIDS myopathy. HIV-antigens are detectable in macrophages in muscle inflammatory infiltrates but are absent in muscle fibers. The inflammatory myopathy associated with early HIV infection usually responds to glucocorticoids. Polymyositis also occurs in patients displaying the spectrum of diseases associated with human T lymphotropic virus type I (HTLV-I) infection, especially in the Caribbean islands and Japan.

AZT myopathy is dose related and usually improves upon discontinuation of the drug or after reduction of the dose. Structural and functional mitochondrial abnormalities are usually associated with AZT myopathy.

INCLUSION BODY MYOSITIS The clinical features of this typically sporadic, but rarely familial disorder, are similar to those of chronic idiopathic polymyositis, except that onset is at an older age, focal and distal muscle involvement are more frequent, and disease duration is longer. Muscle biopsy shows interstitial and occasional perivascular inflammatory infiltrates, necrosis, and regeneration of muscle fibers, but in addition there are "rimmed vacuoles" in the fibers that stain positively with Congo-red, like amyloid. Electron microscopy reveals paramyxovirus-like 15- to 18-nm filaments in the nuclei and sarcoplasm that show immunoreactivity to ubiquitin and β-amyloid protein. The nature of the inflammatory infiltrate and the mechanism of muscle fiber damage are similar to that in polymyositis. Recent immunocytochemical and in-situ hybridization studies suggest that a previously reported etiologic link with the mumps virus seems unlikely. This disorder usually responds poorly to glucocorticoids and immunosuppressive therapy, and the prognosis is for a chronically progressive disorder with loss of ambulation about 5 to 10 years after presentation.

Eosinophilic myositis This rare disease probably represents one manifestation of the spectrum of hypereosinophilic syndrome. There are a number of subtypes. Subacute onset of muscle pain and proximal weakness, elevated serum CK, myopathic features on electromyogram, and histologic appearances of a myositis with an eosinophilic inflammatory infiltrate are characteristic. Some patients may respond to glucocorticoids, methotrexate, or leukapheresis.

EOSINOPHILIA-MYALGIA SYNDROME A syndrome that is more common in women has recently been associated with ingestion of the essential amino acid L-tryptophan. Fever, rash, arthralgia, cough, dyspnea, and edema are commonly accompanied by eosinophilia (more than 1000 cells per microliter), peripheral neuropathy and myositis with endomysial, perimysial, and fascial infiltration of lymphocytes and eosinophils. A di-L-tryptophan aminal of acetaldehyde, a contaminating by-product of the manufacture of some batches of L-tryptophan, has been incriminated. Cell-mediated immunologic muscle damage produced by cytotoxic T cells alone or with accompanying macrophages has been reported.

EOSINOPHILIC FASCIITIS This disorder is characterized by painful swelling and thickening of the skin in the extremities, limitation of movement due to contractures, and mild muscle weakness. Raised sedimentation rate, peripheral eosinophilia, hypergammaglobulinemia, and mildly elevated CK are seen. The EMG may show myopathic features. Histologically there is marked thickening and infiltration of the deep fascia with mononuclear cells and eosinophils, some involvement of the epimysium and perimysium, and varying but not striking degeneration of muscle. Most patients respond to treatment with glucocorticoids.

RELAPSING EOSINOPHILIC PERIMYOSITIS In this disease there are recurrent painful and tender areas in the neck or lower extremities, but without muscle weakness. Raised sedimentation rate and peripheral eosinophilia are frequent, serum CK is sometimes raised, and pathologically there is eosinophilic infiltration of the perimysium. Response to glucocorticoids is usually good.

LABORATORY FINDINGS In all forms of polymyositis there may be elevated serum levels of the enzymes present in skeletal muscle, such as CK, aldolase, serum glutamic oxaloacetic transaminase (SGOT), lactic acid dehydrogenase (LDH), and serum glutamic pyruvate transaminase (SGPT). The degree of rise decreases from the first to the last in this series of enzymes, and the pattern is the reverse of that seen in liver disease. The erythrocyte sedimentation rate is elevated in about two-thirds of cases. Tests for circulating rheumatoid factor are positive in less than one-half and antinuclear antibodies in about three-quarters of the cases. Several autoantibodies seem to be associated with clinically distinct groups of patients. Anti-Jo-1 antibodies are more common in polymyositis, especially in patients with interstitial lung disease, and anti-nRNP antibodies are often associated with polymyositis seen in lupus erythematosus. Other antibodies seen in patients with dermatomyositis and polymyositis in association with connective tissue diseases include anti-Scl-70 (progressive systemic sclerosis), anti-Sm (lupus erythematosus), anti-Ro and anti-La (Sjögren's syndrome and lupus erythematosus), and anti-ENA (mixed connective tissue disease). Myoglobin can be found in the urine when muscle destruction is acute and extensive; rarely, acute polymyositis causes the full syndrome of rhabdomyolysis and myoglobinuria. Most other hematologic indexes are normal. In about 40 percent of cases the electromyogram reveals a markedly increased insertional activity (muscle irritability), together with the typical myopathic triad of motor unit action potentials which are of low amplitude, are polyphasic, and have an abnormally early recruitment. In a further 40 percent of the patients only myopathic changes are present. The ECG is abnormal in about 5 to 10 percent of the cases at presentation. Since the pathologic process in myositis is patchy,

greater diagnostic yield is obtained by taking the biopsy from two clinically affected muscles and by skip serial sectioning of all specimens. Magnetic resonance imaging may serve to identify sites of muscle involvement. Muscles recently used for EMG or intramuscular injection must be avoided as these procedures can produce inflammatory changes and muscle fiber damage, leading to false-positive results. In about two-thirds of cases, the biopsies will demonstrate the typical pathologic changes of myositis, but despite following the above recommendations, about 10 percent of cases have normal muscle biopsy.

Skeletal muscle pathology The principal changes in muscle consist of infiltrates of inflammatory cells (lymphocytes, macrophages, plasma cells, and rare eosinophils and neutrophils) and destruction of muscle fibers with a phagocytic reaction. Perivascular (usually perivenular) inflammatory cell infiltration is the hallmark of polymyositis. Interstitial inflammatory cell infiltration is also a prominent feature of the disease, but lesser degrees of it may be seen in other conditions as a secondary reaction (e.g., in facioscapulohumeral and Becker's muscular dystrophy). Evidence of muscle fiber degeneration and regeneration is almost invariably present. Many of the residual muscle fibers are small, with increased numbers of sarcolemmal nuclei. Either the degeneration of muscle fibers or the infiltration of inflammatory cells may predominate in any given biopsy specimen. Blood vessel changes and perifascicular atrophy are prominent in childhood dermatomyositis, but less so in adult dermatomyositis and polymyositis. Capillary loss due to endothelial cell necrosis occurs particularly in the periphery of fascicles and may explain the perifascicular atrophy. Other features include reduplication of capillary basement membrane and the presence of tubular inclusions within endothelial cells. Type II muscle fiber atrophy and muscle infarcts also may be found. Vasculitis is also seen in polymyositis or dermatomyositis associated with connective tissue disorders.

DIAGNOSIS Patients with dermatomyositis showing the characteristic skin rash, muscle weakness, and evidence of muscle damage by EMG and elevation of serum CK may not require a muscle biopsy to confirm the diagnosis. In the case of idiopathic polymyositis, however, a firm diagnosis must be based on the presence of a typical clinical picture, a typical EMG, elevation of serum CK, and a diagnostic muscle biopsy. All four criteria are required to be certain of the diagnosis, since inflammatory changes may occasionally occur in other myopathies (e.g., facioscapulohumeral muscular dystrophy) and in other connective tissue disorders without clear muscle weakness. However, in less than one-third of cases of polymyositis are *all* these criteria satisfied. It may be particularly difficult to obtain a diagnostic muscle biopsy because of the patchy nature of the disease. Thus, a therapeutic trial of glucocorticoids should be given when full investigation of a patient with significant disability leaves a diagnosis of "possible polymyositis," usually because of a nondiagnostic muscle biopsy.

DIFFERENTIAL DIAGNOSIS The clinical picture of skin rash and proximal or diffuse muscle weakness has few causes other than dermatomyositis. However, proximal muscle weakness without skin involvement can be due to many conditions other than polymyositis and necessitates detailed investigation to establish the correct diagnosis.

Subacute or chronic progressive muscle weakness This may be due to denervating conditions such as the spinal muscular atrophies or amyotrophic lateral sclerosis. Upper motor neuron signs in the latter in addition to the muscle weakness aid in the diagnosis. The muscular dystrophies, such as those of Duchenne and Becker and the limb-girdle and facioscapulohumeral types, may appear similar to polymyositis (Chap. 385). However, the muscular dystrophies usually develop more slowly, rarely present after the age of 30, usually involve the pharyngeal and posterior neck muscles only in their later course, and have a pattern of muscle involvement which is selective, involving some muscles, such as the biceps and brachioradialis, early in the course of the disease, and sparing others, such as the deltoid. Nevertheless, in rare patients it may be difficult, even with a muscle biopsy, to distinguish chronic polymyositis from a rapidly advancing muscular dystrophy. This is particularly true of facioscapulohumeral muscular dystrophy, where interstitial inflammatory cell infiltration is commonly found early in the disease. Such doubtful cases should always be given an adequate trial of glucocorticoid therapy. Dystrophia myotonica produces a characteristic facies with ptosis, facial myopathy, temporalis muscle wasting, and grip myotonia (Chap. 385). Some of the metabolic myopathies, including glycogen storage disease due to myophosphorylase deficiency and the lipid storage diseases due to carnitine and carnitine palmityltransferase deficiency, produce exertional cramps, rhabdomyolysis, and muscle weakness; diagnosis rests upon biochemical studies of the muscle biopsy (Chap. 385). Glycogen storage disease due to acid maltase deficiency also requires muscle biopsy for diagnosis. The endocrine myopathies such as those due to hypercorticosteroidism, hyper- and hypothyroidism, and hyper- and hypoparathyroidism require the appropriate laboratory investigations for diagnosis. Muscle wasting in patients with an underlying neoplasm may be true polymyositis, but it can be due to a protein-wasting state (cachexia), a paraneoplastic neuropathy, or type II fiber atrophy.

Muscle weakness with marked exercise-induced fatigue Fatigue without much muscle wasting may be due to the neuromuscular junction disorders, myasthenia gravis, or the Lambert-Eaton syndrome. Repetitive nerve stimulation studies aid in the diagnosis of these conditions (Chap. 386).

Acute muscle weakness This may be caused by an acute neuropathy such as that due to the Guillain-Barré syndrome or a neurotoxin. When combined with painful muscle cramps, rhabdomyolysis, and myoglobinuria, it may be due to known metabolic disorders including some of the glycogen storage diseases such as myophosphorylase deficiency (McArdle's disease), carnitine palmityltransferase deficiency, and myoadenylate deaminase deficiency. Acute viral infections may cause a similar syndrome. Chronic alcoholics may develop a painful myopathy with myoglobinuria after a bout of heavy drinking or may present with a painless acute hypokalemic myopathy which is completely reversible, or may show an asymptomatic elevation of serum CK and myoglobin. Acute muscle weakness with myoglobinuria may occur in prolonged severe hypokalemia due to potassium loss, or with hypophosphatemia and hypomagnesemia, often seen in chronic alcoholics and in patients on nasogastric suction receiving parenteral hyperalimentation. An acute necrotizing myopathy with myoglobinuria can rarely accompany hypernatremia and hyponatremia.

Drug-induced myopathies Rhabdomyolysis and myoglobinuria have been associated with intake of amphotericin B, ϵ-aminocaproic acid, fenfluramine, heroin, and phencyclidine. A predominantly hypokalemic myopathy may result from prolonged use of diuretics, carbenoxolone, and azathioprine. Penicillamine has been reported to produce a myositis. The use of clofibrate, cimetidine, chloroquine, colchicine, carbimazole, cyclosporine, emetine, lovastatin, phenytoin, and, recently, AZT has been associated with a myopathy. Toxic myopathies usually have a different pathology from polymyositis and require a careful drug history for diagnosis. In other cases investigation reveals no etiology, and these may be due to a true acute autoimmune polymyositis or to an as yet undiscovered metabolic defect.

Pain on movement and muscle tenderness Patients with muscle pain and little or no weakness may be thought to be neurotic or hysterical. A number of conditions including *polymyalgia rheumatica* (Chap. 291) and arthritic disorders of adjacent joints enter into the differential diagnosis of polymyositis. The muscle biopsy either is normal or discloses type II fiber atrophy, but in polymyalgia rheumatica the temporal artery biopsy may show giant cell arteritis (Chap. 291). *Fibrositis* and *fibromyalgia* are syndromes which frequently enter into the differential diagnosis of polymyositis. Patients complain of focal or diffuse muscle tenderness, aching, and weakness, which is sometimes poorly separated from joint pain. In other patients there may be minor signs of a collagen vascular disorder, such as an increased erythrocyte sedimentation rate, antinuclear antibody (ANA),

or rheumatoid factor, and occasionally there is slight elevation of the serum CK. The muscle biopsy occasionally shows a few interstitial inflammatory cells. Where there is a focal "trigger point," biopsy may show inflammatory infiltration of the connective tissue. Rarely does this syndrome develop into frank polymyositis, and the prognosis is therefore more benign than that of polymyositis (see below). Many such patients show some response to nonsteroidal anti-inflammatory agents, though most continue to have indolent complaints.

TREATMENT Glucocorticoids in high dosage are the accepted treatment for severe dermatomyositis-polymyositis, though there is no controlled trial to prove their effectiveness. The best results are obtained from the use of prednisone, starting at a dose of 1 to 2 mg/ kg body weight per day (60 to 100 mg/d for adults). Improvement may begin within 1 to 4 weeks, though in some patients treatment may need to be continued for 3 months before improvement occurs. When there is significant improvement in the weakness, the daily dose may be reduced by 5 mg every 4 weeks. Repeated manual muscle testing and serum CK determinations should be performed to ensure that the myositis does not relapse. At about 40 mg/d, the schedule is changed gradually to 80 mg every other day in order to reduce the incidence of glucocorticoid side effects. There is some evidence that the use of alternate-day glucocorticoids from the outset may be effective, particularly in patients with milder disease. Children and patients with acute to subacute dermatomyositis-polymyositis tend to improve more rapidly than those with chronic polymyositis. If the dose is reduced too rapidly, or to too low a level, relapse will occur, necessitating return to high dosage. Prednisone therapy may have to be continued for several years, but an attempt should be made every year to withdraw the therapy from patients who are clinically stable in order to determine if the disease is still active.

Cytotoxic drugs should be tried when the disease is severe, when the response to glucocorticoids is inadequate after 1 to 3 months, or when relapses are frequent. Azathioprine (2.5 to 3.5 mg/kg body weight per day in divided doses) is the most commonly used cytotoxic drug in this disease, and in combination with glucocorticoids in preliminary studies has shown a better response than glucocorticoids alone. Cyclophosphamide, methotrexate, and cyclosporine also have been used with benefit in uncontrolled reports. The aim of cytotoxic therapy with azathioprine or cyclophosphamide (usual dose about 2 mg/kg body weight per day) is to lower the total lymphocyte count to about 750 per microliter, while maintaining the hemoglobin level above 12 g/dL, the total white cell count above 3000 per microliter, and the platelet count about 125,000 per microliter. Weekly blood counts are required to monitor the cytotoxic drug therapy. Methotrexate is effective at doses that do not produce lymphopenia (usual dose about 0.5 mg/kg body weight per week, attained by slowly increasing to that dose). The combined use of prednisone and a cytotoxic drug usually allows a lower dose of prednisone to be used. In preliminary studies total-body irradiation has been successfully used in some patients with disease refractory to glucocorticoids and immunosuppressants, but long-term follow-up and controlled studies are lacking for this potentially dangerous therapy. A recent controlled trial of plasma exchange and leukapheresis in a small number of patients with dermatomyositis-polymyositis resistant to glucocorticoids showed no benefit over sham pheresis. High-dose intravenous immunoglobulin therapy has produced improvement in patients otherwise refractory to glucocorticoids, immunosuppressive drugs, and plasma exchange, but controlled trials need to be undertaken. Bed rest has been recommended in the acute phase of the disease but is harmful in the long term. Physiotherapy and rehabilitative devices are important in the long-term treatment of patients with dermatomyositis-polymyositis.

Elderly patients, particularly those with dermatomyositis, should be followed closely for the possibility of malignant disease, and any new symptoms or signs must be appropriately investigated by a directed approach. If a malignant lesion is found, it should be treated, since the muscle weakness may disappear if the neoplasm is eradicated. However, a response to glucocorticoids can usually be obtained even in patients with dermatomyositis-polymyositis associated with a malignancy.

The serum CK activity is useful for following patients during reduction of immunosuppressive therapy, since a rise in level generally indicates an incipient clinical relapse. However, it cannot be used to indicate initial response in patients being treated with prednisone for dermatomyositis-polymyositis, since this drug lowers the serum CK activity in a way which is not fully understood, but which is not related to the suppression of muscle inflammation.

Side effects of high-dose daily glucocorticoid therapy (see Chap. 335) are relatively common in patients treated for polymyositis, and these may limit therapy. However, these can be minimized by appropriate use of alternate-day therapy. When patients who have been stable on a static dose of prednisone develop increasing muscle weakness, this may be due to either a relapse of the myositis or to glucocorticoid myopathy. An EMG, serum CK measurement, and, rarely, muscle biopsy may help in differentiating these two conditions if the changes of myositis are present. However, often the only way to separate them is to reduce the dose of prednisone slowly; if glucocorticoid myopathy is the cause of the weakness, it will improve as the dose is reduced; if a relapse of the myositis is responsible, the weakness will increase with reduction in the dose.

Side effects of cytotoxic drugs include marrow suppression, alopecia, gastrointestinal tract disorders, damage to the testes and ovaries (including potential genetic damage), disorders of chronic immunosuppression, and potential for malignancy.

PROGNOSIS The overall mortality rate of individuals with dermatomyositis-polymyositis is about four times that of the general population; death is due usually to pulmonary, renal, and cardiac complications. Females, blacks, and those severely affected at presentation or treated after long delays have a worse prognosis. Unfavorable outcome is also seen in patients with significant dysphagia, associated cancer or connective tissue diseases, and serum antibodies to Jo-1 and SRP. Evidence from several series suggests that patients seen at tertiary referral centers may have less favorable outcome when compared with patients seen at smaller community hospitals, probably because they represent a population with more severe disease which shows poorer response to therapy. Nevertheless, the 5-year survival rate is about 75 percent overall, and is better than this in children. The majority of patients improve with therapy. Many patients make a full functional recovery, though some weakness of the shoulders and hips, usually not disabling, remains at the conclusion of treatment. Relapse may occur at any time. Glucocorticoids should not be discontinued too soon, for the relapse which may follow is often more difficult to treat than the original presentation. About one-half of the patients with this disease recover and can discontinue therapy within 5 years after the onset of the symptoms; about 20 percent still have active disease requiring continued therapy. The remaining 30 percent have inactive disease but residual muscle weakness.

REFERENCES

BANKER BQ, ENGEL AG: The polymyositis and dermatomyositis syndromes, in *Myology*, 2d ed, AG Engel, Franzini-Armstrong C (eds). New York, McGraw-Hill, 1994

BOHAN A et al: A computer-assisted analysis of 153 patients with polymyositis and dermatomyositis. Medicine 56:255, 1977

BRADLEY WG, TANDAN R: Inflammatory diseases of muscle, in *Textbook of Rheumatology*, 3d ed, WN Kelly et al (eds). Philadelphia, Saunders, 1988, chap 72

CACCAMO DV et al: Fulminant rhabdomyolysis in a patient with dermatomyositis. Neurology 43:844, 1993

CARPENTER S, KARPATI G: *Pathology of Skeletal Muscle*. New York, Churchill Livingstone, 1984, pp 515–592

DALAKAS MC: Polymyositis, dermatomyositis and inclusion-body myositis. N Engl J Med 325:1487, 1991

DEVERE R, BRADLEY WG: Polymyositis: Its presentation, mortality, and morbidity. Brain 98:637, 1975

EMSLIE-SMITH AM, ENGEL AG: Microvascular changes in early and advanced dermatomyositis: A quantitative study. Ann Neurol 27:343, 1990

LEONMONZON M et al: Search for HIV proviral DNA and amplified sequences in the muscle biopsies of patients with HIV polymyositis. Muscle Nerve 16:408, 1993

MARTIN RW et al: The clinical spectrum of the eosinophilia-myalgia syndrome associated with L-tryptophan ingestion. Ann Intern Med 113:124, 1990

MILLER FW: Myositis-specific autoantibodies: Touchstones for understanding the inflammatory myopathies. JAMA 270:1846, 1993

SIGURGEIRSSON B et al: Risk of cancer in patients with dermatomyositis or polymyositis: A population-based study. N Engl J Med 326:363, 1992

385 INHERITED, METABOLIC, ENDOCRINE, AND TOXIC MYOPATHIES

JERRY R. MENDELL / ROBERT C. GRIGGS

The muscle disorders discussed in this chapter include diseases that cause acute, subacute, or chronic muscle weakness. Some also cause pain in addition to or instead of weakness. The differential diagnosis of neuromuscular disease is discussed in Chap. 382. Dermatomyositis and polymyositis are discussed in Chap. 384 and periodic paralysis in Chap. 387.

HEREDITARY MYOPATHIES

Muscular dystrophy refers to a group of hereditary progressive diseases. Each type of muscular dystrophy has unique phenotypic and genetic features (Table 385-1).

DUCHENNE MUSCULAR DYSTROPHY This X-linked recessive disorder, sometimes also called *pseudohypertrophic muscular dystrophy*, occurs with an incidence of about 30 per 100,000 live born males. The disease bears the name of the French neurologist Duchenne because he established criteria for diagnosis and accurately described muscle biopsies.

Clinical features Duchenne dystrophy is present at birth, but the disorder usually becomes apparent between ages 3 and 5. The boys fall frequently and have difficulty keeping up with their friends when playing. Running, jumping, and hopping are invariably abnormal. By age 5, muscle weakness is obvious by muscle testing. On getting up from the floor, the patient uses his hands to climb up himself (Gowers' maneuver). In younger children, the calf muscles may feel firm and rubbery and are usually enlarged from true muscle hypertrophy; later calf enlargement is appropriately called *pseudohypertrophy* since muscle is replaced by fat and connective tissue. Contractures of the heel cords and iliotibial bands become apparent by age 6, when toe walking is associated with a lordotic posture. Loss of muscle strength is progressive, with predilection for proximal limb muscles and the neck flexors; leg involvement is more severe than arm involvement. Between ages 8 and 10 walking may require the use of braces; joint contractures and limitations of hip flexion, knee, elbow, and wrist extension are made worse by prolonged sitting. By age 12, most patients are confined to a wheelchair. Contractures become fixed and a progressive scoliosis often develops which may be associated with considerable discomfort. The chest deformity associated with scoliosis impairs the pulmonary function already diminished by muscle weakness. By age 16 to 18, patients are predisposed to serious, sometimes fatal pulmonary infections. Other causes of death include aspiration of food and acute gastric dilatation.

A cardiac cause of death is uncommon despite the existence of a cardiomyopathy in almost all patients. Congestive heart failure seldom occurs except with severe stress such as pneumonia. Cardiac arrhythmias are rare. The typical ECG shows an increase net RS in lead V_1; deep narrow Q waves in the precordial leads; and RSR' or polyphyasic R waves in V_1. Intellectual impairment in Duchenne dystrophy is common; the average intelligent quotient (IQ) is approximately one standard deviation below the mean. Impairment of

TABLE 385-1   Progressive muscular dystrophies

Type	Genetics	Clinical features	Other organ system involvement
Duchenne	X-linked recessive mutation of dystrophin gene	Onset before age 5 Progressive weakness of girdle muscles Inability to walk after age 12 Kyphoscoliosis Respiratory failure in second to third decade	Cardiomyopathy Mental impairment
Becker	X-linked recessive mutation of dystrophin gene	Onset in early to late childhood Slowly progressive weakness of girdle muscles Ability to walk after age 15 Respiratory failure after fourth decade	Cardiomyopathy
Myotonic	Autosomal dominant Expansion of unstable region of DNA at chromosome 19q13.3	Onset any decade Slowly progressive weakness of eyelids, face, neck, distal limb muscles Myotonia	Cardiac conduction defects Mental impairment Cataracts Frontal baldness Gonadal atrophy
Facioscapulohumeral	Autosomal dominant Frequent mutations at chromosome 4q35	Onset before age 20 Slowly progressive face, shoulder girdle, foot dorsiflexion weakness	Hypertension Deafness
Limb-girdle (may include several disorders)	Autosomal recessive or autosomal dominant	Onset in early childhood to adulthood. Slowly progressive weakness of shoulder and hip girdle muscles	Cardiomyopathy
Oculopharyngeal	Autosomal dominant (French-Canadian or Hispanic background)	Onset fifth to sixth decade Slowly progressive weakness of extraocular, eyelid, face, and pharyngeal muscles Cricopharyngeal achalasia	
Congenital (includes several disorders including Fukuyama and cerebro-ocular-dysplasia types)	Autosomal recessive	Onset at birth Hypotonia, contractures, and delayed milestones Early respiratory failure in some, static course in others	Cerebral Eye

intellectual function appears to be nonprogressive and affects verbal ability more than performance. IQs of Duchenne patients are lower than children with comparably disabling and chronic disorders, indicating mental subnormality in Duchenne dystrophy is not solely the reflection of physical limitations. The basis for intellectual impairment in Duchenne dystrophy has not been established.

Laboratory investigation   Serum CK levels are invariably elevated between 20 and 100 times normal. The levels are abnormal at birth but decline late in the disease because of inactivity and loss of muscle mass.

Electromyography (EMG) demonstrates features typical of myopathy. The muscle biopsy shows muscle fibers of varying size as well as small groups of necrotic and regenerating fibers. Connective tissue and fat replace lost muscle fibers. A definitive diagnosis of Duchenne dystrophy can be established on the basis of dystrophin deficiency in biopsied muscle tissue or mutation analysis on peripheral blood leukocytes as discussed below.

Genetics   Duchenne dystrophy, inherited as an X-linked recessive trait, is caused by a mutation of the gene responsible for producing dystrophin. The latter is a 427 kDa protein localized to the inner surface of the sarcolemma of the muscle fiber. The dystrophin gene, an estimated 2000 kb in size, is one of the largest identified human genes. It is localized to the short arm of the X chromosome at the Xp21 site. At the present time, mutations of the gene can be identified (in approximately two-thirds of Duchenne patients) using a battery of cDNA probes. Deletions are not uniformly distributed over the gene, but rather occur with a higher frequency near the middle of the gene. Deletion size does not correlate with severity of disease. Gene duplication represents another type of mutation, although less common, leading to Duchenne dystrophy. Identification of a specific mutation provides for an unequivocal diagnosis and makes possible accurate testing of potential carriers and for use of amniotic fluid cells or chorionic villi in prenatal diagnosis. In families without deletions or duplications, linkage analysis using probes recognizing restriction fragment length polymorphisms is also available.

Dystrophin determination of muscle tissue represents an accurate method of diagnosis of Duchenne dystrophy. The amount and alteration in the size of dystrophin can be determined by western blot analysis of muscle biopsy specimens. In addition, immunocytochemical staining of muscle, using antibodies raised against dystrophin, can be used to demonstrate absence or deficiency of dystrophin localizing to the sarcolemmal membrane. Carriers of the disease may demonstrate a mosaic pattern, but dystrophin analysis of muscle biopsies for carrier detection is not reliable.

Treatment   Prednisone in a dose of 0.75 mg/kg per day has been shown to significantly alter the progression of Duchenne dystrophy for up to 3 years. Despite these favorable results, there are patients who clearly cannot tolerate glucocorticoid therapy. The weight gain represents a significant deterrent for some boys. Treatment must be tailored to the individual.

BECKER MUSCULAR DYSTROPHY   This less severe form of X-linked recessive muscular dystrophy was described by Becker and Keiner in 1955. It is often called the benign form of pseudohypertrophic muscular dystrophy. Until recently it was not known whether Duchenne and Becker muscular dystrophies represented genetically distinct disorders. Molecular genetic studies now indicate that Duchenne and Becker dystrophies result from allelic defects of the same gene. Becker muscular dystrophy is approximately 10 times less frequent than Duchenne, with an incidence of about 3 per 100,000.

Clinical features   The pattern of muscle wasting in Becker muscular dystrophy closely resembles that seen in Duchenne. Proximal muscles, especially of the lower extremities, are prominently involved. As the disease progresses, weakness becomes more generalized. Significant facial muscle weakness is not a feature. Hypertrophy of muscles, particularly the calves, is an early and prominent finding.

The majority of Becker patients first experience difficulties between ages 5 and 15 years, although an onset in the third or fourth decade or even later can occur. By definition, Becker patients ambulate beyond age 15, allowing for a clinical distinction between Becker and Duchenne dystrophy. Becker dystrophy patients have a reduced life expectancy, but the majority survive into the fourth or fifth decade.

Mental retardation may be seen in Becker dystrophy, but not as frequently as in Duchenne. Cardiac involvement occurs in Becker dystrophy and may result in heart failure.

Laboratory features The serum CK, EMG, and muscle biopsy features closely resemble Duchenne dystrophy. The diagnosis of Becker muscular dystrophy requires western blot analysis of muscle biopsy samples demonstrating dystrophin of reduced amount or abnormal size. In addition, in Becker dystrophy mutation analysis of DNA from peripheral blood leukocytes recognizes deletions and duplications of the dystrophin gene in approximately the same number (65 percent) as seen in Duchenne. In both Becker and Duchenne, the size of the DNA deletion does not predict clinical severity; however, in about 95 percent of Becker dystrophy patients DNA deletions do not alter the translational reading frame of messenger RNA. This "in-frame" mutation allows for production of some dystrophin, and accounts for the presence of altered rather than absent dystrophin on western blot analysis.

Phenotypic variations on dystrophin deficiency The preceding discussion implies a clear delineation between typical Duchenne and Becker patients, but in actuality there is a spectrum of muscle weakness ranging from very severe to very mild. A well-recognized subgroup of patients have clinical characteristics intermediate between Duchenne and Becker dystrophy patients. On western blot studies of muscle biopsy, intermediate phenotypic patients show dystrophin of reduced amounts or abnormal size similar to Becker dystrophy.

Treatment The use of prednisone has not been adequately studied in Becker dystrophy and other mild dystrophin-deficiency disorders.

MYOTONIC DYSTROPHY This condition was originally described by Steinert in 1909 and represents the most common adult muscular dystrophy. This disorder has an incidence of 13.5 per 100,000 live births and involves an equal proportion of males and females.

Clinical features The clinical expression of myotonic dystrophy varies widely and affects many systems other than muscle. Myotonic dystrophy patients have a typical "hatchet-faced" appearance due to temporalis, masseter, and facial muscle atrophy and weakness. Men have frontal baldness and women often have a balding hair pattern. Neck muscles, including the flexors and sternocleidomastoids, become involved early as do distal limb muscles. Weakness of wrist extensors, finger extensors, and intrinsic hand muscles impairs function. Ankle dorsiflexor weakness may cause footdrop. Proximal muscles remain stronger throughout the course, although preferential atrophy and weakness of quadriceps muscles occurs in many patients. Palatal, pharyngeal, and tongue involvement produces a dysarthric speech, nasal voice, and swallowing problems. Some patients have diaphragm and intercostal muscle weakness, resulting in respiratory insufficiency.

Myotonia, which usually appears by age 5, is demonstrable by percussion of thenar eminence, tongue, and wrist extensor muscles. Myotonia causes a slow relaxation of hand grip following a forced voluntary closure. Advanced muscle wasting makes myotonia more difficult to detect.

Congenital myotonic dystrophy is a more severe form of the disease occurring in approximately 25 percent of infants of affected mothers. It is characterized by severe facial and bulbar weakness and neonatal respiratory insufficiency. Most patients will recover from respiratory distress. Congenital myotonic dystrophy patients usually have impaired intelligence.

Cardiac disturbances occur in the majority of patients with myotonic dystrophy. Electrocardiographic abnormalities are common, including first degree heart block or more extensive conduction system involvement. Complete heart block and sudden death can occur. Congestive heart failure occurs infrequently, but may result from cor pulmonale secondary to respiratory failure. Mitral valve prolapse also occurs commonly in myotonic dystrophy patients.

Other features associated with myotonic dystrophy include intellectual impairment, hypersomnia, posterior subcapsular cataracts, gonadal atrophy, insulin resistance and decreased esophageal and colonic motility.

Laboratory features The diagnosis of myotonic dystrophy can usually be made on clinical grounds alone and seldom requires laboratory studies. Serum CK levels may be normal or mildly elevated. EMG evidence of myotonia will be found readily in most cases by EMG. Muscle biopsy shows muscle atrophy, selectively involving type 1 fibers in 50 percent of cases. Typically, increased numbers of central nuclei can be seen. Necrosis of muscle fibers and increased connective tissue, common in other muscular dystrophies, do not usually occur in myotonic dystrophy.

Genetics Myotonic dystrophy is an autosomal dominant disorder. Evidence indicates that new mutations do not contribute to the pool of affected individuals. The disorder is transmitted by a mutant gene on the long arm of chromosome 19. Studies now indicate that, at 19q13.3, patients with myotonic dystrophy demonstrate an unstable region of DNA characterized by an increased number of trinucleotide CTG repeats. An increase in the severity of the disease phenotype in successive generations (genetic anticipation) is accompanied by an increase in the number of trinucleotide repeats. A similar type of mutation has been identified in fragile X syndrome (see Chap. 378). The unstable triplet repeat in myotonic dystrophy can be used for prenatal diagnosis. The greater severity of disease in the affected infants of mothers with myotonic dystrophy remains unexplained.

The protein encoded by the myotonic dystrophy gene has an amino acid composition homologous to a protein kinase (referred to as myotonin-protein kinase).

Treatment Myotonia in other forms of myotonic disorders such as myotonia congenita responds well to treatment. Myotonia in myotonic dystrophy, however, rarely warrants treatment. Phenytoin represents the preferred agent for the occasional patient who requires an antimyotonia drug; other agents, particularly quinine and procainamide may worsen cardiac conduction. Cardiac pacemaker insertion should be considered for patients with unexplained syncope or advanced conduction system abnormalities with evidence of second degree heart block or trifascicular conduction disturbances with marked prolongation of the PR interval.

Molded ankle-foot orthoses, for controlling footdrop and stabilizing the ankle, will help prevent patients with distal lower extremity weakness from falling.

FACIOSCAPULOHUMERAL MUSCULAR DYSTROPHY This form of muscular dystrophy, also called *Landouzy-Dejerine dystrophy*, has an incidence of approximately 1 in 20,000.

Clinical features The condition typically has an onset in childhood and young adult years. In most cases, facial weakness represents the initial manifestation, appearing as an inability to smile, whistle, or fully close the eyes. Weakness of the shoulder girdles, rather than facial muscles, usually brings the patient to medical attention. Loss of scapular stabilizer muscles makes arm elevation difficult. Scapular winging becomes apparent with attempts at abduction and forward movement of the arms. Biceps and triceps muscles may be severely affected with relative sparing of the deltoid muscles. Weakness of wrist extension invariably exceeds that of wrist flexion and weakness of the anterior compartment muscles of the legs may lead to footdrop.

In the majority of patients, the weakness remains restricted to facial, upper extremity, and distal lower extremity muscles. In 20 percent of cases, weakness progresses to involve the pelvic girdle muscles and severe functional impairment and possible wheelchair confinement result.

Characteristically, patients with facioscapulohumeral dystrophy do not have involvement of other organ systems, although labile hypertension is common and there is an increased incidence of nerve deafness.

Laboratory features Serum CK may be normal or mildly elevated. EMG usually indicates a myopathic pattern. The muscle biopsy shows nonspecific features of a myopathy. A prominent inflammatory infiltrate, which is often multifocal in distribution, is present in some biopsies. The cause or significance of this finding is unknown.

Genetics An autosomal dominant inheritance pattern with almost complete penetrance has been established, but requires examination of each family member for confirmation since approximately 30 percent of those affected will be unaware of involvement. The gene for facioscapulohumeral dystrophy is on the distal long arm of chromosome 4. A genetic probe localized to the site of the gene has been found so that carrier detection and prenatal diagnosis are possible. Studies with this probe indicate that most sporadic cases represent new mutations.

Treatment No specific treatment is available; ankle-foot orthoses are helpful for those with footdrop. Scapular stabilization procedures improve scapular winging, but may not improve function.

LIMB-GIRDLE DYSTROPHY This term which encompasses more than one disorder, is used to describe muscle weakness occurring in both males and females with onset ranging from late in the first decade to the fourth decade. Both autosomal recessive and autosomal dominant inheritance are found, and variable rates of progression occur. From a practical viewpoint, limb-girdle dystrophy groups together patients who defy classification into one of the better defined groups.

Clinical features In limb-girdle dystrophy, the initial symptoms of weakness of the proximal leg muscles usually begin in the second or third decade. Upper limb involvement with scapular winging appears later. The onset may be delayed until the third or fourth decade. Respiratory insufficiency from diaphragm weakness may occur. Distribution of weakness and rate of progression varies from family to family.

In some patients, cardiac involvement results in congestive heart failure or arrhythmias; occasional patients may present with a cardiomyopathy. Intellectual function remains normal.

Laboratory features Elevated serum CK, a myopathic EMG, and muscle biopsy features indicative of myopathy represent the characteristic changes in limb-girdle dystrophy. Careful attention to exclude phenotypically similar disorders such as spinal muscular atrophy and metabolic and inflammatory myopathies is required. The availability of western blot analysis for dystrophin allows for definite distinction of limb-girdle dystrophy from Becker muscular dystrophy.

Genetics Autosomal recessive or autosomal dominant inheritance may occur, depending on individual families. One variety of autosomal dominant limb-girdle dystrophy has been linked to chromosome 5. In another, inherited as a childhood autosomal recessive condition, a deficiency has been identified in one of the dystrophin-associated glycoproteins, which are a large complex of sarcolemmal glycoproteins linking dystrophin to the extracellular matrix.

Treatment No specific treatment can be offered.

OCULOPHARYNGEAL DYSTROPHY The term *progressive external ophthalmoplegia* (PEO) describes disorders characterized by slowly progressive ptosis and limitation of eye movements with sparing of pupillary reactions for light and accommodation. Patients usually do not complain of diplopia, in contrast to conditions with a more acute onset of ocular muscle weakness (e.g., myasthenia gravis). Oculopharyngeal muscular dystrophy represents one of the distinct disorders presenting with PEO. Two other disorders, centronuclear myopathy and mitochondrial myopathies with PEO, are discussed below.

Clinical features Oculopharyngeal muscular dystrophy usually presents with ptosis and/or dysphagia in the fourth to sixth decade. The swallowing problem may become debilitating and result in pooling of secretions and repeated episodes of aspiration. Mild neck and extremity weakness also occur.

Laboratory features The serum CK may be 2 to 3 times normal. A myopathic EMG is typical. On biopsy muscle fibers contain vacuoles, which by electron microscopy are shown to contain membranous whorls, accumulation of glycogen, and other nonspecific debris related to lysosomes. A distinct feature of oculopharyngeal dystrophy is the presence of tubular filaments, 8.5 nm in diameter, within muscle nuclei.

Genetics Oculopharyngeal dystrophy has an autosomal dominant inheritance pattern with complete penetrance. French-Canadians repre-

sent a commonly affected ethnic group. The disorder also occurs with increased frequency in Spanish-American families of the southwest United States. A large Jewish kindred of eastern European background has been reported.

Treatment Dysphagia can cause inanition and makes oculopharyngeal muscular dystrophy a potentially life-threatening disease. Cricopharyngeal myotomy may improve swallowing, although it does not prevent aspiration. Eyelid crutches can improve vision in patients in whom ptosis obstructs vision; candidates for ptosis surgery must be carefully selected; those with severe facial weakness are not suitable.

CONGENITAL MUSCULAR DYSTROPHY This rare disorder includes one or more genetic diseases; clinically, cases can be divided into a group having associated central nervous system involvement and one with only skeletal muscle disease.

Clinical features One form of congenital muscular dystrophy presents at birth or in the first few months of life with hypotonia, proximal limb weakness, and joint contractures at the elbows, hips, knees, and ankles. Contractures present at birth are referred to as *arthrogryposis*. Weakness of facial muscles may occur, but other cranial nerve musculature is spared. Severity varies greatly, but about half of the affected never achieve the ability to stand independently. Death may ensue because of respiratory insufficiency early in life. Some patients learn to walk, although difficulty in motor activities (e.g., running) persist.

In other forms of congenital muscular dystrophy patients have CNS involvement. A well-defined type is *Fukuyama congenital muscular dystrophy* associated with generalized tonic-clonic seizures and developmental delay in both verbal and mental spheres. Microcephaly and enlarged ventricles occur. A third variant, *cerebro-ocular-dysplasia muscular dystrophy*, has corneal abnormalities, cataracts, retinal dysplasia, and hypoplasia of the optic nerve. Hypomyelination of the cerebral white matter may be seen in patients with congenital muscular dystrophies.

Laboratory features Serum CK elevations range from normal to 20 times normal. The EMG shows a myopathic pattern and muscle biopsy features are nonspecific but demonstrate dystrophic features. Dystrophin analysis must be done on all cases of congenital muscular dystrophy to permit distinction from early-onset Duchenne muscular dystrophy.

Genetics Sporadic occurrences account for most of the cases of congenital muscular dystrophy without CNS involvement. Autosomal recessive inheritance has been established as the major mode of transmission for Fukuyama congenital muscular dystrophy and cerebro-ocular-dysplasia muscular dystrophy. In the Fukuyama-type, there is abnormal expression of dystrophin-associated proteins.

Treatment Supportive care and especially stretching to improve joint range of motion is important for congenital muscular dystrophies. Infants and very young children require special wheelchair modifications and adaptive seating to maximize functional capabilities.

DISTAL MYOPATHIES Patients with predominantly distal weakness and histologic evidence favoring muscular dystrophy are difficult to classify. Four of these disorders fulfill the definition of "muscular dystrophy" because of their hereditary nature and progressive course, although in the literature they are referred to as distal myopathies.

These distal myopathies can be separated into two late adult-onset types and two early adult-onset types.

The most familiar late-onset form was described by Welander. This disorder is seen predominantly in Scandinavian families. It is inherited as an autosomal dominant condition with onset in the fifth decade. Weakness begins in the hands with distal leg muscle involvement occurring later in the course. The lower extremity involvement begins in muscles of the distal anterior compartment (anterior tibial and peroneal muscle groups). The serum CK is either normal or mildly increased in this condition. Muscle biopsy changes are myopathic with some muscle fibers showing vacuoles.

Another late adult-onset form of distal myopathy is also inherited as an autosomal dominant trait but occurs in non-Scandinavian patients. Weakness begins in the anterior compartment of the distal lower extremities. Serum CK is normal or mildly elevated. Muscle biopsies from these patients reveal a myopathy with many fibers showing vacuoles.

Both of the early adult-onset distal myopathies have autosomal recessive inheritance. In one type, the weakness begins in the anterior compartment of the distal lower extremities, although in some cases it may begin in the hands. The serum CK is moderately elevated (less than 10 times normal) and muscle biopsies reveal a myopathy with many fibers showing vacuoles. The other form of early adult-onset distal myopathy is distinguished by weakness beginning in the posterior compartment, i.e., the gastrocnemius muscle. Serum CK is markedly elevated in this latter form (greater than 10 times normal) and biopsy shows a myopathy without vacuolated fibers. This condition with predilection for gastrocnemius weakness has been referred to as *Miyoshi myopathy*.

CONGENITAL MYOPATHIES

These rare disorders are distinguished from muscular dystrophies by the presence of specific histochemical and structural abnormalities in muscle. The description was originally introduced to distinguish nonprogressive muscle disease present at birth from muscular dystrophy which is progressive. Congenital myopathies can be severe and even fatal. Three major types are described: *central core disease, nemaline (rod) myopathy,* and *centronuclear (myotubular) myopathy.* Other rare types such as multicore disease, fingerprint body myopathy, and sarcotubular myopathy are not discussed here (see Banker).

CENTRAL CORE DISEASE   Clinical features Patients with central core disease may have decreased fetal movements and breech presentation. Skeletal abnormalities include congenital hip dislocation, scoliosis, and pes cavus; clubbed feet also occur. Hypotonia and delayed motor milestones, particularly walking, occur. Later in childhood, patients develop problems with stair climbing, running, and getting up from the floor. On examination there is mild facial and neck flexor weakness as well as weakness of the proximal extremity muscles, particularly in the legs. Most cases are nonprogressive but exceptions are well documented.

Laboratory features Serum CK is usually normal. Needle EMG demonstrates a myopathic pattern. The muscle biopsy is diagnostic, showing fibers with single or multiple central or eccentric discrete zones (cores) devoid of oxidative enzymes, and diminished PAS staining.

Genetics Autosomal dominant inheritance is characteristic; sporadic cases also occur. The gene for central core disease has been localized to the long arm of chromosome 19.

Treatment Patients with central core disease usually do not require specific treatment; however, recognition of the disease is important since there is a well-established predisposition for malignant hyperthermia during general anesthesia.

NEMALINE MYOPATHY The term *nemaline* refers to the distinctive presence of rods or coils of thread-like structures (*nema* = thread in Greek) in muscle fibers.

Clinical features Severe neonatal hypotonia with early respiratory distress may occur. A delay in motor milestones is common. The physical appearance may be striking because of the long, narrow facies or head, high arched palate, and open-mouthed appearance due to a prognathous jaw. Other skeletal abnormalities include pectus excavatum, kyphoscoliosis, pes cavus, and clubbed foot deformities. Facial and generalized muscle weakness commonly occur. The course is variable; some exhibit a static or nonprogressive course while others progress to wheelchair confinement. The disease may be fatal in infancy or childhood.

Myocardial involvement represents an unusual manifestation of nemaline myopathy which has been associated with an adult-onset form of the disease.

Laboratory features Serum CK is usually normal or slightly elevated. The EMG in weak muscles demonstrates a myopathic pattern with occasional fibrillation potentials. The muscle biopsy is diagnostic, demonstrating clusters of small rods or nemaline bodies. Rods occur preferentially, but not exclusively, in type 1 muscle fibers and the biopsies often show type 1 muscle fiber predominance. Rods originate from the Z disk material of the muscle fiber.

Genetics Evidence favors autosomal dominant inheritance with incomplete penetrance; sporadic cases also occur.

Treatment No specific treatment exists for this condition; some patients require bracing or surgery for the scoliosis as well as ankle-foot orthoses for distal lower extremity weakness.

CENTRONUCLEAR MYOPATHY   Clinical features Three distinct variants of the disease occur. *A neonatal form of centronuclear myopathy* presents with severe hypotonia and weakness at birth. Respiratory assistance may be required and swallowing difficulties may necessitate a feeding tube. This form of the disease carries a poor prognosis, often with a fatal outcome. The *late infantile–early childhood form of centronuclear myopathy* presents without difficulty at birth, but delayed motor milestones, especially walking, occur. Later, difficulty with running and stair climbing become apparent. Ptosis and varying degrees of ophthalmoplegia represent important distinguishing features of this congenital myopathy. A marfanoid appearance, slender body habitus, long narrow face, and high arched palate are typical. Scoliosis and clubbed feet may be present. The condition may be static or progress to weakness, requiring a wheelchair. A third rare variant, the *late childhood–adult type of centronuclear myopathy* has an onset in the second or third decade. Patients have full extraocular muscle movements and rarely exhibit ptosis. Patients have mild, nonprogressive limb weakness and no associated skeletal abnormalities.

Laboratory features Normal or slightly elevated CK levels occur in each of the forms of centronuclear myopathy. EMG studies are distinctive, showing positive sharp waves and fibrillation potentials, complex and repetitive discharges and myotonic discharges. Muscle biopsy in longitudinal section demonstrates rows of central nuclei, often surrounded by a halo. In transverse sections, central nuclei are found in 25 to 80 percent of muscle fibers.

Genetics Indisputable evidence for X-linked recessive inheritance exists in the neonatal form of centronuclear myopathy. The gene for the X-linked form has been localized to Xq28 allowing for identification of carriers. In the late infantile–early childhood disorder evidence favors autosomal recessive inheritance, and the late childhood–adult form of centronuclear myopathy has an autosomal dominant inheritance pattern.

Treatment Patients with a neonatal form of centronuclear myopathy require careful management for respiratory support and gastric feeding. For patients with the late infantile–early childhood disorder, ambulatory aids and orthotic devices and less often wheelchairs may be necessary. Occasional patients benefit from scoliosis surgery.

DISORDERS OF MUSCLE ENERGY METABOLISM

Skeletal muscle utilizes two principal sources of energy—fatty acids and glucose. Abnormalities in either glucose or lipid utilization can be associated with distinct clinical presentations. The clinical presentation can range from an acute painful syndrome with rhabdomyolysis and myoglobinuria to a chronic progressive muscle weakness simulating muscular dystrophy.

GLYCOGEN STORAGE AND GLYCOLYTIC DEFECTS There are four major disorders of glycogen metabolism (types II, III, IV, and V) and four disorders of glycolysis (types VII, IX, X, and XI) associated with significant skeletal muscle manifestations (see Chap. 350).

ACID MALTASE DEFICIENCY (TYPE II GLYCOGENOSIS) Acid maltase is an acid hydrolase lysosomal enzyme, with α-1,4- and α-1,6- glucosidase activity that breaks down glycogen to glucose.

Clinical features Three clinical forms of acid maltase deficiency can be distinguished. *Infantile acid maltase deficiency* is the most common, with onset of symptoms in 3 months of life. Infants develop severe muscle weakness, cardiomegaly, hepatomegaly, and respiratory insufficiency. Glycogen accumulation in motor neurons of the spinal cord and brainstem contributes to muscle weakness. Death usually occurs by 1 year of age. In *childhood acid maltase deficiency* the picture resembles muscular dystrophy. Delayed motor milestones result from proximal limb muscle weakness and involvement of respiratory muscles. The heart may be involved, but the liver and brain are unaffected. The *adult form of acid maltase deficiency* begins in the third or fourth decade. Respiratory failure and diaphragmatic weakness are often initial manifestations heralding progressive proximal muscle weakness. The heart and liver are not involved.

Laboratory findings Serum CK is usually elevated (2 to 10 times normal). EMG examination demonstrates a myopathic pattern, but other features are especially distinctive including: myotonic discharges; trains of fibrillation and positive waves; and complex repetitive discharges. At times, these special EMG discharges are very prominent in the lumbosacral paraspinal muscles. The muscle biopsy shows vacuoles containing glycogen and the lysosomal enzyme acid phosphatase. By electron microscopy, membrane-bound and free tissue glycogen are found. Definitive diagnosis is established by enzyme determination in muscle.

Genetics The three forms of acid maltase deficiency are all transmitted as an autosomal recessive trait. The gene, localized to the long arm of chromosome 17, has been isolated and sequenced making possible prenatal diagnosis for acid maltase deficiency.

Treatment No adequate method of replacing enzyme has been established, nor is dietary treatment of proven efficacy.

DEBRANCHER ENZYME (TYPE III GLYCOGENOSIS) The complete degradation of glycogen via the phosphorylytic pathway requires debranching enzyme. Absence of this enzyme results in a lesser proportion of muscle glycogen availability.

Clinical features The most common presentation of debrancher enzyme deficiency is the appearance of hepatomegaly, growth retardation, and hypoglycemia. Muscle involvement is often inconspicuous, although hypotonia and delayed motor milestones may be present. These findings usually diminish or disappear after puberty and a slowly progressive form of muscle weakness can develop in adult life. Rarely, myoglobinuria may be seen.

Laboratory features Serum CK is elevated. Forearm exercise test shows no rise in venous lactate. The muscle biopsy demonstrates subsarcolemmal and intermyofibrillar accumulation of glycogen. The definitive diagnosis is established by enzyme analysis of muscle (or liver).

Genetics Debrancher enzyme deficiency is inherited as an autosomal recessive trait.

Treatment No specific form of treatment for debrancher enzyme deficiency has been identified. Avoidance of hypoglycemia during episodes of intercurrent infection is necessary. Occasional patients require treatment for congestive heart failure.

BRANCHING ENZYME DEFICIENCY (TYPE IV GLYCOGENOSIS) This is a rare and fatal glycogen storage disease.

Clinical features This disorder is characterized by failure to thrive and hepatomegaly. Hypotonia and muscle wasting may be present, but the skeletal muscle manifestations are relatively minor compared to liver failure.

Laboratory features Diagnosis is usually established by demonstrating branching enzyme deficiency in skin fibroblasts or peripheral blood leukocytes.

Genetics The disorder is inherited as an autosomal recessive trait.

Treatment One patient has been successfully treated by liver transplantation.

MUSCLE PHOSPHORYLASE DEFICIENCY (TYPE V GLYCOGENOSIS) The clinical description of myophosphorylase defi-

ciency, in 1951 by McArdle, led to later identification of enzyme defect.

Clinical features Exercise intolerance is the dominant feature of the disorder. Symptoms usually occur first in adolescence with muscle pain and fatigue following intense exercise such as running or lifting heavy objects. Many patients report a "second-wind phenomenon" if they rest briefly or reduce intensity during the exercise, allowing them to continue activities for a longer period of time. Overexertion may lead to rhabdomyolysis and myoglobinuria, and renal failure can result. Variance of the classic presentation occurs, with some patients reporting only fatigability, others, having progressive weakness, and rare patients presenting with severe weakness and respiratory failure in infancy.

In the usual patients with McArdle's disease, examination between attacks is normal. Other organs are not affected.

Laboratory findings Serum CK levels fluctuate widely and may be elevated even during symptom-free periods. The forearm exercise test shows no rise in lactic acid; such testing is an important part of the evaluation of patients with myoglobinuria. The EMG is often normal except when taken after an episode of rhabdomyolysis, when muscle irritability (fibrillation potentials and positive waves) may be present. Muscle biopsy often shows subsarcolemmal blebs, containing glycogen, and absence of histochemical myophosphorylase staining; findings should be confirmed biochemically.

Genetics Myophosphorylase deficiency is usually inherited as an autosomal recessive trait with an unexplained predilection for men. The gene for muscle phosphorylase has been localized to the long arm of chromosome 11.

Treatment Patients can remain moderately active once they establish their limitations. Dietary supplementation with either glucose or fructose has not alleviated symptoms.

PHOSPHORYLASE b KINASE DEFICIENCY Muscle phosphorylase exists in two forms: phosphorylase a, the active enzyme initiating glycogen breakdown; and the inactive form, phosphorylase b. Phosphorylase b kinase converts inactive to active phosphorylase. Phosphorylase b kinase deficiency is a rare disorder with heterogeneous presentations. Children have weakness and liver enlargement and adults may have exercise intolerance and myoglobinuria. The inheritance pattern of muscle phosphorylase b kinase deficiency has not been established.

PHOSPHOFRUCTOKINASE DEFICIENCY (TYPE VII GLYCOGENOSIS) This condition is less common than McArdle's disease but has similar manifestations.

Clinical features Myalgias and fatigue occur following exercise and represent the predominant clinical manifestations. Unlike McArdle's disease, patients with phosphofructokinase (PFK) deficiency may worsen with carbohydrate ingestion. Patients present with rhabdomyolysis and myoglobinuria. Permanent limb weakness is less common than in McArdle's disease. Because of erythrocyte deficiency of PFK, a mild hemolytic anemia often occurs and may be useful in diagnosis.

Laboratory findings Elevated serum CK is often found. Reticulocytosis is a common feature, as is slight anemia and elevated bilirubin. The muscle biopsy shows subsarcolemmal blebs containing glycogen. A histochemical stain for phosphofructokinase can demonstrate the deficiency, but the definitive diagnosis requires biochemical analysis of muscle.

Genetics PFK deficiency is transmitted as an autosomal recessive trait. The disorder has an unusually strong male predominance and has an over representation in Ashkenazic Jews.

Treatment The anemia of PFK deficiency usually requires no treatment. Dietary manipulation does not alter muscle symptoms.

PHOSPHOGLYCERATE KINASE DEFICIENCY (TYPE IV GLYCOGENOSIS) **Clinical features** The clinical features of phosphoglycerate kinase (PGK) deficiency usually manifest as a nonspherocytic hemolytic anemia. Central nervous system dysfunction with mental retardation and seizures has been described. A rare variant of

PGK deficiency can also present with exercise intolerance and myoglobinuria.

Laboratory features Serum CK levels can be elevated. The forearm exercise test shows reduced levels of venous lactate compared to controls. The muscle biopsy shows a mild increase in glycogen. Muscle biochemistry confirms the diagnosis.

Genetics PGK deficiency is transmitted as an X-linked recessive trait. The gene is located on the short arm of the X chromosome.

Treatment No specific treatment is available. In patients with hemolytic anemia, splenectomy may be beneficial.

PHOSPHOGLYCERATE MUTASE DEFICIENCY (TYPE X GLYCO-GENOSIS) Clinical features In this rare disorder, patients present with myalgia, muscle cramping, and myoglobinuria following intense exercise. No other organ system involvement occurs.

Laboratory findings Serum CK levels are elevated and the forearm exercise test reveals a reduced rise in venous lactate.

Genetics The inheritance pattern is probably autosomal recessive, although no multigeneration families or sibs have yet been described.

Treatment No specific treatment is available.

LACTIC DEHYDROGENASE DEFICIENCY (GLYCOGENOSIS TYPE XI) Lactic dehydrogenase (LDH) is a tetrameric enzyme composed of two subunits, M and H. M-subunit isoenzymes predominate in skeletal muscle, while H-subunit–containing isoenzymes are the main components of LDH in heart.

Clinical features Patients with LDH-M deficiency have exercise intolerance, muscle pain, and myoglobinuria in the teenage years. No other organ system is involved.

Laboratory findings Serum CK is expectedly high during myoglobinuria, but there is a failure of serum LDH to rise. This corresponds to the defect of LDH-M. Forearm exercise test produces a minimal rise of lactic acid, but serum pyruvate rises substantially, pointing to the defect involved in conversion of pyruvate to lactate. The diagnosis can be confirmed by the biochemical analysis of muscle tissue showing markedly decreased LDH-M subunit. The M subunit can also be shown to be decreased in erythrocytes and leukocytes, although these other tissues are composed of combinations of the two subunits, M and H of LDH.

Genetics The disease appears to be inherited as an autosomal recessive trait. The M subunit of LDH is localized to chromosome 11. A deficiency of the H subunit of LDH, the cardiac isoform, has been described but is not associated with skeletal muscle symptoms.

Treatment Currently no treatment is available for this disorder.

DISORDERS OF LIPID METABOLISM

Lipid is an important muscle energy source during rest and prolonged, submaximal exercise. Fatty acids are derived from circulating very low density lipoprotein (VLDL) in the blood or from triglycerides stored in muscle fibers. Oxidation of fatty acids occurs in the mitochondria. In order to enter the mitochondria, fatty acids must first be converted to an "active fatty acid," acyl-CoA. The fatty acid acyl-CoA must be linked with carnitine by the enzyme carnitine palmityoltransferase 1 (CPT 1) for transport into the mitochondria. CPT 1 is present on the inner side of the outer mitochondrial membrane. Carnitine is removed by CPT 2, an enzyme attached to the inside of the inner mitochondrial membrane, allowing transport of acyl-CoA into the mitochondrial matrix for β-oxidation.

CARNITINE DEFICIENCY Deficiency of this important substrate results in a myopathic and systemic disorder.

Myopathic carnitine deficiency is associated with generalized muscle weakness, usually beginning in childhood. The clinical features overlap with muscular dystrophy and polymyositis. Patients develop progressive, painless proximal weakness. A severe cardiomyopathy may be present. Serum CK levels may be mildly to markedly (greater than 10 times) elevated. The muscle biopsy shows striking lipid accumulation. Serum carnitine is normal. The cause for decreased muscle carnitine is not understood. Most cases are sporadic, but the inheritance pattern is thought to be autosomal recessive. Some patients respond to oral carnitine supplement; this should be tried in all cases. Other patients have responded to prednisone, riboflavin, or propranolol. A diet substituting medium-chain for long-chain triglycerides has been helpful in some cases.

Systemic carnitine deficiency usually presents in infancy and early childhood and is characterized by progressive weakness and episodes of hepatic encephalopathy with nausea, vomiting, confusion, coma, and early death. Carnitine levels are reduced in muscle, liver, kidney, and heart, but the low serum carnitine levels are especially useful in distinguishing this condition from the myopathic form. No single cause has been identified to explain the low serum carnitine levels. Decreased hepatic synthesis explains some cases, while increased urinary excretion is seen in others. Serum CK levels may be slightly elevated. The muscle biopsy may show lipid storage. In some cases, the liver, heart, and kidney will show increased lipid. Treatment with oral carnitine supplements or glucocorticoid has helped some, but not all, patients.

Secondary carnitine deficiency accompanies a variety of disorders in which carnitine deficiency is accounted for by decreased synthesis (cirrhosis), insufficient intake (parenteral nutrition), and excessive loss (renal dialysis, Fanconi's syndrome, or organic acidemia). Carnitine deficiency may also be seen in the muscular dystrophies, thought to be a nonspecific result of loss of muscle tissue. Carnitine treatment has not been shown to clearly benefit patients with these secondary syndromes.

CARNITINE PALMITYOLTRANSFERASE DEFICIENCY (CPT) This disorder is the most common recognizable cause of recurrent myoglobinuria, more common than the glycolytic defects.

Clinical features This disorder usually has its onset in teenage years or in the early twenties. Muscle pain and myoglobinuria occur after prolonged exercise. Fasting predisposes to the development of symptoms. In contrast to defects in glycolysis where muscle cramps follow short intense bursts of exercise, the muscle pain in CPT deficiency does not occur until the limits of utilization have been exceeded and muscle breakdown has already begun. Episodes of rhabdomyolysis may produce severe weakness. In contrast to carnitine deficiency, strength is normal between attacks.

Laboratory findings Serum CK and EMG are both usually normal between episodes. Normal rise of venous lactate during forearm exercise distinguishes this condition from glycolytic defects, especially phosphorylase deficiency. The muscle biopsy does not show lipid accumulation and is usually normal between attacks. The diagnosis requires direct measurement of muscle CPT.

Genetics CPT deficiency is most commonly a sporadic condition of men although the disorder is thought to be transmitted as an autosomal recessive trait.

Treatment It has been suggested that frequent meals and a low-fat, high-carbohydrate diet can prolong exercise tolerance. Others suggest substituting medium-chain triglycerides in the diet. Neither approach has proven benefits.

MYOADENYLATE DEAMINASE DEFICIENCY The muscle enzyme myoadenylate deaminase converts 5′ adenosine monophophosphate (5′AMP) to inosine monophosphate (IMP) with liberation of ammonia. Myoadenylate deaminase may play a role in regulating adenosine triphophosphate (ATP) levels in muscle. In 1978, a group of patients with myalgias and exercise intolerance were found to be deficient in myoadenylate deaminase. The deficiency, however, has been found to occur as an incidental finding in as many as 1 percent of muscle biopsies detected by histochemical staining of muscle tissue. Muscle ammonia production is decreased following forearm exercise in patients deficient in myoadenylate deaminase.

Most subjects with myoadenylate deaminase deficiency have no symptoms. In patients with myalgia and fatigue associated with myoadenylate deaminase deficiency, the cause-and-effect relationship between muscle symptoms and enzyme deficiency remains unclear. There have been numerous questions raised about the clinical effects of myoadenylate deaminase deficiency and specifically the relationship to exertional myalgia and fatigability. No consistent agreement exists. There have been a few patients described with myoglobinuria and a report of two brothers with exercise-exacerbated myalgia and myoglobinuria. At present, it can only be concluded that the full clinical significance of myoadenylate deaminase deficiency has not been established.

MITOCHONDRIAL MYOPATHIES

The mitochondrial myopathies represent a heterogeneous group of diseases recognized by abnormal muscle fibers, called *ragged red fibers*, which have accumulations of abnormal mitochondria. The name "ragged red fiber" is derived from characteristics observed in modified trichrome staining of fresh frozen muscle in which mitochondria accumulations appear red. By electron microscopy, the mitochondria in ragged red fibers are enlarged, often bizarre-shaped, and have distorted cristae and crystalline inclusions.

Mitochondria play a key role in energy production. Oxidation of the major food stuffs derived from carbohydrate, fat, and protein leads to the generation of reducing equivalents (2H). The latter are transported through the respiratory chain in the process known as oxidative phosphorylation, responsible for the generation of ATP. The respiratory chain is composed of four multienzyme complexes: complex I (NADH, coenzyme Q oxidoreductase); complex II (succinate, coenzyme Q oxidoreductase); complex III (coenzyme Q, cytochrome c oxidoreductase); and complex IV (cytochrome c oxidase). In addition, there are two low molecular weight redox carriers, coenzyme Q and cytochrome c. The energy generated by the oxidation-reduction reactions of the respiratory chain is stored in an electrochemical gradient coupled to ATP synthesis from ADP by the enzyme ATP synthetase or complex V.

A novel feature of mitochondria is their genetic composition. Each mitochondrion possesses DNA genomes that are distinct from nuclear DNA. Mitochondrial DNA (mtDNA) consists of a double-stranded, circular DNA molecule composed of 16,569 base pairs. mtDNA codes for 22 transfer RNAs, 2 ribosomal RNAs, and 13 polypeptides of the respiratory chain enzymes. Complex I, made up of 25 polypeptides, has 7 encoded by mtDNA; complex III has 1 of 11 encoded from mtDNA; complex IV includes 13 polypeptides, 3 derived from mtDNA; 2 of the 12 polypeptides of complex V arise from mtDNA. Only polypeptides of complex II have no mtDNA contribution.

The genetics of mitochondrial diseases differ from those of chromosomal disorders. The DNA of mitochondria is directly inherited from the cytoplasm of germline cells, mainly the oocyte. The sperm contributes very little of its mitochondria to the offspring at the time of fertilization. Thus, mitochondrial genes are derived almost exclusively from the mother, accounting for maternal inheritance of mitochondrial disorders.

PROGRESSIVE EXTERNAL OPHTHALMOPLEGIA (PEO) SYNDROMES AND RAGGED RED FIBERS Most patients with fixed, nonfluctuating, insidiously progressive ptosis and ophthalmoplegia have a mitochondrial myopathy.

Kearns-Sayre syndrome This disorder has its onset before age 20, and importantly, has no family history. The characteristic findings are a triad of clinical features: PEO, pigmentary degeneration of the retina, and heart block. The Kearns-Sayre syndrome may also include other features: ataxia, hearing loss, dementia, short stature, delayed secondary sexual characteristics, hypoparathyroidism, hypothyroidism, and peripheral neuropathy.

The diagnosis is established by muscle biopsy which demonstrates ragged red fibers. In addition, the mtDNA extracted from the muscle may demonstrate two populations (heteroplasmy): one demonstrates variable size mtDNA deletions and the other is normal in size. The size of the mtDNA deletions do not correlate with clinical manifestations.

Kearns-Sayre syndrome represents a sporadic, noninherited disease. Mutations leading to an affected individual are thought to take place in the fertilized ovum.

Familial PEO syndrome The clinical features of this disorder, in contrast to the Kearns-Sayre syndrome, are restricted to muscle without other organ system involvement. Varying degrees of PEO and proximal limb weakness occur. Rarely, the weakness may advance to wheelchair confinement. Mutations of mtDNA responsible for this condition have not as yet been identified.

A rare form of familial PEO has been found to be inherited as an autosomal dominant trait. The patients have ragged red fibers on muscle biopsy and multiple mtDNA deletions. The mutation accounting for the autosomal dominant inheritance occurs in a *nuclear* gene that encodes a protein involved in the control of mtDNA replication. A failure or disruption of binding of this nuclear-encoded protein during mtDNA replication results in multiple deletions.

MYOCLONIC EPILEPSY AND RAGGED RED FIBERS This disorder, called the *MERRF syndrome*, consists of mitochondrial myopathy, myoclonus, generalized seizures, intellectual deterioration, ataxia, and hearing loss. PEO does not occur in MERRF. As with other mitochondrial disorders, individuals display varying manifestations of the disease. MERRF syndrome is maternally inherited. In most patients, a defect in mtDNA has been identified as a point mutation in the transfer RNA gene for lysine (tRNA^{lys}) of mtDNA. This abnormality can be detected in mtDNA isolated from peripheral blood leukocytes or skeletal muscle and is useful for clinical diagnosis and genetic counseling.

MITOCHONDRIAL MYOPATHY, ENCEPHALOPATHY, LACTIC ACIDOSIS, AND STROKE-LIKE EPISODES This disorder is usually referred to by the acronym MELAS. It is a multisystem mitochondrial encephalomyopathy that begins in childhood after normal birth and early development. Patients have stunted growth and recurrent stroke-like episodes manifesting as hemiparesis, hemianopsia, or cortical blindness. Episodic vomiting may occur and some patients have hearing loss. Focal or generalized seizures and myoclonic epilepsy may be present. Full expression of the disease leads to dementia, a bedridden state, and death often before age 20. MELAS may be maternally inherited, but sporadic cases are more common. No large pedigrees have been reported. In most patients, a point mutation of the transfer RNA gene for leucine (tRNA^{leu}) of mtDNA has been identified. Mutation analysis provides a specific diagnostic test that can be performed on peripheral blood leukocytes or skeletal muscle.

SUCCINIC DEHYDROGENASE (COMPLEX II) DEFICIENCY This disorder presents in childhood with exercise intolerance. Physical exertion, even of a modest degree, causes exhaustion associated with shortness of breath and palpitations. If physical activity persists, rhabdomyolysis may occur with painful, stiff and swollen muscles associated with myoglobinuria. Physical examination is usually normal, although some patients may have enlarged calf muscles. Exercise-induced dyspnea and tachycardia can be demonstrated by having patients climb a flight of stairs. The diagnosis is established by muscle biopsy which shows ragged red fibers and deficiency of succinic dehydrogenase in muscle fibers. Biochemical analysis of muscle reveals markedly impaired succinate oxidation.

Complex II of the respiratory chain is encoded for entirely by nuclear DNA. The disease is inherited as an autosomal recessive trait.

CYTOCHROME C OXIDASE (COMPLEX IV DEFICIENCY) There are three established clinical syndromes of cytochrome c oxidase (COX) deficiency: two infantile myopathies and a disorder predominantly affecting the brain (subacute necrotizing encephalopathy, also referred to as Leigh disease). A fatal form of COX deficiency inherited as an autosomal recessive trait presents clinically as a myopathy in the neonatal period with respiratory failure. No CNS involvement is seen. These patients have a renal tubular defect leading to aminoaciduria (DeToni-Fanconi-Debré syndrome). Muscle biopsy demonstrates

COX deficiency by histochemistry and biochemistry. Antibodies to the subunits of COX show a selective loss of subunit 7a,b of COX representing a defect in a nuclear-encoded polypeptide of the respiratory chain.

A benign form of infantile myopathy due to COX deficiency is initially indistinguishable from the fatal form of COX deficiency. Patients with the benign form have no renal tubular defect. Spontaneous recovery often occurs during the first year of life, and the child is normal by age 2 to 3.

The muscle biopsy changes during the neonatal period resemble those of fatal COX deficiency. Immune staining, however, demonstrates that in addition to the absence of nuclear-encoded subunit 7a,b of COX, there is a loss of subunit 2 of mtDNA. Immune staining of these subunits returns to normal as the clinical condition improves. Recognition of this distinction on immune staining between the fatal and benign forms of COX deficiency is of great importance in diagnosis.

Leigh disease This disease, also known as *subacute necrotizing encephalomyelopathy,* has more than one cause. At least one form, however, is caused by COX deficiency. A typical presentation occurs in the neonatal period with hypotonia and recurrent vomiting. Later visual and hearing loss occurs and seizures develop. In some cases, the onset of Leigh disease may be delayed until walking begins. In these patients, ataxia and loss of intellectual development accompanies muscle weakness. Patients with Leigh disease have elevated lactate and pyruvate levels in cerebrospinal fluid and blood. COX deficiency can be recognized on muscle biopsy. In addition, immune staining demonstrates that all subunits of COX, both mitochondrial- and nuclear-encoded polypeptides are absent.

Most cases of Leigh disease are sporadic, but the disorder also occurs in siblings suggesting autosomal recessive inheritance.

ENDOCRINE AND METABOLIC MYOPATHIES

Many endocrine disorders cause weakness. Muscle fatigue is more common than true weakness. The cause of weakness in these disorders is not well defined. It is not even clear that weakness results from disease of muscle as opposed to another part of the motor unit since the serum CK level is often normal (except for hypothyroidism), and the muscle histology is characterized by atrophy rather than destruction of muscle fibers. Nearly all endocrine myopathies respond to treatment.

THYROID DISORDERS (See Chap. 334) Abnormalities of thyroid function can cause a wide array of muscle disorders. These conditions relate to the important role of thyroid hormones in the metabolism of carbohydrates and lipids as well as in accelerating protein synthesis and enzyme production. Thyroid hormones also stimulate calorigenesis in muscle, increase muscle demand for vitamins, and enhance muscle sensitivity to circulating catacholamines.

Hypothyroidism Hypothyroid patients have frequent muscle complaints, but definite muscle weakness occurs in only about one-third of patients. Weakness when present, is predominantly proximal. Muscle cramps, pain, and stiffness occur commonly. The so-called myotonoid features characterized by slow muscle contraction and relaxation occur in 25 percent of patients and are often accompanied by myoedema (local contraction produced by tapping or pinching the muscle). The relaxation phase of muscle stretch reflexes is characteristically prolonged. The serum CK levels are often elevated (up to 10 times normal) even with minimal clinical evidence of muscle disease.

In both children and adults, a distinct syndrome has been described. Severe hypothyroid children, especially boys, may have the Debré-Kocher-Sémélaigne syndrome, characterized by weakness, slowness of movement, and striking muscle hypertrophy, causing an "infant Hercules appearance." In adult hypothyroidism, Hoffman's syndrome results in prominent muscle enlargement and weakness with muscle stiffness. The cause of muscle enlargement in these two syndromes

has not been determined. The muscle biopsy shows only muscle atrophy.

Hyperthyroidism Thyrotoxic patients commonly have muscle weakness on clinical examination, but rarely complain of the deficit. Proximal weakness and atrophy with preserved and often brisk muscle stretch reflexes characterize thyrotoxic myopathy. Prominent shoulder-girdle atrophy associated with scapular winging can occur. Bulbar, respiratory and even esophageal muscles may occasionally be affected, causing dysphagia, dysphonia, and aspiration. When bulbar involvement occurs, it is usually accompanied by chronic proximal limb weakness, but may occasionally present in the absence of generalized thyrotoxic myopathy. Other neuromuscular disorders occur in association with hyperthyroidism and include periodic paralysis (see Chap. 387), myasthenia gravis, and a progressive ocular myopathy associated with proptosis (Graves' ophthalmopathy). Serum CK levels are low in thyrotoxic myopathy. The muscle histology usually shows only atrophy of muscle fibers.

PARATHYROID DISORDERS (See Chap. 357) **Hyperparathyroidism** Muscle weakness is an integral part of primary and secondary hyperparathyroidism. Proximal muscle weakness, muscle wasting, and brisk muscle stretch reflexes are the main features of this endocrinopathy. Serum CK levels are usually normal or slightly elevated. Serum calcium and phosphorus levels show no correlation with the clinical neuromuscular manifestations. Muscle biopsies show only varying degrees of atrophy without muscle fiber degeneration.

Hypoparathyroidism An overt myopathy due to hypocalcemia is rarely seen. Neuromuscular symptoms are usually related to localized or generalized tetany. Serum CK levels may be increased secondary to muscle damage following tetany. Hyporeflexia or areflexia is usually present and contrasts with hyperreflexia seen in hyperparathyroidism.

ADRENAL DISORDERS (See Chap. 335) Conditions associated with glucocorticoid excess cause a myopathy and, in fact, steroid myopathy is the most commonly diagnosed endocrine muscle disease. Steroid excess, either endogenous or exogenous, produces varying degrees of proximal limb weakness. Muscle wasting may be striking. A cushingoid appearance invariably precedes or accompanies clinical signs of myopathy. Serum CK level is normal in steroid myopathy. The muscle biopsy shows atrophy predominantly affecting type 2 fibers. Muscle fiber degeneration is usually not seen.

Adrenal insufficiency commonly causes muscle fatigue. Objective weakness occurs less commonly and is typically only mild. Patients with myopathy and adrenal insufficiency usually have hypo- or hyperkalemia. In some cases this may result from adrenal gland destruction, affecting both glucocorticoid and mineralocorticoid production.

In primary hyperaldosteronism or Conn's syndrome, neuromuscular complications are due to potassium depletion. The clinical picture is one of persistent muscle weakness. Long-standing hyperaldosteronism may lead to proximal limb weakness and wasting. Serum CK may be elevated and a muscle biopsy may demonstrate degenerating fibers, some with vacuoles. These changes relate to hypokalemia and are not a direct effect of aldosterone on skeletal muscle.

PITUITARY DISORDERS (See Chap. 331) Muscle weakness and acromegaly develop insidiously and represent a relatively late manifestation of endocrinopathy. Patients usually show mild proximal weakness without muscle atrophy. Muscles often appear enlarged, but have decreased forced generation. The duration of acromegaly, rather than the serum growth hormone levels, correlates with the degree of myopathy.

DIABETES MELLITUS (See Chap. 337) Neuromuscular complications of diabetes mellitus are most often related to neuropathy with cranial and peripheral nerve palsies or distal sensorimotor polyneuropathy. "Diabetic amyotrophy" is sometimes thought to be a primary muscle complication, but there is overwhelming evidence that this is a type of neuropathy affecting the proximal major nerve trunks and lumbosacral plexus. More appropriate terms for this disorder include diabetic proximal neuropathy, lumbosacral plexopathy, or the eponymic designation Bruns-Garland syndrome.

The most notable myopathy of diabetes mellitus is ischemic infarction of thigh muscles. This condition occurs in poorly controlled diabetics and presents with acute onset of pain, tenderness, and edema of one thigh with a palpable mass. Muscles most often affected include the vastus lateralis, thigh adductors, and biceps femoris. Computed tomography or magnetic resonance imaging can demonstrate focal abnormalities in the affected muscle. Imaging of the muscle may avoid muscle biopsy.

VITAMIN DEFICIENCY Vitamin D offers the best evidence that a myopathy occurs as an integral part of vitamin deficiency. Vitamin D deficiency (see Chaps. 77 and 356) from either decreased intake or decrease absorption, as well as impaired vitamin D metabolism as it occurs in renal disease, may lead to chronic muscle weakness. Pain reflects the underlying bone disease (osteomalacia).

It has not been established that deficiency of other vitamins causes a myopathy.

MYOPATHIES OF SYSTEMIC ILLNESS Systemic illnesses such as chronic respiratory, cardiac, or hepatic failure are frequently associated with severe muscle wasting and complaints of weakness. Strength testing often demonstrates mild weakness in such patients. Lack of endurance is a more significant problem.

Myopathy may be a manifestation of chronic renal failure, separate and distinct from the better known uremic polyneuropathy. Abnormalities of calcium and phosphorus homeostasis and bone metabolism in chronic renal failure result from a reduction in 1,25-dihydroxyvitamin D leading to decreased intestinal absorption of calcium. Hypocalcemia, further accentuated by hyperphosphatemia due to decreased renal phosphate clearance, leads to secondary hyperparathyroidism. Renal osteodystrophy results from the compensatory hyperparathyroidism leading to osteomalacia from reduced calcium availability, and to osteitis fibrosa from the parathyroid hormone excess. The clinical picture of the myopathy of chronic renal failure is identical to that of primary hyperparathyroidism and osteomalacia. There is proximal limb weakness with bone pain.

Gangrenous calcification represents a separate, rare, and sometimes fatal complication of chronic renal failure. In this condition widespread arterial calcification occurs and results in ischemia. Extensive skin necrosis may occur along with painful myopathy and even myoglobinuria.

The term *carcinomatous myopathy* has been used to explain the frequent occurrence of muscle atrophy in patients with malignancy. In the usual patient with cancer, weakness is mild. In patients with severe weakness, other disorders should be considered and include: inflammatory myopathies, hormone-producing tumors resulting in hypercalcemia, ectopic ACTH production, or Eaton-Lambert syndrome. The last is caused by a defect in release of acetylcholine from the neuromuscular junction and is not a myopathy (see Chaps. 328 and 386).

TOXIC MYOPATHIES

The classification of toxic myopathies is shown in Table 385-2. Drugs and chemicals may produce focal or generalized damage of skeletal muscle.

The most common cause of focal damage is the injection of narcotic analgesics. Three agents in particular, pentazocine, meperidine, and heroin, may cause a severe fibrotic reaction in muscle. Common injection sites include deltoid, triceps, gluteus maximus, and quadriceps muscles. The muscles become indurated and may have local abscess formation. Cutaneous ulcerations and depressions may occur. Severe joint contractures may develop.

Other drugs may induce generalized muscle weakness, particularly affecting the proximal muscles. In most cases the exact mechanism of drug toxicity is poorly understood. D-Penicillamine induces a condition simulating the clinical and pathologic picture of polymyo-

TABLE 385-2 Toxic myopathies

Focal myopathies: Pentazocine, meperidine, heroin
Generalized myopathies
A Inflammatory: cimetidine, D-penicillamine, procainamide
B Muscle weakness and myalgias: zidovudine, chloroquine, clofibrate, colchicine, glucocorticoids, emetine, ε-aminocaproic acid, labetalol, perhexilene, propranolol, vincristine, niacin, cyclosporine
C Rhabdomyolysis and myoglobinuria: alcohol, heroin, amphetamine, clofibrate, lovastatin, gemfibrozil, ε-aminocaproic acid, phencyclidine, barbiturates, cocaine
D Malignant hyperthermia: halothane, ethylene, diethyl ether, methoxylflurane, ethyl chloride, trichloroethylene, gallamine, succinylcholine, lidocaine, mepivacaine

sitis. A similar condition has been reported with cimetidine. Procainamide may cause myositis as part of a systemic lupus-like reaction.

Zidovudine, used in the treatment of AIDS, produces proximal weakness and pain. On muscle biopsy, zidovudine demonstrates a distinctive pathologic alteration of skeletal muscle resembling ragged red fibers. In some patients, reintroduction of zidovudine in lower doses may be tolerated.

Chloroquine administration may cause a vacuolar myopathy.

The cholesterol-lowering agents including clofibrate, lovastatin, gemfibrozil, and niacin have all been implicated as causes of myopathy. Lovastatin alone or in combination with gemfibrozil has caused rhabdomyolysis and myoglobinuria. Emetine hydrochloride (used for treatment of amebiasis) ε-aminocaproic acid (an antifibrinolytic agent), and perhexilene (used for angina pectoris) have all been observed to cause muscle weakness and muscle fiber necrosis following several weeks of therapy.

Drug-induced myopathy accompanied by proximal weakness occurs with glucocorticoid therapy. Those fluorinated in the 9α-position, such as triamcinolone, dexamethasone, and betamethasone, are most likely to cause weakness, but chronic administration of all glucocorticoids including prednisone causes weakness. Divided-dose as opposed to single-morning-dose therapy produces more severe weakness. A single-dose, alternate-day regimen is still less toxic. The clinical diagnosis of steroid-induced muscle weakness can be difficult if medication is being used to treat an underlying inflammatory myopathy. The presence of a normal serum CK level, minimal or no changes of myopathy on EMG, and type 2 muscle fiber atrophy on biopsy are helpful in suggesting steroid-induced weakness.

Alcohol causes acute muscle weakness with rhabdomyolysis and myoglobinuria by several different mechanisms including prolonged obtundation, seizures, hypokalemia, and hypophosphatemia. Chronic myopathy causing slowly progressive weakness is controversial. Alcoholics are often weak, but the clinical picture usually results from neuropathy, poor nutrition, and other processes.

A very serious drug-induced condition, *malignant hyperthermia* (Chap. 398), occurs in susceptible individuals following exposure to certain general anesthetic and depolarizing muscle relaxants (Table 385-2). The local anesthetic, amides including lidocaine, and mepivacaine have been implicated as precipitating agents.

REFERENCES

BANKER BQ: The congenital myopathies, in *Myology* AG Engel, BQ Banker (eds). New York, McGraw-Hill, 1986, vol. 2

BAROHN RJ et al: Autosomal recessive distal dystrophy. Neurology 41:1365, 1991

BROOKE MH: *A Clinician's View of Neuromuscular Disease*, 2d ed. Baltimore, Williams & Wilkins, 1985

CARROLL JE: Myopathies caused by disorders of lipid metabolism. Neurol Clinics, 6:563, 1988

DALAKAS MC et al: Mitochondrial myopathy caused by long-term zidovudine therapy. N Engl J Med 332:1098, 1990

DIMAURO S et al: Disorders of lipid metabolism in muscle. Muscle Nerve 3:369, 1980

ENGEL AG: Acid maltase deficiency, in *Myology*, AG Engel, BQ Banker (eds). New York, McGraw-Hill, 1986, vol. 2

GRIGGS RC, MOXLEY RT (eds): Metabolic myopathies. Semin Neurol 3:225, 1985

KOENIG M et al: Complete cloning of the Duchenne muscular dystrophy (DMD) cDNA and preliminary genomic organization of the DMD gene in normal and affected individuals. Cell 50:509, 1987

LACOMIS D et al: Myopathy in the elderly. Evaluation of the histopathologic spectrum and the accuracy of clinical diagnosis. Neurology 43:825, 1993

MATSAMURA K et al: Abnormal expression of dystrophin-associated proteins in Fukuyama-type congenital muscular dystrophy. Lancet 341:521, 1993

MORAES CT et al: Mitochondrial DNA deletions in progressive external ophthalmoplegia and Kearns-Sayre syndrome. N Engl J Med 320:1293, 1989

RIGGS JE (ed): *Muscle Disease,* in Neurologic Clinics, vol. 6. Philadelphia, Saunders, 1988

SIMPSON DM et al: Myopathies associated with human immunodeficiency virus and zidovudine. Can their effects be distinguished? Neurology 43:971, 1993

386 MYASTHENIA GRAVIS

DANIEL B. DRACHMAN

Myasthenia gravis (MG) is a neuromuscular disorder characterized by weakness and fatigability of skeletal muscles. The underlying defect is a decrease in the number of available acetylcholine receptors (AChRs) at neuromuscular junctions due to an antibody-mediated autoimmune attack. Treatment now available for MG is highly effective, although a specific cure has remained elusive.

PATHOPHYSIOLOGY To diagnose and manage patients with MG, it is essential to understand the basic function of the neuromuscular junction and the changes that occur as a result of the disease process (see Fig. 386-1). Acetylcholine (ACh) is synthesized in the motor nerve terminal and stored in vesicles (quanta) containing approximately 10,000 molecules each. Quanta of ACh are released spontaneously, giving rise to miniature end-plate potentials. When an action potential reaches the nerve terminal, ACh from 150 to 200 vesicles is released and combines with AChRs that are densely packed at the peaks of postsynaptic folds. Channels in the AChRs are opened, permitting the rapid entry of cations, chiefly sodium, which produces depolarization at the end-plate region of the muscle fiber. If the depolarization is sufficiently large, it initiates an action potential that is propagated along the muscle fiber, triggering muscle contraction. This process is rapidly terminated by diffusion of ACh away from the receptor and hydrolysis of ACh by acetylcholinesterase (AChE).

In MG, the fundamental defect is a decrease in the number of available AChRs at the postsynaptic muscle membrane. In addition, the postsynaptic folds are flattened, or "simplified" (Fig. 386-1*B*). These changes result in decreased efficiency of neuromuscular transmission. Therefore, although ACh is released normally, it

produces small end-plate potentials which may fail to trigger muscle action potentials. Failure of transmission at many neuromuscular junctions results in weakness of muscle contraction.

The amount of ACh released per impulse *normally* declines on repeated activity (termed *presynaptic rundown*). In the myasthenic patient, decreased efficiency of neuromuscular transmission combined with the normal rundown results in the activation of fewer and fewer muscle fibers by successive nerve impulses and hence increasing weakness, or *myasthenic fatigue*. This mechanism also accounts for the decremental response to repetitive nerve stimulation seen on electrodiagnostic testing.

The neuromuscular abnormalities in MG are brought about by an autoimmune response mediated by specific anti-AChR antibodies. The anti-AChR antibodies reduce the number of available AChRs at neuromuscular junctions by three distinct mechanisms: (1) AChRs may be degraded at an accelerated rate by a mechanism involving cross-linking and rapid endocytosis of the receptors; (2) the active site of the AChR, i.e., the site that normally binds ACh, may be blocked by the antibodies; and (3) the postsynaptic muscle membrane may be damaged by the antibody in collaboration with complement.

How the autoimmune response is initiated and maintained in MG is not completely understood. However, the thymus appears to play a role in this process. The thymus is abnormal in approximately 75 percent of patients with MG; in about 65 percent of patients the thymus is "hyperplastic," with the presence of active germinal centers, while 10 percent of patients have thymic tumors (thymomas). Muscle-like cells within the thymus (myoid cells), which bear AChRs on their surface, may serve as a source of autoantigen and trigger the autoimmune reaction within the thymus gland.

CLINICAL FEATURES Myasthenia gravis is not rare, with a prevalence rate of at least 1 in 10,000. It may affect individuals in any age group, but there are peaks of incidence in women in their twenties and thirties and in men in their fifties and sixties. Overall, women are affected more frequently than men, with a ratio of approximately 3:2. The cardinal features are *weakness* and *fatigability* of muscles. The weakness increases during repeated use (fatigue) and may improve following rest or sleep. The course of MG is often variable. Exacerbations and remissions may occur, particularly during the first few years after the onset of the disease. Remissions are rarely complete or permanent. Unrelated infections or systemic disorders often lead to increased myasthenic weakness and may precipitate so-called crisis (see below).

The distribution of muscle weakness has a characteristic pattern. The cranial muscles, particularly the lids and extraocular muscles, are often involved early, and diplopia and ptosis are common initial complaints. Facial weakness produces a "snarling" expression when the patient attempts to smile. Weakness in chewing is most noticeable after prolonged effort, as in chewing meat. Speech may have a nasal timbre caused by weakness of the palate or a dysarthric "mushy" quality due to tongue weakness. Difficulty in swallowing may occur as a result of weakness of the palate, tongue, or pharynx, giving rise to nasal regurgitation or aspiration of liquids or food. In approximately 85 percent of patients, the weakness becomes generalized, affecting the limb muscles as well. The limb weakness in MG is often proximal and may be asymmetric. Despite the muscle weakness, deep tendon reflexes are preserved. If weakness of respiration or swallowing becomes so severe as to require respiratory assistance or intubation, the patient is said to be in *crisis*.

DIAGNOSIS AND EVALUATION The diagnosis is suspected on the basis of weakness and fatigability in the typical distribution described above, without loss of reflexes or impairment of sensation or other neurologic function. The suspected diagnosis should always be confirmed definitively before treatment is undertaken; this is essential because (1) other treatable conditions may closely resemble MG and (2) the treatment of MG may involve surgery and the prolonged use of drugs with adverse side effects.

Anticholinesterase test Drugs that inhibit the enzyme AChE allow ACh to interact repeatedly with the limited number of AChRs,

FIGURE 386-1 Diagrams of (*A*) normal and (*B*) myasthenic neuromuscular junctions. V = vesicles; M = mitochondria. See text for description of normal neuromuscular transmission. The MG junction shows reduced number of AChRs (stippling); flattened, simplified postsynaptic folds; a widened synaptic space; and a normal nerve terminal.

producing improvement in the strength of myasthenic muscles. Edrophonium is used most commonly, because of the rapid onset (30 s) and short duration (about 5 min) of its effect. It is essential that an objective endpoint be used to evaluate the effect of edrophonium. The examiner should focus on one or more unequivocally weak muscle groups and evaluate their strength objectively. For example, weakness of extraocular muscles, impairment of speech, or the length of time that the patient can maintain the arms in forward abduction may be useful measures. An initial dose of 2 mg edrophonium is given intravenously. If definite improvement occurs, the test is considered positive and terminated. If there is no change, the patient is given an additional 8 mg intravenously. The dose is administered in two parts because some patients react to edrophonium with unpleasant side effects such as nausea, diarrhea, salivation, fasciculations, and rarely syncope. Atropine (0.6 mg) should be at hand for intravenous administration if these symptoms become troublesome.

False-positive tests occur in occasional patients with other neurologic disorders, such as amyotrophic lateral sclerosis, and in placebo-reactors. False-negative or equivocal tests also may occur. In some cases it is helpful to use a longer-acting drug such as neostigmine, given orally, since this permits more time for detailed evaluation of strength. In virtually all instances, it is desirable to carry out further testing to establish the diagnosis of MG definitively.

Electrodiagnostic testing   *Repetitive nerve stimulation* often provides helpful diagnostic evidence of MG. Anticholinesterase medication should be stopped at least 6 h prior to testing. It is best to test weak muscles or proximal muscle groups. Electric shocks are delivered at a rate of 2 or 3 per second to the appropriate nerves, and action potentials are recorded from the muscles. In normal individuals, the amplitude of the evoked muscle action potentials does not change at these rates of stimulation. However, in myasthenic patients there is a rapid reduction in the amplitude of the evoked responses of more than 10 to 15 percent. As a further test, a single dose of edrophonium may be given to prevent or diminish this decremental reaction.

Antiacetylcholine receptor antibody   As noted above, anti-AChR antibodies are detectable in the serum of approximately 80 percent of all myasthenic patients, but in only about 50 percent of patients with weakness confined to the ocular muscles. The presence of anti-AChR antibodies is virtually diagnostic of MG, but a negative test does not exclude the disease. The measured level of anti-AChR antibody does not correspond well with the severity of MG in different patients. However, in an individual patient, a treatment-induced fall in the antibody level often correlates with clinical improvement.

Differential diagnosis   Several other conditions that cause weakness of the cranial and/or somatic musculature must be considered in the differential diagnosis of MG; these include drug-induced myasthenia, Lambert-Eaton myasthenic syndrome, neurasthenia, hyperthyroidism, botulism, intracranial mass lesions, and progressive external ophthalmoplegia. Treatment with *penicillamine* (used for scleroderma or rheumatoid arthritis) may result in true MG, but the weakness is mild, and recovery occurs within weeks or months after discontinuing its use. Other drugs such as *aminoglycoside antibiotics* in very large doses and *procainamide* can cause neuromuscular weakness in normal individuals or exacerbation of weakness in myasthenic patients.

The *Lambert-Eaton myasthenic syndrome* is a presynaptic disorder of the neuromuscular junction that can cause weakness similar to that of MG. The proximal muscles of the lower limbs are most commonly affected, but other muscles may be involved as well. Cranial nerve findings, including ptosis of the eyelids and diplopia, occur in up to 70 percent of patients and resemble features of MG. However, the two conditions are readily distinguished, since patients with Lambert-Eaton syndrome have depressed or absent reflexes, autonomic changes such as dry mouth and impotence, and show incremental responses on repetitive nerve stimulation. It is now known that Lambert-Eaton syndrome is caused by an autoantibody directed against calcium channels on the motor nerve terminals, resulting in impaired release of ACh. A majority of patients with this syndrome have an associated malignancy, most commonly small cell carcinoma of the lung, which is thought to trigger the autoimmune response. The diagnosis of Lambert-Eaton syndrome may signal the presence of the tumor long before it would otherwise be detected, permitting early removal. Treatment of the neuromuscular disorder involves plasmapheresis and immunosuppression, as for MG.

Neurasthenia may present with weakness and fatigue, but muscle testing usually reveals the "jerky release" characteristic of nonorganic disorders, and the complaint of fatigue in these patients means tiredness or apathy rather than decreasing muscle power on repeated effort. *Hyperthyroidism* is readily diagnosed or excluded by tests of thyroid function, which should be carried out routinely in patients with suspected MG. It is worth noting that abnormalities of thyroid function (hyper- or hypothyroidism) may increase myasthenic weakness. *Botulism* can cause myasthenic-like weakness, but the pupils are often affected and repetitive nerve stimulation gives an *incremental*, rather than decremental, response. Diplopia that mimics the symptoms of MG may occasionally be due to *intracranial mass lesions* that compress nerves to the extraocular muscles (e.g., sphenoid ridge meningioma), but computed tomography (CT) or magnetic resonance imaging (MRI) scanning of the head and orbits usually reveals the lesion.

Progressive external ophthalmoplegia is a rare condition resulting in weakness of the extraocular muscles, which may be accompanied by weakness of the proximal muscles of the limbs, and a variety of other systemic features that are beyond the scope of this chapter. Most patients with this condition have mitochondrial disorders that can be detected on muscle biopsy (see Chap. 385).

Search for associated conditions   Myasthenic patients have an increased incidence of several associated disorders. *Thymic abnormalities* occur in approximately 75 percent of patients, as noted above. Neoplastic change (thymoma) may produce enlargement of the thymus, which is best detected by CT or MRI scanning of the anterior mediastinum. Enlargement of the thymus in a patient over 40 years of age is highly suspicious of thymoma. *Hyperthyroidism* may occur in 3 to 8 percent of patients and may aggravate the myasthenic weakness. Tests of thyroid function should be obtained. Because of the *association with other autoimmune disorders*, blood tests for rheumatoid factor and antinuclear antibodies should be carried out in all patients. Chronic infection of any kind can exacerbate MG and should be sought carefully. Finally, measurements of *ventilatory function* are valuable because of the frequency and seriousness of respiratory impairment in myasthenic patients.

Because of the side effects of glucocorticoids and other immunosuppressive agents used in the treatment of MG, a thorough medical investigation should be made, searching specifically for evidence of chronic or latent infection (such as tuberculosis or hepatitis), hypertension, diabetes, renal impairment, and glaucoma.

MEDICAL AND SURGICAL THERAPY   The prognosis has improved strikingly as a result of advances in treatment; virtually all myasthenic patients can be returned to full productive lives with proper therapy. The most important methods used in the treatment of myasthenia gravis include anticholinesterase medications, immunosuppressive agents, thymectomy, and plasmapheresis.

Anticholinesterase medications   Most myasthenic patients can be improved, but few can be brought completely to normal by anticholinesterase medication. There is no substantial difference in efficacy among the various anticholinesterase drugs; oral pyridostigmine is most widely used in the United States. As a rule, the beneficial action of oral pyridostigmine begins within 15 to 30 min and lasts for 3 to 4 h, but the individual response may vary. Treatment is begun with a moderate dose, e.g., 60 mg three to five times daily. Adjustment of the dosage, i.e., frequency and amount, should be tailored to the patient's individual requirements throughout the day. For example, patients with weakness in chewing and swallowing may benefit by taking the medication before meals so that optimal strength coincides with mealtime. Long-acting pyridostigmine tablets may be helpful to get the patient through the night but should never be used for daytime medication because of their variable absorption. The maximum useful dose of pyridostigmine rarely exceeds 120 mg every 3 h during daytime. Overdosage with anticholinesterase medication may cause increased weakness and other side effects. In some patients, muscarinic side effects of the anticholinesterase medication (diarrhea, abdominal cramps, salivation, nausea) may limit the dosage tolerated. In these cases, propantheline bromide may be used to block the autonomic side effects without altering the beneficial effects on skeletal muscle. Loperamide is useful for the treatment of diarrhea.

Thymectomy Two separate issues should be distinguished: surgical removal of thymoma, and thymectomy as a treatment for myasthenia gravis. In the case of thymoma, surgical removal is necessary because of the possibility of local tumor spread, although most thymomas are benign. In the absence of a tumor, the available evidence suggests that up to 85 percent of patients improve after thymectomy, and of these, about 35 percent may achieve drug-free remission. However, the improvement is typically delayed for months to years. The advantage of thymectomy is that it offers the possibility of long-term benefit, in some cases diminishing or eliminating the need for continuing medical treatment. In view of these potential benefits and of the negligible risk in skilled hands, thymectomy has gained widespread acceptance in the treatment of MG. It is the consensus that thymectomy should be carried out in all patients with generalized MG between the ages of puberty and at least 55. Whether thymectomy should be recommended as a rule in children, in adults over 55 years of age, and in patients with weakness limited to the ocular muscles is still a matter of debate. Thymectomy must be carried out in a hospital where this procedure is performed regularly and where the staff is experienced in the pre- and postoperative management, anesthesia, and surgical techniques of total thymectomy.

Immunosuppression Immunosuppression using glucocorticoids, azathioprine, and other drugs is effective in nearly all patients with MG. The choice of which drugs to use should be guided by their relative benefits and risks for the individual patients. In general, clinical improvement begins somewhat more rapidly with steroid treatment than with the other immunosuppressive agents. The side effects of each drug may preclude its use in some patients, as indicated below.

STEROID THERAPY Glucocorticoids, when used properly, produce improvement in myasthenic weakness in the great majority of patients. The initial dose of prednisone should be relatively low (15 to 25 mg/d) to avoid the early weakening that occurs in about one-third of patients treated initially with a high-dose regimen. The dose is increased stepwise, as tolerated by the patient (usually 5 mg/d at 2- to 3-day intervals), until there is marked clinical improvement or the dose of 50 mg/d is reached. This dose is maintained for 1 to 3 months and then is gradually modified to an alternate-day regimen over the course of an additional 1 to 2 months, until the dosage of 100 mg on alternate days is reached. Generally, patients begin to improve within a few months after reaching the maximum dose, and improvement continues to progress for months or years. The prednisone dosage may gradually be reduced, but usually months or years may be needed to determine the minimum effective dose and close monitoring is required by patient and doctor. *Few patients are able to do without prednisone entirely.* Patients on long-term glucocorticoid therapy must be followed carefully to prevent or treat adverse side effects. The most common errors in the steroid treatment of myasthenic patients include:

1 Insufficient persistence; improvement may be delayed and gradual.
2 Too early, too rapid, or excessive tapering of steroid dosage.
3 Lack of attention to prevention and treatment of side effects.

The management of patients treated with glucocorticoids is discussed in Chap. 335.

OTHER IMMUNOSUPPRESSIVE DRUGS Azathioprine, cyclosporine (ciclosporin), or occasionally cyclophosphamide is effective in many patients, either alone or in combination with glucocorticoid therapy. Azathioprine is the most widely used because of its relative safety in most patients. Its therapeutic effect may add to that of glucocorticoids

and/or allow the steroid dose to be reduced. However, up to 10 percent of patients are unable to tolerate azathioprine because of idiosyncratic reactions consisting of flulike symptoms of fever and malaise, bone marrow depression, or abnormalities of liver function. An initial dose of 50 mg/d should be used to test for adverse side effects. If this is tolerated, the dose is gradually increased until the white blood count falls to approximately 3000. In patients who are concomitantly receiving steroids, leukocytosis precludes the use of this measure. A reduction of the lymphocyte count below 1000 per microliter and/or an increase of the mean corpuscular volume may be used as indications of adequacy of azathioprine dosage. The typical dosage range is 2 to 3 mg/kg total body weight. The beneficial effect of azathioprine takes at least 3 to 6 months to begin and even longer to reach a maximum level.

Cyclosporine is approximately as effective as azathioprine and is being used increasingly in the management of MG. Its beneficial effect occurs more rapidly than that of azathioprine. It may be used alone but is used most commonly as an adjunct to steroids, in order to reduce the steroid dosage required. The usual dose of cyclosporine is 4 to 5 mg/kg per day, given in two divided doses (so as to minimize side effects). Side effects of cyclosporine include hypertension and nephrotoxicity, which must be closely monitored. "Trough" blood levels of cyclosporine are measured 12 hours after the evening dose. The therapeutic range, as measured by radioimmunoassay, is 150 to 200 ng/L. Cyclophosphamide is reserved for patients refractory to the other drugs because of the relatively high risk of adverse side effects, including late development of malignancies.

Plasmapheresis In view of the antibody-mediated pathogenesis of MG, plasmapheresis has been used therapeutically. The plasma, which contains the pathogenic antibodies, is mechanically separated from the blood cells, which are returned to the patient in a suitable fluid medium. Plasmapheresis produces a short-term reduction in anti-AChR antibodies, with clinical improvement in many patients. Thus it is useful as a temporary expedient in seriously affected patients or to improve the patient's condition prior to surgery (e.g., thymectomy). The long-term treatment of myasthenic patients requires other methods of therapy outlined in this chapter.

Management of myasthenic crisis Myasthenic crisis is defined as an exacerbation of weakness sufficient to endanger life. The usual serious threats to life are respiratory failure, caused by diaphragmatic and intercostal weakness, and aspiration, secondary to pharyngeal weakness. Treatment should be carried out in an intensive care unit staffed with physicians experienced in the management of myasthenia gravis, respiratory insufficiency, infectious disease, and fluid and electrolyte therapy. The possibility that the deterioration could be due to excessive anti-ChE medication ("cholinergic crisis") is best excluded by temporarily stopping anti-ChE drugs. The most common cause of crisis is intercurrent infection. This should be treated immediately, because the mechanical and immunologic defenses of the patient can be assumed to be compromised. The myasthenic patient with fever and early infection should be treated like other immunocompromised patients. Early and effective antibiotic therapy, respiratory assistance, and pulmonary physiotherapy are essentials of the treatment program. As discussed above, plasmapheresis is frequently helpful in hastening recovery.

REFERENCES

ANDREWS PI et al: Acetylcholine receptor antibodies in juvenile myasthenia gravis. Neurology 43:977, 1993

DRACHMAN DB: Biology of myasthenia gravis. Ann Rev Neurosci 4:195, 1981
——— (ed): Myasthenia gravis: Biology and treatment. Ann NY Acad Sci 505:1, 1987

ENGEL AG et al: The motor endplate in myasthenia gravis and in experimental autoimmune myasthenia gravis: A quantitative ultrastructural study. Ann NY Acad Sci 274:60, 1976

FAMBROUGH DM et al: Neuromuscular junction in myasthenia gravis: Decreased acetylcholine receptors. Science 182:293, 1973

LINDSTROM J et al: Myasthenia gravis. Advances in Immunol 42:233, 1988

PENN AS et al (eds): Myasthenia gravis and related disorders: Experimental and clinical aspects. Ann NY Acad Sci 505:1, 1993

Somnier FE, Trojaborg W: Neurophysiological evaluation in myasthenia gravis—A comprehensive study of a complete patient population. Electroencephalogr Clin Neurophysiol 89:73, 1993

Toyka KV et al: Myasthenia gravis: Study of humoral immune mechanisms by passive transfer to mice. N Engl J Med 296:125, 1977

387 PERIODIC PARALYSIS

LOUIS J. PTACEK / ROBERT C. GRIGGS

Disorders that cause patients of normal strength to become weak intermittently are not common. In contrast, the complaint of intermittent weakness is frequently encountered. The evaluation of such symptoms is challenging because the examination is often normal between attacks and because reliance on history is crucial for diagnosis. This chapter considers the primary periodic paralyses. Recent discoveries of the molecular defects in some of the periodic paralyses have provided insight into their pathogenesis and forms the basis for their classification. Other disorders that cause episodic weakness are considered elsewhere (see Chap. 23).

All primary periodic paralyses have some features in common. In most patients the disorders are inherited as autosomal dominant traits. Symptoms usually begin early in life and rarely commence after age 25. Attacks typically follow rest or sleep and almost never occur in the midst of vigorous activity, although antecedent exercise frequently provokes weakness. Patients remain alert during the attacks. Early in the course of these disorders interattack strength is normal but after years of attacks progressive weakness may develop. All forms of periodic paralysis are amenable to treatment and progressive weakness can be prevented and even reversed.

Diagnosis is based upon patient history and confirmed by appropriate evaluation of serum electrolytes during attacks and by evaluating the response of strength to provocative testing with glucose, insulin, potassium, and cold. Since the genetic defects of certain periodic paralyses have been defined, diagnosis will soon be possible by routine molecular DNA studies.

HYPOKALEMIC PERIODIC PARALYSIS   This disorder occurs as an autosomal dominant condition in two-thirds of cases and as sporadic cases in one-third. Males are more frequently and more severely affected. Attacks of weakness characteristically begin in adolescence but may commence in the first decade. Onset after age 25 is rare; the new onset of episodic paralysis in older individuals is almost never due to periodic paralysis.

Attack frequency varies from daily to yearly. Attacks last from 3 to 4 h to as long as a day or more. Meals high in carbohydrate or high in sodium may provoke attacks. Paralysis involves limb muscles, usually proximal more than distal; rarely ocular, bulbar, or respiratory muscles are weakened, and bulbar and respiratory involvement may prove fatal. Reflexes become hypoactive, and cardiac arrhythmias may occur during attacks. Patients may develop persistent proximal weakness after years of attacks. Examination during attack-free intervals is otherwise normal except for the frequent presence of eyelid myotonia.

Diagnosis is established by demonstrating a low serum potassium during a paralytic attack and by excluding secondary causes of hypokalemia (Chap 23). Electrocardiograms during attacks show characteristic features of hypokalemia. Routine electromyography is not helpful in diagnosis, but muscle biopsy often shows the presence of single or multiple centrally placed vacuoles. Patients whose attacks are so infrequent as to preclude the study of a spontaneous attack require provocative testing with glucose and insulin administration. Such tests are potentially hazardous, and patients must be carefully monitored during their performance. Since these disorders are rare such testing is most appropriately carried out in referral centers.

Pathogenesis   The pathogenesis of paralytic attacks is incompletely understood. There is evidence for an abnormality of muscle membrane. The contractile apparatus is normal. Distinctive abnormalities in potassium regulation occur in hypokalemic periodic paralysis. Patients with hypokalemic periodic paralysis often have a decrease in total body potassium but this may reflect muscle wasting. There is no increased excretion of potassium in the urine before or during attacks, but there is excessive flux of potassium from blood into muscle, possibly owing to an abnormality of muscle membrane that causes muscle to become electrically inexcitable. Muscle from these patients is abnormally sensitive to the effect of insulin on potassium uptake; the significance of this increased sensitivity is not known since weakness is often severe at levels of serum potassium that do not affect normal individuals. Moreover, attacks may occur when insulin levels are low. Therefore, factors other than hypokalemia per se are important in the induction of weakness.

Treatment   ACUTE ATTACKS   The acute paralysis improves following the administration of potassium salts. Oral KCl (0.2 to 0.4 mmol/kg) should be given to patients with severe weakness and repeated at 15 to 30 min intervals depending on the response of the ECG, serum potassium, and muscle strength. Milder attacks usually resolve spontaneously; resolution of weakness is hastened by exercising affected muscles. When patients are unable to swallow or are vomiting, intravenous therapy may be necessary. Small, repeated bolus therapy with KCl (0.1 mmol/kg) may be administered over 5 to 10 min with careful monitoring of the ECG and serum potassium. If potassium is administered as a dilute solution (20 to 40 mmol/L) in 5% glucose or in physiologic saline solution, serum potassium may decline, and weakness may worsen.

PREVENTION OF ATTACKS   The goal of therapy is the elimination of attacks, which also prevents interattack weakness and may improve interattack weakness after it has developed. Prior to availability of effective means of attack prevention, chronic progressive interattack weakness frequently caused serious disability. Prophylactic administration of potassium salts, even in large dosage, does not prevent attacks but acetazolamide (125 to 1000 mg/d in divided dosage) abolishes attacks in the majority of cases. The mechanism of action of acetazolamide is not fully understood, but it may block the flux of potassium from blood into muscle. The metabolic acidosis that it produces may underlie its beneficial effect. Paradoxically, acetazolamide lowers serum potassium; to achieve an adequate response in some patients it may be necessary to give supplementary potassium along with acetazolamide and to avoid high-carbohydrate meals. Chronic acetazolamide treatment may be associated with renal calculi, and patients should be monitored for this complication. In occasional patients attacks may not respond to or may even be worsened by acetazolamide. In such patients triamterene (25 to 100 mg/d or spironolactone 25 to 100 mg/d) may prevent attacks.

THYROTOXIC PERIODIC PARALYSIS   Attacks of hypokalemic periodic paralysis can occur in subjects with thyrotoxicosis, most commonly in Latin American or oriental men where up to 10 percent of thyrotoxic patients may have periodic paralysis. In many patients thyrotoxicosis has been overlooked for many months; periodic paralysis can occur with any cause of hyperthyroidism, including that induced by exogenous thyroid hormone administration. The usual age of onset of the disorder is that of thyrotoxicosis; otherwise the clinical features resemble familial hypokalemic periodic paralysis. Acute attacks respond to potassium administration. Treatment of underlying thyrotoxicosis abolishes attacks and β-adrenergic blocking agents reduce the frequency and severity of attacks while measures to control thyrotoxicosis are being instituted. Acetazolamide is not helpful in preventing attacks. The pathogenesis of thyrotoxic periodic paralysis is uncertain but there is evidence for a decrease in the activity of the calcium pump. The pathogenesis of thyrotoxic periodic paralysis may be different from that of nonthyrotoxic periodic paralysis since thyroid hormone does not worsen the latter.

PERIODIC PARALYSES CAUSED BY DISORDERS OF THE SKELETAL MUSCLE SODIUM CHANNEL   These disorders differ from hypokalemic periodic paralysis in that attacks are usually brief

(1 to 2 h) and more frequent; clinical or electromyographic myotonia is often demonstrable. Disease onset is usually at an earlier age than for hypokalemic periodic paralysis; attacks of myotonia may be evident in the first year of life. The disorder is usually transmitted as an autosomal dominant defect; rare sporadic cases occur. Attacks are usually precipitated by fasting, potassium loading, muscle cooling, or by rest following exercise: the particular precipitant of the attacks allows clinical subclassification of these disorders into *hyperkalemic periodic paralysis, normokalemic periodic paralysis,* and *paramyotonia with periodic paralysis.* These three disorders were recognized historically as overlapping, but distinct, clinical entities and are now known to result from allelic defects in the skeletal-muscle sodium channel α subunit. Specific mutations have recently been defined; the correlation of site of sodium channel mutation with clinical phenotype is under study.

Hyper- and normokalemic periodic paralysis   The name "hyperkalemic" is misleading since potassium levels are frequently normal in patients during attacks. The disorder is best defined by the fact that attacks are precipitated by potassium administration. "Potassium-sensitive" periodic paralysis is probably preferable terminology. Moreover, serum potassium is often slightly elevated when patients are not having attacks of weakness. Attacks are characterized by limb weakness. Only rarely are cranial and respiratory muscle involvement found. Cardiac arrhythmias occur occasionally. Paresthesias and muscle pain are frequently present during an attack.

Diagnosis of the hyperkalemic form is suggested by a modest elevation of serum potassium during attacks in nearly half of patients; at times, however, the serum potassium is normal or even low. Intravenous glucose-insulin loading does not precipitate weakness but potassium-loading tests (0.05 to 0.15 g/kg) will provoke weakness in such patients. Myotonia may be increased. Potassium-loading tests are potentially hazardous and are contraindicated in patients with renal disease and diabetes. Random serum potassium measurements may suggest the diagnosis since potassium elevations are frequent during attack-free intervals. Electromyographic evidence of myotonia and the finding of vacuoles on muscle biopsy provide supporting data.

Most subjects with periodic paralysis in whom potassium is normal during attacks behave like those with typical "hyperkalemic" periodic paralysis, since they are similarly sensitive to potassium administration. In fact, genetic linkage data suggest that the so-called hyperkalemic and normokalemic forms of this disorder are allelic disorders resulting from mutations of a single gene. Treatment is the same as for hyperkalemic periodic paralysis. Rare patients with episodic normokalemic paralysis are not potassium sensitive, but they usually show evidence of muscle destruction or other features suggesting that they should not be classified as having a primary periodic paralysis.

Paramyotonia congenita with periodic paralysis   Attacks of paralysis may occur in the paramyotonias, either provoked by cold or spontaneously. Paramyotonia congenita is characterized by paradoxical myotonia (i.e., worsening with activity), cold provocation, spontaneous attacks, and family history compatible with an autosomal dominant defect. The cold provocation of weakness and muscle stiffness distinguishes this disease from other periodic paralyses. A therapeutically useful subclassification of the paramyotonias has been proposed: (1) paramyotonia congenita in which spontaneous attacks of weakness are associated with a lowering of serum potassium and in which measures that decrease serum potassium provoke weakness; and (2) paralysis periodica paramyotonia in which spontaneous attacks may be associated with hyperkalemia and may be provoked by oral potassium administration. This potassium sensitivity has led in the past to the classification of this disorder as a variant of hyperkalemic or normokalemic periodic paralysis. Identification of mutations in these patients has demonstrated that these disorders are allelic defects in the adult skeletal muscle sodium channel α-subunit.

Clinical diagnosis depends upon the provocation of weakness and stiffness with cold. Glucose and insulin loading and potassium challenges aid in the subclassification of the disorder and provide assistance in the choice of medication for treatment. The molecular defect can be determined by appropriate studies of peripheral blood DNA.

Pathogenesis   Patch-clamp recordings from cultured hyperkalemic periodic paralysis myotubes have demonstrated a defect in the voltage-dependent inactivation of a small fraction of sodium channels. Such abnormal inactivation in a subpopulation of channels may cause persistent membrane depolarization, inactivation of normal sodium channels and, ultimately, the membrane inexcitability known to be present in paralyzed patients. Recordings from muscle cells from patients with hyperkalemic and normokalemic periodic paralysis have shown abnormal regulation of skeletal muscle sodium channels. Two distinct sodium channel mutations have now been identified in hyperkalemic periodic paralysis patients (Fig. 387-1).

The two types of paramyotonia probably have different causes. In paramyotonia congenita, cooling of muscle results in an abnormal depolarization, leading first to myotonia and then to inexcitability. Sodium conductance becomes abnormal with cooling of muscle. Five distinct mutations have now been identified in patients with this form of the disorder (Fig. 387-1). It remains to be determined if the site

FIGURE 387-1   The sodium channel is depicted here as a molecule containing four homologous domains. Each domain contains six putative membrane spanning segments. The fourth segment of each domain is thought to act together as the "voltage sensor" for the channel and is cross-hatched in the figure. The tertiary structure of the protein in the membrane and the association of these segments is thought to form a pore through which ions could pass. Mutations that have been identified are shown along with the phenotype that they confer.

of the sodium channel mutations accounts for the clinical findings of the different forms of paramyotonia.

Treatment In hyperkalemic periodic paralysis, attacks of weakness are seldom severe enough to require emergency treatment and are never fatal. Oral glucose or other carbohydrate hastens recovery. Since interattack weakness may develop after repeated attacks, prophylactic treatment may be indicated. Remarkably, acetazolamide (125 to 1000 mg/d), the treatment of choice for hypokalemic periodic paralysis, was first found to be beneficial for hyperkalemic periodic paralysis, possibly because of its kaliopenic effect. Thiazide diuretics (e.g., chlorothiazide 250 to 1000 mg/d) are often effective and may have fewer side effects.

Spontaneous attacks of periodic paralysis in paramyotonia congenita are relatively infrequent. Many patients do not require prophylactic treatment for prevention. In the case of paramyotonia congenita, patients with severe and frequent attacks of weakness may respond to spironolactone, and subjects with paralysis periodica paramyotonica may respond to acetazolamide or thiazides. Acetazolamide may provoke weakness in paramyotonia congenita. Myotonia in both types of paramyotonia improves with mexiletine hydrochloride (150 to 900 mg/d). This antiarrhythmic agent may improve myotonia by blocking abnormal sodium channels; mexiletine also improves weakness and decreases the abnormal uptake of potassium by muscles.

REFERENCES

CANNON SC, STRITTMATTER SM: Functional expression of sodium channel mutations identified in families with periodic paralysis. Neuron 10:317, 1993

ENGEL AG: Periodic paralysis, in *Myology*, 2d ed, AG Engel, Franzini-Armstrong C (eds), New York, McGraw Hill, vol 2, 1994

FEERO WG et al: Hyperkalemic periodic paralysis—Rapid molecular diagnosis and relationship of genotype to phenotype in 12 families. Neurology 43:668, 1993

FONTAINE B et al: Hyperkalemic periodic paralysis and the adult muscle sodium channel gene. Science 250:1000, 1990

OBER KP: Thyrotoxic periodic paralysis in the United States: Report of 7 cases and review of the literature. Medicine 71:169, 1992

PTACEK LJ et al: Current concepts: Genetics of the myotonic muscle disorders. N Engl J Med 328:482, 1993

————: Mutations in an S4 segment of the adult skeletal muscle sodium channel cause paramyotonia congenita. Neuron 8:891, 1992

————: Sodium channel mutations in paramyotonia congenita and hyperkalemic periodic paralysis. Ann Neurol 33:300, 1993

RESNICK JS et al: Acetazolamide prophylaxis in hypokalemic periodic paralysis. N Engl J Med 278:582, 1968

ROJAS CV et al: A met-to-val mutation in the skeletal muscle Na+ channel α-subunit in hyperkalaemic periodic paralysis. Nature 354:387, 1991

STREIB EW: Paramyotonia congenita: Successful treatment with tocainide. Clinical and electrophysiological findings in seven patients. Muscle Nerve 10:155, 1987

section 3 Chronic fatigue syndrome

388 CHRONIC FATIGUE SYNDROME

STEPHEN E. STRAUS

DEFINITION *Chronic fatigue syndrome* is the current name for a disorder characterized by debilitating fatigue and a variety of associated physical, constitutional, and neuropsychological complaints (Table 388-1). The medical literature of the past three centuries informs us that this is not a new type of syndrome. Certain individuals who had been labeled in the past with diagnoses such as the vapors, neurasthenia, effort syndrome, hyperventilation syndrome, chronic brucellosis, epidemic neuromyasthenia, myalgic encephalomyelitis, hypoglycemia, multiple chemical sensitivity syndrome, chronic candidiasis, chronic mononucleosis, chronic Epstein-Barr virus infection, and postviral fatigue syndrome probably had what we are now calling chronic fatigue syndrome. For research purposes, the U.S. Centers for Disease Control and Prevention (CDC) has developed a case definition based predominantly on symptoms and the exclusion of other illnesses (Table 388-2).

EPIDEMIOLOGY Patients with chronic fatigue syndrome are twice as likely to be women as men and are generally 25 to 45 years old, although cases in childhood and in middle age have been described.

Cases are recognized in many developed countries. Most arise sporadically, but over 30 clusters of similar illness have been reported. The most famous of such "outbreaks" occurred in Los Angeles County Hospital in 1934; in Akureyri, Iceland, in 1948; in the Royal Free Hospital, London, in 1955; in Punta Gorda, Florida, in 1956; and in Incline Village, Nevada, and surrounding communities in 1985. While these clustered cases suggest a common environmental or infectious cause, none has been identified.

The prevalence of chronic fatigue syndrome is difficult to ascertain, since its estimate is entirely dependent on case definition. Chronic fatigue itself is a ubiquitous symptom, occurring in as many as 20 percent of patients attending a general medical clinic; the chronic fatigue syndrome is far less common. On the basis of one case definition for the syndrome, an estimate of 37 cases per 100,000 population was obtained in a survey of one rural Australian province. The CDC is currently studying the prevalence of illness meeting its case definition in four U.S. cities.

PATHOGENESIS The diverse names for the syndrome reflect the equally numerous and controversial hypotheses about its etiology. There are several common themes underlying attempts to understand the disorder: It is often postinfectious, it is associated with immunologic disturbances, and it is commonly accompanied by depression.

Some contemporary workers in the field espouse one or more of

TABLE 388-1 The approximate percentage of patients with the chronic fatigue syndrome reporting the indicated symptoms

Symptom	Percentage
Fatigue	100
Difficulty concentrating	90
Headache	90
Sore throat	85
Tender lymph nodes	80
Muscle aches	80
Joint aches	75
Feverishness	75
Difficulty sleeping	70
Psychiatric problems	65
Allergies	55
Abdominal cramps	40
Weight loss	20
Rash	10
Rapid pulse	10
Weight gain	5
Chest pain	5
Night sweats	5

SOURCE: *Straus.*

TABLE 388-2 Summary of the working definition of chronic fatigue syndrome

Both major criteria and either ≥6 minor symptom criteria plus ≥2 minor physical criteria or ≥8 symptom criteria must be present to fulfill the case definition.

Major criteria

1 Persistent or relapsing fatigue or easy fatigability that
   a Does not resolve with bed rest
   b Is severe enough to reduce average daily activity by ≥ 50%
2 Satisfactory exclusion of other chronic conditions, including preexisting psychiatric diseases

Minor criteria

Symptoms:

1 Mild fever (37.5–38.6°C oral if documented by the patient) or chills
2 Sore throat
3 Lymph node pain in anterior or posterior cervical or axillary chains
4 Unexplained generalized muscle weakness
5 Muscle discomfort, myalgia
6 Prolonged (≥24 h), generalized fatigue following previously tolerable levels of exercise
7 New, generalized headaches
8 Migratory noninflammatory arthralgia
9 Neuropsychological symptoms: photophobia, transient visual scotomata, forgetfulness, excessive irritability, confusion, difficulty thinking, inability to concentrate, or depression
10 Sleep disturbance
11 Patient's description of initial onset of symptoms as acute or subacute

Physical findings (documented by a physician on at least two occasions at least 1 month apart):

1 Low-grade fever (37.6–38.6°C oral or 37.8–38.8°C rectal)
2 Nonexudative pharyngitis
3 Palpable or tender anterior or posterior cervical or axillary lymph nodes (<2 cm in diameter)

SOURCE: *Adapted from GP Holmes, Rev Infect Dis 13(suppl 1):S53, 1991.*

several viruses as potential etiologic agents. Among these are lymphotropic herpesviruses, retroviruses, and enteroviruses. The data on which these presumptions rest are as follows: First, chronic fatigue syndrome can be precipitated by acute infections with Epstein-Barr virus, cytomegalovirus, and other agents. Some of these have the ability to persist in humans and cause chronic illness. Second, titers of antibodies to many infectious agents are elevated in patients with chronic fatigue. Included are antibodies to most herpesviruses, measles virus, rubella virus, and coxsackie virus B. Third, there are claims of increased levels of some viral antigens and nucleic acids in patients, but these assertions are not based on firm experimental evidence. While experience suggests that viruses can precipitate the syndrome, it is presently uncertain whether they actually contribute to its long-term features. Common, persisting viruses may simply have a greater likelihood to reactivate because of inadequate immune restraints on them, while causing no symptoms.

Numerous, subtle immunologic disturbances have been reported in patients with chronic fatigue syndrome. In addition to the elevated viral antibody titers mentioned above, there are also mild, nonspecific elevations in titers of antinuclear antibodies, modest immunoglobulin subclass reductions, mild deficiencies in mitogen-induced lymphocyte proliferation in vitro and in ensuing cytokine release, reduced natural killer cell activity, and shifts in lymphocyte phenotypes to greater than normal proportions of T cells expressing activation or differentiation markers. None of the immune findings appear in all patients, nor have any been correlated, as yet, with the severity of illness. None are specific for chronic fatigue syndrome; thus they remain nondiagnostic. An immune disturbance of some type, though, is in line with one favored theory that many of the symptoms of chronic fatigue syndrome derive from excessive cytokine release.

Recent controlled studies of patients with chronic fatigue syndrome documented abnormalities in endocrine function consistent with reduced production of corticotropin-releasing hormone in the hypothalamus. Mean serum cortisol concentrations were lower in patients than

in controls; ACTH levels were correspondingly high. Hypothetically, these neuroendocrine abnormalities could contribute to the impaired energy and mood of patients. Whatever their importance, these changes further indicate the complex and multifactorial nature of chronic fatigue syndrome.

Mild to moderate depression is evident in about two-thirds of patients. Much of this depression may be reactive, but the prevalence exceeds that seen in other chronic medical illnesses. Thus some propose that chronic fatigue syndrome is fundamentally a psychiatric disorder and that the various neuroendocrine and immune disturbances arise secondarily.

MANIFESTATIONS The typical case of chronic fatigue syndrome arises suddenly in a previously active individual. An otherwise unremarkable flulike illness or some other acute stress is recalled with great clarity as the triggering event. Unbearable exhaustion is left in the wake of this incident. Other symptoms, such as headache, sore throat, tender lymph nodes, muscle and joint aches, and frequent feverishness, lead to the belief that an infection persists, and medical attention is sought. Over several weeks, the impact of reassurances proffered during that initial evaluation fades as other features of the syndrome become evident—disturbed sleep, difficulty in concentration, and depression (see Table 388-1).

Depending on the dominant symptoms and the beliefs of the patient, additional consultations may be sought from allergists, rheumatologists, infectious disease specialists, psychiatrists, ecologic therapists, homeopaths, or other professionals, frequently with unsatisfactory results. Once the pattern of illness is established, the symptoms may fluctuate somewhat. Many patients report that diverse complaints are linked—that during periods of greatest fatigue they perceive the most pain and difficulty with concentration. Patients also commonly assert that excessive physical or emotional stress may exacerbate their symptoms.

Most patients remain capable of balancing their limited resources to accommodate the obligations of family, work, or community. The discretionary activities are abandoned first. Some feel unable to engage in any gainful employment. A minority of individuals require help with the activities of daily living.

Ultimately, isolation, pathetic resignation, and frustration can mark the protracted course of illness. Patients may become angry at physicians for failing to acknowledge or resolve their plight. Fortunately, the chronic fatigue syndrome does not appear to progress. On the contrary, many patients experience gradual improvement and eventual recovery.

DIAGNOSIS Physical examination and routine laboratory tests are required to rule out other possible causes of the patient's symptoms. Prominent findings argue strongly in favor of other processes. No laboratory test, however esoteric or exotic, can diagnose this condition or measure its severity. Elaborate, expensive workups should therefore be avoided except in research settings. The great dilemma for patient and clinician alike is that chronic fatigue syndrome has no pathognomonic features and remains a constellation of symptoms and a diagnosis of exclusion. The case definition developed at the CDC for research purposes is cumbersome and imprecise (see Table 388-2). Nevertheless, it is increasingly used in the community for lack of suitable alternatives.

An important deficiency of the CDC case definition is its lack of clarity with regard to the impact of psychiatric illness on eligibility. As originally crafted, the criteria excluded any coexisting or past psychiatric problem. A modification was quickly proposed to allow mild to moderate current depression, recognizing that this condition could be situational. It remains uncertain as to whether an acute psychiatric problem long predating the onset of chronic fatigue should exclude the diagnosis.

MANAGEMENT The primary responsibility of a physician confronted with a chronically fatigued patient is to address the cause by taking a thorough history, conducting a complete physical examination, judiciously using the laboratory, and, throughout this process, considering the differential diagnosis. If other illnesses are excluded, there are several points to address in the long-term care of a patient with chronic fatigue.

First, the patient should be informed about the illness and what is truly known of its pathogenesis; its potential impact on the physical, psychological, and social dimensions of life; and its prognosis. Patients are relieved when their complaints are taken seriously.

Second, periodic reassessment is appropriate to identify an underlying process that is late in declaring itself and to address intercurrent problems that must not be neglected as yet another subjective complaint.

Third, many symptoms of chronic fatigue syndrome respond to treatment. Nonsteroidal anti-inflammatory drugs alleviate headache, diffuse pain, and feverishness. Allergic rhinitis and sinusitis are common in patients with chronic fatigue syndrome; antihistamines or decongestants may be helpful. Although patients are often averse to psychiatric diagnoses, depression is a prominent symptom that should be confronted. Expert psychiatric assessment is sometimes advisable. Nonsedating antidepressants improve mood and disordered sleep and thereby attentuate the fatigue somewhat. Even modest improvements in symptoms can make an important difference in the patient's degree of self-sufficiency and ability to appreciate life's pleasures.

Fourth, practical advice should be given regarding lifestyle. The consumption of heavy meals with alcohol and caffeine at night can make it harder to sleep, compounding fatigue. Total rest is harmful. It leads to further deconditioning and the self-image of being an invalid. Exacerbation of exhaustion by strenuous exertion leads to total avoidance of exercise, so a moderate, carefully graded regimen needs to be encouraged.

Fifth, unproven treatments should be avoided. Controlled trials have established that acyclovir and intramuscular liver extract–folic acid–cyanocobalamin injections are of no value. There are conflicting claims regarding the efficacy of high-dose intravenous immunoglobulin therapy. One study documented no benefit; a second reported transient improvement in some patients. Given the considerable cost of this treatment and its side effects, there is little to recommend immunoglobulin therapy at this time. Countless anecdotes circulate regarding other traditional or nontraditional therapies. It is important to guide patients, flexibly, away from those therapeutic modalities which are most toxic, expensive, and unreasonable.

The physician should promote the patient's efforts toward improvement. A clinical trial in England showed behavioral therapy to be helpful. The therapy was aimed at dispelling cognitive distortions that lead to inactivity and despair. For chronic fatigue syndrome, as for many conditions, a comprehensive approach to physical, psychological, and social aspects is in order.

REFERENCES

ACHESON ED: The clinical syndrome variously called benign myalgic encephalomyelitis, Iceland disease and epidemic neuromyasthenia. Am J Med 26:569, 1959

HOLMES GP et al.: Chronic fatigue syndrome: A working case definition. Ann Intern Med 108:387, 1988

SCHLEUDERBERG A et al (eds): Considerations in the design of studies of chronic fatigue syndrome (monograph). Rev Infect Dis 13(suppl 1):S1, 1991

STRAUS SE: The chronic mononucleosis syndrome. J Infect Dis 157:405, 1988

——— et al.: Acyclovir treatment of the chronic fatigue syndrome: Lack of efficacy in a placebo-controlled trial. N Engl J Med 319:1692, 1988

section 4   Psychiatric disorders

389   MENTAL DISORDERS

LEWIS L. JUDD / KAREN THATCHER BRITTON / DAVID L. BRAFF

INTRODUCTION

Lewis L. Judd

Remarkable scientific progress in the understanding, accurate diagnosis, and successful treatment of the mental disorders has occurred in the last two decades. Fueled by the explosion of research emerging from modern neuroscience, it has been firmly established that the major mental disorders are diseases of the brain. Furthermore, there is unequivocal evidence that the mental disorders result from abnormal brain mechanisms that, with sophisticated neurobiologic techniques, can be characterized at cellular and molecular levels. The progressive unfolding of the pathophysiologic mechanisms in the brain that underlie the mental disorders has led to more rational, specific, and successful treatments for these disorders.

These rapidly accumulating discoveries, together with the development of a scientific, standardized, reliable, and clinically valid classification system for the mental disorders, the *Diagnostic, Statistical Manual of Mental Disorders,* Third Edition-Revised (DSM-III-R), has made it possible for clinicians to routinely identify and diagnose mental disorders that require treatment. Thus the focus of modern psychiatric clinical practice, like that of internal medicine, relies primarily on diagnosis, which in turn dictates the type of treatment prescribed and is highly predictive of clinical outcome.

The primary focus of this chapter is to highlight the most prevalent mental disorders that are of high relevance to the internal medicine and primary care physician. These are the mood and anxiety disorders, which at any one point in time, afflict about 10 percent of the U.S. population. Mood and anxiety disorders are central, or at least important, features in the clinical picture of approximately 25 percent of the patients who present in standard internal medicine practices. The last portion describes current understanding of the disease schizophrenia, which is included because of its prevalence in the general population and the highly disabling nature of its lifetime course. This aspect of the chapter focuses on issues of diagnoses, emphasizing the ability of the internist to differentiate the clinical features of schizophrenia from those of other brain diseases.

MOOD DISORDERS

Lewis L. Judd

The mood disorders are characterized by pervasive, prolonged, and disabling exaggerations of mood and affect that are associated with behavioral, physiologic, cognitive, neurochemical, and psychomotor dysfunctions. The major mood syndromes are *major depressive disorder* (also called unipolar disorder), *bipolar disorder* (also called manic depressive illness or bipolar depression), and *dysthymic disorder.* The classification of mood disorders into the unipolar and bipolar categories is useful clinically because these entities, although closely related mood disorders, are psychobiologically different with somewhat different clinical characteristics, disease patterns, and treatments.

EPIDEMIOLOGY OF MOOD DISORDERS AND RELEVANCE TO INTERNAL MEDICINE   Mood disorders are the second most common mental disorder, afflicting 5.1 percent of the U.S. population over 18 years of age at any one point in time (1-month prevalence). The 1-month prevalence for major depressive disorder is 2.2, for bipolar disorder 0.4, and for dysthymic disorder 3.3 percent. The 1-year prevalence for all mood disorders is 9.5 percent, making these diseases among the most common that people experience.

Clinical studies indicate that nonpsychiatric physicians frequently fail to accurately recognize or diagnose patients with mood disorders. Prevalence of mood disorders among primary care outpatients ranges from 4.8 to 8.6 percent for major depressive disorder, and 2.1 to 8.7 percent for dysthymic disorder. An additional 3.4 to 4.7 percent of patients who experience significant depressive symptoms do not reach the threshold criteria for a formal diagnosis of major depressive disorder or dysthymic disorder.

Therefore, 10.2 to 21 percent of primary care outpatients are suffering from clinically significant mood disorders. This is consistent with observations that patients with mood disorders are very high users of nonpsychiatric medical and primary care and emergency services. A presentation with depressive symptoms is the fourth most common complaint that patients report in primary care settings. The effective practice of internal medicine now requires that practitioners be thoroughly familiar with the accurate diagnosis of mood disorders in their patients. Mood disorders should always be a part of the differential diagnosis whenever patient complaints involve any symptoms in the depressive spectrum (e.g., low energy, difficulty with memory or concentration, impotence).

CLASSIFICATION Mood disorders are usually chronic in nature with a marked tendency to remission and exacerbation throughout the patient's lifetime. Remissions may last for weeks, months, or years (euthymia).

The diagnosis of a mood disorder should be based on the presence of signs and symptoms as defined in the DSM-III-R. Two general types of mood episodes may occur: major depressive episodes (sustained for at least 2 weeks) and manic episodes (sustained for at least 1 week). The diagnostic criteria for major depressive episodes and manic episodes are shown in Table 389-1 and 389-2.

Major depressive disorder may occur rarely as a single episode, but usually is recurrent (recurrent unipolar depression). Patients with the disorder manifest only a single extreme of pathologic mood, that of depression. In *bipolar disorder* both major depressive and manic episodes occur. Bipolar disorders are diagnosed as bipolar disorder, manic, if the current episode meets criteria for a manic episode and as bipolar disorder, depressed, if the episode meets criteria for a major depressive episode. Bipolar patients who have depressive and manic features simultaneously are classified as bipolar disorder, mixed.

Dysthymic disorder (dysthymia) is a chronic, less intense form of depression in which depressive symptoms persist for at least 2 years (see Table 389-3). Clinical studies have found that dysthymic disorder occurs together with major depressive disorder in about 25 percent of patients. This combined condition, called ''double-depression,'' has a much more grave prognosis with substantially higher risks for recurrence and resistance to treatment.

The signs and symptoms of *atypical depression* match those of major depressive disorder, but are distinguished from the latter by the following: reverse vegetative symptoms (e.g., overeating and hypersomnia), sensitivity to interpersonal rejection, a sense of ''leaden paralysis,'' the presence of a significant amount of pathologic anxiety, and/or unusual responsiveness to environmental changes. Distinguishing between atypical and typical major depressive disorder is useful because this disorder is often more responsive to monoamine oxidase (MAO) inhibitor antidepressants.

Other subgroups of mood disorders have been identified that are clinically less common and have less relevance to the internist. These include the following: *major depressive disorder, psychotic; major depressive disorder, melancholic; major depressive disorder, seasonal pattern; postpartum depression; brief recurrent depression; late luteal phase dysphoric disorder (premenstrual dysphoria); and cyclothymic*

TABLE 389-1 Diagnostic criteria for major depressive episode*

A At least five of the following symptoms have been present during the same 2-week period and represent a change from previous functioning; at least one of the symptoms is either (1) depressed mood, or (2) loss of interest or pleasure. (Do not include symptoms that are clearly due to a physical condition, mood-incongruent delusions or hallucinations, incoherence, or marked loosening of associations.)

 1 Depressed mood (or can be irritable mood in children and adolescents) most of the day, nearly every day, as indicated either by subjective account or observation by others

 2 Markedly diminished interest or pleasure in all, or almost all, activities most of the day, nearly every day (as indicated either by subjective account or observation by others of apathy most of the time)

 3 Significant weight loss or weight gain when not dieting (e.g., more than 5% of body weight in a month), or decrease or increase in appetite nearly every day (in children, consider failure to make expected weight gains)

 4 Insomnia or hypersomnia nearly every day

 5 Psychomotor agitation or retardation nearly every day (observable by others, not merely subjective feelings of restlessness or being slowed down)

 6 Fatigue or loss of energy nearly every day

 7 Feelings of worthlessness or excessive or inappropriate guilt (not merely self-reproach or guilt about being sick)

 8 Diminished ability to think or concentrate, or indecisiveness, nearly every day (either by subjective account or as observed by others)

 9 Recurrent thoughts of death (not just fear of dying), recurrent suicidal ideation without a specific plan, or a suicide attempt or a specific plan for committing suicide

B 1 It cannot be established that an organic factor initiated and maintained the disturbance.

 2 The disturbance is not a normal reaction to the death of a loved one (uncomplicated bereavement)[†]

C At no time during the disturbance have there been delusions or hallucinations for as long as 2 weeks in the absence of prominent mood symptoms (i.e., before the mood symptoms developed or after they have remitted).

D Not superimposed on schizophrenia or schizophreniform, delusional, or psychotic disorders.

---

* A major depressive syndrome is defined as criterion *A* above.

† Morbid preoccupation with worthlessness, suicidal ideation, marked functional impairment or psychomotor retardation, or prolonged duration suggest bereavement complicated by major depression.

SOURCE: Adapted from DSM-III-R.

TABLE 389-2 Diagnostic criteria for manic episode*

A A distinct period of abnormal and persistently elevated, expansive, or irritable mood.

B During the period of mood disturbance, at least three of the following symptoms have persisted (four if the mood is only irritable) and have been present to a significant degree:

 1 Inflated self-esteem or grandiosity

 2 Decreased need for sleep, e.g., feels rested after only 3 h of sleep

 3 More talkative than usual or pressure to keep talking

 4 Flight of ideas or subjective experience that thoughts are racing

 5 Distractibility, i.e., attention too easily drawn to unimportant or irrelevant external stimuli

 6 Increase in goal-directed activity (either socially, at work or school, or sexually) or psychomotor agitation

 7 Excessive involvement in pleasurable activities that have a high potential for painful consequences, e.g., the person engages in unrestrained buying sprees, sexual indiscretions, or foolish business investments

C Mood disturbance sufficiently severe to cause marked impairment in occupational functioning or in usual social activities or relationships with others, or to necessitate hospitalization to prevent harm to self or others.

D At no time during the disturbance have there been delusions or hallucinations for as long as 2 weeks in the absence of prominent mood symptoms (i.e., before the mood symptoms developed or after they have remitted).

E Not superimposed on schizophrenia or schizophreniform, delusional, or psychotic disorders.

F It cannot be established that an organic factor initiated and maintained the disturbance.[†]

---

* A manic syndrome is defined as including criteria *A*, *B*, and *C* above. A hypomanic syndrome is defined as including criteria *A* and *B*, but not *C*, i.e., no marked impairment.

† Somatic antidepressant treatment (e.g., drugs, electroconvulsive therapy) that apparently precipitates a mood disturbance should not be considered an etiologic organic factor.

SOURCE: Adapted from DSM-III-R.

TABLE 389-3 Diagnostic criteria for dysthymia

A Depressed mood (or can be irritable mood in children and adolescents) for most of the day, more days than not, as indicated either by subjective account or observation by others, for at least 2 years (1 year for children and adolescents).
B Presence, while depressed, of at least two of the following:
  1 Poor appetite or overeating
  2 Insomnia or hypersomnia
  3 Low energy or fatigue
  4 Low self-esteem
  5 Poor concentration or difficulty making decisions
  6 Feelings of hopelessness
C During a 2-year period (1 year for children and adolescents) of the disturbance, never without the symptoms in A for more than 2 months at a time.
D No evidence of an unequivocal major depressive episode during the first 2 years (1 year for children and adolescents) of the disturbance.*
E Has never had a manic episode or an unequivocal hypomanic episode (see Table 389-2).
F Not superimposed on a chronic psychotic disorder, such as schizophrenia or delusional disorder.
G It cannot be established that an organic factor initiated and maintained the disturbance, e.g., prolonged administration of an antihypertensive medication.

* There may have been a previous major depressive episode, provided there was a full remission (no significant signs or symptoms for 6 months) before development of the dysthymia. In addition, after these 2 years (1 year in children and adolescents) of dysthymia, there may be superimposed episodes of major depression, in which case both diagnoses are given.
SOURCE: DSM-III-R.

disorder. The interested reader should refer to a standard textbook of psychiatry for further information on these diagnostic subgroups.

COURSE OF ILLNESS Major depressive disorder Although major depressive episodes can occur at any age, the peak age of onset for the first episode is 25 years. Major depressive disorders occur twice as frequently in women as in men. Symptoms may develop over days, weeks, or occasionally months, and an untreated episode lasts on average 10 to 12 months (range 6 to 24 months). Major depressive disorder is a chronic disease with marked tendencies to relapse and over 80 percent of patients have at least one more episode. On average patients experience two to three episodes in their lifetime, and 20 to 35 percent of patients manifest a chronic course with considerable interepisode symptomatology and disability. Two-thirds of the cases remit completely between episodes and functioning returns to the premorbid level.

Bipolar disorder The age of risk for bipolar disorders is broad, from 6 or 7 years to over 65 years; the peak age onset for a first episode is 19 years. Bipolar disorders are slightly more frequent in women than men (1.3 : 1). Men have more manic than depressive episodes; women have more depressive episodes. Onset of symptoms can be over hours but is usually over days or weeks and can begin with either a manic or depressive episode. Over half of first episodes are manic and approximately 60 percent of these patients have a predominantly manic course, while the remaining one-third manifest primarily depressive episodes. Clinical studies of untreated bipolar patients show an average of 9 diagnosable manic and depressive episodes during a lifetime (range 2 to more than 20). The typical pattern is that the cycle length, which is measured from the onset of one episode to the onset of the next, decreases and the number of episodes increases over time. For example, in untreated bipolar patients the time between the first and second episode averages from 3.5 to 4 years, between the second and third episodes about 2 years, and between episodes three and four somewhere between 12 and 18 months. Untreated episode duration is from 4 to 13 months, and the average is about 8.5 months, but may be shorter during manic phases (i.e., the untreated illness tends to worsen over time, highlighting the importance of intervention).

A small subgroup of bipolar patients manifest very rapid cycling patterns, with from four episodes per year up to episodes every 24 h. Eighty percent of rapid cyclers are women, and a relationship to impaired thyroid function has been suggested. Although still controversial, there is evidence that in some patients rapid cycling may be related to previous treatment with tricyclic antidepressants and that the condition can only be controlled effectively after tricyclics are discontinued and treatment with thyroid supplement and lithium is begun.

The life-long intensity of illness in all bipolar disorders is greater than in major depressive disorder, recurrent; prior to the discovery of lithium the long-term prognosis was very grim. Bipolar patients have significantly more episodes of illness, require more hospitalizations, spend more time in the hospital during their lifetimes, are more likely to divorce, lose their jobs, and, if left untreated, are at significantly higher risk for suicide.

Dysthymic disorder This disorder is characterized by chronic, mild depressive symptoms manifested over many years. A significant number of dysthymic disorders progress to a major depressive episode within 1 year. Twenty percent or more develop double depression (e.g., combined dysthymic disorder and major depressive disorder), which is a much more malignant form of mood disorder.

MORBIDITY, MORTALITY, AND COMORBIDITY Morbidity There is strong evidence that mood disorders have a major impact on health status and quality of life. In a large sample of medical outpatients (over 22,000 subjects) major depressive and dysthymic disorders were shown to contribute greater disability in physical, social, and occupational functioning than hypertension, diabetes, chronic lung disease, or arthritis. Only patients with acute coronary artery disease had more bed days during the previous month than depressive disorders.

Mortality There are over 32,000 suicides each year in the United States. Suicide is the eighth leading cause of death for adults in this country. It has been estimated that 80 percent of the completed suicides are related to mood disorders. Lifetime suicide attempt rate in major depressive disorders is 14.3 percent and for dysthymic disorders is 14.1 percent. Approximately 15 percent of patients with recurrent major depressive disorders die by suicide.

Patients with bipolar disorders have increased death rate by suicide amounting to 15 to 20 times that of the general population. Fifteen to 20 percent of affected patients attempt suicide, more often women than men, although men are more likely to succeed. Prior to lithium, over 20 percent of manic patients died in the hospital, with about two-thirds of these dying from "exhaustion."

Comorbidity with substance abuse disorders The high prevalence of mood disorders combined with a failure to recognize and treat them probably contribute to the inordinately high rates at which alcohol and/or drug abuse are concurrent with mood disorders. Thirty-two percent of all mood disorder patients also are substance dependent or substance abusers in their lifetime. Lifetime rates for this combination are 60.7 percent for bipolar disorder, 27.2 percent for major depressive disorder, and 31.4 percent for dysthymic disorder. There is growing evidence that concurrent substance abuse significantly worsens the prognosis and treatability of mood disorders.

Comorbidity with medical conditions Many medical illnesses may be associated with mood disorders, including autoimmune disease, neurologic disease (stroke, demyelinative, degenerative, traumatic disorders), metabolic disease, cardiovascular disease, endocrinopathies, and specific malignancies (pancreas, lung, kidney, G.I., brain). The clinical manifestations and the diagnosis of mood disorder that is concurrent with medical disease are based on the same criteria as the pure *primary* mood disorders.

Even though mood disorders may be associated with an extraordinarily large array of nonpsychiatric illnesses, several, because of their importance, should be noted. For example, major depressive episodes have been described in 25 to 55 percent of *poststroke* patients, especially with strokes affecting the left anterior frontal lobe. These episodes, if untreated, can persist for up to 12 months. Major depressive disorder has been found to occur in 8.5 to 60 percent of patients with *diabetes mellitus,* with the mean prevalence being about 30 percent.

About one quarter of patients with *malignancies* experience a clinically significant mood disorder, and 46 to 75 percent of patients with *chronic fatigue syndrome* are found to have a background of major depressive disorder. An even more substantial association between mood disorder and medical illness occurs in patients with *coronary artery disease.* Reports indicate that between 18 and 25 percent of patients after myocardial infarction experience a major depressive disorder that should be treated.

In addition, the chronic administration of the following medications may precipitate a major depressive episode: glucocorticoids, α-methyldopa, propranolol, benzodiazepines, reserpine derivatives, levodopa, neuroleptics, cimetidine, indomethacin, cycloserine, and anticancer drugs. Withdrawal from CNS stimulants such as amphetamines or drugs of abuse like cocaine may also be a precipitating factor.

It is important to recognize that these major depressive episodes occurring either in conjunction with a medical illness or the administration of a specific medication can often be the most important and disabling aspect of a patient's clinical picture and require immediate and specific treatment (e.g., some studies of transplant patients demonstrate the importance of treating depression before surgery to enhance postoperative recovery).

Two strategies can be used for treatment of a mood disorder concurrent with medical illness. First, if the symptoms are due to a primary "pure" mood disorder, the treatment should be initiated in a regimen identical to that used without a concomitant medical illness, unless the medical condition necessitates a modification, such as lowering the dosage because of impaired hepatic metabolism. When it is judged that the depressive symptoms are caused by the medical condition, it should be treated aggressively; at least one half of such patients show remission of depressive symptoms with effective treatment of the underlying medical illness. Often, however, treatment of the major depressive episode may need to be initiated in these patients to facilitate return to normal health.

ETIOLOGY AND PATHOPHYSIOLOGY OF THE MOOD DISORDERS Considerable scientific progress has been made in identifying and characterizing the etiologic factors in mood disorders. Several leads for focused scientific inquiry into the causes of these disorders have emerged; these leads have led to the development of more specific and effective treatments.

Genetic factors Mood disorders, like many other human diseases, result from complex interactions between the patient's genetic makeup and the environment. Genetic factors are particularly significant in bipolar disorders, although genetic components alone are probably insufficient to cause illness in the absence of environmental challenges. In general, the cause of a major mood episode can be conceptualized by two intersecting continua both with progressive intensities. One involves the patient's inherited constitutional vulnerability to develop mood disorder; this interacts with the second continuum of the environmental stresses and life events to which the patient is exposed. Some individuals with high genetic predisposition for mood disorder develop symptoms with minor precipitating events. Others with lower genetic vulnerability develop a mood disorder only when exposed to serious precipitating events and cumulative life stresses.

Data from numerous human genetic studies indicate significant genetic influences in the mood disorders, but as yet the mode of genetic transmission has not been established. The degree of genetic expression varies from one mood disorder to the other and from patient to patient. Twin studies of mood disorders report concordance rates among monozygotic (MZ) twins ranging from 33.3 to 75 percent, and for dizygotic (DZ) twins from 9 to 23 percent. This difference in concordance rates between MZ and DZ twins strongly suggests inherited genetic vulnerability. The concordance rate is highest for recurrent mood disorders (over three episodes). Although no definitive studies have been reported with identical twins reared apart, there are trends in such studies to suggest that adoptees have the higher incidence of affective illness of their biologic parents rather than of their adoptive parents.

Family studies of the mood disorders that include first-degree relatives show that the morbidity risk in relatives of bipolar patients is 2.8 to 17.7 percent and for major depressive disorders up to 22.4 percent. The first-degree relatives of major depressive disorder patients have a risk of 6.4 to 17.0 percent for major depressive episodes and of 0.3 to 29.0 percent for bipolar disorder. Thus bipolar patients have increased prevalence of both bipolar and major depressive disorders in their blood relatives, whereas major depressive disorder patients have increased prevalence of major depressive episodes, but not bipolar disorders, in their relatives.

There are several large ongoing studies combining careful diagnostic and family pedigree studies with molecular genetics in an attempt to identify linkage between specific gene(s) or DNA probes and mood disorder. Linkage on the X chromosome has been reported for bipolar disorder in an Israeli pedigree, as yet unconfirmed by others. In addition, a small subgroup of bipolar families has been found to have a linkage between protan-deutan (red-green) color blindness and glucose-6-phosphate dehydrogenase deficiency.

Neurotransmitter dysregulation The earliest investigations of etiologic mechanisms in the mood disorders involved studies of various neurotransmitter systems in the CNS. The *biogenic amine hypothesis* focused on the neurotransmitters norepinephrine, serotonin, and dopamine, attributing depression and mania, respectively, to the deficiency or excess of these neurotransmitters at important synaptic sites in the brain. This hypothesis continues as a subject of clinical research, and data both consistent and inconsistent with the hypothesis continue to emerge. Urinary and cerebrospinal fluid (CSF) studies of norepinephrine, its metabolite 3-methoxy-4-hydroxyphenethyleneglycol (MHPG), and the catalytic enzyme dopamine β-hydroxylase reported fluctuations in a predictable direction during major depressive and manic episodes. More recently, however, increases in norepinephrine have been described in *both* mania and depression. Studies have identified alterations in serotonin metabolism, with 5-hydroxyindoleacetic acid (5-HIAA), a metabolite, being reported to be reduced in the CSF of patients who make frequent impulsive, violent, and aggressive suicide attempts. However, this observation lacks specificity since similar changes have been observed in other mental disorders, including schizophrenia and antisocial personality disorders. Dopamine and gamma-aminobutyric acid (GABA) functions have also been reported to be abnormal in some patients with major depressive disorder; a cholinergic hypothesis which postulates increased central cholinergic tone in depression, decreased cholinergic tone in mania, and an imbalance between cholinergic and adrenergic neurotransmitter systems also has been proposed with inconclusive results.

More recently, with definition of receptor subtypes in the brain (see Chap. 364), there is growing interest in the possibility that postsynaptic receptor kinetics and activities may be altered during mood disorder episodes and that the psychotropic medications known to ameliorate these disorders may alter receptor functions. The role of postsynaptic receptor systems and especially the cascade of intraneuronal molecular and biochemical events in the postsynaptic neuron following the binding of the neurotransmitter to the receptor are currently under intensive study.

Environmental factors There are data on the type of stresses that are the most significant causes of major mood episodes. The data are inconsistent when efforts are made to relate early childhood loss and parental separation as predisposing factors for the development of a mood disorder. There is, not surprisingly, an overall temporal relationship between stressful and negative life events (e.g., spousal bereavement, a death of a child, job loss, marked change in social status, and severe assaults on self-esteem) and subsequent development of episodes of mood disorder. Research attempting to characterize qualitative differences in the impact of life stress have been disappointing.

Support for the idea of an influence of environmental events has been derived in experiments with subhuman primates. In these studies, phenomena that resemble or are analogous to depressive states in humans are seen in monkeys using mother/infant and peer separation paradigms. Interestingly, the monkey's "despair" response to the separation can be predictably altered (worsened or improved) by drugs known to specifically alter central concentrations and metabolites of several relevant CNS neurotransmitters (e.g., norepinephrine, dopamine), consistent with the view that psychosocial and CNS biochemical factors interact in the genesis of mood disorders.

Brain-environmental interactions   One of the brain's most important and central functions is to receive incoming stimuli from the environment for purposes of storage, integration, and interpretation, which in turn provides the basis for an appropriate behavioral and cognitive response. Thus it should not be surprising to find that environmental events do exert consistent and powerful influences on brain function. Testable hypotheses are beginning to be developed. The learned helplessness paradigm of Seligman has been a very useful strategy in creating and studying depressive-like states in various animal models. These studies have been able to reduce brain 5-OH tryptamine (5HT) levels in response to behavioral stressors, which can be reversed by tricyclic antidepressants. Another exception is the CNS "kindling" hypothesis of Post and colleagues. From the data based in animal studies, including stimulant-induced behavioral sensitization and electrophysiologic kindling (increased sensitivity to electrically induced seizures), the suggestion has been made that a similar sensitization process may be involved in the recurrent episodes characteristic of the bipolar disorders. This hypothesis is consistent with the observations that spontaneous recurrences of affective episodes late in the progression of the illness seem, at times, to occur without precipitating factors; patients respond differently to pharmacotherapies at different stages of the disorder; there is frequently an increased sensitivity to anticonvulsant medications (i.e., carbamazepine combined with lithium) in some patients at late stages; and there is an increased rate of cycling as the disease progresses. One implication of this line of research is that prophylactic maintenance of pharmacotherapy may be justifiable early in the treatment of major depressive and bipolar mood disorders.

Biologic rhythms   Major mood disorders show a marked tendency to periodic manifestation and to seasonal variation. This has stimulated hypotheses to explore dysregulation of biologic rhythms as a mechanism involved in the pathophysiology of some mood disorders. There are reports of desynchronization of circadian rhythms with some bipolar patients manifesting both rapid free-running circadian rhythms (e.g., 23- versus 24-h rhythms) and a phase delay in their rhythms.

There is also a special subgroup of patients with major depression in which the depressive episodes are manifested at specific seasons of the year. The most consistently studied groups are those with so-called "winter" depression (also called *seasonal affective disorder*). These patients, while residing in more northern latitudes, experience major depressive episodes during the winter when days are significantly shorter and periods of darkness more prolonged; conversely, there is a marked reduction or absence of depressive episodes in latitudes where the environmental light/dark cycles are not as extreme. Controlled treatment studies, using intense white light (>2000 lux) presented at a specified time during the day and for a precise period of time, have proven to be therapeutically effective in some patients with this syndrome. Finally, the consistent antidepressant effects of specific forms of sleep deprivation in major depressive disorders also provides support for this hypothesis.

BIOLOGIC CORRELATES AND LABORATORY STUDIES   Neurohormonal correlates   For a number of years, probes into the pathophysiologic mechanisms of the mood disorders have used various neurohormones whose secretion is regulated by one or more of the CNS neurotransmitter pathways (e.g., dopamine, norepinephrine, serotonin). One consistent finding from these studies has been that a significant subpopulation of patients with major depressive disorder hypersecrete cortisol and have abnormal cortisol circadian secretion patterns. Recent investigations with corticotropin-releasing hormone (CRH) stimulation have yielded blunted adrenocorticotropic hormone (ACTH) responses, suggesting that the corticosteroid abnormality is

of central origin. In addition, even though it is now controversial, the dexamethasone suppression test (DST) has been used in both diagnosis and monitoring of treatment in research settings. It has virtually no utility clinically because approximately 50 percent of patients with major depression do not have this abnormality. The standard DST used in psychiatry involves the administration of 1 mg of dexamethasone at 2300 hours with subsequent cortisol determinations at 1600 and 2300 hours the following day. The nonsuppression of cortisol is an abnormal or positive response [>140 nmol/L (>5 µg/dL) cortisol concentration in the 1600 or 2300 sample]. Initial studies reported that up to 50 percent of patients with serious major depressive episodes were nonsuppressors on the DST. Further investigations indicate that DST nonsuppression is a state marker, positive during the depressive episode, with return to normal after successful resolution of the episode. False-positives on the DST occur in patients with alcoholism, malnutrition, obesity, pregnancy, major physical illnesses, anticonvulsant use, excessive caffeine intake, and in patients over 65 years. This has eroded the usefulness of the test. In addition, more recently a number of studies have appeared in the literature reporting a much smaller percentage of DST nonsuppressors associated with major depressive episodes and an increased percentage in many other psychiatric illnesses. DST nonsuppression among depressed patients has now been reported as low as 10 to 15 percent, especially among depressed outpatients, making this test of no value as a screening test for depression. While the status of this diagnostic marker is still controversial, some clinicians advocate monitoring treatment efficacy in DST-positive depressives, since the DST response reverts to normal when the episode remits. Failure of DST to normalize despite apparent clinical recovery has, in some studies, been associated with suicide.

Other neuroendocrine markers have also been explored, but none as widely as the DST. In major depression, between 25 and 30 percent of patients respond to thyrotropin-releasing hormone (TRH) with blunted thyroid-stimulating hormone (TSH) responses. TSH blunting is not specific to depressive episodes, but an exaggerated TSH response is useful in identifying those refractory or rapid-cycling bipolar patients who would benefit from thyroid supplementation (e.g., T_3 or T_4). Small subgroups of depressed patients have manifested blunted growth hormone responses to the following challenge agents: clonidine, amphetamine, levodopa, 5-hydroxytryptophan, and hypoglycemia (insulin tolerance test). Even though 15 to 25 percent of depressed patients have blunted growth hormone responses, it has not been proved to be diagnostically useful. More recently, blunted prolactin responses to both TRH and opiate alkaloid challenges have also been reported in subpopulations of depressed patients; while these findings may be of interest in probing pathophysiologic mechanisms, they are not useful diagnostically.

Sleep studies   The disruption of sleep patterns is present in virtually every patient with mood disorder, and polysomnographic studies of sleep in these patients have proved to be of importance. In approximately 60 percent of cases of major depressive disorder there is a significantly shortened time period between the onset of sleep and the appearance of the first rapid eye movement (REM) (i.e., *decreased REM latency*). In addition, the density of the REM epoch, measured by the number of eye movements, is increased; there is a tendency for the REM epoch to last longer, and there is a shift of REM activity to an earlier part of the night. *These findings from all-night EEG sleep recordings have remained among the most consistent biologic markers for major depressive episodes, although they lack specificity, since short REM latency has also been reported in anorexia nervosa, obsessive-compulsive disorders, sleep apnea, and narcolepsy.*

Neurotransmitter metabolites and enzymes   The neurotransmitter hypotheses of mood disorders have stimulated a number of studies correlating biogenic amine metabolites with manic and depressive episodes. The data are inconclusive and have not been consistently useful either diagnostically or therapeutically. The one possible exception is MHPG, a metabolite of norepinephrine. Some workers have reported low MHPG excretion as predicting a positive therapeutic response to the "norepinephrine" antidepressants such as desipramine, and high MHPG excretion as predicting a response to serotoninergic agents like amitriptyline. While these data are of interest and with further study may result in the identification of biochemical subtypes in major depression, these findings have not been regularly replicated in other laboratories.

Investigators who have examined the levels of the enzyme MAO in platelets report it to be low in bipolar disorders and high in subjects with anxiety disorder. Further, ^{3}[H]imipramine-binding studies in platelets also have been found to be low in major depressives who were suicidal. Again, these findings, although of interest, lack specificity, since similar results have been reported in other psychiatric conditions such as alcoholism, anorexia and bulimia, and impulse control disorders.

GENERAL PRINCIPLES IN THE TREATMENT OF MOOD DISORDERS The prevalence of mood disorders is estimated to be as high as 20 percent in general medical and primary care settings. The first step in the treatment of any mood disorder is recognition. The primary care physician should be aware that a mood disorder may be present in patients exhibiting certain symptoms, although they may be somewhat vague, nonspecific, and of little consequence (e.g., low energy, easy fatigability, loss of interest in every day and pleasurable activities, dysphoria, insomnia, impotence). However, there are some clinical clues that should raise the index of suspicion, such as the presence of treatment for previous major depressive episodes, history of suicide attempts, family history of depression or of suicide attempts, or alcoholism or drug abuse.

Important advances have been made in the treatment of the mood disorders, and the vast majority of these patients can now be treated with a high degree of specificity and success. The most important discoveries have been made in the development of potent psychotropic medications for both major depression and bipolar disorders. The central therapeutic tools in the treatment of the major affective disorders are the antidepressants and lithium and to a lesser extent certain anticonvulsants (e.g., carbamazepine, sodium valproate) (see below).

Because mood disorders have strong tendencies for recurrence, an important aspect of the patient's treatment is the comprehensive education of patients and their families about the disorder. It should be emphasized to the patient that these are psychobiologic disorders that involve altered biochemical states in the brain, and that episodes can be triggered by adverse events and stresses in the environment but may occur spontaneously as well. As with any chronic disease, each patient should be urged to become an expert on his or her own disorder, concentrating on how it manifests itself and what early signs and symptoms may herald a manic or depressive episode. The patient and the family must be urged to take on the responsibility for the early recognition of the impending episode, since the earlier a patient presents for treatment, the easier it is to treat. The absolute necessity of medication compliance must be emphasized, and the patient must understand thoroughly the need to take the medications precisely as prescribed and to be aware of side effects and of the potential medical sequelae of the medications.

With the emergence of new evidence indicating that the mood disorders are chronic lifelong diseases, there has been an increasing emphasis on maintenance treatment strategies whose goals are to keep the patient free of symptoms throughout their lifetime. There is emerging support for the view that maintaining patients with recurrent major depressive disorder on an antidepressant medication at the same dosage that proved to be effective in the original acute episode may prevent relapse. There is an increasing acceptance that the disease model for treatment of the mood disorders more closely resembles diabetes mellitus than lobar pneumonia. The physician's therapeutic approach to patients who are suffering acute mood episodes is simple and straightforward. During the acute phase of these episodes, patients respond better to short (10 to 20 min) visits one to three times per week. During these visits the general focus is on monitoring the medication and side effects, but it is also essential that the physician be very informative, reassuring, and supportive.

Because patients are functioning essentially in an altered state secondary to the depressive or manic episode, the treatment must be sustained by the physician's optimism and knowledge that, with time, these episodes will abate if the proper medication and dose are prescribed. Virtually all the antidepressants and mood-stabilizing medications have a significant delay between when the drug is first taken and when full therapeutic benefits appear. It is during this time that supportive reassurance and encouragement from the physician is particularly important in sustaining the patient in treatment.

It bears repeating that there are approximately 32,000 suicides a year in this country, and clinical surveys indicate that approximately 80 percent of these patients have mood disorders. Suicidal ideation is one of the important symptoms that accompany major depressive episodes, in both bipolar and unipolar disorders; considerations of suicidal lethality are central in the management of these patients. Although it is not possible to distinguish precisely between patients who will attempt suicide and those who will not, there are some factors which should be considered. Generally speaking, it is agreed that patients who have developed a specific plan of suicide, who have concomitant alcoholism or drug abuse, and who are socially isolated with few (if any) social supports have a greater potential risk for suicide. The patient's level of hopefulness also tends to correlate with risk. In addition, elderly males and patients with terminal medical illnesses have a greater risk. Unfortunately, each of the above characteristics lacks specificity in the assessment of suicidal risk. Perhaps the most important of all risk factors is the presence of an undiagnosed and untreated mood disorder.

It is recommended that nonpsychiatric physicians rely primarily on the antidepressants or lithium (depending on the disorder treated) in combination with educational and supportive psychotherapeutic approaches in the management of patients with mood disorders. Specific psychotherapies (cognitive/behavioral psychotherapy and interpersonal psychotherapy of depression) can be used successfully in the treatment of mild to moderate major depressive episodes. It is, however, recommended that the nonpsychiatric physician not experiment with these techniques since competency in these forms of psychotherapy requires considerable training and experience to achieve results comparable to those obtained with the relatively simple administration of an appropriate antidepressant medication.

If the physician assesses the suicide risk to be high, the patient requires psychiatric consultation. High-risk patients may require a supervised environment such as a hospital, although in some instances involved family and friends may serve to monitor the patient.

Patients who have complicated psychiatric histories or fail to respond to the initial medication trial should be referred for psychiatric consultation. This may lead to medication combination (augmentations) or other sophisticated treatment such as electroconvulsive therapy (ECT). The latter remains a potent tool for refractory patients or those who cannot tolerate medication side effects.

ANTIDEPRESSANT MEDICATIONS An almost bewildering array of specific and effective antidepressant drugs is currently available, with new medications appearing with great frequency. The first-generation medications include the tricyclic (TCA) and the MAO inhibitor antidepressants. The main benefit of the newer antidepressants is that they have provided the physician with an expanded range of pharmacologic options for the treatment of patients who cannot tolerate or who do not respond to the older drugs. The MAO inhibitors are clinically effective, but the problems of drug-drug and drug-food interactions have made these a second-choice medication in the treatment of depressive disorders. However, the MAO inhibitors appear to be especially effective for depression accompanied by panic attacks or prominent anxiety. The TCAs imipramine and amitriptyline remain the standards for antidepressant efficacy, although newer drugs are equally effective with fewer side effects.

No antidepressant is ideal, and currently available drugs have at least one of the following undesirable characteristics: delayed onset of therapeutic action (7 to 28 days), significant anticholinergic side effects, sedation, agitation, cardiotoxicity, weight gain, the possible induction of manic or hypomanic episodes in patients with bipolar disorders, or other equally problematic adverse reactions. The search for new medications may yet yield a superior antidepressant, one with a consistently high rate of improvement, rapid onset of action, and fewer side effects.

Mechanisms of action TCAs were originally hypothesized to increase synaptic concentrations of central nervous system monoaminergic neurotransmitter substances (e.g., norepinephrine, serotonin, and dopamine) by blocking their reuptake by presynaptic monoaminergic neurons. While this assumption is still valid, the focus now is on the regulation of postsynaptic receptor activity of monoaminergic neurons and the down-regulation of neurotransmitter receptors that have been associated with an antidepressant effect. These mechanisms have been hypothesized to account for the activity of most of the established antidepressants, but not some of the newer antidepressants. At present, therefore, there is a great deal of information available about how antidepressants may ameliorate the pathophysiologic processes associated with depressive disorders, but no precise central mechanism(s) has been identified by which all drugs with antidepressant properties work.

Clinical conditions for use Antidepressants are very effective in treatment of the clinical syndrome of major depression but do not affect normal mood changes. Chronic low-grade depression or dysthymic disorders have generally not responded well to antidepressants alone, although more recent data indicate promising results from the newer selective serotoninergic antidepressants.

There is growing evidence that antidepressants are effective in the treatment of some anxiety disorders. TCAs and the MAO inhibitor antidepressants are the drugs of choice for agoraphobia and panic disorder. Patients with panic disorders have concomitant anxiety about the recurrence of these attacks; this "anticipatory" anxiety may not respond to antidepressants but may benefit from concomitant treatment with antianxiety medication or behavioral approaches such as desensitization. There is a definitive role for the antidepressants in the management of pure anxiety disorders and mixed depressed and anxious states.

Clinical use of antidepressants Table 389-4 lists the more commonly used first-generation antidepressants and the oral doses needed for therapeutic efficacy in the typical patient. Currently imipramine and amitriptyline are the standards for antidepressant potency. Amitriptyline tends to have sedative effects, while imipramine is more energizing. Because of the undesirable side effects observed in these original TCAs, during the past decade growing numbers of experienced clinical psychopharmacologists have gradually selected the secondary tricyclic amines desipramine and nortriptyline as the antidepressant drugs of choice. Both desipramine and nortriptyline have fewer anticholinergic side effects and are less

sedating. Nortriptyline appears to have a clear relationship between plasma levels and clinical efficacy.

Before antidepressants are prescribed, a patient's physical health must be evaluated by a physical examination. The patient should show normal values on baseline complete blood count (CBC), urinalysis, liver function tests, and (if over 45 years) electrocardiogram (ECG). Patients are usually started on low doses (e.g., 25 mg desipramine qhs) and checked for side effects (e.g., postural hypotension). The dose is then raised over a few days to that needed for a full therapeutic response. The minimum daily dose for clinical response is the low figure in the ranges listed in Table 389-4, but often higher doses are needed. However, dose schedules in the elderly should be reduced 30 to 50 percent. Physicians inexperienced in psychopharmacology should not exceed the upper dosage limits listed in the table. Treatment from 7 to 28 days is required to achieve a full therapeutic effect. Changes in the depressive symptoms are often noted by friends and family before the patient reports feeling better. A therapeutic trial of an antidepressant requires at least 28 days at the upper end of the dose range. Patients are usually maintained on antidepressants for approximately 9 to 12 months after the depressive symptoms disappear, to reduce the possibility of relapse resulting from premature withdrawal of medication. Highest relapse rates occur during the first 2 months after medication is discontinued, and patients and clinicians should be especially watchful during this time period.

Medications can be given in a single dose an hour before bedtime once an appropriate dose has been established. This procedure improves medication compliance, and sedative side effects are likely to induce sleep in depressed patients, who are often insomniac. Further, if troublesome side effects occur, they do so while the patient is asleep. For patients who cannot tolerate the single bedtime dose, a daytime twice daily or thrice daily schedule is necessary. Tests for plasma levels of the tricyclic antidepressants are routinely available, but unfortunately the relationship of plasma levels to clinical response has been inconsistent. For imipramine, desipramine, and amitriptyline, the relationship is linear, but nortriptyline may have a curvilinear plasma level-response relationship, implying a therapeutic window. Plasma levels at steady state after 5 days of a given dose may be useful in treatment-resistant patients to evaluate compliance and to see if the dose is sufficient to maintain concentrations above the threshold necessary for response (e.g., imipramine, >180 ng/mL; desipramine, >125 ng/mL; amitriptyline, >95 ng/mL; and nortriptyline, 50 to 150 ng/mL).

After about 10 to 12 months of treatment with an antidepressant, the drug should be withdrawn gradually over a 3- to 4-week period rather than suddenly stopped. Should depressive symptoms reemerge, antidepressant treatment should be restored and maintained for several more months before the withdrawal attempt is repeated.

Side effects and interactions Listed in Table 389-5 are some of the more common side effects from the tricyclic antidepressants. They include dry mouth, sedation, a fine tremor of the hands, and mild constipation. More serious are the effects on the cardiovascular system, of which tachycardia and postural hypotension are the most common. The TCAs, especially imipramine, have a quinidine-like action, can induce cardiac arrhythmias, and have been associated with sudden death in a few patients (see section below on overdose). For patients with preexisting cardiac illness, especially those with heart conduction defects, TCAs should be used cautiously; drugs with milder cardiac effects should be considered. In some instances, however, the quinidine-like effect can be used to advantage, i.e., to produce a significant antiarrhythmic effect with once-daily dosing. Imipramine has been used as a comparison drug for other type 1-A antiarrhythmics. The most bothersome symptoms are from the anticholinergic effects; while rarely serious, they do cause discomfort and compliance problems.

Some preexisting medical conditions increase the risks associated with using TCAs in certain depressed patients. Tricyclics can produce tachycardia, which may push some patients from asymptomatic congestive failure into symptomatic heart failure. TCAs also lower

TABLE 389-4 Commonly used first-generation antidepressants	
Antidepressant	Daily oral therapeutic dose range, mg
TRICYCLIC DERIVATIVES	
Amitriptyline	150–300
Nortriptyline	50–150
Imipramine	150–300
Desipramine	150–250
Doxepin	150–300
Trimipramine	100–250
MONOAMINE OXIDASE INHIBITORS	
Phenelzine	15–60
Tranylcypromine	20–30
Isocarboxazid	10–30

TABLE 389-5   Common side effects of tricyclic antidepressants

Anticholinergic (atropine-like) responses:
  Dry mouth
  Nausea and vomiting*
  Constipation
  Urinary retention
  Blurred vision (mydriasis and cycloplegia)
Cardiovascular effects:
  Postural hypotension*
  Tachycardia
  Cardiac conduction disturbances
Obstructive jaundice—more rare—is reversible when drug is removed
Drowsiness and sleepiness—may want to avoid driving a car until this
  diminishes*
Fine rapid tremor*
Dizziness, ataxia
Hematologic effects:
  Leukopenia
Endocrine effects:
  Syndrome of inappropriate ADH secretion

*Side effects seen most commonly

the seizure threshold and should be used cautiously in patients with seizures. The anticholinergic effects preclude TCA treatment in patients with narrow-angle glaucoma and pose a problem for men with mild to moderate prostatic hypertrophy, who may develop urinary retention. Finally, the use of tricyclic antidepressants in patients with bipolar disorders may shorten the cycle length between affective episodes, may induce an acute manic episode in some patients, and has been related to the phenomenon of rapid cycling.

The tricyclics, especially amitriptyline, imipramine, and doxepin, potentiate the effects of other CNS-depressant medications (e.g., ethanol, benzodiazepines), and patients should be cautioned about ethanol use while on antidepressants. Patients should either not drink or reduce their usual ethanol dose by one-half during tricyclic treatment. Cimetidine elevates tricyclic levels. Other drug interactions include the potentiation of other anticholinergic agents (e.g., antihistamines, antiparkinsonian agents), which can result in severe constipation, urinary retention, and even paralytic ileus. This combination in the elderly, which can produce a serious anticholinergic blockade (e.g., paralytic ileus, fecal impaction), often has been the cause of frank delirium and confusional states in geriatric patients; it is to be avoided in older patients.

Despite the problems, the risk-benefit ratio is overwhelmingly in favor of the antidepressants, and literally hundreds of thousands of patients have been treated with these compounds safely and effectively.

NEWER ANTIDEPRESSANTS   Table 389-6 lists the more promising second-generation drugs for which evidence of antidepressant efficacy exists. Already they have expanded the physicians' therapeutic choices in the treatment of depressive disorders. These agents, particularly fluoxetine, bupropion, sertraline, and paroxetine offer significant advantages: no anticholinergic side effects, no weight gain, and no cardiac conduction effects.

Amoxapine is a tricyclic derivative with clinical efficacy equal to that of the original antidepressants. An early onset of action (within the first week) has been claimed by the manufacturer, although its clinical efficacy at the endpoint of treatment is identical to that of the

TABLE 389-6   Selected second-generation antidepressants

Antidepressant	Daily oral therapeutic dose range, mg
Fluoxetine	10–40
Bupropion	200–300
Paroxetine	20–40
Sertraline	50–200
Clomipramine	150–300
Amoxapine	150–300
Trazodone	100–600
Maprotiline	100–225

original TCAs. One of its metabolites (7-hydroxyamoxapine) is a neuroleptic, which accounts for the extrapyramidal side effects seen, including tardive dyskinesia and parkinsonism. The neuroleptic component, however, has made amoxapine a drug to be considered in depressed patients who show psychotic features. Other side effects appear to be similar to those of the original tricyclics, although a disproportionate number of seizures was found in some retrospective studies.

Clomipramine, a tricyclic that inhibits serotonin reuptake, commonly used worldwide, is now approved for use in the United States. It has been shown in controlled studies to be an effective drug in the treatment of depression and currently is the drug of choice in obsessive-compulsive disorder, which is frequently disabling and resistant to treatment.

Fluoxetine is a relatively selective serotonin-uptake inhibitor with antidepressant efficacy comparable to imipramine. Side effects similar to those observed with other serotonin-uptake blockers include nausea, diarrhea, tremor, headache, agitation, and weight loss, and range from mild to moderate severity. Administration may also be associated with akathisia, which may be related to controversial reports of suicidal ideas. Akathisia can be treated with a decreased dosage of benzodiazepines or with propranalol. The recommended dose of 20 mg/d is adequate for most patients, but both lower and higher doses may be needed (e.g., 10–40 mg/d). Fluoxetine is now available in elixir form for doses less than 20 mg/d. Patients show few signs of cardiac conduction effects. There are also reports of successful treatment of obsessive-compulsive disorder with fluoxetine in controlled studies. Fluoxetine is one of the first of a series of highly specific and potent serotonin-uptake inhibitors to be marketed in the United States. Sertraline is available in the United States. It is a potent serotonin receptor blocker that may cause less agitation than fluoxetine. It has a much shorter half-life (24 h) and no active metabolite as compared to fluoxetine (7 to 14 days). Paroxetine was approved for use in the United States in 1993. Others are still in clinical trial (e.g., fluroxamine, indalpine).

Maprotiline is a tetracyclic derivative that is equal in antidepressant potency to the original tricyclics and reportedly has fewer anticholinergic side effects. Originally it was offered as a promising drug for use in patients with cardiovascular problems, but this has not been established and it is not recommended for this purpose. It has been reported to cause seizures at two to four times the rate at which the TCAs induce seizures, and a lower dosage schedule is now recommended. Moreover, its use has been asssociated with more than the expected incidence of blood dyscrasia.

Trazodone is a triazolopyridine derivative originally introduced for use as an antidepressant. There remains controversy around whether it has significant antidepressant properties. The drug produces a high level of sedation and is useful as a hypnotic. It has few, if any, cardiotoxic effects but is associated with increased risk of priapism.

Bupropion was withdrawn from the market because it produced a high rate of seizures in a subpopulation of bulimic patients. It was subsequently re-released when the seizure rate was found to be no greater than that produced by the TCAs (estimated at about 0.4 percent) and is currently used for treating major depression. A role for bupropion in combination with lithium in stabilizing patients with rapid-cycling disorders has also been proposed. The mechanism of action may be related to dopamine-reuptake inhibition, although this is not fully established. Bupropion has energizing properties and consequently is less sedating, with mild side effects including headache, agitation, and some anticholinergic effects. It must be given in divided daytime dose to avoid increased seizure frequency.

TRICYCLIC OVERDOSAGE   Antidepressants are the fourth most common cause of drug overdose seen in emergency departments in the United States and the third most frequent cause of drug-related death (after alcohol-drug combinations and heroin). Of the antidepressants, tricyclics are the most frequent cause of death. In a California study (Callaham and Kassel) the annual frequency of fatal tricyclic overdose was 1.3 per 100,000 population; more than two-thirds of the victims were women. Amitriptyline, desipramine, and nortriptyline were the most frequently implicated.

The first 6 h after an overdose of a tricyclic antidepressant are crucial. CNS depression and seizures, respiratory arrest, and cardiovascular arrhythmias are the principal causes of death. ECG changes showing QRS prolongation are early signs of toxicity, and ventricular fibrillation is a common complication. ECG changes are a more sensitive measure for monitoring patients than are blood levels of the drug.

LITHIUM AND OTHER MOOD-NORMALIZING MEDICATIONS

The most important psychotropic medication in this group is lithium. Although lithium possesses some antidepressant properties, it is not, strictly speaking, an antidepressant. Its effectiveness in treating patients with bipolar disorders and other disorders of mood has revolutionized the practice of psychiatry. Lithium's approval by the U.S. Food and Drug Administration in 1970 for the treatment of acute mania and in 1975 for the maintenance treatment of manic-depressive disorder generated an explosion of basic and clinical research focused on its pharmacologic mechanisms and clinical use.

Mechanism of action The central mechanisms by which lithium exerts its clinical effects on extremes of mood are not fully understood. Lithium affects the brain's monoaminergic neurotransmitter concentrations at the synapse, has strong effects on biologic membranes, and intracellularly inhibits the conversion of inositol monophosphate to free inositol. This latter effect may, in turn, reduce neuronal excitability.

Clinical conditions for use Lithium is the drug of choice for treating acute manic/hypomanic episodes and for prevention of recurrent episodes of mania and depression in bipolar illness. Recent studies suggest that the relapse rate among lithium-treated bipolar patients is about one-half that of control patients receiving a placebo. It may also be an effective agent in the prophylaxis of recurrent unipolar depressive disorders. Lithium also has antidepressant properties, especially in depressions seen in bipolar disorders; however, it is not a drug of choice for major depression per se. Lithium also is used to augment TCA and other antidepressants; i.e., to enhance response in nonresponders. It has also been successfully used in conjunction with neuroleptics in schizoaffective disorders; there may be a subpopulation of schizophrenics responsive to lithium, although most workers feel that such lithium responders are atypical bipolar patients and not schizophrenics. Finally, there are some reports that lithium may be useful in treating alcoholism, a possibility requiring further study.

Clinical use of lithium Lithium is a very safe drug with an excellent risk-benefit ratio when it is used knowledgeably. The only genuine contraindication to lithium's use is seriously compromised renal function. The following baseline studies should be obtained before prescribing lithium: CBC, routine urinalysis with a concentration test, thyroxine (T_4), free T_4 index, thyroid-stimulating hormone (TSH), serum creatinine, electrolytes, and (for those over 40) an ECG.

Serum lithium levels peak 1 to 3 h after an oral dose, and the biologic half-life, which averages 24 h, varies with age. Elderly patients frequently have a drug half-life over 30 h, often requiring lower doses. Lithium is monitored by serum levels, which are most informative approximately 10 h after the last dose. Therapeutic efficacy in acute mania is achieved at levels between 0.8 and 1.4 mmol/L. Patients rarely require treatment at serum levels above 1.5 mmol/L. Lithium is always administered orally. Dose ranges are from 600 mg to 3000 mg daily, unless the patient is elderly. A general rule of thumb equates a 0.2 mmol/L rise in serum level with each additional 300-mg tablet of lithium. Unless sustained-release tablets are used, lithium is usually administered twice or three times daily, allowing for smooth, sustained 24-h serum levels. Because there is a 7- to 10-day delay in achieving full therapeutic effects, the addition of antipsychotic medications or clonazepam is often needed during the early phase of treating a manic patient. During acute manic

TABLE 389-7 Common lithium side effects

Severity	Side effect
SIDE EFFECTS COMMONLY SEEN	
Very mild	Thirst
	Nausea (particularly during first few days of treatment)
	Fine tremor of hand
Mild to moderate	Anorexia
	Vomiting
	Diarrhea
	"Upset stomach" or "abdominal pain"
	Polydipsia and/or polyuria
	Muscular weakness and fatigue
SIDE EFFECTS INDICATING TOXICITY	
	Muscle hyperirritability with twitching, muscle fasciculation, or chronic movements
	Sedation, sluggishness, languidness, drowsiness, giddiness
	Coarse tremor
	Ataxia
Moderate to severe	Hypertonic muscles
	Hyperactive deep tendon reflexes
	Hyperextension of arms and legs with grunts and gasping
	Chorea, athetotic movements
	Impairment of consciousness
	Somnolence, confusion, stupor
	Seizures
Very severe	Coma
	Complications of coma
	Death

episodes patients often tolerate relatively higher doses of lithium, but once the manic episode remits, it is necessary to reduce the dose.

The current maintenance treatment strategy is to prevent future recurrent episodes of mania and depression in patients with bipolar disorders. Clinicians are advised to seek the lowest possible serum levels in the range from 0.6 to 1.0 mmol/L that will prevent relapse. Lithium's excretion rate is very stable within each patient; as a result patients can be maintained on the same dose day in and day out, with relative certainty that stable levels are present. During maintenance patients are seen every 3 to 6 months, and serum lithium, sodium, potassium, T_4, free T_4 index, TSH, and creatinine are monitored along with urinalysis with a concentration test. The lithium excretion pattern is altered by conditions that change sodium concentrations, and patients on thiazide diuretics or low-salt diets should be warned and monitored more frequently.

Side effects and interactions Lithium's side effects are listed in a continuum ranging from those seen relatively commonly to those indicating lithium toxicity (see Table 389-7). Many of these are minor side effects, which appear early and disappear as time passes, but some may persist throughout treatment. Because the rapid escalation of serum levels often induces side effects, especially those involving the gastrointestinal tract, smoother, more gradual serum lithium increases are desirable.

Some of the first signs of lithium toxicity are coarsening of tremor, increases in the deep tendon reflexes, and muscle fasciculations. Unusual degrees of sedation and cognitive disruption also may herald lithium toxicity. Lithium toxicity mimics barbiturate intoxication, and when death occurs it is secondary to respiratory depression and its complications. The treatment of lithium toxicity involves good supportive care and excellent hydration. Administration of normal saline is helpful in increasing lithium excretion. Since lithium's half-life is 24 h, this treatment sustains the patient until the kidneys eliminate the medication. Various methods to improve the treatment of lithium toxicity, such as increasing lithium excretion by aminophylline or alkalinizing the urine, have all been disappointing. For life-threatening cases, the last resort is renal dialysis, but toxicity does not commonly progress to the point where this intervention is needed.

There is some evidence that lithium is a teratogen, particularly when administered during the first trimester of pregnancy. Cardiovascular and valve abnormalities have been detected in 18-week-old fetuses. While there is little evidence for teratogenesis during the second and third trimesters other mood-stabilizing medications can be considered in pregnant women and weighed against the risk of untreated bipolar disorder.

Lithium's interactions with other drugs primarily involve its reciprocal relationship with the sodium ion. Diuretics, which increase sodium excretion, can increase lithium toxicity. There have also been reports that combined neuroleptic and lithium therapy has resulted in an irreversible neurotoxicity in a small number of middle-aged and older patients. Clinical observations indicate that this combination is safe and effective provided that both drugs are used in low to moderate doses, carefully monitored, and discontinued as soon as the lithium effect is sufficiently present for the patient to be managed without the neuroleptic.

Medical sequelae of lithium's use Several medical complications can develop during lithium treatment. Because of its effect on adenylate cyclase activity, lithium inhibits the thyroid gland's secretory function; nontoxic goiters and hypothyroidism can develop, which can be readily corrected during lithium therapy by thyroid supplement. Lithium may induce the following ECG changes especially in older patients: T-wave depression, sinus node dysfunctions, and, very rarely, sinoatrial block and ventricular irritability.

The most important sequelae are the renal complications. About 25 percent of patients develop some degree of vasopressin-resistant nephrogenic diabetes insipidus with polyuria and polydipsia. The lithium inhibition of adenylate cyclase activity is responsible for the disruption of renal tubular transport. These symptoms are usually completely reversible by lithium withdrawal and often can be ameliorated by a reduction in dosage. The most economic and accurate method of monitoring changes in renal function during lithium treatment is by the urine concentration test and serum creatinine level. Consistent urine concentration levels below a specific gravity of 1.025 indicate an early renal effect, and a creatinine clearance test should be obtained. If creatinine clearance is abnormal, the patient's clinical condition should be reevaluated and termination of the lithium treatment considered. There have been reports of renal focal necrosis and interstitial fibrosis in a few long-term lithium patients, and there is evidence, by biopsy, for an increased basal rate of renal pathology among patients with affective disorders. Nonetheless, this nonspecific renal lesion does appear more frequently in patients receiving long-term lithium.

Evidence has emerged linking the more serious renal complications to increased episodes of lithium toxicity and possibly to prolonged combined use of lithium and neuroleptics. While good clinical practice should obviate lithium toxicity, it may be equally important to avoid extremes of high and low serum lithium levels during the day. Despite these concerns, lithium remains one of the most important and effective psychotropic agents and its risk-benefit ratio is excellent.

Carbamazepine and valproic acid The anticonvulsant carbamazepine has, in controlled trials, been used successfully in the treatment of manic and, to a lesser extent, depressive episodes in bipolar patients. There is also growing evidence that some bipolar patients (15 to 60 percent) who do not respond to lithium benefit from carbamazepine treatment, and that the combination of lithium and carbamazepine may be therapeutically additive. The drug regimen for bipolar disorders is initiated with 200 mg bid administered orally, increasing to 600 to 1600 mg daily in divided doses and, although not well-correlated with therapeutic response, blood levels may range from 8 to 12 mg/dL.

Carbamazepine is not a completely benign drug; side effects include nausea, blurred vision, and ataxia, and more importantly there have been cases of fatal leukopenia and aplastic anemia reported (incidence ≤ 1 in 20,000). Patients treated with carbamazepine must be monitored for renal, liver, and bone marrow functions while they are on the medication. There are also reports of reversible CNS

toxicity when this drug is combined with lithium. Therefore patients on this combination should be monitored carefully. Valproic acid, the drug of choice in certain seizure disorders, has also been reported to prevent recurrence of manic episodes in a number of bipolar patients. The development of this new class of psychotropic compounds is very promising and may herald the future development of a new and useful group of medications.

ANXIETY DISORDERS IN A MEDICAL SETTING

Karen Thatcher Britton

Anxiety symptoms are common in medically ill patients. Five to 20 percent of medical inpatients and 4 to 14 percent of general medical outpatients suffer from anxiety states. Patients with anxiety disorders are more likely to seek help for their emotional problems from general medical physicians than patients with other psychiatric disorders, and are more likely to use emergency room services. In a recent study, 29 percent of patients with panic disorder used an emergency service for treatment of emotional problems in the preceding year. Furthermore, antianxiety medications have consistently been among the most frequently prescribed medications in the United States over the past 15 years, and more than 80 percent of these prescriptions are written by primary care physicians. Anxiety may occur as a manifestation of a primary psychiatric disorder or secondarily to either the medical illness or the medications prescribed for treatment. It is important for the clinician to be familiar with the diagnosis of anxiety and the role it plays in the patient's illness.

Anxiety appears in several clinically recognizable forms. Distinctions are made between patients who complain of constant, unremitting nervousness, tension, and worry and patients who are relatively symptom free until an acute anxiety or panic attack arises. Further distinctions are made among patients with anxiety due to posttraumatic stress disorder, obsessive-compulsive disorder and the phobic disorders.

PANIC DISORDER **Definition and clinical manifestations** The cardinal feature of panic disorder is the sudden, unexpected, and often overwhelming feeling of terror and apprehension accompanied by somatic symptoms in multiple organ systems such as dyspnea, palpitations, and faintness. The symptoms and signs of panic disorder are similar to those occurring during intense physical exertion or in a life-threatening situation.

A typical panic attack often begins abruptly and without warning when a patient is involved in a relatively nonthreatening and nonstressful activity, like entering a store, driving a car, or sitting at a desk working. The patient becomes lightheaded and sweaty and is overwhelmed by feelings of terror, apprehension, and impending doom. Dyspnea may occur with a subjective sense of choking or smothering, and palpitations or chest pain are often so severe that patients believe they are having a heart attack or are dying. The symptoms of panic attacks usually peak in less than 10 min and resolve in 20 to 30 min. Most frequently the first attack occurs away from home, often in a setting in which the person feels trapped or concerned about attracting attention. The usual response is to obtain help, sometimes going to a doctor's office or emergency room, but the fear has usually subsided by this time. Fatigue or exhaustion frequently follows a panic attack, and the patient may sleep. The DSM-III-R criteria for diagnosis of panic disorder are listed in Table 389-8.

Panic disorder is estimated to occur in 1 to 2 percent of the population and is a relapsing, remitting illness. The most frequent age of onset is the late teen years and early twenties. Panic disorders tend to be familial, and both panic disorders and affective disorders often coexist in the same family. If an individual has a diagnosed panic disorder, up to 18 percent of first-degree relatives also will have panic disorder. Furthermore, twin studies demonstrate a greater incidence in monozygotic twins, suggesting that panic anxiety may have a genetic basis.

Complications After repeated panic attacks, some patients develop anticipatory anxiety and try to avoid those situations that have

TABLE 389-8   Diagnosis of panic disorder

A At some time during the disturbance, one or more panic attacks (discrete periods of intense fear or discomfort) have occurred that were (1) unexpected and (2) not triggered by situations in which the person was the focus of others' attention.

B Either four attacks have occurred within a 4-week period or one or more attacks have been followed by a period of at least a month of persistent fear of having another attack.

C At least four of the following symptoms developed during at least one of the attacks.
  1 Shortness of breath (dyspnea) or smothering sensations
  2 Dizziness, unsteady feelings, or faintness
  3 Palpitations or accelerated heart rate
  4 Trembling or shaking
  5 Sweating
  6 Choking
  7 Nausea or abdominal distress
  8 Depersonalization or derealization
  9 Numbness or tingling sensations (paresthesias)
  10 Flushes or chills
  11 Chest pain or discomfort
  12 Fear of dying
  13 Fear of going crazy or of doing something uncontrolled

D During at least some of the attacks, at least four of the symptoms in C developed suddenly and increased in intensity within 10 min of the beginning of the first C symptom noticed in the attack.

E It cannot be established that an organic factor initiated and maintained the disturbance, e.g., amphetamine or caffeine intoxication or hyperthyroidism.

SOURCE: Adapted from DSM-III-R.

---

been paired with panic attacks in the past. Many patients, particularly females by a two to one ratio to men, develop *agoraphobia*—an irrational fear of being alone or in public places (see Table 389-9). Without effective treatment, the course of panic attacks and agoraphobia may lead to an increasingly restricted life-style marked by preoccupation with avoiding those situations that might trigger an attack. Patients often dramatically increase their use of health services when this complication develops, seeking help from multiple physicians with one or more frightening somatic complaints. Accurate diagnosis and treatment are important because cases of severe panic disorder with agoraphobia have been reported in which patients remain house-bound for one or more decades, convinced that leaving the house will induce an attack. Primary care physicians should ask whether the patient has begun to avoid any situations, especially social situations, since the attacks began, e.g., fear of crowds, public transportation, closed-in spaces like elevators, movie theaters, driving alone, etc. It is important to inquire whether the patient has become fearful of entering these situations *alone,* since many agoraphobic patients will enter fearful situations if accompanied by a spouse or friend.

Other complications of panic disorder are major depression and substance abuse. Approximately 60 to 90 percent of patients with panic disorder develop a major depression at some time in their lives, and 20 percent make a suicide attempt. Patients with panic disorder

TABLE 389-9   Panic disorder with agoraphobia

A Meets criteria for panic disorder

B Agoraphobia: Fear of being in places or situations from which escape might be difficult (or embarrassing) or in which help might not be available in the event of a panic attack. As a result of this fear, the person either restricts travel or endures agoraphobic situations despite intense anxiety. Common agoraphobic situations include being outside the home alone, being in a crowd or standing in line, being on a bridge, and traveling in a bus, train, or car.

Measuring severity of agoraphobic avoidance:
  Mild: Some avoidance (or endurance with distress), but relatively normal life-style.
  Moderate: Avoidance results in constricted life-style, e.g., the person is able to leave the house alone, but not to go more than a few miles unaccompanied.
  Severe: Avoidance results in being nearly or completely housebound or unable to leave the house unaccompanied.

SOURCE: Adapted from DSM-III-R.

---

may also attempt self-medication with alcohol and/or benzodiazepines. These agents have a short anxiolytic action, but the rapid drop in blood levels may then cause an exacerbation of anxiety. In addition, many of the symptoms of alcohol and drug withdrawal are similar to those of panic and therefore may present difficulty in differential diagnosis. Nearly 30 percent of patients with panic disorder experience, at some time in their lives, alcohol problems meeting DSM criteria for alcohol abuse. If alcohol or substance abuse is present, that disorder should be treated first and the patient reassessed after detoxification and treatment.

Differential diagnosis   Once the presence of anxiety is established, the clinician must attempt to rule out an organic anxiety disorder. Medical disorders and medications known to be associated with anxiety are listed in Table 389-10. Thyroid dysfunction and cardiac disorders are the most common differential diagnoses to rule out. The patient's medical history and physical examination guide the clinician in this workup. For example, mitral valve prolapse should be investigated because there may be an increased prevalence of this condition in patients with panic disorder. Some studies have suggested an association between panic disorder and increased cardiovascular morbidity and mortality. Both pulmonary and gastrointestinal disorders also tend to evoke anxiety in many patients, and stress is often linked to exacerbations in these conditions. The physician must also review all pharmacologic agents that the patient is taking that could cause anxiety. For example, a patient with a toxic aminophylline level may have symptoms that mimic anxiety attacks.

Etiology, pathophysiology, and treatment   The etiology of panic disorders is uncertain and involves an interplay of multiple psychological and biologic determinants.

Clinical and experimental evidence point to the involvement of noradrenergic neurons, particularly those projecting rostrally from the locus coeruleus in the upper brainstem in the pathophysiology of panic disorder. Three lines of evidence suggest that hyperactivity of noradrenergic pathways may play a role in the pathogenesis of panic. First, the clinical manifestations of panic attacks are similar to those induced by sudden, massive stimulations of beta-adrenergic receptors. Second, isoproterenol hydrochloride, a beta agonist, and yohimbine,

TABLE 389-10   Medical conditions and drugs associated with anxiety

MEDICAL CONDITIONS

Anemia	Hypothyroidism
Angina pectoralis	Insulinoma
Asthma	Menopausal symptoms
Carcinoid	Mitral valve prolapse
Cardiac arrhythmias	Mass lesion
Cardiomyopathies	Pheochromocytosis
Cushing's syndrome	Porphyria
Chronic obstructive pulmonary disease (COPD)	Pneumothorax
	Pulmonary edema
Electrolyte abnormalities	Pulmonary embolus
Hyperparathyroidism	Temporal lobe epilepsy
Hyperthyroidism	Vertigo
Hypoglycemia	

DRUGS

Alcohol	Glucocorticoids
Amphetamine	Hallucinogens
Aminophylline	Lidocaine
Anticholinergics	Methylphenidate
Antihistamines	Metrizamide
Antihypertensives	Monosodium glutamate
Antituberculous agents	Pentazocine
Bromocriptine	Phenylephrine
Caffeine	Pseudoephedrine
Cocaine	Salicylates
Digitalis (toxicity)	Sedative hypnotics (withdrawal)
Dopamine	Theophylline
Ephedrine	Thyroid agents
Epinephrine	

SOURCE: Adapted from DSM-III-R.

an alpha-adrenergic receptor antagonist that increases noradrenergic function, produce signs and symptoms that mimic panic attacks. Third, clinical studies support a role for noradrenergic beta blockers, such as propranolol, in successful treatment of pathologic anxiety.

Another avenue of investigation is based on the finding that infusions of sodium lactate into patients with a history of panic disorder often provoke a panic attack indistinguishable from a spontaneous one. Normal subjects without a history of panic disorder are unaffected. In addition, patients whose panic attacks are controlled by antidepressants are protected against lactate-induced panic attacks. Inhalation of CO_2 by susceptible persons also precipitates anxiety and panic. Although the mechanism of lactate's effect is unclear, the findings appear to have diagnostic usefulness and provide a good model of anxiety for further clinical investigation.

Overall, the evidence suggests that the main contribution to panic may be a genetic vulnerability to a biologic disease state. Over time, panic attacks may become associated with environmental events that by themselves are able to elicit symptoms. The particular constellation of environmental stimuli that precipitates panic attacks may be influenced by past experience or particular psychological conflicts. A full understanding of the etiology of anxiety probably will require knowledge of a combination of genetic, biologic, and psychological factors.

A comprehensive treatment program combines both pharmacologic and psychotherapeutic approaches. The first step is to block the attacks pharmacologically. Three classes of medication are effective for the treatment of panic disorder: TCAs, MAO inhibitors, and high-potency benzodiazepines (alprazolam or clonazepam). The usual first drug used is a tricyclic in low doses of 10 to 25 mg with increase in small (10- to 25-mg) increments to avoid precipitating panic. In some instances alprazolam or preferably clonazepam (which has a longer half-life) is used to cover panic episodes while a tricyclic is being increased over 1 to 2 weeks. These drugs are 80 to 90 percent effective in the treatment and prevention of spontaneous panic attacks. Beta blockers may block the peripheral manifestations of the panic attacks but have proved ineffective in preventing the psychic fear or panic. They also may predispose to or worsen depressive symptoms. Clonidine has been shown to block panic manifestations, but its efficacy is usually only transient. More recently, beneficial results have been reported for the serotonin uptake inhibitor fluoxetine.

For some patients with panic disorder, particularly those with debilitating agoraphobia, psychotherapy is indicated. The exact form of psychotherapy is controversial, but approaches that seek to understand the anxiety and encourage the patient to confront the feared situations are the most effective.

GENERALIZED ANXIETY DISORDER Unlike patients with panic disorder whose symptoms come on suddenly, patients with generalized anxiety disorder experience persistent diffuse anxiety without the specific symptoms that characterize phobic disorders, panic disorders, or obsessive-compulsive disorders. Although the symptoms and signs of anxiety vary from individual to individual, common signs are motor tension, autonomic hyperactivity, apprehensive expectation, and vigilance. Patients with generalized anxiety disorder do not report acute fluctuations in anxiety level and autonomic arousal characteristic of panic disorder.

The prevalence of generalized anxiety disorder has been estimated at 2 to 3 percent, but precise epidemiologic data are lacking because of variations in definition and case acquisition. In patients who seek professional help for anxiety, women outnumber men by two to one. There is no evidence to support the popular belief that anxiety is related to the stresses of modern society. In contrast to panic disorder, studies showing a familial or genetic basis for generalized anxiety disorder are inconclusive. Although generalized anxiety disorder tends to have a more favorable outcome than panic disorder, the symptoms are persistent and can lead to secondary depression and alcohol and drug abuse.

Etiology, pathophysiology, and treatment One approach to understanding the etiology of anxiety has been to delineate the mechanisms by which antianxiety drugs exert their effects. High-affinity, stereospecific receptors for benzodiazepines have been discovered which appear to be coupled to the receptor for the inhibitory neurotransmitter gamma-aminobutyric acid (GABA). Considerable evidence supports the hypothesis that the anxiolytic actions of the benzodiazepines are mediated through this receptor.

These findings have several implications. First, the characterization of a benzodiazepine receptor complex implies the existence of a natural (endogenous) ligand for the receptor. Conceivably, the levels of this substance might correlate with individual differences in anxiety or emotionality or tolerance to stress. Second, pharmacologic antagonists of this receptor block the effectiveness of benzodiazepines and may induce anxiety, a finding which implicates these mechanisms in pathologic anxiety. Third, new anxiolytic compounds that influence benzodiazepine receptor binding are being discovered that have fewer and potentially less serious side effects. The possibility exists that anxiogenic substances may also be found in the brain. Though major questions remain to be answered, these advances have opened new avenues for understanding the origins and management of anxiety.

Because feelings of anxiety are normal human emotions with adaptive value, a decision must be made before any treatment or medication is considered concerning whether or not the manifestations of anxiety are within the normal range. There is no justification for the use of anxiolytic drugs if anxiety is appropriate to the fear or threat. On the other hand if certain situations produce fear in which the feelings are disproportional to the threat, then treatment should be considered.

Once a decision is made to treat, consideration should be given first to modalities of nonpharmacologic intervention, including supportive or intensive psychotherapy. These approaches may modify maladaptive life-styles, cognition, and avoidance behaviors. Behavior therapy aims at teaching the patient practical techniques like relaxation training, biofeedback, and desensitization. These techniques are of at least temporary benefit for many people.

When generalized anxiety is severe enough to warrant treatment with drugs, benzodiazepines are the agents of choice. In many patients, short courses of anxiolytic drugs (5 to 7 days) are effective, following which the drug should be discontinued. Patients should be warned about the possibility of dependence with long-term use, and the physician should make regular assessments of the need for continuation of medications. Buspirone, a nonbenzodiazepine anxiolytic, may become a drug of first choice for these patients. Although it has a delayed onset of action of about one week, it lacks many of the problems associated with the benzodiazepines such as psychomotor impairment, physicial dependence, or withdrawal symptoms. (See also "Newer Anxiolytic Medications," below.)

POSTTRAUMATIC STRESS DISORDER The diagnostic criteria for posttraumatic stress disorders (PTSD) are listed in Table 389-11. PTSD is classified as either acute or chronic (or delayed). In the former, onset of symptoms begin within 6 months of the trauma, or the duration of the symptoms persist less than 6 months. In the latter, symptoms persist more than 6 months (chronic) or start more than 6 months after the trauma (delayed). Patients with PTSD have experienced a severe catastrophic event that is outside the range of normal human experience and would be distressing to anyone. The patient persistently reexperiences the event by having recurrent dreams or nightmares, or suddenly feels as if the event were recurring. In primary care, patients with PTSD are occasionally seen following trauma precipitated by automobile or industrial accidents or natural disasters such as flood, hurricane, or fire.

Etiology and treatment Whether or not PTSD develops appears to depend upon the nature of the trauma, the characteristics of the individual, and the context in which these events take place. The trauma can be anticipated or not, acute or chronic, constant or repetitive, or due to natural events or malevolence. PTSD can develop in individuals who were apparently healthy, successful, and well-adjusted prior to the traumatic experience. Among the factors which influence the development of PTSD are: (1) the extent to which the

TABLE 389-11 Diagnosis of posttraumatic stress disorder

A The person has experienced an event that is outside the range of usual human experience and that would be markedly distressing to almost anyone.
B The traumatic event is persistently reexperienced in at least one of the following ways.
  1 Recurrent and intrusive distressing recollections of the event
  2 Recurrent distressing dreams of the event
  3 Sudden acting or feeling as if the traumatic event were recurring
  4 Intense psychological distress at exposure to events that symbolize or resemble an aspect of the traumatic event
C Persistent avoidance of stimuli associated with the trauma or numbing of general responsiveness, as indicated by at least three of the following:
  1 Efforts to avoid thoughts or feelings associated with the trauma
  2 Efforts to avoid activities or situations that arouse recollections of the trauma
  3 Inability to recall an important aspect of the trauma
  4 Markedly diminished interest in significant activities
  5 Feeling of detachment or estrangement from others
  6 Restricted range of affect, e.g., unable to have loving feelings
  7 Sense of a foreshortened future, e.g., does not expect to have a career, marriage, children or a long life
D Persistent symptoms of increased arousal, as indicated by at least two of the following:
  1 Difficulty falling or staying asleep
  2 Irritability or outbursts of anger
  3 Difficulty concentrating
  4 Hypervigilance
  5 Exaggerated startle response
  6 Physiologic reactivity upon exposure to events that symbolize or resemble an aspect of the traumatic event
E Duration of the disturbance of at least 1 month (specify delayed onset if the onset of symptoms is at least 6 months after the trauma).

SOURCE: Adapted from DSM-III-R.

individual's life-space is affected; (2) the duration of the impact; (3) the extent to which the individual perceived human malevolence behind the traumatic event (e.g., a fire attributed to arson will probably be more traumatic than one attributed to lightning); and (4) social isolation. It is difficult to gauge the prevalence of PTSD following a traumatic event because studies that have been done often have followed subjects for only a short period of time, and the nature of the events is often very situation-specific. Following a major natural disaster, about 15 percent or more of the civilian population may experience mental distress severe enough to require treatment.

The treatment goals of PTSD are reduction of target symptoms, prevention of chronic disability, and occupational and social rehabilitation. Recent reports suggest both the TCAs and MAO inhibitors may be effective.

OBSESSIVE-COMPULSIVE DISORDER Idiosyncratic rituals and odd personal habits are commonplace. Only when they cause marked anxiety and personal distress, occupy more than an hour a day, and cause significant social or vocational dysfunction do they indicate obsessive-compulsive disorder. The major characteristics of this disorder are recurrent *obsessions,* i.e., persistent, intrusive thoughts, impulses, or urges that are troublesome to the person. Typical examples are thoughts of violence or fears of germs or contamination. Obsessions produce a great amount of anxiety. *Compulsions* are repetitive behaviors performed in response to an obsession, according to specific rules or in a stereotyped fashion. They are designed to neutralize the occurrence of the dreaded or feared event. Typical examples are repetitive handwashing, checking an item repeatedly, or always counting a particular number. As with obsessions, compulsions are recognized by the individual with obsessive-compulsive disorder as being senseless. A consequence of this is that reassurance by a friend, physician, or therapist does not help reduce the behavior's occurrence.

Obsessive-compulsive disorders usually begin in adolescence or young adulthood with about 65 percent of cases beginning before age 25. They are seen less often in children. Clear precipitants are reported in up to 60 percent of cases. Long-term prognosis appears to be variable. Some patients, perhaps 10 percent, show a chronic, unremitting course, but the majority of patients show an episodic course with periods of incomplete remissions.

Etiology and treatment The majority of individuals with obsessive-compulsive disorder are not recognized by primary care physicians because of the generally private nature of their rituals and because they are aware of the irrationality of their compulsions and are ashamed to admit their symptoms. The cause of obsessive-compulsive disorder is unknown, but there are associated changes in brain function. Positron-emission tomography studies have shown abnormalities in the prefrontal cortex that are reversed by chlorimipramine.

Clomipramine appears to be the most effective pharmacologic treatment for obsessive-compulsive disorder. The beneficial effects of clomipramine may be delayed 6 to 8 weeks, and it is most effective when specific compulsions are present. Recent reports suggest that fluoxetine, which has a similar effect on the serotoninergic neurotransmitter system, is also successful in the treatment of some patients with obsessive-compulsive disorder.

Obsessive-compulsive patients also may respond to psychotherapeutic intervention. However, in the absence of adequate studies of psychotherapy in obsessive-compulsive disorder, it is hard to make a valid generalization about its effectiveness. Behavioral therapy can be helpful in this disorder. Desensitization, flooding, implosion therapy, and aversive conditioning have all been used with variable success.

PHOBIC DISORDERS Phobic disorders comprise a group of disorders having in common persistently recurring, irrational severe anxiety of specific objects, activities or situations with secondary avoidance of the phobic stimulus. Phobias are relatively commonplace, and the diagnosis of a phobic disorder is made only when fear or avoidance behavior is a significant source of distress to the individual or when it interferes with social or occupational functioning. Treatment, if required, is behavioral using relaxation therapy or systematic desensitization.

Agoraphobia, the fear of being alone or in public places, may occur rarely in the absence of panic disorder (see "Panic Disorders," above).

Social phobias are persistent irrational fears and the need to avoid any situation where one might be exposed to scrutiny by others and potentially embarrassed or humiliated. Even the possibility of such a situation evokes anticipatory anxiety. The individual is aware that this fear is excessive. Common examples are excessive fear of public speaking, being unable to urinate in a public restroom, and anxiety induced by eating in restaurants or by any public performance. The resulting anxiety may actually impair performance and thereby potentiate the phobic disorder.

Simple phobias are persistent irrational fears and avoidance of specific objects or situations. Common examples include fear of heights (acrophobia), fear of closed spaces (claustrophobia), and fear of animals. Systematic desensitization and in vivo exposure are the most effective treatments for the simple phobias, and no real benefit has been shown from medication.

ANXIETY DISORDERS AND THEIR RELEVANCE TO INTERNAL MEDICINE Unrecognized anxiety disorders are common in both outpatient and inpatient clinical practices. Panic disorder is a relatively new concept in medicine, and many physicians are unfamiliar with its diagnosis and natural history. Physicians in emergency room settings and cardiology clinics should be especially alert to the hidden patient with undiagnosed panic disorder.

A notable feature of many patients is an intense fear of having a heart attack during a panic episode. Because panic attacks often present with such alarming physical symptoms, it is usually the primary care physician who first sees these patients. The problem of chest pain in panic disorder warrants special mention. There is recent evidence that the presentation of chest pain in patients with panic attacks is leading to expensive cardiac workups. Several recent studies have found that 30 to 50 percent of chest pain patients with angiographically normal coronary arteries have panic disorder. In those with diseased coronary arteries, there is no higher than expected rate of panic disorder.

Although patients with panic disorder are frequently hypochondriacal about having heart disease and need reassurance, there is some evidence of increased cardiovascular morbidity and mortality associated with the disease. Higher rates of hypertension, hyperlipidemia, smoking, physical inactivity, and alcohol abuse have been reported in such patients. At this time there are no good guidelines to assist physicians in routine cardiovascular screening of panic disorder patients.

Anxiety also can play an important role in the clinical picture of a patient with documented medical illness and contribute to the distress experienced by the patient as well as influence the outcome of the disorder. Recognition of the presence of anxiety and its part in the symptoms will greatly improve the doctor's ability to provide comprehensive care for the patient. Anxiety can both increase vulnerability to exacerbations of some diseases and adversely affect the course of the disease process by increasing symptoms and impeding recovery. In spite of this, failure to recognize and treat anxiety disorders in the medically ill is common.

Anxiety and panic are frequently associated with pulmonary conditions such as COPD and asthma in an interactive way, thus worsening the attack. Similarly, heightened anxiety is a common response to myocardial infarction and bypass surgery, and has been negatively correlated with many postrecovery variables (e.g., return to work). Stress also has been implicated in the development of gastrointestinal disorders (irritable bowel syndrome, peptic ulcer, colitis), and subsequent anxiety has been linked to exacerbations of the condition. Psychiatric referral may be clinically beneficial in the management of such patients by reframing the medical illness as a condition that worsens with stress and providing treatment of maladaptive illness behavior.

There are a number of reasons why anxiety disorders are frequently unrecognized in the medical setting. A major obstacle is the overlapping of physical and psychological signs or symptoms. Nervousness, trembling, dizziness, tachycardia, chest pain and shortness of breath are symptoms of anxiety; however, each also may be produced by an enormous number of physical disorders and commonly used drugs (Table 389-10). Furthermore, even when anxiety symptoms are recognized by staff, they may be considered as relatively unimportant in comparison with profound medical illness or a natural reaction to illness (e.g., "anyone would feel anxious in his condition"). In addition, the demanding, irritable, hypervigilant nature of the patient with an anxiety symptom may be perceived by staff as negativistic and uncooperative and sometimes evoke anger.

MEDICAL TREATMENT OF ANXIETY DISORDERS

Lewis L. Judd

The development of the benzodiazepines has been a great advance in the pharmacologic management of anxiety. They have also replaced barbiturates as the sedative-hypnotic drugs of choice. The benzodiazepines, unlike the barbiturates, are partial CNS depressants and thus, even at high doses, are rarely associated with lethal respiratory depression or vasomotor collapse. In addition, depending upon the dose, benzodiazepines possess anticonvulsant and muscle relaxant properties.

MECHANISMS OF ACTION There is growing evidence that GABA plays a central role in the brain mechanism(s) of anxiety. Benzodiazepines selectively, but indirectly, enhance GABA neurotransmission, possibly by increasing neuronal receptor sensitivity to GABA. Also, a close interaction has been described between GABA and benzodiazepine receptor binding, leading to an increase in neuronal chloride conductance. Despite these observations, the specific mechanism by which benzodiazepines mediate their clinical effects is not completely understood.

CLINICAL CONDITIONS FOR USE The benzodiazepines are most effective in the management of relatively short-lived reactive states of tension and anxiety and are the drugs of choice in the treatment of generalized anxiety disorders. Although alprazolam at high doses (4 to 10 mg) can block panic attacks, the TCAs and MAO inhibitors are the drugs of choice for treating panic disorders. Recent studies have demonstrated that the MAO inhibitor phenelzine is effective in the treatment of social phobia. Furthermore, there is emerging evidence that short-acting, high-potency benzodiazepines such as clonazepam are also effective in this disorder. In addition, the benzodiazepines may have a role in the treatment of anticipatory anxiety, which is almost always present in patients with panic disorders. Sometimes, both a TCA and a benzodiazepine anxiolytic may be necessary in the treatment of panic disorder. The anxiolytics are also useful in treating anxiety symptoms that accompany phobic disorders.

CLINICAL USE OF ANTIANXIETY MEDICATIONS The benzodiazepines have been most frequently prescribed as anxiolytics. The shorter-acting benzodiazepines, however, are also effective sedative-hypnotics. The more commonly prescribed drugs are listed in Table 389-12 along with the usual oral dose ranges. The pharmacokinetic characteristics of many of the benzodiazepines are complicated by long drug elimination half-lives and the metabolic conversion of parent compounds to active metabolites (see Table 389-12). Diazepam is converted to the active metabolite desmethyldiazepam (nordiazepam) which, in turn, can be hydroxylated to yield oxazepam, also a potent benzodiazepine. This metabolic pathway extends the activity half-life of diazepam threefold. The hypnotic flurazepam is converted to active metabolite *N*-1-desalkylflurazepam, which has a half-life of more than 48 h; hence, repetitive daily doses given in excess of a week or two can result in the accumulation of the active metabolites of the drug. Prazepam has metabolic breakdown products identical to those of diazepam and has a similar drug elimination half-life. Oxazepam and lorazepam, both of which undergo glucuronide conjugation, have no active metabolites and therefore have the advantage of a shorter half-life. The benzodiazepines temazepam, triazolam, and alprazolam also have the advantage of shorter half-lives and to date, no long-acting active metabolites have been identified. Triazolam, however, has such a short half-life that it has been known to produce rebound withdrawal anxiety. For this reason it should be used with caution and only for short intervals (less than 7 days).

Diazepam has been the standard against which all anxiolytic drugs are measured, and no other anxiolytics have demonstrated better antianxiety efficacy. The newly developed benzodiazepines appear equally effective and have eliminated certain of the undesirable side effects. Specifically, lorazepam, oxazepam, and alprazolam are without active metabolites and, with proper dosage, cumulative effects of daytime sedation are less noticeable.

TABLE 389-12 Commonly used benzodiazepines

Benzodiazepine	Daily oral dose range, mg	Half-life, h*
ANXIOLYTICS		
Chlordiazepoxide	20–100[d]	7–28*
Clonazepam	1–20	18–50
Diazepam	5–40[d]	20–90*
Lorazepam	1–10‡	10–12
Oxazepam	30–120‡	3–20
Prazepam	20–60[d]	40–70*
Alprazolam	0.75–10.0‡	12–15
SEDATIVE-HYPNOTICS		
Flurazepam	15–30[t]	24–100*
Temazepam	30[t]	8–10
Triazolam	0.125–0.5[t]	2–5

* Indicates long-acting active metabolites.
[d] Prescribed in a daily or twice daily regimen.
‡ Prescribed in a three or four times daily regimen.
[t] Prescribed in a daily or bedtime regimen.

Treatment regimens usually last 4 weeks or less, and medications are prescribed continually for 7 to 10 days followed by a 2- to 3-day drug holiday; then this sequence is repeated. This schedule helps avoid the development of tolerance to the anxiolytic effects. The shorter-acting medications (e.g., lorazepam, alprazolam, clonazepam) are prescribed in a three or four times daily regimen, and the longer-acting drugs (e.g., diazepam) are given in a single dose or a twice daily regimen. For example, it is common practice to prescribe one dose of diazepam at bedtime, since it will both promote sleep and reduce anxiety levels the following day.

In prescribing the anxiolytic benzodiazepines clinicians should avoid the possibility of habituating patients to chronic benzodiazepine use. One of the earliest signs is the development of tolerance in which the patient repeatedly requests escalations in drug dose. Since benzodiazepines do produce mild euphoria and a sense of well-being, anxious patients often want to preserve this feeling and request additional medication. However, clinical surveys of prescription practices have shown that clinicians are aware of the problems of benzodiazepine habituation and sometimes respond by being too cautious and by unnecessarily undertreating patients. The use of the drug holiday treatment regimen described above and the physician's resistance to repetitively increasing dosage will help to minimize the problem of drug habituation.

In addition to its role as an anxiolytic, diazepam is also the drug of choice in this class for muscle relaxation and for the treatment of alcohol withdrawal syndromes. It is the benzodiazepine of choice for intractable seizures. Oxazepam, because of the nonaccumulation of active metabolites, is a good choice for anxiolysis in the elderly.

Finally, the physician should be aware that during the last decade, there have been multiple controlled studies describing effective treatment strategies in the management of panic disorder. This common subtype of the anxiety disorders has proven to be amenable to treatment with tricyclic antidepressants, MAO inhibitor depressants, and high-potency, short-acting benzodiazepines (alprazolam, clonazepam, etc.). Further, there is now some indication that the selective serotonin reuptake inhibitor antidepressants (fluoxetine, sertraline, paroxetine, etc.) are also effective in panic disorder. However, longitudinal studies of medication treatment have identified high relapse rates (30 to 80 percent) when patients are removed from medications.

These observations have contributed significantly to our understanding of panic disorder; it is a chronic life-long illness which requires maintenance treatment. In addition, promising data are emerging from the empirical testing of a new type of psychotherapy, cognitive behavioral panic control, which has been designed specifically as a short-term, targeted disorder-specific psychotherapy. This type of psychotherapy shows promise in both the acute management of panic disorder and in the maintenance of therapeutic gains and significantly reduced relapse rates post treatment (10 percent or less). Evolving treatments promise new, more effective, and more lasting benefits in the management of panic disorder, which are likely to involve an integration of both medication and specific targeted psychotherapeutic techniques.

SIDE EFFECTS AND INTERACTIONS The most important adverse effect of the benzodiazepines is the discomfort caused by the withdrawal syndrome, which can occur after chronic treatment. There is little risk of debilitating addiction to these drugs when used appropriately. However, physical dependence does occur since withdrawal symptoms are seen in a high percentage of patients after cessation of chronic benzodiazepine treatment. Motivation to sustain mild feelings of well-being and avoid the discomfort of withdrawal symptoms may contribute to psychological dependence. Withdrawal symptoms include muscle aches, agitation, restlessness, insomnia, and generalized anxious dysphoria. In some patients, more commonly those taking short-acting benzodiazepines, more serious CNS withdrawal symptoms may appear, including confusional and delirium states and, more rarely, grand mal seizures. Rebound anxiety can also be seen in patients with anxiety disorders but is less prevalent

when benzodiazepines with long-acting metabolites are used and if medication is gradually discontinued. Risk for withdrawal symptoms increases with the length of treatment; they occur with much greater frequency (e.g., more than 90 percent) among patients who have been treated for 1 year or more. Withdrawal symptoms occur within the first 24 to 48 h after treatment with short-acting benzodiazepines ceases, but for those benzodiazepines with long-acting metabolites (e.g., diazepam, chlordiazepoxide) the withdrawal symptoms can occur 4 to 6 days and even longer after drug cessation. With the usual recommended dosage regimens and the gradual withdrawal technique (e.g., over 3 to 4 weeks), the appearance of a withdrawal syndrome in patients can be minimized significantly. While there is little true addiction potential, patients should be on these medications for only as long as necessary.

The most common minor side effects are daytime sedation, mild cognitive impairment, motor clumsiness, and (e.g., lorazepam, triazolam) specific memory decrements. Another rare but troublesome side effect from some benzodiazepines is paradoxical emotional responses, primarily manifested as aggressive and impulsive behavior.

Unlike barbiturates, the benzodiazepines do not noticeably induce hepatic microsomal enzyme activity and therefore do not affect the metabolism of other medications. The benzodiazepines potentiate the CNS depressant effects of other drugs including barbiturates, general anesthetics, and alcohol. The cross-tolerance with ethanol has made the benzodiazepines ideal medications for the treatment of alcohol withdrawal syndromes. Patients should be cautioned that ethanol's effects are potentiated by benzodiazepines and this combination should be avoided.

NEWER ANXIOLYTIC MEDICATIONS It has been established that certain beta-adrenergic blocking agents, such as *propranolol*, can dampen the peripheral physiologic symptoms of anxiety. Initially, it was felt that these drugs might be better nonsedative anxiolytic compounds, but this promise has not been fulfilled in controlled studies. While propranolol does attenuate somatic manifestations of anxiety (e.g., palpitations, tremor), it appears to have lesser effects on the psychological components (e.g., intense fearfulness). Although propranolol has been used for treating patients extremely fearful of speaking or performing in public (oral dose 40 to 320 mg daily), it is not a comprehensively effective anxiolytic. With additional study, other potentially peripheral blocking agents may prove to be more effective.

A new class of anxiolytic drugs, the azaspirodecanediones, which act on the serotoninergic system, has been developed. One of the first compounds studied clinically is *buspirone*, a compound that acts selectively on the serotonin$_{1A}$ receptor. It has no structural similarity to other anxiolytics or even to other psychotropics. It is not anticonvulsant, does not interact with the benzodiazepine receptor, is not cross-tolerant with other CNS depressants, and no abstinence syndrome has yet been described. In several controlled trials it has proved to be an effective anxiolytic with significantly less sedation and decrements in psychomotor performance, although it is not effective in panic disorder. Because of the near absence of sedation and motor impairment and the relatively long latency for anxiolytic effects to appear (i.e., days to weeks), patients occasionally report that the drug is ineffective. This is most common in individuals who have previously received benzodiazepines such as diazepam. Studies are currently being conducted with buspirone to determine possible side effects.

In addition to the efficacy of TCAs in panic and phobic disorders, there are controlled studies reporting that they are anxiolytics as effective as the benzodiazepines in generalized anxiety disorders. It is possible that continued investigations will identify a broader role for TCAs in the treatment of the full spectrum of anxiety disorders.

SCHIZOPHRENIC DISORDERS

David L. Braff

Schizophrenic disorders are serious mental illnesses characterized by hallucinations, delusions, and disorganized thought and behavior.

They last 6 months or more and cause significant social, vocational, and personal disability, and suffering. The schizophrenic patient may present to the emergency department in crisis with overtly bizarre and obviously psychotic complaints. Alternatively, schizophrenic patients may present more subtly to the primary care physician with strange complaints or ideas which, on close questioning, are related to delusions or thought disorder. Despite its frequently dramatic presentation, perhaps no other psychiatric disorder has proved as vexing and difficult to define, identify, and treat.

Schizophrenia has a lifetime prevalence rate of about 1 percent across all cultures. In the United States alone there are perhaps 2 million affected individuals who often become ill in their late teenage years and in the third decade of life. Poor outcome frequently leads to extensive and long-term disability, and schizophrenia accounts for an estimated 20 billion dollars or more per year of lost productivity. Most patients with schizophrenic disorders also cause major perturbations for family and social support systems, adding to the economic losses and the toll of human misery. Up to 25 percent of hospital beds in the United States may be occupied by schizophrenic patients at any one time. Cumulatively, these factors make schizophrenia one of the most costly and vexing health problems.

DEFINITION AND CLINICAL MANIFESTATIONS In 1919, Emil Kraepelin first made the distinction between dementia praecox, a psychotic illness with progressive deterioration, and manic depressive psychosis. Kraepelin noted, however, that about 13 percent of patients with dementia praecox did not have an inevitably deteriorating outcome, and the size of the group with a favorable outcome has significantly increased largely because of antipsychotic medications, discussed in detail in the section that follows. Eugene Bleuler concentrated on the putative underlying psychological splitting of personality functions in his classic work on the "group of schizophrenias." Bleuler's emphasis was on the "four A's" of schizophrenia: *a*utism, flattened *a*ffect, loose *a*ssociations, and *a*mbivalence. Other authors have focused on specific symptoms of schizophrenia such as the sense of being influenced by others and feelings of being controlled by outside forces. To date, research has yet to identify specific and inevitably pathognomonic signs or symptoms of the schizophrenic disorders since mania, drug-induced psychosis, and other states also present with prominent hallucinations, delusions, and agitated behavior.

According to the DSM-III-R, after the first and most central criterion of psychotic symptoms is met (see Table 389-13), the schizophrenic individual must show deterioration from a previous level of functioning in such areas as work, social relations, and self-care. The disorder is not attributable to other diagnoses such as mood disorder with psychotic features or organic-induced (e.g., drug-induced) syndromes. Finally, continuous signs of the illness should be present for 6 months at some point during the individual's life with some signs of illness at the time of diagnosis. There may be prodromal, active, and/or residual phases of the illness that are not always clearly demarcated. Prodromal or residual symptoms are somewhat nonspecific and may consist of isolation; marked psychosocial impairment; peculiar behavior; impaired personal hygiene and grooming; blunted, flat, or inappropriate affect; digressive, vague, overelaborate, circumstantial, or metaphorical speech; odd or bizarre ideation or magical thinking; and unusual perceptual experiences.

The DSM-III-R lists four major schizophrenic disorders:

1 *Catatonic*—stupor, rigidity, excitement, or posturing; relatively rare.
2 *Disorganized*—incoherence and flat or grossly disorganized affect.
3 *Paranoid*—preoccupation with suspiciousness and one or more systematized delusions.
4 *Undifferentiated*—prominent delusions, hallucinations, incoherence, or disorganized behavior, not meeting the criteria for the other three types (see DSM-III-R for more detailed descriptions).

This emphasis on subtypes carries forward Bleuler's notion of the "group of schizophrenias." There is moderate support for a paranoid/

TABLE 389-13 Diagnosis of schizophrenic disorders
A Presence of characteristic psychotic symptoms in active phase, either *1*, *2*, or *3* for at least 1 week (unless symptoms are successfully treated):
1 Two of the following:
Delusions
Prominent hallucinations
Incoherence or marked loosening of associations
Catatonic behavior
Flat or grossly inappropriate affect
2 Bizarre delusions
3 Prominent hallucinations of a voice with content having no apparent relation to depression or elation, or a voice keeping up a running commentary on the person's behavior or thoughts, or two or more voices conversing with each other
B During the course of disturbance, functioning in areas such as work, social relations, and self-care markedly below highest level achieved before onset of disturbance.
C Schizoaffective disorder and mood disorder with psychotic features have been ruled out.
D Continuous signs of disturbance for at least 6 months. This period must include an active phase (of at least 1 week, or less if symptoms have been successfully treated) during which they were psychotic symptoms characteristic of schizophrenia (see *A* above), with or without a prodromal or residual phase.
E It cannot be established that an organic factor initiated and maintained the disturbance.
F If a history of autistic disorder exists, the additional diagnosis of schizophrenia can be made only if prominent delusions or hallucinations are also present.

SOURCE: Adapted from DSM-III-R.

nonparanoid dichotomy as being important in schizophrenia. In an attempt to reduce diagnostic heterogeneity, researchers have identified as "type I" schizophrenic patients those with a predominance of "positive" symptoms (e.g., hallucinations, paranoid ideation), normal cerebral ventricular size, and symptoms that respond to the hypothesized dopaminergic blocking effects of antipsychotic drugs. In contrast, "type II" schizophrenic patients seem similar to Kraepelin's dementia praecox patients. Type II patients show a predominance of "negative" symptoms (e.g., anhedonia, social withdrawal, asociality), neuropsychological impairment, and possibly increased cerebral ventricular volume; they do not respond well to antipsychotic medications, but seem to display a "deficit" state. Their course of the illness is variable, from "in remission" to "chronic."

DIFFERENTIAL DIAGNOSIS Schizophrenic patients have no unique or pathognomonic signs and symptoms. At times, this makes the diagnosis difficult. DSM-III-R separates psychotic illnesses by a durational criterion into *brief reactive psychoses* lasting 2 weeks or less, *schizophreniform disorders* lasting between 2 weeks and 6 months, and *schizophrenic disorders* lasting more than 6 months. While these distinctions are practical, the scientific basis for such a durational criterion is poorly documented. In addition, an acute manic patient may be difficult to distinguish from the schizophrenic patient, especially on a cross-sectional as opposed to longitudinal basis. To complicate matters further, the initial clinical appearance of a patient intoxicated with phencyclidine (PCP) or amphetamines may be indistinguishable from that of the paranoid schizophrenic patient. It appears then that many functional and organic states may lead to a final common pathway of psychotic symptoms. The diagnosis can only be established reliably by a broad-based multifactorial approach utilizing neurobiologic data (e.g., toxicologic screens, genetic history) and psychosocial data (e.g., premorbid adjustment status) obtained both for the present and across time. Despite these problems, the DSM-III-R criteria for schizophrenic disorders have undergone extensive and successful field trials for reliability and validity. In general, clinicians using the DSM-III-R criteria can accurately and consistently diagnose schizophrenia.

PREDISPOSING, PRECIPITATING, AND SUSTAINING FACTORS These factors may be analyzed in terms of neuroanatomic, biochemical, neurophysiologic, psychophysiologic, intrapsychic, interpersonal, social, and socioeconomic contributors. In a complex, multifactorial disorder such as schizophrenia, neurobiologic and psychosocial factors should be seen as interactive rather than as competing or mutually exclusive. This approach is analogous to comprehensive analyses of diabetes mellitus or hypertension according to the contributions of genetics, receptor physiology, and physiologic, familial, psychosocial, and myriad other conceptually diverse factors. Within this context, predisposing factors are linked to etiologic variables, precipitating factors are related to onset of pathophysiology, and sustaining factors are linked to outcome variables.

ETIOLOGY   Genetic factors   It is clear from twin, family, and adoptive studies that schizophrenia has a significant genetic basis. Monozygotic twins have roughly a 65 percent or greater concordance rate for schizophrenia, whereas dizygotic twins have a 12 percent concordance rate. Other family studies show that the morbid risk for developing schizophrenia is 5 to 10 percent if one parent is schizophrenic. This figure rises to 46 percent or more if both parents are schizophrenics. Second-degree relatives of schizophrenics run a 2 to 4 percent risk of developing the illness compared to a risk of 1 to 2 percent in the general population.

Adoption studies reveal that these risk factors are largely genetically linked and are not primarily due to the "schizophrenogenic" psychosocial environment of certain families. Still, these genetic analyses are fraught with methodologic difficulties. For example, reflecting the probable complex mode of inheritance, 89 percent of schizophrenics do not have a parent who is schizophrenic. Eighty-one percent of schizophrenics do not have either a schizophrenic sibling or parent. The appropriate model with which to explain these figures is complex and may include a weighted polygenic model or other sophisticated interpretations of the available data. Most recently, there has been an explosion of new knowledge about the genetics of schizophrenia featuring molecular studies and linkages to chromosome 5 and possibly X (see the entire volume 15, no. 3, of *Schizophrenia Bulletin*, 1989, and Crow et al.).

The stress-diathesis model hypothesizes that there is a vulnerability which is inherited in schizophrenia-prone individuals. These vulnerable individuals are at high risk for developing schizophrenia under certain stressful circumstances. Studies of high-risk children with one or two schizophrenic parents indicate that such children may have a significantly increased incidence of morbidity in utero, at birth, and in the perinatal period. In addition, these infants and children may have psychophysiologic lability, attentional dysfunction, and specific motor disturbances. A number of human and animal model studies suggest that such labile attentional mechanisms may result partly or largely from instabilities and increased activity of the mesolimbic dopaminergic system and associated decreased frontal lobe activity (hypofrontality). The literature on neurophysiologically labile and vulnerable children seems to tie the genetic, dopaminergic, and attentional dysfunction hypotheses together.

According to the stress-diathesis model, a host of stressful factors may precipitate a psychotic state in a high-risk individual. These factors include intoxication with PCP or amphetamines as well as more nonspecific factors such as medical illnesses and psychosocial life events with concomitant general stress. Further, specific hallucinogens such as LSD may precipitate a rather long-lasting psychotic episode that is ultimately indistinguishable from a schizophrenic disorder. Lastly, there have been a dramatically increasing number of hypotheses that a viral vector or early developmental abnormalities may be important as etiologic agents in at least some cases of schizophrenic disorders.

Psychosocial factors   Empirical support for psychosocial hypotheses concerning the creation of a vulnerability to developing schizophrenia is variable, far from definitive, and interacts strongly with neurobiologic factors.

In the vulnerable individual, schizophrenia often has its onset in a critical developmental period. The teenager may attempt to leave home and separate from family members for school or work reasons. The onset is often, but not invariably, insidious. In terms of psychosocial approaches to schizophrenia, there is felt to be a developmental or intrapsychic deficit in the vulnerable individual.

Once set into motion, the disturbance passes through a series of stages leading to the final common pathway of a psychotic state.

Despite much theorizing, there is no inevitable schizophrenia-prone personality type, although at least a small but significant percentage of individuals with schizoid (withdrawn), paranoid (suspicious), and schizotypal (odd, eccentric) personality disorder do seem to be vulnerable to developing schizophrenic disorders. In the 1960s, a more family-systems–oriented view emerged. An example of this approach is the "double-bind" hypothesis of Bateson and coworkers (1956) who analyzed the formal communications patterns in "schizophrenogenic" families. In this view, communications content is less important than the frequently conflicting and self-contradictory form of communication style of schizophrenic patients' families. It remains unclear whether these familial factors are a cause or result of having a schizophrenic child in the family. As the importance of biologic factors in schizophrenia have become clearer, family psychosocial factors have been seen more as secondary or epiphenomenal factors.

Psychosocial researchers have also examined the importance of socioeconomic factors in schizophrenia. Lower socioeconomic status correlates with a higher incidence of schizophrenia. There are two possible interpretations of this data. First, there may be a "social drift" of vulnerable individuals to lower socioeconomic status. The second hypothesis is more etiologic, as socieconomic stressors may precipitate schizophrenic episodes, especially in vulnerable individuals.

PATHOPHYSIOLOGY   Neurotransmitters and neuropeptides Neurobiologic factors have been correlated with schizophrenic episodes. The predominant neurotransmitter hypothesis involves dopaminergic overactivity. Evidence supporting this hypothesis comes from several sources. First, the potency of all traditional antipsychotic medications can be roughly predicted by their dopaminergic blocking capacity. Second, mesolimbic dopamine plays a role in attentional mechanisms and stimulus filtering. When stimulus filtering mechanisms break down, there is a collapse of the information processing capacity of the individual with resulting sensory inundation, cognitive fragmentation, and symptoms of thought disorder.

Despite this support, the dopamine hypothesis is fraught with difficulties when compared with the catecholamine theory of the affective disorders. Affective disorders hypothetically (and simplistically) reflect a decrease in norepinephrine tone in hypothalamic nuclei leading to a final common pathway of neurovegetative symptoms. In schizophrenia, there seems to be increased dopamine tone in critical subcortical pathways leading to cognitive fragmentation, thought disorder, and clinical symptoms that are quite complex and highly variable. In this framework, affective disorders may be seen as impinging on the diencephalic "core" of the brain, whereas schizophrenia is conceptualized as a disorder of the mesolimbic-frontal cortical mantle. It is doubtful if a "one neurotransmitter" or "one locus" theory can explain any psychiatric disorder, given the interactive complexity of neurobiologic and psychosocial systems, although such theories may be useful.

The hypothesis of dopamine overactivity in schizophrenia is generally characterized as a static theory. In reality, dopamine tone is related in a dynamic and variable manner to GABA, serotonin, and other neurotransmitters that are functionally arrayed in a cascade of important brain systems, such as the dorsolateral prefrontal cortex, mesial temporal cortex, nucleus accumbens, ventral pallidum, and the hippocampus. Longer-term correlates of schizophrenia may also involve alterations of neuropeptides, with their long latency and response effects on behavior. At an electrophysiologic level, it has been hypothesized that the initial disturbance in schizophrenia is an aberrant (perhaps excitotoxic-induced) temporal lobe focus that ultimately perturbs the homeostasis of the dopamine system. More recent evidence implicates a second trimester viremia as a possible early precursor of schizophrenia. According to this theory, the temporal lobes are damaged during fetal development and this deficit is "unmasked" in late adolescence by a failure to prune excess neurons or to down-regulate frontotemporal activity. All of these areas are receiving critical experimental scrutiny.

Neuropathologic factors   The use of computed tomography (CT) and magnetic resonance imaging (MRI) has been widely employed in studies of schizophrenic patients. Initial reports indicated that a minority of schizophrenic patients have abnormally increased ventricular brain ratios, reflecting increased ventricular fluid volume associated with brain atrophy. Subsequent studies in identical twins discordant for schizophrenia have confirmed increased ventricular size and neuropsychologic deficits in schizophrenic patients and perhaps in their "unaffected" co-twin, supporting the contention that schizophrenia is accompanied by brain dysfunction. It is quite possible that type II patients have a disorder that is distinct and associated with poor medication response and poor clinical outcome. Positron emission tomography (PET) data reveal patterns of decreased frontal lobe activity in schizophrenia (hypofrontality) that seem important, especially in view of the close relationship of dopamine activity, frontal lobe function, and mesolimbic activity levels. Future PET studies utilizing new ligands will undoubtedly clarify the role of dopamine and other neurotransmitters in the schizophrenic disorders.

Psychophysiology and information processing   Important insights into the pathophysiology of schizophrenia have also been generated by psychophysiologic and information processing studies. Individuals at high risk for developing schizophrenia and patients with a schizophrenic disorder are frequently psychophysiologically labile and vulnerable to being inundated by stimuli. The proposed mechanism for such vulnerability is an impairment in an individual's ability to screen out irrelevant stimuli and an associated inability to habituate to externally and internally generated cues. Ultimately, this dysfunction, which has been linked to dopamine overactivity in humans and animals, leads to an information processing overload. The affected person becomes inundated with stimuli and displays cognitive fragmentation and thought disorder. It is this fragmented thinking and lapses in speech which sometimes serve as an important clue to the primary care physician that the patient is experiencing serious psychiatric problems. Using attentional tasks, skin conductance habituation, and other measures, investigators have increasingly underscored the importance of these dysfunctions in the schizophrenic disorders. New techniques, such as magnetoencephalography (MEG) also offer exciting possibilities for specifying the possible frontal, temporal, and subcortical locus and type of brain disturbance characteristic of the various types of schizophrenic disorders.

TREATMENT AND OUTCOME Neurobiologic factors   Five-year follow-up studies show that 60 percent of schizophrenic individuals have social recovery and half of those are employed. Some 30 percent are seriously and permanently handicapped, and 10 percent remain chronically hospitalized. This pattern of outcome seems still to be generally accurate across numerous studies. Which factors determine the outcome of the schizophrenic disorders are not clear. It is commonly stated that the outcome of schizophrenia is better when disorientation, affective symptoms, and acute onset are present. The outcome of schizophrenic disorders is thought to be poorer when the patient is well oriented and has fewer affective symptoms, and when the onset is insidious.

The outcome of schizophrenic disorders has been greatly improved by the use of potent and efficacious antipsychotic medications, such as the phenothiazines. Studies indicate that antipsychotic medications (often expressed in terms of chlorpromazine equivalents) act selectively against specific target symptoms that are similar to the "positive" symptoms of type I schizophrenia which include hallucinations and psychotic agitation. In contrast to these responsive target symptoms, antipsychotic medications may not necessarily improve "negative" symptoms such as anhedonia and social withdrawal. The primary modalities for treatment of the acute schizophrenic disorders are antipsychotic medication along with psychosocial therapies. The typical schizophrenic patient usually requires at least the equivalent of 600 to 800 mg/d of chlorpromazine administered for 4 to 6 weeks, although higher doses are frequently necessary. Maintenance doses

of antipsychotic medications in lower doses and given on a continuous or intermittent basis are often required to prevent relapse.

The primary care physician sees two main types of schizophrenic patients. First, there is the acute, psychotically agitated patient with poor behavioral control. These patients need to be referred to an emergency room or other acute care facility, often for rapid neuroleptic medication treatment on an out- or inpatient basis. It is quite important to determine if the psychotic state is of recent onset (which may need a careful differential diagnostic workup to rule out organic, drug-induced, or manic disorders, or an exacerbation of a chronic condition). The second type of schizophrenic patient has more subtle signs and symptoms of psychosis and, though not an emergency case, needs a rapid referral to a psychiatrist for appropriate care.

Antipsychotic medications alter dopaminergic-cholinergic balance in nigrostriatal structures (via dopamine blockade) so that acute extrapyramidal side effects are induced (e.g., dystonia, motor restlessness). These side effects can be treated with anticholinergic medications that restore dopaminergic-cholinergic balance. Aliphatic phenothiazines (such as chlorpromazine) with inherent anticholinergic properties cause fewer extrapyramidal side effects but induce more anticholinergic side effects such as hypotension or blurred vision. Additionally, blood dyscrasias, liver toxicity, and other idiosyncratic reactions occur. Also, the long-term use of antipsychotic medications may induce nigrostriatal damage and tardive dyskinesia, a long-lasting and potentially disabling motor syndrome (see Chap. 21). Thus, the search for new antipsychotic medications with more selective (i.e., nonnigrostriatal) sites of action is important for the pharmacologic treatment of schizophrenia. (See "Antipsychotic or Neuroleptic Medications," below.)

Psychosocial factors   The outcome of schizophrenic patients can be divided into semi-independent axes of symptoms, social function, and vocational function. It is possible to treat the specific psychotic symptoms of a schizophrenic individual (affecting the symptomatic axis of outcome), but the patient may be left with major psychosocial deficits (the social axis of outcome). Antipsychotic medications should thus be combined with sensitive psychosocial management including, where appropriate, individual and group psychotherapy, family counseling, and vocational rehabilitation in order to maximize therapeutic outcome and to restore the patient to the premorbid level of adjustment. For example, returning an acutely treated schizophrenic patient to a home filled with hostility, criticisms, and emotional overinvolvement (the so-called high-expressed-emotion family) without the benefit of family education and therapy is poor psychosocial management and may lead to relapse. Along with appropriate use of antipsychotic medications, family counseling and education is often a critical determinant of therapeutic outcome in the schizophrenic disorders.

ANTIPSYCHOTIC OR NEUROLEPTIC MEDICATIONS
Lewis L. Judd

The antipsychotics have the capacity to sedate, tranquilize, blunt emotional expression, attenuate aggressive and impulsive behavior, and cause lack of initiative and loss of interest in the environment. Unique features of the drugs are that they leave higher intellectual functions relatively intact yet specifically ameliorate the agitation and bizarre behavior and thinking of psychotic patients. Unfortunately no antipsychotic medication currently available even approaches ideal in this respect. Virtually all have prominent anticholinergic side effects and produce a wide variety of dystonias and extrapyramidal symptoms. Of greater concern is the fact that long-term administration of these agents can cause tardive dyskinesia in some patients (see Chap. 21), a seriously disabling movement disorder that is often irreversible. Nonetheless, the antipsychotics, primarily used in schizophrenia, have helped to reduce enormously the patient populations in mental hospitals and have allowed chronic mentally ill patients who previously would have been lifelong residents of hospitals to live in the community.

MECHANISM OF ACTION   With few exceptions, antipsychotic neuroleptics have notable effects on the brain's dopaminergic neurotransmitter system. Specifically, these medications antagonize the effects of the neurotransmitter dopamine in the basal ganglia and in the limbic portions of the forebrain. Since the central characteristic of neuroleptics is their capacity to block dopaminergic neurotransmission, this has led researchers to postulate that an abnormality in the CNS dopaminergic neurotransmitter system is one of the key pathophysiologic mechanisms in the etiology of schizophrenia. Many effects of antipsychotic medications on the brain have been well-described, but the underlying mechanism by which these drugs achieve their antipsychotic efficacy is not yet fully understood.

CLINICAL CONDITIONS FOR USE   Because the overall risk of tardive dyskinesia is estimated at 20 to 40 percent with chronic treatment, antipsychotics should only be used when necessary and in those conditions for which they are the drug of choice: in treating schizophrenic disorders; in combination with lithium for acute manic episodes; and in combination with antidepressants for psychotic and agitated depressions. They are also used in treating Tourette's syndrome and Huntington's disease. Although the antipsychotics should be used with only a relatively narrow spectrum of mental disorders, patients with these disorders make up a significant majority of all patients with serious and chronic mental illness.

CLINICAL USE OF ANTIPSYCHOTICS   The more commonly used antipsychotics from each pharmacologic class and their average daily oral doses are given in Table 389-14. Chlorpromazine, one of the first drugs of this class to be developed, is the prototypic antipsychotic drug and the potency standard for the others. Dose equivalence for an antipsychotic drug is calculated in comparison with the effect of 100 mg of chlorpromazine. For example, 5 mg of trifluoperazine or 2 mg of haloperidol is equivalent in potency to 100 mg of chlorpromazine. Using this ratio as a reference point, acutely psychotic patients usually require an accumulated dose of 500 to 800 mg orally of a chlorpromazine equivalent during the first 24 to 36 h. Following control of the acute agitation, the oral dose is increased over the next week to the chlorpromazine equivalent of between 600 and 1500 mg/d in divided doses. It is uncommon for therapeutic benefits to be measurably increased by exceeding the daily dose equivalent of 1500 mg of chlorpromazine, although it may be necessary to go to two and three times this level in some patients.

Because schizophrenia is a chronic disorder, patients need long-term maintenance on antipsychotics to prevent relapse. In controlled studies as many as 60 percent of schizophrenics relapse within 6 months after discontinuing drug therapy. Patients are maintained on the lowest dose possible that will prevent reemergence of symptoms. This is usually in the range of 20 percent of the peak dose level needed to ameliorate the acute phase of the psychotic symptoms. Compliance is difficult to achieve in this chronically disordered group of patients, and it is often therapeutically advantageous for the clinician to use parenteral long-acting fluphenazine enanthate or decanoate, which can be administered by injection every week or two. Previously it was recommended that drug holidays be used, but this practice has not prevented tardive dyskinesia, and there are few if any advantages to this technique, which is now rarely used.

SIDE EFFECTS AND INTERACTIONS   Initially patients are sedated, lethargic, and drowsy, but within days they develop tolerance to these effects. All of the antipsychotics have anticholinergic action, which may produce dry mouth, cycloplegia, postural hypotension, constipation, and urinary retention. Obstructive jaundice, retinal pigmentation (thioridazine), lenticular opacities, skin pigmentation and hypersensitivity to sunlight, and male impotence are also side effects seen with antipsychotics.

The extrapyramidal side effects are the most troublesome, however. During the first five days of treatment, patients may develop acute muscular dystonic reactions but the extrapyramidal Parkinson-like syndrome is the most common. Both the dystonia and the parkinsonism respond well to antiparkinsonian medications (e.g., benztropine mesylate, 1 to 2 mg bid or tid; trihexyphenidyl, 2 to 5 mg bid or tid). Another common side effect is akathisia, a motor restlessness in which patients feel compelled to move their extremities and to move about. It is not uncommon to mistake akathisia for psychotic agitation and increase the antipsychotic dose, exacerbating the problem. Akathisia may respond to beta blockers and antiparkinsonian agents but more often requires decreasing the dose of the antipsychotic. It is rarely necessary to continue antiparkinsonian drug treatment beyond the first 3 months of antipsychotic maintenance.

The most serious side effect of the antipsychotics is tardive dyskinesia, which has been seen with virtually every neuroleptic. The specter of tardive dyskinesia has altered the risk-benefit ratio of the antipsychotics; they should only be used for those disorders in which they are clearly the drugs of choice. Usually the symptoms of tardive dyskinesia appear late in treatment and consist of involuntary, repetitive movements of the lips, tongue (e.g., tongue thrusting, lip smacking), and not infrequently of the extremities and trunk. Patients over 60 and those with preexisting CNS pathology are at a higher risk for this disorder (up to 70 percent), but other risk factors have not been confirmed. Although tardive dyskinesia cannot be prevented or reversed once it has developed, antipsychotic medications such as clozapine, which can attenuate some of the symptoms, may be substituted for the neuroleptic being used. However, it is too early to determine whether tardive dyskinesia is reduced with some of the newer antipsychotic medications.

The neuroleptic malignant syndrome, a rare complication of neuroleptic drugs, is discussed in Chap. 398.

NEWER ANTIPSYCHOTIC MEDICATIONS (ATYPICAL NEURO-LEPTICS)   Although development of new antipsychotic medications has lagged significantly behind that of the antidepressants and anxiolytic drugs, some promising medications have appeared recently.

Clozapine is a dibenzodiazepine that binds to serotonin and alpha-adrenergic, histaminergic, and dopaminergic receptors. It has been approved by the FDA for use in treatment-refractory psychotic patients and in those who have intolerable side effects with their current medications. Its antipsychotic activity is comparable to the traditional neuroleptics, and it is also effective in attenuating anxiety and tension. Clozapine has proven effective in 30 to 40 percent of treatment-resistant schizophrenics. Often the full therapeutic effects of clozapine may not appear until at least 6 months of treatment. The drug produces some sedation and muscle relaxation but few extrapyramidal symptoms. It is not known to cause tardive dyskinesia and may, in high doses, attenuate it. Clozapine's side effects include orthostatic hypotension, sinus tachycardia, hypersalivation, temperature eleva-

---

TABLE 389-14   Some commonly used antipsychotic medications

	Average daily oral dose range, mg	Potency ratio compared to 100 mg of chlorpromazine
Phenothiazines		
Aliphatics:		
Chlorpromazine	400–800	1:1
Piperazines:		
Fluphenazine	4–20	1:50
Fluphenazine enanthate or decanoate	25–100*	
Perphenazine	8–32	1:10
Trifluoperazine	6–20	1:20
Piperidines:		
Thioridazine	200–600	1:1
Butyrophenones		
Haloperidol	8–32	1:50
Thioxanthenes		
Chlorprothixene	400–800	1:1 (approx)
Thiothixene	15–30	1:25
Oxoindoles		
Molindone	40–200	1:10
Dibenzoxazepines		
Loxapine	60–100	1:10

* For intramuscular injection only.

tion, lowered seizure threshold, and constipation. A 1 to 2 percent incidence of potentially fatal agranulocytosis has been reported but this may be considerably higher in eastern European and Jewish subpopulations. Frequent (e.g., weekly) CBCs should be obtained and medication discontinued if the WBC count begins to decrease.

Sulpiride, which is available in Europe, is a substituted benzamide that selectively binds to presynaptic, sodium-dependent, D-2 receptors. Its antipsychotic efficacy is comparable to traditional neuroleptics. Moreover, it may cause fewer cases of tardive dyskinesia and extrapyramidal syndrome. This novel structure may herald the development of new classes of safer and better antipsychotics.

The success of clozapine has fueled the search for new antipsychotic medications and there are a number of new compounds under active study (e.g., Remoxipride, respiridone, etc.).

REFERENCES

MICHAELS R, MARZUK PM: Progress in psychiatry (first of two parts). N Engl J Med 329:552, 1993

————: Medical progress: Progress in psychiatry (second of two parts). N Engl J Med 329:628, 1993

Mood disorders

ALLEN JM et al: Depressive symptoms and family history in seasonal and nonseasonal mood disorders. Am J Psychiatry 150:443, 1993

BALDESSARINI RJ: Biological hypothesis in psychiatry, in *Chemotherapy in Psychiatry,* Cambridge, Mass, Harvard, 1985, pp 9–12

————: *Biomedical Aspects of Depression.* Washington, DC, APA Press, 1982, pp 1–83

BARON M, RISCH N: X-linkage and genetic heterogeneity in bipolar-related major affective illness: Reanalysis of linkage data. Ann Hum Genet 46 (pt 2):153, 1982

BURKE KC et al: Age at onset of selected mental disorders in five community populations. Arch Genl Psychiat, 47:511, 1990

CALLAHAM M, KASSEL D: Epidemiology of fatal tricyclic antidepressant ingestion: Implications for management. Ann Emerg Med 14:1, 1985

CARNEY RM et al: Major depressive disorder in coronary artery disease. Am J Cardiol 60(16):1273, 1987

CLAYTON PJ, BARRETT JE (eds): *Treatment of Depression: Old Controversies and New Approaches.* New York, Raven, 1983

DEVEAUGHGEISS J: Diagnosis and treatment of obsessive compulsive disorder. Annu Rev Med 44:53, 1993

Diagnostic and Statistical Manual of Mental Disorders, 3d ed. Washington, DC, American Psychiatric Association, 1980

Diagnostic and Statistical Manual of Mental Disorders, 3d ed, revised. Washington, DC, American Psychiatric Association, 1987

Drugs that cause psychiatric symptoms. Med Lett Drugs Ther 35:65, 1993

ELKIN I et al: National Institute of Mental Health Treatment of Depression Collaborative Research Program. General Effectiveness of Treatments. Arch Gen Psychiatry 46:971, 1989

FAEDDA GL et al: Seasonal mood disorders. Patterns of seasonal recurrrence in mania and depression. Arch Gen Psychiatry 50:17, 1993

FRANK E et al: Early recurrence in unipolar depression. Arch Gen Psychiatry 46:397, 1989

————: Conceptualization and rationale for consensus definitions of terms in major depressive disorder: Response, remission, recovery, relapse, and recurrence. Arch Gen Psychiatry 48(9):851, 1991

FRIIS R, NANJUNDAPPA G: Diabetes, depression, and employment status. Soc Sci Med 23(5):471, 1986

GOODWIN FK, JAMISON KR: *Manic-Depressive Illness.* New York, Oxford University Press, 1990

HARDMAN A et al: The recognition of psychiatric morbidity on a medical oncology ward. J Psychosom Res 33(2):235-9, 1989

KELSOE JR et al: Re-evaluation of the linkage relationship between chromosome 11p loci and the gene for bipolar affective disorder in the Old Order Amish. Nature 342:328, 1989

KLERMAN GL: History and development of modern concepts of affective illness, in *Neurobiology of Mood Disorders,* RM Post, RC Ballenger (eds). Baltimore, Williams & Wilkins, 1984, pp 1–19

MARTIN JB, REICHLIN S: *Clinical Neuroendocrinology,* 2d ed. Philadelphia, Davis 1987

OSSER DN: A systematic approach to the classification and pharmacotherapy of nonpsychotic major depression and dysthymia. J Clin Psychopharmacol 13:133, 1993

POST RM, BALLENGER JC (eds): *Neurobiology of Mood Disorders.* Baltimore, Williams & Wilkins, 1984, vol 1

————, WEISS SRB: Kindling and manic depressive illness, in *The Clinical Relevance of Kindling,* TB Bolwigm, MR Trimble (eds). Chichester, England, Wiley, 1989, pp 209–230

REGIER et al: Comorbidity of mental disorders with alcohol and other drug abuse. Results from the Epidemiologic Catchment Area (ECA) Study. JAMA 264(19):2511, 1990

————: One-month prevalence of mental disorders in the United States based on five Epidemiologic Catchment Area Sites. Arch Gen Psychiatry 45:977, 1988

ROBINSON RG et al: Two-year longitudinal study of poststroke mood disorders: Diagnosis and outcome at one and two years. Stroke 18(5):837, 1987

————, et al: Depression and diabetes. Diabetic Med 5(3):268, 1988

ROSENTHAL NE et al: Seasonal affective disorder: A description of the syndrome and preliminary findings with light therapy. Arch Gen Psychiatry 41:72, 1984

SELIGMAN MEP, BEAGLEY G: Learned helplessness in the rat. J Comp Physiol Psychol 88:534, 1975

STEWART AL et al: Functional status and well-being of patients with chronic conditions. Results from the Medical Outcomes Study. JAMA 262(7):907, 1989

WELLS KB et al: The functioning and well-being of depressed patients. Results from the Medical Outcomes Study. JAMA 262(7):914, 1989

WILLNER P: The validity of animal models of depression. Psychopharmacology 83:1, 1984

Anxiety disorders

AGRAS WS: The diagnosis and treatment of panic disorder. Annu Rev Med 44:39, 1993

CHARNEY DS et al: Noradrenergic function in panic anxiety. Arch Gen Psychiatry 41:75, 1984

———— et al: Psychobiologic mechanisms for posttraumatic stress disorder. Arch Gen Psychiatry 50:294, 1993

DIAMOND EL, GRAUER K: The spectrum of anxiety disorders in family practice. Am Fam Physician 36:167, 1987

GOLDBERG J et al: A twin study of the effects of the Vietnam war on posttraumatic stress disorder. JAMA 263:1227, 1990

HORWATH E et al: Epidemiology of panic disorder in African-Americans. Am J Psychiatry 150:465, 1993

KATON W: Panic disorder in the medical setting. Washington, DC, National Institute of Mental Health, Department of Health and Human Services publication (ADM), 1989

KECK PE et al: Valproate treatment of panic disorder and lactate-induced panic attacks. Biol Psychiatry 33:542, 1993

KELLER MB, HANKS DL: Course and outcome in panic disorder. Prog Neuropsychopharmacol Biol Psychiatry 17:551, 1993

KUSHNER MG et al: The relation between alcohol problems and anxiety disorders. Am J Psychiatry 47:685, 1990

MCGLYNN TJ, METCALF HL (eds): *Diagnosis and Treatment of Anxiety Disorders: A Physicians Handbook.* Washington DC, American Psychiatric Press, 1989, pp 43–48

MARKOWITZ JS et al: Quality of life in panic disorder. Arch Gen Psychiatry 46:984, 1989

SHADER RI, GREENBLATT DJ: Drug therapy. Use of benzodiazepines in anxiety disorders. N Engl J Med 328:1398, 1993

YEHUDA R et al: Psychoneuroendocrine assessment of posttraumatic stress disorder. Current progress and new directions. Prog Neuropsychopharmacol Biol Psychiatry 17:541, 1993

Schizophrenic disorders

ALVIR JMJ et al: Clozapine-induced agranulocytosis. Incidence and risk factors in the United States. N Engl J Med 329:162, 1993

BRAFF DL: Attention, information processing, and habituation in psychiatric disorders. Psychiatry, III. Philadelphia, Lippincott, 1985

————, GEYER MA: Sensorimotor gating in schizophrenia. Arch Gen Psychiatry 47:181, 1990

BROWN GW et al: Influence of family life on the course of schizophrenic disorders: A replication. Br J Psychiatry 11:241, 1972

CARLSON G, GOODWIN F: The stages of mania. Arch Gen Psychiatry 28:221, 1973

CHRISTISON GW et al: The quantitative investigation of hippocampal pyramidal cell size, shape and variability of orientation in schizophrenia. Arch Gen Psychiatry 46:1027, 1989

CROW TJ: Molecular pathology of schizophrenia: More than one disease process? Br Med J 280:66, 1980

DOCHERTY JP et al: Stages of onset of schizophrenic psychosis. Am J Psychiatry 135:420, 1978

GERSON SL: Clozapine. Deciphering the risks. N Engl J Med 329:204, 1993

JESTE DV, LOHR JB: Hippocampal pathologic findings in schizophrenia. Arch Gen Psychiatry 46:1019, 1989

ROSENBAUM CP: *The Meaning of Madness.* New York, Science House, 1970

ROSENTHAL D, KETY S: *The Transmission of Schizophrenia.* New York, Pergamon, 1968

SHANER A et al: Unrecognized cocaine use among schizophrenic patients. Am J Psychiatry 150:758, 1993

SHENTON ME et al: Abnormalities of the left temporal lobe and thought disorder in schizophrenia. N Engl J Med 327:604, 1993

SIRIS SG et al: Histories of substance abuse, panic and suicidal ideation in schizophrenic patients with histories of post-psychotic depressions. Prog Neuropsychopharmacol Biol Psychiatry 17:609, 1993

Special Issue: Negative symptoms in schizophrenia. Schizophr Bull 11, 1985

Special Issue: Advances in the genetics of schizophrenia. Schizophr Bull 15(3), 1989

Special Issue: The cost of schizophrenia. Schizophr Bull 17, 1991

STRAUSS JS, CARPENTER WT: *Schizophrenia.* New York, Plenum, 1981

WALKER E et al: Environmental factors related to schizophrenia in psychophysiologically labile high-risk males. J Abnorm Psychol 90:313, 1981

WEINBERGER DR: Implications of normal brain development for the pathogenesis of schizophrenia. Arch Gen Psychiatry 44:660, 1987

WETZEL H, BENKERT O: Dopamine autoreceptor agonists in the treatment of schizophrenic disorders. Prog Neuropsychopharmacol Biol Psychiatry 17:525, 1993

WYSOWSKI DK, BAUM C: Antipsychotic drug use in the United States, 1976–1985. Arch Gen Psychiatry 46:929, 1989

section 5 Alcoholism and drug dependency

390 ALCOHOL AND ALCOHOLISM

MARC A. SCHUCKIT

Ninety percent of people drink alcohol, 40 to 50 percent of men have temporary alcohol-induced problems, and 10 percent of men and 3 to 5 percent of women develop pervasive and persistent alcohol-related problems (alcoholism). The usual alcoholic has a family and a job; only about 5 percent fit the skid row stereotype. Even light drinking may adversely interact with other medications, temporary heavier drinking can exacerbate most medical illnesses, and alcoholism can masquerade as many different medical disorders and psychiatric syndromes. The following sections describe the pharmacology and clinical effects of alcohol and identify circumstances where drinking may cause a major medical or psychiatric problem or exacerbate a preexisting disorder. While these comments apply to the hypothetical "average" person, there is considerable individual variability depending on genetic vulnerability, concomitant drug use, and prior unrelated pathology or disease.

PHARMACOLOGY OF ETHANOL: ABSORPTION AND METABOLISM Ethanol is a weakly charged molecule that moves easily through cell membranes, rapidly equilibrating between blood and tissues. The effects of drinking depend in part on the amount of ethanol consumed per unit of body weight; the level of alcohol in the blood is expressed as milligrams or grams of ethanol per deciliter (e.g., 100 mg/dL or 0.1000 g/dL). In round figures, 340 mL (12 oz) of beer, 115 mL (4 oz) of nonfortified wine, and 43 mL (1.5 oz) (a shot) of 80-proof beverage each contain approximately 10 g of ethanol; 1 pint of 86-proof beverage contains approximately 160 g and 1 L of wine contains approximately 80 g of ethanol. Congeners found in alcohol beverages may contribute to body damage with heavy drinking; these include low-molecular-weight alcohols (e.g., methanol and butanol), aldehydes, esters, histamine, phenols, tannins, iron, lead, and cobalt.

Ethanol is a central nervous system (CNS) depressant that decreases activity of neurons, although some behavioral stimulation is observed at low blood levels. This drug has cross-tolerance and shares a similar pattern of behavioral problems with other brain depressants, including the benzodiazepines, barbiturates, and other sedatives and hypnotics. Alcohol is absorbed from mucous membranes of the mouth and esophagus (in very small amounts), from the stomach and large bowel (in modest amounts), and from the proximal portion of the small intestine (the major site). The rate of absorption *increases* with: rapid gastric emptying; the absence of proteins, fats, or carbohydrates (which interfere with absorption); the absence of congeners; dilution to a modest percentage of ethanol (maximum absorption is seen at about 20 percent by volume); and carbonation (champagne).

Between 2 percent (at low blood alcohol concentrations) and about 10 percent (at high blood alcohol concentrations) of ethanol is excreted directly through the lungs, urine, or sweat, but the greater part is metabolized to acetaldehyde in the liver. At least two metabolic routes, each with different optimal concentrations of ethanol (K_m), result in the metabolism of approximately one drink per hour. The *first* and clinically most important pathway occurs in the cell cytosol via alcohol dehydrogenase (ADH) with a K_m of about 2 mmol. This reaction produces acetaldehyde, which is then rapidly destroyed by aldehyde dehydrogenase (ALDH) in the cytosol and mitochondria.

Each of these steps requires nicotinamide adenine dinucleotide (NAD) as a cofactor, and it is the increased ratio of the reduced cofactor (NADH) to NAD (NADH:NAD) that is responsible for many of the metabolic derangements observed after drinking. *Second*, microsomes of the smooth endoplasmic reticulum (the microsomal ethanol-oxidizing system or MEOS) with a K_m of about 10 mmol may be responsible for 10 percent or more of ethanol oxidation at high blood alcohol concentrations. Increased activity of this system can be induced after repeated exposure to ethanol.

All pathways result in the production of acetaldehyde, which is oxidized to acetate. The specific clinical significance of acetaldehyde is not fully known, but low levels of this substance may cause stimulation and behavioral reinforcement. Accumulation of higher levels in liver, brain, or other body tissues may cause organ damage.

BEHAVIORAL EFFECTS, TOLERANCE, AND DEPENDENCE The behavioral and physiologic effects of any drug depend on the dose, its rate of increase in plasma, the concomitant presence of other drugs or medical problems, and the past experience with the agent. With alcohol, one also must consider whether observation is during rising (where the effects are more intense) or falling blood alcohol levels.

Even though "legal intoxication" requires a blood alcohol concentration of at least 80 to 100 mg/dL (0.1 g/dL), behavioral, psychomotor, and cognitive changes are seen at levels as low as 20 to 30 mg/dL (i.e., after one to two drinks). Narcosis or deep sleep is induced in many people at twice the legal intoxication level, and even in the absence of concomitant medications, death can occur with levels between 300 and 400 mg/dL. Ethanol, either alone or in combination with agents such as benzodiazepines, is probably responsible for more toxic overdose deaths than any other agent.

The mechanisms of action of ethanol on nervous tissues are not fully understood because even modest doses simultaneously change many neurotransmitters and increase the fluidity of neuronal cell membranes. After repeated exposure to the drug, the body compensates in at least three ways to tolerate higher ethanol levels. *First*, after 1 to 2 weeks of daily drinking the liver can increase the metabolic rate of ethanol by as much as 30 percent; i.e., there is *metabolic or pharmacokinetic tolerance*, an alteration that disappears almost as rapidly as it develops. *Second, cellular or pharmacodynamic tolerance* probably occurs through complex neurochemical changes in cell membranes with subsequent altered ion flow—adjustments that may contribute to physical dependence. *Third*, even at the same blood alcohol concentrations and neuronal adaptation, organisms can learn to adapt behavior and to function better than expected under drug influence (*behavioral tolerance*). For example, practicing driving while intoxicated might result in a psychomotor performance which (*while still impaired*) is better than that observed before practice.

Once the cells have adapted to chronic ethanol exposure, the structural or biochemical changes may not return to normal for several weeks or more. In the face of these adjustments, the neurons require ethanol to function optimally; i.e., the person is physically addicted or drug-dependent. This physical condition is distinct from psychological dependence, a poorly defined concept indicating that the person is psychologically uncomfortable without the drug.

NUTRITIONAL FACTORS One gram of ethanol has approximately 29.7 kJ (7.1 kcal), and a drink contains between 293.0 and 418.6 kJ (70 and 100 kcal) from ethanol and other carbohydrates. Therefore, 8 to 10 drinks can yield over 4186 kJ (1000 kcal) per day, but these are "empty" of nutrients such as minerals, proteins, and vitamins.

Any vitamin absorbed through the small intestine by active transport or stored in the liver may be deficient in alcoholics. These include folate (folacin or folic acid), pyridoxine (B_6), thiamine (B_1), nicotinic acid or niacin (B_3), and vitamin A. Thiamine deficiency causes Wernicke's and Korsakoff's syndromes (see Chap. 377).

Low blood potassium, magnesium, calcium, zinc, and phosphorus can occur as a consequence of dietary deficiency and acid-base imbalances during excess alcohol ingestion or withdrawal. Hypokalemia can lead to periodic muscle paralysis and areflexia. Deficiencies in magnesium can add to a clouded sensorium and other neurologic symptoms; hypocalcemia can cause tetany and weakness; low levels of zinc are speculated to contribute to gonadal dysfunction, anorexia, problems with wound healing, and immune deficiencies; and low phosphate levels can contribute to myocardial failure, brain dysfunction, weakness of muscles (including those of respiration), and white blood cell and platelet dysfunction.

An ethanol load in a fasting, healthy individual is likely to produce transient hypoglycemia within 6 to 36 h, secondary to the acute actions of ethanol on gluconeogenesis. This impairment is exacerbated by poor diet and by liver and pancreatic disease. As a result, glucose intolerance may be marked until the alcoholic has been abstinent for 2 to 4 weeks. Alcohol ketoacidosis, probably reflecting a decrease in fatty acid oxidation coupled with poor diet or recurrent vomiting, should not be misdiagnosed as diabetic ketosis. With the former, patients show an increase in serum ketones along with a mild increase in glucose but a large anion gap, a mild to moderate increase in serum lactate, and a β-hydroxybutyrate/lactate ratio of between 2:1 and 9:1 (with normal being 1:1).

THE EFFECTS OF ETHANOL ON BODY SYSTEMS

This overview of acute and chronic effects of alcohol on body systems outlines signs and symptoms that can aid in the recognition of the hidden alcoholic. It emphasizes the interactions between drinking and medications and the effects of alcohol on chronic medical conditions, factors that are also important in helping the clinician to understand the effects of alcohol on nonalcoholic patients.

CENTRAL NERVOUS SYSTEM In addition to acute behavioral effects, an evening of heavy drinking can result in an alcoholic *blackout*, i.e., an episode of forgetting all or part of what occurred during drinking. This problem is experienced by 30 to 40 percent of men in their late teens and early 20s, most of whom do not go on to develop more serious and pervasive alcohol-related problems. Even after only a few drinks, alcohol acutely decreases *sleep* latency (helping people to fall asleep) and depresses rapid eye movement (REM) sleep early in the night, sometimes followed by later REM rebound associated with bad dreams. The consequence is to "fragment" sleep, causing a more rapid than normal alternation between sleep stages and a deficiency in deep sleep. The overall effect is likely to be repeated awakenings and a sense of restless sleep.

Chronic intake of high doses of ethanol can cause *peripheral neuropathy* in 5 to 15 percent of alcoholics (see Chaps. 377 and 383). This syndrome probably results from both thiamine deficiency and direct effects of ethanol and/or acetaldehyde. Patients complain of bilateral limb numbness, tingling, and parasthesias, more pronounced distally than proximally. Although these symptoms can be incapacitating, more often the pain and numbness are mild to moderate in severity. The treatment is abstinence and thiamine supplementation.

Wernicke's and Korsakoff's syndromes are important problems in alcoholics (see Chap. 377). Thiamine deficiency is the major cause in vulnerable individuals (possibly interacting with a genetic transketolase deficiency). Classically, patients with Korsakoff's syndrome present with profound anterograde (unable to learn new material) and retrograde amnesia along with possible impairment in visuospatial, abstract, and conceptual reasoning but with a normal intelligence

quotient (IQ). In general, the level of recent memory loss is out of proportion to the global level of cognitive impairment. While most patients demonstrate an acute onset of Korsakoff's syndrome in association with the neurologic stigmata seen with Wernicke's syndrome (e.g., sixth nerve palsy and ataxia), some individuals may have a more gradual development of symptoms probably secondary to repeated bouts of thiamine deficiency. Wernicke's syndrome responds rapidly to oral thiamine replacement of 50 to 100 mg followed by 50 to 100 mg/d. However, only one-quarter of Korsakoff's patients are likely to achieve full recovery, one-half experience partial recovery, and one-quarter show no improvement with thiamine even after many months of supplementation.

About 1 percent of alcoholics with long histories of associated malnutrition develop *cerebellar degeneration*, a syndrome of progressive unsteady stance and gait often accompanied by mild nystagmus (see Chap. 377). Cerebellar atrophy is seen on CT scan or MRI, but the cerebrospinal fluid is usually normal. While ethanol or acetaldehyde may contribute to the problem, the major cause is probably nutritional, and identical symptoms can be seen with some forms of severe malnutrition alone. Treatment consists of abstinence and multiple vitamin supplementation, although improvement is often minimal.

Alcoholics can show severe *cognitive* problems and impairment in recent and remote memory for weeks to months after an alcoholic binge. Cortical functioning (e.g., psychomotor performance and short-term memory) tends to improve with abstinence, but long-term memory problems, perhaps reflecting subcortical damage, may persist. Increased size of the brain ventricles and cerebral sulci are seen in up to 50 percent of chronic alcoholics. These changes are partially reversible, returning toward normal after a year or more of abstinence. Permanent CNS impairment (*alcoholic dementia*) may supervene. Up to 20 percent of chronically demented patients may have had prior alcoholism. There is no single alcoholic dementia syndrome; rather, this label is used to describe patients who have apparently irreversible cognitive changes (possibly from diverse causes) in the midst of chronic alcoholism (see also Chap. 377).

Finally, to borrow a phrase from the past, alcohol could be termed "the great mimicker" because almost every psychiatric syndrome can be seen during heavy drinking or subsequent withdrawal. These include intense *sadness* lasting for days to weeks in the midst of heavy drinking, a problem that can be viewed as a "normal" effect of alcohol; severe *anxiety* during alcoholic withdrawal, often remaining for many months after cessation of drinking; *psychoses* during the severe form of the alcohol abstinence syndrome; and auditory *hallucinations* and/or *paranoid delusions* in the absence of any obvious signs of withdrawal—a state called *alcoholic hallucinosis* or *alcoholic paranoia*. Whatever the cause, the treatment of alcohol-induced psychopathology includes abstinence and supportive care, with the likelihood of full recovery within several days to 6 weeks. Alcohol intake is an important part of the differential diagnosis of *any* patient with one of these psychological symptoms. Another alcohol-related psychiatric syndrome is *pathologic intoxication* or alcohol idiosyncratic intoxication, a state of severe agitation, confusion, and violence lasting minutes to hours that is seen after a very low dose of ethanol (e.g., one to two drinks) and for which the individual is amnestic. This extremely rare phenomenon, seen almost exclusively in individuals with severe preexisting brain damage, is sometimes invoked erroneously for the purposes of legal defense.

THE GASTROINTESTINAL SYSTEM Esophagus and stomach Acute alcoholic intake can result in inflammation of the esophagus (possibly secondary to reflux of gastric contents) and stomach (resulting from damage to the gastric mucosal barrier). Esophagitis can cause epigastric distress, and gastritis, the most frequent cause of gastrointestinal bleeding in heavy drinkers, can present with anorexia and abdominal pain. Chronic heavy drinking, if associated with violent vomiting, can produce a longitudinal tear in the mucosa at the gastroesophageal junction—a Mallory-Weiss lesion. Although many gastrointestinal problems are reversible, two complications of chronic alcoholism, esophageal varices secondary to cirrhosis-induced portal hypertension and atrophy of gastric cells, may be irreversible (see Chaps. 251 and 253).

Small bowel The greater part of the ethanol is absorbed from the proximal small bowel, where it may interfere with absorption of B vitamins and other nutrients. Acutely, ethanol can cause hemorrhagic lesions of the duodenal villi and diarrhea secondary to increased small-bowel motility and decreased water and electrolyte absorption. Chronic alcoholism can contribute to diarrhea through its effects on the pancreas (see Chaps. 254 and 274).

Pancreas Alcoholics commonly develop acute or chronic pancreatitis (see Chap. 274).

Liver Ethanol absorbed from the small bowel is carried directly to the liver, where it becomes the preferred fuel; NADH accumulates and oxygen utilization escalates, gluconeogenesis is impaired (with a resulting fall in the amount of glucose produced from glycogen), lactate production increases, and there is a decreased oxidation of fatty acids in the citric cycle with an increase in fat accumulation within liver cells. In the healthy individual taking no medications, these changes are reversible, but with repeated exposure to ethanol more severe changes in liver functioning are likely to occur. These include, in overlapping stages, fatty accumulation, alcohol-induced hepatitis, and cirrhosis (see Chap. 268).

Increased cancer risk Cancer is the second leading cause of death in alcoholics (after cardiovascular disease), who have a rate of carcinoma 10 times higher than that expected in the general population. The sites with the greatest increase over expected rates include the head and neck, esophagus, cardia of the stomach, liver, pancreas, and, according to recent data, breast.

HEMATOPOIETIC SYSTEM Ethanol exerts multiple reversible acute and chronic effects on all blood cells. Alcohol alters acutely the production of red blood cells (RBC), and this reaches clinical significance after days to weeks of heavy drinking. The most common finding is an increase in RBC size (mean corpuscular volume, MCV) with a mild anemia. If this is accompanied by folic acid deficiency, there also can be hypersegmented neutrophils, reticulocytopenia, and hyperplastic bone marrow. Other forms of anemia, including sideroblastic changes, can occur concomitantly, especially in the presence of severe malnutrition.

Chronic heavy drinking also can decrease production of most white blood cells (WBC), decrease granulocyte mobility and adherence, and impair the delayed hypersensitivity response to new antigens (with a possible false-negative tuberculin skin test). While the changes in WBCs themselves are usually temporary, they may contribute to the risk of infections and liver damage and perhaps to the increased risk of cancers in alcoholics. Alcohol also can cause toxic granulocytosis.

Many alcoholics present with mild thrombocytopenia (rarely associated with hemorrhage) due to a decrease in platelet survival and altered function; hypersplenism may occur as a complication of cirrhosis. Alcohol may decrease platelet aggregation and inhibit release of thromboxane A_2. These problems usually return toward normal within a week of abstinence.

CARDIOVASCULAR SYSTEM Modest doses of alcohol can have both deleterious and beneficial effects in individuals with normal cardiovascular status who take no medications. Ethanol decreases myocardial contractility and causes peripheral vasodilatation, resulting in a mild drop in blood pressure and a compensatory increased heart rate and cardiac output. Exercise-induced increases in cardiac oxygen consumption are higher after alcohol. On the other hand, a maximum of one to two drinks per day over long periods may decrease the risk of cardiovascular death, perhaps through an increase in high-density lipoprotein (HDL) cholesterol or changes in clotting mechanisms.

Although ethanol in low doses causes a mild acute drop in blood pressure, the consumption of three or more drinks per day results in a dose-dependent increase in blood pressure which returns to normal within weeks of abstinence. As a result, heavy drinking is an important contributor to reversible causes of mild to moderate hypertension. Chronic heavy drinking can cause cardiomyopathy with symptoms

ranging from unexplained arrhythmias in the presence of left ventricular impairment to heart failure with dilatation of all four heart chambers and hypocontractility of heart muscle. Mural thrombi can form in the left atrium or ventricle, while heart enlargement exceeding 25 percent can cause mitral regurgitation. Finally, there is an association between cerebrovascular accidents and alcoholism, especially within 24 h of heavy drinking. Atrial or ventricular arrhythmias, especially paroxysmal tachycardia, also can occur after a binge in individuals showing no other evidence of heart disease—a syndrome known as the "holiday heart."

GENITOURINARY SYSTEM CHANGES, SEXUAL FUNCTIONING, AND FETAL DEVELOPMENT Acutely, modest ethanol doses (e.g., blood alcohol concentrations of 100 mg/dL or even less) increase sexual drive in men. However, modest ethanol doses may simultaneously decrease erectile capacity. Even in the absence of liver impairment, a significant minority of chronic alcoholic men may show irreversible testicular atrophy with concomitant shrinkage of the seminiferous tubules and loss of sperm cells (see Chap. 339).

The repeated ingestion of high doses of ethanol by women can result in amenorrhea, a decrease in ovarian size, an absence of corpora lutea with associated infertility, and spontaneous abortions. Heavy drinking during pregnancy results in the rapid placental transfer of both ethanol and acetaldehyde, which may have serious consequences for fetal development. The *fetal alcohol syndrome* can include a mixture of any of the following: facial changes with epicanthal eye folds, poorly formed concha, and small teeth with faulty enamel; cardiac atrial or ventricular septal defects; an aberrant palmar crease and limitation in joint movement; and microcephaly with mental retardation (see Chap. 378). The specific amount of ethanol and/or specific time of vulnerability during pregnancy have not been defined, making it advisable for pregnant women to abstain completely.

OTHER EFFECTS OF ETHANOL Heavy drinking can produce an acute *alcoholic myopathy* characterized by painful and swollen muscles, high levels of serum creatine phosphokinase (CK), and, rarely, myoglobinemia and myoglobinuria. Effects on the *skeletal system* include alterations in calcium metabolism with an increased risk for fractures and osteonecrosis of the femoral head. *Hormonal* changes include an increase in cortisol levels, which can remain elevated during heavy drinking; inhibition of vasopressin secretion at rising blood alcohol concentrations and the opposite at falling blood alcohol concentrations, with the final result that most alcoholics are likely to be slightly overhydrated; a modest and reversible decrease in serum thyroxine (T_4); and a more marked decrease in serum triiodothyronine (T_3).

ALCOHOLISM (ALCOHOL DEPENDENCE)

Because many drinkers occasionally imbibe to excess, temporary alcohol-related pathology is common in nonalcoholics. The time of heaviest drinking is usually the late teens to the late twenties, when between one-third and one-half of male drinkers experience some isolated (although potentially dangerous) alcohol-related social, occupational, or driving difficulty. These include alcohol-related blackouts, a single drunk driving arrest, arguments with friends, and so on. This prevalent alcohol-related morbidity, however, is temporary and a separate problem from alcohol dependence. The following sections describe diagnostic criteria for alcoholism, offer suggestions for identifying the usual (i.e., middle-class) alcoholic in everyday medical practice, review evidence that alcoholism is a biologic and genetically influenced disorder, and offer advice on confrontation, detoxification, and rehabilitation of alcoholics.

DEFINITIONS AND EPIDEMIOLOGY The most recent revised version of the *Third Diagnostic and Statistical Manual* of the American Psychiatric Association (DSM-IIIR) divides alcoholism into alcohol abuse and alcohol dependence. *Alcohol abuse* indicates alcohol-related life impairment interfering with functioning. *Alcohol dependence* encompasses similar impairment *along with* evidence of a strong compulsion to use alcohol accompanied by increased ethanol tolerance or physical signs on withdrawal from alcohol. The dependence criteria require that three of nine items be met and describe what many clinicians would label alcoholism.

A modified approach to a definition of alcoholism is easier to apply in clinical settings. The diagnosis of *alcoholism* is made when an individual ignores the early warning signs that alcohol is causing problems in marriage and goes on to an alcohol-related marital separation or divorce; *or* when alcohol-related problems on the job actually result in the patient being fired or laid off; *or* when there are two or more arrests related to alcohol; *or* when there is physical evidence that alcohol has harmed health (e.g., cardiomyopathy, cirrhosis, alcoholic hepatitis), including signs of alcoholic withdrawal.

It is important to distinguish between *primary* and *secondary alcoholism*. For example, serious alcohol-related problems occurring during the course of mania or a preexisting antisocial personality disorder (i.e., secondary alcoholism) might be symptomatic of the primary diagnosis, and the course is likely to be that of the primary disorder, not alcoholism. The information on alcoholism offered in this chapter is relevant for *primary alcoholism*. This diagnosis applies to the majority of alcoholics (70 to 80 percent) who develop major life problems from alcohol *before* they fulfill criteria for any other major psychiatric illness.

Using this or similar criteria, the lifetime risk for primary alcoholism in most western countries is about 10 percent for men and 3 to 5 percent for women. When less stringent criteria are used, the rates are substantially higher, but the clinical syndrome is not likely to accurately predict future problems. Alcoholism is seen in all races, ethnic groups, and socioeconomic strata, and therefore, the average alcoholic (just as the average person) is a blue-collar or white-collar worker or housewife. The homeless or skid row alcoholic represents only 5 percent or less of alcoholics.

GENETICS OF ALCOHOLISM There is strong evidence that alcoholism is a multifactorial disorder in which biologic and genetic factors interact. The importance of genetic factors in alcoholism is supported by family, twin, and adoption studies. Close relatives of primary alcoholics have an approximately fourfold increased risk for the disorder but are not significantly more vulnerable for other psychiatric illnesses. The probability that the familial nature of the problem is in part a consequence of genetic factors is supported by twin research, where the risk for the identical twin of an alcoholic is much higher than for the fraternal twin of an alcohol abuser. Finally, adoption studies reveal that the fourfold increased risk for children of alcoholics is true even if they were adopted away at birth and raised without knowledge of the problems of their biologic parents.

The evidence supporting genetic influences in alcoholism has stimulated numerous studies of children of alcoholics. The goal is to identify possible trait markers of a vulnerability toward the disorder before alcoholism appears. For example, some studies suggest that these children become significantly less intoxicated at a given blood alcohol concentration than do controls, even before alcoholism develops. After modest alcohol doses, the sons of alcoholics report less intense subjective feelings of intoxication, show less alcohol-related impairment in cognitive and psychomotor tests, and have less intense changes in prolactin and cortisol secretion than do controls. These data may indicate that men at high future risk for alcoholism may be less able than controls to tell when they are beginning to become intoxicated. Taken as a whole, these data underscore the probability that alcoholism is biologically influenced and not related to a lack of "moral fiber." It is not surprising that the average alcoholic may continue to work, has a family, and may be difficult to identify if the physician persists with old stereotypes.

NATURAL HISTORY For the "average" alcoholic, the age of first drink and first minor problems (e.g., an argument with a friend while drunk or an alcoholic blackout) are similar to those in the general population. However, by the middle to late twenties, most men and women moderate their drinking (perhaps learning from minor problems), whereas difficulties for alcoholics are likely to escalate,

with the first major life problem from alcohol appearing in the late twenties to early forties. Once established, the course of alcoholism is likely to be one of exacerbations and remissions; the alcoholic becomes frightened when a problem develops and abstains for a period of days to months before experimenting with controlled drinking; this step almost inevitably results in escalation of drinking and problems. The course is not hopeless because a fifth or more achieve permanent abstinence without formal treatment or aid from self-help groups such as Alcoholics Anonymous (AA). However, should the alcoholic continue to drink, the life span is shortened by an average of 15 years, with the leading causes of death, in decreasing order, being heart disease, cancer, accidents, and suicide.

IDENTIFICATION AND CONFRONTATION OF THE ALCOHOLIC The physician should recognize that any patient may have alcoholism and must therefore pay attention to physical findings and laboratory tests that are likely to be abnormal in the alcoholic. These include a high normal or slightly elevated MCV, γ-glutamyl transferase (GGT) (35 or more units), serum uric acid [greater than 416 µmol/L (7 mg/dL)], and triglycerides [2.0 mmol/L (180 mg/dL) or more]. Mild and fluctuating levels of hypertension (e.g., 140/95), repeated infections such as pneumonia, and otherwise unexplained cardiac arrhythmias all suggest that the patient might be an alcoholic. Certain specific clinical findings also should raise suspicions, including cancer of the head and neck, esophagus, or cardia of the stomach as well as cirrhosis, unexplained hepatitis, pancreatitis, bilateral parotid gland swelling, and peripheral neuropathy.

Once the likelihood of alcoholism is established, only a few moments are needed to gather the history of alcohol-related life problems. The patient *and spouse* should be asked about patterns of accidents, marital difficulties, problems on the job, and driving-related difficulties, after which the role played by alcohol should be identified. All physicians should be able to take the time needed to gather such information. In addition, a simple 25-item form to be answered by the patient, the Michigan Alcohol Screening Test (MAST), is available to aid in identifying the alcoholic. However, this is only a screening tool, and a careful face-to-face interview is still required for a meaningful diagnosis.

After an alcoholic is identified, he or she should be confronted with the diagnosis. The presenting complaint can be used as an entrée to the alcohol problem. For instance, the patient complaining of insomnia or hypertension could be told that these are clinically important symptoms and that laboratory tests and physical findings indicate that alcohol appears to have contributed to the complaints and is increasing the risk for further medical and psychological problems. The physician should share information about the course of alcoholism and explore possible avenues of attacking the problem.

The process of confrontation is rarely accomplished in one session. It is helpful to let patients know that they are responsible for their own actions and that the decision to quit drinking rests with them. For the person who refuses to stop drinking at the first confrontation, a logical step is to "keep the door open," establishing future meetings so that help is available as problems escalate. In the meantime the family may benefit from counseling or referral to self-help group such as Alanon (the Alcoholics Anonymous group for family members) and Alateen (for teenage children of alcoholics).

Those patients who refuse to stop but who want to "cut down" should be reminded that the average alcoholic successfully cuts back scores of times but that sooner or later drinking again escalates. The patient who refuses to stop might be offered a guideline of drinking no more than two drinks [115 mL (4 oz) of wine, 340 mL (12 oz) of beer, or 43 mL (1.5 oz) of 80-proof beverage amounts to one drink] in any 24-h period, but it is very unlikely that this will be effective for an extended period of time. This is another way of keeping the door open in the hope that the patient will return as drinking escalates.

TREATMENT OF THE ALCOHOL-RELATED WITHDRAWAL SYNDROME The clinical syndrome In the presence of ethanol-induced cellular tolerance, any sudden decrease in ethanol may lead to symptoms of withdrawal from the CNS depressant effects. As with most syndromes, most patients do not develop every symptom, and the usual clinical picture is mild. Features include a tremor of the hands (shakes or jitters); autonomic nervous system dysfunction such as increases in pulse, respiratory rate, and body temperature; insomnia, possibly accompanied by bad dreams; feelings of generalized anxiety or panic attacks; and gastrointestinal upset. Symptoms begin within 5 to 10 h of decreasing ethanol intake (addicted patients are likely to awaken in the morning with some signs of withdrawal), peak in intensity on day 2 or 3, and improve by day 4 or 5. Anxiety, insomnia, and mild levels of autonomic dysfunction may persist for 6 months or more as a protracted abstinence syndrome that may contribute to the tendency to return to drinking.

About 5 percent of alcoholics show evidence of severe withdrawal symptoms. These include a state of confusion sometimes accompanied by visual, tactile, or auditory hallucinations. These psychotic symptoms are likely to disappear as the mental state becomes clearer over a period of several days and are distinct from the chronic alcoholic auditory hallucinosis with a clear sensorium described earlier in this chapter. A small percentage of alcoholics also demonstrate one or two generalized seizures (''rum fits''), usually within 48 h of stopping drinking. These are rarely focal in nature (unless there is underlying neuropathology), and electroencephalographic abnormalities are mild and usually return to normal within several days. There is no evidence that withdrawal seizures represent ''latent'' epilepsy.

The diagnosis of delirium tremens (DTs) is made when the course progresses beyond the usual symptoms of withdrawal to include confusion (with associated delusions and hallucinations), severe agitation, and generalized seizures. The likelihood of developing severe withdrawal symptoms increases with concomitant infections or medical problems, a prior history of withdrawal seizures or DTs, and higher quantity and frequency of drinking. Most periods of severe withdrawal begin and end abruptly, rarely lasting longer than 3 to 5 days. The mortality risk for DTs is quite low but increases with preexisting medical illnesses or organ system failure.

Treatment of withdrawal   The *first* and most important step is to perform a *thorough* physical examination in all alcoholics who are considering stopping drinking and in those patients who might be undergoing withdrawal. It is necessary to evaluate organ systems likely to be impaired by heavy drinking, including searching for evidence of liver failure, gastrointestinal bleeding, cardiac arrhythmia, and glucose or electrolyte imbalance.

The *second* step in treating withdrawal is to give patients adequate nutrition and rest. All patients should be administered multiple B vitamins, including 50 to 100 mg of thiamine daily for a week or more. Most patients enter withdrawal with normal levels of body water or mild levels of overhydration, and intravenous fluids should be avoided unless there is evidence of hypotension or a history of recent excessive bleeding, vomiting, or diarrhea. Usually medications can be administered orally.

The *third* step in treatment is to recognize the CNS symptoms caused by removal of the brain-depressant effects of ethanol. Symptoms can be alleviated by administering another CNS depressant and gradually decreasing the levels of the drug over a 3- to 5-day period. While many CNS depressants are effective, the *benzodiazepines* have the highest margin of safety and are, therefore, the preferred class of drugs in the treatment of alcohol withdrawal. Benzodiazepines with short half-lives (see Chap. 389) are especially useful for patients with serious liver impairment or evidence of preexisting encephalopathy or brain damage. On the other hand, short-half-life benzodiazepines, e.g., oxazepam or lorazepam, result in rapidly changing drug blood levels; administration every 4 h is required to avoid abrupt fluctuations in blood levels that may increase the risk for seizures. Therefore, most clinicians use drugs with longer half-lives, such as diazepam or chlordiazepoxide. The goal is to administer sufficient drug on day 1 to alleviate most of the symptoms of withdrawal and then to decrease the dose by 20 percent on successive days over a period of 3 to 5 days. The dose is increased if signs of withdrawal escalate, and the medication is withheld if the patient is sleeping or shows signs of

increasing orthostatic hypotension. The average patient requires 25 to 50 mg of chlordiazepoxide or 10 mg of diazepam given orally every 4 to 6 h on the first day.

The most effective treatment of *severe withdrawal* including delirium tremens remains controversial. Most clinicians use benzodiazepines, but despite as much as 300 mg or more per day of chlordiazepoxide, the patient may still remain awake and agitated. Since it is probable that the confused, agitated state will persist for 3 to 5 days regardless of the pharmacologic intervention used, drugs are given to control behavior rather than to change the course of the syndrome. Antipsychotic medications such as thioridazine or haloperidol are sometimes used for these delirium tremens (DTs), although they must be prescribed with care because they might lower the seizure threshold. The antipsychotic drugs, however, have no place in the treatment of mild withdrawal symptoms.

The generalized seizures or ''rum fits'' rarely require aggressive pharmacologic intervention beyond that given to the usual patient undergoing withdrawal, i.e., adequate doses of benzodiazepines. There is little evidence that phenytoin is effective in drug-withdrawal seizures, and the risk of seizures usually has passed by the time effective drug levels are reached. The rare patient with status epilepticus can be treated initially with intravenous diazepam. If anticonvulsants are used for alcohol-withdrawal seizures, they should be stopped within 5 to 7 days unless a cause for a persisting seizure disorder is documented.

While alcohol withdrawal is often treated in a hospital, efforts at reducing costs have resulted in experimentation with outpatient detoxification for alcoholics with mild abstinence syndromes. This outpatient approach is appropriate for patients in good physical condition who demonstrate mild signs of withdrawal despite low blood alcohol concentrations and for those without prior history of DTs or withdrawal seizures. Such individuals still require careful physical examination, evaluation of blood tests, and treatment with vitamin supplementation, and appropriate doses of benzodiazepines also might be used. The latter are given *in a 1- to 2-day supply* to be administered to the patient by a spouse four times a day. Patients are asked to *return daily* for evaluation of vital signs, and the patient's family or friends are told to bring him or her to the emergency room if signs and symptoms of withdrawal escalate.

THE TREATMENT OR REHABILITATION OF ALCOHOLICS

After completing alcoholic rehabilitation, 60 percent or more of middle-class alcoholics maintain abstinence for at least a year, many for a lifetime. There is no single best way to rehabilitate the alcoholic, and therapeutic approaches center on general supports that meet commonsense guidelines. Considering the lack of evidence for superiority of any specific treatment type, it is best to keep interventions as simple, safe, and inexpensive as possible.

Maneuvers in rehabilitation fall into two general categories. *First* are attempts to help the alcoholic achieve and maintain a high level of motivation toward abstinence. These include educating the patient about alcoholism, and teaching the family and/or friends to stop protecting the alcoholic from the problems caused by alcohol. The *second* series of maneuvers helps the patient to readjust to life without alcohol and to reestablish a functional lifestyle through personal counseling, vocational rehabilitation, family support, and sexual counseling.

There is no convincing evidence that inpatient rehabilitation is always more effective for the average primary alcoholic than is outpatient care. The decision to hospitalize can be made if (1) the patient has medical problems that are difficult to treat outside a hospital, (2) depression, confusion, or psychosis interfere with outpatient care, (3) the patient has such a severe life crisis that it is difficult to get his or her attention as an outpatient, (4) outpatient treatment has failed, or (5) the patient lives too far from the treatment center. If inpatient care is needed, free-standing treatment programs, units that are divisions of general hospitals, and those in psychiatric hospitals are equally effective. The characteristics of the patient predict outcome more than any specific attribute of the program.

Whether the treatment begins in an inpatient or an outpatient setting, subsequent contact should be maintained for a minimum of 6 months and preferably a full year after abstinence is achieved. Counseling with an individual physician or through groups focuses on day-to-day living—emphasizing areas of improved functioning in the absence of alcohol (i.e., why it is a good idea to continue to abstain) and helping the patient to deal with free time without alcohol, develop a nondrinking peer group, and handle stresses on the job without alcohol.

The physician serves an important role in identifying the alcoholic, treating medical or psychiatric syndromes associated with alcoholism, carrying out detoxification, referring to rehabilitation programs, and counseling alcoholics in an inpatient or outpatient setting. The physician also must regulate drug treatment during alcoholism rehabilitation. Once acute detoxification is complete (an average of 3 to 5 days), there is *no place* for hypnotics or antianxiety drugs in the treatment of most alcoholics. The patient has already demonstrated an inability to moderate the use of one brain depressant, alcohol, and is at considerable risk for abusing sleeping pills or tranquilizers. Anxiety and insomnia can be treated with behavior modification such as relaxation training, meditation, and exercise or through increased activity in hobbies or religion. For example, regarding insomnia, patients should be reassured that this is normal after alcohol withdrawal and will improve over the subsequent weeks and months. They should then follow a rigid bedtime and awakening schedule, avoiding any naps or use of caffeine in the evenings. The sleep pattern will improve rapidly.

One medication that has been used in alcohol rehabilitation is disulfiram, usually given as 250 mg/d. This drug inhibits aldehyde dehydrogenase, causing very high levels of acetaldehyde to accumulate after alcohol is consumed. The disulfiram-ethanol reaction includes tremor, hypertension or hypotension, nausea and possibly severe vomiting, and diarrhea. Disulfiram must not be given to persons for whom such a reaction could be dangerous, including patients with portal hypertension, diabetes mellitus, heart disease, or a history of stroke. All drugs have their dangers, and the physician is advised to read carefully about disulfiram and be fully aware of the potential, although rare, serious adverse reactions that can occur. Unfortunately, there is little convincing evidence from carefully controlled studies that the effectiveness of disulfiram is significantly greater than placebo. As result, this drug should not be routinely prescribed.

Finally, an inexpensive, readily available, and dedicated additional support for all alcoholics is available in almost every community. Alcoholics Anonymous is a self-help group of recovering alcoholics (men and women who have stopped drinking, perhaps many years ago) that offers an effective model showing that abstinence can be achieved, provides a sober peer group, and makes crisis intervention available when the drive to drink escalates. No matter what type of rehabilitation program is planned, the alcoholic should be offered the option of joining Alcoholics Anonymous.

REFERENCES

BLUM K et al: Allelic association of human dopamine D₂ receptor gene in alcoholism. JAMA 263:2055, 1990

CRIQUI MH: Alcohol consumption, blood pressure, lipids, and cardiovascular mortality. Alc Clin Exp Res 10:564, 1986

DONAHUE RP et al: Alcohol and hemorrhagic stroke. JAMA 255:2311, 1986

FULLER RK et al: Disulfiram treatment of alcoholism. JAMA 256:1449, 1986

GOODWIN DW, GUZE SB: *Psychiatric Diagnosis*, 4th ed. New York, Oxford University Press, 1989

GRANT I: Alcohol and the brain. JCCP 55:310, 1987

GREENSPON AJ, SCHAAL SF: The "holiday heart": Electrophysiologic studies of alcohol effects in alcoholics. Ann Intern Med 98:135, 1983

HARPER C et al: Are we drinking our neurones away? Br Med J 294:534, 1987

IRWIN M et al: Monitoring heavy drinking. Am J Psychiatry 145:595, 1988

ISHAK KG et al: Alcoholic liver disease: Pathologic, pathogenetic and clinical aspects. Alc Clin Exp Res 15:45, 1991

JERNIGAN TL et al: Reduced cerebral gray matter observed in alcoholics using magnetic resonance imaging. Alc Clin Exp Res 15:418, 1991

LIEBER C: *Metabolic Aspects of Alcoholism*. Lancaster, England, MTP Press, 1987

————: To drink (moderately) or not to drink? N Engl J Med 310:846, 1984

LISKOW BI, GOODWIN DW: Pharmacological treatment of alcohol intoxication, withdrawal, and dependence. J Stud Alcohol 48:356, 1987

LITTEN RZ et al: Pharmacotherapies for alcoholism. Alc Clin Exp Res 15:620, 1991

MAHESWARAN R et al: High blood pressure due to alcohol: A rapidly reversible effect. Hypertension 17:787, 1991

MEAGHER RC et al: Suppression of hematopoietic-progenitor-cell proliferation by ethanol and acetaldehyde. N Engl J Med 307:845, 1982

MELLO NK, BREE MP: Alcohol self-administration disrupts reproductive function in female macaque monkeys. Science 221:677, 1983

MENDELSON JH, MELLO NK: Biologic concomitants of alcoholism. N Engl J Med 301:912, 1979

MUKHREJEE AB et al: Transketolase abnormality in fibroblasts from chronic alcoholics. J Clin Invest 79:1039, 1987

ÖJEHAGEN A et al: Long-term use of aversive drugs in outpatient alcoholism treatment. Acta Psychiatr Scand 84:185, 1991

PFEFFERBAUM A et al: Brain CT changes in alcoholics. Alc Clin Exp Res 12:81, 1988

POTTER JF, BEEVERS DG: Pressor effect of alcohol in hypertension. Lancet 1:119, 1984

RUSSELL M et al: Measures of maternal alcohol use as predictors of development in early childhood. Alc Clin Exp Res 15:991, 1991

SCHUCKIT MA et al: A simultaneous evaluation of multiple markers of ethanol response in sons of alcoholics. Arch Gen Psychiatry 45:211, 1988

————: Genetic and clinical implications of alcoholism and affective disorder. Am J Psychiatry 143:140, 1986

————: *Drug and Alcohol Abuse: A Clinical Guide to Diagnosis and Treatment*, 3d ed. New York, Plenum, 1989

SCHUCKIT MA: *Alcohol Patterns and Problems*. New Brunswick, NJ, Rutgers Press, 1985

————: Genetics and the risk for alcoholism. JAMA 254:2614, 1985

SELLERS EM, KALANT H: Alcohol intoxication and withdrawal. N Engl J Med 294:757, 1976

VAILLANT GE: *The Natural History of Alcoholism*. Cambridge, Mass., Harvard University Press, 1983

VAN THIEL DH: Gastrointestinal and hepatic manifestations of chronic alcoholism. Gastroenterology 81:594, 1981

VICTOR M, ADAMS RD: *The Wernicke-Korsakoff Syndrome*, 2d ed. Philadelphia, Davis, 1989

WALSH DC et al: Treatment options for alcohol abusing workers. N Engl J Med 325:775, 1991

WALSH JK et al: Sedative effects of ethanol at night. J Stud Alcohol 52:597, 1991

391 OPIOID DRUG USE

MARC A. SCHUCKIT / DAVID S. SEGAL

The principal effects of the opioids (opiate-like drugs) are a significant damping of pain perception along with modest levels of sedation and euphoria. Drugs in this category range from heroin, morphine, and codeine to many nonsteroidal prescription analgesics and many antitussive agents. Thus comments made in this section have wide application in medicine and go far beyond the classical street addict.

Tolerance to any one opioid is likely to generalize to the others (i.e., cross-tolerance is likely), and all share a similar pattern of drug-related problems. Each of these substances is capable of producing physical addiction (and thus they all have some legal restrictions), and the abstinence syndrome from any one of the substances can be treated with administration of any of the others.

PHARMACOLOGY The prototypic opiates, morphine and codeine (3-methoxymorphine), are taken directly from the milky juice of the poppy, *Papaver somniferum*. The semisynthetic drugs produced from the morphine or thebane molecules include hydromorphone, codeine, diacetylmorphine (heroin), and oxycodone. The purely synthetic opioids, sharing many of the basic properties of opium and morphine, include meperidine, propoxyphene, diphenoxylate, buprenorphine, methadone, and pentazocine. Despite claims to the contrary, all these substances (including almost all prescription analgesics) are capable of producing euphoria as well as psychological and physical dependence when taken in high enough doses over prolonged periods of time.

The opioids produce their effects by binding to different types of opioid receptors throughout the body, including the central nervous system. Endogenous opioid peptides (i.e., enkephalins, endorphins, dynorphin, and others) have been identified that appear to be natural ligands for opioid receptors. These peptides have a distinct distribution in the CNS. Recent evidence suggests that the receptors with which opioid peptides interact may be differentially engaged in production of the various opiate effects such as analgesia, respiratory depression, constipation, and euphoria. Substances capable of antagonizing one or more of these actions include nalorphine, levallophan, cyclazocine, buprenorphine, and pentazocine, each of which has mixed agonist and antagonist properties, as well as naloxone and naltrexone, which are pure opiate antagonists. Mixed agonist-antagonist drugs (e.g., pentazocine), if administered to a patient addicted to other narcotics, may precipitate opiate withdrawal symptoms. The availability of relatively specific antagonists has helped identify different receptor subtypes, including the μ_1 and μ_2 subtypes, which affect some of the more classical opioid actions such as pain control and respirations; *kappa* receptors, with similar functions along with sedation and effects on hormones; *sigma* receptors, which have an impact on mood, hallucinations and delusions; and *delta* receptors, thought to respond preferentially to endogenous opiates.

Opiate tolerance, dependence, and withdrawal are considered to be related phenomena and may share some common underlying mechanisms. A number of neurochemical systems and psychological processes appear to be implicated in these effects that emerge with chronic administration of morphine or related opiates. Perhaps reflecting the actions of different classes of receptors, tolerance to various opiate actions may develop at different rates, and these same mechanisms may contribute to the diverse signs and symptoms characteristic of withdrawal. Other biochemical systems that may contribute to the development of tolerance and dependence include changes in intracellular modulators such as adenyl nucleotides, calcium, and related substances, as well as alterations in neurotransmitters, including acetylcholine, serotonin, and the catecholamines norepinephrine and dopamine. Evidence also implicates environmental and learning factors. For example, clinical observations suggest that classic conditioning plays a role in maintaining dependence in at least some addicts and that conditioning extinction procedures may be useful when integrated into a comprehensive treatment program for opioid addiction. Further research into these phenomena and efforts to elucidate neurochemical mechanisms could significantly facilitate the development of more effective approaches to treatment and prevention.

All the opioid drugs are easily absorbed from the gastrointestinal system, the lungs, and/or the muscles. The most rapid and pronounced effects occur following intravenous administration, with only slightly less efficient absorption after smoking or after inhaling the vapor (''chasing the dragon''), and the least intense actions are seen after absorption from the digestive tract, at least in part because some of the oral drug is metabolized before it passes into the general circulation. Most of the metabolism of opiates occurs in the liver, primarily through conjugation with glucuronic acid, and only small amounts are excreted directly in the urine or feces. The plasma half-lives of these drugs range from 2.5 to 3 h for morphine to more than 22 h for methadone and even longer for methadyl acetate.

Street heroin typically contains only 5 to 10 percent of the opiate. The remainder consists of materials such as lactose and fruit sugars, quinine, powdered milk, phenacetin, caffeine, antipyrine, and strychnine which are used to ''cut'' the drug and increase the margin of profit. Any marked unexpected increase in the purity of street drugs is likely to cause unintentional lethal overdoses in addicts expecting less effect from a ''hit.''

THE ACUTE AND CHRONIC EFFECTS OF OPIOID DRUGS ON BODY SYSTEMS With the exception of overdose conditions and changes associated with physical addiction, most opiate actions are relatively benign and rapidly reversible.

Effects on body systems Acute changes in the *gastrointestinal system* are the result of decreased GI motility with resulting constipation and anorexia. Chronic GI problems in opiate addicts typically occur as a consequence of impaired liver function resulting from concomitant administration of other drugs and from the development of hepatitis B from shared ''dirty'' needles.

The direct effects on opiate receptors in the *central nervous system* can result in nausea and vomiting (medulla), decreased pain perception (spinal cord, thalamus, and periaqueductal gray region), euphoria (limbic system), and sedation (reticular activating system and striatum). The adulterants added to street drugs may contribute to some of the more permanent nervous system damage, including peripheral neuropathy, amblyopia, myelopathy, and leukoencephalopathy, while use of contaminated needles can produce abscesses in the CNS and transmit AIDS. The latter has become a major health problem contributing significantly to the spread of this lethal disease among addicts and their sexual partners. Whether from the opiate, adulterants, or the consequences of dirty needles, at least one recent study revealed CNS defects in both cognition and CT evaluations of addicts. Acute opiate administration results in decreases in luteinizing hormone (LH), with a subsequent decrease in testosterone, which might contribute to the decreased sex drive reported by most opiate addicts. Other hormonal changes include a decrease in the release of thyrotropin as well as increases in prolactin and possibly in growth hormone (see Chap. 331).

Acute changes in the *respiratory system* include respiratory depression, which results from a decreased response of the brainstem to carbon dioxide tension, a component of the drug overdose syndrome described below. At even low drug doses, this effect can be clinically significant in individuals with compromised lung activity. *Cardiovascular* changes tend to be relatively mild, with no direct opiate effect on heart rhythm or myocardial contractility, but there is a potential problem from orthostatic hypotension, probably secondary to dilatation of peripheral vessels. Bacterial infections of both the lungs and heart valves can occur from contaminated needles, with the latter capable of producing emboli and a subsequent enhanced risk for stroke.

The toxic reaction or overdose syndrome High doses of opiates taken intentionally (in a suicide attempt) or by the street user who has misjudged the potency of the injected substance can result in a toxic reaction or overdose syndrome with a potentially lethal consequence. The typical syndrome, which occurs immediately with intravenous (IV) overdose, includes shallow respirations of two to four per minute, pupillary miosis (with mydriasis once brain anoxia develops), bradycardia, a decrease in body temperature, and a general absence of responsiveness to external stimulation. If this medical emergency is not treated rapidly, symptoms can progress to cyanosis, and death can ensue from respiratory depression and cardiorespiratory arrest. Postmortem examination reveals few specific changes except for diffuse cerebral edema. An ''allergic-like'' reaction, apparently at least in part related to adulterants, also can occur and is characterized by decreased alertness, a frothy pulmonary edema, and an elevation in the blood eosinophil count.

The first step in treating any overdose is to support the vital signs through a respirator and other emergency procedures. The preferred more definitive treatment for the typical opiate overdose is the narcotic antagonist naloxone given in an initial dose of 0.4 mg (1 mL) or 0.01 mg/kg intramuscularly (IM) or IV, which can be repeated in 3 to 10 min if no response occurs. Because the effects of this drug diminish within 2 to 3 h, it is important to monitor the individual for at least 24 h after a heroin overdose and 72 h after an overdose of longer-acting drugs such as methadone. Patients who are also physically addicted to an opioid are likely to experience a precipitous onset of an abstinence syndrome within 2 to 8 h after administration of the opioid antagonist, but aggressive treatment of this syndrome is not appropriate until all vital signs are relatively stable.

As with any drug overdose, treatment of either the typical or the ''allergic'' type of opiate toxic reaction often requires continued support of vital signs until the body detoxifies the substance. Patients may require a respirator (especially one using oxygen and positive-pressure breathing for the ''allergic'' type of overdose), IV fluids perhaps accompanied by pressor agents to support blood pressure, and gastric lavage to remove any remaining drug, with care taken to use a cuffed endotracheal tube to prevent aspiration if the patient is not alert. Cardiac arrhythmias and/or convulsions, especially likely to be seen with codeine, propoxyphene, or meperidine, also need to be treated.

THE OPIATE ABUSER   The medical abuser   Two groups of individuals are at high risk for abusing analgesics. First, evidence suggests that a majority of people with *chronic pain syndromes* (e.g., back, joint, and muscle disorders) may misuse their prescribed drugs at various times. If physical dependence is established, abstinence syndromes can then intensify the pain, promoting continued drug intake. A few precautions can help the physician to avoid contributing to physical dependence in chronic pain patients, particularly those who have demonstrated a history of misusing opioids: (1) the goal is to minimize the debilitating effects of pain with the understanding that discomfort may not be completely eliminated (see Chap. 11); (2) all possible efforts must be taken to reinforce the need for the patient to become actively involved in and committed to improvement; (3) analgesic medication should be only one component of treatment and limited to oral administration of the least potent analgesic required to take the "edge off" the pain (e.g., ibuprofen or, if needed, propoxyphene); all such drugs should be coordinated through one physician; (4) behavior modification techniques can include muscle relaxation and meditation, while carefully selected exercises can help increase function and decrease pain; and (5) nonmedicinal approaches including electrical transcutaneous neurostimulation for muscle and joint disease can be applied (see also Chap. 11).

The second group at high risk are *physicians*, *nurses*, and *pharmacists*, primarily because of their easy access to substances of abuse. Physicians may begin to use opiates to help them sleep or to reduce stress or physical aches and pains. While all physicians are at risk, a family history of substance abuse (including alcoholism) probably helps to identify the physician at exceptionally high risk. Because of the growing awareness of these problems, impaired physician programs have been established in many hospitals and by most state medical societies. These groups attempt to identify and aid substance-impaired physicians, giving them peer support and education so as to achieve abstinence before problems escalate to the point of licensure revocation. In general, doctors are advised never to prescribe opiates for themselves or for members of their family— physicians deserve the same level of care and protection from future problems as their patients.

The street abuser   Some opiate addicts satisfy criteria for the antisocial personality disorder as evidenced by serious antisocial problems in most life areas beginning prior to age 15 and before the first major life problem from drugs (see Chap. 389). However, the majority of opiate addicts have a relatively high level of premorbid functioning. The usual street abuser begins using opiates occasionally, often after experimenting with tobacco, then alcohol, then marijuana, and then brain depressants or stimulants. Occasional opiate use, or "chipping," might continue for some time, and some individuals probably never escalate their intake to the point of developing serious problems. Another pattern of temporary or intermittent abuse is represented by the experiences of Vietnam soldiers, most of whom had little or no prior experience with opiates and who found themselves in a situation of high stress and readily available drugs. Under these circumstances, as many as one-half tried opiates and, although many became physically addicted, those who had not misused drugs before Vietnam tended to return to drug-free status when back in their home communities.

Of course, opiate-addicted individuals are likely to continue to have experience with many other drugs. At least two of these often remain as problems during the course of opiate addiction. First, alcohol intake is classically used to moderate withdrawal problems, to enhance the opiate high, and as a substitute when the preferred drug is not readily available, including during methadone and other treatments. This pattern of problematic drinking, often meeting criteria for alcohol dependence, is seen in the course of perhaps 50 percent of opiate addicts. The second drug, cocaine, appears to be taken for many of the same reasons as alcohol and is often administered IV concomitantly with the opiate in a mixture known as a "speedball." Dependence on these as well as other drugs must be addressed during opiate detoxification and rehabilitation.

Once persistent opiate use is established, the outcome is often extremely serious. At least 25 percent of such opiate abusers are likely to die within 10 to 20 years of active abuse, with death from suicide, homicide, accidents, and infectious diseases such as tuberculosis, serum hepatitis, or AIDS. The mortality rate has escalated in recent years in response to the epidemic of AIDS among IV drug abusers, with an estimated 60 percent of these men and women carrying the HIV virus (see Chap. 279). As many as 50 percent of male and 25 percent of female addicts turn to alcohol when their primary drug is not available, and many of these people meet the criteria for secondary alcohol abuse. The prevalence of alcohol misuse is higher in drug treatment dropouts than in those who stay with therapy, and abuse is more likely in individuals with a history of alcohol problems before they developed opiate-related difficulties.

PHYSICAL ADDICTION AND THE OPIATE ABSTINENCE SYNDROME   The symptoms of withdrawal   The time to onset as well as the intensity and duration of the acute abstinence syndrome are influenced by a number of factors, including the drug's half-life, its dose, and the chronicity of administration. The withdrawal symptoms tend to be opposite to the acute effects of the drug and include nausea and diarrhea, coughing, lacrimation, rhinorrhea, profuse sweating, twitching muscles, and piloerection, or "goose bumps"; mild elevations in body temperature, respiratory rate, and blood pressure are also observed. In addition, sensations of diffuse body pain, insomnia, and yawning occur with intense drug craving. Drugs with a short half-life, such as morphine or heroin, cause symptoms typically within 8 to 16 h of the last dose (thus many addicts awake in mild withdrawal every morning); peak symptom intensity is apparent within 36 to 72 h after discontinuation of the drug, and the acute syndrome disappears within 5 to 8 days. However, a protracted abstinence phase of mild symptoms (e.g., slight changes in pupillary size, autonomic dysfunction, changes in sleep pattern) may persist for 6 or more months. These lingering symptoms, which can be relieved by administering an opiate, probably contribute to relapse.

Treatment of the withdrawal syndrome   Patients *must* receive a thorough physical examination, which includes an assessment of liver and neurologic function as well as identification of local and systemic infections, especially abscesses. Proper nutrition and rest must be initiated as soon as possible.

Effective treatment of withdrawal, however, also requires readministration of sufficient opiate medication on day 1 to decrease symptoms, followed by a more gradual withdrawal of the drug, usually over 5 to 10 days. Any opiate will work (they all have some level of cross-tolerance), but for ease of administration, many physicians prefer to use a long-acting drug such as methadone. In estimating the first day's dose from the patient's history, 1 mg of methadone is approximately equivalent to 3 mg of morphine, 1 mg of heroin, or 20 mg of meperidine. Most patients require between 10 and 25 mg of methadone orally given twice on day 1, with higher doses given if prominent symptoms of withdrawal are not damped. After several days of a stabilized drug dose, the opiate is then decreased by 10 to 20 percent of the original day's dose each day.

Most states have restrictions on the prescription of opiates to addicts, and in the absence of special permits, detoxification with opiates is often proscribed or limited to 1 month or less. Thus pharmacologic treatments are often limited to symptomatic medication of diarrhea with kaopectate or a similar nonopiate, "sniffles" with decongestants, and pain with nonopiate analgesics (e.g., ibuprofen). Another relatively successful nonopiate approach to the treatment of withdrawal is the use of the alpha$_2$-adrenergic agonist clonidine, used in part to decrease sympathetic nervous system overactivity. Given at doses of approximately 5 µg/kg (up to 0.3 mg given two to four times a day), clonidine causes most patients undergoing opiate withdrawal to experience a decrease in autonomic nervous system dysfunction. Opiates, however, are more effective in relieving discomfort and pain, and clonidine is often not well tolerated because it produces high levels of sedation and orthostatic hypotension. Therefore, under most circumstances opiates are the treatment of choice.

A special case of opiate withdrawal is seen in the newborn passively addicted by the mother's drug misuse during pregnancy. Some level of addiction develops in 50 to 90 percent of children of heroin-dependent mothers, and the withdrawal syndrome carries a mortality of between 3 and 30 percent if not treated when prominent signs are apparent. In distinction to street addicts, as few as 25 percent of infants of methadone maintenance–addicted mothers show clinically relevant withdrawal symptoms. The syndrome consists of irritability, crying, a tremor (in 80 percent), increased reflexes, increased respiratory rate, diarrhea, hyperactivity (in 60 percent), vomiting (40 percent), and sneezing/yawning/hiccuping (in 30 percent). The child usually has a low birth weight but may be otherwise unremarkable until the second day, when symptoms are likely to begin.

The treatment follows the same general steps used in the treatment of the physically addicted adult. The child must be carefully evaluated to rule out medical problems such as hypoglycemia, hypocalcemia, infections, and trauma; general supports in a warm, quiet environment and regulation of electrolytes and glucose are also required. The infant with moderate to severe symptoms can be treated with any of the following: paregoric (0.2 mL orally every 3 to 4 h), methadone (0.1 to 0.5 mg/k per day), phenobarbital (8 mg/kg per day), or diazepam (1 to 2 mg/kg every 8 h). Medication should be given in decreasing levels for 10 to 20 days. It is also possible to help treat the addicted infants of mothers on methadone maintenance by having them breast feed while the mothers continue to take methadone.

REHABILITATION OF OPIATE ADDICTS   Despite some differences in demographics, the same general rules for rehabilitation apply to the opiate abuser and to the alcoholic. The basic strategy includes beginning detoxification and general family support. It is also important to establish realistic patient goals and a program of counseling and education to increase motivation toward abstinence. A long-term commitment to rebuilding a lifestyle without the substance is essential for preventing recidivism.

Identifying and confronting the patient   The first step in treatment requires identification of the opiate abuser—an especially difficult problem with the middle-class street abuser and the medical patient or physician with an iatrogenic addiction. An important step is to take the time with *every* patient, especially those with complaints of pain, to gather a clinical history that includes the patterns of opiate usage and the list of doctors and clinics from which they have received prescriptions. If the chronic use of opiates is suspected, gathering additional data from a resource person such as a spouse can be essential. Another indicator of an enhanced risk for opiate dependence is the history of pervasive antisocial problems beginning in the preteen years. Blood and urine screens can be used to identify opiates in patients in whom misuse is suspected, and clinicians should search for physical stigmata of misuse (e.g., needle marks). One potentially important diagnostic procedure (which should be used carefully because it can precipitate an intense withdrawal) is the opiate antagonist challenge. A 0.4-mg dose of naloxone is given subcutaneously or slowly IV over a 5-min period, and the patient is observed for signs of withdrawal over the next several hours. This challenge test should only be carried out in the presence of a physician, and it is important to be prepared to begin treating withdrawal if needed.

After identifying the opiate addict, the next step is confrontation. The need for active treatment of the abstinence syndrome can be presented, and the availability of help in establishing a drug-free lifestyle can be emphasized. The final decision, of course, rests with the patient. Much of this approach of confrontation is presented in the chapter on alcoholism (see Chap. 390).

Rehabilitation   Most rehabilitation approaches have common elements. Patients are educated about their responsibility for improving their lives, and *motivation for abstinence* is increased by providing information about the medical and psychological problems that can be expected if addiction continues. Patients and families are helped to *establish an opiate-free lifestyle* by being educated about dealing with chronic pain and developing realistic vocational planning (e.g., this applies to pharmacists, physicians, and nurses). The addict also should be encouraged to establish a drug-free peer group and to participate in self-help groups such as Narcotics Anonymous. Much of this advice and counseling can be given by the physician, but many clinicians refer patients to more formal drug programs, including methadone maintenance clinics, programs using narcotic antagonists, and therapeutic communities. Long-term follow-up of treated patients shows that approximately one-third of addicts are completely drug free in the year before the follow-up interview and that a total of 60 percent are off opiates, although some may be abusing other substances. Individuals who stay in methadone maintenance or in therapeutic communities show significant decreases in police and social problems and increases in job functioning. In general, the best prognosis for rehabilitation is for those who are employed, who have higher levels of school completion, and who remain in treatment for at least 2 months. Addiction among health care deliverers, such as physicians, is treated with similar approaches. In addition, a closely supervised "diversion" procedure is usually instituted and carried out for 1 to 2 years or more.

METHADONE MAINTENANCE   Methadone and methadyl acetate maintenance should only be used along with education and counseling. It is important to note that drug maintenance is not aimed at "curing" opiate addiction; rather, it provides a substitute drug that is legally accessible, safer, can be taken orally, and has a long half-life so that it can be taken once a day. The goal is to help the addict who has repeatedly failed in drug-free programs to improve functioning within the family and job, to decrease legal problems, and to improve health.

Methadone is a long-acting opiate that possesses almost all the physiologic properties of heroin. The addict who has been carefully screened to rule out prior psychiatric disorders may be maintained on a relatively low dose (e.g., 30–40 mg/d); a better approach is to use a higher dosage schedule (100–120 mg/d), which may be more effective in blocking heroin-induced euphoria. Although the results are not definite, there is some evidence that the higher methadone doses may result in greater retention in treatment and consequently lower levels of arrest and readdiction to street drugs. Especially following the higher doses, three-quarters or more of addicts are likely to remain heroin-free for 6 months or longer. Methadone is administered in an oral liquid given once a day at the program center, with weekend portions taken by the patient at home. The longer-acting analogues, such as methadyl acetate, can be given in lower doses (e.g., 20–30 mg) two or three times a week, with levels increased to as high as 80 mg three times a week if needed. After a period of maintenance (usually 6 months to 1 year or longer), the clinician should work closely with the patient to regulate the rate of drug decrease (by about 5 percent per week).

In the past, the British have used heroin maintenance with similar goals and following similar guidelines as those used for methadone. There is no evidence that heroin maintenance has any advantages over methadone maintenance, but the heroin approach does add the risk that the drug will be sold on the streets. These factors have contributed to the virtual abandonment of the heroin maintenance approach. Treatment with mixed agonists-antagonists such as buprenorphine has been proposed, especially to help the individual who is also using cocaine. However, at present these must be considered experimental.

OPIATE ANTAGONISTS   The opiate antagonists (e.g., naloxone) compete with heroin and other opiates for opioid receptors, reducing the effects of the opiate agonists. Administered over long periods of time in order to block the "high" produced if the patient takes opiates, these drugs can be useful as part of an overall treatment approach that includes counseling and support. Cyclazocine was the first antagonist tested, but its blockade of receptors is incomplete, and the level of side effects (including an intoxicated feeling) is unacceptable. Naloxone is an excellent narcotic antagonist with no agonistic properties, but it has such a short period of action (2–3 h) that it is of little use in rehabilitation. The most widely used antagonist in rehabilitation is naltrexone, which is effective for about 24 h with few side effects. A dose of 50 mg of naltrexone per day will block 15 mg of heroin for 24 h, and higher doses (125–150 mg) are capable of blocking the effects of 25 mg of IV heroin for up to 3 days. Naltrexone is free of agonist properties, there are no known withdrawal symptoms when the medication is stopped, and side effects tend to be mild. Patients started on this antagonist should be free of opiates for a minimum of 5 days to avoid precipitating a withdrawal syndrome. In addition, they must be given a thorough physical examination and should be challenged with 0.4 or 0.8 mg of the shorter-acting naloxone to be certain that they are able to tolerate the long-acting antagonist. Following this procedure, a test dose of 10 mg of naltrexone can be given, with the expectation that any withdrawal symptoms will be seen in $\frac{1}{2}$ to 2 h. Several variations of this approach can be used with methadone maintenance, including a fairly rapid, medically supervised scheme. Over the next 10 days, the daily dose should be increased to about 100 mg on Mondays and Wednesdays and 150 mg on Fridays. Unfortunately, despite the apparent advantages of this treatment approach, patients demonstrate great resistance to continuing care. In one study, only about 60 percent of the patients completed 6 days of naltrexone induction, and only 10 percent remained in the program at the end of 6 months.

DRUG-FREE PROGRAMS   Most existing half-way houses and recovery centers for the opiate abuser utilize the therapeutic community approach. This is an exception to the general preference for short-term inpatient rehabilitation, since care lasts up to a year while the addict is taken out of the street culture and given a new life within the group. In this structure members, including addict leaders, frequently confront participants in an attempt to help them gain insights into more successful lifestyles for coping with problems.

As is true for treatments of all substance use disorders, it is likely that counseling, behavioral treatments, and relatively simple approaches at psychotherapy add significantly to a positive outcome. Most approaches focus on better handling of stress and enhanced understanding of personality attributes, improving cognitive styles, and addressing problems with interpersonal skills that might have contributed to either the initiation or progression of the substance-abuse problem. It appears as if the combination of these therapies with the approaches described above generates the best results.

Finally, a number of other nonpharmacologic approaches are being evaluated. These include some potentially promising results with acupuncture and transcranial electrostimulation. Efforts to help minimize consequences of opiate dependence, including syringe exchange schemes, are also of great potential importance but are beyond the scope of this chapter.

REFERENCES

BALL J, ROSS A: *The Effectiveness of Methadone Maintenance Treatments*. New York, Springer-Verlag, 1991

FINNEGAN L: Neonatal abstinence syndrome, in *Neonatal Therapy*, F Rubatelli (ed). New York, Elsevier, 1986

FRIEDLAND GH et al: Transmission of the human immunodeficiency virus. N Engl J Med 317:1125, 1987

JAFFE JH, MARTIN WR: Opiate analgesics and antagonists, in *Goodman and Gilman's The Pharmacological Basis of Therapeutics*, 7th ed, AG Gilman et al (eds). New York, Macmillan, 1985

JASINSKI D et al: Clonidine in morphine withdrawal. Arch Gen Psychiatry 42:1063, 1985

KAKU DA, LOWENSTEIN DH: Emergence of recreational drug abuse as a major risk factor for stroke in young adults. Ann Intern Med 113:821, 1990

KERR B et al: Concentration-related effects of morphine on cognition and motor control in human subjects. Neuropsychopharmacology 5:157, 1991

KLEBER HK, RIORDAN CE: The treatment of narcotic withdrawal: A historical review. J Clin Psychiatry 43:30, 1982

KOOB GF: Neural mechanisms of drug reinforcement. Ann NY Acad Sci 654:171, 1992

LEHMAN WEK et al: Alcohol use by heroin addicts 12 years after drug abuse treatment. J Stud Alcohol 51:233, 1990

LOIMER N et al: Similar efficacy of abrupt and gradual opiate detoxification. Am J Drug Alcohol Abuse 17:307, 1991

LONDON ED et al: Morphine-induced metabolic changes in human brain. Arch Gen Psychiatry 47:73, 1990

MCAULIFFE WE et al: Psychoactive drug use among physicians and medical students. N Engl J Med 315:805, 1986

MCKNIGHT AT, REES DC: Opioid receptors and their ligands. Neurotransmissions 7:1, 1991

O'BRIEN CP, WOODY GE: Long-term consequences of opiate dependence. N Engl J Med 304:1098, 1981

OLIVERIO A et al: Psychobiology of opioids. Int Rev Neurobiol 25:277, 1984

PASTERNAK GW: Multiple morphine and enkephalin receptors and the relief of pain. JAMA 259:1362, 1988

PHILIP P et al: Efficiency of transcranial electrostimulation on anxiety and insomnia symptoms during a washout period in depressed patients: A double-blind study. Biol Psychiatry 29:451, 1991

SAN L et al: Assessment and management of opioid withdrawal symptoms in buprenorphine-dependent subjects. Br J Addict 87:55, 1992

———: Follow-up after a six-month maintenance period on naltrexone versus placebo in heroin addicts. Br J Addiction 86:983, 1991

SCHUCKIT MA: *Drug and Alcohol Abuse: A Clinical Guide to Diagnosis and Treatment*, 3d ed. New York, Plenum, 1989

SIMPSON DD et al: Six-year follow-up of opioid addicts after admission to treatment. Arch Gen Psychiatry 39:1318, 1982

STIMSON GV et al: The pilot syringe-exchange project in England and Scotland: A summary of the evaluation. Br J Addiction 81:1283, 1989

STRANG J, GURLING H: Computerized tomography and neuropsychological assessment in long-term high-dose heroin addicts. Br J Addiction 84:1011, 1989

VAILLANT GE: A 20-year follow-up of New York narcotic addicts. Arch Gen Psychiatry 29:237, 1973

WALLOT H, LAMBERT J: Characteristics of physician addicts. Am J Drug Alcohol Abuse 10:53, 1984

---

392   COCAINE AND OTHER COMMONLY ABUSED DRUGS

JACK H. MENDELSON / NANCY K. MELLO

Although there has been a decline in the occurrence of drug abuse–related problems, particularly among youth, the prevalence of drug abuse in the United States remained at epidemic levels during the early 1990s and is believed to exceed that of other industrial nations. The primary data resources for assessing the scope and extent of drug abuse in the United States are the High School Senior Survey, The National Household Survey, and the Drug Abuse Warning Network (DAWN) supported by the National Institute on Drug Abuse (NIDA). During 1991, the High School Senior Survey involved 15,483 senior students from public and private schools, plus 18,000 eighth and 16,000 tenth grade students. The High School Survey revealed that 1.4 percent of students used cocaine within 30 days of their interview and that 0.9 percent of all students had used cocaine at least once in their life. The National Household Survey on drug abuse involved 32,594 randomly selected respondents throughout the United States and also included persons who lived in college dormitories and in homeless shelters. This survey revealed that marijuana continues to be the most commonly used illicit drug in the United States. During 1991, 5.3 million Americans used the drug on a weekly basis, and 3.1 million persons used marijuana daily. Approximately 0.9 percent of Americans over the age of 12 reported use of cocaine within 30 days of the survey interview. The Drug Abuse Warning Network revealed that drug-related emergency room episodes increased from 89,325 incidents in the fourth quarter of 1990 to 100,381 during the second quarter of 1991. Cocaine-related emergency room episodes increased from 19,381 during the fourth quarter of 1990 to 25,370 in the second quarter of 1991.

Chronic drug abuse may be associated with a number of adverse health consequences ranging from pulmonary disease to reproductive dysfunctions. Preexisting disorders such as hypertension and cardiac disease may be exacerbated by drug abuse, and the combined use of two or more drugs may accentuate medical complications associated with abuse of a single drug. The adverse health consequences of drug abuse are further complicated by AIDS, and drug abuse also increases the risk for HIV exposure. Drug abuse contributes to the recent AIDS epidemic through HIV infection transmitted by needle-sharing by intravenous drug users and by direct immunosuppressive and immuno-modulatory effects of abused drugs. In 1992 persons who self-administer drugs intravenously represented the largest single group with HIV infection in several major metropolitan areas in the United States as well as urban areas in Scotland, Italy, Spain, Thailand, and China. Over 30 countries throughout Europe, North America, South America, Asia, Australia, and Africa have reported AIDS or HIV infection among intravenous drug abusers.

The initiation and continuation of drug abuse is determined by a complex interaction of the pharmacologic properties and relative availability of each drug, the personality and expectancy of the user, and the environmental context in which the drug is used. Polydrug abuse, the concurrent use of several drugs with different pharmacologic effects, is increasingly common among individuals from all socioeconomic strata. There has been an alarming increase in a particularly dangerous form of polydrug abuse, the combined use of both heroin and cocaine intravenously, called "speedballing." There is no simple explanation for this change in polydrug use patterns. Sometimes drug abusers attempt to attenuate one drug effect with another, e.g., heroin or alcohol is used to modulate the cocaine high. Sometimes one drug is used to enhance the effects of another, as with benzodiazepines and methadone, or cocaine plus heroin in methadone-maintained patients. Toxic drug interactions associated with polydrug abuse also contribute to the adverse health consequences of drug abuse. This chapter discusses cocaine, marijuana, two hallucinogens (PCP and LSD), and polydrug abuse. Alcohol abuse is discussed in Chap. 390 and opioid abuse in Chap. 391.

COCAINE Cocaine is a stimulant and a local anesthetic with potent vasoconstrictor properties. The leaves of the coca plant (*Erythroxylon coca*) contain approximately 0.5 to 1 percent cocaine. The drug produces physiologic and behavioral effects when administered orally, intranasally, intravenously, or via inhalation following pyrolysis (smoking). It is now recognized that cocaine has potent pharmacologic effects on dopamine, norepinephrine, and serotonin neurons in the central nervous system. These effects include alteration and blockade of cellular membrane transport and prevention of the reuptake of biogenic amines. It has been postulated that cocaine-induced euphoria is due to cocaine-induced blockade of dopamine reuptake, but chronic cocaine use may cause dopamine depletion and destruction of dopaminergic pathways in the brain.

Prevalence of cocaine use Cocaine has become more widely available throughout the United States since its cost (relative to disposable income) has decreased considerably. Cocaine is no longer considered a "status" drug since cocaine abuse occurs in virtually all social and economic strata of society. The prevalence of cocaine abuse in the general population has also been associated with an increase in cocaine abuse by heroin-dependent persons, including those in methadone maintenance programs. Intravenous cocaine is often used concurrently with intravenous heroin (the speedball)—a combination that purportedly attenuates the postcocaine "crash" and substitutes a cocaine "high" for the heroin "high" blocked by methadone. Intravenous use of cocaine plus heroin may further increase risk for HIV infection, both through needle sharing and through the combined immunosuppressive effects of both drugs.

Acute and chronic cocaine intoxication Although cocaine is commonly self-administered by inhalation (snorting), there has been a dramatic increase in both intravenous administration and inhalation of pyrolyzed material via smoking. Following intranasal administration, changes in mood and feeling states are perceived within 3 to 5 min and peak effects occur at 10 to 20 min. Duration of cocaine effects rarely exceed 1 h following intranasal administration. Inhalation of pyrolyzed materials include smoking coca paste, a product produced by extracting cocaine preparations with flammable solvents, and cocaine free-base smoking. Coca paste is frequently contaminated with toxic solvents used in its preparation. Cocaine free-base, including the free-base prepared with sodium bicarbonate (crack), is becoming increasingly popular because of the relative high potency of the compounds and their rapid onset of action (8 to 10 s following smoking).

Cocaine produces a brief, dose-related stimulation and enhancement of mood and dose-related increases in cardiac rate and blood pressure. Body temperature usually increases following cocaine administration, and high doses of cocaine may induce lethal pyrexia or hypertension. Because cocaine inhibits reuptake of catecholamines at adrenergic nerve endings, the drug potentiates sympathetic nervous system activity. Cocaine has a short plasma half-life of approximately 1 h. In humans, cocaine is primarily metabolized by plasma esterases, and cocaine metabolites are excreted in urine. The very short duration of euphorigenic effects of cocaine observed in chronic abusers is probably due to both acute and chronic tolerance. Frequent self-administration of the drug (two to three times per hour) is often reported by chronic cocaine abusers. Alcohol is used to modulate both the cocaine "high" and the dysphoria associated with the abrupt disappearance of cocaine's effects. A metabolite of cocaine, ethylcocaine, has been detected in blood and urine of persons who concurrently abuse alcohol and cocaine. Ethylcocaine induces changes in cardiovascular function similar to those of cocaine alone, and the pathophysiologic consequences of alcohol abuse plus cocaine abuse may be additive when both are self-administered together.

The prevalent assumption that cocaine use is relatively safe is challenged by reports of death from respiratory depression, cardiac arrhythmias, and convulsions after cocaine snorting and intravenous administration. Disorders of cerebral blood flow and perfusion in cocaine dependent persons have been detected with SPECT studies. These brain perfusion abnormalities are very similar to those which have been observed in patients with early HIV dementia. Severe pulmonary disease may develop in individuals who smoke coca paste; this is attributed both to the direct effects of cocaine and to residual solvent contaminants in the smoked material. Hepatic necrosis has also been reported to occur in coca paste smokers. Although men and women who abuse cocaine may report that the drug enhances libidinal drive, chronic cocaine use causes significant loss of libido and adversely affects reproductive function. Impotence and gynecomastia have been observed in male cocaine abusers, and these abnormalities often persist for long periods following drug abstinence. Women who abuse cocaine have reported major derangements in menstrual cycle function including galactorrhea, amenorrhea, and infertility. Chronic cocaine abuse may cause persistent hyperprolactinemia as a consequence of cocaine-induced disorders of dopaminergic regulation of prolactin secretion by the pituitary. Cocaine abuse also may adversely affect pregnancy. Infants exposed to cocaine in utero have an increased risk for congenital malformations as well as perinatal cardiovascular and cerebrovascular disease.

Numerous clinical reports, dating from the late nineteenth century, strongly suggest that protracted cocaine abuse may cause paranoid ideation and visual and auditory hallucinations, a state which resembles alcoholic hallucinosis. Psychological dependence upon cocaine, as manifested by inability to abstain from frequent compulsive use, also has been reported. Although occurrence of withdrawal syndromes involving psychomotor agitation and autonomic hyperactivity remains controversial, severe depression ("crashing") following cocaine intoxication may be a concomitant of drug withdrawal.

Treatment of cocaine intoxication and abuse Treatment of cocaine overdose is a medical emergency that involves resuscitation in an intensive care unit. Cocaine toxicity produces hypertension, tachycardia, tonic-clonic seizures, dyspnea, and ventricular arrhythmias. Intravenous diazepam in doses up to 0.5 mg/kg administered over an 8-h period has been shown to be effective for control of seizures. The systemic concomitants of a hypermetabolic state produced by cocaine toxicity with concurrent ventricular arrhythmias have been managed successfully by administration of 0.5 to 1.0 mg of propranolol intravenously. Since many instances of cocaine-related mortality have also been associated with concurrent use of other illicit drugs (particularly heroin), the physician must be prepared to institute effective emergency treatment for multiple drug toxicity.

Treatment of chronic cocaine abuse requires combined efforts by family physicians, psychiatrists, and psychosocial care providers. Early abstinence from cocaine use is often complicated by symptoms of depression and guilt, insomnia, and anorexia, which may be as severe as those observed in major affective disorders. Individual and group psychotherapy, family therapy, and peer group assistance programs are often useful for inducing prolonged remission from drug use. Preliminary reports suggest that tricyclic antidepressant medication (desipramine) may be of value in the treatment of cocaine abuse, even when affective disorder or depression is not present. In fact, depressive illness does not appear to be a frequent antecedent of cocaine abuse.

MARIJUANA AND CANNABIS COMPOUNDS   *Cannabis sativa* contains over 400 compounds in addition to the psychoactive substance, delta-9-tetrahydrocannabinol (THC). Marijuana cigarettes are prepared from the leaves and flowering tops of the plant, and a typical marijuana cigarette contains 0.5 to 1 g of plant material. Although the usual THC concentration varies between 5 and 20 mg, concentrations as high as 100 mg per cigarette have been detected. Hashish is prepared from concentrated resin of *Cannabis sativa* and contains a THC concentration of between 8 to 12 percent by weight. "Hash oil," a lipid-soluble plant extract, may contain a THC concentration of 25 to 60 percent, and it may be added to marijuana or hashish to enhance their THC concentration. Smoking is the most common mode of marijuana or hashish self-administration. During pyrolysis, over 150 compounds in addition to the THC are released in the smoke. Although most of these compounds do not have psychoactive properties, they do have potential physiologic effects.

THC is quickly absorbed from the lungs into blood and is then rapidly sequestered in tissues. It is metabolized primarily in the liver where it is converted to 11-hydroxy-THC, a psychoactive compound, and more than 20 other metabolites. Most THC metabolites are excreted through the feces at a rate of clearance that is relatively slow in comparison to that of most other psychoactive drugs.

Prevalence of marijuana use   The National Institute on Drug Abuse's 1991 National Household Survey on Drug Abuse revealed that over one-third of all men and women surveyed had used marijuana or hashish at least once in their lifetime, and that 5 percent of the survey population reported using the drug at least once during the month prior to the survey. One encouraging datum is a continued trend in the decrease of marijuana use by high-school students. The annual use of marijuana decreased to 24 percent between 1990 and 1991 and was half the rate of marijuana use reported during 1980.

Acute and chronic marijuana intoxication   Acute intoxication from marijuana and cannabis compounds is related to both the dose of THC and the route of administration. THC is absorbed more rapidly from marijuana smoking than from orally ingested *Cannabis* compounds. Acute marijuana intoxication usually consists of a subjective perception of relaxation and mild euphoria resembling mild to moderate alcohol intoxication. This condition is usually accompanied by some impairment in thinking, concentration, and perceptual and psychomotor functions. Higher doses of *Cannabis* may produce behavioral effects analogous to severe alcohol intoxication. Although the effects of acute marijuana intoxication are relatively benign in normal users, the drug can precipitate severe emotional disorders in individuals who have antecedent psychotic or neurotic problems. As with other psychoactive compounds, both set (user's

expectation) and setting (environmental context) are important determinants of the type and severity of behavioral intoxication.

As is true of alcoholics, chronic marijuana abusers may lose interest in common socially desirable goals and devote progressively more time to drug acquisition and use. However, it should be emphasized that THC does not cause a specific and unique "amotivational syndrome." The range of symptoms sometimes attributed to marijuana use are difficult to distinguish from mild depression and the maturational dysfunctions often associated with protracted adolescence. Chronic use of marijuana has also been reported to increase the probability of exacerbation of psychotic symptoms in individuals with a past history of schizophrenia.

Physical effects of marijuana   Conjunctival injection and tachycardia are the most frequent immediate physical concomitants of smoking marijuana. Tolerance for marijuana-induced tachycardia develops rapidly among regular users; angina may be precipitated by marijuana smoking in persons with a history of coronary insufficiency. Exercise-induced angina may be increased after marijuana use to a greater extent than after tobacco cigarette smoking. Patients with cardiac disease should be strongly advised not to smoke marijuana or use *Cannabis* compounds.

Significant decrements in pulmonary vital capacity have been found in regular daily marijuana smokers. Because marijuana smoking typically involves deep inhalation and prolonged retention of marijuana smoke, marijuana smokers may develop pulmonary disease such as chronic bronchial irritation. Impairment of single-breath carbon monoxide diffusion capacity (DL_{co}) is greater in persons who smoke both marijuana and tobacco than in tobacco smokers. Despite the well-documented association between tobacco smoking and lung cancer, at present there is no direct evidence that marijuana smoking induces lung cancer. However, it should be emphasized that heavy marijuana use among Americans may be too recent to permit detection of this problem.

Although marijuana has also been associated with adverse effects on a number of other systems, many of these studies await replication and confirmation. For example, the reported correlation between marijuana use and decreased testosterone levels in males has not been confirmed. Decreased sperm count and motility and abnormalities of morphology of spermatozoa following marijuana use have also been reported. Administration of high doses of marijuana to female rhesus monkeys has revealed significant marijuana-induced suppression of pituitary gonadotropins and gonadal steroids. Carefully conducted prospective studies demonstrated a significant correlation between impaired fetal growth and development and heavy marijuana use during pregnancy. Marijuana also has been implicated in derangements of the immune response system, in chromosomal abnormalities, and in inhibition of DNA, RNA, and protein synthesis, but these findings have not been confirmed or related to any specific physiologic effect in humans. One report of *Cannabis*-induced brain atrophy in young adults has not been confirmed in computed tomography studies of young men who had documented histories of heavy marijuana smoking.

Tolerance and physical dependence   Habitual marijuana users rapidly develop tolerance to the psychoactive effects of marijuana and often smoke more frequently and try to secure more potent *Cannabis* compounds. Tolerance for physiologic effects of marijuana develops at different rates; e.g., tolerance for marijuana-induced tachycardia develops rapidly, but tolerance for marijuana-induced conjunctival injection develops more slowly. Tolerance to both behavioral and physiologic effects of marijuana decreases rapidly upon cessation of marijuana use.

Withdrawal signs and symptoms have been reported in chronic *Cannabis* users, with severity of symptoms related to dosage and duration of use. These include tremor, nystagmus, sweating, nausea, vomiting, diarrhea, irritability, anorexia, and sleep disturbances. Withdrawal signs and symptoms observed in chronic marijuana users are usually relatively mild in comparison to those observed in heavy opiate or alcohol users and rarely require medical or pharmacologic intervention. Somewhat more severe and protracted abstinence syndromes may occur after sustained use of high-potency *Cannabis* compounds for long periods.

LYSERGIC ACID DIETHYLAMIDE (LSD) The serendipitous discovery of psychedelic effects of LSD in 1947 culminated in an epidemic of LSD abuse during the 1960s. Imposition of stringent legal and regulatory constraints on the manufacture and distribution of LSD (classified as a Schedule I substance by the FDA), as well as public recognition that psychedelic experiences induced by LSD were a health hazard, has resulted in a significant reduction in LSD abuse. During 1991, relatively few instances of LSD abuse were reported, but the drug still retains some popularity among adolescents and young adults. Almost 2 percent of high school students reported using LSD within 30 days of the 1991 High School Survey. There are recent indications that the prevalence of LSD use among young persons has been accelerating in some communities in the United States.

LSD is a very potent drug; oral doses as low as 20 μg may induce profound psychological and physiologic effects. Tachycardia, hypertension, pupillary dilation, tremor, and hyperpyrexia occur within minutes following LSD in oral doses of 0.5 to 2 μg/kg. A variety of bizarre and often conflicting perceptual and mood changes, including visual illusions, synesthesias, and extreme lability of mood, usually occur within one-half hour after LSD intake. The action of LSD may persist for 12 to 18 h even though the half-life of the drug is only 3 h.

Tolerance develops rapidly for LSD-induced changes in psychological function when the drug is used one or more times per day over a course of 4 days or more. Abrupt abstinence following continued use does not produce withdrawal signs or symptoms. To date there have been no clinical reports of death caused by the direct effects of LSD.

The most frequent acute medical emergency associated with LSD use is panic episodes, which may persist up to 24 h (the "bad trip"). Management of this problem is best accomplished by supportive reassurance ("talking down") and, if necessary, administration of small doses of anxiolytic drugs. Adverse consequences of chronic LSD use include enhanced risk for schizophreniform psychosis and derangements in memory function, problem solving, and abstract thinking. Treatment of these disorders is best carried out in specialized psychiatric facilities.

PHENCYCLIDINE (PCP) Phencyclidine, a cyclohexylamine derivative, is widely used in veterinary medicine to briefly immobilize large animals and is sometimes described as a dissociative anesthetic. PCP is easily synthesized and its abusers are primarily young people and polydrug users. The true extent of PCP abuse is unknown, but recent national surveys indicate an increase in frequency of use.

Phencyclidine is taken orally, by smoking, or by intravenous injection. It is also used as an adulterant in illicit sales of THC, LSD, amphetamine, or cocaine. The most common street preparation, "angel dust," is a white granular powder which contains 50 to 100 percent of the drug. Low doses (5 mg) produce agitation, excitement, impaired motor coordination, dysarthria, and analgesia. Users may have horizontal or vertical nystagmus, flushing, diaphoresis, and hyperacusis. Behavioral changes include distortions of body image, disorganization of thinking, and feelings of estrangement. Higher doses of PCP (5 to 10 mg) may produce hypersalivation, vomiting, myoclonus, fever, stupor, or coma. PCP doses of 10 mg or more cause convulsions, opisthotonus, and decerebrate posturing which may be followed by prolonged coma.

The diagnosis of PCP overdose is difficult because the patient's initial symptoms may suggest an acute schizophrenic reaction. Confirmation of PCP use is possible by determination of PCP levels in serum or urine. PCP analysis is currently available at most toxicologic centers. Large quantities of PCP remain in urine for 1 to 5 days following high-dosage PCP intake.

PCP overdose requires prompt life support measures including treatment of coma, convulsions, and respiratory depression in a hospital intensive care unit. There is no specific antidote or antagonist for PCP. PCP excretion from the body can be enhanced by acidification of urine and gastric lavage. Death from PCP overdose may occur as a consequence of some combination of pharyngeal hypersecretion, hyperthermia, respiratory depression, severe hypertension, seizures, hypertensive encephalopathy, and intracerebral hemorrhage.

Acute psychosis associated with PCP use should be considered a psychiatric emergency since patients may be at high risk for suicide or extreme violence toward others. Phenothiazines should not be used for treatment of acute PCP psychosis because these drugs potentiate PCP's anticholinergic effects. Haloperidol (5 mg intramuscularly) has been administered on an hourly basis to induce suppression of psychotic behavior. PCP, like LSD and mescaline, produces vasospasm of cerebral arteries at relatively low doses. Chronic PCP use has been shown to induce insomnia, anorexia, severe social and behavioral changes, and, in some cases, chronic schizophrenia.

POLYDRUG ABUSE Although drug abusers often report a preference for a particular drug, such as alcohol or opiates, the concurrent use of other drugs is common. Multiple drug use often involves substances which may have different pharmacologic effects from the preferred drug. Concurrent use of such dissimilar compounds as stimulants and opiates or stimulants and alcohol is not unusual. The diversity of reported drug use combinations suggests that achieving some perceptible change in state, rather than any particular direction of change (stimulation or sedation), may be the primary reinforcer in polydrug use and abuse. There is also evidence that intoxication with alcohol or opiates is associated with increased tobacco smoking, but marijuana smoking does not increase during alcohol intoxication. At present, there is relatively little systematic information available about drug interactions. However, it is known that the combined use of cocaine, heroin, and alcohol increases the risk for toxic effects and adverse medical consequences over risks associated with use of a single drug.

A practical determinant of polydrug use patterns is the relative availability and cost of the drugs. There are many examples of situationally determined drug use patterns, including the fact that soldiers who became dependent on heroin in Vietnam seldom continued heroin use after separation from military service. However, a significant number of men who were heroin addicts in Vietnam abused alcohol and became alcohol-dependent when they returned to the United States. Alcohol abuse, with its attendant medical complications, is one of the most serious problems encountered in former heroin addicts participating in methadone maintenance programs.

The physician must recognize that perpetuation of polydrug abuse and drug dependence is not necessarily a symptom of an underlying emotional disorder. Neither alleviation of anxiety nor reduction of depression accounts for initiation and perpetuation of polydrug abuse. Severe depression and anxiety are as frequently the consequences of polydrug abuse as they are the antecedents. There is also evidence that some of the most adverse consequences of drug use may be reinforcing and contribute to the continuation of polydrug abuse.

Adequate treatment of polydrug abuse, as well as other forms of drug abuse, requires innovative and eclectic programs of intervention. The first step in successful treatment is detoxification, a process which may be difficult because the patient has abused several drugs with different pharmacologic actions (e.g., alcohol, opiates, and cocaine). Since patients may not recall or may deny simultaneous multiple drug use, diagnostic evaluation should always include urinalysis for qualitative detection of psychoactive substances and their metabolites. Treatment of polydrug abuse requires hospitalization or inpatient residential care during detoxification and the initial phase of drug abstinence. When possible, specialized facilities for the care and treatment of chemically dependent persons should be used. Outpatient detoxification of polydrug abuse patients is likely to be ineffective and may be dangerous.

As in the treatment of alcohol abuse, no single therapeutic modality has been shown to be uniquely effective in inducing remission.

Polydrug abuse is a chronic disorder with an unpredictable pattern of remission and recrudescence. Therapeutic management of chronic disorders such as cardiac or neoplastic disease should serve as a model for helping the person with polydrug abuse problems. Even temporary remissions with attendant physical, social, and psychological improvements are preferable to the continuation or progressive acceleration of polydrug abuse and its related adverse medical and interpersonal consequences. In polydrug abuse, as in most chronic disorders, definitive ''cures'' rarely occur. The concerned physician should continue to assist polydrug abuse patients throughout the cyclic oscillations of this complex behavior disorder, recognizing that resumption of drug use may be the rule rather than the exception.

REFERENCES

CHO AK et al: A pharmacokinetic study of phenylcyclohexyldiethylamine—An analog of phencyclidine. Drug Metab Dispos 21:125, 1993

CREGLER LL, MARK H: Medical complications of cocaine abuse. N Engl J Med 315:1495, 1986

DAS G: Cocaine abuse in North America—A milestone in history. J Clin Pharmacol 33:296, 1993

GAWIN FH: Cocaine addiction: Psychology and neurophysiology. Science 251:1580, 1991

———, ELLINWOOD EH JR: Cocaine and other stimulants. Actions, abuse, and treatment. N Engl J Med 318:1173, 1988

———, ———: Cocaine dependence. Ann Rev Med 40:149, 1989

HOLMAN BL et al: Brain perfusion is abnormal in cocaine-dependent polydrug users: A study using Technetium-99m-HMPAO and ASPECT. J Nucl Med 32:1206, 1991

JAFFE JH: Drug addiction and drug abuse, in Goodman and Gilman's The Pharmacological Basis of Therapeutics, 8th ed., AG Gilman et al (eds). New York, Pergamon, 1990, p 522

JOHANSON CE, FISCHMAN MW: The pharmacology of cocaine related to its abuse. Pharmacol Rev 41:3, 1989

JONES RT: The pharmacology of cocaine smoking in humans, in Research Findings on Smoking of Abused Substances, NIDA Research Monograph vol. 99, CN Chiang, RL Hawks (eds). Washington, DC, U.S. Government Printing Office, 1990, pp 30–41

KREEK MJ: Multiple drug abuse patterns and medical consequences, in Psychopharmacology: The Third Generation of Progress, HY Meltzer (ed). New York, Raven Press, 1987, pp 1597–1604

MENDELSON JH: Marijuana, in Psychopharmacology: The Third Generation of Progress, HY Meltzer (ed). New York, Raven Press, 1987, pp 1565–1571

———, MELLO NK (eds): Medical Diagnosis and Treatment of Alcoholism. New York, McGraw-Hill, 1992

——— et al: Human studies on the biological basis of reinforcement, in Addictive States, CP O'Brien, JH Jaffe (eds). New York, Raven Press, 1992, pp 131–155

OM A et al: Management of cocaine-induced cardiovascular complications. Am Heart J 125:469, 1993

WEISS RD, MIRIN SM: Cocaine. Washington, American Psychiatric Press, 1987

WOODS JH, WINGER G: Phencyclidine and related substances, in Drug Abuse and Drug Abuse Research: The Third Triennial Report to Congress from the Secretary, Department of Health and Human Services. Washington, DC: U.S. Government Printing Office, 1991, p 145

393 NICOTINE ADDICTION

JOHN H. HOLBROOK

Cigarette smoking is the principal cause of preventable disease, disability, and premature death in the United States. Nonetheless, each year more than one million American children and teenagers start smoking, and most established smokers have great difficulty in quitting. The addictive effects of nicotine account for most of this persistent personal and public health dilemma. Recognition of tobacco use as an addiction and of nicotine as the addictive drug is essential for effective patient management.

The primary criteria for defining drug addiction are: compulsive use, psychoactive effects, and drug-reinforced behavior. Nicotine use fulfills these criteria because it produces a compelling urge to smoke, provides pleasurable alterations in mood, and motivates chronic tobacco-seeking and tobacco-using behavior. Tolerance and physical dependence, manifested by an abstinence-mediated withdrawal syn-

drome, contribute to the strong control exerted by nicotine on smoking behavior.

Smokers regulate their nicotine dose to obtain desired effects; these include both intrinsic positive effects, such as pleasure and enhanced performance, and avoidance of the withdrawal syndrome. This syndrome is characterized by anger, anxiety, craving for tobacco products, difficulty concentrating, hunger, impatience, and restlessness. Most of these symptoms peak in 1 to 2 days and return to baseline within 3 to 4 weeks of quitting; however, craving for tobacco products and hunger may persist for extended periods.

The use of tobacco products is a complex, learned behavior that is woven into the fiber of daily living and is linked to how the smoker deals with the world. Numerous daily activities, thoughts, and emotions serve as powerful cues to smoke. Such conditioned ties become paired with positive neuroregulatory effects of nicotine to reinforce the addictive process. Personal characteristics such as educational level, belief in one's ability to change, and coping skills are determinants of tobacco use. Similarly, environmental factors such as the level of acceptance of smoking in the home, peer group, workplace, and community norms influence smoking behavior.

PHYSICOCHEMICAL PROPERTIES OF CIGARETTE SMOKE
Cigarette smoke is a heterogeneous aerosol produced by incomplete combustion of the tobacco leaf. It is composed of a gas phase in which particulate matter is dispersed. Mainstream smoke emerges from the mouthpiece during puffing. Sidestream smoke is emitted between puffs at the burning cone and from the mouthpiece. The composition of the smoke is influenced by several factors including type of tobacco, temperature of combustion, length of the cigarette, porosity of the paper, additives, and filters. Cigarette temperatures vary greatly, from 30°C at the mouthpiece to 900°C at the burning cone. In the presence of intense heat some tobacco constituents undergo thermic decomposition (pyrolysis). Volatile substances are distilled directly into the smoke. Unstable molecules recombine to generate new compounds (pyrosynthesis). Concentration of smoke constituents occurs as the smoke is filtered by unburnt tobacco and is redistilled by the burning cone. Some substances found in tobacco pass unchanged into cigarette smoke.

Approximately 92 to 95 percent of the total weight of mainstream smoke is present in the gas phase. Nitrogen, oxygen, and carbon dioxide account for 85 percent of the smoke's weight. The remaining gases and particulate matter are the substances of medical importance (Table 393-1).

PHARMACOLOGY OF CIGARETTE SMOKE More than 4000 substances have been identified in cigarette smoke, including some that are pharmacologically active, antigenic, cytotoxic, mutagenic, and carcinogenic; these diverse biologic effects provide a framework for understanding the adverse consequences of smoking. A pack-a-day cigarette smoker puffs more than 70,000 times a year, and the membranes of the mouth, nose, pharynx, and tracheobronchial tree are exposed repetitively to tobacco smoke. Some constituents act directly on the membranes, while others are absorbed into the blood or are dissolved in saliva and swallowed.

Tissue and organ system responses to cigarette smoke inhalation are multiple and complex. Most studies in humans have dealt with exposure to whole smoke or to selected constituents thought to pose the greatest risk to health, such as nicotine and carbon monoxide. Relatively little is known about the individual effects and interactions of other potentially toxic smoke constituents that are present in low concentrations.

Nicotine is a highly toxic alkaloid that is both a ganglionic stimulant and depressant. Many of its complex effects are mediated by catecholamine release. Acute cardiovascular responses to nicotine observed in normal smokers include increases in systolic and diastolic blood pressure, heart rate, force of myocardial contraction, myocardial oxygen consumption, coronary artery blood flow, myocardial excitability, and peripheral vasoconstriction. Nicotine has also been shown to increase serum concentrations of glucose, cortisol, free fatty acids, vasopressin, and β-endorphin.

TABLE 393-1 Selected cigarette smoke constituents

Substance	Effect(s)
PARTICULATE PHASE	
"Tar"*	Carcinogen
Polynuclear aromatic hydrocarbons	Carcinogens
Nicotine	Neuroendocrine stimulant and depressant; addicting drug
Phenol	Cocarcinogen and irritant
Cresol	Cocarcinogen and irritant
β-Naphthylamine	Carcinogen
N-Nitrosonornicotine	Carcinogen
Benzo[a]pyrene	Carcinogen
Trace metals (e.g., nickel, arsenic, polonium 210)	Carcinogens
Indole	Tumor accelerator
Carbazole	Tumor accelerator
Catechol	Cocarcinogen
GAS PHASE	
Carbon monoxide	Impairs oxygen transport and utilization
Hydrocyanic acid	Ciliotoxin and irritant
Acetaldehyde	Ciliotoxin and irritant
Acrolein	Ciliotoxin and irritant
Ammonia	Ciliotoxin and irritant
Formaldehyde	Ciliotoxin and irritant
Oxides of nitrogen	Ciliotoxin and irritant
Nitrosamines	Carcinogen
Hydrazine	Carcinogen
Vinyl chloride	Carcinogen

* The aggregate of particulate matter in cigarette smoke after subtracting nicotine and moisture.

Carbon monoxide is a toxic gas that interferes with oxygen transport and utilization. Because cigarette smoke contains 2 to 6 percent carbon monoxide, smokers inhale concentrations as high as 400 parts per million (ppm) and develop elevated carboxyhemoglobin (COHb) levels. The range of COHb found in smokers is 2 to 15 percent, while levels for nonsmokers are near 1 percent. The average COHb level of moderate cigarette smokers is 5 percent. Carbon monoxide produces its adverse effects by reducing the amount of available oxyhemoglobin and myoglobin, and by displacing the oxygen-hemoglobin dissociation curve to the left. Chronic, mild elevations of COHb due to smoking are a common cause of mild polycythemia and may produce subtle impairment of central nervous system function.

Cigarette smoke and its condensate are carcinogenic in several species of animals. The major identified carcinogens in cigarette smoke are polynuclear aromatic hydrocarbons, aromatic amines, and nitrosamines (Table 393-1). Cocarcinogens present in cigarette smoke, such as catechol, greatly enhance its carcinogenicity.

Potent pulmonary irritants and ciliotoxins are found in cigarette smoke (Table 393-1). These substances increase bronchial mucous secretion and mediate acute and chronic decreases in pulmonary and mucociliary function.

EPIDEMIOLOGY Data from large prospective studies of populations in several countries have shown that cigarette-smoking men have 70 percent higher overall death rates than nonsmokers. The effect on mortality is proportionately greatest in younger age groups. The excess mortality of female smokers has been somewhat less than that of male smokers, but it has increased. Cigarette smoking is the largest single health risk in the United States and is responsible for an estimated 390,000 premature deaths each year; this is equivalent to more than one out of every six deaths. Coronary heart disease (CHD) and lung cancer are the chief contributors to smoking-related excess mortality. In the United States, cigarette smokers also experience more disability due to chronic illness and report significantly more days absent from work than do nonsmokers.

A strong dose-response relationship exists between cigarette smoking and excess mortality, as measured by the age at onset of smoking, the number of cigarettes smoked, the number of years of smoking, and the depth of inhalation. Cessation of smoking is associated with a decrease in the excess mortality. These observations together with clinical, experimental, and pathologic studies indicate that smoking, per se, causes the excess mortality.

CHARACTERISTICS OF SMOKERS Demographic, anthropometric, physiologic, and laboratory features which distinguish cigarette smokers from nonsmokers are due both to baseline differences between these groups and to the effects of smoking. Smokers drink more alcohol, coffee, and tea than do nonsmokers. Their weight and blood pressure are slightly less and their heart rate is slightly faster than those of nonsmokers. In women the menopause comes earlier in smokers than in nonsmokers. Smokers have impaired maximum exercise performance and impaired immune systems compared to nonsmokers. A markedly increased number of pulmonary alveolar macrophages is present in smokers, and the function and metabolism of these cells are abnormal. When compared with nonsmokers, smokers show small increases in hematocrit, total white blood cell count, and platelet count, as well as small decreases in leukocyte vitamin C levels, serum uric acid, and albumin. In smokers, the ratio of high-density lipoprotein cholesterol to low-density lipoprotein cholesterol is reduced.

CLINICAL CORRELATIONS Large population studies have shown a strong association between cigarette smoking and several diseases. Atherosclerotic cardiovascular disease, cancer, and chronic obstructive pulmonary disease account for most of the excess mortality and morbidity due to smoking.

Individual patient risks due to cigarette smoking vary widely. Factors which influence these risks include the duration, intensity, and type of smoke exposure; genetically mediated susceptibility; occupational and environmental exposures; use of medication; and coexisting risk factors and diseases.

Cardiovascular disease Cigarette smoking is a major cause of coronary heart disease (CHD), and premature CHD is one of its most important medical consequences. Approximately 20 percent of the 500,000 CHD deaths occurring each year in the United States is attributable to smoking. Cigarette smoking, hypertension, and hypercholesterolemia are the three major CHD risk factors. Smoking acts both independently of and synergistically with these other CHD risk factors. Two risk factors may produce a fourfold increase in CHD risk and three risk factors may produce an eightfold increase in CHD risk. There is a dose-response relationship between CHD risk and cigarette smoking. CHD death rates are 60 to 70 percent greater in male smokers than nonsmokers. Sudden death may be the first manifestation of CHD, and it is two to four times more likely to occur in younger male cigarette smokers than in nonsmokers. Women cigarette smokers are also at greater risk of developing CHD than nonsmokers, and the use of both cigarettes and oral contraceptives increases this risk approximately tenfold. Those who continue to smoke after an acute myocardial infarction are more likely to die from CHD than are those who quit smoking. Smokers who undergo coronary artery bypass surgery have increased perioperative mortality compared to nonsmokers. Cigarette smoking contributes to both coronary atherosclerosis and acute ischemic, thrombotic, and arrhythmic coronary events. Cigarette smoking may interfere with the efficacy of medication used to treat CHD, such as propranolol.

Cigarette smoking is an important cause of cerebrovascular disease and accounts for an estimated 18 percent of the 150,000 stroke deaths that occur each year in the United States. Large epidemiologic studies in men and women have shown an increased risk of stroke among smokers compared to nonsmokers, a dose-response relationship between smoking and stroke risk, and a decrease in stroke risk with smoking cessation. Among women, subarachnoid hemorrhage is more likely to occur in smokers than nonsmokers, and the use of both cigarettes and oral contraceptives greatly increases this risk.

Cigarette smoking is the most powerful risk factor for arteriosclerosis obliterans and thromboangiitis obliterans. It also aggravates peripheral ischemia and may adversely affect peripheral bypass grafts. The mortality rate for atherosclerotic aortic aneurysm is greater in male smokers than nonsmokers.

Cigarette smoking is not a risk factor for the development of hypertension; however, hypertensives who smoke are at a greater risk to develop malignant hypertension and to die from hypertension. Because of the association with chronic obstructive pulmonary disease, cigarette smoking is an important factor leading to chronic pulmonary heart disease.

Cancer Cigarette smoking is the single most important cause of cancer mortality in the United States, accounting for 30 percent of all cancer deaths. In spite of the well-documented cause-and-effect relationship between cigarette smoking and lung cancer, more Americans continue to die from this cancer than from any other tumor (see Chap. 227). In 1991 an estimated 143,000 lung cancer deaths occurred in the United States; 85 percent of these deaths were attributable to cigarette smoking. The risk of developing lung cancer is quantitatively related to cigarette smoke exposure. Men who smoke one pack a day increase their risk tenfold compared with nonsmokers; men who smoke two packs a day may increase their risk more than 25 times compared with nonsmokers. Asbestos workers who smoke cigarettes are at especially high risk for developing lung cancer. Cigarette consumption by women increased rapidly in the United States during the past 50 years, and lung cancer mortality among smokers is currently increasing at a faster rate in women than in men. Lung cancer has become the leading cause of cancer death among American women.

Cigarette smoking is a cause of laryngeal, oral, esophageal, and bladder cancer in men and women. Cigarette smoking is an important contributory factor for the development of kidney and pancreatic cancer; it is also associated with cancer of the stomach and uterine cervix and with myelocytic leukemia.

Respiratory disease Cigarette smoking is the major cause of chronic obstructive pulmonary disease (COPD), that is, chronic bronchitis and emphysema (see Chap. 223). Of the estimated 70,000 deaths from COPD in the United States in 1988, 82 percent were attributable to smoking and many of these deaths were preceded by prolonged respiratory disability. There is a dose-response relationship between COPD death rates and cigarette smoking. Depending upon the extent of smoke exposure, male cigarette smokers experience from 4 to 25 times higher mortality secondary to COPD than do nonsmokers. Although the death rate from COPD among female smokers is somewhat lower than among male smokers, it is increasing much more rapidly in female than in male smokers. Chronic cough, sputum production, and breathlessness are much more common in smokers. Smokers are more likely than nonsmokers to show abnormalities in a number of pulmonary function tests including measurements of elastic recoil, airflow in large and small airways, and diffusing capacity. Mild airflow obstruction in small airways may be present even in teenage smokers.

Cigarette smoking has been associated with an increased incidence of respiratory infections and deaths from pneumonia and influenza. Postoperative respiratory complications and spontaneous pneumothorax are also more common in smokers. Because tobacco smoke may increase airway obstruction, asthmatics should be urged not to smoke. Chronic stomatitis and chronic laryngitis occur more frequently in smokers than in nonsmokers.

Pregnancy Smoking may delay conception, and smoking during pregnancy may affect the fetus adversely. Infants whose mothers smoked during pregnancy weigh, on average, 170 g less than infants whose mothers did not smoke. This effect probably results from impaired uteroplacental circulation. Maternal smoking during pregnancy increases the risk of spontaneous abortion, fetal death, neonatal death, and the sudden infant death syndrome. This increased risk may be much greater in pregnancies already at high risk due to other factors. Smoking during pregnancy may also adversely affect the long-term physical growth and intellectual development of the child.

Gastrointestinal disorders Gastric and duodenal ulcer disease is more prevalent in male and female cigarette smokers than in nonsmokers and causes more deaths in male smokers than in nonsmokers. Smoking impairs spontaneous and drug-induced healing of peptic ulcers, increases the likelihood of duodenal ulcer recurrence, inhibits pancreactic bicarbonate secretion, and decreases the pressure of esophageal and pyloric sphincters. Histamine-2-receptor antagonist inhibition of nocturnal gastric secretion is also prevented by smoking.

Depression Recent studies indicate that the prevalence of cigarette smoking is increased among those who have had a major depressive disorder. Furthermore, smoking cessation rates are lower among depressed smokers, compared to nondepressed smokers. What role antidepressants could play in such individuals who are attempting to quit smoking remains to be determined.

Involuntary smoke inhalation Indoor atmospheres and other confined spaces are often contaminated by tobacco smoke which is inhaled involuntarily by both smokers and nonsmokers. Most of the atmospheric pollutants arise from sidestream smoke. It contains greater concentrations of many smoke constituents than does mainstream smoke, but since sidestream smoke is diluted in a large volume of air, the smoke exposure from involuntary inhalation is less than that associated with smoking.

Initially, involuntary or passive smoking was thought to cause primarily an irritant effect such as ocular burning. It is now recognized as a cause of lung cancer in nonsmokers. Parental smoking in the home is associated with an increased risk of acute respiratory illnesses, middle-ear effusions, chronic respiratory symptoms, and slightly impaired lung function in children. Involuntary smoke inhalation may also cause coronary heart disease.

Drug effects Tobacco smoke constituents induce hepatic microsomal enzyme systems that are important in the metabolism of several drugs. For example, cigarette smoking increases the metabolism of propranolol, propoxyphene, and theophylline. Hence, changes in smoking behavior may cause significant alterations of serum drug levels that may result in either drug toxicity or failure of drug treatment.

TYPES OF SMOKING During the past 20 years the amount of tar and nicotine delivered by cigarettes made in the United States has decreased by more the 50 percent. Filter-tipped cigarettes and lower-tar and -nicotine cigarettes now account for more than 95 and 55 percent of sales, respectively. Lung cancer and laryngeal cancer are the only tobacco-related diseases for which the use of lower-tar and -nicotine cigarettes has been shown to result in risk reduction, compared with the use of higher-tar and -nicotine cigarettes; however, compared with not smoking or quitting, the benefits are minimal. Consumers who choose lower-tar and -nicotine cigarettes and then smoke a larger number of cigarettes or inhale more frequently or deeply may actually increase their exposure to harmful substances. There is also concern because unidentified flavoring agents are added to these cigarettes to enhance consumer acceptance.

Cigar and pipe smokers usually inhale less smoke than cigarette smokers, presumably because the alkaline pH of cigar and pipe tobacco makes it more irritating to the respiratory tract. The smoke exposure and overall mortality rates of pipe and cigar smokers in the United States are substantially less than those of cigarette smokers; however, death rates of cigarette, cigar, and pipe smokers are approximately equal for carcinoma of the oral cavity, larynx, and esophagus, sites where exposures to cigarette, cigar, and pipe smoke are similar. The mortality rates of most cigar and pipe smokers for cancer at other sites, CHD, and COPD are not greatly elevated above the rates of nonsmokers, but cigar and pipe smokers who inhale consistently may experience adverse health effects comparable with those of cigarette smokers.

The use of chewing tobacco and snuff may produce plasma nicotine levels comparable to those of cigarette smokers and lead to nicotine dependence or addiction. The use of such smokeless tobacco products also increases the risk for oral cancer.

CESSATION OF SMOKING In the United States between 1965 and 1990, the prevalence of smoking in adults declined from 52 to 28 percent of men and 34 to 23 percent of women. In 1990 there were an estimated 45.8 million current adult smokers and 44.1 million former smokers; approximately one-half of living Americans who had ever smoked had successfully quit. In recent years, the smoking prevalence among senior high school students has leveled off at about 20 percent. The rate of decline in smoking prevalence among the least educated Americans lags behind other groups.

Benefits Smoking cessation produces immediate and long-term physical, psychological, and economic benefits. Within days of quitting the sense of smell and taste may improve. One year after quitting there is a substantial decrease in risk for a myocardial infarction. When chronic smoking produces permanent damage, as it does in the case of emphysema, the benefits of cessation are more modest such as slowing of the rate of decline of pulmonary function. The U.S. Surgeon General recently summarized the major and immediate health benefits of cessation that are valid for men and women of all ages and for those with and without smoking-related disease. Former smokers live, on the average, longer than continuing smokers. For example those who quit prior to the age of 50 have one-half the risk of dying in the next 15 years, compared to continuing smokers. Cessation reduces the risk for tobacco-related cancers, myocardial infarction, cerebrovascular disease, and chronic obstructive pulmonary disease. Women who quit smoking prior to pregnancy, or during the first trimester, eliminate the risk of delivering a low birth weight baby. The health benefits of quitting smoking far exceed the risks of the average 5-pound weight gain or any adverse psychological effects that may occur after quitting.

Cessation process Most American smokers would like to quit. 80 percent have attempted to stop smoking during their lifetime, and 30 percent have stopped for at least one day during the previous year. Most of these attempts to quit are only temporarily successful. Smoking cessation is a dynamic, cyclic process that leads to overcoming an addictive behavior. Smokers move through a series of stages in their attempts to quit including thinking about quitting, deciding to quit, attempting to quit, and maintaining the ex-smoker status. Most successful quitters relapse and recycle through these stages three or four times before attaining long-term abstinence. Less than 5 percent of smokers move directly to the confirmed ex-smoker status without experiencing relapses. Factors encouraging long-term cessation include decreased social acceptability of smoking, increased concern about the health consequences of active and passive smoking, and increased costs of tobacco products. Factors contributing to relapse include craving for nicotine, weight gain, social pressures, and attempts to cope with negative feelings and interpersonal conflicts.

Cessation methods More than 90 percent of confirmed ex-smokers quit without formal assistance. Quitting "cold turkey" is the method used by more than 80 percent of successful ex-smokers. However, heavy smokers and those most addicted to nicotine may benefit from participation in a cessation program. Organized programs employ a variety of approaches including: self-help, physician advice and counseling, use of medication, group therapy, behavioral training, hypnosis, and acupuncture. With such methods 20 to 30 percent 1-year abstinence rates are commonly reported. Controlled trials have shown significantly greater cessation rates for smokers receiving interventions, compared to control groups. The most effective programs offer multiple treatment modalities, involvement of physician and nonphysician health personnel, and a clear nonsmoking message presented in a variety of formats over time.

Physician guidelines Physicians have unique opportunities and effective tools to promote smoking cessation. Seventy percent of American smokers visit a physician at least once a year. Some of these visits occur when the patient is experiencing symptomatic illness. In such settings patients may be especially responsive to cessation messages, and quit rates may be substantially enhanced. Even brief, physician-delivered stop-smoking messages may double the spontaneous smoking cessation rate. Treatment of nicotine addic-

TABLE 393-2   Physician guidelines for managing nicotine addiction
Assessment
A Smoking history
B Level of nicotine addiction
C Health status
D Quitting experience
E Interest in quitting
Intervention
A Teach
1 Benefits of cessation
2 Cessation process
3 Withdrawal syndrome
B Advise to quit
1 Personalized message
2 Quit date
3 "Cold turkey"
C Select cessation method(s)
1 Self-help
2 Physician-assisted
3 Nicotine replacement
4 Behavioral training
5 Group therapy
D Implement method
E Meet special needs
Follow-up
A Measure progress
B Provide support
C Deal with relapse
D Consider alternative methods
E Consider referral

tion is at least as cost-effective as treating other common medical problems such as hypertension and hypercholesterolemia.

Nicotine addiction should be viewed as a chronic medical problem requiring long-term commitment and management skills. The primary goal for each clinic visit should be to assist the smoker to move one step closer to quitting. The three essential phases for physician management include assessment, intervention, and follow-up (Table 393-2). During the assessment phase data are collected on health status, nicotine addiction, quitting experience, and interest in quitting. If the patient doesn't want to stop smoking, the clinician should review the risks of smoking, recommend quitting, and defer further action until the next clinic visit. Most patients are interested in quitting and progress to the intervention phase. Smokers are taught about the benefits of quitting and the cyclical cessation process. The smoker is advised to choose a quit date and to go "cold turkey." A cessation method(s) is chosen and implemented. Physicians often provide educational material, counseling, and, recently, nicotine replacement therapy. Both nicotine chewing gum and transdermal patches improve cessation rates when used in combination with other interventions. The proper uses, contraindications, and side effects of these products should be understood. For example, nicotine replacement therapy should not be used when the patient is still smoking. The likelihood of success with any cessation method is enhanced when the clinician responds to individual concerns such as weight gain and helps the smoker to develop practical strategies to avoid relapse. The final phase, follow-up, involves assessing progress, providing support, and dealing with relapse. The last should not be viewed as failure but as part of the cyclic process leading to cessation. Follow-up discussions may focus on alternative cessation methods or referral to a smoking cessation specialist.

Political, social, and cultural forces play a critical role in the individual decision to start or stop smoking. For this reason, physicians should lead and support efforts to increase tobacco excise taxes, to eliminate all tobacco advertisements and promotional activities, and to ban smoking in public places.

PREVENTION Ultimately, primary smoking prevention in the pediatric and adolescent age groups may be the most effective program. Young people who have been trained to resist social pressures, who understand the health consequences of smoking, and who appreciate the difficulty of quitting are less likely to start smoking.

REFERENCES

Fiore MC (ed): Cigarette smoking: A clinical guide to assessment and treatment. Med Clinic North Am 76:289, 1992

Lesmes GR (ed): The effects of cigarette smoking: A global perspective. Am J Med 93(1A):1S, 1992

U.S. Department of Health and Human Services: The health consequences of involuntary smoking. A report of the Surgeon General. DHHS(CDC) Publication no 87-8398, 1986

U.S. Department of Health and Human Services: The health consequences of smoking: Nicotine addiction. A report of the Surgeon General. DHHS(CDC) Publication no 88-8406, 1988

U.S. Department of Health and Human Services: Reducing the health consequences of smoking: 25 years of progress. A report of the Surgeon General. DHHS(CDC) Publication no 89-8411, 1989

U.S. Department of Health and Human Services: The health benefits of smoking cessation. A report of the Surgeon General. DHHS(CDC) Publication no 90-8416, 1990

PART FIFTEEN

ENVIRONMENTAL AND OCCUPATIONAL HAZARDS

394 PHYSICIANS AND HAZARDS OF THE ENVIRONMENT AND WORKPLACE

HOWARD HU / FRANK E. SPEIZER

The term *hazards* encompasses chemical hazards as well as other risks posed by the physical environment (changes in temperature or altitude/pressure, exposures to ionizing and nonionizing radiation) and selected natural phenomena (venoms and stings). Unless otherwise defined, *toxins* and *toxic exposures* are synonymous with *hazards*. These hazards may occur in the general environment or in the workplace. Strictly speaking, smoking, alcohol ingestion, poor nutrition, and infectious diseases also could be considered chemical or environmental hazards.

While the identification and control of hazards often lie in the domain of public health, there are a number of compelling reasons for all physicians to become acquainted with both the hazards themselves and the basic precepts of environmental/occupational medicine:

1 Millions of people are exposed to hazards at levels sufficient to result in demonstrable health problems. Public awareness of these hazards has grown, as has the expectation that physicians can diagnose and treat associated disorders.
2 Specialists in occupational/environmental health are few in number.
3 Many manifestations of exposure-related illnesses are nonspecific (e.g., dizziness, headache) or present as commonly encountered problems of general practice (e.g., myocardial infarction, cancer). The establishment of a connection with a hazard requires a high index of suspicion and application of fundamental concepts of environmental/occupational medicine.
4 Early recognition by physicians of unusual patterns of illness or asymptomatic exposure to toxins with low-level effects (e.g., an elevated blood lead level) can alert health officials to the need for control measures.
5 Physicians can contribute to toxicologic knowledge by reporting reactions to new chemicals (similar to the reporting of adverse drug effects). Case reports in the literature often prompt epidemiologic studies.
6 In many states and countries, the reporting by physicians of occupational/environmental diseases is mandatory. For instance, since 1992, physicians in Massachusetts have been required to report cases of pneumoconiosis, occupational asthma, carpal tunnel syndrome, carbon monoxide poisoning, and others.
7 Identification of an environmental/occupational etiology of an illness may have important economic ramifications for the patient (e.g., worker's compensation, which pays for medical bills as well as lost wages). Physicians are frequently asked to provide expert medical testimony on the causal relationship between toxic exposures and diseases during the course of litigation.

For any given physician, it is difficult to estimate the fraction of disease that is likely to be attributable to environmental and occupational factors. A summary of diagnoses based on referral visits to a clinic specializing in environmental/occupational disorders (Table 394-1) revealed a wide variety of disorders, asbestos-related pulmonary disorders being the most common. Whether recognized as hazard-associated illnesses or not, a similarly wide spectrum is probably seen by internists, although variations can be expected due to regional differences in hazardous exposures and referral patterns.

Clinical effects of chemical and environmental hazards are discussed in chapters devoted to the specifically involved organ (Chap. 219) or to specific exposures (Chaps. 395 to 401). To list the vast array of environmental hazard–disease relationships is beyond the scope of this chapter. Utilizing additional references (see "General References" at end of this chapter) is important when considering an environmental/occupational etiology.

THE ILL PATIENT: RECOGNIZING A CHEMICAL OR OTHER ENVIRONMENTAL ETIOLOGY

THE ENVIRONMENTAL/OCCUPATIONAL HISTORY Taking an appropriate environmental/occupational history as part of the medical workup is critical for recognizing these disorders. The level of detail that is called for depends on the clinical situation. *Always obtain information on the current and major past occupations for all patients seen.* When confronted by an illness of uncertain etiology or by an

TABLE 394-1 Most common disorders related to patient visits, 1987–1991[a]

Diagnoses	Average no. of visits per year[b]
Asbestos-related disease	
Pleural disease	220
Asbestosis	68
Mesothelioma	2
Lung cancer and heavy asbestos exposure	2
Unexplained pleural effusion	3
Pneumoconioses (other than asbestos)	3
Chemical bronchitis/tracheitis[c]	4
Occupational/environmental asthma	35
Chemical dermatitis	2
Low back strain	3
Carpal tunnel syndrome	6
Other cumulative trauma disorder	5
Toxic hepatitis[d]	4
Toxic encephalopathy[e]	9
Toxic peripheral neuropathy	5
Lead poisoning/over-exposure	7
Poisoning (miscellaneous)[f]	5
Multiple chemical sensitivity syndrome	5
Tight building syndrome	4
Symptoms, suspected but unproven link to occupational or environmental factors	41

[a] At the Harvard School of Public Health–affiliated Massachusetts Respiratory Hospital Center for Occupational/Environmental Medicine, Braintree, MA, between 1987 and 1991.
[b] Routine visits for screening exams have been excluded. Cases of contact dermatitis, low-back strain, and carpal tunnel syndrome are probably underrepresented because of referral bias.
[c] From welding fumes, chlorine vapors, and other irritants.
[d] Usually from exposure to solvents.
[e] Usually from solvents or carbon monoxide.
[f] From arsenic, mercury, vanadium, pesticides, PCBs, cyanide, ozone, carbon disulfide, etc.

illness for which an environmental/occupational source has not been entertained, these factors should be explored in detail, beginning with an environmental/occupational history.

The identification of potential chemical exposures can be difficult. Household products must list chemical ingredients on their labels. For workplace exposures, the Occupational Safety and Health Administration (OSHA) requires chemical suppliers to provide material safety data sheets (MSDS) with their products and requires employers to retain them and make them available to employees. They can be obtained by the physician or employee by a telephone or written request; failure of an employer to provide them within 30 days of such a request is a violation of OSHA regulations and punishable by fines. In addition to providing information on chemical ingredients and percent composition, the MSDS provides basic information on toxicity. This information is seldom adequate from a clinical perspective but may indicate the general type of toxicity that may be anticipated.

EVALUATING POSSIBLE CHEMICAL OR ENVIRONMENTAL HAZARDS   Given the wide variety of toxic exposures that may be uncovered during a workup, a clinician should routinely consult additional reference material to evaluate whether particular hazards may be associated with the illness at hand.

Many sources of information exist. Some regional poison control centers have extensive information on hazards that can be transmitted by telephone or facsimile. Other resources, depending on the area, may include county and state health departments, regional offices of the National Institute for Occupational Safety and Health (NIOSH) and the Environmental Protection Agency (EPA), the Centers for Disease Control and Prevention (CDC) in Atlanta, the Consumer Products Safety Commission (CPSC) in Washington, D.C., academic institutions, and individual toxicologists, occupational/environmental medicine specialists, or industrial hygienists.

Sophisticated computerized databases are also available, including detailed listings on CD-ROM information systems and MEDLARS, an electronic database maintained by the National Library of Medicine and accessible by modem. In addition to MEDLINE, the on-line bibliographic database familiar to many physicians, MEDLARS has other files that provide specific toxicity information on chemicals and that include toxicologic references not covered by MEDLINE.

As with any other illness, laboratory investigation may be crucial. For example, tests of carboxyhemoglobin level to document carbon monoxide exposure or of serum anticholinesterase level to document organophosphate pesticide absorption should be performed within hours of exposure. As with acute drug overdoses, it is useful to freeze urine and serum samples from any patient suspected of suffering from an acute chemical exposure; such specimens can be analyzed at a later date using sensitive methods of detection. Use of other tests must rely on knowledge of the specific hazard or illness in question.

SUSPICIOUS SCENARIOS   Some medical problems or clinical scenarios demand a particularly high degree of suspicion for occupational or environmental factors as causative or contributing agents of disease.

Respiratory disease   The contribution of occupational/environmental factors to respiratory disease is generally underrecognized, particularly among patients who smoke and the elderly (see Chap. 219). For instance, asthma related to chemical exposure may be treated without regard to cause or erroneously diagnosed as acute tracheobronchitis. Shortness of breath from asbestosis may be attributed to chronic obstructive pulmonary disease. Chemical pneumonitis may be misdiagnosed as a bacterial infection.

Cancer   Many cancers are thought to be causally related to occupational and environmental factors in addition to tobacco. Some are particularly likely to have a chemical or other environmental etiology, including cancers of the skin (solar radiation, arsenic, coal tar, soot), lung (asbestos, arsenic, nickel, radon), pleura (almost exclusively asbestos), nasal cavity and sinuses (chromium, nickel, wood and leather dusts), liver (arsenic, vinyl chloride), bone marrow (benzene, ionizing radiation), and bladder (aromatic amines).

Coronary disease   Carbon monoxide exposure is common, particularly in homes with malfunctioning furnaces or in workplaces close to motor vehicle exhaust. By reducing oxygen transport by hemoglobin and inhibiting mitochondrial metabolism, carbon monoxide can aggravate coronary disease. Methylene chloride, a solvent used in paint stripping, is converted to carbon monoxide and thus poses the same risk. Exposure to carbon disulfide, a chemical used in the production of rayon, accelerates the rate of atherosclerotic plaque formation.

Hepatitis/chronic liver disease   In the absence of evidence that a virus, alcohol ingestion, or drug is the main cause of hepatitis (see Chaps. 266 and 267), a toxin must be considered. Toxin-induced hepatic injury may be cytotoxic, cholestatic, or both. The list of hepatotoxic agents is long, but common ones include organic synthetic compounds such as carbon tetrachloride (used in solvents and cleaning fluids) and methylene diamine (a resin hardener), pesticides such as chlordecone (Kepone), metals, particularly arsenic (used in pesticides and paints and found in well water), and natural toxins such as the pyrrolidizine alkaloids.

Kidney disease   Many chemical and environmental factors can cause renal injury (see Chap. 236). The etiology of much chronic kidney disease, however, remains unknown. An increasing body of evidence now links chronic renal failure with hypertension to lead exposure. Some studies suggest that chronic exposure to hydrocarbons (e.g., gasoline, paints, solvents) may lead to various types of glomerulonephritis, including Goodpasture's syndrome.

Peripheral neuropathy   Organic solvents such as n-hexane, heavy metals such as lead and arsenic, and some organophosphate compounds can damage the axons of peripheral nerves. Dimethylaminopropionitrile (DMAPN), an industrial catalyst, causes bladder neuropathy. Nerve entrapment syndromes of the upper extremity, such as carpal tunnel syndrome, may be caused by jobs that involve repetitive motion, especially those which involve maintenance of awkward positions.

Neuropsychiatric symptoms   Fatigue, memory loss, difficulty in concentration, and emotional lability have been linked to chronic exposure to solvents such as toluene and perchlorethylene. Painters, metal degreasers, plastics workers, and cleaners are commonly exposed to solvents and develop these symptoms at a high rate. Characteristic patterns on formal neurobehavioral testing and stabilization of symptoms with gradual improvement following removal from exposure are among the features that distinguish these patients. Other substances associated with neurobehavioral dysfunction include metals, particularly lead, mercury, arsenic, and manganese; carbon monoxide; and pesticides, such as organophosphates and organochlorines.

Teratogenesis and reproductive problems   Toxins can impair successful reproduction at a variety of levels. Examples include insecticides and herbicides, PCBs and PBBs (polychlorinated and polybrominated biphenyls, see below), ethylene oxide (a sterilizing gas used in hospitals), metals (lead, arsenic, cadmium, mercury), and solvents. Dibromochloropropane (DBCP), a nematocide, suppresses spermatogenesis. Some toxins, such as PCBs, PBBs, and chlorinated pesticides, are concentrated in milk.

Immunosuppression, autoimmunity, and hypersensitivity   Evidence is increasing that exposures to some chemical agents can compromise the immune system, thereby leading to a generalized increased incidence of tumors (e.g., exposure to PBBs) or infections (e.g., respiratory infections after exposure to common air pollutants). Mercury, dieldrin, and methylcholanthrene are known to elicit autoimmune responses. Some chemicals are potent allergic sensitizers that cause dermal and respiratory problems (see Chaps. 53 and 219).

MANAGING A HAZARD-RELATED ILLNESS

Once a chemical or other environmental hazard has been identified as an important contributor to an illness, the next step is to prevent

TABLE 394-2   Environmental/occupational medicine: Examples of unsolved concerns for the 1990s

Topic	Summary of issues involved
Dioxin	(aka TCDD, or 2,3,7,8-tetrachlorodibenzo-*p*-dioxin) Chief ingredient of agent orange and a major contaminant of hazardous waste sites; potent animal carcinogen; most recent epidemiologic studies suggest that it conveys mild risk of soft tissue sarcomas in humans.
PCBs	(aka polychlorinated biphenyls, Arachlor) A mixture of synthetic compounds formerly used to insulate transformers and capacitors; potent animal liver carcinogen; consequences of human exposure unclear, but may involve cancer, reproductive, and neurologic effects.
Multiple chemical sensitivity	Nonspecific symptoms (e.g., headache, dizziness, fatigue, irritability, loss of memory or concentration) in relation to exposure to a wide variety of chemicals at extremely low levels (e.g., formaldehyde vapor from new carpets; solvents found in perfumes, glues, photocopy machines, dry-cleaned clothes); no laboratory abnormalities are found; incidence appears to be increasing; mechanism under investigation.
Hazardous waste	Exposure can occur through direct contact at abandoned or unsecured sites; volatilization or conversion to dust carried in air; seepage into groundwater used by wells; contamination of the food chain through marine organisms living in polluted waters and plants and animals living on contaminated soil; and dissemination by fire and explosion; nausea, headache, nose and throat irritation, and increased respiratory morbidity are common complaints of those residing near chemical waste dumps; the risk of cancer posed by exposure to part-per-billion concentrations of pollutants from such contamination is of continuing concern.
Global climatic change	Stratospheric depletion of ozone is leading to increased exposure to solar ultraviolet radiation (UVR); in addition to increasing the risk of skin cancers, UVR is a risk factor for cataractogenesis and may impair cellular immunity; global warming will lead to increased heat exposure and is also likely to have an indirect effect on health by altering the distribution of communicable disease vectors and exacerbating problems of crop growth and food availability.

further exposure. For chronic diseases such as cancer, this step is irrelevant; the illness remains when the exposure has come and gone. For others, the physician *must be willing to become an active advocate for the patient.* This may involve writing a letter stating that the patient should no longer be exposed to a hazard or should remain out of work, or it may involve contacting appropriate officials in government, industry, or labor or other advocates who can deal with a hazardous exposure. Treatment is dependent on the specific hazard.

In few areas of medicine does a physician deal with more scientific uncertainty. Comprehensive information on toxicants is available for only a small percentage of chemicals. In general, the physician should take a conservative approach (i.e., advise avoidance of a hazard if it is likely to have contributed to the illness) and to use common sense and up-to-date information to evaluate causal relationships.

LOW-LEVEL EXPOSURES AND THEIR EFFECTS

The subclinical effects of toxins that are widespread in our environment and workplaces are of increasing concern. Given the absence of any demonstrable effect threshold, low-level exposure to carcinogens should be avoided. Equally important are the noncarcinogenic effects of chronic low-level exposures such as lead.

Multiple pathways of exposure, including the combustion of leaded gasoline, the use of lead-based paints and solder, and the lead in cans containing food, have contributed to exposure of the entire population. Such low-level exposures can impair neurobehavioral development in infants and children (see Chap. 378) and raise blood pressure in adults. Furthermore, absorbed lead is stored in the skeleton and may reenter the circulation at times of heightened bone turnover (e.g., pregnancy, lactation, osteoporosis, hyperthyroidism).

Subclinical toxic effects can be prevented if chronic low-level exposure is detected early and curtailed. In the case of lead, this takes the form of a test of blood lead level, performed regularly in small children living in old neighborhoods, and as a precautionary measure in adults with a history of lead exposure.

UNSOLVED CONCERNS FOR THE 1990s

Examples of issues in this field, not mentioned elsewhere in this book, that are either of emerging concern or the sources of unresolved controversies are given in Table 394-2. The challenge is to remain abreast of developments in these areas, particularly when confronted by a relevant case.

SPECIFIC REFERENCES

Bailar J: How dangerous is dioxin? N Engl J Med 324:260, 1991
Fiedler N et al: Evaluation of chemically sensitive patients. J Occup Med 34:529, 1992
Freund E et al: Mandatory reporting of occupational diseases by clinicians. JAMA 262:3041, 1989
Goldman RH, Peters JM: The occupational and environmental health history. JAMA 246:2831, 1981
Haines A: Global warming and health. Br Med J 302:669, 1991
Himmelstein JS, Frumkin H: The right to know about toxic exposures: Implications for physicians. N Engl J Med 312:687, 1985
Paul M (ed): *Occupational/Environmental Hazards and Reproductive Health: A Guide for Clinicians.* Baltimore, Williams & Wilkens, 1992
White RF et al: Neurobehavioral effects of toxicity due to metals, solvents, and insecticides. Clin Neuropharmacol 13:392, 1990

GENERAL REFERENCES

Bezman Tarcher A (ed): *Principles and Practice of Environmental Medicine.* New York, Plenum, 1992
Cullen MR et al: Occupational medicine—Medical progress. N Engl J Med 322:594, 1990
LaDou J (ed): *Occupational Medicine.* Norwalk: Appleton & Lange, 1990
National Institute for Occupational Safety and Health: *Pocket Guide to Chemical Hazards.* Cincinnati, National Institute for Occupational Safety and Health, DHHS(NIOSH) Publ No 90-117, 1990.
Rom WN (ed): *Environmental and Occupational Medicine,* 2d ed. Boston, Little, Brown, 1992
Sullivan JB Jr, Krieger GR (eds): *Hazardous Materials Toxicology—Clinical Principles of Environmental Health.* Baltimore, Williams & Wilkins, 1992
Upton AC (ed): Environmental medicine. Med Clin North Am Volume 74: XXX, 1990

395   ACUTE POISON AND DRUG OVERDOSAGE

FREDERICK H. LOVEJOY, JR. / CHRISTOPHER H. LINDEN

A poison (toxin) is a substance capable of producing adverse effects in a living organism. Poisons may be divided into those intended for human use (foods and their additives, pharmaceuticals, toiletries, cosmetics) and those that are not (household products, industrial chemicals, nonfood nondrug botanicals). An overdose implies exposure to excessive amounts of the former and any amount of the latter; it may or may not result in harmful effects (poisoning).

Poisoning may be local (limited to the eyes, skin, lungs, or gastrointestinal tract), systemic, or both, depending on dose, absorption, distribution, potency, and host susceptibility. Absorption and distribution are influenced by properties of the chemical itself (molecular size, degree of ionization, lipid and water solubility, protein binding) and of the biologic barriers (membrane composition, pore size, chemical transport systems) through which it penetrates.

Local effects are due to nonspecific chemical reactions such as oxidation, protein denaturation, desiccation, and solvent activity. The severity and reversibility depend on the dose (concentration), contact time, potency of the chemical, and type and condition of the exposed surface. The nature, extent, severity, and reversibility of systemic effects depend on the dose, potency, and metabolic disposition of the chemical, the functional reserve of the individual, and the presence of secondary complications (shock, hypoxia). Other variables that influence toxicity include coexisting illnesses, previous chemical exposure (e.g., enzyme induction or inhibition, tolerance), and individual differences in biologic response, tissue concentration (pharmacodynamics), and/or absorption, distribution, metabolism, and elimination (pharmacokinetics). When compared with therapeutic dosing, effects of an overdose begin sooner, peak later, and last longer.

EPIDEMIOLOGY

In the United States, potential poisoning (exposures) result in an estimated 5 million requests for medical advice or treatment each year. The common routes of exposure are ingestion (79 percent), dermal (7 percent), ophthalmic (6 percent), inhalation (5 percent), bites and stings (3 percent), and parenteral injections (0.3 percent). Prescribed drugs are involved in 40 percent of exposures. Frequently involved substances include cleaning agents, analgesics, cosmetics, plants, cough and cold preparations, and hydrocarbons. Most exposures are acute, accidental, occur in the home, result in minor or no toxicity, and involve children under 6 years of age.

Accidental exposures can result from the improper use of chemicals at work or play, product mislabeling, label misreading, mistaken identification of unlabeled chemicals, uninformed self-medication, and dosing errors by nurses, parents, pharmacists, physicians, and the elderly. Excluding the recreational use of ethanol, attempted suicide is the most common reason for intentional exposure. Unintended poisonings may result from use of drugs for psychotropic effects (abuse) or excessive self-dosing (misuse).

Although only 4 percent of victims of chemical exposure require hospitalization, they account for roughly 5 percent of intensive care unit admissions and up to 30 percent of psychiatric admissions. Suicide attempts account for most (60 to 90 percent) serious or fatal poisonings. Deaths are most common from carbon monoxide poisoning and occur prior to arrival at a hospital. Antidepressants, analgesics, stimulants and street drugs, cardiovascular agents, sedative-hypnotics, and asthma medications are responsible for most drug-related fatalities. Nonpharmaceutical agents implicated in fatal poisoning include inorganic chemicals, alcohols and glycols, cleaning agents, and hydrocarbons.

DIAGNOSIS OF POISONING

Although poisoning can mimic other illnesses, the correct diagnosis usually can be established by the history, physical examination, routine and toxicologic laboratory evaluations, and clinical course. The history should include the time, route, duration, and circumstances (location, surrounding events, intent) of exposure; the name and amount of each drug, chemical, or ingredient involved; the time of onset, nature, and severity of symptoms; the time and type of first aid measures provided; and the past medical and psychiatric history.

In many cases the victim is confused, comatose, unaware of an exposure, or unable or unwilling to admit to one. Suspicious circumstances include unexplained illness in a previously healthy person; history of psychiatric problems (particularly depression); recent changes in health, economic status, or social relationships; and onset of illness while working with chemicals or after ingesting food, drink (especially ethanol), or medications. Patients who become ill soon after arriving from a foreign country or after arrest for criminal activity should be suspected of having illicit drugs concealed in body cavities (the gastrointestinal tract). Family, friends, paramedics, police, pharmacists, physicians, and employers may provide information regarding habits, hobbies, behavior changes, available medications, and antecedent events. A search of the clothes and place of discovery may reveal a suicide note or empty container of drugs or chemicals. The imprint code on pills and the label on chemical products may be used to identify the ingredients and potential toxicity of a suspected poison by consulting a reference text, a computerized chemical database, the manufacturer, or a regional poison information center.

The physical examination should initially focus on the vital signs and cardiopulmonary and neurologic status to assess the need for immediate supportive treatment. Since the clinical picture can usually be characterized by either physiologic stimulation or depression, these parameters also provide the most important diagnostic clues in poisoning of unknown etiology (Table 395-1). Examination of the eyes (for nystagmus, pupil size, and reactivity), abdomen (for bowel activity and bladder), and skin (for burns, bullae, color, warmth, moisture, pressure sores, and puncture marks) may narrow the diagnosis to a particular syndrome. Grading the severity of poisoning (Table 395-2) is useful for assessing prognosis and the clinical course.

The patient also should be examined for evidence of trauma and underlying illnesses. Except with carbon monoxide, theophylline, and drugs that cause hypoglycemia and hypoxia, seizures and neurologic dysfunction due to poisoning are almost never focal. Hence focal findings should prompt evaluation for a structural central nervous system (CNS) lesion. When the history is unclear, all orifices should be examined for the presence of chemical burns and drug packets. The odor of breath or vomitus and the color of nails, skin, or urine may provide diagnostic clues.

TABLE 395-1   Differential diagnosis of poisoning based on vital signs and CNS activity

Stimulant poisoning	Depressant poisoning
Sympathomimetic syndrome	**Sympatholytic syndrome**
Amphetamines	Adrenergic blockers
Caffeine	Antiarrhythmics
Cocaine	Antidepressants (tricyclic)
Decongestants	Antihypertensives
Ergot alkaloids	Calcium channel blockers
MAO inhibitors	Digoxin
Theophylline	**Cholinergic syndrome**
Anticholinergic syndrome	Bethanecol
Antidepressants (tricyclic)	Carbamate insecticides
Antihistamines	Organophosphate insecticides
Antiparkinsonian agents	Myasthenia gravis drugs
Antipsychotics	(e.g., pyridostigmine)
Antispasmodics (GI, GU)	Physostigmine
Belladonna alkaloids	**Narcotic syndrome**
Cyclobenzaprine	Analgesics
Mydriatics (topical)	Antispasmodics (GI)
Plants/mushrooms	**Sedative-hypnotic syndrome**
Hallucinogenic syndrome	Alcohol
LSD and synthetic analogues	Antiepileptics
Marijuana	Barbiturates
Mescaline and synthetic	Benzodiazepines
analogues	Ethchlorvynol
Phencyclidine	Hydrocarbons
Withdrawal syndrome	Glutethimide
Alcohol	Methyprylon
Antidepressants	
Beta-blockers	
Clonidine	
Narcotics	
Sedative-hypnotics	

TABLE 395-2 Severity of stimulant and depressant poisoning and drug withdrawal

Severity	Signs and symptoms
STIMULANT POISONING	
Grade 1	Diaphoresis, flushing, hyperreflexia, irritability, mydriasis, tremors
Grade 2	Confusion, fever, hyperactivity, hypertension, tachycardia, tachypnea
Grade 3	Delirium, mania, hyperpyrexia, tachyarrhythmias
Grade 4	Coma, convulsions, cardiovascular collapse
DEPRESSANT POISONING	
Grade 1	Lethargic but arousable; able to answer questions and follow commands
Grade 2	Comatose; withdraws from pain; brainstem and deep tendon reflexes intact
Grade 3	Comatose; no response to pain; most reflexes absent; respiratory depression
Grade 4	Comatose; no response to pain; reflexes absent; respiratory and cardiovascular depression

An anion gap metabolic acidosis is characteristic of methanol, ethylene glycol, and salicylate intoxication and may occur in any poisoning that results in hypoxia, hypotension, or seizures. The serum lactate concentration is low (less than the anion gap) in the former nd high (nearly equal to the anion gap) in the latter. An osmolal gap, the difference between the measured serum osmolality (freezing point depression, not the vapor pressure method) and the calculated osmolality (from the serum sodium, glucose, and BUN), of more than 10 mmol/L indicates the presence of a low-molecular-weight solute such as acetone, ethanol, ethylene glycol, isopropyl alcohol, or methanol or an unmeasured electrolyte (magnesium) or sugar (mannitol). An increased anion gap metabolic acidosis with respiratory alkalosis, ketosis, and tinnitus suggests salicylate poisoning; an increased osmolal gap accompanied by back pain, hypocalcemia, and crystalluria suggests ethylene glycol intoxication, and an increased osmolal gap accompanied by visual symptoms suggests methanol poisoning. Poisons that cause specific signs, symptoms, and other laboratory abnormalities are listed in the references cited.

Pulmonary edema (ARDS) can occur with carbon monoxide, cyanide, narcotic, paraquat, phencyclidine, sedative-hypnotic, and salicylate poisoning; inhalation of irritant gases, fumes, or vapors (ammonia, metal oxides, mercury); or prolonged anoxia, hyperthermia, or shock. Aspiration pneumonia is common in patients with coma, seizures, and petroleum distillate ingestion. Radiopaque densities may be visible on abdominal x-rays following the ingestion of calcium salts, chloral hydrate, chlorinated hydrocarbons, enteric-coated tablets, heavy metals, illicit drug packets, iodinated compounds, lithium, phenothiazines, and salicylates.

Bradycardia and AV block may occur in patients poisoned by antiarrhythmic agents, beta blockers, calcium channel blockers, cholinergic agents (carbamate and organophosphate insecticides), digitalis, lithium, phenylpropanolamine, and tricyclic antidepressants. QRS- and QT-interval prolongation may be caused by amantidine, antiarrhythmics, tricyclic antidepressants, fluorides, heavy metals (arsenic, thallium), lithium, magnesium, meperidine metabolites, neuroleptics, and potassium. Ventricular tachyarrhythmias may be seen in poisoning with sympathomimetics and agents that cause QRS and QT prolongation.

Analysis of urine and blood (and occasionally gastric contents and chemical samples) may be useful to confirm or rule out suspected poisoning. Interpretation of laboratory data requires knowledge of the tests used for screening and confirmation (thin-layer, gas-liquid, high-performance liquid chromatography; colorimetric and fluorometric assays; enzyme-multiplied and radioimmunoassays; gas chromatography; mass spectrometry), their sensitivity (limit of detection) and specificity, and the best type and time of sampling of biologic specimens for analysis. Personal communication with the laboratory is essential. A negative screen may mean the poison is not detectable by the test used or its concentration is too low for detection at the time of sampling. In the latter instance, repeating the test at a later time may yield positive results.

Since screening tests require 2 to 6 h for completion, immediate management must be based on the history, physical examination, and routine ancillary tests. When the patient is asymptomatic, or when the clinical picture is consistent with the reported history, qualitative screening is neither clinically useful nor cost-effective. It is of greatest value in patients with severe or unexplained toxicity such as coma, seizures, cardiovascular instability, metabolic or respiratory acidosis, and nonsinus cardiac rhythms. Quantitative analysis is useful for acetaminophen, acetone, alcohol (including ethylene glycol), antiarrhythmic, antiepileptic, barbiturate, digoxin, heavy metal, lithium, salicylate, and theophylline poisoning and in carboxyhemoglobinemia and methemoglobinemia. Results can often be available within an hour.

Response to antidotes also may be used for diagnostic purposes. Resolution of altered mental status and abnormal vital signs within minutes of intravenous dextrose, naloxone, or flumazenil administration is virtually diagnostic of hypoglycemia, narcotic poisoning, and benzodiazepine intoxication, respectively. The prompt reversal of acute dystonic (extrapyramidal) reactions following an intravenous dose of benztropine or diphenhydramine confirms the diagnosis of a drug etiology. *Vin rosé* urine color following a diagnostic dose of deferoxamine can be used to confirm iron poisoning when serum iron and total iron-binding capacity levels are not immediately available. Although reversal of both central and peripheral manifestations of anticholinergic poisoning by physostigmine is diagnostic, physostigmine may cause arousal in patients with CNS depression of any etiology.

The absence of signs and symptoms soon after an overdose does not rule out a poisoning. Common poisons whose effects are delayed in onset include acetaminophen, cancer chemotherapeutic agents, carbamazepine, carbon tetrachloride, colchicine, digoxin, disulfiram, ethylene glycol, heavy metals, lithium, methanol, monoamine oxidase inhibitors, mushrooms, some plants, narcotics, phenytoin, podophylline, salicylate, and enteric-coated, slow- or sustained-released medications.

TREATMENT

Treatment goals include support of vital signs, prevention of further poison absorption, enhancement of poison elimination, administration of specific antidotes, and prevention of reexposure (Table 395-3). Treatment depends on the identity of the poison, the route and amount of exposure, the time of presentation relative to the time of exposure, and the severity of poisoning. Knowledge of toxin pharmacokinetics and pharmacodynamics is essential.

For patients who present prior to the onset of manifestations (preclinical phase) decontamination is the highest priority, and treatment is based solely on the history. The maximum potential toxicity based on the greatest possible exposure should be assumed. When appropriate, gastrointestinal decontamination to minimize absorption and decrease the severity of toxicity is the first priority. Since decontamination is more effective the sooner performed, the history and physical examination should be brief. It is also advisable to establish intravenous access and initiate cardiac monitoring, particularly in patients with potentially serious ingestions or unclear histories. The choice of decontamination procedure depends on the predicted toxicity; the availability, efficacy, and contraindications of the procedure; and the nature, severity, and risk of complications. For the home management of patients with accidental ingestions, reliable histories, and mild predicted toxicity, emesis can be induced with ipecac syrup. For patients treated in medical facilities, activated

TABLE 395-3 Fundamentals of poisoning management

SUPPORTIVE CARE

A Airway protection
B Oxygenation/ventilation
C Treatment of arrhythmias
D Hemodynamic support
E Treatment of seizures
F Correction of temperature abnormalities
G Correction of metabolic derangements
H Prevention of secondary complications

PREVENTION OF FURTHER POISON ABSORPTION

A Gastrointestinal decontamination
  1 Syrup of ipecac–induced emesis
  2 Gastric lavage
  3 Activated charcoal
  4 Whole bowel irrigation
  5 Catharsis
  6 Dilution
  7 Endoscopic/surgical removal
B Decontamination of other sites
  1 Eye decontamination
  2 Skin decontamination
  3 Body cavity evacuation

ENHANCEMENT OF POISON ELIMINATION

A Multiple-dose activated charcoal
B Forced diuresis
C Alteration of urinary pH
D Chelation (see heavy metal section)
E Extracorporal removal
  1 Peritoneal dialysis
  2 Hemodialysis
  3 Hemoperfusion
  4 Hemofiltration
  5 Plasmapheresis
  6 Exchange transfusion
F Hyperbaric oxygenation

ADMINISTRATION OF ANTIDOTES

A Neutralization by antibodies
B Neutralization by chemical binding
C Metabolic antagonism
D Physiologic antagonism

PREVENTION OF REEXPOSURE

A Adult education
B Child-proofing
C Notification of regulatory agencies
D Psychiatric referral

charcoal has comparable or greater efficacy, fewer contraindications and complications, and is less invasive than ipecac or gastric lavage. Alternative methods should be used if the ingested agent is not well absorbed by activated charcoal. Unless there has been a witnessed ingestion of a potentially severe overdose, the use of a large-bore gastric lavage tube is rarely indicated in an asymptomatic patient, since serious complications (aspiration or esophageal perforation) may result from the forcible use of a lavage tube in an uncooperative patient.

When an accurate history is not obtainable and a poison causing delayed toxicity or irreversible damage is suspected, blood and urine should be sent for toxicologic screening and, if indicated, for quantitative analysis. Due to continuing absorption and distribution, blood levels may be greater than those in tissue and may not correlate with toxicity. However, high blood levels of agents whose metabolites are more toxic than the parent compound (acetaminophen, ethylene glycol, or methanol) may indicate the need for additional interventions (antidotes, dialysis).

After evaluation and decontamination, some patients may be sent home because the predicted toxicity is minimal or the time of expected maximal toxicity has passed without incident. Observation for at least

4 to 6 h after gastrointestinal tract decontamination ensures that most patients who remain asymptomatic can be discharged safely. However, patients ingesting agents that slow gastric emptying and intestinal motility (anticholinergics, narcotics, sedative hypnotics, salicylates), have slow dissolution and absorption characteristics (carbamazepine, phenytoin, enteric-coated tablets, lithium, salicylate, and sustained-release preparations), or tend to form bezoars or concretions (enteric-coated tablets, meprobamate, salicylate) may require longer observation. In such patients, documentation of a charcoal stool prior to discharge should prevent delayed absorption and subsequent toxicity.

From the time of onset of poisoning to the time of peak effects (the toxic phase), management is based primarily on clinical and laboratory findings. Resuscitation and stabilization are the first priority. All symptomatic patients should have an intravenous line, supplemental oxygen, cardiac monitoring, continuous observation, and baseline laboratory, ECG, and x-ray evaluation. Patients with altered mental status, particularly those with coma or seizures, should be given an intravenous bolus of glucose, naloxone, and thiamine and additional antidotes as indicated. Decontamination measures should be initiated as soon as possible. Further absorption of ingested poisons should be limited by administering activated charcoal or gastric lavage. Since aspiration is a hazard, ipecac syrup should be used with caution. Patients may be given charcoal by mouth or by a stomach tube. Administering a dose of charcoal both before and after gastric lavage may be more effective than giving charcoal only after lavage. An initial dose of charcoal can be given by small-bore (no. 18 French or less) nasogastric tube while monitoring and supportive measures are being initiated. Once the patient is stable, lavage with a large-bore orogastric tube can be followed with a second dose of charcoal. The rare patient who deteriorates after this regimen should be lavaged and given another dose of charcoal.

Measures that enhance poison elimination may shorten the duration of toxicity and lessen its severity. However, the risks must be weighed against the benefits. Diagnostic certainty (usually via laboratory confirmation) is generally a prerequisite. Intestinal dialysis using activated charcoal is safe and effective in enhancing the elimination of many poisons. Diuresis and chelation therapy are effective in enhancing the elimination of a relatively small number of poisons, and their use is associated with potential complications. Extracorporal methods are effective in removing many poisons, but the expense and risk make their use reasonable only in patients who would otherwise not have a favorable outcome.

Patients with severe poisoning (coma, respiratory depression, hypotension, cardiac conduction abnormalities, cardiac arrhythmias, hypothermia or hyperthermia, seizures), those needing close monitoring or antidotes or enhanced elimination therapy, those showing progressive clinical deterioration, and those with significant underlying medical problems should be admitted to an intensive care unit. Patients with mild to moderate toxicity can be managed on a general medical service, intermediate care unit, or emergency department observation area depending on the anticipated duration and level of monitoring needed (intermittent clinical observation versus continuous clinical, cardiac, and respiratory monitoring). Patients who have attempted suicide require continuous observation until they seem unlikely to make further attempts.

Between peak toxicity and full recovery (the resolution phase of poisoning), supportive care should continue until the patient is alert and laboratory and ECG abnormalities are resolved. Repeat charcoal dosing may prevent rebound toxicity when depressed gastrointestinal function improves and the poison still in the gut is absorbed or additional active metabolites are formed. Since poison is eliminated from the blood before tissues, blood levels are generally lower than tissue levels during this phase and once again may not correlate with toxicity. This is particularly true when extracorporal elimination procedures are used. Because of redistribution of poison, a rebound increase in blood level and clinical relapse may occur after the termination of such procedures. When a metabolite is responsible for toxic effects, continued treatment of an asymptomatic patient may be necessary because of a previous or present toxic blood level (acetaminophen, ethylene glycol, and methanol).

Prior to discharge, patients with accidental ingestions (and/or the caregivers) should be instructed about preventive measures, and suicidal patients should receive appropriate psychiatric assessment, disposition, and follow-up.

SUPPORTIVE CARE

The goal of supportive therapy is to maintain physiologic homeostasis until detoxification is accomplished and to prevent and treat secondary complications such as aspiration, bed sores, cerebral and pulmonary edema, pneumonia, rhabdomyolysis, sepsis, renal failure, and generalized organ dysfunction due to prolonged hypoxia or shock.

In addition to those needing urgent endotracheal intubation, many poisoned patients require semielective endotracheal intubation for protection of the airway against aspiration of gastrointestinal contents and of the poison itself. The gag reflex alone is not a reliable indicator of the need for intubation. Since patients may maintain airway patency while being stimulated but not if left unattended, those who cannot respond to voice or who are unable to sit and drink fluids without assistance are best managed by prophylactic intubation. Patients with severe excitation also may require intubation for airway protection (due to the risk or existence of seizures) and sedation or paralysis for control of agitation and prevention of hyperthermia, acidosis, and rhabdomyolysis. Since clinical assessment is often inaccurate, the need for oxygenation and ventilation is best determined by analyses of arterial blood gases.

Drug-induced pulmonary edema is usually noncardiac rather than cardiac in nature. Profound CNS depression and cardiac conduction abnormalities suggest the latter etiology. Measurement of pulmonary artery pressure may be necessary to establish etiology and direct appropriate therapy. Arrhythmias can result from direct cardiotoxicity, abnormal cardiovascular reflexes, or metabolic derangements. Supraventricular tachycardia associated with hypertension and CNS excitation is almost always due to sympathetic, anticholinergic, or hallucinogenic stimulation or to drug withdrawal (see Table 395-1). Most cases are mild or moderate in severity and require only observation or nonspecific sedation with a benzodiazepine. If severe or associated with hemodynamic instability, chest pain, or ECG evidence of ischemia, specific therapy is indicated. Hypoxia, hypoglycemia, and other metabolic causes of sympathetic stimulation also should be ruled out. For patients with sympathetic hyperactivity, treatment with a combined alpha and beta blocker (labetalol) or a combination of beta blocker and vasodilator (esmolol and nitroprusside) is preferred. For those with anticholinergic poisoning, physostigmine is the treatment of choice. Supraventricular tachycardia without hypertension is generally secondary to vasodilation or hypovolemia and responds to fluid administration.

Ventricular tachyarrhythmias may be caused by sympathetic stimulation, myocardial membrane destabilization, or metabolic derangements. Lidocaine and phenytoin are generally safe, but beta blockers can be hazardous unless the arrhythmia is clearly from sympathetic hyperactivity. In tricyclic antidepressant poisoning, quinidine and procainamide are contraindicated (because of similar electrophysiologic effects), but sodium bicarbonate may be therapeutic. Magnesium sulfate and overdrive pacing (by isoproterenol or a pacemaker) may be useful in patients with torsades de pointes and prolonged QT intervals. Magnesium and antidigoxin antibodies are used in patients with severe digitalis poisoning. Invasive (esophageal or intracardiac) ECG recording may sometimes be necessary to determine the origin (ventricular or supraventricular) of wide-complex tachycardias (see Chap. 198). If the patient is hemodynamically stable, however, it may be prudent to observe rather than to treat with a potentially harmful cardioactive agent. Arrhythmias may be resistant to drug therapy until underlying acid-base and electrolyte derangements, hypoxia, and hypothermia are corrected.

Bradyarrhythmias associated with hypotension generally should be treated as described in Chap 197. In beta blocker and calcium channel blocker poisoning, the administration of calcium and glucagon, respectively, may be effective. Antibody therapy may be indicated for digitalis poisoning. The management of hypotension is described in Chap. 34. If hypotension is unresponsive to volume expansion, norepinephrine or high-dose dopamine may be indicated.

Drug-induced seizures may be due to direct or indirect CNS neuroreceptor stimulation (or inhibition), neuronal membrane destabilization, ischemia, edema, or metabolic abnormalities. Seizures due to excessive stimulation of catecholamine receptors (sympathomimetic or hallucinogen poisoning and drug withdrawal) or decreased activity of gamma-aminobutyric acid (GABA) (isoniazid poisoning) or glycine (strychnine poisoning) are best treated with GABA agonists such as benzodiazepines or barbiturates. Seizures caused by isoniazid, which inhibits the synthesis of GABA, may not respond to agonist therapy until GABA synthesis is restored, because agonists act, at least partially, by promoting the release of GABA from presynaptic vesicles. High doses of pyridoxine, which is necessary for the synthesis of GABA, are often necessary to terminate such seizures. For poisons with central dopaminergic effects (phencyclidine), an agent with opposing activity, such as haloperidol, may be useful. Seizures resulting from membrane destabilization (beta blocker, cyclic antidepressant poisoning) may require a membrane-active agent such as phenytoin as well as a GABA agonist. In rare cases (anticholinergic or cyanide poisoning), specific antidotal therapy may be necessary.

The treatment of seizures secondary to ischemia, edema, or metabolic abnormalities should include correction of the underlying cause. Since prolonged convulsions can lead to rhabdomyolysis and severe acidosis, neuromuscular paralysis is indicated in refractory cases. EEG monitoring and continuing treatment of seizures are necessary to prevent permanent neurologic damage.

Invasive interventions, such as extracorporal membrane oxygenation, intraaortic balloon pump counterpulsation, and partial (femoral) cardiopulmonary bypass pump circulatory support, should be considered in severe but reversible poisoning. Temperature extremes; metabolic, hepatic, and renal abnormalities; and secondary complications should be treated by standard measures.

PREVENTION OF POISON ABSORPTION

GASTROINTESTINAL DECONTAMINATION *Syrup of ipecac* is administered orally in a dose of 30 mL for adults, 15 mL for children, and 10 mL for small infants. Clear liquids also should be given. Ipecac irritates the stomach and stimulates the central chemoreceptor trigger zone. Vomiting usually occurs approximately 22 min following administration. The dose may be repeated if vomiting does not occur. Experimentally, ipecac decreases chemical absorption by an average of 57 percent (range 28 to 73 percent) if given within 5 min of ingestion and about 30 percent (range 2 to 45 percent) if given within half an hour. Because there are no suitable control groups, its efficacy in overdose patients is not established. Side effects include lethargy in children (12 percent) and protracted vomiting (8 to 17 percent). Chronic ipecac use (by patients with anorexia nervosa or bulimia) may cause electrolyte and fluid abnormalities, cardiac toxicity, and myopathy. Except for aspiration, serious complications are rare. Isolated cases of gastric and esophageal tears and perforations and stroke have been reported. Ipecac is contraindicated in patients with recent gastrointestinal surgery, CNS depression, seizures, and ingestions of corrosives and rapidly acting CNS poisons (camphor, cyanide, tricyclic antidepressants, propoxyphene, strychnine).

Gastric lavage is performed using a no. 28 French orogastric tube in children and a no. 40 French tube in adults with volumes of about 5 mL fluid per kilogram of body weight. Except for infants, tap water is acceptable. The patient should be placed in Trendelenburg and left lateral decubitus positions to prevent aspiration (even if an endotracheal tube is in place). Experimentally, lavage decreases chemical absorption by an average of 69 percent (range 54 to 84 percent) if performed within 5 min of ingestion, 31 percent (range 26 to 38 percent) if performed at 30 min, and 11 percent (range 8 to 13 percent) if performed at 60 min. Its efficacy is similar to that of ipecac. Significant amounts of ingested drug are recovered in a tenth of patients. As with ipecac, its effect on the clinical outcome of poisoned patients is not known. Aspiration is a common complication (up to 10 percent), especially when lavage is improperly performed. Serious complications (tracheal lavage, esophageal and gastric perforation) occur in approximately 1 percent of patients. For this reason, only a physician should insert the lavage tube, and the patient must be restrained (with pharmacologic sedation if necessary) during the procedure. Gastric lavage is contraindicated in patients with ingestion of corrosives and petroleum distillate hydrocarbons because of the risk of aspiration-induced hydrocarbon pneumonia and gastroesophageal perforation.

Activated charcoal, as a suspension in water alone or with a cathartic, is given orally via a nippled bottle (for infants), cup, straw, or small-bore nasogastric tube (for uncooperative patients). The recommended dose is 1 to 2 g/kg of body weight, using 8 mL of diluent per gram of charcoal, if a premixed formulation is not available. Palatability may be increased by adding a sweetener (sorbitol) or a flavoring agent (cherry, chocolate, or cola syrup) to the suspension. Charcoal adsorbs ingested poisons within the gut lumen, allowing the charcoal-toxin complex to be evacuated with stool. The complex also can be removed from the stomach by induced emesis or lavage. In vitro, charcoal adsorbs 90 percent or more of most poisons when given in a ratio 10 times that of the toxin. Superactivated charcoal (SuperChar) is two to three times more effective than standard charcoal. Charged (ionized) chemicals such as mineral acids, alkalis, and highly dissociated salts of cyanide, fluoride, iron, lithium, and other inorganic compounds are not well adsorbed by charcoal. Experimentally, charcoal decreases the absorption of other chemicals by an average of 80 percent when given within 5 min of administration, 59 percent when given at 30 min, and 33 percent at 60 min. Charcoal is of equal or greater efficacy than ipecac syrup or gastric lavage. Lavage followed by charcoal is more effective than charcoal alone, and charcoal before and after lavage is more effective than charcoal alone or charcoal after lavage. In general, the clinical outcome after treatment with charcoal alone is more favorable than in those given ipecac followed by charcoal and those treated with lavage followed by charcoal. In comatose patients treated within 1 h of ingestion, however, the combination of lavage and charcoal may be more effective than charcoal alone. Side effects of charcoal include nausea, vomiting, and diarrhea or constipation. Charcoal also may prevent the absorption of orally administered therapeutic agents. Complications include mechanical obstruction of the airway, aspiration, vomiting, and bowel obstruction by inspissated charcoal. Charcoal is contraindicated in patients with corrosive ingestion because it obscures endoscopy.

Whole-bowel irrigation is performed by administering a bowel cleansing solution containing electrolytes and polyethylene glycol (Golytely, Colyte) orally or by gastric tube at a rate of up 0.5 L/h in children and 2.0 L/h in adults until rectal effluent is clear. The patient must be in a sitting position. Although data are limited, whole-bowel irrigation may be as or more effective than the previously discussed procedures, particularly in patients with foreign body, drug packet, and slow-release medication ingestions.

Cathartic salts (disodium phosphate, magnesium citrate and sulfate, sodium sulfate) or *saccharides* (mannitol, sorbitol) promote the rectal evacuation of gastrointestinal contents. The most effective cathartic is sorbitol in a dose of 1 to 2 g/kg of body weight. Alone, cathartics do not prevent poison absorption, except perhaps for the agents noted under whole-bowel irrigation. Their primary use is to prevent constipation following charcoal administration. Abdominal

cramps, nausea, and occasional vomiting are side effects. Complications of repeated dosing include hypermagnesemia and excessive diarrhea. The agents are contraindicated in patients who have ingested corrosives and in those with preexisting diarrhea. Magnesium-containing cathartics should not be used in patients with renal failure.

Dilution is accomplished by having the patient drink 5 mL/kg of body weight of water or other clear liquid as soon as possible after the ingestion of a corrosive (acids, alkali). Dilution also may be used as an adjunct to ipecac syrup. Otherwise, it is not indicated because it may increase the dissolution rate (and hence absorption) of capsules, tablets, and other solids.

Endoscopic or surgical removal of poisons may be useful in rare situations such as ingestion of a potentially toxic foreign body that fails to transit the gastrointestinal tract, a potentially lethal amount of a heavy metal (arsenic, iron, mercury, thallium), or large concretions of pills. Patients who ingest packets of drugs (cocaine) and then become toxic due to packet leakage or rupture require immediate surgical intervention.

DECONTAMINATION OF OTHER SITES Immediate copious flushing with water, saline, or other available clear drinkable liquid is the initial treatment of topical exposures (particularly with corrosives and solvents). Saline is preferred for eye irrigation. A triple wash (water then soap then more water) may be optimal for dermal decontamination. Inhalational exposures should be treated initially with fresh air or oxygen. The removal of liquid poisons from body cavities such as the vagina or rectum is best accomplished by irrigation. Solid poisons (drug packets, pills) should be manually removed with visual guidance.

ENHANCEMENT OF POISON ELIMINATION

Although the elimination of most poisons can be accelerated by therapeutic interventions, pharmacokinetic efficacy (removal of drug at a rate greater than that accomplished by intrinsic elimination) and the clinical benefits (shortened duration of toxicity, improved outcome) are often more theoretical than proven. Hence the decision to use a procedure should be based on the actual or predicted toxicity and the potential efficacy, cost, and risks of therapy.

MULTIPLE-DOSE ACTIVATED CHARCOAL Repeated oral dosing with charcoal (with sorbitol as needed to enhance gastrointestinal motility) enhances the elimination of some poisons. A dose of 1 g/kg of body weight every 2 to 4 h, adjusted downward to avoid regurgitation in patients with decreased gastrointestinal motility, is generally recommended. Experimentally, this treatment enhances the elimination of most drugs and chemicals tested (carbamazepine, dapsone, diazepam, digoxin, glutethimide, meprobamate, methotrexate, phenobarbital, phenytoin, salicylate, theophylline, valproic acid). Efficacy approaches that of hemodialysis for some agents (theophylline). Multiple-dose therapy is not effective in accelerating elimination of chlorpropamide, imipramine, or agents poorly adsorbed to charcoal.

FORCED DIURESIS AND ALTERATION OF URINARY pH Diuresis and ion trapping via alteration of urine pH may prevent the renal reabsorption of poisons that undergo excretion by glomerular filtration and active tubular secretion. Since membranes are more permeable to nonionized molecules than to their ionized counterparts, acidic (low pK_a) poisons are ionized and trapped in an alkaline urine, and basic poisons are ionized and trapped in an acid urine. Alkaline diuresis (a urine pH of 7.5 or greater and a urine output of 3 to 6 mL/kg of body weight per hour) enhances the elimination of chlorphenoxyacetic acid herbicides, chlorpropamide, diflunisal, fluoride, methotrexate, phenobarbital (and probably other long-acting barbiturates), and salicylates. Contraindications include congestive heart failure, renal failure, and cerebral edema. Acid-base, fluid, and electrolyte parameters should be carefully monitored. Saline diuresis may enhance the excretion of bromide, calcium, fluoride, lithium, meprobamate, potassium, and isoniazid. Acid diuresis enhances the renal elimination of amphetamines, chloroquine, cocaine, local anesthetics, phencyclidine, quinidine, quinine, sympathomimetics, strychnine, and tocainide. Its use, however, has been largely abandoned because risks are significant and clinical efficacy has not been established.

EXTRACORPORAL REMOVAL Peritoneal dialysis, hemodialysis, charcoal or resin hemoperfusion, hemofiltration, plasmapheresis, and exchange transfusion are capable of removing any toxin from the bloodstream. Toxins most amenable to enhanced elimination by dialysis have low molecular mass (<500 Da), high water solubility, low protein binding, small volumes of distribution (<1 L/kg of body weight), prolonged elimination (long half-life), and high dialysis clearance relative to total-body clearance. The efficacy of the other forms of extracorporal removal is not limited by molecular weight, water solubility, or protein binding. Dialysis should be considered in severe poisoning due to bromide, chloral hydrate, ethanol, ethylene glycol, isopropyl alcohol, lithium, methanol, salicylate, and possibly heavy metals. Although hemoperfusion may be more effective in removing some of these poisons, it does not correct associated acid-base and electrolyte abnormalities.

Hemoperfusion should be considered in severe poisoning due to chloramphenicol, disopyramide, and hypnotic-sedatives (barbiturates, ethchlorvynol, glutethimide, meprobamate, methaqualone, phenytoin, procainamide, and theophylline). Both techniques require central venous access and systemic anticoagulation and often result in transient hypotension. Hemoperfusion also may cause hemolysis, hypocalcemia, and thrombocytopenia. Peritoneal dialysis and exchange transfusion are less effective but may be used when other procedures are not available, are contraindicated, or are technically difficult (in infants). Exchange transfusion removes poisons affecting red blood cells (e.g., methemoglobinemia or arsine-induced hemolysis). The efficacy of other extracorporal elimination procedures has not been defined.

Candidates for these invasive treatments include patients with severe toxicity who deteriorate despite aggressive supportive therapy; those with potentially prolonged, irreversible, or fatal toxicity; and those with dangerous blood levels of toxins, those who lack the capacity for self-detoxification because of liver or renal failure, and those with serious underlying illnesses or complications that adversely affect recovery.

OTHER TECHNIQUES The elimination of heavy metals can be enhanced by chelation and urinary excretion of the metal-chelator complex, and the elimination of carbon monoxide can be increased by hyperbaric oxygenation, as discussed with the specific poisons.

ADMINISTRATION OF ANTIDOTES

Antidotes counteract the effects of poisons by neutralizing them (antibody-antigen reactions, chelation, chemical binding) or by antagonizing their physiologic effects (activation of opposing nervous system activity, provision of competitive metabolic or receptor substrate). Antidotes can significantly reduce morbidity and mortality, but most antidotes are potentially toxic. Poisons or conditions with specific antidotes include acetaminophen, anticholinergic agents, anticoagulants, benzodiazepines, beta blockers, calcium channel blockers, carbon monoxide, cholinergic agents, cyanide, digitalis, drugs that cause dystonic reactions, ethylene glycol, fluoride, heavy metals, hydrogen sulfide, hypoglycemic agents, isoniazid, methemoglobinemia, narcotics, sympathomimetics, and vacor. Since the safe use of antidotes requires correct identification of a specific poisoning or syndrome, antidotal therapy is discussed with the conditions for which they are indicated.

PREVENTION OF REEXPOSURE

Poisoning is a preventable illness. Unfortunately, some adults and children are poison-prone, and recurrences are common. Adults with accidental exposures should be instructed regarding the safe use of medications and chemicals (according to labeling instructions). Confused patients may need assistance with the administration of medications. Errors in dosing by health care providers require special educational efforts. Patients should be advised to avoid circumstances that result in chemical exposure or poisoning. Appropriate agencies and health departments should be notified in cases of environmental or workplace exposure. The best approach with young children and patients with intentional overdose is to limit access to poisons. In households where children live or visit, alcoholic beverages, medications, household products (automotive, cleaning, fuel, petcare, toiletry products), nonedible plants, and vitamins should be kept out of reach or in locked or child-proof cabinets. Depressed or psychotic patients should be given prescriptions for a limited supply of drugs and with a limited number of refills. All patients should be monitored for compliance and response to therapy.

SPECIFIC POISONS

The poisons discussed in this section are common, produce life-threatening toxicity, or require unique therapeutic interventions. Poisons not mentioned here are described in the referenced texts. Drug and alcohol abuse are discussed in Chaps. 390 to 392. Heavy metal poisoning is discussed in Chap. 396.

ACETAMINOPHEN At therapeutic doses, acetaminophen is metabolized to sulfate and glucuronide conjugates that are excreted in the urine. Minor amounts are excreted unchanged or as mercapturic acid after conjugation with hepatic glutathione. Following an acute overdose of 140 mg/kg of body weight or more, the sulfate and glucuronide pathways become saturated, resulting in an increased fraction of acetaminophen metabolized to mercapturic acid. Once hepatic glutathione is depleted, reactive metabolites are formed that bind covalently to hepatocytes and cause cell lysis. Acetaminophen is rapidly absorbed from the stomach and small bowel and has a volume of distribution of 1 L/kg of body weight. Plasma concentrations range from 160 to 660 μmol/L (0.5 to 2.0 mg/dL) following therapeutic doses. The plasma half-life is usually 2 to 4 h but may be prolonged following overdose.

Clinical toxicity Early manifestations of poisoning are nonspecific and not predictive of subsequent hepatotoxicity. Within 2 to 4 h of ingestion, nausea, vomiting, diaphoresis, and pallor develop. CNS depression is absent unless depressant drugs are coingested. Within 24 to 48 h, hepatotoxicity is evidenced by right upper quadrant tenderness and mild hepatomegaly and followed by the appearance of jaundice, clotting abnormalities, and hepatic encephalopathy. Renal function also may be impaired. Laboratory evidence of hepatic toxicity includes elevation in serum transaminase activity (AST, ALT). With severe poisoning, prolongation of the prothrombin time, elevation of serum bilirubin, and ultimately hyperammonemia may occur. A twofold prolongation of prothrombin time and/or serum bilirubin greater than 68 μmol/L (4 mg/dL) on the third to fifth day after ingestion indicate hepatotoxicity. Histologic evidence of liver damage varies from cytolysis to centrilobular necrosis. In patients who recover, liver function returns to normal within 1 week, and liver histology returns to normal within 3 months.

Diagnosis A serum acetaminophen level should be determined between 4 and 24 h after ingestion and compared against the Rumack-Matthew nomogram (Fig. 395-1). A level above the lower line on the nomogram indicates possible hepatotoxicity and the need for antidotal therapy.

Treatment In patients who present within 4 h of ingestion, initial treatment involves gastrointestinal decontamination. Activated charcoal should be administered. (Charcoal does not significantly interfere with acetylcysteine therapy.) In patients with a potentially toxic acetaminophen level, acetylcysteine is given at a loading dose of 140 mg/kg of body weight, followed by a maintenance dose of 70 mg/kg of body weight every 4 h for 17 doses. Treatment is most

FIGURE 395-1 Nomogram to define risk according to initial plasma acetaminophen concentration. (*After BH Rumack, H Matthew, Pediatrics 55:871, 1975.*)

effective if started within 8 to 10 h but may have some benefit up to 24 h following ingestion. Side effects include nausea, vomiting, and epigastric discomfort. If treatment is started prior to availability of the serum level and if the level is subsequently shown to be below the toxic level, therapy may be discontinued.

ACIDS AND ALKALI Common alkaline products include industrial-strength bleach, drain cleaners (sodium hydroxide), surface cleaners (ammonia, phosphates), laundry and dishwasher detergents (phosphates, carbonates), disk batteries, denture cleaners (borates, phosphates, carbonates), and Clinitest tablets (sodium hydroxides). Acids are used in toilet bowl cleaners (hydrofluoric, phosphoric, sulfuric acids), soldering fluxes (hydrochloric acid), antirust compounds (hydrofluoric, oxalic acids), automobile battery fluid (sulfuric acid), and slate cleaners (hydrofluoric acid).

Alkalies produce liquefactive necrosis with rapidly penetrating tissue burns and higher risk of perforation of the esophagus and stomach than do acids. Acids produce coagulative necrosis. Both burn the mouth, esophagus, and stomach. The lack of oral involvement does not rule out esophageal or gastric injury, however. Liquids tend to produce superficial, often circumferential burns over a larger surface area, while solids and tablets cause localized deeper burns. The severity of the burn relates to the contact time, amount ingested, and the pH (especially <2, >12) of the ingested product.

Clinical toxicity Burns of the mouth result in excess salivation, pain, dysphonia, and dysphagia. Examination of the mouth shows erythema, edema, ulceration, and necrosis. Deep burns may destroy mucosal nerve endings and produce anesthesia. Esophageal symptoms and signs include drooling, painful swallowing, retrosternal pain, and neck tenderness. Vomiting of blood and mucus may occur. Perforation following alkali ingestion is suggested by increased severity of chest pain, often with respiratory distress. Epigastric pain, vomiting, and tenderness may occur with burns to the stomach. Aspiration of acids and alkalis results in fulminant tracheitis and bronchial pneumonia. In severe cases, hypotension, shock, metabolic acidosis, liver and renal dysfunction, hemolysis, and disseminated intravascular coagula-

tion may be seen. Edema, erythema, and ulceration of the esophagus may be followed by fibrosis with stricture formation and obstruction of the esophagus (in the case of alkalis) or of the gastric outlet (in the case of acids).

Diagnosis A careful history will suggest the ingestion of an acid or an alkali. Endoscopy should be safe within 48 h (optimally 12 to 24 h) of the ingestion in all symptomatic patients. It will document the anatomic site and often the severity but not the depth of the injury. Residual effects of the ingestion can be assessed by barium swallow. Chest and abdominal x-rays and routine laboratory values should be obtained to evaluate for aspiration, perforation, and organ dysfunction.

Treatment Treatment consists of immediate dilution. Weak acid or basic solutions should not be used because the heat of neutralization may cause thermal burns and increase tissue injury. Glucocorticoids have traditionally been used for alkali burns to prevent stricture formation. Controlled clinical data, however, have failed to show efficacy in preventing stricture formation following transmucosal (third-degree) injury, and first- and second-degree injuries do not result in stricture formation. Animal studies suggest that therapy should be initiated immediately on presentation. If used, a dose of 1 to 2 mg prednisone per kilogram every 4 to 6 h for at least 2 weeks is suggested. Prophylactic broad-spectrum antibiotic use is controversial. Glucocorticoids are not useful for acid burns. Antacids should be used for burns of the stomach. Esophageal stricture or gastric outlet obstruction may require subsequent dilation and bouginage or surgical reconstruction.

ANTIARRHYTHMIC DRUGS Only drugs that act by blocking myocardial cell membrane sodium channels are discussed here. These agents can be divided into three subclasses: class IA (disopyramide, procainamide, quinidine, and moricizine), class IB (lidocaine, mexiletine, phenytoin, and tocainide), and class IC (encainide, ethmozine, propafanone, and flecainide). The pharmacology is presented in Chap. 198. Because of toxicity, some agents have been withdrawn from the market. These agents are rapidly absorbed (except for disopyramide and sustained-release formulations), have volumes of distribution ranging from 1 to 10 L/kg, have half-lives of 3 to 11 h, and are predominantly eliminated by hepatic metabolism.

Clinical toxicity The acute ingestion of more than twice the usual daily dose is potentially toxic. Onset of toxicity occurs within 1 h, and peak effects are demonstrable within several hours. Toxicity also may develop during chronic therapeutic use. Manifestations include nausea, vomiting, and diarrhea, followed by lethargy, confusion, ataxia, bradycardia, hypotension, and cardiovascular collapse. Anticholinergic effects (blurred vision, dry mucosa) may be seen in disopyramide poisoning. Quinidine and class IB agents may cause agitation, dysphoria, and seizures. Nonspecific ECG findings include bradycardia with AV block and QRS-interval prolongation. Ventricular tachycardia, ventricular fibrillation (including the polymorphous form, torsades de pointes), and QT-interval prolongation are characteristics of poisoning due to class IA and IC drugs. Depressed myocardial contractility and arrhythmias may lead to decreased cardiac output and pulmonary edema. Hypoglycemia and mild hypokalemia may be seen with disopyramide and quinidine intoxication, respectively. Toxicology screening will detect most of these agents. Measurement of serum levels may confirm an overdose and indicate the need for monitoring.

Treatment Treatment consists of gastrointestinal decontamination and supportive therapy. Hypotension, bradyarrhythmias, and seizures are treated with standard measures. Patients with persistent hypotension and bradycardia require monitoring of pulmonary arterial pressure. Cardiac pacing, intraaortic balloon pump counterpulsation, and cardiopulmonary bypass may be necessary. Ventricular tachyarrhythmias that cause hemodynamic instability should be treated with lidocaine, phenytoin, and bretylium. Sodium bicarbonate or sodium lactate (1 mmol/kg by intravenous bolus) may be effective for tachyarrhythmias due to class IA or IC agents. Mild hypokalemia may be protective, and potassium levels that do not fall below 3.0 mmol/L may be best treated by close monitoring. For torsades de pointes (polymorphous or atypical ventricular tachycardia), magnesium sulfate (4 g or 40 mL of a 10% solution intravenously as an initial dose) and overdrive pacing (with isoproterenol or electricity) may be effective. Hemodialysis and hemoperfusion may enhance the elimination of disopyramide, the active procainamide metabolite *N*-acetylprocainamide, and possibly other agents. However, clinical experience is inadequate to support routine use.

BARBITURATES   Barbiturates are GABA receptor agonists and inhibit excitable cells of the CNS and other tissues. Long-acting barbiturates include mephobarbital, barbital, phenobarbital, and primidone. Short-acting agents include those with intermediate, short, and ultrashort durations of action such as amobarbital, aprobarbital, butabarbital, butalbital, pentobarbital, and secobarbital.

Barbiturates are well absorbed from the stomach and the small bowel. Peak plasma concentrations generally occur at a therapeutic dose within 1 to 4 h, with short-acting agents peaking earlier than long-acting ones. Barbiturates are weak acids with pK_a values ranging from 7.2 to 8.5, volumes of distribution of 0.8 to 1.5 L/kg of body weight, and 45 to 70 percent protein binding in the plasma. Most barbiturates are primarily eliminated by hepatic metabolism. Some long-acting agents are converted to active metabolites: mephobarbital to barbital and primidone to phenobarbital and phenylethylmalonanide (PEMA). In contrast to short-acting agents, long-acting ones also undergo significant renal excretion: 95 percent for barbital, 25 to 33 percent for phenobarbital, 15 to 42 percent for primidone, and 95 percent for PEMA. The half-life ranges from 1 to 6 days for long-acting agents and 3 to 48 h for short-acting ones.

Clinical toxicity   Barbiturates cause CNS depression ranging from confusion and lethargy to deep coma. Hypothermia, hypotension, pulmonary edema, and cardiac arrest may occur in severe cases. Pupils are generally constricted but may dilate in terminal phases. Pressure sores can develop with prolonged coma. Bullous skin lesions are seen in severe barbiturate overdose. Signs of toxicity usually appear when serum concentrations of long-acting barbiturates exceed 170 μmol/L (4 mg/dL) and short-acting barbiturates exceed 88 μmol/L (2 mg/dL). Maximal toxicity occurs within 4 to 6 h after short-acting barbiturate but may be delayed 10 h or more after overdosage with long-acting barbiturates. Because of tolerance, the degree of CNS depression relative to ingested dose is dependent on prior exposure to the drug.

Treatment   Initial management involves prompt gastrointestinal decontamination. Barbiturates are well adsorbed by activated charcoal. In the case of phenobarbital (and probably other long-acting barbiturate) poisoning, repetitive administration of activated charcoal every 2 to 4 h enhances elimination threefold and decreases half-life by approximately 50 percent. For all barbiturates, attention should be given to hemodynamic and respiratory support, correction of temperature and electrolyte derangements, and monitoring for pulmonary complications. Since short-acting barbiturates are predominantly metabolized by the liver, diuresis is ineffective. Renal elimination of phenobarbital (and probably other long-acting agents) is significantly enhanced by alkalinization of urine to a pH of 8 (by giving intravenous sodium bicarbonate) and by saline diuresis. Hemodialysis and hemoperfusion are effective in removing both long- and short-acting barbiturates, their use being reserved for severely intoxicated patients with high blood levels.

BENZODIAZEPINES   Benzodiazepines potentiate the inhibitory effect of GABA on the CNS by binding to receptors at polysynaptic terminals where GABA is released, principally in the limbic system and the reticular formation of the midbrain.

Long-acting benzodiazepines include diazepam, chlordiazepoxide, clonazepam, flurazepam, clorazepate, quazepam, and prazepam. Short-acting agents include alprazolam, lorazepam, and oxazepam; ultra-short-acting agents include estrazolam, midazolam, temazepam, and triazolam. All benzodiazepines are well absorbed from the gastrointestinal tract, exhibit 85 to 99 percent protein binding in the plasma, are lipid soluble, and have an apparent volume of distribution of approximately 1.1 L/kg of body weight. They are weak acids with

pK_a values ranging from 1.3 to 6.2. Benzodiazepines are mainly eliminated by hepatic metabolism, and in the case of some (diazepam), the metabolites are pharmacologically active. Metabolites are generally excreted in the urine, whereas only a small amount of the parent compound is excreted unchanged by the kidneys. Long-acting benzodiazepines have half-lives of 1 to 8 days, short-acting agents have half-lives of 6 to 24 h, and ultra-short-acting agents have half-lives of 3 to 12 h.

Clinical toxicity   Effects are evident within 30 min of an overdose and include weakness, ataxia, drowsiness, and in severe cases, coma and respiratory depression. Paradoxical excitation may occur early in the course of poisoning. Pupils are generally constricted. Ethanol enhances the absorption of benzodiazepine and potentiates the CNS depression. Confirmation of the diagnosis is made by identification of the metabolites in urine.

Treatment   Initial management includes prompt gastrointestinal decontamination. Single-dose as well as repeated-dose activated charcoal is indicated. Respiratory support is rarely needed except in the case of ultra-short-acting agents, massive overdose, or the coingestion of other sedative drugs. Flumazenil, a competitive benzodiazepine receptor antagonist, can reverse CNS and respiratory depression and obviate the need for endotracheal intubation. It is administered intravenously in incremental doses of 0.2, 0.3, and 0.5 mg at 1-min intervals until the desired effect is achieved or a cumulative dose of 3 to 5 mg has been given. Since flumazenil has a relatively short duration of action, patients must be monitored carefully for relapse. Should this occur, treatment can be repeated (at intervals of 20 min with a maximum dose of 3 mg/h). Failure to respond to flumazenil suggests that benzodiazepines are not the cause of poisoning. Flumazenil can cause seizures in patients who have coingested stimulants and tricyclic antidepressants and should not be used in these situations. It also can cause seizures (withdrawal syndrome) in patients who are physically dependent on benzodiazepines as a result of chronic high-dose use. The lowest effective dose should be used in these patients. High protein binding of benzodiazepines limits efficacy of hemodialysis.

BETA-ADRENERGIC BLOCKING AGENTS   Beta-adrenergic blocking agents include acebutolol, atenolol, betaxolol, carteolol, esmolol, labetalol, metoprolol, nadolol, penbutolol, pindolol, propranolol, sotalol, and timolol. These drugs act by competitively blocking beta-adrenergic neurohumoral receptors in the bronchial and vascular smooth muscle and mycardium. At therapeutic doses, some beta blockers act predominantly on beta$_1$ receptors and are "cardioselective" (acebutolol, atenolol, betaxolol, metoprolol), some have partial agonist or sympathomimetic activity (acebutolol, carteolol, pindolol, timolol, and possibly penbutol), and some have quinidine-like myocardial membrane stabilizing effects (acebutolol, metoprolol, pindolol, propranolol, sotalol, and possibly betaxolol). Antiarrhythmic effects are due to a reduction of sodium and calcium influx during membrane depolarization (phase 0) as a consequence of decreased production of cyclic AMP by adenylate cyclase. This activity defines beta blockers as class II antiarrhythmics. Beta blockers decrease cardiac contractility by directly inhibiting the release of calcium from sarcoplasmic reticulum. Following overdose, cardioselectivity is often lost, and all beta blockers may cause membrane depressant effects.

Beta blockers are rapidly and well absorbed, exhibit variable protein binding (5 to 93 percent), and have low water solubility and variable volumes of distribution (0.23 to 10.0 L/kg of body weight). Most beta blockers are eliminated predominantly by hepatic metabolism. Atenolol, carteolol, nadolol, and sotalol are primarily eliminated by renal excretion, and esmolol is metabolized by serum esterases.

Clinical toxicity   Effects usually begin within 1/2 h following an overdose and become maximal within 2 h. Common findings include nausea, vomiting, and diarrhea, followed by bradycardia, hypotension, and CNS depression. However, agents with sympathomimetic activity can cause hypertension and tachycardia. CNS effects vary from lethargy and confusion to coma and seizures and tend to be more pronounced with highly lipophilic agents (acebutolol, metoprolol, pindolol, propranolol, and timolol). The skin is often pale and cool. Bronchospasm and pulmonary edema are uncommon unless there is a history of asthma, chronic obstructive pulmonary disease, or congestive heart failure. Metabolic abnormalities include hyperkalemia and hypoglycemia (as a direct result of beta-adrenergic receptor blockade) and metabolic acidosis (due to seizures, shock, or respiratory depression). ECG manifestations include all degrees of AV block, bundle branch block, prolonged QRS duration, and asystole. Sotalol poisoning also may cause QT-interval prolongation with ventricular tachycardia, ventricular fibrillation, and torsades de pointes. Patients with mild poisoning usually recover within 6 to 12 h, whereas those with severe poisoning may be symptomatic for 24 to 48 h. A toxicology screen may identify the presence of beta blockers, but blood levels are not generally available nor helpful in guiding therapy.

Treatment Treatment includes gastrointestinal decontamination, nonspecific supportive measures, and the administration of calcium and glucagon. Because gastric emptying procedures may produce vagal stimulation and exacerbate bradyarrhythmias, monitoring should be instituted first. Treatment of bradycardia and hypotension should begin with atropine, isoproterenol, and vasopressors (dopamine, dobutamine, epinephrine, and norepinephrine have been used with variable success, alone or in combination). With severe poisoning, these agents may be ineffective, and glucagon, calcium, cardiac pacing (external or internal), and intraaortic balloon pump support may be necessary. Glucagon, which stimulates adenylate cyclase by a nonadrenergic mechanism, should be given at an initial dose of 5 to 10 mg for adults. Patients who respond favorably should then be given an infusion of 1 to 5 mg/h. Calcium, which may reverse nonadrenergic negative inotropic effects, should be given in the same initial dose as described for calcium channel blocker poisoning. Patients with altered mental status or abnormal vital signs also should be given an intravenous bolus of glucose. Bronchospasm may be treated with inhaled beta agonist, subcutaneous epinephrine, and intravenous aminophylline. Lidocaine, magnesium (as for antiarrhythmic poisoning), or overdrive pacing may be used for sotalol-induced ventricular tachyarrhythmias. Extracorporal elimination procedures are probably not of benefit, with the possible exceptions of atenolol, carteolol, metoprolol, nadolol, and sotalol.

BLEACH Bleach (Clorox) solutions for home use generally contain 3 to 6% sodium hypochlorite, and industrial bleaches may have higher concentrations. These solutions have a pH or 10.5 to 11.0 and contain free chlorine, which gives the compound its characteristic odor.

Sodium hypochlorite decomposes to hypochloric acid on contact with moisture and is irritating but not caustic. Sodium hypochlorite mixed with acid releases chlorine gas and, when mixed with ammonia, produces chloramine gas. Both these gases are highly irritating.

Clinical toxicity Sodium hypochlorite is irritating to the gastrointestinal mucosa and to mucous membranes of the lips, mouth, and eyes. Household bleach causes only superficial injury to the esophagus, but industrial bleaches cause deep burns of the esophagus with the potential for stricture formation. Chemical pneumonia and pulmonary edema may result from the aspiration of bleach or inhalation of chlorine and chloramine.

Treatment Ingestion of small quantities of household bleach should be treated only by dilution. Large ingestions of sodium hypochlorite may require gastric lavage. When concentrated solutions have been ingested, therapy should be similar to that for acids and alkali. Neutralization is not necessary, and activated charcoal and cathartics are not indicated. Exposed skin and eyes also should be decontaminated. Treatment of pulmonary toxicity is symptomatic and supportive.

CALCIUM CHANNEL BLOCKERS Calcium channel blocking agents include bepridil, felodipine, isradipine, diltiazem, nicardipine, nifedipine, nimodipine, and verapamil. These agents act by decreasing the influx of calcium across slow calcium channels in the membranes of myocardial and vascular smooth-muscle cells during phases 2

(plateau) and 4 (spontaneous depolarization) of the action potential. Electrophysiologic effects include decreased cardiac contractility, heart (SA nodal) rate, AV nodal conduction, and vascular tone. These actions define calcium channel blockers as class IV antiarrhythmics. Bepridil also has class I antiarrhythmic activity.

Calcium channel blockers are rapidly absorbed, exhibit high (80 to 99 percent) protein binding in the plasma, and have large volumes of distribution ranging from 0.6 to 10.0 L/kg of body weight. They are predominantly eliminated by hepatic metabolism, and their half-lives range from 1 to 24 h.

Clinical toxicity Effects begin within 1/2 to 1 h of ingestion of amounts 5 to 10 times the usual therapeutic dose. Toxicity may be delayed following overdoses of sustained-release preparations. Clinical manifestations include bradycardia, hypotension, and CNS depression. Mental status changes range from confusion and drowsiness to coma and seizures and are due both to direct membrane effects and to cerebral hypoperfusion. Hypotension may precipitate myocardial ischemia, and depression of cardiac function may lead to pulmonary edema. ECG findings include all degrees of AV block, prolonged QRS and QT intervals (mainly with verapamil), evidence of ischemia or infarction, and asystole. Metabolic acidosis (secondary to shock) and hyperglycemia (resulting in the inhibition of insulin release) may be present. Serum calcium levels, however, remain normal.

Treatment Gastrointestinal tract decontamination should be accomplished as soon as possible. Symptomatic bradycardia should be treated with atropine, calcium, isoproterenol, glucagon, and electrical (external or internal) pacing. Calcium, as the 10% chloride or gluconate salt solution, is given in a dose of 0.2 mL/kg of body weight (up to 10 mL) intravenously over 5 min. This dose may be repeated up to four times in patients with a partial, transient, or absent response, provided that serum calcium levels are monitored. A continuous calcium infusion (0.2 mL/kg of body weight per hour up to a maximum of 10 mL/h) may be appropriate when relapse occurs after an initial bolus. Although electrical pacing is often required, glucagon, in the same dose as for beta-blocker poisoning, should be tried first. Hypotension that persists despite resolution of bradycardia should be treated with fluids and vasopressors. Amrinone, dopamine, dobutamine, glucagon, and norepinephrine, alone or in combination, have been used. The benefit of restored perfusion is particularly important in patients with organ ischemia. Intraaortic balloon pump support should be used in patients unresponsive to the preceding measures. Patients with mild toxicity usually recover within a few hours, whereas those with severe toxicity or overdose with sustained-release preparations may remain symptomatic for 24 h or longer. Extracorporal removal techniques are unlikely to be of benefit.

CARBON MONOXIDE Carbon monoxide is produced in large amounts in industry as well as by gasoline engines, home appliances, and the incomplete combustion of wood, natural gas, and tobacco products. In addition, methylene chloride, a solvent in paint removers, is metabolized to carbon monoxide.

Carbon monoxide is rapidly absorbed through the lungs and binds to hemoglobin (forming carboxyhemoglobin) with an affinity 210 times that of oxygen. This limits oxygen-carrying by hemoglobin and also decreases the release of oxygen to tissues (the oxygen dissociation curve shifts to the left). Carbon monoxide also binds to myoglobin, decreasing its oxygen-carrying capacity, and to mitochondrial cytochrome oxidase, thereby inhibiting cellular respiration. The net effect is profound tissue hypoxia, anaerobic metabolism, and lactic acidosis. Once carbon monoxide exposure is discontinued, dissociation of the hemoglobin–carbon monoxide complex occurs, and carbon monoxide is excreted through the lungs. In room air, the carbon monoxide half-life is 4 to 6 h; the half-life decreases to 40 to 80 min when breathing 100% oxygen and to 15 to 30 min with hyperbaric oxygen therapy. The apparent half-life after methylene chloride exposure is considerably longer.

Clinical toxicity Manifestations of carbon monoxide poisoning include shortness of breath, dyspnea, tachypnea, headache, emotional lability, confusion, impaired judgment, clumsiness, and syncope. Nausea, vomiting, and diarrhea also may occur. Cerebral edema, coma, respiratory depression, and pulmonary edema occur with severe poisoning. Cardiovascular manifestations include ischemic chest pain, arrhythmias, heart failure, and hypotension. Blisters and bullae may develop over pressure points. Myoglobinuria secondary to muscle necrosis may result in renal failure. The "cherry red" color of skin and mucous membranes is rare, and cyanosis is usual. Visual field defects, blindness, and venous engorgement with papilledema or optic atrophy may be noted. Arterial blood gases reveal metabolic acidosis, a normal P_{O_2}, decreased oxygen saturation (by direct CO-oximetry measurement rather than a calculated or pulse oximetry value), and normal or slightly decreased P_{CO_2}.

Traditionally, levels of 20 to 30 percent are associated with mild symptoms, 30 to 50 percent with moderate symptoms, 50 to 60 percent with severe symptoms, and levels above 60 percent are often fatal. While elevated carboxyhemoglobin levels document carbon monoxide exposure, they do not necessarily correlate with the severity of the poisoning. Serum creatine phosphokinase (CPK) and lactate dehydrogenase (LHD) levels may be elevated.

Up to the 30 percent of patients with loss of consciousness develop persistent neuropsychiatric sequelae evident 1 to 3 weeks after exposure. Manifestations vary from subtle personality changes and intellectual impairment to gross neurologic deficits such as blindness, deafness, incoordination, and parkinsonism.

Treatment The patients should be removed from the site of exposure. In conscious patients, oxygen (100%) should be administered by a non-rebreather mask at 10 L/min until carbon monoxide levels are less than 10 percent and all symptoms have resolved. Infants and pregnant women require treatment for several more hours because fetal hemoglobin has a high affinity for carbon monoxide. Endotracheal intubation and mechanical ventilation with 100% oxygen are indicated in patients with coma, significant CNS dysfunction, or cardiovascular instability. Hyperbaric oxygen at 2 to 3 atm decreases the half-life of carbon monoxide to 15 to 30 min and produces sufficient dissolved oxygen to prevent tissue hypoxia. Arrhythmias and hypotension are treated by usual measures. Patients with coma, syncope, or seizures and those with signs or symptoms of neurologic or cardiovascular dysfunction that do not resolve with oxygen and supportive therapy are candidates for hyperbaric oxygen therapy. Hyperbaric oxygenation shortens the duration of coma and may prevent delayed sequelae.

COCAINE See Chap. 392.

CYANIDE Hydrogen cyanide is used as a fumigant rodenticide and in chemical syntheses. Cyanide salts are used in photography, metallurgy, electroplating, metal cleaning, and ore refining. Organic cyanide compounds (nitriles) are used in the synthetic rubber industry, artificial nail removers, and rodenticides. Cyanogenic glycosides are present in the seeds of the chokeberry, cherry, plum, peach, apricot, pear, bean, apple, and crabapple.

Cyanide inhibits mitochondrial ferricytochrome oxidase and hence blocks electron transport, resulting in decreased oxidative metabolism and oxygen utilization. Lactic acidosis occurs as a consequence of anaerobic metabolism. Cyanide is rapidly absorbed from the stomach, lungs, mucosal surfaces, and unbroken skin. In the stomach it reacts with hydrochloric acid, liberating hydrocyanic acid, which is absorbed as cyanide ion. Cyanide is 60 percent protein-bound, is concentrated in red cells, and has a volume of distribution of 1.5 L/kg of body weight. Cyanide is metabolized by the mitochondrial enzyme rhodanase, which mediates the transfer of sulfur from thiosulfate to the cyanide ion producing thiocyanate, which in turn is excreted in the urine.

Clinical toxicity The lethal dose of potassium or sodium cyanide is 200 to 300 mg and of hydrocyanic acid is 50 mg. Effects begin within seconds of inhalation and within 30 min of ingestion. Initial manifestations of cyanide poisoning include headache, faintness, vertigo, excitement, anxiety, burning sensation in the mouth and throat, and dyspnea. Cardiovascular effects include tachycardia and

hypertension. Nausea, vomiting and diaphoresis are common. A bitter almond odor may be detected on the breath. Later effects include coma, convulsions, opisthotonus, trismus, paralysis, respiratory depression, pulmonary edema, arrhythmias, bradycardia, and hypotension. Variable correlation exists between blood cyanide levels and symptoms: Levels less than 8 μmol/L (0.02 mg/L) are associated with no symptoms, 20 to 40 μmol/L (0.05 to 0.1 mg/dL) with flushing and tachycardia, 40 to 100 μmol/L (0.1 to 0.25 mg/dL) with obtundation, 100 to 200 μmol/L (0.25 to 0.3 mg/dL) with coma and respiratory depression, and levels greater than 120 μmol/L (0.3 mg/dL) with death. Other laboratory abnormalities include lactic acidosis and narrowing of the arteriovenous oxygen saturation difference. ECG abnormalities include both tachyarrhythmias and bradyarrhythmias such as nodal or idioventricular rhythm, AV dissociation, and progressive slowing of heart rate.

Treatment Initial management involves general supportive measures and gastrointestinal decontamination. Since blood cyanide measurements are difficult to obtain, antidotal therapy using amyl nitrite, sodium nitrite, and sodium thiosulfate (the Lilly cyanide antidote kit) coupled with high-dose oxygen must be initiated on the basis of the history and clinical findings. Amyl nitrite is administered for 30 s of each minute. The ampule is broken between two pads of gauze and placed over the airway while the patient breathes spontaneously or is ventilated by a bag-mask unit. A new ampule should be used every 3 min. This process is continued while sodium nitrite is being prepared but may be omitted if endotracheal intubation has been performed or if sodium nitrite is available. Sodium nitrite is administered intravenously as a 3% solution at a rate of 2.5 to 5.0 mL/min up to a total dose of 10 to 15 mL (300 to 450 mg). The dose in children is 0.33 mL/kg of body weight (10 mg/kg of body weight). Sodium thiosulfate is then administered intravenously as a 25% solution at a dose of 50 mL (12.5 g) given over 1 to 2 min. The dose in children is 0.33 mL/kg of body weight (10 mg/kg of body weight). Sodium thiosulfate is then administered intravenously as a 25% solution at a dose of 50 mL (12.5 g) given over 1 to 2 min. The dose in children is 1.65 mL/kg of body weight (0.5 g/kg of body weight). With recurrent or persistent symptoms, half or full doses of both sodium nitrite and sodium thiosulfate are administered. The rationale for antidotal therapy is as follows: Nitrites induce methemoglobinemia; methemoglobin has a higher affinity for cyanide than does cytochrome oxidase, thereby promoting its dissociation from this enzyme; thiosulfate reacts with the cyanide that is slowly released from cyanomethemoglobin, forming the relatively nontoxic thiocyanate, which is excreted in the urine. Oxygen reverses the binding of cyanide to cytochrome oxidase sites and enhances the efficacy of sodium nitrite and sodium thiosulfate, in addition to acting as a substrate for metabolism. The value of hyperbaric oxygen therapy, however, has not been proven.

DIGOXIN Digitalis (cardiac glycoside) poisoning occurs most frequently as overdosage during therapeutic or suicidal use of digoxin and on occasion with plant (oleander) ingestion. Cardiac glycosides act by inhibiting the enzyme sodium-potassium ATPase, leading to increased intracellular Na^+ and Ca^{2+} and decreased K^+. Digoxin is slowly absorbed and slowly distributed. Serum levels may not correlate with pharmacologic effects for up to 8 h following a therapeutic oral dose. Digoxin is 25 to 30 percent protein-bound in the plasma, has a large volume of distribution of 5 to 6 L/kg of body weight, and is localized in skeletal muscle, liver, and heart. Elimination is primarily by renal excretion. The half-life ranges between 36 and 45 h, is prolonged in hepatic failure and in renal failure, and may be shortened in overdose. Approximately 60 percent of a dose is excreted unchanged by the kidneys, and the remainder is metabolized by the liver to inactive metabolites. The mean therapeutic serum concentration ranges from 0.6 to 2.5 nmol/L (0.5 to 2.0 ng/mL).

Clinical toxicity Symptoms of toxicity include vomiting, confusion, delirium, and occasionally hallucinations, blurred vision, photophobia, scotomata, and disturbed color perception. Cardiac manifestations include sinus arrhythmia, sinus bradycardia, and all degrees of atrioventricular block. Premature ventricular contractions, bigeminy, ventricular tachycardia, and fibrillation also occur. The combination of supraventricular tachyarrhythmia and AV block is highly suggestive of digitalis toxicity. While bradyarrhythmias and hypokalemia are common with chronic intoxication, tachyarrhythmias and hyperkalemia are generally seen with acute poisoning. Similarly, serum digoxin levels may be minimally elevated or even therapeutic in chronic toxicity, whereas they are usually markedly elevated following acute overdose. Clinical toxicity occurs with digoxin levels in excess of 3.8 to 6.4 nmol/L (3 to 5 ng/mL), and levels as high as 64 to 77 nmol/L (50 to 60 ng/mL) have been seen in the overdose setting. Levels measured sooner than 8 h after ingestion may not reflect complete tissue distribution.

Treatment Gastrointestinal decontamination should be accomplished as soon as possible, since emesis and gastric intubation may cause vagal stimulation, which may worsen existing conduction block. Activated charcoal is preferred. Repeated doses should be administered because this therapy also can enhance elimination of digoxin metabolites. Diuresis, hemodialysis, and hemoperfusion are ineffective, however. Potassium, magnesium, and calcium abnormalities should be corrected. Electrical pacing may be necessary when sinus bradycardia and second- and third-degree heart block result in hypotension and fail to respond to atropine and isoproterenol. Magnesium sulfate (as for antiarrhythmia poisoning), as well as phenytoin and lidocaine, may be useful in the treatment of ventricular tachyarrhythmias. Digoxin-specific Fab fragment antibodies are also available for the treatment of potentially life-threatening intoxication not immediately responsive to the above. Each 40-mg vial can neutralize 0.6 mg digoxin. Fab fragment antibodies are appropriate for patients with refractory arrhythmias and significantly elevated serum digoxin concentrations. Following their administration, cardiac arrhythmias and hyperkalemia are generally corrected within an hour; the antibodies are given intravenously over 30 min, unless cardiac arrest has occurred, in which case the solution is given as a bolus. The drug-antibody complex is excreted in the urine with a half-life of 16 to 20 h. In patients with renal failure, the drug-antibody complex is metabolized over a period of days to weeks. Although free digoxin levels rapidly decrease to zero following antibody administration, routine methods used to measure digoxin do not differentiate between bound and unbound drug and will have no correlation with toxicity after such therapy. Antibodies cross-react with other cardiac glycosides, but larger doses may be needed for toxicity not involving digoxin.

Formulas and tables for calculating the dose of antibody based on body weight and post-distribution serum digoxin level or the amount of drug acutely ingested are available in the package insert. Unfortunately, toxicity may occur before distribution is complete or before levels are available, the amount of an acute overdose may be unknown, the antibody is expensive, and calculated doses often exceed the effective dose. The following approach is therefore suggested. In patients with chronic digoxin intoxication, whose total-body drug load only slightly exceeds the therapeutic amount and who may be dependent on digoxin for its inotropic effects, begin with a dose of 1 to 2 vials. In acute digoxin overdose, begin with a dose of 5 to 10 vials. These doses may be repeated if necessary, but they will be effective in all but the most severe cases.

ETHANOL See Chap. 390.

ETHYLENE GLYCOL Ethylene glycol is a colorless, odorless, sweet-tasting, water-soluble liquid that is used as a solvent for paints, plastics, and pharmaceuticals and in the manufacture of explosives, fire extinguishers, foams, hydraulic fluids, windshield cleaners, radiator antifreeze, and de-icer preparations.

Ethylene glycol is rapidly absorbed. Peak levels occur approximately 2 h following ingestion. Ethylene glycol has a volume of distribution of 0.6 to 0.8 L/kg of body weight. It is oxidized by alcohol dehydrogenase to glycoaldehyde, which is then metabolized to glycolic acid, glyoxylic acid, and oxalic acid. As much as 20

percent is excreted unchanged in the urine. The half-life ranges from 3 to 8 h. Since alcohol dehydrogenase has a higher affinity for ethanol than ethylene glycol, ethanol is preferentially metabolized when both alcohols are present. Ethanol inhibits metabolism of ethylene glycol and prolongs its half-life to about 17 h. Ethylene glycol and its metabolites produce CNS depression in overdose. Ethylene glycol is more intoxicating than ethanol in this respect. Glycolic acid is responsible for decreased serum bicarbonate, metabolic acidosis, and increased anion gap, as well as for interstitial and tubular damage to the kidney. Glyoxylic acid is more toxic than glycolic acid, but because it is oxidized so rapidly to oxalic acid, glycolic acid contributes little to the toxicity of ethylene glycol. Oxalic acid may precipitate as calcium oxalate crystals in the brain, heart, kidney, lung, pancreas, and urine and may result in hypocalcemia.

Clinical toxicity As little as 120 mg/kg of body weight or 0.1 mL/kg of body weight (one swallow) of pure ethylene glycol can result in a potentially toxic blood concentration of 3 mmol/L (20 mg/dL). Effects begin 30 min following ingestion and include nausea, vomiting, slurred speech, ataxia, nystagmus, and lethargy. A faint, sweet aromatic odor may be detected on the breath. Coma, seizures, respiratory depression, cardiovascular collapse, and death may occur. Effects caused by metabolites begin 4 to 12 h following ingestion. At this stage the patient appears more ill than intoxicated. Manifestations include tachypnea, hypotension, agitation, confusion, lethargy, coma, and seizures. Hypocalcemia occurs in a third of patients. Leukocytosis is present in the majority. In severe cases, adult respiratory distress syndrome, cyanosis, pulmonary edema, and cardiomegaly may be seen. In this stage the diagnosis is suggested by metabolic acidosis, an increased anion gap (low bicarbonate and chloride), and an abnormal urinalysis (crystalluria). In patients who survive the early stages, acute tubular necrosis manifested by proteinuria, oliguria, and anuria ensues 12 to 24 h following ingestion. Renal failure may be permanent but typically lasts days to weeks. In early intoxication, osmolality is elevated. Later, an elevated anion gap and decreased serum bicarbonate and chloride are observed. Signs of alcohol-like intoxication suggest a serum ethylene glycol level greater than 8 to 16 mmol/L (50 to 100 mg/dL). Survival has been reported with levels as high as 100 mmol/L (650 mg/dL).

Diagnosis Diagnosis is suggested by a history of exposure to antifreeze in association with CNS depression, an elevated serum osmolality, and a large anion gap. Ethylene glycol and glycolic acid levels should be measured along with routine laboratory tests. Oxalate crystals in the urine suggest the diagnosis.

Treatment Gastrointestinal lavage and activated charcoal should be administered. Supportive measures include protection of the airway and ventilatory and circulatory support. Seizures should be treated with phenytoin, a short-acting barbiturate, or a benzodiazepine. Hypocalcemia is treated with intravenous calcium salts at a dose of 7 to 14 mL (a 10% solution diluted 10 to 1 with intravenous fluids and given at a rate of 1 mL/min). Metabolic acidosis should be corrected with sodium bicarbonate. Large doses are often required. Fluids and diuretics may reverse oliguria but do not enhance the elimination rate of ethylene glycol. Indications for ethanol therapy include a history or strong suspicion of ethylene glycol ingestion, an ethylene glycol concentration greater than 3 mmol/L (20 mg/dL), and acidosis regardless of the absolute ethylene glycol concentration. A serum ethanol level of at least 20 mmol/L (100 mg/dL) is required to inhibit alcohol dehydrogenase (higher levels may be needed with very high ethylene glycol concentrations). The loading and maintenance doses of ethanol are the same as for methanol poisoning. Serum ethanol and ethylene glycol concentrations should be monitored frequently. Hemodialysis reduces ethylene glycol half-life from 17 h on ethanol therapy to 3 h and enhances the elimination of toxic metabolites. Indications for hemodialysis include metabolic acidosis not readily correctable with bicarbonate and ethanol therapy, failure to improve despite treatment, ethylene glycol concentrations greater than 8 mmol/L (50 mg/dL), or renal failure. Supplemental thiamine and pyridoxine also may be beneficial.

HALLUCINOGENS   (See also Chap. 392) Hallucinogens belong to three chemical classes, phenylalkylamines, tryptamines, and ergolines, with mescaline, psilocybin, and lysergic acid diethylamide (LSD) being the prototype for each. Large numbers of synthetic analogues exist in each class. Mescaline is a derivative of the peyote cactus which grows in the southwestern United States. Psilocybin is derived from mushrooms. Lysergic acid is found in the fungus *Claviceps purpurea*, which grows as a contaminant on rye and wheat and in morning glory seeds. Hallucinogens act by altering the function of the central (and peripheral) neurotransmitter serotonin.

Hallucinogens are well absorbed from the gastrointestinal tract. Mescaline is also rapidly absorbed through the nasal mucosa. Mescaline has an apparent volume of distribution of 2 to 3 L/kg of body weight and is eliminated by hepatic metabolism. Psilocybin itself is inactive but is converted to the active metabolite psilocin. LSD is rapidly absorbed by both the nasal mucosa and gastrointestinal tract. Peak levels of LSD are achieved within 1 to 2 h following ingestion. LSD is protein-bound (80 to 90 percent) and has an apparent volume of distribution of 0.8 L/kg of body weight and is metabolized to inactive metabolites with a half-life of 3 h.

Clinical toxicity   Hallucinogens produce disordered thought, mood changes, and sensory misperceptions (auditory, gustatory, olfactory, and visual dysesthesias). The physiologic effects of LSD last for 4 to 6 h and include mydriasis, conjunctival injection, piloerection, hypertension, tachycardia, tachypnea, anorexia, tremors, and hyperreflexia. Psychological effects include loss of body image, visual illusions, and alteration of the senses. The psychological effects ("trip") generally last for 6 to 12 h and can be pleasant or alarming. The EEG may show paroxysmal discharges, and seizures may occur. Flashbacks or recurrences of visual images may appear up to 18 months after ingestion. The effects of mescaline include nausea, vomiting, and mild physiologic stimulation (see Table 395-2). Psilocybin has effects similar to those of LSD, with unique features including fever, hypotonia, and seizures.

Diagnosis   Identification of LSD in serum is difficult because of its low concentration. In urine, LSD can be detected for up to 5 days following ingestion, and mescaline can be detected for up to 24 h. Psilocybin is not detected in the routine toxic screens.

Treatment   Gastrointestinal decontamination is not useful once symptoms are present and may lead to further exacerbation of symptoms. The mainstay of therapy is prevention of physical injury by calming in a quiet room with low lights. Physical restraint may cause hyperthermia, rhabdomyolysis, and acute renal failure. Benzodiazepines are effective for acute panic reaction, and butyrephenones (haloperidol in particular) may be indicated for severe psychotic reactions (see Chap. 392).

HYDROCARBONS   Hydrocarbons exist in a number of forms, including aromatic hydrocarbons, such as xylene and toluene, halogenated hydrocarbons, such as carbon tetrachloride and trichlorethane, and petroleum distillate hydrocarbons, such as gasoline, lacquer thinner, mineral seal oil, kerosene, and lighter fluid.

All hydrocarbons are CNS depressants. They are rapidly absorbed following inhalation or pulmonary aspiration. Aromatic and halogenated hydrocarbons are also absorbed following ingestion and are toxic to the gastrointestinal tract, heart, lung, liver, and kidneys. Aromatic hydrocarbons also can cause bone marrow suppression and skeletal muscle damage. Petroleum distillate hydrocarbons are poorly absorbed following ingestion but are toxic to the gastrointestinal tract, CNS and lungs. Lung involvement is predominantly due to aspiration pneumonitis.

Clinical toxicity   Hydrocarbons produce excitation in low dose and depression of the CNS in high dose. Rarely, coma and seizures may occur. Psychosis, cerebral and cerebellar atrophy, encephalopathy, and peripheral neuropathy can result from chronic exposure. Other effects include nausea, vomiting, abdominal pain, hepatitis, renal tubular acidosis, acute hepatic or renal failure, and rhabdomyolysis. Sudden death due to myocardial irritability and ventricular fibrillation may occur following hydrocarbon sniffing. Petroleum distillate hydrocarbons cause burning of the mouth and throat with subsequent nausea, vomiting, and diarrhea. Respiratory effects include cough, dyspnea, tachypnea, wheezing, rhonchi, rales, hypoxia, and cyanosis. Lethargy is the most prominent CNS manifestation. Coma and convulsions are rare. Following aspiration, chest x-ray abnormalities include infiltrates, atelectasis, effusions, pneumothorax, and pneumatoceles. Metabolic acidosis with decreased serum calcium chloride phosphate and potassium may result from aromatic hydrocarbon poisoning. Laboratory diagnosis of aromatic, halogenated, or petroleum distillate hydrocarbon poisoning is not available at present.

Treatment   The ingestion of aromatic and halogenated hydrocarbons requires prompt gastric lavage. Ipecac-induced emesis is contraindicated, and activated charcoal is ineffective. Supportive therapy includes oxygen, respiratory support, and monitoring of liver, renal, and myocardial function. In the case of petroleum distillate hydrocarbons, unless very large amounts (greater than 18 mL/kg of body weight) are ingested, gastric lavage and ipecac-induced emesis are contraindicated. Activated charcoal is both ineffective and hazardous because it may induce emesis. Pulmonary aspiration is treated by supportive therapy and by monitoring for superimposed bacterial infection. Glucocorticoids are ineffective. CNS effects are relatively short-lived and require careful monitoring and respiratory support.

HYDROGEN SULFIDE   Hydrogen sulfide is a rapidly acting malodorous ("rotten eggs"), colorless, irritating gas that gains access to the blood through the mucous membranes of the tracheobronchial tree. It is encountered in the petroleum and mining industry, tanning of leather, vulcanization of rubber, production of synthetic fabrics, metal refining, production of heavy water for atomic reactors, and glue and felt manufacturing. It is also found in sewers, sulfur springs, the holds of fishing vessels, and as a by-product of manure storage.

The hydrogen sulfide anion inhibits electron transport in the cytochrome oxidase system, thereby inhibiting aerobic metabolism with resultant cellular anoxia and lactic acidosis. Hydrogen sulfide is detoxified to sulfate products that are principally excreted by the kidneys.

Clinical toxicity   Hydrogen sulfide is highly irritating, resulting in rhinitis, conjunctivitis, and pharyngitis. Systemic effects include headache, vertigo, nausea, vomiting, confusion, seizures, and coma. It also produces hypoventilation, hypoxia, cyanosis, metabolic acidosis, pneumonia, and pulmonary edema. There is no readily available laboratory test, and the diagnosis is based on history and clinical features.

Treatment   Treatment begins with prompt removal of the victim from the site of exposure. The airway should be cleared, ventilation should be assisted when indicated, and 100% oxygen should be administered. Nitrites (see "Cyanide" above) bind the sulfide ion by removing it from cytochrome oxidase sites, thereby forming a sulfide-methemoglobin complex (sulfmethemoglobin). They also enhance detoxification by acting as a catalyst for sulfide oxidation. Except for cardiac arrest, no clear-cut indications for nitrite administration exist. For optimal effectiveness, they must be utilized immediately in symptomatic patients (sulfide oxidation is so rapid that the amount of sulfide bound to cytochrome is minimal by the time the patient presents for treatment). The dosage schedule is the same as for cyanide poisoning (thiosulfate is not necessary). Hyperbaric oxygen should be considered in patients who do not respond to the preceding measures.

IRON   Iron preparations contain ferrous salts that vary in elemental iron content (20 percent in the sulfate salt, 33 percent in the fumarate, and 12 percent in the gluconate). Ingestion of more than 20 mg/kg of body weight of elemental iron produces gastrointestinal toxicity and of more than 60 mg/kg of body weight results in systemic toxicity.

Ferrous iron is absorbed into mucosal cells of the duodenum and jejunum and is oxidized to ferric iron, where it is bound to ferritin. It is slowly released from ferritin into the plasma, where it is bound to transferrin, an iron-specific binding globulin, and transported to tissues for use in hemoglobin, cytochrome, and myoglobin synthesis. Approximately 70 percent of total-body iron is present as hemoglobin,

25 percent is stored in liver and spleen as ferritin and hemosiderin, and 5 percent is present in myoglobin and tissue enzymes. Iron bound to transferrin is nontoxic. Free iron that exceeds the iron-binding capacity and high ferritin levels are toxic to the vasculature and lead to the release of vasoactive substances such as serotonin and histamine. Increased capillary permeability, vasodilation, and fluid loss result in hypotension and metabolic acidosis. Free iron also injures mitochondria, causes lipid peroxidation, and results in renal, tubular, and hepatic necrosis and on occasion in myocardial and pulmonary injury. In overdose, iron is deposited in liver, spleen, and kidneys and causes fatty degeneration and necrosis in hepatocytes, renal tubules, and myocardial cells.

Clinical toxicity Initial manifestations include vomiting and diarrhea (often bloody). X-rays may reveal iron tablets in the stomach or small bowel. A positive x-ray, fever above 101°F (38.5° C), hyperglycemia greater than 8.5 mmol/L (150 mg/dL), and leukocytosis white blood cell count (greater than 15,000 cells per cubic millimeter) are associated with serum iron levels above 50 μmol/L (300 μg/dL) and the potential for systemic toxicity. Systemic effects include lethargy, hypotension, and metabolic acidosis and, with severe poisoning, seizures, coma, pulmonary edema and vascular collapse. Jaundice, elevated hepatic enzymes, prolongation of prothrombin time, and hyperammonemia are indicative of liver injury. Proteinuria and cells in urine indicate renal injury. Pulmonary edema and hemorrhage are seen with severe overdose. In the recovering patient, gastric ulcerations and scars may cause outlet obstruction. Overgrowth of *Yersinia enterocolitica* with sepsis is a rare complication of iron overload.

Diagnosis A serum iron concentration above the iron-binding capacity [a serum level generally greater than 50 μmol/L (300 μg/dL)] suggests serious poisoning. A positive urine deferoxamine provocative challenge test (a *vin rosé* color) indicating the presence of ferrioxamine (the complex of free iron bound to deferoxamine) is diagnostic and indicates an iron level greater than the iron-binding capacity.

Treatment Removal of ingested iron is best accomplished with either ipecac-induced emesis or a large orogastric tube. An x-ray film following gastric lavage will define the success of the decontamination procedure. Whole-bowel irrigation, endoscopic removal, or gastrostomy may be necessary for concretion formation or large quantities of iron tablets. Activated charcoal is ineffective. Bicarbonate lavage (50 to 100 mL 1% solution) has been advocated in an effort to form insoluble ferrous carbonate salt. Oral deferoxamine is administered to complex iron remaining in the stomach into an insoluble, iron-deferoxamine complex (ferrioxamine). Since the amount of the deferoxamine required is large, and since iron is rapidly absorbed, these therapies are rarely used. Serum iron and total iron-binding capacity should be measured. Intravenous sodium bicarbonate should be used to correct metabolic acidosis. Hypotension may respond to volume expansion. Coagulation abnormalities should be treated with vitamin K or blood products.

When the serum iron level indicates potential systemic toxicity or exceeds the iron-binding capacity, parenteral deferoxamine should be administered. If levels are not immediately available, or if the patient has mild clinical toxicity, deferoxamine can be given intramuscularly in a challenge dose of 50 mg/kg up to 2 g. A *vin rosé* urine color indicates a positive test for free iron and the need for intravenous therapy. In those with a positive challenge test or with significant clinical toxicity, deferoxamine should be infused at a rate of 10 to 15 mg/kg per hour. Once the serum iron is less than the iron-binding capacity or the urine color has returned to normal, deferoxamine therapy can be discontinued. When iron levels exceed 180 μmol/L (1000 μg/dL), larger doses (up to 30 mg/kg per hour) of deferoxamine can be given. Exchange transfusion or plasmapheresis to remove the iron-desferal (ferrioxamine) complex should be reserved for patients with renal failure or for those who fail to respond to the preceding therapy.

ISONIAZID Toxic doses of isoniazid decrease the synthesis of the inhibitory neurotransmitter GABA by inhibiting the pyridoxal phosphate–dependent enzyme glutamic acid decarboxylase. The consequence can be CNS stimulation or depression. Isoniazid is rapidly absorbed mainly from the small intestine. Peak serum concentrations occur within 1 to 2 h. The volume of distribution is approximately 0.6 L/kg of body weight. Serum protein binding is small. Isoniazid is primarily eliminated by acetylation to acetyl-isoniazid and then hydrolysis to isonicotinic acid. Approximately 15 percent of an ingested dose of isoniazid is excreted unchanged by the kidneys. The serum half-life of isoniazid in overdose is approximately 1 to 4 h.

Clinical toxicity Effects begin within 30 min of ingestion of doses of greater than 20 mg/kg of body weight. Symptoms include nausea, vomiting, dizziness, slurred speech, lethargy, and confusion. The major manifestations include coma, respiratory depression, generalized seizures, and lactic acid acidosis. Seizures are protracted and relatively unresponsive to standard anticonvulsant therapy. Acidosis does not occur when seizures are prevented. Diagnosis is confirmed by identification of isoniazid in urine or blood. Toxicity occurs with concentrations as low as 15 μmol/L (2 mg/L). Significant symptoms are seen with serum concentrations greater than 30 to 35 μmol/L (4 to 5 mg/L).

Treatment Initial therapy consists of prompt gastrointestinal decontamination and supportive measures. Ipecac-induced vomiting should be avoided because of the high incidence of seizures. Isoniazid is well adsorbed by activated charcoal. Seizures can sometimes be treated with benzodiazepines, barbiturates, and phenytoin but may be refractory to these agents. Pyridoxine (vitamin B6), however, is a cofactor for GABA synthesis and is efficacious in preventing and treating seizures. Diazepam is synergistic with pyridoxine. Bicarbonate may be necessary to correct acidosis. Pyridoxine should be given slowly intravenously in an amount equal to the ingested dose of isoniazid. When the ingested dose is not known, 5 g of pyridoxine should be administered. Pyridoxine should be given over 5 min to patients with seizures but over 30 min in the absence of seizures as a 5% to 10% concentration. Cessation of seizures and correction of metabolic acidosis are prompt. The dose may be repeated with partial response or when symptoms recur. Due to its low protein binding and small volume of distribution, isoniazid is efficiently removed by hemodialysis, but dialysis is rarely necessary because of the efficacy of pyridoxine.

ISOPROPYL ALCOHOL Isopropyl alcohol is a component of rubbing alcohol, solvents, after-shave lotions, antifreeze, and window cleaners. Its metabolite, acetone, is found in cleaners, solvents, and nail polish removers.

Isopropyl alcohol and acetone are about twice as potent, as CNS depressants, as ethanol. Isopropyl alcohol is rapidly absorbed from the stomach and the lungs but only minimally through skin. It is distributed in body water and has a volume of distribution of 0.6 L/kg of body weight. Its half-life ranges from 3 to 6 h. Isopropyl alcohol is metabolized in the liver by the enzyme alcohol dehydrogenase to acetone, which is excreted by the kidneys and lungs with a half-life of 20 to 30 h. Up to 20 percent of isopropyl alcohol is excreted unchanged through the kidneys.

Clinical toxicity Effects begin within 30 min of ingestion and include vomiting, abdominal discomfort, and hematemesis. A characteristic smell of rubbing alcohol may be noted. CNS manifestations include headache, dizziness, confusion, and excitation. With severe ingestion, obtundation, coma, respiratory depression, hypothermia, and hypotension may occur. Hypoglycemia may be seen. Isopropyl alcohol can cause a falsely elevated serum creatinine. A mild anion gap acidosis may be seen as well as an increase in the serum osmolality. Myopathy and hemolytic anemias are occasionally present. Concentrations of 8 to 17 mmol/L (50 to 100 mg/dL) produce lethargy, concentrations greater than 25 to 33 mmol/L (150 to 200 mg/dL) are associated with coma, and concentrations greater than 66 to 84 mmol/L (400 to 500 mg/dL) are potentially fatal.

Treatment Gastrointestinal decontamination must be instituted soon following ingestion. Activated charcoal is ineffective in significantly adsorbing isopropyl alcohol. The diagnosis is confirmed by elevated isopropyl alcohol (early) and acetone (late) levels. Supportive measures should include intravenous fluids and bicarbonate to correct dehydration, shock, and acidosis. Isopropyl alcohol and acetone are efficiently removed by hemodialysis. The procedure should be considered in patients with levels in the potentially lethal range [greater than 66 mmol/L (400 mg/dL)] or in patients inadequately managed by conservative therapy.

LITHIUM Lithium is most commonly available as the carbonate or the citrate salt. Lithium may substitute for cellular cations (K$^+$ and Na$^+$), thereby interfering with adenylate cyclase activation, inhibiting neurotransmitter (norepinephrine) release, and reducing sodium potassium ATPase activity.

The drug is rapidly absorbed from the gastrointestinal tract and reaches peak levels within 2 to 4 h of ingestion (later with overdosage and with sustained-release preparations). It has negligible plasma protein binding and a volume of distribution of approximately 0.6 L/kg of body weight. Removal from the body is primarily (95 percent) by glomerular filtration, with significant reabsorption (80 percent) by the proximal tubules. Lithium clearance is increased by alkalinization of the urine and decreased by hypovolemia and hyponatremia. Serum half-life ranges from 18 to 36 h; therapeutic levels range from 0.6 to 1.2 mmol/L.

Clinical toxicity Effects begin 1 to 4 h after ingestion. Gastrointestinal effects include nausea, vomiting, and diarrhea; neuromuscular effects include weakness, fasciculations, and twitching; CNS effects include ataxia, tremor, myoclonus, choreoathetosis, seizures, confusion, and coma; and cardiovascular effects include arrhythmias and hypotension. Hyperthermia may occur. Laboratory abnormalities include leukocytosis, hyperglycemia, albuminuria, glycosuria, and nephrogenic diabetes insipidus. ECG changes include sinus tachycardia or bradycardia, flattened or inverted T waves, atrioventricular block, and prolonged QT interval. In chronic intoxication, signs and symptoms occur at lower serum levels than with acute intoxication. In chronic poisoning, concentrations between 3 and 4 mmol/L may be associated with severe toxicity. In acute poisoning, serum levels may exceed 8 mmol/L despite minimal symptoms.

Treatment Within 2 to 4 h following ingestion, gastrointestinal decontamination is indicated. Lithium is poorly adsorbed by activated charcoal. Serial lithium levels should be measured until the peak level is achieved because both absorption and tissue distribution occur slowly in the overdose setting. Supportive therapy includes standard treatments for seizures, hypotension, and arrhythmias. Symptomatic patients with serum concentrations greater than 2 mmol/L require intravenous saline to correct dehydration and achieve a normal urine output. Diuresis and alkalinization of the urine are recommended to enhance renal excretion of lithium. Hemodialysis is indicated for severe intoxication and is frequently recommended in symptomatic patients with serum levels above 4.0 mmol/L. Hemodialysis may be indicated in chronic toxicity in patients with serum levels less than 4.0 mmol/L. It may need to be repeated or prolonged due to rebound in serum levels upon cessation of hemodialysis.

MONOAMINE OXIDASE (MAO) INHIBITORS MAO inhibitors include tranylcypromine, phenelzine, and isocarboxazid. These agents block monoamine oxidase, thus inhibiting a major pathway for catabolism of neurotransmitters such as dopamine, norepinephrine, and 5-hydroxytryptamine. Toxicity results from neurotransmitter accumulation and hence from potentiation of their actions.

MAO inhibitors are absorbed efficiently from the gastrointestinal tract. The volume of distribution is not known but is probably large. The drugs are eliminated predominantly by hepatic metabolism, and less than 5 percent is excreted unchanged in the urine. Plasma half-life of phenelzine and tranylcypromine at therapeutic doses is 24 h.

Clinical toxicity Effects may not begin until 6 to 12 h after ingestion and may not peak until 24 h following ingestion. Initial CNS effects include dilated pupils, hyperpyrexia, tachycardia, hypertension, and tachypnea (see Table 395-2). Nausea and vomiting also may occur. Agitation, hyperactivity, and confusion may be coupled with fasciculations, twitching, tremor, and rigidity. Cardiovascular collapse and CNS depression are late effects in severe poisoning. Toxic levels of MAO inhibitors have not been established, and no assay methods are commonly available.

Treatment Gastrointestinal decontamination should be performed as soon as possible. Hyperthermia should be treated with external cooling and sedation and in severe cases with neuromuscular paralysis. Dantrolene (2.5 mg/kg of body weight by mouth or intravenously every 6 h) may be effective for hyperthermia. Severe hypertension and tachycardia may require treatment with nitroprusside and propranolol, respectively. Hypotension should be treated with volume expanders, and pressor therapy should be administered with caution and at lower than normal initial doses because of the possibility of an exaggerated response. In fact, before any drug is given, potential adverse interactions should be investigated. Seizures and neuromuscular hyperactivity should be treated with benzodiazepines and barbiturates. Arrhythmias can be treated by usual measures. Diuresis, hemodialysis, and hemoperfusion are not effective. No specific antidote exists. Because of persistence of MAO inhibition, drug therapy and diet should be carefully controlled for 7 to 10 days after stopping the agents.

METHANOL Methanol is a component of shellacs, varnishes, paint removers, Sterno, windshield-washer solutions, and copy machine fluid. It is also a denaturant to make ethanol unfit for consumption.

Methanol, a slightly less potent CNS depressant than ethanol, is metabolized to formaldehyde and formic acid, which in turn causes metabolic acidosis and injury to the retina.

Methanol is rapidly and completely absorbed from the gastrointestinal tract, and peak levels occur within 1 to 2 h of ingestion. It is distributed throughout body water with a volume of distribution of 0.7 L/kg of body weight. Its protein binding is negligible. Elimination occurs predominantly by hepatic metabolism, with up to 10 percent excreted unchanged by the kidneys. Elimination follows first-order kinetics with a half-life of about 3 h at low serum levels (less than about 15 mmol/L or 50 mg/dL) and converts to zero-order kinetics with an elimination rate of 3 mmol/L per hour (8.5 mg/dL per hour) at higher levels. The rate of elimination at low overdose is approximately 14 to 20 h and at high overdose is 24 to 30 h. Inhibition of alcohol dehydrogenase by ethanol [20 to 30 mmol/L (100 to 150 mg/dL)] increases the elimination time to 30 to 35 h.

Clinical toxicity Onset is variable and may be delayed. Absence of signs and symptoms soon after ingestion should not be equated with absence of subsequent toxicity. Early manifestations are caused by methanol, and late manifestations are due to the metabolite formic acid. Methanol produces nausea, vomiting, abdominal pain, headache, vertigo, and confusion at low overdose. In large overdose [levels greater than 60 mmol/L (200 mg/dL)], obtundation, convulsions, coma, and an increased osmolal gap may be noted. Late manifestations include an increased anion gap, metabolic acidosis, and retinal injury and are due to acidosis secondary to accumulation of formic acid, lactic acid (the result of poor tissue perfusion), and ketones. Ophthalmologic manifestations occur 15 to 19 h or later following ingestion and include clouding and diminished vision, dancing and flashing spots, dilated or fixed pupils, hyperemia of the disk, retinal edema, and blindness. These changes are potentially reversible with prompt institution of therapy. With severe poisoning, myocardial depression, bradycardia, and shock may occur. Anuria predicts a poor prognosis.

Diagnosis Early diagnosis is suggested by ethanol-like signs of intoxication and an elevated serum osmolality and is confirmed by measurement of serum methanol [usually greater than 6 mmol/L (20 mg/dL)] 12 to 48 h following ingestion. The diagnosis of methanol-derived formic acidosis is suggested by a large anion gap, a low serum bicarbonate, an elevated serum formate level, and an elevated blood methanol. The diagnosis is confirmed by elevated serum methanol levels (early), elevated serum formate levels (late), or both.

Treatment Gastrointestinal decontamination is indicated soon after ingestion. Activated charcoal is not effective. Renal clearance is not increased by diuresis. Systemic acidosis should be corrected with sodium bicarbonate. Seizures should be treated with diazepam and phenytoin. Ethanol therapy is indicated in patients who are symptomatic or have a methanol level exceeding 6 to 9 mmol/L (20 to 30 mg/dL). The loading and maintenance doses of ethanol are as follows: loading dose—10 mL/kg of body weight of 10% ethanol intravenously or 1 mL/kg of body weight of 95% ethanol by mouth; maintenance dose—1.5 mL/kg of body weight per hour of 10% ethanol intravenously and 3.0 mL/kg of body weight per hour of 10% ethanol intravenously during dialysis. Therapy should be continued until the serum methanol level falls below 6 mmol/L (20 µg/dL) and all signs of toxicity are resolved. Hemodialysis is indicated when methanol levels exceed 15 mmol/L (50 mg/dL), for patients with visual signs, and when clinical or metabolic abnormalities are unresponsive to the preceding therapy. For patients seen late (12 to 24 h or more) after ingestion, ethanol should be used to block further conversion of methanol to formic acid, and sodium bicarbonate should be given to correct metabolic acidosis. Elimination of formic acid is enhanced by alkalization of the urine and by hemodialysis.

METHEMOGLOBINEMIA Methemoglobinemia results from exposure to chemicals that oxidize the iron in hemoglobin from its ferrous (Fe^{2+}) to its ferric (Fe^{3+}) state. Concomitant oxidation of hemoglobin protein may cause its precipitation (as Heinz bodies) and a hemolytic anemia (with bite cells seen on peripheral blood smear). Oxidizing agents include aniline and its derivates, aminophenols, aminophenones, chlorates, nitrites, nitrates, naphthalene, nitrobenzene and related chemicals, sulfonamides, phenazopyridine, dapsone, primaquine, lidocaine, and benzocaine.

Methemoglobin (ferric hemoglobin) cannot carry oxygen and results in a functional anemia, the shift of the oxygen dissociation curve to the left limiting the release of oxygen to tissues. Symptoms are due to hypoxia and anaerobic metabolism.

Various systems operate normally to keep methemoglobin at normal physiologic levels (1 percent of the total hemoglobin concentration). Oxidant inactivation systems include ascorbic acid and sulfhydryl agents such as glutathione, which combine with oxidizing agents and transform them to less toxic compounds. Mechanisms for reducing methemoglobin to oxyhemoglobin include NADH–methemoglobin reductase (responsible for 95 percent of activity), NADPH–methemoglobin reductase, reduced glutathione, methylene blue, and ascorbic acid.

Clinical toxicity Cyanosis, which is unresponsive to oxygen and may have a gray-brown hue, occurs with methemoglobin levels greater than 15 percent (15 g/L or 1.5 g/dL absolute methemoglobin). Patients are asymptomatic, however, until methemoglobin levels exceed 20 to 30 percent, at which point fatigue, headache, tachycardia, dizziness, and weakness develop. At levels greater than 55 percent, dyspnea, bradycardia, hypoxia, acidosis, seizures, coma, and cardiac arrhythmias may occur. Levels greater than 70 percent are rapidly fatal. Hemolytic anemia may cause hyperkalemia and renal failure within 1 to 3 days.

Diagnosis The diagnosis should be suspected in the presence of respiratory distress, brown or gray cyanosis unresponsive to oxygen, and absence of significant CNS depression. Arterial blood gases reveal a normal P_{O_2} and decreased oxygen saturation (measured by CO-oximeter rather than derived). Oxygen saturation by pulse oximetry may be falsely normal. Blood with high levels of methemoglobin is chocolate colored when placed on filter paper and compared with normal blood. The chocolate color does not revert to pink when oxygen is bubbled through a tube of blood but does return to normal when 10% potassium cyanide is added. Methemoglobin is identified by its absorption at a frequency of 630 nm on light spectrometry. Finally, the toxic screen on blood or urine may identify the drug or chemical that serves as the oxidizing agent.

Treatment The toxin, if recently ingested, should be removed by gastrointestinal decontamination. Most oxidizing agents are metabolized rapidly, making diuresis ineffective. Dialysis may be effective, depending on the specific compound. Methylene blue is indicated for methemoglobin levels above 30 g/L (cyanosis alone is not an indication for methylene blue therapy) or methemoglobinemia with hypoxia. In the patient with anemia or cardiovascular disease, methylene blue may be indicated at lower levels due to a greater risk from tissue hypoxia. Methylene blue is given at a dose of 1 to 2 mg/kg of body weight as a 1% solution over 5 min. If a clinical response is not observed within 1 h, the dose may be repeated. A methemoglobin level of 40 g/L can be expected to decrease by half in 1 to 2 h. As long as the oxidizing agent remains in the body, methemoglobin will be generated, and additional doses may be necessary. Side effects of methylene blue include precordial pain, dyspnea, restlessness, apprehension, and tremor; a transient blue color to the skin and urine; and the enhancement of methemoglobin levels at high doses (greater than 7 mg/kg of body weight). Methylene blue is contraindicated in patients with deficiency of glucose-6-phosphate dehydrogenase. Additional treatments include transfusion with packed red cells optimally to a hemoglobin of 150 g/L to increase oxygen-carrying capacity and administration of 100% oxygen or hyperbaric oxygen to enhance oxygen delivery to tissues. If the methemoglobin level is very high or the patient is deficient in glucose-6-phosphate dehydrogenase, exchange transfusion may be indicated.

MUSCLE RELAXANTS Muscle relaxants include orphenadrine, methocarbamol, baclofen, chlorphenesin, cyclobenzaprine, chlorzoxazone, and carisoprodol. Muscle relaxants exert some direct muscle activity but predominantly act as CNS depressants (see Table 395-2). They also depress spinal synaptic reflexes, prolong synaptic recovery time, and reduce repetitive discharges. Baclofen is a GABA agonist, and cyclobenzoprine and orphenadrine have anticholinergic activity. Muscle relaxants are rapidly and completely absorbed, and peak blood levels occur 1 to 2 h following ingestion. The half-lives are variable, with most between 2 and 6 h. The majority are metabolized by the liver to derivatives that are generally inactive and are excreted by the kidneys. Baclofen, an exception, is largely excreted unchanged in the urine.

Clinical toxicity Effects of carisoprodol, chlorphenesin, chlorzoxazone, and methocarbamol include nausea, vomiting, dizziness, headache, nystagmus, hypotonia, and central nervous system depression. Cyclobenzaprine and orphenadrine may cause agitation, hallucinations, tachycardia, mydriasis, hyperthermia, and dry skin and mucosa. Baclofen causes CNS depression, hypothermia, excitability, delirium, myoclonus, seizures, conduction abnormalities, tachycardia, bradycardia, and hypotension. The drugs may be identified in blood or urine by toxic screen.

Treatment Initial management includes prompt gastrointestinal decontamination. Muscle relaxants are well adsorbed by single-dose activated charcoal. Repetitive charcoal may be used for baclofen. Diuresis is ineffective. The efficacy of hemodialysis or hemoperfusion is not established. Physostigmine (1 to 2 mg intravenously over 2 to 5 min) will reverse the anticholinergic effects of orphenadrine and cyclobenzaprine but should be reserved for patients with severe hallucinations and hyperactivity.

NARCOTICS See Chaps. 391 and 392.

NONSTEROIDAL ANTI-INFLAMMATORY DRUGS Nonsteroidal anti-inflammatory drugs (NSAIDs) include diclofenac, diflunisal, fenoprofen, flurbiprofen, ibuprofen, indomethacin, ketoprofen, ketorolac, mefanamic acid, meclofenamate, naproxine, phenylbutazone, piroxicam, phenylbutazone, sulindac, and tolmetin. NSAIDs inhibit prostaglandin synthesis by blocking cyclooxygenase. They are rapidly absorbed, with peak blood concentrations achieved within 1 to 2 h following ingestion. They are highly bound (greater than 90 percent) to plasma protein and have volumes of distribution of less than 1.0 L/kg of body weight. The pK_a ranges from 3.5 to 6.3. They are predominantly metabolized by conjugation, oxidation, and hydroxylation. A small portion (1 to 15 percent) is eliminated unchanged by the kidneys. Half-lives vary from 1 to 16 h, with the exception of phenylbutazone, which has a half-life of 2 to 4 days.

Clinical toxicity Effects are usually mild and include nausea, vomiting, abdominal pain, drowsiness, headache, glycosuria, hematuria, and proteinuria. Acute renal failure and hepatitis are rare. Diflunisal may produce hyperventilation, tachycardia, and sweating. Ibuprofen can sometimes cause metabolic acidosis, coma, and seizures. Seizures are relatively common in mefenamic acid and phenylbutazone poisoning but rare with ketoprofen and naproxen. Coma, respiratory depression, and cardiovascular collapse or arrest may be caused by mefenamic acid and phenylbutazone. Metabolic acidosis occurs often in phenylbutazone poisoning and rarely with naproxen.

Diagnosis Toxicology testing will identify these drugs in the urine, but quantitative analysis is not useful.

Treatment Therapy for NSAID poisoning includes gastrointestinal decontamination and supportive care. Repeated doses of activated charcoal may be of benefit for indomethacin, phenylbutazone, and piroxicam. Renal excretion is not increased by diuresis, and protein binding limits efficacy of hemodialysis. Although experience is limited, hemoperfusion might be useful in patients with hepatic or renal failure and severe clinical toxicity.

ORGANOPHOSPHATE AND CARBAMATE INSECTICIDES Organophosphorus insecticides include malathion, parathion, dichlorvos, and diazinon. Carbamate insecticides include carbaryl, aldicarb, baygon, ficam, and propoxur. Ambenonium, neostigmine, physostigmine, and pyriodostigmine are related agents. Organophosphorus insecticides irreversibly inhibit acetylcholinesterase and cause accumulation of acetylcholine at muscarinic and nicotinic synapses. Carbamates reversibly inhibit this enzyme. The mechanism by which these insecticides affect the CNS is unclear. Organophosphates are absorbed through the skin, lungs, and gastrointestinal tract, are distributed widely in tissues, and are slowly eliminated by hepatic metabolism. The oxidative metabolites (paroxon, maloxone) are active. Subsequent hydrolysis produces inactive metabolites. Carbamates are rapidly eliminated by serum cholinesterases and by hepatic metabolism.

Clinical toxicity Organophosphorus compounds and carbamates produce muscarinic, nicotinic, and CNS effects. Manifestations occur 30 min to 2 h following exposure. Muscarinic effects include nausea, vomiting, abdominal cramps, urinary and fecal incontinence, increased bronchial secretions, cough, dyspnea, sweating, salivation, lacrimation, and urinary frequency and incontinence. Miosis is usual, and blurring of vision may occur. In severe poisoning, bradycardia, conduction block, hypotension, and pulmonary edema may occur. Nicotinic signs include twitching, fasciculations, weakness, hypertension, tachycardia, and in severe cases hypoventilation with respiratory failure. CNS effects include anxiety, restlessness, tremor, convulsions, confusion, weakness, and coma. Toxicity due to carbamates is shorter in duration and usually less severe than with organophosphates. Most patients recover within 24 to 48 h, but long-acting organophosphates may cause effects for weeks to months. Death is most often due to increased pulmonary secretions and inadequate ventilation.

In acute poisoning, cholinesterase activity in plasma and in red blood cells is reduced to less than 50 percent of normal. A reduction in red blood cell cholinesterase activity is more specific but less readily available, and some organophosphates may inhibit only one cholinesterase. Without treatment, blood cholinesterase activity returns to normal in 4 to 5 weeks.

With carbamate insecticides, depression in plasma or red blood cell cholinesterase levels is rare because of the rapid reversibility of the inhibition. Since cholinesterase assays are not routinely or rapidly available, the initial diagnosis is clinical. Insecticides may be identified in urine on toxic screen.

Treatment Contaminated clothing should be removed, and the skin should be washed with soap and water. The patient should be removed from the site of inhalation exposure, and in the case of ingestion, gastrointestinal decontamination should include activated charcoal. Atropine, a muscarinic receptor antagonist, should be administered for muscarinic effects. A dose of 0.5 to 2 mg atropine is given intravenously every 15 to 20 min until atropinization is adequate (drying of bronchial and mucous membrane secretions). Pupil size and heart rate cannot be used as end points. Repeated doses or a constant atropine drip may be necessary for several days. Atropine is less effective for CNS toxicity and ineffective for nicotinic effects. Pralidoxime (2-PAM), an oxime that reactivates cholinesterases, is indicated for nicotinic symptoms in organophosphate poisoning. The dose is 1 to 2 g intravenously over 5 to 20 minutes. The dose may be repeated every 4 to 6 h until nicotinic signs resolve. Like atropine, its ability to reverse CNS effects is less pronounced. In carbamate poisoning, controversy exists over the use of pralidoxime. It should probably not be used in carbaryl poisoning, and with other carbamates it should only be administered in conjunction with atropine.

PHENOTHIAZINE Phenothiazines include aliphatic (chlorpromazine, promethazine, promazine), piperidine (mesoridazine, thioridazine), and piperazine (perphenazine, fluphenazine, prochlorperazine, trifluoperazine) derivatives. Haloperidol, loxapine, pimozide, and thiothixene differ structurally but have similar pharmacologic activity. These agents block postsynaptic dopamine receptors, exhibit anticholinergic activity, and inhibit reuptake of norepinephrine and 5-hydroxytryptamine in the CNS. They also have peripheral alpha-adrenergic blocking and anticholinergic activity and lower the seizure threshold. Some phenothiazines have a quinidine-like effect on the heart. These agents are efficiently absorbed from the gastrointestinal tract, exhibit 90 to 95 percent protein binding, and have large apparent volumes of distribution (10 to 40 L/kg of body weight). They are slowly eliminated by hepatic metabolism with half-lives of 20 to 40 h. Only 1 percent is excreted unchanged in the urine. The majority of metabolites are inactive.

Clinical toxicity Effects begin within 30 to 60 min of ingestion and include lethargy, obtundation, respiratory depression, hypotension, hypothermia, and coma. Pupils are often constricted, and the skin is usually warm and dry. Cardiac effects include supraventricular tachycardia, atrioventricular block, and atrial and ventricular arrhythmias. Torsades de pointes, prolonged PR, QRS, and QT intervals, and U- and T-wave abnormalities may be seen, especially with thioridazine and its metabolite mesoridazine. The neuroleptic malignant syndrome rarely, if ever, occurs following acute overdose. The neuroleptic malignant syndrome is characterized by hyperthermia, extrapyramidal findings (rigidity, muscle spasms, posturing), autonomic instability (diaphoresis, incontinence, and bouts of hypertension, tachycardia, and tachypnea), altered mental status (confusion, delirium, coma), leukocytosis (white blood cell count >15,000 cells per milliliter), and an elevated creatinine kinase. In acute dystonic reactions, sustained muscle contractions may result in abnormal posturing of the eyes, face, tongue, jaw, neck, back, abdomen, and pelvis, but the patient remains alert. These reactions are idiosyncratic rather than dose-related. The diagnosis is established by toxic screen on blood and urine. Quantitative levels are not helpful.

Treatment Gastrointestinal decontamination should be accomplished as soon as possible. Treatment is supportive. Diuresis and dialysis are ineffective. Seizures should be treated with anticonvulsants, and hypotension should be managed with volume expanders and alpha agonists. Arrhythmias are treated by standard agents. Quinidine and procainanide, however, should be avoided. Sodium bicarbonate and magnesium may be useful for ventricular tachyarrhythmias associated with intraventricular conduction or repolarization abnormalities.

Dantrolene and bromocryptine may be useful in treatment of the neuroleptic malignant syndrome if symptoms cannot be controlled with benzodiazepines. In rare cases, neuromuscular paralysis may be indicated. Acute dystonic reactions respond rapidly to intravenous diphenhydramine (1 mg/kg of body weight) given over 2 min or benztropine (1 to 2 mg). Doses may be repeated in 20 min if the response is incomplete. Treatment is generally continued with an oral formulation for 2 to 3 days to prevent recurrence of symptoms.

SALICYLATES   Salicylates increase the sensitivity of respiratory centers in the brain to changes in P_{O_2} and P_{CO_2} resulting in an increased rate and depth of respiration early in the course of poisoning. Later, salicylates uncouple oxidative phosphorylation and produce increases in metabolic rate, oxygen consumption, glucose utilization, and heat production. They also inhibit the Krebs tricarboxylic cycle and block carbohydrate and lipid metabolism, resulting in metabolic acidosis and ketonemia. Salicylates produce hepatocyte damage, resulting in increased plasma enzyme activity and prolongation of prothrombin time. Salicylates decrease platelet aggregation.

Salicylates are well absorbed both from the stomach and the small bowel, but absorption may continue for 24 h or longer following overdose. Therapeutic blood levels range from 0.7 to 1.4 mmol/L (10 to 20 mg/dL). In the plasma, 50 to 80 percent is bound to albumin. Because salicylate is a weak acid with a pK_a of 3, the unbound portion in the plasma exists mainly in an ionized state. It has a small volume of distribution (0.2 L/kg of body weight) which increases with chronic poisoning and with increasing doses. Acidosis increases distribution of salicylate into brain, liver, and other tissues. Salicylates are eliminated by both hepatic metabolism and renal excretion. The half-life is 2 to 3 h after a single therapeutic dose. Saturation of hepatic metabolic pathways results in a prolonged half-life (20 to 36 h) following overdose. By alkalinizing the urine to a pH of 8, the drug in the renal tubules is maintained in an ionized state, cannot be reabsorbed, and is excreted.

Clinical toxicity   Manifestations of mild poisoning include vomiting, tachycardia, hyperpnea, fever, tinnitus, lethargy, confusion, respiratory alkalosis, and an alkaline urine (pH > 6). In severe poisoning, convulsions, coma, and respiratory and cardiovascular failure may occur. Vomiting, poor intake, and hyperventilation may cause severe dehydration, acute renal failure, and acidosis. An increased anion gap metabolic acidosis with an acidic urine (pH < 6) may be compounded by respiratory acidosis. Other complications include cerebral and pulmonary edema and myocardial or renal failure. An elevated hematocrit, white blood cell count, and platelet count; hypernatremia; hyperkalemia; and hypoglycemia may be seen. Respiratory alkalosis is commonly coupled with metabolic acidosis (40 to 50 percent), but respiratory alkalosis (20 percent), metabolic acidosis (20 percent), and mixed respiratory and metabolic acidosis (5 to 10 percent) also may be present. Lactic and other organic acids are responsible for an increased anion gap. Prothrombin time may be prolonged. Salicylates are identified by a positive ferric chloride test on either blood or urine. In the case of an acute single ingestion, a peak level less than 3 mmol/L (40 mg/dL) is associated with no symptoms, 3 to 7 mmol/L (40 to 100 mg/dL) with mild to moderate manifestations, and greater than 7 mmol/L (100 mg/dL) with severe toxicity. In chronic poisoning, symptoms may occur at levels only slightly above the therapeutic range.

Treatment   Gastrointestinal decontamination is indicated if an ingested dose is greater than 150 mg/kg of body weight. Concretions may delay absorption, and decontamination may be helpful 12 to 24 h after ingestion. Elimination may be increased by repeated administration of activated charcoal. Parenteral fluids should be given to replace fluid losses and to produce a brisk urine flow. Supplemental glucose and oxygen should be given. Electrolyte and metabolic abnormalities should be corrected. Prolongation of prothrombin time should be corrected with intravenous vitamin K. Seizures should be controlled with intravenous phenobarbital or diazepam. Myocardial failure should be treated with standard therapy. Cerebral edema, pulmonary edema, and renal failure require fluid restriction and urgent hemodialysis. Sodium bicarbonate should be administered in the presence of acidosis and thus limit tissue distribution of salicylates. In patients without these complications, treatment should include saline diuresis and alkalinization of the urine to a pH of 8 to enhance urinary excretion. Depending on severity, one to three ampules (44 to 131 mmol) of bicarbonate and 20 to 60 mmol of potassium should be added to a liter of intravenous fluid containing dextrose and administered at a rate of 2 to 6 mL/kg per hour. Electrolytes, calcium,

acid-base status, urine pH, and fluid balance must be monitored carefully during such therapy. Salicylates are effectively removed by hemodialysis, which should be considered with severe overdose, cerebral edema, failure of conventional therapy, or compromised renal or hepatic function.

STIMULANTS   Amphetamines, bronchodilators such as albuterol and metaproterenol, and decongestants such as ephedrine, pseudoephedrine, phenylephrine, and phenylpropanolamine stimulate receptors of the central and sympathetic nervous systems (see Table 395-1).

Amphetamines stimulate both alpha- and beta-adrenergic receptors, whereas bronchodilators are primarily beta agonists and decongestants are primarily alpha agonists. These agents are rapidly absorbed from the gastrointestinal tract, reaching peak levels 1 to 2 h following ingestion. They are weak bases with pK_a values ranging from 8 to 10 and a volume of distribution of 2 to 6 L/kg of body weight. These agents are eliminated by a combination of hepatic metabolism and renal excretion of unchanged drug. Excretion is enhanced in an acid urine and slowed in an alkaline urine. Half-lives range from 2 to 8 h to 6 to 34 h depending on urine flow and pH.

Clinical toxicity   Effects are seen within 30 to 60 min following ingestion and include nausea, vomiting, diarrhea, and abdominal cramps. Talkativeness, irritability, confusion, delirium, headache, combativeness, auditory and visual hallucinations, tremors, tachycardia, palpitations, hypertension, and hyperreflexia are common. Other findings may include dilated pupils, dry mouth, pallor, flushing of the skin, and tachypnea. Hyperpyrexia, seizures, rhabdomyolysis, hypertensive crisis, intracranial hemorrhage, cardiac arrhythmias, and cardiovascular collapse may occur in severe overdose. Bronchodilators may cause hypotension as a result of beta-mediated vasodilatation, and decongestants may cause reflex bradycardia secondary to alpha-mediated hypertension. These agents may be identified in the urine by toxicology screening, but quantitative levels are not useful.

Treatment   Gastrointestinal decontamination should be accomplished as soon as possible. Supportive care includes treatment of seizures with benzodiazepines, barbiturates, and phenytoin; hypertension with labetalol, nifedipine, or phentolamine; hyperpyrexia with cooling blankets, salicylates, and acetaminophen; and agitation with sedatives, and, if necessary, with paralyzing agents. Lidocaine and propranolol are preferred for the treatment of ventricular tachyarrhythmias. Although theoretically effective, acid diuresis is not recommended due to lack of documented efficacy and risks such as worsening acidosis and precipitation of myoglobinuric renal failure.

THEOPHYLLINE   Theophylline causes the release of endogenous catecholamines and prolongs their effects by inhibiting the degradation of cyclic AMP by phosphodiesterase. Theophylline is rapidly absorbed from the stomach and upper small bowel. Following overdose, peak levels are achieved 1 to 2 h after ingestion of liquid preparations, by 2 to 4 h with tablets, and in 6 to 24 h with sustained-release preparations. Theophylline is approximately 60 percent bound to albumin and has a low volume of distribution (0.6 L/kg of body weight). Therapeutic serum levels are 55 to 110 μmol/L (10 to 20 mg/L). Theophylline is primarily eliminated by hepatic metabolism, which is saturable at levels in the high therapeutic range. The serum half-life, normally 4 to 6 h, is therefore prolonged in overdoses to 10 to 12 h. Only 5 percent of the theophylline is excreted unchanged by the kidneys. Theophylline elimination is also decreased with impaired liver function, congestive heart failure, viral infections, and concomitantly administered drugs such as cimetidine, erythromycin, and quinolone antibiotics.

Clinical toxicity   Effects begin 30 min to 2 h following overdose and include nausea, vomiting, restlessness, irritability, agitation, tachypnea, tachycardia, and muscle tremors. Coma, hypotension, respiratory depression, generalized tonic-clonic and focal convulsions, and rhabdomyolysis may occur in severe poisoning. Convulsions are often protracted, repetitive, and resistant to therapy. Cardiovascular effects include atrial arrhythmias, multifocal premature ventricular contractions, idioventricular rhythms, ventricular tachycardia, and ventricular fibrillation. Metabolic abnormalities include ketosis, metabolic acidosis, increased serum amylase, hyperglycemia, and decreased serum potassium, calcium, and phosphorus. Toxicity occurs at lower theophylline levels with chronic than with acute poisoning. Mortality rates are higher after chronic ingestion. Cardiac arrhythmias and seizures occur following chronic ingestion at serum levels of 200 to 300 μmol/L (40 to 60 mg/L). Similar toxicity, along with hypotension, hypokalemia, and metabolic abnormalities, generally occurs at levels above 400 to 500 μmol/L (80 to 100 mg/L) following acute overdose. Serial levels should be measured to determine the peak concentration (serving as an important indicator for hemodialysis).

Treatment   Initial therapy involves prompt gastrointestinal decontamination. Theophylline is well adsorbed by activated charcoal. With sustained-release forms, decontamination should be considered up to 12 to 24 h following ingestion. Repeated doses of charcoal shorten the serum half-life by approximately 50 percent. Metaclopramide is useful in controlling theophylline-induced vomiting. Extreme tachycardia should be treated with propranolol or esmolol, and hypotension is treated with volume expansion. Propranolol is also effective in reversing hypotension. Benzodiazepines and barbiturates are useful for convulsions and hyperactivity. Phenytoin is ineffective. Treatment of ventricular tachyarrhythmias should include propranolol as well as standard antiarrhythmics. Diuresis is ineffective for enhancing removal of theophylline. Hemodialysis and hemoperfusion are effective in removing theophylline and are indicated in patients with severe toxicity or after acute ingestion with a serum level greater than 440 μmol/L (80 mg/L). With chronic ingestion, hemodialysis or hemoperfusion is indicated with serum levels greater than 200 to 300 μmol/L (40 to 60 mg/L).

TRICYCLIC ANTIDEPRESSANTS   Commonly available tricyclic compounds include amitriptyline, imipramine, chlomipramine, desipramine, doxepin, nortriptyline, protriptyline, and trimipramine. Related agents include amoxapine, bupropion, maprotiline, and trazodone. These agents block reuptake of synaptic transmitters such as norepinephrine, dopamine, and serotonin in the CNS. In addition, they have central and peripheral anticholinergic activity, peripheral alpha-blocking activity, and quinidine-like effects on the heart. Fluoxetine is unique in that it selectively inhibits the reuptake of serotonin.

Tricyclics are well absorbed from the gastrointestinal tract, and peak levels are reached within 2 to 6 h of overdose. In some cases, anticholinergic effects may predominate, resulting in prolonged absorption and delayed peak levels (6 to 12 h following ingestion). Tricyclics exhibit high protein binding in the plasma. They have large volumes of distribution in the range of 20 to 40 L/kg of body weight. Elimination is predominantly by hepatic metabolism with an initial demethylation generating pharmacologically active metabolites. These metabolites generally undergo enterohepatic circulation. Subsequent steps of metabolism result in increasing polarity of metabolites that are then excreted by the kidneys. Less than 5 percent of the parent compound is excreted unchanged in urine. The half-lives of tricyclics and their demethylated metabolites range from 25 to 30 h but may be longer in the overdose setting.

Clinical toxicity   Effects generally develop within 30 min of overdose but may be delayed for up to 6 h. In low overdose, anticholinergic effects predominate and are manifest by agitation, myoclonus, mydriasis, urinary retention, confusion, hallucinations, mild fever, hypertension, and tachycardia. In high overdose, marked CNS depression is coupled with cardiotoxicity, seizures, and hypotension. Cardiovascular toxicity is not a feature of fluoxetine overdose, however. Ventricular tachyarrhythmias, atrioventricular and intraventricular conduction delays, terminal bradycardia, and decreased cardiac output occur with high overdose. Aspiration pneumonia and pulmonary edema also may develop. Death occurs usually within the first 2 to 6 h following ingestion. Prolongation of the QRS complex (greater than 100 ms) in severe overdose correlates with an increased risk of cardiac arrhythmias and seizures. Serum levels are diagnostic and generally correlate with severity. Metabolites as well as the parent

compound levels should be summed when estimating the total serum concentration. Levels less than about 1000 nmol/L (300 ng/mL) are therapeutic. Levels over 3300 nmol/L (1000 ng/mL) indicate serious poisoning and are associated with QRS complexes wider than 100 ms.

Treatment   Ipecac-induced emesis is contraindicated with tricyclic ingestions. Gastric lavage is indicated for comatose patients with recent ingestions. Activated charcoal in single and repeated doses should be administered. Treatment includes support of respiration and volume expansion and norepinephrine or high-dose dopamine for hypotension. Hypertension is generally limited and does not require specific therapy. Seizures should be treated with phenytoin or diazepam. Treatment of ventricular tachyarrhythmias should include sodium bicarbonate (0.5 to 1 mmol/kg of body weight), lidocaine, and phenytoin. Beta-adrenergic blockers and class 1A antiarrhythmics (quinidine, procainamide, and disopyramide) should be avoided. Cardiac pacing may be necessary for the severely depressed myocardium and bradycardia. Correction of acidosis is an important component of the treatment of cardiac arrhythmias and seizures. Physostigmine (1 to 2 mg intravenously over 2 to 5 min) will reverse low-dose anticholinergic effects and may be administered in mild poisoning if deterioration has been excluded by a suitable period of observation. Physostigmine can cause asystole in severe poisoning and should not be used in this situation. Physostigmine is absolutely contraindicated in patients with arrhythmias or cardiac conduction disturbances.

REFERENCES

General aspects

AMDUR MO et al (eds): *Casarett and Doull's Toxicology: The Basic Science of Poisons,* 4th ed. New York, Pergamon Press, 1991

BRANCATA DJ, NELSON RC: Poisoning mortality in the United States 1980. Vet Hum Toxicol 26:273, 1984

LITOVITZ TL et al: 1987 Annual report of the American Association of Poison Control Centers National Data Collection System. Am J Emerg Med 6:479, 1988

McCARRON MM: Current trends in drug overdose. West J Med 141:98, 1984

Diagnosis

BRETT AS: Implication of discordance between clinical impression and toxicology analysis in drug overdose. Arch Intern Med 148:437, 1988

COUNCIL OF SCIENTIFIC AFFAIRS, AMERICAN MEDICAL ASSOCIATION: Scientific issues in drug testing. JAMA 257:3110, 1987

GLASSER L et al: Serum osmolality and its applicability to drug overdose. Am J Clin Pathol 60:695, 1973

HEPLER BR et al: Role of the toxicology lab in the treatment of acute poisoning. Med Toxicol 1:61, 1986

JAEGER RW et al: Radiopacity of drugs and plants in vivo—limited usefulness. Vet Hum Toxicol 23(Suppl 1):2, 1981

KELLERMANN AL et al: Impact of drug screening in suspected overdose. Ann Emerg Med 16:1206, 1987

OLSON KR et al: Physical assessment and differential diagnosis of the poisoned patient. Med Toxicol 2:52, 1987

OSTER JR et al: Use of the anion gap in clinical medicine. South Med J 81:229, 1988

ROBERTS JR et al: The body stuffer syndrome: A clandestine form of drug overdose. Am J Emerg Med 4:24, 1986

SCHERZ RG: The differential diagnosis of coma due to poisoning and exogenous toxins. Pediatrician 6:190, 1977

SMITHLINE N, GARDNER KD JR: Gaps—anionic and osmolal. JAMA 236:1594, 1976

Treatment

ALBERTSON TE et al: Superiority of activated charcoal alone compared with ipecac and activated charcoal in the treatment of acute toxic ingestions. Ann Emerg Med 18:56, 1989

BRETT AS et al: Predicting the clinical course of intentional drug overdose: Implications for utilization of the intensive care unit. Arch Intern Med 147:133, 1987

BURTON BT et al: Comparison of activated charcoal and gastric lavage in the prevention of aspirin absorption. J Emerg Med 1:411, 1984

CURTIS RA et al: Efficacy of ipecac and activated charcoal/cathartic: Prevention of salicylate absorption in a simulated overdose. Arch Intern Med 144:48, 1984

GARRETTSON LK, GELLER RJ: Acid and alkaline diuresis: When are they of value in the treatment of poisoning? Drug Safety 5:220, 1990

GOLDBERG MJ et al: An approach to the management of the poisoned patient. Arch Intern Med 146:1381, 1986

GOLDFRANK L et al: Newer antidotes and controversies in antidotal therapy, in *Emergency Medicine Annual,* DA Rund, BW Wolcott (eds). Norwalk, Conn, Appleton-Century-Crofts, 1984, vol 3, pp 223–266.

KING WD: Syrup of ipecac: A drug review. Clin Toxicol 17:353, 1980

KORNBERG AE, DOLGIN J: Pediatric ingestions: Charcoal alone versus ipecac and charcoal. Ann Emerg Med 20:648, 1991

KRENZELOK EP et al: Gastrointestinal transit times of cathartics combined with charcoal. Ann Emerg Med 14:1152, 1985

KULIG K et al: Management of acutely poisoned patients without gastric emptying. Ann Emerg Med 14:562, 1985

LITOVITZ TL: The anecdotal antidotes. Emerg Med Clin North Am 2:145, 1984

MANNO BR, MANNO JE: Toxicology of ipecac: A review. Clin Toxicol 10:221, 1977

McCARRON MM, WOOD JD: The cocaine "body packer" syndrome: Diagnosis and treatment. JAMA 250:1417, 1983

MERRIGIAN KS et al: Prospective evaluation of gastric emptying in the self-poisoned patient. Am J Emerg Med 8:479, 1990

MINOCHA A, SPYKER DA: Acute overdose with sustained-release drug formulations: Perspectives in treatment. Med Toxicol 1:300, 1986

NEUVONEN PJ: Clinical pharmacokinetics of oral activated charcoal in acute intoxications. Clin Pharmacokinet 7:465, 1982

———, OLKKOLA KT: Oral activated charcoal in the treatment of intoxications: Role of single and repeated doses. Med Toxicol 3:33, 1988

PARK GD et al: Expanded role of charcoal in the poisoned and overdosed patient. Arch Intern Med 146:969, 1986

PETERSON RG, PETERSON LN: Cleansing the blood: Hemodialysis, peritoneal dialysis, exchange transfusion, charcoal hemoperfusion, forced diuresis. Pediatr Clin North Am 33:675, 1986

POND SM: Diuresis, dialysis and hemoperfusion: Indications and benefits. Emerg Med Clin North Am 2:29, 1984

ROSENBERG J et al: Pharmacokinetics of drug overdose. Clin Pharmacokinet 6:161, 1981

SHANNON M et al: Cathartics and laxatives: Do they still have a place in management of the poisoned patient? Med Toxicol 1:247, 1986

SPYKER DA, MINOCHA A: Toxicodynamic approach to the management of the poisoned patient. J Emerg Med 6:117, 1988

STEAD AH, MOFFAT AC: A collection of therapeutic, toxic and fatal blood drug concentrations in man. Hum Toxicol 3:437, 1983

STEWART JJ: Effects of emetic and cathartic agents on the gastrointestinal tract and the treatment of toxic ingestion. Clin Toxicol 20:199, 1983

TENEBEIN M: Whole bowel irrigation as a gastrointestinal decontamination procedure after acute poisoning. Med Toxicol 3:77, 1988

——— et al: Efficacy of ipecac-induced emesis, orogastric lavage, and activated charcoal for acute drug overdose. Ann Emerg Med 16:838, 1987

WHEELER-USHER DH et al: Gastric emptying: Risk versus benefit in the treatment of acute poisoning. Med Toxicol 1:142, 1986

ZACCARA G et al: Clinical features, pathogenesis, and management of drug-induced seizures. Drug Safety 5:109, 1990

Reference texts

ARENA JM, DREW RH: Poisoning: Toxicology, Symptoms, Treatments, 5th ed. Springfield, Ill, Charles C Thomas, 1986

BASET RC: Disposition of Toxic Drugs and Chemicals in Man, 2d ed. Davis, Calif, Biomedical Publications, 1982

BLOCK JB: The Signs and Symptoms of Chemical Exposure. Springfield, Ill, Charles C Thomas, 1980

BRYSON PD: Comprehensive Review in Toxicology. Rockville, Md, Aspen, 1989

CLAYTON GD, CLAYTON FE (eds): Patty's Industrial Hygiene and Toxicology, 3d ed. New York, Wiley, 1978

DANGAARD J: Symptoms and Signs in Occupational Disease: A Practical Guide, Copenhagen, Year Book Medical Publishers, 1978

ELLENHORN MJ, BARCELOUX DG: Medical Toxicology: Diagnosis and Treatment of Human Poisoning. New York, Elsevier, 1988

FINKEL AJ: Hamilton and Hardy's Industrial Toxicology, 4th ed. Boston, John Wright, 1983

GOLDFRANK LR et al (eds): Goldfrank's Toxicologic Emergencies, 3d ed. Norwalk, Conn, Appleton-Century-Crofts, 1986

GOSSELIN RE: Clinical Toxicology of Commercial Products: Acute Poisoning, 5th ed. Baltimore, Williams & Wilkins, 1984

HADDAD LM, WINCHESTER JF: Clinical Management of Poisoning and Drug Overdose 2d ed. Philadelphia, Saunders, 1990

HAYES WJ, LAW ER: Handbook of Pesticide Toxicology. San Diego, Academic Press, 1991

KLASSEN CD et al (eds): Casarett and Doull's Toxicology: The Basic Science of Poisons, 3d ed. New York, Macmillan, 1986

LAMPE KF, McCANN MA (eds): AMA Handbook of Poisonous and Injurious Plants. Chicago, American Medical Association, 1985

RUMACK BH (eds): Poisindex Information System (updated quarterly). Denver, Micromedex

Specific poisons

Acetaminophen

FLANAGAN RJ: The role of acetylcysteine in clinical toxicology. Med Toxicol 2:93, 1987

PRESCOTT LF: Paracetamol overdose. Drugs 25:290, 1983

SMILKSTEIN MJ et al: Efficacy of oral N-acetylcysteine in the treatment of acetaminophen overdose. N Engl J Med 319:1558, 1988

Acids and alkali

ANDERSON KD et al: Controlled trial of corticosteroids in children with corrosive injury of the esophagus. N Engl J Med 323:637, 1990

FRIEDMAN EM, LOVEJOY FH JR: The emergency management of caustic ingestions. Emerg Med Clin North Am 2:77, 1984

HOWELL JM et al: Steroids for the treatment of corrosive esophageal injury: A statistical analysis of past studies. Am J Emerg Med 10:421, 1992

WASON S: The emergency management of caustic ingestions. J Emerg Med 2:175, 1984

Antiarrhythmic drugs

DUNBAR DN, PENTEL PR: Antiarrhythmic drug toxicity, in Intensive Care Medicine, JM Rippe et al (eds). Boston, Little, Brown, 1991, p 1174

FREEDMAN MD et al: Extracorporeal pump assistance—a novel treatment for acute lidocaine poisoning. Eur J Clin Pharmacol 22:129, 1982

HRUBY K, MISSLIVETZ J: Poisoning with oral antiarrhythmic drugs. Int J Clin Pharmacol 23:253, 1985

STRATMAN HG, KENNEDY HL: Torsade de pointes associated with drugs and toxins: Recognition and management. Am Heart J 113:1470, 1987

Barbiturates

BOLDY DAR et al: Treatment of phenobarbitone poisoning with repeat oral administration of activated charcoal. Q J Med 235:997, 1986

MATTHEW H: Barbiturates. Clin Toxicol 8(5):495, 1975

McCARRON MM et al: Short-acting barbiturate overdosage: Correlation of intoxication score with serum barbiturate concentration. JAMA 248:55, 1982

Benzodiazepines

DIVOLL M et al: Benzodiazepine overdosage: Plasma concentrations and clinical outcome. Psycho Pharmacol 73:381, 1981

GREENBLATT DJ et al: Acute overdosage with benzodiazepine derivatives. Clin Pharmacol Ther 21:497, 1977

PRISCHL F et al: Value of flumazenil in benzodiazepine self-poisoning. Med Toxicol 3:334, 1988

Beta blockers

CRITCHLEY JA, UNGAR A: The management of acute poisoning due to beta-adrenoreceptor antagonists. Med Tox Adverse Drug Exp 4:32, 1989

HEATH A: β-Adrenoceptor blocker toxicity: Clinical features and therapy. Am J Emerg Med 2:518, 1984

WEINSTEIN RS: Recognition and management of poisoning with beta-adrenergic blocking agents. Ann Emerg Med 13:1123, 1984

Bleach

GAPAY-GAPANAVICIUS M: Chloramine-induced pneumonitis from mixing household cleaning agents. Br Med J 288:1086, 1982

GAUDREAULT P et al: Predictability of esophageal injury from signs and symptoms. Pediatrics 71:767, 1983

LANDAU GD, SAUNDERS WH: The effect of chlorine bleach on the esophagus. Arch Otolaryngol 80:174, 1964

Calcium channel blockers

HERRINGTON DM et al: Nifedipine overdose. Am J Cardiol 81:344, 1986

McMILLAN R: Management of acute severe verapamil intoxication. J Emerg Med 6:193, 1988

SNOVER SW, BOCCHINO V: Massive diltiazem overdose. Ann Emerg Med 15:1221, 1986

Carbon monoxide

DOLAN MC: Carbon monoxide poisoning. Can Med Assoc J 133:392, 1985 Symposium—carbon monoxide poisoning—mechanism of damage, late sequelae and therapy. Clin Toxicol 23:247, 1985

MOFENSON HC et al: Carbon monoxide poisoning. Am J Emerg Med 2:254, 1984

Cyanide

CARAVETI M, LITOVITZ T: Pediatric cyanide intoxication and death from acetonitrile-containing cosmetic. JAMA 260:3740, 1988

GRAHAM DL et al: Acute cyanide poisoning complicated by lactic acidosis and pulmonary edema. Arch Intern Med 137:1051, 1977

HALL AH et al: Clinical toxicology of cyanide: North American clinical experiences, in Clinical and Experimental Toxicology of Cyanides, B Ballantyne, TC Marrs (eds). Bristol, Wright, 1987, p 312

Digoxin

SMITH TW et al: Digitalis glycosides: Mechanisms and manifestations of toxicity. Prog Cardiovasc Dis 26:413, 1984 (part I); 26:495, 1984 (part II); 27:26, 1984 (part III).

——— et al: Treatment of life-threatening digitalis intoxication with digoxin-specific FAB antibody fragments. N Engl J Med 307:1357, 1982

WANGER TL et al: Treatment of 63 severely digitalis-toxic patients with digoxin-specific antibody fragments. J Am Coll Cardiol 5:118A, 1985

Ethanol

GABOW PA et al: Organic acids in ethylene glycol intoxication. Ann Intern Med 105:16, 1986

DAVID DJ, SPYKER DA: The acute toxicity of ethanol: Dosage and kinetic nomograms. Vet Hum Toxicol 21:272, 1979

ECKARDT MJ et al: Health hazards associated with alcohol consumption. JAMA 246:648, 1981

HALPERIN ML et al: Metabolic acidosis in the alcoholic: A pathophysiologic approach. Metabolism 32:308, 1983

Ethylene glycol

JACOBSEN D, MCMARTIN KE: Methanol and ethylene glycol poisonings: Mechanism of toxicity, clinical course, diagnosis and treatment. Med Toxicol 1:309, 1986
PARRY MF, WALLACH R: Ethylene glycol poisoning. Am J Med 57:143, 1974

Hallucinogens

BROWN RT, BRADEN NJ: Hallucinogens. Pediatr Clin North Am 34:341, 1987
COHEN S: The hallucinogens and the inhalents. Psych Clin North Am 7:681, 1984

Hydrocarbons

ANAS N et al: Criteria for hospitalizing children who have ingested products containing hydrocarbons. JAMA 246:840, 1981
STREICHEN M et al: Syndromes of solvent sniffing in adults. Ann Intern Med 94:785, 1981
TRUEMPIER E et al: Clinical characteristics, pathophysiology and management of hydrocarbon ingestion: Case report and review of the literature. Pediatr Emerg Care 3:187, 1987

Hydrogen sulfide

HOIDAL CR et al: Hydrogen sulfide poisoning from toxic inhalations of roofing fumes. Ann Emerg Med 15:826, 1986
SMITH RP: Management of acute sulfide poisoning. Arch Environ Health 31:166, 1976
WHITECRAFT DD et al: Hydrogen sulfide poisoning treated with hyperbaric oxygen. J Emerg Med 3:23, 1985

Iron

BANNER W et al: Iron poisoning. Pediatr Clin North Am 33:393, 1986
PROUDFOOT AT et al: Management of acute iron poisoning. Med Toxicol 1:83, 1986
TENEBEIN M et al: Myocardial failure and shock in iron poisoning. Hum Toxicol 7:281, 1988

Isoniazid

ORLOWSKI JP et al: Treatment of potentially lethal dose isoniazid ingestion. Ann Emerg Med 17:73, 1988
WASON S et al: Single high-dose pyridoxine treatment for isoniazid overdose. JAMA 246:1102, 1981
YARBROUGH B, WOOD J: Isoniazid overdose treated with high-dose pyridoxine. Ann Emerg Med 12:303, 1983

Isopropyl alcohol

LACOUTURE PG et al: A review of acute isopropyl alcohol intoxication: Diagnosis and management. Am J Med 75:680, 1983
NATOWICZ M et al: Pharmacokinetic analysis of a case of isopropyl intoxication. Clin Chem 31:326, 1985

Lithium

AMDISEN A: Clinical features and management of lithium poisoning. Med Toxicol 3:18, 1988
DYSON EH et al: Self-poisoning and therapeutic intoxication with lithium. Human Toxicol 6:326, 1987

MAO inhibitors

KAPLAN RF et al: Phenelzine overdose treated with dantrolene sodium. JAMA 255:642, 1986
LINDEN CH: Monoamine oxidase inhibitor overdose. Ann Emerg Med 13:1137, 1984

Methanol

JACOBSEN D, MCMARTIN KE: Methanol and ethylene glycol poisoning: Mechanism of toxicity, clinical course, diagnosis and treatment. Med Toxicol 1:309, 1986
OSTERLOH JD et al: Serum formate concentrations in methanol intoxication as a criterion for hemodialysis. Ann Intern Med 104:200, 1986
SWARTZ RD et al: Epidemic methanol poisoning: Clinical and biochemical analysis of a recent episode. Medicine 60:373, 1981

Methemoglobinemia

CURRY S: Methemoglobinemia. Ann Emerg Med 11:214, 1982
HALL AH et al: Drug and chemical-induced methaemoglobinaemia. Med Toxicol 1:253, 1986
HARVEY JW, KEITT AS: Studies of the efficacy and potential hazards of methylene blue therapy in aniline-induced methaemoglobinaemia. Br J Haematol 53:29, 1983

Muscle relaxants

BAILEY DN: Meprobamate ingestion: A five-year review of cases with serum concentrations and clinical findings. Am J Clin Pathol 75:102, 1981
COHEN MD et al: Atropine in the treatment of baclofen overdose. Am J Emerg Med 4:552, 1986

Narcotics

CUDDY P: Management of acute opioid intoxication. Crit Care Q 4:65, 1982
FORD M et al: Opioids and designer drugs. Emerg Med Clin North Am 8:495, 1990
LAWSON AAH, NORTHRIDGE DB: Dextropropoxyphene overdose. Med Toxicol 2:430, 1987

Nonsteroidal anti-inflammatory drugs

COURT H, VOLANS GN: Poisoning after overdose with nonsteroidal anti-inflammatory drugs. Adverse Drug React Acute Poisoning Rev 3:1, 1984
HALL AH et al: Ibuprofen overdose: 126 cases. Ann Emerg Med 15:1308, 1986
VALE JA, MEREDITH TJ: Acute poisoning due to nonsteroidal anti-inflammatory drugs: Clinical features and management. Med Toxicol 1:11, 1986

Organophosphate and carbamate insecticides

MINTON NA, MURRAY VSG: A review of organophosphate poisoning. Med Toxicol 3:350, 1988
NAMBA T et al: Poisoning due to organophosphate insecticides. Am J Med 50:475, 1971
SENANAYAKE N, KARALLIEDDE L: Neurotoxic effects of organophosphorus insecticides: An intermediate syndrome. N Engl J Med 316:761, 1987

Phenothiazines

BARRY D et al: Phenothiazine poisoning: A review of 48 cases. Calif Med 118:1, 1983
BENOWITZ NL et al: Cardiopulmonary catastrophes in drug-overdosed patients. Med Clin North Am 63:267, 1979
BORYS DJ et al: Acute fluoxetine overdose: A report of 234 cases. Am J Emerg Med 10:115, 1992
LEE A: Treatment of drug-induced dystonic reactions. J Am Coll Emerg Phys 8:453, 1979
POPE HG et al: Frequency and presentation of neuroleptic malignant syndrome in a large psychiatric hospital. Am J Psychiatry 143:1227, 1986

Salicylates

BRENNER BE, SIMON RR: Management of salicylate intoxication. Drugs 24:335, 1987
GAUDREAULT P et al: The relative severity of acute vs chronic salicylate poisoning in children: A clinical comparison. Pediatrics 70:566, 1982
TEMPLE AR: Acute and chronic effects of aspirin toxicity and their treatment. Arch Intern Med 141:364, 1981
THISTED B et al: Acute salicylate poisoning in 177 consecutive patients treated in an ICU. Acta Anaesthesiol Scand 31:312, 1987

Stimulants

AARO CK: Sympathomimetics. Emerg Med Clin North Am 8:513, 1990
LINDEN CH et al: Amphetamines. Top Emerg Med 7:18, 1985
PENTEL P: Toxicity of over-the-counter stimulants. JAMA 252:1898, 1984

Theophylline

GAUDREAULT P, GUAY J: Theophylline poisoning. Med Toxicol 1:169, 1986
OLSON KR et al: Theophylline overdose: Acute single ingestion versus chronic repeated overmedication. Am J Emerg Med 3:386, 1985
PARK GD et al: Use of hemoperfusion for treatment of theophylline intoxication. Am J Med 74:961, 1983
SHANNON MW, LOVEJOY FH JR: The influence of age versus peak concentration on life-threatening events after chronic theophylline intoxication. Arch Intern Med 150:2045, 1990

Tricyclic antidepressants

BOEHNERT MT, LOVEJOY FH JR: Value of QRS duration versus the serum drug level in predicting seizures and ventricular arrhythmias after an acute overdose of tricyclic antidepressants. N Engl J Med 313:474, 1985
CROME P: Poisoning due to tricyclic antidepressant overdose. Med Toxicol 1:261, 1986
FROMMER DA et al: Tricyclic antidepressant overdose; A review. JAMA 257:521, 1987

396 HEAVY METAL POISONING

JOHN W. GRAEF

ARSENIC

SOURCE Inorganic arsenic compounds such as arsenic trioxide, arsenic pentoxide, and sodium and potassium arsenite and arsenate are found in insecticides, rodenticides, fungicides, wood preservatives, herbicides, and compounds used in glass manufacturing. Organic arsenic is widely distributed in the environment. Arsine gas is produced in the smelting and refining of metals, in galvanizing and etching, in lead plating, and in making silicon microchips. Historically, organic arsenical compounds have been used in the treatment of syphilis, epilepsy, psoriasis, and amebiasis. Currently, acute toxicity is encountered following accidental ingestion, industrial accidents, or suicidal or homicidal intoxications. Chronic exposures occur most commonly following low-dose exposure in industry or chronic consumption of contaminated food, water, or medications. Arsenic toxicity is a common cause of death in children after pesticide ingestion.

METABOLISM Arsenic is absorbed through the skin, lungs, and gastrointestinal tract. Inorganic (trivalent) compounds are absorbed more readily than organic (pentavalent) forms, with greater than 80 percent of an ingested dose absorbed by the gastrointestinal tract. Arsine gas is absorbed through the lungs. Arsenic is distributed from blood to liver, kidney, lung, spleen, and intestine within 24 h of ingestion and to skin, hair, and bone within 2 weeks. Inorganic arsenic compounds are found in high concentrations in leukocytes. Inorganic arsenic does not cross the blood-brain barrier but does cross the placenta. Between 5 and 10 percent is excreted in feces, and 90 to 95 percent is excreted in the urine. Small amounts are recovered in bile, feces, saliva, and breast milk. Arsenic may be detected in urine for at least 10 days following an overdose and detected in the serum for a shorter period of time.

CLINICAL TOXICOLOGY Arsine gas combines with the globin chain of hemoglobin in red blood cells to produce severe hemolysis with anemia, hemoglobinuria, and hematuria within 3 to 4 h of ingestion. Subsequent jaundice may be severe. Signs and symptoms of toxicity include nausea, vomiting and diarrhea, apprehension and malaise, tachycardia, and dyspnea. Acute renal failure is frequent and often fatal.

The reported lethal dose for arsenic ranges from 120 to 200 mg. As little as 2 mg/kg of body weight can be lethal for children. Manifestations of acute toxicity include for the gastrointestinal tract—burning in the throat, difficulty swallowing, nausea, vomiting, diarrhea, abdominal pain, and a garlic odor on the breath; for the cardiovascular system—cyanosis, difficulty breathing, and hypotension with myocardial depression and rare arrhythmias; for the central nervous system—delirium, coma, and seizures; for the kidneys—acute tubular necrosis and oliguria; and for the hematologic system—hemolysis, eosinophilia, and, rarely, bone marrow depression. Manifestations of chronic arsenic poisoning occur 2 to 8 weeks following ingestion and include for the skin and nails—erythroderma, hyperkeratosis, hyperpigmentation, exfoliative dermatitis, and Aldrich-Mees lines (transverse white striae of the fingernails); for the mucous membranes—laryngitis, tracheitis, and bronchitis; and for the peripheral nervous system—polyneuritis (sensory and motor). Basal cell carcinomas, squamous cell carcinomas, Bowen's disease of the skin (see Chap. 54), and lung carcinomas have been associated with chronic arsenic exposure. With chronic exposure, the risk of cancer of the bladder, kidney, and liver may be comparable to that for lung cancer in cigarette smokers.

Arsenic produces its toxicity by binding with tissue sulfhydryl groups. Arsenic also binds to enzymes in the Krebs tricarboxylic acid cycle, thereby interfering with oxidative phosphorylation. Other effects include capillary injury and direct toxic effects on large organs. Pathologic findings include necrosis of the stomach, small bowel, and vasculature and degenerative changes in the liver and kidneys.

LABORATORY FINDINGS Arsenic is radiopaque and is seen on x-ray of the abdomen. It also may be detected in hair and nails for months following exposure. Specific organ effects include abnormal liver function tests; Q-T prolongation and T-wave inversion; anemia, leukocytosis, leukopenia, and hemoglobinemia; and proteinuria, hematuria, hemoglobinuria, and cellular casts in the urine. Urine arsenic (As) levels are normally less than 67 nmol/d (5 µg/d).

TREATMENT Acute ingestion should be treated by inducing vomiting with ipecac syrup if the patient is alert. Gastric lavage is preferable if the patient is obtunded or the ingestion is severe. Activated charcoal and cathartics are of unclear benefit. Dimercaprol chelates arsenic by producing an insoluble complex that is excreted by the kidneys. For mild symptoms and elevated serum or urinary levels, 3 to 5 mg/kg of body weight per dose is given intramuscularly every 4 h for 24 h and then every 12 to 24 h for 7 to 10 days.

Adequacy of urinary mobilization of arsenic is confirmed and followed during treatment by measurement of serum and urinary levels. Treatment should be continued until 24-h urine As levels are less than 67 nmol/d (5 µg/d). Toxic manifestations of dimercaprol (increased blood pressure, tachycardia, nausea, vomiting, headache, burning sensation in the lips, mucous membrane irritation, coma, and convulsions) occur with increasing doses. The water-soluble analogue of dimercaprol, succimer (DMSA), may be more effective and is less toxic than dimercaprol.

Penicillamine has been used successfully in acute and chronic poisoning, administered orally at a dose of 10 mg/kg of body weight per day (the maximum dose not to exceed 1 g/d) in four divided doses for 5 days. Side effects of penicillamine include rash, leukopenia, thrombocytopenia, and nephrotoxicity. Hemodialysis removes arsenic (24 to 100 mg in 24 h) with a clearance of 80 to 90 mL/min and is indicated if renal failure occurs. Hemodialysis early in the clinical course in conjunction with dimercaprol may limit arsenic's distribution phase and enhance clearance of free and complexed arsenic.

Exchange transfusion is the preferred treatment for arsine gas poisoning. Dimercaprol affords no protection against red cell destruction.

CADMIUM

SOURCE Exposure to cadmium is usually occupational or via pollution from mining or smelting operations. Cadmium is produced commercially as a by-product of copper and lead or zinc smelting and is used in the manufacture of batteries, in ceramics, in textiles, in soldering, in electroplating, and as a pigment in paints and plastics. In contaminated areas, high concentrations may be found in shellfish and foodstuffs.

METABOLISM Absorption occurs via ingestion or inhalation. Normal daily oral intake is up to 200 µg, with an estimated mean of 20 to 40 µg/d. Only 5 to 10 percent of this is absorbed, although, like lead, absorption may be increased in the presence of calcium and iron deficiency. About 5 percent of inhaled cadmium is absorbed depending on particle size. Small, highly soluble particles are absorbed at a rate of 25 to 50 percent.

About 50 percent of absorbed cadmium is concentrated in the liver and kidneys. In erythrocytes and soft tissues, cadmium is bound to metallothionein, a low-molecular-weight polypeptide containing a large number of available sulfhydryl groups that exert a protective effect. With large single-dose cadmium exposures, saturation of the protein may result in loss of protective effect. Cadmium does not pass the placenta and gradually accumulates in the body with age. In limited studies, small amounts are found in breast milk. Biologic half-life has been estimated at more than 20 years, except in the presence of kidney damage, when urinary excretion is increased. In the kidney, metallothionein-bound cadmium is filtered at the glomerulus and is then reabsorbed by the proximal tubules. The urinary excretion rarely exceeds 5 nmol/d (0.5 µg/d).

CLINICAL TOXICOLOGY Acute cadmium intoxication may occur after either ingestion or inhalation. Ingestion of water containing concentrations of 15 mg/L or foods containing as little as 30 mg cadmium can induce vomiting, abdominal pain, and severe diarrhea. Shock may ensue. Acute inhalation of cadmium dust produces dyspnea, weakness, chest pain, shortness of breath, and cough. A chemical pneumonitis produces pulmonary edema and respiratory failure. Clinical symptoms may occur with air exposure as low as 1 mg/m² of surface area over 8 h. During the same time period, inhalation of 5 mg/m² of surface area may be fatal. A latent period of 4 to 24 h from exposure to onset of symptoms may complicate accurate diagnosis. Death usually occurs in 5 to 10 days. Chemical pneumonitis may continue for several months, and pulmonary function can be abnormal for longer than 1 year after exposure.

Chronic intoxication usually occurs by industrial inhalation and produces emphysema and characteristic renal tubular damage with proteinuria and increased urinary excretion of beta$_2$ microglobulin. Cadmium's inhibitory effect on α_1-antitrypsin may be responsible for cadmium-induced emphysema. Relatively minor changes in liver function, a microcytic, hypochromic anemia unresponsive to iron therapy, and hypertension are associated findings. Chronic oral intake of contaminated rice and drinking water has produced a syndrome in Japan called *itai-itai* (ouch-ouch) disease with manifestations that include renal tubular damage and osteomalacia. Cadmium is probably a carcinogen for lung cancer, although a suggested association with cancer of the prostate has not been confirmed.

LABORATORY FINDINGS Measurement of blood cadmium levels is not useful. Urinary cadmium excretion exceeding 0.1 μmol/L (10 μg/L) is associated with renal tubular damage, especially when accompanied by elevated urinary beta$_2$ microglobulin and metallothionein levels. Kidney cadmium content obtained by renal biopsy can be assessed by neutron activation analysis. A renal cadmium concentration exceeding 2 μmol/g (200 μg/g) of wet weight is associated with renal disease.

TREATMENT Treatment is controversial. Although chelating agents bind cadmium, they may effectively shift cadmium to the kidney, where further damage can occur. In acute exposure, ethylenediaminetetraacetic acid (edetate) in a dose of 1.5 g/m^2 of surface area in a slow intravenous infusion daily can be beneficial. Dimercaprol is not effective. However, its water-soluble oral congener, succimer appears promising, although experience in cadmium poisoning is limited. Acute inhalation pneumonitis should be treated with glucocorticoids and diuretics. Itai-itai disease appears to respond to large doses of vitamin D. Long-term sequelae of chronic cadmium exposure include emphysema and chronic renal insufficiency.

LEAD

SOURCE Lead is a normal constituent of the earth's crust and is found throughout nature. The increased use of lead during the Industrial Revolution caused extensive disease among lead workers; the addition of lead salts to paints as coloring agents and stabilizers set the stage for the largest epidemic of lead poisoning in history, that of childhood plumbism. As many as 12 million preschool children in the United States may be affected annually by this syndrome, caused by ingestion of lead from paint, soil, household dust, and infrequently, drinking water. Evidence of permanent neurologic sequelae from levels of lead previously thought to be safe has raised fears of possible damage to the fetus and newborn as well. The nature of this epidemic has forced prohibition against the addition of organic lead salts to gasoline as well as extensive prohibitions against the use of lead in consumer products. These efforts have reduced the mean blood lead level in the United States from 0.8 μmol/L (16 μg/dL) in 1978 to less than 0.3 μmol/L (6 μg/dL) in 1990.

METABOLISM Inorganic lead salts are absorbed through ingestion or inhalation. Organic lead salts also may be absorbed through the skin. Generally, gastrointestinal absorption is about 10 percent of an ingested dose, but in children it may be as high as 50 percent. It is enhanced by deficiency of iron, calcium, and zinc. Absorption through the lung varies with tidal volume and particle size. Particles smaller than 1 μm may be absorbed if they reach the alveoli. Adults may ingest up to 0.5 μmol/d (100 μg/d) of lead from normal exposure to food and drinking water. Positive lead balance may occur at these levels, since renal excretion normally does not exceed 0.4 μmol/d (80 μg/d). In children, no more than 0.02 μmol/kg (5 μg/kg) of body weight is tolerated without increasing the body lead burden. Infants are a particular risk through consumption of formula reconstituted with contaminated tap water.

Under steady state conditions, 5 to 10 percent of ingested lead may be found in blood; 95 percent of that fraction is associated with the erythrocyte. In adults, up to 80 to 90 percent is taken up by bone and incorporated into hydroxyapatite crystals, where it is relatively

inactive. The remainder is found in soft tissues, principally the kidneys and brain. The principal route of excretion is stool (80 to 90 percent), and the remainder is found in the urine (10 percent). Small amounts are excreted in hair, nails, sweat, and saliva. Lead passes the placenta and blood-brain barrier and may be found in human milk. The half-life of lead in blood and soft tissues is 24 to 40 days, and in bone, 10^4 days.

Lead is a poison of enzymes, binding to the sulfhydryl groups of proteins. It also interferes with Ca^{2+} transport, synthesis and release of neurotransmitters, and activation of protein kinase C. In high concentration, lead alters the tertiary structure of intracellular proteins, denaturing them and causing cell death and tissue inflammation.

CLINICAL TOXICOLOGY The toxic effects of lead differ between children and adults. The adult form is generally characterized by abdominal pain, anemia, renal disease, headache, peripheral neuropathy with demyelination of long neurons, ataxia, and memory loss. Symptoms are usually associated with prolonged elevation of lead levels above 4 to 5 μmol/L (80 to 100 μg/dL) of whole blood. A subclinical form in adults affects primarily the peripheral nervous system and the kidneys. A linear association between hypertension and elevated lead levels [i.e., greater than 1.5 μmol/L (30 μg/dL)] has been reported. Encephalopathy is rare in adults.

Childhood lead poisoning is manifested by abdominal pain and anemia, but the central nervous system effects are most important. As an enzymatic poison, lead affects developing tissues more than tissues with slow turnover. Hence subclinical lead poisoning is most dangerous to children because its effects emerge without associated symptoms that bring the victim to medical attention. In the acute clinical form, signs and symptoms reflect both the direct effect of high concentrations of lead [i.e., blood lead greater than 4 μmol/L (80 μg/dL)] and consequent severe alterations in porphyrin synthesis. Signs and symptoms include abdominal pain and irritability, followed by lethargy, anorexia, pallor (anemia), ataxia, and slurred speech. In severe cases, convulsions, coma, and death are usually due to severe generalized cerebral edema and renal failure. A history of "high-dose" exposure to lead (usually paint chips), pica (the ingestion of nonfood substances), and malnutrition (iron, calcium, and zinc deficiency) almost always is associated with this syndrome.

The subclinical form of childhood plumbism is associated with elevated blood lead with or without increased erythrocyte protoporphyrin when the blood lead level exceeds 1.5 μmol/L (30 μg/dL). However, no symptoms are usually detected. The syndrome is widespread, and its effects on the developing central nervous system are largely irreversible. These include mental retardation and selective deficits in language, cognitive functions, and behavior, depending on the age and duration of exposure. These latter factors are more important than the height of the lead level. Elevated lead levels at or about 2 years of age are predictive of neurodevelopmental outcome.

LABORATORY FINDINGS Laboratory abnormalities include blood lead levels greater than 0.5 μmol/L (10 μg/dL). Biochemical and neurodevelopmental abnormalities may occur in association with blood lead levels as low as 0.7 μmol/L (15 μg/dL), particularly in very young children. Although a hemolytic anemia is associated with acute plumbism, chronic plumbism is associated with iron deficiency. Other heme precursors are increased in plasma and urine (e.g., delta aminolevulinic acid).

Renal abnormalities include pyuria, the Fanconi syndrome, and azotemia. In plumbism, urinary excretion of lead exceeds 4 μmol/d (80 μg/d). In adults, demyelination of long nerves produces prolonged nerve conduction time and subsequent paralysis of extensor muscles with atrophy (wrist drop or foot drop). While slight prolongation of nerve conduction can be seen in children, it is clinically evident only in those with sickle cell disease. Abnormalities of cardiac, thyroid, and hepatic function occur in adults. In children, a characteristic finding is increased density at the metaphyseal plate of growing long bones, so-called lead lines. These are generally seen in association with levels greater than 2.4 μmol/L (50 μg/dL) of whole blood for a prolonged period. They are not seen in adults.

TREATMENT   The *sine qua non* of treatment is removal of the source of exposure. Cases of industrial lead poisoning should be reported to the Occupational Safety Health Administration (OSHA). Cases of childhood plumbism should be reported to the local board of health to initiate examination of housing for sources of lead.

Reduction of the body burden of lead is accomplished by use of chelating agents, principally edetate calcium disodium (EDTA), dimercaprol, penicillamine, and succimer. The lead mobilization test may be used to determine the size of the "chelatable" pool of lead in patients with moderately elevated levels [i.e., 1.7 to 2.2 μmol/L (35 to 45 μg/dL)]. In this test, administration of a calculated dose of chelating agent, usually edetate, induces a lead diuresis that is then compared with the dose of chelating agent. The test is positive when greater than 2.5 nmol (0.5 μg) lead is excreted per milligram of chelating agent administered per 6 to 8 h. The use of x-ray fluorescence of bone to determine the lead burden is under investigation as an alternative to the lead mobilization test.

In acute encephalopathy, double therapy (dimercaprol and edetate) is used until blood lead levels are less than 2 μmol/L (40 μg/dL). Urine flow must be established, and even in the presence of cerebral edema, fluids must be sufficient to produce a lead diuresis. Cerebral edema should be managed in an intensive care setting, but removal of the metal is essential. In symptomatic adults and children, therapy with both dimercaprol and edetate should be used for 5 days at edetate doses of up to 1.5 g/m² of surface area daily and dimercaprol doses of 12 to 24 mg/kg of body weight per day. If further chelation is required, a minimum interval of 48 to 72 h should intervene between courses of therapy. The penicillamine dose is 20 to 40 mg/kg of body weight per day, not to exceed 1 g/d. Adverse effects, particularly allergy, may be reduced by beginning therapy with one-quarter of the total dose for 1 week and then doubling and redoubling the dose until full dose is reached. Penicillamine can be administered for 3 to 6 months until the body lead burden is depleted. Only penicillamine and, to a lesser extent, edetate remove lead directly from bone. If edetate is indicated, as many separate 5-day courses as are needed may be given provided that the total safe dose is not exceeded and proper intervals between courses are observed.

Succimer is licensed by the Food and Drug Administration for oral treatment of children with Pb levels of 2.2 μmol/L (45 μg/dL). Current recommendations for therapy are 5 days at 30 μg/kg per day in three divided doses, followed by 14 days at 20 μg/kg per day in two divided doses. Side effects include occasional vomiting and transient elevations in hepatic enzymes. "Rebound" in Pb levels as high as 80 percent of the original value necessitates repeat courses for effective reduction in lead burden.

MERCURY

SOURCE   Humans may encounter mercury in an inorganic (elemental or mercuric salt) or an organic (usually methyl) form. All three are toxic, but organic mercury is most widespread and potentially dangerous. Elemental mercury is used in thermometers, sphygmomanometers, dental amalgams, and some disk batteries. It is volatile at room temperature and rapidly oxidizes to mercuric mercury when exposed to oxygen. Toxicity usually occurs from inhalation of mercury vapor during industrial exposure, although elevated mercury levels have been reported in neonates exposed to faulty mercury switches in incubators. Mercuric salts are found in topical medicines, in catalytic agents in the manufacture of plastics, in cathartics (e.g., Calomel), and in foodstuffs. Toxicity occurs usually as a result of gastrointestinal exposure. Organic mercury is found in paints, fungicides, seeds, foods, medicines, cosmetic agents, and wood preservatives. Large amounts of methyl mercury are formed by methylation of mercury salt wastes, as occurred in the mercury epidemic in Minamata Bay, Japan.

METABOLISM   Elemental mercury is poorly absorbed by the gastrointestinal tract but is absorbed efficiently as vapor through the lungs, with 80 to 100 percent of inhaled mercury entering the bloodstream through the alveoli. Absorbed mercury vapor is lipid-soluble and readily crosses the blood-brain barrier and the placenta. It is rapidly oxidized to its mercuric form and combines with sulfhydryl groups. Excretion is via the urine and feces. The half-life of elemental mercury is approximately 60 days.

Inorganic mercury salts are absorbed through the gastrointestinal tract and skin. Large overdoses may produce corrosive effects on the gastrointestinal tract with consequent increased absorption. Normal uptake is less than 10 percent of an ingested dose. Ingestion of disk batteries with consequent decomposition in the gastrointestinal tract has resulted in elevated mercury levels without gastrointestinal symptoms. Mercuric salts accumulate primarily in the kidney but are distributed to the liver, erythrocytes, bone marrow, spleen, lung, intestine, and skin. Little, if any, crosses the blood-brain barrier. Excretion is via the urine and feces. The half-life of inorganic mercury is approximately 40 days.

Organic (methyl) mercury is readily absorbed through the intestines and the skin. Short-chain alkyl and methyl mercury penetrate the erythrocyte membrane and bind to hemoglobin. Because of its high lipid solubility, methyl mercury freely passes the placenta and blood-brain barrier and enters breast milk. Organic mercury also concentrates in the kidneys and the central nervous system. Metallothionein synthesis is induced by mercury, and the augmented concentration of the protein exerts a partial protective effect against tissue damage. Excretion is complex. About 1 percent of organic mercury is excreted in urine directly. Methyl mercury is acetylated in the liver or may be conjugated with cysteine or glutathione. The *N*-acetyl-homocysteine–methyl mercury complex then enters the enterohepatic circulation and is ultimately excreted in the urine. The half-life of organic mercury in humans is about 70 days. Phenyl mercuric compounds are excreted more rapidly.

CLINICAL TOXICOLOGY   Acute metallic mercury (vapor) poisoning causes inflammation of large and small airways and interstitial pneumonitis. The rapid uptake of mercury vapor into the central nervous system produces tremor and increased excitability. Both acute and chronic mercury vapor poisoning primarily affects the central nervous system. Acute mercury vapor poisoning can cause acute inorganic mercury toxicity with consequent possibly irreversible neurologic sequelae. Initial symptoms include lassitude, anorexia, weight loss, and gastrointestinal disturbances. Increasing exposure produces the characteristic intention tremor of mercury poisoning and is accompanied by mercurial *erethism* (timidity, memory loss, insomnia, excitability, and, in severe cases, delirium). This neurologic picture in felt-hat workers exposed to mercury vapor and mercuric salts led to the phrase "mad as a hatter." Intravenous elemental mercury administration can produce symptomatic mercury granulomas in the lung but with little apparent consequence. A contribution of dental amalgams to toxicity has not been demonstrated.

Chronic inorganic mercury poisoning produces the preceding neurologic findings as well as excessive salivation, loosening of the teeth, gingivitis, and stomatitis. When applied to the skin, mercuric salts may cause hypersensitivity reactions ranging from mild erythema to exfoliative dermatitis. Acrodynia, or Pink's disease, occurs in young children and may be mistaken for Kawasaki's disease. Symptoms include generalized rash, irritability, photophobia, hypertrichosis, profuse perspiration, and swelling and desquamation of the feet and hands.

Acute inorganic mercury poisoning is characterized by corrosive effects on the gastrointestinal tract, including nausea, vomiting, hematemesis, and abdominal pain followed by tenesmus, bloody diarrhea, and necrosis of intestinal mucosa. Acute fluid redistribution in massive overdose can produce shock and death. Acute inorganic mercury poisoning causes acute tubular necrosis, while chronic inorganic mercury poisoning produces a nephrotic syndrome.

Acute and chronic organic mercury poisonings are indistinguishable. Prenatal poisoning produces cerebral palsy as a result of cortical and cerebellar atrophy. Postnatal poisoning causes paresthesias, headache, pain, visual, hearing, and speech disorders, neurasthenia, loss of memory, incoordination, erethism, spasticity, paralysis, stupor, and coma. These neurologic abnormalities are often permanent.

The daily intake of methyl mercury should not exceed 100 parts per billion. Blood mercury levels above 180 nmol/L (3.5 μg/dL) and urine mercury levels above 0.7 μmol/L (150 μg/L) are abnormal. Symptoms may be seen with blood mercury levels above 1 μmol/L (20 μg/dL) and urine mercury levels above 3 μmol/L (600 μg/L). Clinical findings may be associated with somewhat lower concentrations depending on when exposure occurred.

TREATMENT Treatment is aimed at reducing the absorption of mercury, protecting susceptible tissues, and enhancing elimination. In the case of ingestion of mercuric salts, initial treatment consists of removing mercury from the stomach by inducing emesis or by gastric lavage. Polythiol resins are effective in binding mercury in the gastrointestinal tract. Activated charcoal, however, does not bind metals.

Generally, chelation therapy is indicated when elevated urine or blood mercury levels are present. Chelating agents with active mono- or dithiol groups are most effective. These include dimercaprol and the oral chelators penicillamine and succimer.

In acute inorganic mercury poisoning, dimercaprol should be used at a dose not exceeding 24 mg/kg of body weight per 24 h, intramuscularly, in divided doses. Generally, therapy should not exceed 5 days at a time but can be reinstituted after a suitable rest period. Penicillamine can be used in the treatment of inorganic mercury poisoning but N-acetyl-DL-penicillamine is equally effective and less toxic. The dose is 30 mg/kg of body weight per day in two to three divided doses. Peritoneal dialysis and hemodialysis also have been used with some success, as has succimer in combination with extracorporeal regional complexing hemodialysis (ERCH) in patients with renal failure. Neither is as effective as chelation therapy, but they may be useful in the presence of renal failure, and neither has been shown to reverse the neurologic sequelae of inorganic mercury poisoning.

In chronic inorganic mercury poisoning, dimercaprol is ineffective. Penicillamine is the drug of choice. The investigational drug N-acetyl-DL-penicillamine is more effective than either dimercaprol or edetate. Succimer may enhance urinary mercury excretion without influencing clinical outcome.

THALLIUM

SOURCE Thallium is used as an insecticide, as a catalyst in fireworks, in manufacturing imitation jewelry and optical lenses, in industry as an alloy, and in cardiac perfusion imaging. It was banned in the United States as a rodenticide in 1972. Accidental as well as intentional ingestions of thallium occur. Epidemic poisoning has followed the ingestion of grain impregnated with thallium. Thallium is available as iodide, sulfate, acetate, carbonate, and nitrate salts.

METABOLISM Thallium is absorbed percutaneously, by inhalation, and by oral ingestion. It has a large volume of distribution of 4 to 6 L/kg of body weight with distribution to body organs including kidney, pancreas, spleen, liver, lung, muscles, and brain. It crosses the placenta. Thallium is bound to sulfhydryl groups on mitochondrial membranes at intracellular sites. The elimination half-life is variable, ranging from 3 to 15 days. The major pathway of elimination is in the urine; 3 percent of a dose is eliminated per day, or 75 mL/min total-body clearance.

Thallium is soluble at physiologic pH and interferes with oxidative phosphorylation by inhibition of ATPase. It substitutes for potassium in many physiologic reactions. Pathologic findings at postmortem include cerebral edema, loss of myelin in peripheral nerves, fatty infiltration of the liver, and degenerative changes in the myocardium.

CLINICAL TOXICOLOGY Severe poisoning occurs following a single ingested dose greater than 1 g or 8 mg/kg of body weight.

Death has occurred following an ingested dose of 15 mg/kg of body weight.

Immediate signs and symptoms (occurring within 3 to 4 h of ingestion) include nausea and vomiting, abdominal pain, diarrhea, hematemesis, and hematochezia. Intermediate manifestations (within 1 week of ingestion) include involvement of the central nervous system with confusion, psychosis, choreoathetosis, organic brain syndrome, convulsions, and coma. Peripheral neurologic involvement is both motor and sensory and includes paresthesias, myalgias, weakness, tremor, and ataxia. Autonomic manifestations are less common and include tachycardia, hypertension, and salivation. Ophthalmologic abnormalities are neuritis, ophthalmoplegia, ptosis, strabismus, and cranial nerve palsies. Late manifestations (occurring 2 to 4 weeks after ingestion) include diffuse hair loss (with sparing of pubic and body hair and the lateral one-third of the eyebrows) with regrowth occurring as body burden decreases over time. Residual effects include memory loss, ataxia, tremor, and foot drop.

LABORATORY FINDINGS Thallium is radiopaque and is evident on an abdominal x-ray. Thallium levels with severe ingestion range, in serum, from 1.5 to 30 μmol/L (30 to 600 μg/dL) and, in urine, from 0.05 to 600 μmol/d (10 to 120,000 μg/d). The electroencephalogram (EEG) is diffusely abnormal, and peripheral nerve conduction may be delayed.

TREATMENT Therapeutic modalities include gastrointestinal decontamination, enhanced renal excretion, and dialysis. Gastric lavage or ipecac syrup is indicated within 4 to 6 h of acute ingestion. Adequacy of removal of thallium can be documented by follow-up abdominal x-ray. Prussian blue absorbs thallium in the gastrointestinal tract by exchanging potassium for thallium on its crystal lattice network, thereby preventing absorption. The oral dose is 250 mg/kg of body weight, administered in three to four divided doses. Activated charcoal is as effective as Prussian blue in increasing fecal elimination by interrupting the enterohepatic circulation of thallium. Mannitol or magnesium citrate is used as a laxative to enhance gastrointestinal removal.

Forced diuresis is the oldest technique in use and increases urinary excretion by 50 to 100 percent. Potassium chloride promotes renal excretion of thallium through the exchange of potassium for thallium, thereby releasing thallium from tissue sites into blood and augmenting urinary excretion two- to threefold. This therapy shortens thallium half-life in humans but may aggravate neurologic symptoms by redistributing thallium into the brain. The amount of thallium removed as compared with the total ingested dose of potassium is small. Diuretics (furosemide) also increase urinary elimination of thallium. Peritoneal dialysis removes 15 to 20 mg thallium per day and hemodialysis 8 mg for each 8 h of dialysis. Prolonged hemodialysis can remove up to 25 mg thallium per day, the total amount removed being relatively small. Charcoal hemoperfusion achieves average blood clearance values of 100 mL/min at a blood flow rate of 300 mL/min. Thus the combination of forced diuresis, diuretic therapy, and hemoperfusion will most effectively enhance total-body clearance of thallium. This therapy should be combined with oral administration of Prussian blue or activated charcoal plus cathartics.

Ditiocarb has been advocated for early use in overdose because it leads to increased thallium blood levels and a two- to threefold increase in thallium excretion. However, ditiocarb-thallium complexes diffuse into the brain with subsequent clinical and EEG worsening; therefore, ditiocarb is contraindicated in thallium intoxication.

CHELATING AGENTS

Chelating agents are used to bind toxic metals in stable, cyclic compounds with relatively low toxicity and enhanced renal and fecal excretion.

DIMERCAPROL (BRITISH ANTI-LEWISITE, BAL) Dimercaprol was first developed as an antidote for the arsenical war gas lewisite; its chelating property is due to its four sulfhydryl groups which bind in a complex to polyvalent metal ions. Its affinity for metals is strong enough to reverse a significant portion of toxic metal enzyme binding. Dimercaprol diffuses into erythrocytes and enhances fecal as well as urinary metal excretion. It is given intramuscularly in peanut oil every 4 to 8 h in a dose of 12 to 24 mg/kg of body weight per 24 h. Toxicity includes mild febrile reactions, nausea, headache, lacrimation, conjunctivitis, salivation, and rhinorrhea. The drug emits a strong sulfide odor, and patients may complain of metallic taste. Contraindications to dimercaprol include glucose-6-phosphate dehydrogenase deficiency, allergy to peanut oil, and concurrent use of medicinal iron, which forms a toxic complex with dimercaprol.

EDETATE (EDTA)   Because the sodium salt of edetate can produce profound hypocalcemia, only the calcium disodium salt should be used in therapy of metal poisoning. Calcium edetate forms a complex with divalent cations, exchanging one atom of calcium for each metal ion. It enhances urinary excretion of lead 20- to 50-fold and also increases excretion of zinc and, to a lesser extent, other metals. It does not enter the erythrocyte but removes metals from the extracellular sites. Oral administration is contraindicated because it is variably absorbed and it enhances absorption of metals from the gastrointestinal tract. The drug is given parenterally either by constant intravenous infusion or intramuscular injection in a dose of 500 to 1000 mg/m^2 of surface area per day. The drug can be used safely in conjunction with other chelating agents. Toxicity increases after 4 to 5 days of administration with concomitant reduction in metal excretion; as a consequence, the drug is given for several "courses" of from 3 to 5 days each.

Toxicity is principally renal, dose-related, and usually reversible. It can be reduced by maintaining adequate urine flow. During treatment renal function should be carefully monitored.

SUCCIMER   Succimer (DMSA, di-mercapto-succinic acid) is a water-soluble oral congener of dimercaprol. It is licensed by the Food and Drug Administration for the treatment of children with blood lead levels exceeding 2.2 μmol/L (45 μg/dL) and is investigational for uses in children with lower lead levels and for treatment of arsenic and mercury poisoning. It is the only drug licensed exclusively for pediatric use to avoid its misuse in occupational exposures. Unlike D-penicillamine, it permits concomitant administration of iron when iron deficiency complicates childhood plumbism, as it often does. Enhancement of renal excretion appears to be comparable with that induced by parenteral edetate, but the relatively high "rebound" values usually necessitate multiple courses of administration. The current dosage regimen is 10 mg/kg of body weight tid for 5 days, followed by 10 mg/kg of body weight bid for 14 days. Rebound values should be measured within 2 weeks of therapy. Side effects include usually mild, apparently transient elevations in hepatic transaminases and cutaneous reactions, usually in adults receiving multiple courses. The drug has an unpleasant sulfurous odor, and vomiting of single doses is common. Because the dramatic but transient depression of blood lead can "mask" active ingestion of lead, its use should be deferred in children with ongoing exposure to lead hazards.

PENICILLAMINE   Penicillamine is the only commercially available oral chelating agent. Not presently approved by the Food and Drug Administration for treatment of lead poisoning, it is licensed for use in the treatment of rheumatoid arthritis, Wilson's disease, and cystinuria. Nevertheless, there is extensive experience in its use in chelation of other metals. The N-acetyl form is particularly helpful in the treatment of inorganic and organic mercury poisoning.

Penicillamine enhances excretion of heavy metals in the urine by an unclear mechanism. The drug is given orally in a dose of 40 mg/kg of body weight per day. By initiating therapy at low doses (usually 25 percent of the anticipated maximum dose) and gradually increasing the dose, the frequency of side effects can be reduced substantially.

Side effects may be seen in up to 20 to 30 percent of patients receiving penicillamine and resemble penicillin hypersensitivity, including rash, fever, thrombocytopenia, and leukopenia. Rare side effects include autoimmune hemolytic anemia and Stevens-Johnson

syndrome. Anorexia, nausea, sleep disturbances, and urinary frequency may be seen occasionally. Nephrotoxicity is reported in adults receiving large doses and in one case has been reported in a child. Patients receiving penicillamine should, therefore, be carefully monitored for signs of renal, hematologic, or allergic side effects.

REFERENCES

Arsenic

BATES MN et al: Arsenic ingestion and internal cancers: A review. Am J Epidemiol 135:462, 1992

ELLENHORN MJ, BARCELOUX DG: *Medical Toxicology*, New York, Elsevier, 1988

FESMIRE FM et al: Survival following massive arsenic ingestion. Am J Emerg Med 6:603, 1988

HUTTON JT et al: Arsenic poisoning. N Engl J Med 307:1080, 1982

MATHIES D et al: Massive arsenic poisoning: Effects of hemodialysis and dimercaprol on arsenic kinetics. Intensive Care Med 18(1):47, 1992

Cadmium

DUNPHY B: Acute occupational cadmium poisoning. J Occup Med 9:22, 1967

FRIBERG L et al: *Cadmium in the Environment*, 2d ed. Cleveland, CRC Press, 1974

LAUWERYS RR et al: Health risk assessment of long-term exposure to chemicals: Applications to cadmium and manganese. Arch Toxicol Suppl 15:97, 1992

WAALKES MP et al: Toxicological principles of metal carcinogenesis with special emphasis on cadmium. Crit Rev Toxicol 22(3–4):175, 1992

Lead

AGENCY FOR TOXIC SUBSTANCES DISEASE REGISTRY: *The Nature and Extent of Lead Poisoning in Children in the United States: A Report to Congress*. Washington, US Department of Health and Human Services, Public Health Service, July 1988

CARNOW B (ed): *Health Effects of Occupational Lead and Arsenic Exposure: A Symposium*. Washington, US Department of Health, Education, and Welfare, 1976

CENTERS FOR DISEASE CONTROL AND PREVENTION: *Preventing Lead Poisoning in Young Children*. Atlanta, CDCP, 1991

GRAEF J: Lead poisoning, parts I, II, and III. Clin Toxicol Rev 14(8, 9, 10), 1992

KEHOE RA: The metabolism of lead in man in health and disease. The Harben Lectures, 1960. J. Inst Public Health 24:101, 1961

SMITH MA et al: *Lead Exposure and Childhood Development: An International Assessment for the Commission of the European Communities and the US Environmental Protection Agency*. Norwell, MA, Kluwer Academic Publishers, 1989.

Mercury

ELHASSANI SB: The many faces of methylmercury poisoning. J Toxicol Clin Toxicol 19:875, 1982–83

GRAEF J: Mercury, parts I and II. Clin Toxicol Rev 2(7, 8), 1980

KOSTYNIAK PJ et al: Extracorporeal regional complexing hemodialysis treatment of acute inorganic mercury intoxication. Hum Exp Toxicol 9(3):137, 1990

NATIONAL ACADEMY OF SCIENCES: *An Assessment of Mercury in the Environment*. Washington, NAC, 1978

THORP JM JR et al: Elemental mercury exposure in early pregnancy. Obstet Gynecol 79(5):874, 1992

Thallium

DAVIS LE et al: Acute thallium poisoning: Toxicological and morphological studies of the nervous system. Ann Neurol 10(1):38, 1981

DEGROOT G: et al: The evaluation of the efficacy of charcoal hemoperfusion in the treatment of three cases of thallium poisoning. Arch Toxicol 57:61, 1985

DESENCLOS JC et al: Thallium poisoning: An outbreak in Florida, 1988. South Med J 85(12):1203, 1992

LOVEJOY FH JR: Thallium. Clin Toxicol Rev 4(5), 1982

VILLANOVA E et al: Poisoning by thallium: A study of five cases. Drug Safety 5(5):384, 1990

WAINWRIGHT AP et al: Clinical features and therapy of acute thallium poisoning. Q J Med 69(258):939, 1988

Chelating Agents

APOSHIAN HV et al: Meso-2,3-dimercaptosuccinic acid: Chemical, pharmacological and toxicological properties of an orally effective metal chelating agent. Annu Rev Pharmacol Toxicol 30:279, 1990

CHISOLM JJ JR: The use of chelating agents in the treatment of acute and chronic lead intoxication in childhood. J Pediatr 73:1, 1968

GRAZIANO JH et al: Dose-response study of oral 2,3-dimercaptosuccinic acid in children with elevated blood level concentrations. J Pediatr 113:751, 1988

HRUBY R et al: 2,3-Dimercapto-1-propanesulphonate in heavy metal poisoning. Med Toxicol 2:317, 1987

SHANNON M: Efficacy and toxicity of D-penicillamine in low-level lead poisoning. J Pediatr 112:799, 1988

ZHENG W et al: Determination and metabolism of dithiol chelating agents: VII. Biliary excretion of dithiols and their interactions with cadmium and metallothionein. Fund Appl Toxicol 14(3):598, 1990

397 DISORDERS CAUSED BY VENOMS, BITES, AND STINGS

JAMES F. WALLACE

Humans come into contact with a great variety of venomous animals, including snakes, lizards, sea animals, spiders, scorpions, and numerous species of insects. In general three types of injuries result: infections, those due to the direct effect of venom on the victim, as exemplified in snakebite, and those due to indirect effects of the poison, as in hypersensitivity reaction to bee stings. Each year in the United States at least 50 persons die as the result of venomous injuries. Hymenopterous insects, snakes, and spiders account for over 90 percent of the fatalities. In addition, there is considerable morbidity and loss in economic productivity from the many nonfatal envenomations.

SNAKEBITE

EPIDEMIOLOGY Fewer than one-tenth of the nearly 3500 known species of snakes are venomous. The poisonous varieties belong to five families: Elapidae (cobras, kraits, mambas, and coral snakes), found in all parts of the world except Europe; Viperidae, (true vipers) found in all parts of the world except the Americas; Hydrophidae (sea snakes); Crotalidae (pit vipers), found in Asia and the Americas; and Colubridae (boomslangs, bird snakes), of the African continent. The poisonous varieties of the United States, with the exception of the coral snake, are pit vipers and include rattlesnakes, the water moccasin, and the copperhead. Although this discussion centers around these species, most of the therapeutic measures are applicable to snakes in all parts of the world.

About 8000 individuals are bitten by poisonous snakes in the United States each year, with a large number occurring in the southeastern and Gulf states. Deaths number fewer than 20 per year, and most are due to rattlesnake bites. In many European countries, deaths from snakebite are unusual, but the annual deaths from snakebite throughout the world are between 30,000 and 40,000, with the largest number in Burma and Brazil, where 2000 deaths are estimated to occur each year.

ETIOLOGY The *coral snake* is found in the southern states from Florida to Arizona. It is usually marked by alternating red and black bands separated by yellow rings; however, black and albino forms exist. Coral snakes are generally nocturnal in their activities, shy and elusive, and rarely bite humans. The fangs are short and permanently erect; the highly toxic venom is injected into multiple puncture wounds produced by a series of chewing movements.

The *pit vipers* are so named because of a small pit between the eye and the nostril. Large venom glands in the temporal regions give the head a triangular appearance. They are generally aggressive and likely to strike if disturbed. The fangs are long and hinged, folding posteriorly when the mouth is closed. Pit vipers strike suddenly with a forward thrust of the head. The instant that the erect fangs make contact, venom is expressed by sudden muscular contraction.

The *rattlesnakes*, recognized by the horny rattle on the tail which buzzes when the snake is disturbed, are widely distributed. The diamondbacks (*Crotalus adamanteus* in the Southeast and *C. atrox* in the Southwest) are the largest and most dangerous snakes in this country. Others include the prairie rattler (*C. confluentus*), the timber rattler (*C. horridus*), and the pigmy rattlers.

The *water moccasin* or cottonmouth (*Agkistrodon piscivorus*) is found in swampy areas or along the banks of streams. It is a strong swimmer and can bite under water. This snake is notorious for inflicting severe facial bites when disturbed in the branches of small trees. The copperhead or highland moccasin (*A. mokasen*) is a closely related species. Its bite is painful but rarely fatal.

PATHOGENESIS Snake venoms The venoms of most species contain mixtures of many toxic proteins and enzymes that have diversified and complicated pharmacologic effects. As an example, the venom of the Indian cobra (*Naja naja*) contains a neurotoxin, a hemolysin, a cardiotoxin, a cholinesterase, at least three phosphatases, a nucleotidase, and a potent inhibitor of cytochrome oxidase. Several venoms, including those of the pit vipers, contain hyaluronidase and proteolytic enzymes. Although the exact roles of these components in toxicity are incompletely understood, the venom of a given species is usually predominantly neurotoxic or necrotizing and is frequently associated with hemolysis, abnormalities of blood coagulation, changes in cardiac dynamics, and alterations in vascular resistance. Venoms of elapids, including the coral snake, are neurotoxic, and death results from respiratory paralysis due to central nervous system damage and interference with transmission at the neuromuscular junction. Venoms of crotalid snakes produce local tissue injury, hemorrhage, and hemolysis. Death is often preceded by circulatory collapse associated with a marked fall in circulating blood volume resulting from pooling of blood in the microcirculation and loss of plasma due to increased capillary permeability. Systemic absorption of venom occurs through the lymphatics, and therapeutic measures designed to reduce lymphatic function are helpful in controlling symptoms.

Factors affecting severity of snake bite Several factors affect the outcome of snake bite:

1 The age, size, and health of the patient. A fatal outcome is more likely in children because a relatively large dose of poison is injected into a small victim.
2 Location of bite. Bites on extremities or into adipose tissue are less dangerous than those on the trunk or face or directly into a blood vessel. A direct strike of the fangs is more dangerous than a scratch, a glancing blow, or one hitting a bone. The discharge orifice of a fang is well above its tip so that the point of the fang can penetrate the skin without envenomation; even a thin layer of clothing may afford great protection. Because of the superficial nature of the wound, as many as one-fifth of patients bitten by venomous snakes have no evidence of envenomation, even though the fangs have penetrated the skin.
3 The size of the snake (a large pit viper can inject over 1000 mg of venom, six times a lethal dose for an adult), the extent of its anger or fear (if hurt, it may inject a larger amount of venom), the condition of the fangs (broken or recently renewed), and the state of the venom glands (recently discharged or full). Contrary to popular belief, the bite of a snake that has recently fed is not necessarily less venomous for humans; the snake usually does not exhaust its venom in a single bite.
4 The presence of various bacteria, particularly clostridia and other anaerobic organisms, in the mouth of the snake or on the skin of the victim. This may lead to serious infection in the necrotic tissues at the local site.
5 Exercise or exertion, such as running, immediately after the bite. This speeds systemic absorption of toxin.

MANIFESTATIONS Following the bite of a pit viper, severe burning pain develops within a few minutes at the site of the wound. Local swelling develops rapidly and spreads in all directions, accompanied by the appearance of ecchymoses and bullae over the involved area. As the edema spreads, serosanguineous fluid oozes from the puncture wounds. Gangrene of the skin and subcutaneous tissues may develop. Systemic effects from the absorption of venom and local tissue destruction may include fever, nausea and vomiting, circulatory collapse, bleeding into the skin and from all body orifices, low-grade jaundice, muscle cramping, pupillary constriction, disorientation, delirium, and convulsions. Death may occur in 6 to 48 h. Survival may be attended by massive local tissue loss from gangrene or secondary infection or complicated by acute renal failure secondary to disseminated intravascular clotting and cortical necrosis or by tubular necrosis following circulatory collapse.

The bite of the coral snake causes little pain and local swelling. There are usually multiple fang marks. Within 10 to 15 min, numbness and weakness begin in the region of the bite, followed by ataxia, ptosis, pupillary dilatation, palatal and pharyngeal paralysis, slurring of speech, salivation, and occasionally nausea and vomiting. The patient becomes comatose, develops respiratory paralysis and seizures, and dies within 8 to 72 h.

Cobra bites are painful and are often accompanied by severe hemolysis, local necrosis, and sloughing in addition to their neurotoxic effects. There is little pain and no edema at the site of a sea snake bite. Symptoms of systemic envenomation follow a latent period which may vary from 15 min to 8 h. Although the venom is both myotoxic and neurotoxic, the injury to skeletal muscle is most prominent and is characterized by generalized muscle pain, weakness, and myoglobinuria. Hemorrhagic manifestations predominate following envenomation by colubrids (boomslangs and bird snakes) and many pit vipers, including certain species of rattlesnake.

LABORATORY ABNORMALITIES Laboratory abnormalities may include progressive anemia, polymorphonuclear leukocytosis, thrombocytopenia, hypofibrinogenemia, disordered tests of coagulation, proteinuria, and azotemia.

TREATMENT An attempt should be made to determine with certainty that the patient has been bitten by a poisonous snake. Absence of distinct fang punctures and failure of local pain, edema, numbness, or weakness to appear within 20 min are strong evidence against envenomation. The approximate size of the snake should be noted, since larger snakes usually cause more severe envenomation. If the species is not known, the offending snake should be killed to allow identification.

First aid The victim should be reassured and calmed, measures should be instituted to retard the absorption of venom and to remove it from the tissues as quickly as possible after the bite, and arrangements should be made for transportation to the nearest hospital. The patient should be promptly placed at rest, and the bitten extremity should be immobilized to reduce the rate of spread of the venom. This is best achieved by splinting. If anatomically feasible, a wide constriction band should be placed a few centimeters above the bite and made tight enough to allow one finger to pass beneath with difficulty. The purpose is to impede lymph flow; it is not necessary to obstruct venous return. The band should be loosened and moved proximally when local swelling causes it to tighten. Since there is no evidence that incision and suction of the wound improve outcome in humans, and since incision in the field can cause secondary infection and traumatize tendons, nerves, and blood vessels, this procedure is no longer recommended.

To assess the severity of envenomation, the level of swelling should be marked on the skin every 15 min while the patient is being transported to a hospital. Ice packs relieve pain and slow lymphatic drainage but do not neutralize venom, and even a small amount of cooling may worsen damage to injured tissues by causing ischemia. For this reason, it is recommended that no form of cooling be used.

Immediate hospital care This should include appropriate treatment for shock and respiratory difficulty, antivenin, measures to combat infection, and general supportive care. Initial laboratory studies in a patient with obvious crotalid envenomation should include blood typing and cross-matching, coagulation screening tests, and an electrocardiogram. None of these tests is particularly helpful in the initial evaluation of a patient with a coral snake bite.

Antivenin is the only specific treatment of snake venom poisoning, and its use in severe bites is vital. In the United States, polyvalent crotaline antivenin effective against all American pit vipers and antivenin for North American coral snake poisoning are commercially available. Both products are a lyophilized powder of refined horse serum. Kits contain antivenin powder (reconstituted by diluting with water to 10 mL per vial), syringe, normal horse serum for prior sensitivity testing of the patient, and detailed instructions. Intravenously administered antivenin leads to the most rapid and effective response. It is not advisable to infiltrate antivenin at the local site. The initial dose should depend on an estimate of the amount of envenomation. For pit viper bites accompanied by progressive local swelling but no systemic symptoms, 5 vials (50 mL) are usually sufficient. When swelling has progressed beyond the site of the bite and mild systemic symptoms and/or hematologic and coagulation abnormalities are present, initial treatment should be 5 to 15 vials (50 to 150 mL). For severe poisonings associated with rapidly progressive and extensive local effects as well as systemic symptoms and evidence of hemolysis or coagulopathy, 15 to 20 vials (150 to 200 mL) or more should be administered. Up to 50 percent more antivenin should be given to children or small adults to neutralize the higher venom concentrations. Reconstituted antivenin is diluted in 500 mL of intravenous fluid and administered as rapidly as tolerated over 1 to 2 h. Additional infusions containing 5 to 10 vials (50 to 100 mL) should be repeated every 2 h until the progression of swelling in the bitten part ceases and systemic signs and symptoms disappear. When an adequate dose has been achieved, improvement in the clinical signs may be rapid.

If *any* evidence of envenomation appears within several hours following a coral snake bite, antivenin should be given without waiting for systemic manifestations. Four vials of antivenin should be given intravenously for bites associated with minimal swelling and/or local paresthesias. If evidence of a bite is more definitive, particularly if there was initial pain, 6 to 10 vials of antivenin should be given as soon as possible. Larger doses should be used in severe bites from large snakes, if the snake bite was prolonged for more than a few seconds, or if the victim is a child.

In the patient with severe envenomation who is allergic to horse serum, the relative risk of death from anaphylaxis rather than from venom poisoning should be weighed before undertaking desensitization with small doses of diluted horse serum.

No antivenin for other snakes is manufactured in the United States, but antiserum of various types is usually kept on hand at large zoos all over the world. A national antivenin index is maintained by the Oklahoma Poison Information Center in cooperation with the Oklahoma City Zoo [(405) 271-5454] and provides 24-h telephone consultation service for physicians needing advice in handling snake-bite accidents.

Respiration should be maintained by mechanical or other means. In patients bitten by elapid snakes, respiratory failure is usually reversible. *Tetanus toxoid* or *tetanus immune globulin* of human origin should be given (see Chap. 106). If wound infections appear, antibiotics should be used with the knowledge that the predominant microorganisms in the mouths of snakes are gram-negative pathogens. Treatment should be preceded by appropriate aerobic and anaerobic cultures. *Fasciotomy* may be necessary to minimize ischemic injury to a massively swollen limb. Whenever possible, intracompartmental tissue pressures should be monitored, with surgical decompression undertaken only if pressure exceeds 30 to 40 mmHg. Vesicles and superficial necrotic tissue should be debrided surgically near the end of the first week following the bite. *Relief of pain* with salicylates or meperidine, moderate sedation, maintenance of fluid balance, measures to combat shock and hemorrhage, and appropriate management of coma or convulsions are all important.

Glucocorticoids do not prevent tissue damage or systemic intoxication but may be of value in the management of shock associated with envenomation and for allergic reactions, such as serum sickness, following the administration of antivenin.

PREVENTION In snake-infested regions, long trousers, high shoes, boots, or leggings, and gloves should be worn. Most important of all is to look where one steps or reaches. A constriction band and antiseptic usually suffice for an emergency kit, but in inaccessible areas antivenin also should be carried.

POISONOUS LIZARD BITE

Only 2 of the nearly 3000 species of lizard in the world are venomous: the Gila monster (*Heloderma suspectum*) of the arid southwestern United States and the Mexican beaded lizard (*H. horridum*) of western Mexico. These reptiles are not aggressive, and virtually every instance of their attacking a human has resulted from teasing or handling the animals in captivity. The venom is elaborated in eight glands in the floor of the mouth and secreted directly into the oral cavity, where it bathes the teeth, which are grooved posteriorly. The lizard clings tenaciously and is often dislodged only after considerable effort; envenomation occurs by contamination of the wound. The venom contains a potent neurotoxin that rarely kills humans. Most often, bites in humans cause tissue injury, excruciating pain, massive edema, and erythema. Acute systemic symptoms may last for 3 to 4 days and include nausea, vomiting, hematemesis, blurred vision, dyspnea, dysphonia, and profound weakness. Intense hyperesthesia of the bitten extremity may persist for weeks. There is no antivenin available. Treatment should consist of constriction band, cooling of the bitten area, measures to prevent or combat infection, including tetanus, and supportive measures. Parenteral meperidine or infiltration of local anesthetic around the bite may be necessary to relieve pain.

SPIDER BITES

The bite of many spiders is locally irritating, and several species can cause severe, even fatal systemic poisoning in humans. In North America, two spiders are of medical importance: the widow spiders (*Latrodectus* species) and the recluse spiders (*Loxosceles* species).

WIDOW SPIDER BITE The most numerous and important of the venomous spiders are members of the genus *Latrodectus*. In the United States and Canada, *L. mactans*, the black widow or show-button spider, causes a majority of clinical arachnidism. In Florida, *L. bishopi*, the red-legged widow spider, can cause similar effects.

It is the female *L. mactans*, the black widow, that bites humans. She is glossy black with a body 1 cm in diameter, a leg span of 5 cm, and a characteristic red hourglass mark on the abdomen. She spins her web in woodpiles, sheds, basements, or outdoor privies, is aggressive, and bites on slight provocation. The venom produces diffuse central and peripheral nervous excitement, autonomic activity, muscle spasm, hypertension, and vasoconstriction.

In the United States, most black widow bites occur between April and October. After a momentary sharp pain at the site, there is cramping pain that begins locally within 15 to 60 min and may spread to involve all extremities and the trunk. The abdomen is boardlike, and the waves of pain become excruciating, causing the patient to turn, toss, and cry out. Respirations are often labored and grunting. There are also nausea, vomiting, headache, sweating, salivation, hyperactive reflexes, twitching, tremor, paresthesias of the hands and feet, and occasionally, systolic hypertension. Leukocytosis is usual, and many patients have fever. After several hours, the pains subside, although mild recurrences for 2 or 3 days are common. It may be a week before well-being is restored. Deaths due to cardiac or respiratory failure have occurred, mostly in children and the aged.

Because the bite itself is not prominent, victims are often thought to have some abdominal catastrophe such as perforated ulcer, pancreatitis, or appendicitis. Renal colic, myocardial infarction, tetanus, strychnine poisoning, lead colic, and porphyria are other conditions to be ruled out. The abdomen is not tender to palpation in arachnidism, and pains in the extremities are not typical of most of these other disorders.

Treatment consists of pain relief and administration of antivenin. Initial treatment should include a hot tub bath which affords prompt, although temporary, relief. The administration of a vial (10 mL) of 10% calcium gluconate intravenously over 10 to 20 min usually produces transient cessation of cramps. The administration of 10%

methocarbamol intravenously also may relieve muscle spasms. Opiates are sometimes necessary. When symptoms are severe or when the patient is a small child or at special risk due to other associated medical problems, *Latrodectus* antivenin should be administered. An intravenous injection of 1 vial (2.5 mL) diluted in 50 mL of saline and administered over a 15-min period is usually effective within a few hours and can be repeated if symptoms recur. Since the antivenin is prepared from horse serum, appropriate testing for hypersensitivity should be undertaken prior to its administration.

LOXOSCELES SPIDER BITE Bites due to *Loxosceles* spiders can cause severe necrosis of tissue. Originally thought to be a problem only in the midwestern states and associated only with the brown recluse spider, necrotic arachnidism also occurs in the southern and southwestern states and in California and has been attributed to at least six species of *Loxosceles* spider. The bite of these spiders may initially produce only a mild stinging discomfort. In severe bites, intense local pain appears within 2 to 8 h, accompanied by bullae formation and erythema at the site of the wound. Subsequently, ischemic necrosis causes a deep ulcer with a necrotic base. The pathogenesis of the local reaction is not completely understood but is thought to involve complement-activated tissue damage. Some patients also experience a systemic reaction characterized by fever, myalgias, and a morbilliform rash 24 to 48 h after the bite. Intravascular hemolysis, hemoglobinuria, and acute renal failure may occur. Fatalities have been reported, mostly in children.

Treatment depends on the severity of the bite. If bullae formation, intense pain, and signs of rapidly progressing ischemic necrosis do not appear within the first 6 to 8 h, the bite is probably not severe, and treatment is unnecessary. When symptoms of more serious local reaction are present, the parenteral use of glucocorticoids within the first 24 h following a bite has been advocated by some to retard progression of the lesion. Dapsone and/or brown recluse antivenin have been reported to prevent extensive ulceration in rapidly progressing *Loxosceles* spider bites. However, use of these forms of therapy should be considered experimental. Other therapeutic measures consist mainly of local wound care, including cool compresses, elevation of the bitten extremity, timely surgical debridement, and treatment of secondary infection. The ulcer usually heals spontaneously, although skin grafting may be required. Patients with systemic loxoscelism should be hospitalized and monitored closely for hemolysis, disseminated intravascular coagulation, and acute renal failure. Although of unproven efficacy, systemic glucocorticoids are usually given for the duration of the acute phase of the illness, which lasts 2 to 4 days. The treatment of renal failure is described in Chap. 236.

SCORPION STING

Glands in the terminal segments of scorpions produce venom, which is injected into the victim by a stinger located on the tip of the tail. Scorpions often enter dwellings. During the day they retreat into crevices; emerging at night, they often get into shoes and clothing and even into bedding. They do not deliberately attack humans, but accidental contact results in a sting.

Of about 650 species, roughly 40 occur in the United States, distributed over three-fourths of the nation. The only dangerous species, *Centruroides exilicauda* (also known as *C. sculpturatus*), is limited to Arizona, New Mexico, southern California, parts of Texas, and northern Mexico. This species reaches a maximal length of about 7 cm. The sting may be fatal to young children or old people but seldom to a healthy adult.

Most of the nonlethal species of scorpions in the United States cause only minor reactions, like a bee sting. Some produce local edema and ecchymosis, with burning pain. In contrast, species whose venom has potentially lethal systemic effects, including the Arizona *Centruroides*, may evoke little or no visible reaction at the site of the sting. There is an immediate burning sensation, followed by local paresthesia ("pins and needles"), hyperesthesia, or numbness. These sensations spread to involve the whole extremity, followed within an hour or two by malaise, restlessness, neurologic hyperexcitability, lacrimation, rhinorrhea, salivation, perspiration, nausea, priapism, and vomiting.

The patient may pass from an agitated state with hyperactive reflexes into coma; convulsions follow, and pleocytosis of the cerebrospinal fluid may be present. Release of catecholamines may result in tachycardia, various arrhythmias, and hypertension. Myocarditis and pancreatitis also have been reported, and cardiomyopathy may be a late complication. Death may occur within 2 days of the sting.

TREATMENT   Despite the reputation for lethality associated with envenomation by *C. sculpturatus*, most often the pain and paresthesias last less than 4 h. These patients can be treated at home with cold compresses and mild analgesics. There is no clear consensus on the management of more severe envenomations. Although the use of constriction bands as in the treatment of snakebite has been recommended, the amount of venom is minute, produces no local necrotizing effect, and is absorbed very rapidly.

Specific antivenin, reconstituted from lyophilized goat serum, is available in some areas but is associated with toxicity and should be considered only if the victim develops signs of cranial nerve dysfunction and increased involuntary activity in skeletal muscles other than those innervated by cranial nerves. An intravenous injection of 1 or 2 vials (5.0 or 10.0 mL) administered over 15 to 30 min usually reverses the severe neurologic symptoms within minutes. Supportive therapy is directed at combating shock and dehydration. Diazepam or phenobarbital is useful in reducing restlessness, and adrenergic blockers may relieve symptoms secondary to catecholamine release. Cardiovascular manifestations can be controlled with channel blocking agents and peripheral vasodilators such as prazosin or isosorbide.

PREVENTION   This depends on alertness in avoiding contact with scorpions in infested areas. Clothing and shoes should be well shaken before being put on in the morning. Towels and bedclothes should be inspected. A house infested with scorpions can in time be rid of them by closing all obvious ways of ingress; picking up debris in the environment, such as piles of brush, logs, and stones; introducing a mixture of fuel oil or kerosene, containing a small amount of creosote, between the earth and the house foundation; and spraying with a mixture of 2% chlordane and 0.2% pyrethrins in an oil base.

HYMENOPTERA STINGS

Each year in the United States, nearly twice as many people die as a result of bites by hymenopterous insects (including bees, wasps, hornets, yellowjackets, and fire ants) as from poisonous snake bites. Occasionally, multiple stings in enormous numbers (500 to 1000) are the cause of death, but most systemic reactions and deaths are due to allergic reactions to the venoms.

Hymenoptera venoms contain many nonallergenic amines and peptides such as histamine and various kinins which contribute to the local sting reaction through their inflammatory and vasoactive properties. The allergenic venom proteins, which elicit an IgE antibody response in those who are stung, include phospholipases, hyaluronidases, acid phosphatases, and melittin. Venoms are distinctly different for each of the three genera capable of causing allergic sting reactions: Apidae (various species of bees), Vespidae (hornets, yellowjackets, and wasps), and *Solenopsis* (fire ants).

The usual reaction to a single bee or wasp sting is sharp pain, which lasts for several minutes, local wheal and erythema, followed by intense itching. All signs of the sting normally subside within a few hours. In the rare case when a bee is swallowed or inhaled, edema of the laryngopharynx or glottis may be life-threatening. A sting directly into a peripheral nerve can destroy its function for a time, and Bell's palsy can result from a sting into the trunk of the

facial nerve. Unusual reactions such as optic neuritis, generalized polyneuropathy, and myasthenia gravis may follow a sting. The etiology of these reactions is unknown. Acute renal failure may occur following multiple bee stings, probably the consequence of venom-induced rhabdomyolysis and renal ischemia.

In hypersensitive individuals, the response to a single sting may vary from an exaggerated local reaction, unassociated with systemic symptoms, to anaphylaxis with urticaria, nausea, abdominal or uterine cramps, bronchospasm, edema of the face and glottis, dyspnea, cyanosis, hypotension, coma, and death. These symptoms usually appear within a few minutes of the sting. Other patients may experience delayed reactions of the serum-sickness type 10 to 14 days after envenomation. Sensitization is usually the result of previous stings. It has been estimated that 10 to 15 percent of the general population is allergic to hymenoptera venom. Those who have experienced a previous systemic allergic reaction to a sting, such as respiratory difficulty, hypotension, or generalized urticaria, are at greatest risk for serious reactions if stung again by the same type of insect.

Since being accidentally introduced into southern Brazil in 1957, Africanized bees have gradually spread through South and Central America and into Texas. Although widely touted as a human health problem, the actual risk is difficult to estimate because of a lack of reliable medical statistics. Africanized bee venom appears to be similar to that of European bees. The real danger from Africanized bees may be that they tend to be aggressive, and multiple stings are common.

Many species of ant can produce stinging bites with local redness and swelling. The most notorious of these are the fire ants (*Solenopsis*), particularly two "imported" South American species (*S. invicta* and *S. richteri*). The *invicta* species is found in many southern states and has largely supplanted other domestic species. In addition to being a major agricultural pest, fire ants, whose bites may result in extensive vesiculation and skin necrosis or cause serious hypersensitivity reactions, constitute a significant health hazard. Unlike other hymenoptera venoms, fire ant venom is mostly a simple insoluble alkaloid, but it may cause life-threatening allergic reactions of the type seen with IgE-mediated immediate hypersensitivity. There is limited cross-sensitivity between fire ant venom and the venoms of bees, wasps, hornets, and yellowjackets.

TREATMENT   The wound site should be examined for a stinger, which, if present, should be removed to prevent further envenomation from the attached gland. The local reaction is treated by local cool application and antipruritic lotions or oral antihistamines. Fire ant stings, which are frequently multiple, should be thoroughly cleaned with soap and water. Secondary bacterial infection is common and should be anticipated and treated promptly. Epinephrine, 0.3 to 0.5 mL of a 1:1000 aqueous solution subcutaneously repeated every 20 to 30 min, may be lifesaving in patients with an anaphylactic reaction to a sting. A tourniquet slows the absorption of venom, and ice packs may relieve pain. Oxygen, endotracheal intubation, vasopressors and other supportive measures should be used as needed. In addition, glucocorticoids should be employed in severe cases.

PREVENTION   Allergic persons should make every effort to avoid contact with these insects, including wearing shoes when outside and not wearing perfumes or bright colors which may attract them. In addition, such persons should keep epinephrine readily available for immediate use in case of a sting, without waiting for symptoms to develop. Sting kits containing premeasured doses of 1:1000 epinephrine in disposable syringes, tourniquets, and antihistamine tablets are available, and patients should be carefully instructed in their use.

IMMUNOTHERAPY   Desensitization by injection of venom of the specific insect has long been recommended for any person who has had a systemic or generalized reaction to hymenopterous insect stings. Purified hymenopterous venoms are used for the diagnosis of sting allergy by skin testing. In addition, venom immunotherapy stimulates production of circulating venom-specific IgG antibodies and provides protection against insect allergy. These venoms are the materials of choice for diagnosis and immunotherapy of high-risk patients, those who have had previous systemic sting reactions and who have positive venom skin tests. The optimal duration of immunotherapy remains to be defined.

TICK BITE

Although ticks may be vectors for such serious diseases as Rocky Mountain spotted fever, Q fever, tularemia, borreliosis, human babesiosis, and Lyme disease, the local reaction to the bite of a tick may be nothing more than an itching papule that subsides within a few days unless there is secondary bacterial infection. However, incomplete removal of a tick, with retention of the mouthparts, may result in the local formation of a pruritic nodule. The definitive treatment is surgical excision of the nodule. Histologically, the nodule is a granuloma, but the inflammatory response is sometimes so bizarre and changes in the overlying epithelium are so striking that, in the absence of a history of tick bite, a mistaken diagnosis of malignancy may be made.

Ticks should always be removed intact using gentle, steady traction. Fine tweezers or blunt forceps should be employed if possible. When fingers are used instead, they should be protected with facial tissue and washed afterwards. Application of a drop of oil, petrolatum, nail polish, or other organic solvent may facilitate removal without leaving embedded remnants. However, touching with a hot object such as a glowing cigarette should be discouraged because of the likelihood of injuring the patient.

TICK PARALYSIS A progressive, ascending, flaccid paralysis, acute ataxia, or a combination of both sometimes develops in humans while a tick is engorging on them. Human cases have most frequently been reported from the northwestern United States and western Canada, where the wood tick, *Dermacentor andersoni* Stiles, is responsible. *D. variabilis* Say, the dog tick, *Amblyomma americanum*, the Lone Star tick, *A. maculatum*, the Gulf Coast tick, and *Ixodes scapularis*, the black-legged deer tick, also have been incriminated.

This disorder is caused by a neurotoxin secreted in the saliva of the engorging tick which acts on spinal and bulbar nuclei, slowing motor nerve conduction without affecting neuromuscular transmission. The tick must feed for several days before symptoms develop.

Most human cases occur in children, generally in young girls. The tick is usually attached to the scalp and hidden by the hair but may be found on any part of the body, including the ear, axilla, groin, vulva, or popliteal region.

The patient may be irritable or restless for up to 24 h before frank motor involvement appears. Weakness usually is noted first in the distal muscles of the lower extremities, progressing over the next 24 to 48 h to flaccid paralysis, which may extend to involve the trunk, arms, neck, tongue, pharynx, and bulbar centers. Sensory changes are typically absent, and there is little or no fever unless a secondary infection is present. Results of routine laboratory tests, including cerebrospinal fluid examination, are normal. Nerve conduction studies may reveal decreased velocities and compound action potentials of nerves and their corresponding muscles.

Among diseases to be considered in the differential diagnosis are diphtheritic polyneuropathy, transverse myelitis, the Guillain-Barré syndrome, myasthenia gravis, the Eaton-Lambert syndrome, botulism, and poliomyelitis.

Definitive treatment requires removal of the tick, including any mouthparts retained in the skin. After this is done, there is striking improvement of motor function within a few hours and complete recovery within 48 h.

The patient should be observed until the recovery trend is established, because if other ticks or retained mouthparts are overlooked, the paralysis may progress. Bulbar or respiratory paralysis may cause death if the tick is not removed in time. The mortality rate is 10 percent; nearly all who die are children.

OTHER ARTHROPOD BITES AND ENVENOMATIONS

FLEA BITE Many fleas attack humans, including *Pulex irritans* and chicken fleas. In sensitive individuals, the salivary secretion of these bloodsuckers produces large, itching papules. Much of the papular urticaria of children is probably due to flea bites. Treatment is symptomatic. Elimination of fleas from the environment may be very difficult, but persistent treatment of animals and of premises with appropriate insecticides is usually successful.

CENTIPEDE BITE The giant desert centipede, which reaches 15 cm in length, is responsible for most centipede bites in the United States. It is capable of inflicting an intensely painful bite, associated with erythema, edema, and sometimes regional lymphangitis. Rhabdomyolysis and acute renal failure have occurred following the bite of this arthropod. Pain usually disappears within a few hours but may require oral or parenteral analgesics. The wound should be washed well with soap and water to help prevent secondary infection.

CATERPILLAR RASH Contact with the early larval or caterpillar stage of several species of moth produces irritation of skin and mucous membranes resulting in a pruritic, erythematous rash, occasionally accompanied by urticaria and bullae. Symptoms come on rapidly after direct contact with caterpillars, after handling cocoons, or on being exposed to windblown fuzz. The pathogenesis is thought to be due to the direct irritant effects of insect hairs or appendages, although other mechanisms, including intracutaneous injection of toxins or hypersensitivity to insect antigens, have been suggested. The symptoms usually subside within a few days. Local soaks and oral antihistamines are often indicated.

BEDBUG BITE Members of the genus *Cimex* inflict bites that leave reactions varying from a simple puncture to large urticarial lesions, apparently depending on the sensitivity of the bitten individual. There is no specific treatment.

KISSING BUG BITE Of the many species of true bugs, those in the family Reduviidae are relatively commonly associated with severe bite reactions. The most important reduviid bug in this country is the kissing bug (genus *Triatoma*), which is found throughout the southern crescent of the United States. The bites of this bug, which is a nocturnal feeder, are characteristically inflicted in multiple groups. Reactions are thought to be allergic in nature and may include intensely pruritic and painful papules with a central punctum, grouped vesicles with moderate swelling and redness but no central lesions, giant urticaria, generalized allergic reactions, including systemic anaphylaxis, and hemorrhagic nodular to bullous lesions on a hand or foot appearing several days after the bite. These may be confused with necrotizing spider bites or with erythema multiforme. However, the former are usually single lesions, and the latter rarely has a unilateral distribution. The possibility of kissing bug bites should be considered in patients who awaken in the middle of the night with intense itching, hives, and other signs of a systemic allergic reaction.

Treatment of the local reaction is symptomatic. More severe reactions should be managed similarly to other allergic sting reactions. Patients who have had accelerated reactions to reduviid bites should be provided with sting kits and instructions in their use. Immunotherapy with whole-body extracts of kissing bugs has been attempted but is unproven.

CHIGGERS OR REDBUGS These tiny mites are found in foliage or grass in many parts of the world. In the United States, the larval form of *Eutrobicula alfreddugesi* attacks the skin by secreting a substance that digests tissue, creating a red papule that itches intensely. The tiny reddish larva can be seen in the center of the lesion. Treatment is palliative and consists of antipruritic agents. The use of insect repellents, protective clothing, and prompt bathing after exposure reduce the risk of infestation.

BLOODSUCKING-FLY BITE Many species of flies, particularly the horsefly and the deerfly, attack and feed on warm-blooded animals, including humans. Transmission of diseases such as anthrax, tularemia, loiasis, and trypanosomiasis has been attributed to horseflies and deerflies. More commonly in North America, however, the bites are responsible for painful, intensely pruritic cutaneous lesions which may be followed by delayed localized allergic reactions characterized by erythema, edema, and urticaria. Treatment should include thorough cleaning of the bite sites, topical glucocorticoids, and oral antihistaminics for severe itching. Antibiotics may be necessary for secondary infections.

MARINE ANIMAL VENOM DISEASES

The venoms of certain marine animals can cause illness in humans after injection or inoculation under naturally occurring conditions. Information concerning these toxins is limited; most appear to be composed of proteins, peptides, and other substances. Although probably less complex than the venoms of reptiles, many marine animal venoms can cause several pathologic effects including neurotoxicity and local necrosis.

PORTUGUESE MAN-OF-WAR AND JELLYFISH STINGS   The burning discomfort induced by contact with sea nettles or jellyfish is familiar to most surf bathers. Contact with the tentacles of the colorful Portuguese man-of-war (*Physalia* species), which is found mainly in or near the Gulf of Mexico, or the more toxic jellyfish (*Chiropsalmus* of the Indian Ocean and *Rhizostoma* of the Atlantic) is followed by burning pain, swelling, and erythema. Severe, generalized muscular cramps, nausea, vomiting, and pulmonary edema may occur. Victims can die as a result of jellyfish stings, sometimes within minutes after contact. In nonfatal cases, systemic symptoms usually subside within several hours. Treatment consists of bathing the wound in saltwater, taking care not to rub the area of the sting. Any tentacles still clinging to the skin should be scraped off after first inactivating any remaining nematocysts to prevent discharge of additional venom into the victim. This can be done by sprinkling baking soda over the wound to form a slurry for sea nettle stings or by bathing with vinegar for man-of-war stings. Rinsing with freshwater, isopropyl alcohol, or household ammonia or rubbing with sand are not recommended because these measures may actually cause nematocysts to discharge. Analgesics should be used for pain control, and antihistamines should be given for pruritus. Severe envenomations may require advanced life-support measures. Glucocorticoids may be helpful in these cases. An antivenin is available for treatment of stings by the highly lethal Australian sea wasp, *Chironex fleckeri*.

CORAL WOUNDS AND STINGS   The colorful structures known as coral are composed of thousands of small marine animals of the coelenterate phylum surrounded by a stony exoskeleton of calcium carbonate. Several species, including the fire coral, contain microscopic nematocysts capable of producing painful stings similar to those caused by jellyfish. Often more serious are wounds resulting from abrasions and cuts by the sharp edges of the outer skeleton. These frequently contain small pieces of animal protein and skeletal material that act as foreign bodies and may lead to chronic, suppurative wound infections if not debrided promptly and adequately.

SEA ANEMONE STING ("SPONGE DIVER'S DISEASE")   Contact with certain sea anemones (especially *Sargatia elegans*) in Mediterranean and African waters produces extensive dermatitis with chronic ulceration. Occasionally, especially during August and September, systemic symptoms include headache, sneezing, nausea, chills, fever, and collapse. Rare fatalities have occurred. Application of vinegar may inactivate nematocyst discharge. No other specific therapy is known; symptomatic treatment with topical steroids or oral antihistaminics may provide temporary relief.

CONE SHELL POISONING   Many species of cone shells in the Pacific are venomous, a great danger to unwary hobbyists who pick them up. The poison, a neurotoxin, is delivered into a wound inflicted by pointed hollow teeth resembling darts in the long proboscis of the animal. Local manifestations include sudden intense pain, followed by swelling and numbness, which may persist for several days. Symptoms of serious poisoning include muscular incoordination and

weakness progressing to respiratory paralysis. Death may occur within 3 to 6 h, but recovery within 24 h is the rule. There is no specific therapy; recommended treatment is the use of tourniquet, incision, and suction and supportive measures which may include artificial respiration and administration of oxygen.

SPONGE DERMATITIS   Direct contact with several species of sponge results in a painful dermatitis which may persist for several weeks. The lesions appear to be caused by mechanical irritation from the exoskeleton of the sponge as well as by toxins within its tissues. Delayed hypersensitivity reactions also may occur. Topical glucocorticoids or oral antihistamines may provide relief from the pruritus; dilute acetic acid ameliorates local pain, while alkali will intensify it. The lesions are self-limited.

SEA URCHIN WOUNDS AND STINGS   Contact with the spines of some species of sea urchin results in painful erythema and ulceration, occasionally accompanied by neurotoxic symptoms of weakness and frank paralysis of lips, tongue, and face lasting for several hours. Treatment is purely symptomatic and supportive. The toxins isolated from sea urchins have produced paralysis in animals and are notably resistant to heat. Deaths from paralysis and drowning have been reported. Occasionally, fragments of sea urchin spines may remain in the skin, leading to granulomatous reactions, or they may migrate into a joint or lodge against a nerve, causing intractable pain. Treatment of these complications is surgical.

PARALYTIC AND NEUROTOXIC SHELLFISH POISONING   Certain dinoflagellates, which make up part of the marine phytoplankton, elaborate a potent neurotoxin. Occasionally, conditions in coastal waters become favorable for the growth of excessive numbers of these organisms, causing the water to develop an amber appearance termed *red tide* and killing massive numbers of fish by exhausting their oxygen supply. When humans ingest shellfish which have themselves ingested toxic dinoflagellates, manifestations include paresthesias of the face and extremities, dysphonia, and generalized muscular weakness, often accompanied by nausea, vomiting, and diarrhea and occasionally by paralysis and respiratory arrest. The more severe syndrome, known as *paralytic shellfish poisoning*, is encountered along the Pacific northwest and New England coasts. A milder form, not associated with paralysis in humans, is seen along the Gulf and Atlantic coasts of Florida. Treatment should include induced emesis and purgation to remove unabsorbed toxin from the gastrointestinal tract and whatever additional supportive measures are necessary. Spontaneous recovery usually takes place within 24 h.

VENOMOUS FISH INJURIES   The dorsal fins or spines of bullhead sharks, dogfish, and ratfish and the dorsal and other fins of the lionfish, weeverfish, toadfish, and catfish are grooved and contain venom glands at the base. Little is known of the venoms involved except that they contain proteins and are capable of causing toxic as well as allergic reactions.

Envenomation results in immediate, severe local pain and edema which, if untreated, reaches greatest intensity in 60 to 90 min and resolves within 8 to 12 h. Local necrosis may occur, particularly following lionfish and catfish stings. Systemic reactions, including cardiac arrhythmias, hypotension, muscular weakness, seizures, and paralysis, have been attributed to the effects of the venom.

Treatment should be immediate immersion of the wound in water as hot as the patient can stand for at least 1 h or until symptoms subside. The venoms are extremely heat labile, accounting for the usefulness of this procedure. Although rarely needed, an antivenin for patients with severe systemic reactions from stonefish envenomation can be obtained from the Health Services Department, Sea World of San Diego [(619) 222-0411]. Tetanus prophylaxis should be given as needed. Narcotics may be required to control pain. Secondary pyogenic infection is a frequent complication.

Probably the most frequent type of fish envenomation in the United States is that produced by the lashing tail of the stingray of the California coast (*Urobatis halleri*). The bony spine is encased in a sheath of epithelial cells containing venom which is expressed into the puncture wound. The wound may be several centimeters deep;

portions of the bony spine may break off in it, or more often, the integumentary sheath remains in the wound. The venom is a circulatory depressant in animals, but local injury predominates in humans. Severe pain and blanching are followed by erythema and edema. Symptoms due to systemic absorption of venom are infrequent but may include salivation, muscle cramps and weakness, cardiac arrhythmias, seizures, and death. Treatment consists of application of a constriction band (the vast majority of these injuries occur on the legs) and copious syringing of the wound with saltwater to remove fragments of sheath. Additional therapeutic measures are the same as for other fish envenomations, including immersion of the injured area in hot water for up to 1 h.

REFERENCES

Snake and lizard bites

GOLD BS, BARISH RA: Venomous snakebites: Current concepts in diagnosis, treatment, and management. Emerg Med Clin North Am 10:249, 1992

JURKOVICH GL et al: Complications of Crotalidae antivenin therapy. J Trauma 28:1032, 1988

KITCHENS CS, VAN MIEROP LHS: Envenomation by the eastern coral snake (*Micrurus fulvius fulvius*): A study of 39 victims. JAMA 258:1615, 1987

LOPRINZI CL et al: Snake antivenin administration in a patient allergic to horse serum. South Med J 76:501, 1983

MITRAKUL C, DHAMKROGN A: Clinical features of neurotoxic snake bite and response to antivenom in 47 children. Am J Trop Med Hyg 33:1258, 1984

RUSSELL FE: *Snake Venom Poisoning*. New York, Scholium International, 1983

———, BOGERT CM: Gila monster: Its biology, venom and bite: A review. Toxicon 19:341, 1981

WINGERT WA, CHAN L: Rattlesnake bites in southern California and rationale for recommended treatment. West J Med 148:37, 1988

Spider bite

ALLEN C: Arachnid envenomations. Emerg Med Clin North Am 10:269, 1992

CLARK RF et al: Clinical presentation and treatment of black widow spider envenomation review of 163 cases. Ann Emerg Med 21:782, 1992

FUTRELL JM: Loxoscelism. Am J Med Sci 304:261, 1992

WILSON DC, KING LE JR: Spiders and spider bites. Dermatol Clin 8:277, 1990

Scorpion sting

BERG RA, TARATINO MD: Envenomation by the scorpion *Centruroides exilicauda* (*C. sculpturatus*): Severe and unusual manifestations. Pediatrics 87:930, 1991

BOND GR: Antivenin administration for centruroides scorpion sting: Risks and benefits. Ann Emerg Med 21:788, 1992

GUERON M, SOFER S: Vasodilators and calcium blocking agents as treatment of cardiovascular manifestations of human scorpion envenomation. Toxicon 28:127, 1990

KUMAR EB et al: Scorpion venom cardiomyopathy. Am Heart J 123:725, 1992

Hymenoptera stings

DESHAZO RD et al: Reactions to the stings of the imported fire ant. N Engl J Med 323:462, 1990

ELGART GW: Ant, bee, and wasp stings: Dermatol Clin 8:229, 1990.

GOLDEN DBK et al: Discontinuing venom immunotherapy (VIT): Immunologic and clinical criteria. J Allergy Clin Immunol 79:126, 1987

MEJIA G et al: Acute renal failure due to multiple stings by Africanized bees. Ann Intern Med 104:210, 1986

REISMAN RE: Stinging insect allergy. Med Clin North Am 76:883, 1992

RHOADES RB et al: Survey of fatal anaphylactic reactions to imported fire ant stings. J Allergy Clin Immunol 84:159, 1989

TAYLOR OR JR: Health problems associated with African bees (editorial). Ann Intern Med 104:267, 1986

VALENTINE MD et al: The value of immunotherapy with venom in children with allergy to insect stings. N Engl J Med 323:1601, 1990

VAN DER LINDEN PWG et al: Insect-sting challenge in 138 patients: Relation between clinical severity of anaphylaxis and mast cell activation. J Allergy Clin Immunol 90:110, 1992

Tick bite and tick paralysis

GOTHE R et al: The mechanism of pathogenicity in the tick paralysis. J Med Entomol 16:357, 1979

KINCAID JC: Tick bite paralysis. Semin Neurol 10:32, 1990

NEEDHAM GR: Evaluation of 5 popular methods for tick removal. Pediatrics 75:997, 1985

SPIELMAN A: How to diagnose and treat tick and mite infestations. Drug Ther 11:77, 1981

Other arthropod bites and envenomations

FRAZIER CA: *Insect Allergy: Allergic and Toxic Reactions to Insects and Other Arthropods*. St. Louis, Grace, 1969

HUNT GR: Bites and stings of uncommon arthropods: Postgrad Med 70:107, 1981

LOGAN JL, OGDEN DA: Rhabdomyolysis and acute renal failure following the bite of the giant desert centiped *Scolopendra heros*. West J Med 142:549, 1985

PINSON RT, MORGAN JA: Envenomation by the puss caterpillar (*Megalopyge opercularis*). Ann Emerg Med 126:562, 1991

ROSEN T: Caterpillar dermatitis. Dermatol Clin 8:245, 1990

SHELLEY ED et al: The diagnostic challenge of non-burrowing mite bites. JAMA 251:2690, 1984

WIRTZ RA: Allergic and toxic reactions to non-stinging arthropods. Annu Rev Entomol 29:47, 1984

Marine animal venom diseases

AUERBACH PS, HALSTEAD BW: Hazardous marinelife, in *Management of Wilderness and Environmental Emergencies*, PS Auerbach, HR Gee (eds). New York, Macmillan, 1983

BROWN CK, SHEPHERD SM: Marine trauma, envenomations, and intoxications. Emerg Med Clin North Am 10:385, 1992

HUGHES JM, MERSON MH: Fish and shellfish poisoning. N Engl J Med 295:1117, 1976

McGOLDRICK J, MARX JA: Marine envenomations: 1. Vertebrates. J Emerg Med 9:497, 1991

———, ———: Marine envenomations: 2. Invertebrates. J Emerg Med 10:71, 1992

ROSSON CL, TOLLE SW: Management of marine stings and scrapes. West J Med 150:97, 1989

ZERMAN MG: Catfish stings: A report of 3 cases. Ann Emerg Med 18:211, 1989

---

398 HYPOTHERMIA AND HYPERTHERMIA

ROBERT G. PETERSDORF

CONTROL OF BODY TEMPERATURE

Normal body temperature in humans is maintained within a narrow range despite extremes in environmental conditions and physical activity. A common accompaniment of systemic illness is a disturbance in temperature regulation, usually an abnormal elevation, or *fever*. Even in the absence of a frank febrile response, interference with body temperature regulation by disease is evident. This may take the form of flushing, pallor, sweating, shivering, and abnormal sensations of cold or warmth, or it may consist of erratic fluctuations of body temperature. The pathogenesis, diagnosis, and treatment of fever are discussed in Chap. 16.

HEAT PRODUCTION The major sources of basal heat production are through thyroid hormone thermogenesis and the action of adenosine triphosphatase (ATPase) on the sodium pump of all membranes. The muscles are most important in promoting increased heat production through increased shivering. The quantity of heat production can be varied according to the need. This variation ranges from small increases and decreases of nerve impulses to the muscles with inapparent tensing or relaxing to shivering or even a generalized rigor. During digestion of food, gastrointestinal production of heat is significant.

HEAT LOSS Heat is lost from the body by *convection, conduction, radiation,* and *evaporation*. Small amounts are used in warming food or drink and in the evaporation of moisture from the respiratory tract. Heat loss by convection results from a temperature gradient between the body surface and the ambient air. Conduction heat loss occurs with direct contact of the body surface. The major loss occurs through radiation, defined as an exchange of electromagnetic energy between the body and the radiant environment. Evaporation is the fourth major mechanism for dissipating heat and is particularly important when the ambient temperature exceeds that of the body or when core temperatures are increased by vigorous exercise. The degree to which each of these four mechanisms contributes to heat loss depends on ambient temperature, wind, solar radiation, and body immersion.

The principal method of regulating heat loss is by varying the volume of blood flowing to the surface of the body. A rich circulation in the skin and subcutaneous tissues carries heat to the surface, where it can escape. In addition, sweating increases heat loss by providing water to be vaporized. The sweat, or eccrine, glands are under the control of cholinergic sympathetic nerves. Heat loss by sweating may be tremendous, and as much as 1 L/h of sweat may be evaporated. The amount of heat loss through sweating is also dependent on the humidity in the air. The greater the humidity, the less the ability to lose heat through sweat.

When there is need for conservation of heat, adrenergic autonomic stimuli cause a sharp reduction in the blood flow to the surface. This causes vasoconstriction and transforms the skin and subcutaneous tissue into layers of insulation.

HEAT TRANSFER WITHIN THE BODY   This depends on conduction, i.e., the transfer of heat between adjacent organs, and on *circulatory convection*, which is governed by bulk movement of body fluids and which is responsible for the transfer of heat between the cells and the bloodstream. It is useful, although oversimplified, to visualize the body as a central core at uniform temperatures surrounded by an insulating shell. The role of the shell as a mediator for heat conservation and heat loss is determined in part by its blood supply and by vasoconstriction or vasodilatation. Although insulation is relatively uniform throughout the body, some parts, such as the digits, are particularly susceptible to cold because of the increased surface-to-volume ratio. Moreover, blood that reaches the digits has already been cooled on the way. Insulation may be enhanced by the addition of clothing.

NEURAL CONTROL OF TEMPERATURE   The control of body temperature, integrating the various physical and chemical processes for heat production or heat loss, is a function of the hypothalamus. The temperature-regulating system is a negative feedback control system and possesses three elements essential to such a system: (1) receptors that sense the existing central temperatures, (2) effector mechanisms, consisting of the vasomotor, sudomotor, and metabolic effectors, and (3) integrative structures that determine whether the existing temperature is too high or too low and that activate the appropriate motor response. A rise in central temperature initiates mechanisms for losing heat, while a fall in central temperature activates mechanisms for heat production and heat conservation. The activation of these effector responses is governed by a central integrative mechanism that may be compared with a thermostat and that responds to a variety of stimuli, such as the sensory impulses engendered in flushing or sweating, behavioral impulses, exercise, endocrine influences, and probably the temperature of the blood circulating through the hypothalamic centers. In a sense, all these stimuli reset the thermostat, thereby activating compensatory heat loss or heat conservation mechanisms.

NORMAL BODY TEMPERATURE   It is not practical to designate an exact upper level of normal body temperature because there are small differences among normal persons. There are rare individuals whose temperatures are always elevated slightly above accepted "normal" levels, and there is considerable variation in temperature in a given individual. In general, however, it is safe to regard an oral temperature above 37.7°C (99.9°F) in a person at bed rest as probable indication of disease. The temperature may be as low as 35.8°C (96.5°F) in healthy persons. Rectal temperature is usually 0.3 to 0.6°C (0.5 to 1.0°F) above oral temperature. In very hot weather, the body temperature may be elevated by the same amounts.

There is a distinct diurnal variation in body temperature in healthy human beings. Oral readings of 36.1°C (97°F) are relatively common on arising in the morning. Body temperature rises steadily through the day, reaches a peak of 37.2°C (99°F) or greater between 6 P.M. and 10 P.M., and then drops slowly to reach a minimum at 2 A.M. to 4 A.M. Although it has been postulated that this diurnal variation is dependent on increasing activity during the day and rest at night, the pattern is not reversed in individuals who work at night and sleep during the day. The variation is now attributed to a circadian rhythm

driven by the hypothalamus (see Chap. 16). The febrile patterns of most human diseases also tend to follow this normal circadian variation. Fevers tend to be higher, i.e., to "spike," in the evening, and many patients with febrile disease have relatively normal temperatures in the early morning hours.

Body temperature is more labile in young children, and transient elevations after relatively slight exertion in warm weather are frequently observed.

Severe or prolonged exercise can produce considerable elevation in body temperature. For example, marathon runners may develop temperatures between 39 and 41°C (103.2 and 105.8°F). Although heat loss may be increased by cutaneous vasodilatation and by hyperventilation, these compensatory mechanisms may fail, leading to hyperpyrexia and, if uncontrolled, to heat stroke. Many of the adverse effects of long-distance running can be prevented by holding races only if the ambient temperature is below 27.8°C (82°F), preferably in the early morning or early evening, and by ensuring ample fluid intake both before and during a race.

DISORDERED THERMOREGULATION   In exercise, there is a temporary imbalance between heat production and heat loss with prompt reestablishment of normal temperatures at rest due to continuing activation of heat loss mechanisms. In prolonged exercise cutaneous vasodilatation in response to an increase in central body temperature ceases in order to preserve central temperature. Less adaptation occurs in fever because once a stable body temperature is reached, heat production equals heat loss, but both are greater than in the basal state. Cutaneous blood flow plays a greater role in controlling heat production and heat loss in fever than does sweating. At the beginning of fever, the body temperature as sensed by the thermoreceptors is low, and the individual responds physiologically as if he or she were cold. *Heat production* is increased by shivering, and *heat loss* is decreased by vasoconstriction. These events explain the sensation of cold or chills that characterizes the beginning of fever. Conversely, when the cause of fever is removed, the temperature returns to normal, and the individual responds as if warm. Cutaneous vasodilation, sweating, and inhibition of shivering are the compensatory responses.

Deviations of ±3°C (approximately 5°F) from the normal body temperature do not interfere appreciably with most bodily functions. Convulsions are common at temperatures higher than 41.1°C (106°F) in children, and irreversible brain damage is common when temperatures of 42.2°C (108°F) are reached. Oral temperatures above 41.1°C (106°F) are relatively rare in humans. Conversely, when temperatures are lowered to 32.8°C (91°F) or below, confusion and loss of consciousness occur; at 30°C (86°F) and below, slow atrial fibrillation supervenes. Ventricular fibrillation occurs at extremely hypothermic temperatures and is often a terminal event.

Disease of the regulatory centers in the hypothalamus may affect body temperature. Destruction of the posterior hypothalamic centers controlling heat-conserving mechanisms results in hypothermia. Cerebral lesions also may cause hyperthermia; they include tumors, degenerative diseases, vascular accidents, particularly cerebral hemorrhage, or infections involving the hypothalamus, such as encephalitis. Central fever is accompanied by lack of a circadian variation, absence of sweating, resistance to antipyretic drugs, excessive response to external cooling, and loss of consciousness.

DISORDERS ASSOCIATED WITH HIGH TEMPERATURES

HEAT SYNDROMES   Four clinical syndromes are associated with high environmental temperature: *heat cramps, heat exhaustion, exertional heat injury*, and *heat stroke*. Although each of these entities may be separated from the others on clinical grounds, there is considerable overlap between them, and they may be considered as a series of syndromes along a single spectrum. The incidence of heat syndromes is unknown, but during an ordinary summer about 200 cases of heat stroke are reported. During the heat wave of June 1984, there was a 35 percent increase in mortality in New York City almost exclusively due to a rise in deaths in elderly persons living at home. Heat syndromes occur primarily at elevated ambient temperatures [>32°C (>90°F)] and at high relative humidities (>60%) in elderly individuals, particularly those with mental illness or alcoholism or who receive antipsychotic drugs, diuretics, and anticholinergics, or those who reside in poorly ventilated places without air conditioning. Heat syndromes are especially prevalent during the first days of a heat wave before effective acclimatization can occur. Prophylaxis by augmenting fluid intake prior to exposure and by ensuring that susceptible individuals, particularly the elderly or the very young, wear light clothing, use fans, take frequent cool baths, remain in a cool environment, and avoid strenuous physical activity can help prevent the full-blown syndrome, especially heat stroke.

Acclimatization The mechanisms by which humans accommodate to excessive temperatures remain unclear. Acclimatization requires 7 to 14 days of exposure. Acclimatization lowers the threshold for sweating; i.e., sweating occurs at a lower core temperature. However, sweating is the most effective natural means of combating heat stress and can occur with little or no change in the core temperature of the body. As long as sweating continues, humans can withstand remarkably high temperatures, provided water and sodium chloride, the most important physiologic constituents of sweat, are replaced. The concentration of sodium chloride varies between very low concentrations and that of interstitial fluid. The sodium concentration in sweat may fall from 65 mEq/L to as low as 5 mEq/L after acclimatization, and the volume may increase from 1 L/h to as much as 4 L/h. Dilatation of the peripheral blood vessels in an attempt to dissipate heat is another major way for the body to acclimatize to hot temperatures. After acclimatization occurs, there is a decreased heart rate at a given temperature, and heat stress is accompanied by an increased stroke volume with no change in cardiac output. These changes occur because of a 10 to 25 percent increase in plasma volume. Other alterations include a decrease in renal blood flow and an increase of antidiuretic hormone (ADH), growth hormone, and aldosterone secretion. The hyperaldosteronism may result in potassium loss, which may be aggravated by replacement of sodium without concomitant repletion of potassium. As heat stress persists, venous return diminishes and cardiac output may fall. If environmental temperatures in excess of the body's temperature persist, heat is retained and hyperpyrexia develops.

Heat cramps Heat cramps are the most benign heat syndrome. They are characterized by brief, intermittent, and often excruciating cramping pain and usually follow strenuous exercise in the muscles that have been subjected to extensive work. They may develop in nonacclimatized laborers or in conditioned athletes. External temperatures do not usually exceed the body temperature, and direct exposure to the sun is not necessary. The body temperature is usually normal, and the victim sweats normally or excessively. Heat cramps may even be precipitated by strenuous exercise in cold environments in untrained persons who are heavily clothed. Muscles of the extremities bear the brunt of physical activity and hence show the highest incidence of cramps. Treatment consists of rest in a cool environment and replacement of sodium, potassium, and fluid. This syndrome may be prevented by liberal salting of food and ample intake of water. Salt tablets are gastric irritants and should not be given. Isotonic electrolyte solutions are recommended by some authors.

Heat exhaustion This is also called *heat prostration* or heat collapse and is probably the most common heat syndrome. Heat exhaustion occurs in two forms, one due to water depletion and the other due to salt depletion. The symptoms arise from a failure of cardiovascular responses to high external temperatures. Water depletion is common in elderly individuals who are receiving diuretics or in anyone who has inadequate water intake in a hot environment. Body temperature elevation is common. Salt depletion occurs with inadequate salt replacement, does not cause hyperthermia, and is accompanied by hyponatremia and hypochloremia. Both forms of heat exhaustion cause weakness, anxiety, fatigue, thirst, vertigo, headache, anorexia, nausea, vomiting, and the urge to defecate, and faintness may precede collapse. There may be hyperventilation, muscular incoordination, agitation, impaired judgment, and confusion. Heat collapse (heat syncope) occurs in both physically active and sedentary individuals. The onset is usually sudden and the duration of collapse brief. During the acute stage, the patient looks ashen-gray. The skin is cold and clammy. The pupils are dilated. Orthostatic hypotension is common, and the pulse rate is elevated. The duration of exposure and the extent to which sweat is lost determine the treatment, which consists of removing the patient to a cool area and placing him or her in the recumbent position. Spontaneous recovery then usually takes place. Intravenous administration of saline solution is sometimes recommended, administered slowly over 48 h, although oral replacement of water and electrolytes may be sufficient.

Heat stroke Heat stroke occurs when body thermal regulation is unable to dissipate adequate amounts of heat with rise in body temperature, often to greater than 41°C (106°F). This results in multiple organ system failure. Heat stroke often begins suddenly with central nervous system (CNS) signs, including headache, slurred speech, vertigo, faintness, hallucinations, seizures, confusion, delirium, or coma. Focal neurologic signs are unusual and should prompt aggressive evaluation of the patient for other causes of CNS abnormalities.

Heat stroke can be divided into *exertional* and *classic forms*. Exertional heat stroke occurs in healthy, young individuals and is usually sporadic. The patient sweats normally. Classic heat stroke occurs in older individuals in epidemic form during heat waves. Patients do not sweat normally. Many persons with classic heat stroke have preexisting chronic disease, including arteriosclerosis and congestive heart failure (particularly when such patients receive diuretics), diabetes mellitus, or alcoholism, or have received one of several drugs that interfere with heat loss. Excessive exertion leads initially to symptoms of headache, piloerection (gooseflesh), chills, hyperventilation, nausea, vomiting, muscle cramps, ataxia, unsteady gait, and incoherent speech. With progression, loss of consciousness may occur. Physical examination shows tachycardia, hypotension, and evidence of low peripheral resistance. Laboratory data show hemoconcentration, hypernatremia, abnormal liver and muscle enzymes, hypocalcemia, hypophosphatemia, and, in some instances, hypoglycemia. As the syndrome progresses after exertion, thrombocytopenia, hemolysis, disseminated intravascular coagulation, rhabdomyolysis, myoglobinuria, and acute tubular necrosis may ensue. Multiple organ failure may occur.

Exertional heat stroke can be prevented by (1) running races early in the morning when the temperature and humidity are likely to be low, (2) educating runners to enter a race well hydrated by drinking 300 mL of water 10 min before a race and 250 mL every 3 to 4 km (salt and glucose solutions should be avoided), (3) placing aid stations at 5-km intervals, (4) instructing runners not to increase their pace after most of the race has been run, and (5) avoiding alcohol before a race.

Classic heat stroke may develop rapidly with few premonitory symptoms, and loss of consciousness may be an early sign. Patients may complain of headache, vertigo, faintness, abdominal distress, confusion, or hyperpnea. Pyrexia and prostration are the most significant findings on physical examination. Rectal temperature greater than 41.1°C (106°F) is common, and internal body temperatures as high as 44.4°C (112 to 113°F) have been recorded. Skin is hot and dry, the pulse rate is rapid, and respirations are weak. The blood pressure is usually low. The muscles are flaccid, and tendon reflexes may be diminished. Lethargy, stupor, or coma, depending on the severity, is present. Shock is common in fatal cases. Coma, hypotension, disseminated intravascular coagulation, and the necessity for intubation are bad prognostic indicators.

Major organ system failure includes right-sided cardiac failure with tachycardia, elevated cardiac index, and elevated central venous pressure. Hepatic damage is common. Jaundice may occur 1 to 2 days after admission. Acute oliguric renal failure may occur. Urinalysis may reveal concentrated urine and proteinuria with granular casts and red blood cells. Rhabdomyolysis and myoglobinuria may contribute to renal failure. Any evidence of bleeding should suggest disseminated intravascular coagulation, which always carries a poor prognosis.

DIFFERENTIAL DIAGNOSIS   The presence of an extremely high core temperature (41°C or higher) with exposure to heat stress, CNS dysfunction, and elevation of liver enzymes are generally required to make the diagnosis of heat stroke. Other illnesses that may mimic the condition are cerebral malaria, meningitis, encephalitis, and rarely, stroke, particularly brainstem hemorrhage. Thyrotoxicosis, delirium tremens, anticholinergic poisoning, and a number of other systemic infectious diseases also may mimic heat stroke.

TREATMENT   Heat stroke is a medical emergency, and immediate heroic emergency measures are required. In hot climates, ambulances should be air-conditioned. Once the patient is in the emergency room, time is of the essence. All clothing should be removed. The patient should be wheeled into a shower on a gurney. At the same time, ice should be applied to the lateral aspects of the trunk while the patient is sprayed with tepid water from the shower. A fan should be directed on the patient to accelerate heat dissipation by convection. Intravenous solutions should be chilled before administration.

After immediate evaluation and measurement of vital signs, the temperature should be measured continuously with an equilibrated thermocouple. Immersion of the patient in an ice-water bath is a time-honored treatment, but it creates difficulties in medical care if resuscitation is required. It should only be used in centers with written protocols and experience with this form of treatment. Other adjunctive forms of cooling include cooling blankets and gastric and rectal lavage. Massage of the skin may be employed along with cooling because it may stimulate return of the cool peripheral blood to the brain and viscera.

Hydration should be done carefully because in most patients fluid requirement over the first 12 h is only 1000 to 1200 mL. If hypotension persists despite successful cooling, central venous pressure should be monitored and further intravenous therapy given. Establishment of a proper airway, avoidance of aspiration, treatment of convulsions, and watching for arrhythmias will lead to survival of most patients, particularly if they are young and were previously well. Unfortunately, the poor, ill, and elderly, who are often not discovered until heat hyperpyrexia has been present for some hours, have a much less favorable outcome.

MALIGNANT HYPERTHERMIA   Etiology and epidemiology
Malignant hyperthermia (MH) consists of a group of inherited disorders that are characterized by a rapid increase in temperature to 39 to 42°C (102.2 to 107.6°F) in response to inhalational anesthetics such as halothane, methoxyflurane, cyclopropane, and ethyl ether or muscle relaxants, notably succinylcholine. In one form of the disease in which the mechanism of inheritance is autosomal dominant, the individuals are normal between attacks, although some have an elevation in creatine phosphokinase (CPK), and in 90 percent of such cases, biopsied muscle from susceptible individuals contracts on exposure to caffeine or halothane at concentrations that do not alter normal muscle contraction.

Interval CPK screening is not useful in detection of susceptible patients. Muscle biopsy followed by the halothane-caffeine contraction reaction is accurate but tedious. A careful history from the patient, including questioning about abnormal reactions during surgery suggestive of MH in relatives, is the most accurate way to detect and prevent MH. The incidence of the autosomal dominant form is 1 in 50,000 to 1 in 100,000 persons. MH occurs in 1 in 40,000 adult and 1 in 15,000 pediatric surgical cases. A linkage to mutations in the skeletal muscle ryanodine receptor (RYR1) has been established in some families with the autosomal dominant disorder. However, not all families have mutations in RYR1.

A second, recessive, form occurs in young boys and, less commonly, girls with a number of congenital abnormalities, including short stature, undescended testes, lumbar lordosis, thoracic kyphosis, pectus carinatum, webbed neck, winged scapulae, small chin, low-set ears, and an antimongoloid obliquity of the palpebral fissures. This form is called the *King syndrome*. MH also has been described in several other myopathies, including myotonia congenita, central core disease, and Duchenne's muscular dystrophy, and in patients with osteogenesis imperfecta.

Pathogenesis   The triggering anesthetic releases calcium from the membrane of the muscle cell's sarcoplasmic reticulum, which is defective in storing this ion. The result is a sudden increase in myoplasmic calcium. The calcium activates myosin ATPase, which converts adenosine triphosphate to adenosine diphosphate, phosphate, and heat. There are also inhibition of troponin, uncoupling of oxidative phosphorylation, activation of phosphorylase kinase, and increased glycolysis. Muscular contraction occurs, and it, as well as the chemical events, leads to production of heat.

Manifestations   Existence of malignant hyperthermia can be suspected if diminished relaxation is noted during induction of anesthesia and muscle fasciculations become evident when succinylcholine is given. In some patients, trismus during intubation is the first sign of a muscle disorder. Although the elevation in temperature is the result of muscular contraction, it may rise very rapidly, and if the temperature is not monitored, the first signs may be a hot skin and tachycardia or a cardiac arrhythmia. During anesthesia, an increase in end-tidal CO_2, unexplained tachycardia, and an increase in core temperature provide early clues to the syndrome. In addition to the high fever, muscle rigidity, hypotension, and mottled cyanosis are present.

Early laboratory abnormalities include respiratory and metabolic acidosis, hyperkalemia and hypermagnesemia, and elevation in blood lactate and pyruvate. Late complications include massive skeletal muscle swelling, pulmonary edema, disseminated intravascular coagulation, acute renal failure, cerebral edema, and seizures.

Treatment   MH is a medical emergency. The treatment protocol prescribed by the American Society of Anesthesiologists should be followed. It includes prompt interruption of surgery, cessation of the inhalational anesthetic, changing rubber tubing on the anesthesia machine, and external cooling. One hundred percent oxygen should be given, along with sodium bicarbonate (1 to 2 mg/kg), to combat the severe metabolic acidosis. A diuresis should be induced with fluids and diuretics to reduce myoglobinemia and hyperkalemia. Specific treatment consists of dantrolene sodium, 1 mg/kg, by rapid intravenous infusion. The drug should be continued until symptoms have begun to subside or up to a maximum single dose of 10 mg/kg. The regimen can be repeated if symptoms recur. Drugs to combat arrhythmias should be administered under ECG monitoring (see Chap. 198).

Prevention   Because of the tendency of this syndrome to run in families, its detection is essential. This can be achieved by monitoring the temperature of all patients under anesthesia; the best way to avert it altogether is to take a thorough family history. However, up to 50 percent of affected patients give a history of prior uneventful anesthetic procedures. Examining patients preoperatively is often not helpful because between attacks persons susceptible to MH are usually entirely normal. In susceptible patients, dantrolene should be given prophylactically. The dose is 4 to 8 mg/kg by mouth for 1 to 2 days prior to surgery; the last dose should be administered 3 to 4 h prior to anesthesia. Some favor an additional dose of 2 to 5 mg/kg intravenously immediately prior to induction of anesthesia.

NEUROLEPTIC MALIGNANT SYNDROME (NMS)   This syndrome is characterized by autonomic dysfunction, extrapyramidal dysfunction, and hyperthermia. Autonomic dysfunction is characterized by tachycardia, labile blood pressure (range 40 to 180 mmHg systolic), profuse diaphoresis, dyspnea, and urinary incontinence. Extrapyramidal dysfunction is manifested by catatonic behavior, dystonia, generalized muscular rigidity, and pseudoparkinsonism (ptyalism, masked facies, tremors, and brady- or akinesia). The temperature may be as high as 41°C (106°F). Consciousness fluctuates from alertness to coma. Laboratory abnormalities consist of leukocytosis (15,000 to 30,000 per microliter) and elevation in CK. The syndrome occurs after use of potent neuroleptics in therapeutic doses. Most cases have been reported after use of haloperidol, thiothixene, or piperazine phenothiazines. Concomitant use of other psychotropic drugs, including lithium, antidepressants, and benzodiazepines, occurs in over half of reported cases of NMS. Young adult males with affective disorders predominate. The NMS lasts 5 to 10 days after administration of oral neuroleptics is discontinued and longer after depot injection. These drugs are not dialyzable, hence the long period necessary for their excretion. The overall mortality is 20 percent, and fatalities have occured as late as 30 days after onset and have been due to renal failure, arrhythmias, pulmonary emboli, or aspiration pneumonia.

The mechanism of action is presumed to be due to blockade of the dopaminic pathways in the basal ganglia and the hypothalamus. Because neuroleptic drugs block dopamine receptors, NMS is attributed to dopamine depletion, and this is the rationale for treatment with bromocriptine (a dopamine agonist) in dosage of 7.5 to 60 mg/d divided into 3 daily doses. Dantrolene sodium (as described above for oral prophylaxis of MH) has been successful occasionally, as has amantadine. Supportive measures, including cooling and drug withdrawal, are the *sine qua non* of treatment.

DISORDERS ASSOCIATED WITH LOW TEMPERATURES

HYPOTHERMIA *Hypothermia* is defined as a central or core temperature of 35°C (95°F) or lower. The central (core) temperature is maintained at the expense of the periphery. During cold weather, blood is shunted away from the skin and the extremities to preserve, protect, and maintain core temperatures. Although far less common than is elevation in temperature, hypothermia is of considerable importance because it can represent a medical emergency.

Accidental hypothermia This is a well-known complication of exposure to cold and has been reported frequently during the winter months. It usually occurs after prolonged exposure, not necessarily to excessively low external temperatures. The diagnosis of hypothermia may prove elusive because clinical thermometers do not record temperatures below 35°C (95°F). Whenever a patient presents with a temperature below this level, the true temperature should be determined with an incubator thermometer or a thermocouple. Accidental hypothermia has been found in association with sepsis, hypothyroidism, pituitary insufficiency, adrenal insufficiency, hypoglycemia, cerebrovascular disease, Wernicke's encephalopathy, myocardial infarction, cirrhosis, pancreatitis, and ingestion of drugs—most particularly alcohol. Alcohol increases heat loss by peripheral dilatation and interferes with thermogenesis by inhibiting shivering. From 1976 to 1985, 7450 deaths in the United States were caused by exposure to cold. Most had core temperatures <35°C (<95°F), and individuals older than age 60 were at greatest risk. In 428 cases reported from 13 emergency departments, there was a direct correlation between lower body temperatures and outcome.

These patients usually appear cold and pale and, when their temperatures are very low, give the appearance of having rigor mortis, so stiff is their musculature. Patients with temperatures less than 26.7°C (90°F) are usually unconscious. The pupils are usually miotic, respiration tends to be shallow and slow, there is bradycardia, and most patients are hypotensive. Generalized edema is often present. When the temperature falls below 25°C (77°F), coma, areflexia, and lack of pupillary response supervene.

Laboratory data tend to show hemoconcentration, mild azotemia, and metabolic acidosis. The acidosis is due to lactic acidemia, which in turn is a consequence of decreased perfusion and hypoxemia in peripheral tissues. At cold temperatures, the hemoglobin dissociation

curve is shifted to the left, and there is decreased unloading of oxygen in the peripheral tissues. Some patients have hypoglycemia, while others have hyperglycemia. Thyroid function tests may give results typical of myxedema. Some patients have elevations in serum amylase, and a few show pancreatitis at autopsy. The electrocardiogram is distorted by muscular tremors and may show bradycardia or slow atrial fibrillation and a characteristic J wave (occurring at the junction of the QRS complex and ST segment). Other arrhythmias are common; ventricular fibrillation is usually a terminal event. The mortality rate is five times higher in people over age 75.

TREATMENT Hypothermia is a medical emergency, and therapy should be instituted at once. The following steps are indicated:

1 An airway must be established and maintained, and the patient should be well oxygenated. Warmed oxygen may be helpful. Tracheal intubation of these patients poses no undue risk.
2 Blood gases should be monitored.
3 Blood volume should be expanded with warmed glucose in saline. Maintenance of blood volume is necessary to prevent the infarctions which have been a hallmark in fatal cases and to avert "rewarming shock." If the patient has persistent hypotension, respiratory failure, or unexplained oliguria, hemodynamic monitoring with Swan-Ganz catheterization may be necessary.
4 Because of the tendency to arrhythmias, the serum potassium level should be monitored carefully; a transvenous pacemaker may be indicated.
5 Although external rewarming with heating blankets or placing the patient in a warm room is appropriate in patients with mild hypothermia, active external rewarming (AER) is the treatment of choice. A source of heat (warm blanket, heating pad, or radiant source) is applied to the thorax only. The extremities are left vasoconstricted to prevent sudden vasodilation and blood pressure fall, which may be accompanied by recirculation of accumulated lactic acid from the periphery to the core. Moderate to severe hypothermia should be treated with active core rewarming (ACR). Humidified warm air administered by endotracheal ventilation, peritoneal dialysis with warmed fluid, heated fluid irrigation of the stomach via gastric lavage, or cardiopulmonary bypass with externally warmed blood have been used. For patients with intractable ventricular fibrillation, mediastinal irrigation and direct mediastinal lavage via left thoracotomy may be the fastest method for rewarming the myocardium.
6 Many of these patients have systemic infections including sepsis (see Chap. 83); cultures of the blood, urine, and other suspected sites should be obtained and broad-spectrum antibiotic therapy initiated and continued until infection has been excluded. Sepsis should be considered strongly in patients on hemodynamic monitoring who are found to have a lowered systemic vascular resistance and elevated cardiac index.
7 Resuscitative efforts should be vigorous and prolonged despite the poor prognosis, which is related primarily to advanced age and associated debilitating disease. In younger individuals, some remarkable rescues have been recorded. Authorities agree that hypothermia victims without vital signs (prolonged asystole) should not be pronounced dead until they have been rewarmed to 36°C (96.8°F) and remain unresponsive to CPR at that temperature. "No one is dead until warm and dead." Mild hypothermia [above 32.2°C (90°F)] has a 25 percent mortality; in moderate hypothermia [26.6 to 32.2°C (80 to 90°F)], the mortality is 50 percent; and below 26.6°C (80°C), it is 60 percent.

Hypothermia secondary to acute illness There is a group of patients who develop moderate hypothermia in association with acute diseases, including congestive heart failure, uremia, diabetes mellitus, drug overdose, acute respiratory failure, and hypoglycemia. These patients are generally elderly and upon admission to the hospital are found to have temperatures of 33.3 to 34.4°C (92 to 93.9°F). They also have a severe metabolic acidosis, due to increased production of lactic acid, and cardiac arrhythmias. Most of these patients are comatose. This entity differs from accidental hypothermia only in the absence of exposure; these cases have all occurred at normal ambient temperatures. The mechanism appears to be an acute failure of thermoregulation; shivering did not occur in any of these patients. Usually these patients have been rewarmed within a few hours. Upon return to normal temperature, cardiac arrhythmias, which were present in most of these patients, responded to treatment, and the sensorium returned to normal. With the exception that core rewarming is established by external means, other facets of therapy should follow the steps outlined above. In addition, treatment of the underlying disease, such as diabetes with insulin, uremia with dialysis, or congestive heart failure with appropriate cardiac drugs and diuretics, is essential. The prognosis is good provided the syndrome is recognized early and treatment is instituted at once. In general, patients under age 60 have the most favorable outcome.

Immersion hypothermia The treatment of immersion hypothermia is essentially identical to that of accidental hypothermia.

LOCAL COLD INJURIES Mechanisms of freezing Injury These can be divided into phenomena that affect cells and extracellular fluids (direct effects) and those which disrupt the function of organized tissues and the integrity of the circulation (indirect effects).

When tissue freezes, ice crystals form and, concomitantly, solutes in the residual liquid become concentrated. The physical dislocation during slow freezing is extreme. Ice crystals many times the size of individual cells form but are confined to the extracellular spaces. Large ice crystals can develop between cells in soft tissue without producing irreversible injury as long as the percentage of water frozen does not exceed a critical amount. A major source of damage to living cells during freezing and thawing appears to be the strong salt solutions which develop during formation and dissolution of ice; changes in the proportions of lipids and phospholipids in the cell membrane are also of great importance.

The fulminating vascular reaction and stasis that supervene are associated with production of histamine-like substances which increase the permeability of the capillary bed. Within blood vessels, cellular elements aggregate. Irreversible occlusion of small blood vessels by cell masses has been demonstrated in thawed tissue following freezing injury. The damaged frozen tissue simulates tissue damage produced by burns.

Manifestations The mildest form of cold injury is called *frostnip* and tends to occur in organs farthest removed from the core of the body such as the earlobes, nose, cheeks, fingers and toes, and hands and feet. Frostnip represents reversible damage that is characterized by discomfort and blanching of the skin and numbness. It can be prevented by warm clothing and treated with simple rewarming. More consequential local cold injuries may be divided into freezing (frostbite) and nonfreezing (immersion foot) injuries. The two types may be observed in the same extremity or in different extremities in the same individual. The diagnosis of freezing versus nonfreezing injury generally can be made on the basis of the history and clinical manifestations.

Immersion foot is an entity observed in shipwreck survivors or in soldiers (trench foot) whose feet have been wet but not freezing cold for prolonged periods. There is primarily injury to nerve and muscle tissue, but no gross or irreparable pathologic changes occur in the blood vessels and skin. Symptoms include numbness, painful paresthesias and leg cramping. The clinical picture reflects primary hypoxic trauma giving rise to three clearly recognizable states: (1) *ischemia*, denoted by a pale, pulseless extremity, (2) *hyperemia*, characterized by a bounding pulsatile circulation in red, swollen, painful feet, and (3) the *posthyperemic* or recovery period. The initial cold-induced vasoconstriction, increased blood viscosity, and impaired oxygen transport in the ischemic state are aggravated by such factors as malnutrition, general hypothermia, dehydration, and trauma from relatively fixed, pendant extremities. The problem of rewarming is critical in these patients during the stage of ischemia, when overheating of tissue may lead to gangrene. In the state of hyperemia, the red, swollen feet require judicious cooling. Severe cases may show muscular weakness, atrophy, ulceration, and gangrene of superficial areas. Sensitivity to cold and pain on weight bearing, which may cause discomfort for many years, are sequelae even of milder injuries.

Frostbite, in contrast to immersion foot, is primarily a vascular problem because the blood vessels may be severely and irreparably injured. The circulation of blood ceases, and the vascular bed of the frozen tissue is occluded by agglutinated cell aggregates and thrombi. The cutaneous injury consists in part of separation of the epidermal-dermal interface. Early the intravascular clumping is reversible. However, with the passage of time, clumped red blood cells within vessels in injured tissue lose their morphologic identity and take on the appearance of a homogeneous, hyalinaceous plug. It has been shown in some, but not all, experimental studies that much of the intravascular aggregation following freezing injury can be reversed and microcirculatory perfusion improved if low-molecular-weight dextran is given intravenously shortly after injury, but the data in humans are less convincing. Tissue damage can be aggravated by trauma to insensitive and friable limbs and by refreezing. Moreover, frostbitten tissues are often neglected and with thawing become macerated. It is important, therefore, not to walk, bear weight, or put excessive pressure on a thawed frostbitten area. Thawing followed by refreezing is particularly harmful. There are four degrees of frostbite. First degree is accompanied by erythema and edema; second degree, by vesiculation, blistering, and eschar formation; third degree, by hemorrhagic blistering and bluish gray discoloration; and fourth degree, by injury to subcutaneous tissue muscle, tendon, and bone leading to mottled, dry, black, and necrotic changes.

The method of rewarming has been a matter of controversy. It seems most rational to warm the core of the body before treating the local area of frostbite. Following restoration of the core temperature to normal, warming of a frostbitten limb should begin in water at 10 to 15°C (50 to 59°F), which is then increased 5°C (9°F) every 5 min to a maximum of 40°C (104°F). Once the frostbitten limb has been rewarmed, treatment of the areas of tissue damage should be conservative and consist of bed rest, elevation of the injured part, tetanus toxoid administration, and use of antibiotics if infection is present; aseptic early drainage of blebs and bullae; daily washes with chlorhexidine or an iodophor; and early institution of physiotherapy. Alcohol and cigarettes are strongly contraindicated. Parenteral analgesics and nonsteroidal anti-inflammatory drugs are usually required for pain. Except for compartment syndromes that may occur as a result of massive swelling in the early postthaw period and that may require surgical release, surgical amputation and reconstruction are usually not necessary. In fact, 3 to 6 months may be required to determine the true level of tissue loss, contraindicating aggressive surgery.

Some patients with frostbite have residua consisting of excessive sweating, pain, cold insensitivity, numbness, abnormal color, dry and cracking skin, arthralgias, and degenerative arthritis. The symptoms are generally worse in the winter and following exposure to cold. These patients also often show abnormal nails, discoloration and pigmentation, hyperhidrosis, and, by x-ray, osteoporosis and cystic defects near the joints. These abnormalities tend to be milder in patients who have had sympathetic blockade. Most cold injuries are preventable by graded exposure to cold, as well as by appropriate clothing in freezing temperatures.

REFERENCES

General

MITCHELL D, LABURN HP: Pathophysiology of temperature regulation. Physiologist 28:507, 1985

MACKOWIAK P et al: A critical appraisal of 98.6°F, the upper limit of the normal body temperature, and other legacies of Carl Reinhold August Wunderlich. JAMA 268:1578, 1992

Heat syndromes

YARBROUGH B: Heat illness, in *Emergency Medicine: Concepts and Clinical Practice*, P Rosen (ed). St. Louis, Mosby, 1992, vol 1

———, HUBBARD R: Heat-related illnesses, in *Management of Wilderness and Environmental Emergencies*, P Auerbach, E Geehr (eds). St. Louis, Mosby, 1989

Malignant hyperthermia

HEIMAN-PATTERSON T: Malignant hyperthermia. Semin Neurol 11:3:220, 1991
LEVITT R: Prospects for the diagnosis of malignant hyperthermia susceptibility using molecular genetic approaches. Anesthesiology 76:1039, 1992
MACLENNAN D, PHILLIPS M: Malignant hyperthermia. Science 256:789, 1992

Neuroleptic malignant syndrome

ADDONIZIO G et al: Neuroleptic malignant syndrome: Review and analysis of 115 cases. Biol Psychol 22:1004, 1987
CAROFF S et al: Neuroleptic malignant syndrome. Med Clin North Am 77:185, 1993

Hypothermia

DANZL D: Accidental hypothermia, in *Emergency Medicine: Concepts and Clinical Practice*, P Rosen (ed). St. Louis, Mosby, 1992, vol 1
——— et al: Accidental hypothermia, in *Management of Wilderness and Environmental Emergencies*, P Auerbach, E Geehr (eds). St. Louis, Mosby, 1989
DELANEY KA et al: Assessment of acid-base disturbances in hypothermia and their physiologic consequences. Ann Emerg Med 18:72, 1989
JOLLY T et al: Accidental hypothermia. Emerg Med Clin North Am 10:311, 1992

Cold injury

DANZL D: Frostbite, in *Emergency Medicine: Concepts and Clinical Practice*, P Rosen (ed). St. Louis, Mosby, 1992, vol 1
SMITH D et al: Frostbite and other cold-induced injuries, in *Management of Wilderness and Environmental Emergencies*, P Auerbach, E Geehr (eds). St. Louis, Mosby, 1989

399 DROWNING AND NEAR-DROWNING

JEROME H. MODELL

It is an unexpected tragedy when a previously healthy person dies or is exposed to severe cerebral hypoxia and suffers permanent brain damage. For many years, drowning was considered a "fight for survival": a person who could not swim, arms flailing and screaming for help, struggled to remain on the surface of the water to reach safety. This situation is rarely reported by persons at the scene of aquatic emergencies. Thus no single set of circumstances comprises drowning or near-drowning. Furthermore, it may be a secondary event following such precursors as head or spinal trauma, hypoxic-induced unconsciousness, or unconsciousness due to preexisting cardiovascular disease, sudden cardiac death, or myocardial infarction. The initiating event is usually unknown, however, and the drowned or near-drowned victim must be treated based on probable physiologic effects of the near-drowning itself. If survival with normal brain function is to occur, a thorough understanding of the pathophysiology of drowning and an organized approach to therapy are imperative.

PATHOPHYSIOLOGY OF DROWNING Approximately 90 percent of drowning victims aspirate fluid into their lungs. In those who do not aspirate fluid, hypoxemia results simply from apnea. In those who do aspirate, the volume and the composition of the fluid determine the physiologic basis of the hypoxemia. Freshwater aspiration alters the surface tension properties of pulmonary surfactant and makes alveoli unstable, which causes a decreased ventilation/perfusion ratio. Some alveoli collapse and become atelectatic, which produces a true or absolute intrapulmonary shunt, while others are poorly ventilated and produce a relative shunt; in either case, significant pulmonary venous admixture occurs. Freshwater in the alveoli is hypotonic and is rapidly absorbed and redistributed throughout the body. While some have proposed that water continues to enter the lungs after death, at autopsy, the lungs of victims who died in the water frequently contain little water. These findings support the premise that active respiration determines the volume of water aspirated. Hypertonic seawater pulls additional fluid from the plasma into the lungs, and thus the alveoli are fluid-filled, but perfused, which causes substantial

pulmonary venous admixture. With both types of water, pulmonary edema may occur and add to the ventilation/perfusion abnormality.

Water that is grossly contaminated with particulate matter or bacteria may complicate the picture. Particulate matter can obstruct the smaller bronchi and respiratory bronchioles. Grossly contaminated water increases the risk of severe pulmonary infection. Neither problem is sufficiently common, however, to recommend specific routine therapy for all victims.

At least 85 percent of near-drowned victims are thought to aspirate 22 mL/kg of water or less, which does not significantly affect blood volume and serum electrolyte concentrations. After resuscitation, by the time blood is analyzed, serum electrolyte concentrations usually are normal or close to normal. Significant changes are documented in only approximately 15 percent of those who cannot be resuscitated and only rarely in those who are resuscitated. This suggests either a small amount of water was aspirated or fluid was rapidly redistributed. Therefore, electrolyte disturbance rarely needs treatment. When a large quantity of water is aspirated, seawater causes hypovolemia, which concentrates extracellular electrolytes, and freshwater causes acute hypervolemia. If enough water is aspirated that plasma becomes severely hypotonic and the patient is hypoxemic, red cell membranes can rupture and plasma hemoglobin and serum potassium concentrations increase significantly. However, this has been reported only on rare occasion. With rapid redistribution of fluid and development of pulmonary edema, even freshwater victims frequently demonstrate hypovolemia by the time they reach the hospital.

Hypercarbia, which is associated with apnea and/or hypoventilation, is less often documented by blood gas analysis than is hypoxemia. While hypoxemia due to pulmonary venous admixture persists in all near-drowned victims who aspirate water, hypercarbia is usually corrected sooner with artificial mechanical ventilation and improved minute ventilation, and thus is reported in a small percentage of victims evaluated at the hospital. Besides hypoxemia, metabolic acidosis also persists in the majority of patients. Abnormal cardiovascular function, usually ascribed to hypoxemia, is brief with effective, timely therapy. Abnormality in renal function is uncommon, but when it does occur, it too is secondary to hypoxemia, alterations in renal perfusion, or, in extremely rare circumstances, significant hemoglobinuria.

TREATMENT OF NEAR-DROWNING The first step is retrieving the victim from the water, and, if necessary, performing artificial ventilation and circulation. According to the American Heart Association recommendation an abdominal thrust should not be used routinely in victims of submersion but rather should be reserved for when the airway is obstructed with a foreign body or when the victim fails to respond to mouth-to-mouth ventilation. Furthermore, an abdominal thrust may lead to regurgitation and pulmonary aspiration of gastric contents and may delay ventilatory or circulatory resuscitation.

Because emergency services and intensive pulmonary and cardiovascular care have improved during the past two decades, central nervous system depression now presents the major therapeutic challenge. The rate of survival with normal cerebral function varies considerably in retrospective studies. Some factors that adversely influence survival are prolonged submersion, delay in initiation of effective cardiopulmonary resuscitation, severe metabolic acidosis (pH <7.1), asystole upon arrival to a medical facility, fixed dilated pupils, and low Glasgow coma score (<5). None of these predictors is absolute, however, and normal survivors have been reported in all of the above categories. In a comparison of outcomes between one institution that added brain preservation techniques to intensive pulmonary and circulatory treatment and another institution that did not add brain preservation techniques, outcome data did not differ significantly.

Hypothermia appears to be protective, but only if it occurs at the time of the accident. This permits the victim a greater chance of cerebral salvage after longer periods of acute hypoxia and cardiac arrest than might be expected with normothermia. The diving reflex produces bradycardia, breath-holding, and circulatory redistribution when the face is submerged in cold water. However, its protective effect in explaining cerebral recovery after prolonged immersion has not been specifically documented.

Significant pulmonary venous admixture usually persists even after successful resuscitation; therefore, supplemental oxygen should be administered until arterial blood gas analysis confirms that oxygen is no longer needed. Intravenous access should be established as soon as possible. Endotracheal intubation should be performed if required for airway maintenance or to facilitate mechanical ventilatory support. Electrocardiographic monitoring will facilitate prompt treatment of cardiac arrhythmias.

Victims should be transported to a hospital where they can receive definitive testing for adequacy of ventilation and blood gas exchange, cardiac activity, and effective circulating blood volume. Analysis of other parameters such as serum electrolyte concentrations, renal function, and cerebral status should be performed as indicated.

The single, most effective treatment for hypoxemia, regardless of its cause, is mechanical ventilatory support including continuous positive airway pressure (CPAP). After freshwater aspiration, improvement in ventilation/perfusion matching is more consistent when CPAP is combined with mechanical inflation of the lung than with spontaneous respiration. The application of CPAP with spontaneous respiration versus its combination with mechanical ventilation should be determined by whether the specific patient can perform the necessary work of breathing, adequately eliminate carbon dioxide, and adequately match ventilation/perfusion ratios. Positive airway pressure should be withdrawn gradually as the lungs stabilize and ventilation/perfusion ratio returns toward normal.

The pH in near-drowned victims is commonly significantly acidotic, which, in turn, can depress cardiac function. This should be corrected pharmacologically, although there is some disagreement on this point. With cardiovascular instability, cannulation of the pulmonary artery with a Swan Ganz catheter or evaluation of the patient with transesophageal echocardiography is indicated. Many patients will be hypovolemic from loss of fluid into the lung as pulmonary edema or from decreased venous return secondary to increased intrathoracic pressure during mechanical ventilatory support.

Body temperature should be taken into account before a decision is made to terminate therapy of individuals submerged under frigid conditions because recovery after long periods of such submersion has been reported. The body temperature of victims depends not only on the temperature of the water from which they are retrieved, but also on the degree of insulation they have from that temperature with body clothing. The volume of water actually aspirated is also important, because a large volume, if distributed before cardiac arrest occurs, can produce rapid central cooling. Thus, cold water can be protective when it produces total body hypothermia, which decreases metabolic oxygen requirement. On the other hand, cold water may also contribute to the accident if hypothermia occurs before total submersion, resulting in severe, or even fatal, cardiac arrhythmia. Several methods of rewarming hypothermic victims have been advocated, but any technique that increases oxygen utilization, such as shivering, should be avoided.

Regardless of the conditions surrounding a drowning or near-drowning, treatment should follow a sequence of priorities:

1 Remove the victim from the water as soon as possible and stabilize the patient's head and neck if trauma is suspected.
2 Immediately follow the ABCs of cardiopulmonary resuscitation—even in the water if this does not endanger the rescuer.
3 If the patient is unconscious, protect the airway as needed with endotracheal intubation.
4 Establish venous access as soon as possible.
5 Provide supplemental oxygen and ventilatory support until each is no longer needed. This can be judged from analysis of arterial blood for oxygen tension, carbon dioxide tension, and pH.
6 Monitor cardiac rhythm with an electrocardioscope as soon as possible.

7 Monitor body temperature and restore it to normal.
8 If the patient has persistent respiratory insufficiency, provide intensive pulmonary support with CPAP and mechanical ventilation therapy as necessary.
9 If the patient has cardiovascular instability, evaluate cardiac output and effective circulatory volume, by invasive monitoring, and measure serum electrolyte concentrations.
10 Renal function and cerebral status should be evaluated as indicated.

Monitoring of intracranial pressure, routine glucocorticoid therapy, and prophylactic antibiotic therapy are no longer recommended.

ACCIDENT PREVENTION Because drowning begins as an accident that results in a medical problem, the definitive strategy is to prevent the accident. For those victims in whom the accident is secondary to a medical condition rather than the primary event, such as persons susceptible to syncope or seizure, the only way to prevent the accident is to identify those who ought to avoid the water or encourage them to use the buddy system. For young children, early swimming lessons, vigilant caretakers, and stringent laws governing pool enclosures are needed. Those who teach parenting classes should routinely warn parents about the risk of toddlers' drowning in such household fixtures as toilets, buckets of water, and even washing machines. Preventing accidents during boating, athletics, and other water-related recreational activities requires public education. Rules associated with these activities to maximize safety and judicious, responsible behavior should be portrayed as life-saving measures. Similarly, alcohol, a "ubiquitous catalyst" to drowning, should be portrayed as life-threatening whenever water is nearby.

REFERENCES

AMERICAN HEART ASSOCIATION: Guidelines for cardiopulmonary resuscitation and emergency cardiac care. JAMA 268:2171, 1992

BOHN DJ et al: Influence of hypothermia, barbiturate therapy, and intracranial pressure monitoring on morbidity and mortality after near-drowning. Crit Care Med 14:529, 1986

FULLER RH: The 1962 Welcome Prize Essay. Drowning and the postimmersion syndrome. A clinicopathologic study. Milit Med 128:22, 1963

GONZALEZ-ROTHI RJ: Near-drowning: Consensus and controversies in pulmonary and cerebral resuscitation. Heart Lung 16:474, 1987

MODELL JH: Drowning. N Engl J Med 328:253, 1993

———— : Pathophysiology and treatment of drowning and near-drowning. Springfield, IL, Charles C Thomas, 1971

————, CONN AW: Current neurological considerations in near-drowning, editorial. Can Anaesth Soc J 27:197, 1980

———— et al: Clinical course of 91 consecutive near-drowning victims. Chest 70:231, 1976

———— et al: Near-drowning: Correlation of level of consciousness and survival. Can Anaesth Soc J 27:211, 1980

ORNATO JP: The resuscitation of near-drowning victims. JAMA 256:75, 1986

400 ELECTRICAL INJURIES

ALAN R. DIMICK

EPIDEMIOLOGY The exact incidence of electrical injury is unknown. Each year in the United States approximately 1000 deaths constituting roughly 1 percent of all accidental deaths are attributed to electric current. The prevalence of electrical technology in modern society has resulted in more people experiencing electrical injury. The current treatment of electrical injury has resulted in a low mortality, ranging from 3 to 15 percent, but the amputation rate remains high, and disfigurement due to extensive soft tissue destruction is frequent. More than 60 percent of the electricity-related fatalities occur in males, with the highest incidence among those 20 to 34 years of age. Approximately one-third of *high-voltage* injuries occur in electrical workers, one-third in construction workers, and the remainder from non-work-related events. One-half of *low-voltage* injuries occur at home, the majority of them to young children. Burn center referral is usually necessary for electrical burns.

PATHOPHYSIOLOGY Electrical burns result from the conversion of electrical energy into heat. Factors that determine the severity and distribution of injury include the type of current (direct or alternating), the quantity of the current (amperage), the potential of the current (voltage), the resistance offered by the body, the pathway of the current, and the duration of contact. These variables are interrelated, and their interactions produce the varied spectrum of injury seen clinically.

Direct and alternating current have different effects. At low voltages (less than 1000 V), the low-frequency (40 to 150 Hz) alternating current range, which is used almost exclusively for incandescent lighting and appliances, is three times more dangerous than direct current. Immediate death can result from ventricular fibrillation, central respiratory arrest, or asphyxia due to tetanic respiratory muscle contractions. Tetanic muscle spasms, which freeze the contact point to the power source, tend to increase the flow of current and the severity of injury. Cutaneous burns may be entirely absent or minimal. In contrast, at high voltages, high-frequency alternating current and direct current are equally lethal.

Survivals from electric shocks of greater than 100,000 V and deaths from as little as 50 V have occurred, which underscores the interplay of the variables already noted. Clinically, the severity of injury relates primarily to the voltage. Low-voltage contact, while potentially lethal, does not result in the magnitude of tissue necrosis seen with high-voltage injury. Tissue resistance is an important factor in determining both the initiation of current flow and its subsequent path. A person completing a circuit between two contact points has a resistance that is the sum of the skin resistances at both contact points plus the internal body resistance. If skin resistance is high, there will be considerable local tissue destruction. Conversely, if skin resistance is low, systemic effects such as those on the heart and brain predominate. Skin resistance varies widely according to the thickness, cleanliness, and wetness of the skin. The resistance of skin in water is only about 0.1 percent of the resistance of dry skin. The extent of tissue damage can be explained by the differing resistances of various tissues. Listed in the order of increasing magnitude of resistance are nerves, blood vessels, muscle, skin, tendon, fat, and bone.

All tissues and organs can be affected by electrical injury. The cutaneous burns are often limited, with variable deep tissue damage. Appreciation of this special property of electrical wounds is critical in their management. Skin wounds are typically leathery or charred areas of full-thickness skin loss. The entry and exit sites are usually depressed, giving the appearance that current exploded the tissues. The arc burn is produced by current coursing external to the body from contact to ground, favoring a path of least resistance. The flexor surfaces of the wrist, elbow, and axilla are most often involved, because the hand is the most commonly involved body part. After several days, the demarcation between viable and nonviable tissue becomes more obvious. Flame burns of the skin may result from ignition of clothing by electrical arcing and may be full-thickness burns because of the prolonged exposure of the dazed victim to the flame.

The most severe cardiopulmonary manifestations occur at the time of the injury. These include anoxia and ventricular fibrillation, which may cause immediate death due to respiratory or cardiac arrest. Major electrical injury is accompanied by a 3 to 15 percent incidence of acute renal failure, which is greater than the incidence after thermal burns.

Nervous tissue is highly susceptible to electrical injury because of its low resistance. Neurologic deficits can be seen up to 3 years after the initial injury, and neurologic aberrations are the most frequent nonfatal sequelae of electrical injury. Lesions of the central nervous system may cause varying levels of consciousness, respiratory, and motor paralysis, which are usually transient; recovery is the rule. If

the effects are permanent, they often assume the character of cortical encephalopathy or hemiplegia with or without aphasia. Spinal cord damage is the most common permanent sequelae of electrical injury and is seldom complete. Many deficits seen initially resolve spontaneously; others may not develop until 6 to 9 months after the electrical injury. Permanent deficits may not be seen for days to months, are of gradual onset, and progress slowly. Often these disturbances are not noted until the rehabilitative phase of recovery, when gait abnormalities become evident. Peripheral nerves may be burned directly or may be compressed by surrounding edema or scar. Neuropathies also can develop in unburned limbs. Autonomic nervous system dysfunction may be seen in both the acute and recovery phases. Reflex sympathetic dystrophy or causalgia can occur. Late onset of burning pain, frequently associated with vasomotor, trophic, and dermal changes, is characteristic.

Cataracts characteristically occur following high-tension injuries. The incidence of these lesions, which are usually bilateral, may be as great as 30 percent when electrical contact is made above the clavicles, particularly when the entry wound is on the head. The latent period between the accident and the onset of blurred vision averages 6 months but ranges from a few weeks to 3 years.

Direct vascular injury is more common after electrical injury than after any other type of burn. The blood flow in large arteries and veins is usually sufficient to dissipate the heat generated by the electric current. However, smaller vessels may experience significant heat-related damage resulting in thrombosis. Direct vascular injury probably contributes to the high amputation rate after high-tension electrical injury. Delayed hemorrhage from mural necrosis of large blood vessels also may occur.

Associated injury in electrical accidents can be due to falls of considerable distance or to the explosive effects of the current. Fractures of the vertebrae and long bones and dislocations also may result from the violent tetanic muscle contractions.

TREATMENT At the scene of the accident, the patient must be separated immediately from the electric current, but rescuers must not touch or approach the patient until the current has been shut off to avoid injury to themselves. Flames should then be extinguished.

Cardiopulmonary support must be initiated if necessary and maintained during transport. Aggressive life support is essential because victims of high-voltage electrical injury may be resuscitated successfully without permanent neurologic damage even after a prolonged cessation of vital functions. Because blunt trauma and skeletal injury may both coexist, a thorough history and careful physical examination are essential. Accurate assessment of the extent and nature of the burns is essential to the determination of subsequent therapy. Neurologic status must be evaluated repeatedly during convalescence because it changes frequently.

Fluid replacement is essential in the initial management. Hypovolemia results from the rapid loss of fluid into damaged tissues. Small entry and exit wounds may lead to underestimation of the underlying injury, so fluid requirements may be grossly underestimated. Normal saline should be infused rapidly (0.5 to 1 mL/kg per hour) as necessary to correct hypovolemia and to maintain urinary output. Large volumes of fluid are necessary in high-voltage injury because the fluid and electrolyte needs are much greater than in patients with thermal burns of equivalent surface area. The adequacy of resuscitation is monitored, with urinary output being the single most reliable indicator of circulatory status. The presence of urinary hemoglobin and myoglobin may necessitate treatment with mannitol to prevent acute renal failure. When hemoglobinuria and/or myoglobinuria is present, the rate and volume of crystalloid infused must be sufficient to maintain a minimum urine output of 100 mL/h. This infusion is continued until the urine is grossly clear of pigment. Acute renal failure, if it occurs, is treated as described in Chap. 236. Red blood cell transfusion, plasma, dextran, or other plasma expanders are unnecessary during the acute resuscitative phase.

Low-voltage injury Injuries resulting from low-voltage current, such as those related to household appliances, are usually small and limited to the area of contact. These burns frequently involve the hands, feet, or, in children, the corners of the mouth, lips, and tongue. The evolution of tissue injury and vascular necrosis from the current itself are complete within 7 to 10 days. During this time, the wounds are allowed to slough and heal by contracture. Small but deep contact injuries on the trunk and extremities may be excised and grafted as necessary when the extent of the slough is evident. Early excision and local flap repair are rarely indicated. Delayed bleeding from the lip, seen in one-quarter of these injuries, is usually readily controlled by direct pressure.

High-voltage injury High-voltage injuries with devitalized skin, fat, and muscle are fundamentally surgical problems. They usually involve a limited amount of the total body surface, have upper extremity contact points, and require amputation or other surgical procedures. They may affect any organ system. The ultimate treatment goals are stabilization of the patient, salvage of the limb, debridement of devitalized tissue, wound coverage, and rehabilitation. Prolonged expectant nonsurgical therapy only increases the risk of invasive infection.

The timing of surgical debridement and its aggressiveness are controversial issues. Opinions range from early total excision with primary wound closure to the now outmoded expectant nonsurgical approach. Most surgeons favor an intermediate approach, individualizing according to the amount of tissue destruction and location and type of injury. Major amputations and surgical debridement are usually performed 2 to 4 days following injury when the extent of necrosis is reasonably well defined but the risk of significant infection is small. High-voltage electrical burns frequently produce muscle compartment syndromes requiring fasciotomy. Circumferential deep limb burns due to associated flame or arc burns also may require escharotomy or fasciotomy. Indications for surgical decompression include loss of distal pulses, impaired capillary filling, paresthesia, and rigid muscle compartments.

Debridement When possible, formal amputation and major debridement are delayed for 2 to 4 days following injury. During this interval, neurologic and cardiopulmonary abnormalities usually have stabilized or resolved, and demarcation between viable and nonviable tissues is more evident. Because these wounds are prone to anaerobic infection, particularly myonecrosis with clostridia, aqueous penicillin is given prophylactically from admission until debridement is complete. Antibiotic administration should be further guided by identification of infecting organisms. Local wound care is started immediately and includes mechanical cleansing followed by the application of topical antibacterial agents and cotton gauze dressings. Silver sulfadiazine cream has excellent antibacterial activity but penetrates only a few millimeters into the tissues. Sulfamylon, a burn cream containing mafenid (a carbonic anhydrase inhibitor which readily penetrates soft tissue), may be advantageous in deep injuries and, therefore, is the topical agent of choice in the prevention and/or treatment of deep-seated infections. However, when absorbed, this drug causes a bicarbonate diuresis resulting in systemic acidosis.

Coverage of open wounds usually requires skin grafting. Deep electrical injuries frequently result in complex soft tissue wounds which may require skin flaps for coverage. Nutritional support is essential and should be instituted early. As with other types of burns, appropriate splints should be fashioned and applied, and an aggressive program of physical therapy should be formulated and instituted. Psychological counseling is usually beneficial for patients who require major amputation or other mutilating surgical procedures.

LIGHTNING INJURY

When the difference in potential between the undersurface of a cloud which progressively become more negative and the surface of the earth which is positive exceeds the insulator strength of air, electrical energy discharges as lightning. There are four mechanisms of lightning strike: direct strike, flashover phenomenon, side flash, and stride

potential. Direct strike consists of a major current flow directly through the victim. It is the most serious type of strike and is facilitated by metal objects such as golf clubs, umbrellas, or tools carried during a thunderstorm. In flashover, the lightning travels on the outside of the body and is facilitated by wet garments and sweat. Side flash occurs when the current splashes from a building, tree, or other person and then travels to the victim. Stride potential occurs when the lightning strikes the ground close to a victim with one foot touching the ground closer to the point of the lightning strike. In this position there will be a potential electrical difference between the legs called *stride potential*. The lightning current may enter one leg and pass up through the victim's body and exit through the other leg. Stride potential and side-flash strikes can involve several individuals at once and may contribute to the multiple casualties often associated with lightning strike.

The pathophysiology of lightning injury is similar to that described for other electrical injuries. Lightning is direct current. The voltage of lightning may range from 3 million to 200 million volts and may carry a current of between 2000 and 3000 A. Lightning victims have a very short exposure to current because of the brief duration of lightning strike, which usually lasts only 1 to 100 ms. The majority of lightning current may flash over the outside of the body. In contrast, the duration of current contact with high-voltage electrical injuries may be prolonged, since the victim may become frozen to the current source. The resulting injuries with lightning strikes are similar to those with both direct current and alternating current, as described above. Thus treatment is essentially the same as for other types of electrical injury. The best form of treatment is prevention by avoiding dangerous situations during rainstorms and electrical storms, such as standing near tall structures and metal poles or beneath metal shelters. It is erroneous to assume that once lightning strikes it is safe to venture into the open, because another strike may occur in the same location. Many towers and churches have sustained multiple strikes.

REFERENCES

Boozalis GT et al: Ocular changes from electrical burn injuries. J Burn Care Rehabil 12:458, 1991

Fontanarosa PB: Electrical shock and lightning strike. Ann Emerg Med 22:378, 1993

Grube BJ et al: Neurologic consequences of electrical burns. J Trauma 30:254, 1990

Hammond JS, Ward CG: High-voltage electrical injuries: Management and outcome of 60 cases. South Med J 81:1351, 1988

Hanumadass ML et al: Acute electrical burns: A 10-year clinical experience. Burns 12:427, 1986

Lee RC, Kolodney MS: Electrical injury mechanisms: Electrical breakdown of cell membranes. Plast Reconstr Surg 80:672, 1987

Lichtenberg R et al: Cardiovascular effects of lightning strikes. J Am Coll Cardiol 21:531, 1993

Lifschultz BD, Donoghue ER: Deaths caused by lightning. J Forensic Sci 38:353, 1993

Rosenberg DB, Nelson M: Rehabilitation concerns in electrical burn patients: A review of the literature. J Trauma 28:808, 1988

401　RADIATION INJURY

STUART C. FINCH

Throughout life human beings are continuously exposed to many types of radiation, some harmless and some harmful. The most harmful is *ionizing radiation*, which damages tissue through the action of charged particles. More is known about the acute and late somatic, teratogenic, and genetic effects of ionizing radiation than about any other environmental, physical, or chemical agent or force, yet many gaps remain in our knowledge concerning its effects. Most important and least well understood are the late effects of chronic low-dose radiation exposure. There is little reliable direct information, based on studies for which there are good quantitative radiation dose estimates and high statistical power, so virtually all estimates of low-dose exposure risks are obtained by means of extrapolations from high-dose exposure results.

There are two types of ionizing radiation. The first consists of high-frequency electromagnetic waves of relatively short wavelength, such as naturally occurring gamma rays or machine-made x-rays. These waves are capable of deep tissue penetration and moderate ionization of the tissues along their pathways by indirect mechanisms. Their interactions with the atoms and molecules of tissue structures result in the release of orbital electrons and the formation of ions and reactive radicals that damage cell components and disrupt biologic processes. The second type of ionizing radiation consists of a variety of subatomic particles, the most important of which are electrically charged alpha particles, protons, electrons, and electrically uncharged neutrons. The charged particles densely ionize structures along their pathways in tissues. The depth of penetration is quite limited and varies as a function of mass, charge, and velocity. Tissue damage is due to the direct ionization of water, oxygen, and other molecules with the formation of free hydroxyl radicals and highly reactive oxygen species. Neutrons penetrate tissues much more deeply than charged particles of equivalent size (such as protons). They indirectly ionize through their interactions with the nuclei of atoms, resulting in the release of protons, alpha particles, and other nuclear fragments that damage other tissues.

The longer-wavelength waves of the electromagnetic spectrum do not ionize, but some may damage tissues by other mechanisms. For example, ultraviolet light penetrates very little, but repeated acute exposures induce photochemical cellular damage that is cumulative and irreversible, predisposing the development of melanomas, basal cell cancers, altered cell-mediated immunity, and other systemic effects. Infrared, radio, and microwave electromagnetic waves are capable of deep tissue penetration with the generation of heat, the effects of which are largely reversible. Weak, low frequency electromagnetic waves have been shown to modulate ion flow and to interfere with both RNA transcription and DNA synthesis at the cellular level. Reports of increased leukemia, brain tumors, and other neoplasms, especially in children, following prolonged exposure to various types of low-frequency electromagnetic waves remain to be confirmed. The controversial medical effects in humans of exposure to electromagnetic radiation are in sharp contrast to the well-established acute and late effects of exposure to ionizing radiation, which is the only subject considered in this chapter.

TERMINOLOGY AND DEFINITIONS Some familiarity with radiation terminology and units is essential for an understanding of the effects of ionizing radiation. An early term for the quantitation of exposure was the *roentgen* (R), which represents the amount of radiation-induced ionization in a standard volume of air. Much more important is the *rad* (radiation absorbed dose), which represents a unit of absorbed dose in tissue. One rad corresponds to the absorption of 100 ergs of energy (or about 1 R) in 1 g of tissue. Since the same dose in rads of different kinds of ionizing radiation can produce different biologic effects, the term *rem* (roentgen equivalent man) was introduced. It is the product of the rad multiplied by its relative biologic effectiveness (RBE), a factor that represents the biologic potency of one type of radiation as compared with another to produce the same biologic effect. The usual standard of comparison used for the RBE is 200-kV x-rays, which are similar in energy to gamma rays. Gamma radiation, therefore, has an RBE of about 1, and 1 rad of gamma exposure is roughly equal to 1 rem. Neutrons and some charged particles may have an RBE of 5 to 20 or greater. The terms *gray* (Gy), 1 unit of which is the equivalent of 100 rad, and *sievert* (Sv), 1 unit of which is equal to 100 rem, have been adopted to replace the terms *rad* and *rem,* respectively. One-thousandth of a gray is written as 10^{-3} Gy or 1 mGy, equivalent to 0.1 rad (10^{-1} rad) or 100 millirad (100 mrad). Similarly, one-thousandth of a sievert is written as 10^{-3} or 1 mSv, equivalent to 0.1 rem (10^{-1} rem) or 100 millirem (100 mrem).

The density of tissue ionization produced per unit length along the pathway of ionizing radiation is expressed as its *linear energy transfer* (LET). In general, electrically charged particles or particles of relatively high mass (alpha particles, protons, and neutrons) have a high energy transfer (high LET), resulting in relatively large amounts of tissue damage. In contrast, electromagnetic forms of ionizing radiation (gamma rays or x-rays) or charged particles of small mass (electrons) transfer less energy per unit length of travel (have low LET) and produce less tissue damage. There is quite a good correlation between LET and RBE.

The *threshold dose* for a specific biologic effects is the minimum radiation dose that will produce the effect. Radiation effects that vary in frequency with dose but not in severity are called *stochastic* effects. Examples of these are radiation-induced carcinogenic, mutagenic, and teratogenic effects. *Nonstochastic* effects vary in severity above a threshold dose depending on the number of cells injured. Examples of such effects are radiation-induced cataracts of the eye or fibrosis of the bone marrow. The interval of time between exposure and the occurrence of a radiation effect is identified as its *latent period*. The *maximum permissible* dose is that dose of ionizing radiation which, in the light of present knowledge, is not expected to cause any appreciable bodily injury to any person at any time during a lifetime. Recommended annual limits by most U.S. radiation regulatory agencies for absorbed whole-body radiation dose are 0.05 Sv for occupationally exposed persons and 0.001 Sv for the general public.

TYPES AND SOURCES OF IONIZING RADIATION Most of a person's lifetime radiation exposure is from low-dose background radiation. The average annual background dose for each person in the United States is quite variable but is estimated to be from 3 to 3.6 mSv. About 80 percent or four-fifths of this radiation is from natural sources, of which radon, cosmic rays, radionuclides in the earth, and radioactive elements in the body are the major contributors.

Radon now is believed to contribute about half of a person's total background radiation exposure. This represents about 1.5 to 2 mSv of exposure per year. Radon is a colorless, odorless, and tasteless alpha-particle-emitting radioactive gas which is derived from naturally occurring uranium deposits in the earth. It seeps up through soil into the air, where it and its decay products attach to dust, aerosols, or droplets that are inhaled and retained in bronchial epithelium and adjacent structures. The greatest exposures occur in certain indoor areas and mines where there are high adjacent rock concentrations of phosphates, granite, and black shale. Radon itself is not particularly harmful, but some of its alpha-emitting polonium radioactive decay products may heavily irradiate bronchial epithelial cells for many months or years.

Cosmic radiation accounts for about 0.3 mSv of background radiation per year at sea level. It is composed of protons, neutrons, and heavy nuclei from galactic sources and low-energy charged particles from the sun that interact with atmospheric nuclei to produce small secondary particles and electrons that enter the body and ionize tissue. The earth's atmosphere acts as a shield so that the dose is about doubled with every 1500 m of increase in altitude. Radioactive potassium and carbon and other radionuclides within the body contribute about another 0.3 to 0.4 mSv to the average person's annual background radiation exposure. Radioactive decay of thorium and uranium radionuclides in the earth's crust constitutes the major source of terrestrial radiation, which, in most areas, is about 0.3 mSv per year. Amounts of terrestrial radiation, however, may vary by a factor of 4 to 6 or more in different geographic locations.

The remaining background radiation exposure is from man-made sources. Diagnostic x-ray and nuclear medicine account for most of the average estimated annual total of from 0.4 to 1 mSv. Exposure from these sources has doubled in the United States and many other countries during the past 20 years. Contributions from nuclear explosions, nuclear power, and all other sources account for less than 1 percent of background radiation.

Most acute or intermittent excessive exposures to ionizing radiation occur in association with radiation diagnosis and therapy, nuclear weapon detonations, radiation device and nuclear reactor accidents, or improper use of radionuclides. Most of such exposures are to low-LET x-rays or gamma rays, but direct exposure to nuclear weapon detonations or fallout or the excessive ingestion, inhalation, or injection of certain radionuclides may result in significant exposures to neutrons, and alpha and beta particles, and high-LET gamma radiation.

PATHOGENESIS OF RADIATION INJURY   There are many types of cellular injury following exposure to ionizing radiation. Most important is damage to the genetic apparatus of the nucleus due to structural alterations of DNA and chromosomes.

Many types of DNA damage may occur, but most common with low-LET radiation are single-strand breaks and base alterations. High-LET radiation produces more double-strand breaks and more complex types of DNA base damage. In both instances, the free radicals generated by ionizing radiation are largely responsible for the DNA and chromosomal alterations. The extent to which damaged DNA will be responsible for cell death or will become a permanent mutation depends on the ability of the cells to repair the damage. Repair of DNA damage from low-LET radiation is much more efficient than it is from high-LET radiation. This is extremely important because most of the somatic mutational and late neoplastic effects in replicating cells probably are due to the persistence of radiation-induced unrepaired or misrepaired DNA bases.

Chromosomal damage of many types as a function of unrepaired DNA constitutes the other major type of radiation-induced injury to the genetic apparatus of the cell. Chromosomal breaks with rearrangements associated with loss of considerable amounts of chromosomal mass usually are responsible for cell death at the first or one of the first few postirradiation mitotic divisions. Consequently, the number of chromosomal aberrations present at any one time during the postirradiation period will depend on both the number induced and the rate of cell turnover. Unbalanced chromosomal rearrangements usually disappear rapidly. Balanced chromosomal rearrangements involving little loss of chromosomal material may persist as stable intracellular markers of radiation injury for many years. There is strong evidence that chromosomal rearrangements involving breaks near proto-oncogenes play an important role in the process of radiation-induced malignant transformation (see Chap. 63).

Repair of radiation-induced DNA and chromosomal damage is inversely related to the rate at which the radiation is absorbed. This is particularly true for low-LET radiation, where a high rate of radiation absorption may increase residual tissue damage by factors of 2 to 10 times that experienced with a low rate of radiation absorption. Thus a risk reduction factor of 2 or more may be applied to the estimation of risk of a biologic effect from exposure to low-LET radiation delivered at a low dose rate in comparison with the risk estimate for the same effect from similar radiation delivered at a high dose rate.

Large doses of radiation may produce direct cell death due to membrane or cytoplasmic structural damage. This type of interphase cell death of autonomic nerve cells, lymphocytes, and capillaries is responsible for most of the early severe clinical manifestations of partial- or whole-body high-dose acute radiation exposure. Direct cell killing from large radiation doses to localized areas also accounts for the late occurrence of tissue hypoplasia or fibrosis rather than the development of cancer.

HISTORY   Most of our knowledge concerning the *late* effects of ionizing radiation exposure for humans has been derived from a series of unfortunate accidents and errors during the past 75 years. In the early 1920s and 1930s, about 2000 luminous dial workers, mostly young women in the United States, inadvertently ingested large amounts of radium 226 by means of absorption from their tongues and lips. Many later developed carcinomas of the paranasal sinuses and osteosarcomas. In Germany in the mid-1940s, a number of children with bone tuberculosis and many adults with rheumatoid arthritis were injected with radium 224. Between 5 and 10 years later,

many of them also developed osteosarcomas. Increased mortality from leukemia and multiple myeloma was reported for radiologists during the early years of the use of medical x-ray equipment. In the 1930s and through the early 1950s, thorium dioxide (Thorotrast) was employed as a contrast medium in a number of medical clinics throughout the world. Many injected persons developed hepatic tumors, leukemia, or aplastic anemia in later years. Increased rates of thyroid cancer and leukemia have been reported in children treated with x-rays in the 1940s and 1950s for tinea capitis and presumed thymus enlargement. Radiation therapy between the years 1935 and 1954 to over 14,000 persons with ankylosing spondylitis in England and Northern Ireland resulted in increased leukemia and several other types of cancer. Survivors of the atomic bomb detonations in 1945 in Hiroshima and Nagasaki are most noted for the subsequent occurrence of leukemia and multiple-site malignant tumors. Fallout from weapons testing in the Marshall Islands in 1954 appears to have been responsible for a small number of cases of hypothyroidism, benign thyroid nodules, and thyroid cancer. An increased incidence of lung cancer has been recognized in uranium miners. Three incidents of industrial radioactive contamination in the Chelyabinsk region in Russia in the 1950s have resulted in an excess of leukemia. The late effects of the Chernobyl reactor accident in the Ukraine in 1986 are largely undetermined but appear to include increased thyroid cancer in exposed children.

Most information concerning the *acute effects* of excessive exposure to ionizing radiation derives from two sources: the many worldwide acute radiation accidents since 1901 and the atomic bomb explosions of 1945 in Japan. There were approximately 110,000 to 120,000 acute civilian deaths from the Japanese atomic bomb explosions, about one-third of which are believed to have been caused by radiation exposure. The Radiation Accident Registry at Oak Ridge, Tennessee, has identified 340 major worldwide radiation accidents between 1944 and 1991 involving 132,928 people. There were 3037 significant exposures and 116 fatalities (including the 32 at Chernobyl) due to either acute radiation effects or physical trauma.

The most extensive and reliable information concerning the *late effects* of excessive exposure to ionizing radiation originate from three sources: the Japanese atomic bomb survivors and patients treated with radiation therapy for either cervical cancer or ankylosing spondylitis.

CLINICAL EFFECTS OF RADIATION EXPOSURE   *Acute* or *early clinical effects* are those which occur within the first few minutes and up to about 2 months following exposure to large amounts of ionizing radiation delivered over a short period of time. They are due to cell killing, impairment of cell function, inflammation, infection, and hemorrhage. *Intermediate effects* occur after the first few months and up to a few years following exposure. *Late effects* are the radiation-related diseases and disorders that develop anytime after the first few years following previous acute or chronic ionizing radiation exposure.

Acute radiation effects   The early systemic manifestations of acute exposure to excessive amounts of ionizing radiation constitute the *acute radiation syndrome*. Survivors of the complete syndrome will experience four classical clinical stages that vary considerably in time of onset, severity, and duration, depending on the quality, quantity, and extent of the radiation exposure. The earliest phase is the prodrome, which consists of anorexia, nausea, and vomiting but also may include diarrhea, increased salivation, abdominal cramps, and dehydration. It commences within minutes to hours of exposure and lasts from a few hours to 1 or 2 days. This phase usually is followed by a relatively asymptomatic second stage of a few days' to a few weeks' duration. The third stage usually begins during the second to fifth weeks following exposure with the abrupt onset of moderate to severe gastrointestinal tract disturbances and manifestations of bone marrow depression. The fourth stage involves recovery, which may take weeks to months.

Persons who receive whole-body radiation in the range of 50 Gy or more invariably will die within 24 to 48 h from complications associated with the *neurovascular syndrome*. This is characterized by the rapid onset of apathy, lethargy, and prostration, frequently followed by seizures ranging from muscle contractions to grand mal convulsions, ataxia, and death. The early occurrence of severe central nervous system problems frequently yields to manifestations of the *cardiovascular syndrome*, characterized by intractable hypotension, arrhythmias, and shock before death occurs.

A significant prodrome also develops rapidly in persons exposed to whole-body radiation in the range of 10 to 50 Gy. Following a latent period of a few days, the *gastrointestinal syndrome* develops as the result of intestinal tract ulceration, infection, and hemorrhage secondary to mucosal cell atrophy and bone marrow depression. Its clinical manifestations are associated with massive fluid, protein, and electrolyte loss. Death almost always supervenes within a few more days.

Whole-body exposures in the range of 2 to 10 Gy are characterized by manifestations of the *bone marrow syndrome* due to a loss of marrow stem cells. Following a prodrome of 1 to 3 days and a relatively asymptomatic period of 1 to 3 weeks, buccal and pharyngeal ulcerations, localized and systemic forms of infection, cutaneous petechiae, and possibly generalized bleeding may develop secondary to thrombocytopenia and agranulocytosis. Concomitant loss of gastrointestinal epithelium often results in persistent diarrhea, abdominal distention, dehydration, circulatory collapse, and death. Survivors will experience rapid clinical improvement following partial return of peripheral blood granulocytes and platelets in 6 to 8 weeks, but full recovery may take several months. Epilation usually commences 1 to 2 weeks following exposure and is greatest at 5 to 7 weeks. Regrowth of new hair may take 4 to 6 months or more.

Mild gastrointestinal symptoms are experienced by 25 to 75 percent of persons exposed to less than 2 Gy of whole-body radiation. Hematologic complications rarely develop, because there is only moderate depression of the formed blood elements. Complete recovery of almost everyone in this exposure category is expected within 2 to 5 weeks.

Peripheral blood lymphopenia invariably develops during the first 12 to 48 h following any significant exposure. The rate and magnitude of the drop in the lymphocyte counts are related to radiation exposures up to about 5 to 6 Gy. At higher levels of exposure, lymphopenia is extreme, so correlations with exposure dose are poor. Reduced lymphocyte levels usually persist for 6 to 8 weeks. There often is a modest increase in the number of peripheral blood granulocytes during the first 1 to 2 days in response to exposure of more than 2 Gy, followed by a continual decline to maximum granulocytopenia in 2 to 5 weeks. The rate of granulocyte decline and the severity of granulocytopenia are functions of the bone marrow exposure dose. The peripheral blood platelet count responses are similar to those of the granulocytes, except that early thrombocytosis is rare and rates of both decline and recovery usually are slower. Reversible dose-dependent reticulocytopenia and mild anemia may develop up to radiation doses of about 5 to 6 Gy. Higher exposures may result in variable amounts of irreversible bone marrow damage, although some stem cells may survive acute exposure of 10 Gy or more.

Early radiation-induced chromosomal aberrations observed in peripheral blood lymphocytes include dicentrics, rings, deletions, translocations, inversions, and other types of rearrangements. Several dose-related somatic mutations observed following acute or chronic exposure to ionizing radiation include the induction of hypoxanthine-guanine phosphoribosyl transferase (HPRT)–deficient lymphocytes, alteration of lymphocyte T cell antigen receptors (TCR), and loss of erythrocyte membrane glycophorin A. Ionizing radiation also may induce lymphocyte micronuclei and structural changes in bone and tooth enamel, resulting in dose-related alteration of electron spin resonance (ESR).

Reproductive system disturbances are other important early clinical sequelae of acute whole-body radiation exposure. Male oligospermia or aspermia usually is temporary for weeks or months following exposures of 1.5 to 4 Gy, but permanent sterility usually develops at exposures of 5 to 9 Gy or greater. Sterility may be temporary in females exposed to 1.5 to 6.5 Gy and permanent at higher levels.

Intermediate and late radiation effects Bilateral posterior-central dotlike opacities with surrounding granules and vacuoles may develop in the *lens* of the eye within weeks or months following low-LET gamma radiation exposure. More heavily irradiated persons may have lateral extension of these tiny opacities with central clearing and anterior extension to the anterior surface of the lens. The lesions are defined as cataracts, but they rarely impair vision or progress over the years. Children are more prone to develop radiation-induced lenticular damage than are adults. The lenticular changes induced by radiation are nonstochastic, with a threshold dose of about 0.3 and 1 Gy for low-LET gamma radiation induction of minimal lesions and cataracts, respectively.

The most important *late effect* of exposure to ionizing radiation is an increased incidence of many different types of cancer. Reliable lifetime risk estimates for cancers due to low-dose radiation exposure are not available, but it is estimated that 3 to 5 percent of all human cancers are due to radiation from all sources. Risks usually are expressed in either *absolute* (additive) or *relative* (multiplicative) terms. The absolute risk is independent of natural incidence and represents the expected number of dose-related cancers above the baseline level. The relative risk represents the dose-released percentage increase above the natural or baseline level.

The earliest and most predictable type of cancer increased from excessive acute or chronic whole-body exposure to low-LET radiation is leukemia. An increased incidence first was observed in Japanese atomic bomb survivors within 2 to 3 years following exposure. Peak rates occurred about 7 to 8 years after the bombings. The types of leukemia which have demonstrated a significant relationship between incidence and radiation exposure dose are acute lymphocytic (ALL), acute myelogenous (AML), and chronic myelogenous (CML). The highest leukemia risks and shortest latent periods to maximum rates were in exposed children: CML for males and AML and ALL for both sexes. The initially high leukemia rates in exposed persons in most age groups have decreased in almost an exponential fashion to near baseline levels at the present time. The AML rate in the older exposed persons, however, has remained constant or has increased over the years. The overall male-to-female ratio for leukemia in exposed atomic bomb survivors was about 2:1. The leukemia response to radiation therapy in the other major worldwide experiences has been very similar to that of the Japanese except for a paucity of ALL in the spondylitis series and a virtual cessation of the leukemogenic response in the cervical irradiation series after 10 years. There is no evidence from any studies of human radiation effects that chronic lymphocytic leukemia is radiation-related. The excess number of deaths from leukemia from low-LET radiation exposure to the bone marrow from study of the atomic bomb survivors was 2.9 per 10^4 person-year-gray (Table 401-1). This risk was five to six times higher than that observed for the x-ray therapy–induced leukemias, probably due to the younger age of the atomic bomb survivors and their rapid rate of exposure. The dose-response curve for atomic bomb–induced leukemia is linear or linear-quadratic in configuration.

Increased incidence of thyroid cancer, benign thyroid adenomas, and hypothyroidism may occur following either external or internal exposure of the thyroid gland to ionizing radiation. The risk of developing thyroid cancer from external irradiation during childhood is about twice that for exposure during adulthood. The female-to-male ratio for radiation-induced thyroid cancer is uncertain and ranges from 4:1 to 1:1 in adults and children, respectively, with latent periods ranging from 4 to 30 years or longer. Persons of Jewish descent appear to be at higher risk than are those of other ethnic backgrounds who have been studied. The incidence of low-LET radiation-induced thyroid cancer is quite uncertain and depends on many factors. Reports range from 0.6 to 12.5 excess cases per 10^4 person-year-gray. The induction rate for benign adenomas is at least 30 to 50 percent greater than it is for thyroid cancer. Radioiodine therapy with thyroid gland doses greater than 40 to 50 Gy destroys parenchymal cells and almost invariably results in hypothyroidism rather than cancer. Radioiodine used for diagnostic thyroid studies increases the incidence of benign adenomas but does not increase the incidence of thyroid cancer.

A significant linear relationship between radiation exposure and the frequency of death from multiple myeloma and cancers of the female breast, esophagus, stomach, colon, lung, ovary, and urinary bladder has been reported in atomic bomb survivors (see Table 401-1). No increases in mortality with increased dose have been observed for lymphomas, bone tumors, and cancers of the larynx, upper respiratory track, rectum, gallbladder, pancreas, uterus, and prostate in this population. Atomic bomb and other studies of ionizing radiation from external sources also suggest radiation-related increases in the incidence of salivary and parathyroid gland tumors and possibly cancers of the skin, kidney, and central nervous system, other than brain. Most of the radiation-induced solid tumors have appeared at their usual ages of occurrence, with minimum latent periods ranging from 15 to 35 years, in marked contrast to the short latent period for leukemia. This suggests that the increased risk for cancer from radiation exposure lasts a lifetime. Children exposed under the age of 10 have shorter cancer latent periods and significantly higher cancer risks than do persons exposed at an older age. Excess deaths for radiation-induced non-sex-related solid tumors are about equal in males and females. The radiation response for the induction of tumors is believed to be stochastic, but organ-absorbed doses in the range of 0.2 to 0.49 Gy for leukemia, lung cancer, and several other cancers are the lowest levels for which a significant increase in cancer mortality has been observed in atomic bomb survivors (see Table 401-1). Excess deaths from low-LET radiation for cancers other than leukemia are estimated on the basis of atomic bomb survivor air dose information to be about 5.8 in males and 8.8 in females per 10^4 person-year-gray. Mortality on the basis of organ-exposed dose for sexes combined is 10.1 deaths per 10^4 person-year-gray (see Table 401-1).

Other late effects of whole-body exposure in atomic bomb survivors include accelerated decline in cell-mediated immunity with aging and an increased occurrence of hyperparathyroidism. On the other hand, the exposed populations have not experienced evidence of accelerated aging, increased infections, increased sterility, or consistent evidence of increased mortality from nonneoplastic diseases.

A radiation dose-response relationship for the occurrence of small head size has been observed in newborn infants following in utero exposure of the fetus to atomic bomb radiation during the first weeks of pregnancy. It has been observed in 40 to 50 percent of these infants following exposures of 1 Gy or more. A dose-related risk of mental retardation also has been observed in children following in utero exposure between the eighth and fifteenth weeks of gestation to greater than 0.4 Gy of low-LET radiation. A lower risk of mental retardation also exists for exposure between the sixteenth and twenty-fifth weeks of gestation with an apparent threshold at about 0.7 Gy. Exposure during the eighth to fifteenth weeks of gestation and, to a lesser extent, between the sixteenth and twenty-eighth weeks also is dose-related to an increased incidence of reduced school achievement, lower intelligence test scores, and unprovoked seizures later in life. Dose-related increased childhood cancer and leukemia have been related to in utero diagnostic x-ray exposure. In utero atomic bomb exposure studies, however, have not confirmed these relationships but have shown a dose-related increase in adult-type cancers with rates comparable with those of exposed children. Prenatal or early childhood whole-body atomic bomb radiation exposures in the range of 1 Gy or more also have resulted in slight reductions in maximum height.

No human studies to date have demonstrated a statistically significant genetic radiation risk in humans. It is believed, however, that there is a linear dose-response relationship without a threshold and that the overwhelming majority of induced mutations are damaging. Although atomic bomb survivor studies have failed to demonstrate a statistically significant increase in genetic effects in the children of exposed persons, the cumulative data from many measurements suggest that the amount of acute low-LET parental radiation required to double the spontaneous mutation rate (doubling dose) is about 2 Sv. The Japanese data also suggest a doubling dose for intermittent or long-term low-level parental radiation exposure between 3.4 and 4.5 Sv, in comparison with other estimates from mouse data ranging from 0.5 to 2.5 Sv. All these estimates have considerable uncertainty. Evidence suggesting that preconceptual parental radiation exposure increases childhood leukemia and possibly other cancers has not been confirmed in the large F_1 atomic bomb survivor populations.

The early radiation-induced dicentric and ring-form chromosomal aberrations in blood lymphocytes disappear with the first mitosis, so few remain in later years, but many of the radiation-induced balanced structural rearrangements persist as dose-related and age-independent biologic radiation markers throughout life. Reciprocal translocations and inversions predominate. The early radiation-induced dose-related structural alterations of glycophorin A in erythrocyte membranes and ESR of tooth enamel also persist for many years, but the lymphocyte micronuclei and other lymphocyte mutations (HPRT and TCR) disappear to virtually undetectable levels over a period of 1 to 5 years.

Many types of cancer and other late effects have been related to exposure to ionizing radiation from internally deposited radioisotopes (Table 401-2). The only clearly recognized late effect from radon exposure is lung cancer. The risk of death in the United States from indoor radon exposure is estimated to be about 0.4 percent. This would result in the development of 6000 to 25,000 lung cancers per year. The risks of radon exposure and smoking for lung cancer are at least additive and may be multiplicative.

TREATMENT There is no specific therapy for tissue radiation injury, but much can be done to reduce morbidity and mortality for persons who have been acutely exposed to excessive amounts of whole-body ionizing radiation.

Persons with possible surface contamination from radioactive substances must be evacuated promptly, monitored for external contamination, and decontaminated if necessary. It is extremely important to estimate the dose of radiation exposure as early as possible for any acute exposure in order to determine the need for various types of therapy. This may be very difficult even under the best of circumstances. The most reliable early indicators of dose in the absence of an actual dosimeter measurement are the exposure history, the severity of clinical symptoms, and the frequency of

---

TABLE 401-1 Significant radiation-induced cancer information for atomic bomb survivors, 1950–1985 (radiation exposure expressed as organ-absorbed dose)

Type of cancer	Excess relative risk at 1 Gy*	Excess deaths per 10^4 person-year-gray	Minimum dose for increased mortality, Gy	Minimum latent period to death, years
Leukemia	5.2	2.9	0.2–0.5	3–5
Multiple myeloma	2.3	0.3	—	30–34
Ovary	1.3	0.7	0.2–0.3	25–29
Urinary tract	1.3	0.7	—	30–34
Female breast	1.2	1.2	0.5–1.0	20–24
Colon	0.9	0.8	1.0–1.9	30–34
Lung	0.6	1.7	0.2–0.5	20–24
Esophagus	0.6	0.5	—	—
All (except leukemia)	0.4	10.1	0.2–0.5	—
Stomach	0.3	2.4	0.5–1.0	15–19

* Rates from UNSCEAR and Radiation Effects Research Foundation reports have been rounded to the nearest tenth.

TABLE 401-2 Late effects of some common radionuclide exposures

Radionuclide	Route of administration	Late effects
^{232}Thorium dioxide (Thorotrast)	Intravenous	Liver angiosarcoma, hemangioendothelioma, hepatic cell carcinoma and cirrhosis. Bile duct carcinoma, kidney cancer, leukemia, splenic atrophy and fibrosis, and aplastic anemia.
^{224,226,227}Radium	Intravenous and oral	Osteosarcoma, chondroblastic sarcoma, cataracts, leukemia, and paranasal, mastoid, and colon cancers
^{222}Radon	Inhalation	Lung cancer
^{125,131}Iodine	External, oral and intravenous	Hypothyroidism, thyroid adenomas, and thyroid cancer.
^{90}Strontium	Topical and inhalation	Anterior lenticular cataracts from eye applications, and beta skin burns with eventual scarring
^{32}Phosphorous	Topical and intravenous	Beta skin burns with eventual scarring and leukemia

certain radiation-induced biologic markers in blood cells. The severity and rapidity of the development of lymphopenia may give some early index of exposure dose, but much more reliable is the radiation-induced frequency of dicentric chromosomal aberrations in mitogen-stimulated and spontaneously dividing peripheral blood lymphocytes. The rate of granulocyte decline also is a very reliable and practical early biologic radiation dosimeter, but it may take 3 to 5 days or more before the rate is determined accurately. Bone marrow aspirations have limited quantitative relationships to exposure, but if performed in various sites, they may indicate the extent of marrow damage. Reliable estimates of radiation dose by means of other biologic dosimeters such as ESR of tooth enamel, loss of lymphocyte T cell receptors, or quantitation of lymphocyte micronuclei may be very difficult to obtain on short notice for acute radiation exposures. These measurements, however, along with determination of the loss of HPRT in lymphocytes or glycophorin A in red cells, may be very useful for intermediate- or late-exposure dosimetry.

Persons with few symptoms probably are exposed to less than 2 Gy and will require little or no therapy but should be kept under close observation with at least daily blood counts for a few days. Persons with estimated exposures in the range of 2 to 5 or 6 Gy require hospitalization for vigorous supportive therapy. Intravenous fluids and broad-spectrum antibiotic coverage should be instituted if either bacterial infections or severe agranulocytosis develops. Other supportive measures may include the administration of immunoglobulin, antifungal and antiviral agents, and antibiotics for the reduction of intestinal tract bacterial flora. Platelet transfusions should be administered for either bleeding due to thrombocytopenia or platelet counts below 20×10^9 per liter. Blood transfusions may be administered if anemia is severe, but granulocyte transfusions are of no value. Bone marrow transfusions are not indicated for persons in this group, but the early and continuous administration of molecularly cloned hematopoietic growth factors, especially granulocyte-macrophage colony stimulating factor (GM-CSF) or granulocyte colony stimulating factor (GSF), may be important adjuncts to the other forms of supportive therapy.

If the level of granulocytes falls during the first week to 0.25×10^9 per liter or less and the level of platelets to less than 30×10^9 per liter in 10 days, the total-body exposure probably is in the range of 5 to 15 Gy. Survival of persons exposed to whole-body irradiation in the range of 7 to 10 or 12 Gy with supportive therapy alone usually is not possible, so the addition of bone marrow transplantation and the concomitant administration of molecularly cloned hematopoietic growth factors may offer the best hopes for survival (see Chap. 313). Bone marrow transplantations probably are most effective if performed within the first 3 to 5 days of exposure, so early radiation dose estimates are very important. Peripheral blood lymphocytes should be collected as early as possible for histocompatibility testing, since they disappear rapidly from circulation. Platelets and blood should be irradiated with about 20 Gy prior to transfusion to reduce recipient alloantigen sensitization. Preparatory immunosuppression probably is not advisable prior to bone marrow transfusion, since permanent engraftment may not be necessary. Furthermore, it will contribute considerably to the severity of the overall illness. Persons with acute exposure to more than 15 to 20 Gy should be admitted to the hospital for supportive therapy only.

It is recommended that persons exposed to fallout in contaminated areas be treated as early as possible with 130 mg/d of potassium iodide for 10 days in order to prevent the accumulation of radioiodine in the thyroid gland. Consumption of all local produce, especially milk and vegetables, should be avoided.

PROGNOSIS Prognosis for survival from acute whole-body exposure to ionizing radiation alone depends almost entirely on tissue dose and therapy. Mortality without any therapy is negligible at 1 Gy or less and is virtually 100 percent above 15 Gy despite optimal therapy. About 50 percent of persons exposed to between 2 and 3 Gy will succumb without therapy, but most will survive with vigorous support. The LD$_{50}$ with optimal therapy is about 4.5 Gy. There is a very high probability of death, even with vigorous general support therapy, at exposures between 5 and 15 Gy, but it seems likely that some people exposed in the 7- to 10-Gy range will survive with bone marrow transplantation and other forms of supportive therapy. At levels of whole-body radiation exposure to 12 to 15 Gy or greater, bone marrow and other modalities of treatment are of little value because death ensues from extensive tissue damage of many other types. Prognosis at any level of exposure may be reduced if associated with thermal or radiation burns, trauma, or underlying illness.

There are no known forms of therapy for prevention of the late effects of ionizing radiation exposure. They are influenced by type of radiation, tissue dose, dose rate, extent of exposure, age at time of exposure, gender, inherent repair mechanisms, subsequent exposure to other carcinogens, and many other unknown constitutional and environmental factors. The clinical courses and responses to therapy of radiation-induced leukemias and solid tumors are not significantly different from those which are not radiation-related.

REFERENCES

BENGTSSON G, MOBERG L: What is a reasonable cost for protection against radiation and other risks. Health Phys 64:661, 1993

COMMITTEE ON THE BIOLOGICAL EFFECTS OF IONIZING RADIATION, NATIONAL RESEARCH COUNCIL: *Health Effects of Exposure to Low Levels of Ionizing Radiation* (BEIR V). Washington, D.C., National Academy Press, 1990

METTLER FA JR et al: The 1986 and 1988 UNSCEAR reports: Findings and implications. Health Phys 58:241, 1990

NEEL JV, SCHULL WJ: *The Children of Atomic Bomb Survivors: A Genetic Study*. Washington, D.C., National Academy Press, 1991

SHIMUZU Y et al: Studies of the mortality of A-bomb survivors: 9. Mortality, 1950–85, part 2: Cancer mortality based on the recently revised doses (DS 86). Radiat Res 121:120, 1990

UNITED NATIONS SCIENTIFIC COMMITTEES ON THE EFFECTS OF ATOMIC RADIATION: *Sources, Effects and Risks of Ionizing Radiation* (Report No. 88, IX, 7). New York, United Nations, 1988

APPENDIX: LABORATORY VALUES OF CLINICAL IMPORTANCE

INTRODUCTORY COMMENTS

All laboratory appendices should be interpreted with caution because normal values differ widely among clinical laboratories. The values given in this appendix are meant primarily for use with this text. In preparing this Appendix, the editors have taken into account the fact the system of international units (SI, système international d'unités) is now used in most countries and in virtually all medical and scientific journals, including most in the United States.[1] However, most clinical laboratories in the United States continue to report values in traditional units. Therefore, a system has been adopted that utilizes both systems for this Appendix and for the text itself. Values in SI units appear first, and *traditional units appear in parentheses* after the SI units. This dual system is also used for the most part in the text. In those instances in which the numbers remain the same but only the terminology is changed (mmol/L for meq/L or IU/L for mIU/L, only the SI units are given. In all other instances in the text the SI unit is followed by the traditional unit in parentheses. The SI base units, SI derived units, other units of measure referred to in this Appendix and SI prefixes are listed in Tables A-1 to A-3 at the end of this Appendix. Conversions from one system to another can be made as follows:

$$\text{mmol/L} = \frac{\text{mg/dL} \times 10}{\text{atomic weight}}$$

$$\text{mg/dL} = \frac{\text{mmol/L} \times \text{atomic weight}}{10}$$

ASCITIC FLUID

See Chapter 43.

BODY FLUIDS AND OTHER MASS DATA

Body fluid, total volume: 50 percent (in obese) to 70 percent (lean) of body weight
  Intracellular: 0.3–0.4 of body weight
  Extracellular: 0.2–0.3 of body weight
Blood:
  Total volume:
    Males: 69 mL/kg of body weight
    Females: 65 mL/kg of body weight
  Plasma volume:
    Males: 39 mL/kg of body weight
    Females: 40 mL/kg of body weight
  Red blood cell volume:
    Males: 30 mL/kg of body weight (1.15–1.21 L/m² of body surface area)
    Females: 25 mL/kg of body weight (0.95–1.00 L/m² of body surface area)

[1] Young DS: Implementation of SI units for clinical laboratory data. Ann Intern Med 106:114–129, 1987

CEREBROSPINAL FLUID[2]

		Conversion Factor (CF) C × CF = SI
Osmolarity	292–297 mmol/kg water (292–297 mOsmol/L)	—
Electrolytes:		
Sodium	137–145 mmol/L (137–145 meq/L)	—
Potassium	2.7–3.9 mmol/L (2.7–3.9 meq/L)	—
Calcium	1–1.5 mmol/L (2.1–3.0 meq/L)	0.5
Magnesium	1–1.2 mmol/L (2.0–2.5 meq/L)	0.5
Chloride	116–122 mmol/L (116–122 meq/L)	—
CO_2 content	20–24 mmol/L (20–24 meq/L)	—
P_{CO_2}	6–7 kPa (45–49 mmHg)	0.1333
pH	7.31–7.34	
Glucose	2.2–3.9 mmol/L (40–70 mg/dL)	0.05551
Lactate	1–2 mmol/L (10–20 mg/dL)	0.1110
Total protein:	0.2–0.5 g/L (20–50 mg/dL)	0.01
Prealbumin	2–6 percent	—
Albumin	56–75 percent	—
Alpha₁ globulin	2–7 percent	—
Alpha₂ globulin	4–12 percent	—
Beta globulin	8–16 percent	—
Gamma globulin	3–12 percent	—
IgG	0.01–0.014 g/L (1–1.4 mg/dL)	0.01
IgG index[3]	<0.65	
IgA	0.001–0.003 g/L (0.1–0.3 mg/dL)	0.01
IgM	0.0001–0.00012 g/L (0.01–0.012 mg/dL)	0.01
Ammonia	15–47 μmol/L (25–80 μg/dL)	0.05872
Creatinine	44–168 μmol/L (0.5–1.9 mg/dL)	88.40
Myelin basic protein	<4 μg/L	—
CSF pressure	50–180 mmH₂O	
CSF volume (adult)	100–160 mL	
Leukocytes:		
Total	<4 per mL	—
Differential:		
Lymphocytes	60–70 percent	—

[2] Since cerebrospinal fluid concentrations are equilibrium values, measurements of the same parameters in blood plasma obtained at the same time is recommended. However, there is a time lag in attainment of equilibrium, and cerebrospinal levels of plasma constituents that can fluctuate rapidly (such as plasma glucose) may not achieve stable values until after a significant lag phase.

[3] $\text{IgG index} = \dfrac{\text{CSF IgG (mg/dL)} \times \text{serum albumin (g/dL)}}{\text{Serum IgG (g/dL)} \times \text{CSF albumin (mg/dL)}}$

		Conversion Factor (CF) $C \times CF = SI$
Monocytes	30–50 percent	—
Neutrophils	None	—

CHEMICAL CONSTITUENTS OF BLOOD

See also function tests, especially metabolic and endocrine.

	CF
Acetoacetate, plasma: <100 μmol/L (<1 mg/dL)	97.95
Albumin, serum: 35–55 g/L (3.5–5.5 g/dL)	10
Aldolase: 0–100 nkat/L (0–6 U/L)	16.67
Alpha$_1$ antitrypsin, serum: 0.8–2.1 g/L (85–213 mg/dL)	0.01
Alpha fetoprotein (adult), serum: <30 μg/L (<30 ng/mL)	—
Aminotransferases, serum:	
Aspartate (AST, SGOT): 0–0.58 μkat/L (0–35 U/L)	0.01667
Alanine (ALT, SGPT): 0–0.58 μkat/L (0–35 U/L)	0.01667
Ammonia, whole blood, venous: 47–65 μmol/L (80–110 μg/dL)	0.5872
Amylase, serum: 0.8–3.2 μkat/L; 60–180 U/L	0.01667
Arterial blood gases:	
[HCO$_3^-$]: 21–28 mmol/L (21–30 meq/L)	—
P$_{CO_2}$: 4.7–5.9 kPa (35–45 mmHg)	0.1333
pH: 7.38–7.44	—
P$_{O_2}$: 11–13 kPa (80–100 mmHg)	0.1333
Ascorbic acid (vitamin C), serum: 23–57 μmol/L (0.4–1.0 mg/dL)	56.78
Barbiturates, serum: normal, nondetectable	
Phenobarbital, "potentially fatal" level: approximately 390 μmol/L (9 mg/dL)	43.06
Most short-acting barbiturates, "potentially fatal" levels: approximately 150 μmol/L (35 mg/dL)	4.419
Base, total, serum: 145–155 mmol/L (145–155 meq/L)	—
β-Hydroxybutyrate, plasma: <300 μmol/L (<3 mg/dL)	96.05
Bilirubin, total, serum (Malloy-Evelyn): 5.1–17 μmol/L (0.3–1.0 mg/dL)	17.10
Direct, serum: 1.7–5.1 μmol/L (0.1–0.3 mg/dL)	17.10
Indirect, serum: 3.4–12 μmol/L (0.2–0.7 mg/dL)	17.10
Bromides, serum: nondetectable	
Toxic levels: >17 mmol/L (>17 meq/L)	—
Calciferols (vitamin D), plasma:	
1,25-Dihydroxyvitamin D [1,25(OH)$_2$D]: 40–160 pmol/L (16 to 65 pg/mL)	0.2400
25-Hydroxyvitamin D [25(OH)D]: 20–200 nmol/L (8–80 ng/mL)	2.496
Calcium, ionized: 1.1–1.4 mmol/L (4.5–5.6 mg/dL)	0.2495
Calcium, plasma: 2.2–2.6 mmol/L (9–10.5 mg/dL)	0.2495
Carbon dioxide content, plasma (sea level): 21–30 mmol/L (21–30 meq/L)	—
Carbon dioxide tension (P$_{CO_2}$), arterial blood (sea level): 4.7–6.0 kPa (35–45 mmHg)	0.1333
Carbon monoxide content, blood: symptoms with over 20 percent saturation of hemoglobin	
Carotenoids, serum: 0.9–5.6 μmol/L (50–300 μg/dL)	0.01863

	CF
Ceruloplasmin, serum: 270–370 mg/L (27–37 mg/dL)	10
Chlorides, serum (as Cl$^-$): 98–106 mmol/L (98–106 meq/L)	—
Cholesterol: see Table A-4	
Complement, serum:	
C3: 0.55–1.20 g/L (55–120 mg/dL)	0.01
C4: 0.20–0.50 g/L (20–50 mg/dL)	0.01
Copper, serum: 11–22 μmol/L (70–140 μg/dL)	0.1574
Creatine phosphokinase, serum (total):	
Females: 0.17–1.17 μkat/L (10–70 U/L)	0.01667
Males: 0.42–1.50 μkat/L (25–90 U/L)	0.01667
Creatinine, serum: <133 μmol/L (<1.5 mg/dL)	88.40
Digoxin serum:	
Therapeutic level: 0.6–2.8 nmol/L (0.5–2.2 ng/mL)	1.281
Toxic level: >3.1 nmol/L (>2.4 ng/mL)	1.281
Ethanol, blood:	
Mild to moderate intoxication: 17–43 mmol/L (80–200 mg/dL)	0.2171
Marked intoxication: 54–87 mmol/L (250–400 mg/dL)	0.2171
Severe intoxication: >87 mmol/L (>400 mg/dL)	0.2171
Fatty acids, free (nonesterified), plasma: <180 mg/L (<18 mg/dL)	10
Ferritin, serum:	
Women: 10–200 μg/L (10–200 ng/ml)	
Men: 15–400 μg/L (15–400 ng/ml)	
Fibrinogen, plasma: see "Hematologic Evaluations: Platelets and Coagulation"	
Fibrinogen split products: see "Hematologic Evaluations: Platelets and Coagulation"	
Folic acid, red cell: 340–1020 nmol/L cells (150–450 ng/mL cells)	2.266
Gastrin, serum: 40–200 ng/L (40–200 pg/mL)	—
Globulins, serum: 20–30 g/L (2.0–3.0 g/dL)	10
Glucose (fasting), plasma:	
Normal: 4.2–6.4 mmol/L (75–115 mg/dL)	0.05551
Diabetes mellitus: >7.8 mmol/L on more than than one occasion (>140 mg dL)	0.05551
Glucose, 2 h postprandial, plasma:	
Normal: <7.8 mmol/L (<140 mg/dL)	0.05551
Impaired glucose tolerance: 7.8–11.1 mmol/L (140–200 mg/dL)	0.05551
Diabetes mellitus: >11.1 mmol/L on more than one occasion (>200 mg/dL)	0.05551
Hemoglobin, blood (sea level):	
Male: 140–180 g/L (14–18 g/dL)	10
Female: 120–160 g/L (12–16 g/dL)	10
Hemoglobin A$_{1c}$: up to 6 percent of total hemoglobin	—
Immunoglobulins, serum:	
IgA: 0.9–3.2 g/L (90–325 mg/dL)	0.01
IgD: 0–0.08 g/L (0–8 mg/dL)	0.01
IgE: <0.00025 g/L (<0.025 mg/dL)	0.01
IgG: 8.0–15.0 g/L (800–1500 mg/dL)	0.01
IgM: 0.45–1.5 g/L (45–150 mg/dL)	0.01
Iron, serum: 9–27 μmol/L (50–150 μg/dL)	0.01791
Iron-binding capacity, serum: 45–66 μmol/L (250–370 μg/dL)	0.01791
Saturation: 0.2–0.45 (20–45 percent)	
Lactate dehydrogenase, serum:	
200–450 units/mL (Wrobleski)	—
60–100 units/mL (Wacker)	—

	Conversion Factor (CF) C × CF = SI
0.4–1.7 μkat/L (25–100 units/L)	0.01667

Lactic dehydrogenase isoenzymes, serum (agarose):

Fraction 1 (of total): 0.14–0.25 (14–26 percent)	0.01
Fraction 2: 0.29–0.39 (29–39 percent)	0.01
Fraction 3: 0.20–0.25 (20–26 percent)	0.01
Fraction 4: 0.08–0.16 (8–16 percent)	0.01
Fraction 5: 0.06–0.16 (6–16 percent)	0.01
Lactate, venous plasma: 0.6–1.7 mmol/L (5–15 mg/dL)	0.1110
Lead, serum: <1.0 μmol/L (<20 μg/dL)	0.04826
Lipids: see Table A-4	—
Lipids, triglyceride, serum: see "Triglycerides"	—
Lipoprotein: see Table A-4	—

Lithium, serum:

Therapeutic level: 0.6–1.2 mmol/L (0.6–1.2 meq/L)	—
Toxic level: >2 mmol/L (2 meq/L)	—
Magnesium, serum: 0.8–1.2 mmol/L (2–3 mg/dL)	0.4114

Osmolality, plasma: 285–295 mmol/kg serum water (285–295 mosmol/kg serum water)

Oxygen content:

Arterial blood (sea level): 17–21 volume percent

Venous blood, arm (sea level): 10–16 volume percent

Oxygen percent saturation (sea level):

Arterial blood: 0.97 mol/mol (97 percent)	0.01
Venous blood, arm: 0.60–0.85 mol/mol (60–85 percent)	0.01
Oxygen tension (P_{O_2}) blood: 11–13 kPa (80–100 mmHg)	0.1333
pH, blood: 7.38–7.44	—

Phenytoin, plasma:

Therapeutic level: 40–80 μmol/L (10–20 mg/L)	3.964
Toxic level: >120 μmol/L (>30 mg/L)	3.964
Phospatase, acid, serum: 0.90 nkat/L (0–5.5 U/L)	—
Phosphatase, alkaline, serum: 0.5–2.0 μkat/L (30–120 U/L)	—
Phosphorus, inorganic, serum: 1.0–1.4 mmol/L (3–4.5 mg/dL)	0.3229
Potassium, serum: 3.5–5.0 mmol/L (3.5–5.0 meq/L)	—
Proteins, total, serum: 55–80 g/L (5.5–8.0 g/dL)	10

Protein fractions, serum:

Albumin: 35–55 g/L [3.5–5.5 g/dL (50–60 percent)]	10
Globulin: 20–35 g/L [2.0–3.5 g/dL (40–50 percent)]	10
Alpha₁: 2–4 g/L [0.2–0.4 g/dL (4.2–7.2 percent)]	10
Alpha₂: 5–9 g/L [0.5–0.9 g/dL (6.8–12 percent)]	10
Beta: 6–11 g/L [0.6–1.1 g/dL (9.3–15 percent)]	10
Gamma: 7–17 g/L [0.7–1.7 g/dL (13–23 percent)]	10
Pyruvate, venous, plasma: 60–170 μmol/L (0.5–1.5 mg/dL)	113.6

Quinidine, serum:

Therapeutic range: 4.6–9.2 μmol/L (1.5–3 mg/L)	3.082
Toxic range: 15.4–18.5 μmol/L (5–6 mg/L)	3.082

	Conversion Factor (CF) C × CF = SI
Salicylate, plasma: 0 mmol/L	—
Therapeutic range: 1.4–1.8 mmol/L (20–25 mg/dL)	0.07240
Toxic range: >2.2 mmol/L (>30 mg/dL)	0.07240
Sodium, serum: 136–145 mmol/L (136–145 meq/L)	—
Steroids: see "Metabolic and Endocrine Tests"	—
Triglycerides: <1.8 mmol/L (<160 mg/dL)	0.01129
Urea nitrogen, serum: 3.6–7.1 mmol/L (10–20 mg/dL)	0.3570

Uric acid, serum:

Men: 150–480 μmol/L (2.5–8.0 mg/dL)	59.48
Women: 90–360 μmol/L (1.5–6.0 mg/dL)	59.48
Vitamin A, serum: 0.7–3.5 μmol/L (20–100 μg/dL)	0.03491
Vitamin B₁₂, serum: 148–443 pmol/L (200–600 pg/mL)	0.7378
Zinc, serum: 11.5–18.5 μmol/L (75–120 μg/dL)	0.1530

CIRCULATION FUNCTION TESTS

Arteriovenous oxygen difference: 30–50 mL/L

Cardiac output (Fick): 2.5–3.6 L/m² of body surface area per minute

Contractility indexes:

Maximum left ventricular dp/dt: 1650 ± 300 mmHg/s

Maximum $(dp/dt)/p$: 44 ± 8.4 s⁻¹

$(dp/dt)/DP$ at DP = 40 mmHg: 37.6 ± 12.2 s⁻¹ (DP = diastolic press.)

Mean normalized systolic ejection rate (angiography): 3.32 ± 0.84 end-diastolic volumes per second

Mean velocity of circumferential fiber shortening (angiography) 1.66 ± 0.42 circumferences per second

Ejection fraction, stroke volume/end-diastolic volume (SV/EDV):

Normal range: 0.55–0.78; average: 0.67

End-diastolic volume: 75 ± 15 mL/m²

End-systolic volume: 25 ± 8 mL/m²

Left ventricular work:

Stroke work index: 30–110 (g·m)/m²

Left ventricular minute work index: 1.8–6.6 [(kg·m)/m²]/min

Oxygen consumption index: 110–150 mL

Pulmonary vascular resistance: 20–120 (dyn·s)/cm⁵ (2–12 kPa·s/L)

Systemic vascular resistance: 770–1500 (dyn·s)/cm⁵ (77–150 kPa·s/L)

GASTROINTESTINAL TESTS

See also "Stool Analysis."

Absorption tests:

D-Xylose absorption test: After an overnight fast, 25 g xylose is given in aqueous solution by mouth. Urine collected for the following 5 h should contain 5–8 g (33–53 mmol) (or >20 percent of ingested dose). Serum xylose should be 25–40 mg/100 mL 1 h after the oral dose (1.7–2.7 mmol/L).

Vitamin A absorption test: A fasting blood specimen is obtained and 200,000 units of vitamin A in oil is given by mouth. Serum vitamin A levels should rise to twice fasting level in 3–5 h.

Bentiromide test (pancreatic function): 500 mg bentiromide (chymex) orally; p-aminobenzoic acid (PABA) measured in plasma and/or urine

Plasma: >3.6 (±1.1) μg/mL at 90 min

Urine: >50 percent recovered as PABA in 6 h

Gastric juice:

Volume:

24 h: 2–3 L

Nocturnal: 600–700 mL

Basal, fasting: 30–70 mL/h

	Conversion Factor (CF) C × CF = SI
Reaction: pH: 1.6–1.8	
Titratable acidity of fasting juice: 4–9 μmol/s (15–35 meq/h)	0.261
Acid output: Basal:	
Females (mean ± 1 SD): 0.6 ± 0.5 μmol/s (2.0 ± 1.8 meq/h)	0.2778
Males (mean ± 1 SD): 0.8 ± 0.6 μmol/s (3.0 ± 2.0 meq/h)	0.2778

Maximal (after subcutaneous histamine acid
  phosphate 0.004 mg/kg body weight and
  preceded by 50 mg promethazine or after
  betazole 1.7 mg/kg body weight or
  pentagastrin 6 μg/kg body weight):	

Females (mean ± 1 SD): 4.4 ± 1.4 μmol/s (16 ± 5 meq/h)	0.2778
Males (mean ± 1 SD): 6.4 ± 1.4 μmol/s (23 ± 5 meq/h)	0.2778
Basal acid output/maximal acid output ratio: 0.6 or less	
Gastrin, serum: 40–200 ng/L (40–200 pg/mL)	—
Secretin test (pancreatic exocrine function: 1 unit/kg of body weight, intravenously	
Volume (pancreatic juice): >2.0 mL/kg in 80 min	—
Bicarbonate concentration: >80 mmol/L (>80 meq/L)	—
Bicarbonate output: >10 mmol in 30 min (>10 meq in 30 min)	—

METABOLIC AND ENDOCRINE TESTS

	Conversion Factor (CF) C × CF = SI
Adrenocorticotropin (ACTH) plasma, 8 A.M.: <18 pmol/L (<80 pg/mL)	0.2202
Adrenal cortex function tests: see Chap. 335	—
Adrenal medulla function tests: see Chap 336	—
Adrenal steroids, plasma:	

Aldosterone, 8 A.M.: <220 pmol/L (patient su-
  pine, 100 meq Na and 60–100 meq K intake)
  (<8 ng/dL)
	27.74

Cortisol:	
8 A.M.: 140–690 nmol/L (5–25 μg/dL)	27.59
4 P.M.: 80–330 nmol/L (3–12 μg/dL)	27.59
Dehydroepiandrosterone (DHEA): 7–31 nmol/L (2–9 μg/L)	3.467
Dehydroepiandrosterone sulfate (DHEA sul- fate): 1.3–6.7 μmol/L (500–2500 μg/L)	0.002714
11-Deoxycortisol (compound S): <30 nmol/L (<1 μg/dL)	28.86
17-Hydroxyprogesterone:	

Women: follicular phase, 0.6–3 nmol/L
    (0.20–1 μg/L); luteal phase, 1.5–10.6 nmol/
    L (0.5–3.5 μg/L)
	3.026

Men: 0.2–9 nmol/L (0.06–3 μg L)	3.026
Adrenal steroids, urinary excretion:	
Aldosterone: 14–53 nmol/d (5–19 μg/d)	2.774
Cortisol, free: 55–275 nmol/d (20–100 μg/d)	2.759
17-Hydroxycorticosteroids: 5.5–28 μmol/d (2– 10) mg/d)	2.759
17-Ketosteroids:	
Men: 24–88 μmol/d (7–25 mg/d)	3.467
Women: 14–52 μmol/d (4–15 mg/d)	3.467
Angiotensin II, plasma, 8 A.M.: 10–30 nmol/L (10–30 pg/mL)	—

	Conversion Factor (CF) C × CF = SI

Arginine vasopressin (AVP), plasma:
  Random fluid intake: 1.5–5.6 pmol/L (1.5–6
  ng/L)
	0.92

Calcitonin, plasma: <50 ng/L (<50 pg/mL)	—
Catecholamines, urinary excretion:	
Free catecholamines: <590 nmol/d (<100 μg/ d)	5.911
Epinephrine: <275 nmol/d (<50 μg/d)	5.458
Metanephrines: <7 μmol/d (<1.3 mg/d)	5.458
Vanillylmandelic acid (VMA): <40 μmol/d (<8 mg/d)	5.046
Glucagon, plasma: 50–100 ng/L (50–100 pg/mL)	—
Gonadal function tests: see Chaps. 339 and 340	—
Gonadal steroids, plasma:	
Androstenedione:	
Women: 3.5–7.0 nmol/L (1–2 ng/ml)	3.492
Men: 3.0–5.0 nmol/L (0.8–1.3 ng/ml)	3.492
Estradiol:	
Women: 70–220 pmol/L (20–60 pg/mL), higher at ovulation	3.671
Men: <180 pmol/L (<50 pg/mL)	3.671
Progesterone:	
Women: luteal peak >16 nmol/L (>5 ng/mL)	3.180

Men, prepubertal girls, preovulatory women,
    and postmenopausal women: <6 nmol/L
    (<2 ng/mL)
	3.180

Testosterone:	
Women: <3.5 nmol/L (<1 ng/mL)	3.467
Men: 10–35 nmol/L (3–10 ng/mL)	3.467
Prepubertal boys and girls: 0.17–0.7 nmol/L (0.05–0.2 ng/mL)	3.467
Gonadotropins, plasma:	
Women, mature, premenopausal, except at ovu- lation:	
FSH: 5–20 IU/L (5–20 mIU/mL)	—
LH: 5–25 IU/L (5–25 mIU/mL)	—
Ovulatory surge:	
FSH: 12–30 IU/L (12–30 mIU/mL)	—
LH: 25–100 IU/L (25–100 mIU/mL)	—
Postmenopausal:	
FSH: 12–30 IU/L (12–30 mIU/mL)	—
LH: >50 IU/L (>50 mIU/mL)	—
Men, mature:	
FSH: 5–20 IU/L (5–20 mIU/mL)	—
LH: 5–20 IU/L (5–20 mIU/mL)	—
Children of both sexes, prepubertal:	
FSH: <5 IU/L (<5 mIU/mL)	—
Growth hormone, after 100 g glucose by mouth: <5 μg/L (<5 ng/mL)	
Human chorionic gonadotropin, β subunit (β- hCG), plasma:	
Men and nonpregnant women: <3 IU/L (<3 mIU/mL)	—
Insulin, serum or plasma, fasting: 43–186 pmol/L (6–26 μU/mL)	7.175
Insulin-like growth factor 1 (somatomedin C, IGF- 1/SM-C): see Chap. 332	—
Oxytocin: random 1–4 pmol/L (1.25–5 ng/L)	0.80
Ovulatory peak in women: 4–8 pmol/L (5–10 ng/L)	—
Pancreatic islet function tests: see Chap. 337	—
Parathyroid function tests: see Chap. 357	—
Pituitary function tests: see Chaps. 331 to 333	—
Pregnancy tests: see Chap. 340	—

	Conversion Factor (CF) C × CF = SI
Prolactin, serum: 2–15 μg/L (2–15 ng/mL)	—
Renin-angiotensin function tests: see Chap. 335	—
Semen analysis: see Chap. 339	—
Thyroid function tests:	
Dynamic tests of thyroid function: see Chap. 334	—
Radioactive iodine uptake, 24 h: 5–30 percent (range varies in different areas due to variations in iodine intake)	—
Resin T_3 uptake: 0.25–0.35 (25–35 percent) (varies among laboratories; for calculation of indexes of resin T_3 uptake, see Chap. 334)	0.01
Reverse triiodothyronine (rT_3), plasma: 0.15–0.61 nmol/L (10–40 ng/dL)	0.01536
Thyroid-stimulating hormone (TSH): 0.4–5 mU/L (0.4–5 μU/mL)	—
Thyroxine (T_4), serum radioimmunoassay: 64–154 nmol/L (5–12 μg/dL)	12.86
Triiodothyronine (T_3), plasma: 1.1–2.9 nmol/L (70–190 ng/dL)	0.01536

PULMONARY FUNCTION TESTS

See Table A-7.

RENAL FUNCTION TESTS

	Conversion Factor (CF) C × CF = SI
Clearances (corrected to 1.72 m² of body surface area):	
Measures of glomerular filtration rate:	
Inulin clearance (C1):	
Males (mean ± 1 SD): 2.1 ± 0.4 mL/s (124 ± 25.8 mL/min)	0.01667
Females (mean ± 1 SD): 2.0 ± 0.2 mL/s (119 ± 12.8 mL/min)	0.01667
Endogenous creatinine clearance: 1.5–2.2 mL/s (91–130 mL/min)	0.01667
Urea: 1.0–1.7 mL/s (60–100 mL/min)	0.01667
Measures of effective renal plasma flow and tubular function:	
p-Aminohippuric acid clearance (Cl_{PAH}):	
Males (mean ± 1 SD): 10.9 ± 2.7 mL/s (654 ± 163 mL/min)	0.01667
Females (mean ± 1 SD): 9.9 ± 1.7 mL/s (594 ± 102 mL/min)	0.01667
Concentration and dilution test:	
Specific gravity of urine:	
After 12-h fluid restriction: 1.025 or more	—
After 12-h deliberate water intake: 1.003 or less	—
Protein excretion, urine: <0.15 g/d (<150 mg/d)	0.01
Males: 0–0.06 g/d (0–60 mg/d)	0.01
Females: 0–0.09 g/d (0–90 mg/d)	0.01
Specific gravity, maximal range: 1.002–1.028	—
Tubular reabsorption, phosphorus: 79–94 percent of filtered load	—

HEMATOLOGIC EVALUATIONS

	Conversion Factor (CF) C × CF = SI
See also "Chemical Constituents of Blood."	—
Bone marrow See Table A-6.	—

	Conversion Factor (CF) C × CF = SI
Carboxyhemoglobin:	
Nonsmoker: 0–0.023 (0–2.3 percent)	0.01
Smoker: 0.021–0.042 (2.1–4.2 percent)	0.01
Erythrocyte:	
Count: 4.15–4.90 × 10¹²/L (4.15–4.90 × 10⁶/mm³)	—
Distribution width (Coulter): 0.13–0.15 (13–15 percent)	—
Glucose-6-phosphate dehydrogenase: 12.1 ± 2 IU/gHb (WHO)	
Life span:	
Normal survival: 120 days	
Chromium-labeled, half-life ($t\frac{1}{2}$): 28 days	
Mean corpuscular hemoglobin (MHC): 28–33 pg/cell (28–33 pg/cell)	
Mean corpuscular hemoglobin concentration (MCHC): 320–360 g/L (32–36 g/dL)	
Mean corpuscular volume (MCV): 86–98 fL (86–98 mm³)	
Ham's test (acid serum): negative	—
Haptoglobin, serum: 0.5–2.2 g/L (50–220 mg/dL)	0.01
Hematocrit:	
Males: 0.42–0.52 (42–52 percent)	—
Females: 0.37–0.48 (37–48 percent)	—
Hemoglobin:	
Plasma: 0.6–3 μmol/L (1–5 mg/dL)	0.6206
Whole blood:	
Males: 8.1–11.2 mmol/L (13–18 g/dL)	0.6206
Females: 7.4–9.9 mmol/L (12–16 g/dL)	0.6206
Hemoglobin A_2 (HbA₂): 0.015–0.035 (1.5–3.5 percent)	0.01
Hemoglobin, fetal (HbF): <0.02 (<2 percent)	0.01
Hemoglobin H prep: negative	—
Leukocytes:	
Alkaline phosphatase (LAP): 0.2–1.6 μkat/L (13–100 U/L)	
Count: 4.3–0.3X10⁹/L (4.3–10.8 × 10³/mm³)	
Differential:	
Neutrophils: 0.45–0.74 (45–74 percent)	
Bands: 0–0.04 (0–4 percent)	
Lymphocytes: 0.16–0.45 (16–45 percent)	
Monocytes: 0.04–0.10 (4–10 percent)	
Eosinophils: 0–0.07 (0–7 percent)	
Basophils: 0–0.02 (0–2 percent)	
Lysozyme (muramidase):	
Serum: 5–25 mg/L (5–25 μg/mL)	—
Urine: <2 mg/L (<2 μg/mL)	—
Methemoglobin: <0.017 mg/L (<1.70 μg/mL)	—
Osmotic fragility:	
Slight hemolysis: 0.45–0.39 percent	—
Complete hemolysis: 0.33–0.30 percent	—
Plasma iron turnover: 20–42 mg/d or 0.45 mg/kg of body weight per day	
Platelets and coagulation parameters:	
Alpha₂ antiplasmin: 70–130 percent	
Antithrombin III: 80–120 percent	
Bleeding time:	
Duke method: <4 min	
Simplate: <7 min	
Clot retraction, qualitative: apparent in 60 min, complete <24 h, usually <6 h	
Euglobulin lysis time: >2 h	
Factor II: 60–100 percent	

	Conversion Factor (CF) C × CF = SI

Factor V: 60–100 percent
Factor VII: 60–100 percent
Factor IX: 60–100 percent
Factor X: 60–100 percent
Factor XI: 60–100 percent
Factor XII: 60–100 percent
Factor XIII: 60–100 percent
Fibrinogen: 200–400 mg/dL
Fibrin split products: <10 μg/mL
Plasminogen: 2.4–4.4 CTA U/mL
Protein C (antigenic assay): 58–148 percent
Protein S (antigenic assay): 58–148 percent
Partial thromboplastin time (activated PTT): comparable with control
Prothrombin time (quick one-stage): control ± 1 s
Protamine paracoagulation (3P) test: negative
Platelets: 130,000–400,000 per microliter
Thrombin time: control ± 3 s
von Willebrand's antigen: 60–150 percent

Protoporphyrin, free erythrocyte (FEP): 0.28–0.64 μmol/L of red blood cells (16–36 μg/dL of red blood cells)	0.0177

Red cells: see "Erythrocytes"
Schilling test: 7–40 percent of orally administered vitamin B_{12} excreted in urine
Sedimentation rate:
   Westergren, <50 years of age:
     Males: 0–15 mm/h
     Females: 0–20 mm/h
   Westergren, >50 years of age:
     Males: 0–20 mm/h
     Females: 0–30 mm/h
Sucrose hemolysis: negative
Viscosity
   Plasma: 1.7–2.1
   Serum: 1.4–1.8
White blood cells: see "Leukocytes"

STOOL ANALYSIS

	Conversion Factor (CF) C × CF = SI
Bulk:	
Wet weight: <197.5 (115 ± 41) g/d	—
Dry weight: <66.4 (34 ± 15) g/d	—
Alpha₁ antitrypsin: 0.98 (±0.17) mg/g dry weight stool	—
Coproporphyrin: 600–1500 nmol/d (400–1000 μg/d)	1.527
Fat (on diet containing at least 50 g fat): <6.0 (4.0 ± 1.5) g/d when measured on a 3-day (or longer) collection	
Percent of dry weight: 0.30 (<30.4 percent)	0.01
Coefficient of fat absorption: >0.95 (>95 percent)	0.01
Fatty acid:	
Free: 0.01–0.10 (1–10 percent of dry matter)	0.01
Combined as soap: 0.005–0.12 (0.5–12 percent of dry matter)	0.01
Nitrogen: <1.7 (1.4 ± 0.2) g/d	—
Protein content: minimal	—
Urobilinogen: 68–470 μmol/d (40–280 mg/d)	1.693
Water: 0.65 (approximately 65 percent)	0.01

URINE ANALYSIS

See also "Metabolic and Endocrine Tests"

	Conversion Factor (CF) C × CF = SI
Acidity, titratable: 20–40 mmol/d (20–40 meq/d)	—
Ammonia: 30–50 mmol/d (30–50 meq/d)	—
Amylase: 35–260 Somogyi units/h	—
Amylase/creatinine clearance ratio [(Cl_{am}/Cl_{cr}) × 100]: 1–5	—
Bentiromide (pancreatic function): 50 percent excreted in 6 h as p-amino benzoic acid (PABA) after 500 mg oral bentiromide	—
Calcium (10 meq/d or 200-mg/d calcium diet): <3.8 mmol/d (<7.5 meq/d)	0.5
Catecholamines: <600 nmol/d (<100 μg/d)	5.911
Copper: 0–0.4 μmol/d (0–25 μg/d)	0.01574
Coproporphyrins (types I and III): 150–460 nmol/d (100–300 μg/d)	1.527
Creatine, as creatinine:	
Adult males: <380 pmol/d (<50 mg/d)	7.625
Adult females: <760 pmol/d (<100 mg/d)	7.625
Creatinine: 8.8–14 mmol/d (1.0–1.6 g/d)	8.840
Glucose, true (oxidase method): 0.3–1.7 mmol/d (50–300 mg/d)	0.5551
5-Hydroxyindoleacetic acid (5-HIAA): 10–47 μmol/d (2–9 mg/d)	5.230
Lead: <0.4 μmol/d (<80 μg/d)	0.004826
Protein: <0.15 g/d (<150 mg/d)	0.1
Porphobilinogen: none	—
Potassium: 25–100 mmol/d [25–100 meq/d (varies with intake)]	—
Sodium: 100–260 mmol/d [100–260 meq/d (varies with intake)]	—
Urobilinogen: 1.7–5.9 μmol/d (1–3.5 mg/d)	1.693
Vanillylmandelic acid (VMA): <40 μmol/d (<8 mg/d)	5.046
D-Xylose excretion: 5 to 8 g within 5 h after oral dose of 25 g	—

TABLE A-1 SI and other units

Quantity	Name of unit	Symbol for unit	Derivation of units
SI BASE UNITS			
Length	meter	m	
Mass	kilogram	kg	
Time	second	s	
Thermodynamic temperature	Kelvin	K	
Amount of substance	mole	mol	
SI DERIVED UNITS			
Area	square meter	m^2	
Force	newton	N	$(m \cdot kg)/s^2$
Pressure	pascal	Pa	$N \cdot m^2$
Work, energy	joule	J	$N \cdot m$
Celsius temperature	degree Celsius	°C	K
OTHER UNITS RETAINED FOR USE			
Time	minute	min	
	hour	h	
	day	d	
Volume	liter	L	

TABLE A-3 SI prefixes and their symbols

Factor	Prefix	Symbol for prefix
10^9	giga	G
10^6	mega	M
10^3	kilo	k
10^2	hecto	h
10^1	deka	da
10^{-1}	deci	d
10^{-2}	centi	c
10^{-3}	milli	m
10^{-6}	micro	μ
10^{-9}	nano	n
10^{-12}	pico	p
10^{-15}	femto	f
10^{-18}	alto	a

TABLE A-4 Classification of total cholesterol and LDL-cholesterol values

	Total plasma cholesterol	LDL-cholesterol	Conversion factor (C to SI)
Desirable	<5.20 mmol/L (<200 mg/dL)	<3.36 mmol/L (<130 mg/dL)	0.02586
Borderline high	5.20–6.18 mmol/L (200–239 mg/dL)	3.36–4.11 mmol/L (130–159 mg/dL)	0.02586
High	≥6.21 mmol/L (≥240 mg/dL)	≥4.14 mmol/L (≥160 mg/dL)	0.02586

SOURCE: The Expert Panel. Report of the National Cholesterol Education Program Expert Panel on Detection, Evaluation, and Treatment of High Blood Cholesterol in Adults. Arch Intern Med 148:36, 1988

TABLE A-2 Radiation derived units

Quantity	Old unit	SI unit	Name for SI unit (and abbreviation)	Conversion
Activity	curie (Ci)	Disintegrations per second (dps)	becquerel (Bq)	1 Ci = 3.7 × 10¹⁰ Bq 1 mCi = 37 mBq 1 μCi = 0.037 MBq or 37 GBq 1 Bq = 2.703 × 10⁻¹¹ Ci
Absorbed dose	rad	joule per kilogram (J/kg)	gray (Gy)	1 Gy = 100 rad 1 rad = 0.01 Gy 1 mrad = 10⁻³ cGy
Exposure	roentgen (R)	coulomb per kilogram (C/kg)	—	1 C/kg = 3876 R 1 R = 2.58 × 10⁻⁴ C/kg 1 mR = 258 pC/kg
Dose equivalent	rem	joule per kilogram (J/kg)	sievert (Sv)	1 Sv = 100 rem 1 rem = 0.01 Sv 1 mrem = 10 μSv

TABLE A-5 Normal values of echocardiographic measurements in adults

	Range, cm	Mean, cm	Number of subjects
Age (years)	13 to 54	26	134
Body surface area (m²)	1.45 to 2.22	1.8	130
RVD—flat	0.7 to 2.3	1.5	84
RVD—left lateral	0.9 to 2.6	1.7	83
LVID—flat	3.7 to 5.6	4.7	82
LVID—left lateral	3.5 to 5.7	4.7	81
Posterior LV wall thickness	0.6 to 1.1	0.9	137
Posterior LV wall amplitude	0.9 to 1.4	1.2	48
IVS wall thickness	0.6 to 1.1	0.9	137
Mid IVS amplitude	0.3 to 0.8	0.5	10
Apical IVS amplitude	0.5 to 1.2	0.7	38
Left atrial dimension	1.9 to 4.0	2.9	133
Aortic root dimension	2.0 to 3.7	2.7	121
Aortic cusps' separation	1.5 to 2.6	1.9	93
Percentage of fractional shortening‡	34 to 44%	36%	20
Mean rate of circumferential shortening (Vcf)‡, or mean normalized shortening velocity	1.02 to 1.94 circ/s	1.3 circ/s	38

* RVD = right ventricular dimension; LVID = left ventricular internal dimension; d = end diastole; s = end systole; LV = left ventricle; IVS = interventricular septum.

† $\dfrac{LVIDd - LVIDs}{LVIDd}$

‡ $\dfrac{LVIDd - LVIDs}{LVIDd \times \text{ejection time}}$

SOURCE: From H. Feigenbaum, Echocardiography, in *Heart Disease*, 4th ed, E Braunwald (ed). Philadelphia, Saunders, 1992.

TABLE A-6 Differential nucleated cell counts of bone marrow

	Normal, mean%*	Range, %†		Normal, mean%*	Range, %†
Myeloid:	56.7		Erythroid:	25.6	
Neutrophilic series:	53.6		Pronormoblasts	0.6	0.2–1.3
Myeloblast	0.9	0.2–1.5	Basophilic normoblasts	1.4	0.5–2.4
Promyelocyte	3.3	2.1–4.1	Polychromatophilic	21.6	17.9–29.2
Myelocyte	12.7	8.2–15.7	normoblasts		
Metamyelocyte	15.9	9.6–24.6	Orthochromatic normoblasts	2.0	0.4–4.6
Band	12.4	9.5–15.3	Megakaryocytes	<0.1	
Segmented			Lymphoreticular	17.8	
Eosinophilic series	3.1	1.2–5.3	Lymphocytes	16.2	11.1–23.2
Basophilic series	<0.1	0–0.2	Plasma cells	2.3	0.4–3.9
			Reticulum cells	0.3	0–0.9

* From MM Wintrobe et al, *Clinical Hematology*, 8th ed. Philadelphia, Lea & Febiger, 1981.
† Range observed in 12 healthy men.

TABLE A-7 Summary of values useful in pulmonary physiology

	Symbol	Typical values	
		Men	Women

PULMONARY MECHANICS

Spirometry—volume-time curves:			
Forced vital capacity	FVC	≥4.0 L	≥3.0 L
Forced expiratory volume in 1 s	FEV$_1$	>3.0 L	>2.0 L
FEV$_1$/FVC	FEV$_1$%	>60%	>70%
Maximal midexpiratory flow	MMF (FEF 25–27)	>2.0 L/s	>1.6 L/s
Maximal expiratory flow rate	MEFR (FEF 200–1200)	>3.5 L/s	>3.0 L/s
Spirometry—flow-volume curves:			
Maximal expiratory flow at 50% of expired vital capacity	V$_{max}$ 50 (FEF 50%)	>2.5 L/s	>2.0 L/s
Maximal expiratory flow at 75% of expired vital capacity	V$_{max}$ 75 (FEF 75%)	>1.5 L/s	>1.0 L/s
Resistance to airflow:			
Pulmonary resistance	RL (R$_L$)	<3.0 (cmH$_2$O/s)/L	
Airway resistance	Raw	<2.5 (cmH$_2$O/s)/L	
Specific conductance	SGaw	>0.13 cmH$_2$O/s	
Pulmonary compliance:			
Static recoil pressure at total lung capacity	Pst TLC	25 ± 5 cmH$_2$O	
Compliance of lungs (static)	CL	0.2 L/cmH$_2$O	
Compliance of lungs and thorax	C(L + T)	0.1 L/cmH$_2$O	
Dynamic compliance of 20 breaths per minute	C dyn 20	0.25 ± 0.05 L/cmH$_2$O	
Maximal static respiratory pressures:			
Maximal inspiratory pressure	MIP	>90 cmH$_2$O	>50 cmH$_2$O
Maximal expiratory pressure	MEP	>150 cmH$_2$O	>120 cmH$_2$O

LUNG VOLUMES

Total lung capacity	TLC	6–7 L	5–6 L
Functional residual capacity	FRC	2–3 L	2–3 L
Residual volume	RV	1–2 L	1–2 L
Inspiratory capacity	IC	2–4 L	2–4 L
Expiratory reserve volume	ERV	1–2 L	1–2 L
Vital capacity	VC	4–5 L	3–4 L

GAS EXCHANGE (SEA LEVEL)

Arterial O$_2$ tension	Pa$_{O_2}$	12.7 ± 0.7 kPa (95 ± 5 mmHg)	
Arterial CO$_2$ tension	Pa$_{CO_2}$	5.3 ± 0.3 kPa (40 ± 2 mmHg)	
Arterial O$_2$ saturation	Sa$_{O_2}$	0.97 ± 0.02 (97 ± 2%)	
Arterial blood pH	pH	7.40 ± 0.02	
Arterial bicarbonate	HCO$_3^-$	24 + 2 meq/L	
Base excess	BE	0 ± 2 meq/L	
Diffusing capacity for carbon monoxide (single breath)	DL$_{CO}$	0.42 mLCO/s/mmHg (25 mL CO/min/mmHg)	
Dead space volume	V$_D$	50 ± 25 mL	
Physiologic dead space; dead space-tidal volume ratio	V$_D$/V$_T$	≤35% V$_T$	
(rest)			
(exercise)		≤20% V$_T$	
Alveolar-arterial difference for O$_2$	A-aD$_{O_2}$	≤2.7 kPa ≤20 kPa (≤20 mmHg)	

INDEX

(Note: Page numbers in **boldface** indicate major topics or principal discussions; numbers preceded by A indicate Atlas plates.)

TOPICAL TABLE OF CONTENTS